Consulta Veterinária em 5 Minutos: Espécies Canina e Felina

5ª EDIÇÃO

Consulta Veterinária em 5 Minutos: Espécies Canina e Felina

5ª EDIÇÃO

Larry Patrick Tilley, DVM
Diplomate, American College of Veterinary
Internal Medicine (Internal Medicine)
President, VetMed Consultants
Consultant, New Mexico Veterinary Referral Center
Sante Fe, New Mexico

Francis W. K. Smith, Jr., DVM
Diplomate, American College of Veterinary
Internal Medicine (Internal Medicine & Cardiology)
Vice President, VetMed Consultants
Lexington, Massachusetts
Clinical Assistant Professor, Department of Medicine
Tufts University, School of Veterinary Medicine
North Grafton, Massachusetts

Manole

Título original em inglês: *Blackwell's Five-Minute Veterinary Consult: Canine and Feline, 5th edition*
A edição original foi publicada em 2011 © 2011 by John Wiley & Sons, Inc.
Primeira edição, © 1997 Lippincott Williams & Wilkins
Segunda edição, © 2000 Lippincott Williams & Wilkins
Terceira edição, © 2004 Lippincott Williams & Wilkins
Quarta edição, © 2007 Blackwell Publishing Professional

Todos os direitos reservados. Tradução do original em inglês publicada mediante acordo com a John Wiley & Sons Limited. A Editora Manole é responsável exclusiva pela tradução desta obra. Nenhuma parte do livro poderá ser reproduzida, por qualquer processo, sem a permissão por escrito da John Wiley & Sons Limited, detentora dos direitos autorais originais.

Este livro contempla as regras do Novo Acordo Ortográfico da Língua Portuguesa.

Editor gestor: Walter Luiz Coutinho
Editora de traduções: Denise Yumi Chinem
Produção editorial: Priscila Pereira Mota Hidaka e Cláudia Lahr Tetzlaff
Assistência editorial: Gabriela Rocha Ribeiro, Michel Arcas Bezerra e Vinicius Asevedo Vieira

Tradução das atualizações da 5ª edição: Dra. Fabiana Buassaly Leistner (parte pós-textual, verbetes e índice remissivo)
Médica veterinária e tradutora

Tradução dos apêndices: Carlos Artur Lopes Leite (parte dos apêndices IX e X)
Doutor em Medicina Veterinária pela FMVZ/Unesp

Thaís Spacov Camargo Pimentel (apêndices I a VIII)
Mestre em Medicina Veterinária pela FMVZ/USP

Fernando Gomes do Nascimento (parte do apêndice IX)
Médico veterinário e tradutor

Tradução da 3ª edição: Prof. Dr. Cid Figueiredo, Dra. Fabiana Buassaly Leistner e Dra. Idília Ribeiro Vanzellotti
Revisão científica da 3ª edição: Prof. Dr. Cid Figueiredo – Professor Titular (aposentado) da FMVZ/Unesp–Botucatu
Revisão de tradução e revisão de prova: Depto. editorial da Editora Manole
Diagramação: Estúdio Asterisco Ltda.
Adaptação da capa para a edição brasileira: Depto. de arte da Editora Manole

Dados Internacionais de Catalogação na Publicação (CIP)
(Câmara Brasileira do Livro, SP, Brasil)

Tilley, Larry Patrick
    Consulta veterinária em 5 minutos: espécies canina e felina /
Larry Patrick Tilley, Francis W. K. Smith Junior;
[tradução Fabiana Buassaly Leistner... [et. al.]. --
5. ed. -- Barueri, SP : Manole, 2015.

    Título original: Blackwell's Five-Minute Veterinary Consult :
Canine and Feline
    Outros tradutores: Carlos Artur Lopes Leite, Fernando
Gomes do Nascimento, Thaís Spacov Camargo Pimentel.
    Bibliografia.
    ISBN 978-85-204-3462-8

    1. Cães - Doenças - Manuais, etc 2. Cães - Doenças -
Diagnóstico 3. Cães - Doenças - Tratamento 4. Gatos -
Doenças - Manuais, etc. 5. Gatos - Doenças - Diagnóstico
6. Gatos - Doenças - Tratamento 7. Medicina veterinária -
Manuais, guias etc. I. Smith Junior., Francis W. K.
II. Título.

	CDD–636.70896
14-12245	-636.80896

Índices para catálogo sistemático:
1. Cães: Doenças : Diagnóstico e tratamento :
Medicina veterinária 636.70896
2. Gatos: Doenças : Diagnóstico e tratamento :
Medicina veterinária 636.80896

A Editora Manole é filiada à ABDR – Associação Brasileira de Direitos Reprográficos.

Edição brasileira – 2015

Direitos em língua portuguesa adquiridos pela:
Editora Manole Ltda.
Av. Ceci, 672 – Tamboré
06460-120 – Barueri – SP – Brasil
Tel. (11) 4196-6000 – Fax (11) 4196-6021
www.manole.com.br | https://atendimento.manole.com.br/
Impresso no Brasil | *Printed in Brazil*

Para minha esposa, Jeri, meu filho, Kyle,
e meu neto, Tucker, em homenagem "à relação
e ao amor secretos" existentes dentro de
nossos corações; para a família e os animais
que representam a pureza da vida.

Larry Patrick Tilley

Para minha esposa, May, meu filho, Ben,
e minha filha, Jade, pois me lembro com grande
estima de nosso tempo juntos, bem como do
amor e apoio constantes. Para meu pai, Frank,
obrigado por ser meu maior exemplo.

Francis W.K. Smith, Jr.

PREFÁCIO

É extremamente difícil se manter a par dos avanços na medicina veterinária, sobretudo para o clínico geral tão ocupado. É impossível se manter atualizado de todos os periódicos durante o exercício da medicina veterinária. No ambiente clínico, o veterinário pode ficar sobrecarregado com todos os achados e conclusões de milhares de estudos conduzidos por especialistas veterinários. A obra *Consulta veterinária em 5 minutos* foi elaborada para fornecer ao clínico que dispõe de pouco tempo e ao estudante de medicina veterinária revisões práticas e concisas de quase todas as doenças e condições clínicas que acometem os cães e gatos. Nosso objetivo ao produzir este livro também foi fornecer informações atualizadas em um formato de fácil acesso. Uma ênfase especial foi dada ao diagnóstico e tratamento de problemas e doenças provavelmente observados pelos veterinários.

Nosso maior sonho foi realizado quando estudantes de veterinária, clínicos veterinários e acadêmicos escolheram e definiram as quatro primeiras edições deste livro como uma fonte de referência abrangente e completa em medicina canina e felina. O formato do livro tem se mostrado de fácil utilização, tornando-se bastante popular entre os clínicos atarefados. O escopo do livro, bem como o número de consultores editoriais e de autores, foi ampliado. Também aumentamos o número de autores estrangeiros (ou seja, de fora da América do Norte) para proporcionar a melhor orientação em âmbito mundial. O número de tópicos aumentou e cada tópico foi atualizado para fornecer ao leitor as informações mais atuais possíveis contidas em um livro. Os apêndices também foram expandidos de modo a incluir tabelas mais úteis e proveitosas, ao mesmo tempo em que o formulário de medicamentos também foi atualizado e ampliado.

Existem vários livros bons de medicina interna veterinária disponíveis. A exclusividade e o valor de *Consulta veterinária em 5 minutos* como uma fonte de rápida referência se devem à consistência e à coerência da apresentação, à amplitude da cobertura, à contribuição de um grande número de especialistas e à preparação do texto em tempo viável. O formato de cada tópico é idêntico, o que facilita o encontro imediato das informações. Uma lista extensa de títulos garante a cobertura completa de cada tópico.

Para a quinta edição, removemos a divisão de tópicos em diferentes seções (i. e., Problemas Apresentados, Diagnóstico – Testes Laboratoriais, Diagnóstico – ECG, e Doenças), pois alguns tópicos não se prestavam a essa classificação; além disso, o sistema induzia à confusão ao se tentar encontrar determinados tópicos. Como resultado dessa mudança, trocamos os nomes dos tópicos relacionados aos testes laboratoriais, de modo a refletir a síndrome clínica e não o nome do teste (p. ex., Cálcio, Hipercalcemia passou a ser chamado apenas Hipercalcemia). Alguns nomes de tópicos também foram alterados de acordo com a terminologia da Nomenclatura Sistematizada de Medicina Humana e Veterinária (SNOMED).

Como o próprio título diz, um dos objetivos deste livro é tornar as informações rapidamente disponíveis. Para tal finalidade, organizamos os tópicos em ordem alfabética. A maioria dos tópicos pode ser encontrada sem utilizar o índice. Há um sumário dividido por sistemas orgânicos, além de um índice remissivo detalhado. Uma grande quantidade de informações úteis se encontra resumida em quadros nos Apêndices, onde também estão incluídos um extenso e detalhado formulário de medicamentos, tabelas de toxicologia, protocolos de testes endócrinos, valores laboratoriais normais e tabelas de conversão.

Foi um grande prazer e privilégio termos contado com a assistência de muitos especialistas em medicina interna veterinária, provenientes de todas as partes do mundo. Mais de 300 especialistas veterinários contribuíram para a elaboração deste livro, o que permitiu que cada capítulo fosse escrito por um especialista no assunto. Além de fornecer informações excepcionais e notáveis, esse amplo grupo de especialistas nos permitiu publicar este importante livro em tempo oportuno.

Muitos livros volumosos levam vários anos para ser redigidos, o que faz com que algumas de suas informações fiquem desatualizadas no momento de sua publicação. Dessa forma, agradecemos aos inúmeros colaboradores e consultores editoriais, cujo trabalho árduo nos permitiu escrever, editar e publicar este livro em dois anos, sendo que a maior parte dos capítulos foi finalizada um ano antes da publicação da obra.

A quinta edição deste livro constitui uma fonte de referência médica atualizada e importante para a clínica e a formação clínica. Esforçamo-nos para torná-la completa e, ao mesmo tempo, prática e de fácil utilização. Nossos sonhos se concretizarão se este livro ajudar o leitor a localizar as informações com rapidez e a utilizar os dados "momentaneamente relevantes" e essenciais para o exercício de uma medicina veterinária de alta qualidade. Apreciaríamos sua opinião a respeito deste livro, pois isso nos ajudará a tonar as edições futuras ainda mais úteis. Se o leitor quiser informações a respeito de qualquer alteração em termos de conteúdo ou formato, acréscimos ou supressões desta edição, por gentileza entre em contato conosco. Envie seus comentários (em inglês) para o seguinte endereço:

Drs. Larry Tilley & Frank Smith
c/o Wiley-Blackwell
Blackwell Publishing Professional
2121 State Avenue
Ames, IA 50014, EUA

AGRADECIMENTOS

A conclusão deste livro oferece uma excelente oportunidade para prestar um reconhecimento por escrito a todos aqueles que nos ajudaram ao longo desta jornada. Os editores estão extremamente gratos aos consultores editoriais e aos colaboradores que, por meio de sua especialização, aperfeiçoaram a qualidade deste livro de forma incontestável.

Também gostaríamos de reconhecer e agradecer aos nossos familiares pelo apoio a este projeto e pelos sacrifícios pelas quais passaram para nos dispensar o tempo necessário para a conclusão deste livro.

Além de agradecer aos veterinários que nos encaminharam seus pacientes, gostaríamos de expressar nossa gratidão a cada estudante e residente de veterinária, de cuja formação nós tivemos o privilégio de fazer parte. A curiosidade e o estímulo intelectual desses estudantes nos fizeram crescer como profissionais e nos impeliram a assumir a tarefa de escrever este livro.

Por fim, um agradecimento especial vai para todos da Wiley-Blackwell. Os departamentos de marketing e vendas também merecem reconhecimento por gerarem tamanho interesse por este livro. Todos eles, sem exceção, são profissionais dedicados e pessoas cordiais que tornaram as etapas finais de preparação deste livro uma tarefa inspiradora e divertida. Um agradecimento especial vai para Janis Cleland, que editou os folhetos de orientação ao proprietário disponíveis neste livro. Um importante objetivo de nossas vidas foi cumprido: fornecer o conhecimento e disponibilizar a experiência na área de medicina interna de pequenos animais em termos mundiais, além de ensinar os princípios contidos neste livro a veterinários e estudantes em todas as partes do mundo.

CONSULTORES EDITORIAIS

STEPHEN C. BARR, BVSc, MVS, PhD
Diplomate ACVIM (Small Animal)
Professor of Medicine
Department of Clinical Sciences
College of Veterinary Medicine
Cornell University
Ithaca, New York, USA
Especialidade: Doença infecciosa

SHARON A. CENTER, DVM
Diplomate ACVIM
Professor
Department of Clinical Sciences
Cornell University
Cornell University Hospital for Animals
Ithaca, New York, USA
Especialidade: Hepatologia/Imunologia

TIMOTHY M. FAN, DVM, PhD
Diplomate ACVIM (Internal Medicine,
Oncology)
Assistant Professor (Medical Oncology)
Department of Veterinary Clinical Medicine
Veterinary Teaching Hospital
College of Veterinary Medicine
University of Illinois at Urbana-Champaign
Urbana, Illinois, USA
Especialidade: Oncologia

DEBORAH S. GRECO, DVM, PhD
Diplomate ACVIM
Senior Research Scientist Petcare
Nestle Purina
New York, New York, USA
Especialidade: Endocrinologia/Metabolismo

DEBRA F. HORWITZ, DVM
Diplomate ACVB
Owner
Veterinary Behavior Consultations
St. Louis, Missouri, USA
Especialidade: Comportamento

ALBERT E. JERGENS, DVM, PhD
Diplomate ACVIM (Internal Medicine)
Professor
Department of Veterinary Clinical Sciences
Internist, Lloyd Veterinary Medical Center
College of Veterinary Medicine
Iowa State University
Ames, Iowa, USA
Especialidade: Gastrenterologia

LYNELLE R. JOHNSON, DVM, PhD
Diplomate ACVIM (Internal Medicine)
Associate Professor
Department of Veterinary Medicine and
Epidemiology
University of California—Davis
Davis, California, USA
Especialidade: Sistema respiratório

HEIDI B. LOBPRISE, DVM
Diplomate American Veterinarian
Dental College
Virbac Corporation
Fort Worth, Texas, USA
Especialidade: Odontologia

SARA K. LYLE, DVM, MS
Diplomate American College of
Theriogenologists
Clinical Instructor
Veterinary Clinical Sciences
School of Veterinary Medicine
Louisiana State University
Baton Rouge, Louisiana, USA
Especialidade: Teriogenologia

PAUL E. MILLER, DVM
Diplomate ACVO
Clinical Professor of Comparative Opthalmology
Department of Surgical Sciences
School of Veterinary Medicine
University of Wisconsin–Madison
Madison, Wisconsin, USA
Especialidade: Oftalmologia

CARL A. OSBORNE, DVM, PhD
Diplomate AVCIM
Professor
Veterinary Clinical Sciences Department
University of Minnesota
St. Paul, Minnesota, USA
Especialidade: Nefrologia/Urologia

GARY D. OSWEILER, DVM, PhD
Diplomate American Board of Veterinary
Toxicology
Professor
Veterinary Diagnostic and Production Animal
Medicine
Veterinary Diagnostic Laboratory
College of Veterinary Medicine
Iowa State University
Ames, Iowa, USA
Especialidade: Toxicologia

JOANE M. PARENT, DVM, MVetSc
Diplomate ACVIM (Neurology)
Professor
Sciences Cliniques
Centre Hospitalier Universitaire Vétérinaire
Université de Montréal
St. Hyacinthe, Quebec, Canada
Especialidade: Neurologia

A.H. REBAR, DVM, PhD
Diplomate ACVP
Senior Associate VP for Research
Executive Director—Discovery Park and
Professor of Clinical Pathology
Office of the Vice President for Research
Purdue University
West Lafayette, Indiana, USA
Especialidade: Hematologia/Imunologia

PETER K. SHIRES, BVSc, MS
Diplomate ACVS
Principal Scientist
Scientific Affairs
Ethicon Endo-Surgery
Cincinnati, Ohio, USA
Especialidade: Sistema musculoesquelético

FRANCIS W.K. SMITH, Jr., DVM
Diplomate ACVIM (Small Animal Internal
Medicine & Cardiology)
Clinical Assistant Professor
Department of Medicine
Cummings School of Veterinary Medicine
Tufts University
North Grafton, Massachusetts, USA
Vice President, VetMed Consultants
Lexington, Massachusetts, USA
Especialidade: Cardiologia

LARRY P. TILLEY, DVM
Diplomate ACVIM (Internal Medicine)
President, VetMed Consultants
Consultant, New Mexico Veterinary Referral
Center
Sante Fe, New Mexico, USA
Especialidade: Cardiologia

ALEXANDER H. WERNER, VMD
Diplomate ACVD
Staff Dermatologist
Animal Dermatology Center
Studio City, California, USA
Especialidade: Dermatologia

COLABORADORES

JONATHAN A. ABBOTT, DVM
Diplomate ACVIM (Cardiology)
Associate Professor of Cardiology
Department of Small Animal Clinical Sciences
Virginia-Maryland Regional College of
Veterinary Medicine
Virginia Polytechnic Institute and State
University
Blacksburg, Virginia
USA

ANTHONY C.G. ABRAMS-OGG, DVM,
DVSc
Diplomate ACVIM (Small Animal Internal
Medicine)
Associate Professor
Department of Clinical Studies
Ontario Veterinary College, University of Guelph
Guelph, Ontario
Canada

LARRY G. ADAMS, DVM, PhD
Diplomate ACVIM (Small Animal Internal
Medicine)
Professor
Department of Veterinary Clinical Sciences
Purdue University
West Lafayette, Indiana
USA

HASAN ALBASAN, DVM, MS, PhD
Assistant Professor, Veterinary Internal Medicine
Faculty of Veterinary Medicine
Erciyes University
Kayseri, Turkey
Research Associate, Department of Veterinary
Clinical Sciences
College of Veterinary Medicine
University of Minnesota
St. Paul, Minnesota
USA

A. RICK ALLEMAN, DVM, PhD
Diplomate ABVP; Diplomate ACVP
Professor, Service Chief, Resident
Co-ordinator, Director of Laboratories
Department of Physiological Sciences
College of Veterinary Medicine
University of Florida
Gainesville, Florida
USA

JAMES M.G. ANTHONY, DVM, BSc (Agr),
MRCVS, P.AG
Fellow Academy of Veterinary Dentistry,
Diplomate AVDC, Diplomate EVDC
Associate Professor
Small Animal Clinical Sciences
Western College of Veterinary Medicine
University of Saskatchewan
Saskatoon, Saskatchewan
Canada

JULIE ARMSTRONG, DVM, MVSc
Diplomate ACVIM (Small Animal Internal
Medicine)
Consultant
Animal Emergency Clinic of the Fraser Valley
Langley, British Columbia
Canada

RODNEY S. BAGLEY, DVM
Diplomate ACVIM (Neurology and Internal
Medicine)
Professor and Chair
Department of Clinical Sciences
College of Veterinary Medicine
Iowa State University
Ames, Iowa
USA

DENNIS B. BAILEY, DVM
Diplomate ACVIM (Oncology)
Staff Oncologist
Oradell Animal Hospital
Paramus, New Jersey
USA

E. MURL BAILEY, DVM, MS, PhD
Diplomate ABVT
Professor
Department of Veterinary Physiology and
Pharmacology
College of Veterinary Medicine
Texas A & M University
College Station, Texas
USA

MELISSA BAIN, DVM, MS
Diplomate ACVB
Assistant Professor of Clinical Animal Behavior
Veterinary Medicine and Epidemiology
University of California
Davis, California
USA

LARRY BAKER, DVM
Diplomate American Veterinary Dentistry
College, Fellow Academy of Veterinary Dentistry
Owner
Northgate Veterinary Dentistry
Decatur, Illinois
USA

TOMAS W. BAKER, MS
Ultrasonographer
Department of Surgical and Radiological Sciences
University of California, Davis
Davis, California
USA

CHERYL E. BALKMAN, DVM
Diplomate ACVIM (Small Animal Internal
Medicine)
Lecturer
Department of Clinical Sciences
College of Veterinary Medicine
Cornell University
Ithaca, New York
USA

MARGARET C. BARR, DVM, PhD
Professor, Virology and Immunology
College of Veterinary Medicine
Western University of Health Sciences
Pomona, California
USA

STEPHEN C. BARR, BVSc, MVS, PhD
Diplomate ACVIM (Small Animal)
Professor of Medicine
Department of Clinical Sciences
College of Veterinary Medicine
Cornell University
Ithaca, New York
USA

JOSEPH W. BARTGES, DVM, PhD
Diplomate ACVIM; Diplomate ACVN
Professor of Medicine and Nutrition, The Acree
Endowed Chair of Small Animal Research
Department of Small Animal Clinical Sciences
Internist and Nutritionist
Small Animal Teaching Hospital
College of Veterinary Medicine
University of Tennessee
Knoxville, Tennessee
USA

ANDREW BEARDOW, BVM&S, MRCVS
Diplomate ACVIM (Cardiology)
Idexx Laboratories Inc.
Westbrook, Maine
USA

ELLEN N. BEHREND, VMD, PhD
Diplomate ACVIM (Small Animal Internal Medicine)
Professor
Clinical Sciences
Auburn University
Auburn, Alabama
USA

JAN BELLOWS, DVM
Diplomate American Veterinary Dental College,
Fellow Academy of Veterinary Dentistry,
Diplomate American Board of Veterinary
Practitioners
All Pets Dental Clinic
Weston, Florida
USA

ELLISON BENTLEY, DVM
Diplomate ACVO
Clinical Assistant Professor
Department of Surgical Sciences
School of Veterinary Medicine
University of Wisconsin–Madison
Madison, Wisconsin
USA

ALLYSON C. BERENT, DVM
Diplomate ACVIM
Director of Interventional Endoscopy
Staff Doctor Internal Medicine
The Animal Medical Center
New York, New York
USA

LAURIE BERGMAN, VMD
Diplomate ACVB
Metropolitan Veterinary Associates
Norristown, Pennsylvania
USA

PHIL J. BERGMAN, DVM, MS, PhD
Diplomate ACVIM (Oncology)
Chief Medical Officer
BrightHeart Veterinary Center
Armonk, New York
USA

CHRISTINE BERTHELIN-BAKER, DVM,
MRCVS
Diplomate ACVIM (Neurology); Diplomate
European College of Veterinary Neurology
Neurologist
All Animal Neurology
Atlanta, Georgia
USA

ADAM J. BIRKENHEUER, DVM, PhD
Diplomate ACVIM
Assistant Professor
Department of Clinical Sciences
North Carolina State University
Raleigh, North Carolina
USA

KARYN BISCHOFF, DVM, MS
Diplomate American Board of Veterinary
Toxicology
Assistant Professor
Population Medicine and Diagnostic Sciences
Diagnostic Toxicologist
New York Animal Health Diagnostic Center
College of Veterinary Medicine
Cornell University
Ithaca, New York
USA

BONNIE C. BLOOM, DVM
Veterinary Dental Resident
Dallas Dental Service Animal Clinic
Dallas, Texas
USA

JOHN D. BONAGURA, DVM, MS
Diplomate ACVIM (Cardiology, Internal
Medicine)
Professor, Veterinary Clinical Sciences Head,
Cardiology Service
Ohio State University Veterinary Hospital
Ohio State University
Columbus, Ohio
USA

DWIGHT D. BOWMAN, MS, PhD
Professor
Department of Microbiology and Immunology
College of Veterinary Medicine
Cornell University
Ithaca, New York
USA

RANDI BRANNAN, DVM
Fellow Academy of Veterinary Dentistry,
Diplomate American Veterinary Dental College
Owner
Animal Dental Clinic
Portland, Oregon
USA

JANICE MCINTOSH BRIGHT, BSN, MS,
DVM
Diplomate ACVIM (Cardiology, Internal
Medicine)
Professor of Cardiology
Department of Clinical Sciences
Cardiologist, Veterinary Medical Center
James L. Voss Veterinary Teaching Hospital
Colorado State University
Fort Collins, Colorado
USA

MARJORY BROOKS, DVM
Diplomate ACVIM
Comparative Coagulation Section
Animal Health Diagnostic Center
Cornell University
Ithaca, New York
USA

DONALD J. BROWN, DVM, PhD
Diplomate ACVIM (Cardiology)
Vermont Veterinary Cardiology Services
Waterbury Center, Vermont
USA

JÖRG BUCHELER, DVM, PhD, FTA
Diplomate ACVIM (Internal Medicine);
Diplomate ECVIM-CA
Chief of Staff
Veterinary Specialty Hospital of South Florida
Palm Beach, Florida
USA

NAOMI L. BURTNICK, MT (ASCP)
Owner and Ultrasonographer
New Mexico Veterinary Specialty Referral Center
Santa Fe, New Mexico
USA

CLAY A. CALVERT, DVM
Diplomate ACVIM (Internal Medicine)
Professor
Department of Small Animal Medicine/Surgery
University of Georgia
Athens, Georgia
USA

KAREN L. CAMPBELL, DVM, MS
Diplomate ACVIM; Diplomate ACVD
Professor and Section Head, Specialty Medicine
Department of Veterinary Clinical Medicine
College of Veterinary Medicine
University of Illinois
Urbana, Illinois
USA

LARRY CARPENTER, DVM, MS
Diplomate ACVS
Surgeon
Veterinary Surgical Service
Sturgis, South Dakota
USA

RENEE T. CARTER, DVM
Diplomate ACVO
Assistant Professor
Department of Veterinary Clinical Sciences
School of Veterinary Medicine
Louisiana State University
Baton Rouge, Louisiana
USA

SHARON A. CENTER, DVM
Diplomate ACVIM
Professor
Department of Clinical Sciences
Cornell University
Cornell University Hospital for Animals
Ithaca, New York
USA

ERIN S. CHAMPAGNE, DVM
Diplomate ACVO
Staff Ophthalmologist
Veterinary Specialists of Western New York
Buffalo, New York
USA

LEEAH R. CHEW, DVM
Resident, Theriogenology
Large Animal Clinical Sciences
Virginia-Maryland Regional College of
Veterinary Medicine
Virginia Tech
Blacksburg, Virginia
USA

DEIRDRE CHIARAMONTE, DVM
Diplomate ACVIM
Staff Internist, Director of Rehabilitation and
Fitness Service Medicine, Rehabilitation
The Animal Medical Center
New York, New York
USA

GEORGINA CHILD, BVSc
Diplomate ACVIM (Neurology) Consultant
Veterinary Teaching Hospital, Sydney
University of Sydney
Specialist Neurologist
Small Animal Specialist Hospital
Camperdown and North Ryde, New South Wales
Australia

E'LISE CHRISTENSEN BELL, DVM
Diplomate ACVB
Veterinary Behaviorist
NYC Veterinary Specialists
New York, New York
USA

JOHN A. CHRISTIAN, DVM, PhD
Associate Professor
Comparative Pathobiology
School of Veterinary Medicine
Purdue University
West Lafayette, Indiana
USA

RUTHANNE CHUN, DVM
Diplomate ACVIM (Oncology)
Clinical Associate Professor
Department of Medical Sciences
Oncology Section Head, Veterinary Medical
Teaching Hospital
School of Veterinary Medicine
University of Wisconsin–Madison
Madison, Wisconsin
USA

**DAVID CHURCH, BVSc, PhD, MRCVS
FHEA, MACVSc**
Vice Principal (Academic and Clinical Affairs)
Veterinary Clinical Sciences
The Royal Veterinary College
Hatfield
United Kingdom

JOHN J. CIRIBASSI, DVM
Diplomate ACVB
Owner
Chicagoland Veterinary Behavior Consultants
Carol Stream, Illinois
USA

JESSIE M. CLEMANS, DVM
Head Internist
Sugar Land Veterinary Specialists
Sugar Land, Texas
USA

CÉCILE CLERCX, DVM, PhD
Dipomate ECVIM-CA
Professor
Equine and Companion Animal Clinical
Sciences, Companion Animal Internal Medicine
University of Liège
Liège
Belgium

CRAIG CLIFFORD, DVM, MS
Diplomate ACVIM (Oncology)
Director of Clinical Research Oncology
Red Bank Veterinary Hospital
Tinton Falls, New Jersey
USA

JOAN R. COATES, BS, DVM, MS
Diplomate ACVIM (Neurology)
Associate Professor, Veterinary Medicine and
Surgery
Neurologist, Service Chief, Neurology/
Neurosurgery
Veterinary Medical Teaching Hospital
College of Veterinary Medicine
University of Missouri
Columbia, Missouri
USA

**SUSAN M. COCHRANE, BSc, MSc, DVM,
DVSc**
Diplomate ACVIM (Neurology)
Clinical Neurologist
Veterinary Emergency Clinic/Referral Centre
Toronto, Ontario
Canada

STEVEN M. COGAR, DVM
Resident
Small Animal Surgery
College of Veterinary Medicine
University of Georgia
Athens, Georgia
USA

CARMEN M.H. COLITZ, DVM, PhD
Diplomate ACVO
Adjunct Associate Professor
Veterinary Clinical Sciences
Ohio State University
Columbus, Ohio
Molecular Biomedical Sciences
North Carolina State University
Raleigh, North Carolina
USA

LESLIE LARSON COOPER, DVM
Diplomate ACVB
Animal Behavior Counseling and Therapy
Davis, California
USA

RHIAN COPE, BVSc, BSC, PhD, MRCVS
Diplomate American Board of Toxicology,
cGLPCP, ERT
Consultant Toxicologist
The Hague
The Netherlands

LARRY D. COWGILL, DVM, PhD
Diplomate ACVIM (Internal Medicine)
Professor and Associate Dean
Department of Medicine and Epidemiology
School of Veterinary Medicine
University of California, Davis
Davis, California
Head, Hemodialysis/Nephrology Services
VMTH and UCVMC-SD and Director
School of Veterinary Medicine
University of California
Veterinary Medical Center–San Diego
San Diego, California
USA

JOHN M. CRANDELL, DVM
Diplomate ACVIM (Internal Medicine)
Staff Internist
Akron Veterinary Referral and Emergency Center
Akron, Ohio
USA

MITCHELL A. CRYSTAL, DVM
Diplomate ACVIM (Internal Medicine)
Chief of Medicine
North Florida Veterinary Specialists, P.A.
Jacksonville and Orange Park, Florida
USA

PAUL A. CUDDON, BVSc
Diplomate ACVIM (Neurology)
Associate Professor
Department of Clinical Sciences
College of Veterinary Medicine and Biomedical
Sciences
Colorado State University
Fort Collins, Colorado
USA

SUZANNE M. CUNNINGHAM, DVM
Diplomate ACVIM (Cardiology)
Assistant Professor
Clinical Sciences, Cummings School of
Veterinary Medicine
Tufts University
Foster Hospital for Small Animals
North Grafton, Massachusetts
USA

ELIZABETH A. CURRY-GALVIN, DVM
Assistant Director, Scientific Activities
American Veterinary Medical Association
Schaumburg, Illinois
USA

TERRY MARIE CURTIS, DVM, MS
Diplomate ACVB
Clinical Behaviorist
Small Animal Clinical Sciences
College of Veterinary Medicine
University of Florida
Gainesville, Florida
USA

RONALDO CASIMIRO DA COSTA, DVM,
MSc, PhD
Diplomate ACVIM (Neurology)
Assistant Professor and Service Head
Neurology and Neurosurgery Department of
Veterinary Clinical Sciences
Ohio State University
Columbus, Ohio
USA

SHEILA D'ARPINO, DVM
Diplomate ACVB
Senior Applied Animal Behaviorist Center for
Shelter Dogs
Animal Rescue League of Boston
Boston, Massachusetts
USA

TANIA N. DAVEY, BVM&S
MACVSc (Canine Medicine) Internist
Queensland Veterinary Specialists
Stafford Heights, Queensland
Australia

AUTUMN P. DAVIDSON, DVM, MS
Diplomate ACVIM
Clinical Professor, Departments of Medicine and
Epidemiology
University of California, Davis
Staff Internist, Internal Medicine, VCA
Animal Care Center of Sonoma
Davis, California
USA

THOMAS KEVIN DAY, DVM, MS
Diplomate ACVA; Diplomate ACVECC, CVA,
DAAPM
Founder, Medical Director
Louisville Veterinary Specialty and Emergency
Services
Louisville, Kentucky
USA

ALEXANDER DE LAHUNTA, DVM, PhD
Diplomate ACVIM, Diplomate ACVP
James Law Professor of Anatomy—Emeritus
Biomedical Sciences
College of Veterinary Medicine
Cornell University
Ithaca, New York
USA

LOUIS-PHILIPPE DE LORIMIER, Dr. med.
vet Diplomate ACVIM (Oncology)
Staff Medical Oncologist
Hôpital Vétérinaire Rive-Sud
Brossard, Quebec
Canada

HELIO AUTRAN DE MORAIS, DVM, MS,
PhD Diplomate ACVIM (Internal Medicine and
Cardiology)
Associate Professor
Department of Clinical Sciences
College of Veterinary Medicine
Oregon State University
Corvallis, Oregon
USA

TERESA C. DeFRANCESCO, DVM
Diplomate ACVIM (Cardiology); Diplomate
ACVECC
Associate Professor in Cardiology and Critical
Care
Department of Clinical Sciences
College of Veterinary Medicine
North Carolina State University
Raleigh, North Carolina
USA

KRYSTA DEITZ, DVM, MS
Diplomate ACVIM (Small Animal)
Assistant Professor
Veterinary Clinical Sciences
College of Veterinary Medicine, Iowa State
University
Ames, Iowa
USA

SAGI DENENBERG, DVM
North Toronto Animal Clinic
Thornhill, Ontario
Canada

NISHI DHUPA, BVM, MRCVS
Diplomate ACVIM (Internal Medicine);
Diplomate ACVECC
Director, Professional Services
Cornell University Hospital for Animals
Ithaca, New York
USA

STEPHEN P. DiBARTOLA, DVM
Diplomate ACVIM (Internal Medicine)
Professor, Department of Veterinary Clinical
Sciences
Clinician, Veterinary Teaching Hospital
College of Veterinary Medicine
Ohio State University
Columbus, Ohio
USA

DAVID C. DORMAN, DVM, PhD
Diplomate American Board of Veterinary
Toxicology; Diplomate American Board of
Toxicology
Associate Dean
College of Veterinary Medicine
North Carolina State University
Raleigh, North Carolina
USA

EDWARD J. DUBOVI, PhD
Professor of Virology, Director—Virology Section
Animal Health Diagnostic Center
Department of Population Medicine and
Diagnostic Sciences
College of Veterinary Medicine
Cornell University
Ithaca, New York
USA

DAVID DUCLOS, DVM
Diplomate ACVD
Clinician
Animal Skin and Allergy Clinic
Lynnwood, Washington
USA

ERIC K. DUNAYER, MD, VMD
Diplomate American Board of Toxicology;
Diplomate American Board of Veterinary
Toxicology
Adjunct Instructor
Department of Veterinary Biosciences
College of Veterinary Medicine
University of Illinois
Senior Toxicologist
ASPCA Animal Poison Control Center
Urbana, Illinois
USA

CAROLINA DUQUE, DVM, MSc, DVSc
Diplomate ACVIM (Neurology)
Head of Department
Neurology
Mississauga Oakville Veterinary Emergency
Hospital and Referral Group
Oakville, Ontario
Canada

MARC ELIE, DVM
Diplomate ACVIM (Internal Medicine)
Staff Internist
Small Animal Internal Medicine
Michigan Veterinary Specialists
Southfield, Michigan
USA

TIMOTHY M. FAN, DVM, PhD
Diplomate ACVIM (Internal Medicine,
Oncology)
Assistant Professor (Medical Oncology)
Department of Veterinary Clinical Medicine
Veterinary Teaching Hospital
College of Veterinary Medicine
University of Illinois at Urbana-Champaign
Urbana, Illinois
USA

RICHARD A. FAYRER-HOSKEN, BVSc, PhD,
MRCVS
Diplomate American College of
Theriogenologists; Diplomate ECAR
Professor
Department of Large Animal Medicine
College of Veterinary Medicine
University of Georgia
Athens, Georgia
USA

ANDREA M. FINNEN, DVM
Senior Resident in Neurology, Départment de
Sciences Cliniques Veterinarian, Clinique des
Animaux de Compagnie
Centre Hospitalier Universitaire
Vétérinaire
Faculté de Médecine Vétérinaire
Université de Montréal
St. Hyacinthe, Quebec
Canada

KEVIN FINORA, DVM
Diplomate ACVIM (Small Animal Internal
Medicine and Oncology)
Staff Oncologist/Staff Internist
Veterinary Emergency Clinic & Referral Centre
Toronto, Ontario
Canada

SCOTT D. FITZGERALD, DVM, PhD
Diplomate ACVP; Diplomate ACPV
Professor
Department of Pathology and Diagnostic
Investigation
College of Veterinary Medicine
Michigan State University
East Lansing, Michigan
USA

GERRARD FLANNIGAN, BSc, DVM, MSc
Diplomate ACVB
Associate Veterinary Behaviorist
Carolina Veterinary Specialists
Greensboro, North Carolina
USA

S. DRU FORRESTER, DVM, MS
Diplomate ACVIM
Associate Director, Scientific Affairs
Hill's Pet Nutrition
Topeka, Kansas
Adjunct Faculty
Department of Clinical Sciences
College of Veterinary Medicine
Kansas State University
Manhattan, Kansas
USA

THERESA FOSSUM, DVM, MS, PhD
Diplomate ACVS
Director, Professor of Surgery
Texas A&M Institute for Preclinical Studies
Texas A&M University
College Station, Texas
USA

LINDA A. FRANK, DVM, MS
Diplomate ACVD
Professor
Small Animal Clinical Sciences
College of Veterinary Medicine
University of Tennessee
Knoxville, Tennessee
USA

JONI L. FRESHMAN, DVM, MS
Diplomate ACVIM (Internal Medicine)
Owner
AcuPets Mobile Veterinary Acupuncture and
Canine Consultations
Colorado Springs, Colorado
USA

VIRGINIA LUIS FUENTES, MA, VetMB,
PhD, MRCVS
Diplomate ACVIM (Cardiology); Diplomate
ECVIM-CA (Cardiology)
Senior Lecturer
Department of Veterinary Clinical Sciences
Royal Veterinary College
Hatfield
United Kingdom

LUIS GAITERO, DVM
Diplomate European College of Veterinary
Neurology
Assistant Professor
Department of Clinical Studies
Ontario Veterinary College
University of Guelph
Guelph, Ontario
Canada

JOAO FELIPE DE BRITO GALVAO, MV
Resident
Department of Veterinary Clinical Sciences
Veterinary Teaching Hospital
College of Veterinary Medicine
Ohio State University
Columbus, Ohio
USA

TAM GARLAND, DVM, PhD
Diplomate American Board of Veterinary
Toxicology
Section Head
Toxicology and Drug Testing
Texas Veterinary Medical Diagnostic Laboratory
Texas A&M University
College Station, Texas
USA

LAURENT GAROSI, DVM, MRCVS
Diplomate European College of Veterinary
Neurology
Head of Neurology/Neurosurgery
Davies Veterinary Specialists
Higham Gobion, Hertfordshire
United Kingdom

LAURA D. GARRETT, DVM
Diplomate ACVIM (Oncology)
Clinical Assistant Professor
Department of Veterinary Clinical Medicine
College of Veterinary Medicine
University of Illinois
Urbana, Illinois
USA

CATHY GARTLEY, DVM, DVSc
Diplomate American College of
Theriogenologists
Assistant Professor, Theriogenology
Department of Population Medicine
Ontario Veterinary College
University of Guelph
Guelph, Ontario
Canada

LORI GASKINS, DVM
Diplomate ACVB
Assistant Professor
Clinical Sciences
School of Veterinary Medicine
St. Matthew's University
Grand Cayman
Cayman Islands

ANNA R.M. GELZER, Dr. med. vet.
Diplomate ACVIM (Cardiology)
Assistant Professor
Department of Clinical Sciences
College of Veterinary Medicine
Cornell University
Ithaca, New York
USA

ANNE GEMENSKY METZLER, DVM, MS
Diplomate ACVO
Associate Professor
Veterinary Clinical Sciences
College of Veterinary Medicine
Ohio State University
Columbus, Ohio
USA

BRIAN C. GILGER, DVM, MS
Diplomate ACVO; Diplomate ABT
Professor
Department of Clinical Sciences
North Carolina State University
Raleigh, North Carolina
USA

MARGI A. GILMOUR, DVM
Diplomate ACVO
Associate Professor
Veterinary Clinical Sciences
Oklahoma State University
Stillwater, Oklahoma
USA

ERIC GLASS, DVM
Diplomate ACVIM (Neurology)
Section Head
Neurology and Neurosurgery
Red Bank Veterinary Hospital
Tinton Falls, New Jersey
USA

MATHIEU M. GLASSMAN, VMD, DACVS
Senior Small Animal Surgery Resident
College of Veterinary Medicine
University of Georgia
Athens, Georgia
Friendship Animal Hospital
Washington, DC
USA

CECILIA GORREL, BSc, MA, DDS, Vet MB,
MRCVS
Diplomate European Veterinary Dental College,
Hon Fellow Academy of Veterinary Dentistry
Director
Petdent Ltd.
Hampshire
United Kingdom

SHARON FOOSHEE GRACE, MS, M.Agric.,
DVM
Diplomate ABVP (Canine/Feline); Diplomate
ACVIM (Small Animal)
Clinical Professor
Department of Clinical Sciences
College of Veterinary Medicine
Mississippi State University
Mississippi State, Mississippi USA

W. DUNBAR GRAM, DVM, MRCVS
Diplomate ACVD
Lecturer in Veterinary Dermatology
The Royal (Dick) School of Veterinary Studies
The University of Edinburgh
Roslin
Scotland
Dermatologist, Dermatology Department
Animal Allergy and Dermatology
Virginia Beach, Virginia
USA

GREGORY F. GRAUER, DVM, MS
Diplomate ACVIM
Professor and Jarvis Chair of Small Animal
Internal Medicine
Department of Clinical Sciences
Veterinary Teaching Hospital
College of Veterinary Medicine
Kansas State University
Manhattan, Kansas
USA

THOMAS K. GRAVES, DVM, PhD
Diplomate ACVIM
Assistant Professor of Small Animal Medicine,
Assistant Department Head
Department of Veterinary Clinical Medicine
College of Veterinary Medicine
University of Illinois at Urbana-Champaign
Chief of Small Animal Internal Medicine
Veterinary Teaching Hospital
University of Illinois
Urbana, Illinois
USA

DEBORAH S. GRECO, DVM, PhD
Diplomate ACVIM
Senior Research Scientist Petcare
Nestle Purina
New York, New York
USA

JEAN S. GREEK, DVM
Diplomate ACVD
Dermatology and Allergy Clinic for Animals
Santa Barbara, California
USA

KURT A. GRIMM, DVM, MS, PhD
Diplomate ACVA; Diplomate ACVCP
Anesthesiologist
Veterinary Specialist Services, PC
Conifer, Colorado
USA

AMY GROOTERS, DVM
Diplomate ACVIM
Professor
Department of Veterinary Clinical Sciences
School of Veterinary Medicine
Louisiana State University
Baton Rouge, Louisiana
USA

SOPHIE A. GRUNDY, BVSc (Hons), MACVSc
Diplomate ACVIM
Internist
Northern California Veterinary Specialists
Sacramento, California
USA

NITA KAY GULBAS, DVM
Private Practice
Phoenix, Arizona
USA

SHARON GWALTNEY-BRANT, DVM, PhD
Diplomate American Board of Veterinary
Toxicology, Diplomate American Board of
Toxicology
Vice President and Medical Director, ASPCA
Animal Poison Control Center Adjunct
Instructor, Department of Veterinary Biosciences
College of Veterinary Medicine
University of Illinois
Urbana, Illinois
USA

TIM B. HACKETT, DVM, MS
Diplomate American College of Veterinary
Emergency and Critical Care Associate Professor,
Department of Clinical Sciences
Small Animal Chief of Staff, James L. Voss
Veterinary Teaching Hospital
Colorado State University
Fort Collins, Colorado
USA

DEBORAH J. HADLOCK, VMD
Diplomate American Board of Veterinary
Practitioners (Canine and Feline); Certified
Veterinary Acupuncturist (CVA)
Senior Veterinarian
Telemedicine
Idexx Laboratories Inc.
Totowa, New Jersey
USA

FRASER A. HALE, DVM
Fellow Academy of Veterinary Dentistry,
Diplomate American Veterinary Dental College
Owner
Hale Veterinary Clinic
Guelph, Ontario
Canada

BARRON P. HALL, DVM
Diplomate American Veterinary Dental College,
Fellow Academy of Veterinary Dentistry
Owner
Animal Dental Clinic
Vienna, Virginia
USA

JEFFERY O. HALL, DVM, PhD
Diplomate American Board of Veterinary
Toxicology
Professor, Head of Diagnostic Veterinary
Toxicology
Animal, Dairy and Veterinary Sciences
Department
Utah State University
Logan, Utah
USA

ROBERT L. HAMLIN, DVM, PhD
ACVIM (Cardiology, Internal Medicine)
Professor
Department of Veterinary Biosciences, Exercise
Physiology and Biomedical Engineering
College of Veterinary Medicine
Ohio State University
Columbus, Ohio
USA

STEVEN R. HANSEN, DVM, MS, MBA
Diplomate American Board of Veterinary
Toxicology
Senior Vice President, ASPCA, Animal Health
Services
Adjunct Professor, Department of Veterinary
Biosciences
University of Illinois
Urbana and Champaign, Illinois
USA

TISHA A.M. HARPER, DVM, MS
Diplomate ACVS
Assistant Professor
Department of Small Animal Clinical Sciences
Virginia-Maryland Regional College of
Veterinary Medicine
Virginia Tech University
Blacksburg, Virginia
USA

JOHN W. HARVEY, DVM, PhD
Diplomate ACVP
Executive Associate Dean
Department of Physiological Sciences
College of Veterinary Medicine
University of Florida
Gainesville, Florida
USA

ELEANOR C. HAWKINS, DVM
Diplomate ACVIM (Small Animal Internal
Medicine)
Professor
Department of Clinical Sciences
College of Veterinary Medicine
North Carolina State University
Raleigh, North Carolina
USA

CRISTINE L. HAYES, DVM
Consulting Veterinarian in Clinical Toxicology
ASPCA Animal Poison Control Center
Urbana, Illinois
USA

KAREN HELTON RHODES, DVM
Diplomate ACVD
Owner
Riverdale Veterinary Dermatology
Riverdale, New Jersey
USA

ROSEMARY A. HENIK, DVM, MS
Diplomate ACVIM (Small Animal Internal
Medicine)
Mobile Veterinary Echocardiography
New Smyrna Beach, Florida
USA

MELISSA A. HERRERA, DVM
Diplomate ACVIM (Internal Medicine)
Ventura Medical and Surgical Group
Ventura, California
USA

IAN P. HERRING, DVM, MS
Diplomate ACVO
Associate Professor
Department of Small Animal Clinical Sciences
Virginia-Maryland Regional College of
Veterinary Medicine
Virginia Tech
Blacksburg, Virginia
USA

MILAN HESS, DVM, MS
Diplomate American College of
Theriogenologists
Staff Theriogenologist
Colorado Veterinary Specialists
Centennial, Colorado
USA

LORA S. HITCHCOCK, DVM
Diplomate ACVIM (Cardiology)
Cardiologist
Ohio Veterinary Cardiology, Ltd.
Metropolitan Veterinary Hospital
Akron, Ohio
USA

MARK E. HITT, DVM, MS
Diplomate ACVIM (Internal Medicine)
Chief of Medicine
Atlantic Veterinary Internal Medicine, LLC
Annapolis, Maryland
USA

JUDY HOLDING, DVM, BS, RN
Consulting Veterinarian in Clinical Toxicology
ASPCA Animal Poison Control Center
Urbana, Illinois
USA

STEPHEN B. HOOSER, DVM, PhD
Diplomate American Board of Veterinary
Toxicology
Professor, Comparative Pathology Director,
Indiana Animal Disease Diagnostic Laboratory
School of Veterinary Medicine
Purdue University
West Lafayette, Indiana
USA

KATE HOPPER, BVSc, MVS
Diplomate ACVECC
Assistant Professor
Veterinary Surgical and Radiological Sciences
University of California, Davis
Davis, California
USA

DEBRA F. HORWITZ, DVM
Diplomate ACVB
Owner
Veterinary Behavior Consultations
St. Louis, Missouri
USA

JOHNNY D. HOSKINS, DVM, PhD
Diplomate ACVIM (Internal Medicine)
Small Animal Consultant
DocuTech Services, Inc.
Choudrant, Louisiana
USA

KATHERINE A. HOUPT, VMD, PhD
Diplomate ACVB
Professor
Department of Clinical Sciences
College of Veterinary Medicine
Cornell University
Ithaca, New York
USA

WAYNE HUNTHAUSEN, DVM
Director
Animal Behavior Consultations
Westwood, Kansas
USA

KAREN DYER INZANA, DVM, PhD
Diplomate ACVIM (Neurology)
Professor
Department of Small Animal Clinical Sciences
Virginia-Maryland Regional College of
Veterinary Medicine
Virginia Tech
Blacksburg, Virginia
USA

JULIE ANN JARVINEN, MA, PhD, DVM
Associate Professor
Department of Veterinary Pathology
College of Veterinary Medicine
Iowa State University
Ames, Iowa
USA

ALBERT E. JERGENS, DVM, PhD
Diplomate ACVIM (Internal Medicine)
Professor, Department of Veterinary Clinical
Sciences
Internist, Lloyd Veterinary Medical Center
College of Veterinary Medicine
Iowa State University
Ames, Iowa
USA

LYNELLE R. JOHNSON, DVM, MS, PhD
Diplomate ACVIM (Internal Medicine)
Associate Professor
Department of Veterinary Medicine and
Epidemiology
University of California, Davis
Davis, California
USA

SPENCER A. JOHNSTON, VMD
Diplomate ACVS
Edward H. Gunst Professor of Small Animal
Surgery
Small Animal Medicine and Surgery
College of Veterinary Medicine
University of Georgia
Athens, Georgia
USA

RICHARD J. JOSEPH, DVM
Diplomate ACVIM (Neurology)
Neurologist, President
Animal Specialty Center
Yonkers, New York
USA

BRUCE W. KEENE, DVM, MSc
Diplomate ACVIM (Cardiology)
Professor, Clinical Sciences
Attending Cardiologist, Veterinary Teaching
Hospital
College of Veterinary Medicine
North Carolina State University
Raleigh, North Carolina
USA

MARC KENT, DVM
Diplomate ACVIM (Internal Medicine,
Neurology)
Associate Professor
Small Animal Medicine and Surgery
College of Veterinary Medicine
University of Georgia
Athens, Georgia
USA

RICHARD D. KIENLE, DVM
Diplomate ACVIM (Cardiology)
Owner/Cardiologist
Mission Valley Veterinary Cardiology
Gilroy, California
USA

LESLEY G. KING, MVB
Diplomate ACVECC; Diplomate ACVIM
Professor, Critical Care
Department of Clinical Studies—Philadephia
School of Veterinary Medicine
Director, Intensive Care Unit
Ryan Veterinary Hospital
University of Pennsylvania
Philadelphia, Pennsylvania
USA

PETER P. KINTZER, DVM
Diplomate ACVIM
Internal Medicine Consultant
Idexx Laboratories Inc.
Westbrook, Maine
USA

REBECCA KIRBY, DVM
Diplomate ACVIM (Internal Medicine);
Diplomate ACVECC
Executive Director
Animal Emergency Center
Glendale, Wisconsin
USA

MARK D. KITTLESON, DVM, PhD
Diplomate ACVIM (Cardiology)
Professor, Medicine and Epidemiology
William R. Pritchard Veterinary Medical
Teaching Hospital
School of Veterinary Medicine
University of California, Davis
Davis, California
USA

JEFFREY S. KLAUSNER, DVM, MS
Diplomate, ACVIM (Internal Medicine, Oncology)
Dean
College of Veterinary Medicine
University of Minnesota
St. Paul, Minnesota
USA

THOMAS KLEIN, DVM
Adjunct Professor of Veterinary Dentistry
Department of Small Animal Medicine, The Ohio State University
Owner, East Hilliard Veterinary Services
Columbus and Hilliard, Ohio
USA

MARY P. KLINCK, DVM
Diplomate ACVB
Faculté de Médecine Vétérinaire
Université de Montréal
St. Hyacinthe, Quebec
Canada

MARGUERITE KNIPE, DVM
Diplomate ACVIM (Neurology)
Health Sciences Assistant
Clinical Professor, Neurology/Neurosurgery
Department of Surgical and Radiological Sciences
William R. Pritchard Veterinary Medical Teaching Hospital
University of California, Davis
Davis, California
USA

JOYCE S. KNOLL, VMD, PhD
Diplomate ACVP (Clinical Pathology)
Associate Professor
Department of Biomedical Sciences
Cummings School of Veterinary Medicine
Tufts University
North Grafton, Massachusetts
USA

BARBARA KOHN, Dr. med. vet., Prof
Diplomate ECVIM-CA (Internal Medicine)
Professor and Head, Small Animal Medicine
Faculty of Veterinary Medicine
Freie Universität Berlin
Berlin
Germany

ANITA M. KORE, DVM, PhD
Diplomate American Board of Veterinary Toxicology
Lead Toxicology Specialist
Medical Department
3M Company
St. Paul, Minnesota
USA

MARC S. KRAUS, DVM
Diplomate ACVIM (Cardiology, Internal Medicine)
Senior Lecturer
Department of Clinical Sciences
College of Veterinary Medicine
Cornell University
Ithaca, New York
USA

ANNEMARIE T. KRISTENSEN, DVM, PhD
Diplomate ACVIM-SA; Diplomate ECVIM-CA & Oncology
Professor
Department of Small Animal Clinical Sciences
Faculty of Life Sciences
University of Copenhagen
Copenhagen
Denmark

JOHN M. KRUGER, DVM, PhD
Diplomate ACVIM
Professor
Small Animal Clinical Sciences
Veterinary Teaching Hospital
Michigan State University
East Lansing, Michigan
USA

NED F. KUEHN, DVM, MS
Diplomate ACVIM (Small Animal Internal Medicine)
Chief of Internal Medicine Services
Department of Internal Medicine
Michigan Veterinary Specialists
Southfield, Michigan
USA

KAREN A. KUHL, DVM
Diplomate ACVD
Midwest Veterinary Dermatology Center
Buffalo Grove, Illinois
USA

DOROTHY P. LAFLAMME, DVM, PhD
Diplomate ACVN
Veterinary Nutritionist
Research
Nestle Purina Petcare
St. Louis, Missouri
USA

LEIGH A. LAMONT, DVM, MS
Diplomate ACVA
Associate Professor of Anesthesiology
Department of Companion Animals
Atlantic Veterinary College
University of Prince Edward Island
Charlottetown, Prince Edward Island
Canada

GARY LANDSBERG, BSc, DVM, MRCVS
Diplomate ACVB; Diplomate ECVBM-CA
Adjunct Professor
University of Guelph
Guelph, Ontario
Veterinary Behaviorist
North Toronto Animal Clinic
Thornhill, Ontario
Canada

OTTO I. LANZ, DVM
Diplomate ACVS
Associate Professor
Department of Small Animal Clinical Sciences
Virginia-Maryland Regional College of Veterinary Medicine
Virginia Tech
Blacksburg, Virginia
USA

KENNETH S. LATIMER, DVM, PhD
Diplomate ACVP (Clinical Pathology)
Professor
Department of Pathology
College of Veterinary Medicine
University of Georgia
Athens, Georgia
USA

SUSANNE K. LAUER, Dr. med. vet.
Diplomate ACVS: CCRP
Associate Professor
Department of Veterinary Clinical Sciences
School of Veterinary Medicine
Louisiana State University
Baton Rouge, Louisiana
USA

MYLÈNE-KIM LECLERC, DVM
Neurology Clinician
Départment de Sciences Cliniques
Clinique des Animaux de Compagnie
Centre Hospitalier Universitaire Vétérinaire
Faculté de Médecine Vétérinaire
Université de Montréal
St. Hyacinthe, Quebec
Canada

RICHARD A. LeCOUTEUR, BVSc, PhD
Professor
Department of Surgical and Radiological Sciences
University of California, Davis
Davis, California
USA

GEORGE E. LEES, DVM, MS
Diplomate ACVIM (Small Animal Internal Medicine)
Professor
Small Animal Clinical Sciences
College of Veterinary Medicine
Texas A&M University
College Station, Texas
USA

ALFRED M. LEGENDRE, DVM, MS
Diplomate ACVIM (Internal Medicine and Oncology)
Professor of Medicine and Oncology
Department of Small Animal Clinical Sciences
College of Veterinary Medicine
University of Tennessee
Knoxville, Tennessee
USA

JOSE A. LEN, DVM, MS
Diplomate American College of Theriogenologists
Clinical Instructor, Theriogenology Veterinary Clinical Sciences
School of Veterinary Medicine
Louisiana State University
Baton Rouge, Louisiana
USA

MICHAEL B. LESSER, DVM
Diplomate ACVIM (Cardiology); Diplomate
ECVIM-CA (Cardiology)
Hospital Director
Advanced Veterinary Care Center
Lawndale, California
USA

EMILY D. LEVINE, DVM, MRCVS
Diplomate ACVB
Animal Emergency Referral Associates
Fairfield, New Jersey
USA

JONATHAN M. LEVINE, DVM
Diplomate ACVIM (Neurology)
Assistant Professor, Neurology/Neurosurgery
Fellow, Texas Brain and Spine Institute
Department of Small Animal Clinical Sciences
College of Veterinary Medicine and Biomedical
Sciences
Texas A&M University
College Station, TX
USA

STEVEN A. LEVY, VMD
President
Veterinary Clinical and Consulting Services LLC
Kansas City, Missouri
USA

ELLEN M. LINDELL, VMD
Diplomate ACVB
Practice Owner
Veterinary Behavior Consultations
Pleasant Valley, New York
USA

DAVID LIPSITZ, DVM
Diplomate ACVIM (Neurology)
Veterinary Specialty Hospital
San Diego, California
USA

HEIDI B. LOBPRISE, DVM
Diplomate American Veterinarian Dental College
Virbac Corporation
Fort Worth, Texas
USA

DAWN E. LOGAS, DVM
Diplomate ACVD
Owner/Staff Dermatologist
Veterinary Dermatology Center
Maitland, Florida
USA

KATHRYN M. LONG, DVM
Diplomate American College of Veterinary
Emergency/Critical Care
Colorado Veterinary Specialists and Emergency
Services
Littleton, Colorado
USA

CHERYL LOPATE, DVM, MS
Diplomate American College of
Theriogenologists
President and Veterinarian
Reproductive Revolutions, Inc.
Aurora, Oregon
USA

CARROLL LOYER, DVM
Diplomate ACVIM (Cardiology)
Cardiologist
Veterinary Heart & Lung Specialists
Englewood, Colorado
USA

JODY P. LULICH, DVM, PhD
Diplomate ACVIM (Internal Medicine)
Professor
Department of Veterinary Clinical Sciences
College of Veterinary Medicine
University of Minnesota
St. Paul, Minnesota
USA

SARA K. LYLE, DVM, MS
Diplomate American College of
Theriogenologists
Clinical Instructor
Veterinary Clinical Sciences
School of Veterinary Medicine
Louisiana State University
Baton Rouge, Louisiana
USA

CATRIONA MacPHAIL, DVM, PhD
Diplomate ACVS
Associate Professor of Small Animal Surgery
Department of Clinical Studies
Colorado State University
Fort Collins, Colorado
USA

PETER MacWILLIAMS, DVM, PhD
Diplomate ACVP
Emeritus Professor
Department of Pathobiological Sciences
School of Veterinary Medicine
University of Wisconsin–Madison
Madison, Wisconsin
Clinical Pathologist
Marshfield Clinic Veterinary Laboratory
Marshfield, Wisconsin
USA

GUILLERMINA MANIGOT
Diplomate UBA Veterinary Medicine
(Universidad de Buenos Aires)
Director—Dermatologist
Dermlink Buenos Aires
Buenos Aires
Argentina

KATIA MARIONI-HENRY, DVM, PhD,
MRCVS
Diplomate ACVIM (Neurology); Diplomate
European College of Veterinary Neurology
Neurologist
Neurology/Neurosurgery
Southern Counties Veterinary Specialists
Ringwood, Hampshire
United Kingdom

STEVEN L. MARKS, BVSc, MS, MRCVS
Diplomate ACVIM (Internal Medicine)
Clinical Associate Professor
Department of Clinical Sciences
College of Veterinary Medicine
North Carolina State University
Raleigh, North Carolina
USA

KENNETH V. MASON, Bsc, MVSc FACVSc
(Veterinary Dermatology)
Adjunct Professor
Veterinary Science
University of Queensland
Brisbane
Australia

CHRISTIANE MASSICOTTE, DVM, MS,
PhD
Diplomate ACVIM (Neurology)
Neurologist, Department of Neurology
Animal Emergency and Referral Associates
Fairfield, New Jersey
Adjunct Faculty, Clinical Studies
University of Pennsylvania
Philadelphia, Pennsylvania
USA

ELIZABETH R. MAY, DVM
Diplomate ACVD
Assistant Professor
Veterinary Clinical Sciences
Iowa State University
Ames, Iowa
USA

ELISA M. MAZZAFERRO, MS, DVM, PhD
Diplomate American College of Veterinary
Emergency and Critical Care
Director of Emergency Services
Wheat Ridge Animal Hospital
Wheat Ridge, Colorado
USA

TERRI L. McCALLA, DVM, MS
Diplomate ACVO
Practice Owner
Animal Eye Care, LLC
Bellingham, Washington
USA

PATRICK L. McDONOUGH, MS, PhD
Associate Professor
Population Medicine and Diagnostic Sciences
Animal Health Diagnostic Center
College of Veterinary Medicine
Cornell University
Ithaca, New York
USA

BRENDAN C. McKIERNAN, DVM
Diplomate ACVIM (Small Animal Internal
Medicine)
Staff Internist
Southern Oregon Veterinary Specialty Center
Medford, Oregon
USA

RON M. McLAUGHLIN, DVM, DVSc
Diplomate ACVS
Professor and Chief, Small Animal Surgery
Head, Department of Clinical Sciences
College of Veterinary Medicine
Mississippi State University
Mississippi State, Mississippi
USA

CHARLOTTE MEANS, DVM, MLIS
Diplomate American Board of Veterinary
Toxicology
Senior Toxicologist
ASPCA Animal Poison Control Center
Urbana, Illinois
USA

DONNA MENSCHING, DVM, MS
Diplomate American Board of Veterinary
Toxicology; Diplomate American Board of
Toxicology
Senior Toxicologist
ASPCA Animal Poison Control Center
Urbana, Illinois
USA

JOANNE B. MESSICK, VMD, PhD
Diplomate ACVP
Associate Professor
Comparative Pathobiology
Purdue University
West Lafayette, Indiana
USA

KATHRYN M. MEURS, DVM, PhD
Diplomate ACVIM (Cardiology)
Professor
North Carolina State
College of Veterinary Medicine
Raleigh, North Carolina
USA

CARRIE J. MILLER, DVM
Diplomate ACVIM
Internist
Internal Medicine
Wheat Ridge Veterinary Specialists
Wheat Ridge, Colorado
USA

MATTHEW W. MILLER, DVM, MS
Diplomate ACVIM (Cardiology)
Professor of Cardiology/Senior Staff Cardiologist
Veterinary Small Animal Clinical Sciences
Veterinary Teaching Hospital
Texas A&M University
College Station, Texas
USA

PAUL E. MILLER, DVM
Diplomate ACVO
Clinical Professor of Comparative
Ophthalmology
Department of Surgical Sciences
School of Veterinary Medicine
University of Wisconsin–Madison
Madison, Wisconsin
USA

KELLY MOFFAT, DVM
Diplomate ACVB
Medical Director
VCA Mesa Animal Hospital
Mesa, Arizona
USA

N. SYDNEY MOISE, DVM, MS
Diplomate ACVIM (Cardiology and Internal
Medicine)
Professor
Clinical Sciences
College of Veterinary Medicine
Cornell University
Ithaca, New York
USA

LISA E. MOORE, DVM
Diplomate ACVIM (Small Animal Internal
Medicine)
Internist
Affiliated Veterinary Specialists
Maitland, Florida
USA

DANIEL O. MORRIS, DVM, MPH
Diplomate ACVD
Associate Professor of Dermatology
Department of Clinical Studies
School of Veterinary Medicine
University of Pennsylvania
Philadelphia, Pennsylvania
USA

JoANN MORRISON, DVM, MS
Diplomate ACVIM (Internal Medicine)
Clinician
Veterinary Clinical Sciences
College of Veterinary Medicine
Iowa State University
Ames, Iowa
USA

WALLACE B. MORRISON, DVM, MS
Diplomate ACVIM (Small Animal)
Professor
Department of Veterinary Clinical Sciences
Veterinary Teaching Hospital
School of Veterinary Medicine
Purdue University
West Lafayette, Indiana
USA

BRADLEY L. MOSES, DVM
Diplomate ACVIM (Cardiology)
Senior Clinician
VCA Roberts Animal Hospital
VCA South Shore Animal Hospital
Hanover and South Weymouth, Massachusetts
USA

JOCELYN MOTT, DVM
Diplomate ACVIM (Small Animal Internal
Medicine)
Internist
Pasadena Veterinary Specialists
South Pasadena, California
USA

KAREN R. MUÑANA, DVM, MS
Diplomate ACVIM (Neurology)
Associate Professor
Department of Clinical Sciences
College of Veterinary Medicine
North Carolina State University
Raleigh, North Carolina
USA

MICHAEL J. MURPHY, DVM, PhD, JD
Diplomate American Board of Veterinary
Toxicology; Diplomate American Board of
Toxicology
U.S. Food and Drug Administration
Washington, DC
USA

ANTHONY J. MUTSAERS, DVM
Diplomate ACVIM (Oncology)
NCIC—Terry Fox Foundation Fellow Molecular
and Cellular Biology
Sunnybrook Health Sciences Centre Medical
Biophysics
University of Toronto
Toronto, Ontario
Canada

KRISTINA NARFSTRÖM, DVM, PhD
Diplomate ECVO
Professor, Department of Veterinary Medicine &
Surgery, College of Veterinary Medicine
Professor, Department of Ophthalmology, Mason
Eye Institute University of Missouri
Columbia, Missouri
USA

REGG D. NEIGER, DVM, PhD
Professor
Department of Veterinary Science
South Dakota State University
Brookings, South Dakota
USA

REBECCA G. NEWMAN, DVM, MS
Diplomate ACVIM (Oncology)
Medical Oncologist
Pittsburgh Veterinary Specialty and Emergency
Center
Pittsburgh, Pennsylvania
USA

RHETT NICHOLS, DVM
Diplomate ACVIM (Internal Medicine)
Consultant
Internal Medicine
Antech Diagnostics
Lake Success, New York
USA

GARY D. NORSWORTHY, DVM
Diplomate ABVP (Feline)
Owner and Chief of Staff
Alamo Feline Health Center
San Antonio, Texas
Adjunct Professor
Department of Clinical Sciences
College of Veterinary Medicine
Mississippi State University
Mississippi State, Mississippi
USA

DENNIS P. O'BRIEN, DVM, PhD
Diplomate ACVIM (Neurology)
Professor of Neurology
Department of Veterinary Medicine & Surgery
Neurologist
Neurology and Neurosurgery, Veterinary Medical
Teaching Hospital
College of Veterinary Medicine
University of Missouri
Columbia, Missouri
USA

FREDERICK W. OEHME, DVM, PhD
Diplomate American Board of Veterinary
Toxicology
Professor of Toxicology, Pathobiology, Medicine
and Physiology
Comparative Toxicology Laboratories
Departments of Diagnostic Medicine and
Pathobiology
College of Veterinary Medicine
Kansas State University
Manhattan, Kansas
USA

NATASHA J. OLBY, VetMB, PhD
Diplomate ACVIM (Neurology)
Associate Professor (Neurology/Neurosurgery)
Department of Clinical Sciences
College of Veterinary Medicine
North Carolina State University
Raleigh, North Carolina
USA

GAVIN L. OLSEN, DVM
Resident
Adjunct Instructor
Veterinary Clinical Sciences
College of Veterinary Medicine
Iowa State University
Ames, Iowa
USA

CARL A. OSBORNE, DVM, PhD
Diplomate AVCIM
Professor
Veterinary Clinical Sciences Department
University of Minnesota
St. Paul, Minnesota
USA

GARY D. OSWEILER, DVM, PhD
Diplomate American Board of Veterinary
Toxicology
Professor
Veterinary Diagnostic and Production Animal
Medicine
Veterinary Diagnostic Laboratory
College of Veterinary Medicine
Iowa State University
Ames, Iowa
USA

JENNIFER L. OWEN, DVM, PhD
Clinical Pathology Resident
Department of Physical Sciences
College of Veterinary Medicine
University of Florida
Gainesville, Florida
USA

MARK PAPICH, DVM, MS
Professor of Clinical Pharmacology
Department of Molecular Biomedical Sciences
College of Veterinary Medicine
North Carolina State University
Raleigh, North Carolina
USA

JOANE M. PARENT, DVM, MVetSc
Diplomate ACVIM (Neurology)
Professor
Sciences Cliniques
Centre Hospitalier Universitaire Vétérinaire,
Universitéde Montréal
St. Hyacinthe, Quebec
Canada

MARLENE PARISER, DVM
Animal Allergy and Dermatology
Chesapeake, Virginia
USA

JOHN S. PARKER, BVM&S, PhD
Associate Professor
Baker Institute for Animal Health
College of Veterinary Medicine
Cornell University
Ithaca, New York
USA

VALERIE J. PARKER, DVM
Internal Medicine Resident
Small Animal Internal Medicine
College of Veterinary Medicine
Iowa State University
Ames, Iowa
USA

ALLAN J. PAUL, DVM, MS
Professor
Department of Pathobiology
College of Veterinary Medicine
University of Illinois
Urbana, Illinois
USA

R. MICHAEL PEAK, DVM
Diplomate American Veterinary Dental College
Chief of Dentistry
Tampa Bay Veterinary Specialists
Largo, Florida
USA

DOMINIQUE PEETERS, DVM, PhD
Diplomate ECVIM-CA
Assistant Professor
Equine and Companion Animal Clinical Sciences
Companion Animal Internal Medicine
University of Liège
Liège
Belgium

MICHAEL E. PETERSON, DVM, MS
Instructor, Toxicology
College of Veterinary Medicine
Oregon State University
Corvallis, Oregon
Associate Veterinarian
Reid Veterinary Hospital
Albany, Oregon
USA

J. PHILLIP PICKETT, DVM
Diplomate ACVO
Professor
Department of Small Animal Clinical Sciences
Virginia-Maryland Regional College of
Veterinary Medicine
Virginia Tech
Blacksburg, Virginia
USA

CARLOS R.F. PINTO, MedVet, PhD
Diplomate American College of
Theriogenologists
Associate Professor
Department of Veterinary Clinical Sciences
Ohio State University
Columbus, OH
USA

KONNIE H. PLUMLEE, DVM, MS
Diplomate ACVIM; Diplomate American Board
of Veterinary Toxicology
Laboratory Director
Veterinary Diagnostic Laboratory
AR Livestock & Poultry Commission
Little Rock, Arkansas
USA

DAVID J. POLZIN, DVM, PhD
Diplomate ACVIM (Internal Medicine)
Professor
Department of Veterinary Clinical Sciences
University of Minnesota
St. Paul, Minnesota
USA

ROBERTO POMA, Dr. med. vet., DVSc
Diplomate ACVIM (Neurology)
Assistant Professor
Department of Clinical Studies
Veterinary Teaching Hospital
Ontario Veterinary College
University of Guelph
Guelph, Ontario
Canada

JILL S. POMRANTZ, DVM
Diplomate ACVIM
Director of Internal Medicine
ASPCA—Bergh Memorial Animal Hospital
New York, New York
USA

ERIC R. POPE, DVM, MS
Diplomate ACVS
Professor, Small Animal Surgery
Clinical Sciences
School of Veterinary Medicine
Ross University
St. Kitts
West Indies

ROBERT H. POPPENGA, DVM, PhD
Diplomate American Board of Veterinary
Toxicology
Professor of Clinical Veterinary Toxicology
California Animal Health and Food Safety
Laboratory
School of Veterinary Medicine
University of California, Davis
Davis, California
USA

ERIN PORTILLO, DVM, MS
Diplomate ACVIM (Small Animal Internal
Medicine)
Medical Director
Mangrove Veterinary Hospital
Chico, California
USA

SIMON A. POT, DVM
Assistant Professor, Veterinary Ophthalmology
Equine Clinic
University of Zurich
Zurich
Switzerland

MICHELLE PRESSEL, DVM
Diplomate ACVIM (Internal Medicine)
Internist
Pacific Veterinary Specialists
Capitola, California
USA

BARRAK M. PRESSLER, DVM, PhD
Diplomate ACVIM
Assistant Professor
Veterinary Clinical Sciences
School of Veterinary Medicine
Purdue University
West Lafayete, Indiana
USA

JAMES C. PRUETER, DVM
Diplomate ACVIM
Director
Shaker Animal Clinic
Shaker Heights, Ohio
USA

DAVID A. PUERTO, DVM
Diplomate ACVS
Chief of Surgery
Center for Animal Referral and Emergency
Services (CARES)
Langhorne, Pennsylvania
USA

BEVERLY J. PURSWELL, DVM, PhD
Diplomate American College of Therigenologists
Professor
Large Animal Clinical Sciences
Virginia-Maryland Regional College of
Veterinary Medicine
Virginia Tech
Blacksburg, Virginia
USA

LISA RADOSTA, DVM
Diplomate ACVB
Florida Veterinary Behavior Service
West Palm Beach, Florida
USA

MERL F. RAISBECK, DVM, PhD
Diplomate American Board of Veterinary
Toxicology
Professor
Wyoming State Veterinary Laboratory
Department of Veterinary Sciences
University of Wyoming
Laramie, Wyoming
USA

ROSE E. RASKIN, DVM, PhD
Diplomate ACVP
Professor of Clinical Pathology
Department of Veterinary Pathobiology
School of Veterinary Medicine
Purdue University
West Lafayette, Indiana
USA

KENNETH M. RASSNICK, DVM
Diplomate ACVIM (Oncology)
Assistant Professor
Department of Clinical Sciences
College of Veterinary Medicine
Cornell University
Ithaca, New York
USA

ALAN H. REBAR, DVM, PhD
Diplomate ACVP
Senior Associate VP for Research
Executive Director—Discovery Park and
Professor of Clinical Pathology
Office of the Vice President for Research
Purdue University
West Lafayette, Indiana
USA

MARSHA R. REICH, DVM
Diplomate ACVB
Veterinary Behaviorist
Maryland-Virginia Veterinary Behavioral
Consulting
Silver Spring, Maryland
USA

S. BRENT REIMER, DVM
Diplomate ACVS
Iowa Veterinary Specialties
Ames, Iowa
USA

ILANA R. REISNER, DVM, PhD
Diplomate ACVB
Assistant Professor, Behavioral Medicine
Department of Clinical Studies—Philadelphia
School of Veterinary Medicine
University of Pennsylvania
Philadelphia, Pennsylvania
USA

ALEXANDER M. REITER, Dr. med. vet
Diplomate, AVDC, EVDC, Tzt
Assistant Professor of Dentistry and Oral Surgery
Head of the Dentistry and Oral Surgery Service
University of Pennsylvania School of Veterinary
Medicine
Philadelphia, Pennsylvania
USA

WESLEY J. ROACH, DVM
Resident
Small Animal Surgery
College of Veterinary Medicine
University of Georgia
Athens, Georgia
USA

MARGARET V. ROOT KUSTRITZ, DVM,
PhD
Diplomate American College of Therigenologists
Associate Professor, Assistant Dean of Education
Department of Veterinary Clinical Sciences
College of Veterinary Medicine
University of Minnesota
St. Paul, Minnesota
USA

SHERI J. ROSS, BSc, DVM, PhD
Diplomate ACVIM (Internal Medicine)
Clinical Specialist
Nephrology, Urology, Hemodialysis
University of California Veterinary Medical
Center—San Diego
San Diego, Califormia
USA

PHIL ROUDEBUSH, DVM
Diplomate ACVIM (Small Animal Internal
Medicine)
Adjunct Professor
Department of Clinical Sciences
College of Veterinary Medicine
Kansas State University
Manhattan, Kansas
Director of Scientific Affairs
Hill's Pet Nutrition, Inc.
Topeka, Kansas
USA

ELIZABETH A. ROZANSKI, DVM
Diplomate ACVIM (Small Animal Internal
Medicine), Diplomate ACVECC
Assistant Professor
Department of Clinical Sciences
Cummings School of Veterinary Medicine
Tufts University
North Grafton, Massachusetts
USA

WILSON K. RUMBEIHA, BVM, PhD
Diplomate American Board of Toxicology;
Diplomate American Board of Veterinary
Toxicology
Associate Professor, Clinical Toxicologist
Diagnostic Center for Population and Animal
Health
Department of Pathobiology and Diagnostic
Investigation
Michigan State University
Lansing, Michigan
USA

CLARE RUSBRIDGE, BVMS, PhD, MRCVS
Diplomate European College of Veterinary
Neurology
Consultant Neurologist
Stone Lion Veterinary Centre
London
United Kingdom

JOHN E. RUSH, DVM, MS
Diplomate ACVIM (Cardiology); Diplomate
American College of Veterinary Emergency/
Critical Care Professor
Clinical Sciences
Cummings School of Veterinary Medicine
Tufts University
North Grafton, Massachusetts
USA

SHERISSE A. SAKALS, DVM
Resident—Surgery
Small Animal Medicine and Surgery
College of Veterinary Medicine
University of Georgia
Athens, Georgia
USA

CARL D. SAMMARCO, BVSc, MRCVS
Diplomate ACVIM (Cardiology)
Cardiologist
Cardiology
Red Bank Veterinary Hospital
Tinton Falls, New Jersey
USA

SHERRY L. SANDERSON, BS, DVM, PhD
Diplomate ACVIM; Diplomate ACVN
Associate Professor
Department of Physiology and Pharmacology
College of Veterinary Medicine
University of Georgia
Athens, Georgia
USA

SCOTT J. SCHATZBERG, DVM, PhD
Diplomate ACVIM (Neurology)
VESC Sante Fe
Sante Fe, New Mexico
USA

THOMAS SCHERMERHORN, VMD
Diplomate ACVIM (Small Animal Internal
Medicine)
Associate Professor
Department of Clinical Sciences
College of Veterinary Medicine
Kansas State University
Manhattan, Kansas
USA

GRETCHEN LEE SCHOEFFLER, DVM
Diplomate American College of Veterinary
Emergency/Critical Care Chief, Emergency and
Critical Care
Department of Clinical Sciences
College of Veterinary Medicine
Cornell University
Ithaca, New York
USA

DONALD P. SCHROPE, DVM
Diplomate ACVIM (Cardiology)
Staff Cardiologist
Cardiology
Oradell Animal Hospital
Paramus, New Jersey
USA

FRED W. SCOTT, DVM, PhD
Professor Emeritus
Department of Veterinary Microbiology and
Immunology
Director—Retired, Cornell Feline Health Center
College of Veterinary Medicine, Cornell
University
Ithaca, New York
USA

J. CATHARINE SCOTT-MONCRIEFF, Vet
MB, MA, MS
Diplomate ACVIM (Small Animal); Diplomate
ECVIM-CA
Professor and Assistant Department Head,
Veterinary Teaching Hospital Department of
Veterinary Clinical Sciences
Purdue University
West Lafayette, Indiana
USA

LYNNE M. SEIBERT, DVM, MS, PhD
Diplomate ACVB
Veterinary Behavior Consultants
Suwanee, Georgia
USA

KIM A. SELTING, DVM, MS
Diplomate ACVIM (Oncology)
Assistant Teaching Professor
Department of Veterinary Medicine and Surgery
University of Missouri
Columbia, Missouri
USA

LINDA G. SHELL, DVM
Diplomate ACVIM (Neurology)
Veterinary Neurology and Internal Medicine
Educating and Consulting
Pilot, Virginia
Veterinary Information Network
Davis, California
Antech Diagnostics
Irvine, California
USA

G. DIANE SHELTON, DVM, PhD
Diplomate ACVIM
Professor
Department of Pathology
University of California—San Diego
LaJolla, California
USA

BARBARA L. SHERMAN, DVM, MS, PhD
Diplomate ACVB; ABS—Certified Applied
Animal Behaviorist
Clinical Associate Professor
Department of Clinical Sciences
College of Veterinary Medicine
North Carolina State University
Raleigh, North Carolina
USA

PETER K. SHIRES, BVSc, MS
Diplomate ACVS
Principal Scientist
Scientific Affairs
Ethicon Endo-Surgery
Cincinnati, Ohio
USA

DEBORAH C. SILVERSTEIN, DVM
Diplomate ACVECC
Assistant Professor of Critical Care
Department of Clinical Studies
Veterinary Teaching Hospital
University of Pennsylvania
Philadelphia, Pennsylvania
USA

ALLEN SISSON, DVM, MS
Diplomate ACVIM (Neurology)
Staff Neurologist
Department of Neurology
Angell Animal Medical Center—Boston
Boston, Massachusetts
USA

D. DAVID SISSON, DVM
Diplomate ACVIM (Cardiology)
Professor
Department of Clinical Sciences
College of Veterinary Medicine
Oregon State University
Corvallis, Oregon
USA

JO SMITH, MA, Vet MB, PhD
Diplomate ACVIM (Small Animal Internal
Medicine)
Assistant Professor
College of Veterinary Medicine
University of Georgia
Athens, Georgia
USA

MARY O. SMITH, BVMS, PhD
Diplomate ACVIM (Neurology)
Staff Neurologist
Affiliated Veterinary Specialists
Maitland, Florida
USA

PATRICIA J. SMITH, MS, DVM, PhD
Diplomate ACVO
Ophthalmologist
Animal Eye Care
Fremont, California
USA

FRANCIS W.K. SMITH, JR., DVM
Diplomate ACVIM (Small Animal Internal
Medicine & Cardiology)
Clinical Assistant Professor
Department of Medicine
Cummings School of Veterinary Medicine
Tufts University
North Grafton, Massachusetts
Vice President
VetMed Consultants
Lexington, Massachusetts
USA

PAUL W. SNYDER, DVM, PhD
Diplomate ACVP
Professor
Comparative Pathobiology
Purdue University
West Lafayette, Indiana
USA

MITCHELL D. SONG, DVM
Diplomate ACVD
Chief of Staff
Animal Dermatology Service
Phoenix, Arizona
USA

JÖRG M. STEINER, med. vet., Dr. med. vet,
PhD
Diplomate ACVIM; Diplomate ECVIM
Associate Professor of Small Animal Internal
Medicine, Department of Small Animal Clinical
Sciences
Director, Gastrointestinal Laboratory
College of Veterinary Medicine and Biomedical
Sciences
Texas A&M University
College Station, Texas
USA

REBECCA L. STEPIEN, DVM, MS
Diplomate ACVIM (Cardiology)
Clinical Professor—Cardiology
Department of Medical Sciences
School of Veterinary Medicine
Staff Cardiologist
Cardiopulmonary Service
UW Veterinary Care
University of Wisconsin–Madison
Madison, Wisconsin
USA

MEREDITH E. STEPITA, DVM
Clinical Behavior Service Resident
Behavior Science
Veterinary Medical Teaching Hospital
University of California, Davis
Davis, California
USA

REINHARD K. STRAUBINGER, Prof. Dr.
med. vet., PhD
Professor
Institute for Infectious Diseases and Zoonoses
Department of Veterinary Sciences
Faculty of Veterinary Medicine
Ludwig-Maximilians-Universität
München
Munich
Germany

ELIZABETH M. STREETER, DVM
Diplomate ACVECC
Clinician
USA

JAN S. SUCHODOLSKI, med. vet., Dr. med.
vet, PhD
Research Assistant Professor, Department of
Small Animal Clinical Sciences
Associate Director, Gastrointestinal Laboratory
College of Veterinary Medicine and Biomedical
Sciences
Texas A&M University
College Station, Texas
USA

STEFFEN D. SUM, DVM
Medical Instructor
Department of Small Animal Medicine and
Surgery
College of Veterinary Medicine
University of Georgia
Athens, Georgia
USA

CHERYL L. SWENSON, DVM, PhD
Diplomate ACVP (Clinical Pathology)
Associate Professor
Department of Pathobiology and Diagnostic
Investigation
College of Veterinary Medicine
Michigan State University
East Lansing, Michigan
USA

JOSEPH TABOADA, DVM
Diplomate ACVIM (Small Animal Internal
Medicine)
Professor and Associate Dean
Department of Veterinary Clinical Studies
School of Veterinary Medicine
Louisiana State University
Baton Rouge, Louisiana
USA

PATRICIA A. TALCOTT, DVM, PhD
Diplomate American Board of Veterinary
Toxicology
Associate Professor
Department of Veterinary Comparative Anatomy
Pharmacology and Physiology Toxicologist
Washington Animal Disease Diagnostic
Laboratory
College of Veterinary Medicine
Washington State University
Pullman, WA
USA

INGE TARNOW, DVM, PhD
Associate Professor
Department of Small Animal Clinical Sciences
Faculty of Life Sciences
University of Copenhagen
Copenhagen
Denmark

SUSAN M. TAYLOR, DVM
Diplomate ACVIM (Small Animal Internal
Medicine)
Professor, Department of Small Animal Clinical
Sciences
Staff Internist, Small Animal Clinic, Veterinary
Teaching Hospital
Western College of Veterinary Medicine
University of Saskatchewan
Saskatoon, Saskatchewan
Canada

JENNIFER S. THOMAS, DVM, PhD
Diplomate ACVP
Associate Professor
Pathobiology and Diagnostic Investigation
Michigan State University
East Lansing, Michigan
USA

JUSTIN D. THOMASON, DVM
Diplomate, ACVIM
Clinical Instructor
Small Animal Medicine and Surgery
University of Georgia
Athens, Georgia
USA

CRAIG A. THOMPSON, DVM
Diplomate ACVP
Clinical Assistant Professor—Clinical Pathology
Comparative Pathobiology
School of Veterinary Medicine
Purdue University
West Lafayette, Indiana
USA

MARY F. THOMPSON, BVSc (Hons)
Diplomate ACVIM (Small Animal Internal
Medicine); MACVSc (Associate)
Lecturer in Companion Animal Medicine
Veterinary Teaching Hospital
The University of Queensland
Brisbane
Australia

JERRY A. THORNHILL, DVM
Diplomate ACVIM (Internal Medicine)
Director
Chicago Veterinary Kidney Center
Veterinary Specialty Center
Buffalo Grove, Illinois
USA

MARY ANNA THRALL, DVM, MS
Diplomate ACVP
Professor
Department of Microbiology, Immunology and
Pathology
Colorado State University
Fort Collins, Colorado
USA
Department of Pathobiology
Ross UniversIty
St. Kitts
West Indies

LARRY P. TILLEY, DVM
Diplomate ACVIM (Internal Medicine)
President, VetMed Consultants Consultant, New
Mexico Veterinary Referral Center
Sante Fe, New Mexico
USA

ANDREA TIPOLD, Prof. Dr.
Diplomate European College of Veterinary
Neurology
Professor of Neurology
Department of Small Animal Medicine and
Surgery
University for Veterinary Medicine, Hannover
Hannover
Germany

SHEILA TORRES, DVM, MS, PhD
Diplomate ACVD
Associate Professor
Veterinary Clinical Sciences
College of Veterinary Medicine
University of Minnesota
St. Paul, Minnesota
USA

WILLIAM J. TRANQUILLI, DVM, MS, BS in
Ed.
Diplomate ACVA
Professor Emeritus
Department of Veterinary Clinical Medicine
College of Veterinary Medicine
University of Illinois
Urbana, Illinois
USA

DAVID C. TWEDT, DVM
Diplomate ACVIM
Professor
Clinical Sciences
College of Veterinary Medicine and Biomedical
Sciences
Colorado State University
Fort Collins, Colorado
USA

VALARIE VAUGHN TYNES, DVM
Diplomate ACVB
Premier Veterinary Behavior Consulting
Forth Worth, Texas
USA

LISA K. ULRICH, CVT
Certified Veterinary Technician
Principal Veterinary Technician
Minnesota Urolith Center
College of Veterinary Medicine
University of Minnesota
St. Paul, Minnesota
USA

SHELLY L. VADEN, DVM, PhD
Diplomate ACVIM
Professor, Internal Medicine
Department of Clinical Sciences
College of Veterinary Medicine
North Carolina State University
Raleigh, North Carolina
USA

MARIA L. VIANNA, DVM
Surgeon
Veterinary Specialty Hospital of South Florida
Palm Beach, Florida
USA

LORI S. WADDELL, DVM
Diplomate ACVECC
Adjunct Assistant Professor, Critical Care
Department of Clinical Studies
University of Pennsylvania
Philadelphia, Pennsylvania
USA

LIORA WALDMAN, BVM&S, MRCVS, Cert
SAD
Dermatologist
Dermatology, Allergy and Ear Clinic
Haifa
Israel

KIRSTEN E. WARATUKE, DVM
Consulting Veterinarian in Clinical Toxicology
ASPCA Animal Poison Control Center
Urbana, Illinois
USA

CRAIG B. WEBB, DVM, PhD
Diplomate ACVIM
Associate Professor
Department of Clinical Sciences
Veterinary Teaching Hospital
Colorado State University
Fort Collins, Colorado
USA

MIKE WEH, DVM
Diplomate ACVS
Assistant Professor of Orthopedic Surgery
Small Animal Medicine and Surgery
Veterinary Teaching Hospital College of
Veterinary Medicine
University of Georgia
Athens, Georgia
USA

GLADE WEISER, DVM
Diplomate ACVP
Professor, Special Appointment
Department of Microbiology, Immunology, and
Pathology
Colorado State University
Fort Collins, Colorado
USA

ALEXANDER H. WERNER, VMD
Diplomate ACVD
Staff Dermatologist
Animal Dermatology Center
Studio City, California
USA

ROBERT B. WIGGS, DVM
Diplomate American Veterinary Dental College,
Fellow Academy of Veterinary Dentistry
Owner
Dallas Dental Service Animal Clinic
Dallas, Texas
USA

HEATHER M. WILSON, DVM
Diplomate ACVIM (Oncology)
Assistant Professor
Department of Veterinary Small Animal Clinical
Sciences
College of Veterinary Medicine
Texas A&M University
College Station, Texas
USA

TINA WISMER, DVM
Diplomate American Board of Veterinary
Toxicology, Diplomate American Board of
Toxicology
Senior Director of Veterinary Outreach and
Education
ASPCA Animal Poison Control Center
Urbana, Illinois
USA

DARREN WOOD, DVM, DVSc
Diplomate ACVP
Associate Professor
Department of Pathobiology
Ontario Veterinary College
University of Guelph
Guelph, Ontario
Canada

J. PAUL WOODS, DVM, MS
Diplomate ACVIM (Internal Medicine,
Oncology)
Professor
Department of Clinical Studies
Ontario Veterinary College
University of Guelph
Guelph, Ontario
Canada

JACKIE M. WYPIJ, DVM, MS
Diplomate ACVIM (Oncology)
Assistant Professor
Department of Veterinary Clinical Medicine
University of Illinois, Urbana-Champaign
Urbana, Illinois
USA

HANY YOUSSEF, BVSc, MS, DVM
Consulting Veterinarian in Clinical Toxicology
ASPCA Animal Poison Control Center
Urbana, Illinois
USA

DEBRA L. ZORAN, DVM, PhD
Diplomate ACVIM
Associate Professor and Chief of Medicine
Department of Veterinary Small Animal Clinical
Sciences
College of Veterinary Medicine and Biomedical
Sciences
Texas A&M University
College Station, Texas
USA

SUMÁRIO

Abdome Agudo	2
Abortamento Espontâneo (Perda Gestacional Precoce) — Cadelas	5
Abortamento Espontâneo (Perda Gestacional Precoce) — Gatas	7
Abortamento, Interrupção da Gestação	9
Abscedação	11
Abscesso da Raiz Dentária (Abscesso Apical)	13
Ácaros Otológicos	14
Acasalamento, Momento Oportuno	15
Acidente Vascular Cerebral (AVC)	17
Acidose Láctica	19
Acidose Metabólica	21
Acidose Tubular Renal	23
Acne — Cães	24
Acne — Gatos	25
Acromegalia — Gatos	26
Actinomicose	27
Adenite Sebácea Granulomatosa	28
Adenocarcinoma da Próstata	29
Adenocarcinoma da Tireoide — Cães	30
Adenocarcinoma das Glândulas Ceruminosas, Orelha	32
Adenocarcinoma das Glândulas Salivares	33
Adenocarcinoma das Glândulas Sebáceas e Sudoríferas	34
Adenocarcinoma do Estômago, Intestinos Delgado, Grosso e Reto	35
Adenocarcinoma do Pâncreas	36
Adenocarcinoma dos Pulmões	37
Adenocarcinoma dos Sacos Anais	38
Adenocarcinoma Nasal	39
Adenocarcinoma Renal	40
Adenoma Hepatocelular	41
Afogamento (Afogamento por um Triz)	42
Agressividade — Visão Geral — Cães	43
Agressividade — Visão Geral — Gatos	46
Agressividade Canina contra Crianças	49
Agressividade contra Pessoas Familiares — Cães	50
Agressividade Defensiva Induzida pelo Medo — Cães	52
Agressividade entre os Cães	54
Agressividade entre os Gatos	56
Agressividade por Medo — Gatos	58
Agressividade Possessiva, Territorial e Induzida pelo Alimento — Cães	59
Alcalose Metabólica	61
Alopecia — Cães	63
Alopecia — Gatos	65
Alopecia Não Inflamatória — Cães	67

Alopecia Paraneoplásica Felina	69
Alopecia Simétrica Felina	70
Amebíase	71
Ameloblastoma	72
Amiloide Hepático	73
Amiloidose	74
Anafilaxia	76
Ancilostomíase	78
Anemia Aplásica	79
Anemia Arregenerativa	80
Anemia de Doença Renal Crônica	82
Anemia Imunomediada	84
Anemia Metabólica (Anemia com Hemácias Espiculadas)	87
Anemia por Corpúsculo de Heinz	88
Anemia por Defeitos de Maturação Nuclear (Anemia Megaloblástica)	89
Anemia por Deficiência de Ferro	90
Anemia Regenerativa	91
Anisocoria	93
Anomalia de Ebstein	95
Anomalia de Pelger-Huët	96
Anomalia do Olho do Collie	97
Anomalia Vascular Portossistêmica Congênita	98
Anomalias do Anel Vascular	101
Anomalias Oculares Congênitas	102
Anorexia	104
Anormalidades dos Espermatozoides	106
Antidepressivos — Toxicose por Antidepressivos Tricíclicos (ATC)	107
Antidepressivos — Toxicose por Inibidor Seletivo de Recaptação da Serotonina (ISRS)	109
Apudoma	110
Arritmia Sinusal	111
Arritmias Ventriculares e Morte Súbita em Pastor Alemão	113
Artrite (Osteoartrite)	114
Artrite Séptica	116
Ascite	118
Asma, Bronquite — Gatos	120
Aspergilose Disseminada	122
Aspergilose Nasal	124
Astrocitoma	126
Ataxia	127
Aterosclerose	129
Atrofia da Íris	130
Avulsão do Plexo Braquial	131
Azotemia e Uremia	132
Babesiose	134
Bailisascaríase	136
Bartonelose	137
Bexiga Pélvica	138
Blastomicose	139
Blefarite	141
Bloqueio Atrioventricular Completo (Terceiro Grau)	143
Bloqueio Atrioventricular de Primeiro Grau	145

Bloqueio Atrioventricular de Segundo Grau — Mobitz Tipo I	147
Bloqueio Atrioventricular de Segundo Grau — Mobitz Tipo II	149
Bloqueio do Ramo Direito do Feixe de His	151
Bloqueio do Ramo Esquerdo do Feixe de His	153
Bloqueio Fascicular Anterior Esquerdo	155
Bordetelose — Gatos	157
Borreliose de Lyme	158
Botulismo	160
Bradicardia Sinusal	161
Bronquiectasia	163
Bronquite Crônica	164
Brucelose	166
Campilobacteriose	168
Candidíase	169
Capilaríase (Pearsonema)	170
Carcinoide e Síndrome Carcinoide	171
Carcinoma de Células de Transição	172
Carcinoma de Células Escamosas da Língua	174
Carcinoma de Células Escamosas da Pele	175
Carcinoma de Células Escamosas da Tonsila	177
Carcinoma de Células Escamosas das Gengivas	178
Carcinoma de Células Escamosas das Orelhas	179
Carcinoma de Células Escamosas do Plano Nasal	180
Carcinoma de Células Escamosas dos Dedos	181
Carcinoma de Células Escamosas dos Pulmões	182
Carcinoma de Células Escamosas dos Seios Nasais e Paranasais	183
Carcinoma de Ducto Biliar	184
Carcinoma Hepatocelular	185
Cáries Dentárias	186
Carrapatos e seu Controle	188
Cataratas	190
Caxumba	192
Celulite Juvenil	193
Ceratite Eosinofílica — Gatos	194
Ceratite Não Ulcerativa	195
Ceratite Ulcerativa	197
Ceratoconjuntivite Seca	199
Choque Cardiogênico	200
Choque Hipovolêmico	202
Choque Séptico	204
Cianose	206
Cilindrúria	208
Cinomose	209
Cirrose e Fibrose do Fígado	211
Cisticercose	213
Cistite Polipoide	214
Cisto Dentígero	216
Cisto Quadrigeminal	217
Cistos Prostáticos	218
Cistos Subaracnoi	219
Citauxzoon	221
Clamidi	222

Claudicação	224
Coagulação Intravascular Disseminada	225
Coagulopatia por Hepatopatia	227
Coccidioidomicose	228
Coccidiose	230
Colapso da Traqueia	231
Colecistite e Coledoquite	233
Colelitíase	234
Colesteatoma	236
Colibacilose	237
Colite e Proctite	239
Colite Ulcerativa Histiocítica	241
Complexo Granuloma Eosinofílico	242
Complexos Atriais Prematuros	244
Complexos Ventriculares Prematuros	246
Comportamento de Marcação Territorial e Errático — Cães	248
Comportamento de Marcação Territorial e Errático — Gatos	250
Comportamentos Destrutivos	252
Comportamentos Indisciplinados: Saltos, Escavação, Perseguição, Furto	254
Compressão Cefálica	256
Condrossarcoma — Boca	258
Condrossarcoma — Laringe e Traqueia	259
Condrossarcoma — Osso	260
Condrossarcoma — Seios Nasais e Paranasais	261
Conjuntivite — Cães	262
Conjuntivite — Gatos	264
Constipação e Obstipação	266
Contusões Pulmonares	268
Coprofagia e Pica	269
Coriorretinite	271
Corpos Estranhos Esofágicos	273
Corrimento Vaginal	275
Criptococose	277
Criptorquidismo	279
Criptosporidiose	280
Crises Convulsivas (Convulsões, Estado Epiléptico) — Cães	281
Crises Convulsivas (Convulsões, Estado Epiléptico) — Gatos	283
Cristalúria	285
Cuterebrose	287
Defeito do Septo Atrial	288
Defeito do Septo Ventricular	289
Deficiência da Fosfofrutoquinase	291
Deficiência da Piruvato Quinase	292
Deficiência de Carnitina	293
Deficiência de Taurina	294
Deficiência dos Fatores de Coagulação	295
Deformidades do Crescimento Antebraquial	297
Degeneração Cerebelar	299
Degeneração da Retina	300
e Hipoplasia Testiculares	303
Infiltrações da Córnea	304
	305

Dentes Decíduos, Persistentes (Retidos)	307
Dentes Manchados	308
Dermatite Acral por Lambedura	310
Dermatite Atópica	311
Dermatite de Contato	313
Dermatite Necrolítica Superficial	314
Dermatite por Malassezia	315
Dermatofilose	316
Dermatofitose	317
Dermatomiosite	319
Dermatoses e Distúrbios Despigmentantes	321
Dermatoses Erosivas ou Ulcerativas	323
Dermatoses Esfoliativas	325
Dermatoses Nasais — Cães	327
Dermatoses Neoplásicas	329
Dermatoses Nodulares/Granulomatosas Estéreis	331
Dermatoses Papulonodulares	333
Dermatoses Vesiculopustulares	335
Dermatoses Virais	337
Descolamento da Retina	338
Desvio Portossistêmico Adquirido	340
Diabetes Insípido	342
Diabetes Melito com Cetoacidose	343
Diabetes Melito com Coma Hiperosmolar	345
Diabetes Melito sem Complicação — Cães	347
Diabetes Melito sem Complicação — Gatos	349
Diarreia Aguda	351
Diarreia Crônica — Cães	353
Diarreia Crônica — Gatos	355
Diarreia Responsiva a Antibióticos	357
Dioctophyma Renale (Também Conhecido como Verme Renal Gigante)	358
Dirofilariose — Cães	360
Dirofilariose — Gatos	362
Disautonomia (Síndrome de Key-Gaskell)	363
Disbiose do Intestino Delgado	364
Discinesia Ciliar Primária	366
Discopatia Intervertebral — Gatos	367
Discopatia Intervertebral Cervical	368
Discopatia Intervertebral Toracolombar	370
Discospondilite	372
Disfagia	374
Displasia Coxofemoral	376
Displasia das Valvas Atrioventriculares	378
Displasia do Cotovelo	380
Displasia Microvascular Hepatoportal	382
Dispneia e Angústia Respiratória	384
Disquezia e Hematoquezia	386
Disrafismo Espinal	387
Distocia	388
Distrofia Neuroaxonal	391
Distrofias da Córnea	392
Distúrbios da Articulação Temporomandibular	393

Distúrbios da Imunodeficiência Primária	394
Distúrbios da Motilidade Gástrica	395
Distúrbios da Unha e do Leito Ungueal	397
Distúrbios do Desenvolvimento Sexual	398
Distúrbios dos Cílios (Triquíase, Distiquíase/Cílios Ectópicos)	400
Distúrbios dos Sacos Anais	401
Distúrbios Mieloproliferativos	402
Disúria e Polaciúria	403
Divertículos Esofágicos	405
Divertículos Vesicouracais	406
Doença da Aglutinina Fria	407
Doença de Chagas (Tripanossomíase Americana)	408
Doença de Legg-Calvé-Perthes	409
Doença de Tyzzer	411
Doença de von Willebrand	412
Doença do Armazenamento de Glicogênio	414
Doença do Ligamento Cruzado Cranial	415
Doença Idiopática do Trato Urinário Inferior dos Felinos	417
Doença Periodontal	419
Doença Renal Policística	421
Doenças do Armazenamento Lisossomal	422
Doenças Endomiocárdicas — Gatos	423
Doenças Orbitais (Exoftalmia, Enoftalmia, Estrabismo)	425
Doenças Renais de Natureza Congênita e de Desenvolvimento	427
Dor Aguda, Crônica e Pós-operatória	429
Dor no Pescoço e no Dorso	433
Eclâmpsia	435
Ectrópio	436
Edema Periférico	437
Edema Pulmonar Não Cardiogênico	439
Efusão Pericárdica	441
Efusão Pleural	443
Encefalite	445
Encefalite Necrosante	447
Encefalite Secundária à Migração Parasitária	448
Encefalitozoonose	449
Encefalopatia Hepática	450
Encefalopatia Isquêmica Felina	452
Endocardiose das Valvas Atrioventriculares	454
Endocardite Infecciosa	457
Enteropatia Causada pelo Glúten no Setter Irlandês	459
Enteropatia com Perda de Proteínas	460
Enteropatia Imunoproliferativa de Basenjis	462
Enteropatia Inflamatória	463
Enterotoxicose Clostrídica	465
Entrópio	467
Envenenamento (Intoxicação)	468
Envenenamento por Arsênico	470
Envenenamento por Cogumelo	471
Envenenamento por Rodenticidas Anticoagulantes	475
Epididimite/Orquite	476
Epífora	477

Epilepsia Idiopática (Genética)	479
Episclerite	481
Epistaxe	482
Epúlide	484
Erliquiose	485
Erupções Medicamentosas Cutâneas	487
Esofagite	488
Espermatocele/Granuloma Espermático	490
Espirro, Espirro Reverso, Ânsia de Vômito	491
Esplenomegalia	493
Espondilomielopatia Cervical (Síndrome de Wobbler)	495
Espondilose Deformante	497
Esporotricose	498
Esquistossomíase Canina (Heterobilharzíase)	499
Esteatite	500
Estenose Aórtica	501
Estenose das Valvas Atrioventriculares	503
Estenose Esofágica	505
Estenose Lombossacra e Síndrome da Cauda Equina	507
Estenose Nasofaríngea	509
Estenose Pulmonar	510
Estenose Retal	512
Estertor e Estridor	513
Estomatite	515
Estrongiloidíase	517
Estupor e Coma	518
Evacuação e Micção Domiciliares pelos Cães	520
Evacuação e Micção Domiciliares pelos Gatos	522
Falha Ovulatória	525
Febre	526
Febre Familiar do Shar-Pei	528
Febre Maculosa das Montanhas Rochosas	530
Febre Q	532
Fenômeno de Schiff-Sherrington	533
Feocromocitoma	534
Fibrilação e Flutter Atriais	536
Fibrilação Ventricular	539
Fibrossarcoma da Gengiva	541
Fibrossarcoma de Osso	542
Fibrossarcoma dos Seios Nasais e Paranasais	543
Fisalopterose	544
Fístula Arteriovenosa	545
Fístula Oronasal	546
Fístula Perianal	547
Flatulência	548
Flebite	550
Fobias a Trovões e Relâmpagos	552
Fobias, Medo e Ansiedade — Cães	553
Fobias, Medo e Ansiedade — Gatos	555
Formação e Estrutura Anormais do Dente	557
Fraqueza e Colapso Induzidos por Exercício em Labradores Retrievers	558
Fratura Dentária	560

Fraturas Maxilares e Mandibulares	562
Gastrenterite Eosinofílica	564
Gastrenterite Hemorrágica	566
Gastrenterite Linfoplasmocitária	568
Gastrite Atrófica	570
Gastrite Crônica	571
Gastropatia Pilórica Hipertrófica Crônica	573
Giardíase	575
Glaucoma	576
Glicosúria	578
Glomerulonefrite	580
Glucagonoma	582
Granulomatose Linfomatoide	584
Halitose	585
Hemangiopericitoma	586
Hemangiossarcoma Cutâneo	587
Hemangiossarcoma do Baço e do Fígado	588
Hemangiossarcoma do Coração	590
Hemangiossarcoma do Osso	591
Hematêmese	592
Hematopoiese Cíclica	594
Hematúria	595
Hemoglobinúria e Mioglobinúria	597
Hemorragia da Retina	599
Hemotórax	601
Hepatite Crônica Ativa	602
Hepatite Granulomatosa	605
Hepatite Infecciosa Canina	607
Hepatite Supurativa e Abscesso Hepático	609
Hepatomegalia	611
Hepatopatia Diabética	613
Hepatopatia Fibrosante Juvenil	614
Hepatopatia por Armazenamento de Cobre	616
Hepatopatia Vacuolar	619
Hepatotoxinas	621
Hepatozoonose	623
Hérnia de Hiato	624
Hérnia Diafragmática	625
Hérnia Diafragmática Peritoneopericárdica	626
Hérnia Perineal	627
Hidrocefalia	628
Hidronefrose	630
Hifema	631
Hiperadrenocorticismo (Síndrome de Cushing) — Cães	633
Hiperadrenocorticismo (Síndrome de Cushing) — Gatos	637
Hiperandrogenismo	638
Hipercalcemia	640
Hipercalemia	642
Hipercapnia	644
Hipercloremia	646
Hipercoagulabilidade	647
Hiperestrogenismo (Toxicidade do Estrogênio)	648

Hiperfosfatemia	650
Hiperglicemia	652
Hiperlipidemia	654
Hipermagnesemia	656
Hipermetria e Dismetria	658
Hipernatremia	659
Hiperosmolaridade	660
Hiperparatireoidismo	662
Hiperparatireoidismo Secundário Renal	664
Hiperplasia das Glândulas Mamárias — Gatas	666
Hiperplasia e Prolapso Vaginais	667
Hiperplasia Gengival	668
Hiperplasia Hepática Nodular	669
Hiperplasia Prostática Benigna	670
Hipersensibilidade à Picada de Pulga e Controle de Pulgas	671
Hipertensão Portal	673
Hipertensão Pulmonar	675
Hipertensão Sistêmica	678
Hipertireoidismo	681
Hipoadrenocorticismo (Doença de Addison)	683
Hipoalbuminemia	685
Hipoandrogenismo	687
Hipocalcemia	688
Hipocalemia	690
Hipocloremia	692
Hipofosfatemia	693
Hipoglicemia	695
Hipomagnesemia	697
Hipomielinização	699
Hiponatremia	700
Hipoparatireoidismo	701
Hipópio e Depósito Lipídico	704
Hipopituitarismo	705
Hipoplasia Cerebelar	706
Hipoplasia/Hipocalcificação do Esmalte	707
Hipostenúria	708
Hipotermia	709
Hipotireoidismo	711
Hipoxemia	714
Histiocitoma	716
Histiocitoma Fibroso Maligno (Tumor de Células Gigantes)	717
Histiocitose — Cães	718
Histoplasmose	720
Icterícia	722
Íleo Paralítico	724
Inalação de Fumaça	725
Inclinação da Cabeça	726
Incontinência Fecal	728
Incontinência Urinária	730
Inércia Uterina	732
Infarto do Miocárdio	733
Infecção Bacteriana do Trato Urinário Inferior	735

Infecção Fúngica do Trato Urinário Inferior	737
Infecção pelo Calicivírus Felino	738
Infecção pelo Poxvírus — Gatos	740
Infecção pelo Vírus da Imunodeficiência Felina	741
Infecção pelo Vírus da Leucemia Felina	743
Infecção pelo Vírus da Pseudorraiva	745
Infecção pelo Vírus Formador de Sincício Felino	746
Infecção pelo Vírus Oeste do Nilo	747
Infecção por Astrovírus	748
Infecção por Coronavírus — Cães	749
Infecção por Helicobacter	750
Infecção por Herpes-Vírus — Cães	752
Infecção por Herpes-Vírus — Gatos	753
Infecção por Ollulanis	755
Infecção por Reovírus	756
Infecções Anaeróbias	757
Infecções Bacterianas pelas Formas L	758
Infecções por Estafilococos	759
Infecções por Estreptococos	760
Infecções por Micobactérias	761
Infecções por Rotavírus	763
Infertilidade das Cadelas	764
Infertilidade dos Cães Machos	766
Infestação por Trematódeos	768
Inflamação Orofaríngea Felina	770
Influenza — Cães	771
Instabilidade Atlantoaxial	772
Insuficiência Cardíaca Congestiva Direita	774
Insuficiência Cardíaca Congestiva Esquerda	776
Insuficiência Hepática Aguda	778
Insuficiência Pancreática Exócrina	780
Insuficiência Renal Aguda	782
Insuficiência Renal Crônica	785
Insulinoma	788
Intermação e Hipertermia	790
Intoxicação Alimentar pelo Salmão	792
Intoxicação pelo Chumbo	793
Intoxicação pelo Lírio	795
Intoxicação por Ácido Acetilsalicílico	796
Intoxicação por Estricnina	797
Intoxicação por Etanol	798
Intoxicação por Etilenoglicol	799
Intoxicação por Metaldeído	801
Introdução de Novos Animais de Estimação na Família	802
Intussuscepção	804
Laceração da Parede Atrial	806
Lacerações da Córnea e Esclera	808
Laringopatia	810
Leiomioma do Estômago e dos Intestinos Delgado e Grosso	812
Leiomiossarcoma do Estômago e dos Intestinos Delgado e Grosso	813
Leishmaniose	814
Leptospirose	815

Lesão Cerebral	817
Lesão por Mordedura de Fio Elétrico	819
Leucemia Linfoblástica Aguda	820
Leucemia Linfocítica Crônica	821
Leucoencefalomielopatia no Rottweiler	822
Linfadenite	823
Linfadenopatia	825
Linfangiectasia	827
Linfedema	829
Linfoma — Cães	830
Linfoma — Gatos	832
Linfoma Cutâneo Epiteliotrópico	834
Lipidose Hepática	835
Lipoma	837
Lipoma Infiltrativo	838
Lúpus Eritematoso Cutâneo (Discoide)	839
Lúpus Eritematoso Sistêmico	840
Luxação do Cristalino	842
Luxação ou Avulsão dos Dentes	843
Luxação Patelar	844
Luxações Articulares	846
Má-Absorção da Cobalamina	848
Má-Formação Arteriovenosa do Fígado	849
Maloclusão Esquelética e Dentária	851
Más-Formações Congênitas Espinais e Vertebrais	853
Más-Formações Vaginais e Lesões Adquiridas	855
Massas Bucais	857
Mastite	860
Mastocitomas	861
Mediastinite	863
Megacólon	864
Megaesôfago	866
Melanoma Uveal em Cães	868
Melanoma Uveal em Gatos	869
Melena	870
Meningioma	871
Meningite-Arterite Responsivas a Esteroides — Cães	873
Meningite/Meningoencefalite/Meningomielite Bacterianas	874
Meningoencefalomielite Eosinofílica	876
Meningoencefalomielite Granulomatosa	877
Mesotelioma	879
Metemoglobinemia	880
Metrite	882
Miastenia Grave	883
Micoplasmose	885
Micoplasmose Hemotrópica (Hemoplasmose)	887
Micotoxicose — Aflatoxina	888
Micotoxicose — Desoxinivalenol	889
Micotoxicose — Toxinas Tremorgênicas	890
Mieloma Múltiplo	891
Mielomalacia (Aguda, Ascendente, Descendente)	893
Mielopatia — Paresia/Paralisia — Gatos	894

Mielopatia Degenerativa	896
Mielopatia Embólica Fibrocartilaginosa	898
Miocardiopatia — Boxer	900
Miocardiopatia Dilatada — Cães	901
Miocardiopatia Dilatada — Gatos	904
Miocardiopatia Hipertrófica — Cães	906
Miocardiopatia Hipertrófica — Gatos	907
Miocardiopatia Restritiva — Gatos	909
Miocardite	911
Miocardite Traumática	913
Mioclonia	914
Miopatia Inflamatória — Polimiosite e Dermatomiosite	915
Miopatia Inflamatória Focal — Miosite dos Músculos Mastigatórios e Extraoculares	917
Miopatia Não Inflamatória — Câibra Hereditária do Terrier Escocês	919
Miopatia Não Inflamatória — Distrofia Muscular Hereditária Ligada ao Cromossomo X	920
Miopatia Não Inflamatória — Endócrina	921
Miopatia Não Inflamatória — Hereditária no Labrador Retriever	923
Miopatia Não Inflamatória — Metabólica	924
Miopatia Não Inflamatória — Miotonia Hereditária	926
Mixedema e Coma Mixedematoso	927
Mortalidade Neonatal (Síndrome do Definhamento)	928
Mucocele da Vesícula Biliar	930
Mucocele Salivar	932
Mucopolissacaridose	934
Narcolepsia e Cataplexia	935
Nefrolitíase	936
Nefrotoxicidade Induzida por Medicamentos	938
Nematódeos (Ascaríase)	940
Neosporose	941
Neurite Idiopática do Trigêmeo	942
Neurite Óptica	943
Neuropatias Periféricas (Polineuropatias)	944
Neutropenia	946
Nistagmo	948
Nocardiose	950
Obesidade	951
Obstrução do Ducto Biliar	953
Obstrução do Trato Urinário	956
Obstrução Gastrintestinal	958
Oftalmia Neonatal	960
Olho Cego "Silencioso"	961
Olho Vermelho	963
Oligúria e Anúria	965
Oncocitoma	967
Osteocondrodisplasia	968
Osteocondrose	969
Osteodistrofia Hipertrófica	971
Osteomielite	973
Osteopatia Craniomandibular	975
Osteopatia Hipertrófica	976

Osteossarcoma	977
Otite Externa e Média	979
Otite Média e Interna	982
Pancitopenia	984
Pancreatite	986
Paniculite	988
Panleucopenia Felina	989
Panosteíte	991
Papiledema	993
Papilomatose	994
Parada Atrial	995
Parada Cardiopulmonar	997
Parada Sinusal e Bloqueio Sinoatrial	999
Parada Ventricular (Assistolia)	1001
Parafimose, Fimose e Priapismo	1003
Paralisia	1004
Paralisia do Carrapato	1006
Paralisia do Coonhound (Polirradiculoneurite Idiopática)	1008
Paraproteinemia	1010
Parasitas Respiratórios	1011
Paresia e Paralisia do Nervo Facial	1013
Parto Prematuro	1015
Parvovirose Canina	1016
Peito Escavado	1018
Pênfigo	1019
Perda de Peso e Caquexia	1021
Perfuração da Traqueia	1024
Pericardite	1025
Peritonite	1027
Peritonite Biliar	1029
Peritonite Infecciosa Felina	1030
Persistência do Ducto Arterioso	1032
Peste	1035
Petéquia, Equimose, Contusão	1036
Pielonefrite	1038
Piodermite	1040
Piometra e Hiperplasia Endometrial Cística	1042
Piotórax	1044
Pitiose	1046
Piúria	1048
Placenta Retida	1050
Plasmocitoma Mucocutâneo	1051
Pneumocistose	1052
Pneumonia Bacteriana	1053
Pneumonia Eosinofílica	1055
Pneumonia Fúngica	1057
Pneumonia Intersticial	1059
Pneumonia por Aspiração	1061
Pneumotórax	1062
Pododermatite	1064
Poliartrite Erosiva Imunomediada	1066
Poliartrite Não Erosiva Imunomediada	1068

Policitemia	1070
Policitemia Vera	1073
Polifagia	1074
Polioencefalomielite — Gatos	1076
Pólipos Nasais e Nasofaríngeos	1077
Pólipos Retoanais	1078
Poliúria e Polidipsia	1079
Problemas Comportamentais Maternos	1081
Problemas Comportamentais Pediátricos — Cães	1083
Problemas Comportamentais Pediátricos — Gatos	1085
Problemas do Ombro, Ligamento e Tendão	1087
Prolapso da Glândula da Terceira Pálpebra (Olho de Cereja)	1089
Prolapso Retal e Anal	1090
Prolapso Uretral	1091
Proptose	1093
Prostatite e Abscesso Prostático	1094
Prostatomegalia	1096
Prostatopatia no Cão Macho Reprodutor	1097
Proteinúria	1099
Prototecose	1101
Protrusão da Terceira Pálpebra	1102
Prurido	1104
Pseudociese	1106
Pseudocistos Perirrenais	1108
Ptialismo	1109
Queiletielose	1111
Quilotórax	1112
Quimiodectoma	1114
Rabdomioma	1115
Rabdomiossarcoma	1116
Rabdomiossarcoma da Bexiga Urinária	1117
Raiva	1118
Reabsorção dos Dentes em Felinos (Reabsorção Odontoclástica)	1120
Reações Alimentares (Gastrintestinais) Adversas	1121
Reações Alimentares Dermatológicas	1123
Reações à Transfusão Sanguínea	1125
Realojamento Bem-Sucedido de Cães e Gatos de Abrigo	1126
Refluxo Gastresofágico	1128
Regurgitação	1129
Renomegalia	1131
Respiração Ofegante e Taquipneia	1133
Retenção Urinária Funcional	1135
Rinite e Sinusite	1137
Rinosporidiose	1139
Ritmo Idioventricular	1140
Ruptura Muscular (Laceração Muscular)	1142
Salmonelose	1144
Sarcoma Associado à Vacina	1146
Sarcoma de Células Sinoviais	1148
Sarna Notoédrica	1149
Sarna Sarcóptica	1150
Schwanoma	1151

Secreção Nasal	1152
Seminoma	1154
Sepse e Bacteremia	1155
Sequestro de Córnea — Gatos	1157
Sertolinoma	1158
Síncope	1159
Síndrome Braquicefálica das Vias Aéreas	1161
Síndrome Colangite e Colangio-Hepatite	1163
Síndrome da Angústia Respiratória Aguda (SARA)	1166
Síndrome da Fragilidade Cutânea Felina	1168
Síndrome de Ansiedade da Separação	1169
Síndrome de Chediak-Higashi	1171
Síndrome de Dilatação e Vólvulo Gástricos	1172
Síndrome de Disfunção Cognitiva	1174
Síndrome de Fanconi	1176
Síndrome de Hiperestesia Felina	1177
Síndrome de Hiperviscosidade	1178
Síndrome de Horner	1179
Síndrome de Tremor Generalizado (Síndrome do Cão Tremedor)	1180
Síndrome de Wolff-Parkinson-White	1181
Síndrome do Intestino Irritável	1183
Síndrome do Nó Sinusal Doente	1184
Síndrome do Vômito Bilioso	1186
Síndrome dos Ovários Remanescentes	1187
Síndrome Hipereosinofílica	1189
Síndrome Nefrótica	1190
Síndrome Tipo-Sjögren	1192
Síndrome Uveodermatológica	1193
Síndromes Mielodisplásicas	1194
Síndromes Paraneoplásicas	1195
Siringomielia e Má-Formação Tipo Chiari	1198
Sopros Cardíacos	1199
Subinvolução dos Sítios Placentários	1201
Surdez	1202
Taquicardia Sinusal	1203
Taquicardia Supraventricular	1205
Taquicardia Ventricular	1207
Tênias (Cestodíase)	1210
Tétano	1211
Tetralogia de Fallot	1212
Timoma	1213
Torção de Lobo Pulmonar	1214
Torção Esplênica	1215
Tosse	1216
Toxicidade da Digoxina	1218
Toxicidade da Vitamina D	1219
Toxicidade das Piretrinas e dos Piretroides	1222
Toxicidade do Paracetamol	1223
Toxicidade do Rodenticida Brometalina	1225
Toxicidade do Veneno de Lacertílios	1226
Toxicidade do Xilitol	1227
Toxicidade do Zinco	1228

Toxicidade dos Agentes Anti-Inflamatórios Não Esteroides	1229
Toxicidade pela Ivermectina	1231
Toxicidade pelo Ferro	1232
Toxicose por Amitraz	1233
Toxicose por Anfetamina	1235
Toxicose por Benzodiazepínicos e Soníferos	1237
Toxicose por Beta-2 Agonistas Inalatórios	1239
Toxicose por Chocolate	1240
Toxicose por Metformina	1243
Toxicose por Monóxido de Carbono	1244
Toxicose por Organofosforado e Carbamato	1245
Toxicose por Pseudoefedrina	1247
Toxicose por Uvas e Passas	1248
Toxicose por Veneno de Aranha — Família da Reclusa-Castanha	1249
Toxicose por Veneno de Aranha — Viúva-Negra	1250
Toxicose por Veneno de Cobra — Corais	1251
Toxicose por Veneno de Cobra — Víboras	1252
Toxicose por Veneno de Sapo	1253
Toxicoses por Hidrocarboneto de Petróleo	1254
Toxoplasmose	1256
Transtornos Compulsivos — Cães	1258
Transtornos Compulsivos — Gatos	1260
Traqueobronquite Infecciosa Canina (Tosse dos Canis)	1262
Traumatismo da Coluna Vertebral	1264
Tremores	1266
Tricomoníase	1268
Tricuríase	1269
Triquinose	1270
Trombocitopatias	1271
Trombocitopenia	1272
Trombocitopenia Imunomediada Primária	1274
Tromboembolia Aórtica	1276
Tromboembolia Pulmonar	1279
Tularemia	1281
Tumor das Células Basais (Basalioma)	1282
Tumor de Células Intersticiais do Testículo	1283
Tumor Venéreo Transmissível	1284
Tumores Cerebrais	1285
Tumores da Bainha Nervosa	1287
Tumores das Glândulas Mamárias — Cadelas	1288
Tumores das Glândulas Mamárias — Gatas	1291
Tumores dos Folículos Pilosos	1292
Tumores Malignos Indiferenciados da Cavidade Bucal	1293
Tumores Melanocíticos Bucais	1294
Tumores Melanocíticos da Pele e dos Dedos	1295
Tumores Miocárdicos	1297
Tumores Ovarianos	1298
Tumores Uterinos	1299
Tumores Vaginais	1300
Úlcera Gastroduodenal	1301
Ulceração Bucal	1303
Ureter Ectópico	1305

Ureterolitíase	1306
Urolitíase por Cistina	1308
Urolitíase por Estruvita — Cães	1309
Urolitíase por Estruvita — Gatos	1311
Urolitíase por Fosfato de Cálcio	1313
Urolitíase por Oxalato de Cálcio	1314
Urolitíase por Urato	1316
Urolitíase por Xantina	1318
Uveíte Anterior — Cães	1319
Uveíte Anterior — Gatos	1321
Vaginite	1323
Vasculite Cutânea — Cães	1325
Vasculite Sistêmica	1326
Vestibulopatia Geriátrica — Cães	1327
Vestibulopatia Idiopática — Gatos	1329
Vocalização Excessiva	1330
Vômito Agudo	1331
Vômito Crônico	1333

Apêndice I — Valores de Referência para Testes Laboratoriais	1338
Tabela I-A — Valores Hematológicos Normais	1338
Tabela I-B — Valores Bioquímicos Normais	1338
Tabela I-C — Tabela de Conversão para Unidades Hematológicas	1339
Tabela I-D — Tabela de Conversão para Unidades Bioquímicas Clínicas	1340

Apêndice II — Testes Endócrinos	1341
Tabela II-A — Protocolos para Testes da Função Endócrina	1341
Tabela II-B — Testes do Sistema Endócrino	1342
Tabela II-C — Tabela de Conversão para Unidades de Análise Hormonal	1343

Apêndice III — Valores Normais Aproximados para Mensurações Comuns em Cães e Gatos	1344

Apêndice IV — Valores Normais para o Eletrocardiograma Canino e Felino	1345

Apêndice V — Toxicoses Clínicas — Sistemas Acometidos e Efeitos Clínicos	1346

Apêndice VI — Agentes Tóxicos e seus Antídotos Sistêmicos — Dosagens e Métodos Terapêuticos	1348

Apêndice VII — Riscos de Intoxicação Provenientes de Casa ou do Jardim, para Animais de Companhia	1351
Tabela VII-A — Plantas Tóxicas — Sinais Clínicos, Antídotos e Tratamentos	1351
Tabela VII-B — Toxicidade Relacionada a Ervas Medicinais	1355
Tabela VII-C — Produtos de Limpeza e seus Sinais Clínicos — Antídotos e Tratamentos	1357

Apêndice VIII — Manejo da Dor	1361
Tabela VIII-A — Dosagens Recomendadas e Indicações de Opioides Parenterais	1361

Tabela VIII-B — Dosagens Recomendadas e Indicações
de Opioides Receitáveis — 1361

Tabela VIII-C — Dosagens Recomendadas e Indicações
de AINE Parenterais — 1361

Tabela VIII-D — Dosagens Recomendadas e Indicações
de AINE Receitáveis — 1362

Tabela VIII-E — Dosagens e Indicações de Medicamentos Selecionados
Utilizados para o Tratamento da Dor Neuropática — 1362

Apêndice XIX — Formulário de Medicamentos para Consulta em 5 Minutos — 1363

Apêndice X — Tabelas de Conversão — 1442

Tabela X-A — Tabela de Conversão do Peso para Área de
Superfície Corporal (em Metros Quadrados) para Cães — 1442

Tabela X-B — Valores Equivalentes Aproximados para Graus
Fahrenheit e Celsius — 1443

Tabela X-C — Fatores de Conversão das Unidades de Peso — 1443

Índice Remissivo — 1445

SUMÁRIO POR ESPECIALIDADE

CARDIOLOGIA

Anomalia de Ebstein	95
Anomalias do Anel Vascular	101
Arritmia Sinusal	111
Arritmias Ventriculares e Morte Súbita em Pastor Alemão	113
Ascite	118
Aterosclerose	129
Bloqueio Atrioventricular Completo (Terceiro Grau)	143
Bloqueio Atrioventricular de Primeiro Grau	145
Bloqueio Atrioventricular de Segundo Grau — Mobitz Tipo I	147
Bloqueio Atrioventricular de Segundo Grau — Mobitz Tipo II	149
Bloqueio do Ramo Direito do Feixe de His	151
Bloqueio do Ramo Esquerdo do Feixe de His	153
Bloqueio Fascicular Anterior Esquerdo	155
Bradicardia Sinusal	161
Choque Cardiogênico	200
Choque Hipovolêmico	202
Choque Séptico	204
Complexos Atriais Prematuros	244
Complexos Ventriculares Prematuros	246
Defeito do Septo Atrial	288
Defeito do Septo Ventricular	289
Deficiência de Carnitina	293
Deficiência de Taurina	294
Dirofilariose — Cães	360
Dirofilariose — Gatos	362
Displasia das Valvas Atrioventriculares	378
Doenças Endomiocárdicas — Gatos	423
Edema Periférico	437
Efusão Pericárdica	441
Efusão Pleural	443
Endocardiose das Valvas Atrioventriculares	454
Endocardite Infecciosa	457
Estenose Aórtica	501
Estenose das Valvas Atrioventriculares	503
Estenose Pulmonar	510
Febre	526
Fibrilação e Flutter Atriais	536
Fibrilação Ventricular	539
Fístula Arteriovenosa	545
Flebite	550
Hérnia Diafragmática Peritoneopericárdica	626
Hipertensão Pulmonar	675
Hipertensão Sistêmica	678

Hipotermia	709
Infarto do Miocárdio	733
Insuficiência Cardíaca Congestiva Direita	774
Insuficiência Cardíaca Congestiva Esquerda	776
Intermação e Hipertermia	790
Laceração da Parede Atrial	806
Lesão por Mordedura de Fio Elétrico	819
Linfedema	829
Miocardiopatia — Boxer	900
Miocardiopatia Dilatada — Cães	901
Miocardiopatia Dilatada — Gatos	904
Miocardiopatia Hipertrófica — Cães	906
Miocardiopatia Hipertrófica — Gatos	907
Miocardiopatia Restritiva — Gatos	909
Miocardite	911
Miocardite Traumática	913
Parada Atrial	995
Parada Cardiopulmonar	997
Parada Sinusal e Bloqueio Sinoatrial	999
Parada Ventricular (Assistolia)	1001
Pericardite	1025
Persistência do Ducto Arterioso	1032
Ritmo Idioventricular	1140
Síncope	1159
Síndrome de Wolff-Parkinson-White	1181
Síndrome do Nó Sinusal Doente	1184
Sopros Cardíacos	1199
Taquicardia Sinusal	1203
Taquicardia Supraventricular	1205
Taquicardia Ventricular	1207
Tetralogia de Fallot	1212
Toxicidade da Digoxina	1218
Tromboembolia Aórtica	1276
Tromboembolia Pulmonar	1279
Vasculite Sistêmica	1326

COMPORTAMENTO

Agressividade — Visão Geral — Cães	43
Agressividade — Visão Geral — Gatos	46
Agressividade Canina contra Crianças	49
Agressividade contra Pessoas Familiares — Cães	50
Agressividade Defensiva Induzida pelo Medo — Cães	52
Agressividade entre os Cães	54
Agressividade entre os Gatos	56
Agressividade por Medo — Gatos	58
Agressividade Possessiva, Territorial e Induzida pelo Alimento — Cães	59
Comportamento de Marcação Territorial e Errático — Cães	248
Comportamento de Marcação Territorial e Errático — Gatos	250
Comportamentos Destrutivos	252
Comportamentos Indisciplinados: Saltos, Escavação, Perseguição, Furto	254
Coprofagia e Pica	269
Evacuação e Micção Domiciliares pelos Cães	520
Evacuação e Micção Domiciliares pelos Gatos	522

	Fobias a Trovões e Relâmpagos	552
	Fobias, Medo e Ansiedade — Cães	553
	Fobias, Medo e Ansiedade — Gatos	555
	Introdução de Novos Animais de Estimação na Família	802
	Polifagia	1074
	Problemas Comportamentais Maternos	1081
	Problemas Comportamentais Pediátricos — Cães	1083
	Problemas Comportamentais Pediátricos — Gatos	1085
	Realojamento Bem-Sucedido de Cães e Gatos de Abrigo	1126
	Síndrome de Ansiedade da Separação	1169
	Síndrome de Disfunção Cognitiva	1174
	Transtornos Compulsivos — Cães	1258
	Transtornos Compulsivos — Gatos	1260
	Vocalização Excessiva	1330

DERMATOLOGIA

Ácaros Otológicos	14
Acne — Cães	24
Acne — Gatos	25
Adenite Sebácea Granulomatosa	28
Alopecia — Cães	63
Alopecia — Gatos	65
Alopecia Não Inflamatória — Cães	67
Alopecia Paraneoplásica Felina	69
Alopecia Simétrica Felina	70
Carrapatos e seu Controle	188
Celulite Juvenil	193
Complexo Granuloma Eosinofílico	242
Demodicose	305
Dermatite Acral por Lambedura	310
Dermatite Atópica	311
Dermatite de Contato	313
Dermatite Necrolítica Superficial	314
Dermatite por Malassezia	315
Dermatofilose	316
Dermatofitose	317
Dermatomiosite	319
Dermatoses e Distúrbios Despigmentantes	321
Dermatoses Erosivas ou Ulcerativas	323
Dermatoses Esfoliativas	325
Dermatoses Nasais — Cães	327
Dermatoses Neoplásicas	329
Dermatoses Nodulares/Granulomatosas Estéreis	331
Dermatoses Papulonodulares	333
Dermatoses Vesiculopustulares	335
Dermatoses Virais	337
Distúrbios da Unha e do Leito Ungueal	397
Distúrbios dos Sacos Anais	401
Erupções Medicamentosas Cutâneas	487
Esporotricose	498
Hipersensibilidade à Picada de Pulga e Controle de Pulgas	671
Infecções por Micobactérias	761
Linfoma Cutâneo Epiteliotrópico	834

	Lúpus Eritematoso Cutâneo (Discoide)	839
	Otite Externa e Média	979
	Paniculite	988
	Papilomatose	994
	Pênfigo	1019
	Piodermite	1040
	Pododermatite	1064
	Prototecose	1101
	Prurido	1104
	Queiletielose	1111
	Reações Alimentares Dermatológicas	1123
	Sarna Notoédrica	1149
	Sarna Sarcóptica	1150
	Síndrome da Fragilidade Cutânea Felina	1168
	Síndrome Uveodermatológica	1193
	Vasculite Cutânea — Cães	1325

DOENÇA INFECCIOSA

Abscedação	11
Actinomicose	27
Amebíase	71
Ancilostomíase	78
Aspergilose Disseminada	122
Babesiose	134
Bailisascaríase	136
Bartonelose	137
Blastomicose	139
Borreliose de Lyme	158
Brucelose	166
Campilobacteriose	168
Candidíase	169
Caxumba	192
Cinomose	209
Cisticercose	213
Citauxzoonose	221
Clamidiose — Gatos	222
Coccidioidomicose	228
Colibacilose	237
Criptococose	277
Criptosporidiose	280
Cuterebrose	287
Doença de Chagas (Tripanossomíase Americana)	408
Doença de Tyzzer	411
Encefalitozoonose	449
Erliquiose	485
Esquistossomíase Canina (Heterobilharzíase)	499
Estrongiloidíase	517
Febre Maculosa das Montanhas Rochosas	530
Febre Q	532
Fisalopterose	544
Giardíase	575
Hepatozoonose	623
Histoplasmose	720

Infecção pelo Calicivírus Felino	738
Infecção pelo Poxvírus — Gatos	740
Infecção pelo Vírus da Imunodeficiência Felina	741
Infecção pelo Vírus da Leucemia Felina	743
Infecção pelo Vírus da Pseudorraiva	745
Infecção pelo Vírus Formador de Sincício Felino	746
Infecção pelo Vírus Oeste do Nilo	747
Infecção por Astrovírus	748
Infecção por Coronavírus — Cães	749
Infecção por Herpes-Vírus — Cães	752
Infecção por Herpes-Vírus — Gatos	753
Infecção por Ollulanis	755
Infecção por Reovírus	756
Infecções Anaeróbias	757
Infecções Bacterianas pelas Formas L	758
Infecções por Estafilococos	759
Infecções por Estreptococos	760
Infecções por Rotavírus	763
Influenza — Cães	771
Intoxicação Alimentar pelo Salmão	792
Leishmaniose	814
Leptospirose	815
Micoplasmose	885
Mortalidade Neonatal (Síndrome do Definhamento)	928
Nematódeos (Ascaríase)	940
Neosporose	941
Nocardiose	950
Panleucopenia Felina	989
Peritonite	1027
Peritonite Infecciosa Felina	1030
Peste	1035
Pneumocistose	1052
Raiva	1118
Rinosporidiose	1139
Salmonelose	1144
Sepse e Bacteremia	1155
Tênias (Cestodíase)	1210
Tétano	1211
Toxoplasmose	1256
Tricomoníase	1268
Tricuríase	1269
Triquinose	1270
Tularemia	1281

ENDOCRINOLOGIA E METABOLISMO

Acidose Láctica	19
Acromegalia — Gatos	26
Apudoma	110
Carcinoide e Síndrome Carcinoide	171
Diabetes Insípido	342
Diabetes Melito com Cetoacidose	343
Diabetes Melito com Coma Hiperosmolar	345
Diabetes Melito sem Complicação — Cães	347

Diabetes Melito sem Complicação — Gatos	349
Esteatite	500
Feocromocitoma	534
Glucagonoma	582
Hiperadrenocorticismo (Síndrome de Cushing) — Cães	633
Hiperadrenocorticismo (Síndrome de Cushing) — Gatos	637
Hiperandrogenismo	638
Hipercalcemia	640
Hipercloremia	646
Hiperestrogenismo (Toxicidade do Estrogênio)	648
Hiperfosfatemia	650
Hiperglicemia	652
Hiperlipidemia	654
Hipermagnesemia	656
Hipernatremia	659
Hiperosmolaridade	660
Hiperparatireoidismo	662
Hipertireoidismo	681
Hipoadrenocorticismo (Doença de Addison)	683
Hipoandrogenismo	687
Hipocalcemia	688
Hipocalemia	690
Hipocloremia	692
Hipofosfatemia	693
Hipoglicemia	695
Hipomagnesemia	697
Hiponatremia	700
Hipoparatireoidismo	701
Hipopituitarismo	705
Hipostenúria	708
Hipotireoidismo	711
Insulinoma	788
Mixedema e Coma Mixedematoso	927

GASTRENTEROLOGIA

Abdome Agudo	2
Anorexia	104
Coccidiose	230
Colite e Proctite	239
Colite Ulcerativa Histiocítica	241
Constipação e Obstipação	266
Corpos Estranhos Esofágicos	273
Diarreia Aguda	351
Diarreia Crônica — Cães	353
Diarreia Crônica — Gatos	355
Diarreia Responsiva a Antibióticos	357
Disbiose do Intestino Delgado	364
Disfagia	374
Disquezia e Hematoquezia	386
Distúrbios da Motilidade Gástrica	395
Divertículos Esofágicos	405
Enteropatia Causada pelo Glúten no Setter Irlandês	459
Enteropatia com Perda de Proteínas	460

Enteropatia Imunoproliferativa de Basenjis	462
Enteropatia Inflamatória	463
Enterotoxicose Clostrídica	465
Esofagite	488
Estenose Esofágica	505
Estenose Retal	512
Fístula Perianal	547
Flatulência	548
Gastrenterite Eosinofílica	564
Gastrenterite Hemorrágica	566
Gastrenterite Linfoplasmocitária	568
Gastrite Atrófica	570
Gastrite Crônica	571
Gastropatia Pilórica Hipertrófica Crônica	573
Hematêmese	592
Hérnia de Hiato	624
Hérnia Perineal	627
Íleo Paralítico	724
Incontinência Fecal	728
Infecção por Helicobacter	750
Insuficiência Pancreática Exócrina	780
Intussuscepção	804
Linfangiectasia	827
Má-absorção da Cobalamina	848
Megacólon	864
Megaesôfago	866
Melena	870
Mucocele Salivar	932
Obesidade	951
Obstrução Gastrintestinal	958
Pancreatite	986
Parvovirose Canina	1016
Perda de Peso e Caquexia	1021
Pitiose	1046
Pólipos Retoanais	1078
Prolapso Retal e Anal	1090
Ptialismo	1109
Reações Alimentares (Gastrintestinais) Adversas	1121
Refluxo Gastresofágico	1128
Regurgitação	1129
Síndrome da Dilatação e Vólvulo Gástricos	1172
Síndrome do Intestino Irritável	1183
Síndrome do Vômito Bilioso	1186
Úlcera Gastroduodenal	1301
Vômito Agudo	1331
Vômito Crônico	1333

HEMATOLOGIA / IMUNOLOGIA

Anafilaxia	76
Anemia Aplásica	79
Anemia Arregenerativa	80
Anemia Imunomediada	84
Anemia Metabólica (Anemia com Hemácias Espiculadas)	87

Anemia por Corpúsculo de Heinz	88
Anemia por Defeitos de Maturação Nuclear (Anemia Megaloblástica)	89
Anemia por Deficiência de Ferro	90
Anemia Regenerativa	91
Anomalia de Pelger-Huët	96
Coagulação Intravascular Disseminada	225
Deficiência da Fosfofrutoquinase	291
Deficiência da Piruvato Quinase	292
Deficiência dos Fatores de Coagulação	295
Distúrbios da Imunodeficiência Primária	394
Doença da Aglutinina Fria	407
Doença de von Willebrand	412
Febre Familiar do Shar-Pei	528
Hematopoiese Cíclica	594
Hipercoagulabilidade	647
Histiocitose — Cães	718
Linfadenite	823
Linfadenopatia	825
Lúpus Eritematoso Sistêmico	840
Metemoglobinemia	880
Micoplasmose Hemotrópica (Hemoplasmose)	887
Mucopolissacaridose	934
Neutropenia	946
Pancitopenia	984
Paraproteinemia	1010
Petéquia, Equimose, Contusão	1036
Policitemia	1070
Reações à Transfusão Sanguínea	1125
Síndrome de Chediak-Higashi	1171
Síndrome de Hiperviscosidade	1178
Síndrome Hipereosinofílica	1189
Síndrome Tipo-Sjögren	1192
Torção Esplênica	1215
Trombocitopatias	1271
Trombocitopenia	1272
Trombocitopenia Imunomediada Primária	1274

HEPATOLOGIA

Amiloide Hepático	73
Anomalia Vascular Portossistêmica Congênita	98
Cirrose e Fibrose do Fígado	211
Coagulopatia por Hepatopatia	227
Colecistite e Coledoquite	233
Colelitíase	234
Desvio Portossistêmico Adquirido	340
Displasia Microvascular Hepatoportal	382
Doença do Armazenamento de Glicogênio	414
Encefalopatia Hepática	450
Esplenomegalia	493
Hepatite Crônica Ativa	602
Hepatite Granulomatosa	605
Hepatite Infecciosa Canina	607
Hepatite Supurativa e Abscesso Hepático	609

Hepatomegalia		611
Hepatopatia Diabética		613
Hepatopatia Fibrosante Juvenil		614
Hepatopatia por Armazenamento de Cobre		616
Hepatopatia Vacuolar		619
Hepatotoxinas		621
Hiperplasia Hepática Nodular		669
Hipertensão Portal		673
Hipoalbuminemia		685
Icterícia		722
Infestação por Trematódeos		768
Insuficiência Hepática Aguda		778
Lipidose Hepática		835
Má-formação Arteriovenosa do Fígado		849
Mucocele da Vesícula Biliar		930
Obstrução do Ducto Biliar		953
Peritonite Biliar		1029
Síndrome Colangite e Colangio-Hepatite		1163

NEFROLOGIA / UROLOGIA

Acidose Metabólica	21
Acidose Tubular Renal	23
Alcalose Metabólica	61
Amiloidose	74
Anemia de Doença Renal Crônica	82
Azotemia e Uremia	132
Bexiga Pélvica	138
Capilaríase (Pearsonema)	170
Cilindrúria	208
Cistite Polipoide	214
Cistos Prostáticos	218
Cristalúria	285
Dioctophyma Renale (Também Conhecido como Verme Renal Gigante)	358
Disúria e Polaciúria	.403
Divertículos Vesicouracais	406
Doença Idiopática do Trato Urinário Inferior dos Felinos	417
Doença Renal Policística	421
Doenças Renais de Natureza Congênita e de Desenvolvimento	427
Glicosúria	578
Glomerulonefrite	580
Hematúria	595
Hemoglobinúria e Mioglobinúria	597
Hidronefrose	630
Hiperparatireoidismo Secundário Renal	664
Hiperplasia Prostática Benigna	670
Incontinência Urinária	730
Infecção Bacteriana do Trato Urinário Inferior	735
Infecção Fúngica do Trato Urinário Inferior	737
Insuficiência Renal Aguda	782
Insuficiência Renal Crônica	785
Nefrolitíase	936
Nefrotoxicidade Induzida por Medicamentos	938
Obstrução do Trato Urinário	956

	Oligúria e Anúria	965
	Pielonefrite	1038
	Piúria	1048
	Poliúria e Polidipsia	1079
	Prolapso Uretral	1091
	Prostatite e Abscesso Prostático	1094
	Prostatomegalia	1096
	Proteinúria	1099
	Pseudocistos Perirrenais	1108
	Renomegalia	1131
	Retenção Urinária Funcional	1135
	Síndrome de Fanconi	1176
	Síndrome Nefrótica	1190
	Ureter Ectópico	1305
	Ureterolitíase	1306
	Urolitíase por Cistina	1308
	Urolitíase por Estruvita — Cães	1309
	Urolitíase por Estruvita — Gatos	1311
	Urolitíase por Fosfato de Cálcio	1313
	Urolitíase por Oxalato de Cálcio	1314
	Urolitíase por Urato	1316
	Urolitíase por Xantina	1318

NEUROLOGIA

Acidente Vascular Cerebral (AVC)	17
Ataxia	127
Avulsão do Plexo Braquial	131
Botulismo	160
Cisto Quadrigeminal	217
Cistos Subaracnoides	219
Compressão Cefálica	256
Crises Convulsivas (Convulsões, Estado Epiléptico) — Cães	281
Crises Convulsivas (Convulsões, Estado Epiléptico) — Gatos	283
Degeneração Cerebelar	299
Disautonomia (Síndrome de Key-Gaskell)	363
Discopatia Intervertebral — Gatos	367
Disrafismo Espinal	387
Distrofia Neuroaxonal	391
Doenças do Armazenamento Lisossomal	422
Dor Aguda, Crônica e Pós-operatória	429
Dor no Pescoço e no Dorso	433
Encefalite	445
Encefalite Necrosante	447
Encefalite Secundária à Migração Parasitária	448
Encefalopatia Isquêmica Felina	452
Epilepsia Idiopática (Genética)	479
Espondilomielopatia Cervical (Síndrome de Wobbler)	495
Espondilose Deformante	497
Estenose Lombossacra e Síndrome da Cauda Equina	507
Estupor e Coma	518
Fenômeno de Schiff-Sherrington	533
Fraqueza e Colapso Induzidos por Exercício em Labradores Retrievers	558
Hidrocefalia	628

Hipermetria e Dismetria	658
Hipomielinização	699
Hipoplasia Cerebelar	706
Inclinação da Cabeça	726
Lesão Cerebral	817
Leucoencefalomielopatia no Rottweiler	822
Más-formações Congênitas Espinais e Vertebrais	853
Meningioma	871
Meningite-Arterite Responsivas a Esteroides — Cães	873
Meningite/Meningoencefalite/Meningomielite Bacterianas	874
Meningoencefalomielite Eosinofílica	876
Meningoencefalomielite Granulomatosa	877
Mielomalacia (Aguda, Ascendente, Descendente)	893
Mielopatia — Paresia/Paralisia — Gatos	894
Mielopatia Degenerativa	896
Mielopatia Embólica Fibrocartilaginosa	898
Mioclonia	914
Narcolepsia e Cataplexia	935
Neurite Idiopática do Trigêmeo	942
Neuropatias Periféricas (Polineuropatias)	944
Nistagmo	948
Otite Média e Interna	982
Paralisia	1004
Paralisia do Carrapato	1006
Paralisia do Coonhound (Polirradiculoneurite Idiopática)	1008
Paresia e Paralisia do Nervo Facial	1013
Polioencefalomielite — Gatos	1076
Síndrome da Hiperestesia Felina	1177
Síndrome de Tremor Generalizado (Síndrome do Cão Tremedor)	1180
Siringomielia e Má-Formação Tipo Chiari	1198
Surdez	1202
Traumatismo da Coluna Vertebral	1264
Tremores	1266
Tumores Cerebrais	1285
Tumores da Bainha Nervosa	1287
Vestibulopatia Geriátrica — Cães	1327
Vestibulopatia Idiopática — Gatos	1329

ODONTOLOGIA

Abscesso da Raiz Dentária (Abscesso Apical)	13
Cáries Dentárias	186
Cisto Dentígero	216
Dentes Decíduos, Persistentes (Retidos)	307
Dentes Manchados	308
Distúrbios da Articulação Temporomandibular	393
Doença Periodontal	419
Epúlide	484
Estomatite	515
Fístula Oronasal	546
Formação e Estrutura Anormais do Dente	557
Fratura Dentária	560
Fraturas Maxilares e Mandibulares	562
Halitose	585

	Hiperplasia Gengival	668
	Hipoplasia/Hipocalcificação do Esmalte	707
	Inflamação Orofaríngea Felina	770
	Luxação ou Avulsão dos Dentes	843
	Maloclusão Esquelética e Dentária	851
	Massas Bucais	857
	Reabsorção dos Dentes em Felinos (Reabsorção Odontoclástica)	1120
	Ulceração Bucal	1303
OFTALMOLOGIA	Anisocoria	93
	Anomalia do Olho do Collie	97
	Anomalias Oculares Congênitas	102
	Atrofia da Íris	130
	Blefarite	141
	Cataratas	190
	Ceratite Eosinofílica — Gatos	194
	Ceratite Não Ulcerativa	195
	Ceratite Ulcerativa	197
	Ceratoconjuntivite Seca	199
	Conjuntivite — Cães	262
	Conjuntivite — Gatos	264
	Coriorretinite	271
	Degeneração da Retina	300
	Degenerações e Infiltrações da Córnea	304
	Descolamento da Retina	338
	Distrofias da Córnea	392
	Distúrbios dos Cílios (Triquíase, Distiquíase/Cílios Ectópicos)	400
	Doenças Orbitais (Exoftalmia, Enoftalmia, Estrabismo)	425
	Ectrópio	436
	Entrópio	467
	Epífora	477
	Episclerite	481
	Glaucoma	576
	Hemorragia da Retina	599
	Hifema	631
	Hipópio e Depósito Lipídico	704
	Lacerações da Córnea e Esclera	808
	Luxação do Cristalino	842
	Melanoma Uveal em Cães	868
	Melanoma Uveal em Gatos	869
	Neurite Óptica	943
	Oftalmia Neonatal	960
	Olho Cego "Silencioso"	961
	Olho Vermelho	963
	Papiledema	993
	Prolapso da Glândula da Terceira Pálpebra (Olho de Cereja)	1089
	Proptose	1093
	Protrusão da Terceira Pálpebra	1102
	Sequestro de Córnea — Gatos	1157
	Síndrome de Horner	1179
	Uveíte Anterior — Cães	1319
	Uveíte Anterior — Gatos	1321

ONCOLOGIA

Adenocarcinoma da Próstata	29
Adenocarcinoma da Tireoide — Cães	30
Adenocarcinoma das Glândulas Ceruminosas, Orelha	32
Adenocarcinoma das Glândulas Salivares	33
Adenocarcinoma das Glândulas Sebáceas e Sudoríferas	34
Adenocarcinoma do Estômago, Intestinos Delgado, Grosso e Reto	35
Adenocarcinoma do Pâncreas	36
Adenocarcinoma dos Pulmões	37
Adenocarcinoma dos Sacos Anais	38
Adenocarcinoma Nasal	39
Adenocarcinoma Renal	40
Adenoma Hepatocelular	41
Ameloblastoma	72
Astrocitoma	126
Carcinoma de Células de Transição	172
Carcinoma de Células Escamosas da Língua	174
Carcinoma de Células Escamosas da Pele	175
Carcinoma de Células Escamosas da Tonsila	177
Carcinoma de Células Escamosas das Gengivas	178
Carcinoma de Células Escamosas das Orelhas	179
Carcinoma de Células Escamosas do Plano Nasal	180
Carcinoma de Células Escamosas dos Dedos	181
Carcinoma de Células Escamosas dos Pulmões	182
Carcinoma de Células Escamosas dos Seios Nasais e Paranasais	183
Carcinoma de Ducto Biliar	184
Carcinoma Hepatocelular	185
Colesteatoma	236
Condrossarcoma — Boca	258
Condrossarcoma — Laringe e Traqueia	259
Condrossarcoma — Osso	260
Condrossarcoma — Seios Nasais e Paranasais	261
Distúrbios Mieloproliferativos	402
Fibrossarcoma da Gengiva	541
Fibrossarcoma de Osso	542
Fibrossarcoma dos Seios Nasais e Paranasais	543
Granulomatose Linfomatoide	584
Hemangiopericitoma	586
Hemangiossarcoma Cutâneo	587
Hemangiossarcoma do Baço e do Fígado	588
Hemangiossarcoma do Coração	590
Hemangiossarcoma do Osso	591
Histiocitoma	716
Histiocitoma Fibroso Maligno (Tumor de Células Gigantes)	717
Leiomioma do Estômago e dos Intestinos Delgado e Grosso	812
Leiomiossarcoma do Estômago e dos Intestinos Delgado e Grosso	813
Leucemia Linfoblástica Aguda	820
Leucemia Linfocítica Crônica	821
Linfoma — Cães	830
Linfoma — Gatos	832
Lipoma	837
Lipoma Infiltrativo	838
Mastocitomas	861

Mesotelioma	879
Mieloma Múltiplo	891
Oncocitoma	967
Osteossarcoma	977
Plasmocitoma Mucocutâneo	1051
Policitemia Vera	1073
Quimiodectoma	1114
Rabdomioma	1115
Rabdomiossarcoma	1116
Rabdomiossarcoma da Bexiga Urinária	1117
Sarcoma Associado à Vacina	1146
Sarcoma de Células Sinoviais	1148
Schwanoma	1151
Seminoma	1154
Sertolinoma	1158
Síndromes Mielodisplásicas	1194
Síndromes Paraneoplásicas	1195
Timoma	1213
Tumor das Células Basais (Basalioma)	1282
Tumor de Células Intersticiais do Testículo	1283
Tumor Venéreo Transmissível	1284
Tumores das Glândulas Mamárias — Cadelas	1288
Tumores das Glândulas Mamárias — Gatas	1291
Tumores dos Folículos Pilosos	1292
Tumores Malignos Indiferenciados da Cavidade Bucal	1293
Tumores Melanocíticos Bucais	1294
Tumores Melanocíticos da Pele e dos Dedos	1295
Tumores Miocárdicos	1297
Tumores Ovarianos	1298
Tumores Uterinos	1299
Tumores Vaginais	1300

SISTEMA MUSCULOESQUELÉTICO

Artrite (Osteoartrite)	114
Artrite Séptica	116
Claudicação	224
Deformidades do Crescimento Antebraquial	297
Discopatia Intervertebral Cervical	368
Discopatia Intervertebral Toracolombar	370
Discospondilite	372
Displasia Coxofemoral	376
Displasia do Cotovelo	380
Doença de Legg-Calvé-Perthes	409
Doença do Ligamento Cruzado Cranial	415
Instabilidade Atlantoaxial	772
Luxação Patelar	844
Luxações Articulares	846
Miastenia Grave	883
Miopatia Inflamatória — Polimiosite e Dermatomiosite	915
Miopatia Inflamatória Focal — Miosite dos Músculos Mastigatórios e Extraoculares	917
Miopatia Não Inflamatória — Cãibra Hereditária do Terrier Escocês	919

Miopatia Não Inflamatória — Distrofia Muscular Hereditária Ligada ao Cromossomo X	920
Miopatia Não Inflamatória — Endócrina	921
Miopatia Não Inflamatória — Hereditária no Labrador Retriever	923
Miopatia Não Inflamatória — Metabólica	924
Miopatia Não Inflamatória — Miotonia Hereditária	926
Osteocondrodisplasia	968
Osteocondrose	969
Osteodistrofia Hipertrófica	971
Osteomielite	973
Osteopatia Craniomandibular	975
Osteopatia Hipertrófica	976
Panosteíte	991
Poliartrite Erosiva Imunomediada	1066
Poliartrite Não Erosiva Imunomediada	1068
Problemas do Ombro, Ligamento e Tendão	1087
Ruptura Muscular (Laceração Muscular)	1142

SISTEMA RESPIRATÓRIO

Afogamento (Afogamento por um Triz)	42
Asma, Bronquite — Gatos	120
Aspergilose Nasal	124
Bordetelose — Gatos	157
Bronquiectasia	163
Bronquite Crônica	164
Cianose	206
Colapso da Traqueia	231
Contusões Pulmonares	268
Discinesia Ciliar Primária	366
Dispneia e Angústia Respiratória	384
Edema Pulmonar Não Cardiogênico	439
Epistaxe	482
Espirro, Espirro Reverso, Ânsia de Vômito	491
Estenose Nasofaríngea	509
Estertor e Estridor	513
Hemotórax	601
Hérnia Diafragmática	625
Hipercapnia	644
Hipoxemia	714
Inalação de Fumaça	725
Laringopatia	810
Mediastinite	863
Parasitas Respiratórios	1011
Peito Escavado	1018
Perfuração da Traqueia	1024
Piotórax	1044
Pneumonia Bacteriana	1053
Pneumonia Eosinofílica	1055
Pneumonia Fúngica	1057
Pneumonia Intersticial	1059
Pneumonia por Aspiração	1061
Pneumotórax	1062
Pólipos Nasais e Nasofaríngeos	1077

Quilotórax	1112
Respiração Ofegante e Taquipneia	1133
Rinite e Sinusite	1137
Secreção Nasal	1152
Síndrome Braquicefálica das Vias Aéreas	1161
Síndrome da Angústia Respiratória Aguda (SARA)	1166
Torção de Lobo Pulmonar	1214
Tosse	1216
Traqueobronquite Infecciosa Canina (Tosse dos Canis)	1262

TERIOGENOLOGIA

Abortamento Espontâneo (Perda Gestacional Precoce) — Cadelas	5
Abortamento Espontâneo (Perda Gestacional Precoce) — Gatas	7
Abortamento, Interrupção da Gestação	9
Acasalamento, Momento Oportuno	15
Anormalidades dos Espermatozoides	106
Corrimento Vaginal	275
Criptorquidismo	279
Degeneração e Hipoplasia Testiculares	303
Distocia	388
Distúrbios do Desenvolvimento Sexual	398
Eclâmpsia	435
Epididimite/Orquite	476
Espermatocele/Granuloma Espermático	490
Falha Ovulatória	525
Hiperplasia das Glândulas Mamárias — Gatas	666
Hiperplasia e Prolapso Vaginais	667
Inércia Uterina	732
Infertilidade das Cadelas	764
Infertilidade dos Cães Machos	766
Más-formações Vaginais e Lesões Adquiridas	855
Mastite	860
Metrite	882
Parafimose, Fimose e Priapismo	1003
Parto Prematuro	1015
Piometra e Hiperplasia Endometrial Cística	1042
Placenta Retida	1050
Prostatopatia no Cão Macho Reprodutor	1097
Pseudociese	1106
Síndrome dos Ovários Remanescentes	1187
Subinvolução dos Sítios Placentários	1201
Vaginite	1323

TOXICOLOGIA

Antidepressivos — Toxicose por Antidepressivos Tricíclicos (ATC)	107
Antidepressivos — Toxicose por Inibidor Seletivo de Recaptação da Serotonina (ISRS)	109
Envenenamento (Intoxicação)	468
Envenenamento por Arsênico	470
Envenenamento por Cogumelo	471
Envenenamento por Rodenticidas Anticoagulantes	475
Intoxicação pelo Chumbo	793
Intoxicação pelo Lírio	795
Intoxicação por Ácido Acetilsalicílico	796

Intoxicação por Estricnina	797
Intoxicação por Etanol	798
Intoxicação por Etilenoglicol	799
Intoxicação por Metaldeído	801
Micotoxicose — Aflatoxina	888
Micotoxicose — Desoxinivalenol	889
Micotoxicose — Toxinas Tremorgênicas	890
Toxicidade da Vitamina D	1219
Toxicidade das Piretrinas e dos Piretroides	1222
Toxicidade do Paracetamol	1223
Toxicidade do Rodenticida Brometalina	1225
Toxicidade do Veneno de Lacertílios	1226
Toxicidade do Xilitol	1227
Toxicidade do Zinco	1228
Toxicidade dos Agentes Anti-Inflamatórios Não Esteroides	1229
Toxicidade pela Ivermectina	1231
Toxicidade pelo Ferro	1232
Toxicose por Amitraz	1233
Toxicose por Anfetamina	1235
Toxicose por Benzodiazepínicos e Soníferos	1237
Toxicose por Beta-2 Agonistas Inalatórios	1239
Toxicose por Chocolate	1240
Toxicose por Metformina	1243
Toxicose por Monóxido de Carbono	1244
Toxicose por Organofosforado e Carbamato	1245
Toxicose por Pseudoefedrina	1247
Toxicose por Uvas e Passas	1248
Toxicose por Veneno de Aranha — Família da Reclusa-Castanha	1249
Toxicose por Veneno de Aranha — Viúva-Negra	1250
Toxicose por Veneno de Cobra — Corais	1251
Toxicose por Veneno de Cobra — Víboras	1252
Toxicose por Veneno de Sapo	1253
Toxicoses por Hidrocarboneto de Petróleo	1254

Consulta Veterinária em 5 Minutos: Espécies Canina e Felina

5ª Edição

Abdome Agudo

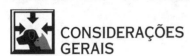

CONSIDERAÇÕES GERAIS

DEFINIÇÃO
Um quadro emergencial caracterizado pelo encontro de um abdome tenso e dolorido na anamnese e no exame físico. O abdome agudo pode representar um quadro com risco de vida.

FISIOPATOLOGIA
- Um paciente com abdome agudo apresenta dor associada à distensão de órgão, inflamação, tração exercida no mesentério ou no peritônio ou isquemia.
- Como as vísceras abdominais são esparsamente inervadas, muitas vezes é necessário o envolvimento visceral difuso para a indução da dor; também existem terminações nervosas nas camadas submucosa e muscular da parede intestinal.
- Qualquer processo que provoque distensão líquida ou gasosa (i. e., obstrução intestinal, dilatação-vólvulo gástricos e íleo paralítico) pode causar dor.
- A inflamação gera dor abdominal pela liberação de substâncias vasoativas, que estimulam as terminações nervosas por via direta.
- Muitos nervos presentes no peritônio são sensíveis à resposta inflamatória difusa.

SISTEMA(S) ACOMETIDO(S)
- Comportamental — tremor, inapetência, vocalização, letargia, depressão e mudanças posturais anormais, como a posição típica de oração, para obter certo conforto e alívio da dor.
- Cardiovascular — inflamação, isquemia e sepse graves podem levar a colapso circulatório agudo (choque).
- Gastrintestinal — vômito, diarreia, inapetência, íleo paralítico funcional generalizado; inflamação, necrose e abscesso pancreáticos podem levar à dor da porção abdominal cranial, vômito e íleo paralítico.
- Hepatobiliar — icterícia associada à colestase extra-hepática decorrente de obstruções biliares (incluindo pancreatite) e peritonite biliar.
- Renal/urológico — a azotemia pode ocorrer por causas pré-renais (desidratação, hipovolemia e choque), renais (pielonefrite aguda e insuficiência renal aguda) e pós-renais (obstrução uretral e uroperitônio decorrente de ruptura vesical).
- Respiratório — aumento na frequência respiratória em função da dor ou de distúrbios metabólicos.

IDENTIFICAÇÃO
- Cães e gatos.
- Os cães costumam ser mais acometidos.
- Os animais mais jovens tendem a ter uma incidência mais alta de problemas relacionados com traumatismo, intussuscepções, além de doenças adquiridas relacionadas com dieta e infecção; já os animais idosos apresentam uma frequência maior de malignidades.
- Cães e gatos machos têm maior risco de obstrução uretral.
- Os cães machos da raça Dálmata particularmente exibem um risco mais elevado de obstrução uretral, em virtude da alta incidência de cálculos urinários de urato.
- Os cães da raça Pastor alemão com atrofia pancreática possuem um risco mais alto de vólvulo mesentérico.
- Os pacientes tratados com corticosteroides e medicamentos anti-inflamatórios não esteroides (AINE) estão sob maior risco de ulceração e perfuração gastrintestinais (GI).

SINAIS CLÍNICOS
Comentários Gerais
Os sinais clínicos variam bastante, dependendo do tipo e da gravidade da doença indutora do abdome agudo.

Achados Anamnésicos
- Tremor, relutância em se mover, inapetência, vômito, diarreia, vocalização e posturas anormais (posição encolhida ou típica de oração) — sinais que podem ser observados pelo proprietário.
- Questionar o proprietário com rigor para determinar qual o sistema acometido; por exemplo, a presença de hematêmese associada à histórico de tratamento com AINE sugere ulceração da mucosa GI.

Achados do Exame Físico
- As anormalidades incluem dor abdominal, enrijecimento da musculatura abdominal, órgãos abdominais preenchidos com gás ou líquido, massa abdominal, ascite, pirexia ou hipotermia, taquicardia e taquipneia.
- Assim que a dor abdominal for confirmada, tentar situá-la na região abdominal cranial, média ou caudal.
- Realizar o exame retal para avaliar o cólon, os ossos pélvicos, a uretra e a próstata, bem como a presença de melena.
- Descartar as causas extra-abdominais de dor por meio da palpação rigorosa dos rins e das vértebras toracolombares.
- A dor associada à discopatia intervertebral frequentemente provoca enrijecimento abdominal referido que, muitas vezes, é confundido com dor abdominal verdadeira. A dor nos rins pode estar associada à pielonefrite.

CAUSAS
Trato gastrintestinal
- Estômago — gastrite, úlceras, perfuração, corpos estranhos, dilatação-vólvulo gástricos.
- Intestino — obstrução (corpos estranhos, intussuscepção, hérnias), enterite, úlceras, perfurações.
- Ruptura após obstrução, ulceração, traumatismo rombo ou perfurante ou decorrente de crescimento tumoral.
- Comprometimento vascular em virtude de infarto, vólvulo mesentérico ou torção.

Pâncreas
- Dor associada à inflamação, a abscesso, à isquemia nesse órgão.
- A presença de massas ou inflamações pancreáticas responsáveis pela obstrução do ducto/papila biliares causará icterícia.

Sistema Hepatobiliar
- A distensão abrupta do fígado e de sua cápsula pode causar dor.
- Obstruções, rupturas ou necrose da vesícula biliar podem levar ao extravasamento de bile e à ocorrência de peritonite.
- Abscesso hepático.

Baço
- Torção, massas, trombo ou abscesso esplênicos.

Trato Urinário
- A distensão representa a principal causa de dor no trato urinário.
- A obstrução do trato urinário inferior pode ser atribuída a tumores na área do trígono vesical ou da uretra, cálculos urinários ou uretrite granulomatosa.
- As rupturas traumáticas dos ureteres ou da bexiga associam-se a traumatismo rombo e pressão intra-abdominal elevada.
- As lacerações uretrais podem estar relacionadas com fraturas pélvicas decorrentes de traumatismo agudo.
- A presença de urina livre na cavidade peritoneal leva à peritonite química.
- Os quadros de pielonefrite aguda, insuficiência renal aguda, nefrólitos e ureterólitos são causas incomuns de abdome agudo.

Trato Genital
- Prostatite e abscesso prostático, piometra; a ruptura da piometra ou de abscesso prostático pode causar endotoxemia, sepse e colapso cardiovascular.
- As causas raras incluem rupturas de útero prenhe após traumatismo abdominal rombo, torção uterina, torção ou tumor ovarianos e torção testicular intra-abdominal (criptorquidismo).

Parede Abdominal/Diafragma
- Hérnias umbilicais, inguinais, escrotais, abdominais ou peritoneais com estrangulamento de vísceras.
- Traumatismo ou defeitos congênitos indutores do deslocamento ou do encarceramento de órgãos na hérnia levarão à dor abdominal em caso de diminuição ou isquemia do aporte vascular dos órgãos envolvidos.

FATORES DE RISCO
- Exposição aos AINE ou à corticoterapia — úlceras gástricas, duodenais ou colônicas.
- Ingestão de lixo ou alimento inconveniente — pancreatite.
- Ingestão de corpo(s) estranho(s) — obstruções intestinais.
- Traumatismo abdominal — ruptura de víscera oca.
- Hérnias — obstrução/estrangulamento intestinal.

DIAGNÓSTICO

DIAGNÓSTICO DIFERENCIAL
- As dores renais, retroperitoneais, espinais ou paraespinais, bem como os distúrbios indutores de mialgia difusa, podem mimetizar a dor abdominal; por isso, a anamnese rigorosa e o exame físico detalhado são essenciais na busca do problema pertinente.
- A enterite por parvovírus pode se apresentar igual à enteropatia obstrutiva; assim, o ensaio para pesquisa do antígeno fecal do parvovírus e o hemograma completo (leucopenia) são úteis nos testes diagnósticos diferenciais.

HEMOGRAMA/BIOQUÍMICA/URINÁLISE
- A inflamação ou a infecção podem estar relacionadas com leucocitose ou leucopenia.
- É possível observar anemias em casos de perda sanguínea associada à ulceração GI.
- A azotemia associa-se a causas pré-renais, renais e pós-renais.
- As anormalidades eletrolíticas podem ajudar a avaliar gastrenteropatia (i. e., alcalose metabólica hipoclorêmica com obstrução ao fluxo de

ABDOME AGUDO

esvaziamento gástrico) e nefropatia (i. e., hipercalemia com insuficiência renal aguda ou obstrução pós-renal).
• A hiperbilirrubinemia e a elevação das enzimas hepáticas ajudam a situar o problema no fígado ou no trato biliar.
• A obtenção da densidade urinária (antes da fluidoterapia) é imprescindível para diferenciar os problemas pré-renais, renais e pós-renais.
• O sedimento urinário pode ser útil em casos de insuficiência renal aguda, intoxicação pelo etilenoglicol e pielonefrite.

OUTROS TESTES LABORATORIAIS
• A imunorreatividade semelhante à da tripsina pode ser útil na avaliação de pancreatite felina.
• A imunorreatividade da lipase pancreática canina é um teste benéfico para o diagnóstico de pancreatite nessa espécie.

DIAGNÓSTICO POR IMAGEM
Radiografia Abdominal
• É possível observar a presença de massas abdominais ou alterações no formato ou desvio de órgãos abdominais.
• A perda do contorno abdominal com acúmulo de líquido no abdome é uma indicação para a realização de abdominocentese.
• A existência de gases livres no abdome é compatível com ruptura de víscera GI ou infecção por bactérias produtoras de gases, além de ser uma indicação de cirurgia em caráter emergencial.
• Deve-se ter cuidado ao se interpretar as radiografias após abdominocentese com punção aberta, em virtude da possibilidade de introdução de gases livres por essa técnica.
• É preciso ter cautela ao se avaliar as radiografias pós-operatórias, pois a presença de gases livres é um achado normal no período após a cirurgia.
• O íleo paralítico é um sinal compatível com a peritonite.
• Caracterizar o íleo paralítico como funcional (atribuído a causas metabólicas ou infecciosas) ou mecânico (gerado por obstrução).
• Os corpos estranhos podem ser radiopacos.
• As radiografias contrastadas (com bário) do trato GI superior são úteis na avaliação desse órgão, particularmente para a determinação de obstrução GI.
• Em caso de inflamação pancreática, pode haver perda de contraste na área referente ao pâncreas.

Ultrassonografia Abdominal
• Uma das ferramentas diagnósticas mais sensíveis para a detecção de massas abdominais, líquido abdominal, abscessos, cistos, linfadenopatia e cálculos biliares ou urinários.

MÉTODOS DIAGNÓSTICOS
Abdominocentese/Análise do Líquido Abdominal
• Efetuar a abdominocentese em todos os pacientes que apresentarem abdome agudo. A coleta de líquido frequentemente é possível para proceder à avaliação diagnóstica, mesmo na presença de pequena quantidade de líquido abdominal livre, bem antes da sensibilidade radiográfica detectável. Embora a ultrassonografia seja muito mais sensível do que a radiografia para a detecção de líquido, a falta de tal detecção não descarta a necessidade da abdominocentese. A análise do líquido abdominal com contagem leucocitária elevada, neutrófilos degenerados e bactérias intracelulares é compatível com peritonite séptica, além de ser uma indicação de cirurgia em caráter emergencial.
• A lavagem peritoneal diagnóstica pode ser efetuada pela introdução de soro fisiológico estéril (10-20 mL/kg) e realização da abdominocentese.
• A mensuração da concentração de glicose na efusão abdominal pode ajudar no diagnóstico de abdome séptico.
• Os pacientes com pancreatite podem exibir uma efusão abdominal, caracterizada como peritonite asséptica (estéril).
• Uma concentração de creatinina no líquido abdominal mais elevada que no soro indica a ocorrência de extravasamento do trato urinário.
• Do mesmo modo, uma concentração de bilirrubina no líquido abdominal mais alta que no soro sugere peritonite biliar.

Sedação e Palpação Abdominal
• Em virtude do enrijecimento abdominal associado à dor, a palpação abdominal minuciosa muitas vezes não é possível sem sedação; esse exame é particularmente útil para detectar corpos estranhos intestinais que não aparecem nas radiografias simples.

Laparotomia Exploratória
• A cirurgia pode ser útil do ponto de vista diagnóstico (bem como terapêutico) em caso de indisponibilidade da ultrassonografia ou do não estabelecimento de uma causa definitiva para o abdome agudo com metodologias diagnósticas apropriadas.

TRATAMENTO
• O tratamento é feito em esquema de internação com a provisão de cuidados de suporte até que se decida entre o tratamento clínico ou cirúrgico.
• É muito importante que a causa subjacente seja identificada imediatamente e submetida a tratamento rigoroso.
• Muitas causas de dor abdominal aguda necessitam de intervenção cirúrgica em caráter de emergência.

CUIDADO(S) DE SUPORTE
• Manter o paciente em jejum (i. e., com nada por via oral) na presença de vômito, até que se determine e se aponte a causa definitiva.
• A fluidoterapia intravenosa costuma ser necessária, em virtude da grande perda líquida associada ao abdome agudo; o objetivo é restabelecer o volume sanguíneo circulante normal.
• Caso haja um comprometimento circulatório grave (choque), suplementar o paciente em princípio com fluidos cristaloides isotônicos (90 mL/kg, cães; 70 mL/kg, gatos) durante 1-2 h; os fluidos hipertônicos ou os coloides também podem ser benéficos.
• Avaliar o estado de hidratação e os níveis de eletrólitos (com ajustes terapêuticos apropriados) frequentemente após o início do tratamento.

CONSIDERAÇÕES CIRÚRGICAS
• Há muitas causas distintas de abdome agudo (com tratamentos tanto clínico como cirúrgico); sempre que possível, é fundamental formular o diagnóstico definitivo antes da intervenção cirúrgica.
• Isso pode evitar não só procedimentos cirúrgicos potencialmente desnecessários e caros, mas também a morbidade e a mortalidade associadas.
• O diagnóstico também permitirá que o cirurgião se prepare para a intervenção e oriente o proprietário acerca do prognóstico e dos custos envolvidos.

MEDICAÇÕES
MEDICAMENTO(S)
Analgésicos
• Tais agentes podem ser indicados para o controle do desconforto abdominal.
• Opioides, como hidromorfona a 0,05-0,1 mg/kg, costumam ser ótimas escolhas.

Antagonistas Histaminérgicos H_2
• Diminuem a produção de ácido gástrico.
• Famotidina a 0,1-0,2 mg/kg IV, SC ou IM a cada 12 h.
• Ranitidina a 2 mg/kg IV a cada 8 h.

Inibidores da Bomba de Prótons
• Pantoprazol a 0,5-1 mg/kg IV sob infusão em velocidade constante durante 24 h.

Protetores da Mucosa Gástrica
• Sucralfato a 0,25-1 g VO a cada 8 h.

Antieméticos
• Metoclopramida a 0,2-0,4 mg/kg IV a cada 6-8 h (ou sob infusão em velocidade constante por 24 h).
• Maropitant a 1 mg/kg SC (cães) e 0,5 mg/kg SC (gatos).
• Ondansetrona a 0,5-1 mg/kg IV lentamente a cada 6-12 h.
• Dolasetrona a 1 mg/kg IV a cada 24 h.

Antibióticos
• Tais agentes poderão ser indicados se houver sinais de infecção (febre, contagem leucocitária elevada, resultados positivos em cultura).
• De amplo espectro contra bactérias Gram-positivas, Gram-negativas e anaeróbias.
• Se possível, efetuar a coloração de Gram e a realização de culturas antes do tratamento.

CONTRAINDICAÇÕES
Não empregar a metoclopramida na suspeita de obstrução GI.

PRECAUÇÕES
A gentamicina e grande parte dos AINEs podem ser nefrotóxicas e devem ser utilizadas com cautela em pacientes hipovolêmicos e naqueles com dano renal.

ACOMPANHAMENTO
MONITORIZAÇÃO DO PACIENTE
Os pacientes costumam necessitar de cuidado clínico intensivo, além de avaliação frequente dos sinais vitais e parâmetros laboratoriais.

DIVERSOS
SINÔNIMO(S)
Cólica.

VER TAMBÉM
• Úlcera Gastroduodenal.
• Intussuscepção.
• Obstrução do Trato Urinário.

ABDOME AGUDO

- Obstrução Gastrintestinal.
- Pancreatite.
- Prostatite e Abscesso Prostático.
- Síndrome da Dilatação e Vólvulo Gástricos.

ABREVIATURAS

- AINE = anti-inflamatório não esteroide.
- GI = gastrintestinal.

Sugestões de Leitura

Beal MW. Approach to the acute abdomen. Vet Clin North Am Small Anim Pract 2005, 35:375-396.

Heeren V, Edwards L, Mazzaferro EM. Acute abdomen: Diagnosis. Compend Contin Educ Pract Vet 2004, 26:350-363.

Heeren V, Edwards L, Mazzaferro EM. Acute abdomen: Treatment. Compend Contin Educ Pract Vet 2004, 26:3566-3673.

Mazzaferro EM. Triage and approach to the acute abdomen. Clin Tech Small Anim Pract 2003, 18:1-6.

Autor Steven L. Marks
Consultor Editorial Albert E. Jergens

Abortamento Espontâneo (Perda Gestacional Precoce) — Cadelas

CONSIDERAÇÕES GERAIS

DEFINIÇÃO
Perda de feto em virtude de reabsorção nas fases precoces ou expulsão nas fases tardias da gestação.

FISIOPATOLOGIA
• Causas diretas — anormalidade congênita, doença infecciosa, traumatismo. • Causas indiretas — placentite infecciosa, função ovariana anormal, ambiente uterino anormal.

SISTEMA(S) ACOMETIDO(S)
• Reprodutivo. • Qualquer disfunção de sistema corporal importante pode comprometer adversamente a gestação.

GENÉTICA
• Não há base genética para grande parte das causas de abortamento • Hipotireoidismo linfocítico — traço genético recessivo isolado (ou seja, de um único gene) em Borzói.

INCIDÊNCIA/PREVALÊNCIA
• Incidência real desconhecida. • Reabsorção estimada entre 11-13%, com algumas estimativas de até 30% de, no mínimo, uma única reabsorção. • Incidência de natimortos relatada como 2,2-4,4%; aumentos em casos de distocia de até 22,3%.

IDENTIFICAÇÃO

Espécies
Cadelas.

Raça(s) Predominante(s)
• Hipotireoidismo linfocítico familiar relatado em Borzói — intervalo prolongado entre os estros (cios), baixos índices de concepção, abortamento na metade da gestação, natimortos. • Muitas raças são consideradas sob risco de hipotireoidismo familiar (ver Hipotireoidismo).

Idade Média e Faixa Etária
• Causas infecciosas, agentes farmacológicos indutores de abortamento, defeitos fetais — observados em todas as idades. • Hiperplasia endometrial cística — geralmente em idade acima de 6 anos.

Sexo Predominante
Cadelas intactas.

SINAIS CLÍNICOS

Achados Anamnésicos
• Falha em dar à luz na hora certa. • Expulsão de fetos ou tecidos placentários identificáveis. • Redução do volume abdominal; perda de peso. • Anorexia. • Vômito, diarreia • Mudanças comportamentais.

Achados do Exame Físico
• Corrimento vulvar sanguinolento ou purulento. • Desaparecimento de vesículas ou fetos previamente confirmados por meio de palpação, ultrassonografia ou radiografia. • Esforço abdominal, desconforto. • Depressão. • Desidratação. • Febre em algumas pacientes.

CAUSAS

Infecciosas
• *Brucella canis*. • Herpes-vírus canino. • *Toxoplasma gondii*, *Neospora caninum*. • *Mycoplasma* e *Ureaplasma*. • Diversas bactérias — *E. coli*, *Streptococcus*, *Campylobacter*, *Salmonella*. • Diversos vírus — vírus da cinomose, parvovírus, adenovírus.

Uterinas
• Hiperplasia endometrial cística e piometra. • Traumatismo — agudo e crônico. • Neoplasia. • Medicamentos embriotóxicos. • Agentes quimioterápicos. • Estrogênios. • Glicocorticoides — altas dosagens.

Ovarianas
• Prostaglandinas — lise de corpos lúteos. • Agonistas dopaminérgicos — lise de corpos lúteos via supressão da prolactina; bromocriptina, cabergolina. • Hipoluteoidismo — anormalidade da função luteal na ausência de doença fetal, uterina ou placentária; concentrações de progesterona <1-2 ng/mL, observadas com maior frequência em gestação de 40-45 dias.

Disfunção Hormonal
• Hipotireoidismo; dados recentes revelam que isso é menos comum do que se acreditava. • Hiperadrenocorticismo. • Fatores ambientais — contaminantes que atacam o sistema endócrino foram relatados em casos de perda fetal em seres humanos e animais silvestres.

Defeitos Fetais
• Anormalidade cromossômica letal. • Defeitos orgânicos letais.

FATORES DE RISCO
• Exposição da cadela reprodutora a animais portadores. • Idade avançada. • Fatores hereditários.

DIAGNÓSTICO

DIAGNÓSTICO DIFERENCIAL
• Diferenciar causas infecciosas de não infecciosas — a *B. canis* é de preocupação zoonótica e imediata. • Diferenciar reabsorção de infertilidade — auxiliada pelo diagnóstico precoce de gestação. • Histórico de uso de medicamentos durante a gestação — particularmente durante o primeiro trimestre ou uso de medicamentos (p. ex., dexametasona, prostaglandinas, cetoconazol, griseofulvina, doxiciclina, tetraciclina, dantroleno, entre outros) sabidamente causadores de morte fetal. • Corrimentos vulvares durante o diestro — podem mimetizar o abortamento; avaliar o corrimento e a origem para diferenciar uteropatias de doença do trato reprodutivo distal. • Necropsia de fetos abortados, filhotes caninos natimortos e placenta — aumenta as chances de obtenção do diagnóstico definitivo; refrigerar, mas não congelar antes do envio. • Histórico de doença sistêmica ou endócrina — pode indicar problemas com o ambiente materno.

HEMOGRAMA/BIOQUÍMICA/URINÁLISE
• Geralmente normais. • Doença sistêmica, infecção uterina, infecção viral ou anormalidades endócrinas — podem produzir alterações nos exames de hemograma completo, bioquímica ou urinálise.

OUTROS TESTES LABORATORIAIS
• Teste sorológico — para detecção de *B. canis*, herpes-vírus canino, *Toxoplasma*, neóspora; coletar o soro o mais rápido possível após a ocorrência do abortamento; repetir o teste em busca de títulos crescentes para herpes-vírus canino, *Toxoplasma* e neóspora. • Teste em lâmina para a *B. canis* — bastante sensível; os resultados negativos são confiáveis; a prevalência de resultados falso-positivos chega até 60%; o diagnóstico definitivo é obtido por meio de cultura. • Teste de aglutinação em tubo para a *B. canis* — fornece os títulos; títulos >1:200 são considerados positivos; títulos de 1:50-1:200 são considerados suspeitos. • Teste de imunodifusão em ágar-gel para a *B. canis* — diferencia com eficácia resultados falso-positivos e positivos verdadeiros nos testes de aglutinação; detecta antígenos de superfície citoplasmática e celular. • Concentração sérica basal do T_4 (quando nenhum agente infeccioso é identificado) — o hipotireoidismo é uma endocrinopatia comum e foi sugerido como uma causa de perda fetal; no entanto, desempenha papel incerto na perda gestacional; concentrações de T_4 abaixo do normal indicam a necessidade de testes adicionais (ver "Hipotireoidismo"). • Concentração sérica da progesterona (quando nenhum agente infeccioso é identificado) — o hipoluteoidismo pode causar perda fetal; as cadelas dependem da produção ovariana de progesterona durante toda a gestação (são necessários, no mínimo, 2 ng/mL para a manutenção da gestação); coletar amostra e determinar a concentração o mais rápido possível após o abortamento; nas gestações subsequentes, é preciso iniciar a monitorização na 3ª semana, ou seja, possivelmente antes que a gestação possa ser revelada pela ultrassonografia; iniciar a amostragem quinzenal perto da idade gestacional da última perda. A perda gestacional tipicamente ocorre durante a 7ª semana de gestação (ver "Parto Prematuro"). • Cultura vaginal — para *B. canis* com teste sorológico positivo; *Mycoplasma*, *Ureaplasma*, outros agentes bacterianos; todos, exceto a *B. canis*, podem pertencer à flora bacteriana normal; portanto, o diagnóstico a partir de culturas vaginais isoladas é uma tarefa difícil; *Salmonella* associada à doença sistêmica na cadela.

DIAGNÓSTICO POR IMAGEM
• Radiografia — identifica estruturas fetais após 45 dias da gestação; em uma fase mais precoce, esse exame é capaz de determinar o aumento de volume uterino, mas não consegue avaliar o seu conteúdo.
• Ultrassonografia — identifica o volume e o conteúdo uterinos; avalia a presença de líquido e sua consistência; examina os resquícios fetais ou a viabilidade fetal pela observação dos batimentos cardíacos (normal, >200 bpm; estresse, <150 ou >280 bpm).

MÉTODOS DIAGNÓSTICOS
• Vaginoscopia — identifica a origem de corrimentos vulvares e lesões vaginais; utilizar um espéculo suficientemente longo (16-20 cm) para examinar toda a extensão da vagina.
• Exame citológico e cultura bacteriana — a vagina pode revelar a presença de processo inflamatório (p. ex., infecção uterina); técnica para cultura: utilizar um *swab* protegido a fim de garantir a obtenção de amostra anterior (o trato reprodutivo distal costuma se apresentar intensamente contaminado por bactérias) ou coleta de secreções via cateterização transcervical.

ACHADOS PATOLÓGICOS
Exame histológico e cultura de tecido fetal e placentário — podem revelar a presença de microrganismos infecciosos; cultura tecidual, particularmente de conteúdo gástrico, para identificar microrganismos bacterianos infecciosos.

Abortamento Espontâneo (Perda Gestacional Precoce) — Cadelas

TRATAMENTO

CUIDADO(S) DE SAÚDE ADEQUADOS(S)
• A maioria das cadelas deve ficar confinada e isolada até o estabelecimento do diagnóstico. • É preferível a hospitalização de pacientes com infecção. • *B. canis* — agente altamente infeccioso para os cães; eliminado em grande quantidade durante o abortamento; os casos sob suspeita devem ser isolados. • Tratamento clínico em esquema ambulatorial — recomendado para pacientes clinicamente estáveis com causas não infecciosas de perda gestacional, endocrinopatias ou doença endometrial. • Abortamento parcial — na possível tentativa de salvar os fetos vivos; administrar antibióticos mediante identificação de componente bacteriano.

CUIDADO(S) DE ENFERMAGEM
Desidratação — utilizar fluidos de reposição suplementados com eletrólitos, caso sejam identificados desequilíbrios por meio de análises bioquímicas séricas.

ATIVIDADE
Abortamento parcial — o repouso em gaiola geralmente é recomendado, embora o efeito positivo dessa medida sobre a redução de abortamentos futuros não seja conhecido.

DIETA
Não há considerações nutricionais específicas para os casos sem complicação.

ORIENTAÇÃO AO PROPRIETÁRIO
• Crítica em caso de *B. canis* — se confirmada, recomenda-se a eutanásia pela falta de tratamento bem-sucedido e como medida de segurança para evitar a disseminação da infecção; a ovário-histerectomia e a antibioticoterapia a longo prazo podem ser experimentadas; discutir os programas de vigilância no caso das seguintes situações de canis: sorologia mensal para todos os animais, abatendo qualquer animal positivo, até que três testes negativos consecutivos sejam obtidos; discutir o potencial zoonótico. • Doença uterina primária — a ovário-histerectomia é indicada em pacientes sem valor reprodutivo; a hiperplasia endometrial cística é uma alteração irreversível. • Infertilidade ou perda gestacional — podem apresentar recidiva nos ciclos estrais subsequentes, apesar da instituição de tratamento imediato bem-sucedido. • Tratamento com prostaglandina — debater os efeitos colaterais (ver "Abortamento, Interrupção da Gestação"). • Doenças infecciosas — estabelecer medidas de vigilância e controle.

CONSIDERAÇÕES CIRÚRGICAS
A ovário-histerectomia é preferencialmente recomendada para pacientes estáveis sem valor reprodutivo.

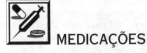

MEDICAÇÕES

MEDICAMENTO(S) DE ESCOLHA
• $PGF_{2\alpha}$ (Lutalyse®, trometamina de dinoprosta) — para a remoção do conteúdo uterino após o abortamento; 0,05-0,1 mg/kg SC a cada 8-24 h; cloprostenol (Estrumate®, cloprostenol) — 1-5 mg/kg SC a cada 24 h; não aprovados para uso em cães, mas a documentação adequada legaliza seu emprego; utilizar apenas se todos os fetos vivos foram expulsos. • Antibióticos — em caso de doenças bacterianas; instituir inicialmente um agente de amplo espectro; a escolha do agente específico depende da cultura e do antibiograma do tecido vaginal ou da necropsia fetal.
• Progesterona (Regu-mate®) na dose de 0,088 mg/kg (1 mL/25 kg VO) ou progesterona em veículo oleoso na dose de 2 mg/kg IM a cada 48-72 h — somente para hipoluteoidismo documentado, visando a manutenção da gestação; no entanto, é imprescindível ter a data prevista exata para saber o momento de interrupção da terapia, pois a gestação inadvertidamente prolongada resultará em morte fetal.

CONTRAINDICAÇÕES
Suplementação de progesterona — contraindicada em cadelas com afecção do endométrio ou das glândulas mamárias.

PRECAUÇÕES
$PGF_{2\alpha}$ — metabolizada no pulmão; os efeitos colaterais, que diminuem a cada injeção, estão relacionados à contração da musculatura lisa e à dose; respiração ofegante, salivação, vômito e defecação são comuns; a dosagem é crítica (DL_{50} da dinoprosta é de 5 mg/kg).

MEDICAMENTO(S) ALTERNATIVO(S)
Ocitocina —1 U/5 kg SC a cada 6-24 h para remoção do conteúdo uterino; mais eficaz nas primeiras 24-48 h após o abortamento.

ACOMPANHAMENTO

MONITORIZAÇÃO DO PACIENTE
• Abortamento parcial — monitorar a viabilidade dos fetos remanescentes por meio da ultrassonografia; monitorar a saúde sistêmica da fêmea durante o resto da gestação. • Corrimentos vulvares — monitorar diariamente quanto à redução na quantidade, no odor e no componente inflamatório, bem como quanto à consistência (o aumento do conteúdo mucoide tem prognóstico bom) • $PGF_{2\alpha}$ — deve ser mantida por 5 dias ou até a interrupção de grande parte do corrimento (3-15 dias). • *B. canis* — monitorizar após a castração e a antibioticoterapia; efetuar testes sorológicos anuais para identificar a ocorrência de recidiva. • Hipotireoidismo — tratar de forma adequada; a castração é recomendável (natureza hereditária); ver "Hipotireoidismo".

PREVENÇÃO
• Brucelose e outros agentes infecciosos — programas de vigilância para evitar a introdução em canis. • Ovário-histerectomia — para cadelas sem valor reprodutivo. • Uso de vacinas vivas modificadas (p. ex., algumas vacinas contra cinomose, parvovírus, etc.).

COMPLICAÇÕES POSSÍVEIS
• Piometra não tratada — septicemia, toxemia, morte. • Brucelose — discospondilite, endoftalmite, uveíte recidivante.

EVOLUÇÃO ESPERADA E PROGNÓSTICO
• Piometra — a taxa de recidiva durante o ciclo subsequente é alta (até 70%) a menos que a gestação esteja estabelecida. • HEC — a recuperação da fertilidade é improvável; a piometra é uma complicação comum. • Disfunção hormonal — frequentemente tratável; os aspectos familiares devem ser levados em consideração. • Brucelose — prognóstico reservado; é extremamente difícil eliminar a infecção de forma bem-sucedida mesmo se associada à castração.

DIVERSOS

FATORES RELACIONADOS COM A IDADE
É mais provável que cadelas com idade mais avançada sofram HEC.

POTENCIAL ZOONÓTICO
B. canis — pode ser transmitida aos seres humanos, especialmente ao manipular a cadela em processo de abortamento expelindo tecidos; é expelida uma quantidade maciça de microrganismos durante o abortamento. Os patologistas devem ser alertados na suspeita de *B. canis*. Indivíduos imunocomprometidos estão sob alto risco de infecção.

VER TAMBÉM
• Brucelose.
• Hipotireoidismo.
• Infertilidade na Fêmea — Cães.
• Parto Prematuro.
• Piometra e Hiperplasia Endometrial Cística.

ABREVIATURA(S)
• HEC = hiperplasia endometrial cística.
• $PGF_{2\alpha}$ = prostaglandina $F_{2\alpha}$.

RECURSOS DA INTERNET
Root-Kustritz MV. Use of supplemental progesterone in management of canine pregnancy. In: Concannon PW, England G, Verstegen III J, Linde-Forsberg C, eds., Recent Advances in Small Animal Reproduction. International Veterinary Information Service, Ithaca NY, www.ivis.org, 2001; A1220.0401

Autor Beverly J. Purswell
Consultor Editorial Sara K. Lyle

Abortamento Espontâneo (Perda Gestacional Precoce) — Gatas

CONSIDERAÇÕES GERAIS

DEFINIÇÃO
• Abortamento espontâneo — expulsão natural de feto(s) antes do momento em que eles sejam capazes de manter a vida fora do útero. • Perda gestacional precoce — termo generalizado para qualquer perda de concepto, incluindo morte e reabsorção embrionárias precoces.

FISIOPATOLOGIA
• As causas infecciosas resultam em perda gestacional por afetar diretamente o embrião, o feto ou as membranas fetais ou indiretamente por criar doença sistêmica debilitante na gata. • As causas não infecciosas de perda gestacional originam-se de qualquer fator que não envolva infecção e que leve à morte ou expulsão prematura do concepto (p. ex., nutrição materna inadequada, disfunção endócrina, toxicidade, defeitos genéticos).

SISTEMA(S) ACOMETIDO(S)
• Endócrino. • Reprodutor. • Outros sistemas — qualquer doença debilitante pode resultar em perda gestacional.

GENÉTICA
Os defeitos genéticos são mais prevalentes em animais altamente endogâmicos; a hereditariedade da suscetibilidade ao vírus da peritonite infecciosa felina (FIPV) é muito alta.

INCIDÊNCIA/PREVALÊNCIA
Desconhecidas — gestação frequentemente não confirmada; os proprietários podem não identificar a perda gestacional tardia se a gata for fastidiosa; não é fácil documentar morte embrionária precoce; as anormalidades genéticas respondem por ~15% da perda gestacional em gatas, incluindo abortamento.

IDENTIFICAÇÃO
Espécies
Gatos.

Raça(s) Predominante(s)
Gatos de raça pura — incidência mais alta de abortamento não infeccioso; a endogamia aumenta o risco de doença genética; o abortamento é uma consequência de certas formas de doenças hereditárias (defeito genético letal, erro cromossômico fatal).

Idade Média e Faixa Etária
O abortamento infeccioso é observado em todas as idades, enquanto o não infeccioso, em gatas jovens e idosas com maior frequência.

SINAIS CLÍNICOS
Comentários Gerais
Morte e reabsorção embrionárias precoces frequentemente não têm sinais clínicos; pode ocorrer qualquer combinação de achados do histórico e do exame físico, sendo que algumas gatas não exibem quaisquer sintomas.

Achados Anamnésicos
Falha em expulsar a ninhada no momento esperado, retorno ao estro mais rápido que o esperado, redução do diâmetro abdominal e perda de peso, descoberta de material fetal, mudança de comportamento, anorexia, vômito, diarreia.

Achados do Exame Físico
Corrimento vaginal purulento, mucoide, aquoso, ou sanguinolento; desidratação, febre, esforço/desconforto abdominais.

CAUSAS
Infecciosas
• Bacterianas — *Salmonella* spp., *Chlamydia*, *Brucella*; os microrganismos envolvidos em abortamento via infecção ascendente incluem *Escherichia coli*, *Staphylococcus* spp., *Streptococcus* spp., *Pasteurella* spp., *Klebsiella* spp., *Pseudomonas* spp., *Salmonella* spp., *Mycoplasma* spp., *Ureaplasma* spp. • Protozoárias — *Toxoplasma gondii* — incomuns. • Virais — FHV-1; FIV; FIPV; FeLV; FPLV — os vírus constituem as causas mais relatadas de abortamento infeccioso na gata.

Não Infecciosas
• Uterinas — complexo HEC-piometra, endometrite crônica, traumatismo mecânico ao útero ou feto. • Ovarianas — hipoluteoidismo; defeitos genéticos são mais prevalentes; interrupção precoce da função do corpo lúteo provoca um declínio nas concentrações séricas de progesterona, resultando em parto prematuro (abortamento). • Fetais — anormalidades cromossômicas que resultam em desenvolvimento anormal ou bloqueio do desenvolvimento, além de morte embrionária ou fetal. • Sistêmicas — deficiência da taurina; deficiência ou toxicidade da vitamina A; desnutrição; doença não reprodutiva grave; administração exógena de medicamentos, como estrogênios, glicocorticoides, prostaglandina $F_{2\alpha}$, e agonistas dopaminérgicos (cabergolina, bromocriptina), interrompe a função normal do corpo lúteo; medicamentos fetotóxicos ou teratogênicos: agentes quimioterápicos, agentes antifúngicos (griseofulvina), esteroides, alguns antibióticos (trimetoprima-sulfonamidas, quinolonas, tetraciclinas, gentamicina), medicamentos anticonvulsivantes (fenitoína); vacinas vivas modificadas.

FATORES DE RISCO
• Histórico prévio de perda gestacional. • Doença sistêmica concomitante. • Traumatismo recente. • Gato de raça pura com alto grau de endogamia. • Gata muito jovem ou idosa. • Desnutrição. • Superlotação ou condições ambientais sanitárias insatisfatórias.

DIAGNÓSTICO

DIAGNÓSTICO DIFERENCIAL
• Perda gestacional precoce:
  ◦ Falha de concepção.
  ◦ Ciclo anovulatório.
• Corrimento vulvar:
  ◦ Piometra, mucometra, piometra do coto uterino.
  ◦ Vaginite, metrite, cistite.
  ◦ Parto iminente ou distocia.
  ◦ Neoplasia ou traumatismo de órgãos como bexiga urinária, uretra, vagina ou útero.
  ◦ Estro — tipicamente se observa pouquíssimo corrimento.
• Esforço ou desconforto abdominal. • Obstrução da uretra. • Corpo estranho intestinal, pancreatite, peritonite. • Traumatismo.

HEMOGRAMA/BIOQUÍMICA/URINÁLISE
• Podem permanecer normais. • Leucograma inflamatório ou leucograma de estresse, dependendo da resposta à doença sistêmica. • Hemoconcentração e azotemia em caso de desidratação.

OUTROS TESTES LABORATORIAIS
Causas Infecciosas
• Citologia e cultura bacteriana de corrimento vaginal, feto, membranas fetais ou conteúdo uterino (cultura aeróbia, anaeróbia e micoplasmática). • FeLV — teste para detecção de antígenos em gatas com o uso de ELISA ou IFA. • FHV-1 — IFA ou PCR de swabs corneanos ou conjuntivais, isolamento viral de swabs conjuntivais, nasais ou faríngeos. • FIPV — PCR para detecção do RNAm do gene M do coronavírus felino (Molecular Diagnostics, College of Veterinary Medicine, Auburn University, http://www.vetmed.auburn.edu/feline_infectious_peritonitis_virus2). • FIV — ELISA — confirmar os resultados positivos com a técnica de *Western blot**. • FPLV — isolamento viral de fetos enviados para necropsia; documentar a soroconversão na gata.

Causas Não Infecciosas
• Hipoluteoidismo — níveis séricos de progesterona; baixos níveis não indicam uma causa primária a menos que registrada antes do abortamento. • Para descartar ciclo anovulatório, confirmar o aumento da progesterona acima de 1,5 ng/mL 1 semana após o acasalamento. • A evidência comportamental de estro (cio) e o exame de citologia vaginal podem confirmar o estro; a obtenção repetida e frequente de amostras de citologia vaginal pode induzir a ovulação.

DIAGNÓSTICO POR IMAGEM
• Ultrassonografia abdominal — confirma a gestação; permite a triagem em busca de indícios de reabsorção; avalia a saúde e a viabilidade do(s) feto(s) e das membranas e líquidos associados; determina a presença de acúmulo anormal de líquido uterino e doença não reprodutiva.
• Radiografia — avalia o tamanho, a posição e o número relativos dos esqueletos fetais; pode ser usada para fazer a triagem de monstros fetais, má apresentação fetal, e doença não reprodutiva.

MÉTODOS DIAGNÓSTICOS
• Defeitos genéticos — necropsia do(s) feto(s) abortado(s); enviar amostrar de fetos abortados e natimortos ao laboratório para cariotipagem.
• Nutrição — enviar amostra da dieta para análise nutricional se houver preocupação com os níveis de taurina ou vitamina A na dieta, de particular importância quando a gata está se alimentando de dieta caseira. • Obtenção do histórico completo e avaliação do pedigree — para calcular o coeficiente de endogamia. • Avaliar o gatil em termos de protocolos de vacinação, regime alimentar, procedimentos sanitários gerais e procedimentos de quarentena para gatas prenhes e recém-chegados.
• Enviar amostras do trato reprodutor (útero, ovários, tubas uterinas) ao patologista especialista na avaliação desses órgãos para avaliar a presença de alterações anatomopatológicas. • Evitar feto(s) abortado(s), natimorto(s), mumificado(s) e membranas fetais (frescas, refrigeradas, ou congeladas úmidas) ao patologista especialista em órgãos reprodutores para os exames de necropsia,

---

* N. T.: Também conhecida como "mancha ocidental".

Abortamento Espontâneo (Perda Gestacional Precoce) — Gatas

histopatologia, culturas e isolamento viral; soro da mãe/progenitora da ninhada; conteúdo estomacal e sangue do feto são úteis.

TRATAMENTO

CUIDADO(S) DE SAÚDE ADEQUADO(S)
- Tratamento ambulatorial:
  - Tipicamente não há necessidade de tratamento médico para gatas estáveis não infecciosas; as gatas com doença infectocontagiosa devem ser isoladas e tratadas de forma pertinente.
  - Hipoluteoidismo — pode ser tratado em um esquema ambulatorial com o uso de agentes tocolíticos em combinação com tocodinamometria se o valor da gata superar o potencial de perpetuar essa condição possivelmente hereditária.
- Tratamento médico-hospitalar:
  - Necessário para doença sistêmica e tratamento com prostaglandina $F_{2\alpha}$.
- Tratamento cirúrgico:
  - Ovário-histerectomia para gatas com doença grave causada por piometra ou metrite.

ATIVIDADE
- Isolamento de gatas com suspeita de doença infectocontagiosa. • Não há restrições de atividade para a maioria das perdas gestacionais não infecciosas. • Restrição da atividade, conforme indicado, para perda gestacional provocada por traumatismo.

DIETA
Corrigir as dietas com concentrações inadequadas de taurina ou vitamina A.

ORIENTAÇÃO AO PROPRIETÁRIO
- Doenças infectocontagiosas — verificar se o proprietário está não só adotando bons protocolos de vacinação e medidas de vigilância de doenças, mas também utilizando instalações de quarentena para gatas prenhes e recém-chegados. • Manejo reprodutivo — abordar o comportamento reprodutivo normal e o bom manejo reprodutivo; orientar os proprietários a manter registros detalhados em relação ao desempenho reprodutivo, análise do pedigree, e comportamento social de gatas dentro do gatil. • Nutrição — discutir as recomendações nutricionais de rotina para gatas em reprodução; aconselhar a análise nutricional de dietas caseiras. • Doença genética — aumenta em indivíduos endogâmicos; muitos traços reprodutivos são hereditários. • Abordagem médica — abordar os efeitos colaterais da prostaglandina $F_{2\alpha}$ ($PGF_{2\alpha}$); o tratamento médico deve ser tentado para gatas jovens às de meia-idade com inestimável valor reprodutivo. • Debater o risco de doença zoonótica por *Toxoplasma gondii*.

MEDICAÇÕES

MEDICAMENTO(S) DE ESCOLHA
- Depende(m) da etiologia. • Amoxicilina-ácido clavulânico na dose de 13,75 mg/kg VO a cada 12 h ou enrofloxacino na dose de 5 mg/kg/dia VO, dependendo dos resultados da cultura bacteriana. • Trometamina de dinoprosta ($PGF_{2\alpha}$) na dose de 0,05-0,2 mg/kg SC a cada 6-12 horas para remoção do conteúdo uterino; continuar até o completo esvaziamento uterino com base na avaliação ultrassonográfica. • Terbutalina na dose de 0,08-1,0 mg VO, conforme a necessidade, com base na tocodinamometria; 0,03 mg/kg VO a cada 8 h se a tocodinamometria não estiver disponível. • Progesterona em veículo oleoso — 2,0-3,0 mg/kg IM, conforme a necessidade, com base na tocodinamometria; a cada 72 h se a tocodinamometria não estiver disponível.

CONTRAINDICAÇÕES
- $PGF_{2\alpha}$ — gestação pretendida (desejada), comprometimento respiratório, comprometimento renal, doença uterina grave. • Terbutalina — doença cardíaca ou respiratória, piometra, doença infectocontagiosa, hipertensão. • Progesterona em veículo oleoso — diabetes, piometra, doença infectocontagiosa, HEC.

PRECAUÇÕES
- As gatas são mais toleráveis ao tratamento com $PGF_{2\alpha}$ que as cadelas, mas os proprietários devem assinar um termo de consentimento informado antes da instituição da terapia; os efeitos colaterais do tratamento com $PGF_{2\alpha}$ incluem respiração ofegante, salivação, inapetência, micção, diarreia, vocalização (grito), formação de ninhos, taquipneia, vômito, inquietação, e higiene pessoal excessiva. Os efeitos colaterais diminuem com injeções repetidas. • O uso de tocolíticos para manter a gestação requer o registro preciso das datas de acasalamento para saber o momento em que a terapia deve ser interrompida; os tocolíticos são utilizados com maior sucesso em combinação com a tocodinamometria para estabelecer o intervalo posológico desejado com base no aumento da atividade uterina pré-termo. • A terbutalina pode causar hipertensão, levando ao aumento da hemorragia proveniente dos sítios placentários durante o parto ou no momento da cesariana.

INTERAÇÕES POSSÍVEIS
- A administração de progesterona durante a gestação é associada à masculinização de fetos do sexo feminino; não administrar na primeira metade da gestação e utilizar com a assinatura do termo de consentimento informado. • O uso de tocolíticos para manter a gestação é associado ao aumento no risco de distocia, falha de separação normal da placenta no momento do parto, falta de desenvolvimento das glândulas mamárias e da produção de leite, e comportamento materno deficiente nos primeiros dias após o parto.

MEDICAMENTO(S) ALTERNATIVO(S)
- Altrenogeste (Regu-Mate®, Hoechst-Roussel) na dose de 0,088 mg/kg VO a cada 24 h — capacidade imprevisível em manter a gestação na gata. • É recomendável evitar o uso de análogos da prostaglandina em função de sua margem estreita de segurança e da falta de informações posológicas eficazes no gato.

ACOMPANHAMENTO

MONITORIZAÇÃO DO PACIENTE
- Avaliação ultrassonográfica seriada a cada 5 dias em gatas tratadas com prostaglandina $F_{2\alpha}$ para determinar o momento de interrupção. • Avaliação ultrassonográfica seriada a cada 5-7 dias para avaliar a viabilidade fetal em gatas submetidas a tocolíticos se a monitorização diária com tocodinamometria não estiver disponível.

PREVENÇÃO
- Instituir um plano de prevenção, controle e vigilância de doença infectocontagiosa. • Substituir gatas inférteis por animais mais qualificados em termos reprodutivos. • Evitar a exposição a agentes abortivos, teratogênicos ou fetotóxicos.

COMPLICAÇÕES POSSÍVEIS
- Dependem da etiologia. • Metrite, endometrite, ruptura uterina, sepse, choque. • Diabetes, HEC, masculinização de fetos do sexo feminino em caso de tratamento com progesterona.

EVOLUÇÃO ESPERADA E PROGNÓSTICO
- Doença infectocontagiosa — é possível a constatação de gestação normal, abortamento frequente ou infertilidade em caso de doença viral. • Prognóstico mau quanto à possibilidade de gestação normal nas gatas com HEC grave. • Prognóstico bom para uma gestação bem-sucedida com o tratamento para hipoluteoidismo; é necessária uma monitorização significativa para obtenção dos melhores resultados. • É provável a recorrência de perda gestacional por anormalidades genéticas se a gata for acasalada com um gato do mesmo pedigree.

DIVERSOS

FATORES RELACIONADOS COM A IDADE
- Gatas com >6 anos de idade têm maior incidência de infertilidade. • A perda gestacional é observada com maior frequência em gatas muito jovens e idosas.

POTENCIAL ZOONÓTICO
Toxoplasma gondii.

VER TAMBÉM
- Acasalamento, Momento Oportuno.

ABREVIATURAS
ELISA = ensaio imunoadsorvente ligado à enzima.
FeLV = vírus da leucemia felina.
FHV-1 = herpes-vírus felino tipo 1.
FIPV = vírus da peritonite infecciosa felina.
FIV = vírus da imunodeficiência felina.
FPLV = vírus da panleucopenia felina.
HEC = hiperplasia endometrial cística.
IFA = anticorpo fluorescente indireto.
$PGF_{2\alpha}$ = prostaglandina $F_{2\alpha}$.

RECURSOS DA INTERNET
www.theriojournal.com
www.whelpwise.com

Autor Milan Hess
Consultor Editorial Sara K. Lyle

ABORTAMENTO, INTERRUPÇÃO DA GESTAÇÃO

CONSIDERAÇÕES GERAIS

DEFINIÇÃO
Interrupção de gestação indesejada. Pode ser concluída por meio de medicamentos que alteram o transporte do embrião no oviduto, impedindo o estabelecimento de uma gestação, e/ou causam regressão luteal, interrompendo uma gestação estabelecida. Em função dos possíveis efeitos colaterais (HEC, anemia aplásica e mielossupressão), os medicamentos que prejudicam o trânsito embrionário pelo oviduto (estrogênios) não são comumente utilizados nem recomendados.

FISIOPATOLOGIA
Após a fertilização, o embrião percorre o oviduto em tempo oportuno antes de ingressar no útero. O comprometimento no transporte do embrião pelo oviduto leva a anormalidades de degeneração e implante embrionários. No cão e gato, a manutenção gestacional depende da produção de progesterona pelo corpo lúteo. Em cães, a manutenção do corpo lúteo durante a segunda metade da gestação também é amparada pela prolactina. Os medicamentos que causam regressão luteal, antagonizam a prolactina e/ou competem com os receptores da progesterona promoverão interrupção da gestação.

SISTEMA(S) ACOMETIDO(S)
• Cardiovascular. • Digestório. • Neurológico (causado por medicamentos utilizados para o tratamento). • Reprodutor. • Respiratório.

GENÉTICA
N/D.

INCIDÊNCIA/PREVALÊNCIA
N/D.

DISTRIBUIÇÃO GEOGRÁFICA
N/D.

IDENTIFICAÇÃO
Espécies
Cães e gatos.
Raça(s) Predominante(s)
Não há predileção racial.
Idade Média e Faixa Etária
N/D.
Sexo Predominante
Fêmea.

SINAIS CLÍNICOS
• Dependem da fase da gestação:
  ◦ Nenhum.
  ◦ Corrimento vaginal.
  ◦ Expulsão fetal.

CAUSAS
• Transporte prejudicado pelo oviduto. • Regressão luteal. • Antagonismo dos receptores de progesterona.

FATORES DE RISCO
N/D.

DIAGNÓSTICO

DIAGNÓSTICO DIFERENCIAL
• Averiguar se o acasalamento ocorreu; formação de trava na cadela e reação "pós-coito" na gata.
• Determinar a fase do ciclo estral por meio de citologia vaginal e concentração sérica da progesterona (ver Acasalamento, Momento Oportuno). • Avaliar a presença de espermatozoides na citologia vaginal; no entanto, a ausência de esperma não descarta um acasalamento prévio.
• Diagnóstico de gestação:
  ◦ Palpação abdominal (cadela: 31-33 dias após o pico de LH; gata: 21-25 dias após o acasalamento).
  ◦ Ultrassonografia transabdominal (cadela: >25 dias após o pico de LH; gata: >16 dias após o acasalamento).
  ◦ Radiografias abdominais (cadela: >45 dias após o pico de LH; gata: >38 dias após o acasalamento).
  ◦ Concentração sérica de relaxina na cadela (>28 dias após o pico de LH) (Witness® Relaxin, Synbiotics Corp., http://synbiotics.com/index.html).

HEMOGRAMA/BIOQUÍMICA/URINÁLISE
• Dentro dos limites de normalidade durante a primeira metade da gestação em pacientes saudáveis. • O declínio do volume globular durante a segunda metade da gestação em cadelas e gatas é normal. • Recomendados como testes de triagem antes do tratamento em pacientes com suspeita de doença subjacente.

OUTROS TESTES LABORATORIAIS
• Teste de citologia vaginal — determina a fase do ciclo estral e a presença de espermatozoides.
• Concentração sérica de progesterona — determina se a fêmea está em diestro e monitoriza a regressão luteal durante o tratamento.

DIAGNÓSTICO POR IMAGEM
• Ultrassonografia transabdominal (método de escolha): possibilita o diagnóstico de gestação e monitoriza a remoção do conteúdo uterino durante o tratamento. • Radiografias abdominais.

ACHADOS PATOLÓGICOS
N/D.

TRATAMENTO

CUIDADO(S) DE SAÚDE ADEQUADO(S)
• Exame físico antes do início do tratamento.
• Monitorizar a paciente 30-60 minutos depois do tratamento quanto à ocorrência de efeitos colaterais (vômito, defecação, hipersalivação, hiperpneia, micção, taquicardia). • É recomendada a confirmação da gestação antes do início do tratamento; mais de 60% das cadelas erroneamente acasaladas podem não engravidar.
• O status da gestação no início do diestro é desconhecido; a confirmação ultrassonográfica da gestação não é possível até 4-5 semanas após o acasalamento. • Tratamento no dia 6-10 do diestro — pode ter eficácia reduzida em comparação ao tratamento no meio da gestação, mas pode ser menos desagradável ao proprietário (menor quantidade de corrimento e ausência de eliminação de fetos identificáveis). • $PGF_{2\alpha}$ e bromocriptina — a combinação aumenta a eficácia de qualquer um dos medicamentos administrados isoladamente.

CUIDADO(S) DE ENFERMAGEM
N/D.

ATIVIDADE
Normal.

DIETA
Evitar a alimentação antes de cada tratamento e por 1-2 horas depois dos tratamentos (diminui os sintomas de náusea e vômito).

ORIENTAÇÃO AO PROPRIETÁRIO
• Discutir o futuro reprodutivo do paciente com o proprietário. Se nenhuma ninhada for desejável, o procedimento de ovário-histerectomia será a melhor opção. • Abordar os efeitos colaterais potenciais das opções terapêuticas junto ao proprietário; chegar a um acordo mútuo sobre o plano terapêutico.

CONSIDERAÇÕES CIRÚRGICAS
A ovário-histerectomia é recomendada aos pacientes sem valor reprodutivo ou cujos proprietários não desejam ninhadas futuras.

MEDICAÇÕES

MEDICAMENTO(S) DE ESCOLHA
• É recomendável a confirmação da gestação antes de iniciar qualquer um dos protocolos terapêuticos sugeridos adiante. A duração do tratamento sugerido pode variar; no entanto, os tratamentos devem ser mantidos até a conclusão do abortamento. ◦ $PGF_{2\alpha}$: provoca regressão luteal com subsequente declínio na concentração de progesterona, relaxamento da cérvix uterina, e contrações uterinas; cadelas: 100 mg/kg SC a cada 8 h por 2 dias, depois 200 mg/kg SC a cada 8 h até a interrupção da gestação; gatas: 0,5-1 mg/kg SC a cada 12 h em dias alternados depois do dia 40, ou 2 mg/gata IM a cada 24 h por 5 dias depois do dia 33. ◦ Cloprostenol (análogo da prostaglandina): cadelas: 2,5 mg/kg SC a cada 8 h ou a cada 12 h a cada 48 horas até a interrupção da gestação (~6 dias depois do início do tratamento). ◦ Dexametasona: o modo de ação é desconhecido; cadelas: 0,2 mg/kg VO a cada 12 h por 7 dias, com subsequente redução de 0,16 para 0,02 mg/kg nas últimas 5 administrações; as falhas do tratamento não são incomuns. ◦ Cabergolina (antagonista da prolactina): provoca regressão luteal; cadelas: 1,65 mg/kg SC a cada 24 h por 5 dias ou 5 mg/kg VO a cada 24 h por 5 dias depois do dia 40; gatas: 0,825 mg/kg SC a cada 12 h por 5 dias depois do dia 30 ou 5-15 mg/kg VO a cada 24 h por 5 dias depois do dia 25. ◦ Bromocriptina (antagonista da prolactina): provoca regressão luteal; cadelas: 62,5 mg/kg VO a cada 12 h por até 6 dias depois do dia 43. ◦ Combinação de cloprostenol e cabergolina: cadelas: cabergolina 5 mg/kg VO a cada 24 h por 10 dias mais cloprostenol 2,5 mg/kg SC a cada 24 h no início do tratamento, ou 1 mg/kg SC a cada 24 h no início do tratamento e no dia 5 do tratamento; o tratamento deve ser iniciado 28 dias depois do pico de LH; gata: cabergolina 5 mg/kg VO a cada 24 h mais cloprostenol 5 mg/kg SC a cada 48 h (>30 dias depois do acasalamento) até a conclusão do abortamento (~9 dias). ◦ Combinação de cloprostenol e bromocriptina; cadelas: bromocriptina 30 mg/kg a cada 8 h VO por 10 dias mais cloprostenol 2,5 mg/kg SC a cada 24 h ou 1 mg/kg SC no início do tratamento e no dia 5 do tratamento; o tratamento deve ser iniciado 28 dias depois do pico de LH.

Abortamento, Interrupção da Gestação

CONTRAINDICAÇÕES
- $PGF_{2\alpha}$ e análogos: animais com doença respiratória (broncoconstrição); não administrar por via IV. • Cabergolina e bromocriptina: animais hipersensíveis a alcaloides de Ergot; esses medicamentos devem ser administrados com cuidado em pacientes com comprometimento da função hepática. • Estrogênios — podem causar hiperplasia endometrial cística, piometra e mielossupressão, levando à pancitopenia.

PRECAUÇÕES
- $PGF_{2\alpha}$ e análogos: os efeitos colaterais são dose-dependentes e incluem vômito, defecação, dispneia, taquicardia, salivação, inquietação e ansiedade; os efeitos colaterais desaparecem em até 60 minutos; a gravidade dos efeitos pode ser atenuada por meio de pré-medicação (>15 minutos) com uma combinação de atropina (0,025 mg/kg); ter extremo cuidado em cães e gatos com doenças cardiopulmonares, hepáticas e renais preexistentes. • Dexametasona: polidipsia, poliúria e polifagia são os efeitos colaterais relatados. A administração prolongada é associada a hiperadrenocorticismo. • Cabergolina e bromocriptina: os efeitos colaterais podem incluir vômito e anorexia; o uso prolongado (>2 semanas) pode provocar alteração na cor da pelagem.

INTERAÇÕES POSSÍVEIS
- $PGF_{2\alpha}$ e análogos: o efeito pode ser reduzido pela administração concomitante de progestinas; o uso pode acentuar os efeitos da ocitocina.
- Cabergolina e bromocriptina: os efeitos da cabergolina podem ser diminuídos com a administração concomitante de antagonistas dopaminérgicos (D_2); evitar o tratamento concomitante com medicamentos hipotensores.

MEDICAMENTO(S) ALTERNATIVO(S)
- Os medicamentos expostos a seguir são recomendados para o uso em cadelas, mas não estão disponíveis nos Estados Unidos:
  ◦ É recomendável o uso da mifepristona (RU486®; antagonista dos receptores de progestina e glicocorticoide): 2,5 mg/kg VO a cada 12 h por 4 dias e meio depois do 32º dia da gestação; não há relatos de efeitos colaterais.
  ◦ Aglepristona (antagonista dos receptores de progestina e glicocorticoide): 10 mg/kg SC a cada 24 h por 2 dias 32 dias depois do pico de LH; a gestação é interrompida em 4-7 dias; não há relatos de efeitos colaterais; pode ser observado um leve corrimento vaginal.
  ◦ Antagonistas do GnRH (bloqueiam os receptores desse hormônio na hipófise, provocando um declínio na concentração de gonadotropinas): é aconselhável um único tratamento com 110-330 mg/kg SC; a gestação é interrompida em até 6-10 dias depois do tratamento; foi observado um comportamento tipo pré-parto; o abortamento pode ser acompanhado por corrimento vaginal serossanguinolento por 2-3 dias.

ACOMPANHAMENTO

MONITORIZAÇÃO DO PACIENTE
Exames ultrassonográficos transabdominais devem ser realizados para monitorizar a remoção completa do conteúdo uterino.

PREVENÇÃO
• Ovário-histerectomia para cadelas e gatas sem intenção reprodutiva. • Supressão do estro ou confinamento de cadelas e gatas com intenção reprodutiva durante um ciclo subsequente para evitar acasalamento malsucedido.

COMPLICAÇÕES POSSÍVEIS
A interrupção da gestação pode não ser concluída após um único protocolo terapêutico, podendo haver a necessidade de manutenção ou modificação desse protocolo.

EVOLUÇÃO ESPERADA E PROGNÓSTICO
• O intervalo interestro em cadelas tratadas com prostaglandinas e inibidores da prolactina pode ser abreviado (~1 mês). As gatas podem retomar o comportamento estral 7-10 dias após a interrupção da gestação. • A fertilidade do estro subsequente não é afetada.

DIVERSOS

DISTÚRBIOS ASSOCIADOS
N/D.

FATORES RELACIONADOS COM A IDADE
N/D.

POTENCIAL ZOONÓTICO
N/D.

GESTAÇÃO/FERTILIDADE/REPRODUÇÃO
N/D.

SINÔNIMO(S)
Abortamento induzido.

VER TAMBÉM
Acasalamento, Momento Oportuno.

ABREVIATURAS
GnRH = hormônio liberador de gonadotropina.
HEC = hiperplasia endometrial cística.
LH = hormônio luteinizante.
$PGF_{2\alpha}$ = prostaglandina $F_{2\alpha}$.

RECURSOS DA INTERNET
Wanke MM, Romangnoli S, Verstegen J, Concannon PW. Pharmacologic approaches to pregnancy termination in dogs and cats including the use of prostaglandins, dopamine agonists, and dexamethasone. In: Concannon PW, England G, Verstegen III J, Linde-Forsberg C, eds., Recent Advances in Small Animal Reproduction. International Veterinary Information Service, Ithaca NY, www.ivis.org, 2001.

Sugestões de Leitura
Corrada Y, Klima L, De la Sota RL, Rodriguez R. Use of prostaglandins and bromocriptine mesylate for pregnancy termination in bitches. JAVMA 2002, 220(7):1017-1019.
Eilts BE Pregnancy termination in the bitch and queen. Clin Tech Small Anim Pract 2002, 17:116-123.
Fieni F, Dumon C, Tainturier D, Bruyas JF. Clinical protocol for pregnancy termination in bitches using prostaglandin $F_{2\alpha}$. J Repro Fert 1997, 51:245-250.
Johnston SD, Root Kustritz MV, Olson PNS. Prevention and termination of canine pregnancy. In: Canine and Feline Theriogenology. Philadelphia: Saunders, 2001, pp. 168-192.
Johnston SD, Root Kustritz MV, Olson PNS. Prevention and termination of feline pregnancy. In: Canine and Feline Theriogenology. Philadelphia: Saunders, 2001, pp. 447-452.

Autor Jose A. Len
Consultor Editorial Sara K. Lyle

ABSCEDAÇÃO

CONSIDERAÇÕES GERAIS

DEFINIÇÃO
Abscesso corresponde a uma coleção localizada de exsudato purulento contido dentro de uma cavidade.

FISIOPATOLOGIA
• As bactérias são frequentemente inoculadas sob a pele por meio de ferida perfurante; em seguida, ocorre o fechamento da superfície da ferida.
• Quando há persistência de bactérias e/ou corpos estranhos no tecido, ocorrem a formação e o acúmulo do exsudato purulento. • Acúmulo de exsudato purulento — caso não ocorra a rápida reabsorção ou a secreção do material para alguma superfície externa, esse acúmulo estimula a formação de cápsula fibrosa, podendo finalmente levar à ruptura do abscesso. • Atraso prolongado de eliminação — pela formação de parede fibrosa; para haver a cicatrização, a cavidade deverá ser preenchida por tecido de granulação; nesse caso, o agente causal pode não ser totalmente eliminado; isso pode levar à secreção crônica ou intermitente de exsudato a partir de trajeto sinuoso drenante.

SISTEMA(S) ACOMETIDO(S)
• Cutâneo/Exócrino — percutâneo (gatos > cães); sacos anais (cães > gatos). • Gastrintestinal — pâncreas (cães > gatos). • Reprodutivo — próstata (cães > gatos); glândula mamária. • Oftalmológico — tecidos periorbitais. • Hepatobiliar — parênquima hepático.

GENÉTICA
N/D.

INCIDÊNCIA/PREVALÊNCIA
N/D.

DISTRIBUIÇÃO GEOGRÁFICA
N/D.

IDENTIFICAÇÃO
Espécies
Cães e gatos.
Raça(s) Predominante(s)
N/D.
Idade Média e Faixa Etária
N/D.
Sexo(s) Predominante(s)
Glândulas mamárias (fêmeas); próstata (machos).

SINAIS CLÍNICOS
Comentários Gerais
• Determinados pelo sistema orgânico e/ou tecido acometido. • Associados a uma combinação de inflamação (dor, tumefação, rubor, calor e perda da função), destruição tecidual e/ou disfunção orgânica causada pelo acúmulo de exsudatos.
Achados Anamnésicos
• Histórico de lesão traumática ou infecção prévia.
• Tumefação dolorosa de aparecimento rápido com ou sem secreção, se a área acometida estiver visível.
Achados do Exame Físico
• Determinados pelo sistema orgânico ou tecido acometido. • Pode ser detectável a presença de massa discreta. • Se o abscesso for superficial e tiver sofrido ruptura para alguma superfície externa, poderão ser visíveis o processo inflamatório e a secreção a partir de trajeto fistuloso. • Pode ser palpável a existência de massa dolorosa de tamanho variável e consistência flutuante a firme aderida aos tecidos circunjacentes. • Se o abscesso não sofrer ruptura nem drenagem, haverá o aparecimento de febre.
• Ocasionalmente, ocorre sepse, sobretudo no caso de ruptura interna do abscesso.

CAUSAS
• Corpos estranhos. • Bactérias piogênicas — *Staphylococcus* spp.; *Escherichia coli*; *Streptococcus* spp. β-hemolíticos; *Pseudomonas*; *Mycoplasma* e microrganismos semelhantes ao *Mycoplasma* (formas-L); *Pasteurella multocida*; *Corynebacterium*; *Actinomyces* spp.; *Nocardia*; *Bartonella*. • Anaeróbios obrigatórios — *Bacteroides* spp.; *Clostridium* spp.; *Peptostreptococcus*; *Fusobacterium*.

FATORES DE RISCO
• Sacos anais — impactação; saculite anal.
• Cérebro — otite interna; sinusite; infecção bucal. • Fígado — onfaloflebite; sepse. • Pulmão — pneumonia bacteriana por aspiração de corpo estranho. • Glândulas mamárias — mastite.
• Região periorbital — odontopatias; mastigação de madeira ou outro material vegetal. • Região percutânea — brigas. • Próstata — prostatite bacteriana. • Imunossupressão — infecção pelo FeLV/FIV; quimioterapia imunossupressora; disfunções adquiridas ou hereditárias do sistema imune; doença predisponente subjacente (p. ex., diabetes melito, insuficiência renal crônica, hiperadrenocorticismo).

DIAGNÓSTICO

DIAGNÓSTICO DIFERENCIAL
Lesões Expansivas Tipo Massa
• Cisto — menos ou apenas transitoriamente doloroso; crescimento mais lento. • Tecido cicatricial fibroso — firme; indolor. • Granuloma — menos doloroso; crescimento mais lento; geralmente mais firme, sem centro flutuante.
• Hematoma/seroma — dor variável (depende da causa); não encapsulado; crescimento inicial rápido, mas aumento lento uma vez atingido o volume total; não aderido aos tecidos circunjacentes; inicialmente, apresenta-se flutuante e preenchido por líquido, porém mais firme com o processo de organização. • Neoplasia — crescimento variável; consistente; doloroso.
Trajetos Drenantes
• Micobacteriose. • Micetoma — botriomicose, micetoma actinomicótico, micetoma eumicótico.
• Neoplasias.
• Feoifomicose. • Esporotricose. • Infecção fúngica sistêmica — blastomicose, coccidioidomicose, criptococose, histoplasmose, tricosporose.

HEMOGRAMA/BIOQUÍMICA/URINÁLISE
• Hemograma completo — permanece normal ou exibe neutrofilia com ou sem desvio regenerativo à esquerda. Na presença de sepse, há neutropenia e desvio degenerativo à esquerda. • Urinálise e perfil químico sérico — dependem do sistema acometido. • Infecção prostática — piúria.
• Exame das funções hepática e/ou pancreática — altos níveis das enzimas hepáticas e/ou da bilirrubina total. • Função pancreática (cães) — amilase/lipase elevadas. • Diabetes melito — hiperglicemia e glicosúria persistentes.

OUTROS TESTES LABORATORIAIS
• FeLV e FIV — para gatos com abscessos de caráter recidivante ou de cicatrização lenta.
• Avaliação do LCS — aumento esperado na celularidade e no teor proteico em caso de abscesso cerebral. • Função adrenal — para pesquisar hiperadrenocorticismo.

DIAGNÓSTICO POR IMAGEM
• Radiografia — constatação de massa com densidade de tecido mole na área acometida; pode revelar a presença de corpo estranho.
• Ultrassonografia — determina se a massa está preenchida por material líquido ou sólido; define o sistema orgânico acometido; revela o líquido de aspecto floculento característico de pus; pode demonstrar a presença de corpo estranho.
• Ecocardiografia — útil para o diagnóstico de abscesso pericárdico. • TC e RM — exames proveitosos para o diagnóstico de abscesso cerebral.

MÉTODOS DIAGNÓSTICOS
Aspirado
• Revela um líquido de coloração vermelha, branca, amarela ou verde. • Teor proteico >2,5-3,0 g/dL.
• Contagem de células nucleadas — 3.000-100.000 (ou mais) células/µL; compõem-se principalmente de neutrófilos degenerados com menor número de macrófagos e linfócitos.
• Bactérias piogênicas — podem ser observadas em células e livres dentro do líquido. • Se o agente causal não for prontamente identificado por meio de corante do tipo Romanovsky, as amostras deverão ser coradas com corante acidorresistente para detectar micobactérias ou *Nocardia* e corante de PAS para detectar fungos.
Biopsia
• A mesma amostra deve conter tecidos, que se apresentam tanto normais como anormais.
• Esfregaços por impressão (decalque) — corados e examinados. • Tecidos — enviar para exame histopatológico e cultura. • Entrar em contato com o laboratório diagnóstico em busca de orientações específicas.
Cultura
• Tecido acometido e/ou exsudato — para pesquisa de bactérias aeróbias/anaeróbias e fungos.
• Sangue e/ou urina — isolar a bactéria responsável pela possível sepse. • Sensibilidade bacteriana (antibiograma).

ACHADOS PATOLÓGICOS
• Lesão expansiva tipo massa com pus, acompanhada por inflamação. • Abscesso palpável — massa variavelmente firme ou flutuante.
• Abscesso rompido — pode-se observar a drenagem de pus diretamente a partir da massa ou de trajeto adjacente. • Exsudato — grande quantidade de neutrófilos em diversas fases de degeneração; outras células inflamatórias; tecido necrótico. • Tecido circunjacente — congesto; fibrina; grande quantidade de neutrófilos; número variável de linfócitos; plasmócitos; macrófagos.
• Agente causal inconstantemente detectável.

TRATAMENTO

CUIDADO(S) DE SAÚDE ADEQUADO(S)
• Depende da localização do abscesso e do tratamento exigido. • Pacientes ambulatoriais — abscessos induzidos por mordidas. • Pacientes

ABSCEDAÇÃO

internados — sepse; procedimentos cirúrgicos extensos; tratamento que exige internação prolongada. • Estabelecer e manter drenagem adequada. • Promover a remoção cirúrgica do foco de infecção ou de corpo(s) estranho(s), se necessário. • Proceder à instituição de antibioticoterapia adequada.

CUIDADO(S) DE ENFERMAGEM
• Depende da localização do abscesso. • Aplicar compressas quentes sobre a área inflamada, conforme a necessidade. • Utilizar bandagem protetora e/ou colar elizabetano, se necessário. • Acúmulo de exsudato — efetuar a drenagem do abscesso; manter a drenagem por meios clínicos e/ou cirúrgicos. • Sepse ou peritonite — fluidoterapia e suporte rigorosos.

ATIVIDADE
Restringir a atividade física até o desaparecimento do abscesso e a cicatrização adequada dos tecidos.

DIETA
• Aporte nutricional suficiente para promover um balanço nitrogenado positivo. • Depende da localização do abscesso e do tratamento exigido.

ORIENTAÇÃO AO PROPRIETÁRIO
• Discutir a necessidade de corrigir ou evitar os fatores de risco. • Debater a necessidade de drenagem apropriada e da continuidade da antibioticoterapia por período de tempo adequado.

CONSIDERAÇÕES CIRÚRGICAS
• Debridamento e drenagem suficientes — pode haver a necessidade de deixar a ferida aberta para uma superfície externa; além disso, pode ser necessária a aplicação de drenos cirúrgicos.
• Drenagem precoce — para evitar maiores danos teciduais e formação de parede no abscesso.
• Remover qualquer corpo estranho, tecido necrótico ou foco infeccioso.

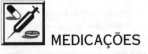
MEDICAÇÕES
MEDICAMENTO(S) DE ESCOLHA
• Antibióticos — eficazes contra o agente infeccioso; ganham acesso ao local da infecção.
• Agente de amplo espectro — com ação bactericida e atividade tanto aeróbia como anaeróbia; utilizado até que os resultados da cultura e do antibiograma sejam conhecidos. Cães e gatos: amoxicilina (11-22 mg/kg VO a cada 8-12 h); amoxicilina/ácido clavulânico (12,5-25 mg/kg VO a cada 12 h); clindamicina (5 mg/kg VO a cada 12 h); e trimetoprima/sulfadiazina (15 mg/kg VO ou IM a cada 12 h). Gatos com *Mycoplasma* e formas-L: doxiciclina (3-5 mg/kg VO a cada 12 h). • Antibioticoterapia rigorosa — para sepse ou peritonite.

CONTRAINDICAÇÕES
N/D.

PRECAUÇÕES
N/D.

INTERAÇÕES POSSÍVEIS
N/D.

MEDICAMENTO(S) ALTERNATIVO(S)
N/D.

ACOMPANHAMENTO
MONITORIZAÇÃO DO PACIENTE
Monitorizar quanto à redução progressiva do abscesso na drenagem, ao desaparecimento da inflamação e à melhora dos sinais clínicos.

PREVENÇÃO
• Abscessos percutâneos — evitar brigas.
• Abscessos dos sacos anais — evitar impactação; considerar o procedimento de saculectomia anal em casos recidivantes. • Abscessos prostáticos — a castração possivelmente é útil. • Mastite — evitar a lactação (castração). • Abscessos periorbitais — não permitir a mastigação de corpo(s) estranho(s).

COMPLICAÇÕES POSSÍVEIS
• Sepse. • Peritonite/pleurite em caso de ruptura de abscesso intra-abdominal e intratorácico.
• Comprometimento da função orgânica. • A demora na remoção do abscesso pode levar à formação de trajetos fistulosos de drenagem crônica.

EVOLUÇÃO ESPERADA E PROGNÓSTICO
Dependem do sistema orgânico envolvido e do nível de destruição tecidual.

DIVERSOS
DISTÚRBIOS ASSOCIADOS
• Infecção pelo FeLV ou FIV. • Imunossupressão.

FATORES RELACIONADOS COM A IDADE
N/D.

POTENCIAL ZOONÓTICO
• Mínimo em relação às bactérias piogênicas.
• Micobactérias e infecções fúngicas sistêmicas carreiam certo potencial.

GESTAÇÃO/FERTILIDADE/REPRODUÇÃO
Agentes teratogênicos — evitar o uso em animais prenhes.

VER TAMBÉM
• Actinomicose. • Colibacilose. • Infecções Anaeróbias. • Micoplasmose. • Nocardiose. • Sepse e Bacteremia.

ABREVIATURA(S)
• FeLV = vírus da leucemia felina. • FIV = vírus da imunodeficiência felina. • LCS = líquido cerebrospinal. • PAS = ácido periódico de Schiff. • RM = ressonância magnética. • TC = tomografia computadorizada.

Sugestões de Leitura
Birchard SJ, Sherding RG, eds. Saunders manual of small animal practice. Philadelphia: Saunders, 1994.
DeBoer DJ. Nonhealing cutaneous wounds. In: August JR, ed. Consultations in feline internal medicine. Philadelphia: Saunders, 1991:101-6.
McCaw D. Lumps, bumps, masses, and lymphadenopathy. In: Ettinger SJ, Feldman EC, eds. Textbook of veterinary internal medicine. 4th ed. Philadelphia: Saunders, 1995:219-22.

Autor Johnny D. Hoskins
Consultor Editorial Stephen C. Barr

Abscesso da Raiz Dentária (Abscesso Apical)

CONSIDERAÇÕES GERAIS

REVISÃO
• O abscesso consiste no acúmulo localizado de pus em uma cavidade formada pela desintegração de tecidos. • Pode se dividir em fases aguda e crônica, com base na gravidade da dor e na presença ou ausência de sinais e sintomas sistêmicos. • Acúmulo de células inflamatórias no ápice de um dente desvitalizado — abscesso periapical. • A exacerbação aguda de um abscesso periapical crônico recebe o nome de *abscesso fênix*. • Um abscesso dissemina-se ao longo das vias de menor resistência a partir do ápice dentário, resultando em osteomielite e, se perfurado através do córtex, em celulite, que pode irromper através da pele, criando um trajeto cutâneo. • A disseminação sistêmica de bactérias (bacteremia e piemia) pode comprometer outros órgãos e sistemas. • A doença periodontal pode se estender para a região apical do dente, resultando em envolvimento endodôntico (lesão periendodôntica). • Pode envolver qualquer dente; os dentes caninos e os carniceiros são os mais comumente acometidos. • Pode surgir sem a presença de bactérias (abscesso estéril).

IDENTIFICAÇÃO
• Cães e gatos. • Pode ocorrer na dentição decídua e na permanente em qualquer idade. • Costuma ocorrer em animais ativos que mordem ou mastigam muito.

SINAIS CLÍNICOS
• O dente encontra-se visivelmente quebrado ou quase exibe exposição da polpa — 90% dos casos. • O dente pode parecer manchado. • O dente não se mostra sensível à percussão nem a líquidos ou alimentos quentes ou frios. Nota: a fratura dentária aguda com exposição da polpa apresenta sensibilidade. • Tumefação facial: geralmente localizada, mas pode se espalhar, resultando em celulite. • Exsudação de pus por trajeto sinuoso cutâneo — periodontite apical supurativa. • Pode haver uma leve sensibilidade facial, que pode se estender se não houver drenagem. • O animal recusa-se a mastigar, especialmente do lado acometido (pode ocorrer o acúmulo de placa e cálculo dentários) ou, então, ele morde o alimento, mas rapidamente o libera em vez de segurá-lo. • O dente pode permanecer assintomático por muito tempo, mas será acometido mais cedo ou mais tarde. • O dente possivelmente permanece assintomático do ponto de vista clínico, embora possa haver outros problemas como bacteremia. • Uma bolsa periodontal profunda pode se estender até o ápice do dente acometido. • Odor pútrido. • É possível que o dente esteja frouxo e dolorido à palpação. • Pode ocorrer linfadenite facial. • Sinusite — o seio maxilar costuma ser o mais acometido. • O olfato pode ser acometido, especialmente com cães farejadores de drogas, bombas ou alimentos.

CAUSAS E FATORES DE RISCO
• Qualquer traumatismo pulpar; trauma direto, indutor de fratura da coroa dentária; defesa (brigas — dentes caninos); mastigação de objetos duros (dentes carniceiros); traumatismo por má oclusão; brincadeiras com filhotes de cães, arrastando e puxando trapos de panos de sua boca; aplicação de placas ósseas para o reparo de raízes lesionadas. • Bactérias — a polpa pode ser acometida por bactérias provenientes de cáries dentárias, túbulos dentinários expostos ou extensão para o sistema endodôntico. • Calor térmico que resulta em necrose pulpar — queimaduras por fio elétrico, iatrogênico causado por polimento excessivo durante procedimento de higiene bucal ou uso de brocas rotativas. • Bolsa periodontal profunda, especialmente na raiz palatina de cão de pequeno porte, pode envolver o ápice, local onde as bactérias podem ingressar no sistema pulpar.

DIAGNÓSTICO

DIAGNÓSTICO DIFERENCIAL
• Reabsorção dentária — as radiografias não revelam qualquer radiotransparência ou abscedação apical. • Carcinoma de células escamosas e fibrossarcoma — tumores invasivos de crescimento rápido; deslocam os dentes e aumentam sua mobilidade. • Cementomas — as radiografias demonstram aumento nas raízes apicais, com uma zona radiotransparente delgada, em continuidade com o ligamento periodontal. • Ameloblastoma — desloca os dentes e aumenta sua mobilidade; expande-se lentamente. • Cistos — as radiografias costumam mostrar uma área lítica bastante ampla; podem mimetizar os abscessos apicais, que podem se tornar císticos (cistos radiculares, granulomas periodontais apicais); o tratamento endodôntico convencional não é bem-sucedido; no local de ausência congênita de um dente, desenvolvem-se cistos primordiais, que apresentam radiotransparência oval arredondada com margem radiopaca delgada nas radiografias. • Cisto dentígero — ocorre a partir do cisto folicular de um dente impactado ou incrustado (em geral, os primeiros pré-molares nos cães); as radiografias revelam um dente dentro do cisto. • Cicatriz periapical — ocorre geralmente em um dente submetido a tratamento endodôntico, onde não houve nenhum aumento adicional na radiotransparência apical após 6 meses do tratamento. • Anatomia normal — os forames mentuais podem ser confundidos com transparências apicais na interpretação radiográfica (o forame mental médio encontra-se imediatamente abaixo do segundo pré-molar).

HEMOGRAMA/BIOQUÍMICA/URINÁLISE
O hemograma completo pode exibir leucocitose e/ou leve anemia regenerativa.

DIAGNÓSTICO POR IMAGEM
• Auxílio diagnóstico fundamental — demonstra o espessamento do ligamento periodontal apical; radiotransparência pouco definida; revela perda óssea no ápice à medida que a lesão se torna crônica. • Conforme a lesão evolui, ocorrem lesões radiográficas compatíveis com osteomielite e celulite. • Se ocorreu fistulação, pode-se aplicar um cone de guta-percha no trajeto fistuloso e obter radiografias para identificar o dente acometido.

MÉTODOS DIAGNÓSTICOS
• Remoção cirúrgica do local do abscesso (cirurgia endodôntica) ou extração. • Avaliação do tratamento endodôntico em 6 meses a 1 ano. • A transiluminação com fibra óptica de luz intensa pode ajudar o clínico na distinção entre polpas viáveis e necróticas.

ACHADOS PATOLÓGICOS
• A região apical apresenta uma área central de necrose de liquefação, contendo neutrófilos em processo de desintegração e debris celulares, circundados por macrófagos, linfócitos e plasmócitos; podem-se observar bactérias. • A extensão da lesão para o osso esponjoso resulta em inflamação do osso periapical e reabsorção. • Nas alterações crônicas, pode ocorrer o desenvolvimento de trajetos, que podem ter revestimento epitelial; lesões de osteomielite ou celulite podem se tornar fibróticas com cápsula (cisto radicular e/ou granuloma periodontal periapical).

TRATAMENTO

• Drenagem e eliminação do foco de infecção. • Extração do dente envolvido e curetagem da área infectada apical. • Tratamento endodôntico do dente acometido (cirúrgico em caso de ampla lesão apical). • As condições crônicas exigem a remoção cirúrgica do tecido de granulação e a curetagem do trajeto fistuloso. • Após o tratamento, a aplicação de compressas frias (i. e., bolsas de gelo) sobre a área ajudará a reduzir a inflamação. • Repouso total por alguns dias. • Por alguns dias, não se deve fornecer nenhum objeto ou material duro para ser mastigado.

MEDICAÇÕES

MEDICAMENTO(S)
• Antibióticos no pré-operatório para evitar a disseminação sistêmica da infecção. • Antibióticos de amplo espectro por 7-10 dias do pós-operatório. • Analgésicos nos períodos pré, intra e pós-operatórios por 3-4 dias. • Caso se efetuem cirurgias endodônticas ou extrações, poderá ser necessário o uso de colar protetor.

ACOMPANHAMENTO

• Reavaliar em 10 dias do pós-operatório. • Exame geral da área; teste de percussão quanto à sensibilidade, à cicatrização do local da extração ou da cirurgia endodôntica e à integridade dos preenchimentos de acesso endodôntico. • Reavaliar em 6 meses a 1 ano; repetir as radiografias para verificar se a lesão desapareceu (em casos de tratamento endodôntico). • Evitar lesões traumáticas (p. ex., deixar os cães correrem atrás de carros, mastigar objetos/brinquedos duros, parar de brigar). • Restringir as mordidas — evitar mangas de adestradores que estejam rasgadas ou furadas e evitar movimentos de torção. • Examinar a boca regularmente em busca de dentes quebrados ou manchados.

Autor James M. G. Anthony
Consultor Editorial Heidi B. Lobprise

ÁCAROS OTOLÓGICOS

CONSIDERAÇÕES GERAIS

REVISÃO
Os ácaros *Otodectes cynotis* causam uma reação de hipersensibilidade que resulta em irritação intensa da orelha externa de cães e gatos.

IDENTIFICAÇÃO
- Comuns em cães e gatos jovens, embora possam ocorrer em qualquer idade.
- Não há predileção racial nem sexual.

SINAIS CLÍNICOS
- Prurido localizado principalmente em torno das orelhas, na cabeça e no pescoço; ocasionalmente, generalizado.
- Crostas espessas de coloração vermelho-acastanhada ou negra — observadas comumente na face externa da orelha.
- Pode ocorrer a formação de crostas e escamas no pescoço, no quarto posterior e na cauda.
- Com frequência, ocorrem escoriações na superfície convexa dos pavilhões auriculares, por conta do prurido intenso.

CAUSAS E FATORES DE RISCO
Otodectes cynotis.

DIAGNÓSTICO

DIAGNÓSTICO DIFERENCIAL
- Hipersensibilidade à picada de pulga.
- Pediculose.
- Dermatite (rabdítica) por *Pelodera*.
- Sarna sarcóptica.
- Sarna notoédrica.
- Ácaros trombiculídeos.
- Otite externa alérgica.

HEMOGRAMA/BIOQUÍMICA/URINÁLISE
Normais.

OUTROS TESTES LABORATORIAIS
N/D.

DIAGNÓSTICO POR IMAGEM
N/D.

MÉTODOS DIAGNÓSTICOS
- Raspados cutâneos — identificam os ácaros se os sinais forem generalizados.
- *Swabs* otológicos colocados em óleo mineral — geralmente constituem um meio de identificação bastante eficaz.
- Os ácaros podem ser observados no canal auditivo externo com o auxílio do otoscópio.
- Em animais hipersensíveis, o diagnóstico pode ser feito por meio da resposta ao tratamento.

TRATAMENTO
- Em esquema ambulatorial.
- Dieta e atividade — não há necessidade de nenhuma modificação.
- Sarna muito contagiosa — é imprescindível o tratamento dos animais em contato com o animal acometido.
- Limpar e tratar o ambiente totalmente.

MEDICAÇÕES

MEDICAMENTO(S)
- As orelhas devem ser completamente limpas com uma solução otológica comercial.
- É recomendável utilizar parasiticidas otológicos por 7 a 10 dias para erradicar os ácaros e os ovos. Os produtos comerciais tópicos eficazes contêm piretrinas, tiabendazol, ivermectina, rotenona; também é sugerido que o tratamento durante semanas alternadas por 2 a 3 ciclos terapêuticos previna a reinfestação por ovos.
- Selamectina (Revolution®, Pfizer) — aplicada por via tópica na base do pescoço a cada 2-4 semanas.
- Imidacloprida/moxidectina (Advantage Multi/Advocate®) — combinação aplicada por via tópica a cada 2-4 semanas.
- Moxidectina — 0,2-0,4 mg/kg SC a cada 1-2 semanas durante 4 tratamentos; uso não aprovado pela FDA.
- Ivermectina — 300 µg/kg SC a cada 1-2 semanas por 4 vezes: uso não aprovado pela FDA.
- Milbemicina — 1-2 mg/kg VO a cada 24 h em semanas alternadas por 2 a 3 ciclos terapêuticos; uso não aprovado pela FDA.
- É aconselhável aplicar tratamentos contra as pulgas aos animais para eliminação de ácaros ectópicos.
- Os ácaros podem persistir no ambiente, a menos que eles sejam completamente removidos.

CONTRAINDICAÇÕES/INTERAÇÕES POSSÍVEIS
- Ivermectina e moxidectina — não usar por via oral nem injetável em cães das raças Collie, Sheltie e seus mestiços ou em outras raças de pastoreio; empregar apenas se for absolutamente necessário em animais com <6 meses de vida; em filhotes de gatos, há relatos de um número crescente de reações tóxicas.
- Ivermectina e milbemicina — provocam aumento nos níveis de metabólitos de neurotransmissores monoaminicos, o que pode resultar em interações medicamentosas adversas com amitraz e benzodiazepínicos.

ACOMPANHAMENTO
- O *swab* otológico e o exame físico devem ser feitos 1 mês após o início da terapia.
- O prognóstico é bom.
- Raras vezes, a infestação será removida apenas para se constatar uma alergia subjacente que mantém a otite externa ativa.
- A infestação repetida indica a existência de uma fonte não controlada de ácaros.

DIVERSOS

POTENCIAL ZOONÓTICO
Dermatite papular transitória em seres humanos.

Sugestões de Leitura
Medleau LA, Hnilica KA. Small Animal Dermatology: A Color Atlas and Therapeutic Guide. St. Louis; Saunders Elsevier, 2006.
Scott DW, Miller WH, Griffin CE. Muller & Kirk's Small Animal Dermatology, 6th ed. Philadelphia: Saunders, 2001.

Autor Karen A. Kuhl
Consultor Editorial Alexander H. Werner

ACASALAMENTO, MOMENTO OPORTUNO

CONSIDERAÇÕES GERAIS

DEFINIÇÃO
Momento oportuno de inseminações durante o estro para maximizar a fertilidade e o tamanho da ninhada.

FISIOPATOLOGIA
Cadelas
• Necessário para determinar o momento da ovulação, para que a reprodução (acasalamento) ocorra no momento adequado apesar do estro prolongado. • Sêmen fresco, resfriado ou congelado — limita-se, em geral, a uma ou duas inseminações; exige a sincronização da inseminação com a ovulação para a obtenção da máxima fertilidade. • A ovulação pode variar em relação ao início do cio (estro) permanente; efetuar a citologia vaginal. • Hormônio luteinizante (LH) — controla a ovulação; atinge seu pico no mesmo dia ou após a observação da cornificação completa; a ovulação ocorre aproximadamente 2 dias após o pico; são necessários mais 2-3 dias (48-54 horas) para a maturação dos oócitos; oócitos maduros tornam-se viáveis em mais outros 2-3 dias; dessa forma, o período fértil fica entre 4-8 dias após o pico desse hormônio e a fertilidade atinge o máximo 5-6 dias também depois desse pico; a análise hormonal constitui um método exato para determinar o dia desse pico. • Sinais físicos isolados — podem não ser confiáveis para a determinação precisa do período fértil. • Início do estro — geralmente associado a uma alteração no corrimento vaginal de sanguinolento para um pouco vermelho e uma redução da intumescência vulvar; o corrimento sanguinolento pode continuar durante o estro e cessar apenas no início do diestro (nessa fase, o período fértil já passou e a cadela não se mostra mais receptiva). • Receptividade — pode ser detectada por carícias próximas à região do períneo em qualquer um dos lados da vulva; se estiver receptiva, a fêmea elevará sua cauda em bandeira para um lado. • Exame citológico vaginal — melhor indicador do período fértil, quando comparado com os sinais comportamentais ou físicos; a cornificação do epitélio vaginal é controlada pelo estrogênio; a cornificação plena com um fundo claro costuma coincidir com a receptividade sexual; a estimativa do dia da ovulação não é exata com base no exame da citologia vaginal. • Progesterona sérica — elevação estritamente associada ao pico do LH; útil para estimar a ovulação e, consequentemente, o período fértil; concentração <1 ng/mL (3,18 nmol/L) antes do pico de LH, 1,5-4 ng/mL (4,8-12,7 nmol/L) no dia do pico, 4-10 ng/mL (12,7-31,8 nmol/L) no momento da ovulação; continua subindo durante o diestro ou a gestação. Vários laboratórios comerciais utilizam diversos métodos de mensuração da concentração de progesterona, pois os valores indicativos do LH e da ovulação variam entre os laboratórios. O registro de uma rápida elevação na progesterona subsequente ao aumento inicial é um indicador mais confiável de ovulação do que a mensuração isolada do pico de LH ou a elevação inicial da progesterona.

Gatas
• Ovulação — normalmente induzida; o momento do coito/acasalamento não é tão crítico quanto nas cadelas; depende da liberação adequada do LH, deflagrada pela estimulação da vagina. • Estimulação adequada — caracterizada por um gemido (choro) copulatório e uma reação pós-coito; a frequência de estímulos do coito é importante na determinação da adequação do contato sexual. • LH — o pico da concentração e a duração da elevação determinam a ovulação; concentração plasmática mais elevada com múltiplas cópulas; a resposta à cópula depende do dia do estro (maior liberação no 3º dia do estro do que no 1º); a liberação parcial depende da duração de exposição ao estrogênio.

SISTEMA(S) ACOMETIDO(S)
Reprodutor.

SINAIS CLÍNICOS
Comentários Gerais
Cadelas
• Cadela normal — o corrimento vulvar sanguinolento durante o proestro torna-se menor em termos de quantidade e mais claro em relação à cor durante o estro; a intumescência vulvar do proestro diminui levemente durante o estro; mostra-se receptiva aos machos no período do estro. • Em caso de número limitado de cruzamentos disponíveis — é imprescindível conhecer o dia da ovulação.

Gatas
• Resposta do LH a um único acasalamento — pode variar substancialmente.

Achados Anamnésicos
Cadelas
• Recusa em aceitar o macho no momento esperado. • Corrimento vulvar sanguinolento durante o estro.

Gatas
• Retorno ao estro em <30 dias — pode indicar falha na ovulação; o interestro costuma ser de 8-10 dias, mas altamente variável até mesmo na própria gata; algumas gatas também acasalarão enquanto estiverem prenhes.

Achados do Exame Físico
Cadelas
• Epitélio vaginal completamente cornificado. • Manifestação de interesse pelo macho. • Vulva menos intumescida (túrgida). • Corrimento vaginal — coloração e quantidade reduzidas. • Elevação da cauda em bandeira.

Gatas
• Epitélio vaginal completamente cornificado. • Manifestação de interesse pelo macho. • Sem alterações na genitália externa. • Vocalização e fricção sobre objetos. • Postura em lordose ("postura arrastada").

CAUSAS
Cadelas
• Número limitado de acasalamentos. • Não receptivas ao macho. • Reprodução por meio de inseminação artificial (sêmen fresco, resfriado ou congelado).

Gatas
• Coito — muito precoce ou muito tardio no estro; pouquíssimas vezes. • Reprodução por meio de inseminação artificial.

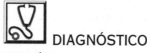

DIAGNÓSTICO

DIAGNÓSTICO DIFERENCIAL
• Corrimento vaginal — proestro ou estro; vaginite; neoplasia; piometra, infecção do trato urinário. • Recusa em permitir a penetração peniana — problema anatômico de estenose ou resquício do hímen ou hiperplasia vaginal, além de problema comportamental.

OUTROS TESTES LABORATORIAIS
Cadelas
• Teste semiquantitativo da progesterona na clínica — como adjuvante ao exame citológico vaginal; para estabelecer uma linha basal, iniciar a mensuração quando a citologia vaginal revelar 60-75% de células epiteliais cornificadas. • Teste quantitativo da progesterona — mais preciso; exame preferido quando a reprodução é feita com sêmen congelado; particularmente útil na cadela ou no macho com fertilidade reduzida. • Teste do LH — é imprescindível a coleta de amostras diárias para se observar o pico do LH; pode-se usar o nível sérico da progesterona para sinalizar o momento de início do teste ou como um indicador substituto do pico de LH.

Gatas
Para verificar a ovulação, submeter as amostras ao teste da progesterona.

DIAGNÓSTICO POR IMAGEM
Ultrassonografia dos ovários — pode ajudar a determinar a ovulação; não é confiável como método isolado de verificação da ovulação; precisa ser realizada diariamente pelo menos uma vez, melhor se várias vezes ao dia.

MÉTODOS DIAGNÓSTICOS
Cadelas
• Comportamento — cauda em bandeira, extremo interesse pelo macho, fêmeas que montam uma nas outras. • Corrimento vaginal muito menos hemorrágico, vulva mais macia e menos intumescida. • Palpação digital da vagina pode ser ressentida pela cadela no proestro com melhora ao longo do proestro até o estro. Pode ser palpada a presença de massa edematosa no assoalho da porção caudal da vagina, imediatamente cranial ao osso da uretra. Essa massa deve diminuir conforme o período fértil ideal se aproxima. • Exame citológico vaginal — no início do proestro (na linguagem de criadores: no "dia 1" ao primeiro sinal de corrimento vaginal hemorrágico); a maioria das células epiteliais não se encontra cornificada (o núcleo aparece pontilhado como uma célula viável normal); a porcentagem de células cornificadas (células com citoplasma angular e núcleos picnóticos ou núcleos que falham em absorver o corante) aumenta durante o proestro, chegando muitas vezes a 90% ou mais próximo ao estro (há variação individual). Os criadores referem-se a esse estágio pelo dia, em vez de usar o termo "estro"; isso costuma ser em torno do dia 10-18 em termos reprodutivos. O fundo da lâmina é livre (isento) de debris durante o estro. No início do diestro, ocorre um declínio abrupto na porcentagem de células cornificadas (20-50%) em um único dia; o primeiro dia de declínio notável na cornificação é definido como o dia 1 do diestro (D1); é normal observar a presença de neutrófilos nos dias 1-4 do diestro. • Vaginoscopia — pregas vaginais edematosas até o pico de LH e, depois, leve enrugamento à medida que o edema diminui com o declínio no estradiol; por volta do período fértil ideal, formam-se rugas evidentes (crenulação) até o diestro quando as pregas ficam muito achatadas e o edema desaparece. • Teste sorológico para pesquisa de *B. canis* (cadelas) — o teste de aglutinação rápida em lâmina é utilizado como triagem; exame

ACASALAMENTO, MOMENTO OPORTUNO

sensível, mas inespecífico (D-Tec CB, Synbiotics Corp.); reavaliar os testes positivos das lâminas por meio do exame de imunodifusão em ágar gel (Cornell University Diagnostic Laboratory) ou cultura bacteriana de sangue total ou aspirado de linfonodos.

TRATAMENTO

CUIDADO(S) DE SAÚDE ADEQUADO(S)

Cadelas
• Sêmen fresco: múltiplos acasalamentos — inseminar três vezes por semana após observar a elevação inicial na progesterona até o D1. • Dois acasalamentos — inseminar nos dias 3 e 5 ou nos dias 4 e 6 após o pico do LH ou a elevação inicial na progesterona. • Sêmen congelado ou fresco resfriado — o congelado é menos viável do que o fresco resfriado; dessa forma, o momento oportuno para a inseminação é mais crítico; uma ou duas inseminações intrauterinas são mais comuns: inseminar no dia 5 ou 6 após o pico do LH ou a elevação inicial da progesterona (dia 0) ou 3 dias após um nível de progesterona ≥5 ng/mL (16 nmol/L); a inseminação intrauterina transcervical via endoscopia ou cateter Norueguês ou inseminação cirúrgica. • A progesterona no dia da inseminação deve estar ≥12 ng/mL (38 nmol/L). • O momento oportuno da inseminação com base no nível da progesterona aumenta as chances de concepção e o tamanho da ninhada. • São adequadas consultas em dias alternados para coleta de sangue e exame da citologia vaginal.

Gatas
• Aumentar a probabilidade de ovulação e o tamanho da ninhada, maximizando o número de acasalamentos; cruzar em dias sucessivos. • Cruzar pelo menos 4 vezes ao dia com intervalo de no mínimo 2-3 horas nos dias 2 e 3 do estro para maximizar a liberação do LH. • Pode-se induzir à ovulação por meio da administração de hormônios exógenos — GnRH ou hCG após o acasalamento.

ATIVIDADE
• Não há necessidade de nenhuma mudança na atividade. • É imprescindível manter as fêmeas estritamente distantes de machos sexualmente intactos indesejáveis.

ORIENTAÇÃO AO PROPRIETÁRIO
Orientar o proprietário quanto às alterações físicas, comportamentais e endocrinológicas durante o ciclo estral, bem como no que diz respeito à possível variação do momento dessas alterações de um animal para outro — isso pode aumentar a confiança e a satisfação do proprietário.

CONSIDERAÇÕES CIRÚRGICAS
A inseminação artificial cirúrgica exige cuidados pós-operatórios padrão.

MEDICAÇÕES

MEDICAMENTO(S) DE ESCOLHA
Gatas — hCG (100-500 UI, IM); GnRH (25-50 µg, IM).

ACOMPANHAMENTO

MONITORIZAÇÃO DO PACIENTE
• Cadelas — continuar obtendo amostras vaginais após o cruzamento para determinar o D1; a estimativa retrospectiva do dia da ovulação é de 6 dias antes do D1. • A gestação das cadelas é de 65 dias a partir do pico de LH, 63 dias a partir da ovulação ou 57 dias a partir do D1. Para uso de sêmen fresco, resfriado ou congelado: repetir a análise quantitativa da progesterona após a elevação inicial desse hormônio ou o pico de LH até verificar um nível >5 ng/mL (16 nmol/L). • Gatas — utilizar o ensaio de progesterona para verificar a ovulação. • A gestação das gatas é de 62-71 dias a partir do primeiro acasalamento.

COMPLICAÇÕES POSSÍVEIS

Cadelas
• Exame citológico vaginal — compara o D1 com a estimativa prospectiva, com base no nível da progesterona; se as estimativas diferirem, os índices de gestação serão reduzidos. • Kits para o teste semiquantitativo da progesterona — devem estar à temperatura ambiente antes do uso; a obtenção de valores falsamente elevados é comum ao se utilizar um kit frio. • Progesterona sérica — permitir a coagulação sanguínea em temperatura fria; separar as células a partir do soro ou do plasma em até 20 minutos da coleta; ao se empregar soro misturado com hemácias, ocorrerão valores falsamente baixos, pois a progesterona estará conjugada (ligada) a essas células. • Amostra hemolisada ou lipêmica — pode gerar um valor falsamente baixo da progesterona em alguns ensaios. • Ensaio quantitativo da progesterona (quimioluminescência, fluorescência, ensaio imunoenzimático) — mais preciso quando realizado por um laboratório comercial do que os kits semiquantitativos; preferível em casos de fertilidade questionável; os períodos de oscilação hormonal podem dificultar seu emprego na determinação prospectiva do momento oportuno para o acasalamento. • Não utilizar tubos de separação do soro — podem gerar uma falsa elevação quando a progesterona é mensurada por ensaio quimioluminescente; o tipo de anticoagulante pode afetar o valor (valor: soro > plasma heparinizado > plasma com EDTA). • LH sérico — fatores não identificados no soro de algumas cadelas interferem nos kits de LH; deve-se contar, assim, com a progesterona sérica.

DIVERSOS

DISTÚRBIOS ASSOCIADOS
Estenoses vulvovestibulares, estenoses vestibulovaginais e resquícios do hímen.

FATORES RELACIONADOS COM A IDADE
Cios divididos em cadelas jovens — tipificados por um período de proestro (pode ser prolongado para 6 semanas ou mais), seguido pela interrupção dos sinais e subsequente retomada do ciclo estral (1-3 semanas mais tarde); no primeiro proestro/estro, não ocorre nenhuma elevação inicial nos níveis da progesterona ou do LH; o estro subsequente costuma ser normal.

GESTAÇÃO/FERTILIDADE/REPRODUÇÃO
Fazer o exame de gestação — os conceptos podem ser detectados pela primeira vez 19-20 dias após o pico do LH (isso requer um exame de alta resolução e alta frequência); no entanto, os exames são comumente realizados 30 dias após o pico de LH; é recomendável o exame mais precoce em cadelas com histórico de perda gestacional ou infertilidade.

VER TAMBÉM
• Corrimento Vaginal. • Infertilidade na Fêmea.

ABREVIATURA(S)
• D1= 1º dia do diestro. • GnRH = hormônio liberador da gonadotrofina. • hCG = gonadotrofina coriônica humana. • LH = hormônio luteinizante.

RECURSOS DA INTERNET
Root Kustritz MV. Use of commercial luteinizing hormone and progesterone assay kits in canine breeding management. In: Concannon PW, England G, Verstegen III J, Linde-Forsberg C, eds., Recent Advances in Small Animal Reproduction. International Veterinary Information Service, Ithaca NY, www.ivis.org, 2001; A1202.0500.

Sugestões de Leitura
De Gier J, Kooistra HS, Djajadiningrat-Laanen SC, et al. Temporal relations between plasma concentrations of luteinizing hormone, estradiol-17B, progesterone, prolactin, and α-melanocyte-stimulating hormone during the follicular, ovulatory, and early luteal phase in the bitch. Theriogenology 2006, 65:1346-1359.
Fontbonne A, Malandain E. Ovarian ultrasonography and follow-up of estrus in the bitch and queen. Waltham Focus 2006,16(2):22-29, available at www.ivis.org.
Johnston SD, Root Kustritz MV, Olson PN. Vaginal cytology. In: Canine and Feline Theriogenology. Philadelphia: Saunders, 2001, pp. 32-40.
Johnston SD, Root Kustritz MV, Olson PN. Breeding management, artificial insemination, in vitro fertilization, and embryo transfer in the queen. In: Canine and Feline Theriogenology. Philadelphia: Saunders, 2001, pp. 406-413.
Reynaud K, Fontbonne A, Marseloo N, Viaris de Lesegno C, Saint-Dizier M, Chastant-Maillard S. In vivo canine oocyte maturation, fertilization and early embryogenesis: A review. Theriogenology 2006, 66:1685-1693.
Volkmann D. The effects of storage time and temperature and anticoagulant on laboratory measurements of canine blood progesterone concentrations. Theriogenology 2006, 66:1583-1586.

Autor Cathy Gartley
Consultor Editorial Sara K. Lyle
Agradecimento A autora e a editora agradecem a contribuição prévia de Dale Paccamonti.

ACIDENTE VASCULAR CEREBRAL (AVC)

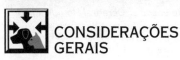

CONSIDERAÇÕES GERAIS

DEFINIÇÃO
- Acidente vascular cerebral refere-se ao início súbito de sinais cerebrais focais não progressivos, secundários à vasculopatia cerebral.
- Os sinais devem permanecer por mais de 24 horas para um diagnóstico de AVC.
- Em geral, o AVC resulta em dano cerebral permanente.
- O episódio recebe o nome de ataque isquêmico transitório ou "AIT" se os sinais clínicos desaparecerem em até 24 horas.

FISIOPATOLOGIA
- As vasculopatias cerebrais constituem a causa subjacente de AVC.
- Anormalidade cerebral resultante de um processo patológico que compromete a irrigação sanguínea ao cérebro.
- As lesões que afetam os vasos sanguíneos cerebrais são divididas em duas amplas categorias:
  ○ Acidente vascular cerebral hemorrágico — ruptura de vaso sanguíneo que resulta em hemorragia intracerebral ou em torno do cérebro.
  ○ Acidente vascular cerebral isquêmico — interrupção abrupta do fluxo sanguíneo em direção ao cérebro, causada por obstrução de alguma artéria com consequente privação de oxigênio e glicose ao tecido cerebral.

SISTEMA(S) ACOMETIDO(S)
- Nervoso.
- Multissistêmico — na presença de causa subjacente.

INCIDÊNCIA/PREVALÊNCIA
Desconhecidas; supostamente baixas em comparação às de seres humanos.

IDENTIFICAÇÃO
Espécies
Cães e gatos.

Raça(s) Predominante(s)
- Acidente vascular cerebral isquêmico — as raças Cavalier King Charles spaniel e Galgo parecem predispostas; é mais provável que raças de pequeno (≤15 kg) e grande (>15kg) porte sofram de infarto cerebelar e infarto mesencefálico ou talâmico, respectivamente.
- Acidente vascular cerebral hemorrágico — desconhecida.

Idade Média e Faixa Etária
Desconhecidas

Sexo Predominante
Desconhecido.

SINAIS CLÍNICOS
Achados Anamnésicos
- Acidente vascular cerebral isquêmico — sinais cerebrais focais não progressivos, superagudos a agudos.
- Acidente vascular cerebral hemorrágico — sinais cerebrais focais ou multifocais, agudos a subagudos, que podem evoluir por um curto período de tempo.

Achados do Exame Físico
- Exame de fundo do olho — pode revelar vasos tortuosos (hipertensão sistêmica), hemorragia (coagulopatia ou hipertensão sistêmica) ou papiledema (PIC elevada).
- Defeitos de coagulação — podem constituir a base do acidente vascular cerebral hemorrágico e causar hemorragia em qualquer tecido ou órgão, além de anemia.

Achados do Exame Neurológico
- Acidente vascular cerebral isquêmico — os sinais dependem da localização do insulto vascular (prosencéfalo, mesencéfalo, ponte, medula oblonga, cerebelo).
- Acidente vascular cerebral hemorrágico — os sinais relacionam-se com o aumento da PIC em caso de distúrbio inespecífico do prosencéfalo e/ou do tronco encefálico.

CAUSAS
Acidente Vascular Cerebral Isquêmico
Cães
- Desconhecidas em 50% dos casos.
- Endocrinopatias — hiperadrenocorticismo, hipotireoidismo, diabetes.
- Embolia, tromboembolia — neoplásica (hemangiossarcoma, linfoma), infecciosa (associada à endocardite bacteriana ou a outras fontes de infecção), e aórtica ou cardíaca.
- Hipertensão sistêmica.
- Embolia fibrocartilaginosa.
- Linfoma intravascular.
- Migração (*Cuterebra*) ou embolia (*Dirofilaria immitis*) parasitária.

Gatos
- Migração parasitária (*Cuterebra*).
- Hipertensão sistêmica — hipertireoidismo, doença renal crônica, cardiopatia.
- Embolia neoplásica.

Acidente Vascular Cerebral Hemorrágico
Cães
- Ruptura de aneurismas congênitos.
- Tumores cerebrais primários e secundários.
- Doença inflamatória de artérias e veias (vasculite).
- Linfoma intravascular.
- Infarto hemorrágico cerebral.
- Distúrbio de coagulação.

Gatos
- Tumores cerebrais primários e secundários.
- Doença inflamatória de artérias e veias (vasculite).
- Infarto hemorrágico cerebral.
- Distúrbio de coagulação.
- Hipertensão sistêmica.

FATORES DE RISCO
- Acidente vascular cerebral isquêmico — hipertensão sistêmica, distúrbio sistêmico associado à síndrome de hipercoagulabilidade.
- Acidente vascular cerebral hemorrágico — hipertensão sistêmica.

DIAGNÓSTICO

DIAGNÓSTICO DIFERENCIAL
- Traumatismo craniencefálico — achados anamnésicos e físicos sugestivos de traumatismo.
- Descompensação de tumor cerebral primário ou metastático — os sinais são progressivos.
- Encefalite infecciosa e não infecciosa — sinais clínicos agudos a subagudos que pioram gradativamente.
- Neurotoxicidade — déficits neurológicos simétricos e bilaterais.

HEMOGRAMA/BIOQUÍMICA/URINÁLISE
Normais com maior frequência; podem revelar alterações que refletem a causa subjacente.

OUTROS TESTES LABORATORIAIS
- Líquido cerebrospinal — é improvável que o exame desse líquido confirme o AVC, mas pode ajudar a descartar doença inflamatória do SNC. Achados variáveis; achados normais ou leve pleocitose mononuclear ou neutrofílica; concentração proteica ocasionalmente elevada.
- Tempo de protrombina — teste de triagem para defeitos dos mecanismos extrínsecos.
- Tempo de tromboplastina parcial ativada — teste de triagem para defeitos dos mecanismos intrínsecos.
- Tempo de sangramento — prolongado em pacientes com doença de von Willebrand; normal em muitos outros defeitos de coagulação, exceto em coagulação intravascular disseminada.
- Tromboelastografia, ensaio de D-dímeros e antitrombina III — testes de triagem para síndrome de hipercoagulabilidade como possível causa de acidente vascular cerebral isquêmico.
- Teste endócrino — hiperadrenocorticismo, doença da tireoide, e feocromocitoma.

DIAGNÓSTICO POR IMAGEM
Acidente Vascular Cerebral Isquêmico
- TC — frequentemente normal durante a fase aguda.
- RM — realizada dentro de 12-24 horas do início para distinguir hemorragia de infarto. As imagens ponderadas em T2 e as imagens líquido-atenuadas da recuperação da inversão (FLAIR, sigla em inglês) são particularmente úteis. As imagens ponderadas em T2* (ecogradiente) são usadas para demonstrar ou excluir a presença de hemorragia intracraniana. As imagens ponderadas em difusão são utilizadas como uma sequência ideal para identificação de acidente vascular cerebral hiperagudo, excluindo *stroke mimics* (sinais e sintomas que mimetizam o diagnóstico clínico de AVC). As imagens ponderadas em perfusão podem ser empregadas para retratar as regiões cerebrais de hipoperfusão e auferir o tecido sob risco, comparando os resultados com os achados obtidos nas imagens ponderadas em difusão. A angiografia por ressonância magnética com tempo de voo e a angiografia por ressonância magnética contrastada podem ser usadas para avaliar o estado vascular intracraniano de pacientes com AVC.

Acidente Vascular Cerebral Hemorrágico
- TC — exame muito sensível para detecção de hemorragia aguda; hiperdensidade por hiperatenuação do feixe de raios X pela porção de globina do sangue. A atenuação diminui até que o hematoma fique isodenso em aproximadamente 1 mês do início. O contraste da periferia do hematoma acentua-se de 6 dias a 6 semanas após o início devido à revascularização.
- RM — a intensidade do sinal de hemorragia intracraniana é influenciada por vários fatores intrínsecos (tempo de ocorrência do *ictus*, origem, tamanho e localização da hemorragia) e extrínsecos (sequência de pulso e força do campo magnético). À medida que o hematoma envelhece, a oxiemoglobina no sangue degrada-se sequencialmente em vários produtos paramagnéticos (desoxiemoglobina, metemoglobina, hemossiderina), sendo que cada um deles apresenta diferentes intensidades de sinal de RM. Em comparação com outras sequências

Acidente Vascular Cerebral (AVC)

convencionais, as imagens ponderadas em T2* (ecogradiente) demonstram hipointensidade facilmente detectável, independentemente do tempo de ocorrência do *ictus*, da origem e do local da hemorragia ou da força do campo magnético.

MÉTODOS DIAGNÓSTICOS
• Diagnóstico das causas subjacentes potenciais.

Acidente Vascular Cerebral Isquêmico
• Avaliar o paciente quanto à presença de hipertensão (e causas subjacentes potenciais), endocrinopatia (hiperadrenocorticismo, hipotireoidismo, hipertireoidismo, diabetes melito), doença renal crônica (especialmente nefropatia com perda de proteínas), cardiopatia e doenças metastáticas (particularmente hemangiossarcoma).

Acidente Vascular Cerebral Hemorrágico
• Avaliar o paciente quanto à presença de coagulopatia (e causas subjacentes potenciais), hipertensão (e causas subjacentes potenciais) e doenças metastáticas (particularmente hemangiossarcoma).

ACHADOS PATOLÓGICOS

Acidente Vascular Cerebral Isquêmico
• Necrose isquêmica concentrada na substância cinzenta em função de vulnerabilidade seletiva.
• Lesões restritas à área cerebral vascularizada pelo vaso acometido com bordas nitidamente delimitadas; tecido cerebral circunjacente normal; efeito de massa ou expansivo mínimo a ausente.
• Isquemia cerebral global costuma afetar uma área densa de neurônios seletivamente vulneráveis. Regiões anatômicas específicas, incluindo córtex cerebral, hipocampo, certos núcleos basais (p. ex., núcleos caudados), tálamo e camadas de células de Purkinje do cerebelo são mais suscetíveis à lesão hipóxica.
• Ocorrem alterações celulares isquêmicas precoces com rapidez, como resultado da privação de energia com tumefação da mitocôndria e do retículo endoplasmático, o que causa microvacuolização citoplasmática. As lesões mais crônicas são caracterizadas por atrofia pós-necrótica do parênquima cerebral, proliferação endotelial em capilares viáveis e acúmulo de células de Gitter.

Acidente Vascular Cerebral Hemorrágico
• O sangramento do parênquima origina-se de ruptura das pequenas artérias cerebrais penetrantes. A maioria dos casos agudos revela hemorragia recente e necrose neuronal aguda que é lentamente removida pelos macrófagos, deixando com o passar do tempo uma cavidade cística revestida por astrócitos fibrilares.
• A histologia é caracterizada pela presença de edema, dano neuronal, macrófagos e neutrófilos na região que circunda o hematoma.
• Embora algumas hemorragias cerebrais cessem rapidamente como resultado dos processos de coagulação e tamponamento pelas regiões circunjacentes, outras tendem a se expandir com o passar do tempo. Estas hemorragias resultam do sangramento contínuo a partir da fonte primária e estão relacionadas com a ruptura mecânica de vasos circunjacentes. A hemorragia dissemina-se entre os planos de clivagem da substância branca com destruição mínima, deixando ninhos de tecido neural intacto dentro e em torno do hematoma.

TRATAMENTO

CUIDADO(S) DE SAÚDE ADEQUADO(S)
• Qualquer doença subjacente identificada deve ser tratada.
• O tratamento visa fornecer os cuidados de suporte, manter a oxigenação adequada dos tecidos e controlar as complicações neurológicas e não neurológicas.
• Terapias mais específicas são direcionadas à prevenção de deterioração neurológica futura.

CUIDADO(S) DE ENFERMAGEM

Acidente Vascular Cerebral Isquêmico
• Monitorização e correção de variáveis fisiológicas básicas (p. ex., nível de oxigênio, equilíbrio hídrico, pressão arterial, temperatura corporal).
• Manutenção da pressão arterial sistêmica dentro da faixa fisiológica; é recomendável evitar a redução agressiva da pressão arterial durante os estágios agudos a menos que o paciente esteja sob alto risco de dano a órgãos-alvo (pressões arteriais sistólicas que permanecem acima de 180 mmHg).
• Não há evidência de que o glicocorticoide confira neuroproteção benéfica; a maioria dos agentes neuroprotetores testados até o momento não se mostrou eficaz em ensaios clínicos ou está aguardando investigação adicional.

Acidente Vascular Cerebral Hemorrágico
• Estabilização do paciente (proteção das vias aéreas, monitorização e correção dos sinais vitais).
• Avaliação e monitorização do estado neurológico.
• Determinação e tratamento das causas subjacentes potenciais de hemorragia.
• Avaliação do paciente quanto à necessidade de medidas terapêuticas específicas, incluindo controle da PIC elevada, o que gira em torno da redução do edema cerebral, otimização do volume sanguíneo cerebral e eliminação da massa ocupadora de espaço.
• O risco de deterioração neurológica e instabilidade cardiovascular é mais alto durante as primeiras 24 horas após o início da hemorragia intracraniana à medida que a lesão ocupadora de espaço lentamente se expande e o edema vasogênico cerebral se desenvolve.

MEDICAÇÕES

MEDICAMENTO(S) DE ESCOLHA

Acidente Vascular Cerebral Isquêmico
• Anti-hipertensivo — considerar em caso de pressão arterial sistêmica >180 mmHg sob avaliação seriada e/ou manifestações oculares graves de hipertensão.
• Inibidor da ECA — enalapril (0,25-0,5 mg/kg a cada 12 h) ou benazepril (0,25-0,5 mg/kg a cada 12 h) e/ou bloqueadores dos canais de cálcio como anlodipino (0,1-0,25 mg/kg a cada 24 h).
• Prevenção da formação de coágulo — considerar em casos de origens cardíacas comprovadas de embolia; terapia antiplaquetária com baixas doses de ácido acetilsalicílico (0,5 mg/kg VO a cada 24 h) ou clopidogrel (2-4 mg/kg VO a cada 24 h) e heparina de baixo peso molecular pode ser usada para fins profiláticos.

Acidente Vascular Cerebral Hemorrágico
• Manitol — na suspeita de PIC elevada irresponsiva às medidas de estabilização extracranianas (0,25-1 g/kg IV durante 10-20 minutos).

ACOMPANHAMENTO

MONITORIZAÇÃO DO PACIENTE
Avaliações neurológicas frequentes nas primeiras 48-72 horas para monitorizar a evolução.

COMPLICAÇÕES POSSÍVEIS
Recidiva de acidente vascular cerebral isquêmico

EVOLUÇÃO ESPERADA E PROGNÓSTICO
• A gravidade máxima dos sinais costuma ser atingida em até 24 horas do acidente vascular cerebral isquêmico.
• Resolução dos sinais — gradual dentro de 2-10 semanas. Alguns cães e gatos podem ficar com sinais neurológicos permanentes em virtude de dano cerebral irreversível.
• Há uma probabilidade significativamente maior de que os cães com distúrbio clínico causal sofram recidiva e tenham um tempo de sobrevida mais curto que aqueles sem distúrbio clínico identificável.
• É difícil predizer o prognóstico de isquemia cerebral global, pois não há estudos controlados.

DIVERSOS

SINÔNIMO(S)
AVC.

ABREVIATURAS
• AVC = acidente vascular cerebral.
• ECA = enzima conversora de angiotensina.
• PIC = pressão intracraniana.
• RM = ressonância magnética.
• SNC = sistema nervoso central.
• TC = tomografia computadorizada.

Sugestões de Leitura
Garosi LS, McConnell JF. Ischemic stroke in dogs and humans: A comparative review. J Small Anim Pract 2005, 46:521-529.
Garosi LS, McConnell JF, Platt SR, et al. Clinical characteristics and topographical magnetic resonance of suspected brain infarction in 40 dogs. J Vet Intern Med 2006, 20:311-321.
Garosi LS, McConnell JF, Platt SR, et al. Results of investigations and outcome of dog brain infarcts. J Vet Intern Med 2005, 19:725-731.
Garosi LS, Platt SR. Treatment of cerebrovascular disease. In: Bonagura JD, Twedt DC, ed., Current Veterinary Therapy XIV. St. Louis: Saunders Elsevier, 2009, pp. 1074-1077.

Autor Laurent Garosi
Consultor Editorial Joane M. Parent

Acidose Láctica

CONSIDERAÇÕES GERAIS

DEFINIÇÃO
• Hiperlactatemia — concentração do lactato sérico >1,5 mmol/L para cães e filhotes com >70 dias de vida e >1,8 mmol/L para gatos. • Acidose láctica — hiperlactatemia com pH arterial abaixo da faixa normal.

FISIOPATOLOGIA
• O ácido láctico é o produto final do metabolismo tanto aeróbio como anaeróbio da glicose; sob pH fisiológico, o ácido láctico imediatamente se dissocia em lactato e íon hidrogênio. Pequenas quantidades do lactato se formam diariamente nos indivíduos sadios, porém o acúmulo clinicamente significativo do lactato provém da glicólise anaeróbia. O ácido láctico é produzido durante processos fisiológicos (p. ex., exercício) e durante processos patológicos (p. ex., choque, crises convulsivas). • Normalmente, o metabolismo hepático e renal de lactato mantém o equilíbrio entre a produção e a depuração desse elemento, ao mesmo tempo em que fornece uma fonte regular de glicose para o cérebro e as hemácias, os quais preferencialmente utilizam esse açúcar; importante na manutenção do equilíbrio acidobásico, já que o íon hidrogênio produzido durante a dissociação do ácido láctico é usado na gliconeogênese. • Na maior parte dos pacientes críticos ou lesados, a hiperlactatemia e a acidose láctica são atribuídas a condições que induzem à hipoxia tecidual, com desvio para a glicólise anaeróbia. • Perfusão inadequada, hipoxemia grave, demandas aumentadas de oxigênio, concentração reduzida de hemoglobina ou combinações desses fatores provocam hipoxia tecidual. • Dependendo da duração e da gravidade da hipoxia, pode ocorrer o desenvolvimento de hiperlactatemia e, possivelmente, de acidose láctica. • A hiperlactatemia geralmente se desenvolve quando a perfusão tecidual é adequada e os sistemas de tamponamento acidobásico estão intactos. • Em geral, não ocorre hipoperfusão tecidual clinicamente evidente nos pacientes apenas com hiperlactatemia; no entanto, pode haver hipoperfusão "oculta" não detectável por meio de monitorização de rotina; tal hipoperfusão "oculta" pode representar uma fase precursora da hipoperfusão manifesta. • A acidose láctica costuma estar presente em associação com regulação metabólica anormal secundária à hipoxia tecidual acentuada, determinados medicamentos ou toxinas ou defeitos congênitos no metabolismo dos carboidratos; em geral, os sistemas de tamponamento não conseguem lidar com a acidose em desenvolvimento. • A gravidade da hiperlactatemia e da acidose que se desenvolve nos pacientes criticamente enfermos ou lesados reflete a gravidade da hipoxia tecidual; portanto, a avaliação dos níveis de lactato nesses pacientes ajuda a avaliar o grau de hipoperfusão e hipoxia teciduais. • Estudos em pacientes humanos com traumatismo e choque demonstram que o lactato prevê o desfecho clínico e que a mortalidade se correlaciona com a gravidade da acidose láctica: quanto mais elevado o nível do lactato, maior a mortalidade. • A mensuração do lactato possibilita uma estimativa confiável da resposta pelas pessoas criticamente doentes ou lesadas à terapia de ressuscitação inicial e contínua. • As concentrações do lactato estão aumentadas nos cães criticamente enfermos e lesados; existe uma aparente associação entre a gravidade das concentrações elevadas do lactato e o desfecho clínico e as diferenças nas concentrações do lactato entre os vários estados mórbidos e tipos de lesão (crises convulsivas, intoxicação pelo etilenoglicol e pelo ácido acetilsalicílico, além de trauma maior). • Inúmeros estudos experimentais e clínicos em pacientes humanos criticamente doentes e resultados recentes em cães criticamente enfermos e lesados demonstram com clareza que a mensuração do lactato sanguíneo é uma ferramenta útil para avaliar a gravidade da hipoxia tecidual e a resposta ao tratamento, além de ser uma ferramenta prognóstica em termos de desfecho clínico.

SISTEMA(S) ACOMETIDO(S)
• Acidose láctica persistente pode gerar complicações cardiovasculares graves, incluindo diminuição da contratilidade cardíaca, resposta pressora comprometida às catecolaminas, aumento da sensibilidade do miocárdio a arritmias ventriculares e débito cardíaco reduzido. Essas alterações aumentam a probabilidade de hipoperfusão orgânica, acentuando ainda mais a hipoxia tecidual. • À medida que a acidose e a hipoxia tecidual se tornam mais graves, podem ocorrer falência múltipla de órgãos e até mesmo morte.

IDENTIFICAÇÃO
Cão e gato.

SINAIS CLÍNICOS

Comentários Gerais
Em geral, relacionam-se mais com o distúrbio subjacente indutor da acidose do que com os efeitos diretos da acidose em si. Conforme a hipoperfusão tecidual, a hipoxia e a acidose se agravam, podem ocorrer sinais de disfunção em qualquer sistema orgânico.

Achados Anamnésicos
Os distúrbios que provocam acidose láctica são comuns; portanto, fatos do histórico devem incitar a suspeita de alguma acidose subjacente.

Achados do Exame Físico
• Nesses pacientes, costuma haver taquipneia à medida que tentam a compensação respiratória. • A maior parte dos pacientes com acidose encontra-se hipovolêmica e, portanto, demonstra indícios de má perfusão tecidual ou desidratação — mucosas escurecidas, tempo de preenchimento capilar prolongado e turgor cutâneo aumentado. • Pacientes gravemente acidóticos podem apresentar disritmias cardíacas e contratilidade deficiente.

CAUSAS
• Dois tipos, A e B, com base na presença ou ausência clínica de hipoperfusão ou hipoxia tecidual. • Acidose láctica tipo A — mais comum; atribuída à distribuição diminuída ou inadequada do oxigênio e consumo desse gás (i. e., má perfusão tecidual e hipoxia tecidual). • As causas do tipo A incluem choque, hipoperfusão regional, obstrução arterial, hipoxemia grave, anemia grave, intoxicação por monóxido de carbono, asma grave e crises convulsivas motoras graves. • Acidose láctica do tipo B — inclui todas as outras causas de acidose láctica; subdivide-se em três subgrupos (B_1, B_2 e B_3); caracteriza-se pela ausência de hipoxemia ou má perfusão tecidual. • Muitas causas de acidose láctica do tipo B podem ser hipoperfusão "oculta" não detectável pelos parâmetros de monitorização de rotina ou possivelmente combinações de acidose láctica dos tipos A e B. • As causas mais comuns de acidose láctica do tipo B na medicina veterinária incluem neoplasia, alcalose, sepse, insuficiência renal, hepatopatia, uso de catecolaminas (noradrenalina, adrenalina) e intoxicações (estricnina, cianeto, etilenoglicol, salicilatos, paracetamol, propilenoglicol). • Em pacientes com linfoma e meningioma, já se observaram níveis sanguíneos elevados de lactato. Embora o tipo e a causa dos altos níveis de lactato nesses animais não sejam claramente compreendidos, a presença de hiperlactatemia deve alertar o clínico para a avaliação de outros marcadores de perfusão (frequência cardíaca, coloração das mucosas, qualidade do pulso, preenchimento capilar, creatinina sérica) antes de se tentar uma ressuscitação hídrica rigorosa.

FATORES DE RISCO
• Os fatores de risco para o desenvolvimento da hiperlactatemia e da acidose láctica relacionam-se diretamente com os fatores de risco para os distúrbios específicos que causam a hipoxia tecidual subjacente. • Em geral, animais jovens estão sob maior risco de choque traumático e de intoxicações. • É mais provável que animais idosos desenvolvam neoplasia, insuficiência renal, insuficiência cardíaca, hepatopatia, anemias graves e distúrbios vasculares; consultar as seções "Fatores de Risco" desses distúrbios específicos.

DIAGNÓSTICO

DIAGNÓSTICO DIFERENCIAL
• Os diagnósticos diferenciais para hiperlactatemia e acidose láctica incluem aqueles distúrbios descritos sob o título "Causas". • Todo animal gravemente doente ou lesado é suspeito de acidose subjacente; por esse motivo, a avaliação da concentração do lactato pode auxiliar no diagnóstico.

ACHADOS LABORATORIAIS

Medicamentos Capazes de Alterar os Resultados Laboratoriais
• Uso de carvão ativado, catecolaminas, salicilatos, paracetamol, terbutalina, nitroprusseto, halotano, bicarbonato e propilenoglicol, sem exceção, podem provocar aumentos leves a moderados nas concentrações do lactato na ausência de hipoperfusão e hipoxia tecidual verdadeira. • Concentrações mais baixas do lactato são mais encontradas nas amostras com o anticoagulante citrato de sódio do que naquelas contendo heparina e EDTA. • Até mesmo pequenas quantidades de fluidos intravenosos contendo lactato (p. ex., solução de Ringer lactato) podem causar aumentos falsos na concentração do lactato circulante em amostra de sangue, não adequadamente retirada do cateter ou do tubo pelo qual a administração do fluido intravenoso foi iniciada.

Distúrbios Capazes de Alterar os Resultados Laboratoriais
• Estresse, tremores, resistência à contenção, agitação e estase venosa podem aumentar o lactato para 2,5-5,0 mmol/L, mas o lactato geralmente se normaliza em ≤2 h. • Crises convulsivas ou esforço

Acidose Láctica

muscular extremo podem aumentar o lactato para 4-10 mmol/L, mas o lactato costuma se normalizar em ≤2 h. • Diversos tipos de neoplasia aumentam as concentrações do lactato, porque as células tumorais preferencialmente utilizam o metabolismo anaeróbio da glicose como parte da síndrome de caquexia cancerosa. • Alcalose, sepse, hepatopatia e insuficiência renal também podem aumentar as concentrações do lactato por outros mecanismos que não a má perfusão tecidual e hipoxia. • A falha em detectar concentrações elevadas do lactato não garante a perfusão adequada para todos os órgãos; talvez exista hipoperfusão orgânica significativa que finalmente acaba levando à falência múltipla de órgãos. • Hipoperfusão regional, especialmente esplâncnica, ocorre na ausência, ou antes, de aumentos no lactato sistêmico e na acidose metabólica e quase sempre a despeito do tratamento que mantenha com êxito a pressão arterial, o débito cardíaco, a frequência cardíaca, a oferta de oxigênio (DO_2) e seu consumo (VO_2), bem como os parâmetros respiratórios.

Os Resultados Serão Válidos se os Exames Forem Realizados em Laboratório Humano?
• Sim, técnicas semiautomáticas e automáticas estão disponíveis para a rápida mensuração da concentração do lactato em amostras de microlitro de sangue total, de soro e de plasma. • A concentração do lactato é idealmente mensurada na amostra arterial; entretanto, não há diferença significativa entre os locais de amostragem do ponto de vista clínico; manter a constância dos locais de mensuração seriada.

HEMOGRAMA/BIOQUÍMICA/URINÁLISE
• Poucos achados específicos do hemograma completo sugeririam as causas da hiperlactatemia e da acidose láctica. • Achados da bioquímica e da urinálise ajudam a determinar a causa subjacente; os exemplos incluem azotemia renal e osmolalidade sérica acentuadamente aumentada observada na intoxicação pelo etilenoglicol; azotemia renal, hipercalcemia e cilindros tubulares observados na insuficiência renal aguda; e concentração aumentada do lactato, proteína total elevada e hematócrito aumentado na desidratação e má perfusão tecidual no paciente em choque.

OUTROS TESTES LABORATORIAIS
• Gasometria sanguínea arterial pode ajudar a definir a extensão de distúrbio respiratório concomitante e de distúrbio acidobásico misto. • Testes adicionais (p. ex., etilenoglicol, glicose sérica e urinária, bem como cetonas urinárias) podem ser valiosos, dependendo da causa sob suspeita.

TRATAMENTO
• A hiperlactatemia isolada raramente é significativa o suficiente a ponto de incitar tratamento específico, sendo mais importante como marcador de possíveis problemas sistêmicos graves ou em desenvolvimento. Ressuscitação hídrica rigorosa não será indicada se a acidose não acompanhar altos níveis sanguíneos de lactato. • Como a acidose láctica quase sempre é grave, fica geralmente indicado o tratamento rigoroso para corrigir a(s) causa(s) subjacente(s) e tratar a acidose de forma específica. • A detecção da hiperlactatemia, com ou sem acidose, deve induzir o clínico a procurar por causas de hipoperfusão e ainda deve ditar as intervenções terapêuticas precoces para melhorar a distribuição de oxigênio tecidual a fim de interromper a isquemia orgânica e evitar a evolução para o choque circulatório.

MEDICAÇÕES
MEDICAMENTO(S) DE ESCOLHA
• O uso de medicações e fluidos específicos depende da causa subjacente. • Muitas causas de hiperlactatemia e acidose láctica caracterizam-se por déficits de volume hídrico; portanto, a fluidoterapia rigorosa tradicionalmente é a primeira etapa no tratamento. • Apesar de controversa, a terapia com bicarbonato de sódio para corrigir o pH sanguíneo abaixo de 7,2 pode ser indicada quando o pH não aumentar em resposta à ressuscitação hídrica rigorosa.

PRECAUÇÕES
• O bicarbonato de sódio fica reservado para os pacientes com pH abaixo de 7,2 com o objetivo de evitar os efeitos cardiovasculares da acidose grave. O bicarbonato deve ser utilizado apenas para corrigir o pH até 7,2. Isso pode ser alcançado, calculando-se o déficit de bicarbonato ou administrando-se pequenas doses empíricas de 1-2 mEq/kg com subsequente avaliação do pH sanguíneo. • É provável que o bicarbonato de sódio seja mais eficaz em pacientes com acidose metabólica de hiato aniônico normal (lactato normal) do que naqueles com acidose metabólica de hiato aniônico elevado, pois os últimos podem desenvolver uma alcalose metabólica quando os ânions orgânicos (lactato ou cetoácidos) são convertidos em bicarbonato durante a recuperação hemodinâmica. • Com a conversão imediata de 10-15% do bicarbonato em CO_2, é importante que a ventilação dos pacientes aumente para evitar uma queda maior no pH. • As possíveis complicações da terapia com bicarbonato de sódio incluem sobrecarga volêmica pelo sódio em excesso, acidose paradoxal do SNC, tetania hipocalcêmica e desvio da curva de dissociação de oxigênio-hemoglobina para a esquerda por alcalose iatrogênica.

ACOMPANHAMENTO
MONITORIZAÇÃO DO PACIENTE
• Determinações seriadas do lactato são mais valiosas do que uma única mensuração (internamento, máximo) dos níveis de lactato; monitorizar o lactato com o passar do tempo em pacientes críticos. • A capacidade de um paciente depurar o lactato prediz a resposta ao tratamento e a sobrevida. • Continuar verificando outros parâmetros que ajudam a avaliar a resposta ao tratamento da causa subjacente.

PREVENÇÃO
Os proprietários devem conhecer os sinais precoces de alerta da(s) condição(ões) que induziu(ram) à acidose láctica em seus animais de estimação, com instruções para procurar atendimento médico imediato se ela(s) recidivar(em).

COMPLICAÇÕES POSSÍVEIS
• As pessoas com acidose láctica estão sob maior risco de desenvolvimento de falência múltipla de órgãos e apresentam taxa de mortalidade mais elevada do que os pacientes sem acidose láctica. • Cães e cavalos com concentrações elevadas do lactato e acidose láctica também apresentam desfechos clínicos piores. • Lactato >6-6,5 mmol/L sugere hipoperfusão tecidual (p. ex., choque) ou isquemia local (p. ex., necrose gástrica em pacientes com dilatação e vólvulo gástricos).

EVOLUÇÃO ESPERADA E PROGNÓSTICO
• Uma acidose láctica que rapidamente é corrigida com terapia de suporte indica resolução do problema primário, enquanto uma acidose láctica que não responde ao tratamento é um indicador prognóstico grave. • Concentrações sanguíneas seriadas de lactato e pH serão mais prognósticas que uma única mensuração, para que os clínicos avaliem a resposta ao tratamento.

DIVERSOS
DISTÚRBIOS ASSOCIADOS
• Acidose láctica pode ser encontrada juntamente com qualquer condição indutora de hipoxia tecidual. • Níveis sanguíneos elevados de lactato já foram observados em pacientes com linfoma e meningioma. Esses pacientes podem ou não ter acidose concomitante. Nesses pacientes, é recomendável o uso de outros parâmetros para avaliar a perfusão tecidual, já que o lactato sanguíneo pode permanecer elevado apesar da ressuscitação adequada.

VER TAMBÉM
Acidose Metabólica.

ABREVIATURA(S)
• EDTA = etilenodiaminotetracético.

Sugestões de Leitura
DiBartola SP. Metabolic acid-base disorders. In: DiBartola SP, ed., Fluid, Electrolyte and Acid-Base Disorders in Small Animal Practice, 3rd ed. Philadelphia: Elsevier, 2006, pp. 263–269.
Karagiannis M, Reniker A, Kerl M, et al. Lactate measurement as an indicator of perfusion. Compend Contin Educ Pract Vet 2006, 28:287–300.
Sullivan LA, Campbell VL, Klopp LS, Rao S. Blood lactate concentrations in anesthetized dogs with intracranial disease. J Vet Intern Med 2009, 23:488–492.

Autor Tim B. Hackett
Consultor Editorial Deborah S. Greco
Agradecimento O autor gostaria de agradecer o trabalho feito por Dr. Michael S. Lagutchik nas edições prévias deste capítulo.

ACIDOSE METABÓLICA

CONSIDERAÇÕES GERAIS

DEFINIÇÃO
Diminuição no pH plasmático associada ao declínio na concentração de bicarbonato ([HCO_3^-]; (cães, <18 mEq/L; gatos, <16 mEq/L) e à redução compensatória na tensão do dióxido de carbono (PCO_2).

FISIOPATOLOGIA
• A acidose metabólica pode se desenvolver secundariamente à hiperfosfatemia (acidose hiperfosfatêmica), à hipercloremia corrigida (acidose hiperclorêmica) e ao acúmulo de ânions fortes metabolicamente produzidos (acidose com hiato aniônico forte ou elevado).
• Acidose hiperfosfatêmica:
  ○ O aumento nos ácidos fracos do plasma (p. ex., fosfato inorgânico) é associado à acidose metabólica e ao aumento do hiato aniônico. Em pH de 7,4, o aumento de 1 mg/dL na concentração de fosfato é associado à redução de 0,58 mEq/L na [HCO_3^-] e à elevação de 0,58 mEq/L no hiato aniônico.
• Acidose hiperclorêmica:
  ○ A acidose hiperclorêmica pode ser causada pela retenção de cloreto (p. ex., insuficiência renal, acidose tubular renal), perda excessiva de sódio em relação ao cloreto (p. ex., diarreia) ou administração de substâncias contendo mais cloreto do que sódio em comparação com a composição do líquido extracelular normal (p. ex., administração de cloreto de potássio, cloreto de sódio a 0,9%).
  ○ A acidemia não costuma ser grave em pacientes com acidose hiperclorêmica.
• Acidose com hiato aniônico elevado:
  ○ Aumento na concentração de outros ânions fortes por adição (p. ex., toxicidade pelo etilenoglicol), produção excessiva (p. ex., lactato produzido por metabolismo anaeróbio prolongado) ou retenção renal (p. ex., insuficiência renal) de outros ânions fortes que causam acidose metabólica, sem aumentar a concentração do cloreto (a assim denominada acidose metabólica normoclorêmica ou com hiato aniônico elevado).

SISTEMA(S) ACOMETIDO(S)
• Cardiovascular — uma queda no pH resulta em um aumento na descarga simpática, mas simultaneamente provoca um declínio na sensibilidade dos miócitos cardíacos e da musculatura lisa vascular aos efeitos das catecolaminas. Em condições levemente acidêmicas (pH acima de 7,2), os efeitos de estimulação simpática elevada predominam, resultando em um leve aumento na frequência cardíaca e no débito cardíaco. Uma acidemia mais intensa (pH abaixo de 7,1), especialmente se aguda, pode diminuir a contratilidade cardíaca e predispor o coração a arritmias ventriculares e fibrilação ventricular.
• Respiratório — o aumento na [H^+] estimula os quimiorreceptores periféricos e centrais a aumentar a ventilação alveolar; a hiperventilação diminui a PCO_2, o que compensa os efeitos da baixa concentração plasmática do HCO_3^- sobre o pH. Nos cães, espera-se um declínio de aproximadamente 0,7 mmHg na PCO_2 para cada redução de 1 mEq/L na [HCO_3^-] plasmática.

Pouco se sabe a respeito da compensação nos gatos, mas parece ser quase inexistente.
• Renal/Urológico — os rins aumentam a excreção ácida líquida, principalmente por aumentar a excreção de NH_4^+ e cloreto. Esse mecanismo compensatório não é muito eficaz em gatos.

IDENTIFICAÇÃO
Qualquer raça, idade ou sexo de cães e gatos.

SINAIS CLÍNICOS
Achados Anamnésicos
• Processos patológicos crônicos que induzem à acidose metabólica (p. ex., insuficiência renal, diabetes melito e hipoadrenocorticismo), exposição a toxinas (p. ex., etilenoglicol, salicilato e paraldeído), diarreia e administração de inibidores da anidrase carbônica (p. ex., acetazolamida e diclorfenamida).

Achados do Exame Físico
• Em geral, relacionam-se com a doença subjacente.
• Depressão em pacientes gravemente acidóticos.
• Em alguns pacientes, observa-se taquipneia resultante do aumento compensatório na ventilação.
• Em cães e gatos, não é comum observar a respiração de Kussmaul, geralmente observada em seres humanos com acidose metabólica.

CAUSAS
Associadas à Hipercloremia (Acidose Metabólica Hiperclorêmica)
• Diarreia.
• Acidose tubular renal.
• Administração de inibidores da anidrase carbônica, espironolactona, cloreto de potássio ou NH_4Cl.
• Fluidoterapia com fluidos ricos em cloreto (p. ex., cloreto de sódio a 0,9%, fluidos suplementados com cloreto de potássio).
• Nutrição parenteral total com fluidos que contenham aminoácidos catiônicos: lisina, arginina e histidina.
• Correção rápida de hipocapnia (alcalose respiratória crônica).

Associadas à Normocloremia (Acidose Metabólica com Hiato Aniônico Elevado)
• Acidose urêmica.
• Cetoacidose diabética.
• Acidose láctica.
• Intoxicação por etilenoglicol, salicilato, paraldeído e metanol.
• Hiperfosfatemia.

FATORES DE RISCO
• Pacientes com insuficiência renal crônica, diabetes melito e hipoadrenocorticismo estão sob alto risco de desenvolverem acidose metabólica como uma complicação do processo patológico crônico.
• Pacientes com má perfusão ou hipoxia teciduais também apresentam alto risco de desenvolverem acidose láctica.

DIAGNÓSTICO

DIAGNÓSTICO DIFERENCIAL
A baixa [HCO_3^-] plasmática e a hipercloremia também podem ser compensatórias em animais com alcalose respiratória crônica, que exibem PCO_2 baixa e pH alto ou próximo ao normal, apesar da [HCO_3^-] reduzida e do aumento na concentração de cloreto. Para a diferenciação, é necessária a determinação da gasometria sanguínea.

ACHADOS LABORATORIAIS
Medicamentos Capazes de Alterar os Resultados Laboratoriais
• O brometo de potássio é mensurado como cloreto em grande parte dos analisadores, de modo que a administração de brometo de potássio promove artificialmente a diminuição do hiato aniônico.

Distúrbios Capazes de Alterar os Resultados Laboratoriais
• Grande quantidade de heparina (>10% da amostra) diminui a [HCO_3^-].
• As amostras sanguíneas armazenadas à temperatura ambiente por mais de 20 minutos apresentam um pH baixo, em decorrência do aumento na PCO_2.
• Hipoalbuminemia reduz o hiato aniônico; cargas negativas de albumina constituem o principal componente do hiato aniônico.

Os Resultados Serão Válidos se os Exames Forem Realizados em Laboratório Humano?
Sim.

HEMOGRAMA/BIOQUÍMICA/URINÁLISE
• CO_2 total baixo — CO_2 total em amostras séricas manipuladas em meio aeróbio aproxima-se da concentração sérica de HCO_3^-; infelizmente, os pacientes com alcalose respiratória crônica também exibem CO_2 total baixo; assim, não é possível fazer a distinção entre os dois casos sem análise da gasometria.
• Tradicionalmente, as acidoses metabólicas são divididas nas de fundo hiperclorêmico e nas com hiato aniônico elevado, por meio do hiato aniônico. O hiato aniônico (HA), que corresponde à diferença entre os cátions e os ânions mensurados, é calculado como $HA = [Na^+] - ([HCO_3^-] + [Cl^-])$ ou $HA = ([Na^+] + [K^+]) - ([HCO_3^-] + [Cl^-])$, dependendo da preferência do clínico ou do laboratório. Os valores normais com a inclusão de potássio no cálculo costumam ser de 12-24 mEq/L nos cães e 13-27 mEq/L nos gatos. As cargas negativas da albumina representam os principais fatores que contribuem para o hiato aniônico normal; dessa forma, isso deve ser levado em consideração ao se avaliar o hiato aniônico em pacientes com hipoalbuminemia. Em pH de 7,4 nos cães, um declínio de 1 g/dL na albumina é associado a uma queda de 4,1 mEq/L no hiato aniônico.
• Hiato aniônico normal (i. e., acidose metabólica hiperclorêmica) — a diarreia é a causa mais comum; além disso, considera-se o quadro de hipoadrenocorticismo.
• Hiato aniônico elevado (i. e., acidose metabólica normoclorêmica) — as causas mais comuns são insuficiência renal, diabetes melito, acidose láctica (causada por hipoperfusão tecidual) e hipoadrenocorticismo (causado por acidose láctica). A hiperfosfatemia também eleva o hiato aniônico. Em pH de 7,4, cada aumento de 1 mg/dL na concentração de fosfato está associado a uma elevação de 0,58 mEq/L no hiato aniônico.
• Hiperglicemia — considerar diabetes melito.
• Azotemia — considerar insuficiência renal.
• Hiperfosfatemia — considerar insuficiência renal, toxicidade por enema hipertônico de fosfato

Acidose Metabólica

de sódio e toxicidade a acidificantes urinários que contenham fosfato em sua composição.
• Concentração elevada de lactato — considerar acidose láctica por má perfusão tecidual ou metabolismo deficiente de lactato (p. ex., hepatopatia e linfoma).
• Hipercalemia — comumente associada a, mas quase nunca causada por, acidose. Só a acidose hiperclorêmica aguda pode levar à translocação de potássio grave o suficiente a ponto de causar hipercalemia. Do contrário, a hipercalemia origina-se do processo patológico indutor da acidose metabólica (p. ex., insuficiência renal e diabetes melito), e não da acidose propriamente dita. Não é recomendável o uso de fórmulas de correção para ajustar a concentração de potássio com base nas alterações do pH.

OUTROS TESTES LABORATORIAIS
A análise da gasometria sanguínea revela HCO_3 baixa, PCO_2 baixa e pH baixo.

DIAGNÓSTICO POR IMAGEM
Nenhum.

MÉTODOS DIAGNÓSTICOS
Nenhum.

TRATAMENTO
• Distúrbios acidobásicos são fenômenos secundários; a resolução bem-sucedida depende do diagnóstico e do tratamento do processo mórbido subjacente.
• Tratar de forma rigorosa os pacientes com pH sanguíneo ≤7,1, enquanto se busca o diagnóstico definitivo.
• Interromper os medicamentos que possam causar acidose metabólica.
• Cuidado(s) de enfermagem — a solução de Ringer lactato constitui o fluido de escolha para os pacientes com acidose metabólica leve e função hepática normal.

MEDICAÇÕES
MEDICAMENTO(S) DE ESCOLHA
• $NaHCO_3$ pode ajudar os pacientes com acidose hiperclorêmica, hiperfosfatêmica ou urêmica, mas não aqueles com acidose láctica ou cetoacidose diabética.
  ○ Estimativa da dose de HCO_3^-: cães, 0,3 × peso corporal (kg) × (21 − [HCO_3^-] do paciente); gatos, 0,3 × peso corporal (kg) × (19 − [HCO_3^-] do paciente). Fornecer metade dessa dose lentamente por via IV e reavaliar os gases sanguíneos antes de decidir sobre a necessidade de administrações adicionais. Uma dose empírica de 1-2 mEq/kg, acompanhada pela reavaliação do nível dos gases sanguíneos, é segura na maioria dos pacientes.
  ○ Complicações potenciais da administração de $NaHCO_3$: sobrecarga volêmica decorrente da administração do sódio, tetania resultante da baixa concentração de cálcio ionizado, aumento na afinidade da hemoglobina pelo oxigênio, acidose paradoxal do SNC, excesso de alcalose metabólica e hipocalemia.
• Acidose hiperclorêmica: o $NaHCO_3$ é eficaz e deve ser considerado sempre que o pH estiver abaixo de 7,2.
• Acidose urêmica: a eficácia do $NaHCO_3$ na terapia aguda de acidose urêmica está relacionada com o desvio de fosfato para dentro das células e consequente melhora da acidose hiperfosfatêmica.
• Acidose láctica: o $NaHCO_3$ aumenta a produção de lactato e, portanto, é de pouco a nenhum valor em casos de acidose láctica. A terapia deve ser direcionada ao aumento da distribuição tecidual de oxigênio e ao restabelecimento do débito cardíaco. Pequenas doses tituladas de $NaHCO_3$ podem se utilizadas como uma medida temporária para manter a [HCO_3^-] acima de 5 mEq/L, se necessário.
• Cetoacidose diabética: o $NaHCO_3$ afeta adversamente o desfecho em seres humanos com cetoacidose diabética quando o pH se encontra abaixo de 7,0.
• A administração de $NaHCO_3$ a pacientes cetoacidóticos não pode ser recomendada em qualquer pH. A terapia deve ser direcionada à administração de insulina e fluidos. O restabelecimento do volume plasmático e da perfusão renal permitirá a excreção de cetoânions pelos rins, substituindo-os por cloreto.

CONTRAINDICAÇÕES
• Evitar o $NaHCO_3$ em pacientes com acidose respiratória, pois ele gera CO_2.
• Os pacientes com acidose respiratória não conseguem excretar o CO_2 de forma adequada; além disso, o aumento na PCO_2 diminuirá ainda mais o pH.
• Evitar o uso de diuréticos com ação no néfron distal (p. ex., espironolactona).
• Evitar os inibidores da anidrase carbônica (p. ex., acetazolamida e diclorfenamida).

PRECAUÇÕES
Utilizar o $NaHCO_3$ com cuidado em pacientes com insuficiência cardíaca congestiva, visto que a carga de sódio pode causar descompensação da insuficiência cardíaca.

INTERAÇÕES POSSÍVEIS
Nenhuma.

MEDICAMENTOS(S) ALTERNATIVO(S)
Nenhum.

ACOMPANHAMENTO
MONITORIZAÇÃO DO PACIENTE
Reavaliar o estado acidobásico; a frequência é ditada pela doença subjacente e pela resposta do paciente ao tratamento.

COMPLICAÇÕES POSSÍVEIS
• Hipercalemia em acidose hiperclorêmica aguda.
• Depressão miocárdica e arritmias ventriculares.

DIVERSOS
DISTÚRBIOS ASSOCIADOS
• Hipercalemia.
• Hipercloremia.

FATORES RELACIONADOS COM A IDADE
Nenhum.

POTENCIAL ZOONÓTICO
Nenhum.

GESTAÇÃO/FERTILIDADE/REPRODUÇÃO
N/D.

SINÔNIMO(S)
• Acidose dilucional — acidose metabólica decorrente do aumento de água livre no plasma.
• Acidose hiperclorêmica — acidose com hiato aniônico normal.
• Acidose hiperfosfatêmica — acidose metabólica resultante da alta concentração de fosfato.
• Acidose não respiratória.
• Acidose normoclorêmica — acidose com hiato aniônico elevado.
• Acidose orgânica — acidose metabólica causada pelo acúmulo de ânions orgânicos (p. ex., cetoacidose, acidose urêmica e acidose láctica).

VER TAMBÉM
• Diabetes Melito com Cetoacidose.
• Hipercalemia.
• Hipercloremia.

ABREVIATURA(S)
• H^+ = íon de hidrogênio.
• HA = hiato aniônico.
• HCO_3^- = bicarbonato.
• $NaHCO_3$ = bicarbonato de sódio.
• O_2 = oxigênio.
• PCO_2 = tensão do dióxido de carbono.
• SNC = sistema nervoso central.

Sugestões de Leitura
de Morais HSA, Constable PD. Strong ion approach to acid-base disorders. In: DiBartola SP, ed., Fluid, Electrolyte and Acid-Base Disorders, 3rd. ed. Philadelphia: Saunders, 2006, pp. 310-321.
de Morais HA, Leisewitz Al. Mixed acid-base disorders. In: DiBartola SP, ed., Fluid, Electrolyte and Acid-Base Disorders, 3rd. ed. Philadelphia: Saunders, 2006, pp. 296-309.
DiBartola SP. Metabolic acid-base disorders. In: DiBartola SP, ed. Fluid, Electrolyte and Acid-Base Disorders, 3rd. ed. Philadelphia: Saunders, 2006, pp.251-283.

Autor Helio Autran de Morais
Consultor Editorial Carl A. Osborne

ACIDOSE TUBULAR RENAL

CONSIDERAÇÕES GERAIS

REVISÃO
- Síndrome caracterizada por acidose metabólica hiperclorêmica em virtude da reabsorção diminuída de bicarbonato pelo túbulo renal proximal (acidose tubular renal proximal ou do tipo 2) ou secreção reduzida de íons hidrogênio no túbulo distal (acidose tubular renal distal clássica ou do tipo 1) em pacientes com taxa de filtração glomerular normal ou próxima do normal e ausência de diarreia.
- Em seres humanos, a deficiência de aldosterona ou a resistência a esse hormônio podem provocar acidose tubular renal distal do tipo 4, levando à hipercalemia; essa síndrome não foi descrita na medicina veterinária. A acidose tubular renal proximal não foi registrada como uma entidade isolada em cães, mas foi observada como parte da síndrome de Fanconi.
- A discussão a seguir está limitada à acidose tubular renal distal clássica. Na acidose tubular renal distal, a urina não pode ser acidificada ao máximo apesar da concentração plasmática de bicarbonato moderada a acentuadamente diminuída como consequência da secreção prejudicada de hidrogênio nos ductos coletores. O pH urinário tipicamente se encontra acima de 6,0 (normalmente, o pH urinário deve estar entre 4,5-5,0 na presença de acidose sistêmica).

IDENTIFICAÇÃO
- Relatada em 5 cães e 3 gatos.
- Sem predileção racial ou sexual aparente.
- Faixa etária no momento do diagnóstico, 1-8 anos.

SINAIS CLÍNICOS
- Associados à acidemia, podendo incluir fraqueza muscular (pode estar relacionada com hipocalemia), inapetência, náusea, perda de peso, retardo do crescimento e sinais neurológicos.
- Outros sinais dependem da presença ou da ausência de doenças associadas (p. ex., pielonefrite).
- Respiração ofegante.
- Poliúria e polidipsia (associadas, em geral, à hipocalemia ou calciurese).
- Vômito.
- Hematúria e disúria (secundárias à urolitíase).
- Osteomalacia associada à acidose metabólica crônica (ainda não foi relatada em cães e gatos).

CAUSAS E FATORES DE RISCO
- Podem ser primários (i. e., hereditários) ou secundários a hipercalciúria, toxinas, medicamentos (p. ex., anfotericina B), metabolismo alterado do cálcio com indução de nefrocalcinose (p. ex., hipervitaminose D, hiperparatireoidismo primário), doença autoimune (p. ex., lúpus eritematoso sistêmico, rejeição de transplante renal), distúrbios hipergamaglobulinêmicos (p. ex., mieloma múltiplo, lúpus eritematoso sistêmico) e nefropatias tubulointersticiais.
- Nos gatos, a acidose tubular renal distal foi associada à pielonefrite (dois casos) e lipidose hepática (um caso).
- Nos cães, todos os relatos clínicos de acidose tubular renal distal pareceram ser idiopáticos; ocorreu urolitíase por estruvita (em um caso) secundária à acidose tubular renal distal; a acidose tubular renal distal também foi provocada por isquemia renal induzida experimentalmente.

DIAGNÓSTICO

DIAGNÓSTICO DIFERENCIAL
Considerar outras causas de acidose metabólica hiperclorêmica (hiato aniônico normal) (p. ex., diarreia, inibidores da anidrase carbônica, cloreto de amônio, aminoácidos catiônicos, acidose metabólica pós-hipocápnica, acidose dilucional, hipoadrenocorticismo). Diarreia do intestino delgado é o diagnóstico diferencial mais importante.

HEMOGRAMA/BIOQUÍMICA/URINÁLISE
- Os resultados variam, dependendo das doenças associadas.
- Hipocalemia (por causa da excreção renal aumentada) em alguns animais; pode ser grave o suficiente a ponto de provocar fraqueza muscular.
- Urina alcalina — pH >6; descartar infecção do trato urinário por microrganismos urease-positivos (p. ex., *Staphylococcus aureus*, *Proteus sp.*) como uma causa de urina alcalina.

OUTROS TESTES LABORATORIAIS
Avaliação dos gases sanguíneos (gasometria) e eletrólitos séricos indica acidose metabólica hiperclorêmica (hiato aniônico normal). O pH urinário é >6,0 em acidose tubular renal distal versus <5,5 em acidose tubular renal proximal.

DIAGNÓSTICO POR IMAGEM
Radiografias — pode detectar a presença de urólitos ou osteomalacia (incomum).

MÉTODOS DIAGNÓSTICOS
- A principal característica diagnóstica é acidose metabólica com hiato aniônico normal, acompanhada por pH urinário inapropriadamente alcalino (>6).
- Teste de tolerância ao cloreto de amônio — administrar 200 mg/kg VO em cães; medir o pH urinário antes do teste e de hora em hora por 5 h; esvaziar a bexiga urinária também de hora em hora. O pH urinário em cães normais diminui para <5,5 em até 4 h. Evitar a realização desse teste na presença de acidose grave.
- Acidose tubular renal do tipo 1 e 2 pode ser diferenciada com base na resposta ao $NaHCO_3$ infundido a 0,5-1,0 mEq/kg/h. A excreção fracional de bicarbonato aumentará acentuadamente em casos de acidose tubular renal do tipo 2.

TRATAMENTO
- Individualizar, na dependência da natureza e da gravidade dos distúrbios associados.
- Tipicamente, há necessidade de menos bicarbonato para resolver a acidose metabólica associada à acidose tubular renal distal do que é necessário para resolver a acidose associada à acidose tubular renal proximal.
- A hipocalemia pode se resolver apenas com a administração de bicarbonato ou citrato ou, então, pode haver a necessidade de suplementação adicional de potássio.

MEDICAÇÕES

MEDICAMENTO(S)
- Citrato de potássio isoladamente ou em combinação com citrato de sódio (dependendo da concentração sérica de potássio) em uma dose total de 1-5 mEq/kg/dia VO, divididos em duas doses, ou bicarbonato de sódio a 10-50 mg/kg a cada 8-12 h VO (1-3 mEq/kg/dia).
- Suplementação de potássio — gliconato de potássio; gatos: 2-8 mEq/dia divididos a cada 12 h VO; cães (dependendo do porte): 2-44 mEq/dia divididos a cada 12 h VO, se necessária.

CONTRAINDICAÇÕES/INTERAÇÕES POSSÍVEIS
É recomendável evitar o uso de citrato em pacientes com insuficiência renal submetidos a hidróxido de alumínio, porque o citrato aumenta a permeabilidade intestinal e pode levar à absorção excessiva de alumínio.

ACOMPANHAMENTO
- Gasometria sanguínea seriada (p. ex., a cada 3-5 dias) até que o estado acidobásico esteja normalizado.
- Monitorizar os eletrólitos séricos, particularmente o potássio, conforme a necessidade.
- O prognóstico a longo prazo depende da natureza e da gravidade dos distúrbios associados; pode ser razoavelmente bom nos pacientes sem outras doenças, embora haja poucas informações sobre a evolução dessa doença a longo prazo em cães e gatos.

DIVERSOS

VER TAMBÉM
- Acidose Metabólica.
- Hipocalemia.
- Síndrome de Fanconi.

ABREVIATURA(S)
- $NaHCO_3$ = bicarbonato de sódio.

Sugestões de Leitura
Kerl ME. Renal tubular diseases. In: Ettinger SJ, Feldman EC, eds., Textbook of Veterinary Internal Medicine, 7th ed. St. Louis: Elsevier Saunders, 2010, pp. 2062-2068.

Autores João Felipe de Brito Galvão e Stephen P. DiBartola
Consultor Editorial Carl A. Osborne

ACNE — CÃES

CONSIDERAÇÕES GERAIS

REVISÃO
- Distúrbio inflamatório crônico do queixo e dos lábios de animais jovens.
- Caracterizado por foliculite e furunculose.
- Identificado quase exclusivamente em raças de pelo curto.
- A predisposição genética pode desempenhar um papel mais relevante do que os efeitos hormonais.

IDENTIFICAÇÃO
- Cães.
- Raças predispostas de pelo curto — Boxer, Doberman pinscher, Buldogue inglês, Dogue alemão, Weimaraner, Mastim, Rottweiler, Pointer alemão de pelo curto e Pit Bull terrier.

SINAIS CLÍNICOS
- As margens ventrais no queixo e no lábio podem estar mínima a acentuadamente inchadas, com inúmeras pápulas e pústulas eritematosas.
- Estágios avançados — as lesões podem ser exsudativas, indicando foliculite-furunculose bacteriana profunda secundária.
- As lesões podem ser dolorosas à palpação; a maioria não é dolorosa nem pruriginosa.
- As lesões de resolução crônica podem exibir formação cicatricial e liquenificação.

CAUSAS E FATORES DE RISCO
Determinadas raças de pelo curto parecem ser geneticamente predispostas à hiperqueratose folicular e infecção bacteriana secundária.

DIAGNÓSTICO

DIAGNÓSTICO DIFERENCIAL
- Dermatofitose.
- Demodicose.
- Corpo estranho.
- Dermatite de contato.

HEMOGRAMA/BIOQUÍMICA/URINÁLISE
N/D.

OUTROS TESTES LABORATORIAIS
N/D.

DIAGNÓSTICO POR IMAGEM
N/D.

MÉTODOS DIAGNÓSTICOS
- Cultura bacteriana e antibiograma — em pacientes com foliculite e furunculose supurativas não responsivas à escolha antibiótica inicial.
- Biopsia — confirmação histológica para os casos de diagnóstico questionável.
- Raspados cutâneos — demodicose.
- Cultura para dermatófitos — dermatofitose.

ACHADOS PATOLÓGICOS
- Os sinais clínicos e os achados histopatológicos são diagnósticos.
- Lesões iniciais — pápulas foliculares sem pelos; caracterizadas no exame histopatológico por ceratose folicular acentuada, formação de tampões, dilatação e perifoliculite.
- Bactérias — nos estágios precoces: não são observadas nem podem ser isoladas a partir das lesões.
- À medida que a doença evolui, as pápulas aumentam e se rompem, promovendo o aparecimento de foliculite e furunculose supurativas.

TRATAMENTO

- Depende da gravidade e da cronicidade da doença.
- Reduzir o traumatismo comportamental ao queixo (p. ex., esfregar-se sobre o tapete e mastigar ossos que aumentam a salivação).
- Promover a limpeza frequente com xampu ou gel de peróxido de benzoíla.
- Aplicar pomada de mupirocina a 2% para diminuir a quantidade de bactérias sobre a superfície da pele.
- Orientar os proprietários a não espremer as lesões, o que pode causar a ruptura interna da pápula e levar a uma inflamação maciça.

MEDICAÇÕES

MEDICAMENTO(S)
Tópicos
- Xampu ou gel de peróxido de benzoíla (antibacteriano).
- Pomada de mupirocina a 2% (agente antiestafilocócico).
- Isotretinoína (vitamina A) ou tretinoína (Retin-A®) — podem diminuir a ceratose folicular.
- Corticosteroides — podem ser necessários para reduzir a inflamação; limitar a frequência de uso para evitar efeitos locais e sistêmicos.

Sistêmicos
- Antibióticos adequados para infecção bacteriana profunda — particularmente as cefalosporinas (cefalexina, 22 mg/kg VO a cada 8 h durante 6-8 semanas).
- Talvez seja necessária a realização de cultura bacteriana e antibiograma.
- Corticosteroides orais: reduzir as dosagens da prednisolona gradativamente (dose inicial de 0,5 mg/kg/dia) para diminuir inflamação significativa; não utilizados para uso contínuo.

CONTRAINDICAÇÕES/INTERAÇÕES POSSÍVEIS
- Peróxido de benzoíla — pode manchar tapetes e tecidos, além de ser irritante.
- Pomadas de mupirocina — são oleosas.
- Retinoides tópicos — podem ressecar e irritar a pele.
- Esteroides tópicos — podem causar supressão da adrenal com o uso frequente.
- Isotretinoína — pode causar ceratoconjuntivite seca, hiperatividade, prurido auricular, junção mucocutânea eritematosa, letargia com vômito, distensão abdominal e eritema, anorexia com letargia, colapso e língua inchada; as anormalidades do hemograma completo e da bioquímica sérica incluem contagem elevada de plaquetas, hipertrigliceridemia, hipercolesterolemia, e atividade elevada da alanina transaminase.

ACOMPANHAMENTO

MONITORIZAÇÃO DO PACIENTE
- Manter os antibióticos até a cicatrização das lesões.
- Repetir os exames de cultura bacteriana e antibiograma em caso de piora das lesões.
- Interromper os corticosteroides tópicos sempre que possível.

EVOLUÇÃO ESPERADA E PROGNÓSTICO
- Pode ser necessário o tratamento tópico a longo prazo.
- A terapia precoce e rigorosa pode evitar a formação cicatricial crônica.

DIVERSOS

GESTAÇÃO/FERTILIDADE/REPRODUÇÃO
Retinoides sintéticos — teratogênicos; não utilizar em animais prenhes, outros com intenção reprodutiva ou em fêmeas intactas; não devem ser manipulados por mulheres em idade fértil.

Sugestões de Leitura
Scott DW, Miller WH, Griffin CE. Bacterial skin diseases. In: Kirk's small animal dermatology. 5th ed. Philadelphia: Saunders, 1995:304-305.

Autor Karen Helton Rhodes
Consultor Editorial Alexander H. Werner

ACNE — GATOS

CONSIDERAÇÕES GERAIS

REVISÃO
• Dermatite inflamatória que afeta o queixo e os lábios.
• Os sintomas podem ser recorrentes ou persistentes.
• A etiologia exata não é conhecida.

IDENTIFICAÇÃO
• Gatos.
• Não há relatos de prevalência sexual, etária ou racial.

SINAIS CLÍNICOS
• Os gatos podem ter um único episódio, um problema recorrente vitalício, ou uma doença contínua.
• A frequência e a gravidade de cada ocorrência variam com o animal individualmente.
• Comedões, pápulas eritematosas leves, crostas serosas e debris de queratina escuros desenvolvem-se no queixo e, menos comumente, nos lábios.
• Tumefação (inchaço) do queixo.
• Casos graves — nódulos, crostas hemorrágicas, pústulas, cistos, fístulas, eritema intenso, alopecia, e dor.
• Dor frequentemente associada à furunculose bacteriana.

CAUSAS E FATORES DE RISCO
A etiologia exata é desconhecida; pode envolver fatores como distúrbio de queratinização, prática insatisfatória de higiene e embelezamento, produção anormal de sebo, imunossupressão, infecção viral, ou estresse.

DIAGNÓSTICO

DIAGNÓSTICO DIFERENCIAL
• Foliculite bacteriana.
• Demodicose.
• Infecção por Malassezia.
• Lepra felina.
• Dermatofitose.
• Neoplasia de glândulas sebáceas ou apócrinas.
• Granuloma eosinofílico.
• Hipersensibilidade de contato.

HEMOGRAMA/BIOQUÍMICA/URINÁLISE
N/D.

OUTROS TESTES LABORATORIAIS
N/D.

DIAGNÓSTICO POR IMAGEM
N/D.

MÉTODOS DIAGNÓSTICOS
• Raspados cutâneos — demodicose.
• Cultura fúngica — dermatofitose.
• Citologia — bactérias, *Malassezia*.
• Biopsia — raramente exigida; necessária em casos selecionados para caracterizar alterações como folículos císticos, diferenciar acne de outras doenças como demodicose, infecções (por bactérias, leveduras ou dermatófitos) ou diagnosticar neoplasia.

ACHADOS PATOLÓGICOS
• Doença leve — distensão folicular com queratina (comedo), hiperqueratose, e tampão folicular.
• Doença grave — foliculite e perifoliculite leves a graves com formação de pústula folicular.
• A ruptura folicular libera queratina, pelo e ácaros *Demodex* na derme; induz à furunculose, caracterizada por neutrófilos e inúmeros macrófagos que circundam debris de queratina.
• Bactérias e *Malassezia* nessas lesões são consideradas como microrganismos invasores secundários e não como agentes causais.
• Ácaros *Demodex* podem ser agentes primários dessa doença.

TRATAMENTO

• Tratamento inicial — utilizar um único medicamento ou uma combinação dos medicamentos listados abaixo até que todas as lesões desapareçam.
• Interromper o tratamento, reduzindo gradativamente a medicação em um período de 2 a 3 semanas.
• Episódios recorrentes — assim que a taxa de recorrência for determinada, pode-se traçar um protocolo de manutenção adequado para cada animal individualmente.
• Episódios contínuos — nesse caso, há necessidade de tratamento de manutenção vitalício.

MEDICAÇÕES

MEDICAMENTO(S)
• Antibióticos sistêmicos — amoxicilina com clavulanato, uma cefalosporina, ou uma fluoroquinolona.
• Os casos graves podem justificar o tratamento com isotretinoína (Accutane®) ou ciclosporina modificada (Atopica®).
• Demodicose — ivermectina oral na dose de 400 mg/kg diariamente até que os ácaros sejam eliminados.
• Xampu — aplicação de xampu antisseborreico (enxofre-ácido salicílico, peróxido de benzoíla, ou lactato de etila) 1 ou 2 vezes por semana.
• Agentes tópicos de limpeza — peróxido de benzoíla, ácido salicílico, clorexidina-fitosfingosina.
• Pomada antibiótica tópica — mupirocina a 2%.
• Outros agentes tópicos — solução ou pomada de clindamicina ou eritromicina.
• Agentes tópicos combinados — géis de peróxido de benzoíla com antibióticos (p. ex., Benzamycin®).
• Retinoides tópicos — Tretinoína (gel de Retin-A® a 0,01%).

CONTRAINDICAÇÕES/INTERAÇÕES POSSÍVEIS
• Peróxido de benzoíla e ácidos salicílicos — podem ser irritantes para a pele.
• Isotretinoína sistêmica — utilizar com cuidado se o animal não permitir a aplicação de medicamentos tópicos; advertência: potenciais efeitos colaterais deletérios em seres humanos (interações medicamentosas e teratogenicidade); o recipiente deve ser rotulado para uso veterinário apenas e mantido distante dos medicamentos humanos para evitar o uso acidental; atualmente, não é fácil obter essa medicação para os pacientes veterinários.

ACOMPANHAMENTO

• Monitorizar as recidivas.
• Programas de manutenção de limpeza podem ser utilizados para reduzir as recidivas.

DIVERSOS

GESTAÇÃO/FERTILIDADE/REPRODUÇÃO
Não é recomendável o uso da isotretinoína sistêmica nos animais em reprodução.

Sugestões de Leitura

Jazic E, Coyner KS, Loeffler DG, Lewis TP. An evaluation of the clinical, cytological, infectious and histopathological features of feline acne. Vet Dermatol 2006, 17(2):134-140.

Rosencrantz WS. The pathogenesis, diagnosis, and management of feline acne. Vet Med 1993, 5:504-512.

Scott DW, Miller WH, Griffin CE. Keratinization defects. In: Muller & Kirk's Small Animal Dermatology, 6th ed. Philadelphia: Saunders, 2001, pp. 1042-1043.

Werner AH, Power HT. Retinoids in veterinary dermatology. Clin Dermatol 1994, 12(4):579-586.

White SD. Feline acne and results of treatment with mupirocin in an open clinical trial: 25 cases (1994-96). Vet Dermatol 1997, 8:157.

Autor David Duclos
Consultor Editorial Alexander H. Werner

Acromegalia — Gatos

CONSIDERAÇÕES GERAIS

REVISÃO
• Síndrome que resulta de hipersecreção do hormônio de crescimento (somatotropina) por somatótrofos tumorais ou hiperplásicos no lobo anterior da hipófise. • Os sinais clínicos são atribuídos aos efeitos catabólicos/diabetogênicos diretos do hormônio de crescimento e seus efeitos anabólicos indiretos mediados pelo fator de crescimento insulinossímile I (IGF-1), que é secretado pelo fígado em resposta à estimulação do hormônio de crescimento. • A atividade elevada do IGF-1 induz a crescimento excessivo dos tecidos moles, organomegalia visceral, remodelagem e espessamento ósseos (especialmente em ossos formados por ossificação membranosa), resultando em artropatia, características faciais amplas e baqueteamento digital acentuado. • Em muitos gatos, ocorre hipertrofia do miocárdio, embora o desenvolvimento de insuficiência cardíaca seja incomum. • As ações catabólicas do GH originam-se de antagonismo insulínico, induzindo finalmente à exaustão das células β pancreáticas e ao desenvolvimento de diabetess melito. Entre 25 e 33% dos gatos diabéticos podem ter acromegalia. • Como ocorre na maioria dos gatos diabéticos, o potencial de remissão permanece caso se normalize a produção excessiva de GH; a probabilidade de remissão é inversamente relacionada com a duração do diabetes melito.

IDENTIFICAÇÃO
• Gatos. • Idade média — 11 anos (faixa etária de 6-17 anos). • Aproximadamente 80% são machos.

SINAIS CLÍNICOS
• Os sinais clínicos iniciais relacionam-se com diabetes melito desregulado na grande maioria dos casos, apresentando-se com poliúria, polidipsia e, frequentemente, polifagia acentuada acompanhada por ganho de peso concomitante (também há relatos de perda de peso). • Muitos pacientes ganham peso e exibem um porte corporal maior em função do aumento da massa de tecido mole e ósseo, e não por incremento do tecido adiposo. O ganho de peso em um gato diabético desregulado é fortemente sugestivo de acromegalia. • Alargamento das características faciais, prognatia inferior e aumento do tamanho das patas refletem doença antiga (ou seja, existente há algum tempo) ou grave. • Organomegalia — mais comumente reno/hepatomegalia bilateral. • Ocasionalmente, há sopro e/ou ritmo de galope; os sinais de insuficiência cardíaca são incomuns. • Pode ocorrer o desenvolvimento de claudicação. • São possíveis sinais neurológicos atribuíveis à doença intracraniana por meio de lesão hipofisária expansiva tipo massa. • Relatos recentes sugerem que a maioria dos gatos com acromegalia é indistinguível do ponto de vista fenotípico daqueles diabéticos sem acromegalia.

CAUSAS E FATORES DE RISCO
• Hipersecreção de GH. • Progestinas não causam secreção de GH e acromegalia em gatos como nos cães.

DIAGNÓSTICO

DIAGNÓSTICO DIFERENCIAL
• Diabetes melito sem complicação ou secundário a hiperadrenocorticismo. • Hiperadrenocorticismo hipófise-dependente e acromegalia podem produzir diabetes melito insulinorresistente com lesão hipofisária tipo massa associada. A diferenciação pode exigir o uso do teste de supressão com baixas doses de dexametasona para descartar hiperadrenocorticismo hipófise-dependente. • Podem ocorrer acromegalia e hiperadrenocorticismo hipófise-dependente concomitantemente. • Outros distúrbios causadores de perda de peso com polifagia, poliúria e polidipsia, como hipertireoidismo, não costumam ser associados à intolerância significativa à glicose. • Em todos os gatos com acromegalia, espera-se o quadro de diabetes melito insulinorresistente (>2,0 U de insulina/kg/12 h); a dosagem tende a aumentar com o passar do tempo, com doses não raras de 12-50 U/gato/12 h. • Em qualquer gato diabético que demonstre sinais de insulinorresistência inexplicável, deve-se suspeitar de acromegalia.

HEMOGRAMA/BIOQUÍMICA/URINÁLISE
• A maioria das anormalidades é atribuída ao controle insatisfatório do diabetes melito — hiperglicemia, glicosúria e níveis elevados de frutosamina são achados compatíveis em grande parte dos gatos com acromegalia. • Hiperproteinemia. • As anormalidades são tradicionalmente associadas à insuficiência renal e hipertensão, embora estudos mais recentes sugiram que este não seja o caso.

OUTROS TESTES LABORATORIAIS
• IGF1 — gatos diabéticos submetidos à insulina podem ter níveis mais altos de IGF1 que o normal; por essa razão, existe um potencial significativo de sobreposição entre gatos diabéticos com e sem acromegalia; no entanto, níveis de IGF1 drasticamente elevados (p. ex., >1.000 ng/mL) são fortemente sugestivos de acromegalia. • Como o IGF1 se mantém bem preservado entre as espécies, comumente existem ensaios válidos disponíveis. • GH — níveis séricos basais elevados são diagnósticos. Contudo, como o GH não é bem preservado entre as espécies, um ensaio de fGH validado tem disponibilidade limitada.

DIAGNÓSTICO POR IMAGEM
• Obtenção de imagem intracraniana para demonstrar a presença de lesão hipofisária tipo massa; o exame de RM é mais sensível que a TC contrastada, embora a diferença seja modesta e, do ponto de vista de custo-benefício, a TC geralmente constitui o método preferido. • As anormalidades ecocardiográficas podem incluir aumento de volume do átrio esquerdo, espessamento assimétrico do septo e da parede livre do ventrículo esquerdo, movimento anterior sistólico da valva atrioventricular esquerda (mitral) e disfunção diastólica. • As alterações radiográficas abrangem aumento dos tecidos moles orofaríngeos, artropatia degenerativa com osteofitose periarticular, espondilose deformante espinal, e organomegalia abdominal variável.

TRATAMENTO

RADIOTERAPIA
• A radioterapia constitui o único meio atualmente disponível de se reduzir a hiperprodução autônoma de GH pelo lobo anterior da hipófise. Infelizmente, a radioterapia é mais adequada para reduzir o tamanho do tumor do que para atingir reduções clinicamente significativas na secreção de GH. • Com frequência, sugere-se uma dose total entre 3.500 e 5.500 cGy*, administrada em doses variavelmente fracionadas. Relatos recentes sugerem que o maior êxito pode ser alcançado com uma dose total de 3.700 cGy, administrada sob a forma de um protocolo incremental de radioterapia hipofracionada de 10 doses. Com o uso desse método, 13 de 14 gatos com acromegalia exibiram um controle acentuadamente melhor do diabetes.

HIPOFISECTOMIA
• Em seres humanos com acromegalia, a remoção cirúrgica de pequenos adenomas hipofisários não invasivos frequentemente induz a cura; a maioria dos gatos acometidos apresenta grandes tumores, diminuindo acentuadamente as chances de remoção cirúrgica bem-sucedida; além disso, a hipofisectomia em gatos é associada a altos níveis de complicações pós-operatórias. • O procedimento de crio-hipofisectomia foi descrito em dois gatos — um sofreu uma crise hipoglicêmica e cegueira permanente 2 meses depois da cirurgia, enquanto o outro teve um resultado mais bem-sucedido.

MEDICAÇÕES

• Análogos de somatostatina de ação prolongada — são uniformemente malsucedidos em gatos. • Pegvisomanto, um antagonista dos receptores de GH, foi utilizado de forma eficaz em seres humanos. No entanto, a eficácia em gatos não foi avaliada. • Como o controle médico da hiperprodução de GH não é possível, o objetivo da terapia médica consiste no controle do diabetes melito insulinorresistente para limitar o nível de hiperglicemia e evitar a ocorrência de cetoacidose. É essencial uma posologia de 2 vezes ao dia com doses de 3-5 U/kg (nenhum limite superior à dose requerida).

ACOMPANHAMENTO

• Os sinais clínicos que podem ser atribuídos ao controle diabético insatisfatório (p. ex., polifagia acentuada) não melhoram com o controle diabético eficiente; dessa forma, os níveis de proteínas glicosiladas ou os níveis de glicose sanguínea são indicadores mais eficientes do controle diabético que os sinais clínicos. • Os níveis séricos de IGF1 não são adequados para monitorização da terapia, pois eles não se alteram durante ou após a radioterapia. • Os tempos de sobrevida relatados variam enormemente — de alguns meses a muitos anos, além de mortes por causas improvavelmente relacionadas com acromegalia.

ABREVIATURA(S)
• fGH = forma livre do hormônio de crescimento

Autor David Church
Consultor Editorial Deborah S. Greco

---

* N. T.: Centigray = unidade de radiação.

ACTINOMICOSE

CONSIDERAÇÕES GERAIS

REVISÃO
- Doença infecciosa causada por bactérias em forma de bastão (bastonetes), pleomórficas, ramificadas e Gram-positivas do gênero *Actinomyces*.
- *A. viscosus* e *A. hodeovulneris* — isolamentos mais comumente identificados (embora a maioria dos isolamentos não seja identificada ao nível de espécie); sobrevive em condições microaerófilas ou anaeróbias.
- Raramente encontrado como o único agente bacteriano em uma lesão; costuma ser um componente de uma infecção microbiana múltipla.
- Pode haver um sinergismo entre os *Actinomyces* e outros microrganismos. • Os sistemas orgânicos acometidos podem incluir: ○ Cutâneo; ○ Respiratório; ○ Cardiovascular; ○ Musculoesquelético; ○ Nervoso.

IDENTIFICAÇÃO
- Cães e gatos (incomum). • Mais comum em cães machos jovens de raças esportivas.

SINAIS CLÍNICOS
- Infecções — geralmente localizadas; podem ser disseminadas; a área cervicofacial costuma estar envolvida.
- Tumefações ou abscessos cutâneos com trajetos drenantes — podem ser observados grânulos amarelos ("grânulos de enxofre") nos exsudatos associados.
- Dor, febre e perda de peso.
- Efusões pleurais ou peritoneais exsudativas; ocasionalmente se observam efusões pericárdicas.
- Tosse, dispneia, ruídos pulmonares ventrais diminuídos (empiema). • Retroperitonite — lombalgia; paresia ou paralisia dos membros pélvicos. • Osteomielite de vértebras ou ossos longos — provavelmente secundária à expansão da infecção cutânea; pode desenvolver claudicação ou tumefação das extremidades. • Déficits sensório-motores — relatados em casos de compressão da medula espinal por granulomas.
- Piotórax e feridas subcutâneas por mordeduras constituem os sinais clínicos mais comumente apresentados em gatos.

CAUSAS E FATORES DE RISCO
- *Actinomyces spp.* — residentes normais da cavidade bucal de cães e gatos.
- Perda das barreiras protetoras normais (mucosa, pele), imunossupressão ou mudança no microambiente bacteriano podem predispor os animais à infecção; acredita-se que a actinomicose ocorra como uma infecção oportunista.
- Fatores de risco específicos — traumatismo (feridas provocadas por mordedura), migração de corpos estranhos (espinhos/farpas de gramíneas ou capim rabo-de-raposa no oeste dos EUA) e doença periodontal.

DIAGNÓSTICO

DIAGNÓSTICO DIFERENCIAL
- Nocardiose — principal diagnóstico diferencial; o *Actinomyces* não é diferenciado das espécies de *Nocardia* de forma confiável por meio da coloração de Gram, da citologia ou dos sinais clínicos.
- Devem ser avaliadas outras causas de trajetos drenantes crônicos e efusões pleurais ou peritoneais.

HEMOGRAMA/BIOQUÍMICA/URINÁLISE
- Alterações inespecíficas. • Leucocitose com desvio à esquerda e monocitose — são relatados.
- Anemia arregenerativa — pode se desenvolver.
- Hipoglicemia e hiperglobulinemia — são relatados.

DIAGNÓSTICO POR IMAGEM
- Radiografias de osso infectado — neoformação óssea periosteal, osteosclerose reativa e osteólise.
- Radiografias torácicas — padrões pulmonares alveolointersticiais com possível consolidação do pulmão; efusão pleural; efusão pericárdica; massas subcutâneas na parte lateral do tórax.
- Radiografias abdominais — efusão peritoneal; efeito de massa no abdome. • Radiografias da coluna vertebral — neoformação óssea periosteal, especialmente na região de T13-L3.

MÉTODOS DIAGNÓSTICOS
- Amostras de pus ou fragmentos ósseos osteolíticos enviadas em recipientes para a realização de cultura anaeróbia (ver "Infecções Anaeróbias") podem fornecer o diagnóstico definitivo; notificar o laboratório para pesquisa de actinomicose; também é aconselhável o envio de amostra para cultura aeróbia.
- Esfregaços frescos — coloração de Gram, citologia e coloração acidorresistente; a coloração não descarta a necessidade da cultura; o *Actinomyces* não se cora com os corantes acidorresistentes; já a *Nocardia* é variável.

ACHADOS PATOLÓGICOS
Exame histopatológico — como o encontro dos grânulos de enxofre não é uma tarefa fácil, é recomendável o envio de múltiplos cortes de tecido; corantes especiais podem realçar a visualização dos microrganismos; ferramenta diagnóstica útil, especialmente na presença de grânulos; celulite piogranulomatosa ou granulomatosa com colônias de bactérias filamentosas é característica.

TRATAMENTO

- O líquido exsudativo (tórax, abdome, tecido subcutâneo) deve ser submetido à drenagem e lavagem.
- Em gatos com piotórax, há necessidade de tubo torácico com sucção contínua; os cães respondem melhor à exploração cirúrgica do tórax antes da colocação de tubo para identificar e remover qualquer espinho ou farpa de gramínea.
- Talvez haja necessidade de remoção dos lobos pulmonares acometidos.
- Os cães com massas solitárias envolvendo a parede torácica ou abdominal podem ser curados por meio de excisão cirúrgica radical.

MEDICAÇÕES

MEDICAMENTO(S)
- É importante distinguir entre *Actinomyces* e *Nocardia* para a seleção adequada de antibiótico.
- Antibióticos — um estudo retrospectivo sugere a administração desses agentes por no mínimo 3-4 meses após a resolução de todos os sinais; talvez seja preciso direcioná-los contra outros microrganismos associados.
- Penicilina — considerada como o medicamento de escolha; na maioria dos casos, pode-se iniciar a terapia oral, não havendo necessidade de terapia parenteral; a amoxicilina deve ser administrada na dose de 20-22 mg/kg a cada 8 h VO.

CONTRAINDICAÇÕES/INTERAÇÕES POSSÍVEIS
- Metronidazol — evitar seu uso; é improvável que a actinomicose responda a esse agente.
- Aminoglicosídeos — não utilizar; são ineficazes contra infecções anaeróbias. • *A. hordeovulneris* — variante com deficiência da parede celular (fase L); não costuma responder de forma satisfatória à penicilina; considerar o emprego de clindamicina, eritromicina e cloranfenicol.

ACOMPANHAMENTO

MONITORIZAÇÃO DO PACIENTE
Monitorizar os pacientes atentamente quanto à recidiva nos meses subsequentes à interrupção da terapia.

PREVENÇÃO
Evitar o contato com espinhos e farpas de gramíneas, bem como feridas por mordeduras.

COMPLICAÇÕES POSSÍVEIS
Doença ou terapia imunossupressora concomitante pode complicar o tratamento.

EVOLUÇÃO ESPERADA E PROGNÓSTICO
Pode-se esperar o reaparecimento da infecção no local inicial em cerca da metade dos casos.

DIVERSOS

FATORES RELACIONADOS COM A IDADE
Cães jovens com acesso à rua.

POTENCIAL ZOONÓTICO
Não há relatos de casos de transmissão de actinomicose dos animais para o homem; como é possível a transmissão via feridas provocadas por mordeduras, tais feridas merecem uma atenção especial.

Sugestões de Leitura
Edwards DF. Actinomycosis and nocardiosis. In: Greene CE, ed. Infectious diseases of the dog and cat, 3rd ed. St. Louis: Saunders Elsevier, 2006, pp. 451-461.
Thomovsky E, Kerl ME. Actinomycosis and nocardiosis. Compend Contin Educ Pract Vet 2008, 10:4-10.

Autor Sharon Fooshee Grace
Consultor Editorial Stephen C. Barr

Adenite Sebácea Granulomatosa

CONSIDERAÇÕES GERAIS

REVISÃO
- Processo mórbido inflamatório destrutivo direcionado contra estruturas dos anexos cutâneos (glândulas sebáceas).
- Pode ser geneticamente hereditária, imunomediada ou metabólica.
- Defeito inicial — distúrbio de queratinização ou disfunção do metabolismo lipídico (acúmulo de metabólitos intermediários tóxicos).

SISTEMA(S) ACOMETIDO(S)
Cutâneo/exócrino.

IDENTIFICAÇÃO
- Cães jovens adultos aos de meia-idade.
- Duas formas — uma em raças de pelo longo e outra em raças de pelo curto.
- Raças predispostas — Poodle standard (padrão), Akita, Samoieda e Vizsla.

SINAIS CLÍNICOS
Raças de Pelo Longo
- Alopecia simétrica parcial.
- Pelagem quebradiça e sem brilho (opaca).
- Caspas branco-prateadas firmemente aderidas.
- Moldes ou cilindros foliculares ao redor da haste do pelo ("colarete de queratina").
- Pequenos tufos de pelos emaranhados.
- Lesões — frequentemente observadas no início ao longo da linha média dorsal e dorso da cabeça.
- Grave — foliculite bacteriana secundária, prurido e odor fétido.
- Cães da raça Akita — quase sempre são acometidos de forma relativamente grave; morbidade associada a infecções bacterianas secundárias profundas.
- Cães da raça Poodle standard — os animais acometidos são frequentemente descritos com pelagens excelentes antes do desenvolvimento das lesões; é raro o aparecimento de foliculite bacteriana secundária; a maior parte dos pacientes não exibe doença sistêmica.

Raças de Pelo Curto
- Alopecia — com aspecto roído por traça, circular ou difuso.
- Leve descamação.
- Com frequência, as lesões são semelhantes a placas.
- Acomete o tronco, a cabeça e os pavilhões auriculares.
- É rara a presença de foliculite bacteriana secundária.
- As lesões podem produzir uma formação cicatricial significativa.

CAUSAS E FATORES DE RISCO
- O modo de herança está sendo estudado, mas foi registrado um modo de herança autossômica recessiva em Poodle standard e há suspeitas desse tipo de herança em Akita.
- Especula-se o envolvimento de múltiplas causas fisiopatológicas, incluindo autoimunidade contra as glândulas sebáceas e/ou extravasamento do conteúdo dessas glândulas para a derme circunjacente, causando reação inflamatória e consequente destruição das glândulas.

DIAGNÓSTICO

DIAGNÓSTICO DIFERENCIAL
- Seborreia primária — distúrbio de queratinização.
- Foliculite bacteriana.
- Demodicose.
- Dermatofitose.
- Pênfigo foliáceo.
- Dermatopatia endócrina.

HEMOGRAMA/BIOQUÍMICA/URINÁLISE
N/D.

OUTROS TESTES LABORATORIAIS
N/D.

DIAGNÓSTICO POR IMAGEM
N/D.

MÉTODOS DIAGNÓSTICOS
- Raspados cutâneos — normais.
- Cultura para dermatófitos — negativa.
- Testes de função endócrina — normais.
- Biopsias cutâneas.

ACHADOS PATOLÓGICOS
- Reação inflamatória granulomatosa a piogranulomatosa nodular na altura das glândulas sebáceas.
- Hiperqueratose ortoqueratótica e formação de moldes/cilindros foliculares; mais proeminentes nas raças de pelagem longa.
- Avançada — perda completa das glândulas sebáceas; fibrose em torno dos anexos.
- É rara a destruição de toda a unidade pilossebácea formada pelo folículo piloso e anexos.

TRATAMENTO
- Os sinais clínicos podem aparecer e desaparecer independentemente do tratamento.
- Não foram realizados estudos controlados para comprovar a eficácia de nenhum tratamento.
- Os resultados são extremamente variáveis; a resposta pode depender da gravidade da doença no momento do diagnóstico.
- Raça Akita — raça mais refratária ao tratamento.

MEDICAÇÕES

MEDICAMENTO(S)
- Propilenoglicol e água — mistura em uma proporção de 50-75%; borrifar a cada 24 h nas áreas acometidas.
- Óleo de bebê — embeber as áreas acometidas durante 1 h; acompanhar com a aplicação de xampus diversos para remover o óleo e as caspas.
- Banhos frequentes com xampus queratolíticos (duas vezes por semana).
- Suplementação de ácidos graxos essenciais e óleo de prímula (500 mg) — VO a cada 12 h; os possíveis efeitos colaterais incluem vômito, diarreia e flatulência.
- Isotretinoína (Accutane®) — 1 mg/kg VO a cada 12 h; reduzir para 1 mg/kg a cada 24 h depois de 1 mês e para 1 mg/kg a cada 48 h depois de 2 meses; continuar, conforme a necessidade, para manutenção.
- Ciclosporina — 5 mg/kg VO a cada 12-24 h; os efeitos colaterais incluem vômito, diarreia, hiperplasia gengival, hirsutismo, lesões cutâneas papilomatosas, incidência elevada de infecções, nefro e hepatotoxicidade.
- Tetraciclina e niacinamida (<10 kg = 250 mg de cada VO a cada 8 h; >10 kg = 500 mg de cada VO a cada 8 h) com a vitamina E.
- Antibióticos bactericidas para foliculite bacteriana secundária.

CONTRAINDICAÇÕES/INTERAÇÕES POSSÍVEIS
Isotretinoína (Accutane®) — teratógeno conhecido; não usar em cadelas prenhes; orientar os proprietários sobre o risco.

ACOMPANHAMENTO
Incentivar o registro dos animais acometidos por parte dos proprietários, para que o modo de herança possa ser determinado.

DIVERSOS
Sugestões de Leitura
Rosser EJ. Sebaceous adenitis. In: Griffin CE, Kwochka KW, MacDonald JM, eds., Current Veterinary Dermatology. St. Louis: Mosby, 1993, pp. 211-214.

Autor Karen Helton Rhodes
Consultor Editorial Alexander H. Werner

Adenocarcinoma da Próstata

CONSIDERAÇÕES GERAIS

REVISÃO
- Um tumor maligno que se desenvolve tanto em cães machos castrados como nos intactos.
- Embora essa neoplasia represente <1% de todas as malignidades caninas, o adenocarcinoma da próstata corresponde ao distúrbio mais comum dessa glândula em cães machos castrados.
- É comum a ocorrência de metástases para linfonodos regionais, pulmões e coluna lombossacra.

IDENTIFICAÇÃO
- Cães e, raramente, gatos.
- Cães machos castrados ou intactos de médio a grande porte.
- Idade média, 9-10 anos.

SINAIS CLÍNICOS
Achados Anamnésicos
- Tenesmo — com a produção de fezes semelhantes a fitas.
- Perda de peso.
- Estrangúria e disúria.
- Claudicação dos membros posteriores.
- Letargia.
- Intolerância ao exercício.

Achados do Exame Físico
- Próstata firme, assimétrica e imóvel.
- A prostatomegalia é comum, mas nem sempre está presente.
- Dor — pode ser eliciada em resposta à palpação abdominal ou retal.
- Também é possível identificar massa abdominal caudal, caquexia, pirexia e dispneia.

CAUSAS E FATORES DE RISCO
Cães machos castrados têm alto risco de neoplasia prostática.

DIAGNÓSTICO

DIAGNÓSTICO DIFERENCIAL
- Outra neoplasia primária — carcinoma de células escamosas, carcinoma de células de transição.
- Neoplasia metastática ou localmente invasiva — carcinoma de células de transição.
- Prostatite aguda ou crônica, hipertrofia prostática benigna e cistos prostáticos — possíveis diferenciais em cães machos intactos, mas altamente improváveis nos castrados.

HEMOGRAMA/BIOQUÍMICA/URINÁLISE
- Um leucograma inflamatório é possível.
- A atividade da fosfatase alcalina pode estar elevada.
- Pode haver azotemia pós-renal em caso de obstrução uretral.
- É prudente avaliar amostras urinárias obtidas por técnicas de cistocentese e micção espontânea, pois podem ser observadas alterações como hematúria, piúria e células epiteliais malignas nas amostras coletadas por micção espontânea; esses sinais, no entanto, não são usuais nas amostras obtidas por cistocentese.

OUTROS TESTES LABORATORIAIS
Os marcadores plasmáticos séricos e seminais (p. ex., fosfatase ácida, antígeno prostático específico e esterase prostática canina específica) não estão elevados em cães com adenocarcinoma da próstata.

DIAGNÓSTICO POR IMAGEM
- Radiografia torácica — as metástases podem aparecer como nódulos pulmonares ou padrões intersticiais acentuados.
- Radiografia abdominal — podem ser observadas linfadenomegalia sublombar, mineralização prostática e lesões líticas nas vértebras lombares ou na pelve.
- Ultrassonografia abdominal — hiperecogenicidade focal a multifocal com assimetria e contorno prostático irregular, com ou sem mineralização da próstata.
- Cistografia contrastada — pode ajudar na diferenciação entre prostatopatia e vesicopatia.

MÉTODOS DIAGNÓSTICOS
- Exame de aspirado prostático (percutâneo ou transretal) ou lavado prostático.
- Biopsia prostática com a coleta de amostras por via percutânea ou durante a cirurgia.
- A biopsia percutânea foi associada à disseminação do tumor ao longo do trajeto da agulha.

TRATAMENTO

- Prostatectomia — em caso de doença local; o êxito desse procedimento depende da habilidade do cirurgião e da extensão da doença.
- Radioterapia — pode aliviar os sinais e prolongar a sobrevida.
- Castração — no entanto, grande parte dos tumores não é responsiva aos hormônios androgênios.

MEDICAÇÕES

MEDICAMENTO(S)
- Quimioterapia — carboplatina, cisplatina ou doxorrubicina; pode ter benefícios a curto prazo.
- Alívio da dor — AINEs e medicamentos derivados de morfina.
- Amolecedor de fezes — para alívio do tenesmo.

CONTRAINDICAÇÕES/INTERAÇÕES POSSÍVEIS
N/D.

ACOMPANHAMENTO

MONITORIZAÇÃO DO PACIENTE
- Capacidade de micção e defecação.
- Dor secundária a metástases ósseas.
- Qualidade de vida.

PREVENÇÃO
Manter os cães sexualmente intactos pode diminuir o risco.

COMPLICAÇÕES POSSÍVEIS
- Obstrução uretral.
- Metástase para linfonodos regionais, ossos e pulmões.

EVOLUÇÃO ESPERADA E PROGNÓSTICO
Prognóstico reservado a mau, com sobrevida de 2-6 meses, dependendo dos sintomas clínicos apresentados.

DIVERSOS

DISTÚRBIOS ASSOCIADOS
Nenhum.

FATORES RELACIONADOS COM A IDADE
Nenhum.

POTENCIAL ZOONÓTICO
Nenhum.

GESTAÇÃO/FERTILIDADE/REPRODUÇÃO
N/D.

ABREVIATURA(S)
- AINE = anti-inflamatório não esteroide.

Sugestões de Leitura
Bryan JN, et al. A population study of neutering status as a risk factor for canine prostate cancer. Prostate 2007, 67:1174-1181.

Autor Ruthanne Chun
Consultor Editorial Timothy M. Fan

Adenocarcinoma da Tireoide — Cães

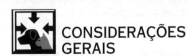

CONSIDERAÇÕES GERAIS

DEFINIÇÃO
Tumor maligno que se origina de células foliculares ou parafoliculares (medulares/células-C) da glândula tireoide.

FISIOPATOLOGIA
• Cerca de 60% dos pacientes são eutireóideos, 30%, hipotireóideos e 10%, hipertireóideos.
• Tipicamente, os tumores são muito invasivos com alto índice metastático (pulmões, linfonodos retrofaríngeos, fígado), sendo que até 35-40% dos cães apresentam metástase no momento do diagnóstico.
• Os animais com tumores bilaterais têm um risco 16 vezes maior de desenvolver doença metastática que aqueles com tumores unilaterais.

SISTEMA(S) ACOMETIDO(S)
• Cardiovascular — os cães hipertireóideos costumam ser taquicárdicos e podem exibir hipertensão sistêmica; em casos de doença avançada, é possível observar anemia e CID.
• Endócrino/metabólico — os cães acometidos podem ser hipotireóideos, eutireóideos ou hipertireóideos; a hipercalcemia pode ser observada como síndrome paraneoplásica ou secundária à hiperplasia paratireoide ou a adenocarcinoma paratireoide concomitante.
• Respiratório — os cães podem ficar dispneicos pela presença de massa expansiva adjacente à traqueia; é comum a ocorrência de metástase para os pulmões.

GENÉTICA
Desconhecida.

INCIDÊNCIA/PREVALÊNCIA
Responde por 1,2-3,8% de todos os tumores em cães, mas representa 10-15% de todos os tumores primários da cabeça e do pescoço.

DISTRIBUIÇÃO GEOGRÁFICA
Pode ser mais comum em áreas onde há deficiência de iodo.

IDENTIFICAÇÃO
Espécies
Cães.

Raça(s) Predominante(s)
Boxer, Golden retriever e Beagle — apresentam risco elevado embora possa ser observado em qualquer raça.

Idade Média e Faixa Etária
Cães mais idosos (média, 9-11 anos; faixa etária, 4-18 anos).

Sexo(s) Predominante(s)
Sem predileção sexual.

SINAIS CLÍNICOS
Comentários Gerais
• Não costuma ser diagnosticado até que uma massa volumosa seja palpável.
• Aproximadamente 65% são unilaterais, enquanto 35%, bilaterais.

Achados Anamnésicos
• Massa/tumefação palpáveis na região cervical, tosse, dispneia, disfagia, disfonia, edema facial, cervicalgia.
• Em caso de tumor funcional da tireoide, podem-se observar poliúria, polidipsia, polifagia, perda de peso, comportamento inquieto, diarreia.
• No animal hipotireoide, podem-se verificar mau aspecto da pelagem, ganho de peso e letargia.

Achados do Exame Físico
• Massa cervical livremente móvel ou fixa, uni ou bilateral.
• Raramente se pode observar síndrome de Horner ou síndrome da veia cava cranial.
• No paciente hipertireóideo, observam-se arritmias ou sopros cardíacos.

CAUSAS
Desconhecidas.

FATORES DE RISCO
• Foi demonstrado que o hipotireoidismo sem tratamento é um fator de risco em uma colônia de Beagles.
• Predisposição racial.
• Deficiência de iodo.

DIAGNÓSTICO

DIAGNÓSTICO DIFERENCIAL
• Outras neoplasias primárias — linfoma; sarcoma dos tecidos moles; adenocarcinoma das glândulas salivares; carcinoma das glândulas paratireoides; tumor do corpo carotídeo.
• Tumores secundários — carcinoma bucal metastático de células escamosas; melanoma bucal.
• Inflamatório — abscesso ou granuloma.
• Mucocele salivar.

HEMOGRAMA/BIOQUÍMICA/URINÁLISE
• Em geral, permanecem normais.
• Pode-se observar anemia normocítica normocrômica arregenerativa típica de doença crônica, além de leucocitose.
• Alterações raras — hipercalcemia; isostenúria; CID.

OUTROS TESTES LABORATORIAIS
Hormônios tireoidianos (níveis de T_4 e/ou T_4 livre) e níveis do TSH endógeno.

DIAGNÓSTICO POR IMAGEM
• Radiografias torácicas (três projeções) — possibilitam a avaliação dos pulmões e de outras estruturas torácicas para pesquisa de metástase.
• Ultrassonografia e tomografia computadorizada da região cervical — permitem a avaliação do tecido de origem, da vascularidade, do grau de invasão e dos linfonodos cervicais.
• Cintilografia com tecnécio-99m — para avaliar o paciente em busca de tecido tireóideo ectópico ou lesões metastáticas.
• Estudos com iodo radioativo — podem fornecer informações a respeito da capacidade de produção dos hormônios tireoidianos pelo tumor.

MÉTODOS DIAGNÓSTICOS
Biopsia
Não é recomendável o uso da agulha Tru-Cut®, em virtude do alto risco de hemorragia grave; em geral, há necessidade de biopsia aberta.

Citologia
• Exame de aspirado (por agulha fina) coletado a partir do tumor e dos linfonodos regionais palpáveis.
• A amostra quase sempre vem a ser maciçamente contaminada com sangue, em decorrência da natureza altamente vascularizada do tumor.
• População homogênea de células epiteliais, algumas vezes com grânulos contendo coloide e/ou tirosina.
• Não é capaz de diferenciar células tireóideas malignas *versus* benignas; no entanto, quase todas as neoplasias das tireoides são malignas em cães.

ACHADOS PATOLÓGICOS
Macroscópicos
• Caracterizados por alta vascularidade, com áreas de hemorragia e necrose.
• Em geral, pouco encapsulados; muitas vezes, invadem os tecidos adjacentes (p. ex., traqueia e esôfago, além da vasculatura circundante); podem se aderir à veia jugular, à artéria carótida e ao tronco vagossimpático.

Histopatológicos
• Três tipos principais — folicular, papilar e compacto (maciço); em cães, são mais comuns os tumores foliculares e maciços mistos.
• São menos comuns os carcinomas de células C (p. ex., parafoliculares e medulares).

TRATAMENTO

CUIDADO(S) DE SAÚDE ADEQUADO(S)
• O tratamento definitivo depende do estágio tumoral (tamanho e mobilidade do tumor, bem como indícios de doença metastática).
• A excisão cirúrgica completa é recomendada para tumores livremente móveis da tireoide.
• É aconselhável um curso completo de radioterapia de feixe externo no pré-operatório para tumores volumosos, como monoterapia para tumores não ressecáveis ou no pós-operatório para tumores submetidos à excisão cirúrgica incompleta.
• Radio e/ou quimioterapia paliativas são recomendadas para tumores metastáticos à apresentação.
• Também se pode fazer uso do iodo-131, embora as doses sejam muito altas (60-100 mCi); por essa razão, há poucas instituições que oferecem esse tipo de terapia.

CUIDADO(S) DE ENFERMAGEM
Varia de acordo com os sinais observados ao exame clínico.

ATIVIDADE
Restringir a atividade física se o animal estiver dispneico.

DIETA
N/D.

ORIENTAÇÃO AO PROPRIETÁRIO
• Alertar os proprietários sobre a importância do controle da frequência e do ritmo cardíacos em pacientes hipertireóideos e a possibilidade de episódios de colapso.
• Advertir os donos dos animais quanto à possível paralisia pós-operatória da laringe e a ocorrência intraoperatória de hemorragia.
• Prevenir os proprietários sobre os efeitos tóxicos agudos da radioterapia — descamação úmida, laringite, traqueíte, esofagite.

CONSIDERAÇÕES CIRÚRGICAS
Ver a seção "Cuidado(s) de Saúde Adequado(s)".

Riscos
• Hemorragia acentuada — tumores altamente vascularizados e invasivos para estruturas circunjacentes, incluindo a vasculatura; pode haver a necessidade de transfusões sanguíneas e cuidados pós-operatórios intensivos.

ADENOCARCINOMA DA TIREOIDE — CÃES

- Paralisia da laringe — em função do traumatismo ao nervo laríngeo recorrente.
- Dano às glândulas paratireoides — possível ocorrência durante a cirurgia.

MEDICAÇÕES

MEDICAMENTO(S) DE ESCOLHA
- Agentes quimioterápicos:
  - A quimioterapia é recomendada como tratamento isolado ou em combinação com a cirurgia e/ou a radioterapia.
  - Cisplatina (60 mg/m^2 a cada 3 semanas) ou doxorrubicina (30 mg/m^2 a cada 3 semanas) — há relatos de remissão parcial em aproximadamente 50% dos casos.
  - Cisplatina — nefrotóxica; é imprescindível utilizá-la com diurese salina (18,3 mL/kg/h IV durante 6 h; administrar a cisplatina após 4 h).
- Antieméticos para a terapia com cisplatina:
  - Maropitanto — 1 mg/kg SC antes da cisplatina, ou
  - Dolasetrona — 0,6-1 mg/kg IV ou VO a cada 24 h, ou
  - Butorfanol — 0,4 mg/kg IM, antes e depois da cisplatina.
- Tratamento da tireoide:
  - Tiroxina — são recomendadas doses de manutenção para diminuir a produção de TSH; alguns tumores possuem receptores para o TSH; ainda não está determinado o valor da terapia de reposição hormonal em cães acometidos.
  - Metimazol — 5 mg VO a cada 8 h para cães de médio a grande porte; pode ser benéfico em pacientes hipertireóideos.
  - β-bloqueadores — podem ser indicados em casos de taquicardia ou hipertensão nos pacientes hipertireóideos.

CONTRAINDICAÇÕES
- Doxorrubicina — é cumulativamente tóxica para os miócitos cardíacos, provocando declínio na função do miocárdio. Não administrar a animais com disfunção cardíaca ou miocardiopatia dilatada.
  - Cisplatina — é nefrotóxica; não fornecer a pacientes com nefropatia.

PRECAUÇÕES
A quimioterapia pode causar toxicidades em órgãos como trato gastrintestinal, medula óssea, coração e outros — buscar orientação de veterinário especialista em oncologia caso não se esteja familiarizado com o uso de agentes citotóxicos.

INTERAÇÕES POSSÍVEIS
Verapamil — pode potencializar a cardiotoxicidade induzida pela doxorrubicina.

MEDICAMENTO(S) ALTERNATIVO(S)
N/D.

ACOMPANHAMENTO

MONITORIZAÇÃO DO PACIENTE
- Concentração sérica de cálcio — mensurar caso tenha sido efetuada uma tireoidectomia bilateral; podem ser observados sinais de hipocalcemia (agitação, respiração ofegante, tremores musculares, tetania e crises convulsivas).
  - Tratar com gliconato de cálcio a 10% (1,0-1,5 mL/kg IV durante 10-20 min).
  - Manter o nível sérico de cálcio com diidrotaquisterol (vitamina D) por via oral.
- Hormônios tireoidianos — talvez haja necessidade de suplementação com tiroxina após tireoidectomia bilateral.
- Concentração do TSH — um dos objetivos da suplementação de tiroxina é sub-regular a secreção corporal do TSH.
- Local do tumor primário — exame físico e ultrassom cervical; radiografias torácicas a cada 3 meses para detectar metástases pulmonares.

PREVENÇÃO
Desconhecida.

COMPLICAÇÕES POSSÍVEIS
- Tumor — anemia; trombocitopenia; hipercalcemia; CID; angústia respiratória.
- Quimioterapia — miocardiopatia dilatada; insuficiência renal; pancreatite; sepse; desarranjo gastrintestinal.
- Cirurgia — hemorragia; hipotireoidismo; hipocalcemia secundária a hipoparatireoidismo; paralisia da laringe.
- Radioterapia — efeitos colaterais agudos — descamação úmida; mucosite na faringe; esofagite; traqueíte; efeitos colaterais tardios — alopecia ou mudança de coloração da pele ou da pelagem (no local submetido à radiação).

EVOLUÇÃO ESPERADA E PROGNÓSTICO
- Prognóstico — relaciona-se com o estágio da doença (tamanho e mobilidade do tumor, bem como indícios de doença metastática), sendo que os tumores pequenos, unilaterais, não aderidos e não metastáticos possuem o melhor prognóstico.
- O tempo médio de sobrevida após remoção cirúrgica de tumor da tireoide livremente móvel é >36 meses.
- Para os animais tratados com curso completo de radioterapia de feixe externo — a sobrevida livre de progressão foi de 80 e 72% em 1 e 3 anos, respectivamente; em outro estudo, o tempo médio de sobrevida foi de 24,5 meses.
- Radioterapia paliativa em 13 cães — tempo médio de sobrevida de 24 meses.
- Terapia com iodo (^{131}I) isolado ou em combinação com cirurgia — os tempos médios de sobrevida foram de 30 e 34 meses, respectivamente.
- Animais tratados apenas com a cisplatina (13 cães) — a taxa de resposta global foi de 53%, com intervalo médio livre de progressão para os responsivos de 202 dias e tempo médio de sobrevida global de 98 dias.

DIVERSOS

DISTÚRBIOS ASSOCIADOS
- As malignidades não tireóideas são comuns.
- Há relatos de neoplasias endócrinas múltiplas.

FATORES RELACIONADOS COM A IDADE
Nenhum.

POTENCIAL ZOONÓTICO
N/D.

GESTAÇÃO/FERTILIDADE/REPRODUÇÃO
Não é recomendável acasalar os animais com câncer. A quimioterapia é teratogênica — portanto, não se deve administrá-la a fêmeas prenhes.

SINÔNIMO(S)
Carcinoma tireóideo.

ABREVIATURA(S)
- CID = coagulação intravascular disseminada.
- TSH = hormônio tireostimulante.

Sugestões de Leitura
Bailey DB, Page RL. Tumors of the endocrine system. In: Withrow SJ, Vail DM, eds., Small Animal Clinical Oncology, 4th ed. Philadelphia: Saunders, 2007, pp. 591-596.
Klein MK, Powers BE, Withrow SJ, et al. Treatment of thyroid carcinoma in dogs by surgical resection alone: 20 cases (1981-1989). JAVMA 1995, 206:1007-1009.
Liptak JM. Canine thyroid carcinoma. Clin Tech Small Anim Pract 2007, 22(2):75-81.
Pack L, Roberts RE, Davson SD, Dookwah HD. Definitive radiation therapy for infiltrative thyroid carcinoma in dogs. Vet Radiol Ultrasound 2001, 42:471-474.
Walers CB, Scott-Moncrieff JCR. Cancer of endocrine origin. In: Morrison WB, ed.,
Cancer in Dogs and Cats: Medical and Surgical Management, 2nd ed. Jackson, WY: Teton NewMedia, 2002, pp. 573-580.

Autor Rebecca G. Newman
Consultor Editorial Timothy M. Fan
Agradecimento O autor e os editores agradecem a colaboração prévia de Linda S. Fineman.

Adenocarcinoma das Glândulas Ceruminosas, Orelha

CONSIDERAÇÕES GERAIS

REVISÃO
- Tumor maligno primário mais comum do meato acústico externo, originário a partir das glândulas sudoríferas apócrinas modificadas (p. ex., glândulas ceruminosas).
- Embora seja localmente invasivo, é associado a uma baixa taxa metastática.

IDENTIFICAÇÃO
- Apesar de raro, trata-se do tumor maligno mais comum do canal auditivo em cães e gatos, seguido pelo carcinoma de células escamosas.
- A raça Cocker spaniel pode ser super-representada.
- Idade média — cães, 10 anos; gatos, 11 anos.
- Não há predisposição sexual conhecida.

SINAIS CLÍNICOS
- Semelhantes aos de otite externa crônica e recorrente.
- Aspecto inicial — massa(s) nodular(es) hemorrágica(s), ulcerativa(s), friável(is) e rosa pálida(s).
- Aspecto final — preenchimento do canal auditivo e invasão de estruturas circunjacentes através da parede desse canal por grande(s) massa(s).
- Linfadenomegalia regional.
- Pode haver sinais neurológicos (sinais vestibulares, síndrome de Horner).
- Sinais de dor e desconforto; dor à abertura da boca.

CAUSAS E FATORES DE RISCO
O processo de inflamação crônica e a ocorrência de hiperplasia/displasia das glândulas ceruminosas parecem desempenhar um papel no desenvolvimento tumoral.

DIAGNÓSTICO

DIAGNÓSTICO DIFERENCIAL
- Otite externa crônica proliferativa.
- Hiperplasia nodular.
- Pólipos inflamatórios (gatos).
- Outros tumores, incluindo carcinoma de células escamosas, tumor de células basais (basalioma), mastocitoma, papiloma, tumor das glândulas sebáceas, adenoma das glândulas ceruminosas.

HEMOGRAMA/BIOQUÍMICA/URINÁLISE
Costumam permanecer normais.

OUTROS TESTES LABORATORIAIS
- Citologia otológica por *swab* para pesquisa de bactérias e leveduras.
- Cultura bacteriana e antibiograma, conforme a necessidade.

DIAGNÓSTICO POR IMAGEM
- Radiografias do crânio — determinam o envolvimento potencial da bula timpânica.
- Radiografias torácicas — avaliam a ocorrência de metástase pulmonar.
- TC ou RM — muito úteis para estadiamento locorregional e antes de cirurgia e radioterapia; fornecem mais detalhes do que as radiografias.

MÉTODOS DIAGNÓSTICOS
- Exame citológico de aspirado obtido dos linfonodos regionais.
- Biopsia e histopatologia.

ACHADOS PATOLÓGICOS
- Características histopatológicas — diferenciação apócrina das glândulas ceruminosas e invasão local no estroma.
- Células tumorais — revelam atipia nuclear moderada a acentuada, com mitoses frequentes.

TRATAMENTO
- Ablação total do canal auditivo e osteotomia lateral da bula timpânica — métodos cirúrgicos preferidos à ressecção auricular lateral.
- Radioterapia pode ser considerada para massas grandes (intenção paliativa) ou parcialmente excisadas (intenção curativa).

MEDICAÇÕES

MEDICAMENTO(S)
- A quimioterapia não foi avaliada, mas ocasionalmente é considerada com base nas informações do exame histológico e nos resultados do estadiamento clínico.
- Uso de múltiplas modalidades terapêuticas que incorporam medicamentos anti-inflamatórios e outros analgésicos.
- Antibioticoterapia com base nos resultados da cultura e do antibiograma.

CONTRAINDICAÇÕES/INTERAÇÕES POSSÍVEIS
N/D.

ACOMPANHAMENTO

MONITORIZAÇÃO DO PACIENTE
- A realização do exame físico e a obtenção de radiografias torácicas são recomendáveis em intervalos regulares após o tratamento (a cada 2-4 meses).
- Pode ser recomendada a realização de TC ou RM seriada para monitorar a ocorrência de novo crescimento local do tumor.

COMPLICAÇÕES POSSÍVEIS
- Síndrome de Horner transitória ou permanente, secundária à cirurgia.
- Paralisia facial transitória ou permanente após a cirurgia (mais frequente em gatos).

EVOLUÇÃO ESPERADA E PROGNÓSTICO
- Sobrevida média após ressecção auricular lateral gira em torno de 10 meses tanto para cães como para gatos.
- Sobrevida média após ablação do canal auditivo e osteotomia lateral da bula timpânica é superior a 3 anos em cães e gatos.
- Sobrevida média após radioterapia é superior a 3 anos, mas as informações publicadas são apenas em pequeno número.
- Prognóstico mau associado ao extenso envolvimento tumoral (estágio avançado), aos sinais neurológicos pré-operatórios e à terapia conservativa (p. ex., ablação lateral do canal auditivo apenas).

DIVERSOS

DISTÚRBIOS ASSOCIADOS
- Otite externa.
- Vestibulopatia periférica, síndrome de Horner.
- Dor crônica.

ABREVIATURA(S)
- RM = ressonância magnética.
- TC = tomografia computadorizada.

Sugestões de Leitura
Bacon NJ, Gilbert RL, Bostock DE, White RA. Total ear canal ablation in the cat: Indications, morbidity and long-term survival. J Small Anim Pract 2003, 44:430-434.
Fan TM, de Lorimier LP. Inflammatory polyps and aural neoplasia. Vet Clin North Am Small Anim Pract 2004, 34:489-509.
London CA, Dubilzieg RR, Vail DM, et al. Evaluation of dogs and cats with tumors of the ear canal: 145 cases (1978-1992). JAVMA 1996, 208:1413-1418.
Moisan PG, Watson GL. Ceruminous gland tumors in dogs and cats: A review of 124 cases. JAAHA 1996, 32:448-452.
Théon AP, Barthez PY, Madewell BR, Griffey SM. Radiation therapy of ceruminous gland carcinomas in dogs and cats. JAVMA 1994, 205:566-569.

Autor Louis-Philippe de Lorimier
Consultor Editorial Timothy M. Fan
Agradecimento O autor e os editores agradecem a colaboração prévia de Joanne C. Graham.

ADENOCARCINOMA DAS GLÂNDULAS SALIVARES

CONSIDERAÇÕES GERAIS

REVISÃO
- Tumor originário de glândulas salivares maiores (p. ex., parótidas, mandibulares, sublinguais ou zigomáticas) ou menores.
- As glândulas mandibulares ou parótidas constituem 80% dos casos.
- A glândula mandibular é a mais frequentemente acometida nos cães.
- Maior acometimento da glândula parótida nos gatos.
- Localmente invasivo.
- Os gatos tipicamente apresentam a doença mais avançada do que os cães no momento do diagnóstico.
- Metástase — para linfonodo regional em 39% dos gatos e 17% dos cães no ato do diagnóstico; relato de metástase à distância em 16% dos gatos e 8% dos cães por ocasião do diagnóstico, mas pode exibir um desenvolvimento lento.
- Outras neoplasias das glândulas salivares — carcinoma; carcinoma de células escamosas; neoplasia mista.
- As malignidades epiteliais representam aproximadamente 85% dos tumores das glândulas salivares.
- Fibrossarcomas, lipomas, mastocitomas e linfomas envolvem as glândulas salivares por extensão e invasão diretas. Também foram descritos histiocitoma fibroso maligno (tipo de células gigantes) e tumor misto maligno (provavelmente de origem ductal) concomitantes dentro das glândulas salivares.
- Os adenomas compreendem apenas 5% dos tumores salivares.

IDENTIFICAÇÃO
- Cães e gatos.
- Idade média, 10-12 anos.
- Gatos Siameses — podem apresentar um risco relativamente mais alto.
- Na espécie felina, os machos são duas vezes mais acometidos do que as fêmeas.
- Ainda não foi determinada nenhuma outra predileção racial ou sexual.

SINAIS CLÍNICOS
- Tumefação unilateral, firme, indolor na região cervical superior (mandibulares e sublinguais), na base auricular (parótidas), no lábio superior ou no maxilar (zigomáticas) ou na mucosa labial (acessórias ou tecido salivar secundário).
- Outros sinais podem incluir halitose, perda de peso, anorexia, disfagia, exoftalmia, síndrome de Horner, espirros e disfonia.

CAUSAS E FATORES DE RISCO
Desconhecidos.

DIAGNÓSTICO

DIAGNÓSTICO DIFERENCIAL
- Carcinoma de células escamosas.
- Mucocele.
- Abscessos.
- Sarcoma de tecidos moles, p. ex., histiocitoma fibroso maligno ou fibrossarcoma.
- Linfoma.

HEMOGRAMA/BIOQUÍMICA/URINÁLISE
Os resultados frequentemente permanecem normais.

OUTROS TESTES LABORATORIAIS
N/D.

DIAGNÓSTICO POR IMAGEM
- Radiografias regionais — costumam permanecer normais; pode-se observar reação periosteal nos ossos adjacentes ou deslocamento de estruturas circunjacentes.
- RM ou TC — possibilita a discriminação superior do tumor para planejamento terapêutico de cirurgia e/ou radioterapia.
- Radiografias torácicas — são indicadas para a pesquisa de metástases pulmonares.

MÉTODOS DIAGNÓSTICOS
- Exame citológico de aspirado — pode diferenciar adenocarcinoma salivar de mucocele e abscesso.
- Biopsia do núcleo do tumor com agulha ou em cunha — fornece o diagnóstico definitivo.

TRATAMENTO

- Ressecção cirúrgica rigorosa — sempre que possível; grande parte desses tumores é invasiva e de difícil excisão completa.
- Radioterapia — controle local satisfatório e sobrevida prolongada em três casos relatados.
- A ressecção local rigorosa (em geral, incompleta do ponto de vista histológico), acompanhada por radiação adjuvante, pode proporcionar um controle local e uma sobrevida a longo prazo; no entanto, ainda são necessários outros estudos para determinar o tratamento mais eficaz, inclusive o possível papel da quimioterapia.

MEDICAÇÕES

MEDICAMENTO(S)
A eficácia da quimioterapia basicamente não é relatada; entretanto, pode ser indicada para tratamento/alívio de doença metastática.

CONTRAINDICAÇÕES/INTERAÇÕES POSSÍVEIS
N/D.

ACOMPANHAMENTO

MONITORIZAÇÃO DO PACIENTE
Avaliações — exame físico e radiografias torácicas a cada 3 meses são medidas razoáveis se for efetuada cirurgia rigorosa e/ou radioterapia.

COMPLICAÇÕES POSSÍVEIS
Com a radioterapia, esperam-se efeitos colaterais agudos temporários (p. ex., dermatite úmida e alopecia).

EVOLUÇÃO ESPERADA E PROGNÓSTICO
- Melhoria no tempo de sobrevida em cães, sem indícios de metástase aos nodos ou à distância no ato do diagnóstico; o estágio clínico não é prognóstico para os gatos.
- Sobrevida média de 550 dias para os cães e 516 dias para os gatos em um estudo retrospectivo.
- O controle local por meio de radiação ou múltiplas cirurgias continua crucial.

DIVERSOS

ABREVIATURA(S)
- RM = ressonância magnética.
- TC = tomografia computadorizada.

Sugestões de Leitura
Hammer A, Getzy D, Ogilvie G, et al. Salivary gland neoplasia in the dog and cat: Survival times and prognostic factors. JAAHA 2001, 37:478-482.

Autor Anthony J. Mutsaers
Consultor Editorial Timothy M. Fan

Adenocarcinoma das Glândulas Sebáceas e Sudoríferas

CONSIDERAÇÕES GERAIS

REVISÃO
Crescimento maligno que se origina das glândulas sebáceas ou sudoríferas apócrinas da pele.

IDENTIFICAÇÃO
- Adenocarcinoma das glândulas sudoríferas apócrinas — raro em cães, porém incomum em gatos.
- Adenocarcinoma das glândulas sebáceas — raro tanto em cães como em gatos.
- Acomete animais de estimação de meia-idade a mais idosos.
- As cadelas foram super-representadas para o adenocarcinoma das glândulas sudoríferas apócrinas em um estudo.

SINAIS CLÍNICOS
- Pode aparecer como lesões cutâneas superficiais maciças, firmes e salientes (ou seja, em relevo).
- Pode exibir ulceração e sangramento, além de ser acompanhado por inflamação do tecido circunjacente.
- Adenocarcinoma das glândulas sudoríferas apócrinas — muitas vezes pouco circunscrito; ulcerado; bastante invasivo nos tecidos subjacentes; pode ocorrer em qualquer lugar do corpo, afetando com frequência o tronco em cães.
- Adenocarcinoma das glândulas sebáceas — lesão frequentemente ulcerada e inflamada, com risco moderado de envolvimento de linfonodos.

CAUSAS E FATORES DE RISCO
Desconhecidos.

DIAGNÓSTICO

DIAGNÓSTICO DIFERENCIAL
- Outros tumores cutâneos mais frequentes.
- Doenças histiocíticas cutâneas.
- Doenças cutâneas imunomediadas.
- Infecções bacterianas/fúngicas.

HEMOGRAMA/BIOQUÍMICA/URINÁLISE
Normais.

OUTROS TESTES LABORATORIAIS
N/D.

DIAGNÓSTICO POR IMAGEM
É recomendável a obtenção de radiografias torácicas no momento do diagnóstico para avaliar a presença de metástases à distância.

MÉTODOS DIAGNÓSTICOS
- Biopsia para a realização de exame histopatológico e obtenção do diagnóstico definitivo.
- Exame citológico ou biopsia de linfonodos regionais.

ACHADOS PATOLÓGICOS
- Carcinomas das glândulas sudoríferas apócrinas são tipicamente invasivos no estroma e nos vasos sanguíneos subjacentes, mas com frequência exibem margens pouco delimitadas e índice mitótico elevado.
- Adenocarcinomas das glândulas sebáceas frequentemente revelam invasão dos vasos linfáticos.

TRATAMENTO

- Para ambos os tipos, recomenda-se a excisão cirúrgica rigorosa em bloco, incluindo a ressecção dos linfonodos drenantes. A análise histopatológica dos linfonodos ajuda na determinação do prognóstico e no estabelecimento de plano terapêutico adjuvante.
- É imprescindível examinar as margens de toda a amostra tecidual por meio de exame histopatológico para avaliar se a ressecção foi completa.
- Radioterapia pode ser recomendada para o tratamento de linfonodos drenantes após ressecção para evitar a recidiva e o desenvolvimento de metástase regional; o tratamento do tumor primário é recomendável sempre que a ressecção ampla e completa não for possível.

MEDICAÇÕES

MEDICAMENTO(S)
- Múltiplos agentes quimioterápicos foram utilizados para o tratamento de ambos os tipos de tumor, em ambas as espécies, com certo benefício (incluindo a cisplatina, a carboplatina, a mitoxantrona e a gencitabina).
- É recomendável o contato com veterinário especialista em oncologia em busca de quaisquer tratamentos atualizados que possam estar disponíveis.
- Os anti-inflamatórios não esteroides e outros analgésicos são recomendados, conforme indicação, para o controle da dor.

CONTRAINDICAÇÕES/INTERAÇÕES POSSÍVEIS
Não há.

ACOMPANHAMENTO

- Adenocarcinoma das glândulas sebáceas — pouco se sabe a respeito do potencial metastático dessa malignidade, embora ela possa sofrer rápida metástase aos linfonodos regionais em alguns pacientes; o prognóstico a longo prazo parece muito bom quando se combina uma cirurgia rigorosa com quimio e radioterapia.
- Adenocarcinoma das glândulas apócrinas — associado a um prognóstico razoável a bom a longo prazo; o achado histológico de invasão vascular constitui um fator prognóstico negativo de metástases sistêmicas; a ressecção cirúrgica rigorosa (controle tumoral local e regional) acompanhada por quimioterapia adjuvante é recomendável para aumentar a sobrevida. Um estudo relatou um tempo médio de sobrevida pós-excisão de 30 meses em cães.

DIVERSOS

Sugestões de Leitura

Carpenter JL, Andrews LK, Holzworth J. Tumors and tumor like lesions. In: Holzworth J, ed., Diseases of the Cat: Medicine and Surgery. Philadelphia: Saunders, 1987, pp. 406-596.

Pakhrin B, Kang MS, Bae IH, et al. Retrospective study of canine cutaneous tumors in Korea. J Vet Sci 2007, 8:229-236.

Simko E, Wilcock BP, Yager JA. A retrospective study of 44 canine apocrine sweat gland adenocarcinomas. Can Vet J 2003, 44(1):38-42.

Thomas RC, Fox LE. Tumors of the skin and subcutis. In: Morrison WB, ed., Cancer in Dogs and Cats: Medical and Surgical Management. Jackson, WY: Teton NewMedia, 2002, pp. 469-488.

Autor Louis-Philippe de Lorimier
Consultor Editorial Timothy M. Fan
Agradecimento O autor e os editores agradecem a colaboração prévia de Phyllis Glawe.

Adenocarcinoma do Estômago, Intestinos Delgado, Grosso e Reto

CONSIDERAÇÕES GERAIS

REVISÃO
- Tumor incomum, que se origina do revestimento epitelial do trato gastrintestinal.
- O prognóstico é reservado a mau.

IDENTIFICAÇÃO
- Os cães costumam ser mais acometidos do que os gatos.
- Animais de meia-idade a mais idosos (>6 anos); faixa etária de 3-13 anos.
- Não há raça predominante.
- Mais comum em machos do que em fêmeas.

SINAIS CLÍNICOS
Achados Anamnésicos
- Sinais relacionados com o trato gastrintestinal.
- Estômago — vômito, anorexia, perda de peso, hematêmese e melena.
- Intestino delgado — vômito, perda de peso, borborigmo, flatulência e melena.
- Intestino grosso e reto — fezes mucosas, hematoquezia e tenesmo.

Achados do Exame Físico
- Estômago — inespecíficos.
- Intestino delgado — pode-se palpar massa em região mesogástrica; distensão abdominal e sensibilidade das alças do intestino delgado à palpação; melena ao exame retal.
- Intestino grosso e reto — massa palpável por via retal, podendo formar uma espécie de "argola para guardanapo" ou protrusão de múltiplas lesões nodulares para o interior do cólon; presença de sangue vivo nas fezes.

CAUSAS E FATORES DE RISCO
- Desconhecidos.
- Nitrosaminas — relatadas como agentes causais na literatura experimental.
- Possível causa genética — adenocarcinomas gástricos no Pastor belga e em cães aparentados (Tervuren).

DIAGNÓSTICO

DIAGNÓSTICO DIFERENCIAL
- Corpo estranho.
- Enteropatia inflamatória.
- Linfoma.
- Parasitas.
- Leiomioma.
- Leiomiossarcoma.
- Pancreatite.

HEMOGRAMA/BIOQUÍMICA/URINÁLISE
- Estômago e intestino delgado — pode-se observar anemia microcítica hipocrômica (anemia ferropriva [ou seja, por deficiência de ferro]).
- Intestino grosso e reto — sem alterações características.

OUTROS TESTES LABORATORIAIS
Sangue oculto nas fezes pode ser positivo; a dieta pode afetar os resultados — pode-se confirmar após alimentação vegetariana (sem carne) por 3 dias.

DIAGNÓSTICO POR IMAGEM
- Ultrassonografia — pode revelar o espessamento da parede gástrica ou intestinal; é possível a observação de massa no trato gastrintestinal e enfartamento dos linfonodos.
- Radiografia com contraste positivo — pode mostrar a presença de defeito de preenchimento (estômago) do meio de contraste; constrição anular ou expansiva intraluminal (intestino delgado); as neoplasias gástricas são encontradas mais frequentemente nos dois terços distais do estômago.
- Radiografia com contraste duplo — intestino grosso e reto; pode detectar massas expansivas polipoides ou anulares.

MÉTODOS DIAGNÓSTICOS
- Aspirado de massa intestinal ou de linfonodo infartado com agulha fina guiada por ultrassom pode revelar células de carcinoma à citologia, o que pode ser útil para descartar linfoma.
- Biopsia por via endoscópica pode não ser diagnóstica, pois muitas vezes os tumores ficam situados em níveis profundos na superfície mucosa; assim, a biopsia cirúrgica é frequentemente necessária.

TRATAMENTO

- Ressecção cirúrgica — tratamento de escolha; raramente curativa.
- Tumor gástrico — geralmente não ressecável.
- Intestino delgado — remover o tumor por meio de ressecção e anastomose; é comum a ocorrência de metástase para linfonodos regionais e fígado.
- Intestino grosso e reto — ocasionalmente, podem ser submetidos à ressecção por meio de um procedimento cirúrgico de tração completa; é comum a existência de metástase; o debridamento do tumor por via transcolônica pode conferir o alívio da obstrução.

MEDICAÇÕES

MEDICAMENTO(S)
- Quimioterapia — há apenas relatos breves; em geral, não é bem-sucedida.
- Piroxicam — 0,3 mg/kg VO a cada 24 h pode representar um tratamento paliativo para os tumores do intestino grosso e do reto.

CONTRAINDICAÇÕES/INTERAÇÕES POSSÍVEIS
Antes de iniciar o tratamento com medicamentos citotóxicos, deve-se buscar orientação especializada.

ACOMPANHAMENTO

Exame físico, radiografias torácicas e ultrassonografia abdominal — em 1, 3, 6, 9 e 12 meses após a cirurgia.

EVOLUÇÃO ESPERADA E PROGNÓSTICO
Cães
- No geral, o prognóstico é mau; tumores retais pedunculados têm um prognóstico melhor; a maioria dos casos apresenta recidiva local, desenvolve metástase ou sofre ambos os processos com rapidez.
- Sobrevida média do adenocarcinoma no estômago — 2 meses.
- Sobrevida média do adenocarcinoma no intestino delgado — 10 meses.
- Sobrevida média do adenocarcinoma no intestino grosso — 1,6 meses (anular) *versus* 32 meses (pedunculado).

Gatos
- Prognóstico reservado.
- Há poucos casos relatados; no entanto, eles podem exibir sobrevida prolongada (>1 ano).

DIVERSOS

Sugestões de Leitura

Crawshaw J, Berg J, Sardinas JC, et al. Prognosis for dogs with nonlymphomatous small intestinal tumors treated by surgical excision. JAAHA 1998, 34:451-456.

Lubbes D, Mandigers PJ, Heuven HC, et al. [Incidence of gastric carcinoma in Dutch Tervueren shepherd dogs born between 1991 and 2002]. Tijdschr Diergeneeskd 2009, 134:606-610.

Morrison WB. Nonlymphomatous cancers of the esophagus, stomach, and intestines. In: Morrison WB, ed., Cancer in Dogs and Cats: Medical and Surgical. Jackson, WY: Teton NewMedia, 2002, pp. 527-534.

Swann HM, Holt DE. Canine gastric adenocarcinoma and leiomyosarcoma: A retrospective study of 21 cases (1986-1999) and literature review. JAAHA 2002, 38:157-164.

Takiguchi M, Yasuda J, Hashimoto A, et al. Esophageal/gastric adenocarcinoma in a dog. JAAHA 1997, 33:42-44.

Autor Laura D. Garrett
Consultor Editorial Timothy M. Fan

Adenocarcinoma do Pâncreas

CONSIDERAÇÕES GERAIS

REVISÃO
- Tumor maligno de origem ductal ou acinar, originário do pâncreas exócrino.
- Costuma ter sofrido metástase até o momento do diagnóstico.

IDENTIFICAÇÃO
- Raro em cães — 0,5-1,8% de todos os tumores.
- Raro em gatos — 2,8% de todos os tumores.
- As cadelas com idade mais avançada e a raça Airedale terrier exibem um risco mais elevado do que outros animais.
- Idade média (cães) — 9,2 anos.

SINAIS CLÍNICOS
- Inespecíficos — febre; vômito; fraqueza; anorexia; icterícia; má digestão; perda de peso.
- Dor abdominal — variável.
- É comum a ocorrência de metástases para tecidos ósseos e moles.
- Há relatos de fraturas patológicas secundárias à metástase.
- Massa abdominal.
- Pode haver síndromes paraneoplásicas de necrose epidérmica, hiperinsulinemia e hiperglucagonemia.

CAUSAS E FATORES DE RISCO
Desconhecidos.

DIAGNÓSTICO

DIAGNÓSTICO DIFERENCIAL
- Pancreatite primária; pode ser um quadro concomitante e complicar ou retardar o diagnóstico precoce.
- Pseudocisto pancreático.
- Hiperplasia nodular pancreática.
- Neoplasia hepática.
- Outras causas de vômito e icterícia.

HEMOGRAMA/BIOQUÍMICA/URINÁLISE
- Em geral, as alterações são inespecíficas (p. ex., anemia branda e neutrofilia).
- A hiperamilasemia é menos confiável do que a hiperlipasemia.
- Com frequência, a concentração da lipase encontra-se acentuadamente elevada e pode ser de origem tumoral; portanto, essa mensuração pode servir como um marcador bioquímico não invasivo de neoplasia do pâncreas e do fígado em cães.

OUTROS TESTES LABORATORIAIS
Raramente, pode haver alterações metabólicas significativas que afetam as concentrações do glucagon, da insulina e de aminoácidos.

DIAGNÓSTICO POR IMAGEM
- Radiografias abdominais podem revelar a presença de massa ou perda de detalhes da serosa associadas à pancreatite concomitante.
- Ultrassonografia pode demonstrar a existência de massa ou pancreatite concomitante (ecogenicidade mista, pâncreas aumentado de volume, gordura peripancreática hiperecoica). Podem ser identificadas alterações como espessamento pancreático, efusão abdominal e nódulos isolados a múltiplos de tamanho variado. Pode ser impossível diferenciar os achados sonográficos de adenocarcinoma do pâncreas com hiperplasia nodular pancreática. Raras vezes, o ultrassom do pâncreas pode parecer normal, exceto pela dilatação do ducto pancreático.

MÉTODOS DIAGNÓSTICOS
- Biopsia cirúrgica — diagnóstico definitivo.
- Citologia de aspirado por agulha fina — diagnóstico de apoio.

TRATAMENTO

- Não há relato de nenhum tratamento curativo bem-sucedido.
- Alívio da dor, bem como de obstrução intestinal e biliar — cirurgia, em caso de necessidade.
- Pancreatectomia parcial ou total.
- Tratar a pancreatite concomitante.
- Antieméticos e cuidados de suporte (hidratação e necessidades calóricas).

MEDICAÇÕES

MEDICAMENTO(S)
- A gencitabina é utilizada em seres humanos para o tratamento de carcinoma pancreático; apesar de ser usado em cães, esse agente não foi estabelecido como o padrão de cuidado em animais dessa espécie com adenocarcinoma pancreático.
- Sempre se deve consultar um veterinário especialista em oncologia em busca das atualizações no tratamento dessa rara neoplasia.

CONTRAINDICAÇÕES/INTERAÇÕES POSSÍVEIS
N/D.

ACOMPANHAMENTO

COMPLICAÇÕES POSSÍVEIS
Obstrução intestinal
- Obstrução biliar.
- Abscesso pancreático.
- Peritonite.
- Metástase.

EVOLUÇÃO ESPERADA E PROGNÓSTICO
A evolução ao óbito é frequentemente rápida em virtude da indisponibilidade de qualquer tratamento curativo bem-sucedido.

DIVERSOS

DISTÚRBIOS ASSOCIADOS
Carcinoma pancreático secretor de gastrina (gastrinoma) foi relatado em cães e gatos. Os sinais clínicos são associados à hipergastrinemia, o que resulta em secreção inadequada de ácido clorídrico pelo estômago, levando à gastroduodenite.

Sugestões de Leitura

Cave T, Evans H, Hargreavest J, et al. Metabolic epidermal necrosis in a dog associated with pancreatic adenocarcinoma, hyperglucagonaemia, hyperinsulinaemia, and hypoaminoacidaemia. J Small Anim Pract 2007, 48:522-526.

Hecht S, Penninck DG, Keating JH. Imaging findings in pancreatic neoplasia and nodular hyperplasia in 19 cats. Vet Radiol Ultrasound 2006, 48:45-50.

Lurcye JC, Behrend EN. Endocrine tumors. Vet Clin North Am Small Anim Pract 2001, 31:1083-1110.

Morrison WB. Primary cancers and cancer-like lesions of the liver, biliary epithelium, and exocrine pancreas. In: Morrison WB, ed., Cancer in Dogs and Cats: Medical and Surgical Management. Jackson, WY: Teton NewMedia, 2002, pp. 535-544.

Newman SJ, Steiner JM, Woosley K, et al. Correlation of age and incidence of pancreatic exocrine nodular hyperplasia in the dog. Vet Pathol 2005, 42:510-513.

Quigley KA, Jackson ML, Haines DM. Hyperlipasemia in 6 dogs with pancreatic or hepatic neoplasia: Evidence for tumor lipase production. Vet Clin Pathol 2001, 30:114-120.

Autor Wallace B. Morrison
Consultor Editorial Timothy M. Fan

Adenocarcinoma dos Pulmões

CONSIDERAÇÕES GERAIS

REVISÃO
- Compreende 75% dos tumores pulmonares primários em cães e gatos. • São tumores pulmonares primários raros em cães e gatos. • Os indicadores mais fortes do desfecho incluem o grau do tumor, o envolvimento dos nodos e os sinais clínicos do paciente. • Pode sofrer metástase. • Pode ser associado à osteopatia hipertrófica.

IDENTIFICAÇÃO
Cães
- Representa 1% de todos os tumores. • A idade média dos animais acometidos é de 10 anos, embora a maioria seja mais idosa. • Não há sexo predominante, embora haja o envolvimento de mais fêmeas em alguns relatos. • Os cães da raça Boxer ou as raças braquicefálicas podem ser predispostos. • As raças de médio a grande porte são super-representadas.

Gatos
- Mais raro do que nos cães. • A idade média dos animais acometidos é de 11 anos. • Não há raça predominante. • Alguns estudos sugerem uma super-representação das fêmeas.

SINAIS CLÍNICOS
Achados Anamnésicos

Relacionados com a Presença de Massa Pulmonar
- Tosse improdutiva (>50% dos cães). • Dispneia (pode estar relacionada com pneumotórax). • Taquipneia. • Perda de peso. • Hemoptise. • Dor — envolvimento pleural.

Sinais Paraneoplásicos
- Claudicação — metástase óssea ou osteopatia hipertrófica (cães ou gatos), metástase lítica dos dedos de sustentação do peso (gatos). • Poliúria ou polidipsia — hipercalcemia ou hiperadrenocorticismo decorrente da produção ectópica do ACTH. • Fraqueza ou emaciação muscular — polineuropatia; polimiopatia.

Achados do Exame Físico
- O animal pode permanecer assintomático. • Taquipneia e dispneia. • Febre. • Tumefação dos membros. • Efusão pleural. • Síndrome da veia cava.

CAUSAS E FATORES DE RISCO
- Potencial risco de ambiente urbano. • Potencial exposição passiva à fumaça de cigarro.

DIAGNÓSTICO

DIAGNÓSTICO DIFERENCIAL
- Lesão granulomatosa (por fungo, corpo estranho, parasita). • Granulomatose linfomatoide ou eosinofílica. • Abscesso pulmonar. • Outro tumor pulmonar primário. • Tumor pulmonar metastático. • Pneumonia. • Asma. • Tromboembolia pulmonar. • Cisto congênito. • Torção ou hematoma pulmonares.

HEMOGRAMA/BIOQUÍMICA/URINÁLISE
Não há anormalidades específicas.

OUTROS TESTES LABORATORIAIS
- Gasometria arterial. • Os tempos de coagulação devem ser mensurados antes da obtenção de aspirado ou da realização de biopsia.

DIAGNÓSTICO POR IMAGEM
- Radiografia torácica — costuma revelar a presença de massa focal, solitária e bem circunscrita; deve ser obtida em gatos que se apresentam com múltiplos tumores nos dedos para fazer a triagem de tumor pulmonar primário (síndrome do baqueteamento digital por tumor nos pulmões). • Ultrassonografia — pode ajudar não só na obtenção de material aspirado ou amostra de biopsia, mas também na avaliação do abdome. • TC — avaliação mais precisa para determinar a viabilidade da cirurgia e identificar a presença de linfadenopatia (precisão de 93%) e doença metastática.

MÉTODOS DIAGNÓSTICOS
- Toracocentese com exame citológico — em caso de efusão pleural. • Citologia — aspirado transtorácico por agulha fina (concordância de 83% com a histopatologia); o exame citológico pode ser guiado por técnicas de diagnóstico por imagem como TC ou fluoroscopia; em caso de localização periférica do tumor contra a parede torácica, pode-se usar o ultrassom. • Biopsia tecidual percutânea — utilizar o instrumento do tipo Tru-Cut®. • Biopsia pulmonar aberta — obtenção de amostra via toracoscopia minimamente invasiva ou toracotomia.

ACHADOS PATOLÓGICOS
- Adenocarcinoma — classificado de acordo com a localização (bronquial, bronquiolar, bronquíolo-alveolar ou alveolar) e o grau de diferenciação. • Positividade do fator de transcrição da tireoide-1 — pode distinguir carcinoma primário de metastático. • Tumores indiferenciados — maior invasividade e maior probabilidade de metástase, em comparação aos tumores bem diferenciados; os locais de metástase incluem linfonodos, ossos, pleura, olhos (coroide) e SNC. • Os gatos tendem a ter tumores pouco diferenciados, correspondendo a um comportamento mais agressivo.

TRATAMENTO

- Cirurgia — representa a base do tratamento; lobectomia parcial ou completa com biopsia ou remoção dos linfonodos traqueobrônquicos. • Radioterapia — embora os relatos não tenham comprovação científica nem verificação experimental, determinados pacientes podem se beneficiar desse tratamento. • Quimioterapia — deve ser considerada após a cirurgia para tumores de alto grau, indiferenciados e/ou com envolvimento nodal. Centros cirúrgicos seletos podem oferecer quimioterapia inalatória para se obter concentrações locais mais elevadas com poucos efeitos colaterais sistêmicos. • Quimioterapia intracavitária — pode ser usada para tratar a efusão pleural.

MEDICAÇÕES

MEDICAMENTO(S)
- A vinorelbina concentra-se nos pulmões e, por isso, foram observadas respostas clínicas. • Doxorrubicina, cisplatina, carboplatina, mitoxantrona, vinorelbina e/ou vindesina — escolhas racionais para o tratamento paliativo.

CONTRAINDICAÇÕES/INTERAÇÕES POSSÍVEIS
- Doxorrubicina — monitorizar rigorosamente os pacientes com cardiopatia subjacente; considerar o pré-tratamento com difenidramina e a obtenção de ecocardiogramas e ECGs seriados. • Cisplatina — não fornecer aos gatos (fatal); não usar em cães com nefropatia preexistente; nunca utilizar esse medicamento sem uma diurese apropriada e concomitante.

ACOMPANHAMENTO

MONITORIZAÇÃO DO PACIENTE
- Radiografias torácicas seriadas — considerar esse exame a cada 3 meses; administrar no mínimo dois ciclos de quimioterapia antes de avaliar a resposta ao tratamento. • Efetuar os exames de hemograma completo (com qualquer quimioterapia) e perfil da função renal (cisplatina) antes de cada tratamento quimioterápico.

COMPLICAÇÕES POSSÍVEIS
Pneumotórax ou hemotórax.

EVOLUÇÃO ESPERADA E PROGNÓSTICO
- Metástase para os linfonodos traqueobrônquicos — o único indicador prognóstico mais satisfatório; a sobrevida média sem metástase chega a 1 ano e, com metástase, a 60 dias. • A sobrevida pós-operatória em cães (~1 ano) é melhor que em gatos (~4 meses), mas gira em torno de 2 anos em qualquer uma das espécies se houver fatores prognósticos positivos. • Outros fatores (relacionados com o paciente, o tumor e o tratamento) que influenciam o prognóstico — excisão cirúrgica completa; tamanho do tumor primário (<5 cm tem prognóstico melhor); metástase (prognóstico melhor na ausência de metástase); grau de diferenciação celular (escore histológico; prognóstico melhor se bem diferenciado), ausência de sinais clínicos antes da cirurgia.

DIVERSOS

GESTAÇÃO/FERTILIDADE/REPRODUÇÃO
A quimioterapia não é aconselhável em animais prenhes.

ABREVIATURA(S)
- ACTH = hormônio adrenocorticotrófico.
- ECG = eletrocardiograma.
- SNC = sistema nervoso central.
- TC = tomografia computadorizada.

Sugestões de Leitura
Paoloni MC, Adams WM, Dubielzig RR, et al. Comparison of results of computed tomography and radiography with histopathologic findings in tracheobronchial lymph nodes in dogs with primary lung tumors: 14 cases (1999-2002). JAVMA 2006, 228(11):1718-1722.
Rissetto KC, Lucas P, Fan TM. An update on diagnosing and treating primary lung tumors. Vet Med 2008, 103(3):154.

Autor Kim A. Selting
Consultor Editorial Timothy M. Fan
Agradecimento Renee Al-Saraff

Adenocarcinoma dos Sacos Anais

CONSIDERAÇÕES GERAIS

REVISÃO
- Neoplasia maligna rara derivada de glândulas apócrinas dos sacos anais.
- Localmente invasiva.
- Alto índice metastático, muitas vezes para os linfonodos sublombares.
- Frequentemente associado à hipercalcemia, em decorrência da secreção do peptídeo relacionado com o paratormônio (PTHrP) pelas células tumorais.
- Prognóstico reservado a mau.

IDENTIFICAÇÃO
- Cães com idade mais avançada; extremamente raro em gatos.
- As fêmeas são super-representadas em alguns estudos de pequeno porte, mas não em estudos mais amplos.
- Pode haver um risco elevado em caso de castração (particularmente nos machos).
- Os cães da raça Cocker spaniel são significativamente super-representados; as raças Springer spaniel e Cavalier King Charles spaniel também são super-representadas.

SINAIS CLÍNICOS
Achados Anamnésicos
Podem ser decorrentes do tumor primário (massa retal, tenesmo), da metástase aos linfonodos locais (tenesmo, constipação, estrangúria) ou da hipercalcemia (anorexia, poliúria/polidipsia, letargia).

Achados do Exame Físico
- Massa associada aos sacos anais; pode ser muito pequena apesar da doença metastática maciça.
- Linfadenopatia sublombar — à palpação retal ou abdominal.

CAUSAS E FATORES DE RISCO
Suposto papel hormonal.

DIAGNÓSTICO

DIAGNÓSTICO DIFERENCIAL
- Abscesso dos sacos anais.
- Adenoma/adenocarcinoma perianais.
- Mastocitoma.
- Linfoma.
- Carcinoma de células escamosas.
- Hérnias perineais.

HEMOGRAMA/BIOQUÍMICA/URINÁLISE
- Hipercalcemia — 25-50% dos casos.
- É possível o desenvolvimento de insuficiência renal secundária.

OUTROS TESTES LABORATORIAIS
Níveis do paratormônio (PTH) e do PTHrP — os níveis elevados do último ajudarão a confirmar a neoplasia como a causa da hipercalcemia.

DIAGNÓSTICO POR IMAGEM
- Radiografia abdominal — para avaliar os linfonodos sublombares, bem como os ossos lombares e pélvicos.
- Radiografia torácica — para pesquisar a presença de metástase pulmonar.
- Ultrassonografia abdominal — além de nódulos no fígado/baço, esse exame pode identificar os linfonodos sublombares levemente infartados não visualizados por meio radiográfico.

MÉTODOS DIAGNÓSTICOS
- Aspirado (por agulha fina) de massa dos sacos anais para descartar outras condições, que não sejam adenocarcinoma; a diferenciação entre neoplasia benigna *versus* maligna das massas perianais não é uma tarefa fácil.
- Aspirado (por agulha fina) de linfonodos infartados, fígado ou nódulos esplênicos para confirmar a ocorrência de metástase.
- Há necessidade de biopsia incisional com exame histopatológico para a formulação do diagnóstico definitivo, embora a biopsia excisional possa ser adequada se a localização da massa e o exame de citologia apoiarem uma neoplasia das glândulas anais.

TRATAMENTO
- Ressecção cirúrgica — tratamento de escolha.
- A cura é possível se detectado precocemente.
- A ressecção do tumor primário e dos linfonodos infartados pode prolongar a sobrevida.
- Se a massa for volumosa e regionalmente invasiva no momento do diagnóstico, a cirurgia será muitas vezes paliativa e não curativa.
- O debridamento de todo o tecido acometido pode controlar a hipercalcemia até que ocorra a recidiva do tumor.
- Se a hipercalcemia for grave, efetuar a diurese salina (200-300 mL/kg/dia) no pré-operatório.
- A radioterapia pode ajudar a retardar a recidiva local e controlar o crescimento das metástases sublombares — os efeitos colaterais agudos e crônicos da radiação podem ser moderados a graves.

MEDICAÇÕES

MEDICAMENTO(S)
- Há relatos limitados de respostas parciais aos compostos de platina em cães —cisplatina (70 mg/m^2 IV administrada com diurese salina em um período de 6 horas — 18,3 mL/kg/h), carboplatina (300 mg/m^2 IV administrada lentamente sob a forma de bólus) a cada 3 semanas.
- Mitoxantrona (5 mg/m^2 IV a cada 3 semanas por 5 tratamentos) em combinação com radioterapia foi usada em uma pequena série de casos.
- Possível papel da melfalana (7 mg/m^2 VO diariamente por 5 dias a cada 3 semanas) após a cirurgia de debridamento.

CONTRAINDICAÇÕES/INTERAÇÕES POSSÍVEIS
- Evitar agentes quimioterápicos de platina em cães com insuficiência renal.
- Não usar a cisplatina em gatos.

ACOMPANHAMENTO

MONITORIZAÇÃO DO PACIENTE
- Ressecção completa — exame físico, radiografia torácica, ultrassonografia abdominal e bioquímica sérica em 1, 3, 6, 9 e 12 meses do pós-operatório.
- Ressecção parcial — monitorizar o volume do tumor, bem como os valores sanguíneos do cálcio e a função renal.

EVOLUÇÃO ESPERADA E PROGNÓSTICO
- Prognóstico reservado com ocorrência tanto de invasão local como de metástase.
- Poderão ocorrer curas se o tumor for detectado no início e tratado de forma rigorosa.
- Como o crescimento do tumor pode ser lento, o debridamento da doença metastática em linfonodos pode significativamente prolongar a sobrevida.
- A hipercalcemia é variavelmente associada a um prognóstico mau.
- Quatro trabalhos (envolvendo 200 cães) revelaram tempos médios de sobrevida de 6 a 20 meses, dependendo do estágio tumoral e do tratamento.
- Um relato recente sobre 16 cães sem metástase revelou um tempo médio de sobrevida incompatível com um acompanhamento de 33 meses.
  ○ Os cães com metástase para linfonodos viviam significativamente mais se os nodos fossem extirpados.
- Por fim, os cães não submetidos à excisão completa de seus tumores sucumbem às complicações relacionadas com a hipercalcemia ou ao efeito expansivo do tumor primário ou de metástases nodais sublombares.

DIVERSOS

DISTÚRBIOS ASSOCIADOS
Hipercalcemia como uma síndrome paraneoplásica.

ABREVIATURA(S)
- PTHrP = peptídeo relacionado com o paratormônio.

Sugestões de Leitura
Anderson CR, McNeil EA, Gillette EL, et al. Late complications of pelvic irradiation in 16 dogs. Vet Radiol Ultrasound 2002, 43:187-192.
Emms SG. Anal sac tumours of the dog and their response to cytoreductive surgery and chemotherapy. Australian Vet J 2005, 83:340-343.
Polton GA, Brearley MJ. Clinical stage, therapy, and prognosis in canine anal sac gland carcinoma. J Vet Intern Med 2007, 21:274-280.
Turek MM, Forrest LJ, Adams WM, et al. Postoperative radiotherapy and mitoxantrone for anal sac adenocarcinoma in the dog: 15 cases (1991-2001). Vet Comp Onc 2003, 1:94-104.
Williams LE, Gliatto JM, Dodge RK, et al. Carcinoma of the apocrine glands of the anal sac in dogs: 113 cases (1985-1995). JAVMA 2003, 223:825-831.

Autor Laura D. Garrett
Consultor Editorial Timothy M. Fan

Adenocarcinoma Nasal

CONSIDERAÇÕES GERAIS

REVISÃO
• Representa menos de 5% de todos os tumores em cães e gatos. • Invasão local e regional progressiva da cavidade nasal, dos seios paranasais e dos tecidos circunjacentes por células epiteliais neoplásicas e glandulares. • Frequentemente já evoluiu para envolvimento bilateral no momento do diagnóstico. • Muitos se originam dos seios frontais. • Em cães, o adenocarcinoma nasal é mais comum que carcinoma de células escamosas, condrossarcoma e outros tumores. • Em gatos, o tumor mais comum dos seios nasais é o linfoma, seguido por adenocarcinoma e outros.

IDENTIFICAÇÃO
• Cães e gatos. • A idade média em cães é de 10 anos, mas de 13 anos para os gatos. • Os cães de médio a grande porte são mais comumente acometidos, com possível super-representação de raças mesocefálicas e dolicocefálicas.

SINAIS CLÍNICOS
Achados Anamnésicos
• Histórico intermitente e progressivo de epistaxe uni a bilateral e/ou secreção mucopurulenta (duração média, 3 meses). • Epífora. • Espirros e aumento dos ruídos respiratórios superiores. • Respiração de boca aberta. • Halitose. • Anorexia (mais frequente nos gatos). • Crises convulsivas (secundárias à invasão da abóbada craniana).

Achados do Exame Físico
• Secreção nasal (sanguinolenta, mucopurulenta). • Deformidade facial, exoftalmia. • Massa orbital invasiva (impossibilidade de retropulsão ocular). • Dor à palpação da cavidade nasal ou dos seios paranasais ou à abertura da boca. • Fluxo de ar (uni ou bilateral) diminuído ou ausente nas vias nasais. • Linfadenomegalia regional. • Atividade mental anormal ou outros achados neurológicos.

CAUSAS E FATORES DE RISCO
A morfologia dolicocefálica, o ambiente urbano e o tabagismo passivo podem desempenhar algum papel.

DIAGNÓSTICO

DIAGNÓSTICO DIFERENCIAL
• Outros tumores dos seios nasais (p. ex., carcinoma de células escamosas, linfoma, sarcomas). • Infecção viral — gatos. • Infecções fúngicas, incluindo aspergilose (cães) e criptococose (gatos). • Corpo(s) estranho(s). • Traumatismo. • Abscesso radicular dentário e fístula oronasal. • Coagulopatias. • Parasitas (p. ex., ácaros nasais). • Erliquiose, leishmaniose. • Hipertensão sistêmica. • Sinusite bacteriana — rara.

HEMOGRAMA/BIOQUÍMICA/URINÁLISE
• Costumam permanecer normais. • Ocasionalmente, há anemia por perda de sangue.

OUTROS TESTES LABORATORIAIS
• Exame citológico — ocasionalmente útil (p. ex., aspirados da massa subcutânea em caso de deformidade facial). • Perfil de coagulação.

DIAGNÓSTICO POR IMAGEM
• Radiografia simples do crânio — pode revelar a destruição assimétrica dos ossos turbinados, acompanhada por efeito expansivo de massa dos tecidos moles; pode-se observar densidade líquida nos seios frontais, secundariamente à obstrução ao fluxo de saída das secreções. • Radiografia torácica — pesquisar a presença de metástase pulmonar (incomum). • TC ou RM — melhor método para efetuar o estadiamento local e inspecionar a integridade da placa cribriforme ou a ocorrência de invasão orbital; tais técnicas também são usadas para planejamento terapêutico.

MÉTODOS DIAGNÓSTICOS
• Mensuração da pressão arterial. • Exame bucal completo sob anestesia. • Rinoscopia — permite uma inspeção direta da massa; evitar o avanço caudal do rinoscópio em direção à placa cribriforme. Esse procedimento pode ser dispensado em caso de massa confirmada por técnicas avançadas de diagnóstico por imagem ou mediante a identificação de deformidade facial. • Biopsia tecidual — necessária para a formulação do diagnóstico definitivo. As biopsias podem ser realizadas às cegas, após técnicas avançadas de diagnóstico por imagem, com o uso de pinça de biopsia, cânula (sucção fechada) ou hidropulsão. • Avaliação citológica de linfonodos regionais — para detectar doença metastática.

TRATAMENTO

• A cirurgia isolada é ineficaz em virtude da extensão e da invasividade da doença. • Turbinectomia — pode ser efetuada antes ou depois de irradiação. • Radioterapia — constitui o tratamento-padrão, conferindo os melhores resultados clínicos em cães e gatos.

MEDICAÇÕES

MEDICAMENTO(S)
• A quimioterapia pode ser benéfica em alguns pacientes. Foram descritos vários medicamentos, incluindo cisplatina (apenas nos cães), carboplatina, doxorrubicina e piroxicam. Consultar um veterinário especialista em oncologia em busca de mais detalhes. • É recomendável o emprego de terapia analgésica adequada, conforme a necessidade, em pacientes que sofrem de doença invasiva com destruição óssea, sinais de dor e efeitos colaterais dolorosos da radioterapia. • Terapias recentes podem ser consideradas em casos irresponsivos à terapia-padrão.

CONTRAINDICAÇÕES/INTERAÇÕES POSSÍVEIS
Cisplatina — jamais utilizar em gatos.

ACOMPANHAMENTO

MONITORIZAÇÃO DO PACIENTE
Radiografia simples do crânio ou, de preferência, TC/RM mediante a recidiva dos sinais clínicos ou de forma periódica.

EVOLUÇÃO ESPERADA E PROGNÓSTICO
• Adenocarcinoma nasal não tratado — sobrevida média de 3-4 meses. • Radioterapia — tempos médios de sobrevida em torno de 12-18 meses em cães e 10-18 meses em gatos; taxa de sobrevida de 20-57% em 1 ano (cães e gatos); taxa de sobrevida de 20-48% em 2 anos (cães e gatos). • Presença de envolvimento cerebral ou doença metastática (estágio avançado) — indicador de prognóstico mau. • Complicações oftalmológicas decorrentes da radioterapia — mais prováveis em cães do que em gatos. • A ocorrência de rinite crônica é comum após radioterapia de tumores dos seios nasais, podendo necessitar de terapia sintomática.

DIVERSOS

ABREVIATURA(S)
• RM = ressonância magnética. • TC = tomografia computadorizada.

Sugestões de Leitura
Adams WA, Bjorling DE, McAnulty JF, et al. Outcome of accelerated radiotherapy alone or accelerated radiotherapy followed by exenteration of the nasal cavity in dogs with intranasal neoplasia: 53 cases (1990-2002). JAVMA 2005, 227:936-941.

Hahn KA, Knapp DW, Richardson RC, Matlock CL. Clinical response of nasal adenocarcinoma to cisplatin chemotherapy in 11 dogs. JAVMA 1992, 200:355-357.

Henry CJ, Brewer WG, Tyler JW, et al. Survival in dogs with nasal adenocarcinoma: 64 cases (1981-1995). J Vet Intern Med 1998, 12:436-439.

LaDue TA, Dodge R, Page RL, et al. Factors influencing survival after radiotherapy of nasal tumors in 130 dogs. Vet Radiol Ultrasound 1999, 40:312-317.

Langova V, Mutsaers AJ, Phillips B, Straw R. Treatment of eight dogs with nasal tumours with alternating doses of carboplatin and doxorubicin in conjunction with oral piroxicam. Australian Vet J 2004, 82:676-680.

Rassnick KM, Goldkamp CE, Erb HN, et al. Evaluation of factors associated with survival in dogs with untreated nasal carcinomas: 139 cases (1993-2003). JAVMA 2006, 229:401-406.

Autor Louis-Philippe de Lorimier
Consultor Editorial Timothy M. Fan

Adenocarcinoma Renal

CONSIDERAÇÕES GERAIS

REVISÃO
• Responde por <1% de todas as neoplasias relatadas em cães.
• Os tumores renais tendem a ser altamente metastáticos, localmente invasivos e muitas vezes bilaterais.
• Em cães da raça Pastor alemão, foi descrito o cistoadenocarcinoma renal, uma síndrome hereditária rara com comportamento menos agressivo e prognóstico melhor a longo prazo do que o adenocarcinoma renal.

IDENTIFICAÇÃO
• Adenocarcinoma — cães mais idosos (8-9 anos); proporção de machos:fêmeas, 1,6:1; não há raça predominante.
• Cistoadenocarcinoma — Pastor alemão, frequentemente as fêmeas.

SINAIS CLÍNICOS
• Adenocarcinoma — pode ser insidioso, com sinais inespecíficos (p. ex., perda de peso, inapetência, letargia, hematúria e mucosas pálidas).
• Cistoadenocarcinoma — pode estar associado a uma dermatofibrose nodular (síndrome de lesões fibrosas, firmes, indolores da pele e dos tecidos subcutâneos).

CAUSAS E FATORES DE RISCO
• Adenocarcinoma — desconhecidos.
• Cistoadenocarcinoma — hereditário em cães Pastor alemão.

DIAGNÓSTICO

DIAGNÓSTICO DIFERENCIAL
• Outra neoplasia primária — linfoma; nefroblastoma.
• Neoplasia metastática — hemangiossarcoma.
• Adenoma ou cisto renais.
• Pielonefrite.

HEMOGRAMA/BIOQUÍMICA/URINÁLISE
• Hemograma completo pode exibir policitemia, leucocitose ou anemia paraneoplásicas.
• Bioquímica pode permanecer normal ou revelar azotemia.
• Urinálise pode demonstrar hematúria, proteinúria, bacteriúria ou cilindros.

OUTROS TESTES LABORATORIAIS
Cultura e antibiograma urinários.

DIAGNÓSTICO POR IMAGEM
• Radiografias torácicas — doença metastática relatada em até 16% dos pacientes.
• Radiografias abdominais — massa observada em 81% dos pacientes.
• Ultrassonografia abdominal, TC ou radiografia contrastada — úteis para identificação e estadiamento da doença.

MÉTODOS DIAGNÓSTICOS
Biopsia renal (guiada por ultrassom ou cirúrgica) para obtenção do diagnóstico definitivo.

TRATAMENTO

• A excisão cirúrgica rigorosa é o tratamento de escolha para doença unilateral.
• Não foi descrito tratamento quimioterápico bem-sucedido para adenocarcinoma ou cistoadenocarcinoma.
• Talvez haja necessidade de cuidados de suporte para os pacientes com insuficiência renal.

MEDICAÇÕES

MEDICAMENTO(S)
Nenhum.

CONTRAINDICAÇÕES/INTERAÇÕES POSSÍVEIS
N/D.

ACOMPANHAMENTO

MONITORIZAÇÃO DO PACIENTE
• Insuficiência renal — mensurar os níveis séricos de ureia e creatinina; urinálise.
• Qualidade de vida — avaliar nos animais com doença bilateral ou sem possibilidade de tratamento cirúrgico.

PREVENÇÃO
N/D.

COMPLICAÇÕES POSSÍVEIS
• Insuficiência renal.
• Doença metastática.
• Invasão de estruturas vitais locais — veia cava; aorta.

EVOLUÇÃO ESPERADA E PROGNÓSTICO
• Adenocarcinoma — a sobrevida média relatada de 49 cães foi de 16 meses (variação de 0-59 meses).
• Cistoadenocarcinoma — há poucos estudos de grande escala sobre essa doença rara; sobrevida média relatada de 12 meses ou mais, sem nenhum tratamento definitivo.

DIVERSOS

DISTÚRBIOS ASSOCIADOS
• Há relatos de síndromes paraneoplásicas de osteopatia hipertrófica, policitemia e leucocitose neutrofílica em casos isolados
• Insuficiência renal.
• Dermatofibrose nodular e leiomioma uterino são comumente associados ao cistoadenocarcinoma.

ABREVIATURA(S)
• TC = tomografia computadorizada.

Sugestões de Leitura
Bryan JN, et al. Primary renal neoplasia of dogs. J Vet Intern Med 2006, 20:1155-1160.
Knapp DW. Tumors of the urinary system. In: Withrow SJ, Vail DM, eds., Small Animal Clinical Oncology, 4th ed. Philadelphia: Saunders, 2007, pp. 649-658.

Autor Ruthanne Chun
Consultor Editorial Timothy M. Fan

ADENOMA HEPATOCELULAR

CONSIDERAÇÕES GERAIS

REVISÃO
• Tumor hepático benigno de origem epitelial.
• Mais comum que tumores hepáticos malignos primários.

IDENTIFICAÇÃO
• Raro em cães e muito raro em gatos. • Os cães acometidos costumam ter mais de 10 anos de idade. • Predisposições raciais desconhecidas.

SINAIS CLÍNICOS
• Em geral, o quadro permanece assintomático; quando presentes, no entanto, os sinais podem ser inespecíficos. • A ruptura aguda do tumor pode ocasionar hemoperitônio, resultando em fraqueza. • Ocasionalmente, os tumores podem causar dor abdominal cranial, vômitos e inapetência.

CAUSAS E FATORES DE RISCO
Não se conhece a causa exata para o desenvolvimento do tumor; entretanto, a tumorigênese pode ser associada à inflamação crônica ou a insulto hepatotóxico.

DIAGNÓSTICO

DIAGNÓSTICO DIFERENCIAL
• Adenocarcinoma hepático. • Abscesso hepático.
• Massa abdominal. • Esplenomegalia.
• Hiperplasia nodular.

HEMOGRAMA/BIOQUÍMICA/URINÁLISE

Hemograma Completo
• Geralmente normal. • Anemia — regenerativa se o tumor estiver sangrando. • Leucocitose com desvio à esquerda — tumores com centros necróticos.

Bioquímica
• Níveis de atividade variáveis das enzimas hepáticas. • Fosfatase alcalina, ALT, AST — normais ou leve a acentuadamente elevadas.
• Valores séricos de bilirrubina total — geralmente normais.

Urinálise
• Sem anormalidades significativas.

OUTROS TESTES LABORATORIAIS
• Ácidos biliares séricos costumam permanecer normais a menos que o crescimento do tumor comprometa a perfusão hepática e o fluxo de bile na porta hepática. • Raramente, ocorrem anormalidades de coagulação compatíveis com CID associadas a grandes tumores necróticos e hemorrágicos.

DIAGNÓSTICO POR IMAGEM

Radiografia
• Pode demonstrar uma única lesão expansiva tipo massa ou assimetria aparente da silhueta hepática.
• Raramente, observa-se a presença de gás no centro necrótico do tumor.

Ultrassonografia Abdominal
• Pode identificar leve efeito de massa com ecogenicidade variável, ditado pela presença de necrose intratumoral, hemorragia, gás ou cavidades císticas. • A massa tumoral primária pode ser tão volumosa a ponto de dificultar a obtenção de medidas precisas. • Padrão ecogênico misto — mais comum.

Tomografia Computadorizada Abdominal
• Pode permitir uma avaliação mais aprimorada quanto à viabilidade da cirurgia. • Pode detectar áreas necróticas e/ou hemorragia intraparenquimatosa.

MÉTODOS DIAGNÓSTICOS
• Citologia hepática por aspiração com o uso de agulha de calibre 22 e 4 cm de comprimento sob orientação ultrassonográfica permite a identificação de hepatócitos normais ou células com leve atipia. • Biopsia hepática com agulha; por haver a necessidade de várias biopsias do centro para obtenção de tecido suficiente para caracterização histopatológica, ela não é recomendada (uma quantidade insuficiente de tecido pode prejudicar a caracterização precisa); o adenoma hepatocelular costuma ser confundido com nódulos regenerativos ou hiperplásicos; a histopatologia de massa submetida à ressecção constitui o método diagnóstico preferível; é recomendável uma ressecção ampla, pois a massa pode ser um carcinoma hepatocelular.

ACHADOS PATOLÓGICOS

Macroscópicos
• Em geral, apresenta-se como nódulos isolados bem circunscritos com menos de 10 cm de diâmetro. • Podem ser amarelo-acastanhados.
• Com frequência, os nódulos são moles, altamente vasculares e friáveis. • Ocasionalmente, múltiplos. • Eventualmente, muito grandes (com mais de 20 cm).

Microscópicos
• Pode ser difícil distinguir de hiperplasia nodular ou tecido hepático normal; pode ser formulado um diagnóstico errôneo de carcinoma hepatocelular. • Em geral, exibe um padrão trabecular bem definido; não necessariamente encapsulado. • É comum a compressão de parênquima hepático adjacente. • Figuras mitóticas são pouco frequentes. • As células hepáticas acometidas lembram hepatócitos normais, mas geralmente são maiores e têm citosol transparente. • Ausência visível de tratos portais.
• Padrão de reticulina normal ajuda a diferenciar adenomas de nódulos regenerativos e carcinoma hepatocelular.

TRATAMENTO
• Cuidados sintomáticos para minimizar o desconforto. • Ambulatorial — apropriado a menos que o pós-operatório de intervenção cirúrgica necessite de cuidados críticos.
• Sangramento tumoral — requer transfusão de sangue; é aconselhável a excisão cirúrgica.
• Atividade — normal a menos que o aumento maciço de lobo hepático provoque desconforto ou hemorragia; internar em caso de sangramento ativo. • Recentemente, foi descrita a técnica de embolização transarterial com mistura de óleo iodado mais quimioterapia para tratar tumores amplos e não ressecáveis.

CONSIDERAÇÕES CIRÚRGICAS
• A excisão é recomendada para grandes lesões isoladas em forma de massa. • Entre 60-70% do fígado poderão ser submetidos à ressecção se o paciente receber cuidados críticos adequados.
• Efetuar biopsia de linfonodos locais e do fígado normal para avaliação histológica e comparação.

MEDICAÇÕES
Nenhuma.

ACOMPANHAMENTO

MONITORIZAÇÃO DO PACIENTE
• Palpação abdominal — a cada 3-4 meses; avaliar a ocorrência de recidiva (método de avaliação pouco produtivo). • Enzimas hepáticas — avaliação sequencial; avaliar a recidiva da liberação de enzimas associada à massa. • Ultrassonografia abdominal — a cada 3-4 meses no primeiro ano; método preferível de reavaliação.

COMPLICAÇÕES POSSÍVEIS
Risco de necrose tumoral e hemorragia abdominal maciça se não for submetido à ressecção.

EVOLUÇÃO ESPERADA E PROGNÓSTICO
Em geral, bons.

DIVERSOS

SINÔNIMO(S)
Hepatoma — termo confuso que deve ser evitado; diz respeito a carcinoma hepatocelular na medicina humana, embora seja considerado como sinônimo de adenoma hepatocelular na medicina veterinária.

VER TAMBÉM
Carcinoma Hepatocelular.

ABREVIATURA(S)
• ALT = alanina aminotransferase.
• AST = aspartato aminotransferase.
• CID = coagulação intravascular disseminada.

Sugestões de Leitura
Cave TA, Johnson V, Beths T, et al. Treatment of unresectable hepatocellular adenoma in dogs with transarterial iodized oil and chemotherapy with and without an embolic agent: A report of two cases. J Vet Comp Oncology 2004, 1:191-199.

Morrison WB. Primary cancers and cancer-like lesions of the liver, biliary epithelium, and exocrine pancreas. In: Morrison WB, ed., Cancer in Dogs and Cats: Medical and Surgical Management. Jackson, WY: Teton NewMedia, 2002, pp. 535-544.

Autor Wallace B. Morrison
Consultor Editorial Timothy M. Fan

Afogamento (Afogamento por um Triz)

CONSIDERAÇÕES GERAIS

REVISÃO
- Submersão na água, acompanhada pela sobrevida por no mínimo 24 h (i. e., afogamento por um triz). • Após a submersão, as elevações nos níveis de dióxido de carbono na corrente sanguínea estimulam a respiração e a subsequente aspiração de água. As quatro fases são as seguintes: (1) o animal prende a respiração e começa a nadar; (2) ocorrem a aspiração de água, a asfixia e o esforço de se debater; (3) vômito; e (4) interrupção do movimento seguida pelo óbito. • A aspiração de água doce dilui o surfactante pulmonar e leva ao colapso alveolar ± à pneumonia infecciosa. Já a aspiração de água salgada hipertônica (i. e., do mar) leva à difusão de água intersticial para os alvéolos. Tipicamente, não são aspirados grandes volumes de água; no entanto, independentemente da quantidade de água aspirada, ocorre um desequilíbrio entre os processos de ventilação e perfusão, conduzindo à hipoxemia e acidose metabólica. • O tempo de submersão, a temperatura da água e o tipo de água (doce *versus* salgada *versus* química) alterarão significativamente o desenvolvimento de dano orgânico. • Pode afetar os sistemas respiratório e cardiovascular em primeiro lugar e, depois, os sistemas neurológico, gastrintestinal, hêmico, renal e hepático.

IDENTIFICAÇÃO
Cães e gatos. Aproximadamente metade dos animais envolvidos em acidentes de imersão possui menos de 4 meses de vida.

SINAIS CLÍNICOS
- Observados agudamente após exposição à água.
- Cianose, apneia, angústia respiratória. • Tosse ± expectoração, de clara a vermelha espumosa.
- Vômito. • Embotamento até o estado de coma.
- Auscultação torácica de crepitações ou sibilos.
- Taquicardia ou bradicardia, assistolia.

CAUSAS E FATORES DE RISCO
- Maior risco próximo a reservatórios de água (inclusive piscinas), embora o afogamento dentro de casa seja comum (baldes, banheiras).
- Negligência do proprietário. • Precauções inadequadas de segurança. • Animais jovens (<4 meses de vida). • Os animais que se encontram na água ou próximos a ela no momento de crises convulsivas, traumatismos cranianos, eventos hipoglicêmicos, arritmias cardíacas ou síncopes estão sob risco de afogamento.

DIAGNÓSTICO

DIAGNÓSTICO DIFERENCIAL
- É recomendável descartar hipotermia, traumatismo cervical e meningite. • Na ocorrência de afogamento secundário a crises convulsivas, traumatismos cranianos, eventos hipoglicêmicos, arritmias cardíacas ou síncopes, devem-se realizar testes diagnósticos apropriados. Muitas vezes, a anamnese obtida no momento da consulta fornece diversas informações.

HEMOGRAMA/BIOQUÍMICA/URINÁLISE
- A inalação ou a ingestão de grandes quantidades de água doce pode levar à hemodiluição e hemólise, além de diminuir os níveis de sódio/cloreto e a densidade urinária. • A inalação ou a ingestão de água salgada hipertônica pode levar à hemoconcentração, mas aumentar os níveis de sódio/cloreto e a densidade urinária.

OUTROS TESTES LABORATORIAIS
A gasometria arterial revela hipoxemia (PaO_2<80 mmHg), hipoventilação ($PaCO_2$>50 mmHg) e distúrbios acidobásicos, como acidose respiratória ou metabólica (HCO_3<18 mEq/L).

DIAGNÓSTICO POR IMAGEM
- As alterações radiográficas podem não ser detectáveis por 24-48 h. • Há um padrão alveolar focal ou difuso, decorrente de pneumonia por aspiração ou edema pulmonar não cardiogênico.
- Pode haver padrões brônquicos, alveolares e intersticiais mistos, bem como um preenchimento das vias aéreas por material radiopaco ("broncograma aéreo"). • A inalação de corpos estranhos pode produzir atelectasia segmentar. • A evolução da lesão pulmonar para SARA é possível, podendo aparecer como infiltrados alveolares bilaterais, difusos e simétricos.

MÉTODOS DIAGNÓSTICOS
- Se o animal estiver estabilizado, indica-se a obtenção de lavado endotraqueal ou transtraqueal, com avaliação citológica e cultura/antibiograma.
- Também se recomenda a monitorização eletrocardiográfica. • Em casos selecionados, as radiografias da região cervical, a TC ou a RM do cérebro e a avaliação da RAETC podem ser úteis.

TRATAMENTO
- No local de ocorrência do afogamento, iniciar a reanimação com a respiração boca a focinho. • Há necessidade de uma internação de emergência. • A desobstrução das vias aéreas é prioridade, se estiverem obstruídas. • A ressuscitação cardiopulmonar pode ser necessária. • Deve-se proporcionar a suplementação de oxigênio. • Em animais com hipoxemia grave, hipercapnia ou fadiga respiratória iminente, poderá haver a necessidade de entubação e ventilação mecânica com pressão expiratória final positiva. • Não se recomendam a drenagem gravitacional ou as compressões abdominais (manobra de Heimlich) na ausência de obstrução das vias aéreas, por conta do alto risco de regurgitação e subsequente aspiração de conteúdo gástrico. • A fluidoterapia e a terapia acidobásica/eletrolítica são decisivas.
- Reaquecer os animais hipotérmicos gradativamente (em 2-3 h).

MEDICAÇÕES

MEDICAMENTO(S) DE ESCOLHA
- A terapia com manitol, 0,5 g/kg IV durante 20 min, pode ser benéfica em animais com suspeita de edema cerebral e pressões intracranianas elevadas.
- Em casos de pneumonia por aspiração, pode ser indispensável a administração de antibióticos de amplo espectro (p. ex., ampicilina, 22 mg/kg IV a cada 8 h, e enrofloxacino, 10-20 mg/kg IV a cada 24 h nos cães ou 5 mg/kg IV a cada 24 h nos gatos). • Em animais com suspeita de broncospasmo, os β-2 agonistas podem ser úteis.

CONTRAINDICAÇÕES
- Não se indica a terapia com corticosteroides em vítimas de afogamentos; além disso, o uso desses agentes pode ser nocivo em animais com pneumonia por aspiração. • O emprego de enrofloxacino em animais jovens pode causar erosão cartilaginosa.

ACOMPANHAMENTO

MONITORIZAÇÃO DO PACIENTE
- Efetuar a monitorização frequente ou contínua de alguns itens, como: frequência e ritmo cardíacos, frequência respiratória, coloração das mucosas e tempo de preenchimento capilar, débito urinário, pressão sanguínea arterial, temperatura retal, estado neurológico, ± pressão venosa central.
- Conforme a necessidade, é recomendável a avaliação de gasometria sanguínea arterial, hemograma completo, perfil bioquímico, coagulograma e estado acidobásico.

PREVENÇÃO
Monitorização rigorosa dos animais (especialmente os jovens), que se encontram próximos a reservatórios de água.

COMPLICAÇÕES POSSÍVEIS
Pneumonia por aspiração, edema pulmonar não cardiogênico, SARA, sangramento gastrintestinal, diarreia, vômito, insuficiência renal aguda, distúrbios neurológicos permanentes, CID, diabetes insípido central.

EVOLUÇÃO ESPERADA E PROGNÓSTICO
Relacionados diretamente com o estado do animal no momento da admissão hospitalar: os pacientes que se apresentam comatosos, estão gravemente acidóticos (pH <7,0) ou necessitam de ressuscitação cardiopulmonar ou ventilação mecânica exibem prognóstico mau. Os animais que se mostram conscientes têm prognóstico bom caso não ocorra nenhuma complicação.

DIVERSOS

ABREVIATURA(S)
- CID = coagulação intravascular disseminada.
- RAETC = resposta auditiva evocada do tronco cerebral.
- RM = ressonância magnética.
- SARA = síndrome da angústia respiratória aguda.
- TC = tomografia computadorizada.

Sugestões de Leitura
Powell LL. Accidental drowning and submersion injury. In: King LG, ed., Textbook of Respiratory Disease in Dogs and Cats. St. Louis: Saunders, 2004, pp. 484-486.

Autor Deborah C. Silverstein
Consultor Editorial Lynelle R. Johnson

AGRESSIVIDADE — VISÃO GERAL — CÃES

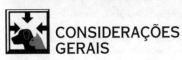

CONSIDERAÇÕES GERAIS

DEFINIÇÃO
• Ação produzida por um cão e direcionada contra outro organismo vivo, resultando em dano, limitação ou privação desse ser.
• Existem inúmeros tipos funcionais. Nesse caso, a agressividade é classificada com base em duas categorias: ofensiva ou defensiva.
• A agressividade ofensiva é uma reação não provocada, mas direcionada contra um indivíduo a fim de controlar o acesso a algum recurso à custa desse indivíduo; inclui agressividade por domínio/*status* social, agressividade possessiva, agressividade entre machos ou entre fêmeas e agressividade predatória. Os alvos comuns são pessoas familiares.
• A agressividade defensiva é direcionada contra um indivíduo encarado como um instigador ou uma ameaça; compreende as agressividades motivadas por medo, por defesa territorial, por proteção e por irritação (associada à dor ou relacionada com frustração), bem como as maternas. Os alvos comuns são pessoas não familiares.
• A probabilidade de agressividade manifesta pode ser influenciada por motivação, agitação e ansiedade. Os incidentes específicos podem envolver componentes ofensivos e defensivos.
• Em todos os casos, é imprescindível descartar as explicações médicas (inclusive a dor).

FISIOPATOLOGIA
• A agressividade é uma forma normal de comunicação nos cães.
• Alguns estados patológicos são associados a um aumento na agressividade, em decorrência dos efeitos gerados sobre o SNC.
• Síndrome de raiva/agressividade impulsiva, direcionada geralmente contra indivíduos familiares; foram implicadas anormalidades no sistema neurotransmissor serotoninérgico do SNC.
• A agressividade pode ter um componente aprendido, levando a um aumento nesse comportamento com o passar do tempo.
• Exceto nos casos de autodefesa real, as técnicas de confronto não devem ser usadas para controlar a agressividade. Apesar de serem amplamente promovidas, as técnicas de controle por confronto aumentam a probabilidade de agressão defensiva motivada pelo medo, induzindo a um incremento na frequência desse comportamento com o passar do tempo.

SISTEMA(S) ACOMETIDO(S)
Comportamental.

GENÉTICA
• Algumas tendências agressivas específicas à raça e estilos de mordida foram selecionadas para programas reprodutivos, embora isso não possa predizer o comportamento de cada cão.
• Um único estudo relacionou cães agressivos da raça Springer spaniel inglês a um único macho reprodutor, implicando um componente hereditário.

INCIDÊNCIA/PREVALÊNCIA
• A agressividade canina é a categoria diagnóstica mais comum observada pelos veterinários especialistas em comportamento nos EUA.
• De acordo com o Centro Norte-americano de Controle e Prevenção de Doenças (2009), cerca de 4,7 milhões de pessoas são mordidas por cães todo ano nos EUA.
• Quase 1 dentre 5 pessoas que são mordidas (um total de 885.000) necessita de atendimento médico para lesões relacionadas com mordidas de cães.
• Entre adultos e crianças, é mais provável que indivíduos do sexo masculino sejam mordidos em comparação aos do sexo feminino.
• A taxa de lesões relacionadas com mordidas de cães é mais alta para crianças de 5-9 anos de idade.

DISTRIBUIÇÃO GEOGRÁFICA
Mundial.

IDENTIFICAÇÃO
Espécies
Cães.

Raça(s) Predominante(s)
• Qualquer raça.
• As raças Pit bull e Rottweiler são as mais comumente implicadas em mordidas caninas fatais nos EUA, embora não haja a disponibilidade de frequências comparativas de agressividade com base na ocorrência racial.
• A reprodução seletiva para traços comportamentais pode predispor os cães a tipos específicos de agressividade; por exemplo, as raças caninas selecionadas para brigas entre cães podem ser agressivas contra outros cães.
• Os cães da raça Springer spaniel inglês parecem sob risco de agressividade impulsiva ("raiva").

Idade Média e Faixa Etária
• Qualquer idade.
• A agressividade comumente se torna mais problemática na maturidade social, 1-2 anos de idade.

Sexo(s) Predominante(s)
Machos — intactos ou castrados costumam ser os mais implicados em mordidas de cães.

SINAIS CLÍNICOS

Comentários Gerais
• Os sinais de alerta comportamental incluem imobilidade, rosnados ou abocanhadas.
  ◦ Ofensiva — cabeça ereta, cauda erguida e rígida, olhar fixo e direto, imobilidade na face.
  ◦ Defensiva — cabeça baixa, cauda abaixada, recuo do corpo, pata dianteira suspensa.
• Histórico — constitui a base para a análise do risco e os detalhes do programa terapêutico. Questões relevantes: em que circunstâncias ocorre a agressividade? Para quem é direcionada a agressão? Qual a gravidade das lesões resultantes?

Achados Anamnésicos
Variam de acordo com a situação e o tipo funcional da agressividade.

Agressividade Ofensiva
• Frequentemente direcionada contra os membros da família.
• Deflagradores (direcionados contra seres humanos): ao chegar perto do animal de estimação, passar a mão na cabeça, abordar ou deslocar o animal quando ele se encontra em locais elevados de repouso ou se aproximar de alimentos, brinquedos ou objetos furtados.

Agressividade Defensiva
• Direcionada com frequência contra seres humanos ou cães não familiares que se aproximam ou supervisionam o comportamento. Certas pessoas familiares podem ficar imunes.
• Pode ser específica ao local, como nos casos em que estranhos se aproximam da casa, do jardim ou do carro.
• Pode ser exacerbada se o animal for contido.
• À medida que a distância do estímulo diminui, a reação pode mudar para agitação, latido, bote e exibição dos dentes.
• O comportamento de aproximação e fuga é comum.
• A agressividade materna é direcionada contra indivíduos que se aproximam da área do parto ou dos filhotes.

Achados do Exame Físico
• Em geral, não são dignos de nota; não há sinais específicos universalmente associados a esse problema.
• As agressividades ofensivas e defensivas podem ser observadas durante o exame físico.
• É preciso ter extrema cautela ao manipular cães agressivos; utilizar focinheiras e outros dispositivos de contenção para evitar lesões ao examinador.
• Anormalidades no exame neurológico podem sugerir algum processo patológico orgânico (p. ex., raiva).

CAUSAS
• Está dentro dos limites de normalidade do comportamento; é fortemente influenciada por alguns fatores, como raça, sexo, socialização precoce, manipulação, temperamento individual e outras variáveis.
• Manifestação de uma condição orgânica — possível, mas rara.
• Em todos os casos, é fundamental descartar as causas clínicas de agressividade.

FATORES DE RISCO
• Machos, intactos.
• Socialização inadequada durante um período crítico (3-14 semanas).
• Experiência(s) traumática/negativa(s).
• Condições ambientais predisponentes — associação com outros cães em uma matilha; frustrações causadas por obstáculos ou correntes; crueldades e abusos, bem como provocações e brigas entre cães.
• Histórico prévio de agressividade/mordida (número de incidentes, alvo, gravidade da agressão); citação legal da mordida.
• Imprevisibilidade de incidentes agressivos sem sinais de alerta.
• Incapacidade do proprietário em confinar ou controlar o cão com segurança para evitar futuros incidentes. Os métodos envolvem o uso de cercas, focinheiras, coleiras ou cabrestos e guias.
• Crianças, idosos e outros humanos ou animais que vivem ou visitam essa casa estão sob alto risco.

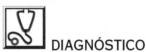

DIAGNÓSTICO

DIAGNÓSTICO DIFERENCIAL
• Identificar as condições patológicas associadas à agressividade antes de se formular um diagnóstico puramente comportamental.
• Em todos os casos de agressividade, é recomendável a condução de uma avaliação clínica completa.
• É fundamental descartar anormalidades relacionadas com o desenvolvimento (hidrocefalia, lissencefalia, desvios hepáticos), distúrbios metabólicos (hipoglicemia, encefalopatia hepática, diabetes), neuroendocrinopatias (hipotireoidismo, hiperadrenocorticismo), dermatopatia, condições neurológicas (neoplasia intracraniana, crises convulsivas), toxinas, doenças inflamatórias

AGRESSIVIDADE — VISÃO GERAL — CÃES

(encefalite, raiva), disfunção cognitiva, dor aguda ou crônica e causas iatrogênicas, como administração de glicocorticoides.

HEMOGRAMA/BIOQUÍMICA/URINÁLISE
- Costumam permanecer normais.
- As anormalidades podem sugerir causas metabólicas ou endócrinas subjacentes ou outras condições clínicas.

OUTROS TESTES LABORATORIAIS
Realizados conforme indicação (p. ex., função da tireoide ou teste de estimulação com ACTH, além de outros testes pertinentes).

DIAGNÓSTICO POR IMAGEM
- Pode ser indicado para identificar as origens de dor ou doenças.
- Se houver suspeita de neoplasia cerebral, obter imagens por RM ou TC.

MÉTODOS DIAGNÓSTICOS
Teste de anticorpo fluorescente após o óbito — indicado para quaisquer cães agressivos com suspeita de raiva como diagnóstico diferencial, inclusive para aqueles não submetidos à quarentena por 10 dias após mordida a algum ser humano ou outro animal.

ACHADOS PATOLÓGICOS
Nenhum a menos que haja suspeita de etiologia clínica subjacente.

TRATAMENTO

CUIDADO(S) DE SAÚDE ADEQUADO(S)
- O sucesso terapêutico depende de uma combinação de múltiplas modalidades: controle ambiental, modificação comportamental e farmacoterapia.
- É recomendável a consulta com veterinário experiente, além de adestramento para o controle da agressividade.
- A eutanásia deve ser recomendada quando o risco de lesão é alto. Anote a recomendação no prontuário médico.

CUIDADO(S) DE ENFERMAGEM
Um hotelzinho para cães capaz de controlá-los com segurança pode ser útil até que um plano terapêutico seguro possa ser implementado ou até que uma decisão seja tomada.

ATIVIDADE
Como a frustração e a agitação podem aumentar a incidência de agressividade, é recomendável a incorporação de um esquema seguro e adequado de exercícios ao programa terapêutico.

DIETA
Existem provas modestas de que uma dieta com baixo teor de proteína possa reduzir a agressividade territorial em cães — um efeito que pode ser intensificado pela suplementação com o triptofano.

ORIENTAÇÃO AO PROPRIETÁRIO
- Práticas seguras devem ditar a tomada de todas as decisões. Essas práticas incluem confinamento seguro, barreiras físicas, cabrestos, controle com guia, uso de focinheiras e supervisão por algum adulto competente.
- O proprietário deve ser orientado a considerar os riscos de responsabilidade pessoal e legal de manter o cão. A agressividade canina pode resultar em lesões de seres humanos, processos judiciais relacionados com mordidas e perda de seguros residenciais. Tal avaliação de risco pode ajudar o proprietário a avaliar a situação de forma objetiva.
- As situações que levaram à agressividade devem ser listadas e um plano específico desenvolvido para evitar essas situações e os locais associados no futuro.
- É recomendável evitar a punição, pois ficou demonstrado que isso aumenta a agitação, o medo e o comportamento defensivo.
- As técnicas de confronto, como rolamentos, aumentam a probabilidade de resposta agressiva defensiva, podem levar à lesão de seres humanos e devem ser estritamente evitadas.
- É aconselhável o uso de técnicas que não utilizam o confronto, mas empregam recursos e ensinam os cães a terem respostas adequadas.
- O cão deve ser tranquilamente afastado de situações que provoquem a agressividade.
- A eutanásia deverá ser considerada caso não se consiga efetuar um controle seguro ou quando o risco de lesão é elevado.

CONSIDERAÇÕES CIRÚRGICAS
Castração de machos.

MEDICAÇÕES

MEDICAMENTO(S) DE ESCOLHA
- Não há nenhum agente aprovado pela FDA para o tratamento de agressividade.
- Nenhum medicamento eliminará a probabilidade de agressão.
- Fazer uso de medicações apenas quando um plano seguro de controle foi implementado.
- Informar ao proprietário a respeito da natureza experimental desses tratamentos e do risco envolvido; registrar a discussão no prontuário médico e obter assinatura de termo de consentimento informado.
- Os medicamentos que aumentam os níveis da serotonina (neurotransmissor) podem ser benéficos para diminuir os comportamentos de ansiedade, agitação e impulsividade.
- Duração do tratamento: mínimo de 4 meses e, no máximo, pelo resto da vida.
- Ver Tabela 1 em busca dos medicamentos utilizados para facilitar o tratamento de agressividade em combinação com um plano seguro de controle.

CONTRAINDICAÇÕES
- A fluoxetina é contraindicada em casos de hepatopatia e crises convulsivas.
- A clomipramina é contraindicada em casos de distúrbios de condução cardíaca ou crises convulsivas; em um único estudo, esse agente não é mais eficaz que o controle nos casos de agressividade direcionada contra o proprietário.
- A amitriptilina é contraindicada em pacientes com distúrbios de condução cardíaca, glaucoma ou hepatopatia.

PRECAUÇÕES
Evitar o uso de benzodiazepínicos (p. ex., diazepam) em cães agressivos por causa do risco de desinibição comportamental. A agressividade pode aumentar quando os cães perdem o medo das repercussões da mordida.

INTERAÇÕES POSSÍVEIS
Não utilizar os ISRSs nem os ATCs com inibidores da MAO, incluindo o amitraz e o L-deprenyl, ou entre si por causa do risco de síndrome serotoninérgica.

MEDICAMENTO(S) ALTERNATIVO(S)
- L-triptofano — 10 mg/kg VO a cada 12 h.
- Acetato de megestrol — 1 mg/kg VO a cada 24 h durante 2 semanas; em seguida, reduzir gradativamente para a dosagem mais baixa, porém eficaz; último recurso terapêutico em casos de agressividade relacionada com domínio e entre os machos; os efeitos colaterais incluem obesidade, discrasias sanguíneas, piometra, poliúria/polidipsia, diabetes melito, hiperplasia mamária e câncer de mama (carcinoma).

ACOMPANHAMENTO

MONITORIZAÇÃO DO PACIENTE
- O contato semanal a quinzenal é recomendado nas fases iniciais.
- Os proprietários frequentemente necessitam de retorno e assistência com os programas de

Tabela 1

Medicamentos e dosagens utilizados para controlar a agressividade canina				
Agente	Classe Medicamentosa	Dosagem Oral no Cão (mg/kg)	Frequência de Dosagem
Fluoxetina	ISRS	1-2 mg/kg	a cada 24 h
Paroxetina	ISRS	1-2 mg/kg	a cada 24 h
Sertralina	ISRS	2-4 mg/kg	a cada 24 h
Clomipramina	ATC	1-2 mg/kg	a cada 12 h
Amitriptilina	ATC	1-2 mg/kg	a cada 12 h

AGRESSIVIDADE — VISÃO GERAL — CÃES

mudança comportamental e o controle terapêutico.

PREVENÇÃO
• Para evitar incidentes agressivos, evitar todas as situações que já induziram à agressividade, fazendo uso de confinamento seguro, portões, cabrestos, coleiras, guias e focinheiras.
• Diminuir o risco de agressividade nos cães jovens com um programa de socialização positiva (3-14 semanas); evitar as técnicas de intimidação e situações negativas indutoras de medo.

COMPLICAÇÕES POSSÍVEIS
• Lesão a seres humanos ou animais.
• Nos casos de agressividade entre os cães, os seres humanos que interferem na briga costumam ser seriamente feridos por acidente ou por agressão redirecionada, apesar de não serem o alvo pretendido; os proprietários não devem se aproximar de uma briga entre cães, mas afastá-los com o uso das guias.
• Responsabilidade do proprietário e do veterinário.

EVOLUÇÃO ESPERADA E PROGNÓSTICO
• Os cães agressivos que pesam mais de 18,5 kg estão sob risco de sofrerem eutanásia comportamental.
• Os cães explicitamente agressivos nunca são curados, embora o comportamento possa ser controlado com êxito, dependendo do caso.
• O prognóstico depende do caso em função dos fatores de risco e das características de controle de cada situação.

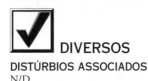

DIVERSOS

DISTÚRBIOS ASSOCIADOS
N/D.

FATORES RELACIONADOS COM A IDADE
A agressividade de início no adulto sugere alguma causa clínica; avaliar de forma minuciosa a acuidade sensorial e a função cognitiva, bem como as origens da dor.

POTENCIAL ZOONÓTICO
• As mordidas de cães constituem um risco significativo à saúde pública.
• A raiva é uma causa de agressividade em potencial.

GESTAÇÃO/FERTILIDADE/REPRODUÇÃO
Os antidepressivos tricíclicos (ATCs) são contraindicados em machos reprodutores e fêmeas prenhes.

VER TAMBÉM
• Agressividade Defensiva Induzida pelo Medo — Cães.
• Agressividade Possessiva, Territorial e pelo Alimento — Cães.
• Agressividade entre os Cães.
• Agressividade contra Pessoas Familiares — Cães.

ABREVIATURA(S)
• ACTH = hormônio adrenocorticotrófico.
• ATC = antidepressivo tricíclico.
• FDA = U.S. Food and Drug Administration (agência norte-americana de controle de alimentos e medicamentos).
• ISRS = inibidor seletivo de recaptação da serotonina.
• MAO = monoamina oxidase.
• RM = ressonância magnética.
• SNC = sistema nervoso central.
• TC = tomografia computadorizada.

RECURSOS DA INTERNET
• American Veterinary Medical Association Dog Bite Prevention: http://www.avma.org/public health/dogbite/default.asp.
• ASPCA Aggression in Dogs: http://www.aspcabehavior.org/articles/49/Aggression-in-Dogs.aspx.
• Centers for Disease Control and Prevention Dog Bite Prevention: http://www.cdc.gov/homeandrecreationalsafety/dog-bites/biteprevention.html.
• University of California-Davis, Companion Animal Behavior Program, Dog Aggression: http://www.vetmed.ucdavis.edu/CCAB/aggression.html.

Sugestões de Leitura
Bain M. Aggression toward unfamiliar people and animals. In: Horwitz DF, Mills D, eds., BSAVA Manual of Canine and Feline Behavioural Medicine, 2nd ed. Gloucestershire, UK: BSAVA, 2009, pp. 211-222.
deKeuster T, Jung H. Aggression toward familiar people and animals. In: Horwitz DF, Mills D, eds. BSAVA Manual of Canine and Feline Behavioural Medicine, 2nd ed. Gloucestershire, UK: BSAVA, 2009, 182-210.
Herron ME, Shofer FS, Reisner IR. Survey of the use and outcome of confrontational and non-confrontational training methods in client-owned dogs showing undesired behaviors. Appl Anim Behav Sci 2009, 117(1-2):47-54.
Luescher AU, Reisner IR. Canine aggression toward familiar people: A new look at an old problem. Vet Clin North Am Small Anim Pract 2008, 38:1107-1130.
Reisner, IR. Differential diagnosis and management of human-directed aggression in dogs. Vet Clin North Am Small Anim Pract 2003, 33:303-320.

Autor Barbara L. Sherman
Consultor Editorial Debra F. Horwitz

Agressividade — Visão Geral — Gatos

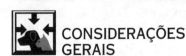

CONSIDERAÇÕES GERAIS

DEFINIÇÃO
Agressividade
- Uma estratégia comportamental utilizada para controlar situações aversivas.
- Pode ser normal e adequada em certos contextos.
- Pode ser anormal com graves efeitos deletérios sobre o bem-estar físico e emocional do gato.
- Agressividade: descreve traços tanto de humor como de temperamento relacionados à propensão de demonstrar agressividade quando circunstâncias ambientais ditam que ela pode ser usada.

PANORAMA GERAL DOS TIPOS

Agressividade por Brincadeira (Contra Pessoas)
- Tipicamente se refere a um gato que arranha e morde os proprietários durante brincadeiras.
- Não constitui uma agressão verdadeira, mas sim brincadeiras exageradas sem controle adequado dos impulsos em virtude da falta de adestramento ou *feedback* social intraespecífico apropriado.
- A intenção do gato não é machucar a pessoa.
- Comportamento incentivado e recompensado pelos proprietários por brincadeiras grosseiras e brutas com um filhote; quando o animal fica maior e mais forte, a brincadeira já é vista como uma agressão e não como uma atividade lúdica demasiada.

Comportamento Predatório (Contra Pessoas ou Outros Animais)
- Os gatos possuem um instinto inato para "caçar" ou exibir comportamento predatório, que envolve os atos de espreitar, se esconder e atacar.
- A predação não ocorre diretamente em função da fome.
- Além de ser tipicamente estimulado por movimentos rápidos, esse comportamento pode evoluir até que o gato se esconda e espere por um animal ou pessoa para andar por eles.
- A atividade lúdica é um meio comum para que gatos jovens aperfeiçoem as habilidades predatórias; as agressividades por brincadeira e predação podem se sobrepor.

Agressividade Redirecionada (Contra Pessoas ou Outros Animais)
- Gatos que veem, ouvem ou sentem um comportamento agressivo direto e deflagrador contra o espectador inocente mais próximo.
- Em alguns casos, uma pessoa ou animal na casa torna-se a vítima designada, mas o gato pode desviar de um indivíduo próximo e procurar pela vítima preferida.
- Alguns gatos podem ficar agitados por 24-72 h após um evento deflagrado.
- Um deflagrador comum que incita a agressividade redirecionada ocorre quando o gato vê outro gato ou vida silvestre do lado de fora da casa.

Agressividade Defensiva Induzida pelo Medo (Contra Pessoas ou Outros Animais)
- O gato exibirá posturas corporais indicativas de medo/ansiedade e pode usar a agressividade como uma estratégia para controlar essa situação aversiva.
- Os comportamentos típicos exibidos incluem uma combinação de qualquer um dos expostos a seguir: sibilos, salivação, piloereção, coluna arqueada, afastamento, corrida, acuamento, rolamento sobre seu dorso e patada (posição defensiva, não submissa) se encurralado.

Agressividade Territorial (Contra Pessoas ou Outros Animais)
- Alguns gatos, particularmente os machos, demonstram comportamentos territoriais nos ambientes domésticos em virtude do tamanho e da presença de mais recursos (p. ex., pessoas, alimentos, áreas de repouso, áreas de alimentação, locais de evacuação, etc.) para se defenderem em uma área menor.
- Os comportamentos territoriais incluem marcação com urina, fezes ou odores (como a fricção das bochechas em superfícies para o depósito de feromônios) e arranhões (que também depositam feromônios e deixam marcas visuais) e podem estar associados à agressividade.
- Em casos graves, o agressor pode procurar por outros indivíduos e atacar.
- A postura corporal com agressão territorial é assertiva, firme e confiante.

Agressividade por Dor (Contra Pessoas e Animais)
Os gatos com dor podem exibir agressividade (sibilos, rosnados, arranhaduras e mordidas) quando são fisicamente manipulados ou, então, antes ou depois de movimentos como saltos para dentro ou fora de um móvel.

Agressividade Materna
Uma fêmea pode revelar comportamentos agressivos contra indivíduos que se aproximam de seus filhotes.

Agressividade por Falta de Controle dos Impulsos
Os gatos que mostram reações agressivas intensas a estímulos brandos sem muito ou qualquer sinal de alerta podem ter deficiência de serotonina, conhecida muitas vezes como transtorno do controle de impulsos.

Agressividade Induzida por Frustração (Contra Pessoas e Outros Animais)
Alguns gatos têm personalidades muito extrovertidas e sociáveis, mas exibirão agressividade se a vida doméstica não suprir suas necessidades comportamentais.

Agressividade por Carícias ou Induzida pelo Contato (Contra Pessoas)
- Os gatos revelarão sinais precoces de aversão quando as pessoas os acariciarem no momento em que eles se encontram com as orelhas para trás e a cauda abanando.
- Se o contato físico continuar, os gatos tipicamente morderão.
- Com frequência, os proprietários passam despercebidos pelos sinais de alerta precoces.
- Quando os gatos lambem outro, é típico que eles limitem a higienização à região da cabeça.
- Para alguns gatos, pode ser anormal e indesejável ser acariciado ao longo do dorso, método comumente usado pelos proprietários.

Agressividade entre os Gatos dentro de Casa
- Cinquenta por cento dos proprietários de gatos relatam brigas (arranhões e mordidas) depois de introduzir um novo gato em casa.
- O número de gatos, o sexo e a idade não são fatores significativos para predizer quais gatos exibirão agressividade.
- Qualquer uma das categorias de agressividade citadas anteriormente, sem exceção, são possibilidades de brigas entre os gatos.
- Medo/ansiedade constitui a causa mais comum de agressividade intraespecífica.

FATORES QUE CONTRIBUEM PARA A FISIOPATOLOGIA
Os problemas comportamentais são tipicamente de etiologia multifatorial; apesar disso, segue um diagrama ilustrando alguns dos componentes mais comuns que precisam ser avaliados com precisão para o diagnóstico e o tratamento dos casos de agressividade.

SISTEMA(S) ACOMETIDO(S)
- Comportamental — variam com o tipo de agressão, ocorrendo de forma isolada ou em combinação: atos de abanar/torcer a cauda, virar as orelhas para os lados ou nivelá-las, enrijecer os ombros/membros, agachar, sibilar, salivar, rosnar, perseguir, atacar, espreitar ou dar o bote, além de exibir dilatação das pupilas, piloereção ou olhar fixo.

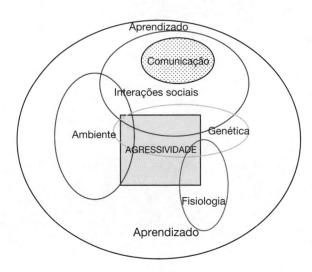

Figura 1

ESPÉCIES CANINA E FELINA

AGRESSIVIDADE — VISÃO GERAL — GATOS

- Cardiovascular — sinais associados à ativação da via simpática e do eixo hipotalâmico-hipofisário-adrenal.
- Endócrino/metabólico — agressividade a longo prazo associada a medo/estresse/ansiedade, sintomas vinculados à ativação prolongada do eixo hipotalâmico-hipofisário-adrenal.
- Gastrintestinal — com a estimulação crônica do eixo hipotalâmico-hipofisário-adrenal, pode-se observar um gato mais propenso a úlceras GI. Em casos de agressividade aguda por medo, observam-se evacuação intestinal e possível diarreia. A enteropatia inflamatória é possível em estresse crônico.
- Sanguíneo/linfático/imune — resposta imunológica diminuída com a estimulação crônica do eixo hipotalâmico-hipofisário-adrenal; leucograma de estresse.
- Musculoesquelético — uma agressão pode resultar em dano à pele e aos músculos pelas unhas e pelos dentes.
- Tanto a vítima como o agressor podem sofrer lesões. Com a ativação crônica do eixo hipotalâmico-hipofisário-adrenal, pode-se observar emaciação muscular.
- Nervoso — reatividade aumentada por até 72 h após um ataque agressivo. Pode-se observar um aumento na agressividade com declínio na provocação, pois as sinapses na tonsila ficam sensibilizadas. Alguns animais podem exibir uma queda dos níveis de serotonina, provocando ataques agressivos. Dependendo do tipo de agressão, pode haver padrões motores ritualizados, como sacudidas ou tremores.
- Oftálmico — pupilas dilatadas com a estimulação simpática.
- Renal/urológico — podem-se observar jatos ou pequenas quantidades de urina em superfícies horizontais. O gato pode exibir sinais compatíveis com doença do trato urinário inferior dos felinos atribuída a estresse/ansiedade/medo.
- Respiratório — taquipneia em casos agudos ou sob estresse.
- Cutâneo/exócrino — dano gerado por brigas. Dano devido à higienização excessiva associada a agressão/ansiedade/angústia induzidas por medo.

IDENTIFICAÇÃO
- Existem provas preliminares de que os traços comportamentais em gatos variem de acordo com a raça e o sexo.
- É mais provável que os machos exibam agressividade contra machos do que as fêmeas.
- As raças Abissínio, Azul da Rússia, Somali, Siamês e Chinchilla revelaram maior agressividade.
- Já as raças Maine Coon, Ragdoll e Fold escocês demonstraram menor agressividade.

SINAIS CLÍNICOS
- Podem aparecer na maturidade social (2-4 anos de idade), exceto para agressividade relacionada com brincadeiras, e devem ocorrer em interações/contextos sociais específicos. Se a idade de início ocorrer em um gato mais idoso, as causas clínicas deverão ser descartadas em primeiro lugar.
- Comentários gerais: a maioria dos proprietários é capaz de detectar sinais manifestos de agressão (ou seja, os atos de morder, sibilar e rosnar), mas pode passar despercebida pelos sinais mais sutis que tipicamente ocorrem entre os gatos (como olhar fixo) e pelos comportamentos ansiosos resultantes que podem culminar em agressão (colocar-se em posição fetal, desviar o olhar, etc.). Os videoteipes das interações entre os gatos permitem que o clínico avalie o comportamento.

CAUSAS
- Problemas clínicos subjacentes podem causar agressividade.
- O temperamento (comportamento) é influenciado por fatores como: genética, criação, socialização, ambiente onde o gato vive e tipos de interações do gato com as pessoas.

DIAGNÓSTICO
DIAGNÓSTICO DIFERENCIAL
- Doenças do SNC (infecções, toxinas, tumores, etc.).
- Hipertireoidismo.
- Encefalopatia hepática.
- Qualquer condição indutora de dor (artrite, pancreatite, doença dentária, saculite anal, etc.).
- Intoxicação pelo chumbo.
- Raiva.
- Neuropatia diabética (agressividade induzida por dor ao tocar nas patas).

HEMOGRAMA/BIOQUÍMICA/URINÁLISE
Todos esses exames devem ser feitos.

OUTROS TESTES LABORATORIAIS
- Qualquer gato que morda ou arranhe pessoas deve ser submetido ao teste em busca de *Bartonella*.
- Níveis dos hormônios tireoidianos.
- Urinálise =/– cultura se a evacuação domiciliar fizer parte do problema de agressividade.
- Sorologia felina para calicivírus felino, FeLV, FIV.

TRATAMENTO
- Nunca usar correção/punição física, pois isso pode aumentar a agressividade.
- Jamais tentar manipular ou manusear um gato fisicamente em um estado agressivo.
- Evitar deflagradores conhecidos.
- Identificar os deflagradores, dessensibilizando e contracondicionando o gato a esses deflagradores.
- Implementar medidas de segurança (protetores de garras, uso de calças compridas/mangas longas, manutenção de caixas de papelão dobradas em torno da casa entre o dono e o gato, redirecionamento do comportamento na fase inicial de agitação).
- Implantar modificações comportamentais para redirecionar o gato e diminuir a agitação (planos específicos dependem da peculiaridade de cada caso).
- Adestrar o gato a comandos como "sentar" (*sit*), vá para o lugar (*go to place*) etc.
- Efetuar o enriquecimento do ambiente.
- Orientar os proprietários a identificar os sinais precoces de agitação, para que o gato possa ser redirecionado ou para que eles consigam evitá-lo.
- Após um ataque muito agressivo, manter o agressor isolado em um cômodo por pelo menos 24 h (se este animal for um gato que permanece agitado depois de um ataque).
- Feromônios.
- Agentes terapêuticos.

MEDICAÇÕES
MEDICAMENTO(S)
- ISRSs: fluoxetina e paroxetina a 0,5 mg/kg VO a cada 24 h.
- ATCs: clomipramina a 0,5 mg/kg VO a cada 24 h.
- Amitriptilina a 0,5-1,0 mg/kg VO a cada 12-24 h.
- Buspirona a 0,5-1,0 mg/kg VO a cada 8-24 h.
- Benzodiazepínicos: oxazepam a 0,2-0,5 mg/kg a cada 12-24 h.
- SAMe: 90 mg VO a cada 24 h.

CONTRAINDICAÇÕES
- Gatos com nefro ou hepatopatia.
- Cuidado com o uso de ATCs e ISRSs em diabéticos.
- ATCs em pacientes com anormalidades cardíacas.

INTERAÇÕES POSSÍVEIS
- Não é recomendável a utilização concomitante de ATCs e ISRSs.
- Determinadas coleiras antipulgas.
- Certas ervas.
- A mirtazapina não deve ser usada em combinação com ATC ou ISRS.
- O clínico deve avaliar se qualquer outra medicação à qual o gato está sendo submetido utiliza o sistema enzimático do fígado no metabolismo para maximizar a segurança ao combinar os medicamentos.

ACOMPANHAMENTO
MONITORIZAÇÃO DO PACIENTE
- Telefonar para os proprietários uma vez a cada 1-2 semanas nos 2 primeiros meses após a recomendação de um plano terapêutico. Determinar a implementação das recomendações de segurança e o plano de intervenção comportamental.
- Se medicações estiverem envolvidas na agressividade, a dose deverá se reavaliada a cada 3-4 semanas.
- A frequência de acompanhamento será ditada pela gravidade do caso e pela obediência do proprietário.
- Obter hemograma completo, bioquímica sérica, perfil de T_4 antes da medicação. Reavaliar os valores hepáticos e renais 2-3 semanas depois de iniciar os medicamentos. Avaliar novamente a função sanguínea uma vez por ano em pacientes saudáveis jovens, mas semestralmente em pacientes mais idosos.
- Repetir os exames físicos em pacientes mais idosos em intervalos semestrais, pois condições indutoras de dor podem começar a contribuir para a agressividade ou exacerbar esse comportamento.

EVOLUÇÃO ESPERADA E PROGNÓSTICO
- A evolução e o prognóstico dependem basicamente do tipo específico de agressão e da obediência dos proprietários em relação ao plano terapêutico sugerido.
- A maioria dos casos de agressividade necessita da combinação de mudança comportamental, modificação ambiental, adestramento e, quando

AGRESSIVIDADE — VISÃO GERAL — GATOS

necessário, medicação para maximizar as chances de melhora.
• Alguns tipos de agressividade podem desaparecer ou melhorar dentro de algumas semanas, enquanto outros podem levar vários meses ou mais.
• Algumas formas de agressão têm prognóstico mau.

DIVERSOS
FATORES RELACIONADOS COM A IDADE
• Gatos mais idosos — declínio cognitivo, doença do SNC, artrite, meningioma, outros problemas clínicos.
• Idade (2-4 anos) — maturidade social, período durante o qual os gatos podem começar a demonstrar certos tipos de agressividade.

ABREVIATURA(S)
• ATC = antidepressivo tricíclico.
• FeLV = vírus da leucemia felina.
• FIV = vírus da imunodeficiência felina.
• GI = gastrintestinal.
• ISRS = inibidor seletivo de recaptação da serotonina.
• SAMe = S-adenosil-L-metionina.
• SNC = sistema nervoso central.

Sugestões de Leitura
Crowell-Davis SL, Murray T. Veterinary Psychopharmacology. Ames, IA: Blackwell, 2006.
Levine ED. Feline fear and anxiety. Vet Clin North Am Small Anim Pract 2008, 38:1065-1079.
Levine ED, Perry P, Scarlett J, et al. Intercat aggression in households following the introduction of a new cat. Appl Anim Behav Sci 2004, 90:325-336.

Autor Emily D. Levine
Consultor Editorial Debra F. Horwitz
Agradecimento Karen L. Overall

AGRESSIVIDADE CANINA CONTRA CRIANÇAS

CONSIDERAÇÕES GERAIS

REVISÃO
O problema abrange tanto a medicina veterinária como a saúde pública. As crianças representam as vítimas mais frequentes de mordidas relatadas e tendem a sofrer lesões mais graves que os adultos.

IDENTIFICAÇÃO
Cães de qualquer raça, idade, sexo e castrados são capazes de morder uma criança.

Raça
- Os relatos de raças são inconsistentes e variam com a demografia da população de estudo. • As raças que se apresentaram em um serviço de encaminhamento para distúrbios comportamentais incluíam Springer spaniel inglês, Pastor alemão, Labrador retriever, Golden retriever e Cocker spaniel americano. • A maioria dos ataques fatais (raros) é atribuído a Rottweiler, Pit bull e seus cruzamentos. • Talvez seja mais provável que as raças de porte maior e mistas provoquem lesões graves. • As raças de porte menor também podem ser perigosas.

Sexo/Castração
- A agressividade, em geral, é mais frequente em machos que em fêmeas, mas ambos os sexos podem morder. • A castração sozinha não reduzirá significativamente o risco de mordida.

Idade
- A agressividade é observada com maior frequência em cães socialmente maduros. • O comportamento agressivo é possível em cães de qualquer idade, inclusive filhotes. • O risco pode aumentar em cães mais idosos por causa de dor crônica ou irritabilidade.

CAUSAS E FATORES DE RISCO

Categorias Clínicas/Motivações para Agressividade
- Agressividade relacionada com medo.
- Agressividade relacionada com dor. • Proteção de recursos (alimentos). • Agressividade relacionada com brincadeiras. • Agressividade relacionada com conflito. • Comportamento predatório.
- Agressividade territorial.

Fatores de Risco Associados ao Cão
- Doença e irritabilidade associada. • Dor.
  ◦ Agressividade relacionada com dor e proteção de recursos (alimentos) são os motivos mais comuns de mordidas em crianças familiares com menos de 6 anos de idade.
- Ansiedade generalizada. • Comportamento de medo. • Cães que se deitam, adormecem ou acordam, particularmente embaixo ou sobre uma mobília. • Ansiedade ou agressividade de qualquer progenitor ou dos companheiros da ninhada.

Fatores de Risco Ambientais/Sociais
- Presença de um cão na casa; crianças menores são mais provavelmente mordidas pelo animal de estimação da família ou outros cães familiares.
- Presença de bebês (risco de ataques predatórios).
- Presença de crianças pequenas. • Presença de alimentos, brinquedos comestíveis.
- Adestramento inadequado à base de punição.
- Supervisão inadequada ou compreensão indevida de supervisão por pais/responsáveis. • Histórico de rosnar, estalar do maxilar, morder (não necessariamente). • Abraçar, beijar ou se deitar sobre um cão ansioso, medroso ou agressivo.

DIAGNÓSTICO

DIAGNÓSTICO DIFERENCIAL
Ver "Categorias Clínicas/Motivações para Agressividade".

HEMOGRAMA/BIOQUÍMICA/URINÁLISE
Achados compatíveis com o estado de saúde do cão, podendo ou não ser significativos. O comportamento de mordedura ocorre em cães clinicamente saudáveis ou pode aumentar em caso de doença/mal-estar/dor.

OUTROS TESTES LABORATORIAIS
- Uma evidência qualitativa, empírica e incidental (apenas) correlaciona o hipotireoidismo canino com agressividade acentuada, mas não há evidências dessa correlação com base em dados científicos. • A suplementação desnecessária com hormônios tireoidianos pode provocar uma agitação ou agressividade elevada.

MÉTODOS DIAGNÓSTICOS
Obter um histórico detalhado do evento da mordida e do comportamento tanto do cão como da criança para determinar a motivação da mordida.

TRATAMENTO

SEGURANÇA COM CÃES FAMILIARES
- Nunca deixe bebês ou crianças pequenas sem supervisão juntamente com cães. Separe os bebês dos cães quando sozinhos, ainda que seja momentaneamente, mesmo se ambos estiverem adormecidos. • Na presença de um único adulto, separe o cão das crianças pequenas. • Se houver mais de um adulto presente, atribuir a responsabilidade do cuidado do cão para um dos adultos e da criança para o outro. • Não permita que as crianças se aproximem ou interajam com o cão quando ele estiver deitado. • Não deixe que as crianças removam qualquer objeto do cão. • Não permita também que as crianças abracem, beijem, se inclinem sobre nem se deitem ao lado do cão.
- Isole o cão quando ele estiver comendo. • Separe o cão quando ele estiver mastigando objetos valiosos.

SEGURANÇA COM CÃES NÃO FAMILIARES
- Não prenda nem amarre os cães sem supervisão.
- Não permita que crianças pequenas interajam com cães não familiares (ou seja, desconhecidos).
- Feche as portas com segurança em jardins ou quintais com cercas. • Evite cercas elétricas subterrâneas para permitir o acesso ao jardim.

MUDANÇA DE COMPORTAMENTO POR MEIO DE APRENDIZADO E ADESTRAMENTO
- Redirecionar a atenção do cão: ensinar dicas de "olhar" ou "toque". • Estabelecer um "porto seguro" separado para o cão. • Restringir o contato, se necessário, quando crianças pequenas estiverem presentes. • Prender o cão medroso ou reativo com coleira e oferecer o alimento a uma distância segura das crianças, transformando uma situação negativa em uma positiva.

MEDICAÇÕES

MEDICAMENTOS
Agentes ansiolíticos podem ser indicados para cães com comportamento de ansiedade ou medo generalizado ou circunstancial.

Inibidores Seletivos de Recaptação da Serotonina (ISRS)
- Fluoxetina 0,5-2,0 mg/kg a cada 24 h.
- Sertralina 0,5-3 mg/kg a cada 24 h.

Antidepressivos Tricíclicos (ATC)
- Clomipramina 1-3 mg/kg a cada 12 h.

CONTRAINDICAÇÕES/INTERAÇÕES POSSÍVEIS
- Os medicamentos psicotrópicos podem aumentar os comportamentos de agitação e ansiedade ou desinibir a agressividade. Utilizar com cuidado e com as recomendações de segurança mencionadas anteriormente para evitar a ocorrência de mordidas.
- É recomendável evitar as seguintes combinações: ◦ SRS + ATC. ◦ ISRS ou ATC + tramadol. ◦ ISRS ou ATC + inibidor da MAO, incluindo amitraz (ingrediente ativo presente em coleiras contra carrapatos e preventivos contra pulgas e carrapatos). ◦ ISRS + AINE (a combinação pode ser usada com cuidado, mas o risco de hemorragia GI ou em outro órgão aumenta).

ACOMPANHAMENTO

PREVENÇÃO
- Não contar apenas com o adestramento para eliminar a agressividade. • As medidas preventivas são muito importantes no manejo da agressividade canina contra crianças. Até mesmo os cães satisfatoriamente adestrados podem morder.

COMPLICAÇÕES POSSÍVEIS
- A família pode não admitir nem reconhecer os riscos. • Estados patológicos podem piorar a agressividade. • A família pode não ser obediente às medidas de segurança. • Os medicamentos psicotrópicos podem não ser realisticamente confiáveis nem eficazes. • Crianças pequenas podem ser impulsivas e difíceis de controlar.

EVOLUÇÃO ESPERADA E PROGNÓSTICO
- O comportamento agressivo frequentemente pode ser reduzido e controlado. Contudo, há necessidade de obediência pelo resto da vida. • O prognóstico será mau se o ambiente social/físico não puder ser controlado. • Em alguns casos, pode ser necessário orientar os proprietários a submeter os cães a realojamento ou à eutanásia, enquanto em outros o comportamento do cão pode melhorar à medida que as crianças ficam mais velhas.

DIVERSOS

ABREVIATURA(S)
- AINE = anti-inflamatório não esteroide. • ATC = antidepressivo tricíclico. • GI = gastrintestinal. • ISRS = inibidor seletivo de recaptação da serotonina. • MAO = monoamina oxidase.

Sugestões de Leitura
Herron ME, Shofer FS, Reisner IR. Survey of the use and outcome of confrontational and non-confrontational training methods in client-owned dogs showing undesired behaviors. Appl Anim Behav Sci 2009, 117:47-54.
Reisner IR, Shofer FS, Nance ML. Behavioral assessment of child-directed canine aggression. Inj Prev 2007, 13:348-351.

Autor Ilana R. Reisner
Consultor Editorial Debra F. Horwitz

Agressividade contra Pessoas Familiares — Cães

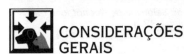

CONSIDERAÇÕES GERAIS

DEFINIÇÃO
Agressividade (com rosnadas, elevação labial, latidos, abocanhadas, botes, mordidas) direcionada geralmente contra os membros da casa ou pessoas com quem o cão tem uma relação estabelecida, em situações que envolvam o acesso a recursos estimados. Também é denominada agressividade por domínio, agressividade relacionada com o *status*, agressividade por conflito ou competição.

FISIOPATOLOGIA
Antigamente, acreditava-se que esse tipo de agressividade era um comportamento social canino normal direcionado contra as pessoas. No entanto, esses cães podem exibir ansiedade ou ser impulsivos e imprevisíveis.

SISTEMA(S) ACOMETIDO(S)
Comportamental.

GENÉTICA
Embora existam predileções raciais, as análises de *pedigree* demonstraram uma ocorrência elevada em cães aparentados. O modo de herança não é conhecido.

INCIDÊNCIA/PREVALÊNCIA
20-40% dos casos de referência comportamental.

DISTRIBUIÇÃO GEOGRÁFICA
Há diferenças raciais regionais.

IDENTIFICAÇÃO
Espécies
Cães.

Raça(s) Predominante(s)
Spaniel (Springer e Cocker spaniel), Terrier, Lhasa apso e Rottweiler, mas pode ser exibida por qualquer raça.

Idade Média e Faixa Etária
Geralmente se manifesta no início da maturidade social (12-36 meses de idade). Pode ser observada em cães jovens.

Sexo(s) Predominante(s)
Os machos (castrados e intactos) são mais comumente representados do que as fêmeas.

SINAIS CLÍNICOS
Comentários Gerais
A obtenção de histórico meticuloso se faz necessária para a determinação do diagnóstico, a avaliação dos riscos envolvidos na posse do cão aos proprietários e à saúde pública, bem como para a formulação de um plano terapêutico seguro e realista. Os proprietários podem não identificar nem dar crédito aos sinais comportamentais mais brandos de agressividade, como olhar fixo, rosnadas, exibição dos dentes ou abocanhadas que, muitas vezes, podem estar presentes antes da ocorrência de mordidas. Os detalhes de episódios agressivos precoces são decisivos para o estabelecimento do diagnóstico e a definição do prognóstico. O clínico deve estar ciente de que nem toda a agressividade direcionada contra o proprietário é motivada pelo desejo de domínio, mas frequentemente é baseada na ansiedade ou no medo.

Achados Anamnésicos
• Com frequência, esse tipo de agressividade é observado em torno das áreas de repouso/descanso, do alimento e dos brinquedos, bem como com a manipulação (incluindo carícias e aproximações) e perto dos pertences favoritos, envolvendo pessoas. A agressividade costuma ser direcionada contra os membros da casa ou pessoas que possuem uma relação firmada com o cão. Os comportamentos agressivos podem ser constatados em outros contextos, incluindo, mas não se limitando à defesa do território, quando os cães são repreendidos ou têm o acesso negado a itens ou atividades, e contra pessoas não familiares. A coleta do histórico deve tentar estabelecer os deflagradores da agressividade, a frequência dos episódios agressivos e sua gravidade. • O comportamento agressivo pode não ser verificado toda vez que o cão estiver em certa situação nem ser direcionado de maneira uniforme contra cada pessoa da casa. • Os sinais de postura corporal rígida, olhar fixo e atento, cabeça erguida, orelhas eretas e voltadas para a frente ou cauda elevada costumam acompanhar o comportamento agressivo. Os proprietários podem relatar uma combinação dessas posturas com posturas mais submissas (p. ex., cauda elevada, mas orelhas encolhidas, e olhos desviados), que podem representar um elemento de conflito, ansiedade ou medo na motivação do cão. • Os proprietários frequentemente descrevem esses cães como "mal-humorados" e podem ser capazes de julgar o momento em que o cão provavelmente estará agressivo. Nos episódios iniciais, o cão pode revelar comportamentos de medo, como desvio do olhar, encolhimento da cauda e fuga, que podem diminuir à medida que o animal se torna mais convencido de que essa agressividade modificará as consequências. • A ansiedade pode ser notada em interações entre o animal doméstico e o proprietário, bem como em outras circunstâncias, como afastamentos desse dono por viagem ou abandono ou situações novas. Determinados cães têm domínio de seu ambiente, fazendo uso da agressividade somente por ela se mostrar eficaz; tais cães, no entanto, encontram-se ansiosos em qualquer encontro, enquanto outros cães parecem confiantes e seguros.

Achados do Exame Físico
• Não costumam ser dignos de nota. • As condições clínicas, particularmente as dolorosas, podem contribuir para a manifestação de agressividade. Esses cães podem não revelar a agressividade contra um examinador confiante, mas não ameaçador. Contudo, é preciso ter extrema cautela ao examinar os cães que manifestarem agressividade, abrangendo o uso de focinheiras ou outros dispositivos humanos de contenção.

CAUSAS
• Pode ser na verdade parte de um repertório comportamental social canino normal, mas seu caráter é influenciado por certos fatores, como ambiente, aprendizado e genética. • A manifestação da agressividade pode ser influenciada por condições clínicas subjacentes, experiências anteriores (pelo aprendizado de que a agressividade influi e ajuda no controle de situações), inconstância ou falta de regras claras e objetivas, bem como de uma rotina, dentro de casa e nas interações entre o homem e o animal.
• Raramente essa agressividade representa um sintoma de condições clínicas; entretanto, é preciso descartar doenças concomitantes, já que enfermidade e/ou dor podem influenciar a tendência a comportamentos agressivos.

FATORES DE RISCO
Fatores como punição física inconsequente ou inconveniente e interações incompatíveis com o proprietário podem contribuir para o desenvolvimento de comportamento divergente, conflitante e/ou agressivo.

DIAGNÓSTICO

DIAGNÓSTICO DIFERENCIAL
• Agressividade baseada no medo. • Condições promotoras de ansiedade. • Distúrbios patológicos associados à agressividade (p. ex., condições indutoras de dor e endocrinopatias).

HEMOGRAMA/BIOQUÍMICA/URINÁLISE
Em geral, não são dignos de nota; se encontradas, as anormalidades podem indicar algum distúrbio clínico subjacente ou colaborador.

OUTROS TESTES LABORATORIAIS
Efetuados conforme indicação para descartar doenças subjacentes.

DIAGNÓSTICO POR IMAGEM
Obter imagens por RM na suspeita de envolvimento do SNC; tais imagens são obtidas, conforme a necessidade, para descartar distúrbios clínicos subjacentes; podem ser úteis para excluir as origens da dor.

TRATAMENTO

CUIDADO(S) DE SAÚDE ADEQUADO(S)
Modificação comportamental como paciente de ambulatório; tratamento clínico, conforme a necessidade.

ATIVIDADE
A atividade física adequada pode ajudar a diminuir as incidências de agressividade.

DIETA
As dietas com baixo teor de proteína e alto conteúdo de triptofano podem auxiliar a reduzir a agressividade, mas é improvável que elas façam uma diferença significativa sem a mudança comportamental.

ORIENTAÇÃO AO PROPRIETÁRIO
Comentários Gerais
• O tratamento bem-sucedido, que resulta em um declínio nos incidentes agressivos, depende sobretudo do comportamento social canino básico julgado pelo proprietário e dos riscos envolvidos na posse de um cão agressivo, bem como da implementação de recomendações relativas à segurança e ao manejo. • O tratamento visa o controle do problema, e não a "cura". • Os proprietários devem estar cientes de que a única forma de prevenção de lesões futuras é a realização da eutanásia. • É muito importante que os proprietários sejam orientados sobre os riscos do uso das técnicas de punição física e adestramento que se apoiam no "domínio" de seus cães por esses donos. Nos últimos anos, tem se observado o ressurgimento dessas técnicas. O uso inadequado e impróprio das técnicas de domínio/punições físicas, que variam desde correções com enforcadores até os chamados "*alpha-rolls*" (manobras de luta livre) para iniciar situações que provoquem a agressividade para depois corrigi-la, pode induzir a lesões em seres humanos, intensificação do comportamento agressivo, aumento na ansiedade e ruptura do elo homem-animal.

Agressividade contra Pessoas Familiares — Cães

Recomendações de Segurança
• Se os proprietários não optarem pela eutanásia, eles deverão estar cientes de que sua principal responsabilidade será prevenir lesões em seres humanos, evitando de forma consciente situações capazes de evocar uma reação agressiva, inclusive aquelas que tenham resultado em um cão medroso, ainda que ele não seja agressivo. Utilizar informações obtidas na anamnese do paciente para ajudar os proprietários a identificar situações específicas a serem evitadas. Não permitir que o cão suba na mobília. Não fornecer petiscos ou brinquedos estimados (p. ex., como aqueles de couro cru). Recolher os brinquedos e fazer com que os donos tenham controle sobre os momentos de brincadeiras e atividades. Limitar o contato físico com o cão, incluindo carícias. Não punir nem repreender o cão fisicamente. • É mais provável que o tratamento seja bem-sucedido se for instituído um período para evitar a exposição a estímulos indutores de agressividade antes da modificação comportamental. • O adestramento do cão para que ele se adapte a uma espécie de cabresto (Gentle Leader®) com uma guia de 2,5 a 3 m e uma focinheira tipo cesta, sempre que o animal estiver em contato com pessoas, torna mais fácil e mais seguro o controle de situações potencialmente perigosas. • Utilizar guias compridas para afastar o cão de situações que possam eliciar o comportamento agressivo; não abordar o cão diretamente.

Terapia Comportamental
• Modificação comportamental — utilizar métodos não confrontacionais para adestrar os cães a encararem as pessoas como líderes. Além disso, usar técnicas de adestramento baseadas em recompensas para orientar os cães a obedecer aos comandos provenientes de humanos, sem gerar conflito ou agressividade. • Controle da afeição — faz o cão obedecer a um comando antes de ele receber qualquer coisa que deseja do homem (isso também é conhecido como "Nada na vida é de graça" ou "Aprender a ouvir"). Por exemplo, o cão deve se sentar ou deitar antes de ser alimentado e acariciado, bem como antes de brincar ou sair para passear. Por um período inicial de 2-3 semanas, os proprietários devem dar atenção ao cão apenas durante breves períodos estruturados (p. ex., comando-resposta-recompensa). Em outros momentos, eles devem ignorar o cão, especialmente se ele estiver solicitando atenção. A interação é iniciada por um comando transmitido pelo proprietário e finalizada antes que o cão esteja preparado. • Contracomando ou substituição de resposta — utilizar reforço positivo (p. ex., alimentos, brinquedos, jogos e carícias) para ensinar comportamentos contrários àqueles que resultaram em agressividade no passado. Por exemplo, ensinar o comando "fora!" para sair dos móveis ou o comando "solte!" para largar os brinquedos.
• Dessensibilização e contracondicionamento — técnica utilizada para diminuir a responsividade a situações que culminaram em agressividade no passado. Como segurança, pode haver a necessidade do uso de focinheira. Essa técnica não deve ser instituída até que o proprietário tenha assumido um nível maior de controle sobre o cão pelos métodos de controle da afeição e adestramento com base em recompensas. O cão é ensinado primeiramente a se sentar e relaxar sob um comando verbal em locais neutros, utilizando recompensas de alimentos. Para que nenhuma reação de medo e/ou agressividade seja eliciada, tenta-se a exposição gradativa do cão a um estímulo bastante reduzido. O comportamento não agressivo e sem medo é, então, recompensado. O nível de estimulação é gradativamente aumentado, permanecendo abaixo do limiar que resultaria em medo e/ou agressão. A evolução do método é lenta e cautelosa. É essencial a monitorização das respostas.

CONSIDERAÇÕES CIRÚRGICAS
• Castrar machos intactos. • As fêmeas que começam a demonstrar agressividade por domínio em uma idade inferior a 6 meses de vida podem ser menos agressivas quando estiverem na idade adulta se não forem castradas.

MEDICAÇÕES

MEDICAMENTO(S) DE ESCOLHA
• Não há medicamentos aprovados para o tratamento da agressividade canina. Os proprietários devem estar cientes de que o uso de medicamento está fora da indicação aprovada pela FDA. Em virtude de questões relativas à responsabilidade, é preciso anotar na ficha do paciente o fato de que os proprietários foram informados sobre os riscos e os efeitos colaterais em potencial. É recomendável, portanto, a assinatura de termos de consentimento informado. NUNCA usar medicações sem a modificação comportamental. Antes de prescrever o medicamento, ter a certeza de que os proprietários não só compreenderam os riscos envolvidos na posse de um cão agressivo, mas também que eles adotarão os procedimentos de segurança e não contarão com o medicamento para promover a segurança de outras pessoas. O medicamento pode não ser apropriado em algumas circunstâncias familiares, como as que envolvem crianças pequenas, membros da família portadores de deficiências ou indivíduos imunocomprometidos.
• Em casos de agressividade por domínio, o único estudo medicamentoso duplo-cego controlado por placebo revelou um efeito intenso do placebo e não constatou qualquer diferença entre esse placebo e o medicamento na redução dos comportamentos agressivos.

Inibidores Seletivos de Recaptação da Serotonina (ISRSs)
• Fluoxetina a 0,5-2 mg/kg VO a cada 24 h (cães).
• Paroxetina a 0,5-1 mg/kg VO a cada 24 h (cães).
• Sertralina a 1-3 mg/kg VO a cada 24 h (cães).
• Efeitos colaterais: sedação, irritabilidade, efeitos GI; a anorexia é comum, mas costuma ser transitória.

Antidepressivos Tricíclicos (ATCs)
• Clomipramina a 2-4 mg/kg VO a cada 24 h ou divididos a cada 12 h (cães) (bula restrita para agressividade). • Efeitos colaterais: sedação, efeitos GI, efeitos anticolinérgicos, possíveis distúrbios de condução cardíaca em animais predispostos.

CONTRAINDICAÇÕES
Ter cautela ao prescrever os benzodiazepínicos, pois eles poderão desinibir a agressividade se diminuírem a inibição (baseada no medo) contra mordidas.

PRECAUÇÕES
Qualquer medicamento psicotrópico pode aumentar, em vez de diminuir, a agressividade. Os corticosteroides são contraindicados se o cão se mostrar agressivo diante do alimento; a polifagia pode levar a aumentos na frequência e intensidade do comportamento agressivo.

INTERAÇÕES POSSÍVEIS
Não associar ISRSs ou ATCs com inibidores da MAO (p. ex., amitraz e selegilina) e tramadol — essas combinações podem resultar em síndrome serotoninérgica potencialmente fatal.

ACOMPANHAMENTO

MONITORIZAÇÃO DO PACIENTE
Com frequência, os proprietários precisam de assistência contínua em problemas comportamentais, especialmente em casos de agressividade. É aconselhável, no mínimo, dar um telefonema de acompanhamento nas primeiras 1-3 semanas após a consulta. Nesse momento, devem ser previstos os acompanhamentos futuros por telefone ou pessoalmente.

PREVENÇÃO
As recomendações terapêuticas são para toda a vida — a recidiva da agressividade pode ser observada com lapsos do tratamento. Talvez seja necessário evitar os fatores desencadeantes de agressividade de forma contínua.

COMPLICAÇÕES POSSÍVEIS
Lesões em seres humanos; eutanásia ou abandono do paciente.

EVOLUÇÃO ESPERADA E PROGNÓSTICO
Não há cura. O prognóstico quanto à melhora é mais satisfatório se o comportamento agressivo for de baixa intensidade e ocorrer apenas em algumas situações relativamente previsíveis. O prognóstico é altamente dependente da obediência do proprietário ao tratamento.

DIVERSOS

DISTÚRBIOS ASSOCIADOS
Outras formas de agressividade, especialmente aquelas por disputa territorial e outras entre os cães. Os cães agressivos costumam ter uma ansiedade subjacente.

FATORES RELACIONADOS COM A IDADE
As cadelas com menos de 6 meses de vida que manifestam agressividade por domínio podem revelar um declínio no nível desse comportamento se não forem castradas.

POTENCIAL ZOONÓTICO
Lesão em seres humanos por feridas causadas por mordeduras.

GESTAÇÃO/FERTILIDADE/REPRODUÇÃO
Não acasalar cães agressivos.

SINÔNIMO(S)
• Agressividade por domínio. • Agressividade por conflito. • Síndrome de raiva. • Agressividade por competição. • Agressividade por *status*.

ABREVIATURA(S)
• ATC = antidepressivo tricíclico. • GI = gastrintestinal. • ISRS = inibidor seletivo de recaptação da serotonina. • MAO = monoamina oxidase. • RM = ressonância magnética. • SNC = sistema nervoso central.

Autores Laurie Bergman e Meredith Stepita
Consultor Editorial Debra F. Horwitz

Agressividade Defensiva Induzida pelo Medo — Cães

CONSIDERAÇÕES GERAIS

REVISÃO
Esse tipo de agressividade ocorre quando o cão encara uma situação como ameaçadora. Pode estar dentro dos limites de normalidade para o comportamento, embora o medo (fobia) excessivo também seja possível.

SISTEMA(S) ACOMETIDO(S)
- Comportamental.
- Sinais de estimulação simpática (p. ex., taquipneia, taquicardia).

IDENTIFICAÇÃO
- Cão.
- Não há um sexo predominante; comportamento não influenciado pela castração.
- Pode ocorrer em qualquer idade. Os sinais frequentemente se desenvolvem à medida que os filhotes caninos deixam o período de pico para a socialização (cerca de 12-16 semanas de vida) e novamente aos 6-9 meses.

SINAIS CLÍNICOS
- Sinais de agressividade (como rosnadas, elevação labial, latidos, abocanhadas, botes, mordidas) acompanhados por posturas corporais submissas ou amedrontadas/expressões faciais (cabeça baixa, agachamento, recuo, orelhas voltadas para trás, cauda encolhida, olhar distante, lambedura dos lábios).
- O histórico pode incluir o sofrimento de uma lesão pelo cão ou de um susto em uma situação semelhante.
- Muitas vezes, essa agressividade é direcionada contra pessoas não familiares.
- Pode ocorrer quando o cão está encurralado ou não consegue escapar.
- Pode ser pior quando preso à coleira do que solto.

CAUSAS E FATORES DE RISCO
- Pode ser um comportamento canino normal, dependendo das circunstâncias.
- Fortemente influenciado por experiências anteriores (p. ex., socialização prévia inadequada, condições dolorosas, manipulação grosseira e punição imprópria).
- Condições clínicas subjacentes, especialmente aquelas indutoras de dor, podem aumentar a intensidade da resposta agressiva.

DIAGNÓSTICO

DIAGNÓSTICO DIFERENCIAL
- Agressividade por domínio ou *status* social.
- Agressividade por conflito.
- Outros, dependendo das circunstâncias.

HEMOGRAMA/BIOQUÍMICA/URINÁLISE
Em geral, não são dignos de nota. As anormalidades sugerem uma condição clínica subjacente ou colaboradora.

OUTROS TESTES LABORATORIAIS
Não costumam ser dignos de nota.

DIAGNÓSTICO POR IMAGEM
Obter imagem por RM na suspeita de envolvimento do SNC. Outras imagens devem ser obtidas, conforme a necessidade, para descartar condições clínicas subjacentes.

MÉTODOS DIAGNÓSTICOS
N/D.

TRATAMENTO

ORIENTAÇÃO AO PROPRIETÁRIO
- O tratamento visa o controle do problema, e não a "cura". O tratamento bem-sucedido, conforme é mensurado por um declínio nos incidentes agressivos, depende sobretudo do comportamento social canino básico julgado pelo proprietário, dos riscos envolvidos na posse de um cão agressivo, da adoção de recomendações relativas à segurança e ao manejo, bem como da identificação correta dos estímulos indutores do medo.
- Os proprietários devem ter a consciência de que a única forma de prevenção de todas as lesões futuras é a realização de eutanásia.
- Se os proprietários não optarem pela eutanásia, eles deverão estar cientes de que sua principal responsabilidade será prevenir lesões em seres humanos, evitando de forma consciente situações capazes de evocar uma reação agressiva, inclusive aquelas que tenham resultado em um cão medroso, ainda que ele não seja agressivo.
- Os proprietários poderão ser mais obedientes às recomendações de prevenção se compreenderem que, em muitas jurisdições, os donos de cães são responsáveis pelas mordidas e poderão enfrentar processos civis/criminais se uma pessoa sofrer algum tipo de lesão.
- É mais provável que o tratamento seja bem-sucedido se for instituído um período para evitar a exposição a estímulos indutores do medo antes da modificação comportamental.

Recomendações de Segurança
- Confinar o cão distante de vítimas em potencial ou submetê-lo a controle físico direto de um adulto responsável, sempre que possa surgir uma situação indutora de agressividade (p. ex., em qualquer local público, em passeios ou quando há visitas em casa).
- Adestrar o cão para que ele se adapte a uma espécie de cabresto (Gentle Leader®) e uma focinheira tipo cesta para um controle mais fácil e mais seguro.
- Em virtude do ressurgimento atual na popularidade das técnicas de adestramento baseadas em punição e domínio, os proprietários deverão ser orientados sobre a etiologia (i. e., medo) da agressividade de seus cães. O emprego dessas técnicas pode resultar em comportamento agressivo acentuado, medo, agitação e/ou lesões.

Terapia Comportamental
- Controle da afeição: empregado para aumentar a previsibilidade da vida do cão e para diminuir a ocorrência de situações indutoras do medo (ver "Agressividade contra Pessoas Familiares — Cães").
- Modificação comportamental: dessensibilização e contracondicionamento sistemáticos a estímulos específicos indutores de medo e agressividade (ver "Agressividade contra Pessoas Familiares — Cães").
- Adestrar o cão a se sentar e relaxar a um comando verbal em locais neutros, utilizando alimentos como recompensas.
- A exposição gradativa do cão a um estímulo bastante reduzido é a próxima tentativa, para que nenhuma reação de medo seja eliciada.
- O comportamento isento de medo é, então, recompensado.
- O nível de estimulação é aumentado gradativamente, ficando abaixo do limiar que resultaria em medo e/ou agressividade.
- Embora a evolução seja lenta, é essencial o monitoramento rigoroso das respostas.
- As recidivas são comuns e, por essa razão, os proprietários sempre devem estar vigilantes e no controle do comportamento do cão.

MEDICAÇÕES

MEDICAMENTO(S)
- Não existem medicamentos aprovados para o tratamento da agressividade canina. Os proprietários devem estar cientes de que o uso de medicamento está fora da indicação aprovada pela FDA. Em virtude de questões relativas à responsabilidade, é preciso anotar na ficha do paciente o fato de que os proprietários foram informados sobre os riscos potenciais e os efeitos colaterais. É recomendável, portanto, a assinatura de um termo de consentimento informado.
- NUNCA usar medicamentos sem modificação comportamental.
- Antes de prescrever o medicamento, ter a certeza de que os proprietários não só compreenderam os riscos envolvidos na posse de um cão agressivo, mas também que eles adotarão os procedimentos de segurança e não contarão com o medicamento para promover a segurança de outras pessoas.
- O medicamento pode não ser apropriado em certas situações familiares, como na existência de crianças, membros da família portadores de deficiências ou indivíduos imunocomprometidos.
- Pesquisas confirmaram o intenso efeito exercido por placebo ao utilizar medicações para o tratamento da agressividade canina. Estudos não demonstraram um efeito substancial da terapia medicamentosa sobre o comportamento agressivo.

Inibidores Seletivos de Recaptação da Serotonina (ISRSs)
- Fluoxetina a 0,5-2 mg/kg VO a cada 24 h (cães).
- Paroxetina a 0,5-1 mg/kg VO a cada 24 h (cães).
- Sertralina a 1-3 mg/kg VO a cada 24 h (cães).
- Efeitos colaterais: sedação, irritabilidade, efeitos GI; a anorexia é comum, mas costuma ser transitória.

Antidepressivos Tricíclicos (ATCs)
- Clomipramina a 2-4 mg/kg VO a cada 24 h ou divididos a cada 12 h (cães) (bula restrita para agressividade).
- Efeitos colaterais: sedação, efeitos GI, efeitos anticolinérgicos, possíveis distúrbios de condução cardíaca em animais predispostos.

Benzodiazepínicos
- Alprazolam a 0,05-0,1 mg/kg VO a cada 12 h ou prescrito conforme a necessidade.

PRECAUÇÕES
- Qualquer medicação psicotrópica pode aumentar e não diminuir a agressividade.
- Ter cautela ao prescrever os benzodiazepínicos, pois eles poderão desinibir a agressividade se diminuírem a inibição (baseada no medo) contra mordidas.
- Não associar ISRSs ou ATCs com inibidores da MAO (p. ex., amitraz e selegilina) ou tramadol — essas combinações podem resultar em síndrome serotoninérgica fatal.

AGRESSIVIDADE DEFENSIVA INDUZIDA PELO MEDO — CÃES

ACOMPANHAMENTO

MONITORIZAÇÃO DO PACIENTE
- Com frequência, os proprietários precisam de assistência contínua e devem receber no mínimo um telefonema de acompanhamento nas primeiras 1-3 semanas após a consulta. Nesse momento, deverão ser previstos os acompanhamentos futuros. A comunicação contínua aumenta a obediência do proprietário ao tratamento.

PREVENÇÃO
- As recomendações terapêuticas são para toda a vida — a recidiva da agressividade pode ser observada com lapsos do tratamento e exposição contínua a estímulos indutores do medo. Os proprietários sempre devem estar vigilantes e no controle do comportamento do cão.
- A socialização e a habituação precoces satisfatórias podem ajudar a evitar os comportamentos tardios baseados no medo. Isso envolve a inscrição do filhote canino em aulas bem estruturadas de reforço positivo, começando durante o período de pico para a socialização.

COMPLICAÇÕES POSSÍVEIS
Lesões em seres humanos; eutanásia ou abandono do paciente.

EVOLUÇÃO ESPERADA E PROGNÓSTICO
Não há cura. O prognóstico quanto à melhora será melhor se o comportamento agressivo for de baixa intensidade e ocorrer apenas em algumas situações previsíveis. O prognóstico é altamente dependente da obediência do proprietário ao tratamento.

DIVERSOS

DISTÚRBIOS ASSOCIADOS
Outras condições baseadas no medo ou na ansiedade podem ser observadas (p. ex., fobias a ruídos e ansiedade da separação).

POTENCIAL ZOONÓTICO
Lesões em seres humanos e feridas causadas por mordeduras.

GESTAÇÃO/FERTILIDADE/REPRODUÇÃO
Não acasalar cães com comportamento extremamente medroso ou com medo/agressividade.

VER TAMBÉM
Agressividade contra Pessoas Familiares — Cães.

ABREVIATURA(S)
- ATC = antidepressivo tricíclico.
- GI = gastrintestinal.
- ISRS = inibidor seletivo de recaptação da serotonina.
- MAO = monoamina oxidase.
- RM = ressonância magnética.
- SNC = sistema nervoso central.

Sugestões de Leitura
Herron ME, Shofer SS, Reisner IR. Survey of the use and outcome of confrontational and non-confrontational training methods in client-owned dogs showing undesired behaviors. Appl Anim Behav Sci 2009, 177:47-54.
Moffat K. Addressing canine and feline aggression in the veterinary clinic. Vet Clin North Am Small Anim Pract 2008, 38(5):983-1003.
Virga V, Houpt KA, Scarlett JA. Efficacy of amitriptyline as a pharmacological adjunct to behavioral modification in the management of aggressive behaviors in dogs. JAAHA 2001, 37:325-330.

Autores Laurie Bergman e Meredith Stepita
Consultor Editorial Debra F. Horwitz

Agressividade entre os Cães

CONSIDERAÇÕES GERAIS

REVISÃO
• Existem duas formas básicas de agressividade: uma direcionada a outros cães dentro de uma residência e outra voltada a cães estranhos. Há várias motivações distintas, que incluem medo, territorialidade e *status* social. Em geral, tais comportamentos estão dentro dos limites de normalidade, embora a agressividade excessiva atribuída ao aprendizado ou em virtude da genética (cão criado especificamente para briga) também seja possível.

SISTEMA(S) ACOMETIDO(S)
Comportamental.

IDENTIFICAÇÃO
• Cão.
• Mais comum em machos intactos.
• Há predisposição racial em "cães de briga" (p. ex., Pit bull terriers) e Terriers.
• Os sinais costumam se desenvolver na puberdade (entre os 6-9 meses de vida) ou na maturidade social (entre os 18-36 meses de idade).

SINAIS CLÍNICOS
• Agressividade (rosnadas, elevação labial, latidos, abocanhadas, botes, mordidas) direcionada a outros cães. Isso pode ser acompanhado por posturas corporais submissas ou amedrontadas/expressões faciais (agachamento, recuo, orelhas voltadas para trás, cauda encolhida, olhar distante, lambedura dos lábios) ou por posturas corporais confiantes/dominantes (posição ereta, aproximação ao outro cão, contato direto com outro cão, elevação da cauda, orelhas voltadas para a frente).
• O histórico pode incluir o cão ter sido vítima de agressividade por outros cães (particularmente se a agressividade for direcionada a cães estranhos).
• Quando a briga ocorre dentro de casa, o histórico antes do início das brigas pode incluir sinais sutis de controle/domínio social (p. ex., olhar fixo, repousar nas portas para obstruir o acesso de outros cães a algum cômodo) e submissão (p. ex., desviar do olhar fixo do cão ou não entrar na mesma sala que o outro cão).
• Em casos de briga dentro de casa, os cães podem se sair bem dessa situação, exceto em situações específicas.

CAUSAS E FATORES DE RISCO
• Pode ser um comportamento canino normal; fortemente influenciado por experiências anteriores (p. ex., socialização prévia inadequada, encontros agressivos com outros cães, punição imprópria na presença de outros cães).
• Predileções raciais em virtude do acasalamento seletivo para agressividade entre os cães.
• É provável que a agressividade seja pior em cães do mesmo sexo.
• Em casos de agressividade dentro de casa, pode haver histórico de interferência nos métodos normais de comunicação canina pelos proprietários, sobretudo quando um cão parece negar o acesso de outro cão a algo que os proprietários consideram que eles deveriam "compartilhar". Essa mudança pode, na verdade, apoiar um cão no que seria considerado um comportamento "canino" inadequado e resultar na intensificação da agressividade entre os cães. Por exemplo, um proprietário que chama o cão "A" para uma sala quando o outro cão "B" teve seu acesso bloqueado ainda que o cão "A" estivesse disposto a permanecer fora da sala ou o proprietário que pune o cão "B" por bloquear o acesso do cão "A". Ambas as situações minam o cão "B" em sua posição hierárquica, ao mesmo tempo em que sutilmente reafirma o controle de que o cão "A" estava disposto a respeitar.
• Condições clínicas subjacentes, especialmente as indutoras de dor, podem aumentar o nível da agressividade.

DIAGNÓSTICO

DIAGNÓSTICO DIFERENCIAL
• Brincadeiras ou excitação não agressiva.
• Outros, dependendo das circunstâncias.

HEMOGRAMA/BIOQUÍMICA/URINÁLISE
Em geral, não são dignos de nota. As anormalidades sugerem alguma condição clínica subjacente ou colaboradora.

OUTROS TESTES LABORATORIAIS
Não costumam ser dignos de nota.

DIAGNÓSTICO POR IMAGEM
Obter imagem por RM na suspeita de envolvimento do SNC. Outras imagens devem ser obtidas, conforme a necessidade, para descartar condições clínicas subjacentes.

MÉTODOS DIAGNÓSTICOS
N/D.

TRATAMENTO

ORIENTAÇÃO AO PROPRIETÁRIO
• O tratamento visa o controle do problema, e não a "cura". O tratamento bem-sucedido, conforme é mensurado por um declínio nos incidentes agressivos, depende do comportamento social canino básico julgado pelo proprietário, dos riscos envolvidos na posse de um cão agressivo e da adoção de recomendações relativas à segurança e ao manejo.
• Os proprietários devem ter a consciência de que a única forma de prevenir lesões futuras é mudar de casa (se a agressividade ocorrer dentro do lar) ou efetuar a eutanásia.
• Se os proprietários não optarem pela eutanásia, eles deverão estar cientes de que sua principal responsabilidade será prevenir lesões em seres humanos, evitando de forma consciente situações capazes de evocar uma reação agressiva, inclusive aquelas que tenham resultado em um cão medroso, ainda que ele não seja agressivo. Talvez seja necessário que os cães dentro de uma casa sejam mantidos separados para evitar o contato e possíveis brigas.
• Se houver necessidade, os proprietários deverão ser orientados quanto aos métodos de separar as brigas entre cães com segurança.
• Os proprietários poderão ser mais obedientes às recomendações de prevenção se compreenderem que, em muitas jurisdições, os donos de cães são responsáveis pelas mordidas e poderão enfrentar processos civis/criminais se uma pessoa sofrer algum tipo de lesão.
• É mais provável que o tratamento seja bem-sucedido se for instituído um período para evitar a exposição a estímulos indutores da agressividade antes da modificação comportamental.
• O cão deve ficar confinado longe de vítimas em potencial ou sob o controle físico direto de um adulto responsável sempre que possa surgir uma situação indutora de agressividade (p. ex., em qualquer local público, em passeios, em torno de alimentos ou outros recursos estimados).
• O adestramento dos cães para que eles se adaptem a uma espécie de cabresto (Gentle Leader®) e uma focinheira tipo cesta torna mais fácil e mais seguro o controle de situações potencialmente perigosas.
• Tratando-se de agressividade dentro de casa, determinar qual é o cão mais dominante/controlador e reforçar esse domínio, fazendo com que o cão possa ter acesso a coisas que ele valoriza ou estima (p. ex., alimento, brinquedos, áreas de repouso e atenção humana).
• Ter consciência de que tanto os "agressores" como o acesso a recursos entre os cães da casa podem ser dependentes do contexto.

Terapia Comportamental
• Dessensibilização e contracondicionamento sistemáticos a estímulos específicos indutores de agressividade.
• JAMAIS permitir que os cães "cedam a brigas" (ver "Agressividade contra Pessoas Familiares — Cães").
• Controle da afeição: especialmente para os casos de agressividade entre os cães dentro de uma casa. Para aumentar a liderança dos proprietários sobre os cães e a previsibilidade da vida desses cães (ver "Agressividade Contra Pessoas Familiares — Cães").

MEDICAÇÕES

MEDICAMENTO(S)
• Não há medicamentos aprovados para o tratamento da agressividade canina. Os proprietários devem estar cientes de que o uso de medicamento está fora da indicação aprovada pela FDA. Em virtude de questões relativas à responsabilidade, é preciso anotar na ficha do paciente o fato de que os proprietários foram informados sobre os riscos e os efeitos colaterais em potencial.
• É recomendável, portanto, a assinatura de um termo de consentimento informado.
• NUNCA usar medicamentos sem modificação comportamental.
• Antes de prescrever o medicamento, ter a certeza de que os proprietários não só compreenderam os riscos da posse de um cão agressivo, mas também que adotarão os procedimentos de segurança e não contarão com o medicamento para garantir a segurança pública.
• O medicamento pode não ser apropriado em certas situações familiares, como na existência de crianças, membros da família portadores de deficiências ou indivíduos imunocomprometidos.
• Pesquisas confirmaram o intenso efeito exercido por placebo ao utilizar medicações para o tratamento da agressividade canina. Estudos não demonstraram um efeito substancial da terapia medicamentosa sobre o comportamento agressivo.
• É mais provável que os medicamentos sejam benéficos em situações nas quais há um forte componente de medo/ansiedade, exatamente o contrário daquelas que utilizam a agressividade

AGRESSIVIDADE ENTRE OS CÃES

para o estabelecimento de domínio entre cães intimamente agrupados.

Inibidores Seletivos de Recaptação da Serotonina (ISRSs)
- Fluoxetina a 0,5-2 mg/kg VO a cada 24 h (cães).
- Paroxetina a 0,5-1 mg/kg VO a cada 24 h (cães).
- Sertralina a 1-3 mg/kg VO a cada 24 h (cães).
- Efeitos colaterais: sedação, irritabilidade, efeitos GI; a anorexia é comum, mas costuma ser transitória.

Antidepressivos Tricíclicos (ATCs)
- Clomipramina a 2-4 mg/kg VO a cada 24 h ou divididos a cada 12 h (cães) (bula restrita para agressividade).
- Efeitos colaterais: sedação, efeitos GI, efeitos anticolinérgicos, possíveis distúrbios de condução cardíaca em animais predispostos.

Benzodiazepínicos
- Alprazolam a 0,05-0,1 mg/kg VO a cada 12 h ou prescrito conforme a necessidade.

CONTRAINDICAÇÕES/INTERAÇÕES POSSÍVEIS
- Qualquer medicação psicotrópica pode aumentar e não diminuir a agressividade.
- Ter cautela ao prescrever os benzodiazepínicos, pois eles poderão desinibir a agressividade se diminuírem a inibição (baseada no medo) contra mordidas.
- Não associar ISRSs ou ATCs com inibidores da MAO (p. ex., amitraz e selegilina) ou tramadol — essas combinações podem resultar em síndrome serotoninérgica potencialmente fatal.

ACOMPANHAMENTO

MONITORIZAÇÃO DO PACIENTE
Com frequência, os proprietários precisam de assistência contínua e devem receber no mínimo um telefonema de acompanhamento nas primeiras 1-3 semanas após a consulta. Nesse momento, deverão ser previstos os acompanhamentos futuros.

PREVENÇÃO
As recomendações terapêuticas são para toda a vida — a recidiva da agressividade pode ser observada com lapsos do tratamento e exposição contínua a fatores desencadeantes de agressividade.

COMPLICAÇÕES POSSÍVEIS
Lesões aos cães e seres humanos envolvidos; eutanásia ou abandono do paciente.

EVOLUÇÃO ESPERADA E PROGNÓSTICO
Não há cura. O prognóstico quanto à melhora é mais satisfatório se a agressividade for relativamente de baixa intensidade e ocorrer apenas em algumas situações previsíveis. O prognóstico é altamente dependente da obediência do proprietário ao tratamento.

DIVERSOS

DISTÚRBIOS ASSOCIADOS
Outras condições baseadas no medo ou na ansiedade podem ser observadas (p. ex., fobias a ruídos e ansiedade da separação); agressividade territorial.

POTENCIAL ZOONÓTICO
Ao separar brigas de cães, serão geradas lesões em seres humanos e feridas por mordeduras.

GESTAÇÃO/FERTILIDADE/REPRODUÇÃO
Não acasalar cães com agressividade extrema entre animais da mesma espécie.

VER TAMBÉM
- Agressividade contra Pessoas Familiares — Cães.
- Agressividade Defensiva Induzida pelo Medo — Cães.

ABREVIATURA(S)
- ATC = antidepressivo tricíclico.
- GI = gastrintestinal.
- ISRS = inibidor seletivo de recaptação da serotonina.
- MAO = monoamina oxidase.
- RM = ressonância magnética.
- SNC = sistema nervoso central.

Sugestões de Leitura

deKeuster T, Jung H. Aggression toward familiar people and animals. In: Horwitz DF, Mills D, eds., BSAVA Manual of Canine and Feline Behavioural Medicine, 2nd ed. Gloucestershire, UK: BSAVA, 2009, pp. 182-210.

Herron ME, Shofer SS, Reisner IR. Survey of the use and outcome of confrontational and non-confrontational training methods in client-owned dogs showing undesired behaviors. Appl Anim Behav Sci 2009, 177:47-54.

Mertens PA. Canine aggression. In: Horwitz D, Mills D, Heath S, eds., BSAVA Manual of Canine and Feline Behavioural Medicine. Gloucestershire, UK: BSAVA, 2002, pp. 195-215.

Autores Laurie Bergman e Meredith Stepita
Consultor Editorial Debra F. Horwitz

Agressividade entre os Gatos

CONSIDERAÇÕES GERAIS

REVISÃO
• Olhar fixo, deslocamento, vocalização (rosnados, uivos e gritos), salivação, sibilos, golpes, botes, caça/perseguição e/ou mordida de outros gatos. Existem múltiplas motivações.

SISTEMA(S) ACOMETIDO(S)
• Comportamental. • Sanguíneo/linfático/imune. • Nervoso.

IDENTIFICAÇÃO
• Não se observa distribuição etária, sexual ou racial. • Pode ocorrer em qualquer idade como uma manifestação crônica de agressividade redirecionada ou quando o ambiente social sofre mudanças (por exemplo, a adição de um novo gato, retorno de um gato do veterinário etc.).
• Relações felinas previamente estáveis podem se desintegrar à medida que os gatos atingem a maturidade social.

SINAIS CLÍNICOS
Agressor
• Sinais velados: olhar fixo, deslocamento de outros gatos, linguagens/movimentos corporais rígidos enquanto se aproxima de outro gato.
• Sinais evidentes: rosnados, uivos, salivação, sibilos, golpes, botes, caça/perseguição e/ou mordidas de outros gatos, além de pupilas dilatadas; podem ser acompanhados por linguagem corporal de medo (como a postura clássica de gato do Halloween — piloereção, dorso arqueado, cauda elevada) ou linguagem corporal mais ofensiva (músculos rígidos, extremidade da cauda elevada e restante rebaixado, dorso reto ou levemente inclinado em direção à cabeça, orelhas voltadas para a frente ou para o lado), expressões faciais excessivas e, talvez, marcação com urina.

Vítima
• Sinais velados: evitar o agressor, esconder-se, mudar os hábitos de auto-higienização e alimentação, mostrar-se hipervigilante e exibir pupilas dilatadas. • Sinais evidentes: sibilos, golpes, corrida, vocalização (inclusive rosnados), postura de gato de Halloween, que podem aumentar para um ataque defensivo se o animal se sentir ou for encurralado.

Evacuação Domiciliar Fora da Bandeja Sanitária
• Os agressores podem obstruir o acesso à área da bandeja sanitária, forçando as vítimas a escolherem locais alternativos de evacuação; podem surgir preferências por outros substratos e/ou locais, além de aversões. • Tanto as vítimas como os agressores podem marcar o território com eliminação de urina tanto horizontal como vertical. • Gatos extremamente medrosos podem urinar ou defecar durante eventos agressivos.

CAUSAS E FATORES DE RISCO
• Limitação de recursos (espaço vertical e/ou horizontal insuficiente, falta de áreas adequadas de esconderijo e acesso limitado a alimento, água e bandejas sanitárias, etc.) • Instabilidade social e ambiental, como a adição de um novo gato, perda de um gato residente, alteração nos odores (retorno de um gato do veterinário ou dar banho em um gato), envelhecimento ou doença de um ou ambos os gatos, um ou múltiplos gatos em maturidade social, mudanças, troca ou movimentação da mobília ou outras áreas de repouso, etc. • Exposição a estímulos indutores de agitação (gatos intrusos no jardim, visitantes, ruídos, odores, etc.) pode gerar comportamentos agressivos redirecionados que, possivelmente, evoluem para interações agressivas persistentes.
• Falta de socialização apropriada com outros gatos como um filhote. • É mais provável que gatos geneticamente não aparentados e aqueles que passaram a morar recentemente juntos demonstrem comportamentos agressivos entre si.
• Problemas clínicos indutores de dor ou irritabilidade acentuada. • Certa agressividade entre os gatos é um comportamento normal nos sistemas de socialização felina. • Os gatos residentes costumam adotar uma exposição prolongada a novos gatos antes de estarem dispostos a aceitá-los em um grupo, sem exibir comportamentos defensivos ou ofensivos.

DIAGNÓSTICO

DIAGNÓSTICO DIFERENCIAL
Diferenciais Comportamentais
• Agressividade relacionada com medo, agressividade vinculada ao *status* social, agressividade territorial, agressividade redirecionada, falha de reconhecimento (mais provavelmente em virtude de mudanças no odor da vítima), agressividade materna, agressividade entre os machos, agressividade sexual, comportamento predatório.

Diferenciais Clínicos
• Qualquer doença indutora de mal-estar, dor ou irritabilidade acentuada (hipertensão, artrite, abscesso, doença dentária). • Endócrinos: hipertireoidismo. • Neurológicos: lesões expansivas (meningioma, linfoma), encefalite, crises convulsivas, encefalopatia isquêmica felina, traumatismo, déficit sensorial ou cognitivo.
• Infecciosos: raiva, toxoplasmose, migrações parasitárias aberrantes (como cuterebríase), FIV, FeLV. • Iatrogênicos: administração de medicamentos que possam aumentar a irritabilidade ou desinibir o comportamento agressivo (como mirtazapina, benzodiazepínicos, buspirona). • Tóxicos: chumbo, ingestão de substâncias ilícitas.

HEMOGRAMA/BIOQUÍMICA/URINÁLISE
• Obter esses exames na consulta inicial ou antes do encaminhamento para especialistas a fim de descartar quaisquer problemas clínicos que estejam contribuindo para o quadro. • Se o paciente estiver sendo submetido à medicação psicotrópica, repetir tais exames a cada 6 meses a 1 ano, dependendo da idade e do estado geral de saúde do animal de estimação.

OUTROS TESTES LABORATORIAIS
• Gatos com >6 anos de idade precisam ser submetidos à mensuração dos níveis de T_4/T_4 livre.
• Deverão ser obtidos exames de urocultura e antibiograma de gatos que estejam urinando fora da bandeja sanitária a menos que haja um diagnóstico claro de marcação territorial com urina para todas as micções feitas fora dessa bandeja.

DIAGNÓSTICO POR IMAGEM
Em casos de evacuação domiciliar imprópria por gatos, é recomendável a obtenção de imagens por radiografias e/ou ultrassonografias.

MÉTODOS DIAGNÓSTICOS
• Obter histórico detalhado por comunicação oral ou por escrito. • Identificar o número, a localização e os tipos de bandejas sanitárias, bem como os locais onde cada um dos gatos gasta a maior parte de seu tempo. • Se houver múltiplos gatos dentro da casa, tentar determinar que gatos gastam grande parte do tempo juntos e quais se evitam, bem como as áreas de alimentação, brincadeiras e repouso, além dos locais de qualquer evacuação domiciliar ou marcação territorial. • Caso não seja possível uma visita em domicílio, fazer com que os proprietários desenhem uma planta baixa com os detalhes descritos anteriormente. • A obtenção de videoteipes e fotografias da interação dos gatos pode trazer informações valiosas. • Anotar quaisquer outras alterações no comportamento e na rotina, bem como nos hábitos de alimentação e auto-higienização, de todos os envolvidos.

TRATAMENTO
• Para casos graves e crônicos ou para agressividade irresponsiva ao tratamento, os proprietários poderão eleger a separação permanente, mudando um dos gatos de casa ou dividindo a residência. O veterinário deve estar preparado para fornecer recomendações sobre esse processo. • Castrar os machos intactos.

PARA OS CASOS COM BAIXA FREQUÊNCIA DE ATAQUES AGRESSIVOS NOCIVOS E INTENSOS
• Separar os gatos quando a supervisão direta não for possível (criar "zonas de segurança"). • Manter os mesmos espaços todos os dias na tentativa de produzir um território central separado para cada gato ou "compartilhar" os espaços entre os gatos a fim de evitar que cada um deles explore apenas uma pequena área durante um período prolongado. • Caso se opte em manter as mesmas zonas de segurança para cada gato, deixar para o agressor a área menor (manter a área central do agressor pequena). • Para múltiplos gatos, separar de acordo com a estabilidade de relação entre os gatos. Quaisquer gatos despóticos/agressores devem ser confinados isoladamente.
• Recompensar os gatos com alimentos, brincadeiras e/ou atenção por estarem no mesmo ambiente ou espaço juntos, sem quaisquer eventos agressivos. Os gatos devem permanecer a uma distância que permita um envolvimento calmo e tranquilo. • Engajar os gatos em sessões diárias de atividades prazerosas (brincadeiras, adestramento, petiscos palatáveis, etc.) a distâncias que tenham uma probabilidade muito baixa de gerar eventos agressivos. Aproxime gradativamente as sessões de divertimento. • O objetivo das medidas de manejo e segurança é evitar a ocorrência de eventos agressivos. Em uma emergência, o uso criterioso de interruptores (como pistolas d'água, cobertores atirados sobre os gatos, etc.) pode interromper os eventos em andamento, mas não deve ser considerado a base da terapia. Tais recursos só devem ser usados quando o comportamento agressivo estiver começando a ficar mais efetivo. Se isso puder ser feito com segurança, o agressor deverá ser colocado em sua zona de segurança ou atraído para ela ao primeiro sinal de qualquer comportamento ameaçador. O emprego de

Agressividade entre os Gatos

dispositivos para interrupção e punição do comportamento pode aumentar a agressividade em alguns gatos e as associações negativas com outros gatos; por essa razão, tais dispositivos devem ser utilizados com cuidado. • Elementos de distração, como ponteiras a laser, brinquedos lançados e outros ativados por controle remoto, podem ser usados para redirecionar os agressores no início da sequência do comportamento agressivo (olhar fixo, contorção da cauda e dilatação das pupilas) sem correr o risco de criar associações negativas entre os gatos. • Colocar uma espécie de sino ou campainha no agressor tipo coleira de segurança ou de rápida liberação, para que o proprietário e a vítima possam identificar com rapidez a localização do animal. • Aumentar o número de recursos em toda a residência. • Adquirir um número a mais de bandejas sanitárias em relação a cada gato (ou seja, três bandejas para dois gatos). • Acrescentar bandejas sanitárias em diferentes locais, de modo que um gato não consiga impedir o acesso de outros gatos; os locais com mais de uma entrada/saída são ideais. • Aumentar o número e os locais das áreas destinadas ao alimento e à água. • Ampliar os locais de esconderijo e as áreas confortáveis de repouso; concentrar-se especialmente no aumento dos espaços verticais (i. e., áreas de descanso em prateleiras, soleiras de janelas, etc.). • Incrementar as atividades lúdicas e adicionar brinquedos dispensadores de alimentos. • Não é recomendável a introdução de novos gatos à casa.

PARA OS CASOS EM QUE OS GATOS NÃO CONSEGUEM FICAR NO MESMO AMBIENTE SEM FICAREM IMEDIATAMENTE AGITADOS

• Separar os gatos completamente quando estiverem sem supervisão. • Atender às necessidades de cada gato por brincadeiras, bandejas sanitárias, alimentos, água e atenção. • Iniciar sessões diárias de dessensibilização e contracondicionamento sistemáticos; em princípio, utilizar barreiras físicas e visuais. • Adestrar ambos os gatos a tolerar o uso de coleiras e peitorais, para que elas possam ser utilizadas durante as sessões de adestramento. Isso é particularmente valioso para o agressor. • Quando for permitido que os gatos tenham mais liberdade entre si, seguir as instruções expostas anteriormente em casos de agressividade menos grave entre os gatos.

MEDICAÇÕES

MEDICAMENTO(S)

Azapirona
• Buspirona a 0,5-1 mg/kg VO a cada 8-24 h (dose para gatos). • Reservada para as vítimas em virtude do potencial de aumento na confiança social e, possivelmente, como auxílio na interrupção do ciclo de corrida/perseguição; além disso, esse agente terapêutico pode melhorar os casos de marcação territorial com urina. • É necessária a atualização por parte do proprietário a cada 2 semanas. Planeje usar por, no mínimo, 4-6 semanas após a resolução dos sinais. • Os efeitos colaterais incluem o possível aumento na agressividade entre os gatos, pois a vítima agora pode reagir e ceder à briga.

Benzodiazepínicos
• Lorazepam a 0,125-0,25 mg/gato VO até a cada 12-24 h. • Oxazepam a 0,2-0,5 mg/kg VO a cada 12-24 h (dose para gatos). • Para gatos assustados agressivos. • Os efeitos colaterais compreendem intensificação na sociabilidade, diminuição no ato de se esconder, aumento no apetite e desinibição do comportamento agressivo, além de ataxia. • Podem-se observar os efeitos clínicos em até 1 h. • Nota: substância controlada, capaz de causar dependência. • É imprescindível a atualização por parte do proprietário por não mais do que 48 h depois de iniciar a medicação.

Inibidores Seletivos de Recaptação da Serotonina (ISRSs)
• Fluoxetina a 0,5-1 mg/kg VO a cada 24 h (dose para gatos). • Paroxetina a 0,5-1 mg/kg VO a cada 24 h (dose para gatos). • Indicados para comportamento agressivo, ansiedade e/ou marcação territorial com urina, podendo diminuir a impulsividade. • É indispensável a atualização por parte do proprietário a cada 2 semanas. Planeje usar por, no mínimo, 4-6 semanas após a resolução dos sinais. • Os efeitos colaterais dos ISRSs abrangem sedação, retenção urinária, desarranjo gastrintestinal (incluindo diarreia, constipação, vômito, anorexia), agitação/irritabilidade acentuadas.

Antidepressivos Tricíclicos (ATCs)
• Amitriptilina a 0,5-1 mg/kg VO a cada 12-24 h (dose felina): para gatos ansiosos com sintomas comórbidos, recidivantes e graves de cistite idiopática felina/doença do trato urinário inferior dos felinos. • Clomipramina a 0,3-0,5 mg/kg VO a cada 24 h (dose felina): para gatos ansiosos e/ou agressivos, com ou sem componentes de marcação territorial com urina. • É essencial a atualização por parte do proprietário a cada 2 semanas. Planeje utilizar por, no mínimo, 4-6 semanas após a resolução dos sinais. • Os efeitos colaterais dos ATCs envolvem sedação, aumento na sede, retenção urinária, constipação e diminuição do limiar convulsivo. Não usar em pacientes com arritmias ou cardiopatias.

Feromônios
• Os feromônios Feliway® e Felifriend® (duas frações diferentes de feromônio facial felino) podem ser úteis nos casos de agressividade entre os gatos quando utilizados com um plano terapêutico multimodal.

CONTRAINDICAÇÕES/INTERAÇÕES POSSÍVEIS

• Os ISRSs e ATCs devem ser usados com cuidado em pacientes com históricos de anormalidades cardíacas, histórico epiléptico e/ou hepatopatia, além de não ser recomendável o uso concomitante desses agentes. • Em virtude do potencial de indução de hepatopatias, os benzodiazepínicos devem ser utilizados com cautela em gatos. • Os medicamentos que alteram os níveis de serotonina podem sofrer importantes interações com outros agentes terapêuticos (como selegilina e amitraz). • Nos EUA, todas as medicações para problemas comportamentais em gatos estão fora da indicação do rótulo até o momento.

ACOMPANHAMENTO

MONITORIZAÇÃO DO PACIENTE

• Os clínicos devem ser atualizados a cada 2 semanas após o início do tratamento por telefone ou pessoalmente. É recomendável a realização de *check-ups* antes de 8 semanas do tratamento. • Reavaliar os exames laboratoriais a cada 6 meses a 1 ano, dependendo do estado de saúde e da idade dos pacientes para gatos submetidos à medicação a longo prazo.

PREVENÇÃO

A socialização apropriada pode ajudar a diminuir a probabilidade de comportamento agressivo entre os gatos em alguns animais dessa espécie. A introdução gradativa é mais parecida com o processo natural, por meio do qual novos gatos são admitidos a um grupo existente; por essa razão, esse método é preferido ao se introduzir novos gatos. Pode ser menos provável que gatos geneticamente aparentados sofram agressões intensas entre eles. Em casas estáveis, deve-se evitar a adição de outros gatos.

EVOLUÇÃO ESPERADA E PROGNÓSTICO

• Casos recentes e leves (lesões raras/brandas de baixa intensidade e baixa frequência) parecem ter um desfecho melhor a longo prazo. • O prognóstico é complicado por duração prolongada, alta gravidade, distúrbios clínicos subjacentes e obediência parcial do proprietário ao tratamento.

DIVERSOS

ABREVIATURA(S)

• ATC = antidepressivo tricíclico. • FeLV = vírus da leucemia felina. • FIV = vírus da imunodeficiência felina. • ISRS = inibidor seletivo de recaptação da serotonina. • T_4 = tiroxina.

Sugestões de Leitura

Amat M, et al. Evaluation of inciting causes, alternative targets, and risk factors associated with redirected aggression in cats. JAVMA 2008, 233(4):586-589.

Curtis TM, Knowles RJ, Crowell-Davis SL. Influence of familiarity and relatedness on proximity and allogrooming in domestic cats (Felis catus). Am J Vet Res 2003, 64:1151-1154.

Heath S. Feline aggression. In: Horwitz DF, Mills D, Heath, S, eds., BSAVA Manual of Canine and Feline Behavioral Medicine. Gloucestershire, UK: BSAVA, 2002, pp. 216-228.

Landsberg G, Hunthausen W, Ackerman L. Feline aggression. In: Handbook of Behavior Problems of the Dog and Cat, 2nd ed. Philadelphia: Elsevier Saunders, 2003, pp. 427-453.

Autor E'Lise Christensen Bell
Consultor Editorial Debra F. Horwitz

Agressividade por Medo — Gatos

CONSIDERAÇÕES GERAIS

REVISÃO
Agressividade felina direcionada ao ser humano e motivada pelo medo.

SISTEMA(S) ACOMETIDO(S)
• Comportamental. • Gastrintestinal — diminuição do apetite (hiporexia). • Sanguíneo/linfático/imune — efeitos de estresse crônico sobre a função imunológica. • Oftálmico — pupilas dilatadas (midríase) em resposta à estimulação do sistema nervoso autônomo. • Cutâneo/exócrino — pode revelar um problema comportamental secundário, como auto-higienização excessiva.

IDENTIFICAÇÃO
Gatos de qualquer idade, sexo ou estado reprodutivo (intacto ou não).

SINAIS CLÍNICOS
Manifestação do comportamento pelos gatos: orelhas para trás, corpo e cauda rebaixados/encolhidos, piloereção, dilatação pupilar; pode sibilar e rosnar. Evita a(s) pessoa(s) que elicia(m) a agressividade. Possíveis ataques se abordado e/ou encurralado. Casos extremos: liberação de secreção das glândulas anais, micção e/ou defecação. Comportamento de refúgio.

CAUSAS E FATORES DE RISCO
Socialização insatisfatória com seres humanos e/ou vida selvagem, evento aversivo associado a uma pessoa ou a pessoas em geral.

DIAGNÓSTICO

DIAGNÓSTICO DIFERENCIAL
• Agressividade motivada pela dor. • Agressividade motivada por brincadeiras. • Intolerância a afagos/carícias. • Agressividade redirecionada.

HEMOGRAMA/BIOQUÍMICA/URINÁLISE
Utilizados para descartar problemas médicos que contribuem para o quadro. Efetuar a urinálise em caso de micção inadequada e/ou marcação territorial com urina.

OUTROS TESTES LABORATORIAIS
Gatos idosos: função completa da tireoide.

DIAGNÓSTICO POR IMAGEM
Solicitados com base no exame clínico e/ou no componente de dor sob suspeita.

MÉTODOS DIAGNÓSTICOS
Histórico comportamental completo, incluindo uma descrição das posturas do gato durante a agressão e as lesões infligidas, uso de bandeja sanitária, consumo alimentar e comportamentos de refúgio.

TRATAMENTO

ORIENTAÇÃO AO PROPRIETÁRIO

Evitar Situações Indutoras de Medo
• A exposição contínua a situações indutoras de medo pode agravar os sinais, provocar estresse intenso e comprometer o bem-estar do animal.
• Exposição aos estímulos apenas sob exercícios controlados descritos adiante.

Proceder a Exercícios de Modificação do Comportamento

Dessensibilização e Contracondicionamento
• Dessensibilização: expor o gato ao estímulo indutor de medo (pessoa medrosa/assustada) a um nível baixo, de modo que o gato NÃO reaja com medo ou agressividade. Com o passar do tempo, a intensidade do estímulo é aumentada (ou seja, diminui-se a distância entre o gato e o estímulo) sem causar reações indutoras de medo.
• Contracondicionamento: recompensar o gato com algum petisco, brinquedo, higienização/embelezamento ou carícia especial para relaxamento.

CONDICIONAMENTO CLÁSSICO
• Condicionamento clássico: emparelhar o estímulo (pessoa que ameaça o gato) com algum petisco saboroso, brinquedo ou carícia. Exemplo: colocar a pessoa medrosa ao lado de um peixe de atum. À medida que o gato relaxa na presença da pessoa, o relaxamento é recompensado.

MEDICAÇÕES
Pode haver a necessidade de medicação para diminuir os níveis gerais de ansiedade e reatividade.

MEDICAMENTO(S)

Azapironas
• Buspirona 0,5-1,0 mg/kg a cada 12 h. Muito útil para gatos medrosos e retraídos. Diminui a ansiedade e pode aumentar a "autoconfiança". Relatos não publicados de "aumento na afeição" e possível incremento na agressividade quando administrado ao agressor. A resposta é observada em 1-2 semanas.

Inibidores Seletivos de Recaptação da Serotonina
• Fluoxetina, paroxetina, sertralina 0,5-1,5 mg/kg a cada 24 h.

Antidepressivos Tricíclicos
• Amitriptilina 0,5-2,0 mg/kg a cada 12-24 h.
• Clomipramina 0,25-1,3 mg/kg a cada 24 h.
• Inibidores seletivos de recaptação da serotonina e antidepressivos tricíclicos devem ser administrados diariamente. Pode levar de 4-8 semanas para atingir os efeitos máximos.

Benzodiazepínicos
• Alprazolam 0,125-0,25 mg/gato a cada 8-24 h.
• Diazepam 0,1-1,0 mg/kg a cada 12-24 h (raramente utilizado em virtude do potencial de hepatopatias). • Os benzodiazepínicos podem ser administrados "conforme a necessidade" para encontros específicos com pessoas que induzem à resposta de medo e durante as sessões de dessensibilização/contracondicionamento e condicionamento clássico. Tais agentes podem ser utilizados em conjunto com azapironas, inibidores seletivos de recaptação da serotonina e antidepressivos tricíclicos.

Feromônios
• Feliway® — disponível em difusor e *spray*.
• Utilizados para ajudar a acalmar o gato durante situações indutoras de estresse.

CONTRAINDICAÇÕES/INTERAÇÕES POSSÍVEIS
• Nenhuma das medicações listadas são aprovadas para uso em gatos. • Todos os medicamentos devem ser administrados por via oral, pois não há provas de que eles sejam eficazes por via transdérmica.
• Azapironas: os efeitos colaterais são raros, embora ocasionalmente se observe agitação. Não devem ser administradas em combinação com inibidores da monoamina oxidase. Evitar o uso no gato agressor; pode aumentar algum comportamento de "intimidação". • Inibidores seletivos de recaptação da serotonina e antidepressivos tricíclicos não devem ser combinados nem utilizados em combinação com inibidores da monoamina oxidase.
• Inibidores seletivos de recaptação da serotonina: os efeitos colaterais incluem leve sedação e hiporexia (diminuição do apetite), constipação e retenção urinária. Promovem inibição competitiva das enzimas hepáticas do sistema citocromo P450; quando administrados concomitantemente com medicamentos que fazem uso desse sistema enzimático, os níveis plasmáticos desses medicamentos podem aumentar, gerando níveis tóxicos. • Antidepressivos tricíclicos: os efeitos colaterais abrangem sedação, constipação, diarreia, retenção urinária, alterações do apetite, ataxia, produção lacrimal reduzida, midríase, arritmias cardíacas, taquicardia e alterações na pressão arterial.
• Benzodiazepínicos: os efeitos colaterais englobam sedação, ataxia, relaxamento muscular, aumento do apetite, excitação paradoxal e aumento da afabilidade. Há relatos de necrose hepática idiopática em gatos. • Recomendações específicas para o uso de diazepam: exame físico basal, hemograma completo e perfis bioquímicos sanguíneos para confirmar o bom estado de saúde. Repetir o exame bioquímico sanguíneo em 3-5 dias. Em caso de elevação das enzimas alanina aminotransferase ou aspartato aminotransferase, interromper a medicação.

ACOMPANHAMENTO

MONITORIZAÇÃO DO PACIENTE
É recomendável o acompanhamento semanal, especialmente quando o animal estiver sob medicamento(s). Para os gatos submetidos à medicação, é aconselhável a avaliação do exame de sangue a cada 6-12 meses.

PREVENÇÃO
Sempre que possível, evitar os estímulos indutores de medo. A socialização precoce com pessoas e eventos pode ajudar a evitar algumas ocorrências de respostas relacionadas com medo em direção às pessoas.

COMPLICAÇÕES POSSÍVEIS
Possível lesão em seres humanos — especialmente se o gato for abordado ou encurralado.

EVOLUÇÃO ESPERADA E PROGNÓSTICO
A evolução ocorre de forma lenta. O reaprendizado é um processo e cada caso é um caso. Se houver indicação de medicamentos, iniciar com uma dose baixa e proceder à avaliação conforme a necessidade. Para interromper a medicação, aguardar até que o novo comportamento se estabilize (8-12 semanas) e retirar lentamente, em geral em algumas semanas. Se o comportamento de medo recidivar, retornar à última dose que controlou a ansiedade e manter o tratamento.

DIVERSOS

POTENCIAL ZOONÓTICO
As pessoas que sofrem lesões durante algum ataque motivado por medo devem procurar atendimento médico imediato. A arranhadura ou mordedura de gatos pode resultar em infecção por *Bartonella henselae*.

Autor Terry Marie Curtis
Consultor Editorial Debra F. Horwitz

Agressividade Possessiva, Territorial e Induzida pelo Alimento — Cães

CONSIDERAÇÕES GERAIS

REVISÃO
- Agressividade possessiva por alimento — proteção agressiva ao alimento (p. ex., comedouros, materiais de couro cru, ossos de verdade e itens furtados ou encontrados) ou a objetos (p. ex., brinquedos e objetos furtados).
- Agressividade territorial — defesa agressiva por um território, que pode ser um local fixo (p. ex., casinha, jardim, carro, cama ou área de repouso). A agressividade pode não ser evidente em outros locais. Em outros casos, o território é móvel e fica em torno do cão; assim, as respostas agressivas podem ocorrer em qualquer momento. A agressividade territorial poderá ser exacerbada se o animal for contido.
- Em geral, tais comportamentos estão dentro dos limites de normalidade; no entanto, o aprendizado pode contribuir para a manifestação excessiva de agressividade.

SISTEMA(S) ACOMETIDO(S)
Comportamental.

IDENTIFICAÇÃO
Não há predileções raciais ou sexuais para agressividade alimentar/possessiva. A agressividade territorial é mais comum em machos intactos e os sinais clínicos costumam estar presentes por volta de 1 ano de idade.

SINAIS CLÍNICOS
- Alimentar/possessiva — agressividade (rosnadas, elevação labial, latidos, abocanhadas, botes, mordidas) contra pessoas ou outros cães na presença de itens alimentares ou objetos estimados.
- Territorial — agressividade em defesa de um local ou espaço.

CAUSAS E FATORES DE RISCO
- Pode fazer parte de um repertório comportamental canino normal. Fortemente influenciado por experiências prévias de êxito na defesa de alimentos, objetos ou território por meio da agressividade.
- Condições clínicas subjacentes e medicamentos, especialmente aqueles indutores de polifagia, ou dietas com restrição calórica podem aumentar o nível de agressividade pelo alimento.

DIAGNÓSTICO

DIAGNÓSTICO DIFERENCIAL
- Agressividade por medo.
- Agressividade por domínio/*status* social ou por conflito.
- Outros, dependendo das circunstâncias.

HEMOGRAMA/BIOQUÍMICA/URINÁLISE
Em geral, não são dignos de nota. As anormalidades sugerem alguma condição clínica subjacente ou colaboradora.

OUTROS TESTES LABORATORIAIS
Não costumam ser dignos de nota.

DIAGNÓSTICO POR IMAGEM
Obter imagem por RM na suspeita de envolvimento do SNC. Outras imagens devem ser obtidas, conforme a necessidade, para descartar condições clínicas subjacentes.

MÉTODOS DIAGNÓSTICOS
N/D.

TRATAMENTO

ORIENTAÇÃO AO PROPRIETÁRIO

Recomendações de Segurança
- Confinar o cão distante de vítimas em potencial ou submetê-lo a controle físico direto de um adulto responsável, sempre que possa surgir uma situação indutora de agressividade.
- Alimentar os cães confinados e distantes de pessoas; evitar o acesso a itens capazes de evocar a agressividade.
- Confinar os cães em locais onde eles não consigam ver/ouvir as pessoas que se aproximam de seu território antes que eles fiquem agressivamente agitados.
- Adestrar o cão para que ele se adapte a uma espécie de cabresto (Gentle Leader®) e uma focinheira tipo cesta a fim de facilitar o controle de situações potencialmente perigosas.
- O tratamento visa o controle do problema, e não a "cura".
- O tratamento bem-sucedido, mensurado por um declínio nos incidentes agressivos, depende do comportamento social canino básico julgado pelo proprietário, dos riscos envolvidos na posse de um animal agressivo e da adoção de recomendações relativas à segurança e ao manejo.
- O único meio de evitar lesões futuras é a realização de eutanásia.
- Se o cão permanecer na casa, a principal responsabilidade será prevenir lesões em seres humanos, evitando de forma consciente situações capazes de evocar uma reação agressiva.
- Para auxiliar na obediência ao tratamento, é preciso ajudar os proprietários a compreenderem que os donos de cães são frequentemente responsáveis pelas mordidas e poderão enfrentar processos civis/criminais se uma pessoa sofrer algum tipo de lesão.
- O ato de evitar a exposição a estímulos indutores da agressividade por um período antes da modificação comportamental pode auxiliar no êxito da terapia.
- Em virtude do ressurgimento atual na popularidade das técnicas de adestramento baseadas em punição e domínio, os proprietários deverão ser orientados sobre a etiologia (i. e., medo) da agressividade de seus cães. O emprego dessas técnicas pode resultar em comportamento agressivo acentuado, medo, agitação e/ou lesões.

Modificação Comportamental
- Controle da afeição: empregado para aumentar a liderança dos proprietários sobre os cães (ver "Agressividade contra Pessoas da Família — Cães").
- Dessensibilização e contracondicionamento sistemáticos a estímulos específicos indutores de agressividade. Utilize pedaços de comida do tamanho de uma ervilha para diminuir a probabilidade de o cão se tornar agressivo durante a modificação comportamental (ver "Agressividade contra Pessoas Familiares — Cães").
- Adestrar o cão a executar comportamentos alternativos (p. ex., um comando verbal para ficar quieto [*quiet*], outro para abandonar objetos [*drop*] ou ainda outro para sair da mobília [*off*]) sob recompensas. Com frequência, isso recebe o nome de contracomando ou substituição de resposta.

MEDICAÇÕES

MEDICAMENTO(S)
- Não existem medicamentos aprovados para o tratamento da agressividade canina. Os proprietários devem estar cientes de que o uso de um medicamento está fora da indicação aprovada pela FDA. Em virtude de questões relativas à responsabilidade, é preciso anotar na ficha do paciente o fato de que os proprietários foram informados sobre os riscos e os efeitos colaterais em potencial. É recomendável, portanto, a assinatura de um termo de consentimento informado. NUNCA usar medicamentos sem modificação comportamental. Antes de prescrever o medicamento, ter a certeza de que os proprietários não só compreenderam os riscos da posse de um cão agressivo, mas também que adotarão as recomendações de segurança e não contarão com o medicamento para garantir a segurança pública. O medicamento pode não ser apropriado em certas situações familiares, como na existência de crianças, membros da família portadores de deficiências ou indivíduos imunocomprometidos.
- Pesquisas confirmaram o intenso efeito exercido por placebo ao utilizar medicações para o tratamento da agressividade canina. Estudos não demonstraram um efeito substancial da terapia medicamentosa sobre o comportamento agressivo.

Inibidores Seletivos de Recaptação da Serotonina (ISRSs)
- Fluoxetina a 0,5-2 mg/kg VO a cada 24 h (cães).
- Paroxetina a 0,5-1 mg/kg VO a cada 24 h (cães).
- Sertralina a 1-3 mg/kg VO a cada 24 h (cães).
- Efeitos colaterais: sedação, irritabilidade, efeitos GI; a anorexia é comum, mas costuma ser transitória.

Antidepressivos Tricíclicos (ATCs)
- Clomipramina a 2-4 mg/kg VO a cada 24 h ou divididos a cada 12 h (cães) (bula restrita para agressividade).
- Efeitos colaterais: sedação, efeitos GI, efeitos anticolinérgicos, possíveis distúrbios de condução cardíaca em animais predispostos.

CONTRAINDICAÇÕES/INTERAÇÕES POSSÍVEIS
- Qualquer medicação psicotrópica pode aumentar e não diminuir a agressividade.
- Ter cautela ao prescrever os benzodiazepínicos, pois eles poderão desinibir a agressividade se diminuírem a inibição (baseada no medo) contra mordidas.
- Não associar ISRSs ou ATCs com inibidores da MAO (p. ex., amitraz e selegilina) e tramadol — essas combinações podem resultar em síndrome serotoninérgica potencialmente fatal.

ACOMPANHAMENTO

MONITORIZAÇÃO DO PACIENTE
Com frequência, os proprietários precisam de assistência contínua e devem receber no mínimo um telefonema de acompanhamento nas primeiras 1-3 semanas após a consulta. Nesse momento, deverão ser previstos os acompanhamentos futuros.

Agressividade Possessiva, Territorial e Induzida pelo Alimento — Cães

PREVENÇÃO
As recomendações terapêuticas são para toda a vida — a recidiva da agressividade pode ser observada com lapsos do tratamento e exposição contínua a fatores desencadeantes de agressividade.

COMPLICAÇÕES POSSÍVEIS
Lesões em seres humanos; eutanásia ou abandono do paciente.

EVOLUÇÃO ESPERADA E PROGNÓSTICO
Não há cura. O prognóstico quanto à melhora será mais favorável se o comportamento agressivo for de baixa intensidade e ocorrer apenas em algumas situações previsíveis. O prognóstico é altamente dependente da obediência do proprietário ao tratamento.

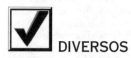
DIVERSOS
DISTÚRBIOS ASSOCIADOS
Agressividade por medo e domínio/conflito.

POTENCIAL ZOONÓTICO
Lesão em seres humanos e feridas causadas por mordeduras.

GESTAÇÃO/FERTILIDADE/REPRODUÇÃO
Não acasalar os cães com agressividade extrema.

VER TAMBÉM
- Agressividade contra Pessoas da Família — Cães.
- Agressividade Defensiva Induzida pelo Medo — Cães.

ABREVIATURA(S)
- ATC = antidepressivo tricíclico.
- GI = gastrintestinal.
- ISRS = inibidor seletivo de recaptação da serotonina.
- MAO = monoamina oxidase.
- RM = ressonância magnética.
- SNC = sistema nervoso central.

Sugestões de Leitura
deKeuster T, Jung H. Aggression toward familiar people and animals. In: Horwitz DF, Mills D, eds., BSAVA Manual of Canine and Feline Behavioural Medicine, 2nd ed. Gloucestershire, UK: BSAVA, 2009, pp. 182-210.

Herron ME, Shofer SS, Reisner IR. Survey of the use and outcome of confrontational and non-confrontational training methods in client-owned dogs showing undesired behaviors. Appl Anim Behav Sci 2009, 177:47-54.

Landsberg G, Hunthausen W, Ackerman L. Handbook of Behavior Problems of the Dog and Cat. Oxford: Butterworth-Heinemann, 1997.

Mertens PA. Canine aggression. In: Horwitz D, Mills D, Heath S, eds., BSAVA Manual of Canine and Feline Behavioural Medicine. Gloucestershire, UK: BSAVA, 2002, pp. 195-215.

Autores Laurie Bergman e Meredith Stepita
Consultor Editorial Debra F. Horwitz

ALCALOSE METABÓLICA

CONSIDERAÇÕES GERAIS

DEFINIÇÃO
Aumento no pH associado à elevação na concentração plasmática de bicarbonato (HCO_3^-) (cães, >24 mEq/L; gatos, >22 mEq/L) e aumento compensatório na tensão de dióxido de carbono (PCO_2).

FISIOPATOLOGIA
• A alcalose metabólica pode se desenvolver secundariamente à hipocloremia corrigida (alcalose hipoclorêmica) ou à hipoalbuminemia (alcalose hipoalbuminêmica).
• Alcalose hipoclorêmica:
  ○ Perda de líquido rico em cloreto e íons hidrogênio (H^+) pelo trato digestório ou pelos rins. A perda de cloreto e H^+ é associada a um aumento na concentração plasmática de HCO_3^-. Com a perda de cloreto e a depleção de volume, os rins reabsorvem o sódio com o HCO_3^- no lugar do cloreto, perpetuando a alcalose metabólica.
  ○ A administração crônica de álcalis (fluidos com alta concentração de sódio e baixa de cloreto) também pode resultar em alcalose metabólica transitória. A excreção renal de álcalis administrados por via exógena é eficaz, embora seja difícil criar uma alcalose metabólica, aumentando-se a ingestão de HCO_3^- a menos que o paciente tenha disfunção renal.
• Alcalose hipoalbuminêmica:
  ○ Diminuição nos ácidos fracos do plasma — a perda de albumina, um ácido fraco, é associada à alcalose metabólica.

SISTEMA(S) ACOMETIDO(S)
• Nervoso — raramente ocorrem espasmos musculares e crises convulsivas em cães. A alcalose metabólica e a hipocalemia associada podem precipitar a ocorrência de encefalopatia hepática em pacientes com insuficiência hepática.
• Renal/urológico — os rins excretam com rapidez e eficácia os álcalis em excesso. Em pacientes com deficiência de cloreto (e, com menor importância, depleção de volume), os rins não conseguem excretar os álcalis em excesso, dando continuidade à alcalose metabólica. Nesses pacientes, a administração de cloreto é necessária para que ocorra a compensação renal, enquanto a expansão de volume acelerará a compensação. Os pacientes com excesso de mineralocorticoide apresentam perda excessiva de cloreto, mas a administração desse componente não leva à hipercloremia nem à correção da alcalose metabólica (a chamada alcalose metabólica resistente ao cloreto).
• Respiratório — a baixa concentração de H^+ diminui a ventilação alveolar. A hipoventilação aumenta a PCO_2 e ajuda a compensar os efeitos da alta concentração plasmática do HCO_3^- sobre o pH. Em cães, pode-se esperar um aumento de aproximadamente 0,7 mmHg na PCO_2 para cada incremento de 1 mEq/L na concentração plasmática do HCO_3^-. Embora haja dados limitados para os gatos, o grau de compensação respiratória parece semelhante.

IDENTIFICAÇÃO
Cães e gatos de qualquer raça, idade ou sexo.

SINAIS CLÍNICOS
Achados Anamnésicos
• Administração de diuréticos de alça (p. ex., furosemida) ou tiazídicos.
• Vômito.

Achados do Exame Físico
• Sinais relacionados com a doença subjacente ou a depleção concomitante de potássio (p. ex., fraqueza, arritmias cardíacas e íleo paralítico).
• Espasmos musculares causados pela baixa concentração de cálcio ionizado.
• Desidratação em pacientes com depleção volêmica.
• Espasmos musculares e crises convulsivas em pacientes com envolvimento neurológico (raro).

CAUSAS
• Alcalose metabólica responsiva ao cloreto — administração de diuréticos, vômito de conteúdo gástrico e correção rápida de hipercapnia crônica (acidose respiratória).
• Alcalose metabólica resistente ao cloreto — hiperadrenocorticismo e hiperaldosteronismo primário.
• Administração oral de álcalis — fornecimento de bicarbonato de sódio ou outros ânions orgânicos com sódio (p. ex., lactato, acetato e gliconato); administração de resina de troca catiônica com álcalis não absorvíveis (p. ex., quelantes de fósforo).
• Hipoalbuminemia.

FATORES DE RISCO
• Administração de diuréticos de alça ou tiazídicos.
• Vômito.
• Drenagem gástrica.
• Doenças associadas à hipoalbuminemia (p. ex., síndrome nefrótica, insuficiência hepática).

DIAGNÓSTICO

DIAGNÓSTICO DIFERENCIAL
Nos animais, a alta concentração plasmática de HCO_3^- e a hipocloremia também podem ser compensatórias em casos de acidose respiratória crônica, na qual a PCO_2 se apresenta elevada e o pH se encontra baixo apesar da alta concentração do HCO_3^- e da baixa concentração de cloreto; a diferenciação exige a determinação da gasometria sanguínea.

ACHADOS LABORATORIAIS
Medicamentos Capazes de Alterar os Resultados Laboratoriais
Nenhum.

Distúrbios Capazes de Alterar os Resultados Laboratoriais
• Grande quantidade de heparina (>10% da amostra) diminui a concentração do HCO_3^-.
• Amostras sanguíneas armazenadas em temperatura ambiente por mais de 20 minutos apresentam um pH baixo, em função da PCO_2 elevada.

Os Resultados Serão Válidos se os Exames Forem Realizados em Laboratório Humano?
Sim.

HEMOGRAMA/BIOQUÍMICA/URINÁLISE
• CO_2 total elevado (o CO_2 total em amostras manipuladas em meio aeróbio aproxima-se bastante da concentração de HCO_3^-).
• Concentração sanguínea baixa de cálcio ionizado.
• Os distúrbios eletrolíticos séricos variam com a causa subjacente.
• Hipocloremia — considerar uma alcalose metabólica hipoclorêmica, a razão mais comum para alcalose metabólica em cães e gatos, que resulta geralmente da administração de diuréticos ou de vômitos de conteúdo gástrico.
• Concentração alta de sódio, porém normal de cloreto — levar em consideração a alcalose metabólica resistente ao cloreto (p. ex., hiperadrenocorticismo ou hiperaldosteronismo primário) ou a administração de álcalis.
• Hipoalbuminemia — contemplar uma alcalose metabólica hipoalbuminêmica (p. ex., insuficiência hepática, enteropatia ou nefropatia com perda de proteínas). *In vitro*, uma diminuição de 1 g/dL na concentração de albumina é associada com um aumento no pH de 0,093 em gatos e 0,047 em cães.
• Hipocalemia — esse distúrbio eletrolítico provavelmente se origina da alcalose metabólica ou do problema subjacente (p. ex., vômito de conteúdo gástrico ou administração de diuréticos de alça); em cães e gatos, não ocorre a alcalose metabólica induzida pela hipocalemia.

OUTROS TESTES LABORATORIAIS
A gasometria sanguínea revela alta concentração de HCO_3^-, bem como PCO_2 e pH elevados.

DIAGNÓSTICO POR IMAGEM
Nenhum.

MÉTODOS DIAGNÓSTICOS
Nenhum.

TRATAMENTO
• O diagnóstico e o tratamento do processo mórbido subjacente são partes integrantes da resolução bem-sucedida dos distúrbios acidobásicos, que correspondem a fenômenos secundários.
• Apesar de incomum, a alcalemia grave pode ser potencialmente letal. Os pacientes com doença respiratória crônica e alcalose respiratória estão sob risco de desenvolvimento de alcalemia grave se começarem a vomitar ou receberem diuréticos.
• Interromper o fornecimento de medicamentos capazes de causar alcalose metabólica.

CUIDADO(S) DE ENFERMAGEM
Os fluidos de escolha contêm cloreto; em pacientes com depleção de volume, administrar uma infusão intravenosa de NaCl a 0,9% suplementada com KCl; os pacientes com hipocalemia podem necessitar de altas doses de KCl (ver "Hipocalemia").

MEDICAÇÕES

MEDICAMENTO(S) DE ESCOLHA
Alcalose Hipoclorêmica
• Se houver indícios de depleção volêmica, o déficit deverá ser corrigido com fluido que contenha cloreto (p. ex., NaCl a 0,9%).
• Caso não seja possível a correção da causa subjacente (p. ex., pacientes com insuficiência cardíaca crônica submetidos a diuréticos), pode-se

Alcalose Metabólica

lançar mão de compostos orais que contenham cloreto sem sódio (p. ex., KCl e NH_4Cl); considerar também o uso simultâneo de bloqueadores dos túbulos distais (p. ex., espironolactona).
- Os bloqueadores dos receptores histaminérgicos H_2 como ranitidina ou famotidina diminuem a secreção ácida gástrica e podem ser considerados como terapia adjuvante em caso de perdas gástricas contínuas.
- A alcalose metabólica resistente ao cloreto pode ser corrigida apenas por meio da resolução da doença subjacente; nesses pacientes, a alcalose metabólica costuma ser branda.
- Se a alcalose metabólica estiver associada à hipocalemia e a déficits corporais totais de potássio, a correção desse déficit com KCl é um meio particularmente eficaz de reverter a alcalose.

Alcalose Hipoalbuminêmica
- O tratamento para alcalose hipoalbuminêmica deve ser direcionado à causa subjacente e à redução da pressão oncótica coloidal.

CONTRAINDICAÇÕES
- Evitar os fluidos isentos de cloreto — podem corrigir a depleção volêmica, mas não corrigirão a alcalose hipoclorêmica.
- Evitar o uso de sais de potássio sem cloreto (p. ex., fosfato de potássio) — o potássio será excretado na urina e não corrigirá a alcalose nem o déficit desse elemento.

PRECAUÇÕES
Não empregar os bloqueadores dos túbulos distais (p. ex., espironolactona) em pacientes com depleção volêmica.

INTERAÇÕES POSSÍVEIS
Nenhuma.

MEDICAMENTO(S) ALTERNATIVO(S)
Nenhum.

ACOMPANHAMENTO
MONITORIZAÇÃO DO PACIENTE
Status acidobásico — a frequência é ditada pela doença subjacente e pela resposta do paciente ao tratamento.

COMPLICAÇÕES POSSÍVEIS
- Hipocalemia.
- Sinais neurológicos.

DIVERSOS
DISTÚRBIOS ASSOCIADOS
- Hipocalemia.
- Hipocloremia.

FATORES RELACIONADOS COM A IDADE
Nenhum.

POTENCIAL ZOONÓTICO
Nenhum.

GESTAÇÃO/FERTILIDADE/REPRODUÇÃO
N/D.

SINÔNIMO(S)
- Alcalose não respiratória.
- Alcalose metabólica responsiva ao cloreto — tipo de alcalose que responde à administração de cloreto.
- Alcalose metabólica resistente ao cloreto — tipo de alcalose que é secundária ao aumento na atividade mineralocorticoide e não responde à administração de cloreto.
- Alcalose metabólica hipoclorêmica — tipo de alcalose causada pela baixa concentração de cloreto.
- Alcalose hipoalbuminêmica — alcalose metabólica provocada pela baixa concentração de albumina.
- Alcalose por concentração — alcalose metabólica resultante da redução na água livre no plasma.
- Alcalose por contração — alcalose metabólica atribuída antigamente a uma contração volêmica; hoje em dia, no entanto, sabe-se que ela é causada pela depleção de cloreto. A depleção de volume é uma característica comum, mas não essencial.

VER TAMBÉM
- Hipocalemia.
- Hipocloremia.

ABREVIATURA(S)
- H^+ = íon(s) hidrogênio.
- HCO_3^- = bicarbonato.
- KCl = cloreto de potássio.
- PCO_2 = tensão de dióxido de carbono.

Sugestões de Leitura
de Morais HA. Chloride ion in small animal practice: The forgotten ion. J Vet Emerg Crit Care 1992, 2:11-24.
de Morais HA, Constable PD. Strong ion approach to acid-base disorders. In: DiBartola SP, ed., Fluid, Electrolyte and Acid-Base Disorders, 3rd. ed. Philadelphia: Saunders, 2006, pp. 310-321.
de Morais HA, Leisewitz AL. Mixed acid-base disorders. In: DiBartola SP, ed., Fluid, Electrolyte and Acid-Base Disorders, 3rd. ed. Philadelphia: Saunders, 2006, pp. 296-309.
DiBartola SP. Metabolic acid-base disorders. In: DiBartola SP, ed., Fluid, Electrolyte and Acid-Base Disorders, 3rd. ed. Philadelphia: Saunders, 2006, pp. 251-283.
Robinson EP, Hardy RM. Clinical signs, diagnosis, and treatment of alkalemia in dogs: 20 cases (1982-1984). JAVMA 1988, 192:943-949.

Autores Hélio Autran de Morais e Stephen P. DiBartola
Consultor Editorial Carl A. Osborne

ALOPECIA — CÃES

CONSIDERAÇÕES GERAIS

DEFINIÇÃO
- Distúrbio comum.
- Caracterizada por ausência completa ou parcial de pelo em áreas onde ele costuma estar presente.
- Pode estar associada a múltiplas causas, constituir o distúrbio primário ou ser secundária a alguma causa subjacente.

FISIOPATOLOGIA
- Causas multifatoriais.
- Todos os distúrbios representam uma interrupção no crescimento dos folículos pilosos por infecção, traumatismo, ataque imunológico, "tamponamento" mecânico, anormalidades endócrinas, neoplasia e/ou bloqueio dos sítios de receptores para a estimulação do ciclo de crescimento dos pelos.

SISTEMA(S) ACOMETIDO(S)
- Cutâneo/exócrino.
- Endócrino/metabólico.
- Sanguíneo/linfático/imunológico.

IDENTIFICAÇÃO
A predileção racial está listada abaixo.

SINAIS CLÍNICOS
- Pode ter início agudo ou ser lentamente progressiva.
- Placas multifocais de alopecia circular — muito frequentemente associadas à foliculite por infecção bacteriana e demodicose.
- Áreas alopécicas amplas e mais difusas — podem indicar uma displasia folicular ou um componente metabólico.
- O padrão e o grau da perda de pelo são importantes para o estabelecimento de um diagnóstico diferencial.

CAUSAS

Multifocais
- Demodicose localizada — alopecia parcial a completa, com eritema e leve descamação; as lesões podem ficar inflamadas e crostosas.
- Dermatofitose — alopecia parcial a completa, com formação de escamas; com ou sem eritema; nem sempre anular.
- Foliculite estafilocócica — padrões circulares de alopecia, com formação de colaretes epidérmicos, eritema, crostas e máculas hiperpigmentadas.
- Reações à injeção — inflamação com alopecia e/ou atrofia cutânea decorrente da formação cicatricial.
- Vasculite secundária à vacina antirrábica — placa alopécica bem delimitada observada 2-3 meses após a vacinação.
- Esclerodermia localizada — placa espessa, alopécica, lisa, brilhante e bem delimitada.
- Alopecia areata — áreas não inflamatórias de alopecia completa.
- Adenite sebácea (raças de pelo curto) — áreas anulares a policíclicas de alopecia e descamação.

Simétricas
- Hiperadrenocorticismo — alopecia do tronco, associada à atrofia cutânea, a comedões e à piodermite.
- Hipotireoidismo — a alopecia é uma manifestação incomum.
- Alopecia não inflamatória (alopecia X) — alopecia simétrica do tronco associada à hiperpigmentação; a alopecia frequentemente começa ao longo da região cervical correspondente ao local de aplicação da coleira; as raças Pomerânia, Chow chow, Akita, Samoieda, Keeshonden, Malamute do Alasca e Husky siberiano são acometidas.
- Hiperestrogenismo (fêmeas) — alopecia simétrica dos flancos, bem como das regiões perineal e inguinal, com aumento de volume da vulva e das glândulas mamárias.
- Hipogonadismo em fêmeas intactas — alopecia das regiões do períneo, flanco e tronco.
- Dermatose responsiva à testosterona em machos castrados — alopecia lentamente progressiva do tronco.
- Feminização masculina decorrente de sertolinoma — alopecia do períneo e da região genital, com ginecomastia.
- Dermatose responsiva à castração — perda de pelo na área correspondente à coleira, na garupa, no períneo e nos flancos.
- Dermatose responsiva aos estrogênios em cadelas castradas — alopecia das regiões do períneo e genital.
- Alopecia sazonal/cíclica do flanco — alopecia serpiginosa do flanco, com hiperpigmentação; as raças acometidas incluem Boxer, Buldogue inglês e Airedale terrier.

Irregulares a Difusas
- Demodicose — frequentemente associada a eritema, foliculite e hiperpigmentação.
- Foliculite bacteriana — varia desde uma área multifocal de alopecia circular até amplas áreas coalescentes de perda de pelo; presença de colaretes epidérmicos.
- Dermatofitose — muitas vezes acompanhada pela formação de escamas.
- Adenite sebácea — alopecia com formação de escamas espessas e aderentes; ocorre predominantemente sobre o dorso, abrangendo a cabeça e as extremidades.
- Alopecia do mutante da cor/alopecia por diluição da cor — adelgaçamento da pelagem, com foliculite secundária.
- Displasia folicular — alopecia lentamente progressiva.
- Defluxos anagênico e telogênico — início agudo de alopecia.
- Hipotireoidismo — adelgaçamento difuso da pelagem.
- Hiperadrenocorticismo — alopecia do tronco, com adelgaçamento da pele e formação de comedões.
- Linfoma epiteliotrópico — alopecia generalizada e difusa do tronco, com formação de escamas e eritema e, posteriormente, de nódulos e placas.
- Pênfigo foliáceo — perda de pelo associada à formação de escamas e crostas.
- Distúrbios de queratinização — alopecia associada à formação excessiva de escamas e a uma textura oleosa da superfície cutânea.

Localizações Específicas
- Alopecia do pavilhão auricular/calvície padrão — miniaturização dos pelos e surgimento de alopecia progressiva; as raças Dachshund, Galgo, Water spaniel americano, Water spaniel português, Boston terrier, Manchester terrier, Whippet, Galgo italiano, Chihuahua podem ser acometidas.
- Alopecia por tração — perda de pelo na parte superior e na face lateral do crânio, secundariamente à aplicação de presilhas/fivelas ou elásticos ao pelo.
- Alopecia pós-tosa — falha de repilação após a tosa; pode estar associada à interrupção no ciclo de crescimento dos pelos.
- Melanoderma (alopecia do Yorkshire terrier) — alopecia simétrica dos pavilhões auriculares, da ponte nasal, da cauda e dos pés.
- Alopecia sazonal/cíclica do flanco — alopecia serpiginosa do flanco, com hiperpigmentação; as raças Boxer, Buldogue inglês e Airedale terrier são predispostas.
- Displasia folicular dos pelos negros — alopecia exclusiva das áreas com pelos negros.
- Dermatomiosite — alopecia da face, da ponta das orelhas, da cauda e dos dedos; associada à formação de escamas, crostas e cicatrizes.

Alopecia Relacionada com a Raça
- Raças alopécicas por natureza: Cão de crista chinês (Chinese crested), Pelado mexicano, Pelado hinca, Pelado peruano (Peruvian Inca Orchid), Terrier americano sem pelo ou Pelado americano (frequentemente associado a comedões, foliculite e furunculose).
- Hipotricose congênita: Cocker spaniel, Pastor belga, Poodle, Whippet, Beagle, Buldogue francês, Yorkshire terrier, Labrador retriever, Bichon frisé, Lhasa apso, Basset hound.
- Alopecia por diluição da cor: Doberman pinscher azul ou castanho-amarelado, Labrador prata, Chow chow creme, Setter irlandês dourado, Pit bull terrier azul, bem como outras raças com colorações diluídas de suas pelagens.
- Melanoderma com alopecia em Yorkshire terrier.
- Alopecia sazonal/cíclica do flanco — alopecia serpiginosa do flanco com hiperpigmentação; Boxer, Buldogue inglês e Airedale terrier.
- Alopecia do pavilhão auricular/calvície padrão — miniaturização dos pelos e surgimento de alopecia progressiva; Dachshund, Galgo, Water spaniel americano, Water spaniel português, Boston terrier, Manchester terrier, Whippet, Galgo italiano, Chihuahua.
- Alopecia não inflamatória (alopecia X) — alopecia simétrica do tronco associada à hiperpigmentação; a alopecia frequentemente começa ao longo da região cervical correspondente ao local de aplicação da coleira; as raças Pomerânia, Chow chow, Akita, Samoieda, Keeshonden, Malamute do Alasca e Husky siberiano são acometidas.

FATORES DE RISCO
N/D.

DIAGNÓSTICO

DIAGNÓSTICO DIFERENCIAL
- Padrão e grau — aspectos importantes na formulação do diagnóstico diferencial.
- Presença de inflamação, escamas, crostas e colaretes epidérmicos — relevante na determinação do diagnóstico.

HEMOGRAMA/BIOQUÍMICA/URINÁLISE
Descartam as causas metabólicas, como o hiperadrenocorticismo.

OUTROS TESTES LABORATORIAIS
- Teste de função da tireoide — permite o diagnóstico do hipotireoidismo.
- Teste de resposta ao ACTH, TSDBD e TSDAD — avalia a existência do hiperadrenocorticismo.

ALOPECIA — CÃES

- Perfis dos hormônios sexuais (validade questionável).

DIAGNÓSTICO POR IMAGEM
Ultrassonografia — avalia as glândulas adrenais em busca de indícios de hiperadrenocorticismo.

MÉTODOS DIAGNÓSTICOS
- Resposta à terapia como um teste.
- Cultura fúngica.
- Raspado cutâneo.
- Citologia.
- Biopsia cutânea.

TRATAMENTO
- Demodicose — amitraz, ivermectina, milbemicina.
- Dermatofitose — griseofulvina, cetoconazol, itraconazol, banhos de imersão com enxofre, terbinafina.
- Foliculite estafilocócica — xampu e antibioticoterapia.
- Adenite sebácea — xampu queratolítico, suplementação de ácidos graxos essenciais, retinoides, ciclosporina.
- Distúrbios de queratinização — xampus, retinoides, vitamina D, ciclosporina.
- Disfunções endócrinas — ovário-histerectomia, castração, Lysodren®, trilostano, adrenalectomia.

MEDICAÇÕES

MEDICAMENTO(S) DE ESCOLHA
Varia com a causa específica; ver a seção "Tratamento".

CONTRAINDICAÇÕES
N/D.

PRECAUÇÕES
Toxicidade com griseofulvina, retinoides, ivermectina, trilostano, Lysodren®, ciclosporina.

INTERAÇÕES POSSÍVEIS
Nenhuma.

MEDICAMENTO(S) ALTERNATIVO(S)
Nenhum.

ACOMPANHAMENTO

MONITORIZAÇÃO DO PACIENTE
Varia com a causa.

COMPLICAÇÕES POSSÍVEIS
N/D.

DIVERSOS

DISTÚRBIOS ASSOCIADOS
N/D.

FATORES RELACIONADOS COM A IDADE
N/D.

POTENCIAL ZOONÓTICO
A dermatofitose pode causar lesões cutâneas em seres humanos.

GESTAÇÃO/FERTILIDADE/REPRODUÇÃO
Evitar o uso de retinoides e griseofulvina em animais prenhes.

VER TAMBÉM
- Alopecia Não Inflamatória — Cães.
- Demodicose.
- Dermatomiosite.
- Dermatofitose.
- Hiperadrenocorticismo (Síndrome de Cushing) — Cães.
- Hipotireoidismo.
- Pênfigo.
- Adenite Sebácea Granulomatosa.
- Sertolinoma.

ABREVIATURA(S)
- ACTH = hormônio adrenocorticotrófico.
- TSDAD = teste de supressão com dexametasona em altas doses.
- TSDBD = teste de supressão com dexametasona em baixas doses.

Sugestões de Leitura
Helton-Rhodes KA. Cutaneous manifestations of canine and feline endocrinopathies. Probl Vet Med 1990, 12:617-627.
Schmeitzel LP. Growth hormone responsive alopecia and sex hormone associated dermatoses. In: Birchard SJ, Sherding RG, eds., Saunders Manual of Small Animal Practice. Philadelphia: Saunders, 1994, pp. 326-330.
Scott DW, Griffin CE, Miller BH. Acquired alopecia. In: Muller & Kirk's Small Animal Dermatology, 5th ed. Philadelphia: Saunders, 1995, pp. 720-735.
Scott DW, Griffin CE, Miller BH. Endocrine and metabolic diseases. In: Muller & Kirk's Small Animal Dermatology, 5th ed. Philadelphia: Saunders, 1995, pp. 627-719.
Scott DW, Griffin CE, Miller BH. Keratinization defects. In: Muller & Kirk's Small Animal Dermatology, 5th ed. Philadelphia: Saunders, 1995, pp. 736-805.

Autor Karen Helton Rhodes
Consultor Editorial Alexander H. Werner

Alopecia — Gatos

CONSIDERAÇÕES GERAIS

DEFINIÇÃO
- Distúrbio comum.
- Padrão da perda de pelo — variável ou simétrico.
- Causas — multifatoriais.

FISIOPATOLOGIA
Específica e exclusiva para cada causa.

SISTEMA(S) ACOMETIDO(S)
- Cutâneo/exócrino.
- Endócrino/metabólico.
- Sanguíneo/linfático/imune.

IDENTIFICAÇÃO
- Não há idade, raça nem sexo predominante.
- Alopecias associadas a neoplasias e síndromes paraneoplásicas — identificadas geralmente em gatos idosos.

SINAIS CLÍNICOS
Dependem do diagnóstico específico.

CAUSAS
- Neurológicas/comportamentais — transtorno obsessivo-compulsivo.
- Endócrinas — alopecia responsiva aos hormônios sexuais, hipertireoidismo, hiperadrenocorticismo, diabetes melito.
- Imunológicas — dermatite alérgica, alopecia areata, alopecia mucinosa, foliculite mural linfocítica, pseudopelado.
- Parasitárias — demodicose, queiletielose.
- Infecciosas — dermatofitose.
- Fisiológicas/metabólicas — adenite sebácea.
- Neoplásicas — dermatite paraneoplásica, carcinoma de células escamosas *in situ*, linfoma epiteliotrópico, timoma com dermatite esfoliativa.
- Idiopáticas/hereditárias — alopecia universal, hipotricose, alopecia auricular espontânea, defluxo anagênico e telogênico.
- Reação no local da injeção.
- Efeito de medicamentos — corticosteroides.
- Virais — doença associada a FeLV e FIV (dermatose de células gigantes).

FATORES DE RISCO
FeLV/FIV — em casos de demodicose.

DIAGNÓSTICO

DIAGNÓSTICO DIFERENCIAL

Alopecia Endócrina/Responsiva aos Hormônios Sexuais
- Raramente representa uma anormalidade hormonal.
- Causas hormonais — ocorre principalmente em machos castrados; caracterizada por alopecia ao longo da face caudal dos membros posteriores, que pode se estender junto ao períneo.
- Administração excessiva de corticosteroide.
- Acetato de megestrol — pode produzir lesões semelhantes ou associadas ao diabetes melito ou hiperadrenocorticismo.

Transtorno Obsessivo-Compulsivo
- Incomum como única fonte dos sintomas.
- Com frequência, é erroneamente diagnosticado em casos de dermatite alérgica.
- Frequentemente diagnosticado de forma incorreta como alopecia endócrina.
- O padrão de alopecia é muitas vezes simétrico, sem inflamação associada.

Dermatite Alérgica
- Varia desde uma alopecia parcial branda com pouca inflamação até escoriação e ulceração graves.
- É frequente o corte da pelagem clandestinamente, levando ao diagnóstico errado de alopecia endócrina.
- Distribuição — variável; muitas vezes, as regiões cefálica e cervical são as mais gravemente acometidas.
- Alergia alimentar, atopia/dermatite de contato e hipersensibilidade a ectoparasitas.

Hipertireoidismo
- Alopecia parcial a completa por autoaparamento de pelos.
- Padrão variável.
- Gatos de meia-idade a idosos.
- Com frequência, diagnosticado erroneamente em casos de dermatoses alérgicas, transtorno obsessivo-compulsivo ou outra alopecia hormonal.

Diabetes Melito
- Alopecia parcial com pelagem descuidada e descamação excessiva.
- Cicatrização deficiente de feridas.
- Aumento na suscetibilidade a infecções.
- Xantomatose cutânea secundária à hiperlipidemia (placas alopécicas nodulares a lineares de coloração amarelo-rosada, que tendem a ulcerar).

Hiperadrenocorticismo
- Raro; caracterizado por alopecia e fragilidade cutânea.
- Alopecia do tronco, com ou sem rabo pelado e pontas enroladas dos pavilhões auriculares.
- A fragilidade extrema da pele é observada em aproximadamente 70% dos casos.
- Ocorre secundariamente a tumores hipofisários ou adrenais.
- A forma iatrogênica é menos comum em gatos do que em cães.

Alopecia Paraneoplásica
- A maioria dos casos está associada a adenocarcinomas pancreáticos exócrinos, carcinomas dos ductos biliares, dermatite esfoliativa com timoma.
- Gatos de meia-idade a idosos (9-16 anos).
- Carcinoma pancreático/carcinoma dos ductos biliares: início agudo, evolução rápida, distribuição bilateral simétrica e ventral (também se localiza ao longo da ponte nasal e na região periocular), fácil epilação (ou seja, os pelos se destacam com facilidade), prurido raro, eritema com fissuras e ressecamento nos coxins podais, pele alopécica com aspecto brilhante, pele frequentemente delgada e hipotônica, rápida perda de peso.
- Timoma com dermatite esfoliativa: dermatite escamosa não pruriginosa que começa na cabeça e no pescoço.

Adenite Sebácea
- Alopecia parcial lentamente progressiva associada à formação de escamas ao longo do dorso e das extremidades.
- As glândulas sebáceas são seletivamente destruídas por meio de metabólitos intermediários tóxicos ou mecanismos imunológicos.
- Há um possível acúmulo drástico de pigmento junto às margens palpebrais.
- Associação questionável com doença sistêmica (p. ex., enteropatia inflamatória, síndromes semelhantes ao lúpus e infecções do trato respiratório superior).

Carcinoma de Células Escamosas in Situ
- Dermatose pré-maligna multicêntrica em gatos idosos.
- Associado ao papilomavírus; carcinoma bowenoide *in situ*.
- Lesões levemente salientes, muitas vezes pigmentadas, semelhantes a placas ou papiladas, com formação de escamas e superfícies parcialmente alopécicas.
- Com frequência, é erroneamente diagnosticada como seborreia antes do desenvolvimento de lesões distintas.
- Cerca de 25% dos casos podem se converter em carcinoma de células escamosas com lesões *in situ* ao longo das bordas (do ponto de vista histológico).

Linfoma Epiteliotrópico
- Estágios precoces — graus variados de alopecia associados à formação de escamas e eritema.
- Estágios mais tardios — placas e nódulos.
- Gatos idosos.

Alopecia Areata/Pseudopelado/Foliculite Mural Linfocítica
- Esse grupo de diagnósticos diferenciais é frequentemente considerado como uma lesão pré-neoplásica com alguma causa imunológica incitante.
- Alopecia areata — rara e completa, em uma distribuição irregular sem inflamação; cabeça, pescoço, orelhas; acúmulo histológico de linfócitos em torno do bulbo piloso.
- Foliculite mural linfocítica — alopecia difusa da face, das pálpebras e do focinho; a pele tem aparência cerosa espessa à palpação; invasão histológica de linfócitos na bainha radicular externa do folículo piloso e na epiderme.
- Pseudopelado — alopecia bem circunscrita não pruriginosa que frequentemente começa na face; as unhas podem se esfacelar.

Alopecia Universal (Gato Sphinx [Esfinge])
- Hereditária.
- Ausência completa dos pelos primários; redução dos pelos secundários.
- Espessamento da epiderme; normalidade da derme.
- Desembocadura dos ductos sebáceos e apócrinos diretamente na superfície cutânea; oleosidade da pele ao toque.
- Enrugamento da fronte; olhos dourados; ausência de vibrissas*; penugem macia nas patas, na extremidade da cauda e no escroto.
- Comedões com ou sem foliculite secundária.

Hipotricose Felina
- Gatos das raças Siamês e Devon Rex (alopecia autossômica recessiva).
- Desenvolvimento deficiente dos folículos pilosos telogênicos primários.
- O animal nasce com uma pelagem normal, que se torna delgada e esparsa no gato jovem adulto.

Alopecia Auricular Espontânea
- Predisposição dos gatos da raça Siamês.
- Pode representar uma forma de alopecia areata ou de calvície-padrão.

Defluxo Anagênico e Telogênico
- Perda aguda de pelos, em função da interferência no ciclo de crescimento.
- Causas — estresse, infecção, distúrbio endócrino ou metabólico, febre, cirurgia, anestesia, prenhez, terapia medicamentosa.

---

* N. T.: Também conhecidas como suíças ou bigodes.

Alopecia — Gatos

Demodicose
- Rara nos gatos.
- Alopecia multifocal parcial a completa da área correspondente às pálpebras, bem como das regiões periocular, cefálica e cervical.
- Além de otite externa ceruminosa, há um prurido variável com eritema e formação de escamas e crostas.
- O *Demodex cati* (formato alongado) frequentemente está associado à doença metabólica (p. ex., FIV, lúpus eritematoso sistêmico e diabetes melito).
- O ácaro *D. gatoi* curto/rombo raramente constitui um marcador de doença metabólica; essa forma está associada a prurido e pode ser transmissível de um gato a outro.

Queiletielose
- Prurido variável com formação de escamas.
- Nem todos os animais da casa podem ser acometidos.

Dermatofitose
- Inúmeras manifestações clínicas; sempre associadas à alopecia.

HEMOGRAMA/BIOQUÍMICA/URINÁLISE
Pode-se observar a presença de anormalidades nos casos de diabetes melito, hiperadrenocorticismo e hipertireoidismo.

OUTROS TESTES LABORATORIAIS
- FeLV e FIV — fatores de risco de demodicose.
- Hormônios tireoidianos — verifica o hipertireoidismo.
- Título do ANA — pesquisa o lúpus eritematoso sistêmico.
- Teste de resposta ao ACTH, TSDBD e TSDAD — diagnostica o hiperadrenocorticismo.

DIAGNÓSTICO POR IMAGEM
- Ultrassonografia abdominal — avalia as adrenais em casos de hiperadrenocorticismo e pesquisa a existência de câncer em animais com síndrome paraneoplásica.
- Varredura por TC — procura por tumores hipofisários em animais com hiperadrenocorticismo.

MÉTODOS DIAGNÓSTICOS
- Biopsia cutânea.
- Raspado cutâneo.
- Cultura fúngica para dermatófitos.
- Uso de camisetas ou colares elizabetanos para demonstrar o autotraumatismo.
- Ensaios com dietas de eliminação.
- Teste cutâneo intradérmico de alergia.

TRATAMENTO
- A terapia é limitada para muitos desses distúrbios.
- A mudança de comportamento ou o uso de uma camiseta podem ajudar a evitar o autoaparamento dos pelos.
- A remoção de um item agressor da dieta pode aliviar os sintomas de alergia alimentar.
- Se o animal de estimação for obediente, o uso de xampus e outras terapias tópicas poderão ajudar em distúrbios secundários (como hiperqueratose na adenite sebácea, formação de crostas na demodicose, infecções bacterianas secundárias e odor desagradável nas condições oleosas).

MEDICAÇÕES

MEDICAMENTO(S)
- Transtorno obsessivo-compulsivo — amitriptilina (10 mg/gato/dia), bem como outros agentes modificadores do comportamento.
- Alopecia endócrina (machos) — suplementação de testosterona.
- Dermatite alérgica — anti-histamínicos, dieta com restrição de ingrediente, corticosteroides, imunoterapia alérgeno-específica, controle de ectoparasitas.
- Hipertireoidismo — medicamentos orais (como o metimazol [Tapazol®]) ou terapia com iodo radioativo.
- Diabetes melito — regulação dos níveis de glicose (insulina).
- Hiperadrenocorticismo — cirurgia; nenhuma terapia clínica conhecida é eficaz.
- Alopecia paraneoplásica — não há terapia; frequentemente fatal.
- Linfoma epiteliotrópico — retinoides (isotretinoína), corticosteroides, interferona, ciclosporina, lomustina.
- Adenite sebácea — retinoides, corticosteroides, ciclosporina.
- Carcinoma de células escamosas *in situ* — excisão cirúrgica, retinoides (tópicos e orais), creme de uso tópico que contenha o medicamento imiquimode.
- Alopecia areata — não há terapia; possivelmente contra irritantes.
- Demodicose — banhos de imersão com enxofre em intervalos semanais, por 4-6 vezes.
- Queiletielose — antiparasitários tópicos e controle ambiental.
- Dermatofitose — griseofulvina (**CUIDADO:** toxicidade idiossincrática), itraconazol, terbinafina.

PRECAUÇÕES
Toxicidade pela griseofulvina e pelo itraconazol (ver "Dermatofitose").

INTERAÇÕES POSSÍVEIS
N/D.

MEDICAMENTO(S) ALTERNATIVO(S)
N/D.

ACOMPANHAMENTO

MONITORIZAÇÃO DO PACIENTE
Depende do diagnóstico específico.

PREVENÇÃO
Depende do diagnóstico específico.

COMPLICAÇÕES POSSÍVEIS
Depende do diagnóstico específico.

EVOLUÇÃO ESPERADA E PROGNÓSTICO
Depende do diagnóstico específico.

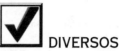

DIVERSOS

POTENCIAL ZOONÓTICO
- Dermatofitose — pode causar lesões cutâneas em seres humanos.
- Queiletielose — pode provocar irritação em seres humanos.

GESTAÇÃO/FERTILIDADE/REPRODUÇÃO
Não se devem administrar retinoides nem griseofulvina em animais prenhes.

VER TAMBÉM
- Adenite Sebácea Granulomatosa.
- Alopecia Paraneoplásica Felina.
- Demodicose.
- Dermatofitose.
- Diabetes Melito sem Complicação — Gatos.
- Hipertireoidismo.
- Queiletielose.

ABREVIATURA(S)
- ACTH = hormônio adrenocorticotrófico.
- ANA = anticorpo antinuclear.
- FeLV = vírus da leucemia felina.
- FIV = vírus da imunodeficiência felina.
- TC = tomografia computadorizada.
- TSDAD = teste de supressão com dexametasona em altas doses.
- TSDBD = teste de supressão com dexametasona em baixas doses.

Sugestões de Leitura
Baer KE, Helton KA. Multicentric squamous cell carcinoma in situ resembling Bowens' disease in cats. Vet Pathol 1993, 30:535–543.
Helton Rhodes KA, Wallace M, Baer KE. Cutaneous manifestations of feline hyperadrenocorticism. In: Ihrke PJ, Mason IS, White SD. Advances in Veterinary Dermatology. New York: Pergamon, 1993.
Scott DW, Griffin CE, Miller BH. Acquired alopecia. In: Muller & Kirk's Small Animal Dermatology, 5th ed. Philadelphia: Saunders, 1995, pp. 720–735.
Scott DW, Griffin CE, Miller BH. Congenital and hereditary defects. In: Muller & Kirk's Small Animal Dermatology, 5th ed. Philadelphia: Saunders, 1995, pp. 736–805.
Scott DW, Griffin CE, Miller BH. Endocrine and metabolic diseases. In: Muller & Kirk's Small Animal Dermatology, 5th ed. Philadelphia: Saunders, 1995, pp. 627–719.

Autor Karen Helton Rhodes
Consultor Editorial Alexander H. Werner

Alopecia Não Inflamatória — Cães

CONSIDERAÇÕES GERAIS

DEFINIÇÃO
- Distúrbios alopécicos incomuns que são associados ao ciclo anormal dos folículos pilosos.
- Tanto as doenças endócrinas como as não endócrinas podem ser associadas à alopecia.
- O diagnóstico definitivo frequentemente exige a exclusão das alopecias endócrinas mais comuns.
- A alopecia X também é conhecida como alopecia responsiva ao hormônio de crescimento, alopecia responsiva à castração, síndrome tipo hiperplasia adrenal, entre outros.

FISIOPATOLOGIA
- Existem muitos fatores que afetam o ciclo piloso, tanto hormonais como não hormonais.
- O aumento dos hormônios sexuais pode afetar o ciclo piloso. O estrogênio é um inibidor conhecido da fase de crescimento anagênica do folículo piloso.
- O mecanismo por meio do qual a alopecia X influencia o ciclo piloso não é conhecido.

SISTEMA(S) ACOMETIDO(S)
- Comportamental.
- Endócrino/Metabólico.
- Hematológico/Linfático/Imune.
- Cutâneo/Exócrino.

GENÉTICA
Existem predisposições raciais para a alopecia X; no entanto, o modo de herança é desconhecido.

INCIDÊNCIA/PREVALÊNCIA
- Hiperestrogenismo e hiperandrogenismo são causas incomuns a raras de alopecia.
- Alopecia X é relativamente comum em raças predispostas.

DISTRIBUIÇÃO GEOGRÁFICA
Nenhuma.

IDENTIFICAÇÃO
Espécies
Cães.

Raça(s) Predominante(s)
- Hiperestrogenismo e hiperandrogenismo — não há predileções raciais.
- Alopecia X — Poodle miniatura e raças de pelagem felpuda, como Pomerânia, Chow chow, Akita, Samoieda, Keeshonden, Malamute do Alasca e Husky siberiano.

Idade Média e Faixa Etária
- Hiperestrogenismo e hiperandrogenismo — cães intactos de meia-idade a idosos.
- Alopecia X — 1-5 anos de idade; contudo, os cães mais idosos podem desenvolver o problema.

Sexo Predominante
- Hiperandrogenismo, principalmente machos intactos.
- Hiperestrogenismo, sobretudo fêmeas intactas.
- Alopecia X, cães castrados ou intactos de qualquer um dos sexos.

SINAIS CLÍNICOS
Achados Anamnésicos
- Alteração geral na pelagem — ressecada ou esbranquiçada porque os pelos não estão sendo trocados; falta de muda normal.
- Machos com hiperestrogenismo podem atrair outros cães machos.

Achados do Exame Físico
- Alopecia — geralmente difusa com alopecia bilateral simétrica do tronco que poupa a cabeça e as extremidades distais. Incomum com hiperandrogenismo.
- Pelagem — pode ficar ressecada ou esbranquiçada.
- Seborreia, prurido, piodermite, comedões, otite externa ceruminosa, e hiperpigmentação secundários — variáveis.
- Aumento do volume de mamilos, glândulas mamárias, vulva, prepúcio — pode estar associado a hiperestrogenismo.
- Melanose macular e dermatite prepucial linear — podem estar associados a hiperestrogenismo.
- Testículos de tamanho anormal — podem estar associados a hiperestrogenismo ou hiperandrogenismo.
- Os testículos também podem aparecer de tamanho normal.
- Hiperplasia da glândula da cauda e hiperplasia das glândulas perianais — geralmente associadas a hiperandrogenismo.
- Sinais sistêmicos (PU/PD/polifagia) NÃO costumam estar presentes.

CAUSAS
Hiperestrogenismo — Fêmeas
- Excesso de estrogênio associado a ovários císticos, tumores ovarianos (raros) ou suplementação exógena de estrogênio.
- Os animais com concentrações séricas normais de estrogênio podem ter números elevados de receptores estrogênicos na pele (não documentados).

Hiperestrogenismo — Machos
- O excesso de estrogênio causado por sertolinoma (mais comum), seminoma ou tumor de células intersticiais (raro).
- Associado a pseudo-hermafroditismo do macho em Schnauzers miniaturas.

Hiperandrogenismo — Machos
Tumores testiculares produtores de androgênio (especialmente tumores de células intersticiais).

Alopecia X
Embora haja uma falha no ciclo do folículo piloso, ainda não foi identificada uma causa endócrina subjacente.

FATORES DE RISCO
- Cães machos e fêmeas intactos estão sob alto risco de desenvolvimento de tumores testiculares e cistos/tumores ovarianos, respectivamente.
- Os machos criptorquídicos também apresentam risco elevado de desenvolvimento de tumores testiculares.
- Suplementação exógena de estrogênio.
- Não há fatores de risco conhecidos para alopecia X, exceto a predisposição racial.

DIAGNÓSTICO

DIAGNÓSTICO DIFERENCIAL
- Causas inflamatórias de alopecia (piodermite, demodicose e dermatofitose) — devem ser descartadas; essas doenças geralmente provocam um padrão de alopecia irregular e não difuso.
- Hipotireoidismo e hiperadrenocorticismo — é crítico descartá-las, pois essas doenças podem causar um padrão muito semelhante de alopecia difusa associado à falta de ciclo do folículo piloso.
- Displasias foliculares, incluindo alopecia por diluição da cor e displasia folicular do pelo preto — a alopecia deve ser restrita à cor.
- Alopecia padronizada de várias raças (Dachshund, Boston terrier, Galgo, Spaniel d'água, e outras) — alopecias específicas às raças de causa desconhecida.
- Alopecia cíclica do flanco — alopecia do flanco e dorso, padrões frequentemente bizarros com hiperpigmentação, com maior frequência em raças de pelo curto (Boxer, Buldogue inglês, Airedale) e pode exibir recorrência sazonal.
- Alopecia pós-tricotomia — falha de repilação após tricotomia; contudo, ocorre repilação em até 1 ano.
- Defluxo telogênico — a alopecia ocorre 1-2 meses após uma doença ou episódio grave de estresse e o início costuma ser mais súbito com relativa facilidade de epilação.

HEMOGRAMA/BIOQUÍMICA/URINÁLISE
- Geralmente, não são dignos de nota.
- Anemia e/ou hipoplasia ou aplasia de medula óssea podem estar associadas a hiperestrogenismo.

OUTROS TESTES LABORATORIAIS
- Concentrações séricas dos hormônios sexuais — frequentemente normais; tratar de acordo com a suspeita diagnóstica com base nos sinais clínicos e descartar outros distúrbios.
- Concentrações séricas de estradiol — algumas vezes elevadas em cães machos com tumores testiculares ou cadelas com cistos ovarianos; no entanto, ocorre oscilação normal do estradiol ao longo do dia, dificultando a interpretação das concentrações desse hormônio.

DIAGNÓSTICO POR IMAGEM
Radiografia, ultrassonografia e laparoscopia — para identificar ovários císticos, tumores ovarianos, tumores testiculares (escrotais ou abdominais), linfadenopatia sublombar e possíveis metástases torácicas de tumores malignos.

MÉTODOS DIAGNÓSTICOS
- Citologia prepucial — pode revelar cornificação de células nos machos com hiperestrogenismo (similar a uma cadela no cio).
- Biopsia cutânea.

ACHADOS PATOLÓGICOS
As alterações histológicas associadas a dermatoses endócrinas (pelos telógenos, ceratoses foliculares, hiperceratose, queratinização triquilemal excessiva [folículos em chama], adelgaçamento da epiderme e da derme) também podem ser observadas em casos de alopecias não inflamatórias, incluindo hiperestrogenismo e alopecia X. A histopatologia ajudará a descartar causas inflamatórias de alopecia e alguns dos outros diagnósticos diferenciais listados anteriormente.

TRATAMENTO

CUIDADO(S) DE SAÚDE ADEQUADO(S)
N/D.

CUIDADO(S) DE ENFERMAGEM
N/D.

ATIVIDADE
Nenhuma.

DIETA
Nenhuma.

Alopecia Não Inflamatória — Cães

ORIENTAÇÃO AO PROPRIETÁRIO
Alopecia X é um problema estético que resulta apenas em perda da pelagem, embora não haja uma cura definitiva para a perda de pelo. O risco do tratamento deve ser ponderado com esses fatos. A repilação ocorrerá somente em uma parte dos cães, independentemente do tratamento escolhido, e a perda de pelo pode recorrer meses a anos depois apesar da manutenção do tratamento.

CONSIDERAÇÕES CIRÚRGICAS
Hiperestrogenismo/Hiperandrogenismo
• Castração — para tumores testiculares escrotais.
• Laparotomia exploratória — para diagnóstico e remoção cirúrgica (ovário-histerectomia e castração) de cistos e tumores ovarianos, bem como de tumores testiculares abdominais.

Alopecia X
• Castração de animais intactos — um certo número apresentará repilação após a castração. A repilação pode levar até 3 meses para se tornar evidente.

MEDICAÇÕES
MEDICAMENTO(S) DE ESCOLHA
Tratamentos Gerais
• Xampus antisseborreicos tópicos — para comedões e seborreia associados à alopecia.
• Antibióticos — para infecções cutâneas secundárias associadas à alopecia.

Alopecia X
Melatonina — 3 mg e 6-12 mg a cada 12 h para raças de pequeno e grande porte, respectivamente; a repilação pode levar até 3 meses para se tornar evidente. Esse tratamento funciona em quase 40% dos casos. Como esse tratamento é o mais benigno, ele é considerado o tratamento de escolha após a castração. Assim que ocorrer a repilação, deve-se interromper o tratamento.

CONTRAINDICAÇÕES
Nenhuma.

PRECAUÇÕES
A melatonina em altas doses pode causar insulinorresistência; portanto, deve-se ter cuidado no tratamento de cães com diabetes melito.

INTERAÇÕES POSSÍVEIS
Nenhuma.

MEDICAMENTO(S) ALTERNATIVO(S)
• Mitotano — 15-25 mg/kg — 1 vez ao dia como indução por 5-7 dias, seguido de tratamento de manutenção 2 vezes por semana; a repilação ocorre em uma parte dos cães tratados, o que pode levar até 3 meses para se tornar evidente. O uso desse medicamento pode resultar em uma crise addisoniana e outros efeitos colaterais observados no tratamento da síndrome de Cushing. É recomendável a monitorização regular dos níveis de eletrólitos e do cortisol pelo teste de estimulação com ACTH.
• Trilostano — dosagens semelhantes àquelas descritas para o tratamento da síndrome de Cushing; a repilação ocorre em uma parte dos cães tratados, o que pode levar até 3 meses para se tornar evidente. O uso desse medicamento pode resultar em uma crise addisoniana e outros efeitos colaterais observados no tratamento da síndrome de Cushing. É recomendável a monitorização regular dos níveis de eletrólitos e do cortisol pelo teste de estimulação com ACTH.
• A administração do hormônio de crescimento e o uso de metiltestosterona podem resultar em repilação. O hormônio de crescimento pode causar diabetes melito, enquanto a metiltestosterona pode culminar em aumento da agressividade, colangioepatite e seborreia oleosa. Portanto, esses medicamentos não são recomendados.

ACOMPANHAMENTO
MONITORIZAÇÃO DO PACIENTE
• Mitotano — mensuração regular dos níveis de eletrólitos e do cortisol pelo teste de estimulação com ACTH.
• Trilostano — mensuração regular dos níveis de eletrólitos e do cortisol pelo teste de estimulação com ACTH.

PREVENÇÃO
Nenhuma.

COMPLICAÇÕES POSSÍVEIS
Nenhuma.

EVOLUÇÃO ESPERADA E PROGNÓSTICO
• Hiperestrogenismo da fêmea — a melhora deve ocorrer em até 3-6 meses após o procedimento de ovário-histerectomia.
• Tumores secretores de estrogênio e androgênio — a resolução dos sinais deve ocorrer em até 3-6 meses após a castração.
• Alopecia X — a repilação ocorrerá apenas em uma parte dos cães, independentemente do tratamento escolhido, e a perda de pelo pode recorrer apesar da manutenção do tratamento. Portanto, se a repilação ocorrer, dever-se-á interromper o tratamento para preservá-lo em caso de futura recorrência da alopecia. O risco do tratamento deve ser ponderado com o fato de ser um problema estético.

DIVERSOS
DISTÚRBIOS ASSOCIADOS
• Piodermite, seborreia, comedões podem estar associados à alopecia.
• Comportamentais — mudanças associadas ao hiperestrogenismo ou hiperandrogenismo.

FATORES RELACIONADOS COM A IDADE
Nenhum.

POTENCIAL ZOONÓTICO
Nenhum.

GESTAÇÃO/FERTILIDADE/REPRODUÇÃO
N/D — a castração costuma ser recomendada para o tratamento desses distúrbios.

SINÔNIMOS
Alopecia X — alopecia responsiva ao hormônio de crescimento, alopecia responsiva à castração, síndrome tipo hiperplasia adrenal, entre outros.

ABREVIATURA(S)
• ACTH = hormônio adrenocorticotrófico.
• PU/PD = poliúria/polidipsia.

RECURSOS DA INTERNET
http://www.vet.utk.edu/hairloss/.

Sugestões de Leitura
Frank LA. Sex hormone and endocrine look-alike dermatoses. In: Birchard SJ, Sherding RG, eds., Saunders Manual of Small Animal Practice, 3rd ed. Philadelphia: Saunders, 2006, p. 517.

Autor Linda A. Frank
Consultor Editorial Alexander H. Werner

Alopecia Paraneoplásica Felina

CONSIDERAÇÕES GERAIS

REVISÃO
- Distúrbio raro caracterizado por lesões cutâneas, que servem como marcadores de neoplasia interna.
- Grande parte dos gatos acometidos sofre de adenocarcinoma pancreático com metástase para órgãos com fígado, pleura e/ou peritônio; também há relatos de carcinoma dos ductos biliares e carcinoma hepatocelular.
- A ligação entre processos neoplásicos internos e lesões cutâneas é desconhecida; pode envolver citocinas que produzem atrofia dos folículos pilosos.

IDENTIFICAÇÃO
- Há relatos de casos apenas em gatos domésticos de pelo curto.
- Idade média de 13 anos; faixa etária de 7-16 anos.

SINAIS CLÍNICOS
- Diminuição do apetite, seguida por perda de peso rápida e eliminação excessiva.
- Prurido — variável; às vezes com excesso de lambedura.
- Perda de pelos — rapidamente progressiva.
- Alguns gatos acometidos podem exibir relutância em andar, em virtude de fissuras dolorosas nos coxins palmoplantares.
- Os pelos se soltam com facilidade.
- Alopecia grave — na parte ventral do pescoço, no abdome e na parte medial das coxas.
- O estrato córneo pode "esfolar", conferindo aspecto brilhante à pele.
- A pele alopécica é brilhante, inelástica e delgada, mas não frágil.
- Podem surgir lentigos acinzentados nas áreas de alopecia.
- Podem surgir fissuras e/ou descamação nos coxins palmoplantares; frequentemente dolorosas.

CAUSAS E FATORES DE RISCO
- A maioria dos casos está associada a adenocarcinoma pancreático subjacente.
- Outros carcinomas internos, como os dos ductos biliares e os hepatocelulares, são possíveis causas.

DIAGNÓSTICO

DIAGNÓSTICO DIFERENCIAL
- Hiperadrenocorticismo — poliúria, polidipsia e fragilidade cutânea.
- Hipertireoidismo — polifagia.
- Hipotireoidismo — condição espontânea rara em gatos; não associado à pele brilhante.
- Alopecia simétrica felina — perda de pelos autoinduzida; não está associada à epilação fácil.
- Demodiciose — os ácaros não estão associados à alopecia paraneoplásica.
- Dermatofitose — perda de pelos, associada, em geral, à quebra, e não à queda espontânea; inapetência e perda de peso são raras.
- Alopecia areata — raramente envolve toda a superfície ventral; inapetência e perda de peso são raras.
- Eflúvio telogênico — não está associado à miniaturização dos folículos pilosos.
- Síndrome de fragilidade cutânea — pele frágil não associada à alopecia paraneoplásica.
- Dermatite necrolítica superficial — não associada à esfoliação acentuada e miniaturização dos folículos pilosos.

HEMOGRAMA/BIOQUÍMICA/URINÁLISE
N/D.

OUTROS TESTES LABORATORIAIS
- Endócrinos (provas de função da tireoide e teste de supressão com dexametasona) — descartam endocrinopatias.
- Raspados de pele — excluem demodiciose.
- Exame dos pelos com hidróxido de potássio (também conhecido como potassa) e/ou cultura de fungos — descartam dermatofitose.
- Citologia de pele — avalia possível infecção secundária por *Malassezia* (indutora de prurido).

DIAGNÓSTICO POR IMAGEM
- Ultrassonografia — massa pancreática e/ou lesões nodulares no fígado ou na cavidade peritoneal; a falha na demonstração de nódulos não exclui o diagnóstico, porque eles podem ser muito pequenos para serem detectados.
- Radiografias torácicas — lesões metastáticas nos pulmões ou na cavidade pleural.

MÉTODOS DIAGNÓSTICOS
- Biopsias cutâneas.
- Laparoscopia ou laparotomia exploratória — para identificar tumores primários e metastáticos.

ACHADOS PATOLÓGICOS
- Exame histopatológico da pele — alopecia não cicatricial; atrofia intensa dos folículos pilosos e anexos cutâneos; miniaturização dos bulbos pilosos; leve acantose; ausência variável de estrato córneo; infiltrados perivasculares superficiais mistos variáveis de neutrófilos, eosinófilos e células mononucleares; alguns pacientes exibem infecções secundárias por *Malassezia*.
- Tumor primário — em geral, adenocarcinoma pancreático; raramente carcinomas primários dos ductos biliares ou carcinomas hepatocelulares.
- Nódulos metastáticos — comuns no fígado, nos pulmões, na pleura e no peritônio.

TRATAMENTO

- A remoção do tumor via pancreatectomia parcial pode ser curativa; no entanto, o prognóstico é reservado, pois a maioria dos gatos tem doença metastática.
- Quimioterapia ou outros medicamentos — nenhuma resposta relatada.
- Os animais acometidos deterioram rapidamente; a eutanásia deve ser sugerida como intervenção humanitária.
- Cuidados de suporte — apenas se os proprietários se recusarem a considerar a eutanásia; alimentos altamente palatáveis ricos em nutrientes e/ou sonda de alimentação.

MEDICAÇÕES

MEDICAMENTO(S)
N/D.

CONTRAINDICAÇÕES/INTERAÇÕES POSSÍVEIS
N/D.

ACOMPANHAMENTO

- Deterioração progressiva.
- Cuidados de suporte — ultrassonografia e radiografias torácicas podem demonstrar a evolução de doença metastática.
- O animal frequentemente vem a óbito em 2-20 semanas após o início das lesões cutâneas.

DIVERSOS

VER TAMBÉM
Adenocarcinoma Pancreático.

Sugestões de Leitura
Brooks DG, Campbell KL, Dennis JS, et al. Pancreatic paraneoplastic alopecia in three cats. JAAHA 1994, 30:557-562.
Marconato L, Albanese F, Viacava P, Marchetti V, Abramo F. Paraneoplastic alopecia associated with hepatocellular carcinoma in a cat. Vet Dermatol 2007, 18:267-271.
Pascal-Tenorio A, Olivry T, Gross TL, et al. Paraneoplastic alopecia associated with internal malignancies in the cat. Vet Dermatol 1997, 8:47-52.
Tasker S, Griffon D, Nutall T, et al. Resolution of paraneoplastic alopecia following surgical removal of a pancreatic carcinoma in a cat. J Small Anim Pract 1999, 40:16-19.
Turek MM. Cutaneous paraneoplastic syndromes in dogs and cats: A review of the literature. Vet Dermatol 2003, 14:279-296.

Autor Karen L. Campbell
Consultor Editorial Alexander H. Werner

Alopecia Simétrica Felina

CONSIDERAÇÕES GERAIS

REVISÃO
- Alopecia em um padrão simétrico sem alterações visíveis na pele.
- Manifestação clínica comum em gatos.
- Manifestação de vários distúrbios subjacentes.

IDENTIFICAÇÃO
Sem predominância etária, racial ou sexual.

SINAIS CLÍNICOS
- Perda de pelos parcial ou total; mais frequentemente simétrica embora possa ocorrer em uma distribuição irregular.
- As regiões corporais comumente acometidas são o ventre, a parte caudal do dorso, bem como as partes lateral e caudal das coxas.
- Às vezes, áreas dispersas de perda de pelos (assimétricas) nas partes distais dos membros ou do tronco.

CAUSAS E FATORES DE RISCO
- Hipersensibilidade cutânea — dermatite alérgica à pulga, hipersensibilidade alimentar, atopia.
- Ectoparasitas — dermatite alérgica à pulga, queiletielose.
- Infecções — dermatofitose.
- Neurológicos ou comportamentais — "alopecia psicogênica".
- Estresse ou metabólicos — eflúvio telogênico.
- Neoplasia — pancreática (alopecia paraneoplásica).
- Hiperadrenocorticismo.
- Alopecia areata.
- Estado hipertireóideo (sinal precoce).

DIAGNÓSTICO

DIAGNÓSTICO DIFERENCIAL
Ver a seção "Causas e Fatores de Risco".

HEMOGRAMA/BIOQUÍMICA/URINÁLISE
Eosinofilia em alguns gatos alérgicos.

OUTROS TESTES LABORATORIAIS
Tiroxina sérica — hipertireoidismo.

DIAGNÓSTICO POR IMAGEM
N/D.

MÉTODOS DIAGNÓSTICOS
- Uso de pente antipulga — para identificar as pulgas, seus excrementos ou ambos.
- Exame microscópico do pelo — a perda de pelos autoinduzida resulta em extremidades quebradiças, enquanto a perda endógena culmina em extremidades afuniladas.
- Exame coprológico (fezes) — excesso de pelos, ácaros e ovos (*Cheyletiella*), tênias ou pulgas.
- Dieta hipoalergênica (teste de eliminação alimentar) — reações adversas aos alimentos.
- Teste cutâneo intradérmico — atopia.
- Biopsia cutânea — confirma a causa subjacente (p. ex., dermatite por hipersensibilidade, alopecia psicogênica ou, raramente, doença sistêmica).
- Citologia de pápulas ou crostas, se presentes, pode exibir uma grande quantidade de eosinófilos.
- O exame microscópico de raspados cutâneos ou pelos arrancados pode revelar a presença de artrósporos de dermatófitos ou ácaros de *Demodex*.

ACHADOS PATOLÓGICOS
- Achados histopatológicos — variam dependendo da causa.
- Alopecia psicogênica felina — folículos pilosos e pele normais.
- Números elevados de mastócitos, eosinófilos, linfócitos ou macrófagos sugerem dermatite alérgica.
- Alopecia areata — inflamação linfocítica que circunda a porção bulbar dos folículos pilosos; rara.

TRATAMENTO
- É importante o tratamento eficaz da doença subjacente.
- Informar ao proprietário sobre o plano diagnóstico e o momento em que se deve observar uma resposta (novo crescimento da pelagem, no caso).

MEDICAÇÕES

MEDICAMENTO(S)
- Anti-histamínicos — por exemplo, clorfeniramina, 0,5 mg/kg VO a cada 8 h.
- Glicocorticosteroides — 0,5 mg/kg VO, em dias alternados.
- Amitriptilina — 1-2 mg/kg VO diariamente.
- Cloridrato de clomipramina — 0,5 mg/kg a cada 24 h.
- Ciclosporina modificada — 5 mg/kg VO 1 vez ao dia.

CONTRAINDICAÇÕES/INTERAÇÕES POSSÍVEIS
- Glicocorticosteroides — podem causar alopecia, diabetes melito, polidipsia, poliúria, polifagia e ganho de peso; podem suprimir o prurido, dificultando a determinação da causa subjacente.
- Retirada de medicações antipruriginosas (inclusive os glicocorticosteroides) quando os exames diagnósticos estiverem quase concluídos (p. ex., pesquisa de reações de hipersensibilidade alimentar com a dieta de eliminação).

ACOMPANHAMENTO
- Exames frequentes são indispensáveis para confirmar os diagnósticos diferenciais.
- A identificação bem-sucedida da causa subjacente proporcionará o melhor prognóstico caso seja possível o controle da causa (p. ex., picadas de pulgas ou hipersensibilidade alimentar).

DIVERSOS

Sugestões de Leitura
Mertens PA, Torres S, Jessen C. The effects of clomipramine hydrochloride in cats with psychogenic alopecia: A prospective study. JAAHA 2006, 42(5):336-343.
O'Dair HA, Foster AP. Focal and generalized alopecia. Vet Clin North Am Small Anim Pract 1995, 25(4):851-870.
Sawyer LS, Moon-Fanelli AA, Dodman NH. Psychogenic alopecia in cats: 11 cases (1993-1996). JAVMA 1999, 214(1):71-74.
Swanepoel N, Lee E, Stein DJ. Psychogenic alopecia in a cat: Response to clomipramine. J S Afr Vet Assoc 1998, 69(1):22.
Waisglass SE, Landsberg GM, Yager JA, Hall JA. Underlying medical conditions in cats with presumptive psychogenic alopecia. JAVMA 2006, 228(11):1705-1709.

Autor David Duclos
Consultor Editorial Alexander H. Werner

AMEBÍASE

CONSIDERAÇÕES GERAIS

REVISÃO
- Ameba parasitária facultativa que infecta pessoas e primatas não humanos, incluindo cães e gatos.
- Encontrada principalmente em regiões tropicais em todo o mundo, inclusive América do Norte.

IDENTIFICAÇÃO
- Cães e gatos.
- Acomete, sobretudo, animais jovens e/ou imunossuprimidos.

SINAIS CLÍNICOS
Cães
- Infecções por *Entamoeba histolytica* geralmente são assintomáticas.
- Infecções graves — resultam em colite ulcerativa até causar disenteria (pode ser fatal).
- Disseminação hematógena — resulta em falências dos órgãos (invariavelmente fatais).
- Meningoencefalite amebiana granulomatosa (causada por *Acanthamoeba* spp.) — provoca sinais clínicos semelhantes à cinomose (anorexia, febre, letargia, secreção oculonasal, angústia respiratória, e anormalidades neurológicas difusas).
- Há relatos da síndrome de secreção inadequada do hormônio antidiurético em um cão jovem com acantamebíase causadora de meningoencefalite granulomatosa com invasão do hipotálamo.

Gatos
- Colite — causadora de diarreia intratável crônica (de acordo com os cães).
- Amebíase sistêmica ou *Acanthamoeba* — não há relatos em gatos.

CAUSAS E FATORES DE RISCO
- *Entamoeba histolytica* — a infecção ocorre pela ingestão de cistos provenientes de fezes humanas.
- Como é rara a ocorrência de encistamento de trofozoítas em cães ou gatos, esses animais não constituem uma fonte de infecção.
- Um dos poucos microrganismos transmitidos do homem para os animais domésticos, mas raramente dos animais domésticos para o homem.
- Trofozoítas (o estágio patogênico) — habitam o lúmen do cólon como microrganismos comensais ou invadem a parede do cólon, mas podem se disseminar para outros órgãos (raro), incluindo pulmões, fígado, cérebro e pele.
- Os trofozoítas lesionam as células epiteliais do intestino, secretando enzimas responsáveis pela lise celular e ruptura das junções intercelulares.
- Certas bactérias e uma dieta deficiente em proteína aumentam a virulência da ameba.
- A resposta imune do hospedeiro à invasão exacerba a doença.
- A ulceração colônica ocorre quando os trofozoítas na submucosa invadem a mucosa.
- *Acanthamoeba castellani* e *A. culbertsoni* — espécies de vida livre encontradas em água doce, água salgada, solo e esgoto; podem infectar os cães.
- *Acanthamoeba* spp. — acredita-se que a infecção ocorra por inalação de microrganismos provenientes de água contaminada ou colonização da pele ou córnea; pode ocorrer disseminação hematógena ou disseminação direta a partir da cavidade nasal através da placa cribriforme até o sistema nervoso central, resultando em uma meningoencefalite amebiana granulomatosa.

DIAGNÓSTICO

DIAGNÓSTICO DIFERENCIAL
Cães
- Causas de diarreia sanguinolenta ou tenesmo, inclusive constipação; intolerância/alergia alimentares; parasitismo (tricúris, leishmaniose, balantidíase); gastrenterite hemorrágica; corpo estranho; síndrome do intestino irritável; enteropatia inflamatória; divertículos; infecções (parvovírus, enterite clostrídica, proliferação bacteriana e outras causas bacterianas, fúngicas como histoplasmose ou blastomicose); neoplasia; colite ulcerativa; endocrinopatia (doença de Addison); tóxicas (chumbo, fungo ou planta); ocasionalmente, comprometimento de órgãos importantes causando ulceração colônica, como insuficiência renal.
- Outras causas de doença neurológica difusa em animais jovens, incluindo infecciosas (cinomose, fúngicas como *Cryptococcus*, *Blastomyces*, *Histoplasma*, bactérias, protozoários como *Toxoplasma* e *Neospora*); tóxicas (chumbo, organofosforados); traumatismo; meningoencefalopatia granulomatosa; extracranianas (hipoglicemia; encefalopatia hepática); epilepsia hereditária; neoplasia.

Gatos
- Outras causas de diarreia, incluindo intolerância/alergia alimentares; enteropatia inflamatória; parasitismo (giardíase, parasitas como ancilóstomos, nematódeos, tritrichomonas); infecciosas (panleucopenia, FIV, síndrome tipo leucopenia causada pelo FeLV, bacterianas incluindo *Salmonella*, raramente *Campylobacter*); medicamento (paracetamol); neoplasia; pancreatite; e disfunção de órgãos importantes.

HEMOGRAMA/BIOQUÍMICA/URINÁLISE
Normais; podem refletir a diarreia grave.

OUTROS TESTES LABORATORIAIS
- Exame microscópico — as biopsias colônicas (H&E) obtidas via endoscopia constituem o método mais confiável.
- Detecção de trofozoítas nas fezes — muito difícil; o corante azul de metileno aumenta as chances.
- Coloração tricrômica e ferro-hematoxilina — embora sejam os corantes fecais ideais, há necessidade de um laboratório de referência para a realização.
- Técnicas de concentração fecal — não têm utilidade.
- LCS — contagem elevada de leucócitos (70% de células mononucleares), presença de proteína e xantocromia em cães com meningoencefalite amebiana granulomatosa causada por *Ancathamoeba*.

DIAGNÓSTICO POR IMAGEM
RM — revela os granulomas cerebrais.

MÉTODOS DIAGNÓSTICOS
Biopsia cerebral — necessária para a obtenção do diagnóstico definitivo das formas neurológicas antes do óbito.

TRATAMENTO
- Colite (causada por *E. histolytica*) — responde ao metronidazol, embora os cães continuem eliminando os microrganismos nas fezes.
- Formas sistêmicas (em particular a doença neurológica) — invariavelmente fatal apesar do tratamento.

MEDICAÇÕES

MEDICAMENTO(S)
- Tinidazol (44 mg/kg VO a cada 24 h por 6 dias) em cães — mais eficaz do que o metronidazol para o tratamento de amebíase em pessoas.
- Metronidazol (20 mg/kg VO a cada 12 h por 7 dias).

CONTRAINDICAÇÕES/INTERAÇÕES POSSÍVEIS
Altas doses de metronidazol (em geral >30 mg/kg) por períodos prolongados podem causar sinais neurológicos em cães.

ACOMPANHAMENTO
Os animais domésticos costumam adquirir as infecções da mesma fonte que seus proprietários; os veterinários devem alertar os proprietários sobre o possível risco.

DIVERSOS

ABREVIATURA(S)
- FeLV = vírus da leucemia felina.
- FIV = vírus da imunodeficiência felina.
- H&E = hematoxilina e eosina.
- LCS = líquido cerebrospinal.
- RM = ressonância magnética.

Sugestões de Leitura
Brofman PJ, Knostman KAB, Dibartola SP. Granulomatous amebic meningoenchephalitis causing the syndrome of inappropriate secretion of antidiuretic hormone in a dog. J Vet Intern Med 2003, 17:230–234.
Fung HB, Doan TL. Tinidazole: A nitroimidazole antiprotozoal agent. Clin Ther 2005, 27:1859–1884.

Autor Stephen C. Barr
Consultor Editorial Stephen C. Barr

Ameloblastoma

CONSIDERAÇÕES GERAIS

REVISÃO
- Tumor bucal comum de origem ectodérmica odontogênica (estruturas dentárias).
- Do ponto de vista biológico, esses tumores são benignos ao exame histológico, embora possuam propriedades localmente invasivas.
- Foi descrita uma forma maligna rara (altamente invasiva).
- Os tumores podem surgir em qualquer lugar dentro de arcada dentária.
- Existem vários subtipos histológicos, mas todos têm comportamento invasivo semelhante.

IDENTIFICAÇÃO
- Cães de meia-idade e idosos.
- Raro nos gatos.

SINAIS CLÍNICOS
Os cães podem se apresentar com massa gengival firme e lisa, em geral não ulcerada.

CAUSAS E FATORES DE RISCO
N/D.

DIAGNÓSTICO

DIAGNÓSTICO DIFERENCIAL
- Epúlide.
- Tumor bucal maligno.
- Hiperplasia gengival.
- Outros tumores relacionados com o aparelho odontogênico.

HEMOGRAMA/BIOQUÍMICA/URINÁLISE
Sem alterações.

OUTROS TESTES LABORATORIAIS
N/D.

DIAGNÓSTICO POR IMAGEM
- As radiografias do crânio frequentemente revelam lise óssea em localização profunda à massa superficial.
- Não foram descritas metástases regionais e à distância.
- O exame de tomografia computadorizada pode ser útil para o planejamento da cirurgia ou da radioterapia.

MÉTODOS DIAGNÓSTICOS
Biopsias teciduais profundas são necessárias e recomendadas para o diagnóstico definitivo.

TRATAMENTO

- É recomendável a excisão cirúrgica radical, como mandibulectomia ou maxilectomia, com margens de segurança de, no mínimo, 1-2 cm, para garantir a excisão completa.
- A radioterapia pode ser curativa, sem o desfiguramento associado à cirurgia.

MEDICAÇÕES

MEDICAMENTO(S)
N/D.

CONTRAINDICAÇÕES/INTERAÇÕES POSSÍVEIS
N/D.

ACOMPANHAMENTO

É aconselhável o exame bucal rigoroso em 1, 3, 6, 9 e 12 meses após o tratamento definitivo para monitorizar o resultado terapêutico.

DIVERSOS

Sugestões de Leitura

Gelberg HB. Alimentary system. In: McGavin MD, Carlton WW, Zachary JF, eds., Thompson's Special Veterinary Pathology. St. Louis: Mosby, 2001, pp. 1-79.

Morrison WB. Cancers of the head and neck. In: Morrison WB, ed., Cancer in Dogs and Cats: Medical and Surgical Management. Jackson, WY: Teton NewMedia, 2002, pp. 489-496.

Walsh KM, Denholm LJ, Cooper BJ. Epithelial odontogenic tumors in domestic animals. J Comp Pathol 1987, 97:503-521.

Autor Wallace B. Morrison
Consultor Editorial Timothy M. Fan

Amiloide Hepático

CONSIDERAÇÕES GERAIS

REVISÃO
• Amiloidose — distúrbios de etiologia diversa, que compartilham a característica comum do depósito patológico de matriz proteinácea β-preguada fibrilar extracelular insolúvel com propriedades distintas de coloração e ultraestrutura fibrilar.
• Em animais, o amiloide acumula-se como um processo focal ou sistêmico secundário a distúrbios inflamatórios ou linfoproliferativos ou como um distúrbio genético familiar.
• Amiloidose familiar — descrita em certos parentes de gatos, afetando determinadas raças; parentes de cães com distúrbios inflamatórios singulares são predispostos ao depósito de amiloide.
• Múltiplos órgãos costumam ser envolvidos.
• Acúmulo hepático de amiloide — é insidioso; pode ser associado a atividade normal ou elevada das enzimas hepáticas, hepatomegalia grave, coagulopatias, ruptura hepática com consequente hemoabdome (gatos) e/ou insuficiência hepática.

IDENTIFICAÇÃO
• Cães — certos Shar-peis chineses com febres cíclicas (síndrome da febre do Shar-pei), Akitas com febre cíclica e poliartropatia, bem como Collies com a "síndrome do Collie cinza" são predispostos; em geral, desenvolvem sinais renais, embora alguns desenvolvam sinais de insuficiência hepática.
• Gatos — as raças Oriental de pelo curto e Siamês são predispostas; também relatado em Devon rex e doméstico de pelo curto; em geral, os animais têm menos de 5 anos de idade quando se encontram sintomáticos (os sinais hepáticos e as coagulopatias predominam); distúrbio familiar em Abissínio (nesse caso, os sinais renais predominam). Infecção viral do trato respiratório superior pode deflagrar o desenvolvimento de amiloidose em Siamês.

SINAIS CLÍNICOS
Achados Anamnésicos
• Febre episódica e jarretes tumefatos — Shar-pei.
• Poliartropatia episódica, dor e sinais de meningite — Akita. • Letargia aguda e cíclica.
• Anorexia episódica. • Poliúria e polidipsia.
• Vômitos.

Achados do Exame Físico
• Palidez. • Efusão abdominal — hemorragia ou ascite. • Icterícia: incomum. • Hepatomegalia com o depósito de amiloide. • Edema: causado por hipoalbuminemia secundária à proteinúria patológica. • Dor articular: Akita e síndromes do Shar-pei. • Dor não localizada, dor meníngea e desconforto abdominal: com diferentes distúrbios inflamatórios primários que promovem o depósito de amiloide.

CAUSAS E FATORES DE RISCO
• Distúrbios imunorreguladores familiares — parentes de cães e gatos predispostos. • Infecção crônica — coccidioidomicose; blastomicose; doenças transmitidas por carrapatos.
• Neutropenia cíclica — síndrome do Collie cinza.
• Endocardite bacteriana. • Inflamação crônica (p. ex., LES). • Neoplasia.

DIAGNÓSTICO

DIAGNÓSTICO DIFERENCIAL
• Inflamação hepática crônica. • Neoplasia hepática infiltrativa. • Coagulopatia primária ou induzida por rodenticidas. • Glomerulonefrite.
• Pielonefrite. • LES. • Traumatismo abdominal.
• Peritonite. • Meningite.

HEMOGRAMA/BIOQUÍMICA/URINÁLISE
• Anemia secundária à hemorragia hepática ou ruptura ou inflamação crônica de lobo hepático.
• Leucocitose com desvio à esquerda durante episódios febris nas raças Shar-pei e Akita.
• Enzimas hepáticas, bilirrubina total e ácidos biliares séricos normais ou elevados em caso de depósito hepático grave de amiloide.
• Azotemia em caso de infiltração renal grave: os glomérulos constituem o alvo de depósito em cães (proteinúria), enquanto o interstício renal representa o alvo em gatos (azotemia).
• Proteinúria: atribuída ao depósito de amiloide glomerular em cães.
• Urina diluída — com acometimento ou insuficiência renal.
• Amiloidose sistêmica felina — envolve múltiplos sistemas orgânicos, incluindo tireoide, coração, rins, intestinos, pâncreas, medula óssea, linfonodos, adrenais.

OUTROS TESTES LABORATORIAIS
• Provas de coagulação — tempos de coagulação normais a prolongados, além de hiperfibrinogenemia.
• Líquido sinovial — em cães com tumefação ou dor articular: revela inflamação asséptica supurativa.
• LCS — em caso de dor meníngea, exibe aumento do conteúdo de proteína e inflamação supurativa.

DIAGNÓSTICO POR IMAGEM
• Radiografia abdominal — hepatomegalia; tamanho variável dos rins; efusão.
• Ultrassonografia abdominal — hepatomegalia; parênquima hipoecoico com amiloide difuso; tamanho variável dos rins com parênquima normal ou equivocadamente hipoecoico; linfadenopatia mesentérica inconsistente; parede intestinal espessada em virtude do depósito de amiloide; efusão abdominal.

MÉTODOS DIAGNÓSTICOS
• Citologia de aspirado por agulha fina — pode revelar a presença de material fibrilar amorfo.
• Biopsia do fígado ou de outro tecido.
• Abdominocentese — hemorrágica ou transudativa em pacientes com envolvimento hepático difuso.

ACHADOS PATOLÓGICOS
Macroscópicos
• Fígado — coloração normal a pálida; grande, firme a friável; hemorragias (hematomas subcapsulares, lacerações capsulares) até franca ruptura.

Microscópicos
• Fígado — material amorfo acelular depositado de forma difusa no espaço de Disse, associado à atrofia dos cordões hepáticos; pode envolver principalmente os vasos sanguíneos na tríade portal (gatos Abissínios) (ver "Amiloidose").

TRATAMENTO
• Ditado pela gravidade dos sinais clínicos. • Não há tratamento curativo; tratar a doença subjacente quando identificada; a colchicina, conforme descrito adiante, pode reduzir o depósito orgânico de amiloide. • Fluidos — para a desidratação.
• Transfusões de sangue — para perda sanguínea aguda; importante para gatos com ruptura de lobo hepático induzida por amiloide hepático. • Dieta — adaptada individualmente à função do órgão do paciente. • Insuficiência hepática — considerar a tomada de medidas apropriadas para encefalopatia hepática quando for conveniente.
• Proteinúria patológica — ver "Síndrome Nefrótica". • Alertar o proprietário sobre a dificuldade de tratamento da amiloidose hepática; além disso, tem prognóstico reservado a mau.
• Considerações cirúrgicas — ressecção do lobo hepático como medida de emergência para sangramento catastrófico decorrente de fratura de lobo hepático em gatos.

MEDICAÇÕES

MEDICAMENTO(S)
• Colchicina — cães: 0,03 mg/kg VO a cada 24 h; pode interromper o depósito de amiloide no início da doença ou controlar o depósito em distúrbios mais crônicos; modula a expressão de moléculas de adesão e fatores quimiotáticos; provoca polimerização de microtúbulos ao se ligar à tubulina, o que interrompe a mitose em células como os neutrófilos. Os efeitos atenuam as respostas inflamatórias que deflagram a produção de proteína de fase aguda (precursor de amiloide). Monitorizar o hemograma quanto à ocorrência de mielotoxicidade; observar o paciente em busca de efeitos colaterais gastrintestinais (vômito, diarreia sanguinolenta). Utilizar a colchicina sem a adição de probenecida. Experiência limitada em gatos.
• DMSO — usar apenas em gradação médica; cães: 80 mg/kg em solução a 18% em água estéril administrados por via SC 3 vezes por semana; pode promover dissolução de fibrilas de amiloide ou ter um efeito anti-inflamatório ou antiamiloide.

INTERAÇÕES POSSÍVEIS
A colchicina combinada com probenecida pode causar vômito.

ACOMPANHAMENTO
• Shar-pei — os cães dessa raça com amiloide hepático podem sobreviver por mais de 2 anos; a maioria terá episódios de febre e colestase; em alguns, haverá resolução dos sinais clínicos e diminuição do amiloide hepático com a terapia com colchicina. • Akita com sinais clínicos cíclicos — prognóstico grave. • Gatos que sobrevivem à hemorragia hepática acabam sucumbindo por insuficiência hepática causada pelo depósito de amiloide.

Autor Sharon A. Center

Amiloidose

CONSIDERAÇÕES GERAIS

DEFINIÇÃO
Um grupo de condições de etiologia diversificada, nas quais a deposição extracelular de proteínas fibrilares insolúveis (amiloide) em diversos órgãos e tecidos compromete sua função normal.

FISIOPATOLOGIA
• Os pacientes costumam ser acometidos por amiloidose reativa sistêmica; os depósitos teciduais contêm proteína amiloide A, que corresponde a um fragmento de reagente de fase aguda, denominada proteína amiloide A sérica.
• Fases de deposição de amiloide.
  ○ *Fase de Pré-deposição:* a concentração da proteína amiloide A sérica apresenta-se elevada, mas não ocorrem depósitos de amiloide; a administração de colchicina durante essa fase pode evitar o desenvolvimento da doença. ○ *Fase de Deposição (Fração Rápida):* os depósitos de amiloide aumentam com rapidez; a administração da colchicina retarda, mas não evita a deposição tecidual de amiloide; o DMSO pode promover a dissolução dos depósitos de amiloide e um declínio persistente na concentração da proteína amiloide A sérica.
  ○ *Fase de Deposição (Fração de Platô):* a deposição real de amiloide sofre pouca alteração; nessa fase, nem o DMSO nem a colchicina são benéficos.
• Em cães e gatos, os sinais clínicos costumam estar associados à deposição de amiloide nos rins.
• Cães — os depósitos de amiloide são comumente encontrados nos glomérulos, levando à proteinúria e à síndrome nefrótica. • Gatos — os depósitos de amiloide são, em geral, encontrados no interstício medular, mas podem ocorrer nos glomérulos. • Alguns cães da raça Shar-pei chinês com amiloidose familiar apresentam amiloidose medular, sem envolvimento glomerular. • Os gatos da raça Oriental de pelo curto e Siamês com amiloidose familiar exibem amiloidose hepática.
• Um tipo diferente de amiloide, o polipeptídeo amiloide das ilhotas pancreáticas, ou amilina, deposita-se no pâncreas de gatos idosos. A amilina é um hormônio secretado juntamente com a insulina pelas células β do pâncreas. O estímulo acentuado e crônico para a secreção de amilina por essas células (p. ex., estados de insulinorresistência) leva à amiloidose das ilhotas pancreáticas.

SISTEMA(S) ACOMETIDO(S)
Renal/Urológico — predileção para deposição renal de proteína amiloide A; órgãos como fígado, baço, adrenais, pâncreas, árvore traqueobrônquica e trato gastrintestinal também podem ser acometidos.

GENÉTICA
Ainda não se determinou claramente qualquer envolvimento genético; a amiloidose familiar ocorre no Shar-pei chinês, Foxhound inglês e Beagle, bem como em gatos das raças Abissínio, Oriental de pelo curto e Siamês.

INCIDÊNCIA/PREVALÊNCIA
Ocorre principalmente em cães; rara em gatos, exceto no Abissínio.

IDENTIFICAÇÃO
Espécies
Cães e gatos.

Raça(s) Predominante(s)
• Cães — Shar-pei chinês, Beagle, Collie, Pointer, Foxhound inglês e Walker hound; o Pastor alemão e as raças mestiças exibem um risco menor.
• Gatos — Abissínio, Oriental de pelo curto e Siamês.

Idade Média e Faixa Etária
• Grande parte dos cães e gatos acometidos tem mais de 5 anos de idade. • Cães — a idade média ao diagnóstico é de 9 anos; variação, 1-15 anos.
• Gatos — a idade média ao diagnóstico é de 7 anos; variação, 1-17 anos. • A prevalência aumenta com a idade. • Gato Abissínio — variação <1-17 anos. • Cães da raça Shar-pei chinês — geralmente apresentam <6 anos de idade quando se desenrolam os sinais de insuficiência renal; variação, 1,5-6 anos. • Gatos da raça Siamês com amiloidose familiar hepática e tireóidea costumam desenvolver sinais de hepatopatia quando estão com 1-4 anos de idade.

Sexo(s) Predominante(s)
Cães e gatos da raça Abissínio — as fêmeas parecem exibir um risco levemente mais alto (<2:1). A relação de fêmeas:machos é mais alta em cães da raça Shar-pei chinês (~2,5:1).

SINAIS CLÍNICOS
Comentários Gerais
• Dependem dos órgãos acometidos, da quantidade de amiloide e da reação dos órgãos envolvidos aos depósitos de amiloide. • Costumam ser causados pelo envolvimento renal; ocasionalmente, o envolvimento hepático pode gerar sinais no Shar-pei chinês, bem como nos gatos das raças Oriental de pelo curto e Siamês.

Achados Anamnésicos
• Na maioria dos casos (~75%), não há um histórico claro de distúrbio predisponente.
• Anorexia, letargia, poliúria e polidipsia, perda de peso, vômito e diarreia (incomum). • Ascite e edema periférico em animais com síndrome nefrótica. • Os cães da raça Shar-pei chinês podem ter um histórico prévio de tumefação articular e febre alta episódicas, que desaparecem espontaneamente em alguns dias. • Os cães da raça Beagle com poliartrite juvenil podem exibir um histórico de febre e dor no pescoço (cervicalgia), que persistem por 3-7 dias. • Os gatos das raças Oriental de pelo curto e Siamês podem se apresentar com hemorragia hepática espontânea, que leva ao colapso agudo e hemoabdome.

Achados do Exame Físico
• Relacionados com insuficiência renal — ulceração bucal, emaciação, vômito e desidratação; os rins geralmente se encontram pequenos, firmes e irregulares nos gatos acometidos; podem estar pequenos, normais ou levemente aumentados de volume nos cães acometidos. • Sinais de síndrome nefrótica (p. ex., ascite e edema subcutâneo).
• Relacionados com o processo patológico primário inflamatório ou neoplásico. • Fenômenos tromboembólicos — podem ocorrer em até 40% dos cães acometidos; os sinais variam com a localização do trombo; os pacientes podem desenvolver tromboembolia pulmonar (p. ex., dispneia) ou tromboembolia arterial ilíaca ou femoral (p. ex., paresia caudal). • Os cães da raça Shar-pei chinês e os gatos das raças Oriental de pelo curto e Siamês podem apresentar sinais de hepatopatia (p. ex., icterícia, caquexia e ruptura hepática espontânea com hemorragia intraperitoneal).

CAUSAS
• Em 30-50% dos cães com amiloidose reativa, podem-se constatar condições inflamatórias crônicas infecciosas e não infecciosas, além de neoplasia. • Inflamações crônicas — micoses sistêmicas (p. ex., blastomicose e coccidioidomicose), infecções bacterianas crônicas (p. ex., osteomielite, broncopneumonia, pleurite, esteatite, piometra, pielonefrite, dermatite supurativa crônica, artrite supurativa crônica, peritonite crônica, nocardiose e estomatite crônica), infecções parasitárias (p. ex., dirofilariose, leishmaniose e hepatozoonose) e doenças imunomediadas (p. ex., lúpus eritematoso sistêmico). • Neoplasias (p. ex., linfoma, plasmocitoma, mieloma múltiplo, tumores mamários e tumores testiculares). • Familiares (p. ex., Shar-pei chinês, Foxhound inglês e Beagle; gatos das raças Abissínio, Siamês e Oriental de pelo curto). • Outras — hematopoiese cíclica em Collie de pelagem cinza, poliartrite juvenil em Beagle.

FATORES DE RISCO
• Inflamação crônica ou neoplasia. • Histórico familiar em determinadas raças.

DIAGNÓSTICO

DIAGNÓSTICO DIFERENCIAL
• Cães — a glomerulonefrite constitui o principal diagnóstico diferencial; o sinal de proteinúria tende a ser mais grave em cães com amiloidose glomerular, em comparação àqueles com glomerulonefrite, embora haja uma notável sobreposição. • Gatos e cães da raça Shar-pei chinês com amiloidose medular — considerar outras causas de nefropatia medular (p. ex., pielonefrite e doença intersticial crônica).

HEMOGRAMA/BIOQUÍMICA/URINÁLISE
• Em alguns cães e gatos com insuficiência renal induzida por amiloide, verifica-se uma anemia arregenerativa. • Cães — podem-se observar hipercolesterolemia (>85%), azotemia (>70%), hipoalbuminemia (70%), hiperfosfatemia (>60%), hipocalcemia (50%) e acidose metabólica.
• Hipercolesterolemia — achado comum em gatos com distúrbios renais (>70% de gatos com nefropatia em um único estudo), mas não prediz com segurança a presença de glomerulopatia.
• Hipoproteinemia — mais comum do que a hiperproteinemia (24 *versus* 8,5%) em cães com amiloidose; a hiperglobulinemia é comum em gatos. • Proteinúria — com sedimento inativo é comum em cães; leve ou ausente em animais com amiloidose medular sem envolvimento glomerular (grande parte dos gatos de raças mestiças, pelo menos 25% dos gatos da raça Abissínio e no mínimo 33% dos cães da raça Shar-pei chinês).
• Em alguns pacientes, observam-se cilindros hialinos, granulares e céreos, além de isostenúria.

OUTROS TESTES LABORATORIAIS
Proteinúria — mensurar a relação de proteína:creatinina urinárias para estimar a gravidade.

DIAGNÓSTICO POR IMAGEM
Achados Radiográficos Abdominais
• Rins usualmente pequenos nos gatos acometidos; rins pequenos, normais ou aumentados de volume nos cães acometidos.

AMILOIDOSE

Achados Ultrassonográficos Abdominais
• Os rins costumam aparecer hiperecoicos e pequenos nos gatos acometidos; podem se apresentar pequenos, normais ou aumentados de volume nos cães acometidos.

MÉTODOS DIAGNÓSTICOS
É necessária a realização de biopsia renal para diferenciar os quadros de amiloidose e glomerulonefrite. Nos cães não pertencentes à raça Shar-pei chinês, a amiloidose corresponde primariamente a uma glomerulopatia e a biopsia do córtex renal possibilita a obtenção do diagnóstico. Em grande parte dos gatos domésticos, em alguns gatos da raça Abissínio e em determinados cães da raça Shar-pei chinês, pode ocorrer a amiloidose medular sem envolvimento glomerular; para a formulação do diagnóstico, é imprescindível obter amostra de tecido medular dos rins.

ACHADOS PATOLÓGICOS
• Rins pequenos nos gatos; rins pequenos, normais ou aumentados de volume nos cães. • Os depósitos de amiloide aparecem homogêneos e eosinofílicos quando corados pela hematoxilina-eosina e observados por meio da microscopia óptica convencional. Tais depósitos demonstram uma birrefringência verde após a coloração com o vermelho-congo quando vistos sob luz polarizada. A avaliação dos cortes histológicos corados pelo vermelho-congo antes e depois da oxidação com o permanganato permite o diagnóstico presuntivo da amiloidose por proteína amiloide A (*versus* outros tipos), já que esse tipo de amiloidose perde sua afinidade pelo corante mencionado após a oxidação com o permanganato. • O fígado apresenta-se bastante friável e geralmente contém extensos depósitos de amiloide em gatos com hemorragia hepática aguda.

TRATAMENTO

CUIDADO(S) DE SAÚDE ADEQUADO(S)
• Internar os pacientes com insuficiência renal crônica e desidratação para o tratamento clínico inicial. • É possível tratar os pacientes estáveis e aqueles com proteinúria assintomática em um esquema ambulatorial.

CUIDADO(S) DE ENFERMAGEM
Corrigir a desidratação com soro fisiológico a 0,9% ou solução de Ringer lactato; os pacientes com acidose metabólica grave podem necessitar da suplementação de bicarbonato (ver "Acidose Metabólica").

ATIVIDADE
Normal.

DIETA
• Pacientes com insuficiência renal crônica — restrição de fósforo e moderadamente de proteínas. • Pacientes com hipertensão — restrição de sódio.

ORIENTAÇÃO AO PROPRIETÁRIO
• Discutir a evolução da doença. • Abordar a predisposição familiar em raças suscetíveis. • Debater as complicações potenciais (p. ex., hipertensão e tromboembolia).

MEDICAÇÕES

MEDICAMENTO(S) DE ESCOLHA
• Identificar os processos subjacentes inflamatórios e neoplásicos e tratá-los, se possível. • Tratar a insuficiência renal de acordo com os princípios do tratamento clínico conservativo (ver "Insuficiência Renal Aguda e Crônica"). • Normalizar a pressão sanguínea em pacientes com hipertensão (ver "Hipertensão Sistêmica"). • Os pacientes com síndrome tromboembólica e síndrome nefrótica causada pela amiloidose glomerular costumam apresentar uma concentração plasmática baixa de antitrombina; assim, a heparina é relativamente ineficaz. Para cães com glomerulopatia, sugere-se a administração do ácido acetilsalicílico (0,5 mg/kg VO a cada 12 h); essa dosagem baixa é tão eficiente para evitar a agregação plaquetária quanto a dose de 10 mg/kg VO a cada 24 h. • DMSO — pode ajudar os pacientes a dissolver as fibrilas de amiloide e diminuir a concentração sérica da proteína amiloide A sérica, além de reduzir a inflamação e a fibrose intersticiais nos rins acometidos; pode causar opacificação do cristalino em cães. Em caso de administração intravenosa do DMSO não diluído, podem ocorrer inflamação perivascular e trombose local. A aplicação subcutânea de DMSO não diluído pode ser dolorosa. Os autores têm utilizado o DMSO a 90% na diluição de 1:4 com água esterilizada, em uma dose de 90 mg/kg SC três vezes por semana nos cães. Ainda é controverso se o tratamento com o DMSO beneficia ou não os cães com amiloidose renal. • Metilsulfonilmetano — é um metabólito ativo do DMSO que pode ser administrado por via oral e não possui o odor do DMSO. Esse metabólito foi usado de forma empírica em cães com amiloidose, mas não há provas de que ele seja benéfico em animais dessa espécie com amiloidose renal. • Colchicina — diminui a liberação da proteína amiloide A sérica pelos hepatócitos; evita o desenvolvimento de amiloidose em seres humanos com febre familiar do Mediterrâneo (uma amiloidose familiar) e estabiliza a função renal em pacientes com síndrome nefrótica, mas sem insuficiência renal manifesta; não há indícios de benefícios, uma vez que o paciente desenvolve insuficiência renal; pode causar vômito, diarreia e neutropenia idiossincrática nos cães. A colchicina (0,01-0,04 mg/kg VO a cada 24 h) é utilizada particularmente em cães da raça Shar-pei chinês com febre ou poliartrite episódicas antes do desenvolvimento de insuficiência renal.

CONTRAINDICAÇÕES
Evitar o uso de medicamentos nefrotóxicos.

PRECAUÇÕES
• Em pacientes com insuficiência renal, podem ser necessários ajustes na dosagem de medicamentos excretados pelos rins. • Em pacientes com amiloidose medular, utilizar os medicamentos anti-inflamatórios não esteroides com cautela; além disso, tais medicamentos podem reduzir o fluxo sanguíneo renal em pacientes desidratados.

ACOMPANHAMENTO

MONITORIZAÇÃO DO PACIENTE
• Monitorização diária do apetite e do nível de atividade por parte do proprietário; monitorização semanal do peso corporal. • Concentrações séricas de albumina, creatinina e ureia a cada 2-6 meses em pacientes estáveis. • Pela mensuração das relações de proteína:creatinina urinárias, torna-se possível a avaliação seriada do grau de proteinúria.

PREVENÇÃO
Não acasalar os animais acometidos.

COMPLICAÇÕES POSSÍVEIS
• Insuficiência renal. • Síndrome nefrótica. • Hipertensão sistêmica. • Hemorragia intraperitoneal induzida por ruptura hepática. • Doença tromboembólica.

EVOLUÇÃO ESPERADA E PROGNÓSTICO
A amiloidose é uma doença progressiva, que costuma estar avançada no momento do diagnóstico. O prognóstico exibirá uma melhora se a doença imunológica, inflamatória ou neoplásica subjacente for detectada e tratada com êxito. Em um único estudo, a sobrevida de cães com amiloidose glomerular variou de 3 a 20 meses; ocasionalmente, alguns cães podem ter uma vida mais longa. Em geral, os gatos com insuficiência renal decorrente da amiloidose sobrevivem <1 ano. Os gatos levemente acometidos podem não desenvolver a insuficiência renal e exibir uma expectativa de vida quase normal.

DIVERSOS

DISTÚRBIOS ASSOCIADOS
• Infecção do trato urinário. • Poliartrite no Shar-pei chinês. • Poliarterite no Beagle.

GESTAÇÃO/FERTILIDADE/REPRODUÇÃO
Alto risco em animais acometidos.

VER TAMBÉM
• Glomerulonefrite. • Insuficiência Renal Aguda. • Insuficiência Renal Crônica. • Proteinúria. • Síndrome Nefrótica.

ABREVIATURA(S)
• DMSO = dimetilsulfóxido.

Sugestões de Leitura
DiBartola SP. Renal amyloidosis. In: Osborne CA, Low D, Finco DR, eds., Canine and Feline Urology, 2nd ed. Philadelphia: Saunders, 1995, pp. 400-415.

Autores Hélio Autran de Morais e Stephen P. DiBartola
Consultor Editorial Carl A. Osborne

ANAFILAXIA

CONSIDERAÇÕES GERAIS

DEFINIÇÃO
- Manifestação aguda de reação de hipersensibilidade do tipo I, mediada pela rápida introdução de antígeno em hospedeiro portador de anticorpos antígeno-específicos da subclasse IgE.
- A ligação do antígeno aos mastócitos sensibilizados com a IgE resulta na liberação de mediadores químicos pré-formados e recém-sintetizados.
- As reações anafiláticas podem ser localizadas (atopia) ou sistêmicas (choque anafilático).
- A anafilaxia não mediada pela IgE é designada como uma reação anafilactoide e não será discutida neste capítulo.

FISIOPATOLOGIA
- A primeira exposição do paciente a um determinado antígeno (alérgeno) provoca uma resposta humoral e resulta na produção de IgE, que se liga à superfície dos mastócitos; o paciente, então, passa a ser considerado um indivíduo sensibilizado a esse antígeno.
- A segunda exposição ao antígeno culmina na ligação cruzada de duas ou mais moléculas de IgE sobre a superfície celular, o que resulta na degranulação e na ativação dos mastócitos; a liberação dos grânulos contidos nos mastócitos desencadeia uma reação anafilática.
- Os principais mediadores derivados dos mastócitos incluem: a histamina, o fator quimiotático eosinofílico, o ácido araquidônico, os metabólitos inflamatórios (p. ex., prostaglandinas, leucotrienos e tromboxanos), o fator ativador de plaquetas e as proteases; tais mediadores geram uma resposta inflamatória, que consiste em um aumento na permeabilidade vascular, na contração da musculatura lisa, no influxo de células inflamatórias e no dano tecidual.
- As manifestações clínicas dependem da via de exposição ao antígeno, da dose do antígeno e da intensidade de resposta da IgE.

SISTEMA(S) ACOMETIDO(S)
- Cutâneo/exócrino — prurido, urticária e edema.
- Respiratório (gatos) — dispneia e cianose.
- Gastrintestinal — salivação, vômito e diarreia.
- Hepatobiliar (cães) — em função da hipertensão portal e vasoconstrição.

GENÉTICA
Há relatos de uma base familiar para a reação de hipersensibilidade do tipo I em cães.

INCIDÊNCIA/PREVALÊNCIA
- As reações localizadas de hipersensibilidade do tipo I não são incomuns.
- As reações sistêmicas de hipersensibilidade do tipo I são raras.

DISTRIBUIÇÃO GEOGRÁFICA
Nenhuma.

IDENTIFICAÇÃO
Espécies
Cães e gatos.

Raça(s) Predominante(s)
- Cães — inúmeras raças são registradas com uma predisposição ao desenvolvimento de atopia.
- Gatos — não há raças registradas com predisposição à atopia.

Idade Média e Faixa Etária
- Cães — a idade de início clínico varia de 3 meses a alguns anos de idade; a maioria dos animais acometidos tem 1-3 anos de idade.
- Gatos — a idade de início clínico varia de 6 meses a 2 anos.

Sexo(s) Predominante(s)
- Cães — a atopia é mais comum em fêmeas.
- Gatos — não há relato de predisposição sexual.

SINAIS CLÍNICOS
Comentários Gerais
- Os sinais clínicos iniciais variam, dependendo da via de exposição ao antígeno desencadeante (alérgeno).
- Choque — corresponde ao resultado final de uma reação anafilática grave.
- Órgão de choque — cães, fígado; gatos, sistemas respiratório e gastrintestinal.
- Podem ficar restritos ao local de exposição, embora possam evoluir para uma reação sistêmica.

Achados Anamnésicos
- Início imediato dos sinais (geralmente em minutos).
- Cães — prurido, urticária, vômito, defecação e micção.
- Gatos — prurido intenso na cabeça, dispneia, salivação e vômito.

Achados do Exame Físico
- Edema cutâneo localizado no local de exposição.
- Hepatomegalia em alguns cães.
- Possível hiperexcitabilidade nos estágios precoces.
- Depressão e colapso nos estágios terminais.

CAUSAS
Praticamente qualquer agente; os mais comumente relatados incluem venenos, produtos derivados do sangue, vacinas, alimentos e medicamentos.

FATORES DE RISCO
A exposição prévia (sensibilização) aumenta a possibilidade de desenvolvimento de uma reação pelo animal.

DIAGNÓSTICO

DIAGNÓSTICO DIFERENCIAL
- Outros tipos de choque.
- Traumatismo.
- Depende do principal sistema orgânico envolvido ou de uma reação localizada ou não; o diagnóstico pode ser feito essencialmente com base na anamnese e nos sinais clínicos.

HEMOGRAMA/BIOQUÍMICA/URINÁLISE
Em virtude do início agudo da doença, não há testes disponíveis que predizem com segurança a suscetibilidade individual.

OUTROS TESTES LABORATORIAIS
- Teste cutâneo intradérmico para identificar os alérgenos.
- Teste radioalergoabsorvente para quantificar a concentração sérica de IgE específica para um determinado antígeno.

DIAGNÓSTICO POR IMAGEM
N/D.

MÉTODOS DIAGNÓSTICOS
São limitados, em decorrência do possível desenvolvimento de uma reação anafilática por animal gravemente alérgico quando exposto a quantidades até mesmo pequenas de antígeno.

ACHADOS PATOLÓGICOS
- As lesões variam, dependendo da gravidade da reação, desde edema cutâneo localizado até edema pulmonar grave (em gatos) e represamento sanguíneo visceral (em cães).
- Outros achados inespecíficos variam e são característicos de choque.
- São características inespecíficas de reações localizadas: edema, vasculite e tromboembolia.

TRATAMENTO

CUIDADO(S) DE SAÚDE ADEQUADO(S)
Em animal acometido de forma aguda, a reação é considerada uma emergência clínica que exige internação.

CUIDADO(S) DE ENFERMAGEM
Eliminação do antígeno desencadeante, se possível.

Anafilaxia Sistêmica
- Objetivo — suporte vital de emergência por meio de manutenção de via aérea desobstruída, prevenção de colapso circulatório e restabelecimento dos parâmetros fisiológicos.
- Fluidoterapia intravenosa em doses de choque para neutralizar a hipotensão.

Anafilaxia Localizada
Objetivo — limitar a reação e evitar a evolução para uma reação sistêmica.

ATIVIDADE
N/D.

DIETA
Na suspeita de algum alérgeno de base alimentar (incomum), evitar os alimentos associados à reação de hipersensibilidade.

ORIENTAÇÃO AO PROPRIETÁRIO
- Debater a natureza imprevisível da doença.
- Discutir a necessidade de se identificar a presença de alguma condição alérgica, que possa exigir o atendimento clínico imediato do animal.

CONSIDERAÇÕES CIRÚRGICAS
Nenhuma.

MEDICAÇÕES

MEDICAMENTO(S) DE ESCOLHA
Anafilaxia Sistêmica
- Cloridrato de epinefrina [adrenalina] (na diluição de 1:1.000; 0,01 mL/kg) administrado por via parenteral em casos de choque.
- Corticosteroides contra o choque — succinato sódico de prednisolona (2 mg/kg IV a cada 8 h) ou fosfato sódico de dexametasona (0,25 mg/kg IV a cada 12 h).
- Sulfato de atropina (0,04 mg/kg IM) para neutralizar os sinais de bradicardia e hipotensão.
- Aminofilina (10 mg/kg IM ou lentamente IV) em pacientes gravemente dispneicos.

Anafilaxia Localizada
- Cloridrato de difenidramina (1-2 mg/kg IV ou IM).
- Prednisolona (2 mg/kg VO).
- Cloridrato de epinefrina [adrenalina] (0,15 mL SC no local do desencadeamento).
- Em caso de desenvolvimento do choque, instituir o tratamento da anafilaxia sistêmica.

ANAFILAXIA

CONTRAINDICAÇÕES
Nenhuma.

PRECAUÇÕES
A reação localizada pode evoluir para uma reação sistêmica.

INTERAÇÕES POSSÍVEIS
N/D.

MEDICAMENTO(S) ALTERNATIVO(S)
N/D.

 ACOMPANHAMENTO

MONITORIZAÇÃO DO PACIENTE
Durante um período de 24-48 h, monitorizar de perto os pacientes internados.

PREVENÇÃO
Caso se consiga identificar o antígeno desencadeante (alérgeno), eliminar ou reduzir a exposição.

COMPLICAÇÕES POSSÍVEIS
Nenhuma.

EVOLUÇÃO ESPERADA E PROGNÓSTICO
• Se a reação localizada for tratada precocemente, o prognóstico será bom.
• Se o animal estiver em choque ao exame, o prognóstico será reservado a mau.

 DIVERSOS

DISTÚRBIOS ASSOCIADOS
Nenhum.

FATORES RELACIONADOS COM A IDADE
Nenhum.

POTENCIAL ZOONÓTICO
Nenhum.

GESTAÇÃO/FERTILIDADE/REPRODUÇÃO
N/D.

VER TAMBÉM
• Choque Cardiogênico.

RECURSOS DA INTERNET
Manual Merck de Veterinária: www.merckvetmanual.com.

Sugestões de Leitura
Mueller DL, Noxon JO. Anaphylaxis: Pathophysiology and treatment. Compend Contin Educ Pract Vet 1990, 12:157-170.

Autor Paul W. Snyder
Consultor Editorial A.H. Rebar

Ancilostomíase

CONSIDERAÇÕES GERAIS

REVISÃO
• Parasitas nematoides do intestino delgado; *Ancylostoma caninum* em cães; *A. tubaeforme* em gatos; *A. braziliense* e *Uncinaria stenocephala* em cães e gatos. • Nos EUA, o *A. braziliense* é encontrado nos estados do sul; os outros também são encontrados na zona temperada. • Adultos hematófagos vorazes e larvas de quarto estágio de *A. caninum* e *A. tubaeforme* provocam anemia por perda sanguínea e enterite; vermes ativos deixam os locais da mordida com drenagem contínua de sangue. • Doença superaguda a crônica; a forma superaguda em neonatos origina-se de infecção transmamária; doença aguda em filhotes caninos com mais idade; em adultos, a infecção pode ser aguda, compensatória crônica, ou crônica sem compensação em cães imunossuprimidos ou debilitados. • *Uncinaria* tem pouca importância clínica. • *A. braziliense* é a principal causa de larva migrans cutânea. • A tosse pode resultar da migração de larvas nos pulmões após a penetração na pele. • *A. caninum* é transmitido via colostro/leite para os filhotes de cães; todas as espécies são transmitidas pela ingestão de larvas infectantes no alimento, na água ou nos hospedeiros de transporte ou por penetração cutânea.

IDENTIFICAÇÃO
• Doença superaguda a aguda em animais jovens, mas assintomática ou crônica em cães e gatos maduros. • A gravidade clínica é maior em cães que em gatos.

SINAIS CLÍNICOS
Achados Anamnésicos
• Mucosas pálidas. • Fezes escuras alcatroadas (melena); diarreia; constipação. • Perda da condição. • Falta de apetite. • Tosse seca. • Morte súbita.

Achados do Exame Físico
• Má condição do corpo e mal aspecto da pelagem. • Mucosas pálidas. • Lesões pruriginosas e eritematosas, além de pápulas nos pés, especialmente nos "dedões".

CAUSAS E FATORES DE RISCO
• Cadela ou gata infectada. • Ambiente contaminado com fezes de cães ou gatos infectados por ancilóstomos. • Infecções entéricas concomitantes. • Outras condições comprometedoras (p. ex., prenhez, desnutrição).

DIAGNÓSTICO

DIAGNÓSTICO DIFERENCIAL
• Outras causas de destruição eritrocitária ou perda sanguínea que resultem em anemia. • Ascaridíase (infecção por nematoide grande), coccidiose e estrongiloidíase podem causar sinais clínicos semelhantes, sem anemia significativa. • Podem ocorrer melena e anemia leve em fisalopterose; o principal sinal clínico é a ocorrência de vômito crônico.

HEMOGRAMA/BIOQUÍMICA/URINÁLISE
• Eosinofilia. • Anemia geralmente regenerativa normocítica normocrômica aguda; pode ser microcítica hipocrômica em virtude da deficiência crônica de ferro.

MÉTODOS DIAGNÓSTICOS
• Flutuação fecal para detectar ovos morulados típicos de estrongiloides; há pequenas diferenças de tamanho entre as espécies; os ovos de *Uncinaria* são um pouco maiores que os de *Ancylostoma*.
• Necropsia de ninhadas que tenham morrido depois do aparecimento de sinais clínicos semelhantes.

ACHADOS PATOLÓGICOS
• Macroscópicos: visualização de ancilóstomos aderidos à mucosa do intestino delgado; constatação de ulcerações hemorrágicas multifocais ("locais da mordida") na mucosa; presença de sangue no lúmen intestinal. • Microscópicos: enterite eosinofílica atribuída à atividade de larvas na parede do intestino delgado.

TRATAMENTO

• Casos superagudos e agudos graves são tratados com internação; agente anti-helmíntico, fluidoterapia e transfusão sanguínea, além de suplementação de oxigênio, conforme indicado pela gravidade da anemia e pelos sinais clínicos.
• Alertar o proprietário sobre a possibilidade de morte súbita apesar do tratamento em casos superagudos e agudos graves. • Casos crônicos compensatórios: uso de anti-helmíntico; em casos não compensatórios, fornecer suporte nutricional (suplemento de ferro).

MEDICAÇÕES

MEDICAMENTO(S)
Anti-helmínticos com Atividade Adulticida e Larvicida
• Fembendazol — 50 mg/kg VO a cada 24 h por 3 dias consecutivos em cães. • Milbemicina oxima — 0,5 mg/kg (cães) ou 2 mg/kg (gatos) VO a cada 30 dias. • Emodepsida (3 mg/kg)/praziquantel (12 mg/kg) por via tópica uma única vez em gatos.
• Moxidectina — 0,17 mg/kg SC a cada 6 meses em cães. • Moxidectina 2,5 mg/kg (cães) ou 1,0 mg/kg (gatos)/imidoclopramida 10 mg/kg, por via tópica a cada 30 dias. • Ivermectina — 24 µg/kg VO a cada 30 dias em gatos.

Anti-helmínticos com Atividade Adulticida
• Pamoato de pirantel — dose da bula em cães; 10-20 mg/kg VO em gatos (fora da indicação da bula). • Praziquantel/pamoato de pirantel/febantel — dose da bula em cães. • Praziquantel/pamoato de pirantel — dose da bula em gatos.
• Ivermectina/pamoato de pirantel ou ivermectina/pamoato de pirantel/praziquantel — dose da bula em cães. • Selamectina, 6 mg/kg por via tópica uma única vez a cada 30 dias em gatos.

ACOMPANHAMENTO

• Monitorizar as contagens de ovos nas fezes após o tratamento. • Monitorizar o hematócrito em pacientes anêmicos.

PREVENÇÃO
• Eliminar os estágios intestinais e as larvas "dormentes" (latentes) ativadas na cadela reprodutora: fembendazol na dose de 50 mg/kg/dia a partir do 40º dia de gestação até o 14º dia de lactação ou ivermectina na dose de 0,5 mg/kg 4-9 dias antes de dar cria e novamente 10 dias depois.
• Iniciar o tratamento anti-helmíntico quinzenal de filhotes caninos com 2 semanas de vida; continuar até o desmame, especialmente em filhotes sob alto risco de infecção a partir da cadela ou do ambiente; tratar mensalmente após o desmame. • Tratar a gata com anti-helmíntico adulticida/larvicida antes do acasalamento e depois de dar cria. • Iniciar o tratamento anti-helmíntico de filhotes felinos com 3-4 semanas de vida; tratar mensalmente depois disso. • Remover e descartar as fezes imediatamente para evitar a contaminação do ambiente com larvas. • Evitar a caça ou o consumo de alimentos em putrefação (lixo, p. ex.) para impedir a ingestão de hospedeiros de transporte potenciais.

EVOLUÇÃO ESPERADA E PROGNÓSTICO
• Os filhotes caninos com infecção superaguda ou aguda por *A. caninum* podem vir a óbito apesar do tratamento. • Espera-se uma recuperação completa em grande parte dos outros casos com tratamento anti-helmíntico e suporte nutricional. • O tratamento anti-helmíntico de cães adultos com larvas "dormentes" (latentes) em seus tecidos pode resultar na ativação das larvas e repopulação do intestino delgado.

DIVERSOS

FATORES RELACIONADOS COM A IDADE
• Doença mais aguda em animais jovens e crônica em adultos. • A transmissão de larvas de *A. caninum* da cadela para a prole via colostro/leite resulta em alta taxa de infecção nos filhotes.

POTENCIAL ZOONÓTICO
• Todos os ancilóstomos, especialmente o *A. braziliense*, provocam larva migrans cutânea quando as larvas infectantes penetram na pele humana; a migração na derme gera lesões pruriginosas e serpiginosas. • As larvas de *A. caninum* podem causar larva migrans visceral ou migrar para o trato GI, ocasionando dor abdominal e eosinofilia sem se tornar patente.

ABREVIATURA(S)
• GI = gastrintestinal.

RECURSOS DA INTERNET
• www.capcvet.org. • www.cdc.gov.

Sugestões de Leitura
Bowman DD. Georgis' Parasitology for Veterinarians, 9th ed. St. Louis: Saunders, 2008, pp. 179-185.

Autor Julie Ann Jarvinen
Consultor Editorial Stephen C. Barr

ANEMIA APLÁSICA

CONSIDERAÇÕES GERAIS

REVISÃO
- Um distúrbio de células precursoras hematopoiéticas, caracterizado pela substituição da medula óssea normal por tecido adiposo e pelo declínio na produção de granulócitos, eritrócitos e plaquetas, resultando em pancitopenia no sangue periférico. Algumas vezes, a doença recebe o nome de pancitopenia aplásica.
- Na forma aguda, há um predomínio de neutropenia e trombocitopenia em virtude do curto período de vida dessas células; na forma crônica, também ocorre anemia arregenerativa. Em ambas as formas, a medula óssea exibe graus variados de pan-hipoplasia.
- Há muitas causas precipitantes de hematopoiese deficiente, como doenças infecciosas, efeitos de medicamentos, inanição e exposição a toxinas; com frequência, suspeita-se do envolvimento de mecanismos imunomediados.
- Acomete os sistemas sanguíneo/linfático/imunológico.

IDENTIFICAÇÃO
Cães e gatos, sem predileção racial ou sexual aparente. Em um único estudo, a idade média de 9 cães acometidos foi de 3 anos.

SINAIS CLÍNICOS
- Forma aguda: sinais atribuídos à neutropenia e à trombocitopenia (i. e., febre, hemorragias petequiais, epistaxe, hematúria e melena).
- Forma crônica: sinais atribuíveis à anemia (i. e., mucosas pálidas, fraqueza e letargia), além daqueles observados nas formas agudas.

CAUSAS E FATORES DE RISCO
Muitas vezes não são identificados.

Agentes Infecciosos
- FeLV, FIV.
- Parvovírus canino e felino.
- Microrganismos riquetsiais (p. ex., *Ehrlichia* spp.).

Medicamentos e Substâncias Químicas
- Estrogênios (administração exógena, sertolinomas e tumores de células intersticiais).
- Metimazol (gatos).
- Quimioterápicos, como azatioprina, ciclofosfamida, citosina-arabinosídeo, doxorrubicina, vimblastina e hidroxiureia.
- Antibióticos, como trimetoprima-sulfadiazina, cefalosporinas e cloranfenicol.
- Griseofulvina.
- AINEs, como fenilbutazona e ácido meclofenâmico.
- Fembendazol, albendazol.
- Captopril.
- Quinidina.
- Tiacetarsamida.
- Radiação ionizante.
- Micotoxinas (gatos).

DIAGNÓSTICO

DIAGNÓSTICO DIFERENCIAL
Causas de pancitopenia associada à normo ou hipercelularidade da medula óssea (p. ex., distúrbios mielodisplásicos, leucemias e mielofibrose).

HEMOGRAMA/BIOQUÍMICA/URINÁLISE
- Leucopenia, caracterizada por neutropenia com ou sem linfopenia.
- Anemia normocítica, normocrômica, arregenerativa.
- Trombocitopenia.

OUTROS TESTES LABORATORIAIS
- Testes imunológicos em busca de doenças infecciosas (p. ex., títulos sorológicos, ELISA e AIF).
- PCR para os agentes infecciosos.
- Teste sorológico para a pesquisa de anticorpos antieritrocitários (teste de Coombs).

DIAGNÓSTICO POR IMAGEM
N/D.

MÉTODOS DIAGNÓSTICOS
- Aspirado da medula óssea — com frequência, coleta-se uma amostra inadequada ou gordurosa, em decorrência da redução do tecido hematopoiético e da substituição por lipócitos.
- Biopsia central da medula óssea — permite não só a avaliação da arquitetura do órgão, mas também revela a hipoplasia das linhagens celulares e a substituição por tecido adiposo.

TRATAMENTO
Cuidados de suporte, antibióticos, terapia à base de constituintes hematológicos, todos ditados pela condição clínica do paciente.

MEDICAÇÕES

MEDICAMENTO(S) DE ESCOLHA
- Ciclosporina A — 10-25 mg/kg VO a cada 12 h (cães), 4-5 mg/kg VO a cada 12 h (gatos).
- Fatores de crescimento hematopoiéticos recombinantes (p. ex., rhG-CSF: 5 µg/kg/dia SC).
- As administrações de androgênios e corticosteroides não são largamente bem-sucedidas.

CONTRAINDICAÇÕES/INTERAÇÕES POSSÍVEIS
N/D.

OUTROS MEDICAMENTOS
- Na presença de febre e neutropenia, indica-se o uso de antibióticos para o tratamento de infecções secundárias.
- Se houver indicação, realizar transfusões de sangue total ou de componentes sanguíneos.

ACOMPANHAMENTO

MONITORIZAÇÃO DO PACIENTE
- Exame físico diário.
- Hemograma completo a cada 3-5 dias até intervalos semanais.
- Repetir a avaliação da medula óssea se houver necessidade.

PREVENÇÃO
- Castração de machos criptorquídicos.
- Vacinação contra doenças infecciosas.
- Monitorização frequente do hemograma completo em pacientes com câncer submetidos à quimio ou radioterapia.

COMPLICAÇÕES POSSÍVEIS
- Sepse.
- Hemorragia.

EVOLUÇÃO ESPERADA E PROGNÓSTICO
- Reservado a mau.
- Se ocorrer, a recuperação da hematopoiese pode levar semanas a meses.
- Ocasionalmente, ocorre a recuperação espontânea, sobretudo em animais jovens.

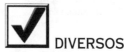

DIVERSOS

VER TAMBÉM
Pancitopenia.

ABREVIATURA(S)
- AIF = anticorpo imunofluorescente.
- AINE = anti-inflamatório não esteroide.
- ELISA = ensaio imunoabsorvente ligado à enzima.
- FeLV = vírus da leucemia felina.
- FIV = vírus da imunodeficiência felina.
- PCR = reação em cadeia da polimerase.
- rhG-CSF = fator estimulador das colônias de granulócitos humano recombinante.

Sugestões de Leitura
Brazzell JL, Weiss DJ. A retrospective study of aplastic pancytopenia in the dog: 9 cases (1996-2003). Vet Clin Path 2006, 35:413-417.
Weiss DJ. Aplastic anemia. In: Weiss DJ, Wardrop KJ, eds., Schalm's Veterinary Hematology, 6th ed. Ames, IA: Blackwell Publishing Ltd., 2010, pp. 256-260.

Autor Darren Wood
Consultor Editorial A.H. Rebar

Anemia Arregenerativa

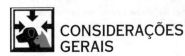

CONSIDERAÇÕES GERAIS

DEFINIÇÃO
Massa eritrocitária baixa sem indícios de resposta regenerativa (policromasia acentuada ou reticulocitose) no sangue periférico.

FISIOPATOLOGIA
• A característica-chave consiste em uma produção ou liberação baixa ou inadequada de células eritroides. • O início de anemia e de seus sinais relacionados é insidioso a menos que o tempo de sobrevida das hemácias seja concomitantemente abreviado por hemorragia ou hemólise. • Pode ser causada por alteração seletiva na eritropoiese ou lesão generalizada da medula óssea que também comprometa os leucócitos e as plaquetas. • Os mecanismos de alteração seletiva na eritropoiese incluem estimulação hormonal deficiente, deficiência nutricional, sequestro de ferro mediado por citocinas e distúrbio do metabolismo ou destruição de precursores; a lesão generalizada da medula óssea costuma ser causada por toxinas, infecções ou processos infiltrativos.

SISTEMA(S) ACOMETIDO(S)
• Cardiovascular — sopro cardíaco associado à baixa viscosidade sanguínea. • Hepatobiliar — degeneração centrolobular associada à lesão hipóxica. • Sanguíneo/linfático/imunológico.

IDENTIFICAÇÃO
• Varia com a causa primária. • Cães: Schnauzer gigante, Border collie e Beagle — má absorção congênita de cobalamina.

SINAIS CLÍNICOS

Comentários Gerais
• Em geral, é uma condição secundária. • Os sinais associados à doença primária muitas vezes antecedem os sinais atribuídos à anemia.

Achados Anamnésicos
• Falta de vigor, intolerância ao exercício, inapetência e intolerância ao frio. • Outros achados refletem a condição primária, como poliúria e polidipsia (p. ex., insuficiência renal crônica), exposição à tinta proveniente de casas antigas em reforma (p. ex., intoxicação pelo chumbo), habitação em ambientes domésticos com muitos gatos (p. ex., FeLV) e tratamento de cadelas contra acasalamentos indesejáveis ou incontinência urinária, além de feminização em machos caninos (p. ex., hiperestrogenismo).

Achados do Exame Físico
• Palidez, sopro cardíaco (anemia grave) e, possivelmente, taquicardia ou polipneia. • Os sinais que refletem a condição primária compreendem hálito urêmico e ulcerações bucais (p. ex., insuficiência renal crônica), caquexia (p. ex., câncer), linfadenopatia e/ou esplenomegalia (p. ex., linfoma), sinais gastrintestinais ou neurológicos (SNC) (p. ex., intoxicação pelo chumbo), alopecia simétrica (p. ex., hipotireoidismo e hiperestrogenismo).

CAUSAS

Anemia Arregenerativa sem Outras Citopenias
• Anemia de doença inflamatória — a causa mais comum de anemia arregenerativa leve; a anemia pode ser observada dentro de 3 a 10 dias de infecção, inflamação, lesão tecidual, processos imunomediados e neoplasia local ou disseminada; o aumento na produção hepática de hepcidina, juntamente com a liberação de IL-1, interferona e TNF de linfócitos-T e macrófagos, levam ao sequestro de ferro dentro dos macrófagos teciduais, à diminuição na absorção intestinal de ferro, à redução nos níveis séricos de ferro e transferrina, ao aumento na concentração de ferritina nos macrófagos (e no soro), à queda na produção de eritropoietina, à diminuição na resposta medular à anemia e ao tempo de vida abreviado das hemácias. • Insuficiência renal crônica — os rins não conseguem produzir uma quantidade adequada de eritropoietina; as toxinas urêmicas abreviam o tempo de vida das hemácias e prejudicam a resposta à eritropoietina. • Hepatopatia crônica — alterações morfológicas eritrocitárias (células-alvo e acantócitos) e encurtamento do tempo de sobrevida das hemácias causados por alterações nos lipídios da membrana eritrocitária; a diminuição na síntese de transferrina e o comprometimento na mobilização de ferro hepático contribuem para a deficiência funcional de ferro. • Endocrinopatia — os hormônios tireoidianos e o cortisol estimulam a eritropoiese e facilitam o efeito da eritropoietina; uma anemia leve costuma estar associada ao hipotireoidismo e, ocasionalmente, pode ser observada em pacientes com hipoadrenocorticismo e hipopituitarismo. • Destruição imunomediada de precursores — aplasia pura de hemácias. • Destruição infecciosa de precursores, embora, em geral, haja o envolvimento de mais de uma linhagem celular (p. ex., FeLV e erliquiose, *Citauxzoon felis*).

Deficiência Nutricional ou Mineral
• Deficiência de ferro — costuma ser causada por perda sanguínea externa crônica; inicialmente regenerativa; no entanto, à medida que a gravidade aumenta, a anemia torna-se arregenerativa.
• Deficiências de cobalamina (vitamina B$_{12}$) e/ou folato — raras em cães e gatos, mas podem ser causadas por insuficiência alimentar, má absorção ou administração crônica de medicamentos que inibam o folato (p. ex., metotrexato, sulfas e anticonvulsivantes); há relatos de um defeito congênito na absorção de cobalamina em Schnauzer gigante, Border collie e Beagle; ocasionalmente, pode causar anemia normocítica ou macrocítica; podem ser observadas alterações megaloblásticas na medula óssea. • Interrupção do metabolismo de precursores — a intoxicação crônica pelo chumbo e, possivelmente, as concentrações elevadas de alumínio e cádmio inibem a síntese da molécula heme; também se relata que o cádmio promove toxicidade renal e diminuição na produção da eritropoietina.

Anemia Arregenerativa com Outras Citopenias
• Toxicidades — medicamentos ou substâncias químicas (p. ex., quimioterápicos contra o câncer, cloranfenicol, fenilbutazona, sulfadiazina-trimetoprima, zonisamida, fenobarbital, griseofulvina, metimazol, fembendazol, albendazol e benzeno), hormônios (p. ex., toxicidade estrogênica secundária à terapia com abortivos e sertolinomas). • Infecções — FeLV, FIV, erliquiose, babesiose e parvovirose (embora a recuperação geralmente anteceda o desenvolvimento da anemia). • Processos infiltrativos — mielodisplasia, doença mieloproliferativa, doença linfoproliferativa, neoplasia metastática, mielofibrose e osteosclerose.

FATORES DE RISCO
• Insuficiência renal. • Processo patológico inflamatório ou crônico. • Insuficiência hepática. • Sertolinoma. • Câncer. • Perda sanguínea crônica. • Gatos oriundos de ambientes domésticos com muitos felinos (FeLV). • Exposição ao chumbo — crônica.

DIAGNÓSTICO

DIAGNÓSTICO DIFERENCIAL
No início, a anemia regenerativa pode parecer arregenerativa; o início súbito dos sinais é mais compatível em casos de anemia regenerativa do que nos de anemia arregenerativa; no entanto, a última aparentemente poderá ter um início agudo se estiver associada a uma exacerbação abrupta da condição primária crônica.

ACHADOS LABORATORIAIS

Distúrbios Capazes de Alterar os Resultados Laboratoriais
• Os fatores indutores de turbidez (lipemia) podem elevar falsamente os valores da hemoglobina e da CHCM. • Em casos de intoxicação pelo chumbo, o aumento das hemácias nucleadas pode gerar uma falsa elevação da contagem leucocitária.

Os Resultados Serão Válidos se os Exames Forem Realizados em Laboratório Humano?
• Cães — sim. • Gatos — sim se os equipamentos hematológicos do laboratório utilizarem parâmetros específicos para a espécie; entretanto, o uso de equipamentos destinados estritamente para a análise de amostras humanas pode subestimar as pequenas hemácias felinas.

HEMOGRAMA/BIOQUÍMICA/URINÁLISE

Hemograma Completo e Esfregaço Sanguíneo
• Baixos níveis do hematócrito, da contagem eritrocitária e da hemoglobina. • Anemia geralmente normocítica e normocrômica, com VCM e CHCM normais. • Macrocitose (VCM alto) — sem policromasia, sugere um defeito de maturação nuclear (as células pulam uma etapa da divisão celular); observada em gatos com FeLV; causada ocasionalmente por deficiências da vitamina B$_{12}$ ou do folato. • Microcitose (VCM baixo) — indica um defeito de maturação citoplasmática (as células sofrem uma divisão extra); a deficiência de ferro é a causa mais habitual; nos estágios tardios, uma hipocromasia concomitante (CHCM baixa) é comum em cães, mas não em gatos; observada também em cerca de um terço dos pacientes com insuficiência hepática ou desvio vascular. • Morfologias eritrocitárias específicas — os esquistócitos são comuns em casos de deficiência de ferro; os acantócitos associam-se à hepatopatia colestásica; as células-alvo estão relacionadas com deficiência de ferro, hepatopatia e hipotireoidismo. • Um leucograma inflamatório apoia a presença de anemia de doença inflamatória. • A trombocitose muitas vezes acompanha a deficiência de ferro.
• Em animais com intoxicação pelo chumbo, observa-se uma grande quantidade de hemácias nucleadas sem policromasia ou desproporcional ao grau de anemia e policromasia; hematopoiese extramedular, internação e lesão ao estroma da

ANEMIA ARREGENERATIVA

medula óssea por endotoxemia ou hipoxia são outras fontes de hemácias nucleadas circulantes.
• Precursores eritrocitários ou leucocitários no sangue periférico sem uma evolução ordenada para formas mais maduras apontam para mielodisplasia ou doença mieloproliferativa (leucemia).
• Citopenia concomitante em outras linhagens celulares sem indícios de responsividade medular (p. ex., neutrófilos em banda e macroplaquetas) indica lesão generalizada da medula óssea.

Bioquímica Sérica e Urinálise
• Altos níveis da ureia e creatinina com uma concentração urinária inadequada (cães, <1,030; gatos, <1,035) apoiam anemia de doença renal crônica. • Atividade elevada da ALT e da bilirrubina total sugerem hepatopatia. • Alta concentração sérica do colesterol (>500 mg/dL) é fortemente sugestiva de hipotireoidismo. • Relação de sódio:potássio <23, linfocitose e eosinofilia em cães doentes sugerem hipoadrenocorticismo.

OUTROS TESTES LABORATORIAIS
• Contagem de reticulócitos — um valor de <60.000/μL em cães ou <50.000/μL em gatos, acompanhado por hematócrito baixo, confirma a anemia arregenerativa. • Teste direto das antiglobulinas (teste de Coombs) — a destruição imunomediada de precursores eritroides pode levar à anemia sem reticulocitose; esferocitose, autoaglutinação ou teste de Coombs positivos sustentam anemia imunomediada. • Perfil sérico de ferro — indicado para pacientes com anemia microcítica; em pacientes com deficiência de ferro, observam-se baixa concentração sérica desse elemento, variação na capacidade de ligação do ferro total e baixo nível sérico da ferritina; em pacientes com anemia de doença inflamatória, o ferro sérico encontra-se baixo, mas a ferritina sérica mostra-se elevada (VCM e CHCM costumam permanecer normais). • Mensuração dos ácidos biliares — pode ser indicada para avaliação de anemia microcítica e confirmação de insuficiência hepática ou desvio vascular.
• Mensuração sérica do chumbo — indicada na presença de hemácias nucleadas, sobretudo quando o paciente apresenta sinais gastrintestinais ou neurológicos (SNC) concomitantes; um valor >30 μL/dL (0,3 ppm) apoia fortemente uma intoxicação pelo chumbo. • Testes sorológicos — pesquisa do FeLV em qualquer gato com anemia arregenerativa; talvez haja indicação de mensuração dos títulos para *Ehrlichia canis*, *Anaplasma phagocytophilia* (*E. equi*) e *Babesia* ou ensaios de PCR em cães com anemia inexplicável, especialmente quando ela for acompanhada com trombocitopenia ou hiperglobulinemia. • Testes endócrinos — indicados quando os sinais clínicos e os testes laboratoriais sugerirem um possível distúrbio endócrino; tireoide: concentrações de T_4, T_4 livre e TSH; adrenal: teste de supressão com dexametasona em baixas doses e teste de estimulação com ACTH.

MÉTODOS DIAGNÓSTICOS
Exame Citológico da Medula Óssea e Biopsia Central
• Indica-se o exame citológico de aspirado em todos os pacientes a menos que se evidencie a causa primária com facilidade (p. ex., anemia de doença inflamatória e insuficiência renal crônica).
• Biopsia da medula óssea — útil na avaliação da arquitetura e da celularidade global dessa medula; importante para o diagnóstico de medula aplásica ou mielofibrose. • A constatação de hipoplasia ou aplasia eritroides confirma o problema, embora o histórico e outros testes, conforme indicação acima, possam ser necessários para determinar a etiologia subjacente. • A presença de hiperplasia mieloide e as altas reservas de ferro suportam a anemia de doença inflamatória. • A ausência das reservas de ferro na medula óssea canina (mas não na felina), que ocorre antes da microcitose, apoia a deficiência desse elemento; classicamente, essa deficiência associa-se a uma expansão do éritron e alta quantidade de metarrubrícitos. • O aumento na eritrofagocitose sugere dano celular (p. ex., doença imunomediada e tóxica). • Uma sequência incompleta de maturação indica lesão em algum estágio específico de maturação (p. ex., causas imunomediadas e tóxicas) ou, possivelmente, recuperação parcial a partir de uma lesão prévia (reavaliar em 3-5 dias). • Uma sequência desordenada de maturação e uma morfologia atípica das células indicam síndrome mielodisplásica. • Uma medula hipercelular com quantidade elevada de blastócitos (>20% de células nucleadas) aponta para neoplasia hematopoiética; imunofenotipagem e colorações citoquímicas são utilizadas para identificar a(s) linhagem(ns) celular(es) acometida(s); podem-se ou não observar células neoplásicas circulantes.
• Células não medulares indicam neoplasia metastática.

TRATAMENTO
• A anemia arregenerativa costuma desaparecer com a resolução da doença subjacente. • As condições associadas à anemia ou pancitopenia graves muitas vezes exibem um prognóstico reservado a mau e podem envolver um tratamento a longo prazo, sem a resolução completa. • Em casos de anemia arregenerativa de desenvolvimento lento, ocorrerá uma compensação metabólica; assim, uma anemia leve a moderadamente grave (hematócrito >15%) geralmente não necessita de nenhuma intervenção de suporte. • Em pacientes com anemia grave (hematócrito <10-15%), o grau de hipoxia provavelmente exigirá uma restrição da atividade física, a prática de transfusões ou ambas as medidas. • Se o volume sanguíneo e a perfusão tecidual forem comprometidos por perda sanguínea ou choque concomitantes, administrar soluções de Ringer lactato ou coloides.

MEDICAÇÕES
MEDICAMENTO(S)
• Eritropoietina em pacientes com anemia por insuficiência renal crônica (ver "Anemia de Doença Renal Crônica"). • Suplementação de ferro em pacientes com anemia por deficiência desse elemento (ver "Anemia por Deficiência de Ferro"). • Pode-se suplementar com ácido fólico a uma dose de 4-10 mg/kg/dia. • Também é permitida a suplementação com cobalamina (vitamina B_{12}) a uma dose de 100-200 mg/dia VO (cães) ou 50-100 mg/dia VO (gatos); os cães das raças Schnauzer gigante, Beagle ou Border collie com má absorção hereditária de cobalamina necessitam da administração parenteral dessa vitamina (0,5-1 mg IM uma vez por semana ou em pequenos intervalos mensais).

PRECAUÇÕES
Monitorizar a ocorrência de reações transfusionais em pacientes submetidos a múltiplas transfusões.

ACOMPANHAMENTO
MONITORIZAÇÃO DO PACIENTE
• Em pacientes com anemia grave, efetuar a avaliação do hematócrito e o exame do esfregaço sanguíneo a cada 1-2 dias. • Em animais estabilizados com evolução crônica ou recuperação lenta da doença, reavaliar a cada 1-2 semanas.

DIVERSOS
GESTAÇÃO/FERTILIDADE/REPRODUÇÃO
Em alguns animais prenhes, pode-se observar o hematócrito levemente baixo causado pela expansão do volume sanguíneo.

SINÔNIMO(S)
Anemia não responsiva.

ABREVIATURA(S)
• ACTH = hormônio adrenocorticotrópico. • ALT = alanina aminotransferase. • CHCM = concentração de hemoglobina corpuscular média.
• FeLV = vírus da leucemia felina. • FIV = vírus da imunodeficiência felina. • IL-1 = interleucina-1.
• PCR = reação em cadeia da polimerase. • SNC = sistema nervoso central. • TNF = fator de necrose tumoral. • TSH = hormônio tireostimulante.
• VCM = volume corpuscular médio.

RECURSOS DA INTERNET
Erythrocytes: Overview, Morphology, Quantity; A.H. Rebar, P.S. MacWilliams, B.F. Feldman, et. al.: http://www.ivis.org/advances/Rebar/Chap4/chapter.asp?LA = 1

Sugestões de Leitura
Feldman BF. Nonregenerative anemia. In: Ettinger SJ, Feldman EC, eds., Textbook of Veterinary Internal Medicine: Diseases of the Dog and Cat, 6th ed. Philadelphia: Elsevier Saunders, 2005, pp. 1908-1917.

Autor Joyce S. Knoll
Consultor Editorial A.H. Rebar

Anemia de Doença Renal Crônica

CONSIDERAÇÕES GERAIS

DEFINIÇÃO
Declínios progressivos do hematócrito, da contagem eritrocitária e da hemoglobina, bem como hipoplasia dos elementos eritroides da medula óssea, são características previsíveis de anemia renal crônica progressiva. A anemia é normocítica, normocrômica, arregenerativa e proporcional ao estágio da doença renal crônica. A principal causa corresponde à insuficiência da medula óssea secundariamente à produção inadequada de eritropoietina pelos rins. O encurtamento do tempo de vida das hemácias, os inibidores urêmicos da eritropoiese, a perda sanguínea, as deficiências nutricionais e a fibrose medular podem contribuir para o quadro.

IDENTIFICAÇÃO
Acomete principalmente cães e gatos de meia-idade a idosos; esse tipo de anemia é observado em animais jovens com doença renal crônica hereditária, congênita ou adquirida.

SINAIS CLÍNICOS
• A anemia contribui para o desenvolvimento de anorexia, perda de peso, fadiga, letargia, depressão, fraqueza, apatia, intolerância ao frio, assim como para mudanças de comportamento e de personalidade características de doença renal crônica.
• Palidez das mucosas.
• Taquipneia.
• Taquicardia.
• Sopro sistólico.
• Síncope e crises convulsivas (raros).

CAUSAS E FATORES DE RISCO
• Todas as formas hereditárias, congênitas e adquiridas de doença renal crônica (p. ex., pielonefrite, glomerulonefrite, amiloidose, nefropatia policística e linfoma).
• Exacerbados por deficiência de ferro, doença inflamatória ou neoplásica, perda sanguínea gastrintestinal, hemólise e distúrbios mieloproliferativos.

DIAGNÓSTICO

DIAGNÓSTICO DIFERENCIAL
• Anemia de doença crônica infecciosa, inflamatória ou neoplásica; doença mieloproliferativa; perda sanguínea crônica; anemia aplásica; endocrinopatia; reação a medicamentos; e anemia crônica imunomediada, tóxica, viral, riquetsiana ou parasitária; hemodiluição.
• Uma anemia regenerativa exclui o diagnóstico de anemia de doença renal crônica.
• Geralmente mascarada até que haja doença renal crônica avançada.

HEMOGRAMA/BIOQUÍMICA/URINÁLISE
• Anemia normocítica, normocrômica e hipoproliferativa (progressiva; a anemia pode ser mascarada pela desidratação).
• Reticulócitos — redução dos índices corrigidos e das contagens absolutas (≤10.000/μL).
• Doença renal crônica moderada a avançada — altos níveis de ureia, creatinina e fósforo; concentração variavelmente alta do cálcio, mas irregularmente baixa de bicarbonato e potássio.
• Uma relação elevada de ureia:creatinina pode predizer uma perda sanguínea gastrintestinal concomitante.
• Capacidade baixa de concentração urinária, proteinúria leve a moderada e sedimento variavelmente ativo.

OUTROS TESTES LABORATORIAIS
• Ferro sérico — normal ou variavelmente baixo.
• Saturação da transferrina — normal ou variavelmente baixa (<20%).
• Testes sorológicos para FeLV e FIV ou hemobartonela (gatos) ou títulos riquetsiais ou PCR (cães) para excluir mielodiscrasia induzida por agentes infecciosos.
• Eritropoietina sérica — normal (inapropriadamente) ou baixa.

DIAGNÓSTICO POR IMAGEM
• Rins pequenos e irregulares, com perda ou desorganização da arquitetura renal observada em radiografias ou ultrassonografias.
• Rins aumentados de volume, policísticos, hiponefróticos, infiltrativos.

MÉTODOS DIAGNÓSTICOS
Exame citológico da medula óssea — hipoplasia eritroide; relação mieloide:eritroide normal ou elevada; ferro corável normal ou variavelmente baixo.

TRATAMENTO

• Aumentar a massa eritrocitária se o paciente estiver sintomático para anemia (cães, hematócrito ≤25%; gatos, hematócrito ≤23).
• Nos pacientes com crise urêmica, estabilizar a azotemia.
• Estabelecer uma ingestão apropriada de nitrogênio, calorias, fosfato, vitaminas e ferro não só para reduzir os inibidores urêmicos e a tendência ao sangramento, mas também para estender o tempo de vida das hemácias.
• Garantir a não deficiência do ferro.
• Corrigir a ulceração e a perda sanguínea gastrintestinais, administrando-se famotidina, ranitidina, omeprazol ou sucralfato.
• Corrigir a hipertensão sistêmica.

MEDICAÇÕES

MEDICAMENTO(S) E FLUIDO(S)

Reposição de Eritropoietina
• Alfaepoetina (EPOHu-r) — proteína sintética original estimulante da eritropoiese; uma réplica da eritropoietina humana (Epogen® e Procrit®); proporciona uma correção constante, rápida e de longo prazo para a anemia em cães e gatos com doença renal crônica; há potencial de produção de anticorpos anti-EPOHu-r e aplasia pura de hemácias.
• Alfadarbepoetina (Aranesp®), um novo análogo hiperglicosilado de EPOHu-r com meia-vida prolongada e efeitos contínuos; parece ser equipotente à EPOHu-r e, com a experiência atual, tem pouca tendência à indução de anticorpos; deve ser utilizada preferencialmente no lugar da alfaepoetina.
• Hematócrito-alvo — cães, 37-45%; gatos, 30-40%.
• Dosagem inicial — alfadarbepoetina — 0,45-0,6 mcg/kg (2,5-5 mcg para cães de pequeno porte e gatos), SC 1 vez por semana, até que o hematócrito atinja o extremo inferior do alvo e, em seguida, diminuir para a cada 2 semanas. Alfaepoetina —50-100 U/kg 3 vezes por semana até o extremo inferior do alvo do hematócrito e, depois, reduzir para 2 vezes por semana. Ao converter a alfaepoetina para darbepoetina, dividir as unidades semanais por 400 para estabelecer a dose em mcg a ser administrada 1 vez por semana.
• Dosagem de manutenção — alfadarbepoetina — 2,5-5 mcg a cada 2-3 semanas. Alfaepoetina — 50-100 U/kg SC 1 ou 2 vezes por semana, para manter o hematócrito-alvo. Tratar cada paciente individualmente; há necessidade de tratamento vitalício. Se a alfaepoetina for administrada 1 vez por semana, administrar a alfadarbepoetina a cada 2 semanas com a conversão.
• Se o hematócrito exceder o alvo, interromper a transfusão até que se atinja o limite superior do alvo e depois diminuir a dosagem prévia em 25-50% ou aumentar o intervalo entre as doses.
• O nível sérico do ferro e a saturação da transferrina devem ser normalizados antes de iniciar o fornecimento da EPOHu-r e durante essa administração. O ferro injetável (50 mg/kg IM a cada 4-8 semanas) é preferível e mais bem tolerado que as preparações orais.
• Eritropoietinas espécie-específicas para cães e gatos, bem como tratamentos alternativos estimulantes da eritropoietina, estão sob desenvolvimento como alternativas às proteínas estimulantes da eritropoiese.

Transfusão Sanguínea
• Correção rápida ou a curto prazo (hematócrito ≤20%) — fornecer sangue total ou papa de hemácias compatíveis.
• O hematócrito-alvo é de 25-30%.
• Em casos de tratamento prolongado, a transfusão poderá ser feita de forma intermitente.

Esteroides Anabólicos
• Pouca ou nenhuma eficácia ou indicação de uso.

ACOMPANHAMENTO

MONITORIZAÇÃO DO PACIENTE
• Hematócrito — em intervalos semanais a quinzenais durante 3 meses, depois mensais a bimestrais.
• Pressão sanguínea — em intervalos quinzenais a mensais.
• Nível sérico de ferro e saturação da transferrina — com 1, 3 e 6 meses, depois semianual.
• Interromper a eritropoietina se o paciente desenvolver indícios de eritrocitemia, sensibilidade local ou sistêmica, formação de anticorpos anti-EPOHu-r, aplasia pura de hemácias ou hipertensão refratária.

COMPLICAÇÕES POSSÍVEIS

Relacionadas com a Eritropoietina
• Desenvolvimento de eritrocitemia, crises convulsivas, hipertensão, depleção de ferro, dor no local da injeção e reações mucocutâneas.
• O desenvolvimento de aplasia pura de hemácias durante o tratamento com a alfaepoetina sugere a formação de anticorpos contra essa substância; tais anticorpos neutralizam a alfaepoetina e a

ANEMIA DE DOENÇA RENAL CRÔNICA

eritropoietina nativa, gerando uma anemia grave em 20-30% dos animais; isso é frequentemente reversível com a interrupção do tratamento.
• Os sinais associados à produção de anticorpos anti-EPOHu-r enquanto o paciente estiver recebendo a alfaepoetina incluem hematócrito diminuído, hipoplasia eritroide, contagem reticulocitária absoluta próxima ao zero e relação mieloide:eritroide ≥8. Esses sinais também devem ser monitorizados no tratamento com a alfadarbepoetina.
• Utilizar as reposições de eritropoietina com cautela ou suspendê-las caso ocorra o desenvolvimento de hipertensão ou deficiência de ferro; o tratamento poderá ser reinstituído assim que a hipertensão e a deficiência de ferro forem corrigidas.

Relacionadas com a Transfusão
• Reação de incompatibilidade.
• Sobrecarga circulatória ou férrica.
• Hipertensão sistêmica.
• Transmissão de infecções.

EVOLUÇÃO ESPERADA E PROGNÓSTICO
• A correção da anemia aumenta o apetite, a atividade, a higienização, o afeto e a atividade lúdica, o ganho de peso e a tolerância ao frio e diminui o sono.
• O uso da reposição de eritropoietina em cães e gatos exige a avaliação cuidadosa dos riscos e dos benefícios para cada paciente em particular.
• O prognóstico a curto prazo depende da gravidade da insuficiência renal. O prognóstico a longo prazo é de reservado a mau, em decorrência da insuficiência renal crônica subjacente.

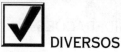

DIVERSOS

ABREVIATURA(S)
• EPOHu-r = eritropoietina humana recombinante.
• FeLV = vírus da leucemia felina.
• FIV = vírus da imunodeficiência felina.
• PCR = reação em cadeia da polimerase.

Sugestões de Leitura
Cowgill LD, et al. Use of recombinant human erythropoietin for management of anemia in dogs and cats with renal failure. JAVMA 1998, 212:521-528.

Autor Larry D. Cowgill
Consultor Editorial Carl A. Osborne

Anemia Imunomediada

CONSIDERAÇÕES GERAIS

DEFINIÇÃO
Destruição ou remoção aceleradas de hemácias, em decorrência de uma reação de hipersensibilidade do tipo II.

FISIOPATOLOGIA
- Os anticorpos antieritrocitários são formados contra antígenos de superfície inalterados endógenos (AHIM primária) ou antígenos da membrana eritrocitária alterados (AHIM secundária).
- Microrganismos infecciosos, medicamentos, exposição a antígenos não expostos previamente ou adsorção de complexos antígeno-anticorpo pré-formados à membrana eritrocitária podem alterar os antígenos constituintes dessa membrana.
- A imunoglobulina (IgG ou IgM, com ou sem complemento) deposita-se sobre a membrana eritrocitária, provocando hemólise intravascular direta ou remoção acelerada pelo sistema reticuloendotelial composto por monócitos e macrófagos (hemólise extravascular).
- Quando os anticorpos adsorvidos (em geral, a IgG) ativam o complemento, ocorre a hemólise intravascular.
- Quando a IgM ou títulos elevados das moléculas de IgG formam pontes com as hemácias, ocorre a aglutinação eritrocitária *in vivo*.
- A remoção extravascular das hemácias ocorre em órgãos como baço, fígado, medula óssea ou outro local de atividade macrofágica.
- Acredita-se que uma forma de AHIM arregenerativa seja causada pela destruição imunomediada de precursores eritrocitários na medula óssea.
- Raramente, anticorpos reativos ao frio causam hemólise *in vivo* e aglutinação eritrocitária na vasculatura periférica.

SISTEMA(S) ACOMETIDO(S)
- Sanguíneo/linfático/imune — destruição imunomediada das hemácias, elaboração de mediadores pró-inflamatórios (p. ex., citocinas e substâncias derivadas do endotélio), CID.
- Hepatobiliar — a hemólise leva à hiperbilirrubinemia e icterícia, bem como bilirrubinúria, quando a função hepática é sobrepujada; a hipoxia pode causar necrose centrolobular.
- Cardiovascular — a hipoxia induz a taquicardia; a viscosidade sanguínea baixa e o fluxo sanguíneo turbulento provocam sopros cardíacos de baixa intensidade.
- Respiratório — a hipoxia produz taquipneia. A ocorrência de tromboembolia pulmonar pode ser o resultado de um estado hipercoagulável por aumento na atividade de fatores pró-coagulantes, presença de hemoglobina livre, concentração reduzida de fatores fibrinolíticos e anticoagulantes, vasculite e reatividade aumentada das plaquetas.
- Cutâneo — raramente, a AHIM do tipo frio pode causar necrose de extremidades e pontas das orelhas, em virtude da aglutinação eritrocitária nos vasos periféricos.

GENÉTICA
Os cães da raça Cocker spaniel estão sob alto risco. A ausência de antígeno eritrocitário canino 7 é associada a um aumento no risco nessa raça.

DISTRIBUIÇÃO GEOGRÁFICA
A AHIM secundária pode ter prevalência mais alta em áreas endêmicas para doenças infecciosas associadas.

IDENTIFICAÇÃO
Espécies
Cães e gatos.

Raça(s) Predominante(s)
- O Cocker spaniel é a raça sob maior risco. Outras raças comumente acometidas incluem Poodle miniatura, Setter irlandês, Springer spaniel inglês, Old English sheepdog, Doberman, Collie, Bichon frisé, Pinscher miniatura e Finnish spitz.
- Gatos domésticos de pelo curto.

Idade Média e Faixa Etária
- Em cães, a idade média é de 5-6 anos, com faixa etária relatada de 1-13 anos.
- Em gatos, a idade média é de 2 anos, com faixa etária relatada de 0,5-9 anos.

Sexo(s) Predominante(s)
- As cadelas podem ter um risco mais alto.
- Na espécie felina, os machos são super-representados.

SINAIS CLÍNICOS
Achados Anamnésicos
- Letargia/fraqueza/colapso.
- Anorexia.
- Intolerância ao exercício/dispneia.
- Taquipneia.
- Vômito e/ou diarreia.
- Urina de cor vermelho-escura.
- Pica ou "apetite depravado" (gatos).

Achados do Exame Físico
- Mucosas pálidas, taquicardia e taquipneia.
- Esplenomegalia e hepatomegalia.
- Icterícia e pigmentúria (hemoglobina ou bilirrubina).
- Febre e linfadenomegalia.
- Sopro sistólico.
- Petéquias, equimoses ou melena em animais com trombocitopenia ou CID concomitantes.
- Outros achados do exame físico (p. ex., artralgia e glomerulonefrite) se a AHIM for um componente do LES.
- Necrose de extremidades e pontas auriculares em AHIM do tipo frio (rara).

CAUSAS
AHIM Primária
Anemia hemolítica autoimune (idiopática) em virtude de desregulação imune pouco caracterizada.

AHIM Secundária
- Causas infecciosas (p. ex., *Mycoplasma* spp. hemotrópicos, *Ehrlichia canis*, *Anaplasma phagocytophilum*, *Babesia* spp., *Leishmania*, *Dirofilaria immitis*, *Ehrlichia*, FeLV, PIF, infecção bacteriana crônica).
- Neoplasia (linfoma, leucemia linfoide, hemangiossarcoma, sarcoma histiocítico hemofágico).
- Medicamentos (p. ex., antibióticos beta-lactâmicos, propiltiouracila, metimazol, sulfonamidas).

CAUSAS DIVERSAS
- LES.
- Isoeritrólise neonatal.
- Hemólise gerada por transfusão sanguínea com antígeno eritrocitário canino incompatível.

FATORES DE RISCO
Há hipóteses de que fatores como exposição a agentes infecciosos, vacinação, substâncias químicas ou medicamentos, cirurgia, alteração hormonal ou outro evento indutor de estresse sejam possíveis deflagradores da AHIM.

DIAGNÓSTICO

DIAGNÓSTICO DIFERENCIAL
Cães
- Deficiência da piruvato quinase.
- Deficiência da fosfofrutoquinase.
- Intoxicação (zinco, cebolas, alho, brócolis, cobre, naftaleno, odor de gambá).
- Envenenamento por cobra/aranha (cobras corais, aranhas reclusas).
- Hipofosfatemia grave.
- Anemia gerada por hemorragia (trombocitopenia imunomediada, toxicose por rodenticida).
- Anemia microangiopática gerada por neoplasia esplênica, CID, torção esplênica.

Gatos
- Intoxicação (paracetamol, zinco, cebolas, alho).
- Hipofosfatemia grave.
- Porfiria felina congênita.
- Fragilidade osmótica aumentada (raças Abissínio e Somali).

HEMOGRAMA/BIOQUÍMICA/URINÁLISE
- Hemograma completo — anemia, VCM alto (3-5 dias após o episódio hemolítico), esferócitos, anisocitose, policromasia, hemácias nucleadas, aumento na amplitude de distribuição eritrocitária, leucocitose acentuada com neutrofilia e desvio à esquerda. Anemia arregenerativa em 30% dos cães e 50% dos gatos.
- Bioquímica sérica — hiperbilirrubinemia, hemoglobinemia, atividade elevada da ALT.
- Urinálise — hemoglobinúria, bilirrubinúria.

OUTROS TESTES LABORATORIAIS
- Teste de aglutinação espontânea em salina — antes e depois da lavagem das hemácias.
- Antiglobulina direta positiva (teste de Coombs) — positiva em até 75% dos animais com AHIM.
- Detecção de imunoglobulina e complemento ligados à membrana por citometria de fluxo.
- Reticulocitose — contagem absoluta >60.000/μL nos cães e >50.000/μL nos gatos em AHIM regenerativa.
- Trombocitopenia em 60% dos cães. Essa anormalidade bioquímica pode ser grave nos animais com síndrome de Evans e CID.
- TTPA e TP prolongados, aumento dos produtos de degradação da fibrina, D-dímero e redução da antitrombina em pacientes com CID.
- Aumento na concentração de fibrinogênio.
- Positividade no título do ANA e na pesquisa das células do lúpus eritematoso em animais com LES.
- Resultados positivos nos títulos serológicos ou no método de PCR em AHIM secundária a causas infecciosas.
- Encontro de hemoparasitas em esfregaços sanguíneos do sangue capilar em AHIM secundária a causas infecciosas.
- Aumento na fragilidade osmótica eritrocitária.

DIAGNÓSTICO POR IMAGEM
- Achados radiográficos — hepatomegalia e esplenomegalia; o tórax costuma estar dentro dos limites de normalidade; podem-se observar

indícios de tromboembolia pulmonar em cães com AHIM (padrão alveolar irregular, padrão intersticial e líquido pleural); no entanto, os cães com embolia pulmonar podem exibir radiografias torácicas normais.
• Achados ultrassonográficos — hepatomegalia e esplenomegalia; o fígado e o baço podem exibir aspecto mosqueado e estar hiper ou hipoecoicos.

MÉTODOS DIAGNÓSTICOS
• O exame do aspirado da medula óssea costuma revelar hiperplasia da série eritroide.
• Nos animais com AHIM arregenerativa, pode-se observar a interrupção da maturação ou a presença de hipoplasia eritroide.
• Nos animais com AHIM crônica, pode-se constatar mielofibrose.

ACHADOS PATOLÓGICOS
• Hepatosplenomegalia, necrose hepática centrolobular.
• Hematopoiese extramedular esplênica e hepática.
• Linfadenomegalia reativa.
• Tromboembolia pulmonar e CID.

TRATAMENTO

CUIDADO(S) DE SAÚDE ADEQUADO(S)
• Internação durante a crise hemolítica aguda; tratamento ambulatorial após a estabilização do hematócrito, o controle da hemólise contínua e a resolução dos sinais clínicos da anemia.
• Lançar mão da internação caso o animal apresente complicações como CID, tromboembolia pulmonar, trombocitopenia, sangramento gastrintestinal ou necessite de múltiplas transfusões.
• A hemólise extravascular crônica de baixo grau poderá ser tratada em um esquema ambulatorial se o paciente não estiver exibindo sinais clínicos secundários à anemia.

CUIDADO(S) DE ENFERMAGEM
• Fluidoterapia para manter o volume vascular e corrigir a desidratação.
• Monitorização rigorosa de complicações como tromboembolia pulmonar, sangramento (sobretudo gastrintestinal), CID, infecção.
• Repouso em gaiola.

ORIENTAÇÃO AO PROPRIETÁRIO
• A AHIM e suas complicações (p. ex., CID e tromboembolia pulmonar) podem ser fatais.
• Pode haver a necessidade de tratamento pelo resto da vida; além disso, pode ocorrer recidiva da doença.
• Os efeitos colaterais do tratamento podem ser graves.

CONSIDERAÇÕES CIRÚRGICAS
• A esplenectomia poderá ser considerada em caso de falha do tratamento clínico no controle da doença.
• Considerar o fornecimento de produtos derivados do sangue no período pré-operatório.

MEDICAÇÕES

MEDICAMENTO(S) DE ESCOLHA
• Papa de hemácias tipadas ou compatíveis para receptor *naive* (aquele que nunca recebeu uma transfusão). O sangue deve ser compatível para receptores que já receberam transfusões prévias.
• Volume de transfusão = peso do receptor (kg) × 85 (cão) ou 50 (gato) × hematócrito desejado – hematócrito atual/hematócrito do doador.
• Velocidade de transfusão = 0,25 mL/kg/h nos primeiros 30 min e, em seguida, 5-10 mL/kg/h.
• Corticosteroides — prednisona a 1-2 mg/kg/dia a cada 12 h por 2-4 semanas.
• Assim que o hematócrito aumentar acima de 30%, diminuir a dose para 1 mg/kg a cada 12 h.
• Subsequentemente, a dose é reduzida de forma gradual por uma taxa máxima de 25-50% por mês em um período de 3 a 6 meses, dependendo do valor do hematócrito e da gravidade dos efeitos colaterais. Se após 6 meses a dose da prednisona tiver sido reduzida para uma dosagem baixa em dias alternados e a doença estiver em remissão, deve-se tentar a descontinuação do medicamento.
• Adicionar azatioprina (cães) em caso de resposta insatisfatória à prednisona após 5-7 dias ou se houver indicadores prognósticos maus (p. ex., hemólise intravascular, bilirrubina sérica >8-10 mg/dL, autoaglutinação persistente, síndrome de Evans).
• A dose da azatioprina é de 2 mg/kg/dia, podendo ser reduzida para 2 mg/kg em dias alternados em caso de supressão da medula óssea. Monitorizar o animal quanto à ocorrência de imunossupressão, hepatotoxicose, pancreatite.
• Para a prevenção de tromboembolia (cães), considerar o uso de heparina não fracionada a 300 U/kg SC a cada 6-8 h (dose ajustada com base no prolongamento do TTPA) ou ácido acetilsalicílico com doses ultrabaixas de 0,5-1,0 mg/kg/dia ou enoxaparina (heparina de baixo peso molecular) a 0,8 mg/kg a cada 6 h ou 1,5 mg/kg a cada 12 h.
• Tratar a causa subjacente (p. ex., infecção e medicamentos) em caso de AHIM secundária.

CONTRAINDICAÇÕES
• Não usar heparina, enoxaparina ou ácido acetilsalicílico em cães com trombocitopenia grave (<80.000/μL).
• Não utilizar múltiplos agentes citotóxicos concomitantemente.

PRECAUÇÕES
• Não administrar azatioprina a gatos por causa do risco de toxicidade da medula óssea.
• A prednisona pode gerar sinais de síndrome de Cushing e potencialmente aumentar o risco de tromboembolia pulmonar, pancreatite, infecção secundária e úlceras gástricas (considerar o fornecimento de protetores gástricos).
• Os medicamentos citotóxicos podem causar supressão da medula óssea, infecção secundária, pancreatite (azatioprina), cistite (ciclofosfamida) e infertilidade.

INTERAÇÕES POSSÍVEIS
Tanto a azatioprina como a prednisona são associadas ao desenvolvimento de pancreatite.

MEDICAMENTO(S) ALTERNATIVO(S)
• Dexametasona (0,25-0,5 mg/kg/dia IV) — pode ser usada no lugar da prednisona em animais intolerantes a medicamentos orais até que a ingestão por via oral seja possível.
• Clorambucila — para os gatos, 0,1-0,2 mg/kg VO a cada 24 h inicialmente e, em seguida, a cada 48 h.
• Ciclosporina — microemulsão (p. ex., Atopica®) — cães, 5-10 mg/kg/dia VO divididos 2 vezes ao dia; gatos, 0,5-3 mg/kg a cada 12 h.
• Ciclofosfamida — cães, 50 mg/m^2/dia VO por 4 de 7 dias ou 200 mg/m^2 IV 1 vez por semana (apenas em cães intolerantes à azatioprina ou ciclosporina); gatos, 2,5 mg/kg/dia VO por 4 de 7 dias ou 7 mg/kg IV 1 vez por semana.
• Gamaglobulina humana — 0,5-1,5 g/kg ao longo de 12 h em uma única infusão IV.

ACOMPANHAMENTO

MONITORIZAÇÃO DO PACIENTE
• Durante a internação, sempre monitorar as frequências cardíaca e respiratória, bem como a temperatura corporal.
• Controlar as reações adversas ao tratamento (p. ex., reações transfusionais e super-hidratação).
• Se houver suspeita de tromboembolia pulmonar, efetuar a monitorização frequente das radiografias torácicas e da gasometria sanguínea arterial.
• No primeiro mês de tratamento, checar o hematócrito semanalmente até sua estabilização e depois a cada 2 semanas por 2 meses; se ainda permanecer estável, reavaliá-lo mensalmente por 6 meses e, então, por 2-4 vezes ao ano; as reavaliações talvez tenham de ser mais frequentes se o paciente estiver sob uma terapia a longo prazo.
• Durante o tratamento, é recomendável a reavaliação, no mínimo, mensal do hemograma completo e da contagem de reticulócitos, especialmente no uso de medicamentos citotóxicos; se a contagem neutrofílica cair para <3.000 células/mL, partir para a interrupção desses agentes terapêuticos até que a contagem se restabeleça; reinstituí-los em uma dosagem mais baixa.
• O teste de Coombs pode ser monitorizado para ajudar na redução gradativa dos medicamentos.

PREVENÇÃO
Considerar a necessidade de aplicação de vacinas caso a caso em cães, cuja AHIM se desenvolveu após a vacinação.

COMPLICAÇÕES POSSÍVEIS
• Tromboembolia nos pulmões e em múltiplos órgãos (até 80% de todos os casos à necropsia).
• CID.
• Necrose hepática centrolobular e necrose tubular renal secundária à hipoxia.
• Infecção secundária à terapia imunossupressora.
• Ulceração gastrintestinal causada por altas doses de glicocorticoides.
• Hiperadrenocorticismo iatrogênico.

EVOLUÇÃO ESPERADA E PROGNÓSTICO
• A mortalidade varia de 30 a 80% em cães, mas é de 25% em gatos.
• As causas de óbito incluem tromboembolia, infecção por imunossupressão, CID, anemia persistente.
• Hiperbilirrubinemia >5 mg/dL, autoaglutinação, hemólise intravascular, trombocitopenia grave, hipoalbuminemia são associadas a um prognóstico pior.
• A resposta terapêutica pode levar de semanas a meses; a AHIM arregenerativa pode ter um início mais gradativo do que a AHIM típica e exibir uma resposta mais lenta ao tratamento.
• Apesar da terapia prévia ou atual, poderá ocorrer a recidiva da AHIM.

Anemia Imunomediada

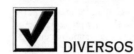

DIVERSOS

SINÔNIMO(S)
- Anemia hemolítica autoimune.
- Anemia imunomediada.

VER TAMBÉM
- Anemia Regenerativa.
- Coagulação Intravascular Disseminada.
- Doença da Aglutinina Fria.
- Os capítulos referentes às diversas causas de AHIM secundária.

ABREVIATURA(S)
- AHIM = anemia hemolítica imunomediada.
- ALT = alanina aminotransferase.
- ANA = anticorpo antinuclear.
- CID = coagulação intravascular disseminada.
- FeLV = vírus da leucemia felina.
- FIV = vírus da imunodeficiência felina.
- LES = lúpus eritematoso sistêmico.
- PCR = reação em cadeia da polimerase.
- TP = tempo de protrombina.
- TTPA = tempo de tromboplastina parcial ativada.
- VCM = volume corpuscular médio.

Sugestões de Leitura
Kohn B, Weingart C, Eckmann V, et al. Primary immune-mediated hemolytic anemia in 19 cats: Diagnosis, therapy, and outcome (1998-2004). J Vet Intern Med 2006, 20:159-166.
Piek CJ, Dekker JA, Slappendel RJ, Teske E. Idiopathic immune-mediated hemolytic anemia: Treatment outcome and prognostic factors in 149 dogs. J Vet Intern Med 2008, 22:366-373.

Autores J. Catharine Scott-Moncrieff e Rose E. Raskin
Consultor Editorial A.H. Rebar

Anemia Metabólica (Anemia com Hemácias Espiculadas)

CONSIDERAÇÕES GERAIS

REVISÃO
• Algumas vezes, ocorre concomitantemente com doenças difusas do fígado ou dos rins e, raras vezes, do baço.
• Na maioria dos animais com hepatopatias, as células espiculadas possuem 2-10 projeções digitiformes, rombas e alongadas a partir de suas superfícies, sendo classificadas como acantócitos.
• As anemias acantocíticas podem estar associadas a doenças renais; as anemias decorrentes dessa condição patológica exibem muitas vezes hemácias ovais com membranas irregulares ou franzidas (células crenadas).
• Raramente, as anemias acantocíticas podem ser observadas em associação com doença esplênica isolada.
• A patogenia não está totalmente esclarecida; com maior frequência, implica-se como a causa o metabolismo lipídico anormal com transporte de colesterol livre das membranas eritrocitárias.
• Muitas vezes, os cães com hemangiossarcoma abdominal disseminado com envolvimento hepático apresentam acantócitos.

IDENTIFICAÇÃO
Cães e gatos (raramente).

SINAIS CLÍNICOS
• Ausentes em grande parte dos animais (em geral, é uma condição leve a moderada).
• A detecção de hemácias espiculadas no esfregaço do sangue periférico pode ser o primeiro marcador de doença hepática, renal ou esplênica.
• Em cães de grande porte com sinais vagos ou esplenomegalia, sugere-se a possibilidade de hemangiossarcoma esplênico ou hepático.

CAUSAS E FATORES DE RISCO
• Qualquer doença hepática, renal ou, possivelmente, esplênica.
• A probabilidade de anormalidades morfológicas eritrocitárias corre paralelamente com a gravidade do envolvimento orgânico.
• O hemangiossarcoma com envolvimento hepático é uma causa frequente.
• Observada em gatos com síndrome do fígado gorduroso.

DIAGNÓSTICO

DIAGNÓSTICO DIFERENCIAL
A determinação de causas renais ou hepáticas baseia-se nos resultados do perfil bioquímico e da urinálise.

HEMOGRAMA/BIOQUÍMICA/URINÁLISE
• Níveis leves a moderadamente baixos do hematócrito, da contagem de eritrócitos e da hemoglobina.
• Na maioria dos animais, observam-se resultados normais no volume corpuscular médio e na concentração de hemoglobina corpuscular média.
• Anemia normocítica, normocrômica e arregenerativa.
• Nos esfregaços sanguíneos, haverá policromasia apenas com perda sanguínea concomitante (como ocorre em casos de hemangiossarcoma hepático).
• As alterações leucocitárias são variáveis, com base na causa subjacente de doença hepática ou renal.
• É provável que as condições inflamatórias sejam acompanhadas por leucograma inflamatório.
• Achados variáveis nos testes de função hepática e renal (bioquímica sérica e urinálise).

Doenças Hepáticas
• Atividade elevada da ALT, fosfatase alcalina e gamaglutamil transferase.
• Níveis altos dos ácidos biliares e da amônia sérica.
• Concentração sérica possivelmente baixa da albumina e da ureia.
• Bilirrubinúria e cristais de bilirrubina na urina.

Doenças Renais
• Concentração sérica elevada de ureia, creatinina e fósforo.
• Achados altamente variáveis da urinálise, incluindo isostenúria (densidade urinária de 1,008-1,025 nos cães; de 1,008-1,035 nos gatos).
• Cilindros tubulares e/ou proteicos.
• Piúria.
• Proteinúria.
• Hematúria.

OUTROS TESTES LABORATORIAIS
Nenhum.

DIAGNÓSTICO POR IMAGEM
Radiografias e ultrassonografias abdominais — avaliam as estruturas hepáticas, renais e esplênicas.

MÉTODOS DIAGNÓSTICOS
Biopsia hepática ou renal, se indicada.

TRATAMENTO

Concentrar o tratamento no diagnóstico e na terapia de doença hepática, renal ou esplênica subjacente.

MEDICAÇÕES

MEDICAMENTO(S)
Variáveis, de acordo com a causa subjacente.

CONTRAINDICAÇÕES/INTERAÇÕES POSSÍVEIS
Variáveis, de acordo com a causa subjacente.

ACOMPANHAMENTO

Monitorizar o hemograma completo periodicamente enquanto se trata a condição subjacente.

DIVERSOS

VER TAMBÉM
• Anemia de Doença Renal Crônica.
• Hemangiossarcoma do Baço e do Fígado.

ABREVIATURA(S)
• ALT = alanina aminotransferase.

Sugestões de Leitura
Harvey JW. Atlas of Veterinary Hematology, Blood and Bone Marrow of Domestic Animals. Philadelphia: Saunders, 2001, p. 29.
Rebar AH. Hemogram Interpretation for Dogs and Cats. Wilmington, DE: Gloyd Group for Ralston Purina Co., 1998, pp. 22-23.
Rebar AH, Lewis HB, DeNicola DB, Halliwell WH, Boon GD. Red blood cell fragmentation in the dog: An editorial review. Vet Pathol 1981, 18:415-426.
Rebar AH, MacWilliams PS, Feldman BF, Metzger FL, Pollock RVH, Roche J. A Guide to Hematology in Dogs and Cats. Jackson, WY: Teton NewMedia, 2002, p. 36.
Thrall MA, Campbell TW, DeNicola D, Fettman MJ, Lassen ED, Rebar A, Weiser G. Veterinary Hematology and Clinical Chemistry. Baltimore: Lippincott Williams & Wilkins, 2004, p. 96.
Weiser EG. Erythrocyte responses and disorders. In: Ettinger SJ, Feldman EC, eds. Textbook of Veterinary Internal Medicine, 4th ed. Philadelphia: Saunders, 1995, pp. 1864-1891.

Autor Alan H. Rebar
Consultor Editorial A.H. Rebar

Anemia por Corpúsculo de Heinz

CONSIDERAÇÕES GERAIS

REVISÃO
• Os corpúsculos de Heinz causam anemia hemolítica e indicam dano oxidativo às hemácias.
• Tais corpúsculos se formam quando os oxidantes superam as vias redutoras de proteção nas hemácias e provocam desnaturação irreversível da hemoglobina (grupos sulfidrila e/ou hemicromos), precipitação e fixação da hemoglobina alterada à membrana celular, aglomerados da banda 3 e alteração dos antígenos de superfície.
• As hemácias são menos deformáveis, direcionadas à remoção por macrófagos no baço, e podem sofrer lise intravascular.
• A função de "fossa" do baço pode remover os corpúsculos de Heinz, resultando no surgimento de esferócitos.
• Os corpúsculos de Heinz costumam ser causados por exposição a oxidantes químicos ou alimentares.
• Os gatos são particularmente suscetíveis à formação de corpúsculos de Heinz, porque a hemoglobina dessa espécie é rica em grupos sulfidrila e o baço felino não é sinusoidal com função limitada de "fossa".
• Os gatos saudáveis podem ter corpúsculos de Heinz sem anemia.
• Com frequência, encontram-se corpúsculos de Heinz em gatos com hipertireoidismo, linfoma e diabetes melito (em particular se houver cetoacidose), possivelmente em virtude do aumento de oxidantes endógenos (p. ex., β-hidroxibutirato). Pode ou não haver anemia.
• Os corpúsculos de Heinz podem ser acompanhados por metemoglobinemia (hemoglobina que contém Fe^{3+}) e/ou excentrócitos (dano oxidativo às membranas eritrocitárias com deslocamento da hemoglobina para um lado). Os fatores que controlam o(s) tipo(s) de dano oxidativo não estão claros.

IDENTIFICAÇÃO
• Cães e gatos.
• Não há predisposição sexual, racial ou etária.

SINAIS CLÍNICOS
Achados Anamnésicos
• Exposição a oxidantes.
• Início súbito de fraqueza, letargia ou anorexia.
• Urina de coloração castanho-avermelhada (hemoglobinúria) em caso de hemólise intravascular grave.
• Sinais relacionados com a doença subjacente em gatos com doença sistêmica e corpúsculos de Heinz.

Achados do Exame Físico
• Mucosas pálidas ou ictéricas.
• Sangue de cor escura ou chocolate em caso de metemoglobinemia.
• Taquipneia, taquicardia.

CAUSAS E FATORES DE RISCO
• Alimentares: cebolas (i. e., cruas, cozidas, desidratadas e pulverizadas [em pó]), alho (cães), propilenoglicol (gatos), cebolinha chinesa (cães).
• Medicamentosos: paracetamol, fenacetina (gatos), fenazopiridina (gatos), azul de metileno, vitamina K_1 ou K_3 (cães), DL-metionina (gatos), benzocaína (tópica), fenil-hidrazina (cães), propofol (gatos).
• Diversos: zinco (porcas, parafusos, moedas, cremes dermatológicos), naftaleno (ingestão de bola de naftalina por cães), exposição a gambás (cães).

DIAGNÓSTICO

DIAGNÓSTICO DIFERENCIAL
• Outras causas de anemia hemolítica regenerativa (p. ex., mecanismo imunomediado e hemoparasitas).
• Os corpúsculos de Heinz podem ser encontrados em gatos saudáveis ou enfermos sem anemia. O diagnóstico de anemia por corpúsculo de Heinz requer o registro de anemia regenerativa, apoiando os indícios de um processo hemolítico (p. ex., hiperbilirrubinemia), a identificação dos corpúsculos de Heinz em esfregaço e a eliminação de outras causas de hemólise ou perda sanguínea.

HEMOGRAMA/BIOQUÍMICA/URINÁLISE
• Anemia regenerativa (hematócrito diminuído, policromasia, hemácias nucleadas) será esperada se houver tempo suficiente para uma resposta da medula óssea; a gravidade da anemia depende da dose do oxidante e do tempo de exposição.
• A concentração da hemoglobina e o valor da CHCM podem estar falsamente elevados em virtude da interferência corporal pelos corpúsculos de Heinz.
• Os corpúsculos de Heinz são visíveis em um esfregaço sanguíneo de rotina como pequenas inclusões arredondadas de cor vermelho-pálido que podem se projetar a partir da superfície eritrocitária. Na presença de pecilocitose acentuada, pode ser difícil identificá-los.
• Pequenos corpúsculos de Heinz isolados (<0,5 μm) podem ser constatados nas hemácias de gatos sem anemia.
• Grandes e/ou múltiplos corpúsculos de Heinz em gato anêmico são sugestivos de anemia hemolítica causada por esses corpúsculos.
• Os cães podem ter excentrócitos concomitantes no esfregaço sanguíneo.
• Hiperbilirrubinemia e bilirrubinúria são possíveis anormalidades.
• Em casos de hemólise intravascular grave, ocorrem hemoglobinemia e hemoglobinúria apesar de incomuns.
• Podem ocorrer neutrofilia e monocitose.

OUTROS TESTES LABORATORIAIS
• O novo azul de metileno cora os corpúsculos de Heinz de azul, facilitando sua identificação e quantificação, mesmo na presença de pecilocitose acentuada.
• Efetuar teste de metemoglobina se a cor do sangue estiver escura ou chocolate.
• Mensurar a concentração sérica de zinco se houver indicação.

DIAGNÓSTICO POR IMAGEM
As radiografias abdominais podem revelar objetos metálicos no trato gastrintestinal em casos de intoxicação por zinco.

TRATAMENTO

• A identificação e a remoção imediatas do oxidante podem ser suficientes embora possa levar alguns dias para que a gravidade da anemia atinja o nadir (ponto mais baixo).
• Os cuidados de suporte dependem da gravidade da crise hemolítica, incluindo fluidos IV, transfusões de hemácias, oxigênio e restrição da atividade física.
• Endoscopia ou cirurgia para remover itens metálicos no trato gastrintestinal.

MEDICAÇÕES

MEDICAMENTO(S) DE ESCOLHA
• Metemoglobinemia grave — azul de metileno (0,2 mg/kg IV, em dose única, lentamente).
• Intoxicação pelo paracetamol em gatos — N-acetilcisteína (140 mg/kg VO ou IV, seguido por 7 tratamentos adicionais de 70 mg/kg a cada 8 h).

CONTRAINDICAÇÕES/INTERAÇÕES POSSÍVEIS
O azul de metileno pode agravar a hemólise induzida por oxidante.

MEDICAMENTO(S) ALTERNATIVO(S)
O uso de antioxidantes na dieta (vitamina C, vitamina E, bioflavonoides) é controverso, mas pode ajudar a evitar a formação adicional de corpúsculos de Heinz.

ACOMPANHAMENTO

MONITORIZAÇÃO DO PACIENTE
Obtenção de hemogramas completos seriados e reavaliação de esfregaços sanguíneos são recomendadas para avaliar a regeneração das hemácias e o desaparecimento dos corpúsculos de Heinz.

PREVENÇÃO
Orientar os proprietários a evitarem a exposição de seus animais a oxidantes.

COMPLICAÇÕES POSSÍVEIS
N/D.

EVOLUÇÃO ESPERADA E PROGNÓSTICO
O prognóstico é bom com a remoção do oxidante e os cuidados de suporte assim que a crise hemolítica tiver acabado.

DIVERSOS

VER TAMBÉM
• Anemia Regenerativa.
• Metemoglobinemia.
• Toxicidade do Paracetamol.
• Toxicidade do Zinco.

ABREVIATURA(S)
• CHCM = concentração de hemoglobina corpuscular média.

Sugestões de Leitura
Andrews D. Disorders of red blood cells. In: Handbook of Small Animal Practice, 5th ed. St. Louis: Saunders, 2008, pp. 632-635.
Stockham SL, Scott MA. Erythrocytes. In: Fundamentals of Veterinary Clinical Pathology, 2nd ed. Ames, IA: Blackwell, 2008, pp. 186-187.

Autor Jennifer S. Thomas
Consultor Editorial A.H. Rebar

Anemia por Defeitos de Maturação Nuclear (Anemia Megaloblástica)

CONSIDERAÇÕES GERAIS

REVISÃO
- Anemia arregenerativa caracterizada por interrupção no desenvolvimento dos núcleos de precursores eritrocitários (como resultado da interferência na síntese do DNA), enquanto o citoplasma se desenvolve normalmente (assincronia nucleocitoplasmática).
- Os precursores eritrocitários acometidos não conseguem se dividir normalmente e, dessa forma, ficam maiores do que os precursores normais correspondentes com o mesmo grau de maturidade citoplasmática (hemoglobinização); por serem deficientes em cromatina (DNA), seus núcleos têm uma aparência exposta e pontilhada distinta; esses precursores gigantes com núcleos imaturos e atípicos são conhecidos como megaloblastos.
- Embora essas alterações assincrônicas sejam mais proeminentes em precursores eritrocitários, também se observa um acometimento semelhante de precursores leucocitários e plaquetários.

IDENTIFICAÇÃO
- Cães e gatos.
- Ocorrência espontânea e clinicamente sem importância em cães da raça Poodle toy (ocasional).
- Raça(s) predominante(s): Schnauzer gigante com má absorção hereditária da cobalamina.
- Defeito geralmente adquirido.

SINAIS CLÍNICOS
- Em cães, o problema consiste, em geral, em uma leve anemia, que não costuma ter importância do ponto de vista clínico.
- Em gatos com anemia por defeito de maturação nuclear associada ao FeLV, pode-se esperar pelos sinais relacionados com essa infecção viral. A anemia pode ser leve a grave.

CAUSAS E FATORES DE RISCO
- Infecciosos — FeLV; a infecção por retrovírus corresponde à causa mais comum de anemia megaloblástica em gatos.
- Nutricionais — deficiências de ácido fólico e vitamina B_{12}.
- Tóxicas — toxicidade da fenitoína (Dilantin®) e do metotrexato (antagonista de folato).
- Congênitos — cães da raça Poodle toy.

DIAGNÓSTICO

DIAGNÓSTICO DIFERENCIAL
- Em cães, todas as outras anemias arregenerativas leves a moderadas, inclusive as anemias por doença inflamatória, nefropatia e intoxicação pelo chumbo.
- A diferenciação é feita com base nos achados peculiares do hemograma completo e da medula óssea, já listados.
- Em gatos, a infecção por FeLV constitui o principal diferencial.

HEMOGRAMA/BIOQUÍMICA/URINÁLISE
- Em cães, anemia leve a moderada (hematócrito: 30-40%).
- Em gatos, a anemia pode ser leve a grave.
- Anemia tipicamente macrocítica (volume corpuscular médio elevado) e normocrômica (concentração normal de hemoglobina corpuscular média).
- Hemácias grandes e completamente hemoglobinizadas; megaloblastos ocasionais a numerosos, particularmente na chanfradura; policromasia mínima a ausente.
- Em gatos com FeLV, pode ocorrer anemia em associação com alguma síndrome mielodisplásica ou em conjunto com leucemia de linhagem celular distinta.

OUTROS TESTES LABORATORIAIS
FeLV.

DIAGNÓSTICO POR IMAGEM
N/D.

MÉTODOS DIAGNÓSTICOS
Biopsia da Medula Óssea
- Em cães, a medula costuma se apresentar hiperplásica, frequentemente em todas as linhagens celulares.
- Em gatos, os achados medulares são altamente variáveis, podendo exibir hiper a hipocelularidade.
- Interrupção da maturação com assincronia nuclear e citoplasmática em todas as linhagens celulares.
- Podem-se observar muitos precursores eritrocitários megaloblásticos.
- Hiperplasia macrofágica com fagocitose ativa de hemácias nucleadas e megaloblastos (comum).

TRATAMENTO
- Tratar o quadro com vistas à causa subjacente, se possível.
- Exceto nos casos de anemia associada ao FeLV em gatos, a anemia megaloblástica é uma condição relativamente branda.
- Tratar a maioria dos pacientes em um esquema ambulatorial.

MEDICAÇÕES

MEDICAMENTO(S)
- Em animais com intoxicação por medicamentos, interromper a administração do agente agressor.
- Em todos os animais, considerar a suplementação com ácido fólico (4-10 mg/kg/dia) ou vitamina B_{12} (cães, 100-200 mg/dia VO; gatos, 50-100 mg/dia VO).
- O Schnauzer gigante com má absorção hereditária de cobalamina necessita de tratamento parenteral com vitamina B_{12} (0,5-1,0 mg IM uma vez por semana ou em pequenos intervalos mensais).

CONTRAINDICAÇÕES/INTERAÇÕES POSSÍVEIS
Em pacientes com condições resultantes de outras causas, é recomendável evitar o uso de medicamentos sabidamente indutores de anemia megaloblástica (p. ex., metotrexato e fenitoína).

ACOMPANHAMENTO
- Monitorizar a resposta ao tratamento por meio do hemograma completo (semanalmente), bem como pela coleta e avaliação ocasionais da medula óssea.
- Monitorizar de perto os gatos positivos para o FeLV em busca de indícios do início de outros sinais clínicos de discrasia hematopoiética no sangue periférico e na medula óssea.
- Prognóstico — depende da causa subjacente; em gatos positivos para o FeLV, o prognóstico é reservado; em animais com anemia associada a medicamentos, o prognóstico torna-se bom quando se interrompe o uso do agente agressor.

DIVERSOS

VER TAMBÉM
- Anemia Arregenerativa.
- Infecção pelo Vírus da Leucemia Felina (FeLV).

ABREVIATURA(S)
- DNA = ácido desoxirribonucleico.
- FeLV = vírus da leucemia felina.

Sugestões de Leitura
Harvey JW. Atlas of Veterinary Hematology, Blood and Bone Marrow of Domestic Animals. Philadelphia: Saunders, 2001, pp. 135-137.
Rebar AH. Hemogram Interpretation for Dogs and Cats. Wilmington, DE: Gloyd Group for Ralston Purina Co., 1998, p. 23.
Rebar AH, MacWilliams PS, Feldman BF, Metzger FL, Pollock RVH, Roche J. A Guide to Hematology in Dogs and Cats. Jackson, WY: Teton NewMedia, 2002, pp. 57-58.
Thrall MA, Campbell TW, DeNicola D, Fettman MJ, Lassen ED, Rebar A, Weiser G. Veterinary Hematology and Clinical Chemistry. Baltimore: Lippincott Williams & Wilkins, 2004, pp. 161-162.
Weiser EG. Erythrocyte responses and disorders. In: Ettinger SJ, Feldman EC, eds. Textbook of Veterinary Internal Medicine, 4th ed. Philadelphia: Saunders, 1995, pp. 1864-1891.

Autor Alan H. Rebar
Consultor Editorial A.H. Rebar

Anemia por Deficiência de Ferro

CONSIDERAÇÕES GERAIS

REVISÃO
• Adultos — causada por hemorragia externa crônica.
• Surge quando as hemácias são produzidas sob a condição de disponibilidade limitada de ferro.
• As alterações características incluem microcitose eritrocitária, aspecto hipocrômico gerado pelo adelgaçamento da geometria celular, além da formação de queratócitos e esquistócitos.
• A identificação é importante, pois leva o clínico ao processo patológico subjacente, que corresponde a uma perda sanguínea externa crônica.

IDENTIFICAÇÃO
• Razoavelmente comum em cães adultos.
• Rara em gatos adultos.
• Uma anemia transitória neonatal por deficiência de ferro ocorre com 5-10 semanas de vida em cerca de 50% dos filhotes felinos.

SINAIS CLÍNICOS
• Sinais de anemia (p. ex., letargia, depressão, fraqueza, anorexia e taquipneia) e da doença subjacente.
• Melena intermitente com perda sanguínea gastrintestinal.
• Possível carga maciça de parasitas hematófagos (p. ex., pulgas e ancilóstomos).

CAUSAS E FATORES DE RISCO
• Qualquer forma de perda sanguínea externa crônica.
• A perda sanguínea ocorre mais frequentemente pelo trato gastrintestinal.
• Causas comuns — linfoma GI, ancilostomíase, neoplasia gástrica ou intestinal.
• Locais menos comuns — pele (p. ex., infestação intensa por pulgas) e trato urinário.
• Uso abusivo de doadores de sangue.

DIAGNÓSTICO

DIAGNÓSTICO DIFERENCIAL
• Qualquer causa de anemia, particularmente hemorragia.
• Anemia microcítica em casos de desvio portossistêmico pode ou não ser atribuída à deficiência de ferro.
• Anemia de doença inflamatória crônica.

HEMOGRAMA/BIOQUÍMICA/URINÁLISE
• O hematócrito costuma estar baixo (mas nem sempre), geralmente 10-40% nos cães.
• A anemia pode ser regenerativa ou arregenerativa.
• Microcitose — indicada por VCM normal baixo ou baixo, acompanhado muitas vezes por uma heterogeneidade de alto volume, detectada pelo alargamento do histograma eritrocitário ou pelo alto valor de amplitude de distribuição eritrocitária.
• Índices eritrocitários mais recentes, como volume reticulocitário médio e conteúdo de hemoglobina dos reticulócitos, são sensíveis para a detecção de eritropoiese com deficiência de ferro; exame disponível atualmente apenas em um único sistema de hematologia laboratorial central: ver a seção "Sugestões de Leitura" dos autores Steinberg e Olver ou Fry e Kirk.
• Alterações eritrocitárias podem ser observadas no esfregaço sanguíneo — hipocromia (indicada por palidez central acentuada), lesões oxidativas (p. ex., queratócitos), fragmentação.
• O declínio do CHCM não é sensível nem específico para deficiência de ferro.
• Pode ocorrer trombocitose.
• Hipoproteinemia — achado compatível apenas se a perda sanguínea for contínua; ambas as frações de albumina e globulina encontram-se em um nível normal baixo ou baixo.

OUTROS TESTES LABORATORIAIS
• Hipoferremia (ferro sérico <70 μg/dL) e baixa saturação de transferrina (<15%) apoiam o diagnóstico.
• Os valores séricos de ferro podem permanecer normais, mesmo em animais com características hematológicas de deficiência desse íon, se a perda sanguínea tiver cessado e o animal estiver sendo submetido à repleção de ferro.
• Exame de flutuação fecal para descartar a suspeita clínica de ancilostomíase.
• Pesquisa de sangue oculto nas fezes ou de melena macroscópico para detectar sangramento gastrintestinal.

DIAGNÓSTICO POR IMAGEM
Estudos de diagnóstico por imagem — avaliar gastrenteropatias responsáveis pela perda sanguínea.

MÉTODOS DIAGNÓSTICOS
O hemograma completo e as mensurações de ferro estão detalhados acima.

TRATAMENTO

• Identificar e corrigir a causa da perda sanguínea externa crônica.
• Administrar o ferro até que as características hematológicas de deficiência desse elemento desapareçam.
• Em caso de anemia excepcionalmente grave (i.e., hematócrito <15%), poderá haver a necessidade de transfusão para tratar a condição que represente um risco de vida; administrar sangue total (10-20 mL/kg IV) ou papa de hemácias.

MEDICAÇÕES

MEDICAMENTO(S)
Suplementação de Ferro

Suplementação Parenteral
• A terapia de reposição do ferro deve ser iniciada com a formulação injetável desse elemento.
• Ferrodextrana — formulação de ferro injetável de liberação lenta; 1 aplicação (10-20 mg/kg IM) acompanhada pela suplementação oral.

Suplementação Oral
• Os animais com deficiência grave de ferro apresentam uma redução na absorção intestinal desse íon, tornando a suplementação oral de pouco valor até que ocorra a repleção parcial desse elemento.
• Acompanhar a aplicação parenteral de ferro com a suplementação oral desse íon por 1-2 meses ou até que as características de deficiência de ferro desapareçam.
• Os filhotes felinos sofrem recuperação espontânea e a repleção do ferro começa com 5-6 semanas de vida, coincidindo com a ingestão de alimento sólido.

Suplementos Orais de Ferro
• Sulfato ferroso em pó — colocar no alimento ou na água de bebida (100-300 mg VO a cada 24 h).
• Gliconato ferroso — 1 comprimido de 325 mg VO a cada 24 h.
• Ferro e vitaminas — qualquer ferro adequado com suplemento multivitamínico; conforme recomendação ou 1 vez ao dia.

CONTRAINDICAÇÕES/INTERAÇÕES POSSÍVEIS
A suplementação oral de ferro é associada a óbitos inexplicáveis em filhotes felinos e, por essa razão, é recomendável evitá-la.

ACOMPANHAMENTO

• Monitorizar o hemograma completo a cada 1-4 semanas; em caso de anemia grave, recomenda-se a monitorização mais frequente para acompanhar a recuperação total do animal de condições com risco de vida.
• Um tratamento eficaz é associado ao aumento no VCM e no volume reticulocitário.
• Histograma eritrocitário — o tratamento bem-sucedido está relacionado com o deslocamento do gráfico para a direita à medida que ocorre a produção de novas células normais; a subpopulação de micrócitos produzidos sob condições de deficiência de ferro desaparece lentamente conforme essas células completam seu tempo de sobrevida; o restabelecimento de um histograma normal pode levar alguns meses em determinados animais.

DIVERSOS

ABREVIATURA(S)
• CHCM = concentração de hemoglobina corpuscular média.
• GI = gastrintestinal.
• VCM = volume corpuscular médio.

Sugestões de Leitura
Fry MM, Kirk CA. Reticulocyte indices in a canine model of nutritional iron deficiency. Vet Clin Path 2006, 35:172-181.
Steinberg JD, Olver CS. Hematologic and biochemical abnormalities indicating iron deficiency are associated with decreased reticulocyte hemoglobin content (CHr) and reticulocyte volume (rMCV) in dogs. Vet Clin Path 2005,34:23-27.
Thrall MA. Regenerative anemias. In: Thrall MA, et al., Veterinary Hematology and Clinical Chemistry. Baltimore: Lippincott Williams & Wilkins, 2004, pp. 95-98.

Autor Glade Weiser
Consultor Editorial A.H. Rebar

ANEMIA REGENERATIVA

CONSIDERAÇÕES GERAIS

DEFINIÇÃO
Caracterizada por queda na massa eritrocitária circulante (conforme indicada por baixos níveis do hematócrito, da hemoglobina e da contagem eritrocitária total), acompanhada pelo aumento compensatório pertinente na produção de hemácias pela medula óssea (p. ex., reticulocitose no sangue periférico e hiperplasia eritrocitária na medula óssea).

FISIOPATOLOGIA
- A anemia regenerativa é causada por perda sanguínea ou hemólise. • Hemólise — ocasionada por defeitos eritrocitários intrínsecos (p. ex., defeitos congênitos da membrana eritrocitária ou deficiências enzimáticas) ou fatores extrínsecos como hemoparasitas, lesão oxidativa, hemolisinas, alterações osmóticas, destruição eritrocitária imunomediada, intermação e hipofosfatemia grave. • A hemólise intravascular pode levar ao desenvolvimento de CID e ao aparecimento de hemoglobinúria. • A anemia hemolítica costuma ser mais regenerativa do que a anemia por perda de sangue; a perda sanguínea externa promove a depleção corporal tanto de células como de ferro; a hemólise preserva o ferro, que fica prontamente disponível para uma reutilização na produção de hemácias; a disponibilidade desse elemento torna a anemia hemolítica geralmente mais responsiva.

SISTEMA(S) ACOMETIDO(S)
- Cardiovascular — sopros em casos de anemia acentuada; taquicardia em casos de anemias graves de aparecimento súbito. • Sanguíneo/linfático/imune — hiperplasia eritrocitária acentuada na medula óssea; hematopoiese extramedular no baço; a esplenomegalia atribuída à hematopoiese extramedular e à hiperplasia histiocítica pode ser uma característica de anemia hemolítica extravascular. • Hepático — a anoxia provoca degeneração centrolobular do fígado. • Renal — hemólise intravascular grave (raramente) levar à necrose tubular renal e insuficiência renal aguda.

IDENTIFICAÇÃO
- Não há predisposição racial, sexual nem etária para a ampla categoria de anemia regenerativa.
- Deficiência da piruvato quinase — cães das raças Basenji, Beagle, Cairn terrier, Chihuahua, Dachshund, Poodle miniatura, Pug, West Highland white terrier e Esquimó americano, além de gatos das raças Somali, Abissínio e doméstico de pelo curto. • Deficiência da fosfofrutoquinase — cães das raças Springer spaniel inglês, Cocker spaniel americano e outros mestiços com parentesco spaniel. • Em cães da raça Golden retriever, foi relatada uma deficiência de espectrina. • Fragilidade osmótica eritrocitária acentuada — cães da raça Springer spaniel inglês, além de gatos das raças Abissínio, Somali, Siamês e doméstico de pelo curto. • Porfiria congênita felina — gatos das raças Siamês e doméstico de pelo curto. • Algumas raças de cães apresentam uma predisposição genética para certas coagulopatias hereditárias, como deficiência do fator VIII e doença de von Willebrand. • As cadelas de meia-idade, particularmente das raças Cocker spaniel americano, Springer spaniel inglês, Setter irlandês, Old English sheepdog, Poodle e Pastor de Shetland, exibem predisposição a síndromes imunomediadas, como anemia hemolítica imunomediada e LES.

SINAIS CLÍNICOS
- Palidez. • Fraqueza, intolerância ao exercício. • Anorexia. • Possível sopro cardíaco, com taquicardia e pulsos saltitantes. • Possíveis icterícia e hemoglobinúria. • Petéquias, epistaxe, melena sugerem perda sanguínea atribuída à vasculite ou problema de plaquetas. • Hematomas ou sangramentos cavitários são sugestivos de coagulopatia. • Os sinais clínicos dependem do grau de anemia e da rapidez de início. • A perda súbita de 15-25% do volume sanguíneo ou a ocorrência de hemólise aguda resulta em choque e, possivelmente, em óbito. • Em pacientes com anemia crônica, os aumentos compensatórios na frequência cardíaca e, finalmente, no tamanho cardíaco diminuem o tempo de circulação das hemácias; a hemoglobina pode cair até 50% do valor normal mínimo, sem gerar sinais evidentes de hipoxia.

CAUSAS

Imunomediadas
- A presença de anticorpos, imunocomplexos e/ou complemento na superfície eritrocitária abrevia o tempo de vida das hemácias. Os anticorpos podem ter como alvo os componentes da membrana eritrocitária ou ser direcionados contra antígenos tumorais, agentes infecciosos, vacinas ou medicamentos (p. ex., sulfonamidas, penicilinas, cefalosporinas, metimazol, amiodarona) diretamente aderidos à superfície eritrocitária ou parte de imunocomplexos aderidos às hemácias.
- Hemólise — pode ser intra ou extravascular. As hemácias revestidas por IgG são tipicamente fagocitadas por macrófagos esplênicos, enquanto aquelas revestidas por IgM são frequentemente destruídas por ativação do complemento. • Em geral, os anticorpos hemolíticos ficam reativos à temperatura corporal; raramente, os antígenos que agem no frio causam hemólise e/ou aglutinação eritrocitária *in vivo* na vasculatura periférica mais fria. • A transfusão de sangue tipo A em gato de tipo sanguíneo B pode resultar em hemólise intravascular súbita e grave; observa-se isoeritrólise neonatal em filhotes felinos nascidos de uma gata pertencente ao tipo sanguíneo B, acasalada com um macho do tipo sanguíneo A. • O sangue canino tipo DEA* 1.1 pode gerar hemólise em cão negativo para esse antígeno, embora uma única transfusão incompatível possa ser tolerada. • Os tipos sanguíneos recém-identificados *Mik* (gatos) e *Dal* (cães) podem causar reações transfusionais hemolíticas significativas em animais que carecem desses antígenos eritrocitários comuns.

Lesão Oxidativa
- Oxidantes podem induzir à formação de corpúsculos de Heinz (agregados de hemoglobina oxidada), excentrócitos (lesão oxidativa às membranas eritrocitárias) e metemoglobinemia.
- As hemácias lesionadas são prematuramente removidas da circulação (hemólise extravascular). A desestabilização das membranas eritrocitárias provoca hemólise intravascular. • Seguem alguns oxidantes: cebolas e alho, paracetamol (particularmente em gatos), toxicidade do zinco (decorrente da ingestão de moedas cunhadas após 1982, pomada de óxido de zinco e parafusos de zinco), toxicose aguda por cobre, benzocaína, vitamina K_3 (cães), propofol, DL-metionina (gatos), compostos fenólicos (bolas de naftalina) e fenazopiridina (gatos). • Em gatos, algumas doenças sistêmicas (p. ex., diabetes melito, hipertireoidismo e linfoma) intensificam a formação dos corpúsculos de Heinz, mas não necessariamente causam anemia.

Hemoparasitas
- *Mycoplasma haemofelis* (antigamente conhecido como *Haemobartonella felis*); *M. haemominutum, M. turicensis* e *M. haemotoparvum* (gatos).
- *Mycoplasma haemocanis* (antigamente conhecido como *H. canis*; cães). • *Babesia canis* e *B. gibsoni* (cães). • *Cytauxzoon felis* (doméstico de pelo curto e Bobcat).

Fragmentação Eritrocitária Mecânica
- Doença tromboembólica (p. ex., CID).
- Dirofilariose. • Vasculite. • Hepato, nefro ou cardiopatias. • Neoplasia (p. ex., hemangiossarcoma). • Torção esplênica.
- Síndrome hemolítico-urêmica.

Anormalidades Eritrocitárias Hereditárias
- Deficiência da piruvato quinase — provoca uma diminuição no uso da glicose pelo eritrócito e na formação de ATP, levando à destruição prematura das hemácias; traço autossômico recessivo.
- Deficiência da fosfofrutoquinase — gera uma fragilidade alcalina acentuada, induzida pelo dano à síntese de 2,3-difosfoglicerato; episódios hemolíticos são deflagrados por alcalemia induzida por hiperventilação, tal como ocorre após exercícios vigorosos. • O aumento na fragilidade osmótica eritrocitária leva à anemia grave recidivante e esplenomegalia. No entanto, não foi identificado o defeito eritrocitário responsável. • A deficiência de espectrina induz à desestabilização das membranas eritrocitárias, levando ao aumento na fragilidade osmótica das hemácias; traço autossômico dominante; não se sabe se isso resulta em anemia hemolítica. • Porfiria congênita felina — a deficiência da uroporfirinogênio III cossintase em gatos da raça Siamês leva a uma incapacidade na produção de quantidades normais de hemoglobina; consequentemente, há um acúmulo de coproporfirina e uroporfirina, gerando manchas de coloração castanho-avermelhada nos dentes e nos ossos, além de fotossensibilidade e anemia hemolítica grave; um traço autossômico dominante secundário e menos grave em gatos domésticos de pelo curto provoca manchas nos tecidos, sem anemia ou fotossensibilidade.

Perda Sanguínea
- Traumatismo. • Neoplasias hemorrágicas (p. ex., hemangiossarcoma, adenocarcinoma intestinal).
- Coagulopatia (p. ex., intoxicação pela varfarina, hemofilia e trombocitopenia). • Parasitas hematófagos (p. ex., pulgas, carrapatos e *Ancylostoma*). • Úlceras gastrintestinais.

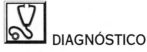

DIAGNÓSTICO

DIAGNÓSTICO DIFERENCIAL
Diferenciada da anemia arregenerativa pela alta contagem de reticulócitos.

---

* N. T.: De *Dog Erythrocyte Antigen* = antígeno eritrocitário canino.

ANEMIA REGENERATIVA

ACHADOS LABORATORIAIS

Distúrbios Capazes de Alterar os Resultados Laboratoriais
• A presença de lipemia na amostra pode causar leve hemólise *in vitro*, sem anemia apreciável, além de CHCM falsamente alta. • A autoaglutinação pode diminuir falsamente a contagem de eritrócitos.

Os Resultados Serão Válidos se os Exames Forem Realizados em Laboratório Humano?
• Cães — sim. • Gatos — sim se os equipamentos hematológicos do laboratório utilizarem parâmetros específicos para a espécie; entretanto, o uso de equipamentos destinados estritamente para a análise de amostras humanas pode subestimar as pequenas hemácias felinas. • Os laboratórios humanos podem não estar familiarizados com os reticulócitos pontilhados encontrados em gatos e podem incluí-los na contagem reticulocitária, superestimando com isso a resposta regenerativa.

HEMOGRAMA/BIOQUÍMICA/URINÁLISE
• Baixos níveis do hematócrito, da contagem eritrocitária e da hemoglobina. • A proteína total encontra-se frequentemente baixa em casos de anemia por perda sanguínea e pode ser o único sinal de hemorragia em cães com perda aguda de sangue; o hematócrito normal pode ser mantido por contração esplênica transitória. • A gravidade da perda sanguínea aguda pode ser subestimada até que o volume plasmático seja restabelecido pela administração de fluidos e/ou por desvios internos de líquido. • Os índices eritrocitários variam, dependendo da causa da anemia e do grau de resposta regenerativa: VCM, normal a alto; CHCM, normal a baixo em grande parte dos pacientes; CHCM, artificialmente alto com hemólise intravascular e hemoglobinemia. • Os cães com deficiência de ferro decorrente de perda sanguínea crônica podem exibir baixos níveis de VCM, HCM e CHCM; já os gatos com deficiência de ferro apresentam VCM baixo, mas HCM e CHCM normais. • Morfologias eritrocitárias específicas podem apontar uma causa de hemólise: uma esferocitose acentuada indica doença imunomediada; os corpúsculos de Heinz ou excentrócitos sugerem lesão oxidativa; e inúmeros esquistócitos lembram microangiopatia. • Em gatos, não se conseguem detectar com facilidade os esferócitos (formados por fagocitose eritrocitária incompleta), em função da ausência de palidez central das hemácias. • As hemácias aglutinadas indicam uma anemia imunomediada; é imprescindível a distinção entre a autoaglutinação e a formação de *rouleaux***, por meio da diluição generosa da amostra com solução salina. • A hemólise pode gerar leucograma inflamatório (neutrofilia com desvio à esquerda e monocitose). A perda sanguínea aguda pode ser associada a leucograma de estresse (neutrofilia e linfopenia leves). • A perda sanguínea pode ser acompanhada por trombocitose de rebote ou trombocitopenia; a deficiência de ferro é muitas vezes seguida por trombocitose. • As anormalidades de hiperbilirrubinemia e bilirrubinúria acompanham uma hemólise acentuada; em caso de hemólise intravascular, observam-se hemoglobinemia e hemoglobinúria.

** N. T.: Hemácias em forma de pilhas lineares (semelhante a uma pilha de moedas).

OUTROS TESTES LABORATORIAIS
• Em animais anêmicos, uma contagem absoluta de reticulócitos (contagem eritrocitária × % de reticulócitos) de >50.000/μL (gatos) ou >60.000/μL (cães) sugere anemia regenerativa. • A % de reticulócitos deve ser corrigida para o grau de anemia; fórmula = % de reticulócitos × (hematócrito/hematócrito normal); hematócrito normal: 45%, cães; 37%, gatos; a contagem reticulocitária corrigida de >1% indica uma resposta regenerativa. • Leva-se de 3 a 5 dias para que a medula óssea monte uma resposta regenerativa máxima à anemia; portanto, uma reticulocitose pode estar ausente no início de perda sanguínea aguda ou hemólise. • Na suspeita de anemia hemolítica imunomediada, indica-se um teste direto de antiglobulinas (teste de Coombs); um resultado positivo no teste, bem como indícios de esferocitose e policromasia no sangue periférico, são características confirmatórias; tanto os resultados falso-negativos como os falso-positivos são possíveis; dessa forma, é preciso ter cuidado ao se interpretar o teste em questão.

MÉTODOS DIAGNÓSTICOS
• Aspirado da medula óssea — esse teste faz-se necessário apenas quando não houver indícios de responsividade eritrocitária no sangue periférico (i. e., sem reticulocitose); a hiperplasia eritrocitária confirma uma resposta regenerativa; a ausência de hiperplasia eritrocitária indica anemia arregenerativa. • Biopsia da medula óssea — útil na avaliação tanto da arquitetura como da celularidade global dessa medula; importante para a confirmação de um processo arregenerativo.

TRATAMENTO
• Em caso de anemia grave e de rápido surgimento, o tratamento torna-se emergencial. • Uma hemorragia maciça leva ao choque hipovolêmico e à anoxia; já uma hemólise aguda induz à anoxia. • Ficam indicados o repouso em gaiola e a inspeção rigorosa do animal, dependendo da gravidade dos sinais clínicos.

ANEMIAS POR PERDA SANGUÍNEA
• Em caso de perda sanguínea traumática importante indutora de choque, os fluidos cristaloides podem corrigir rapidamente a hipovolemia e restabelecer a circulação. As soluções coloides (p. ex., dextrana 70) podem produzir uma expansão volêmica levemente maior. • A reposição de hemácias (papa de hemácias ou sangue total) ficará indicada em casos de hematócrito <15-20% e se houver sinais graves de hipoxia (i. e., mucosas extremamente pálidas, fraqueza, taquicardia e taquipneia) ou, então, a oxiemoglobina (30 mL/kg a uma velocidade de 10 mL/kg/h; OPK Biotech, Cambridge, MA) pode tanto gerar uma pressão oncótica como representar um carreador de oxigênio. • Os animais com perda sanguínea crônica são normovolêmicos com débito cardíaco elevado e, por essa razão, os volumes e as velocidades de transfusão devem ser conservativos para evitar insuficiência cardíaca. Os gatos são propensos à sobrecarga volêmica.

ANEMIAS HEMOLÍTICAS
Podem ser indicadas as práticas de transfusão sanguínea, bem como o fornecimento de oxiemoglobina; em pacientes com processo imunomediado, as hemácias provavelmente sobrevivem do mesmo modo que as próprias hemácias do paciente; dessa forma, não se deve suspender a transfusão na presença de sinais acentuados de anemia.

MEDICAÇÕES
MEDICAMENTO(S)
• Anemias por perda sanguínea — a administração de ferro pode ser benéfica em animais com anemia por perda crônica de sangue (ver "Anemia por Deficiência de Ferro"). • Anemias hemolíticas — o tratamento varia com a causa da hemólise.

ACOMPANHAMENTO
MONITORIZAÇÃO DO PACIENTE
• No início, proceder à mensuração da massa eritrocitária (p. ex., hematócrito, contagem eritrocitária e hemoglobina) e à avaliação morfológica de esfregaço do sangue periférico (i. e., policromasia) a cada 24 h para monitorar a eficácia do tratamento e a responsividade da medula óssea. • À medida que a regeneração se torna evidente (indicada pela elevação dos valores eritrocitários e pela policromasia), os pacientes deverão ser examinados a cada 3-5 dias; o retorno aos valores normais deve ocorrer em cerca de 14 dias após o episódio de hemorragia aguda, embora possa demorar mais diante de processo imunomediado.

DIVERSOS
VER TAMBÉM
• Anemia Imunomediada. • Anemia por Corpúsculo de Heinz. • Anemia por Deficiência de Ferro. • Babesiose. • Bartonelose. • Citauxzoonose. • Lúpus Eritematoso Sistêmico. • Toxicidade do Zinco.

ABREVIATURA(S)
• ATP = trifosfato de adenosina. • CHCM = concentração de hemoglobina corpuscular média. • CID = coagulação intravascular disseminada. • HCM = hemoglobina corpuscular média. • LES = lúpus eritematoso sistêmico. • VCM = volume corpuscular médio.

RECURSOS DA INTERNET
Erythrocytes: Overview, Morphology, Quantity; A.H. Rebar, P.S. MacWilliams, B.F. Feldman, et al.: http://www.ivis.org/advances/Rebar/Chap4/chapter.asp?LA = 1.

Sugestões de Leitura
Giger U. Regenerative anemias caused by blood loss or hemolysis. In: Ettinger SJ, Feldman EC, eds., Textbook of Veterinary Internal Medicine: Diseases of the Dog and Cat, 6th ed. Philadelphia: Elsevier Saunders, 2005, pp. 1886-1907.

Autor Joyce S. Knoll
Consultor Editorial A.H. Rebar

ANISOCORIA

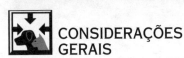

CONSIDERAÇÕES GERAIS

DEFINIÇÃO
Desigualdade do tamanho da abertura pupilar.

FISIOPATOLOGIA
- Interrupção da inervação simpática ou parassimpática da pupila — provoca alteração no tamanho da abertura pupilar.
- Oftalmopatia.

SISTEMA(S) ACOMETIDO(S)
- Nervoso.
- Oftálmico.

IDENTIFICAÇÃO
Cães e gatos.

SINAIS CLÍNICOS
Pupilas desiguais.

CAUSAS

Neurológicas
- Ver Tabela 1.
- Doenças com envolvimento do nervo óptico, trato óptico, nervo oculomotor ou cerebelo.

Oculares
- Ver Tabela 2.
- Uveíte anterior.
- Glaucoma.
- Atrofia ou hipoplasia da íris.
- Sinequia posterior.
- Bloqueio farmacológico.
- Neoplasia.
- Síndrome da pupila espástica.

FATORES DE RISCO
N/D.

DIAGNÓSTICO

DIAGNÓSTICO DIFERENCIAL
- É preciso determinar qual pupila se encontra anormal — ver Figura 1.
- Distinguir entre causas neurológicas e oculares.

HEMOGRAMA/BIOQUÍMICA/URINÁLISE
N/D.

OUTROS TESTES LABORATORIAIS
N/D.

DIAGNÓSTICO POR IMAGEM
- Ver Tabela 1.
- Ultrassonografia — identificação de lesões oculares e retrobulbares.
- TC e RM — localização e identificação de lesões no SNC.

MÉTODOS DIAGNÓSTICOS
- Ver Tabela 1.
- Punção do LCS — avalia a presença de doenças no SNC.
- Eletrorretinograma — examina a função da retina.
- Potencial evocado visual — avalia a função do nervo óptico.
- Testes farmacológicos — ver Figura 1; as lesões pós-ganglionares geram uma supersensibilidade por denervação; os medicamentos (para) simpaticomiméticos de ação direta induzem à constrição ou dilatação da pupila.
- Lesões pré-ganglionares — respondem aos (para) simpaticomiméticos de ação indireta.

TRATAMENTO
Depende da doença subjacente.

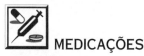

MEDICAÇÕES

MEDICAMENTO(S) DE ESCOLHA
Dependem da doença subjacente.

CONTRAINDICAÇÕES
N/D.

Tabela 1

Lesões Neurológicas Indutoras de Anisocoria

Lesão	Sinais Neurológicos	Diagnóstico Diferencial	Plano Diagnóstico
Nervo óptico	Midríase ipsilateral Anopsia* monocular ipsilateral (cegueira total em um dos olhos) Ausência de reflexo pupilar à luz direta no olho acometido Reflexo pupilar à luz consensual no olho acometido	Neurite óptica, neoplasia Doença infecciosa/inflamatória	TC/RM LCS Eletrorretinograma (ERG)
Nervo oculomotor	Pupila ipsilateral dilatada Visão normal/ausência de reflexo pupilar à luz direta	Neoplasia	TC/RM
III par de nervos cranianos do núcleo parassimpático	Ausência de reflexo pupilar à luz consensual do olho oposto Ptose da pálpebra superior Estrabismo ventrolateral	Doença infecciosa/inflamatória Traumatismo Herniação cerebral Massa retrobulbar	LCS Ultrassonografia da órbita
Doença cerebelar	Midríase contralateral Reflexo pupilar à luz normal/visão normal Ausência ipsilateral de resposta à ameaça Outros sinais cerebelares	Neoplasia Doença infecciosa/inflamatória Traumatismo	TC/RM LCS

* N. T.: Desuso ou perda da visão em um olho, como ocorre na catarata congênita ou no estrabismo muito acentuado; sinônimo de anopia.

Tabela 2

Doenças Oculares Indutoras de Anisocoria

Lesão	Sinais Associados	Causas
Uveíte anterior	Miose, rubor aquoso, edema de córnea, hiperemia conjuntival	Doença infecciosa/inflamatória, traumatismo, neoplasia
Glaucoma	Midríase Reflexo pupilar à luz vagaroso/ausente, pressão intraocular aumentada, edema de córnea	Glaucoma primário, glaucoma secundário
Neoplasia	Miose/midríase, alteração na cor da íris	Linfoma, melanoma
Sinequia posterior	Formato variável da pupila, reflexo pupilar à luz vagaroso/ausente, uveíte anterior	Secundária à uveíte anterior
Atrofia da íris	Formato variável da pupila, adelgaçamento da íris	Alteração etária antiga
Hipoplasia da íris	Reflexo pupilar à luz vagaroso/ausente, margem pupilar irregular, outras anormalidades oculares	Congênita
Bloqueio farmacológico	Midríase Reflexo pupilar à luz direta/consensual ausente Visão normal	Atropina
Síndrome da pupila espástica	Miose, visão normal	FeLV

ANISOCORIA

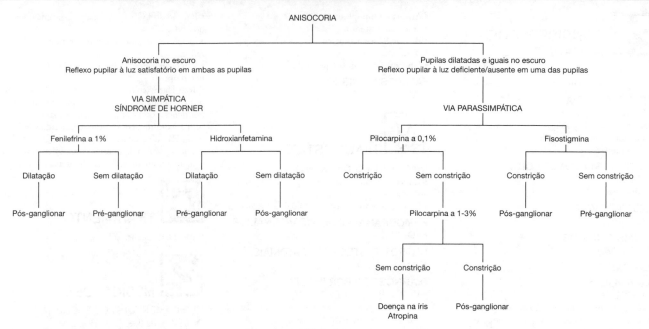

Figura 1

PRECAUÇÕES
N/D.

INTERAÇÕES POSSÍVEIS
N/D.

MEDICAMENTO(S) ALTERNATIVO(S)
N/D.

ACOMPANHAMENTO

MONITORIZAÇÃO DO PACIENTE
N/D.

COMPLICAÇÕES POSSÍVEIS
N/D.

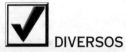

DIVERSOS

DISTÚRBIOS ASSOCIADOS
N/D.

FATORES RELACIONADOS COM A IDADE
N/D.

POTENCIAL ZOONÓTICO
N/D.

GESTAÇÃO/FERTILIDADE/REPRODUÇÃO
N/D.

VER TAMBÉM
- Atrofia da Íris.
- Glaucoma.
- Neurite Óptica.
- Síndrome de Horner.
- Uveíte Anterior — Cães.
- Uveíte Anterior — Gatos.

ABREVIATURA(S)
- FeLV = vírus da leucemia felina.
- LCS = líquido cerebrospinal.
- RM = ressonância magnética.
- SNC = sistema nervoso central.
- TC = tomografia computadorizada.

RECURSOS DA INTERNET
http://www.emedicine.com/oph/topic160.htm.

Sugestões de Leitura
Neer TM, Carter JD. Anisocoria in dogs and cats. Ocular and neurologic causes. Compend Contin Educ Pract Vet 1987, 9:817-824.
Scagliotti RH. Comparative neuro-ophthalmology. In: Gelatt KN, ed., Veterinary Ophthalmology, 3rd ed. Philadelphia: Lippincott Williams & Wilkins, 1999, pp. 1307-1400.

Autor David Lipsitz
Consultor Editorial Paul E. Miller

ANOMALIA DE EBSTEIN

CONSIDERAÇÕES GERAIS

REVISÃO
- Atrialização do ventrículo direito — deslocamento apical do aparato da valva atrioventricular direita (tricúspide) em direção ao ventrículo direito.
- Acompanhada por graus variados de insuficiência ou estenose da valva atrioventricular direita.
- Fisiopatologia importante relacionada ao grau de insuficiência ou estenose da valva atrioventricular direita.
- Uma via acessória anormal pode conduzir a taquicardias supraventriculares.

IDENTIFICAÇÃO
- Muito rara — encontrada ocasionalmente em cães e gatos.
- Não há predileção racial nem sexual.
- Auscultação de sopro em uma idade jovem, embora possa ser muito difícil auscultá-lo em caso de estenose.

SINAIS CLÍNICOS
- Os animais com leve insuficiência ou estenose da valva atrioventricular direita permanecem assintomáticos.
- Com frequência, os animais com insuficiência ou estenose moderada são intolerantes ao exercício.
- Os animais com insuficiência ou estenose grave apresentam ICCD com efusão pleural e/ou ascite.

DIAGNÓSTICO

DIAGNÓSTICO DIFERENCIAL
Displasia da valva atrioventricular direita.

HEMOGRAMA/BIOQUÍMICA/URINÁLISE
Os resultados costumam permanecer normais.

OUTROS TESTES LABORATORIAIS
N/D.

DIAGNÓSTICO POR IMAGEM
Radiografia Torácica
- Aumento de volume do átrio e do ventrículo direitos.
- Hepatomegalia.

Ecocardiografia
- A ecocardiografia bidimensional revela o deslocamento apical da valva atrioventricular direita com aumento de volume do átrio e do ventrículo direitos.
- O Doppler colorido revela insuficiência e/ou estenose da valva atrioventricular direita.
- O Doppler espectral confirma a presença de estenose da valva atrioventricular direita e estima a pressão do ventrículo direito.

OUTROS MÉTODOS DIAGNÓSTICOS
Eletrocardiografia
- A obtenção simultânea da pressão intracardíaca e de traçados eletrocardiográficos pode ser necessária para confirmar o diagnóstico.
- Via de condução acessória (pré-excitação ventricular) ou taquicardia supraventricular.

TRATAMENTO

- Atualmente, o tratamento clínico constitui a única abordagem praticável.
- A substituição cirúrgica da valva atrioventricular direita pode ser efetuada de forma bem-sucedida em algumas instituições veterinárias.
- Em caso de desenvolvimento de insuficiência cardíaca direita, restringir o consumo de sódio.

MEDICAÇÕES

MEDICAMENTO(S)
- Pacientes com ICCD — instituir a furosemida (2-4 mg/kg a cada 6-12 h) e o enalapril (0,5 mg/kg a cada 12 h).
- Pacientes com estenose da valva atrioventricular direita — aumentar gradativamente a dose do atenolol (0,1-1 mg/kg a cada 12 h) para obter uma frequência cardíaca normal baixa e, consequentemente, facilitar o enchimento ventricular.
- Pacientes com taquicardia supraventricular (síndrome de Wolff-Parkinson-White) — iniciar com a procainamida (15 mg/kg a cada 8 h).
- Se a síndrome de Wolff-Parkinson-White persistir, considerar a administração de algum bloqueador dos canais de cálcio (i. e., verapamil ou diltiazem) ou de algum β-bloqueador (i. e., propranolol ou atenolol).

CONTRAINDICAÇÕES/INTERAÇÕES POSSÍVEIS
Não utilizar os bloqueadores dos canais de cálcio e os β-bloqueadores concomitantemente.

ACOMPANHAMENTO

Monitorizar com ecocardiografia seriada.

DIVERSOS

VER TAMBÉM
Displasia da Valva Atrioventricular.

ABREVIATURA(S)
- ECG = eletrocardiografia.
- ICCD = insuficiência cardíaca congestiva direita.

Sugestões de Leitura
Bonagura JD, Lehmkuhl LB. Congenital heart disease. In: Fox PR, Sisson D, Moise NS, eds., Textbook of Canine and Feline Cardiology, 2nd ed. Philadelphia: Saunders, 1999, pp. 471-535.
Friedman WF. Congenital heart disease in infancy and childhood. In: Braunwald E, ed., Heart Disease, 4th ed. Philadelphia: Saunders, 1992.

Autor Carroll Loyer
Consultores Editoriais Larry P. Tilley e Francis W.K. Smith, Jr.

Anomalia de Pelger-Huët

CONSIDERAÇÕES GERAIS

REVISÃO
- Distúrbio hereditário congênito observado em diversas raças de cães e gatos domésticos de pelo curto.
- É provável um padrão de herança autossômico dominante.
- É observada hipossegmentação nuclear de muitos a todos os granulócitos (neutrófilos, eosinófilos e basófilos) e monócitos.
- Os padrões da cromatina de leucócitos são normocromáticos ou ocasionalmente hipercromáticos.
- O citoplasma das células não é notável (ou seja, nenhuma alteração tóxica é observada).
- A função celular permanece normal em heterozigotos.
- Os animais heterozigotos são assintomáticos.
- É preciso tomar cuidado para não interpretar erroneamente o leucograma como um grave desvio à esquerda.

IDENTIFICAÇÃO
- Cães — a anomalia de Pelger-Huët foi relatada em cães de raças mistas, bem como em inúmeros animais de raças puras. De modo geral, a incidência é baixa; no entanto, foi demonstrado que os cães da raça Pastor australiano têm uma taxa de incidência de 9,8%.
- Gatos — há relatos da anomalia de Pelger-Huët apenas em gatos domésticos de pelo curto. A incidência global em animais dessa espécie é desconhecida; entretanto, é provavelmente rara quando comparados aos cães.
- É provável um modo de herança autossômico dominante; todavia, foi observada uma penetrância incompleta no Pastor australiano.

SINAIS CLÍNICOS
- Nenhum sinal clínico é associado a animais heterozigotos, pois os leucócitos permanecem completamente funcionais.
- Os animais homozigotos sofrem morte intrauterina ou são natimortos com alterações condrodisplásicas significativas.

CAUSAS E FATORES DE RISCO
Os cães da raça Pastor australiano podem ter uma incidência mais alta da anomalia do que outras raças; contudo, as taxas de incidência em outras raças não foram completamente investigadas.

DIAGNÓSTICO

DIAGNÓSTICO DIFERENCIAL
- O principal diagnóstico diferencial a ser descartado é um desvio à esquerda regenerativo ou degenerativo grave, indicando inflamação grave e/ou endotoxemia.
- Um leucograma inflamatório pode revelar leucocitose ou leucopenia. Os leucócitos imaturos exibem um padrão de cromatina pálida aberta.
- Com frequência, observam-se alterações tóxicas (corpúsculos de Döhle, citoplasma espumoso azul, granulação tóxica etc.) em casos de inflamação e/ou endotoxemia grave.
- As células de Pelger-Huët são dotadas de núcleo com padrão de cromatina condensada madura e não exibem alterações tóxicas.
- Os animais com anomalia de Pelger-Huët apresentam-se clinicamente bem, enquanto aqueles com desvios à esquerda graves tendem a exibir doença sistêmica.
- No entanto, sempre é preciso lembrar que os animais com anomalia de Pelger-Huët podem sofrer doença inflamatória grave com características de toxicidade de granulócitos.

HEMOGRAMA/BIOQUÍMICA/URINÁLISE
- O esfregaço sanguíneo revela hipossegmentação variada de todos os granulócitos e frequentemente dos monócitos.
- Os núcleos dos granulócitos podem ser arredondados, ovais ou bilobados ou, então, em formato de amendoim, haltere ou ferradura.
- Um achado-chave é o padrão de cromatina condensada madura.
- O perfil da bioquímica sérica e o exame de urina (urinálise) não são dignos de nota em casos de anomalia de Pelger-Huët.
- Na presença de desvio à esquerda grave, os testes laboratoriais frequentemente estarão anormais, de acordo com a doença subjacente.

OUTROS TESTES LABORATORIAIS
Não há nenhum outro teste indicado para o diagnóstico da anomalia de Pelger-Huët.

DIAGNÓSTICO POR IMAGEM
- As técnicas de diagnóstico por imagem não são úteis para diagnosticar a anomalia de Pelger-Huët.
- Na presença de alguma doença subjacente capaz de estimular um desvio à esquerda acentuado, as alterações das técnicas de diagnóstico por imagem serão compatíveis com a doença em questão.

MÉTODOS DIAGNÓSTICOS
- Não há nenhum outro método diagnóstico indicado para diagnosticar anomalia de Pelger-Huët.
- Métodos diagnósticos adicionais serão justificáveis na suspeita de alguma doença subjacente capaz de causar um desvio à esquerda grave.

TRATAMENTO

Nenhum tratamento é indicado para a anomalia de Pelger-Huët.

ACOMPANHAMENTO

Não há necessidade de acompanhamento.

DIVERSOS

Sugestões de Leitura
Latimer KS. Pelger-Huët anomaly. In: Feldman BF, Zinkle JG, Jain NC, eds., Schalm's Veterinary Hematology, 5th ed. Philadelphia: Lippincott Williams & Wilkins, 2000, pp. 976-983.
Schalm's Veterinary Hematology, 6th ed. Ames, IA: Wiley-Blackwell, 2006, pp. 277-278, 325-326, 824, 338.

Autor Craig A. Thompson
Consultor Editorial A.H. Rebar

Anomalia do Olho do Collie

CONSIDERAÇÕES GERAIS

REVISÃO
- Distúrbio congênito, presumivelmente autossômico recessivo, que consiste, no mínimo, em hipoplasia temporal ou superotemporal da coroide até a cabeça do nervo óptico.
- Colobomas do nervo óptico — segunda anormalidade primária que também pode estar presente em cães acometidos.
- Como possíveis defeitos concomitantes, indicativos de manifestações mais graves, destacam-se estafiloma; descolamento da retina; hemorragia intraocular; neovascularização da retina.
- Sempre bilateral; pode-se observar gravidade discrepante entre os olhos.
- Em função do descolamento da retina e da hemorragia intraocular recorrente, há potencial para cegueira.
- Como anomalias associadas, que não fazem parte diretamente da síndrome, temos — enoftalmia; microftalmia; pregas retinianas; mineralização do estroma anterior da córnea.
- Aproximadamente 70-97% dos cães da raça Collie de pelo áspero e liso nos Estados Unidos e Grande britânico são acometidos.
- Cerca de 68% dos cães da raça Collie de pelo áspero na Suécia são afetados.
- Pode afetar até 2-3% da raça Border collie.
- Há mutação genética identificada.

IDENTIFICAÇÃO
- Collie de pelo áspero e liso, Border collie, Pastor de Shetland, Pastor australiano, Boykin spaniel, Lancashire heeler, Whippet de pelo longo, Nova Scotia duck tolling retriever.
- Presente ao nascimento.
- Uma deleção homozigota de 7,8 kb no gene NHEJ1 no cromossomo canino 37 está presente em todos os cães acometidos.
- Os cães de várias outras raças em que essa mutação genética não foi comprovada podem se apresentar com hipoplasia da coroide e colobomas do nervo óptico.

SINAIS CLÍNICOS
- A cegueira pode variar de nula (ausente) a parcial ou completa.
  - Achados oftalmoscópicos mínimos necessários para o diagnóstico — hipoplasia da coroide (uma área focal a difusa da coroide em que o número de vasos coroidais é reduzido e seu arranjo, irregular); o padrão vascular irradiado é normal para a coroide.
  - Localizados na região temporal ou superotemporal ao disco óptico; em casos graves, a lesão pode se estender mais no sentido nasal.
  - O tapete sobrejacente costuma estar ausente no plano focal ("defeito de janela"), permitindo a visualização dos vasos coroidais e da esclera subjacentes.
- Também se pode observar coloboma do nervo óptico (depressão da cabeça desse nervo).
- Descolamento da retina e hemorragia intraocular geralmente são secundários à presença de coloboma.
- Os vasos retinianos podem ficar tortuosos, mas costumam permanecer normais.
- "Os cães seguem normais" — a hipoplasia da coroide pode estar presente em cães jovens (<8 semanas de vida), mas desaparece à medida que o cão envelhece. Isso presumivelmente resulta do desenvolvimento do tapete sobrejacente, que obscurece as alterações mais profundas da coroide. Esses cães são denominados como "normais", mas são geneticamente acometidos.

CAUSAS E FATORES DE RISCO
- Mutação no cromossomo 37 do cão. Penetrância de quase 100%; é possível a penetrância parcial em heterozigoto.
- Hipoplasia da coroide e coloboma do nervo óptico são provavelmente transmitidos por mutações genéticas separadas.
- Ocorre somente a partir da reprodução de animais acometidos ou portadores.
- Um ou mais genes modificadores podem estar envolvidos. Esses genes podem explicar a variabilidade na gravidade do distúrbio e o fenômeno de "normalidade".

DIAGNÓSTICO

DIAGNÓSTICO DIFERENCIAL
- Tortuosidade excessiva dos vasos retinianos sem morfologia anormal dos vasos coroidais subjacentes — não se classifica como anomalia do olho do Collie.
- Colobomas do nervo óptico e descolamento da retina, não acompanhados por hipoplasia da coroide — não se classificam como anomalia do olho do Collie.
- Falta de pigmento na camada epitelial pigmentada da retina, permitindo a visualização da vasculatura normal da coroide; diferenciada pelos vasos coroidais irradiados, regulares e normais.
- Disgenesia ocular do Merle.

OUTROS TESTES LABORATORIAIS
O laboratório Optigen (EUA) oferece testes genéticos *on-line* para todas as raças acometidas.

TRATAMENTO
- Não há nenhum tratamento para a reversão do distúrbio.
- Criocirurgia ou cirurgia a *laser* na área circunjacente ao coloboma do nervo óptico — podem evitar o descolamento da retina e a hemorragia intraocular, mas também podem ser utilizadas para ajudar na refixação da retina.

ACOMPANHAMENTO

MONITORIZAÇÃO DO PACIENTE
Pacientes com colobomas — monitorizar durante o primeiro ano de vida quanto ao descolamento secundário da retina; depois de 1 ano, raramente ocorrerão descolamentos retinianos.

PREVENÇÃO
- O traço pode ser eliminado apenas por meio do acasalamento de cães normais no aspecto genotípico.
- O acasalamento de cães pouco acometidos com cadelas na mesma condição ou portadoras pode resultar em envolvimento mínimo da ninhada; entretanto, tais acasalamentos podem gerar qualquer nível de gravidade. É bastante provável que a reprodução de cães mais gravemente acometidos também produza uma ninhada com o mesmo nível de acometimento.
- Um único estudo cuidou de 8.204 cães da raça Collie de pelo áspero na Suécia durante um período de 8 anos (76% de todos os Collies registrados nesse país). Os criadores tinham a tendência de selecionar contra os cães com colobomas, mas continuavam a acasalar cães com hipoplasia da coroide. Essa estratégia resultou em um aumento significativo na prevalência de hipoplasia da coroide de 54 para 68% de 1989 a 1997 e não reduziu a prevalência de colobomas (8,3 *vs.* 8,5%).

EVOLUÇÃO ESPERADA E PROGNÓSTICO
- Não evolui, exceto quando um coloboma leva ao descolamento da retina e/ou hemorragia intraocular após o nascimento.
- Alguns pacientes com áreas menores de hipoplasia da coroide podem ficar "normais"; por essa razão, o exame precoce (nas primeiras 6-8 semanas de vida) é altamente recomendável.

DIVERSOS

DISTÚRBIOS ASSOCIADOS
- Microftalmia.
- Enoftalmia.
- Pregas retinianas.
- Mineralização do estroma anterior da córnea.
- O tamanho da ninhada é significativamente reduzido se pelo menos um dos progenitores for acometido por coloboma.

SINÔNIMO(S)
Síndrome de ectasia escleral.

VER TAMBÉM
- Descolamento da Retina.
- Hemorragia da Retina.

RECURSOS DA INTERNET
http://www.optigen.com/.

Sugestões de Leitura
Lowe JK, Kukekova AV, Kirkness EF, et al. Linkage mapping of the primary disease locus for collie eye anomaly. Genomics 2003, 82:86-95.
Narfström K, Petersen-Jones SM. Diseases of the canine ocular fundus. In: Gelatt KN, ed. Veterinary Ophthalmology, 4th ed. Ames, IA: Blackwell, 2007, pp. 944-1025.
Parker HG, Kukekova AV, Akey DT, et al. Breed relationships facilitate fine-mapping studies: A 7.8-kb deletion cosegregates with Collie eye anomaly across multiple dog breeds. Genome Res 2007, 17:1562-1571.
Roberts SR. The collie eye anomaly. JAVMA 1969, 155:859-865.
Wallin-Hakanson B, Wallin-Hakanson N, Hedhammar A. Collie eye anomaly in the rough collie in Sweden: Genetic transmission and influence on offspring vitality. J Small Anim Pract 2000, 41:254-258.

Autor Simon A. Pot
Consultor Editorial Paul E. Miller
Agradecimento Stephanie L. Smedes

Anomalia Vascular Portossistêmica Congênita

CONSIDERAÇÕES GERAIS

DEFINIÇÃO
- Anomalia vascular portossistêmica congênita — más-formações venosas (em geral, de um único vaso) que unem as circulações portal e sistêmica, fazendo com que o sangue portal se desvie do fígado (circulação hepatofugal).
- Pode ser extra-hepática (mais comum em cães de pequeno porte e gatos) ou intra-hepática (mais comum em cães de grande porte).
- Muitas raças caninas de pequeno porte com anomalia vascular portossistêmica também apresentam anormalidades vasculares envolvendo a microvasculatura intra-hepática (ver "Displasia Microvascular Hepatoportal").

FISIOPATOLOGIA
- Sinais clínicos — a gravidade reflete o grau de desvio; causados pela circulação hepatofugal; impede a remoção de toxinas entéricas e das substâncias nitrogenadas derivadas do alimento pelo sangue portal.
- Priva o fígado dos fatores hepatotróficos de origem intestinal, causando micro-hepatia.
- Encefalopatia hepática episódica — associada à ingestão de alimento rico em proteína, sangramento gastrintestinal, desidratação, azotemia, alcalose, distúrbios eletrolíticos, transfusão sanguínea, hemólise, infecções, catabolismo e certos medicamentos.
- Hiperamonemia e transformação prejudicada do ácido úrico em alantoína hidrossolúvel provocam cristalúria ou cálculos de biurato de amônio; pode ser o principal problema apresentado.

SISTEMA(S) ACOMETIDO(S)
- Nervoso — encefalopatia hepática episódica (comum).
- Gastrintestinal — inapetência intermitente; vômito; diarreia; pica ("apetite depravado"); ptialismo (gatos).
- Urogenital — rins grandes (especialmente nos cães); urolitíase por urato de amônio; 50% dos machos caninos criptorquídicos em um único relato.

GENÉTICA
- Raças acometidas — p. ex., mas não exclusivas, Yorkshire terrier, Cairn terrier, Maltês, Spaniel tibetano, Schnauzer miniatura, Norfolk terrier, Pug, Shih tzu, Havanês, Wolfhound irlandês, Old English sheepdog.
- Suspeita de traço autossômico dominante com penetrância incompleta.

INCIDÊNCIA/PREVALÊNCIA
0,2-0,6% de grande parte da população clínica de encaminhamento.

DISTRIBUIÇÃO GEOGRÁFICA
Mundial.

IDENTIFICAÇÃO
Espécies
Os cães são mais comumente acometidos que os gatos.

Raça(s) Predominante(s)
- Maior risco — raças caninas puras; cães de raças mistas pertencentes à linhagem de pequenos terriers; gatos mestiços.
- Ver a seção "Genética".

Idade Média e Faixa Etária
Em geral, é identificada pela primeira vez em animais jovens; no entanto, os cães podem ter até 13 anos no diagnóstico inicial.

Sexo Predominante
Nenhum.

SINAIS CLÍNICOS
Achados Anamnésicos
- Retardo do crescimento — comum.
- Os sinais frequentemente começam com o desmame do filhote canino ou felino e a transição para a ração comercial.
- Sinais gastrintestinais — inapetência; vômito; diarreia; pica.
- Acredita-se que os gatos tenham infecção respiratória superior inicialmente, pois exibem ptialismo.
- Encefalopatia hepática episódica — os episódios melhoram transitoriamente com fluidoterapia, antibióticos de amplo espectro e lactulose.
- Sinais do SNC — fraqueza; andar compassado; ataxia; desorientação; compressão da cabeça contra objetos; cegueira; mudanças comportamentais: agressividade (gatos), vocalização, alucinações; crises convulsivas; coma.
- Sinais urinários — poliúria e polidipsia; cristalúria por biurato de amônio: polaciúria, disúria; hematúria; obstrução uretral (raramente ureteral) por urólito.
- Alguns cães carecem de sinais clínicos: ~20%.

Achados do Exame Físico
- Aparência normal; estatura mal desenvolvida; micro-hepatia; encefalopatia hepática; coloração dourada ou cor de cobre das íris nos gatos que não possuem olhos azuis (nota: as raças Persa, Azul da Rússia e algumas outras têm normalmente íris cor de cobre; a coloração não muda com a ligadura da anomalia vascular portossistêmica).
- Sinais neurológicos (ver anteriormente).
- Ascite ou edema: raros.

CAUSAS
- Más-formações congênitas.
- Desvio portossistêmico adquirido nos animais com anomalia vascular portossistêmica congênita — subsequente à atresia portal congênita rara (gatos > cães) ou hipertensão portal induzida por via cirúrgica.

FATORES DE RISCO
- Anomalia vascular portossistêmica — cães de raças puras, especialmente raças pequenas tipo Terrier.
- A raça Wolfhound irlandês parece sofrer um fechamento lento do ducto venoso; uma triagem precoce pode identificar erroneamente os cães como acometidos.

DIAGNÓSTICO

DIAGNÓSTICO DIFERENCIAL
- Sinais do SNC — distúrbios infecciosos (p. ex., PIF, cinomose, toxoplasmose, infecções relacionadas com FeLV ou FIV); intoxicações (p. ex., chumbo, cogumelos e substâncias psicoativas); hidrocefalia; epilepsia idiopática; distúrbios metabólicos (p. ex., hipoglicemia, hipo ou hipercalcemia, hipocalcemia graves).
- Sinais gastrintestinais — obstrução intestinal; imprudência alimentar; ingestão de corpo estranho; enteropatia inflamatória.
- Sinais do trato urinário — infecção bacteriana do trato urinário; urolitíase.
- Poliúria e polidipsia — distúrbios da concentração de urina (p. ex., diabetes insípido, função adrenal anormal, hipercalcemia e polidipsia primária); atribuídas à alta taxa de filtração glomerular na anomalia vascular portossistêmica.
- Hepatopatia primária — distinguida pelas técnicas de diagnóstico por imagem e pela biopsia do fígado.
- Função hepática anormal (ácidos biliares séricos totais elevados) sugestiva de anomalia vascular portossistêmica, mas sem desvio macroscópico — displasia microvascular hepatoportal.
- Desvio portossistêmico adquirido — muitos diferenciais; ver "Desvio Portossistêmico Adquirido".

HEMOGRAMA/BIOQUÍMICA/URINÁLISE
- Hemograma completo — microcitose; anemia arregenerativa leve; pecilocitose (gatos); células em alvo (cães).
- Bioquímica — é comum, mas inconsistente, a constatação de níveis baixos de ureia, creatinina, glicose e colesterol; atividade variável das enzimas hepáticas (fosfatase alcalina geralmente elevada nos pacientes jovens [isoenzima óssea]); bilirrubina normal, mas hipoalbuminemia inconsistente e leve.
- Urinálise — urina diluída; cristalúria por biurato de amônio, hematúria, piúria e proteinúria: inflamação e infecção secundárias a cálculos metabólicos.

OUTROS TESTES LABORATORIAIS
- Ácidos biliares séricos totais — indicadores sensíveis de desvio portossistêmico; valores mensurados em jejum e obtidos ao acaso podem estar dentro da faixa normal de referência; valores medidos 2 h depois das refeições (i. e., pós-prandiais) encontram-se acentuadamente elevados (em geral, >100 μmol/L).
- Valores sanguíneos de amônia — menos confiáveis do que os ácidos biliares séricos totais na prática clínica, porque as amostras não podem ser refrigeradas nem enviadas para análise; teste de tolerância à amônia — demonstra intolerância a essa substância, mas pode provocar encefalopatia hepática.
- Testes de coagulação — anormais em alguns cães; não costumam estar associados a sangramento.
- Proteína C — valores baixos ajudam a diferenciar anomalia vascular portossistêmica de displasia microvascular; observam-se níveis baixos em anomalia vascular portossistêmica, porém normais na displasia microvascular; reflete a gravidade do desvio, mas pode permanecer normal em cães assintomáticos com anomalia vascular portossistêmica; utilizada para avaliar a influência da ligadura desse tipo de anomalia, já que os ácidos biliares séricos totais frequentemente permanecem anormais.
- Efusão abdominal — complicação pós-cirúrgica; em geral, constitui transudato puro ou modificado.

DIAGNÓSTICO POR IMAGEM
Radiografia Abdominal
- Micro-hepatia — cães > gatos.
- Renomegalia.
- Efusão abdominal (desvio portossistêmico adquirido) — após ligação cirúrgica; se preceder a cirurgia, será sugestiva de fístula AV, hipertensão

ANOMALIA VASCULAR PORTOSSISTÊMICA CONGÊNITA

portal não cirrótica, hipertensão portal idiopática ou atresia portal.
• Urolitíase por urato de amônio — radiotransparente a menos que combinada com envoltório mineral radiodenso.

Portovenografia Radiográfica
• Portografia mesentérica — delimita a circulação portal e verifica o local do desvio: a localização extra-hepática é sugerida pela extensão caudal de anomalia vascular portossistêmica caudal à vértebra T_{13}; intra-hepática em caso de extensão caudal de anomalia vascular portossistêmica cranial à vértebra T_{13}.

Ultrassonografia Abdominal
• Avaliações subjetivas; micro-hepatia; hipovascularidade; pode ser difícil a identificação da anomalia vascular portossistêmica.
• Doppler de fluxo colorido — ajuda na localização do desvio; examinar a veia cava cranial à veia frenicoabdominal e a junção com a veia cava (uma turbulência nesse local apoia a presença de anomalia vascular portossistêmica extra-hepática).
• Desvios intra-hepáticos — facilmente observados em técnicas de diagnóstico por imagem.
• Renomegalia, além de urólitos (císticos, pélvicos e, raramente, ureterais) comuns.

Cintilografia Colorretal
• Teste não invasivo sensível — confirma o desvio.
• Não é capaz de diferenciar anomalia vascular portossistêmica e desvio portossistêmico adquirido ou anomalia vascular portossistêmica intra e extra-hepática.
• Administrar pertecnetato de tecnécio-99m por via retal; obter a imagem com câmara gama para determinar o aparecimento do isótopo no coração antes do fígado; fração de desvio <15% é normal; frações de desvio da anomalia vascular portossistêmica costumam ser >60%.
• Cintilografia esplenoportal: requer injeção de contraste no baço; não há vantagens com esse método.

TC Multissetorial
• Técnica de diagnóstico por imagem com padrão de excelência: demonstra a vasculatura portal e o vaso do desvio.
• Teste não invasivo: administração de contraste por via IV e anestesia geral a curto prazo.

MÉTODOS DIAGNÓSTICOS
• Citologia de aspirado obtido por agulha fina — não é capaz de diagnosticar anomalia vascular portossistêmica; é comum o encontro de pequenos hepatócitos binucleados.
• Biopsia do fígado — há necessidade de biopsia cirúrgica aberta em cunha ou amostragem laparoscópica (pinça de biopsia em cálice), com a obtenção de tecido de diversos lobos hepáticos (evitar o lobo caudado, pois contém menos lesões); biopsia central com agulha pode ser inadequada para o diagnóstico definitivo de hipoperfusão portal.

ACHADOS PATOLÓGICOS
• Macroscópicos — fígado pequeno com superfície lisa; pode ser difícil verificar a anomalia vascular portossistêmica na autopsia; animais jovens com atresia portal podem apresentar desvio portossistêmico adquirido.
• Microscópicos — pequenas vênulas portais não perfundidas ou ausentes; distensão linfática; múltiplos cortes transversais de arteríolas portais; tríades portais juvenis, atrofia lobular, lipogranulomas variáveis dispersos contendo hemossiderina; musculatura estrangulada proeminente espessa de vênulas hepáticas (perfis longitudinais anormais dessas vênulas); alguns cães apresentam vacuolização lipídica e inflamação não supurativa graves na zona 3, que colidem com as vênulas hepáticas.
• Displasia microvascular — apresenta características histopatológicas idênticas, mas carece de anomalia vascular portossistêmica macroscópica.

TRATAMENTO

CUIDADO(S) DE SAÚDE ADEQUADO(S)
Paciente internado — no caso de sinais graves de encefalopatia hepática; fornecimento de cuidados de suporte para encefalopatia hepática antes da biopsia do fígado e da ligadura da anomalia vascular portossistêmica.

CUIDADO(S) DE ENFERMAGEM
Ver "Encefalopatia Hepática".

DIETA
• Suporte nutricional — essencial para manter a condição corporal, já que a musculatura serve como um importante local de desintoxicação temporária da amônia.
• Dieta balanceada com restrição proteica — recomendada; daí em diante, a porção de proteína é titulada de acordo com a resposta em combinação com tratamentos que melhoram a encefalopatia hepática; conforme a tolerância, adicionar 0,5 g/kg de proteína (utilizar queijo *cottage* ou caseinato de cálcio para os cães): observar em intervalos de 5 a 7 dias (ver "Encefalopatia Hepática").
• Animais assintomáticos ou minimamente sintomáticos podem sobreviver bem apenas com a intervenção na dieta.

ORIENTAÇÃO AO PROPRIETÁRIO
• Explicar todas as opções: médica *versus* cirúrgica.
• Ligadura cirúrgica — esperar a melhora, mas não a cura; pode não ser necessária para todos os cães (ver a seção "Dieta").
• Sinais clínicos — podem persistir apesar da ligadura do ducto, exigindo tratamento nutricional e clínico por tempo prolongado.
• Riscos cirúrgico-anestésicos — 5-25% de mortalidade; dependem da experiência do cirurgião, do tipo de anomalia vascular portossistêmica, da existência de lesões microscópicas hepáticas e dos cuidados críticos de suporte.
• Se a cirurgia não for levada a cabo ou se a ligadura não for tolerada, monitorar o paciente quanto à presença de uropatias obstrutivas por biurato de amônio que podem exigir uretrostomia permanente.

CONSIDERAÇÕES CIRÚRGICAS
• Ligadura cirúrgica da anomalia vascular portossistêmica — o objetivo ideal consiste na ligadura total; pode não ser tolerada, levando a desvio portossistêmico adquirido (especialmente com constritor ameroide ou bandagem de celofane).
• Ligadura parcial: restabelece a saúde do paciente.
• O grau de tolerância ao fechamento da anomalia vascular portossistêmica é avaliado no momento da cirurgia: resposta fisiológica à oclusão temporária do desvio (mudança na pressão portal ou na circulação esplâncnica); avaliações intraoperatórias podem ser imprecisas em termos prognósticos.
• Constritor ameroide — diminui os riscos cirúrgicos imediatos da ligadura; pode resultar mais tarde em desvio portossistêmico adquirido em alguns pacientes (sobretudo nos cães da raça Yorkshire terrier).
• Encefalopatia hepática — deve ser aliviada com o tratamento clínico antes da cirurgia.
• Anomalia vascular portossistêmica intra-hepática — ligadura mais difícil; apesar de ser um procedimento alternativo, a taxa de êxito da embolectomia com espiral ainda não foi bem estabelecida.
• Portografia intraoperatória é aconselhada para todos os pacientes — para verificar a ligadura apropriada do vaso.
• Complicações pós-operatórias — hipertensão portal grave aguda; trombos venosos portais; isquemia mesentérica; endotoxemia; crises convulsivas; sepse; pancreatite aguda; hemorragia; desvio portossistêmico adquirido — desenvolvem-se subsequentemente à hipertensão portal e podem ocorrer após a aplicação de constritores ameroides, ligadura cirúrgica com seda ou bandagem de anomalia vascular sistêmica com celofane.
• Hipotermia intraoperatória e pós-operatória — em pacientes muito pequenos; prolonga o tempo de recuperação.
• Cirurgia de emergência — raramente necessária para remoção da ligadura; a retirada de constritores ameroides não é uma tarefa fácil.
• Efusão abdominal — comum após a ligadura do desvio; isoladamente, não indica hipertensão portal patológica intolerável, que causará desvio portossistêmico adquirido; ficar atento para os sinais clínicos de isquemia mesentérica (diarreia sanguinolenta, dor abdominal, falha na recuperação da cirurgia/anestesia, taquicardia inexplicável, hipertermia ou hipotermia); monitorizar a circunferência abdominal e o peso corporal.
• Coloides sintéticos aumentam os riscos de sangramento.
• Terapia com componente sanguíneo contendo o anticoagulante citrato de sódio pode provocar hipocalcemia e coagulopatia (hipercitratemia) em pacientes com <5 kg.
• Monitorização na UTI — recomendada no pós-operatório por 72-96 h.
• Crises convulsivas intratáveis em <5% dos cães após a ligadura; causa desconhecida; tratamento para edema cerebral e necessidade de sedação; não há provas de que o brometo de potássio profilático seja benéfico; a infusão em velocidade constante de propofol ou flumazenil (0,005-0,01 mg/kg em bólus IV) não é confiável para o controle das crises.

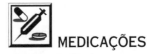

MEDICAÇÕES

MEDICAMENTO(S)
Ver "Encefalopatia Hepática".

PRECAUÇÕES
Tomar cuidado com o metabolismo alterado dos medicamentos.

ANOMALIA VASCULAR PORTOSSISTÊMICA CONGÊNITA

ACOMPANHAMENTO

MONITORIZAÇÃO DO PACIENTE
- Reavaliar — o comportamento do paciente em casa; averiguar a condição corporal, a circunferência abdominal (no pós-operatório) e o peso corporal; avaliar o hemograma completo (resolução da microcitose), a bioquímica (resolução dos níveis baixos de colesterol, ureia e creatinina) e urinálise (resolução da cristalúria por biurato de amônio).
- Ácidos biliares séricos totais (raças caninas de pequeno porte) — valores persistentemente elevados não corroboram com a falha cirúrgica em função da coexistência comum de displasia microvascular.
- Proteína C — normaliza ou aumenta após cirurgia bem-sucedida.

COMPLICAÇÕES POSSÍVEIS
Ver a seção "Considerações Cirúrgicas".

PREVENÇÃO
Múltiplos desvios portossistêmicos — devem ser detectados por meio de ultrassom e sugerem desvio portossistêmico adquirido; não prosseguir com a ligadura cirúrgica; implica atresia portal ou alguma outra hepatopatia subjacente ou distúrbio indutor de hipertensão portal; a anomalia vascular portossistêmica tipicamente não é associada à hipertensão portal ou ao desvio portossistêmico adquirido.

EVOLUÇÃO ESPERADA E PROGNÓSTICO
- Resposta imprevisível à cirurgia.
- Cães — a ligadura melhora os sinais clínicos em 70-80% dos pacientes sintomáticos.
- Gatos — podem desenvolver desvio portossistêmico adquirido.
- Após a cirurgia — continuar o tratamento da encefalopatia hepática (especialmente a dieta) até a reavaliação do paciente.
- Alguns pacientes — necessitam de tratamento por tempo indefinido.
- Ligadura parcial — pode resultar em atenuação completa do desvio (reação de granulação à ligadura).
- Constritor ameroide — pode resultar em ligadura completa dentro de alguns dias (torção após a colocação, formação de trombos); pode provocar desvio portossistêmico adquirido.
- Aumento no risco de desfechos cirúrgicos insatisfatórios em determinados cães de pequeno porte (amplas lesões na zona 3 que atenuam a vênula hepática) e nos gatos.
- Apesar da resposta inicial satisfatória, pode ocorrer a recidiva do desvio 3 anos após a ligadura.
- Os cães assintomáticos não submetidos à ligadura da anomalia vascular portossistêmica podem ter uma expectativa de vida normal.

DIVERSOS

DISTÚRBIOS ASSOCIADOS
- Urolitíase por urato de amônio.
- Íris cor de cobre (gatos).
- Criptorquidismo (cães).
- Encefalopatia hepática.

FATORES RELACIONADOS COM A IDADE
Os cães com anomalia vascular portossistêmica identificados em idades mais avançadas costumam ser assintomáticos para encefalopatia hepática e frequentemente são submetidos à atenuação dos desvios com facilidade (desconexão ázigo-portal).

GESTAÇÃO/FERTILIDADE/REPRODUÇÃO
- Cadelas assintomáticas podem levar a gestação a termo.
- Cães assintomáticos já foram utilizados como reprodutores.
- Não é aconselhável o acasalamento de cães com anomalia vascular portossistêmica, por conta da base genética.

SINÔNIMO(S)
Desvio portocaval.

VER TAMBÉM
- Desvio Portossistêmico Adquirido.
- Displasia Microvascular Hepatoportal.
- Encefalopatia Hepática.
- Hepatopatia Fibrosante Juvenil.

ABREVIATURA(S)
- AV = arteriovenosa.
- FeLV = vírus da leucemia felina.
- FIV = vírus da imunodeficiência felina.
- GI = gastrintestinal.
- PIF = peritonite infecciosa felina.
- SNC = sistema nervoso central.
- TC = tomografia computadorizada.

Sugestões de Leitura

Center SA. Hepatic vascular diseases. In: Guilford WG, Center SA, Strombeck DR, et al., eds. Strombeck's Small Animal Gastroenterology, 3rd ed. Philadelphia: Saunders, 1996, pp. 802-846.

MehlML, Kyles AE, Hardie EM, et al. Evaluation of ameroid ring constrictors for treatment for single extrahepatic portosystemic shunts in dogs: 168 cases (1995-2001). JAVMA 2005, 226:2020-2030.

Autor Sharon A. Center
Consultor Editorial Sharon A. Center

ANOMALIAS DO ANEL VASCULAR

CONSIDERAÇÕES GERAIS

REVISÃO
Arco Aórtico Direito
- Encarceramento do esôfago por persistência do 4° arco aórtico (aorta dextroposicionada) à direita e dorsalmente, com a base cardíaca e a artéria pulmonar ventralmente e o ducto ou ligamento arterioso à esquerda e dorsalmente.
- Causa megaesôfago cranialmente à obstrução na base do coração.

Arco Aórtico Duplo
- Encarceramento do esôfago por arco aórtico funcional à direita, arco aórtico atrésico à esquerda, com a base cardíaca e a artéria pulmonar ventralmente e o ducto ou ligamento arterioso à esquerda e dorsalmente.
- Causa megaesôfago cranialmente à obstrução na base do coração; também provoca certa compressão da traqueia.

IDENTIFICAÇÃO
- Cães e gatos.
- Observadas mais comumente em Pastor alemão, Setter irlandês e Boston terrier.

SINAIS CLÍNICOS
- Regurgitação de alimento sólido não digerido em animais com menos de 6 meses de vida.
- Desnutrição em muitos animais.
- O tempo entre a alimentação e a regurgitação é variável.
- Sinais de pneumonia por aspiração (p. ex., tosse, taquipneia ou dispneia) em alguns animais.

CAUSAS E FATORES DE RISCO
N/D.

DIAGNÓSTICO

DIAGNÓSTICO DIFERENCIAL
- Megaesôfago congênito.
- Estenose, divertículo ou corpo estranho esofágico.
- Distúrbio da motilidade esofágica em Shar-pei.

HEMOGRAMA/BIOQUÍMICA/URINÁLISE
- Os resultados costumam permanecer normais.
- Leucograma elevado em alguns animais com pneumonia por aspiração.

OUTROS TESTES LABORATORIAIS
N/D.

DIAGNÓSTICO POR IMAGEM
- Radiografia torácica — revela a porção cranial do esôfago repleta de alimento ou sinais de pneumonia por aspiração em alguns animais.
- Esofagografia contrastada — confirma a presença de megaesôfago, que se estende até a base do coração.
- Fluoroscopia — pode ser utilizada para diferenciar os distúrbios da motilidade esofágica.
- Angiografia — possivelmente necessária para distinguir as anomalias específicas do anel vascular.

OUTROS MÉTODOS DIAGNÓSTICOS
A esofagoscopia pode ser usada na diferenciação dos distúrbios da motilidade esofágica.

TRATAMENTO

- Em casos de encarceramento vascular, fica indicada a correção cirúrgica.
- O tratamento clínico dos casos de pneumonia por aspiração, concomitantes à anomalia do anel vascular, pode ser indispensável.
- Em casos de megaesôfago, os procedimentos relacionados com a alimentação também podem ser imprescindíveis por períodos de tempo prolongados.
- Os animais com pneumonia por aspiração podem exigir cuidados de suporte com o fornecimento de oxigênio.

MEDICAÇÕES

MEDICAMENTO(S)
Em animais com pneumonia por aspiração, é recomendável a instituição de antibióticos de amplo espectro, como enrofloxacino (2,5 mg/kg a cada 12 h) e amoxicilina (10-15 mg/kg a cada 12 h).

CONTRAINDICAÇÕES/INTERAÇÕES POSSÍVEIS
N/D.

ACOMPANHAMENTO

EVOLUÇÃO ESPERADA E PROGNÓSTICO
- O prognóstico quanto à resolução do problema é de reservado a mau, mesmo depois da cirurgia.
- As complicações de desnutrição e pneumonia por aspiração são comuns e graves.
- A função esofágica, muitas vezes, sofre comprometimento permanente.

Sugestões de Leitura
Bonagura JD, Lehmkuhl LB. Congenital heart disease. In: Fox PR, Sisson D, Moise NS, eds., Textbook of Canine and Feline Cardiology, 2nd ed. Philadelphia: Saunders, 1999, pp. 471-535.
Goodwin J. Double aortic arch. In: Tilley LP, Smith FWK, eds., The 5-Minute Veterinary Consult, 2nd ed. Philadelphia: Lippincott Williams & Wilkins, 2000, p. 636.

Autor Carroll Loyer
Consultores Editoriais Larry P. Tilley e Francis W.K. Smith, Jr.

Anomalias Oculares Congênitas

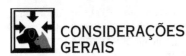

CONSIDERAÇÕES GERAIS

DEFINIÇÃO
Anormalidades solitárias ou múltiplas, que comprometem o bulbo ocular ou seus anexos e podem ser observadas em cães e gatos jovens ao nascimento ou nas primeiras 6-8 semanas de vida.

FISIOPATOLOGIA
• Defeitos hereditários relacionados com a raça. • Más-formações espontâneas. • Infecções e inflamações sistêmicas intrauterinas, exposição a compostos tóxicos e falta de nutrientes específicos em gatas ou cadelas prenhes.

SISTEMA(S) ACOMETIDO(S)
Oftálmico — o olho inteiro ou qualquer parte dele; uni ou bilateral.

GENÉTICA
• Modo de herança conhecido, suspeito ou desconhecido. • Membrana pupilar persistente (MPP) em Basenji — traço dominante. • Túnica vascular do cristalino hiperplásica persistente (TVCHP) e vítreo primário hiperplásico persistente (VPHP) em Doberman pinscher — alelo dominante com expressão variável. • Displasia multifocal da retina em Springer spaniel inglês — traço recessivo. • Anomalia do olho do Collie — traço recessivo. • Distrofia da retina em Briard — alelo recessivo. • Displasia de bastonetes e cones em Collie, Setter irlandês, Cardigan Welsh corgi e Sloughi — traço recessivo; doença não alélica. • Distrofia de cones e bastonetes em Pit bull terrier e em Dachshund de pelo longo e curto — traço recessivo; doença não alélica. • Displasia de fotorreceptores em gatos das raças Abissínio, Persa e doméstico de pelo curto — traço dominante em Abissínio e gato doméstico de pelo curto, mas recessivo em Persa.

INCIDÊNCIA/PREVALÊNCIA
• Incidência em cães e gatos — baixa na população em geral; um pouco mais alta na espécie canina do que na felina. • Anomalia do olho do Collie — 50% em Collies, porém mais baixa em outras raças.

IDENTIFICAÇÃO
Espécies
• Cães e gatos.
Raça(s) Predominante(s)
Ver a seção "Genética".
Idade Média e Faixa Etária
Ver a seção "Definição".

SINAIS CLÍNICOS
Comentários Gerais
• Dependem do defeito. • Podem não causar nenhum sinal de doença; frequentemente representam um achado incidental. • Pode ser uma doença congênita indutora de cegueira.
Achados Anamnésicos
Variam desde a ausência de achados até uma diminuição grave na acuidade visual ou cegueira.
Achados do Exame Físico
• Microftalmia — um olho pequeno de natureza congênita; associada frequentemente a outros defeitos hereditários. • Anoftalmia — falta congênita do bulbo ocular; associada a outros defeitos hereditários. • Criptoftalmia — bulbo ocular pequeno, ocultado por outros defeitos nos anexos. • Agenesia ou coloboma palpebrais — podem resultar em pálpebras abertas de natureza congênita; afeta a porção temporal da pálpebra superior; podem causar blefarospasmo e epífora. • Dermoides — ilhotas de tecido cutâneo aberrante, que envolvem as pálpebras, a conjuntiva ou a córnea; podem causar blefarospasmo e epífora. • Atresia e orifícios imperfurados do sistema lacrimal — comuns em raças caninas; resultam em vestígios lacrimais no canto nasal; costumam não estar associados a outros achados oculares. • Ceratoconjuntivite seca congênita — pode ocorrer de forma esporádica em qualquer raça canina ou felina; geralmente unilateral; o olho acometido parece menor do que o normal; apresenta secreção mucoide espessa proveniente de um olho vermelho e irritado. • MPP — resquícios da membrana pupilar, que se estendem desde o colarete da íris até o endotélio da córnea, a cápsula anterior do cristalino ou imediatamente através da pupila; pode coexistir com outros defeitos; documentada em inúmeras raças caninas, especialmente Basenji. • Cistos da íris — estruturas esféricas, pigmentadas ou não, que oscilam livremente na câmara anterior do olho ou podem ficar aderidas à íris ou ao endotélio corneano. • Glaucoma congênito — acomete cães e gatos; raro; observam-se intensificação no lacrimejamento e olho aumentado de volume, vermelho e sensível. • Anormalidades pupilares — policoria (mais de uma pupila); acoreia ou ancoria (ausência de pupila); aniridia (falta da íris); discoria (pupila de formato anormal). • Cataratas congênitas — primárias, frequentemente hereditárias ou secundárias a outros defeitos de desenvolvimento; associadas a outras anomalias do cristalino, incluindo microfacia (cristalino pequeno), lenticone ou lentiglobo (protrusão da cápsula do cristalino, geralmente no sentido posterior) e coloboma (incisura no equador do cristalino, que também pode incluir defeitos nas zônulas e no corpo ciliar); associadas comumente à leucoria (pupila branca). • TVCHP e VPHP — defeitos hereditários, que acometem as raças Doberman pinscher e Staffordshire bull terrier; persistência de partes da vasculatura hialoide; aberrações de desenvolvimento do humor vítreo, do cristalino e da cápsula lenticular; podem-se notar as seguintes alterações: catarata, leucoria e/ou reflexo (brilho) avermelhado proveniente da área pupilar, em conjunto com sangramento intralenticular. • Displasia da retina — acomete diversas raças caninas; ocorrência esporádica em gatos; o efeito sobre a estrutura da retina depende da gravidade; varia desde pregas focais, passando por descolamento focal geográfico, até o descolamento completo da retina. • Coloboma do segmento posterior — encontrado em conjunto com a anomalia do olho do Collie; observado tipicamente na cabeça do nervo óptico; em geral na posição correspondente às 6 horas; também pode ser vista em outros locais do fundo ocular, próximos à cabeça do nervo óptico. • Displasia de bastonetes e cones em cães — acomete as raças Setter irlandês e Collie; displasia de bastonetes e degeneração precoce de bastonetes comprometem a raça Elkhound norueguês; degeneração de cones ou hemeralopia afeta a raça Malamute do Alasca. • Distrofia de cones e bastonetes em cães da raça Pit bull terrier — revela dilatação pupilar e dificuldades visuais com 6-7 semanas de vida, além de respostas reduzidas ao exame de ERG a partir desses fotorreceptores. • Distrofia de cones e bastonetes em cães da raça Dachshund de pelo curto — déficit visual em luz intensa com 6-7 semanas de vida; 60% dos cães acometidos exibem pupilas acentuadamente mióticas à luz. Os ERGs adaptados à luz revelam respostas reduzidas ou não registráveis dos cones. • Distrofia de cones e bastonetes em cães da raça Dachshund de pelo longo — grande variação dos sinais clínicos; desde cegueira no início do dia (madrugada) até leve déficit visual na luz do dia com 6-7 semanas de vida e respostas não registráveis dos cones e respostas reduzidas dos bastonetes ao exame de ERG. • Displasia de bastonetes e cones em gatos — acomete as raças Persa e Abissínio; revela dilatação pupilar com 2-3 semanas, nistagmo com 4-5 semanas, sinais oftalmoscópicos de degeneração da retina com 8 semanas e, mais tarde, cegueira diurna e noturna. • Distrofia da retina — acomete cães da raça Briard; mutação nula no gene RPE65; causa cegueira noturna congênita; ERGs não registráveis adaptados ao escuro; nistagmo e pupilas dilatadas; fundo ocular normal até a meia-idade. • Descolamento da retina — observado em conjunto com outras doenças hereditárias (p. ex., displasia da retina); verificado nas raças Labrador retriever, Bedlington terrier e Sealyham terrier, bem como em casos de anomalia do olho do Collie; frequentemente constatado com outros defeitos oculares; os sinais incluem pupilas amplamente dilatadas, irresponsivas aos estímulos luminosos; o descolamento completo resulta em cegueira. • Hipoplasia do nervo óptico — ocorrência esporádica como um defeito ocular congênito em cães e gatos; fundo hereditário em Poodle miniatura e toy; pode resultar em cegueira.

CAUSAS
• Genéticas. • Más-formações espontâneas. • Infecções e inflamações durante a prenhez. • Toxicidade durante a prenhez. • Deficiências nutricionais.

FATORES DE RISCO
É fator de risco acasalar cães ou gatos que sejam homozigotos ou heterozigotos para uma doença hereditária com herança recessiva ou animais acometidos cuja doença exibe um modo de herança dominante.

DIAGNÓSTICO

DIAGNÓSTICO DIFERENCIAL
• Processos infecciosos e inflamatórios nos anexos — podem mimetizar e mascarar anormalidades congênitas. • Cataratas induzidas em uma idade precoce e especialmente aquelas com evolução rápida — podem parecer congênitas. • Lesões oftálmicas pós-inflamatórias com sinequias — facilmente confundidas com MPP. • Tumores do segmento anterior ocular — podem ser confundidos com cistos da íris. • Retinopatia generalizada de origem inflamatória — pode se parecer com displasia de fotorreceptores associada à atrofia da retina; geralmente unilateral. • Descolamento da retina como resultado de traumatismo ou uveíte em cães jovens — pode parecer uma anormalidade congênita da retina neural. • Atrofia do nervo óptico causada por processo inflamatório — pode ser difícil diferenciar de uma hipoplasia congênita do nervo óptico.

DIAGNÓSTICO POR IMAGEM
• Tomografia de coerência óptica — para visualização *in vivo* das camadas da retina; recomendada em casos de descolamento da retina e distrofias de bastonetes/cones ou cones/bastonetes. • Ultrassonografia — possibilita o diagnóstico de anormalidades do cristalino e do segmento posterior ocular.

Anomalias Oculares Congênitas

MÉTODOS DIAGNÓSTICOS
• Exame com foco luminoso — permite o diagnóstico de anomalias dos anexos oculares, bem como dos segmentos anterior e posterior.
• Avaliação da produção lacrimal (uso de fitas do teste de lágrima de Schirmer) — realizar como rotina em casos de processos inflamatórios e infecciosos crônicos nos anexos. • Tonometria — indicada na suspeita de glaucoma. • Oftalmoscopia direta e/ou indireta e biomicroscopia — exames necessários para diagnosticar anormalidades de estruturas internas; examinar após a dilatação das pupilas; exames de difícil execução em pacientes com menos de 5 semanas de vida.
• Eletrorretinografia e potenciais evocados visuais — avaliação objetiva das funções da retina e dos trajetos visuais; exames efetuados em pacientes com 7-12 semanas de vida; a eletrorretinografia é diagnóstica em casos de displasias de bastonetes/cones e distrofias da retina do cão Briard.
• Angiografia — método diagnóstico de anomalias vasculares e outros distúrbios do segmento posterior ocular; a fluoresceína é utilizada por via IV para obtenção de imagens detalhadas da vasculatura retiniana e a indocianina verde para aquisição de informações sobre os vasos coroidais.

ACHADOS PATOLÓGICOS
• Ceratoconjuntivite seca congênita — consiste geralmente em uma ceratite com neovascularização, formação cicatricial e pigmentação corneanas; alterações inflamatórias conjuntivais; além disso, pode-se notar o desenvolvimento anormal ou a atrofia das glândulas lacrimais. • Glaucoma congênito — a buftalmia é comum, algumas vezes com luxação secundária do cristalino e adelgaçamento neurorretiniano; colapso do ângulo de filtração iridocorneano. • TVCHP e VPHP — variação de defeitos, desde pontos e placas retrolenticulares pigmentados até filamentos de tecido vascular, que passam pela cabeça do nervo óptico até à cápsula posterior do cristalino; com frequência, há defeitos da cápsula posterior do cristalino e formação de catarata. • Displasia da retina — pregueamento anormal da neurorretina; defeitos multifocais, muitas vezes, ao longo dos principais vasos sanguíneos no fundo tapetal central; em casos de defeito geográfico, verifica-se em geral uma área ampla e anormal, onde a retina se encontra saliente e o tecido circunjacente se apresenta hiperpigmentado e escoriado; algumas vezes, há descolamento completo da retina.
• Displasia de bastonetes e cones — anormalidades nos bastonetes e/ou nos cones nos segmentos interno e externo; degeneração de núcleos dos fotorreceptores. • Distrofia da retina em Briard — corpúsculos de inclusão lipoides e amplos no epitélio pigmentar retiniano, bem como desorganização e degeneração dos fotorreceptores com o passar do tempo. • Colobomas — incisura no tecido acometido com defeitos do segmento anterior; adelgaçamento da retina neural, na região da cabeça do nervo óptico ou próximo à sua borda em casos de defeitos do segmento posterior.
• Descolamento da retina — retina neural descolada a partir do epitélio pigmentar retiniano.
• Hipoplasia do nervo óptico — a cabeça desse nervo encontra-se avascular, escura, anormalmente pequena e circular.

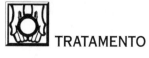 TRATAMENTO

CUIDADO(S) DE SAÚDE ADEQUADO(S)
• Os pacientes costumam ser encaminhados a um oftalmologista. • Não há nenhum tratamento clínico para grande parte das anormalidades congênitas, exceto tratamento sintomático ou cirurgia.

CUIDADO(S) DE ENFERMAGEM
• Em casos de ceratoconjuntivite seca — remoção das secreções e irrigação com soro fisiológico. • Os animais cegos não devem ter acesso à rua sem coleira e sem supervisão.

ATIVIDADE
Os animais cegos ou com diminuição da acuidade visual necessitam de níveis adequados de exercício.

DIETA
Fornecer uma dieta adequada em termos de vitaminas, antioxidantes e ácidos graxos ômega-3, especialmente em casos de degenerações de fotorreceptores.

ORIENTAÇÃO AO PROPRIETÁRIO
• Depende da anormalidade. • Discutir a capacidade visual, a possível evolução e as sequelas.

CONSIDERAÇÕES CIRÚRGICAS
• Dependem da anormalidade específica.
• Anormalidades dos anexos — efetuar a cirurgia o mais rápido possível. • Orifícios imperfurados — correção cirúrgica assim que a anestesia for segura.
• Ceratoconjuntivite seca congênita — transposição do ducto parotídeo. • Extração de catarata — a catarata congênita pode exibir outras anomalias indutoras de complicações cirúrgicas; há necessidade de avaliação pré-cirúrgica cuidadosa com a obtenção de imagens e exames de ERG.
• Glaucoma congênito — o procedimento de enucleação ou a aplicação de prótese intraesclerar constituem os tratamentos de escolha; em casos bilaterais, considerar a eutanásia.

 MEDICAÇÕES

MEDICAMENTO(S) DE ESCOLHA
• Ceratoconjuntivite seca congênita — substitutos lacrimais; aplicação frequente dos medicamentos; podem ser adicionados antibióticos ao tratamento; pomada oftálmica de ciclosporina a cada 12 h.
• Cataratas congênitas — quando envolver apenas a região nuclear do cristalino, pode-se lançar mão dos midriáticos para aumentar a capacidade visual.

PRECAUÇÕES
Os gatos são sensíveis à administração sistêmica de enrofloxacino (Baytril®) — é comprovado que esse medicamento provoca degeneração retiniana e cegueira nessa espécie quando administrado 10 vezes a dose normal.

MEDICAMENTO(S) ALTERNATIVO(S)
Uma alternativa ao uso de Optimmune® administrado a cada 12 h em casos de ceratoconjuntivite seca consiste na administração frequente de substitutos lacrimais.

 ACOMPANHAMENTO

MONITORIZAÇÃO DO PACIENTE
• Depende do defeito. • Ceratoconjuntivite seca congênita — requer monitorização frequente da produção lacrimal e do estado das estruturas oculares externas. • Cataratas congênitas e TVCHP/VPHP graves — avaliações regulares, geralmente a cada 6 meses; monitorizar a evolução. • Amplos defeitos colobomatosos do fundo ocular e displasia geográfica da retina — avaliações regulares para monitorizar possível descolamento da retina.

PREVENÇÃO
Restringir a reprodução de animais acometidos e de portadores conhecidos com defeitos hereditários registrados; notar que os testes à base de DNA estão disponíveis para certos defeitos de bastonetes, cones e epitélio pigmentar retiniano.

COMPLICAÇÕES POSSÍVEIS
• A cirurgia de catarata pode resultar em glaucoma, descolamento da retina e formação cicatricial na córnea em filhotes caninos e felinos; a cirurgia raramente é recomendada antes de 8-12 semanas de vida. • Na presença de más-formações graves das partes externas do olho, ficará difícil a correção total dos defeitos. • Em casos de ceratoconjuntivite congênita com transposição do ducto parotídeo, podem ocorrer ceratite e dermatite em função do depósito excessivo de minerais provenientes da saliva.

EVOLUÇÃO ESPERADA E PROGNÓSTICO
• A maioria das anormalidades que afetam os anexos oculares pode ser corrigida em cães e gatos jovens. • Em casos de ceratoconjuntivite seca congênita com transposição do ducto parotídeo, o prognóstico é bom. • O prognóstico em casos de glaucoma é mau.

 DIVERSOS

DISTÚRBIOS ASSOCIADOS
Displasia da retina — descrita em casos de anormalidades esqueléticas condrodisplásicas nas raças Labrador e Samoieda em experimentos a campo.

FATORES RELACIONADOS COM A IDADE
• Pequenos defeitos podem não necessitar de cirurgia; em alguns casos, é melhor esperar até que o filhote canino ou felino atinja a fase adulta, já que alguns defeitos podem sofrer correção espontânea. • Estar ciente de que o filhote canino ou felino crescerá e, consequentemente, todo o olho e seus anexos.

GESTAÇÃO/FERTILIDADE/REPRODUÇÃO
• Depende do defeito. • Os cães e gatos acometidos por anomalias oculares congênitas com cegueira e/ou dor não devem ser utilizados para fins reprodutivos. • Como muitas anomalias oculares congênitas são hereditárias, o uso dos animais acometidos na reprodução deve ser proibido ou submetido à restrição rigorosa. É recomendável a busca por orientação reprodutiva em canis ou associações de criadores.

ABREVIATURA(S)
• ERG = eletrorretinografia. • VPHP = vítreo primário hiperplásico persistente. • TVCHP = túnica vascular do cristalino hiperplásica persistente. • MPP = membranas pupilares persistentes.

Autor Kristina Narfström
Consultor Editorial Paul E. Miller

Anorexia

CONSIDERAÇÕES GERAIS

DEFINIÇÃO
Trata-se da falta ou perda do apetite pelo alimento; o apetite é psicológico e sua existência em animais é hipotética. Do ponto de vista fisiológico, a fome é estimulada pela necessidade corporal de alimento. A anorexia pode ser parcial ou completa. Além disso, a anorexia resulta em diminuição na ingestão alimentar, o que induz à perda de peso. A pseudoanorexia é associada mais à incapacidade de preensão ou deglutição do alimento e não à perda real do apetite.

FISIOPATOLOGIA
- O controle do apetite corresponde a uma interação complexa entre o sistema nervoso central e o periférico.
- O hipotálamo e o tronco encefálico contêm neurônios peptidérgicos reguladores da ingestão de alimento, que atuam como pontos de entrada para informações hormonais e gastrintestinais. Essas populações celulares projetam-se em diversas regiões cerebrais e sofrem uma extensa conexão.
- Os sinais periféricos que influenciam o apetite incluem a palatabilidade, a textura e a quantidade do alimento recém-consumido.
- A saciedade é influenciada pela distensão gástrica e duodenal, bem como pela presença de nutrientes no trato gastrintestinal.
- A fome é afetada pelas concentrações plasmáticas de glicose e ácidos graxos, em decorrência da interação com receptores específicos aos nutrientes, existentes no fígado e no trato gastrintestinal.
- A redução e o aumento no metabolismo oxidativo efetuado pelo fígado conduzem à fome e à saciedade, respectivamente.
- O comportamento aprendido e os ritmos circadianos modulam o apetite e podem sobrepujar outros sinais da saciedade e da fome.
- A leptina é produzida principalmente pelos adipócitos e atua sobre receptores hipotalâmicos específicos de modo a diminuir tanto o metabolismo como o apetite.
- O neuropeptídeo Y liberado a partir do trato gastrintestinal induz à fome e à hiperfagia, além de reduzir o gasto de energia após a restrição alimentar.
- A colecistocinina (CCK) e a bombesina liberadas a partir do trato gastrintestinal diminuem o apetite.
- A grelina produzida pelo estômago é um agente procinético, que diminui a produção de leptina e aumenta a produção do neuropeptídeo Y.
- A serotonina, um importante mediador da saciedade, possivelmente o último, atua por via central pelo trato serotoninérgico, que passa próximo ao hipotálamo ventromedial.
- Os tratos dopaminérgicos existentes no hipotálamo ajudam a regular a ingestão de alimento e estão intimamente associados ao hipotálamo lateral (centro clássico de controle da alimentação).
- O apetite é estimulado pela aldosterona e corticosterona, mas suprimido pelo glucagon e pela somatostatina.
- As doenças inflamatórias e neoplásicas podem levar à anorexia, pela liberação de citocinas pró-inflamatórias, como a interleucina-1, o fator de necrose tumoral e a interferona.
- Em pacientes com câncer, há uma perda frequente da suprarregulação esperada de ingestão alimentar em resposta ao gasto energético elevado.
- A queda no apetite associada ao envelhecimento, a assim denominada anorexia do envelhecimento, predispõe os pacientes mais idosos à desnutrição proteico-energética, sendo provavelmente mediada pela CCK e por um efeito acentuado de saciedade promovido pelos carboidratos no intestino delgado.
- As toxinas exógenas e endógenas (p. ex., insuficiência renal e hepática) causam anorexia.
- Qualquer distúrbio que diminua a excitabilidade cerebral reduzirá potencialmente a ingestão de alimento.
- A gastroparesia, associada à neoplasia, a distúrbios metabólicos e à doença gastrintestinal primária, está relacionada com redução no apetite.
- Medo, dor e estresse podem diminuir o apetite.

SISTEMA(S) ACOMETIDO(S)
Todos os sistemas corporais.

IDENTIFICAÇÃO
Espécies
Cães e gatos.
Raça(s) Predominante(s)
N/D.
Idade Média e Faixa Etária
N/D.
Sexo(s) Predominante(s)
N/D.

SINAIS CLÍNICOS
Achados Anamnésicos
- A recusa em se alimentar é uma queixa comum apresentada pelos proprietários de pequenos animais, pois o apetite reduzido está fortemente associado a doenças.
- Os pacientes com distúrbios indutores de disfunção ou dor em regiões como face, pescoço, orofaringe e esôfago podem exibir interesse pelo alimento, mas não conseguem se alimentar. Esses pacientes são denominados como pseudoanoréticos.
- Os animais com perda do olfato (anosmia) muitas vezes não demonstram o sinal de farejamento.
- Pode-se notar a perda de peso.

Achados do Exame Físico
- Na anorexia, os sinais clínicos variam dependendo da causa subjacente, mas incluem febre, palidez, icterícia, dor, alterações no volume do órgão, anormalidades oculares, distensão abdominal, dispneia, sons cardíacos e ruídos pulmonares abafados, ruídos pulmonares adventícios (casuais), sopros cardíacos e massas.
- Os pacientes pseudoanoréticos costumam exibir perda de peso, halitose, salivação excessiva, dificuldade de preensão e mastigação do alimento, além de odinofagia (dor à deglutição).

CAUSAS
Anorexia
- Quase todo processo patológico sistêmico pode causar anorexia.
- Psicológica — dieta não palatável, aversão ao alimento, estresse, alterações na rotina e no ambiente.
- Distúrbios acidobásicos.
- Insuficiência cardíaca.
- Intoxicações e medicamentos.
- Dor.
- Endocrinopatia e doença metabólica.
- Neoplasia.
- Doença infecciosa.
- Doença imunomediada.
- Doença respiratória.
- Gastrenteropatia.
- Doença musculoesquelética.
- Doença neurológica.
- Anorexia do envelhecimento.
- Diversas; por exemplo, doença do movimento (cinetose) e temperatura ambiente elevada.

Pseudoanorexia
- Qualquer doença indutora de dor ou disfunção na preensão, mastigação e deglutição.
- Estomatite, glossite, gengivite, faringite e esofagite (p. ex., agentes físicos, substâncias cáusticas, infecções bacterianas ou virais, corpos estranhos, doenças imunomediadas e uremia).
- Distúrbios retrofaríngeos (p. ex., linfadenopatia, abscesso, hematoma e sialocele).
- Doença dentária ou doença periodontal.
- Abscesso retrobulbar.
- Neoplasia bucal, glossal, faríngea ou esofágica.
- Distúrbios neurológicos (p. ex., raiva; neuropatias dos V, VII, IX, X e XII pares de nervos cranianos e lesões do sistema nervoso central).
- Lesões musculoesqueléticas (p. ex., miosite mastigatória, artropatia temporomandibular, fraturas, osteopatia craniomandibular, miastenia grave, botulismo e acalasia cricofaríngea).
- Neoplasia ou inflamação das glândulas salivares.

FATORES DE RISCO
N/D.

DIAGNÓSTICO

DIAGNÓSTICO DIFERENCIAL
- Questionar os proprietários a respeito do interesse do paciente pelo alimento, bem como da capacidade de preensão, mastigação e deglutição do alimento.
- Efetuar exame oftalmológico, dentário, orofaríngeo, facial e cervical completo (para tanto, talvez haja necessidade de sedação ou anestesia), além de inspecionar a ingestão de alimento pelo paciente para descartar a pseudoanorexia.
- Trazer à tona um histórico detalhado, considerando itens como: ambiente, dieta, mudanças na rotina, presença de pessoas ou existência de outros animais domésticos, para ajudar a identificar as etiologias psicológicas em potencial.
- Para determinar a presença de doença sistêmica, há necessidade de um exame físico completo.
- Para a formulação do diagnóstico definitivo, com frequência é imprescindível a coleta de um banco de dados, incluindo hemograma completo, perfil bioquímico sérico, urinálise, sorologia para dirofilariose e para retrovírus, estudos conduzidos com base na obtenção de imagens torácica e abdominal, além de endoscopia e histologia/citologia de amostras teciduais/celulares.
- É recomendável a abstenção de uma conduta diagnóstica extra apenas se a anamnese, o exame físico e o banco de dados forem fortemente sugestivos de anorexia psicológica; em tais casos, o contato diário com o proprietário do animal de estimação é essencial até que a anorexia desapareça.

HEMOGRAMA/BIOQUÍMICA/URINÁLISE
• As anormalidades variam com diferentes doenças subjacentes e causas de pseudoanorexia e anorexia.
• Podem permanecer normais em pacientes com causas clínicas, bem como psicológicas, de anorexia.

OUTROS TESTES LABORATORIAIS
Pode haver a necessidade de testes diagnósticos especiais para descartar doenças específicas sugeridas pela anamnese, pelo exame físico e por testes preliminares.

DIAGNÓSTICO POR IMAGEM
• Com frequência, os estudos (radiográficos e ultrassonográficos) para a obtenção de imagens torácicas e abdominais são incluídos no banco de dados mínimo com o objetivo de detectar as anormalidades anatômicas.
• A fluoroscopia pode ser indicada para avaliar especificamente a função faríngea e esofágica.

MÉTODOS DIAGNÓSTICOS
• Variam com a condição subjacente sob suspeita.
• A endoscopia pode ser útil para a visualização das estruturas faríngeas e esofágicas.

TRATAMENTO
• A base do tratamento visa identificar e corrigir a doença subjacente.
• A terapia sintomática envolve uma atenção especial para os distúrbios hidreletrolíticos, a redução de fatores ambientais indutores de estresse e a mudança da dieta para melhorar a palatabilidade.
• A palatabilidade pode ser melhorada, adicionando-se flavorizantes (como caldos de galinha ou de carne bovina), temperando-se com condimentos como alho em pó, aumentando-se o teor lipídico ou proteico do alimento e aquecendo o alimento à temperatura corporal.
• Como regra geral, cães e gatos com doença debilitante não devem ficar sem alimento por mais de 3-5 dias antes de se utilizar uma alimentação enteral ou parenteral.
• A decisão de instituir a alimentação enteral ou parenteral pode ser influenciada por vários fatores. Em animais com perda de peso ≥10%, hipoalbuminemia, linfopenia, escore de condição corporal mais baixo e processos patológicos crônicos, deve-se considerar a suplementação nutricional.
• As técnicas de fornecimento de nutrição enteral incluem alimentação forçada e colocação de sondas nasoesofágicas ou via esofagostomia, gastrostomia ou jejunostomia.

MEDICAÇÕES
MEDICAMENTO(S) DE ESCOLHA
• O diazepam é um estimulante do apetite, de curta ação, com propriedades sedativas, utilizado na dose de 0,1 mg/kg IV diariamente ou 1 mg VO uma vez ao dia em gatos.
• O oxazepam (2 mg/gato VO a cada 12 h) é um estimulante do apetite e sedativo, de curta ação.
• A ciproeptadina, um anti-histamínico com propriedades antisserotoninérgicas, foi utilizada como estimulante de apetite com sucesso variável em uma dosagem de 0,2-0,4 mg/kg VO, 10-20 min antes da refeição.
• Os analgésicos podem estimular o apetite em condições dolorosas.
• A metoclopramida (0,2-0,4 mg/kg SC ou VO), a ranitidina (2 mg/kg SC, IV ou VO) ou a eritromicina (0,5-1,0 mg/kg VO) serão úteis se a anorexia estiver associada à gastroparesia ou ao íleo.
• Os antieméticos, como a proclorperazina (0,1-0,5 mg/kg VO) ou a metoclopramida, são benéficos para diminuir a anorexia associada à náusea.

CONTRAINDICAÇÕES
• Evitar os antieméticos na suspeita ou existência de obstrução gastrintestinal.
• Os medicamentos com propriedades sedativas devem ser usados com cuidado em animais gravemente debilitados.

PRECAUÇÕES
N/D.

INTERAÇÕES POSSÍVEIS
N/D.

MEDICAMENTO(S) ALTERNATIVO(S)
N/D.

ACOMPANHAMENTO
MONITORIZAÇÃO DO PACIENTE
• Mensuração do peso corporal, avaliação do escore da condição corporal e determinação da hidratação.
• Retorno do apetite.

PREVENÇÃO
Fornecer uma dieta altamente palatável.

COMPLICAÇÕES POSSÍVEIS
• Desidratação, desnutrição e caquexia são as mais prováveis; essas complicações exacerbam a doença subjacente.
• Uma perda de mais de 25-30% da proteína corporal compromete o sistema imune e a força muscular, resultando no óbito por infecção e/ou insuficiência pulmonar.
• A lipidose hepática felina é uma possível complicação de anorexia em gatos obesos.
• A ruptura da barreira da mucosa intestinal é preocupante em pacientes debilitados.

EVOLUÇÃO ESPERADA E PROGNÓSTICO
Variam com a causa subjacente.

DIVERSOS
DISTÚRBIOS ASSOCIADOS
N/D.

FATORES RELACIONADOS COM A IDADE
Pode haver a necessidade de suporte nutricional e/ou do fornecimento de fluidos que contenham glicose para tratar ou evitar a hipoglicemia em filhotes caninos e felinos anoréticos.

POTENCIAL ZOONÓTICO
N/D.

GESTAÇÃO/FERTILIDADE/REPRODUÇÃO
N/D.

SINÔNIMO(S)
N/D.

VER TAMBÉM
Ver a seção "Causas".

ABREVIATURA(S)
• CCK = colecistocinina.

Sugestões de Leitura
Guilford WG. Nutritional management of gastrointestinal diseases. In: Guilford WG, Center SA, Strombeck DR, et al., eds., Strombeck's Small Animal Gastroenterology, 3rd ed. Philadelphia: Saunders, 1996, pp. 889-910.
Hoover JP, Monroe WE. Anorexia. In: Ettinger SJ, Feldman EC, eds., Veterinary Internal Medicine, 6th ed. Philadelphia: Elsevier Saunders, 2005, pp. 117-119.
Monroe WE. Anorexia and polyphagia. In: Ettinger SJ, Feldman EC, eds., Veterinary Internal Medicine, 5th ed. Philadelphia: Saunders, 2000, pp. 102-104.
Remillard RL, Armstrong PJ, et al. Assisted feeding in hospitalized patients: Enteral and parenteral nutrition. In: Hand MS, Thatcher CD, Remillard RL, et al., eds., Small Animal Clinical Nutrition, 4th ed. Topeka, KS: Mark Morris Institute, 2000, pp. 351-399.

Autor Elizabeth M. Streeter
Consultor Editorial Albert E. Jergens

Anormalidades dos Espermatozoides

CONSIDERAÇÕES GERAIS

REVISÃO
• Teratozoospermia — presença de quantidades significativas de anormalidades dos espermatozoides; considera-se a existência desse distúrbio quando as anormalidades dos espermatozoides forem iguais ou superiores a 40% no ejaculado; o efeito de anormalidades específicas sobre a fertilidade é basicamente desconhecido.
• Espera-se uma fertilidade ideal nos cães com, no mínimo, 80% de espermatozoides morfologicamente normais. • Elevada porcentagem de anormalidades nos espermatozoides pode causar infertilidade; espera-se um declínio na fertilidade nos cães com ≥40% de anormalidades no ejaculado. • Alguns gatos férteis inerentemente apresentam ≥40% de anormalidades nos espermatozoides. • As anormalidades dos espermatozoides, às vezes, são classificadas em defeitos primários e secundários; os defeitos primários ocorrem durante a espermatogênese, enquanto os secundários durante o transporte e o armazenamento dentro do epidídimo ou por manipulação inadequada do sêmen.

IDENTIFICAÇÃO
• Cães e gatos de qualquer idade; é mais provável que cães e gatos mais idosos tenham outras doenças ou condições relacionadas com a idade acometendo a qualidade geral do esperma. • Não há nenhuma predileção racial nos cães nem nos gatos; relata-se que os cães da raça Wolfhound irlandês possuem qualidade do sêmen significantemente mais baixa do que os cães de outras raças. • Cães da raça Springer spaniel inglês acometidos com fucosidose. • Cães acometidos com discinesia ciliar primária.

SINAIS CLÍNICOS
• Constatação de infertilidade após acasalamento sincronizado de forma adequada com diversas cadelas comprovadamente férteis. • Encontro de anormalidades dos espermatozoides durante avaliação reprodutiva de rotina.

CAUSAS E FATORES DE RISCO
Congênitas
• Cães com fucosidose — doença do armazenamento lisossomal provocada pela deficiência da enzima α-L-fucosidase; os processos de espermatogênese (defeitos acrossômicos) e maturação espermática (retenção de gotículas proximais) ficam comprometidos; cães da raça Springer spaniel inglês — padrão de herança autossômica recessiva. • Discinesia ciliar primária — anormalidade ultraestrutural dos cílios, provocando ausência de motilidade ou motilidade anormal das células ciliadas; os animais acometidos são inférteis; relatada em muitas raças; provável herança autossômica recessiva. • Idiopática — nos cães, além de gatos com morfologia espermática inerente ruim. • Hipoplasia testicular — machos felinos com pelagem casco de tartaruga ou *calico*.
• Consanguinidade excessiva — a consanguinidade em gatos domésticos gerou uma redução significativa na porcentagem de células morfologicamente normais dentro de uma única geração; as espécies de gatos selvagens com perda da diversidade genética sofrem aumento na teratozoospermia e declínio na fertilidade.

Adquiridas
• Condições que interrompem a termorregulação testicular normal — traumatismo; hematocele; hidrocele; orquite; epididimite; febre prolongada secundária a infecções sistêmicas; obesidade (aumento da gordura escrotal); animal não adaptado a temperaturas ambientais elevadas; exaustão pelo calor induzida por exercício; época do ano (meses do verão). • Infecções do trato reprodutivo — prostatite; brucelose; orquite; epididimite. • Medicamentos — esteroides anabolizantes; androgênios; estrogênios; progestogênios; corticosteroides; agentes quimioterápicos; cetoconazol; anfotericina B; cimetidina; fitoestrogênio (coumestrol); análogos do GnRH (acilina); injeções intratesticulares de arginina zíncica. • Neoplasia testicular.
• Abstinência sexual prolongada. • Utilização exagerada. • Degeneração testicular.

DIAGNÓSTICO

DIAGNÓSTICO DIFERENCIAL
Número excessivo de caudas torcidas ou espiraladas dos espermatozoides pode representar artefatos iatrogênicos provocados pela coloração; reavaliar a amostra em microscópio de contraste de fase após a diluição com solução salina tamponada com fosfato de formalina.

OUTROS TESTES LABORATORIAIS
• Perfil hormonal — as concentrações de gonadotropina (FSH) e de hormônios esteroides no plasma ou no soro devem ser determinadas para descartar endocrinopatias. • Ejaculados azoospérmicos (ausência de células espermáticas) — devem ser examinados quanto à presença de fosfatase alcalina para confirmar a azoospermia; ejaculados completos possuem >5.000 U/L de fosfatase alcalina. • Teste de aglutinação rápida em lâmina para pesquisa de brucelose — utilizado como um método de triagem; sensível, porém inespecífico (D-Tec CB®, Synbiotics Corp.); é recomendável reavaliar os cães que exibem resultados positivos na lâmina com o teste de imunodifusão em ágar gel (Cornell University Diagnostic Laboratory) ou, então, com a cultura bacteriana do sangue total ou o aspirado de linfonodo.

DIAGNÓSTICO POR IMAGEM
Ultrassonografia — valiosa para diagnosticar condições que possam afetar a morfologia do esperma, como tumores testiculares, orquite, hidrocele, hematocele, espermatocele.

MÉTODOS DIAGNÓSTICOS
• Avaliação à microscopia óptica de lâmina montada a seco — coloração com eosina-nigrosina (corante da Society for Theriogenology; Lane Manufacturing, Denver, CO) ou coloração de Giemsa modificada (Diff-Quik®; Baxter Healthcare, Deerfield, IL) são utilizadas para corar os espermatozoides; recomendam-se o uso de corante preaquecido e o preparo das lâminas sobre uma lâmina mais quente; a secagem mais rápida diminui a incidência de artefatos como caudas torcidas ou espiraladas; uma quantidade de, no mínimo, 100 (de preferência, 200) células espermáticas é contada com aumento de 1.000 ×.
• Coloração do acrossomo — o dano a essa estrutura pode ser avaliado com a coloração azul de Coomassie ou a coloração Spermac (Conception Technologies, San Diego, CA), comercializadas para esperma humano, embora funcionem muito bem para esperma canino. • Microscopia óptica de contraste de fase ou de contraste por interferência diferencial de lâmina preparada em câmara úmida — amostras diluídas com solução salina tamponada com fosfato de formalina; verificar se a alta porcentagem de caudas torcidas ou espiraladas observadas na lâmina corada se deve a algum artefato na coloração.

ACHADOS PATOLÓGICOS
• Biopsia — biopsia incisional ou aspirado testicular obtido por agulha fina para determinar o estado da espermatogênese. • Ausência de espermátides ou de espermatócitos — espermatogênese comprometida. • Neoplasia.
• Inflamação — acúmulo linfocitário peritubular.
• Alterações degenerativas. • Hipoplasia.

TRATAMENTO
• Não existe tratamento específico para as anormalidades dos espermatozoides; quando aplicável, a doença ou condição subjacente deve ser tratada de acordo. • Antibióticos e agentes anti-inflamatórios nas doenças infecciosas.
• Orquiectomia unilateral para tumores testiculares unilaterais ou orquite grave. • Repouso sexual em caso de edema ou hematocele associados a traumatismo. • Coleta frequente do sêmen pode melhorar temporariamente a qualidade do esperma nos cães ou gatos com teratozoospermia idiopática. • Remover o cão ou o gato dos ambientes que causem estresse pelo calor extremo.
• Alterar o programa de exercícios para reduzir o estresse pelo calor.

MEDICAÇÕES

CONTRAINDICAÇÕES
• Hormônios exógenos — esteroides anabolizantes; estrogênios; testosterona; progestogênios. • Glicocorticoides. • Agentes quimioterápicos. • Cetoconazol; anfotericina B.
• Cimetidina.

ACOMPANHAMENTO

MONITORIZAÇÃO DO PACIENTE
• Caso se identifique e trate alguma causa subjacente, a avaliação espermática deverá ser realizada 30 e 70 dias após a resolução do problema. • Nos casos atribuídos a causas reversíveis, a melhora completa na morfologia espermática não ocorre antes dos 70 dias (aproximadamente a duração de um completo ciclo espermatogênico).

PREVENÇÃO
• Ambiente com clima controlado para os animais não adaptados a temperaturas ambientais elevadas.
• Evitar a exaustão pelo calor durante a prática de exercício ou banho e tosa.

DIVERSOS

ABREVIATURA(S)
• FSH = hormônio foliculoestimulante.
• GnRH = hormônio liberador de gonadotropina.

Autor Carlos R. F. Pinto
Consultor Editorial Sara K. Lyle

Antidepressivos — Toxicose por Antidepressivos Tricíclicos (ATC)

CONSIDERAÇÕES GERAIS

DEFINIÇÃO
- Toxicidade secundária à ingestão aguda ou crônica de algum antidepressivo tricíclico.
- Os ATC incluem amitriptilina, amoxapina, clomipramina, desipramina, doxepina, imipramina, maprotilina (antidepressivo tetracíclico), nortriptilina, protriptilina, e trimipramina.

FISIOPATOLOGIA
- Os ATC bloqueiam a recaptação de norepinefrina, dopamina e serotonina na membrana neuronal. Além de possuírem atividade anticolinérgica, acredita-se que os ATC exerçam efeitos estabilizantes de membrana sobre o miocárdio (particularmente inibindo os canais rápidos de sódio no miocárdio ventricular). Também podem ter leve atividade de bloqueio alfa-adrenérgico e efeitos anti-histamínicos.
- Os ATC são rapidamente e bem absorvidos pelo trato digestório. Tais agentes podem diminuir a motilidade GI e retardar o esvaziamento gástrico, resultando em absorção medicamentosa tardia.
- Esses antidepressivos são lipofílicos, ligados a proteínas e bem distribuídos por todos os tecidos.
- São metabolizados pelo fígado e sofrem recirculação enteroepática. Os metabólitos inativos são eliminados na urina.

SISTEMA(S) ACOMETIDO(S)
- Cardiovascular — os efeitos anticolinérgicos e a inibição da recaptação de norepinefrina contribuem para a taquicardia; o bloqueio alfa-adrenérgico, a estabilização da membrana cardíaca e a diminuição da contratilidade cardíaca contribuem para o desenvolvimento de hipotensão e arritmias.
- Gastrintestinal — os efeitos anticolinérgicos podem causar íleo paralítico e retardo do esvaziamento gástrico.
- Nervoso — o aumento dos níveis de dopamina, serotonina e norepinefrina no SNC contribui para os sinais neurológicos.
- Oftálmico — os efeitos anticolinérgicos podem causar dilatação pupilar.
- Renal/Urológico — os efeitos anticolinérgicos podem provocar retenção urinária.

GENÉTICA
Diferenças individuais e entre as espécies em termos de absorção, metabolismo e eliminação podem ser significativas.

INCIDÊNCIA/PREVALÊNCIA
A incidência é desconhecida.

DISTRIBUIÇÃO GEOGRÁFICA
N/D.

IDENTIFICAÇÃO
Espécies
Cães e gatos.

Raça(s) Predominante(s)
Nenhuma.

Idade Média e Faixa Etária
Nenhuma.

Sexo Predominante
Nenhum.

SINAIS CLÍNICOS
Comentários Gerais
- É possível a observação dos sinais com doses terapêuticas.
- Os sinais de toxicidade podem ser observados em até 30-60 minutos ou adiados por várias horas.

Achados Anamnésicos
- Evidência de consumo acidental do medicamento do proprietário ou de algum outro animal de estimação.
- Depressão do SNC (letargia, ataxia).
- Vocalização.
- Vômito ou hipersalivação.
- Respiração ofegante.
- Agitação ou inquietação.
- Taquipneia ou dispneia.
- Tremores.
- Crises convulsivas.

Achados do Exame Físico
- Depressão ou estimulação do SNC.
- Taquicardia.
- Midríase.
- Hipotermia.
- Hipertensão.
- Palidez.
- Cianose.
- Hipertermia.
- Arritmias.
- Hipotensão.
- Retenção urinária.
- Constipação.

CAUSAS
Exposição acidental, administração inadequada, ou uso terapêutico.

FATORES DE RISCO
- Uso concomitante de outros medicamentos antipsicóticos.
- Cardiopatia preexistente.

DIAGNÓSTICO

DIAGNÓSTICO DIFERENCIAL
- Toxicidade causada por outros medicamentos antipsicóticos, substâncias estimulantes (p. ex., anfetaminas, cocaína, metilxantinas, ou pseudoefedrina) ou substâncias capazes de causar arritmias cardíacas (p. ex., quinidina, propranolol, albuterol, digoxina).
- Os diferenciais não toxicológicos incluem hipercalemia, isquemia cardíaca, miocardiopatia e outros distúrbios de condução cardíaca.

HEMOGRAMA/BIOQUÍMICA/URINÁLISE
Supostamente normais.

OUTROS TESTES LABORATORIAIS
- Gasometria sanguínea — pode-se observar acidose metabólica.
- Triagem de medicamentos de venda livre na urina para detecção de ATC — pode ser usada para determinar a ocorrência de exposição.
- Níveis séricos de ATC — podem ser mensurados para determinar a ocorrência de exposição; não é útil para determinar o grau de toxicidade.

DIAGNÓSTICO POR IMAGEM
N/D

MÉTODOS DIAGNÓSTICOS
- ECG para monitorizar a presença de arritmias.
- Monitorização da pressão arterial.

ACHADOS PATOLÓGICOS
Não se esperam lesões específicas.

TRATAMENTO

CUIDADO(S) DE SAÚDE ADEQUADO(S)
- Tratamento ambulatorial — não recomendado para os pacientes sintomáticos, cardiopatas ou aqueles que ingeriram uma dose de ATC maior que a terapêutica.
- Tratamento hospitalar — em pacientes assintomáticos:
  ○ Descontaminação com êmese (menos de 15 minutos da exposição), lavagem gástrica em exposições volumosas, e carvão ativado.
  ○ Monitorizar em uma clínica por, no mínimo, 6 horas após a exposição.
- Tratamento hospitalar — em pacientes sintomáticos — estabilizar os sistemas cardiovascular e neurológico (SNC), além de fornecer cuidados de suporte.

CUIDADO(S) DE ENFERMAGEM
- Fluidoterapia — restabelecer a hidratação em virtude do vômito e regular a pressão arterial na presença de hipotensão.
- Termorregulação, conforme a necessidade.
- Enema com água tépida (morna) se o animal não defecar em até 6-12 horas.

ATIVIDADE
N/D.

DIETA
Nada por via oral na presença de vômito.

ORIENTAÇÃO AO PROPRIETÁRIO
- Com um ATC de prescrição médica, orientar o proprietário a monitorizar a ocorrência de efeitos adversos ou idiossincráticos, bem como a interromper a medicação e entrar em contato com o médico se eles ocorrerem.
- Evitar a exposição a medicamento de venda livre, ou seja, adquiridos sem prescrição médica.

CONSIDERAÇÕES CIRÚRGICAS
N/D.

MEDICAÇÕES

MEDICAMENTO(S) DE ESCOLHA
Descontaminação
- Êmese dentro de 15 minutos da ingestão *somente em paciente assintomático*; induzir à êmese com peróxido de hidrogênio ou apomorfina.
- A lavagem gástrica sob anestesia pode ser considerada em caso de grandes exposições.
- Após a êmese (ou se transcorridos >15 minutos da exposição), administrar carvão ativado (1-2 g/kg VO) com um catártico como sorbitol (sorbitol a 70% na dose de 3 mL/kg) ou sulfato de sódio (0,25 colher das de chá/5 kg) na ausência de diarreia.
- Repetir metade da dose do carvão ativado em 4-6 horas se o paciente ainda estiver sintomático.

Outros
- Ciproeptadina: cães, 1,1 mg/kg a cada 6 h VO ou por via retal; gatos, 2-4 mg/gato a cada 6 h VO ou por via retal; usada para o tratamento de síndrome serotoninérgica.
- Bicarbonato de sódio — utilizado para manter o pH sanguíneo a 7,55; sem a monitorização do estado acidobásico, começar com 2-3 mEq/kg IV durante 15-30 minutos em um paciente sintomático.

Antidepressivos — Toxicose por Antidepressivos Tricíclicos (ATC)

- Diazepam 0,5-1 mg/kg IV, repetir se houver necessidade; para agitação ou crises convulsivas.
- Acepromazina 0,02 mg/kg IV, repetir se houver necessidade; para agitação ou leve hipertensão.
- Fenobarbital — conforme a necessidade para controle das crises convulsivas.

CONTRAINDICAÇÕES
- Não é recomendável o uso da atropina, pois os ATC possuem efeitos anticolinérgicos que são exacerbados por esse medicamento.
- O sulfato de magnésio não deve ser usado como um catártico. A presença de íleo paralítico ou a redução da motilidade gástrica aumentará a absorção do magnésio, podendo resultar em toxicidade por esse elemento químico.
- β-bloqueadores (p. ex., propranolol, atenolol) não devem ser usados para taquicardia por causa de seu potencial de exacerbação da hipotensão.
- Não induzir à êmese em paciente que já está exibindo sinais clínicos.

PRECAUÇÕES
N/D.

INTERAÇÕES POSSÍVEIS
- Os ATC aumentam o risco de hipertermia, crises convulsivas e morte com o uso de inibidores da MAO.
- Medicamentos simpaticomiméticos e anticolinérgicos aumentam o risco de arritmias ou efeitos cardíacos pelos ATC.
- A levotiroxina aumenta o risco de arritmias quando utilizada com ATC.

MEDICAMENTO(S) ALTERNATIVO(S)
N/D.

ACOMPANHAMENTO

MONITORIZAÇÃO DO PACIENTE
- Estado acidobásico — monitorizar o paciente quanto à ocorrência de acidose e em caso de implementação da terapia com bicarbonato de sódio.
- Pressão arterial — monitorizar até que o paciente se torne assintomático.
- ECG — monitorizar até que o paciente fique assintomático.

PREVENÇÃO
Manter os medicamentos fora do alcance dos animais de estimação.

COMPLICAÇÕES POSSÍVEIS
Pode ocorrer edema pulmonar secundário à fluidoterapia rigorosa.

EVOLUÇÃO ESPERADA E PROGNÓSTICO
- Em virtude da variação da meia-vida dos diferentes ATC, os sinais podem durar 24 horas ou mais.
- O prognóstico é geralmente bom em pacientes que exibem sinais leves a moderados.
- O prognóstico é reservado em pacientes que exibem sinais graves, como crises convulsivas, arritmias, ou hipotensão pouco responsivas à terapia.

DIVERSOS

DISTÚRBIOS ASSOCIADOS
Pode ocorrer síndrome serotoninérgica como resultado da ingestão de ATC.

FATORES RELACIONADOS COM A IDADE
Nenhum.

POTENCIAL ZOONÓTICO
Nenhum.

GESTAÇÃO/FERTILIDADE/REPRODUÇÃO
Os ATC atravessam a placenta e podem ser encontrados no leite materno; até o momento, o significado disso não é conhecido.

VER TAMBÉM
- Antidepressivos — Toxicose por Inibidores Seletivos de Recaptação da Serotonina (ISRS).
- Envenenamento (Intoxicação).

ABREVIATURA(S)
- ATC = antidepressivo tricíclico.
- ECG = eletrocardiograma.
- GI = gastrintestinal.
- MAO = monoamina oxidase.
- SNC = sistema nervoso central.

RECURSOS DA INTERNET
http://www.aspcapro.org/animal-poison-control-center-articles.php.

Sugestões de Leitura
Gwaltney-Brant S. Antidepressants: Tricyclic antidepressants. In: Plumlee KH, ed., Clinical Veterinary Toxicology. St. Louis: Mosby, 2004, pp. 286-288.
Johnson LR. Tricyclic antidepressant toxicosis. Vet Clin North Am Small Anim Pract 1990, 20:393-403.
Volmer PA. "Recreational" drugs: Tricyclic antidepressants. In: Peterson ME, Talcott PA, eds., Small Animal Toxicology, 2nd ed. St. Louis: Saunders Elsevier, 2006, pp. 303-306.
Wismer TA. Antidepressant drug overdoses in dogs. Vet Med 2000, 95:520-525.

Autor Cristine L. Hayes
Consultor Editorial Gary D. Osweiler

Antidepressivos — Toxicose por Inibidor Seletivo de Recaptação da Serotonina (ISRS)

CONSIDERAÇÕES GERAIS

DEFINIÇÃO
- Toxicidade secundária à dosagem excessiva de algum inibidor seletivo de recaptação da serotonina (ISRS) ou coingestação de dois tipos de medicamentos serotoninérgicos. • Os ISRSs incluem citalopram (Celexa®), escitalopram (Lexapro®), fluoxetina (Prozac®), fluvoxamina (Luvox®), paroxetina (Paxil®), sertralina (Zoloft®)

FISIOPATOLOGIA
- Os ISRSs constituem uma classe de antidepressivos que inibem a recaptação de serotonina, um neurotransmissor envolvido em agressividade, ansiedade, apetite, depressão, enxaqueca, dor e sono. • A estimulação excessiva de receptores serotoninérgicos pode ocorrer por intensificação da síntese de serotonina, aumento da liberação pré-sináptica de serotonina, inibição da captação de serotonina pelo neurônio pré-sináptico, inibição do metabolismo de serotonina ou agonismo da serotonina. A síndrome serotoninérgica é caracterizada em seres humanos como uma combinação de sintomas que incluem, pelo menos, três dos itens a seguir: mioclonia, aberração mental, agitação, hiper-reflexia, tremores, diarreia, ataxia, ou hipertermia. • As dosagens tóxicas variam muito entre os ISRSs comumente disponíveis e não são bem definidas na medicina veterinária.

SISTEMA(S) ACOMETIDO(S)
- Cardiovascular — diminuição do tônus vascular (hipotensão), aumento da frequência cardíaca e do volume sistólico (taquicardia). • Gastrintestinal — aumento da contratilidade dos músculos lisos (vômito, diarreia). • Nervoso — estimulação (agitação, inquietação, crises convulsivas) e alteração do estado mental (vocalização, desorientação). • Neuromuscular — disfunção autonômica (hiperatividade) e hiperatividade neuromuscular (hiper-reflexia, mioclonia, tremores). • Oftálmico — aumento da função autonômica (midríase). • Respiratório — aumento da contração da musculatura lisa dos brônquios (dispneia).

INCIDÊNCIA/PREVALÊNCIA
Aumento na incidência em virtude do uso crescente de medicamentos serotoninérgicos.

IDENTIFICAÇÃO
Espécies
Cães e gatos.

Idade Média e Faixa Etária
Qualquer idade pode ser acometida.

SINAIS CLÍNICOS
Achados Anamnésicos
- Agitação ou letargia. • Pupilas dilatadas. • Vômito. • Tremores. • Hipersalivação. • Diarreia. • Crises convulsivas. • Nistagmo.

Achados do Exame Físico
- Agitação. • Ataxia. • Midríase. • Tremores. • Vômito. • Desorientação. • Hipertermia. • Vocalização. • Depressão. • Taquicardia. • Hipotensão. • Diarreia. • Cegueira. • Crises convulsivas. • Hipersalivação. • Morte.

CAUSAS
- Dosagem excessiva de ISRS — exposição acidental, administração inadequada, ou uso terapêutico. • Ingestão de algum ISRS juntamente com alguma outra classe de medicamentos que aumente a serotonina (ATCs, IRSNs, inibidores da MAO, antidepressivos recentes, tramadol, fentanila, meperidina, anfetaminas, cocaína, dextrometorfano, 5-HTP, buspirona, bupropiona, triptanas, LSD).

FATORES DE RISCO
- Animais sob algum medicamento serotoninérgico. • Doença renal ou hepática subjacente.

DIAGNÓSTICO

DIAGNÓSTICO DIFERENCIAL
- Toxicológico: ATCs, IRSNs, inibidores da MAO, metaldeído, chumbo, etileno glicol, lúpulo, anticolinérgicos, anti-histamínicos. • Não toxicológico: meningite (p. ex., raiva, cinomose canina), neoplasia, intermação, hipertermia maligna.

HEMOGRAMA/BIOQUÍMICA/URINÁLISE
- Hemograma e bioquímica: não se esperam quaisquer alterações. • Urinálise: pode ser observada mioglobinúria secundária à rabdomiólise.

OUTROS TESTES LABORATORIAIS
- Gasometria sanguínea: pode ser observada acidose metabólica. • Podem ser realizados testes para detecção de ISRSs, mas esses testes não são clinicamente úteis.

MÉTODOS DIAGNÓSTICOS
Não há testes diagnósticos para confirmar a síndrome serotoninérgica.

TRATAMENTO

CUIDADO(S) DE SAÚDE ADEQUADO(S)
- Êmese (em casos assintomáticos e ingestão recente) ou lavagem gástrica (na ingestão de grande número de comprimidos). • Carvão ativado com catárticos (talvez haja necessidade de repetição em função da meia-vida longa de grande parte desses medicamentos).

CUIDADO(S) DE ENFERMAGEM
Fluidos IV não só para ajudar a manter a pressão arterial e a temperatura corporal, mas também para proteger os rins contra mioglobinúria.

ORIENTAÇÃO AO PROPRIETÁRIO
Se o animal aparecer cego, a visão deve retornar ao normal.

MEDICAÇÕES

MEDICAMENTO(S) DE ESCOLHA
- Agitação:
  ◦ Fenotiazinas (acepromazina 0,025-0,05 mg/kg IV, titular a dose para cima conforme a necessidade).
  ◦ Ciproeptadina (cão, 1,1 mg/kg; gato, 2-4 mg VO a cada 4-6 h ou pode ser administrada por via retal na presença de vômito).
  ◦ Benzodiazepínicos (diazepam 0,5-2 mg/kg IV) (ver "Precauções").
- Tremores:
  ◦ Metocarbamol (50-150 mg/kg IV, titular a dose para cima, mas sem exceder 330 mg/kg/dia).

CONTRAINDICAÇÕES
- Alto risco de síndrome serotoninérgica: outros ISRSs, inibidores da MAO, ATCs, anfetaminas, 5-HTP, claritromicina, dextrometorfano, lítio, erva-de-são-joão. • Baixo risco de síndrome serotoninérgica: tramadol, fentanila, amantadina, bupropiona, carbamazepina, codeína.

PRECAUÇÕES
Os benzodiazepínicos (p. ex., diazepam) são relatados por algumas fontes por exacerbar a síndrome serotoninérgica; sendo assim, o uso desses agentes para toxicose por ISRS não é universalmente recomendado.

INTERAÇÕES POSSÍVEIS
- Diminuição do metabolismo de ISRSs: cimetidina, diuréticos, quinidina, lítio. • Aumento dos níveis dos medicamentos (metabolismo reduzido): teofilina, coumadina, digoxina.

ACOMPANHAMENTO

MONITORIZAÇÃO DO PACIENTE
Pressão arterial, frequência cardíaca, coloração da urina: monitorizar de hora em hora e, depois, com menor frequência à medida que o animal permanece estável.

PREVENÇÃO
- Manter os medicamentos fora do alcance dos animais. • Seguir as instruções do rótulo e da bula durante a administração de medicamentos serotoninérgicos aos animais.

COMPLICAÇÕES POSSÍVEIS
Insuficiência renal secundária à mioglobinúria produzida por rabdomiólise. CID secundária à hipertermia.

EVOLUÇÃO ESPERADA E PROGNÓSTICO
- O prognóstico é bom na maioria dos casos, com recuperação em 12-24 horas. • Os pacientes que se apresentam em estado epiléptico ou com hipertermia grave apresentam um prognóstico reservado.

DIVERSOS

FATORES RELACIONADOS COM A IDADE
Animais jovens e idosos estão sob maior risco de desenvolvimento de toxicose grave.

GESTAÇÃO/FERTILIDADE/REPRODUÇÃO
Os ISRSs podem causar aumento da mortalidade da ninhada e possíveis defeitos congênitos.

ABREVIATURA(S)
- 5-HTP = 5-hidroxitriptofano. • ATC = antidepressivo tricíclico. • IRSN = inibidor da recaptação de serotonina e norepinefrina. • ISRS = inibidor seletivo de recaptação da serotonina. • MAO = monoamina oxidase.

Autor Tina Wismer
Consultor Editorial Gary D. Osweiler

APUDOMA

CONSIDERAÇÕES GERAIS

REVISÃO
- O apudoma refere-se a tumores de células endócrinas, capazes de realizar a captação e a descarboxilação de precursores amínicos (APUD), bem como a secreção de hormônios peptídicos; os tumores são nomeados de acordo com os hormônios secretados por eles.
- As células APUD geralmente são encontradas no trato gastrintestinal e no SNC.
- Esse tópico trata dos tumores secretores da gastrina e do polipeptídeo pancreático; já o insulinoma e o glucagonoma serão discutidos separadamente.
- A hipergastrinemia decorrente dos tumores secretores da gastrina provoca gastrite e hiperacidez duodenal, que podem levar à ulceração gástrica, disfunção esofágica por refluxo crônico e atrofia das vilosidades intestinais.
- A concentração elevada do polipeptídeo pancreático também causa hiperacidez gástrica e suas consequências.

IDENTIFICAÇÃO
- Gastrinoma — raro em cães e gatos; faixa etária de 3-12 anos; média de 7,5 anos (cães).
- Polipeptídeo pancreático — extremamente raro em cães.

SINAIS CLÍNICOS
- Vômito.
- Perda de peso.
- Anorexia.
- Diarreia.
- Letargia, depressão.
- Polidipsia.
- Melena.
- Dor abdominal.
- Hematêmese.
- Hematoquezia.
- Febre.

CAUSAS E FATORES DE RISCO
Não são conhecidos.

DIAGNÓSTICO

DIAGNÓSTICO DIFERENCIAL
- Outras condições associadas à hipergastrinemia, hiperacidez gástrica e ulceração gastrintestinal.
- Uremia.
- Insuficiência hepática.
- Ulceração induzida por medicamentos (p. ex., AINEs ou esteroides).
- Gastrite inflamatória.
- Ulceração induzida por estresse.
- Mastocitopatia.

HEMOGRAMA/BIOQUÍMICA/URINÁLISE
- Permanecem normais ou refletem os efeitos crônicos da doença geral.
- Anemia por deficiência de ferro (ferropriva), secundariamente a sangramento gastrintestinal.
- Aumento nos níveis da ureia, secundariamente a sangramento gastrintestinal.
- Hipoproteinemia.
- Distúrbios eletrolíticos na presença de vômitos crônicos.

OUTROS TESTES LABORATORIAIS
- A concentração sérica da gastrina permanece normal ou normal a elevada em pacientes com gastrinoma.
- Teste provocativo da secreção de gastrina — o aumento na concentração desse hormônio após a administração intravenosa de gliconato de cálcio ou de secretina sugere a presença de gastrinoma; ver os protocolos e as interpretações no Apêndice II deste livro.

DIAGNÓSTICO POR IMAGEM
Ocasionalmente, a ultrassonografia abdominal demonstra a existência de massa pancreática, mas em geral não exibe anormalidades.

MÉTODOS DIAGNÓSTICOS
- Endoscopia associada a biopsias gástrica e duodenal.
- Na suspeita de mastocitopatia, obter aspirado de qualquer massa detectável.
- Na ausência de massas detectáveis, examinar um esfregaço de camada leucocitária em busca de mastócitos.

ACHADOS PATOLÓGICOS
- A biopsia endoscópica revela ulceração gastrintestinal.
- O exame histopatológico de tumores pancreáticos demonstra achados compatíveis com tumores das ilhotas pancreáticas, mas é inespecífico quanto ao tipo hormonal.
- A coloração imunocitoquímica pode auxiliar no diagnóstico específico.
- O exame histopatológico ainda pode evidenciar a ocorrência de metástases no fígado e nos linfonodos regionais.

TRATAMENTO

- Avisar ao proprietário sobre o caráter maligno de grande parte dos apudomas, a possível presença de metástases no momento do diagnóstico e a dificuldade de controle da condição a longo prazo.
- Ocasionalmente, o tratamento clínico rigoroso pode aliviar os sinais durante meses a anos.
- A exploração cirúrgica e a biopsia excisional de massa pancreática são importantes tanto em termos diagnósticos como terapêuticos.
- O tratamento clínico é útil em casos de hiperacidez gástrica.

MEDICAÇÕES

MEDICAMENTO(S)
- Antagonistas dos receptores histaminérgicos H_2 — cimetidina, ranitidina e famotidina; diminuem a secreção ácida pelas células parietais gástricas.
- Omeprazol — inibidor da bomba de prótons; é o inibidor da secreção ácida gástrica mais potente disponível; altamente eficaz e caro.
- Sucralfato — adere-se à mucosa gástrica ulcerada e a protege contra o ataque ácido; promove a cicatrização não só pela ligação à pepsina e aos ácidos biliares, mas também pela estimulação das prostaglandinas locais.

CONTRAINDICAÇÕES/INTERAÇÕES POSSÍVEIS
Como o sucralfato pode ser menos eficaz em um ambiente alcalino e pode reduzir a absorção de outros medicamentos, ele deve ser administrado 1-2 h antes de agentes antiácidos.

ACOMPANHAMENTO

MONITORIZAÇÃO DO PACIENTE
- O exame físico e os sinais clínicos são as medidas mais úteis para avaliar a eficácia do tratamento e a evolução da doença.
- A gastroscopia é capaz de monitorizar a evolução da gastrite, embora não seja necessária.
- As radiografias ou as ultrassonografias abdominais podem detectar o desenvolvimento de massas abdominais.

EVOLUÇÃO ESPERADA E PROGNÓSTICO
- Difícil previsão.
- O tratamento clínico possibilita o controle dos pacientes com gastrinoma durante meses a anos.
- Não há cura disponível.

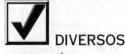

DIVERSOS

VER TAMBÉM
Úlcera Gastroduodenal.

ABREVIATURA(S)
- AINE = anti-inflamatório não esteroide.
- APUD = captação e descarboxilação de precursores amínicos.
- SNC = sistema nervoso central.

Sugestões de Leitura
Lurye JC, Behrend EN. Endocrine tumors. Vet Clin North Am Small Anim Pract 2001, 31(5):1083-1110, ix-x.
Zerbe CA. Islet cell tumors secreting insulin, pancreatic polypeptide, gastrin, or glucagon. In: Kirk RW, Bonagura JD, eds., Current Veterinary Therapy XI. Philadelphia: Saunders, 1992, pp. 368-375.

Autor Thomas K. Graves
Consultor Editorial Deborah S. Greco

ARRITMIA SINUSAL

CONSIDERAÇÕES GERAIS

DEFINIÇÃO
• Formação de impulso sinusal normal, caracterizada por variação fásica na duração do ciclo sinusal. O intervalo R-R irregular está presente com mais de 10% de variação na duração do ciclo sinusal (ou variabilidade de 0,12 s [cão], 0,10 s [gato] ou maior variação entre ondas P sucessivas).
• Existem duas formas básicas — arritmia sinusal respiratória: o intervalo P-P encurta-se de forma cíclica durante a inspiração, principalmente em virtude da inibição reflexa do tônus vagal, mas alonga-se durante a expiração; arritmia sinusal não respiratória: variação fásica no intervalo P-P não relacionada com o ciclo respiratório.

Características do ECG
• Exceto pelo ritmo irregular, todos os outros critérios de ritmo sinusal estão presentes.
• Frequência cardíaca normal.
• Onda P positiva nas derivações I, II, III e aVF a menos que um marca-passo migratório esteja presente; nesse caso, as ondas P podem ser positivas, difásicas ou negativas temporariamente.
• Uma onda P está presente para cada complexo QRS.
• Um complexo QRS está presente para cada onda P.
• O intervalo PR é relativamente constante.

FISIOPATOLOGIA
A velocidade de descarga do nó sinusal depende de duas influências antagônicas do sistema nervoso autônomo. O estímulo vagal diminui a velocidade de descarga espontânea do nó sinusal e predomina sobre o estímulo simpático. Durante a inspiração, a retroalimentação (*feedback*) dos centros respiratório e cardíaco na medula oblonga produz aceleração cardíaca por diminuir o controle vagal sobre o nó sinusal; ocorre o oposto durante a expiração. A gênese da arritmia sinusal também depende dos reflexos que envolvem os receptores de estiramento no pulmão, os receptores sensoriais de pressão-volume no coração (*Bainbridge*, barorreceptor), os vasos sanguíneos e fatores químicos do sangue.

SISTEMA(S) ACOMETIDO(S)
Cardiovascular — geralmente sem consequência hemodinâmica, embora a arritmia sinusal acentuada possa produzir uma pausa sinusal longa o suficiente a ponto de provocar síncope se não for acompanhada por um ritmo de escape.

GENÉTICA
N/D.

INCIDÊNCIA/PREVALÊNCIA
Forma mais frequente de arritmia no cão.

IDENTIFICAÇÃO
Espécies
• A arritmia sinusal respiratória é um achado normal frequente nos cães.
• Incomum, geralmente anormal em gatos sem relação com as fases da respiração.

Raça(s) Predominante(s)
• Raças braquicefálicas são predispostas.
• Cães — raças: Buldogue, Lhasa apso, Pequinês, Pug, Shar-pei, Shih tzu, Boxer.
• Gatos — raças: Persa, Himalaio.

Idade Média e Faixa Etária
N/D.

Sexo Predominante
N/D.

SINAIS CLÍNICOS
Comentários Gerais
• Apesar de incomum, pode ocorrer o desenvolvimento de fraqueza caso as pausas entre os batimentos sejam excessivamente prolongadas; pode ocorrer síncope quando se desenvolvem arritmia sinusal acentuada e bradicardia sinusal.
• Em geral, os sintomas são mais comuns na forma não respiratória que na respiratória.

Achados Anamnésicos
• Arritmia sinusal respiratória — nenhum.
• Arritmia sinusal não respiratória — podem ser achados relacionados com a causa subjacente.

Achados do Exame Físico
• Podem estar normais.
• Ritmo irregular à auscultação.
• Podem ser achados relacionados com a doença específica que acentua o tônus vagal (p. ex., estertor e estridor em paciente com síndrome braquicefálica das vias aéreas).

CAUSAS
• Alteração cíclica normal no tônus vagal associada à respiração no cão; a frequência cardíaca aumenta com a inspiração e diminui com a expiração.
• Condições subjacentes que aumentam o tônus vagal — pressão intracraniana elevada, doença gastrintestinal, doença respiratória, distúrbios cerebrais, intoxicação por digitálicos.
• Massagem no seio carotídeo ou compressão no globo ocular (manobra vagal) podem acentuar.

FATORES DE RISCO
• Conformação braquicefálica.
• Tratamento com digoxina.
• Qualquer doença que aumente o tônus vagal.

DIAGNÓSTICO

DIAGNÓSTICO DIFERENCIAL
• Com frequência, a auscultação de arritmia sinusal é confusa; o ECG ajuda a diferenciar arritmia sinusal normal da verdadeira arritmia patológica.
• Marca-passo sinusal migratório frequentemente associado e uma variante da arritmia sinusal. O local de formação do impulso muda dentro do nó sinoatrial ou se desvia para um foco atrial ou nó AV, alterando a configuração da onda P.
• É importante diferenciar arritmia sinusal normal de arritmias patológicas, incluindo complexos atriais prematuros, síndrome do nó sinusal doente, fibrilação atrial lenta e dissociação AV.

HEMOGRAMA/BIOQUÍMICA/URINÁLISE
N/D.

OUTROS TESTES LABORATORIAIS
Gatos com doença respiratória crônica podem estar positivos para o vírus da leucemia felina ou para o vírus da imunodeficiência felina.

DIAGNÓSTICO POR IMAGEM
Radiografias da cabeça e do pescoço para avaliar a conformação anatômica anormal que pode predispor a problemas das vias aéreas.

MÉTODOS DIAGNÓSTICOS
• Faringoscopia/laringoscopia na suspeita de doença das vias aéreas superiores.
• Teste de desafio da atropina (administrar esse medicamento na dose de 0,04 mg/kg IM seguida pelo ECG em 30 min ou 0,04 mg/kg IV acompanhada pelo ECG em 10 min) se associada à bradicardia sinusal e se houver suspeita de disfunção primária do nó sinusal.

ACHADOS PATOLÓGICOS
Ver a doença específica.

TRATAMENTO

CUIDADO(S) DE SAÚDE ADEQUADO(S)
Em geral, o tratamento específico só é necessário em casos de arritmia sinusal associada à bradicardia sinusal sintomática; se não relacionada com a respiração, a causa subjacente deverá ser tratada. Se o paciente estiver sofrendo de angústia respiratória, ficará indicado o tratamento apropriado com internação do paciente até sua estabilização.

CUIDADO(S) DE ENFERMAGEM
Nenhum a menos que associada à doença subjacente (ver adiante).

ATIVIDADE
Sem restrição a menos que associada à doença específica (p. ex., os animais braquicefálicos podem necessitar de limitação do exercício, sobretudo em ambientes de temperaturas elevadas).

DIETA
Restrição calórica para os animais obesos com comprometimento das vias aéreas.

ORIENTAÇÃO AO PROPRIETÁRIO
Nenhuma a menos que associada à doença específica.

CONSIDERAÇÕES CIRÚRGICAS
Nenhuma a menos que associada à doença específica.

MEDICAÇÕES

MEDICAMENTO(S) DE ESCOLHA
• Em geral, não há indicação de terapia; a arritmia sinusal é um ritmo normal.
• Doenças respiratórias infecciosas necessitam de antibioticoterapia apropriada.
• Se associada à bradicardia sinusal sintomática ou parada ou bloqueio sinusais, o uso de anticolinérgicos poderá ser indicado — atropina (0,04 mg/kg IV, IM, SC) ou glicopirrolato (0,01 mg/kg IM, SC).

CONTRAINDICAÇÕES
Interromper a administração da digoxina caso a intoxicação seja problema.

PRECAUÇÕES
Evitar a atropina em pacientes com doença respiratória; um efeito adverso é o ressecamento das secreções.

INTERAÇÕES POSSÍVEIS
N/D.

ARRITMIA SINUSAL

MEDICAMENTO(S) ALTERNATIVO(S)
N/D.

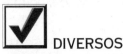
ACOMPANHAMENTO
MONITORIZAÇÃO DO PACIENTE
Apenas quando associada à doença específica.
PREVENÇÃO
N/D.
COMPLICAÇÕES POSSÍVEIS
N/D.
EVOLUÇÃO ESPERADA E PROGNÓSTICO
N/D.

DIVERSOS
DISTÚRBIOS ASSOCIADOS
- Síndrome do nó sinusal doente.
- Síndrome braquicefálica das vias aéreas.
- Asma.
- Doença pulmonar obstrutiva crônica.

FATORES RELACIONADOS COM A IDADE
Geralmente mais pronunciada nos jovens adultos.
POTENCIAL ZOONÓTICO
N/D.
GESTAÇÃO/FERTILIDADE/REPRODUÇÃO
Incidência aumentada de arritmias.
SINÔNIMO(S)
- Arritmia sinusal respiratória = arritmia sinusal fásica.
- Arritmia sinusal não respiratória = arritmia sinusal não fásica; irregularidade sinusal.
- Arritmia sinusal ventriculofásica — forma de arritmia sinusal não fásica na qual os ciclos atriais contendo complexos ventriculares são mais curtos do que aqueles nos quais estão ausentes. Ou seja, o intervalo P-P que inclui o complexo QRS é mais curto que o intervalo P-P sem um complexo QRS. Isso pode ser observado em bloqueio AV de segundo grau, bloqueio AV completo ou na presença de complexos ventriculares prematuros com uma pausa compensatória completa.

VER TAMBÉM
- Parada Sinusal e Bloqueio Sinoatrial.
- Síndrome Braquicefálica das Vias Aéreas.
- Síndrome do Nó Sinusal Doente.

ABREVIATURA(S)
- AV = atrioventricular.
- bpm = batimentos por minuto.
- ECG = eletrocardiograma.

Sugestões de Leitura
Hamlin RL, Smith CR, Smetzer DL. Sinus arrhythmia in the dog. Am J Physiol 1966, 210:321-328.
Hayano J, Yasuma F. Hypothesis: Respiratory sinus arrhythmia is an intrinsic resting function of cardiopulmonary system. Cardiovasc Res 2003, 58(1):1-9.
Libby P, Bonow R, Mann D, Zipes D. Braunwald's Heart Disease: A Textbook of Cardiovascular Medicine, 8th ed. Philadelphia: Saunders, 2008.
Tilley LP. Essentials of Canine and Feline Electrocardiography, 3rd ed. Baltimore: Williams & Wilkins, 1992.
Yasuma F, Hayano J. Respiratory sinus arrhythmia: Why does the heartbeat synchronize with respiratory rhythm? Chest 2004, 125:683.

Autor Deborah J. Hadlock
Consultores Editoriais Larry P Tilley e Francis W.K. Smith, Jr.

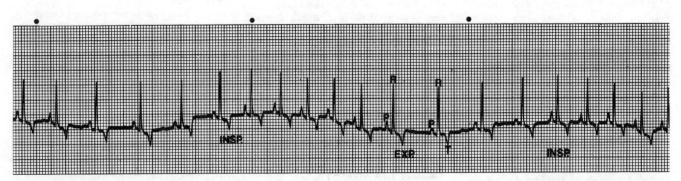

Figura 1 Arritmia sinusal respiratória com frequência média de 120 bpm (velocidade do papel, 25 mm/s; 6 complexos entre 1 conjunto de linhas do tempo '20). A frequência aumenta durante a inspiração (*INSP*) e diminui durante a expiração (*EXP*). A oscilação da linha de base correlaciona-se com o deslocamento dos eletrodos pela cavidade torácica. (De: Tilley LP: *Essentials of canine and feline electrocardiography*. 3. ed. Baltimore: Williams & Wilkins, 1992, com permissão.)

Arritmias Ventriculares e Morte Súbita em Pastor Alemão

CONSIDERAÇÕES GERAIS

REVISÃO
Distúrbio hereditário que resulta em arritmias ventriculares em cães Pastores alemães jovens e saudáveis sob outros aspectos. O espectro fenotípico é amplo, sendo que alguns cães acometidos apresentam complexos ventriculares prematuros isolados infrequentes enquanto outros sofrem de taquicardia ventricular frequente e rápida associada à morte súbita. O padrão de herança é complexo, dependendo fortemente da genética de base. Irmãos de cães da raça Pastor alemão que morreram subitamente devem ser avaliados quanto à presença desse distúrbio.

IDENTIFICAÇÃO
• A maioria dos cães desenvolve arritmias com aproximadamente 12 semanas de vida (identificadas com apenas 6 semanas de vida). O número e a gravidade das arritmias tendem a atingir o pico entre os 5 e 9 meses de vida. Em torno de 18-24 meses de vida, grande parte dos cães sofre apenas algumas arritmias.
• Machos e fêmeas são igualmente afligidos.

SINAIS CLÍNICOS
• Os sinais clínicos são muito raros (p. ex., em >500 cães examinados, apenas 1 teve síncope), porque a taquicardia ventricular perigosa é do tipo não sustentada até se degenerar em alguns cães em fibrilação ventricular, resultando em morte (geralmente entre 5 e 9 meses de vida).
• As arritmias são frequentemente detectadas durante o exame de rotina antes de castração.
• A morte é associada a sono, repouso após exercício, ou agitação depois do sono, particularmente no início da manhã.

CAUSAS E FATORES DE RISCO
• A(s) mutação(ões) genética(s) responsável(is) por esse distúrbio não foi(ram) identificada(s).
• Foram identificadas múltiplas anormalidades eletrofisiológicas — pós-despolarizações precoces e tardias, duração do potencial de ação heterogênea e alterada, densidade da corrente dos canais iônicos, ciclagem de cálcio, e inervação simpática.
• A taquicardia ventricular tende a ser mais frequente com frequências cardíacas lentas (induzidas por medicamento [p. ex., fenilefrina, fentanila], ou durante o sono).

DIAGNÓSTICO

DIAGNÓSTICO DIFERENCIAL
Descartar miocardite.

HEMOGRAMA/BIOQUÍMICA/URINÁLISE
Os resultados dos exames laboratoriais de rotina encontram-se dentro dos limites de normalidade.

OUTROS TESTES LABORATORIAIS
Concentração de troponina — para descartar miocardite. Os cães com arritmias hereditárias apresentam níveis normais dessa proteína.

DIAGNÓSTICO POR IMAGEM
• Radiografias torácicas normais.
• Ecocardiografia — os ecocardiogramas de cães individuais costumam permanecer normais.

MÉTODOS DIAGNÓSTICOS
Eletrocardiograma Ambulatorial de 24 Horas (Registro com Holter)
• Necessário para o diagnóstico e a classificação da gravidade.
• As arritmias identificadas com maior frequência são taquicardia ventricular polimórfica, que é rápida (frequências >400 bpm) com complexos prematuros isolados, mais comumente de origem ventricular esquerda (negativa na derivação II). Embora a taquicardia ventricular polimórfica rápida não sustentada seja a arritmia mais característica, cerca de 15% dos cães terão taquicardia ventricular monomórfica mais lenta e mais sustentada.
• Alguns cães terão milhares de arritmias isoladas sem taquicardia ventricular; foram encontrados extensos períodos de bigeminia ventricular em outros.
• Depois de 6 meses de vida, as séries de taquicardia ventricular são mais comuns após pausas.

ACHADOS PATOLÓGICOS
O exame macroscópico e histopatológico de rotina encontra-se dentro dos limites de normalidade.

TRATAMENTO

• Estudos limitados demonstraram que o estabelecimento do ritmo do coração para manter a frequência cardíaca acima de 120 bpm diminuía a frequência das arritmias; no entanto, não impedia a morte súbita.
• O implante de desfibriladores de cardioversão pode ser útil, mas a programação adequada desses dispositivos em cães jovens é complicada.
• Evitar medicamentos que retardam a frequência cardíaca.
• A anestesia não é contraindicada nesses cães contanto que os agentes anticolinérgicos sejam usados para evitar bradicardia durante a faixa etária em que existem as arritmias.
• O tratamento é necessário apenas para os cães com taquicardia ventricular. Os cães acometidos apenas por complexos ventriculares prematuros não vêm a óbito. No entanto, se um cão jovem for identificado com esse distúrbio, é aconselhável repetir a monitorização com Holter para garantir que o fenótipo desse cão em particular não inclui taquicardia ventricular (p. ex., os efeitos de pico desse cão ainda não ocorreram).

MEDICAÇÕES

MEDICAMENTO(S)
• As arritmias ventriculares costumam ser facilmente suprimidas com lidocaína na dose de 2 mg/kg IV.
• O controle das arritmias com medicação oral é mais problemático.
• Sotalol sozinho pode ser pró-arrítmico e não deve ser utilizado isoladamente.
• O sotalol na dose de 2-3 mg/kg VO a cada 12 h combinado com mexiletina na dose de 4-8 mg/kg VO a cada 8 h suprime as arritmias ventriculares, mas a resposta em cada cão é altamente variável.

CONTRAINDICAÇÕES/INTERAÇÕES POSSÍVEIS
• Evitar os medicamentos que retardam a frequência cardíaca até que os cães tenham mais de 18-24 meses de vida.
• Os medicamentos que retardam ou prolongam a duração do potencial de ação, como sotalol, fenilefrina ou fentanila, são pró-arrítmicos.

ACOMPANHAMENTO

MONITORIZAÇÃO DO PACIENTE
• É altamente aconselhável repetir a monitorização com Holter para avaliar a eficácia dos medicamentos.
• Após 18-24 meses de vida, a monitorização com Holter é repetida. Se o número de complexos ventriculares ectópicos for <2.000 complexos isolados sem taquicardia ventricular, o risco de morte do cão é muito baixo e os medicamentos podem ser interrompidos.
• Embora alguns cães tenham uma queda drástica na contagem e gravidade das arritmias durante o tratamento, a maioria não apresenta essa queda. Portanto, a ausência de arritmias nos registros de Holter após 18-24 meses de vida indica uma alteração no distúrbio e não um efeito antiarrítmico.
• Não há necessidade de tratamento vitalício.

EVOLUÇÃO ESPERADA E PROGNÓSTICO
• Cerca de 50% dos cães acometidos com >10 séries de taquicardia ventricular em um período de 24 horas sofrerão morte súbita antes de 1 ano de idade. Se um cão não tiver taquicardia ventricular identificada por monitorização eletrocardiográfica de 24 horas, a probabilidade de óbito será muito baixa.
• Se um Pastor alemão jovem com taquicardia ventricular frequente não morrer, ele permanecerá vivo. Embora essa afirmação seja irônica na melhor das hipóteses, até mesmo os cães gravemente acometidos que atingiram os 2 anos de idade com ausência documentada de arritmia terão uma vida normal >12 anos.

DIVERSOS

DISTÚRBIOS ASSOCIADOS
Nenhum.

FATORES RELACIONADOS COM A IDADE
Como a identificação dos cães acometidos depende da determinação de arritmias antes de 1 ano de idade (idealmente 4-9 meses) até 2 anos (no máximo), os cães acometidos podem facilmente passar despercebidos, já que o único sinal clínico é a morte súbita sem evidência de uma causa encontrada no exame pós-morte de rotina.

GESTAÇÃO/FERTILIDADE/REPRODUÇÃO
N/D.

Autor N. Sydney Moise
Consultor Editorial Larry P. Tilley e Francis W.K. Smith, Jr.

Artrite (Osteoartrite)

CONSIDERAÇÕES GERAIS

DEFINIÇÃO
Osteoartrite ou artropatia degenerativa refere-se à deterioração progressiva e permanente da cartilagem articular de articulações diartrodiais (sinoviais) por causas primárias (idiopáticas) e secundárias.

FISIOPATOLOGIA
• A artropatia degenerativa é desencadeada por estresse (tensão) mecânico — lesão traumática, instabilidade, conformação anormal, atividade anormal etc.
• As enzimas metaloproteinases, serina protease e cisteína protease são liberadas de condrócitos lesionados, provocando degradação do colágeno e perda da ligação cruzada dessa proteína na cartilagem.
• A síntese do colágeno é alterada, resultando em declínio na interação entre colágeno/proteoglicano e diminuição nas propriedades da matriz hidrofílica.
• A matriz cartilaginosa é ainda mais comprometida pelo aumento na degradação dos proteoglicanos e na produção de proteoglicanos de qualidade inferior.
• O óxido nítrico é liberado, sendo mediador da degradação da cartilagem e manutenção da inflamação crônica. A apoptose do condrócito é facilitada pela enzima ciclo-oxigenase-2.
• A inflamação da membrana sinovial leva à diminuição na viscosidade do líquido sinovial, reduzindo a lubrificação.
• O líquido sinovial de qualidade inferior diminui o aporte de oxigênio e nutrientes para os condrócitos.
• O osso subcondral torna-se esclerótico, agravando as qualidades da carga imposta sobre o osso e a cartilagem sobrejacente.
• A dor da artropatia degenerativa origina-se da estimulação de receptores da dor existentes em tendões, ligamentos, ossos subcondrais e cápsulas articulares.
• O resultado desses processos é a degradação progressiva da cartilagem, variando desde uma fibrilação até a formação de fissuras profundas. Finalmente, pode ocorrer a perda de toda a espessura da cartilagem.
• Para diminuir o movimento articular (e a dor), ocorre fibrose periarticular, induzindo a uma vascularidade deficiente da membrana sinovial.
• Para aumentar a área de superfície responsável pela sustentação da carga, desenvolvem-se osteófitos e entesiófitos em torno e dentro da articulação.
• Essas alterações diminuem a funcionalidade e acabam levando à anquilose.

SISTEMA(S) ACOMETIDO(S)
Musculoesquelético — articulações diartrodiais.

GENÉTICA
• A artropatia degenerativa primária é rara — foi associada a uma colônia de cães da raça Beagle.
• Cães — as causas de artropatia degenerativa secundária são variadas, incluindo displasia do quadril e do cotovelo, osteocondrose dissecante, luxação patelar, luxação congênita do ombro, doença de Legg-Perthes e ruptura do ligamento cruzado cranial.
• Gatos — as causas de artropatia degenerativa secundária são luxação patelar, displasia coxofemoral e artropatia.

INCIDÊNCIA/PREVALÊNCIA
• Cães — muito comum; 20% dos cães com mais de 1 ano de idade possuem certo grau de artropatia degenerativa.
• Gatos — 90% dos animais dessa espécie com mais de 12 anos de idade tinham indícios de artropatia degenerativa ao exame radiográfico.
• Os problemas clínicos são mais prevalentes em animais muito ativos, acima do peso ideal e de porte maior.
• A artropatia degenerativa primária é rara.

IDENTIFICAÇÃO
Espécies
Cães e gatos.

Idade Média e Faixa Etária
• Artropatia degenerativa secundária atribuída a distúrbios congênitos (osteocondrodisplasia, displasia do coxal) — observada em animais imaturos; alguns se apresentam com sinais de artropatia degenerativa quando se encontram mais velhos (displasia do coxal e do cotovelo).
• Secundária a traumatismo — qualquer idade.

SINAIS CLÍNICOS
Achados Anamnésicos
• Cães — redução no nível de atividade ou na disposição na execução de determinadas tarefas; claudicação intermitente ou marcha rígida que evolui lentamente; possível histórico de traumatismo articular, osteocondrodisplasia ou distúrbios do desenvolvimento; pode ser exacerbada por exercício, longos períodos de decúbito e clima frio.
• Gatos — pode não se notar claudicação evidente. Podem ter dificuldade de realizar a auto-higienização, de saltar sobre os móveis ou de entrar na bandeja sanitária e de sair dela; aumento na irritabilidade.

Achados do Exame Físico
• Rigidez na marcha ou alteração na marcha (p. ex., saltos de coelho na displasia do coxal) ou não utilização do membro.
• Diminuição na amplitude de movimentos.
• Crepitação.
• Tumefação articular (efusão e/ou espessamento da cápsula articular).
• Artralgia (dor articular).
• Instabilidade articular.
• Deformidade articular macroscópica.

CAUSAS
• Primária — sem causa conhecida.
• Secundária — origina-se de uma causa desencadeante: desgaste anormal sobre a cartilagem normal (p. ex., instabilidade articular, incongruência articular, traumatismo à cartilagem ou aos tecidos moles de sustentação) ou desgaste normal sobre a cartilagem anormal (p. ex., defeitos osteocondrais).

FATORES DE RISCO
• Cães ativos, atléticos e obesos aplicam maior tensão sobre suas articulações.
• Cães com distúrbios que afetam o colágeno ou a cartilagem (síndrome de Cushing, diabetes melito, hipotireoidismo, hiperfrouxidão, administração prolongada de esteroides).

DIAGNÓSTICO

DIAGNÓSTICO DIFERENCIAL
• Artrite neoplásica (sarcoma de células sinoviais; raramente, condrossarcoma; osteossarcoma).
• Artrite infecciosa (causada por bactérias; espiroquetas; formas L em gatos; *Mycoplasma*; *Rickettsia*; *Ehrlichia*; bem como por agentes virais, como o calicivírus felino; além de fungos e protozoários).
• Artrite imunomediada (erosiva *versus* não erosiva).

OUTROS TESTES LABORATORIAIS
• O teste de Coombs, o título do ANA e a pesquisa do fator reumatoide podem ajudar a descartar a artrite imunomediada.
• Os títulos séricos para *Borrelia*, *Ehrlichia* e *Rickettsia* ajudam a avaliar a presença de artrite infecciosa.

DIAGNÓSTICO POR IMAGEM
• Alterações radiográficas — incluem distensão da cápsula articular, osteofitose, entesiofitose, espessamento dos tecidos moles e estreitamento dos espaços articulares; em pacientes gravemente acometidos: esclerose subcondral, cistos ósseos subcondrais, atrito do osso subcondral, mineralização dos tecidos moles articulares e corpos calcificados intra-articulares (articulação de camundongo).
• A gravidade radiográfica muitas vezes não se correlaciona com a gravidade clínica.
• A radiografia obtida sob estresse pode identificar a instabilidade subjacente e acentuar a incongruência articular (p. ex., o índice de distração, que detecta frouxidão passiva da articulação coxofemoral, é preditivo de artropatia degenerativa do coxal).
• A cintilografia nuclear óssea pode ajudar a localizar artropatia degenerativa sutil.

MÉTODOS DIAGNÓSTICOS
• Artrocentese e análise do líquido sinovial — a contagem celular permanece normal ou levemente aumentada (<2.000-5.000 células/mL); é predominantemente mononuclear (macrófagos), embora ocasionalmente haja células do revestimento sinovial.
• Cultura bacteriana do líquido sinovial — negativa.
• Biopsia do tecido sinovial — para descartar neoplasias ou artrites imunomediadas, como sinovite linfocítica plasmocitária ou LES.
• Aplicação de placa de força ou sustentação de carga estática — possibilita a quantificação da diminuição na carga imposta sobre o membro.

ACHADOS PATOLÓGICOS
• Fibrilação ou erosão da cartilagem articular.
• Eburnação* e esclerose do osso subcondral.
• Espessamento e fibrose da cápsula articular.
• Do ponto de vista macroscópico, o líquido sinovial apresenta-se normal a fino e aquoso, mas costuma exibir aumento de volume.
• Hipertrofia e hiperplasia vilosa da membrana sinovial.
• Osteófitos e entesiófitos nas inserções da cápsula articular e adjacentes à articulação.
• Em casos graves, observa-se neovascularização ou pano sobre as superfícies articulares.

---

* N. T.: Ossificação das cartilagens articulares.

ARTRITE (OSTEOARTRITE)

TRATAMENTO

CUIDADO(S) DE SAÚDE ADEQUADO(S)
- Clínico — colocado em prática geralmente como uma tentativa inicial.
- Opções cirúrgicas — para melhorar a geometria articular ou remover as áreas de contato entre os ossos.

CUIDADO(S) DE ENFERMAGEM
- Fisioterapia — muito benéfica.
- Manutenção ou aumento do movimento articular — exercícios passivos com amplitude de movimentos, massagem, cavalete, natação.
- Controle da dor — combinação de termoterapia e crioterapia.
- Fortalecimento do tônus muscular — natação com exercícios aeróbios e mínima sustentação do peso; passeios controlados e guiados por coleiras em montes ou superfícies fofas, como areia ou esteira seca ou subaquática.

ATIVIDADE
Restrita até um nível que minimize o agravamento dos sinais clínicos.

DIETA
- Redução de peso em pacientes obesos — diminui a tensão aplicada sobre as articulações artríticas.
- Ácidos graxos ômega-6 e 3 — diminuem a produção de certas prostaglandinas e modulam a inflamação.

ORIENTAÇÃO AO PROPRIETÁRIO
- Informar ao proprietário sobre o caráter paliativo da terapia clínica e a probabilidade de evolução da condição.
- Discutir as opções terapêuticas, o nível de atividade e a dieta.

CONSIDERAÇÕES CIRÚRGICAS
- Artrotomia — usada para remover as causas agravantes (p. ex., fragmentação do processo coronoide, não união do processo ancôneo e retalhos osteocondrais).
- Artroscopia — técnica empregada para diagnosticar e remover as causas agravantes; a irrigação da articulação pode ser benéfica.
- Procedimentos reconstrutivos — utilizados para eliminar a instabilidade articular e corrigir os problemas anatômicos (p. ex., luxação patelar, deformidade angular).
- Remoção da articulação — ostectomia da cabeça e do colo femorais, artroplastia da articulação temporomandibular.
- Substituição da articulação — a substituição total do quadril é amplamente utilizada; já a reposição total do cotovelo ainda é experimental.
- Fusão da articulação (artrodese) — em casos crônicos selecionados e para instabilidade articular, parcial ou completa; carpo: resultado geralmente excelente; ombro, cotovelo, soldra e jarrete: resultado menos previsível.

MEDICAÇÕES

MEDICAMENTO(S) DE ESCOLHA
AINEs
- Atuam inibindo a síntese de prostaglandina por meio da enzima ciclo-oxigenase.
- Deracoxibe (3-4 mg/kg VO a cada 24 h, mastigável).
- Carprofeno (2,2 mg/kg VO a cada 12 ou 24 h).
- Etodolaco (10-15 mg/kg VO a cada 24 h).
- Meloxicam (dose de ataque de 0,2 mg/kg VO e, em seguida, 0,1 mg/kg VO a cada 24 h: formulação líquida).
- Tepoxalina (dose de ataque de 20 mg/kg e, em seguida, 10 mg/kg VO a cada 24 h).
- Gatos — meloxicam (0,1 mg/kg VO a cada 24 h: formulação líquida).

Suplementos Condroprotetores/Regenerativos
- Fornecem glicosaminoglicanos polissulfatados para o reparo e a regeneração da cartilagem.
- Existe uma variedade de produtos, muitos com pouca supervisão de produção; por essa razão, os efeitos são amplamente variáveis.
- Glicosamina e sulfato de condroitina — Adequan® injetável, Cosequin® oral, MSM® oral, misturas (Glycoflex II®, SynFlex® etc.).
- Adequan® — estudo clínico em cães com displasia do coxal; a dose de 4,4 mg/kg IM a cada 3-5 dias por 8 injeções teve um efeito temporário positivo.
- Cosequin® — os ensaios revelaram efeitos positivos.

CONTRAINDICAÇÕES
- Os AINEs não devem ser administrados com esteroides.
- O paracetamol não deve ser fornecido aos gatos.

PRECAUÇÕES
- AINEs — podem causar ulceração gástrica.
- Anti-inflamatórios inibidores seletivos da ciclo-oxigenase 2 — podem interferir na função hepática.
- Ao fazer a troca de AINEs — aguardar 3 dias para a eliminação do agente antes de iniciar novo medicamento.

INTERAÇÕES POSSÍVEIS
Esteroides e AINEs.

MEDICAMENTO(S) ALTERNATIVO(S)
- Varredores de radicais livres.
- Glicocorticoides — inibem os mediadores inflamatórios e as citocinas; no entanto, o uso crônico retarda a cicatrização e desencadeia danos à cartilagem articular; são descritos efeitos colaterais sistêmicos potenciais; a meta terapêutica consiste em fornecer uma dose baixa (cães, 0,5-2,0 mg/kg; gatos, 2,0-4,0 mg/kg) em dias alternados.
- Prednisona — dose inicial de 1-2 mg/kg VO a cada 24 h para cães e 4 mg/kg VO a cada 24 h para gatos.
- Hexacetonida de triancinolona — a injeção intra-articular de 5 mg em cães revelou um efeito protetor e terapêutico em um único modelo animal.

ACOMPANHAMENTO

MONITORIZAÇÃO DO PACIENTE
Deterioração clínica — indica a necessidade de modificar a escolha terapêutica ou a dosagem; pode sugerir a necessidade de intervenção cirúrgica.

PREVENÇÃO
A identificação precoce de causas predisponentes e o tratamento imediato ajudam a reduzir a evolução de condições secundárias, como, por exemplo, remoção cirúrgica de lesões osteocondrais.

EVOLUÇÃO ESPERADA E PROGNÓSTICO
- É provável uma evolução lenta da doença.
- Determinadas modalidades de tratamento clínico ou cirúrgico geralmente conferem uma boa qualidade de vida.

DIVERSOS

SINÔNIMO(S)
- Osteoartrite.
- Osteoartrose.
- Artropatia degenerativa.
- Artrite degenerativa.

ABREVIATURA(S)
- ANA = anticorpo antinuclear.
- AINE = anti-inflamatório não esteroide.
- LES = lúpus eritematoso sistêmico.

Sugestões de Leitura

Aragon CL, Hofmeister EH, Budsberg SC. Systematic review of clinical trials of treatments for osteoarthritis in dogs. JAVMA 2007, 230(4):514-521.

Baime MJ. Glucosamine and chondroitin sulphate did not improve pain in osteoarthritis of the knee. Evid Based Med 2006, 11(4):115.

Beale BS, Goring RL. Degenerative joint disease. In: Bojrab MJ, ed., Disease Mechanisms in Small Animal Surgery. Philadelphia: Febiger, 1993, pp. 727-736.

Budsberg SC, Bartges JW. Nutrition and osteoarthritis in dogs: Does it help? Vet Clin North Am Small Anim Pract 2006, 36(6):1307-1323.

Glass GG. Osteoarthritis. Dis Mon 2006, 52(9):343-362 (human review). Hampton T. Efficacy still uncertain for widely used supplements for arthritis. JAMA 2007 297(4):351-352.

Herrero-Beaumont G, Ivorra JA, et al. Glucosamine sulfate in the treatment of knee osteoarthritis symptoms: A randomized, double-blind, placebo-controlled study using acetaminophen as a side comparator. Arthritis Rheum 2007, 56(2):555-567.

Johnston SJ. Osteoarthritis joint anatomy, physiology and pathobiology. Vet Clin North Am 1997, 27:699-723.

Mlacnik E, Bockstahler BA, Muller M, Tetrick MA, Nap RC, Zentek J. Effects of caloric restriction and a moderate or intense physiotherapy program for treatment of lameness in overweight dogs with osteoarthritis. JAVMA 2006, 229(11):1756-1760.

Pederson NC. Joint diseases of dogs and cats. In: Ettinger SJ, ed., Textbook of Veterinary Internal Medicine, 5th ed. Philadelphia: Saunders, 2000, pp. 1862-1886.

Van Der Kraan PM, Van Den Berg WB. Osteophytes: Relevance and biology. Osteoarthritis Cartilage 2007, 15(3):237-244.

Autor Peter K. Shires
Consultor Editorial Peter K. Shires
Agradecimento O autor e os editores agradecem as colaborações de Brian S. Beale e Jennifer J. Warnock em uma edição mais antiga.

Artrite Séptica

CONSIDERAÇÕES GERAIS

DEFINIÇÃO
Microrganismos patogênicos presentes dentro do espaço fechado de uma ou mais articulações sinoviais.

FISIOPATOLOGIA
• Causada geralmente por contaminação associada a lesões traumáticas (p. ex., lesão penetrante direta, como ferimentos provocados por mordeduras, projéteis balísticos ou corpos estranhos); sequela de cirurgia, artrocentese ou injeção intra-articular; disseminação hematógena de microrganismos a partir de focos sépticos distantes ou extensão de osteomielite primária.
• Fontes primárias de infecção hematógena — sistemas urogenital, cutâneo (incluindo orelhas e sacos anais), respiratório, cardíaco e gastrintestinal.

SISTEMA(S) ACOMETIDO(S)
Sistema musculoesquelético — costuma acometer uma única articulação.

GENÉTICA
N/D.

INCIDÊNCIA/PREVALÊNCIA
Representa uma causa relativamente incomum de artrite monoarticular em cães e gatos.

DISTRIBUIÇÃO GEOGRÁFICA
Pode exibir um aumento na incidência em áreas endêmicas para a doença de Lyme.

IDENTIFICAÇÃO
Espécies
• Mais comum em cães.
• Rara em gatos.

Raça(s) Predominante(s)
Raças de médio a grande porte — mais comumente em Pastor alemão, Doberman e Labrador retriever.

Idade Média e Faixa Etária
Qualquer idade; geralmente entre 4 e 7 anos.

Sexo Predominante
Macho.

SINAIS CLÍNICOS
Comentários Gerais
O clínico sempre deve considerar o diagnóstico em pacientes com claudicação monoarticular associada aos sinais de tumefação, calor e dor em tecidos moles.

Achados Anamnésicos
• Claudicação — o início agudo é mais comum, mas pode se apresentar na forma crônica.
• Letargia.
• Anorexia.
• Pode haver o relato de traumatismo prévio — mordeduras provocadas por cães, lesões penetrantes, cirurgia prévia ou outro procedimento invasivo na articulação.

Achados do Exame Físico
• Claudicação monoarticular, raramente com envolvimento oligoarticular ou pauciarticular (quatro ou poucas articulações) ou poliarticular (cinco ou mais articulações).
• Artralgia e tumefação articular — costuma acometer as articulações do carpo, da soldra, do jarrete, do ombro ou do cotovelo.
• Calor articular localizado.
• Diminuição na amplitude de movimentos.
• Febre.

CAUSAS
• Microrganismos bacterianos aeróbios — mais comuns: estafilococos, estreptococos, coliformes e *Pasteurella*.
• Microrganismos anaeróbios — mais comuns: *Propionibacterium*, *Peptostreptococcus*, *Fusobacterium* e *Bacteroides*.
• Espiroqueta — *Borrelia burgdorferi*.
• *Mycoplasma*.
• Agentes fúngicos — *Blastomyces*, *Cryptococcus* e *Coccidiodes*.
• *Ehrlichia*.
• *Leishmania*.
• Calicivírus felino.

FATORES DE RISCO
• Fatores predisponentes à infecção hematógena — diabetes melito; hipoadrenocorticismo (doença de Addison); imunossupressão.
• Traumatismo penetrante na articulação, incluindo cirurgia.
• Osteoartrite ou outro dano articular existente.
• Injeção intra-articular, particularmente no caso de aplicação de esteroides.

DIAGNÓSTICO

DIAGNÓSTICO DIFERENCIAL
• Osteoartrite.
• Traumatismo.
• Artropatia imunomediada.
• Poliartrite transitória pós-vacinal.
• Poliartrite dos Galgos.
• Poliartrite progressiva felina.
• Artropatia induzida por cristais.
• Sarcoma de células sinoviais.

HEMOGRAMA/BIOQUÍMICA/URINÁLISE
• Hemograma — desvio inflamatório à esquerda em alguns casos.
• Outros resultados permanecem normais.

OUTROS TESTES LABORATORIAIS
Testes sorológicos em busca de patógenos específicos.

DIAGNÓSTICO POR IMAGEM
Radiografia
• Doença precoce — pode revelar tecidos periarticulares espessos e densos; pode-se observar a presença de indícios de efusão articular. Muitas vezes, o diagnóstico de doença precoce por via radiográfica não é uma tarefa fácil.
• Doença tardia — revela destruição óssea, osteólise, espaço articular irregular, erosões discretas e osteofitose periarticular.

MÉTODOS DIAGNÓSTICOS
Análise do Líquido Sinovial
• Aumento de volume.
• Líquido turvo.
• Viscosidade diminuída.
• Diminuição da reação do coágulo de mucina.
• Fazer lâminas imediatamente; caso se obtenha uma quantidade extra de líquido, colocá-lo em tubo de EDTA.
• Contagem leucocitária elevada — >80% de neutrófilos com >40.000/mm^3 (líquido articular normal <10% de neutrófilos e <3.000/mm^3).
• Os neutrófilos no líquido sinovial podem revelar alterações degenerativas (cromatólise, vacuolização, tumefação nuclear, perda de segmentação). Contudo, a presença de neutrófilos tóxicos não é necessária para o diagnóstico.
• Diagnóstico definitivo — neutrófilos com bactérias fagocitadas (observados em aproximadamente metade dos casos) ou bactérias no líquido sinovial.

Cultura do Líquido Sinovial
• Resultados positivos em cultura são definitivos, mas dispensáveis, para o diagnóstico.
• É imprescindível a coleta asséptica; requer sedação intensa ou anestesia geral.
• Depositar a amostra do líquido em Culturettes® aeróbico e anaeróbico, bem como em um meio de hemocultura.
• Utilizar a diluição de 1:9 (líquido sinovial:meio de hemocultura).
• Amostras de Culturette® — submetidas imediatamente à cultura na chegada ao laboratório.
• Meio de hemocultura — a repetição da cultura após 24 h de incubação aumenta a precisão do método por volta de 50%; por essa razão, constitui-se o método de preferência.
• *Mycoplasma*, formas L-bacterianas e protozoários necessitam de procedimentos específicos de cultura — entrar em contato com o laboratório antes da coleta da amostra.

Outros
• Biopsia sinovial — para descartar artropatia imunomediada; não é mais eficaz do que o meio de hemocultura incubado para o crescimento de microrganismos bacterianos.
• Se houver suspeita de fonte hematógena, fazer culturas do sangue e da urina.

ACHADOS PATOLÓGICOS
• Sinóvia — espessa; coloração alterada; frequentemente bastante proliferativa.
• Histologia — evidência de sinoviócitos hiperplásicos.
• Número elevado de neutrófilos, macrófagos e debris fibrinosos.
• Cartilagem — perda de proteoglicanos, destruição da superfície articular, formação de pano.

TRATAMENTO

CUIDADO(S) DE SAÚDE ADEQUADO(S)
• Internação — estabilização inicial; instituir antibioticoterapia sistêmica imediatamente após a coleta do líquido para a realização de cultura bacteriana; considerar a drenagem/lavagem articular o mais rápido possível para minimizar a lesão intra-articular.
• Na suspeita de disseminação hematógena, identificar e tratar a fonte.
• Esquema ambulatorial — tratamento a longo prazo.

CUIDADO(S) DE ENFERMAGEM
• Compressas quentes e frias alternadas — são benéficas para estimular o aumento do fluxo sanguíneo e a diminuição da tumefação.
• A imobilização articular pode aumentar o conforto do paciente, mas não deve ser prolongada em função do risco de agravamento no dano articular.

ATIVIDADE
Restrita até a resolução dos sintomas.

ARTRITE SÉPTICA

DIETA
N/D.

ORIENTAÇÃO AO PROPRIETÁRIO
- Discutir a causa provável.
- Alertar o proprietário sobre a necessidade de antibióticos a longo prazo e a probabilidade de artropatia degenerativa residual.

CONSIDERAÇÕES CIRÚRGICAS
- Doença aguda com alterações radiográficas mínimas — recomendação geral para descompressão articular inicial via artrocentese e, possivelmente, lavagem articular via artrocentese com agulha, lavagem artroscópica ou artrotomia. Nas articulações mais amplas, pode-se inserir um cateter de irrigação (entrada/saída). Existe um debate considerável a respeito da superioridade dos procedimentos de artrocentese repetida com agulha, lavagem artroscópica ou lavagem aberta.
- Doença crônica — pode necessitar de artroscopia ou artrotomia com debridamento da sinóvia e lavagem abundante; se pertinente, pode-se aplicar um cateter de irrigação (entrada/saída) para lavar a articulação no período pós-operatório.
- Lavagem — utilizar o soro fisiológico ou a solução de Ringer lactato, ambas aquecidas (2-4 mL/kg a cada 8 h), até que o efluente esteja límpido. Não adicionar iodopovidona ou clorexidina para promover a lavagem do líquido.
- Líquido efluente — monitorizado diariamente por meio citológico quanto à existência e à natureza de bactérias e neutrófilos.
- Remoção dos cateteres — na ausência de bactérias no líquido efluente e na presença de neutrófilos sãos (sadios) do ponto de vista citológico.
- Artroscopia — possibilita a inspeção visual de cartilagem articular, a lavagem e a biopsia, além de ser um método menos invasivo de lavagem articular em comparação à artrotomia.
- Relatos recentes sugerem que possa não haver qualquer diferença entre o tratamento clínico e cirúrgico combinado e o tratamento clínico isolado.

MEDICAÇÕES

MEDICAMENTO(S) DE ESCOLHA
- Na espera dos resultados da cultura e do teste de suscetibilidade (antibiograma) — optar pelos antibióticos bactericidas, como a cefalosporina de primeira geração ou a associação amoxicilina-ácido clavulânico, de preferência.
- Escolha de medicamentos antimicrobianos — depende principalmente da determinação *in vitro* da suscetibilidade dos microrganismos; fatores como a toxicidade, a frequência, a via de administração e os custos também são levados em consideração; a maioria desses medicamentos penetra satisfatoriamente na sinóvia; no entanto, é necessário administrá-los por, no mínimo, 4-8 semanas.
- AINE e outros analgésicos — pode ajudar a diminuir a dor e a inflamação.

CONTRAINDICAÇÕES
Evitar o uso de quinolonas fluoradas em pacientes pediátricos, pois esses medicamentos induzem a lesões cartilaginosas por via experimental.

PRECAUÇÕES
Falha de resposta à antibioticoterapia convencional — pode ser sugestiva de doença anaeróbia ou outra causa não usual (fúngica, espiroqueta).

INTERAÇÕES POSSÍVEIS
N/D.

MEDICAMENTO(S) ALTERNATIVO(S)
N/D.

ACOMPANHAMENTO

MONITORIZAÇÃO DO PACIENTE
- Observação do animal quanto à presença dos sinais clínicos de artralgia (dor articular) e tumefação.
- Citologia repetida do líquido sinovial para avaliar a resposta ao tratamento.
- Duração da antibioticoterapia — 2 semanas após a resolução dos sinais clínicos. O tratamento total pode ser de 4-8 semanas ou mais, dependendo dos sinais clínicos e do microrganismo patogênico.
- Inflamação sinovial persistente sem microrganismos bacterianos viáveis (cães) — pode ser causada por fragmentos bacterianos antigênicos ou depósito de complexo antígeno anticorpo.
- Fisioterapia — pode ser necessária para evitar a contratura dos músculos, manter a integridade da cartilagem e maximizar a dinâmica normal da articulação.

PREVENÇÃO
Em caso de recidiva dos sinais clínicos, o tratamento precoce (dentro de 24-48 h) trará maiores benefícios.

COMPLICAÇÕES POSSÍVEIS
- Doença crônica — artropatia degenerativa grave.
- Recidiva da infecção.
- Limitação da amplitude dos movimentos articulares.
- Sepse generalizada.
- Osteomielite.

EVOLUÇÃO ESPERADA E PROGNÓSTICO
- A doença diagnosticada de forma aguda (dentro de 24-48 h) responde satisfatoriamente à antibioticoterapia.
- A formulação tardia do diagnóstico ou a presença de microrganismos resistentes ou altamente virulentos implicam um prognóstico reservado a mau.

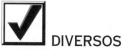

DIVERSOS

DISTÚRBIOS ASSOCIADOS
N/D.

FATORES RELACIONADOS COM A IDADE
N/D.

POTENCIAL ZOONÓTICO
N/D.

GESTAÇÃO/FERTILIDADE/REPRODUÇÃO
N/D.

SINÔNIMO(S)
- Artrite infecciosa.
- Artrose.

VER TAMBÉM
- Osteomielite.
- Poliartrite Erosiva Imunomediada.
- Poliartrite Não Erosiva Imunomediada.

ABREVIATURA(S)
- AINE = anti-inflamatório não esteroide.
- EDTA = ácido etilenodiaminotetracético.

Sugestões de Leitura
Bennett D, Taylor DJ. Bacterial infective arthritis in the dog. J Small Anim Pract 1988, 29:207-230.
Benzioni H, Shahar R, Yudelevitch S, Milgram J. Bacterial infective arthritis of the coxofemoral joint in dogs with hip dysplasia. Vet Comp Orthop Traumatol 2008, 21:262-266.
Clements DN, Owen MR, Mosely JR, et al. Retrospective study of bacterial infective arthritis in 31 dogs. J Small Anim Pract 2005, 46:171-176.
Ellison RS. The cytologic examination of synovial fluid. Semin Vet Med Surg Small Anim 1988, 3:133-139.
Fitch RB, Hogan TC, Kudnig ST. Hematogenous septic arthritis in the dog: Results of five patients treated nonsurgically with antibiotics. JAAHA 2003, 39:563-566.
Hodgin EC, Michaelson F, Howerth EW. Anaerobic bacterial infections causing osteomyelitis/arthritis in a dog. JAVMA 1992, 201:886-888.
Luther JF, Cook JL, Stoll MR. Arthroscopic exploration and biopsy for diagnosis of septic arthritis and osteomyelitis of the coxofemoral joint in a dog. Vet Comp Orthop Traumatol 2005, 18:47-51.
Machevsky AM, Read RA. Bacterial septic arthritis in 19 dogs. Australian Vet J 1999, 77:233-237.
MacWilliams PS, Friedrichs KR. Laboratory evaluation and interpretation of synovial fluid. Vet Clin North Am Small Anim Pract 2003, 33:153-178.

Autores Sherisse A. Sakals e Spencer A. Johnston
Consultor Editorial Peter K. Shires

ASCITE

CONSIDERAÇÕES GERAIS

DEFINIÇÃO
O escape de líquido, transudato ou exsudato, para o interior da cavidade abdominal entre os peritônios parietal e visceral.

FISIOPATOLOGIA
A ascite pode ser causada por:
- ICC e interferência associada no retorno venoso.
- Depleção de proteínas plasmáticas, associada à perda inapropriada de proteínas por doença renal ou gastrintestinal — nefropatias ou enteropatias com perda proteica, respectivamente.
- Obstrução da veia cava ou da veia porta, bem como da drenagem linfática, decorrente de oclusão neoplásica.
- Efusão neoplásica manifesta.
- Peritonite — infecciosa ou inflamatória.
- Desequilíbrio eletrolítico, especialmente hipernatremia.
- Cirrose hepática.

SISTEMA(S) ACOMETIDO(S)
- Cardiovascular.
- Gastrintestinal.
- Renal/urológico.
- Sanguíneo/linfático/imune.

IDENTIFICAÇÃO
- Cães e gatos.
- Não há predisposição de espécie ou raça.

SINAIS CLÍNICOS
- Fraqueza episódica.
- Letargia.
- Repleção abdominal.
- Desconforto abdominal à palpação.
- Dispneia decorrente de distensão abdominal ou efusão pleural associada.
- Anorexia.
- Vômito.
- Ganho de peso.
- Edema escrotal ou peniano.
- Gemidos ao se deitar.

CAUSAS
- Síndrome nefrótica.
- Cirrose hepática.
- ICC direita.
- Hipoproteinemia.
- Ruptura vesical.
- Peritonite.
- Neoplasia abdominal.
- Hemorragia abdominal.

FATORES DE RISCO
N/D.

DIAGNÓSTICO

DIAGNÓSTICO DIFERENCIAL
Diferenciação de Distensão Abdominal sem Efusão
- Organomegalia — hepatomegalia, esplenomegalia, renomegalia e hidrometra.
- Neoplasia abdominal.
- Gestação.
- Distensão vesical.
- Obesidade.
- Dilatação gástrica.

Diferenciação de Doenças
- Transudato — síndrome nefrótica, cirrose hepática, ICC direita, hipoproteinemia e ruptura vesical.
- Exsudato — peritonite, neoplasia abdominal e hemorragia.

HEMOGRAMA/BIOQUÍMICA/URINÁLISE
- Em pacientes com infecção sistêmica, ocorre leucocitose neutrofílica.
- O nível da albumina encontra-se baixo em pacientes com síntese hepática prejudicada ou com perda gastrintestinal ou renal.
- A concentração do colesterol apresenta-se baixa em pacientes com síntese hepática comprometida.

Enzimas Hepáticas
- Atividade reduzida a normal em pacientes com síntese hepática prejudicada.
- Atividade elevada em pacientes com hepatite, hiperadrenocorticismo, obstrução da vesícula biliar e congestão passiva crônica.

Bilirrubina Total e Direta
- Nível baixo a normal em pacientes com síntese hepática comprometida.
- Nível elevado em pacientes com obstrução biliar causada por tumor, distensão da vesícula biliar ou obstrução.

Ureia e Creatinina
- Concentrações altas em pacientes com insuficiência renal.
- Nível baixo de ureia em pacientes com síntese hepática prejudicada ou hiperadrenocorticismo.

Glicose
- Concentração baixa em pacientes com síntese hepática comprometida.

OUTROS TESTES LABORATORIAIS
- Para detectar hipoproteinemia — eletroforese proteica e perfil imunológico.
- Para revelar proteinúria — relação de proteína:creatinina urinárias (normal <0,5:1).

DIAGNÓSTICO POR IMAGEM
- Algumas vezes, as radiografias torácicas e abdominais são úteis.
- As ultrassonografias hepáticas, esplênicas, pancreáticas, renais, vesicais e abdominais frequentemente podem determinar a causa.
- Estágios de ascite:
  - Estágio I: ascite mínima. Detectado apenas por meio de ultrassom.
  - Estágio II: ascite moderada. Distensão abdominal visível e/ou observada ao balotamento*.
  - Estágio III: ascite significativa. Distensão abdominal acentuada. Paciente desconfortável, possivelmente com respiração laboriosa.

MÉTODOS DIAGNÓSTICOS
Avaliação do Líquido Ascítico
Exame citológico esfoliativo, além de cultura bacteriana e antibiograma — retirar aproximadamente 3-5 mL de líquido abdominal por meio de técnica asséptica.

Transudato
- Límpido e incolor.
- Proteína <2,5 g/dL.
- Densidade específica <1,018.

---

* N. T.: Técnica palpatória de exame físico, destinada à comprovação de existência da presença de líquido ou de objeto flutuante em cavidade corporal.

- Células <1.000/mm³ — neutrófilos e células mesoteliais.

Transudato Modificado
- Vermelho ou rosa; pode se apresentar levemente turvo.
- Proteína 2,5-5,0 g/dL.
- Densidade específica >1,018.
- Células <5.000/mm³ — neutrófilos, células mesoteliais, eritrócitos e linfócitos.

Exsudato (Não Séptico)
- Rosa ou branco; turvo.
- Proteína 2,5-5,0 g/dL.
- Densidade específica >1,018.
- Células 5.000-50.000/mm³ — neutrófilos, células mesoteliais, macrófagos, eritrócitos e linfócitos.

Exsudato (Séptico)
- Vermelho, branco ou amarelo; turvo.
- Proteína >4,0 g/dL.
- Densidade específica >1,018.
- Células 5.000-100.000/mm³ — neutrófilos, células mesoteliais, macrófagos, eritrócitos, linfócitos e bactérias.

Hemorragia
- Vermelho; sobrenadante centrifugado límpido e sedimento vermelho.
- Proteína >5,5 g/dL.
- Densidade específica 1,007-1,027.
- Células compatíveis com sangue periférico.
- Não coagula.

Quilo
- Rosa, amarelo palha ou branco.
- Proteína 2,5-7,0 g/dL.
- Densidade específica 1,007->1,040.
- Células <10.000/mm³ — neutrófilos, células mesoteliais e grande população de linfócitos pequenos.
- Outros — quando refrigerado, o líquido no tubo separa-se em uma camada semelhante a um creme; as gotículas de gordura coram-se pelo Sudan III.

Pseudoquilo
- Branco.
- Proteína >2,5 g/dL.
- Densidade específica 1,007-1,040.
- Células <10.000/mm³ — neutrófilos, células mesoteliais e linfócitos pequenos.
- Outros — quando refrigerado, o líquido no tubo não se separa em uma camada semelhante a um creme; além disso, não se cora pelo Sudan III.

Urina
- Amarela clara a pálida.
- Proteína >2,5 g/dL.
- Densidade específica 1,000->1,040.
- Células 5.000-50.000/mm³ — neutrófilos, eritrócitos, linfócitos e macrófagos.
- Outros — em caso de ruptura vesical <12 h antes da coleta, os níveis urinários de glicose e proteína podem estar negativos; em caso de ruptura vesical >12 h antes da coleta, a urina torna-se um meio de diálise com ultrafiltrado de plasma e contém glicose e proteína.

Bile
- Levemente turva e amarela.
- Proteína >2,5 g/dL.
- Densidade específica >1,018.
- Células 5.000-750.000/mm³ — neutrófilos, eritrócitos, macrófagos e linfócitos.
- Outros — a presença de bilirrubina é confirmada pelo uso de fitas urinárias de imersão; o paciente não ictérico pode apresentar ruptura da vesícula

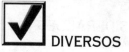

biliar, extravasamento da árvore biliar ou ruptura da porção proximal do intestino.

TRATAMENTO

• Pode-se planejar o tratamento em um esquema ambulatorial, com acompanhamento ou cuidados de internação, dependendo da condição física do paciente e da causa subjacente do quadro.
• Se os pacientes ficarem acentuadamente desconfortáveis em decúbito ou mais dispneicos com o estresse, considerar a remoção de uma quantidade suficiente do líquido ascítico para reverter esses sinais.
• A restrição de sal na dieta pode ajudar a controlar o acúmulo de transudato, em virtude de ICC, cirrose ou hipoproteinemia.
• Para o controle de ascite por exsudato, deve-se tratar a causa subjacente; com frequência, indica-se a cirurgia corretiva, acompanhada por uma conduta terapêutica específica (p. ex., paciente com tumor esplênico: remoção do tumor, controle do sangramento abdominal e realização de transfusões sanguíneas).

PARACENTESE DE GRANDES VOLUMES
• Tratamento de ascite no estágio III.
• Tratar o paciente antes com hetamido (6%) a 1-2 mL/kg por 2 h.
• Punção abdominal (paracentese) até que a velocidade de drenagem diminua.
• Tratar o paciente depois com hetamido (6%) a 1-2 mL/kg por 4 h.

MEDICAÇÕES

MEDICAMENTO(S) DE ESCOLHA
• Pacientes com insuficiência hepática ou ICC — restringir o sódio e administrar uma combinação diurética de hidroclorotiazida (2-4 mg/kg a cada 12 h VO) e espironolactona (1-2 mg/kg a cada 12 h VO); caso o controle se mostre inadequado, a tiazida poderá ser substituída pela furosemida (1-2 mg/kg a cada 8 h VO), com manutenção da espironolactona; deve-se monitorizar a concentração sérica de potássio para evitar os desequilíbrios desse íon.
• Animais com hipoproteinemia, síndrome nefrótica e acúmulo de líquido ascítico associado — é possível tratá-los conforme indicado anteriormente, com a adição de hetamido (hetamido a 6% em solução de NaCl a 0,9%); administrar um bólus IV (cães, 20 mL/kg; gatos, 10-15 mL/kg) lentamente durante ~1 hora; o hetamido aumenta a pressão oncótica do plasma e atrai líquido para dentro do espaço intravascular por até 24-48 h.
• A antibioticoterapia sistêmica é ditada pela identificação bacteriana e pelo antibiograma em pacientes com ascite por exsudato séptico.

CONTRAINDICAÇÕES
N/D.

ACOMPANHAMENTO

MONITORIZAÇÃO DO PACIENTE
• Varia com a causa subjacente.
• Se o paciente for mantido sob terapia diurética, torna-se fundamental a avaliação periódica dos níveis de sódio, potássio, ureia e creatinina, bem como das oscilações de peso.

COMPLICAÇÕES POSSÍVEIS
A administração diurética intensiva pode causar hipocalemia, o que possivelmente predispõe o paciente à alcalose metabólica e à exacerbação da encefalopatia hepática nos animais com hepatopatia subjacente; a alcalose, por sua vez, provoca a transformação de NH_4 em NH_3.

DIVERSOS

DISTÚRBIOS ASSOCIADOS
N/D.

FATORES RELACIONADOS COM A IDADE
N/D.

POTENCIAL ZOONÓTICO
N/D.

GESTAÇÃO/FERTILIDADE/REPRODUÇÃO
N/D.

SINÔNIMO(S)
Efusão abdominal.

VER TAMBÉM
• Cirrose e Fibrose do Fígado.
• Insuficiência Cardíaca Congestiva Direita.
• Hipoalbuminemia.
• Síndrome Nefrótica.

ABREVIATURA(S)
• ICC = insuficiência cardíaca congestiva.

Sugestões de Leitura
Kramer RE, Sokol RJ, Yerushalmi B, Liu E, MacKenzie T, Hoffenberg EJ, Narkewicz MR. Large-volume paracentesis in the management of ascites in children. J Ped Gastro Nutr 2001; 33:245-249.
Lewis LD, Morris ML Jr,, Hand MS. Small Animal Clinical Nutrition, 3rd ed. Topeka, KS: Mark Morris Associates, 1987.
Li MK. Management of ascites. Hong Kong Med Di 2009, 14:27-29.
Runyon BA. Management of adult patients with ascites due to cirrhosis. Hepatol 2004, 39:1-16.

Autor Jerry A. Thornhill
Consultores Editoriais Larry P. Tilley e Francis W.K. Smith, Jr.

Asma, Bronquite — Gatos

CONSIDERAÇÕES GERAIS

DEFINIÇÃO
• Bronquite crônica — inflamação nas vias aéreas (brônquios e bronquíolos), caracterizada por tosse diária crônica de mais de 2 meses de duração.
• Asma — inflamação aguda ou crônica das vias aéreas associada a um aumento na responsividade dessas vias a diversos estímulos, estreitamento das vias aéreas por hipertrofia ou constrição da musculatura lisa, reversibilidade dessa constrição e presença de eosinófilos, linfócitos e mastócitos no interior das vias aéreas.
• O termo bronquite ou doença broncopulmonar felina é usado para descrever a síndrome clínica de tosse e/ou sibilo agudos ou crônicos atribuídos à inflamação das vias aéreas inferiores.

FISIOPATOLOGIA
• Estímulos nocivos ou alérgicos deflagram um processo inflamatório dentro das vias aéreas inferiores. • Constrição da musculatura lisa bronquiolar — reversível de forma espontânea ou com o tratamento. • A hipertrofia da musculatura lisa implica a cronicidade do quadro — geralmente irreversível. • Ocorre um aumento nas células caliciformes da mucosa e na produção de muco, além da formação de edema na parede brônquica.
• O muco excessivo pode causar obstrução bronquiolar, atelectasia ou bronquiectasia. • A inflamação crônica pode levar à fibrose.

SISTEMA(S) ACOMETIDO(S)
• Respiratório.
• Cardíaco — raramente hipertensão pulmonar.

DISTRIBUIÇÃO GEOGRÁFICA
Mundial. As causas parasitárias são mais comuns nos estados do sul e do meio-oeste dos Estados Unidos. O *Paragonimus kellicotti* é encontrado na região dos Grandes Lagos. A dirofilariose é a doença mais prevalente nos estados norte-americanos do sul.

IDENTIFICAÇÃO
Espécies
Gatos.

Raça(s) Predominante(s)
O gato Siamês é super-representado.

Idade Média e Faixa Etária
Qualquer idade; mais comum entre 2-8 anos.

Sexo(s) Predominante(s)
Um único estudo revela a super-representação de fêmeas.

SINAIS CLÍNICOS
Achados Anamnésicos
• Tosse (80%), espirro (60%), respiração laboriosa ou sibilo (40%).
• Os sinais são tipicamente episódicos e podem ser agudos ou crônicos.

Achados do Exame Físico
• Os gatos gravemente acometidos podem apresentar uma respiração com a boca aberta, taquipneia e cianose. • É comum o aumento na sensibilidade traqueal. A auscultação torácica pode revelar crepitações e/ou sibilos expiratórios ou, então, permanecer normal. • Respiração laboriosa tipicamente associada a um aumento no esforço expiratório com pressão abdominal à expiração.

CAUSAS
Os deflagradores de inflamação das vias aéreas são desconhecidos.

FATORES DE RISCO
• A exposição à fumaça de cigarros, bandeja sanitária de gatos empoeirada, *spray* de cabelo e ar-condicionado possivelmente exacerbam a doença. • As infecções pulmonares parasitárias são mais comuns em gatos de rua em determinadas localizações geográficas. • O uso do brometo de potássio foi apontado como a causa dos sinais de bronquite ou de asma em alguns gatos.

DIAGNÓSTICO

DIAGNÓSTICO DIFERENCIAL
• Descartar pneumonia infecciosa (*Mycoplasma*, *Toxoplasma*, pneumonia bacteriana ou fúngica), *Dirofilaria immitis* (dirofilariose) e parasitas pulmonares primários (*Aelurostrongylus abstrusus*, *Capillaria aerophilia* e *Paragonimus kellicotti*).
• As neoplasias primárias ou metastáticas podem ter aspecto clínico e radiográfico semelhante.
• O quadro de fibrose pulmonar idiopática pode se assemelhar com bronquite felina.

HEMOGRAMA/BIOQUÍMICA/URINÁLISE
Frequentemente normais; ~40% dos gatos com doença brônquica apresentam eosinofilia periférica.

OUTROS TESTES LABORATORIAIS
• Exames de fezes — flutuação para pesquisa de *Capillaria*; sedimentação para *Paragonimus*; técnica de Baermann para *Aelurostrongylus*. É comum a obtenção de resultados falso-negativos.
• Teste da dirofilariose — recomenda-se a pesquisa tanto do antígeno como do anticorpo.
• Teste radioalergosorvente (RAST) ou teste cutâneo intradérmico — atualmente, não há registros de uma correlação entre alergias cutâneas e respiratórias.

DIAGNÓSTICO POR IMAGEM
Radiografia
• Classicamente, há um espessamento difuso da parede brônquica; é possível a observação de um padrão intersticial ou alveolar irregular. • A gravidade das alterações radiográficas pode não se correlacionar com a gravidade ou a duração clínicas. • Hiperinsuflação dos campos pulmonares — caracteriza-se por achatamento e deslocamento caudal do diafragma, aumento na distância entre o coração e o diafragma ou expansão dos pulmões até as primeiras vértebras lombares. • A ocorrência de colapso do lobo pulmonar médio direito é relatada em 11% dos casos. • Há suspeitas de dirofilariose em caso de dilatação da artéria lobar pulmonar.

Ecocardiografia
Exame útil para o registro de dirofilariose ou hipertensão pulmonar secundária.

MÉTODOS DIAGNÓSTICOS
Lavado Traqueal Transbucal
• Uso de sonda endotraqueal estéril e cateter de polipropileno para coleta de líquidos das vias aéreas ao nível da carina traqueal.

Broncoscopia/Lavado Broncoalveolar
• Permite a inspeção da traqueia e dos brônquios. Em casos de bronquite, é comum a observação de quantidades excessivas de muco espesso. A mucosa das vias aéreas tipicamente se encontra hiperêmica e edematosa.
• É recomendável a realização do lavado broncoalveolar para coleta de líquidos das vias aéreas das áreas mais gravemente acometidas.

Citologia
• Os eosinófilos e os neutrófilos são os tipos celulares mais proeminentes. Em cerca de 21% dos gatos, ocorre uma população celular mista.
• Em gatos normais, é possível encontrar até 20% de eosinófilos na citologia do lavado broncoalveolar.

Culturas Bacterianas
• Recomenda-se a realização de culturas quantitativas; são incomuns contagens de colônias bacterianas >100-300 UFC/mL.
• Talvez haja necessidade de cultura específica para *Mycoplasma*.

Biopsia
• Biopsia com a remoção de amostra em forma de buraco de fechadura — é capaz de diferenciar entre fibrose pulmonar idiopática e bronquite.

ACHADOS PATOLÓGICOS
Hiperplasia/hipertrofia das células caliciformes, hipertrofia da musculatura lisa das vias aéreas, erosão epitelial e infiltrados inflamatórios.

TRATAMENTO

CUIDADO(S) DE SAÚDE ADEQUADO(S)
• Afastar o paciente de desencadeantes ambientais.
• Internar o paciente em caso de crise respiratória aguda.

CUIDADO(S) DE ENFERMAGEM
Oxigenoterapia e uso de sedativos em casos de crise aguda. Minimizar a manipulação para diminuir o estresse e as necessidades de oxigênio pelo animal.

ATIVIDADE
Em geral, é autolimitada pelo paciente.

DIETA
Restrição calórica para gatos obesos.

ORIENTAÇÃO AO PROPRIETÁRIO
• Grande parte das causas de bronquite refere-se a doenças progressivas crônicas.
• Não interromper a terapia clínica após a resolução dos sinais clínicos — a inflamação subclínica é comum e pode levar à evolução da doença. Geralmente, há necessidade de medicação pelo resto da vida e mudanças ambientais.
• Alguns proprietários podem ser orientados a aplicar injeções subcutâneas de terbutalina e corticosteroide em situações de crise.

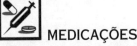

MEDICAÇÕES

MEDICAMENTO(S) DE ESCOLHA
Tratamento de Emergência
• Combinar o uso do oxigênio e de algum broncodilatador parenteral. Terbutalina injetável (0,01 mg/kg IV ou SC); se não houver melhora clínica (diminuição na frequência ou no esforço respiratórios) em 20-30 minutos, pode-se repetir a dose.

ASMA, BRONQUITE — GATOS

- Um sedativo pode ajudar a diminuir a ansiedade (tartarato de butorfanol a 0,2-0,4 mg/kg IV ou IM, buprenorfina a 0,01 mg/kg IV ou IM, ou acepromazina a 0,01-0,05 mg/kg SC).
- Também pode ser imprescindível a administração parenteral de corticosteroide a curto prazo. Fosfato sódico de dexametasona (0,25-0,5 mg/kg IV ou SC). Caso não se observe melhora dentro de 20-30 min, pode-se repetir a dose. Succinato sódico de prednisolona (Solu-Delta-Cortef®) também pode ser usado (50-100 mg IV).

Tratamento a Longo Prazo
Corticosteroides
- Diminuem a inflamação.
- Para monitorização mais rigorosa da dose e da duração da terapia, prefere-se o tratamento oral ao injetável.
- Prednisolona: 0,5-1 mg/kg VO a cada 12 h. Na melhora dos sinais clínicos, iniciar a redução gradativa da dose (50% a cada semana) após 1-2 semanas. Terapia de manutenção = 0,5-1 mg/kg VO a cada 24-48 h.
- Os esteroides parenterais de ação mais prolongada (Vetalog® ou Depomedrol®) devem ficar reservados somente para situações em que os proprietários se mostrem incapazes de administrar o medicamento oral de forma rotineira.

Corticosteroides Inalados
- Requer uma máscara facial de formato anatômico e ajustável, um espaçador e um inalador dosimetrado. As marcas veterinárias incluem Aerokat® (Trudell medical) ou Nebulair® (DVM pharmaceuticals).
- O corticosteroide mais comumente utilizado sob a forma de inalador dosimetrado é o propionato de fluticasona (Flovent®). É recomendável o uso de Flovent® de 220 ou 110 mg (1-2 acionamentos, 7-10 respirações a cada 12 h), juntamente com broncodilatadores e corticosteroides orais, dependendo da gravidade dos sinais clínicos. Em um único estudo, o uso de Flovent® de 44 mg diminuiu a contagem de eosinófilos do lavado broncoalveolar em gatos experimentais.
- Para o controle a longo prazo de inflamação das vias aéreas, também se emprega o Flovent®. Tomar por 10-14 dias até atingir o efeito máximo; durante esse período, é aconselhável o uso concomitante de esteroides orais.
- Resulta em certa supressão do eixo hipotalâmico-hipofisário, mas os efeitos colaterais sistêmicos parecem ser reduzidos.

Broncodilatadores
- Metilxantinas — são recomendadas as formulações de teofilina de liberação sustentada, mas a farmacocinética pode variar bastante. Atualmente, apenas a formulação genérica está disponível. Dose de 10-20 mg/kg VO a cada 24 h à noite.
- Beta-2 agonistas (terbutalina, albuterol) — inibem a constrição da musculatura lisa. A dose da terbutalina oral é 1/4 de um comprimido de 2,5 mg a cada 12 h. A dose inicial do albuterol é de 20 µg/kg VO a cada 12 h; pode-se aumentá-la em até 50 µg/kg VO a cada 8 h.

Broncodilatadores Inalados
- Albuterol — broncodilatador inalatório preferido; o efeito dura menos de 4 h. O uso a longo prazo de formulação racêmica tradicional de albuterol inalado (enantiômeros R e S) foi associado ao agravamento da inflamação das vias aéreas. O enantiômero-R específico do albuterol deve ser usado se o medicamento for necessário em gatos moderada a gravemente acometidos (a cada 12-24 h) ou durante angústia respiratória.
- Brometo de ipratrópio — anticolinérgico inalado; pode conferir broncodilatação e agir de modo sinérgico com o albuterol para produzir broncodilatação máxima.

Anti-helmínticos
- Terapia empírica é indicada para gatos com sinais clínicos de doença broncopulmonar felina e citologia eosinofílica das vias aéreas em uma localização geográfica apropriada.
- Considerar o uso de fembendazol, ivermectina ou praziquantel.

Antibióticos
- O emprego desses agentes deve ser feito com base na cultura quantitativa e no antibiograma.

CONTRAINDICAÇÕES
Em virtude de sua capacidade de bloqueio da broncodilatação mediada por via simpática, os antagonistas dos receptores beta-2 (p. ex., propranolol) são contraindicados.

PRECAUÇÕES
- O uso de esteroides a longo prazo aumenta o risco do desenvolvimento de diabetes melito e predispõe o animal à imunossupressão.
- O emprego de corticosteroides em gatos pode precipitar insuficiência cardíaca congestiva.
- Os broncodilatadores podem exacerbar a cardiopatia subjacente.

INTERAÇÕES POSSÍVEIS
As fluoroquinolonas diminuem o metabolismo das metilxantinas em cães, embora esse efeito não tenha sido pesquisado em gatos.

MEDICAMENTO(S) ALTERNATIVO(S)
Ciproeptadina
Antagonista serotoninérgico. Esse medicamento inibe a constrição da musculatura lisa das vias aéreas *in vitro*, embora os efeitos sejam desconhecidos em gatos com asma/bronquite.

Ciclosporina (Neoral® ou Gengraf®)
- Administrar 2,5-5,0 mg/kg a cada 12 h — monitorizar seus níveis. Pode ser útil em pacientes refratários à terapia com broncodilatadores e corticosteroides.

Inibidores de Leucotrienos ou Bloqueadores dos Receptores de Leucotrienos
Não há indícios que apoiem o uso desses medicamentos na asma felina.

ACOMPANHAMENTO
MONITORIZAÇÃO DO PACIENTE
- Os proprietários devem relatar qualquer intensificação nos sinais de tosse, espirro, sibilo ou angústia respiratória. As medicações devem ser aumentadas de forma pertinente em caso de piora dos sinais clínicos.
- As radiografias de acompanhamento podem ser úteis para avaliar a resposta à terapia clínica.
- O proprietário deverá ficar atento ao aparecimento de PU/PD como possíveis indicadores de diabetes melito ou nefropatia. Monitorizar a glicemia e as uroculturas.

PREVENÇÃO
- Eliminar quaisquer fatores ambientais capazes de deflagrar uma situação de crise (ver a seção "Fatores de Risco").
- Fazer a troca periódica dos filtros de ar-condicionado e sistemas de calefação. Considerar o uso de bandejas sanitárias limpas sem poeira.

COMPLICAÇÕES POSSÍVEIS
- Os episódios agudos podem ser potencialmente letais.
- Como resultado de bronquite crônica, pode-se desenvolver uma cardiopatia direita.

EVOLUÇÃO ESPERADA E PROGNÓSTICO
- Deve-se esperar uma terapia a longo prazo.
- Se a recidiva dos sinais clínicos for monitorizada com rigor e a terapia clínica convenientemente ajustada, a maioria dos gatos responderá de forma satisfatória.
- Alguns gatos serão refratários ao tratamento, carreando dessa forma um prognóstico muito pior.

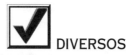

DIVERSOS
DISTÚRBIOS ASSOCIADOS
A *cor pulmonale* pode ser uma sequela de doença crônica das vias aéreas.

GESTAÇÃO/FERTILIDADE/REPRODUÇÃO
Os glicocorticoides são contraindicados no animal prenhe. Os broncodilatadores, por sua vez, devem ser utilizados com cautela.

SINÔNIMO(S)
Bronquite alérgica, doença pulmonar obstrutiva crônica, bronquite asmática, doença das vias aéreas inferiores dos felinos, asma extrínseca, bronquite eosinofílica, doença imunomediada das vias aéreas.

VER TAMBÉM
- Dirofilariose — Gatos.
- Parasitas Respiratórios.

ABREVIATURA(S)
- PU/PD = poliúria/polidipsia.

RECURSOS DA INTERNET
- www.aerokat.com: para pedidos de máscaras faciais e espaçadores para terapia inalatória.
- www.fritzthebrave.com: fonte de pesquisa sobre o uso de medicações inalatórias.

Sugestões de Leitura
Cohn LA, DeClue AE, Cohen RL, Reinero CR. Effects of fluticasone propionate dosage in an experimental model of feline asthma. J Feline Med Surg 2010, 12(2):91-96.

Dye JA, McKiernan BC, Rozanski EA, et al. Bronchopulmonary disease in the cat: Historical, physical, radiographic, clinicopathologic, and pulmonary functional evaluation of 24 affected and 15 healthy cats. J Vet Intern Med 1996, 10:385-399.

Kirschvink J, Leemans J, Delvaux F, et al. Inhaled fluticasone reduces bronchial responsiveness and airway inflammation in cats with mild chronic bronchitis. J Feline Med Surg 2006, 8(1):45-54.

Reinero CR, Delgado C, Spinka C, DeClue AE, Dhand R. Enantiomer-specific effects of albuterol on airway inflammation in healthy and asthmatic cats. Int Arch Allergy Immunol 2009, 150(1):43-50.

Autor Carrie J. Miller
Consultor Editorial Lynelle R. Johnson

ASPERGILOSE DISSEMINADA

CONSIDERAÇÕES GERAIS

REVISÃO
- Uma infecção fúngica oportunista causada pelo *Aspergillus* spp., bolores comuns e ubíquos no meio ambiente, que produzem inúmeros esporos na poeira, na palha, no capim aparado e no feno.
- A doença disseminada não parece estar relacionada com a forma nasal da doença, embora um único relato de um cão que desenvolveu osteomielite fúngica 6 meses após o tratamento de aspergilose nasal levante a possibilidade.
- Doença disseminada — em geral, o *A. terreus*; também se associam o *A. deflectus* e o *A. fumigatus*; ainda não se determinou a porta de entrada de forma definitiva, mas a infecção possivelmente se dá pelo trato respiratório ou gastrintestinal, com subsequente disseminação hematógena.

IDENTIFICAÇÃO
Cães
- Mais comum em cães do que em gatos.
- Os cães da raça Pastor alemão são super-representados, embora haja relatos esporádicos em muitas raças; a idade média é de 3 anos (faixa de 1-9 anos); leve inclinação para as fêmeas.

Gatos
- Persas — incidência marginalmente elevada.
- Os casos disseminados afetam principalmente os pulmões e/ou o trato gastrintestinal.

SINAIS CLÍNICOS
Cães
- Pode se desenvolver de forma aguda ou lenta por um período de vários meses.
- Frequentemente associada à dor espinal por discospondilite fúngica ou à claudicação por osteomielite fúngica.
- Neurológica — dano à medula espinal.
- SNC — sinais vestibulares, crises convulsivas, hemiparesia, embotamento mental, ataxia, paraparesia, déficit visual, andar em círculo.
- Poliúria/polidipsia e hematúria — envolvimento renal.
- Uveíte — envolvimento ocular.
- Inespecíficos — febre, perda de peso, vômito, linfadenopatia e anorexia.

Gatos
- Em geral, os sinais são inespecíficos (p. ex., letargia, depressão, vômito e diarreia).
- Ocular — exoftalmia.

CAUSAS E FATORES DE RISCO
- Causada por espécies de *Aspergillus*, mais comumente *A. terreus*, *A. deflectus* e, menos comumente, *A. fumigatus*, *A. niger*, *A. flavipes*.
- Os cães da raça Pastor alemão estão sob maior risco.
- Imunodeficiência — pode desempenhar um fator-chave para a disseminação do microrganismo, embora a doença seja rara; sugere-se um defeito imunológico relacionado com a raça Pastor alemão e seus mestiços.
- Condições geográficas/ambientais — podem representar um fator, já que algumas regiões apresentam uma incidência mais elevada do que outras (p. ex., Califórnia, Louisiana, Michigan, Geórgia, Flórida e Virgínia nos Estados Unidos; região ocidental da Austrália; Barcelona e Milão).
- Gatos — associada a PIF, vírus da panleucopenia felina, FeLV, diabetes melito e administração crônica de corticosteroides e antibióticos.

DIAGNÓSTICO

DIAGNÓSTICO DIFERENCIAL
Osteomielite/discospondilite bacteriana; neoplasias espinais; discopatia intervertebral; neoplasias esqueléticas; pielonefrite bacteriana; pneumonia bacteriana; outras causas de sinais vestibulares/crises convulsivas; outras causas de uveíte (ver "Uveíte Anterior — Gatos" e "Uveíte Anterior — Cães").

HEMOGRAMA/BIOQUÍMICA/URINÁLISE
- Inespecíficos.
- Cães — com frequência, apresentam leucocitose neutrofílica madura e linfopenia.
- Gatos — podem exibir anemia arregenerativa e leucopenia.
- Alterações bioquímicas — pode-se verificar uma elevação nas concentrações de globulinas, creatinina, fosfato, ureia e cálcio.
- Urinálise — podem-se observar isostenúria, hematúria, piúria e possíveis hifas fúngicas no sedimento; pode-se melhorar a detecção dessas hifas fúngicas, incubando-se a amostra à temperatura ambiente por 24-48 h; é possível examinar as amostras de sedimento não coradas e na forma de preparações úmidas ou secas ao ar e coradas com Diff-Quick (as hifas que se ramificam a 45° coram-se de púrpura).

OUTROS TESTES LABORATORIAIS
- Sorologia fúngica positiva (difusão dupla em ágar gel, contraimunoeletroforese e ELISA) — apoiam o diagnóstico; há relatos de resultados falso-negativos com imunodifusão em ágar gel; também se relatam resultados falso-positivos e reatividade cruzada com *Penicillium* spp.
- Interpretar a sorologia em conjunto com outros testes diagnósticos.
- Gatos — testes para FeLV e FIV, uma vez que tais agentes virais influenciam o prognóstico.
- Cultura fúngica positiva de líquidos e tecidos corporais normalmente estéreis; p. ex., urina, osso, LCS, sangue, linfonodo, efusões pleurais, aspirados de disco intervertebral, rim, baço.

DIAGNÓSTICO POR IMAGEM
Achados Radiográficos
- As projeções radiográficas da coluna vertebral podem revelar lise da placa terminal, tentativa de formação de ponte intervertebral óssea e lise dos corpos vertebrais compatíveis com discospondilite; lesões produtivas e destrutivas dos corpos vertebrais.
- Proliferação e lise ósseas, bem como reação periosteal, típicas de osteomielite da região diafisária dos ossos longos.
- Raro envolvimento pulmonar, com padrão intersticial/alveolar misto, linfonodos esternais e/ou traqueobrônquicos enfartados, efusão pleural; lesões produtivas e destrutivas das esternébras.

Achados Ultrassonográficos
- Rins — local mais comum para detectar alterações; as alterações observadas incluem dilatação da pelve renal ± debris ecogênicos dentro da pelve; perda da distinção corticomedular; distorção renal e aspecto mosqueado do parênquima; dilatação da porção proximal do ureter; renomegalia; nódulos ou massas; hidronefrose.
- Baço — áreas hipoecoicas, rendadas e nitidamente demarcadas sem sinal de Doppler sugestivas de infarto constituem o achado mais significativo no baço; outros achados incluem nódulos/massas, parênquima mosqueado, trombose venosa esplênica.
- Outros — linfadenomegalia abdominal; hipoecogenicidade hepática difusa.

Achados da RM
Útil para definir ainda mais as lesões cerebrais em animais com sinais do SNC; alterações semelhantes a outras doenças cerebrais inflamatórias infecciosas e não infecciosas.

MÉTODOS DIAGNÓSTICOS
A escolha do procedimento diagnóstico é feita conforme indicado pela apresentação clínica, mas pode incluir punção do LCS, aspirados das articulações, aspirados do espaço de disco intervertebral, abdomino/toracocentese, aspirado de vários órgãos (baço, fígado, rins).

ACHADOS PATOLÓGICOS
Histopatologia — com esse exame, torna-se mais provável a obtenção do diagnóstico definitivo; pode haver a necessidade de corantes especiais; na doença disseminada (rins, fígado, baço e vértebras), observam-se granulomas e infartos em múltiplos órgãos.

TRATAMENTO

CÃES
- O tratamento raramente é curativo; pode deter a evolução dos sinais clínicos.
- Fluidoterapia — indicada pelo grau de comprometimento renal e azotemia.

GATOS
- Disseminada — é provavelmente difícil de tratar; além disso, os dados são limitados.

MEDICAÇÕES

MEDICAMENTO(S)
- Itraconazol, 5-10 mg/kg VO a cada 24 h (pode ser dividido) — medicamento de escolha; os cães dificilmente são curados, embora a doença possa ser contida com o uso contínuo desse antifúngico.
- Embora haja descrição de combinações medicamentosas, nenhuma delas resultou em cura relatada da doença. Algumas das combinações relatadas incluem:
  ○ Complexo lipídico de anfotericina B (cães, 2-3 mg/kg IV 3 dias por semana por um total de 9-12 tratamentos, até uma dose cumulativa de 24-27 mg/kg) + itraconazol (5 mg/kg VO a cada 24 h).
  ○ Itraconazol (5 mg/kg VO a cada 24 h) + terbinafina (5-10 mg/kg VO a cada 24 h).
  ○ Novos agentes triazóis, voriconazol (5 mg/kg VO a cada 12 h) e posaconazol (5 mg/kg VO a cada 24 h), são alternativas potenciais para os casos pouco responsivos ao itraconazol. Uso relatado em combinação com o complexo lipídico de anfotericina B.
  ○ Inibidores da β-glucana sintase, como caspofungina, micafungina, anidulafungina

— podem vir a ser úteis, apesar das informações clínicas muito limitadas.
◦ Terapia combinada com flucitosina (25-50 mg/kg VO a cada 6 h, cães) e anfotericina B pode vir a ser bem-sucedida, mas não há relatos publicados.

CONTRAINDICAÇÕES/INTERAÇÕES POSSÍVEIS
• Anfotericina B — contraindicada em cães com comprometimento ou insuficiência renais preexistentes; o complexo lipídico de anfotericina B diminui significativamente a nefrotoxicidade.
• Azóis orais — náusea, anorexia intermitente, elevação das enzimas hepáticas.
• Combinação de flucitosina e anfotericina B — erupções medicamentosas cutâneas em cães.
• Evitar o midazolam e a cisaprida com os antifúngicos azóis — reações medicamentosas fatais são observadas em seres humanos.
• O itraconazol em altas doses (10 mg/kg) é associado à dermatite ulcerativa em 5-10% dos cães — identificar precocemente e interromper e, em seguida, reinstituir com uma dose reduzida; caso contrário, pode ocorrer esfacelamento cutâneo e subcutâneo grave.

ACOMPANHAMENTO
Disseminada — monitorizar radiografias seriadas a cada 1-2 meses, testes de função renal e uroculturas; prognóstico mau, especialmente em cães da raça Pastor alemão.

DIVERSOS
POTENCIAL ZOONÓTICO
Nenhum.

ABREVIATURA(S)
• ELISA = ensaio imunoabsorvente ligado à enzima.
• FeLV = vírus da leucemia felina.
• FIV = vírus da imunodeficiência felina.
• LCS = líquido cerebrospinal.
• PIF = peritonite infecciosa felina.
• RM = ressonância magnética.
• SNC = sistema nervoso central.

Sugestões de Leitura
Maddison JE, Page SW, Church DB. Small Animal Clinical Pharmacology, 2nd ed. Edinburgh: Saunders, 2008, pp. 186-197.
Schultz RM, Johnson EG, Wisner ER, Brown NA, Byrne BA, Sykes JE. Clinicopathologic and diagnostic imaging characteristics of systemic aspergillosis in 30 Dogs. J Vet Intern Med 2008, 22:851-859.

Autor Tania N. Davey
Consultor Editorial Stephen C. Barr

Aspergilose Nasal

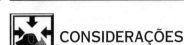

CONSIDERAÇÕES GERAIS

REVISÃO
- Doença nasal causada por *Aspergillus* spp., principalmente o *A. fumigatus*.
- Fungo saprófito e ubíquo no ambiente.
- Patógeno oportunista.

FISIOPATOLOGIA
- A inalação do fungo induz à doença na cavidade nasal com destruição dos ossos turbinados e produção excessiva de muco, provocando sinais clínicos de doença nasal.
- Raramente pode estar associada a corpo estranho subjacente ou traumatismo prévio.
- Provoca doença localmente agressiva e invasiva, mas não resulta em micose sistêmica.
- Confinada às regiões da cavidade nasal e do seio frontal — forma sinonasal (mais comum em cães).
- Também pode se estender para a órbita em gatos e raramente em cães — forma sino-orbital.

SISTEMA(S) ACOMETIDO(S)
Respiratório — cavidade nasal, seios nasais, órbita (em gatos, mas rara em cães).

GENÉTICA
Desconhecida.

INCIDÊNCIA/PREVALÊNCIA
Desconhecidas, embora seja um diagnóstico comum em cães com secreção nasal em muitos locais.

DISTRIBUIÇÃO GEOGRÁFICA
Mundial.

IDENTIFICAÇÃO
Espécies
Cães e gatos (menos comum).

Raça(s) Predominante(s)
- Cães — raças dolicocefálicas e mesocefálicas.
- Gatos — raças braquicefálicas podem ser super-representadas.

Idade Média e Faixa Etária
- Cães — predominantemente jovens aos de meia-idade.
- Gatos — sem predileção etária.

Sexo Predominante
Nenhum identificado.

SINAIS CLÍNICOS
Achados Anamnésicos
- Secreção nasal uni ou bilateral — tipicamente mucoide, mucopurulenta ou serossanguinolenta, embora possa haver epistaxe.
- Espirro.
- Sinais tipicamente crônicos — vários meses.
- Muitos pacientes foram tratados com antibióticos por uma possível infecção bacteriana antes da manifestação com resposta variável.

Achados do Exame Físico
- Secreção nasal uni ou bilateral.
- Aumento no fluxo de ar nasal no lado acometido.
- Despigmentação com ulceração do plano nasal — ~40% dos cães.
- Dor facial.
- Linfadenopatia mandibular ipsilateral.
- Estertor, exoftalmia, ulceração do palato duro, perda do fluxo de ar nasal — gatos.

CAUSAS
- Não se identificou qualquer causa subjacente, embora corpo estranho ou traumatismo preexistente seja ocasionalmente implicado.
- Provavelmente atribuída à inalação de grande bolo de fungo, ubíquo no ambiente.
- Espécies — mais comumente *A. fumigatus*; outros — *A. niger*, *A. flavus*.

FATORES DE RISCO
Desconhecidos.

DIAGNÓSTICO

DIAGNÓSTICO DIFERENCIAL
- Corpo estranho.
- Fístula oronasal.
- Rinite linfoplasmocitária.
- Neoplasia.
- Pólipo nasofaríngeo, tumor nasal ou criptococose — apenas nos gatos.

HEMOGRAMA/BIOQUÍMICA/URINÁLISE
- Frequentemente normais.
- Possível leucograma inflamatório.

OUTROS TESTES LABORATORIAIS
Sorologia
- Detecta anticorpos séricos específicos para o fungo.
- Imunodifusão em ágar gel — disponível no mercado; especificidade de 98%; sensibilidade de 67% em cães; a sorologia seriada não parece se correlacionar com o estado clínico.
- ELISA — sensibilidade de 88%, especificidade de 96,8%.
- Contraimunoeletroforese — especificidade de 85% em cães.
- Galactomanana sérica — não se mostrou confiável.

Cultura
- Cultura fúngica tecidual da área acometida; a obtenção de amostra de biopsia visualizada de uma região sob suspeita de crescimento fúngico revelou especificidade de 100% e sensibilidade de 81%.
- A cultura da secreção nasal é menos específica e insensível.

DIAGNÓSTICO POR IMAGEM
Tomografia Computadorizada
- Método de escolha para obtenção de imagem.
- Lise do tipo cavitária dos ossos turbinados.
- Espessamento da mucosa ao longo dos turbinados nasais.
- Efeito expansivo proliferativo no seio frontal.
- Massa de tecido mole nas coanas nasais ou na nasofaringe — gatos.
- Necessária para avaliação da placa cribriforme antes do tratamento antifúngico tópico.

Radiografia do Crânio
- Radiografia dorsoventral intrabucal da cavidade nasal revela lise dos ossos turbinados.
- Projeção rostrocaudal ou tipo *skyline* (tangencial) do seio frontal pode demonstrar o aumento na densidade dos tecidos moles nesse seio nasal.
- Esse exame não é capaz de avaliar a placa cribriforme.

MÉTODOS DIAGNÓSTICOS
Rinoscopia
- A rinoscopia flexível em cães permite o exame da nasofaringe e, possivelmente, do seio frontal se a abertura do ducto nasofrontal estiver destruída pela infecção fúngica.
- A rinoscopia rígida possibilita apenas o exame da cavidade nasal; é possível uma visualização satisfatória em virtude dos grandes espaços aéreos gerados pela lise dos ossos turbinados; a quantidade excessiva de muco e a ocorrência de sangramento podem dificultar o exame completo.
- A visualização de placas fúngicas (brancas, amarelas, negras ou verde-claras) na mucosa da cavidade nasal e/ou do seio nasal confirma a infecção fúngica.

ACHADOS PATOLÓGICOS
- Biopsias obtidas da área acometida sob inspeção rinoscópica direta com o uso de instrumentos para biopsia em cálice.
- As amostras são fixadas por imersão em formalina tamponada a 10% e processadas de forma habitual.
- Indícios que apoiam o diagnóstico de aspergilose — identificação de hifas e conídios ramificados e septados ao exame histopatológico. A inflamação circunjacente costuma ser neutrofílica ou linfoplasmocitária, raramente eosinofílica.
- Biopsias feitas às cegas em área não acometida da cavidade nasal podem resultar no diagnóstico falso de inflamação.

TRATAMENTO

CUIDADO(S) DE SAÚDE ADEQUADO(S)
É necessária a hospitalização durante a noite após tratamento tópico ou cirurgia.

CUIDADO(S) DE ENFERMAGEM
Manter as narinas livres de secreção nasal.

ATIVIDADE
Não há necessidade de restrição da atividade física.

DIETA
N/D.

ORIENTAÇÃO AO PROPRIETÁRIO
- Cães — informar ao cliente sobre a necessidade habitual de múltiplos tratamentos tópicos para se obter a cura da doença; o acompanhamento com rinoscopia é altamente recomendado para garantir a resolução.
- Não há protocolos terapêuticos estabelecidos para gatos.

CONSIDERAÇÕES CIRÚRGICAS
Trepanação do Seio Frontal
- Recomendada para cães com envolvimento do seio frontal.
- Realizada com o uso de mandril de Jacob e pino intramedular.
- Possibilita a inspeção direta do seio frontal com rinoscópio rígido e debridamento local de placas fúngicas.
- Permite a lavagem e o tratamento tópico da área, utilizando um cateter de borracha vermelha.

Debridamento Cirúrgico e Exenteração
- Procedimentos usados em alguns gatos com doença sino-orbital.

Debridamento Endoscópico
- A curetagem e a remoção extensivas de material fúngico do nariz e do seio frontal são essenciais para permitir a eficácia da medicação tópica.

ASPERGILOSE NASAL

MEDICAÇÕES

MEDICAMENTO(S) DE ESCOLHA

Terapia Tópica com Clotrimazol ou Enilconazol
- Infusão de 1 h na cavidade nasal sob anestesia.
- O tratamento costuma ser realizado durante a mesma anestesia utilizada no diagnóstico.
- Tratamento de escolha em cães; eficácia relatada de 85-89% com múltiplos tratamentos.
- Cateteres de Foley são usados para ocluir as narinas e a nasofaringe.
- Dose — clotrimazol: 1 g desse agente em 100 mL de polietilenoglicol 200 (solução a 1%) uniformemente dividida entre duas seringas de 60 mL e aplicadas sob a forma de infusão lenta em 1 h em cada lado para cães de grande porte; caso se faça uso da trepanação, dividir a quantidade entre a cavidade e o seio nasal do mesmo lado; usar um volume menor em cães de pequeno porte. Enilconazol: 100 mL de solução a 1, 2 ou 5%.
- O cão é colocado em decúbito dorsal com a cabeça virada para cada lado a cada 15 min durante a infusão.
- No final do procedimento, o cão é colocado em decúbito esternal com a cabeça virada para baixo para permitir a drenagem de toda a medicação.
- Essa terapia foi usada em gatos sem envolvimento orbital em combinação com terapia antifúngica oral com sucesso variado.

Terapia Sistêmica
- Os agentes triazóis antifúngicos devem ser considerados se a placa cribriforme não estiver intacta; também são usados como a terapia primária em alguns gatos.
- Também pode ser utilizada em combinação com a terapia tópica.
- Pode ser muito cara em termos de custo.
- Itraconazol a 5 mg/kg VO a cada 12 h em cães, com eficácia relatada de 60-70%; 10 mg/kg VO a cada 24 h em gatos.
- Voriconazol a 5 mg/kg VO a cada 12 h; a eficácia como monoterapia não foi estabelecida.
- Posaconazol a 5 mg/kg VO a cada 24 h; a eficácia como monoterapia não foi estabelecida.
- Anfotericina B (desoxicolato) a 0,8 mg/kg SC em 400 mL de dextrose a 2,5%/salina a 0,45% aquecida a cada 3-4 dias; dose cumulativa de 10-14 mg/kg em combinação com agentes triazóis.
- Fluconazol não é recomendado por conta da resistência.

CONTRAINDICAÇÕES
- A ruptura na placa cribriforme pode permitir o contato da medicação antifúngica com o cérebro, resultando em sinais neurológicos e possível óbito.
- A doença sino-orbital necessita do emprego da terapia sistêmica.

PRECAUÇÕES
- O clotrimazol e o enilconazol tópicos são agentes cáusticos para todas as superfícies mucosas — vestes protetoras como luvas e óculos de proteção devem ser usadas por toda a equipe que estiver em contato estrito com o animal.
- O enilconazol pode ser associado à tumefação (inchaço) dos tecidos e obstrução das vias aéreas superiores.

INTERAÇÕES POSSÍVEIS
N/D.

MEDICAMENTO(S) ALTERNATIVO(S)

Enilconazol
- Também é ativo na fase de vapor.

Irritação de Clotrimazol e Terapia de Depósito Combinadas
- O clotrimazol (a 1%) é irrigado por meio do orifício do trépano no seio frontal por 5 minutos; 50 mL de cada lado em cães com >10 kg; 25 mL de cada lado naqueles com menos de 10 kg.
- Em seguida, o clotrimazol em creme (a 1%) é introduzido nos seios frontais; 20 g de cada lado em cães com >10 kg; 10 g de cada lado naqueles com <10 kg.
- A eficácia relatada é semelhante ao uso tópico isolado de clotrimazol ou enilconazol (86%).

ACOMPANHAMENTO

MONITORIZAÇÃO DO PACIENTE

Cães
- Monitorizar os sinais clínicos, embora a redução desses sinais não estabeleça a resolução da doença.
- Em todos os casos, é recomendável a rinoscopia de acompanhamento para determinar a resposta terapêutica, independentemente dos sinais clínicos — os exames de histopatologia e cultura podem ajudar a definir a resposta.
- A sorologia seriada (imunodifusão em ágar gel) parece não se correlacionar com o estado clínico.
- A repetição da varredura por TC deve ser considerada para a reavaliação da placa cribriforme antes de se repetir o tratamento tópico caso se observe a piora dos sinais clínicos.
- Monitorizar a atividade das enzimas hepáticas em animais sob terapia triazólica.

Gatos
- Monitorizar os sinais clínicos quanto à melhora ou resolução.
- Proceder à monitorização das enzimas hepáticas em animais sob terapia triazólica.
- Efetuar o monitoramento dos parâmetros renais em animais sob anfotericina B.

PREVENÇÃO
N/D.

COMPLICAÇÕES POSSÍVEIS
- Terapia tópica — monitorar o animal depois do tratamento de quaisquer complicações, como tumefação da orofaringe, sinais neurológicos, infecção/tumefação do local de inserção do trépano.
- Os agentes triazóis podem causar anorexia e ser hepatotóxicos.
- A anfotericina B pode ser nefrotóxica.

EVOLUÇÃO ESPERADA E PROGNÓSTICO
- Estudos demonstraram uma taxa de reposta de 87% à terapia tópica em cães após 1 a 3 tratamentos.
- Um estudo mais recente revelou que a recidiva ou a reinfecção é mais comum do que se acreditava e pode ocorrer anos após terapia supostamente bem-sucedida.
- O prognóstico para gatos com aspergilose sinonasal é melhor do que para aqueles com a forma sino-orbital.

DIVERSOS

DISTÚRBIOS ASSOCIADOS
N/D.

FATORES RELACIONADOS COM A IDADE
N/D.

POTENCIAL ZOONÓTICO
Não há casos registrados de infecção em seres humanos a partir de cão ou gato acometido.

GESTAÇÃO/FERTILIDADE/REPRODUÇÃO
N/D.

ABREVIATURA(S)
- ELISA = ensaio imunoabsorvente ligado à enzima.
- TC = tomografia computadorizada.

Sugestões de Leitura

Barrs VR. Feline sino-orbital aspergillosis: An emerging clinical syndrome. ACVIM Forum Proceedings 2009, pp. 395-397.

Friend E, Anderson DM, White RAS. Combined clotrimazole irrigation and depot therapy for canine nasal aspergillosis. J Small Anim Pract 2006, 47(6):312-315.

Mathews KG, Davidson AP, Koblik PD, et al. Comparison of topical administration of clotrimazole through surgically placed versus nonsurgically placed catheters for treatment of nasal aspergillosis in dogs: 60 cases (1990-1996). JAVMA 1998, 213:501-506.

McLellan GJ, Aquino SM, Mason DR, Myers RK. Use of posaconazole in the management of invasive orbital aspergillosis in a cat. JAAHA 2006, 42:302-307.

Pomrantz JS, Johnson LR, Nelson RW, Wisner ER. Comparison of serologic evaluation via agar gel immunodiffusion and fungal culture of tissue for diagnosis of nasal aspergillosis in dog. JAVMA 2007, 230:1319-1323.

Autor Jill S. Pomrantz
Consultor Editorial Lynelle R. Johnson

Astrocitoma

CONSIDERAÇÕES GERAIS

REVISÃO
- Categorizado como neoplasia de células gliais, que costuma afetar o cérebro, mas raras vezes a medula espinal. • As células neoplásicas são de origem astrocitária. • Esse tumor é a neoplasia intracraniana intra-axial (situada dentro do parênquima cerebral) mais comum de cães, mas raramente diagnosticado em gatos. • Os tumores estão frequentemente localizados na área piriforme do lobo temporal, nos hemisférios cerebrais, no tálamo, hipotálamo ou mesencéfalo. • O comportamento biológico desse tumor é ditado pelo grau de anaplasia (grau I-IV, do melhor ao pior prognóstico). • Tipicamente, os tumores não penetram no sistema ventricular ou sofrem metástase para fora da abóbada craniana.

IDENTIFICAÇÃO
- Cães — com frequência, acomete raças braquicefálicas com >5 anos de idade; não há relato de predisposição sexual. • Gatos — em geral, ocorre em animais idosos (>9 anos); não há relato de predisposição sexual ou racial.

SINAIS CLÍNICOS
- Dependem da localização do tumor e da cinética do crescimento. • Crises convulsivas. • Mudanças comportamentais. • Desorientação. • Perda da propriocepção consciente. • Anormalidades dos nervos cranianos. • Tetraparesia atribuível à lesão do neurônio motor superior.

CAUSAS E FATORES DE RISCO
Desconhecidos.

DIAGNÓSTICO

DIAGNÓSTICO DIFERENCIAL
- Outros tumores primários que surgem de tecidos do SNC. • Neoplasia metastática com tropismo cerebral. • Meningoencefalite granulomatosa. • Traumatismo. • Infarto cerebrovascular. • Meningite.

HEMOGRAMA/BIOQUÍMICA/URINÁLISE
Em geral, permanecem normais.

OUTROS TESTES LABORATORIAIS
Análise do LCS — pode revelar uma dissociação albuminocitológica (alto nível proteico com poucas células). A análise deve compreender a caracterização do líquido, incluindo aspectos como cor, turbidez, concentração de proteína, contagem total de células nucleadas, avaliação citológica e títulos de anticorpos contra agentes infecciosos, além da realização de cultura.

DIAGNÓSTICO POR IMAGEM
- RM do cérebro é ideal para a confirmação de lesão expansiva. Ao contrário da varredura por TC, não ocorrem artefatos de endurecimento do feixe originários de osso compacto espesso com a RM; portanto, o exame de RM é superior à TC para a detecção de lesões nas fossas médias e caudais. Além disso, a RM é mais sensível que a TC para a detecção de alterações sutis nas propriedades químicas do tecidos moles; portanto, é possível detectar infartos e edema em um estágio mais precoce. • TC do cérebro com ou sem contraste pode ser útil para a confirmação de lesão, mas não é tão sensível para a obtenção de imagem de lesão dos tecidos moles quanto à RM.

MÉTODOS DIAGNÓSTICOS
- Exame neurológico. • Exame oftalmológico. • Técnicas avançadas de diagnóstico por imagem, como RM ou TC. • Análise do LCS. • Raramente se faz biopsia do cérebro por causa da morbidade induzida pelo procedimento; no entanto, esse tipo de exame pode não só fornecer o diagnóstico definitivo, mas também ajudar no planejamento da terapia e no estabelecimento do prognóstico.

TRATAMENTO
- Cirurgia. • Quimioterapia. • Radioterapia pode ser muito eficaz em alguns casos; entretanto, é recomendável a consulta com um veterinário especialista em oncologia e radiação.

MEDICAÇÕES

MEDICAMENTO(S)

Controle das Crises Convulsivas
- Estado epiléptico — diazepam (0,5-1,0 mg/kg IV, administrados por até 3 vezes para atingir o efeito desejado); na ausência de resposta a esse medicamento, utilizar o pentobarbital (5-15 mg/kg IV lentamente até se obter o efeito esperado). • Tratamento a longo prazo — fenobarbital (1-4 mg/kg VO a cada 12 h) com ou sem brometo de potássio como adjuvante (20 mg/kg VO a cada 24 h).

Controle do Tumor
- Embora a radioterapia possa ser eficaz, é aconselhável a consulta com um veterinário especialista em oncologia e radiação. A radiocirurgia estereotáxica ou a radioterapia de intensidade modulada devem ser consideradas como opções terapêuticas de primeira linha. • A quimioterapia pode ser eficaz para o tratamento de cães. Os agentes quimioterápicos potenciais que podem exercer efeitos antineoplásicos mensuráveis incluem a lomustina (70 mg/m^2 VO a cada 3 semanas) ou a carmustina (50 mg/m^2 IV a cada 6 semanas). • Apesar de a prednisona (0,5-1,0 mg/kg a cada 24 h) não ser citotóxica para as células cancerígenas, esse medicamento pode ser eficaz no controle do edema peritumoral e na melhora dos sinais clínicos.

CONTRAINDICAÇÕES/INTERAÇÕES POSSÍVEIS
- Prednisona e fenobarbital podem causar polifagia, polidipsia e poliúria. • Fenobarbital pode provocar sedação por até 2 semanas após o início do tratamento; além disso, pode gerar um aumento nas enzimas hepáticas em um perfil bioquímico sérico. • Hemograma completo e contagem plaquetária são recomendados 7-10 dias após a quimioterapia e imediatamente antes de cada aplicação quimioterápica, a fim de monitorizar a mielossupressão. • Carmustina tem o potencial de causar toxicidade pulmonar em doses cumulativas de 1.400 mg/m^2. • A quimioterapia pode ser tóxica; portanto, é recomendável a busca por orientação de um veterinário especialista em oncologia antes de se iniciar o tratamento.

ACOMPANHAMENTO

MONITORIZAÇÃO DO PACIENTE
- Concentração sanguínea do fenobarbital deve ser avaliada após 7-10 dias de tratamento, com modificações da dosagem para atingir as concentrações plasmáticas-alvo. • TC ou RM seriadas podem ser consideradas para registrar a resposta do paciente se houver indicação clínica e se for viável em termos econômicos. • É recomendável a avaliação seriada do hemograma completo e das contagens plaquetárias para registrar a mielotoxicidade associada à quimioterapia.

EVOLUÇÃO ESPERADA E PROGNÓSTICO
- Prognóstico a longo prazo — reservado. • O tempo de sobrevida sem nenhum tratamento é variável e depende de fatores relacionados com o tumor e o hospedeiro. • O tempo médio de sobrevida após a quimioterapia associada ao tratamento clínico pode ser de até 7 meses. • Há relatos de que o tempo médio de sobrevida após a radioterapia seja de até 12 meses.

DIVERSOS

GESTAÇÃO/FERTILIDADE/REPRODUÇÃO
Não acasalar os animais submetidos à quimioterapia.

VER TAMBÉM
- Crises Convulsivas (Convulsões, Estado Epiléptico) — Cães. • Crises Convulsivas (Convulsões, Estado Epiléptico) — Gatos.

ABREVIATURA(S)
- LCS = líquido cerebrospinal. • RM = ressonância magnética. • SNC = sistema nervoso central. • TC = tomografia computadorizada.

Sugestões de Leitura
Bley CR, Sumova A, Roos M, Kaser-Hotz B. Irradiation of brain tumors in dogs with neurologic disease. J Vet Intern Med 2005, 19:849-854.
Meyerholz DG, Haynes JS. Solitary retinal astrocytoma in a dog. Vet Pathol 2004, 41:177-178.
Morrison WB. Cancer affecting the nervous system. In: Morrison WB, ed., Cancer in Dogs and Cats: Medical and Surgical Management. Jackson, WY: Teton NewMedia, 2002, pp. 631-640.
Snyder JM, Shofer FS, Van Winkle TJ, et al. Canine intracranial primary neoplasia: 173 cases (1986-2003). J Vet Intern Med 2006, 20:669-675.
Troxel MT, Vite CH, Van Winkle TJ, et al. Feline intracranial neoplasia: Retrospective review of 160 cases (1985-2001). J Vet Intern Med 2003, 17:850-859.

Autor Wallace B. Morrison
Consultor Editorial Timothy M. Fan

Ataxia

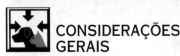

CONSIDERAÇÕES GERAIS

DEFINIÇÃO
- Um sinal de disfunção sensorial que produz incoordenação dos membros, da cabeça e/ou do tronco.
- Há três tipos clínicos — sensorial (proprioceptiva), vestibular e cerebelar; todos eles produzem alterações na coordenação dos membros, mas as ataxias vestibulares e cerebelares também geram alterações nos movimentos da cabeça e do pescoço.

FISIOPATOLOGIA

Sensorial (Proprioceptiva)
- As vias proprioceptivas na medula espinal (i. e., fascículo grácil, fascículo cuneado e tratos espinocerebelares) retransmitem as posições dos membros e do tronco ao cérebro.
- Quando a medula espinal é lentamente comprimida, os déficits proprioceptivos costumam ser os primeiros sinais observados, pois essas vias se encontram mais superficialmente na substância branca e seus axônios mais calibrosos se mostram mais suscetíveis à compressão do que outros tratos.
- Em geral, essa ataxia é acompanhada por fraqueza em virtude do envolvimento precoce concomitante do neurônio motor superior; a fraqueza nem sempre é evidente no início do curso da doença.
- Pode ocorrer ataxia em lesões na medula espinal, no tronco cerebral e no cérebro; leve com lesões unilaterais do tronco cerebral, mas sutil a ausente com lesão unilateral do cérebro.

Vestibular
- As mudanças de posição da cabeça e do pescoço são retransmitidas por meio do nervo vestibulococlear até o tronco cerebral.
- Os receptores vestibulares ou o nervo vestibular na orelha interna são considerados parte do sistema nervoso periférico, enquanto os núcleos no tronco cerebral constituem parte integrante do sistema nervoso central.
- É fundamental situar os sinais vestibulares ao sistema nervoso vestibular central ou periférico, já que o prognóstico e os diagnósticos de exclusão diferem para essas duas localizações.
- Ambas as localizações da vestibulopatia geram diversos graus de desequilíbrio, com consequente ataxia vestibular.
- O animal acometido se inclina, tomba, cai ou, até mesmo, rola em direção ao lado da lesão; tais sinais são acompanhados por inclinação da cabeça.
- Os sinais vestibulares centrais costumam apresentar tipos variados de nistagmo ou nistagmo vertical; sonolência, estupor ou coma (em função do envolvimento do sistema de ativação reticular adjacente); múltiplos sinais atribuídos aos nervos cranianos; déficits proprioceptivos e quadriparesia ou hemiparesia.
- Os sinais vestibulares periféricos não incluem alterações no estado mental, nistagmo vertical, déficits proprioceptivos, quadriparesia ou hemiparesia.

Cerebelar
- O cerebelo regula, coordena e modula a atividade motora.
- A propriocepção permanece normal, já que as vias proprioceptivas ascendentes em direção ao córtex continuam intactas; em virtude da persistência na integridade dos neurônios motores superiores, não se observa sinal de fraqueza.
- Inadequação no desempenho da atividade motora; conservação da força; ausência de déficits proprioceptivos.
- O animal acometido revela incoordenação na atividade motora dos membros, da cabeça e do pescoço; hipermetria; dismetria; tremores cefálicos; tremores intencionais; e oscilação do tronco.

SISTEMA(S) ACOMETIDO(S)
Nervoso — medula espinal (além do tronco e córtex cerebrais), cerebelo, sistema vestibular.

IDENTIFICAÇÃO
Qualquer idade, raça ou sexo.

SINAIS CLÍNICOS
- É importante definir o tipo de ataxia para localizar o problema.
- Apenas um membro envolvido — considerar um problema de claudicação.
- Apenas os membros pélvicos acometidos — provável presença de distúrbio medular, com acometimento dos tratos espinocerebelares.
- Todos ou ambos os membros ipsilaterais acometidos — lesão cerebelar.
- Inclinação da cabeça — lesão vestibular.

CAUSAS

Neurológicas

Cerebelar
- Degenerativas — abiotrofia (Kerry blue terrier, Setter gordon, Collie de pelo áspero, Kelpie australiano, Airedale, cães Montanhês de Berna, Finnish harrier, Spaniel britânico, Border collie, Beagle, Samoieda, Fox terrier de pelo duro, Labrador retriever, Dogue alemão, Chow chow, Rhodesian ridgeback, gatos domésticos de pelo curto); com frequência, as doenças de armazenamento apresentam um envolvimento cerebelomedular.
- Anômalas — hipoplasia secundária à infecção perinatal pelo vírus da panleucopenia (gatos); má-formação cerebelar decorrente de infecção pelo herpes-vírus (filhotes caninos recém-nascidos); cisto aracnoide ou epidermoide localizado próximo ao quarto ventrículo.
- Neoplásicas — qualquer tumor (primário ou secundário) do SNC localizado no cerebelo.
- Infecciosas — vírus da cinomose; PIF; e qualquer outra infecção no SNC com acometimento do cerebelo.
- Inflamatórias, idiopáticas, imunomediadas — meningoencefalomielite granulomatosa.
- Tóxicas — metronidazol.

Vestibular — SNC
- Infecciosas — PIF; vírus da cinomose; riquetsioses.
- Inflamatórias, idiopáticas, imunomediadas — meningoencefalomielite granulomatosa.
- Nutricional — deficiência da tiamina.
- Tóxicas — metronidazol.

Vestibular — SNP
- Infecciosas — otite média interna; granuloma por *Cryptococcus* (gatos).
- Idiopáticas — vestibulopatia geriátrica (cães); síndrome vestibular idiopática (gatos); pólipos (orelha média) nasofaríngeos (gatos).
- Metabólicas — hipotireoidismo.
- Neoplásicas — carcinoma de células escamosas; tumores ósseos.
- Traumáticas.

Medula Espinal
- Degenerativas — mielopatia degenerativa (Pastor alemão idoso, Welsh corgi).
- Vasculares — mielopatia embólica fibrocartilaginosa.
- Anômalas — hemivértebras; hipoplasia do processo odontoide com subluxação-luxação atlantoaxial; má-formação semelhante à de Chiari; outras más-formações da medula espinal e das vértebras; cisto aracnoide espinal.
- Neoplásicas — tumores ósseos primários; mieloma múltiplo e tumores metastáticos com infiltração no corpo vertebral; meningioma; outros.
- Infecciosas — discoespondilite; mielite.
- Traumáticas — herniação do disco intervertebral; fratura ou luxação; espondilomielopatia cervical; subluxação-luxação atlantoaxial.

Metabólicas
- Anemia.
- Policitemia.
- Distúrbios eletrolíticos — especialmente hipocalemia, hipocalcemia e hipoglicemia.

Diversas
- Medicamentos — acepromazina; anti-histamínicos; anticonvulsivantes.
- Comprometimento respiratório.
- Comprometimento cardíaco — ducto arterioso persistente reverso, tromboembolia aórtica.

FATORES DE RISCO
- Discopatia intervertebral — Dachshund, Poodle, Cocker spaniel e Beagle.
- Espondilomielopatia cervical — Doberman e Dogue alemão.
- Embolia fibrocartilaginosa — cães jovens de grande porte e Schnauzer miniatura.
- Hipoplasia do processo odontoide e luxação atlantoaxial — cães de pequeno porte, Poodle.
- Má-formação semelhante à de Chiari — Cavalier King Charles spaniel, raças caninas de pequeno porte.

DIAGNÓSTICO

DIAGNÓSTICO DIFERENCIAL
- Diferenciar os tipos de ataxia.
- Diferenciar de outros processos patológicos capazes de comprometer a marcha — distúrbios musculoesqueléticos, metabólicos, cardiovasculares, respiratórios.
- Distúrbios musculoesqueléticos — tipicamente produzem claudicação, dor e relutância ao movimento; a artropatia degenerativa frequentemente melhora com incremento nos movimentos.
- Doença sistêmica, endocrinopatias, bem como distúrbios cardiovasculares e metabólicos — podem causar ataxia intermitente, sobretudo dos membros pélvicos; os sinais de febre, perda de peso, sopros, arritmias, perda de pelos ou colapso com a prática de exercícios levantam a suspeita de uma causa não neurológica; obter um banco de dados mínimo, constituído por hemograma, análise bioquímica e urinálise.
- Inclinação da cabeça ou nistagmo — lesão provavelmente vestibular.
- Tremores intencionais da cabeça ou hipermetria — lesão provavelmente cerebelar.

ATAXIA

- Todos os quatro membros acometidos: a lesão encontra-se na região cervical ou apresenta-se multifocal a difusa; apenas os membros pélvicos acometidos: a lesão situa-se em qualquer região caudal à segunda vértebra torácica.

HEMOGRAMA/BIOQUÍMICA/URINÁLISE
Normais a menos que haja uma causa metabólica (p. ex., hipoglicemia, desequilíbrio eletrolítico, anemia, policitemia).

OUTROS TESTES LABORATORIAIS
- Hipoglicemia — determinar a concentração sérica de insulina na mesma amostra (para descartar insulinoma).
- Anemia — diferenciar em arregenerativa ou regenerativa, com base na contagem de reticulócitos.
- Distúrbio eletrolítico — corrigir o problema; observar se a ataxia desaparece.
- Medicamentos anticonvulsivantes — se forem administrados, avaliar a concentração sérica quanto à ocorrência de toxicidade.

DIAGNÓSTICO POR IMAGEM
- Radiografias da coluna, mielografia, TC ou RM — na suspeita de disfunção da medula espinal.
- Radiografia das bulhas timpânicas — na suspeita de vestibulopatia periférica; TC ou RM são exames superiores às radiografias; a RM é superior à TC em caso de doença da orelha interna.
- Radiografias torácicas — no caso de pacientes idosos e naqueles sob suspeita de neoplasia ou infecção fúngica sistêmica.
- TC ou RM — na suspeita de doença cerebelar; avaliam uma doença craniana em potencial; a RM é superior à TC.
- Ultrassonografia abdominal — na suspeita de disfunções hepáticas, renais, adrenais ou pancreáticas.

MÉTODOS DIAGNÓSTICOS
LCS — ajuda a confirmar as causas do sistema nervoso.

TRATAMENTO
- Feito geralmente em um esquema ambulatorial, dependendo da gravidade e da intensidade dos sinais clínicos.
- Exercícios — diminuir ou restringir se houver a suspeita de mielopatia.
- O proprietário deve monitorizar a marcha quanto à presença de disfunção ou fraqueza progressivas; em caso de agravamento da paresia ou desenvolvimento de paralisia, justifica-se a realização de outros testes.
- Evitar o uso de medicamentos que possam contribuir para o problema; no entanto, isso pode não ser possível em pacientes sob efeito de medicamentos anticonvulsivantes para o controle de crises convulsivas.

MEDICAÇÕES
MEDICAMENTO(S) DE ESCOLHA
Não recomendados até que se identifique a origem ou a causa do problema.

ACOMPANHAMENTO
MONITORIZAÇÃO DO PACIENTE
Exames neurológicos periódicos para avaliar a condição.

COMPLICAÇÕES POSSÍVEIS
- Medula espinal — evolução para fraqueza e, possivelmente, paralisia.
- Hipoglicemia — crises convulsivas.
- Doença cerebelar — tremores e oscilações da cabeça.
- Doença do tronco cerebral — estupor, coma, óbito.

DIVERSOS
FATORES RELACIONADOS COM A IDADE
N/D.

VER TAMBÉM
- Degeneração Cerebelar.
- Inclinação da Cabeça.
- Paralisia.
- Ver causas específicas.

ABREVIATURA(S)
- LCS = líquido cerebrospinal.
- PIF = peritonite infecciosa felina.
- RM = ressonância magnética.
- SNC = sistema nervoso central.
- SNP = sistema nervoso periférico.
- TC = tomografia computadorizada.

RECURSOS DA INTERNET
IVIS: www.ivis.org

Sugestões de Leitura
Davies C, Shell L. Neurological problems. In: Common Small Animal Medical Diagnoses: An Algorithmic Approach. Philadelphia: Saunders, 2002, pp. 36-59.
Lorenz MD, Kornegay JN. Handbook of Veterinary Neurology, 4th ed. Philadelphia: Saunders, 2004, pp. 219-244.
Thomas WB. Vestibular dysfunction. Vet Clin North Am Small Anim Pract 2000, 30:227-249.

Autor Linda G. Shell
Consultor Editorial Joane M. Parent

ATEROSCLEROSE

CONSIDERAÇÕES GERAIS

REVISÃO
Espessamento da parede arterial interna, associado a depósitos lipídicos. Corresponde a uma alteração arterial crônica, caracterizada por perda da elasticidade e estreitamento do lúmen, bem como por lesões proliferativas e degenerativas das túnicas íntima e média.

IDENTIFICAÇÃO
- Rara em cães.
- Não descrita em gatos.
- Prevalência mais elevada em Schnauzer miniatura, Doberman, Poodle e Labrador retriever.
- Pacientes geriátricos (>9 anos de idade).

SINAIS CLÍNICOS
Achados Anamnésicos
- Ausentes em alguns animais.
- Letargia.
- Anorexia.
- Fraqueza.
- Dispneia.
- Colapso.
- Vômito.
- Diarreia.

Achados do Exame Físico
- Dispneia.
- Ritmo irregular.
- Insuficiência cardíaca.
- Desorientação.
- Cegueira.
- Andar em círculos.
- Coma.
- Claudicação episódica.

CAUSAS E FATORES DE RISCO
- Hipotireoidismo grave.
- Idade avançada.
- Hiperlipidemia em Schnauzer miniatura.
- Sexo masculino (os machos caninos podem exibir predisposição).
- Altos níveis do colesterol total.
- Diabetes.
- Glomerulonefrite.

DIAGNÓSTICO

DIAGNÓSTICO DIFERENCIAL
Arteriosclerose.

HEMOGRAMA/BIOQUÍMICA/URINÁLISE
- Hipercolesterolemia.
- Hiperlipidemia.
- Altos níveis de ureia e creatinina.
- Atividade elevada das enzimas hepáticas.

OUTROS TESTES LABORATORIAIS
- Baixos níveis de T_3 e T_4.
- Valores elevados das frações alfa-2 e beta na eletroforese proteica.

DIAGNÓSTICO POR IMAGEM
Radiografia
As radiografias torácicas e abdominais podem revelar cardiomegalia e hepatomegalia.

MÉTODOS DIAGNÓSTICOS
Eletrocardiografia
- Anormalidades da condução cardíaca e chanfradura dos complexos QRS.
- Fibrilação atrial.
- Elevação ou depressão do segmento ST em casos de infarto do miocárdio.

TRATAMENTO

- Tratar o distúrbio subjacente e os sinais clínicos (p. ex., dispneia caso se desenrole uma insuficiência cardíaca congestiva).
- Dieta — dieta com baixo teor de gordura, programa de perda de peso e consumo elevado de fibras solúveis para o controle da hiperlipidemia.

MEDICAÇÕES

MEDICAMENTO(S)
- Tratar os distúrbios de condução cardíaca e as arritmias, se houver indicação clínica.
- Na confirmação de hipotireoidismo, efetuar a reposição dos hormônios tireoidianos.
- Caso se constate uma hipertensão, lançar mão de terapia anti-hipertensiva.
- Se o animal estiver hiperlipidêmico, fornecer medicamentos redutores do colesterol sanguíneo.
- Tratar o diabetes.

CONTRAINDICAÇÕES/INTERAÇÕES POSSÍVEIS
N/D.

ACOMPANHAMENTO

- Monitorizar a concentração do T_4, 4-6 horas após a administração depois das primeiras 6 semanas de tratamento e ajustar a dosagem de acordo com essa monitorização.
- Monitorizar os níveis sanguíneos de triglicerídeos e colesterol.
- Monitorizar o ECG quanto à presença de distúrbios de condução cardíaca e alterações do segmento ST.

DIVERSOS

DISTÚRBIOS ASSOCIADOS
- Hipotireoidismo.
- Diabetes.
- Valvulopatia mitral (mixomatosa).
- Glomerulonefrite.

FATORES RELACIONADOS COM A IDADE
Pacientes geriátricos (>9 anos de idade).

VER TAMBÉM
Infarto do Miocárdio.

RECURSOS DA INTERNET
www.vetgo.com/cardio.

Sugestões de Leitura

Drost WT, Bahr RJ, Henay GA, Campbell GA. Aortoiliac thrombus secondary to a mineralized arteriosclerotic lesion. Vet Radiol Ultrasound 1999, 40:262-266.

Hamlen HJ. Sinoatrial node arteriosclerosis in two young dogs. JAVMA 1994, 204:751.

Hess RS, Kass PH, Van Winkle JV. Association between diabetes mellitus, hypothyroidism or hyperadrenocorticism and atherosclerosis in dogs. J Vet Intern Med 2003, 17:489-494.

Kidd L, Stepien RL, Amrheiw DP. Clinical findings and coronary artery disease in dogs and cats with acute and subacute myocardial necrosis: 28 cases. JAAHA 2000, 36:199-208.

Liu SK, Tilley LP, Tappe JP, Fox PR. Clinical and pathologic findings in dogs with atherosclerosis: 21 cases (1970-1983). JAVMA 1986, 189:227-232.

Autor Larry P. Tilley
Consultores Editoriais Larry P. Tilley e Francis W.K. Smith, Jr.

ATROFIA DA ÍRIS

CONSIDERAÇÕES GERAIS

REVISÃO
• Degeneração dos tecidos da íris; tanto o estroma como o epitélio posterior da íris podem ser acometidos, resultando em perda de função do esfíncter e do músculo dilatador da íris, atrofia dos vasos da íris e perda do pigmento da íris.
• Tanto a margem pupilar como as porções mais periféricas da íris podem ser acometidas, resultando em uma íris delgada ou dotada de áreas de perda tecidual de espessura completa.
• Alteração senil ou secundária.
• Atrofia secundária da íris costuma ser o resultado de inflamação crônica (uveíte).
• Com frequência, o músculo esfíncter da íris é acometido, culminando em constrição pupilar incompleta e, possivelmente, configuração anormal da pupila (discoria).
• Margem pupilar irregular, com aspecto roído por traça e em concha, constitui uma manifestação comum.
• A margem pupilar pode permanecer inalterada; a perda periférica do tecido da íris pode produzir grandes "buracos" na íris que se assemelham a múltiplos orifícios pupilares.
• A visão basicamente permanece inalterada.
• Pode causar desconforto em ambientes com luz intensa.

IDENTIFICAÇÃO
• Cães — modificação comum da idade; embora possa acometer todas as raças, é mais comum naquelas de pequeno porte (p. ex., Poodle toy e miniatura, Schnauzer miniatura e Chihuahua).
• Gatos — rara; mais comum quando a íris é azul.
• Secundária — qualquer raça canina ou felina.

SINAIS CLÍNICOS
Achados Anamnésicos
• Pupila grande ou discórica em um ou ambos os olhos.
• Fotofobia.
• Episódios prévios de uveíte.

Achados do Exame Físico
• Reflexo pupilar incompleto ou ausente à luz, acompanhado pela resposta normal à ameaça e reflexo de ofuscamento.
• Pode haver anisocoria com apresentação unilateral ou assimétrica.
• Margem pupilar com borda irregular e em concha; discoria.
• Reflexo tapetal visível por meio de áreas finas ou ausentes da íris à transiluminação: manchas ou orifícios translúcidos dentro do estroma da íris — podem se assemelhar a pupilas adicionais.

• Os filamentos da íris ocasionalmente permanecem, estendendo-se sobre partes da pupila.
• Secundária — pode ser acompanhada por qualquer sinal associado à uveíte crônica.

CAUSAS E FATORES DE RISCO
• Normal com a idade.
• Uveíte.
• Glaucoma.

DIAGNÓSTICO

DIAGNÓSTICO DIFERENCIAL
• É imprescindível diferenciar de anomalias congênitas da íris.
  ○ Aplasia da íris — rara nos cães e gatos.
  ○ Hipoplasia da íris — diferenciar com base na idade à primeira manifestação dos sinais clínicos.
  ○ Coloboma da íris — área completa de espessura total da falta de desenvolvimento de todas as camadas da íris; frequentemente associada à condição da pelagem cinza-azulada, com pontilhado preto no fundo (melro ou merle); também pode estar associada à falta de zônulas do cristalino e à indentação do cristalino profundamente à área do coloboma; diferenciar com base na idade e na presença de anormalidades associadas.
  ○ Policoria — mais de uma pupila, sendo que cada uma delas possui a capacidade de efetuar a constrição em virtude da presença do esfíncter da íris.
  ○ Membranas pupilares persistentes — emergem do colarete (porção média) da íris, não da margem pupilar livre.
• Dilatação da pupila causada por glaucoma — pode haver pressão intraocular elevada, edema de córnea, congestão conjuntival +/− escleral, aumento do bulbo ocular; também pode estar cego.
• Aderências da íris ao cristalino ou à córnea (sinéquia posterior ou anterior) como resultado de uveíte ou traumatismo — diferenciar com base nas anormalidades associadas compatíveis com uveíte ou traumatismo perfurante (p. ex., cicatriz corneana de espessura completa).

HEMOGRAMA/BIOQUÍMICA/URINÁLISE
N/D.

OUTROS TESTES LABORATORIAIS
N/D.

DIAGNÓSTICO POR IMAGEM
N/D.

MÉTODOS DIAGNÓSTICOS
Tonometria — possivelmente pressão intraocular baixa quando secundária à uveíte; pressão intraocular elevada se secundária a glaucoma ou se a uveíte também causou um glaucoma secundário; pressão intraocular normal em caso de atrofia primária senil da íris.

TRATAMENTO
• Quadro irreversível.
• Secundária — tratamento direcionado ao controle da doença subjacente. Pode interromper a evolução do distúrbio.
• O paciente pode exibir fotofobia por causa da incapacidade de promover a constrição pupilar; fornecer sombreamento adequado.

MEDICAÇÕES

MEDICAMENTO(S)
• Senil — nenhum.
• Secundária — depende da causa subjacente.

CONTRAINDICAÇÕES/INTERAÇÕES POSSÍVEIS
Atropina tópica — exacerba a fotofobia e a dilatação pupilar.

ACOMPANHAMENTO
• Senil — pode continuar evoluindo com a idade.
• Secundária — geralmente não evolui uma vez controlada a doença primária.

DIVERSOS

VER TAMBÉM
• Glaucoma.
• Uveíte Anterior — Cães.
• Uveíte Anterior — Gatos.

RECURSOS DA INTERNET
http://www.vetmed.ucdavis.edu/courses/vet_eyes/conotes/con_chapter_11.html.

Sugestões de Leitura
Hendrix DVH. Diseases and surgery of the canine anterior uvea. In: Gelatt KN, ed., Veterinary Ophthalmology, 4th ed. Ames, IA: Blackwell, 2007, pp. 812-858.

Autor Simon A. Pot
Consultor Editorial Paul E. Miller
Agradecimento Stephanie L. Smedes

Avulsão do Plexo Braquial

CONSIDERAÇÕES GERAIS

REVISÃO
- O traumatismo com tração c/ou abdução do membro torácico causa avulsão das raízes nervosas a partir de suas inserções na medula espinal.
- As raízes (motoras) ventrais são mais suscetíveis que as raízes (sensoriais) dorsais.
- É fundamental descartar avulsão das raízes nervosas em animais traumatizados incapazes de sustentar seu peso em um membro torácico, especialmente antes do reparo cirúrgico de lesões ortopédicas.

IDENTIFICAÇÃO
- Cães e gatos.
- Não há predisposição etária, sexual ou racial.

SINAIS CLÍNICOS
- Dependem do grau e da distribuição do dano radicular.
- Sinais motores — desde fraqueza (dano parcial) até paralisia (avulsão das raízes ventrais).
- Sinais sensoriais — desde diminuição até ausência da percepção à dor (avulsão das raízes dorsais).
- Atrofia muscular — inicia-se em uma semana após a lesão.
- Avulsão completa — nervos espinais de C5 a T2; muito comum; associa déficits por avulsões cranial e caudal.
- Avulsão cranial — nervos espinais de C5 a C7; causa perda dos movimentos do ombro, flexão do cotovelo (cotovelo caído), bem como analgesia da porção craniodorsal da escápula e da face medial do antebraço. Pode-se observar hemiplegia do diafragma por meio do exame de fluoroscopia (raízes dos nervos frênicos de C5 a C7). Se as raízes de C8 a T2 forem preservadas, a sustentação do peso permanecerá quase normal.
- Avulsão caudal — nervos espinais de C7 a T2; leva à incapacidade de sustentação do peso, com apoio sobre o dorso das patas. Se as raízes de C5 a C7 forem poupadas, o membro será mantido em uma posição fletida e haverá analgesia distal ao cotovelo (exceto em uma pequena área na face medial do antebraço). O envolvimento de T1 a T2 gera uma síndrome de Horner ipsolateral parcial (apenas anisocoria) e perda da contração ipsilateral do reflexo cutâneo do tronco* (contração presente no sentido contralateral).
- Bilateral — raramente encontrada, ocorrendo após queda significativa com pouso esternal e abertura (expansão) dos membros.

CAUSAS E FATORES DE RISCO
Traumatismo — acidentes automobilísticos; suspensão pelos pés; quedas.

DIAGNÓSTICO

DIAGNÓSTICO DIFERENCIAL
- Traumatismo do plexo braquial sem avulsão — raro; déficit temporário em decorrência da contusão radicular.
- Tumor do plexo braquial — geralmente de início crônico, progressivo.
- Neurite do plexo braquial ou neuropatia — rara, déficits bilaterais. Início agudo, mas sem traumatismo.
- Mielopatia por êmbolos fibrocartilaginosos — geralmente ocorrem déficits do membro pélvico ipsilateral e déficits leves dos membros torácico e pélvico contralaterais.
- Paralisia pura do nervo radial causada por fratura do úmero ou da primeira costela — nenhum sinal de envolvimento radicular.

HEMOGRAMA/BIOQUÍMICA/URINÁLISE
Em geral, permanecem normais.

DIAGNÓSTICO POR IMAGEM
TC ou RM — permitem a visualização da lesão; exames raramente necessários para o diagnóstico.

MÉTODOS DIAGNÓSTICOS
- Clínicos — histórico de traumatismo com início súbito de déficits neurológicos típicos.
- Definir as raízes nervosas espinais envolvidas — mapear os déficits motores e sensoriais; verificar os sinais da síndrome de Horner; determinar a presença do reflexo cutâneo do tronco.
- Eletrofisiologia (EMG) e estudos de condução nervosa — a EMG demonstra a desnervação nos músculos acometidos 5–7 dias após a lesão. A EMG e os estudos de condução nervosa podem ajudar a definir ainda mais os déficits e detectar os sinais de recuperação.

ACHADOS PATOLÓGICOS
- Avulsões das raízes ventrais e dorsais — intradural na altura da junção raiz-medula espinal (área mais frágil pela falta do perínio protetor).
- Formação de neuroma — na superfície da pia-máter da medula espinal.

TRATAMENTO

CUIDADO(S) DE SAÚDE ADEQUADO(S)
- Não há tratamento específico.
- O resultado depende do dano inicial.
- Amputação do membro — pode ser necessária em pacientes que exibem complicações e não manifestam nenhuma melhora.
- Fusão dos carpos (artrodese) e transposição do tendão do músculo bíceps — considerar essa técnica apenas em casos de funcionamento adequado do músculo tríceps e do nervo musculocutâneo.

CUIDADO(S) DE ENFERMAGEM
- Utilizar bandagens ou botas protetoras quando o paciente caminhar em superfícies ásperas, em virtude do aumento na fragilidade cutânea e da ausência dos reflexos protetores no membro acometido.
- Fisioterapia — decisiva para manter a mobilidade das articulações e dos músculos durante a recuperação de lesões reversíveis; promover a amplitude passiva de movimento e a massoterapia.
- Monitorar os casos não complicados por 4–6 meses antes de se considerar a amputação.

MEDICAÇÕES

MEDICAMENTO(S)
Prednisolona (prednisona) — dose anti-inflamatória inicial por 1 semana pode diminuir o edema e favorecer a cicatrização de componentes reversíveis da lesão.

---

* N. T.: Também conhecido como panículo.

ACOMPANHAMENTO

MONITORIZAÇÃO DO PACIENTE
Monitorização clínica e eletrofisiológica seriada — avaliar a melhora do paciente e a gravidade do quadro.

PREVENÇÃO
Evitar o comportamento errático.

COMPLICAÇÕES POSSÍVEIS
- Escoriação cutânea e infecção secundária — por traumatismo pelo fato de a pata estar desprotegida.
- Úlceras tróficas — na pele delgada e traumatizada, especialmente sobre os locais de artrodese.
- Parestesia — pode levar à automutilação.

EVOLUÇÃO ESPERADA E PROGNÓSTICO
- Sensibilidade preservada à dor (raízes dorsais intactas) — sugere lesão menos grave às raízes nervosas ventrais.
- Avulsão cranial — o prognóstico é melhor, já que a sensibilidade na porção distal do membro e a capacidade de sustentação do peso são poupadas.
- Avulsão completa — prognóstico mau quanto à recuperação, sendo provável a amputação.
- Raramente, os casos leves podem se resolver após 2–3 meses.

DIVERSOS

VER TAMBÉM
Neuropatias Periféricas (Polineuropatias).

ABREVIATURA(S)
- EMG = eletromiografia.
- RM = ressonância magnética.
- TC = tomografia computadorizada.

RECURSOS DA INTERNET
Braund KG. Neuropathic Disorders (Acesso em 6 de fevereiro de 2003): http://www.ivis.org/advances/Vite/braund20b/chapter frm.asp.

Sugestões de Leitura
Bailey CS. Patterns of cutaneous anesthesia associated with brachial plexus avulsions in the dog. JAVMA 1984, 185:889–899.
Cuddon PA, Delauche AJ, Hutchison JM. Assessment of dorsal nerve root and spinal cord dorsal horn function in clinically normal dogs by determination of cord dorsum potentials. Am J Vet Res 1999, 60(2):222–226.
Moissonnier P, Duchossoy Y, Lavieille S, et al. Evaluation of ventral root reimplantation as a treatment of experimental avulsion of the cranial brachial plexus in the dog. Revue de Médecine V'et'erinaire 2001, 152:587–596.
Munoz A, Mateo I, Lorenzo V, et al. Imaging diagnosis: Traumatic dural tear diagnosed using intrathecal gadopentate dimeglumine. Vet Radiol Ultrasound 2009, 50(5):502–505.

Autor Christine Berthelin-Baker
Consultor Editorial Joane M. Parent

Azotemia e Uremia

CONSIDERAÇÕES GERAIS

DEFINIÇÃO
- A azotemia corresponde ao excesso de ureia, creatinina ou outras substâncias nitrogenadas não proteicas no sangue, plasma ou soro.
- A uremia refere-se à síndrome tóxica polissistêmica, resultante de perda acentuada nas funções renais. Nos animais, ela ocorre simultaneamente com quantidades elevadas de constituintes urinários no sangue.

FISIOPATOLOGIA
- A azotemia pode ser causada por: 1) alta produção de substâncias nitrogenadas não proteicas, 2) baixa taxa de filtração glomerular ou 3) reabsorção de urina que extravasou do trato urinário para a corrente sanguínea. A produção elevada de substâncias residuais nitrogenadas não proteicas pode se originar do alto consumo de proteínas (dieta ou sangramento gastrintestinal) ou do catabolismo acelerado de proteínas endógenas. A taxa de filtração glomerular pode declinar em virtude de queda na perfusão renal (azotemia pré-renal), doença renal aguda ou crônica (azotemia renal) ou obstrução urinária (azotemia pós-renal). A reabsorção de urina para a circulação sistêmica pode resultar do extravasamento de urina a partir das vias excretoras (também denominada azotemia pós-renal).
- Fisiopatologia da uremia — parcialmente compreendida; pode estar relacionada com: 1) efeitos sistêmicos metabólicos e tóxicos de produtos residuais retidos por falha na função excretora dos rins, 2) desarranjo na regulação renal de líquidos e eletrólitos, bem como no equilíbrio acidobásico e 3) dano à produção e degradação renais de hormônios e outras substâncias (p. ex., eritropoietina e 1,25-diidroxicolecalciferol).

SISTEMA(S) ACOMETIDO(S)
- A uremia afeta praticamente qualquer sistema orgânico.
- Cardiovascular — hipertensão arterial, hipertrofia do ventrículo esquerdo, sopro cardíaco, cardiomegalia, distúrbios do ritmo cardíaco.
- Endócrino/metabólico — hiperparatireoidismo secundário renal, produção inadequada de 1,25-diidroxicolecalciferol e eritropoietina, hipergastrinemia, perda de peso.
- Gastrintestinal — anorexia, náusea, vômito, diarreia, estomatite urêmica, xerostomia, hálito urêmico, constipação.
- Sanguíneo/linfático/imune — anemia e imunodeficiência.
- Neuromuscular — embotamento, entorpecimento/sonolência, letargia, fadiga, irritabilidade, tremores, desequilíbrio da marcha, flacidez muscular, mioclonia, mudanças comportamentais, demência, déficits de nervos cranianos isolados, crises convulsivas, estupor, coma, termorregulação comprometida.
- Oftálmico — congestão escleral e conjuntival, retinopatia, cegueira de início agudo.
- Respiratório — dispneia.
- Cutâneo/exócrino — palidez, equimose, aumento na queda natural de pelos, aparência descuidada, perda do brilho normal da pelagem.

IDENTIFICAÇÃO
Cães e gatos.

SINAIS CLÍNICOS
Comentários Gerais
A azotemia pode ou não estar associada a anormalidades anamnésicas ou físicas. A menos que o paciente apresente uremia, os achados clínicos limitam-se à doença responsável pela azotemia. Os achados descritos aqui pertencem à uremia.

Achados Anamnésicos
- Perda de peso.
- Diminuição do apetite (hiporexia) ou anorexia.
- Nível reduzido de atividade.
- Depressão.
- Fadiga.
- Fraqueza.
- Vômito.
- Diarreia.
- Halitose.
- Constipação.
- Alterações no volume urinário (aumento ou diminuição).
- Pelagem em más condições ou aparência descuidada.

Achados do Exame Físico
- Emaciação muscular: caquexia.
- Depressão mental.
- Desidratação.
- Fraqueza.
- Palidez.
- Petéquias e equimoses.
- Pelagem opaca e descuidada.
- Hálito urêmico.
- Estomatite urêmica.
- Congestão escleral e conjuntival.
- Hipotermia relativa.

CAUSAS
Azotemia Pré-renal
- Queda na perfusão renal, em virtude de hipovolemia ou hipotensão.
- Produção acelerada de produtos residuais nitrogenados, em função do catabolismo tecidual acentuado em associação com infecção, febre, traumatismo, excesso de corticosteroides ou queimaduras.
- Aumento nos processos de digestão e absorção gastrintestinais de fontes proteicas (dieta ou hemorragia gastrintestinal).

Azotemia Renal
- Doenças renais agudas ou crônicas (nefropatia primária com acometimento de glomérulos, túbulos renais, interstício renal ou vasculatura renal) que comprometa pelo menos 75% da função renal.

Azotemia Pós-renal
- Obstrução urinária; ruptura das vias excretoras.

FATORES DE RISCO
- Condições clínicas — doença renal, hipoadrenocorticismo, baixo débito cardíaco, hipotensão, febre, sepse, poliúria, hepatopatia, piometra, hipoalbuminemia, desidratação, acidose, exposição a substâncias químicas nefrotóxicas, hemorragia gastrintestinal, urolitíase, tampões uretrais em gatos, traumatismo uretral e neoplasia.
- A idade avançada pode ser um fator de risco.
- Medicamentos — agentes potencialmente nefrotóxicos, AINEs, diuréticos, medicamentos anti-hipertensivos; a falha em ajustar a dosagem de agentes terapêuticos eliminados principalmente pelos rins corresponde ao declínio na função renal.
- Toxinas — etilenoglicol, uvas (cães), lírios (gatos).

DIAGNÓSTICO

DIAGNÓSTICO DIFERENCIAL
- Desidratação, má perfusão periférica, baixo débito cardíaco, histórico de perda hídrica recente, dieta rica em proteínas ou fezes hipercólicas (alcatroadas) e negras — descartar azotemia pré-renal.
- Início recente de alteração no débito urinário (alto ou baixo), sinais clínicos compatíveis com uremia, exposição a possíveis agentes nefrotóxicos ou lesão renal isquêmica ou rins normais ou aumentados de volume — excluir insuficiência renal aguda.
- Perda progressiva de peso, poliúria, polidipsia, rins pequenos, palidez e sinais de uremia que se desenvolveram em algumas semanas a meses — descartar insuficiência renal crônica.
- Declínio abrupto no débito urinário e início dos sinais de uremia; ocasionalmente, disúria, estrangúria e hematúria; bexiga distendida ou abdome preenchido com líquido — excluir azotemia pós-renal.

HEMOGRAMA/BIOQUÍMICA/URINÁLISE
Hemograma completo
- Anemia arregenerativa (normocítica, normocrômica) — presença constante em casos de insuficiência renal crônica.
- Hemoconcentração — ocorrência frequente em casos de azotemia pré-renal; também pode ser observada em casos de insuficiência renal aguda e azotemia pós-renal.

Bioquímica
- Determinações seriadas das concentrações séricas de ureia e creatinina podem ajudar a diferenciar a causa da azotemia. Em pacientes com azotemia pré-renal, uma terapia apropriada para restabelecer a perfusão renal tipicamente produz uma redução drástica na azotemia (em geral, dentro de 24-48 h). A correção da obstrução ao fluxo urinário ou a abertura nas vias excretoras tipicamente confere um declínio rápido na magnitude da azotemia.
- Hipercalemia concomitante pode ser compatível com azotemia pós-renal, azotemia renal primária por insuficiência renal oligúrica ou azotemia pré-renal associada ao hiperadrenocorticismo.
- O aumento na concentração sérica de albumina e globulina sugere azotemia pré-renal ou algum componente pré-renal.

Urinálise
- Densidade urinária ≥1,030 em cães e ≥1,035 em gatos apoia o diagnóstico de azotemia pré-renal. A fluidoterapia antes da coleta de urina pode interferir na interpretação de valores baixos na densidade urinária.
- Os pacientes azotêmicos que não foram tratados com fluidos e exibem densidades urinárias <1,030 (cães) e <1,035 (gatos) tipicamente apresentam azotemia renal primária. Uma exceção notável a essa regra corresponde à glomerulopatia em cães e gatos. Essa doença glomerular caracteriza-se algumas vezes por um desequilíbrio glomerulotubular, no qual a capacidade de concentração urinária pode persistir apesar de danos glomerulares renais suficientes a ponto de causar azotemia renal primária; esses pacientes são identificados por proteinúria moderada a acentuada na ausência de hematúria e piúria.
- A densidade urinária não é útil na identificação de azotemia pós-renal.

OUTROS TESTES LABORATORIAIS
Para confirmar a azotemia causada pela diminuição na taxa de filtração glomerular, pode-se lançar mão dos testes de depuração de creatinina, ioexol ou inulina endógenos ou exógenos ou de outros testes específicos para essa taxa de filtração.

DIAGNÓSTICO POR IMAGEM
• Radiografias abdominais — utilizadas para determinar o tamanho renal (rins pequenos são compatíveis com doença renal crônica; aumento de volume leve a moderado dos rins pode ser compatível com insuficiência renal aguda ou obstrução urinária) e para descartar a presença de obstrução urinária (dilatação acentuada da bexiga e densidades minerais no interior das vias excretoras).
• Ultrassonografia — pode detectar alterações na ecogenicidade do parênquima renal, bem como no tamanho e no formato dos rins, que apoiem o diagnóstico de azotemia renal primária; útil para descartar azotemia pós-renal, caracterizada pela distensão das vias excretoras e existência de urólitos ou massas dentro dessas vias ou colidindo com essas vias e ainda pelo acúmulo de líquido intra-abdominal (em casos de ruptura das vias excretoras).
• Urografia excretora, pielografia ou cistouretrografia — podem ajudar a estabelecer o diagnóstico de azotemia pós-renal em caso de obstrução urinária ou ruptura das vias excretoras.

MÉTODOS DIAGNÓSTICOS
Pode-se empregar a biopsia renal para confirmar o diagnóstico de doença renal primária, diferenciar as doenças renais aguda e crônica e também tentar definir o processo mórbido subjacente responsável pela doença renal primária.

TRATAMENTO
• Azotemia pré-renal causada por dano à perfusão renal — a terapia visa à correção da causa subjacente de hipoperfusão renal; a intensidade do tratamento depende da gravidade da condição subjacente e da probabilidade de indução de lesão ou insuficiência renal primária por hipoperfusão renal persistente.
• Azotemia renal primária e uremia associada — 1) a terapia específica visa interromper ou reverter o processo mórbido primário com envolvimento dos rins e 2) além da terapia de suporte, devem-se instituir tratamentos sintomáticos e paliativos que amenizem os sinais clínicos da uremia, minimizem o impacto clínico exercidos pelos déficits e excessos nos equilíbrios hidreletrolítico e acidobásico, reduzam os efeitos da biossíntese renal inadequada de hormônios e outras substâncias e mantenham uma nutrição adequada.
• Azotemia pós-renal — visa eliminar a obstrução urinária ou reparar as rupturas nas vias excretoras; a suplementação de fluidos frequentemente é necessária para evitar a desidratação, que pode se desenvolver durante a diurese por solutos após a correção da azotemia pós-renal.
• Fluidoterapia — indicada para a maioria dos pacientes azotêmicos; as escolhas preferidas de fluidos incluem o soro fisiológico a 0,9% ou a solução de Ringer lactato. Estima-se a quantidade de fluido a ser administrada com base na gravidade da desidratação ou na depleção de volume. Sem a evidência de qualquer desidratação clínica, admite-se com prudência que o paciente tenha menos de 5% de desidratação e administra-se um volume correspondente de fluido. Via de regra, 50 a 75% da reposição volêmica devem ser fornecidos durante 2-6 h, exceto em pacientes com suspeita ou manifestação de insuficiência cardíaca.
• Manitol (0,5-1 g/kg IV a cada 8 h ou 0,25-0,5 mg/kg/h sob infusão em velocidade constante) pode ser utilizado em pacientes poliúricos para promover a diurese e estimular a eliminação de resíduos nitrogenados.
• Tratar os pacientes em choque de forma apropriada.
• Considerar o fornecimento de dietas formuladas para doença renal a fim de reduzir a magnitude de anormalidades como azotemia, hiperfosfatemia e acidose.

MEDICAÇÕES
MEDICAMENTO(S) DE ESCOLHA
• Para uremia em pacientes com doença renal, pode-se indicar a terapia sintomática.
• Famotidina (0,5-1,0 mg/kg VO, SC, IM, IV a cada 12-24 h) ou outros antagonistas dos receptores histaminérgicos H_2 podem ser usados para reduzir os sintomas de hiperacidez gástrica e náusea.
• Antieméticos como maropitanto (1 mg/kg a cada 24 h VO ou SC por 5 dias).

CONTRAINDICAÇÕES
Administração de medicamentos nefrotóxicos.

PRECAUÇÕES
• É preciso ter cautela ao se administrar medicamentos que exijam a excreção renal. Consultar referências adequadas a respeito dos esquemas de redução das doses ou quanto aos ajustes dos intervalos de manutenção.
• Ter prudência também ao se fornecer fluidos a pacientes oligúricos ou anúricos. Durante a fluidoterapia, é preciso monitorizar a taxa de produção urinária e o peso corporal para minimizar a probabilidade de indução de super-hidratação.
• Ter cuidado ao se aplicar medicamentos que possam promover hipovolemia ou hipotensão (p. ex., diuréticos); monitorizar com rigor a resposta a tais medicamentos, estimando-se o estado de hidratação, a perfusão periférica e a pressão sanguínea, com avaliações seriadas dos testes de função renal.
• Os corticosteroides podem agravar a azotemia por meio do aumento no catabolismo de proteínas endógenas.

MEDICAMENTO(S) ALTERNATIVO(S)
Azodyl®, um probiótico, pode intensificar a excreção gastrintestinal de resíduos nitrogenados, reduzindo com isso a magnitude da azotemia e possivelmente melhorando alguns sinais urêmicos.

ACOMPANHAMENTO
MONITORIZAÇÃO DO PACIENTE
Mensurar as concentrações séricas de ureia e creatinina 24 h após a instituição da fluidoterapia; verificar também a produção de urina e o estado de hidratação, bem como o peso corporal.

COMPLICAÇÕES POSSÍVEIS
• A falha na correção da azotemia pré-renal causada por hipoperfusão renal pode resultar rapidamente em doença renal primária isquêmica.
• A azotemia renal primária pode evoluir para uremia.
• Em pacientes com azotemia pós-renal, o insucesso no restabelecimento do fluxo urinário normal pode culminar em danos renais progressivos ou em óbitos por hipercalemia e uremia.

DIVERSOS
DISTÚRBIOS ASSOCIADOS
Em gatos, pode haver uma associação entre hipocalemia e azotemia. Os achados preliminares sugerem que a hipocalemia possa estar associada a alterações renais funcionais ou estruturais, indutoras de azotemia.

FATORES RELACIONADOS COM A IDADE
Embora a insuficiência renal primária possa ocorrer em animais de qualquer idade, os cães e gatos geriátricos parecem exibir um risco substancialmente mais alto tanto de doença renal aguda como da crônica. Não se admite, no entanto, que a azotemia em cães e gatos geriátricos indique uma doença renal primária, já que esses pacientes também apresentam risco mais elevado de causas pré e pós-renais de azotemia.

POTENCIAL ZOONÓTICO
Leptospirose.

GESTAÇÃO/FERTILIDADE/REPRODUÇÃO
• Os dados a respeito de azotemia e gestação em cadelas e gatas são bastante limitados. Os seres humanos podem exibir uma tolerância satisfatória em caso de doença renal mínima durante a gestação; entretanto, a capacidade de manter a viabilidade gestacional diminui à medida que a função renal declina.
• Animais azotêmicos prenhes — preferem-se os agentes farmacológicos excretados por vias não renais.

VER TAMBÉM
• Capítulos sobre doença renal aguda e crônica.
• Obstrução do Trato Urinário.

RECURSOS DA INTERNET
International Renal Interest Society (IRIS): www.iris-kidney.com.

Sugestões de Leitura
Polzin D. Chronic kidney disease. In: Ettinger SJ, Feldman EC, eds., Textbook of Veterinary Internal Medicine, 7th ed. Philadelphia: Saunders, 2010, pp. 2036-2067.
Ross L. Acute renal failure. In: Bonagura JD, Twedt DC, Kirk's Veterinary Therapy XIV. Philadelphia: Saunders, 2009, pp. 879-882.

Autor David J. Polzin
Consultor Editorial Carl A. Osborne

BABESIOSE

CONSIDERAÇÕES GERAIS

REVISÃO
- Babesiose é a doença causada pelos parasitas protozoários do gênero *Babesia*. Os merozoítos ou os piroplasmas correspondem ao estágio infectante das hemácias dos mamíferos.
- *B. canis* — é um piroplasma amplo (4-7 μm), que infecta os cães. Além de ter distribuição mundial, existem três subespécies, classificadas com base em dados genéticos, biológicos e geográficos. Há relatos da *B. canis vogeli* nos Estados Unidos, bem como na África, Ásia e Austrália. A *B. canis rossi* é a cepa mais virulenta e está presente na África, enquanto a *B. canis canis* foi relatada na Europa.
- Alguns propuseram que esses microrganismos sejam, de fato, de três espécies distintas: *B. vogeli*, *B. rossi* e *B. canis*.
- Estudos recentes identificaram pelo menos três piroplasmas pequenos (2-5 μm) geneticamente distintos, capazes de infectar os cães:
  ○ *B. gibsoni* (também conhecido como *B. gibsoni* [Ásia]) — piroplasma pequeno que infecta os cães; distribuição mundial; doença emergente nos Estados Unidos.
  ○ *B. conradae* (também conhecido como *B. gibsoni* [EUA/Califórnia]) — piroplasma pequeno que acomete os cães; relatado apenas na Califórnia.
  ○ Babesia (*Theileria*) *annae* (também conhecido como piroplasma canino da Espanha e parasita semelhante à *B. microti*) — piroplasma pequeno que também infecta os cães; descrito na Espanha, em outras partes da Europa e, mais recentemente, nos Estados Unidos.
- *Babesia* sp. (Coco) — piroplasma grande identificado em cães esplenectomizados e imunossuprimidos nos Estados Unidos.
- Foram publicados vários outros relatos de caso único de novas espécies de *Babesia* e outros piroplasmas (ou seja, *T. equi*).
- *B. felis* — piroplasma pequeno (2-5 μm) que infecta os gatos; relatado na África.
- *Cytauxzoon felis* — piroplasma pequeno que infecta os gatos; relatado nos Estados Unidos.
- A infecção pode ocorrer por transmissão pelo carrapato, transmissão direta via transferência sanguínea durante mordidas de cachorro; transfusão sanguínea ou por meio da placenta.
- O período de incubação gira em torno de 2 semanas, mas alguns casos não são clinicamente diagnosticados durante meses a anos.
- Os piroplasmas infectam e replicam-se nas hemácias, resultando em anemia hemolítica tanto direta como imunomediada.
- É provável que a anemia hemolítica imunomediada seja mais importante do ponto de vista clínico do que a hemólise induzida pelo parasita, já que a gravidade dos sinais não depende do grau de parasitemia.

SISTEMA(S) ACOMETIDO(S)
- Sanguíneo/linfático/imune — anemia, trombocitopenia (as tendências ao sangramento parecem raras), febre, esplenomegalia, linfadenomegalia, vasculite (apenas experimental).
- Hepatobiliar — aumento na atividade das enzimas hepáticas (de leve a moderado, mas não constitui a única anormalidade detectada).
- Nervoso — babesiose cerebral, fraqueza, desorientação, colapso (mais comum em infecção por *B. canis rossi*).
- Renal/urológico — insuficiência renal (*B. canis rossi* e *B. annae*).

IDENTIFICAÇÃO
- Qualquer idade ou raça de cão pode ser infectada.
- As infecções pela *B. canis* são mais prevalentes em cães galgos.
- As infecções pela *B. gibsoni* (Ásia) são mais prevalentes na raça Pit bull terrier americano.
- Qualquer idade ou raça de gato pode ser infectada, mas até o momento há relatos apenas do *C. felis* nos Estados Unidos.

SINAIS CLÍNICOS
- Os sinais são semelhantes em cães e gatos.
- Podem ser superagudos, agudos ou crônicos.
- Alguns animais portadores não apresentam quaisquer sinais clínicos detectáveis.
- Cães — letargia, anorexia, mucosas pálidas, febre, esplenomegalia, linfadenomegalia, pigmentúria, icterícia, perda de peso, fezes com coloração alterada.
- Gatos — letargia, anorexia, mucosas pálidas, icterícia.

CAUSAS E FATORES DE RISCO
- Histórico de infestação por carrapatos.
- Os animais esplenectomizados desenvolvem uma doença clínica mais grave.
- Histórico de esplenectomia ou quimioterapia parece ser fatores de risco para *Babesia* sp. (Coco).
- A imunossupressão pode gerar sinais clínicos e parasitemia acentuada em cães com infecção crônica.
- Histórico de feridas recentes ocasionadas pela mordedura de cães é um risco de infecção pela *B. gibsoni* (Ásia).
- Transfusão sanguínea recente de doador com infecção subclínica.

DIAGNÓSTICO

DIAGNÓSTICO DIFERENCIAL
- Qualquer causa de anemia hemolítica ou trombocitopenia imunomediadas, incluindo anemia hemolítica ou trombocitopenia imunomediadas idiopáticas, erliquiose, febre maculosa das Montanhas Rochosas, lúpus eritematoso sistêmico, neoplasia, endocardite, micoplasmose hemotrópica (hemobartonelose) e citauxzoonose.
- O teste positivo de Coombs não descarta a babesiose, pois muitos animais acometidos por essa hemoparasitose também manifestam positividade nesse teste.
- Anemia hemolítica não mediada pelo sistema imune, incluindo anemia microangiopática, síndrome da veia cava, torção esplênica, CID, anemia por corpúsculo de Heinz, deficiência da piruvato quinase, deficiência da fosfofrutoquinase.
- Icterícia hepática e pós-hepática.

HEMOGRAMA/BIOQUÍMICA/URINÁLISE
- Anemia — de leve a grave; geralmente regenerativa (reticulocitose) a menos que os sinais se mostrem bastante agudos; pode ser grave em alguns casos (VG <10%), mas não está presente em todos os casos.
- Trombocitopenia — costuma ser de moderada a grave; alguns animais apresentam trombocitopenia sem anemia.
- As respostas leucocitárias são variáveis, com relatos tanto de leucocitose como de leucopenia.
- Hiperbilirrubinemia pode estar presente, dependendo da taxa de hemólise.
- Hiperglobulinemia é comum em infecções crônicas e pode ser a única anormalidade bioquímica constatada em alguns animais.
- Em virtude da anemia/hipoxia, a atividade das enzimas hepáticas apresenta-se levemente elevada.
- Já foram relatados casos de insuficiência renal e acidose metabólica em infecções pela *B. canis rossi* e *B annae*.
- É comum a presença de bilirrubinúria.
- A detecção da hemoglobinúria é menos habitual nos Estados Unidos do que na África.

OUTROS TESTES LABORATORIAIS
- Exame microscópico de esfregaços sanguíneos delgados ou espessos corados — pode fornecer o diagnóstico definitivo; a sensibilidade depende da experiência do examinador e da técnica de coloração; tem-se obtido o máximo êxito com o uso do corante de Wright modificado rápido; o sangue capilar pode acentuar a sensibilidade; no entanto, a microscopia pode não ser capaz de diferenciar as espécies ou as subespécies com precisão.
- IFA — testes séricos para detecção de anticorpos que reagem contra a *Babesia*; a reatividade cruzada pode impedir a diferenciação entre as espécies e as subespécies; alguns animais infectados, particularmente os cães jovens, podem não ter anticorpos detectáveis.
- PCR — teste para determinação da presença de DNA da *Babesia* em amostra biológica (em geral, sangue total com EDTA como anticoagulante); esse teste mostra-se capaz de diferenciar as subespécies e as espécies, sendo mais sensível do que a microscopia.

TRATAMENTO
- Pode exigir a internação ou o cuidado ambulatorial do paciente, dependendo da gravidade da doença.
- Os animais hipovolêmicos devem ser submetidos à fluidoterapia rigorosa.
- Os pacientes gravemente anêmicos podem necessitar de transfusões sanguíneas.

MEDICAÇÕES

MEDICAMENTO(S) DE ESCOLHA
- O dipropionato de imidocarbe (aprovado pela FDA; 6,6 mg/kg SC ou IM a cada 1-2 semanas) e o aceturato de diminazeno (sem aprovação pela FDA; 3,5-7 mg/kg SC ou IM a cada 1-2 semanas) diminuem a morbidade e a mortalidade em animais acometidos. Esses agentes terapêuticos podem eliminar completamente as infecções pela *B. canis*, mas não aquelas provocadas pela *B. gibsoni* (Ásia).
- A terapia de combinação com azitromicina (10 mg/kg VO 1 vez ao dia por 10 dias) e atovaquona (13,5 mg/kg VO 3 vezes ao dia por 10 dias) é o tratamento de escolha e o único tratamento capaz de eliminar potencialmente as infecções por *B.*

gibsoni (Ásia) em cães. Em um estudo controlado, 85% dos cães ficaram livres da infecção após o tratamento.
- Uma combinação de clindamicina (25 mg/kg VO a cada 12 h), metronidazol (15 mg/kg VO a cada 12 h) e doxiciclina (5 mg/kg VO a cada 12 h) foi associada à eliminação ou redução dos parasitas abaixo do limite de detecção no teste de PCR. Infelizmente, ainda não foi estabelecido um curso terapêutico bem definido, com períodos variando de 24 a 92 dias.
- Há relatos de que o metronidazol (25-50 mg/kg VO a cada 24 h por 7 dias), a clindamicina (12,5-25 mg/kg VO a cada 12 h por 7-10 dias) ou a doxiciclina (10 mg/kg VO a cada 12 h por 7-10 dias) isoladamente diminuem os sinais clínicos, mas não eliminam as infecções.
- O fosfato de primaquina (1 mg/kg IM em uma única injeção) é o tratamento de escolha contra a *B. felis*.
- Como a anemia e a trombocitopenia são frequentemente imunomediadas, podem-se indicar os agentes imunossupressores, como a prednisona (2,2 mg/kg/dia VO), em alguns casos. A terapia imunossupressora prolongada ANTES da terapia antiprotozoária específica é contraindicada.
- O uso de uma solução de hemoglobina polimerizada de origem bovina pode melhorar a capacidade carreadora de oxigênio em animais gravemente anêmicos, mas parece não ser superior à transfusão de papa de hemácias.
- Os medicamentos contra a babesiose (imidocarbe e diminazeno) são capazes de gerar sinais colinérgicos, que podem ser minimizados pela administração de atropina (0,02 mg/kg SC, 30 minutos antes da aplicação desses medicamentos).

CONTRAINDICAÇÕES
Altas doses de medicamentos contra a babesiose (imidocarbe e diminazeno) resultam em insuficiência hepática e renal.

ACOMPANHAMENTO
- Reavaliar o hemograma completo e o perfil bioquímico, conforme a necessidade, para monitorizar a resolução da anemia, trombocitopenia, icterícia e de outros sinais.
- A maior parte dos pacientes apresenta uma resposta clínica dentro de 1-2 semanas do tratamento.
- Devem ser realizados 2-3 testes consecutivos negativos de PCR, começando 2 meses depois do tratamento, para descartar falha terapêutica e parasitemia persistente. Os títulos de IFA não são recomendados para o acompanhamento, porque podem persistir por anos.
- Não há relatos a respeito do acompanhamento pós-terapêutico a longo prazo das infecções por *B. conradae* e *B. annea* ou *B. felis*.
- Quando um cão hospedado em um canil for diagnosticado com a babesiose, todos os cães presentes nesse alojamento deverão ser submetidos à triagem, pois existe uma alta porcentagem de animais portadores em ambientes como esse.
- Deve ser considerada a coinfecção por outros patógenos (p. ex., *Erhlichia*, *Mycoplasma* hemotrópico e *Leishmania*) transmitidos por vetores, especialmente em animais não responsivos ao tratamento.

PREVENÇÃO
Existem vacinas contra a *B. canis canis* e a *B. canis rossi* disponíveis na Europa, mas que não oferecem proteção contra outras espécies de *Babesia*. Sendo assim, o controle parasitário dos carrapatos torna-se importante para a prevenção da doença. Alguns estudos recentes sugerem que o uso de acaricidas pode prevenir a infecção por *Babesia* spp. Todos os carrapatos aderidos à pele devem ser removidos dentro de 24 h após sua fixação/infestação.

DIVERSOS
Todos potenciais doadores de sangue devem ser negativos quanto à presença da doença (preferencialmente em 2-3 testes consecutivos negativos de PCR) antes de seu emprego como doador.

POTENCIAL ZOONÓTICO
N/D.

GESTAÇÃO/FERTILIDADE/REPRODUÇÃO
Transmissão transplacentária.

ABREVIATURA(S)
- CID = coagulação intravascular disseminada.
- EDTA = ácido etilenodiaminotetracético.
- FDA = Food and Drug Administration (repartição do governo norte-americano que testa, controla e inspeciona alimentos e medicamentos).
- IFA = imunofluorescência indireta.
- PCR = reação em cadeia da polimerase.
- VG = volume globular (hematócrito).

Sugestões de Leitura
Birkenheuer AJ, Correa MT, Levy MG, Breitschwerdt EB. Geographic distribution of babesiosis among dogs in the United States and association with dog bites: 150 cases (2000-2003). JAVMA 2005, 227(6):942-947.
Irwin PJ. Canine babesiosis: From molecular taxonomy to control. Parasites & Vectors 2009, 2(Suppl 1):S4.

Autor Adam J. Birkenheuer
Consultor Editorial Stephen C. Barr

Bailisascaríase

CONSIDERAÇÕES GERAIS

REVISÃO
- Em cães, há relatos de duas formas de bailisascaríase: uma infestação intestinal, com ocorrência em adultos; e visceropatia causada pela migração larval em filhotes caninos.
- A doença é causada pelo nematódeo *Baylisascaris procyonis* no guaxinim. A infecção dos guaxinins ocorre pela ingestão de ovos ou de larvas em tecidos do hospedeiro paratênico mamífero.
- Os cães são infectados pela ingestão de ovos infectantes ou hospedeiros paratênicos e desenvolvem infecções patentes por vermes adultos no intestino delgado. Os filhotes caninos, possivelmente infectados pela ingestão de ovos, desenvolvem a visceropatia como a maioria dos outros mamíferos.
- Os cães acometidos pela infestação intestinal tipicamente não exibem sinais clínicos. Os filhotes caninos com a bailisascaríase larval manifestam sinais de doença neurológica.

IDENTIFICAÇÃO
- Cães.
- Forma intestinal — relatada a partir de animais adultos.
- Forma larval — descrita em dois filhotes; suspeita-se que somente os casos graves foram relatados; a infecção apenas por algumas larvas provavelmente não gera uma doença grave em grande parte dos filhotes caninos.

SINAIS CLÍNICOS
- Forma intestinal — nenhum.
- Forma larval — fraqueza, ataxia, disfagia, andar em círculo, decúbito.

CAUSAS E FATORES DE RISCO
Compartilhar o espaço com áreas frequentadas por guaxinins.

DIAGNÓSTICO

DIAGNÓSTICO DIFERENCIAL
- Forma intestinal — nas fezes, é possível distinguir os ovos de *Baylisascaris* dos de *Toxocara* ou de *Toxascaris*.
- Forma larval — raiva, cinomose, defeito neurológico congênito.

HEMOGRAMA/BIOQUÍMICA/URINÁLISE
Em geral, permanecem normais.

OUTROS TESTES LABORATORIAIS
N/D.

DIAGNÓSTICO POR IMAGEM
Formal larval — com base nas lesões de toxocaríase ou bailisascaríase em seres humanos, as lesões podem aparecer na ultrassonografia abdominal ou nas varreduras por TC como lesões pequenas, pouco definidas isoladas ou múltiplas, ovais ou alongadas, de baixa atenuação no parênquima hepático. Em lesões neurológicas, a RM revela comprometimento difuso da substância branca periventricular com atrofia.

MÉTODOS DIAGNÓSTICOS
- Forma intestinal — esfregaço fecal direto ou flutuação fecal.
- Forma larval — o exame oftalmoscópico pode revelar trajetos migratórios na retina; podem ser utilizadas técnicas de diagnóstico por imagem para visualizar lesões nos tecidos moles ou no cérebro.

TRATAMENTO

- Forma intestinal — pode ser desejável a internação do paciente para evitar a contaminação ambiental por ovos e garantir o descarte (em consequência do risco biológico) ou a destruição (incineração) adequado de material fecal e dos vermes após o tratamento.
- Forma larval — não há terapia até o momento.

ORIENTAÇÃO AO PROPRIETÁRIO
Alertar o proprietário sobre o risco potencial aos seres humanos que possam frequentar habitats semelhantes aos dos guaxinins.

MEDICAÇÕES

MEDICAMENTO(S)
Forma Intestinal
- Pamoato de pirantel (5 mg/kg) (Nemex®).
- Febantel (25-35 mg/kg), pamoato de pirantel (5-7 mg/kg), praziquantel (5-7 mg/kg) (Drontal Plus®).
- Ivermectina (0,005 mg/kg), pamoato de pirantel (5 mg/kg) (Heartgard Plus®).
- Milbemicina (0,5 mg/kg) (Interceptor®).

Forma Larval
Os corticosteroides e o albendazol a longo prazo (25-50 mg/kg/dia por 10 dias) podem vir a ser benéficos.

CONTRAINDICAÇÕES/INTERAÇÕES POSSÍVEIS
N/D.

ACOMPANHAMENTO

- Forma intestinal — examinar as fezes duas semanas após a vermifugação e, novamente, 1 mês depois.
- Forma larval — a doença tem se mostrado fatal.

DIVERSOS

POTENCIAL ZOONÓTICO
- Forma intestinal — os ovos não se mostram infectantes ao serem eliminados nas fezes, mas podem se desenvolver no ambiente em alguns dias; a ingestão de ovos contendo larvas infectantes pelos seres humanos pode gerar uma doença grave, isto é, a bailisascaríase larval.
- Forma larval — os filhotes caninos infectados não representam nenhuma ameaça zoonótica; em um único caso, um filhote manifestou a forma típica da bailisascaríase larval, durante a ocupação dos animais em áreas previamente habitadas por um guaxinim.
- Alertar os proprietários a respeito do risco zoonótico em potencial, especialmente das pessoas que possam frequentar os mesmos habitats dos guaxinins.

ABREVIATURA(S)
- RM = ressonância magnética.
- TC = tomografia computadorizada.

Sugestões de Leitura
Chang S, Lim JH, Choi D, et al. Hepatic visceral larva migrans of *Toxocara canis*: CT and sonographic findings. Am J Roentgenology 2006, 187:W622-W629.
Kazacos KR. *Baylisascaris procyonis* and related species. In: Samuel WM, Pybus MJ, Kocan AA, eds., Parasitic Diseases of Wild Mammals, 2nd ed. Ames: Iowa State University Press, 2001, pp. 301-341.
Rowley HA, Uht RM, Kazacos KR, et al. Radiologic-pathologic findings in raccoon roundworm (*Baylisascaris procyonis*) encephalitis. Am J Neuroradiol 2000, 21:415-420.

Autor Dwight D. Bowman
Consultor Editorial Stephen C. Barr

BARTONELOSE

CONSIDERAÇÕES GERAIS

REVISÃO
- Agentes infecciosos emergentes altamente adaptados a hospedeiros reservatórios preferenciais, nos quais estabelecem uma bacteremia intraeritrocitária crônica.
- Agentes — bactérias (bacilos) bastonetes Gram-negativas hemotrópicas argirofílicas intracelulares fastidiosas facultativas curvas e pequenas.
- Transmitida por vetores (pulgas, carrapatos).
- Síndrome humana — ampla variedade de síndromes clínicas, incluindo, mais comumente, doença da arranhadura do gato, caracterizada por linfadenopatia regional após arranhão ou mordedura por essa espécie de animal, distal ao linfonodo envolvido; ocorrência mundial; estimada >25.000 casos/ano nos Estados Unidos; >2.000 casos necessitam de internação; quase não há óbitos.
- Gatos — geralmente permanecem assintomáticos.
- Cães — síndrome clínica emergente.
- Sazonal; maior quantidade de casos relatados entre os meses de julho e janeiro*.

IDENTIFICAÇÃO
- Cães e gatos.
- A maioria dos pacientes humanos (80%) tem <21 anos de idade; acomete mais machos do que fêmeas (1,2:1).

SINAIS CLÍNICOS

Seres Humanos
- Pápula eritematosa no local da inoculação (arranhão, mordedura); a seguir, aparece linfadenopatia regional unilateral (dolorosa e, muitas vezes, supurativa) em 3-10 dias (>90% dos casos).
- Febre leve.
- Calafrios — pouco frequentes.
- Mal-estar.
- Anorexia.
- Mialgia.
- Náusea.
- Manifestações atípicas (em até 25% dos casos) — encefalopatia (1-7%); conjuntivite palpebral (3-5%); meningite; lesões osteolíticas; hepatite granulomatosa; esplenite granulomatosa; pneumonia.

Gatos
- Sem sinais de doença.
- Entre 5 e 60% de soropositivos, dependendo da área geográfica.
- Hiperplasia linfoide (ocasionalmente), uveíte, endocardite (rara), febre autolimitante.

Cães
Espectro expansivo de doenças, incluindo endocardite, miocardite, linfadenite granulomatosa, rinite, vasculite, uveíte, coriorretinite, artrite, meningoencefalite.

CAUSAS E FATORES DE RISCO
- Contato com filhotes felinos e gatos domésticos (>90%), particularmente gatos jovens infestados com pulgas.
- Arranhaduras provocadas por gatos — até 83%.

---

* N. T.: Informação referente aos países do hemisfério norte.

- Até 95% dos gatos que residem em lares de seres humanos acometidos são soropositivos.
- Infecções localizadas em indivíduos imunocompetentes; infecções sistêmicas em indivíduos imunocomprometidos.
- Cães: os fatores de risco incluem exposição a pulgas e carrapatos e ambiente rural.

DIAGNÓSTICO

DIAGNÓSTICO DIFERENCIAL
- Adenopatia benigna em crianças e jovens adultos humanos — causa mais comum.
- Histórico de contato com gato.
- Formação de pápula no local da inoculação primária (arranhão ou mordedura).
- Quadro clínico compatível — linfadenite regional unilateral.
- Exclusão de outras causas identificáveis.
- Achados histopatológicos característicos.
- Testes sorológicos — imunofluorescência indireta contra a *B. henselae*.
- Não se emprega mais o teste cutâneo positivo.
- Outras causas de linfadenopatia — linfogranuloma venéreo; sífilis; tuberculose típica ou atípica; outras formas de adenite bacteriana; esporotricose; tularemia; brucelose; histoplasmose, sarcoidose; toxoplasmose; mononucleose infecciosa; e tumores benignos ou malignos.
- Cães: coinfecções com outras doenças originárias de carrapatos (*Ehrlichia*, *Babesia*).

HEMOGRAMA/BIOQUÍMICA/URINÁLISE
Não colaboram com o diagnóstico.

OUTROS TESTES LABORATORIAIS
- Imunofluorescência indireta.
- Imunoensaio enzimático — anticorpos IgG contra a *B. henselae* (Specialty Laboratories, Valencia, CA).
- Cultura — em meios enriquecidos (contendo sangue) na presença de dióxido de carbono a 5% a 35-37°C; crescimento fastidioso e lento; requer 14-30 dias.
- Amplificação do DNA bacteriano a partir das lesões por meio do teste de PCR (Galaxy Diagnostics, Research Triangle Park, NC).

ACHADOS PATOLÓGICOS
- Histopatologia de linfonodos — reação inflamatória inespecífica, incluindo granuloma, microabscesso e necrose.
- Coloração com prata de Warthin-Starry — cora bacilos.

TRATAMENTO

- Tratamento de suporte — repouso em cama; aplicação de calor sobre os linfonodos edemaciados; aspiração por agulha dos nodos supurativos.
- Limpeza meticulosa de todos os arranhões e mordeduras por gatos.
- Evitar o contato dos gatos com feridas abertas.

MEDICAÇÕES

MEDICAMENTO(S)
- Antibióticos específicos — sem eficácia.

- A maioria dos casos manifesta resolução espontânea em algumas semanas ou meses.
- Casos graves — pode ser adequada a antibioticoterapia (gentamicina, doxiciclina, eritromicina, azitromicina), selecionada com base na suscetibilidade antimicrobiana da *B. henselae*.
- Cães: a terapia ideal não foi estabelecida, mas provavelmente envolve a administração de antibióticos a longo prazo (4-6 semanas) consistindo em macrolídeos (eritromicina, azitromicina).

ACOMPANHAMENTO

PREVENÇÃO
As pessoas imunocomprometidas devem evitar o contato com gatos jovens.

COMPLICAÇÕES POSSÍVEIS
São incomuns.

DIVERSOS

- Um único episódio parece conferir imunidade vitalícia.
- Angiomatose bacilar — dermatopatia proliferativa vascular; também pode ser causada pela *B. henselae*; responde aos antibióticos, o que raramente a bartonelose faz.
- Não se conhece o hospedeiro natural da *B. henselae*; uma espécie relacionada, a *B. quintana*, dissemina-se em piolhos e causa a febre das trincheiras** em seres humanos.

POTENCIAL ZOONÓTICO
- O risco da transmissão de microrganismos de cães e gatos infectados a seres humanos é desconhecido, embora os gatos infectados provavelmente sirvam como fonte de microrganismos para pulgas que, supostamente, transmitem a infecção para os seres humanos por meio de feridas contaminadas por fezes de pulgas infectadas (ou seja, doença da arranhadura do gato).
- Os cães também podem servir como reservatórios sanguíneos cronicamente infectados para espécies de *Bartonella*, que podem se disseminar por vetores artrópodes aos seres humanos.

ABREVIATURA(S)
- PCR = reação em cadeia da polimerase.

Sugestões de Leitura
Breitschwerdt EB. Feline bartonellosis and cat scratch disease. Vet Immunol Immunopathol 2008, 123:167-171.
Guptill-Yoran L, Breitschwerdt EB, Chom BB. Bartonellosis. In: Greene CE, ed., Infectious Diseases of the Dog and Cat, 3rd ed. Philadelphia: Saunders Elsevier, 2006, pp. 510-524.
Lamps LW, Scott MA. Cat-scratch disease: Historic, clinical, and pathologic perspectives. Am J Clin Pathol 2004, 121:S71-S80.

Autor J. Paul Woods
Consultor Editorial Stephen C. Barr

** N. T.: Também conhecida como tifo exantemático.

Bexiga Pélvica

CONSIDERAÇÕES GERAIS

REVISÃO
Também conhecida como "bexiga intrapélvica", pois o colo vesical urinário se encontra caudal ao osso púbico, fazendo com que grande parte da uretra e uma porção variável da bexiga urinária permaneçam dentro da pelve óssea. É comum a associação de uretra curta e incompetência no mecanismo do esfíncter uretral.

IDENTIFICAÇÃO
- Cães e, raramente, gatos.
- Acomete principalmente cadelas jovens (<1 ano de idade); a incontinência frequentemente piora após ovariectomia/ovário-histerectomia.
- Em geral, é detectada em cães machos depois da castração.

SINAIS CLÍNICOS
- Pode permanecer assintomática.
- A incontinência pode ser contínua ou intermitente.
- Com frequência, há padrões conscientes de micção.
- Urgência miccional com eliminação de pequeno volume de urina.
- Períneo manchado/encharcado com urina; queimadura por escaldagem de urina; vulva/prepúcio úmidos.

CAUSAS E FATORES DE RISCO
Foi demonstrado que a posição da bexiga urinária em cadelas incontinentes é mais intrapélvica e associada a uma uretra mais curta, sugerindo que a combinação de colo vesical intrapélvico e uretra curta estimula a incontinência urinária.

DIAGNÓSTICO

DIAGNÓSTICO DIFERENCIAL
- Incontinência urinária — ureter ectópico, incompetência no mecanismo do esfíncter uretral, micção inapropriada, incontinência de urgência, infecção do trato urinário, incontinência neurogênica (doença do neurônio motor inferior).
- O grau de incontinência frequentemente excede aquele observado em incompetência no mecanismo do esfíncter uretral, mas não é tão grave quanto aquele visto em ureteres ectópicos.

HEMOGRAMA/BIOQUÍMICA/URINÁLISE
- Os exames de hemograma completo e bioquímica tipicamente não são dignos de nota.
- A urinálise pode revelar indícios de infecção do trato urinário (incluindo piúria, hematúria e bacteriúria) ou poliúria (p. ex., densidade urinária <1,035).
- É recomendável a realização de urocultura e antibiograma via cistocentese. Os resultados da urocultura são frequentemente positivos.

DIAGNÓSTICO POR IMAGEM
- Radiografias abdominais podem revelar o deslocamento caudal da bexiga urinária, embora isso deva ser interpretado com cuidado sem distensão vesical controlada.
- A urografia excretora também pode permitir a observação dos rins, das terminações ureterais, da bexiga urinária e da uretra. Sem distensão vesical adequada, a interpretação do local do colo da bexiga deve ser feita com cuidado.
- Vaginouretrografia ou uretrocistografia retrógrada permite a observação da cúpula vaginal, da uretra, do comprimento da uretra, da próstata, do formato da bexiga urinária e da localização do colo vesical.
- Se a bexiga urinária e a uretra estiverem dentro da pelve óssea, o exame de cistouretrografia de duplo contraste pode ser necessário para a observação completa dessas estruturas. Após a máxima dilatação com infusão de dióxido de carbono ou meio de contraste, grande parte da bexiga urinária, o colo vesical e toda a uretra permanecem dentro do canal pélvico, caudalmente ao cíngulo pélvico ósseo. Com frequência, há uma uretra larga e curta.
- A ultrassonografia dos rins, dos ureteres e da bexiga urinária pode auxiliar na confirmação de anomalias urológicas concomitantes, hidronefrose, pielonefrite concomitante ou ureteres ectópicos concomitantes.
- A combinação diagnóstica de escolha consiste no uso de uretrocistoscopia e cistouretrografia. Essa combinação permite a investigação meticulosa de defeitos uretrais, ureterais, císticos, vaginais e vestibulares. Também possibilita a mensuração mais precisa do comprimento e da largura da uretra, além de ajudar na formulação da terapia.

MÉTODOS DIAGNÓSTICOS
- Exame neurológico deve permanecer normal.
- Procedimentos urodinâmicos — considerar o emprego de cistometrografia e perfilometria da pressão uretral para avaliar a função vesical e uretral, bem como o comprimento funcional da uretra. A função do músculo detrusor geralmente se encontra normal; entretanto, pressões limiares mais elevadas podem ser geradas com volumes menores. O comprimento uretral funcional está encurtado e a pressão intrauretral quase sempre, reduzida, resultando em incompetência no mecanismo do esfíncter uretral.

TRATAMENTO

- Identificar e tratar a infecção do trato urinário de modo apropriado.
- O objetivo é aumentar a resistência uretral (esfíncteres uretrais artificiais, injeções intrauretrais de agentes formadores de volume etc.), ampliar o comprimento da uretra (reconstrução do colo vesical) e/ou reposicionar o colo vesical para uma posição intra-abdominal (colpossuspensão, uretropexia, prostatopexia ou deferentopexia).
- Foi sugerido o relaxamento do músculo detrusor para tratar os cães com incontinência refratária.
- O tratamento clínico de incompetência tradicional no mecanismo do esfíncter uretral é tipicamente bem-sucedido em 75-90% das cadelas.

CONSIDERAÇÕES CIRÚRGICAS
- Colpossuspensão é a abordagem cirúrgica mais altamente recomendada. Há relatos de uma taxa de cura de 53%.
- A colocação de esfíncter uretral artificial ou oclusor hidráulico foi bem-sucedida, constituindo o tratamento cirúrgico de escolha se outras intervenções médicas ou minimamente invasivas falharem. No entanto, a experiência com esse procedimento é limitada.

TRATAMENTO MINIMAMENTE INVASIVO
A terapia submucosa transuretral com agente formador de volume (p. ex., implante de colágeno) foi descrita para o tratamento de pacientes refratários à terapia clínica e está associada a um sucesso relativamente satisfatório. Esse tipo de procedimento é efetuado com orientação cistoscópica.

MEDICAÇÕES

MEDICAMENTO(S)
- Fenilpropranolamina: um agonista α-adrenérgico (1-1,5 mg/kg VO a cada 8 h) que melhora a continência em incompetência no mecanismo do esfíncter uretral na maioria dos casos.
- Dietilestilbestrol (DES): inicialmente 0,1-0,3 mg/kg a cada 24 h por 7 dias e, depois, 1 vez por semana; 0,1-1 mg VO por 3-5 dias e, depois, 1 mg por semana. Reduzir gradativamente para a dose mais baixa, porém ainda eficaz. O DES é tóxico para a medula óssea em cães e gatos, podendo causar discrasias sanguíneas. Isso pode evoluir, em casos raros, para anemia aplásica fatal. Em alguns cães, uma combinação de estrogênio e fenilpropanolamina pode ser mais eficaz.

ACOMPANHAMENTO

MONITORIZAÇÃO DO PACIENTE
- A cada 3-6 meses para infecção do trato urinário.
- Os pacientes submetidos a algum agonista α-adrenérgico devem passar por avaliações seriadas da pressão arterial, pois esse tipo de medicamento é contraindicado em pacientes hipertensos ou naqueles com doença cardíaca ou renal.
- Os pacientes submetidos ao DES devem passar por avaliações seriadas do hemograma completo para monitorizar a ocorrência de discrasia da medula óssea.
- Utilizar todos os medicamentos na dose mais baixa, porém ainda eficaz.

COMPLICAÇÕES POSSÍVEIS
- Incontinência refratária.
- Infecção do trato urinário recidivante e pielonefrite.
- Queimadura por escaldagem de urina e dermatite perivulvar.

DIVERSOS

ABREVIATURA(S)
- DES = dietilestilbestrol.

Sugestões de Leitura
Crawford JT, Adams WM. Influence of vestibulovaginal stenosis, pelvic bladder, and recessed vulva on response to treatment for clinical signs of lower urinary tract disease in dogs: 38 cases (1990-1999). JAVMA 2002, 221(7):995-999.

Autor Allyson C. Berent
Consultor Editorial Carl A. Osborne

BLASTOMICOSE

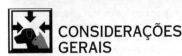

CONSIDERAÇÕES GERAIS

DEFINIÇÃO
Infecção micótica sistêmica, causada pelo microrganismo *Blastomyces dermatitidis* presente no solo.

FISIOPATOLOGIA
• Um esporo pequeno (conídios) é liberado no solo a partir da fase micelial de crescimento do microrganismo e depois inalado, penetrando nas vias aéreas terminais.
• À temperatura corporal, o esporo transforma-se em uma levedura, o que desencadeia a infecção nos pulmões.
• A partir desse foco de pneumonia micótica, a levedura dissemina-se por via hematógena por todo o corpo.
• A resposta imune contra o microrganismo invasor produz um infiltrado piogranulomatoso para controlar e conter tal agente.
• O resultado disso corresponde a uma disfunção orgânica.

SISTEMA(S) ACOMETIDO(S)
• Respiratório — 85% dos cães acometidos apresentam pneumopatia.
• Olhos, pele, sistema linfático e ossos — são comumente acometidos.
• Cérebro, testículos, próstata, glândula mamária, cavidade nasal, nasofaringe, gengiva, coração e vulva — são acometidos com menor frequência.

INCIDÊNCIA/PREVALÊNCIA
Depende das condições do ambiente e do solo que favoreçam o crescimento do *Blastomyces*.

DISTRIBUIÇÃO GEOGRÁFICA
Mais comum junto às bacias dos rios Mississipi, Ohio e Tennessee. Também é encontrada na região dos Grandes Lagos e do rio São Lourenço nos Estados Unidos, sul do Canadá e fora da área endêmica no Colorado.

IDENTIFICAÇÃO
Espécies
• Cães
• Ocasionalmente, gatos.

Raça(s) Predominante(s)
Cães de grande porte, com peso ≥25 kg, especialmente as raças atléticas; pode refletir o aumento da exposição, em vez de suscetibilidade.

Idade Média e Faixa Etária
• Cães — mais comum com 2-4 anos de idade; incomum após os 7 anos de idade.
• Gatos — jovens aos de meia-idade.

Sexo Predominante
Cães — machos em grande parte dos estudos.

SINAIS CLÍNICOS
Achados Anamnésicos
• Perda de peso.
• Diminuição do apetite (hiporexia).
• Tosse e dispneia.
• Inflamação e secreção oculares.
• Claudicação.
• Lesões cutâneas drenantes.
• Síncope se houver envolvimento cardíaco.

Achados do Exame Físico
Cães
• Febre de até 40°C — aproximadamente 50% dos pacientes.
• Ruídos pulmonares secos e ásperos, associados a um aumento no esforço respiratório — comuns.
• Linfadenopatia generalizada ou regional, com ou sem lesões cutâneas.
• Uveíte com ou sem glaucoma secundário, além de conjuntivite, exsudatos oculares e edema corneano.
• Claudicação — comum em função da osteomielite fúngica.
• Aumento de volume testicular e prostatomegalia — ocasionalmente observados.
• Sopro e bloqueio AV — em caso de endocardite e miocardite.

Gatos
• Aumento no esforço respiratório.
• Lesões cutâneas granulomatosas.

FATORES DE RISCO
• Ambiente úmido — promove o crescimento do fungo; margens de rios, correntezas e lagos ou pântanos; a maior parte dos cães acometidos vive a uma distância de até 400 m da água.
• Exposição a áreas recém-escavadas.
• A blastomicose também pode ocorrer em gatos que vivem só dentro de casa.

DIAGNÓSTICO

DIAGNÓSTICO DIFERENCIAL
• Sinais respiratórios — pneumonia bacteriana, neoplasia, insuficiência cardíaca ou outras infecções fúngicas.
• Enfartamento dos linfonodos — similar ao quadro de linfoma.
• A combinação de doença respiratória com envolvimento ocular, ósseo ou cutâneo em cães jovens é sugestiva do diagnóstico.

HEMOGRAMA/BIOQUÍMICA/URINÁLISE
• As alterações do hemograma completo refletem uma inflamação leve a moderada.
• Em cães com infecções crônicas, observam-se níveis séricos elevados das globulinas com concentrações da albumina no limite inferior.
• Em alguns cães, observa-se hipercalcemia secundária a alterações granulomatosas.
• Em cães com envolvimento prostático, podem-se encontrar leveduras de *Blastomyces* na urina.

OUTROS TESTES LABORATORIAIS
• Teste antigênico na urina — útil para a formulação do diagnóstico caso não se consiga encontrar os microrganismos nos exames citológicos ou histopatológicos; o resultado positivo sugere fortemente o diagnóstico, com sensibilidade >90%.
• O teste antigênico na urina exibe reação cruzada com algumas outras infecções fúngicas, como histoplasmose.
• IDAG — esse exame não é sensível no início da doença, mas muito específico para infecção fúngica.

DIAGNÓSTICO POR IMAGEM
Radiografias
• Pulmões — as radiografias pulmonares são essenciais para o diagnóstico e o prognóstico.
• Infiltrado generalizado intersticial a nodular, embora possa se observar uma distribuição não uniforme das lesões.
• Linfadenopatia traqueobrônquica — comum.
• Alterações — incompatíveis com pneumonia bacteriana; podem se assemelhar a tumores metastáticos, especialmente hemangiossarcoma.
• Nos cães, pode ocorrer quilotórax secundário à blastomicose.
• Lesões ósseas focais — líticas e proliferativas; podem ser confundidas com osteossarcoma.

MÉTODOS DIAGNÓSTICOS
• Citologia de aspirados de linfonodos ou de pulmões, líquido de lavado traqueal ou esfregaços por impressão (decalques) de lesões cutâneas drenantes — melhor método para o diagnóstico.
• Histopatologia de biopsias ósseas ou olhos cegos enucleados — identifica o microrganismo.
• Microrganismos — geralmente abundantes nos tecidos; podem ser escassos em lavados traqueais na ausência de tosse produtiva.

ACHADOS PATOLÓGICOS
• Lesões — piogranulomatosas, com muitas leveduras de parede espessa em brotamento; ocasionalmente, as lesões são bastante fibrosas, com poucos microrganismos.
• Os pulmões com grande quantidade de infiltrado inflamatório não sofrem colapso à abertura do tórax.
• Corantes especiais para fungos — facilitam o encontro dos microrganismos.

TRATAMENTO

CUIDADO(S) DE ENFERMAGEM
Cães gravemente dispneicos — necessitam de gaiola de oxigênio por no mínimo 1 semana, antes que o restabelecimento dos pulmões seja suficiente para proporcionar certo alívio ao ar ambiente; cerca de 25% dos cães exibem uma piora da pneumopatia durante os primeiros dias do tratamento, atribuída ao aumento na resposta inflamatória após a morte do *Blastomyces* e à liberação do conteúdo desses microrganismos.

ATIVIDADE
É imprescindível restringir a atividade física em pacientes com comprometimento respiratório.

DIETA
Fornecer uma dieta palatável de alta qualidade para estimular o apetite.

ORIENTAÇÃO AO PROPRIETÁRIO
Informar ao proprietário que o tratamento é caro e dura no mínimo 60-90 dias.

CONSIDERAÇÕES CIRÚRGICAS
Quando o tratamento clínico não for capaz de solucionar a infecção, poderá ser necessária a remoção de algum lobo pulmonar abscedado.

MEDICAÇÕES

MEDICAMENTO(S) DE ESCOLHA
Itraconazol
• Cães — 5 mg/kg VO a cada 12 h com uma refeição rica em gordura (tal como as rações caninas enlatadas), durante os primeiros 3 dias, para se atingir uma concentração sanguínea terapêutica o mais rapidamente possível; em seguida, reduzir para 5 mg/kg a cada 24 h.
• Gatos — 5 mg/kg VO a cada 12 h; abrir as cápsulas de 100 mg com péletes em sua composição e misturar com um alimento palatável. Evitar qualquer medicamento antiácido que possa diminuir a absorção do itraconazol.

BLASTOMICOSE

- Tratar o animal por no mínimo 60 dias ou por 1 mês após o desaparecimento de todos os sinais clínicos da doença.
- Tomar cuidado com o itraconazol manipulado, pois a absorção do medicamento não é confiável nesse caso.
- Os cães com sinais neurológicos devem ser tratados com a anfotericina B.
- Olhos cegos devem ser submetidos à enucleação para remover os locais potenciais de infecção residual.

CONTRAINDICAÇÕES/INTERAÇÕES POSSÍVEIS

Corticosteroides — geralmente contraindicados, pois seus efeitos anti-inflamatórios permitem a proliferação desenfreada e descontrolada dos microrganismos; os pacientes com histórico de esteroidoterapia prévia necessitam de tratamento antifúngico mais prolongado; para os cães dispneicos com risco de morte, a dexametasona (0,2 mg/kg diariamente) por 2-3 dias pode salvá-los quando administrada em conjunto com o itraconazol; interromper os esteroides assim que for possível.

PRECAUÇÕES

Toxicidade do Itraconazol
- Anorexia — sinal mais comum; atribuído à hepatotoxicidade; monitorizar mensalmente a concentração sérica da ALT durante todo o tratamento ou na ocorrência da anorexia; interromper temporariamente a administração em pacientes com anorexia e atividades da ALT >200; após o restabelecimento do apetite, reiniciar a terapia com a metade da dose previamente utilizada.
- Dermatite ulcerativa — observada em alguns cães; o resultado de vasculite; condição relacionada à dose; efetuar também a suspensão temporária do medicamento; ao desaparecimento das úlceras, reiniciar a terapia utilizando a metade da dose anterior.

MEDICAMENTO(S) ALTERNATIVO(S)
- Anfotericina B — 0,5 mg/kg IV em dias alternados em cães intolerantes aos medicamentos orais ou irresponsivos ao itraconazol (ver "Histoplasmose"); utilizar o complexo lipídico para cães com disfunção renal que não conseguem tomar o itraconazol.
- Fluconazol — 5 mg/kg VO a cada 12 h; alternativa mais barata, quando comparada ao itraconazol; no entanto, a resposta é inferior e o índice de recidiva, mais alto.

ACOMPANHAMENTO

MONITORIZAÇÃO DO PACIENTE
Perfil bioquímico sérico — mensal, para monitorizar a ocorrência de hepatotoxicidade ou diante do desenvolvimento de anorexia.

Radiografias Torácicas
- Determinam a duração do tratamento.
- Após a resolução da infecção, ainda podem ocorrer consideráveis alterações permanentes nos pulmões, dificultando a determinação da doença ativa persistente.
- Aos 60 dias do tratamento — caso se observe pneumopatia ativa, prosseguir o tratamento por 30 dias.
- Se os pulmões estiverem normais, interromper o tratamento e obter radiografias novamente em 30 dias.
- Aos 90 dias do tratamento — se a situação dos pulmões for a mesma no 60º dia, as alterações serão residuais. Fibrose — indica doença inativa; se a condição estiver melhor que no 60º dia, continuar o tratamento por mais um mês; se as lesões estiverem significativamente piores do que aos 60 dias, alterar o tratamento para a anfotericina B e então tirar novas radiografias.
- Aos 120 dias do tratamento — efetuar outras radiografias. Manter a terapia, contanto que haja uma melhora nos pulmões. Na ausência de melhora adicional e na falta de indicação de doença ativa, as lesões provavelmente serão cicatriciais.

PREVENÇÃO
- Não se conhece o local de crescimento ambiental dos microrganismos *Blastomyces*; assim, fica difícil evitar a exposição; a restrição da exposição a lagos e riachos é possível, mas isso não é muito prático.
- Os cães que se recuperam da infecção ficam provavelmente imunes à reinfecção.

EVOLUÇÃO ESPERADA E PROGNÓSTICO
- Óbito — 25% dos cães morrem durante a primeira semana de tratamento; o diagnóstico precoce aumenta as chances de sobrevida.
- A gravidade do envolvimento pulmonar e a invasão cerebral influenciam o prognóstico.
- Recidiva — cerca de 20% dos cães; em geral, dentro de 3-6 meses após o término do tratamento, mesmo com a terapia de 60-90 dias; pode ocorrer até 15 meses após o tratamento; um segundo curso terapêutico com o itraconazol levará à cura de grande parte dos pacientes; ainda não se observou a resistência a esse antifúngico.
- Com a descoberta precoce da blastomicose, o prognóstico nos gatos parece ser o mesmo dos cães.

DIVERSOS

POTENCIAL ZOONÓTICO
- Não se dissemina dos animais ao ser humano, exceto por feridas provocadas por mordeduras; já ocorreu a inoculação de microrganismos a partir de mordeduras de cães.
- Evitar cortes durante a necropsia de cães infectados e picadas de agulha ao se aspirar as lesões.
- Alertar os proprietários quanto à aquisição da blastomicose a partir de uma fonte ambiental; ainda existe a possibilidade de que eles tenham sido expostos ao mesmo tempo que o paciente; já se registrou uma fonte comum de exposição em caçadores de patos e guaxinins; a incidência nos cães é 10 vezes maior que nos seres humanos.
- Estimular os proprietários com lesões respiratórias e cutâneas a informar seus médicos sobre a provável exposição à blastomicose.

GESTAÇÃO/FERTILIDADE/REPRODUÇÃO
Não há efeitos teratogênicos do itraconazol em doses terapêuticas em ratos e camundongos; constatação de embriotoxicidade em altas doses; não há estudos em cães ou gatos; uma cadela submetida ao itraconazol na metade de sua gestação pariu uma ninhada normal.

ABREVIATURA(S)
- ALT = alanina aminotransferase.
- AV = atrioventricular.
- IDAG = imunodifusão em ágar gel.

RECURSOS DA INTERNET
Informações sobre o teste antigênico: www.miravistalabs.com.

Sugestões de Leitura

Arceneaux KA, Taboada J, Hosgood G. Blastomycosis in dogs: 115 cases (1980-1995). JAVMA 1998, 213:658-664.

Crews LJ, Feeney DA, Jessen CR, et al. Radiographic findings in dogs with pulmonary blastomycosis: 125 cases (1989-2006). JAVMA 2008, 232:215-221.

Gilor C, Graves TK, Barger AM, et al. Clinical aspects of natural infection with Blastomyces dermatitidis in cats: 8 cases. JAVMA 2006, 229:96-99.

Krawiec DR, McKiernan BC, Twardock AR, et al. Use of amphotericin B lipid complex for treatment of blastomycosis in dogs. JAVMA 1996, 209:2073-2075.

Legendre AM. Blastomycosis. In: Greene CE, ed., Infectious Diseases of the Dog and Cat, 3rd ed. St. Louis: Saunders Elsevier, 2006, pp. 569-576.

Legendre AM, Rohrbach BW, Toal RL, et al. Treatment of blastomycosis with itraconazole in 112 dogs. J Vet Intern Med 1996, 10:365-371.

Mazepa AS, Trepanir LA, Fox DS. Retrospective comparison of the efficacy of fluconazole or itraconazole for the treatment of systemic blastomycosis in dogs. J Vet Intern Med 2011, epub.

Spector D, Legendre AM, Wheat J, et al. Antigen and antibody testing for the diagnosis of blastomycosis in dogs. J Vet Intern Med 2008, 22:839-843.

Autor Alfred M. Legendre
Consultor Editorial Stephen C. Barr

BLEFARITE

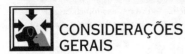

CONSIDERAÇÕES GERAIS

DEFINIÇÃO
• Inflamação das porções externa (pele) e média (musculatura, tecido conjuntivo e glândulas) das pálpebras, geralmente associada à inflamação secundária da conjuntiva palpebral. • Crônica — anterior ou posterior, com base no local de envolvimento predominante. • Anterior — mais comumente associada à infecção bacteriana ou autotraumatismo. • Posterior — distúrbios das glândulas meibomianas.

FISIOPATOLOGIA
• Semelhante à praticamente qualquer condição que comprometa a pele em geral. • Mecanismos da inflamação — imunomediado, infeccioso, mediado por via endócrina, autotraumatismo e traumatismo externo, parasitário, radiação e nutricional. • A resposta inflamatória mostra-se frequentemente exagerada, já que a conjuntiva palpebral é rica em mastócitos e densamente vascularizada. • Disfunção da glândula meibomiana — comum; as lipases bacterianas alteram os lipídios meibomianos, promovendo o entupimento da glândula com um tampão; essas lipases também produzem ácidos graxos irritantes, estimulam o crescimento bacteriano e desestabilizam o filme lacrimal.

SISTEMA(S) ACOMETIDO(S)
Oftálmico.

IDENTIFICAÇÃO
Ver a seção "Causas".

SINAIS CLÍNICOS
• Secreção ocular serosa, mucoide ou mucopurulenta. • Blefarospasmo. • Hiperemia, edema e espessamento palpebrais. • Prurido. • Escoriação. • Despigmentação — pele; pelos. • Alopecia. • Glândulas meibomianas intumescidas de coloração creme. • Orifícios das glândulas meibomianas elevados e puntiformes. • Abscessos. • Escamas e crostas. • Pápulas ou pústulas. • Tumefações hiperêmicas nodulares isoladas ou múltiplas. • Conjuntivite e/ou ceratite concomitantes. • Em gatos da raça Siamês com manchas coloridas, a blefarite crônica frequentemente causa clareamento dos pelos sobre as pálpebras acometidas em função do aumento da temperatura da pele.

CAUSAS

Congênitas
• Anormalidades palpebrais — podem promover autotraumatismo ou dermatite úmida. • Pregas nasais proeminentes, triquíase medial e entrópio da pálpebra inferior — cães das raças Shih tzu, Pequinês, Buldogue inglês, Lhasa apso, Pug, bem como gatos das raças Persa e Himalaio. • Distiquíase — cães das raças Shih tzu, Pug, Golden retriever, Labrador retriever, poodle, Buldogue inglês. • Cílios ectópicos. • Entrópio palpebral lateral — cães das raças Shar pei, Chow chow, Labrador retriever, Rottweiler; gatos adultos (raro). • Lagoftalmia — cães braquicefálicos; gatos das raças Persa, Himalaio e Birmanês. • Bolsas profundas no canto medial dos olhos — cães dolicocefálicos. • Dermoides — cães das raças Rottweiler, Dachshund e outros; gato Birmanês.

Alérgicas
• Do tipo I (imediatas) — atopia; hipersensibilidade alimentar; picada de insetos; inalantes; hipersensibilidade ao *Staphylococcus*. • Do tipo II (citotóxicas) — pênfigo; penfigoide; erupção medicamentosa. • Do tipo III (por imunocomplexos) — LES; hipersensibilidade ao *Staphylococcus*; erupção medicamentosa. • Do tipo IV (mediadas por células) — hipersensibilidade de contato e à picada de pulgas; erupção medicamentosa.

Bacterianas
• Hordéolo — abscesso localizado das glândulas palpebrais, geralmente estafilocócico; pode ser externo (terçol em cães jovens, com o envolvimento das glândulas de Zeis) ou interno (em cães idosos, envolve uma ou mais glândulas meibomianas). • Blefarite e meibomianite bacterianas generalizadas — causadas em geral por *Staphylococcus* ou *Streptococcus*. • Piogranulomas. • Hipersensibilidade ao *Staphylococcus* — cães jovens e idosos.

Neoplásicas
• Adenomas e adenocarcinomas sebáceos — originam-se da glândula meibomiana. • Carcinoma de células escamosas — gatos brancos. • Mastocitoma — pode ser mascarado como uma lesão intumescida e hiperêmica.

Outras
• Traumatismo externo — lacerações palpebrais; queimaduras térmicas ou químicas. • Micóticas — dermatofitose; granulomas fúngicos sistêmicos. • Parasitárias — demodicose; sarna sarcóptica; *Cuterebra* e *Notoedres cati. Nota:* o ácaro *Demodex injai* tem propensão à infestação das glândulas sebáceas e pode ser associado à disfunção das glândulas sebáceas em cães, incluindo calázio e blefarite granulomatosa. • Calázio(s) — tumefações estéreis, amarelo-esbranquiçadas e indolores das glândulas meibomianas, causadas por uma resposta inflamatória granulomatosa ao escape de secreção glandular para o tecido palpebral circunjacente. • Nutricionais — dermatose responsiva ao zinco (raças Husky siberiano, Malamute do Alasca e filhotes caninos); deficiência de ácidos graxos. • Endócrinas — hipotireoidismo (cães); hiperadrenocorticismo (cães); dermatose diabética. • Virais — blefarite crônica em gatos secundária ao FHV-1. • Irritantes — reação a medicamentos oculares tópicos; fumaça de cigarro (nicotina) no ambiente; ou como um quadro subsequente à transposição do ducto parotídeo. • Dermatomiosite canina familiar — Collie e Pastor de shetland. • Episcleroceratite granulomatosa nodular — histiocitoma fibroso e granuloma do Collie; pode acometer as pálpebras, a córnea ou a conjuntiva. • Granuloma eosinofílico — gatos; pode afetar as pálpebras, as córneas ou as conjuntivas. • Contato das pálpebras com fluxo lacrimal excessivo e exsudato purulento (queimadura lacrimal). • Conjuntivite. • Ceratite. • Ressecamento ocular. • Dacriocistite. • Doença orbitária. • Radioterapia. • Contato com irritantes medicamentosos — qualquer medicamento, frequentemente a neomicina. • Idiopáticas — particularmente em gatos com conjuntivite idiopática crônica.

FATORES DE RISCO
• Predisposição racial a anormalidades palpebrais congênitas (p. ex., entrópio, ectrópio etc.). • Animais de rua — risco de traumatismos. • Hipotireoidismo — pode promover doença bacteriana crônica em cães. • Seborreia canina — pode favorecer a meibomianite generalizada crônica, com predisposição para infecção por *Demodex injai*.

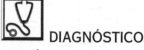

DIAGNÓSTICO

DIAGNÓSTICO DIFERENCIAL
Os sinais clínicos são diagnósticos.

HEMOGRAMA/BIOQUÍMICA/URINÁLISE
Em geral, não são diagnósticos, a menos que haja uma causa metabólica (p. ex., dermatose diabética).

OUTROS TESTES LABORATORIAIS
• Indicados na suspeita de distúrbio sistêmico. • Considerar os testes endócrinos para pesquisa do hipotireoidismo.

MÉTODOS DIAGNÓSTICOS
• Se possível, evitar a instilação tópica de anestésicos ou fluoresceína antes de se obter as amostras para cultura. • Citologia — raspados cutâneos profundos; raspados conjuntivais; extração manual de exsudato das glândulas meibomianas e de pústulas. • Cultura para dermatófitos — raspados cutâneos profundos. • Avaliação com a lâmpada de Wood — pele. • Preparação com hidróxido de potássio (KOH) — raspados cutâneos. • Cultura bacteriana aeróbia e antibiograma — exsudato proveniente da pele; conjuntiva; extração manual de exsudato das glândulas meibomianas e de pústulas; com frequência, não se recuperará o microrganismo *Staphylococcus* de pacientes com meibomianite crônica e suspeita de hipersensibilidade estafilocócica. • IFI ou PCR em busca do FHV-1 e da *Chlamydia* — raspados conjuntivais de gatos com conjuntivite ou ceratite primárias. • Exame ocular — buscar a causa desencadeante potencial; úlcera de córnea; corpo(s) estranho(s); distiquíase; cílios ectópicos; ressecamento ocular. • Testes oculares complementares — aplicação de fluoresceína; teste lacrimal de Schirmer. • Anamnese e exame dermatológico completos — ajudam a identificar uma dermatopatia generalizada. • Biopsia palpebral cuneiforme de espessura completa — avaliação histológica. • Imunofluorescência direta em busca de doenças autoimunes; teste cutâneo intradérmico, RAST, ELISA e dieta de eliminação (hipoalergênica) em casos de doença induzida por hipersensibilidade.

ACHADOS PATOLÓGICOS
• Em doenças crônicas, a histopatologia de rotina muitas vezes não é diagnóstica. • Biopsia em cunha — pode ser frustrante; selecionar cuidadosamente os pacientes, com base na anamnese, no exame oftálmico e na resposta à terapia clínica.

TRATAMENTO

CUIDADO(S) DE SAÚDE ADEQUADO(S)
Ver a seção "Cuidado(s) de Enfermagem".

CUIDADO(S) DE ENFERMAGEM
• Doença secundária — tratar a doença primária. • Suspeita de autotraumatismo — usar colar elizabetano. • Medicamentos antivirais tópicos de

BLEFARITE

gentamicina, neomicina, terramicina (p. ex., solução de trifluridina) e grande parte das pomadas oftálmicas — podem causar uma blefaroconjuntivite irritante (rara); a suspensão do agente terapêutico pode solucionar o problema.
• Limpeza das pálpebras — para remover as crostas; aplicação de compressas mornas por 5-15 minutos, 3-4 vezes ao dia, evitando-se as superfícies oculares; utilizar soluções fisiológica, Ringer lactato ou agentes comerciais de limpeza ocular (p. ex., Eye Scrub®); é imprescindível aparar os pelos da região periocular.

DIETA
Apenas em casos de doença induzida por alergia alimentar.

ORIENTAÇÃO AO PROPRIETÁRIO
• Em gatos com blefarite relacionada com infecção por FHV-1, alertar o proprietário sobre a impossibilidade de cura da maioria dos pacientes e o possível controle clínico da condição. • Informar aos proprietários a ausência de cura para o FHV-1 e a frequente recidiva dos sinais clínicos no animal sob estresse. • Orientar os proprietários a manterem o colar elizabetano durante todo o tempo.

CONSIDERAÇÕES CIRÚRGICAS
• Suturas temporárias de pálpebras invertidas — em casos de entrópio espástico; ou em filhotes caninos antes da correção cirúrgica permanente.
• Reparo das lacerações palpebrais.
• Lancetamento — apenas em abscessos amplos; incisar com lanceta e fazer a curetagem dos hordéolos resistentes ao tratamento clínico e dos calázios endurecidos e puntiformes indutores de ceratite; promover a extração manual das secreções das glândulas meibomianas infectadas.

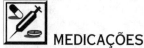

MEDICAÇÕES
MEDICAMENTO(S)
Antibióticos
• Sistêmicos — em geral, necessários para um tratamento eficaz contra infecções palpebrais bacterianas; pode-se tentar a combinação de amoxicilina-ácido clavulânico ou a cefalexina; 20 mg/kg a cada 8 h. • Tópicos — pode-se experimentar a neomicina, a polimixina B, a combinação de bacitracina ou o cloranfenicol. Evitar a neomicina na suspeita de irritação como a causa.

Forma Congênita
• Pomada antibiótica tópica — a cada 6-12 h; aplicada até que se efetue a cirurgia, para evitar o atrito friccional de pelos ou cílios palpebrais sobre a superfície ocular. • Soluções fisiológica, Ringer lactato ou de irrigação ocular — para remover regularmente os debris (fragmentos) presentes em bolsas profundas dos cantos mediais.

Traumatismo Externo
• Pomada antibiótica tópica — a cada 6-12 horas; em casos de entrópio espástico secundário à dor e ao blefaroespasmo para reduzir a fricção até que o entrópio seja aliviado por meio cirúrgico.
• Também fica indicado o uso de antibióticos sistêmicos.

Alérgicos
• Blefarite por hipersensibilidade ao *Staphylococcus* — antibióticos sistêmicos de amplo espectro e corticosteroides sistêmicos (prednisolona, 0,5 mg/kg a cada 12 h por 3-5 dias; em seguida, reduzir a dose gradativamente); muitos pacientes respondem drasticamente aos corticosteroides sistêmicos isolados. Utilizar ciclosporina sistêmica em casos refratários a corticosteroides (5 mg/kg VO a cada 24 h até a remissão e, depois, a cada 48-72 h).
• Glândulas meibomianas infectadas — tetraciclina (15-20 mg/kg VO a cada 8 h) ou doxiciclina (3-5 mg/kg VO a cada 12 h) ou cefalexina (22 mg/kg a cada 8 h) por no mínimo 3 semanas (os dois primeiros são lipofílicos e causam declínio na produção de lipases bacterianas e ácidos graxos irritantes); aplicação ocular tópica de polimixina B e neomicina com dexametasona a 0,1% (a cada 6-8 h) ou pomada tópica manipulada de tacrolimo a 0,02% (a cada 8-12 h). Nota: Alguns cães acometidos também podem ter infecção concomitante por *Demodex injai* e necessitam de tratamento acaricida contra demodecose. • Em casos de falha terapêutica — pode-se tentar a aplicação de injeções de bacterinas homólogas ou comerciais do *Staphylococcus aureus* (Staphage Lysate®). • Imunoterapia com o *Propionibacterium acnes* — sob pesquisa; de valor desconhecido. • Lesões palpebrais associadas à piodermite de filhotes caninos — em geral, beneficiam-se com o tratamento da condição generalizada.

Bacterianos
• Com base na cultura e no antibiograma. • Na pendência dos resultados — aplicar polimixina B e neomicina tópicas com pomada de dexametasona a 0,1% (a cada 4-6 h); associar um antibiótico sistêmico de amplo espectro.

Micóticos
• Infecção pelo *Microsporum canis* — geralmente autolimitante; o tratamento inclui creme de miconazol a 2%, creme de clotrimazol a 1% ou solução diluída de iodopovidona (1 parte para 300 partes de solução fisiológica), aplicados a cada 12-24 h por no mínimo 6 semanas; não utilizar loções.

Parasitários
• Demodicose — doença localizada, tratada com amitraz diluído (1 parte de amitraz para 9 partes de óleo mineral; Mitaban®) uma vez ao dia a cada 3 dias por 4-8 semanas; razoavelmente segura em torno dos olhos (ver "Demodicose"). Alguns cães necessitam de tratamento sistêmico com moxidectina, ivermectina, ou milbemicina oxima.
• Infecção por *Notoedres* — banhos de imersão com soluções sulfuradas. • Sarna sarcóptica — tratamento similar aos casos de doença generalizada.

Idiopáticos
• Os sinais clínicos frequentemente são controlados com a aplicação tópica de polimixina B e neomicina associadas à dexametasona a 0,1% (a cada 8-24 h ou conforme a necessidade); ocasionalmente, pode necessitar também de prednisolona sistêmica (0,5 mg/kg a cada 12 h por 3-5 dias; com subsequente redução gradativa da dose) e/ou de um antibiótico sistêmico.

CONTRAINDICAÇÕES
• Corticosteroides tópicos — não utilizar em casos de úlcera de córnea. • Gatos — muitos pacientes com suposta blefaroconjuntivite idiopática, na verdade, apresentam infecção pelo FHV-1; os corticosteroides tópicos e sistêmicos podem exacerbar a infecção. • Tetraciclina e doxiciclina orais — não usar em filhotes caninos e felinos.
• Neomicina — evitar o uso tópico caso se suspeite desse medicamento como o agente causal da blefarite.

PRECAUÇÕES
Ectoparasitismo — usar luvas; não permitir o contato do medicamento com as superfícies oculares; aplicar lágrima artificial para proteção dos olhos.

INTERAÇÕES POSSÍVEIS
Bacterina estafilocócica em casos de hipersensibilidade ao *Staphylococcus* — reação anafilática (rara).

ACOMPANHAMENTO
MONITORIZAÇÃO DO PACIENTE
• Depende da causa e da forma de terapia.
• Bacteriana — tratada por vias tópica e sistêmica por no mínimo 3 semanas; deve-se notar uma melhora dentro de 10 dias. • Causas mais comuns de falha terapêutica — uso de concentrações inibitórias de antibióticos abaixo do ideal; falha na correção de um ou mais fatores predisponentes; interrupção precoce dos medicamentos.

PREVENÇÃO
Depende da causa.

COMPLICAÇÕES POSSÍVEIS
• Contratura cicatricial com consequente retração palpebral — resulta em triquíase, ectrópio ou lagoftalmia. • Entrópio espástico — decorrente de blefaroespasmo e dor. • Impossibilidade de abertura das pálpebras — em virtude de um emaranhado de secreção e pelos. • Deficiência qualitativa do filme lacrimal — origina-se da perda de secreção adequada das glândulas meibomianas. • Recidiva da infecção bacteriana ou da blefaroconjuntivite por FHV-1.

EVOLUÇÃO ESPERADA E PROGNÓSTICO
Dependem da causa.

DIVERSOS
POTENCIAL ZOONÓTICO
• Dermatofitose. • Sarna sarcóptica.

VER TAMBÉM
• Ceratite Não Ulcerativa. • Ceratite Ulcerativa.
• Conjuntivite — Cães. • Conjuntivite — Gatos.
• Epífora. • Olho Vermelho.

ABREVIATURA(S)
• ELISA = ensaio imunoabsorvente ligado à enzima. • FHV-1 = herpes-vírus felino do tipo 1.
• IFI = imunofluorescência indireta. • LES = lúpus eritematoso sistêmico. • PCR = reação em cadeia da polimerase. • RAST = teste radioalergossorvente.

Sugestões de Leitura
Maggs D. Eyelids. In: Maggs DJ, Miller PE, Ofri R, Slatter's Fundamentals of Veterinary Ophthalmology, 4th ed. St. Louis: Saunders, 2008, pp. 107-134.

Autor Terri L. McCalla
Consultor Editorial Paul E. Miller

BLOQUEIO ATRIOVENTRICULAR COMPLETO (TERCEIRO GRAU)

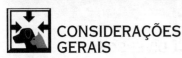

CONSIDERAÇÕES GERAIS

DEFINIÇÃO
- Todos os impulsos atriais são bloqueados na junção AV; além disso, os batimentos atriais e ventriculares são independentes. Um marca-passo com ritmo secundário de "escape" (juncional ou ventricular) estimula os ventrículos.
- A frequência atrial permanece normal.
- O ritmo de escape idioventricular apresenta-se lento.

Características do ECG
- Frequência ventricular mais lenta do que a atrial (mais ondas P do que complexos QRS) — ritmo de escape ventricular (idioventricular) geralmente <40 bpm; ritmo de escape juncional (idiojuncional) de 40-60 bpm em cães e 60-100 bpm em gatos.
- Ondas P — costumam exibir configuração normal (Fig. 1).
- Complexo QRS — apresenta-se amplo e bizarro quando o marca-passo se localiza no ventrículo ou na junção AV inferior em paciente com bloqueio de ramo do feixe de His; permanece normal quando o marca-passo de escape se encontra na junção AV inferior (acima da bifurcação do feixe de His) em animal sem bloqueio de ramo desse feixe.
- Não há nenhuma condução entre os átrios e os ventrículos; as ondas P não apresentam uma relação constante com os complexos QRS; os intervalos P-P e R-R permanecem relativamente constantes (exceto em casos de arritmia sinusal).

FISIOPATOLOGIA
Os ritmos lentos de escape ventricular (<40 bpm) resultam em baixo débito cardíaco e consequente insuficiência cardíaca, muitas vezes quando o animal se encontra agitado ou se exercita, uma vez que a demanda por um aumento no débito cardíaco não é satisfeita. À medida que o coração entra em insuficiência, os sinais aumentam mesmo com atividades leves.

SISTEMA(S) ACOMETIDO(S)
Cardiovascular.

GENÉTICA
Pode ser um defeito congênito isolado.

INCIDÊNCIA/PREVALÊNCIA
Não há registros.

DISTRIBUIÇÃO GEOGRÁFICA
N/D.

IDENTIFICAÇÃO
Espécies
Cães e gatos.

Raça(s) Predominante(s)
- Cocker spaniel — pode ter fibrose idiopática.
- Pug e Doberman pinscher — podem apresentar quadros associados de morte súbita, defeitos de condução AV e lesões do feixe de His.

Idade Média e Faixa Etária
Acomete animais geriátricos, exceto pacientes com cardiopatia congênita. A idade média para gatos é de 14 anos.

Sexo(s) Predominante(s)
Cadelas intactas.

SINAIS CLÍNICOS
Achados Anamnésicos
- Intolerância ao exercício.
- Fraqueza ou síncope.
- Ocasionalmente, ICC.

Achados do Exame Físico
- Bradicardia.
- Sons variáveis da terceira e quarta bulhas cardíacas.
- Variação na intensidade da primeira bulha cardíaca.
- Sinais de ICC.
- Ondas A intermitentes "em canhão" nos pulsos venosos jugulares.

CAUSAS E FATORES DE RISCO
- Defeito congênito isolado.
- Fibrose idiopática.
- Miocardiopatia infiltrativa (amiloidose ou neoplasia).
- Miocardiopatia hipertrófica em gatos.
- Toxicidade dos digitálicos.
- Miocardite.
- Endocardite.
- Distúrbio eletrolítico.
- Infarto do miocárdio.
- Outros defeitos cardíacos congênitos.
- Doença de Lyme.
- Doença de Chagas.

DIAGNÓSTICO

DIAGNÓSTICO DIFERENCIAL
- Bloqueio AV avançado de segundo grau.
- Parada atrial.
- Ritmo idioventricular acelerado.

HEMOGRAMA/BIOQUÍMICA/URINÁLISE
- É possível a constatação de níveis séricos anormais dos eletrólitos (p. ex., hipercalemia e hipocalemia).
- Leucograma elevado com desvio à esquerda em animais com endocardite bacteriana.

OUTROS TESTES LABORATORIAIS
- Em caso de bloqueio AV secundário à intoxicação por digoxina, haverá uma concentração elevada desse medicamento no soro.
- Em caso de bloqueio AV atribuído à doença de Lyme, haverá títulos séricos quanto à presença da *Borrelia* e sinais clínicos concomitantes.

DIAGNÓSTICO POR IMAGEM
Para avaliar a estrutura e a função cardíacas, efetuam-se a ecocardiografia e a ultrassonografia Doppler.

MÉTODOS DIAGNÓSTICOS
- Eletrocardiografia.
- Eletrograma do feixe de His para determinar o local do bloqueio AV.
- Registro eletrocardiográfico ambulatorial contínuo (com Holter) a longo prazo em caso de bloqueio AV intermitente.

ACHADOS PATOLÓGICOS
Degeneração ou fibrose do nó AV e de seus ramos, associada à fibrose endomiocárdica e endomiocardite organizada.

TRATAMENTO

CUIDADO(S) DE SAÚDE ADEQUADO(S)
- Marca-passo cardíaco temporário ou permanente — único tratamento eficaz em pacientes sintomáticos.
- Animais assintomáticos sem marca-passo — monitorização meticulosa quanto ao desenvolvimento de sinais clínicos.

CUIDADO(S) DE ENFERMAGEM
Repouso em gaiola antes do implante do marca-passo; quando o gerador de pulso for introduzido em uma bolsa subcutânea, será necessária a aplicação de uma bandagem não compressiva em torno da porção ventral do pescoço ou do abdome por 3-5 dias para evitar a formação de seroma ou o deslocamento do marca-passo.

ATIVIDADE
Restringir a atividade física no animal sintomático.

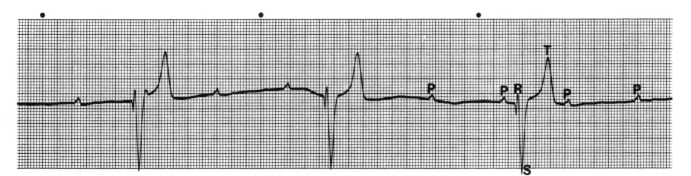

Figura 1 Bloqueio cardíaco completo. As ondas P ocorrem na frequência de 120 bpm, independentemente da frequência ventricular de 50 bpm. A configuração do QRS corresponde a um padrão de bloqueio de ramo direito do feixe de His. A frequência cardíaca regular e o QRS estável indicam que o foco de escape provavelmente se encontra próximo à junção AV. (De: Tilley LP. *Essentials of canine and feline electrocardiography*, 3.ed. Blackwell Publishing, 1992, com permissão.)

Bloqueio Atrioventricular Completo (Terceiro Grau)

DIETA
Sem mudanças a menos que solicitadas para o tratamento da condição subjacente (p. ex., dieta com baixo teor de sal).

ORIENTAÇÃO AO PROPRIETÁRIO
• Marca-passo cardíaco temporário ou permanente — representa o único tratamento eficaz em pacientes sintomáticos.
• Animais assintomáticos sem marca-passo — é imprescindível uma monitorização meticulosa quanto ao desenvolvimento de sinais clínicos.

CONSIDERAÇÕES CIRÚRGICAS
• A maioria dos pacientes encontra-se sob alto risco cardiopulmonar anestésico; em geral, o ritmo cardíaco é regularizado no período pré-operatório com um sistema de marca-passo externo temporário.
• O pequeno porte dos gatos dificulta ainda mais o implante do marca-passo, quando comparado com os cães.

MEDICAÇÕES

MEDICAMENTO(S) DE ESCOLHA
• Tratamento com medicamentos — em geral, não tem nenhum valor. Utilizado tradicionalmente para tratar o bloqueio AV completo: atropina, isoproterenol, corticosteroides e dobutamina.
• A infusão intravenosa de isoproterenol pode ajudar a aumentar a frequência do ritmo de escape ventricular para estabilizar a hemodinâmica.
• Em caso de ICC — pode haver a necessidade de terapia diurética e vasodilatadora antes do implante do marca-passo.

CONTRAINDICAÇÕES
Evitar o uso de digoxina, xilazina, acepromazina, β-bloqueadores (p. ex., propranolol e atenolol) e bloqueadores dos canais de cálcio (p. ex., verapamil e diltiazem); os agentes antiarrítmicos ventriculares são perigosos, pois suprimem os focos inferiores de escape.

PRECAUÇÕES
Vasodilatadores — podem causar hipotensão em animais com bloqueio AV completo; monitorizar o paciente de perto, como de costume, especialmente antes do implante do marca-passo.

INTERAÇÕES POSSÍVEIS
N/D.

MEDICAMENTO(S) ALTERNATIVO(S)
N/D.

ACOMPANHAMENTO

MONITORIZAÇÃO DO PACIENTE
• Monitorização do funcionamento do marca-passo com ECGs seriados.
• Obtenção de radiografias — após o implante do marca-passo para confirmar o posicionamento da derivação e do gerador.

PREVENÇÃO
N/D.

COMPLICAÇÕES POSSÍVEIS
Geradores de pulso — ampla variação na expectativa de vida; a substituição do marca-passo será necessária em caso de esgotamento da bateria, mau funcionamento do gerador de pulso ou desenvolvimento de bloqueio de saída do próprio dispositivo; as derivações do marca-passo podem vir a ser desalojadas e infectadas.

EVOLUÇÃO ESPERADA E PROGNÓSTICO
Se nenhum marca-passo cardíaco for implantado, o prognóstico a longo prazo será mau, especialmente quando o animal apresentar sinais clínicos. Algumas vezes, os gatos podem sobreviver por >1 ano.

DIVERSOS

DISTÚRBIOS ASSOCIADOS
Nenhum.

FATORES RELACIONADOS COM A IDADE
N/D.

POTENCIAL ZOONÓTICO
N/D.

GESTAÇÃO/FERTILIDADE/REPRODUÇÃO
N/D.

ABREVIATURA(S)
• AV = atrioventricular.
• bpm = batimentos por minuto.
• ECG = eletrocardiograma.
• ICC = insuficiência cardíaca congestiva.

RECURSOS DA INTERNET
www.vetgo.com/cardio.

Sugestões de Leitura
Bright JM. Pacemaker therapy. In: Tilley LP, Smith FWK, Oyama MA, Sleeper MM, eds., Manual of Canine and Feline Cardiology, 4th ed. St. Louis: Saunders Elsevier, 2008, pp. 386-397.
Kellum HB, Stepien RL. Third-degree atrioventricular block in 21 cats (1997-2004). J Vet Intern Med 2006, 20:97-103.
Schrope DP, Kelch WJ. Signalment, clinical signs, and prognostic indicators associated with high-grade second or third-degree atrioventricular block in dogs: 124 cases (January 1, 1997-December 31, 1997). JAVMA 2006, 228:1710-1717.

Autores Larry P. Tilley e Naomi L. Burtnick
Consultores Editoriais Larry P. Tilley e Francis W.K. Smith, Jr.

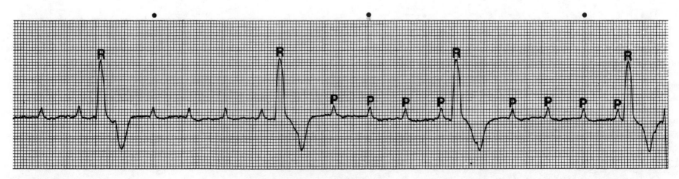

Figura 2 Bloqueio cardíaco completo em um gato. A frequência das ondas P é de 240/min, independentemente da frequência ventricular de 48/min. A configuração do QRS corresponde a um padrão de bloqueio de ramo esquerdo do feixe de His. (De: Tilley LP. *Essentials of canine and feline electrocardiography*, 3.ed. Blackwell Publishing, 1992, com permissão.)

BLOQUEIO ATRIOVENTRICULAR DE PRIMEIRO GRAU

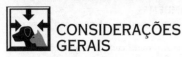

CONSIDERAÇÕES GERAIS

DEFINIÇÃO
Refere-se a um atraso na condução cardíaca, que ocorre entre as ativações atrial e ventricular.

Características do ECG
- Frequência e ritmo — em geral, normais.
- Ocorrência regular de ondas P e complexos QRS normais (Figs. 1 e 2).
- Intervalos PR consistentes e prolongados — cães >0,13 s; gatos, >0,09 s (Figs. 1 e 2).

FISIOPATOLOGIA
- Quase nunca gera sinais clínicos.
- Em alguns animais, pode se tornar um distúrbio de condução AV mais grave.
- Normalmente, o intervalo PR tende a se encurtar em casos de frequência cardíaca elevada.
- Pode ser o resultado de atraso na condução intra-atrial (prolongamento do intervalo PA* no ECG de superfície e eletrograma simultâneo do feixe de His) ou atraso na condução dentro do nó AV em si (prolongamento do intervalo AH** no eletrograma do feixe de His).

SISTEMA(S) ACOMETIDO(S)
Cardiovascular.

GENÉTICA
N/D.

INCIDÊNCIA/PREVALÊNCIA
Comum.

DISTRIBUIÇÃO GEOGRÁFICA
Nenhuma.

IDENTIFICAÇÃO
Espécies
Cães e gatos.

---

* N. T.: O intervalo PA é medido do começo da onda P do ECG de superfície à inscrição do eletrograma atrial direito, registrado com o cateter intracardíaco, fornecendo uma avaliação da condução intra-atrial durante o ritmo sinusal normal.
** N. T.: O intervalo AH é uma medida do tempo de condução do átrio direito baixo pelo nó atrioventricular (AV) ao feixe de His, sendo uma aproximação do tempo de condução do nó AV.

Raça(s) Predominante(s)
Raças Cocker spaniel americano e Dachshund, além de cães braquicefálicos e gatos da raça Persa.

Idade Média e Faixa Etária
- Pode ocorrer em cães jovens e saudáveis de modo geral, como uma manifestação de tônus vagal elevado.
- O atraso na condução intra-atrial envolvendo o átrio direito pode ser observado em casos de cardiopatia congênita, sobretudo defeitos do septo atrioventricular.
- Pode ser notado em pacientes idosos com comprometimento degenerativo no sistema de condução, particularmente nas raças caninas Cocker spaniel e Dachshund.
- Constatado também em gatos de qualquer idade com tônus vagal elevado e naqueles de qualquer idade com miocardiopatia hipertrófica.

SINAIS CLÍNICOS

Achados Anamnésicos
- A maioria dos animais apresenta-se assintomática.
- Em caso de indução por medicamentos, pode haver histórico de sinais clínicos relacionados com intoxicação medicamentosa — anorexia, vômito e diarreia com o uso da digoxina; fraqueza com o emprego de bloqueadores dos canais de cálcio ou antagonistas β-adrenérgicos.

Achados do Exame Físico
- Normais — a menos que também haja sinais de miocardiopatia, toxicidade medicamentosa ou doença extracardíaca mais generalizada.

CAUSAS
- Pode ocorrer em animais normais.
- Estimulação vagal acentuada resultante de doenças extracardíacas — acompanhada, em geral, por arritmia sinusal, parada sinusal e/ou bloqueio AV de segundo grau Mobitz tipo I.
- Agentes farmacológicos (p. ex., digoxina, antagonistas β-adrenérgicos, bloqueadores dos canais de cálcio, propafenona, amiodarona, agonistas α₂-adrenérgicos, agentes parassimpaticomiméticos [betanecol, fisostigmina, pilocarpina] e intoxicação grave por procainamida ou quinidina).
- Doença degenerativa do sistema de condução.
- Miocardiopatia hipertrófica.
- Miocardite (especialmente *Trypanosoma cruzi*, *Borrelia burgdorferi* e *Rickettsia rickettsii*).
- Doenças infiltrativas (tumores, amiloide).

- A administração de atropina por via IV pode transitoriamente prolongar o intervalo PR.

FATORES DE RISCO
Qualquer condição ou intervenção que eleve o tônus vagal.

DIAGNÓSTICO

DIAGNÓSTICO DIFERENCIAL
As ondas P sobrepostas nas ondas T prévias em função do bloqueio AV de primeiro grau devem ser diferenciadas de ondas T bífidas.

HEMOGRAMA/BIOQUÍMICA/URINÁLISE
- Eletrólitos séricos — hipocalemia e hipercalemia podem predispor o animal a distúrbios de condução AV.
- Leucocitose — pode ser observada em casos de endocardite ou miocardite bacteriana.

OUTROS TESTES LABORATORIAIS
- Concentração sérica da digoxina — pode estar alta.
- Títulos para *T. cruzi*, *B. burgdorferi* e *R. rickettsii* — podem estar elevados.
- T_4 — pode estar alta em gatos se associado à miocardiopatia tireotóxica.

DIAGNÓSTICO POR IMAGEM
Exame ecocardiográfico — pode revelar distúrbio miocárdico hipertrófico ou infiltrativo.

MÉTODOS DIAGNÓSTICOS
Pode ser necessária a identificação das causas de elevação do tônus vagal — doença das vias aéreas superiores, massas cervicais e torácicas, distúrbios gastrintestinais e pressão intraocular elevada.

ACHADOS PATOLÓGICOS
Variáveis — dependem da causa subjacente.

TRATAMENTO

CUIDADO(S) DE SAÚDE ADEQUADO(S)
- Remover ou tratar a(s) causa(s) subjacente(s).
- A internação pode ser indispensável para o tratamento da causa subjacente (p. ex., miocardiopatia, gastrenteropatia e doença das vias aéreas).

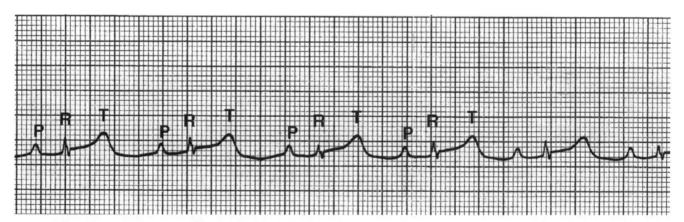

Figura 1 Registro eletrocardiográfico na derivação II de gato com miocardiopatia hipertrófica. Observam-se bradicardia sinusal (120 bpm) e bloqueio de condução atrioventricular de primeiro grau. O intervalo PR é de 0,12 segundo (velocidade do papel = 50 mm/s).

BLOQUEIO ATRIOVENTRICULAR DE PRIMEIRO GRAU

CUIDADO(S) DE ENFERMAGEM
N/D.

ATIVIDADE
Sem restrição a menos que exigida pela condição subjacente.

DIETA
Sem mudanças nem restrições a menos que solicitadas para o tratamento da condição subjacente.

ORIENTAÇÃO AO PROPRIETÁRIO
Geralmente desnecessária.

CONSIDERAÇÕES CIRÚRGICAS
Nenhuma a menos que requeridas para o tratamento da condição subjacente.

MEDICAÇÕES
MEDICAMENTO(S) DE ESCOLHA
Os medicamentos serão utilizados apenas se forem imprescindíveis para o tratamento da condição subjacente.

CONTRAINDICAÇÕES
• Evitar hipocalemia — aumenta a sensibilidade ao tônus vagal; é capaz de potencializar o atraso na condução AV.
• Evitar medicamentos que provavelmente prejudicam ainda mais a condução do impulso (bloqueadores dos canais de cálcio, antagonistas β-adrenérgicos, agonistas α$_2$-adrenérgicos, amiodarona, propafenona).

PRECAUÇÕES
Os medicamentos com ação vagomimética (p. ex., digoxina, betanecol, fisostigmina e pilocarpina) podem potencializar o bloqueio de primeiro grau.

INTERAÇÕES POSSÍVEIS
N/D.

MEDICAMENTO(S) ALTERNATIVO(S)
N/D.

ACOMPANHAMENTO
MONITORIZAÇÃO DO PACIENTE
Exceto em animais jovens saudáveis, é fundamental monitorizar o ECG para detectar qualquer evolução no distúrbio de condução.

PREVENÇÃO
N/D.

COMPLICAÇÕES POSSÍVEIS
N/D.

EVOLUÇÃO ESPERADA E PROGNÓSTICO
• Dependem da causa subjacente.
• O prognóstico costuma ser excelente na ausência de doença subjacente significativa.

DIVERSOS
DISTÚRBIOS ASSOCIADOS
Nenhum.

FATORES RELACIONADOS COM A IDADE
Intervalo PR — tende a se prolongar com o avanço da idade.

POTENCIAL ZOONÓTICO
Nenhum.

GESTAÇÃO/FERTILIDADE/REPRODUÇÃO
N/D.

VER TAMBÉM
• Bloqueio Atrioventricular Completo (Terceiro Grau).
• Bloqueio Atrioventricular de Segundo Grau — Mobitz Tipo I.
• Bloqueio Atrioventricular de Segundo Grau — Mobitz Tipo II.

ABREVIATURA(S)
• AV = atrioventricular.
• bpm = batimentos por minuto.
• ECG = eletrocardiograma.
• T_4 = tiroxina.

Sugestões de Leitura
Miller MS, Tilley LP, Smith FWK, Fox PR. Electrocardiography. In: Fox PR, Sisson D, Moise NS, eds., Textbook of Canine and Feline Cardiology. Philadelphia: Saunders, 1999, pp. 67-106.
Podrid PJ, Kowey PR. Cardiac arrhythmia — mechanisms, diagnosis, and management. Baltimore: Williams & Wilkins, 1995.
Tilley LP. Essentials of Canine and Feline Electrocardiography, 3rd ed. Baltimore: Williams & Wilkins, 1992.
Tilley LP, Smith FWK Jr. Electrocardiography. In: Tilley LP, Smith FWK, Oyama MA, Sleeper MM, eds., Manual of Canine and Feline Cardiology, 4th ed. St. Louis: Saunders Elsevier, 2008, pp. 49-77.

Autor Janice McIntosh Bright
Consultores Editoriais Larry P. Tilley e Francis W.K. Smith, Jr.

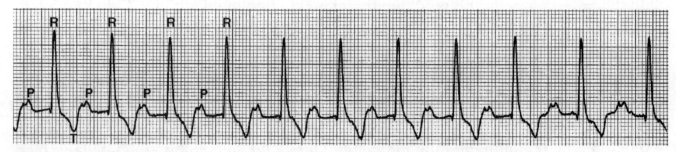

Figura 2 Registro eletrocardiográfico na derivação II de cão com taquicardia sinusal (175 bpm) e bloqueio de condução atrioventricular de primeiro grau. Como a frequência cardíaca se encontra rápida, as ondas P ficam sobrepostas sobre a curva descendente das ondas T prévias. O intervalo PR excede 0,16 segundo (velocidade do papel = 50 mm/s).

Bloqueio Atrioventricular de Segundo Grau — Mobitz Tipo I

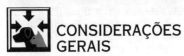

CONSIDERAÇÕES GERAIS

DEFINIÇÃO
Bloqueio AV de segundo grau refere-se à falha de uma ou mais ondas P, mas nem todas as ondas P são conduzidas. O bloqueio AV de segundo grau Mobitz tipo I ocorre quando a transmissão AV é progressivamente adiada antes de uma onda P não conduzida.

Características do ECG
- Intervalo PR — torna-se progressivamente mais prolongado antes do aparecimento de uma onda P não seguida por um complexo QRS (Fig. 1).
- Frequência cardíaca e morfologia do QRS — em geral, permanecem normais.
- Frequentemente cíclico.

FISIOPATOLOGIA
- Associada muitas vezes a um elevado tônus vagal em repouso e arritmia sinusal em cães.
- Não costuma ter importância do ponto de vista patológico ou hemodinâmico.
- Esse tipo de bloqueio AV geralmente resulta de atraso na condução dentro do nó AV em si (e não do atraso em outros segmentos do sistema de condução AV), sendo caracterizado por aumento progressivo no intervalo AH com consequente bloqueio entre as deflexões A e H no registro do feixe de His.

SISTEMA(S) ACOMETIDO(S)
Cardiovascular.

GENÉTICA
N/D.

INCIDÊNCIA/PREVALÊNCIA
Os estudos conduzidos com base em radiotelemetria revelaram que essa arritmia ocorre em 64% dos cães jovens adultos e 100% dos filhotes caninos saudáveis com 8-12 semanas de vida.

DISTRIBUIÇÃO GEOGRÁFICA
N/D.

IDENTIFICAÇÃO
Espécies
Cães; incomum em gatos.

Raça(s) Predominante(s)
N/D.

Idade Média e Faixa Etária
- Costuma ocorrer em cães jovens saudáveis de modo geral, como uma manifestação de tônus vagal elevado.
- Ocasionalmente ocorre em cães mais idosos com tônus vagal anormalmente forte.
- Raramente observado em cães idosos com comprometimento degenerativo no sistema de condução.

SINAIS CLÍNICOS
Achados Anamnésicos
- A maioria dos animais apresenta-se assintomática.
- Em caso de indução por medicamentos, o proprietário pode relatar sinais de intoxicação medicamentosa — anorexia, vômito e diarreia com o uso da digoxina; fraqueza com o emprego de bloqueadores dos canais de cálcio ou antagonistas β-adrenérgicos.
- Se a frequência cardíaca estiver anormalmente lenta, poderá ocorrer síncope ou fraqueza.

Achados do Exame Físico
- Podem permanecer normais a menos que haja sinais de miocardiopatia ou doença extracardíaca mais generalizadas.
- Pausas intermitentes no ritmo cardíaco.
- A primeira bulha cardíaca pode se tornar progressivamente mais tênue, seguida por uma pausa.
- Uma quarta bulha cardíaca S4 audível não acompanhada por S1 e S2 pode ser auscultada quando ocorre o bloqueio.

CAUSAS
- Ocasionalmente, constatado em animais normais.
- Estimulação vagal acentuada resultante de doenças extracardíacas — acompanhadas geralmente por arritmia sinusal e parada sinusal.
- Agentes farmacológicos — digoxina, antagonistas β-adrenérgicos, bloqueadores dos canais de cálcio, propafenona, amiodarona, agonistas α_2-adrenérgicos, opioides.

FATORES DE RISCO
Qualquer condição ou intervenção que intensifique o tônus vagal.

DIAGNÓSTICO

DIAGNÓSTICO DIFERENCIAL
- As ondas P não conduzidas decorrentes de impulsos supraventriculares prematuros ou taquicardias supraventriculares devem ser distinguidas de bloqueio AV de segundo grau.
- Bloqueio AV de segundo grau Mobitz tipo II (sem variação nos intervalos PR).

HEMOGRAMA/BIOQUÍMICA/URINÁLISE
A hipocalemia pode predispor o animal a distúrbios de condução AV.

OUTROS TESTES LABORATORIAIS
Concentração sérica da digoxina — pode estar elevada.

DIAGNÓSTICO POR IMAGEM
N/D.

MÉTODOS DIAGNÓSTICOS
- Pode ser necessária a identificação das causas específicas de intensificação do tônus vagal (p. ex., doença das vias aéreas superiores, massas cervicais e torácicas, distúrbios gastrintestinais e pressão intraocular elevada).
- Teste de resposta à atropina — administrar 0,04 mg/kg desse medicamento por via IM e repetir o ECG em 20-30 minutos; esse teste pode ser utilizado para determinar se o bloqueio AV se deve ou não ao tônus vagal; a resolução do bloqueio AV com a aplicação de atropina confirma a etiologia vagal.
- Estudos eletrofisiológicos não costumam ser necessários, mas confirmarão esse tipo de bloqueio AV de segundo grau se o ECG de superfície for duvidoso.

ACHADOS PATOLÓGICOS
Em geral, não há achados macroscópicos ou histopatológicos.

TRATAMENTO

CUIDADO(S) DE SAÚDE ADEQUADO(S)
- Geralmente, não há necessidade de tratamento.
- Tratar ou remover a(s) causa(s) subjacente(s).

CUIDADO(S) DE ENFERMAGEM
Em geral, desnecessário(s).

ATIVIDADE
Sem restrição.

DIETA
Recomendam-se mudanças ou restrições apenas para o tratamento da condição subjacente.

ORIENTAÇÃO AO PROPRIETÁRIO
Explicar ao proprietário o fato de que qualquer tratamento deve ser direcionado à reversão ou à eliminação da causa subjacente.

CONSIDERAÇÕES CIRÚRGICAS
N/D exceto para tratar a condição subjacente.

MEDICAÇÕES

MEDICAMENTO(S)
Conforme a necessidade, apenas para tratar a condição subjacente.

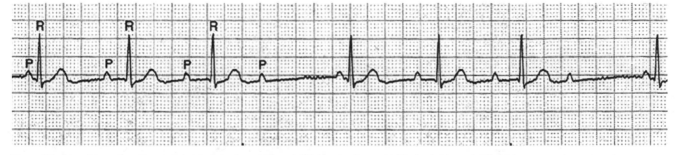

Figura 1 Registro eletrocardiográfico na derivação II de cão com bloqueio AV de segundo grau Mobitz tipo I. O intervalo PR torna-se progressivamente mais prolongado, sendo que os intervalos PR mais longos antecedem as ondas P não conduzidas [fenômeno típico de Wenckebach (velocidade do papel = 50 mm/s)].

BLOQUEIO ATRIOVENTRICULAR DE SEGUNDO GRAU — MOBITZ TIPO I

CONTRAINDICAÇÕES
Os medicamentos com ação vagomimética (p. ex., digoxina, betanecol, fisostigmina e pilocarpina) podem potencializar o bloqueio.

PRECAUÇÕES
A hipocalemia aumenta a sensibilidade ao tônus vagal e pode potencializar o atraso na condução AV.

INTERAÇÕES POSSÍVEIS
N/D.

ACOMPANHAMENTO

MONITORIZAÇÃO DO PACIENTE
Tipicamente desnecessária.

PREVENÇÃO
N/D.

COMPLICAÇÕES POSSÍVEIS
N/D.

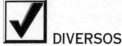

DIVERSOS

DISTÚRBIOS ASSOCIADOS
N/D.

FATORES RELACIONADOS COM A IDADE
N/D.

GESTAÇÃO/FERTILIDADE/REPRODUÇÃO
N/D.

SINÔNIMO(S)
• Fenômeno de Wenckebach.
• Periodicidade de Wenckebach.

VER TAMBÉM
• Bloqueio Atrioventricular Completo (Terceiro Grau).
• Bloqueio Atrioventricular de Primeiro Grau.
• Bloqueio Atrioventricular de Segundo Grau — Mobitz Tipo II.

ABREVIATURA(S)
• AV = atrioventricular.
• ECG = eletrocardiograma.

Sugestões de Leitura

Branch CE, Robertson BT, Williams JC. Frequency of second-degree atrioventricular heart block in dogs. Am J Vet Res 1975, 36:925-929.
Mangrum JM, DiMarco JP. The evaluation and management of bradycardia. N Engl J Med 2000, 342:703-709.
Podrid PJ, Kowey PR. Cardiac Arrhythmia — Mechanisms, Diagnosis, and Management. Baltimore: Williams & Wilkins, 1995.
Tilley LP, Smith FWK Jr. Electrocardiography. In: Tilley LP, Smith FWK, Oyama MA, Sleeper MM, eds., Manual of Canine and Feline Cardiology, 4th ed. St. Louis: Saunders Elsevier, 2008, pp. 49-77.
Tilley LP. Essentials of Canine and Feline Electrocardiography, 3rd ed. Baltimore: Williams & Wilkins, 1992.

Autor Janice McIntosh Bright
Consultores Editoriais Larry P. Tilley e Francis W.K. Smith, Jr.

BLOQUEIO ATRIOVENTRICULAR DE SEGUNDO GRAU — MOBITZ TIPO II

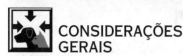

CONSIDERAÇÕES GERAIS

DEFINIÇÃO
O bloqueio AV de segundo grau refere-se à falha de uma ou mais ondas P, mas nem todas as ondas P são conduzidas. O bloqueio AV de segundo grau Mobitz tipo II ocorre quando uma ou mais ondas P são bloqueadas sem um atraso progressivo prévio na transmissão AV.

Características do ECG
- Uma ou mais ondas P não acompanhadas por um complexo QRS; os intervalos PR são constantes, mas podem ser normais ou consistentemente prolongados (Fig. 1).
- Frequência ventricular — geralmente lenta.
- Pode ocorrer uma relação fixa entre as ondas P e os complexos QRS (p. ex., bloqueio AV de 2:1, 3:1 e 4:1).
- O bloqueio AV de segundo grau de alta intensidade (avançado) é caracterizado por uma ou mais ondas P bloqueadas consecutivas.
- No bloqueio AV de segundo grau com relação de condução de 2:1 ou mais alta, é impossível observar o prolongamento do intervalo PR antes do bloqueio; dessa forma, uma designação de Mobitz não é apropriada.
- Os complexos QRS podem parecer normais, mas também podem ser largos ou exibir morfologia anormal em virtude da condução intraventricular aberrante ou do aumento de volume do ventrículo.
- Os complexos QRS anormalmente largos podem indicar cardiopatia grave e extensa.

FISIOPATOLOGIA
- Raro em animais saudáveis.
- Pode ter significado hemodinâmico quando a frequência ventricular se encontra anormalmente lenta.
- Muitas vezes, evolui para um bloqueio AV completo, particularmente quando acompanhado por complexos QRS largos.
- Tipicamente, esse tipo de bloqueio AV resulta de atraso na condução dentro do nó AV em si (e não do atraso em outro segmento do sistema de condução AV), caracterizado por intervalos AH normais ou prolongados com bloqueio intermitente entre as deflexões A e H no eletrograma do feixe de His.

SISTEMA(S) ACOMETIDO(S)
- Cardiovascular.
- Sistema nervoso central ou musculoesquelético em caso de débito cardíaco inadequado.

GENÉTICA
Pode ser hereditário em cães da raça Pug.

INCIDÊNCIA/PREVALÊNCIA
Desconhecidas.

DISTRIBUIÇÃO GEOGRÁFICA
N/D.

IDENTIFICAÇÃO
Espécies
Cães e gatos.

Raça(s) Predominante(s)
Cocker spaniel americano, Pug, Dachshund, Airedale terrier, Doberman pinscher.

Idade Média e Faixa Etária
Geralmente ocorre em animais mais idosos.

Sexo Predominante
N/D.

SINAIS CLÍNICOS
Achados Anamnésicos
- A queixa apresentada pode ser síncope, colapso, fraqueza ou letargia.
- Alguns animais permanecem assintomáticos.
- Os animais podem revelar sinais do processo patológico subjacente.

Achados do Exame Físico
- Pode ou não demonstrar fraqueza.
- É comum a constatação de bradicardia.
- Pode exibir pausas intermitentes no ritmo cardíaco.
- Quando ocorre o bloqueio, uma quarta bulha cardíaca S4 poderá ser auscultada no lugar das bulhas cardíacas normalmente esperadas (i. e., S1 e S2).
- Se associado à intoxicação por digoxina, poderá haver vômito, anorexia e diarreia.
- Pode haver outras anormalidades que refletem a etiologia subjacente.

CAUSAS
- Bloqueio hereditário em cães da raça Pug.
- Estimulação vagal acentuada decorrente de doenças extracardíacas.
- Alteração degenerativa dentro do sistema de condução cardíaca — substituição das células do nó AV e/ou fibras de Purkinje por tecido fibrosado e adiposo em cães e gatos idosos.
- Agentes farmacológicos (p. ex., digoxina, antagonistas β-adrenérgicos, bloqueadores dos canais de cálcio, propafenona, agonistas α_2-adrenérgicos, agonistas colinérgicos muscarínicos ou intoxicação grave por procainamida ou quinidina).
- Distúrbios miocárdicos infiltrativos (neoplasia, amiloide).
- Endocardite (particularmente com envolvimento da válvula aórtica).
- Miocardite (viral, bacteriana, parasitária, idiopática).
- Miocardiopatia (sobretudo em gatos).
- Traumatismo.
- A administração intravenosa de atropina pode causar bloqueio cardíaco transitório de primeiro ou segundo grau antes do aumento da frequência cardíaca.

FATORES DE RISCO
Qualquer condição ou intervenção que intensifique o tônus vagal.

DIAGNÓSTICO

DIAGNÓSTICO DIFERENCIAL
- Forma de alta intensidade (avançada) deve ser distinguida do bloqueio AV completo.
- Ondas P não conduzidas, originárias da refratariedade do sistema de condução durante as taquicardias supraventriculares, precisam ser diferenciadas de bloqueio patológico de condução cardíaca.

HEMOGRAMA/BIOQUÍMICA/URINÁLISE
- Eletrólitos séricos — a hipocalemia e a hipercalemia podem predispor o animal a distúrbios de condução AV.
- Leucocitose — pode ser observada em casos de endocardite ou miocardite bacteriana.
- Anormalidades eletrolíticas (p. ex., hipocalemia, hipercalemia ou hipercalcemia grave) podem predispor o paciente a bloqueio AV.

OUTROS TESTES LABORATORIAIS
- Concentração sérica da digoxina — pode estar elevada.
- Altos níveis de T_4 em gatos — se associado a hipertireoidismo.
- Hipertensão arterial — se relacionado com cardiopatia hipertensiva.
- Títulos positivos para *Borrelia*, *Rickettsia* ou *Trypanosoma cruzi* — se associado a um desses agentes infecciosos.
- As hemoculturas podem ficar positivas em pacientes com endocardite vegetativa.

DIAGNÓSTICO POR IMAGEM
O exame ecocardiográfico pode revelar cardiopatia estrutural (p. ex., endocardite, neoplasia ou miocardiopatia).

MÉTODOS DIAGNÓSTICOS
- Teste de resposta à atropina — administrar 0,04 mg/kg desse medicamento por via IM e repetir o ECG em 20-30 minutos; esse teste pode ser utilizado para determinar se o bloqueio AV se deve ou não ao tônus vagal elevado.
- Teste eletrofisiológico — em geral, não é necessário, mas pode ser feito para confirmar esse

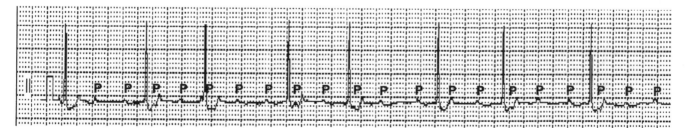

Figura 1 Ritmo eletrocardiográfico na derivação II de cão com bloqueio atrioventricular de primeiro e segundo graus. O bloqueio AV de segundo grau é de alta intensidade com bloqueio 2:1 e 3:1, resultando em variação nos intervalos RRs. O intervalo PR para os batimentos conduzidos é prolongado, mas constante (0,28 segundo) (velocidade do papel = 25 mm/s).

BLOQUEIO ATRIOVENTRICULAR DE SEGUNDO GRAU — MOBITZ TIPO II

tipo de bloqueio AV se os achados eletrocardiográficos de superfície forem duvidosos.

ACHADOS PATOLÓGICOS
• Variáveis — dependem da causa subjacente.
• Os animais idosos com alteração degenerativa do sistema de condução cardíaca podem apresentar mineralização focal da crista do septo interventricular visível macroscopicamente; no exame histopatológico, observam-se metaplasia condroide do corpo fibroso central e aumento do tecido conjuntivo fibroso no feixe AV.

TRATAMENTO

CUIDADO(S) DE SAÚDE ADEQUADO(S)
• Tratamento — poderá não ser necessário se a frequência cardíaca mantiver um débito cardíaco adequado.
• Para pacientes sintomáticos, indicam-se as intervenções dromotrópicas* positivas.
• Tratar ou remover a(s) causa(s) subjacente(s).

CUIDADO(S) DE ENFERMAGEM
Geralmente desnecessários.

ATIVIDADE
Para pacientes sintomáticos, é aconselhável o repouso em gaiola.

DIETA
Recomendam-se mudanças ou restrições apenas para o tratamento da condição subjacente.

ORIENTAÇÃO AO PROPRIETÁRIO
• É imprescindível procurar e tratar a causa subjacente de forma específica.
• Os agentes farmacológicos podem não ser eficazes a longo prazo.

CONSIDERAÇÕES CIRÚRGICAS
Para o tratamento prolongado de pacientes sintomáticos, poderá ser indispensável a implantação de marca-passo permanente.

MEDICAÇÕES

MEDICAMENTO(S) DE ESCOLHA
• Em caso de resposta positiva à atropina, pode-se fazer uso desse medicamento (0,02-0,04 mg/kg IV,

---

* N. T.: Referente ou inerente à condutividade da excitação de uma fibra nervosa ou muscular. Diz-se da ação que modifica a condutibilidade das fibras do miocárdio.

IM) ou do glicopirrolato (0,005-0,01 mg/kg IV, IM) para tratamentos a curto prazo.
• Terapia crônica com anticolinérgicos (propantelina 0,5-2 mg/kg VO a cada 8-12 h ou hiosciamina 0,003-0,006 mg/kg a cada 8 h) — indicada para pacientes sintomáticos se houver melhora na condução AV com o teste de resposta à atropina.
• Em situações agudas com risco de vida, pode-se lançar mão do isoproterenol (0,04-0,09 µg/kg/min IV até fazer efeito) ou da dopamina (2-5 µg/kg/min IV até fazer efeito) para estimular a condução AV e/ou acelerar um foco de escape.

CONTRAINDICAÇÕES
• Os medicamentos com ação vagomimética (p. ex., digoxina, betanecol, fisostigmina e pilocarpina) podem potencializar o bloqueio.
• Evitar os medicamentos que provavelmente prejudicam ainda mais a condução do impulso cardíaco ou deprimem um foco de escape ventricular (p. ex., procainamida, quinidina, lidocaína, bloqueadores dos canais de cálcio e bloqueadores β-adrenérgicos).

PRECAUÇÕES
Hipocalemia — aumenta a sensibilidade ao tônus vagal e pode potencializar o atraso na condução AV.

INTERAÇÕES POSSÍVEIS
N/D.

MEDICAMENTO(S) ALTERNATIVO(S)
N/D.

ACOMPANHAMENTO

MONITORIZAÇÃO DO PACIENTE
É recomendável o ECG frequente, pois esse distúrbio muitas vezes evolui para um bloqueio AV completo (terceiro grau).

PREVENÇÃO
N/D.

COMPLICAÇÕES POSSÍVEIS
A bradicardia prolongada pode causar insuficiência cardíaca congestiva secundária ou perfusão renal inadequada.

EVOLUÇÃO ESPERADA E PROGNÓSTICO
• Variáveis — dependem da causa.
• Em caso de doença degenerativa do sistema de condução cardíaca, esse distúrbio frequentemente evolui para um bloqueio AV completo (terceiro grau).

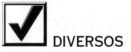

DIVERSOS

DISTÚRBIOS ASSOCIADOS
Pode ser observado em gatos com miocardiopatia primária ou secundária.

FATORES RELACIONADOS COM A IDADE
N/D.

POTENCIAL ZOONÓTICO
N/D.

GESTAÇÃO/FERTILIDADE/REPRODUÇÃO
N/D.

VER TAMBÉM
• Bloqueio Atrioventricular Completo (Terceiro Grau).
• Bloqueio Atrioventricular de Segundo Grau — Mobitz Tipo I.

ABREVIATURA(S)
• AV = atrioventricular.
• ECG = eletrocardiograma.
• T_4 = tiroxina.

Sugestões de Leitura
Kittleson MD. Electrocardiography. In: Kittleson MD, Kienle RD, eds., Small Animal Cardiovascular Medicine. St. Louis: Mosby, 1998, pp. 72-94.
Mangrum JM, DiMarco JP. The evaluation and management of bradycardia. N Engl J Med 2000, 342:703-709.
Podrid PJ, Kowey PR. Cardiac Arrhythmia— Mechanisms, Diagnosis, and Management. Baltimore: Williams & Wilkins, 1995.
Tilley LP, Smith FWK Jr. Electrocardiography. In: Tilley LP, Smith FWK, Oyama MA, Sleeper MM, eds., Manual of Canine and Feline Cardiology, 4th ed. St. Louis: Saunders Elsevier, 2008, pp. 49-77.
Tilley LP. Essentials of Canine and Feline Electrocardiography, 3rd ed. Baltimore: Williams & Wilkins, 1992.

Autor Janice McIntosh Bright
Consultores Editoriais Larry P. Tilley e Francis W.K. Smith, Jr.

BLOQUEIO DO RAMO DIREITO DO FEIXE DE HIS

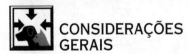 **CONSIDERAÇÕES GERAIS**

DEFINIÇÃO
Retardo ou bloqueio da condução cardíaca no ramo direito do feixe de His, resultando na ativação tardia do ventrículo direito; o bloqueio pode ser completo ou incompleto.

Características do ECG
• Desvio do eixo para a direita e QRS amplo (≥0,08 s em cães; ≥0,06 s em gatos) na maior parte dos pacientes.
• Ondas S grandes e largas nas derivações I, II, III e aVF.
• O bloqueio incompleto do ramo direito do feixe de His apresenta desvio do eixo para a direita com complexos QRS de amplitude normal.

FISIOPATOLOGIA
• O ramo direito do feixe de His é anatomicamente vulnerável à lesão, porque se trata de um filamento delgado de tecido e possui trajeto longo e sem divisão.
• Não há comprometimento hemodinâmico.

SISTEMA(S) ACOMETIDO(S)
Cardiovascular.

GENÉTICA
N/D.

INCIDÊNCIA/PREVALÊNCIA
• Cães — é a forma mais frequente de defeito da condução intraventricular.
• Gatos — não é tão frequente quanto o bloqueio fascicular anterior esquerdo.

DISTRIBUIÇÃO GEOGRÁFICA
N/D.

IDENTIFICAÇÃO
Espécies
Cães e gatos.

Raça(s) Predominante(s)
Em cães da raça Beagle, o bloqueio incompleto do ramo direito do feixe de His pode resultar de uma variação localizada geneticamente determinada na espessura da parede do ventrículo direito.

Sexo Predominante
N/D.

SINAIS CLÍNICOS
Achados Anamnésicos
• Geralmente se trata de um achado incidental do ECG — não provoca anormalidades hemodinâmicas.
• Os sinais observados estão, em geral, associados à condição subjacente.

Achados do Exame Físico
• Desdobramento das bulhas cardíacas por causa da ativação assincrônica dos ventrículos em alguns pacientes.
• Não provoca sinais de comprometimento hemodinâmico.

CAUSAS
• Ocasionalmente observado em cães e gatos normais e saudáveis.
• Cardiopatia congênita.
• Fibrose valvular crônica.
• Após a correção cirúrgica de defeito cardíaco.
• Traumatizado provocado pela punção cardíaca por agulha para obtenção de amostra de sangue.
• Traumatismo gerado por outras causas.
• Infecção crônica por *Trypanosoma cruzi* (doença de Chagas).
• Neoplasia.
• Dirofilariose.
• Tromboembolia aguda.
• Miocardiopatia.
• Hipercalemia (mais comumente em gatos com obstrução uretral).

FATORES DE RISCO
N/D.

 DIAGNÓSTICO

DIAGNÓSTICO DIFERENCIAL
• Aumento de volume do ventrículo direito — a ausência de aumento ventricular direito nas radiografias torácicas ou ao ecocardiograma garante o diagnóstico de bloqueio do ramo direito do feixe de His.
• Também pode ser confundido com batimentos ectópicos ventriculares (especialmente se o bloqueio for intermitente), embora haja intervalos PR constantes e ausência de déficits de pulso em casos de bloqueio do ramo direito do feixe de His.

HEMOGRAMA/BIOQUÍMICA/URINÁLISE
• Nada específico.
• O potássio sérico pode estar extremamente elevado nos gatos com obstrução uretral.

OUTROS TESTES LABORATORIAIS
• Teste para dirofilariose oculta pode ser positivo em cães ou gatos.
• Teste do anticorpo fluorescente indireto para Chagas, hemaglutinação direta e teste de fixação do complemento podem ser positivos nos cães.

DIAGNÓSTICO POR IMAGEM
• O ecocardiograma pode demonstrar cardiopatia estrutural; a ausência de aumento de volume do lado direito do coração garante o diagnóstico.
• Radiografias toracoabdominais podem revelar massas ou lesões metastáticas pulmonares; as lesões traumáticas podem causar densidades pulmonares localizadas ou difusas.

MÉTODOS DIAGNÓSTICOS
• Eletrocardiografia.
• Ecocardiografia.

ACHADOS PATOLÓGICOS
Possíveis lesões ou formação cicatricial na superfície endocárdica no trajeto dos ramos do feixe de His; a aplicação de iodo lugol à superfície do endocárdio dentro de 2 h após a morte proporciona uma clara visualização do sistema de condução cardíaca.

 TRATAMENTO

CUIDADO(S) DE SAÚDE ADEQUADO(S)
Direcionar o tratamento à causa subjacente.

CUIDADO(S) DE ENFERMAGEM
N/D.

ATIVIDADE
Sem restrição.

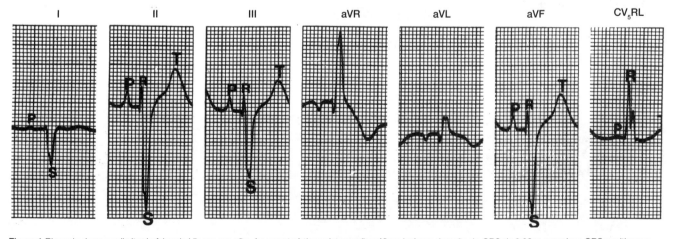

Figura 1 Bloqueio do ramo direito do feixe de His em um cão. As características eletrocardiográficas incluem duração do QRS de 0,08 s; complexo QRS positivo nas derivações aVR, aVL e CV₅RL (forma de M); além disso, há ondas S grandes e largas nas derivações I, II, III e aVF. Existe um desvio do eixo para a direita (aproximadamente -110°) (50 mm/s, 1 cm = 1 mV). (De: Tilley LP. *Essentials of canine and feline electrocardiography*. 3. ed. Baltimore: Lippincott Williams & Wilkins, 1992, com permissão.)

BLOQUEIO DO RAMO DIREITO DO FEIXE DE HIS

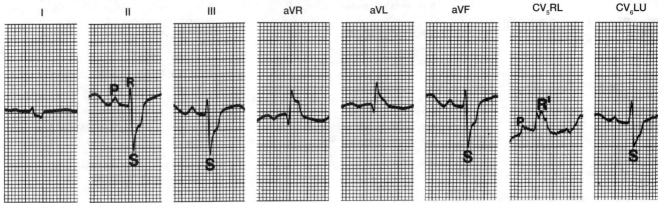

Figura 2 Bloqueio do ramo direito do feixe de His em um gato com a forma dilatada da miocardiopatia. A duração do QRS é de 0,08 s (4 quadrados). Ondas S grandes e largas estão presentes nas derivações I, II, III, aVF e CV$_6$LU. O QRS em CV$_5$RL apresenta onda R larga (forma de M). Existe um acentuado desvio do eixo (aproximadamente –90°). (De: Tilley LP: *Essentials of canine and feline electrocardiography*. 3. ed. Baltimore: Lippincott Williams & Wilkins, 1992, com permissão.)

DIETA
Sem modificações a menos que sejam necessárias para tratar a condição subjacente.

ORIENTAÇÃO AO PROPRIETÁRIO
• Não provoca anormalidades hemodinâmicas em si.
• A lesão indutora do bloqueio pode evoluir, levando a arritmias mais sérias ou ao bloqueio cardíaco completo.

CONSIDERAÇÕES CIRÚRGICAS
N/D.

MEDICAÇÕES

MEDICAMENTO(S) DE ESCOLHA
Não são necessários, exceto para o tratamento da condição subjacente.

CONTRAINDICAÇÕES
N/D.

PRECAUÇÕES
N/D.

INTERAÇÕES POSSÍVEIS
N/D.

MEDICAMENTO(S) ALTERNATIVO(S)
N/D.

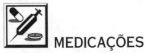

ACOMPANHAMENTO

MONITORIZAÇÃO DO PACIENTE
ECG seriado pode demonstrar resolução da lesão ou evolução para bloqueio cardíaco completo.

PREVENÇÃO
N/D.

COMPLICAÇÕES POSSÍVEIS
• A lesão causal pode evoluir, levando à arritmia mais séria ou bloqueio cardíaco completo.
• Bloqueio AV de primeiro ou de segundo grau pode indicar o envolvimento do ramo esquerdo do feixe de His.

EVOLUÇÃO ESPERADA E PROGNÓSTICO
Nenhum comprometimento hemodinâmico.

DIVERSOS

DISTÚRBIOS ASSOCIADOS
N/D.

FATORES RELACIONADOS COM A IDADE
N/D.

POTENCIAL ZOONÓTICO
N/D.

GESTAÇÃO/FERTILIDADE/REPRODUÇÃO
N/D.

VER TAMBÉM
• Bloqueio Atrioventricular Completo (Terceiro Grau).
• Bloqueio Atrioventricular de Primeiro Grau.
• Bloqueio Atrioventricular de Segundo Grau — Mobitz Tipo I.
• Bloqueio Atrioventricular de Segundo Grau — Mobitz Tipo II.
• Bloqueio do Ramo Esquerdo do Feixe de His.
• Bloqueio Fascicular Anterior Esquerdo.

ABREVIATURA(S)
• AV = atrioventricular.
• ECG = eletrocardiograma.

RECURSOS DA INTERNET
www.vetgo.com/cardio.

Sugestões de Leitura
Tilley LP. Essentials of Canine and Feline Electrocardiography, 3rd ed. Baltimore: Williams & Wilkins, 1992.
Tilley LP, Smith FWK, Jr. Electrocardiography. In: Tilley LP, Smith FWK, Oyama MA, Sleeper MM, eds., Manual of Canine and Feline Cardiology, 4th ed. St. Louis: Saunders Elsevier, 2008, pp. 72-73.

Autores Larry P. Tilley e Naomi L. Burtnick
Consultores Editoriais Larry P. Tilley e Francis W.K. Smith, Jr.

BLOQUEIO DO RAMO ESQUERDO DO FEIXE DE HIS

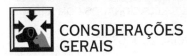

CONSIDERAÇÕES GERAIS

DEFINIÇÃO
Atraso ou bloqueio de condução nos fascículos anterior e posterior esquerdos do ramo esquerdo do feixe de His (Figs. 1 e 2); um impulso supraventricular ativa primeiro o ventrículo direito por meio do ramo direito do feixe de His; o ventrículo esquerdo é ativado mais tarde, fazendo com que o QRS se torne largo e bizarro.

Características do ECG
- QRS prolongado — cães, >0,08 s, gatos, >0,06 s.
- QRS amplo e positivo nas derivações I, II, III e aVF.
- O bloqueio pode ser intermitente ou constante.

FISIOPATOLOGIA
- Como o ramo esquerdo do feixe de His é espesso e extenso, a lesão indutora do bloqueio deve ser ampla.
- Geralmente, trata-se de um achado acidental ao ECG — não provoca anormalidades hemodinâmicas.

SISTEMA(S) ACOMETIDO(S)
Cardiovascular.

GENÉTICA
N/D.

INCIDÊNCIA/PREVALÊNCIA
Raro em cães e gatos. Nos gatos com miocardiopatia hipertrófica, o bloqueio do ramo esquerdo do feixe de His não é tão comumente observado quanto o bloqueio fascicular anterior esquerdo.

DISTRIBUIÇÃO GEOGRÁFICA
N/D.

IDENTIFICAÇÃO
Espécies
Cães e gatos.
Raça(s) Predominante(s)
N/D.
Idade Média e Faixa Etária
N/D.
Sexo Predominante
N/D.

SINAIS CLÍNICOS
Achados Anamnésicos
- Em geral, constitui um achado acidental ao ECG — não provoca anormalidades hemodinâmicas.
- Os sinais costumam estar associados à condição subjacente.

Achados do Exame Físico
Não provoca sinais ou comprometimento hemodinâmico.

CAUSAS
- Miocardiopatia.
- Traumatismo cardíaco direto ou indireto (p. ex., atropelamento por automóvel e punção cardíaca por agulha).
- Neoplasia.
- Estenose aórtica subvalvular.
- Fibrose.
- Miocardiopatia isquêmica (p. ex., arteriosclerose das artérias coronárias, infarto do miocárdio e hipertrofia miocárdica com obstrução das artérias coronárias).

FATORES DE RISCO
N/D.

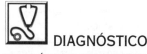

DIAGNÓSTICO

DIAGNÓSTICO DIFERENCIAL
- Aumento do ventrículo esquerdo.
- A ausência de aumento do ventrículo esquerdo na radiografia torácica ou em estudos ecocardiográficos apoia o diagnóstico de bloqueio isolado do ramo esquerdo do feixe de His.
- Também pode ser confundido com batimentos ectópicos ventriculares, embora o intervalo PR geralmente seja constante e o bloqueio do ramo esquerdo do feixe de His não apresente déficits de pulso.

HEMOGRAMA/BIOQUÍMICA/URINÁLISE
N/D.

OUTROS TESTES LABORATORIAIS
N/D.

DIAGNÓSTICO POR IMAGEM
- A ecocardiografia pode revelar cardiopatia estrutural; ausência de aumento do ventrículo esquerdo apoia o diagnóstico de bloqueio do ramo esquerdo do feixe de His.
- Radiografias toracoabdominais podem demonstrar a presença de massas ou lesões

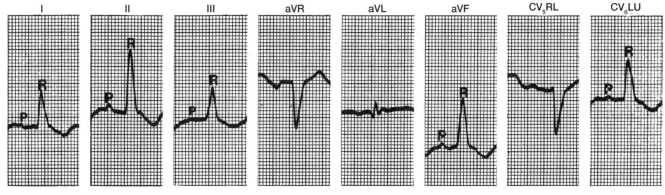

Figura 1 Bloqueio do ramo esquerdo do feixe de His em gato com miocardiopatia hipertrófica. O complexo QRS tem duração de 0,07 s, sendo positivo nas derivações I, II, III e aVF. Nessas derivações, não ocorrem ondas Q nem S. O complexo QRS está invertido na derivação aVR. (De: Tilley LP. *Essentials of canine and feline electrocardiography*. 3.ed. Baltimore: Williams & Wilkins, 1992, com permissão.)

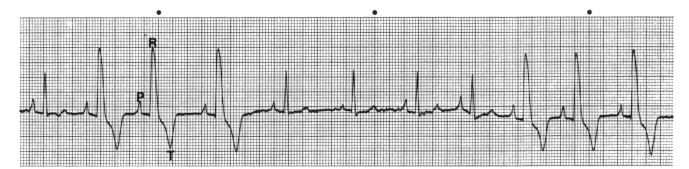

Figura 2 Bloqueio intermitente do ramo esquerdo do feixe de His em Chihuahua. Os complexos QRS são mais amplos (0,07-0,08 s) no segundo, no terceiro e no quarto complexos e nos três últimos complexos. O intervalo PR constante confirma a origem sinusal dos complexos QRS de aspecto anormal (derivação II, 50 mm/s, 1 cm = 1 mV). (De: Tilley LP. *Essentials of canine and feline electrocardiography*. 3.ed. Baltimore: Williams & Wilkins, 1992, com permissão.)

BLOQUEIO DO RAMO ESQUERDO DO FEIXE DE HIS

metastáticas pulmonares; lesões traumáticas podem resultar em densidades pulmonares localizadas ou difusas.

MÉTODOS DIAGNÓSTICOS
- Eletrocardiografia.
- Monitorização eletrocardiográfica ambulatorial a longo prazo com Holter pode revelar bloqueio intermitente do ramo esquerdo do feixe de His.

ACHADOS PATOLÓGICOS
Possíveis lesões ou formações cicatriciais na superfície endocárdica no trajeto dos ramos do feixe de His; a aplicação de Lugol (uma combinação de iodo e iodeto de potássio) à superfície endocárdica dentro de 2 h após a morte permite a visualização clara do sistema de condução cardíaca.

TRATAMENTO

CUIDADO(S) DE SAÚDE ADEQUADO(S)
Direcionado à causa subjacente.

CUIDADO(S) DE ENFERMAGEM
Geralmente, não há necessidade desse tipo de cuidado.

ATIVIDADE
Irrestrita a menos que seja necessária para o tratamento da condição subjacente.

DIETA
Sem modificação a menos que exigida para o tratamento da condição básica.

ORIENTAÇÃO AO PROPRIETÁRIO
- O bloqueio do ramo esquerdo do feixe de His, por si só, não provoca anormalidades hemodinâmicas.
- A lesão indutora do bloqueio pode evoluir, levando a arritmias mais graves ou a bloqueio cardíaco completo.

CONSIDERAÇÕES CIRÚRGICAS
N/D.

MEDICAÇÕES

MEDICAMENTO(S) DE ESCOLHA
N/D a menos que seja(m) necessário(s) para o tratamento da condição subjacente.

CONTRAINDICAÇÕES
N/D.

PRECAUÇÕES
N/D.

INTERAÇÕES POSSÍVEIS
N/D.

MEDICAMENTO(S) ALTERNATIVO(S)
N/D.

ACOMPANHAMENTO

MONITORIZAÇÃO DO PACIENTE
ECG seriados podem demonstrar a compensação ou a evolução para bloqueio cardíaco completo.

PREVENÇÃO
N/D.

COMPLICAÇÕES POSSÍVEIS
- A lesão causal pode evoluir, levando a arritmias mais graves ou a bloqueio cardíaco completo.
- Bloqueio AV de primeiro ou de segundo grau pode indicar o envolvimento do ramo direito do feixe de His.

EVOLUÇÃO ESPERADA E PROGNÓSTICO
Sem comprometimento hemodinâmico.

DIVERSOS

DISTÚRBIOS ASSOCIADOS
N/D.

FATORES RELACIONADOS COM A IDADE
N/D.

POTENCIAL ZOONÓTICO
N/D.

GESTAÇÃO/FERTILIDADE/REPRODUÇÃO
N/D.

VER TAMBÉM
- Bloqueio Atrioventricular Completo (Terceiro Grau).
- Bloqueio Atrioventricular de Primeiro Grau.
- Capítulos sobre Bloqueio Atrioventricular de Segundo Grau.
- Bloqueio Fascicular Anterior Esquerdo.
- Bloqueio do Ramo Direito do Feixe de His.

ABREVIATURA(S)
- AV = atrioventricular.
- ECG = eletrocardiograma.

RECURSOS DA INTERNET
www.vetgo.com/cardio.

Sugestões de Leitura
Tilley LP. Essentials of Canine and Feline Electrocardiography, 3rd ed. Baltimore: Williams & Wilkins, 1992.
Tilley LP, Smith FWK, Jr. Electrocardiography. In: Tilley LP, Smith FWK, Oyama MA, Sleeper MM, eds., Manual of Canine and Feline Cardiology, 4th ed. St. Louis: Saunders Elsevier, 2008, p. 72.

Autores Larry P. Tilley e Naomi L. Burtnick
Consultores Editoriais Larry P. Tilley e Francis W.K. Smith, Jr.

BLOQUEIO FASCICULAR ANTERIOR ESQUERDO

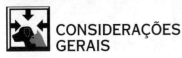

CONSIDERAÇÕES GERAIS

DEFINIÇÃO
• Atraso ou bloqueio de condução no fascículo anterior do ramo esquerdo do feixe de His (Figs. 1 e 2).
• A ativação do ventrículo esquerdo, em seguida, sofre alteração ou atraso no sentido do fascículo bloqueado e músculo papilar correspondente.

Características do ECG
• Complexo QRS — duração normal.
• Desvio do eixo para a esquerda — cães, <+40°; gatos, <0°.
• Ondas q pequenas e ondas R altas nas derivações I e aVL — onda q pequena não é essencial.
• Ondas S profundas (ultrapassando as ondas R) nas derivações II, III e aVF.

FISIOPATOLOGIA
• Base anatômica ainda especulativa — o fascículo anterior é vulnerável, porque, além de ser longo e fino, possui um único suprimento sanguíneo e está localizado no fluxo turbulento do trato de saída do ventrículo esquerdo.
• Sem comprometimento hemodinâmico.

SISTEMA(S) ACOMETIDO(S)
Cardiovascular.

GENÉTICA
N/D.

INCIDÊNCIA/PREVALÊNCIA
• Forma mais comumente descrita de bloqueio de ramo do feixe de His nos gatos.
• Raro em cães.

DISTRIBUIÇÃO GEOGRÁFICA
N/D.

IDENTIFICAÇÃO
Espécies
Cães e gatos.
Raça(s) Predominante(s)
N/D.
Idade Média e Faixa Etária
N/D.
Sexo Predominante
N/D.

SINAIS CLÍNICOS
Achados Anamnésicos
• Os sinais costumam estar associados à causa subjacente.
• Em geral, trata-se de um achado acidental ao ECG.
Achados do Exame Físico
Nenhum sinal ou comprometimento hemodinâmico associado.

CAUSAS
• Miocardiopatia hipertrófica (gatos).
• Hipertrofia do ventrículo esquerdo (p. ex., insuficiência mitral, estenose aórtica, tumor do corpo aórtico, hipertensão e hipertireoidismo).
• Hipercalemia (p. ex., obstrução uretral, insuficiência renal aguda e doença de Addison).
• Miocardiopatia isquêmica (p. ex., arteriosclerose das artérias coronárias, infarto do miocárdio e hipertrofia miocárdica com obstrução das artérias coronárias).

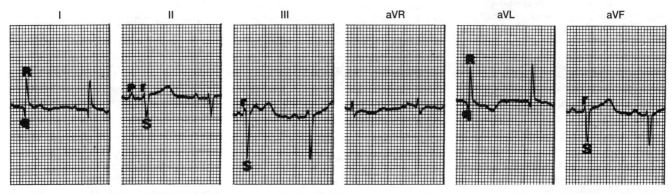

Figura 1 Bloqueio fascicular anterior esquerdo em gato com miocardiopatia hipertrófica. Desvio grave do eixo para a esquerda (-60°) com padrão qR nas derivações I e aVL e padrão rS nas derivações II, III e aVF. Os complexos QRS são de duração normal. (De: Tilley LP. *Essentials of canine and feline electrocardiography*. 3.ed. Baltimore: Williams & Wilkins, 1992, com permissão.)

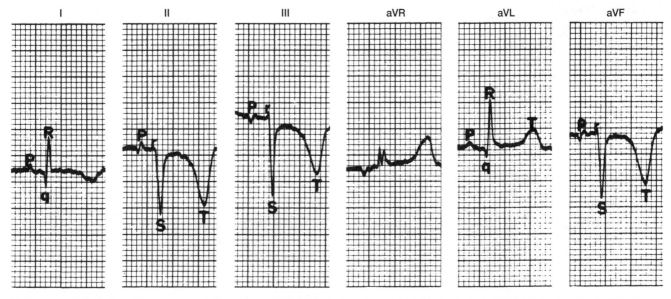

Figura 2 Bloqueio fascicular anterior esquerdo em cão com hipercalemia (potássio sérico, 5,3 mEq/L). Existe desvio anormal do eixo para a esquerda (-60°) com padrão qR nas derivações I e aVL e padrão rS nas derivações II, III e aVF. As grandes ondas T são compatíveis com hipercalemia. (De: Tilley LP. *Essentials of canine and feline electrocardiography*. 3.ed. Baltimore: Williams & Wilkins, 1992, com permissão.)

Bloqueio Fascicular Anterior Esquerdo

- Reparo cirúrgico de defeito cardíaco (p. ex., defeito do septo ventricular ou valvulopatia aórtica).
- Miocardiopatia restritiva (gatos).
- Fibrose.

FATORES DE RISCO
N/D.

DIAGNÓSTICO

DIAGNÓSTICO DIFERENCIAL
- Aumento do ventrículo esquerdo — a ausência desse aumento na radiografia torácica ou à ecocardiografia apoia o diagnóstico de bloqueio fascicular anterior esquerdo.
- Bloqueio do ramo direito do feixe de His — ondas S profundas e amplas nas derivações I, II, III e aVF, provocando o desvio do eixo para a direita; nos pacientes com bloqueio fascicular anterior esquerdo, as derivações I e aVL são positivas, enquanto as derivações II, III e aVF possuem ondas S profundas, resultando no desvio do eixo para a esquerda.
- Posição alterada do coração dentro do tórax — as radiografias torácicas ajudam a identificar a presença de massa ou corpo estranho, que pode estar deslocando o coração.
- Suspeitar de hipercalemia se houver sinais de obstrução uretral, insuficiência renal ou hipoadrenocorticismo (doença de Addison); determinar a concentração do potássio sérico.

HEMOGRAMA/BIOQUÍMICA/URINÁLISE
Possível hipercalemia.

OUTROS TESTES LABORATORIAIS
N/D.

DIAGNÓSTICO POR IMAGEM
- Ecocardiograma pode revelar cardiopatia estrutural.
- Radiografias toracoabdominais podem demonstrar a existência de massa, lesão metastática pulmonar, corpo estranho ou posição cardíaca anormal.

MÉTODOS DIAGNÓSTICOS
- Eletrocardiografia.
- Monitorização eletrocardiográfica ambulatorial a longo prazo com Holter pode revelar bloqueio intermitente de ramo do feixe de His.

ACHADOS PATOLÓGICOS
Possíveis lesões ou formações cicatriciais na superfície endocárdica no trajeto dos ramos do feixe de His; a aplicação de Lugol (uma combinação de iodo e iodeto de potássio) à superfície endocárdica dentro de 2 h após a morte permite a visualização clara do sistema de condução cardíaca.

TRATAMENTO

CUIDADO(S) DE SAÚDE ADEQUADO(S)
- Não há necessidade de tratamento.
- Tratar a causa subjacente.

CUIDADO(S) DE ENFERMAGEM
Desnecessário(s).

ATIVIDADE
Irrestrita a menos que a limitação seja indicada pela condição subjacente.

DIETA
Nenhuma mudança a menos que indicada pela condição subjacente.

ORIENTAÇÃO AO PROPRIETÁRIO
O bloqueio fascicular, por si só, não provoca o comprometimento hemodinâmico; quando combinado com o bloqueio do ramo direito do feixe de His, pode evoluir para bloqueio AV de segundo ou de terceiro grau, tornando o tratamento essencial; é necessário tratar a causa subjacente.

CONSIDERAÇÕES CIRÚRGICAS
N/D.

MEDICAÇÕES

MEDICAMENTO(S) DE ESCOLHA
Tratamento direcionado à doença primária subjacente (p. ex., medicamentos para reduzir o potássio sérico em caso de hipercalemia).

CONTRAINDICAÇÕES
N/D.

PRECAUÇÕES
N/D.

INTERAÇÕES POSSÍVEIS
N/D.

MEDICAMENTO(S) ALTERNATIVO(S)
N/D.

ACOMPANHAMENTO

MONITORIZAÇÃO DO PACIENTE
ECG regularmente.

PREVENÇÃO
N/D.

COMPLICAÇÕES POSSÍVEIS
A lesão causal pode evoluir e levar a arritmias mais graves ou a bloqueio cardíaco completo.

EVOLUÇÃO ESPERADA E PROGNÓSTICO
Sem comprometimento hemodinâmico.

DIVERSOS

DISTÚRBIOS ASSOCIADOS
N/D.

FATORES RELACIONADOS COM A IDADE
N/D.

POTENCIAL ZOONÓTICO
N/D.

GESTAÇÃO/FERTILIDADE/REPRODUÇÃO
N/D.

VER TAMBÉM
- Bloqueio Atrioventricular Completo (Terceiro Grau).
- Bloqueio Atrioventricular de Primeiro Grau.
- Capítulos sobre Bloqueio Atrioventricular de Segundo Grau.
- Bloqueio do Ramo Direito do Feixe de His.
- Bloqueio do Ramo Esquerdo do Feixe de His.

ABREVIATURA(S)
- AV = atrioventricular.
- ECG = eletrocardiograma.

RECURSOS DA INTERNET
www.vetgo.com/cardio.

Sugestões de Leitura
Tilley LP. Essentials of Canine and Feline Electrocardiography, 3rd ed. Baltimore: Williams & Wilkins, 1992.

Autores Larry P. Tilley e Naomi L. Burtnick
Consultores Editoriais Larry P. Tilley e Francis W.K. Smith, Jr.

BORDETELOSE — GATOS

CONSIDERAÇÕES GERAIS

REVISÃO
• Doença bacteriana contagiosa de gatos, indutora principalmente de anormalidades respiratórias.
• Os gatos alojados em populações de alta densidade têm o maior risco de infecção.

IDENTIFICAÇÃO
• Mais grave em filhotes felinos com <6 semanas de vida e naqueles residentes em condições higiênicas abaixo do ideal.
• Ocorre em todas as idades e, frequentemente, está associada à doença subclínica preexistente das vias aéreas (p. ex., herpes-vírus e calicivirose felinas).
• Ainda não se identificou nenhuma predisposição racial ou sexual.

SINAIS CLÍNICOS
• Podem ser inexistentes, leves ou graves (p. ex., filhotes felinos acometidos por pneumonia com risco de morte); costumam ter início em torno de 5 dias após a exposição ao agente infeccioso.
• Agente bacteriano — dissemina-se com rapidez, a partir de gatos aparentemente saudáveis para outros situados no mesmo ambiente.
• Febre, espirros, corrimento nasal, linfadenopatia mandibular e tosse espontânea ou induzida — são característicos de doença não complicada.

Doença Grave
• Pode-se notar uma febre constante, de grau baixo ou oscilante (39,4-40°C).
• Tosse — pode ser observada; úmida e produtiva.
• Corrimento nasal.
• Letargia.
• Anorexia.
• Dificuldade ou angústia respiratória.
• Ruídos pulmonares — frequentemente permanecem normais; pode-se detectar aumento na intensidade de ruídos normais, crepitações ou (com menor frequência) sibilos.

CAUSAS E FATORES DE RISCO
• *Bordetella bronchiseptica* — cocobacilo pequeno, aeróbio e Gram-negativo.
• Doença subclínica coexistente das vias aéreas — anomalias congênitas; bronquite crônica.

DIAGNÓSTICO

DIAGNÓSTICO DIFERENCIAL
• O diagnóstico específico não é uma tarefa fácil; os sinais clínicos mimetizam aqueles observados com outros agentes causais de doença respiratória.
• Diversos agentes podem estar envolvidos de forma concomitante, o que aumenta a confusão dos sinais clínicos.
• Ver "Tosse".

HEMOGRAMA/BIOQUÍMICA/URINÁLISE
• Leucocitose neutrofílica com desvio à esquerda — frequentemente encontrada em casos de pneumonia grave.
• Perfil bioquímico sérico e urinálise — costumam permanecer normais.

OUTROS TESTES LABORATORIAIS
• Amostras de *swab* nasal ou orofaríngeo para cultura ou PCR — para identificar os microrganismos *B. bronchiseptica*.
• Isolamento da bactéria — relativamente fácil em casos de doença clínica ativa; com frequência, poucos microrganismos são eliminados no estado de portador crônico.

DIAGNÓSTICO POR IMAGEM
Radiografias torácicas — não são dignas de nota em casos de doença não complicada; úteis para descartar causas não infecciosas; podem revelar o padrão pulmonar intersticial e alveolar com distribuição cranioventral típica de pneumonia bacteriana, o padrão pulmonar intersticial difuso típico de pneumonia viral ou o padrão pulmonar misto (combinação de padrões pulmonares alveolar, intersticial e peribrônquico).

MÉTODOS DIAGNÓSTICOS
Lavado endotraqueal ou traqueobrônquico obtido por broncoscopia na suspeita de doença grave; identificam os padrões de sensibilidade antimicrobiana — ajudam a desenvolver um plano terapêutico eficaz.

TRATAMENTO
• Ambulatorial — fortemente recomendado em caso de doença não complicada.
• Internação — intensamente indicada em caso de doença não complicada e/ou pneumonia.
• Fluidoterapia — em caso de doença complicada e/ou pneumonia.
• Repouso forçado — por pelo menos 14-21 dias em caso de doença não complicada; no mínimo, durante os indícios radiográficos de pneumonia.

MEDICAÇÕES

MEDICAMENTO(S)
• Tetraciclina (10 mg/kg VO a cada 8 h), doxiciclina (3-5 mg/kg VO, IV a cada 12 h ou 10 mg/kg VO a cada 24 h) ou amoxicilina/ácido clavulânico (62,5 mg/gato VO a cada 12 h) por 10-14 dias.
• Antibioticoterapia — pode continuar por pelo menos 10 dias depois da resolução radiográfica.

CONTRAINDICAÇÕES/INTERAÇÕES POSSÍVEIS
Tetraciclina e medicamentos relacionados — podem induzir à febre medicamentosa.

ACOMPANHAMENTO

MONITORIZAÇÃO DO PACIENTE
• Doença não complicada — deve responder ao tratamento em 10-14 dias; questionar o diagnóstico de doença não complicada na existência de sinais respiratórios 14 dias ou mais após a instituição do tratamento.
• Doença grave — repetir as radiografias torácicas por no mínimo 14 dias após a resolução de todos os sinais clínicos.

PREVENÇÃO
• Eliminação da *B. bronchiseptica* nas secreções respiratórias de portadores subclínicos — responsável pela persistência da doença em gatos, abrigos de animais, hotéis e hospitais veterinários.
• Há vacinas disponíveis.

COMPLICAÇÕES POSSÍVEIS
N/D.

EVOLUÇÃO ESPERADA E PROGNÓSTICO
• Doença não complicada sem tratamento — evolução natural, 10-14 dias.
• Doença grave — evolução típica, 2-6 semanas.
• Óbito — pneumonia grave, que acomete múltiplos lobos pulmonares.
• Soroconversão de filhotes felinos em ambientes infectados — com 7-10 semanas de vida.
• Os gatos acometidos podem eliminar a *B. bronchiseptica* por pelo menos 19 semanas após a infecção.

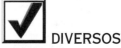

DIVERSOS

ABREVIATURA(S)
• PCR = reação em cadeia da polimerase.

RECURSOS DA INTERNET
www.nobivacbb.com.

Sugestões de Leitura
Egberink H, Addie D, Belák S, et al. Bordetella bronchiseptica infection in cats. ABCD guidelines on prevention and management. J Feline Med Surg 2009, 11(7):610-614.
Jacobs AA, Chalmers WS, Pasman J, et al. Feline bordetellosis: Challenge and vaccine studies. Vet Record 1993, 133:260-263.
Veir JK, Ruch-Gallie R, Spindel ME, Lappin MR. Prevalence of selected infectious organisms and comparison of two anatomic sampling sites in shelter cats with upper respiratory tract disease. J Feline Med Surg 2008, 10(6):551-557.

Autor Johnny D. Hoskins
Consultor Editorial Lynelle R. Johnson

Borreliose de Lyme

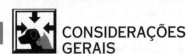

CONSIDERAÇÕES GERAIS

DEFINIÇÃO
- Uma das doenças zoonóticas mais comuns transmitidas por carrapatos no mundo.
- No homem, é causada por espécie de espiroqueta do grupo *lato sensu Borrelia burgdorferi* (p. ex., *B. burgdorferi stricto sensu, B. afzelli, B, garinii* e outros).
- Característica clínica dominante (cães) — claudicação recidivante atribuída à artrite; algumas vezes, anorexia e depressão; pode desenvolver doenças renais e, raramente, cardíacas ou neurológicas.
- Relatada em seres humanos, cães, cavalos e, esporadicamente, gatos.

FISIOPATOLOGIA
- Artrite — causada pela presença de espiroquetas migratórias nos tecidos e pelas subsequentes respostas imunes celulares e humorais do hospedeiro.
- Infecção cutânea local após a picada do carrapato é seguida uma semana a meses depois por infecção generalizada de tecido predominantemente conjuntivo em articulações, tendões, músculos e linfonodos.
- Embora um eritema migratório possa ser observado no local de inoculação da *B. burgdorferi*, essa lesão é exclusiva de seres humanos. O eritema migratório não é observado em cães.
- Foram demonstrados imunocomplexos com antígenos específicos da *B. burgdorferi* em cães; tais imunocomplexos podem se depositar nos rins; no entanto, não são encontrados microrganismos viáveis da *B. burgdorferi* nos rins.
- O período de incubação em cães infectados por via experimental é de 2 a 5 meses.

SISTEMA(S) ACOMETIDO(S)
- *B. burgdorferi* persistente — encontrada em tecidos com alto conteúdo de colágeno (pele, articulações, tendões, pericárdio, peritônio, meninges, músculo, coração e linfonodos); raramente encontrada em líquidos corporais (sangue, LCS e líquido sinovial).
- Alterações patológicas — com raras exceções, ficam restritas às articulações e aos linfonodos regionais; em casos raros, envolvimento dos rins.

GENÉTICA
Há relatos de que determinadas raças caninas desenvolvem insuficiência renal grave (p. ex., Montanhês de Berna, além de Labrador e Golden retrievers).

INCIDÊNCIA/PREVALÊNCIA
- A soroprevalência em cães dentro de uma população é extremamente variável com exposição a carrapatos infectados em áreas endêmicas; nas porções superiores das regiões meio-oeste e nordeste dos EUA e na região central da Europa, a soroprevalência é de 2-10%.
- A borreliose de Lyme clinicamente aparente se desenvolve em uma parcela de indivíduos infectados; o mecanismo é incerto.

DISTRIBUIÇÃO GEOGRÁFICA
- Hemisfério norte (América do Norte, Europa, Ásia).
- Estados Unidos — a maioria dos casos é relatada nos estados do Meio Atlântico até os estados costeiros da Nova Inglaterra, além dos estados norte-americanos do nordeste e meio-oeste superior. Existem condições ecológicas que apoiam a existência da borreliose de Lyme em estados adjacentes e também na costa oeste.
- Europa — ausente ou menos frequente em áreas limítrofes à bacia do Mediterrâneo.

IDENTIFICAÇÃO
Espécies
Cães e, raramente, gatos.

Idade Média e Faixa Etária
Do ponto de vista experimental, os cães jovens (filhotes) parecem ser mais suscetíveis que os adultos.

SINAIS CLÍNICOS
- Claudicação recidivante atribuída à artrite.
- Experimentalmente, a forma aguda dura apenas 3-4 dias; ocorre recidiva dias a semanas depois no mesmo membro ou em outros membros (claudicação com desvio); uma ou mais articulações podem estar intumescidas (inchadas) e quentes; uma resposta à dor é eliciada por palpação; responde bem à antibioticoterapia.
- Os cães acometidos podem se recusar a caminhar ou ficar em estação ou, então, apresentar marcha rígida com dorso arqueado e podem ser sensíveis ao toque.
- Poliartrite crônica não erosiva é encontrada em animais com infecção prolongada sem tratamento adequado; pode persistir apesar do tratamento com antimicrobianos.
- Os sinais de febre, anorexia e depressão podem acompanhar o quadro de artrite.
- Os linfonodos superficiais próximos à picada infectante do carrapato podem estar infartados.
- Rins — relatos de glomerulonefrite por depósito de imunocomplexos nos glomérulos, levando à nefropatia fatal; os pacientes podem se apresentar com insuficiência renal (vômito, diarreia, anorexia, perda de peso, poliúria/polidipsia, edema periférico ou ascite); perda proteica (nefropatia com perda de proteínas); hipoalbuminemia.
- Sinais cardíacos — relatados, porém raros; incluem bloqueio cardíaco completo.
- Complicações neurológicas — raras.

CAUSAS
- *B. burgdorferi* — transmitida por espécies de carrapato de repasto lento e carapaça dura do gênero *Ixodes* (p. ex., *I. scapularis, I. pacificus, I. ricinus, I. persulcatus*).
- Infecção — ocorre somente depois da fixação do carrapato (ninfa ou fêmea adulta) ao hospedeiro por, no mínimo, 18 horas.

Carrapatos Ixodes
- Possuem ciclo vital de 2 a 3 anos, dependendo da disponibilidade de hospedeiros.
- Ovos não infectados são depositados no solstício de verão.
- Larvas — eclodem algumas semanas depois; tornam-se infectadas, fazendo o repasto em pequenos mamíferos ou pássaros que carreiam a *B. burgdorferi*.
- Ninfas — as larvas passam pela muda (ecdise), transformando-se em ninfas na primavera do ano seguinte; permanecem infectadas ou ficam infectadas ao se alimentar novamente em mamíferos, pássaros ou lagartos.
- Adultos — as ninfas sofrem muda para adultos no verão e permanecem infectadas; as fêmeas acasalam e se alimentam de mamíferos maiores (p. ex., cervídeos); caem e se escondem sob as folhas até o próximo verão, quando cada uma delas deposita cerca de 2.000 ovos; os machos não costumam se aderir ao hospedeiro e nem se alimentam dele.

FATORES DE RISCO
A borreliose de Lyme canina é uma doença peridoméstica em virtude da expansão de ambientes para o habitat de carrapatos; caminhadas ou viagens para áreas endêmicas colocam os cães sob risco.

DIAGNÓSTICO

O diagnóstico da borreliose de Lyme é uma conclusão clínica tirada com base em sinais clínicos compatíveis, resposta à antibioticoterapia, exclusão de outros diagnósticos, dados laboratoriais apropriados (particularmente teste de anticorpos) e histórico de exposição a ambiente epidemiológico que confira a oportunidade de infecção por *B. burgdorferi*.

DIAGNÓSTICO DIFERENCIAL
- Artrite de Lyme — diferenciar de outras artrites inflamatórias.
- Bactérias — anaplasmose; erliquiose; febre maculosa das Montanhas Rochosas, outras.
- Doenças imunomediadas — idiopáticas, lúpus eritematoso, artrite reumatoide.
- Doenças específicas a determinadas raças — artrite do Akita, febre do Shar-pei.
- Descartar outros distúrbios com ensaios sorológicos e testes imunológicos (anticorpos antinucleares; preparações para lúpus eritematoso).

HEMOGRAMA/BIOQUÍMICA/URINÁLISE
- Apenas artrite — nada digno de nota.
- Na presença de glomerulopatia com perda de proteínas — geralmente ocorrem uremia, proteinúria, hipercolesterolemia, hiperfosfatemia e hipoalbuminemia.

OUTROS TESTES LABORATORIAIS
- Líquido coletado das articulações acometidas — contagens elevadas de leucócitos (até 75.000/µL; até 97% de polimorfonucleares).
- Sorologia positiva por ELISA e *Western blot** — indica exposição a antígenos da *B. burgdorferi*; o teste ELISA habitual não pode ser usado para diferenciar entre vacinação e infecção, mas o *Western blot* possibilita essa diferenciação; a reação cruzada com anticorpos induzidos por outras infecções bacterianas é mínima e específica ao fabricante.
- O teste ELISA em membrana feito na clínica (Snap 3Dx ou 4Dx®, IDEXX Labs, Westbrook, ME) detecta um subgrupo de anticorpos contra a proteína de superfície externa VlsE da *B. burgdorferi* com o uso do peptídeo C6; teste conveniente que só indica a infecção, mas não responde aos anticorpos induzidos pela vacina — os anticorpos C6-específicos normalmente declinam e até podem desaparecer cerca de 4-6 meses após a antibioticoterapia. Níveis pré-terapêuticos baixos a moderados não sofrem uma queda drástica.

DIAGNÓSTICO POR IMAGEM
Radiografias — ajudam a identificar efusões na articulação; podem ajudar a distinguir doença articular erosiva da não erosiva; descartam traumáticas.

---

* N. T.: Teste também conhecido como mancha ocidental.

BORRELIOSE DE LYME

MÉTODOS DIAGNÓSTICOS
• Os microrganismos podem ser demonstrados regularmente em amostras teciduais obtidas de pele ou da sinóvia após infecções experimentais por meio de PCR ou cultura; no entanto, sob condições a campo, esses testes são demorados, caros e não confiáveis (e, portanto, não recomendados). • As amostras de sangue, em particular, são tipicamente negativas quando testadas por PCR ou cultura.

ACHADOS PATOLÓGICOS
Macroscópicos
• Articulações tumefatas com excesso de líquido sinovial. • Às vezes, linfonodos infartados.

Histopatologia
• Artrite aguda clinicamente aparente — sinovite fibrinopurulenta. • Outras articulações — pode haver sinovite branda com infiltração de linfócitos e plasmócitos. • Linfonodos — podem apresentar hiperplasia cortical com múltiplos folículos aumentados e áreas parafoliculares expandidas. • Pele próxima ao local da picada do carrapato — revela infiltrados perivasculares de plasmócitos, linfócitos e alguns mastócitos na derme superficial. • Lesões renais — glomerulonefrite, necrose tubular difusa com regeneração e inflamação intersticial.

TRATAMENTO

CUIDADO(S) DE SAÚDE ADEQUADO(S)
Paciente de ambulatório.

CUIDADO(S) DE ENFERMAGEM
Manter o paciente quente e seco.

ATIVIDADE
Atividade reduzida até que os sinais clínicos apresentem melhora.

DIETA
Não há necessidade de modificação.

ORIENTAÇÃO AO PROPRIETÁRIO
• Informar o proprietário sobre a importância da aplicação regular de antibióticos, conforme a prescrição. • Um caso de borreliose de Lyme canina diagnosticada deve incitar uma discussão sobre o risco a seres humanos que vivem na mesma área que o cão.

CONSIDERAÇÕES CIRÚRGICAS
Aspirado do líquido sinovial — pode ser considerado para fins diagnósticos.

MEDICAÇÕES

MEDICAMENTO(S) DE ESCOLHA
• Antibióticos mais comumente utilizados — doxiciclina (5-10 mg/kg VO a cada 12 h; juntamente com o alimento; possível ocorrência de vômito e gastrite), amoxicilina (20 mg/kg VO a cada 8-12 h) ou azitromicina (25 mg/kg VO a cada 24 h). • Doxiciclina — agente de escolha quando ocorre coinfecção por *Anaplasma phagocytophilum*. • Antibióticos — não eliminam a infecção por completo; consequentemente, permanece uma infecção persistente com carga bacteriana muito baixa; o tratamento melhora os sinais clínicos e a doença de forma expressiva. • Período terapêutico recomendado — 4 semanas.

CONTRAINDICAÇÕES
Considerar os efeitos colaterais potenciais dos medicamentos aplicados.

PRECAUÇÕES
Não tratar animais jovens com tetraciclinas.

MEDICAMENTO(S) ALTERNATIVO(S)
• Corticosteroides — em princípio, podem melhorar os sinais clínicos; mascaram os efeitos dos antibióticos para fins diagnósticos; intensificam os sinais clínicos mais tarde por imunossupressão. • Analgésicos (não esteroides) — utilizar com bom senso para não mascarar os sinais.

ACOMPANHAMENTO

MONITORIZAÇÃO DO PACIENTE
• Melhora — observada dentro de 2-5 dias do tratamento com antibióticos em casos de artrite de Lyme aguda. • Na ausência de melhora ou na exacerbação dos sinais clínicos — considerar o diagnóstico diferencial.

PREVENÇÃO
• Remoção mecânica dos carrapatos — escovação diária dos animais. • Prevenção da fixação de carrapatos — acaricidas e repelentes (não usar permetrina em gatos) sob a forma de *spot-on*, *sprays* ou coleiras. • Vacinas — todas as vacinas disponíveis atualmente dependem, sobretudo, do efeito de anticorpos contra a proteína A de superfície externa (OspA) das espiroquetas. Esses anticorpos impedem a migração das espiroquetas dentro do carrapato do intestino para as glândulas salivares. As vacinas disponíveis no mercado para cães contêm OspA recombinante como adjuvante ou OspA e inúmeros antígenos (p. ex., OspC) com adjuvantes (bacterinas) produzidos a partir da *B. burgdorferi* inativada em cultura. Estudos demonstraram que a taxa de proteção melhora com o passar do tempo em função das imunizações de reforço que induzem a títulos de anticorpos vacinais mais altos e mais duradouros. • Controle da população de carrapatos no ambiente — restrito a pequenas áreas; sucesso limitado, reduzindo a população de cervídeos e/ou roedores.

COMPLICAÇÕES POSSÍVEIS
• Insuficiência renal fatal.

EVOLUÇÃO ESPERADA E PROGNÓSTICO
• Espera-se a recuperação da claudicação aguda 2-5 dias após o início do tratamento com antibióticos. • A doença pode ser recidivante com intervalos de semanas a meses; responde novamente ao tratamento com antibióticos.

DIVERSOS

FATORES RELACIONADOS COM A IDADE
• Os cães jovens (filhotes) parecem ser mais suscetíveis que os adultos sob condições experimentais. • A doença pode ocorrer em cães de todas as idades.

POTENCIAL ZOONÓTICO
• Ocorre em seres humanos; carrapatos infectados constituem a fonte de infecção. • Os cães podem transportar carrapatos não aderidos que, mais tarde, se fixam em seres humanos — no entanto, os carrapatos ixodídeos não são hematófagos intermitentes e se aderem com rapidez; assim que o carrapato inicia o repasto sanguíneo no cão, esse ectoparasita se alimenta até a repleção e não troca de hospedeiro. • A borreliose de Lyme não pode ser transmitida diretamente dos cães para os seres humanos.

GESTAÇÃO/FERTILIDADE/REPRODUÇÃO
• Apesar de possível, não existem provas convincentes de que a infecção por *B. burgdorferi* seja transmitida *in utero* nos cães. • Animais prenhes toleram tratamento com antibiótico; não utilizar tetraciclinas. • Anticorpos maternos C6-específicos podem ser transmitidos de cadelas para seus filhotes.

SINÔNIMO(S)
• Doença de Lyme.
• Artrite de Lyme.

ABREVIATURA(S)
• ELISA = ensaio imunoabsorvente ligado à enzima. • LCS = líquido cerebrospinal. • PCR = reação em cadeia da polimerase.

RECURSOS DA INTERNET
• Centers for Disease Control and Prevention: www.cdc.gov/ncidod/dvbid/lyme/index.htm.
• European Centre of Disease Prevention and Control: alturl.com/m9emd.
• European Union Concerted Action on Lyme Borreliosis: meduni09.edis.at/eucalb/cms/index.php.
• National Institutes of Health: health.nih.gov/topic/LymeDisease.

Sugestões de Leitura
Greene CE, Straubinger RK. Borreliosis. In: Greene CE, ed., Infectious Diseases of the Dog and Cat, 3rd ed. St. Louis: Saunders Elsevier, 2006, pp. 417–435.
Liang ET, Jacobson RH, Straubinger RK, et al. Characterization of Borreliam burgdorferi VIsE invariable region useful in canine Lyme disease serodiagnosis by enzyme-linked immunosorbent assay. J Clin Microbiol 2000, 38:4160–4166.
Littman MP, Goldstein RE, Labato MA, et al. ACVIM small animal consensus statement on Lyme disease in dogs: Diagnosis, treatment, and prevention. J Vet Intern Med 2006, 20;422–434.
Straubinger RK, Straubinger AF, Summers BA, et al. Status of Borrelia burgdorferi infection after antibiotic treatment and the effects of corticosteroids: An experimental study. J Infect Dis 2000, 181:1069–1081.
Töpfer KH, Straubinger RK. Characterization of the humoral immune response in dogs after vaccination against the Lyme borreliosis agent. A study with five commercial vaccines using two different vaccination schedules. Vaccine 2007, 25:314–326.

Autor Reinhard K. Straubinger
Consultor Editorial Stephen C. Barr

BOTULISMO

CONSIDERAÇÕES GERAIS

REVISÃO
• Doença paralítica causada pela neurotoxina pré-formada produzida pela bactéria *Clostridium botulinum* contida em alimento malcozido, carcaça e silagem contaminada ou inadequadamente armazenada.
• A maioria dos casos em cães é causada pela neurotoxina botulínica sorotipo C produzida pelo *Clostridium botulinum*. A neurotoxina interfere na liberação de acetilcolina na junção neuromuscular, resultando em sinais difusos atribuídos ao neurônio motor inferior.

IDENTIFICAÇÃO
Cães (naturalmente infectados) e gatos (experimentalmente infectados exceto por um único relato de caso de toxicose natural por *Clostridium botulinum* tipo C).

SINAIS CLÍNICOS
Achados Anamnésicos
• Os sinais aparecem algumas horas a 6 dias depois da ingestão de toxina.
• Outros cães da casa, vizinhança ou canil podem ser acometidos.
• Ocorre o desenvolvimento de fraqueza progressiva aguda, começando nos membros posteriores e subindo para as regiões de tronco, membros anteriores, pescoço e músculos inervados pelos nervos cranianos. Isso resulta em tetraparesia ou tetraplegia grave.

Achados do Exame Neurológico
• Nervo craniano — pode revelar reflexos pupilares lentos à luz, diminuição dos reflexos palpebrais, redução do tônus da mandíbula, declínio do reflexo do vômito, salivação e disfonia.
• Marcha e postura — inicialmente se observa uma marcha rígida de passadas curtas (sem ataxia) até o desenvolvimento de decúbito (geralmente em até 12-24 horas).
• Reflexos espinais — diminuídos a ausentes com queda do tônus muscular (até atonia) e atrofia dos músculos. A morte pode ser causada por insuficiência dos músculos respiratórios; ocasionalmente se observam megaesôfago e regurgitação.
• Sinais autonômicos — midríase com reflexos pupilares diminuídos à luz, redução do lacrimejamento, íleo paralítico e retenção de urina ou micção frequente de pequenos volumes de urina.

DIAGNÓSTICO

DIAGNÓSTICO DIFERENCIAL
Polirradiculoneurite canina aguda (paralisia do Coonhound), miastenia grave, paralisia por picada de carrapatos, toxicidade do veneno de cobra coral, forma silenciosa da raiva.

HEMOGRAMA/BIOQUÍMICA/URINÁLISE
Geralmente normais.

OUTROS TESTES LABORATORIAIS
• O diagnóstico definitivo é formulado com base na detecção de toxina botulínica em amostras de soro, fezes, vômito ou alimento ingerido; por teste de neutralização em pequenos roedores; ou por teste *in vitro* que mede a antigenicidade da toxina e não a toxicidade.
• A detecção de anticorpos antineurotoxina botulínica C pode ajudar a apoiar o diagnóstico clínico.

DIAGNÓSTICO POR IMAGEM
Radiografias do tórax podem revelar a presença de megaesôfago e/ou pneumonia por aspiração.

MÉTODOS DIAGNÓSTICOS
• O exame de eletromiografia pode revelar potenciais de fibrilação e ondas agudas positivas nos músculos acometidos.
• A velocidade de condução dos nervos motores pode permanecer normal ou sofrer declínio com amplitude reduzida dos potenciais evocados das unidades motoras.

TRATAMENTO

• Os cães levemente acometidos recuperam-se em alguns dias com tratamento de suporte, incluindo fisioterapia passiva e ativa, mudança frequente de posição, uso de uma boa cama acolchoada (para evitar úlceras de decúbito), cuidados vesicais (compressão ou cateterização) e alimentação em uma posição elevada (na presença de megaesôfago).
• Os cães com dificuldades respiratórias necessitam de cuidados intensivos com monitorização da gasometria arterial, sucção esofágica intermitente, alimentação por tubo nasogástrico ou gastrotomia e, finalmente, suporte ventilatório.

MEDICAÇÕES

MEDICAMENTO(S)
• Antitoxina tipo C (10.000-15.000 U IV ou IM 2 vezes em intervalos de 4 h) ou antitoxina polivalente tipo C (5 mL IV ou IM; Statens Serum Institute, Copenhagen, Dinamarca) — pode não estar disponível; pode causar anafilaxia; é recomendada a realização de teste intradérmico (0,1 mL 20 minutos antes da administração sistêmica); sem eficácia quando a toxina já está fixada na terminação nervosa pré-sináptica, mas benéfica para inativar a toxina circulante não ligada (se a absorção ainda estiver ocorrendo).
• Laxantes e enemas em caso de ingestão recente ou constipação.
• A aplicação de pomada oftálmica evita úlcera de córnea por exposição na presença de ceratoconjuntivite seca.
• Antibióticos orais não são recomendados, pois podem agravar a doença por promover a liberação de mais toxinas por meio de lise bacteriana ou a ocorrência de infecção intestinal. Serão utilizados apenas em caso de infecções secundárias (respiratórias, urinárias).

CONTRAINDICAÇÕES/INTERAÇÕES POSSÍVEIS
É recomendável evitar o uso de aminoglicosídeos, penicilina procaína, tetraciclinas, fenotiazinas, agentes antiarrítmicos e magnésio, pois tais medicamentos têm o potencial de bloquear a transmissão neuromuscular.

ACOMPANHAMENTO

MONITORIZAÇÃO DO PACIENTE
Monitorizar os pacientes quanto à ocorrência de insuficiência respiratória, pneumonia por aspiração, e sinais progressivos atribuídos ao neurônio motor inferior.

PREVENÇÃO
• Evitar não só o acesso a carcaças, mas também a alimentação dos cães com comida malcozida.
• Evitar o contato com carne crua estragada.

COMPLICAÇÕES POSSÍVEIS
• Insuficiência respiratória e morte em casos graves.
• Pneumonia por aspiração decorrente de megaesôfago e regurgitação.
• Ceratoconjuntivite seca e ulceração corneana.
• Atelectasia e infecção pulmonares associadas a decúbito prolongado; úlceras de decúbito; queimadura por escaldagem de urina.

EVOLUÇÃO ESPERADA E PROGNÓSTICO
• A gravidade máxima dos sinais clínicos costuma ser atingida em até 12-24 horas.
• Os sinais neurológicos desaparecem na ordem inversa de aparecimento. A recuperação completa do paciente geralmente ocorre em até 1-3 semanas, mas necessita da formação de terminações nervosas novas e junções neuromusculares funcionais.

DIVERSOS

VER TAMBÉM
• Paralisia do Coonhound (Polirradiculoneurite Idiopática).
• Paralisia pelos Carrapatos.
• Toxicose por Veneno de Cobra — Corais.
• Miastenia Grave.

Sugestões de Leitura
Barsanti JA, Greene CE, eds. Infectious Diseases of the Dog and Cat, 3rd ed. St. Louis: Saunders Elsevier, 2006, pp. 389-394.
Bruchim Y, Steinman A, Markovitz M, et al. Toxicological, bacteriological and serological diagnosis of botulism in a dog. Vet Record 2006, 158:768-769.
Elad D, Yas-Natan E, Aroch I, et al. Natural Clostridium type C toxicosis in a group of cats. J Clin Microbiol 2004, 42(11):5406-5408.

Autor Roberto Poma
Consultor Editorial Joane M. Parent

BRADICARDIA SINUSAL

CONSIDERAÇÕES GERAIS

DEFINIÇÃO
Ritmo sinusal no qual os impulsos emergem do nó sinoatrial em velocidade mais lenta que a normal.

CARACTERÍSTICAS DO ECG
- Cães — frequência sinusal <70 bpm (<60 bpm nas raças de porte gigante).
- Gatos — frequência sinusal <120 bpm em casa ou <140 bpm na clínica.
- Ritmo regular, quase sempre com leve variação no intervalo R-R; pode ser irregular caso haja bradicardia atribuída a tônus vagal elevado; frequentemente coexiste com arritmia sinusal.
- Onda P normal para cada complexo QRS.
- Intervalo P-R constante.

FISIOPATOLOGIA
- Pode ser um achado incidental em animais saudáveis ou durante o sono.
- Pode representar a resposta fisiológica ao treinamento atlético; pode resultar de aumento no tônus parassimpático cardíaco ou diminuição no tônus simpático cardíaco, bem como de alterações intrínsecas no nó sinusal; as alterações na frequência de descarga do nó sinoatrial costumam ser produzidas pelos nervos autonômicos cardíacos.
- Pode representar a resposta fisiopatológica gerada por tônus vagal elevado, alteração no pH, PCO_2, PO_2 sanguíneos ou distúrbios eletrolíticos séricos, hipotireoidismo, pressão intracraniana elevada, toxinas e certos medicamentos.
- Pode ser o resultado de síndrome do nó sinusal doente.

SISTEMA(S) ACOMETIDO(S)
Cardiovascular — a maior parte dos casos consiste em arritmia benigna e pode ser benéfica por produzir um período mais prolongado de diástole e um tempo aumentado de enchimento ventricular; pode estar associada à síncope quando atribuída a reflexo anormal (neurocardiogênico) ou doença intrínseca do nó sinusal.

GENÉTICA
Fêmeas de Schnauzer miniatura predispostas à síndrome do nó sinusal doente, o que pode provocar bradicardia.

INCIDÊNCIA/PREVALÊNCIA
- Comum no cão, menos comum no gato.
- A interpretação da frequência do nó sinusal também depende do ambiente e do tipo de paciente. Por exemplo, uma frequência sinusal pode ser de até 20 bpm em um cão normal que esteja dormindo.

IDENTIFICAÇÃO
Espécies
Cães e gatos.

Raça(s) Predominante(s)
Bradicardia associada à síndrome do nó sinusal doente: Schnauzer miniatura, Cocker spaniel, Dachshund, Pug e West Highland white terrier.

Idade Média e Faixa Etária
- Prevalência diminuída com o avanço da idade a menos que associada à doença intrínseca do nó sinoatrial.
- Síndrome do nó sinusal doente tipicamente observada em pacientes geriátricos.

Sexo Predominante
Na síndrome do nó sinusal doente, fêmeas idosas.

SINAIS CLÍNICOS
Comentários Gerais
- A importância depende da causa.
- Pode ser insignificante ou grave, dependendo dos sinais e da causa subjacente.

Achados Anamnésicos
- Frequentemente assintomáticos. • Letargia.
- Intolerância ao exercício. • Síncope. • Ataxia episódica. • Crises convulsivas.

Achados do Exame Físico
- Frequência de pulso lenta. • Pode haver hipotermia. • Má perfusão. • Síncope. • Nível reduzido de consciência.

CAUSAS
Fisiológicas
- Condicionamento atlético.
- Hipotermia.
- Entubação.
- Sono.

Fisiopatológicas
- Aumento no tônus vagal associado a doenças gastrintestinais, respiratórias, neurológicas e faríngeas.

Patológicas
- Pressão intracraniana elevada. • Hipercalcemia.
- Hipercalcemia. • Hipocalcemia.
- Hipermagnesemia. • Hipoxemia.
- Hipotireoidismo. • Hipoglicemia. • Pode preceder a parada cardíaca. • Síndrome do nó sinusal doente. • Miocardiopatia dilatada felina.
- Bloqueio sinoatrial. • Neurocardiogênica.
- Vasovagal. • Hiperatividade do seio carotídeo.
- Situacional (micção, defecação, tosse, deglutição). • Miocardite viral.

Farmacológicas
- Anestesia geral. • Fenotiazínicos.
- β-bloqueadores. • Glicosídeos digitálicos.
- Bloqueadores dos canais de cálcio. • Agonistas $α_2$-adrenérgicos. • Ampla variedade de outros medicamentos, incluindo fentanila e amiodarona.

FATORES DE RISCO
- Qualquer situação ou doença que possa aumentar o tônus parassimpático. • Sedação exagerada. • Hipoventilação sob anestesia.

DIAGNÓSTICO

DIAGNÓSTICO DIFERENCIAL
- Bradicardia sinusal persistente e acentuada deve elevar a possibilidade de síndrome do nó sinusal doente. • Os sinais clínicos podem mimetizar disfunção cerebral.

HEMOGRAMA/BIOQUÍMICA/URINÁLISE
- Possível hipercalemia, hipercalcemia, hipocalcemia ou hipermagnesemia. • Hemograma completo e perfil bioquímico sérico podem revelar alterações associadas à doença metabólica, como a insuficiência renal.

OUTROS TESTES LABORATORIAIS
- Ensaios de T_3 e T_4 séricas, T_4 livre (T_4L) e TSH na suspeita de hipotireoidismo. • Mensuração da concentração da digoxina sérica, se aplicável, 6-8 h depois da última dose; a concentração sérica terapêutica normal deve ser de 0,8-1,5 ng/mL.
- Triagem toxicológica.

DIAGNÓSTICO POR IMAGEM
Se houver indicações específicas, os exames de radiografias simples e ultrassom podem revelar indícios de anormalidades cardíaca, renal ou de outros órgãos.

MÉTODOS DIAGNÓSTICOS
- Teste de resposta provocativa à atropina para avaliar a função do nó sinusal — administrar esse medicamento na dose de 0,04 mg/kg IV, esperar 10-15 min e, depois, registrar o ECG ou administrar a mesma dose IM, aguardar 30 min e, em seguida, rodar o ECG; uma taquicardia sinusal persistente >140 bpm é a resposta esperada. Doses mais baixas da atropina têm uma tendência elevada a provocar acentuação inicial da bradicardia sinusal e bloqueio AV de primeiro ou de segundo graus por causa do aumento no tônus vagal mediado por via central.
- Monitoramento de 24 h com Holter ou registro de evento no ECG (dispositivo acionado pelo

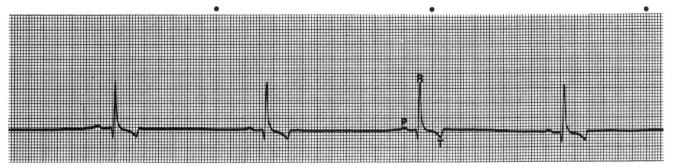

Figura 1 Bradicardia sinusal na frequência de 75 bpm em gato por complicações anestésicas durante cirurgia. Note as ondas R altas. (De: Tilley LP: *Essentials of canine and feline electrocardiography*, 3. ed. Baltimore: Williams & Wilkins, 1992, com permissão.)

BRADICARDIA SINUSAL

proprietário) serão valiosos se a bradiarritmia transitória for a causa sob suspeita dos sinais clínicos.

ACHADOS PATOLÓGICOS
Dependem da doença primária, se houver alguma.

TRATAMENTO

CUIDADO(S) DE SAÚDE ADEQUADO(S)
• Muitos animais não apresentam sinais clínicos e não necessitam de tratamento. Nos cães sem cardiopatia estrutural, frequências cardíacas tão baixas quanto 40-50 bpm, em geral, produzem um débito cardíaco normal em repouso.
• Abordagens terapêuticas — variam de modo acentuado; dependem do mecanismo da bradicardia sinusal, da frequência ventricular e da gravidade dos sinais clínicos.
• Tratamento como paciente de ambulatório ou internado — depende da causa subjacente e do estado clínico do paciente.

CUIDADO(S) DE ENFERMAGEM
• Fornecer terapia de suporte geral, incluindo fluidoterapia intravenosa para os pacientes hipotérmicos e hipovolêmicos.
• Interromper qualquer agente terapêutico causal.
• Corrigir qualquer desequilíbrio eletrolítico sério com fluidoterapia apropriada.

ATIVIDADE
Sem restrições a menos que o paciente apresente bradicardia sinusal sintomática relacionada com cardiopatia estrutural; nesse caso, a restrição ao exercício é recomendada até a intervenção clínica e/ou cirúrgica.

DIETA
Considerações especiais poderão ser indicadas se a causa estiver associada a distúrbio eletrolítico secundário à nefropatia.

ORIENTAÇÃO AO PROPRIETÁRIO
• Discutir a importância de obedecer ao tratamento clínico diário ao se tratar a doença subjacente.
• Orientar sobre o fato de que a bradicardia sintomática persistente pode necessitar do implante de marca-passo permanente para o tratamento confiável a longo prazo.

CONSIDERAÇÕES CIRÚRGICAS
• Se a bradicardia progressiva ocorrer durante a anestesia e for atribuída à hipoventilação, interromper imediatamente o anestésico inalatório e fornecer ventilação adequada; geralmente, a atropina é ineficaz nessa situação.
• Se a manipulação cirúrgica que deflagra os reflexos vagais (olho, nervo vago, laringe) for prevista, o tratamento prévio com atropina (0,04 mg/kg IM, SC) ou o glicopirrolato (0,005-0,01 mg/kg IM, SC) poderá evitar a bradicardia.
• A bradicardia grave pode precipitar a parada cardiopulmonar; identificar o agente ou o problema causais para o tratamento eficaz.

MEDICAÇÕES

MEDICAMENTO(S) DE ESCOLHA
• Se o paciente apresentar hipotireoidismo, suplementar com L-tiroxina.
• Na hipocalcemia grave (<6 mg/dL), administrar gliconato de cálcio a 10% (0,5-1,5 mL/kg IV) lentamente por 15-30 min; monitorizar com ECG.
• Nos casos de bradicardias sintomáticas induzidas por medicamento, distúrbios indutores de tônus vagal excessivo e tratamento inicial da bradicardia associada à síndrome do nó sinusal doente, administrar atropina (0,04 mg/kg IV) ou glicopirrolato (0,005-0,01 mg/kg IV); o tratamento anticolinérgico pode ser mantido a curto prazo com o uso de atropina (0,04 mg/kg IM, SC a cada 6-8 h) ou glicopirrolato (0,01 mg/kg IM, SC a cada 6-8 h). Considerar o brometo de propantelina (0,25-0,5 mg/kg VO a cada 8-12 h) ou a hiosciamina (0,003-0,006 mg/kg VO a cada 8 h [Levsin®]), a teofilina (10 mg/kg VO a cada 12 h, cães; 12,5 mg VO a cada 24 h no final da tarde, gatos [Theochron® ou Theocap®]) e/ou a terbutalina (0,2 mg/kg VO a cada 8 h, cães; 0,625 mg/gato VO, gatos) para tratar bradicardia sintomática associada à doença do nó sinoatrial.
• Para o tratamento temporário da bradicardia persistente sintomática até que o implante de marca-passo possa ser efetuado, considerar a infusão IV contínua de isoproterenol (1-2 µg/min ou até fazer efeito) ou a dobutamina (2,5-20 µg/kg/min sob infusão IV, cães; 1-5 µg/kg/min sob infusão IV, gatos). Contudo, se o implante de marca-passo temporário estiver disponível, este será o procedimento inicial de escolha.

CONTRAINDICAÇÕES
• Para bradicardia induzida por hipotermia com pulso, medidas de reaquecimento e de suporte devem ser a base do tratamento. Agentes parassimpaticolíticos geralmente não são recomendados.
• Agentes parassimpaticolíticos são contraindicados nos pacientes em acidose e com hipercarbia sob anestesia (hipoventilação); a bradicardia nesse quadro pode proteger o miocárdio por diminuir o consumo de oxigênio.

PRECAUÇÕES
• É recomendável a monitorização rigorosa do ECG quando se administram soluções de cálcio para o tratamento da hipocalcemia; na ocorrência de encurtamento do intervalo QT ou de bradicardia, interromper a administração temporariamente.
• Nos pacientes com cardiopatia, aconselha-se uma dose inicial mais baixa de L-tiroxina para permitir a adaptação à taxa metabólica mais elevada.
• Administrar a atropina seletivamente; a administração IV rápida pode predispor o paciente a arritmias ventriculares por alterar o equilíbrio autonômico.

MEDICAMENTO(S) ALTERNATIVO(S)
• Bradicardia associada à cardiopatia estrutural é tratada de forma mais confiável pelo implante de marca-passo permanente.
• O glicopirrolato pode apresentar efeito de bloqueio vagal mais prolongado e gerar batimentos ectópicos ventriculares menos frequentes do que a atropina.

ACOMPANHAMENTO

MONITORIZAÇÃO DO PACIENTE
• Avaliar a T_4 sérica 4-6 h após a dosagem de L-tiroxina, 30 e 60 dias após o início do tratamento.
• Doença de Addison — avaliar os eletrólitos a cada 3-4 meses após a estabilização do paciente.
• É recomendável verificar a função do marca-passo pelo ECG e a frequência desse aparelho durante cada exame de acompanhamento.

PREVENÇÃO
• Manter a PaO_2 normal durante a anestesia com ventilação apropriada; monitorizar com oxímetro de pulso ou gasometria sanguínea.
• Evitar a hipotermia no intraoperatório.

COMPLICAÇÕES POSSÍVEIS
Mau funcionamento do marca-passo.

EVOLUÇÃO ESPERADA E PROGNÓSTICO
• Os sinais, quando presentes, devem desaparecer com a correção do problema metabólico ou endócrino causal.
• O tratamento da bradicardia sinusal sintomática com o marca-passo permanente geralmente oferece prognóstico bom quanto ao controle do ritmo cardíaco. O prognóstico global varia com a natureza da cardiopatia estrutural, se presente.

DIVERSOS

DISTÚRBIOS ASSOCIADOS
• Síndrome do nó sinusal doente. • Bloqueio cardíaco. • Arritmia sinusal.

GESTAÇÃO/FERTILIDADE/REPRODUÇÃO
Hipocalcemia puerperal geralmente se desenvolve 1-4 semanas após o parto, embora possa ocorrer na gestação a termo, antes do parto ou no final da lactação.

VER TAMBÉM
• Eclâmpsia. • Hipercalcemia. • Hipercalemia. • Hipermagnesemia. • Hipocalcemia. • Hipotermia. • Hipotireoidismo. • Toxicidade dos Organofosforados e Carbamatos. • Síndrome do Nó Sinusal Doente. • Toxicidade da Digoxina.

ABREVIATURA(S)
• AV = atrioventricular. • bpm = batimento por minuto. • ECG = eletrocardiograma. • T_3 = tri-iodotironina. • T_4 = tiroxina. • TSH = hormônio tireostimulante.

Autor Deborah J. Hadlock
Consultores Editoriais Larry P. Tilley e Francis W.K. Smith, Jr.

BRONQUIECTASIA

CONSIDERAÇÕES GERAIS

REVISÃO
• Condição clínica observada principalmente em cães, que se caracteriza por uma dilatação irreversível dos brônquios; causada por doença infecciosa ou inflamatória crônica das vias aéreas ou associada à discinesia ciliar primária.
• Ocasionalmente ocorre em gatos como uma sequela de pneumopatia inflamatória de longa duração ou neoplasia. • A produção de citocinas e enzimas destrutivas por leucócitos ou bactérias e o contato prolongado de mediadores inflamatórios com o tecido pulmonar levam ao dano das estruturas de sustentação dentro do pulmão. • As vias aéreas são mantidas abertas pelo tecido pulmonar circunjacente; ocorre o acúmulo de secreções, o que perpetua o dano pulmonar e permite a colonização por bactérias. • Pode ser cilíndrica ou sacular, focal ou difusa.

IDENTIFICAÇÃO
• Principalmente cães e, raramente, gatos. • As raças Cocker spaniel e, talvez, West Highland white terrier são predispostas. • Animais jovens (<1 ano) com discinesia ciliar primária. • Cães de meia-idade a idosos com pneumopatia crônica.

SINAIS CLÍNICOS
• Tosse crônica — costuma ser úmida e produtiva; os proprietários atentos podem notar hemoptise.
• Febre recorrente. • Intolerância ao exercício.
• Taquipneia ou angústia respiratória.
• Crepitações inspiratórias ásperas e úmidas, bem como ruídos pulmonares expiratórios sonoros ou sibilos. • Hipersensibilidade traqueal. • Secreção nasal ou sinusite crônicas, particularmente em casos de discinesia ciliar primária.

CAUSAS E FATORES DE RISCO
• Discinesia ciliar primária. • Condições pulmonares infecciosas ou inflamatórias tratadas de forma inadequada. • Inalação de fumaça e toxinas ambientais, pneumonia por aspiração, lesão por radiação — predispõem o animal à lesão das vias aéreas e à colonização por bactérias.
• Obstrução brônquica crônica ou pneumonia por corpo(s) estranho(s) — é comum o desenvolvimento de bronquiectasia distalmente à região obstruída. • Os sinais relacionados com bronquiectasia podem não ser identificados até muito tempo depois da lesão primária.

DIAGNÓSTICO

DIAGNÓSTICO DIFERENCIAL
• Broncopneumonia bacteriana recorrente.
• Pneumonia fúngica. • Bronquite crônica.
• Bronquite infecciosa ou parasitária. • Pneumonia por corpo(s) estranho(s) • Neoplasia.

HEMOGRAMA/BIOQUÍMICA/URINÁLISE
• Neutrofilia e monocitose. • Hiperglobulinemia.
• Proteinúria — pode ser observada em casos de amiloidose, glomerulonefrite ou sepse secundárias.

OUTROS TESTES LABORATORIAIS
Gasometria sanguínea arterial — hipoxemia; aumento no gradiente alveoloarterial de oxigênio.

DIAGNÓSTICO POR IMAGEM
• Radiografia — exame insensível para o diagnóstico. As anormalidades visíveis no final da evolução da doença incluem dilatação dos brônquios lobares com falta do afunilamento (estreitamento) normal na periferia; espessamento difuso das paredes brônquicas; padrão brônquico, intersticial e alveolar misto. • As alterações podem ser focais ou difusas. • TC — diâmetro do brônquio 2 vezes maior que a largura da artéria pulmonar adjacente, brônquios anormalmente dilatados próximos à periferia do pulmão; espessamento das vias aéreas; dilatações císticas dos brônquios com ou sem acúmulo de líquido.

MÉTODOS DIAGNÓSTICOS
• Broncoscopia — dilatação sacular ou tubular das vias aéreas; perda do formato cilíndrico do lúmen.
• Amostragem das vias aéreas — exame citológico de amostras obtidas por lavados broncoalveolar ou transtraqueal; culturas bacterianas aeróbia e anaeróbia e para pesquisa de *Mycoplasma*; tipicamente se verifica uma inflamação supurativa, com alta quantidade de neutrófilos e monócitos ou pode ser observado o aumento no número de eosinófilos; pode-se obter uma população mista de bactérias ao exame de cultura; *Pseudomonas* spp. parece ser a mais comum; talvez pareça ter uma inflamação estéril.

ACHADOS PATOLÓGICOS
• Inflamação e fibrose peribrônquicas e alveolares difusas. • Metaplasia escamosa do epitélio brônquico. • Obliteração bronquiolar.

TRATAMENTO

• Internação — em casos graves: fluidos e antibióticos intravenosos; administração de oxigênio. • A maior parte dos pacientes beneficia-se de certos procedimentos, como a umidificação e a tapotagem das vias aéreas, para facilitar a remoção de secreções pulmonares viscosas.
• Estimular a atividade física leve e suave — o máximo que o estado do paciente permitir — aumenta a depuração das secreções.
• Administração de antibióticos. • Enfatizar ao proprietário a importância dos cuidados adequados de acompanhamento. • Acometimento de um único lobo pulmonar ou obstrução brônquica — podem necessitar de lobectomia pulmonar.

MEDICAÇÕES

MEDICAMENTO(S)
• Antibióticos intravenosos — podem ser necessários inicialmente; boas escolhas: ampicilina (10-20 mg/kg IV a cada 6-8 h) e enrofloxacino (5-10 mg/kg a cada 24 h). • Agentes de amplo espectro com eficácia contra microrganismos aeróbios e anaeróbios, além de boa penetração no tecido pulmonar — são os medicamentos preferidos; a combinação de enrofloxacino (5-20 mg/kg VO a cada 24 h) e clindamicina (5-11 mg/kg VO a cada 12 h) é frequentemente eficaz. • Uso de antibióticos a longo prazo (dos 2 meses de vida até o resto da vida) — com base nos resultados da cultura bacteriana e do antibiograma; podem ser indispensáveis mesmo na ausência de qualquer crescimento na cultura de amostras das vias aéreas.
• Em alguns cães, pode haver a necessidade de rodízio mensal dos antibióticos.
• Broncodilatadores — podem ser benéficos, embora os animais costumem apresentar restrição irreversível do fluxo de ar nas vias aéreas; teofilina, terbutalina ou albuterol de liberação estendida.
• Pneumopatia eosinofílica necessita de tratamento com glicocorticoides.

CONTRAINDICAÇÕES/INTERAÇÕES POSSÍVEIS
• Derivados teofilínicos e fluoroquinolonas — o emprego concomitante gera concentração plasmática alta e, possivelmente, tóxica da teofilina. • Furosemida — evitar; provoca o ressecamento das secreções das vias aéreas.
• Supressores da tosse — evitar; promovem o encarceramento de secreções e bactérias nas vias aéreas inferiores e perpetuam o dano.

ACOMPANHAMENTO

MONITORIZAÇÃO DO PACIENTE
• Temperatura corporal — mensuração em um esquema ambulatorial. • Obtenção seriada de hemograma completo, gasometria sanguínea e radiografias torácicas.

PREVENÇÃO
• Antibióticos — concluir o curso terapêutico completo em pacientes que parecem ter infecção parenquimatosa; as terapias a curto prazo (10-14 dias) podem predispor o paciente à infecção por bactérias resistentes. • Identificação e resolução precoces de pneumonia por corpo(s) estranho(s).
• Tratamento adequado de pneumonia eosinofílica.

COMPLICAÇÕES POSSÍVEIS
É provável uma infecção pulmonar recorrente crônica.

EVOLUÇÃO ESPERADA E PROGNÓSTICO
• São esperados sinais clínicos crônicos e recorrentes; certo grau de tosse sempre estará presente. • Os animais podem viver por anos com bronquiectasia se forem tratados de forma adequada. • O paciente pode sucumbir à insuficiência respiratória. • Podem ocorrer hipertensão pulmonar e cor pulmonale. • Caso ocorra o desenvolvimento de bacteremia ou glomerulonefrite, outros órgãos poderão entrar em falência.

DIVERSOS

DISTÚRBIOS ASSOCIADOS
• Discinesia ciliar primária. • Sinusite crônica.
• Bronquite crônica. • Pneumonia — bacteriana, eosinofílica, por aspiração de corpo(s) estranho(s).
• Inalação de fumaça.

Autor Lynelle R. Johnson
Consultor Editorial Lynelle R. Johnson

BRONQUITE CRÔNICA

CONSIDERAÇÕES GERAIS

DEFINIÇÃO
• Tosse crônica por mais que 2 meses consecutivos, não atribuível a outra causa (p. ex., neoplasia, insuficiência cardíaca congestiva, pneumonia eosinofílica, ou bronquite infecciosa). • Condição parcialmente irreversível e, muitas vezes, lentamente progressiva, em virtude de alterações patológicas concomitantes das vias aéreas.

FISIOPATOLOGIA
• Raramente se determina a causa específica, mas há suspeitas de inflamação recorrente das vias aéreas. • Irritação traqueobrônquica persistente — causa tosse crônica; leva a alterações no epitélio traqueobrônquico e na submucosa. • Inflamação, edema e espessamento epiteliais das vias aéreas — proeminentes. • A produção excessiva de muco é uma característica típica. • Em casos graves muito crônicos — provável aumento da resistência pulmonar; diminuição do fluxo de ar expiratório, especialmente em gatos.

SISTEMA(S) ACOMETIDO(S)
• Respiratório. • Cardiovascular — hipertensão pulmonar, cor pulmonale. • Nervoso — síncope (pouco frequente).

INCIDÊNCIA/PREVALÊNCIA
Comum em cães e gatos.

DISTRIBUIÇÃO GEOGRÁFICA
Mundial.

IDENTIFICAÇÃO

Espécies
Cães e gatos.

Raça(s) Predominante(s)
• Cães — comum em raças pequenas e toys; quadro também observado em raças de grande porte. • Cocker spaniel — a bronquiectasia é comum após histórico prolongado de bronquite crônica. • Gatos siameses e domésticos de pelo curto também são acometidos.

Idade Média e Faixa Etária
Acomete mais frequentemente os animais de meia-idade e idosos.

Sexo Predominante
N/D, embora fêmeas castradas sejam frequentemente super-representadas.

SINAIS CLÍNICOS

Achados Anamnésicos
• Tosse — indicação de irritação traqueobrônquica; geralmente áspera e seca; é comum uma espécie de engasgo ou náusea após a tosse (os proprietários podem interpretar erroneamente como vômito, sobretudo em cães). • Intolerância ao exercício, dificuldade respiratória, sibilos (em gatos). • Cianose e até mesmo síncope — podem ser observadas em casos graves.

Achados do Exame Físico
• Os pacientes costumam permanecer espertos, alertas e afebris. • Palpação da traqueia — tipicamente resulta em tosse, em função do aumento da sensibilidade nessa estrutura. • Comprometimento das vias aéreas de pequeno calibre — admitido quando se detecta esforço abdominal expiratório (durante a respiração tranquila) ou sibilo término-expiratório. • Possivelmente, auscultam-se ruídos pulmonares broncovesiculares, crepitações terminoinspiratórias e sibilos (como resultado do fluxo de ar pelas vias aéreas obstruídas). • Estalido terminoexpiratório sonoro, sugestivo de colapso concomitante das vias aéreas. • Auscultação cardíaca — são comuns, em cães, sopros secundários à insuficiência valvar, mas nem sempre eles estão associados à insuficiência cardíaca congestiva; a bronquite crônica geralmente culmina em uma frequência cardíaca normal ou mais lenta que o normal em repouso e arritmia sinusal pronunciada. Em gatos, é possível a presença de taquicardia. • Obesidade — comum; importante fator de complicação. • Odontopatia grave pode predispor à colonização das vias aéreas inferiores e possível infecção (cães).

CAUSAS
Inflamação crônica das vias aéreas, desencadeada por múltiplas causas, embora uma causa específica raramente seja identificada.

FATORES DE RISCO
• Exposição prolongada a irritantes inalados. • Obesidade. • Infecção bacteriana recorrente. • Odontopatia e laringopatia — resultam na exposição das vias aéreas inferiores a bactérias.

DIAGNÓSTICO

DIAGNÓSTICO DIFERENCIAL
• Bronquiectasia. • Pneumopatia alérgica ou eosinofílica. • Corpos estranhos. • Dirofilariose. • Pneumonia bacteriana ou fúngica. • Neoplasias — as metastáticas são mais comuns do que as primárias. • Parasitas pulmonares ou migração parasitária larval. • Fibrose pulmonar — em gatos e cães. • Granulomatose pulmonar. • Insuficiência cardíaca congestiva — tipicamente associada a alta frequência cardíaca em repouso e aumento de volume do átrio esquerdo, o que pode levar a colapso do brônquio principal esquerdo.

HEMOGRAMA/BIOQUÍMICA/URINÁLISE
• Raramente são diagnósticos. • É comum a constatação de leucocitose neutrofílica. • Eosinofilia absoluta — sugestiva, mas não diagnóstica, de bronquite alérgica. • Policitemia secundária à hipoxia crônica — possível constatação possível. • As enzimas hepáticas e os ácidos biliares podem estar elevados, em virtude da congestão passiva.

OUTROS TESTES LABORATORIAIS
• Exames de fezes e testes de dirofilariose — excluem os parasitas pulmonares. • Oximetria de pulso — útil para detecção de dessaturação de hemoglobina. • Gasometria sanguínea arterial — coletar, refrigerar e analisar em um hospital local; em casos graves, é comum PaO_2 leve a moderadamente baixa, auxilia no estabelecimento do prognóstico e na monitorização do tratamento. • Como o hiperadrenocorticismo pode ser responsável pela obesidade e/ou aumento de volume do abdome/fígado, deve-se considerar o teste para pesquisa dessa endocrinopatia se houver indicação clínica.

DIAGNÓSTICO POR IMAGEM

Radiografia Torácica
Características comuns (em ordem decrescente de frequência) — espessamento brônquico (classicamente, em formato de rosquinhas e trilhos de trem); padrões intersticiais; consolidação do lobo pulmonar médio (gatos); atelectasia; hiperinsuflação e achatamento diafragmático (principalmente gatos).

Ecocardiografia
• Pode revelar aumento de volume do lado direito do coração com hipertensão pulmonar. • Ajuda a descartar cardiopatia como causa da tosse. • Avalia a presença de hipertensão pulmonar por meio da ecocardiografia Doppler.

MÉTODOS DIAGNÓSTICOS

Eletrocardiografia (Cães)
Marca-passo atrial migratório, arritmia sinusal acentuada, P *pulmonale* e, ocasionalmente, indícios de aumento de volume do ventrículo direito.

Avaliação de Secreções das Vias Aéreas
• Provenientes obrigatoriamente das vias aéreas inferiores — ajudam a estabelecer a causa subjacente, se presente, ou a determinar a gravidade da inflamação. • Culturas de *swab* da orofaringe (garganta) — não são representativas da flora das vias aéreas inferiores. • Aspirado traqueal ou lavado broncoalveolar (LBA) — coletar amostras para exame citológico e cultura bacteriana/micoplasmal. • As culturas aeróbias quantitativas do LBA ajudam a diferenciar infecção *vs.* colonização das vias aéreas; relata-se uma margem de corte ≥$1,7 \times 10^3$ UFC para infecção em cães. Culturas anaeróbias e *Mycoplasma* também são recomendadas. • Citologia — inflamação como o principal achado; constituída principalmente por neutrófilos, eosinófilos ou macrófagos; pesquisar bactérias, parasitas, células neoplásicas e contaminação com materiais estranhos. • Infecções recorrentes — envolvidas na patogenia de bronquite; no entanto, não há relatos frequentes de culturas positivas; o envolvimento do *Mycoplasma* é discutível, mas raramente confirmado como uma causa.

Broncoscopia
• Teste preferido para avaliar as vias aéreas inferiores. • Permite a inspeção direta das alterações estruturais e funcionais (dinâmicas) encontradas; possibilita a amostragem de via aérea selecionada (p. ex., biopsia e lavado). • Alterações macroscópicas — secreções mucoides a mucopurulentas em excesso; edema ou espessamento epiteliais associados a embotamento (obstrução) das bifurcações brônquicas; mucosa irregular ou granular; proliferações polipoides da mucosa podem indicar bronquite crônica ou pneumonia eosinofílica crônica. • Alterações de calibre das vias aéreas calibrosas (p. ex., colapso estático ou dinâmico das vias aéreas e bronquiectasia) — podem ser detectadas como complicações.

ACHADOS PATOLÓGICOS
Ver o item "Broncoscopia" em "Métodos Diagnósticos".

TRATAMENTO

CUIDADO(S) DE SAÚDE ADEQUADO(S)
• Geralmente em um esquema ambulatorial — em casos crônicos, o oxigênio pode ser fornecido em casa. • Internação — necessita de oxigenoterapia, medicamentos parenterais e terapia com aerossol; recomendada aos pacientes que não conseguem se

BRONQUITE CRÔNICA

manter calmos no ambiente doméstico durante a recuperação.

CUIDADO(S) DE ENFERMAGEM
Considerar a nebulização com soro fisiológico (acompanhada de tapotagem ou exercícios suaves) para estimular a remoção das secreções nas vias aéreas.

ATIVIDADE
• Exercícios — moderados (jamais forçados) são úteis na remoção das secreções; auxiliam também na perda de peso. • Restringir se o esforço físico resultar em tosse excessiva. • Utilizar uma coleira peitoral em vez da coleira comum.

DIETA
A perda de peso é crítica — restabelece a PaO_2, melhora a postura do animal, aumenta a tolerância ao exercício em pacientes obesos; também diminui a frequência da tosse.

ORIENTAÇÃO AO PROPRIETÁRIO
• Orientar o proprietário de que a bronquite crônica constitui uma doença incurável e a supressão completa de toda a tosse representa um objetivo inatingível. • Enfatizar que o tratamento rigoroso — incluindo controle do peso, afastamento dos fatores de risco e uso de terapia clínica — minimiza a gravidade da tosse e retarda a evolução da doença em grande parte dos pacientes.

CONSIDERAÇÕES CIRÚRGICAS
Tratar a odontopatia grave para minimizar as complicações bacterianas secundárias.

MEDICAÇÕES

MEDICAMENTO(S) DE ESCOLHA

Corticosteroides
• Diminuem a inflamação das vias aéreas e a tosse, independentemente da causa subjacente.
• Indicados em condições não infecciosas. • Em casos de reações alérgicas ou hipersensibilidade — é necessária a administração a longo prazo; tentar retirar os esteroides gradativamente ou determinar a dosagem eficaz mais baixa. • A prednisolona é o medicamento preferido em gatos.
• Prednisona ou prednisolona costumam ser iniciadas a 0,5-1,0 mg/kg VO a cada 12 h por um período de tempo variável, com redução gradativa da dose com base nos sinais clínicos.
• Corticosteroides inalados são frequentemente eficazes e podem ser usados para diminuir os efeitos colaterais sistêmicos de corticosteroides.

Broncodilatadores
• Efeitos benéficos (dependem do medicamento) — broncodilatação; aumento na depuração mucociliar; melhora na contratilidade diafragmática; diminuição na pressão arterial pulmonar; ampliação na sensibilidade do SNC à $PaCO_2$; e estabilização dos mastócitos.
• β-agonistas — terbutalina (1,25-5 mg/cão VO a cada 8-12 h; 0,625 mg/gato VO a cada 12 h) e albuterol (0,02-0,05 mg/kg VO a cada 8-12 h em cães). • Teofilina de liberação sustentada — administração oral; atualmente, apenas os produtos genéricos de liberação sustentada estão disponíveis. Considerar a administração de 10 mg/kg VO a cada 12 h em cães e 15-20 mg/kg/diariamente, às noites, nos gatos. • Aminofilina — comprimidos de liberação imediata ou formulações injetáveis não são recomendados.

Antibióticos
• Selecionar com base nos resultados da cultura e do antibiograma. • Na indisponibilidade dos resultados da cultura bacteriana — escolher um agente com amplo espectro contra Gram-negativos, boa penetração nos tecidos e nas secreções e efeito bactericida com mínima toxicidade (p. ex., sulfa potencializada pela trimetoprima, amoxicilina/ácido clavulânico, ou enrofloxacino). • Aspiração crônica ou odontopatia associadas — pode-se dar preferência a um antibiótico de espectro contra microrganismos anaeróbios e Gram-positivos.

Antitussígenos
• Indicados em casos de tosse improdutiva, paroxística, contínua ou debilitante. • Cães — butorfanol (0,55 mg/kg VO a cada 6-12 h; 0,055-0,11 mg/kg SC); hidrocodona (2,5-5 mg/cão a cada 6-24 h VO); codeína (0,1-0,3 mg/kg a cada 6-8 h VO).

CONTRAINDICAÇÕES
Lasix® e atropina — não utilizar em função dos efeitos de ressecamento sobre as secreções traqueobrônquicas.

PRECAUÇÕES
• β-agonistas (p. ex., terbutalina e albuterol) — podem causar taquicardia, nervosismo e tremores musculares; efeitos tipicamente transitórios.
• Teofilina — podem ocasionar taquicardia, inquietação, excitabilidade, vômito e diarreia; avaliar uma amostra de plasma com EDTA quanto ao pico da concentração plasmática (idealmente 5-20 μg/mL). Toxicidade pode ser mais comum com formulações genéricas.

INTERAÇÕES POSSÍVEIS
As fluoroquinolonas diminuem a depuração da teofilina nos cães e, consequentemente, podem resultar em intoxicação.

MEDICAMENTO(S) ALTERNATIVO(S)
• Inaladores dosimetrados (esteroides pouco metabolizados — fluticasona ou budesonida; broncodilatadores — albuterol) e antibióticos aerossolizados (gentamicina) estão sendo utilizados em muitos casos. Esses agentes devem ser administrados apenas via máscara facial e câmara de espaçamento. • Bloqueio serotoninérgico (mas não bloqueadores de leucotrieno) — poucas provas para recomendar esse medicamento na prática clínica. • Imunossupressão induzida pela ciclosporina — poucas provas para recomendar esse medicamento na prática clínica.

ACOMPANHAMENTO

MONITORIZAÇÃO DO PACIENTE
• Acompanhar as anormalidades reveladas pelo exame físico e por testes diagnósticos selecionados — determinar a resposta ao tratamento.
• Monitorizar o peso; a gasometria sanguínea arterial costuma melhorar após perda de peso acentuada.

PREVENÇÃO
Evitar e tratar os fatores de risco (ver a seção "Fatores de Risco").

COMPLICAÇÕES POSSÍVEIS
• Síncope — complicação frequente de tosse crônica, particularmente em cães de raças toys.
• Hipertensão pulmonar e cor pulmonale — complicações mais graves.
• Bronquiectasia e remodelagem das vias aéreas.

EVOLUÇÃO ESPERADA E PROGNÓSTICO
• Alterações progressivas das vias aéreas — são comuns episódios de síncope, hipoxia crônica, hipertrofia do ventrículo direito e hipertensão pulmonar. • Exacerbações agudas — comuns em casos de mudanças sazonais, alterações na qualidade do ar, agravamento da inflamação e, potencialmente, desenvolvimento de infecção secundária.

DIVERSOS

DISTÚRBIOS ASSOCIADOS
• Síncope — secundária à tosse crônica ou desenvolvimento de hipertensão pulmonar.
• Aumento na suscetibilidade à infecção das vias aéreas, hipoxia crônica, hipertensão pulmonar e cor pulmonale.

GESTAÇÃO/FERTILIDADE/REPRODUÇÃO
Ainda não se estabeleceu a segurança em animais prenhes para grande parte dos medicamentos recomendados.

SINÔNIMO(S)
• Bronquiolite, comprometimento das vias aéreas de pequeno calibre. • Bronquite crônica.
• Pneumopatia obstrutiva crônica (POC).
• Doença pulmonar obstrutiva crônica (DPOC).

VER TAMBÉM
• Asma e Bronquite — Gatos. • Bronquiectasia.
• Colapso da Traqueia — Cães. • Hipoxia. • Tosse.
• Traqueobronquite Infecciosa Canina (Tosse dos Canis).

ABREVIATURA(S)
• EDTA = ácido etilenodiaminotetracético. • LBA = lavado broncoalveolar. • SNC = sistema nervoso central. • UFC = unidade formadora de colônia.

Sugestões de Leitura
Bay JD, Johnson LR. Feline bronchial disease/asthma. In: King LG, ed., Textbook of Respiratory Disease in Dogs and Cats. St. Louis: Saunders, 2004, pp. 388-396.
Kuehn NE. Chronic bronchitis in dogs. In: King LG, ed., Textbook of Respiratory Disease in Dogs and Cats. St. Louis: Saunders, 2004, pp. 379-387.

Autores Cécile Clercx e Brendan C. McKiernan
Consultor Editorial Lynelle R. Johnson

BRUCELOSE

CONSIDERAÇÕES GERAIS

DEFINIÇÃO
- Doença contagiosa de cães causada pela *Brucella canis*, um microrganismo pequeno, intracelular e Gram-negativo.
- Caracterizada por abortamento e infertilidade em cadelas, bem como por epididimite e atrofia testicular em machos caninos.

FISIOPATOLOGIA
B. canis — um parasita intracelular; tem propensão ao crescimento nos tecidos linfáticos, placentários e genitais masculinos (epidídimo e próstata).

SISTEMA(S) ACOMETIDO(S)
- Sanguíneo/linfático/imune — linfonodos e baço; medula óssea; leucócitos mononucleares.
- Reprodutivo — tecidos-alvo de esteroides gonadais (útero prenhe, feto, testículos [epidídimos], próstata).
- Outros tecidos — discos intervertebrais, úvea anterior, meninges (incomum).

GENÉTICA
- Não há predisposição genética conhecida.
- Ocorre mais comumente em Beagles.

INCIDÊNCIA/PREVALÊNCIA
- Incidência desconhecida.
- Taxas de soroprevalência — não definidas com precisão; nos testes de aglutinação, são comuns resultados falso-positivos.
- Prevalência — relativamente baixa (1-18%) nos EUA e no Japão; nos EUA, mais alta nas áreas rurais do sul; em países como México e Peru, 25-30% em cães errantes.

DISTRIBUIÇÃO GEOGRÁFICA
Cães errantes, animais de estimação e canis — EUA (principalmente Beagle), México, Japão e diversos países sul-americanos; observada também na Espanha, Tunísia, China e Bulgária; surtos individuais na Alemanha e na antiga Tchecoslováquia (alguns surtos rastreados da importação de cães).

IDENTIFICAÇÃO
Espécies
Acomete cães e, com menor frequência, seres humanos.

Raça(s) Predominante(s)
- Sem indícios de suscetibilidade racial, embora haja uma prevalência excepcionalmente alta em Beagle.
- Encontro de cães infectados da raça Labrador retriever e de diversas outras raças em canis comerciais (de "adestramento de filhotes caninos").

Idade Média e Faixa Etária
- Não há preferência etária.
- Mais comum em cães sexualmente maduros.

Sexo(s) Predominante(s)
- Acometimento de ambos os sexos.
- Mais comum nas cadelas.

SINAIS CLÍNICOS
Comentários Gerais
Suspeitar sempre que as cadelas sofrerem abortamentos ou falhas reprodutivas ou se os machos tiverem doenças genitais.

Achados Anamnésicos
- Os animais acometidos, especialmente as cadelas, podem parecer saudáveis ou apresentar sinais vagos de doença.
- Letargia.
- Perda da libido.
- Linfonodos enfartados.
- Dorsalgia (dor no dorso).
- Abortamento — comumente com 6-8 semanas após a concepção, embora o término da gestação possa ocorrer em qualquer estágio.

Achados do Exame Físico
- Machos — bolsas escrotais intumescidas, frequentemente com dermatite escrotal; epidídimos aumentados de volume e firmes.
- Infecção crônica — atrofia testicular uni ou bilateral; dor na coluna vertebral, fraqueza posterior; ataxia.
- Uveíte anterior unilateral crônica e recorrente sem outros sinais sistêmicos de doença; também inclui hiperpigmentação da íris, infiltrados vítreos, e coriorretinite multifocal.
- Febre — achado raro.
- É comum o enfartamento dos linfonodos superficiais (p. ex., retrofaríngeos e inguinais externos).
- O corrimento vaginal pode perdurar por algumas semanas após o abortamento.

CAUSAS
B. canis — cocobacilo Gram-negativo; do ponto de vista morfológico, é indistinguível de outros membros do gênero; ao contrário de outras espécies de *Brucella* (p. ex., *B. abortus*, *B. suis* e *B. melitensis*), a *B. canis* pode resultar em uma taxa elevada (50%) de reações falso-positivas nos testes comumente utilizados.

FATORES DE RISCO
- Canis de reprodução e matilhas de caça.
- Aumento do risco em casos de infecção de animais reprodutores.
- Contato com cães errantes em áreas endêmicas.

DIAGNÓSTICO

DIAGNÓSTICO DIFERENCIAL
- Abortamentos — anormalidades maternas, fetais ou placentárias.
- Infecções sistêmicas — cinomose, infecção por herpes-vírus canino, infecção por *B. abortus*, estreptococos hemolíticos, *E. coli*, leptospirose e toxoplasmose.
- Hérnias inguinais — podem ser provocadas por epididimite e edema escrotal; causadas também por blastomicose e outras infecções granulomatosas, bem como por febre maculosa das Montanhas Rochosas.
- Discospondilite — infecções fúngicas, actinomicose, infecções estafilocócicas, nocardiose, estreptococos ou *Corynebacterium diphtheroids*.

HEMOGRAMA/BIOQUÍMICA/URINÁLISE
- Em geral, permanecem normais em casos não complicados.
- Os cães com infecção crônica podem exibir hiperglobulinemia (com hipoalbuminemia concomitante).
- LCS — pleocitose que consiste, principalmente, em neutrófilos, e teor proteico elevado em meningoencefalite, mas normal em discospondilite.
- A urinálise costuma permanecer normal mesmo se houver bactérias na cultura de urina.

OUTROS TESTES LABORATORIAIS
Teste sorológico — método diagnóstico mais comumente utilizado; sujeito a erros; costumam ocorrer reações falso-positivas aos antígenos lipopolissacarídeos de diversas espécies de bactérias no TARL e no teste de aglutinação em tubo com mercaptoetanol.

TARL
- Disponível no mercado; método simples e rápido.
- Detecta cães infectados 3-4 semanas após a infecção; teste preciso na identificação de cães não infectados ("negativos").
- Sofre uma taxa elevada (50%) de reações falso-positivas.
- Os resultados devem ser confirmados por outros testes.

Teste de Aglutinação em Tubo com Mercaptoetanol
- Semiquantitativo.
- Realizado geralmente por laboratórios diagnósticos comerciais.
- Fornece informações semelhantes ao TARL.
- Padece da falta de especificidade; representa um bom teste de triagem.

Testes de IDAG
- Teste para detecção do antígeno da parede celular — emprega um antígeno lipopolissacarídeo derivado das paredes celulares da *B. canis*; altamente sensível; condições de teste ainda não padronizadas; resultados falso-positivos frequentes; não recomendado.
- Teste de aglutinação com antígeno solúvel — utiliza antígenos solúveis que consistem em proteínas extraídas do citoplasma bacteriano; antígenos altamente específicos para os anticorpos contra as espécies de *Brucella* (incluindo *B. canis*, *B. abortus* e *B. suis*); os anticorpos reativos aparecem 4-12 semanas após a infecção e persistem por um período de tempo prolongado; pode gerar linhas de precipitina após outros testes questionáveis ou negativos; altamente recomendado.
- ELISA — realizado com o uso de antígenos citoplasmáticos purificados. Disponível apenas em laboratórios especializados.
- PCR — é comprovadamente mais sensível que os exames de hemocultura e sorologia na detecção de infecção em pacientes humanos.

DIAGNÓSTICO POR IMAGEM
- Indícios radiográficos de discospondilite — teste para brucelose.
- As alterações radiográficas são de desenvolvimento lento e podem não estar presentes mesmo na existência de dor na coluna vertebral.

MÉTODOS DIAGNÓSTICOS
Isolamento do Microrganismo
- Hemoculturas — quando os achados clínicos e sorológicos são sugestivos do diagnóstico; as espécies de *Brucella* serão facilmente isoladas a partir do sangue de cães infectados se eles não foram submetidos a antibióticos; o início da bacteremia ocorre 2-4 semanas depois da exposição oronasal e pode persistir por 8 meses a 5 anos e meio.
- Culturas de líquidos vaginais — após o abortamento; em geral, fornecem resultados positivos.
- Culturas do sêmen ou da urina — método impraticável no diagnóstico de rotina, já que o crescimento excessivo de contaminantes é comum.
- Amostras contaminadas — os meios de cultura com antibióticos em sua composição (p. ex., meio Thayer-Martin®) têm utilidade comprovada.

BRUCELOSE

Qualidade do Sêmen
- Motilidade dos espermatozoides, espermatozoides imaturos, células inflamatórias (neutrófilos) — em casos de epididimite.
- Anormalidades — evidenciadas geralmente em torno de 5-8 semanas após a infecção; notáveis por volta de 20 semanas.
- Aspermia sem células inflamatórias — comum em casos de atrofia testicular bilateral.

Biopsia de Linfonodo
- Revela hiperplasia linfoide associada a grande quantidade de plasmócitos.
- Se efetuada de modo asséptico, os tecidos deverão ser submetidos à cultura em meios adequados.
- Bactérias intracelulares — podem ser observadas dentro de macrófagos com o uso de colorações especiais (p. ex., corante de Brown-Brenn).
- Exame histopatológico dos testículos — com frequência, exibe vasculite necrosante, infiltração de células inflamatórias e lesões granulomatosas.

ACHADOS PATOLÓGICOS
- Macroscópicos — enfartamento dos linfonodos; esplenomegalia; machos caninos: epidídimos aumentados de volume e firmes, edema escrotal, ou atrofia de um ou ambos os testículos; infecção crônica: uveíte anterior e discospondilite.
- Microscópicos — relativamente compatíveis; hiperplasia linforreticular difusa; infecção crônica: sinusoides dos linfonodos com abundância de plasmócitos e macrófagos contendo bactérias; infiltrado linfocitário difuso e lesões granulomatosas em todos os órgãos geniturinários (especialmente próstata, epidídimo, útero e escroto); pode haver um extenso infiltrado de células inflamatórias e necrose do parênquima prostático e dos túbulos seminíferos.
- Alterações oculares — iridociclite granulomatosa; retinite exsudativa; exsudatos leucocitários na câmara anterior.

TRATAMENTO

CUIDADO(S) DE SAÚDE ADEQUADO(S)
Em um esquema ambulatorial.

ATIVIDADE
Restringir a atividade de cães ativos de trabalho.

ORIENTAÇÃO AO PROPRIETÁRIO
- O proprietário deve estar ciente de que o objetivo do tratamento consiste na erradicação da *B. canis* a partir do animal (constatação de soronegatividade e ausência de bacteremia por pelo menos 3 meses), mas algumas vezes o resultado corresponde a títulos de anticorpos persistentemente baixos sem nenhuma infecção sistêmica.
- Informar o proprietário sobre o fato de que o tratamento com antibióticos, especialmente minociclina e doxiciclina, é caro, demorado e controverso (em virtude dos resultados incertos).
- Não se recomenda o tratamento em canis reprodutores ou comerciais; dessa forma, ele é indicado apenas para cães sem fins reprodutivos ou aqueles já submetidos à castração.
- Antes de se tentar o tratamento em um animal doméstico intacto ou um cão reprodutor, é imprescindível que o proprietário esteja totalmente de acordo com a castração ou a eutanásia do animal em caso de falha terapêutica.

CONSIDERAÇÕES CIRÚRGICAS
Castração associada ao tratamento — quando a eutanásia for inaceitável para o proprietário.

MEDICAÇÕES

MEDICAMENTO(S) DE ESCOLHA
- Foram avaliados diversos esquemas terapêuticos, mas os resultados são duvidosos.
- Esquemas de maior êxito — combinação de alguma tetraciclina (cloridrato de tetraciclina, clortetraciclina ou minociclina a 25 mg/kg VO a cada 8 h por 4 semanas) ou doxiciclina (10 mg/kg VO a cada 12 h por 4 semanas) e diidroestreptomicina (10 mg/kg IM a cada 8 h durante a 1ª e a 4ª semana).
- Enrofloxacino (5 mg/kg VO a cada 24 h por 4 semanas).

CONTRAINDICAÇÕES
- Tetraciclinas — não utilizar em filhotes caninos prematuros.
- Gentamicina — contraindicada em casos de nefropatias.

PRECAUÇÕES
Gentamicina — monitorizar a função renal com rigor.

MEDICAMENTO(S) ALTERNATIVO(S)
Gentamicina — 3 mg/kg a cada 12 h; sucesso limitado; dados insuficientes sobre a eficácia quando associada à tetraciclina.

ACOMPANHAMENTO

MONITORIZAÇÃO DO PACIENTE
- Testes sorológicos — mensalmente por no mínimo 3 meses após o término do tratamento; o declínio contínuo e persistente no nível dos anticorpos até a negatividade indica o sucesso do tratamento.
- Infecções recrudescentes (elevação nos níveis dos anticorpos e recorrência da bacteremia após a terapia) — tratar novamente, castrar e repetir o tratamento ou submeter o animal à eutanásia.
- Hemoculturas — negativas por pelo menos 3 meses após o término do tratamento.

PREVENÇÃO
- Vacina — nenhuma; seu uso complicaria os testes sorológicos.
- Testes — testar todas as cadelas de uma linhagem, antes de entrarem no cio caso se planeje o cruzamento; testar em intervalos frequentes os machos utilizados como reprodutores.
- Efetuar a quarentena e testar todos os novos cães em intervalos quinzenais antes de permitir seu ingresso em um canil reprodutor.

COMPLICAÇÕES POSSÍVEIS
- Os proprietários podem se mostrar relutantes em autorizar a castração ou a eutanásia de cães valiosos, independentemente da falha terapêutica.
- Lembrar os proprietários sobre as ponderações éticas e sua obrigação de não comercializar nem distribuir cães infectados.

EVOLUÇÃO ESPERADA E PROGNÓSTICO
- Prognóstico reservado.
- Para cães infectados por <3-4 meses — a resposta terapêutica é provável.
- Infecções crônicas — os machos podem não responder à terapia.
- Casos de discospondilite — talvez haja necessidade de repetição do tratamento farmacológico, mas raramente há necessidade de intervenção cirúrgica.
- A combinação de múltiplos medicamentos como gentamicina ou estreptomicina, doxiciclina, enrofloxacino e rifampicina é bem-sucedida no tratamento de doença ocular em cães.
- Cães tratados (soronegativos) com êxito — são completamente suscetíveis à reinfecção.

DIVERSOS

POTENCIAL ZOONÓTICO
- Infecções em seres humanos — relatadas; geralmente brandas; respondem prontamente às tetraciclinas.
- Contudo, foi relatado um surto em 6 membros de uma família que vivia em contato estreito com uma cadela infectada.

GESTAÇÃO/FERTILIDADE/REPRODUÇÃO
- Os abortamentos com 45-60 dias de gestação são típicos.
- Os filhotes caninos gerados por cadelas infectadas podem ser acometidos pela infecção ou permanecer normais.

SINÔNIMO(S)
Abortamento canino contagioso.

ABREVIATURA(S)
- ELISA = ensaio imunoabsorvente ligado à enzima.
- IDAG = imunodifusão em ágar gel.
- LCS = líquido cerebrospinal.
- PCR = reação em cadeia da polimerase.
- TARL = teste de aglutinação rápida em lâmina com 2-mercaptoetanol.

Sugestões de Leitura
Carmichael LE, Greene CE. Canine brucellosis. In: Greene CE, ed., Infectious Diseases of the Dog and Cat, 3rd ed. St. Louis: Saunders Elsevier, 2006, pp. 369-381.
Ledbetter EC, Landry MP, Stokol T, et al. Brucella canis endophthalmitis in 3 dogs: Clinical features, diagnosis, and treatment. Vet Ophthalmology 2009, 12:183-191.
Keid LB, Soares RM, Vasconcellos SA, et al. Comparison of agar gel immunodiffusion test, rapid slide agglutination test, microbiological culture, and PCR for the diagnosis of canine brucellosis. Res Vet Sci 2009, 86:22-26.
Lucero NE, Corazza R, Almuzara MN, et al. Human Brucella canis outbreak linked to infection in dogs. Epidemiol Infect 2009, 5:1-6.
Wanke MM, Delpino MV, Baldi PC. Use of enrofloxacin in the treatment of canine brucellosis in a dog kennel (clinical trial). Theriogenology 2006, 66:1573-1578.

Autor Stephen C. Barr
Consultor Editorial Stephen C. Barr

Campilobacteriose

CONSIDERAÇÕES GERAIS

REVISÃO
• *Campylobacter jejuni* — bactéria Gram-negativa, curvilínea, microaerófila e fastidiosa; frequentemente isolada a partir do trato gastrintestinal de cães, gatos e outros mamíferos saudáveis; pode causar enterocolite erosiva superficial. • Infecção — via orofecal a partir da contaminação de alimento, água, carne fresca (ave, bovina) e do ambiente; localizada nas criptas intestinais preenchidas por muco; a motilidade rápida (flagelos) é essencial para a colonização; produz enterotoxina, citotoxina, toxina distensora citoletal e invasina. • Invasão da mucosa gastrintestinal — hematoquezia; leucócitos nas fezes; ulceração; edema; congestão intestinal; bacteremia; ocasionalmente, septicemia; bactérias eliminadas nas fezes por semanas a meses. • Até 49% dos cães sem diarreia e 45% dos gatos normais são portadores do *C. jejuni* e o eliminam pelas fezes. • Em cães mais jovens (mas não em gatos), maior quantidade de animais com diarreia elimina o *Campylobacter*, em comparação a controles diarreicos. • *Campylobacter* spp. (e *Salmonella* spp.) são frequentemente encontrados em dietas à base de carne crua (especialmente frango) fornecidas a cães e gatos.

IDENTIFICAÇÃO
• Cães e, menos comumente, gatos. • Prevalência — mais alta em filhotes caninos e felinos, desde o nascimento até os 6 meses de vida. • Pode resultar em doença crônica.

SINAIS CLÍNICOS
• Diarreia — varia desde o aspecto mucoso e aquoso até sanguinolento ou com estrias de bile; achado comum; pode ser crônica. • O tenesmo é comum. • Os sinais de febre (branda ou ausente), anorexia e vômito intermitente (duração de 3-15 dias) podem acompanhar a diarreia. • Animais jovens (até 6 meses de vida) — sinais clínicos mais graves; atribuíveis à enterocolite/diarreia. • Adultos — em geral, são portadores assintomáticos.

CAUSAS E FATORES DE RISCO
• *C. jejuni*, *C. coli*, *C. upsaliensis*, *C. gracilis*, *C. concisus*, *C. showae*, e *C. helveticus*. • Canis com má higiene e acúmulo fecal no ambiente. • Animais jovens — debilitados, imunossuprimidos ou parasitados (p. ex., *Giardia*, *Toxocara* e *Isospora*). • Em pacientes internados, pode ocorrer o desenvolvimento de infecção nosocomial. • Adultos — infecções gastrintestinais concomitantes (p. ex., *Salmonella*, parvovírus e anciló́stomos).

DIAGNÓSTICO

DIAGNÓSTICO DIFERENCIAL
• A identificação do animal, a anamnese e os exames físico e fecal (esfregaço direto e cultura bacteriana) possibilitam o diagnóstico em grande parte dos casos. • Diferenciar de outras causas de enterocolite aguda. • Enterocolite bacteriana — *Salmonella*, *Yersinia enterocolitica*, *Clostridium difficile* e *Clostridium perfringens*. • Enterocolite parasitária — helmintos (particularmente *Trichuris*) e protozoários (p. ex., *Giardia* e *Isospora*). • Enterocolite viral — parvovírus; os sinais frequentemente são mais graves do que em casos de *Campylobacter*. • Imprudência ou intolerância alimentar. • Medicamentos e toxinas. • Pancreatite aguda. • Pacientes gravemente acometidos — considerar também gastrenterite viral, intussuscepção e outras causas de dor abdominal. • Distinguir de outras causas de diarreia crônica. • Enteropatia primária.

HEMOGRAMA/BIOQUÍMICA/URINÁLISE
• Leucocitose — caso a cepa seja invasiva e ocorra bacteremia. • Anormalidades bioquímicas — efeitos da diarreia e da desidratação (p. ex., azotemia e distúrbios eletrolíticos).

MÉTODOS DIAGNÓSTICOS
• Leucócitos fecais — no trato gastrintestinal e nas fezes. • Coprocultura — microaerófila a aproximadamente 42°C por 48 horas em placas de ágar sangue especiais para o *Campylobacter*. • PCR quantitativa espécie-específica (PCRq) — exame cujo alvo é o gene da chaperonina de 60 kDa (cpn60) de diferentes espécies de *Campylobacter*.

Exame Fecal Direto
• Coloração de Gram — fazer um esfregaço das fezes aquosas sobre uma lâmina de vidro; fixar pelo calor; utilizar o corante de Gram; deixar o neutralizador (safranina) por mais tempo que o normal. • Câmara úmida — gotejar uma pequena quantidade de fezes (se não estiverem aquosas, misturá-las com um pouco de solução salina) em uma lâmina de vidro; cobrir com lamínula; examinar em objetiva de fase ou de campo escuro (× 40); observar uma grande quantidade de bactérias curvilíneas e altamente móveis (motilidade rápida característica).

ACHADOS PATOLÓGICOS
• Macroscópicos — espessamento e congestão/edema difusos do cólon; hiperemia do intestino delgado; enfartamento dos linfonodos mesentéricos.
• Em gatos infectados, foi descrito espessamento da musculatura lisa do intestino.

TRATAMENTO

ENTEROCOLITE LEVE
• Em esquema ambulatorial. • Geralmente autolimitante.

ENTEROCOLITE GRAVE
• Internação, especialmente de pacientes neonatais e imaturos. • Doença neonatal grave — isolar o paciente; confinar em gaiola; monitorizar; incentivar o repouso. • Não fornecer nada por via oral durante 24 h; em seguida, oferecer uma dieta leve. • Desidratação branda — fluidoterapia oral com solução de reposição hídrica entérica. • Desidratação grave — fluidoterapia intravenosa com solução isotônica poliônica balanceada. • Se a albumina sérica estiver abaixo de 2 g/dL, poderá ser necessária a realização de transfusões de plasma. • Adsorventes e protetores intestinais de ação local.

MEDICAÇÕES

MEDICAMENTO(S)
• Antibióticos — recomendados na presença de sinais de doença sistêmica (p. ex., febre alta ou desidratação) quando a diarreia ou os sinais clínicos anormais persistem por mais de 7 dias e em pacientes imunossuprimidos. • Eritromicina — 10-20 mg/kg VO a cada 8 h por 5 dias; medicamento de escolha. • Enrofloxacino: cão, 5-20 mg/kg a cada 24 h VO, IV, IM. Efeito adverso de artropatia em cães com 4-28 semanas de vida. Gato, 5 mg/kg a cada 24 h VO, IM. • Tilosina — 11 mg/kg VO a cada 8 h por 7 dias; pode ser eficaz. • Neomicina — 10-20 mg/kg VO a cada 6-12 h por 5 dias; pode ser eficiente. • Penicilinas e ampicilina — potencialmente ineficazes. • Septicemia — pode-se instituir a administração de antibióticos parenterais com algum aminoglicosídeo (p. ex., amicacina) e alguma cefalosporina.

CONTRAINDICAÇÕES/INTERAÇÕES POSSÍVEIS
• Ficam contraindicados os medicamentos antidiarreicos que diminuem a motilidade intestinal.
• Enrofloxacino — pode induzir à artropatia se administrado a cães com menos de 28 semanas de vida. Não administrar a gatos doses >5 mg/kg nem administrar por via IV.

ACOMPANHAMENTO

MONITORIZAÇÃO DO PACIENTE
Repetir a coprocultura após o término do tratamento.

PREVENÇÃO
• Boa higiene (lavagem das mãos). • Limpar e desinfetar com certa rotina as instalações e os corredores de passagem dos animais, bem como os comedouros e os bebedouros. • Não fornecer dietas à base de carne crua aos animais de companhia.

EVOLUÇÃO ESPERADA E PROGNÓSTICO
• Adultos — geralmente autolimitante. • Jovens com enterocolite grave ou persistente — tratar com antibióticos.

DIVERSOS

DISTÚRBIOS ASSOCIADOS
Infecção concomitante pelo *Campylobacter* e por outras bactérias patogênicas, parasitas entéricos ou agentes virais.

POTENCIAL ZOONÓTICO
Alto potencial de infecção em seres humanos (especialmente *C. jejuni*, *C. coli*, *C. upsaliensis*, *C. gracilis*, *C. concisus*, *C. showae*).

GESTAÇÃO/FERTILIDADE/REPRODUÇÃO
• Eritromicina — antibiótico seguro para uso no início da gestação. • Cloranfenicol e gentamicina — não utilizar em animais prenhes.

ABREVIATURAS
• PCR = reação em cadeia da polimerase.

Autor Patrick L. McDonough
Consultor Editorial Stephen C. Barr

CANDIDÍASE

CONSIDERAÇÕES GERAIS

REVISÃO
• *Candida* — parte integrante da flora normal da boca, do nariz, das orelhas, bem como dos tratos gastrintestinal e genital de cães e gatos; seu isolamento a partir das superfícies mucosas não implica a existência de doença; microrganismo oportunista que coloniza tecidos lesionados ou invade tecidos normais de animais imunossuprimidos; seu papel patogênico é determinado pela identificação do fungo no sangue (fungemia), pela infiltração do microrganismo nos tecidos ou por indícios desse agente em locais supostamente estéreis (p. ex., bexiga urinária).
• Isolamento — as condições supressoras do sistema imunológico aumentam a probabilidade de isolamento do microrganismo em animais assintomáticos; isolado a partir de culturas orofaríngeas (garganta) em uma frequência cinco vezes maior em gatos infectados pelo FIV do que naqueles assintomáticos não infectados por esse vírus, de idade e sexo semelhantes.
• Infecção — rara; associada a neutropenia, infecção pelo parvovírus, diabetes melito, imunossupressão induzida por retrovírus, glicocorticoterapia crônica, hiperadrenocorticismo, antibioticoterapia prolongada, tubos inseridos via gastrotomia, sondas urinárias de demora, uretrostomia, cateteres IV, e esvaziamento vesical incompleto. Cistite bacteriana e cálculos urinários podem predispor o paciente à infecção fúngica.
• Ocasionalmente se observa infecção local ou sistêmica por *Candida* em animais sem condições predisponentes.

IDENTIFICAÇÃO
Cães e gatos de qualquer idade e raça.

SINAIS CLÍNICOS
• Envolvimento da bexiga urinária — cistite.
• Otite — meneios da cabeça e arranhadura.
• Envolvimento da cavidade bucal — salivação.
• Inflamação em torno dos cateteres IV ou dos tubos inseridos via gastrotomia e possível febre.
• Lesões cutâneas eritematosas e ulcerativas.
• Pode ser observada uma doença sistêmica com pericardite, espondilite, e sinais neurológicos.

CAUSAS & FATORES DE RISCO
• Pele lesionada por queimaduras, traumatismos ou dermatite necrosante.
• Trato urinário — local preferido em cães e gatos diabéticos e naqueles com retenção urinária decorrente de estenoses secundárias à uretrostomia; sondas de demora.
• Neutropenia secundária à infecção por parvovírus, FeLV ou FIV, ou à mielossupressão por quimioterapia.
• Cateteres IV.

DIAGNÓSTICO

DIAGNÓSTICO DIFERENCIAL
A candidíase é considerada sempre que o distúrbio primário não responder conforme o esperado.

HEMOGRAMA/BIOQUÍMICA/URINÁLISE
• Refletem o distúrbio subjacente.

• Urinálise — pode revelar a fase leveduriforme ou aglomerados de elementos miceliais (pseudo-hifas), acompanhados por um aumento nas células inflamatórias; com frequência, ocorre infecção bacteriana do trato urinário juntamente com a infecção fúngica.
• Pacientes neutropênicos — pode não ocorrer uma resposta inflamatória.

OUTROS TESTES LABORATORIAIS
Piúria sem crescimento bacteriano — solicitar cultura para fungos e *Mycoplasma*.

MÉTODOS DIAGNÓSTICOS
• Lesões — biopsia para estudo histopatológico a fim de determinar se a *Candida*, de fato, está atuando como patógeno; exige a demonstração da penetração tecidual pelos microrganismos. Podem ser observadas hifas em tecidos profundos e leveduras na superfície.
• Amostra urinária — coletar por meio de cistocentese e submeter à cultura; a obtenção de muitas colônias de *Candida* é fortemente sugestiva do diagnóstico; esperar por infecção bacteriana concomitante.
• Otite (cães) — a cultura da *Candida* ou a identificação de leveduras ou elementos miceliais na citologia otológica sugere o diagnóstico.
• Em pacientes febris, submeter as pontas de cateteres à cultura para pesquisa de bactérias e fungos.
• Hemocultura pode identificar os microrganismos fúngicos.

ACHADOS PATOLÓGICOS
• Pode ser observada a presença de focos caseosos brancos no tecido infectado.
• Em geral, observa-se uma grande quantidade tanto de leveduras como de pseudo-hifas nos tecidos, circundadas por necrose e reação inflamatória supurativa.
• Em locais mais crônicos de infecção, a resposta pode ser piogranulomatosa.

TRATAMENTO

• Estabilizar os casos de diabetes melito e controlar o hiperadrenocorticismo.
• Remover as sondas de demora.
• Se possível, melhorar o estado imunológico contra a imunossupressão.

MEDICAÇÕES

MEDICAMENTO(S)
• Fluconazol — 5 mg/kg VO a cada 12 h (cães e gatos); muito eficaz; excretado de forma inalterada na urina, atingindo alta concentração nos locais comumente infectados.
• Itraconazol — eficaz; utilizar se o microrganismo se tornar resistente ao fluconazol; não é recomendado em casos de infecção do trato urinário por não ser excretado na urina.
• Nas infecções do trato urinário pela *Candida* resistentes ao fluconazol, infundir 10 a 30 mL de clotrimazol a 1% na bexiga urinária em dias alternados por 3 vezes.
• A *Candida* pode desenvolver resistência medicamentosa. Se a infecção persistir, entrar em contato com Fungus Testing Lab para a realização de teste de sensibilidade.

ACOMPANHAMENTO

MONITORIZAÇÃO DO PACIENTE
• Fluconazol e itraconazol — hepatotoxicidade; monitorizar os níveis séricos da ALT mensalmente e avaliar se o paciente se torna anoréxico; suspender o medicamento se a ALT ficar acima de 200 UI ou em casos de anorexia.
• Subsequente ao desaparecimento dos sinais — solicitar novas culturas das áreas infectadas; continuar o tratamento por mais 2 semanas; repetir as culturas 2 semanas após o término do tratamento e, novamente, em caso de recidiva dos sinais.

EVOLUÇÃO ESPERADA E PROGNÓSTICO
• O quadro deve desaparecer dentro de 2-4 semanas de tratamento se a imunossupressão for corrigida.
• Para evitar as recidivas, faz-se necessário o controle da doença subjacente.
• Pode apresentar resolução espontânea se o distúrbio subjacente for corrigido.

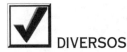

DIVERSOS

POTENCIAL ZOONÓTICO
Similaridades genéticas entre isolamentos do microrganismo em seres humanos e animais sugerem um potencial de transmissão da *C. albicans* entre as espécies.

ABREVIATURA(S)
• ALT = alanina aminotransferase.
• FIV = vírus da imunodeficiência felina.
• FeLV = vírus da leucemia felina.

Sugestões de Leitura
Forward ZA, Legendre AM, Khalsa HDS. Use of intermittent bladder infusion with clotrimazole for treatment of candiduria in a dog. JAVMA 2002, 220:1496-1498.
Greene CE, Chandler FW. Candidiasis and rhodotorulosis. In: Greene CE, ed., Infectious Diseases of the Dog and Cat, 3rd ed. St. Louis: Saunders Elsevier, 2006, pp. 627-633.
Jin Y, Lin D. Fungal urinary tract infections in the dog and cat: A retrospective study (2001-2004). JAAHA 2005, 41:373-381.
Pressler BM, Vaden SL, Lane IF, et al. Candida spp. urinary tract infections in 13 dogs and seven cats: Predisposing factors, treatment, and outcome. JAAHA 2003, 39:263-270.

Autor Alfred M. Legendre
Consultor Editorial Stephen C. Barr

Capilaríase (Pearsonema)

CONSIDERAÇÕES GERAIS

REVISÃO
- *Pearsonema* e *Capillaria* são nomes empregados de forma intercambiável e parecem ser idênticos em termos de taxonomia e comportamento biológico.
- *Pearsonema* (*Capillaria*) *plica* são parasitas pequenos, amarelos e filiformes que invadem a mucosa ou a submucosa da bexiga urinária e, raramente, da pelve renal e do ureter, provocando uma resposta inflamatória leve.
- A *P. plica* em cães e gatos e a *P. feliscati* em gatos raramente se associam a sinais de doença do trato urinário inferior.
- A *P. plica* elimina ovos bioperculados na urina. Após a ingestão de ovos embrionados por minhocas, o parasita evolui para o estágio infectante. A ingestão de minhocas infectadas resulta na infecção patente dos cães em 58-88 dias. Alguns pesquisadores forneceram provas de um ciclo biológico direto.
- O ciclo vital da *P. feliscati* é pouco compreendido.

IDENTIFICAÇÃO
- Cães — não há relatos de predisposição. Relatada em cães, raposas, coiotes, guaxinins, martens, martas, texugos, lontras, linces, doninhas/fuinhas, lobos.
- Gatos — os animais acometidos quase sempre têm mais de 8 meses de vida.

SINAIS CLÍNICOS
- Em geral, ausentes.
- Polaciúria, hematúria, estrangúria e disúria em alguns animais intensamente infectados.

CAUSAS E FATORES DE RISCO
Cães
- A alta prevalência de infecção (até 50%) nos hospedeiros naturais (p. ex., raposas e guaxinins) no sudeste dos Estados Unidos pode predispor os animais dessa região geográfica.
- Em canis, as altas taxas de infecção associam-se a solos contaminados.

Gatos
Rara nos Estados Unidos; na Austrália, relata-se uma prevalência de 18-34% da infecção.

DIAGNÓSTICO

DIAGNÓSTICO DIFERENCIAL
Considerar outras causas mais comuns de doença do trato urinário inferior, como urolitíase, infecção do trato urinário, traumatismo e neoplasia.

HEMOGRAMA/BIOQUÍMICA/URINÁLISE
- A presença de ovos incolores bioperculados com leve depressão no sedimento urinário é diagnóstica.
- Considerar a possibilidade de contaminação fecal da urina por ovos de *Trichuris vulpis* ou outros ovos morfologicamente similares ao se utilizar amostras urinárias obtidas por micção espontânea ou caso ocorra uma punção retal inadvertida e aspiração de fezes com *T. vulpis* durante a cistocentese.
- Alternativamente, a contaminação das fezes por urina pode produzir achados falsos no exame fecal do animal acometido.
- Infecções sintomáticas costumam ser associadas a indícios de inflamação (hemácias, leucócitos e proteinúria). As culturas urinárias bacterianas são tipicamente estéreis.

OUTROS TESTES LABORATORIAIS
N/D.

DIAGNÓSTICO POR IMAGEM
N/D.

MÉTODOS DIAGNÓSTICOS
N/D.

TRATAMENTO

- A infecção costuma ser autolimitante em ambas as espécies.
- Os ovos não serão mais detectáveis no sedimento urinário de cães infectados em 10-12 semanas se esses animais forem isolados.
- A substituição dos pisos de terra por areia, cascalho ou concreto pode reduzir a prevalência da infecção em canis contaminados por *P. plica* e *P. feliscati*.

MEDICAÇÕES

MEDICAMENTO(S)
- Considerar a terapia anti-helmíntica na presença de sinais clínicos; monitorar o sucesso terapêutico pelo exame do sedimento urinário em busca de ovos e pela observação dos sinais clínicos.
- Pode haver a necessidade de múltiplos cursos terapêuticos para eliminar a infecção.
- Há relatos de que o fembendazol (50 mg/kg VO a cada 24 h durante 3 dias) resulte no desaparecimento dos ovos do sedimento urinário em cães e gatos.
- Sugere-se a ivermectina (0,2 mg/kg SC em dose única) como uma terapia alternativa; no entanto, há poucas informações objetivas a respeito de sua eficácia nessa doença.
- Há relatos de que o tratamento oral com albendazol (50 mg/kg VO a cada 12 h por 30 dias) seja eficaz em cães.

CONTRAINDICAÇÕES/INTERAÇÕES POSSÍVEIS
N/D.

ACOMPANHAMENTO

- Monitorizar o sucesso terapêutico, por meio da avaliação do sedimento urinário em busca de ovos do parasita e da observação dos sinais clínicos do paciente.
- Na ausência de reinfecção, a capilaríase urinária pode ser autolimitante. Portanto, o isolamento de cães e gatos das minhocas deve ser suficiente para eliminar uma infecção vesical por *Capillaria* em 90 dias.

DIVERSOS

SINÔNIMOS
Pearsonema.

RECURSOS DA INTERNET
Companion Animal Parasite Council: http://www.capcvet.org.

Sugestões de Leitura
Brown SA, Prestwood KA. Parasites of the urinary tract. In: Kirk RW, ed. Current veterinary therapy IX. Philadelphia: Saunders, 1986:1153-1155.

Autor Carl A. Osborne
Consultor Editorial Carl A. Osborne
Agradecimento O autor e o editor agradecem a contribuição prévia de Susan E. Little.

Carcinoide e Síndrome Carcinoide

CONSIDERAÇÕES GERAIS

REVISÃO
- Siegfried Oberndorfer criou o termo carcinoide ("semelhante a carcinoma") em 1907 para descrever um tumor gastrintestinal em ser humano, com a característica peculiar de comportamento semelhante a um tumor benigno. Os tumores carcinoides são tumores neuroendócrinos que surgem de células do sistema APUD (sistema de captação e descarboxilação de aminas precursoras).
- Os carcinoides originam-se mais comumente das células enterocromafins e células tipo-enterocromafins do trato gastrintestinal, mas também podem ser encontrados em órgãos como fígado, árvore traqueobronquial, pâncreas e sistema geniturinário em função das origens embriológicas.
- Os carcinoides podem secretar uma variedade de aminas, como histamina, serotonina, e peptídeos como bradicininas e taquicininas. Em seres humanos, essas substâncias secretoras podem causar uma "síndrome carcinoide" e/ou "crise carcinoide" bem identificada em aproximadamente 5-10% dos pacientes acometidos por carcinoides uma vez que a metástase tenha ocorrido no fígado e a degradação hepática de tais substâncias seja desviada. A síndrome carcinoide humana é mais comumente caracterizada por rubor, dor abdominal, diarreia, broncospasmo, e cianose. Até o momento, não há relatos de que os pequenos animais domésticos demonstrem esses sinais clínicos, embora um cão tenha sido recentemente relatado por ter colapso episódico e melena em associação a um carcinoide ileocecal. As taxas de morbidade e mortalidade dependem com maior frequência do tamanho do tumor e da obstrução do trato gastrintestinal em cães e gatos com carcinoide.
- Foram relatados tumores carcinoides primários em órgãos como estômago, intestino delgado, cólon, pulmão, vesícula biliar e fígado em cães. Em gatos, os carcinoides foram encontrados no estômago, intestino delgado, fígado e coração.

IDENTIFICAÇÃO
- Cão — raro, geralmente >8-9 anos de idade.
- Gato — raro, geralmente >7-8 anos de idade.

SINAIS CLÍNICOS
- Os sinais clínicos dependem geralmente da localização do tumor primário e/ou da ocorrência de metástases, podendo incluir:
  - Anorexia. ○ Vômito. ○ Disquesia. ○ Melena.
  - Colapso episódico. ○ Ascite. ○ Perda de peso.
  - Sinais de insuficiência hepática.
- Cardiopatia carcinoide é uma síndrome em seres humanos com síndrome carcinoide avançada que ocorre em virtude do desenvolvimento de placas endocárdicas fibróticas e disfunção valvar secundária em resposta ao excesso de secreção de serotonina.

DIAGNÓSTICO

DIAGNÓSTICO DIFERENCIAL
Os diagnósticos diferenciais variam dependendo da queixa apresentada e incluem doenças gastrintestinais primárias, como outras neoplasias, infecções, inflamações, parasitas, ingestão de corpo estranho, alimentação inadequada ou imprudência alimentar, ou doença hepática/biliar.

HEMOGRAMA/BIOQUÍMICA/URINÁLISE
- Os resultados podem aparecer normais, exceto por uma anemia leve geralmente arregenerativa.
- Anormalidades eletrolíticas e enzimas hepáticas elevadas podem estar presentes, dependendo da localização e da apresentação clínica.

OUTROS TESTES LABORATORIAIS
- Serotonina sérica, cromogranina A sérica e ácido 5-hidroxindolacético urinário são mensurados em seres humanos com suspeita de tumores carcinoides. Esses testes parecem mais diagnósticos do que a mensuração direta dos níveis séricos de aminas e peptídeos.
- Foram constatados níveis séricos elevados de serotonina (10 vezes maior) em um cão com carcinoide intestinal com múltiplas metástases. Não foram documentados outros testes séricos e urinários em animais com tumores carcinoides.

DIAGNÓSTICO POR IMAGEM
- A ultrassonografia é usada para identificar tanto os tumores primários como as metástases no abdome e tórax de cães e gatos.
- As imagens de TC e RM são utilizadas com sucesso leve a moderado para a localização de carcinoides em seres humanos.
- Modalidades de imagem molecular mais recentes e mais sensíveis incluem o uso de (1) cintilografia para receptores de somatostatina e octreotida radiomarcada ("OctreoScan"), (2) imagem com metaiodobenzilguanidina (MIBG) radiomarcada com iodo e (3) imagens obtidas por PET.

MÉTODOS DIAGNÓSTICOS
- A biopsia do tecido acometido com exame histopatológico frequentemente confirma o diagnóstico. • Se os resultados histopatológicos forem duvidosos, podem ser usados os exames de microscopia eletrônica e/ou imuno-histoquímica (para pesquisa da expressão de cromogranina A e/ou sinaptofisina) para determinar as aminas e os peptídeos ativamente secretados com o objetivo de auxiliar na confirmação do diagnóstico de carcinoide.

ACHADOS PATOLÓGICOS
Esses tumores tipicamente possuem um estroma fibrovascular fino com pleomorfismo celular mínimo a moderado. O citoplasma é eosinofílico e, em geral, contém grânulos secretores que frequentemente são argirofílicos e/ou argentafina-positivos.

TRATAMENTO

Em muitos casos, a excisão cirúrgica pode ser curativa, especialmente quando não houver evidência de metástase. A ressecção pode diminuir a secreção de hormônio em seres humanos e pode aliviar os sinais gastrintestinais em animais que estão obstruídos por causa do tamanho do tumor.

MEDICAÇÕES

MEDICAMENTO(S)
- Octreotida, um análogo da somatostatina, é frequentemente usada em seres humanos como terapia paliativa quando a cirurgia não constitui uma opção terapêutica. A octreotida inibe a secreção de hormônio das células tumorais. Como a síndrome carcinoide não parece ser o principal mecanismo da doença nos animais com relatos de tumores carcinoides, a octreotida pode ser de pouco benefício em pacientes veterinários com carcinoides.
- Altas doses de MIBG radiomarcada com iodo estão sendo utilizadas com sucesso moderado em seres humanos com carcinoide não ressecável e/ou metastático.
- As interferonas têm demonstrado um êxito limitado em seres humanos com tumores carcinoides. Até o momento, não foi relatado o uso de interferonas para o tratamento de cães ou gatos com carcinoide.
- Há relatos de que a quimiorradioterapia tenha uma eficácia mínima em seres humanos com tumores carcinoides, pois se acredita que os carcinoides sejam relativamente resistentes à quimiorradioterapia.
- O uso de carboplatina adjuvante foi recém-relatado em um cão com carcinoide jejunal não metastático submetido à excisão completa.

ACOMPANHAMENTO

- O exame de sangue deve ser monitorado de forma seriada no pós-operatório para delinear a metástase hepática destrutiva.
- Também é recomendável a realização de ultrassonografia abdominal e radiografias torácicas (em três projeções) seriadas no pós-operatório para delinear a metástase para o fígado e/ou outros órgãos.

DIVERSOS

ABREVIATURAS
- TC = tomografia computadorizada.
- MIBG = metaiodobenzilguanidina.
- RM = ressonância magnética.
- PET = tomografia por emissão de pósitrons.

RECURSOS DA INTERNET
- www.cancer.gov/cancertopics/types/gastrointestinalcarcinoid.
- www.carcinoid.com.
- www.carcinoid.org.

Sugestões de Leitura
Rossmeisl JH Jr., Forrester SD, Robertson JL, Cook WT. Chronic vomiting associated with a gastric carcinoid in a cat. JAAHA 2002, 38(1):61-66.
Sugnini EP, Gargiulo M, Assin R, D'Avino A, Mellone P, Citro G, Cardelli P, Baldi A. Adjuvant carboplatin for the treatment of intestinal carcinoid in a dog. In Vivo 2008, 22(6):759-761.

Autor Phil Bergman
Consultor Editorial Deborah Greco

Carcinoma de Células de Transição

CONSIDERAÇÕES GERAIS

DEFINIÇÃO
Malignidade originária do epitélio de transição renal, ureteral, vesical, uretral, prostático ou vaginal.

FISIOPATOLOGIA
A etiologia subjacente do carcinoma de células de transição ainda permanece incerta. É possível que algum carcinógeno ambiental possa desencadear ou promover a transformação maligna do epitélio de transição. Os possíveis agentes etiológicos investigados incluem produtos utilizados para o controle de pulgas à base de organofosforados e carbamatos, além da ciclofosfamida.

SISTEMA(S) ACOMETIDO(S)
- Rins — acometidos com menor frequência; possível local de carcinoma primário de células de transição.
- Bexiga (pode ou não incluir os ureteres) — o trígono vesical é o local mais comumente envolvido em cães. A invasão local da porção distal do ureter também é comum e pode levar à azotemia pós-renal. O ápice da bexiga urinária é muito mais acometido em gatos, embora toda a bexiga frequentemente esteja envolvida no momento do diagnóstico em virtude da detecção tardia do tumor.
- Uretra — constitui o segundo local mais comum em cães; alguns pacientes apresentam obstrução uretral e azotemia pós-renal.
- Vagina — costuma ser menos acometida; representa um possível local de carcinoma primário de células de transição.
- Próstata — pode ser envolvida por invasão local ou como o local primário do carcinoma de células de transição.
- Locais de metástases — os linfonodos regionais e os pulmões são os mais comuns; outros locais incluem ossos, cérebro e olhos.
- Envolvimento paraneoplásico de órgãos — há relatos de casos de osteopatia hipertrófica secundária ao carcinoma de células de transição da bexiga.

GENÉTICA
N/D.

INCIDÊNCIA/PREVALÊNCIA
- Representa menos de 1% de todas as malignidades relatadas em cães.
- Raro em gatos.

DISTRIBUIÇÃO GEOGRÁFICA
N/D.

IDENTIFICAÇÃO
As cadelas castradas de pequeno porte, de meia-idade a idosas, costumam ser mais descritas com a doença.

Espécies
- Cães e gatos.

Raça(s) Predominante(s)
- Os cães da raça Terrier escocês têm um risco 18 vezes maior em comparação a outras raças.
- As raças West Highland white terrier, Pastor de shetland, Esquimó americano e Dachshund também podem ser acometidas.
- Pode ocorrer em qualquer raça.
- Não há predisposição racial em gatos.

Idade Média e Faixa Etária
- Cães — 8 anos; faixa, 1-15 anos de idade ou mais.

Sexo Predominante
- Fêmea.

SINAIS CLÍNICOS

Comentários Gerais
- Semelhantes aos sinais de infecção bacteriana do trato urinário ou urolitíase.
- Considerar o carcinoma de células de transição em pacientes que exibem uma resposta temporária ou nula à antibioticoterapia adequada.

Achados Anamnésicos
- Queixas de estrangúria, polaciúria, hematúria, disúria, incontinência urinária recidivantes ou qualquer combinação dos sinais mencionados anteriormente devem incitar a pesquisa por carcinoma de células de transição.
- Os sinais podem responder temporariamente à antibioticoterapia.

Achados do Exame Físico
- Com frequência, permanecem normais.
- Ocasionalmente, há massa palpável na região hipogástrica/vesical.
- O carcinoma de células de transição da uretra/vagina/próstata pode ser palpável ao exame retal.
- Enfartamento dos linfonodos intrapélvicos ou sublombares é raramente palpável ao exame retal.

CAUSAS
- Cães — os fatores de risco relatados incluem obesidade, carcinógenos ambientais, exposição crônica a organofosforados ou carbamatos e, (raramente), ciclofosfamida sob altas doses em bólus ou a longo prazo.
- Gatos — desconhecidas.

FATORES DE RISCO
Cães — raça Terrier escocês, obesidade, exposição a organofosforados ou carbamatos, terapia com ciclofosfamida.

DIAGNÓSTICO

DIAGNÓSTICO DIFERENCIAL
- Condições não neoplásicas — infecção bacteriana do trato urinário, urolitíase, uretrite, vaginite, prostatite.
- Condições neoplásicas — outras neoplasias primárias (p. ex., carcinoma de células escamosas) ou metastáticas (p. ex., carcinoma prostático localmente invasivo).

HEMOGRAMA/BIOQUÍMICA/URINÁLISE
- Hemograma completo e perfil bioquímico — costumam permanecer dentro dos limites de normalidade.
- Bioquímica — pode exibir sinais de azotemia renal e/ou pós-renal em caso de obstrução ureteral ou uretral.
- Urinálise — pode revelar células epiteliais com múltiplos critérios de malignidade; se a amostra apresentar células inflamatórias, será preciso interpretar o exame citológico com cautela, pois as células epiteliais podem exibir critérios de malignidade na presença de inflamação.

OUTROS TESTES LABORATORIAIS
- Cultura urinária e antibiograma — são indicados, em virtude do achado habitual de infecção concomitante do trato urinário; no entanto, é preciso ter cuidado ao se realizar a cistocentese em pacientes com suspeita de carcinoma de células de transição, pois pode ocorrer a disseminação das células tumorais ao longo do trajeto da agulha.
- Biopsia (cirúrgica, traumática por cateter ou cistoscópica) — constitui o método com padrão de excelência para o diagnóstico definitivo. Mesmo com uma baixa recuperação de amostras teciduais de algumas cateterizações traumáticas, é obtida uma quantidade tipicamente suficiente de células para a formulação de um diagnóstico citológico.

DIAGNÓSTICO POR IMAGEM

Radiografias Torácicas
- Padrões metastáticos incluem múltiplos nódulos intersticiais bem-definidos, padrão intersticial elevado e infiltrados alveolares.

Radiografias Abdominais
- Provavelmente não revelarão doença vesical específica a menos que a massa esteja mineralizada (raro).
- Podem revelar linfadenomegalia sublombar ou metástase óssea.

Cistografia com Duplo Contraste
- Cães — lesão expansiva, geralmente no trígono vesical.
- Gatos — lesão expansiva, que pode estar no ápice da bexiga urinária.
- Dependendo do local primário, os exames de pielografia intravenosa, uretrograma miccional ou vaginograma podem ser indicados.

Ultrassonografia
- Técnica altamente sensível de diagnóstico por imagem, útil na identificação do local e da extensão da doença; contudo, não constitui um método confiável para monitorizar a resposta à terapia.

OUTROS MÉTODOS DIAGNÓSTICOS

Laparotomia Exploratória
- Usada para obter amostras de biopsias do tumor primário e dos linfonodos regionais.
- A cura cirúrgica é muito improvável em função da natureza infiltrativa do tumor.
- Como a disseminação tumoral é admitida nos casos de carcinoma de células de transição, é preciso trocar as luvas e os instrumentos cirúrgicos após a manipulação do tumor.

Cistoscopia
- Representa o meio menos invasivo para a identificação e a biopsia do carcinoma de células de transição dentro da bexiga ou da uretra.

Cateterização Traumática
- Utilizar um cateter de polipropileno para obtenção traumática de pequenas amostras teciduais para o diagnóstico histológico ou citológico.

Biopsia Guiada por Ultrassom
- Não é recomendável, pois a disseminação de células tumorais viáveis pelo trajeto da agulha de biopsia é uma sequela altamente possível.

ACHADOS MACROSCÓPICOS E HISTOPATOLÓGICOS
- Espessamento irregular a difuso da mucosa vesical.
- Possível metástase a linfonodos regionais, pulmões e ossos (ou seja, vértebra, pelve).

TRATAMENTO
É provável que a radioterapia venha a ser a opção terapêutica mais comum com aparelhos modulados por intensidade ou de tomoterapia.

Carcinoma de Células de Transição

INTERNAÇÃO VERSUS TRATAMENTO AMBULATORIAL
- A avaliação inicial e o diagnóstico levam 1-2 dias.
- Os pacientes estáveis não necessitam de internação.

ATIVIDADE
Normal.

DIETA
Normal a menos que haja insuficiência renal concomitante.

ORIENTAÇÃO AO PROPRIETÁRIO
- Prognóstico mau a longo prazo.
- É frequentemente possível o tratamento paliativo.
- A doença não costuma ser passível de ressecção cirúrgica em cães.

CONSIDERAÇÕES CIRÚRGICAS
- O carcinoma de células de transição é altamente esfoliativo e transplantável — há múltiplos relatos de disseminação de células tumorais induzida por via cirúrgica.
- É recomendável a substituição de todos os instrumentos cirúrgicos e luvas depois de entrar em contato com o tumor.
- Até 50% da bexiga urinária pode ser submetida à ressecção com perda mínima da função.
- A colocação de sonda via cistostomia pode prolongar o tempo de sobrevida, por desviar a obstrução uretral.
- A colocação de *stent** uretral também pode prolongar a sobrevida, por aliviar a obstrução temporariamente.

MEDICAÇÕES

MEDICAMENTO(S) DE ESCOLHA
- Piroxicam (0,3 mg/kg VO a cada 24 h juntamente com o alimento); há relatos de que esse medicamento tenha efeito em cerca de 15% dos casos com sobrevida média de 180 dias.
- Convencionalmente, emprega-se a cisplatina (50-70 mg/m² IV a cada 3 semanas em cães); contudo, a atividade relatada não é superior a 20% dos casos.
- Terapia combinada de mitoxantrona (5 mg/m² IV a cada 3 semanas) e piroxicam apresenta uma taxa de resposta relatada de 35% com sobrevida média de 291 dias.

---
* N. T.: Dispositivo metálico, utilizado com a finalidade de manter o lúmen de artéria ou trajeto permeável, com seu calibre próximo do normal, formando uma nova "parede" para o vaso ou ducto.

- Outros agentes quimioterápicos como doxorrubicina (utilizada isoladamente ou em combinação com ciclofosfamida) podem ter ação contra esse tipo de tumor.

CONTRAINDICAÇÕES
- Piroxicam — não utilizar em animais com erosões ou úlceras gastrintestinais conhecidas; não usar em pacientes com insuficiência renal.
- Piroxicam — não combinar com a cisplatina.
- A terapia com piroxicam parece ser tolerada em gatos, mas em uma frequência posológica reduzida (a cada 48 h) em comparação aos cães.
- Cisplatina — não é recomendada em gatos; não empregar em animais com insuficiência renal.

PRECAUÇÕES
- Animais com carcinoma de células de transição podem ter dano renal causado por hidroureter, hidronefrose ou pielonefrite, secundariamente à infecção crônica do trato urinário associada ao tumor.
- Os cães submetidos à quimioterapia devem ser monitorizados quanto à ocorrência de mielossupressão.
- Buscar orientação especializada antes de iniciar o tratamento caso não se esteja familiarizado com o uso dos medicamentos citotóxicos.

INTERAÇÕES POSSÍVEIS
Não é recomendável o uso concomitante da cisplatina com outros agentes nefrotóxicos (p. ex., antibióticos aminoglicosídeos).

MEDICAMENTO(S) ALTERNATIVO(S)
Antibióticos — a antibioticoterapia deve ser administrada conforme a necessidade.

ACOMPANHAMENTO

MONITORIZAÇÃO DO PACIENTE
- Cistografia contrastada ou ultrassonografia — a cada 6-8 semanas para avaliar o estado da doença.
- Radiografias torácicas — a cada 2-3 meses para detectar a presença de metástases.

PREVENÇÃO
Orientar o proprietário sobre a necessidade de micção frequente após a terapia com ciclofosfamida para minimizar o tempo de contato com a mucosa vesical.

COMPLICAÇÕES POSSÍVEIS
- Obstrução uretral ou ureteral e insuficiência renal.
- Metástase para linfonodos regionais, pulmões ou ossos.
- Infecção recidivante do trato urinário.
- Incontinência urinária.
- Mielossupressão ou toxicidade gastrintestinal secundárias à quimioterapia.
- Ulceração gastrintestinal secundária à terapia com piroxicam.

EVOLUÇÃO ESPERADA E PROGNÓSTICO
- Prognóstico grave a longo prazo.
- Doença provavelmente progressiva.
- Sobrevida média — sem tratamento, 4-6 meses; com tratamento, 6-12 meses.

DIVERSOS

DISTÚRBIOS ASSOCIADOS
- Infecções recidivantes do trato urinário.
- Azotemia pós-renal.
- Osteopatia hipertrófica paraneoplásica.

FATORES RELACIONADOS COM A IDADE
Nenhum.

POTENCIAL ZOONÓTICO
Nenhum.

GESTAÇÃO/FERTILIDADE/REPRODUÇÃO
N/D.

SINÔNIMOS
Nenhum.

VER TAMBÉM
N/D.

Sugestões de Leitura

Glickman LT, Schofer FS, McKee LJ. Epidemiologic study of insecticide exposures, obesity, and risk of bladder cancer in household dogs. J Toxicol Environ Health 1989, 28:407-414.

Henry CJ, McCaw DL, Turnquist SE, et al. Clinical evaluation of mitoxantrone and piroxicam in a canine model of human invasive urinary bladder carcinoma. Clin Cancer Res 2003, 9:906-911.

Knapp DW, Richardson RC, Chan TCK, et al. Piroxicam therapy in 34 dogs with transitional cell carcinoma of the urinary bladder. J Vet Intern Med 1994, 8:273-278.

Smith JD, Stone EA, Gilson SD. Placement of a permanent cystostomy catheter to relieve urine outflow obstruction in dogs with transitional cell carcinoma. JAVMA 1995, 206:496-499.

Weisse C, Berent A, Todd K, et al. Evaluation of palliative stenting for management of malignant urethral obstructions in dogs. JAVMA 2006, 229:226-234.

Autor Ruthanne Chun
Consultor Editorial Timothy M. Fan

Carcinoma de Células Escamosas da Língua

CONSIDERAÇÕES GERAIS

REVISÃO
- Tumor maligno do epitélio escamoso.
- Tumor raro que ocorre mais comumente nos gatos do que nos cães.
- Em geral, cresce com rapidez.
- Gatos — neoplasia lingual mais comum, localizada geralmente na base ventral da língua na altura do frênulo; é mais frequente a evolução local antes dos indícios clínicos de metástase.
- Cães — segunda neoplasia lingual maligna mais comum (25%); altamente metastático via vasos linfáticos para os linfonodos regionais e para os pulmões (37-43% no momento do exame).
- Sistema orgânico acometido: gastrintestinal.

IDENTIFICAÇÃO
- Gatos — meia-idade ou idosos (>7 anos).
- Cães — idade média de 10-11 anos; as fêmeas são mais comumente acometidas; também é mais comum em raças de grande porte, sobretudo Poodle standard, Labrador retriever e Samoieda.

SINAIS CLÍNICOS

Achados Anamnésicos
- Salivação excessiva.
- Halitose.
- Disfagia ou dificuldade de preensão do alimento.
- Secreção bucal sanguinolenta.
- Apetite reduzido (hiporexia).
- Perda de peso.
- Higienização pessoal insatisfatória (no caso dos gatos).

Achados do Exame Físico
- Achado incidental.
- Massa lingual — aspecto variável, frequentemente nodular e ulcerada.
- Tumefação ou deformidade facial.
- Intumescimento intramandibular (gatos).
- Linfadenomegalia cervical — ocasionalmente.

CAUSAS E FATORES DE RISCO
Há um risco potencial elevado de carcinoma felino de células escamosas da cavidade bucal associado a coleiras antipulgas, comida enlatada (atum em particular) e possivelmente exposição à fumaça de cigarro.

DIAGNÓSTICO

DIAGNÓSTICO DIFERENCIAL
- Outras malignidades linguais (melanoma, sarcoma).
- Traumatismo.
- Glossite ulcerativa.
- Lesão benigna (papiloma).
- Infecção/abscesso.

HEMOGRAMA/BIOQUÍMICA/URINÁLISE
Geralmente normais.

OUTROS TESTES LABORATORIAIS
Exame físico completo da região cervical para detectar linfadenomegalia (linfonodos mandibulares e retrofaríngeos) com citologia e/ou biopsia dos linfonodos para avaliar a presença de metástases; mais comuns em cães.

DIAGNÓSTICO POR IMAGEM
- Radiografia do crânio — de utilidade limitada, já que o envolvimento ósseo é raro.
- Radiografias do tórax — há necessidade de três projeções para avaliar os pulmões quanto à existência de metástases (em geral, nodulares); mais comuns em cães.

MÉTODOS DIAGNÓSTICOS
- Citologia — esfregaço por impressão (decalque) obtido a partir de amostra de biopsia incisional (em cunha); pode estabelecer o diagnóstico; no entanto, a presença de ulceração, inflamação e infecção secundária pode limitar a utilidade diagnóstica.
- Biopsia tecidual profunda — necessária para o diagnóstico definitivo.

TRATAMENTO

- Cirúrgico — a maior parte deles é inoperável, sobretudo em gatos; pode ser justificável a excisão rigorosa; em geral, a função da língua após a recuperação é aceitável.
- Quase sempre há necessidade de cuidados pós-cirúrgicos (p. ex., sonda de esofagostomia ou gastrotomia) pelo proprietário.
- Glossectomia parcial — pode ser realizada na metade rostral (língua móvel) ou na metade longitudinal da língua (remoção de 40-60%); mais de 50% dos pacientes apresentam margens cirúrgicas incompletas.
- Glossectomia subtotal pode ser considerada em casos selecionados.
- Outros métodos cirúrgicos (p. ex., eletrocautério e criocirurgia) não oferecem nenhuma vantagem adicional à excisão convencional.
- Linfadenectomia cervical — raramente curativa; realizar apenas para obtenção do diagnóstico ou antes da terapia adjuvante.
- Resposta à radioterapia — insatisfatória (<7 semanas); pode ser utilizada de forma adjuvante na presença de doença microscópica no pós-operatório.
- Quimioterapia — não existem agentes eficazes disponíveis para o controle local ou sistêmico; segundo relatos breves, os agentes quimioterápicos úteis em carcinoma de células escamosas da cavidade bucal foram usados em carcinoma de células escamosas da língua.
- Piroxicam — pode ter atividade antineoplásica em alguns pacientes.
- Deve-se considerar o uso de medicamentos de suporte/paliativos para analgesia e antibióticos para infecções bacterianas secundárias.

MEDICAÇÕES

MEDICAMENTO(S)
Piroxicam (cão) — 0,3 mg/kg VO a cada 24 h; as doses não foram estabelecidas para os gatos; no entanto, foi utilizada a dosagem de 0,3 mg/kg VO a cada 48 h sem comprovação científica ou verificação experimental.

CONTRAINDICAÇÕES/INTERAÇÕES POSSÍVEIS
A quimioterapia pode ser tóxica; buscar por orientação de veterinário especialista em oncologia antes de iniciar o tratamento caso não esteja familiarizado com o uso de agentes citotóxicos.

ACOMPANHAMENTO

MONITORIZAÇÃO DO PACIENTE
Após a ressecção cirúrgica completa, reavaliar em 1 mês e, depois, a cada 3 meses com exame físico e avaliação em busca de metástases.

COMPLICAÇÕES POSSÍVEIS
Possíveis complicações no pós-operatório — dificuldade de preensão do alimento e recidiva local a longo prazo.

EVOLUÇÃO ESPERADA E PROGNÓSTICO
- Prognóstico — grave, em função da doença local extensa (gato) e da taxa moderada de metástase (cão).
- Sobrevida após a excisão cirúrgica (cães) — <25% sobrevivem 1 ano.
- Fatores prognósticos negativos (cães): localização caudal, excisão incompleta, recidiva, volume maior; grau histológico (a sobrevida média dos tumores de grau I é de 16 meses em comparação àqueles de graus II-III, com sobrevida média de 3-4 meses).
- Piroxicam — taxa de resposta de 17% em carcinoma de células escamosas da cavidade bucal com intervalo médio livre de progressão de 3,5-6 meses; foi observada uma única resposta parcial em três cães com carcinoma de células escamosas da língua.
- O prognóstico em gatos é semelhante ao de carcinoma de células escamosas em outros locais da cavidade bucal.
- Causa do óbito — secundária à recidiva local, disfagia e subsequente caquexia.

DIVERSOS

VER TAMBÉM
- Carcinoma de Células Escamosas das Gengivas.
- Carcinoma de Células Escamosas da Tonsila.

Sugestões de Leitura
Syrcle JA, Bonczynski JJ, Monette S, Bergman PJ. Retrospective evaluation of lingual tumors in 42 dogs: 1999-2005. JAAHA 2008, 44(6):308-319.

Autor Jackie M. Wypij
Consultor Editorial Timothy M. Fan

Carcinoma de Células Escamosas da Pele

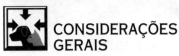

CONSIDERAÇÕES GERAIS

DEFINIÇÃO
- Tumor maligno do epitélio escamoso.
- Carcinoma multicêntrico *in situ* de células escamosas — também conhecido como tumor semelhante à doença de Bowen ou carcinoma bowenoide *in situ* (gatos).

FISIOPATOLOGIA
- A doença local pode evoluir de carcinoma *in situ* para carcinoma invasivo.
- A ocorrência de metástase é rara; os locais mais comuns são linfonodos regionais e pulmões.

SISTEMA(S) ACOMETIDO(S)
Pele/exócrino — pele e sítios metastáticos.

GENÉTICA
Desconhecida.

INCIDÊNCIA/PREVALÊNCIA
Representa 9-25% de todos os tumores cutâneos nos gatos e 4-18% nos cães.

DISTRIBUIÇÃO GEOGRÁFICA
O carcinoma de células escamosas (actínico) induzido pela luz solar é mais prevalente em climas ensolarados e altitudes elevadas (alta exposição à luz ultravioleta).

IDENTIFICAÇÃO
Espécies
Cães e gatos.

Raça(s) Predominante(s)
- Gatos — nenhum relato; os pacientes quase sempre possuem pele clara ou despigmentada; os gatos Siameses são sub-representados para carcinoma de células escamosas induzido pela luz solar, provavelmente em virtude de seu pigmento protetor.
- Cães — pode haver predisposição nas raças Terrier escocês, Pequinês, Boxer, Poodle, Elkhound norueguês, Dálmata, Beagle, Whippet e Bull terrier inglês branco.

Idade Média e Faixa Etária
- Cães — 8 anos.
- Gatos — 9 anos (2-16) para a forma actínica; 10 anos (7-17) para o carcinoma multicêntrico *in situ* de células escamosas.

Sexo Predominante
Nenhum.

SINAIS CLÍNICOS
Achados Anamnésicos
- Crostas, úlceras ou massas possivelmente presentes há meses e irresponsivas a tratamento conservativo.
- Carcinoma multicêntrico *in situ* de células escamosas (gatos) — a pele fica pigmentada; formam-se úlceras no centro; acompanhada por lesão crostosa dolorida que pode se expandir perifericamente.
- Envolvimento dos lábios, do nariz e do pavilhão auricular — pode começar como lesão crostosa superficial que evolui para úlcera profunda.
- Envolvimento da pele da face (gatos).

Achados do Exame Físico
- Lesões cutâneas proliferativas ou erosivas; as lesões erosivas são mais comuns no gato.
- Gatos — os locais mais comuns de lesões induzidas pela luz solar são o plano nasal, as pálpebras, os lábios e o pavilhão auricular.
- O carcinoma multicêntrico *in situ* de células escamosas pode ocorrer em qualquer local, não relacionado com a exposição solar ou a pigmentação cutânea; podem-se notar 2 a >30 lesões nas regiões de cabeça, dedos, pescoço, tórax, ombros e abdome ventral; o pelo na lesão epila-se com facilidade; as crostas grudam à haste pilosa epilada.
- Cães — afeta mais comumente os dedos, o escroto, o nariz, as pernas e o ânus.
- Envolvimento do flanco e do abdome em alguns casos.

CAUSAS
- Exposição à radiação ultravioleta (forma actínica).
- Estudos recentes revelam uma associação com os papilomavírus em carcinoma de células escamosas no gato em cerca de 50% das amostras testadas; também foi demonstrado que os cães apresentam carcinoma de células escamosas positivo para papilomavírus; em seres humanos, os papilomavírus contribuem para o desenvolvimento de carcinoma de células escamosas na pele exposta à luz solar.

FATORES DE RISCO
- Exposição prolongada à luz ultravioleta.
- Pele clara ou despigmentada.
- Lesão térmica anterior — cicatriz da queimadura.
- Fatores de risco para carcinoma multicêntrico *in situ* de células escamosas são indeterminados, mas podem ser associados à imunossupressão.

DIAGNÓSTICO

DIAGNÓSTICO DIFERENCIAL
- Infecção/abscesso.
- Dermatofitose.
- Traumatismo.
- Dermatite alérgica.
- Outras dermatites.
- Complexo granuloma eosinofílico.
- Doença imunomediada.
- Linfoma cutâneo.
- Mastocitoma.

HEMOGRAMA/BIOQUÍMICA/URINÁLISE
Geralmente normais; podem exibir alterações do hemograma completo, compatíveis com inflamação crônica, como leve leucocitose neutrofílica.

OUTROS TESTES LABORATORIAIS
- Exame citológico — o aspirado da lesão primária obtido por agulha fina pode confirmar o diagnóstico; no entanto, a presença de ulceração, inflamação e infecção secundária pode limitar a utilidade diagnóstica.
- Exame citológico de linfonodos — deve ser realizado para identificar metástases.

DIAGNÓSTICO POR IMAGEM
- Radiografia torácica — a obtenção de três projeções pode detectar metástase pulmonar (rara).
- Radiografia ou ultrassonografia abdominal — avalia e monitoriza os linfonodos sublombares se a dermatopatia envolver a metade caudal do paciente.

MÉTODOS DIAGNÓSTICOS
Biopsia e histopatologia — a realização de biopsia profunda em cunha é frequentemente necessária para obtenção do diagnóstico definitivo de carcinoma de células escamosas da pele.

ACHADOS PATOLÓGICOS
Macroscópicos
- Tumores ulcerativos — mais comuns; podem aparecer superficiais e com crostas, mas evoluir para crateras profundas.
- Tumores proliferativos — podem apresentar aspecto de couve-flor; podem ulcerar e sangrar com facilidade.
- Carcinoma multicêntrico *in situ* de células escamosas — múltiplas úlceras dolorosas que formam crostas e se expandem perifericamente até atingirem mais de 4 cm de diâmetro.

Histopatológicos
- Cordões ou massas irregulares de células epidérmicas, que se infiltram na derme e no subcutâneo.
- Grande número de pérolas córneas (queratina) nos tumores bem diferenciados.
- É comum o encontro de desmossomas e figuras mitóticas.
- Carcinoma multicêntrico *in situ* de células escamosas — queratinócitos displásicos e altamente ordenados se proliferam, substituindo a epiderme normal; no entanto, esses queratinócitos não penetram na membrana basal em direção à derme subjacente.

TRATAMENTO

CUIDADO(S) DE SAÚDE ADEQUADO(S)
- Tumores superficiais supostamente induzidos pela luz solar — a realização de ampla excisão cirúrgica pode ser localmente curativa; outras opções terapêuticas incluem criocirurgia, terapia fotodinâmica ou radiação (plesioterapia com estrôncio).
- Tumores invasivos — necessitam de excisão cirúrgica rigorosa; a aplicação de terapia fotodinâmica e a plesioterapia com estrôncio-90 têm pouca eficácia; a radioterapia com feixe externo demonstrou eficácia no pós-operatório ou isoladamente para tumores não passíveis de ressecção.
- Carcinoma multicêntrico *in situ* de células escamosas pode ser tratado por meio de cirurgia com intenção de cura para o controle local; no entanto, a maioria dos gatos desenvolve novas lesões em outros locais; portanto, o tratamento com agentes imunomoduladores (imiquimode) pode ser mais eficaz para doença multicêntrica.
- Retinoides sintéticos tópicos — podem ser valiosos para lesões superficiais precoces induzidas pela luz solar.
- Radioterapia com feixe externo — recomendada para tumores inoperáveis ou como adjuvante à cirurgia.
- Quimioterapia adjuvante — recomendada em casos de excisão cirúrgica incompleta, massa não ressecável e metástase; há relatos de que a cisplatina (para os cães somente), a carboplatina e a mitoxantrona induzam à remissão parcial e completa; geralmente de curta duração; pequeno número de pacientes; em alguns casos, a quimioterapia intralesional pode ser eficaz.
- Eletroquimioterapia (bleomicina) mostra-se promissora em um estudo-piloto; não disponível de forma rotineira na prática clínica.

Carcinoma de Células Escamosas da Pele

CUIDADO(S) DE ENFERMAGEM
- Considerar o uso de analgésicos conforme a necessidade.
- Infecções cutâneas secundárias podem se beneficiar com antibioticoterapia.
- Nutrição parenteral intervencionista (por meio de sonda) — em casos de ressecção do plano nasal.

ATIVIDADE
- Ditada pela localização do tumor e pelo tipo de tratamento.
- Restrita, em geral, até que as suturas sejam removidas, caso a cirurgia tenha sido executada.

DIETA
Normal.

ORIENTAÇÃO AO PROPRIETÁRIO
- Informar o proprietário sobre o benefício do diagnóstico e do tratamento precoces.
- Discutir os fatores de risco associados ao desenvolvimento do tumor (exposição à luz ultravioleta).
- A maioria dos gatos (75%) com carcinoma multicêntrico *in situ* de células escamosas desenvolverá novas lesões em outros locais.

CONSIDERAÇÕES CIRÚRGICAS
- Excisão cirúrgica ampla — tratamento de escolha para tumores invasivos e induzidos pela luz solar; às vezes, há necessidade da aplicação de retalhos cutâneos e reconstrução da parede corporal.
- Talvez haja necessidade de terapia clínica adjuvante.

MEDICAÇÕES

MEDICAMENTO(S) DE ESCOLHA
- Imiquimode a 5% sob a forma de creme para carcinoma multicêntrico *in situ* de células escamosas — aplicar por via tópica sobre as lesões acometidas a cada 24-48 h; a maioria dos gatos responde a esse tratamento, mas desenvolve novas lesões em outros locais; com frequência, essas lesões respondem subsequentemente à terapia tópica.
- Cisplatina — apenas para os cães, na dose de 60 mg/m^2 IV a cada 3 ou 4 semanas por 4 tratamentos; por ser um agente nefrotóxico, é imprescindível o uso com diurese salina (18,3 mL/kg/h IV por 6 h; administrar a cisplatina depois de 4 h); efetuar tratamento prévio com algum antiemético.
- Carboplatina — cães, 300 mg/m^2 IV a cada 3 semanas; gatos, 200–250 mg/m^2 IV a cada 3–4 semanas por 4 a 5 tratamentos.
- Mitoxantrona — cães e gatos, 5–6 mg/m^2 IV a cada 3 semanas por 4 a 5 tratamentos.

CONTRAINDICAÇÕES
Cisplatina — não utilizar em gatos, pois provoca hidrotórax grave, edema pulmonar e morte; não usar em cães com nefropatia concomitante, por ser potencialmente nefrotóxica; não empregar em conjunto com AINEs.

PRECAUÇÕES
- Quimioterápicos — seguir as diretrizes e os protocolos publicados para uso com segurança; o clínico deve se familiarizar com os efeitos colaterais potenciais; podem ser tóxicos; por essa razão, é preciso buscar orientação de veterinário especialista em oncologia antes de iniciar o tratamento caso não se esteja familiarizado com os agentes citotóxicos.
- Imiquimode — aproximadamente 25% dos gatos desenvolvem eritema local; <10% dos gatos desenvolvem elevação das enzimas hepáticas, neutropenia ou desarranjo gastrintestinal; a maioria dos gatos desenvolve novas lesões que, subsequentemente, respondem ao tratamento com o imiquimode.

INTERAÇÕES POSSÍVEIS
Nenhuma.

MEDICAMENTO(S) ALTERNATIVO(S)
Retinoides sintéticos tópicos (p. ex., tretinoína) — podem ser úteis para lesões superficiais precoces induzidas pela luz solar; podem ser irritantes para a pele.

ACOMPANHAMENTO

MONITORIZAÇÃO DO PACIENTE
- Hemograma completo e perfil bioquímico sérico de rotina devem ser avaliados durante a terapia clínica com o uso de quimioterapia ou creme de imiquimode.
- Exame físico em 1 mês após a resolução do tumor e, depois, a cada 3 meses após o tratamento ou se o proprietário achar que o tumor está recidivando.
- Radiografia do tórax e avaliação dos linfonodos na reavaliação a cada 3 meses; radiografia ou ultrassonografia abdominal se a lesão estiver na porção caudal do paciente.

PREVENÇÃO
- Limitar a exposição ao sol, especialmente entre 10 e 15 h.
- A realização de tatuagens nas áreas despigmentadas pode ser útil.
- Filtros solares — costumam ser removidos por lambedura pelo paciente; podem ser valiosos em algumas áreas (p. ex., pavilhão auricular).

COMPLICAÇÕES POSSÍVEIS
N/D.

EVOLUÇÃO ESPERADA E PROGNÓSTICO
Prognóstico — bom nas lesões superficiais que receberem tratamento adequado; reservado em casos de lesões invasivas, estágio avançado da doença ou lesões recidivantes.

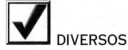

DIVERSOS

DISTÚRBIOS ASSOCIADOS
Nenhum.

FATORES RELACIONADOS COM A IDADE
Nenhum.

POTENCIAL ZOONÓTICO
Nenhum.

GESTAÇÃO/FERTILIDADE/REPRODUÇÃO
N/D.

SINÔNIMO(S)
Carcinoma multicêntrico *in situ* de células escamosas — também conhecido como tumor semelhante à doença de Bowen ou carcinoma bowenoide *in situ* (gatos).

VER TAMBÉM
Carcinoma de Células Escamosas — Plano Nasal.

ABREVIATURA(S)
- AINE = anti-inflamatório não esteroide.

Sugestões de Leitura
Gill VL, Bergman PJ, Baer KE, Craft D, Leung C. Use of imiquimod 5% cream (Aldara) in cats with multicentric squamous cell carcinoma in situ: 12 cases (2002-2005). J Vet Comp Oncology 2008, 6(1):55-64.

Marks SL, Song MD, Stannard AA, et al. Clinical evaluation of etretinate for the treatment of canine solar-induced squamous cell carcinoma and preneoplastic lesions. J Am Acad Dermatol 1992, 27(1):11-16.

Munday JS, Dunowska M, De Grey S. Detection of two different papillomaviruses within a feline cutaneous squamous cell carcinoma: Case report and review of the literature. N Z Vet J 2009, 57(4):248-251.

Ruslander D, Kaser-Hotz B, Sardinas JC. Cutaneous squamous cell carcinoma in cats. Compendium Contin Educ Small Anim Compend Contin Educ Pract Vet 1997, 19:1119-1129.

Vail DM, Withrow SJ. Tumors of the skin and subcutaneous tissues. In: Withrow SJ, Vail DM, eds., Small Animal Clinical Oncology, 4th ed. St. Louis: Saunders Elsevier, 2007, pp. 375-401.

Autor Jackie M. Wypij
Consultor Editorial Timothy M. Fan

Carcinoma de Células Escamosas da Tonsila

CONSIDERAÇÕES GERAIS

REVISÃO
- Invasão local rápida e progressiva por cordões de epitélio escamoso neoplásico que surgem da fossa tonsilar para dentro do tecido linfoide tonsilar.
- Mais comum em cães que em gatos; compreende 9% dos tumores bucais caninos.
- Invasividade local elevada para os tecidos moles.
- Metástase precoce; considerada uma doença sistêmica ao diagnóstico, já que 70-90% acabam sofrendo metástase, independentemente do controle local (linfonodos, pulmões, outros órgãos distantes).
- Comumente unilateral; pode ser bilateral.
- Sistema orgânico acometido: gastrintestinal.

IDENTIFICAÇÃO
- Cães e gatos de meia-idade ou idosos (faixa, 2,5-17 anos).
- Sem predileção racial ou sexual conhecida.

SINAIS CLÍNICOS
Achados Anamnésicos
- Salivação excessiva.
- Halitose.
- Disfagia.
- Secreção bucal sanguinolenta.
- Aumento dos ruídos respiratórios.
- Perda de peso.

Achados do Exame Físico
- Tonsila anormalmente grande (massa bucal).
- Possível linfadenomegalia cervical.
- Dor à abertura da mandíbula.

CAUSAS E FATORES DE RISCO
A causa exata é desconhecida; no entanto, é dez vezes mais comum nos animais que vivem em ambiente urbano do que naqueles que vivem em ambiente rural.

DIAGNÓSTICO

DIAGNÓSTICO DIFERENCIAL
- Linfoma (geralmente associado à linfadenomegalia e doença bilateral).
- Abscesso.
- Neoplasia metastática (melanoma bucal, sarcoma).
- Tonsilite.
- Corpo estranho na cripta tonsilar.
- Tumor das glândulas salivares.
- Mastocitoma.

HEMOGRAMA/BIOQUÍMICA/URINÁLISE
Geralmente normais.

OUTROS TESTES LABORATORIAIS
Citologia e/ou biopsia dos linfonodos regionais (mandibulares, retrofaríngeos) para avaliar a presença de doença metastática; em cães, 20% já se apresentam com metástases ao diagnóstico e 75% à necropsia.

DIAGNÓSTICO POR IMAGEM
- Radiografia torácica — três projeções para detectar metástases pulmonares; 10-20% são positivas para metástase à apresentação; 60-85% de metástase à necropsia.
- Tomografia computadorizada — avalia a extensão local de tumor primário, bem como o envolvimento de linfonodos mandibulares e retrofaríngeos; recomendada antes do planejamento terapêutico (ou seja, antes de cirurgia ou radioterapia).
- Ultrassonografia abdominal — avalia os órgãos abdominais; em cães, 20% exibem metástase disseminada para múltiplos órgãos à necropsia.

MÉTODOS DIAGNÓSTICOS
- Avaliação citológica de lesão — as amostras de aspirado por agulha fina frequentemente não são diagnósticas; obter esfregaço por impressão (decalque) a partir de amostra de biopsia incisional (em cunha); a presença de ulceração, inflamação e infecção secundária pode limitar a utilidade diagnóstica.
- Ampla biopsia tecidual profunda com exame histopatológico — necessária para diferenciar de outras malignidades bucais.

TRATAMENTO

- Cirurgia — a maior parte é inoperável; pode ser justificável a excisão rigorosa nos pacientes com obstrução das vias aéreas; a tonsilectomia, quando realizada, deve ser bilateral.
- Quase sempre, há necessidade de cuidados pós-operatórios (p. ex., sonda de esofagostomia ou gastrotomia) pelo proprietário.
- Outros métodos cirúrgicos (p. ex., eletrocautério e criocirurgia) — sem vantagem sobre a excisão convencional.
- Linfadenectomia cervical — raramente curativa; realizar apenas para a obtenção do diagnóstico ou antes da terapia adjuvante.
- Radioterapia regional — é eficaz para o controle local e alívio dos sinais clínicos.
- Quimioterapia — há relatos breves do uso de cisplatina, carboplatina ou doxorrubicina com sucesso limitado.
- Piroxicam — pode ter efeitos antineoplásicos em alguns cães.
- Talvez haja indicação de analgésicos para o controle da dor e antibióticos para o tratamento de infecções bacterianas secundárias.

MEDICAÇÕES

MEDICAMENTO(S)
- Cisplatina (cães) — 60-70 mg/m^2 IV uma vez a cada 3-4 semanas por 4 tratamentos; confere alívio acentuado dos sinais clínicos; a resposta depende da gravidade da lesão localizada ou metastática; agente nefrotóxico — é imprescindível o uso com diurese salina (18,3 mL/kg/h IV por 6 h; administrar a cisplatina depois de 4 h); efetuar tratamento prévio com algum antiemético.
- Carboplatina — cães, 300 mg/m^2 IV a cada 3 semanas; gatos, 200-250 mg/m^2 IV a cada 3-4 semanas por 4 a 5 tratamentos.
- Piroxicam (cães) — 0,3 mg/kg VO a cada 24 h; as doses em gatos não foram bem estabelecidas; entretanto, foi utilizada a dosagem de 0,3 mg/kg VO a cada 48 h sem comprovação científica ou verificação experimental.
- Doxorrubicina — cães com >10 kg, 30 mg/m^2 IV; cães com <10 kg e gatos, 1 mg/kg uma vez a cada 2-3 semanas por 5 tratamentos.

CONTRAINDICAÇÕES/INTERAÇÕES POSSÍVEIS
A quimioterapia pode ser tóxica; procurar por orientação de veterinário especialista em oncologia antes de iniciar o tratamento caso não esteja familiarizado com o uso de agentes citotóxicos.

ACOMPANHAMENTO

MONITORIZAÇÃO DO PACIENTE
A maioria dos pacientes é submetida à eutanásia dentro de meses por conta da evolução local ou de metástase; os pacientes submetidos a terapias com intenção de cura devem ser reavaliados com exame físico e quanto à ocorrência de metástase em 1 mês e, depois, a cada 3 meses. O novo crescimento local pode ser avaliado por TC seriada.

COMPLICAÇÕES POSSÍVEIS
Complicações pós-operatórias — recidivas do tumor; podem exigir a colocação de sondas de alimentação no pós-operatório, sobretudo em gatos (a longo prazo); alimentos pastosos para minimizar a ulceração e após a cirurgia bucal.

EVOLUÇÃO ESPERADA E PROGNÓSTICO
- Prognóstico — grave em função de doença local extensa e da elevada taxa de recidiva (língua, faringe, linfonodos) e metástase; poucos pacientes sobrevivem >6 meses depois do diagnóstico.
- Sobrevida (cães) — sobrevida média de 2 meses, com taxa de sobrevida <10% em 1 ano.
- Cirurgia e radioterapia (cães) — sobrevida média de 110 dias, com taxa de sobrevida de 22% em 1 ano.
- Cirurgia e quimioterapia (cães) — sobrevida média de 105 dias.
- Cirurgia, radioterapia e quimioterapia sistêmica (cães) — sobrevida média de 270 dias.
- Radioterapia regional — controle local raro em 75% dos casos, respostas parciais observadas (24-63 Gy) e alívio dos sinais (3-9 meses).
- Quimioterapia sistêmica (cães) — sobrevida de 60-130 dias.
- Piroxicam — apresenta taxa de resposta de 17% em carcinoma de células escamosas da cavidade bucal com intervalo médio livre de progressão de 3,5-6 meses; três de cinco cães com carcinoma de células escamosas da tonsila exibiram remissão parcial ou doença estável.
- Há pouquíssimas informações para os gatos; entretanto, eles parecem ter um prognóstico grave.

DIVERSOS

VER TAMBÉM
- Carcinoma de Células Escamosas das Gengivas.
- Carcinoma de Células Escamosas da Língua.

Sugestões de Leitura
Murphy S, Hayes A, Adams V, Maglennon G, Neath P, Ladlow J, Brearley MJ. Role of carboplatin in multi-modality treatment of canine tonsillar squamous cell carcinoma—a case series of five dogs. J Small Anim Pract 2006, 47(4):216-220.

Autor Jackie M. Wypij
Consultor Editorial Timothy M. Fan

Carcinoma das Células Escamosas das Gengivas

CONSIDERAÇÕES GERAIS

REVISÃO
• Tumor maligno do epitélio escamoso.
• Evolução rápida (semanas); localmente invasivo, com alta invasividade óssea (77%).
• Malignidade bucal mais comum nos gatos; segundo relatos, segunda malignidade bucal mais comum nos cães.
• Metástases — raras nos gatos; os linfonodos constituem o local mais comum de metástases; aproximadamente 10-20% de metástases nos cães (linfonodos, pulmões), taxa metastática mais baixa para lesões rostrais.

IDENTIFICAÇÃO
• Cães e gatos.
• Idade média (cães e gatos) — 10,5 anos (faixa etária, 3-15 anos).
• Mais comum em raças caninas de médio e grande portes.

SINAIS CLÍNICOS
Achados Anamnésicos
• Massa. • Salivação excessiva. • Disfagia.
• Halitose. • Secreção bucal sanguinolenta. • Perda de peso.

Achados do Exame Físico
• Lesão eritematosa e ulcerada com aspecto de couve-flor. • A mandíbula rostral constitui o local mais comum. • Dentes frouxos. • Tumefação ou deformidade faciais. • Exoftalmia. • Dor à abertura da mandíbula.

CAUSAS E FATORES DE RISCO
Os fatores de risco potenciais nos gatos incluem coleiras antipulgas, ração enlatada, atum e, possivelmente, fumaça de cigarro.

DIAGNÓSTICO

DIAGNÓSTICO DIFERENCIAL
• Outra malignidade bucal — fibrossarcoma nos gatos; melanoma, fibrossarcoma, osteossarcoma nos cães. • Epúlide. • Abscesso da raiz dentária.
• Crescimento ou pólipo benigno. • Hiperplasia gengival. • Complexo granuloma eosinofílico.

HEMOGRAMA/BIOQUÍMICA/URINÁLISE
Geralmente normais.

DIAGNÓSTICO POR IMAGEM
• Radiografia do crânio — avaliar o envolvimento ósseo profundo à massa; requer 40-50% de destruição óssea antes de se tornar evidente ao exame radiográfico.
• Radiografia dos dentes — pode aumentar a capacidade de avaliação das lesões.
• TC — ideal para avaliar a extensão de acometimento dos tecidos moles, a invasão do tecido ósseo e o envolvimento dos linfonodos regionais antes do planejamento cirúrgico.
• Radiografias do tórax — três projeções para detectar a presença de metástases pulmonares (desenvolvem-se em 3-36% dos cães, mas são raras nos gatos).

MÉTODOS DIAGNÓSTICOS
• Avaliação citológica da lesão — as amostras de aspirado obtido por agulha fina frequentemente não são diagnósticas; fazer esfregaço por decalque (impressão) de amostra obtida por biopsia incisional (em cunha); ulceração, inflamação e infecção secundária podem limitar a utilidade diagnóstica.
• Biopsia grande e profunda do tecido (abaixo do osso) — necessária para diferenciar o suficiente de outras malignidades bucais via histopatologia.
• Citologia e/ou biopsia de linfonodos regionais (mandibulares, retrofaríngeos) para avaliar a ocorrência de metástases (desenvolvem-se em cerca de 10-30% dos cães, porém são raras nos gatos).

TRATAMENTO

CÃES
• Excisão cirúrgica radical — necessária (p. ex., hemimandibulectomia ou maxilectomia parcial); em geral, é bem tolerada pelo paciente; são necessárias margens de no mínimo 2 cm.
• Criocirurgia — indicada para pequenas lesões sem envolvimento ósseo.
• Terapia fotodinâmica — técnica que é adjuvante à cirurgia e pode ser eficaz para o controle local de pequenos tumores; sobrevida média de 17 meses em oito cães que responderam a esse tratamento.
• Radioterapia — eficaz para o controle a longo prazo; tratamento com intenção de cura utilizado isoladamente ou em combinação com cirurgia ou quimioterapia.
• Quimioterapia — isolada ou em combinação com outras modalidades terapêuticas; carboplatina, cisplatina.
• Piroxicam pode ter alguns efeitos antineoplásicos.
• Talvez haja indicação de analgésicos para o controle da dor e antibióticos para o tratamento de infecções bacterianas secundárias.

GATOS
• Cirurgia — a maioria dos tumores é passível de ressecção; pequenas lesões rostrais podem ser excisadas com margens amplas de 2-3 cm (hemimandibulectomia); os gatos não toleram cirurgia bucal rigorosa tão bem quanto os cães.
• Os tratamentos paliativos incluem radioterapia de fracionamento de forma grosseira (resposta <50%).
• Bisfosfonatos — utilizados como tratamento paliativo para dor associada à invasão óssea.
• Pode haver indicação de analgésicos para o controle da dor e antibióticos para o tratamento de infecções bacterianas secundárias.

MEDICAÇÕES

MEDICAMENTO(S)
• Cisplatina (cães) 60-70 mg/m^2 IV uma vez a cada 3-4 semanas por 4 tratamentos; confere alívio acentuado dos sinais clínicos; a resposta depende da gravidade da lesão localizada ou metastática; nefrotóxica — deve ser utilizada com diurese salina (18,3 mL/kg/h IV durante 6 h; administrar a cisplatina depois de 4 h); efetuar pré-tratamento com algum antiemético.
• Carboplatina — cães, 300 mg/m^2 a cada 3 semanas IV; gatos, 200-250 mg/m^2 a cada 3-4 semanas por 4 a 5 tratamentos.
• Mitoxantrona (gatos) — 5-6 mg/m^2 a cada 3 semanas IV por 4 a 5 tratamentos.
• Piroxicam (cães) — 0,3 mg/kg VO diariamente; pode ser valioso para induzir à remissão parcial em alguns pacientes; as dosagens em gatos ainda não foram bem estabelecidas; no entanto, foi utilizada a dose de 0,3 mg/kg VO a cada 48 h sem comprovação científica ou verificação experimental.

CONTRAINDICAÇÕES/INTERAÇÕES POSSÍVEIS
• Cisplatina — jamais utilizar nos gatos.
• Não administrar a cisplatina com AINEs; há relatos de grave nefrotoxicidade nos cães.

ACOMPANHAMENTO

MONITORIZAÇÃO DO PACIENTE
Reavaliar com exame físico completo do paciente, avaliação dos linfonodos e obtenção de radiografias em três projeções em 1 mês e, depois, a cada 3 meses após excisão completa/terapia adjuvante.

COMPLICAÇÕES POSSÍVEIS
Complicações pós-operatórias — recidiva do tumor, ptialismo, desvio da mandíbula com consequente má oclusão, dificuldade de preensão do alimento, incapacidade de auto-higienização.

EVOLUÇÃO ESPERADA E PROGNÓSTICO
Cães
• Fatores prognósticos negativos — localização caudal ou maxilar, diâmetro >2 cm, idade mais avançada, excisão incompleta. • Excisão cirúrgica — sobrevida média de 15-16 meses, mas de 34 meses quando combinada com radioterapia; resultados melhores com mandibulectomia do que com maxilectomia. • Combinação de carboplatina e piroxicam com ou sem cirurgia — proporciona um tempo médio de sobrevida >18 meses.
• Piroxicam — taxa de resposta de 17% com intervalo médio livre de evolução de 3,5-6 meses.

Gatos
• Excisão cirúrgica — sobrevida média de 1 ano para tumores passíveis de ressecção; a radioterapia adjuvante pode prolongar a sobrevida.
• Radioterapia paliativa — sobrevida média de 2-4 meses; 10 meses caso se atinja a remissão completa.

DIVERSOS

VER TAMBÉM
• Carcinoma de Células Escamosas da Língua.
• Carcinoma de Células Escamosas da Tonsila.

ABREVIATURA(S)
• AINE = anti-inflamatório não esteroide.

Sugestões de Leitura
de Vos JP, Burm AG, Focker AP, Boschloo H, Karsijns M, Van Der Waal I. Piroxicam and carboplatin as a combination treatment of canine oral non-tonsillar squamous cell carcinoma: A pilot study and a literature review of a canine model of human head and neck squamous cell carcinoma. J Vet Comp Oncology 2005, 3(1):16-24.

Autor Jackie M. Wypij
Consultor Editorial Timothy M. Fan

Carcinoma de Células Escamosas das Orelhas

CONSIDERAÇÕES GERAIS

REVISÃO
- Tumor maligno do epitélio escamoso, que ocorre no pavilhão auricular, na orelha externa e/ou na orelha média. • Pavilhão auricular — localização mais comum nos gatos; os tumores do pavilhão auricular nos cães raramente correspondem a carcinoma de células escamosas. • Canal auditivo externo e orelha média — localizações incomuns nos cães e gatos. • Sistema orgânico acometido: cutâneo/exócrino.

IDENTIFICAÇÃO
- Gatos e cães. • Tumores do pavilhão auricular — comum nos gatos com pigmentação clara, média de 12 anos. • Tumores do canal auditivo — observados em cães e gatos mais idosos. • Sem predileção sexual. • Os cães da raça Cocker spaniel foram super-representados para tumores benignos e malignos do canal auditivo em um único estudo.

SINAIS CLÍNICOS
- Tumores do pavilhão auricular: ◦ Lesões de desenvolvimento lento da margem do pavilhão auricular. ◦ Estágio pré-canceroso — caracteriza-se por lesões eczematosas crostosas (dermatite actínica). ◦ Estágio canceroso — evolui para proliferação e/ou ulceração. ◦ Múltiplas lesões cutâneas (cerca de 15% dos gatos). • Tumores do canal auditivo: ◦ Geralmente unilaterais. ◦ Lesão expansiva tipo massa (em relevo, com ulceração e em base larga). ◦ Secreção otológica de odor fétido. ◦ Prurido. ◦ Dor. ◦ Sinais vestibulares/síndrome de Horner (paralisia do nervo facial, inclinação da cabeça, andar em círculo). ◦ Dificuldade de abertura da mandíbula. ◦ Linfadenomegalia cervical (retrofaríngea, mandibular).

CAUSAS E FATORES DE RISCO
- Tumores do pavilhão auricular — exposição crônica à luz solar nos gatos com pelagem branca e pigmentação clara da pele. • Tumores do canal auditivo — inflamação crônica pode ser um fator de risco.

DIAGNÓSTICO

DIAGNÓSTICO DIFERENCIAL
- Pavilhão auricular (gatos) — lesões causadas por vasculite ou crioglobulinemia. • Pavilhão auricular (cães) — mastocitoma, histiocitoma, traumatismo, tumor das glândulas sebáceas. • Canal auditivo/orelha média (gatos) — pólipo inflamatório/nasofaríngeo (orelha média); praticamente todos os tumores da orelha externa são malignos (adenocarcinoma das glândulas ceruminosas, outros). • Canal auditivo/orelha média (cães) — otite crônica; 60% dos tumores do canal auditivo externo são malignos (adenoma ou adenocarcinoma das glândulas ceruminosas, papiloma).

HEMOGRAMA/BIOQUÍMICA/URINÁLISE
Geralmente normais.

OUTROS TESTES LABORATORIAIS
Exame físico completo e citologia e/ou biopsia dos linfonodos regionais (mandibulares, retrofaríngeos) para avaliar a ocorrência de metástases (raras para lesões do pavilhão auricular).

DIAGNÓSTICO POR IMAGEM
- Radiografias do tórax — é necessária a obtenção de três projeções para avaliar a presença de metástases pulmonares (raras com lesões do pavilhão auricular). • Radiografias do crânio — podem identificar as estruturas de tecido mole e a lise óssea da bula timpânica em caso de tumores do canal auditivo/orelha média. • Tomografia computadorizada — ideal para avaliação do envolvimento de tecidos moles e ósseos antes do planejamento da ressecção cirúrgica de tumores que envolvem o canal auditivo; 57-67% dos tumores são localmente invasivos para os tecidos circundantes.

MÉTODOS DIAGNÓSTICOS
- Para o exame dos tumores que envolvem o canal auditivo, geralmente há necessidade de sedação e/ou anestesia. • Citologia da lesão primária pode confirmar o diagnóstico; no entanto, a presença de ulceração, inflamação e infecção secundária pode limitar a utilidade diagnóstica. • Biopsia do pavilhão auricular ou da massa auricular para confirmar o diagnóstico via exame histopatológico; o exame de vídeo-otoscopia pode ajudar na realização da biopsia.

ACHADOS PATOLÓGICOS
Diferenciado ao exame microscópico por grupos característicos de células epiteliais e células queratinizantes formando pérolas de queratina.

TRATAMENTO

- Tumores do pavilhão auricular: ◦ Excisão cirúrgica rigorosa pode necessitar de remoção do pavilhão auricular e, possivelmente, ablação da porção vertical do canal auditivo; é preciso remover a lesão com margem de tecido normal que circunda qualquer epitélio anormal. ◦ As alternativas incluem terapia fotodinâmica (menos previsível; com frequência, há necessidade de mais de um tratamento), criocirurgia (bem-sucedida para pequenas lesões superficiais) ou plesioterapia com estrôncio (radioterapia superficial). • Tumores do canal auditivo/orelha média: ◦ Excisão cirúrgica rigorosa com ablação total do canal auditivo e osteotomia da bula timpânica costuma ser necessária para obter a excisão completa; a ressecção da porção lateral do canal auditivo raramente alcança margens cirúrgicas completas. ◦ Segundo relatos casuais, a radioterapia pode ser utilizada como tratamento paliativo de tumores não passíveis de ressecção ou no pós-operatório para doença microscópica.

MEDICAÇÕES

MEDICAMENTO(S)
- Tumores do pavilhão auricular (gatos):
  ◦ Imiquimode sob a forma de creme a 5% — aplicar por via tópica a cada 24 h.
  ◦ Etretinato — 0,75-1 mg/kg a cada 24 h; utilizado com sucesso para prevenir a evolução das lesões pré-cancerosas; não disponível no mercado nos EUA nem no Canadá.
  ◦ Acitretina (1 mg/kg VO a cada 24 h) pode ser usada no lugar do etretinato.
  ◦ Vitamina E — 400-600 UI VO a cada 12 h; pode ser benéfica para prevenir ou retardar a evolução das lesões pré-cancerosas.
  ◦ Quimioterapia — benefício ainda não estabelecido; entrar em contato com veterinário especialista em oncologia em busca das recomendações quimioterápicas mais recentes.
- Tumores do canal auditivo:
  ◦ Quimioterapia — benefício ainda não determinado; entrar em contato com veterinário especialista em oncologia em busca das recomendações quimioterápicas mais recentes.

CONTRAINDICAÇÕES/INTERAÇÕES POSSÍVEIS
Mulheres que estão grávidas ou pretendem engravidar não devem manipular a acitretina.

ACOMPANHAMENTO

MONITORIZAÇÃO DO PACIENTE
Reavaliar com exame físico completo do paciente, radiografias do tórax e avaliação dos linfonodos em 1 mês e, depois, a cada 3 meses após o tratamento (excisão cirúrgica completa).

PREVENÇÃO
- Limitar a exposição ao sol, sobretudo entre as 10 h da manhã e as 15 h da tarde. • Pode ser útil a realização de tatuagens nas áreas despigmentadas. • Filtros solares podem ser úteis, mas frequentemente são retirados com a pata e, posteriormente, lambidos pelo paciente.

EVOLUÇÃO ESPERADA E PROGNÓSTICO
- Tumores do pavilhão auricular — o prognóstico é bom em caso de excisão cirúrgica completa; sobrevida >1,5 anos com a remoção completa dessa estrutura auricular. • Tumores do canal auditivo são muitas vezes localmente invasivos (57-67%) e exibem recidiva local apesar da cirurgia; o prognóstico é reservado. • Cães — sobrevida média de 5,3 meses com envolvimento da bula timpânica em comparação a >58 meses sem esse tipo de acometimento. • Gatos — sobrevida média de 3,8 meses; prognóstico pior com envolvimento da bula timpânica; sobrevida média de 1,5 meses na presença de sinais neurológicos.

DIVERSOS

VER TAMBÉM
- Carcinoma das Glândulas Ceruminosas das Orelhas. • Carcinoma de Células Escamosas do Plano Nasal. • Carcinoma de Células Escamosas da Pele.

Sugestões de Leitura
Fan TM, de Lorimier LP. Inflammatory polyps and aural neoplasia. Vet Clin North Am Small Anim Pract 2004, 34(2):489-509.

Autor Jackie M. Wypij
Consultor Editorial Timothy M. Fan

Carcinoma de Células Escamosas do Plano Nasal

CONSIDERAÇÕES GERAIS

REVISÃO
- Tumor maligno das células epiteliais escamosas do plano nasal.
- Localmente invasivo e raramente sofre metástase.
- Sistemas orgânicos acometidos: cutâneo/exócrino, respiratório.

IDENTIFICAÇÃO
- Comum em gatos; raro em cães.
- Idade média — gatos, 8,5-12,1 anos; cães, 9-10 anos.
- É mais provável que esse tipo de carcinoma se desenvolva em animais com nariz pouco pigmentado (gatos).
- Não há relatos de predileção sexual ou racial nos gatos.
- Cães — super-representação de machos e da raça Labrador retriever em um único estudo.

SINAIS CLÍNICOS
- Gatos — lesão lentamente progressiva; pode ser benigno sob a forma de crostas e cascas superficiais, evolui para carcinoma *in situ* e desenvolve-se em carcinoma superficial e depois erosivo invasivo; outras regiões cutâneas podem ser acometidas (gatos — carcinoma de células escamosas multicêntrico *in situ*).
- Cães — espirros; epistaxe; tumefação e ulceração do plano nasal, lesão proliferativa.
- Linfadenomegalia cervical — ocasionalmente nos cães, mas rara nos gatos.

CAUSAS E FATORES DE RISCO
- Exposição à luz ultravioleta.
- Ausência de pigmento protetor (gatos).

DIAGNÓSTICO

DIAGNÓSTICO DIFERENCIAL
- Infecção/abscesso.
- Traumatismo.
- Dermatite alérgica.
- Outras dermatites.
- Complexo granuloma eosinofílico (gatos).
- Doença imunomediada.
- Linfoma cutâneo.
- Mastocitoma.

HEMOGRAMA/BIOQUÍMICA/URINÁLISE
Geralmente normais.

OUTROS TESTES LABORATORIAIS
Exame citológico e/ou biopsia de linfonodos regionais devem ser realizados para identificar a presença de metástases (ocasionalmente nos cães, mas raras nos gatos).

DIAGNÓSTICO POR IMAGEM
- Radiografias torácicas — três projeções para avaliar a ocorrência de metástases (raras).
- TC — avalia a extensão de acometimento dos tecidos moles e a invasão de tecido ósseo antes do planejamento cirúrgico; exame essencial para tumores caninos em que amplas estruturas subjacentes são frequentemente envolvidas.

MÉTODOS DIAGNÓSTICOS
- Exame citológico — aspirado por agulha fina da lesão primária pode confirmar o diagnóstico; no entanto, a presença de ulceração, inflamação e infecção secundária pode limitar a utilidade diagnóstica desse exame.
- Biopsia e histopatologia — a realização de biopsia profunda em cunha é frequentemente necessária para o diagnóstico definitivo de carcinoma de células escamosas.

ACHADOS PATOLÓGICOS
- Lesões — podem variar em termos de aspecto, dependendo do estágio da doença nos gatos; tipicamente ulcerativas nos gatos; mais provavelmente proliferativas nos cães.
- Histopatológicos — caracterizados por massas irregulares ou cordões de células epidérmicas que se proliferam para baixo dentro da derme.
- Formação de queratina, pérolas córneas, desmossomas, figuras mitóticas e atipia celular — frequentes.

TRATAMENTO
- Tumores superficiais — cirurgia, criocirurgia, irradiação (plesioterapia com estrôncio-90) ou terapia fotodinâmica.
- Tumores invasivos — necessitam de excisão cirúrgica radical e radioterapia adjuvante por feixe externo (gatos); os cães não são tão responsivos à radioterapia.
- Talvez haja necessidade de suporte nutricional pós-operatório imediato, especialmente para os gatos.
- Pode haver indicação de analgésicos para o controle da dor e antibióticos para o tratamento de infecções bacterianas secundárias.

MEDICAÇÕES

MEDICAMENTO(S)
- Quimioterapia — ainda não foi bem avaliada.
- Etretinato — 0,75–1 mg/kg VO a cada 24 h; retinoide sintético; pode ser útil para lesões pré-cancerosas precoces; não está disponível no mercado nos EUA ou no Canadá.
- Acitretina (1 mg/kg VO a cada 24 h) pode ser utilizada no lugar do etretinato.
- Imiquimode a 5% sob a forma de creme para lesões do plano nasal associadas a carcinoma de células escamosas multicêntrico *in situ* — aplicar por via tópica nas lesões acometidas a cada 24-48 h; a maioria dos gatos responde a esse medicamento, mas desenvolve novas lesões em outros locais; muitas vezes, tais lesões respondem subsequentemente à terapia tópica.

CONTRAINDICAÇÕES/INTERAÇÕES POSSÍVEIS
Mulheres que estão grávidas ou pretendem engravidar não devem manipular a acitretina.

ACOMPANHAMENTO

MONITORIZAÇÃO DO PACIENTE
- Exame físico e radiografia torácica — em 1 mês e, depois, a cada 3 meses após o tratamento.
- Biopsia — qualquer lesão nova sob suspeita.

PREVENÇÃO
- Limitar a exposição ao sol, sobretudo entre as 10 h da manhã e as 15 h da tarde.
- Pode ser útil a realização de tatuagens nas áreas despigmentadas.
- Filtros solares são geralmente ineficazes.

EVOLUÇÃO ESPERADA E PROGNÓSTICO
- Prognóstico — bom para pequenos tumores não invasivos; reservado para tumores invasivos.
- Sobrevida apenas com a radioterapia (gatos) — média, 17,7 meses; 1 ano, 61,5%, com recidiva de 81,8%.
- Sobrevida média apenas com a cirurgia (rinectomia nos gatos) — mais de 22 meses.
- Plesioterapia com estrôncio-90 (gatos, tumores superficiais) — taxa de resposta de 98%; intervalo médio livre de evolução de 4,5 anos; sobrevida média >8 anos.
- Terapia fotodinâmica (gatos, tumores superficiais) — taxa de resposta de 96%; com frequência, há necessidade de múltiplos tratamentos; não parece ser tão eficaz quanto outras terapias a longo prazo.
- Cães (tumores superficiais) — apenas a cirurgia poderá ser curativa.
- Cães (tumores invasivos) — em um único estudo de 8 cães, o tempo médio de sobrevida foi de 5,4 meses; em outro estudo de 17 cães tratados com cirurgia e/ou radioterapia, 70% dos tumores recidivaram com tempo médio de sobrevida de 3–6 meses.

DIVERSOS

ABREVIATURA(S)
- TC = tomografia computadorizada.

VER TAMBÉM
- Carcinoma de Células Escamosas das Orelhas.
- Carcinoma de Células Escamosas da Pele.

Sugestões de Leitura
Hammond GM, Gordon IK, Theon AP, Kent MS. Evaluation of strontium Sr 90 for the treatment of superficial squamous cell carcinoma of the nasal planum in cats: 49 cases (1990-2006). JAVMA 2007, 231(5):736-741.

Autor Jackie M. Wypij
Consultor Editorial Timothy M. Fan

Carcinoma de Células Escamosas dos Dedos

CONSIDERAÇÕES GERAIS

REVISÃO
- Tumor maligno localmente invasivo que costuma surgir do epitélio subungueal.
- Gatos — metástase para um ou mais dedos a partir de sítio pulmonar primário relatado.
- Cães — tumor mais comum dos dedos (cerca de 50% dos tumores desse local).
- Os membros torácicos são mais comumente acometidos que os pélvicos.
- Sistemas orgânicos acometidos: cutâneo/exócrino, musculoesquelético.

IDENTIFICAÇÃO
- Cães e, raramente, gatos.
- Idade média — cães e gatos: 10 anos; relatado em cães de até 3 anos de idade.
- Não há predileção sexual nos cães; em um pequeno estudo de gatos, as fêmeas foram mais comumente acometidas.
- Cães pertencentes a raças de grande porte e de pelagem negra são predispostos; as raças relatadas incluem Poodle standard, Labrador retriever, Schnauzer gigante, Rottweiler, Dachshund, Retriever de pelagem plana.

SINAIS CLÍNICOS
- Tumefação do dedo ou massa tumoral no dedo.
- Claudicação.
- Ulceração.
- Unha fraturada ou ausente.
- Múltiplos dedos raramente são acometidos nos cães (6-10%, relatos frequentes em cães de grande porte e pelagem negra).
- O envolvimento de inúmeros dedos costuma ser observado nos gatos (30%); em geral, faz parte de um processo metastático; pode ser difícil distinguir isso em termos clínicos.
- Linfadenomegalia regional (incomum no momento do diagnóstico).
- Tosse ou sinais respiratórios compatíveis com doença pulmonar metastática (rara no momento do diagnóstico) ou neoplasia pulmonar primária (gatos).

CAUSAS E FATORES DE RISCO
- Causa — desconhecida.
- Fatores de risco (cães) — hereditário; pigmentação negra da pele.

DIAGNÓSTICO

DIAGNÓSTICO DIFERENCIAL
- Infecção do leito ungueal (paroníquia).
- Traumatismo.
- Outros tumores (cães) — melanoma; sarcomas de tecido mole; mastocitoma; osteossarcoma.
- Outros tumores (gatos) — fibrossarcoma; adenocarcinoma; osteossarcoma.
- Lesões benignas — cisto de inclusão epitelial; queratoacantoma.

HEMOGRAMA/BIOQUÍMICA/URINÁLISE
Geralmente normais.

OUTROS TESTES LABORATORIAIS
N/D.

DIAGNÓSTICO POR IMAGEM
- Radiografias do tórax — é importante a obtenção de três projeções para descartar doença metastática (desenvolve-se em cerca de 15-25% dos cães) e excluir carcinoma pulmonar primário (gatos).
- Radiografias dos membros — lise da terceira falange do dedo acometido em 80% dos pacientes.
- Ultrassonografia do abdome — para lesões dos membros pélvicos, avaliar os linfonodos intra-abdominais quanto à presença de doença metastática.

MÉTODOS DIAGNÓSTICOS
- Citologia — utilidade diagnóstica limitada se houver inflamação grave, infecção secundária ou tumor bem diferenciado.
- Biopsia da lesão em cunha — necessária para confirmar o diagnóstico via exame histopatológico.
- Citologia e/ou biopsia dos linfonodos regionais — indicada(s) para avaliar a presença de doença metastática.

TRATAMENTO

- Amputação do dedo acometido na altura da articulação falângica do metacarpo (ou do metatarso).
- Em gatos com tumor pulmonar primário, a amputação de um único dedo pode ser considerada como um tratamento paliativo.
- Em gatos com múltiplos dedos acometidos em virtude de metástases, a cirurgia não constitui uma opção terapêutica porque os dedos de múltiplos membros estão geralmente acometidos.
- Pode haver indicação de analgésicos para o controle da dor e antibióticos para o tratamento de infecções bacterianas secundárias.
- O benefício da quimioterapia ainda não foi estabelecido; no entanto, em pacientes com estágio avançado da doença, pode-se considerar a quimioterapia conforme aquela utilizada para carcinoma de células escamosas de outros locais.

MEDICAÇÕES

MEDICAMENTO(S)
Piroxicam (cães) — 0,3 mg/kg VO a cada 24 h para analgesia; (gatos) dosagens não estabelecidas; entretanto, a dose de 0,3 mg/kg VO a cada 48 h foi utilizada sem comprovação científica ou verificação experimental.

CONTRAINDICAÇÕES/INTERAÇÕES POSSÍVEIS
Nenhuma.

ACOMPANHAMENTO

MONITORIZAÇÃO DO PACIENTE
- Excisão cirúrgica completa da lesão primária e sem indícios de metástase — pode não haver necessidade de tratamento adicional.
- Reavaliar com exame físico do paciente, radiografias do tórax, avaliação dos linfonodos ± ultrassonografia do abdome em 1 mês e, em seguida, a cada 3 meses após o tratamento (excisão cirúrgica completa).

EVOLUÇÃO ESPERADA E PROGNÓSTICO
- Tempo de sobrevida após a excisão cirúrgica completa depende da localização do tumor no dedo — carcinoma de células escamosas que se origina do epitélio subungueal: sobrevida de 95% e 74% em 1 e 2 anos, respectivamente; carcinoma de células escamosas que se origina de outras partes do dedo: sobrevida de 60% e 44% em 1 e 2 anos, respectivamente.
- Em um único relato recente, a sobrevida em 1 e 2 anos foi de 50% e 18%, respectivamente, enquanto em outro estudo retrospectivo recente menos da metade dos cães morreu por carcinoma de células escamosas e o tempo médio de sobrevida não foi atingido.
- A cirurgia para amputar o dedo acometido, independentemente da presença de metástases, exerce um impacto positivo na sobrevida do cão; em um pequeno estudo, entretanto, era mais provável que os cães com doença metastática no momento da consulta apresentassem recidiva local.
- O prognóstico para gatos é mau, com tempos médios de sobrevida de 2-3 meses e índices de metástases de aproximadamente 25%; os tempos de sobrevida são semelhantes nos gatos com carcinoma de células escamosas primário e metastático.

DIVERSOS

VER TAMBÉM
- Tumores Melanocíticos da Pele e dos Dedos.
- Carcinoma de Células Escamosas da Pele.

Sugestões de Leitura
Wobeser BK, Kidney BA, Powers BE, Withrow SJ, Mayer MN, Spinato MT, Allen AL. Diagnoses and clinical outcomes associated with surgically amputated canine digits submitted to multiple veterinary diagnostic laboratories. Vet Pathol 2007, 44(3):355-361.

Autor Jackie M. Wypij
Consultor Editorial Timothy M. Fan

Carcinoma de Células Escamosas dos Pulmões

CONSIDERAÇÕES GERAIS

REVISÃO
- Tumor primário raro de origem epitelial brônquica com metaplasia escamosa (carcinoma epidermoide).
- Desenvolve-se comumente nos lobos pulmonares caudais.
- Elevado potencial metastático para os linfonodos regionais e o parênquima pulmonar.
- Sistema orgânico acometido: respiratório.

IDENTIFICAÇÃO
- Cães e gatos.
- Animais mais idosos, idade média — cães, 11 anos; gatos, 12 anos.
- Sem predileção racial.

SINAIS CLÍNICOS
Achados Anamnésicos
- Achado acidental.
- Tosse áspera, não produtiva.
- Dispneia.
- Letargia ou intolerância ao exercício.
- Caquexia e perda de peso.
- Claudicação (possível metástase ou osteopatia hipertrófica).

Achados do Exame Físico
- Taquipneia.
- Sibilo.
- Ruídos pulmonares anormais à auscultação.
- Hemoptise.
- Osteopatia hipertrófica.
- Lesões digitais isoladas ou múltiplas (metástase) nos gatos.
- Neuromiopatia (como megaesôfago) e paraplegia (rara).

CAUSAS E FATORES DE RISCO
- Há suspeitas de que o ambiente urbano e a inalação passiva de fumaça de cigarro promovam o desenvolvimento de câncer de pulmão, mas não foi demonstrada uma correlação definitiva em diversos estudos.

DIAGNÓSTICO

DIAGNÓSTICO DIFERENCIAL
- Outra neoplasia pulmonar primária (p. ex., adenocarcinoma).
- Neoplasia pulmonar metastática.
- Cisto broncogênico.
- Bolhas.
- Abscesso.
- Pneumonia por aspiração.
- Paragonimíase.
- Doença pulmonar eosinofílica.

HEMOGRAMA/BIOQUÍMICA/URINÁLISE
- Leucocitose neutrofílica.
- Hipercalcemia (rara).

DIAGNÓSTICO POR IMAGEM
- Radiografia torácica:
  ○ Três projeções, muito comumente demonstram a presença de massa solitária com margem bem circunscrita.
  ○ Com frequência, afeta os lobos pulmonares caudais; lobo caudal direito nos cães e caudal esquerdo nos gatos.
  ○ Pode deslocar ou comprimir a traqueia ou os brônquios principais.
  ○ Pode resultar em obstrução parcial ou completa das vias aéreas e atelectasia periférica.
  ○ Pode identificar linfadenomegalia traqueobrônquica (baixa sensibilidade) ou lesões metastáticas pulmonares.
- Tomografia computadorizada:
  ○ Ideal para avaliar a possibilidade de ressecção cirúrgica.
  ○ Exame mais preciso do que as radiografias para detectar metástases nos pulmões e linfonodos; praticamente todos os casos (90%) acabam sofrendo metástases.
- Radiografia dos membros:
  ○ Raramente, identificam-se metástases isoladas ou múltiplas nos dedos em gatos; pode identificar lise óssea na falange distal.

MÉTODOS DIAGNÓSTICOS
- Citologia via aspirado transtorácico por agulha fina de lesões periféricas pode fornecer um diagnóstico presuntivo; a orientação ultrassonográfica pode ajudar a obter amostras de aspirado por agulha fina.
- As amostras citológicas obtidas via escovação brônquica endoscópica frequentemente não são diagnósticas, mas podem ser úteis para lesões de localização central.
- Os lavados broncoalveolares e transtraqueais raramente são diagnósticos.
- A realização de biopsia tecidual é necessária para o diagnóstico definitivo, podendo ser obtida via biopsia com agulha em buraco de fechadura, toracoscopia ou toracotomia (biopsia excisional).
- As complicações potencialmente letais dos procedimentos de aspiração/biopsia incluem pneumotórax, hemotórax, efusão pleural, infecção e, raramente, disseminação iatrogênica do tumor.

TRATAMENTO

- Cirurgia (toracotomia e lobectomia pulmonar) — a ressecção ampla e completa do lobo pulmonar acometido proporciona uma melhor oportunidade para controle a longo prazo; palpar manualmente todos os lobos pulmonares remanescentes; examinar os linfonodos traqueobrônquicos; é aconselhável a biopsia dos linfonodos, mesmo se estiverem aparentemente normais; apesar de ser ideal a extirpação do linfonodo, isso frequentemente não é realizado por ser um procedimento difícil.
- Quimioterapia — pode-se administrar antes ou depois da cirurgia; a aplicação de quimioterapia intracavitária pode ser útil para carcinomatose e efusão pleural.

MEDICAÇÕES

MEDICAMENTO(S)
- Cisplatina (apenas para os cães) — 60 mg/m² IV a cada 3 ou 4 semanas por 4 tratamentos; por ser um agente nefrotóxico, deve ser utilizado com diurese salina (18,3 mL/kg/h IV durante 6 h; administrar a cisplatina depois de 4 h).
- Doxorrubicina — cães com >10 kg: 30 mg/m² IV uma vez a cada 2-3 semanas por 5 tratamentos; cães com <10 kg e gatos: 1 mg/kg na mesma posologia; proporciona alívio acentuado.
- Carboplatina — cães, 300 mg/m² IV a cada 3 semanas; gatos, 200-250 mg/m² IV a cada 3-4 semanas por 4 a 5 tratamentos.
- Mitoxantrona (efusão pleural) — cães e gatos, 5-6 mg/m² a cada 3 semanas; é possível a administração intracavitária e/ou a aplicação IV por 4 a 5 tratamentos.

CONTRAINDICAÇÕES/INTERAÇÕES POSSÍVEIS
- Cisplatina — jamais utilizar nos gatos.
- Quimioterapia pode ser tóxica; portanto, deve-se buscar orientação de veterinário especialista em oncologia antes de iniciar o tratamento se o clínico não estiver familiarizado com medicamentos citotóxicos.

ACOMPANHAMENTO

MONITORIZAÇÃO DO PACIENTE
Após excisão completa, considerar as opções quimioterápicas; reavaliar com radiografias torácicas em três projeções e/ou TC em 1 mês e, depois, a cada 3 meses.

EVOLUÇÃO ESPERADA E PROGNÓSTICO
- Sobrevida se deixado sem tratamento ou com evidência de doença metastática — em geral, <3 meses.
- Sobrevida média com a excisão completa do tumor primário e linfonodos traqueobrônquicos negativos para células neoplásicas (cães e gatos) — >300 dias.
- Sobrevida média com excisão cirúrgica incompleta do tumor primário ou linfonodos traqueobrônquicos positivos para células neoplásicas (cães e gatos) — <75 dias.
- Fatores prognósticos negativos para tumores pulmonares primários: tumor de grande volume, localização central *versus* periférica, metástase, efusão pleural.

DIVERSOS

DISTÚRBIOS ASSOCIADOS
Osteopatia hipertrófica paraneoplásica.

ABREVIATURA(S)
- TC = tomografia computadorizada.

Sugestões de Leitura
Paoloni MC, Adams WM, Dubielzig RR, Kurzman I, Vail DM, Hardie RJ. Comparison of results of computed tomography and radiography with histopathologic findings in tracheobronchial lymph nodes in dogs with primary lung tumors: 14 cases (1999-2002). JAVMA 2006, 228(11):1718-1722. Erratum in: JAVMA 2006, 229(5):710.

Autor Jackie M. Wypij
Consultor Editorial Timothy M. Fan

Carcinoma de Células Escamosas dos Seios Nasais e Paranasais

CONSIDERAÇÕES GERAIS

REVISÃO
• Invasão local progressiva do epitélio escamoso neoplásico queratinizante e não queratinizante que surge de dentro dos seios nasais e paranasais.
• Lentamente progressivo (meses) e costuma ser bilateral.
• Prevalência — 15-17% das neoplasias nasais em cães e gatos.

IDENTIFICAÇÃO
• Mais comum nos cães do que nos gatos.
• Cães — idade média, 9-10 anos (faixa etária, 3-16 anos); a forma queratinizante tem predileção por macho (3,4:1); gatos — idade média de 10 anos.
• Cães — predileção para tumores sinonasais em raças de médio e grande portes.

SINAIS CLÍNICOS
Achados Anamnésicos
• Epistaxe intermitente e progressiva uni a bilateral e/ou secreção mucopurulenta. • Epífora.
• Espirros. • Halitose. • Anorexia. • Dispneia.
• Crises convulsivas secundárias à invasão do crânio (relatadas em até 35% dos cães).

Achados do Exame Físico
• Secreção nasal (epistaxe, mucopurulenta, serossanguinolenta e/ou sanguinolenta).
• Deformidade facial.
• Anormalidades oculares: epífora, retropulsão diminuída, elevação da terceira pálpebra, exoftalmia ou tumefação facial periorbital.
• Dor ao exame dos seios nasais ou paranasais.
• Obstrução do fluxo de ar nasal (uni ou bilateral).

CAUSAS E FATORES DE RISCO
• Desconhecidos.
• Especula-se que os cães dolicocefálicos, aqueles que vivem em ambiente urbano e em outros expostos à fumaça de cigarro estejam sob risco mais elevado.

DIAGNÓSTICO

DIAGNÓSTICO DIFERENCIAL
• Outras neoplasias malignas intranasais — adenocarcinoma, carcinoma indiferenciado, linfoma (gatos), sarcomas (cães). • Abscesso da raiz dentária.
• Infecção viral — gatos. • Criptococose — gatos.
• Aspergilose; outra infecção fúngica. • Corpo estranho. • Traumatismo. • Fístula oronasal.
• Coagulopatia. • Hipertensão. • Sinusite bacteriana — rara. • Rinite linfocítica-plasmocitária. • Pólipos inflamatórios (gatos). • Parasitas.

HEMOGRAMA/BIOQUÍMICA/URINÁLISE
Geralmente normais; pode apresentar anemia em caso de epistaxe crônica e/ou grave.

OUTROS TESTES LABORATORIAIS
• Citologia e/ou biopsia dos linfonodos regionais — detectam doença metastática (até 10% no momento do diagnóstico).
• Epistaxe — avaliar o perfil de coagulação e a pressão arterial para descartar hipertensão e coagulopatia; essa avaliação deve ser efetuada antes da realização de biopsia intranasal.

DIAGNÓSTICO POR IMAGEM
• Radiografias do crânio — revelam destruição assimétrica dos turbinados caudais; sobreposição de massa de tecido mole; densidade líquida nos seios frontais; perda dos dentes; deslocamento de estruturas da linha média; envolvimento do palato duro.
• Radiografias do tórax — detectam metástases pulmonares (raras).
• TC ou RM — permitem a identificação de massa com densidade de tecido mole, perda de detalhes dos turbinados, opacidade de líquido/tecido mole dos seios nasais; método mais eficiente para avaliar a invasividade tumoral, incluindo invasão de tecido ósseo, da placa cribriforme ou da órbita.

MÉTODOS DIAGNÓSTICOS
• Rinoscopia — revela massa amolecida, friável, carnosa; tumor frequentemente mascarado por exsudatos.
• Biopsia tecidual profunda com exame histopatológico — necessária para o diagnóstico definitivo; os métodos incluem rubor nasal intenso, biopsia através das narinas às cegas com pinça ou cureta óssea, biopsia guiada por fibra óptica, biopsia ou aspirado percutâneo de grandes deformidades faciais, biopsia pelo local de extração dentária, rinotomia.
• Devem ser tomadas precauções na biopsia para minimizar o risco de penetração da placa cribriforme.

TRATAMENTO

• Apenas a cirurgia — não costuma ser curativa; não melhora os resultados em grande parte dos estudos; os procedimentos de exenteração e radioterapia podem trazer benefícios em casos selecionados.
• Radioterapia com o paciente internado — 36-60 Gy; com ou sem cirurgia; melhor controle clínico nos cães e gatos; foi demonstrado que a radioterapia de fracionamento grosseiro também é benéfica nos cães.
• Quimioterapia adjuvante — relatos de respostas casuais em cães para os agentes à base de platina e a mitoxantrona; recomendada para massa não passível de ressecção, como tratamento paliativo dos sinais clínicos e na presença de metástases.
• Analgésicos para controle da dor.

MEDICAÇÕES

MEDICAMENTO(S)
• Cisplatina (apenas para os cães) — 60-70 mg/m^2, IV uma vez a cada 3 semanas por 4 tratamentos; pode ser uma boa opção; por ser nefrotóxica, deve ser utilizada com diurese salina (18,3 mL/kg/h IV durante 6 h; administrar a cisplatina depois de 4 h); fornecer algum antiemético antes da quimioterapia.
• Carboplatina — cães, 300 mg/m^2 IV a cada 3 semanas; gatos, 200-250 mg/m^2 IV a cada 3-4 semanas por 4 a 5 tratamentos.
• Mitoxantrona (cães) — 5-6 mg/m^2 IV a cada 3 semanas por 4 a 5 tratamentos.

CONTRAINDICAÇÕES/INTERAÇÕES POSSÍVEIS
Cisplatina — jamais utilizar em gatos.

ACOMPANHAMENTO

MONITORAÇÃO DO PACIENTE
Reavaliar com exame físico do paciente, radiografias do tórax, avaliação dos linfonodos ± varredura por TC a cada 3 meses após o tratamento ou mediante a recidiva dos sinais clínicos.

COMPLICAÇÕES POSSÍVEIS
• Rinite — após a radioterapia; geralmente desaparece em 1-2 meses; no entanto, pode ser crônica.
• Osteomielite, fístula oronasal.

EVOLUÇÃO ESPERADA E PROGNÓSTICO
• Carcinomas sinonasais não tratados (todos os tipos) — sobrevida média de 3 meses; a epistaxe carreia um prognóstico ruim.
• Radioterapia de curso completo (carcinomas sinonasais) — sobrevida média de aproximadamente 12-18 meses (cães e gatos); taxa de sobrevida de 30-48% em 2 anos (cães); sobrevida média de 8-25 meses (cães); média, 1-36 meses (gatos).
• Radioterapia de fracionamento grosseiro (todos os tipos de tumor) — melhora dos sinais clínicos em > dois terços dos cães; sobrevida média de 4,8-7 anos.
• Exenteração cirúrgica e radioterapia (todos os tipos de tumor) — sobrevida de aproximadamente 4 anos (cães).
• Há relatos de que o carcinoma de células escamosas carreia um prognóstico pior em comparação a outros tumores nasais; tempos médios de sobrevida de 6-9,4 meses com radioterapia em dois relatos; tempo médio de sobrevida de 2 meses em oito cães (com ou sem terapia); outros estudos não demonstram qualquer diferença significativa com o subtipo histológico.
• Recidiva local com extensão para o cérebro — comum; o envolvimento cerebral é um sinal prognóstico mau.

DIVERSOS

VER TAMBÉM
• Adenocarcinoma Nasal.
• Condrossarcoma dos Seios Nasais e Paranasais.

ABREVIATURA(S)
• TC = tomografia computadorizada.
• RM = ressonância magnética.

Sugestões de Leitura
Correa SS, Mauldin GN, Mauldin GE, Patnaik AK. Efficacy of cobalt-60 radiation therapy for the treatment of nasal cavity nonkeratinizing squamous cell carcinoma in the dog. JAAHA 2003, 39(1):86-89.

Autor Jackie M. Wypij
Consultor Editorial Timothy M. Fan

Carcinoma de Ducto Biliar

CONSIDERAÇÕES GERAIS

DEFINIÇÃO
Processo maligno de ducto biliar ou da vesícula biliar. Os nomes utilizados para classificação histológica dessa neoplasia incluem colangiocarcinoma ou cistoadenocarcinoma do ducto biliar.

FISIOPATOLOGIA
Neoplasia epitelial que se desenvolve a partir das células que revestem o(s) ducto(s) biliar(es) ou a vesícula biliar.

SISTEMA(S) ACOMETIDO(S)
• A origem neoplásica em ducto biliar intra-hepático é mais comum, enquanto os tumores de ducto biliar extra-hepático ou da vesícula biliar são raros.
• Os focos comuns de metástases incluem pulmões, linfonodos hepáticos e peritônio.
  ○ Outros focos metastáticos envolvem outros linfonodos, diafragma, intestinos, pâncreas, coração, baço, rins, medula espinal, bexiga urinária e ossos.
  ○ Alopecia paraneoplásica foi associada a carcinoma de ducto biliar em gatos, enquanto miastenia grave adquirida, relatada em cão com carcinoma colangiocelular.

INCIDÊNCIA/PREVALÊNCIA
• Neoplasia hepatobiliar mais comum em gatos.
• Segunda neoplasia hepática mais comum em cães, representando de 22 a 41% de todos os tumores malignos no fígado desses animais.

IDENTIFICAÇÃO
Espécies
Cães e gatos.
Raça(s) Predominante(s)
Possivelmente o Labrador retriever.
Idade Média e Faixa Etária
Acima de 10 anos de idade.
Sexo Predominante
Pode haver predisposição das fêmeas.

SINAIS CLÍNICOS
Achados Anamnésicos
• Frequentemente vagos e inespecíficos.
• Anorexia.
• Letargia.
• Polidipsia e poliúria.
• Vômito.
• Icterícia.
• Ascite.
Achados do Exame Físico
• Hepatomegalia (massa abdominal ± palpável).
• Ascite.
• Distensão abdominal.
• Icterícia.

CAUSAS
• Associação potencial entre colangiocarcinoma e infecção por ancilóstomos e/ou tricúris em cães.
• Carcinoma experimental do trato biliar canino foi induzido por N-etil-N'-nitro-N-nitrosoguanidina.

FATORES DE RISCO
Exposição ambiental aos carcinógenos envolvidos.

DIAGNÓSTICO

DIAGNÓSTICO DIFERENCIAL
• Achados macroscópicos — adenoma hepatocelular, adenocarcinoma hepatocelular, adenoma colangiocelular, hiperplasia nodular, cirrose, hepatite crônica ativa, mielolipoma hepático, cistoadenoma hepatobiliar e carcinoide.
• Histopatologia — facilmente distinguido de adenocarcinoma hepatocelular; no entanto, a imuno-histoquímica (para detecção de anticorpo monoclonal anti-hepatócito embebido em parafina 1) é capaz de distinguir entre neoplasias hepatocelulares e biliares.

HEMOGRAMA/BIOQUÍMICA/URINÁLISE
• A atividade sérica enzimática elevada (p. ex., fosfatase alcalina, ALT e AST) é inespecífica para neoplasias e provavelmente reflete dano hepático e estase biliar.
• O nível sérico alto da fosfatase alcalina é menos comum em gatos, em função da meia-vida enzimática curta nessa espécie.
• Relação de AST:ALT < 1 é compatível com carcinoma de ducto biliar ou carcinoma hepatocelular *versus* tumores neuroendócrinos hepáticos ou sarcoma (geralmente > 1).
• Leucocitose e bilirrubinemia são achados inconsistentes.

OUTROS TESTES LABORATORIAIS
• Alfafetoproteína (uma glicoproteína oncofetal) é elevada em 55% dos cães com carcinoma de ducto biliar e pode diferenciar as lesões neoplásicas daquelas não neoplásicas.
• Antes da biopsia ou de qualquer procedimento cirúrgico, é recomendável a obtenção do perfil de coagulação.

DIAGNÓSTICO POR IMAGEM
• Radiografias abdominais — podem situar a presença de massa no fígado, demonstrar deslocamento do estômago ou, então, revelar a perda dos detalhes entre os órgãos em pacientes com ascite.
• Radiografias torácicas — podem identificar a ocorrência de metástases pulmonares.
• Ultrassonografias abdominais — determinam a localização da lesão, a ecogenicidade do fígado remanescente e a presença de efusão e ainda orientam a biopsia.
• TC e RM são técnicas de diagnóstico por imagem mais sensíveis, capazes de identificar o tipo histológico do tumor em seres humanos; além disso, é mais provável que essas técnicas detectem lesões menores não observadas à ultrassonografia.

MÉTODOS DIAGNÓSTICOS
• Na presença de líquido ascítico, efetuar a abdominocentese e a avaliação citológica.
• Obtenção de amostras por meio de orientação ultrassonográfica para os exames de citologia ou biopsia aspirativa por agulha fina.
• Amostras obtidas por laparoscopia ou laparotomia ajudam na formulação do diagnóstico definitivo.

ACHADOS PATOLÓGICOS
• Os tipos morfológicos incluem neoplasia maciça (37-46%), nodular (0-21%) ou difusa (17-54%).
• Lesões benignas — geralmente císticas e multinodulares. • Lesões malignas — frequentemente envolvem múltiplos lobos.
• Classificação histológica — não é um indicador prognóstico.

TRATAMENTO

• A excisão cirúrgica é o tratamento de escolha, especialmente se a ressecção completa for viável e praticável. • Até 80% do fígado podem ser submetidos à ressecção se o tecido hepático remanescente permanecer funcional. • Não existe tratamento cirúrgico eficaz em caso de neoplasia nodular ou difusa.

MEDICAÇÕES

MEDICAMENTO(S)
É improvável que a quimioterapia seja eficaz.

CONTRAINDICAÇÕES/INTERAÇÕES POSSÍVEIS
• Medicamentos que sofrem metabolismo hepático devem ser utilizados com cuidado se houver indícios de disfunção desse órgão. • Também é recomendável cautela para o uso de medicamentos que dependem da depuração entero-hepática.

ACOMPANHAMENTO

MONITORIZAÇÃO DO PACIENTE
• Mensuração da atividade enzimática hepática e realização de exame físico a cada 3 meses.
• Ultrassonografia abdominal e radiografia torácica a cada 3 meses.

PREVENÇÃO
É justificável a terapia anti-helmíntica de rotina em virtude da associação potencial entre carcinoma de ducto biliar e infecção por ancilóstomos ou tricúris em cães.

COMPLICAÇÕES POSSÍVEIS
Ruptura/hemorragia tumoral, especialmente em caso de neoplasia maciça.

EVOLUÇÃO ESPERADA E PROGNÓSTICO
• Natureza agressiva; prognóstico de reservado a mau; alto índice de metástases (67-88%). • A maioria dos pacientes vem a óbito 6 meses após a cirurgia por causa de recorrência local ou metástase.

DIVERSOS

GESTAÇÃO/FERTILIDADE/REPRODUÇÃO
Os medicamentos quimioterápicos podem ser carcinogênicos e mutagênicos.

ABREVIATURA(S)
• ALT = alanina aminotransferase. • AST = aspartato aminotransaminase. • TC = tomografia computadorizada. • RM = ressonância magnética.

Autor Craig Clifford
Consultor Editorial Timothy M. Fan
Agradecimento Contribuição prévia de Sue Downing.

Carcinoma Hepatocelular

CONSIDERAÇÕES GERAIS

REVISÃO
- Tumor maligno do fígado de origem epitelial.
- Menos comum que os tumores hepáticos benignos em cães, mas é responsável por mais de 50% dos tumores hepáticos malignos. • Muito raramente, ocorrem as formas extra-hepáticas em cães e gatos. • A ocorrência de metástase para linfonodos regionais, pulmões e cavidade peritoneal em cães é mais comum com as formas nodulares e difusas do carcinoma hepatocelular.

IDENTIFICAÇÃO
- Raro em cães e muito raro em gatos. • Os cães acometidos costumam ter mais de 10 anos de idade. • Não há predisposição racial, embora as raças Golden retriever e Schnauzer miniatura, bem como os cães machos, sejam super-representados em alguns estudos.

SINAIS CLÍNICOS
- Tipicamente ausentes até que a doença esteja em um grau avançado. • Letargia. • Fraqueza.
- Anorexia. • Perda de peso. • Polidipsia.
- Diarreia. • Vômitos. • Hepatomegalia (assimétrica) — achado compatível; antecede o desenvolvimento de sinais clínicos francos.
- Hemorragia abdominal.

CAUSAS E FATORES DE RISCO
- Desconhecidos. • Podem estar associados à inflamação crônica ou hepatotoxicidade. • Toxinas — induzem ao surgimento de tumor em animais experimentais (p. ex., aflatoxina, dimetilnitrosamina e CCl_4) e em seres humanos (p. ex., vírus da hepatite crônica).

DIAGNÓSTICO

DIAGNÓSTICO DIFERENCIAL
- Adenoma hepático. • Abscesso hepático. • Massa abdominal. • Esplenomegalia. • Hiperplasia nodular. • Cistadenoma biliar. • Adenoma/carcinoma do ducto biliar. • Neoplasia metastática.
- Doença hepática policística — forma menos comum; hiperplasia fibrosa do estroma com células ductais anaplásicas; poucos cistos.
- Linfoma hepático. • Hemangiossarcoma hepático. • Carcinoide hepático.

HEMOGRAMA/BIOQUÍMICA/URINÁLISE

Hemograma Completo
- Geralmente normal. • Foi detectada anemia em >50% dos casos com carcinoma hepatocelular maciço em um único estudo. • A anemia pode ser regenerativa se o tumor for hemorrágico.
- Leucocitose com desvio à esquerda — tumores com centros necróticos. • Em alguns casos, há relatos de trombocitose.

Bioquímica
- Níveis de atividade variáveis das enzimas hepáticas. • ALT, AST, fosfatase alcalina e GGT — em geral, muito altas; sugerem um processo patológico mais grave que o indicado pelos sinais clínicos. • Valores séricos de bilirrubina total — geralmente normais. • É possível a constatação de hipoalbuminemia, hiperglobulinemia, hipoglicemia e hipercolesterolemia.

OUTROS TESTES LABORATORIAIS
- Ácidos biliares séricos — normais a menos que o tumor diminua estrategicamente a perfusão hepática e o fluxo de bile na porta hepática.
- Parâmetros de coagulação — podem ser observadas anormalidades compatíveis com CID em pacientes com tumores maciços ou necróticos ou sangramento abdominal.

DIAGNÓSTICO POR IMAGEM

Radiografia
- Pode demonstrar uma única lesão em massa ou assimetria aparente da silhueta hepática associada a um único lobo. • Deslocamento caudolateral do estômago causado pela hepatomegalia acentuada.
- Raramente, revela a presença de gás no centro necrótico do tumor.

Ultrassonografia Abdominal
- Lesão em massa discreta com ecogenicidade variável, dependendo da presença de necrose intratumoral, hemorragia, gás ou cavidades císticas.
- Ocasionalmente, observa-se um aumento de volume maciço de um único lobo hepático.
- Padrão ecogênico misto — mais comum.

TC/RM
- Métodos preferidos para a formulação do diagnóstico e o estadiamento dos tumores hepáticos em seres humanos; entretanto, esses exames não foram avaliados para o estadiamento em cães e gatos. • As imagens de TC de tumores maciços podem fazer com que eles pareçam não ressecáveis quando, na verdade, eles podem ser.

MÉTODOS DIAGNÓSTICOS
- Citologia do aspirado hepático — em geral, reflete displasia e aspectos malignos francos; ocasionalmente, recuperam-se apenas células necróticas. • Biopsia hepática cirúrgica para confirmação — biopsia com agulha não é recomendada por causa do pequeno tamanho da amostra.

ACHADOS PATOLÓGICOS
- São descritos três subtipos morfológicos desse tumor — maciço, nodular e difuso. • As formas nodulares são responsáveis por 29%, enquanto os tipos difusos respondem por 10% de todos os carcinomas hepatocelulares relatados em cães; além disso, ambos os tipos envolvem múltiplos lobos hepáticos. • A forma maciça que está confinada a um único lobo responde por 61% dos casos de carcinoma hepatocelular canino em um único relato. • Pode ser friável. • A cor varia de quase branco à cor normal do fígado. • O centro necrótico pode ser evidente. • Tumores com infiltração difusa podem não ser macroscopicamente visíveis, além da hepatomegalia (dos lobos acometidos).

TRATAMENTO

NUTRIÇÃO
Considerar o emprego de estratégias apropriadas para neoplasia — refeições frequentes em pequenas quantidades; aumento do consumo de calorias; desvio do consumo de energia para proteína e gordura em vez de carboidrato (se a assimilação de gordura estiver normal).

CONSIDERAÇÕES CIRÚRGICAS
- A excisão é recomendada sempre que possível.
- A forma maciça é frequentemente acessível à ressecção cirúrgica. • Com frequência, as formas nodulares e difusas não são acessíveis à cirurgia.
- Entre 60-70% dos lobos hepáticos poderão ser ressecados se o paciente receber os cuidados críticos apropriados.

MEDICAÇÕES

MEDICAMENTO(S)
Quimioterapia — nenhuma geralmente é eficaz.

ACOMPANHAMENTO

MONITORIZAÇÃO DO PACIENTE
- Ultrassonografia abdominal — a cada 2-4 meses no primeiro ano. • TC e/ou RM abdominais são mais sensíveis que a ultrassonografia para detecção de pequenas lesões recidivantes. • Monitorizar as enzimas hepáticas.

COMPLICAÇÕES POSSÍVEIS
Risco de necrose tumoral e hemorragia abdominal maciça se não for submetido à ressecção.

EVOLUÇÃO ESPERADA E PROGNÓSTICO
- Prognóstico variável; a classificação histológica não é prognóstica. • As formas maciças apresentam um prognóstico melhor do que as nodulares ou difusas. • Em um único estudo, a sobrevida média de cães acometidos pela forma maciça e tratados por meio de cirurgia foi >1.460 dias.

DIVERSOS

DISTÚRBIOS ASSOCIADOS
- Hepatite crônica. • Colangio-hepatite. • Doença hepática policística. • Ingestão crônica de toxina.

ABREVIATURA(S)
- ALT = alanina aminotransferase. • AST = aspartato aminotransferase. • CCl_4 = tetracloreto de carbono. • CID = coagulação intravascular disseminada. • GGT = gama-glutamil transferase.
- RM = ressonância magnética. • TC = tomografia computadorizada.

Sugestões de Leitura
Liptak JM, Dernell WS, Monnet E, et al. Massive hepatocellular carcinoma in dogs: 48 cases (1992-2002). JAVMA 2004, 225(8):1225-1230.
Liptak JM, Dernell WS, Withrow SJ. Liver tumors in cats and dogs. Compend Contin Educ Pract Vet 2004, 26:50-56.

Autor Wallace B. Morrison
Consultor Editorial Timothy M. Fan

CÁRIES DENTÁRIAS

CONSIDERAÇÕES GERAIS

REVISÃO
- A cárie corresponde à deterioração dos tecidos dentários firmes (esmalte, cimento e dentina), em virtude dos efeitos de bactérias bucais sobre os carboidratos fermentáveis presentes na superfície dos dentes.
- O termo *caries* vem do latim e significa podridão, destruição ou putrefação.
- As bactérias da cavidade bucal fermentam os carboidratos presentes na superfície dos dentes, resultando na produção de ácidos; tais ácidos, por sua vez, levam à desmineralização dos tecidos firmes, permitindo a digestão bacteriana e leucocitária da matriz orgânica do dente.
- A cárie é muito comum em seres humanos em sociedades "ocidentais", onde as dietas ricas em carboidratos altamente refinados constituem o padrão. Orientações públicas e medidas preventivas rigorosas têm resultado em um declínio na incidência de cárie nas últimas décadas.
- Em seres humanos, o microrganismo *Streptococcus mutans* é particularmente implicado no desenvolvimento de cáries.
- Por diversas razões (p. ex., dieta pobre em carboidratos refinados, pH mais alto da saliva, menor quantidade da amilase salivar, formato cônico da coroa, espaçamento interdentário mais amplo e flora bucal nativa distinta), a cárie não é comum no cão doméstico, mas ela ocorre e deve ser pesquisada.
- Um estudo publicado no *Journal of Veterinary Dentistry* [Periódico de Odontologia Veterinária] em 1998 (ver a seção "Sugestões de Leitura") assinalou que 5,3% dos cães com 1 ano de idade ou mais apresentavam uma ou mais lesões de cáries e, dentre eles, 52% exibiam lesões simétricas bilaterais.
- As cáries podem comprometer a coroa ou as raízes dos dentes e são classificadas como cáries do tipo depressão-e-fissura, de superfície lisa ou de raiz.

IDENTIFICAÇÃO
- As cáries ocorrem em cães.
- Descritas em gatos; algumas vezes, lesões reabsortivas odontoclásticas felinas (reabsorção dentária) são erroneamente nomeadas como cáries felinas. Pelo conhecimento do autor, não há relatos publicados quanto à ocorrência de cáries dentárias verdadeiras no gato doméstico, embora isso seja teoricamente possível.
- Não há predileção racial, etária ou sexual conhecida.
- Segundo breves relatos não publicados, o autor observou uma incidência mais alta de lesões do tipo depressão-e-fissura nas plataformas oclusais dos primeiros molares maxilares em cães de grande porte, como Labrador retriever e Pastor alemão.

SINAIS CLÍNICOS
- Cáries incipientes de superfície lisa — aparecem como uma área de esmalte branco glacial e insensível.
- Cáries clínicas — aparecem como um defeito estrutural na superfície da coroa ou na raiz.
- O defeito frequentemente é ocupado ou revestido por dentina necrótica mole e escura. O defeito também pode encarcerar e reter restos de comida.
- A dentina acometida será submetida a um explorador odontológico e poderá ser removida com o auxílio de cureta ou escavador odontológico.

CAUSAS E FATORES DE RISCO
- A cárie é causada por bactérias bucais que fermentam os carboidratos presentes na superfície dentária, levando à produção de alguns ácidos (acético, láctico, propiônico); esses ácidos, por sua vez, promovem a desmineralização do esmalte, do cimento e da dentina, seguida pela digestão da matriz orgânica do dente por bactérias bucais e/ou leucócitos.
- Há uma troca constante de minerais entre as superfícies dentárias (esmalte, qualquer dentina exposta ou cimento radicular) e os líquidos bucais; se houver uma perda real de minerais, ocorrerá o desenvolvimento da cárie.
- As cáries precoces (incipientes) podem ser reversíveis por meio de remineralização.
- Assim que a matriz proteica sofrer colapso, a lesão torna-se irreversível.
- Qualquer fator que permita a retenção prolongada de carboidratos fermentáveis e a formação de placa bacteriana na superfície dentária predispõe o indivíduo ao desenvolvimento de cáries.
- Uma fossa oclusal profunda no 1° dente molar maxilar representa o local mais comum de desenvolvimento das cáries.
- As superfícies dentárias que estão em contato estrito com cáries estabelecidas apresentam risco de surgimento da lesão por extensão.
- As fossas oclusais profundas e os sulcos em desenvolvimento na superfície da coroa predispõem o indivíduo a cáries do tipo depressão-e-fissura.
- Os contatos interdentários estreitos predispõem o indivíduo a cáries de superfície lisa.
- As bolsas periodontais profundas predispõem o indivíduo a cáries de raiz.
- Os animais com esmalte pouco mineralizado, pH salivar mais baixo, dietas ricas em carboidratos fermentáveis e higiene bucal deficiente estão sob risco de desenvolvimento de cáries.
- A perda do esmalte por quaisquer meios (hipocalcificação no estágio de desenvolvimento, desgaste ou atrito abrasivo, fratura traumática) que exponha a dentina subjacente (tecido mais mole) pode aumentar o risco de desenvolvimento de cáries.

DIAGNÓSTICO

DIAGNÓSTICO DIFERENCIAL
- Coroa — fratura, desgaste ou atrito abrasivo com exposição da dentina terciária ou mancha extrínseca.
- Hipocalcificação do esmalte com dentina exposta e corada.
- No passado, as lesões reabsortivas odontoclásticas felinas (reabsorção dentária) foram erroneamente nomeadas como cáries felinas.
- A reabsorção dentária também pode ocorrer em cães, podendo ser confundida com cáries.
- A dentina sadia é firme e não cede ao explorador odontológico, enquanto a dentina cariada é mole e cede a um instrumento penetrante.
- As cáries de raiz podem ser confundidas com reabsorção radicular externa; embora a distinção muitas vezes seja acadêmica, em qualquer um dos casos costuma ser indicado o procedimento de extração.
- A lesão deve ser classificada conforme a profundidade do processo patológico.
- A Tabela 1 abaixo foi adaptada a partir da nomenclatura aprovada para reabsorção dentária pela American Veterinary Dental College (Faculdade Norte-americana de Odontologia Veterinária), conforme publicação em seu site.

HEMOGRAMA/BIOQUÍMICA/URINÁLISE
N/D.

OUTROS TESTES LABORATORIAIS
N/D.

DIAGNÓSTICO POR IMAGEM
Radiografias dentárias intrabucais:
- As áreas de desmineralização e perda tecidual aparecerão como áreas translúcidas, em contraste com os tecidos dentários normais radiodensos.
- Se a lesão tiver penetrado na câmara pulpar, haverá doença endodôntica e poderá haver doença periapical evidente se a lesão for suficientemente antiga.
- Pode ser difícil demonstrar lesões pequenas em virtude da sobreposição de tecidos normais radiodensos (dentários e esqueléticos).

MÉTODOS DIAGNÓSTICOS
- Inspeção — superfície dentária seca e limpa sob iluminação e ampliação satisfatórias.

Tabela 1

Estágio 1	O defeito envolve apenas o esmalte ou o cimento.
Estágio 2	O defeito estende-se para o interior da dentina, mas não envolve o canal pulpar.
Estágio 3	Perda de tecido dentário firme profundo (cimento e/ou esmalte com perda da dentina que se estende até a cavidade pulpar); a maior parte do dente conserva sua integridade.
Estágio 4	Ampla perda do tecido dentário firme (cimento e/ou esmalte com perda da dentina que se estende até a cavidade pulpar); a maior parte do dente perdeu sua integridade.
Estágio 5	Perda de grande parte da coroa; resquícios radiculares.

- Exploração com instrumento dentário penetrante — o explorador penetra e crava na dentina cariada, dando a sensação de "tração ou repuxamento" à retirada.
- Exploração subgengival — revela irregularidades na superfície radicular.
- Os corantes para detecção de cáries são utilizados por dentistas humanos e veterinários para auxiliar na diferenciação entre tecido sadio e cariado da dentina. Contudo, o uso desses corantes pode levar a resultados falso-positivos e tratamentos exagerados por meio da remoção de tecido em excesso. É preferível a confiança nos achados visuais, táteis e radiográficos.

TRATAMENTO

- Foco na prevenção — examinar a dentição permanente (adulta) de cães adolescentes (de 6-8 meses de vida) para identificar áreas anatomicamente comprometidas sob risco do desenvolvimento de cáries. Fossas profundas na superfície oclusal do 1º molar maxilar, por exemplo, podem ser preenchidas com selante de depressão-e-fissura ou agente ligante de dentina liberador de flúor para evitar o desenvolvimento de cáries se identificadas antes do desenvolvimento de qualquer deterioração.
- Cáries incipientes — podem ser interrompidas e, possivelmente, revertidas pela aplicação do verniz com flúor ou de um agente ligante de dentina liberador de flúor e pela modificação dos fatores de risco.
- Lesões resultantes em perda tecidual coronária leve a moderada (estágios 1 ou 2) — remover a dentina cariada e o esmalte sobrejacente sem sustentação com o uso de instrumentos odontológicos manuais e/ou rotativos motorizados e, depois, restaurar a anatomia coronária com amálgama (tradicional), restaurações de resina composta ou restaurações protéticas.
- Lesões que se estendem em direção ao canal pulpar (estágio 3) — o tratamento endodôntico deve preceder a restauração. Alternativamente, pode ser indicada a extração. Como o tecido pulpar nas raízes estará contaminado, torna-se essencial a remoção completa de todos os resquícios radiculares se a extração for realizada.
- Lesões resultantes em perda tecidual coronária extensa (estágios 4 ou 5) — a extração é tipicamente a única opção terapêutica. Como o tecido pulpar nas raízes estará contaminado, torna-se essencial a remoção completa de todos os resquícios radiculares.
- Cáries de raiz — caso se consiga tratar a doença periodontal e aplicar o material restaurativo na área supragengival, haverá possibilidade de restauração; no entanto, a extração será o tratamento de escolha para grande parte dos dentes com cáries radiculares.
- Se apenas uma única raiz de um dente multirradicular estiver cariada — a extração da raiz acometida com o tratamento endodôntico da(s) raiz(es) remanescente(s) também será uma opção.
- Pacientes de alto risco — pode-se considerar a aplicação do selante de depressão-e-fissura e/ou do agente ligante de dentina liberador de flúor sobre os dentes remanescentes com superfícies oclusais.

MEDICAÇÕES

MEDICAMENTO(S)
- Antibióticos de amplo espectro no pós-operatório — poderão ser indicados se houver envolvimento pulpar que necessite de tratamento endodôntico ou extração.
- Analgesia pós-operatória com medicamentos anti-inflamatórios não esteroides e/ou narcóticos — indicada depois de tratamento endodôntico ou exodôntico ou trabalho extenso de restauração de dentes vitais.

CONTRAINDICAÇÕES/INTERAÇÕES POSSÍVEIS
N/D.

ACOMPANHAMENTO

MONITORIZAÇÃO DO PACIENTE
- Examinar e radiografar os dentes tratados 6 meses após a intervenção cirúrgica, depois em intervalos anuais ou diante de qualquer oportunidade.
- Avaliar a integridade das restaurações, estimar a presença de outras deteriorações nas margens ou sob as restaurações e determinar o desenvolvimento de doença endodôntica.
- Como os indivíduos acometidos frequentemente apresentam mais de uma cárie, examinar com cautela todos os dentes por meios clínicos e radiológicos em busca do desenvolvimento de novas lesões em qualquer momento oportuno.

PREVENÇÃO
Evitar o consumo de dietas e petiscos ricos em carboidratos refinados pode reduzir o risco do desenvolvimento de cáries futuras.

EVOLUÇÃO ESPERADA E PROGNÓSTICO
Se uma lesão for adequadamente submetida a debridamento e restauração, ela deverá ter um prognóstico excelente. A seleção e o estadiamento adequados do caso, a remoção completa de todos os tecidos cariados e a adesão aos princípios da restauração são medidas essenciais.

DIVERSOS

SINÔNIMOS
- Cavidades.
- Deterioração dentária.

RECURSOS DA INTERNET
- A respeito de cáries dentárias em cães: http://www.toothvet.ca/PDFfiles/DentalCaries.pdf.
- Sobre o estadiamento de reabsorção dentária: http://www.avdc.org/Nomenclature.html#resorption.
- Referente à reabsorção dentária em gatos: http://www.toothvet.ca/PDFfiles/NewsOnRLs.pdf.
- Com respeito à reabsorção dentária em cães: http://www.toothvet.ca/PDFfiles/RLs in Dogs.pdf.

Sugestões de Leitura

Hale FA. Dental caries (cavities) In: Lobprise HB, ed., Blackwell's Five-Minute Veterinary Consult Clinical Companion—Small Animal Dentistry. Ames, IA: Blackwell, 2007, pp. 212-224.

Hale FA. Dental caries in the dog. J Vet Dent 1998, 15:79-83.

Hale FA. Veterinary Dentistry. Dental caries in the dog. CVJ 2009, 50:1301-1304.

Lobprise HB. Blackwell's Five-Minute Veterinary Consult Clinical Companion—Small Animal Dentistry. Ames, IA: Blackwell, 2007 (em busca de outros assuntos, incluindo métodos diagnósticos e técnicas).

McComb D. Caries-detector dyes—how accurate and useful are they? J Can Dent Assoc 2000, 66:195-198, disponível em http://www.cda-adc.ca/jcda/vol-66/issue-4/195.html.

Autor Fraser A. Hale
Consultor Editorial Heidi B. Lobprise

Carrapatos e seu Controle

CONSIDERAÇÕES GERAIS

DEFINIÇÃO
- Os cães e gatos podem ser parasitados por carrapatos pertencentes às famílias *Ixodidae* e *Argasidae*.
- Ectoparasitas artrópodes que se alimentam exclusivamente do sangue de seus hospedeiros; estreitamente relacionados com escorpiões, aranhas e ácaros.
- Patógenos microbianos transmitidos — protozoários, bactérias, riquétsias e vírus.
- Podem causar toxicose, hipersensibilidade, paralisia e anemia por perda sanguínea.

FISIOPATOLOGIA
- Anemia por perda sanguínea — decorrente de infestações maciças.
- Dano ao tegumento — as peças bucais dos carrapatos penetram na pele do hospedeiro; as picadas costumam ser indolores; podem ocorrer irritação e infecção locais. Existem adaptações dos carrapatos para suprimir a resposta do hospedeiro, permitindo que esses ectoparasitas se alimentem por até 1 semana.
- Secreção salivar de neurotoxinas — pode induzir a sinais sistêmicos (paralisia causada por carrapato); outros compostos provocam danos à hemostasia e imunossupressão na lesão de repasto sanguíneo pelo carrapato.
- Patógenos — são adquiridos quando os carrapatos se alimentam de hospedeiros reservatórios infectados (frequentemente, roedores e pequenos mamíferos selvagens).

BIOLOGIA DO CARRAPATO
- Carrapatos resistentes — apresentam quatro estágios de vida: ovo, larva, ninfa e adulto; as larvas e as ninfas alimentam-se até a repleção antes de eclodir e sofrer ecdise; como as fêmeas adultas dos carrapatos ixodídeos ingurgitam, elas podem aumentar seu peso em mais de 100 vezes; após o descolamento, as fêmeas depositam milhares de ovos e morrem. Vários estágios de carrapatos podem sobreviver durante o inverno e apresentam tolerância prolongada à inanição, mas também toleram baixa umidade e inanição de água.
- Em algumas espécies, os microrganismos disseminam-se para os ovários dos carrapatos, ocorrendo a transmissão transovariana; os ovos infectados eclodem e produzem larvas infectadas. Em outras espécies, ocorre transmissão transestadial; carrapatos imaturos vêm a ser infectados durante o repasto sanguíneo nos hospedeiros reservatórios e mantém a infecção por meio da muda de um estágio de vida para o outro. Ocorre infecção do hospedeiro quando as infecções adquiridas durante um estágio de vida prévio são transmitidas a novos hospedeiros no momento em que o próximo estágio de vida se alimenta.
- A saliva do carrapato contém compostos farmacologicamente ativos que fazem a intermediação da resposta imune do hospedeiro. Os carrapatos mantém as lesões de repasto sanguíneo por suprimir as respostas do hospedeiro e usar anticoagulantes.
- Em geral, os hospedeiros adquirem carrapatos por um processo passivo de emboscada. Quando um hospedeiro adequado roça ou esbarra em uma vegetação com carrapatos, esses ectoparasitas passarão para o hospedeiro. O *Amblyomma americanum* é o único ectoparasita capaz de ser um caçador ativo e atravessar distâncias de até ~18 metros para atacar um hospedeiro adequado.

SISTEMA(S) ACOMETIDO(S)
- Cutâneo/exócrino.
- Hematológico/linfático/imune.
- Nervoso.
- Musculoesquelético.

DISTRIBUIÇÃO GEOGRÁFICA
- Para certas espécies de carrapatos e seus patógenos associados, existem fortes especificidades geográficas; assim, a prevalência geográfica está ligada às doenças associadas.
- As variações de carrapatos estão se expandindo e, por essa razão, a incidência de parasitismo por carrapatos e de infecções transmitidas por diversas espécies desses ectoparasitas também está em expansão.
- Observa-se o surgimento de novas infecções e coinfecções por carrapatos, representando uma forte tendência.
- A incidência de coinfecções em rápida expansão está ocorrendo em virtude de carrapatos vetores coinfectados ou parasitismo de hospedeiros por múltiplos carrapatos de uma ou mais espécies.
- *Ixodes scapularis* e *I. pacificus* — meio-oeste, nordeste, sudeste e centro-sul dos EUA, além da costa ocidental, respectivamente.
- *Rhipicephalus sanguineus* — encontrado em todo o continente norte-americano; o *R. sanguineus* é o único carrapato entre esses ectoparasitas resistentes capaz de sobreviver e estabelecer seu ciclo de vida dentro de residências ou canis sob (baixas) umidades (daí o nome comum "carrapato de canil").
- *Dermacentor variabilis* — costas oriental e ocidental.
- *Amblyomma americanum* — encontrado em todo o meio-oeste, centro-sul, sudeste e partes do nordeste dos EUA com expansão de forte alcance.

IDENTIFICAÇÃO
Espécies
- Cães e gatos.
- Os gatos são muito eficientes na remoção de carrapatos, mas a fixação desses ectoparasitas e as doenças transmitidas por esses vetores, incluindo a doença de Lyme, a anaplasmose e a citauxzoonose, são diagnosticadas nos felinos domésticos.

SINAIS CLÍNICOS
- Podem ser observados os carrapatos aderidos à pele ou nas cavidades de repasto nos locais onde esses ectoparasitas foram removidos.
- Irritação secundária à picada.
- Formação de petéquias secundárias à transmissão de microrganismos infecciosos (o microrganismo *Rickettsia rickettsii* invade o endotélio vascular com consequente vasculite necrosante, enquanto o *Anaplasma platys* provoca trombocitopenia.
- Anemia por perda sanguínea (efeito direto); trombocitopenia, anemia, corpúsculos de inclusão em neutrófilos, monócitos e hemácias, secundários à transmissão de microrganismos infecciosos.
- Alterações em membros e articulações secundárias à transmissão de microrganismos infecciosos (*Borrelia burgdorferi* e outros microrganismos envolvidos em oligo ou poliartrite).
- Anormalidades cardíacas — vários graus de bloqueio cardíaco secundários à transmissão de microrganismos infecciosos (*B. burgdorferi*).
- Paralisia induzida por neurotoxina — sinais atribuídos ao SNC desenvolvem-se secundariamente à transmissão de microrganismos infecciosos (*R. rickettsii*).

CAUSAS
- Carrapatos — são atraídos aos hospedeiros por calor, presença de dióxido de carbono, contato físico e odores associados ao hospedeiro.

FATORES DE RISCO
- Animais domésticos — podem entrar em contato íntimo com carrapatos, em virtude da invasão desses ectoparasitas em ambientes suburbanos e da expansão desse tipo de ambiente em locais como florestas, campinas e áreas costeiras circunjacentes.
- Viagens constituem um fator de risco para exposição a carrapatos fora do ambiente doméstico de um animal de estimação.

DIAGNÓSTICO

DIAGNÓSTICO DIFERENCIAL
- Carrapatos — examinar a pele em busca de carrapatos aderidos ou das cavidades de repasto sanguíneo.
- Doenças transmitidas por carrapatos — avaliar as considerações epidemiológicas para cada doença e o histórico de parasitismo por carrapato, além de realizar o exame clínico completo.

OUTROS TESTES LABORATORIAIS
Snap 4Dx® — testes rápidos efetuados dentro do consultório para pesquisa de infecções por múltiplos vetores. Detectam anticorpos (ELISA realizado com base no peptídeo C_6) induzidos nas infecções por carrapatos com a transmissão de *B. burgdorferi*, *E. canis* e *A. phagocytophilum* (conhecido antigamente como *E. equi*), bem como a *Dirofilaria immitis* oriunda de picada de inseto. Os testes são sensíveis e específicos. O teste para pesquisa de *B. burgdorferi* não sofre reação cruzada com anticorpos induzidos por vacinas.

TRATAMENTO

CUIDADO(S) DE SAÚDE ADEQUADO(S)
- Tratar o paciente em um esquema ambulatorial após a remoção dos carrapatos.
- Remoção — efetuar o mais rápido possível para limitar o tempo disponível de transmissão de neurotoxinas e patógenos; apreender os carrapatos próximos à pele com o auxílio de pinças de ponta fina e tracioná-los delicadamente.

CUIDADO(S) DE ENFERMAGEM
Lavar as cavidades de repasto sanguíneo com água e sabão; em geral, esse procedimento é suficiente para evitar inflamação local ou infecção secundária.

ORIENTAÇÃO AO PROPRIETÁRIO
Informar ao proprietário que a aplicação de palitos de fósforos quentes, vaselina ou outros materiais não só atrapalha a retirada do carrapato, mas também confere períodos mais prolongados de fixação e repasto.

CARRAPATOS E SEU CONTROLE

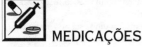

MEDICAÇÕES

MEDICAMENTO(S) DE ESCOLHA
Ver a seção "Prevenção".

ACOMPANHAMENTO

PREVENÇÃO
- Pode não ser uma tarefa fácil evitar os ambientes que albergam carrapatos.
- O controle dos carrapatos nem sempre equivale ao controle das doenças transmitidas por esses ectoparasitas; com frequência, o objetivo consiste na ausência perceptível de carrapatos no animal hospedeiro (repelência clínica).
- Animais de estimação — pode haver certo período de fixação e repasto sanguíneo ou, então, os carrapatos vivos podem ficar algum tempo rastejando sobre o animal após a exposição a níveis letais de algum acaricida; os carrapatos imaturos de determinadas espécies são muito pequenos.
- Patógenos transportados por carrapatos — podem ser transmitidos muito rapidamente (agentes virais) ou necessitar de algumas horas (*R. rickettsii*), menos de 1 dia (*A. phagocytophilum*), 1-2 dias (*B. burgdorferi*), ou 2-3 dias (espécies de *Ehrlichia* e *B. canis*).

Inseticidas e Acaricidas
- Nos EUA, a EPA (Environmental Protection Agency [Agência de Proteção Ambiental]) aprova os pesticidas como substâncias seguras e eficazes.
- Em muitas áreas, há necessidade de controle de carrapatos durante todo o ano.
- Coleiras acaricidas (Preventic®).
- Tratamentos sob a forma de spot-on (Frontline® top spot, K9 Advantix®, Promeris® e Vectra 3D®) — têm conquistado uso disseminado; a facilidade de aplicação e a obediência do proprietário ao tratamento são tão importantes quanto a eficácia do produto.
- Foram publicados estudos sobre a interrupção da transmissão de doenças para os produtos que contenham fipronil, amitraz ou permetrina em sua composição. A destruição rápida e a repelência clínica do ectoparasita são essenciais para evitar ou interromper o repasto sanguíneo. Em aproximadamente 4 semanas após a aplicação do produto, a eficácia na prevenção de transmissão de *B. burgdorferi* a cães foi de 75-87,5% para o fipronil (encontrado no Frontline® top spot) e 100% para a permetrina (encontrada nos produtos K9 Advantix® e Vectra 3D®); o amitraz (encontrado na coleira Preventic® e no produto Promeris®) se mostrou 100% eficaz em 7 dias após a aplicação.

COMPLICAÇÕES POSSÍVEIS
Doenças transmitidas por carrapatos ou paralisia causada por esse ectoparasita.

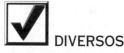

DIVERSOS

DISTÚRBIOS ASSOCIADOS
- Babesiose canina — transmitida pelo *R. sanguineus*; causada pelo protozoário *Babesia canis*, que infecta as hemácias caninas, levando à sedimentação nos capilares e destruição no baço.
- Febre maculosa das Montanhas Rochosas — transmitida pelo *D. variabilis*.
- Erliquiose monocítica canina — transmitida pelo *R. sanguineus*; causada pela *E. canis*, que infecta as células mononucleares e as plaquetas. A *E. chaffeensis* transmitida pelo *A. americanum* infecta as células mononucleares.
- Trombocitopenia cíclica — causada por *A. platys*, o único patógeno intracelular de plaquetas.
- Anaplasmose granulocítica — causada por *A. phagocytophilum* transmitido por *I. scapularis* e *I. pacificus*; infecta os granulócitos; *E. ewingii* transmitido por *A. americanum* também infecta os granulócitos e provoca erliquiose granulocítica.
- Doença de Lyme — transmitida pelo *I. scapularis* e *I. pacificus*; causada pela *B. burgdorferi*; associada à artrite ou a síndromes indutoras de bloqueio cardíaco completo, nefropatia com perda de proteínas e, possivelmente, anormalidades neurológicas.
- Hepatozoonose canina americana — causada pelo protozoário *H. americanum* após o cão ingerir o *A. maculatum* infectado.
- Hepatozoonose canina — causada pelo protozoário *H. canis* após o cão ingerir o *R. sanguineus* infectado.
- Paralisia causada por carrapatos — ocasionada por uma neurotoxina; compromete a síntese e/ou a liberação de acetilcolina na junção neuromuscular do animal hospedeiro; a paralisia flácida ascendente afeta, em princípio, os membros pélvicos 5-9 dias após a fixação do carrapato.

Vacinas
- Atualmente, há vacinas disponíveis para a doença de Lyme; existem dois tipos para cães: bacterina morta de célula inteira (desde 1990) e proteína A de superfície externa [OspA] (desde 1996).
- Segurança e eficácia — foi demonstrado que ambos os tipos de vacinas são seguros. Estudos laboratoriais revelam alta eficácia, mas não são capazes de reproduzir a exposição natural. Em um estudo de exposição natural precoce (1993) da bacterina de célula inteira (LymeVax®), a incidência da doença foi de 1% em 1.969 cães imunizados e 4,7% em 4.498 cães-controle não imunizados. Em estudos mais recentes de exposição natural, foi determinado que a incidência de infecção em cães imunizados com a LymeVax® e a vacina de subunidade OspA Recombitek rLyme® é de 5 e 25%, respectivamente. A bacterina (LymeVax®) tinha uma fração de prevenção de 92,2%, enquanto a vacina de subunidade OspA (rLyme®), de 60,3%. O autor imunizou centenas de cães positivos para Lyme com a LymeVax® e não observou qualquer aumento nos eventos adversos, incluindo doenças autoimunes ou anormalidades renais.
- Quando cães assintomáticos positivos para Lyme foram tratados com doxiciclina ou amoxicilina concomitantemente com a imunização LymeVax® e submetidos a acompanhamento clínico por até 4 anos, não foi observado nenhum episódio de qualquer forma da doença de Lyme.
- Uma lista extensa de referências bibliográficas a respeito dos estudos sobre vacinação pode ser encontrada adiante.

POTENCIAL ZOONÓTICO
- Os carrapatos podem parasitar animais silvestres, domésticos ou seres humanos em diferentes estágios do seu ciclo de desenvolvimento; as infecções adquiridas em estágios de vida precoces podem ser transmitidas quando os carrapatos voltam a se alimentar no estágio seguinte.
- Se forem parasitados, os seres humanos poderão ficar expostos a microrganismos presentes em carrapatos infectados. *B. burgdorferi*, *A. phagocytophilum*, *R. rickettsia* e *E. chaffeensis* também são patógenos de humanos.

SINÔNIMO(S)
Acaríase.

VER TAMBÉM
- Babesiose.
- Borreliose de Lyme.
- Erliquiose.
- Febre Maculosa das Montanhas Rochosas.
- Hepatozoonose.
- Paralisia pelo Carrapato.

ABREVIATURA(S)
- ELISA = ensaio imunoabsorvente ligado à enzima.
- SNC = sistema nervoso central.

RECURSOS DA INTERNET
Stafford KC, III. Tick Management Handbook. The Connecticut Agricultural Experiment Station: http://www.ct.gov/caes/search/search.asp?qu=tick+management&go.x=16&go.y=6.

Sugestões de Leitura

Blagburn BL, Spencer JA, Butler JM, et al. Prevention of transmission of Borrelia burgdorferi and Anaplasma phagocytophilum from ticks to dogs using K9 Advantix and Frontline Plus applied 25 days before exposure to infected ticks. Int J Appl Res Vet Med 2005, 3(2):69-75.

Elfassy OJ, Goodman FW, Levy SA, et al. Efficacy of an amitraz-impregnated collar in preventing transmission of Borrelia burgdorferi by adult Ixodes scapularis to dogs. JAVMA 2001, 219:185-189.

Jacobsen R, McCall J, Hunter J, et al. The ability of fipronil to prevent transmission of Borrelia burgdorferi, the causative agent of Lyme disease to dogs. Int J Appl Res Vet Med 2004, 3(2)39-45.

Levy SA. Use of a C6 ELISA test to evaluate the efficacy of a whole-cell bacterin for the prevention of naturally transmitted canine Borrelia burgdorferi infection. J Vet Ther 2002, 3(4):420-424.

Levy SA, Clark KC, Glickman LT. Infection rates in dogs vaccinated and not vaccinated with an ospA Borrelia burgdorferi vaccine in a Lyme disease endemic area of Connecticut. Int J Appl Res Vet Med 2005, 3(1):1-5.

Levy SA, Lissman BA, Ficke CM. Performance of a Borrelia Burgdorferi bacterin in borreliosis-endemic areas. JAVMA 1993, 202:1834-1838.

Sonenshine D. Biology of Ticks, Volumes 1 and 2. New York: Oxford University Press, 1991, 1993.

Autor Steven A. Levy
Consultor Editorial Alexander H. Werner

CATARATAS

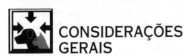

CONSIDERAÇÕES GERAIS

DEFINIÇÃO
• Opacificação do cristalino (focal ou difusa).

FISIOPATOLOGIA
• O cristalino normal é composto de fibras lenticulares perfeitamente alinhadas que criam uma estrutura transparente. Uma cápsula clara envolve o córtex e o núcleo do cristalino. Novas fibras lenticulares são continuamente produzidas na região equatorial do córtex do cristalino durante toda a vida. O humor aquoso fornece nutrição ao cristalino.
• A catarata ocorre quando há um desarranjo das fibras lenticulares em virtude de alterações na nutrição do cristalino, metabolismo de energia, síntese ou metabolismo de proteína, ou equilíbrio osmótico.
• O quadro de uveíte anterior é uma causa comum de alteração da nutrição do cristalino. A genética pode resultar em alteração do metabolismo de proteína e energia, ou na síntese de proteína, no cristalino.
• O diabetes melito afetará o equilíbrio osmótico dentro do cristalino do cão. A hiperglicemia aumenta o nível de glicose no humor aquoso e no cristalino, sobrepujando a via normal de glicólise; a glicose, então, é desviada para a via do sorbitol; ao ser produzido, o sorbitol cria um gradiente osmótico que atrai a água para o cristalino, resultando na rápida formação de catarata por tumefação (inchaço) e desarranjo das fibras lenticulares. Como a via do sorbitol requer a atuação da enzima aldose redutase, quanto mais enzima estiver presente no cristalino, mais rapidamente as cataratas diabéticas se formarão. Os cães possuem mais aldose redutase que os gatos, tornando essa última espécie mais resistente ao desenvolvimento de cataratas diabéticas. Existe certa variabilidade individual entre os cães, o que pode explicar o motivo pelo qual alguns cães diabéticos são mais resistentes ao desenvolvimento de cataratas.

SISTEMA(S) ACOMETIDO(S)
Oftálmico.

GENÉTICA
• Foi estabelecido o modo de herança para muitas raças caninas (ver "Sugestões de Leitura"); o modo de herança mais comum é autossômica recessiva.
• O modo de herança também foi estabelecido no gato Himalaio (autossômica recessiva).

INCIDÊNCIA/PREVALÊNCIA
• Catarata é uma das principais causas de cegueira em cães.
• A prevalência de cataratas genéticas varia significativamente entre as raças; há relatos de até 10% em algumas raças.
• A maioria dos cães diabéticos desenvolverá cataratas, independentemente de seu controle glicêmico.
• As cataratas são raras em gatos.

IDENTIFICAÇÃO
Espécies
Cães e gatos.

Raça(s) Predominante(s)
Suspeita-se que mais de 135 raças caninas sejam predispostas a cataratas hereditárias.

Idade Média e Faixa Etária
As cataratas podem se desenvolver em qualquer idade; as cataratas genéticas podem ocorrer já com 6 meses de vida.

SINAIS CLÍNICOS
Achados Anamnésicos
• O proprietário pode notar o aspecto turvo/branco do cristalino.
• A perda de visão pode ser observada pelo proprietário quando as cataratas são bilaterais, especialmente as diabéticas que apresentam início rápido e bilateral.
• Os sinais de poliúria/polidipsia costumam ser constatados pelo proprietário antes do desenvolvimento da catarata em cães diabéticos.

Achados do Exame Físico
• Achados do exame físico geral: nada digno de nota a menos que o cão seja um animal diabético não diagnosticado.
• Achados do exame oftálmico: opacificação em um ou ambos os cristalinos.
• Estágio incipiente: pequena(s) opacidade(s) focal(is) no cristalino que não interfere na visualização do fundo do olho; ausência de déficits visuais.
• Estágio imaturo: aspecto difusamente turvo do cristalino com reflexo tapetal ainda visível e algumas porções do fundo ocular visíveis por meio da dilatação da pupila; o reflexo à ameaça é positivo, mas o rastreamento pode ser negativo.
• Estágio maduro: cristalino completamente opaco sem reflexo tapetal visível; olho cego.
• Estágio hipermaduro: cápsula lenticular enrugada, áreas de mineralização branca densa, pode ter partes do córtex lenticular liquefeito (branco, brilhante a claro); câmara anterior profunda; olho cego a menos que haja uma ampla área de córtex liquefeito claro.
• Catarata madura intumescente: cristalino opaco e intumescido, geralmente em virtude do efeito hiperosmótico do diabetes; câmara anterior superficial.

CAUSAS
• Hereditária — causa mais comum em cães.
• Diabetes melito.
• Uveíte anterior — por nutrição alterada do cristalino por causa de anormalidade do humor aquoso, ou por sinequias posteriores ou *debris* inflamatórios que causam opacificação da cápsula anterior do cristalino.
• Traumatismo — lesão perfurante que rompe a cápsula anterior do cristalino, causada mais comumente por arranhadura de gato, sobretudo em filhotes caninos e felinos.
• Senil — catarata lentamente progressiva em animais geriátricos que costuma se iniciar como uma esclerose nuclear densa acompanhada por opacidades graduais semelhantes a raios que se estendem para o córtex.
• Congênita — por hereditariedade, lesão intrauterina, ou associada a outras anomalias oculares congênitas, como membranas pupilares persistentes, túnica vascular do cristalino hiperplásica persistente/ vítreo primário hiperplásico persistente, ou fixação da artéria hialoide.
• Cirúrgica — cirurgia por laser transpupilar, traumatismo por instrumento intraocular.
• Tóxica — por terapia prolongada com cetoconazol; suspeita de catarata secundária a subprodutos tóxicos de fotorreceptores em processo de degeneração em cães com atrofia progressiva da retina.
• Radiação — quando o olho está no campo da radiação para tratamento de neoplasia craniencefálica.
• Hipocalcemia — pode causar cataratas puntiformes ou incipientes bilaterais e difusas.
• Nutricional — uso de sucedâneos do leite desbalanceados em filhotes caninos e felinos alimentados com mamadeira.
• Choque elétrico — mastigação de fios elétricos ou queda de raio.

FATORES DE RISCO
• Diabetes melito é um fator de risco importante em cães.
• Uveíte anterior crônica.
• Atrofia progressiva da retina.

DIAGNÓSTICO

DIAGNÓSTICO DIFERENCIAL
• Esclerose nuclear lenticular — alteração normal do envelhecimento no cristalino de cães e gatos, que começa aos 6 anos de idade em virtude da compressão de fibras lenticulares mais velhas no centro do cristalino; gradativamente se torna mais visível com a idade e pode ser confundida com catarata em pacientes geriátricos; o diagnóstico definitivo pode ser feito com o uso de midríase (tropicamida a 1%), a observação de um núcleo perfeitamente redondo, bilateralmente simétrico e homogêneo no centro de cada cristalino e a capacidade de visualizar o fundo ocular por meio do cristalino; a visão raramente é afetada e o tratamento não é indicado.

HEMOGRAMA/BIOQUÍMICA/URINÁLISE
Os cães com cataratas diabéticas podem ter hiperglicemia e glicosúria.

DIAGNÓSTICO POR IMAGEM
Ultrassonografia ocular pode ser usada para avaliar a cápsula posterior do cristalino em busca de qualquer sinal de ruptura, além de ser capaz de avaliar o descolamento da retina antes da cirurgia de catarata.

MÉTODOS DIAGNÓSTICOS
Eletrorretinografia é um exame realizado antes da cirurgia de catarata para avaliar a presença de degeneração da retina quando o fundo ocular não é visualizado por conta da catarata.

TRATAMENTO

ATIVIDADE
Como medida de segurança, não se deve permitir que os animais cegos tenham acesso a piscinas ou decks suspensos com grades abertas; ter cuidado perto de escadas; restringir a atividade fora de casa com quintais cercados ou passeios com coleiras.

ORIENTAÇÃO AO PROPRIETÁRIO
• A cirurgia de catarata é um procedimento de rotina, com taxa de sucesso global de 80-90%.
• Uma vez removidas, as cataratas não conseguem recidivar.
• Os implantes de cristalino artificial basicamente restabelecerão a visão normal.

- A avaliação do paciente para cirurgia deve ser feita no início do desenvolvimento da catarata para evitar complicações que possam resultar em uma catarata inoperável, dar tempo para planejar a cirurgia e, em alguns casos, eliminar a necessidade e o custo extra de ultrassonografia ocular e eletrorretinografia.

CONSIDERAÇÕES CIRÚRGICAS
- Facoemulsificação (remoção da catarata por meio de incisão de 3 mm na córnea com o uso de ondas ultrassônicas para emulsificar e, depois, aspirar o córtex e o núcleo do cristalino) constitui a técnica mais usual para remoção de catarata.
- O momento ideal para cirurgia de catarata é o estágio imaturo/maduro precoce.
- Cataratas hereditárias, diabéticas e senis são candidatos potencialmente bons para cirurgia; cataratas secundárias à uveíte anterior normalmente são maus candidatos cirúrgicos.
- Cristalinos intraoculares artificiais são implantados com certa rotina dentro da cápsula lenticular do paciente; os implantes de cristalino restabelecem o foco normal e ajudam a minimizar a fibrose da cápsula posterior; se o implante de cristalino não for possível (p. ex., em função de instabilidade da cápsula lenticular ou luxação do cristalino), o cão ou o gato ainda terá uma visão bastante funcional.
- Perfuração traumática do cristalino com liberação do córtex lenticular para a câmara anterior exige a remoção imediata do cristalino para evitar o desenvolvimento de uveíte anterior granulomatosa grave e a perda da visão.

MEDICAÇÕES
MEDICAMENTO(S) DE ESCOLHA
- É recomendado o uso de agente anti-inflamatório tópico a cada 6-24 h para ajudar a evitar ou tratar a uveíte induzida pelo cristalino com cataratas imaturas, maduras e hipermaduras; esse agente pode ser um AINE tópico, como flurbiprofeno ou diclofenaco, ou um esteroide tópico, como prednisolona a 1% ou dexametasona a 0,1%; os AINE tópicos são preferidos em pacientes diabéticos a menos que a uveíte seja grave.
- Atropina tópica a cada 8-24 h é indicada para uveíte induzida pelo cristalino; *a atropina é contraindicada na presença de glaucoma.*
- AINE orais (carprofeno, meloxicam, tepoxalina) também são usados para tratar a uveíte induzida pelo cristalino.
- Antioxidantes tópicos são anunciados como agentes capazes de reverter as alterações da catarata; até o momento, não há dados conclusivos publicados que comprovem uma reversão significativa, ou retardo na evolução, de uma catarata com terapia antioxidante; infelizmente, o tempo gasto na tentativa de uma terapia médica atrasará a avaliação cirúrgica, resultando na realização da cirurgia em um estágio fora do ideal ou em complicações advindas de catarata inoperável.
- Inibidores da aldose redutase tópicos estão atualmente sob investigação e podem se mostrar úteis no adiamento do início das cataratas diabéticas em cães no futuro.

ACOMPANHAMENTO
MONITORIZAÇÃO DO PACIENTE
- É recomendável a monitorização regular de cataratas incipientes ou imaturas precoces quanto à evolução para selecionar o momento ideal da cirurgia e evitar complicações associadas às cataratas.
- A monitorização pós-operatória pelo cirurgião é uma medida crítica para o sucesso da cirurgia e deve ser claramente abordada com o proprietário antes do procedimento cirúrgico.
- Itens como incisão da córnea, ocorrência de uveíte pós-operatória, formação de fibrina na câmara anterior, pressão intraocular, posição do implante do cristalino e estado da retina são, sem exceção, monitorizados atentamente.

PREVENÇÃO
Não acasalar os animais com cataratas.

COMPLICAÇÕES POSSÍVEIS
- Uveíte induzida pelo cristalino — associada a cataratas hipermaduras e cataratas de evolução muito rápida; causada por proteínas lenticulares antigênicas que extravasam através da cápsula do cristalino. Os sinais clínicos podem ser muito sutis (p. ex., pressão intraocular baixa) até extremos (uveíte granulomatosa com depósito aquoso denso, miose, sinequia, precipitados ceráticos); a uveíte pré-operatória induzida pelo cristalino aumenta o risco de complicações pós-operatórias.
- Glaucoma secundário — diminuição do fluxo de saída do humor aquoso decorrente de alterações intraoculares associadas à uveíte induzida pelo cristalino ou de catarata intumescente indutora de deslocamento anterógrado da íris com consequente estreitamento do ângulo iridocorneano.
- Descolamento da retina — associado a cataratas hipermaduras e cataratas em cães jovens com início rápido e liquefação cortical.
- Luxação do cristalino — associada a cataratas hipermaduras em que o cristalino e a cápsula se contraem, fazendo com que as zônulas sofram estiramento e ruptura, com subsequente subluxação e luxação do cristalino.

EVOLUÇÃO ESPERADA E PROGNÓSTICO
- Grande parte das cataratas é progressiva, embora a velocidade de evolução possa variar muito, dependendo da idade, da raça e da localização da catarata.
- O prognóstico a longo prazo após cirurgia de catarata é muito bom; no entanto, alguns pacientes têm um risco elevado de complicações pós-operatórias; uveíte anterior preexistente (mesmo quando controlada por meios médicos), predisposição genética para glaucoma, e retina periférica instável ou lacerações retinianas periféricas não detectadas aumentam o risco de uveíte crônica, glaucoma, e descolamento da retina pós-operatórios, respectivamente.

DIVERSOS
DISTÚRBIOS ASSOCIADOS
- Descolamento da retina.
- Uveíte induzida pelo cristalino.
- Anomalias oculares congênitas.

FATORES RELACIONADOS COM A IDADE
- É recomendável o encaminhamento imediato dos casos de cataratas em cães jovens (<2 anos de idade), pois elas podem evoluir muito rapidamente com liquefação cortical parcial seguida de descolamento da retina.
- O quadro de esclerose nuclear é proeminente em animais geriátricos; pode ser necessária a realização de exame com as pupilas dilatadas para a diferenciação definitiva entre esclerose nuclear e catarata.

VER TAMBÉM
- Uveíte Anterior — Cães.
- Uveíte Anterior — Gatos.
- Capítulos sobre Diabetes.

ABREVIATURA(S)
- AINE = anti-inflamatório não esteroide

Sugestões de Leitura

Adkins EA, Hendrix DVH. Cataract evaluation and treatment in dogs. Compend Contin Educ Pract Vet 2003, 25:812-825.

Appel SL, Maggs DJ, Hollingsworth SR, Kass PH. Evaluation of client perceptions concerning outcome of cataract surgery in dogs. JAVMA 2006, 228:870-875.

Gelatt KN. Veterinary Ophthalmology, 4th ed. Ames, IA: Blackwell, 2007, p. 869. Maggs DJ, Miller PE, Ofri R. Slatter's Fundamentals of Vet Ophthalmology, 4th ed. St. Louis: Saunders, 2008, pp. 261-272.

Park SA, Yi NY, Jeong MB, Kim WT, Kim SE, Chae JM, Seo KM. Clinical manifestations of cataracts in small breed dogs. Vet Ophthalmology 2009, 12:205-210.

Sigle KJ, Nasisse MP. Long-term complications after phacoemulsification for cataract removal in dogs: 172 cases (1995-2002). JAVMA 2006, 228:74-79.

Autor Margi A. Gilmour
Consultor Editorial Paul E. Miller

Caxumba

CONSIDERAÇÕES GERAIS

REVISÃO
- Doença comum em seres humanos.
- Os cães contraem a doença a partir de crianças infectadas.
- Incidência (cães) — baixa.

IDENTIFICAÇÃO
- Cães de todas as idades.
- Nenhuma predileção sexual ou racial.

SINAIS CLÍNICOS
- Glândulas salivares parótidas aumentadas de volume.
- Febre.
- Anorexia.

CAUSAS E FATORES DE RISCO
Vírus da caxumba — família Paramyxoviridae; gênero *Paramyxovirus*.

DIAGNÓSTICO

DIAGNÓSTICO DIFERENCIAL
- Aumento de volume benigno da glândula salivar parótida.
- Neoplasia.

HEMOGRAMA/BIOQUÍMICA/URINÁLISE
Sem achados específicos.

OUTROS TESTES LABORATORIAIS
N/D.

DIAGNÓSTICO POR IMAGEM
N/D.

MÉTODOS DE DIAGNÓSTICO
Sorológico — anticorpos virais contra a caxumba.

TRATAMENTO

Geralmente não é necessário.

MEDICAÇÕES

MEDICAMENTO(S)
Nenhum.

CONTRAINDICAÇÕES/INTERAÇÕES POSSÍVEIS
Nenhuma.

ACOMPANHAMENTO

MONITORIZAÇÃO DO PACIENTE
Monitorizar itens como hidratação, nível de eletrólitos, equilíbrio acidobásico e temperatura corporal.

EVOLUÇÃO ESPERADA E PROGNÓSTICO
Os pacientes costumam se recuperar dentro de 5-10 dias da infecção.

DIVERSOS

POTENCIAL ZOONÓTICO
O vírus da caxumba dissemina-se apenas de seres humanos agudamente infectados para cães suscetíveis.

Sugestões de Leitura
Greene CE. Mumps and influenza virus infections. In: Greene CE, ed., Infectious Diseases of the Dog and Cat, 3rd ed. St. Louis: Saunders Elsevier, 2006, pp. 187.

Autor Johnny D. Hoskins
Consultor Editorial Stephen C. Barr

CELULITE JUVENIL

CONSIDERAÇÕES GERAIS

REVISÃO
- Distúrbio granulomatoso e pustular raro dos filhotes caninos.
- Raramente observado em cães adultos.
- Afeta principalmente a face, os pavilhões auriculares e os linfonodos submandibulares.
- Imunopatogenia desconhecida.

IDENTIFICAÇÃO
- Cães.
- Faixa etária — geralmente entre 3 semanas e 4 meses de vida.
- Raças predispostas — Golden retriever, Dachshund e Setter Gordon.

SINAIS CLÍNICOS
- Tumefação (inchaço) aguda da face (pálpebras, lábios e focinho).
- Linfadenopatia submandibular.
- Dermatite pustular e exsudativa acentuada, que frequentemente apresenta fístulas e se desenvolve em 24-48 h.
- Otite externa purulenta.
- As lesões quase sempre formam crostas.
- A pele acometida costuma estar dolorida.
- Letargia — 50% dos casos.
- Anorexia, pirexia e artrite supurativa estéril — 25% dos casos.
- Paniculite piogranulomatosa estéril (rara) sobre o tronco, as regiões prepucial ou perianal; as lesões podem aparecer como nódulos subcutâneos flutuantes que formam fístulas.

CAUSAS E FATORES DE RISCO
- Desconhecidos: suspeita-se de uma disfunção imunológica com causa hereditária.

DIAGNÓSTICO

DIAGNÓSTICO DIFERENCIAL
- Foliculite/furunculose bacteriana.
- Demodicose.
- Erupção medicamentosa.
- Infecção fúngica profunda.
- Hipersensibilidade cutânea.
- Reação a vacinas.
- Intoxicação por *Hymenoptera* ou insetos.

OUTROS TESTES LABORATORIAIS
- Citologia — inflamação piogranulomatosa sem microrganismos; neutrófilos não degenerados.
- Cultura — estéril.

MÉTODOS DIAGNÓSTICOS
Biopsia de pele.

ACHADOS PATOLÓGICOS
- Múltiplos granulomas e piogranulomas isolados ou confluentes — aglomerados de grandes macrófagos epitelioides e neutrófilos.
- Glândulas sebáceas e glândulas apócrinas podem estar obliteradas.
- Alterações supurativas na derme — predominam nos estágios tardios.
- Paniculite.
- Cultura de exsudato: importante para a seleção de antibióticos na suspeita de infecção secundária.

TRATAMENTO

- Há necessidade de tratamento precoce e rigoroso, porque a formação cicatricial pode ser grave.
- Terapia tópica — pode ser suavizante e paliativa; adjuvante dos corticosteroides.

MEDICAÇÕES

MEDICAMENTO(S)
- Corticosteroides — é necessário o uso de doses elevadas; prednisona (2,2 mg/kg divididos 2 vezes ao dia por, no mínimo, 2 semanas).
- Não reduzir muito rapidamente.
- Quimioterapia — casos raros de resistência.
- Cães adultos com paniculite podem necessitar de tratamento mais prolongado.
- Antibióticos — se houver indícios de infecção bacteriana secundária; como terapia adjuvante com doses imunossupressoras de corticosteroides.

ACOMPANHAMENTO

- A maior parte dos casos não apresenta recidiva.
- A cicatrização pode ser problemática, especialmente ao redor dos olhos.

DIVERSOS

Sugestões de Leitura
Scott DW, Miller WH, Griffin CE, eds. Muller & Kirk's Small Animal Dermatology, 5th ed. Philadelphia: Saunders, 1995, pp. 938-941.

Autor Karen Helton Rhodes
Consultor Editorial Alexander H. Werner

CERATITE NÃO ULCERATIVA

CONSIDERAÇÕES GERAIS

DEFINIÇÃO
Distúrbio inflamatório da córnea que não retenha o corante de fluoresceína.

FISIOPATOLOGIA
• Resposta patológica que resulta em diminuição na claridade da córnea, secundariamente a edema, infiltração celular inflamatória, vascularização, pigmentação, depósito de lipídio ou de cálcio ou cicatrização.
• A vascularização da córnea pode ser superficial ou profunda; os vasos corneanos superficiais são dendríticos (aparência de três ramos) e indicam doença ocular externa; já os vasos corneanos profundos são curtos e retos, indicando doença corneana profunda ou intraocular (p. ex., uveíte, glaucoma).

SISTEMA(S) ACOMETIDO(S)
Oftálmico.

GENÉTICA
• Nenhuma base genética comprovada em cães e gatos.
• Ceratite superficial crônica (pano) — predisposição hereditária considerada no Pastor alemão.

INCIDÊNCIA/PREVALÊNCIA
Causa comum de doença ocular em cães e gatos.

DISTRIBUIÇÃO GEOGRÁFICA
A ceratite superficial crônica é mais comum em regiões de altitude elevada (>4.000 pés [1.200 m]).

IDENTIFICAÇÃO
Espécies
• Cães — ceratite superficial crônica (pano); ceratite pigmentar; episcleroceratite granulomatosa nodular (ver "Episclerite"); ceratoconjuntivite seca (ver "Ceratoconjuntivite Seca").
• Gatos — ceratite eosinofílica (ver "Ceratite, Eosinofílica — Gatos") por herpes-vírus (forma estromal); sequestro de córnea; a ceratoconjuntivite seca é incomum e geralmente secundária à infecção crônica por herpes-vírus.

Raça(s) Predominante(s)
Cães
• Ceratite superficial crônica (pano) — pode ocorrer em qualquer raça; prevalência mais alta no Pastor alemão e no Galgo.
• Ceratite pigmentar — acomete notavelmente raças braquicefálicas com ceratopatia por exposição a partir de lagoftalmia, deficiências do filme lacrimal e triquíase secundária a entrópio do canto medial e pregas nasais.
• Episcleroceratite granulomatosa nodular — pode ocorrer em qualquer raça; prevalente nas raças Cocker spaniel, Collie e Pastor de Shetland.
• Ceratoconjuntivite seca — raças braquicefálicas, Cocker spaniel, Buldogue inglês, West Highland white terrier, Cavalier King Charles spaniel, Bloodhound.

Gatos
• Ceratite eosinofílica — mais prevalente em gato doméstico de pelo curto.
• Sequestro de córnea — mais prevalente em Persa, Siamês, Birmanês e Himalaio.

Idade Média e Faixa Etária
• Cães: ceratite superficial crônica — pode ocorrer em qualquer idade; maior risco entre 3 e 6 anos de idade (mais jovem em Galgos); ceratite pigmentar — pode ocorrer em qualquer idade; episcleroceratite granulomatosa nodular — pode ocorrer em qualquer idade; em Collie — jovem a meia-idade (média de 3,8 anos); ceratoconjuntivite seca — geralmente meia-idade a mais idoso.
• Gatos: herpes-vírus — todas as idades; ceratite eosinofílica e sequestro corneano — todas as idades exceto neonatos.

Sexo Predominante
• Cães: há relatos de predisposição de fêmeas para pano e ceratoconjuntivite seca.
• Gatos: predisposição de machos castrados relatada para ceratite eosinofílica.

SINAIS CLÍNICOS
Achados Anamnésicos
Pode provocar coloração corneana variável e desconforto ocular.

Achados do Exame Físico
Cães
• Ceratite superficial crônica — lesões vascularizadas geralmente bilaterais, muitas vezes róseas assimétricas (i. e., tecido de granulação) com pigmentação variável; a maioria dos casos envolve a córnea lateral ou ventrolateral; a evolução da doença leva ao envolvimento de outros quadrantes; as terceiras pálpebras podem estar acometidas e parecer espessadas ou despigmentadas; depósitos brancos (degeneração da córnea) podem estar presentes na borda principal da lesão; pode induzir à cegueira em casos de doença avançada.
• Ceratite pigmentar — aparece como uma coloração castanha, focal a difusa, da córnea; quase sempre associada à vascularização ou cicatrização corneanas.
• Episcleroceratite granulomatosa nodular — massas geralmente bilaterais, elevadas e carnosas que afetam o limbo lateral e a córnea; também podem ocorrer depósitos e edema de córnea no estroma corneano adjacente; terceiras pálpebras lenta a rapidamente progressivas podem aparecer espessadas.
• Ceratoconjuntivite seca — achados variáveis; pode ser uni ou bilateral; secreção ocular mucoide a mucopurulenta, hiperemia conjuntival, vascularização da córnea, pigmentação e cicatrização; pode ocorrer ulceração de córnea.

Gatos
• Herpes-vírus (forma estromal) — pode ser uni ou bilateral; caracterizada por edema estromal, infiltrados, vascularização profunda e cicatrização; frequentemente ocorre com ulceração; poderá comprometer a visão se houver cicatrização grave.
• Ceratite eosinofílica — em geral, unilateral; acomete principalmente a córnea perilimbal lateral ou medial; lesão vascularizada elevada com infiltrados róseos e brancos que formam placas arenosas; pode reter o corante de fluoresceína na periferia da lesão.
• Sequestro de córnea — geralmente unilateral, mas pode ser bilateral; aparece como placas de coloração âmbar, castanha ou negra da córnea central ou paracentral; pode variar em termos de tamanho e profundidade da córnea acometida; as bordas podem parecer elevadas; a vascularização da córnea é variável; pode reter a fluoresceína na periferia da lesão.

CAUSAS
Cães
• Ceratite superficial crônica — presume-se que ela seja imunomediada; altitude elevada e subsequente aumento na exposição à radiação UV aumentam a prevalência e a gravidade da doença.
• Ceratite pigmentar — secundária à irritação crônica da córnea; avaliar o paciente em busca de condições oculares subjacentes primárias; mais frequentemente associada à ceratopatia por exposição e ceratoconjuntivite seca.
• Episcleroceratite granulomatosa nodular — supostamente imunomediada.
• Ceratoconjuntivite seca — bilateral — geralmente imunomediada ou induzida por medicamentos; unilateral — congênita, iatrogênica, neurogênica.

Gatos
• Herpes-vírus (forma estromal) — é mais uma reação imunomediada por linfócitos-T do que um efeito citopático do vírus.
• Ceratite eosinofílica — possível reação de hipersensibilidade; alta incidência de animais PCR-positivos para FHV-1; menos animais positivos para agentes semelhantes a Chlamydia.
• Sequestro de córnea — desconhecido; provavelmente atribuído à irritação ou ulceração crônicas da córnea; relação sugerida com herpes-vírus.

FATORES DE RISCO
Cães — é mais provável que ocorra ceratite superficial crônica em altitudes elevadas secundariamente ao aumento na exposição UV.

DIAGNÓSTICO

DIAGNÓSTICO DIFERENCIAL
Cães
• Ceratite infecciosa, em geral, é ulcerativa e dolorosa; o exame citológico da córnea revela a presença de leucócitos e microrganismos.
• Neoplasia — envolvimento raro da esclera ou da córnea; distinguir com base na cor, na idade do animal, na predileção racial; geralmente unilateral; resposta ao tratamento anti-inflamatório tópico.

Gatos
• Ceratite infecciosa — geralmente ulcerativa e dolorosa; a infecção do estroma por herpes-vírus pode estar associada à ceratite ulcerativa; o exame citológico da córnea revela a presença de leucócitos e microrganismos.
• Neoplasia — muito rara; geralmente envolve a área do limbo.

MÉTODOS DIAGNÓSTICOS
Cães
Ceratite superficial crônica: o exame citológico de raspados da conjuntiva ou da córnea revela linfócitos, plasmócitos e mastócitos; pode ser considerado o procedimento de biopsia; episcleroceratite granulomatosa nodular: biopsia de massa nodular episcleral ou da córnea (ceratectomia superficial); teste lacrimal de Schirmer para ceratite pigmentar, ceratoconjuntivite seca ou qualquer doença da córnea de causa indeterminada; valores normais são ≥15 mm/min; os valores compatíveis com ceratoconjuntivite seca são <10 mm/min; valores entre 10 e 15 mm/min sugerem ceratoconjuntivite seca, porém devem ser interpretados, levando-se a raça e os achados oculares em consideração.

CERATITE NÃO ULCERATIVA

Gatos
Herpes: os raspados da conjuntiva ou da córnea para a realização de PCR são mais bem-sucedidos para o diagnóstico; os exames de IFA ou cultura viral são de valor limitado; a interpretação pode ser difícil; obter amostras para a IFA antes da instilação de fluoresceína; ceratite eosinofílica: a citologia da córnea é positiva para eosinófilos ± mastócitos; a biopsia da córnea (ceratectomia superficial) pode ser considerada para ceratite eosinofílica ou sequestro, porém costuma ser desnecessária.

TRATAMENTO

CUIDADO(S) DE SAÚDE ADEQUADO(S)
- Paciente de ambulatório — em geral é suficiente.
- Paciente internado — casos que justifiquem a cirurgia em virtude da resposta inadequada ao tratamento clínico.

ORIENTAÇÃO AO PROPRIETÁRIO

Cães
Tipicamente há necessidade de tratamento por toda a vida; a doença é mais controlada do que curada; a cirurgia pode ser necessária para ceratite pigmentar ou ceratoconjuntivite seca.

Gatos
- Herpes-vírus — desconforto ocular e ceratite quase sempre recidivantes.
- Ceratite eosinofílica — doença mais controlada do que curada.
- Sequestro de córnea — o sequestro pode esfacelar espontaneamente; a evolução clínica frequentemente é demorada sem cirurgia; a remoção do sequestro por meio de ceratectomia superficial pode ser curativa, embora seja possível a ocorrência de recidiva.

CONSIDERAÇÕES CIRÚRGICAS

Cães
- Ceratite superficial crônica — a ceratectomia superficial pode ser realizada nos casos de doença grave em que a visão se encontra prejudicada em virtude de pigmentação da córnea; os pacientes ainda necessitam de tratamento clínico por tempo indefinido para evitar recidiva; irradiação-β com sonda de estrôncio-90 é um método não invasivo, podendo ser efetuada em casos graves.
- Ceratite pigmentar — a ceratectomia superficial só pode ser realizada após a correção da causa subjacente inicial; apenas em casos graves que coloquem a visão sob risco.
- Episcleroceratite granulomatosa nodular — a ceratectomia superficial é diagnóstica; em geral desnecessária; resolve apenas temporariamente os sinais clínicos; o tratamento clínico ainda é necessário.
- Ceratoconjuntivite seca — transposição do ducto parotídeo ou tarsorrafia parcial permanente para reduzir a exposição.

Gatos
- Ceratite eosinofílica — a ceratectomia superficial é diagnóstica, mas não curativa; o tratamento clínico é o preferido.
- Sequestro de córnea — a ceratectomia superficial pode ser curativa; a recidiva é possível; o desconforto ocular é a principal indicação de cirurgia.

MEDICAÇÕES

MEDICAMENTO(S)

Cães
- Ceratite superficial crônica — corticosteroides tópicos (prednisolona a 1% ou dexametasona a 0,1% a cada 6-12 h); ciclosporina a 0,2-2%, pimecrolimo a 1% ou tacrolimo a 0,03% a cada 8-12 h por via tópica; esses medicamentos podem ser utilizados isoladamente ou em combinação para os casos mais graves; a injeção subconjuntival de corticosteroides pode ser usada como adjuvante ao tratamento tópico nos casos graves (acetonida de triancinolona a 4-8 mg).
- Ceratite pigmentar — tratamento direcionado à causa subjacente; corticosteroides tópicos se a causa primária for inflamatória; lubrificantes e ciclosporina ou tacrolimo se a condição primária for ceratoconjuntivite seca; a ciclosporina ou o tacrolimo pode reduzir a pigmentação em todos os casos.
- Episcleroceratite granulomatosa nodular — corticosteroides e/ou ciclosporina tópicos conforme descrito acima; azatioprina sistêmica (2 mg/kg/dia inicialmente, em seguida reduzir de modo gradual) pode ser eficaz quando utilizada isoladamente ou em combinação com medicações tópicas.
- Ceratoconjuntivite seca — ciclosporina tópica a 0,2-2% ou tacrolimo a 0,02-0,03% a cada 8-12 h (ver Ceratoconjuntivite Seca).

Gatos
- Herpes-vírus — é recomendável o uso de agentes antivirais tópicos: trifluridina (Viroptic®) a cada 4-6 h por 2 dias e, em seguida, reduzir de forma gradual. Alternativamente, foi relatado o uso de idoxuridina a 0,5-1% a cada 6-8 h, vidarabina a 3% a cada 8 h e cidofovir a 0,5% a cada 12 h; para inflamação, podem ser utilizados agentes não esteroides tópicos ou ciclosporina a cada 12 h; lisina por via oral (250 mg a cada 12 h até 500 mg a cada 24 h) também pode ser benéfica; para os casos graves, há relatos do uso de fanciclovir (agente antiviral por via oral).
- Ceratite eosinofílica — corticosteroides tópicos (prednisolona a 1% ou dexametasona a 0,1%) a cada 6-12 h geralmente provoca remissão; os corticosteroides devem ser usados com cautela e o paciente monitorizado em busca de ulceração ou quanto ao agravamento dos sinais clínicos; antivirais tópicos podem ser utilizados em combinação com os corticosteroides na suspeita de infecção por herpes-vírus; o uso de ciclosporina tópica (a 0,2-1,5%) também foi relatado com resultados variáveis; nos casos refratários graves, pode-se considerar o acetato de megestrol (Ovaban® 5 mg VO a cada 24 h durante cinco dias, em seguida 5 mg a cada 48 h por 1 semana e depois 5 mg semanalmente para manutenção).
- Sequestro de córnea — antibiótico triplo tópico a cada 8-12 h na ulceração de córnea associada; a lubrificação com lágrima artificial pode aliviar o desconforto; antivirais tópicos podem ser usados na suspeita de infecção por herpes-vírus; pomada tópica de atropina a 1% 1-2 vezes ao dia para a dor associada a uveíte concomitante se presente.

CONTRAINDICAÇÕES
Corticosteroides tópicos são contraindicados nas úlceras de córnea; a atropina tópica está contraindicada na ceratoconjuntivite seca, no glaucoma ou na luxação do cristalino.

PRECAUÇÕES
- Azatioprina pode provocar sinais gastrintestinais, pancreatite, hepatotoxicidade e mielossupressão.
- Acetato de megestrol — não aprovado pela FDA para utilização nos gatos; os possíveis efeitos colaterais incluem polifagia, diabetes melito, hiperplasia mamária, neoplasia mamária e piometra.
- Fanciclovir — é recomendável a monitorização por meio de hemograma completo e perfil bioquímico; há relatos de anorexia e polidipsia como efeitos colaterais.

ACOMPANHAMENTO

MONITORIZAÇÃO DO PACIENTE
O exame ocular periódico é recomendado para avaliar a eficácia das medicações tópicas e sistêmicas; examinar em intervalos de 1-2 semanas, aumentando gradualmente o intervalo com a remissão ou a resolução dos sinais clínicos; avaliar a resposta ao tratamento e reduzir as medicações de forma gradativa com base na resolução dos sinais clínicos; pode não ocorrer a resolução completa da pigmentação. É recomendável a proteção da luz UV (protetores de olhos) em casos de pano.

COMPLICAÇÕES POSSÍVEIS
Todos os fatos mencionados anteriormente podem levar a desconforto ocular contínuo, defeitos visuais ou cegueira nos casos graves.

DIVERSOS

VER TAMBÉM
- Sequestro de Córnea — Gatos.
- Episclerite.
- Ceratite Eosinofílica — Gatos.
- Ceratite Ulcerativa.
- Ceratoconjuntivite Seca.

ABREVIATURA(S)
- FHV-1 = herpes-vírus felino tipo 1.
- IFA = ensaio imunofluorescente.
- PCR = reação em cadeia da polimerase.

Sugestões de Leitura
Andrew SE. Immune-mediated canine and feline keratitis. Vet Clin Small Anim 2008, 38:269-290.
Chavkin MJ, Roberts SM, Salman MD, et al. Risk factors for development of chronic superficial keratitis in dogs. JAVMA 1994, 204:1630-1634.

Autor Renee T. Carter
Consultor Editorial Paul E. Miller
Agradecimento O autor agradece as contribuições feitas por B. Keith Collins e George Mckie na preparação deste capítulo.

CERATITE ULCERATIVA

CONSIDERAÇÕES GERAIS

DEFINIÇÃO
Inflamação da córnea associada à perda do epitélio corneano (erosão de córnea) e possivelmente perda de quantidades variáveis do estroma corneano subjacente (úlcera de córnea).

FISIOPATOLOGIA
• Pode ser provocada por qualquer condição (traumática ou não) que promova a ruptura do epitélio ou do estroma corneano. • Úlceras — classificadas como superficiais ou profundas, complicadas ou não complicadas. • Superficial — envolve o epitélio e possivelmente o estroma superficial. • Profunda — envolve uma espessura maior do estroma e pode se estender para a membrana de Descemet (descemetocele), levando possivelmente à ruptura do globo. • Complicada — persistência da causa subjacente/incitante, infecção microbiana ou produção de enzimas de degradação. • Cicatrização de ferida epitelial — células epiteliais corneanas adjacentes se desprendem e começam a migração sobre o defeito dentro de algumas horas; ocorre mitose dentro de alguns dias para restaurar a espessura epitelial normal; o processo de cicatrização é concluído em 5-7 dias nas úlceras superficiais não complicadas. • Cicatrização de ferida estromal — mais lenta e mais complexa; pode ocorrer de forma vascular ou avascular; nas feridas superficiais, a migração epitelial e a mitose podem ser suficientes para preencher o defeito; o epitélio pode recobrir algumas úlceras mais profundas mesmo quando o epitélio e a regeneração estromal são insuficientes para restaurar a espessura corneana normal (o defeito desnudado não ulcerado recebe o nome de faceta); o estroma geralmente cicatriza por infiltração fibrovascular, a qual pode demorar várias semanas e quase sempre resulta na perda ou na diminuição da claridade corneana. • Úlceras estromais — frequentemente complicadas por infecção microbiana ou destruição enzimática iniciada por microrganismos microbianos, células inflamatórias do hospedeiro ou por células epiteliais ou estromais da córnea; a destruição enzimática excessiva pode resultar na aparência gelatinosa do estroma corneano, denominada úlcera desnaturada ou colagenase.

SISTEMA(S) ACOMETIDO(S)
Oftálmico.

GENÉTICA
• Nenhuma base genética foi comprovada, apesar de serem observadas algumas predileções raciais.
• Pode ocorrer secundariamente a outras doenças corneanas que apresentam predisposições raciais e presumivelmente uma base genética, como distrofia epitelial corneana no Pastor de Shetland e distrofia endotelial corneana no Boston terrier.

INCIDÊNCIA/PREVALÊNCIA
Comum.

IDENTIFICAÇÃO
Espécies
Cães e gatos.

Raça(s) Predominante(s)
• Cães — as raças braquicefálicas são predispostas. • Defeitos epiteliais crônicos espontâneos da córnea — ocorrem em qualquer raça. • Gatos — Persa, Himalaio, Siamês e Birmanês são predispostos a sequestros de córnea (ver "Sequestro de Córnea — Gatos").

Idade Média e Faixa Etária
• Idade de início — variável; determinada pela causa. • Defeitos epiteliais crônicos espontâneos da córnea — cães de meia-idade e mais idosos.

SINAIS CLÍNICOS
Achados Anamnésicos
• Podem ser agudos ou crônicos (defeitos epiteliais crônicos espontâneos da córnea).
• Lacrimejamento, estrabismo, fricção dos olhos.
• Os proprietários podem relatar o aparecimento de um filme sobre o olho (muitas vezes, edema de córnea); além disso, pode haver prolapso da terceira pálpebra. • Às vezes, há histórico de traumatismo. • Úlceras herpéticas (gatos) — pode haver histórico de doença respiratória.

Achados do Exame Físico
• Inespecíficos — secreção ocular serosa a mucopurulenta; blefarospasmo; fotofobia; prolapso da membrana nictitante; hiperemia conjuntival.
• Superficiais — pode-se notar um ou mais defeitos circunscritos, lineares ou geográficos na córnea.
• Úlcera estromal profunda ou descemetocele — pode aparecer com defeito crateriforme.
• Dependendo da causa e da duração — podem-se observar neovascularização, pigmentação, cicatrização, depósitos lipídicos ou minerais, infiltrado celular inflamatório (opacidade amarelada a cor de creme com margens indistintas, frequentemente circundadas por edema de córnea), atividade colagenolítica (desnaturada) do estroma corneano. • Defeitos epiteliais crônicos espontâneos da córnea — bordas epiteliais frouxas ou redundantes; pode demonstrar a coloração pela fluoresceína, estendendo-se para as áreas com epitélio aparentemente intacto (anel de coloração menos intensa). • Doença corneana ulcerativa geralmente estimula a produção lacrimal; a ausência de lacrimejamento óbvio sugere um componente de olho seco (ceratoconjuntivite seca). • Uveíte anterior reflexa — leve ou grave, secundária à ulceração; a forma grave pode resultar em hipópio e sugere infecção bacteriana concomitante.

CAUSAS
• Traumatismo — contuso (rombo); penetrante; perfurante. • Comprometimento dos anexos oculares — cílios ectópicos, entrópio, ectrópio, massa palpebral, distiquíase. • Lagoftalmia (incapacidade de fechar as pálpebras completamente) — resulta em ceratite por exposição; pode estar relacionada com a raça nos cães braquicefálicos e gatos; pode ser provocada por exoftalmia, buftalmia ou ser neuroparalítica por paralisia do nervo facial. • Anormalidade do filme lacrimal — deficiência quantitativa de lágrimas (ceratoconjuntivite seca); deficiência qualitativa do filme lacrimal provocada por deficiência de mucina ou por alguma outra anormalidade lacrimal não identificada. • Infecção — quase sempre secundária nos cães; pode ser uma infecção primária por herpes-vírus nos gatos.
• Doença corneana primária — distrofia endotelial; outra doença endotelial. • Diversos — corpo estranho (corneano ou conjuntival); queimaduras químicas; ceratite neurotrófica (perda sensorial do trigêmeo); doença imunomediada.

DIAGNÓSTICO

DIAGNÓSTICO DIFERENCIAL
• Retenção do corante fluoresceína — característica diagnóstica. • Outras causas de olho vermelho e doloroso — conjuntivite, uveíte, ceratoconjuntivite seca, glaucoma (ver "Olho Vermelho"). • Pode se desenvolver concomitantemente com outras causas de olho vermelho (p. ex., secundária à ceratoconjuntivite seca).

OUTROS TESTES LABORATORIAIS
• Cultura e antibiograma da córnea — bactérias aeróbicas; particularmente nas úlceras de córnea complicadas, profundas ou rapidamente progressivas. • Herpes-vírus (gatos) — existem exames disponíveis de PCR ou IFA para detecção desse vírus; resultados negativos não descartam infecção por herpes-vírus.

MÉTODOS DIAGNÓSTICOS
Coloração pela Fluoresceína
• Absorção homogênea do corante — úlcera superficial ou estromal; pode variar de circular a geográfica, linear ou uma combinação disso; a localização e a forma podem ajudar a determinar a causa (p. ex., linear pode indicar corpo estranho ou atrito de cílios ectópicos); interpretação subjetiva da profundidade. • Defeitos epiteliais crônicos espontâneos da córnea — pode haver extravasamento do corante sob o epitélio frouxo circundante. • Defeito crateriforme que retém o corante na periferia, mas é claro no centro.
• Descemetocele — pode-se observar a membrana de Descemet, projetando-se para frente em caso de defeitos grandes. • Defeito crateriforme com acúmulo transitório do corante, embora esse corante possa ser facilmente enxaguado — úlcera estromal anterior que foi epitelizada (faceta); deve ser distinguida de descemetocele.

Outros
• Avaliação citológica da córnea e coloração de Gram, Giemsa ou Wright podem não só revelar a presença de microrganismos microbianos ou fúngicos, mas também ajudar a direcionar a terapia antimicrobiana inicial. • Coloração da córnea com rosa bengala (gatos) pode delinear úlceras superficiais, lineares e epiteliais (úlceras dendríticas), as quais são consideradas patognomônicas para infecção por herpes-vírus. • Teste lacrimal de Schirmer pode identificar ulceração associada à ceratoconjuntivite seca; é contraindicado em casos de úlceras muito profundas ou descemetoceles.

ACHADOS PATOLÓGICOS
• Úlceras — inflamação tipicamente supurativa, com possível neovascularização, além de perda do epitélio e da membrana basal; também é possível o encontro de microrganismos. • Defeitos epiteliais crônicos espontâneos da córnea — zona hialinizada superficial no estroma; borda epitelial elevada ao redor das erosões; graus e tipos variáveis de infiltrado leucocitário e fibrose.

TRATAMENTO

CUIDADO(S) DE SAÚDE ADEQUADO(S)
Hospitalizar os animais com úlceras profundas ou rapidamente progressivas; esse tipo de úlcera pode necessitar de cirurgia e/ou tratamentos clínicos frequentes.

CUIDADO(S) DE ENFERMAGEM
Manter os pelos faciais limpos e afastados dos olhos.

ATIVIDADE
• Restringir a atividade em casos de úlcera estromal profunda ou descemetocele para evitar a

CERATITE ULCERATIVA

ruptura. • Evitar o traumatismo autoinfligido com o uso de colar elizabetano.

ORIENTAÇÃO AO PROPRIETÁRIO
• Orientar o proprietário a esperar no mínimo 5 minutos entre as medicações se mais de um colírio for prescrito; aguardar mais tempo entre a aplicação de pomadas. • Aconselhar o proprietário a entrar em contato com o veterinário se o animal estiver aparentemente com mais dor ou se o aspecto do olho tiver sofrido uma alteração acentuada.
• Defeitos epiteliais crônicos espontâneos da córnea — abordar a evolução prolongada com o proprietário; a cicatrização costuma ocorrer dentro de 2-6 semanas, embora possa haver a necessidade de reavaliações semanais e múltiplos procedimentos.

CONSIDERAÇÕES CIRÚRGICAS
• Úlceras superficiais geralmente não necessitam de cirurgia se a causa desencadeante foi eliminada.
• Úlcera que se estende até a metade da espessura corneana ou afeta uma espessura maior dessa estrutura ocular e, particularmente, acomete a membrana de Descemet pode se beneficiar com a cirurgia. • Descemetocele e laceração corneana de espessura completa — considerada como uma emergência cirúrgica para um possível encaminhamento.

Procedimentos
• Defeitos epiteliais crônicos espontâneos da córnea — debridamento do epitélio frouxo com o uso de swab seco, esterilizado e com extremidade de algodão após a aplicação de anestesia tópica (taxa de sucesso de 50%); o procedimento de ceratotomia puntiforme ou em grade é facilmente realizado após o debridamento epitelial com anestesia tópica (taxa de sucesso de 80%); a ceratectomia superficial é mais invasiva e pode provocar maior cicatrização, porém apresenta taxa de sucesso de 100%; aplicação de lente de contato ou retalho da membrana nictitante após qualquer um desses procedimentos irá melhorar o conforto e auxiliar a cicatrização.
• Colocação de lente de contato terapêutica — atua como bandagem para reduzir tanto a irritação friccional das pálpebras como a dor; maior utilidade em defeitos epiteliais crônicos espontâneos da córnea; além de fácil aplicação, ainda permite o exame do olho; a maioria permanece por uma a duas semanas e, em seguida, é removida; lente plana (sem correção) costuma ser mais utilizada; deve-se monitorar o olho quanto ao aumento da dor e do edema de córnea, o que indica falta de acomodação do contato e consequente indução de hipoxia corneana. • Retalho conjuntival de pedículo rotacional, transposição corneoscleral, transplante de córnea — métodos cirúrgicos para úlceras maiores do que 50% da espessura do estroma e para descemetoceles. • Reparo com cianoacrilato (cola de córnea) — pode ser empregada para úlceras profundas; promove vascularização corneana e estabiliza a córnea, mas apresenta uma taxa de sucesso um tanto mais baixa em comparação com outras cirurgias de córnea.

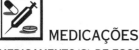

MEDICAÇÕES
MEDICAMENTO(S) DE ESCOLHA
Antibióticos
• Agentes tópicos — indicados para todos os pacientes. • Frequência de aplicação — determinada pela gravidade e pela preparação utilizada; as pomadas possuem um tempo de contato relativamente longo e são aplicadas a cada 6-12 horas; as soluções são aplicadas com maior frequência (4, 6, 8 ou até 12 vezes ao dia) no tratamento inicial de úlceras complicadas; as soluções provavelmente são mais apropriadas nas úlceras profundas. • Agentes comumente usados — oxitetraciclina (gatos); antibiótico triplo, gentamicina e tobramicina. • Úlceras não complicadas ou erosões superficiais — a combinação de neomicina, polimixina B e bacitracina constitui uma primeira escolha excelente; amplo espectro de atividade antimicrobiana; utilizada com frequência 2-3 vezes ao dia como terapia profilática. • Úlceras complicadas — utilizar frequentemente a terapia combinada de cefazolina (utilizar solução IV para perfazer uma solução de 33-50 mg em salina ou lágrimas artificiais para uso tópico) com algum aminoglicosídeo (tobramicina, gentamicina) ou fluoroquinolona (ciprofloxacino, ofloxacino); indicados, em particular, nas úlceras rapidamente progressivas, profundas ou desnaturadas; a frequência depende da gravidade, mas geralmente é a cada 3-4 horas no mínimo.

Atropina
• Pomada ou solução a 1%. • Indicada na uveíte anterior reflexa; frequência — em geral, a cada 8-24 h até fazer efeito (midríase).

Agentes Antivirais
• Indicados para úlceras herpéticas em gatos.
• Solução de trifluridina (Viroptic®) — a cada 4-6 horas até a resposta clínica ser observada; em seguida, reduzir por 1-2 semanas após o desaparecimento dos sinais clínicos.

AINE
• Podem ser indicados pelas propriedades anti-inflamatórias e analgésicas. • Ácido acetilsalicílico (cães) — 10-15 mg/kg VO a cada 12 h.

CONTRAINDICAÇÕES
• Corticosteroides tópicos — contraindicados em qualquer erosão ou úlcera de córnea. • AINEs tópicos — contraindicados nas úlceras herpéticas ou desnaturadas. • Atropina tópica — contraindicada em casos de glaucoma e ceratoconjuntivite seca.

PRECAUÇÕES
• AINEs tópicos (flurbiprofeno, diclofenaco) — podem não só retardar a cicatrização da córnea, mas também potencializar a desnaturação dessa estrutura ocular. • Trifluridina, neomicina — podem ser irritantes. • Ciclosporina tópica — pode ser usada com segurança em úlcera não complicada nos pacientes com ceratoconjuntivite seca.

INTERAÇÕES POSSÍVEIS
Antibióticos combinados em solução podem inativar alguns antibióticos.

MEDICAMENTO(S) ALTERNATIVO(S)
• Acetilcisteína — agente anticolagenolítico utilizado no tratamento das úlceras desnaturadas; a eficácia é controversa; diluir a solução original a 20% para 5-10% com lágrimas artificiais; aplicar a cada 2-4 h. • Soro autólogo — agente anticolagenolítico; manter refrigerado; evitar contaminação; descartar após 48 h.

ACOMPANHAMENTO
MONITORIZAÇÃO DO PACIENTE
• Úlceras superficiais — repetir a coloração com fluoresceína em 3-6 dias; se persistir por 7 dias ou mais, a causa desencadeante não foi eliminada ou o paciente possui defeitos epiteliais crônicos espontâneos da córnea. • Úlceras estromais profundas ou rapidamente progressivas — avaliar inicialmente a cada 24 h no caso de paciente de ambulatório até que se observe a melhora; muitos desses pacientes são internados ou submetidos à cirurgia; diminuir a frequência da antibioticoterapia conforme a condição apresenta melhora.

PREVENÇÃO
• Cães braquicefálicos — administração de pomada lubrificante, cirurgia de tarsorrafia parcial permanente ou as duas medidas podem ajudar a evitar a ocorrência de recidiva da úlcera. • Úlceras relacionadas com ceratoconjuntivite seca — tratamento da ceratoconjuntivite seca por toda a vida (ciclosporina) ou cirurgia de transposição do ducto parotídeo para evitar a ulceração contínua.
• Herpes-vírus (gatos) — pode-se tentar o uso de lisina a 250 mg VO 2 vezes ao dia para evitar a replicação viral; pode diminuir a gravidade e/ou a frequência dos surtos.

COMPLICAÇÕES POSSÍVEIS
Ulceração corneana progressiva — ruptura do globo; endoftalmite; glaucoma secundário; ftise do bulbo; cegueira; olho cego e doloroso (pode necessitar de enucleação).

EVOLUÇÃO ESPERADA E PROGNÓSTICO
• Úlcera superficial não complicada — costuma cicatrizar em 5-7 dias. • Defeitos epiteliais crônicos espontâneos da córnea — pode persistir por semanas a meses; pode necessitar de múltiplos procedimentos. • Úlcera de córnea profunda submetida a tratamento clínico — pode necessitar de várias semanas para o reparo fibrovascular do defeito; nem sempre granula de forma satisfatória; é possível a ocorrência de deterioração contínua da úlcera e ruptura do globo. • Úlcera profunda tratada com retalho conjuntival — frequentemente resulta em mais conforto dentro de alguns dias da cirurgia; o aporte sanguíneo para o retalho pode ser incisado em 4-6 semanas se bem cicatrizado para diminuir a formação de cicatriz.

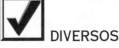

DIVERSOS
ABREVIATURA(S)
• AINE = anti-inflamatório não esteroide. • IFA = ensaio imunofluorescente. • PCR = reação em cadeia da polimerase.

Autor Ellison Bentley
Consultor Editorial Paul E. Miller
Agradecimento a B. Keith Collins pela preparação deste capítulo.

CERATITE EOSINOFÍLICA — GATOS

CONSIDERAÇÕES GERAIS

REVISÃO
- Ceratite/ceratoconjuntivite eosinofílica felina é uma inflamação supostamente imunomediada da córnea, caracterizada por vascularização perilimbal, infiltrado branco a rosa e edema.
- Sinônimo — ceratite proliferativa.

IDENTIFICAÇÃO
Os gatos jovens adultos aos de meia-idade são mais comumente acometidos.

SINAIS CLÍNICOS
- Uni ou bilateral.
- Geralmente pouca a nenhuma dor ocular.
- Secreção ocular serosa a mucoide.
- Vascularização limbal da superfície da córnea, envolvendo 90-360° (em geral, os quadrantes temporal ou nasal inferior são acometidos em primeiro lugar).
- Infiltrado corneano plano ou em relevo de cor branca a rosa que pode ter uma textura granular.
- Pequenos focos multifocais de depósitos arenosos brancos na córnea.
- Edema de córnea.
- Com ou sem ulceração da córnea.
- Hiperemia e espessamento conjuntivais com ou sem textura de paralelepípedo à superfície conjuntival.
- Espessamento e hiperemia da terceira pálpebra.
- Quemose.
- Despigmentação da pele periocular.

CAUSAS E FATORES DE RISCO
- Herpes-vírus felino-1 (FHV-1) pode estar associado à ceratite/ceratoconjuntivite eosinofílica felina, mas o papel exato é incerto.
- 76% das amostras de ceratite/ceratoconjuntivite eosinofílica felina foram FHV-1-positivas no exame de PCR em um único estudo, mas 0% exibiu resultado positivo em outro.
- A etiopatogênese exata é desconhecida, mas as teorias propostas são: (1) hipersensibilidade tipo I com degranulação de mastócitos e eosinófilos mediada por IgE, (2) reação do tipo IV em que linfócitos-T sensibilizados via IL-5 estimulam o dano à córnea mediado por eosinófilos locais.
- Cultura, histopatologia e microscopia eletrônica descartaram infecção bacteriana e fúngica como etiologias compatíveis, embora possa ocorrer ceratite bacteriana secundária.

DIAGNÓSTICO

DIAGNÓSTICO DIFERENCIAL
- Ulceração crônica da córnea com vascularização secundária dessa estrutura ocular (tecido de granulação).
- Ceratite estromal por FHV-1 — parece semelhante a ceratite/ceratoconjuntivite eosinofílica felina, mas não possui o componente proliferativo; na ceratite estromal, também costuma haver sinais de dor ocular e ulceração corneana mais graves.
- Neoplasia da córnea: (1) linfoma — é comum a infiltração conjuntival e/ou uveal concomitante, (2) carcinoma de células escamosas — raramente envolve a córnea em gatos.
- *Chlamydia psittaci* — geralmente causa doença conjuntival apenas; o envolvimento da córnea é raro.
- *Mycoplasma felis* — costuma causar doença conjuntival apenas; o envolvimento da córnea também é raro.

HEMOGRAMA/BIOQUÍMICA/URINÁLISE
Pode estar presente eosinofilia periférica.

OUTROS TESTES LABORATORIAIS
- O exame de citologia da córnea fornece o diagnóstico definitivo e deve ser realizado em primeiro lugar. Nesse exame, observam-se inúmeros eosinófilos, grânulos eosinofílicos e/ou mastócitos livres, neutrófilos, linfócitos e células epiteliais.
- A citologia da secreção ocular também pode revelar a presença de eosinófilos ou grânulos eosinofílicos.
- A citologia ajuda a descartar corpúsculos de inclusão intracitoplasmáticos de *Chlamydia* e corpúsculos cocoides epicelulares de *Mycoplasma*.
- PCR "aninhado" para detecção de FHV-1 — valor diagnóstico limitado, pois gatos saudáveis normais podem carrear esse vírus e exibir resultados positivos no exame de PCR.
- Teste de IFA para pesquisa de *Chlamydia psittaci*.
- Coloração de fluoresceína para avaliar a ulceração da córnea.

MÉTODOS DIAGNÓSTICOS
- Os procedimentos de ceratectomia e histopatologia podem confirmar um diagnóstico em casos crônicos ou irresponsivos.
- As amostras revelam hipertrofia e hiperplasia da camada de células epiteliais, vascularização da córnea, excrescências com *debris* nucleares e material eosinofílico amorfo, inúmeros eosinófilos e grânulos eosinofílicos livres, além de camadas mais profundas de membrana basal espessa e material eosinofílico.
- Também é observado espessamento do estroma com eosinófilos predominantemente e células inflamatórias mistas, além de tecido de granulação.

TRATAMENTO
Geralmente médico em um esquema ambulatorial.

MEDICAÇÕES

MEDICAMENTO(S)
- Corticosteroides tópicos — suspensão oftálmica de acetato de prednisolona a 1% ou solução oftálmica de fosfato sódico de dexametasona a 0,1% (inicialmente a cada 6-12 h por 5-7 dias e, depois, redução gradual para a frequência mais baixa e eficaz de aplicação, a cada 2-7 dias). Por fim, podem ser interrompidos em muitos gatos.
- Terapia antiviral tópica e/ou sistêmica adjuvante pode ser justificável nos casos em que o histórico ou os sinais clínicos são compatíveis com infecção por FHV-1.
- Corticosteroides subconjuntivais — acetonida de triancinolona (0,1-0,2 mL a cada 3-7 dias); utilizar apenas em gatos que são difíceis de tratar com medicamentos tópicos.
- Acetato de megestrol — 2,5 mg VO a cada 24 h por 3-5 dias e, depois, 2,5 mg VO a cada 48 h por 3-5 dias, com subsequente redução gradativa da frequência do tratamento após a cada 3-5 tratamentos para a frequência mais baixa e eficaz de administração (p. ex., 2,5 mg VO a cada 7 dias) ou, finalmente, interromper.
- Ciclosporina A tópica a cada 8-12 h, com subsequente redução gradual para a frequência mais baixa e eficaz de aplicação e/ou interrupção do medicamento. Pode ser usada em gatos nos quais o megestrol e os corticosteroides tópicos são contraindicados (diabetes, FHV-1 etc.). Pode ser irritante.
- Prednisolona sistêmica — começar com 2,2 mg/kg VO a cada 12 h e reduzir gradativamente. Utilizar apenas se o gato não tolerar a terapia tópica com corticosteroide ou ciclosporina A nem o acetato de megestrol.

CONTRAINDICAÇÕES/INTERAÇÕES POSSÍVEIS
- A administração tópica de corticosteroide pode ser associada à recrudescência de ceratoconjuntivite por FHV-1 e, portanto, deve ser utilizada de forma criteriosa e monitorizada com cuidado. É aconselhável que o proprietário relate imediatamente qualquer alteração adversa no estado do olho (blefarospasmo, edema de córnea, aumento da secreção ocular etc.).
- O acetato de megestrol provoca supressão do córtex da adrenal, podendo resultar em diabetes melito, polifagia, mudança de temperamento, hiperplasia da glândula mamária ou neoplasia e piometra. Não deve ser utilizado em gatos com hepatopatia ou outra doença.

ACOMPANHAMENTO
- A resposta à terapia costuma ser muito rápida.
- A resolução completa pode levar alguns dias a meses. Muitos gatos necessitam de terapia prolongada para controlar a doença.
- A vascularização e o infiltrado na córnea podem desaparecer completamente com formação cicatricial mínima nessa estrutura ocular.
- As recorrências são comuns tanto a longo como a curto prazo após a interrupção da terapia.

DIVERSOS
Tipicamente, a ceratite/ceratoconjuntivite eosinofílica felina não é associada ao complexo granuloma eosinofílico dermatológico.

ABREVIATURA(S)
- FHV-1 = herpes-vírus felino-1
- IFA = teste de anticorpo imunofluorescente
- PCR = reação em cadeia da polimerase

Sugestões de Leitura
Morgan RV, Abrams KL, Kern TJ. Feline eosinophilic keratitis: A retrospective study of 54 cases (1989–1994). Vet Ophthalmology 1996, 6(2):131–134.
Stiles J, Townsend WM, Gelatt KN. Feline ophthalmology. In: Gelatt KN, ed., Veterinary Ophthalmology, 4th ed. Ames, IA: Blackwell, 2007, pp. 1095–1164.

Autor Anne Gemensky Metzler
Consultor Editorial Paul E. Miller

Ceratoconjuntivite Seca

CONSIDERAÇÕES GERAIS

REVISÃO
Deficiência do filme lacrimal aquoso, resultando em ressecamento e inflamação da córnea e da conjuntiva.

IDENTIFICAÇÃO
- Muito comum nos cães; muito mais rara nos gatos.
- Raças caninas predispostas — incluem Cocker spaniel, Buldogue, West Highland white terrier, Lhasa apso e Shih-tzu.
- Herança — indefinida.
- Idade de início — depende da causa desencadeante.
- Alguns estudos relatam as fêmeas como predispostas.

SINAIS CLÍNICOS
- Os gatos tendem a ser menos sintomáticos que os cães.
- Blefarospasmo.
- Hiperemia conjuntival.
- Quemose.
- Membrana nictitante proeminente, enoftalmia.
- Secreção ocular mucoide a mucopurulenta.
- Alterações da córnea (doença crônica) — vascularização superficial; pigmentação; ulceração.
- Doença grave — diminuição ou perda da visão.

CAUSAS E FATORES DE RISCO
- Imunológicas — adenite imunomediada mais comum e frequentemente associada a outras doenças imunomediadas (p. ex., atopia).
- Congênitas — Yorkshire terrier, esporadicamente em outras raças.
- Neurogênicas — observada algumas vezes após proptose traumática ou doença neurológica que interrompe a inervação da glândula lacrimal; muitas vezes, exibe ressecamento nasal no mesmo lado que o ressecamento ocular.
- Induzidas por medicamentos — anestesia geral e atropina provocam ceratoconjuntivite seca transitória.
- Intoxicação por medicamentos — alguns agentes terapêuticos contendo sulfa (p. ex., trimetoprima-sulfametoxazol) ou etodolaco podem causar a condição transitória ou permanente.
- Iatrogênicas — remoção da glândula nictitante pode predispor o animal à ceratoconjuntivite seca, especialmente nas raças sob risco.
- Radioterapia — quando a área periocular fica próxima do feixe primário.
- Doença sistêmica — vírus da cinomose; qualquer doença debilitante.
- Conjuntivite crônica (gatos) — herpes crônico ou conjuntivite por *Chlamydia*.
- Blefaroconjuntivite crônica (cães).
- Predisposição relacionada com a raça.

DIAGNÓSTICO

DIAGNÓSTICO DIFERENCIAL
Quase sempre confundida com a conjuntivite bacteriana; a maioria dos cães com ceratoconjuntivite seca crônica exibe proliferação bacteriana secundária; diferenciada pelo uso do teste lacrimal de Schirmer.

MÉTODOS DIAGNÓSTICOS
- Teste lacrimal de Schirmer — resultados diminuídos são diagnósticos; valor normal (cães): no mínimo 15 mm/min de umedecimento da fita; pacientes sintomáticos: geralmente <10 mm/min de umedecimento da fita.
- Coloração com fluoresceína — úlceras de córnea.
- Proceder aos exames de cultura e sensibilidade bacterianas aeróbias se o tratamento inicial não for bem-sucedido; não recomendado rotineiramente, porque a proliferação bacteriana é comum em casos de doença crônica.
- Citologia conjuntival — pode indicar a natureza e o grau da proliferação bacteriana.

TRATAMENTO

- Ambulatorial — a menos que seja identificada uma doença secundária (p. ex., ceratite ulcerativa).
- Aconselhar os proprietários a entrarem em contato com o veterinário se a dor ocular aumentar, já que os pacientes são predispostos à ulceração grave da córnea.
- Transposição do ducto parotídeo — método cirúrgico que redireciona a liberação de saliva pelo ducto parotídeo no fundo de saco inferior; realizada com uma frequência muito menor desde a introdução de terapia lacrimogênica tópica; a saliva pode ser irritante para a córnea; alguns pacientes sentem desconforto após a cirurgia e necessitam de tratamento clínico tópico contínuo.

MEDICAÇÕES

MEDICAMENTO(S)
- Tacrolimo pode ser aviado sob a forma de solução ou pomada a 0,01-0,03% e tem se mostrado mais eficaz no aumento da produção lacrimal em comparação à ciclosporina. É recomendável a terapia a cada 12 h.
- Pomada de ciclosporina a 0,2% — é aconselhável a terapia a cada 12 h.
- Pilocarpina a 0,25% tópica a cada 12 h; alternativamente, pode-se usar 1 gota de pilocarpina a 2%/10 kg de peso corporal a cada 12 h no alimento e aumentar lentamente em incrementos de 1 gota até que se observem lacrimejamento ou efeitos colaterais sistêmicos (anorexia, salivação, vômito, diarreia, bradicardia). Mais eficaz na ceratoconjuntivite seca neurogênica.
- Lágrimas artificiais e pomadas lubrificantes (lacrimomiméticos) — ajudam a umedecer a córnea; devem ser utilizadas com frequência; alívio apenas transitório do ressecamento; as preparações variam muito em sua composição; agentes mais espessos podem ser emolientes para olhos muito ressecados nos pacientes que não respondem ao tratamento com a ciclosporina.
- Antibióticos de amplo espectro — tópicos (soluções ou pomadas); frequentemente indicados na proliferação bacteriana secundária; raramente indicados, uma vez que a proliferação bacteriana esteja controlada e a produção lacrimal seja restabelecida; antibióticos sistêmicos podem ser recomendados em casos refratários.
- Corticosteroides — tópicos; minimizam a inflamação; eficazes na redução da vascularização e pigmentação da córnea; não são utilizados comumente, mas podem ser úteis em alguns pacientes. Interromper caso ocorra o desenvolvimento de ulceração.
- Agentes mucolíticos (p. ex., acetilcisteína) — ocasionalmente utilizados para ajudar a interromper a secreção mucosa persistente; raramente indicados assim que a produção lacrimal se restabelecer.

CONTRAINDICAÇÕES/INTERAÇÕES POSSÍVEIS
- Ciclosporina tópica — raras vezes irritante.
- Corticosteroides tópicos — evitados na ceratite ulcerativa.
- Pilocarpina tópica — inicialmente irritante.
- Tacrolimo tópico — raramente irritante.

ACOMPANHAMENTO

- Reavaliar o animal em intervalos regulares — monitorizar a resposta do paciente e a evolução do quadro.
- Teste lacrimal de Schirmer — realizado 4-6 semanas após iniciar o tratamento com o tacrolimo ou a ciclosporina; avaliar a resposta (o paciente deve ter recebido o medicamento no dia da consulta).
- Doença imunomediada — geralmente requer tratamento por toda a vida.
- Outros tipos de doença — podem ser transitórios (p. ex., tratamento com atropina); necessitam de tratamento somente até que a produção lacrimal retorne ao normal.

DIVERSOS

Sugestões de Leitura
Maggs DJ, Miller PE, Ofri R. Slatter's Fundamentals of Veterinary Ophthalmology, 4th ed. St. Louis: Saunders, 2008, pp. 166-171.

Autor Erin S. Champagne
Consultor Editorial Paul E. Miller

Choque Cardiogênico

CONSIDERAÇÕES GERAIS

DEFINIÇÃO
- O choque cardiogênico consiste em uma manifestação grave de insuficiência cardíaca anterógrada. Resulta do comprometimento profundo da função cardíaca, culminando em baixo débito cardíaco, fluxo sanguíneo anterógrado inadequado e má perfusão tecidual na presença de volume intravascular adequado.
- O comprometimento cardíaco pode se originar de disfunção sistólica (miocardiopatia dilatada, sepse, miocardite e isquemia), disfunção diastólica (miocardiopatia hipertrófica, miocardiopatia restritiva, pneumotórax/mediastino de tensão, pericardite restritiva e tamponamento pericárdico), defeitos de condução cardíaca e arritmias, valvulopatias, doenças obstrutivas, tromboembolia pulmonar e defeitos estruturais. A compreensão do defeito subjacente e de suas consequências hemodinâmicas é imperativa para a instituição de terapia adequada.
- Em casos de insuficiência cardíaca congestiva (ICC), algumas vezes denominada insuficiência cardíaca retrógrada, o ventrículo não bombeia todo o sangue que recebe. Esse aumento nas pressões de enchimento ventricular resulta na formação de edema pulmonar e/ou sistêmico. Isso contrasta com a insuficiência cardíaca anterógrada, quando o coração não bombeia sangue suficiente para suprir as necessidades do corpo. A maioria dos pacientes veterinários, mas nem todos, que se apresenta em choque cardiogênico terá ICC concomitante.

FISIOPATOLOGIA
- Disfunção do miocárdio e declínio do débito cardíaco (diante de volume intravascular adequado) levam à hipotensão arterial e hipoperfusão sistêmica.
- A hipotensão arterial diminui a pressão de perfusão coronária, resultando em isquemia coronária que provoca ainda mais disfunção miocárdica.
- A hipoperfusão sistêmica ativa respostas neuroendócrinas compensatórias que culminam em vasoconstrição periférica. Essa vasoconstrição prejudica ainda mais a perfusão tecidual e aumenta a atividade miocárdica, exacerbando com isso a disfunção do miocárdio.
- A hipoperfusão tecidual causa isquemia de órgãos e depleção de energia, levando à função orgânica anormal. Quando isso ocorre, os sinais de insuficiência de fluxo anterógrado e débito baixo tornam-se evidentes.

SISTEMA(S) ACOMETIDO(S)
- Cardiovascular — a disfunção cardíaca constitui a causa. A hipoperfusão miocárdica resultante leva à isquemia do miocárdio, exacerbando com isso a disfunção cardíaca. • Gastrintestinal — a má perfusão ao trato gastrintestinal resulta em congestão e hemorragia para o lúmen. A perda de função da barreira intestinal pode levar à translocação bacteriana e sepse. • Hematológico — o fluxo sanguíneo reduzido pode resultar em CID. • Hepatobiliar — a hipoperfusão e a consequente hipoxia hepática podem levar ao aumento na concentração sérica de enzimas hepatocelulares. Além disso, a congestão hepática pode resultar de ICC direita. • Musculoesquelético — baixo débito cardíaco e hipoperfusão muscular induzem à fraqueza da musculatura esquelética.
- Nervoso — ocorre depressão do SNC em resposta à hipoperfusão dos órgãos. • Renal — hipotensão sistêmica e hipoperfusão renal podem resultar em oligúria, dano tubular isquêmico e desenvolvimento de insuficiência renal aguda.
- Respiratório — à medida que a disfunção cardíaca evolui e a pressão diastólica final ventricular aumenta, ocorrem o desenvolvimento de efusão pleural e a formação de edema pulmonar. Por fim, a troca gasosa pulmonar fica comprometida, resultando em hipoxemia.

IDENTIFICAÇÃO
- Cães e gatos. • Qualquer raça, idade ou sexo.

SINAIS CLÍNICOS

Achados Anamnésicos
- A descompensação cardíaca pode estar associada a histórico de cardiopatia previamente compensada e administração de medicamento para o coração.
- A suspeita de cardiopatia não diagnosticada anteriormente pode resultar do histórico de tosse, intolerância ao exercício, fraqueza ou síncope.

Achados do Exame Físico
- Indicadores de má perfusão:
  ○ Mucosas pálidas. ○ Tempo de preenchimento capilar prolongado. ○ Pulso femoral fraco.
  ○ Fraqueza muscular. ○ Embotamento mental.
  ○ Extremidades frias e hipotermia. ○ Oligúria.
- Sons cardíacos abafados na presença de efusão pericárdica ou pleural.
- Frequência cardíaca variável com possível arritmia cardíaca, sopro cardíaco ou ritmo de galope.
- Frequência respiratória variável com possíveis ruídos broncovesiculares aumentados, crepitações ou tosse úmida (especialmente se houver ICC concomitante).

CAUSAS

Cardiopatia Primária
- Todos os tipos de miocardiopatias — dilatada, hipertrófica, intermediária e restritiva.
- Insuficiência grave da valva atrioventricular esquerda (mitral) ou outra valvulopatia em estágio terminal. • Taqui ou bradiarritmias. • Miocardite.
- Endomiocardite (gatos). • Defeitos estruturais.

Disfunção Cardíaca Secundária
- Constrição ou tamponamento pericárdico.
- Sepse. • Desarranjo eletrolítico grave (potássio, magnésio e cálcio). • Tromboembolia pulmonar.
- Pneumotórax/mediastino de tensão. • Síndrome das veias cavas.

FATORES DE RISCO
- Cardiopatia subjacente.
- Doença concomitante indutora de hipoxemia, acidose, desequilíbrios eletrolíticos ou liberação de citocinas que podem afetar a função do miocárdio.

DIAGNÓSTICO

DIAGNÓSTICO DIFERENCIAL

Diferenciar Sinais Semelhantes
O choque circulatório ocorre quando a distribuição de oxigênio para os tecidos não supre a demanda, sendo caracterizado por sinais clínicos de má perfusão. O choque cardiogênico é diferenciado de outras causas de choque circulatório quando há indícios de débito cardíaco reduzido e hipoxia tecidual diante de volume intravascular adequado.

HEMOGRAMA/BIOQUÍMICA/URINÁLISE
- Hemograma completo — frequentemente permanece normal, embora possa exibir leucograma de estresse.
- Bioquímica — os pacientes podem ter uma ou mais das seguintes alterações:
  ○ Hiato aniônico elevado (acúmulo de ácido láctico e ácidos renais). ○ Aumento na atividade das enzimas hepatocelulares, secundário à hipoxia hepática (ALT e AST). ○ Níveis aumentados de fósforo em virtude da diminuição na taxa de filtração glomerular.
  ○ Azotemia atribuída à queda na taxa de filtração glomerular e/ou lesão renal induzida por hipoxia. ○ Hiponatremia e leve hipoalbuminemia (mais comum em pacientes com insuficiência cardíaca crônica).
- Urinálise — terapia diurética concomitante ou lesão tubular aguda secundária à hipoxia renal podem resultar em isostenúria.

OUTROS TESTES LABORATORIAIS
- Gasometria arterial pode revelar acidose metabólica e indícios de extração aumentada de oxigênio pelos tecidos (uma diferença arteriovenosa ampliada de oxigênio e/ou uma concentração venosa diminuída desse gás em paciente que não esteja hipoxêmico ou anêmico).
- Hiperlactatemia é frequentemente registrada como um evento secundário à hipoperfusão tecidual.
- Troponina I cardíaca é um marcador altamente sensível e específico de lesão do miocárdio, podendo ser detectada no plasma por meio de técnicas de imunoensaio.

DIAGNÓSTICO POR IMAGEM

Achados Radiográficos
A radiografia torácica pode revelar cardiomegalia, indícios de edema pulmonar (ICC) e/ou efusão pleural (ICC).

Ecocardiografia
Pode registrar e caracterizar miocardiopatia, valvulopatia, contratilidade miocárdica deprimida, doença estrutural, pericardiopatia ou dirofilariose.

MÉTODOS DIAGNÓSTICOS
- A mensuração da pressão arterial pode comprovar a hipotensão.
- A eletrocardiografia pode ajudar na detecção e caracterização de arritmias.
- A oximetria de pulso pode registrar a baixa saturação de oxigênio em pacientes com ICC concomitante.
- A monitorização da pressão venosa central pode auxiliar na avaliação da pré-carga cardíaca e da saturação venosa central de oxigênio.
- Monitorização hemodinâmica para avaliar a saturação venosa mista de oxigênio, o débito cardíaco e a resistência vascular sistêmica.

TRATAMENTO

CUIDADO(S) DE SAÚDE ADEQUADO(S)
Tratar como paciente internado de emergência; o grau de disfunção cardíaca necessita de tratamento clínico intensivo.

CHOQUE CARDIOGÊNICO

CUIDADO(S) DE ENFERMAGEM
• Minimizar o estresse, pois esses pacientes são extremamente frágeis e estão sob risco de parada cardíaca. • É crítica a suplementação de oxigênio.
• A efusão pleural significativa (ICC) deve ser aliviada com o procedimento de toracocentese.
• Os pacientes que exibem insuficiência respiratória secundária à ICC talvez necessitem de entubação e ventilação mecânica. • A maioria dos pacientes em choque cardiogênico NÃO deve receber NENHUMA fluidoterapia até que a etiologia da disfunção cardíaca subjacente seja compreendida e a função cardíaca esteja restabelecida. As exceções a essa regra incluem pacientes em choque cardiogênico secundário a tamponamento pericárdico, pneumotórax/mediastino de tensão e tromboembolia pulmonar.
• O tamponamento pericárdico deve ser aliviado com a pericardiocentese de emergência.

ATIVIDADE
Repouso estrito em gaiola.

DIETA
Livre acesso à água e fornecimento intermitente de alimentos altamente palatáveis.

ORIENTAÇÃO AO PROPRIETÁRIO
Informar ao proprietário sobre o perigo de parada cardíaca iminente nesses animais e abordar o "código do estado" do animal com antecedência, sempre que possível.

CONSIDERAÇÕES CIRÚRGICAS
• A bradiarritmia pode necessitar da implantação de marca-passo.
• O pneumotórax de tensão talvez necessite da colocação de tubo por toracostomia ou toracotomia exploratória.
• A síndrome da veia cava secundária à infecção por *Dirofilaria immitis* exigirá a extração dos vermes pelo trato de entrada do ventrículo direito.

MEDICAÇÕES

MEDICAMENTO(S) DE ESCOLHA
• Utilizar agentes inotrópicos positivos de ação rápida para melhorar a função cardíaca e manter a perfusão de órgãos-alvo em pacientes com contratilidade reduzida do miocárdio (dobutamina na dose de 5-20 µg/kg/min sob infusão em velocidade constante em cães; 2,5-15 µg/kg/min sob infusão em velocidade constante em gatos; pimobendana na dose de 0,25 mg/kg VO a cada 12 h apenas em cães).
• Arritmias e anormalidades de condução podem afetar de forma considerável o débito cardíaco e devem ser corrigidas imediatamente com terapia antiarrítmica, cardioversão ou implantação de marca-passo.
• Taquicardia ventricular:
  ○ Os cães podem responder à lidocaína (2 mg/kg IV como dose de ataque e, depois, 50 µg/kg/min sob infusão em velocidade constante) ou procainamida (10-15 mg/kg IV como dose de ataque e, em seguida, 25-50 µg/kg/min sob infusão em velocidade constante).
  ○ Os cães da raça Boxer com miocardiopatia arritmogênica do ventrículo direito podem responder favoravelmente ao sotalol (2 mg/kg VO a cada 12 h) isolado ou em combinação com mexiletina (5-8 mg/kg VO a cada 8 h).
• Taquiarritmia supraventricular:
  ○ Tratamentos para diminuir a frequência cardíaca em cães com taquiarritmia supraventricular incluem manobras vagais, bloqueadores dos canais de cálcio (diltiazem a 0,125-0,35 mg/kg IV durante 2-3 min ou 0,125-0,35 mg/kg/h sob infusão em velocidade constante), ß-bloqueadores (esmolol a 0,5 mg/kg IV por 1 min) e procainamida (6-8 mg/kg IV durante 5-10 min e, depois, 20-40 µg/kg/min sob infusão em velocidade constante).
  ○ Os pacientes irresponsivos às manobras vagais ou à terapia medicamentosa de emergência podem necessitar de cardioversão por corrente direta ou marca-passo com estimulação programada (*overdrive pacing**).
• Bradiarritmia:
  ○ O tratamento de escolha para cães e gatos com bradiarritmia grave consiste na implantação de marca-passo artificial. Contudo, alguns pacientes podem se beneficiar da terapia com atropina (0,02-0,04 mg/kg IV) ou isoproterenol (0,4 mg em 250 mL de solução de glicose a 5% em água lentamente até fazer efeito).
• ICC concomitante:
  ○ Furosemida para tratar edema pulmonar e intensificar a oxigenação em cães e gatos com ICC (2-8 mg/kg IV ou IM; ou 0,5-1,0 mg/kg/h sob infusão em velocidade constante). A via IV é preferível, embora a IM seja apropriada quando o acesso IV necessitar de contenção manual.
  ○ Alívio da dor ou ansiedade com sulfato de morfina (0,1-0,5 mg/kg/h IV sob infusão em velocidade constante ou 0,2-2 mg/kg IM) pode reduzir a atividade simpática excessiva, mas diminuir a demanda de oxigênio, a pré-carga e a pós-carga.

CONTRAINDICAÇÕES
• Evitar a terapia diurética em pacientes com efusão pericárdica, pneumotórax/mediastino de tensão e tromboembolia pulmonar.
• Evitar β-bloqueadores e bloqueadores dos canais de cálcio em pacientes com contratilidade miocárdica reduzida.

PRECAUÇÕES
• As infusões de catecolaminas precisam ser tituladas com cuidado para maximizar a pressão de perfusão coronária com o menor aumento possível na demanda de oxigênio pelo miocárdio.
• Os redutores da pós-carga e os vasodilatadores (inibidores da enzima conversora de angiotensina, nitroglicerina e nitroprusseto) devem ser usados com cautela por causa do risco de precipitar uma hipotensão adicional e diminuir o fluxo sanguíneo coronário.

MEDICAMENTO(S) ALTERNATIVO(S)
A dopamina pode ser utilizada como alternativa à dobutamina na dose de 5–10 µg/kg/min (cães e gatos) para restabelecer a função sistólica.

ACOMPANHAMENTO

MONITORIZAÇÃO DO PACIENTE
• Avaliação subjetiva e objetiva seriada da perfusão (atividade mental, coloração das mucosas, tempo

---

* N. T.: Corresponde ao processo de aumentar a frequência cardíaca por meio de um marca-passo cardíaco artificial a fim de suprimir certas arritmias.

de preenchimento capilar, qualidade do pulso, força muscular, temperatura, lactato sérico, débito urinário, frequência cardíaca, pressão arterial e índices de oxigenação) é essencial para otimizar a terapia. • Avaliação seriada de frequência e esforço respiratórios, além de auscultação pulmonar.
• Gasometria arterial e oximetria de pulso para acompanhar a oxigenação tecidual, a ventilação e o equilíbrio acidobásico. • Hematócrito, proteína total sérica, eletrólitos séricos, enzimas hepatocelulares, ureia e creatinina sérica para monitorizar os efeitos de hipoxia tecidual sistêmica. • Monitorização diária de troponina I cardíaca para avaliar o nível de lesão do miocárdio.
• Monitorização eletrocardiográfica contínua para detectar arritmia significativa. • Pressão arterial contínua, pressão venosa central ou outra monitorização hemodinâmica seriada.

COMPLICAÇÕES POSSÍVEIS
• ICC. • Arritmias cardíacas. • Síncope.
• Distúrbios acidobásicos. • Disfunção renal.
• Disfunção hepática. • Parada cardíaca.

EVOLUÇÃO ESPERADA E PROGNÓSTICO
Dependem da causa subjacente. Os pacientes com cardiopatia primária, em geral, apresentam prognóstico pior (mau a grave) em comparação àqueles com disfunção cardíaca secundária.

DIVERSOS

DISTÚRBIOS ASSOCIADOS
ICC.

VER TAMBÉM
• Bloqueio Atrioventricular.
• Choque Hipovolêmico.
• Doenças Endomiocárdicas — Gatos.
• Efusão Pericárdica.
• Endocardiose das Valvas Atrioventriculares.
• Insuficiência Cardíaca Congestiva Direita.
• Insuficiência Cardíaca Congestiva Esquerda.
• Miocardiopatia.
• Miocardite.
• Pericardite.
• Pneumotórax.
• Sepse e bacteremia.
• Síndrome do Nó Sinusal Doente.
• Taquicardia Supraventricular.
• Taquicardia Ventricular.
• Tromboembolia pulmonar.

ABREVIATURA(S)
• AST = aspartato aminotransferase.
• ALT = alanina aminotransferase.
• CID = coagulação intravascular disseminada.
• ICC = insuficiência cardíaca congestiva.
• SNC = sistema nervoso central.

Sugestões de Leitura
Brown AJ, Mandell DC. Cardiogenic shock. In: Silverstein DC, Hopper K, ed., Small Animal Critical Care Medicine, 1st ed. St. Louis: Saunders, 2009, pp. 146–150.
Cote E. Cardiogenic shock and cardiac arrest. Vet Clin North Am Small Anim Pract 2001, 31(6):1129–1146.

Autores Gretchen Lee Schoeffler e Nishi Dhupa
Consultores Editoriais Larry P. Tilley e Francis W.K. Smith, Jr.

Choque Hipovolêmico

CONSIDERAÇÕES GERAIS

DEFINIÇÃO
Perda de líquido interno ou externo, que resulta em volume circulante e perfusão tecidual inadequados.

FISIOPATOLOGIA
• Hemorragia ou perda de outro líquido resulta em uma redução crítica no volume intravascular, declínio no retorno venoso e diminuição no débito cardíaco.
• A queda no débito cardíaco ativa respostas neuroendócrinas compensatórias que levam à vasoconstrição periférica, exacerbando a isquemia dos tecidos e a depleção de energia com consequente função anormal dos órgãos.

SISTEMA(S) ACOMETIDO(S)
• Cardiovascular — as respostas compensatórias incluem aumento na frequência e contratilidade cardíacas, além de vasoconstrição periférica. Além disso, o incremento na demanda de oxigênio pelo coração diante de uma distribuição diminuída desse gás pode resultar em arritmia.
• Endócrino — hiperglicemia e insulinorresistência.
• Gastrintestinal — isquemia gastrintestinal leva a necrose e esfacelamento das mucosas, bem como hemorragia e translocação bacteriana.
• Hematológico — desequilíbrios hemostáticos levam à trombose microvascular, além de coagulopatia intravascular disseminada hiper ou hipocoagulável.
• Hepatobiliar — a hipoxia hepática resulta em extravasamento de enzimas hepatocelulares, colestase, depuração reduzida de bactérias e subprodutos bacterianos e função anormal de síntese.
• Musculoesquelético — a hipoperfusão induz à fraqueza da musculatura esquelética.
• Nervoso — ocorre depressão do SNC em resposta à hipoperfusão dos órgãos.
• Renal/urológico — hipotensão sistêmica e hipoperfusão renal podem resultar em dano tubular isquêmico, oligúria e desenvolvimento de insuficiência renal aguda.
• Respiratório — pode ocorrer hiperventilação na tentativa de compensar a acidose metabólica.

GENÉTICA
Desconhecida.

INCIDÊNCIA/PREVALÊNCIA
Desconhecidas.

IDENTIFICAÇÃO
• Cães e gatos.
• Qualquer raça, idade ou sexo.

SINAIS CLÍNICOS
Achados Anamnésicos
Podem estar associados a histórico de traumatismo, fraqueza e colapso, cirurgia, vômito e diarreia, ou poliúria e polidipsia.

Achados do Exame Físico
• O choque compensado também é conhecido como choque térmico ou pré-choque:
  ○ Os mecanismos compensatórios podem fazer com que um cão ou gato saudável sob outros aspectos permaneça relativamente assintomático apesar do declínio de 10% no volume sanguíneo efetivo total. Quando os mecanismos homeostáticos não conseguirem mais compensar, os pacientes manifestarão sinais de choque descompensado.
• Choque hipovolêmico descompensado:
  ○ Marcadores de má perfusão:
    — Mucosas pálidas (podem ser agravadas por anemia).
    — Tempo de preenchimento capilar prolongado.
    — Pulso periférico débil (fraco).
    — Fraqueza muscular.
    — Embotamento mental.
    — Hipotermia e extremidades frias.
    — Oligúria.
  ○ Distensão mínima ou ausente da veia jugular.
  ○ Taquicardia ± arritmia.
  ○ Taquipneia.
  ○ Desidratação clínica, conforme evidenciado por diminuição no turgor da pele, mucosas pegajosas e olhos fundos, é mais comum em pacientes com perda de líquido do que com hemorragia.
  ○ À medida que o choque evolui, os pacientes exibem uma fase hipodinâmica ou terminal caracterizada por bradicardia, colapso circulatório completo, coma e morte.

CAUSAS
Choque Induzido por Hemorragia
• Traumatismo rombo ou penetrante.
• Neoplasia, como ruptura de hemangiossarcoma.
• Sangramento gastrintestinal secundário à doença ulcerativa, neoplasia ou trombocitopenia grave.
• Coagulopatia, como intoxicação por rodenticidas anticoagulantes, falha na síntese hepática, coagulação intravascular disseminada, hemofilia e deficiência significativa do fator de von Willebrand.

Choque Induzido por Perda de Líquido
• Trato gastrintestinal (vômito e diarreia).
• Trato urinário (insuficiência renal, diabetes melito, diabetes insípido, hipercalcemia, doença de Addison, e síndrome de Cushing).
• Queimaduras.
• Perda para o terceiro espaço (sepse, pancreatite, síndrome de resposta inflamatória sistêmica, e cirrose).

FATORES DE RISCO
O choque hipovolêmico origina-se de uma diminuição no volume sanguíneo, causada por alguma outra condição; como tal, esse tipo de choque não tem fatores de risco específicos.

DIAGNÓSTICO

DIAGNÓSTICO DIFERENCIAL
Diferenciar Sinais Semelhantes
• Choque hipovolêmico — o volume circulante inadequado resulta em diminuição do débito cardíaco diante de função cardíaca normal ou aumentada e resistência vascular sistêmica normal ou elevada.
• Choque cardiogênico — o volume circulante adequado com queda no débito cardíaco se deve à função cardíaca insuficiente e resistência vascular sistêmica normal ou aumentada.
• Choque distributivo — volume circulante adequado com função e débito cardíacos normais ou aumentados e resistência vascular sistêmica insuficiente.

HEMOGRAMA/BIOQUÍMICA/URINÁLISE
Hemograma Completo
• Neutrofilia madura e linfopenia, secundárias a estresse.
• Hematócrito, proteína total e contagem plaquetária são variáveis (podem estar diminuídos em casos de hemorragia).

Perfil Bioquímico
• Hiperglicemia secundária a estresse.
• Proteína total e albumina são variáveis (diminuídas com hemorragia e aumentadas em perda de líquido).
• Aumento na atividade das enzimas hepatocelulares (ALT, AST).
• Desarranjos eletrolíticos são variáveis (mais prováveis em perda de líquido).
• Hiato aniônico elevado (acúmulo de ácido láctico e ácidos renais).
• Azotemia atribuída à diminuição na taxa de filtração glomerular.

Urinálise
• A densidade urinária pode estar aumentada; no entanto, lesão tubular aguda secundária à hipoxia renal pode resultar em isostenúria.

OUTROS TESTES LABORATORIAIS
• O teste de coagulação é indicado em pacientes criticamente enfermos e naqueles com indícios de hemorragia significativa.
• A gasometria arterial pode revelar acidose metabólica e indícios de extração aumentada de oxigênio pelos tecidos (uma diferença arteriovenosa ampliada de oxigênio e uma concentração venosa reduzida desse gás em paciente que não esteja hipoxêmico ou anêmico).
• Hiperlactatemia reflete a depuração diminuída e a produção aumentada de lactato.

DIAGNÓSTICO POR IMAGEM
A radiografia torácica pode revelar microcardia e perfusão vascular pulmonar abaixo do ideal.

MÉTODOS DIAGNÓSTICOS
• Toracocentese, abdominocentese e pericardiocentese, quando houver indicação, podem fornecer uma pista da etiologia subjacente.
• Outros testes, conforme for indicado pelos diagnósticos diferenciais da causa subjacente.

TRATAMENTO

CUIDADO(S) DE SAÚDE ADEQUADO(S)
• Existem três objetivos do tratamento de emergência de pacientes com choque hipovolêmico:
  ○ Maximizar o conteúdo de oxigênio no sangue, garantindo a suficiência da ventilação e a saturação sanguínea desse gás, além de corrigir a anemia.
  ○ Restabelecer o fluxo sanguíneo e controlar as perdas adicionais.
  ○ Promover a ressuscitação hídrica.
• Os parâmetros tradicionais de ressuscitação, incluindo restabelecimento dos parâmetros clínicos de perfusão normal (atividade mental, tempo de preenchimento capilar, frequência cardíaca, qualidade do pulso periférico e temperatura retal), pressão arterial e débito urinário continuam sendo os padrões de cuidado. Contudo, foi registrado que até 85% dos pacientes humanos gravemente lesionados apresentam indícios de hipoxia tecidual contínua apesar da

normalização dos sinais vitais, sendo sugestivos de débito oculto de oxigênio e da presença de choque compensado. Há provas de que a normalização dos sinais vitais, do lactato sanguíneo, do déficit de base, das variáveis de transporte de oxigênio como índice cardíaco, distribuição e consumo desse gás, saturação venosa mista e central de oxigênio em conjunto sejam os marcadores mais sensíveis da suficiência de perfusão tecidual do que qualquer uma dessas variáveis isoladas. Até que haja provas mais sólidas para a seleção preferencial de um parâmetro sobre os outros, a utilização do máximo de marcadores disponíveis parece ser aconselhável em qualquer paciente.

CUIDADO(S) DE ENFERMAGEM
- Maximizar o conteúdo de oxigênio no sangue:
  - Avaliar e estabilizar as vias aéreas e a respiração do paciente, conforme a necessidade.
  - Sempre administrar a suplementação de oxigênio em alto fluxo e fornecer suporte ventilatório, quando necessário.
  - Anemia significativa (hematócrito <25-30%) em paciente hipovolêmico é preocupante e deve ser corrigida.
- Controlar a perda adicional de sangue ou líquido:
  - O sangramento externo é frequentemente controlado com compressão direta, enquanto o sangramento interno pode necessitar de intervenção cirúrgica.
  - Uma área de interesse a respeito da ressuscitação em casos de hemorragia está na dúvida de se restabelecer o volume circulante normal e a pressão arterial antes do controle definitivo do sangramento. Embora haja provas de que a ressuscitação hipotensiva possa melhorar o desfecho em alguns modelos de trauma, ainda não sabemos que lesões são mais responsivas a essa estratégia terapêutica ou que pressão arterial deve ser o alvo.
  - O controle de perda adicional de líquido que não seja hemorragia concentra-se no controle dos sintomas (p. ex., antieméticos) e na correção do distúrbio subjacente.
- Ressuscitação com fluido:
  - Assim que o acesso intravenoso ou intraósseo for obtido, a ressuscitação inicial com fluidos será realizada com algum cristaloide isotônico, como solução de Ringer lactato, solução fisiológica, Plasmalyte-A® e Normosol-R® (30 mL/kg por 15 min). Se o paciente não estiver significativamente desidratado, a adição de salina hipertônica a 7,5% (4 mL/kg por 15 min) pode acelerar a ressuscitação.
  - Após a administração do bólus inicial, a resposta do paciente é avaliada. Se os sinais vitais e outros parâmetros de ressuscitação retornarem ao normal, será imprescindível a monitorização do paciente para garantir a estabilidade. Se os sinais vitais e outros parâmetros de ressuscitação apresentarem uma melhora transitória ou se pouca ou nenhuma melhora for observada, outro bólus de cristaloide deverá ser infundido e fluidos como hetamido (5-20 mL/kg, cão: 5-10 mL/kg, gato) ou produtos derivados do sangue (10-20 mL/kg), considerados.
  - Esse processo é repetido até que os parâmetros de ressuscitação do paciente se normalizem. Ao administrar os fluidos em bólus para corrigir os déficits de perfusão, o clínico deverá monitorar não apenas a resposta à terapia, mas também as complicações potenciais.
  - A administração de fluidos em bólus é usada para corrigir os déficits de perfusão. Contudo, à medida que o bólus é administrado e o volume intravascular sobe rapidamente, o fluxo sanguíneo dos rins e a taxa de filtração glomerular também aumentam, resultando em aumento no débito urinário. Em consequência disso, pelo menos parte do bólus será perdida na urina. É por essa razão que os déficits de hidratação precisam ser corrigidos de forma mais lenta, após a perfusão ter se normalizado. Os clínicos devem ter como objetivo a correção dos déficits de hidratação em 12-24 h.

ORIENTAÇÃO AO PROPRIETÁRIO
Informar ao proprietário que seu animal de estimação está sob risco de parada cardíaca. Um "código do estado" deve ser abordado com antecedência sempre que possível.

CONSIDERAÇÕES CIRÚRGICAS
Identificar e reparar a origem da perda de líquido (mais comum em choque hipovolêmico induzido por hemorragia).

MEDICAÇÕES

MEDICAMENTO(S) DE ESCOLHA
- Para os pacientes com choque hipovolêmico refratário, é importante incluir ou excluir perdas contínuas (especialmente a categoria induzida por hemorragia) e administrar produtos derivados do sangue, conforme a necessidade.
- Se o volume circulante adequado for garantido e o paciente ainda estiver exibindo sinais clínicos de choque (não muito comum em pacientes com choque hipovolêmico), considerar:
  - Um agente pressórico como a dopamina (5-20 µg/kg/min), a norepinefrina (0,05-2 µg/kg/min) ou a vasopressina (0,5-2 mU/kg/min). Esses agentes podem ser utilizados para suporte vasopressor tanto em cães como em gatos. Monitorizar o paciente quanto à ocorrência de taquiarritmia e vasoconstrição periférica excessiva.
  - Um agente inotrópico positivo como a dobutamina (2-20 µg/kg/min). A dobutamina pode ser benéfica em pacientes com contratilidade diminuída ou depressão miocárdica. Monitorar o animal quanto à presença de taquiarritmia. Embora a dobutamina possa ser usada com segurança em cães, foram observadas crises convulsivas em alguns gatos sob doses superiores a 5 µg/kg/min.

ACOMPANHAMENTO

MONITORIZAÇÃO DO PACIENTE
- Avaliação subjetiva e objetiva seriada da perfusão (atividade mental, coloração das mucosas, tempo de preenchimento capilar, qualidade do pulso, força muscular, temperatura, lactato sérico, débito urinário, frequência cardíaca, pressão arterial e índices de oxigenação) é essencial para otimizar a terapia:
  - A mensuração da pressão arterial confirma a hipotensão e, muitas vezes, revela uma pressão diastólica desproporcionalmente baixa.
  - Pressão venosa jugular e central reduzida em virtude de hipovolemia e pré-carga diminuída.
- Avaliação seriada da frequência cardíaca, da qualidade do pulso, da frequência e do esforço respiratórios, além de auscultação pulmonar.
- O exame eletrocardiográfico pode ajudar na caracterização das arritmias.
- Um banco de dados mínimo coletado diariamente como hematócrito, proteína total sérica, glicemia, gasometria, eletrólitos séricos, enzimas hepatocelulares, ureia e creatinina sérica para monitorizar os efeitos da hipoxia tecidual sistêmica e orientar o tratamento clínico.
  - Os pacientes com choque hipovolêmico induzido por hemorragia devem ser submetidos a uma avaliação mais frequente do hematócrito e da proteína total.
  - A mensuração diária da pressão oncótica coloidal pode ajudar a guiar a fluidoterapia.

PREVENÇÃO
As estratégias preventivas são direcionadas às várias etiologias subjacentes.

COMPLICAÇÕES POSSÍVEIS
- Podem ocorrer coagulopatia dilucional e baixa pressão oncótica coloidal em pacientes submetidos a volumes muito grandes de ressuscitação (mais de 1-2 volumes sanguíneos). Isso se deve à diluição dos fatores de coagulação e das proteínas, respectivamente, embora seja raro na primeira hora da ressuscitação. Os tempos de coagulação devem ser usados para orientar a administração de plasma fresco congelado. A pressão oncótica coloidal baixa é mais comum, sendo tratada de forma eficiente com a administração de soluções coloides artificiais.
- Sobrecarga volêmica com sinais clínicos de edema pulmonar e/ou periférico.
- Anemia e trombocitopenia.
- Distúrbios acidobásicos.
- Disfunção múltipla de órgãos.
- Parada cardíaca.

EVOLUÇÃO ESPERADA E PROGNÓSTICO
Dependem da causa subjacente e da possibilidade de instituição de terapia adequada.

DIVERSOS

VER TAMBÉM
- Choque Cardiogênico.

ABREVIATURA(S)
- ALT = alanina aminotransferase.
- AST = aspartato aminotransferase.

Sugestões de Leitura
Aldrich J. Shock fluids and fluid challenge. In: Silverstein DC, Hopper K, eds., Small Animal Critical Care Medicine, 1st ed. St. Louis: Saunders, 2009, pp. 276-280.
Boag A, Hughes D. Fluid therapy. In: King L, Boag A, eds. BSAVA Manual of Small Animal Emergency and Critical Care, 2nd ed. Gloucestershire, UK: BSAVA, 2007, pp. 30-45.
Day TK, Bateman S. Shock syndromes. In: Dibartola SP, ed., Fluid Therapy in Small Animal Practice, 3rd ed. Philadelphia: Saunders, 2006, pp. 540-564.

Autores Gretchen Lee Schoeffler e Nishi Dhupa
Consultores Editoriais Larry P. Tilley e Francis W.K. Smith, Jr.

CHOQUE SÉPTICO

CONSIDERAÇÕES GERAIS

DEFINIÇÃO
Trata-se de hipotensão induzida por sepse que persiste apesar de volume intravascular e débito cardíaco adequados, sendo atribuível à baixa resistência vascular sistêmica.

FISIOPATOLOGIA
• Na sepse, um agente infeccioso deflagra a ativação de monócitos, macrófagos e neutrófilos em grande escala; tais células, em seguida, interagem com as células endoteliais, induzindo a uma resposta inflamatória generalizada.
• No subgrupo de pacientes sépticos descritos como tendo choque séptico, a interação elaborada de células e mediadores inflamatórios diminui a resistência vascular sistêmica e provoca má distribuição do fluxo sanguíneo (efeito distributivo). Eles também aumentam a permeabilidade capilar de tal modo que o líquido se desvia para fora do espaço intravascular. Para compensar a queda no volume plasmático, as catecolaminas aumentam o débito cardíaco e a contratilidade miocárdica. Diante de vasodilatação arterial grave, o débito cardíaco não é suficiente para manter a distribuição de oxigênio para os tecidos.
• A distribuição diminuída de oxigênio é agravada pela presença de edema intersticial e esfacelamento microvascular. No devido tempo, a hipoxia tecidual leva à falência de órgãos e ao óbito.

SISTEMA(S) ACOMETIDO(S)
• Cardiovascular — predominam alterações como débito cardíaco elevado, vasodilatação arterial e má distribuição do fluxo sanguíneo. Contudo, é importante notar que a disfunção do miocárdio secundária a fatores depressores circulantes desse músculo cardíaco pode ser uma variável importante (ver "Choque Cardiogênico").
• Endócrino — as anormalidades podem se manifestar sob a forma de hiperglicemia e insulinorresistência ou como produção insuficiente de corticosteroides e vasopressina da adrenal.
• Gastrintestinal — a perda de função da barreira intestinal pode resultar em translocação de bactérias; a má perfusão pode levar à congestão e hemorragia dentro do lúmen gastrintestinal.
• Hematológico — desequilíbrios homeostáticos levam à trombose microvascular, bem como coagulopatia intravascular disseminada hiper e hipocoagulável.
• Hepatobiliar — a lesão do fígado pode resultar em disfunção na síntese hepática, colestase, extravasamento de enzimas hepatocelulares e depuração reduzida de bactérias e subprodutos bacterianos pelo sistema reticuloendotelial.
• Nervoso — estado mental diminuído.
• Renal/urológico — a isquemia renal resulta em necrose tubular aguda e oligúria.
• Respiratório — a permeabilidade microvascular acentuada culmina na formação de edema intersticial e alveolar; a hipercoagulabilidade pode resultar em tromboembolia pulmonar.

GENÉTICA
Desconhecida.

INCIDÊNCIA/PREVALÊNCIA
Desconhecidas.

IDENTIFICAÇÃO
• Cães e gatos.
• Qualquer raça, idade ou sexo.

SINAIS CLÍNICOS
Achados Anamnésicos
Possível histórico de infecção recente, lesão, doença grave, cirurgia ou imunossupressão (doenças associadas à imunossupressão ou iatrogênica).

Achados do Exame Físico
• Os cães podem exibir uma forma hiperdinâmica, caracterizada por estado mental diminuído, letargia e fraqueza, taquicardia, taquipneia, hiperemia, tempo de preenchimento capilar reduzido, qualidade do pulso saltitante e febre. Os gatos raramente demonstram esses sinais hiperdinâmicos.
• À medida que o choque evolui, muitos desses pacientes exibirão uma fase hipodinâmica, caracterizada por bradicardia, estado mental diminuído, fraqueza ou colapso, taquipneia ou dispneia, mucosas pálidas, tempo de preenchimento capilar prolongado, qualidade do pulso fraca e hipotermia.

CAUSAS
• Peritonite séptica — ruptura do trato gastrintestinal ou translocação de bactérias, ferida abdominal penetrante, ruptura infectada do trato urinário, ruptura de abscesso intra-abdominal.
• Respiratório e espaço pleural — pneumonia e piotórax.
• Infecções da pele ou de tecidos moles — especialmente feridas causadas por mordeduras e corpos estranhos.
• Trato urinário — pielonefrite.
• Reprodutivo — prostatite e piometra.
• Cardiovascular — endocardite bacteriana.
• Musculoesquelético — artrite e osteomielite sépticas.
• Fontes iatrogênicas de infecção — cateteres, implantes e feridas cirúrgicas.
• Sistema nervoso central — meningite e encefalite.

FATORES DE RISCO
• Extremos de idade.
• Doenças concomitantes como diabetes melito, hiperadrenocorticismo, processos malignos e doença cardiopulmonar.
• Imunossupressão resultante de neutropenia, medicamentos (corticosteroides e quimioterápicos) e asplenia.
• Cirurgia de grande porte, traumatismo e queimaduras.
• Antibioticoterapia prévia.

DIAGNÓSTICO

DIAGNÓSTICO DIFERENCIAL
• Outras causas de choque distributivo incluem reação a medicamentos ou toxinas, anafilaxia e insuficiência adrenal.
• Choque hipovolêmico.
• Choque cardiogênico.
• Intermação/insolação.

HEMOGRAMA/BIOQUÍMICA/URINÁLISE
• Neutrofilia ou neutropenia com desvio à esquerda e alterações tóxicas concomitantes.
• Linfopenia secundária a estresse.
• Trombocitopenia.
• Hematócrito variável.
• Glicemia variável.
• Hipoalbuminemia.
• Níveis elevados de bilirrubina ou das enzimas hepáticas.
• Desarranjos eletrolíticos.
• Azotemia.
• Isostenúria e sedimento urinário ativo.

OUTROS TESTES LABORATORIAIS
• O perfil da coagulação pode exibir prolongamento dos tempos de tromboplastina parcial ativada e da protrombina, aumento de D-dímeros ou dos produtos de degradação da fibrina e níveis reduzidos da antitrombina e proteína C.
• Gasometria arterial pode revelar hipoxemia e distúrbios acidobásicos.
• Lactato sérico encontra-se elevado quando existe hipoperfusão tecidual significativa.
• Obter amostras de possíveis locais de infecção para citologia, coloração de Gram, além de cultura e antibiograma.
• Outros exames de cultura e antibiograma de urina e/ou do sangue podem ser úteis, particularmente quando a origem da sepse é desconhecida.
• Como a baixa pressão oncótica coloidal é comum, a monitorização é proveitosa para otimizar a fluidoterapia.
• Realizar teste de estimulação com ACTH em pacientes irresponsivos à terapia-padrão, pois pode ocorrer insuficiência adrenal relatava em uma porcentagem muito pequena desses pacientes.

DIAGNÓSTICO POR IMAGEM
• As radiografias torácicas podem revelar algum foco séptico ou uma causa de disfunção respiratória.
• A ecocardiografia pode documentar uma lesão valvular vegetativa e/ou caracterizar a suficiência da função cardíaca.
• A ultrassonografia abdominal pode detectar algum foco séptico.

MÉTODOS DIAGNÓSTICOS
• A mensuração da pressão arterial confirma a hipotensão e, frequentemente, revela uma pressão diastólica desproporcionalmente baixa.
• A eletrocardiografia pode ajudar na detecção e caracterização de arritmias.
• Oximetria de pulso pode registrar a baixa saturação de oxigênio em pacientes com comprometimento respiratório.
• A mensuração da pressão venosa central pode ser feita para avaliar a pré-carga cardíaca e a saturação venosa central de oxigênio.
• A monitorização hemodinâmica é realizada para avaliar a saturação venosa mista de oxigênio, o débito cardíaco e a resistência vascular sistêmica.

TRATAMENTO

CUIDADO(S) DE SAÚDE ADEQUADO(S)
Os pacientes em choque séptico necessitam de cuidados intensivos de emergência. Os objetivos terapêuticos incluem ressuscitação (com o uso de medidas de suporte para corrigir hipoxia, hipotensão e oxigenação tecidual prejudicada), identificação e tratamento da origem da infecção (com o uso de terapia antimicrobiana, cirurgia ou

ambos); e manutenção de função adequada dos órgãos (conforme orientada por monitorização cardiovascular e laboratorial).

CUIDADO(S) DE ENFERMAGEM
- A suplementação de oxigênio é importante em todos os pacientes sépticos.
- Os pacientes sépticos se beneficiarão de uma abordagem metódica para restabelecimento da distribuição sistêmica de oxigênio por meio da manipulação e otimização do volume, da pressão arterial e da contratilidade cardíaca. A normalização ou a melhoria de vários parâmetros de perfusão, incluindo atividade mental, frequência cardíaca, pressão arterial média, coloração das mucosas, preenchimento capilar, lactato sérico, saturação venosa central ou mista de oxigênio e débito urinário; indicam ressuscitação adequada.
- Pacientes sépticos que receberam grandes volumes de fluidos podem atingir um volume circulante adequado sem a normalização da pressão arterial e de outros parâmetros de perfusão. Esses pacientes estão em choque séptico e se beneficiariam de uma avaliação mais objetiva do estado volêmico, utilizando a monitorização da pressão venosa central e do débito cardíaco. É importante reconhecer que a fluidoterapia rigorosa contínua nesses pacientes resultará em sobrecarga volêmica e que os vasopressores e/ou inotrópicos positivos são indicados.
- Os pacientes sépticos que se encontram hipovolêmicos necessitam de ressuscitação hídrica rigorosa. A ressuscitação volêmica é mais comumente alcançada com combinações variáveis de cristaloides, coloides sintéticos e produtos sanguíneos. A fluidoterapia é orientada pela condição geral do paciente, bem como pela avaliação frequente do estado volêmico e cardiovascular:
  - A terapia com cristaloide isotônico para repor o volume intravascular pode exigir ou, em casos raros, exceder 90 mL/kg (cão) ou 60 mL/kg (gato). Comece administrando 30 mL/kg (cão) ou 20 mL/kg (gato) sob a forma de bólus durante 15-20 min, mas reavalie para determinar a necessidade de bólus adicionais. Monitorizar o paciente de perto, pois grandes volumes podem precipitar a formação de edema pulmonar em pacientes com extravasamento capilar ou baixa pressão oncótica coloidal.
  - Hidroxietilamido (coloide sintético) é usado em conjunto com cristaloide isotônico. Esse tipo de coloide ajudará a manter a pressão oncótica coloidal adequada e ainda pode reduzir a quantidade de cristaloide necessária para obter uma ressuscitação efetiva. Os bólus de hidroxietilamido (5-20 mL/kg cão; 5-10 mL/kg gato) são mais bem administrados durante 5-10 minutos e podem exacerbar a coagulopatia em altas doses.
  - Se o paciente não estiver desidratado no meio intersticial, um bólus de salina hipertônica a 7% (4 mL/kg para cão e gato) administrado durante 15 min expandirá com rapidez o volume intravascular e ajudará a obter uma ressuscitação mais rápida.
  - Os produtos sanguíneos devem ser administrados com base na necessidade do paciente. As células de papa de hemácias são administradas em pacientes anêmicos para melhorar a capacidade de transporte do oxigênio. Os produtos de plasma são usados para corrigir os déficits de coagulação, enquanto os produtos concentrados de albumina são mais eficazes, elevando a pressão oncótica coloidal.

DIETA
Nada por via oral.

ORIENTAÇÃO AO PROPRIETÁRIO
Informar ao proprietário que seu animal de estimação está em risco de parada cardíaca iminente. Um "código do estado" do animal deve ser abordado com antecedência, sempre que possível.

CONSIDERAÇÕES CIRÚRGICAS
Identificar e remover a origem da sepse (p. ex., peritonite séptica, abscesso, piotórax, piometra e feridas de tecidos moles).

MEDICAÇÕES
MEDICAMENTO(S) DE ESCOLHA
- Assim que o volume circulante adequado for atingido, a melhora na pressão arterial sistêmica e de outros parâmetros clínicos de ressuscitação pode exigir o uso de um ou mais vasopressores e/ou agentes inotrópicos positivos.
  - Dopamina (5-20 µg/kg/min), norepinefrina (0,05-2 µg/kg/min) e vasopressina (0,5-2 mU/kg/min) podem ser usados para suporte vasopressor (cães e gatos). Monitorizar o paciente quanto à presença de taquiarritmia e vasoconstrição periférica excessiva.
  - Dobutamina (2-20 µg/kg/min) é utilizada principalmente como um agente inotrópico positivo no subgrupo de pacientes caninos em choque séptico com contratilidade diminuída ou depressão miocárdica. Monitorizar o animal quanto à ocorrência de taquiarritmia. Embora a dobutamina possa ser utilizada com segurança em muitos pacientes felinos, foram observadas crises convulsivas em alguns gatos em doses superiores a 5 µg/kg/min.
- É essencial que a antibioticoterapia empírica, intravenosa e de amplo espectro seja instituída precocemente em pacientes sépticos; o espectro deve ser estreitado quando os resultados da cultura estiverem disponíveis. A escolha empírica é formulada com base no estado imunológico subjacente do paciente, na origem sob suspeita e no(s) microrganismo(s) responsável(is), nas propriedades antibióticas específicas (penetração tecidual, atividade bactericida *versus* estática) e nas considerações quanto à resistência (uso prévio de antibióticos, infecção adquirida no hospital [nosocomial] ou na comunidade).
- É racional tratar de forma empírica os pacientes que não estejam respondendo de modo adequado à terapia-padrão com 0,75-1,0 mg/kg a cada 6 h de hidrocortisona intravenosa após um teste de estimulação com ACTH em andamento. A terapia deve ser mantida em pacientes, cuja insuficiência adrenal relativa foi registrada, e naqueles que demonstram melhora significativa no estado cardiovascular após o tratamento.

ACOMPANHAMENTO
MONITORIZAÇÃO DO PACIENTE
- Avaliação subjetiva e objetiva seriada da perfusão (atividade mental, coloração das mucosas, tempo de preenchimento capilar, qualidade do pulso, força muscular, temperatura, lactato sérico, débito urinário, frequência cardíaca, pressão arterial e índices de oxigenação) é essencial para otimizar a terapia.
- A titulação ideal de fluidos e da terapia vasoativa é realizada de forma mais objetiva com monitorização hemodinâmica (pressão arterial direta, pressão venosa central e débito cardíaco).
- ECG contínuo para detectar arritmia significativa.
- Avaliação seriada de frequência e esforço respiratórios, além de auscultação pulmonar.
- Gasometria arterial e oximetria de pulso para acompanhar a oxigenação tecidual, a ventilação e o equilíbrio acidobásico.
- Um banco de dados mínimo deve ser obtido diariamente, incluindo hematócrito, proteína total sérica, glicemia, eletrólitos séricos, enzimas hepatocelulares, ureia e creatinina sérica para monitorizar os efeitos da hipoxia tecidual sistêmica.
- Mensuração diária da pressão oncótica coloidal para orientar a fluidoterapia.

PREVENÇÃO
- Tratamento oportuno e eficaz de feridas.
- Uso adequado de terapia antimicrobiana.

COMPLICAÇÕES POSSÍVEIS
- Sobrecarga volêmica.
- Edema pulmonar.
- Vasculite e edema periférico.
- Hipoglicemia.
- Anemia e trombocitopenia.
- Coagulopatia.
- Falência múltipla de órgãos (cardíaca, respiratória, renal, hepática, gastrintestinal, pancreática, adrenal e neurológica [cérebro]).
- Parada cardíaca.

EVOLUÇÃO ESPERADA E PROGNÓSTICO
Dependem da etiologia subjacente e da possibilidade de instituir a terapia adequada.

DIVERSOS
VER TAMBÉM
- Coagulação Intravascular Disseminada.
- Choque Cardiogênico.
- Choque Hipovolêmico.

ABREVIATURA(S)
- ACTH = hormônio adrenocorticotrópico.
- ECG = eletrocardiograma.

Sugestões de Leitura
Brady CA, Otto CM. Systemic inflammatory response syndrome, sepsis and multiple organ dysfunction. Vet Clin North Am Small Anim Pract 2001, 31(6):1147-1162.
Mittleman Boller E, Otto CM. Sepsis. In: Silverstein DC, Hopper K, ed., Small Animal Critical Care Medicine, 1st ed. St. Louis: Saunders, 2009, pp. 454-458.
Mittleman Boller E, Otto CM. Septic Shock. In: Silverstein DC, Hopper K, ed., Small Animal Critical Care Medicine, 1st ed. St. Louis: Saunders, 2009, pp. 459-463.

Autores Gretchen Lee Schoeffler e Nishi Dhupa
Consultores Editoriais Larry P. Tilley e Francis W.K. Smith, Jr.

Cianose

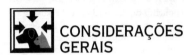

CONSIDERAÇÕES GERAIS

DEFINIÇÃO
Corresponde à coloração azulada da pele e das mucosas, em função do aumento na quantidade de hemoglobina reduzida ou desoxigenada na circulação sanguínea.

FISIOPATOLOGIA
• Concentração da hemoglobina desoxigenada — deve ser >5 g/dL para detectar o problema; consequentemente, uma anemia (hematócrito <15%) pode mascarar sua detecção.
• Central — associada a hipoxemia arterial sistêmica ou anormalidades hemoglobínicas.
• Periférica — limitada a uma ou mais extremidades corporais; associada à diminuição no fluxo sanguíneo periférico; tipicamente, a tensão e a saturação arteriais de oxigênio permanecem normais.

Hipoxemia Arterial
• Declínio na fração de oxigênio inspirado — altitude elevada.
• Hipoventilação — distúrbios obstrutivos das vias aéreas superiores; pneumopatia restritiva ou obstrutiva; distúrbios do espaço pleural; insuficiência neuromuscular.
• Desequilíbrio entre ventilação e perfusão — doenças parenquimatosas ou tromboembólicas pulmonares.
• Dano à difusão — espessamento da barreira alveolar através da qual o oxigênio deve passar para chegar às hemácias.
• Adição de sangue venoso à circulação arterial — defeitos cardíacos congênitos com desvio da direita para a esquerda (p. ex., tetralogia de Fallot e transposição dos grandes vasos); defeitos cardíacos com desvio inverso, causados por uma alta resistência vascular pulmonar (p. ex., persistência do ducto arterioso, defeito do septo atrial e defeito do septo ventricular com desvio da direita para a esquerda).
• Desvios anatômicos — diferenciados de outras causas de hipoxemia pela falha de resposta à suplementação de oxigênio.

Hemoglobina Anormal
• Metemoglobina — pigmento heme anormal mais comum; incapaz de se ligar ao oxigênio; formado normalmente em uma taxa baixa nos eritrócitos.
• NADH-metemoglobina redutase — enzima redutora intracelular; mantém a proporção de metemoglobina:hemoglobina a <2%; a deficiência e/ou a exposição a agentes oxidantes causa metemoglobinemia.
• Hipoxia — quando >20-40% de hemoglobina foram oxidados em metemoglobina.

Outros
• Cianose periférica — origina-se do aumento na extração de oxigênio proveniente do suprimento arterial para uma determinada área, por exemplo, um membro; causada por vasoconstrição intensa, fluxo sanguíneo periférico deficiente, obstrução ao fluxo associada à tromboembolia arterial ou ainda estagnação ou obstrução do fluxo sanguíneo venoso.
• Cianose diferencial — em casos de persistência do ducto arterioso com desvio inverso, a cabeça e o pescoço recebem sangue oxigenado via tronco braquiocefálico e artéria subclávia esquerda, que se origina do arco aórtico; o restante do corpo recebe sangue dessaturado pelo ducto localizado na aorta descendente.

SISTEMA(S) ACOMETIDO(S)
• Central — todos os sistemas acometidos.
• Periféricos — podem diminuir ou abolir a função neuromuscular do(s) membro(s) acometido(s).

IDENTIFICAÇÃO
• Desvios cardíacos da direita para a esquerda em associação com resistência vascular pulmonar elevada e hipertensão pulmonar (fisiologia de Eisenmenger) — cães: Keeshond, Buldogue inglês e Beagle; alguns gatos; geralmente animais jovens.
• Colapso da traqueia — em geral, raças caninas de pequeno porte, jovens ou de meia-idade (p. ex., Pomerânia, Yorkshire terrier e Poodle).
• Paralisia congênita da laringe — animais jovens; descrita em Dálmata, Bouvier de Flandres e Husky siberiano.
• Paralisia adquirida da laringe — mais comum em cães idosos de grande porte (p. ex., as raças de Retrievers).
• Hipoplasia da traqueia — identificada em Buldogue inglês jovem; ocasionalmente, ocorre em outras raças.
• Asma (gatos) — incidência mais alta descrita em Siamês.

SINAIS CLÍNICOS

Achados Anamnésicos
• Centrais — estridor; angústia respiratória; tosse; mudança na vocalização; fraqueza episódica; síncope; exposição a substâncias oxidantes ou medicamentos indutores de metemoglobinemia.
• Periféricos — paresia ou paralisia de membro.

Achados do Exame Físico
• Sopro cardíaco ou desdobramento da segunda bulha cardíaca — em casos de cardiopatia ou hipertensão pulmonar.
• Crepitações ou sibilos pulmonares — em casos de edema pulmonar ou doença respiratória.
• Abafamento dos sons cardíacos — em virtude de doença no espaço pleural ou no pericárdio.
• Estridor das vias aéreas superiores em casos de paralisia laríngea.
• Tosse grasnante — típica de colapso traqueal; pode ser induzida por palpação da traqueia.
• Dispneia — pode ser inspiratória, expiratória ou uma combinação (ver a seção "Diagnóstico Diferencial").
• Membros — podem ficar cianóticos, frios, pálidos, doloridos e edematosos; podem exibir a ausência de pulso em condições indutoras de cianose periférica.
• Fraqueza — pode ser generalizada e persistente em casos de cardiopatias graves; pode se mostrar episódica e particularmente notável com atividade física ou agitação.
• Paresia ou paralisia posterior — pode ser observada em casos de tromboembolia arterial da aorta distal; diferenciada de doença neuromuscular primária pela ausência total ou parcial de pulsos.

CAUSAS

Sistema Respiratório
• Laringe — paralisia (adquirida ou congênita); colapso; espasmo; edema; traumatismo; neoplasia; doença granulomatosa.
• Traqueia — colapso; neoplasia; corpo estranho; traumatismo; hipoplasia.
• Vias aéreas inferiores e parênquima — pneumonia (viral, bacteriana, fúngica, alérgica, micobacteriana, por aspiração); bronquite crônica; broncopatia por hipersensibilidade (alérgica, asmática); bronquiectasia; neoplasia; corpo estranho; parasitas (*Filaroides*, *Paragonimus*, *Pneumocystis jiroveci*, toxoplasmose, *Aelurostrongylus* spp.); contusão ou hemorragia pulmonares; edema não cardiogênico (inalação, picada de cobra, choque elétrico); casos de afogamento por um triz.
• Espaço pleural — pneumotórax; causas infecciosas (bacteriana, fúngica, PIF); quilotórax; hemotórax; neoplasia; traumatismo.
• Parede torácica ou diafragma — casos congênitos (hérnias pericárdica e diafragmática); traumatismo (hérnia diafragmática, costelas fraturadas, tórax frouxo); doença neuromuscular (paralisia por carrapato, paralisia do Coonhound).

Sistema Cardiovascular
• Defeitos congênitos — fisiologia de Eisenmenger (persistência do ducto arterioso, defeito do septo ventricular, defeito do septo atrial com desvio da direita para a esquerda); tetralogia de Fallot; tronco arterioso; ventrículo direito com saída dupla; retorno venoso pulmonar anômalo; atresia das válvulas aórtica ou pulmonar ou da valva atrioventricular direita (tricúspide).
• Doença adquirida — valvulopatia mitral; miocardiopatia.
• Efusão pericárdica — doença idiopática; neoplasia.
• Doença tromboembólica pulmonar — hiperadrenocorticismo; anemia hemolítica imunomediada; nefropatia com perda de proteínas; dirofilariose.
• Hipertensão pulmonar — idiopática; desvios cardíacos da direita para a esquerda.
• Vasculopatia periférica — tromboembolia arterial (miocardiopatias felinas); obstrução venosa; débito cardíaco reduzido; choque, constrição arteriolar.

Sistema Neuromusculosquelético
• Disfunção do tronco encefálico — encefalite; traumatismo; hemorragia; neoplasia; depressão do centro respiratório induzida por medicamentos (morfina, barbitúricos).
• Disfunção da medula espinal — edema; traumatismo; fraturas vertebrais; prolapso de disco.
• Disfunção neuromuscular — superdosagem de agentes paralisantes (succinilcolina, pancurônio); paralisia por carrapato; botulismo; polirradiculoneurite aguda (paralisia do Coonhound); disautonomia; miastenia grave.

Metemoglobinemia
• Congênita — deficiência da NADH-metemoglobina redutase (cães).
• Ingestão de substâncias químicas oxidantes — paracetamol; nitratos; nitritos; fenacetina; sulfonamidas; benzocaína; corantes anilínicos, dapsona.

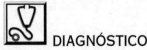

DIAGNÓSTICO

DIAGNÓSTICO DIFERENCIAL
• Cianose generalizada — hipoxemia sistêmica ou anormalidade hêmica.
• Cianose apenas periférica — declínio no fluxo sanguíneo em direção às extremidades.

- Região corporal caudal — persistência do ducto arterioso com desvio da direita para a esquerda.
- Causas cardíacas *versus* causas respiratórias — a diferenciação pode ser difícil; a presença de sopro cardíaco pode sugerir cardiopatia; no entanto, é frequente a auscultação de sopros em pacientes idosos com doença respiratória primária; as radiografias torácicas e a ecocardiografia são úteis para essa distinção.
- Sinais neurológicos centrais ou periféricos — devem incitar a preocupação quanto à hipoxemia arterial decorrente de doença neuromuscular primária.

Padrão Respiratório
- Pode ajudar a definir a causa.
- Dispneia inspiratória — associada frequentemente à doença obstrutiva das vias aéreas superiores ou do espaço pleural; o estridor muitas vezes situa o problema na laringe.
- Dispneia expiratória — observada em geral em casos de doença obstrutiva das vias aéreas inferiores.
- Respiração rápida e superficial (restritiva) — pode se relacionar com doença do espaço pleural ou anormalidades neuromusculares da parede torácica.

HEMOGRAMA/BIOQUÍMICA/URINÁLISE
- Coloração do sangue — pode estar escurecido nessa condição; coloração castanho-chocolate em casos de metemoglobinemia.
- Policitemia — muitas vezes acompanha cardiopatia congênita; pode ocorrer em casos de hipoxemia crônica decorrente de doença respiratória grave.
- Proteinúria — acompanha nefropatias com perda de proteínas, o que pode resultar em tromboembolia pulmonar secundária.
- Pan-hipoproteinemia — acompanha enteropatias com perda de proteínas, o que pode levar à tromboembolia pulmonar.

OUTROS TESTES LABORATORIAIS
- Concentrações da metemoglobina — mensurar em laboratório; alternativamente, pode-se agitar uma amostra de sangue ao ar por 15 minutos: coloração vermelha — hemoglobina reduzida em casos de doença cardíaca ou respiratória; coloração castanho-chocolate — metemoglobinemia.
- Gasometria sanguínea arterial.
- Proporção de proteína:creatinina na urina — na suspeita de tromboembolia pulmonar secundária à nefropatia com perda de proteínas.

DIAGNÓSTICO POR IMAGEM
- Radiografia — essencial para determinar a causa.
- Ecocardiografia com Doppler — auxilia no diagnóstico de cardiopatias congênita ou adquirida, hipertensão pulmonar e tromboembolia pulmonar.
- Tomografia computadorizada torácica — pode definir ainda mais o comprometimento dos pulmões ou do espaço pleural.

MÉTODOS DIAGNÓSTICOS
- Oximetria de pulso — para definir a saturação de oxigênio.
- Exame laringoscópico — avalia a estrutura da laringe e a função da aritenoide.
- Broncoscopia — frequentemente útil no diagnóstico de doença das vias aéreas e dos pulmões.
- Lavado transtraqueal, lavado broncoalveolar ou aspirado pulmonar por agulha fina — necessários muitas vezes para caracterizar as broncopneumopatias.
- Toracocentese — exigida para o diagnóstico e o tratamento de distúrbios do espaço pleural.
- Eletrocardiografia — pode revelar alterações de aumento no volume cardíaco; não é confiável; a ecocardiografia mostra-se mais eficiente.
- Biopsia do pulmão — pode ser necessária para o diagnóstico de pneumopatia intersticial.

TRATAMENTO
- Internação — realização de teste diagnóstico e instituição do tratamento imediatas.
- Terapia de estabilização (p. ex., oxigênio, toracocentese e traqueostomia) — instituída geralmente antes dos testes diagnósticos rigorosos.
- Terapia específica — depende do diagnóstico definitivo; em geral, a restrição de atividade física e a mudança da dieta são imprescindíveis.
- Tratamento cirúrgico — depende do processo patológico primário e do grau de envolvimento cardíaco ou respiratório.
- Ao se admitir o paciente no hospital, alertar o proprietário de que as doenças associadas à cianose podem ter resultados catastróficos.

MEDICAÇÕES
MEDICAMENTO(S) DE ESCOLHA
- Oxigenoterapia — providenciar o mais rápido possível.
- Terapia medicamentosa adicional depende do diagnóstico final.
- Diuréticos (furosemida) — indica-se o emprego rigoroso na suspeita de edema pulmonar cardiogênico.
- Metemoglobinemia como resultado da ingestão de substâncias oxidantes (paracetamol) — administrar, assim que possível, acetilcisteína (140 mg/kg VO ou IV; depois 70 mg/kg a cada 4 h por 5 tratamentos no total); a cimetidina (10 mg/kg VO; depois 5 mg/kg VO a cada 6 h por 48 h) é um adjuvante útil para a acetilcisteína; o ácido ascórbico (30 mg/kg VO a cada 6 h por 7 tratamentos) pode ter algum valor, mas não deve ser usado como agente único.
- Citrato de sildenafila — inibidor da fosfodiesterase tipo 5 utilizado para tratar hipertensão arterial pulmonar a uma dose de 1-3 mg/kg VO a cada 8-12 h.

CONTRAINDICAÇÕES
Evitar o uso de agentes paralisantes (succinilcolina, pancurônio) e agentes indutores de depressão profunda do centro respiratório (morfina, barbitúricos).

ACOMPANHAMENTO
MONITORIZAÇÃO DO PACIENTE
- Os pacientes contidos em gaiola de oxigênio devem ser incomodados o mínimo possível durante a monitorização.
- Avaliar a eficácia da terapia — alterações na profundidade e na frequência respiratórias; coloração das mucosas (deverá retornar à cor rosada normal se a causa não for um desvio anatômico e se o paciente tiver reservas suficientes); oximetria de pulso ou gasometria arterial.
- Instruir o proprietário a monitorizar a coloração da mucosa e o esforço respiratório e aconselhar o fornecimento de cuidados veterinários imediatos em casos de recidiva da condição cianótica.

COMPLICAÇÕES POSSÍVEIS
Doenças avançadas dos pulmões ou das vias aéreas e cardiopatias graves — prognóstico mau a longo prazo.

DIVERSOS
DISTÚRBIOS ASSOCIADOS
- Obesidade — pode complicar ou exacerbar as doenças respiratórias ou cardíacas subjacentes.
- Ascite — pode complicar ou exacerbar o esforço respiratório e reduzir a capacidade pulmonar em função do deslocamento cranial do diafragma.

FATORES RELACIONADOS COM A IDADE
Anormalidades cardíacas congênitas — costumam ser a causa em pacientes jovens.

GESTAÇÃO/FERTILIDADE/REPRODUÇÃO
- A prenhez avançada pode intensificar os sintomas, em virtude da pressão exercida sobre o diafragma e da diminuição na expansão pulmonar.
- É provável que os fetos corram riscos de lesões ou sejam abortados pela hipoxemia associada à cianose.

VER TAMBÉM
- Dispneia e Angústia Respiratória.
- Estertor e Estridor.
- Respiração Ofegante e Taquipneia.

ABREVIATURA(S)
- PIF = peritonite infecciosa felina.
- NADH-metemoglobina redutase = metemoglobina redutase dependente da nicotinamida adenina dinucleotídeo.

Sugestões de Leitura
Krotje LJ. Cyanosis: Physiology and pathogenesis. Compend Contin Educ Pract Vet 1987, 9:271-278.
Lee JA, Drobatz KJ. Respiratory distress and cyanosis in dogs. In: King LG, ed., Textbook of Respiratory Disease in Dogs and Cats. Philadelphia: Saunders, 2004, pp. 1-12.
Petrie JP. Cyanosis. In: Ettinger SJ, Feldman EC, eds., Textbook of Veterinary Internal Medicine, 6th ed. St. Louis: Elsevier, 2005, pp. 219-222.

Autor Ned F. Kuehn
Consultor Editorial Lynelle R. Johnson

Cilindrúria

CONSIDERAÇÕES GERAIS

DEFINIÇÃO
• Quantidade anormalmente alta de cilindros (>2-3 cilindros/campo óptico de baixa luminosidade) no sedimento urinário. Pode se desenvolver em cães ou gatos com nefropatias primárias ou distúrbios sistêmicos que afetam secundariamente os rins.
• O número elevado de cilindros indica degeneração celular renal acelerada, extravasamento glomerular de proteínas, hemorragia ou exsudação para os lumens tubulares renais.

SISTEMA(S) ACOMETIDO(S)
Renal/urológico.

IDENTIFICAÇÃO
Cães e gatos.

CAUSAS E FATORES DE RISCO
Nefrotoxicose
• Toxinas — etilenoglicol, ingestão de uvas/passas (cães), ingestão de lírios (gatos), hipercalcemia.
• Medicamentos nefrotóxicos — aminoglicosídeos, tetraciclinas administradas por via intravenosa, anfotericina B, cisplatina, anti-inflamatórios não esteroides, inibidores da enzima conversora da angiotensina.
• Agentes diagnósticos — meio de contraste radiográfico aplicado por via intravenosa.

Isquemia Renal (Anoxia)
• Desidratação. • Hipovolemia. • Débito cardíaco baixo — insuficiência cardíaca congestiva, arritmias cardíacas ou pericardiopatias. • Trombose venosa renal — êmbolos provenientes de endocardite bacteriana ou CID. • Hemoglobinúria — hemólise intravascular. • Mioglobinúria — rabdomiólise.

Inflamação Renal
• Doenças infecciosas (p. ex., pielonefrite, leptospirose, peritonite infecciosa felina, febre maculosa das Montanhas Rochosas ou erliquiose).

Glomerulopatia
• Glomerulonefrite. • Amiloidose.

DIAGNÓSTICO

DIAGNÓSTICO DIFERENCIAL
• Histórico de exposição potencial a toxinas ou medicamentos nefrotóxicos — descartar necrose tubular aguda.
• Início recente de vômito ou diarreia — excluir isquemia renal causada por desidratação.
• Anestesia inalatória recente — descartar necrose tubular ocasionada por isquemia.
• Potencial de exposição a doenças infecciosas — excluir nefrite.
• Febre — descartar doenças infecciosas, inflamatórias e neoplásicas.
• Sopros cardíacos, especialmente se forem diastólicos e de início recente — excluir endocardite bacteriana.
• Petéquias e equimoses — descartar trombose sistêmica.
• Cilindrúria associada à azotemia e concentração urinária adequada (densidade de 1,030 em cães e 1,040 em gatos) — considerar distúrbios pré-renais, como desidratação.
• Cilindrúria associada à azotemia e concentração urinária inadequada (densidade <1,030 em cães e <1,040 em gatos) — pensar em insuficiência renal.
• Cilindrúria associada à leucocitose — cogitar distúrbios infecciosos e inflamatórios.
• Cilindrúria associada à trombocitopenia — cogitar a presença de CID.
• Cilindrúria associada à glicosúria e proteinúria — levar necrose tubular renal em consideração.

ACHADOS LABORATORIAIS
Distúrbios Capazes de Alterar os Resultados Laboratoriais
• Uma espera de mais de 2 h para a realização da urinálise pode resultar no desaparecimento dos cilindros.
• A urina alcalina causa dissolução dos cilindros.
• A urina diluída (densidade <1,003) provoca dissolução dos cilindros; por essa razão, deve-se interpretar a quantidade de cilindros, levando-se em consideração a densidade urinária.

Os Resultados Serão Válidos se os Exames Forem Realizados em Laboratório Humano?
Sim.

HEMOGRAMA/BIOQUÍMICA/URINÁLISE
• Os cilindros epiteliais, granulosos e/ou céreos indicam doenças indutoras de degeneração e necrose do epitélio tubular renal.
• Os cilindros eritrocitários apontam para glomerulopatia ou hemorragia tubular renal graves.
• Os cilindros leucocitários sugerem inflamação renal, causada com maior frequência por pielonefrite; no entanto, a maioria dos pacientes com pielonefrite não apresenta cilindros leucocitários.
• Cilindros hialinos — associados comumente a distúrbios indutores de proteinúria; também é possível observá-los durante a diurese ou depois de desidratação.
• Em alguns pacientes, observam-se anemia, hemoconcentração, leucocitose ou trombocitopenia.
• Em pacientes com desidratação ou doença renal, verificam-se concentrações séricas elevadas de ureia, creatinina e fósforo.

OUTROS TESTES LABORATORIAIS
• Se o paciente apresentar trombocitopenia ou cilindros eritrocitários, realizar os estudos de coagulação (p. ex., TTP, TP, produtos de degradação da fibrina e D-dímeros) para descartar uma coagulopatia de consumo, como a CID. • Na presença de proteinúria, determinar a proporção de proteína:creatinina na urina para avaliar a magnitude desse achado. • Em casos de piúria ou cilindros leucocitários, submeter a urina à cultura para descartar infecção do trato urinário. • Na suspeita de doenças infecciosas sistêmicas, efetuar testes sorológicos em busca de títulos apropriados.

MÉTODOS DIAGNÓSTICOS
Considerar a realização de biopsia renal se a nefropatia persistir ou evoluir ou caso não se consiga determinar a causa a partir de testes laboratoriais de rotina.

TRATAMENTO

• Tratar em um esquema ambulatorial a menos que o paciente se encontre desidratado ou apresente insuficiência renal descompensada.
• Se o paciente estiver saudável sob outros aspectos, oferecer uma dieta normal e permitir a atividade física regular. Se houver doença renal crônica e a creatinina permanecer >2 mg/dL, é recomendável o uso de uma dieta renal terapêutica para aumentar o tempo de sobrevida e melhorar a qualidade de vida.
• Caso o animal não consiga manter a hidratação, administrar a solução de Ringer lactato ou outro fluido de manutenção por vias intravenosa ou subcutânea.
• Se o paciente exibir desidratação ou perdas hídricas contínuas (como vômito ou diarreia), fornecer fluidos por via intravenosa para corrigir os déficits de hidratação, manter as necessidades hídricas diárias e repor as perdas contínuas.

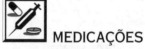

MEDICAÇÕES

CONTRAINDICAÇÕES
Evitar agentes nefrotóxicos.

ACOMPANHAMENTO

MONITORIZAÇÃO DO PACIENTE
Exame físico, incluindo o peso do paciente, para avaliar o estado de hidratação.

PREVENÇÃO
Evitar ou corrigir os fatores de risco que predispõem ao desenvolvimento de exposição dos rins a toxinas e/ou anoxia renal.

COMPLICAÇÕES POSSÍVEIS
Doença renal permanente, dependendo da causa subjacente de cilindrúria.

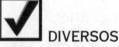

DIVERSOS

POTENCIAL ZOONÓTICO
Possível em pacientes com leptospirose. Nesses casos, deve-se evitar o contato direto com urina infectada.

VER TAMBÉM
Nefrotoxicidade, Induzida por Medicamentos.

ABREVIATURA(S)
• CID = coagulação intravascular disseminada.
• TP = tempo de protrombina.
• TTP = tempo de tromboplastina parcial.

Sugestões de Leitura
DiBartola SP. Clinical approach and laboratory evaluation of renal disease. In: Ettinger SJ, Feldman EC, eds., Textbook of Veterinary Internal Medicine, 7th ed. St. Louis: Elsevier, 2009, pp. 1955-1969.
Osborne CA, Stevens JB. Urinalysis: A Clinical Guide to Compassionate Patient Care. Shawnee Mission, KS: Bayer, 1999, pp. 136-141.

Autor S. Dru Forrester
Consultor Editorial Carl A. Osborne

Cinomose

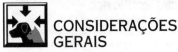

CONSIDERAÇÕES GERAIS

DEFINIÇÃO
• Doença febril, contagiosa, aguda a subaguda e frequentemente fatal, com manifestações respiratórias, urogenitais, gastrintestinais, oculares e neurológicas (SNC).
• Causada pelo vírus da cinomose, um morbilivírus pertencente à família Paramyxoviridae.
• Acomete muitas espécies diferentes da ordem Carnivora; a taxa de mortalidade é bastante variável entre as espécies.

FISIOPATOLOGIA
• Via natural de infecção — aerógena e exposição a gotículas; a partir da cavidade nasal, da faringe e dos pulmões, os macrófagos carreiam o vírus até os linfonodos locais, onde ocorre a replicação viral; dentro de 1 semana, praticamente todos os tecidos linfáticos vêm a ser infectados; a disseminação desse agente ocorre por viremia rumo ao epitélio superficial dos tratos respiratório, gastrintestinal e urogenital, bem como ao SNC.
• A febre por 1-2 dias e a linfopenia podem representar os únicos achados durante a fase inicial do processo patológico; a subsequente evolução da doença depende da cepa viral e da resposta imunológica.
• Respostas imunes celular e humoral intensas — com elas, o quadro pode permanecer subclínico.
• Resposta imune débil — infecção subaguda; o hospedeiro pode sobreviver por mais tempo.
• Falha na resposta imune — morte aguda do hospedeiro em 2-4 semanas após a infecção; as convulsões e outros distúrbios neurológicos (SNC) constituem causas frequentes de óbito.

SISTEMA(S) ACOMETIDO(S)
• Multissistêmico — todos os tecidos linfáticos; epitélio superficial dos tratos respiratório, digestório e urogenital; glândulas endócrinas e exócrinas.
• Nervoso — pele; substâncias cinzenta e/ou branca do cérebro e/ou medula espinal do SNC.

INCIDÊNCIA/PREVALÊNCIA
• Cães — restrita a surtos esporádicos.
• Animais selvagens (guaxinins, gambás, raposas, tigres) — razoavelmente comum.

DISTRIBUIÇÃO GEOGRÁFICA
Mundial.

IDENTIFICAÇÃO
Espécies
• Grande parte das espécies da ordem Carnivora — Canidae, Hyaenidae, Mustelidae, Procyonidae, Viverridae.
• Família Felidae — grandes felinos em zoológicos da Califórnia e na Tanzânia.

Idade Média e Faixa Etária
Os animais jovens, especialmente os não vacinados, são mais suscetíveis que os adultos.

SINAIS CLÍNICOS
• Febre — o primeiro pico se dá em 3-6 dias após a infecção, mas pode passar despercebido; o segundo pico ocorre alguns dias mais tarde (e de forma intermitente depois disso) e costuma estar associado à secreção nasal e ocular, depressão e anorexia.
• Sinais gastrintestinais e/ou respiratórios — ocorrem em seguida; com frequência, são exacerbados por infecção bacteriana secundária.
• SNC — muitos cães infectados; observados frequentemente, mas nem sempre, após uma doença sistêmica; dependem da cepa viral; doença aguda da substância branca ou cinzenta.
• Doença da substância cinzenta: afeta estruturas como córtex cerebral, tronco encefálico e medula espinal, podendo causar meningite não supurativa, crises convulsivas, estupor, histeria, e ataxia. Os cães podem vir a óbito em 2-3 semanas; alguns cães se recuperam (em função da resposta imune humoral e celular imediata), enquanto outros evoluem e desenvolvem doença da substância branca.
• Doença da substância branca: sinais variáveis de doença multifocal, comumente com sinais cerebelovestibulares, paresia e ataxia atribuídas à medula espinal e, ocasionalmente, mioclonia; alguns cães morrem 4-5 semanas após a infecção inicial com doença desmielinizante não inflamatória; outros cães podem se recuperar com lesão mínima do SNC.
• Podem ocorrer neurite óptica e lesões retinianas; algumas vezes, os vasos sanguíneos esclerais são infectados por uveíte anterior.
• Endurecimento dos coxins palmoplantares (hiperceratose) e do nariz — determinadas cepas virais; no entanto, é relativamente incomum.
• Após uma infecção neonatal, é comum a hipoplasia do esmalte dentário.

CAUSAS
• Vírus da cinomose, um morbilivírus enquadrado dentro da família Paramyxoviridae; estritamente relacionado com os vírus do sarampo, da peste bovina e da cinomose de focas e golfinhos.
• Vacinas parcialmente atenuadas (raro).
• As infecções bacterianas secundárias frequentemente envolvem os sistemas respiratório e gastrintestinal.

FATORES DE RISCO
Contato de animais não imunizados com animais infectados pelo vírus da cinomose (cães ou carnívoros selvagens).

DIAGNÓSTICO

DIAGNÓSTICO DIFERENCIAL
• Tosse dos canis — pode mimetizar a doença respiratória.
• Sinais entéricos — diferenciar de parvovirose e coronavirose caninas, parasitismo (giardíase), infecções bacterianas, gastrenterite por ingestão de toxinas, enteropatia inflamatória.
• Forma neurológica (SNC) — diferenciar de meningoencefalite autoimune (meningoencefalomielite granulomatosa, encefalite necrosante), meningoencefalite por protozoários (p. ex., toxoplasmose, neosporose), meningoencefalite por fungos (p. ex., criptococose) e meningoencefalite por riquétsias (p. ex., erliquiose, febre maculosa das Montanhas Rochosas).

HEMOGRAMA/BIOQUÍMICA/URINÁLISE
Linfopenia durante a fase inicial da infecção.

OUTROS TESTES LABORATORIAIS
• Sorologia — valor limitado; os testes sorológicos positivos *não* diferenciam entre a vacinação e a exposição a cepas virulentas; o paciente pode vir a óbito por uma doença aguda antes da geração de anticorpos neutralizantes; pode-se observar a resposta de IgM por até 3 meses após a exposição a cepas virulentas e por até 3 semanas após a vacinação.
• Anticorpos contra o vírus da cinomose no LCS — são sugestivos, mas nem sempre diagnósticos, da encefalite por cinomose.

DIAGNÓSTICO POR IMAGEM
• Radiografias — podem determinar a extensão da pneumonia.
• Tomografia computadorizada (TC) e ressonância magnética (RM) — podem ou não revelar a presença de lesões. A RM é sensível para visualização de desmielinização.

MÉTODOS DIAGNÓSTICOS
• Detecção imuno-histoquímica em pele com pelos, mucosa nasal e epitélio dos coxins palmoplantares.
• Antígenos virais ou corpúsculos de inclusão viral — na camada leucocitária, no sedimento urinário e nos decalques conjuntivais ou vaginais (os resultados negativos não descartam o diagnóstico).
• PCR-RT — na camada leucocitária, nas células do sedimento urinário, nos *swabs* conjuntivais e no LCS.
• LCS — pleocitose moderada de células mononucleares (linfócitos e macrófagos), anticorpo viral específico para cinomose, interferona, e antígeno viral no início da evolução da doença.
• Diagnóstico pós-morte — histopatologia, imunofluorescência e/ou imunocitoquímica, isolamento viral e/ou PCR-RT; os tecidos preferidos são obtidos a partir de órgãos como pulmões, estômago, bexiga urinária, linfonodos e cérebro.

ACHADOS PATOLÓGICOS
Macroscópicos
• Timo — em animais jovens, apresenta-se de tamanho bastante reduzido; algumas vezes, gelatinoso.
• Pulmões — consolidação irregular, em consequência de pneumonia intersticial.
• Coxins palmoplantares e nariz — raramente, hiperceratose.
• Secreções mucopurulentas — oculares e nasais, broncopneumonia, enterite catarral, e pústulas cutâneas; causadas provavelmente por infecções bacterianas secundárias; comumente observadas.

Histológicos
• Corpúsculos de inclusão eosinofílicos e intracitoplasmáticos — encontrados com frequência nos epitélios bronquial, gástrico e vesical; também são observados nas células reticulares e nos leucócitos em tecidos linfáticos.
• Corpúsculos de inclusão no SNC — células gliais e neurônios; frequentemente intranucleares; também podem ser constatados no citoplasma.
• A coloração por meio de anticorpos fluorescentes ou imunoperoxidase pode detectar os antígenos virais em locais onde não se observam os corpúsculos de inclusão.

TRATAMENTO

CUIDADO(S) DE SAÚDE ADEQUADO(S)
Internação e isolamento para evitar a infecção de outros cães.

Cinomose

CUIDADO(S) DE ENFERMAGEM
- Sintomático(s).
- Fluidos intravenosos — em casos de anorexia e diarreia.
- Assim que a febre e as infecções bacterianas secundárias estiverem controladas, os pacientes geralmente começarão a se alimentar de novo.
- Limpar e remover as secreções oculares.

ATIVIDADE
Restrita.

DIETA
Depende do grau de envolvimento gastrintestinal.

ORIENTAÇÃO AO PROPRIETÁRIO
- Informar o proprietário sobre a taxa de mortalidade de aproximadamente 50%.
- Notificar o proprietário de que os cães que parecem se recuperar dos sinais catarrais precoces podem desenvolver sinais neurológicos (SNC) fatais mais tarde.

MEDICAÇÕES

MEDICAMENTO(S) DE ESCOLHA
- Medicamentos antivirais — não se conhece nenhum agente eficaz.
- Antibióticos — para diminuir as infecções bacterianas secundárias, já que o vírus da cinomose é altamente imunossupressor.
- Terapia anticonvulsivante — fenobarbital, brometo de potássio; para controlar as crises convulsivas.

CONTRAINDICAÇÕES
Corticosteroides — utilizar as doses anti-inflamatórias com cautela; podem conferir um controle dos sinais a curto prazo; as doses imunossupressoras podem intensificar a disseminação viral.

PRECAUÇÕES
Tetraciclina e fluoroquinolonas — é melhor evitar esses agentes em animais jovens e em crescimento.

ACOMPANHAMENTO

MONITORIZAÇÃO DO PACIENTE
- Monitorizar quanto à presença de sinais neurológicos (SNC), pois a ocorrência de crises convulsivas geralmente acompanha o quadro.
- Na fase aguda da doença, monitorizar o animal em busca de sinais de pneumonia ou desidratação decorrente da diarreia.

PREVENÇÃO
- A vacinação é a chave da prevenção.
- Evitar a infecção de filhotes caninos por meio do isolamento, impedindo o contágio a partir de animais selvagens (p. ex., guaxinins, raposas, gambás) ou de cães infectados pelo vírus da cinomose.
- Os cães recuperados não se tornam portadores.

Vacinas
- VVM-C — evita a infecção e a doença; há dois tipos disponíveis, cada um deles com suas vantagens e desvantagens.
- Vacinas adaptadas à cultura tecidual canina (p. ex., cepa Rockborn) — induzem à imunidade completa em praticamente 100% dos cães suscetíveis; raramente se desenvolve uma encefalite fatal pós-vacinal 7-14 dias após a vacinação, especialmente em animais imunossuprimidos.
- Vacinas adaptadas ao cultivo de embriões de galinha (p. ex., cepas Onderstepoort e Lederle) — mais seguras; não ocorre a encefalite pós-vacinal; apenas cerca de 80% dos cães suscetíveis exibem soroconversão.
- Outras espécies — pode-se utilizar a vacina adaptada aos embriões de galinha com segurança em diversas espécies de zoológico e de vida selvagem (p. ex., raposas cinzentas); nesses animais, o tipo Rockborn é fatal.
- Vacinas mortas — úteis para espécies nas quais qualquer tipo de VVM-C se mostra fatal (p. ex., pandas vermelhos e furões de pés negros).
- Vacina recombinante de varíola do canário contra o vírus da cinomose.

Anticorpos Maternos
- Importantes.
- A maioria dos filhotes caninos perde a proteção advinda dos anticorpos maternos com 6-12 semanas da vida; durante esse período, é recomendável aplicar 2-3 vacinações.
- Vacinação heterotípica (vírus do sarampo) — recomendada para filhotes caninos que possuem anticorpos maternos; induz à proteção contra a doença, mas não contra a infecção.

COMPLICAÇÕES POSSÍVEIS
A ocorrência de sinais neurológicos (SNC) é possível por 2-3 meses após a diminuição dos sinais catarrais.

EVOLUÇÃO ESPERADA E PROGNÓSTICO
- Dependem da cepa e da resposta individual do hospedeiro — infecções subclínica, aguda, subaguda, fatal ou não fatal.
- Sinais brandos atribuídos ao SNC — o paciente pode se recuperar; a mioclonia pode persistir por alguns meses ou por tempo indefinido.
- Óbito — 2 semanas a 3 meses após a infecção; a taxa de mortalidade chega a aproximadamente 50%.
- Eutanásia — o proprietário poderá optar por essa prática caso se desenvolvam sinais neurológicos ou diante desses sinais; indicada mediante a ocorrência de crises convulsivas não controladas.
- Os cães que se recuperam totalmente não disseminam o vírus da cinomose.

DIVERSOS

DISTÚRBIOS ASSOCIADOS
- Infecções persistentes ou latentes por *Toxoplasma gondii* — reativadas, em virtude do estado imunossupressor.
- Infecções respiratórias pela *Bordetella bronchiseptica* (importante agente causal da tosse dos canis).

FATORES RELACIONADOS COM A IDADE
- Filhotes caninos jovens — mais suscetíveis; a taxa de mortalidade é mais alta.
- Cães idosos não imunizados — altamente suscetíveis à infecção e à doença.

POTENCIAL ZOONÓTICO
- É possível que os seres humanos adquiram a infecção subclínica pelo vírus da cinomose; a imunização contra o vírus do sarampo também protege o homem contra a infecção pelo vírus da cinomose.
- Especula-se que o vírus da cinomose deflagre esclerose múltipla; diversos estudos, no entanto, contestam essa proposta; há muitas provas irrefutáveis: a cinomose tornou-se rara nessa espécie após a introdução das vacinas de VVM-C no início da década de 1960, embora a incidência da esclerose múltipla permaneça inalterada; o período de incubação da esclerose múltipla costuma ser inferior a 30 anos; dessa forma, o vírus da cinomose não pode ser a causa primária.

GESTAÇÃO/FERTILIDADE/REPRODUÇÃO
A infecção intrauterina de fetos ocorre em cadelas soronegativas (isentas de anticorpos); rara; pode levar ao abortamento ou à infecção persistente; os neonatos infectados podem desenvolver uma doença fatal por volta de 4-6 semanas de vida.

SINÔNIMO(S)
- Doença dos coxins ásperos.
- Doença dos quartos caídos.
- Mal de Carré.

VER TAMBÉM
Mioclonia (embora não seja exclusiva para cinomose).

ABREVIATURA(S)
- LCS = líquido cerebrospinal.
- PCR-RT = reação em cadeia da polimerase via transcriptase reversa.
- VVM-C = vírus vivo modificado da cinomose

RECURSOS DA INTERNET
http://www.ivis.org/advances/Vite/braund27/chapter frm.asp?LA = 1#Distemper_Encephalomyelitis.

Sugestões de Leitura
Appel MJG, Summers BA. Pathogenicity of morbilliviruses for terrestrial carnivores. Vet Microbiology 1995, 44:187-191.
Bathen-Noethen A, Stein VM, Puff C, Baumgaertner W, Tipold A. Magnetic resonance imaging findings in acute canine distemper virus infection. J Small Anim Pract 2008, 49(9):460-467.
Greene CE, Appel MJ. Canine distemper. In: Greene CE, ed., Infectious Diseases of the Dog and Cat, 3rd ed. St. Louis: Saunders Elsevier, 2006, pp. 25-41.
Haines DM, Martin KM, Chelack BJ, Sargent RA, Outerbridge CA, Clark EG. Immunohistochemical detection of canine distemper virus in haired skin, nasal mucosa, and footpad epithelium: A method for antemortem diagnosis of infection. J Vet Diagn Invest 1999, 11(5):396-399.

Autor Scott J. Schatzberg
Consultor Editorial Stephen C. Barr

Cirrose e Fibrose do Fígado

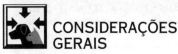
CONSIDERAÇÕES GERAIS

DEFINIÇÃO
• Fibrose hepática — substituição ou extinção do parênquima hepático por matriz extracelular.
• Cirrose — fibrose difusa associada a nódulos regenerativos e desarranjo da arquitetura hepática.

FISIOPATOLOGIA
• Fibrose — desenvolve-se após lesão crônica; associada à liberação de citocinas/mediadores, que estimulam a produção ou o acúmulo de matriz extracelular. • Pode ser idiopática em cães jovens, podendo ocorrer após inflamação intestinal/bacteremia portal. • Cirrose — consequência de fibrogênese crônica e combinada com a tentativa de regeneração hepática; caracterizada pela formação de nódulos regenerativos; redução da massa hepática funcional; depósito de colágeno ao longo dos sinusoides hepáticos e/ou em torno das tríades portais. • Cirrose/fibrose — leva à disfunção hepática associada à hipertensão portal; desvio intra-hepático em sinusoides colagenizados ou em vias vasculares recanalizadas na interface fibrótica entre os nódulos regenerativos.
• Hipertensão portal — induz a (1) DPSA e encefalopatia hepática, (2) coleção esplâncnica de sangue, diminuição do volume sanguíneo efetivo, retenção renal de sódio e água culminando em ascite e (3) vasculopatia intestinal hipertensiva portal associada a sangramento intestinal.

SISTEMA(S) ACOMETIDO(S)
• Endócrino/metabólico — hipoglicemia em casos terminais (ocasionados pelo jejum). • Gastrintestinal — a hipertensão portal leva à ascite e propensão a sangramento intestinal. • Sanguíneo — microcitose eritrocitária com DPSA; tendências hemorrágicas: falha na síntese ou na ativação dos fatores de coagulação ou trombocitopenia. • Neurológico — encefalopatia hepática. • Renal/urológico — cristalúria por biurato de amônio; isostenúria; poliúria/polidipsia; síndrome hepatorrenal (rara).
• Respiratório — taquipneia secundária à ascite e ao enrijecimento abdominal; edema pulmonar (raro).
• Cutâneo — dermatite necrolítica superficial (ver "Hepatopatia Diabética").

GENÉTICA
Predisposição familiar para hepatite crônica — Doberman pinscher, Cocker spaniel, Labrador retriever, outras.

INCIDÊNCIA/PREVALÊNCIA
Alta em cães com hepatopatia necroinflamatória crônica ou animais com OEHDB crônica.

IDENTIFICAÇÃO
Espécies
Cães e gatos.

Raça(s) Predominante(s)
• Qualquer raça ou cães sem raça definida.
• Hepatopatia por armazenamento de cobre — Bedlington terrier; alguns parentes de Dálmata, possivelmente alguns cães da raça Doberman pinscher, além de Labrador retriever. • Fibrose hepática "idiopática" juvenil — Pastor alemão, Poodle standard, outras. • Distúrbios indeterminados — West Highland white terrier, Skye blue terrier, outras.

Idade Média e Faixa Etária
• Cirrose (cães) — qualquer idade; comum em animais de meia-idade e idosos; hepatopatia por armazenamento de cobre e fibrose hepática idiopática — jovens adultos/meia-idade. • Cirrose biliar (gatos) com colangio-hepatite crônica — mais de 7 anos de idade. • Fibrose — gatos com má-formação hepática policística avançada (acúmulo de matriz extracelular).

Sexo Predominante
• Cocker spaniel — predisposição 2-8 vezes maior em machos. • Doberman pinscher e Labrador retriever — pode ser mais comum em fêmeas.

SINAIS CLÍNICOS
Comentários Gerais
• Fase inicial — sinais vagos e inespecíficos. • Fase mais tardia — os sinais relacionam-se com as complicações decorrentes de hipertensão portal (p. ex., encefalopatia hepática, ascite e sangramento gastroduodenal) e comprometimento da função hepática.

Achados Anamnésicos
• Letargia intermitente crônica, anorexia, declínio da condição corporal. • Sinais GI: vômito, diarreia, ou constipação. • Melena: estágio final.
• Polidipsia e poliúria. • Início tardio — ascite, icterícia, sangramento, encefalopatia hepática.
• Gatos — a ocorrência de ascite é incomum; ptialismo em casos de encefalopatia hepática.

Achados do Exame Físico
• Letargia. • Má condição do corpo e da pelagem.
• Icterícia. • Ascite. • Encefalopatia hepática.
• Uropatia obstrutiva por cálculos de biuratos de amônio. • Anasarca — rara; pode se desenvolver com a fluidoterapia exagerada. • Volume do fígado — micro-hepatia em cães; tamanho variável em gatos.
• Tendências hemorrágicas (raras). • Lesões cutâneas com dermatite necrolítica superficial (cirrose não verdadeira; ver "Hepatopatia Diabética").

CAUSAS
• Lesão hepática necroinflamatória, oxidante ou imunomediada crônica — muitas causas (p. ex., subsequente à enteropatia inflamatória crônica ou pancreatite). • Lesão hepática induzida por medicamentos ou toxinas — hepatopatia por armazenamento de cobre; anticonvulsivantes; antifúngicos azólicos; oxibendazol; trimetoprima-sulfametoxazol; AINEs; toxina crônica de origem alimentar (aflatoxinas), outras. • Infecções — leptospirose; adenovírus canino do tipo 1.
• Colangio-hepatite crônica (gatos). • OEHDB crônica (>6 semanas, cães ou gatos). • Episódio isolado de necrose hepática maciça.

FATORES DE RISCO
• Predisposição racial: hepatotoxicidade do cobre ou outras causas ainda mal definidas (ver anteriormente). • Ingestão excessiva de cobre na dieta; acúmulo hepático de cobre ou ferro; a causa ou o efeito podem não estar claros. • Inflamação hepatobiliar crônica. • OEHDB. • Administração crônica de fenobarbital (cães).

DIAGNÓSTICO

DIAGNÓSTICO DIFERENCIAL
• Hepatite crônica — comum em cães. • Colangio-hepatite — comum em gatos. • Hipertensão portal não cirrótica: cães. • OEHDB crônica — cães, gatos. • Pancreatite crônica — cães, gatos.
• Neoplasia hepática. • Neoplasia ou carcinomatose metastáticas. • Anomalia vascular portossistêmica congênita. • Insuficiência cardíaca direita. • Gatos — lipidose hepática; PIF; toxoplasmose. • Anemia hemolítica (causa de icterícia, que pode ser confundida com cirrose/fibrose hepáticas; considerar no diagnóstico diferencial).

HEMOGRAMA/BIOQUÍMICA/URINÁLISE
Hemograma Completo
• Leve anemia microcítica. • Leve trombocitopenia. • Leucograma: variável.

Bioquímica
• Nível variável da bilirrubina. • Atividade das enzimas hepáticas — elevada (principalmente da fosfatase alcalina e ALT); observada antes do aparecimento dos sinais clínicos ou da disfunção hepática; em casos de doença terminal, pode permanecer normal ou exibir apenas um leve aumento. • Hipoalbuminemia. • Níveis normais de globulina a hiperglobulinemia.
• Hipocolesterolemia — hepatopatia terminal e DPSA. • Níveis baixos de ureia — em casos de atividade reduzida do ciclo da ureia, DPSA, dieta pobre em proteínas; poliúria/polidipsia.
• Hipoglicemia — cães; raramente em gatos.
• Hipocalemia — pode predispor o paciente à encefalopatia hepática. • Hiponatremia — doença terminal com ascite.

Urinálise
• Isostenúria — com poliúria e polidipsia.
• Cristalúria por biurato de amônio.
• Bilirrubinúria, cristalúria por bilirrubina.

OUTROS TESTES LABORATORIAIS
• Líquido ascítico — transudato puro ou modificado. • Teste de coagulação — prolongamento inconstante nos TP, TTPA, TCA e/ou no tempo de sangramento da mucosa bucal.
• Baixa atividade da proteína C reflete DPSA.
• Ácidos biliares séricos — elevados.
• Hiperamonemia: deduzida a partir da cristalúria por biurato de amônio.

DIAGNÓSTICO POR IMAGEM
Radiografia
• Abdominais — fígado pequeno (cães); fígado normal a aumentado de volume (gatos); a ascite pode obscurecer os detalhes abdominais da imagem; os cálculos translúcidos de urato ficarão visíveis se estiverem mineralizados com cálcio, ou seja, unidos sob a forma de complexos.

Ultrassonografia
• Abdominal — a imagem hepática pode ficar hiperecoica ou apresentar ecogenicidade mista; além disso, pode-se observar a presença de padrão nodular, efusão abdominal (ascite), esplenomegalia e DPSA; em alguns casos, não há nenhuma alteração parenquimatosa. • Pesquisa da vasculatura portal com Doppler — pode revelar um fluxo sanguíneo portal hepatofugal, que se afasta do fígado, ou ninhos de DPSA (especialmente próximos do rim esquerdo e do baço).

MÉTODOS DIAGNÓSTICOS
• Citologia de aspirado por agulha fina — ajuda a descartar neoplasias; detecta infecção bacteriana; *não é capaz de definir fibrose ou inflamação não supurativa*. • Biopsia hepática — necessária para obtenção do diagnóstico definitivo; as biopsias centrais aspirativas com agulha de calibre 18 são frequentemente imprecisas em função do pequeno tamanho da amostra. • Laparoscopia — melhor método de biopsia; permite a inspeção macroscópica do órgão; registra a presença de DPSA; possibilita o acesso a múltiplos lobos hepáticos e lesões focais.

ACHADOS PATOLÓGICOS
Macroscópicos
• Fibrose — fígado pequeno e firme, com contorno irregular a finamente nodular. • Cirrose — fígado firme, com contorno irregular e micro ou macronódulos proeminentes.

Cirrose e Fibrose do Fígado

TRATAMENTO

CUIDADO(S) DE SAÚDE ADEQUADO(S)
• Esquema ambulatorial — aos pacientes com sintomas mínimos. • Internação — para a realização de testes diagnósticos; tratamento contra desidratação, anorexia, encefalopatia hepática grave ou sangramento intestinal (vasculopatia hipertensiva).

CUIDADO(S) DE ENFERMAGEM
• Fluidos — evitar a solução de lactato em casos de insuficiência hepática; evitar o NaCl a 0,9% na presença de ascite. • Vitaminas do complexo B (especialmente gatos) — recomenda-se a dose de 2 mL/L de fluido; vitamina K_1 na dose de 0,5-1,5 mg/kg SC a cada 12 h por três doses inicialmente; titular com PIVKA ou outro teste de TP. • Glicose — em casos de hipoglicemia; glicose a 2,5-5% em solução poliônica; titular até obtenção da resposta. • Cloreto de potássio — suplementação nos fluidos, conforme a necessidade. • Evitar a ocorrência de alcalose — agrava a encefalopatia hepática. • Em casos de ascite sintomática com enrijecimento abdominal e irresponsiva a tratamentos médicos, efetuar a abdominocentese terapêutica de grandes volumes.

ATIVIDADE
Restrita.

DIETA
• Suspender a alimentação oral se houver encefalopatia hepática grave aguda com estupor ou coma, vômitos associados a sangramento intestinal ou pancreatite; considerar o uso de nutrição parenteral parcial ou total. • Em caso de encefalopatia hepática: restringir a ingestão de proteína; utilizar soja ou fontes proteicas lácteas (cães) combinadas com intervenções médicas para aumentar a tolerância ao nitrogênio; individualizar o consumo proteico para manter a condição do corpo, o nível de albumina e controlar a encefalopatia hepática (ver "Encefalopatia Hepática"). • Restrição de sódio na presença de ascite. • A restrição de gordura raramente é necessária. • Suplementação de vitaminas hidrossolúveis.

ORIENTAÇÃO AO PROPRIETÁRIO
• O tratamento é paliativo e sintomático.
• Atenuar os fatores predisponentes à encefalopatia hepática — (ver "Encefalopatia Hepática").

CONSIDERAÇÕES CIRÚRGICAS
• Cirrose — alto risco anestésico; é preferível o uso de anestésicos inalatórios — isoflurano ou sevoflurano. • Coagulopatia — pode predispor o paciente a sangramentos causados até mesmo por procedimentos cirúrgicos de pequeno porte.
• Cuidado intensivo pós-operatório — é crítico para evitar a encefalopatia hepática; manter a hidratação e a normoglicemia. • Predisposição à translocação bacteriana intestinal — administrar antibióticos adequados de forma empírica.

MEDICAÇÕES

MEDICAMENTO(S) DE ESCOLHA
• Concentrar o tratamento sobre a etiologia específica; promover a quelação de cobre em casos de hepatopatia por armazenamento desse elemento metálico; suspender os medicamentos potencialmente hepatotóxicos. • Não há ensaios clínicos que comprovem a eficácia de esquemas terapêuticos específicos.

Imunomodulação
• Ver "Hepatite Crônica Ativa". • Prednisolona/prednisona —1-4 mg/kg diariamente VO; reduzir gradativamente para a dose eficaz mais baixa (p. ex., 0,25-0,5 mg/kg VO a cada 48 h).
• Azatioprina — em cães: 1 mg/kg VO a cada 48 h; tóxica aos gatos; em cães, é combinada com prednisolona, antioxidantes, PPC antifibrótico.

Antifibróticos
• Ver "Hepatite Crônica Ativa". • Ursodiol (7,5 mg/kg VO a cada 12 h juntamente com o alimento) — utilizar por tempo indefinido.
• Polienilfosfatidilcolina poli-insaturada (25-100 mg/kg/dia) — misturar com o alimento.
• Colchicina — 0,025-0,03 mg/kg VO a cada 24-48 h.

Antioxidantes
• Utilizar os antioxidantes em distúrbios necroinflamatórios. • SAMe: 20 mg/kg/dia VO com o estômago vazio. • Vitamina E: tocoferóis mistos, 10 U/kg/dia VO juntamente com o alimento. • Nota: agentes como prednisona, SAMe, silibinina, vitamina E também são considerados antifibróticos.

Hepatoprotetores
• Ursodesoxicolato, vitamina E, SAMe conferem efeitos hepatoprotetores. • A eficácia da silibinina é incerta; utilizar a forma de complexo da PPC, 2-5 mg/kg VO a cada 24 h. • Zinco elementar: 1,5-3 mg VO a cada 24 h (se o nível hepático de zinco estiver baixo); ajustar a dose com base na mensuração sequencial dos valores plasmáticos desse elemento; evitar >800 µg/dL.

Condições Específicas
• Ascite: ◦ Restringir a atividade e a ingestão de sódio (0,2% com base na matéria seca ou <100 mg/100 kcal). ◦ Diuréticos (ver "Hepatite Crônica Ativa"); mobilizar lentamente a efusão de líquido ascítico: furosemida (0,5-2 mg/kg IV, SC, VO a cada 12 h) com espironolactona (0,5-2 mg/kg VO a cada 12 h); ajustar a dose, reavaliando a resposta do animal a cada 4-7 dias; individualizar o tratamento crônico de acordo com a resposta; os diuréticos podem ser utilizados de forma intermitente para mobilizar a ascite recorrente. ◦ Abdominocentese terapêutica de grandes volumes se a mobilização da ascite não responder em 7-14 dias. • Coagulopatia — ver "Coagulopatia por Hepatopatia". • Encefalopatia hepática — ver o capítulo sobre essa doença.
• Sangramento intestinal — gastroprotetores ou inibidores da acidez gástrica (ver "Hepatite Crônica Ativa"); eliminar os parasitas intestinais.

CONTRAINDICAÇÕES
AINEs — evitar o uso; potencializam o sangramento intestinal; podem agravar a ascite; são potencialmente hepatotóxicos.

PRECAUÇÕES
• Diuréticos — podem agravar a encefalopatia hepática em virtude da possível indução de desidratação, hipocalemia e alcalose.
• Glicocorticoides — aumentam a suscetibilidade a infecções; promovem sangramento intestinal, retenção de água e sódio, catabolismo proteico e encefalopatia hepática. • Evitar ou reduzir a dose dos medicamentos que dependem da extração hepática de primeira passagem e aqueles que necessitam da conjugação ou da biotransformação hepática para sua eliminação; p. ex., metronidazol — reduzir a dose convencional para 7,5 mg/kg VO a cada 12 h (frequentemente utilizado para encefalopatia hepática).

MEDICAMENTO(S) ALTERNATIVO(S)
• Dexametasona — empregar na presença de ascite; utilizar no lugar da prednisona ou prednisolona (isso elimina o efeito mineralocorticoide); utilizar 1/8 a 1/10 da dose da prednisona ou prednisolona; administrar a cada 3-4 dias; reduzir a dose gradativamente até a eficácia. • Micofenolato — medicamento alternativo ao uso da azatioprina.

ACOMPANHAMENTO

MONITORIZAÇÃO DO PACIENTE
• Mensuração dos níveis de enzimas hepáticas, albumina, ureia e colesterol — monitorar em intervalos mensais ou trimestrais, dependendo da condição do paciente. • Monitorização seriada dos valores de ácidos biliares séricos totais — não acrescentam informações prognósticas ou diagnósticas. • Escore da condição corporal e avaliação da massa muscular — refletem a ingestão nutricional adequada e o balanço nitrogenado.
• Medir a cintura/circunferência abdominal — reflete o volume da ascite. • Azatioprina, micofenolato, colchicina — monitorizar quanto à possível toxicidade da medula óssea (por meio de hemogramas completos seriados) e outros efeitos colaterais.

COMPLICAÇÕES POSSÍVEIS
Encefalopatia hepática, septicemia e sangramento — podem ser potencialmente letais; CID — pode ser um evento terminal.

EVOLUÇÃO ESPERADA E PROGNÓSTICO
• As exacerbações ocasionais de encefalopatia hepática e ascite podem necessitar de internações para ajuste das intervenções nutricionais e médicas. A restrição de sódio e o uso de diuréticos podem exigir a titulação para o controle da ascite.
• A evolução natural de hepatopatia fibrótica/cirrótica em cães é mal caracterizada. • A presença de ascite indica doença grave quando associada à hepatite. • Fibrose idiopática juvenil (cães) — sobrevida de até 9 anos após o diagnóstico.
• Cirrose — sobrevida >5 anos com intervenções terapêuticas rigorosas.

DIVERSOS

POTENCIAL ZOONÓTICO
Os cães com hepatopatia crônica associada à leptospirose (rara) podem eliminar os microrganismos no ambiente.

VER TAMBÉM
• Encefalopatia Hepática. • Hepatite Crônica Ativa. • Hepatopatia Diabética. • Hepatopatia Fibrosante Juvenil. • Hepatopatia por Armazenamento de Cobre. • Hipertensão Portal.

ABREVIATURA(S)
• DPSA = desvio portossistêmico adquirido.
• OEHDB = obstrução extra-hepática do ducto biliar. • PIAVK = proteínas invocadas pela ausência ou antagonismo da vitamina K. • PPC = polienilfosfatidilcolina poli-insaturada. • SAMe = dissulfato tosilato de S-adenosil-L-metionina.
• TCA = tempo de coagulação ativada. • TP = tempo de protrombina. • TTPA = tempo de tromboplastina parcial ativada.

Autor Sharon A. Center

CONSIDERAÇÕES GERAIS

REVISÃO
- Doença rara de cães causada pelas larvas de *Taenia crassiceps*; os adultos desse parasita, por sua vez, são encontrados em raposas, coiotes e, algumas vezes, cães domésticos.
- Os ovos liberados no ambiente pelas raposas são consumidos por coelhos ou outros roedores e, nesses animais, desenvolvem-se até o estágio de cisticerco nos tecidos abdominais e subcutâneos. O cisticerco da *Taenia crassiceps* pode sofrer reprodução assexuada e se desenvolver em uma quantidade muito ampla nos tecidos dos hospedeiros intermediários.
- Os cães infectados com o estágio de cisticerco podem desenvolver massas volumosas de cisticercos na cavidade abdominal, nos pulmões, na musculatura e nos tecidos subcutâneos.
- Na Europa e nos EUA, há relatos de casos raros.

IDENTIFICAÇÃO
Cães — mais idosos, bem como em animais imunocomprometidos jovens.

SINAIS CLÍNICOS
- Massas subcutâneas.
- Sinais associados à formação de massas em outros órgãos — insuficiência respiratória (pulmões), efusão pericárdica e colapso circulatório, icterícia (cavidade abdominal), anemia (de doença crônica) e anorexia.

CAUSAS E FATORES DE RISCO
O modo de infecção ainda não está esclarecido, mas há três hipóteses:
- Ingestão de ovos do parasita (provavelmente nas fezes de raposa infectada).
- Autoinfecção com ovos provenientes de uma infecção intestinal com os estágios adultos.
- Ingestão do estágio de cisticerco.

DIAGNÓSTICO

DIAGNÓSTICO DIFERENCIAL
- Infecção pelas larvas de *Mesocestoides* spp.
- Neoplasias, particularmente em animais mais idosos.

HEMOGRAMA/BIOQUÍMICA/URINÁLISE
Não foram descritos.

OUTROS TESTES LABORATORIAIS
N/D.

DIAGNÓSTICO POR IMAGEM
- Radiografias — determinar o grau de disseminação a órgãos internos.
- Ultrassonografia — traçar a natureza cística da massa (no subcutâneo ou na cavidade abdominal), oposta às massas sólidas de neoplasia.

MÉTODOS DIAGNÓSTICOS
- Citologia aspirativa.
- Biopsia cirúrgica.

TRATAMENTO

- Internação se o paciente estiver debilitado.
- Tratar os sinais clínicos, conforme a necessidade.
- Remoção cirúrgica, por meio de biopsia ou laparotomia, da maior quantidade de microrganismos possível.

MEDICAÇÕES

MEDICAMENTO(S)
- Praziquantel — 5 mg/kg VO inicialmente; depois aumentar a dose de forma progressiva em algumas semanas para 50 mg/kg, se for aparentemente tolerável; existe uma preocupação quanto à possibilidade de reação do cão aos cisticercos mortos.
- Albendazol — a dose de 50 mg/kg VO a cada 24 h por 10-20 dias após o término da terapia com o praziquantel pode ajudar a evitar recidivas.
NOTA: Nessa dose, o albendazol pode ser mielossupressor — dessa forma, é recomendável avaliar o hemograma completo.
- Fembendazol — a dose de 50 mg/kg VO a cada 24 h por 30 dias também pode ser utilizada com certa expectativa de êxito na prevenção de recidivas a longo prazo.

ACOMPANHAMENTO

A recidiva das lesões é bastante frequente. Assim, é imprescindível acompanhar o cão de perto para monitorizar a disseminação potencial das lesões e o desenvolvimento de novas lesões em regiões distintas com o auxílio da ultrassonografia abdominal.

DIVERSOS

POTENCIAL ZOONÓTICO
Os estágios indutores dos sinais clínicos em cães não representam qualquer ameaça zoonótica.

Sugestões de Leitura
Hoberg EP, Ebinger W, Render JA. Fatal cysticercosis by *Taenia crassiceps* (Cyclophyllidea: Taeniidae) in a presumed immunocompromised canine host. J Parasitol 2000;85:1174-1180.

Autor Dwight D. Bowman
Consultor Editorial Stephen C. Barr

Cistite Polipoide

CONSIDERAÇÕES GERAIS

REVISÃO
Cistite polipoide é uma condição inflamatória crônica da bexiga urinária, caracterizada por protrusões vilosas ou polipoides da mucosa. Projeções polipoides estão difusamente localizadas sobre a superfície vesical e podem estar presentes na uretra. Se essas projeções vierem a sofrer erosão e ulceração, ocorrerão graus variados de hematúria e disúria. O aspecto macroscópico dos pólipos pode não ser diferenciado daquele de neoplasias vesicais, como os carcinomas de células de transição. A cistite polipoide nos cães parece estar associada à irritação crônica da mucosa por inflamação infecciosa ou não.

IDENTIFICAÇÃO
• Cães com infecções crônicas do trato urinário ou urolitíase.
• Não há relatos de casos em gatos.

SINAIS CLÍNICOS
• Inicialmente, o animal pode permanecer assintomático.
• A hematúria é o sinal clínico mais comum.
• Com frequência, ocorre hematúria macroscópica no jato final da micção.
• Polaciúria e disúria também podem estar presentes e são associadas à irritação mecânica dos pólipos.
• Poderá ocorrer obstrução uretral se houver um número suficiente de pólipos localizados na área do trígono vesical. Os pólipos que se originam na uretra ou estão situados nessa estrutura também podem causar obstrução parcial ou total.
• Pode ocorrer obstrução ureteral se o orifício dos ureteres estiver circundado pelos pólipos.
• Pode haver infecção concomitante do trato urinário, o que pode predispor o animal à infecção do trato urinário superior.

CAUSAS E FATORES DE RISCO
• As causas de cistite polipoide nos cães não foram bem comprovadas, mas esse distúrbio costuma estar associado à infecção do trato urinário ou urolitíase.
• Infecção e inflamação crônicas secundárias à colocação de cateteres urinários transuretrais permanentes* foram relacionadas com casos de cistite polipoide em seres humanos.

DIAGNÓSTICO

DIAGNÓSTICO DIFERENCIAL
• A cistite polipoide deve ser descartada nos casos de hematúria, polaciúria, disúria e infecção recidivante do trato urinário.
• Neoplasias vesicais (como carcinoma de células de transição), infecção do trato urinário e urolitíase são os diagnósticos diferenciais mais comuns.

HEMOGRAMA/BIOQUÍMICA/URINÁLISE
• Os perfis bioquímicos séricos devem permanecer normais em grande parte dos casos de cistite polipoide a menos que haja azotemia como resultado de obstrução ao fluxo de saída da urina e/ou pielonefrite concomitante.
• A urinálise irá revelar hematúria, piúria e células epiteliais de transição.

OUTROS TESTES LABORATORIAIS
• A urina deve ser submetida à cultura por meio de cateterização estéril ou no momento da cistoscopia, mas não por cistocentese até que o carcinoma de células de transição esteja descartado. Isso evitará a disseminação abdominal potencial do carcinoma de células de transição ao longo do trajeto da agulha.
• Os pólipos representativos removidos via cistoscopia ou cistotomia devem ser colocados em formalina para exame sob microscopia óptica.
• Uma amostra adequada de tecido vesical deve ser colocada em meio de cultura apropriado para o crescimento de microrganismos. É recomendável a interrupção do tratamento com antimicrobianos para minimizar a inibição do crescimento de patógenos no tecido vesical.

DIAGNÓSTICO POR IMAGEM
• As radiografias simples podem exibir bexiga urinária normal, espessamento irregular do contorno vesical e/ou urolitíase concomitante.
• Cistografia com duplo contraste ou cistografia com contraste positivo pode revelar massas polipoides irregulares no lúmen vesical e/ou espessamento da parede vesical. A localização mais comum do envolvimento é a parede cranioventral da bexiga urinária. Podem ser observados grandes pólipos isolados com base estreita ou ampla, dispersos ao longo do acúmulo de contraste. Os urólitos irão migrar para a parte pendente do acúmulo de contraste.
• A ultrassonografia pode demonstrar a presença de pólipos espalhados ao longo da superfície da mucosa vesical, sobretudo na face cranioventral.

MÉTODOS DIAGNÓSTICOS
• Biopsia guiada por cistoscopia ou ultrassom pode ser utilizada a fim de obter porções representativas dos pólipos para o exame de cortes corados das lesões sob microscopia óptica.
• Biopsias mais invasivas de espessura completa da parede vesical via cistotomia podem ser necessárias para incluir a base dos pólipos com margem adequada de tecido saudável.

ACHADOS PATOLÓGICOS
• Alterações macroscópicas envolvendo a superfície da mucosa vesical incluem pequenas massas isoladas ou múltiplas, que variam de 1 a 10 mm de tamanho. As massas podem ser nodulares com base ampla ou pedunculadas à parede vesical por um delicado pedículo.
• Alterações histopatológicas revelam projeções polipoides de epitélio hiperplásico que circundam um núcleo de tecido conjuntivo proliferativo, mescladas com inflamação aguda e crônica (congestão e edema, além de células inflamatórias agudas e crônicas). Achados característicos de malignidade (p. ex., expansão desproporcional dos núcleos em relação ao citoplasma; aumento no conteúdo de cromatina, gerando hipercromasia; alterações estruturais, como padrões aberrantes da cromatina, falta de limites celulares distintos, irregularidade dos contornos celulares; ampliação e/ou aumento no número dos núcleos; células multinucleadas com núcleos atípicos; número anormal de figuras mitóticas; inclusões citoplasmáticas e vacuolização; invasão das membranas basais) estão visivelmente ausentes.

Em alguns pacientes, há um predomínio de alterações típicas de inflamação granulomatosa.

TRATAMENTO

• A eliminação de bactérias que constituem uma fonte de irritação crônica é um objetivo terapêutico racional.
• A remoção não cirúrgica de urocistólitos (por uro-hidropropulsão miccional, litotripsia, manejo da dieta) indutores de irritação crônica pode resultar na eliminação de pólipos inflamatórios.
• Os pólipos também podem ser removidos por cistoscopia ou cistotomia.
• Talvez haja necessidade de cistectomia parcial para remover os pólipos que estejam envolvendo grandes porções vesicais. A porção remanescente da bexiga urinária pode sofrer uma compensação, aumentando sua capacidade para conter a urina em 3-6 meses.

MEDICAÇÕES

MEDICAMENTO(S)
• Selecionar o antibiótico com base na cultura da urina e do tecido do pólipo. O paciente deve receber a antibioticoterapia por, no mínimo, 4-6 semanas.
• A administração de piroxicam e o uso de agentes imunossupressores não têm valor comprovado.

CONTRAINDICAÇÕES/INTERAÇÕES POSSÍVEIS
N/D.

ACOMPANHAMENTO

MONITORIZAÇÃO DO PACIENTE
• A urocultura deve ser realizada 7 a 10 dias após o início da terapia antimicrobiana para confirmar a esterilidade da urina. A urinálise e as uroculturas de acompanhamento também devem ser efetuadas por cistocentese 7 dias após a interrupção da terapia antimicrobiana e 1 mês depois do tratamento.
• A reavaliação ultrassonográfica do trato urinário é recomendada em 1, 3 e 6 meses.

PREVENÇÃO
Controle dos fatores predisponentes, como infecção do trato urinário e urolitíase.

COMPLICAÇÕES POSSÍVEIS
• Infecções crônicas do trato urinário.
• Infecção do trato urinário superior.
• Obstrução completa dos ureteres ou da uretra.

EVOLUÇÃO ESPERADA E PROGNÓSTICO
• A evolução esperada será favorável e o prognóstico bom se a causa subjacente for tratada e erradicada.
• Raramente os pacientes com cistite polipoide desenvolvem carcinoma de células de transição vários anos após o diagnóstico inicial. Não se sabe se alguns desses casos podem representar carcinoma precoce *in situ*.

---

* N. T.: Também conhecidos como cateteres de demora.

CISTITE POLIPOIDE

✓ DIVERSOS

DISTÚRBIOS ASSOCIADOS
• Infecção do trato urinário.
• Urolitíase.

FATORES RELACIONADOS COM A IDADE
Não há relatos de nenhum fator relacionado com a idade.

VER TAMBÉM
• Hematúria.
• Carcinoma de Células de Transição.
• Obstrução do Trato Urinário.
• Urolitíase.

Sugestões de Leitura
Cooper JE, Brearley MJ. Urothelial abnormalities in the dog. Vet Record 1986, 118:513-514.
Johnston SD, Osborne CA, Stevens JB. Canine polyploid cystitis. JAVMA 1975, 166:1155-1160.

Martinez I, Matton JS, Eaton KA, et al. Polypoid cystitis in 17 dogs (1978-2001). J Vet Intern Med 2003, 17:499-509.
Tagiguchi M, Inaba M. Diagnostic ultrasound of polypoid cystitis in dogs. J Vet Med Sci 2005, 67(1):57-61.

Autores Carl. A. Osborne e Jody P. Lulich
Consultor Editorial Carl A. Osborne

Cisto Dentígero

CONSIDERAÇÕES GERAIS

REVISÃO
Formação de cisto originário do tecido que circunda a coroa de dente não irrompido.

IDENTIFICAÇÃO
• Qualquer raça que esteja sob alto risco de erupção dentária prejudicada.
• Boxer, Buldogue — primeiros pré-molares mandibulares, frequentemente bilaterais.
• Dentes não irrompidos aos 6-7 meses de idade, embora possa não ocorrer o desenvolvimento cístico até muito tempo depois, se ocorrer.

SINAIS CLÍNICOS
• Em princípio, as alterações císticas podem ser inaparentes.
• Dente "ausente".
• Formação de inchaço macio no local de ausência de um dente, frequentemente flutuante com líquido.
• O paciente pode se apresentar por conta de fratura patológica da mandíbula em virtude da destruição cística do osso circunjacente, sem indicação prévia de algum problema.

CAUSAS E FATORES DE RISCO
Dentes não irrompidos.

DIAGNÓSTICO

DIAGNÓSTICO DIFERENCIAL
• Cisto primordial — degeneração cística de um botão dentário antes da formação de esmalte/dentina (cisto sem a presença de dente).
• Massa bucal — odontoma. Estruturas dentárias (complexas ou compostas) contidas algumas vezes dentro da estrutura cística, mas com diferentes níveis de organização.

HEMOGRAMA/BIOQUÍMICA/URINÁLISE
• Nenhuma anormalidade é tipicamente encontrada.
• Diagnóstico pré-operatório quando adequado.

OUTROS TESTES LABORATORIAIS
N/D.

DIAGNÓSTICO POR IMAGEM
• Diagnóstico definitivo por meio de radiografia.
• As radiografias são essenciais em qualquer caso de dentes ausentes ou não irrompidos.
• Ao exame radiográfico, observa-se cisto radiotransparente que se origina de remanescentes do órgão do esmalte no colo do dente e engloba a coroa (um halo).

MÉTODOS DIAGNÓSTICOS
Avaliação histopatológica se atípico.

TRATAMENTO

• Terapia antimicrobiana pré-operatória adequada e terapia analgésica para controle da dor quando indicadas.
• Monitorização e suporte adequados do paciente durante o procedimento anestésico.
• Na presença de formação cística, considerar a extração cirúrgica, com debridamento completo do revestimento do cisto; considerar também o uso de produtos osteopromotores.
• Se um dente incrustado estiver presente em um animal maduro, avaliá-lo em busca de qualquer estrutura cística ou outras alterações patológicas que envolvam o dente; a monitorização contínua pode ser sensata se a extração cirúrgica lesionar grandes quantidades de osso.
• Se um dente não estratégico puder ser extraído com facilidade, é melhor fazer isso, ainda que não haja alterações císticas.

MEDICAÇÕES

MEDICAMENTO(S)
Analgésicos pós-operatórios, conforme a necessidade.

CONTRAINDICAÇÕES/INTERAÇÕES POSSÍVEIS
N/D.

ACOMPANHAMENTO

COMPLICAÇÕES POSSÍVEIS
• Pode ocorrer fratura patológica se o cisto dentígero não for diagnosticado e tratado.
• Fratura de mandíbula no momento da extração, se comprometida.

EVOLUÇÃO ESPERADA E PROGNÓSTICO
• Bom em caso de detecção e extração precoces.
• Razoável a reservado em caso de destruição óssea extensa ou fratura patológica.

DIVERSOS

RECURSOS DA INTERNET
http://www.avdc.org/Nomenclature.html.

Sugestões de Leitura
Lobprise HB. Blackwell's Five-Minute Veterinary Consult Clinical Companion—Small Animal Dentistry. Ames, IA: Blackwell, 2007 (for additional topics, including diagnostics and techniques).
Regezi JA, Sciubba JJ, Jordan RCK. Oral Pathology Clinical Pathologic Correlations, 4th ed. St. Louis: Saunders, 1999, pp. 246-248.
White SC, Pharoah MJ. Oral Radiology Principles and Interpretation, 5th ed. St. Louis: Mosby, 2004, pp. 388-392.

Autor Heidi B. Lobprise
Consultor Editorial Heidi B. Lobprise

Cisto Quadrigeminal

CONSIDERAÇÕES GERAIS

REVISÃO
O cisto quadrigeminal refere-se a um divertículo preenchido por LCS, dentro do espaço subaracnoide ao nível da cisterna quadrigeminal (dorsal ao mesencéfalo e adjacente ao terceiro ventrículo). Os sinais clínicos podem se desenvolver como resultado de expansão gradual do espaço subaracnoide em virtude do mecanismo valvular associado ao fluxo pulsátil do líquido cerebrospinal. O cisto quadrigeminal também pode representar um achado incidental.

IDENTIFICAÇÃO
Cães e gatos.

Raça(s) Predominante(s)
Pug e Shih tzu são super-representadas.

Idade Média e Faixa Etária
- Média — 5 anos.
- Faixa — 2 meses-10 anos.

SINAIS CLÍNICOS
- Crises convulsivas.
- Comportamento anormal.
- Se associado à hidrocefalia, o cisto quadrigeminal pode se manifestar com desorientação, mudanças comportamentais, cegueira cortical, andar compulsivo em círculos, compressão cefálica.

CAUSAS E FATORES DE RISCO
- Distúrbio da embriogênese em que a divisão da membrana aracnoide primitiva leva ao acúmulo de líquido.
- Distúrbios inflamatórios que afetam as meninges.
- Traumatismo pós-cirúrgico (discopatia intervertebral, tumor espinal).
- Neoplasia e hemorragia.
- Hemorragia intracística secundária a traumatismo pode resultar em expansão do cisto e subsequente compressão do parênquima cerebral adjacente.
- Os cistos quadrigeminais também podem representar um achado incidental.

DIAGNÓSTICO

DIAGNÓSTICO DIFERENCIAL
- Anomalias cerebrais congênitas (anencefalia, hidrocefalia, outras).
- Doença de armazenamento.
- Doenças inflamatórias infecciosas — virais (vírus da cinomose, outros vírus); fúngicas (*Blastomyces dermatidis*, *Coccidioides* spp., *Cryptococcus neoformans*); riquetsianas (*Rickettsia rickettsii*); bacterianas (*Ehrlichia* spp., *E. coli*, *Streptococcus*); protozoárias (*Neospora caninum*, *Toxoplasma gondii*).
- Outra doença inflamatória — encefalite relacionada à raça (encefalite necrosante do Yorkshire terrier, Maltês, e Pug).
- Tumor cerebral — meningioma, glioma, papiloma do plexo coroide, linfoma.

HEMOGRAMA/BIOQUÍMICA/URINÁLISE
Geralmente normais.

OUTROS TESTES LABORATORIAIS
- RM — massa extra-axial preenchida por LCS na cisterna quadrigeminal. Nas imagens ponderadas em T1, a lesão é hipointensa em relação ao tecido cerebral e isointensa em relação ao LCS. Nas imagens ponderadas em T2, a lesão é tipicamente hiperintensa em relação ao tecido cerebral e isointensa em relação ao LCS.
- Nas sequências de imagens líquido-atenuadas da recuperação da inversão (FLAIR, sigla em inglês), o cisto costuma ser hipointenso, confirmando a presença de LCS. A dilatação do sistema ventricular pode ser identificada se o cisto estiver obstruindo o fluxo do LCS.

DIAGNÓSTICO POR IMAGEM
Análise do LCS — para descartar a presença de inflamação concomitante. Caso se registre uma reação inflamatória, o cisto pode representar um achado incidental.

TRATAMENTO
- Terapia médica para controlar as crises convulsivas e tentar reduzir a produção de LCS.
- Se os sinais forem progressivos, a fenestração cirúrgica do cisto através de craniotomia ou craniectomia pode resultar em melhora clínica. Na presença de hidrocefalia, pode-se considerar a aplicação de desvio cirúrgico. Outros processos patológicos devem ser descartados antes de se contemplar a cirurgia. A estrutura cística pode representar apenas um achado incidental.
- Os pacientes estáveis podem receber alta com a terapia médica recomendada.
- Tratamento hospitalar — para cães gravemente acometidos; monitorizar o paciente atentamente para avaliar a evolução dos déficits neurológicos.
- Administração de fluidos intravenosos para o paciente anoréxico.
- Gaiola almofadada para cães com atividade convulsiva.
- A posição dos pacientes em decúbito deve ser trocada com frequência.
- A avaliação sequencial do diâmetro da pupila e da reação pupilar à luz, bem como do estado mental, é útil para determinar o risco de herniação cerebral.

MEDICAÇÕES

MEDICAMENTO(S)
- Glicocorticosteroides — dexametasona na dose de 0,1 mg/kg IV ou VO a cada 24 h por 3 dias, seguida por prednisona na dose de 0,25-0,5 mg/kg VO a cada 24 h por 10 dias e, depois, reavaliar a resposta à terapia para ajustar a dose. Para evitar ulceração gastrintestinal, combinar a esteroidoterapia com famotidina na dose de 0,5-1 mg/kg IV ou VO a cada 12 h.
- Agentes anticonvulsivantes — fenobarbital na dose de 2 mg/kg IV ou VO a cada 12 h ou levetiracetam na dose de 20 mg/kg VO a cada 8-12 h.
- Diurético — acetazolamida na dose de 10 mg/kg a cada 6-8 h como inibidor da anidrase carbônica

que pode ajudar a reduzir a produção de LCS e a pressão intracraniana.

CONTRAINDICAÇÕES/INTERAÇÕES POSSÍVEIS
- Não utilizar a acetazolamida em pacientes desidratados.
- A combinação de glicocorticosteroide e diurético pode causar desidratação acentuada e aumento da viscosidade sanguínea, capazes de resultar em má perfusão cerebral e deterioração neurológica.

ACOMPANHAMENTO

MONITORIZAÇÃO DO PACIENTE
- Repetir o exame neurológico periodicamente (a cada 2-4 semanas).
- A terapia com corticosteroide pode ser necessária por um longo período de tempo ou pelo resto da vida. A dose do esteroide deve ser ajustada de acordo com a resposta ao tratamento e os efeitos colaterais. O objetivo é encontrar a dose que mantém os sinais clínicos sob controle com efeitos colaterais mínimos.
- Avaliar os níveis de fenobarbital após 4-5 semanas do início da terapia.
- Se o fenobarbital for mantido, reavaliar o perfil bioquímico e os ácidos biliares para avaliar a função hepática a cada 6 meses.

COMPLICAÇÕES POSSÍVEIS
- Deterioração dos sinais clínicos apesar do tratamento rigoroso.
- Estado epiléptico, demência, herniação cerebral, e morte.

EVOLUÇÃO ESPERADA E PROGNÓSTICO
- O prognóstico é variável, dependendo da gravidade dos sinais clínicos e da resposta à terapia.
- O cisto quadrigeminal pode ser um achado incidental ou resultar em deterioração neurológica progressiva.

DIVERSOS

DISTÚRBIOS ASSOCIADOS
Hidrocefalia.

GESTAÇÃO/FERTILIDADE/REPRODUÇÃO
Corticosteroides — pode afetar a gestação.

ABREVIATURA(S)
- LCS = líquido cerebrospinal.
- RM = ressonância magnética.

RECURSOS DA INTERNET
IVIS: www.ivis.org.
VIN: www.vin.com.

Sugestões de Leitura
Matiasek LA, Platt SR, Shaw S, Dennis R. Clinical and magnetic resonance imaging characteristics of quadrigeminal cysts in dogs. J Vet Intern Med 2007, 21(5):1021-1026.

Autor Carolina Duque
Consultor Editorial Joane M. Parent

Cistos Prostáticos

CONSIDERAÇÕES GERAIS

REVISÃO
- Os cistos prostáticos no cão incluem aqueles associados a (1) alteração cística epitelial difusa por hipertrofia prostática benigna (HPB) dependente de androgênio, (2) cistos de retenção dentro do parênquima prostático que são lesões cavitárias repletas de líquido com cápsula distinta, e (3) cistos paraprostáticos que são lesões cavitárias repletas de líquido com cápsula distinta localizada fora do parênquima prostático. Os cistos prostáticos podem variar em termos de diâmetro, desde alguns milímetros até mais de 20 cm.
- Os cistos paraprostáticos costumam surgir em posição craniolateral à próstata, deslocando a bexiga urinária nos sentidos cranial e ventral, ou em posição caudal à próstata na pelve. Os cistos prostáticos podem representar resquícios embrionários dilatados dos ductos de Wolff.
- A patogenia é desconhecida, embora haja especulações de que os cistos de retenção nos cães com tumores de células de Sertoli secretores de estrogênio sejam dilatações dos ácinos prostáticos secundárias à metaplasia escamosa induzida pelo estrogênio.

IDENTIFICAÇÃO
- Machos caninos intactos. Ocorrência rara em cães castrados.
- Faixa etária de 2-12 anos, idade média de 8 anos.
- Os cães de grande porte são mais comumente acometidos que os de pequeno porte.

SINAIS CLÍNICOS
- Assintomáticos.
- Letargia e anorexia.
- Distensão abdominal.
- Tenesmo em caso de compressão do reto pelo cisto.
- Disúria em caso de compressão da uretra pelo cisto.
- Secreção uretral sanguinolenta na presença de HPB.

CAUSAS E FATORES DE RISCO
- Hipertrofia prostática benigna.
- Hormônios androgênicos.
- Hormônios estrogênicos.

DIAGNÓSTICO

DIAGNÓSTICO DIFERENCIAL
- HPB — distinguida pela ultrassonografia.
- Abscesso prostático — diferenciado por meio de ultrassonografia e cultura do sêmen.
- Distensão vesical — distinguida por cistocentese e técnicas de diagnóstico por imagem.
- Massa abdominal caudal de origem indeterminada — diferenciada por técnicas de diagnóstico por imagem.

HEMOGRAMA/BIOQUÍMICA/URINÁLISE
Sem anormalidades.

OUTROS TESTES LABORATORIAIS
- Exame do líquido prostático coletado por ejaculação ou massagem prostática confirma a ausência de infecção.
- Cultura e citologia do líquido cístico coletado por meio de aspirado por agulha fina guiado pelo ultrassom ou aspirado durante exploração cirúrgica revela líquido claro ou sanguinolento estéril compatível com o líquido prostático.

DIAGNÓSTICO POR IMAGEM
Uretrocistografia retrógrada com contraste seguida por ultrassonografia prostática não só confirma a presença, a localização, a ecotextura e o tamanho dos cistos prostáticos, mas também diferencia os cistos de retenção dos cistos paraprostáticos.

MÉTODOS DIAGNÓSTICOS
É recomendável a coleta de líquido prostático por ejaculação, seguida pela obtenção de imagem da próstata antes do aspirado por agulha fina do líquido cístico a fim de descartar a presença de infecção bacteriana.

ACHADOS PATOLÓGICOS
Observa-se a ocorrência de cistos epiteliais dentro do parênquima prostático em casos de hipertrofia e hiperplasia do parênquima; pode haver metaplasia escamosa dos ductos e alvéolos. Além de serem revestidos por uma única camada de epitélio prostático ou de tecido conjuntivo fibroso, os cistos de retenção e os paraprostáticos contêm líquido claro a sanguinolento com fibrina.

TRATAMENTO

- Cistos intraprostáticos (epiteliais, de retenção) respondem à involução prostática, a qual pode ser induzida pela castração ou pela finasterida (inibidor da 5-alfa redutase). Cistos volumosos podem ser drenados por via percutânea com orientação ultrassonográfica antes do início da terapia com finasterida.
- Grandes cistos de retenção e paraprostáticos devem ser submetidos à ressecção cirúrgica parcial ou total, dependendo da aderência às estruturas circundantes, ou marsupializados e drenados por 1-2 meses.
- Não é recomendada a simples drenagem do(s) cisto(s), já que a persistência da cápsula pode resultar em recidiva.

MEDICAÇÕES

MEDICAMENTO(S)
- Os cistos epiteliais difusos e parenquimatosos prostáticos involuem depois do tratamento com a finasterida (inibidor da 5-alfa redutase) administrada na dose de 0,1-1 mg/kg VO a cada 24 h durante 2-4 meses. A finasterida impede a conversão da testosterona em di-hidrotestosterona, provocando a involução prostática sem afetar adversamente a libido ou a espermatogênese. Ocorre recidiva da HPB após a interrupção do tratamento com a finasterida. Cistos paraprostáticos não respondem à terapia com a finasterida.

CONTRAINDICAÇÕES/INTERAÇÕES POSSÍVEIS
N/D.

ACOMPANHAMENTO

- Avaliação do tamanho do cisto por meio das técnicas de diagnóstico por imagem em intervalos de 4 semanas depois do tratamento.
- Monitorização pós-operatória padrão do estoma marsupializado, se presente.

DIVERSOS

ABREVIATURA(S)
- HPB = hipertrofia prostática benigna.

Sugestões de Leitura

Johnston SD, Root Kustritz MV, Olson PN. Disorders of the canine prostate. In: Canine and Feline Theriogenology. Philadelphia: Saunders, 2001, pp. 337-355.

Rawlings CA, Mahaffey MB, Barsanti JA, et al. Use of partial prostatectomy for treatment of prostatic abscesses and cysts in dogs. JAVMA 1997, 211:868-871.

Smith J. Canine prostatic disease: A review of anatomy, pathology, diagnosis, and treatment. Theriogenology 2008, 70:375-383.

Stowater JL, Lamb CR. Ultrasonographic features of paraprostatic cysts in nine dogs. Vet Radiol Ultrasound 1989, 30:232-239.

White RAS, Herrtage ME, Dennis R. The diagnosis and management of paraprostatic and prostatic retention cysts in the dog. J Small Anim Pract 1987, 28:551-574.

Autor Margaret V. Root Kustritz
Consultor Editorial Carl A. Osborne

Cistos Subaracnoides

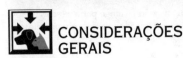

CONSIDERAÇÕES GERAIS

DEFINIÇÃO
Cistos subaracnoides referem-se à dilatação do espaço subaracnoide, com consequente compressão da medula espinal subjacente. O uso do termo "cisto" é equivocado, pois a maioria não tem uma parede cística definida com revestimento epitelial.

FISIOPATOLOGIA
• Há várias etiologias propostas de cistos subaracnoides.
• Qualquer processo patológico indutor de aracnoidite tem o potencial de causar aderências que resultam na formação de válvulas unidirecionais através das quais o LCS flui, mas não consegue retornar, produzindo com isso um "cisto".

SISTEMA(S) ACOMETIDO(S)
Nervoso — medula espinal.

GENÉTICA
Certas raças parecem ser predispostas (p. ex., Pug, Rottweiler), mas não há dados que confirmem a hereditariedade ou um modo de herança.

INCIDÊNCIA/PREVALÊNCIA
Distúrbio raro sem dados específicos sobre incidência/prevalência.

DISTRIBUIÇÃO GEOGRÁFICA
N/D.

IDENTIFICAÇÃO
Espécies
Cães, gatos.
Raça(s) Predominante(s)
Pug, Rottweiler.
Idade Média e Faixa Etária
Qualquer idade, mas os cistos cervicais são mais comuns em cães com <3 anos.
Sexo Predominante
N/D.

SINAIS CLÍNICOS
Achados Anamnésicos
• Os proprietários relatam ataxia e paresia lentamente progressivas envolvendo todos os membros ou apenas os membros pélvicos.
• Incontinência fecal — sinal precoce comum de cistos toracolombares, com desenvolvimento de incontinência urinária logo depois.
• Os proprietários não costumam relatar que o animal de estimação está com dor.
• Pode haver um histórico prévio de lesão traumática da medula espinal.
Achados do Exame Físico
Geralmente normais, embora as possíveis consequências secundárias da mielopatia incluam abrasões da face dorsal dos dedos dos pés, desgaste das unhas e infecções do trato urinário.
Achados do Exame Neurológico
• Os sinais neurológicos refletem a localização da lesão — envolvimento dos membros posteriores para cistos toracolombares e todos os membros para cistos cervicais.
• Ataxia frequentemente caracterizada por hipermetria.
• Paresia.
• Déficits proprioceptivos.
• Incontinência fecal e/ou urinária; retenção de urina (em virtude de micção defeituosa).
• Os reflexos espinais podem estar diminuídos em caso de lesão na intumescência braquial ou lombossacra; do contrário, permanecem normais ou aumentados.
• Raramente, é eliciada dor espinal.

CAUSAS
• Várias etiologias propostas.
• Má-formação congênita da substância aracnoide (*septum posticum* * dilatado; em cães jovens).
• Secundários à lesão traumática da aracnoide, causando aderências e desenvolvimento de válvulas unidirecionais para o fluxo do LCS.
• Secundários à microtraumatismo crônico da aracnoide, causando aderências e desenvolvimento de válvulas unidirecionais para fluxo do LCS. Possíveis fontes de microtraumatismo incluem herniações de disco tipo II.

FATORES DE RISCO
• Lesão traumática da medula espinal que lesiona a substância aracnoide.
• Herniações de disco tipo II são raramente associadas a cistos subaracnoides em certas raças de cães (Pugs).

DIAGNÓSTICO

DIAGNÓSTICO DIFERENCIAL
• Características peculiares — paresia e ataxia, não dolorosas, lentamente progressivas com marcha hipermétrica e presença de incontinência fecal e/ou urinária em animal que ainda exibe deambulação.
• Qualquer causa de mielopatia focal pode provocar a mesma manifestação neurológica.
• Herniação de disco intervertebral.
• Neoplasia.
• Traumatismo.
• Mielite inflamatória ou infecciosa.
• Má-formação vertebral/espinal congênita.
• Má-formação vascular intraespinal.

HEMOGRAMA/BIOQUÍMICA/URINÁLISE
Urinálise pode revelar evidência de infecção do trato urinário (piúria, hematúria, proteinúria, e bacteriúria).

OUTROS TESTES LABORATORIAIS
Cultura urinária aeróbia se houver evidência de infecção do trato urinário.

DIAGNÓSTICO POR IMAGEM
• Radiografia torácica — em pacientes mais idosos para descartar neoplasia metastática.
• Radiografia espinal — deve ser realizada em todos os pacientes; tipicamente, esse exame não se mostra digno de nota em pacientes com cistos subaracnoides. Contudo, alguns pacientes podem ter evidência de fraturas espinais e, ocasionalmente, há evidência de má-formação vertebral (espinha bífida, hemivértebra, ou vértebra em bloco) cossituada com os sinais neurológicos.
• Mielografia — dilatação focal do espaço subaracnoide mais comumente localizada na região dorsal, mas algumas vezes na ventral; a dilatação pode ser multilobada.
• Mielografia por TC — delineia ainda mais o espaço subaracnoide dilatado em corte transversal; sem contraste intratecal, esse exame não demonstrará a lesão.
• RM — revela claramente a dilatação do espaço subaracnoide em corte sagital e transversal nas imagens ponderadas em T2. A presença de aracnoidite ativa pode ser detectada nas imagens ponderadas em T1 antes e depois do contraste.

MÉTODOS DIAGNÓSTICOS
LCS — para descartar um processo inflamatório primário; pode demonstrar inflamação leve como uma consequência secundária do cisto subaracnoide.

ACHADOS PATOLÓGICOS
• Na cirurgia, podem ser evidenciadas aderências no espaço subaracnoide. Ocasionalmente, uma parede cística delgada está aparente (isso não é usual).
• Histopatologia da aracnoide excisada — pode revelar fibrose ou leve inflamação.
• Histopatologia da medula espinal — revela lesão compressiva crônica com perda da substância cinzenta e branca, degeneração walleriana, desmielinização.

TRATAMENTO

CUIDADO(S) DE SAÚDE ADEQUADO(S)
• Os pacientes com sinais leves podem ser submetidos a tratamento médico; a cirurgia é recomendada para cães jovens com sinais progressivos moderados.
• Os pacientes sem deambulação devem ser hospitalizados para avaliação diagnóstica e possível descompressão cirúrgica o mais rápido possível.

CUIDADO(S) DE ENFERMAGEM
• Os pacientes que apresentam micção incompleta devem ser submetidos à compressão manual da bexiga 3 a 4 vezes ao dia. Se isso não for possível, as bexigas desses pacientes devem ser cateterizadas de forma estéril 1 a 2 vezes ao dia.
• É recomendável a administração de fluidos de manutenção adequados no período pós-operatório imediato.
• A presença de dor no pós-operatório deve ser avaliada regularmente (a cada 6 h) e tratada conforme a necessidade com opiáceos e agentes anti-inflamatórios não esteroides.
• É aconselhável a aplicação de compressas frias sobre as incisões cirúrgicas por 5-10 minutos 3 vezes ao dia por 24 horas após a cirurgia e, depois, compressas quentes por um período semelhante por mais 2-5 dias.
• A reabilitação é importante; por essa razão, deve ser desenvolvido um programa de reabilitação específico para o paciente, incluindo adestramento da marcha e restabelecimento da força.

ATIVIDADE
• É necessário restringir os pacientes com paresia e ataxia a superfícies planas não escorregadias para evitar quedas.
• O exercício deve ser limitado a passeios com coleira para evitar quedas, embora o exercício controlado seja importante na manutenção da força muscular e integridade articular.

---

* N. T.: Septo longitudinal, dorsal, mediano, que vai da região cervical à lombar, fenestrado em muitos pontos. Lateralmente existem septos dorsolaterais, também fenestrados. Os septos podem ser completos ou circundar as raízes nervosas posteriores.

CISTOS SUBARACNOIDES

• No pós-operatório, os pacientes devem ficar limitados a um espaço pequeno e bem acolchoado (uma espécie de engradado) para garantir que eles não caiam enquanto o local da laminectomia está cicatrizando. É recomendável a realização de exercício controlado restrito durante esse período.

DIETA
N/D

ORIENTAÇÃO AO PROPRIETÁRIO
• É necessário orientar os proprietários sobre as implicações de um quadro de mielopatia compressiva crônica; nesse caso, o dano permanente à medula espinal já ocorreu e pode não ser reversível. O principal objetivo do tratamento é evitar deterioração adicional, com esperança de se produzir uma melhora clínica.
• Pode haver uma deterioração inicial no período pós-operatório imediato; há uma pequena chance de que essa deterioração possa ser permanente.
• É provável que a incontinência, se presente, seja permanente.
• A doença pode recorrer apesar da terapia cirúrgica.

CONSIDERAÇÕES CIRÚRGICAS
• A descompressão cirúrgica de cistos subaracnoides é recomendada em cães jovens e pode ser tentada em animais mais idosos.
• A marsupialização das meninges pode reduzir as chances de recorrência.

MEDICAÇÕES
MEDICAMENTO(S) DE ESCOLHA
• Doses anti-inflamatórias de prednisona (0,5 mg/kg VO 1 a 2 vezes ao dia) podem melhorar os sinais clínicos e reduzir a inflamação. Se não houver melhora, a prednisona deve ser gradativamente reduzida e interrompida.
• Omeprazol pode diminuir a velocidade de produção do LCS e melhorar os sinais clínicos. Na ausência de melhora, esse medicamento também deve ser interrompido.

CONTRAINDICAÇÕES
N/D

PRECAUÇÕES
Os corticosteroides devem ser utilizados com cuidado se o paciente tiver infecção do trato urinário.

INTERAÇÕES POSSÍVEIS
N/D

MEDICAMENTO(S) ALTERNATIVO(S)
N/D

ACOMPANHAMENTO
MONITORIZAÇÃO DO PACIENTE
• Se a resposta à prednisona estiver sendo avaliada, também é recomendável a reavaliação da marcha e das reações posturais do paciente em 1-2 semanas. A avaliação de continência feita pelo proprietário também é importante.
• Se houver uma resposta positiva ao tratamento médico, o paciente deve ser monitorizado a cada 8-12 semanas para manutenção da melhora durante os próximos 6 meses e, depois, a cada 6-12 meses. O proprietário deve ser orientado a entrar em contato se for detectada uma deterioração nos sinais clínicos.
• Tratamento cirúrgico — paciente reavaliado em 7-10 dias para remover a sutura, avaliar a incisão e garantir que não haja qualquer deterioração na marcha, nível da dor, continência; reavaliação em 1-3 meses e, subsequentemente, a cada 6-12 meses. Acompanhamentos e atualizações por telefone são aceitáveis se o paciente estiver passando bem.

PREVENÇÃO
N/D

COMPLICAÇÕES POSSÍVEIS
• Os proprietários podem se deparar com incontinência fecal e urinária em seus animais.
• Na presença de incontinência, há predisposição a infecções do trato urinário.
• Os sinais podem recorrer em qualquer momento.

EVOLUÇÃO ESPERADA E PROGNÓSTICO
• A descompressão cirúrgica produz um resultado satisfatório a longo prazo (mais de 1 ano) em cerca de 66% dos cães.
• A idade de início dos sinais e a duração dos sinais são associadas ao resultado. É mais provável que os cães com menos de 3 anos de idade e curta duração dos sinais (menos de 4 meses) tenham um resultado satisfatório a longo prazo.
• Não há dados sobre o prognóstico com o tratamento médico; segundo relatos breves e incidentais, no entanto, o autor pode relatar um resultado satisfatório a longo prazo em cães idosos com sinais leves quando tratados com prednisona e reabilitação apenas.

DIVERSOS
DISTÚRBIOS ASSOCIADOS
N/D

FATORES RELACIONADOS COM A IDADE
Os cistos cervicais são mais comuns em cães com menos de 3 anos de idade, enquanto os toracolombares, em Pugs idosos.

POTENCIAL ZOONÓTICO
N/D

GESTAÇÃO/FERTILIDADE/REPRODUÇÃO
N/D

SINÔNIMOS
Divertículos aracnoides, cisto aracnoide, cisto meníngeo ou leptomeníngeo.

ABREVIATURA(S)
• LCS = líquido cerebrospinal.
• TC = tomografia computadorizada.
• RM = ressonância magnética.

RECURSOS DA INTERNET
http://www.ivis.org/advances/Vite/toc.asp.

Sugestões de Leitura
Gnirs K, Ruel Y, Blot S, et al. Spinal subarachnoid cysts in 13 dogs. Vet Radiol Ultrasound 2003, 44:402-408.
Jurina K, Grevel V. Spinal arachnoid pseudocysts in 10 rottweilers. J Small Anim Pract 2004, 45:9-15.
Rylander H, Lipsitz D, Berry WL, et al. Retrospective analysis of spinal arachnoid cysts in 14 dogs. J Vet Intern Med 2002, 16:690-696.
Skeen TM, Olby NJ, Muʻnana KR, Sharp NJ. Spinal arachnoid cysts in 17 dogs. JAAHA 2003, 39:271-282.

Autor Natasha J. Olby
Consultor Editorial Joane M. Parent

Citauxzoonose

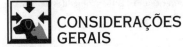

CONSIDERAÇÕES GERAIS

REVISÃO
- Infecção pelo protozoário *Cytauxzoon felis*.
- Acomete o sistema vascular de órgãos como pulmões, fígado, baço, rins e cérebro; a medula óssea; os estágios de desenvolvimento das hemácias.
- Incomum em grande parte das regiões, mas comum durante as épocas de primavera e verão em áreas endêmicas.
- Afeta gatos selvagens e domésticos nas regiões centro-sul, sudeste e mesoatlântica dos EUA.

IDENTIFICAÇÃO
- Gatos selvagens e domésticos de todas as idades.
- Não há predileção racial ou sexual.

SINAIS CLÍNICOS
- Alguns gatos podem ser infectados, mas permanecer assintomáticos.
- Doença grave na consulta.
- Mucosas pálidas.
- Depressão.
- Anorexia.
- Desidratação.
- Febre alta.
- Icterícia.
- Esplenomegalia.
- Hepatomegalia.

CAUSAS E FATORES DE RISCO
- Picada de carrapato ixodídeo infectado.
- Perambulação em áreas compartilhadas por hospedeiros reservatórios em comum (lince, pantera da Flórida).
- Convívio na mesma casa com algum gato diagnosticado com citauxzoonose.

DIAGNÓSTICO

DIAGNÓSTICO DIFERENCIAL
- Outras causas de anemia — diminuição acentuada no volume globular (hematócrito), que começa 5-6 dias após a infecção.
- Outras causas de febre e icterícia, como pancreatite, hepatite e colangite.
- Outras causas de pancitopenia, como sepse e panleucopenia.

HEMOGRAMA/BIOQUÍMICA/URINÁLISE
- Bicitopenia ou pancitopenia constituem os achados mais comuns. A trombocitopenia quase sempre está presente.
- Hiperbilirrubinemia e bilirrubinúria moderadas.
- Atividade normal ou levemente aumentada da ALT.
- Hiperglicemia leve.
- Refletem alterações associadas à anemia grave, causada pela combinação de hemólise e hemorragia.

OUTROS TESTES LABORATORIAIS
- Esfregaço sanguíneo fresco — forma eritrocitária do *Cytauxzoon*; 1-2 μm de diâmetro; possui formato de anel de sinete ou alfinete de segurança ou assemelha-se a pontos diminutos.
- Aspirados de órgãos como baço, linfonodos, fígado ou medula óssea — mais adequados para demonstrar a forma extraeritrocitária.
- Ensaio de PCR está disponível no mercado.

DIAGNÓSTICO POR IMAGEM
N/D.

MÉTODOS DIAGNÓSTICOS
N/D.

ACHADOS PATOLÓGICOS
Microrganismos presentes no interior das células mononucleares no aspirado de medula óssea e em células endoteliais, drasticamente aumentadas de tamanho, de vênulas pulmonares, hepáticas, esplênicas, renais e cerebrais.

TRATAMENTO

- Internação com terapia de suporte rigorosa.
- Transfusão sanguínea.
- Sonda de alimentação para medicamentos e suporte nutricional.

MEDICAÇÕES

MEDICAMENTO(S)
- Combinação de atovaquona (15 mg/kg VO a cada 8 h com refeição gordurosa) e azitromicina (10 mg/kg VO a cada 24 h) com cuidados de suporte é associada com taxas de sobrevida de 60%.
- É recomendável o dipropionato de imidocarbe na dose de 5 mg IM sob a forma de 2 injeções com intervalo de 14 dias, mas seu uso é associado a taxas de sobrevida de aproximadamente 27%.
- Heparina (100-300 U/kg SC a cada 8 h ou 300-900 U/kg/dia sob a forma de infusão contínua) até o momento da alta (por mais tempo caso se desenvolvam problemas significativos de coagulação, como tromboembolia pulmonar).

CONTRAINDICAÇÕES/INTERAÇÕES POSSÍVEIS
N/D.

ACOMPANHAMENTO

EVOLUÇÃO ESPERADA E PROGNÓSTICO
- Com a provisão de cuidados de suporte rigorosos e tratamento agressivo, esperam-se 3-7 dias de internação em casos de doença grave.
- Alguns gatos desenvolvem efusão pleural (presumivelmente secundária à hipertensão pulmonar) e necessitam de toracocentese.
- Contudo, os gatos que sobrevivem retornarão ao normal em até 2-4 semanas da alta hospitalar e aparentemente se tornarão imunes a novas infecções.
- Alguns gatos permanecem persistentemente infectados com a forma intraeritrocitária sem sinais clínicos evidentes.
- Sem tratamento, a maioria dos gatos infectados vem a óbito dentro de 5 dias após a consulta.

DIVERSOS

POTENCIAL ZOONÓTICO
- Não há nenhum risco conhecido aos seres humanos.
- Não há possibilidade de transmissão direta a outro gato, exceto por meio de inoculação de sangue ou tecido.

ABREVIATURA(S)
- PCR = reação em cadeia da polimerase.

RECURSOS DA INTERNET
www.vet.uga.edu/vpp/clerk/Dailey/index.htm.

Sugestões de Leitura
Brown HM, Latimer KS, et al. Detection of persistent Cytauxzoon felis infection by polymerase chain reaction in three asymptomatic domestic cats. J Vet Diagn Invest 2008, 20(4):485-488.
Greene CE, Meinkoth J, Kocan AA. Cytauxzoonosis. In: Greene CE, ed., Infectious Diseases of the Dog and Cat, 3rd ed. St. Louis: Saunders Elsevier, 2006, pp. 716-722.
Haber MD, Tucker MD, et al. The detection of Cytauxzoon felis in apparently healthy free-roaming cats in the USA. Vet Parasitol 2007, 146(3-4):316-320.

Autor Johnny D. Hoskins
Consultor Editorial Stephen C. Barr

Clamidiose — Gatos

CONSIDERAÇÕES GERAIS

DEFINIÇÃO
Infecção respiratória crônica de gatos, causada por uma bactéria intracelular e caracterizada por conjuntivite, sinais respiratórios superiores brandos e pneumonite leve.

FISIOPATOLOGIA
• *Chlamydophila felis* (conhecida antigamente como *Chlamydia psittaci var. felis*) — bactéria intracelular obrigatória; replica-se na mucosa dos epitélios respiratórios superior e inferior; produz uma flora comensal persistente, que causa irritação local com consequentes sinais respiratórios superiores e inferiores brandos; também pode colonizar a mucosa dos tratos gastrintestinal e reprodutivo.
• Período de incubação — 7-10 dias; mais longo do que o de outros patógenos respiratórios comuns dos gatos.

SISTEMA(S) ACOMETIDO(S)
• Gastrintestinal — gato: infecção sem doença clínica; outras espécies: podem apresentar gastrenterite clínica.
• Oftálmico — conjuntivite crônica, frequentemente unilateral, mas pode ser bilateral.
• Reprodutivo — infecção sem doença clínica.
• Respiratório — rinite, bronquite e bronquiolite brandas.

INCIDÊNCIA/PREVALÊNCIA
• Incidência de doença clínica — esporádica; podem ocorrer surtos de doença respiratória, especialmente em instalações com muitos gatos.
• Prevalência da *C. felis* na população felina — não é incomum, 5-10% com infecção crônica.

DISTRIBUIÇÃO GEOGRÁFICA
Mundial.

IDENTIFICAÇÃO
Espécies
• Gatos.
• Seres humanos.

Idade Média e Faixa Etária
Geralmente filhotes felinos com menos de 1 ano de idade; no entanto, pode acometer gatos de qualquer idade.

SINAIS CLÍNICOS
Comentários Gerais
• A infecção muitas vezes é subclínica.
• Doença clínica — comumente como uma infecção concomitante causada por outros microrganismos.

Achados Anamnésicos
• Infecção do trato respiratório superior, com espirros, lacrimejamento e tosse.
• Algumas vezes, há dificuldade respiratória.
• Graus variados de anorexia.

Achados do Exame Físico
• Conjuntivite — frequentemente granular; é unilateral em princípio, mas geralmente evolui e transforma-se em bilateral.
• Lacrimejamento, fotofobia e blefarospasmo.
• Rinite com secreção nasal — costuma ser branda.
• Pneumonite — com o processo inflamatório nos alvéolos; os bronquíolos e as vias aéreas produzem estertores audíveis.

CAUSAS
Chlamydophila felis.

FATORES DE RISCO
• Infecções concomitantes com outros patógenos respiratórios.
• Falta de vacinação.
• Instalações com muitos gatos, especialmente abrigos de adoção ou gatis de reprodução.

DIAGNÓSTICO

DIAGNÓSTICO DIFERENCIAL
• Rinotraqueíte viral felina — período de incubação curto (4-5 dias); conjuntivite bilateral de aparecimento rápido; espirros intensos; e ceratite ulcerativa.
• Calicivirose felina — período de incubação curto (3-5 dias); estomatite ulcerativa; e pneumonia grave.
• Reovirose felina — infecção respiratória superior muito leve; incubação e duração breves.
• Broncopneumonia causada por bactérias como *Bordetella bronchiseptica* — áreas localizadas de radiodensidade nos pulmões.

HEMOGRAMA/BIOQUÍMICA/URINÁLISE
Leucocitose.

DIAGNÓSTICO POR IMAGEM
Radiografias dos pulmões — úteis em casos de pneumonite.

MÉTODOS DIAGNÓSTICOS
• Ensaio de PCR para detecção de *C. felis* — exame preferido; amostras de *swabs* conjuntivais.
• Título de anticorpo sérico — gatos não vacinados; indica infecção.
• Raspados conjuntivais corados pelo corante Giemsa — corpúsculos de inclusão intracitoplasmáticos característicos.
• Amostras de *swabs* conjuntivais — isolamento do microrganismo causal em culturas celulares.

ACHADOS PATOLÓGICOS
• Macroscópicos — evidências de conjuntivite crônica com secreção ocular mucopurulenta; rinite secundária com corrimento nasal; ocasionalmente, há alterações pulmonares indicativas de pneumonite.
• Histopatológicos (conjuntiva) — infiltrado inicial intenso de neutrófilos; mudanças na resposta inflamatória para linfócitos e plasmócitos; corpúsculos de inclusão detectados com corantes especiais; corpúsculos de inclusão invisíveis com os corantes de rotina (H&E).

TRATAMENTO

CUIDADO(S) DE SAÚDE ADEQUADO(S)
Geralmente em esquema ambulatorial.

CUIDADO(S) DE ENFERMAGEM
• Manter as narinas e os olhos limpos de secreções.
• Em geral, não há necessidade de outras terapias de suporte (p. ex., fluidos), a menos que seja complicada por outras infecções concomitantes.

ATIVIDADE
• Os gatos acometidos devem ser mantidos em quarentena, evitando seu contato com outros gatos.
• Não permitir que os gatos acometidos tenham acesso à rua.

DIETA
Normal.

ORIENTAÇÃO AO PROPRIETÁRIO
Orientar o proprietário quanto ao microrganismo causal, à evolução crônica prevista da doença e à necessidade de vacinação de outros gatos antes da exposição.

MEDICAÇÕES

MEDICAMENTO(S) DE ESCOLHA
• Sistêmico(s) — tetraciclina (antibiótico de escolha; 22 mg/kg VO a cada 8 h por 3-4 semanas); doxiciclina (10 mg/kg VO diariamente por 4 semanas para evitar recidivas).
• Ocular(es) — pomadas oftálmicas contendo tetraciclina (a cada 8 h).

CONTRAINDICAÇÕES
Tetraciclina — pode comprometer os dentes em crescimento de filhotes felinos.

PRECAUÇÕES
Colônias/abrigos/gatis reprodutores — talvez todos os gatos tenham de ser tratados; pode ser necessário que o tratamento seja mantido por até 4 semanas.

ACOMPANHAMENTO

MONITORIZAÇÃO DO PACIENTE
Monitorar o animal quanto ao restabelecimento de sua saúde durante a conduta terapêutica.

PREVENÇÃO
Vacinas
• Para reduzir a gravidade da infecção, há vacinas inativadas e vivas modificadas disponíveis.
• As vacinas não evitam a infecção, mas diminuem a gravidade e a duração da doença clínica.
• American Association of Feline Practitioners (Associação Norte-americana de Clínicos Felinos) — classifica tal vacinação como uma prática dispensável ou não essencial; indicada para gatos de alto risco; essa associação recomenda a vacinação única na primeira consulta até 9 semanas de vida e a repetição em 3-4 semanas; aplicação de reforços anuais em áreas onde a *C. felis* é endêmica.

COMPLICAÇÕES POSSÍVEIS
Reações vacinais adversas — doença clínica branda com as vacinas vivas modificadas; pequena porcentagem de gatos vacinados.

EVOLUÇÃO ESPERADA E PROGNÓSTICO
• Tende a ser crônica, com duração de semanas ou meses, a menos que se forneça antibioticoterapia bem-sucedida.
• Prognóstico bom.

DIVERSOS

FATORES RELACIONADOS COM A IDADE
Principalmente uma doença de gatos jovens.

POTENCIAL ZOONÓTICO

A *C. felis* é capaz de infectar o homem, sobretudo indivíduos imunocomprometidos; há um número limitado de relatos de conjuntivite branda em seres humanos, transmitida a partir de gatos infectados.

GESTAÇÃO/FERTILIDADE/REPRODUÇÃO

• Gatis reprodutores endêmicos — tratar todos os gatos com doxiciclina por no mínimo 4 semanas e, depois, vaciná-los.
• Papel patogênico da *C. felis* durante a prenhez — indeterminado; pode colonizar a mucosa reprodutiva; pode ocorrer conjuntivite neonatal grave em neonatos felinos infectados no momento do parto ou logo após o nascimento.

SINÔNIMOS

Pneumonite felina.

ABREVIATURA(S)

• H&E = hematoxilina e eosina.

• PCR = reação em cadeia da polimerase.

Sugestões de Leitura

Gaskell RM. Upper respiratory disease in the cat (including Chlamydia): Control and prevention. Feline Pract 1993, 21:29-34.

Greene CE, Sykes JE. Chlamydial infections. In: Greene CE, ed., Infectious Diseases of the Dog and Cat, 3rd ed. St. Louis: Saunders Elsevier, 2006, pp. 245-252.

Gruffydd-Jones T, Addie D, Belák S, et al. Chlamydophila felis infection: ABCD guidelines on prevention and management. J Feline Med Surg 2009, 11:605-609.

Hoover EA. Viral respiratory diseases and chlamydiosis. In: Holzworth J, ed., Diseases of the Cat. Philadelphia: Saunders, 1987, pp. 214-237.

Richards JR, Elston TH, Ford RB, et al. The 2006 American Association of Feline Practioners Feline Vaccine Advisory Panel Report. JAVMA 2006, 229:1405-1441.

Sykes JE. Feline chlamydiosis. Clin Tech Small Anim Pract 2005, 20:129-134.

Autor Fred W. Scott
Consultor Editorial Stephen C. Barr

CLAUDICAÇÃO

CONSIDERAÇÕES GERAIS

DEFINIÇÃO
Distúrbio na marcha e na locomoção em resposta a dor, problema anatômico ou a lesão.

FISIOPATOLOGIA
• Dor grave e aguda — movimento limitado dos membros durante todas as fases da locomoção, com pouca a nenhuma sustentação do peso em movimento ou em repouso.
• Dor vaga e contínua, porém mais leve — diminuição na sustentação do peso e no contato com o chão durante todas as fases da locomoção.
• Dor produzida apenas durante determinadas fases do movimento — o paciente ajusta seu movimento e sua marcha para minimizar o desconforto.

SISTEMA(S) ACOMETIDO(S)
• Musculoesquelético. • Nervoso.

IDENTIFICAÇÃO
• Qualquer idade ou raça canina.
• Predileção por idade, raça ou sexo — depende da doença específica.

SINAIS CLÍNICOS
Comentários Gerais
• Membro anterior unilateral — compensado pelo movimento da cabeça e do pescoço para cima à medida que o membro acometido toca o solo e para baixo quando o membro sadio suporta o peso.
• Membro posterior unilateral — a pelve abaixa quando o membro acometido sustenta o peso, mas levanta quando deixa de sustentar o peso.
• Membro posterior bilateral — o quarto posterior é rebaixado para desviar o peso para frente.
• Sempre avaliar o estado neurológico do paciente, especialmente na suspeita de lesão proximal.

Achados Anamnésicos
• Anamnese completa — identificar traumatismo conhecido; avaliar alterações no clima, tolerância ao exercício, resposta ao repouso e efeito de tratamentos prévios.
• Determinar a velocidade de início da claudicação.
• Definir a evolução — estática; lenta; rápida.
• Como o paciente manifesta dor?

Achados do Exame Físico
• Realizar o exame clínico de rotina.
• Observar a postura — em estação e ao se levantar, deitar ou sentar.
• Avaliar a marcha — caminhando; trotando; subindo escadas; fazendo o número oito ao caminhar.
• Palpar — assimetria da massa muscular (medir e comparar); proeminências ósseas.
• Manipular ossos e articulações, começando distalmente e seguindo em direção proximal.
• Avaliar — instabilidade; incongruência; dor; amplitude de movimento (medir); sons anormais.
• Examinar a área suspeita de envolvimento por último — começando pelos membros normais, o paciente pode relaxar, permitindo a comparação de reações normais e anormais.

CAUSAS
Membro Anterior
Cão em Crescimento (<12 meses de vida)
• Osteocondrose do ombro. • Luxação ou subluxação do ombro — congênita.
• Osteocondrose do cotovelo. • Não união do processo ancôneo. • Fragmentação do processo coronoide medial. • Incongruência do cotovelo.
• Avulsão ou calcificação dos músculos flexores — cotovelo. • Crescimento assimétrico do rádio e da ulna. • Panosteíte. • Osteodistrofia hipertrófica.
• Traumatismo — tecido mole; osso; articulação.
• Infecção — local; sistêmica. • Desequilíbrios nutricionais. • Anomalias congênitas.

Cão Adulto (>12 meses de vida)
• Artropatia degenerativa. • Tenossinovite bicipital. • Calcificação ou mineralização do tendão supraespinal ou infraespinal. • Contratura do músculo supraespinal ou infraespinal.
• Neoplasia de tecidos moles ou ósseos — primária; metastática. • Traumatismo — tecido mole; osso; articulação. • Panosteíte.
• Poliartropatias. • Polimiosite. • Polineurite.

Membro Posterior
Cão em Crescimento (<12 meses de vida)
• Displasia coxofemoral. • Necrose avascular da cabeça femoral — doença de Legg-Calvé-Perthes.
• Osteocondrite do joelho. • Luxação da patela — medial ou lateral. • Osteocondrite do jarrete.
• Panosteíte. • Osteodistrofia hipertrófica.
• Traumatismo — tecido mole; osso; articulação.
• Infecção — local; sistêmica. • Desequilíbrios nutricionais. • Anomalias congênitas.

Cão Adulto (>12 meses de vida)
• Artropatia degenerativa (displasia coxofemoral).
• Doença do ligamento cruzado. • Avulsão do tendão extensor longo dos dedos. • Neoplasia de tecidos moles ou ósseos — primária; metastática.
• Traumatismo — tecido mole; osso; articulação.
• Panosteíte. • Poliartropatias. • Polimiosite.
• Polineurite.

FATORES DE RISCO
Raça (porte), sobrepeso (ou seja, peso acima do ideal) e atividade vigorosa.

DIAGNÓSTICO

DIAGNÓSTICO DIFERENCIAL
É imprescindível diferenciar causas musculoesqueléticas de causas neurogênicas e metabólicas.

HEMOGRAMA/BIOQUÍMICA/URINÁLISE
A lesão muscular eleva os níveis de creatina fosfoquinase.

OUTROS TESTES LABORATORIAIS
Dependem da causa sob suspeita.

DIAGNÓSTICO POR IMAGEM
• Radiografias — é recomendável a obtenção de duas projeções da região de interesse.
• TC, RM e cintilografia nuclear quando convenientes.

MÉTODOS DIAGNÓSTICOS
• Exame citológico do líquido articular — identificar e diferenciar doença intra-articular.
• EMG — diferençar doença neuromuscular crônica de musculosquelética.
• Biopsia de músculo e/ou de nervo — revela e identifica doença neuromuscular.

TRATAMENTO
Depende da causa subjacente.

MEDICAÇÕES

MEDICAMENTO(S) DE ESCOLHA
• Analgésicos e AINEs — minimizam a dor e diminuem a inflamação; meloxicam (dose de ataque de 0,2 mg/kg VO e, depois, 0,1 mg/kg diariamente VO — na forma líquida), carprofeno (2,2 mg/kg VO a cada 12 h), etodolaco (10-15 mg/kg VO a cada 24 h), deracoxibe (3-4 mg/kg VO a cada 24 h — mastigável) por 7 dias no pós-operatório.
• Corticosteroides — utilizar de modo criterioso, em virtude dos efeitos colaterais a longo prazo e do dano à cartilagem articular.

PRECAUÇÕES
AINEs — a irritação gastrintestinal pode impedir o uso em alguns pacientes.

MEDICAMENTO(S) ALTERNATIVO(S)
Medicamentos condroprotetores (p. ex., glicosaminoglicanos polissulfatados, glicosamina e sulfato de condroitina) — podem ser benéficos para limitar o dano à cartilagem e favorecer a regeneração.

ACOMPANHAMENTO

MONITORIZAÇÃO DO PACIENTE
Depende da causa subjacente.

DIVERSOS

VER TAMBÉM
Capítulos que tratem de distúrbios musculoesqueléticos e neuromusculares.

ABREVIATURA(S)
• AINEs = anti-inflamatórios não esteroides.
• EMG = eletromiografia.
• RM = ressonância magnética.
• TC = tomografia computadorizada.

Sugestões de Leitura
Brinker WO, Piermattei DL, Flo GL. Physical examination for lameness. In: Handbook of Small Animal Orthopedics and Fracture Repair, 3rd ed. Philadelphia: Saunders, 1997, pp. 228-230.

Autor Peter K. Shires
Consultor Editorial Peter K. Shires
Agradecimento O autor e os editores agradecem as colaborações de Peter D. Schwarz, que foi o autor deste capítulo em uma edição mais antiga.

Coagulação Intravascular Disseminada

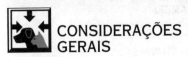

CONSIDERAÇÕES GERAIS

DEFINIÇÃO
Defeito hemostático complexo com acentuação nos processos de coagulação e fibrinólise, secundárias à doença sistêmica grave.

FISIOPATOLOGIA
- A CID começa com um estado hipercoagulável, que leva à formação de microtrombos em muitos vasos de pequeno calibre.
- Diversos distúrbios desencadeiam essa alteração por meio de dois mecanismos principais: (1) aumento maciço do fator tecidual que ativa a via extrínseca de coagulação e/ou (2) dano endotelial disseminado.
- O dano ao endotélio promove a geração de trombina, o que produz a ativação da via intrínseca de coagulação por *feedback* e converte o fibrinogênio em fibrina. Na sequência, ocorre oclusão vascular.
- As plaquetas e os leucócitos contribuem para esses dois mecanismos. Os fagócitos mononucleares expressam grandes quantidades do fator tecidual e produzem TNFα pró-inflamatório; esse mediador, por sua vez, ativa o endotélio. Os neutrófilos e as plaquetas liberam citocinas que ativam o endotélio e provocam agregação, contribuindo para a oclusão vascular e promovendo a inflamação.
- O depósito disseminado de fibrina (microtrombos) consome os fatores de coagulação e as plaquetas, ao mesmo tempo em que desencadeia uma fibrinólise descontrolada. Os subprodutos da fibrinólise (produtos de degradação da fibrina) possuem propriedades anticoagulantes e reduzem a função plaquetária. Ocorre hemorragia em diversos locais.
- A evolução descontrolada leva à hipoxia tecidual disseminada, falência múltipla de órgãos e morte.

SISTEMA(S) ACOMETIDO(S)
Multissistêmico.

GENÉTICA
N/D.

INCIDÊNCIA/PREVALÊNCIA
Associada à doença sistêmica grave, muitas vezes nos estágios terminais.

DISTRIBUIÇÃO GEOGRÁFICA
N/D.

IDENTIFICAÇÃO
Espécies
Cães e gatos, porém é mais diagnosticada na primeira espécie.

Raça(s) Predominante(s)
Nenhuma.

Idade Média e Faixa Etária
Dependem da doença primária.

Sexo Predominante
Nenhum.

SINAIS CLÍNICOS
- Variam com a doença primária e com a disfunção orgânica associada à CID.
- Petéquias e sangramento a partir dos locais de venopunção, bem como em mucosas ou nas cavidades corporais.
- O sangramento é frequente em gatos, levando possivelmente a um subdiagnóstico.

CAUSAS
- Dilatação-vólvulo gástrica.
- Insuficiência cardíaca.
- Dirofilariose.
- Intermação/insolação.
- Hemólise, especialmente imunomediada.
- Gastrenterite hemorrágica.
- Doenças infecciosas sistêmicas (sobretudo endotoxemia).
- Inflamação grave — independentemente da causa subjacente.
- Hepatopatia, se grave (p. ex., hepatite infecciosa canina, toxicidade do xilitol em cães; lipidose em gatos).
- Processos malignos, particularmente hemangiossarcoma, carcinoma mamário e adenocarcinoma pulmonar em cães e linfoma em gatos.
- Síndrome nefrótica.
- Pancreatite.
- Choque, hipoxia, acidose.
- Trombocitopenia, principalmente imunomediada.
- Incompatibilidade na transfusão.
- Traumatismo.
- Veneno.

FATORES DE RISCO
Variam de acordo com a causa.

DIAGNÓSTICO

DIAGNÓSTICO DIFERENCIAL
- Diferenciais-chave: trombocitopenia imunomediada, toxicidade de anticoagulantes, deficiência dos fatores de coagulação, paraproteinemia.
- Suspeitar de CID sempre que a anormalidade de trombocitopenia e os testes de coagulação prolongados forem observados concomitantemente.
- Padrão diagnóstico altamente variável, incluindo trombocitopenia, testes de coagulação prolongados (TP, TTPA), diminuição do fibrinogênio e da antitrombina III, além de aumento da fibrinólise (produtos de degradação da fibrina, D-dímeros). O encontro de no mínimo três alterações em animais acometidos por algum distúrbio predisponente (ver a seção "Causas") é considerado diagnóstico.
- A insuficiência hepática pode mimetizar o padrão da CID. É comum a produção reduzida dos fatores de coagulação. O declínio na depuração dos subprodutos normais de lise da fibrina e do fibrinogênio pode aumentar os valores dos produtos de degradação da fibrina. Também pode ser observada uma leve trombocitopenia idiopática. É rara a ocorrência de sangramento espontâneo a menos que o quadro de CID esteja presente.

HEMOGRAMA/BIOQUÍMICA/URINÁLISE
- Leucograma de estresse e/ou inflamatório.
- Trombocitopenia; a constatação de macroplaquetas em cães indica o aumento na produção dessas células.
- É possível a presença de anemia. A fragmentação eritrocitária (esquistócitos) é um achado que corrobora com o quadro.
- Alterações bioquímicas refletem os órgãos acometidos.

OUTROS TESTES LABORATORIAIS
- Testes de coagulação prolongados (TP, TTPA); o TTPA é mais sensível.
- Hipofibrinogenemia, embora o aumento inflamatório possa mascarar o consumo.
- Aumento dos produtos de degradação da fibrina e D-dímeros. Os D-dímeros são muito sensíveis; dessa forma, se estiverem baixos ou negativos, será improvável o quadro de CID. Nenhum teste isolado é específico o suficiente para o diagnóstico de CID.
- Diminuição da antitrombina III; pode ser um reagente positivo de fase aguda em gatos, mascarando o consumo.
- Segundo relatos, a tromboelastografia identifica os estados hiper e hipocoaguláveis em casos de CID. A taxa de óbito dos casos é significativamente mais alta no estado hipocoagulável.

DIAGNÓSTICO POR IMAGEM
N/D.

MÉTODOS DIAGNÓSTICOS
Nenhum.

ACHADOS PATOLÓGICOS
- Em geral, relacionam-se com a doença primária ou com os órgãos afetados pela CID.
- As petéquias são comuns.

TRATAMENTO

CUIDADO(S) DE SAÚDE ADEQUADO(S)
- Requer tratamento intensivo com internação.
- É essencial o tratamento rigoroso da doença primária.

CUIDADO(S) DE ENFERMAGEM
- Manter a perfusão e a oxigenação teciduais com o uso de fluidos, transfusões e oxigenoterapia.
- Repor os fatores de coagulação depletados por meio de transfusões de sangue/plasma.
- Evitar outras tromboses.

ATIVIDADE
Será restrita em função da gravidade da doença.

DIETA
N/D.

ORIENTAÇÃO AO PROPRIETÁRIO
Informar o proprietário sobre a natureza potencialmente letal dos processos associados.

CONSIDERAÇÕES CIRÚRGICAS
Relacionadas com a doença primária.

MEDICAÇÕES

MEDICAMENTO(S) DE ESCOLHA
- Os protocolos medicamentosos bem-sucedidos basicamente não são publicados ou não têm comprovação científica e tradicionalmente consistem no uso de heparina até a obtenção do efeito desejado (avaliado pela melhora clínica do paciente e pelos resultados dos exames).
- A heparina liga-se à antitrombina-III, potencializando a ação desse inibidor da coagulação. Para que a heparina seja eficaz, com frequência há necessidade de transfusões de plasma ou sangue para repor a antitrombina-III.
- A dose da heparina depende da gravidade dos sinais clínicos e das alterações laboratoriais.
- Doença leve a moderada: heparina na dose de 5-200 U/kg SC a cada 8 h ou IV (a cada 8 h ou sob infusão contínua).

Coagulação Intravascular Disseminada

• Doença grave: heparina na dose de 300-1.000 U/kg SC a cada 8 h ou IV (a cada 8 h ou sob infusão contínua).

CONTRAINDICAÇÕES
Não é recomendável o uso de inibidores da fibrinólise, pois esse processo é importante na remoção dos trombos.

PRECAUÇÕES
• Altas doses de heparina podem causar hemorragia fatal.
• Ficar atento quanto à ocorrência de super-hidratação em casos de comprometimento renal ou pulmonar.
• Os corticosteroides diminuem a função de fagócitos mononucleares, retardando possivelmente a remoção dos fatores de coagulação ativados e dos produtos de degradação da fibrina. Evitar o uso prolongado.

INTERAÇÕES POSSÍVEIS
Nenhuma.

MEDICAMENTO(S) ALTERNATIVO(S)
Heparina de baixo peso molecular: há muitas formulações disponíveis com atividade variável. Embora haja relatos de menos complicações, esse produto é muito caro. A maioria das informações não foi publicada ou não tem comprovação científica.

ACOMPANHAMENTO

MONITORIZAÇÃO DO PACIENTE
• A melhora clínica e a interrupção do sangramento são indicações de uma resposta positiva ao tratamento.

• É justificável a realização de testes diários em casos graves para identificar tendências positivas ou negativas. A execução de testes com menos frequência pode ser suficiente em casos mais leves.
• Os tempos de coagulação e os níveis de fibrinogênio frequentemente retornam ao normal com mais rapidez do que os produtos de degradação da fibrina e as contagens de plaquetas.

PREVENÇÃO
Relacionada com a doença primária.

EVOLUÇÃO ESPERADA E PROGNÓSTICO
Em virtude da natureza grave das doenças primárias, esses animais apresentam alto índice de mortalidade. Os índices de mortalidade para os cães variam de 50 a 77%, enquanto para os gatos podem ser >90%.

DIVERSOS

DISTÚRBIOS ASSOCIADOS
Ver a seção "Causas".

FATORES RELACIONADOS COM A IDADE
N/D.

POTENCIAL ZOONÓTICO
Nenhum.

GESTAÇÃO/FERTILIDADE/REPRODUÇÃO
Ao contrário dos seres humanos, as complicações obstétricas não constituem uma causa comum em cães e gatos.

SINÔNIMO(S)
• Coagulopatia de consumo.
• CID.

VER TAMBÉM
• Deficiência dos Fatores de Coagulação.
• Trombocitopenia.

ABREVIATURA(S)
• CID = coagulação intravascular disseminada.
• TP = tempo de protrombina.
• TTPA = tempo de tromboplastina parcial ativada.
• TNF = fator de necrose tumoral.

Sugestões de Leitura
Estrin MA, Wehausen CE, Jessen CR, Lee JA. Disseminated intravascular coagulation in cats. J Vet InternMed 2006, 20:1334-1339.

Feldman BF, Kirby R, Caldin M. Recognition and treatment of disseminated intravascular coagulation. In: Bonagura JD, ed., Current Veterinary Therapy XIII. Philadelphia: Saunders, 2000, pp. 190-194.

Thomason JD, Calvert CA, Greene CE. DIC: Diagnosis and treating a complex disorder. Vet Med 2005, 100:670-678.

Winberg B, Jensen AL, Johansson PI, Rozanski E, Tranholm M, Kristensen AT. Thromboelastographic evaluation of hemostatic function in dogs with disseminated intravascular coagulation. J Vet Intern Med 2008, 22:357-365.

Autor John A. Christian
Consultor Editorial A.H. Rebar

COAGULOPATIA POR HEPATOPATIA

CONSIDERAÇÕES GERAIS

REVISÃO
• O fígado representa o principal ou único local de síntese dos fatores de coagulação, bem como das proteínas anticoagulantes e fibrinolíticas, exceto os fatores V, VIII, FvW, FT e APt. • Apesar dos defeitos hemostáticos mensuráveis, poucos pacientes exibem sangramento espontâneo. • Causas: (1) síntese ou ativação reduzida de fatores/proteínas; deficiência da vitamina K, (2) disfibrinogenemia associada à polimerização anormal da fibrina, (3) alta concentração de produtos de degradação da fibrina e de anticoagulantes, (4) trombocitopenia ou trombocitopatia, (5) fibrinólise acentuada.
• Deficiência da vitamina K — ligada à colestase intra ou extra-hepática grave ou esteatorreia ou administração prolongada de antibióticos orais.

IDENTIFICAÇÃO
Cães e gatos de qualquer idade, raça ou sexo.

SINAIS CLÍNICOS
• Muitas vezes, não há sinais clínicos evidentes de sangramento. • Melena; hematêmese; hematoquezia; hematúria. • Sangramento prolongado se provocado por venopunção, cistocentese, biopsia, feridas cirúrgicas.
• Contusões/equimoses ou hematomas espontâneos — raros a menos que haja uma deficiência grave de vitamina K_1 ou CID fulminante.

CAUSAS E FATORES DE RISCO
• Insuficiência hepática grave de qualquer etiologia. • Hepatopatia viral aguda. • OEHDB.
• Hepatopatia crônica — especialmente cirrose.
• Doença concomitante do intestino delgado (p. ex., em gatos com o complexo colangio-hepatite) predispõe o paciente à deficiência da vitamina K.
• AVPS: deficiência assintomática de fator e TTPA prolongado; raras tendências hemorrágicas.

DIAGNÓSTICO

DIAGNÓSTICO DIFERENCIAL
• Toxicidades — rodenticidas anticoagulantes, AINEs (lesões GI), causas de insuficiência hepática aguda (p. ex., ingestão de aflatoxina ou cicádea).
• Defeitos hemostáticos hereditários.
• Trombocitopenia. • CID — qualquer causa.
• Distúrbios gastrintestinais infiltrativos.
• Amiloidose hepática (deficiência de fatores, fraturas espontâneas de lobos hepáticos).
• Traumatismos abdominais.

HEMOGRAMA/BIOQUÍMICA/URINÁLISE
• Hemograma completo — pode permanecer normal; anemia regenerativa em casos de sangramento intenso (2-5 dias); microcitose em casos de desvio portossistêmico; trombocitopenia.
• Bioquímica — atividade elevada das enzimas hepáticas; bilirrubinemia; hipoalbuminemia; hipoglobulinemia; hipocolesterolemia. • Urinálise — hematúria; bilirrubinúria.

OUTROS TESTES LABORATORIAIS
Testes hemostáticos — trombocitopenia; prolongamento do TTPA (TCA), TP, TCT e PIAVK; níveis baixos do fibrinogênio e dos fatores de coagulação; níveis baixos dos fatores anticoagulantes (antitrombina, proteína C); elevação dos produtos de degradação da fibrina e de D-dímeros.

DIAGNÓSTICO POR IMAGEM
Ultrassonografia Abdominal
• Efusão (ascite, hemorragia). • As alterações hepáticas variam com os distúrbios. • Motilidade intestinal anormal, espessamento na área de sangramento (vasculopatia hipertensiva portal).

TRATAMENTO
• Não é necessário a menos que se planejem procedimentos invasivos ou se observe hemorragia espontânea. • Sangue total fresco — proporciona a reposição de hemácias, fatores de coagulação, plaquetas funcionais. • Plasma fresco congelado — também fornece fatores de coagulação e diminui o risco de sensibilização das hemácias ou sobrecarga por volume. • Crioprecipitado — em casos de hipofibrinogenemia grave ou sangramento intenso com doença de von Willebrand coexistente.
• Plasma rico em plaquetas — raramente indicado.

BIOPSIA
• Alto risco de sangramento — prolongamento no TCA, TTPA, TP ou PIAVK por volta de >50%; trombocitopenia <50.000/μL; ou tempo prolongado do sangramento de mucosas. • Hemorragia iatrogênica — prognóstico grave em casos de sangramento espontâneo, no qual não se conseguiu identificar a causa. • Suporte à hemostasia — para hemorragia subsequente ao procedimento. • Biopsia aspirativa guiada por ultrassom — risco mais elevado; observar o local por 15 minutos e, novamente, algumas horas após o procedimento. • Laparoscopia — possibilita a inspeção e a hemostasia (aplicação de cautério, Gelfoam® [gelatina absorvível]).
• Laparotomia — biopsia em cunha; pouco aconselhada em casos de sangramento evidente.

MEDICAÇÕES

MEDICAMENTO(S)
• Fornecer tratamento específico, bem como cuidado de suporte, com base na causa da hepatopatia.
• Deficiência da vitamina K — administração parenteral da vitamina K_1 (0,5-1,5 mg/kg a cada 12 h SC por até 3 doses em intervalo de 24 h); administração oral da vitamina K_1 (Mephyton®, 1 mg/kg a cada 24 h) se a absorção dos ácidos biliares intestinais estiver normal. • CID — corrigir a doença primária; considerar a heparina em casos de CID trombótica (heparina não fracionada: 200 U/kg a cada 6-12 h; ou heparina de baixo peso molecular [enoxaparina]: 1 mg/kg a cada 12-24 h), titular a dose com base no estado clínico e na monitorização laboratorial (TCA, TTPa [heparina não fracionada], atividade anti-Xa da heparina [todas as heparinas]). • Produtos sanguíneos — sangue total fresco (hemácias, plaquetas, proteínas hemostáticas): 12-20 mL/kg a cada 24 h; plasma fresco congelado (todas as proteínas hemostáticas): 10-20 mL/kg a cada 12 h; criossobrenadante plasmático (albumina, fatores dependentes da vitamina K): 10-20 mL/kg a cada 12 h; crioprecipitado (fibrinogênio, FvW, fator VIII): 1 U/10 kg ou titular a dose até fazer efeito; plasma rico em plaquetas (plaquetas e proteínas hemostáticas): 6-10 mL/kg. • DDAVP — 0,5-1,0 μg/kg IV diluído em solução salina; pode aumentar os fatores de coagulação, encurtar o tempo de sangramento de mucosas e diminuir as tendências hemorrágicas; utilizado para sangramento induzido por biopsia; pode ser aplicado localmente para fazer efeito.

CONTRAINDICAÇÕES
• Transfusão de sangue total armazenado — pode provocar encefalopatia hepática. • Vitamina K_1 (gatos) — grandes quantidades causam hemólise por corpúsculos de Heinz e dano hepático oxidativo.
• Ácido acetilsalicílico ou outros AINEs — podem predispor o paciente à insuficiência renal, agravar ascite, provocar êmese e sangramento espontâneo.
• Transfusão de altos volumes de sangue em anticoagulantes à base de citrato (particularmente em animais com <5 kg) pode induzir à hipocalcemia sintomática. • Evitar procedimentos provocativos — p. ex., venopunção ou colocação de cateter nas veias jugulares, além de cistocentese, se houver tendências hemorrágicas identificadas.

ACOMPANHAMENTO

MONITORIZAÇÃO DO PACIENTE
• Teste otimizado do TP, PIAVK e fator VII — mais sensíveis para deficiência da vitamina K; se não houver melhora dentro de 48 h de injeção da vitamina K_1, será improvável que as aplicações subsequentes dessa vitamina sejam benéficas.
• Monitorizar a frequência cardíaca, a pressão arterial, a coloração e o preenchimento das mucosas, o volume globular (hematócrito) e os sólidos totais em caso de sangramento ativo. • Local de biopsia — observação imediata e sequencial (ultrassonografia) em busca de evidências de hemorragia. • Amostra de efusão abdominal — para determinar a presença de hemorragia ou ascite.

PREVENÇÃO
• Dieta bem balanceada, repleta de vitaminas.
• Considerar a possibilidade de comprometimento à disponibilidade ou à síntese da vitamina K, ocasionados por antibioticoterapia oral crônica.
• Procedimentos invasivos — prever o sangramento; ficar preparado para a terapia com transfusão; tratar o paciente previamente com a vitamina K_1; administrar o DDAVP dentro de 20 min do procedimento previsto de biopsia ou se houver a persistência de tendências hemorrágicas apesar da terapia com a vitamina K_1; administrar plasma fresco congelado como o tratamento definitivo; a repetição da DDAVP não é de praxe.
• Eliminar o parasitismo intestinal.

COMPLICAÇÕES POSSÍVEIS
Hemorragia, anemia, hipovolemia, encefalopatia hepática.

EVOLUÇÃO ESPERADA E PROGNÓSTICO
Hemorragia espontânea, coagulopatia refratária e CID — prognóstico mau.

DIVERSOS

ABREVIATURA(S)
• AINEs = anti-inflamatórios não esteroides. • APt = ativador do plasminogênio tecidual. • AVPS = anomalia vascular portossistêmica. • CID = coagulação intravascular disseminada. • DDAVP = 1-desamino-8-D-arginina vasopressina. • FT = fator tecidual. • FvW = fator de von Willebrand.
• OEHDB = obstrução extra-hepática do ducto biliar. • PIAVK = proteínas invocadas pela ausência ou antagonismo da vitamina K. • TCA = tempo de coagulação ativada. • TCT = tempo de coagulação da trombina. • TP = tempo de protrombina.
• TTPA = tempo de tromboplastina parcial ativada.

Autor Marjory Brooks

COCCIDIOIDOMICOSE

CONSIDERAÇÕES GERAIS

DEFINIÇÃO
Micose sistêmica causada pela inalação de artroconídios infectantes do fungo *Coccidioides immitis* oriundo do solo.

FISIOPATOLOGIA
• A inalação de artroconídios infectantes representa a via primária de infecção. Podem-se observar os sinais de febre, letargia, inapetência, tosse e artralgia ou rigidez articular. A disseminação pode ocorrer 10 dias após a exposição, resultando em sinais relacionados com o sistema orgânico envolvido. Podem ocorrer infecções assintomáticas, e alguns animais desenvolvem imunidade sem demonstrar sinais clínicos.
• As lesões cutâneas costumam estar associadas à disseminação, mas há relatos raros de feridas penetrantes relacionadas com essas lesões.
• A inalação de uma quantidade inferior a 10 artrósporos é suficiente para causar a doença em animais suscetíveis. O termo "suscetível" refere-se aos animais que sofrem uma disseminação extrapulmonar. Os sinais de disseminação podem não ficar evidentes por alguns meses após a infecção inicial.

SISTEMA(S) ACOMETIDO(S)
• Respiratório — o local de infecção inicial.
• Pode ocorrer a disseminação extrapulmonar em ossos longos e articulações, olhos, pele, fígado, rins, SNC, sistema cardiovascular (pericárdio e miocárdio) e testículos.

INCIDÊNCIA/PREVALÊNCIA
Não é uma doença rara em áreas endêmicas, mas é rara em áreas não endêmicas. Ocorre com maior frequência em cães, mas raramente em gatos.

DISTRIBUIÇÃO GEOGRÁFICA
O *Coccidioides immitis* é encontrado no sudoeste dos Estados Unidos, na região geográfica mais baixa do deserto de Sonora. É mais comum no sul da Califórnia, no Arizona e no sudoeste do Texas, porém menos prevalente no Novo México, em Nevada e em Utah.

IDENTIFICAÇÃO
Espécies
Cães e gatos.

Raça(s) Predominante(s)
Nenhuma.

Idade Média e Faixa Etária
Embora seja diagnosticada com maior frequência em animais jovens (<4 anos de idade), é observada em animais de todas as idades.

Sexo Predominante
Nenhum.

SINAIS CLÍNICOS
Achados Anamnésicos
• Anorexia.
• Tosse.
• Febre irresponsiva a antibióticos.
• Claudicação.
• Fraqueza, paraparesia, dor na coluna vertebral e no pescoço (dorsalgia e cervicalgia).
• Crises convulsivas.
• Alterações visuais.
• Perda de peso.

Achados do Exame Físico
Cães
Sinais com Envolvimento Pulmonar
• Tosse.
• Dispneia.
• Febre.

Sinais na Doença Disseminada
• Tumefação óssea, aumento de volume articular e claudicação.
• Caquexia.
• Letargia.
• Linfadenomegalia.
• Disfunção neurológica, incluindo crises convulsivas, causada pela disseminação ao sistema nervoso tanto central como periférico.
• Úlceras cutâneas e trajetos fistulosos drenantes.
• Uveíte, ceratite, irite.

Gatos
• Caquexia.
• Lesões cutâneas drenantes.
• Dispneia.
• Claudicação causada por envolvimento ósseo.
• Uveíte.

CAUSAS
O *Coccidioides immitis* cresce a muitos centímetros de profundidade no solo, local onde esse fungo sobrevive a altas temperaturas ambientais e a baixa umidade. Após um período de chuvas, o microrganismo retorna à superfície do solo, onde sofre esporulação, liberando muitos artroconídios, que são disseminados pelo vento ou por tempestades de poeira.

FATORES DE RISCO
• O farejamento ativo do solo e da vegetação rasteira pode expor os animais suscetíveis a amplas doses do fungo em solos contaminados.
• Tempestades de poeira após as estações chuvosas.
• Após terremotos, observa-se um aumento na incidência.
• As explorações agrícolas em locais onde ocorrem muita rachadura e destruição do solo podem levar a um aumento na exposição.

DIAGNÓSTICO

DIAGNÓSTICO DIFERENCIAL
• As lesões pulmonares podem lembrar as de outras micoses sistêmicas (p. ex., histoplasmose e blastomicose).
• Em casos de linfoma, outras micoses sistêmicas e infecções bacterianas localizadas, pode-se observar linfadenomegalia.
• As lesões ósseas podem se assemelhar àquelas causadas por tumores ósseos primários ou metastáticos ou osteomielite bacteriana.
• É imprescindível diferenciar as lesões cutâneas de abscessos comuns ou de outros processos patológicos bacterianos.
• Diferenciais de crises convulsivas, incluindo etiologias inflamatórias e oncológicas.

HEMOGRAMA/BIOQUÍMICA/URINÁLISE
• Hemograma — leve anemia arregenerativa, leucocitose neutrofílica, monocitose.
• Perfil bioquímico sérico — hiperglobulinemia, hipoalbuminemia, azotemia em casos de envolvimento renal.
• Urinálise — densidade urinária baixa e proteinúria em casos de glomerulonefrite inflamatória.

OUTROS TESTES LABORATORIAIS
Os testes sorológicos em busca dos anticorpos contra o *C. immitis* em laboratório especializado podem fornecer o diagnóstico presuntivo e auxiliar na monitorização da resposta à terapia.

DIAGNÓSTICO POR IMAGEM
As radiografias dos pulmões (infiltrados intersticiais) e de lesões ósseas (osteólise) podem ajudar no diagnóstico. A RM do cérebro é útil no diagnóstico de granulomas formados no SNC.

MÉTODOS DIAGNÓSTICOS
• Teste sorológico; repetir a mensuração dos títulos séricos em 4-6 semanas quando títulos baixos forem acompanhados por sinais clínicos. A identificação microscópica da forma ampla de esférula do *C. immitis* em lesões ou materiais de biopsia constitui o método definitivo de diagnóstico. Em alguns pacientes, os aspirados de linfonodos e os esfregaços por impressão (decalque) de lesões cutâneas ou exsudatos drenantes podem recuperar os microrganismos.
• É preciso ter cuidado ao se efetuar a cultura de lesões drenantes com suspeita de infecção pelo *C. immitis*, já que a forma micelial é altamente contagiosa. As culturas devem ser feitas por pessoas treinadas, utilizando-se máscaras e gorros protetores.
• Para evitar os resultados falso-negativos, prefere-se muitas vezes a biopsia de tecido infectado. Os tecidos envolvidos, no entanto, podem não estar facilmente acessíveis; nesse caso, o teste sorológico representa a abordagem mais racional e coerente.

ACHADOS PATOLÓGICOS
• Inflamação granulomatosa, supurativa ou piogranulomatosa, presente em muitos tecidos.
• Presença de esférulas características nos tecidos acometidos. Em alguns pacientes, a quantidade de esférulas pode ser pequena.

TRATAMENTO

CUIDADO(S) DE SAÚDE ADEQUADO(S)
• Em geral, o tratamento é feito em um esquema ambulatorial.
• Os sinais clínicos concomitantes (p. ex., crises convulsivas, dor e tosse) devem ser tratados de forma apropriada.

ATIVIDADE
Restringir a atividade física até que os sinais clínicos comecem a diminuir.

DIETA
Fornecer uma dieta palatável de alta qualidade para manter o peso corporal.

ORIENTAÇÃO AO PROPRIETÁRIO
É preciso rever a necessidade e o custo da terapia a longo prazo para uma doença grave com a possibilidade de falha terapêutica. Além disso, o proprietário deve estar ciente dos possíveis efeitos colaterais dos medicamentos utilizados.

CONSIDERAÇÕES CIRÚRGICAS
Em casos de envolvimento granulomatoso focal de órgãos (p. ex., lobos pulmonares consolidados, olhos e rins), pode-se indicar a remoção cirúrgica do órgão acometido.

COCCIDIOIDOMICOSE

MEDICAÇÕES

MEDICAMENTO(S) DE ESCOLHA
A coccidioidomicose é considerada uma das micoses sistêmicas de maior gravidade e maior risco de vida. Com frequência, o tratamento da doença disseminada requer no mínimo um ano de terapia antifúngica rigorosa.

Cães
• Atualmente, há diversos medicamentos orais disponíveis pertencentes à família azólica para o tratamento das coccidioidomicoses.
• Fluconazol — 5 mg/kg VO a cada 12 h; com esse medicamento, observa-se um aumento notável no sucesso terapêutico. Os neurologistas recomendam 10 mg/kg para reforçar a penetração desse antifúngico em casos de infecções neurológicas. O custo desse medicamento foi significativamente reduzido com a disponibilidade de genéricos. Foram observadas falhas terapêuticas com o uso de formulações manipuladas.
• Cetoconazol — 5-10 mg/kg VO a cada 12 h. Pode ser administrado juntamente com alimento: alguns acreditam que a coadministração de altas doses de vitamina C possa aumentar a absorção desse agente. O tratamento deve prosseguir por 1 ano.
• Itraconazol — 5 mg/kg VO a cada 12 h, sendo administrado da mesma forma que o cetoconazol. Há relatos de uma taxa de penetração mais acentuada quando comparado com o cetoconazol, mas ainda não se observou uma resposta clínica mais satisfatória.
• Anfotericina B — raramente recomendada, em função do alto risco de dano renal e da disponibilidade de medicamentos orais eficazes. Esse antifúngico pode ser administrado a 0,5 mg/kg IV (como infusão lenta [em cães gravemente doentes] ou em bólus rápido [em cães razoavelmente saudáveis]) 3 vezes por semana, na dose total cumulativa de 8-10 mg/kg. No caso de infusão lenta, acrescentar a anfotericina B em 250-500 mL de solução de glicose a 5% e administrar sob a forma de gotejamento em um período de 4-6 h. Na aplicação em bólus rápido, adicionar a anfotericina B a 30 mL de solução de glicose a 5% e administrar durante um período de 5 minutos por meio de cateter tipo borboleta. Para diminuir os efeitos renais adversos da anfotericina B, fornecer a solução de NaCl a 0,9% (2 mL/kg/h) durante algumas horas antes de iniciar a terapia antifúngica com esse agente.

Gatos
• Pode-se empregar qualquer um dos antifúngicos azólicos expostos a seguir:
• Cetoconazol — dose total de 50 mg VO a cada 12 h.
• Fluconazol — dose total de 25-50 mg VO a cada 12 h.
• Itraconazol — dose total de 25-50 mg VO a cada 12 h.

CONTRAINDICAÇÕES
• Não é recomendável a administração de medicamentos que sofrem metabolização hepática primária juntamente com o cetoconazol.
• Também não é aconselhável a administração de medicamentos que sofrem metabolização renal primária juntamente com a anfotericina B.

PRECAUÇÕES
• Os efeitos colaterais dos agentes azólicos incluem: inapetência, vômito e hepatotoxicidade. Os medicamentos podem ser interrompidos até a diminuição dos sinais clínicos e reinstituídos em seguida com uma dose mais baixa, que poderá ser lentamente aumentada até a dose recomendada se o animal se mostrar tolerante ao agente. Os antifúngicos azólicos mais recentes (itraconazol e fluconazol) apresentam menos efeitos colaterais.
• Os efeitos colaterais da terapia com a anfotericina B podem ser graves, incluindo disfunção renal, febre, inapetência, vômito e flebite.

ACOMPANHAMENTO

MONITORIZAÇÃO DO PACIENTE
• É recomendável monitorar os títulos séricos a cada 3-4 meses. Os animais devem ser tratados até que seus títulos declinem para <1:4. Os pacientes que exibir uma resposta insatisfatória à terapia devem ser submetidos à mensuração dos níveis plasmáticos do medicamento 2-4 h após sua administração para garantir a absorção medicamentosa adequada.
• Em todos os animais tratados com a anfotericina B, devem-se monitorar a ureia e a urinálise. Se o nível de ureia estiver superior a 50 mg/dL ou caso se observem cilindros granulosos na urina, o tratamento deverá ser temporariamente interrompido.

PREVENÇÃO
• Não há vacina disponível para cães nem para gatos.
• É imprescindível evitar o contato com solos contaminados em áreas endêmicas, particularmente durante tempestades de poeira após as estações chuvosas.

COMPLICAÇÕES POSSÍVEIS
• A pneumopatia que resulta em tosse grave pode se agravar temporariamente após a instituição da terapia, por conta da inflamação nos pulmões. Para o alívio dos sinais respiratórios, poderá ser necessário o uso de prednisona e antitussígenos orais em doses baixas e períodos breves.
• A terapia com o cetoconazol pode resultar em hepatotoxicidade.
• A terapia com a anfotericina B pode culminar em nefrotoxicidade.

EVOLUÇÃO ESPERADA E PROGNÓSTICO
• O prognóstico é reservado a grave. Muitos cães exibirão uma melhora após a terapia oral; entretanto, podem-se observar recidivas, especialmente se a terapia for abreviada. Estima-se uma taxa de recuperação global de 60%, mas alguns autores relatam uma resposta de 90% à terapia com o fluconazol.
• O prognóstico em gatos ainda não está bem registrado, mas deve-se prever uma disseminação rápida que exija terapia a longo prazo.
• Para monitorizar a possibilidade de recidiva, recomenda-se o teste sorológico a cada 3-4 meses após o término da terapia.
• A recuperação espontânea da coccidioidomicose disseminada sem tratamento é extremamente rara.

DIVERSOS

POTENCIAL ZOONÓTICO
• A forma de esférula do fungo, conforme encontrada nos tecidos animais, não é diretamente transmissível a pessoas ou outros animais.
• Sob certas circunstâncias raras, no entanto, pode haver a reversão para o crescimento da forma fúngica infectante de bolor sob ou sobre as bandagens aplicadas em lesões drenantes ou em camas contaminadas. As lesões drenantes podem levar à contaminação do ambiente com artrósporos. É preciso ter cuidado ao manipular uma lesão drenante infectada.
• É fundamental adotar medidas especiais em ambientes domésticos de proprietários que possam estar imunossuprimidos.

GESTAÇÃO/FERTILIDADE/REPRODUÇÃO
• O cetoconazol deve ser utilizado em animais prenhes apenas se o benefício justificar o risco potencial à ninhada.
• Já foram identificados efeitos teratogênicos.

SINÔNIMO(S)
• Febre do Vale do São Joaquim.
• Febre do Vale.
• Reumatismo do Deserto (em seres humanos).

ABREVIATURA(S)
• RM = ressonância magnética.
• SNC = sistema nervoso central.

Sugestões de Leitura
Armstrong PJ, DiBartola SP. Canine coccidioidomycosis: a literature review and report of eight cases. J Am Anim Hosp Assoc 1983;19:937-945.
Greene RT. Coccidioidomycosis. In: Greene CE, ed. Infectious diseases of the dog and cat. 2nd ed. Philadelphia: Saunders, 1998:391-398.
Legendre AM. Coccidioidomycosis. In: Sherding RG, ed. The cat: diseases and clinical management. 2nd ed. New York: Churchill Livingstone, 1994:561.

Autor Nita Kay Gulbas
Consultor Editorial Stephen C. Barr

COCCIDIOSE

CONSIDERAÇÕES GERAIS

REVISÃO
- Infecção intestinal, tradicionalmente associada a *Isospora canis* (cães) e *Isospora felis* (gatos) como patógenos potenciais; outras espécies de *Isospora* também podem estar presentes.
- Estritamente específica ao hospedeiro (i. e., não há transmissão cruzada).
- As espécies de *Eimeria* não são agentes parasitários para cães ou gatos.
- O *Toxoplasma gondii* em gatos e o *Cryptosporidium parvum* em neonatos caninos e felinos são coccídios em um sentido não tradicional.
- A infecção pelo *Toxoplasma* em gatos pode gerar sinais clínicos semelhantes aos das infecções pelo *Isospora*; os oocistos eliminados no ambiente têm o potencial de ocasionar um problema de saúde pública.
- O *Cryptosporidium* ainda está sendo avaliado como agente de coccidiose aguda potencialmente letal (criptosporidiose) de neonatos caninos e felinos.
- Diarreia aquosa abundante é característica; em casos de criptosporidiose, a autoinfecção e a reciclagem contínua no interior do trato intestinal resultam em perda rápida do revestimento da mucosa.

IDENTIFICAÇÃO
Cães e gatos (especialmente os filhotes de ambas as espécies).

SINAIS CLÍNICOS
- Diarreia aquosa a mucoide, algumas vezes com manchas de sangue.
- Fraqueza de filhotes caninos e felinos.
- Animais imunocomprometidos.

CAUSAS E FATORES DE RISCO
- Cães ou gatos infectados que contaminam o ambiente com oocistos de *Isospora* spp. ou *Cryptosporidium*.
- Estresse.

DIAGNÓSTICO

DIAGNÓSTICO DIFERENCIAL
Viroses entéricas e outros parasitas intestinais.

HEMOGRAMA/BIOQUÍMICA/URINÁLISE
Em geral, permanecem normais; em caso de desidratação, pode haver hemoconcentração.

OUTROS TESTES LABORATORIAIS
N/D.

DIAGNÓSTICO POR IMAGEM
N/D.

MÉTODOS DIAGNÓSTICOS
- Exame coprológico (fecal) em busca de oocistos (diferenciar das espécies pseudoparasitárias de *Eimeria*); utilizar o método de flutuação em solução de sacarose (densidade: 1,27); sulfato de zinco (densidade: 1,18) ou corantes especiais como as colorações acidorresistentes para o *Cryptosporidium*.
- Os oocistos de *Isospora* devem ter 40 μm de comprimento, enquanto os cistos de *Cryptosporidium* têm aproximadamente 5 μm de diâmetro.

TRATAMENTO
- Em geral, o paciente é tratado em um esquema ambulatorial.
- Proceder à internação em animais debilitados.
- Fornecer fluidoterapia em casos de desidratação.

MEDICAÇÕES

MEDICAMENTO(S)
- Sulfadimetoxina — 55 mg/kg VO no primeiro dia, depois 25-50 mg/kg 1 vez ao dia por até 10-14 dias ou até o cão se apresentar assintomático quanto à presença de *Isospora* e o exame coprológico ficar negativo quanto aos oocistos.
- Sulfadiazina/trimetoprima — 15-30 mg/kg de sulfadiazina VO diariamente por até 10 dias; para toxoplasmose em gatos 15 mg/kg de sulfadiazina VO a cada 12 h por 28 dias.
- Amprólio (uso fora da indicação da bula) para a prevenção: cães, 30 mL de solução a 9,6% em 1 galão de água de bebida ou 1,25 g de pó a 20% na ração para alimentar quatro filhotes diariamente. Administrar como única fonte de alimento ou água por 7 dias antes de dar alta; as cadelas podem receber uma solução a 9,6% como única fonte de água 10 dias antes de dar à luz; ou para o tratamento: cães, 100 mg a cada 24 h VO por 7 dias; gatos com *Cystoisospora* 60-100 mg da dose total VO 1 vez ao dia por 7 dias.
- Não há nenhum tratamento eficaz ou aprovado contra o *Cryptosporidium*; sugere-se o emprego (fora da indicação da bula) da paromomicina na dose de 165 mg/kg a cada 12 h por 5 dias.
- Tilosina a 10-20 mg/kg VO a cada 12 h por 2-4 semanas.
- Clindamicina a 10 mg/kg VO a cada 12 h por 2-4 semanas para toxoplasmose.

PRECAUÇÕES
- Como acontece com a maioria dos antibióticos, pode-se observar um leve desarranjo gastrintestinal com o uso dos agentes antimicrobianos apresentados aqui.
- Amprólio — seu uso não é recomendável por mais de 12 dias em filhotes caninos; a administração exógena de tiamina em altas doses pode diminuir a eficácia desse medicamento; há relatos de sinais neurológicos em alguns cães — se observados, interromper a medicação e iniciar a suplementação de tiamina.
- Sulfadimetoxina — função renal ou hepática diminuída ou obstrução urinária.
- Sulfadiazina/trimetoprima — combinação potencialmente teratogênica; cão: ceratoconjuntivite seca irreversível, hipersensibilidade tipo 1 ou 3 (especialmente em cães de porte maior); gato: anorexia, leucopenia, anemia, hematúria.

CONTRAINDICAÇÕES
- Medicações à base de sulfa — doença hepática ou renal preexistente.

ACOMPANHAMENTO
Exame coprológico em busca de oocistos 1-2 semanas após o tratamento.

DIVERSOS

FATORES RELACIONADOS COM A IDADE
A doença é mais grave em pacientes jovens.

VER TAMBÉM
- Criptosporidiose.
- Toxoplasmose.

Sugestões de Leitura
Bowman DD, Hendrix CM, Lindsay DS, Barr SC. Feline Clinical Parasitology. Ames: Iowa State University Press, 2002, pp. 5-14.
Bowman DD, Lynn RC, Eberhard ML. Georgis' Parasitology for Veterinarians, 8th ed. St. Louis: Saunders (Elsevier Science), 2003, pp. 92-100.
Dubey JP, Greene CE, Little SE. In: Greene CE, ed., Infectious Diseases of the Dog and Cat, 3rd ed. St. Louis: Saunders Elsevier, 2006, pp. 667-669, 775-791.
Hall EJ, German AJ. In: Ettinger SJ, Feldman EC. Textbook of Veterinary Internal Medicine, 6th ed. St. Louis: Elsevier Saunders, 2005, pp. 1359-1360.
Plumb DC. Veterinary Drug Handbook, 6th ed. Ames, IA: Wiley-Blackwell, 2008.

Autor Gavin L. Olsen
Consultor Editorial Albert E. Jergens

COLAPSO DA TRAQUEIA

CONSIDERAÇÕES GERAIS

DEFINIÇÃO
• Redução dinâmica no diâmetro luminal das vias aéreas calibrosas com a respiração.
• Pode envolver as porções cervical ou intratorácica da traqueia ou ambos os segmentos.
• Broncomalacia é o termo utilizado para se referir ao colapso dos brônquios lobares e das vias aéreas menos calibrosas, o que pode ser observado em conjunto com colapso da traqueia (traqueobroncomalacia) ou sozinho.
• Compressão da traqueia ou dos brônquios como resultado de linfadenopatia hilar ou lesões expansivas externas — não é considerada parte dessa condição.

FISIOPATOLOGIA
• Em alguns cães, identifica-se uma cartilagem traqueal hipocelular na região cervical em termos históricos. • A falta de sulfato de condroitina e/ou a redução das glicoproteínas dentro da matriz cartilaginosa resulta no declínio na ligação de água e perda da turgidez na cartilagem.
• Alternativamente, as anormalidades da cartilagem podem representar defeitos na condrogênese associados a influências genéticas, deficiências nutricionais ou alterações degenerativas causadas por doença crônica das vias aéreas. • Colapso — a cartilagem fraca confere o achatamento da estrutura do anel traqueal; ocorre o colapso da traqueia em uma direção dorsoventral quando há mudança nas pressões no lúmen das vias aéreas. Durante a inspiração, a pressão intrapleural fica mais negativa, levando a uma queda na pressão dentro das vias aéreas. A pressão atmosférica excede a pressão aérea na região cervical e a falta de sustentação da cartilagem resulta em colapso da porção cervical da traqueia. Durante a expiração forçada, a pressão intrapleural fica positiva e excede a pressão dentro das vias aéreas torácicas. Quando as paredes cartilaginosas das vias aéreas são enfraquecidas por broncomalacia, observa-se o colapso das vias aéreas intratorácicas à expiração. • O aumento na tensão sobre o músculo dorsal da traqueia ou a atrofia neurogênica do músculo provoca o estiramento da membrana dorsal da traqueia com protrusão em direção ao lúmen das vias aéreas. • Tosse — o traumatismo mecânico à mucosa traqueal decorrente do colapso da membrana dorsal da traqueia exacerba o edema e a inflamação das vias aéreas. • A obstrução das vias aéreas superiores agrava os sinais clínicos, enquanto o aumento crônico no esforço respiratório pode levar a anormalidades secundárias na estrutura e na função da laringe. • O comprometimento das vias aéreas de pequeno calibre eleva o gradiente de pressão das vias aéreas e potencializa o colapso na região intratorácica.

SISTEMA(S) ACOMETIDO(S)
• Respiratório — irritação crônica das vias aéreas.
• Cardiovascular — hipertensão pulmonar.
• Nervoso — pode estar envolvido quando ocorre o desenvolvimento de síncope por hipoxia ou reflexo vasovagal associado à tosse.

GENÉTICA
Desconhecida.

INCIDÊNCIA/PREVALÊNCIA
Entidade clínica comum.

DISTRIBUIÇÃO GEOGRÁFICA
Mundial.

IDENTIFICAÇÃO
Espécies
Principalmente em cães, mas raras vezes em gatos.
Raça(s) Predominante(s)
Poodle miniatura, Yorkshire terrier, Chihuahua, Pomerânia, além de cães *toys* e outras raças de pequeno porte.
Idade Média e Faixa Etária
• Meia-idade a idosos — início dos sinais clínicos aos 4-14 anos de idade. • Animais gravemente acometidos com <1 ano de idade.

SINAIS CLÍNICOS
Achados Anamnésicos
• Agravados geralmente por excitação (agitação), calor, umidade, exercício ou obesidade. • Tosse seca estridente. • Pode ter histórico crônico de tosse intermitente ou dificuldade respiratória.
• Ânsia de vômito/vômito seco — observado com frequência em virtude das tentativas de remoção das secreções respiratórias da laringe. • Taquipneia, intolerância a exercícios e/ou angústia respiratória — comuns. • Cianose ou síncope — podem ser observadas em indivíduos gravemente acometidos.
Achados do Exame Físico
• Aumento na sensibilidade da traqueia — quase sempre é constatado. • Angústia respiratória — inspiratória em casos de colapso da porção cervical da traqueia; expiratória em casos de colapso das vias aéreas intratorácicas. • Ruídos traqueais sibilantes ou musicais à auscultação sobre a região de estreitamento da traqueia. • Estalido expiratório final — pode ser auscultado quando ocorre o colapso de amplos segmentos das vias aéreas intratorácicas durante a expiração forçada.
• Sibilos ou crepitações — indicativos de comprometimento concomitante das vias aéreas de pequeno calibre. • Sopros cardíacos por insuficiência da valva mitral — muitas vezes, são encontrados concomitantemente em cães de pequeno porte. • Frequência cardíaca normal a baixa e/ou arritmia respiratória acentuada.
• Segunda bulha cardíaca sonora — sugestiva de hipertensão pulmonar. • Hepatomegalia — causa desconhecida.

CAUSAS
• Etiologia desconhecida — suspeita de defeitos congênitos, nutricionais ou familiares de condrogênese.
• Sugere-se que a inflamação crônica das vias aéreas de pequeno calibre contribua para a broncomalacia, embora essa relação não esteja claramente estabelecida.

FATORES DE RISCO
• Obesidade.
• Infecção ou inflamação das vias aéreas.
• Obstrução das vias aéreas superiores.
• Entubação endotraqueal.

DIAGNÓSTICO

DIAGNÓSTICO DIFERENCIAL
• Traqueobronquite infecciosa. • Obstrução ou corpo estranho traqueal ou laríngeo. • Bronquite crônica. • Pneumonia — viral, bacteriana, fúngica, parasitária, eosinofílica. • Bronquiectasia.

HEMOGRAMA/BIOQUÍMICA/URINÁLISE
• Hemograma completo — pode exibir leucograma inflamatório secundário a estresse crônico ou infecção concomitante. • É comum a elevação na atividade das enzimas hepáticas.

OUTROS TESTES LABORATORIAIS
Ácidos biliares elevados — mecanismo incerto.

DIAGNÓSTICO POR IMAGEM
Radiografia Torácica
• O colapso das vias aéreas pode ser evidenciado ao exame radiográfico em uma grande porcentagem de cães. Contudo, o local do colapso em radiografias estáticas é compatível com a área determinada pela fluoroscopia em <50% dos casos. • Radiografias inspiratórias — revelam principalmente o colapso na porção cervical e na entrada torácica da traqueia. • Radiografias expiratórias — demonstram o colapso na porção intratorácica da traqueia; também se podem observar o colapso do brônquio principal e a distensão da porção cervical da traqueia.
• Bronquite, pneumonia ou bronquiectasia — podem ser identificadas. • Aumento de volume do lado direito do coração — pode ser observado secundariamente à pneumopatia crônica ou cor pulmonale ou, então, o aumento do coração pode ser um artefato gerado pela obesidade ou conformação da raça.
Fluoroscopia
• Colapso dinâmico da traqueia cervical ou intratorácica e/ou da membrana traqueal dorsal pode ser visualizado durante as respirações correntes — costuma ser identificado com maior facilidade após a indução de tosse. Em casos graves, observa-se herniação pulmonar cranial por meio da entrada torácica.

MÉTODOS DIAGNÓSTICOS
É preciso ter cautela ao anestesiar e entubar os cães com colapso da traqueia. A irritação promovida pelo tubo endotraqueal pode agravar a doença, enquanto a perda do controle respiratório por anestesia ou excitação (agitação) excessiva na recuperação pode precipitar uma crise.
Lavado Traqueal
• Utilizar entubação oral (em vez de abordagem transtraqueal) com uma sonda endotraqueal de pequeno calibre e um cateter estéril ao se obter amostras para exame citológico, cultura bacteriana e antibiograma.
Broncoscopia
• Avalia os níveis de gravidade do colapso; Grau I — protrusão leve da membrana dorsal da traqueia em direção ao lúmen das vias aéreas; redução do diâmetro em menos de 25%; Grau II — diminuição do lúmen traqueal por volta de 50%; Grau III — redução do lúmen traqueal em torno de 75%; Grau IV — achatamento dos anéis traqueais; é possível observar <10% do lúmen traqueal; pode-se notar a traqueia com lúmen duplo quando o músculo traqueal entra em contato com a superfície ventral da traqueia e os anéis se curvam no sentido dorsal.
• Identifica o comprometimento das vias aéreas de pequeno calibre — enviar as amostras das vias aéreas ao exame citológico, à cultura bacteriana e ao antibiograma; é recomendável a realização de culturas específicas para *Mycoplasma*.
Citologia
• Não é digna de nota em casos não complicados de colapso da traqueia ou das vias aéreas.

Colapso da Traqueia

- Sepse e supuração, juntamente com a proliferação bacteriana acentuada de algum patógeno — sugestivo de infecção pulmonar.
- Neutrófilos sem bactérias intracelulares ou proliferação bacteriana notável — indicativo de inflamação das vias aéreas.

ACHADOS PATOLÓGICOS
- Músculo dorsal da traqueia — alongado.
- Anéis cartilaginosos — achatados.
- Pode-se notar inflamação da traqueia ou formação de pseudomembrana.
- Hipocelularidade da cartilagem com níveis baixos de glicoproteínas ou sulfato de condroitina — pode ser observada por meio de exame histopatológico ou microscopia eletrônica.
- Podem-se observar alterações associadas à doença inflamatória crônica das vias aéreas.

TRATAMENTO

CUIDADO(S) DE SAÚDE ADEQUADO(S)
- Esquema ambulatorial — pacientes estáveis.
- Internação — oxigenoterapia e sedação em casos de angústia respiratória grave. Sedação e supressão da tosse — butorfanol (0,05 mg/kg SC); a adição de acepromazina (0,025 mg/kg SC) pode intensificar os efeitos sedativos e ainda diminuir o reflexo da tosse.

CUIDADO(S) DE ENFERMAGEM
Oxigenoterapia e sedação com butorfanol e/ou acepromazina em pacientes gravemente dispneicos.

ATIVIDADE
- Restrição intensa até a estabilização do paciente.
- Durante o tratamento da doença — recomendam-se exercícios leves para estimular a perda de peso.

DIETA
- A maioria dos cães acometidos melhora após a perda de peso. • Instituir programa de perda de peso com dieta redutora rica em fibras. • Fornecer 80% das necessidades diárias totais de calorias; empregar programa de redução de peso lenta.

ORIENTAÇÃO AO PROPRIETÁRIO
- Alertar o proprietário sobre o fato de que condições como obesidade, excitação/agitação demasiada e umidade podem precipitar uma crise.
- Orientar o proprietário a utilizar uma guia peitoral, em vez de coleira, em seu animal.
- Esclarecer ao proprietário que o colapso da traqueia é um quadro irreversível e que as estratégias terapêuticas são destinadas a diminuir os deflagradores da tosse. • Para os candidatos cirúrgicos, informar o proprietário sobre a probabilidade de complicações após a cirurgia, tais como: tosse persistente, angústia respiratória ou paralisia laríngea; alguns pacientes podem necessitar de traqueostomia permanente. Advertir o proprietário sobre a necessidade de acompanhamento prolongado após a aplicação de *stent** para evitar a fratura e/ou migração desse dispositivo ou a formação de granuloma.

CONSIDERAÇÕES CIRÚRGICAS
- Tratamento de distúrbios obstrutivos das vias aéreas superiores (p. ex., alongamento do palato mole, eversão dos sáculos laríngeos) — pode diminuir os sinais relativos à traqueia.
- Aplicação de *stents* extraluminais em formato de C em pacientes selecionados com colapso da porção cervical da traqueia por cirurgião habilidoso e experiente — melhora a qualidade de vida e diminui os sinais clínicos quando se consegue alcançar estabilização adequada das vias aéreas e quando a broncomalacia não limita a resolução da doença.
- Aplicação de *stents* intraluminais pode poupar a vida em casos selecionados com colapso das vias aéreas intratorácicas, irresponsivo a procedimentos de recuperação com tratamento clínico.

MEDICAÇÕES

MEDICAMENTO(S) DE ESCOLHA
- O aumento do gradiente de pressão dentro das vias aéreas inferiores pode ser útil em cães com colapso das vias aéreas intratorácicas — teofilina de liberação sustentada (10 mg/kg VO a cada 12 h) ou terbutalina (1,25-5 mg/cão VO a cada 8-12 h); os broncodilatadores não exercem efeito sobre o diâmetro da traqueia.
- Embora a ocorrência de infecção bacteriana seja rara, a doxiciclina (3-5 mg/kg VO a cada 12 h) é algumas vezes benéfica, pois esse agente pode diminuir a carga bacteriana nas vias aéreas ou reduzir a inflamação.
- Supressores narcóticos da tosse (butorfanol a 0,5-1 mg/kg VO a cada 4-8 h ou hidrocodona a 0,22 mg/kg VO a cada 4-8 h) são eficazes para o tratamento crônico.
- Redução da inflamação traqueal — a prednisona (0,5 mg/kg VO a cada 12 h; em seguida, 0,25 mg/kg a cada 12 h) por um total de 5-7 dias pode ser útil. Esteroides inalados administrados via máscara facial e câmara de espaçamento são preferíveis para evitar efeitos sistêmicos de respiração ofegante e ganho de peso.

PRECAUÇÕES
Evitar o uso de esteroides a longo prazo em virtude da tendência ao ganho de peso e ao aparecimento de doenças associadas à imunossupressão.

INTERAÇÕES POSSÍVEIS
Metabolismo da teofilina — aumentado pelo tratamento concomitante com cetoconazol ou fenobarbital, o que resulta na concentração plasmática inadequada; diminuído pela administração de fluoroquinolonas (p. ex., enrofloxacino), eritromicina, cimetidina, esteroides, β-bloqueadores, mexiletina e tiabendazol, o que resulta em concentrações plasmáticas tóxicas e desarranjo gastrintestinal, nervosismo ou taquicardia; ajustar as dosagens quando houver a necessidade de uso concomitante.

MEDICAMENTO(S) ALTERNATIVO(S)
Xarope Robitussin® DM — pode proporcionar alívio paliativo.

ACOMPANHAMENTO

MONITORIZAÇÃO DO PACIENTE
- Peso corporal.
- Tolerância a exercícios.
- Padrão respiratório.
- Incidência da tosse.

PREVENÇÃO
- Evitar a obesidade nas raças comumente afligidas.
- Evitar o calor e a umidade.
- Usar guia peitoral em vez de coleira cervical.

COMPLICAÇÕES POSSÍVEIS
Angústia respiratória intratável, que leva à insuficiência respiratória ou à eutanásia.

EVOLUÇÃO ESPERADA E PROGNÓSTICO
- As combinações de medicamentos juntamente com o controle do peso podem reduzir os sinais clínicos, embora seja provável que o paciente exiba tosse pelo resto da vida e possa sofrer exacerbações recidivantes da doença.
- Cirurgia — beneficia alguns cães, principalmente aqueles com colapso da porção cervical da traqueia.
- Aplicação de *stent* — beneficia alguns cães, sobretudo aqueles com colapso das vias aéreas intratorácicas.
- Prognóstico — formulado com base na evidência broncoscópica de obstrução das vias aéreas.

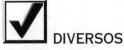

DIVERSOS

DISTÚRBIOS ASSOCIADOS
- Bronquite crônica.
- Paralisia da laringe.
- Eversão dos sacos laríngeos.
- Hipertensão pulmonar.
- As raças caninas que desenvolvem colapso da traqueia também costumam ter insuficiência da valva mitral.

VER TAMBÉM
- Bronquite Crônica.
- Traqueobronquite Infecciosa Canina (Tosse dos Canis).

RECURSOS DA INTERNET
http://www.vet.upenn.edu/RyanHospital/SpecialtyCareServices/InterventionalRadiology/CurrentVeterinaryApplications/TrachealStentingforTrachealCollapse/tabid/945/Default.aspx.

Sugestões de Leitura
Buback JL, Boothe HW, Hobson HP. Surgical treatment of tracheal collapse in dogs: 90 cases (1983-1993). JAVMA 1996, 308:380-384.
Johnson LR, Pollard RE. Tracheal collapse and bronchomalacia in dogs: 58 cases (7/2001-1/2008). J Vet Intern Med 2010, 24(2):298-305.
Macready DM, Johnson LR, Pollard RE. Fluoroscopic and radiographic evaluation of tracheal collapse in dogs: 62 cases (2001-2006). JAVMA 2007, 230(12):1870-1876.
Sura PA, Krahwinkel DJ. Self-expanding nitinol stents for the treatment of tracheal collapse in dogs: 12 cases (2001-2004). JAVMA 2008, 232(2):228-236.

Autor Lynelle R. Johnson
Consultor Editorial Lynelle R. Johnson

---

* N. T.: Dispositivo utilizado para manter o lúmen de vasos e/ou vias aéreas.

COLECISTITE E COLEDOQUITE

CONSIDERAÇÕES GERAIS

REVISÃO
• Inflamação da vesícula biliar, algumas vezes associada à colelitíase ou mucocele biliar; frequentemente associada à obstrução e/ou inflamação do ducto biliar comum e/ou do sistema biliar intra-hepático. • Os casos graves resultam na ruptura da vesícula biliar e subsequente peritonite biliar. • A obstrução do ducto biliar ou a ocorrência de peritonite biliar intensifica a migração transmural de bactérias entéricas pela circulação portal, levando a endotoxemia, bacteremia, sepse e, em caso de peritonite biliar, peritonite séptica.

IDENTIFICAÇÃO
• Cães e gatos. • Não há predileção racial, sexual nem etária. • Colecistite necrosante (cães) — geralmente em animais de meia-idade ou mais idosos.

SINAIS CLÍNICOS
• Início súbito de inapetência, letargia, vômito e dor abdominal vaga. • Doença grave — choque por endotoxemia, bacteremia e hipovolemia. • São comuns os sinais de icterícia leve a moderada e febre. • Massa de tecido mole no quadrante cranial direito do abdome — reflete inflamação e aderências envolvendo a vesícula biliar e os tecidos adjacentes.

CAUSAS E FATORES DE RISCO
• Comprometimento do fluxo biliar no ducto cístico ou na vesícula biliar, distúrbio de motilidade ou lesão isquêmica à parede da vesícula biliar podem preceder a colecistite. • A presença de irritantes na bile (p. ex., sedimentação/deposição biliar, lisolecitina, prostaglandinas, colélitos e trematódeos hepáticos) ou o fluxo retrógrado das enzimas pancreáticas (gatos) podem desencadear ou aumentar a inflamação da vesícula ou do ducto biliar. • Distúrbios entéricos, traumatismos ou cirurgias abdominais prévios — podem ser fatores que contribuem para o quadro. • Desenvolvimento anômalo da vesícula ou do ducto biliar — cisto coledocal (raro, em gatos). • Infecção bacteriana — comum; invasão retrógrada a partir do intestino ou disseminação hematógena. • Toxoplasmose e coccidiose biliar — causas raramente descritas. • Colecistite necrosante (cães) — a ruptura da vesícula biliar e o desenvolvimento de colelitíase são causas comuns; a *Escherichia coli* é a bactéria mais comumente isolada. • Colecistite/coledoquite enfisematosa — associada ao diabetes melito, à isquemia traumática da vesícula biliar e à colecistite aguda (com ou sem colelitíase); recuperação frequente de microrganismos produtores de gases (p. ex., *Clostridia*) e *E. coli* à cultura; a colecistite enfisematosa é rara. • Cães hiperlipidêmicos são predispostos à mucocele da vesícula biliar, levando à colestase e colecistite.

DIAGNÓSTICO

DIAGNÓSTICO DIFERENCIAL
• Pancreatite. • Peritonite focal ou difusa. • Peritonite biliar. • Gastrenterite com envolvimento secundário do trato biliar. • Colelitíase. • Colangio-hepatite. • Necrose hepática. • Abscedação hepática. • Septicemia. • OEHDB. • Mucocele da vesícula biliar.

HEMOGRAMA/BIOQUÍMICA/URINÁLISE
• Leucocitose variável com neutrófilos tóxicos e desvio à esquerda inconsistente. • Hiperbilirrubinemia e bilirrubinúria. • Atividades enzimáticas elevadas da ALT, AST, fosfatase alcalina e GGT. • Hipoalbuminemia em casos de peritonite. • Níveis elevados de colesterol e bilirrubina em casos de OEHDB.

OUTROS TESTES LABORATORIAIS
• Abdominocentese — observação de citologia inflamatória na efusão abdominal (ver Peritonite Biliar). • Cultura da bile (cães) — para detecção de *E. coli*, *Klebsiella* spp., *Pseudomonas* spp., *Clostridium* spp. e outros microrganismos. • Testes de coagulação — anormais em casos de OEHDB crônica decorrente de deficiência da vitamina K (por OEHDB) ou CID por doença grave associada à sepse.

DIAGNÓSTICO POR IMAGEM
• Radiografias abdominais — podem revelar perda de detalhes da região abdominal cranial compatível com peritonite ou efusão focal ou difusa, íleo paralítico, colélitos radiodensos, ou acúmulo de gás nas estruturas biliares; em caso de mineralização distrófica por inflamação crônica, pode-se observar uma vesícula biliar radiodensa (a assim chamada vesícula de porcelana, rara). • Ultrassonografia — parede da vesícula biliar difusamente espessa em caso de hiperecogenicidade segmentar e aspecto laminado da parede em caso de colecistite necrosante; o aspecto de bicamada na parede da vesícula biliar também pode ser observado em casos de colecistite aguda, hepatite, colangio-hepatite, dispersão de líquido para o terceiro espaço, sobrecarga iatrogênica por fluido; lúmen da vesícula biliar preenchido com um padrão estrelado ecogênico amorfo ou finamente estriado, semelhante à fruta kiwi cortada ("sinal de kiwi") em caso de mucocele dessa vesícula; ruptura da vesícula biliar associada à solução de continuidade da parede dessa vesícula, líquido pericolecístico ou efusão generalizada, e hiperecogenicidade de tecidos circunjacentes; a falha na obtenção de imagens da vesícula biliar pode indicar ruptura de estruturas biliares ou parede mineralizada dessa vesícula; os ductos biliares intra-hepáticos podem ser de difícil visualização ou parecer proeminentes (colangite ascendente: paredes espessas, ou OEHDB: ductos dilatados); o encontro de líquido pericístico é sugestivo de colecistite necrosante ou emergência cirúrgica.

ACHADOS PATOLÓGICOS
Aspecto macroscópico — vesícula biliar eritematosa; em casos de lesão necrosante, pode aparecer de coloração verde-enegrecida; colélitos pigmentados em casos de infecção.

TRATAMENTO

• Internação — necessária para o fornecimento de cuidados críticos durante as avaliações diagnósticas e os preparos pré-cirúrgicos. • Colocação de cateter intravenoso em veias periféricas para a administração de fluidos, coloides e componentes sanguíneos. • Restabelecimento do equilíbrio hidroeletrolítico; monitorização frequente do nível dos eletrólitos. • Fluidos poli-iônicos — administração concomitante com coloides. • Plasma — coloide preferido; indicado em casos de hipoalbuminemia e coagulopatia. • Sangue total ou plasma fresco congelado — recomendado em casos cirúrgicos com tendências hemorrágicas. • Hetamido — fluido preferencial em relação à dextrana 70; 10-20 mL/kg/dia por gotejamento lento sob taxa de infusão constante; no entanto, prefere-se o plasma. • Monitorização do débito urinário. • Ao manipular estruturas biliares ou durante o procedimento de colecistocentese, ficar atento ao reflexo vasovagal (bradicardia patológica abrupta, hipotensão, parada cardíaca); estar preparado com anticolinérgicos à mão (p. ex., atropina). • Ressecção da vesícula biliar — é recomendável, embora seja mais eficiente com base na avaliação dessa estrutura no momento da cirurgia.

MEDICAÇÕES

MEDICAMENTO(S)
• Antibióticos — administração *antes da cirurgia*; amplo espectro; as manipulações cirúrgicas facilitam a bacteremia; selecionar os antibióticos contra a flora anaeróbica e Gram-negativa intestinal; refinar o tratamento, utilizando os resultados da cultura e do antibiograma; boas escolhas iniciais: combinação de metronidazol, ticarcilina ou fluoroquinolona. Na ocorrência de colestase e icterícia, reduzir a dose-padrão do metronidazol pela metade. • Ácido ursodesoxicólico — 10-15 mg/kg VO a cada 12 h com alimento. • Antioxidantes: vitamina E — 10 UI/kg (ver Obstrução do Ducto Biliar); *S*-adenosilmetionina (SAMe) — doador de glutationa (20 mg/kg VO a cada 24 h), duas horas antes da refeição. • Vitamina K1 — 0,5-1,5 mg/kg SC ou IM a cada 12 h por 3 doses; **advertência:** em função do risco de reações anafilactoides, jamais administre a vitamina K1 por via intravenosa; instituir tratamento precoce para permitir a resposta antes das manipulações cirúrgicas.

CONTRAINDICAÇÕES
Ácido ursodesoxicólico — contraindicado em casos de OEHDB não corrigida ou peritonite biliar.

ACOMPANHAMENTO

MONITORIZAÇÃO DO PACIENTE
Exame físico e testes diagnósticos pertinentes — a cada 2-4 semanas até a resolução dos sinais clínicos e das anormalidades clinicopatológicas.

COMPLICAÇÕES POSSÍVEIS
Prever a evolução clínica prolongada em casos de ruptura do trato biliar ou na presença de peritonite.

DIVERSOS

DISTÚRBIOS ASSOCIADOS
• Colelitíase. • OEHDB. • Coledoquite. • Mucocele da vesícula biliar. • Peritonite biliar.

POTENCIAL ZOONÓTICO
Os microrganismos *Campylobacter* e *Salmonella* podem causar colecistite em cães.

ABREVIATURA(S)
• ALT = alanina aminotransferase. • AST = aspartato aminotransferase. • CID = coagulação intravascular disseminada. • GGT = γ-glutamiltransferase. • OEHDB = obstrução extra-hepática do ducto biliar.

Autor Sharon A. Center
Consultor Editorial Sharon A. Center

COLELITÍASE

CONSIDERAÇÕES GERAIS

REVISÃO
- Cálculos radiopacos ou radiotransparentes nos ductos biliares, na vesícula biliar ou, raramente, no parênquima hepático (hepatolitíase). A mucocele da vesícula biliar é considerada uma forma de colelitíase (ver "Mucocele da Vesícula Biliar").
- Pode se apresentar como um quadro assintomático ou se associar a sinais atribuídos à sedimentação/deposição de bile, OEHDB, colecistite, colangio-hepatite ou peritonite biliar.
- Constituintes primários de colélitos— mucina, cálcio e pigmentos de bilirrubina; tipicamente, a bile do cão não é litogênica em comparação a de seres humanos (saturação mais baixa de colesterol).
- Em gatos, 50% dos colélitos são mineralizados e podem ser visíveis ao exame radiográfico.
- Tratamento clínico e/ou cirúrgico — não é recomendado na ausência de sinais clínicos ou clinicopatológicos.

IDENTIFICAÇÃO
- Cães e gatos.
- Raças caninas de pequeno porte podem ser predispostas.
- Cães hiperlipidêmicos — predispostos ao desenvolvimento de sedimentação biliar mucinosa espessa, que pode se comportar como colélitos (ver "Mucocele da Vesícula Biliar").

SINAIS CLÍNICOS
- Os animais podem permanecer assintomáticos.
- Quando acompanhada por infecção ou OEHDB (com ou sem peritonite) — há vômito; dor abdominal; febre; icterícia. A dor abdominal pode ocorrer no período pós-prandial, mas ainda permanecer vaga e passageira.

CAUSAS E FATORES DE RISCO
- Fatores predisponentes — condições indutoras de estase do fluxo biliar (distúrbio da motilidade da vesícula biliar, cistos de colédoco [gatos]); formação do ninho (núcleo) do cálculo (debris inflamatórios, infecção, tumor ou esfoliação epitelial); supersaturação de bile (pigmento de bilirrubina, cálcio, mucina, colesterol); a união anatômica dos ductos pancreático e biliar (gatos) pode promover a inflamação do ducto e a estase de bile, causando OEHDB, coledoquite e pancreatite.
- Sedimentação de bile e/ou distensão da vesícula biliar — estimulam o aumento na produção de mucina e a coalescência de partículas biliares.
- Mediadores inflamatórios e enzimas bacterianas associados à colecistite — agravam a precipitação de cálculos (produção de mucina; desconjugação e desidroxilação de bilirrubina com subsequente precipitação de pigmentos biliares).
- Dietas com baixo teor de proteínas, taurina e metionina para cães — são consideradas litogênicas.

DIAGNÓSTICO

DIAGNÓSTICO DIFERENCIAL
- OEHDB — atribuída a distúrbios inflamatórios, infecciosos ou neoplásicos que envolvam o fígado ou os tecidos extra-hepáticos adjacentes à porta hepática; sugerida por aumentos acentuados nos níveis de fosfatase alcalina, GGT e bilirrubina e por aumento modesto nos níveis de colesterol.
- Colangio-hepatite.
- Colecistite.
- Coledoquite.
- Pancreatite.
- Peritonite biliar.
- Mucocele da vesícula biliar.

HEMOGRAMA/BIOQUÍMICA/URINÁLISE
- Hemograma completo — pode permanecer normal; as anormalidades refletem infecção bacteriana, endotoxemia, obstrução biliar ou fatores causais subjacentes; em alguns casos, observa-se leucograma inflamatório.
- Bioquímica — hiperbilirrubinemia, bem como elevações variáveis nas atividades séricas da fosfatase alcalina, GGT, ALT e AST.
- Podem não revelar quaisquer anormalidades clinicopatológicas.

OUTROS TESTES LABORATORIAIS
- Cultura bacteriana — bile: é frequente o envolvimento de bactérias aeróbias e anaeróbias em pacientes sintomáticos. O ninho (núcleo) do cálculo pode albergar bactérias vivas.
- Perfil de coagulação — tempo de coagulação prolongado (especialmente PIAVK e TP); quadro responsivo à administração parenteral da vitamina K_1; em casos de OEHDB crônica, podem ocorrer hemorragias (ver "Obstrução do Ducto Biliar").
- Análise do colélito: salientar que o cálculo é um colélito e enviar para análise própria e equipada para colélitos; a composição habitual inclui carbonato de cálcio unido sob a forma de complexo com mucina e pigmentos de bilirrubina.
- Cultura do ninho (núcleo) do colélito: pode identificar infecção bacteriana associada.

DIAGNÓSTICO POR IMAGEM
- Radiografias abdominais — valor limitado no delineamento da estrutura ou do conteúdo da vesícula biliar; com frequência, os colélitos são pequenos e radiotransparentes; raramente, pode-se confundir o quadro de mineralização distrófica da árvore biliar com colélitos em animais com colangite crônica.
- Ultrassonografia — exame capaz de detectar colélitos bem diminutos de até 2 mm de diâmetro, espessamento da parede da vesícula biliar, distensão do trato biliar, lesões do parênquima hepático (alteração na ecogenicidade pela presença de inflamação, lipídios, glicogênio ou fibrose) e envolvimento de ducto extra-hepático; pode facilitar a coleta de amostras para a realização de cultura, citologia e histopatologia; pode detectar indícios de OEHDB dentro de 72 h. **Cuidado:** a distensão da vesícula biliar com sedimentação/depósito da bile é um achado ultrassonográfico comum em pacientes com anorexia ou em jejum: não confundir com obstrução da vesícula biliar. Hepatolitíase evidente com base na sombra acústica encontrada no parênquima. A obtenção de imagens dos colélitos nos ductos extra-hepáticos pode não ser uma tarefa fácil em função dos gases entéricos que embaçam a "janela" acústica.

MÉTODOS DIAGNÓSTICOS
A avaliação histopatológica do fígado é necessária em pacientes submetidos à remoção cirúrgica do colélito não só para detectar a presença de distúrbios comórbidos, mas também para determinar o tratamento e o prognóstico.

TRATAMENTO

- Controverso se a colerese com ursodesoxicolato for indicada em animais que carecem de sinais clínicos ou clinicopatológicos.
- Fluidos de suporte — administrados em caso de internação e selecionados de acordo com o estado de hidratação, depleção de eletrólitos e equilíbrio acidobásico.
- Hiperlipidemia como fator predisponente — prescrever dieta pobre em gordura e controlar os distúrbios anteriores predisponentes, sobretudo infecção da árvore biliar (com antimicrobianos) e disfunção da motilidade da vesícula biliar (por remoção dessa vesícula).
- Cirurgia exploratória, coledocotomia, colecistotomia e, possivelmente, colecistectomia ou anastomose entérica biliar — indicadas em casos sintomáticos de acordo com as circunstâncias.
- Alertar o proprietário sobre a natureza crônica da colelitíase e a possibilidade de formação de novos cálculos mesmo após a remoção cirúrgica e o tratamento médico.

MEDICAÇÕES

MEDICAMENTO(S)
- Antibióticos — selecionados com base nos resultados da cultura da bile, de tecido e do ninho do colélito ou direcionados contra os microrganismos intestinais oportunistas; o tratamento inicial com ticarcilina/ácido clavulânico (Timentin®) ou metronidazol, combinados com alguma fluoroquinolona costuma ser bem-sucedido.
- Ácido ursodesoxicólico — 10-15 mg/kg/dia VO, divididos a cada 12 h e administrados juntamente com o alimento (a formulação de comprimido possui a melhor biodisponibilidade); esse medicamento não só exerce efeitos coleréticos, hepatoprotetores, antiendotóxicos e antifibróticos, mas também pode facilitar a dissolução dos cálculos; a terapia será mantida pelo resto da vida caso não se identifique nenhuma causa de colelitíase.
- Vitamina K_1 — administração parenteral; 0,5-1,5 mg/kg até, no máximo, 3 doses em 36 h em pacientes ictéricos. Em função do risco de anafilaxia, jamais administrar por via IV.

Antioxidantes
- Vitamina E (acetato de α-tocoferol) — 10 UI/kg/dia para pacientes com atividades enzimáticas hepáticas elevadas ou inflamação hepatobiliar confirmada.
- SAMe (Denosyl-SD4® tem biodisponibilidade e eficácia comprovadas) — é doador de glutationa (importante antioxidante hepatobiliar, a glutationa gera uma força motriz para a produção de bile) e tem potencial colerético para pacientes com atividades enzimáticas hepáticas elevadas e inflamação hepatobiliar confirmada (20-40 mg/kg de comprimido revestido entérico VO a cada 24 h, administrar 2 horas antes das refeições; doses mais altas são associadas à colerese); também pode ter benefícios antifibróticos e anti-inflamatórios.

COLELITÍASE

CONTRAINDICAÇÕES
Ácido ursodesoxicólico — contraindicado em casos de OEHDB até a descompressão biliar.

ACOMPANHAMENTO

MONITORIZAÇÃO DO PACIENTE
• Exame físico e testes diagnósticos pertinentes — a cada 2-4 semanas até a resolução pós-operatória dos sinais clínicos e das anormalidades clinicopatológicas.
• Ultrassonografia periódica — avaliar o estado dos colélitos, a integridade do trato biliar e a alteração do parênquima hepático.

COMPLICAÇÕES POSSÍVEIS
Início súbito de febre, dor abdominal e mal-estar — pode indicar peritonite biliar e/ou sepse por um colapso na contenção da bile.

EVOLUÇÃO ESPERADA E PROGNÓSTICO
• O animal pode permanecer assintomático.
• Doença sintomática — depende da presença de infecção, OEHDB, colecistite ou peritonite biliar.

DIVERSOS

DISTÚRBIOS ASSOCIADOS
• Colecistite.
• Coledoquite.
• Obstrução extra-hepática do ducto biliar.
• Mucocele da vesícula biliar.

ABREVIATURA(S)
• ALT = alanina aminotransferase.
• AST = aspartato aminotransferase.
• GGT = γ-glutamiltransferase.
• OEHDB = obstrução extra-hepática do ducto biliar.
• PIAVK = proteínas invocadas pela ausência ou antagonismo da vitamina K.
• TP = tempo de protrombina.
• SAMe = dissulfato tosilato de S-adenosil-L-metionina.

Sugestões de Leitura
Center SA. Diseases of the gallbladder and biliary tree. Vet Clin North Am Small Anim Pract 2009, 39(3):543-598.

Autor Sharon A. Center
Consultor Editorial Sharon A. Center

Colesteatoma

CONSIDERAÇÕES GERAIS

REVISÃO
- Forma rara de cisto epidermoide encontrado no interior da cavidade auditiva média de cães. O termo é errôneo, pois não corresponde a um granuloma ou uma neoplasia e não contém gordura. A estrutura cística é revestida por epitélio queratinizado escamoso estratificado que repousa sobre um estroma fibroso de tecido de granulação inflamatório e lentamente aumenta de volume em virtude do desprendimento de queratina em direção ao lúmen, o que também incita a resposta inflamatória.
- O colesteatoma pode ser congênito ou adquirido como uma complicação de otite média. A forma congênita desenvolve-se a partir de células embrionárias no interior da cavidade auditiva média e ainda não foi identificada em cães. A forma adquirida desenvolve-se fora do epitélio escamoso estratificado a partir da membrana timpânica ou da orelha externa e também pode envolver uma metaplasia do epitélio respiratório. Além disso, a forma adquirida ainda pode ser primária, como resultado de disfunção crônica do conduto auditivo por otite média, ou secundária à perfuração do tímpano, causada por meios iatrogênicos ou traumáticos.

IDENTIFICAÇÃO
- Acomete cães; a condição ainda não foi descrita em gatos.
- Não há predisposição racial, etária ou sexual aparente, embora as raças caninas predispostas à otite possam ter um risco elevado.
- O colesteatoma foi descrito em cães de 13 meses de vida até 9 anos e meio de idade.

SINAIS CLÍNICOS
- Os cães apresentam-se com sinais de otopatia uni ou, mais frequentemente, bilateral crônica (muitas vezes com duração superior a 1 ano), em geral otite externa com arranhadura/prurido nas orelhas e meneios de cabeça. Em consequência disso, o colesteatoma pode ser subdiagnosticado.
- Pode haver desconforto durante a alimentação, ao abrir a boca (bocejo, por exemplo) ou na manipulação da mandíbula.
- Podem ocorrer anormalidades neurológicas, como inclinação da cabeça, ataxia ou paralisia facial unilateral. Raramente, também pode haver sinais de diminuição da audição ou surdez, nistagmo, andar em círculo ou atrofia unilateral dos músculos temporal e masseter.
- O exame otoscópico frequentemente revela acúmulo intenso de debris e estenose no canal auditivo. Muitas vezes, a inspeção detalhada da membrana timpânica não é possível por conta dessa estenose no canal auditivo ou da obstrução pela massa.

CAUSAS E FATORES DE RISCO
- Otite crônica.
- Congênito (ainda não há relatos em cães).

DIAGNÓSTICO

DIAGNÓSTICO DIFERENCIAL
- Pólipo inflamatório, granuloma por colesterol, ou cisto.
- Otite média crônica.
- Carcinoma ou adenoma das glândulas ceruminosas.
- Carcinoma das células escamosas.

HEMOGRAMA/BIOQUÍMICA/URINÁLISE
Não há anormalidades específicas.

OUTROS TESTES LABORATORIAIS
As culturas aeróbias e anaeróbias de material obtido a partir do conduto auditivo são indicadas, mas muitas vezes os animais já foram tratados com antibióticos e/ou antifúngicos ou estão sendo submetidos a esses agentes terapêuticos.

DIAGNÓSTICO POR IMAGEM
- A radiografia revela estenose do canal auditivo ipsolateral e muitas vezes calcificação/ossificação das cartilagens auricular e anular. O aumento da densidade da orelha média e/ou a ruptura da parede da bula timpânica também estão presentes. Além disso, é possível observar o envolvimento da articulação temporomandibular.
- A TC é um exame superior às radiografias tradicionais, pois ela confere alta resolução de imagem e fornece informações mais precisas sobre o estado da cavidade da orelha média e da espessura do osso. É possível determinar a extensão da massa de tecido mole, a diminuição da aeração e a esclerose da bula timpânica, bem como o envolvimento da membrana timpânica e do canal auditivo.

MÉTODOS DIAGNÓSTICOS
Não é provável que a citologia aspirativa com agulha fina e a biopsia incisional confirmem o diagnóstico, pois uma amostra superficial pode não revelar todas as camadas da lesão.

ACHADOS PATOLÓGICOS
- Do ponto de vista macroscópico, verifica-se uma estrutura cística (0,5-1,5 cm), que ocupa parte do mesotímpano da cavidade da orelha média.
- A análise histológica revela uma estrutura cística epitelial escamosa com o centro constituído por lamelas de queratina envolvidas pela membrana timpânica. Fica evidente a presença de tecido de granulação, mas podem ser encontradas aderências entre esse tecido e a membrana timpânica. Também pode haver alterações no epitélio respiratório.

TRATAMENTO

A extirpação cirúrgica dos tecidos acometidos no interior da orelha média e do canal auditivo externo constitui o tratamento de escolha. Tal intervenção cirúrgica costuma ser efetuada por meio da ablação total do canal auditivo com osteotomia lateral ou ventral da bula timpânica, dependendo da extensão da lesão. Também foi descrita uma abordagem cirúrgica auricular caudal bem-sucedida, com preservação da audição e da aparência externa auricular.

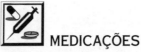

MEDICAÇÕES

MEDICAMENTO(S)
- A terapia clínica visa tratar a infecção concomitante. Em termos ideais, o tratamento antibiótico e antifúngico deve ter como base os resultados da cultura e do antibiograma. Também fica indicada a antibioticoterapia no período perioperatório.
- Dado o papel desempenhado pela infecção e inflamação no processo patológico, é aconselhável a antibioticoterapia prolongada após a cirurgia.

CONTRAINDICAÇÕES/INTERAÇÕES POSSÍVEIS
É preciso ter cautela quanto ao emprego de antibióticos aminoglicosídeos nas orelhas de cães.

ACOMPANHAMENTO

MONITORIZAÇÃO DO PACIENTE
Avaliar o local da cirurgia até que a cicatrização se mostre satisfatória.

PREVENÇÃO
O tratamento precoce bem-sucedido da otite externa pode diminuir as chances de otite média e, consequentemente, o desenvolvimento do colesteatoma; no entanto, ainda não há provas disso.

COMPLICAÇÕES POSSÍVEIS
- Se a doença não for tratada, serão possíveis a ocorrência e a evolução de sinais neurológicos.
- As complicações cirúrgicas podem incluir perda auditiva parcial e/ou dano ao nervo facial.

EVOLUÇÃO ESPERADA E PROGNÓSTICO
- Espera-se a cura clínica apenas com a excisão cirúrgica completa do colesteatoma e o uso de técnica cirúrgica adequada.
- Se o problema não for tratado precocemente, será comum a recorrência.
- Sinais neurológicos, incapacidade de abrir a mandíbula e/ou lise óssea temporal ao exame de TC, sem exceção, indicam doença avançada, maior probabilidade de recorrência e prognóstico mais reservado.
- Embora o colesteatoma seja uma complicação incomum de otite média, é ponderável conferir um prognóstico mau quanto ao tratamento dessa doença.

DIVERSOS

GESTAÇÃO/FERTILIDADE/REPRODUÇÃO
É provável que a cirurgia possa ser adiada até o parto.

VER TAMBÉM
Otite Externa e Média.

Sugestões de Leitura
Hardie EM, Linder KE, Pease AP. Aural cholesteatoma in twenty dogs. Vet Surg 2008, 37:763-770.

Autor Anthony J. Mutsaers
Consultor Editorial Timothy M. Fan

COLIBACILOSE

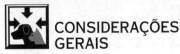

CONSIDERAÇÕES GERAIS

DEFINIÇÃO
• *Escherichia coli* — membro Gram-negativo da família *Enterobacteriaceae*; habitante da flora intestinal de grande parte dos mamíferos; juntamente com outros agentes infecciosos, pode aumentar a gravidade da parvovirose.
• Infecção aguda de filhotes caninos e felinos na primeira semana de vida; caracterizada por septicemia e envolvimento de múltiplos órgãos.
• Isolamento a partir das fezes de animais jovens — indícios não conclusivos de seu potencial patogênico por fazer parte da flora normal.
• Isolamento a partir de hemoculturas ou de órgãos internos — bons indícios de causalidade.
• Infecção de cães e gatos idosos — já existem registros; as cepas individuais são mal caracterizadas em relação aos atributos de virulência.

FISIOPATOLOGIA
• Fatores de virulência — ainda não estão bem definidos; é provável que a *E. coli* como a causa de septicemia em cães e gatos neonatos reflita um equilíbrio entre a imaturidade imunológica e função da barreira intestinal do hospedeiro e a *E. coli* entérica residente, e não a virulência de uma cepa específica.
• Cepas de *E. coli* enterotoxigênica, enteropatogênica (ou seja, com lesão tipo aderência íntima e destruição das microvilosidades), uropatogênica e com FNC+ — recuperadas de cães.
• Cepas de *E. coli* semelhantes — isoladas de gatos (cepas pouco caracterizadas).
• As cepas intestinais colonizam e proliferam-se no intestino delgado; em seguida, a cepa enterotoxigênica elabora adesinas e enterotoxinas não caracterizadas (STa); o fator de aderência íntima e destruição das microvilosidades é elaborado pela cepa enteropatogênica (EAE+).
• Muitas cepas da *E. coli* provenientes de cães e gatos são hemolíticas.
• Um novo tipo de *E. coli* foi encontrado em cães da raça Boxer com enteropatia inflamatória (colite granulomatosa), caracterizada pela capacidade de aderência, invasão e replicação em macrófagos, resultando em uma resposta inflamatória acentuada no interior da parede intestinal.

SISTEMA(S) ACOMETIDO(S)
• Neonatos — intestino delgado (enterite); múltiplos sistemas corporais (septicemia).
• Filhotes caninos/felinos e adultos — intestino delgado (enterite); sistema urogenital (cistite, endometrite, pielonefrite, prostatite); glândula mamária (mastite); intestino grosso (colite).

GENÉTICA
Os cães da raça Boxer podem ser predispostos à colite do intestino grosso.

INCIDÊNCIA/PREVALÊNCIA
• Há poucos dados estatísticos disponíveis.
• É mais comum em neonatos caninos e felinos com menos de 1 semana de vida que não tomaram o colostro ou não o receberam em quantidades adequadas.
• Problema em canis e gatis superlotados.
• Relatos esporádicos em cães e gatos idosos (principalmente com diarreia e problemas urogenitais).
• Piodermatite, bem como otite e meningoencefalomielite purulentas.

Cães
• *E. coli* enterotoxigênica — 2,7-29,5% dos cães diarreicos; cepas: STa/STb +/– e FNC+ isoladas de cães diarreicos, juntamente com hemolisinas.
• *E. coli* (geralmente β-hemolítica) — principal causa de septicemia em filhotes caninos recém--nascidos expostos na vida intrauterina, durante o nascimento ou ao leite contaminado por mastite.

Gatos
• Cepas enteropatogênicas com aderência íntima e destruição das microvilosidades — gatos diarreicos; cepas: EAE+, hemolisinas.
• Cepa patogênica extraintestinal — pneumonia e pleurite necrosantes e hemorrágicas agudas; cepas: FNC-1 mais outras aderências.
• Cepa uropatogênica — cistite; cepas: FNC-1+, P-fímbria, hemolisinas.

DISTRIBUIÇÃO GEOGRÁFICA
Mundial.

IDENTIFICAÇÃO
Espécies
Cães e gatos.

Raça(s) Predominante(s)
Os cães da raça Boxer podem ser predispostos à colite do intestino grosso.

Idade Média e Faixa Etária
• São comuns as infecções (diarreia, septicemia) de neonatos até 2 semanas de vida.
• Filhotes caninos/felinos e animais adultos — doença esporádica associada frequentemente a outros agentes infecciosos.

Sexo Predominante
Nenhum.

SINAIS CLÍNICOS
Comentários Gerais
E. coli — uma das causas mais comuns de septicemia e óbito em filhotes caninos e felinos.

Achados Anamnésicos
• Neonatos — vômito de início súbito, fraqueza/letargia, diarreia, pele fria; acomete um ou mais animais em uma ninhada.
• Filhotes caninos/felinos e animais adultos — vômito e diarreia.

Achados do Exame Físico
• Neonatos — depressão aguda, anorexia, vômito, taquicardia, fraqueza, hipotermia, cianose, diarreia aquosa.
• Filhotes caninos/felinos e animais adultos — *E. coli* enterotoxigênica associada a vômito agudo, diarreia, anorexia, desidratação rápida, febre.

CAUSAS
• *E. coli* — membro da flora microbiana endógena do trato gastrintestinal, do prepúcio e da vagina de animais adultos.
• Muitas cepas isoladas a partir de material de casos clínicos são mal caracterizadas em relação aos fatores de virulência.
• Encontrada com frequência em cães e gatos idosos, concomitantemente com outros agentes infecciosos.

FATORES DE RISCO
Neonatos
• Cadela/gata em más condições de saúde e nutrição — são incapazes de proporcionar cuidados satisfatórios e fornecer quantidades suficientes de colostro à prole.
• Falta ou quantidade insuficiente de colostro.
• Parto em ambiente sujo.
• Nascimento ou trabalho de parto laboriosos ou prolongados.
• Instalações lotadas — o acúmulo de fezes no ambiente aumenta as chances de disseminação orofecal da infecção.

Filhotes Caninos/Felinos e Adultos
• Doença concomitante — parvovirose; parasitismo maciço.
• Antimicrobianos — promovem o desarranjo da flora microbiana do trato gastrintestinal.
• Imunossupressão.
• Mastite pós-parto.
• Cateterização venosa.

DIAGNÓSTICO

DIAGNÓSTICO DIFERENCIAL
• Enterite infecciosa — viral: panleucopenia felina, FeLV, FIV, coronavirose entérica, parvovirose canina, rotavirose, cinomose; bacteriana: *Salmonella, E. coli, Campylobacter jejuni, Yersinia enterocolitica*; síndrome de proliferação bacteriana excessiva, *Clostridium difficile, Clostridium perfringens*; parasitária: ancilóstomos, ascarídeos, tricúris, *Strongyloides, Giardia*, coccídios, *Cryptosporidia*; riquétsias (envenenamento por salmão).
• Enterite induzida pela dieta — alimentação excessiva; mudanças abruptas; inanição; sede; intolerância ou alergia a alimentos; imprudências alimentares ou alimentação inadequada (p. ex., corpo estranho ou lixo).
• Enterite induzida por medicamentos ou toxinas — agentes antimicrobianos; agentes antineoplásicos; anti-helmínticos; metais pesados; organofosforados.
• Distúrbios extraintestinais ou doenças metabólicas — pancreatite aguda; hipoadrenocorticismo; hepatopatia ou doença renal; piometra; peritonite.
• Íleo paralítico funcional ou mecânico — dilatação-vólvulo gástrico; intussuscepção; distúrbio eletrolítico; corpo estranho gastrintestinal.
• Distúrbios neurológicos — vestibulopatia; distúrbios psicogênicos (como medo, agitação, dor).
• Definhamento de neonatos.

HEMOGRAMA/BIOQUÍMICA/URINÁLISE
• Em função da rapidez de óbito em filhotes caninos, observam-se poucas anormalidades.
• Adultos com enterite podem revelar anormalidades bioquímicas, dependendo do estado de desidratação.

MÉTODOS DIAGNÓSTICOS
• Antimicrobianos — produzirão resultados falso-negativos se forem utilizados antes de se obter as culturas bacterianas.
• É imprescindível a realização de cultura bacteriana de rotina e identificação da *E. coli* a partir do sangue (antes do óbito) ou de tecidos obtidos na necropsia (como medula óssea, sangue cardíaco, fígado/baço, cérebro, linfonodos mesentéricos).
• Testes apropriados para identificação das cepas — identificam as adesinas e as toxinas (por meio da hibridização de colônia com sondas de DNA,

COLIBACILOSE

além da técnica de PCR) nas cepas enterotoxigênicas e verocitotoxigênicas.

ACHADOS PATOLÓGICOS
• Enterite aguda.
• Inflamação da mucosa do intestino delgado.
• Petéquias e lesões hemorrágicas na superfície serosa das mucosas gastrintestinais e de todas as cavidades corporais.
• Deposição de fibrina sobre a parede abdominal.
• Necrose hepática/esplênica.

TRATAMENTO

CUIDADO(S) DE SAÚDE ADEQUADO(S)
Filhotes caninos/felinos com a doença aguda — internação; provisão de cuidados satisfatórios de enfermagem.

CUIDADO(S) DE ENFERMAGEM
• Solução isotônica poliônica parenteral balanceada (Ringer lactato) — restabelece o equilíbrio hídrico.
• Solução de glicose hipertônica oral — em casos de diarreia secretória, conforme a necessidade.

ATIVIDADE
Filhotes caninos/felinos imaturos agudamente doentes (bacterêmicos/septicêmicos) — restrição da atividade física, repouso em gaiola para pequenos animais, monitorização e aquecimento.

DIETA
Filhotes caninos — provavelmente ainda estão mamando quando são acometidos; é necessária a alimentação com mamadeira e/ou a aplicação de nutrientes por via intravenosa.

ORIENTAÇÃO AO PROPRIETÁRIO
Neonatos — quadro potencialmente letal, com prognóstico mau.

MEDICAÇÕES

MEDICAMENTO(S) DE ESCOLHA
• Terapia antimicrobiana — em casos de septicemia.
• Orientada por cultura e antibiograma (concentração inibitória mínima) da *E. coli*; terapia empírica até os resultados estarem disponíveis.
• Amicacina: cão e gato, 20 mg/kg IV a cada 24 h.
• Cefazolina: cão e gato, 5-15 mg/kg IV a cada 6-8 h.
• Cefoxitina: cão e gato, 30 mg/kg em dose única e, depois, 15 mg/kg IV a cada 4 h.
• Enrofloxacino: cão, 10 mg/kg IV a cada 24 h; gato, 5 mg/kg IV a cada 24 h; evitar o uso em fêmeas prenhes, neonatos ou animais em fase de crescimento (cães de porte médio <8 meses de vida; raças grandes ou gigantes <12-18 meses de vida) em virtude de lesões cartilaginosas.
• Ticarcilina-clavulanato: cães e gatos, 50 mg/kg VO a cada 6 h.

CONTRAINDICAÇÕES
• Fluoroquinolonas — enrofloxacino: evitar o uso em fêmeas prenhes, neonatos ou animais em fase de crescimento (cães de porte médio <8 meses de vida; raças grandes ou gigantes <12-18 meses de vida) em virtude de lesões cartilaginosas.
• Cloranfenicol e trimetoprima-sulfa — são provavelmente ineficazes contra septicemia por *E. coli*.

PRECAUÇÕES
Garantir a hidratação e a perfusão adequadas ao se utilizar os aminoglicosídeos.

ACOMPANHAMENTO

MONITORIZAÇÃO DO PACIENTE
• Realizar hemocultura — filhotes caninos/felinos com febre e/ou diarreia.
• Monitorizar a temperatura — na presença de sinais de letargia e/ou depressão.
• Monitorizar o comportamento — a ingestão de alimentos, água e/ou leite; nível adequado de ganho de peso.

PREVENÇÃO
• Cadela/gata — boas condições de saúde; vacinadas; estado nutricional satisfatório.
• Limpar e desinfetar o local do parto (água sanitária diluída a 1:32); limpar a cama com frequência após o nascimento dos filhotes.
• Assegurar a ingestão adequada de colostro a toda a ninhada.
• Separar a mãe com a ninhada lactente de outros cães ou gatos.
• Manter a densidade populacional baixa em canis ou gatis.
• Lavar as mãos e trocar de roupas e sapatos após manipular outros cães/gatos e antes de lidar com os neonatos.

EVOLUÇÃO ESPERADA E PROGNÓSTICO
• Neonatos — quadro potencialmente letal; prognóstico frequentemente mau; o neonato pode sucumbir com rapidez; o tratamento imediato com a provisão dos cuidados de suporte é essencial para a sobrevida desses animais.
• Adultos — quadro autolimitante com os cuidados de suporte, dependendo do grau de desidratação e da existência de outras doenças.

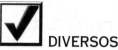
DIVERSOS

FATORES RELACIONADOS COM A IDADE
Neonatos — maior risco de infecção e subsequente septicemia.

POTENCIAL ZOONÓTICO
• Há poucas informações registradas a respeito do potencial de virulência das cepas de *E. coli* de cães ou gatos para os seres humanos, embora, recentemente, já se tenham descoberto similaridades entre a *E. coli* fecal e de infecção do trato urinário canino e a *E. coli* humana associada à infecção do trato urinário, sepse e meningite.
• Em virtude do risco de aquisição de outros agentes infecciosos (p. ex., *Salmonella* e *Giardia*), é fundamental lavar as mãos sempre após a manipulação dos animais (particularmente aqueles com diarreia).
• **CUIDADO:** manter as crianças e as pessoas imunossuprimidas distantes dos animais de estimação com diarreia.

SINÔNIMO(S)
• Enterite neonatal.
• Septicemia por *E. coli*.

ABREVIATURA(S)
• DNA = ácido desoxirribonucleico.
• EAE = encefalomielite autoimune experimental.
• FNC = fator necrosante citotóxico.
• FIV = vírus da imunodeficiência felina.
• FeLV = vírus da leucemia felina.
• PCR = reação em cadeia da polimerase.
• ST = termoestável.

Sugestões de Leitura
Brady CA, Otto CM. Systemic inflammatory response syndrome, sepsis and multiple organ dysfunction. Vet Clin North Am Small Anim Pract 2001, 31:1147-1162.
Johnson JR, Johnston B, Clabots CR, Kuskowski MA, Roberts E, DebRoy C. Virulence genotypes and phylogenetic background of Escherichia coli serogroup O6 isolates from humans, dogs, and cats. J Clin Microbiol 2008, 46:417-422.
Stenske KA, Bemis DA, Gillespie BE, Oliver SP, Draughon FA, Matteson KJ, Bartges JW. Prevalence of urovirulence genes cnf, hlyD, sfa/foc, and papGIII in fecal Escherichia coli from healthy dogs and their owners. Am J Vet Res 2009, 70:1401-1406.

Autor Patrick L. McDonough
Consultor Editorial Stephen C. Barr

COLITE E PROCTITE

CONSIDERAÇÕES GERAIS

DEFINIÇÃO
- Colite — inflamação do cólon.
- Proctite — inflamação do reto.

FISIOPATOLOGIA
- A inflamação do cólon provoca o acúmulo de citocinas inflamatórias, rompe as junções impermeáveis existentes entre as células epiteliais, estimula a secreção colônica, incita a secreção de muco pelas células caliciformes e interrompe a motilidade.
- Esses mecanismos diminuem a capacidade colônica de absorção de água e eletrólitos, bem como de armazenamento das fezes, o que leva a diarreias frequentes, quase sempre com muco e/ou sangue.

SISTEMA(S) ACOMETIDO(S)
Gastrintestinal.

GENÉTICA
- Há uma predisposição racial à colite ulcerativa histiocítica em cães da raça Boxer.
- Possível associação entre colite e fístulas perianais em cães da raça Pastor alemão.

INCIDÊNCIA/PREVALÊNCIA
- Acomete aproximadamente 30% dos cães com diarreia crônica, examinados em um hospital universitário.
- A prevalência não está bem documentada.

DISTRIBUIÇÃO GEOGRÁFICA
Em geral, N/D, exceto para certas doenças infecciosas (pitiose: na Costa do Golfo e no sudeste dos Estados Unidos; histoplasmose: região do Meio-Oeste e na porção oriental dos Estados Unidos).

IDENTIFICAÇÃO
Espécies
Cães e gatos.

Raça(s) Predominante(s)
- Boxer (colite ulcerativa histiocítica).
- Pastor alemão: possivelmente associada com fístulas perianais.

Idade Média e Faixa Etária
Acomete qualquer idade; os cães da raça Boxer costumam ficar sintomáticos por volta dos 2 anos de idade.

SINAIS CLÍNICOS
Achados Anamnésicos
- As fezes variam de semiformadas a líquidas.
- Alta frequência de defecação com pequeno volume de fezes.
- Após a defecação, os cães frequentemente manifestam tenesmo prolongado.
- Diarreia crônica, muitas vezes com muco e/ou sangue; os gatos podem apresentar fezes formadas com hematoquezia.
- Ocasionalmente, há dor durante a defecação.
- Vômito em alguns cães (~30%).
- A perda de peso é rara.

Achados do Exame Físico
- Geralmente normais.
- Os cães com colite ulcerativa histiocítica podem revelar sinais sistêmicos de perda de peso e anorexia.

CAUSAS
- Imprudência ou intolerância alimentar.
- Administração de medicamentos (antibióticos, AINE).
- Infecciosas — *Trichuris vulpis*, *Ancylostoma caninum*, *Entamoeba histolytica*, *Balantidium coli*, *Giardia* spp., *Trichomonas* spp., *Cryptosporidium* spp., *Salmonella* spp., *Clostridium* spp., *Campylobacter* spp., *Yersinia enterocolitica*, *Escherichia coli*, *Prototheca*, *Histoplasma capsulatum* e pitiose/ficomicose.
- Traumáticas — corpo estranho e material abrasivo.
- Uremia.
- Segmentares — secundárias à pancreatite crônica (colite transversa).
- Alérgicas — proteína da dieta e, possivelmente, bactérias.
- Inflamatórias/imunes — linfoplasmocitárias, eosinofílicas, granulomatosas e histiocíticas.

DIAGNÓSTICO

DIAGNÓSTICO DIFERENCIAL
- Neoplasia — linfoma e adenocarcinoma.
- Síndrome do intestino irritável.
- Pólipos retocolônicos.
- Inversão cecal.
- Intussuscepção ileocecocólica.

HEMOGRAMA/BIOQUÍMICA/URINÁLISE
- Os resultados costumam permanecer normais; é possível a presença de neutrofilia com desvio à esquerda; ocasionalmente, observa-se eosinofilia em casos de colite eosinofílica, parasitismo, histoplasmose e pitiose/ficomicose.
- Em alguns pacientes com sangramento persistente, pode ocorrer leve anemia microcítica hipocrômica.
- Em certos pacientes (gatos, em particular) com doença crônica, observa-se hiperglobulinemia.

OUTROS TESTES LABORATORIAIS
- Os exames de flutuação fecal (múltiplos), esfregaço fecal direto, cultura bacteriana ou cultura fúngica (*Pythium*) podem revelar alguma causa infecciosa.
- As fezes podem exibir positividade ao teste da toxina do *Clostridium perfringens* ou *C. difficile*.
- A presença de microrganismos em brotamento (esporos) pode apoiar a existência de toxina clostrídica.
- Citologia retal em busca de microrganismos *Histoplasma*.
- O meio In Pouch TF** para cultura de *Tritrichomonas foetus*.

DIAGNÓSTICO POR IMAGEM
- Radiografias abdominais — geralmente normais.
- Enema baritado — pode revelar irregularidades da mucosa ou defeitos de preenchimento em pacientes gravemente acometidos, mas esse procedimento é demorado e com baixa relação custo-benefício.
- Ultrassonografia abdominal — pode demonstrar massas, espessamento difuso ou arquitetura alterada do cólon, ou enfartamento dos linfonodos associados.

---

* N. T.: Um sistema ou kit que contém um meio de cultivo próprio e consiste em uma espécie de "bolsa plástica" semelhante às de coleta de sangue que contém o meio de cultura.

OUTROS MÉTODOS DIAGNÓSTICOS
- Colonoscopia com biopsia — técnica de escolha para o diagnóstico; possivelmente se observam o desaparecimento de vasos sanguíneos da submucosa, o aspecto granular da mucosa, bem como a presença de hiperemia, muco excessivo, ulceração, hemorragia puntiforme (ulcerações pequenas) ou massa(s).
- Coletar sempre múltiplas amostras de biopsia, já que o grau de alteração da mucosa não reflete necessariamente a gravidade ou a ausência da doença.

ACHADOS PATOLÓGICOS
Os achados histopatológicos dependem do tipo histológico da colite — linfoplasmocitária, eosinofílica, granulomatosa ou histiocítica; pode-se constatar uma mucosa hiperplásica em casos de síndrome do intestino irritável; além disso, podem-se observar diversos agentes infecciosos com o uso de corantes especiais.

TRATAMENTO

CUIDADO(S) DE SAÚDE ADEQUADO(S)
O tratamento clínico é feito em um esquema ambulatorial a menos que a diarreia seja grave o suficiente a ponto de causar desidratação.

CUIDADO(S) DE ENFERMAGEM
Administrar a pacientes desidratados solução eletrolítica balanceada e suplementada com potássio por vias intravenosa, subcutânea ou oral.

DIETA
- Os pacientes com colite aguda podem ficar em jejum por 24-48 h.
- Experimentar uma dieta hipoalergênica ou com nova fonte proteica em pacientes com colite inflamatória; utilizar rações comerciais ou dietas caseiras que contenham uma fonte proteica à qual o cão ou gato ainda não tenham sido expostos.
- Para aumentar o volume fecal, melhorar a contratilidade do músculo colônico e reter a água fecal para produzir fezes formadas, recomenda-se a suplementação da dieta com fibras pouco fermentáveis (p. ex., farelo de cereais e α-celulose).
- Algumas fibras fermentáveis (p. ex., psílio ou uma dieta com polpa de beterraba ou fruto-oligossacarídeos) podem ser benéficas — os ácidos graxos de cadeia curta produzidos pela fermentação podem ajudar a cicatrizar o cólon e a restaurar a flora bacteriana colônica normal.

ORIENTAÇÃO AO PROPRIETÁRIO
- O tratamento pode ser intermitente e prolongado em pacientes com colite inflamatória/imune e, em alguns casos, observam-se recidivas frequentes, especialmente em animais com a forma granulomatosa.
- Os quadros de colite granulomatosa, pitiose/ficomicose e colite prototecal respondem de forma insatisfatória ao tratamento clínico; pode haver a necessidade de cirurgia.

CONSIDERAÇÕES CIRÚRGICAS
Os segmentos colônicos gravemente acometidos por fibrose decorrente de inflamação crônica e subsequente formação de estenose podem necessitar de excisão cirúrgica, sobretudo em pacientes com a forma granulomatosa da doença; os casos de inversão cecal e intussuscepção ileocecocólica também exigem a intervenção

COLITE E PROCTITE

cirúrgica; com frequência, a pitiose/ficomicose requer a excisão ou o debridamento cirúrgicos.

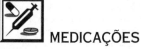

MEDICAÇÕES

MEDICAMENTO(S) DE ESCOLHA

Antimicrobianos
- *Trichuris*, *Ancylostoma* e *Giardia* — fembendazol (50 mg/kg VO a cada 24 h durante 3 dias, repetir após 3 meses).
- *Entamoeba*, *Balantidium* e *Giardia* — metronidazol (25 mg/kg VO a cada 12 h durante 5-7 dias).
- *Tritrichomona foetus* — possivelmente ronidazol (30-50 mg/kg a cada 12 h por 14 dias).
- *Salmonella* — o tratamento é controverso, pois ele pode induzir ao estado de portador; em pacientes com envolvimento sistêmico, selecionar o antibiótico com base nos resultados da cultura bacteriana e do antibiograma (p. ex., enrofloxacino, cloranfenicol ou trimetoprima--sulfa).
- *Clostridium* spp. — metronidazol (10-15 mg/kg VO a cada 12 h por 5-14 dias) ou tilosina (10-15 mg/kg VO a cada 12 h por 7 dias).
- *Campylobacter* spp. — eritromicina (30-40 mg/kg VO a cada 24 h por 5 dias) ou tilosina (45 mg/kg VO a cada 24 h por 5 dias).
- *Yersinia* spp. e *E. coli* — selecionar o medicamento com base nos resultados da cultura bacteriana e do antibiograma.
- *Prototheca* — não há nenhum tratamento conhecido.
- *Histoplasma* — itraconazol (cães, 10 mg/kg VO a cada 24 h; gatos, 5 mg/kg VO a cada 12 h; são necessários vários meses de terapia); em casos avançados, emprega-se a anfotericina B (0,25-0,5 mg/kg lentamente IV a cada 48 h, até uma dose cumulativa de 4-8 mg/kg).
- Pitiose/ficomicose — complexo lipídico de anfotericina B (diluir em solução de glicose a 5% a 1 mg/mL e administrar 3 mg/kg IV nas segundas, quartas e sextas-feiras em um total de 9 tratamentos).

Anti-inflamatórios e Imunossupressores para Colite Inflamatória/Imune
- Sulfassalazina — cães, 25-40 mg/kg VO a cada 8 h por 2-4 semanas; gatos, 20 mg/kg VO a cada 12 h por 2 semanas; pode ser necessário o uso prolongado (com cautela).
- Corticosteroides — prednisona (cães, 2 mg/kg VO a cada 24 h; gatos, 2-4 mg/kg VO a cada 24 h; diminuir a dosagem de forma lenta e gradual em 4-6 meses até se obter a remissão clínica).
- Azatioprina (cães, 2 mg/kg VO a cada 24 h por 2 semanas, seguida por uma redução gradual e, por fim, administração em dias alternados; utilizar em gatos com extrema cautela em virtude da mielossupressão irreversível, 0,3 mg/kg VO a cada 24 h por 3-4 meses; em gatos, considerar a clorambucila, no lugar da azatioprina, a 2 mg em dias alternados até a cada 3 dias).
- Ciclosporina modificada (2-5 mg/kg VO a cada 12 h).
- Sulfassalazina ou outro ácido 5-aminossalicílico — podem ser os medicamentos de escolha para colite linfoplasmocitária.
- A prednisona e a azatioprina ficam indicadas em casos de colite eosinofílica e colite linfoplasmocitária *grave* irresponsiva a outras terapias.
- A colite ulcerativa histiocítica em cães pode responder ao tratamento com enrofloxacino (5-20 mg/kg/dia) isoladamente ou em combinação com metronidazol a 15-20 mg/kg VO a cada 12 h e amoxicilina a 10-20 mg/kg VO a cada 12 h por 6 semanas.
- Reavaliar o diagnóstico com cuidado em cães irresponsivos ao tratamento com o ácido 5-aminossalicílico em 4 semanas; certificar-se que uma causa subjacente (p. ex., infecção pelo *C. perfringens*) não tenha passado despercebida.

Modificadores da Motilidade (Apenas para o Alívio Sintomático)
- Loperamida (0,1 mg/kg VO a cada 8-12 h).
- Difenoxilato (0,1-0,2 mg/kg VO a cada 8 h).
- Brometo de propantelina (0,25-0,5 mg/kg VO a cada 8 h) se o espasmo colônico estiver contribuindo para os sinais clínicos.

CONTRAINDICAÇÕES
Anticolinérgicos.

PRECAUÇÕES
- Monitorizar os pacientes submetidos à sulfassalazina quanto ao aparecimento dos sinais de ceratoconjuntivite seca.
- Monitorizar os pacientes submetidos à azatioprina quanto à ocorrência de mielossupressão — realizar o hemograma completo a cada 2-3 semanas; interromper o tratamento ou administrá-lo em dias alternados se o leucograma declinar abaixo de 3.000 células/μL.
- A anfotericina B e o complexo lipídico de anfotericina B são nefrotóxicos, exigindo a avaliação e a monitorização da função renal.

MEDICAMENTO(S) ALTERNATIVO(S)
Em caso de ineficácia do fembendazol ou do metronidazol, empregar o albendazol (25 mg/kg VO a cada 12 h por 2 dias) para o tratamento da giardíase; monitorizar a ocorrência de mielossupressão.

ACOMPANHAMENTO

MONITORIZAÇÃO DO PACIENTE
Raros exames de reavaliação ou telefonemas do proprietário.

PREVENÇÃO
- Evitar a exposição a agentes infecciosos (p. ex., a outros cães, alimentos contaminados e ambientes úmidos).
- Evitar mudanças bruscas na dieta.

COMPLICAÇÕES POSSÍVEIS
- Observa-se a recidiva dos sinais com a falta de tratamento, a redução gradativa do tratamento ou a evolução da doença.
- Formação de estenose, em virtude da inflamação crônica.

EVOLUÇÃO ESPERADA E PROGNÓSTICO
- Maior parte das infecções — excelentes com a instituição do tratamento (cura).
- *Prototheca* — graves; não há nenhum tratamento conhecido, exceto a excisão.
- *Histoplasma* spp. — maus em casos de doença avançada ou disseminada; os casos leves a moderados geralmente respondem à terapia.
- Pitiose/ficomicose — reservados a maus; pouco responsiva ao tratamento; alguns cães exibem resultados razoáveis com a excisão e o complexo lipídico de anfotericina B.
- Origens traumáticas, urêmicas e segmentares — bons se a causa subjacente for tratável.
- Inversão cecal, intussuscepção ileocecocólica e pólipos — bons com a remoção cirúrgica.
- Causas inflamatórias — bons com o tratamento em pacientes acometidos pela doença linfoplasmocitária, eosinofílica e, possivelmente, histiocítica. Na persistência dos sinais clínicos, reavaliar o diagnóstico; prognóstico mau em pacientes com a doença granulomatosa a curto prazo, que se agrava com a ocorrência de recidiva ou a resposta insatisfatória ao tratamento.

DIVERSOS

DISTÚRBIOS ASSOCIADOS
As doenças inflamatórias/imunes e os agentes infecciosos também podem afetar o intestino delgado.

POTENCIAL ZOONÓTICO
Entamoeba, *Balantidium*, *Giardia*, *Salmonella*, *Clostridium*, *Campylobacter*, *Yersinia*, *E. coli*; *Prototheca* e *Histoplasma* em animais imunossuprimidos.

GESTAÇÃO/FERTILIDADE/REPRODUÇÃO
É preciso ter cautela com o uso de corticosteroides, azatioprina, antifúngicos e antibióticos.

SINÔNIMO(S)
- Diarreia do intestino grosso.
- Enteropatia inflamatória.

VER TAMBÉM
- Capítulos individuais sobre Agentes Infecciosos e Parasitários.
- Colite Ulcerativa Histiocítica.
- Enteropatia Inflamatória.

ABREVIATURA(S)
- AINE = anti-inflamatório não esteroide.

Sugestões de Leitura
Parnell NK. Chronic colitis. In: Bonagura JD, Twedt DC, eds., Current Veterinary Therapy XIV. St. Louis: Elsevier, 2009, pp. 515-520.
Washabau RJ, Holt DE. Diseases of the large intestine. In: Ettinger SJ, Feldman EC, eds., Textbook of Veterinary Internal Medicine, 6th ed. St. Louis: Elsevier, 2005, pp. 1378-1408.

Autor Lisa E. Moore
Consultor Editorial Albert E. Jergens

COLITE ULCERATIVA HISTIOCÍTICA

CONSIDERAÇÕES GERAIS

REVISÃO
- Doença rara caracterizada por ulceração e inflamação da mucosa colônica, com histiócitos (macrófagos) positivos ao ácido periódico de Schiff (PAS).
- Mecanismos etiológico e patogênico desconhecidos; no entanto, foi postulada uma causa infecciosa.

IDENTIFICAÇÃO
- Cães; acomete principalmente Boxer jovem, em geral, com menos de 2-4 anos de idade.
- Há relatos de casos em Buldogue francês, Mastife, Malamute do Alasca e Doberman pinscher; também foi relatada em 1 gato.
- Possível base genética, mas desconhecida.

SINAIS CLÍNICOS
- Diarreia sanguinolenta e mucoide, com aumento na frequência de defecação.
- Tenesmo.
- No final do processo patológico, o animal pode exibir perda de peso e debilidade.

CAUSAS E FATORES DE RISCO
Não há causas ou fatores predisponentes conhecidos, além daqueles relacionados com a raça Boxer.

DIAGNÓSTICO

DIAGNÓSTICO DIFERENCIAL
- Outras causas de colite — enteropatia inflamatória não histiocítica, colite infecciosa, colite parasitária, colite alérgica.
- Inversão cecal.
- Intussuscepção ileocólica.
- Neoplasia — linfoma, adenocarcinoma.
- Corpo estranho.
- Pólipos retocolônicos.
- Síndrome do intestino irritável.
- Diferenciar por meio dos exames de flutuação fecal, esfregaço direto, cultura bacteriana em busca de patógenos, obtenção de imagens abdominais, bem como colonoscopia e biopsia.

HEMOGRAMA/BIOQUÍMICA/URINÁLISE
- Costumam permanecer normais.
- Em alguns pacientes, há neutrofilia, leve anemia e hipoalbuminemia.

OUTROS TESTES LABORATORIAIS
N/D.

DIAGNÓSTICO POR IMAGEM
Na ultrassonografia abdominal, podem ser observadas alterações como parede colônica espessada e linfonodos enfartados.

MÉTODOS DIAGNÓSTICOS
A colonoscopia revela focos avermelhados irregulares (ulcerações puntiformes), ulceração evidente, pregas espessadas da mucosa, áreas de tecido de granulação e estenoses; obter múltiplas amostras de biopsia.

ACHADOS PATOLÓGICOS
- Espessamento e distorção da lâmina própria, além de infiltração da mucosa e da submucosa por histiócitos; no entanto, também podem ser observados linfócitos e plasmócitos; em alguns animais, observam-se perda do epitélio colônico e das células caliciformes, além de ulceração com infiltração neutrofílica.
- Positividade dos histiócitos à coloração com PAS.

TRATAMENTO
- Tratamento clínico em um esquema ambulatorial.
- Mudança na dieta com suplementação de fibras moderadamente fermentáveis.
- Orientar o proprietário sobre a natureza progressiva e a possibilidade de recidiva.

MEDICAÇÕES

MEDICAMENTO(S)
Antimicrobianos — Terapia de Primeira Linha
- Enrofloxacino (5-20 mg/kg/dia) isoladamente ou em combinação com metronidazol e/ou amoxicilina.
- Metronidazol (15 mg/kg VO a cada 12 h).
- Tilosina (45 mg/kg VO a cada 24 h).

Anti-inflamatórios/Imunossupressores (Considerar Apenas se os Antimicrobianos forem Ineficazes; Eficácia Questionável)
- Corticosteroides — prednisona (2 mg/kg VO a cada 24 h até a remissão clínica; em seguida, reduzir a dose de forma gradativa e lenta em 4-6 meses).
- Sulfassalazina (25-40 mg/kg VO a cada 8 h).
- Azatioprina (2 mg/kg a cada 24 h por 2 semanas, seguidos pela administração em dias alternados).

CONTRAINDICAÇÕES/INTERAÇÕES POSSÍVEIS
- Evitar os anticolinérgicos.
- Monitorizar o paciente quanto à ocorrência de ceratoconjuntivite seca, observada algumas vezes com o uso da sulfassalazina.
- Monitorizar também quanto ao desenvolvimento de neutropenia (por meio de hemogramas completos), constatada ocasionalmente com o emprego da azatioprina.

ACOMPANHAMENTO

MONITORIZAÇÃO DO PACIENTE
- Inicialmente, monitorizar os sinais clínicos e o peso corporal em intervalos semanais a quinzenais.
- Talvez haja necessidade de terapia prolongada com o enrofloxacino.

PREVENÇÃO
N/D.

COMPLICAÇÕES POSSÍVEIS
- Pode ser uma doença progressiva e incontrolável.
- Estenose colônica em caso de inflamação não controlada por longos períodos.

EVOLUÇÃO ESPERADA E PROGNÓSTICO
- Relatos recentes indicam que os cães podem ficar livres dos sinais clínicos por até 21 meses após a antibioticoterapia (enrofloxacino).
- Ainda pode haver um subgrupo de cães que respondem inicialmente ao tratamento, seguido por evolução e sinais clínicos irresponsivos.

DIVERSOS

GESTAÇÃO/FERTILIDADE/REPRODUÇÃO
- É preciso ter cautela com o uso de corticosteroides e azatioprina.
- Os pacientes provavelmente não devem ser acasalados em função do potencial de hereditariedade.

VER TAMBÉM
Colite e Proctite.

ABREVIATURA(S)
- PAS = ácido periódico de Schiff.

Sugestões de Leitura
Hostutler RA, Luria BJ, Johnson SE, et al. Antibiotic-responsive histiocytic ulcerative colitis in 9 dogs. J Vet Intern Med 2004, 18:499-504.
Mansfield CS, James FE, Craven M, et al. Remission of histiocytic ulcerative colitis in Boxer dogs correlates with eradication of invasive intramucosal Escherichia coli. J Vet Intern Med 2009, 23:964-969.

Autor Lisa E. Moore
Consultor Editorial Albert E. Jergens

Complexo Granuloma Eosinofílico

CONSIDERAÇÕES GERAIS

DEFINIÇÃO
• Gatos — termo geralmente confuso para quatro síndromes distintas: placa eosinofílica, granuloma eosinofílico, úlcera indolente e dermatite miliar alérgica; agrupadas principalmente de acordo com suas similaridades clínicas, seu desenvolvimento concomitante frequente (e recorrente) e sua resposta positiva aos corticosteroides.
• Cães — os granulomas eosinofílicos caninos são raros; não fazem parte do complexo da doença; diferenças específicas dos gatos são listadas separadamente.

FISIOPATOLOGIA
• Placa eosinofílica — reação de hipersensibilidade, mais frequente a insetos (pulgas, mosquitos); menos frequente a alérgenos alimentares ou ambientais; exacerbada por traumatismo mecânico.
• Granuloma eosinofílico — envolve múltiplas causas, inclusive predisposição genética e possivelmente hipersensibilidade.
• Úlcera indolente — pode ter causas tanto de hipersensibilidade como genéticas.
• Dermatite miliar alérgica — reação de hipersensibilidade muito comum, muito frequentemente a pulgas.
• Eosinófilo — principal célula infiltrativa no granuloma eosinofílico, na placa eosinofílica e na dermatite miliar alérgica, mas não na úlcera indolente; leucócitos localizados em maior número nos tecidos epiteliais; mais frequentemente associado a problemas alérgicos ou parasitários, mas exerce um papel mais genérico na reação inflamatória.
• Granulomas eosinofílicos caninos — pode haver predisposição genética e ter como causa a hipersensibilidade (sobretudo em raças não suscetíveis em termos genéticos).

SISTEMA(S) ACOMETIDO(S)
Pele/exócrino.

GENÉTICA
Vários relatos de indivíduos aparentados acometidos e um estudo do desenvolvimento da doença em uma colônia de gatos livres de patógeno específico indicam que, pelo menos em alguns indivíduos, a predisposição genética (que talvez resulte em uma disfunção hereditária de regulação eosinofílica) é um componente significativo para o desenvolvimento de granuloma eosinofílico e úlcera indolente.

INCIDÊNCIA/PREVALÊNCIA
N/D.

DISTRIBUIÇÃO GEOGRÁFICA
A incidência sazonal em algumas áreas geográficas pode indicar exposição a inseto ou alérgeno do ambiente.

IDENTIFICAÇÃO
Espécies
• Gatos — placa eosinofílica, úlcera indolente e dermatite miliar alérgica.
• Cães e gatos — granuloma eosinofílico.

Raça(s) Predominante(s)
• Gatos — nenhuma.
• Granulomas eosinofílicos caninos — Husky siberiano (76% dos casos), Cavalier King Charles Spaniel, possivelmente Pastor alemão.

Idade Média e Faixa Etária
• Placa eosinofílica — 2-6 anos de idade.
• Granuloma eosinofílico de origem genética — <2 anos de idade.
• Distúrbio alérgico — >2 anos de idade.
• Úlcera indolente — não há relato de predisposição etária.
• Granulomas eosinofílicos caninos — em geral, <3 anos de idade.

Sexo Predominante
• Gatos — predileção relatada por fêmeas.
• Granulomas eosinofílicos caninos — machos (72% dos casos).

SINAIS CLÍNICOS
Comentários Gerais — Gatos
• A distinção entre as síndromes depende dos sinais clínicos e dos achados histopatológicos.
• Podem ocorrer lesões atribuídas a mais de uma síndrome simultaneamente.

Achados Anamnésicos — Gatos
• Lesões de todas as quatro síndromes podem se desenvolver de forma espontânea e aguda.
• O desenvolvimento de placas eosinofílicas pode ser precedido por períodos de letargia.
• É possível uma incidência sazonal.
• É comum haver exacerbação e diminuição dos sinais clínicos em todas as quatro síndromes.

Achados do Exame Físico
• Placas eosinofílicas — manchas alopécicas, eritematosas e erosivas ou placas bem delimitadas e de parede íngreme; em geral, ocorrem nas regiões inguinais, perineal, lateral das coxas, abdominal ventral e axilares; são frequentemente úmidas ou brilhantes; é comum a presença de linfadenopatia.
• Granulomas eosinofílicos — existem cinco tipos, com manifestações ocasionalmente sobrepostas:
  ○ Orientação distintamente linear (granuloma linear) na parte caudal das coxas.
  ○ Placas individuais ou coalescentes em qualquer local do corpo; ulceradas com padrão em "paralelepípedo" ou irregular; brancas ou amarelas, possivelmente representando degeneração do colágeno.
  ○ Margem labial e queixo inchados ("bolsa").
  ○ Coxins palmoplantares tumefatos e dolorosos com claudicação (mais comuns em gatos com menos de 2 anos de idade).
  ○ Ulcerações na cavidade bucal (sobretudo na língua, no palato e nos arcos palatinos); os gatos com lesões bucais podem exibir disfagia, halitose e salivação.
• O desenvolvimento das lesões pode cessar espontaneamente em alguns gatos, em especial na forma hereditária do granuloma eosinofílico.
• Dermatite miliar alérgica — múltiplas pápulas crostosas de cor castanha/escura e eritematosas; as lesões são mais frequentemente palpadas do que visualizadas; pode ser associada à alopecia; vinculada, em geral, com prurido; com frequência, afeta o dorso.
• Úlceras indolentes — ulcerações classicamente côncavas e endurecidas de aspecto granular e cor amarelo-alaranjada, confinadas aos lábios superiores adjacentes ao filtro nasal.
• Granulomas eosinofílicos caninos — placas e massas ulceradas; cor escura ou alaranjada; muito frequente, afetam a língua e os arcos palatinos; há relatos de lesões cutâneas no prepúcio e nos flancos.

CAUSAS
• Alergia — a pulgas ou insetos (picada de mosquito), hipersensibilidade alimentar e atopia.
• Foi proposta uma disfunção hereditária da proliferação de eosinófilos.
• Granulomas eosinofílicos caninos — causas desconhecidas; genética em raças suscetíveis; em geral, suspeita-se de uma reação de hipersensibilidade (a picadas de inseto) em raças não suscetíveis em termos genéticos.

DIAGNÓSTICO

DIAGNÓSTICO DIFERENCIAL
• Inclui as outras doenças do complexo.
• Dermatite por herpes-vírus.
• Infecção por FeLV ou FIV.
• Lesões irresponsivas — excluir pênfigo foliáceo, dermatofitose e infecção fúngica profunda, demodiciose, piodermite e neoplasia (especialmente adenocarcinoma metastático, carcinoma de células escamosas e linfoma epiteliotrópico).
• Granulomas eosinofílicos caninos — neoplasia, histiocitose, granuloma infeccioso e não infeccioso, traumatismo.

HEMOGRAMA/BIOQUÍMICA/URINÁLISE
Hemograma completo — eosinofilia leve a moderada.

OUTROS TESTES LABORATORIAIS
FIV e FeLV — doenças pruriginosas associadas a esses vírus.

MÉTODOS DIAGNÓSTICOS
• Esfregaços por impressão das lesões — grande número de eosinófilos.
• Controle satisfatório e abrangente de pulgas e insetos — ajuda a excluir hipersensibilidade a picadas de pulgas e mosquitos.
• Ensaios de exclusão de alimentos ("dieta de eliminação" ou hipoalergênica) — em todos os casos; fornecer uma fonte proteica nova ou dieta hidrolisada; usar exclusivamente por 8-10 semanas; em seguida, voltar à dieta prévia e observar se surgem novas lesões (reexposição provocativa).
• Atopia — identificada por teste cutâneo intradérmico (de preferência); injetar por via intradérmica pequenas quantidades de alérgenos diluídos; uma reação positiva é indicada pelo desenvolvimento de urticária ou vergão no local da injeção. Também existem testes sorológicos disponíveis para alergia.

ACHADOS PATOLÓGICOS
• Diagnóstico histopatológico — necessário para distinguir as síndromes.
• Placa eosinofílica — espongiose e mucinose foliculares e epidérmicas graves com exocitose eosinofílica; infiltrado eosinofílico dérmico perivascular a difuso intenso; epiderme erodida ou ulcerada.
• Granuloma eosinofílico — focos distintos de degranulação eosinofílica e degeneração do colágeno semelhantemente à formação de granuloma ("figuras em chama"); apoptose dos queratinócitos associada aos eosinófilos; epiderme acantótica erodida, ulcerada e exsudativa.

Complexo Granuloma Eosinofílico

- Úlcera indolente — ulceração grave da epiderme ou da mucosa com degranulação eosinofílica ao nível da necrose; dermatite fibrosante e inflamação neutrofílica; é incomum uma infiltração eosinofílica significativa.
- Dermatite miliar alérgica — focos discretos de erosão e necrose epidérmicas com crostas eosinofílicas brilhantes; infiltrado dérmico perivascular a intersticial rico em eosinófilos.
- Granulomas eosinofílicos caninos — focos de granulomas em paliçada e "figuras em chama" em torno das fibras de colágeno; infiltrado com eosinófilos mesclados com macrófagos, mastócitos, plasmócitos e linfócitos.

TRATAMENTO

CUIDADO(S) DE SAÚDE ADEQUADO(S)
- A maioria dos pacientes pode ser tratada de forma ambulatorial a menos que a doença bucal grave impeça a ingestão adequada de líquido.
- Identificar e eliminar o(s) alérgeno(s) agressor(es) antes da intervenção clínica.
- Hipossensibilização de gatos com teste cutâneo intradérmico positivo — pode ter sucesso na maioria dos casos; preferível à administração prolongada de corticosteroides.

CUIDADO(S) DE ENFERMAGEM
Desestimular o proprietário a escovar muito o paciente para não agravar as lesões.

ATIVIDADE
Sem restrições.

DIETA
Sem restrições a menos que haja suspeita de alergia alimentar.

ORIENTAÇÃO AO PROPRIETÁRIO
- Informar os proprietários sobre as possíveis causas alérgicas ou hereditárias.
- Discutir a natureza flutuante dessas doenças, com exacerbações e melhoras.
- Proprietários responsáveis podem preferir adiar a intervenção clínica a menos que surjam lesões graves.

CONSIDERAÇÕES CIRÚRGICAS
Granulomas eosinofílicos caninos — lesões individuais podem ser excisadas se sofrerem traumatismo mecânico e forem irresponsivas ao tratamento clínico.

MEDICAÇÕES

MEDICAMENTO(S) DE ESCOLHA
Placa e Granuloma Eosinofílicos
- Alguns casos melhoram com antibióticos: trimetoprima-sulfadiazina a 15 mg/kg a cada 12 h, cefalexina a 22 mg/kg a cada 12 h, amoxicilina triidratada-clavulanato a 12,5 mg/kg a cada 12 h, ou clindamicina a 5,5 mg/kg a cada 12 h.
- Metilprednisolona injetável — 20 mg/gato, repetir em 2 semanas (se necessário); tratamento mais comum; é usual a taquifilaxia com injeções repetidas; não é aconselhável para terapia a longo prazo.
- Corticosteroides orais — tratamento contínuo com prednisolona (2-4 mg/kg a cada 48 h) necessário para controlar as lesões; pode ocorrer taquifilaxia esteroide, podendo ser específica para o medicamento administrado; pode ser válido mudar a formulação; outros medicamentos: dexametasona (0,1-0,2 mg/kg a cada 24-72 h) e triancinolona (0,1-0,2 mg/kg a cada 24-72 h); talvez haja necessidade de dosagens maiores para indução, embora elas devam ser diminuídas o mais rapidamente possível.
- Tópicos: fluocinolona/DMSO (Synotic® loção) para lesões individuais; não são práticos e/ou podem causar efeitos sistêmicos em pacientes com grande quantidade de lesões.

Úlcera Indolente
- Corticosteroides injetáveis ou orais — ver o item "Placa e Granuloma Eosinofílicos" (acima).
- Alfainterferona — 30-60 U diárias em ciclos de 7 dias sim, 7 dias não; sucesso limitado; efeitos colaterais raros; não há necessidade de qualquer monitorização terapêutica específica.
- Alguns casos melhoram com antibióticos: trimetoprima-sulfadiazina a 15 mg/kg a cada 12 h, cefalexina a 22 mg/kg a cada 12 h, amoxicilina triidratada-clavulanato a 12,5 mg/kg a cada 12 h, ou clindamicina a 5,5 mg/kg a cada 12 h.

Terapias Alternativas
- Clorambucila a 0,1-0,2 mg/kg a cada 48-72 h.
- Ciclosporina a 5 mg/kg a cada 24-48 h.
- Doxiciclina a 5-10 mg/kg a cada 24 h.
- Alfainterferona a 30-60 UI em ciclos de 7 dias sim, 7 dias não; sucesso limitado.

Granulomas Eosinofílicos Caninos
- Prednisolona oral — 0,5-2,2 mg/kg/dia inicialmente; em seguida, diminuir de forma gradual.
- Corticosteroides intralesionais — 5 mg de metilprednisolona/lesão.
- É comum a interrupção da terapia sem recidiva.

MEDICAMENTO(S) ALTERNATIVO(S)
Acetato de megestrol — 2,5-5 mg a cada 2-7 dias; a incidência significativa de efeitos colaterais (diabetes, câncer de mama) impedem o uso em todos os casos, exceto nos graves e recalcitrantes.

ACOMPANHAMENTO

MONITORIZAÇÃO DO PACIENTE
- Corticosteroides — hemogramas basais e frequentes, perfis bioquímicos séricos e urinálises com cultura.
- Medicamentos imunossupressores seletivos — hemogramas frequentes (primeiro 2 vezes por semana, em seguida 1 ou 2 vezes por mês à medida que a terapia continua) para monitorizar a supressão da medula óssea; perfis bioquímicos séricos rotineiros e urinálises com cultura (primeiro mensalmente, depois a cada 3 meses) para monitorizar complicações (doença renal, diabetes melito e infecção do trato urinário).

EVOLUÇÃO ESPERADA E PROGNÓSTICO
- Se uma causa primária puder ser determinada e controlada, as lesões desaparecerão permanentemente.
- A maioria das lesões apresenta exacerbações e melhoras, com ou sem terapia; portanto, deve-se esperar um esquema de recidiva imprevisível.
- As dosagens dos medicamentos devem ser diminuídas para o menor nível possível (ou interrompidas, se possível) assim que as lesões desaparecerem.
- As lesões em gatos com a doença hereditária podem exibir resolução espontânea depois de alguns anos.
- Granulomas eosinofílicos caninos — as lesões podem ser recalcitrantes à intervenção clínica.

DIVERSOS

GESTAÇÃO/FERTILIDADE/REPRODUÇÃO
Glicocorticoides sistêmicos e agentes imunossupressores não devem ser usados durante a prenhez.

SINÔNIMO(S)
- Dermatopatias eosinofílicas felinas.
- Granuloma eosinofílico — granuloma colagenolítico felino; granuloma linear felino.
- Úlcera indolente — úlcera eosinofílica; úlcera do roedor; dermatite ulcerativa felina do lábio superior.

VER TAMBÉM
- Dermatite Atópica.
- Reações Alimentares (Dermatológicas).

ABREVIATURA(S)
- DMSO = dimetilsulfóxido.
- FIV = vírus da imunodeficiência felina.
- FeLV = vírus da leucemia felina.

Sugestões de Leitura
Power HT, Ihrke PJ. Selected feline eosinophilic skin diseases (eosinophilic granuloma complex). In: Kunkle G, ed. Feline dermatoses. Vet Clin North Am Sm Anim Pract 1995;25:833-850.
Rosenkrantz WS. Feline eosinophilic granuloma complex. In: Griffin CE, Kwochka KW, MacDonald JM, eds. current veterinary dermatology: the science and art of therapy. St. Louis: Mosby, 1993.

Autor Alexander H. Werner
Consultor Editorial Alexander H. Werner

COMPLEXOS ATRIAIS PREMATUROS

CONSIDERAÇÕES GERAIS

DEFINIÇÃO
Correspondem a batimentos atriais prematuros que se originam fora do nó sinoatrial e interrompem o ritmo sinusal fisiológico por um ou mais batimentos.

CARACTERÍSTICAS DO ECG
• A frequência cardíaca costuma permanecer normal; o ritmo apresenta-se irregular em decorrência das ondas P prematuras (denominadas ondas P'), que interrompem o ritmo fisiológico da onda P (Fig. 1).
• Onda P' ectópica — prematura; sua configuração difere das ondas P sinusais e pode ser negativa, positiva, bifásica ou estar sobreposta à onda T anterior.
• Complexo QRS — prematuro; em geral, sua configuração permanece normal (a mesma que a dos complexos sinusais). Se a onda P' aparecer durante o período refratário do nó AV, não ocorrerá a condução ventricular (complexos atriais prematuros não conduzidos), de tal modo que nenhum complexo QRS acompanhará a onda P'. Se houver uma recuperação parcial no nó AV ou nos sistemas de condução intraventricular, a onda P' será conduzida com intervalo P'-R prolongado ou configuração anormal do QRS (condução aberrante). Quanto mais prematuro for o complexo, mais acentuada será a aberração.
• Na relação P-QRS, o intervalo P'-R geralmente se mostra tão longo quanto o intervalo P'-R sinusal, ou até mais prolongado.
• Em geral, uma pausa não compensatória seguirá um complexo atrial prematuro, quando o intervalo R-R dos dois complexos sinusais normais que envolvem um complexo atrial prematuro for menor que os intervalos R-R de três complexos sinusais consecutivos (Fig. 2). O impulso atrial ectópico dispara o nó sinusal e reinicia o ciclo.

FISIOPATOLOGIA
• Mecanismos — aumento na automaticidade das fibras miocárdicas atriais ou existência de um único circuito de reentrada.
• Podem ser um achado normal em cães idosos; comumente observados em cães com aumento de volume atrial, secundário à insuficiência crônica da valva atrioventricular esquerda (mitral); também é possível constatá-los em cães ou gatos com qualquer doença atrial.
• Podem não causar problemas hemodinâmicos; a importância clínica relaciona-se com a frequência, o tempo de regulação do ritmo em relação a outros complexos e os problemas clínicos subjacentes.
• Podem predizer distúrbios rítmicos mais graves (p. ex., fibrilação atrial, *flutter* atrial ou taquicardia atrial).

SISTEMA(S) ACOMETIDO(S)
Cardiovascular.

GENÉTICA
N/D.

INCIDÊNCIA/PREVALÊNCIA
Não há registros.

DISTRIBUIÇÃO GEOGRÁFICA
N/D.

IDENTIFICAÇÃO
Espécies
Cães e gatos.
Raça(s) Predominante(s)
Raças caninas de pequeno porte.
Idade Média e Faixa Etária
Animais geriátricos, exceto aqueles com cardiopatia congênita.
Sexo(s) Predominante(s)
N/D.

SINAIS CLÍNICOS
Achados Anamnésicos
• Ausência de sinais.
• ICC.
• Tosse e dispneia.
• Intolerância ao exercício.
• Síncope.
Achados do Exame Físico
• Ritmo cardíaco irregular.
• Sopro cardíaco.
• Ritmo de galope.
• Sinais de ICC.

CAUSAS E FATORES DE RISCO
• Valvulopatia crônica.
• Cardiopatia congênita.
• Miocardiopatia.
• Miocardite atrial.
• Distúrbios eletrolíticos.
• Neoplasias.
• Hipertireoidismo.
• Toxemias.
• Toxicidade de medicamentos (p. ex., digitálicos).
• Variação normal em animais idosos.

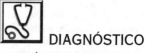

DIAGNÓSTICO

DIAGNÓSTICO DIFERENCIAL
• Arritmia sinusal acentuada.
• Complexos ventriculares prematuros, quando uma condução ventricular aberrante acompanha um complexo atrial prematuro.

HEMOGRAMA/BIOQUÍMICA/URINÁLISE
N/D.

OUTROS TESTES LABORATORIAIS
N/D.

DIAGNÓSTICO POR IMAGEM
A ecocardiografia e a ultrassonografia Doppler podem revelar o tipo e a gravidade da cardiopatia subjacente.

MÉTODOS DIAGNÓSTICOS
Eletrocardiografia.

ACHADOS PATOLÓGICOS
Aumento de volume atrial; outras características variam, dependendo da causa subjacente.

TRATAMENTO

CUIDADO(S) DE SAÚDE ADEQUADO(S)
• Tratar o paciente em regime de internação ou em esquema ambulatorial.
• Tratar a ICC, a cardiopatia ou outras causas subjacentes.

CUIDADO(S) DE ENFERMAGEM
Em geral, não são necessários; variam com a causa subjacente.

ATIVIDADE
Restringir a atividade física no animal sintomático.

DIETA
Sem mudanças a menos que solicitadas para o tratamento da condição subjacente (i. e., dieta com baixo teor de sal [hipossódica]).

ORIENTAÇÃO AO PROPRIETÁRIO
Os complexos atriais prematuros podem não gerar anormalidades hemodinâmicas, mas possivelmente são precursores de arritmias graves.

CONSIDERAÇÕES CIRÚRGICAS
N/D.

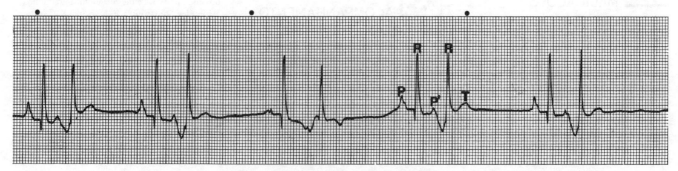

Figura 1 Complexos atriais prematuros em um cão. A onda P' representa o complexo prematuro. O QRS prematuro assemelha-se ao QRS basal. A onda P' vertical encontra-se sobreposta à onda T do complexo anterior. (De: Tilley LP. *Essentials of canine and feline electrocardiography*. 3.ed. Blackwell Publishing, 1992, com permissão.)

COMPLEXOS ATRIAIS PREMATUROS

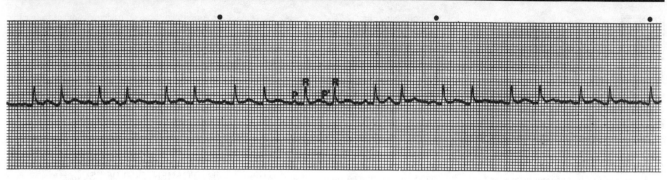

Figura 2 Complexos atriais prematuros em caso de bigeminismo em um gato sob anestesia geral. O segundo complexo de cada par refere-se a um complexo atrial prematuro, no qual o primeiro corresponde a um complexo sinusal. A anormalidade no ritmo desapareceu após a interrupção do anestésico. (De: Tilley LP. *Essentials of canine and feline electrocardiography*. 3.ed. Blackwell Publishing, 1992, com permissão.)

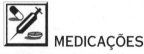
MEDICAÇÕES
MEDICAMENTO(S) DE ESCOLHA
Usados para tratar a ICC e corrigir qualquer desequilíbrio eletrolítico ou acidobásico.
Cães
- Para o tratamento de arritmias significativas do ponto de vista clínico, recomenda-se o uso de digoxina (0,005-0,01 mg/kg VO a cada 12 h, como dose de manutenção), diltiazem (0,5-1,5 mg/kg VO a cada 8 h) ou atenolol (0,25-1 mg/kg VO a cada 12 h).
- Digoxina — terapia de escolha; também é indicada para tratar a descompensação cardíaca normalmente presente.
- A ICC é tratada com dosagens apropriadas de diuréticos e inibidores da enzima conversora da angiotensina; o tratamento adequado da ICC pode reduzir a frequência do complexo atrial prematuro.

Gatos
- Gatos com miocardiopatia hipertrófica — diltiazem (1-2,5 mg/kg VO a cada 8 h) ou atenolol (6,25-12,5 mg VO a cada 12-24 h).
- Gatos com miocardiopatia dilatada — digoxina (1/4 de um comprimido de 0,125 mg a cada 24 ou 48 h).

CONTRAINDICAÇÕES
Em animais com ICC, não é recomendável o emprego dos agentes inotrópicos negativos (p. ex., propranolol).

PRECAUÇÕES
Em animais com bloqueio atrioventricular ou hipotensão subjacente, utilizar com cautela a digoxina, o diltiazem, o atenolol ou o propranolol.

INTERAÇÕES POSSÍVEIS
N/D.

MEDICAMENTO(S) ALTERNATIVO(S)
N/D.

ACOMPANHAMENTO
MONITORIZAÇÃO DO PACIENTE
Monitorizar a frequência e o ritmo cardíacos por meio de ECGs seriados.

PREVENÇÃO
N/D.

COMPLICAÇÕES POSSÍVEIS
Os complexos atriais prematuros frequentes podem diminuir ainda mais o débito cardíaco em pacientes com cardiopatia subjacente e agravar os sintomas clínicos.

EVOLUÇÃO ESPERADA E PROGNÓSTICO
Mesmo em casos de uma terapia antiarrítmica ideal, alguns animais exibem um aumento na frequência de complexos atriais prematuros ou apresentam uma deterioração progressiva para arritmias mais graves à medida que a doença subjacente evolui.

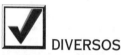
DIVERSOS
DISTÚRBIOS ASSOCIADOS
Nenhum.

FATORES RELACIONADOS COM A IDADE
Ocorrem tipicamente em cães geriátricos.

POTENCIAL ZOONÓTICO
N/D.

GESTAÇÃO/FERTILIDADE/REPRODUÇÃO
N/D.

SINÔNIMO(S)
Extrassístoles atriais, contrações atriais prematuras, impulsos atriais prematuros.

VER TAMBÉM
Taquicardia Supraventricular.

ABREVIATURA(S)
- AV = atrioventricular.
- ICC = insuficiência cardíaca congestiva.

RECURSOS DA INTERNET
www.vetgo.com/cardio.

Sugestões de Leitura
Tilley LP, Smith FWK Jr. Electrocardiography. In: Tilley LP, Smith FWK, Oyama MA, Sleeper MM, eds., Manual of Canine and Feline Cardiology, 4th ed. St. Louis: Saunders Elsevier, 2008, pp. 66-67.

Autores Larry P. Tilley e Naomi L. Burtnick
Consultores Editoriais Larry P. Tilley e Francis W.K. Smith, Jr.

Complexos Ventriculares Prematuros

CONSIDERAÇÕES GERAIS

DEFINIÇÃO
Trata-se de um impulso cardíaco isolado, desencadeado dentro dos ventrículos, e não no nó sinusal.

Características do ECG
- Complexos QRS tipicamente largos e bizarros.
- Ondas P desassociadas dos complexos QRS.

FISIOPATOLOGIA
Os mecanismos incluem aumento na automaticidade, reentrada e pós-despolarizações tardias.

SISTEMA(S) ACOMETIDO(S)
Cardiovascular — efeitos secundários em outros sistemas, decorrentes da má perfusão.

GENÉTICA
Distúrbio poligênico em cães da raça Pastor alemão — arritmia ventricular hereditária.

INCIDÊNCIA/PREVALÊNCIA
Desconhecidas.

IDENTIFICAÇÃO
Espécies
Cães e gatos.

Raça(s) Predominante(s)
- Comuns em cães de grande porte com miocardiopatia, especialmente Boxer e Doberman pinscher.
- Arritmia ventricular hereditária em Pastor alemão.
- Comuns em gatos com miocardiopatia; observados ocasionalmente em gatos com hipertireoidismo.

Idade Média e Faixa Etária
Constatados em todas as faixas etárias.

SINAIS CLÍNICOS
Achados Anamnésicos
- Fraqueza.
- Intolerância a exercícios.
- Síncope.
- Morte súbita.
- Frequentemente assintomáticos.

Achados do Exame Físico
- Ritmo irregular associado a déficits de pulso; pode-se auscultar o desdobramento da primeira ou da segunda bulhas cardíacas.
- Podem se mostrar normais se a arritmia for intermitente e estiver ausente durante o exame.
- Podem-se observar sinais de ICC (p. ex., tosse e dispneia) ou sopro, dependendo da causa da arritmia.

CAUSAS
- Miocardiopatia.
- Defeitos congênitos (sobretudo estenose subaórtica).
- Valvulopatia crônica.
- Dilatação e vólvulo gástricos.
- Miocardite traumática (cães).
- Intoxicação por digitálicos.
- Hipertireoidismo (gatos).
- Neoplasia cardíaca.
- Miocardite.
- Pancreatite.

FATORES DE RISCO
- Hipocalemia.
- Hipomagnesemia.
- Distúrbios acidobásicos.
- Hipoxia.

DIAGNÓSTICO

DIAGNÓSTICO DIFERENCIAL
- Batimentos supraventriculares prematuros com bloqueio de ramo do feixe de His.
- Pesquisar por ondas P associadas a complexos QRS largos; um complexo atrial prematuro com condução aberrante possui onda P associada.
- Um complexo atrial prematuro costuma ser acompanhado por pausa não compensatória, em que o intervalo R-R dos dois complexos sinusais incluindo uma contração atrial prematura é menor que o intervalo R-R de três complexos sinusais consecutivos.
- Um complexo ventricular prematuro, em geral, é acompanhado por pausa compensatória, em que o intervalo R-R de dois complexos sinusais incluindo uma contração ventricular prematura é superior ou igual ao intervalo R-R de três complexos sinusais consecutivos.

HEMOGRAMA/BIOQUÍMICA/URINÁLISE
- A hipocalemia e a hipomagnesemia predispõem os animais a arritmias ventriculares e atenuam a resposta aos antiarrítmicos de classe I (p. ex., lidocaína, procainamida, mexiletina e quinidina).
- Se a condição for secundária à pancreatite, haverá altos níveis de amilase e lipase.

OUTROS TESTES LABORATORIAIS
Se a condição for secundária ao hipertireoidismo, haverá altos níveis de T_4 (gatos).

DIAGNÓSTICO POR IMAGEM
A ecocardiografia pode revelar a presença de cardiopatia estrutural.

MÉTODOS DIAGNÓSTICOS
Registro eletrocardiográfico deambulatório (Holter) a longo prazo para detectar arritmias ventriculares transitórias em pacientes com síncope ou fraqueza inexplicáveis.

ACHADOS PATOLÓGICOS
Variam de acordo com a causa subjacente.

TRATAMENTO

CUIDADO(S) DE SAÚDE ADEQUADO(S)
Em geral, o tratamento é feito em um esquema ambulatorial.

CUIDADO(S) DE ENFERMAGEM
Varia(m) de acordo com a causa subjacente.

ATIVIDADE
Restringir a atividade física se a arritmia for acompanhada por sinais clínicos ou indícios de cardiopatia estrutural.

ORIENTAÇÃO AO PROPRIETÁRIO
Alertar o proprietário quanto ao potencial de agravamento da arritmia e quanto à possível ocorrência de síncope ou morte súbita.

CONSIDERAÇÕES CIRÚRGICAS
- É recomendável a monitorização eletrocardiográfica contínua, enquanto o animal se encontra anestesiado.
- A pré-medicação do paciente com acepromazina (0,02-0,05 mg/kg) eleva o limiar de fibrilação ventricular.
- Não se recomendam as induções com máscaras; a liberação simpática durante esse tipo de indução pode agravar a arritmia.
- Evitar o uso de anticolinérgicos a menos que ocorra o desenvolvimento de bradicardia.

MEDICAÇÕES

MEDICAMENTO(S) DE ESCOLHA
Comentários Gerais
- Corrigir qualquer hipocalemia ou hipomagnesemia.
- Terapia medicamentosa na ausência de sinais clínicos — controversa; os estudos em seres humanos com complexos ventriculares prematuros assintomáticos e infartos do miocárdio demonstraram alta incidência de morte súbita quando o tratamento era iniciado com agentes antiarrítmicos de classe I; não foram conduzidos estudos semelhantes em pacientes veterinários.
- O autor geralmente não prescreve os medicamentos antiarrítmicos a menos que haja indícios de sinais clínicos de baixo débito cardíaco (p. ex., fraqueza episódica ou síncope) ou a crença de que o paciente esteja sob alto risco de morte súbita, com base na presença do fenômeno de R sobre T ou associação racial com complexos ventriculares prematuros e morte súbita (p. ex., Boxer e Doberman pinscher).
- Se a terapia antiarrítmica for instituída na tentativa de reduzir o risco de morte súbita, o autor costuma escolher algum β-bloqueador ou o sotalol; ainda não se realizaram quaisquer estudos para confirmar a eficácia dos β-bloqueadores na prevenção de morte súbita em cães ou gatos.

Cães
- Paciente que não se encontra em ICC ou hipotenso — iniciar a terapia com algum β-bloqueador, como o propranolol (0,2-1 mg/kg VO a cada 8 h), o atenolol (0,2-1 mg/kg a cada 12 h) ou o metoprolol (0,2-1 mg/kg VO a cada 8-12 h) ou com algum agente antiarrítmico de classe III, como o sotalol (1-3,5 mg/kg VO a cada 12 h).
- Paciente em ICC ou hipotenso — iniciar a terapia com algum antiarrítmico de classe I, como a mexiletina (5-8 mg/kg VO a cada 8 h) ou a procainamida (8-20 mg/kg VO a cada 6-8 h).
- Se uma arritmia relevante persistir, deve-se associar algum medicamento antiarrítmico de classe I com algum β-bloqueador ou com o sotalol.

Gatos
- Atenolol (6,25-12,5 mg VO a cada 12 h).

CONTRAINDICAÇÕES
Evitar a administração de atropina e catecolaminas (p. ex., adrenalina e dopamina) até que a arritmia esteja controlada.

PRECAUÇÕES
- Em animais com ICC, devem-se utilizar os β-bloqueadores com cautela; inicialmente, tais agentes deprimem a contratilidade do miocárdio.
- Usar a digoxina com cuidado, pois esse agente pode potencialmente agravar as arritmias ventriculares.

COMPLEXOS VENTRICULARES PREMATUROS

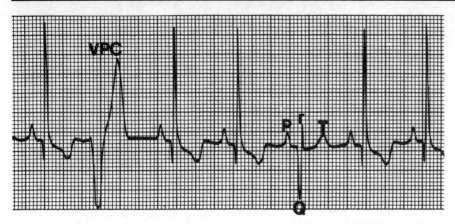

Figura 1 Complexo ventricular prematuro e complexo de fusão (quinto complexo) em cão com miocardite decorrente de pancreatite. O complexo de fusão corresponde à ativação simultânea do ventrículo por impulsos provenientes do nó sinoatrial e dos focos ectópicos ventriculares. O complexo QRS apresenta uma forma intermediária. (De: Tilley LP. *Essentials of canine and feline electrocardiography*. 3.ed., Baltimore: Williams & Wilkins, 1992, com permissão.)

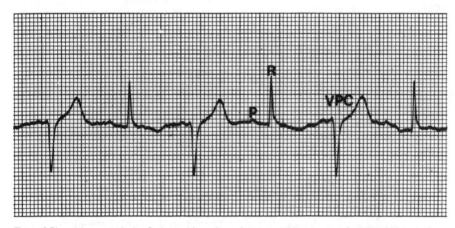

Figura 2 Bigeminismo ventricular. Cada complexo alternado corresponde a um complexo ventricular prematuro proveniente do mesmo foco. Cada um deles está acoplado (o intervalo é o mesmo entre este e o complexo sinusal adjacente) ao complexo normal anterior. (De: Tilley LP. *Essentials of canine and feline electrocardiography*. 3.ed., Baltimore: Williams & Wilkins, 1992, com permissão.)

- Os medicamentos que prolongam o potencial de ação (p. ex., sotalol) podem piorar a arritmia em Pastor alemão com arritmia ventricular hereditária.

INTERAÇÕES POSSÍVEIS
A quinidina e a amiodarona elevam os níveis séricos da digoxina.

MEDICAMENTO(S) ALTERNATIVO(S)
- Considerar a amiodarona (5-10 mg/kg VO a cada 12 h) em casos de arritmias refratárias em cães (medicamento reservado, em geral, para taquicardia ventricular).
- Considerar o sotalol (10-20 mg/gato VO a cada 12 h) ou a procainamida (3-8 mg/kg VO a cada 6-8 h) para gatos intolerantes aos β-bloqueadores.

ACOMPANHAMENTO

MONITORIZAÇÃO DO PACIENTE
- O uso do aparelho Holter é preferível para monitorizar a gravidade da arritmia e a eficácia da terapia antiarrítmica; o objetivo da terapia antiarrítmica é reduzir a frequência de ectopia ventricular em >85%.
- Os ECGs seriados não são tão úteis quanto a monitorização com o Holter — os complexos ventriculares prematuros e a taquicardia ventricular paroxística podem ocorrer esporadicamente ao longo do dia.
- Monitorizar os níveis séricos da digoxina em pacientes submetidos a essa medicação.

PREVENÇÃO
Corrigir os fatores predisponentes, tais como hipocalemia, hipomagnesemia, hipoxia do miocárdio e intoxicação por digoxina.

COMPLICAÇÕES POSSÍVEIS
Síncope e morte súbita.

EVOLUÇÃO ESPERADA E PROGNÓSTICO
- Se a causa for metabólica — a condição pode desaparecer e apresentar um prognóstico bom.
- Se a condição estiver associada à cardiopatia — o prognóstico torna-se reservado; os complexos ventriculares prematuros podem aumentar o risco de morte súbita.

DIVERSOS

VER TAMBÉM
- Doença de Chagas (Tripanossomíase Americana).
- Miocardite.
- Taquicardia Ventricular.
- Toxicidade da Digoxina.

ABREVIATURA(S)
- ECG = eletrocardiograma.
- ICC = insuficiência cardíaca congestiva.
- T_4 = tiroxina.

Sugestões de Leitura

Knight DH. Reason must supersede dogma in the management of ventricular arrhythmias. In: Bonagura JD, ed., Kirk's Current Veterinary Therapy XIII. Philadelphia: Saunders, 2000, pp. 730-733.

Kraus MS, Gelzer ARM, Moise S. Treatment of cardiac arrhythmias and conduction disturbances. In: Tilley LP, Smith FWK, Oyama MA, Sleeper MM, eds., Manual of Canine and Feline Cardiology, 4th ed. St. Louis: Saunders Elsevier, 2008, pp. 315-332.

Tilley LP, Smith FWK, Jr. Electrocardiography. In: Tilley LP, Smith FWK, Oyama MA, Sleeper MM, eds., Manual of Canine and Feline Cardiology, 4th ed. St. Louis: Saunders Elsevier, 2008, pp. 49-77.

Autor Francis W.K. Smith, Jr.
Consultores Editoriais Larry P. Tilley e Francis W.K. Smith, Jr.

Comportamento de Marcação Territorial e Errático — Cães

CONSIDERAÇÕES GERAIS

REVISÃO
- Comportamento de marcação — os cães emitem um sinal para animais da mesma espécie com uma marca visual ou deixam um cheiro (urina, fezes, sacos anais ou glândulas sebáceas) em um objeto ou para delimitar território.
- Comportamento errático — andar errante para exploração ou busca de parceiros potenciais, alimento ou contato social.
- Comportamentos normais com múltiplas causas — pode ser maladaptativo devido a estímulos no ambiente do cão.

IDENTIFICAÇÃO
- Qualquer sexo ou raça.
- Idade de início — maturidade sexual (em torno de 1 ano de idade).
- Sexo — ambos, mas predominantemente em machos.
- Mais comum em machos intactos ou fêmeas intactas no estro (cio).
- Também exibido por machos e fêmeas castrados.

SINAIS CLÍNICOS
- Comportamento de marcação — depósito de urina e/ou material fecal em locais inaceitáveis para os proprietários; ocorre dentro e fora da casa.
- Comportamento errático — comportamento errante que faz o cão sair de sua casa; pode ocorrer secundariamente a outros problemas comportamentais.
- Os achados do exame físico não são dignos de nota a menos que haja uma etiologia médica para o comportamento de marcação.

CAUSAS
- Comportamentos caninos normais. A marcação com urina ocorre mais comumente em áreas novas e não no ambiente doméstico. As cadelas raramente efetuam marcação na casa.
- Regulação hormonal; é provável que os machos intactos tenham um comportamento de marcação territorial e errático.
- Possíveis componentes aprendidos; o estado reprodutivo não é a única variável.

Comportamento Errático
- Ansiedade.
- Curiosidade.
- Reprodução.
- Contato social e atividade lúdica.

Comportamento de Marcação Territorial
- Problema médico.
- Comunicação com animais da mesma espécie; transmite informações como *ranking* social, estado sexual, limites territoriais ou informações gerais, não relacionadas com a necessidade de esvaziar a bexiga urinária ou o intestino.
- Ansiedade.

FATORES DE RISCO
- É mais provável que os machos intactos tenham o comportamento de marcação territorial e errático.
- Marcação durante passeios; comportamento aprendido.
- Cadelas intactas, ou fêmeas castradas após o primeiro cio.

DIAGNÓSTICO

DIAGNÓSTICO DIFERENCIAL
Definir a causa do comportamento como normal ou um sinal de outro diagnóstico.

Comportamento Errático
- Comportamento sexualmente motivado.
- Tumores produtores de testosterona.
- Fome/busca pelo alimento.
- Ansiedade da separação.
- Fobias a ruídos.
- Comportamento territorial.
- Facilitação social.
- Comportamento predatório.
- Escape de algum recinto — comportamento lúdico/investigativo.

Comportamento de Marcação Territorial
- Comportamento sexualmente motivado.
- Tumores produtores de testosterona.
- Comportamento territorial.
- Comportamento de estado social.
- Comportamento de conflito.
- Ansiedade.
- Evacuação domiciliar; adestramento domiciliar incompleto ou perda desse adestramento.
- Doença do trato urinário.
- Qualquer problema médico que cause PU/PD.
- Constipação ou diarreia.
- Doença dos sacos anais.

HEMOGRAMA/BIOQUÍMICA/URINÁLISE
Se anormais, tratar os problemas médicos.

OUTROS TESTES LABORATORIAIS
Conforme indicação:
- Teste de função da tireoide em caso de comportamento errático causado por fome.
- Mensuração dos níveis sanguíneos de testosterona em animais castrados que demonstram comportamentos de macho intacto.
- Cultura e antibiograma da urina.
- Citologia vaginal para determinar o ciclo estral.

DIAGNÓSTICO POR IMAGEM
Radiografias ou ultrassonografia em caso de doença do trato urinário.

TRATAMENTO

COMPORTAMENTO ERRÁTICO
- Castrar os machos intactos.
- Prender o animal para evitar fugas.
- Passear com coleira.
- Providenciar exercício, atenção, supervisão e estimulação adequados.
- Considerar o uso de creches ou hotéis para cães.

COMPORTAMENTO DE MARCAÇÃO
- Castrar os machos intactos. A castração reduzirá a marcação domiciliar em 90% ou mais em 40% dos cães machos, enquanto 80% dos cães diminuirão a marcação em no mínimo 50%. A castração exerce pouco a nenhum efeito sobre a marcação com urina em áreas externas.
- Castrar as fêmeas precocemente — antes do primeiro cio para evitar os efeitos hormonais.
- Restringir o acesso a áreas-alvo específicas e fornecer supervisão domiciliar adequada quando o proprietário estiver em casa.
- Providenciar o confinamento, se tolerado, quando o animal estiver sozinho em casa.
- Remover estímulos ou deflagradores.
- Comprimir os sacos anais, se necessário.
- Utilizar faixa abdominal para os machos (tipo Bellyband®) ou calças higiênicas de filhotes para as fêmeas.
- Limpar as áreas marcadas com detergentes enzimáticos eficazes.
- Promover a interação à base de comando/recompensa com o cão.
- Considerar o contracondicionamento ou a dessensibilização sistemática para deflagrar estímulos ou para problemas de ansiedade.
- Considerar a punição à distância para o comportamento de marcação (como borrifação de água, alarme, spray de citronela).

MEDICAÇÕES

MEDICAMENTO(S)
- Não há necessidade de medicação para o comportamento errático a menos que o problema primário (ansiedade da separação ou fobias a ruídos) justifique seu uso. As etiologias médicas devem ser tratadas de acordo.
- Nenhuma medicação é aprovada para a terapia do comportamento de marcação; é aconselhável a assinatura de termo de consentimento informado pelo proprietário. O uso de medicamentos é adequado *apenas* se houver forte suspeita de ansiedade persistente como uma motivação colaboradora.
- A medicação deve ser utilizada *somente* em combinação com um plano satisfatório de mudança comportamental.

Antidepressivos Tricíclicos
- Amitriptilina 1-3 mg/kg a cada 12 h.
- Clomipramina 1-3 mg/kg a cada 12 h.
- Os efeitos colaterais incluem sedação, efeitos anticolinérgicos, distúrbios de condução cardíaca, e sinais GI.

Inibidores Seletivos de Recaptação da Serotonina
- Fluoxetina 0,5-1 mg/kg a cada 24 h.
- Paroxetina 1-2 mg/kg a cada 24 h.
- Sertralina 1-3 mg/kg a cada 24 h.
- Os efeitos colaterais incluem sedação, inapetência, letargia, irritabilidade, retenção de urina, constipação.

Azapirona
- Buspirona 0,5-2 mg/kg a cada 8-12 horas.
- Efeitos colaterais: sinais GI.

Benzodiazepínicos
- Em cães com diagnósticos de ansiedade concomitante — alprazolam 0,01-0,1 mg/kg a cada 8-12 h.

Acetato de Megestrol
- Tratamento ultrapassado, utilizado apenas como último recurso.
- Os efeitos colaterais incluem obesidade, piometra, PU/PD, diabetes melito, hiperplasia mamária e carcinoma.

CONTRAINDICAÇÕES/INTERAÇÕES POSSÍVEIS
- ATCs são contraindicados em animais com distúrbios de condução cardíaca ou glaucoma.
- ATCs e ISRSs são contraindicados para cães com histórico de crises convulsivas.

COMPORTAMENTO DE MARCAÇÃO TERRITORIAL E ERRÁTICO — CÃES

- ATCs e ISRSs não devem ser utilizados em combinação.
- Há relatos de que os medicamentos clomipramina e fluoxetina causam agressividade em cães.
- Ter cuidado com todos os medicamentos se o cão tiver comprometimento hepático ou renal.
- Utilizar os benzodiazepínicos com cuidado em cães agressivos por causa da desinibição.
- Não usar ATCs ou ISRSs com inibidores da monoamina oxidase, incluindo produtos à base de amitraz e selegilina.

ACOMPANHAMENTO

MONITORIZAÇÃO DO PACIENTE
O acompanhamento é variável, dependendo da gravidade do problema e da prescrição ou não de medicamento. Pode haver a necessidade de ajuda para implementar as mudanças para modificação ambiental e comportamental. Os proprietários devem ser incentivados a manter registros ou diários com detalhes dos episódios de marcação territorial ou comportamento errático para avaliar o sucesso do tratamento ou a ausência de resposta. Se a medicação for prescrita, o acompanhamento e os diários são essenciais para avaliar a resposta. Em caso de marcação com urina, é recomendável que os proprietários supervisionem o cão dentro de casa e inspecionem as áreas diariamente em busca de marcas de urina.

PREVENÇÃO
- A castração de machos e fêmeas diminui a probabilidade dos comportamentos de marcação territorial e errático.
- É útil orientar o proprietário sobre técnicas adequadas de criação.

COMPLICAÇÕES POSSÍVEIS
- Comportamento errático — o animal pode ficar perdido ou ser apanhado pelo centro de controle de zoonoses; possível ocorrência de lesão por acidentes de carro ou briga com outros animais.
- Comportamento de marcação territorial — dano à propriedade quando ocorre dentro de casa.
- Abandono do animal de estimação.

DIVERSOS

FATORES RELACIONADOS COM A IDADE
Animais intactos mais idosos que a maturidade sexual.

POTENCIAL ZOONÓTICO
O comportamento errático expõe o animal de estimação a outros animais, inclusive àqueles de vida selvagem — possível exposição à raiva.

GESTAÇÃO/FERTILIDADE/REPRODUÇÃO
É recomendável evitar os medicamentos listados na gestação.

VER TAMBÉM
Evacuação domiciliar — Cães.

ABREVIATURA(S)
- ATC = antidepressivo tricíclico.
- GI = gastrintestinal.
- ISRS = inibidor seletivo de recaptação da serotonina.
- PU/PD = poliúria/polidipsia.

Sugestões de Leitura
Hopkins SG, Schubert TA, Hart BL. Castration of adult male dogs: Effects on roaming, aggression, urine marking, and mounting. JAVMA 1976, 168:1108–1110.
Neilson JC, Ekstein RA, Hart BL. Effect of castration on behavior of male dogs with reference to the role of age and experience. JAVMA 1997, 211:180–182.

Autor Gerrard Flannigan
Consultor Editorial Debra F. Horwitz
Agradecimento Tracy L. Kroll

Comportamento de Marcação Territorial e Errático — Gatos

CONSIDERAÇÕES GERAIS

REVISÃO

Marcação com Urina
- Depósito de urina em superfícies verticais (jato) ou horizontais (itens novos) para fins de comunicação (territorial, sexual ou situações agonísticas).
- A marcação pode responder por 30% dos problemas comportamentais felinos.

Comportamento Errático
- Escape ou atividade errante com a finalidade de acasalamento, delimitação de território, obtenção de alimento ou estimulação/enriquecimento sensorial.
- Os comportamentos de marcação com urina e errático são comportamentos felinos normais, mas indesejáveis em gatos de companhia.

IDENTIFICAÇÃO
- Comum em machos intactos, especialmente se houver fêmeas no cio.
- Também pode ocorrer em fêmeas intactas ou animais castrados de qualquer sexo.
- Não há predileção etária ou racial para o comportamento de marcação ou errático.

SINAIS CLÍNICOS
- A marcação com urina é caracterizada pelo fato de o gato se voltar para um objeto com a cauda ereta e trêmula e projetar um jato de urina para trás e para cima em direção ao objeto.
- Também pode ocorrer com o gato que assume uma postura agachada e deposita a urina em superfícies horizontais; particularmente sobre itens pessoais ou novos no ambiente.
- Acredita-se que a marcação com urina seja caracterizada pelo depósito de pequenas quantidades de urina, em múltiplos tipos de superfície, em conjunto com o uso normal de bandeja sanitária para eliminação do material fecal e da urina.

CAUSAS E FATORES DE RISCO
- A marcação com urina pode funcionar para delimitação territorial, intenção agressiva ou objetivos reprodutivos entre os gatos ou pode ocorrer como meio de controlar a ansiedade.
- A probabilidade de marcação com urina dentro da casa parece aumentar com a densidade populacional de gatos no ambiente. As pesquisas mais antigas implicam uma chance de 100% da presença de marcação com >10 gatos na casa; contudo, a marcação com urina pode ocorrer em casas com apenas 1-2 gatos.
- As relações agonísticas (agressivas) entre os gatos na mesma casa e a presença de gatos de rua são correlacionadas com um aumento na probabilidade do comportamento de marcação.
- O comportamento errático é um comportamento exploratório felino normal com os gatos que procuram enriquecimento ambiental, alimento ou atividade sexual.
- Essa atividade errante é mais provável em gatos de rua que são abrigados dentro de casa, em machos intactos, e naqueles alojados em ambiente doméstico deserto (o que aumenta a motivação de explorar a rua).

DIAGNÓSTICO

DIAGNÓSTICO DIFERENCIAL
- Descartar causas de doença do trato urinário inferior, como cálculos urinários.
- É imprescindível que a marcação com urina seja diferenciada de micção inadequada com a finalidade de esvaziamento vesical. O último problema é caracterizado pela eliminação de urina sobre uma superfície ou um local constante, pode envolver a eliminação de fezes e, em geral, está associada a uma redução no uso da bandeja sanitária. Os gatos podem continuar usando a bandeja para eliminação fecal, ao mesmo tempo em que evitam a micção; o inverso também é possível. Os gatos com comportamento de marcação com urina continuarão utilizando a bandeja sanitária para evacuação e micção.
- O comportamento errático pode ocorrer em virtude de qualquer processo patológico capaz de fazer com que um gato busque isolamento por causa de doença.

HEMOGRAMA/BIOQUÍMICA/URINÁLISE
Raramente os gatos com comportamento de marcação com urina exibem anormalidades nas avaliações laboratoriais. Os exames de hemograma completo e bioquímica podem fornecer não só informações úteis para descartar problemas coexistentes, mas também dados basais de referência antes do início da terapia farmacológica. Repetir esses exames 3-4 semanas após o início da medicação para descartar efeitos nocivos à função dos órgãos.

OUTROS TESTES LABORATORIAIS
A menos que indicado pelos dados basais de referência, nenhum outro teste laboratorial é necessário.

DIAGNÓSTICO POR IMAGEM
Radiografias e ultrassonografia se os dados laboratoriais indicarem a necessidade de exploração adicional do trato urinário.

MÉTODOS DIAGNÓSTICOS
Nenhum indicado.

TRATAMENTO

PARA COMPORTAMENTO DE MARCAÇÃO COM URINA
- Castrar os animais intactos. Sempre que possível, reduzir o número de gatos na casa para diminuir a densidade populacional em caso de superlotação como fator de risco.
- Fornecer opções alternativas para o comportamento de marcação, como postes de arranhadura, caixas de arranhadura, pentes faciais de marcação (*Cat-A-Comb*). Considerando-se que a marcação com urina é um comportamento normal, o uso de um ponto de marcação para o depósito de urina (por exemplo, uma bandeja sanitária vazia posicionada na vertical no local onde ocorre a marcação) pode ser adequado para alguns gatos.
- Providenciar bandejas sanitárias verticais em múltiplos locais (1 bandeja sanitária por gato mais uma bandeja extra), além de vários comedouros e bebedouros.
- Controlar a higiene da bandeja sanitária, de modo que as caixas sejam esvaziadas todos os dias e completamente limpas 1 vez por semana (bandejas de argila) ou 1 vez por mês (bandejas tipo aglomerado) com o uso de água quente apenas (sem removedores).
- Aumentar as oportunidades de pouso e esconderijo (especialmente locais elevados) em cada ambiente da casa.
- Isolar o gato da área que está sendo marcada.
- Tornar as áreas marcadas com urina locais aversivos, utilizando fita dupla face, bolinhas de naftalina, *scat mat* (tapete sensível ao toque que emite um pequeno choque estático quando o gato pula sobre ele), plástico bolha, etc.
- Tratar os fatores estressantes existentes na casa (alterar a rotina da casa, tratar os problemas de relacionamento entre os gatos na casa, manejar as interações entre os gatos e as pessoas na casa para aumentar as relações positivas, incentivando o adestramento à base de atividade lúdica e reforço positivo).
- Reduzir a exposição a gatos de rua, bloqueando o acesso visual, diminuir o número de gatos no quintal (uso de cercas, instalação de regadores de chão acionados pelo movimento, remoção de alimentadores de pássaros, etc.).
- Aumentar (ou diminuir) o tempo permitido fora de casa.
- Utilizar feromônio facial sintético (fração F3).

PARA COMPORTAMENTO ERRÁTICO
- Proceder à castração em caso de animal intacto.
- Confinar em um ambiente por algumas semanas.
- Alternativamente, permitir o acesso controlado à rua, utilizando áreas com cercas ou telas para gatos ou durante passeio em guia e coleira.
- Utilizar barreiras duplas nas saídas (por exemplo, portas com tela).
- Enriquecer o ambiente doméstico com aumento do acesso aos alimentos, petiscos aleatórios e oportunidades lúdicas. Alimentar o gato apenas quando ele voltar para casa, nunca antes de ele sair.
- Remover os reforços (atrativos) da rua, como a visualização ou o acesso de gatos de rua por meio do uso de cercas e regadores de chão acionados pelo movimento, por exemplo.
- Remover alimentadores de pássaros.
- Utilizar identificação para o gato (etiquetas, tatuagens ou *microchips*).

MEDICAÇÕES

PARA COMPORTAMENTO DE MARCAÇÃO COM URINA
- Fluoxetina 0,5-1,0 mg/kg a cada 24 h.
- Efeitos colaterais: sedação, anorexia, irritabilidade, retenção de urina, constipação.
- Clomipramina 0,5-1,0 mg/kg a cada 24 h
- Efeitos colaterais: sedação, efeitos anticolinérgicos, arritmias e distúrbios GI.

PARA COMPORTAMENTO ERRÁTICO
Nenhuma medicação é recomendada para esse tipo de comportamento.

CONTRAINDICAÇÕES/INTERAÇÕES POSSÍVEIS
- Cuidado em gatos com crises convulsivas.
- Não utilizar com inibidores da MAO, como amitraz ou selegilina.

COMPORTAMENTO DE MARCAÇÃO TERRITORIAL E ERRÁTICO — GATOS

- Cuidado ao utilizar ATCs, como clomipramina, no tratamento de gatos com diabetes, glaucoma ou cardiopatia.
- Não combinar ATC e ISRS; possível síndrome serotoninérgica.

ACOMPANHAMENTO

MONITORIZAÇÃO DO PACIENTE
- Acompanhamento por telefone em até 2 semanas após a consulta, repetir conforme a necessidade para monitorizar a evolução e avaliar a resposta ao tratamento.
- Eletrocardiograma caso haja preocupações quanto ao estado do coração.
- Hemograma completo e perfil bioquímico a cada 6 meses enquanto o gato estiver sob medicação.

EVOLUÇÃO ESPERADA E PROGNÓSTICO
- A resposta à terapia é avaliada pela diminuição da marcação com urina em até 4 semanas.

- Continuar a terapia farmacológica por, no mínimo, 8 semanas caso se observe uma resposta; continuar 1 mês depois da resolução.
- Quando o comportamento permanecer estável, diminuir a dose em 25% por semana.
- Se o comportamento recorrer, reinstituir a dose eficaz e mais baixa.
- Alguns animais talvez necessitem ser mantidos sob medicação por tempo indefinido.

DIVERSOS

ABREVIATURA(S)
- ATC = antidepressivo tricíclico.
- GI = gastrintestinal.
- ISRS = inibidor seletivo de recaptação da serotonina.

Sugestões de Leitura
Hart BL, Barrett RE. Effects of castration on fighting, roaming, and urine spraying in adult male cats. JAVMA 1973, 163:290–292.

Hart BL, Cliff KD, Tynes VV, Bergman L. Control of urine marking by use of long term treatment with fluoxetine or clomipramine in cats. JAVMA 2005, 226(3):378–382.

Landsberg GM, Wilson AL. Effects of clomipramine on cats presented for urine marking. JAAHA 2005, 41(1):3–11.

Ogata N, Takeuchi Y. Clinical trial of a feline pheromone analogue for feline urine marking. J Vet Sci 2001, 63(2):157–161.

Pryor PA, Hart BL, Bain MJ, Cliff KD. Causes of urine marking in cats and the effects of environmental management on the frequency of marking. JAVMA 2001, 219:1709–1713.

Pryor PA, Hart BL, Bain MJ, Cliff KD. Effects of a selective serotonin reuptake inhibitor on urine spraying behavior in cats. JAVMA 2001, 219(11):1557–1561.

Autor John J. Ciribassi
Consultor Editorial Debra F. Horwitz

Comportamentos Destrutivos

CONSIDERAÇÕES GERAIS

REVISÃO
- Comportamento indutor de dano à casa do proprietário ou aos seus pertences.
- O comportamento destrutivo primário constitui uma conduta normal, que inclui o comportamento exploratório e à base de atividades lúdicas, a arranhadura de superfícies durante a auto-higienização felina e a marcação territorial.
- O comportamento destrutivo secundário corresponde a um sinal clínico, que reflete qualquer um dos vários transtornos comportamentais e outros estados patológicos.

SISTEMA(S) ACOMETIDO(S)
- Gastrintestinal — dano aos dentes; vômito e diarreia, obstrução em caso de ingestão de itens-alvo.
- Musculoesquelético — dano traumático causado por arranhadura ou mastigação intensa.
- A ingestão de material tóxico pode comprometer qualquer sistema orgânico.

IDENTIFICAÇÃO
Cães e Gatos
- Qualquer raça ou sexo; provável base genética em raças orientais de gatos que são submetidos à consulta por problemas de sucção ou mastigação de tecido.
- O comportamento destrutivo primário é observado com maior frequência em cães e gatos com menos de 1 ano de idade, enquanto o comportamento destrutivo secundário, em animais adultos.

SINAIS CLÍNICOS
Comportamento Destrutivo Primário
- Ocorre em princípio na presença ou na ausência do proprietário.
- Não é precedido por um deflagrador ambiental específico.
- Ausência de ansiedade ou agressão.
- Os deflagradores usuais são: itens pequenos, artigos maleáveis, beiradas de móveis e plantas domésticas.

Comportamento Destrutivo Secundário
- Comportamento de busca de atenção (cães e gatos) — o comportamento destrutivo ocorre na presença do proprietário.
- Comportamento obsessivo-compulsivo (cães e gatos) — lambedura, mastigação e/ou ingestão de itens não alimentícios; ocorre na presença ou na ausência do proprietário; o tempo despendido, engajado no comportamento, é excessivo.
- Ansiedade relacionada com separação (cães) — o comportamento destrutivo ocorre na ausência do proprietário e, na maioria das vezes, manifesta-se nos afastamentos dos proprietários; os itens-alvo podem incluir pertences pessoais, móveis ou pontos de saída.
- Fobia a tempestades e ruídos (cães) — observa-se comportamento destrutivo e/ou comportamento relacionado à ansiedade (andar compassado, respiração ofegante, tremor) na presença do proprietário; o comportamento destrutivo é intermitente e depende, sobretudo, da presença de deflagrador relevante; com frequência, os pontos de saída constituem os alvos. A intensidade do comportamento pode ser maior durante a ausência do proprietário.
- Agressividade territorial (cães) — nota-se reatividade a estímulos externos na presença do proprietário; o comportamento destrutivo é intermitente, com base na presença de deflagradores; nesse tipo de comportamento, danificam-se armações de janelas e vãos de portas.

CAUSAS E FATORES DE RISCO
- O comportamento destrutivo primário representa um comportamento normal; a supervisão inadequada e o acesso insuficiente a brinquedos mastigáveis ou postes de arranhadura apropriados podem influenciar esse tipo de comportamento.
- Os proprietários reforçam inadvertidamente o comportamento, repreendendo ou perseguindo os animais de estimação com hábitos de mastigação ou arranhadura de itens inadequados.
- Ainda não se identificaram com clareza os fatores de risco dos problemas baseados na ansiedade.
- A agressividade territorial pode ter componentes de base genética e de aprendizagem.

DIAGNÓSTICO

DIAGNÓSTICO DIFERENCIAL
- É imprescindível identificar os problemas patológicos antes de se atribuir um diagnóstico puramente comportamental.
- Se o comportamento de pica (apetite depravado) acompanhar a mastigação destrutiva — descartar condições que comprometam os processos de digestão/absorção e o apetite, incluindo mudança recente de dieta.
- Em caso de início súbito do comportamento destrutivo em animais de estimação adultos na ausência de mudanças ambientais significativas — excluir afecções clínicas associadas à dor ou ansiedade.
- Em caso de comportamento destrutivo de início tardio em cães idosos — descartar a síndrome de disfunção cognitiva.

HEMOGRAMA/BIOQUÍMICA/URINÁLISE
Geralmente permanecem normais.

OUTROS TESTES LABORATORIAIS
Realizados, conforme indicação, para descartar distúrbios clínicos (função da tireoide, teste de resposta ao ACTH).

DIAGNÓSTICO POR IMAGEM
Pode ser indicado em caso de início súbito em animais de estimação adultos.

MÉTODOS DIAGNÓSTICOS
Exame físico com especial atenção à cavidade bucal.

TRATAMENTO

Tratar qualquer doença subjacente.

COMPORTAMENTO DESTRUTIVO PRIMÁRIO
- Supervisionar/confinar até o estabelecimento de padrões comportamentais adequados.
- Garantir o acesso a brinquedos mastigáveis aceitáveis (alternar para assegurar a novidade)/substratos de arranhar (colocar postes em locais proeminentes, selecionar materiais adequados).
- Recompensar os comportamentos apropriados — selecionar brinquedos e postes de arranhadura que dispensem recompensas de alimentos.
- Interromper os comportamentos inconvenientes — puxar delicadamente a coleira ou espécie de cabresto (cães), aplicar produtos atóxicos de sabor amargo sobre os itens-alvo para deter a mastigação e aplicar fita adesiva dupla-face sobre os móveis para impedir a arranhadura dos gatos.
- Providenciar atividades e exercícios alternativos adequados.
- Pode-se lançar mão de dispositivos ativados por controle remoto, destinados a espantar os animais de estimação — orientar os proprietários a empregar tais dispositivos de forma humanitária e cautelosa. Os erros na aplicação de correções podem induzir à ansiedade ou agressão.
- Uma forma de vazão ou escape apropriado para os comportamentos normais deve estar imediatamente acessível.
- Em caso de arranhadura felina normal, não se deve considerar a remoção das garras como a primeira linha terapêutica; enquanto a mudança comportamental estiver sendo implementada, podem-se aplicar os protetores plásticos nas garras para evitar maiores danos.

COMPORTAMENTO DESTRUTIVO SECUNDÁRIO
- Comportamento de busca de atenção — estabelecer interações desencadeadas pelo proprietário; rever os princípios de aprendizado e reforço.
- Transtorno compulsivo — identificar e reduzir as fontes de ansiedade no ambiente; oferecer brincadeiras interativas e itens mastigáveis apropriados; evitar o acesso a itens-alvo para garantir a segurança do animal de estimação.
- Ansiedade relacionada com separação — mudança comportamental para diminuir a ansiedade vinculada à separação, além de enriquecimento do ambiente; a punição é contraindicada. Modificação comportamental (dessensibilização e contracondicionamento) para reduzir a reatividade a deflagradores relevantes.
- Agressividade territorial — mudança comportamental (dessensibilização e contracondicionamento); cães: dieta pobre em proteína. Modificação ambiental (portas e portões seguros, além de supervisão) para garantir a segurança.

MEDICAÇÕES

MEDICAMENTO(S)
- A administração de agentes terapêuticos complementa a mudança comportamental e pode conferir a resolução mais rápida dos sinais clínicos ao se tratar as afecções decorrentes de ansiedade (comportamento obsessivo-compulsivo, ansiedade da separação, fobias) em pacientes selecionados.
- Os medicamentos não costumam ser aconselháveis em casos de comportamentos destrutivos primários ou comportamento de busca de atenção.
- Na prescrição de medicamentos não aprovados para uso em cães ou gatos, deve-se obter um termo de consentimento informado do proprietário.

Antidepressivos Tricíclicos (ATCs)
Clomipramina — cães, 1-3 mg/kg a cada 12 h; gatos, 0,5 mg/kg a cada 24 h.

COMPORTAMENTOS DESTRUTIVOS

Inibidores Seletivos de Recaptação de Serotonina (ISRSs)
Fluoxetina — cães, 0,5-1 mg/kg a cada 24 h; gatos, 0,5 mg/kg a cada 24 h.

Benzodiazepínicos
Alprazolam — cães, 0,01-0,2 mg/kg a cada 12 h (para diminuir a ansiedade situacional).

Nutracêuticos
Novifit® (SAMe): cães e gatos (para reduzir a ansiedade relacionada com declínio cognitivo).

CONTRAINDICAÇÕES/INTERAÇÕES POSSÍVEIS
• Não é indicado o uso de agentes psicotrópicos para tratar o comportamento destrutivo primário.
• Não devem ser utilizados os ATCs nem os ISRSs com os inibidores da monoamina oxidase, incluindo os produtos tópicos com amitraz e selegilina em sua composição.
• Os ATCs e os ISRSs podem interferir no metabolismo de outros medicamentos, inclusive do fenobarbital.
• Os benzodiazepínicos podem desinibir a agressividade; utilizar com cuidado em cães e gatos com histórico de comportamento agressivo.

ACOMPANHAMENTO
MONITORIZAÇÃO DO PACIENTE
Comunicação de acompanhamento semanal durante a fase inicial da terapia.

EVOLUÇÃO ESPERADA E PROGNÓSTICO
• A resolução do comportamento exploratório normal costuma ser rápida.
• As condições decorrentes de ansiedade frequentemente necessitam de tratamento a longo prazo, incluindo o uso prolongado de medicamentos psicotrópicos.

DIVERSOS
FATORES RELACIONADOS COM A IDADE
A idade na consulta pode não ser equivalente à idade de início do comportamento.

GESTAÇÃO/FERTILIDADE/REPRODUÇÃO
Comportamento destrutivo pré-parturiente (ninhada).

VER TAMBÉM
• Agressividade por Alimento, Posse e Território — Cães.
• Transtornos Compulsivos — Gatos.
• Transtornos Compulsivos — Cães.
• Síndrome de Ansiedade da Separação.
• Fobias a Trovões e Relâmpagos.

ABREVIATURA(S)
• ACTH = hormônio adrenocorticotrófico.
• ATC = antidepressivo tricíclico.
• ISRS = inibidor seletivo de recaptação da serotonina.
• SAMe = dissulfato de S-adenosil-L-metionina-tosilato.

Sugestões de Leitura
Casey R. Management problems in cats. In: Horwitz DF, Mills DS, eds., BSAVA Manual of Canine and Feline Behavioural Medicine, 2nd ed. Gloucestershire, UK: BSAVA, 2009, pp. 98-110.
Landsberg G, Hunthausen W, Ackerman L. Handbook of Behavior Problems of the Dog and Cat, 2nd ed. Philadelphia: Elsevier Saunders, 2003, pp. 311-347.
Lindell E. Management problems in dogs. In: Horwitz DF, Mills DS, eds., BSAVA Manual of Canine and Feline Behavioural Medicine, 2nd ed. Gloucestershire, UK: BSAVA, 2009, pp. 83-97.

Autor Ellen M. Lindell
Consultor Editorial Debra F. Horwitz

Comportamentos Indisciplinados: Saltos, Escavação, Perseguição, Furto

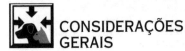

CONSIDERAÇÕES GERAIS

DEFINIÇÃO
• Saltos — manter-se sobre os membros pélvicos, com os membros torácicos apoiados em uma pessoa ou um objeto ou pular no ar, apoiando-se ou não em uma pessoa. • Escavação — usar as patas para raspar uma superfície como se estivesse tentando escavar o substrato. • Perseguição — perseguir uma pessoa, um animal ou um objeto em movimento. • Furto — tomar um item, sem a intenção de uso pelo cão.

FISIOPATOLOGIA
• Todos esses comportamentos estão dentro dos limites de normalidade dos comportamentos caninos. • A atividade insuficiente pode contribuir para o aparecimento de todos eles. • Os saltos que fazem parte de uma saudação excessiva podem estar associados à ansiedade da separação ou ansiedade social. • A escavação pode estar associada a transtornos comportamentais, distúrbios neurológicos ou dor abdominal.

SISTEMA(S) ACOMETIDO(S)
• Comportamental. • Gastrintestinal. • Nervoso.

IDENTIFICAÇÃO
Espécies
Cães.

Raça(s) Predominante(s)
• As raças de pastoreio e de caça podem ser mais propensas a exibir o comportamento de perseguição. • As raças de caça (incluindo as raças Terrier) têm maior probabilidade de manifestar comportamentos de escavação.

Idade Média e Faixa Etária
Mais comuns em cães mais jovens, mas podem ocorrer em qualquer idade.

SINAIS CLÍNICOS
Achados Anamnésicos
• Os saltos em cima das pessoas costumam ocorrer em associação com chegadas ou partidas ou saudações em outras ocasiões; também se associam com a exploração do conteúdo de bancadas ou mesas. • A escavação frequentemente ocorre em áreas ao longo de uma cerca ou naquelas de jardinagem recente, em tocas de roedores e no chão do interior da casa, com ou sem a presença do proprietário. • O deslocamento de objetos ou a ausência de alimentos presentes em superfícies são queixas comuns de furto.

Achados do Exame Físico
• Em geral, não são dignos de nota. • Desgaste das unhas. • A presença de dor à palpação abdominal pode sugerir comprometimento dos órgãos. • O exame neurológico também pode ser sugestivo de acometimento dos órgãos.

CAUSAS
• Os saltos constituem um comportamento normal de saudação e brincadeira. A agitação, a estimulação do comportamento por outros ou a recompensa inadvertida do comportamento perpetuam os saltos. A ansiedade da separação pode resultar em saltos excessivos sobre os proprietários no retorno ao lar ou em partidas. A ansiedade social pode produzir saudações exageradas de visitantes, com saltos. • A escavação é um comportamento normal. A presença de roedores, a ansiedade, a termorregulação corporal, a subestimulação ou a falta de exercícios adequados, o ato de esconder ou recuperar alimentos, a fuga do confinamento, a dor (particularmente abdominal), a ansiedade da separação, o transtorno obsessivo-compulsivo (TOC) e as neuropatias podem, sem exceção, ser as causas de escavação. • O furto, um comportamento adquirido normal, pode ser causado por um cão que busca chamar a atenção do dono ou pelo desejo de um item alimentar ou brinquedo. • A perseguição também é um comportamento normal. As causas incluem pastoreio, caça, divertimento ou defesa.

FATORES DE RISCO
• Exercícios inadequados. • Estímulos abaixo do ideal. • Furto de alimento — dietas com restrição ou para redução do peso, fenobarbital, benzodiazepínicos, glicocorticoides, hiperadrenocorticismo e diabetes melito.
• Perseguição — comum em raças de pastoreio.

DIAGNÓSTICO

DIAGNÓSTICO DIFERENCIAL
Escavação
• Ansiedade da separação — fugas ou tentativas de fuga de áreas confinadas na ausência do proprietário e frequentemente ocorre nas chegadas e em engradados. Presença de outros sinais compatíveis com a ansiedade da separação, incluindo vocalização, micção, defecação, outros comportamentos destrutivos ou salivação, na ausência do proprietário. • Outras ansiedades ou fobias (trovões/relâmpagos ou outro estímulo, como fogos de artifício). • Dor, particularmente abdominal — enrijecimento do abdome, outros sinais gastrintestinais, sinais atribuídos ao trato urinário e dificuldade do cão em se manter confortável. • TOC (como perseguição da luz ou escavação em direção à luz) — esse comportamento costuma ocupar grande parte do tempo do cão, interfere em suas funções normais e pode ser de difícil interrupção. • Neuropatia — presença de outras anormalidades neurológicas, como crises convulsivas.

HEMOGRAMA/BIOQUÍMICA/URINÁLISE
• Não costumam ser dignos de nota. • Pode haver anormalidades compatíveis com o sistema acometido.

OUTROS TESTES LABORATORIAIS
Para descartar a origem da dor ou a presença de doença endócrina ou neurológica (TSDBD, relação de cortisol:creatinina urinários, ácidos biliares, análise do LCS), conforme indicação.

DIAGNÓSTICO POR IMAGEM
Radiografias, ultrassonografia, RM ou TC, conforme indicados pelos achados do exame físico.

TRATAMENTO

CUIDADO(S) DE SAÚDE ADEQUADO(S)
O paciente é tratado em um esquema ambulatorial.

ATIVIDADE
Aumentar os exercícios diários do cão e as oportunidades de estimulação mental.

DIETA
Rever as necessidades calóricas nos casos de furto de alimentos.

ORIENTAÇÃO AO PROPRIETÁRIO
Saltos
• Durante o adestramento, é essencial a prevenção dos comportamentos indesejáveis de saltos. • O uso de coleira e guia facilita o adestramento para afastar o cão delicadamente de saltar. • Receber os visitantes do lado de fora de casa pode diminuir o comportamento de saltos ou, então, o acesso do cão à situação de visita pode ser restrito, colocando-o em outro cômodo da casa até que o visitante se sente. • Ensinar o cão a sentar e permanecer parado com os comandos verbais "*sit*" e "*stay*" em inglês*, respectivamente, como método alternativo de saudação das pessoas. • Quando o cão estiver calmo e dócil, praticar o ato de sentar em troca de uma recompensa de alimento em diferentes áreas da casa. • As sessões devem ser breves — 3-5 minutos com 8-12 repetições por sessão. • É recomendável que o alimento seja altamente palatável e pequeno (0,5 cm^2 ou maior, dependendo do porte e do peso do cão). Em princípio, o alimento deve ser usado de forma constante e regular. • Acrescentar a palavra "fica" ("*stay*") quando o ato de sentar durar alguns segundos; afastar um passo, voltar ao cão e fornecer a recompensa de alimento. Aumentar o tempo distante do cão para 3-5 minutos. • Repetir os exercícios próximos à porta, com o acréscimo de partidas e retornos. • Em seguida, pedir para o cão se sentar em troca de uma recompensa de alimento, ao retornar do trabalho ou em outras ausências de algumas horas de duração. • Os visitantes familiares podem entrar em casa, pedir para o cão se sentar e dar uma recompensa de alimento. • Alternativamente, o proprietário poderá recompensar o cão por este permanecer sentado à medida que as pessoas entrarem em casa. • Por fim, as recompensas de alimento podem ser reduzidas para uso intermitente, porém frequente. • Os cães que gostam de apanhar o objeto e ficam muito agitados por permanecer sentados podem se sentir melhor se uma bola for arremessada conforme um visitante entrar em casa. Isso será mais benéfico se o cão for adestrado a se sentar antes de algum objeto ser arremessado novamente. • O proprietário deve evitar o aumento da agitação do cão, caminhando com tranquilidade em direção à porta e falando com uma voz calma e suave. • As pessoas devem evitar a recompensa de saltos em busca de atenção, como empurrar o cão. Não aceitar nem interagir com o cão; manter os braços junto ao corpo e afastar-se. Alguns cães param de saltar e ignoram a pessoa. • Medidas como pisar sobre os dedos do cão ou esmagar as patas e outras punições semelhantes costumam ser ineficazes e podem induzir à agressão, devendo ser evitadas.

Escavação
• A escavação associada à termorregulação ocorre em climas frio ou quente para ajudar a refrescar o cão ou a conservar o calor do animal. Um abrigo adequadamente aquecido ou fresco deve minimizar esse problema.

---

* N. T.: Muitos adestramentos, se não a maioria, utilizam os comandos verbais em inglês. Por essa razão, esses comandos também foram mantidos em inglês ao longo do texto.

Comportamentos Indisciplinados: Saltos, Escavação, Perseguição, Furto

- A escavação vinculada a roedores pode ocorrer dentro ou fora de casa. É provável que esse comportamento persista mesmo após a remoção dos roedores.
- A escavação relacionada com ansiedade da separação, fuga por um estímulo fóbico ou TOC deve desaparecer com o tratamento dessas condições. Os cães acometidos por ansiedade da separação não devem ser deixados sozinhos no quintal por períodos de tempo prolongados.
- Em relação à escavação na presença do proprietário ou não associada a nenhum dos itens expostos acima, o proprietário deverá aumentar os exercícios e as atividades físicas do cão. É recomendável a prática de exercícios aeróbios antes de se deixar o cão no quintal sem supervisão. O fornecimento de brinquedos interativos, como lançadores automáticos de bolas de tênis ou brinquedos recheados de ração, pode ser útil.
- Se a escavação persistir, criar uma área onde esse comportamento seja aceitável. Para tal finalidade, pode-se lançar mão de um quadrado de madeira com areia (utilizado normalmente para as crianças brincarem); ou, então, pode-se delimitar uma área com madeira e preenchê-la com areia ou solo arável. Inicialmente, enterre brinquedos ou itens alimentares diante do cão, de modo que ele seja conduzido à área específica e recompensado por escavar nela.
- A supervisão é necessária para redirecionar o cão a outra atividade assim que ele começar a escavação. Para interromper a escavação, podem-se utilizar estímulos aversivos (ruídos sonoros, *sprays* com água); no entanto, é possível que tais estímulos não influenciem a escavação na ausência do proprietário. A aplicação de estímulos aversivos ativados por controle remoto (um detector de movimento em um esguicho de jardim), o uso de pedras ou a colocação de água na área escavada podem evitar a escavação nessa área específica, mas possivelmente não influenciam a repetição desse ato em outras áreas; portanto, não são recomendadas.

Perseguição
- Uma coleira cervical ou peitoral que não deixa o cão puxar pode ser extremamente útil para controlar o cão na presença do estímulo de perseguição. As raças de pastoreio exibem um comportamento fenotípico mais responsivo ao controle e manejo do que ao tratamento.
- Os cães com esse comportamento de perseguição precisam ser dessensibilizados (gradativamente expostos) e contracondicionados (adestrados a ter uma resposta diferente) ao estímulo.
- O proprietário deve praticar o mesmo exercício de "senta e fica" ("*sit* e *stay*") conforme foi descrito acima, com o acréscimo de um comando "visual" ("*look*"), usando um petisco conduzido até os olhos do proprietário. Isso ajudará a chamar a atenção do cão e a focalizará de volta ao proprietário quando ele vir o estímulo em movimento.
- As sessões devem durar 3-5 minutos, com inúmeras repetições por sessão. A princípio, deve-se trabalhar com o cão dentro de casa sem distrações, fazendo-o sentar, parar e observar ("*sit*", "*stay*" e "*look*").
- Em seguida, deve-se trabalhar com o cão em um quintal tranquilo, mantendo-o preso a uma coleira e fazendo-o sentar, parar, caminhar, voltar e observar ("*sit*", "*stay*", "*step away*", "*return*" e "*look*"); e, por fim, fornecer a recompensa de alimento. Quando o cão for bem-sucedido, o processo poderá ser repetido em uma parte mais divertida do quintal. Se o cão ainda permanecer muito distraído, o proprietário deverá trabalhar com o animal nas horas do dia em que há poucas distrações (i. e., transeuntes e tráfego).
- O proprietário deve trabalhar com o cão inicialmente sem a presença do estímulo de perseguição. Se o proprietário for capaz de prender a atenção do cão, ele deverá fazer com que o estímulo de perseguição (como uma bicicleta ou a corrida de uma pessoa) passe a uma grande distância do animal, ao mesmo tempo em que trabalha com o cão. Talvez seja preciso que o proprietário aumente a velocidade das repetições e as recompensas.
- Se o cão conseguir ignorar o estímulo de perseguição, o proprietário deverá aproximar o estímulo do animal alguns centímetros todos os dias. Mas, se o cão não se mostrar capaz de ignorar o estímulo de perseguição, a distância deverá ser aumentada. Quando o cão passar despercebido pelo estímulo de perseguição no quintal, o proprietário poderá incorporar o mesmo exercício durante os passeios. Quando o proprietário vir o estímulo indutor de perseguição, ele deverá pedir que o cão se sente, pare e observe ("*sit*", "*stay*" e "*look*"), recompensando-o logo em seguida.

Furto
- As tentativas do cão em iniciar brincadeiras e perseguições podem resultar em furto.
- O fornecimento adequado de atenção, exercícios e brinquedos antes que o proprietário se ocupe com outras atividades (p. ex., fazendo o jantar, trabalhando ou assistindo à TV) ajudará a diminuir a motivação pelo furto.
- Os proprietários não devem se ocupar em correr atrás do cão, mas sim ignorá-lo, seguir adiante, pegar um petisco e chamá-lo próximo a eles. Enquanto o cão estiver no processo de soltar o item, o proprietário poderá dizer "largue" ("*drop*"), complementar com "bom cachorro" e fornecer o petisco ao animal. Dessa forma, o cão está sendo recompensado por renunciar ao item.
- O proprietário poderá fornecer um segundo petisco, para que não haja "competição" pelo item descartado. Algumas vezes, é necessário espalhar uma série de petiscos para o cão apanhar enquanto o item é removido. O item deve ser colocado longe da visão do cão e não ser exposto a este.
- Se o cão se esconder debaixo da mobília, o proprietário não deverá persegui-lo. Se o cão se sentir ameaçado ou encurralado, ele poderá se defender de forma agressiva. Se for imprescindível que o item seja recuperado, talvez haverá necessidade de o proprietário atrair o cão para fora do esconderijo com petiscos valiosos ou oferecer algum passeio ou atividade lúdica.
- Em relação ao furto de alimentos, é indispensável colocá-los fora do alcance do cão, já que sua aquisição é altamente gratificante para o animal. Pode ser necessário afastar o cão das áreas de preparo dos alimentos e dos locais das refeições.
- Os produtos levemente aversivos capazes de interromper o comportamento de furto podem ajudar a corrigir tal conduta. Os detectores de movimento podem ser úteis para deter o comportamento de furto. Os detectores tradicionais emitem sons e alarmes ao detectar um movimento. Um spray de ar comprimido ativado pelo movimento constitui um novo equipamento de detecção de movimentos destinado aos animais de estimação. Se o furto de alimentos ocorrer em função de uma dieta, poderão ser adicionadas fontes proteicas como frango cozido ou outro tipo de carne ou alimentos de baixa caloria, como vegetais crus ou cozidos, à ração canina para reduzir a fome do cão.

MEDICAÇÕES
MEDICAMENTO(S) DE ESCOLHA
Nenhum.

ACOMPANHAMENTO
MONITORIZAÇÃO DO PACIENTE
Inicialmente, a cada 2-3 semanas.

PREVENÇÃO
A supervisão rigorosa, a prática de exercícios e a exposição do cão a diferentes estímulos, ainda quando filhote, podem ajudar a evitar alguns desses comportamentos indisciplinados.

COMPLICAÇÕES POSSÍVEIS
Lesões resultantes de fuga por meio de grades, perseguição a algum estímulo, escavação em substrato impenetrável ou impermeável ou ingestão de item inapropriado.

EVOLUÇÃO ESPERADA E PROGNÓSTICO
Em geral, a resposta terapêutica é boa em casos de salto, escavação e furto se o proprietário colaborar com o adestramento. Os comportamentos de perseguição podem se mostrar mais difíceis e resistentes ao tratamento.

DIVERSOS
FATORES RELACIONADOS COM A IDADE
Os cães mais jovens necessitam de uma quantidade maior de exercícios do que muitos proprietários preveem.

VER TAMBÉM
- Transtornos Compulsivos — Cães.
- Medos, Fobias e Ansiedades — Cães.
- Síndrome de Ansiedade da Separação.

ABREVIATURA(S)
- LCS = líquido cerebrospinal.
- RM = ressonância magnética.
- TC = tomografia computadorizada.
- TOC = transtorno obsessivo-compulsivo.
- TSDBD = teste de supressão com dexametasona em baixas doses.

Sugestões de Leitura
Landsberg G, Hunthausen W, Ackerman, L. Unruly behaviors. In: Handbook of Behavior Problems of the Dog and Cat, 2nd ed. Philadelphia: Elsevier Saunders, 2003, pp. 305-322.
Lindell E. Control problems in dogs In: Horwitz D, Mills D, Heath S, eds., BSAVA Manual of Canine and Feline Behavioural Medicine. Gloucestershire, UK: BSAVA, 2002.

Autor Marsha R. Reich
Consultor Editorial Debra F. Horwitz

Compressão Cefálica

CONSIDERAÇÕES GERAIS

DEFINIÇÃO
Pressão compulsiva da cabeça contra uma parede ou outro objeto sem razão aparente.

FISIOPATOLOGIA
• Mudanças comportamentais — causadas por lesões no prosencéfalo (i. e., cérebro, sistema límbico, tálamo e hipotálamo), particularmente aquelas que acometem o sistema límbico e os córtex frontotemporais.
• As lesões podem resultar em marcha compulsiva; ao atingir um obstáculo (p. ex., uma parede), o animal pode pressionar a cabeça contra ele por longos períodos de tempo, mostrando-se aparentemente incapaz de se voltar e se afastar dali.
• Incapacidade aparente de se afastar voluntariamente — pode refletir integração prejudicada das informações sensoriais, ocasionando comportamento inadequado.

SISTEMA(S) ACOMETIDO(S)
Nervoso.

GENÉTICA
N/D.

INCIDÊNCIA/PREVALÊNCIA
N/D.

DISTRIBUIÇÃO GEOGRÁFICA
N/D.

IDENTIFICAÇÃO
Cães e gatos de qualquer idade, raça e sexo.

SINAIS CLÍNICOS
• Pressão com a cabeça — apenas um sinal de doença do prosencéfalo.
• Marcha compulsiva e em círculos para o lado da lesão.
• Alteração no comportamento de aprendizagem.
• Crises convulsivas.
• Déficits de reações posturais contralaterais.
• Déficits visuais contralaterais com reflexos pupilares normais à luz.
• Hiperalgesia facial contralateral.

CAUSAS E FATORES DE RISCO
• Anatômicos — hidrocefalia, mais comumente em cães jovens de raças *toy*; lissencefalia (Lhasa apso).
• Metabólicos — encefalopatia hepática como resultado de desvio portossistêmico ou hepatopatia grave; hiper ou hiponatremia graves.
• Nutricionais — muito incomuns, pois a maioria dos animais de estimação é alimentada com rações compostas; pode ocorrer deficiência de tiamina em gatos que só ingerem peixe cru ou naqueles com síndromes graves de má absorção; contudo, predominam sinais vestibulares.
• Neoplásicos — tumores primários (p. ex., glioma e meningioma) ou metastáticos (p. ex., hemangiossarcoma) que afetam o cérebro; mais comuns em animais idosos (com mais de 6 anos de idade).
• Imunomediados/inflamatórios — meningoencefalite granulomatosa; encefalites necrosantes (encefalite do Maltês, encefalite do Pug); meningoencefalite de etiologia desconhecida.
• Infecciosos (cães) — virais (vírus da raiva e da cinomose), por riquétsias (*Ehrlichia canis*, febre maculosa das Montanhas Rochosas), protozoários (*Toxoplasma gondii*, *Neospora caninum*) ou fúngicos (*Blastomyces*, *Cryptococcus*); a raiva é de peculiar importância, porque os neurônios no sistema límbico costumam ser infectados em carnívoros.
• Infecciosos (gatos) — virais (raiva, PIF, FeLV [a imunossupressão associada predispõe a outras encefalites e neoplasia], FIV [pode causar encefalopatia a princípio e predispor a outras encefalites e neoplasias em virtude da imunossupressão]); *Bartonella henselae*; migração de *Cuterebra*; toxoplasmose; *Cryptococcus* e outras infecções fúngicas.
• Tóxicos — por exemplo, intoxicação pelo chumbo.
• Traumatismo.
• Vasculares — hemorragia intracraniana como resultado de hipertensão (considerar em gatos idosos com hipertireoidismo ou insuficiência renal crônica); distúrbio hemorrágico (primário ou secundário à toxicidade de rodenticida); acidente vascular cerebral (encefalopatia isquêmica felina ou secundário à doença metabólica, inflamatória ou neoplásica sistêmica).

DIAGNÓSTICO

DIAGNÓSTICO DIFERENCIAL
Um animal que ficou recentemente cego pode se chocar contra objetos, mas a compressão prolongada da cabeça não seria tipicamente associada à perda da visão.

HEMOGRAMA/BIOQUÍMICA/URINÁLISE
• Pode refletir uma causa metabólica ou tóxica.
• Encefalopatia hepática — queda das concentrações séricas de albumina, ureia, colesterol e glicose, com ou sem elevação da fosfatase alcalina, da ALT e da bilirrubina; anemia microcítica pode estar presente; pode haver cristais de biurato de amônio na urina.
• Toxicidade do chumbo — eritrócitos com pontilhado basófilo; presença de reticulócitos e hemácias nucleadas na ausência de anemia.
• Encefalite — os achados, em geral, não revelam nada digno de nota, mas podem refletir um processo inflamatório (p. ex., com infecção fúngica).
• Linfoma do SNC — podem-se observar indícios de acometimento da medula óssea.

OUTROS TESTES LABORATORIAIS
• Tolerância aos ácidos biliares — para diagnosticar encefalopatia hepática; as concentrações sanguíneas de amônia também podem estar elevadas.
• Títulos sorológicos das fases aguda e convalescente — para diagnosticar doenças causadas por riquétsias, protozoários, fungos e vírus; para algumas infecções (p. ex., cinomose, toxoplasmose e criptococose), medir também os títulos de anticorpos ou antígenos (*Cryptococcus*) no LCS.
• PCR no LCS e no soro — para diagnosticar doenças causadas por riquétsias, bactérias, protozoários, fungos e vírus; exame sensível e específico na presença do agente infeccioso no LCS ou no soro.
• Concentração sanguínea de chumbo — para diagnosticar toxicidade por esse metal.

DIAGNÓSTICO POR IMAGEM
• Radiografia torácica — recomendada em pacientes idosos para identificar doença metastática.
• Ultrassonografia abdominal — recomendada em pacientes idosos se houver suspeita de neoplasia intra-abdominal; indicada na suspeita de desvio portossistêmico ou outra hepatopatia.
• Cintilografia retal — pode ser usada para obtenção do diagnóstico definitivo de desvio portossistêmico.
• TC ou RM cerebrais — para identificar massas intracranianas, más-formações, fraturas de crânio, inflamação e hemorragia.
• Ultrassonografia do cérebro via fontanelas persistentes — pode ser empregada para diagnosticar hidrocefalia em cães jovens.

MÉTODOS DIAGNÓSTICOS
• Exame do fundo de olho — para identificar o quadro de coriorretinite (indícios de doença infecciosa/inflamatória) e lesões vasculares.
• Mensuração da pressão arterial — para identificar a presença de hipertensão.
• Análise do LCS — para diagnosticar a existência de encefalite.

ACHADOS PATOLÓGICOS
Os achados à necropsia refletem a etiologia.

TRATAMENTO

CUIDADO(S) DE SAÚDE ADEQUADO(S)
• Sinais clínicos graves — hospitalização para a avaliação diagnóstica e o tratamento.
• Suspeita de raiva — realizar quarentena para o animal errante não vacinado ou com histórico de vacinação desconhecido na presença de sinais neurológicos rapidamente progressivos e se o animal viver em área endêmica para a raiva; minimizar o número de pessoas em contato com ele e fazer uma escala de contato; se os sinais neurológicos se deteriorarem rapidamente, submeter o animal à eutanásia e enviá-lo ao laboratório de saúde pública para exame de raiva.

CUIDADO(S) DE ENFERMAGEM
• Quando hospitalizados, os pacientes devem ser monitorizados de perto quanto à deterioração do estado mental e à ocorrência de crises convulsivas.
• Talvez haja necessidade de fluidos intravenosos de manutenção aos pacientes com síndrome prosencefálica grave.
• A gaiola talvez tenha de ser almofadada para evitar autotraumatismo em caso de compressão constante da cabeça e andar compulsivo.
• É recomendável a monitorização regular dos olhos quanto ao desenvolvimento de úlceras de córnea causadas por traumatismo.
• Cateteres intravenosos centrais devem ser colocados na veia safena e não na veia jugular se possível, para evitar o aumento da pressão intracraniana pela oclusão das veias jugulares.

ATIVIDADE
N/D.

DIETA
• Na suspeita de encefalopatia hepática — dieta apropriada com baixo teor de proteínas.
• A alimentação manual pode ser necessária em pacientes com encefalopatia grave; no entanto, há risco de aspiração se o paciente deixar de preender e engolir corretamente.

COMPRESSÃO CEFÁLICA

ORIENTAÇÃO AO PROPRIETÁRIO
- Específica para a condição subjacente.
- Os proprietários devem ser alertados quanto à possibilidade de crises convulsivas, orientados com a descrição de uma crise e instruídos sobre o que fazer quando elas ocorrerem.
- Também é recomendável o fornecimento de uma descrição dos sinais de descompensação aguda provocada por herniação cerebral aos proprietários.

CONSIDERAÇÕES CIRÚRGICAS
- Se os sinais forem atribuídos à doença intracraniana, será provável a presença de pressão intracraniana elevada e, portanto, haverá risco de herniação durante a anestesia; nesse caso, a indução e a recuperação da anestesia representam o maior risco. Os pacientes devem ser submetidos à ventilação meticulosa para garantir que a pressão parcial de dióxido de carbono permaneça dentro dos limites de normalidade (30-40 mmHg).
- A hidrocefalia pode ser tratada pela colocação de desvio ventriculoperitoneal.
- Neoplasia cerebral, particularmente tumores extra-axiais como meningiomas, pode ser tratada por meio cirúrgico se o local do tumor for acessível.

MEDICAÇÕES
MEDICAMENTO(S)
- Diferentes causas necessitam de diferentes tratamentos; não iniciar a terapia até que o diagnóstico tenha sido estabelecido.
- Se o estado mental do paciente se deteriorar sugerindo uma herniação cerebral iminente, poderá se lançar mão do manitol (0,25-1 g/kg IV durante 10-30 min) para reduzir a pressão intracraniana transitoriamente; o tratamento pode ser repetido, mas o uso recorrente simplesmente resultará em desidratação.
- Furosemida (0,7 mg/kg IV) administrada antes da aplicação do manitol pode complementar o uso deste último agente terapêutico e prolongar seu efeito.

CONTRAINDICAÇÕES
N/D.

PRECAUÇÕES
Os sedativos devem ser utilizados com cautela em pacientes que exibem compressão da cabeça, pois tais agentes impedem a avaliação de alterações no estado mental e podem suprimir o controle respiratório, provocando aumento na pCO_2 e causando por meio disso elevação na pressão intracraniana.

INTERAÇÕES POSSÍVEIS
N/D.

MEDICAMENTO(S) ALTERNATIVO(S)
N/D.

ACOMPANHAMENTO
MONITORIZAÇÃO DO PACIENTE
- Repetir periodicamente o exame neurológico para monitorizar a evolução.
- Ver doenças específicas.

PREVENÇÃO
N/D.

COMPLICAÇÕES POSSÍVEIS
N/D.

EVOLUÇÃO ESPERADA E PROGNÓSTICO
N/D.

DIVERSOS
DISTÚRBIOS ASSOCIADOS
N/D.

FATORES RELACIONADOS COM A IDADE
N/D.

POTENCIAL ZOONÓTICO
- A raiva deve ser considerada em áreas endêmicas.
- Infecções fúngicas podem ser zoonóticas em caso de liberação de esporos no ambiente; é mais provável que isso ocorra se houver lesões cutâneas exsudativas.

GESTAÇÃO/FERTILIDADE/REPRODUÇÃO
N/D.

VER TAMBÉM
- Encefalite.
- Encefalopatia Hepática.
- Hidrocefalia.
- Lesão Cerebral.

ABREVIATURA(S)
- ALT = alanina aminotransferase.
- FeLV = vírus da leucemia felina.
- FIV = vírus da imunodeficiência felina.
- LCS = líquido cerebrospinal.
- PCR = reação em cadeia da polimerase.
- RM = ressonância magnética.
- SNC = sistema nervoso central.
- TC = tomografia computadorizada.

RECURSOS DA INTERNET
http://www.ivis.org/advances/Vite/braund1/chapter frm.asp?LA=1#Cerebral_Syndrome.

Sugestões de Leitura
Bagley RS. Clinical features of important and common diseases involving the intracranial nervous system of dogs and cats. In: Fundamentals of Veterinary Clinical Neurology. Ames, IA: Blackwell, 2005, pp. 134-140.
Dewey CW. Encephalopathies: Disorders of the brain. In: Dewey CW, A Practical Guide to Canine and Feline Neurology, 2nd ed. Ames, IA: Wiley-Blackwell, 2008, pp. 115-220.

Autor Natasha J. Olby
Consultor Editorial Joane M. Parent

Condrossarcoma — Boca

CONSIDERAÇÕES GERAIS

REVISÃO
• Condrossarcoma é um tumor mesenquimal maligno, que produz matriz condroide e fibrilar, mas não osteoide.
• O condrossarcoma responde por 5-10% de todos os tumores ósseos primários. Há relatos de condrossarcoma mandibular e maxilar em cães, mas tais localizações não são comuns para esse tipo de tumor. (Ver "Condrossarcoma, Osso" e "Condrossarcoma, Seios Nasais e Paranasais".)
• Em cães com condrossarcoma envolvendo o maxilar, há necessidade de avaliação completa para garantir que isso não seja um tumor nasal primário com invasão secundária no maxilar.
• Em gatos, o condrossarcoma é raro, embora haja relatos de tumores originários da mandíbula.

IDENTIFICAÇÃO
• Cães e, raramente, gatos.
• Mais comuns em raças caninas de médio a grande porte. Os cães das raças Golden retriever, Boxer e Pastor alemão, bem como aqueles sem raça definida, são super representados.
• A idade média é de 8 anos (faixa etária relatada, 1-15 anos).
• Gatos — não há predileções raciais ou sexuais evidentes.

SINAIS CLÍNICOS
Achados Anamnésicos
• Massa visível envolvendo a mandíbula ou o maxilar. • Halitose. • Sialorreia. • Secreção bucal sanguinolenta. • Disfagia. • Dor bucal — comportamento desconfiado (avesso a afagos e carinhos na cabeça) e/ou ingestão alimentar reduzida apesar de demonstrar interesse pelo alimento. • Perda de peso secundária à diminuição prolongada no consumo alimentar.

Achados do Exame Físico
• O exame da boca do animal sob sedação ou anestesia é frequentemente útil. • Mais comumente, observa-se a existência de massa firme a dura em torno do maxilar ou da mandíbula. • A mucosa gengival sobrejacente costuma permanecer intacta, embora a presença de traumatismo e ulceração causados por maloclusão dentária seja comum com tumores mais volumosos. • Halitose, sialorreia e/ou sangramento bucal. • Dentes frouxos ou ausentes. • Dificuldade ou dor à abertura da boca (especialmente em casos de tumores caudais). • Deformidade facial.
• Linfadenopatia mandibular ipsilateral (hiperplasia reativa ou, menos provavelmente, metástase). • Secreção nasal, epistaxe ou fluxo de ar reduzido por meio das narinas (tumores maxilares).

CAUSAS E FATORES DE RISCO
Não identificados.

DIAGNÓSTICO

DIAGNÓSTICO DIFERENCIAL
• Osteossarcoma. • Osteocondrossarcoma multilobular (tumor multilobular do osso).
• Osteopatia craniomandibular (cães, especialmente as raças West Highland white terrier, Cairn terrier, e Scottish terrier). • Cisto dentígero. • Abscesso radicular dentário.
• Osteomielite. • Carcinoma de células escamosas.
• Fibrossarcoma. • Melanoma amelanótico.
• Ameloblastoma (epúlide acantomatoso).
• Periodontoma fibromatoso ou ossificante (epúlide).

HEMOGRAMA/BIOQUÍMICA/URINÁLISE
Em geral, permanecem normais.

DIAGNÓSTICO POR IMAGEM
• Radiografias cranianas ou dentárias revelarão características de lesão óssea agressiva (lise óssea, destruição cortical, formação óssea não homogênea, zona mal-definida de transição).
• Radiografias dentárias ricas em detalhes podem ser adequadas para a visualização de lesões menores.
• Varredura por TC permite o estadiamento mais preciso de doença local, sendo útil para o planejamento de cirurgia e/ou radioterapia. É particularmente útil para tumores maxilares e tumores mandibulares amplos ou caudais.
• Os exames de radiografia e TC não podem ser utilizados para diferenciar condrossarcoma de outros tumores ósseos primários, tumores que se originam de tecidos moles adjacentes e invadem secundariamente o osso, ou osteomielite. Para obtenção do diagnóstico definitivo, há necessidade de biopsia.
• Radiografias torácicas são recomendadas para exibição de metástases.
• Se o paciente estiver sendo submetido à TC, é recomendável a obtenção concomitante de imagens do tórax como um método mais sensível para exibição de metástases pulmonares.

MÉTODOS DIAGNÓSTICOS
• O exame histopatológico é necessário para obtenção do diagnóstico definitivo. Todo tecido removido deve ser enviado ao patologista. Isso permite não só a formulação de diagnóstico mais preciso, mas também a determinação da margem de segurança para avaliar a plenitude da excisão.
• São recomendados os exames de aspiração e citologia de linfonodo madibular ipsilateral com agulha fina, especialmente em caso de enfartamento.

TRATAMENTO

• Excisão cirúrgica — sempre que possível, é recomendável a remoção do segmento ósseo acometido (maxilectomia ou mandibulectomia) com margem de, no mínimo, 2-3 cm.
• Se a excisão for incompleta, a radioterapia adjuvante pode ajudar a aumentar o controle local, embora haja poucas informações a respeito da eficácia.
• A radioterapia pode ser considerada como uma modalidade terapêutica local única. Embora haja poucas informações sobre sua eficácia para tumores bucais primários, esse tipo de terapia é utilizado com sucesso para condrossarcoma nasal primário.
• Em função da matriz condroide produzida por condrossarcomas, a radioterapia provavelmente estabilizará o tamanho do tumor na melhor das hipóteses e não provocará redução substancial.
• Embora não tenha sido avaliada, acredita-se que a quimioterapia seja eficaz.
• Os cuidados paliativos concentram-se no controle da dor. Os analgésicos orais são abordados adiante. O bloqueio nervoso regional também pode conferir analgesia por até algumas semanas. Também é aconselhável o fornecimento de alimentos pastosos.

MEDICAÇÕES

MEDICAMENTO(S)
• Agentes anti-inflamatórios não esteroides:
  ◦ Ácido acetilsalicílico (10-25 mg/kg VO a cada 8-24 h).
  ◦ Carprofeno (2 mg/kg VO a cada 12 h).
  ◦ Deracoxibe (1-2 mg/kg VO a cada 24 h).
  ◦ Meloxicam (0,1 mg/kg VO a cada 24 h).
  ◦ Firocoxibe (5 mg/kg VO a cada 24 h).
• Tramadol (2-5 mg/kg VO a cada 6-12 h).
• Gabapentina (10-15 mg/kg VO a cada 8-12 h).
• Pamidronato (1-2 mg/kg IV a cada 3-4 semanas) diminui a reabsorção óssea, aumenta a densidade mineral óssea e pode reduzir a dor associada a tumores ósseos.
• Antibioticoterapia empírica pode ser considerada para infecções bacterianas secundárias.

ACOMPANHAMENTO

MONITORIZAÇÃO DO PACIENTE
Realização de exames físicos e obtenção de radiografias torácicas a cada 2-3 meses.

EVOLUÇÃO ESPERADA E PROGNÓSTICO
• A maioria dos pacientes vem a óbito ou é submetida à eutanásia em virtude da doença local.
• O índice metastático global é de 15-30%, sendo os pulmões os órgãos mais comumente acometidos.
• A frequência de metástases chega a 50% para tumores de alto grau.
• O prognóstico depende do tamanho e da localização do tumor, bem como do rigor da cirurgia.
• Com excisão completa, é possível o controle tumoral a longo prazo.
• Com excisão parcial, é provável a recorrência local dentro de 6-12 meses.

DIVERSOS

VER TAMBÉM
• Condrossarcoma, Osso.
• Condrossarcoma, Seios Nasais e Paranasais.

ABREVIATURA(S)
• TC= tomografia computadorizada.

Sugestões de Leitura
Verstraete FJ. Mandibulectomy and maxillectomy. Vet Clin North Am Small Anim Pract 2005, 35(4):1009-1039.
Waltman SS, Seguin B, Cooper BJ, Kent M. Clinical outcome of nonnasal chondrosarcoma in dogs: Thirty-one cases (1986-2003). Vet Surg 2007, 36:266-271.

Autor Dennis B. Bailey
Consultor Editorial Timothy M. Fan

Condrossarcoma — Laringe e Traqueia

CONSIDERAÇÕES GERAIS

REVISÃO
• Condrossarcoma é um tumor mesenquimal maligno que produz uma matriz condroide e fibrilar, mas não um osteoide.
• Osteocondroma é um tumor benigno com uma margem apical de cartilagem hialina e uma base de osso esponjoso.
• Em geral, os tumores da laringe e traqueia são raros tanto em cães como em gatos.

IDENTIFICAÇÃO
• Cães.
• O condrossarcoma origina-se tanto da laringe como da traqueia em cães, sem predileções sexuais ou raciais evidentes.
• Faixa etária de 1 a 10 anos.
• O osteocondroma tipicamente ocorre na traqueia de cães jovens (<1 ano de idade), sem predileções sexuais ou raciais evidentes.
• Não há relatos de condrossarcoma e osteocondroma na laringe ou traqueia de gatos.

SINAIS CLÍNICOS
Achados Anamnésicos
• Mudança na vocalização.
• Respiração sonora ou estertorosa.
• Tosse ou dispneia.
• Intolerância ao exercício.
• Angústia respiratória grave; cianose; e colapso agudo.
• Disfagia.

Achados do Exame Físico
• Estertor inspiratório.
• Estridor respiratório.
• Dispneia, cianose.
• Pode-se observar a presença de massa laríngea ao exame bucal sem sedação.
• Raramente, é possível a detecção de massa laríngea ou traqueal por palpação externa.

CAUSAS E FATORES DE RISCO
Nenhum conhecido.

DIAGNÓSTICO

DIAGNÓSTICO DIFERENCIAL
• Paralisia laríngea.
• Alongamento do palato mole (especialmente raças braquicefálicas).
• Colapso (colabamento) da laringe.
• Colapso (colabamento) da traqueia.
• Espirro reverso.
• Corpo estranho na faringe ou laringe.
• Traumatismo da laringe e inflamação secundária.
• Outros tumores da laringe, incluindo rabdomioma, oncocitoma, carcinoma de células escamosas, adenocarcinoma, mastocitoma, osteossarcoma, fibrossarcoma, plasmocitoma e linfoma.
• Outros tumores da traqueia, incluindo carcinoma de células escamosas, linfoma, mastocitoma, leiomioma, adenocarcinoma e osteossarcoma.
• Adenocarcinoma da tireoide com compressão ou invasão secundária da laringe ou traqueia.

HEMOGRAMA/BIOQUÍMICA/URINÁLISE
Em geral, permanecem normais.

OUTROS TESTES LABORATORIAIS
Oximetria de pulso e/ou realização de gasometria arterial.

DIAGNÓSTICO POR IMAGEM
• Radiografias cervicais são de benefício limitado. Os tumores da laringe são tipicamente visualizados ao exame radiográfico somente quando os tumores se tornam muito grandes.
• Ultrassonografia cervical pode ajudar a identificar a presença de massa laríngea e orientar a aspiração percutânea com agulha fina ou biopsia central com agulha.
• Radiografias torácicas também são recomendadas para fazer a triagem em busca de metástase pulmonar.
• Tomografia computadorizada é indicada para identificar a origem do crescimento neoplásico, bem como a extensão da doença.

MÉTODOS DIAGNÓSTICOS
• Exame da laringe sob sedação — os procedimentos de sedação e anestesia não são isentos de risco; portanto, é preciso estar preparado para entubar o paciente e/ou realizar uma traqueostomia de emergência.
• Laringoscopia e traqueoscopia — estar preparado para efetuar uma traqueostomia de emergência.
• Citologia de amostras coletadas por meio de aspiração com agulha fina ou aspiração com agulha fina guiada por ultrassom.
• Os procedimentos de biopsia tecidual e histopatologia são necessários para obter o diagnóstico definitivo.

TRATAMENTO

• Tratamento da angústia respiratória — manter o paciente calmo, fornecer suporte de oxigênio e administrar medicamentos anti-inflamatórios. Em casos de angústia respiratória grave advinda de uma obstrução quase completa, o clínico deve ficar preparado para a realização de traqueostomia de emergência.
• Tumores laríngeos benignos pequenos podem ser removidos por meio cirúrgico via ressecção submucosa ou laringectomia parcial.
• Cânceres laríngeos invasivos grandes são mais bem tratados com laringectomia total e traqueostomia permanente. Os proprietários devem estar cientes da necessidade de cuidados pós-operatórios extensos a longo prazo e das altas taxas de complicações.
• Tumores traqueais benignos pequenos podem ser submetidos a debridamento via traqueoscopia e eletrocautério.
• Tumores traqueais maiores e malignos devem ser tratados por meio de ressecção — a remoção de toda a espessura do tumor com anastomose terminoterminal pode ser realizada em 20-60% da traqueia, em geral até 4-8 anéis traqueais.
• A radioterapia raramente é utilizada. Em função da matriz condroide e mineral produzida pelos condrossarcomas e osteocondromas, a radioterapia provavelmente estabilizará o tamanho do tumor na melhor das hipóteses e não provocará redução substancial.

MEDICAÇÕES

MEDICAMENTO(S)
• Fosfato sódico de dexametasona (0,1-0,2 mg/kg IV) para ajudar a aliviar a inflamação secundária que contribui para a angústia respiratória aguda.
• Não foi demonstrado que a quimioterapia seja eficaz.

CONTRAINDICAÇÕES/INTERAÇÕES POSSÍVEIS
Linfoma laríngeo e traqueal é observado raramente em cães e ocasionalmente em gatos. Todos os esforços devem ser feitos para descartar a presença de linfoma antes da administração de esteroides.

ACOMPANHAMENTO

MONITORIZAÇÃO DO PACIENTE
• É aconselhável a realização de exames físicos mensais.
• Para tumores laríngeos, deve-se realizar um exame da laringe sob sedação a cada 2-3 meses.
• Para tumores traqueais, é recomendável a obtenção de radiografias da traqueia e/ou a realização de traqueoscopia a cada 2-3 meses.
• Para fazer a triagem em busca de possíveis metástases pulmonares, devem-se obter radiografias torácicas a cada 2-3 meses.

EVOLUÇÃO ESPERADA E PROGNÓSTICO
• O prognóstico de condrossarcoma é reservado, porque a maioria dos cães apresenta doença infiltrativa avançada no momento do diagnóstico. Mesmo quando os tumores podem ser removidos, a excisão costuma ser incompleta, sendo comum a recorrência local.
• O prognóstico de osteocondroma traqueal a longo prazo é bom caso seja possível a ressecção completa da lesão.

DIVERSOS

Sugestões de Leitura
Carlisle CH, Biery DN, Thrall DE. Tracheal and laryngeal tumors in the dog and cat: Literature review and 13 additional patients. Vet Radiol Ultrasound 1991, 5:229-235.

Autor Dennis B. Bailey
Consultor Editorial Timothy M. Fan

Condrossarcoma — Osso

CONSIDERAÇÕES GERAIS

REVISÃO
- Condrossarcoma é um tumor mesenquimal maligno que produz matriz condroide e fibrilar, mas não osteoide.
- Corresponde ao segundo tumor ósseo primário mais comum em cães, respondendo por 5-10% de todos os tumores ósseos primários. Em gatos, os tumores ósseos primários são raros, mas o condrossarcoma é o terceiro em incidência depois do osteossarcoma e fibrossarcoma.
- A maioria dos condrossarcomas origina-se de ossos chatos. Aproximadamente 30% ocorrem na cavidade nasal, respondendo por 15% de todos os tumores nasais; 20% dos condrossarcomas surgem das costelas, respondendo por 30-40% de todos os tumores primários do gradil costal.
- 20% dos condrossarcomas têm origem no esqueleto apendicular, frequentemente (mas nem sempre) nos locais típicos onde ocorre osteossarcoma. O condrossarcoma responde por apenas 3-5% de todos os tumores ósseos primários no esqueleto apendicular.
- Outros locais relatados incluem ossos faciais, crânio, vértebras, pelve, dedos e osso peniano.
- Raramente, os condrossarcomas podem se originar em áreas de tecidos moles (ou seja, extraesqueléticos). Nos gatos, os condrossarcomas podem ter origem nos locais de vacinação prévia.

IDENTIFICAÇÃO
- Cães e gatos (raro).
- Mais comum em raças caninas de médio a grande porte que pesam entre 20 e 40 kg. Os cães das raças Golden retriever, Boxer e Pastor alemão, bem como aqueles sem raça definida, são super-representados.
- A idade média é de 8 anos (faixa etária relatada de 1-15 anos).
- Gatos — não há predileções óbvias.

SINAIS CLÍNICOS
Achados Anamnésicos
- Os pacientes frequentemente se apresentam com massa visível no local acometido.
- O condrossarcoma apendicular costuma estar associado à claudicação.
- Raramente, os tumores das costelas podem estar associados a sinais respiratórios.
- Outros sinais clínicos variam com o local de envolvimento tumoral.

Achados do Exame Físico
- Os achados dependem da localização anatômica.
- Com frequência, mas nem sempre, será palpável a presença de massa firme a dura. A massa é frequentemente dolorosa, mas nem sempre.
- Os condrossarcomas do esqueleto apendicular e dos dedos geralmente estão associados à claudicação.
- Os condrossarcomas das costelas ocorrem com maior frequência na junção costocondral. Qualquer costela pode ser acometida. É raro o sinal de dispneia.

CAUSAS E FATORES DE RISCO
- Etiologia basicamente desconhecida.
- As lesões de osteocondromatose (exostose cartilaginosa múltipla) podem se transformar em condrossarcoma.

DIAGNÓSTICO

DIAGNÓSTICO DIFERENCIAL
- Outros tumores ósseos primários (osteossarcoma, fibrossarcoma, hemangiossarcoma). • Tumores ósseos metastáticos (carcinomas de células de transição, da próstata, das glândulas mamárias, da tireoide, das glândulas apócrinas e dos sacos anais).
- Tumores com invasividade local dos ossos adjacentes (especialmente tumores das cavidades bucal e nasal, dos dedos e das articulações).
- Osteomielite bacteriana ou fúngica.

HEMOGRAMA/BIOQUÍMICA/URINÁLISE
Em geral, permanecem normais.

DIAGNÓSTICO POR IMAGEM
- Radiografias da lesão primária revelam características de lesão óssea agressiva (lise óssea, destruição cortical, formação óssea não homogênea, zona mal-definida de transição).
- Radiografias torácicas são recomendadas para exibição de metástase pulmonar. • Varredura por TC é recomendável em casos de tumores axiais para estadiamento mais preciso de doença local e planejamento de cirurgia e/ou radioterapia. • Se o paciente estiver sendo submetido à TC, é aconselhável a obtenção concomitante de imagens do tórax como um método mais sensível para exibição de metástase pulmonar.

MÉTODOS DIAGNÓSTICOS
- O exame histopatológico é necessário para obtenção do diagnóstico definitivo. • Aspirado citológico de tecido ósseo obtido com agulha fina pode fornecer um diagnóstico presuntivo.

TRATAMENTO

- Amputação é um procedimento recomendado para tumores apendiculares.
- Para tumores axiais, é recomendável a realização de ampla excisão sempre que possível. Se a excisão for parcial, a aplicação de radioterapia adjuvante pode ajudar a melhorar o controle local.
- O tratamento paliativo é aconselhável em pacientes com doença local não ressecável ou metástase macroscópica ou em casos de deterioração da terapia definitiva. Os cuidados paliativos concentram-se no controle da dor.

MEDICAÇÕES

MEDICAMENTO(S)
Controle da Dor
- Seleção e dosagens de medicamentos anti-inflamatórios não esteroides:
  - Ácido acetilsalicílico (10-25 mg/kg VO a cada 8-24 h).
  - Carprofeno (2 mg/kg VO a cada 12 h).
  - Deracoxibe (1-2 mg/kg VO a cada 24 h).
  - Meloxicam (0,1 mg/kg VO a cada 24 h).
  - Firocoxibe (5 mg/kg VO a cada 24 h).
  - Tramadol (2-5 mg/kg VO a cada 6-12 h).
- Gabapentina (10-15 mg/kg VO a cada 8-12 h).
- Pamidronato (1-2 mg/kg IV a cada 3-4 semanas) reduz a reabsorção óssea, aumenta a densidade mineral óssea e pode diminuir a dor associada a tumores ósseos.

Quimioterapia
O papel desempenhado pela quimioterapia não foi definido em oncologia veterinária. Em seres humanos com tumores de alto grau, os protocolos tipicamente incluem doxorrubicina com ou sem cisplatina, ifosfamida e/ou metotrexato.

CONTRAINDICAÇÕES/INTERAÇÕES POSSÍVEIS
- Utilizar os AINE com cuidado em gatos e em cães com insuficiência renal.
- Não combinar AINE com esteroides.

ACOMPANHAMENTO

MONITORIZAÇÃO DO PACIENTE
Realização de exames físicos e obtenção de radiografias torácicas a cada 2-3 meses para monitorizar o controle local do tumor e as metástases à distância, respectivamente.

EVOLUÇÃO ESPERADA E PROGNÓSTICO
- Em geral, 15-30% dos casos desenvolverão doença metastática, sendo os pulmões os órgãos mais comumente acometidos. A frequência de metástases chega a 50% para tumores de alto grau.
- Com a realização de cirurgia rigorosa, a sobrevida média gira em torno de mais de 3 anos e muitos cães gozarão de um controle local a longo prazo. Contudo, dependendo da localização do tumor e da plenitude da excisão, até 40% dos casos desenvolverão recorrência local.
- Apenas com o fornecimento de cuidados paliativos, ainda serão possíveis tempos de sobrevida superiores a 1 ano.

DIVERSOS

VER TAMBÉM
- Condrossarcoma, Laringe e Traqueia.
- Condrossarcoma, Seios Nasais e Paranasais.
- Fibrossarcoma, Osso.
- Osteossarcoma.

ABREVIATURA(S)
- AINE = anti-inflamatórios não esteroides.
- TC = tomografia computadorizada.

Sugestões de Leitura
Farese JP, Kirpensteijn J, Kik M, et al. Biologic behavior and clinical outcome of 25 dogs with canine appendicular chondrosarcoma treated by amputation: A veterinary society of surgical oncology retrospective study. Vet Surg 2009, 38:914-919.

Liptak JM, Kamstock DA, Dernell WS, et al. Oncologic outcome after curative-intent treatment in 39 dogs with primary chest wall tumors (1992-2005). Vet Surg 2008, 37(5):488-496.

Waltman SS, Sequin B, Cooper BJ, et al. Clinical outcome of nonnasal chondrosarcoma in dogs: Thirty-one cases (1986-2003). Vet Surg 2007, 36(3):266-271.

Autor Dennis B. Bailey
Consultor Editorial Timothy M. Fan

CONDROSSARCOMA — SEIOS NASAIS E PARANASAIS

CONSIDERAÇÕES GERAIS

REVISÃO
- Condrossarcoma é um tumor mesenquimal maligno que produz matriz condroide e fibrilar, mas não osteoide.
- Condrossarcoma nasal origina-se mais comumente dos ossos turbinados nasais.
- Em cães, aproximadamente 30% de todos os condrossarcomas ocorrem na cavidade nasal; isso responde por 15% de todos os tumores nasais.

IDENTIFICAÇÃO
- Para os condrossarcomas em geral, os cães das raças Golden retriever, Boxer e Pastor alemão, bem como aqueles sem raça definida, são super-representados.
- A idade média é de 7 anos (faixa etária, 2-11 anos).
- O condrossarcoma tende a se desenvolver em uma idade mais jovem quando comparado com outros tumores nasais.
- Raro em gatos — não há predileções raciais ou sexuais evidentes.

SINAIS CLÍNICOS
Achados Anamnésicos
- Epistaxe uni ou bilateral e/ou secreção mucopurulenta.
- Espirro.
- Respiração estertorosa.
- Deformidade facial.
- Diminuição do apetite e/ou halitose secundárias à invasão da cavidade bucal.
- Crises convulsivas, mudanças comportamentais e/ou obnubilação secundárias à invasão craniana.

Achados do Exame Físico
- Epistaxe e/ou secreção nasal (uni ou bilateral).
- Diminuição do fluxo de ar nasal (uni ou bilateral).
- Dor à palpação ou percussão dos seios nasais ou paranasais.
- Deformidade facial.
- Retropulsão diminuída dos olhos ou exoftalmia.
- Epífora e/ou secreção ocular.
- Efeito de massa visível que se projeta por meio do palato para a cavidade bucal.

CAUSAS E FATORES DE RISCO
Desconhecidos.

DIAGNÓSTICO

DIAGNÓSTICO DIFERENCIAL
- Outros tumores nasais — adenocarcinoma, carcinoma de células escamosas, osteossarcoma, fibrossarcoma, linfoma, tumor venéreo transmissível (cães), pólipo nasofaríngeo (gatos).
- Rinite fúngica — aspergilose e penicilose (cães), criptococose (gatos), esporotricose (ambos).
- Rinosporidiose (cães).
- Rinite viral — herpes-vírus e calicivírus (gatos).
- Corpo estranho.
- Trombocitopenia ou outra coagulopatia.
- Hipertensão.
- Abscesso radicular dentário.
- Rinite alérgica.
- Sinusite bacteriana — incomum.
- Fístula oronasal.

HEMOGRAMA/BIOQUÍMICA/URINÁLISE
Em geral, permanecem normais — avaliar o paciente em busca de trombocitopenia se houver sinais de epistaxe.

OUTROS TESTES LABORATORIAIS
- Exame citológico e cultura bacteriana de irrigação nasal — raramente são úteis.
- Perfil de coagulação.
- Tempo de coagulação da mucosa bucal.

DIAGNÓSTICO POR IMAGEM
- Radiografias simples (crânio) — revelam opacidade de tecidos moles na cavidade nasal e/ou nos seios frontais, bem como destruição de estruturas como ossos turbinados, septo nasal, vômer ou ossos palatinos, maxilares e/ou frontais circunjacentes.
- Radiografias torácicas — detectam metástases pulmonares.
- Varredura por TC — é superior às radiografias para detectar opacidade de tecidos moles dentro da cavidade nasal e dos seios circunjacentes, destruição óssea e extensão do tumor por meio da placa cribriforme para o cérebro. O exame de TC também é usado para o planejamento da radioterapia (ver a seção "Tratamento" adiante).
- Se o paciente estiver sendo submetido à TC, é recomendável a obtenção concomitante de imagens do tórax como um método mais sensível para exibição de metástases pulmonares.

MÉTODOS DIAGNÓSTICOS
- Medição da pressão arterial e exame do fundo ocular.
- Citologia dos linfonodos mandibulares para detecção de possível metástase.
- Rinoscopia pode ocasionalmente ser útil para visualização de massa ou placa fúngica e orientação de biopsias futuras. Para obtenção do diagnóstico definitivo, há necessidade dos exames de biopsia tecidual e histopatologia. Os instrumentos utilizados na biopsia não devem passar caudalmente ao nível do canto medial do olho para evitar a penetração da placa cribriforme.

TRATAMENTO

- A radioterapia é o tratamento de escolha.
- Protocolos definidos comuns:
  - 57 Gy aplicados em 19 frações de 3,0 Gy a cada semana de segunda a sexta-feira.
  - 42 Gy aplicados em 10 frações de 4,2 Gy a cada semana de segunda a sexta-feira.
- Protocolos paliativos (menos tratamentos e menor dose radioativa total) podem ser preferíveis para cães com doença muito avançada.
- A cirurgia isolada é ineficaz, mas há certa evidência de que a exenteração da cavidade nasal após radioterapia aumente o tempo de sobrevida para cães com vários tumores nasais.
- Consultar um médico especialista em oncologia e/ou oncologista especialista em radioterapia em busca das recomendações atuais.

MEDICAÇÕES

MEDICAMENTO(S)
- Prednisona (0,5-1 mg/kg VO a cada 24 h) para ajudar a aliviar a congestão nasal.
- Spray nasal de fenilefrina pode ser usado de forma intermitente para ajudar em casos de epistaxe.
- Antibioticoterapia empírica pode ser considerada para infecções bacterianas secundárias.
- A quimioterapia não foi avaliada para o tratamento de carga patológica mensurável.

CONTRAINDICAÇÕES/INTERAÇÕES POSSÍVEIS
Nenhuma.

ACOMPANHAMENTO

MONITORIZAÇÃO DO PACIENTE
- Realização de exames físicos e obtenção de radiografias torácicas são recomendadas a cada 2-3 meses.
- TC do crânio pode ser considerada em casos de recorrência ou evolução dos sinais clínicos.

EVOLUÇÃO ESPERADA E PROGNÓSTICO
- <10% dos casos desenvolvem metástase (os pulmões são acometidos com maior frequência).
- A sobrevida média apenas com cuidados paliativos é de 3 meses.
- Com radioterapia definida, as taxas de sobrevida livre de recidiva em um período de 1 e 2 anos giram em torno de 50 e 30%, respectivamente.
- Os pacientes com sarcomas nasais têm uma probabilidade 3 vezes menor de sofrerem recorrência local em comparação àqueles com carcinomas nasais.
- Para os pacientes com tumores nasais em geral, a extensão para os seios frontais e/ou a erosão por meio dos ossos das vias nasais está associada a um aumento de 3 vezes no risco de recorrência local.
- O envolvimento do cérebro é um sinal prognóstico mau.
- O envolvimento uni ou bilateral não é um fator prognóstico significativo.

DIVERSOS

VER TAMBÉM
- Adenocarcinoma, Nasal.
- Condrossarcoma, Osso.
- Condrossarcoma, Laringe e Traqueia.
- Epistaxe.

ABREVIATURA(S)
- TC = tomografia computadorizada.

Sugestões de Leitura
Patnaik AK, Lieberman PH, Erlandson RA, et al. Canine sinonasal skeletal neoplasms: Chondrosarcomas and osteosarcomas. Vet Pathol 1984, 21(5):475-482.
Theon AP. Megavoltage irradiation of neoplasms of the nasal and paranasal cavities in 77 dogs. JAVMA 1993, 202:1469-1475.

Autor Dennis B. Bailey
Consultor Editorial Timothy M. Fan

Conjuntivite — Cães

CONSIDERAÇÕES GERAIS

DEFINIÇÃO
Inflamação da conjuntiva, a mucosa vascularizada que recobre a porção anterior do bulbo ocular (porção bulbar) e reveste as pálpebras e a terceira pálpebra (porção palpebral).

FISIOPATOLOGIA
• Primária — alérgica; infecciosa; ambiental; ceratoconjuntivite seca.
• Secundária a doenças oculares ou sistêmicas subjacentes — glaucoma; uveíte; doença imunomediada; neoplasia, outras.

SISTEMA(S) ACOMETIDO(S)
Oftálmico — quadro ocular, com envolvimento ocasional das pálpebras (p. ex., blefaroconjuntivite).

GENÉTICA
N/D.

INCIDÊNCIA/PREVALÊNCIA
Comum.

DISTRIBUIÇÃO GEOGRÁFICA
N/D.

IDENTIFICAÇÃO
Espécies
Cães.

Raça(s) Predominante(s)
As raças predispostas a dermatopatias alérgicas ou imunomediadas (p. ex., atopia) tendem a ter mais problemas com conjuntivite alérgica ou ceratoconjuntivite seca.

Idade Média e Faixa Etária
N/D.

Sexo Predominante
N/D.

SINAIS CLÍNICOS
• Blefarospasmo.
• Hiperemia conjuntival.
• Secreção ocular — serosa, mucoide ou mucopurulenta.
• Quemose.
• Formação de folículos.
• Conjuntivas bulbar ou palpebral — podem ser primariamente envolvidas.

CAUSAS
Bacterianas
• Distúrbios primários (i. e., não secundários a outra afecção, como a ceratoconjuntivite seca) — raros.
• Neonatais — acúmulo de exsudatos, muitas vezes com um componente bacteriano ou viral; observada antes da separação das pálpebras.

Virais
• Vírus da cinomose.
• Herpes-vírus tipo 1.
• Adenovírus tipo 2.

Imunomediadas
• Alérgicas — especialmente em pacientes atópicos.
• Conjuntivite folicular — sobretudo em cães com menos de 18 meses, secundariamente à estimulação antigênica crônica.
• Conjuntivite plasmocitária — particularmente em cães da raça Pastor alemão.
• Relacionadas com doenças imunomediadas sistêmicas (p. ex., pênfigo).

Neoplásicas e Pseudoneoplásicas
• Tumores com envolvimento da conjuntiva — raros; incluem melanomas, hemangiomas, hemangiossarcomas, linfossarcomas, papilomas e mastocitomas.
• Pseudoneoplásicas — episclerite nodular (também conhecida como histiocitoma fibroso, granuloma nodular ocular e pseudotumor conjuntival); observada mais comumente em Collie e mestiços dessa raça; supostamente imunomediada; massa de coloração rósea, localizada geralmente no limbo temporal.

Secundárias a Comprometimento dos Anexos
• Deficiência do filme lacrimal aquoso (ver "Ceratoconjuntivite Seca").
• Blefaropatias (p. ex., entrópio, ectrópio e fundo-de-saco exagerado) e doenças dos cílios (p. ex., distiquíase e cílios ectópicos) — podem levar a sinais clínicos de conjuntivite.
• Secundárias à obstrução da porção de escoamento do sistema nasolacrimal (p. ex., ducto nasolacrimal obstruído e orifício lacrimal imperfurado).

Secundárias a Traumatismo ou Causas Ambientais
• Corpo estranho conjuntival.
• Irritação — poeira, substâncias químicas ou medicamentos oftalmológicos.

Secundárias a Outras Doenças Oculares
• Ceratite ulcerativa.
• Uveíte anterior.
• Glaucoma.

Outras
• Conjuntivite lenhosa — particularmente observada em cadelas jovens da raça Doberman.

FATORES DE RISCO
N/D.

DIAGNÓSTICO

DIAGNÓSTICO DIFERENCIAL
• Primária — deve-se distinguir de condições secundárias a outras doenças oculares.
• Doença intraocular — envolvimento da conjuntiva bulbar, associado a acometimento mínimo ou nulo da conjuntiva palpebral.
• Primária ou alérgica — envolvimento principalmente da conjuntiva palpebral, poupando-se a conjuntiva bulbar; considerar as causas primárias e secundárias se ambas as superfícies estiverem envolvidas.
• É imprescindível diferenciar os vasos conjuntivais (que apresentam mobilidade e ficam pálidos com simpaticomiméticos) e os episclerais (que permanecem imóveis e não ficam pálidos com simpaticomiméticos), pois a congestão episcleral indica doença intraocular, enquanto a hiperemia conjuntival pode ser um sinal de conjuntivite primária ou doença intraocular.

HEMOGRAMA/BIOQUÍMICA/URINÁLISE
Normais, exceto em casos de doença sistêmica.

OUTROS TESTES LABORATORIAIS
N/D.

DIAGNÓSTICO POR IMAGEM
N/D.

MÉTODOS DIAGNÓSTICOS
• Exame oftalmológico completo (teste lacrimal de Schirmer) — excluir ceratoconjuntivite seca.
• Coloração com fluoresceína — descartar ceratite ulcerativa.
• Mensuração da pressão intraocular — excluir glaucoma.
• Exame em busca de sinais de uveíte anterior (p. ex., hipotonia, rubor aquoso e miose).
• Exame detalhado dos anexos — descartar anormalidades das pálpebras e dos cílios, bem como corpos estranhos nos fundos-de-saco (fórnix) conjuntivais ou sob a membrana nictitante.
• Lavagem com irrigação nasolacrimal — considerada para descartar doença nasolacrimal.
• Cultura bacteriana aeróbia e antibiograma — em casos de secreção mucopurulenta; as amostras são idealmente coletadas antes de se instilar qualquer coisa nos olhos (p. ex., anestésico tópico, fluoresceína e irrigação) para evitar a inibição ou a diluição do crescimento bacteriano; exames não indicados com rotina em casos de ceratoconjuntivite seca e secreção mucopurulenta, pois a proliferação bacteriana secundária é quase incontestável.
• Citologia conjuntival — pode revelar a causa (raro); o encontro de eosinófilos e basófilos podem ajudar a diagnosticar conjuntivite alérgica e eosinofílica, mas essas células raramente são observadas em casos de conjuntivite alérgica, exceto à biopsia; como indicadores de infecção bacteriana, podem-se observar neutrófilos degenerados e bactérias intracitoplasmáticas; podem-se verificar corpúsculos de inclusão (intracitoplasmáticos em casos de envolvimento do vírus da cinomose).
• Biopsia conjuntival — pode ser útil em casos de lesões expansivas (tipo massa) e doenças imunomediadas; pode auxiliar na obtenção do diagnóstico definitivo em casos de doença crônica.
• Teste cutâneo intradérmico — pode ter utilidade na suspeita de conjuntivite alérgica.

ACHADOS PATOLÓGICOS
• Biopsia — sinais típicos de inflamação (p. ex., neutrófilos e linfócitos); podem-se notar agentes infecciosos.
• Características histopatológicas de lesões expansivas tipo massa (p. ex., papiloma e mastocitoma) — compatíveis com lesões semelhantes em qualquer outro lugar.
• Conjuntivite lenhosa — material hialino eosinofílico amorfo característico.

TRATAMENTO

CUIDADO(S) DE SAÚDE ADEQUADO(S)
• Conjuntivite primária — frequentemente em um esquema ambulatorial.
• Conjuntivite secundária a outras doenças (p. ex., uveíte e ceratite ulcerativa) — pode necessitar de internação, enquanto se diagnostica e se trata o problema subjacente.

ATIVIDADE
• Conjuntivite primária — não costuma haver restrição.
• Suspeita de contato com irritantes ou doença alérgica aguda — evitar (se possível) o contato com o agente agressor.
• Não expor os pacientes a animais suscetíveis.

DIETA
Suspeita de dermatopatia e/ou alergia alimentar subjacentes — é recomendável o fornecimento de uma dieta de eliminação (hipoalergênica).

ORIENTAÇÃO AO PROPRIETÁRIO
- Caso se observe uma secreção ocular abundante, orientar o proprietário a limpar os olhos antes de administrar o tratamento.
- Na prescrição tanto de soluções como de pomadas, ensinar o proprietário a utilizar a(s) solução(ões) antes da(s) pomada(s).
- Se muitas soluções forem prescritas, instruir o proprietário a esperar alguns minutos entre os tratamentos.
- Instruir o proprietário a buscar esclarecimentos se a condição piorar, o que pode indicar afecção irresponsiva, provável evolução do quadro ou ainda possível reação adversa ao medicamento prescrito.
- Informar o proprietário sobre a necessidade de colocação do colar elizabetano no paciente na ocorrência de autotraumatismo.

CONSIDERAÇÕES CIRÚRGICAS
- Obstrução do ducto nasolacrimal — procedimento trabalhoso; tratamento frequentemente não recomendado (ver "Epífora").
- Neoplasia conjuntival — pode exigir apenas a ressecção local; pode envolver a técnica de excisão, acompanhada por irradiação com raios beta, crioterapia, hipertermia por radiofrequência, enucleação ou exenteração, dependendo do tipo de tumor e do grau de envolvimento.

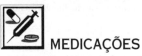
MEDICAÇÕES
MEDICAMENTO(S) DE ESCOLHA
Bacteriana
- Tratamento selecionado com base nos resultados da cultura bacteriana e do antibiograma.
- Tratamento inicial — antibiótico tópico de amplo espectro ou agente específico escolhido com base nos resultados do exame citológico, enquanto se aguardam os resultados da cultura; pode-se tentar um tratamento empírico, efetuando-se a cultura apenas se o paciente se mostrar refratário à terapia.
- Combinação antibiótica tripla ou cloranfenicol tópicos — caso se observem cocos ao exame citológico.
- Gentamicina ou tobramicina — caso se observem bastonetes ao exame citológico.
- Ciprofloxacino ou outras quinolonas — a cada 6-12 h, dependendo da gravidade; resistência bacteriana limitada (alguns estreptococos são resistentes); pode ser útil em casos de conjuntivite bacteriana grave.
- Antibióticos sistêmicos — ocasionalmente indicados, em particular no caso de uma doença mais generalizada (p. ex., piodermite).

Neonatal
- Abrir as margens palpebrais com cuidado (no sentido medial a lateral), instituir drenagem e tratar com antibióticos tópicos.

Imunomediada
- Depende da gravidade.
- Corticosteroides tópicos — dexametasona a 0,1%; melhoram os sinais clínicos de conjuntivites alérgicas, foliculares e plasmocitárias; muitas vezes, a melhora é temporária.
- O tratamento de qualquer doença subjacente (p. ex., atopia) frequentemente melhora os sinais clínicos.

CONTRAINDICAÇÕES
Corticosteroides tópicos — evitar caso se observe ulceração corneana.

PRECAUÇÕES
- Aminoglicosídeos tópicos — podem ser irritantes.
- Corticosteroides tópicos — monitorizar todos os pacientes com rigor em busca de sinais de ulceração corneana; interromper o agente imediatamente se ocorrer esse tipo de ulceração.

INTERAÇÕES POSSÍVEIS
N/D.

MEDICAMENTO(S) ALTERNATIVO(S)
Outros corticosteroides — acetato de prednisolona a 1%; betametasona; hidrocortisona.

ACOMPANHAMENTO
MONITORIZAÇÃO DO PACIENTE
Reavaliar o paciente logo após a instituição do tratamento (em 5-7 dias); em seguida, repetir a avaliação conforme a necessidade.

PREVENÇÃO
Tratar qualquer doença subjacente que possa estar exacerbando a doença ocular (p. ex., dermatopatia alérgica ou imunomediada e ceratoconjuntivite seca).

COMPLICAÇÕES POSSÍVEIS
N/D.

EVOLUÇÃO ESPERADA E PROGNÓSTICO
- Bacteriana — costuma desaparecer com antibióticos apropriados; pode depender da resolução da doença subjacente (p. ex., ceratoconjuntivite seca).
- Doenças imunomediadas — tendem a ser controladas e não curadas; podem necessitar de tratamento crônico no nível mais baixo possível.

DIVERSOS
DISTÚRBIOS ASSOCIADOS
- Atopia.
- Piodermite.

FATORES RELACIONADOS COM A IDADE
N/D.

POTENCIAL ZOONÓTICO
N/D.

GESTAÇÃO/FERTILIDADE/REPRODUÇÃO
- Se forem empregados, usar os antibióticos e os corticosteroides sistêmicos com cautela em fêmeas prenhes.
- Considerar a possibilidade de absorção de medicamentos tópicos e ponderar os benefícios terapêuticos em contraste com as possíveis complicações.

VER TAMBÉM
- Ceratoconjuntivite Seca.
- Epífora.
- Olho Vermelho.

Sugestões de Leitura
Maggs DJ, Miller PE, Ofri R. Slatter's Fundamentals of Veterinary Ophthalmology, 4th ed. St. Louis: Saunders, 2008, pp. 135-150.

Autor Erin S. Champagne
Consultor Editorial Paul E. Miller

CONJUNTIVITE — GATOS

CONSIDERAÇÕES GERAIS

DEFINIÇÃO
Inflamação da conjuntiva, a mucosa vascularizada que recobre a porção anterior do bulbo ocular (porção bulbar) e reveste as pálpebras e a terceira pálpebra* (porção palpebral).

FISIOPATOLOGIA
Pode ser primária (p. ex., infecciosa) ou secundária a doenças oculares ou sistêmicas subjacentes (p. ex., glaucoma, uveíte, doença imunomediada e neoplasia).

SISTEMA(S) ACOMETIDO(S)
Oftálmico — quadro ocular, com envolvimento ocasional das pálpebras (p. ex., blefaroconjuntivite).

GENÉTICA
N/D.

INCIDÊNCIA/PREVALÊNCIA
Comum.

DISTRIBUIÇÃO GEOGRÁFICA
N/D.

IDENTIFICAÇÃO
Espécies
Gatos.
Raça(s) Predominante(s)
Infecciosa — os gatos de raças puras parecem predispostos.
Idade Média e Faixa Etária
Infecciosa — acomete mais comumente animais jovens.
Sexo Predominante
N/D.

SINAIS CLÍNICOS
- Blefarospasmo.
- Hiperemia conjuntival.
- Secreção ocular — serosa, mucoide ou mucopurulenta.
- Quemose.
- Conjuntivas bulbar ou palpebral — podem ser primariamente envolvidas.
- Infecção respiratória superior — possível.

CAUSAS
Virais
- FHV — causa infecciosa mais comum; a única que leva a alterações corneanas (p. ex., úlceras dendríticas ou geográficas).
- Calicivírus.

Bacterianas
- Distúrbios primários (i. e., não secundários a outra afecção, como a ceratoconjuntivite seca) — raros, a não ser em casos de clamídias e micoplasmas.
- Neonatais — acúmulo de exsudatos, muitas vezes com um componente bacteriano ou viral; observada antes da separação das pálpebras.

Imunomediadas
- Eosinofílicas.
- Relacionadas com doenças imunomediadas sistêmicas — pênfigo.

---
* N. T.: Também conhecida como membrana nictitante ou nictante.

Neoplásicas e Pseudoneoplásicas
- Raras; o linfossarcoma e o carcinoma de células escamosas são os mais comuns.

Secundárias a Comprometimento dos Anexos
- Deficiência do filme lacrimal aquoso.
- Possível desenvolvimento de ceratoconjuntivite seca em virtude da formação cicatricial (ver "Ceratoconjuntivite Seca").
- Blefaropatias (p. ex., entrópio) — podem levar a sinais clínicos de conjuntivite.
- Secundárias à obstrução na porção de escoamento do sistema nasolacrimal — ducto nasolacrimal obstruído.

Secundárias a Traumatismo ou Causas Ambientais
- Corpo estranho conjuntival.
- Irritação provocada por poeira, substâncias químicas ou medicamentos oftalmológicos.

Secundárias a Outras Doenças Oculares
- Ceratite ulcerativa.
- Uveíte anterior.
- Glaucoma.

FATORES DE RISCO
N/D.

DIAGNÓSTICO

DIAGNÓSTICO DIFERENCIAL
- Primária — deve-se distinguir de problemas secundários a outras doenças oculares.
- Doença intraocular — envolvimento da conjuntiva bulbar, associado ao acometimento mínimo ou nulo da conjuntiva palpebral.
- Primária ou alérgica — envolvimento principalmente da conjuntiva palpebral, poupando-se a conjuntiva bulbar; considerar as causas primárias e secundárias se ambas as superfícies estiverem envolvidas.
- É imprescindível diferenciar os vasos conjuntivais (que apresentam mobilidade e ficam pálidos com simpaticomiméticos) e os episclerais (que permanecem imóveis e não ficam pálidos com simpaticomiméticos) — a congestão episcleral indica doença intraocular; a hiperemia conjuntival pode ser um sinal de conjuntivite primária ou doença intraocular.

HEMOGRAMA/BIOQUÍMICA/URINÁLISE
Normais, exceto em casos de doença sistêmica.

OUTROS TESTES LABORATORIAIS
Infecciosa — considerar a realização de testes sorológicos para pesquisa de FeLV/FIV; descartar imunocomprometimento subjacente.

DIAGNÓSTICO POR IMAGEM
N/D.

MÉTODOS DIAGNÓSTICOS
- Exame oftalmológico completo — excluir doenças intraoculares subjacentes (p. ex., uveíte e glaucoma).
- Exame detalhado dos anexos — descartar anormalidades palpebrais e corpos estranhos nos fundos-de-saco (fórnix) conjuntivais ou sob a membrana nictitante.
- Irrigação nasolacrimal — considerada para descartar doença nasolacrimal.
- Cultura bacteriana aeróbia e antibiograma — em casos de secreção mucopurulenta; as amostras são idealmente coletadas antes de se instilar qualquer coisa nos olhos (p. ex., anestésico tópico, fluoresceína e irrigação) para evitar a inibição ou a diluição do crescimento bacteriano.
- Citologia conjuntival — pode revelar a causa (raro); o encontro de eosinófilos e basófilos pode ajudar a diagnosticar conjuntivite alérgica e eosinofílica, mas raramente essas células são observadas em casos de conjuntivite alérgica, exceto à biopsia; como indicadores de infecção bacteriana, podem-se observar neutrófilos degenerados e bactérias intracitoplasmáticas; as infecções por clamídias ou micoplasmas podem exibir corpúsculos de inclusão; em casos de FHV, é rara a observação de corpúsculos de inclusão.
- Raspados conjuntivais para pesquisa de FHV — utilizar as técnicas de PCR ou de IFA; no entanto, podem-se verificar resultados falso-positivos em casos de doença crônica; a PCR é a técnica mais sensível e representa o teste de escolha; caso se efetue a coloração com fluoresceína antes do teste de IFA, será possível a constatação de resultados falso-positivos.
- Raspados conjuntivais para pesquisa de *Chlamydia* — empregar corantes especiais, razoavelmente confiáveis.
- Cultura viral — não disponível amplamente, mas pode ajudar a diagnosticar o FHV.
- Biopsia conjuntival — pode ser útil em casos de lesões expansivas (tipo massa) e doenças imunomediadas; pode auxiliar na obtenção do diagnóstico definitivo em casos de doença crônica.

ACHADOS PATOLÓGICOS
- Biopsia — sinais típicos de inflamação (p. ex., neutrófilos e linfócitos); possivelmente há agentes infecciosos.
- Características histopatológicas de lesões expansivas tipo massa (p. ex., carcinoma de células escamosas e linfossarcoma) — compatíveis com lesões semelhantes em qualquer outro lugar.

TRATAMENTO

CUIDADO(S) DE SAÚDE ADEQUADO(S)
- Conjuntivite primária — frequentemente em um esquema ambulatorial.
- Conjuntivite secundária a outras doenças (p. ex., uveíte e ceratite ulcerativa) — pode necessitar de internação, enquanto se diagnostica e se trata o problema subjacente.

ATIVIDADE
- Conjuntivite primária — não há nenhuma restrição para grande parte dos pacientes.
- Suspeita de contato com irritantes ou doença alérgica aguda — evitar (se possível) o contato com o agente agressor.
- Suspeita de FHV — recomenda-se a minimização do estresse.
- Não expor os pacientes a animais suscetíveis.

DIETA
Suspeita de dermatopatia e/ou alergia alimentar subjacentes — é recomendável o fornecimento de dieta de eliminação (hipoalergênica).

ORIENTAÇÃO AO PROPRIETÁRIO
- Caso se observe uma secreção ocular abundante, orientar o proprietário a limpar os olhos antes de administrar o tratamento.
- Na prescrição tanto de soluções como de pomadas, ensinar o proprietário a utilizar a(s) solução(ões) antes da(s) pomada(s).

CONJUNTIVITE — GATOS

• Se muitas soluções forem prescritas, instruir o proprietário a esperar alguns minutos entre os tratamentos.
• Instruir o proprietário a buscar esclarecimentos se a condição piorar, o que pode indicar afecção irresponsiva, provável evolução do quadro ou ainda possível reação adversa ao medicamento prescrito.

CONSIDERAÇÕES CIRÚRGICAS
• Obstrução do ducto nasolacrimal — procedimento trabalhoso; tratamento frequentemente não recomendado (ver "Epífora").
• Neoplasia conjuntival — pode exigir apenas a ressecção local; pode envolver a técnica de excisão, acompanhada por irradiação com raios beta, crioterapia, hipertermia por radiofrequência, enucleação ou exenteração, dependendo do tipo de tumor e do grau de envolvimento.
• Simbléfaro — pode necessitar de ressecção cirúrgica assim que a infecção conjuntival ativa estiver controlada.
• Sequestro corneano — o procedimento de ceratectomia pode ser imprescindível.

MEDICAÇÕES

MEDICAMENTO(S) DE ESCOLHA

Herpética
• A condição costuma ser leve e autolimitante.
• Tratamento antiviral — indicado em casos de ceratite herpética antes de se efetuar a ceratectomia para sequestros corneanos supostamente relacionados com o FHV e para conjuntivite intratável grave; a penetração de medicamentos na conjuntiva (em comparação à córnea) não é satisfatória; portanto, a terapia é opcional; o tratamento pode ser direcionado apenas ao controle da infecção bacteriana secundária.
• Solução de idoxuridina a 0,1% (disponível em farmácias de manipulação) — tópica a cada 6 h em princípio.
• Pomada de vidarabina a 3% — também por via tópica a cada 6 h inicialmente.
• Trifluridina — recomendada de hora em hora no primeiro dia, depois 5 vezes ao dia.
• Lisina — 250-500 mg VO a cada 12 h para gatos adultos (a eficácia é controversa).
• Recentemente, descobriu-se que o fanciclovir por via oral seja eficaz e seguro para utilização em gatos, embora não seja aprovado para uso nessa espécie. A dosagem é controversa — mais comumente utilizado em uma dose de 1/4 do comprimido de 125 mg VO a cada 12 h por 10 dias; no entanto, esse medicamento é frequentemente utilizado sem complicação em doses mais altas e por períodos prolongados.

Clamidial ou Micoplasmal
• Pomada oftálmica de tetraciclina (Terramicina®) — tópica a cada 6 h; continuar por alguns dias após a resolução de todos os sinais clínicos; a recidiva ou a reinfecção são comuns; alguns autores recomendam o tratamento sistêmico em casos difíceis.
• Soluções oftalmológicas tópicas de cloranfenicol ou ciprofloxacino a cada 6-8 h são alternativas ao uso de pomada oftalmológica tópica de oxitetraciclina.
• Azitromicina — 5 mg/kg VO a cada 72 h por 3 semanas.

Bacteriana
• Escolha feita com base nos resultados da cultura bacteriana e do antibiograma.

Neonatal
• Abrir as margens palpebrais com cuidado (no sentido medial a temporal), instituir drenagem e tratar com antibióticos e antivirais (na suspeita de FHV) tópicos.
• Simbléfaro (aderências entre as superfícies conjuntivais e, possivelmente, a córnea) — sequela comum; talvez haja necessidade de intervenção cirúrgica.

Eosinofílica
• Corticosteroides tópicos — tratamento habitual; a dexametasona a 0,1% é geralmente eficaz quando utilizada três ou quatro vezes ao dia; reduzir a dose gradativamente para a dose mais baixa, mas eficiente.
• Acetato de megestrol por via oral — pode ajudar em condições resistentes; considerar os possíveis efeitos colaterais sistêmicos.
• Ciclosporina — um relato recente revelou que a solução tópica desse medicamento a 1,5% seja segura e eficaz.

CONTRAINDICAÇÕES
Corticosteroides tópicos — evitar em casos de conjuntivite herpética conhecida ou sob suspeita; as evidências revelam que esses agentes predispõem o paciente à formação de sequestro corneano; evitar caso se observe ulceração corneana.

PRECAUÇÕES
• Os aminoglicosídeos e os antivirais tópicos podem ser irritantes.
• Monitorizar todos os pacientes tratados com corticosteroides tópicos quanto ao aparecimento de sinais de ulceração corneana; interromper o agente imediatamente se ocorrer esse tipo de ulceração.

INTERAÇÕES POSSÍVEIS
N/D.

MEDICAMENTO(S) ALTERNATIVO(S)
Outros corticosteroides — acetato de prednisolona a 1%; betametasona; hidrocortisona.

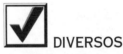

ACOMPANHAMENTO

MONITORIZAÇÃO DO PACIENTE
Reavaliar o paciente logo após a instituição do tratamento (em 5-7 dias); em seguida, repetir a avaliação conforme a necessidade.

PREVENÇÃO
• Tratar qualquer doença subjacente que possa estar exacerbando a doença ocular — dermatopatia alérgica ou imunomediada; ceratoconjuntivite seca.
• Evitar a reexposição à fonte de infecção.
• Minimizar o estresse em pacientes com conjuntivite herpética.
• Isolar os pacientes com conjuntivite infecciosa para impedir a disseminação.
• Vacinação contra causas virais — recomendada; a infecção ainda será possível se o gato for exposto ao agente infeccioso antes de ser vacinado (p. ex., herpes-virose felina proveniente de alguma gata infectada).

COMPLICAÇÕES POSSÍVEIS
• Sequestro corneano.
• Simbléfaro.
• Ceratoconjuntivite seca.

EVOLUÇÃO ESPERADA E PROGNÓSTICO
• FHV — a maioria dos pacientes torna-se portadora crônica; os episódios mostram-se menos comuns à medida que o paciente amadurece; podem-se observar exacerbações repetidas; tende-se a observar sinais clínicos mais graves nos momentos de estresse ou imunocomprometimento.
• Conjuntivite bacteriana — costuma desaparecer com a administração apropriada de antibióticos; caso se descubra alguma doença subjacente (p. ex., ceratoconjuntivite seca), a resolução poderá depender do fornecimento de tratamento adequado e da solução do processo patológico.
• Doenças imunomediadas (p. ex., eosinofílicas) — controle sem cura; podem exigir o tratamento crônico no nível mais baixo possível.

DIVERSOS

DISTÚRBIOS ASSOCIADOS
FeLV e FIV — podem predispor o paciente ao estado de portador crônico da conjuntivite por FHV.

FATORES RELACIONADOS COM A IDADE
FHV — tende a ser mais grave em filhotes felinos e gatos idosos com declínio da imunidade.

POTENCIAL ZOONÓTICO
Chlamydia psittaci — baixo.

GESTAÇÃO/FERTILIDADE/REPRODUÇÃO
• Se forem empregados, usar os antibióticos e os corticosteroides sistêmicos com cautela em fêmeas prenhes.
• É imprescindível considerar a possibilidade de absorção de medicamentos tópicos e ponderar os benefícios terapêuticos em contraste com as possíveis complicações.

VER TAMBÉM
Ceratoconjuntivite Seca.

ABREVIATURA(S)
• FeLV = vírus da leucemia felina.
• FHV = herpes-vírus felino.
• FIV = vírus da imunodeficiência felina.
• IFA = anticorpo imunofluorescente.
• PCR = reação em cadeia da polimerase.

Sugestões de Leitura
Maggs DJ, Miller PE, Ofri R. Slatter's Fundamentals of Veterinary Ophthalmology, 4th ed. St. Louis: Saunders, 2008, pp. 135-150.

Autor Erin S. Champagne
Consultor Editorial Paul E. Miller

Constipação e Obstipação

CONSIDERAÇÕES GERAIS

DEFINIÇÃO
• Constipação — defecação infrequente, incompleta ou dificultosa, com a eliminação de fezes duras ou secas.
• Obstipação — constipação intratável, causada por retenção prolongada de fezes duras e secas; a defecação é impossível no paciente obstipado.

FISIOPATOLOGIA
• A constipação pode se desenvolver em qualquer doença que prejudique a passagem de fezes através do cólon.
• O atraso no trânsito fecal permite a remoção de quantidades adicionais de sal e água, produzindo fezes mais ressecadas.
• As contrações peristálticas podem aumentar durante a constipação, mas a motilidade acaba diminuindo em virtude da degeneração muscular lisa secundária à distensão crônica excessiva.

SISTEMA(S) ACOMETIDO(S)
Gastrintestinal.

GENÉTICA
N/D.

INCIDÊNCIA/PREVALÊNCIA
Problema clínico comum.

DISTRIBUIÇÃO GEOGRÁFICA
N/D.

IDENTIFICAÇÃO
Espécies
• Cães e gatos.
• Mais comum em gatos.

Raça(s) Predominante(s)
N/D.

Idade Média e Faixa Etária
N/D.

Sexo Predominante
N/D.

SINAIS CLÍNICOS
Achados Anamnésicos
• Esforço para defecar com pouco ou nenhum volume fecal.
• Fezes duras e secas.
• Defecação infrequente.
• Quantidade pequena de fezes líquidas e mucoides — algumas vezes com a presença de sangue produzido após tenesmo prolongado.
• Vômitos ocasionais, inapetência e/ou depressão.

Achados do Exame Físico
• Cólon preenchido por fezes duras.
• Outros achados dependem da causa.
• O exame retal pode revelar massa, estenose, hérnia perineal, doença dos sacos anais, corpo ou material estranho, aumento de volume prostático ou estreitamento do canal pélvico.

CAUSAS
Alimentares
• Ossos.
• Pelos.
• Material estranho.
• Quantidade excessiva de fibras.
• Consumo inadequado de água.

Ambientais
• Falta de atividade física.
• Mudança de ambiente — internação, bandeja sanitária suja.
• Incapacidade de deambulação.

Medicamentosas
• Anticolinérgicos.
• Anti-histamínicos.
• Opioides.
• Sulfato de bário.
• Sucralfato.
• Antiácidos.
• Caopectina.
• Suplementos de ferro.
• Diuréticos.

Defecação Dolorosa
• Doença anorretal — saculite anal, abscesso do saco anal, fístula perianal, estenose anal, espasmo anal, corpo estranho retal, prolapso retal, proctite.
• Traumatismo — fratura da pelve, fratura de membros, deslocamento do coxal, ferida ou laceração perianais por mordedura, abscesso perineal.

Obstrução Mecânica
• Extraluminal — consolidação de fratura da pelve com estreitamento do canal pélvico, hipertrofia prostática, prostatite, neoplasia prostática, neoplasia intrapélvica, linfadenopatia sublombar.
• Intraluminal e intramural — neoplasia ou pólipo colônicos ou retais, estenose retal, corpo estranho retal, divertículo retal, hérnia perineal, prolapso retal e defeito congênito (atresia anal).

Doença Neuromuscular
• Sistema nervoso central — paraplegia, mielopatia, discopatia intervertebral, encefalopatia (intoxicação pelo chumbo, raiva).
• Sistema nervoso periférico — disautonomia, neuropatia sacral, traumatismo de nervos sacrais (p. ex., lesão por fratura ou tração da cauda).
• Disfunção da musculatura lisa colônica — megacólon idiopático nos gatos.

Doença Metabólica e Endócrina
• Comprometimento à função da musculatura lisa colônica — hiperparatireoidismo, hipotireoidismo, hipocalemia (insuficiência renal crônica), hipercalcemia.
• Debilidade — fraqueza muscular generalizada, desidratação, neoplasia.

FATORES DE RISCO
• Terapia medicamentosa — anticolinérgicos, narcóticos, sulfato de bário.
• Doença metabólica como causa de desidratação.
• Macho intacto — hérnia perineal, prostatopatia.
• Fístula perianal.
• Pica — material estranho.
• Auto-higienização excessiva — ingestão de pelos.
• Diminuição ou incapacidade de se auto-higienizar — gatos de pelo longo, pseudocoprostase.
• Fratura pélvica.

DIAGNÓSTICO

DIAGNÓSTICO DIFERENCIAL
• Disquezia e tenesmo (p. ex., causados por colite) — diferentemente da constipação, associam-se com frequência elevada de tentativas de defecar e produção frequente de quantidades pequenas de fezes líquidas, contendo sangue e/ou muco; o exame retal revela a presença de diarreia e a ausência de fezes duras.
• Estrangúria (p. ex., causada por cistite/uretrite) — ao contrário da constipação, pode associar-se com hematúria e achados anormais na urinálise (piúria, cristalúria, bacteriúria).

HEMOGRAMA/BIOQUÍMICA/URINÁLISE
• Em geral, permanecem normais.
• Podem detectar hipocalemia, hipercalcemia.
• Aumento do volume globular (hematócrito) e das proteínas totais em pacientes desidratados.
• Elevação no número de leucócitos em pacientes com abscesso, fístula perianal, prostatopatia.
• Piúria e hematúria em casos de prostatite.

OUTROS TESTES LABORATORIAIS
• Se o paciente (cão) estiver hipercolesterolêmico, considerar a avaliação da função da tireoide para descartar o hipotireoidismo.
• Se o paciente estiver hipercalcêmico, considerar a análise do paratormônio.

DIAGNÓSTICO POR IMAGEM
• As radiografias abdominais registram a gravidade da impactação colônica. Outros achados podem incluir corpos estranhos colônicos ou retais, massas colônicas ou retais, aumentos de volume prostático, fraturas da pelve, deslocamentos do coxal ou hérnias perineais.
• Enema baritado para geração de pneumocólon (após a limpeza do cólon com enemas) pode definir ainda mais massas ou estenoses intraluminais.
• A ultrassonografia pode ajudar a delimitar massa extraluminal e prostatopatia.

MÉTODOS DIAGNÓSTICOS
A colonoscopia pode ser necessária para identificar massas, estenoses ou outras lesões colônicas ou retais; sempre devem ser obtidas amostras por biopsia.

TRATAMENTO

CUIDADO(S) DE SAÚDE ADEQUADO(S)
• Remover ou amenizar qualquer causa subjacente, se possível.
• Interromper qualquer medicamento capaz de causar constipação.
• Na presença de obstipação e/ou desidratação, pode haver a necessidade de internação.

CUIDADO(S) DE ENFERMAGEM
Os pacientes desidratados devem ser submetidos à fluidoterapia com soluções eletrolíticas balanceadas por vias SC ou, de preferência, IV (com a suplementação de potássio se indicada).

ATIVIDADE
Estimular a atividade física.

DIETA
A suplementação da dieta com agentes formadores de volume (farelo de cereais, metilcelulose, abóbora enlatada, psílio) é frequentemente útil, embora eles possam algumas vezes agravar a distensão fecal colônica; nesse caso, fornecer dieta que produza pouca quantidade de resíduos.

ORIENTAÇÃO AO PROPRIETÁRIO
Oferecer a dieta apropriada e estimular a atividade física.

CONSIDERAÇÕES CIRÚRGICAS
• Se os enemas e os medicamentos não tiverem êxito, pode ser necessária a remoção manual das

fezes com o animal sob anestesia geral (após reidratação).
• Pode ser imprescindível a colectomia subtotal em casos de obstipação recidivante, que responde de forma insatisfatória à terapia clínica rigorosa.

MEDICAÇÕES

MEDICAMENTO(S) DE ESCOLHA
• Laxantes emolientes — docusato de sódio ou docusato de cálcio (cães, 50-100 mg VO a cada 12-24 h; gatos, 50 mg VO a cada 12-24 h).
• Laxantes estimulantes — bisacodil (5 mg/animal VO a cada 8-24 h).
• Laxantes salinos — mistura isosmótica de polietilenoglicol e sais pouco absorvíveis; costumam ser administrados sob a forma de gotejamento via tubo nasesofágico durante 6-12 horas.
• Laxantes dissacarídeos — lactulose (1 mL/4,5 kg VO a cada 8-12 h, até fazer efeito).
• Talvez haja necessidade de enemas de água morna; pode-se adicionar uma pequena quantidade de sabão neutro ou docusato sódico, mas em geral isso não é necessário; os enemas de retenção de fosfato de sódio (p. ex., Fleet Enema®, C.B. Fleet Co., Inc.) são contraindicados em virtude de sua associação com hipocalcemia grave.
• No lugar dos enemas, pode-se lançar mão dos supositórios; utilizar produtos à base de glicerol, bisacodil ou docusato sódico.
• Pode-se tentar o uso de modificadores da motilidade — a cisaprida (cães, 0,1-0,5 mg/kg VO a cada 8-12 h; gatos, 2,5-10 mg/gato VO a cada 8-12 h) pode estimular a motilidade; indicados no início de megacólon.

CONTRAINDICAÇÕES
• Lubrificantes (como o óleo mineral e a vaselina branca) NÃO são recomendados em função do risco de pneumonia por aspiração lipoide fatal decorrente da falta de paladar.
• Fleet enemas.
• Anticolinérgicos.
• Diuréticos.

PRECAUÇÕES
Metoclopramida, cisaprida e colinérgicos — podem ser utilizados com cautela; contraindicados em processos obstrutivos.

INTERAÇÕES POSSÍVEIS
N/D.

MEDICAMENTO(S) ALTERNATIVO(S)
• A ranitidina provoca contração da musculatura lisa colônica *in vitro*.
• Medicamentos de gerações mais recentes, semelhantes à cisaprida, poderão estar disponíveis em breve.

ACOMPANHAMENTO

MONITORIZAÇÃO DO PACIENTE
Monitorizar a frequência da defecação e a consistência das fezes pelo menos duas vezes por semana no início, depois em intervalos semanais ou quinzenais.

PREVENÇÃO
Manter o animal de estimação ativo e oferecer uma dieta apropriada.

COMPLICAÇÕES POSSÍVEIS
• A constipação crônica ou a obstipação recidivante podem levar ao megacólon adquirido.
• O uso abusivo de laxantes e de enemas pode causar diarreia.
• A mucosa colônica pode ser lesionada por técnica inapropriada de aplicação do enema, fragmentação mecânica frequente e rude das fezes ou necrose isquêmica secundária à compressão de fezes duras.

• A irritação e a ulceração perineais podem induzir à incontinência fecal.

EVOLUÇÃO ESPERADA E PROGNÓSTICO
Variam com a causa subjacente.

DIVERSOS

DISTÚRBIOS ASSOCIADOS
Vômito — em casos de obstipação grave/prolongada.

FATORES RELACIONADOS COM A IDADE
N/D.

POTENCIAL ZOONÓTICO
N/D.

GESTAÇÃO/FERTILIDADE/REPRODUÇÃO
N/D.

SINÔNIMO(S)
• Impactação colônica.
• Impactação fecal.

VER TAMBÉM
Megacólon.

Sugestões de Leitura
Washabau RJ, Holt D. Diagnosis and management of feline idiopathic megacolon. Vet Clin North Am 1999, 29:589-603.
Washabau RJ, Holt D. Diseases of the large intestine. In: Ettinger SJ, Feldman EC, eds., Textbook of Veterinary Internal Medicine, 6th ed. St. Louis: Elsevier, 2005, pp. 1378-1408.

Autores Albert E. Jergens
Consultor Editorial Albert E. Jergens

Contusões Pulmonares

CONSIDERAÇÕES GERAIS

REVISÃO
• Hemorragia no parênquima pulmonar provocada por laceração e esmagamento durante traumatismo direto ao tórax.
• Volumes relativamente pequenos de sangue nos pulmões podem comprometer acentuadamente a função pulmonar.
• Nos pacientes que sofrem contusões pulmonares, a ressuscitação com fluidoterapia para o tratamento de choque pode exacerbar a disfunção pulmonar pela produção de edema.

IDENTIFICAÇÃO
• Cães e gatos. • Sem predileção por raça específica, idade ou sexo.

SINAIS CLÍNICOS
• Achados anamnésicos compatíveis com traumatismo rombo. • Taquipneia. • Esforço respiratório anormal. • Adaptações posturais à angústia respiratória. • Mucosas cianóticas ou pálidas. • Auscultação de ruídos broncovesiculares ásperos ou crepitações. • Expectoração de sangue ou de líquido manchado de sangue.

CAUSAS E FATORES DE RISCO
• Traumatismo rombo.
• Acidentes com veículos motorizados.
• Quedas de locais altos.
• Maltratos — espancamento.

DIAGNÓSTICO

DIAGNÓSTICO DIFERENCIAL
• Hemotórax — pode provocar ruídos pulmonares maciços (efusão pleural nas radiografias torácicas).
• Pneumotórax — pode gerar ruídos pulmonares maciços (ar pleural nas radiografias torácicas).
• Hérnia diafragmática — diferenciada ao exame radiográfico.
• Coagulopatia — pode causar hemorragia pulmonar; identificada por anormalidade nos testes de coagulação ou na contagem das plaquetas.
• Início agudo de hemorragia pulmonar — pode ser característica de algumas neoplasias (p. ex., hemangiossarcoma); ocasionalmente atribuído a infarto pulmonar associado à endocardite bacteriana ou dirofilariose.
• Pode ocorrer expectoração de líquido sanguinolento (não hemorragia franca) em animais com SARA ou insuficiência cardíaca congestiva.

HEMOGRAMA/BIOQUÍMICA/URINÁLISE
• Hemograma completo — pode revelar anemia ou neutrofilia madura.
• Perfil bioquímico sérico — pode demonstrar hipoproteinemia, indicando perda sanguínea; pode revelar lesão a outros sistemas orgânicos.
• Urinálise — geralmente normal.

DIAGNÓSTICO POR IMAGEM
Radiografias Torácicas
• Costumam revelar um padrão alveolar irregular, frequentemente focal ou assimétrico, embora possa ser generalizado.
• Na presença de fraturas concomitantes de costela, as contusões podem ser mais graves na área das fraturas.
• Sempre é recomendável a obtenção de radiografias torácicas em pacientes traumatizados após a estabilização para descartar hemotórax, pneumotórax e hérnia diafragmática.

MÉTODOS DIAGNÓSTICOS
• Testes de coagulação para coagulopatia ou CID.
• Oximetria de pulso ou gasometria sanguínea arterial — pode confirmar a hipoxemia.
• Exame citológico do lavado transtraqueal — pode demonstrar uma quantidade excessiva de eritrócitos e macrófagos; submeter à cultura para monitorizar o desenvolvimento de infecção bacteriana sobreposta.

TRATAMENTO
• O paciente costuma ser internado para estabilização.
• Manter a função respiratória e estabilizar a função cardiovascular.
• Avaliar e tratar as lesões a outros sistemas orgânicos.
• Restringir a atividade, minimizar o estresse e monitorizar cuidadosamente quanto à deterioração da função respiratória durante as primeiras 24 h.
• Suporte respiratório — suplementação de oxigênio para hipoxemia; entubação e ventilação com pressão positiva nos pacientes gravemente acometidos.
• Choque — talvez haja necessidade de fluidoterapia; se possível, manter-se conservador com a administração de fluidos, pois isso pode criar ou exacerbar o edema pulmonar; para minimizar o desenvolvimento do edema, considerar o uso de coloides sintéticos nos animais com hipoproteinemia.
• Transfusão de sangue ou plasma — considerar se a hemorragia tiver resultado em anemia ou em pacientes com coagulopatia.
• Suporte nutricional — para manter a condição corporal e o estado imunológico em caso de necessidade.

MEDICAÇÕES

MEDICAMENTO(S)
• Suplementação de oxigênio com o uso de tubos/cânulas nasais, gaiola ou tenda em animais com dispneia ou hipoxia.
• Diuréticos em doses baixas — furosemida (0,5-2 mg/kg IV, IM); utilizados apenas quando a hemorragia for acompanhada por edema e em caso de grave angústia respiratória. A diurese excessiva pode exacerbar o choque.

CONTRAINDICAÇÕES/INTERAÇÕES POSSÍVEIS
Diuréticos — sem valor nos estágios iniciais das contusões pulmonares e podem até ser nocivos; diminuem o volume intravascular, o que é contraindicado no choque.

ACOMPANHAMENTO

MONITORIZAÇÃO DO PACIENTE
• Monitorizar a frequência e o esforço respiratórios, a coloração das mucosas, a frequência cardíaca e a qualidade do pulso, bem como os ruídos pulmonares.
• Medir o hematócrito e os sólidos totais de forma seriada e efetuar a oximetria de pulso e/ou a gasometria sanguínea arterial, conforme a necessidade, nas primeiras 24 h.
• Monitorizar o ECG frequentemente para detectar arritmias ventriculares associadas a hipoxemia ou miocardite.
• Radiografias — repetidas em 48-72 h para garantir a resolução das contusões.

PREVENÇÃO
Restrição adequada do animal para evitar exposição a traumatismos.

COMPLICAÇÕES POSSÍVEIS
• Pneumonia bacteriana (incomum) — atribuída à imunossupressão sistêmica por traumatismo, choque e defesas pulmonares reduzidas.
• Desenvolvimento de tosse produtiva úmida e ausência de melhora dentro de 48 h — suspeitar de pneumonia.
• Pacientes com choque grave podem desenvolver SARA (menos comum).

EVOLUÇÃO ESPERADA E PROGNÓSTICO
• A função respiratória pode deteriorar nas primeiras 12-24 h após o traumatismo e, em seguida, deve melhorar de forma gradual.
• Uma melhora clínica acentuada no estado respiratório ocorre, em geral, dentro de 48 h, com resolução mais gradativa das lesões radiográficas.
• Se o paciente não melhorar depois de 48 h, avaliar quanto à ocorrência de complicações ou doença concomitante.

DIVERSOS

DISTÚRBIOS ASSOCIADOS
• Pneumotórax. • Fraturas de costelas. • Tórax flácido. • Ruptura da traqueia, dos brônquios ou do esôfago. • Arritmias cardíacas — ventriculares.
• Outras complicações possíveis do traumatismo.

VER TAMBÉM
Pneumotórax.

ABREVIATURA(S)
• CID = coagulação intravascular disseminada.
• ECG = eletrocardiograma.
• SARA = síndrome da angústia respiratória aguda.

Sugestões de Leitura
Campbell VL, King LG. Pulmonary function, ventilator management and outcome of dogs with thoracic trauma and pulmonary contusions: 10 cases (1994-1998). JAVMA 2000, 217:1505-1509.
Powell LL, Rozanski EA, Tidwell AS, Rush JE. A retrospective analysis of pulmonary contusion secondary to motor vehicular accidents in 143 dogs: 1994-1997. J Vet Emerg Crit Care 1999, 9:127-136.
Vnuk D, Pirkic B, Maticic D, Radisic B, Stejskal M, Babic T, Kreszinger M, Lemo N. Feline high-rise syndrome: 119 cases (1998-2001). J Feline Med Surg 2004, 6:5, 305-312.

Autor Lesley G. King
Consultor Editorial Lynelle R. Johnson

CONSIDERAÇÕES GERAIS

DEFINIÇÃO
Pica consiste em um comportamento anormal de ingestão em que se consomem itens não alimentícios. A coprofagia (consumo de fezes) é uma forma de pica.

FISIOPATOLOGIA
• Atualmente, a fisiopatologia da pica é desconhecida. • A coprofagia não é necessariamente um distúrbio patológico. • Qualquer problema clínico que leva a deficiências nutricionais, desequilíbrios eletrolíticos, distúrbios gastrintestinais, polifagia ou transtornos do SNC pode induzir à pica e/ou coprofagia. • Dietas intensamente restritas em termos de calorias ou desbalanceadas indutoras de deficiências podem levar à pica e/ou coprofagia.

SISTEMA(S) ACOMETIDO(S)
Gastrintestinal — obstrução por corpo estranho ou desarranjo GI com consequente vômito e diarreia. Em casos de coprofagia, há chances elevadas de parasitismo GI.

GENÉTICA
Não há nenhuma base genética conhecida.

INCIDÊNCIA/PREVALÊNCIA
Desconhecidas.

IDENTIFICAÇÃO
Espécies
A coprofagia é comum em cães, mas rara em gatos. Entretanto, a pica é observada tanto em cães como em gatos.

Raça(s) Predominante(s)
Raças orientais de gato, como Siamês, podem exibir maior risco de pica.

Idade Média e Faixa Etária
A pica ocorre com maior frequência em filhotes caninos que em cães adultos. Em gatos, é mais provável que a pica comece durante o primeiro ano de vida.

SINAIS CLÍNICOS
Achados Anamnésicos
• Em cães, ingestão de itens não alimentícios inadequados, como pedras, roupas e/ou fezes. • Em gatos, ingestão de tecidos, plásticos ou outros itens não alimentícios inadequados.

Achados do Exame Físico
• Halitose em caso de coprofagia como o problema apresentado. • Traumatismo dentário se o alvo de consumo do cão for objetos duros. • Palidez ou fraqueza na presença de anemia como um fator que contribui para o quadro. • Condição corporal deficiente se os sinais clínicos forem acompanhados por má digestão ou má absorção. • Sinais neurológicos se o comportamento for causado por doença neurológica.

CAUSAS
Causas Comportamentais
• A coprofagia é considerada como um comportamento materno normal. A cadela ou a gata lambe a região anogenital do neonato para estimular a evacuação e, depois, consome os excrementos. • A coprofagia pode ser considerada como um comportamento exploratório normal em filhotes caninos. Foi postulado que os altos níveis de ácido deoxicólico nas fezes podem contribuir

para o desenvolvimento neurológico. • É normal que os cães procurem pelas fezes de gatos, pois elas são ricas em proteínas e, portanto, atrativas. • As fezes de ungulados também são atrativas para os cães, aparentemente em função da matéria vegetal parcialmente digerida. • Os cães submetidos a dietas altamente restritas podem ter um apetite voraz, levando aos comportamentos de coprofagia e pica. • Como as fezes são apetitosas para os cães, o comportamento é autorrecompensador. • Os cães que foram punidos por evacuar em casa podem aprender a comer suas próprias fezes em uma aparente tentativa de evitar a punição. • Os cães também podem comer suas próprias fezes como uma forma de "limpeza do ninho". • A coprofagia pode ocorrer como uma forma de comportamento de busca por atenção se o cão aprender que o comportamento seguramente leva à atenção imediata do proprietário. • A coprofagia também pode se desenvolver como uma resposta à ansiedade. • Os comportamentos de coprofagia e pica podem ser um transtorno compulsivo (ver "Transtornos Compulsivos — Gatos" e "Transtornos Compulsivos — Cães"). • A pica pode ocorrer secundariamente a um comportamento de roubo quando o cão está altamente motivado a impedir que o proprietário recupere o objeto roubado. • A pica pode se desenvolver como um resultado de ansiedade que leva à destruição e, então, ao consumo de um item não alimentício.

Causas Clínicas
• Anemia. • Desnutrição com consequente polifagia. • Endocrinopatias — hipertireoidismo, diabetes melito, hiperadrenocorticismo. • Má digestão/má absorção (p. ex., insuficiência pancreática exócrina). • Enteropatia inflamatória. • Proliferação bacteriana no intestino delgado. • Doença do SNC. • Desvio portossistêmico. • Parasitismo intestinal.

Causas Induzidas por Medicamentos
Administração de medicamentos como corticosteroides, progestinas ou benzodiazepínicos, pode levar à polifagia.

FATORES DE RISCO
• Foi postulado que o desmame precoce de filhotes felinos leva à sucção e ingestão de tecidos. • Gatos alimentados com dietas pobres em fibras e/ou impedidos de terem acesso a fontes de fibras, como gramas. • Os cães privados de um ambiente com estímulos adequados, níveis apropriados de atividade ou interações sociais podem estar sob risco de pica e/ou coprofagia. • Períodos longos de confinamento, especialmente em um ambiente árido e/ou estéril, podem predispor à coprofagia.

DIAGNÓSTICO

DIAGNÓSTICO DIFERENCIAL
• O diagnóstico baseia-se na anamnese obtida a partir dos proprietários e na descrição do comportamento por eles. • Um histórico comportamental completo e detalhado deve incluir: ○ Descrição do problema — quando e onde ele aparece. ○ Idade de início. ○ A reação habitual do proprietário e qualquer correção tentada até o momento, bem como seus resultados. ○ Mudanças e/ou alterações na casa, horários, dieta ou saúde, associadas ao desenvolvimento do problema. ○ Rotina de

alimentação dos animais de estimação — quando, onde e por quem são alimentados. ○ Presença de qualquer outro comportamento oral incomum. ○ Outros problemas comportamentais presentes. ○ Nível de adestramento doméstico — quando e onde o animal de estimação evacua. ○ Como o animal foi adestrado em casa. ○ Relacionamento com outros animais de estimação, se presentes. ○ Ambiente, incluindo os programas diários de atividades lúdicas (brincadeiras), exercícios, atenção ou adestramento. • O problema clínico deve ser avaliado, incluindo apetite e peso, quaisquer sinais de náusea ou desarranjo GI, como lambedura excessiva dos lábios ou de superfície, bem como cor e consistência das fezes. • A pica real/verdadeira também deve ser diferenciada de mastigação destrutiva, em que os itens podem ser despedaçados, mas não consumidos. • Também é imprescindível diferenciar a pica real/verdadeira daqueles casos em que um animal consome um item não alimentício, porque esse item havia tocado previamente em algum alimento e, portanto, tem cheiro e/ou gosto de comida.

HEMOGRAMA/BIOQUÍMICA/URINÁLISE
• Os resultados podem sugerir diabetes melito, hiperadrenocorticismo, hipertireoidismo ou polifagia induzida por medicamentos. • Anemia ou hipoproteinemia. • Os resultados também podem ser sugestivos da presença de desvio portossistêmico — microcitose, células-alvo, hipoalbuminemia, níveis baixos de ureia, cristalúria por biurato de amônio. • Em caso de parasitismo gastrintestinal ou enteropatia inflamatória eosinofílica, pode ocorrer eosinofilia periférica.

OUTROS TESTES LABORATORIAIS
• Imunorreatividade semelhante à da tripsina — pode estar baixa caso haja insuficiência pancreática exócrina. • Níveis séricos de cobalamina e folato para estimar a proliferação bacteriana no intestino delgado e avaliar o comprometimento da mucosa desse segmento intestinal. • Teste de tripsina e gordura fecais pode ajudar a avaliar a presença de insuficiência pancreática exócrina e outros problemas relacionados com má absorção ou má digestão. • Perfil da função tireoide para determinar se o animal sofre de hipertireoidismo. • Exames coprológicos para fazer a triagem em busca de parasitas intestinais. • Mensuração dos ácidos biliares para avaliar a existência de desvio portossistêmico. • Teste de estimulação com ACTH para verificar o quadro de hiperadrenocorticismo.

DIAGNÓSTICO POR IMAGEM
Os exames de radiografias abdominais simples e/ou ultrassonografia abdominal podem ser necessários para descartar obstrução por corpo estranho. Também podem revelar a presença de micro-hepatia se houver algum desvio portossistêmico.

MÉTODOS DIAGNÓSTICOS
Talvez haja necessidade da obtenção de amostras do intestino delgado por biopsia para avaliar a presença de enteropatia infiltrativa. As culturas do intestino delgado servem para estimar a proliferação bacteriana nesse segmento intestinal.

COPROFAGIA E PICA

TRATAMENTO

CUIDADO(S) DE SAÚDE ADEQUADO(S)

Tratamento da Pica
• Impedir o acesso a itens não alimentícios que provavelmente podem ser alvos de pica. ○ Confinar o animal em locais distantes de itens não alimentícios tidos como alvo. ○ Colocar focinheira nos cães; ficar atento ao aquecimento excessivo em climas quentes e quando utilizá-la por períodos de tempo prolongado. ○ Cogitar o uso de armadilhas escondidas para manter o animal de estimação distante de certas áreas e itens. • Proceder à mudança alimentar para uma dieta com maior teor de fibras. • Fornecer brinquedos comestíveis e oportunidades aceitáveis de acesso à forragem (p. ex., plantas verdes como gramínea ou *catnip** para gatos). • Ensinar aos cães os comandos verbais "*Drop it*" ("Pare com isso") ou "*Leave it*" ("Largue isso"), para que o proprietário possa evitar o consumo de itens não alimentícios inadequados.

Tratamento da Coprofagia
• Evitar o acesso às fezes. ○ Passear com o cão na coleira e apanhar as fezes imediatamente. ○ Utilizar focinheira; tomar precauções para evitar o superaquecimento em climas mais quentes. ○ Usar coleira cervical a fim de aumentar a capacidade de guiar o animal de estimação para longe das fezes e recompensar "desviando do local" após a defecação. • Mudar a característica das fezes. ○ Fornecer ForBid*†, amaciadores de carne, etc., que podem tornar as fezes menos palatáveis. ○ Mudar a dieta para uma que produza fezes mais moles e menos formadas a fim de diminuir a atração por elas. • Utilizar uma coleira de citronela‡ ativada por controle remoto para distrair o animal toda vez que ele tentar farejar ou ingerir as fezes. ○ Esse método deve ser empregado toda vez que o animal tiver acesso às fezes para ser eficaz. ○ Os cães devem ser recompensados com algum petisco palatável (saboroso) por se voltarem ao proprietário sob voz de comando. • A aversão ao paladar pode ser ensinada, tratando-se as fezes com uma substância potencialmente aversiva (p. ex., molho picante, pimenta-de-caiena, etc.). ○ Todas as fezes com que o cão possa entrar em contato devem ser tratadas para que isso seja eficaz. ○ Os cães podem aprender a reconhecer o odor das fezes tratadas, evitá-lo e procurar por outras fezes não tratadas. ○ É mais provável que os medicamentos indutores de náusea imediata e desarranjo gástrico sejam eficientes (p. ex., cloreto de lítio, apomorfina).

ATIVIDADE
• Níveis elevados de atividade podem ajudar no tratamento e na prevenção de pica e coprofagia.
• Programas mais regulares e previsíveis de interação e exercício podem não só diminuir a ansiedade, mas também auxiliar no tratamento de pica e coprofagia.

DIETA
As mudanças na dieta podem ser úteis em alguns casos de coprofagia. O uso de dieta de alta digestibilidade ou a adição de suplementos enzimáticos à base de plantas tem tido êxito na redução da coprofagia em certos casos.

ORIENTAÇÃO AO PROPRIETÁRIO
• Os proprietários devem ser orientados sobre o fato de que a coprofagia é, na maioria dos casos, um comportamento canino normal e inofensivo a menos que o cão consuma fezes com parasitas. • É recomendável que os proprietários sejam alertados a evitar o uso de qualquer forma de punição direta ou confronto para os comportamentos de pica ou coprofagia em função do risco de aumento da ansiedade que, possivelmente, agrava o comportamento e/ou induz a outros problemas comportamentais.

MEDICAÇÕES

MEDICAMENTO(S) DE ESCOLHA
Caso se determine que o comportamento seja atribuído a algum transtorno compulsivo ou secundário à ansiedade, pode ser indicado o uso de agentes psicoativos. (Ver "Transtornos Compulsivos" em busca das medicações e dosagens sugeridas).

CONTRAINDICAÇÕES
Sempre que possível, deve-se evitar o uso de qualquer medicamento que possa contribuir para o sinal de polifagia.

PRECAUÇÕES
• Evitar o emprego de antidepressivos tricíclicos em animais com comportamento de agressividade, histórico de crises convulsivas, problemas cardíacos, glaucoma, ou retenção de fezes ou urina. • Os efeitos colaterais anticolinérgicos não são raros. • A clomipramina pode potencializar os efeitos colaterais de alguns depressores do SNC, como benzodiazepínicos, barbitúricos e anestésicos gerais.

INTERAÇÕES POSSÍVEIS
A clomipramina não deve ser administrada em conjunto com inibidores da MAO ou em até 2 semanas após a interrupção desses inibidores. Também não é recomendável a combinação de clomipramina com SSRI.

MEDICAMENTO(S) ALTERNATIVO(S)
SSRI, como a fluoxetina, em comportamentos atribuídos à ansiedade ou a algum transtorno compulsivo.

ACOMPANHAMENTO

MONITORIZAÇÃO DO PACIENTE
• Entrar em contato com o proprietário em 1-2 semanas para confirmar a obediência do animal e determinar a melhora do quadro.
• Na ausência de melhora ou em caso de melhora mínima, devem-se recomendar outros testes diagnósticos.

PREVENÇÃO
• Impedir o acesso a itens não alimentícios inadequados que provavelmente serão consumidos constitui a melhor forma de prevenção.
• A supervisão rigorosa durante o adestramento doméstico pode ajudar a evitar a exploração de fezes e o reforço da coprofagia pelos filhotes caninos.
• A administração de preventivos mensais contra dirofilariose também pode evitar os parasitas GI.

COMPLICAÇÕES POSSÍVEIS
Obstrução por corpo estranho representa a sequela mais comum de pica tanto em cães como em gatos.

EVOLUÇÃO ESPERADA E PROGNÓSTICO
• O prognóstico será reservado se: (1) o problema estiver presente por um longo período de tempo; (2) o proprietário não estiver disposto a fazer a supervisão rigorosa do cão durante a evacuação do animal.
• Se o proprietário estiver disposto a supervisionar o cão e obedecer às recomendações terapêuticas, o prognóstico melhora.

DIVERSOS

FATORES RELACIONADOS COM A IDADE
Problemas clínicos subjacentes primários devem ficar fortemente sob suspeita em casos de início de pica ou coprofagia na fase adulta ou geriátrica.

GESTAÇÃO/FERTILIDADE/REPRODUÇÃO
• O uso de antidepressivos tricíclicos deve ser evitado em fêmeas prenhes e lactantes.
• Os proprietários de gatos com o comportamento de sucção de lã devem ser advertidos sobre o fato de que esse comportamento parece ter uma predisposição racial; dessa forma, pode ser prudente evitar o acasalamento desse animal, além de uma atitude responsável.
• Se o comportamento supostamente for associado a algum transtorno compulsivo, o animal não deverá ser acasalado, pois os transtornos compulsivos parecem ter uma base hereditária.

SINÔNIMO(S)
• Apetite depravado.
• Sucção ou mastigação de lã em gatos.

VER TAMBÉM
• Transtornos Compulsivos — Cães.
• Transtornos Compulsivos — Gatos.

ABREVIATURA(S)
• ACTH = hormônio adrenocorticotrópico.
• GI = gastrintestinal.
• MAO = monoamina oxidase.
• SNC = sistema nervoso central.
• SSRI = inibidor seletivo de recaptação da serotonina.

Sugestões de Leitura
Horwitz DF, Neilson JC. Blackwell's Five-Minute Veterinary Consult Clinical Companion — Canine and Feline Behavior. Ames, IA: Blackwell, 2007, pp. 236-242 and 406-413.
Houpt KA. Domestic Animal Behavior, 4th ed. Ames, IA: Blackwell, 2005, pp. 321-334.
Landsberg G, Hunthausen W, Ackerman L. Handbook of Behavior Problems of the Dog and Cat, 2nd ed. Philadelphia: Elsevier Saunders, 2003, pp. 167-182.

Autor Valarie Vaughn Tynes
Consultor Editorial Debra F. Horwitz
Agradecimento Katherine A. Houpt

---

* N. T.: Também conhecido como "erva do gato", uma planta medicinal e aromática pertencente à família da hortelã.
† N. T.: Substância comercial amarga e picante.
‡ N. T.: Cuidado: a citronela é tóxica para gatos.

CORIORRETINITE

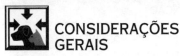

CONSIDERAÇÕES GERAIS

DEFINIÇÃO
- Inflamação da coroide e da retina.
- A coroide também é denominada úvea posterior.
- Uma inflamação difusa pode resultar no descolamento franco da retina (ver "Descolamento da Retina").

FISIOPATOLOGIA
- Causada por agentes infecciosos, células neoplásicas ou imunocomplexos (doenças imunomediadas); são mais comuns fatores patogênicos hematógenos que induzem à inflamação coroidal.
- Coroide e retina — estruturas intimamente justapostas; interdependentes do ponto de vista fisiológico; inflamação de uma delas costuma resultar na inflamação da outra.
- Também pode ocorrer como uma retinocoroidite — inflamação da retina prévia e indutora de inflamação coroidal.

SISTEMA(S) ACOMETIDO(S)
- Nervoso.
- Oftálmico.
- Outros sistemas em caso de doença subjacente sistêmica.

INCIDÊNCIA/PREVALÊNCIA
- Razoavelmente comum.
- Incidência exata desconhecida.

DISTRIBUIÇÃO GEOGRÁFICA
Depende da prevalência da causa infecciosa (p. ex., micoses sistêmicas, riquetsioses).

IDENTIFICAÇÃO
Espécies
Cães e gatos.

Raça(s) Predominante(s)
- Micoses sistêmicas — mais comuns em raças caninas de caça e de grande porte.
- Síndrome uveodermatológica — predisposição das raças Akita, Chow chow e Husky siberiano.
- Raças Borzoi, Border collie, Beagle: coriorretinopatia
- Cães da raça Montanhês de Berna: histiocitose sistêmica.

Idade Média e Faixa Etária
Dependem da causa subjacente.

Sexo Predominante
Síndrome uveodermatológica — mais comum em machos caninos jovens.

SINAIS CLÍNICOS
- Não costuma ser dolorosa, exceto quando houver o envolvimento da úvea anterior.
- Anormalidades vítreas — podem-se observar exsudatos, hemorragias ou sinéreses (liquefação).
- Interrupção ou alteração do trajeto dos vasos sanguíneos retinianos — em virtude da elevação da retina.
- Oftalmomiíase (gatos) — trajetos curvilíneos gerados pela migração das larvas.
- Outros — relacionados com a doença sistêmica subjacente.

Lesões
- Ativas — margens indistintas; hiporrefletividade tapetal; coloração cinza-esbranquiçada; alteração do trajeto dos vasos sanguíneos retinianos.
- Raras e diminutas — pode não se observar nenhum déficit visual aparente.
- Extensas, envolvendo áreas mais amplas da retina — cegueira ou diminuição da visão.
- Inativas (cicatrizes) — margens discretas; hiper-refletividade tapetal, algumas vezes com áreas centrais hiperpigmentadas; despigmentadas na região não tapetal e podem exibir certa hiperpigmentação circunjacente ou central.

CAUSAS
Cães
- Septicemia ou bacteremia — discospondilite; endocardite.
- Virais — cinomose; herpes-virose (rara, geralmente em neonatos); raiva.
- Bacterianas ou riquetsiais — septicemia ou bacteremia; leptospirose; brucelose; piometra (uveíte tóxica); *Borrelia*; erliquiose; febre maculosa das Montanhas Rochosas, bartonelose.
- Fúngicas — aspergilose; blastomicose; coccidioidomicose; histoplasmose; criptococose; acremoniose; um único relato de *Pseudallescheriasis*; geotricose.
- Algas — prototecose.
- Parasitárias — larva migrans ocular (*Strongyles, Ascarids, Baylisascaris*); toxoplasmose; leishmaniose; *Neospora*; toxoplasmose e oftalmomiíase interna (larva migrans de dípteros) podem ocorrer em cães, porém são mais comuns em gatos.

Gatos
- Virais — FeLV; FIV; PIF.
- Bacterianas — septicemia ou bacteremia, bartonelose.
- Fúngicas — criptococose; histoplasmose; blastomicose; outras.
- Parasitárias — toxoplasmose, oftalmomiíase interna (das ordens Diptera e Cuterebra); larva migrans ocular, leishmaniose (um único relato).
- Protozoárias — toxoplasmose.

Idiopáticas
- Comuns.
- Coriorretinite ou coriorretinopatia multifocal em cães da raça Borzoi, Border collie e Beagle — uma síndrome adquirida em que os cães acometidos apresentam edema retiniano multifocal ou atrofia coriorretiniana.
- Cães da raça Montanhês de Berna e outras raças — histiocitose sistêmica ou maligna.

Imunológicas
- Qualquer doença imunomediada pode causar vasculite ou inflamação, resultando em descolamento da retina exsudativo ou coriorretinite; a causa exata é geralmente indeterminada; em casos de trombocitopenia, podem-se constatar hemorragias retinianas e/ou vítreas amplas ou multifocais pequenas com inflamação associada.
- Septicemia ou bacteremia com doença por imunocomplexos associada.
- Cães — a síndrome (uveodermatológica) semelhante à de Vogt-Koyanagi-Harada tem como alvo os grânulos de melanina (pigmento abundante no tecido uveal), o que leva a uma grave inflamação anterior e posterior (os cães acometidos também podem exibir despigmentação da pele, especialmente nas junções mucocutâneas); o LES apresenta os antígenos nucleares como alvo.
- Gatos — periarterite nodosa; LES.

Metabólicas
Retinopatia hipertensiva precoce pode exibir lesões localizadas multifocais.

Neoplásicas
Mieloma múltiplo, linfoma e neoplasia podem sofrer metástase.

Tóxicas
- Etilenoglicol; reações medicamentosas idiossincráticas (p. ex., trimetoprima-sulfa); ivermectina, especialmente em raças predispostas com gene de resistência a múltiplos medicamentos.
- Lesão fótica: a exposição à luz intensa pode queimar a retina, ou seja, manipulação da iluminação de microscópios, exposição à soldagem.

Traumatismo
- Infecções exógenas — traumatismo (ferida perfurante ou migração de corpo estranho).

FATORES DE RISCO
- Leucemia ou imunodeficiência felinas — podem predispor o gato à toxoplasmose ocular e/ou a outras causas infecciosas de coriorretinite/uveíte.
- Cães ou gatos sob terapia imunossupressora para outros problemas.

DIAGNÓSTICO

DIAGNÓSTICO DIFERENCIAL
- Exame oftalmológico — costuma ser suficiente para o diagnóstico; no acometimento de amplas áreas da retina, pode-se notar lentidão no reflexo pupilar à luz.
- Cegueira e diminuição na acuidade visual — neurite óptica; doença no SNC; inflamação retiniana difusa.
- Ver a seção "Causas".
- Displasia da retina — pregas bilaterais simétricas ou aglomerados geográficos de pigmento ou alteração na refletividade do fundo ocular; sem sinais associados de inflamação ocular; os cães das raças Labrador retriever e Springer spaniel são predispostos, mas pode ocorrer em muitas raças.

HEMOGRAMA/BIOQUÍMICA/URINÁLISE
- Normais — em problemas confinados aos olhos.
- Anormais — dependem da doença sistêmica subjacente.

OUTROS TESTES LABORATORIAIS
- Dependem do problema sistêmico sob suspeita.
- Título de AAN para suspeita de LES.
- Eletroforese proteica para pesquisa de mieloma.
- Constatação da proteína de Bence-Jones na urina.
- Biopsia cutânea — LES; síndrome uveodermatológica.
- Perfil de coagulação.
- Cultura bacteriana de líquidos oculares ou corporais.
- Testes sorológicos — doenças infecciosas (ver a seção "Causas").
- Citologia de aspirados de linfonodos.
- Histopatologia de olhos enucleados.

DIAGNÓSTICO POR IMAGEM
- Radiografias torácicas — linfadenopatia; doença metastática; infiltrados compatíveis com os agentes infecciosos.
- Radiografias vertebrais (coluna vertebral) — alterações ósseas compatíveis com discospondilite ou mieloma múltiplo.
- Ultrassonografia ocular — descolamentos da retina; massas intraoculares; exame

CORIORRETINITE

particularmente útil se os meios oculares não se encontrarem translúcidos.
- Ultrassonografia abdominal — exame para triagem de neoplasia primária, envolvimento de outros órgãos.

MÉTODOS DIAGNÓSTICOS
- Oftalmoscopia indireta — exibe uma ampla área da retina.
- Oftalmoscopia direta — facilita o exame de áreas sob suspeita.
- Punção do LCS — indicada na presença de sinais de doença neurológica (SNC) ou de neurite óptica.
- Vitreocentese ou aspirado do líquido sub-retiniano — poderão ser realizados se os outros testes diagnósticos não revelarem um agente causal ou na suspeita de agente infeccioso ou neoplasia; a vitreocentese pode agravar a inflamação ou induzir à hemorragia ou ao descolamento da retina, diminuindo as chances de recuperação da visão.
- Medição da pressão arterial.

ACHADOS PATOLÓGICOS
- Massas ou exsudatos retinianos ou coroidais.
- Microrganismos fúngicos — nos exsudatos e nas células inflamatórias.
- Inflamação perivascular — vasculite; PIF.
- Lesões inativas — atrofias (adelgaçamentos) retinianas e coroidais; é possível observar a hiperpigmentação do epitélio pigmentar retiniano e a destruição do tapete.

TRATAMENTO

CUIDADO(S) DE SAÚDE ADEQUADO(S)
- Depende(m) da condição física do paciente.
- Fornecido(s) geralmente em esquema ambulatorial.

CUIDADO(S) DE ENFERMAGEM
Fluidoterapia ou outra terapia em caso de doença sistêmica.

ORIENTAÇÃO AO PROPRIETÁRIO
- Informar ao proprietário que a coriorretinite pode ser um sinal de doença sistêmica e, nesse caso, a realização de testes diagnósticos é de suma importância.
- Alertar o proprietário sobre a necessidade de terapia vitalícia em casos de doença imunomediada para o controle da inflamação.
- Orientar o proprietário quanto à possível ocorrência de uveíte anterior e glaucoma secundário em cães com síndrome uveodermatológica, quadros que exigem o tratamento. A dermatite também necessita de tratamento.

MEDICAÇÕES

MEDICAMENTO(S) DE ESCOLHA
- Identificar e tratar qualquer doença sistêmica subjacente (p. ex., itraconazol ou fluconazol em casos de micose sistêmica, doxiciclina para *Rickettsia*, azitromicina ou doxiciclina para *Bartonella*).
- Medicamentos tópicos — ineficazes em cães com cristalinos intactos; indicados para tratar qualquer uveíte anterior associada, p. ex., corticosteroides tópicos (acetato de prednisolona a 1% ou dexametasona a 0,1% aplicado a cada 6-8 h) e parassimpatolíticos (atropina a 1% aplicada a uma frequência que dilate a pupila e diminua a dor) — para pan-uveíte (uveíte anterior concomitante). Tratar qualquer glaucoma secundário com medicamentos adequados para essa oftalmopatia (maleato de timolol a 0,5%, dorzolamida a 2%).
- Terapia sistêmica — indispensável.
- Toxoplasmose felina — clindamicina a 12,5 mg/kg VO a cada 12 h por 14-21 dias.
- Prednisona sistêmica em doses anti-inflamatórias — 0,5 mg/kg VO, com redução gradual em seguida; indicada quando já se descartou um quadro de micose sistêmica ou quando essa condição já estiver sendo submetida a tratamento com antifúngico sistêmico adequado; evitar o uso, a menos que exista o acometimento de amplas áreas da retina e haja grave risco de dano à visão.
- Prednisona em doses imunossupressoras — 2 mg/kg, divididos a cada 12 h por 3-10 dias (ideal), com subsequente redução gradual bastante lenta da dose durante meses; indicada em caso de doença imunomediada; pode facilitar a readerência da retina.

CONTRAINDICAÇÕES
Corticosteroides administrados por via sistêmica — não utilizar, a menos que a micose sistêmica já tenha sido descartada ou já esteja sendo submetida a um tratamento definitivo.

PRECAUÇÕES
Em casos de tratamento com a prednisona, considerar o uso concomitante de antiácidos por via oral, como a ranitidina ou a famotidina.

MEDICAMENTO(S) ALTERNATIVO(S)
- Condições neoplásicas (linfossarcoma, MEG ou mieloma múltiplo) — agentes quimioterápicos.
- Síndrome uveodermatológica — pode exigir a administração de azatioprina ou ciclosporina (ver "Descolamento da Retina") e de esteroides para o controle da inflamação.

ACOMPANHAMENTO

MONITORIZAÇÃO DO PACIENTE
- Adequado para a causa subjacente e o tipo de tratamento clínico.
- Hemograma completo, contagem plaquetária e enzimas hepáticas — em caso de fornecimento da azatioprina.
- Medição da PIO — em caso de uveíte anterior.

PREVENÇÃO
Medidas de controle de pulgas e carrapatos.

COMPLICAÇÕES POSSÍVEIS
- Cegueira permanente.
- Cataratas.
- Glaucoma.
- Dor ocular crônica.
- Óbito — secundário a uma doença sistêmica.

EVOLUÇÃO ESPERADA E PROGNÓSTICO
- Prognóstico quanto à visão — de reservado a bom, dependendo da magnitude de envolvimento da retina; na destruição de amplas áreas da retina, haverá déficits visuais ou cegueira; doenças focais e multifocais não prejudicam a visão de forma acentuada, mas deixam cicatrizes.
- Prognóstico quanto à vida — de reservado a bom, dependendo da causa subjacente.

DIVERSOS

DISTÚRBIOS ASSOCIADOS
Diversas doenças sistêmicas.

POTENCIAL ZOONÓTICO
- Toxoplasmose — poderá ser transmitida aos seres humanos se o paciente estiver eliminando oocistos nas fezes.
- Doenças transmitidas por vetores — os animais infectados podem atuar como reservatórios, ou seja, *Bartonella*, *Rickettsia*, outras.

SINÔNIMO(S)
Retinocoroidite.

VER TAMBÉM
- Degeneração da Retina.
- Descolamento da Retina.
- Síndrome Uveodermatológica.

ABREVIATURA(S)
- AAN = anticorpo antinuclear.
- FeLV = vírus da leucemia felina.
- FIV = vírus da imunodeficiência felina.
- LCS = líquido cerebrospinal.
- LES = lúpus eritematoso sistêmico.
- MEG = meningoencefalite granulomatosa.
- PIF = peritonite infecciosa felina.
- PIO = pressão intraocular.
- SNC = sistema nervoso central.

Sugestões de Leitura
Narfström K, Petersen-Jones S. Diseases of the canine ocular fundus. In: Gelatt KN, ed., Veterinary Ophthalmology, 4th ed. Ames, IA: Blackwell, 2007, pp. 989-1025.
Stiles J. Infectious diseases and the eye. Vet Clin North Am Small Anim Pract 2000, 30:971-1167.

Autor Patricia J. Smith
Consultor Editorial Paul E. Miller

CORPOS ESTRANHOS ESOFÁGICOS

CONSIDERAÇÕES GERAIS

DEFINIÇÃO
Ingestão de material estranho ou comestível muito grande para passar pelo esôfago, causando obstrução intraluminal.

FISIOPATOLOGIA
Corpos estranhos esofágicos causam obstrução mecânica, inflamação da mucosa com edema e, possivelmente, necrose isquêmica.

SISTEMA(S) ACOMETIDO(S)
• Gastrintestinal.
• Respiratório — em caso de pneumonia por aspiração.

GENÉTICA
N/D.

INCIDÊNCIA/PREVALÊNCIA
Desconhecida.

DISTRIBUIÇÃO GEOGRÁFICA
N/D.

IDENTIFICAÇÃO
Espécies
Em virtude dos hábitos alimentares indiscriminados de muitos cães, a incidência é maior neles do que em gatos.

Raça(s) Predominante(s)
Mais comuns em cães de pequeno porte; as raças do tipo Terrier são frequentemente super-representadas.

Idade Média e Faixa Etária
Mais comuns em animais jovens a de meia-idade.

Sexo Predominante
N/D.

SINAIS CLÍNICOS
Comentários Gerais
O animal pode ter sido visto ingerindo um corpo estranho.

Achados Anamnésicos
Os mais comuns incluem vômito seco ou ânsia de vômito, engasgo, letargia, anorexia, ptialismo, regurgitação, inquietação, disfagia e tentativa persistente de deglutição.

Achados do Exame Físico
• Na maioria das vezes, não são dignos de nota.
• Ocasionalmente, há desconforto à palpação do pescoço ou da região abdominal cranial (epigástrica).

CAUSAS
Ocorrem mais frequentemente com um objeto, cujo tamanho, formato ou textura não permite sua movimentação livre pelo esôfago, fazendo com que ele fique alojado antes de possibilitar a passagem.

FATORES DE RISCO
N/D.

DIAGNÓSTICO

DIAGNÓSTICO DIFERENCIAL
• Esofagite.
• Estenose esofágica.
• Neoplasia esofágica.
• Megaesôfago.
• Outros distúrbios esofágicos.

HEMOGRAMA/BIOQUÍMICA/URINÁLISE
• Em geral, normais.
• Ocasionalmente, observam-se anormalidades eletrolíticas, leucograma inflamatório e/ou hemoconcentração, dependendo da gravidade dos sinais e do grau de desidratação.

OUTROS TESTES LABORATORIAIS
N/D.

DIAGNÓSTICO POR IMAGEM
Radiografia Torácica
• A maioria dos corpos estranhos esofágicos é radiopaca e facilmente visualizada. Tais objetos costumam ficar alojados em pontos de distensão esofágica mínima, incluindo a entrada torácica, a base do coração e o hiato esofágico.
• Pode-se observar uma distensão esofágica com ar, cranialmente ao corpo estranho.
• É necessária a realização de esofagograma contrastado para identificar objetos radiotransparentes. Na suspeita de perfuração, utilizar um agente de contraste iodado orgânico aquoso para a obtenção das imagens.
• A presença de ar e/ou líquido no mediastino ou no espaço pleural é sugestiva de perfuração esofágica; dependendo da gravidade, isso pode ser indicação para cirurgia em vez de esofagoscopia.
• Infiltrados pulmonares sugerem pneumonia por aspiração.

MÉTODOS DIAGNÓSTICOS
A esofagoscopia proporciona a inspeção direta tanto do corpo estranho como da mucosa esofágica, permitindo a avaliação do grau da lesão esofágica.

ACHADOS PATOLÓGICOS
N/D.

TRATAMENTO

CUIDADO(S) DE SAÚDE ADEQUADO(S)
• Emergências — tratar como pacientes hospitalizados e fazer endoscopia o mais rápido possível depois do diagnóstico.
• Caso se consiga retirar o corpo estranho durante a endoscopia e a lesão esofágica for mínima, o paciente poderá receber alta no mesmo dia.

CUIDADO(S) DE ENFERMAGEM
• Se o procedimento para retirar o corpo estranho for atraumático e o esôfago tiver sofrido lesão mínima, não haverá necessidade de qualquer cuidado especial.
• O traumatismo grave da mucosa pode exigir a colocação de sonda de gastrostomia para fornecimento de nutrição enteral durante a cicatrização do esôfago.

ATIVIDADE
O paciente pode retomar a atividade normal depois da retirada rotineira de um corpo estranho do esôfago.

DIETA
Não há necessidade de qualquer alteração.

ORIENTAÇÃO AO PROPRIETÁRIO
Discutir a possibilidade de complicações e repetição do problema.

CONSIDERAÇÕES CIRÚRGICAS
• A endoscopia é muito menos traumática e invasiva que a cirurgia.
• A cirurgia fica indicada quando (a) não se consegue retirar o corpo estranho durante a endoscopia, (b) esse exame faz com que o objeto avance para o lúmen gástrico, embora ele seja muito grande para passar pelo trato gastrintestinal, ou (c) uma grande perfuração do esôfago ou área de necrose requer ressecção.
• Em geral, é menos traumático avançar um corpo estranho ósseo para o estômago que tentar retirá-lo.
• É possível esperar que a maioria dos corpos estranhos ósseos se dissolva com segurança no estômago sem a necessidade de retirada cirúrgica. Objetos estranhos não digeríveis que passam para o estômago talvez necessitem de remoção por via cirúrgica.

MEDICAÇÕES

MEDICAMENTO(S) DE ESCOLHA
Se houver lesão significativa da mucosa (i. e., esofagite), as recomendações incluirão:
• Antibióticos de amplo espectro como amoxicilina ou Clavamox® por 10-14 dias.
• Papa de sucralfato (0,5-1 g/cão VO a cada 8 h) para citoproteção e cicatrização da mucosa.
• Corticosteroides a curto prazo (prednisona, 1 mg/kg VO a cada 24 h) diminuem o risco da formação de estenose por inibirem os fibroblastos; contraindicados se houver pneumonia por aspiração.
• Antagonistas H_2 (p. ex., ranitidina, 2 mg/kg VO, IV, SC a cada 12 h, ou famotidina, 0,5 mg/kg VO a cada 24 h) para esofagite por refluxo.
• Metoclopramida (0,2-0,5 mg/kg IV, SC, VO a cada 8 h) para minimizar a esofagite por refluxo.
• Colocação percutânea de sonda de gastrostomia para nutrição enteral durante a cicatrização da mucosa.

CONTRAINDICAÇÕES
N/D.

PRECAUÇÕES
N/D.

INTERAÇÕES POSSÍVEIS
N/D.

MEDICAMENTO(S) ALTERNATIVO(S)
N/D.

ACOMPANHAMENTO

MONITORIZAÇÃO DO PACIENTE
• Examinar o esôfago atentamente em busca de lesão da mucosa.
• Eritema/erosões discretas não são raros e tendem a cicatrizar sem complicações.
• Se houver laceração/perfuração esofágica — a nutrição parenteral ou a alimentação com sonda de gastrostomia permite que o esôfago descanse e cicatrize.
• Radiografias torácicas simples são aconselháveis após o procedimento para avaliar a presença de pneumomediastino/pneumotórax.
• Monitorizar por no mínimo 2-3 semanas em busca de indícios de estenose.
• Estenose esofágica — o sinal clínico mais comum é a regurgitação; esofagograma e/ou esofagoscopia podem ser indicados.

CORPOS ESTRANHOS ESOFÁGICOS

PREVENÇÃO
Monitorizar com cuidado o ambiente e o que o animal come.

COMPLICAÇÕES POSSÍVEIS
• Aproximadamente 25% dos pacientes com corpos estranhos desenvolvem complicações.
• As complicações mais frequentemente encontradas incluem perfuração do esôfago, estenoses esofágicas, fístulas esofágicas e esofagite grave. Podem ocorrer distúrbios focais transitórios da motilidade do esôfago, secundários a traumatismo desse órgão.
• Podem ocorrer pneumomediastino, pneumotórax, pneumonia, pleurite, mediastinite e fístulas broncoesofágicas secundários à perfuração.

EVOLUÇÃO ESPERADA E PROGNÓSTICO
• A maioria desses pacientes passa bem e se recupera sem complicações.
• Nas complicações, o prognóstico é reservado.

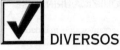

DIVERSOS

DISTÚRBIOS ASSOCIADOS
Nenhum.

FATORES RELACIONADOS COM A IDADE
N/D.

POTENCIAL ZOONÓTICO
Nenhum.

GESTAÇÃO/FERTILIDADE/REPRODUÇÃO
N/D.

VER TAMBÉM
• Divertículos Esofágicos.
• Regurgitação.

RECURSOS DA INTERNET
Rede de Informações Veterinárias: www.vin.com/VIN.plx.

Sugestões de Leitura
Gualtieri M. Esophagoscopy. Vet Clin North Am Small Anim Pract 2001, 31:605-630.
Spielman BL, Shaker EH, Garvey MS. Esophageal foreign body in dogs: A retrospective study of 23 cases. JAAHA 1992, 28:570-574.
Tams TR. Endoscopic removal of gastrointestinal foreign bodies. In: Tams TR, ed., Small Animal Endoscopy, 2nd ed. Philadelphia: Mosby, 1999, pp. 247-295.

Autor Albert E. Jergens
Consultor Editorial Albert E. Jergens

CORRIMENTO VAGINAL

CONSIDERAÇÕES GERAIS

DEFINIÇÃO
Qualquer substância proveniente dos lábios vulvares.

FISIOPATOLOGIA
• Depende da causa subjacente do corrimento vaginal.
• Pode ter origem em órgãos como útero, vagina, vestíbulo, clitóris, seio clitoriano, derme perivulvar ou trato urinário.

SISTEMA(S) ACOMETIDO(S)
• Reprodutor.
• Renal.
• Cutâneo.
• Urinário.

INCIDÊNCIA/PREVALÊNCIA
• Desconhecida por haver muitas causas.
• Quadro considerado como uma razão comum pela busca de atendimento veterinário.

IDENTIFICAÇÃO
• Cadelas saudáveis com <6-12 meses de vida (pré-púberes) — vaginite de filhote canino (juvenil) e anomalias congênitas são mais comuns.
• Cadelas não prenhes que tiveram pelo menos um único ciclo estral — estro normal, estro persistente (doença cística ovariana ou tumor de células da granulosa); piometra; neoplasia.
• Cadelas que cruzaram nos últimos 30-70 dias — parto normal (50-70 dias) ou abortamento (<50 dias).
• Cadelas que pariram recentemente — lóquios normais ou metrite pós-parto são mais comuns; subinvolução dos sítios placentários.
• Cadelas submetidas à ovário-histerectomia — estenose vaginal ou incontinência urinária responsiva a estrogênio são mais comuns; neoplasia.

SINAIS CLÍNICOS
Achados Anamnésicos
• Corrimento proveniente da vulva.
• Lambedura, arrastamento da região perineal no chão e manchas na pele.
• Atração de machos.
• Parto — em casos de corrimento pós-parto.
• Estro recente — em casos de piometra.
• Corrimento hemorrágico ≥8 semanas após o parto — subinvolução dos sítios placentários.
• Vômito, anorexia — podem ser observados com metrite e piometra.

Achados do Exame Físico
• O corrimento vaginal pode ser serossanguinolento, purulento, loquial, hemorrágico, mucoide ou fétido.

CAUSAS
Condições Fisiológicas
• Proestro. • Estro. • Diestro. • Fase final da gestação. • Parto. • Lóquios normais.

Condições Patológicas
• Doença cística ovariana (estro persistente).
• *Brucella canis.*
• Metrite.
• Piometra.
• Placenta ou fetos retidos.
• Subinvolução dos sítios placentários (corrimento hemorrágico ≥8 semanas após o parto).
• Neoplasia — útero, vagina, trato urinário (inclusive o tumor venéreo transmissível), ovário (tumor de células da granulosa/estro persistente).
• Vaginite.
• Incontinência urinária responsiva a estrogênios.
• Coagulopatia.
• Defeitos congênitos do trato genital distal — problemas de intersexo, fusão embrionária imperfeita dos ductos müllerianos (vagina), união das pregas genitais (vestíbulo) e tumefações genitais (lábios vulvares), ureteres ectópicos.

FATORES DE RISCO
• Antibióticos profiláticos — podem alterar a flora vaginal normal e predispor o animal à infecção secundária.
• Administração exógena de estrogênios — predispõe à piometra na cadela intacta.
• Androgênios exógenos — podem causar hipertrofia do clitóris.
• Progesterona exógena ou endógena — predispõe à piometra ou piometra de coto.
• Obesidade — pregas cutâneas excessivas em torno da vulva.

DIAGNÓSTICO

DIAGNÓSTICO DIFERENCIAL
• Cadelas saudáveis com <6-12 meses de vida — vaginite juvenil (pré-púbere), ciclo estral normal, traumatismo ou neoplasia urogenital, corpo estranho, coagulopatia, ureter(es) ectópico(s), anormalidades congênitas do períneo ou trato genital distal, problemas de intersexo, doença do trato urinário.
• Cadelas não prenhes que tiveram pelo menos um único ciclo estral — estro normal, piometra, cio cortado*, corpo estranho, traumatismo urogenital, neoplasia, coagulopatia, doença cística ovariana (cistos foliculares).
• Cadelas que cruzaram nos últimos 30-70 dias — abortamento, piometra, parto normal (>57 dias a partir do acasalamento), morte embrionária/fetal, cio cortado, infecção por *Brucella canis.*
• Cadelas que pariram recentemente — lóquios (normais até 6-8 semanas após o parto), subinvolução dos sítios placentários (corrimento hemorrágico ≥8 semanas após o parto), metrite pós-parto, traumatismo vaginal, placenta ou fetos retidos.
• Cadelas submetidas à ovário-histerectomia — estenose vaginal, corpo estranho, neoplasia, pólipos, piometra de coto gerada por progesterona exógena ou endógena, dermatite perivulvar, síndrome dos ovários remanescentes, incontinência urinária responsiva a estrogênios.

HEMOGRAMA/BIOQUÍMICA/URINÁLISE
• Anemia regenerativa — pode ser normal na prenhez ou durante o estro.
• Leucocitose com desvio à esquerda — em casos de piometra ou metrite pós-parto.
• Níveis elevados de ureia e creatinina — piometra.
• Isostenúria — em casos de poliúria e polidipsia associadas à piometra.
• Urinálise — pode indicar infecção do trato urinário.

---
* N. T.: Também conhecido como cio da loba.

OUTROS TESTES LABORATORIAIS
• Concentração sérica de progesterona — determina se a cadela se encontra na fase lútea, o que aumenta a probabilidade de piometra. Os hormônios progesterona e 17-hidroxiprogesterona podem ser secretados em animais com doença do córtex adrenal (teste de estimulação com ACTH; Clinical Endocrinology Service, University of Tennessee).
• Sorologia para *Brucella canis* — triagem com teste de aglutinação rápida em lâmina (D-Tec CB, Synbiotics Corp.); teste de imunodifusão em ágar gel (Cornell University Diagnostic Laboratory); cultura bacteriana de sangue total ou aspirado de linfonodos.

DIAGNÓSTICO POR IMAGEM
Radiografia
• Exame capaz de detectar aumento de volume do útero ou do ovário, além de confirmar gestação.
• Indícios de morte fetal — presença de gases em torno do feto ou mau alinhamento e/ou colapso do esqueleto fetal.

Ultrassonografia
• Exame apto a determinar o conteúdo do útero — a presença de líquido livre nesse órgão é característica de piometra, hidrometra e mucometra.
• Permite o diagnóstico de gestação e a avaliação do bem-estar embrionário/fetal: o batimento cardíaco pode ser observado já com 20 dias do diestro; uma frequência cardíaca <180-220 bpm indica estresse fetal.
• Possibilita a detecção de massas — neoplasia, granulomas, doença cística ovariana ou tumor de células da granulosa ou corpo estranho; a distensão da vagina com solução fisiológica pode ajudar na visualização.

Radiografia Contrastada — Vaginograma/ Uretrograma/Cistograma/Pielograma intravenoso
• Identifica conformação ou estrutura anormais (i. e., neoplasia ou corpo estranho) dentro da vagina.
• Descarta estenoses vestibulovaginais, além de fístulas retovaginais e uretrovaginais.
• Exclui a lista de diagnósticos diferenciais e ajuda a localizar o problema.
• Pregas (rugas) pronunciadas da vagina durante o estro provocarão defeitos de preenchimento (isso, no entanto, é normal).

MÉTODOS DIAGNÓSTICOS
Citologia Vaginal
• Determina a natureza do corrimento — inflamatório, hemorrágico.
• Avalia as células epiteliais quanto ao processo de cornificação — presença de cornificação sob a influência de estrogênio.
• Sempre é realizada para interpretar culturas vaginais.

Cultura Vaginal e Antibiograma
• Efetuada antes de outros procedimentos diagnósticos.
• Utilizar *swab* protegido para obter amostra da porção cranial da vagina.
• Os microrganismos mais comuns da flora normal incluem *E. coli, Streptococcus* spp., *Pasteurella* spp., e *Staphylococcus* spp.
• Outros microrganismos da flora normal compreendem *Mycoplasma* spp., *Enterobacter* spp., *Pseudomonas* spp., *Klebsiella* spp.
• Lembrete: como a vagina não é um ambiente estéril, a cultura de cadelas normais pode resultar

Corrimento Vaginal

no crescimento da flora vaginal normal; o uso de citologia vaginal e de outras ferramentas diagnósticas é essencial para a interpretação dos resultados da cultura. A flora normal consiste em inúmeros patógenos oportunistas, p. ex., *E. coli* e *Mycoplasma* spp.

Vaginoscopia
- Cistouretroscópio rígido, gastroscópio pediátrico ou proctoscópio; ou endoscópio flexível utilizado para inspecionar a vagina.
- Identifica a origem do corrimento vaginal — uterino, vaginal, vestibular ou uretral.
- Visualiza anomalias, hímen persistente, neoplasia, corpo estranho, traumatismo, abscesso, além de avaliar a mucosa vaginal e vestibular.
- Se houver indicação, pode-se usar um vaginoscópio (espéculo) especializado para irrigar o útero.
- Permite a remoção de corpo estranho ou a biopsia de massa vaginal.

Outros
- Exame digital do vestíbulo, da junção vaginovestibular e da porção distal da vagina.
- Biopsia e exame histopatológico de massa.
- Cistocentese — urocultura e antibiograma.
- Perfil de coagulação.

TRATAMENTO
- O tratamento é feito com base no diagnóstico.
- Não há tratamento para as causas fisiológicas de corrimento vaginal.
- Em geral, o corrimento vaginal é tratado em um esquema ambulatorial, exceto os casos de piometra.
- Recorrer também aos capítulos de cada doença.

CONSIDERAÇÕES CIRÚRGICAS
- A piometra pode ser tratada por meio clínico ou cirúrgico (ovário-histerectomia).
- Ovariectomia ou ovário-histerectomia é o tratamento de escolha em condições neoplásicas.
- Doença cística ovariana pode ser submetida a tratamento clínico ou cirúrgico (ovariectomia/ ovário-histerectomia).
- Remoção de corpo estranho ou excisão cirúrgica de massa(s).
- Excisão cirúrgica ou radioterapia são opções terapêuticas para o tumor venéreo transmissível.

MEDICAÇÕES
MEDICAMENTO(S) DE ESCOLHA
- Prostaglandina $F_{2\alpha}$ para evacuação uterina (contrações do miométrio) e luteólise — Lutalyse® (dinoprosta — $PGF_{2\alpha}$) — 50-100 µg/kg SC 1 a 3 vezes ao dia até que o nível de progesterona decline para <2,0 ng/mL e o útero esteja isento de líquido; Estrumate® (cloprostenol) — 1-5 µg/kg SC 1 vez ao dia.
- Antibiótico — escolha feita com base nos resultados da cultura e do antibiograma de amostra coletada da porção cranial da vagina.
- Agonista dopaminérgico — pode ser usado em adição à $PGF_{2\alpha}$ para luteólise via supressão da prolactina (luteotrófica) — bromocriptina (10 µg/ kg VO) ou cabergolina (5 µg/kg VO) 1 a 3 vezes ao dia até que o nível sérico de progesterona esteja abaixo de 2,0 ng/mL.
- Cuidados de suporte, inclusive fluidos intravenosos, conforme indicação.

CONTRAINDICAÇÕES
Certos antibióticos podem ser contraindicados durante a gravidez e a amamentação.

PRECAUÇÕES
- Prostaglandina $F_{2\alpha}$ — os efeitos colaterais incluem respiração ofegante, vômito, defecação/ diarreia e, possivelmente, hipotensão. Tais efeitos colaterais duram 30-40 minutos e diminuem de forma gradativa com as doses subsequentes, rapidamente metabolizadas nos pulmões.
- Agonistas dopaminérgicos — os efeitos colaterais incluem vômito e náusea; tais efeitos podem ser controlados com antieméticos.
- Monitorização rigorosa das pacientes submetidas a tratamento clínico de piometra, pois esses animais podem ficar endotoxêmicos ou septicêmicos e necessitar de ovário-histerectomia de emergência.
- Estabilização da paciente antes da indução de anestesia para o tratamento cirúrgico de piometra.

MEDICAMENTO(S) ALTERNATIVO(S)
Aglepristona (10 mg/kg SC, 2 doses administradas separadas por um intervalo de 24 h) — antiprogestina que pode ser utilizada isoladamente ou em combinação com a terapia à base de prostaglandina para o tratamento de piometra (atualmente não disponível nos Estados Unidos).

ACOMPANHAMENTO
MONITORIZAÇÃO DA PACIENTE
Piometra
- Reavaliar a progesterona sérica até um nível abaixo de 2,0 ng/mL.
- Averiguar o ultrassom após a queda da progesterona (<2,0 ng/mL) para monitorar a depuração do líquido uterino.
- Verificar o hemograma completo e o perfil bioquímico para monitorizar a saúde sistêmica.

Subinvolução dos Sítios Placentários
- Monitorizar o hematócrito — dependendo da quantidade de perda sanguínea.

PREVENÇÃO
- Vaginite de filhote canino — adiar a ovário-histerectomia eletiva até o primeiro ciclo estral em casos de vaginite juvenil; isso pode evitar vaginite crônica.
- Evitar o uso de esteroides exógenos (estrogênios, progestinas, androgênios) em cadelas intactas.

COMPLICAÇÕES POSSÍVEIS
Em casos de piometra ou metrite, podem ocorrer endotoxemia e septicemia.

DIVERSOS
DISTÚRBIOS ASSOCIADOS
Piometra e hiperplasia endometrial cística.

FATORES RELACIONADOS COM A IDADE
- Aumento no risco de piometra após cada ciclo estral.
- Neoplasia é mais comum em cadelas mais idosas.

POTENCIAL ZOONÓTICO
- *Brucella canis* — os líquidos e o tecido fetal durante o abortamento são altamente contaminados com microrganismos.
- Seres humanos imunocomprometidos estão sob maior risco. Tratadores e patologistas de animais também estão sob risco em virtude da alta exposição.

GESTAÇÃO/FERTILIDADE/REPRODUÇÃO
- Piometra — prognóstico grave quanto à fertilidade futura em cadelas diagnosticadas com piometra em conjunto com hiperplasia endometrial cística; prognóstico melhor (há relatos de gestações bem-sucedidas) se os sinais manifestos de hiperplasia endometrial cística não estiverem presentes e se a cadela for acasalada no próximo ciclo estral.
- Neoplasia — prognóstico mau quanto à fertilidade futura.
- Tumor venéreo transmissível — doença sexualmente transmitida; por essa razão, deve-se evitar o acasalamento.
- *Brucella canis* — doença sexualmente transmitida e prognóstico grave quanto à resolução da doença e fertilidade normal; os animais acometidos não devem ser usados para reprodução.

VER TAMBÉM
- Abortamento Espontâneo (Perda Gestacional Precoce) — Gatas.
- Abortamento Espontâneo (Perda Gestacional Precoce) — Cadelas.
- Brucelose.
- Síndrome dos Ovários Remanescentes.
- Falha Ovulatória.
- Piometra e Hiperplasia Endometrial Cística.
- Placenta retida.
- Distúrbios do Desenvolvimento Sexual.
- Subinvolução dos Sítios Placentários.
- Tumor Venéreo Transmissível.
- Más-formações Vaginais e Lesões Adquiridas.
- Vaginite.

ABREVIATURA(S)
- ACTH = hormônio adrenocorticotrópico.
- bpm = batimentos por minuto.

Sugestões de Leitura
Feldman EC, Nelson RW. Vulvar discharges. In: Canine and Feline Endocrinology and Reproduction. St. Louis: Saunders, 2004, pp. 909-913.
Johnston SD, Root Kustritz MV, Olson PN. Disorders of the canine vagina, vestibule, and vulva. In: Canine and Feline Theriogenology. Philadelphia: Saunders, 2001, pp. 225-242.
Purswell BJ. Vaginal disorders. In: Ettinger SJ, Feldman EC, eds., Textbook of Veterinary Internal Medicine, 6th ed. St. Louis: Elsevier, 2005, pp. 1686-1690.
Purswell BJ. Vaginal disorders. In: Root Kustritz MV, ed., Small Animal Theriogenology. St. Louis: Butterworth Heineman, 2003, pp. 395-419.

Autores Leeah R. Chew, Beverly J. Purswell
Consultor Editorial Sara K. Lyle

CRIPTOCOCOSE

CONSIDERAÇÕES GERAIS

DEFINIÇÃO
Infecção fúngica localizada ou sistêmica, causada pela levedura *Cryptococcus* spp. do ambiente.

FISIOPATOLOGIA
- *C. neoformans* — cresce em excrementos de aves e vegetação em decomposição; problemas no solo aumentam o risco de infecção.
- Os cães e os gatos inalam a levedura, estabelecendo-se um foco de infecção, geralmente nas vias nasais; os microrganismos retraídos, ressecados e menores podem atingir as vias aéreas terminais (incomum). Pode haver colonização ou infecção subclínica das vias nasais com resolução espontânea.
- As infecções gástricas e intestinais sugerem a ocorrência de entrada GI primária.
- Disseminação — por via hematógena a partir das vias nasais até órgãos como cérebro, olhos, pulmões e outros tecidos; por extensão direta até órgãos como pele do nariz, olhos, tecidos retro-orbitais e linfonodos drenantes.

SISTEMA(S) ACOMETIDO(S)
- Gatos — acomete principalmente regiões como nariz e seios nasais; pele facial; plano nasal; nasofaringe; cérebro; olhos.
- Cães — afeta basicamente regiões como cabeça e cérebro, vias e seios nasais; pele sobre as regiões nasais e sinusais; mucosas; linfonodos drenantes; olhos; áreas periorbitais; ocasionalmente, envolve pulmões e órgãos abdominais.

INCIDÊNCIA/PREVALÊNCIA
- Cães — rara nos EUA; prevalência de 0,00013%.
- Gatos — 7-10 vezes mais comum do que nos cães.

DISTRIBUIÇÃO GEOGRÁFICA
- Mundial.
- Algumas áreas do sul da Califórnia e da Austrália apresentam incidência elevada; além disso, já se observou a ocorrência de surto na Ilha de Vancouver em British Columbia, Canadá.
- A espécie *Cryptococcus gattii* cresce satisfatoriamente em árvores de eucalipto.

IDENTIFICAÇÃO
Espécies
Cães e gatos.

Raça(s) Predominante(s)
- Cães — as raças Cocker spaniel americano, Dinamarquês, Doberman pinscher e Boxer são super-representadas.
- Gatos — o Siamês exibe alto risco.

Idade Média e Faixa Etária
- Mais comum com 2-7 anos de idade (cães e gatos).
- Pode ocorrer em qualquer idade, mas é frequentemente observada em cães com menos de 6 meses de vida.

Sexo Predominante
- Cães — nenhum.
- Gatos — os machos podem ser super--representados.

SINAIS CLÍNICOS
Achados Anamnésicos
- Letargia.
- Variam, dependendo dos sistemas orgânicos envolvidos.
- Podem apresentar histórico de problemas por semanas a meses.

Cães
- Neurológicos — crises convulsivas, ataxia, paresia, cegueira.
- Ulceração cutânea.
- Linfadenopatia.
- Vômito e diarreia.

Gatos
- Secreção nasal e sinais oculares.
- Sinais neurológicos — crises convulsivas, desorientação e sinais vestibulares.
- Tecido granulomatoso observado nas narinas.
- Tumefações firmes na ponte nasal.

Achados do Exame Físico
- Febre leve — <50% dos pacientes.
- Cães — anorexia; secreção nasal.
- Gatos — aumento dos ruídos respiratórios; lesões cutâneas crostosas e ulceradas na cabeça; linfadenopatia; achados neurológicos; sinais oculares.

CAUSAS
Exposição a microrganismos criptocócicos e deficiência do sistema imune em evitar a colonização e a invasão tecidual.

FATORES DE RISCO
Exposição a solo contaminado.

DIAGNÓSTICO

DIAGNÓSTICO DIFERENCIAL
Cães
- Outras causas de neuropatia focal ou difusa — cinomose; meningoencefalite bacteriana; tumores cerebrais; riquetsioses; meningoencefalomielite granulomatosa; outras doenças fúngicas.
- Lesões nasais, especialmente na junção mucocutânea — consideradas imunomediadas.
- Linfoma — possível causa da linfadenopatia.
- Em casos de coriorretinite e neurite óptica — considerar outras infecções fúngicas, cinomose e neoplasias.

Gatos
- Lesões nasais — semelhantes a tumores nasais, rinite crônica e sinusite crônica.
- Alterações cutâneas ulcerativas — podem resultar de infecções bacterianas, brigas ou tumores (especialmente carcinoma de células escamosas do plano nasal).
- Sinais oculares e cerebrais — podem ser atribuídos a linfoma, PIF e toxoplasmose.

HEMOGRAMA/BIOQUÍMICA/URINÁLISE
- Leve anemia em alguns gatos.
- Ocasionalmente, observa-se eosinofilia.
- A bioquímica sérica costuma permanecer normal.

OUTROS TESTES LABORATORIAIS
- Teste de aglutinação em látex ou ELISA — detectam o antígeno da cápsula criptocócica no soro; poucos resultados falso-positivos; a maioria dos animais infectados apresenta títulos mensuráveis do antígeno capsular; a magnitude do título correlaciona-se com o grau de infecção.
- O ensaio antigênico talvez seja menos sensível em cães. Pode ser positivo apenas quando há colonização; no entanto, títulos antigênicos iguais ou superiores a 1:32 são observados em casos de invasão fúngica.

DIAGNÓSTICO POR IMAGEM
- Radiografias nasais (gatos) — material com densidade de tecido mole, que preenche as vias nasais; destruição óssea ocasional do dorso nasal.
- TC ou RM contrastados — são os exames mais eficientes para identificar lesões cerebrais e nasais.
- Radiografias torácicas — não são indicadas a menos que haja sinais de doença do trato respiratório inferior.

MÉTODOS DIAGNÓSTICOS
Cães
Doença neurológica — procedimentos extras: o exame citológico e cultura do LCS, bem como a mensuração do antígeno capsular no LCS, frequentemente estabelecem o diagnóstico.

Gatos
- Diagnóstico definitivo — aspirados do material mucoide das vias nasais ou biopsia do tecido granulomatoso, que se projeta a partir das narinas. A irrigação do nariz com solução salina pode desalojar o tecido granulomatoso.
- Pacientes com obstrução respiratória superior ou ruídos respiratórios intensos — indica a presença de granuloma na nasofaringe; identificar por meio da tração do palato mole para frente com um gancho cirúrgico (utilizado em castração de cadela) para expor a massa ou por meio da retroflexão do endoscópio na nasofaringe para examinar e fazer a biopsia da massa na área das coanas.
- Biopsia — lesões cutâneas da cabeça; aspirados dos linfonodos envolvidos; geralmente identifica os microrganismos.
- Culturas — confirmam o diagnóstico; determinam a suscetibilidade do fungo a medicamentos em casos de infecção pouco responsiva.

ACHADOS PATOLÓGICOS
- Lesões macroscópicas — massa gelatinosa de coloração cinza, produzida pela cápsula polissacáride; costumam ser encontradas no nariz, nos seios nasais e na nasofaringe dos gatos. As lesões cutâneas são geralmente ulcerativas.
- Lesões neurológicas — observadas comumente em cães; granulomas difusos ou fúngicos, produtores de massa cerebral.
- Coriorretinite com ou sem descolamento da retina ou neurite óptica — cães e gatos.
- Resposta histológica — em geral piogranulomatosa; o infiltrado de células inflamatórias pode ser leve, pois a cápsula polissacáride interfere na migração neutrofílica.

TRATAMENTO

CUIDADO(S) DE SAÚDE ADEQUADO(S)
- Feito em um esquema ambulatorial se o paciente se encontrar estabilizado.
- Sinais neurológicos — podem exigir terapia de suporte intensiva até a estabilização do animal.

CUIDADO(S) DE ENFERMAGEM
Gatos — a obstrução nasal influencia o apetite; estimular os pacientes a se alimentar, oferecendo alimentos palatáveis.

ATIVIDADE
Sem restrição na maioria dos casos.

CRIPTOCOCOSE

DIETA
• Nenhum alimento especial.
• Pacientes tratados com itraconazol — fornecer a medicação com alimentos gordurosos (p. ex., ração enlatada) para melhorar a absorção.

ORIENTAÇÃO AO PROPRIETÁRIO
• Informar o proprietário sobre a natureza crônica da doença e a necessidade de meses de tratamento.
• Tranquilizar o proprietário a respeito do caráter não zoonótico da infecção.

CONSIDERAÇÕES CIRÚRGICAS
Remover as massas granulomatosas na nasofaringe para diminuir as dificuldades respiratórias.

MEDICAÇÕES
MEDICAMENTO(S) DE ESCOLHA
• Fluconazol — agente preferido em casos de envolvimento ocular ou neurológico (SNC), pois é hidrossolúvel e exibe melhor penetração no sistema nervoso; gatos, 50 mg VO a cada 12 h; cães, 5 mg/kg VO a cada 12 h; constitui a escolha mais econômica.
• Itraconazol sob a forma de cápsulas — administrar juntamente com uma refeição gordurosa para maximizar a absorção; gatos, 10 mg/kg VO diariamente; cães, 5 mg/kg VO a cada 12 h; o conteúdo da cápsula pode ser misturado com o alimento; aparentemente, não tem gosto desagradável. Itraconazol sob a forma de líquido — melhor absorção com o estômago vazio. Itraconazol manipulado — absorção errática (ou seja, que não é fixa).
• Anfotericina B pode ter algumas vantagens em casos graves da doença a uma dose intravenosa de 0,5 mg/kg a cada 48 h, administrada em 3-4 h. Monitorizar a função renal atentamente.
• Terbinafina a uma dose de 5 mg/kg a cada 12 h mostrou-se eficaz no tratamento de gatos com infecções resistentes.

CONTRAINDICAÇÕES
Evitar os esteroides.

PRECAUÇÕES
• Triazóis — hepatotoxicidade; o sinal de anorexia indica problemas; monitorizar as enzimas hepáticas mensalmente.
• Terbinafina — monitorizar quanto à ocorrência de hepatotoxicidade e anorexia.
• Anfotericina B — nefrotoxicidade.

• Itraconazol — dermatite ulcerativa (diferenciar das lesões cutâneas de criptococose); o aparecimento de novas lesões cutâneas após a melhora da doença deve ser considerado como uma reação medicamentosa.

MEDICAMENTO(S) ALTERNATIVO(S)
Os microrganismos criptocócicos são propensos a adquirir resistência ao tratamento antifúngico. Anfotericina B (intravenosa) — cães e gatos irresponsivos aos triazóis; monitorizar os níveis de ureia de perto para evitar danos renais permanentes.

ACOMPANHAMENTO
MONITORIZAÇÃO DO PACIENTE
• Monitorizar as enzimas hepáticas mensalmente em pacientes submetidos a agente antifúngico triazol.
• A melhora dos sinais clínicos, a resolução das lesões, o restabelecimento do bem-estar e o retorno do apetite estimam a resposta terapêutica.
• Títulos do antígeno capsular — após 2 meses de terapia, os títulos deverão diminuir de forma substancial se o tratamento for eficaz; em caso de ineficácia terapêutica, tentar a terbinafina, já que o microrganismo pode se tornar resistente.
• Continuar a monitorização dos títulos antigênicos a cada 1-2 meses durante o tratamento e, após a interrupção do tratamento, identificar a ocorrência de recidiva da doença. Tentam-se atingir títulos iguais a zero. Em alguns animais, baixos títulos antigênicos persistem por um longo período de tempo.

PREVENÇÃO
O microrganismo é ubíquo, sendo impossível evitá-lo.

COMPLICAÇÕES POSSÍVEIS
Os pacientes com a doença neurológica podem apresentar crises convulsivas e alterações neurológicas permanentes.

EVOLUÇÃO ESPERADA E PROGNÓSTICO
Tratamento — duração prevista de 4 meses a 1 ano; os pacientes com doença do SNC podem necessitar de manutenção pelo resto da vida. O tempo médio de um tratamento bem-sucedido com o fluconazol foi de 4 meses, enquanto com o itraconazol, 8 meses.

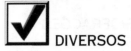
DIVERSOS
DISTÚRBIOS ASSOCIADOS
N/D.

FATORES RELACIONADOS COM A IDADE
N/D.

POTENCIAL ZOONÓTICO
• Embora não seja considerada uma zoonose, há possibilidade de transmissão por meio de feridas ocasionadas por mordeduras.
• Informar o proprietário sobre a aquisição do microrganismo a partir do ambiente, o que aumenta o risco de transmissão, especialmente em estados imunossuprimidos.

GESTAÇÃO/FERTILIDADE/REPRODUÇÃO
N/D.

ABREVIATURA(S)
• ELISA = ensaio imunoabsorvente ligado à enzima.
• LCS = líquido cerebrospinal.
• PIF = peritonite infecciosa felina.
• SNC = sistema nervoso central.
• RM = ressonância magnética.
• TC = tomografia computadorizada.

Sugestões de Leitura
Jacobs GJ, Medleau L, Clavert C, et al. Cryptococcal infection in cats: Factors influencing treatment outcome, and results of sequential serum antigen titers in 35 cats. J Vet Intern Med 1997, 11:1-4.
Malik R, Craig AJ, Wigney DI, et al. Combination chemotherapy of canine and feline cryptococcosis using subcutaneously administered amphotericin B. Australian Vet J 1996, 73:124-128.
Medleau L, Jacobs GJ, Marks A. Itraconazole for the treatment of cryptococcosis in cats. J Vet Intern Med 1995, 9:39-42.
O'Brien CR, Krockenberger MB, Martin P, et al. Long-term outcome of therapy for 59 cats and 11 dogs with cryptococcosis. Australian Vet J 2006, 84:384-392.
O'Brien CR, Krockenberger MB, Wigney DI, et al. Retrospective study of feline and canine cryptococcosis in Australia from 1981 to 2001: 195 cases. Med Mycol 2004, 42:449-460.

Autor Alfred M. Legendre
Consultor Editorial Stephen C. Barr

CRIPTORQUIDISMO

CONSIDERAÇÕES GERAIS

REVISÃO
- A descida incompleta de um ou ambos os testículos para o escroto.
- Inguinal — testículo retido frequentemente palpável.
- Abdominal — dificuldade de palpação ou identificação do testículo por meio da radiologia; a ultrassonografia constitui a melhor opção disponível para determinar o tamanho e a localização do testículo.
- Descida para a posição escrotal final — espera-se que ela seja concluída em 2 meses pós-parto; pode ocorrer mais tarde em algumas raças, mas raramente após 6 meses em qualquer animal específico; presumir o diagnóstico se não houver nenhum testículo palpável em 2 meses.
- Beagle — testículos no anel inguinal exterior em torno do 5º dia pós-parto, entre o anel inguinal e o escroto por volta do 15º dia e no escroto em torno do 40º dia.

IDENTIFICAÇÃO
- Cães — relatado em quase todas as raças; Chihuahua, Poodle *toy*, Pomerânia e Yorkshire terrier; as raças *toy* e miniatura apresentam um risco 2,7 vezes maior de criptorquidismo em comparação àquelas de porte maior; em certas populações, as raças Pastor alemão, Boxer e Staffordshire bull terrier também exibem um risco acentuadamente elevado; o unilateral é mais comum que o bilateral (75:25); nos cães, o testículo direito fica retido em uma frequência duas vezes maior que o esquerdo; nos gatos, os testículos direito e esquerdo ficam retidos em uma frequência equivalente.
- Incidência — cães, relatam-se faixas de 0,8-10%; no entanto, a incidência aumenta com a proporção de cães de raça pura na população; gatos, 1-1,7%; incidência de 50% no Schnauzer miniatura afetado por síndrome de persistência dos ductos mullerianos.
- Genética (cães) — o modo exato de herança é desconhecido; base genética complexa; provavelmente traço poligênico recessivo; provavelmente hereditário.
- Genética (gatos) — pode ser hereditário; no entanto, não há dados que comprovem o defeito hereditário; levantamentos indicam o gato Persa como uma raça super-representada.

SINAIS CLÍNICOS
- Os animais com criptorquidismo bilateral são inférteis, enquanto aqueles com a forma unilateral da doença são tipicamente férteis.
- Raramente associados à dor ou a outros sinais de doença.
- Início agudo de dor abdominal — o cordão espermático dos testículos retidos apresenta alto risco de torção; 36% dos testículos retidos com torção desse cordão eram neoplásicos.
- Síndrome paraneoplásica de feminização — os sertolinomas secretores de estrogênio em testículos retidos produzem sinais de feminização: ginecomastia, alopecia simétrica do tronco e dos flancos, hiperpigmentação da pele inguinal, bainha prepucial pendulosa, metaplasia escamosa prostática.

CAUSAS E FATORES DE RISCO
- Remoção de machos acometidos das linhagens de reprodução — acredita-se que isso ocasione uma redução na frequência do quadro e que a hereditariedade envolva mais de um gene.
- Fatores predisponentes não hereditários (p. ex., peso ao nascimento) — identificados em seres humanos; ainda não foram descritos em cães.

DIAGNÓSTICO

DIAGNÓSTICO DIFERENCIAL
- Castração — diferenciar uma condição bilateral de castração prévia, castração precedente de um único testículo escrotal com testículo abdominal retido, ou anorquidismo (raro).
- Os gatos com criptorquidismo bilateral podem apresentar odor urinário e comportamento de animais intactos.

OUTROS TESTES LABORATORIAIS
Teste de estimulação com hCG — duplica a testosterona sanguínea em caso de afecção bilateral; duplica a testosterona sanguínea em caso de afecção unilateral na qual se removeu apenas o testículo escrotal; diferencia entre criptorquidismo e castração; esse teste consiste na administração de 750 UI de hCG por via IV ou 50 μg de GnRH por via IM, com coleta das amostras sanguíneas pré e 2-3 h pós-injeção; os cães castrados apresentam concentrações de testosterona <0,1 ng/mL e não se estimulam com a administração do hCG ou do GnRH.

DIAGNÓSTICO POR IMAGEM
Ultrassonografia transabdominal — exame muito específico e eficiente para localizar os testículos nas regiões inguinal ou abdominal.

TRATAMENTO
- Nenhum tratamento é recomendado, exceto a castração de ambos os testículos, tanto do retido como do escrotal.
- Orquiopexia — posicionamento cirúrgico de um testículo retido no interior do escroto; intervenção considerada antiética.
- hCG ou GnRH — evidências não publicadas de indução da descida quando administrados aos cães com menos de 4 meses de vida.
- Alertar o proprietário quanto ao risco elevado de neoplasia testicular em cães com testículos retidos; incentivá-lo a castrar seu cão por volta dos 4 anos de idade; 53% dos sertolinomas e 36% dos seminomas ocorrem em testículos retidos.

MEDICAÇÕES

MEDICAMENTO(S)
- hCG (cães) — 100-1.000 UI por via IM, quatro vezes, em um período de 2 semanas antes de 16 semanas de vida (cães); depois de 16 semanas, esse medicamento não costuma ter êxito.
- GnRH (cães) — 50-750 μg, 1-6 vezes, entre 2 e 4 meses de vida.

ACOMPANHAMENTO
- A descida após 4 meses de vida é rara; depois de 6 meses, torna-se improvável.
- Acredita-se que o risco de neoplasia testicular seja aproximadamente 13,6 vezes maior em cães acometidos que nos normais; os testículos retidos exibem maior risco de torção do cordão espermático.

DIVERSOS

DISTÚRBIOS ASSOCIADOS
- Hérnia inguinal, hérnia umbilical.
- Displasia do coxal.
- Luxação patelar.
- Defeitos penianos e prepuciais (p. ex., hipospadias).

VER TAMBÉM
- Seminoma.
- Sertolinoma.
- Distúrbios do Desenvolvimento Sexual.

ABREVIATURA(S)
- GnRH = hormônio liberador de gonadotropina.
- hCG = gonadotropina coriônica humana.

RECURSOS DA INTERNET
Memon M, Tibary A. Canine and feline cryptorchidism. In: Concannon PW, England G, Verstegen III J, Linde-Forsberg C, eds., Recent Advances in Small Animal Reproduction. International Veterinary Information Service, Ithaca NY, www.ivis.org, 2001; A1217.0901.

Sugestões de Leitura
Birchard SJ, Nappier M. Cryptorchidism. Compend Contin Educ Pract Vet 2008, 30(6):325-337.
England GCW, Allen WE, Porter DJ. Evaluation of the testosterone response to hCG and the identification of a presumed anorchid dog. J Small Anim Pract 1989, 30(8):441-443.
Feldman EC, Nelson RW. Canine and Feline Endocrinology and Reproduction. Philadelphia: Saunders, 1987, pp. 697-699.
Hecht S, King R, Tidwell AS, Gorman SC. Ultrasound diagnosis: Intra-abdominal torsion of a non-neoplastic testicle in a cryptorchid dog. Vet Radiol Ultrasound 2004, 45(1):58-61.
Johnston SD, Root Kustritz MV, Olson PNS. Disorders of the canine testes and epididymes. In: Canine and Feline Theriogenology. Philadelphia: Saunders, 2001, pp. 312-332.
Johnston SD, Root Kustritz MV, Olson PNS. Disorders of the feline testes and epididymes. In: Canine and Feline Theriogenology. Philadelphia: Saunders, 2001, pp. 525-536.
Romagnoli SE. Canine cryptorchidism. Vet Clin North Am Small Anim Pract 1991, 21:533-544.
Yates D, Hayes G, Heffernan M, Beynon R. Incidence of cryptorchidism in dogs and cats. Vet Record 2003, 152(16):502-504.

Autor Carlos R.F. Pinto
Consultor Editorial Sara K. Lyle

Criptosporidiose

CONSIDERAÇÕES GERAIS

REVISÃO
- *Cryptosporidium* spp. — protozoário coccídio; causa gastrenteropatia em cães, gatos, seres humanos, bezerros e roedores; microrganismo ubíquo na natureza; distribuição mundial; ciclo vital entérico. • Infecção — ao se ingerir oocistos esporulados, ocorre a liberação de esporozoítos, que penetram no epitélio intestinal; após a reprodução assexuada, liberam-se merozoítos para infectar outras células. • Período pré-patente — gatos, 5-10 dias. • Animais imunocompetentes — enteropatia. • Animais imunocomprometidos — infecções do trato intestinal e respiratório, bem como do fígado, da vesícula biliar e do pâncreas. • Gatos — a sorologia sugere uma exposição de aproximadamente 15% nos animais dessa espécie nos Estados Unidos.

IDENTIFICAÇÃO
- Cães e gatos. • Não há predileção sexual ou racial. • Cães — praticamente todos os casos clínicos ocorrem em animais com ≤6 meses de vida; os cães idosos podem excretar oocistos, sem manifestar sinais clínicos. • Mais comum em filhotes felinos jovens e recém-nascidos com <6 meses de vida.

SINAIS CLÍNICOS
- A maior parte das infecções é subclínica.
- Consistem principalmente em diarreia do intestino delgado. • Há relatos de diarreia proveniente do intestino grosso.

CAUSAS E FATORES DE RISCO
- *C. canis* (cães) e *C. felis* (gatos) — adquiridos por meio da ingestão de água ou fezes contaminadas.
- Em termos morfológicos, as espécies são muito semelhantes. • Algumas espécies são hospedeiro-específicas (*C. canis* e *C. felis*); outras (*C. parvum*) infectam múltiplas espécies. • Praticamente todos os casos clínicos são relatados em gatos imunocomprometidos. • Imunossupressão — principal fator de risco; são causas comuns: FeLV (gatos), vírus da cinomose (cães), parvovírus canino e linfoma intestinal (cães e gatos).
- Animais imunocompetentes — geralmente sofrem infecção intestinal assintomática com liberação de oocistos nas fezes por 2 semanas.
- Animais imunocomprometidos — enterite e, possivelmente, infecções respiratórias, hepáticas, biliares e pancreáticas.

DIAGNÓSTICO

DIAGNÓSTICO DIFERENCIAL
- Imprudência ou intolerância alimentar.
- Medicamentos — antibióticos. • Toxinas — chumbo. • Parasitas — giardíase, tricuríase.
- Agentes infecciosos — parvovírus, coronavírus, PIF, *Salmonella*, *Campylobacter*, *Rickettsia*, *Histoplasma*. • Comprometimento em outros órgãos — insuficiências cardíaca, renal, hepática e pancreática exócrina. • Doenças metabólicas — hipoadrenocorticismo, hipertireoidismo (gatos).
- Neoplasias — linfoma intestinal. • Doenças infiltrativas — por exemplo, enteropatia inflamatória.

HEMOGRAMA/BIOQUÍMICA/URINÁLISE
Costumam permanecer normais a menos que haja uma doença imunossupressora subjacente.

MÉTODOS DIAGNÓSTICOS
- Teste de detecção de antígenos fecais (ProSpecT *Cryptosporidium* Microtiter Assay; Color-Vue *Cryptosporidium*) — disponível.
- Flutuação em açúcar e sulfato de zinco — densidade = 1,18; promove a concentração de oocistos fecais (como os oocistos possuem 5 μm, a flotação rotineira em solução salina frequentemente fracassa); os oocistos são observados de forma mais eficiente após coloração com corante acidorresistente modificado.
- Técnicas de imunofluorescência — disponível em alguns laboratórios (Meridian Diagnostics).
- Envio de fezes a um laboratório — misturar 1 parte de formalina a 100% com 9 partes de fezes para inativar os oocistos e diminuir o risco à saúde dos funcionários do laboratório.
- Técnica de PCR — disponível no laboratório Animal Disease Diagnostic do estado de Michigan nos Estados Unidos; cerca de 10-100 vezes mais sensível para o diagnóstico de criptosporidiose em gatos do que outras técnicas.
- Citometria de fluxo — pode aumentar a sensibilidade de detecção dos oocistos.
- Biopsia intestinal — identificação citológica e histopatológica de microrganismos intracelulares; diagnóstica, mas pouco prática; pode gerar resultados falso-negativos.

ACHADOS PATOLÓGICOS
- Lesões macroscópicas — linfonodos mesentéricos infartados; mucosa intestinal (particularmente do íleo) hiperêmica; fixar as amostras em solução de Bouin ou de formalina dentro de algumas horas após o óbito, pois a autólise provoca a rápida perda da superfície intestinal que contém os microrganismos.
- Lesões microscópicas — atrofia vilosa; tecido linfoide reativo; infiltrados inflamatórios na lâmina própria; é possível encontrar os parasitas por todo o intestino, mas eles costumam ser mais numerosos na porção distal do intestino delgado.

TRATAMENTO
- Esquema ambulatorial.
- Em animais imunocompetentes — a diarreia costuma ser leve e autolimitante.
- Alimento — pode suspendê-lo por 24-48 h até que a diarreia esteja sob controle.
- Diarreia leve — solução glicoeletrolítica oral (Entrolyte®, SmithKline).
- Diarreia grave com desidratação — fluidos parenterais (isotônicos com adição de potássio).

MEDICAÇÕES

MEDICAMENTO(S)
- Paromomicina (Humatin®) — 125-165 mg/kg VO a cada 12 h por 5 dias; antibiótico aminoglicosídeo eficaz no tratamento de pacientes com problemas intestinais agudos; pode causar doença renal em animais jovens com a barreira gastrintestinal lesionada. A toxicidade responde à diurese; monitorizar a toxicidade renal, avaliando-se a urina em busca de cilindros.
- Tilosina — 11 mg/kg VO a cada 12 h por 28 dias; mostrou-se eficiente no tratamento de um gato acometido que também sofria de duodenite linfocítica.
- Nitazoxanida (Alinia®, 25 mg/kg VO a cada 24 h por 7-28 dias) — registrada para o tratamento de criptosporidiose e giardíase em seres humanos; interrompe a liberação de oocistos em gatos; a dosagem costuma ser associada a vômito, que pode ser amenizado com antieméticos (p. ex., clorpromazina). Foi utilizada apenas em um número limitado de gatos com criptosporidiose e, por essa razão, há necessidade de mais avaliações. Poucos efeitos colaterais além do vômito.

ACOMPANHAMENTO
- Monitorizar a melhora clínica quanto à eficácia terapêutica.
- Monitorizar a liberação de oocistos nas fezes 2 semanas após o término do tratamento ou mediante a persistência dos sinais.
- Prognóstico excelente, caso se consiga superar a causa da imunossupressão.

DIVERSOS

POTENCIAL ZOONÓTICO
Alertar os proprietários sobre o potencial de transmissão zoonótica a partir dos microrganismos liberados nas fezes e quanto ao maior risco apresentado por pessoas imunocomprometidas (p. ex., pacientes HIV positivo ou aqueles submetidos à quimioterapia ou corticosteroides sistêmicos). Contudo, há indícios crescentes de que a transmissão de *Cryptosporidia* spp. de cães e gatos para os seres humanos seja extremamente rara em virtude da especificidade ao hospedeiro.

Desinfecção
- Microrganismo resistente a alvejante comercial (hipoclorito de sódio a 5,25%) e cloração da água de bebida.
- Solução de formaldeído a 10% ou de amônia a 5% eliminará os oocistos, mas há necessidade de 18 horas de exposição.
- Concentrações mais altas de amônia (50%) eliminarão os oocistos em 30 minutos.
- Calor úmido (vapor ou pasteurização [>55°C]), congelamento e descongelamento ou secagem minuciosa também são medidas eficazes.

ABREVIATURA(S)
- PIF = peritonite infecciosa felina.
- FeLV = vírus da leucemia felina.
- HIV = vírus da imunodeficiência felina.
- PCR = reação em cadeia da polimerase.

Sugestões de Leitura
Lappin MR. Diagnosis and management of Cryptosporidiosis in dogs and cats. Proc Am Col Vet Int Med 2002, 20:654-656.
Palmer CS, Traub RJ, Robertson ID, et al. Determining the zoonotic significance of Giardia and Cryptosporidium in Australian dogs and cats. Vet Parasitol 2008, 154:142-147.

Autor Stephen C. Barr
Consultor Editorial Stephen C. Barr

CRISES CONVULSIVAS (CONVULSÕES, ESTADO EPILÉPTICO) — CÃES

CONSIDERAÇÕES GERAIS

DEFINIÇÃO
• Epilepsia — recidiva de crises convulsivas de origem cerebral primária. • Epilepsia idiopática — apenas epilepsia, sem lesão cerebral subjacente observável ou outros sinais ou sintomas neurológicos. • Epilepsia sintomática — as crises convulsivas são o resultado de lesões cerebrais estruturais identificáveis. • Epilepsia provavelmente sintomática — quando há suspeita de epilepsia sintomática, mas não se consegue demonstrar uma lesão. • Crises convulsivas aglomeradas — >1 crise/24 horas. • Estado epiléptico — atividade convulsiva contínua ou crises convulsivas repetidas em intervalos breves sem recuperação plena entre as crises. • O estado epiléptico pode ser focal ou generalizado. • As crises convulsivas são classificadas como focais, generalizadas e focais com generalização secundária.

FISIOPATOLOGIA
• Desorganização paroxística de 1 ou várias funções cerebrais que se originam da região corticotalâmica. Qualquer distúrbio ou processo patológico nesse nível pode levar à atividade convulsiva. • Nem todas as regiões corticais têm a mesma propensão para crises convulsivas; seguem as regiões mais prováveis a menos prováveis de causarem crises — lobos temporais, frontais, parietais e occipitais. • Conforme ocorrem mais crises convulsivas, há tendência a dano neuronal e propensão a mais crises ou aumento do estado epiléptico; esse efeito de ativação propagada não ocorre em todas as regiões corticais. • O aspecto clínico da crise convulsiva está relacionado com a localização da hiperatividade neuronal. Se a anormalidade elétrica permanecer regional, as crises convulsivas serão focais. Se houver recrutamento de ambos os hemisférios, as crises convulsivas evoluirão para uma forma generalizada.

SISTEMA(S) ACOMETIDO(S)
Nervoso.

IDENTIFICAÇÃO
Cães de qualquer raça, idade ou sexo.

SINAIS CLÍNICOS
Comentários Gerais
• Pródromo — horas a dias antes da crise convulsiva; sem alterações EEG. • Aura — início de uma crise convulsiva; indica início focal; o cão pode parecer assustado, procurar por assistência do proprietário, etc. • Icto — pode começar com uma aura e evoluir para crises convulsivas generalizadas; decúbito lateral com contrações tônico-clônicas simétricas bilaterais dos músculos dos membros; frequentemente é acompanhado por sinais autonômicos, p. ex., salivação, micção, defecação. • Fase pós-ictal — desorientação, confusão mental, deambulação sem rumo, cegueira, polidipsia, polifagia. • Uma crise convulsiva dura <2 min. • A maioria das crises convulsivas ocorre quando o cão está em repouso ou dormindo. • Em crises convulsivas focais, o cão apresenta-se consciente, mas costuma exibir alteração da atividade mental; indicam lesão cerebral focal; podem se generalizar; a atividade motora frequentemente predomina de 1 lado (o lado oposto à lesão cerebral).

Achados Anamnésicos
• Confirmar no histórico que a crise convulsiva de fato ocorreu. • Padrão das crises convulsivas (idade de início da crise, além do tipo e da frequência das crises) — fator mais importante para definir a lista das possíveis causas. • Doenças metabólicas costumam causar crises convulsivas generalizadas. • Sinais neurológicos assimétricos antes, durante ou depois das crises convulsivas indicam lesão cerebral estrutural. • Presença de alterações comportamentais nos dias/semanas que antecedem o início das crises convulsivas indica doença cerebral estrutural. • O paciente pode ser conhecido como epiléptico.

Achados do Exame Físico
• Animal pós-ictal ou normal à apresentação. • Atividade mental, respostas à ameaça, resposta à estimulação do septo nasal e posicionamento proprioceptivo — testes neurológicos que avaliam o córtex cerebral. A assimetria indica lesão cerebral estrutural. • Estado epiléptico em estágio compensado, nos primeiros 30 min — salivação, hipertermia, taquicardia, arritmia, aumento da pressão arterial. • Estado epiléptico em estágio descompensado — dificuldade respiratória, pulso débil (fraco), hipotensão arterial, preenchimento capilar lento.

CAUSAS
Extracranianas
• Metabólicas — hipoglicemia; hipocalcemia; insuficiência renal aguda; encefalopatia hepática. • Toxinas epileptogênicas (p. ex., metaldeído, piretrinas, chumbo, hexaclorofeno, hidrocarbonetos clorados, organofosforados, micotoxinas).

Intracranianas
• Degenerativas — encefalopatia. • Más-formações. • Metabólicas — doenças de armazenamento celular. • Neoplásicas — primárias (gliomas, meningioma); secundárias (metastática). • Infecciosas inflamatórias — virais (p. ex., cinomose); fúngicas; protozoárias (*Neospora*, *Toxoplasma*); riquetsianas (erliquiose, febre maculosa das Montanhas Rochosas). • Idiopáticas ou imunomediadas — meningoencefalomielite granulomatosa; meningoencefalomielite eosinofílica; encefalite do Pug; meningoencefalite necrosante das raças Maltês e Yorkshire terrier. • Traumáticas. • Vasculares — acidente vascular cerebral. • Epilepsia idiopática. • Epilepsia provavelmente sintomática — cicatriz glial pós-encefalítica, displasia cortical.

DIAGNÓSTICO

DIAGNÓSTICO DIFERENCIAL
• Síncope — o corpo fica mole, com uma fase de recuperação rápida, sem comportamento anormal; ocorre com atividade física, tosse, agitação. • Aparecimento superagudo de crises convulsivas e comportamento anormal — provável AVC. • Transtornos obsessivos-compulsivos ou estereótipos — comportamentos complexos e direcionados a algum alvo; o comportamento pode ser interrompido. • Toxinas epileptogênicas — evolução de tremor em todo o corpo para estado epiléptico e morte se deixado sem tratamento. • Encefalopatia metabólica — crises convulsivas não usuais e acompanhadas por obnubilação e comportamento anormal; sem sinais lateralizantes. • Provável doença cerebral estrutural — em caso de início agudo de >2 crises convulsivas generalizadas dentro da primeira semana de início, início agudo de crises convulsivas focais com evolução gradativa para crises generalizadas ou presença de déficits neurológicos interictais incluindo alterações comportamentais. • Epilepsia idiopática — diferenciada com base na idade, na raça e no padrão das crises convulsivas; início progressivo de crises convulsivas generalizadas com ou sem aura. • Dor/espasmos cervicais — podem ser confundidos com crises convulsivas focais. • Oscilação da cabeça no sentido vertical ou tremor de cabeça idiopático — o cão permanece ativo; consegue comer, beber e andar.

HEMOGRAMA/BIOQUÍMICA/URINÁLISE
• Doenças infecciosas do SNC — podem refletir envolvimento multissistêmico. • Hipoglicemia — raças de porte pequeno/toy durante a ocorrência de estado epiléptico. • Disfunção hepática e renal — estado epiléptico avançado.

OUTROS TESTES LABORATORIAIS
• Gases sanguíneos — é frequente a presença de acidose metabólica com estado epiléptico. • Perfil de coagulação — CID em estado epiléptico avançado. • Ácidos biliares — suspeita de encefalopatia hepática. • Glicemia de jejum e relação alterada de insulina:glicose — cães com >5 anos e crises convulsivas ocasionais durante o exercício. • Sorologia (doenças infecciosas) — se os sinais sistêmicos e as anormalidades laboratoriais sugerirem doença.

DIAGNÓSTICO POR IMAGEM
• Radiografias torácicas e ultrassonografia abdominal — para identificar doença metastática ou sistêmica ou, então, patologia pulmonar decorrente do estado epiléptico. • RM — melhor para definir o local, a extensão e a natureza da lesão.

MÉTODOS DIAGNÓSTICOS
• Exame do LCS — na suspeita de causa estrutural intracraniana; títulos do LCS e do soro, bem como PCR, para diagnosticar doenças infecciosas.

TRATAMENTO

CUIDADO(S) DE SAÚDE ADEQUADO(S)
• Ambulatorial — para crises convulsivas isoladas em um cão saudável sob outros aspectos. • Internação — para crises convulsivas aglomeradas e estado epiléptico.

CUIDADO(S) DE ENFERMAGEM E DE SUPORTE
• Proceder à supervisão constante do paciente. • Resfriar o animal em caso de hipertermia. • Estabelecer via de acesso IV para administração de medicamentos e fluidos. • Coletar o sangue para mensuração rápida dos níveis de gases sanguíneos, glicose, cálcio e medicamentos anticonvulsivantes se pertinentes.

DIETA
Dieta cetogênica — não se mostrou eficaz.

ORIENTAÇÃO AO PROPRIETÁRIO
• Tratar as crises convulsivas aglomeradas e o estado epiléptico generalizado precocemente — quanto mais crises convulsivas em um determinado período, maiores serão a quantidade de medicamentos para controle da crise, o tempo

Crises Convulsivas (Convulsões, Estado Epiléptico) — Cães

para recuperação e o custo do tratamento. • O tratamento anticonvulsivante, em epilepsia sintomática, pode não ajudar até que a causa primária seja tratada. • Manter um calendário das crises convulsivas, anotando a data, o horário, a gravidade e a duração das crises. • Esboçar um plano terapêutico de emergência em casa para crises convulsivas aglomeradas.

CONSIDERAÇÕES CIRÚRGICAS
• Craniotomia — excisão de tumor em caso de meningioma ou outra massa acessível.

MEDICAÇÕES

MEDICAMENTO(S) DE ESCOLHA
O tipo e a frequência das crises convulsivas determinam a abordagem terapêutica.

Crises Convulsivas Aglomeradas ou Estado Epiléptico

Diazepam
• Administrar bólus IV de 0,5-1 mg/kg; repetir 5 min depois se a atividade motora visível não tiver desaparecido; acompanhar com 0,5-1 mg/kg/h sob infusão em velocidade constante adicionada aos fluidos de manutenção em uma bureta embutida na linha de acesso venoso. • Retal — não deve substituir a administração intravenosa em situação de emergência; usar apenas nos casos em que não se consegue obter o acesso IV; pode diminuir ou interromper a atividade convulsiva motora visível para permitir a colocação do cateter IV. • Pode ocorrer o rápido desenvolvimento de refratariedade, exigindo a adição de fenobarbital sob infusão em velocidade constante.

Fenobarbital
• Adicionar caso as crises convulsivas persistam após o segundo bólus de diazepam ou durante a infusão desse medicamento em velocidade constante; administrar o fenobarbital sob infusão em velocidade constante (2-6 mg/cão/h adicionados à infusão de diazepam) se o paciente já estiver sendo tratado com o fenobarbital ou como dose de ataque se o paciente nunca foi submetido a ele. • Dose de ataque (mg totais) = (nível sérico desejado em mg/L) × (peso corporal em kg) × (0,8 L/kg); administrar um quarto da dose de ataque a cada 15 min até se obter o efeito desejado. Faixa terapêutica ideal = 100-120 μmol/L (23-28 mg/L). • Se o paciente já estiver sob efeito do fenobarbital, obter o nível sérico antes de iniciar a infusão desse medicamento em velocidade constante. Pode ser administrada a dose de 2-5 mg/kg em bólus IV enquanto se aguardam os resultados. • Assim que as crises convulsivas estiverem controladas por 4-6 h, desmamar o paciente da infusão de forma gradativa ao longo de muitas horas. • Iniciar ou retomar o tratamento anticonvulsivante de manutenção por via oral, utilizando o fenobarbital e/ou o brometo de potássio e/ou outros agentes anticonvulsivantes para crises generalizadas assim que o paciente for capaz de engolir.

Outros
• Se as crises convulsivas continuarem, o propofol será administrado na dose de 2-8 mg/kg IV lentamente em 60 s, acompanhado por infusão em velocidade constante na dose de 0,1-0,6 mg/kg/min; monitorizar o paciente anestesiado com EEG para avaliar a resposta ao tratamento. • Brometo de potássio — não utilizar para tratar estado epiléptico; meia-vida muito longa; a dose de ataque não é recomendada. • Dexametasona — 0,25 mg/kg a cada 24 h por 1-3 dias; diminui o edema cerebral. • Dexametasona — para tratamento agudo de edema cerebral secundário à doença inflamatória grave do SNC, mesmo se infecciosa.

Estado Epiléptico Focal Agudo
• É importante procurar e tratar a causa primária. • Diazepam e fenobarbital sob infusão em velocidade constante — eficazes para crises focais e generalizadas. • Com frequência, não é fácil controlar esse tipo de estado epiléptico. • Muitos casos de estado epiléptico focal crônico — o proprietário não tem consciência de que ele está ocorrendo (p. ex., encefalopatia senil); se as crises convulsivas permanecerem focais e a qualidade de vida do paciente não sofrer alteração significativa, não haverá necessidade de tratamento. Efetuar o tratamento anticonvulsivante a longo prazo se necessário — fenobarbital (3-5 mg/kg a cada 12 h VO), levetiracetam (20 mg/kg a cada 12-8 h VO) ou zonisamida (5 mg/kg a cada 12 h VO).

CONTRAINDICAÇÕES
• Aminofilina, teofilina — agitação do SNC; podem causar crises convulsivas. • Esteroides — alteram os parâmetros do LCS; evitar caso se contemple a análise desse líquido.

PRECAUÇÕES
• Fenobarbital — ligado à proteína e metabolizado pelo fígado; na hipoalbuminemia ou hepatopatia, reduzir a dose; monitorizar os níveis com rigor; para o estado epiléptico, adicionar o diazepam com cuidado, porque os medicamentos se potencializam, podendo resultar em depressão cardíaca e respiratória. • Esteroides — contraindicados nas doenças infecciosas, mas uma única dose de dexametasona (0,25 mg/kg IV) pode diminuir o edema cerebral em caso de herniação cerebral iminente ou na suspeita de edema potencialmente letal.

INTERAÇÕES POSSÍVEIS
Cimetidina, ranitidina e cloranfenicol — interferem no metabolismo do fenobarbital; podem levar a níveis tóxicos deste último medicamento.

MEDICAMENTO(S) ALTERNATIVO(S)
Pentobarbital — utilizado se o estado epiléptico não responder ao diazepam e fenobarbital sob infusão em velocidade constante; anestesia profunda para obtenção do efeito anticonvulsivante; há necessidade de monitorização EEG e entubação endotraqueal.

ACOMPANHAMENTO

MONITORAÇÃO DO PACIENTE
• Pacientes internados — necessitam de supervisão constante para monitorização das crises convulsivas. • Contração espasmódica das pálpebras ou dos lábios em paciente intensamente sedado é sinal de atividade convulsiva contínua. • Talvez o paciente necessite de 7-10 dias antes de retornar ao normal após o estado epiléptico; a visão retorna por último.

COMPLICAÇÕES POSSÍVEIS
• Fenobarbital — hepatotoxicidade após tratamento a longo prazo com níveis séricos >140 μmol/L (>33 μg/L); neutropenia aguda (rara) nas primeiras semanas de utilização exige a retirada permanente do medicamento. • As crises convulsivas podem continuar a despeito dos níveis séricos adequados do medicamento anticonvulsivante. • Déficits neurológicos permanentes (p. ex., cegueira, comportamento anormal e sinais cerebelares) podem acompanhar o estado epiléptico grave. • O estado epiléptico generalizado pode levar a hipertermia, desequilíbrios acidobásicos e eletrolíticos, edema pulmonar, colapso cardiovascular e morte.

EVOLUÇÃO ESPERADA E PROGNÓSTICO
• Epilepsia idiopática representa uma grande proporção de cães com estado epiléptico generalizado. É recomendável a tomada de medidas de emergência em casa com o uso de diazepam por via retal. • Cães com encefalite e estado epiléptico generalizado — desfecho insatisfatório. • Cães epilépticos sintomáticos recuperados de doença primária (p. ex., *Ehrlichia canis*) — desmamar o paciente lentamente (durante meses) dos medicamentos anticonvulsivantes após 6 meses livres de crises convulsivas; se as crises retornarem, reinstituir o medicamento anticonvulsivante.

DIVERSOS

FATORES RELACIONADOS COM A IDADE
• O cérebro imaturo tem maior propensão a crises convulsivas. • Epilepsia idiopática — 6 meses a 5 anos de idade; frequentemente grave e refratária quando o início ocorre em <2 anos de idade. • Fenobarbital — uma dose mais elevada é necessária nos filhotes (<5 meses de vida) para atingir a faixa terapêutica; dose inicial de 5 mg/kg a cada 12 h; mensuração dos níveis séricos a cada 5 dias até que os níveis terapêuticos sejam atingidos.

VER TAMBÉM
• Epilepsia — Idiopática (Genética). • Ver a seção "Causas".

ABREVIATURA(S)
• AVC = acidente vascular cerebral. • CID = coagulação intravascular disseminada. • EEG = eletroencefalograma. • LCS = líquido cerebrospinal. • PCR = reação em cadeia da polimerase. • RM = ressonância magnética. • SNC = sistema nervoso central.

Sugestões de Leitura

Parent J. Seizures and status epilepticus in dogs. In: Mathews K, ed., Veterinary Emergency and Critical Care Manual, 2nd ed. Guelph, Ontario: Lifelearn, 2006, pp. 460-464.

Parent J, Poma R. Single seizure, cluster seizures, and status epilepticus. In: Wingfield WE, Raffe MR, eds., The Veterinary ICU Book. Jackson, WY: Teton NewMedia, 2002, pp. 871-879.

Platt SR, Haag M. Canine status epilepticus: A retrospective study of 50 cases. J Small Anim Pract 2002, 43(4):151-153.

Saito M, Muñana KR, Sharp NJ, et al. Risk factors for development of status epilepticus in dogs with idiopathic epilepsy and effects of status epilepticus on outcome and survival time: 32 cases (1990-1996). JAVMA 2001, 219(5):618-623.

Autor Joane M. Parent
Consultor Editorial Joane M. Parent

Crises Convulsivas (Convulsões, Estado Epiléptico) — Gatos

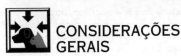

CONSIDERAÇÕES GERAIS

DEFINIÇÃO
• Epilepsia — recidiva de crises convulsivas de origem cerebral primária.
• Epilepsia idiopática — síndrome que se refere apenas à epilepsia, sem lesão cerebral subjacente demonstrável ou outros sinais ou sintomas neurológicos; rara nos gatos.
• Epilepsia sintomática — síndrome em que as crises convulsivas são o resultado de lesões cerebrais estruturais identificáveis; frequente nos gatos.
• Epilepsia provavelmente sintomática — quando há suspeitas de epilepsia sintomática, mas não se consegue demonstrar uma lesão.
• Crises convulsivas aglomeradas — >1 crise/24 h.
• Estado epiléptico — atividade convulsiva contínua ou crises convulsivas repetidas em intervalos breves sem recuperação plena entre as crises. O estado epiléptico pode ser focal ou generalizado. O estado epiléptico convulsivo é uma emergência médica potencialmente letal.

FISIOPATOLOGIA
• Desorganização paroxística de 1 ou várias funções cerebrais que se originam da região corticotalâmica. Qualquer distúrbio ou processo patológico nesse nível pode levar à atividade convulsiva.
• Nem todas as regiões corticais têm a mesma propensão para crises convulsivas; seguem as regiões mais prováveis a menos prováveis de causarem crises — lobos temporais, frontais, parietais e occipitais.
• Conforme ocorrem mais crises convulsivas, há tendência a dano neuronal e propensão a mais crises ou aumento do estado epiléptico; esse efeito de ativação propagada não ocorre em todas as regiões corticais.
• O aspecto clínico da crise convulsiva está diretamente relacionado com a localização da hiperatividade neuronal. Se a anormalidade elétrica permanecer regional, as crises convulsivas serão focais. Se houver recrutamento de ambos os hemisférios, as crises convulsivas evoluirão para uma forma generalizada.
• A grande maioria das crises convulsivas e do estado epiléptico nos gatos é secundária a lesões cerebrais estruturais.

SISTEMA(S) ACOMETIDO(S)
Nervoso.

INCIDÊNCIA/PREVALÊNCIA
Desconhecidas.

DISTRIBUIÇÃO MUNDIAL
Mundial.

IDENTIFICAÇÃO
Gatos de qualquer idade, raça ou sexo.

SINAIS CLÍNICOS
Comentários Gerais
• Crises convulsivas focais com ou sem generalização secundária são as mais frequentes; os movimentos da musculatura facial predominam, como contrações espasmódicas das pálpebras, dos bigodes e das orelhas; podem estar associadas a tremor/agitação de todo o corpo, movimentos unilaterais dos membros, piloereção, pupilas dilatadas, corrida frenética e colisão com objetos. O estado epiléptico focal é frequente.
• Em crises convulsivas motoras tônico-clônicas generalizadas, há contrações tônico-clônicas simétricas bilaterais de músculos dos membros e dorsiflexão da cabeça, associados muitas vezes a sinais autonômicos, como salivação, micção, defecação. No momento da admissão hospitalar, a atividade motora visível pode ter sido interrompida, embora ainda possa haver contrações espasmódicas das pálpebras e movimentos rítmicos do corpo/membro.
• É frequente a automutilação — mordida da língua, avulsão da unha.

Achados Anamnésicos
• Confirmar no histórico que a atividade convulsiva de fato ocorreu.
• Padrão das crises convulsivas (idade de início da crise, além do tipo e da frequência das crises) — fator mais importante na listagem das possíveis causas.
• Doenças metabólicas causam crises convulsivas generalizadas.
• Com a maioria das toxinas epileptogênicas, há um aumento gradual de hiperexcitabilidade, agitação, tremor e, por fim, crises convulsivas generalizadas e óbito.
• A assimetria nos sinais (contrações espasmódicas das pálpebras, movimentos dos membros principalmente de um lado, andar em círculo) antes, durante ou depois da crise convulsiva indica lesão focal do córtex cerebral.
• Fatores como dosagem excessiva de insulina, pós-transplante renal, tireoidectomia bilateral levam a crises convulsivas generalizadas logo após o fato.
• A presença de comportamento anormal nos dias/semanas que antecedem a atividade convulsiva indica doença cerebral estrutural.
• A existência de sinais gastrintestinais, respiratórios ou outros sinais sistêmicos concomitantes sugere doença sistêmica.

Achados do Exame Físico
• Atividade mental, resposta à ameaça, resposta à estimulação do septo nasal e posicionamento proprioceptivo são testes neurológicos que avaliam o córtex cerebral. A assimetria indica lesão cerebral estrutural na face contralateral dos déficits.
• Na presença de coriorretinite, procurar por doenças infecciosas.
• Mucosas de coloração vermelho-escura sugerem policitemia vera.

CAUSAS
Extracranianas
• Metabólicas — hipoglicemia por dosagem excessiva de insulina, hipocalcemia por tireoidectomia bilateral, hipertensão secundária a transplante renal, encefalopatia hepática.
• Toxinas.

Intracranianas
• Anatômicas — má-formação congênita.
• Metabólicas — doença de armazenamento celular (p. ex., lipofuscinose ceroide neuronal relatada em um único gato com mioclonia e atividade convulsiva).
• Neoplásicas — meningioma, glioma, linfoma.
• Infecciosas inflamatórias — viral sem PIF, PIF, toxoplasmose, criptococose.
• Traumáticas.
• Toxicidade — organoclorados, piretrinas e piretroides; as crises convulsivas costumam ser observadas no estágio terminal; clorambucila no tratamento de linfoma.
• Vasculares — policitemia vera secundária à hiperviscosidade, encefalopatia isquêmica felina secundária à larva de *Cuterebra*.

FATORES DE RISCO
• Qualquer lesão do prosencéfalo.
• Tratamento com clorambucila.
• Insuficiência renal.
• Diabetes melito.

DIAGNÓSTICO

DIAGNÓSTICO DIFERENCIAL
• Distúrbios do sono — o gato não acorda ou tem um comportamento de vigília normal após o episódio.
• Síncope — o corpo fica mole, com uma fase de recuperação rápida, sem comportamento anormal.
• Aparecimento superagudo de crises convulsivas e comportamento anormal — provável evento vascular.
• Quando as crises convulsivas são precedidas por doença sistêmica transitória vaga (hiporexia, sinais GI nas semanas que antecedem o aparecimento das crises convulsivas em um gato saudável sob outros aspectos — encefalite viral não relacionada com PIF ou de etiologia desconhecida.
• Quando as crises convulsivas são precedidas por sinais sistêmicos que persistem (>3 semanas) — criptococose, PIF.
• Comportamento anormal insidioso com ou sem andar em círculo em gato com >10 anos de idade que se apresenta com atividade convulsiva sugere meningioma.
• Gatos com encefalopatia hepática exibem salivação excessiva.
• Gatos com policitemia vera apresentam sinais GI e mucosas escuras.
• Estro — fêmeas intactas; comportamento associado ao estro.

HEMOGRAMA/BIOQUÍMICA/URINÁLISE
• Hematócrito elevado (>60%) em casos de policitemia vera.
• Glicemia baixa com dosagem excessiva de insulina.
• Baixos níveis de cálcio em pós-tireoidectomia bilateral.
• Altos níveis de ureia e creatinina com densidade urinária baixa em casos de insuficiência renal aguda.
• Creatina quinase — leve a acentuadamente elevada em gatos com estado epiléptico mesmo não convulsivo; com ou sem mioglobinúria; indica necrose muscular.

OUTROS TESTES LABORATORIAIS
• Teste sorológico — os títulos de FIV e FeLV frequentemente não contribuem para o diagnóstico; os títulos de PIF e *Toxoplasma gondii* não são confiáveis por si só.
• Teste dos ácidos biliares — indicado nos gatos com apresentação característica; não em gatos que se mostram normais no período interictal.

DIAGNÓSTICO POR IMAGEM
• Radiografias torácicas e ultrassonografia abdominal — na suspeita de doença infecciosa; para avaliar patologia pulmonar em caso de estado epiléptico; procurar por neoplasia caso se suspeite de tumor.
• RM — melhor para definir o local, a extensão e a natureza da lesão.

Crises Convulsivas (Convulsões, Estado Epiléptico) — Gatos

MÉTODOS DIAGNÓSTICOS
Exame do LCS — sensível para detectar doença estrutural; inespecífica por si só para obter o diagnóstico, exceto quando se observa o microrganismo causal (p. ex., criptococose).

ACHADOS PATOLÓGICOS
- Os achados refletem a etiologia.
- Pequenas lesões passam despercebidas com facilidade em epilepsia provavelmente sintomática.

TRATAMENTO

CUIDADO(S) DE SAÚDE ADEQUADO(S)
- Ambulatorial — para crises convulsivas recidivantes isoladas em gato saudável sob outros aspectos.
- Internação — para crises convulsivas aglomeradas e estado epiléptico.

CUIDADO(S) DE ENFERMAGEM E DE SUPORTE
- Proceder à supervisão constante do paciente.
- Estabelecer via de acesso IV para administração de medicamentos e fluidos.
- Coletar o sangue para mensuração rápida dos níveis de gases sanguíneos, glicose, cálcio e medicamentos anticonvulsivantes se pertinentes.
- Resfriar o animal em caso de hipertermia.

ORIENTAÇÃO AO PROPRIETÁRIO
O tratamento anticonvulsivante, em epilepsia sintomática, pode não ajudar até que a causa primária seja tratada.

CONSIDERAÇÕES CIRÚRGICAS
Craniotomia — excisão de tumor em caso de meningioma ou outra massa acessível.

MEDICAÇÕES

MEDICAMENTO(S) DE ESCOLHA
O tipo e a frequência das crises convulsivas determinam a abordagem terapêutica.

Crises Convulsivas Generalizadas Recidivantes Isoladas
- Fenobarbital — 7,5 a 15 mg a cada 12 h/gato; níveis séricos terapêuticos ideais de 100-130 µmol/L (23-30 µg/L).
- Diazepam — segunda escolha; 0,5-2,0 mg/kg/dia VO a cada 8-12 h.
- Levetiracetam — como adição ao fenobarbital; 20 mg/kg a cada 8 h.
- Iniciar gradativamente para evitar sedação visível.

Crises Convulsivas Aglomeradas e Estado Epiléptico
- Tratar as crises aglomeradas e o estado epiléptico generalizado precocemente — quanto mais crises convulsivas em um determinado período, maiores serão a quantidade de medicamentos para controle da crise, o tempo para recuperação e o custo do tratamento.
- Ausência de atividade convulsiva contínua à apresentação e paciente que nunca foi submetido à medicação — fenobarbital em bólus IV a 10 mg/kg até, no máximo, 60 mg/gato em 15 min, seguido pela dose de manutenção VO 12 h depois.
- Atividade convulsiva contínua à apresentação — diazepam em bólus IV na dose de 0,5-1 mg/kg, seguido por infusão em velocidade constante a 0,25-0,5 mg/gato/h em uma bureta embutida na linha de acesso venoso com o uso de bomba de fluido; o bólus IV de diazepam pode ser repetido 5 min após o primeiro bólus caso a atividade convulsiva visível persista; nesse caso, adicionar o fenobarbital à infusão em velocidade constante a 4 mg/gato/h.
- Iniciar o fenobarbital por via oral na dose de manutenção assim que o paciente conseguir engolir.
- Depois de 6 h livres de crises convulsivas, desmamar o paciente da infusão de forma gradual em 4-6 h.

Crises Convulsivas Persistentes
- Doses subanestésicas de propofol em bólus IV (1-3,5 mg/kg) e 0,01-0,25 mg/kg/min sob a forma de infusão em velocidade constante titulado até fazer efeito.

Tratamento com Agentes Não Anticonvulsivantes
- Dexametasona a 0,25 mg/kg IV a cada 24 h por 1-3 dias, para melhorar o edema secundário ao estado epiléptico e tratar a causa primária se não houver suspeita de doença infecciosa sistêmica; esse corticosteroide altera os resultados da análise do LCS.

CONTRAINDICAÇÕES
- Não usar o brometo de potássio em gatos, pois os efeitos colaterais incluem doença respiratória potencialmente letal.
- A deficiência de tiamina provoca vestibulopatia bilateral, sem crises convulsivas; não há necessidade de tratamento.
- Evitar a administração de aminofilina, teofilina, cetamina e fentanila aos gatos epilépticos.

PRECAUÇÕES
- O uso prolongado de propofol (>24 h) pode causar anemia por corpúsculo de Heinz em gatos.
- Com frequência, os gatos sob infusão em velocidade constante ficam visivelmente sedados; pode ocorrer depressão cardiovascular e respiratória; há necessidade de monitorização rigorosa; lubrificar os olhos, comprimir a bexiga urinária manualmente e corrigir a hipotermia.
- O monitoramento de perto é necessário para observar se uma leve atividade convulsiva contínua persiste.

INTERAÇÕES POSSÍVEIS
Cloranfenicol, cimetidina, ranitidina — não usar em conjunto com o fenobarbital; inibem o metabolismo desse anticonvulsivante, provocando elevação nos níveis séricos.

MEDICAMENTO(S) ALTERNATIVO(S)
- Gabapentina a 5-10 mg/kg VO a cada 8-12 h.
- Zonisamida a 5-10 mg/kg VO a cada 24 h.

ACOMPANHAMENTO

MONITORIZAÇÃO DO PACIENTE
- Obter hemograma completo e bioquímica antes de iniciar o medicamento anticonvulsivante.
- Mensurar a CK para avaliar a necrose muscular e indiretamente a atividade convulsiva contínua sutil.
- Medir o nível sérico do fenobarbital 2 semanas após o início; corrigir a dose de forma adequada; repetir a mensuração até que a faixa terapêutica seja atingida.
- Repetir o hemograma completo e a bioquímica a cada 6-12 meses.
- Se o paciente com epilepsia sintomática tiver se recuperado da doença primária e permanecer livre das crises por 6 meses, retirar os anticonvulsivantes de forma gradativa ao longo de muitos meses.

COMPLICAÇÕES POSSÍVEIS
- Hipersensibilidade ao fenobarbital — trombocitopenia, neutropenia, prurido e tumefação (inchaço) dos pés; repetir o hemograma completo 4-6 semanas após o início do fenobarbital.
- Diazepam — pode causar necrose hepática aguda: monitorizar as enzimas hepáticas dentro de 5-7 dias após o início do tratamento.
- Colapso cardiovascular e respiratório por dosagem excessiva durante o tratamento de estado epiléptico.

EVOLUÇÃO ESPERADA E PROGNÓSTICO
- Dependem da causa subjacente e da resposta ao tratamento.
- Os gatos com epilepsia provavelmente sintomática têm prognóstico bom a longo prazo.
- Os gatos podem se recuperar apesar do episódio de crises convulsivas aglomeradas graves e do estado epiléptico generalizado.

DIVERSOS

FATORES RELACIONADOS COM A IDADE
Os gatos com início de crises convulsivas antes de 1 ano de idade e diagnosticados com epilepsia provavelmente sintomática apresentam prognóstico reservado quanto ao controle das crises.

VER TAMBÉM
- Encefalopatia Isquêmica Felina.
- Meningioma.

ABREVIATURA(S)
- CK = creatina quinase.
- FeLV = vírus da leucemia felina.
- FIV = vírus da imunodeficiência felina.
- GI = gastrintestinal.
- LCS = líquido cerebrospinal.
- PIF = peritonite infecciosa felina.
- RM = ressonância magnética.
- SNC = sistema nervoso central.

Sugestões de Leitura

Barnes HL, Chrisman CL, Mariani CL, Sims M, Alleman AR. Clinical signs, underlying cause, and outcome in cats with seizures: 17 cases (1997-2002). JAVMA 2004, 225:1723-1726.

Parent J. Seizures and status epilepticus in cats. In: Veterinary Emergency and Critical Care Manual, 2nd ed. Guelph, Ontario: Lifelearn, 2006, pp. 456-459.

Quesnel AD. The cat with seizures, circling and/or changed behavior. In: Rand JS, ed., Problem-Based Feline Medicine. Edinburgh: Elsevier/Saunders 2006, pp. 795-820.

Quesnel AD, Parent JM, McDonell W. Clinical management and outcome of cats with seizure disorders: 30 cases (1991-1993). JAVMA 1997, 210:72-77.

Thomas WB. Idiopathic epilepsy in dogs and cats. Vet Clin North Am Small Anim Pract 2010, 40:161-179.

Autor Joane M. Parent
Consultor Editorial Joane M. Parent

CRISTALÚRIA

CONSIDERAÇÕES GERAIS

DEFINIÇÃO
Aparecimento de cristais na urina.

FISIOPATOLOGIA
• Os cristais formam-se apenas em urina que está ou esteve recentemente supersaturada com substâncias cristalogênicas; dessa forma, a cristalúria representa um fator de risco para urolitíase. Contudo, a detecção de cristais urinários não é sinônimo de urólitos e dos sinais clínicos associados a eles nem mesmo constitui evidência irrefutável de uma tendência à formação de cálculos.
• Determinados tipos de cristais indicam uma doença subjacente. A identificação e a interpretação adequadas dos cristais urinários também são importantes na formulação de protocolos clínicos para dissolver os urólitos. A avaliação dos cristais urinários pode auxiliar na (1) detecção de distúrbios que predispõem os animais à formação de urólitos (2) estimativa da composição mineral dos urólitos; e (3) avaliação da eficácia dos protocolos clínicos instituídos para dissolver ou evitar os urólitos.
• A cristalúria em indivíduos com tratos urinários normais do ponto de vista anatômico e funcional é geralmente inócua, já que os cristais são eliminados antes de se tornarem grandes o suficiente a ponto de interferir na função urinária normal. No entanto, esses cristais representam um fator de risco para urolitíase.
• Os cristais que se formam após a eliminação ou a remoção de urina do paciente frequentemente apresentam pouca relevância clínica. A identificação de cristais que se formam *in vitro* não justifica a terapia.
• A detecção de alguns tipos de cristais (p. ex., cistina e urato de amônio) em pacientes clinicamente assintomáticos, a detecção frequente de amplos agregados de cristais (p. ex., oxalato de cálcio ou fosfato-amônio-magnésio) em indivíduos aparentemente normais ou a detecção de qualquer forma de cristais em urina recém-coletada de pacientes com urolitíase confirmada podem ter importância diagnóstica, prognóstica ou terapêutica.

SISTEMA(S) ACOMETIDO(S)
Renal/urológico.

IDENTIFICAÇÃO
• Oxalato de cálcio — cães das raças Schnauzer miniatura, Yorkshire terrier, Lhasa apso e Poodle miniatura, além de gatos das raças Birmanês, Himalaio e Persa.
• Cistina — cães das raças Dachshund, Buldogue inglês, Terra Nova, Mastife e outros.
• Urato de amônio — cães das raças Dálmata e Buldogue inglês.
• Urólitos de xantina — cães da raça Cavalier King Charles spaniel.

SINAIS CLÍNICOS
Nenhum ou aqueles causados por urolitíase concomitante.

CAUSAS
Variáveis In Vivo
• Concentração de substâncias cristalogênicas na urina (que, por sua vez, é influenciada por sua velocidade de excreção e pela concentração urinária de água).
• pH urinário (os cristais de estruvita e fosfato de cálcio são os mais comuns em urina neutra a alcalina, enquanto os cristais de urato de amônio, urato de sódio, oxalato de cálcio, cistina e xantina são os mais usuais em urina ácida a neutra).
• Solubilidade de substâncias cristalogênicas na urina.
• Excreção de agentes diagnósticos (p. ex., meios de contraste radiopacos) e medicamentos (p. ex., sulfonamidas).
• Influência da dieta — a dieta hospitalar pode diferir da dieta doméstica/caseira; o momento de coleta da amostra (em jejum *versus* pós-prandial) pode influenciar a evidência de cristalúria.

Variáveis In Vitro
• Temperatura.
• Evaporação.
• Alteração do pH após a coleta da amostra.
• Técnica de preparo da amostra — centrifugação *versus* não centrifugação, volume urinário examinado.
• Alterações *in vitro* importantes que ocorrem após a coleta da urina podem acentuar a formação ou a dissolução de cristais. Quando o conhecimento do tipo e da quantidade de cristal urinário *in vivo* for particularmente relevante, devem-se examinar amostras recém-coletadas, idealmente à temperatura corporal. Se isso não for possível, as amostras deverão estar à temperatura ambiente, e não sob refrigeração.

FATORES DE RISCO
Ver discussão prévia sobre as variáveis *in vivo* e *in vitro* na cristalúria.

DIAGNÓSTICO

DIAGNÓSTICO DIFERENCIAL

Cristalúria por Urato de Amônio, Urato de Sódio e Urato Amorfo
• Raramente observada em cães e gatos de aparência saudável.
• Observada com frequência em cães e ocasionalmente em gatos com anomalias vasculares portais, com ou sem urólitos concomitantes de urato de amônio.
• Verificada em alguns cães e gatos com urólitos de urato, causados por outros distúrbios que não sejam anomalias vasculares portais.

Cristalúria por Bilirrubina
• Observada em urina altamente concentrada proveniente de alguns cães saudáveis.
• Grandes quantidades em amostras seriadas devem levantar a suspeita de anormalidade no metabolismo da bilirrubina.
• Costuma estar associada a doenças subjacentes em gatos.

Cristalúria por Oxalato de Cálcio Mono e Di-hidratado
• Pode ser observada em cães e gatos aparentemente saudáveis ou com urólitos compostos principalmente de oxalato de cálcio.
• O oxalato de cálcio di-hidratado é constatado em alguns cães e gatos intoxicados pelo etilenoglicol, mas os cristais de oxalato de cálcio mono-hidratado são mais comuns (a intoxicação pelo etilenoglicol também pode ocorrer sem cristalúria).

Cristalúria por Fosfato de Cálcio
• Observa-se um número abundante de cristais compostos presumivelmente de fosfato de cálcio em cães com aparência saudável, mas também naqueles com urina alcalina persistente, urólitos de fosfato de cálcio e urólitos compostos de uma mistura de fosfato e oxalato de cálcio.
• Também pode ocorrer uma pequena quantidade de cristais de fosfato de cálcio em associação com cristalúria por estruvita induzida por infecção.
• Pode ser observada em cães e gatos com hiperparatireoidismo primário e acidose tubular renal.

Cristalúria por Cistina
• Observada em cães e gatos com erros inatos do metabolismo, caracterizados por transporte anormal de cistina e outros aminoácidos dibásicos.

Cristalúria por Estruvita
• Verificada em cães e gatos aparentemente saudáveis.
• Observada em cães e gatos com urólitos de estruvita induzidos por infecção, urólitos de estruvita estéreis, urólitos sem estruvita e urólitos de composição mista (p. ex., núcleo composto de oxalato de cálcio e invólucro constituído de estruvita).
• Também é constatada em cães e gatos com doença do trato urinário sem urólitos.

Cristalúria por Ácido Úrico
• Rara em cães e gatos.
• Sua importância é a mesma descrita para os uratos de amônio e amorfos.

Cristalúria por Xantina
• Sugere a administração de dosagens excessivas de alopurinol em combinação com o consumo de quantidades relativamente altas de precursores de purina na dieta.
• Observa-se xantinúria primária em cães da raça Cavalier King Charles spaniel.
• Além da xantinúria primária, ocorrem urólitos de xantina em gatos.

Cristalúria Diversa
• Cristais de colesterol — observados em seres humanos com destruição tecidual excessiva, síndrome nefrótica e quilúria; constatados em cães aparentemente saudáveis.
• Cristais de ácido hipúrico — aparentemente raros em cães e gatos; importância desconhecida.
• Cristais de leucina em cães — sua relevância ainda não foi determinada; podem ocorrer em associação com cistinúria.
• Cristais de tirosina — ocorrem em conjunto com hepatopatias graves em seres humanos; raramente observados em cães e gatos com distúrbios hepáticos. Os cristais de urato de sódio semelhantes a agulhas costumam ser erroneamente interpretados como cristais de tirosina de aparência semelhante.

Cristalúria Induzida por Medicamentos
• Pode ser observada após a administração de meios de contraste radiopacos ou depois de tratamentos com sulfadiazina, fluoroquinolonas, primidona e tetraciclina.
• A administração de alopurinol pode ser associada à formação de cristais de xantina.

ACHADOS LABORATORIAIS

Medicamentos Capazes de Alterar os Resultados Laboratoriais
• Acidificantes urinários (p. ex., d,l-metionina e cloreto de amônio).

CRISTALÚRIA

- Alcalinizantes urinários (p. ex., bicarbonato de sódio e citrato de potássio).

Distúrbios Capazes de Alterar os Resultados Laboratoriais
N/D.

Os Resultados Serão Válidos se os Exames Forem Realizados em Laboratório Humano?
Sim.

HEMOGRAMA/BIOQUÍMICA/URINÁLISE
- Os cristais de bilirrubina podem estar associados à bilirrubinemia e a outras anormalidades laboratoriais decorrentes de distúrbios hepáticos.
- A maioria dos cães e gatos com cristalúria por oxalato e fosfato de cálcio permanece normocalcêmica; alguns se apresentam hipercalcêmicos.
- Alguns cães e gatos com cristalúria por oxalato de cálcio podem estar acidêmicos.
- Quando o conhecimento do tipo de cristal urinário *in vivo* for particularmente importante, devem-se efetuar exames seriados de amostras recém-coletadas; avaliar o número, o tamanho e a estrutura dos cristais, bem como sua tendência à agregação.
- A avaliação microscópica do aspecto dos cristais urinários fornece apenas uma indicação presuntiva de sua composição; condições variáveis associadas a sua formação, crescimento e dissolução podem alterar o aspecto desses cristais. A identificação definitiva da composição dos cristais depende de uma ou mais das seguintes técnicas: cristalografia óptica, espectrofotometria de infravermelho, análise térmica, difração de raios X, análise com microssonda eletrônica.

OUTROS TESTES LABORATORIAIS
- Em geral, a cristalúria por cistina é associada a uma reação urinária positiva do cianeto-nitroprussiato.
- A cristalúria por sulfonamidas pode estar associada ao teste positivo de lignina.
- Os cristais de uratos de amônio e amorfos são insolúveis em ácido acético; a adição de ácido acético a 10% ao sedimento urinário que contenha esses cristais produz frequentemente cristais de ácido úrico e, algumas vezes, de urato de sódio.
- Grande parte dos cães e alguns gatos com cristalúria por estruvita apresentam infecções do trato urinário, causadas por bactérias produtoras de urease (especialmente estafilococos e às vezes *Proteus* spp.).
- Os cães e gatos com cristalúria por urato de amônio e desvios portossistêmicos exibem com frequência níveis séricos elevados de ácidos biliares e hiperamonemia.
- Os cães e gatos com cristalúria por oxalato de cálcio secundária à intoxicação pelo etilenoglicol demonstram níveis detectáveis dessa substância tóxica no soro e na urina em até 48 h após a ingestão.

DIAGNÓSTICO POR IMAGEM
A cristalúria pode estar associada a urólitos detectáveis por meios radiográfico ou ultrassonográfico.

MÉTODOS DIAGNÓSTICOS
Micção por uro-hidropropulsão ou aspiração de urina por meio de sonda transuretral para recuperar urocistólitos pequenos.

TRATAMENTO
- Tratar a cristalúria *in vivo* clinicamente importante por meio da eliminação ou do controle da(s) causa(s) subjacente(s) ou dos fatores de risco associados.
- Minimizar a cristalúria relevante em termos clínicos por meio do aumento no volume urinário, do estímulo de micções completas e frequentes, da mudança na dieta, do emprego de terapia medicamentosa apropriada e, em alguns casos, da modificação do pH.

MEDICAÇÕES
MEDICAMENTO(S) DE ESCOLHA
N/D.
CONTRAINDICAÇÕES
N/D.
PRECAUÇÕES
N/D.
INTERAÇÕES POSSÍVEIS
N/D.
MEDICAMENTO(S) ALTERNATIVO(S)
N/D.

ACOMPANHAMENTO
MONITORIZAÇÃO DO PACIENTE
- Reavaliar a urinálise para determinar a presença de cristalúria.
- Ver os capítulos sobre os tipos específicos de urólitos para monitoração da urolitíase.

COMPLICAÇÕES POSSÍVEIS
- A cristalúria persistente pode contribuir para a formação e o crescimento de urólitos.
- A cristalúria pode solidificar tampões de matriz cristalina, resultando em obstrução uretral.

DIVERSOS
DISTÚRBIOS ASSOCIADOS
N/D.
FATORES RELACIONADOS COM A IDADE
N/D.
POTENCIAL ZOONÓTICO
Nenhum.
GESTAÇÃO/FERTILIDADE/REPRODUÇÃO
N/D.
VER TAMBÉM
- Nefrolitíase.
- Urolitíase por Cistina.
- Urolitíase por Estruvita — Cães.
- Urolitíase por Estruvita — Gatos.
- Urolitíase por Fosfato de Cálcio.
- Urolitíase por Urato.
- Urolitíase por Xantina.

Sugestões de Leitura
Osborne CA, Davis LS, Sanna J, et al. Identification and interpretation of crystalluria in domestic animals: A light and scanning electron microscopic study. Vet Med 1990, 85:18-37.
Osborne CA, Lulich JP, Bartges JW, et al. Drug-induced urolithiasis. Vet Clin North Am 1999, 29:251-266.
Osborne CA, Lulich JP, Ulrich LK, et al. Feline crystalluria: Detection and interpretation. Vet Clin North Am 1996, 26369-26391.
Osborne CA, Stevens B. Urinalysis: A Clinical Guide to Compassionate Patient Care. Shawnee Mission, KS: Bayer, 1999.

Autores Carl A. Osborne and Lisa K. Ulrich
Consultor Editorial Carl A. Osborne

CUTEREBROSE

CONSIDERAÇÕES GERAIS

REVISÃO
- As moscas do gênero *Cuterebra* são encontradas nas Américas, local onde elas atuam como parasitas obrigatórios de roedores e lagomorfos. As moscas adultas depositam seus ovos em folhas de gramíneas ou em ninhos e, então, eles eclodem e rastejam em direção à pele do hospedeiro intermediário ou de transporte. As larvas pequenas penetram em um orifício corporal, migram através de vários tecidos internos e, por fim, percorrem seus trajetos cutâneos onde estabelecem um berne. As larvas maduras, que podem ter aproximadamente 2,5 cm de comprimento, abandonam o roedor ou o coelho como hospedeiro e, em seguida, transformam-se na fase de pupa no solo.
- Os cães e gatos são infectados ao passarem por folhas de gramíneas com ovos que contenham larvas infectantes; essas larvas, por sua vez, são estimuladas a eclodir e a saltar no hospedeiro-animal intermediário. As larvas, então, rastejam pelo cão ou gato até que encontrem um orifício por onde penetrar.
- Os cães e gatos podem desenvolver as larvas nos bernes ou sinais associados à migração tecidual das larvas.
- Além disso, os cães e gatos podem se apresentar com sinais respiratórios, sinais neurológicos, lesões oftálmicas ou larvas cutâneas.

IDENTIFICAÇÃO
- Cães e gatos — todas as idades.
- No norte dos EUA, a maioria dos casos ocorre no final do verão e início do outono com base no tempo de surgimento das fêmeas adultas que depositam os ovos na primavera e início do verão.

SINAIS CLÍNICOS
- Respiratórios — doença respiratória eosinofílica.
- Neurológicos — ataxia, andar em círculo, paralisia, cegueira, decúbito.
- Lesões oftálmicas — larvas na conjuntiva.
- Dermatológicos — berne, contendo larvas com espiráculos em protrusão.

CAUSAS E FATORES DE RISCO
- Cães e gatos com acesso à rua, local onde eles entram em contato com os ovos e as larvas.
- Os gatos neonatos são infectados em casa, presumivelmente por larvas trazidas no pelo das gatas.

DIAGNÓSTICO

DIAGNÓSTICO DIFERENCIAL
- Respiratórios — alergias, vermes pulmonares, ascarídeos migratórios ou ancilóstomos.
- Neurológicos — raiva, cinomose, angiostrongilose.
- Lesões oftálmicas — larvas de *Hypoderma* ou de *Oestrus*.
- Dermatológicos — berne adulto inconfundível; o berne jovem pode se apresentar como uma pústula ou pápula.

HEMOGRAMA/BIOQUÍMICA/URINÁLISE
Pode exibir contagem elevada de eosinófilos.

OUTROS TESTES LABORATORIAIS
N/D.

DIAGNÓSTICO POR IMAGEM
A varredura de TC revela lesões nas imagens cranianas de gatos.

MÉTODOS DIAGNÓSTICOS
N/D.

TRATAMENTO
- É possível remover as larvas a partir das lesões subcutâneas, dos olhos ou das narinas.
- As manifestações de migração pulmonar podem ser aliviadas por meio de corticosteroides.
- A doença neurológica pode apresentar prognóstico mau; assim, a eutanásia representa uma opção.

MEDICAÇÕES

MEDICAMENTO(S)
Ivermectina — 0,2 mg/kg SC — deve eliminar as larvas migratórias; pode ser desejável a instituição da corticoterapia antes de sua administração. A ivermectina pode ser aplicada tanto para aliviar os sinais clínicos causados pelas larvas com suspeita de migração pulmonar como para destruir as larvas presentes em outros tecidos, incluindo o SNC.

ACOMPANHAMENTO
Após o tratamento com a ivermectina, é possível o retorno satisfatório à função.

DIVERSOS
- No norte dos EUA, a doença é bastante sazonal e a maioria dos casos ocorre no final do verão e início do outono, momento em que as moscas adultas se encontram ativas. A sazonalidade é menos delimitada em regiões com temperaturas mais quentes e moscas ativas durante os períodos mais longos do ano.
- Aparentemente não há qualquer imunidade prolongada; o mesmo gato pode desenvolver lesões cutâneas alguns anos depois em uma briga.
- A aplicação de preventivos mensais contra dirofilariose (produtos com ivermectina em sua composição), de agentes de controle do desenvolvimento de pulgas (produtos com lufenurona em sua composição) ou de tratamentos tópicos contra pulgas e carrapatos pode evitar o desenvolvimento de larvas em cães e gatos ou eliminá-las antes de ganharem acesso a um orifício de entrada. Com base em informações não publicadas, no entanto, alguns cães e gatos sob esses produtos ainda desenvolverão bernes com larvas.

POTENCIAL ZOONÓTICO
As larvas em cães ou gatos não representam nenhuma ameaça zoonótica.

ABREVIATURA(S)
- SNC = sistema nervoso central.

Sugestões de Leitura
Bordelon JT, Newcomb BT, Rochat MC. Surgical removal of a Cuterebra larva from the cervical trachea of a cat. JAAHA 2009, 45:52-54.
Bowman DD. Georgis' Parasitology for Veterinarians, 9th ed. Philadelphia: Saunders, 2009, pp. 31-33.
Bowman DD, Hendrix CM, Lindsay DS, et al. Feline Clinical Parasitology. Ames: Iowa State University Press, 2002, pp. 430-439.

Autor Dwight D. Bowman
Consultor Editorial Stephen C. Barr

Defeito do Septo Atrial

CONSIDERAÇÕES GERAIS

REVISÃO
• Anomalia cardíaca congênita, que permite a comunicação entre os átrios por meio de um defeito no septo interatrial. • Os defeitos ocorrem em um dos três locais expostos a seguir: defeito do óstio primário, septo atrial inferior; defeito do óstio secundário, próximo à fossa oval; e defeito do seio venoso, craniodorsal à fossa oval. • O sangue costuma sofrer um desvio para o átrio direito, o que ocasiona uma sobrecarga de volume no átrio e no ventrículo direito, bem como na vasculatura pulmonar; ocasionalmente, isso leva à hipertensão pulmonar. • Em caso de pressões elevadas no lado direito do coração, poderá ocorrer um desvio da direita para a esquerda, causando cianose generalizada. • Compreende 0,7% dos defeitos cardíacos congênitos nos cães e 9% desses defeitos nos gatos. Um estudo recente conduzido na França sugere uma incidência mais alta em casos de defeito do septo atrial, respondendo por 37,7% dos defeitos cardíacos congênitos em dados coletados de cães e gatos. • Defeitos tipo óstio secundário são mais comuns (98,7% em um único estudo).

IDENTIFICAÇÃO
• Cães e gatos.
• Os cães das raças Boxer, Poodle standard, Terra Nova, Doberman, Old English sheepdog e Samoieda podem ser super-representados.

SINAIS CLÍNICOS
Comentários Gerais
Se o defeito for pequeno, possivelmente não haverá nenhum sinal. Em um único estudo, 73,7% dos casos apresentaram-se assintomáticos.

Achados Anamnésicos
Graus variáveis de intolerância ao exercício (7%), síncope (5,3%), tosse (2,3%) e dispneia (2,3%).

Achados do Exame Físico
• Em decorrência de uma estenose pulmonar relativa, observa-se um leve sopro sistólico sobre a válvula pulmonar (20%).
• Raramente, há um sopro diastólico sobre a valva atrioventricular direita (tricúspide), em virtude de uma estenose tricúspide relativa.
• Na presença de defeito do coxim endocárdico ou de fenda da valva atrioventricular esquerda (mitral), pode-se auscultar um sopro sistólico mitral.
• Cianose em caso de desvio da direita para a esquerda.
• Ascite no desenvolvimento de insuficiência cardíaca direita.
• Desdobramento fixo da segunda bulha cardíaca.

CAUSAS E FATORES DE RISCO
Desconhecidos; não há registros de uma base genética.

DIAGNÓSTICO

DIAGNÓSTICO DIFERENCIAL
• Estenose da válvula pulmonar — o sopro produzido por essa estenose costuma ser de som áspero e intensamente sonoro.
• Retorno venoso pulmonar anômalo ao átrio direito.

HEMOGRAMA/BIOQUÍMICA/URINÁLISE
Em alguns pacientes com desvio da direita para a esquerda, observa-se policitemia.

DIAGNÓSTICO POR IMAGEM
Achados Radiográficos
• Ausentes em pacientes com defeitos pequenos.
• Aumento de volume do coração direito e dos vasos pulmonares em pacientes com defeitos amplos.

Achados Ecocardiográficos
• Dilatação atrial e ventricular direita.
• Podem demonstrar o defeito — perda de ecos pelo defeito do septo.
• O Doppler é útil na comprovação do fluxo por meio do defeito e da alta velocidade de ejeção através da artéria pulmonar.

OUTROS MÉTODOS DIAGNÓSTICOS
Eletrocardiografia
• Em alguns pacientes com defeitos amplos, verifica-se um padrão de aumento do lado direito do coração (eixo para direita, ondas S profundas na derivação II, ondas P altas) no ECG.
• É possível a constatação de arritmias e distúrbios de condução intraventricular.

TRATAMENTO

• Internar os pacientes com insuficiência cardíaca congestiva (ICC) até sua estabilização.
• Restringir a atividade física.
• Uma dieta com baixo teor de sódio pode ser valiosa se houver ICC.
• O dispositivo Amplatzer® pode ser implantado via colocação transvenosa ou transatrial para fechar alguns defeitos tipo óstio secundário.
• Para grande parte dos proprietários, a correção cirúrgica é extremamente cara, pois exige a cirurgia aberta do coração. Recentemente, foi descrita uma abordagem híbrida, envolvendo a fixação de dispositivo ativo após oclusão venosa temporária após a colocação de dispositivo transatrial.
• Em pacientes com doença grave, a ligadura da artéria pulmonar pode ser uma medida paliativa.

MEDICAÇÕES

MEDICAMENTO(S) E FLUIDO(S)
• ICC — diuréticos; furosemida, 1-2 mg/kg VO a cada 6-12 h. • Os vasodilatadores podem ajudar a diminuir os sinais de ICC (p. ex., enalapril, 0,5 mg/kg VO a cada 12-24 h, ou benazepril, 0,25-0,5 mg/kg VO a cada 24 h).

ACOMPANHAMENTO

MONITORIZAÇÃO DO PACIENTE
Em caso de descompensação ou no desenvolvimento de outros sinais clínicos, o paciente deverá ser reavaliado.

EVOLUÇÃO ESPERADA E PROGNÓSTICO
• Dependem do tamanho do defeito e das anormalidades coexistentes; é improvável que pequenos defeitos isolados produzam sinais ou evoluam. Defeitos tipo óstio primário tipicamente são maiores e apresentam prognóstico pior. Defeitos >12 mm podem desenvolver insuficiência cardíaca. • Se o defeito for amplo ou estiver associado a algum defeito do coxim endocárdico, espera-se uma ICC direita progressiva. • Em gatos, o prognóstico é frequentemente reservado a ruim.

DIVERSOS

DISTÚRBIOS ASSOCIADOS
• Estenose pulmonar e displasia tricúspide.
• Defeitos do coxim endocárdico.

VER TAMBÉM
Insuficiência Cardíaca Congestiva Direita.

ABREVIATURA(S)
• ECG = eletrocardiografia.
• ICC = insuficiência cardíaca congestiva.

Sugestões de Leitura
Bonagura JD, Lehmkuhl LB. Congenital heart disease. In: Fox PR, Sisson D, Moise ND, eds., Textbook of Canine and Feline Cardiology, 2nd ed. Philadelphia: Saunders, 1999, pp. 471-535.
Chetboul V, Charles V, Nicolle A, et al. Retrospective study of 156 atrial septal defects in dogs and cats (2001-2005). J Vet Med A Physiol Pathol Clin Med 2006, 53(4):179-184.
Gordon SG, Miller MW, Roland RM, et al. Transcatheter atrial septal defect closure with the Amplatzer atrial septal occluder in 13 dogs: short- and mid-term outcome. J Vet Intern Med 2009, 23(5):995-1002.
Gordon SG, Nelson DA, Achen SE, et al. Open heart closure of an atrial septal defect by use of an atrial septal occluder in a dog. JAVMA 2010, 236(4):434-439.

Autor Francis W.K. Smith, Jr.
Consultores Editoriais Larry P. Tilley e Francis W.K. Smith, Jr.

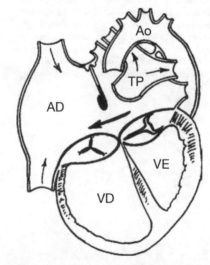

Figura 1 Defeito do septo atrial. O defeito envolve a porção mais inferior do septo atrial, sendo conhecido como defeito do óstio primário. Observar o desvio predominante da esquerda para a direita. VD = ventrículo direito, VE = ventrículo esquerdo, AD = átrio direito, Ao = aorta, TP = tronco pulmonar. (De: Roberts W. *Adult congenital heart disease*. Philadelphia: FA Davis Co., 1987, com permissão.)

Defeito do Septo Ventricular

CONSIDERAÇÕES GERAIS

DEFINIÇÃO
Trata-se de uma comunicação anômala entre os dois ventrículos. O defeito pode estar na entrada, na saída, na camada muscular ou no septo membranoso. A maior parte dos defeitos do septo ventricular em pequenos animais é perimembranosa, de tal modo que o defeito é subaórtico e possui um orifício ventricular direito abaixo do folheto septal da valva tricúspide.

FISIOPATOLOGIA
- O defeito do septo ventricular resulta em desvio sistêmico pulmonar — a direção e o volume do desvio são determinados pelo tamanho do defeito, pela relação das resistências vascular sistêmica e pulmonar, bem como pela presença de outras anomalias.
- Grande parte dos defeitos do septo ventricular em cães e gatos é pequena e, portanto, restritiva (i. e., suficientemente pequena a ponto de a diferença das pressões entre os ventrículos esquerdo e direito ser mantida). Os defeitos do septo ventricular de tamanho moderado são apenas parcialmente restritivos e resultam em vários graus de hipertensão do ventrículo direito. Os defeitos amplos do septo ventricular possuem uma área tão ampla quanto ou maior que a abertura da válvula aórtica; tais defeitos são não restritivos, de tal modo que as pressões dos ventrículos esquerdo e direito se apresentam necessariamente iguais. Apenas os defeitos moderados e amplos impõem uma carga de pressão sobre o ventrículo direito.
- Em um paciente com resistência normal à ejeção do ventrículo direito, a direção do desvio é da esquerda para a direita, o que aumenta o retorno venoso pulmonar e impõe uma sobrecarga de volume sobre o átrio e o ventrículo esquerdos. Em casos de desvios amplos, pode se desenvolver uma insuficiência congestiva do ventrículo esquerdo.
- Em geral, o ventrículo esquerdo descarrega no sistema arterial pulmonar durante a sístole; a menos que o defeito seja de tamanho moderado ou amplo, o ventrículo direito é poupado.

SISTEMA(S) ACOMETIDO(S)
- Respiratório — caso se desenvolva edema pulmonar.
- Cardiovascular — teoricamente, um desvio amplo pode resultar em vasculopatia pulmonar, hipertensão pulmonar e inversão do desvio* (i. e., síndrome de Eisenmenger). Isso é raro em pequenos animais; se houver inversão do desvio, ela ocorrerá em geral no início da vida do paciente.

GENÉTICA
São identificadas predisposições raciais; entretanto, ainda não se estabeleceu nenhuma transmissão genética.

INCIDÊNCIA/PREVALÊNCIA
Em um único estudo, o defeito do septo ventricular correspondeu a uma das más-formações cardíacas congênitas mais comuns em gatos, representando 15% dos casos de defeitos cardíacos congênitos. No entanto, o defeito do septo ventricular é menos comum em cães, ocorrendo em 10% dos casos de defeitos cardíacos congênitos, de acordo com um único estudo.

---

* N. T.: Também conhecido como desvio reverso.

DISTRIBUIÇÃO GEOGRÁFICA
N/D.

IDENTIFICAÇÃO
Espécies
Cães e gatos.

Raça(s) Predominante(s)
Buldogue inglês, Springer spaniel inglês, Basset hound, Akita, West Highland white terrier, Lakeland terrier.

Idade Média e Faixa Etária
A maioria dos defeitos é detectada durante o exame de rotina de filhotes caninos e felinos.

Sexo Predominante
N/D.

SINAIS CLÍNICOS

Achados Anamnésicos
- Geralmente assintomáticos.
- Os sinais clínicos de insuficiência do ventrículo esquerdo incluem dispneia, intolerância a exercícios, síncope e tosse.

Achados do Exame Físico
- O defeito restritivo do septo ventricular resulta em sopro sistólico, que é tipicamente alto, em formato de bandas e mais bem auscultado sobre o hemitórax direito. Pode haver um sopro mesossistólico, mais suave, de estenose pulmonar funcional, auscultado sobre a base cardíaca esquerda. Ocorrerá um sopro diastólico decrescente se o defeito do septo ventricular enfraquecer a sustentação anatômica da válvula aórtica, causando regurgitação aórtica. Em geral, os pacientes com desvios da direita para a esquerda não apresentam sopros.
- Em alguns pacientes, observa-se o desdobramento da segunda bulha cardíaca.
- Os pulsos femorais costumam permanecer normais.
- Mucosas — rosadas a menos que uma hipertensão pulmonar provoque um desvio da direita para a esquerda e hipoxemia arterial.
- Se ocorrer insuficiência do ventrículo esquerdo, os sinais de taquicardia, dispneia e crepitações poderão estar evidentes.

CAUSAS
Congênitas; podem ter base genética.

FATORES DE RISCO
N/D.

DIAGNÓSTICO

DIAGNÓSTICO DIFERENCIAL
- Outras más-formações cardíacas congênitas indutoras de sopros sistólicos incluem displasia das valvas atrioventriculares, estenose aórtica ou pulmonar e más-formações complexas, como a tetralogia de Fallot.
- O sopro tipo "vai e vem" resultante da complicação de um defeito do septo ventricular por regurgitação da válvula aórtica deve ser distinguido do sopro contínuo decorrente da persistência do ducto arterioso.
- Em geral, o diagnóstico de más-formações cardíacas congênitas requer a avaliação ecocardiográfica, incluindo os estudos com Doppler.

HEMOGRAMA/BIOQUÍMICA/URINÁLISE
- Os resultados costumam permanecer normais.
- Os desvios incomuns da direita para a esquerda resultam em eritrocitose compensatória.
- Os pacientes com ICC grave podem ter azotemia pré-renal.

OUTROS TESTES LABORATORIAIS
N/D.

DIAGNÓSTICO POR IMAGEM

Radiografia Torácica
- O aspecto radiográfico é determinado pelo tamanho e pela direção do desvio. As radiografias torácicas poderão permanecer normais se o defeito do septo ventricular for pequeno. Os defeitos mais amplos provocam diversos graus de aumento de volume cardíaco do lado esquerdo ou até mesmo generalizado. A hiperperfusão pulmonar com proeminência do segmento da artéria pulmonar principal pode ser aparente. A ICC manifesta-se como edema pulmonar.
- Os pacientes com desvios da direita para a esquerda apresentam cardiomegalia do lado direito; as artérias pulmonares encontram-se aumentadas no sentido proximal, mas adelgaçadas no sentido distal; já as veias pulmonares apresentam-se pequenas, em virtude da perfusão pulmonar reduzida.

Ecocardiografia
- O estudo ecocardiográfico bidimensional pode demonstrar o aumento de volume do átrio esquerdo, com dilatação e hipertrofia do ventrículo esquerdo. A função sistólica do miocárdio costuma ser preservada. A hipertrofia do ventrículo direito será aparente apenas se o tamanho do defeito for moderado ou grande ou, então, se o defeito do septo ventricular fizer parte de uma má-formação complexa, como a tetralogia de Fallot. O estudo rigoroso geralmente exibirá o defeito. É preciso avaliar as imagens ecocardiográficas de forma crítica; o artefato de "desaparecimento de vista do septo" é bastante comum.
- O diagnóstico é confirmado pela pesquisa do septo interventricular por meio da pesquisa com Doppler. Se o defeito for restritivo, o Doppler espectral revelará um jato sistólico discreto de alta velocidade. O desvio pode ser observado diretamente por meio do Doppler de fluxo colorido. A ecocardiografia contrastada pode ajudar no diagnóstico de um defeito do septo ventricular da direita para a esquerda.
- Raramente, os defeitos do septo ventricular se fecham de forma espontânea. O mecanismo de fechamento envolve, em geral, a aderência de uma parte do folheto septal da valva tricúspide ao septo interventricular, resultando no aspecto ecocardiográfico de "aneurisma septal". Já foi registrado o fechamento espontâneo dos defeitos do septo ventricular. Ocasionalmente, um "aneurisma septal" é um achado ecocardiográfico incidental.

Cateterização Cardíaca
- A cateterização cardíaca seletiva permite a inspeção do defeito por meio da angiocardiografia contrastada e pelo cálculo da fração do desvio (QP/QS) e da resistência vascular pulmonar.

OUTROS MÉTODOS DIAGNÓSTICOS

Achados Eletrocardiográficos
- Evidência de aumento de volume do átrio esquerdo, hipertrofia do ventrículo esquerdo ou até mesmo hipertrofia do ventrículo direito em alguns animais.
- Padrão de aumento de volume do ventrículo direito em grande parte dos animais se o desvio for

Defeito do Septo Ventricular

da direita para a esquerda, em virtude de vasculopatia ou estenose pulmonares.

ACHADOS PATOLÓGICOS
O tamanho do defeito determina o grau de aumento e hipertrofia da câmara cardíaca; em pacientes com ICC, observam-se edema pulmonar e, possivelmente, ascite.

TRATAMENTO

CUIDADO(S) DE SAÚDE ADEQUADO(S)
Os sinais clínicos relacionam-se com a ICC; a maioria dos pacientes pode ser tratada em um esquema ambulatorial.

CUIDADO(S) DE ENFERMAGEM
N/D.

ATIVIDADE
Restringir a atividade física se o animal tiver ICC; não é necessário limitar a atividade de pacientes assintomáticos com defeitos pequenos.

DIETA
Em pacientes com ICC, recomenda-se a restrição moderada de sódio.

ORIENTAÇÃO AO PROPRIETÁRIO
A correção cirúrgica definitiva não se encontra amplamente disponível; em caso de desenvolvimento de ICC, o quadro será terminal, mesmo com a provisão de cuidados paliativos.

CONSIDERAÇÕES CIRÚRGICAS
• Apenas uma minoria dos defeitos do septo ventricular é suficientemente ampla a ponto de justificar o reparo cirúrgico.
• Considerar a realização de reparo cirúrgico definitivo do defeito durante o desvio cardiopulmonar em casos de defeitos associados a um grande desvio. Atualmente, a cirurgia de desvio cardiopulmonar é realizada em um pequeno número de centros veterinários. Ponderar a execução de ligadura da artéria pulmonar como um procedimento paliativo em pacientes com desvios moderados ou amplos e ICC.
• Alguns defeitos do septo ventricular são passíveis de fechamento com o uso de dispositivos oclusivos metálicos designados para essa finalidade.

MEDICAÇÕES

MEDICAMENTO(S) DE ESCOLHA
Furosemida, enalapril, pimobendana e, em algumas circunstâncias, digoxina — recomendados em animais com ICC (ver "Insuficiência Cardíaca Congestiva Esquerda").

CONTRAINDICAÇÕES
Vasodilatadores — são contraindicados ou utilizados com extrema cautela apenas em pacientes com más-formações complexas que envolvem lesões estenóticas.

PRECAUÇÕES
Os inibidores da ECA e a digoxina deverão ser usados com cuidado se o paciente tiver disfunção renal.

INTERAÇÕES POSSÍVEIS
N/D.

MEDICAMENTO(S) ALTERNATIVO(S)
N/D.

ACOMPANHAMENTO

MONITORIZAÇÃO DO PACIENTE
Em pacientes sem sinais clínicos, sugere-se a avaliação radiográfica ou ecocardiografia periódica.

PREVENÇÃO
Não se recomenda a reprodução dos animais acometidos.

COMPLICAÇÕES POSSÍVEIS
• Insuficiência congestiva do ventrículo esquerdo.
• Endocardite bacteriana.
• Hipertensão pulmonar.
• Arritmias.

EVOLUÇÃO ESPERADA E PROGNÓSTICO
• Os pacientes com desvios pequenos podem exibir uma expectativa de vida normal; em geral, os defeitos restritivos e isolados do septo ventricular não provocam sinais clínicos.
• As anomalias concomitantes, como estenose pulmonar ou insuficiência aórtica, agravam o prognóstico.
• Os pacientes com ICC evidente podem viver de 6 a 18 meses com o tratamento clínico.
• O desenvolvimento do quadro de hipertensão pulmonar e de inversão do desvio é incomum, mas costuma estar associado a um prognóstico mau.

DIVERSOS

DISTÚRBIOS ASSOCIADOS
• O defeito do septo ventricular pode ser um componente de más-formações complexas, como a tetralogia de Fallot.
• Grande parte dos defeitos do septo ventricular é perimembranosa e subaórtica. Portanto, a insuficiência da válvula aórtica resultante do suporte valvular aórtico deficiente complica a condição em alguns pacientes.
• Em gatos, o defeito do septo ventricular pode estar associado a defeitos do septo atrial e anormalidades das valvas atrioventriculares, como parte de um defeito completo do septo atrioventricular (defeito do coxim endocárdico).

FATORES RELACIONADOS COM A IDADE
O sopro decorrente de defeito do septo ventricular torna-se aparente logo após o nascimento, quando a resistência vascular pulmonar declina.

POTENCIAL ZOONÓTICO
N/D.

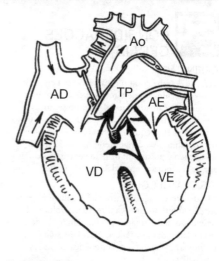

Figura 1 Defeito do septo ventricular. Nesse desenho esquemático, o defeito resulta em uma comunicação desobstruída. A hipertrofia ventricular direita e a hipertensão pulmonar estão associadas. Está ilustrado o desvio da esquerda para a direita. AD = átrio direito, AE = átrio esquerdo, VD = ventrículo direito, VE = ventrículo esquerdo, Ao = aorta, TP = tronco pulmonar. (De Roberts W. *Adult congenital heart disease*. Philadelphia: FA Davis, 1987, com autorização.)

GESTAÇÃO/FERTILIDADE/REPRODUÇÃO
Alto risco em pacientes com defeitos amplos; não é recomendável o acasalamento dos animais acometidos.

SINÔNIMO(S)
Defeito do septo interventricular.

VER TAMBÉM
• Insuficiência Cardíaca Congestiva Esquerda.
• Tetralogia de Fallot.

ABREVIATURA(S)
• ECA = enzima conversora de angiotensina.
• ICC = insuficiência cardíaca congestiva.

Sugestões de Leitura
Bonagura JD, Lehmkuhl LB. Congenital heart disease. In: Fox PR, Sisson D, Moise NS, eds., Textbook of Canine and Feline Cardiology, 2nd ed. Philadelphia: Saunders, 1999, pp. 471-535.
Kittleson MD. Septal defects. In: Small Animal Cardiovascular Medicine. St. Louis: Mosby, 1998, pp. 231-239.

Autor Jonathan A. Abbott
Consultores Editoriais Larry P. Tilley e Francis W.K. Smith, Jr.

DEFICIÊNCIA DA FOSFOFRUTOQUINASE

CONSIDERAÇÕES GERAIS

REVISÃO
- A fosfofrutoquinase é a enzima mais importante responsável pelo controle da velocidade no processo de glicólise, mas as hemácias e os músculos esqueléticos de intensa atividade dependem excessivamente da glicólise anaeróbica para produção de energia.
- Os cães acometidos têm anemia hemolítica compensada e geralmente miopatia leve causada pela atividade acentuadamente reduzida de fosfofrutoquinase total em ambos os tecidos.
- Ocorre o desenvolvimento de anemia por causa da geração insuficiente de ATP para manter a configuração normal, a composição iônica e a deformabilidade das hemácias e também pelo fato de que as hemácias dos cães acometidos são alcalinas frágeis e sofrem lise quando o pH do sangue está levemente elevado.

IDENTIFICAÇÃO
- Springer spaniel inglês, Cocker spaniel americano, Whippet e raças mistas.
- Transmitida como traço autossômico recessivo.
- Os animais homozigotos acometidos geralmente não são identificados como anormais antes de 1 ano de idade.

SINAIS CLÍNICOS
- Alguns animais demonstram sinais clínicos leves que passam despercebidos por anos; outros manifestam regularmente episódios de doença grave.
- Depressão ou fraqueza concomitantes com episódios de pigmentúria vermelha a castanha; é menos provável que a hemoglobinúria seja identificada em cadelas, por causa da diferença sexual no padrão miccional.
- Letargia leve com febre branda durante episódios hemolíticos moderados.
- Letargia acentuada, fraqueza, mucosas pálidas ou ictéricas, hepatosplenomegalia leve, emaciação muscular e febre alta de até 41°C são possíveis durante crises hemolíticas graves.
- A hemólise intravascular pode ser causada por alcalemia induzida por hiperventilação associada a exercício ou agitação.
- Sinais de disfunção muscular — geralmente limitados à intolerância ao exercício e massa muscular levemente diminuída, embora possam ocorrer cãibras musculares e miopatia progressiva grave.
- Dois cães acometidos da raça Whippet tiveram cardiopatia progressiva, além de cãibras musculares após o exercício.
- Os animais portadores heterozigotos parecem clinicamente normais.

CAUSAS E FATORES DE RISCO
Deficiência da subunidade de tipo muscular da fosfofrutoquinase — atividade total acentuadamente reduzida nas hemácias e no músculo esquelético.

DIAGNÓSTICO

DIAGNÓSTICO DIFERENCIAL
- Outras causas de anemia hemolítica — anemia hemolítica imunomediada, micoplasmose hemotrópica, babesiose, anemia hemolítica por corpúsculos de Heinz, anemia hemolítica microangiopática e deficiência da piruvato quinase.
- Cães acometidos — teste de Coombs negativo, sem parasitas ou corpúsculos de Heinz nos esfregaços sanguíneos corados, soronegativos para *Babesia* spp. e sem indícios de CID ou dirofilariose.
- Diferenciado da deficiência de piruvato quinase por ensaios enzimáticos específicos ou teste de DNA.

HEMOGRAMA/BIOQUÍMICA/URINÁLISE
- Anemia hemolítica compensada persistente.
- VCM usualmente de 80-90 fL.
- Contagem de reticulócitos geralmente de 10-30%.
- Os valores do hematócrito são, em geral, de 30-40%; durante as crises hemolíticas, podem diminuir para ≤15%.
- Bilirrubinúria — frequentemente muito alta nos cães machos.
- Hemoglobinúria em associação com episódios de hemólise intravascular.
- Soro — níveis levemente elevados de potássio, magnésio, cálcio, ureia, AST, proteína total e globulina; níveis leve a moderadamente altos de LDH, fosfatase alcalina, ferro e bilirrubina; níveis acentuadamente aumentados de bilirrubina em associação com crise hemolítica; aumento acentuado de ureia e creatinina caso ocorra o desenvolvimento de insuficiência renal secundária a nefrose hemoglobínica ou choque.

OUTROS TESTES LABORATORIAIS
- Mensurar a atividade da fosfofrutoquinase da hemácia — identifica facilmente os animais acometidos com mais de 3 meses de vida; os cães portadores heterozigotos têm aproximadamente metade da atividade normal.
- Realizar teste de DNA pela tecnologia PCR — diferencia claramente os animais normais e portadores em qualquer idade.

TRATAMENTO
- O transplante de medula óssea é a única forma de cura.
- Nos pacientes com hemólise intravascular grave, a fluidoterapia IV minimiza a possibilidade de insuficiência renal aguda.
- As transfusões de sangue geralmente não são necessárias, mas deverão ser administradas se a anemia tiver risco de morte.

MEDICAÇÕES

MEDICAMENTO(S)
Para a febre que frequentemente acompanha a hemólise intravascular e potencializa a crise hemolítica — ácido acetilsalicílico (10 mg/kg VO a cada 12 h) ou dipirona (0,055 mL de solução a 50%/kg SC a cada 8 h).

ACOMPANHAMENTO
- Os cães acometidos raramente morrem durante a crise hemolítica por causa da anemia ou de insuficiência renal.
- Os animais acometidos podem ter uma vida normal se tratados de forma adequada.
- Os proprietários devem evitar colocar os cães acometidos em situações de estresse ou sujeitá-los a exercício extenuante, agitação ou altas temperaturas ambientais.

DIVERSOS

ABREVIATURA(S)
- AST = aspartato aminotransferase.
- ATP = trifosfato de adenosina.
- CID = coagulação intravascular disseminada.
- LDH = lactato desidrogenase.
- PCR = reação em cadeia da polimerase.
- VCM = volume corpuscular (globular) médio.

RECURSOS DA INTERNET
http://research.vet.upenn.edu/penngen

Sugestões de Leitura

Gerber K, Harvey JW, D'Agorne S, Wood J, Giger U. Hemolysis, myopathy, and cardiac diseases associated with hereditary phosphofructokinase deficiency in two whippets. Vet Clin Path 2009, 38:46-51.

Giger U. Erythrocyte phosphofructokinase and pyruvate kinase deficiencies. In: Feldman BF, Zinkl JG, Jain NC, eds., Schalm's Veterinary Hematology, 5th ed. Philadelphia: Lippincott Williams & Wilkins, 2000, pp. 1020-1025.

Harvey JW. Pathogenesis, laboratory diagnosis, and clinical implications of erythrocyte enzyme deficiencies in dogs, cats, and horses. Vet Clin Path 2006, 35:144-156.

———. Red blood cell enzyme activity. In: Vaden SL, Knoll JS, Smith FWK, Tilley LP, eds., Blackwell's Five-Minute Veterinary Consult: Laboratory Tests and Diagnostic Procedures—Canine & Feline. Ames, IA: Wiley-Blackwell, 2009, pp. 520-521.

Autor John W. Harvey
Consultor Editorial A.H. Rebar

Deficiência da Piruvato Quinase

CONSIDERAÇÕES GERAIS

REVISÃO
• As hemácias necessitam de energia sob a forma de ATP para manutenção da forma, deformabilidade, transporte ativo de membrana e atividades sintéticas limitadas; as hemácias maduras carecem de mitocôndrias e dependem da glicólise anaeróbica para a geração do ATP.
• A piruvato quinase catalisa uma importante etapa geradora de ATP e controladora de velocidade na glicólise; em consequência disso, o metabolismo energético fica acentuadamente prejudicado nas hemácias com deficiência da piruvato quinase, resultando em encurtamento na vida útil dessas células e anemia; a medula óssea tenta compensar isso por meio de hiperplasia eritroide, com reticulose acentuada no sangue periférico.

IDENTIFICAÇÃO
• Traço autossômico recessivo identificado nos cães das raças Basenji, Beagle, West Highland white terrier, Cairn terrier, Poodle miniatura, Dachshund, Chihuahua, Pug, cão Esquimó americano e nos gatos das raças Abissínio, Somali e doméstico de pelo curto.
• Em geral, os animais homozigotos acometidos não são identificados como anormais até depois de alguns meses de vida ou na idade adulta.

SINAIS CLÍNICOS
• Os gatos acometidos frequentemente permanecem assintomáticos.
• Letargia ou intolerância ao exercício.
• Mucosas pálidas.
• Com frequência, há esplenomegalia.
• Taquicardia.
• Sopros cardíacos sistólicos relatados em cães.
• Ocasionalmente, observa-se icterícia em gatos, embora esse achado seja raro nos cães.
• Os cães acometidos podem ser levemente menores do que os normais para a raça e a idade e podem apresentar fraqueza e emaciação muscular.
• Os gatos acometidos podem exibir diarreia, inapetência, baixa qualidade da pelagem e perda de peso.

CAUSAS E FATORES DE RISCO
• As hemácias dos cães adultos normais possuem apenas uma única isoenzima da piruvato quinase (o tipo R).
• Defeitos específicos de raças no gene *PKLR* resultam em deficiência de piruvato quinase no eritrócito dos cães.
• Foi descrito um defeito molecular comum nos gatos.

DIAGNÓSTICO

DIAGNÓSTICO DIFERENCIAL
• Outras causas de anemia hemolítica — anemia hemolítica imunomediada, micoplasmose hemotrópica, babesiose, anemia hemolítica por corpúsculos de Heinz, anemia hemolítica microangiopática e deficiência de fosfofrutoquinase (cães).
• Animais acometidos — teste de Coombs negativo, ausência de parasitas ou corpúsculos de Heinz nos esfregaços de sangue corados, soronegativos para *Babesia* spp. e sem indícios de CID ou de dirofilariose.
• Ao contrário da deficiência de fosfofrutoquinase, os cães com deficiência da piruvato quinase não apresentam episódios de hemólise intravascular nem hemoglobinúria; essas deficiências são diferenciadas por ensaios enzimáticos específicos ou por testes de DNA.

HEMOGRAMA/BIOQUÍMICA/URINÁLISE
• Anemia hipocrômica macrocítica persistente com valores de hematócrito de 16-28% e contagens de reticulócitos não corrigidas de 15-50% em cães.
• Anemia intermitente (hematócrito de 13-40%), com contagens de reticulócitos agregados leve a acentuadamente aumentadas em gatos.
• Contagens de leucócitos totais normais ou levemente elevadas.
• Contagem de plaquetas normal a levemente aumentada.
• Policromasia moderada a acentuada, anisocitose e inúmeras hemácias nucleadas nos esfregaços sanguíneos corados.
• Há relatos de pecilocitose em cães esplenectomizados.
• Possíveis achados anormais do exame de bioquímica sérica, como hiperferremia e hiperbilirrubinemia, além de atividades levemente elevadas de ALT e fosfatase alcalina; é comum a constatação de hiperglobulinemia em gatos; cães com insuficiência hepática podem apresentar hipoalbuminemia.
• Urinálise normal, exceto pela bilirrubinúria nos cães.

OUTROS TESTES LABORATORIAIS
• Atividade total da piruvato quinase das hemácias — baixo valor diagnóstico nos gatos e em alguns cães; muitos cães acometidos apresentam atividades normais ou elevadas por causa da expressão de uma isoenzima M_2, que normalmente não ocorre nas hemácias maduras; aproximadamente 50% da atividade normal nos animais heterozigotos.
• Ensaios adicionais (p. ex., teste de estabilidade enzimática ao calor, mensuração dos intermediários glicolíticos das hemácias, eletroforese de isoenzimas e imunoprecipitação enzimática) — para chegar ao diagnóstico nos cães cuja atividade enzimática total não se encontra baixa.
• Testes diagnósticos do DNA — para triagem de várias raças.

DIAGNÓSTICO POR IMAGEM
N/D.

MÉTODOS DIAGNÓSTICOS
N/D.

TRATAMENTO
• Os animais acometidos só podem ser curados mediante transplante de medula óssea.
• O procedimento de esplenectomia pode diminuir a gravidade da anemia em gatos.

MEDICAÇÕES

MEDICAMENTO(S)
Apesar de não adequadamente avaliado, o tratamento a longo prazo com medicamentos quelantes do ferro pode prolongar a expectativa de vida dos animais acometidos.

CONTRAINDICAÇÕES/INTERAÇÕES POSSÍVEIS
Nenhuma.

ACOMPANHAMENTO
• Sobrecarga de ferro hepático — desenvolve-se nos cães acometidos; pode resultar em cirrose e insuficiência hepática.
• Mielofibrose e osteosclerose — desenvolvem-se nos cães acometidos com o avanço da idade; portanto, a maior parte deles morre em torno dos 5 anos de idade como resultado de insuficiência da medula óssea ou do fígado.
• Anemia grave com reticulocitose mínima ou testes anormais de função hepática e ascite secundária à hipoalbuminemia indicam o estágio terminal da doença nos cães.
• Há relatos de obstrução biliar extra-hepática com colelitíase por bilirrubina em dois gatos.

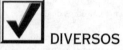

DIVERSOS

ABREVIATURA(S)
• ALT = alanina aminotransferase.
• ATP = trifosfato de adenosina.
• CID = coagulação intravascular disseminada.

RECURSOS DA INTERNET
http://research.vet.upenn.edu/penngen

Sugestões de Leitura
Giger U. Erythrocyte phosphofructokinase and pyruvate kinase deficiencies. In: Feldman BF, Zinkl JG, Jain NC, eds., Schalm's Veterinary Hematology, 5th ed. Philadelphia: Lippincott Williams & Wilkins, 2000, 1020-1025.
Harvey JW. Pathogenesis, laboratory diagnosis, and clinical implications of erythrocyte enzyme deficiencies in dogs, cats, and horses. Vet Clin Path 2006, 35:144-156.
Red blood cell enzyme activity. In: Vaden SL, Knoll JS, Smith FWK, Tilley LP, eds., Blackwell's Five-Minute Veterinary Consult: Laboratory Tests and Diagnostic Procedures — Canine & Feline. Ames, IA: Wiley-Blackwell, 2009, pp. 520-521.

Autor John W. Harvey
Consultor Editorial A.H. Rebar

DEFICIÊNCIA DE CARNITINA

CONSIDERAÇÕES GERAIS

REVISÃO

A L-carnitina é uma amina quaternária, que corresponde a um componente importante dos sistemas enzimáticos transportadores de ácidos graxos para o interior das mitocôndrias, de modo que eles possam ser oxidados, tornando a energia disponível à célula. Também desempenha funções importantes no metabolismo e na varredura celular. No coração e em outros órgãos dependentes da oxidação de ácidos graxos para suprir suas altas exigências energéticas para contração ou outra atividade, a deficiência de L-carnitina resulta na produção inadequada de energia para atender a tais necessidades. A deficiência de carnitina parece complicar alguns casos de miocardiopatia dilatada em cães. A presença da deficiência de L-carnitina em associação com miocardiopatia não significa que a deficiência seja a única causa da miopatia, embora a correção dessa deficiência (se possível) tenha sentido do ponto de vista clínico e fisiológico. A L-carnitina não é sintetizada nas musculaturas cardíaca e esquelética e, por essa razão, é imprescindível transportá-la para o interior dessas células a partir do plasma. No cão, a ingestão de carnitina na dieta influencia de modo significativo as concentrações plasmáticas, mas a suplementação oral desse aminoácido costuma ser um meio eficaz de elevar seus níveis plasmáticos e, subsequentemente, musculares. A FDA aprovou a adição de quantidades fisiológicas de carnitina a rações caninas comerciais para a prevenção da deficiência plasmática (e, subsequentemente, muscular) desse aminoácido. Essa medida é prudente, com base no conhecimento atual em relação à falta de L-carnitina em grande parte das rações caninas comerciais e ao efeito dessas dietas sobre os níveis plasmáticos de carnitina nos cães. Não se sabe se essa medida influenciará a prevalência da miocardiopatia dilatada ou de outras manifestações da deficiência de carnitina.

IDENTIFICAÇÃO

Cães

• As raças Boxer, Doberman pinscher, Dinamarquês, Wolfhound irlandês e outras raças de porte grande e gigante parecem ser mais comumente acometidas pela miocardiopatia dilatada.
• Ao menos alguns cães da raça Cocker spaniel americano com MCD são deficientes em carnitina, e os indícios de um ensaio cego controlado por placebo revelaram que a suplementação da L-carnitina combinada com a suplementação de taurina é benéfica no tratamento clínico desses pacientes.

SINAIS CLÍNICOS

• Os sinais clínicos de deficiência da carnitina podem ser diversos, pois as mitocôndrias em todos os tecidos fazem uso da L-carnitina para produzir energia a partir dos ácidos graxos.
• Os sinais variam desde insuficiência miocárdica e miocardiopatia dilatada (mais frequentemente identificada) até mialgia esquelética, fraqueza, intolerância a exercício e/ou letargia.
• Ver o capítulo "Miocardiopatia Dilatada — Cães".

CAUSAS E FATORES DE RISCO

• Relata-se que alguns cães com miocardiopatia tenham defeitos no transporte de carnitina; nesses casos, os níveis musculares de carnitina encontram-se baixos mesmo diante de concentrações plasmáticas adequadas desse aminoácido. Para transportar os ácidos graxos ou outros compostos (como a acetil Co-A) para dentro ou para fora das mitocôndrias, a L-carnitina livre é esterificada em uma substância, formando um éster de carnitina. Em alguns defeitos enzimáticos mitocondriais (p. ex., múltiplos defeitos da Co-A desidrogenase), a L-carnitina livre é usada para fazer a "varredura" do excesso de metabólitos potencialmente tóxicos, que aparecem de forma inócua na urina sob a forma de ésteres de carnitina. Nesses casos, a quantidade total de carnitina (carnitina livre + aquela esterificada em outras moléculas) no plasma ou na musculatura pode permanecer normal ou até mesmo ficar elevada, mas a proporção da carnitina livre em relação à esterificada diminui. Tal situação é conhecida como insuficiência de carnitina (pois a concentração da carnitina livre é insuficiente para suprir as necessidades corporais patologicamente elevadas para a forma livre desse aminoácido, embora sua concentração possa estar dentro dos limites de normalidade). • Certas famílias de cães da raça Boxer parecem estar sob risco particularmente alto de desenvolvimento de miocardiopatia dilatada sintomática em associação com deficiência de carnitina e provavelmente causada por essa deficiência.

DIAGNÓSTICO

DIAGNÓSTICO DIFERENCIAL

Ver o capítulo "Miocardiopatia Dilatada — Cães".

HEMOGRAMA/BIOQUÍMICA/URINÁLISE

Normais.

OUTROS TESTES LABORATORIAIS

A concentração plasmática de carnitina parece ser um indicador específico, mas insensível, de deficiência desse aminoácido no miocárdio ou na musculatura esquelética. As concentrações plasmáticas de carnitina livre inferiores a 8 μmol/L são consideradas diagnósticas de deficiência sistêmica desse aminoácido. As concentrações plasmáticas dentro do limite de normalidade ou acima do normal não descartam a deficiência ou a insuficiência de carnitina miocárdica.

DIAGNÓSTICO POR IMAGEM

Ver o capítulo "Miocardiopatia Dilatada — Cães".

MÉTODOS DIAGNÓSTICOS

As amostras obtidas por meio de biopsia endomiocárdica devem ser preparadas como blocos secos e congeladas instantaneamente em nitrogênio líquido. A mensuração das concentrações de L-carnitina livre e esterificada normalizadas em relação à quantidade de proteína não colagenosa na biopsia continua sendo o único teste diagnóstico definitivo. As concentrações miocárdicas de carnitina livre abaixo de 3,5 nmol/mg de proteína não colagenosa são consideradas diagnósticas de deficiência desse aminoácido no miocárdio. As proporções de carnitina esterificada em relação à livre superiores a 0,4 são consideradas diagnósticas de insuficiência de carnitina.

TRATAMENTO

O tratamento com a L-carnitina não substitui a terapia convencional para a MCD, mesmo em grande parte dos cães com deficiência de carnitina. Alguns cães, incluindo determinadas famílias de Boxer deficientes em carnitina, não respondem clinicamente à suplementação. Embora a suplementação promova de forma drástica a melhora de uma pequena porcentagem (cerca de 5% na experiência do autor) de cães com miocardiopatia dilatada, ainda não se comprovou a eficácia global da suplementação com a L-carnitina no tratamento desse tipo de miocardiopatia.

MEDICAÇÕES

MEDICAMENTO(S)

Suplementação de Carnitina

• Raças caninas de grande porte — 2 g (cerca 1 colher das de chá de L-carnitina em pó) a cada 8-12 h.
• Cocker spaniel americano (em combinação com a taurina) — 1 g (aproximadamente meia colher das de chá de L-carnitina em pó) a cada 8-12 h.

CONTRAINDICAÇÕES/INTERAÇÕES POSSÍVEIS

• Ainda não se identificou nenhuma contraindicação ou interação possível.
• Em algumas pessoas, associa-se uma leve diarreia a doses altas de carnitina.

ACOMPANHAMENTO

Repetir o ecocardiograma 3-6 meses após o início da suplementação com a L-carnitina para avaliar a eficácia do tratamento.

DIVERSOS

Sugestões de Leitura

Keene BW, Kittleson MD, Rush JE, et al. Myocardial carnitine deficiency associated with dilated cardiomyopathy in Doberman pinschers. J Vet Intern Med 1989, 3:126 (Abstract).
Keene BW, Panciera DP, Atkins CE, et al. Myocardial L-carnitine deficiency in a family of dogs with dilated cardiomyopathy. JAVMA 1991, 201:647-650.
Sanderson SL, Gross KL, Ogburn PN, et al. The effect of dietary fat and L-carnitine on plasma and whole blood taurine concentrations and cardiac function in healthy dogs consuming protein-restricted diets. Am J Vet Res 2001, 62:1616-1623.

Autor Bruce W. Keene
Consultores Editoriais Larry P. Tilley e Francis W. K. Smith Jr.

Deficiência de Taurina

CONSIDERAÇÕES GERAIS

REVISÃO
- A taurina é um aminoácido essencial na dieta dos gatos; os animais dessa espécie precisam conjugar os ácidos biliares com a taurina e não conseguem sintetizá-la o suficiente a ponto de lidar com essa perda obrigatória; por essa razão, dietas deficientes em taurina provocam a deficiência desse aminoácido nos gatos. Todos os fabricantes de rações para gatos adicionam a taurina às suas dietas felinas. A taurina não é um aminoácido essencial nos cães e, dessa forma, a maior parte das dietas caninas não contém a adição desse aminoácido. Contudo, algumas rações caninas para problemas cardíacos e algumas outras rações, especialmente aquelas que contêm carne de cordeiro e arroz, podem ter taurina adicionada a elas.
- A taurina é encontrada por todo o organismo, com concentrações mais altas nos tecidos excitáveis (p. ex., miocárdio, sistema nervoso central e retina), onde sua função exata permanece um mistério. Ela provavelmente ajuda a manter gradientes osmolares e pode ajudar a regular o movimento do cálcio. Ela fica ativamente concentrada nas células miocárdicas por uma bomba de membrana que está sob a influência das catecolaminas.
- A deficiência de taurina resulta em degeneração da retina e insuficiência do miocárdio (i. e., contratilidade miocárdica reduzida), uma condição comumente denominada de miocardiopatia dilatada, que foi identificada em gatos domésticos, raposas e alguns cães. Nesses animais, a insuficiência miocárdica costuma ser completa ou parcialmente reversível com a suplementação de taurina na dieta.

IDENTIFICAÇÃO
- Gatos — a miocardiopatia dilatada atribuída à deficiência de taurina é rara, porque esse aminoácido é adicionado à maioria das rações para gatos.
- Cães — os animais da raça Cocker spaniel americano com miocardiopatia dilatada são quase uniformemente deficientes em taurina. Alguns cães pertencentes a raças gigantes (Terra Nova) com miocardiopatia dilatada, especialmente aqueles sob dieta à base de carne de cordeiro e arroz, exibiram deficiência em taurina. Alguns cães com miocardiopatia dilatada pertencentes a raças que não costumam ter miocardiopatia dilatada ou cães de raças mistas com miocardiopatia dilatada apresentam baixa concentração plasmática de taurina.

SINAIS CLÍNICOS
Ver "Miocardiopatia Dilatada (Gatos e Cães)".

CAUSAS E FATORES DE RISCO
- Gatos alimentados com dietas caseiras (p. ex., dietas vegetarianas ou com carne cozida) estão sob risco; raramente um gato com miocardiopatia dilatada que esteja recebendo alguma ração comercial apresentará baixa concentração plasmática de taurina.
- Cães — predisposição racial (Cocker spaniel americano), porte da raça (p. ex., Terra Nova), dieta e cistinúria são fatores de risco.

DIAGNÓSTICO

DIAGNÓSTICO DIFERENCIAL
Miocardiopatia dilatada idiopática ou insuficiência miocárdica atribuída a alguma outra causa; ver "Miocardiopatia Dilatada (Gatos e Cães)".

HEMOGRAMA/BIOQUÍMICA/URINÁLISE
- Sem anormalidades características.
- Cistinúria em alguns cães.

OUTROS TESTES LABORATORIAIS
- Obter amostra de sangue heparinizado, colocá-la no gelo e centrifugar por 30 min. Não deixar coagular, porque as plaquetas são ricas em taurina. Evitar a ocorrência de hemólise. A concentração de taurina plasmática abaixo de 40-60 nmoles/L é muito baixa nos cães e nos gatos. O sangue total heparinizado também pode ser testado; a concentração no sangue total abaixo de 200 nmoles/L é muito baixa.
- O jejum prolongado nos gatos pode produzir baixa concentração de taurina no plasma; a concentração no sangue total permanece dentro dos limites de normalidade por mais tempo.

DIAGNÓSTICO POR IMAGEM
A insuficiência miocárdica costuma ser diagnosticada pela identificação de aumento no diâmetro sistólico final, em geral com aumento compensatório menor no diâmetro diastólico final e consequente fração de encurtamento reduzida no ecocardiograma.

MÉTODOS DIAGNÓSTICOS
Examinar todo paciente com deficiência de taurina em busca de degeneração central da retina.

TRATAMENTO

- Utilizar o tratamento convencional para insuficiência cardíaca até que a suplementação com taurina tenha induzido a uma melhora ecocardiográfica e clínica significativa; em geral, a terapia medicamentosa pode ser interrompida depois de 3-6 meses de suplementação com taurina, tanto nos cães como nos gatos responsivos à suplementação.
- Praticamente todos os gatos com insuficiência cardíaca ficam melhores quando mandados de volta para casa, desde que o proprietário consiga fornecer cuidados satisfatórios de enfermagem.
- Não há nenhum benefício conhecido à suplementação de taurina em cão ou gato com doença cardíaca além da miocardiopatia dilatada causada por deficiência desse aminoácido.

MEDICAÇÕES

MEDICAMENTO(S)
- Suplemento de taurina (gatos: 250 mg VO a cada 12 h; cães: 250-1.000 mg VO a cada 12 h), em geral por toda a vida.
- Suplementos com taurina — podem ser obtidos de lojas de produtos naturais sem receita; são relativamente baratos.
- Suplementação com carnitina — (1 g VO a cada 12 h) também é recomendada para os animais da raça Cocker spaniel americano, especialmente se eles não forem responsivos à suplementação isolada de taurina.

CONTRAINDICAÇÕES/INTERAÇÕES POSSÍVEIS
Não é conhecido nenhum efeito adverso da suplementação com taurina; o excesso desse aminoácido é excretado na urina.

ACOMPANHAMENTO

Exames de rotina para paciente com insuficiência cardíaca; repetir o ecocardiograma em 3-6 meses para comprovar a melhora. Caso não haja melhora, pode-se interromper a suplementação com taurina.

DIVERSOS

RECURSOS DA INTERNET
http://www.vmth.ucdavis.edu/cardio/cases/case32/case32.htm.

Sugestões de Leitura
Backus RC, Cohen G, Pion PD, Good KL, Rogers QR, Fascetti JR. Taurine deficiency in Newfoundlands fed commercially available complete and balanced diets. JAVMA 2003, 223:1130-1136.
Fascetti AJ, Reed JR, Rogers QR, Backus RC. Taurine deficiency in dogs with dilated cardiomyopathy: 12 cases (1997-2001). JAVMA 2003, 223:1137-1141.
Kittleson MD, Keene B, Pion PD, Loyer CG, and the MUST Study Investigators. Results of the Multicenter Spaniel Trial (MUST): Taurine- and carnitine-responsive dilated cardiomyopathy in American cocker spaniels with decreased plasma taurine concentration. J Vet Intern Med 1997, 11(4):204-211.
Kramer GA, Kittleson MD, Fox PR, et al. Plasma taurine concentrations in normal dogs and in dogs with heart disease. J Vet Intern Med 1995, 9:253-258.
Pion PD, Kittleson MD, Rogers QR, Morris JG. Myocardial failure in cats associated with low plasma taurine: A reversible cardiomyopathy. Science 1987, 237:764-768.
Sanderson SL, Osborne CA, Lulich JP, et al. Evaluation of urine carnitine and taurine excretion in 5 cystinuric dogs with carnitine and taurine deficiency. J Vet Intern Med 2000, 15:94-100.

Autor Mark D. Kittleson
Consultores Editoriais Larry P. Tilley e Francis W.K. Smith, Jr.

DEFICIÊNCIA DOS FATORES DE COAGULAÇÃO

CONSIDERAÇÕES GERAIS

DEFINIÇÃO
Defeitos hemostáticos caracterizados pela falta de um ou mais fatores de coagulação.

FISIOPATOLOGIA
• O mecanismo de coagulação envolve uma série complexa de reações enzimáticas, que levam à geração de trombina (fator II) em locais de lesão vascular. A trombina promove a clivagem do fibrinogênio plasmático em monômeros de fibrina que, subsequentemente, são polimerizados e entrelaçados para formar o coágulo de fibrina insolúvel.
• As deficiências funcionais e/ou quantitativas dos fatores de coagulação causam a falha na formação do coágulo de fibrina.
• O fígado constitui o único ou principal local de síntese de grande parte dos fatores de coagulação. Após a síntese, os fatores II, VII, IX e X necessitam de uma modificação dependente da vitamina K para se tornarem plenamente eficazes.

SISTEMA(S) ACOMETIDO(S)
• Os defeitos dos fatores de coagulação podem ocasionar hemorragia espontânea, hemorragia pós-traumática prolongada e, por fim, anemia por perda sanguínea.
• Hemorragia espontânea — frequentemente se desenvolve nas cavidades corporais ou em espaços potenciais (ou seja, hemotórax, hemoperitônio, hemartrose, hematoma subcutâneo ou intramuscular).

IDENTIFICAÇÃO
• Deficiências adquiridas dos fatores de coagulação — dependem do processo patológico subjacente.
• Deficiências hereditárias dos fatores de coagulação — os defeitos graves manifestam-se por volta de 3-6 meses de idade; no entanto, os defeitos hemostáticos mais brandos manifestam-se após cirurgia ou traumatismo.
• Hemofilia A e B (deficiências dos fatores VIII e IX) — traços recessivos ligados ao cromossomo X (os portadores do sexo masculino manifestam a tendência hemorrágica, enquanto os do sexo feminino permanecem clinicamente normais).
• Hemofilia A — é uma deficiência hereditária comum de fator de coagulação, observada em todas as raças e também em cães e gatos sem raça definida.
• Deficiências de todos os outros fatores — traços autossômicos; machos e fêmeas manifestam os sinais com frequência equivalente. É mais provável que defeitos específicos sejam propagados dentro de uma única raça, embora todas as raças estejam sob risco do desenvolvimento de novas mutações.
• Deficiência do fator XII — é comum em gatos, mas não causa tendência hemorrágica clínica.

SINAIS CLÍNICOS
• Formação de hematoma.
• Hemorragia intracavitária.
• Hemorragia pós-cirúrgica ou pós-traumática prolongada.
• Anemia por perda sanguínea.

CAUSAS
• Adquiridas — falha na síntese (hepatopatia); deficiência de vitamina K (colestase, toxicidade por rodenticida anticoagulante, má absorção, administração prolongada de antibióticos, coumadina); inibição de fator (dosagem excessiva de heparina; envenenamento); consumo e depleção dos fatores (CID); diluição dos fatores (transfusão de altos volumes; expansores de plasma).
• Hereditárias — mutações distintas nos genes responsáveis pela codificação dos fatores de coagulação.

FATORES DE RISCO
Ver o item sobre causas adquiridas (anteriormente).

DIAGNÓSTICO

DIAGNÓSTICO DIFERENCIAL
• A trombocitopenia deve ser o primeiro sinal a ser descartado para qualquer paciente com hemorragia anormal.
• As coagulopatias adquiridas frequentemente se desenvolvem por causa de hepatopatia, ingestão de rodenticida anticoagulante, e CID.
• Hepatopatia é acompanhada por alterações no hemograma completo e nos perfis bioquímicos (ver Coagulopatia por Hepatopatia).
• A toxicidade por rodenticida anticoagulante prolonga os testes de triagem de TTPA e TP, mas não afeta os testes de TCT ou fibrinogênio.
• A CID sempre se desenvolve secundariamente à doença sistêmica (sobretudo sepse ou neoplasia), sendo acompanhada muitas vezes por contagem plaquetária baixa ou em queda.
• Transfusão maciça (>1 volume sanguíneo) com produtos sanguíneos armazenados pode diluir os fatores funcionais, o fibrinogênio e as plaquetas abaixo dos níveis hemostáticos.
• As deficiências hereditárias dos fatores de coagulação geram prolongamento nos testes de triagem de coagulação, enquanto a doença de von Willebrand, não.

ACHADOS LABORATORIAIS

Medicamentos Capazes de Alterar os Resultados Laboratoriais
Dosagens terapêuticas de heparina não fracionada, coumadina e expansores plasmáticos (dextrana, hetamido) prolongam os testes de triagem de coagulação.

Distúrbios Capazes de Alterar os Resultados Laboratoriais
• A coleta inadequada de amostra invalidará os resultados dos testes de coagulação (técnica insatisfatória de venopunção, tubos de coleta parcialmente preenchidos com citrato, uso de tubos heparinizados ou com ativador de coágulo).
• Lipemia, hemoglobinemia ou icterícia extremas podem interferir na detecção de coágulos por alguns analisadores foto-ópticos de coagulação.
• Em virtude da instabilidade de alguns fatores de coagulação, é recomendável analisar as amostras no local ou separar o plasma do restante da amostra e enviá-lo conservado no gelo ao laboratório.

Os Resultados Serão Válidos se os Exames Forem Realizados em Laboratório Humano?
• A interpretação dos resultados dos ensaios de coagulação necessita de faixas de referência da mesma espécie e controles. Por exemplo, os valores de TTPA em seres humanos são geralmente o dobro daqueles de cães e gatos.
• O laboratório deve confirmar a ocorrência de reatividade cruzada dos ensaios antigênicos e a otimização de testes funcionais para os plasmas dos animais.

HEMOGRAMA/BIOQUÍMICA/URINÁLISE
• Ocorre o desenvolvimento de anemia regenerativa após perda sanguínea.
• A contagem plaquetária permanece normal a menos que o paciente apresente CID ou sangramento maciço.
• A reabsorção de sangue proveniente de hematomas extensos pode gerar elevação nos níveis da bilirrubina.

OUTROS TESTES LABORATORIAIS
• Os testes de triagem de coagulação (TCA, TTPA, TP, TCT) são testes funcionais que medem o tempo para a formação de coágulo *in vitro*. As deficiências dos fatores de coagulação e do fibrinogênio prolongam o tempo de coagulação (ver algoritmo, Figura 1).
• O TCA é um teste de triagem realizado no momento da prestação de cuidados que detecta deficiências graves de todos os fatores (exceto do fator VII). O TCA pode ser influenciado por anemia, trombocitopenia e alterações na viscosidade sanguínea.
• O TTPA é um teste de triagem para via de contato (pré-calicreína, cininogênio de alto peso molecular, fator XII), via intrínseca (fatores XI, IX, VIII), via comum (fatores X, V, II) e deficiência grave de fibrinogênio.
• O TP é um teste de triagem para fator VII, via comum e deficiência grave de fibrinogênio.
• O TCT é um teste de triagem de fibrinogênio funcional, sendo sensível à presença de inibidores do fibrinogênio.
• As deficiências adquiridas dos fatores de coagulação geralmente causam prolongamento de mais de um teste de triagem. As deficiências hereditárias mais comuns de fatores (hemofilia e deficiência do fator XII) prolongam especificamente o TTPA.
• Para o diagnóstico definitivo de coagulopatias hereditárias ou complexas, podem ser realizados ensaios de cada fator individualmente.

DIAGNÓSTICO POR IMAGEM
N/D.

MÉTODOS DIAGNÓSTICOS
O tempo de sangramento da mucosa bucal encontra-se prolongado em pacientes com trombocitopenia grave, disfunção plaquetária, doença de von Willebrand e deficiência de fibrinogênio, mas esse tempo é insensível às deficiências dos fatores de coagulação.

TRATAMENTO

• A transfusão de sangue total fresco, plasma fresco e plasma fresco congelado suprirá todos os fatores de coagulação.
• O crioprecipitado é uma fonte específica de fator VIII, fibrinogênio e fator de von Willebrand. O criossobrenadante plasmático fornece todos os outros fatores.
• A terapia com o(s) componente(s) necessário(s) é preferida para profilaxia cirúrgica e em pacientes não anêmicos para evitar a sensibilização das hemácias e a sobrecarga por volume.

Deficiência dos Fatores de Coagulação

- Os pacientes com graves deficiências adquiridas ou hereditárias dos fatores de coagulação podem necessitar de transfusões repetidas (a cada 8-12 h) para controlar ou evitar hemorragia.

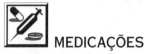

MEDICAÇÕES

MEDICAMENTO(S) DE ESCOLHA
A vitamina K_1 é um tratamento eficaz para pacientes com envenenamentos por rodenticidas anticoagulantes ou outras causas de deficiência de vitamina K.

CONTRAINDICAÇÕES
É recomendável evitar o uso de AINEs, anticoagulantes e expansores plasmáticos para evitar maior comprometimento da hemostasia.

PRECAUÇÕES
- Em virtude do risco de indução de sangramentos extras, é recomendável evitar as injeções intramusculares e a colocação de cateter jugular.
- Da mesma maneira, não se recomenda a administração intravenosa da vitamina K por causa do risco de anafilaxia.

INTERAÇÕES POSSÍVEIS
Nenhuma.

MEDICAMENTO(S) ALTERNATIVO(S)
Alternativas como antifibrinolíticos e fator VIIa recombinante ainda não foram avaliadas em ensaios clínicos veterinários.

ACOMPANHAMENTO

MONITORIZAÇÃO DO PACIENTE
- Em animais com intoxicação por anticoagulantes, pode-se lançar mão dos ensaios de TP, PIVKA ou fator VII para monitorizar a eficácia da administração da vitamina K. Os resultados dos testes devem se normalizar 24-48 horas após o início da terapia.
- O TCA é um substituto menos sensível, porém razoável, para monitorizar a resposta à vitamina K.
- Os defeitos hereditários podem ser monitorizados pela interrupção clínica do sangramento, estabilização do hematócrito, resolução do hematoma e, se necessário, por análises de fatores específicos.

COMPLICAÇÕES POSSÍVEIS
A transfusão representa um risco de reações imunes (p. ex., sensibilização eritrocitária, urticária) e não imunes (p. ex., transmissão de doenças, sobrecarga de volume).

DIVERSOS

DISTÚRBIOS ASSOCIADOS
Nenhuma.

FATORES RELACIONADOS COM A IDADE
Nenhum.

POTENCIAL ZOONÓTICO
Nenhum.

GESTAÇÃO/FERTILIDADE/REPRODUÇÃO
Os pacientes com deficiências hereditárias dos fatores de coagulação não devem ser acasalados.

SINÔNIMO(S)
- Defeitos de coagulação.
- Coagulopatias.

VER TAMBÉM
- Coagulopatia por Hepatopatia.
- Coagulação Intravascular Disseminada.
- Doença de von Willebrand.

ABREVIATURA(S)
- AINEs = anti-inflamatórios não esteroides.
- CID = coagulação intravascular disseminada.
- PIAVK = proteínas induzidas pela ausência ou antagonismo da vitamina K.
- TCA = tempo de coagulação ativada.
- TCT = tempo de coagulação da trombina.
- TP = tempo de protrombina.
- TTPA = tempo de tromboplastina parcial ativada.

RECURSOS DA INTERNET
http://www.labtestsonline.org/understanding/analytes/coagulation_factors/test.html.

Sugestões de Leitura

Brooks M. Coagulopathies and Thrombosis. In: Ettinger SJ, Feldman EC, ed. Textbook of veterinary internal medicine. Philadelphia: Saunders, 2000:1829-1841.

Dodds WJ. Hemostasis. In: Kaneko JJ, Harvey JW, Bruss ML, eds. Clinical biochemistry of domestic animals. New York: Academic Press, 1997:241-283.

Jain NC. Coagulation and its disorders. In: Jain NC, ed. Essentials of veterinary hematology. Philadelphia: Lea & Febiger, 1993:82-104.

Autor Marjory Brooks
Consultor Editorial A. H. Rebar

TESTES DE TRIAGEM DE COAGULAÇÃO: TTPA, TP, TCT

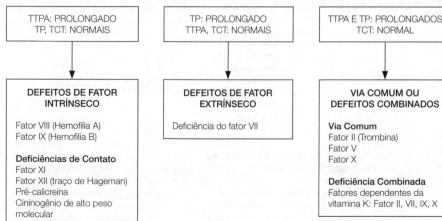

Figura 1 Algoritmo diagnóstico para deficiências dos fatores de coagulação.

Deformidades do Crescimento Antebraquial

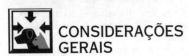

CONSIDERAÇÕES GERAIS

DEFINIÇÃO
Configuração anormal dos membros torácicos e/ou mau alinhamento do cotovelo ou das articulações cárpicas antebraquiais, resultantes do desenvolvimento anormal do rádio ou da ulna no animal em processo de crescimento.

FISIOPATOLOGIA
• Antebraço — predisposto a deformidades resultantes do crescimento contínuo de um único osso após interrupção prematura do crescimento ou redução na taxa de crescimento do osso pareado.
• A taxa reduzida de alongamento em um único osso comporta-se como uma espécie de tira retardadora; o osso pareado em crescimento deve sofrer uma deformação e um arqueamento em direção oposta ao osso curto ou exibir um crescimento exagerado no cotovelo ou no carpo; isso, por sua vez, gera um mau alinhamento articular.
• Crescimento normal — os ossos alongam-se por meio do processo de ossificação endocondral, que ocorre na fise; o fechamento fisário se dá quando a camada de células germinativas interrompe sua produção de cartilagem nova e a cartilagem existente sofre hipertrofia, ossificação e remodelagem em tecido ósseo.
• Hereditária — há relatos de um fechamento prematuro da fise ulnar distal como um traço recessivo no Skye terrier; pode ser um componente de mau alinhamento comum da articulação do cotovelo em muitas raças condrodisplásicas (Basset hound e Lhasa apso).
• Osteocondrose ou suplementação nutricional excessiva — possivelmente associada com o retardo da ossificação endocondral (centros cartilaginosos retidos) em raças caninas de porte gigante.
• Osteodistrofia hipertrófica — síndrome de crescimento juvenil com inflamação da fise e do periósteo que pode impedir o crescimento fisário.
• Traumatismo — a causa mais comum; em caso de compressão da camada condroproliferativa da fise (fratura de Salter Harris do tipo V), ocorrerá a interrupção de nova produção cartilaginosa e do alongamento ósseo.

SISTEMA(S) ACOMETIDO(S)
Musculosquelético.

GENÉTICA
• Cães da raça Skye terrier — descritas como um traço hereditário recessivo.
• Raças condrodisplásicas (cães) — predispostas ao mau alinhamento do cotovelo.

INCIDÊNCIA/PREVALÊNCIA
• Traumática — pode ocorrer após lesões dos membros torácicos em até 10% dos animais em crescimento ativo; incomum em gatos.
• Síndrome de mau alinhamento do cotovelo ± deformidade angular (raças caninas condrodisplásicas) — razoavelmente comum e pode ser bilateral.
• Induzida por fator nutricional — a incidência diminui com a melhoria dos padrões nutricionais.
• Agenesia genética do rádio (gatos e, raramente, cães) — observada ocasionalmente; resulta em uma grave curvatura do antebraço e subluxação do carpo.

DISTRIBUIÇÃO GEOGRÁFICA
N/D.

IDENTIFICAÇÃO
Espécies
Cães e gatos.

Raça(s) Predominante(s)
• Cães da raça Skye terrier — forma hereditária recessiva.
• Raças condrodisplásicas e toys (especialmente Basset hound, Dachshund, Lhasa apso, Pequinês, Jack Russell terrier) — podem ser predispostas a maus alinhamentos do cotovelo.
• Raças gigantes (p. ex., Dogue alemão e Wolfhound) — pode ser induzida pelo crescimento rápido decorrente de uma nutrição excessiva ou desbalanceada, osteocondrodisplasia, osteodistrofia hipertrófica.

Idade Média e Faixa Etária
• Traumática — em qualquer momento durante a fase de crescimento ativo.
• Más articulações do cotovelo — no transcorrer do crescimento; podem não ser identificadas até que as alterações artríticas secundárias se tornem graves, ocasionalmente após alguns anos de idade.

Sexo(s) Predominante(s)
N/D.

SINAIS CLÍNICOS
Comentários Gerais
• Cães de membros mais longos — as deformidades angulares geralmente são mais comuns.
• Cães de membros mais curtos — tendem a desenvolver maus alinhamentos articulares mais graves.
• Idade no momento de fechamento prematuro — acomete o grau relativo de deformidade e má articulação das juntas; talvez em função da variação na rigidez do osso com a idade e da duração de alteração no crescimento até a maturidade.

Achados Anamnésicos
• Traumática — angulação ou claudicação progressivas dos membros em 3-4 semanas após a lesão; o proprietário pode não ter consciência do evento causal.
• Maus alinhamentos evolutivos do cotovelo — início insidioso de claudicação em um ou ambos os membros torácicos; mais evidente após a prática de exercícios.

Achados do Exame Físico
Fechamento Ulnar Distal Prematuro
• Três deformidades da porção distal do rádio — desvio lateral (valgo), arqueamento cranial (curvo) e rotação externa (supinação).
• Encurtamento relativo da extensão do membro, em comparação ao membro contralateral de crescimento normal.
• Subluxação caudolateral da articulação radiocárpica e má articulação do cotovelo — podem ocorrer; provocam claudicação e restrição articular dolorosa.

Fechamento Fisário Radial Prematuro
• Membro acometido — significativamente mais curto do que o contralateral normal.
• Gravidade da claudicação — depende do grau de má articulação da junta.
• Fechamento simétrico completo da fise distal — pode-se observar um membro reto com uma ampliação do espaço articular radiocárpico; além disso, pode-se notar um arqueamento caudal em relação ao rádio e à ulna.
• Fechamento assimétrico da fise distal medial — deformidade angular do tipo varo; ocasionalmente, observa-se uma rotação interna.
• Fechamento da fise distal lateral — deformidade angular do tipo valgo; rotação externa.
• Fechamento da fise radial proximal com crescimento ulnar contínuo — má articulação do cotovelo; ampliação dos espaços entre o rádio e o úmero, bem como entre o úmero e o processo ancôneo.

CAUSAS
• Traumatismo.
• Fundo evolutivo.
• Base nutricional.

FATORES DE RISCO
• Traumatismo dos membros torácicos.
• Suplementação nutricional excessiva.

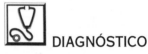

DIAGNÓSTICO

DIAGNÓSTICO DIFERENCIAL
• Displasia do cotovelo.
• Fragmentação do processo coronoide medial.
• Não união do processo ancôneo.
• Panosteíte.
• Contratura do tendão flexor.
• Osteodistrofia hipertrófica.

HEMOGRAMA/BIOQUÍMICA/URINÁLISE
N/D.

OUTROS TESTES LABORATORIAIS
N/D.

DIAGNÓSTICO POR IMAGEM
• Dano ao potencial de crescimento da fise — comumente pode não ser observado no momento do traumatismo; costuma ser notado 2-4 semanas antes de estar evidente no exame radiográfico.
• Projeções radiográficas padrão (craniocaudal e mediolateral) — abrangem toda a articulação do cotovelo; estendem-se desde a porção média do úmero em sentido proximal até os dedos no sentido distal; obter a mesma sequência radiográfica para fins comparativos com o membro contralateral normal.
• Grau de deformidade angular e de encurtamento relativo — determinado pela comparação das extensões relativas do rádio e da ulna dentro do par deformado em relação ao par contralateral normal.
• Grau de deformidade rotacional — determinado pela comparação da posição rotacional do cotovelo e do carpo na mesma projeção, ou seja, as projeções lateral do cotovelo e oblíqua do carpo a 45° registram a deformidade rotatória.
• Articulações do cotovelo e do carpo — avaliar quanto ao grau de mau alinhamento (tratamento cirúrgico) e à existência de artrite (p. ex., osteófitos; influencia o prognóstico).
• Articulação do cotovelo — avaliar quanto à presença de não união do processo ancôneo e fragmentação do processo coronoide medial associados.

MÉTODOS DIAGNÓSTICOS
N/D.

ACHADOS PATOLÓGICOS
A cartilagem de uma oclusão fisária prematura é substituída por osso.

Deformidades do Crescimento Antebraquial

TRATAMENTO

CUIDADO(S) DE SAÚDE ADEQUADO(S)
• Predisposição genética — não acasalar o animal.
• Dano fisário traumático — não é observado no momento da lesão; é revelado 2-4 semanas mais tarde.
• Após o diagnóstico, recomenda-se o tratamento cirúrgico o mais rápido possível.

CUIDADO(S) DE ENFERMAGEM
N/D.

ATIVIDADE
Restrição de exercícios — diminui o dano por mau alinhamento articular; retarda a evolução artrítica.

DIETA
• Reduzir a suplementação nutricional em raças caninas gigantes — lentifica o crescimento rápido; pode diminuir a incidência do quadro.
• Evitar o excesso de peso — ajuda a controlar a artralgia resultante do mau alinhamento e do uso articular excessivo.

ORIENTAÇÃO AO PROPRIETÁRIO
• Discutir a hereditariedade dos cães da raça Skye terrier e, possivelmente, das raças condrodisplásicas.
• Expor a não evidenciação dos danos ao potencial de crescimento fisário no momento do traumatismo aos membros torácicos e a frequente formulação do diagnóstico em 2-4 semanas após a lesão.
• Debater a importância do mau alinhamento articular e da artrite resultante como causas primárias de claudicação.
• Enfatizar a obtenção de um prognóstico mais satisfatório a partir do tratamento cirúrgico precoce.

CONSIDERAÇÕES CIRÚRGICAS
• Fechamento prematuro da fise ulnar distal em paciente com <5-6 meses de vida (potencial significativo de crescimento radial remanescente) — tratado por meio de ostectomia ulnar segmentar; deformidades do tipo valgo ≤25° — muitas vezes exibem correção espontânea e podem não necessitar de cirurgia extra; pacientes jovens e aqueles com deformidades mais graves — frequentemente exigem uma segunda correção definitiva após a maturidade.
• Fechamento da fise radial ou ulnar em paciente adulto (potencial de crescimento limitado ou nulo) requer a correção da deformidade, o realinhamento da articulação ou ambas as medidas.
• Correção da deformidade — pode ser concluída por meio de diversas técnicas de osteotomia; pode ser estabilizada com a utilização de vários dispositivos diferentes de fixação; essa intervenção deve corrigir tanto as deformidades rotacionais como as angulares; efetuada no ponto da curvatura maior.
• Mau alinhamento articular (particularmente do cotovelo) — deve ser corrigido para minimizar o desenvolvimento de lesões artríticas (causa primária de claudicação); obter um alinhamento articular ideal via osteotomia dinâmica da porção proximal da ulna (empregar a tração do músculo tríceps e a compressão da articulação) ou encurtamento de osso mais longo (ostectomia radial ou ulnar, conforme a indicação).
• Discrepâncias significativas de extensão dos membros — osteogênese por distração; a osteotomia do osso encurtado sofre uma separação progressiva na velocidade de 1 mm/dia com um sistema fixador externo, criando um novo comprimento ósseo.

MEDICAÇÕES

MEDICAMENTO(S) DE ESCOLHA
Medicamentos anti-inflamatórios — tratamento sintomático da artrite.

CONTRAINDICAÇÕES
Corticosteroides — não utilizar, por conta dos efeitos colaterais sistêmicos potenciais e dos danos cartilaginosos observados com o uso a longo prazo.

PRECAUÇÕES
Alertar o proprietário quanto aos possíveis desarranjos gastrintestinais associados à terapia anti-inflamatória crônica.

INTERAÇÕES POSSÍVEIS
N/D.

MEDICAMENTO(S) ALTERNATIVO(S)
Nutracêuticos (p. ex., glicosaminas) — podem ajudar a minimizar o dano à cartilagem e o desenvolvimento de artrite; podem ser anti-inflamatórios e analgésicos.

ACOMPANHAMENTO

MONITORIZAÇÃO DO PACIENTE
• Pós-operatória — depende do tratamento cirúrgico.
• Avaliações periódicas — avaliar o estado artrítico e a terapia anti-inflamatória.

PREVENÇÃO
• Acasalamento seletivo de raças suscetíveis.
• Evitar a suplementação nutricional excessiva em raças caninas gigantes de rápido crescimento.

COMPLICAÇÕES POSSÍVEIS
São habitualmente observadas em diversas técnicas de fixação da osteotomia (p. ex., infecção, não união da osteotomia e inflamação do trajeto do pino fixador).

EVOLUÇÃO ESPERADA E PROGNÓSTICO
• Em geral, constatam-se os melhores resultados com diagnóstico e tratamento cirúrgico precoces — minimizam a artrite.
• Fechamento ulnar prematuro — o tratamento tende a ser mais fácil; produz resultados mais satisfatórios.
• Alongamento do membro via osteogênese por distração — exige tratamento pós-operatório extenso tanto por parte do veterinário como do proprietário; alto índice de complicações.

DIVERSOS

DISTÚRBIOS ASSOCIADOS
• Osteocondrose.
• Osteodistrofia hipertrófica.
• Não união do processo ancôneo.

FATORES RELACIONADOS COM A IDADE
Quanto menor for a idade no momento do fechamento fisário induzido por via traumática, mais graves serão a deformidade e a má articulação.

POTENCIAL ZOONÓTICO
N/D.

GESTAÇÃO/FERTILIDADE/REPRODUÇÃO
N/D.

SINÔNIMO(S)
Rádio curvo.

Sugestões de Leitura
Balfour RJ, Boudrieau RJ, Gores BR. T-plate fixation of distal radial closing wedge osteotomies for treatment of angular limb deformities in 18 dogs. Vet Surg 2000, 29:207-217.
Dismukes DI, Fox DB, Tomlinson JL, Essman SC. Use of radiographic measures and three-dimensional computed tomographic imaging in surgical correction of an antebrachial deformity in a dog. JAVMA 2008, 232(1):68-73.
Fox DB, Tomlinson JL, Cook JL, Breshears LM. Principles of uniapical and biapical radial deformity correction using dome osteotomies and the center of rotation of angulation methodology in dogs. Vet Surg 2006, 35(1):67-77.
Henney LH, Gambardella PC. Premature closure of the ulnar physis in the dog: A retrospective clinical study. JAAHA 1989, 25:573-581.
Meola SD, Wheeler JL, Rist CL. Validation of a technique to assess radial torsion in the presence of procurvatum and valgus deformity using computed tomography: A cadaveric study. Vet Surg 2008, 37(6):525-529.
Quinn MK, Erhart N, Johnson AL, Schaeffer DJ. Realignment of the radius in canine antebrachial growth deformities treated with corrective osteotomy and bilateral (Type II) external fixation. Vet Surg 2000, 29:558-563.

Autor Peter K. Shires
Consultor Editorial Peter K. Shires

Degeneração Cerebelar

CONSIDERAÇÕES GERAIS

REVISÃO
- Envelhecimento e morte prematuros de neurônios corticais cerebelares, progressivos, específicos a determinadas raças e geneticamente induzidos, decorrentes de falhas no aporte energético neuronal, excitotoxicidade e inflamação; início na idade neonatal, pós-natal e, raramente, adulta.
- Ocorre após infecções virais intrauterinas ou neonatais em gatos (panleucopenia felina) e cães (herpes-vírus canino) como um distúrbio não progressivo.

IDENTIFICAÇÃO
Não Progressiva
- Cães e gatos.
- Setter irlandês, Fox terrier de pelo duro, Samoieda, Chow chow, Collie de pêlo áspero, Border collie, Bulmastife, Labrador retriever, Beagle — comumente acometidas, embora o quadro possa ser observado em outras raças de cães e gatos.
- Os sinais aparecem quando o paciente se encontra com 3-5 semanas de vida.

Progressiva
- Cães e gatos.
- Kerry blue terrier (sinais entre 12-16 semanas de vida), Collie de pêlo áspero na Austrália, Harrier finlandês, cães de corrida de Berna, Setter irlandês, Pointer inglês, Setter gordon (sinais entre 6-36 meses de vida), Spaniel britânico (sinais entre 7-13 anos), Staffordshire terrier americano (1 ano e meio-6 anos) e Buldogue inglês (5-8 meses).
- Modo de herança autossômica recessiva — provável em Setter gordon, Kerry blue terrier, Collie de pêlo áspero, Old English sheepdog e, possivelmente, gatos.
- Modo de herança ligado ao cromossomo X — provável no Pointer inglês porque só os machos são acometidos.
- Degeneração cerebelar e diluição da cor da pelagem — relatados em uma família de Rhodesian ridgeback.
- Coton de Tulear — início entre 2-6 semanas de vida, provavelmente de base genética.
- No gato doméstico de pelo curto, já foram descritas abiotrofia cortical cerebelar e degeneração retiniana com início na idade adulta.

SINAIS CLÍNICOS
- Dismetria — com frequência, manifesta-se como hipermetria.
- Postura em base larga.
- Movimentos oscilatórios do corpo.
- Tremores intencionais.
- Ausência de respostas à ameaça, com visão e força muscular facial normais.
- Inclinação da cabeça e episódios de ataxia vestibular com nistagmo de repouso ou de posicionamento.
- Hiper-refletividade tapetal difusa à fundoscopia (exame de fundo ocular por oftalmoscopia direta).
- Postura de descerebração — opistótono com rigidez extensora dos membros torácicos e flexão dos membros pélvicos.
- As alterações no estado mental, os déficits proprioceptivos e a paresia não são características desse distúrbio.
- A evolução dos sinais é variável.

CAUSAS E FATORES DE RISCO
- Infecção intrauterina ou neonatal pela panleucopenia felina ou pelo herpes-vírus canino.
- Histórico deficiente de vacinação ou exposição ao vírus vivo modificado durante a gestação.
- Reprodução de animais acometidos ou aqueles com histórico familiar e predisposição à degeneração cerebelar.
- Em uma ninhada de cães da raça Montanhês de Berna, foi descrita uma síndrome de degeneração hepatocerebelar.
- Em seres humanos, há relatos de degeneração cerebelar paraneoplásica.

DIAGNÓSTICO

DIAGNÓSTICO DIFERENCIAL
- Doenças do armazenamento lisossomal — doenças difusas do SNC; diferenciar por meio dos sinais relacionados a outras partes do SNC, além do cerebelo.
- Toxicidade (p. ex., hexaclorofeno) — diferenciar pelo histórico de exposição.
- Doenças inflamatórias (p. ex., cinomose canina e PIF) — frequentemente acompanhadas ou precedidas por sinais sistêmicos de doença; diferenciar pela análise do LCS.
- Cisto cerebelar — diferenciar por técnicas de diagnósticos por imagem (RM ou TC).
- Meduloblastoma (tumor cerebelar) — relatado em cães e gatos com menos de 1 ano de idade; diferenciar por técnicas de diagnósticos por imagem (RM e TC) e análise do LCS.
- Outros tumores primários e metastáticos em cães adultos — diferenciar por técnicas de diagnósticos por imagem (RM e TC) e análise do LCS.

HEMOGRAMA/BIOQUÍMICA/URINÁLISE
Em geral, permanecem normais.

OUTROS TESTES LABORATORIAIS
N/D.

DIAGNÓSTICO POR IMAGEM
RM — o cerebelo pode estar menor que o normal.

MÉTODOS DIAGNÓSTICOS
- Análise do LCS — normal em casos de doença não progressiva; concentração proteica normal ou elevada e contagens celulares normais em casos de doença progressiva.
- Biopsia cerebelar — pode ser o único método diagnóstico definitivo antes do óbito.

TRATAMENTO

- A amantadina tem efeitos potencializadores sobre a neurotransmissão dopaminérgica no SNC e atividade anticolinérgica; a buspirona é um agonista serotoninérgico; modelos de pesquisas demonstram que esses medicamentos são promissores para degeneração cerebelar progressiva.
- Agentes neuroprotetores que podem ter efeitos promissores, como Coenzima Q10 e Acetil-L--Carnitina.
- Tratamento em esquema ambulatorial — a menos que déficits graves impeçam a prestação dos cuidados de enfermagem em casa.
- Restringir a atividade a áreas seguras; evitar escadas, piscinas, etc.
- Dieta — normal; limitar o consumo de alimento se os episódios vestibulares forem acompanhados por êmese (para evitar pneumonia por aspiração).
- Doença não progressiva — o paciente pode exibir certa melhora à medida que ele aprende a compensar suas dificuldades motoras.

MEDICAÇÕES

MEDICAMENTO(S)
N/D.

CONTRAINDICAÇÕES/INTERAÇÕES POSSÍVEIS
N/D.

ACOMPANHAMENTO

- Estado neurológico — examinar em intervalos semanais a mensais se a evolução dos sinais for incerta; considerar a filmagem do paciente para determinar a evolução de forma mais objetiva.
- Evolução dos sinais — a velocidade varia de dias a anos e depende da identificação do animal.
- Não vacinar os animais prenhes com vacinas de vírus vivo modificado.
- Não acasalar os animais com histórico familiar de doença cerebelar.

DIVERSOS

ABREVIATURA(S)
- LCS = líquido cerebrospinal
- PIF = peritonite infecciosa felina
- RM = ressonância magnética
- SNC = sistema nervoso central
- TC = tomografia computadorizada

Sugestões de Leitura
Summers BA, Cummings JF, de Lahunta A. Veterinary neuropathology. St. Louis: Mosby, 1995:301-305.
van der Merwe LL, Lane E. Diagnosis of cerebellar cortical degeneration in a Scottish terrier using magnetic resonance imaging. J Small Anim Pract 2001;42(8):409-412.

Autor Richard J. Joseph
Consultor Editorial Joane M. Parent

Degeneração da Retina

CONSIDERAÇÕES GERAIS

DEFINIÇÃO
• Degeneração da retina por qualquer causa, hereditária ou adquirida.
• Hereditária — APR generalizada; grupo de doenças progressivas da retina; pode ser subdividida em displasias de fotorreceptores (começam antes de a retina se desenvolver completamente, <12 semanas) e degenerações de fotorreceptores (começam após o amadurecimento da retina).

FISIOPATOLOGIA
• Foram identificados vários defeitos genéticos no metabolismo de fotorreceptores.
• Pode ser secundária à doença do epitélio pigmentar retiniano ou da coroide (APR central; cães da raça Briard com cegueira noturna estacionária congênita; deficiência de ornitina; e as mucopolissacaridoses).
• Também pode ser idiopática, secundária à inflamação e cicatrização difusas ou focais (p. ex., coriorretinite), deficiência nutricional ou descolamento prévio da retina.

SISTEMA(S) ACOMETIDO(S)
• Sistema nervoso em doenças do armazenamento lisossomal.
• Oftálmico.

GENÉTICA
Cães
• APR — autossômica recessiva na maior parte das raças, particularmente Collie, Setter irlandês, Poodle miniatura, Cocker spaniel, Briard e Labrador retriever. Dominante em Mastiff, mas ligado ao cromossomo X em Samoieda e Husky siberiano.
• APR central — autossômica dominante com penetrância incompleta na raça Labrador retriever.
• A herança em muitas raças não foi determinada.
• Lipofuscinose ceroide neuronal — autossômica recessiva (comprovada ou presumida) em grande parte das raças.
• Hemeralopia — displasia autossômica recessiva de cones na raça Malamute do Alasca; herança indeterminada na raça Poodle miniatura.

Gatos
• Displasia de bastonetes e cones (os gatos da raça Abissínio apresentam 2 formas) — autossômica dominante: sinais clínicos aos 4 meses de vida; autossômica recessiva: o animal pode ficar cego por volta dos 2 anos de idade.
• Também pode apresentar início tardio aos 2 anos de idade, com problemas de visão em torno dos 4 anos de idade.
• Relatos isolados de herança dominante e recessiva em gatos jovens da raça Persa e Doméstico de pelo curto.
• Atrofia convoluta — autossômica recessiva; deficiência de ornitina aminotransferase.

INCIDÊNCIA/PREVALÊNCIA
• Hereditária — prevalência maior nos cães do que nos gatos.
• Deficiência de taurina — rara nos dias atuais, pois os gatos são suplementados de forma adequada.

DISTRIBUIÇÃO GEOGRÁFICA
APR central — mais comum em cães da Europa do que naqueles dos Estados Unidos.

IDENTIFICAÇÃO
Espécies
Cães e gatos.

Raça(s) Predominante(s)
Hereditária — Cães
• Displasia da retina — raças Bedlington terrier, Sealyham terrier, Springer spaniel inglês, Cocker spaniel e outras.
• APR de início precoce — raças Setter irlandês, Collie, Elkhound norueguês, Schnauzer miniatura, Pastor belga, Mastiff, Cardigan Welsh corgi e Briard; APR de início tardio — raças Poodle toy e miniatura, Cocker spaniel inglês e americano, Labrador retriever, Terrier tibetano, Dachshund miniatura de pelo longo, Akita, Samoieda, Husky siberiano.
• APR central — raças Labrador, Golden retriever, Border collie, Collie, Pastor de shetland, Briard, outras.
• Doença degenerativa dos cones — Pointer alemão de pelo curto e Malamute do Alaska.
• Lipofuscinose ceroide neuronal — raças Setter inglês, Border collie, Buldogue americano, Dálmata, Terrier tibetano, Collie.
• SDSAR — raças Spaniel britânico, Schnauzer miniatura, Dachshund, qualquer raça.

Hereditária — Gatos
• Abissínio e Somali (Abissínio de pelo longo).
• Siamês.
• Persa.

Idade Média e Faixa Etária
• APR e distrofias precoces — 3-4 meses a 2 anos.
• APR tardia — sinais clínicos > 4-6 anos.
• Doença degenerativa dos cones — 3-4 meses.
• SDSAR — meia-idade a idosos.

Sexo Predominante
• APR — condição recessiva ligada ao cromossomo X nas raças Husky siberiano e Samoieda; portanto, é mais provável que esteja presente nos machos.
• SDSAR — 70% são fêmeas.

SINAIS CLÍNICOS
Achados Anamnésicos
• APR (cães) — nictalopia (cegueira noturna) de evolução gradativa, que acaba afetando a visão à luz intensa; podem-se notar pupilas dilatadas ou reflexo tapetal mais brilhante à noite; pode aparecer como cegueira aguda (quando o paciente se torna totalmente cego ou se muda para ambientes desconhecidos).
• Hemeralopia ou doença degenerativa dos cones — rara; degeneração dos cones; perda da visão diurna.
• APR central (cães) — rara nos EUA; perda da visão central; pode nunca ficar completamente cego; acomete sobretudo raças de caça.
• Doença degenerativa dos cones — os filhotes caninos entre 8 e 12 semanas de vida revelam fotofobia e dificuldades de locomoção à luz intensa. Evolui para cegueira diurna total. A visão noturna permanece normal.
• SDSAR — perda da visão em 1-4 semanas; poliúria, polidipsia e polifagia são sinais comuns.

Achados do Exame Físico
• Quando grave — reflexos pupilares à luz consensuais e diretos prejudicados ou quase abolidos.
• Hiper-refletividade do tapete e despigmentação não tapetal ou hiperpigmentação mosqueada; adelgaçamento dos vasos sanguíneos da retina e atrofia do nervo óptico.
• APR (cães) — é comum a presença de cataratas.
• SDSAR (cães) — obesidade; podem-se notar reflexos pupilares à luz lentos ou ausentes.
• Retinopatia por deficiência de taurina (gatos) — começa como uma mancha na área central; em seguida, forma-se uma faixa horizontal superior ao nervo óptico; por fim, ocorrem degeneração difusa e hiper-refletividade.
• Cicatrizes pós-inflamatórias da retina — lesões focais ou multifocais manifestam-se como áreas de hiper-refletividade tapetal ou pigmentação alterada.
• Displasia do esqueleto pode estar associada a cães das raças Samoieda e Labrador retriever (i. e., nanismo).
• Displasia da retina também pode estar associada a outras inúmeras anomalias oculares nas raças Akita e Doberman pinscher.

CAUSAS
Degenerativas
• APR — acomete ambos os olhos de forma simétrica; muitas formas da APR são herdadas de forma recessiva, exceto para a forma dominante de APR em Bullmastiff.
• Glaucoma crônico ou não controlado — atrofia da retina e do nervo óptico.
• Secundária à cicatrização gerada por inflamação ou descolamento multifocais ou difusos prévios da retina.

Anômalas
• Displasias de fotorreceptores de cones e bastonetes — base genética; acometem ambos os olhos; perda da visão.
• Outras displasias — podem ser multifocais e sem cegueira (p. ex., nas raças Springer spaniel inglês e Labrador retriever).
• Displasia oculosquelética em Labrador e Samoieda.

Metabólicas
• Mucopolissacaridoses — cães de raças mistas; gatos das raças Siamês e Doméstico de pelo curto.
• Deficiência de ornitina aminotransferase — enzima mitocondrial; atrofia convoluta progressiva e total da coroide e da retina.

Neoplásicas
• Infiltrado de células neoplásicas pode levar à formação de cicatrizes por descolamento prévio da retina se tratado.

Nutricionais
• Deficiência grave das vitaminas E ou A (cães e gatos) — deficiência experimental ou natural em cães alimentados com dietas pobres nessas vitaminas (porém ricas em gorduras poli-insaturadas) pode provocar degeneração parcial ou completa.
• Deficiência de taurina (gatos) — provoca degeneração da retina e miocardiopatia dilatada.

Infecciosas/Imunes
• A retina sofre degeneração em decorrência de processo inflamatório; pode ser focal, multifocal ou generalizada — ver "Descolamento da Retina; Coriorretinite".

Idiopáticas
• SDSAR — cães; ver "Descolamento da Retina; Coriorretinite".
• Ver "Descolamento da Retina"; "Coriorretinite".

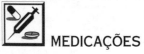

DEGENERAÇÃO DA RETINA

Tóxicas
• Reação idiossincrásica à griseofulvina ou ao enrofloxacino (gatos).
• Radiação — cães ou gatos tratados para neoplasia nasal ou neurológica (SNC).
• Administração concomitante de cloridrato de cetamina e metilnitrosoureia induz à degeneração difusa (gatos).

FATORES DE RISCO
• Doença ocular — cataratas; inflamação do segmento posterior; coriorretinite; descolamento da retina; glaucoma.
• Gatos — a dose de enrofloxacino não deve exceder 5 mg/kg/dia. Observa-se intoxicação com doses menores, especialmente em animais comprometidos (i. e., nefropatas, filhotes doentes, etc.).

DIAGNÓSTICO
DIAGNÓSTICO DIFERENCIAL
• Ver "Olho Cego Silencioso".
• Perda aguda da visão — reflexo pupilar à luz lento ou ausente; SDSAR, neurite óptica, descolamento da retina, APR não identificada ou glaucoma; reflexo pupilar à luz normal: doença do córtex visual ou cataratas diabéticas de rápido desenvolvimento.
• Perda visual lentamente progressiva — APR; cataratas; doença grave da córnea (p. ex., pigmentação, formação cicatricial ou edema); retinite crônica; coriorretinite; inflamação vítrea; diferenciada pelo exame oftalmológico.

HEMOGRAMA/BIOQUÍMICA/URINÁLISE
• Em geral, normais a menos que secundária a alguma doença sistêmica.
• SDSAR (cães) — os resultados podem ser compatíveis com hiperadrenocorticismo, o qual o paciente pode apresentar.

OUTROS TESTES LABORATORIAIS
• Testes de estimulação com ACTH e de supressão com dexametasona, avaliação dos níveis dos hormônios sexuais, mensuração da pressão arterial e determinação de proteinúria — na SDSAR.
• Concentração de taurina (gatos) — degeneração difusa, especialmente na miocardiopatia dilatada.
• Concentrações de ornitina (gatos) no soro e na urina — elevadas na deficiência de ornitina aminotransferase.
• Teste genético em amostras sanguíneas — OptiGen* LLC fornece testes genéticos em amostras sanguíneas para diversas variedades de doenças oculares geneticamente herdadas e algumas outras doenças metabólicas. Novos testes para diversas raças estão sendo continuamente desenvolvidos. Detalhes sobre os testes disponíveis, as amostras necessárias e como interpretar os resultados podem ser encontrados em www.optigen.com. Alguns testes genéticos (nos cães das raças Corgi e Setter irlandês) também estão disponíveis no laboratório VetGen* ou na Universidade do Estado de Michigan. Os resultados do teste frequentemente permitem a identificação dos portadores acometidos, não acometidos e prováveis com boa margem de confiança. Os resultados podem ajudar a direcionar os acasalamentos para evitar a obtenção de cães acometidos.

DIAGNÓSTICO POR IMAGEM
• Radiografias torácicas e ultrassom cardíaco — podem ser indicados em gatos com suspeita de deficiência de taurina.
• Radiografias e ultrassonografias abdominais (cães) — podem ser indicados em casos de SDSAR na suspeita de síndrome de Cushing.
• TC ou RM — utilizadas para descartar causas de cegueira central (p. ex., lesão do nervo óptico, cegueira cortical e SDSAR com adenoma hipofisário).

MÉTODOS DIAGNÓSTICOS
• Exame oftalmológico completo.
• Eletrorretinografia — confirma a cegueira não aparente à oftalmoscopia; resposta mínima ou ausente em casos graves (SDSAR, APR tardia); normal com neurite óptica e cegueira neurológica (SNC).
• Punção do LCS — pode ser realizada nos casos com suspeita de neurite óptica.

ACHADOS PATOLÓGICOS
• Retina delgada.
• Bordas das cicatrizes retinianas focais — nitidamente delineadas; curso inalterado dos vasos sanguíneos.
• Áreas hiperpigmentadas — associadas a cicatrizes pós-inflamatórias ou APR central.
• Características histológicas de degenerações em estágio final — atrofia acentuada de fotorreceptores; redução generalizada na densidade de células da retina.
• Acúmulo de lipopigmento no neuroepitélio — APR central, lipofuscinose ceroide, cegueira noturna estacionária congênita.
• Doenças do armazenamento lisossomal — acúmulo nas camadas neuronais/retinianas.

TRATAMENTO
DIETA
• Gatos — o alimento deve conter 500-750 ppm de taurina.
• Cães — dieta balanceada, evitando todas as carnes ricas em gorduras poli-insaturadas.

ORIENTAÇÃO AO PROPRIETÁRIO
• Informar ao proprietário que os cães são capazes de memorizar seu ambiente e que, a menos que a família se mude de casa ou troque a disposição da mobília, a maioria dos animais cegos vive bem.
• Avisar o proprietário que os cães cegos devem ser observados ou mantidos em coleira quando estiverem fora de casa, mas não devem ficar em jardins cercados ou em área com piscina.
• Sugerir o uso de brinquedos que façam ruídos.
• Alguns animais cegos idosos com outros problemas como perda de audição ou com senilidade podem não se adaptar bem à cegueira.
• Determinados animais cegos sofrem mudanças comportamentais, como aumento da agressividade ou diminuição da atividade.
• Os animais acometidos por um único olho cego podem exercer suas funções normalmente.
• Gatos cegos devem ser mantidos dentro de casa.

CONSIDERAÇÕES CIRÚRGICAS
Não indicada em pacientes com olhos cegos, mas sem dor.

MEDICAÇÕES
MEDICAMENTO(S)
• Atualmente, não há nenhum medicamento eficaz.
• Suplementação com piridoxina (gatos) — na deficiência de ornitina aminotransferase; pode aumentar a atividade da enzima; do ponto de vista clínico, não interrompe nem reverte a degeneração.
• Nível adequado de taurina na dieta — pode interromper a evolução da retinopatia causada por deficiência desse aminoácido.

TERAPIA GENÉTICA
Experimental — alguns centros de pesquisa estão trabalhando em certas retinopatias; i. e., distrofia do epitélio pigmentar retiniano nos cães da raça Briard.

CONTRAINDICAÇÕES
N/D.

PRECAUÇÕES
Cirurgia de catarata — não recomendada em pacientes com degeneração da retina; a eletrorretinografia pré-operatória é valiosa para evitar cirurgia desnecessária.

ACOMPANHAMENTO
MONITORIZAÇÃO DO PACIENTE
• Exames seriados do fundo ocular — confirmam a degeneração progressiva se o diagnóstico for duvidoso; serão observados sinais óbvios de degeneração durante semanas nas retinas dos cães com SDSAR.
• Cataratas em processo de desenvolvimento e evolução — na APR; ficar atento para complicações dolorosas (p. ex., glaucoma e uveíte).

PREVENÇÃO
• Não acasalar os animais com suspeita de APR hereditária.
• Não cruzar portadores conhecidos (p. ex., filho de animal acometido).

COMPLICAÇÕES POSSÍVEIS
• Cataratas.
• Glaucoma.
• Uveíte.
• Traumatismo ocular como resultado de diminuição da acuidade visual.
• Obesidade — secundária à atividade reduzida.

EVOLUÇÃO ESPERADA E PROGNÓSTICO
• APR hereditária — evolui para cegueira completa; a evolução quase sempre é lenta o suficiente para o paciente se adaptar à perda visual; não dolorosa.
• Degeneração causada por inflamação ou traumatismo anteriores — em geral, não evolui, a menos que uma doença sistêmica provoque inflamação ocular persistente (p. ex., síndrome uveodermatológica) ou recidivante.
• SDSAR — cegueira irreversível.
• Deficiência transitória de taurina (gatos) — a degeneração pode parar em qualquer estágio (p. ex., faixa horizontal de hiper-refletividade sobre o nervo óptico).

Degeneração da Retina

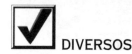

DIVERSOS

DISTÚRBIOS ASSOCIADOS
SDSAR — hiperadrenocorticismo adrenal ou hipofisário, proteinúria, hipertensão, hormônios sexuais elevados.

FATORES RELACIONADOS COM A IDADE
N/D.

POTENCIAL ZOONÓTICO
N/D.

GESTAÇÃO/FERTILIDADE/REPRODUÇÃO
N/D.

SINÔNIMO(S)
• APR — degeneração progressiva de bastonetes e cones; atrofia da retina.
• Retinopatia causada por deficiência de taurina — anteriormente denominada degeneração central da retina felina.

VER TAMBÉM
• Olho Cego "Silencioso".
• Coriorretinite.
• Doenças do Armazenamento Lisossomal.
• Descolamento da Retina.

ABREVIATURA(S)
• ACTH = hormônio adrenocorticotrópico.
• APR = atrofia progressiva da retina.
• LCS = líquido cerebrospinal.
• SDSAR = síndrome de degeneração súbita e adquirida da retina.
• RM = ressonância magnética.
• SNC = sistema nervoso central.
• TC = tomografia computadorizada.

RECURSOS DA INTERNET
Cegueira
www.blinddogs.com.
http://angelvest.homestead.com/.
http://www.pepedog.com/.
http://www.petcarebooks.com/.

Teste Genético e Doenças
http://www.aht.org.uk/genetics tests.html.
http://www.caninegeneticdiseases.net/.
http://www.vetgen.com/research-geneticdisease.html.www.optigen.com.

Sugestões de Leitura
Carter RT, Oliver JW, Stepien RL, et al. Elevations in sex hormones in dogs with acquired sudden acquired retinal degeneration syndrome (SARDs). JAAHA 2009, 45(5):207-214.
Narfström K, Petersen-Jones S. Diseases of the canine ocular fundus. In: Gelatt KN, ed., Veterinary Ophthalmology, 4th ed. Ames, IA: Blackwell, 2007, pp. 944-1025.

Autor Patricia J. Smith
Consultor Editorial Paul E. Miller

Degeneração e Hipoplasia Testiculares

CONSIDERAÇÕES GERAIS

REVISÃO
- Degeneração — alterações histológicas nos testículos após a puberdade; pode ser diferenciada da hipoplasia pela espessura aumentada da membrana basal no testículo degenerado.
- Hipoplasia — uma variedade de lesões histológicas que, supostamente, são congênitas (apesar de nem sempre óbvias até depois da puberdade) ou hereditárias.

IDENTIFICAÇÃO
- Cães e gatos.
- Cães — qualquer idade ou raça; hipoplasia, geralmente no jovem; degeneração, em geral no idoso.
- Gatos com pelagem cor de casco de tartaruga — podem ser férteis; geralmente ligados a anormalidades cromossômicas sexuais (ver "Distúrbios do Desenvolvimento Sexual").

SINAIS CLÍNICOS
- Infertilidade.
- Tamanho reduzido do testículo e perda da turgidez normal.
- Oligospermia (baixos números de espermatozoides no ejaculado) ou azoospermia (sem espermatozoides no ejaculado).
- Hipoplasia (cães) — raramente quaisquer sinais físicos além dos testículos pequenos.
- Degeneração (cães) — qualquer lesão anterior escrotal ou testicular pode estar relacionada.

CAUSAS E FATORES DE RISCO
Degeneração
- Calor.
- Irradiação.
- Metais — sais de chumbo; cádmio; compostos orgânicos de mercúrio.
- Compostos contendo nitrogênio e halogenados.
- Outras toxinas.
- Orquite — infecciosa (como brucelose) ou não infecciosa (autoimune).
- Hormônios esteroides — estrogênio secretado por Sertolinoma.
- Outras anormalidades hormonais — hipotireoidismo; hipocortisolismo; hiperadrenocorticismo.
- Avanço da idade — 6,3% dos cães da raça Beagle conservados até os 7,75 anos apresentavam espermatogênese incompleta.
- Esclerose arterial.
- Alguns agentes quimioterápicos — cimetidina; cetoconazol; nitrofuranos; flutamida.
- Biopsias testiculares incisionais.
- Qualquer lesão escrotal ou testicular anterior pode estar relacionada.
- Oclusão do epidídimo.

Hipoplasia
- Síndrome de Klinefelter (XXY).
- Hipogonadismo hipogonadotrópico — pode ser adquirido por lesão traumática ou neoplásica da hipófise.
- Inversão sexual XX — pseudo-hermafroditismo feminino.

DIAGNÓSTICO

DIAGNÓSTICO DIFERENCIAL
- Degeneração — cães idosos anteriormente férteis, azoospérmicos ou gravemente oligospérmicos, com testículos pequenos.
- Hipoplasia — cães jovens, azoospérmicos, nunca férteis com testículos pequenos.
- Espermatocele.
- Granuloma espermático.
- Orquite.
- Neoplasia.
- Falha na ejaculação — ejaculação retrógrada; ejaculação incompleta.

OUTROS TESTES LABORATORIAIS
- Ensaio do FSH canino — diferenciar de obstrução (espermatocele); concentração elevada indica espermatogênese incompleta associada à hipoplasia ou degeneração.
- Concentração da fosfatase alcalina do plasma seminal — descartar ejaculação incompleta; amostras com níveis de fosfatase alcalina <5.000 U/L são compatíveis com ejaculação completa ou obstrução bilateral do epidídimo.

DIAGNÓSTICO POR IMAGEM
Ultrassonografia — para avaliar o tamanho dos testículos e a homogenicidade do parênquima.

MÉTODOS DIAGNÓSTICOS
- Avaliação do sêmen — método primário de diagnóstico; cão: sempre obtido com a utilização de vagina artificial ou cone de coleta; gato: obtido por eletroejaculação, quando disponível; coletar dois ejaculados em dias separados ou com 1 h de intervalo; definir a presença de azoospermia ou oligospermia.
- Biopsia do testículo (em caso de azoospermia) — agulha fina: identificar espermátides longas e espermatozoides; Tru-Cut® (tampão tecidual): diagnóstico histopatológico mais completo; fixar o tecido para corte histopatológico em fixador de Bouin ou Zenker.
- Cariótipo — identificar o cromossomo X extra ou outra anomalia cromossômica numérica ou estrutural.

ACHADOS PATOLÓGICOS
- Espermatogênese normal — indica obstrução em cães azoospérmicos.
- Espessamento da membrana basal — diferencia hipoplasia da degeneração.

TRATAMENTO

- Degeneração ligada a disfunção hipofisária, adrenal, tireóidea ou outro distúrbio metabólico — o objetivo é corrigir a causa subjacente.
- Nenhum diagnóstico específico — pode-se tentar o uso de hormônios gonadotrópicos; segundo relatos, o sucesso é raro.

MEDICAÇÕES

MEDICAMENTO(S)
- Apesar de nenhum estudo controlado validar um aumento na produção de espermatozoides e da fertilidade com o uso de GnRH ou gonadotropinas, ambos os medicamentos são usados em muitas espécies; muito provavelmente geram melhoras em casos de hipogonadismo hipogonadotrópico, o que é raro nos animais domésticos.
- hCG — 500 UI SC 2 vezes por semana.
- GnRH — 1 µg/kg SC com ou sem hCG (1.600 UI IM).

ACOMPANHAMENTO

MONITORIZAÇÃO DO PACIENTE
Suspeita de degeneração testicular (cães) — é necessária a repetição da análise do sêmen realizada no mínimo 70 dias após a correção de qualquer causa subjacente identificada antes que a reversibilidade possa ser avaliada.

EVOLUÇÃO ESPERADA E PROGNÓSTICO
- Hipoplasia (cães) — prognóstico mau em termos de fertilidade.
- Degeneração (cães) — o prognóstico quanto à fertilidade depende da causa, do local e da extensão da lesão; geralmente reservado a mau.

DIVERSOS

VER TAMBÉM
- Brucelose.
- Distúrbios do Desenvolvimento Sexual.
- Espermatocele/Granuloma Espermático.
- Infertilidade dos Machos — Cães.
- Anormalidades dos Espermatozoides.

ABREVIATURA(S)
- FSH = hormônio foliculoestimulante.
- GnRH = hormônio liberador de gonadotropina.
- hCG = gonadotropina coriônica humana.

RECURSOS DA INTERNET
Gradil CM, Yeager A, Concannon PW. Assessment of reproductive problems in the male dog. In: Concannon PW, England G, Verstegen III J, Linde-Forsberg C, eds., Recent Advances in Small Animal Reproduction. International Veterinary Information Service, Ithaca NY, www.ivis.org, última atualização em 19 de abril de 2006; A1234.0406.

Sugestões de Leitura
Axner E, Strom B, Linde-Forsberg C, et al. Reproductive disorders in 10 domestic male cats. J Small Anim Pract 1996, 37:394-401.
Johnston SD, Root Kustritz MV, Olson PNS. Disorders of the canine penis and prepuce. In: Canine and Feline Theriogenology. Philadelphia: Saunders, 2001, pp. 356-367.
McEntee K. Reproductive Pathology of Domestic Animals. San Diego: Academic, 1990, pp. 262-263.

Autor Carlos R.F. Pinto
Consultor Editorial Sara K. Lyle
Agradecimento O autor e os editores agradecem a colaboração prévia de Rolf E. Larsen.

Degenerações e Infiltrações da Córnea

CONSIDERAÇÕES GERAIS

REVISÃO
Degeneração da córnea — alteração patológica adquirida da córnea, caracterizada por depósito de lipídio ou cálcio. As lesões podem ser uni ou bilaterais, ter margens distintas e ocorrer secundariamente a outros distúrbios oculares ou sistêmicos.

IDENTIFICAÇÃO
A degeneração da córnea ocorre principalmente em cães, mas é rara em gatos. O depósito de lipídio ocorre com maior frequência em cães de meia-idade a idosos com hiperlipoproteinemia sistêmica.

SINAIS CLÍNICOS
- Os sinais clínicos variam com base no tipo predominante de depósito e no distúrbio ocular ou sistêmico associado.
- Depósitos de lipídio — cinzas/brancos ou cristalinos; podem ser irregulares, em formato de bandas, ou circulares. Podem estar presentes em qualquer nível da córnea.
- Depósitos de cálcio — brancos densos a cristalinos; lesões irregulares, puntiformes ou em formato de bandas no estroma superficial.
- Frequentemente associadas a distúrbios inflamatórios, como ceratite ou uveíte.
- Com frequência, há vascularização, edema e pigmentação da córnea.
- Com a evolução do quadro, a córnea pode desenvolver um aspecto rugoso; o epitélio pode vir a sofrer ruptura, levando à ulceração.
- Distúrbios oculares associados que podem levar à alteração degenerativa da córnea — cicatrizes corneanas, ceratoconjuntivite seca, ceratite por exposição, uveíte crônica, episclerite, tísica bulbar (atrofia do bulbo), terapia tópica crônica com esteroides.
- Quando o depósito de lipídio ocorre secundariamente à hiperlipoproteinemia sistêmica, pode-se formar um anel perilimbal (arco lipoide corneano) com uma zona clara entre a córnea e o limbo acometidos; muitas vezes, ocorre envolvimento bilateral, mas assimétrico; a vascularização é variável.

CAUSAS E FATORES DE RISCO
- Depósitos de lipídio — hiperlipoproteinemia: pode aumentar o risco, agravar os depósitos já existentes; ou ser secundária a hipotireoidismo, diabetes melito, hiperadrenocorticismo, imprudência alimentar, pancreatite, síndrome nefrótica, hepatopatia, hiperlipidemia primária dos cães da raça Schnauzer miniatura. • Depósitos de cálcio — hipercalcemia, hiperfosfatemia, hipervitaminose D, hiperadrenocorticismo, uremia. • Ambos — distúrbios oculares listados anteriormente.

DIAGNÓSTICO

DIAGNÓSTICO DIFERENCIAL
- Outras causas de opacidades corneanas.
- Cicatriz corneana — lesão indolor de coloração cinza a branca, dependendo da gravidade; sem retenção do corante de fluoresceína (ou seja, resultado negativo do teste); superfície corneana relativamente lisa.
- Distrofias do estroma corneano — focos bilaterais e frequentemente simétricos de depósitos, com aparência cinza a esbranquiçada e margens distintas; distúrbio hereditário, não associado à inflamação ocular; sem retenção da fluoresceína; muitas vezes, ocorre distante do limbo.
- Edema — coloração azulada a cinza; em geral, mais homogêneo; pode variar de tamanho, dependendo da gravidade; margens indistintas; possível retenção da fluoresceína na presença de erosão/ulceração corneanas.
- Úlcera de córnea — resulta em dor ocular (oftalmalgia); retenção da fluoresceína; graus variados de edema podem circundar a lesão.
- Infiltrados de células inflamatórias — resultam em dor ocular (oftalmalgia); aparecem de coloração cinza a branca, com margens indistintas; o exame citológico da córnea revela a presença de leucócitos e microrganismos.

HEMOGRAMA/BIOQUÍMICA/URINÁLISE
- Depósitos de lipídio — avaliar os níveis de colesterol, triglicerídeos e glicose do paciente em jejum.
- Depósitos de cálcio — avaliar os níveis séricos desse elemento.

OUTROS TESTES LABORATORIAIS
- Depósitos de lipídio — hipotireoidismo: concentrações baixas dos hormônios tireoidianos e diminuição da resposta ao TSH.
- Síndrome de Cushing — teste de estimulação com ACTH.
- Na suspeita de pancreatite — teste de imunorreatividade da lipase pancreática.

DIAGNÓSTICO POR IMAGEM
N/D.

MÉTODOS DIAGNÓSTICOS
Se estiverem em relevo, as lesões poderão reter o corante de fluoresceína em torno das margens do depósito.

TRATAMENTO

- Tratar as doenças oculares primárias, se presentes.
- Em geral, os animais beneficiam-se com uma dieta pobre em gordura em casos de hiperlipoproteinemia; tratar as doenças sistêmicas primárias, se existentes; ambas as condutas podem ajudar a retardar ou interromper a evolução da doença.
- Os depósitos da córnea, responsáveis pela diminuição na acuidade visual ou na produção de desconforto ocular no animal, podem se beneficiar com diversos procedimentos, desde raspado vigoroso dessa estrutura ocular ou ceratectomia superficial até ressecção da lesão, acompanhados por tratamento clínico; no entanto, a recidiva dos depósitos é provável após o tratamento se a causa subjacente não for previamente corrigida.

MEDICAÇÕES

MEDICAMENTO(S)
- Antibióticos tópicos de amplo espectro (i. e., antibiótico triplo) — indicados em casos de úlcera de córnea; a frequência depende da gravidade; em geral, o tratamento de úlceras não complicadas é feito a cada 8-12 h.
- Anti-inflamatórios não esteroides tópicos a cada 8-12 h — indicados caso se observe uveíte.
- Ciclosporina tópica a 0,2% — para melhorar a qualidade do filme lacrimal e reduzir a inflamação.
- Atropina tópica a 1% a cada 8-24 h — indicada para diminuir a dor na presença de uveíte ou ulceração.
- Solução tópica de EDTA a 0,4-1,38% a cada 6 h — pode ajudar a minimizar os depósitos de cálcio; utilizada, em geral, após procedimento de ressecção para melhorar a eficácia do medicamento.
- Pomada de lágrima artificial a cada 6-12 h — pode evitar a ocorrência ou diminuir a frequência de ulceração corneana secundária; confere lubrificação aos olhos e melhora o conforto ocular quando a superfície da córnea se encontra rugosa/irregular.

CONTRAINDICAÇÕES/INTERAÇÕES POSSÍVEIS
- Corticosteroides tópicos — não recomendados; possível aumento na gravidade; contraindicados em casos de ulceração da córnea.
- Atropina tópica — contraindicada em casos de ceratoconjuntivite seca, glaucoma, luxação do cristalino.

ACOMPANHAMENTO

MONITORIZAÇÃO DO PACIENTE
Monitorizar os níveis séricos de colesterol e triglicerídeos para avaliar a eficácia da terapia nutricional; monitorizar o tratamento na presença de doença primária.

EVOLUÇÃO ESPERADA E PROGNÓSTICO
- Ulceração da córnea — pode estar associada ao agravamento da doença.
- Visão — pode vir a ser comprometida em casos de doença avançada; possivelmente grave na existência de doença ocular primária (p. ex., uveíte).
- Após cirurgia de ceratectomia superficial, o paciente poderá exibir recidiva dos depósitos.

DIVERSOS

VER TAMBÉM
- Ceratite Ulcerativa.
- Distrofias Corneanas.

ABREVIATURA(S)
- ACTH = hormônio adrenocorticotrópico.
- EDTA = ácido etilenodiaminotetracético.
- TSH = hormônio tireostimulante.

RECURSOS DA INTERNET
http://dro.hs.columbia.edu/ced1.htm.

Sugestões de Leitura
Crispin SM, Barnett KC. Dystrophy, degeneration and infiltration of the canine cornea. J Small Anim Pract 1983, 24:63-83.

Autor Renee T. Carter
Consultor Editorial Paul E. Miller
Agradecimento O autor deseja agradecer as contribuições feitas por George A. McKie na preparação deste capítulo.

DEMODICOSE

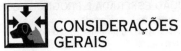

CONSIDERAÇÕES GERAIS

DEFINIÇÃO
- Doença parasitária inflamatória de cães e, raramente, de gatos, caracterizada pelo aumento no número de ácaros nos folículos pilosos e na epiderme, o que muitas vezes leva à furunculose e infecção bacteriana secundária.
- Pode ser localizada ou generalizada.

FISIOPATOLOGIA
Cães
- Foram identificadas três espécies de ácaros no cão:
  - *Demodex canis* — ácaro folicular; parte da flora normal da pele; tipicamente está presente em pequena quantidade; reside nos folículos pilosos e nas glândulas sebáceas da pele; transmitido de mãe para o neonato em 2-3 dias de aleitamento.
  - *Demodex injai* — ácaro grande de corpo alongado, encontrado na unidade pilossebácea; modo de transmissão desconhecido; associado apenas à doença de início na fase adulta, com incidência mais alta observada nas raças do tipo terrier, frequentemente ao longo da linha média dorsal (West Highland white terrier e Fox terrier de pelo duro).
  - *Demodex cornei* — vive no estrato córneo da epiderme; modo de transmissão desconhecido.
- O processo patológico desenvolve-se quando o número de ácaros excede o tolerado pelo sistema imunológico.
- A proliferação inicial dos ácaros pode ser o resultado de um distúrbio genético ou imunológico.

Gatos
- Distúrbio pouco compreendido.
- Os ácaros foram identificados na pele e dentro do canal auditivo externo.
- Foram identificadas duas espécies no gato:
  - *D. gatoi* — é considerado potencialmente contagioso e associado à dermatite pruriginosa.
  - *D. cati* — as infecções por esse ácaro são frequentemente associadas a doenças imunossupressoras e metabólicas.

SISTEMA(S) ACOMETIDO(S)
Cutâneo/exócrino.

GENÉTICA
A proliferação inicial de ácaros pode resultar de um distúrbio genético.

INCIDÊNCIA/PREVALÊNCIA
- Cães — comum.
- Gatos — rara.

IDENTIFICAÇÃO
Espécies
Cães e gatos.

Raça(s) Predominante(s)
- Incidência elevada em potencial nos gatos das raças Siamês e Birmanês.
- West Highland white terrier e Fox terrier de pelo duro — dermatite seborreica oleosa associada ao *D. injai*.

Idade Média e Faixa Etária
- Localizada — geralmente em cães jovens; idade média de 3-6 meses.
- Generalizada — tanto animais jovens como idosos.
- Não há dados coletados para o gato.

SINAIS CLÍNICOS
Cães
Localizada, Início Juvenil
- Lesões — costumam ser brandas; consistem em eritema e descamação leve.
- Placas — podem-se notar várias; o local mais comum é a face, especialmente nas áreas peribucais e perioculares, além dos membros anteriores; também podem ser constatadas no tronco e nos membros posteriores.

Generalizada, Início na Fase Jovem ou Adulta
- Os sinais podem ser disseminados desde o início, com múltiplas placas pouco circunscritas de eritema, alopecia e descamação.
- À medida que os folículos pilosos se distendem com uma grande quantidade de ácaros, as infecções bacterianas secundárias passam a ser comuns, resultando muitas vezes em ruptura do folículo (furunculose).
- Com a evolução da sarna, a pele pode ficar gravemente inflamada, exsudativa e granulomatosa.
- *D. injai* pode estar associado a uma dermatite seborreica oleosa do tronco dorsal, além de comedões, eritema, alopecia e hiperpigmentação.

Gatos
- Caracterizados frequentemente por alopecia multifocal parcial a completa de áreas como pálpebras, região periocular, cabeça, pescoço, flanco e ventre.
- Lesões — variavelmente pruriginosas, com eritema, descamação e crosta; com frequência, as lesões causadas pelo *D. gatoi* são bastante pruriginosas e podem ser contagiosas.
- Também se relata otite externa ceruminosa.
- *D. cati* está associado muitas vezes a doenças imunossupressoras.

CAUSAS
- Cão — *Demodex canis*, *D. injai* e *D. cornei*.
- Gato — *Demodex cati* e *D. gatoi*.

FATORES DE RISCO
Cães
- Não se conhece o mecanismo imunopatológico exato.
- Os estudos indicam que os cães com demodicose generalizada apresentam porcentagem abaixo do normal de receptores da IL-2 em seus linfócitos e produção também subnormal dessa interleucina.
- Fatores genéticos (especialmente para a sarna localizada de início juvenil), imunossupressão e/ou doenças metabólicas podem predispor o animal.

Gatos
- Associados muitas vezes a doenças metabólicas (p. ex., FIV, lúpus eritematoso sistêmico e diabetes melito).
- *D. gatoi* — curto e rombo; raramente constitui um marcador de doença metabólica; pode ser transmissível de um gato para outro dentro do mesmo ambiente doméstico.

DIAGNÓSTICO
DIAGNÓSTICO DIFERENCIAL
Cães
- Foliculite/furunculose bacteriana.
- Dermatofitose.
- Dermatite de contato.
- Complexo pênfigo.
- Dermatomiosite.
- Lúpus eritematoso sistêmico.

Gatos
- Dermatite alérgica.
- Escabiose felina (sarna notoédrica).
- Dermatofitose.
- Dermatite psicogênica.

HEMOGRAMA/BIOQUÍMICA/URINÁLISE
Podem permanecer normais a menos que haja algum processo subjacente.

OUTROS TESTES LABORATORIAIS
- Sorologia para FeLV e FIV, além dos títulos contra toxoplasmose.
- Amostras fecais: é raro o encontro de ácaros nas fezes.

MÉTODOS DIAGNÓSTICOS
- Raspados cutâneos — diagnósticos por encontrar os ácaros na maioria dos casos.
- Tricogramas — podem constituir uma técnica eficaz para a identificação do ácaro.
- Biopsia cutânea — pode ser necessária quando as lesões são crônicas, granulomatosas e fibrosadas (particularmente nos pés).

TRATAMENTO
CUIDADO(S) DE SAÚDE ADEQUADO(S)
- Esquema ambulatorial.
- Localizada — terapia conservativa; grande parte dos casos (90%) exibe resolução espontânea sem nenhum tratamento.
- Avaliar o estado de saúde geral de cães com a forma localizada ou a generalizada.

ORIENTAÇÃO AO PROPRIETÁRIO
- Localizada — a maior parte dos casos apresenta resolução espontânea.
- Generalizada — problema terapêutico frequente; o custo e a frustração com a cronicidade do problema representam pontos de discussão; muitos casos são controlados por meio clínico, mas não têm cura; a sarna de início juvenil é considerada uma predisposição hereditária e, portanto, não se recomenda o acasalamento de animais acometidos.

MEDICAÇÕES
MEDICAMENTO(S) DE ESCOLHA
Amitraz
- Uma formamidina inibidora da monoamina oxidase e da síntese de prostaglandina; um agonista α_2-adrenérgico: utilizar semanalmente ou em semanas alternadas até a resolução dos sinais clínicos e a não constatação de ácaros nos raspados cutâneos; não enxaguar; deixar o animal secar ao ar.
- Tratar por mais 1 mês após a obtenção de raspado cutâneo negativo.
- Aplicar xampu de peróxido de benzoíla antes da aplicação do banho de imersão como terapia bactericida e para aumentar a exposição dos ácaros ao acaricida pela atividade de lavagem folicular.
- A eficácia é proporcional à frequência da administração e à concentração do banho de imersão.
- Raramente utilizado em gatos — 0,015-0,025% aplicado sobre todo o corpo do animal a cada 1-2 semanas (não utilizar em gatos diabéticos).

DEMODICOSE

- Cães — 0,03-0,05% aplicado semanalmente ou em semanas alternadas; tratamentos corporais totais/tópicos adicionais para áreas focais (pododermatite) podem ser empregados a cada 1-3 dias com solução a 0,125%.
- Promeris® — produto tópico aplicado a cada 2-4 semanas.
- Coleira preventiva — relatos não publicados de sucesso; trocar a coleira a cada 2-4 semanas; uso não aprovado pela FDA.
- Não haverá cura de 11-30% dos casos; sendo assim, pode-se tentar uma terapia alternativa ou o controle com banhos de manutenção a cada 2-8 semanas.

Ivermectina
- Uma lactona macrocíclica com atividade GABA-agonista.
- Cão: a administração oral diária de 0,3-0,6 mg/kg é muito eficaz, mesmo quando o amitraz falha (é recomendável iniciar com a metade da dose [ou aproximadamente 0,12 mg/kg] durante a primeira semana para observar quaisquer sinais de toxicidade/efeitos colaterais).
- Tratar por mais 30-60 dias após a obtenção de raspados cutâneos negativos (média, 3-8 meses).
- Relatada como uma opção terapêutica no gato; no entanto, a dose exata é desconhecida (frequentemente dosada a 300 μg/kg).

Milbemicina (Interceptor®)
- Uma lactona macrocíclica com atividade GABA-agonista.
- A dosagem de 1-2 mg/kg VO a cada 24 h cura 50% dos casos, enquanto 2 mg/kg VO a cada 24 h cura 85% dos casos.
- Tratar por mais 30-60 dias após a obtenção de múltiplos raspados cutâneos negativos.
- Muito caro.

Moxidectina (Avermectina)
- Relatos não publicados no cão quando utilizada a 400 μg/kg VO uma vez por semana.
- Não utilizar em raças sensíveis à ivermectina.

Gatos
- Ainda não foram definidos protocolos exatos.
- Os banhos de imersão tópicos com enxofre a cada 3-7 dias por 4 a 8 tratamentos conduzem muitas vezes a uma resolução satisfatória dos sinais clínicos; terapia recomendada em gatos.
- Os estudos com milbemicina e ivermectina estão em falta, embora haja inúmeros relatos não publicados quanto à eficácia.
- Foi relatado que a doramectina seja eficaz na dose de 0,6 mg/kg SC uma vez por semana.

CONTRAINDICAÇÕES
- Ivermectina — contraindicada em cães das raças Collie, Pastor de Shetland, Old English sheepdog, outras raças de pastoreio e mestiços dessas raças; as raças sensíveis parecem tolerar as dosagens acaricidas de milbemicina (ver anteriormente).
- As raças sensíveis podem ter a deficiência de um gene (mutação MDR1/ABCB1), responsável pela codificação de uma glicoproteína-P (bomba de efluxo do medicamento), o que predispõe à toxicidade.

PRECAUÇÕES
Amitraz
- Efeitos colaterais — sonolência, letargia, depressão, anorexia, observados em 30% dos pacientes por 12-36 horas após o tratamento.
- Efeitos colaterais raros — vômito, diarreia, prurido, poliúria, midríase, bradicardia, hipoventilação, hipotensão, hipotermia, ataxia, íleo paralítico, timpanismo, hiperglicemia, convulsões, morte.
- A incidência e a gravidade dos efeitos colaterais não parecem ser proporcionais à dose ou à frequência de uso.
- Os seres humanos podem desenvolver dermatite, cefaleias e dificuldade respiratória após a exposição.
- A ioimbina a 0,11 mg/kg IV constitui um antídoto.

Ivermectina e Milbemicina
- Sinais de toxicidade — salivação, vômito, midríase, confusão mental, ataxia, hipersensibilidade a estímulo sonoro, fraqueza, decúbito, coma e morte.
- Ivermectina — contraindicada em cães das raças Collie, Pastor de Shetland, Old English sheepdog, outras raças de pastoreio e mestiços dessas raças; as raças sensíveis parecem tolerar as dosagens acaricidas de milbemicina (ver anteriormente).
- As raças sensíveis podem ter a deficiência de um gene (mutação MDR1/ABCB1), responsável pela codificação de uma glicoproteína-P (bomba de efluxo do medicamento), o que predispõe à toxicidade.

INTERAÇÕES POSSÍVEIS
- Amitraz — pode interagir com antidepressivos heterocíclicos, xilazina, benzodiazepínicos e lactonas macrocíclicas.
- Ivermectina e milbemicina — geram níveis elevados de metabólitos de neurotransmissores monoamínicos, o que pode resultar em interações medicamentosas adversas com o amitraz e os benzodiazepínicos.
- O uso de espinosade (para controle de pulgas) é contraindicado com a ivermectina.

ACOMPANHAMENTO
MONITORIZAÇÃO DO PACIENTE
Para monitorizar a evolução da doença, empregam-se múltiplos raspados de pele (tricogramas) e indícios da resolução clínica.

PREVENÇÃO
Não acasalar os animais com a forma generalizada.

COMPLICAÇÕES POSSÍVEIS
Foliculite e furunculose bacterianas secundárias.

EVOLUÇÃO ESPERADA E PROGNÓSTICO
- Prognóstico (cães) — depende intensamente da genética, da resposta imunológica e das doenças subjacentes.
- Localizada — a maioria dos casos (90%) apresenta resolução espontânea sem nenhum tratamento; <10% dos casos evoluem para a forma generalizada.
- De início na fase adulta (cães) — é frequentemente grave e refratária ao tratamento.
- Os casos felinos causados pelo D. cati podem ter um prognóstico mau associado à doença subjacente.

DIVERSOS
DISTÚRBIOS ASSOCIADOS
- De início no adulto — a ocorrência súbita associa-se muitas vezes à doença interna, neoplasia maligna e/ou doença imunossupressora; aproximadamente 25% dos casos são idiopáticos em um período de acompanhamento de 1-2 anos.
- O D. cati associa-se a infecções por FeLV ou FIV ou a quadros de toxoplasmose e lúpus eritematoso sistêmico.

FATORES RELACIONADOS COM A IDADE
Os cães jovens são frequentemente predispostos a uma forma localizada.

POTENCIAL ZOONÓTICO
Nenhum.

GESTAÇÃO/FERTILIDADE/REPRODUÇÃO
Não acasalar os animais com a forma generalizada.

SINÔNIMO(S)
- Sarna demodécica.
- Sarna vermelha.

VER TAMBÉM
- Toxicidade pela Ivermectina.
- Toxicose pelo Amitraz.

ABREVIATURA(S)
- FeLV = vírus da leucemia felina.
- FIV = vírus da imunodeficiência felina.
- GABA = ácido gama-aminobutírico.
- IL = interleucina.

Sugestões de Leitura
Scott DW, Miller WH, Griffin CE, eds. Parasitic skin diseases. In: Muller & Kirk's Small Animal Dermatology. 5th ed. Philadelphia: Saunders, 1995, pp. 417-432.

Autor Karen Helton Rhodes
Consultor Editorial Alexander H. Werner

Dentes Decíduos, Persistentes (Retidos)

CONSIDERAÇÕES GERAIS

REVISÃO
- Um dente decíduo persistente (retido) é aquele que ainda está presente quando o dente permanente começa a sofrer erupção ou já sofreu erupção.
- Inúmeros fatores influenciam a esfoliação de dentes decíduos: falta de sucessor permanente; anciolose da raiz decídua em relação ao alvéolo e reabsorção ou esfoliação radicular incompleta; e falha de a coroa permanente entrar em contato com a raiz decídua durante a erupção dentária permanente.

IDENTIFICAÇÃO
- Mais comuns em cães que nos gatos.
- Mais comuns em raças caninas de pequeno porte (p. ex., Maltês, Poodle, Yorkshire terrier).
- Durante a fase de erupção dentária permanente, que começa aos 3 meses para os incisivos e até os 6-7 meses para os dentes caninos e molares.
- Podem passar despercebidos sem diagnóstico até uma idade mais avançada.
- Não há predileção sexual.

SINAIS CLÍNICOS
Comentários Gerais
- Os dentes decíduos persistentes podem fazer com que os dentes permanentes sofram erupção em posições anormais, resultando em maloclusão. São essenciais a identificação e a intervenção precoces.
- Os dentes caninos maxilares sofrem erupção em posição mesial (rostral) aos dentes caninos decíduos persistentes. Isso pode estreitar o espaço (diastema) entre o dente canino maxilar e o terceiro incisivo, não deixando qualquer espaço para o dente canino mandibular ocupar.
- Os dentes caninos mandibulares sofrem erupção em posição lingual (medial) aos dentes decíduos persistentes. Isso pode resultar em um estreitamento do espaço entre os caninos inferiores (estreitamento da base), culminando em impingidela (colisão/impacto) sobre os tecidos moles do palato duro.
- Todos os incisivos sofrem erupção em posição lingual aos incisivos decíduos persistentes. Isso pode resultar em uma mordida cruzada rostral (anterior).

Achados do Exame Físico
- Presença de dente decíduo com dente permanente que está em processo de erupção ou sofreu erupção completa.
- Posição anormal de dente permanente devido à persistência de dente decíduo.
- Odor bucal fétido (halitose) decorrente do acúmulo de debris e placas pelo apinhamento dos dentes decíduos persistentes.
- Gengivite local e doença periodontal causadas pelo apinhamento.
- Fístula oronasal proveniente de dentes caninos permanentes mandibulares de base estreita.
- Presença de dente decíduo sem nenhum sucessor permanente.
- O dente decíduo costuma ser menor que o permanente.
- Sem o dente permanente subjacente, o dente decíduo frequentemente permanecerá intacto e viável, embora possa acabar sofrendo esfoliação.

CAUSAS E FATORES DE RISCO
- Causa desconhecida.
- Predisposição de raças caninas de pequeno porte.

DIAGNÓSTICO

DIAGNÓSTICO DIFERENCIAL
- Dentes supranumerários.
- Geminação da coroa.

HEMOGRAMA/BIOQUÍMICA/URINÁLISE
N/D.

OUTROS TESTES LABORATORIAIS
N/D.

DIAGNÓSTICO POR IMAGEM
Radiografias Intrabucais
- Distinguem entre dentes permanentes e decíduos.
- Fornecem provas quanto à presença de dentes decíduos retidos ou ao grau de reabsorção radicular do dente decíduo.
- Identificam anormalidades dentárias antes da extração, inclusive dente decíduo persistente sem nenhum sucessor permanente, raiz retida com ausência de coroa, e dente permanente não irrompido.

MÉTODOS DIAGNÓSTICOS
- Mapeamento completo da cavidade bucal para indicar a presença de dentes decíduos.
- Métodos diagnósticos pré-operatórios adequados, quando houver indicação.

ACHADOS PATOLÓGICOS
N/D.

TRATAMENTO

ORIENTAÇÃO AO PROPRIETÁRIO
- Iniciar o exame dos dentes na primeira consulta do filhote canino ou felino.
- Informar aos proprietários sobre a avaliação da erupção adequada dos dentes permanentes, bem como da esfoliação dos dentes decíduos.

CONSIDERAÇÕES CIRÚRGICAS
- É ideal realizar a extração assim que o dente permanente sofrer erupção através da gengiva.
- Anestesia geral com colocação de sonda endotraqueal e insuflação de manguito.
- Radiografias intrabucais.

Extração
- É crítica a elevação cuidadosa e delicada da gengiva para extração do dente decíduo. A aplicação de força excessiva pode lesionar o dente permanente em desenvolvimento.
- Se o dente permanente tiver sofrido erupção em uma posição anormal, a extração radicular completa do dente decíduo é essencial. Talvez haja necessidade de remoção de raiz fraturada ou retida com retalho (*flap*) gengival.
- Em alguns casos, a raiz já pode ter sofrido reabsorção, dispensando avaliações futuras (se os dentes permanentes não estiverem com maloclusão).

MEDICAÇÕES

MEDICAMENTO(S)
- Irrigação tópica da cavidade bucal com antimicrobianos antes da extração.
- Analgésicos para controle da dor antes e depois da extração.

CONTRAINDICAÇÕES/INTERAÇÕES POSSÍVEIS
N/D.

ACOMPANHAMENTO

MONITORIZAÇÃO E CUIDADO DOMÉSTICO DO PACIENTE
- Após a cirurgia, restringir a atividade física pelo resto do dia.
- Fornecimento de dieta pastosa por 3-5 dias — ração enlatada ou seca umedecida.
- Analgesia (AINE) por 48 h no pós-operatório.
- Nenhum brinquedo mastigável por 3-5 dias.
- Irrigação com colutórios bucais (clorexidina) por 3-5 dias se houver indicação.
- Manutenção da escovação diária dos dentes após 3-5 dias.

PREVENÇÃO
Podem ser prevalentes em certas raças e linhagens — evitar o acasalamento.

EVOLUÇÃO ESPERADA E PROGNÓSTICO
- Uma vez extraídos, não deve haver quaisquer complicações a menos que a maloclusão resultante necessite de mais atenção.
- Em geral, a gengiva cicatriza-se bem sem intercorrências.
- O prognóstico depende da oclusão depois de a erupção dos dentes permanentes estar concluída.
- Talvez haja necessidade de tratamento da maloclusão dos dentes permanentes.
- Dentes caninos mandibulares de base estreita.
- Mordida cruzada rostral.
- Dentes caninos maxilares com desvio rostral.

DIVERSOS

VER TAMBÉM
Maloclusão — Esquelética e Dentária.

ABREVIATURA(S)
- AINE = anti-inflamatório não esteroide.

Sugestões de Leitura
Wiggs R, Lobprise H. Veterinary dentistry, principles and practice. Philadelphia: Lippincott-Raven, 1997.

Autor Randi Brannan
Consultor Editorial Heidi B. Lobprise

Dentes Manchados

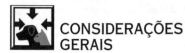
CONSIDERAÇÕES GERAIS

DEFINIÇÃO
• Qualquer alteração da normalidade — a coloração normal varia e depende da tonalidade, translucidez e espessura do esmalte. O esmalte translúcido é branco-azulado, enquanto o opaco, branco-acinzentado.
• Extrínseca — por acúmulo de pigmento exógeno na superfície dentária.
• Intrínseca — secundária a fatores endógenos indutores de manchas na dentina subjacente.

FISIOPATOLOGIA
Manchas Extrínsecas
• Pigmentação de origem bacteriana — bactérias cromogênicas conferem coloração verde, castanho-escura ou laranja, que geralmente se situa 1 mm acima da margem gengival do dente.
• Relacionada com a placa bacteriana — mancha castanho-escura; geralmente secundária à formação de sulfeto férrico decorrente da interação dessa substância bacteriana e do ferro na saliva. A placa sobre a dentição costuma ser branca.
• Alimentos — biscoitos de carvão vegetal e produtos semelhantes penetram nas depressões e fissuras do esmalte; os alimentos que contenham clorofila em abundância podem produzir mancha verde.
• Hemorragia gengival — gera mancha verde resultante do desdobramento da hemoglobina em biliverdina (pigmento verde).
• Materiais de restauração dentária — o amálgama confere coloração cinza-escura.
• Medicamentos — produtos que contenham ferro ou iodo produzem coloração negra; aqueles que contenham sulfetos, nitrato de prata ou manganês conferem mancha cinza-amarelada a castanho-enegrecida; outros que contenham cobre ou níquel geram coloração verde; produtos com cádmio dão origem à mancha amarela a castanho-dourada (p. ex., o fluoreto estanoso a 8% combina-se com sulfetos bacterianos, conferindo mancha negra; a clorexidina gera mancha castanho-amarelada).
• Metais — desgaste decorrente da mordedura de gaiolas ou comedouros metálicos.
• Fragmentos coronários — menor translucidez em virtude da desidratação do fragmento.
• Restaurações manchadas.
• Desgaste do dente com exposição da dentina — dentina terciária, dentina reparadora, dentina secundária.
• Coroa coberta de cálculo dentário — varia em termos de cor, de amarelo-escura a castanho-escura.

Manchas Intrínsecas
• Hiperbilirrubinemia — compromete todos os dentes; ocorre durante os estágios de desenvolvimento da dentição (i. e., no período de formação da dentina); o acúmulo da bilirrubina na dentina ocorre a partir da degradação eritrocitária excessiva; a extensão de mancha nos dentes depende da duração da hiperbilirrubinemia (podem-se observar linhas de resolução sobre os dentes assim que a condição estiver solucionada); confere mancha verde aos dentes.
• Destruição eritrocitária localizada, geralmente em um único dente — costuma acompanhar lesões dentárias traumáticas; a mancha provém da degradação da hemoglobina no interior da polpa por pulpite, e sua liberação secundária nos túbulos dentinários adjacentes; a mancha varia de rósea (pulpite) a cinza (necrose pulpar ou resolução) até negra (necrose de liquefação); os fatores sanguíneos indutores de mancha nos dentes são: hemoglobina, metemoglobina, hematoidina, hemossiderina, hematina, hemina e sulfometemoglobina.
• Amelogênese imperfeita — alteração de desenvolvimento na estrutura do esmalte, que acomete todos os dentes; os dentes apresentam aspecto calcário e tonalidade rosada; pode representar um problema de formação, mineralização ou maturação da matriz orgânica.
• Dentinogênese imperfeita — alteração de desenvolvimento na formação da dentina; o esmalte separa-se facilmente da dentina, resultando em mancha acinzentada.
• Agentes infecciosos (sistêmicos) — parvovírus, vírus da cinomose ou qualquer agente infeccioso que provoque elevação contínua da temperatura corporal; afeta a formação do esmalte; uma linha distinta de resolução fica visível sobre os dentes; compromete todos os dentes; resulta em hipoplasia do esmalte, local onde as áreas erodidas apresentam margens negras e a dentina se encontra acastanhada.
• Fluorose dentária — acomete todos os dentes; o consumo excessivo de fluoreto influencia a maturação do esmalte, resultando em depressões (hipoplasia do esmalte) com margens negras; o esmalte apresenta-se de cor branca opaca e sem brilho, com zonas de tonalidade amarelo-acastanhada.
• Erosão dentária causada por vômitos constantes resulta em depressões no esmalte com manchas escuras.
• Atrito — o desgaste entre os dentes culmina em perda da coroa e formação da dentina reparadora (coloração amarelo-acastanhada).
• Abrasão — desgaste do dente com a superfície de outro; isso ocorre, por exemplo, com a mastigação de bolas de tênis ou a automastigação por algum problema dermatológico. Ocorre a formação de dentina reparadora (coloração amarelo-acastanhada).
• Envelhecimento — a dentição de animais mais idosos é mais amarela e menos translúcida.
• Desnutrição (generalizada, deficiência da vitamina D, deficiência da vitamina A) — pode resultar em opacidades delimitadas no esmalte em casos graves.

Reabsorção Interna/Externa
• Interna — acompanha lesão pulpar (traumatismo) indutora de alterações vasculares com aumento na tensão de oxigênio e diminuição no pH, resultando em destruição (reabsorção) dentária de dentro da polpa por ação de dentinoclastos; o dente apresenta tonalidade rosada; costuma acometer um único dente.
• Externa — muitos fatores podem causar esse tipo de reabsorção, como traumatismo, tratamento ortodôntico, forças oclusais excessivas, doença periodontal, bem como tratamento, tumores e inflamação periapical; a reabsorção pode ocorrer em qualquer área ao longo do ligamento periodontal e pode se estender até a polpa; os osteoclastos reabsorvem a estrutura dentária. Com frequência, a área é reparada por depósito de osteodentina.

Medicamentos e Manchas
• Tetraciclinas — ligam-se ao cálcio, formando um complexo de ortofosfato de cálcio, que se deposita na matriz colágena do esmalte; ocorre em todos os dentes; ocorre apenas quando o esmalte está sendo formado; resulta em mancha amarelo-acastanhada. Com o uso prolongado de tetraciclina e seus derivados em animais maduros, o aparecimento de manchas nos dentes ocorre secundariamente ao envolvimento da formação de dentina secundária subjacente.
• Amálgama (como ocorre em casos de mancha extrínseca).
• Iodo/óleos essenciais.
• Em dentes submetidos a tratamento endodôntico, com a penetração dos medicamentos nos túbulos dentinários.
• Antibióticos macrolídeos (descritos em seres humanos): em virtude do aumento na quantidade de cariopicnose* do ameloblasto no estágio de transição do desenvolvimento, resultando em degeneração vacuolar do ameloblasto e alteração cística à maturação e hipocalcificação, o que confere à lesão uma coloração branca com faixas horizontais sobre o esmalte.
• "Arrastamento" de bactérias (extravasamento) — ocorre em torno das margens de uma restauração e costuma ser de coloração enegrecida.

SISTEMA(S) ACOMETIDO(S)
Gastrintestinal — cavidade bucal.

GENÉTICA
• Tanto a amelogênese como a dentinogênese imperfeitas em seres humanos são distúrbios hereditários que apresentam muitos modos de herança: dominante ligada ao cromossomo X, recessiva ligada ao cromossomo X, autossômica dominante, autossômica recessiva. Ainda não foi estudado o modo de herança nos animais.
• Hipotireoidismo congênito.
• Doenças metabólicas.

INCIDÊNCIA/PREVALÊNCIA
• O aparecimento de manchas nos dentes ou em um único dente é extremamente comum em todos os animais.
• As manchas extrínsecas são bastante usuais, sobretudo as pigmentações de origem bacteriana; os outros tipos são menos comuns.
• Do mesmo modo, as manchas intrínsecas são muito corriqueiras, particularmente os casos de reabsorções interna e externa, acompanhadas por destruição eritrocitária localizada; as outras causas são raras.

DISTRIBUIÇÃO GEOGRÁFICA
• Metais pesados provenientes de atividades de mineração.
• A fluoretação gera áreas com quantidades excessivas de fluoreto na água de bebida.
• Normalmente, não há nenhuma distribuição geográfica.

IDENTIFICAÇÃO
Espécies
Cães e gatos.

Raça(s) Predominante(s)
Nenhuma.

Idade Média e Faixa Etária
Há uma variação na faixa etária descrita — quando o problema acomete o esmalte ou a

---
* N. T.: Retração e aumento nucleares da basofilia.

DENTES MANCHADOS

dentina em processo de maturação, é possível notá-lo pela primeira vez após os 6 meses de vida.

Sexo Predominante
Nenhum.

SINAIS CLÍNICOS

Achados Anamnésicos
O proprietário relata uma variação na coloração de um ou mais dentes.

Achados do Exame Físico
- Coloração anormal de um ou mais dentes.
- Esmalte erodido, com manchas.
- Fratura dentária.
- Anéis ou linhas de manchas em torno de um ou mais dentes.
- Desgaste nas coroas da dentição ou em áreas selecionadas como ocorre em causas comportamentais (mordeduras de gaiolas — acometimento da face distal dos dentes caninos).
- Erosão do esmalte.

CAUSAS E FATORES DE RISCO
- Manchas extrínsecas — pigmentações produzidas por bactérias a partir do depósito de placas bacterianas e cálculos dentários; alimentos; hemorragia gengival; materiais de restauração dentária, medicamentos (clorexidina, fluoreto estanoso a 8%), metais.
- Manchas intrínsecas — reação interna (traumatismo); reabsorção externa (lesões reabsortivas osteoclásticas felinas); destruição eritrocitária localizada no dente (traumatismo); infecções sistêmicas; medicamentos (tetraciclinas); fluorose; hiperbilirrubinemia; amelogênese imperfeita; dentinogênese imperfeita.

DIAGNÓSTICO

DIAGNÓSTICO DIFERENCIAL
- Cálculos dentários.
- Envelhecimento normal do dente — aumento na translucidez.
- Restos de alimentos alojados nos espaços ou nas lacunas entre dois dentes (diastema).

HEMOGRAMA/BIOQUÍMICA/URINÁLISE
- Anemia — distúrbios relacionados com o sangue.
- Bilirrubina — elevada em casos de hepatopatias.

OUTROS TESTES LABORATORIAIS
- T_3/T_4 — baixos em casos de hipotireoidismo congênito.
- Diminuição ou ausência de enzimas metabólicas específicas — tirosinemia.

DIAGNÓSTICO POR IMAGEM
As radiografias dentárias são extremamente úteis na identificação de reabsorções interna ou externa, materiais de restauração ou pigmentação de origem bacteriana decorrente de percolação coronária.

MÉTODOS DIAGNÓSTICOS
- Caso muitos dentes sejam acometidos, um único dente poderá ser extraído e enviado para avaliação histológica (ver adiante).
- A transiluminação com fibra óptica sob luz intensa pode beneficiar o clínico, distinguindo polpas vital e necrosada.
- Métodos diagnósticos pré-operatórios adequados, quando houver indicação.

ACHADOS PATOLÓGICOS
- Um ou mais dentes apresentam-se manchados; o esmalte e/ou a dentina podem estar erodidos ou quebrados, com pigmentação.
- Manchas extrínsecas — toda pigmentação encontra-se no esmalte ou na dentina exposta, mas de modo geral a estrutura dentária permanece normal.
- Manchas intrínsecas — hiperbilirrubinemia; hipoplasia do esmalte; linhas de resolução sobre o dente; todos os dentes acometidos.
- Destruição eritrocitária localizada — mancha nos túbulos dentinários; pulpite/necrose de liquefação da polpa.
- Reabsorção interna — aumento de volume bem circunscrito de uma área do sistema endodôntico, com tecido de granulação contendo muitos odontoclastos.
- Reabsorção externa — estrutura dentária com aspecto corroído em qualquer área ao longo do ligamento periodontal; pode se estender em direção ao sistema endodôntico; as áreas de reabsorção dentária apresentam tecido de granulação com muitos osteoclastos.
- Fluorose — hipoplasia do esmalte; hipocalcificação do esmalte; medicamentos; sistêmica (p. ex., as tetraciclinas provocam formação irregular da matriz do esmalte e da dentina); todos os dentes acometidos.
- Amelogênese imperfeita — formação, mineralização ou maturação irregulares da matriz do esmalte.
- Dentinogênese imperfeita — formação irregular da dentina; o esmalte pode estar separado da dentina.

TRATAMENTO

CUIDADO(S) DE SAÚDE ADEQUADO(S)
- Remoção das manchas extrínsecas — procedimento basicamente estético.
- Tratamento das manchas intrínsecas — de caráter funcional e para alívio da dor.

CUIDADO(S) DE ENFERMAGEM
- Manchas extrínsecas — remover a causa desencadeante.
- Manchas intrínsecas — alimentos moles; remover os brinquedos mastigáveis.

ATIVIDADE
Restringir a atividade ou tratar anormalidades comportamentais específicas (mordedura de gaiolas).

DIETA
Manchas intrínsecas — alimentos moles.

ORIENTAÇÃO AO PROPRIETÁRIO
- Prevenção nos próximos animais ou futuras ninhadas.
- Causas intrínsecas — se o(s) dente(s) não for(em) tratado(s), haverá maior probabilidade do acúmulo de placas bacterianas e cálculos dentários, levando à subsequente doença periodontal; as fraturas dentárias são mais prevalentes, o que pode resultar em abscedação dentária.

CONSIDERAÇÕES CIRÚRGICAS
- Manchas extrínsecas (estéticas) — branqueamento interno e/ou externo; aplicação de vernizes ou jaquetas. O polimento dos dentes acometidos com o uso de peróxido de hidrogênio a 3% e pedra-pomes ajudará a remover as manchas extrínsecas. Além disso, os cuidados satisfatórios de higiene bucal com controle da placa bacteriana realizados em casa permitirão a reavaliação do novo desenvolvimento de algumas manchas (placas/cálculos/pigmentações bacterianas).
- Manchas intrínsecas (de caráter funcional e alívio da dor) — possível tratamento endodôntico (reabsorção interna e destruição eritrocitária localizada).
- Procedimentos de restauração, como jaquetas ou vernizes, para proteger tanto o dente como a polpa.
- Talvez haja necessidade da extração dos dentes acometidos, especialmente com reabsorção externa.

MEDICAÇÕES

MEDICAMENTO(S) DE ESCOLHA
N/D.

ACOMPANHAMENTO

PREVENÇÃO
- Ver a seção "Fisiopatologia".
- Cuidados satisfatórios de higiene bucal em casa ajudarão a evitar a recidiva de certas manchas específicas.

COMPLICAÇÕES POSSÍVEIS
Ver a seção "Orientação ao Proprietário".

EVOLUÇÃO ESPERADA E PROGNÓSTICO
Variam, dependendo da etiologia, desde um simples problema estético até uma dor intensa significativa.

DIVERSOS

DISTÚRBIOS ASSOCIADOS
Púrpura juvenil.

FATORES RELACIONADOS COM A IDADE
Mais comum em cães e gatos jovens.

POTENCIAL ZOONÓTICO
Nenhum.

GESTAÇÃO/FERTILIDADE/REPRODUÇÃO
- A administração de tetraciclina durante a prenhez pode resultar no aparecimento de manchas permanentes nos dentes da ninhada.
- Ver a seção "Genética".

SINÔNIMO(S)
- Pigmentação intrínseca.
- Pigmentação por tetraciclina.
- Pigmentação extrínseca.
- Pigmentação por clorexidina.

Sugestões de Leitura
Harvey CE, Emily PP. Small animal dentistry. Philadelphia: Mosby, 1993.
Wiggs RB, Lobprise HB. Veterinary dentistry: principles and practice. Philadelphia: Lippincott-Raven, 1997.

Autor James M. G. Anthony
Consultor Editorial Heidi B. Lobprise

Dermatite Acral por Lambedura

CONSIDERAÇÕES GERAIS

REVISÃO
Dermatopatia crônica ou recidivante causada diretamente pela lambedura das extremidades. Pode se desenvolver um ciclo de lambedura compulsiva e infecção/prurido secundários.

SISTEMA(S) ACOMETIDO(S)
Cutâneo/Exócrino.

IDENTIFICAÇÃO
• Cães • Mais comum em raças de grande porte — especialmente Doberman pinscher, Labrador retriever, Dogue alemão, Setter irlandês e inglês, Golden retriever, Akita, Dálmata, Shar pei e Weimaraner. • Idade de início — varia com a causa. • Sexo predominante — algumas fontes sugerem maior incidência em machos; outras indicam nenhuma preferência.

SINAIS CLÍNICOS
• Lambedura e mordedura excessivas da área acometida. • Ocasionalmente, há um histórico de traumatismo sobre a área acometida. • Placas firmes alopécicas, ulcerativas, espessadas e salientes, geralmente situadas na face dorsal do carpo, metacarpo, tarso ou metatarso. • As lesões muitas vezes ocorrem de forma isolada, embora possam ocorrer em mais de um local.

CAUSAS E FATORES DE RISCO
Doenças associadas — furunculose estafilocócica, alergia, endocrinopatia, demodicose, dermatofitose, reação a corpos estranhos, neoplasia, artrite, traumatismo e disfunção nervosa psicogênica e sensorial.

DIAGNÓSTICO

DIAGNÓSTICO DIFERENCIAL
• Neoplasia • Furunculose bacteriana
• Demodicose focal • Dermatofitose focal

HEMOGRAMA/BIOQUÍMICA/URINÁLISE
Permanecem normais, exceto em casos de hiperadrenocorticismo.

OUTROS TESTES LABORATORIAIS
• Baixos níveis dos hormônios tireoidianos, TSH elevado — sugere hipotireoidismo.
• Anormalidade no teste de estimulação com ACTH ou no teste de supressão com dexametasona em baixas doses — sugere hiperadrenocorticismo.

DIAGNÓSTICO POR IMAGEM
Radiologia — neoplasia; algumas formas de traumatismo; corpos estranhos radiopacos; é possível observar uma proliferação óssea secundária à irritação crônica.

MÉTODOS DIAGNÓSTICOS
• Raspados cutâneos — demodicose. • Cultura para dermatófitos — infecção fúngica. • Citologia epidérmica — infecção bacteriana. • Cultura bacteriana e antibiograma — o tecido deve ser enviado para os exames de cultura e antibiograma, pois as culturas teciduais frequentemente diferem da cultura de superfície da pele. • Dieta de eliminação — determina alergia alimentar. • Teste alérgico intradérmico — útil em caso de animais atópicos. • Biopsia — para descartar neoplasia e outras infecções. • Histórico comportamental.

ACHADOS PATOLÓGICOS
Histopatologia — acantose, alongamento folicular, inflamação dérmica linfoplasmocitária, foliculite, furunculose, peri-hidradenite, hidradenite e fibrose reticular vertical.

TRATAMENTO

• O animal acometido deve receber bastante atenção e praticar atividades físicas.
• O contracondicionamento pode ser útil.
• Restrições físicas — uso de colares elizabetanos e bandagens a curto prazo.
• Foi proposta a ablação da lesão com terapia a laser, mas atualmente não há publicações que avaliem a eficácia dessa modalidade terapêutica.
• Dieta — sem modificação a menos que haja suspeita de hipersensibilidade alimentar.
• O tratamento é difícil, especialmente se nenhuma outra causa subjacente for encontrada; alertar o proprietário sobre a necessidade de tempo e paciência.
• Cirurgia — não considerar esse procedimento até que todas as outras terapias tenham sido esgotadas; frequentemente causará aumento na lambedura e maior atenção sobre a área acometida, resultando em uma oclusão deficiente da ferida; a recidiva será provável se as causas subjacentes não forem tratadas.

MEDICAÇÕES

MEDICAMENTO(S)

Antibióticos
• Seleção com base nos resultados da cultura e do antibiograma.
• Administrá-los até que a infecção desapareça por completo (com frequência, durante 6 semanas no mínimo).

Sistêmicos
• Anti-histamínicos — p. ex., hidroxizina (1-2 mg/kg VO a cada 12 h); clorfeniramina (4-8 mg/cão VO a cada 12 h; dose máxima de 0,5 mg/kg a cada 12 h).
• ISRS — p. ex., fluoxetina (1 mg/kg VO a cada 24 h); paroxetina (0,5-1 mg/kg VO a cada 24 h)
• Antagonistas dopaminérgicos — p. ex., naltrexona (2,2 mg/kg VO a cada 12-24 h).
• Antidepressivos tricíclicos — p. ex., cloridrato de amitriptilina (1,1-2,2 mg/kg VO a cada 12 h) — utilizar a dose mais baixa por 10 dias e, se não houver melhora, usar a dose mais alta por 10 dias; doxepina (3-5 mg/kg VO a cada 12 h; dose máxima de 150 mg a cada 12 h); clomipramina (1-3,5 mg/kg VO a cada 12 h).
• Combinar e/ou suspender esses medicamentos com cuidado.

Tópicos
• Flunixino meglumina e fluocinolona em dimetilsulfóxido (combinados).
• Mupirocina. • Peróxido de benzoíla tópico a 5%.
• Produtos tópicos contendo capsaicina.
• Os corticosteroides intralesionais foram defendidos, mas raramente são úteis.
• Os medicamentos tópicos devem ser aplicados com o auxílio de luvas.
• É imprescindível impedir a lambedura da área pelos animais por 10-15 minutos.

CONTRAINDICAÇÕES/INTERAÇÕES POSSÍVEIS
• Doxepina — cuidado ao utilizar com inibidores da monoamina oxidase, clonidina, anticonvulsivantes, anticoagulantes orais, hormônios esteroides, anti-histamínicos ou ácido acetilsalicílico.
• Anti-histamínicos — cuidado ao utilizar mais de um por vez • A hidroxizina pode diminuir o limiar convulsivo. Evitar o uso em epilépticos.
• Medicamentos psicotrópicos devem ser combinados e/ou suspensos com cuidado.

ACOMPANHAMENTO

• Monitorizar de perto o grau de lambedura e mordedura.
• Tratar a doença subjacente para evitar recidiva.
• Caso não se detecte nenhuma doença subjacente, suspeitar de causas psicogênicas (transtorno obsessivo-compulsivo ou automutilação); o prognóstico é reservado.
• Em casos raros, há relatos de cardiotoxicidade e hepatotoxicidade em animais submetidos a antidepressivos tricíclicos. Selecionar e monitorizar os pacientes com cautela.

DIVERSOS

FATORES RELACIONADOS COM A IDADE
Cães < 5 anos de idade — fortemente sugestivo de alergia.

POTENCIAL ZOONÓTICO
• Transmitida aos seres humanos apenas se a dermatofitose for a causa subjacente; extremamente raro.
• As espécies de *Staphylococcus* resistentes à meticilina têm implicações zoonóticas.

ABREVIATURA(S)
• ACTH = hormônio adrenocorticotrófico.
• TSH = hormônio tireostimulante.

Sugestões de Leitura
Shumaker AK, Angus JC, et al. Microbiological and histopathological features of canine acral lick dermatitis. Vet Dermatol 2008 19(5):288-98.

Autor Jean S. Greek.
Consultor Editorial Alexander H. Werner.

DERMATITE ATÓPICA

CONSIDERAÇÕES GERAIS

DEFINIÇÃO
• Reação de hipersensibilidade a substâncias normalmente inócuas, como polens (gramíneas, ervas daninhas e arbustos), bolores, ácaros da poeira doméstica, alérgenos epiteliais e outros alérgenos ambientais.
• Manifesta-se como uma dermatopatia inflamatória, recidivante, crônica, pruriginosa e não contagiosa.

FISIOPATOLOGIA
• Animais suscetíveis tornam-se sensibilizados a alérgenos ambientais, produzindo IgE alérgeno-específica (mediada pelas células de Langerhans).
• IgE alérgeno-específica liga-se a sítios de receptores presentes em mastócitos cutâneos.
• A reexposição a algum alérgeno, principalmente por absorção percutânea, provoca a degranulação dos mastócitos (reação de hipersensibilidade imediata tipo I), resultando na liberação de histamina, enzimas proteolíticas, citocinas, quimiocinas e muitos outros mediadores químicos.
• A resposta da citocina do tipo Th2 predomina na fase aguda.
• Em caso de dermatite atópica (intrínseca) crônica, predomina uma resposta da citocina do tipo Th1. Superantígenos bacterianos, autoantígenos liberados pelo dano a queratinócitos, e *Malassezia* podem desempenhar um papel na perpetuação do processo inflamatório.

SISTEMA(S) ACOMETIDO(S)
• Oftálmico.
• Respiratório.
• Cutâneo/Endócrino.

GENÉTICA
• Cães — predisposição hereditária; embora o modo de herança seja desconhecido, as influências ambientais são importantes.
• Gatos — influência genética incerta.

INCIDÊNCIA/PREVALÊNCIA
• Espécie canina — a prevalência real é desconhecida; estimada em 3-15% da população canina; relatada por ser a segunda dermatopatia alérgica mais comum no passado; no entanto, com a disponibilidade de medidas eficazes no controle de pulgas, a dermatite atópica pode ser mais prevalente hoje em dia.
• Espécie felina — desconhecida; em geral, acredita-se que a incidência e a prevalência da dermatite atópica sejam muito mais baixas em comparação aos cães.

DISTRIBUIÇÃO GEOGRÁFICA
Espécie canina — reconhecida mundialmente; fatores ambientais locais (temperatura, umidade e flora) influenciam a sazonalidade, a gravidade e a duração dos sinais clínicos.

IDENTIFICAÇÃO
Espécies
Cães e gatos
Raça(s) Predominante(s)
• Espécie canina — qualquer raça, incluindo os cães sem raça definida; identificado com maior frequência em certas raças ou famílias (pode variar em termos geográficos).
• Estados Unidos — Boston terrier, Cairn terrier, Dálmata, Buldogue inglês, Setter inglês, Setter irlandês, Lhasa apso, Schnauzer miniatura, Pug, Sealyham terrier, Terrier escocês, West Highland white terrier, Fox terrier de pelo duro, e Golden retriever.
• Espécie felina — não há relatos.
Idade Média e Faixa Etária
Espécie canina — a idade média de início é de 1-3 anos; faixa etária: 3 meses-6 anos; os sinais podem ser leves no primeiro ano, mas costumam evoluir e se tornar clinicamente aparentes antes dos 3 anos de idade.
Sexo Predominante
Não há relatos.

SINAIS CLÍNICOS
Comentários Gerais
• Prurido — coceira, arranhadura, fricção, lambedura.
• Grande parte das alterações cutâneas causadas por traumatismo autoinduzido; em geral, as lesões primárias não são identificadas.
Achados Anamnésicos
• Prurido facial, podal ou axilar.
• Idade precoce de início.
• Histórico em indivíduos aparentados.
• Pode ser sazonal em princípio.
• Infecção cutânea ou otológica recorrente.
• Resposta temporária a glicocorticosteroides.
• Os sintomas progressivamente pioram com o tempo.
Achados do Exame Físico
• Regiões mais comumente acometidas — espaços interdigitais, áreas correspondentes aos ossos do carpo e tarso, focinho, região periocular e inguinal, axilas e pavilhões auriculares.
• Lesões — variam desde sua ausência até pelos quebradiços ou manchas de saliva até eritema, reações papulares, crostas, alopecia, hiperpigmentação, liquenificação, seborreia excessivamente oleosa ou seca, e hiperidrose (sudorese apócrina).
• Infecções cutâneas secundárias por bactérias e leveduras (comuns).
• Otite externa recidivante crônica.
• Pode ocorrer conjuntivite.

CAUSAS
• Polens (gramíneas, ervas daninhas e arbustos).
• Esporos de fungos (dentro e fora de casa).
• Malassezia.
• Ácaros da poeira doméstica.
• Descamação da pele e dos pelos (caspas) de animais de estimação.
• Insetos (controversos).
• Desregulação de citocinas.

FATORES DE RISCO
• Ambientes de clima temperado com épocas prolongadas de alergia e altos níveis de polens e esporos de fungos.
• Dermatoses pruriginosas concomitantes, como hipersensibilidade à picada de pulga e reação alimentar adversa (efeito somatório).

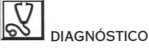
DIAGNÓSTICO

DIAGNÓSTICO DIFERENCIAL
• Reação alimentar adversa — pode causar a mesma distribuição das lesões e os mesmos achados do exame físico, mas não deve ser sazonal; pode ocorrer concomitantemente com dermatite atópica; a diferenciação é feita pela observação da resposta à dieta hipoalergênica.
• Hipersensibilidade à picada de pulga — causa mais comum de prurido sazonal em regiões geográficas propícias; pode ocorrer concomitantemente com dermatite atópica; a diferenciação é feita pela observação da distribuição das lesões, resposta ao controle de pulgas e eliminação de outras causas.
• Sarna sarcóptica — frequentemente ocorre em cães jovens ou errantes; provoca prurido intenso da parte ventral do tórax, lateral dos cotovelos e jarretes, bem como margens do pavilhão auricular; a diferenciação é feita por múltiplos raspados cutâneos e/ou resposta completa a uma tentativa de terapia acaricida.
• Piodermite secundária — geralmente causada por *Staphylococcus pseudointermedius*; caracterizada por pápulas foliculares, pústulas, crostas e colaretes epidérmicos.
• Infecções secundárias por leveduras — causadas por *Malassezia pachydermatis*; caracterizadas por pregas corporais e áreas intertriginosas eritematosas, escamosas, crostosas, oleosas e muito fétidas; a diferenciação é feita pela demonstração de inúmeros microrganismos leveduriformes em brotamento por citologia da pele e obtenção de uma resposta favorável à terapia antifúngica.
• Dermatite de contato (alérgica ou irritante) — pode causar eritema e prurido intensos dos pés e das áreas com poucos pelos do ventre.

HEMOGRAMA/BIOQUÍMICA/URINÁLISE
Eosinofilia — rara em cães sem infestações concomitantes por pulgas; comum em gatos.

OUTROS TESTES LABORATORIAIS
Testes Alérgicos Sorológicos
• Existem testes disponíveis no mercado para medir a quantidade do anticorpo IgE alérgeno-específica no soro do paciente.
• Vantagens sobre o teste intradérmico — disponibilidade; não há necessidade de tricotomia de grandes áreas de pelo; também não há necessidade de sedação.
• Desvantagens — frequentes reações falso-positivas ou falso-negativas; número limitado de alérgenos testados; validação do ensaio, controle de qualidade e confiabilidade inconsistentes (podem variar com o laboratório utilizado).

MÉTODOS DIAGNÓSTICOS
Teste Intradérmico (Preferido)
• O diagnóstico de atopia é feito pelo histórico, exame físico e descarte dos diagnósticos diferenciais.
• O teste intradérmico é usado para formular uma prescrição de imunoterapia.
• Pequenas quantidades do alérgeno testado são injetadas por via intradérmica; a formação de pápulas é mensurada e avaliada de forma subjetiva.
• É mais difícil interpretar os resultados em gatos em virtude da produção de pápulas relativamente pequenas.
• Podem ocorrer reações falso-positivas e falso-negativas.

ACHADOS PATOLÓGICOS
• Lesões macroscópicas — ver "Achados do Exame Físico".
• Biopsia cutânea — pode ajudar a descartar outros diagnósticos diferenciais; os resultados não costumam ser patognomônicos.

DERMATITE ATÓPICA

• Alterações dermato-histopatológicas — acantose, dermatite perivascular superficial mononuclear mista, metaplasia das glândulas sebáceas, com foliculite bacteriana superficial secundária.

TRATAMENTO

CUIDADO(S) DE SAÚDE ADEQUADO(S)
Tratamento ambulatorial.

ATIVIDADE
Evitar os alérgenos ofensores sempre que possível.

DIETA
Dietas ricas em ácidos graxos essenciais podem ser benéficas.

ORIENTAÇÃO AO PROPRIETÁRIO
• Explicar a natureza progressiva do problema.
• Informar ao proprietário que raramente ocorre remissão e que pode não haver cura.
• Comunicar ao proprietário que alguma forma de terapia pode ser necessária para manter a qualidade de vida.

MEDICAÇÕES

MEDICAMENTO(S) DE ESCOLHA

Imunoterapia (Hipossensibilização)
• Administração de injeções subcutâneas de doses gradualmente crescentes dos alérgenos causais para reduzir a sensibilidade.
• Seleção de alérgenos — com base nos resultados dos testes de alergia, no histórico do paciente e/ou no conhecimento de exposição local.
• Os procedimentos de formulação e os protocolos de administração da imunoterapia não são padronizados e variam muito entre os clínicos.
• Indicada quando for desejável evitar ou diminuir a quantidade de corticosteroides necessários para controlar os sinais clínicos, quando os sinais duram mais de 4-6 meses por ano ou quando as formas não esteroides de terapia não são eficazes.
• Reduz com sucesso o prurido em 60-80% dos cães e gatos.
• A resposta costuma ser lenta, necessitando frequentemente de 3-6 meses e até 1 ano, para obtenção do máximo efeito.

Ciclosporina
• A ciclosporina (Atopica® 5 mg/kg/dia) é eficaz no controle de prurido associado à dermatite atópica crônica.
• A resposta é similar àquela obtida com glicocorticosteroides.
• O início de ação é mais lento (tipicamente, 1-4 semanas).
• Muitos pacientes podem ser devidamente controlados a longo prazo com dosagens menos frequentes (a cada 2-4 dias).
• É recomendável a monitorização frequente do paciente.

Corticosteroides
• Podem ser administrados para alívio a curto prazo e para interrupção do ciclo vicioso de prurido-arranhadura.
• Devem ser reduzidos gradativamente até a dose mais baixa e eficaz para controle adequado do prurido.
• Comprimidos de prednisolona ou metilprednisolona (0,2-0,5 mg/kg VO a cada 48 h).
• Gatos — administração pouco frequente de acetato de metilprednisolona injetável (4 mg/kg).

Anti-histamínicos
• Menos eficazes que os corticosteroides.
• É baixa a evidência de eficácia.
• Cães — hidroxizina (1-2 mg/kg VO a cada 12 h), clorfeniramina (0,2-0,4 mg/kg VO a cada 12 h), difenidramina (2,2 mg/kg VO a cada 12 h), e clemastina (0,04-0,10 mg/kg VO a cada 12 h).
• Gatos — clorfeniramina (0,5 mg/kg VO a cada 12 h); a eficácia é estimada em 10-50%.

PRECAUÇÕES
• Corticosteroides — utilizar com bom senso em cães para evitar hiperglicocorticismo iatrogênico e problemas associados, agravamento da piodermite, e indução de demodicose.
• Anti-histamínicos — podem produzir sonolência, anorexia, vômito, diarreia e, até mesmo, aumento do prurido; utilizar com cuidado em pacientes com arritmias cardíacas.

INTERAÇÕES POSSÍVEIS
O uso concomitante de ciclosporina e cetoconazol requer uma redução da dose da ciclosporina.

MEDICAMENTO(S) ALTERNATIVO(S)
• A aplicação de banhos frequentes com água fria e xampus antipruriginosos é muito benéfica.
• Dietas ricas em ácidos graxos podem beneficiar os pacientes com prurido; alguns estudos indicaram que o ácido graxo ômega-3 (ácido eicosapentaenoico 66 mg/kg/dia) pode ser mais eficaz que o ácido graxo ômega-6 (ácido linoleico 130 mg/kg/dia).
• Antidepressivos tricíclicos (doxepina 1-2 mg/kg VO a cada 12 h; ou amitriptilina 1-2 mg/kg VO a cada 12 h) foram administrados a cães como agentes antipruriginosos, mas a eficácia geral desses medicamentos e o modo de ação são incertos; não foram amplamente estudados nos gatos.
• Triancinolona tópica sob a forma de *spray* a 0,015% (Genesis® Virbac) pode ser usada sobre amplas áreas de superfícies corporais para controlar o prurido com mínimos efeitos colaterais.

ACOMPANHAMENTO

MONITORIZAÇÃO DO PACIENTE
• Examinar o paciente a cada 2-8 semanas quando se inicia um novo curso terapêutico.
• Monitorizar os sinais de prurido, autotraumatismo, desenvolvimento de foliculite bacteriana e possíveis reações adversas aos medicamentos.
• Assim que um nível aceitável de controle for atingido, examinar o paciente a cada 3-12 meses.
• Hemograma, bioquímica sérica e urinálise — recomendados a cada 3-12 meses para os pacientes sob terapia crônica com corticosteroide ou ciclosporina.

PREVENÇÃO
• Se os alérgenos ofensores forem identificados por meio dos testes de alergia, o proprietário deverá se esforçar para reduzir a exposição do animal ao máximo possível; raramente isso exerce um impacto significativo sobre o nível do prurido.
• Minimizar outras fontes de prurido (p. ex., infestação de pulga, reação alimentar adversa e infecção cutânea secundária) pode reduzir o nível do prurido.

COMPLICAÇÕES POSSÍVEIS
• Foliculite bacteriana secundária ou dermatite por *Malassezia*.
• Quadros concomitantes de hipersensibilidade à picada de pulga e/ou reação adversa aos alimentos.

EVOLUÇÃO ESPERADA E PROGNÓSTICO
• Não é potencialmente letal a menos que o prurido intratável resulte em eutanásia.
• Sem tratamento, o grau de prurido piora e os sinais duram mais tempo a cada ano.
• Alguns casos exibem resolução espontânea.

DIVERSOS

DISTÚRBIOS ASSOCIADOS
• Hipersensibilidade à picada de pulga.
• Reação alimentar adversa/hipersensibilidade alimentar.
• Foliculite bacteriana.
• Dermatite por *Malassezia*.
• Otite externa.

FATORES RELACIONADOS COM A IDADE
A gravidade piora com o avanço da idade.

GESTAÇÃO/FERTILIDADE/REPRODUÇÃO
• Corticosteroides — contraindicados durante a gestação.
• Os animais acometidos não devem ser usados para fins reprodutivos.

SINÔNIMOS
• Atopia.
• Doença atópica canina.

VER TAMBÉM
• Hipersensibilidade à Picada de Pulga e Controle de Pulga.
• Reações Alimentares, Dermatológicas.
• Otite Externa e Média.
• Piodermite.

Sugestões de Leitura
Reedy LM, Miller WH, Willemse T. Allergic Skin Diseases of Dogs and Cats, 2nd ed. Philadelphia: Saunders, 1997.

Autor Alexander H. Werner
Consultor Editorial Alexander H. Werner

DERMATITE DE CONTATO

CONSIDERAÇÕES GERAIS

REVISÃO
• Dermatite de contato por irritante e dermatite de contato alérgica — duas síndromes fisiopatológicas raras e possivelmente distintas, com sinais clínicos semelhantes; entretanto, a diferenciação pode ser mais conceitual do que prática. • Dermatite de contato por irritante — origina-se do dano direto aos queratinócitos por exposição a algum composto específico; os queratinócitos lesionados induzem a uma resposta inflamatória direcionada contra a pele. • Dermatite de contato alérgica — além de ser classicamente considerada como uma reação de hipersensibilidade do tipo IV (tardia), corresponde a um evento imunológico que requer sensibilização e eliciação: as células de Langerhans interagem com os antígenos que penetram na pele, levando à ativação dos linfócitos-T após reexposição e à liberação de citocinas (mais notavelmente o TNF-α). • Relatos recentes eliminam a distinção entre dermatite de contato por irritante, dermatite de contato alérgica e dermatite atópica.

IDENTIFICAÇÃO
• Cães e gatos. • Dermatite de contato por irritante — ocorre em qualquer idade, como resultado direto da natureza irritante do composto ofensor. • Dermatite de contato alérgica — rara em animais jovens; grande parte dos animais sofre exposição crônica ao antígeno (meses a anos); extremamente rara em gatos, exceto quando expostos aos inseticidas com D-limoneno em sua composição. • Alto risco de dermatite de contato alérgica — Pastor alemão, Poodle, Fox terrier de pelo crespo, Scottish terrier, West Highland white terrier, Labrador e Golden retrievers.

SINAIS CLÍNICOS
Lesões
• A localização é determinada pelo contato com o antígeno; comumente limitada à pele glabra (ou seja, sem pelos) e às regiões que estão em contato frequente com o chão (queixo, porção ventral do pescoço, esterno, face ventral do abdome, região inguinal, períneo, escroto, bem como regiões de contato ventral da cauda e das áreas interdigitais).
• A pelagem espessa dos cães constitui uma barreira física eficiente contra os irritantes de contato.
• A eritrodermia extrema demonstra interrupção abrupta na linha limítrofe do pelo. • Inicialmente, as lesões consistem em eritema e tumefação, levando ao surgimento de pápulas e placas; o aparecimento de vesículas é raro. • A exposição crônica leva à liquenificação e hiperpigmentação.

Outros
• As reações a medicamentos tópicos (mais frequentemente preparações otológicas) costumam ser localizadas.
• As reações generalizadas, resultantes da aplicação de xampus ou sprays inseticidas, são menos comuns.
• Prurido — de moderado a grave (o prurido intenso é mais comum).
• A incidência sazonal pode indicar planta ou elemento ambiental externo como antígeno agressor.

CAUSAS E FATORES DE RISCO
• Dermatite inflamatória — pode aumentar a penetração de antígenos por meio da pele e, consequentemente, facilitar a dermatite de contato alérgica.
• Substâncias ofensoras descritas — plantas, palha radicular, lascas de cedro/madeira; tecidos, tapetes e carpetes, plásticos, borracha, couro, níquel, cobalto, concreto; sabões, detergentes; ceras de piso, desodorizantes (de carpete, lixo e camas dos animais); herbicidas, fertilizantes, inseticidas (incluindo os tratamentos tópicos mais recentes contra pulgas), coleiras antipulgas; preparações tópicas especialmente neomicina.
• Aumento na incidência de dermatite de contato alérgica em animais atópicos.

DIAGNÓSTICO

DIAGNÓSTICO DIFERENCIAL
• Atopia.
• Alergia alimentar.
• Erupções medicamentosas.
• Hipersensibilidade ou infestação parasitárias.
• Picadas de insetos.
• Piodermite.
• Dermatite por *Malassezia*.
• Dermatofitose.
• Demodiciose.
• Lúpus eritematoso.
• Dermatite seborreica.
• Dermatite solar.
• Lesões térmicas.
• Traumatismo decorrente de superfícies ásperas.

MÉTODOS DIAGNÓSTICOS
• Teste de remendo fechado — ocasionalmente útil (é preciso interromper os corticosteroides e os AINEs 3-6 semanas antes do teste); utilizar materiais obtidos diretamente do ambiente ou um kit de teste de remendo padrão para os seres humanos, aplicado à pele sob uma bandagem por 48 h.
• Teste diagnóstico mais eficiente — eliminar o irritante ou o antígeno de contato e prosseguir com o teste de exposição provocativa.
• Se indicadas, podem-se efetuar culturas bacterianas para definir a presença de piodermite secundária.
• A tricotomia de uma pequena porção de pelo em uma região não acometida deve resultar no desenvolvimento de uma reação local por facilitar o contato com o antígeno.
• Biopsia cutânea.

ACHADOS PATOLÓGICOS
• Vesiculação e espongiose intraepidérmicas; edema dérmico superficial, com infiltrado perivascular de células mononucleares tanto na dermatite de contato por irritante como na dermatite de contato alérgica; infiltrado de células polimorfonucleares na dermatite de contato por irritante; é comum a exocitose de leucócitos.
• Na dermatite de contato alérgica canina, observam-se infiltrado espongiótico linfocítico ou eosinofílico e infiltrado espongiótico linfocítico com pústulas eosinofílicas intraepidérmicas.

TRATAMENTO

• Eliminar a(s) substância(s) agressora(s).
• Aplicar banhos com xampus hipoalergênicos para remover o antígeno da pele.
• Criar barreiras mecânicas, se possível — meias, camisetas, restrição de contato com o ambiente, etc.

MEDICAÇÕES

MEDICAMENTO(S)
• Corticosteroides sistêmicos — prednisona (0,25-0,5 mg/kg VO a cada 24 h por 3-5 dias; depois, a cada 48 h por 2 semanas).
• Corticosteroides tópicos em lesões focais.
• Pentoxifilina — 10 mg/kg VO a cada 8-12 h inicialmente; pode ser reduzida para a cada 24 h como manutenção; pode causar irritação gástrica.

CONTRAINDICAÇÕES/INTERAÇÕES POSSÍVEIS
Pentoxifilina — não administrar com agentes alquilantes, cisplatina e anfotericina B; a cimetidina pode aumentar os níveis séricos da pentoxifilina.

ACOMPANHAMENTO

PREVENÇÃO
Remover as substâncias ofensoras oriundas do ambiente.

EVOLUÇÃO ESPERADA E PROGNÓSTICO
Dermatite de contato por irritante
• Condição aguda — pode ocorrer após uma única exposição; pode se manifestar dentro de 24 h da exposição.
• Os corticosteroides raramente são úteis.
• As lesões desaparecem 1-2 dias após a remoção do irritante.

Dermatite de contato alérgica
• Requer meses a anos de exposição para que a hipersensibilidade se desenvolva.
• A reexposição resulta no desenvolvimento de sinais clínicos 3-5 dias após a exposição; os sinais podem persistir por algumas semanas.
• Responde satisfatoriamente aos corticosteroides; no entanto, o prurido retornará após a interrupção desses agentes terapêuticos se o estímulo antigênico não for removido.
• A hipossensibilização não é uma medida eficaz.
• Prognóstico — bom, caso se identifique e se remova o alérgeno; mau, caso não se identifique o alérgeno, o que poderá exigir um tratamento vitalício, ou seja, pelo resto da vida.

DIVERSOS

ABREVIATURA(S)
• AINEs = anti-inflamatórios não esteroides.
• TNF-α = fator de necrose tumoral alfa.

Sugestões de Leitura
Scott DW, Miller WH, Griffin CE. Muller & Kirk's Small Animal Dermatology, 6th ed. Philadelphia: Saunders, 2001, pp. 608-615.

Autores Liora Waldman e Alexander H. Werner
Consultor Editorial Alexander H. Werner

Dermatite Necrolítica Superficial

CONSIDERAÇÕES GERAIS

REVISÃO
- Distúrbio canino incomum; distúrbio felino raro. • Em geral, trata-se de um marcador cutâneo de hepatopatia avançada com ou sem diabetes melito concomitante. • Lesões — patogenia incerta; resultado da degeneração e necrose de queratinócitos, possivelmente em virtude da privação nutricional cutânea; os quadros de hiperglucagonemia, hipoaminoacidemia, deficiências de zinco e de ácido graxo essencial supostamente desempenham um papel direto ou indireto.

SISTEMA(S) ACOMETIDO(S)
- Pele/exócrino. • Hepatobiliar. • Endócrino/metabólico.

IDENTIFICAÇÃO
- Sem predileção racial. • Frequentemente cães idosos. • Machos caninos podem ser predispostos. • Pouquíssimos gatos acometidos para determinar as predileções.

SINAIS CLÍNICOS
- Lesões cutâneas — queixa apresentada usual; as lesões precedem os indícios clínicos de doença interna por semanas a meses; tais lesões consistem em eritema, crostas e erosões ou ulcerações que acometem o focinho, as áreas mucocutâneas da face, o pavilhão auricular, a parte distal dos membros (especialmente cotovelos e jarretes), os pés e a genitália externa, bem como a região perineal ou perianal. • Coxins palmoplantares — hiperqueratóticos com fissuras e ulcerações; dor associada ao caminhar. • O prurido da pele acometida pode ser ausente a intenso. • Infecções bacterianas e/ou leveduriformes secundárias — quase sempre associadas a lesões nos coxins palmoplantares. • Gatos — alopecia e descamação dos membros e do tronco (dois casos); eritema, ulceração, crosta e alopecia dos membros e do tronco (um único caso).

CAUSAS E FATORES DE RISCO
- Causa específica desconhecida.
- Privação nutricional cutânea — provavelmente hipoaminoacidemia e/ou deficiências em ácidos graxos essenciais e de zinco; dermatite atribuída a anormalidades metabólicas provocadas por níveis séricos elevados de glucagon, disfunção hepática ou uma combinação desses.
- Associada, em geral, à hepatopatia avançada com ou sem diabetes melito concomitante.
- Raramente associada a tumor pancreático ou extrapancreático secretor de glucagon ou terapias com fenobarbital ou fenitoína a longo prazo.
- Gatos — associados a um único caso (cada um) de carcinoma pancreático, hepatopatia e carcinoma pancreático, hepatopatia e linfoma intestinal.

DIAGNÓSTICO

DIAGNÓSTICO DIFERENCIAL
- Pênfigo foliáceo.
- Lúpus eritematoso sistêmico.
- Dermatose responsiva ao zinco.
- Necrólise epidérmica tóxica.
- Erupção medicamentosa.
- Dermatopatias esfoliativas felinas: dermatite esfoliativa associada a timoma e linfoma epiteliotrópico cutâneo.
- Eritema das extremidades distais e hiperqueratose dos coxins palmoplantares com fissuras ou ulcerações — aumentam o índice de suspeita para essa condição em cães.

HEMOGRAMA/BIOQUÍMICA/URINÁLISE
- Anemia — achado ocasional; normocítica, normocrômica e arregenerativa.
- Anormalidades eritrocitárias — policromasia; anisocitose; pecilocitose; e células-alvo.
- Fosfatase alcalina, ALT e AST — atividade elevada em casos de hepatopatia avançada.
- Níveis de bilirrubina total — variavelmente elevados.
- Níveis de albumina — frequentemente baixos.
- Anormalidades bioquímicas são incomuns nos cães com tumores secretores de glucagon.
- A maior parte dos pacientes acaba desenvolvendo hiperglicemia franca ou limítrofe.

OUTROS TESTES LABORATORIAIS
- Níveis de ácidos biliares — variavelmente altos.
- Biopsia do fígado — hepatopatia vacuolar com colapso parenquimatoso e hiperplasia nodular.
- Níveis plasmáticos elevados de glucagon — presentes com tumores secretores de glucagon; variáveis com distúrbios hepáticos crônicos.
- Hipoaminoacidemia — comum.
- Podem ser observados altos níveis de insulina.
- Retenção de sulfobromoftaleína — tipicamente aumentada.

DIAGNÓSTICO POR IMAGEM
- Radiografia e ultrassonografia abdominais — é observado o padrão em "favo de mel" à avaliação ultrassonográfica do fígado em casos de hepatopatia avançada.
- Em geral, não há nada digno de nota nos tumores pancreáticos ou raramente extrapancreáticos secretores de glucagon a menos que haja um tumor grande o suficiente para ser visualizado.

MÉTODOS DIAGNÓSTICOS
Biopsias cutâneas — obter amostras de lesões precoces, incluindo crostas e evitando lesões erodidas/ulceradas.

ACHADOS PATOLÓGICOS
- Biopsias cutâneas — hiperqueratose paraqueratótica difusa com edema epidérmico intracelular e intercelular de alta intensidade; hiperplasia epidérmica irregular e dermatite perivascular superficial leve a grave.
- Lesões crônicas — hiperqueratose paraqueratótica acentuada e hiperplasia epidérmica.

TRATAMENTO
- Geralmente como pacientes de ambulatório.
- Cuidados de suporte para sinais sistêmicos.
- Excisão cirúrgica dos tumores secretores de glucagon — poderá ser curativa se o diagnóstico for obtido antes da ocorrência de metástase.
- A maior parte dos casos está associada à hepatopatia irreversível crônica.
- Suporte nutricional por via oral — suplemento ou dieta proteicas de alta qualidade para casos sem encefalopatia; três a seis ovos inteiros ou gemas de ovos cozidos por dia.
- Informar aos clientes que esse distúrbio indica doença interna concomitante com prognóstico mau.
- Hidroterapia e xampus — ajudam a remover as crostas; diminuem o prurido e a dor.

MEDICAÇÕES

MEDICAMENTO(S)
- Tratamento específico — tentar corrigir a doença subjacente se possível.
- Terapia sintomática inespecífica — antibióticos e antifúngicos para infecções cutâneas secundárias.
- Hiperalimentação com aminoácidos — administração intravenosa de solução de aminoácidos cristalinos a 10% (p. ex., Aminosyn®) a aproximadamente 25 mL/kg, administrados em 6-8 h e repetidos a cada 7-10 dias. A terapia com aminoácidos por via oral pode ser benéfica.
- Octreotida (análogo da somatostatina) — 2-3,2 µg/kg por via SC 2 a 4 vezes ao dia como terapia de manutenção para pacientes com tumores secretores de glucagon não passíveis de ressecção.
- Glicocorticoides — podem melhorar as lesões cutâneas; no entanto, seu uso deve ser considerado com cuidado, pois tais agentes podem induzir a diabetes melito.
- Sulfato ou gliconato de zinco (10 e 5 mg/kg/dia, respectivamente); os resultados não são recompensadores como monoterapia.
- Ácidos graxos essenciais — não são benéficos como monoterapia.

ACOMPANHAMENTO

COMPLICAÇÕES POSSÍVEIS
- Insuficiência hepática.
- Infecções cutâneas bacterianas e/ou leveduriformes secundárias.

EVOLUÇÃO ESPERADA E PROGNÓSTICO
- Prognóstico mau; tempo de sobrevida relatado em 5 meses após o desenvolvimento das lesões cutâneas.
- Incidência muito rara de recuperação se o insulto hepático/metabólico desaparecer.

DIVERSOS

DISTÚRBIOS ASSOCIADOS
Diabetes melito — geralmente não cetoacidótico; o desenvolvimento indica piora do prognóstico.

VER TAMBÉM
- Hepatopatia Diabética. • Glucagonoma.

ABREVIATURA(S)
- ALT = alanina aminotransferase.
- AST = aspartato aminotransferase.

Sugestões de Leitura
Byrne KP. Metabolic epidermal necrosis-hepatocutaneous syndrome. Vet Clin North Am Small Anim Pract 2006, 29(6):1337-1354.

Autor Sheila Torres
Consultor Editorial Alexander H. Werner

Dermatite por Malassezia

CONSIDERAÇÕES GERAIS

REVISÃO
• *Malassezia pachydermatis* (sinônimo *Pityrosporum canis*) — levedura; comensal normal da pele, das orelhas e das regiões mucocutâneas; pode se proliferar e causar dermatite, queilite e otite em cães e gatos. • *M. pachydermatis* tem afinidade pelos lipídios, embora várias espécies isoladas do cão e gato sejam dependentes de lipídios. • A quantidade de leveduras nas áreas acometidas costuma ser excessiva, embora este seja um achado variável. • As causas da transformação de comensal inócuo a patógeno são mal compreendidas, porém parecem relacionadas com alergia, condições seborreicas e, possivelmente, fatores congênitos e hormonais.

SISTEMA(S) ACOMETIDO(S)
Cutâneo/exócrino.

IDENTIFICAÇÃO
• Cães — qualquer raça canina; entretanto, as raças West Highland white terrier, Poodle, Basset hound, Cocker spaniel e Dachshund são predispostas. • Gatos — menos comum do que nos cães; especula-se que a doença e as causas predisponentes sejam semelhantes àquelas tanto no cão como em gatos jovens aos de meia-idade; gatos idosos podem ter dermatite por *Malassezia* associada à neoplasia interna; qualquer raça pode ser acometida; todavia, gatos jovens da raça Rex são predispostos. • Nenhuma predileção sexual. • Dermatite canina por *Malassezia* e dermatite seborreica associada com *Malassezia* — comuns em todas as regiões geográficas do mundo.

SINAIS CLÍNICOS
• Prurido — com graus variados de eritema, alopecia, descamação e exsudato gorduroso e fétido; acomete lábios, orelhas, pés, axilas, região inguinal e porção ventral do pescoço. • Hiperpigmentação e liquenificação — casos crônicos. • Cera escura concomitante à otite seborreica — frequentes. • Prurido facial frenético — raro, porém característico. • Com frequência, há um histórico de suspeita de alergia, que piora e parece desenvolver resistência ou ser resistente ao tratamento com glicocorticoides. • Foliculite bacteriana concomitante e hipersensibilidade, além de distúrbios endócrinos e de queratinização.

CAUSAS E FATORES DE RISCO
• Umidade e temperatura elevadas — podem aumentar a frequência. • Reações de hipersensibilidade concomitantes (particularmente atopia, alergia a pulgas e algumas intolerâncias/alergias alimentares) — podem ser um fator predisponente. • Defeitos do processo de cornificação e seborreias (especialmente em cães jovens) — nas raças predispostas. • Endocrinopatias (sobretudo em cães idosos) — há suspeitas de associação com fatores predisponentes. • Fatores genéticos — há suspeitas de início em jovens nas raças caninas predispostas e nos gatos da raça Rex. • Aumento concomitante na população cutânea de *Staphylococcus pseudintermedius* e foliculite bacteriana resultante — achado confirmado; em casos selecionados, sugere-se que a dermatite seborreica canina seja o resultado dessa combinação de proliferação do patógeno; o tratamento de apenas uma delas não resulta na resolução de todos os sinais, mas apenas mascara a outra; somente o tratamento antilevedura resolve todos os sinais de dermatite por *Malassezia*. • Os gatos possuem a doença tanto na idade jovem como na adulta, a qual pode estar associada à alergia. Nos gatos da raça Rex, as características genéticas associadas às características singulares de sua pelagem ou da pele ou ainda sua predisposição à anormalidade dos mastócitos denominada urticária pigmentosa podem ser fatores. Gatos idosos podem apresentar dermatite por *Malassezia* associada a timomas e carcinomas do pâncreas e do fígado.

DIAGNÓSTICO
O diagnóstico é realizado pela demonstração de quantidade excessiva do microrganismo na pele acometida e pela melhora significativa nos sinais clínicos após a remoção da levedura.

DIAGNÓSTICO DIFERENCIAL
• Dermatite alérgica — incluindo alergia a pulgas, atopia e alergia alimentar.
• Foliculite bacteriana superficial.
• Seborreias primária e secundária (defeito de queratinização).
• Acantose nigricante — cães da raça Dachshund.

HEMOGRAMA/BIOQUÍMICA/URINÁLISE
Normais a menos que sejam influenciados pela causa subjacente.

OUTROS TESTES LABORATORIAIS
• Cultura fúngica — utilizar placas de contato (pequenas placas de ágar preparadas a partir de pequenas tampas de frascos e preenchidas com ágar Sabouraud ou, de preferência, ágar Dixon modificado, especialmente no gato); pressionar as placas sobre a superfície da pele acometida; incubar a 32-37°C por 3-7 dias; contar as colônias amarelas ou cor de couro, arredondadas e em forma de cúpula (1-1,5 mm); fornecem dados semiqualitativos.
• Métodos não quantitativos de cultura — sem valor porque a *Malassezia* é um microrganismo comensal normal.

MÉTODOS DIAGNÓSTICOS
• Citologia cutânea — por contato, *swab* de algodão ou preparação com fita de celofane corada com Diff-Quik; aplicar uma gota do corante diretamente na lâmina (a levedura pode ser removida durante a coloração); passar chama sob a lâmina para melhorar a penetração do corante e a visualização do microrganismo.
• É mais provável que as áreas gordurosas e/ou descamadas produzam resultados positivos.

TRATAMENTO
• Identificar e tratar todos os fatores predisponentes ou as doenças.
• Tratamento tópico — a levedura está localizada principalmente no estrato córneo.
• Tratamento com xampu — para remover as escamas e os exsudatos.
• Tratamento tópico (com base em dados de ensaios) — xampus de miconazol e clorexidina são mais eficazes; xampu de sulfeto de selênio é menos eficaz, porém útil; o tratamento deve ser aplicado 2 vezes por semana.
• Outros tratamentos tópicos com xampus antibacterianos e antifúngicos (p. ex., cetoconazol) também são valiosos se realizados com medicamentos sistêmicos apropriados.
• Combinações alternativas — tratamento tópico com xampu queratolítico com medicamentos sistêmicos contra leveduras e bactérias.

MEDICAÇÕES

MEDICAMENTO(S)
• Casos localizados — podem responder a cremes e loções contendo compostos imidazólicos.
• Cetoconazol — 10 mg/kg a cada 24 h por 2-4 semanas nos casos disseminados ou liquenificados crônicos.
• Outros imidazóis também são eficazes.
• Casos liquenificados crônicos — cetoconazol (7-10 mg/kg a cada 24 h) como um método diagnóstico rápido por 7-10 dias com tratamento à base de xampu antimicótico tópico eficaz; uma boa resposta confirma o diagnóstico; a resposta pode ser lenta nos casos crônicos, em que a levedura se enterra profundamente nas dobras epidérmicas.
• Xampu antibacteriano tópico — para manter a remissão nos casos crônicos.

CONTRAINDICAÇÕES/INTERAÇÕES POSSÍVEIS
Cetoconazol — raramente pode provocar reação hepática; mascara os sinais do hiperadrenocorticismo e interfere nos testes de função adrenal em virtude do bloqueio da produção de cortisol (via inibição do citocromo P-450) na glândula adrenal; contraindicado nos gatos com malignidade interna hepática e debilitante grave, já que podem não ser capazes de metabolizar o medicamento.

ACOMPANHAMENTO
• Exame físico e citologia cutânea — após 2-4 semanas para monitorizar o tratamento.
• Tratar até a demonstração de raros microrganismos ou 7 dias após uma resposta completa ser alcançada.
• Prurido e odor — costumam exibir uma melhora notável dentro de 1 semana.
• Recidivas — comuns quando as dermatoses subjacentes não estiverem bem controladas; banho regular com xampu antibacteriano e antifúngico ajuda a reduzir a recidiva.

DIVERSOS

GESTAÇÃO/FERTILIDADE/REPRODUÇÃO
Cetoconazol é contraindicado.

Sugestões de Leitura
Scott DW, Miller WH, Griffin CE. Muller & Kirk's Small Animal Dermatology, 5th ed. Philadelphia: Saunders, 1995.

Autor K.V. Mason
Consultor Editorial Alexander H. Werner

Dermatofilose

CONSIDERAÇÕES GERAIS

REVISÃO
- Também conhecida como "erupção do lodo" ou "febre do lodo", trata-se de uma rara dermatite crostosa em cães e gatos, bem como de uma rara doença subcutânea nodular e bucal em gatos.
- *Dermatophilus congolensis* — agente causal; bactéria Gram-positiva, filamentosa, ramificada, classificada como Actinomiceto; causa muito comum de dermatoses formadoras de crostas em animais ungulados; persiste no ambiente no interior das crostas.
- Raras vezes, cães, gatos e seres humanos podem sofrer infecção secundária.

SISTEMA(S) ACOMETIDO(S)
Cutâneo/exócrino.

IDENTIFICAÇÃO
- Cães e gatos.
- Não há predileção etária, racial ou sexual.

SINAIS CLÍNICOS

Achados Anamnésicos
- Associação com bovinos, ovinos ou equinos.
- Ocasionalmente, acomete cães errantes, ou seja, de vida livre.
- Gatos com a doença subcutânea — episódio de traumatismo; existência de corpo estranho; lesões geralmente crônicas; ausência de sinais clínicos sistêmicos, exceto quando se desenvolvem lesões nos órgãos internos ou lesões amplas na boca.

Achados do Exame Físico
- Cães — lesões: papulares; crostosas; principalmente na pele do tronco e/ou da cabeça; de circulares a coalescentes; semelhantes às decorrentes de piodermite bacteriana superficial causada pelo *Staphylococcus pseudintermedius*; as lesões podem se assemelhar à dermatofilose em equinos (crostas cinza-amareladas, espessas e aderentes, que incorporam os pelos e deixam uma erosão superficial, brilhante e circular quando removidas); o prurido é variável.
- Gatos — nódulos ou abscessos ulcerados e fistulosos subcutâneos, bucais ou internos, semelhantes às lesões causadas por outros actinomicetos nessa espécie; recentemente, relatou-se uma dermatopatia crostosa piogênica superficial da face.

CAUSAS E FATORES DE RISCO
- Cães, gatos e seres humanos — podem ser expostos diretamente a partir de lesões em grandes animais ou de exposição ao meio ambiente.
- Estágio infeccioso — requer umidade para sua ativação; não consegue penetrar no epitélio intacto; a ocorrência de pequeno traumatismo ou transmissão mecânica por meio da picada de ectoparasitas (*Amblyomma variegatum*) pode ajudar a estabelecer a infecção.
- Infecções mais profundas — necessitam de inoculação traumática de material infeccioso.

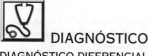

DIAGNÓSTICO

DIAGNÓSTICO DIFERENCIAL

Cães
- Foliculite estafilocócica.
- Dermatite úmida aguda.
- Dermatofitose.
- Pênfigo foliáceo.
- Distúrbio de queratinização.

Gatos
- Actinomicose e nocardiose.
- Granuloma micobacteriano oportunista.
- Esporotricose.
- Criptococose.
- Corpo estranho.
- Abscesso crônico causado por ferida/mordedura.
- Infecção pelas formas L bacterianas.
- Infecção pelo *Rhodococcus equi*.
- Neoplasias cutâneas ou mucosas, particularmente carcinoma de células escamosas.

HEMOGRAMA/BIOQUÍMICA/URINÁLISE
Em geral, permanecem normais; possível leucocitose neutrofílica em gatos.

MÉTODOS DIAGNÓSTICOS

Cães
- Exame citológico das crostas — constitui o procedimento mais importante; permite a diferenciação de piodermites bacterianas mais típicas.
- Microrganismo — morfologia distinta em preparados citológicos e histológicos; assemelha-se a "trilhos de trem", já que a bactéria forma cadeias ramificadas de diplococos pequenos.
- Diagnóstico citológico — a partir de esfregaços por impressão (decalque) feitos de exsudato presente sob as crostas ou por meio de preparados de crostas maceradas; fragmentar as crostas delicadamente em uma gota de água e permitir sua maceração por alguns minutos; em seguida, secar o preparado e corar com corante de Wright--Giemsa.
- Amostras histopatológicas — as crostas contêm os microrganismos; enviar com amostras teciduais.

Gatos
- Exame histopatológico — biopsia de nódulos; método de escolha.
- Exame citológico — exsudato obtido a partir de aspirado de nódulo ou da aplicação de *swab* em trajeto drenante.
- Cultura realizada a partir das amostras de biopsia — pode recuperar o microrganismo; facilitada se o laboratório for alertado quanto ao diagnóstico diferencial de *Dermatophilus* (agente aeróbio de crescimento relativamente lento e facilmente mascarado por contaminação).
- Cultura feita a partir de crostas — requer o uso de meio seletivo especial; o isolamento é possível, mas costuma ser muito difícil.

ACHADOS PATOLÓGICOS
- Cães — dermatite crostosa e pustular superficial; crostas em paliçada com hiperqueratose ortoqueratótica e paraqueratótica; microrganismo observado dentro das crostas.
- Gatos — inflamação piogranulomatosa; necrose central; formação de trajeto fistuloso; microrganismo observado próximo ao centro necrosado dos granulomas, especialmente com o uso do corante de Gram.

TRATAMENTO

- Cães — xampu antibacteriano e remoção delicada (e descarte) das crostas; o xampu pode conter peróxido de benzoíla, lactato de etila, clorexidina ou dissulfeto de selênio; na maioria dos casos, uma ou duas aplicações são suficientes. Também pode ser utilizada solução de iodo ou enxofre.
- Gatos — em casos de piogranulomas e abscessos: debridamento cirúrgico; exploração em busca de corpo estranho; estabelecimento de drenagem para o exsudato.

MEDICAÇÕES

MEDICAMENTO(S)
- Penicilina V — 10 mg/kg VO a cada 12 h por 10-20 dias; medicamento de escolha.
- Tetraciclina 22-30 mg/kg a cada 8 h VO, doxiciclina 5-10 mg/kg a cada 12 h VO ou minociclina 5-12 mg/kg a cada 12 h VO.
- Ampicilina — 10-20 mg/kg VO a cada 12 h por 10-20 dias; alguns isolamentos são resistentes *in vitro*.
- Amoxicilina — 10-20 mg/kg VO a cada 12 h por 10-20 dias; alguns isolamentos também exibem resistência *in vitro*.

CONTRAINDICAÇÕES/INTERAÇÕES POSSÍVEIS
Hipersensibilidade à penicilina e ampicilina.

ACOMPANHAMENTO

MONITORIZAÇÃO DO PACIENTE
- Cães — reavaliar após 2 semanas do tratamento para garantir a resolução completa dos sintomas; fornecer a terapia sistêmica por mais 7 dias se houver indicação.
- Gatos — monitorizar em intervalos quinzenais por 1 mês após a resolução aparente das lesões, dependendo de sua localização.

EVOLUÇÃO ESPERADA E PROGNÓSTICO
- Cães — excelente.
- Gatos — varia com a localização das lesões e a extensão do debridamento cirúrgico; pode-se obter a resolução completa das lesões com a formulação do diagnóstico em tempo oportuno, bem como por meio de terapias clínica e cirúrgica apropriadas.

DIVERSOS

POTENCIAL ZOONÓTICO
- Veterinários e tratadores de animais — são infectados com frequência muito rara, mesmo após exposição traumática, ao lidar com animais pecuários infectados.
- Cães e gatos — é bastante improvável que tais espécies sirvam como fonte de infecção humana; é justificável certa cautela quanto à exposição de indivíduos imunocomprometidos.

Sugestões de Leitura
Greene CE. Dermatophilosis. In: Greene CE, ed., Infectious Diseases of the Dog and Cat, 3rd ed. St. Louis: Saunders Elsevier, 2006, pp. 488-490.

Autor Mitchell D. Song
Consultor Editorial Alexander H. Werner

DERMATOFITOSE

CONSIDERAÇÕES GERAIS

DEFINIÇÃO
- Infecção fúngica cutânea que acomete as regiões cornificadas dos pelos, das unhas e, ocasionalmente, das camadas superficiais da pele.
- Microrganismos isolados com maior frequência — *Microsporum canis*, *Trichophyton mentagrophytes* e *M. gypseum*.

FISIOPATOLOGIA
- A exposição a um dermatófito ou o contato com esse microrganismo não resultam necessariamente em infecção.
- A infecção pode não culminar em sinais clínicos.
- Dermatófitos — crescem nas camadas queratinizadas dos pelos, das unhas e da pele; não se desenvolvem no tecido vivo ou persistem na presença de inflamação grave; período de incubação: 1-4 semanas.
- O animal acometido pode permanecer em um estado de portador (assintomático) inaparente por um período de tempo prolongado; alguns animais nunca se tornam sintomáticos.
- Os corticosteroides podem modular a inflamação e prolongar a infecção.

SISTEMA(S) ACOMETIDO(S)
Cutâneo/exócrino.

INCIDÊNCIA/PREVALÊNCIA
- As lesões podem mimetizar muitos distúrbios dermatológicos; pode ser comum o diagnóstico demasiado.
- As taxas de infecção variam amplamente, dependendo da população estudada.

DISTRIBUIÇÃO GEOGRÁFICA
- Embora seja uma afecção ubíqua, a incidência é mais alta em regiões de clima quente e úmido.
- A incidência dos dermatófitos geofílicos pode variar em termos geográficos.

IDENTIFICAÇÃO
Espécies
Cães e gatos.

Raça(s) Predominante(s)
Gatos — mais comum em raças de pelo longo.

Idade Média e Faixa Etária
Sinais clínicos — mais comuns em animais jovens e mais idosos.

SINAIS CLÍNICOS
Achados Anamnésicos
- As lesões podem começar sob a forma de alopecia ou más condições da pelagem.
- O histórico de infecção ou exposição previamente confirmadas a algum animal infectado ou ambiente contaminado (p. ex., gatil) constitui um achado útil, mas inconsistente.

Achados do Exame Físico
- Variam desde o estado de portador inaparente até alopecia irregular ou circular.
- Alopecia circular clássica — comum em gatos; frequentemente mal-interpretada em cães.
- Escamas, eritema, hiperpigmentação e prurido — variáveis.
- Podem ocorrer paroníquia, lesões granulomatosas ou quérions.

CAUSAS
- Gatos — *M. canis* é o agente mais comum.
- Cães — *M. canis*, *M. gypseum* e *T. mentagrophytes*; a incidência de cada agente varia em termos geográficos.
- Outros microrganismos fúngicos foram identificados com uma frequência significativamente menor.

FATORES DE RISCO
- Imunocomprometimento causado por doenças (FeLV, FIV) ou por medicamentos (corticosteroides).
- Infecção pelo FIV (prevalência 3 vezes maior).
- Densidade populacional elevada.
- Nutrição deficiente.
- Práticas insatisfatórias de manejo.
- Falta de um período adequado de quarentena.

DIAGNÓSTICO

DIAGNÓSTICO DIFERENCIAL
- Gatos — dermatite alérgica e muitas outras dermatoses.
- Cães — foliculite bacteriana (colaretes epidérmicos) e muitas causas de alopecia.
- Demodicose — orifícios/poros foliculares macroscopicamente dilatados com furunculose.
- Dermatopatias imunomediadas/autoimunes — semelhantes à inflamação grave associada à dermatofitose, que acomete a face ou os pés.

MÉTODOS DIAGNÓSTICOS
Exame com Lâmpada de Wood
- Não constitui uma ferramenta de triagem muito útil.
- Muitos dermatófitos patogênicos não emitem fluorescência.
- É comum a obtenção de fluorescência falsa; medicamentos, queratina associada a escamas epidérmicas e sebo podem produzir fluorescência falso-positiva.
- A lâmpada deve ser aquecida por no mínimo 5 minutos e depois ficar exposta às lesões sob suspeita por até 5 minutos.
- Uma reação positiva verdadeira associada ao *M. canis* consiste na fluorescência de coloração verde-maçã na haste pilosa.

Exame Microscópico do Pelo
- O exame dos pelos arrancados após o uso de uma solução clareadora pode ajudar a fornecer o diagnóstico imediato.
- Esse exame é demorado e, muitas vezes, gera resultados falso-negativos.
- Utilizar os pelos que exibem fluorescência sob iluminação com a lâmpada de Wood para aumentar a probabilidade de identificação das hifas fúngicas associadas à haste pilosa.

Cultura Fúngica com Identificação
- Melhor método para obtenção do diagnóstico.
- Os pelos que exibem fluorescência verde-maçã positiva sob exame com a lâmpada de Wood são considerados candidatos ideais para a cultura.
- Arrancar os pelos da periferia de uma área alopécica; não usar um padrão aleatório.
- Para obter os melhores resultados, utilizar uma escova de dentes esterilizada para escovar a pelagem do animal assintomático.
- Meios de cultura para pesquisa de dermatófito — alteram-se para a cor vermelha quando se tornam alcalinos; os dermatófitos produzem essa mudança de coloração durante a fase precoce de crescimento de sua cultura; os saprófitas provocam a mudança de cor após crescimento significativo da colônia; assim, é importante examinar os meios diariamente.
- Exame microscópico do crescimento de microconídios e macroconídios — necessário para confirmar o dermatófito patogênico, bem como para identificar o gênero e a espécie; ajuda a identificar a fonte de infecção.
- Cultura positiva — indica a existência do dermatófito; entretanto, a presença desse microrganismo pode ser apenas transitória, como costuma ocorrer quando se obtém a cultura a partir dos pés, uma região de contato provável com o dermatófito geofílico.

Biopsia Cutânea
- Não costuma ser necessária para obtenção do diagnóstico.
- Pode ser útil na confirmação de invasão e infecção verdadeiras ou para o diagnóstico de casos sob suspeita com cultura fúngica negativa.

ACHADOS PATOLÓGICOS
- Foliculite, perifoliculite ou furunculose são comuns.
- Podem ocorrer hiperqueratose, pústulas intraepidérmicas e padrão reacional piogranulomatoso.
- Nos cortes histológicos corados pela hematoxilina e eosina (H&E), podem-se observar as hifas fúngicas; os corantes especiais permitem a observação mais fácil do microrganismo.

TRATAMENTO

CUIDADO(S) DE SAÚDE ADEQUADO(S)
- A maioria dos animais é tratada em um esquema ambulatorial.
- Em virtude da natureza contagiosa e zoonótica da doença, considerar a prática de quarentena.

DIETA
- Uma refeição rica em gordura melhora a absorção da griseofulvina.
- Uma refeição ácida (adicionar molho de tomate) intensifica a absorção do cetoconazol.

ORIENTAÇÃO AO PROPRIETÁRIO
- Informar ao proprietário que muitos gatos de pelo curto em ambiente com um único gato e muitos cães sofrerão remissão espontânea.
- Os animais de pelo longo deverão ser submetidos à tosa para diminuir a contaminação ambiental.
- Avisar que o tratamento pode ser tanto frustrante como dispendioso, especialmente em ambientes domésticos com múltiplos animais ou em casos recidivantes.
- Instruir o proprietário sobre a importância do tratamento ambiental, inclusive dos fômites, particularmente em casos recidivantes; a água sanitária diluída (os relatos variam quanto a potência/concentração necessária) constitui um meio prático e relativamente eficaz de proporcionar a descontaminação ambiental; a água sanitária concentrada e a formalina (a 1%) são mais eficientes na eliminação dos esporos, mas o uso desses produtos não é tão prático em muitas circunstâncias; em estudos-piloto, a clorexidina não se mostrou eficaz.
- Notificar ao proprietário que o tratamento e o controle podem ser bastante complicados em ambientes com múltiplos animais ou em gatis;

DERMATOFITOSE

deve-se ponderar o encaminhamento a um veterinário especialista nesse tipo de situação.

MEDICAÇÕES

MEDICAMENTO(S) DE ESCOLHA
- Griseofulvina — até pouco tempo, era o medicamento sistêmico mais amplamente prescrito; formulação em micropartículas: 25-60 mg/kg VO a cada 12-24 h por 4-10 semanas; formulação em ultramicropartículas: 2,5-15 mg/kg VO a cada 12-24 h; a absorção é aumentada, dividindo-se a dose para 2 vezes ao dia e administrando-a com uma refeição rica em gordura; as doses mais elevadas associam-se a uma alta probabilidade de toxicidade, devendo ser utilizadas com extremo cuidado; um desarranjo gastrintestinal constitui o efeito colateral mais comum; aliviá-lo por meio da diminuição da dose ou divisão da dose para uma posologia mais frequente.
- Cetoconazol — a eficácia real é desconhecida; dose: 10 mg/kg VO a cada 24 h ou divididos a cada 12 h por 4-8 semanas; a anorexia e o vômito representam os efeitos colaterais mais comuns; não recomendado em gatos; no entanto, constitui o tratamento de escolha de muitos clínicos para cães de médio a grande porte.
- Itraconazol — semelhante ao cetoconazol, mas com menos efeitos colaterais, mais eficaz e mais caro; a dose das cápsulas de itraconazol em cães é de 5-10 mg/kg VO a cada 24 h por 4-8 semanas; a dose em gatos é de 10 mg/kg VO a cada 24 h por 4-8 semanas ou até a cura; a dose de 20 mg/kg a cada 48 h pode ser considerada tanto para os cães como para os gatos. Em alguns gatos, o esquema posológico é alterado após 4 semanas de terapia para um esquema em semanas alternadas por um total de 8-10 semanas de terapia; o esquema alternativo consiste em uma semana com medicamento e outra semana sem medicamento, com eficácia aparente na redução do custo do tratamento; disponível em cápsulas de 100 mg e sob a forma líquida a 10 mg/mL, contendo ciclodextrina; prefere-se a forma líquida às formulações manipuladas em virtude da variabilidade na absorção. O itraconazol tem se tornado a escolha terapêutica preferida dos clínicos para dermatofitose em cães de pequeno porte e gatos (filhotes de até 6 semanas de vida).
- Terapia tópica e tricotomia — uso recomendado com terapia sistêmica concomitante; podem ajudar a evitar a contaminação ambiental; associadas muitas vezes a uma exacerbação inicial dos sinais clínicos após a instituição dos procedimentos; os xampus à base de enxofre (diluição de 1:16), o enilconazol e o miconazol (com ou sem clorexidina) constituem os agentes tópicos generalizados mais eficazes; o enxofre é odorífero e pode manchar; o enilconazol não se encontra disponível nos EUA para uso doméstico. As soluções contendo miconazol estão disponíveis sob a forma de xampus e preparações *leave-on* (ou seja, sem enxágue); o uso do colar elizabetano, particularmente em gatos, é recomendado para evitar a ingestão desses produtos. Também foi demonstrado que a clorexidina sozinha seja ineficaz, embora haja pesquisas recentes que demonstrem uma possível ação sinérgica da clorexidina com o miconazol para aumentar sua eficácia.

CONTRAINDICAÇÕES
- Corticosteroides.
- Griseofulvina em gatos com FeLV ou FIV.

PRECAUÇÕES
Griseofulvina
- Altamente teratogênica.
- Como reação idiossincrásica ou em caso de terapia prolongada, pode ocorrer mielossupressão (anemia, pancitopenia e neutropenia).
- Neutropenia — reação fatal mais comum em gatos; pode persistir após a suspensão do medicamento; pode ser potencialmente letal em gatos com infecção pelo FeLV ou FIV.
- Efeitos colaterais neurológicos.

Cetoconazol
- Há relatos de hepatopatia, possivelmente muito grave.
- Em cães, inibe a produção endógena dos hormônios esteroides.

Itraconazol
- Foram relatados os efeitos de vasculite e lesões cutâneas necroulcerativas em 7,5% dos cães com blastomicose, tratados com doses de 5 mg/kg a cada 12 h. As lesões não foram observadas em pacientes submetidos a 5 mg/kg a cada 24 h.
- Nos cães, há relatos de hepatotoxicidade em aproximadamente 5-10% dos casos tratados para blastomicose.

Solução de Enxofre
- Há relatos não publicados de que a ingestão de enxofre pode levar a erosões bucais.

MEDICAMENTO(S) ALTERNATIVO(S)
- Lufenurona — um inibidor da síntese de quitina, utilizado no controle de pulgas; não é eficaz em estudos controlados.
- Fluconazol — a eficácia não está bem documentada em estudos; mais barato que o itraconazol.
- Terbinafina — pode ser útil em casos resistentes aos agentes azólicos.

ACOMPANHAMENTO

MONITORIZAÇÃO DO PACIENTE
- A cultura de dermatófitos representa o único meio de monitorizar de fato a resposta à terapia; muitos animais apresentarão melhora clínica, mas permanecerão positivos à cultura.
- Repetir as culturas fúngicas próximo ao término do esquema terapêutico e prosseguir com a terapia até a negatividade de pelo menos um resultado de cultura.
- Em casos resistentes, a cultura poderá ser repetida em intervalos semanais, utilizando-se a técnica da escova de dentes; continuar o tratamento até a obtenção de 2-3 resultados negativos consecutivos à cultura.
- Hemograma completo semanal ou quinzenal caso se faça uso da griseofulvina; avaliação periódica das enzimas hepáticas caso se lance mão do cetoconazol ou itraconazol.

PREVENÇÃO
- Para evitar a reinfecção a partir de portadores inaparentes, é recomendável instituir o período de quarentena, bem como obter culturas de dermatófitos, em todos os animais que ingressarem no ambiente doméstico.
- Considerar a possibilidade da participação de roedores na disseminação da doença.
- Caso haja o envolvimento de algum dermatófito geofílico, deve-se evitar o contato com solos contaminados.
- Ponderar o tratamento profilático de animais expostos.

COMPLICAÇÕES POSSÍVEIS
Culturas de dermatófitos falso-negativas.

EVOLUÇÃO ESPERADA E PROGNÓSTICO
- Muitos animais "autoeliminarão" a infecção por dermatófito em alguns meses.
- O tratamento contra a doença acelera a cura clínica e ajuda a diminuir a contaminação ambiental.
- Certas infecções, particularmente em gatos de pelo longo ou em circunstâncias com múltiplos animais, podem ser muito persistentes.

DIVERSOS

POTENCIAL ZOONÓTICO
A dermatofitose é uma zoonose significativa.

GESTAÇÃO/FERTILIDADE/REPRODUÇÃO
- A griseofulvina é teratogênica.
- O cetoconazol pode afetar a síntese dos hormônios esteroides, especialmente da testosterona.

SINÔNIMO(S)
Tinha.

ABREVIATURA(S)
- FeLV = vírus da leucemia felina.
- FIV = vírus da imunodeficiência felina.

Sugestões de Leitura
Colombo S, Cornegliani L, Vercelli A. Efficacy of itraconazole as a combined continuous/pulse therapy in feline dermatophytosis: Preliminary results in nine cases. Vet Dermatol 2001, 12:347-350.
DeBoer DJ, Moriello KA. Cutaneous fungal infections. In: Greene CE, ed., Infectious Diseases of the Dog and Cat, 3rd ed. St. Louis: Saunders Elsevier, 2006, pp. 550-569.
Moriello K. Treatment of dermatophytosis in dogs and cats: Review of published studies. Vet Dermatol 2004, 15:99-107.
Newbury S, Moriello K, Verbrugge M, Thomas C. Use of lime sulphur and itraconazole to treat shelter cats naturally infected with Microsporum canis in an annex facility: An open field trial. VetDermatol 2007, 19:324-331.
Perrins N, Bond R. Synergistic inhibition of the growth in vitro of Microsporum canis by miconazole and chlorhexidine. Vet Dermatol 2003, 14:99-102.
Scott DW, Miller WH, Griffin CE. Muller & Kirk's Small Animal Dermatology, 6th ed. Philadelphia: Saunders, 2001.
Sparkes A, Robinson A, MacKay A, Shau S. A study of the efficacy of topical and systemic therapy for the treatment of feline Microsporum canis infection. J Feline Med Surg 2000, 2:135-142.

Autores W. Dunbar Gram e Marlene Pariser
Consultor Editorial Alexander H. Werner

DERMATOMIOSITE

CONSIDERAÇÕES GERAIS

DEFINIÇÃO
Trata-se de uma doença inflamatória hereditária da pele, dos músculos e da vasculatura, que se desenvolve em cães jovens das raças Collie, Pastor de Shetland e seus cruzamentos aparentados.

FISIOPATOLOGIA
• Não se conhece a patogenia exata da dermatomiosite.
• Há relatos de predisposição familiar em Collie e Pastor de Shetland; no entanto, os possíveis deflagradores dessa doença incluem agentes infecciosos (especialmente virais), vacinas e outros medicamentos, assim como é observado em casos de dermatopatia isquêmica em outras raças.
• Com base em evidências clínicas e histopatológicas, é possível o envolvimento de um processo imunomediado ou autoimune.

SISTEMA(S) ACOMETIDO(S)
• Cutâneo/exócrino.
• Musculosquelético.

GENÉTICA
Herança autossômica dominante, com expressão variável em cães das raças Collie e Pastor de Shetland.

INCIDÊNCIA/PREVALÊNCIA
Não se conhece a prevalência exata.

DISTRIBUIÇÃO GEOGRÁFICA
N/D.

IDENTIFICAÇÃO
Espécies
Cães.

Raça(s) Predominante(s)
• Doença hereditária em Collie, Pastor de Shetland e seus cruzamentos.
• Sintomas semelhantes relatados em outras raças, como Pastor de Beauceron, Welsh corgi, Lakeland terrier, Chow chow, Pastor alemão, Schipperke e Kuvasz.
• Alguns animais em outras raças com sinais clínicos similares são, atualmente, classificados como sofrendo de dermatopatia isquêmica (semelhante à dermatomiosite) e não dermatomiosite conforme descrição prévia.

Idade Média e Faixa Etária
• As lesões cutâneas tipicamente se desenvolvem antes dos 6 meses de vida do cão, mas podem aparecer já com 7 semanas de vida.
• A plenitude das lesões costuma estar presente por volta de 1 ano de idade, mas podem diminuir depois disso.
• Apesar de rara, pode ocorrer dermatomiosite de início no adulto.

Sexo Predominante
Nenhum relatado.

SINAIS CLÍNICOS
Comentários Gerais
Os sinais clínicos variam desde lesões cutâneas sutis e miosite subclínica até lesões cutâneas graves com atrofia muscular generalizada, anormalidade da marcha e megaesôfago.

Achados Anamnésicos
• Aumento e declínio de lesões cutâneas em torno da face, da extremidade da cauda e das proeminências ósseas, bem como ao redor dos olhos, lábios e pavilhões auriculares — observadas geralmente em cães acometidos com <6 meses de vida.
• Formação de cicatriz — constitui frequentemente uma sequela das lesões cutâneas iniciais.
• Atrofia dos músculos masseteres e temporais — pode ficar evidente.
• Os cães mais gravemente acometidos podem apresentar dificuldade de comer, beber e deglutir.
• Marcha rígida ou de passo elevado.
• Várias ninhadas podem ser acometidas, mas a gravidade da doença varia frequentemente de forma significativa entre os cães envolvidos.

Achados do Exame Físico
• Lesões cutâneas — caracterizadas por graus variáveis de erosões crostosas, úlceras e alopecia, com eritema, descamação e formação cicatricial na face, em torno dos lábios e dos olhos, na face interna do pavilhão auricular e na extremidade da cauda; toda a face pode estar envolvida.
• Os pontos de pressão e as áreas expostas da pele sobre proeminências ósseas costumam ser acometidos em primeiro lugar.
• Podem ocorrer úlceras nos coxins palmoplantares e na boca, bem como anormalidades ou perdas ungueais.
• Miosite — os sinais podem estar ausentes ou variam desde a diminuição sutil na massa dos músculos temporais até a atrofia muscular simétrica generalizada e marcha rígida ou de passo elevado.
• Os cães com megaesôfago podem se apresentar com pneumonia por aspiração.

CAUSAS
• Hereditárias em cães das raças Collie, Pastor de Shetland e seus cruzamentos.
• Agentes infecciosos ou medicamentos podem constituir um evento deflagrador.
• Doenças imunomediadas em outras raças.

FATORES DE RISCO
A compressão e o traumatismo mecânicos, bem como a exposição à luz ultravioleta, podem agravar as lesões cutâneas.

DIAGNÓSTICO

DIAGNÓSTICO DIFERENCIAL
• Demodicose.
• Dermatofitose.
• Foliculite bacteriana.
• Celulite juvenil.
• Lúpus eritematoso discoide.
• Lúpus eritematoso sistêmico.
• Polimiosite.
• Dermatopatia isquêmica.
• Epidermólise bolhosa simples.

HEMOGRAMA/BIOQUÍMICA/URINÁLISE
A creatina cinase sérica pode estar elevada em função do dano muscular.

OUTROS TESTES LABORATORIAIS
Títulos de anticorpo antinuclear — para descartar lúpus eritematoso sistêmico.

DIAGNÓSTICO POR IMAGEM
N/D.

MÉTODOS DIAGNÓSTICOS
• Biopsia cutânea — pode ser diagnóstica em casos de dermatomiosite, embora possa ser difícil a obtenção do diagnóstico definitivo dessa doença; evitar as lesões infectadas e cicatrizadas.
• Biopsia muscular — a seleção adequada do músculo pode não ser uma tarefa fácil, pois as alterações patológicas podem ser brandas.
• EMG — idealmente, esse método é empregado para selecionar os músculos acometidos à prática da biopsia; caso a EMG não esteja disponível, os músculos atrofiados deverão ser submetidos à biopsia.

ACHADOS PATOLÓGICOS
Biopsia Cutânea
• Apoptose ou vacuolização disseminadas de células basais individuais — observação possível; podem levar à formação de fendas intrabasais ou subepidérmicas.
• Leve incontinência pigmentar.
• Infiltrados celulares dérmicos e perivasculares superficiais, brandos e difusos — compostos por linfócitos, plasmócitos e histiócitos.
• Atrofia folicular e fibrose perifolicular são comuns.
• Ulceração epidérmica e formação cicatricial dérmica secundárias — podem estar presentes.
• As características histopatológicas podem ser sutis e consistem principalmente em alterações atróficas; no entanto, a combinação de degeneração celular epidérmica e folicular, inflamação perivascular e atrofia folicular com fibrose é altamente sugestiva de dermatomiosite.

Biopsia Muscular
• Acúmulos multifocais variáveis de células inflamatórias, incluindo linfócitos, plasmócitos, macrófagos e neutrófilos.
• Degeneração miofibrilar — caracterizada por fragmentação, vacuolização, atrofia, fibrose e regeneração.

Eletromiografia
Alterações eletromiográficas estão presentes nos músculos acometidos; os achados incluem potenciais de fibrilação, descargas bizarras de alta frequência e ondas pontiagudas positivas.

TRATAMENTO

CUIDADO(S) DE SAÚDE ADEQUADO(S)
• A maioria dos cães pode ser tratada em um esquema ambulatorial.
• Os cães com miosite e megaesôfago graves podem necessitar de internação para a provisão dos cuidados de suporte.
• Os casos graves talvez justifiquem a eutanásia.

CUIDADOS DE ENFERMAGEM
Auxiliar na alimentação se os músculos da mastigação estiverem envolvidos; alimentar o animal em uma posição elevada caso ocorra o desenvolvimento de megaesôfago.

ATIVIDADE
• Evitar atividades que possam traumatizar a pele.
• Manter os animais dentro de casa durante o dia para evitar a exposição à luz solar intensa.

DIETA
N/D.

ORIENTAÇÃO AO PROPRIETÁRIO
• Discutir a natureza hereditária da doença.
• Mencionar que os cães acometidos não devem ser acasalados.

DERMATOMIOSITE

- Informar o proprietário sobre o caráter incurável da doença, embora possa ocorrer resolução espontânea ou aumento e declínio dos sintomas.
- Debater o prognóstico e as possíveis complicações, particularmente em relação aos cães com acometimento grave.

MEDICAÇÕES

MEDICAMENTO(S) DE ESCOLHA
- A terapia sintomática inespecífica inclui a aplicação de banhos com xampu hipoalergênico, o tratamento de foliculite bacteriana e demodicose secundárias, bem como a prevenção de traumatismo e da exposição à luz solar.
- Vitamina E — 200-400 UI VO a cada 12-24 h.
- Suplementação com ácidos graxos essenciais.
- Prednisona — 1-2 mg/kg VO a cada 12-24 h até a remissão, com administração subsequente em dias alternados até duas vezes por semana, utilizando a dose mais baixa possível para o controle a longo prazo.
- Medicamento anti-inflamatório não esteroide.
- Pentoxifilina — 10 mg/kg a cada 8-12 h.
- Pode ser difícil avaliar a eficácia terapêutica do tratamento clínico, pois a doença tende a ser de natureza cíclica e é frequentemente autolimitante.

CONTRAINDICAÇÕES
O uso da pentoxifilina não é recomendável em cães sensíveis aos derivados metilxantínicos.

PRECAUÇÕES
- Pentoxifilina — raramente causa irritação gástrica; pode afetar os tempos de coagulação (prolongamento do TP/TTPA e trombocitopenia); os cães submetidos à terapia anticoagulante devem ser monitorizados com rigor quando tratados com esse medicamento; possíveis, mas raras crises convulsivas ou redução do limiar convulsivo em epilépticos.
- Glicocorticoides — debater os possíveis efeitos colaterais com o proprietário.

INTERAÇÕES POSSÍVEIS
Os glicocorticoides e anti-inflamatórios não esteroides combinados podem causar sangramento GI.

MEDICAMENTO(S) ALTERNATIVO(S)
N/D.

ACOMPANHAMENTO

MONITORIZAÇÃO DO PACIENTE
N/D.

PREVENÇÃO
- Não acasalar os animais acometidos.
- Castrar os animais intactos para reduzir a influência hormonal sobre os sintomas.
- Minimizar o traumatismo e a exposição à luz solar.

COMPLICAÇÕES POSSÍVEIS
- Foliculite bacteriana e demodicose secundárias.
- Os cães acometidos de forma leve a moderada podem exibir formação cicatricial residual.
- Os cães gravemente acometidos poderão ter problemas na mastigação, na ingestão de líquidos e na deglutição se os músculos mastigatórios e esofágicos estiverem envolvidos.
- O desenvolvimento de megaesôfago é possível, predispondo o cão à pneumonia por aspiração.

EVOLUÇÃO ESPERADA E PROGNÓSTICO
- Prognóstico a longo prazo — variável, dependendo da gravidade da doença.
- Doença mínima — prognóstico bom; tende a apresentar resolução espontânea, sem nenhuma evidência de cicatrizes.
- Doença leve a moderada — também tende a desaparecer espontaneamente, mas a formação cicatricial residual é comum.
- Doença grave — prognóstico mau quanto à sobrevida a longo prazo, pois a dermatite e a miosite podem ser vitalícias.

DIVERSOS

DISTÚRBIOS ASSOCIADOS
Lúpus eritematoso cutâneo vesicular de cães das raças Pastor de Shetland e Collie — doença pouco compreendida; descrita em cães adultos das raças mencionadas; caracterizada por úlceras serpiginosas bem delimitadas nas áreas intertriginosas das regiões inguinal e axilar; pode ocorrer de forma isolada ou em associação com dermatomiosite; pode representar um subgrupo de dermatomiosite.

FATORES RELACIONADOS COM A IDADE
- Os sinais clínicos iniciais costumam ocorrer em cães com <6 meses de vida.
- Início na idade adulta — raro; observado mais comumente em cães que tiveram lesões sutis quando filhotes.

POTENCIAL ZOONÓTICO
Nenhum.

GESTAÇÃO/FERTILIDADE/REPRODUÇÃO
- Não acasalar os cães acometidos.
- A prenhez e o estro podem exacerbar os sintomas clínicos.

SINÔNIMO(S)
- Dermatomiosite canina familiar.
- Dermatomiosite familiar canina.
- Dermatopatia isquêmica em cães das raças Collie e Pastor de Shetland.

VER TAMBÉM
- Lúpus Eritematoso Cutâneo (Discoide).
- Lúpus Eritematoso Sistêmico.

ABREVIATURA(S)
- EMG = eletromiografia.
- GI = gastrintestinal.
- TP = tempo de protrombina.
- TPPA = tempo de tromboplastina parcial.

Sugestões de Leitura
Carlotti DN, Grucker S, Germain PA. Dermatomyositis in a four month old schipperke. Pratique Medicale a Chirurgicale de l'Animal de Compagnie 2005, 40(3):141-144.
Gross TL, Ihrike PJ, Walder EJ, Affolter VK. Skin Diseases of the Dog and Cat, 2nd ed. Oxford: Blackwell Science, 2005, pp. 49-52, 503-505.
Hargis AM, Mundell AC. Familial canine dermatomyositis. Compend Contin Educ Pract Vet 1992, 14:855-864.
Scott DW, Miller WH, Griffin CE. Muller & Kirk's Small Animal Dermatology, 6th ed. Philadelphia: Saunders, 2001, pp. 940-946.
Wahl JM, Clark LA, Skalli O, Ambrus A, Rees CA, Mansell JL, Murphy KE. Analysis of gene transcript profiling and immunobiology in Shetland sheepdog with dermatomyositis. Vet Dermatol 2008, 19(2):52-58.

Autores Liora Waldman e Alexander H. Werner
Consultor Editorial Alexander H. Werner

Dermatoses e Distúrbios Despigmentantes

CONSIDERAÇÕES GERAIS

DEFINIÇÃO
• Distúrbios patológicos ou estéticos que envolvem a despigmentação da pele e/ou da pelagem por falta de pigmentação ou dano aos melanócitos.
• Leucotriquia — branqueamento do pelo (localização inespecífica).
• Poliose — branqueamento do pelo sobre a cabeça e a face.
• Leucodermia — branqueamento da pele.

FISIOPATOLOGIA
• Depende da causa.
• Os melanócitos podem ser lesionados ou destruídos por toxinas (incluindo precursores tóxicos da melanina), mediadores inflamatórios, autoanticorpos e/ou inibidores de melanogênese.

SISTEMA(S) ACOMETIDO(S)
• Cutâneo/exócrino.
• Oftálmico.

DISTRIBUIÇÃO GEOGRÁFICA
O lúpus eritematoso discoide e o pênfigo eritematoso são mais comuns em regiões com exposições mais elevadas à luz ultravioleta.

IDENTIFICAÇÃO
• Piodermite mucocutânea — Pastor alemão.
• LES e LED — Collie, Pastor de Shetland, Pastor alemão.
• LED — pode ocorrer com maior frequência em fêmeas.
• Pênfigo foliáceo — Chow chow, Akita.
• Síndrome uveodermatológica — Akita, Samoieda, Husky siberiano.
• Vitiligo — cães: Tervuren Belga, Pastor alemão, Doberman pinscher, Rottweiler, Pointer alemão de pelo curto, Old English sheepdog e Dachshund; geralmente com <3 anos de idade.
• Vitiligo — gatos: Siamês.
• Hipopigmentação nasal sazonal — Husky siberiano, Malamute do Alasca, Labrador retriever amarelo e Golden retriever.
• Linfoma epiteliotrópico (micose fungoide) — tipicamente cães com >10 anos de idade.
• Arterite proliferativa do filtro nasal — São Bernardo, Schnauzer gigante.
• Leucotriquia maculosa.
• Leucotriquia periocular — gatos da raça Siamês.
• Síndrome de Chediak-Higashi — gatos da raça Persa.

SINAIS CLÍNICOS
• Leucotriquia.
• Leucodermia.
• Atenuação da pigmentação da pele (observado com frequência como uma mudança de coloração para "grisalho" ou "castanho" de áreas previamente pigmentadas).
• Eritema.
• Erosão e ulcerações.

CAUSAS
• Piodermite mucocutânea.
• LED.
• LES.
• Pênfigo foliáceo.
• Pênfigo eritematoso.
• Síndrome uveodermatológica.
• Hipersensibilidade por contato.
• Vitiligo.
• Despigmentação nasal sazonal.
• Albinismo.
• Síndrome do Schnauzer dourado.
• Reação medicamentosa.
• Eritema multiforme.
• Arterite proliferativa do filtro nasal.
• Despigmentação pós-inflamatória.
• Incontinência pigmentar imunomediada.

FATORES DE RISCO
• Exposição ao sol — LED, LES, pênfigo eritematoso.

DIAGNÓSTICO

DIAGNÓSTICO DIFERENCIAL

Piodermite Mucocutânea
• Lesões cutâneas — afeta os lábios, a área peribucal e as pregas nasais/alares.
• Semelhante do ponto de vista clínico ao intertrigo (foliculite bacteriana das dobras cutâneas).
• A formação de tumefação e fissura leva a erosões e crostas.
• Com a cronicidade, ocorre o desenvolvimento de despigmentação.
• Biopsia — hiperplasia epidérmica com formação de pústulas superficiais.
• Quadro bastante responsivo a antibióticos.
• A recidiva será frequente se o quadro for atribuído a alguma causa subjacente.

Dermatite Solar Nasal
• Lesões confinadas à região dorsal do focinho e precipitadas por exposição à luz solar intensa.
• Não constitui um distúrbio despigmentante primário.
• Começa na pele pouco pigmentada, na junção do plano nasal e da região dorsal do focinho.
• A despigmentação pode ser uma sequela de inflamação causada por radiação actínica*.
• Negativa quanto à imunofluorescência direta.
• Uma vasculopatia solar pode parecer semelhante.

LED
• Acomete principalmente a região nasal, bem como as margens palpebrais e labiais.
• Exacerbado pela radiação actínica.
• Imunofluorescência direta positiva na zona da membrana basal.
• Biopsia — dermatite de interface.
• Predileção racial — Coolie, Pastor de Shetland, Pastor alemão, Husky siberiano.

LES
• Doença multissistêmica.
• Lesões cutâneas — frequentemente envolvem o nariz, a face e as junções mucocutâneas; multifocais ou generalizadas.
• AAN — positivo.
• Imunofluorescência direta positiva na zona da membrana basal.

Pênfigo Foliáceo
• Lesões — em geral, iniciam-se na face e nas orelhas; costumam envolver os coxins palmoplantares; por fim, acabam se generalizando.
• Ocorre despigmentação secundariamente à inflamação.
• Biopsia — pústulas subcorneais com acantólise.

---
* N. T.: Diz-se das radiações que provocam uma ação química (raios ultravioletas). A luz solar é um tipo de radiação actínica.

• Imunofluorescência direta positiva nos espaços intercelulares da epiderme.

Pênfigo Eritematoso
• Lesões — confinadas principalmente a regiões como face, orelhas, plano nasal e margens labiais.
• A despigmentação é mais notável do que no pênfigo foliáceo e frequentemente precede lesões significativas.
• Exacerbado por radiação actínica.
• Biopsia — pústulas intraepidérmicas com acantólise e dermatite de interface.
• Imunofluorescência direta positiva na zona da membrana basal e nos espaços intercelulares.
• AAN — ocasionalmente positivo.

Síndrome Uveodermatológica
• Acomete raças típicas: Akita, Samoieda, Chow chow, Husky siberiano.
• Uveíte constitui o sintoma mais significativo; muitas vezes, mas nem sempre, antecede a doença dermatológica.
• Despigmentação macular cutânea com inflamação no nariz, nos lábios e nas pálpebras.
• Poliose e leucotriquia notáveis.
• Biopsia de lesões precoces — dermatite de interface, incontinência pigmentar.

Outros
• Dermatite de contato por comedouro/brinquedo de plástico ou borracha (muito rara) — despigmentação e eritema do plano nasal rostral e dos lábios; ausência de ulceração e formação mínima de crostas; histórico de exposição.
• Vitiligo — despigmentação macular cutânea sem inflamação no nariz, nos lábios, nas pálpebras, nos coxins palmoplantares e nas unhas; a leucotriquia pode estar presente em casos de leucodermia.
• Hipopigmentação nasal sazonal — a coloração escura normal do plano nasal desbota gradativamente para castanho-claro ou rosa; costuma ser sazonal ou lentamente progressiva com o avanço da idade.
• Albinismo — falta hereditária de pigmento na pele, na pelagem e na íris (não constitui um processo despigmentante).
• Síndrome do Schnauzer dourado — os cães jovens da raça Schnauzer miniatura podem desenvolver uma coloração dourada idiopática da pelagem, principalmente no tronco.
• Endocrinopatia pode causar alteração na cor da pelagem, principalmente de negra a castanho-avermelhada.
• Reação medicamentosa — pode se assemelhar a vários distúrbios cutâneos, como LED, LES, pênfigo foliáceo e pênfigo eritematoso; o prurido é variável; o início dos sinais clínicos costuma ocorrer dentro de 2 semanas após a administração do medicamento.
• Arterite proliferativa do filtro nasal — ulceração focal acentuada do plano nasal que, frequentemente, resulta em hemorragia aguda e grave. Não se observam lesões cutâneas adicionais. Esse quadro pode se tratar de uma síndrome idiopática associada à alergia.
• Despigmentação pós-inflamatória — uma perda benigna de pigmento, que deverá se resolver quando a causa da inflamação for tratada.
• Dermatofitose — pode ocorrer despigmentação como resultado de inflamação na porção dorsal do focinho e na face. Também pode ocorrer hiperpigmentação, especialmente em casos de infecção por *Trichophyton mentagrophytes*.

Dermatoses e Distúrbios Despigmentantes

- Linfoma epiteliotrópico — ocorre despigmentação em áreas mucocutâneas, nariz e pele.
- Eritema multiforme em cães — lesões anulares clássicas com um centro claro; a despigmentação é com maior frequência secundária à inflamação.
- Deficiência de zinco — esse elemento é necessário para a síntese normal de melanina.
- Síndrome de Chediak-Higashi — gatos jovens da raça Persa (coloração azul esfumaçada); sinais oftalmológicos e sangramento prolongado.
- Neutropenia cíclica em cães jovens da raça Collie de pelagem cinza-prateada com nariz de cor clara.

HEMOGRAMA/BIOQUÍMICA/URINÁLISE
- Em geral, permanecem normais.
- LES — podem-se observar anemia hemolítica, trombocitopenia ou indícios de glomerulonefrite.
- Anormalidades hematológicas em gatos da raça Persa acometidos pela síndrome de Chediak-Higashi.
- Neutropenia cíclica em cães da raça Collie (anomalias hematopoiéticas cíclicas).

OUTROS TESTES LABORATORIAIS
Cultura para dermatófitos.

MÉTODOS DIAGNÓSTICOS
- Citologia — células acantolíticas (pênfigo), linfócitos neoplásicos (linfoma epiteliotrópico).
- Punção articular — indícios de poliartrite em casos de LES.
- AAN — positivo em grande parte dos casos de LES.
- Exame oftalmológico — uveíte em casos de síndrome uveodermatológica.
- Imunofluorescência direta — depósito de imunoglobulinas na zona da membrana basal em casos de LED, LES e pênfigo eritematoso, bem como nos espaços intercelulares da epiderme em casos de pênfigos foliáceo e eritematoso.
- Biopsia cutânea.

ACHADOS PATOLÓGICOS
- Dermatite de interface — LED, LES, síndrome uveodermatológica.
- Incontinência pigmentar — LED, pênfigo eritematoso.
- Pústulas intraepidérmicas com acantólise — pênfigos foliáceo e eritematoso.
- Hipomelanose — vitiligo, síndrome uveodermatológica, hipopigmentação nasal sazonal e síndrome do Schnauzer dourado.
- Apoptose (necrose celular individual de queratinócitos) — reação medicamentosa e eritema multiforme.
- Proliferação de células fusiformes de artérias e arteríolas dérmicas — arterite proliferativa.

- Infiltração de linfócitos neoplásicos — linfoma epiteliotrópico.

TRATAMENTO

- Efetuado em um esquema ambulatorial, exceto em casos de LES, eritema multiforme e linfoma cutâneo, na presença de uma grave disfunção em múltiplos órgãos.
- Diminuir a exposição à luz solar — LED, LES e pênfigo eritematoso.
- Evitar o contato com medicamentos tópicos.
- Substituir os comedouros de plástico ou de borracha — particularmente aqueles de bordas ásperas que provocam abrasões.
- Aplicar pomadas ou géis resistentes à água com fator de proteção solar (FPS) >30 sobre as áreas despigmentadas.
- Utilizar antibióticos adequados nos casos de piodermite.
- Empregar antifúngicos apropriados para dermatofitose.

MEDICAÇÕES

MEDICAMENTO(S) DE ESCOLHA
- LES — terapia imunossupressora com prednisolona ou dexametasona e azatioprina (cães) ou clorambucila (gatos).
- Tetraciclina e niacinamida (cães <10 kg 250 mg a cada 8 h; >10 kg, 500 mg a cada 8 h): pênfigo eritematoso, LED.
- Corticosteroides tópicos — pênfigo eritematoso, LED.
- Vitiligo e despigmentação nasal — não há nenhum tratamento.
- Linfoma epiteliotrópico — existem muitos protocolos de manutenção.

CONTRAINDICAÇÕES
Terapia com a azatioprina — não é recomendada em gatos; pode causar leucopenia ou trombocitopenia fatais.

PRECAUÇÕES
Cetoconazol — pode causar clareamento da pelagem, elevação da fosfatase alcalina e desarranjo gastrintestinal.

MEDICAMENTO(S) ALTERNATIVO(S)
- Ciclosporina modificada — 5 mg/kg/dia para distúrbios autoimunes.

- Tacrolimo — aplicação diária sob a forma de gel a 0,1% nas lesões em combinação com corticosteroides ou como substitutos desses agentes.
- Pimecrolimo — aplicação diária sob a forma de creme a 1% nas lesões em combinação com corticosteroides ou como substitutos desses agentes.
- Imiquimode a 5% — aplicação sob a forma de creme a cada 1-2 dias para queratose actínica.

ACOMPANHAMENTO

MONITORIZAÇÃO DO PACIENTE
Varia com a doença específica e o tratamento prescrito.

COMPLICAÇÕES POSSÍVEIS
- Carcinoma de células escamosas — em casos de dano solar e queratose actínica de áreas despigmentadas.
- LES — formação cicatricial associada em casos de dermatite ulcerativa.

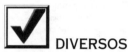

DIVERSOS

POTENCIAL ZOONÓTICO
Dermatofitose — pode causar infecção em seres humanos.

VER TAMBÉM
- Erupções Medicamentosas Cutâneas.
- Lúpus Eritematoso Cutâneo (Discoide).
- Lúpus Eritematoso Sistêmico.
- Linfoma Cutâneo Epiteliotrópico.
- Pênfigo.
- Síndrome Uveodermatológica.

ABREVIATURA(S)
- AAN = anticorpo antinuclear.
- LED = lúpus eritematoso discoide.
- LES = lúpus eritematoso sistêmico.

Sugestões de Leitura
Hill PB. Small Animal Dermatology. Oxford: Butterworth-Heinemann, 2002.
Medleau L, Hnilica KA. Small Animal Dermatology: A Color Atlas and Therapeutic Guide, 2nd ed. St. Louis: Saunders, 2006.

Autores Guillermina Manigot e Alexander H. Werner
Consultor Editorial Alexander H. Werner

Dermatoses Erosivas ou Ulcerativas

CONSIDERAÇÕES GERAIS

DEFINIÇÃO
Correspondem a um grupo heterogêneo de distúrbios cutâneos caracterizados por descontinuidade da epiderme (erosões) ou, se a membrana basal estiver comprometida, da epiderme e da derme (úlceras).

FISIOPATOLOGIA
Varia amplamente, dependendo da causa; pode incluir distúrbios congênitos ou evolutivos, que comprometem a coesão tecidual; lesão mediada por células (inflamatórias ou neoplásicas); lesão anóxica; distúrbios autoimunes antígeno-específicos que rompem a coesão tecidual; e necrose atribuída a traumatismo, toxinas, contactantes (irritantes), microrganismos ou migração parasitária.

SISTEMA(S) ACOMETIDO(S)
Cutâneo/exócrino.

GENÉTICA
Algumas doenças provavelmente são hereditárias em virtude das predileções raciais; no entanto, não há testes genéticos de triagem disponíveis para qualquer uma das doenças listadas.

INCIDÊNCIA/PREVALÊNCIA
• Algumas doenças, como distúrbios bolhosos autoimunes, são extremamente raras. • Outras como demodicose, alergia à picada de pulga e piodermite estafilocócica em cães são comuns.

IDENTIFICAÇÃO
Espécies
Cães e gatos.

Raça(s) Predominante(s)
Algumas causas específicas (ver adiante) apresentam fortes predileções raciais, p. ex., distúrbios lupoides, dermatomiosite familiar e dermatose responsiva ao zinco.

Idade Média e Faixa Etária
• Altamente variáveis de acordo com a etiologia. • Celulite juvenil canina e várias doenças congênitas (ver adiante) são diagnosticadas em animais muito jovens.

Sexo Predominante
As predisposições sexuais podem variar de acordo com a doença em questão.

SINAIS CLÍNICOS
Achados Anamnésicos
• Histórico de prurido que pode resultar em úlceras ou erosões em virtude do autotraumatismo. Isso é especialmente relevante em casos de ectoparasitismo, piodermite superficial e dermatite por *Malassezia*. • Histórico de exposição a substâncias químicas cáusticas, queimaduras, estresse por frio, répteis e insetos venenosos, etc. • Algumas doenças infecciosas (p. ex., pitiose, coccidioidomicose, cowpox felino) apresentam variações muito restritas. • Histórico de doenças ou sintomas sistêmicos prévios ou concomitantes.

Achados do Exame Físico
• A manifestação das lesões pode ser heterogênea em termos macroscópicos. Algumas doenças resultam em erosões eritematosas com formação mínima de crostas ou escamas, enquanto outras provocam formação de crostas ou escamas com consequente erosão quando removidas. • As úlceras podem ser superficiais/rasas ou profundas. A ulceração profunda pode se apresentar sob a forma de trajetos sinusais drenantes, lesões cavitárias com bordas bem-delimitadas ou lesões crostosas exsudativas. • Algumas doenças específicas são tipicamente acompanhadas por febre e mal-estar, sobretudo distúrbios autoimunes e algumas etiologias infecciosas. • Outros achados podem estar associados à doença extracutânea (p. ex., dermatite necrolítica superficial e síndrome hipereosinofílica de gatos).

CAUSAS
Autoimunes
• Pênfigo foliáceo: formação de crostas com erosão. • Pênfigo vulgar: dermatose ulcerativa superficial. • Penfigoide bolhoso: dermatose ulcerativa superficial. • Lúpus eritematoso discoide: dermatose ulcerativa superficial ou erosiva. • Lúpus esfoliativo (Pointer alemão de pelo curto): formação de escamas com erosão. • Lúpus vesicular (Collie de pelo duro e Pastor de Shetland): dermatose ulcerativa superficial. • Doença da aglutinina fria: dermatose ulcerativa profunda.

Imunomediadas
• Eritema multiforme e necrólise epidérmica tóxica (geralmente induzidos por medicamentos): dermatose erosiva a ulcerativa superficial. • Vasculite: dermatose ulcerativa superficial a profunda (pode ser cavitária). • Paniculite idiopática: dermatose ulcerativa profunda (geralmente exsudativa com formação de crostas). • Furunculose eosinofílica canina da face (pode estar relacionada com insetos): dermatose ulcerativa com formação de crostas. • Celulite juvenil canina (piodermite de filhotes caninos): dermatose erosiva a ulcerativa superficial ou profunda. • Úlcera indolente felina (também conhecida como "úlcera do roedor"): dermatose erosiva a ulcerativa superficial ou profunda.

Infecciosas
• Piodermite superficial: dermatite piotraumática úmida aguda (também conhecida como *hot spots* ou manchas quentes): dermatose erosiva. • Foliculite estafilocócica superficial: dermatose erosiva a ulcerativa superficial. • Foliculite/furunculose bacterianas profundas: dermatose ulcerativa profunda (geralmente com formação de crostas, com ou sem trajetos sinusais e drenantes). • Micoses superficiais (dermatite por *Malassezia*, dermatofitose): dermatose erosiva a ulcerativa superficial. • Micoses profundas (p. ex., esporotricose, criptococose, histoplasmose, blastomicose, coccidioidomicose): dermatose ulcerativa profunda com ou seu trajetos sinusais e drenantes. • Micobacteriose oportunista: nódulos ulcerativos profundos com trajetos sinusais e drenantes. • Bactérias actinomicetas (p. ex., *Nocardia* spp., *Actinomyces* spp., *Streptomyces* spp.): nódulos ulcerativos profundos com trajetos sinusais e drenantes. • Pitiose/lagenidiose e prototecose: dermatose ulcerativa e proliferativa com ou sem trajetos drenantes. • Leishmaniose: dermatose erosiva a ulcerativa superficial ou profunda. • Cowpox felino: dermatose ulcerativa profunda. • Relacionadas com FIV/FeLV: dermatose erosiva a ulcerativa superficial. • Associadas ao herpes-vírus felino: dermatose ulcerativa com formação de crostas.

Parasitárias
• Demodicose: dermatose ulcerativa com formação de crostas (especialmente com foliculite bacteriana secundária). • Sarnas sarcóptica/notoédrica: dermatose erosiva ± formação de crostas. • Alergia à picada de pulga: dermatose erosiva a ulcerativa (na presença de infecção secundária). • Hipersensibilidade felina à picada de mosquito: dermatose erosiva a ulcerativa superficial ou profunda. • Migração de *Pelodera* e ancilóstomo: dermatose ulcerativa profunda.

Congênitas/Hereditárias
• Dermatomiosite familiar canina (predominantemente em cães da raça Collie e Pastor de Shetland): dermatose erosiva. • Epidermólise bolhosa juncional: dermatose ulcerativa superficial. • Astenia cutânea (síndrome de Ehlers-Danlos): dermatose ulcerativa profunda (lacerações cutâneas). • Aplasia cutânea (epiteliogênese imperfeita): dermatose ulcerativa profunda (geralmente fatal ao nascimento).

Metabólicas
• Dermatite necrolítica superficial (associada, em geral, a hepatopatia ou glucagonoma): formação de crostas com erosão. • Hiperadrenocorticismo (dermatose erosiva a ulcerativa; quando complicado por infecções secundárias ou calcinose cutânea). • Uremia (mucosas): dermatose ulcerativa superficial.

Neoplásicas
• Carcinoma de células escamosas: dermatose erosiva a ulcerativa com formação de escamas ou crostas. • Carcinoma felino de células escamosas *in situ* (carcinoma bowenoide *in situ*): dermatose erosiva com formação de escamas ou crostas. • Mastocitomas: dermatose ulcerativa superficial a profunda. • Linfoma epiteliotrópico (micose fungoide): dermatose erosiva a ulcerativa superficial. • Dermatose esfoliativa associada a timoma felino: formação de escamas com erosão. • Alopecia paraneoplásica felina: dermatose erosiva.

Nutricionais
• Dermatose responsiva ao zinco: formação de crostas com erosão. • Dermatose alimentar canina genérica: formação de crostas com erosão.

Dermatoses Físicas/Conformacionais
• Úlceras em pontos de compressão: dermatose ulcerativa profunda. • Intertrigo (piodermite das dobras cutâneas): dermatose erosiva. • Autotraumatismo, como resultado de dermatoses pruriginosas: altamente variável.

Idiopáticas
• Úlcera cervical dorsal felina: dermatose ulcerativa profunda. • Acnes canina e felina: dermatose erosiva a ulcerativa com formação de crostas. • Pododermatite plasmocitária felina: dermatose ulcerativa superficial a profunda.

Diversas
• Queimaduras térmicas, elétricas, solares ou químicas: a profundidade das lesões depende da gravidade do insulto. • Crioulceração: a profundidade das lesões depende da gravidade do insulto. • Substâncias químicas irritantes: a profundidade das lesões depende da gravidade do insulto. • Picadas de cobras e insetos venenosos: dermatose ulcerativa profunda (geralmente com necrose evidente).

FATORES DE RISCO
Altamente variável de acordo com a doença (p. ex., imunossupressão subjacente associada a doenças infecciosas secundárias).

Dermatoses Erosivas ou Ulcerativas

DIAGNÓSTICO

DIAGNÓSTICO DIFERENCIAL
Anamnese e exame físico são particularmente importantes em função da extensa lista de diagnósticos diferenciais. Muitas dessas doenças apresentam diferenças sutis em termos de aspecto e distribuição das lesões. Uma atenção especial à natureza e evolução das lesões, bem como ao padrão de distribuição no paciente, pode dar indícios valiosos.

HEMOGRAMA/BIOQUÍMICA/URINÁLISE
Muito úteis na suspeita de doença metabólica ou em qualquer paciente com sinais clínicos de doença sistêmica.

OUTROS TESTES LABORATORIAIS
Ver a seção "Métodos Diagnósticos" (adiante) em busca dos testes de rotina.

DIAGNÓSTICO POR IMAGEM
- Raramente é indicado.
- Radiografias torácicas — em casos de micoses profundas/sistêmicas e neoplasia sistêmica.
- Ultrassonografia abdominal — dermatite necrolítica superficial (cães) ou alopecia paraneoplásica (gatos) sob suspeita ou confirmados por meio de biopsia cutânea.

MÉTODOS DIAGNÓSTICOS
- Raspados cutâneos — na suspeita de parasitismo.
- Citologia por impressão/decalque direto — identifica as células acantolíticas em casos de pênfigo, além de identificar bactérias e leveduras.
- Aspirado por agulha fina com citologia — para lesões endurecidas ou nodulares.
- Culturas bacterianas (aeróbias e anaeróbias), micobacterianas e/ou fúngicas — na suspeita de doença infecciosa (especialmente em gatos com úlceras ou trajetos drenantes).
- Sorologia para fungos, bem como para pitiose e lagenidiose — pode ser indicada caso a caso, dependendo da localização geográfica.
- PCR e imuno-histoquímica — são técnicas adjuvantes para o diagnóstico histológico de dermatite associada ao herpes-vírus felino.

ACHADOS PATOLÓGICOS
- Biopsia cutânea para histopatologia — teste mais informativo.
- Em casos de lesões cavitárias, deve-se coletar a margem principal com o auxílio de uma lâmina de bisturi se o defeito for amplo demais para ser submetido à excisão total.
- A biopsia com saca-bocado (também conhecido como *punch*) é suficiente em lesões erosivas difusas; deve-se obter a pele normal próxima à lesão, além de lesões que estejam tanto no início como no final de seu desenvolvimento.

TRATAMENTO

CUIDADO(S) DE SAÚDE ADEQUADO(S)
- Ambulatorial na maior parte das doenças.
- Varia amplamente, de acordo com a causa.

CUIDADO(S) DE ENFERMAGEM
- Terapia de suporte.
- O controle da dor pode ser uma consideração importante para alguns animais.

ATIVIDADE
Não há necessidade de restrições em grande parte dos distúrbios (exceto em casos de infecções e infestações zoonóticas).

DIETA
- O suporte nutricional pode ser necessário em animais debilitados, especialmente aqueles com dermatite necrolítica superficial.
- A correção de deficiências nutricionais constitui o único tratamento para dermatose alimentar canina genérica.
- A suplementação de zinco é imprescindível em casos de dermatose responsiva a esse elemento.

ORIENTAÇÃO AO PROPRIETÁRIO
Variável por diagnóstico; mais relevante na suspeita ou mediante o diagnóstico de doença zoonótica.

CONSIDERAÇÕES CIRÚRGICAS
- A cirurgia é indicada como tratamento curativo para dermatite esfoliativa associada a timoma felino.
- A intervenção cirúrgica pode ser curativa para tumores pancreáticos ou hepatobiliares não metastáticos causadores de alopecia paraneoplásica.
- Excisão cirúrgica radical de nódulos e trajetos drenantes pode ser uma medida adjuvante à terapia antimicrobiana de infecções causadas por espécies de *Mycobacteria* e *Nocardia* de crescimento rápido em gatos, bem como de pitiose ou lagenidiose em cães.

MEDICAÇÕES

MEDICAMENTO(S) DE ESCOLHA
Variam amplamente, de acordo com a causa.

CONTRAINDICAÇÕES
O diagnóstico definitivo é imperativo, pois alguns casos imunomediados que necessitam de imunossupressão podem mimetizar doenças infecciosas que exigem quimioterapia antimicrobiana específica (e para as quais a imunossupressão poderia ser fatal).

PRECAUÇÕES
Efeitos colaterais — associados a muitos medicamentos antimicrobianos, imunossupressores e antineoplásicos.

INTERAÇÕES POSSÍVEIS
Dependem dos medicamentos administrados.

ACOMPANHAMENTO

MONITORIZAÇÃO DO PACIENTE
Depende do processo patológico, da(s) doença(s) sistêmica(s) concomitante(s), dos medicamentos utilizados e dos efeitos colaterais potenciais esperados.

PREVENÇÃO
- A incidência de muitas doenças infecciosas felinas pode ser minimizada, restringindo-se o acesso dos gatos à rua.
- Algumas doenças autoimunes (p. ex., lúpus eritematoso discoide e pênfigo eritematoso) são agravadas por exposição à luz ultravioleta; nesse caso, é recomendável a restrição da exposição à luz solar durante os horários de pico do dia.

COMPLICAÇÕES POSSÍVEIS
- Determinadas pela causa.
- Algumas doenças são potencialmente letais.
- Determinadas doenças apresentam potencial zoonótico.
- Em casos que necessitem de imunossupressão, é possível a ocorrência de superinfecções e efeitos colaterais medicamentosos.

EVOLUÇÃO ESPERADA E PROGNÓSTICO
- Certas doenças infecciosas (nocardiose, micobacteriose atípica) podem ser controladas com terapia antimicrobiana crônica, mas geralmente não serão passíveis de cura se a evolução da lesão for ampla no momento do diagnóstico.
- Pitiose/lagenidiose: o prognóstico é extremamente mau quanto à resposta à terapia e em termos de sobrevida.

DIVERSOS

POTENCIAL ZOONÓTICO
- Sarna sarcóptica.
- Dermatofitose.
- Esporotricose.
- A fase micelial de alguns fungos (p. ex., *Coccidioides immitis*, *Blastomyces dermatitidis*), quando cultivados em meios de cultura, pode ser contagiosa aos seres humanos via inalação. Não se aconselha a realização de culturas fúngicas no ambiente interno da clínica (exceto em casos de dermatófitos).

GESTAÇÃO/FERTILIDADE/REPRODUÇÃO
- Em função da gravidade potencial das síndromes e dos sinais clínicos, qualquer paciente diagnosticado com alguma doença erosiva/ulcerativa que ocorra com predileções raciais moderadas a intensas não deve ser utilizado para fins reprodutivos.
- Muitos medicamentos utilizados para o tratamento de doenças autoimunes, imunomediadas e infecciosas listadas podem ser teratogênicos.

SINÔNIMO(S)
Dermatite necrolítica superficial = eritema migratório necrolítico, necrose epidérmica metabólica, síndrome hepatocutânea.

VER TAMBÉM
Ver os capítulos específicos dedicados às doenças listadas na seção "Causas".

ABREVIATURA(S)
- FeLV = vírus da leucemia felina.
- FIV = vírus da imunodeficiência felina.
- PCR = reação em cadeia da polimerase.

Sugestões de Leitura
Mason IS. Erosions and ulcerations. In: Ettinger SJ, Feldman EC, eds., Textbook of Veterinary Internal Medicine, 6th ed. St. Louis: Elsevier, 2005, pp. 46-50.
Scott DW, Miller WH, Griffin CE. Muller & Kirk's Small Animal Dermatology, 6th ed. Philadelphia: Saunders, 2001.

Autor Daniel O. Morris
Consultor Editorial Alexander H. Werner

DERMATOSES ESFOLIATIVAS

CONSIDERAÇÕES GERAIS

DEFINIÇÃO
Liberação excessiva ou anormal de células epidérmicas, resultando na apresentação clínica de descamação cutânea.

FISIOPATOLOGIA
• O aumento na produção, o incremento na descamação ou a diminuição na coesão de queratinócitos resultam na liberação anormal de células epidérmicas individualmente (escamas finas) e em lâminas (escamas grossas).
• Distúrbios esfoliativos primários — defeitos de queratinização, nos quais o controle genético da proliferação e maturação das células epidérmicas se encontra anormal.
• Distúrbios esfoliativos secundários — decorrentes dos efeitos de estados patológicos sobre a maturação e a proliferação normais das células epidérmicas.

SISTEMA(S) ACOMETIDO(S)
Cutâneo/exócrino.

IDENTIFICAÇÃO
• Cães e gatos.
• Primárias — aparentes por volta dos 2 anos de idade; características nas raças acometidas (ver a seção "Causas").
• Secundárias — qualquer idade; qualquer raça canina ou felina.

SINAIS CLÍNICOS

Achados Anamnésicos
• Descamação excessiva.
• Pele de odor fétido.
• Prurido.
• Pele e pelagem oleosas.

Achados do Exame Físico
• Acúmulos secos ou oleosos de escamas finas ou blocos grosseiros de células epidérmicas localizadas de forma difusa por toda a pelagem ou focalmente em placas queratináceas.
• É comum o odor de "gordura rançosa".
• Comedões.
• Cilindros foliculares (acúmulo de debris aderentes em torno da haste pilosa).
• Depósitos sobre o pelo, semelhantes à cera de vela.
• Alopecia.
• Prurido.
• Foliculite bacteriana secundária.
• Dermatite secundária por *Malassezia*.

CAUSAS

Primárias
• Seborreia idiopática primária (distúrbio de queratinização primário) — defeito celular primário; epidermopoiese acelerada e hiperproliferação da epiderme, do infundíbulo folicular e da glândula sebácea, identificadas em algumas raças de maior risco: Cocker e Springer spaniels, West Highland white terrier, Basset hound, Doberman pinscher, Setter irlandês e Labrador retriever; existem duas formas (seca e oleosa), mas a determinação do tipo tem pouco valor prognóstico.
• Dermatose responsiva à vitamina A — nutricionalmente responsiva; observada sobretudo em cães jovens da raça Cocker spaniel; os sinais clínicos são semelhantes aos de uma seborreia idiopática grave; identificada por meio da resposta à suplementação oral dessa vitamina.
• Dermatose responsiva ao zinco — nutricionalmente responsiva; resulta em alopecia, descamação seca, formação de crosta e eritema em torno dos olhos, das orelhas, dos pés, dos lábios e de outros orifícios externos; há duas síndromes: cães jovens adultos (especialmente Husky siberiano e Malamute do Alasca) e filhotes caninos de raças de grande porte e de crescimento rápido.
• Defeitos ectodérmicos — displasias foliculares; observados como mutantes de cor ou alopecia por diluição; representam anormalidades na melanização da haste pilosa e no crescimento da estrutura pilosa; especulam-se os defeitos de queratinização como agentes causais de diversas síndromes; raças comumente acometidas: Doberman pinscher, Setter irlandês, Dachshund, Chow chow, Yorkshire terrier, Poodle, Dinamarquês, Whippet, Saluki e Galgo italiano de pelagem azul e castanho-amarelado; os sinais incluem a falha na repilação de pelo azul ou castanho-amarelado com crescimento de pelos "pontudos" normais, descamação excessiva, formação de comedões e piodermite secundária.
• Hiperqueratose nasodigital idiopática — acúmulo excessivo de escamas e crostas no plano nasal e nas margens dos coxins palmoplantares; possivelmente uma alteração senil, observada em cães das raças Spaniel e Labrador; as lesões costumam ser assintomáticas. A formação de rachaduras e a ocorrência de infecção bacteriana secundária podem causar dor intensa.
• Adenite sebácea — doença inflamatória que tem as glândulas e os ductos sebáceos como alvo. São observadas três síndromes específicas: (1) cães de meia-idade das raças Poodle standard e Samoieda: perda de pelo difusa ou irregular e descamação excessiva características; cilindros foliculares bem aderentes; em geral, a maioria dos cães permanece saudável e assintomática; (2) Akita: frequentemente desenvolvem piodermite bacteriana grave e profunda; (3) Vizla: a doença parece claramente distinta e granulomatosa. Outras raças revelam uma incidência mais baixa.
• Displasia epidérmica e ictiose — distúrbio de queratinização congênito raro e grave; descrito em West Highland white terrier e Golden retriever; acúmulos generalizados de escamas e crostas em uma idade precoce; infecções secundárias (por bactérias e leveduras) são comuns.
• Seborreia primária em filhotes felinos recém-nascidos da raça Persa.

Secundárias
• Hipersensibilidade cutânea — atopia, dermatite alérgica à pulga, alergia alimentar e dermatite de contato; prurido e consequente irritação e traumatismo cutâneos.
• Ectoparasitismo — escabiose, demodicose e queiletielose; inflamação e esfoliação.
• Foliculite bacteriana — desprendimento enzimático bacteriano e aumento na esfoliação de queratinócitos na tentativa de eliminar os microrganismos patogênicos.
• Dermatofitose — comumente esfoliativa; o aumento na liberação de queratinócitos acometidos constitui o principal mecanismo cutâneo na resolução de infecções fúngicas.
• Endocrinopatia — hipotireoidismo: anormalidades na queratinização, falha na repilação e produção demasiada de sebo; hiperadrenocorticismo: queratinização anormal e atividade folicular diminuída; a descamação excessiva e a piodermite secundária são comuns em ambas as síndromes; outras anormalidades hormonais (p. ex., distúrbios dos hormônios sexuais, hipertireoidismo e diabetes melito) também podem estar associadas ao excesso de descamação.
• Idade — os animais geriátricos podem apresentar a pelagem opaca, quebradiça e escamosa; essas mudanças podem ser causadas por alterações naturais no metabolismo epidérmico associadas à idade; ainda não se identificou nenhum defeito específico.
• Distúrbios nutricionais — desnutrição e dermatose alimentar canina genérica; resultam em descamação por anormalidades na queratinização.
• Dermatopatias autoimunes — complexo pênfigo: pode parecer esfoliativo; as vesículas tornam-se escamosas e crostosas; lúpus eritematoso cutâneo e sistêmico: os sinais cutâneos frequentemente aparecem como áreas de alopecia e descamação.
• Neoplasia — neoplasia epidérmica primária (linfoma epiteliotrópico): pode produzir alopecia e descamação à medida que as estruturas epidérmicas são lesionadas por infiltração de linfócitos; distúrbios pré-neoplásicos (queratose actínica): parecem esfoliativas no início.
• Diversas — qualquer processo patológico pode resultar em formação excessiva de escamas em função de discrasias metabólicas ou inflamações cutâneas.
• Distúrbios esfoliativos — raros em gatos: hiperplasia da glândula da cauda, dermatite esfoliativo associada a timoma.

DIAGNÓSTICO

DIAGNÓSTICO DIFERENCIAL
• Identificação e anamnese — fundamentais na distinção das possíveis causas de esfoliação.
• Presença de prurido — ajuda a determinar a possibilidade de hipersensibilidade cutânea; os defeitos primários de queratinização são frequentemente não pruriginosos, a menos que se desenvolvam quadros secundários de foliculite bacteriana ou dermatite por *Malassezia*.
• Sinais concomitantes (p. ex., letargia, ganho de peso, poliúria/polidipsia, falha reprodutiva, mudança na conformação corporal e ausência de repilação), com ou sem inflamação, podem auxiliar na diferenciação.

HEMOGRAMA/BIOQUÍMICA/URINÁLISE
• Normais — em casos de distúrbios primários de queratinização.
• Anemia arregenerativa leve e hipercolesterolemia — compatíveis com hipotireoidismo.
• Neutrofilia, monocitose, eosinopenia, linfopenia, fosfatase alcalina sérica elevada, hipercolesterolemia e hipostenúria — sugerem hiperadrenocorticismo.

OUTROS TESTES LABORATORIAIS
Na suspeita de alguma endocrinopatia, efetuar as provas de funções da tireoide (níveis dos hormônios tireoidianos) e adrenal; ver os capítulos específicos em relação às recomendações desses testes.

DIAGNÓSTICO POR IMAGEM
Radiografias torácicas — dermatite esfoliativa associada a timoma felino.

Dermatoses Esfoliativas

MÉTODOS DIAGNÓSTICOS
- Raspados cutâneos — diagnosticam ectoparasitismo.
- Biopsia cutânea — descarta diagnósticos diferenciais específicos; fortemente recomendada na maior parte dos casos.
- Teste alérgico intradérmico — identifica os casos de atopia.
- Tentativa de uma dieta de eliminação com base na restrição de ingrediente — identifica os casos de hipersensibilidade alimentar.
- Citologia da superfície cutânea — identifica as bactérias e/ou as leveduras na pele.
- Exame de pelos arrancados — macromelanossomos e anormalidades estruturais em casos de displasia folicular e alopecia por diluição da cor.

TRATAMENTO
- Terapia tópica frequente e apropriada — representa a base do tratamento adequado.
- Uma menor quantidade de banhos, em vez de uma maior quantidade, constitui um erro comum.
- Diagnosticar e controlar todas as doenças primárias e secundárias tratáveis.
- A recidiva de infecções secundárias pode exigir a repetição da terapia e outros testes diagnósticos.
- A manutenção do controle é frequentemente vitalícia.
- Há uma ênfase recente sobre a restauração da integridade e da função da barreira epidérmica.

MEDICAÇÕES
MEDICAMENTO(S) DE ESCOLHA
Xampus
- Tempo de contato — são necessários 5-15 min; não se incentiva um tempo >15 min, pois isso resulta em maceração e ressecamento/irritação excessivos da epiderme, bem como perda da função de barreira.
- Hipoalergênicos — úteis apenas em casos leves de descamação seca e na manutenção de esfoliação secundária após o controle da doença primária.
- Enxofre/ácido salicílico — queratolítico, queratoplástico e bacteriostático; constitui uma excelente escolha inicial para o paciente com descamação moderada; não provoca ressecamento excessivo.
- Peróxido de benzoíla — intensamente queratolítico, antimicrobiano e desobstruidor de folículos; pode causar irritação e ressecamento intenso; constitui a melhor opção em casos de infecção bacteriana recidivante e/ou oleosidade extrema.
- Lactato de etila — menos eficaz do que o peróxido de benzoíla em termos de lavagem folicular e atividade antimicrobiana, mas não tão irritante ou ressecante; muito útil em casos de foliculite bacteriana moderada e descamação seca.
- Clorexidina — antimicrobiano; leve ressecamento; útil para foliculite bacteriana moderada e dermatite por *Malassezia*.
- Alcatrão — queratolítico, queratoplástico e antipruriginoso; menos desengordurante que o peróxido de benzoíla; utilizado em casos de descamação moderada associada a prurido; pode ser irritante e carcinogênico; não se encontra amplamente disponível em formulações veterinárias.

Hidratantes
- Excelentes no restabelecimento da hidratação da pele (a aplicação frequente de xampus pode resultar em ressecamento e desconforto excessivos) e no aumento da eficácia de xampus subsequentes.
- Umectantes — acentuam a hidratação do estrato córneo pela atração de água a partir da derme; em altas concentrações, podem ser queratolíticos.
- Propilenoglicol sob a forma de *spray* (diluição de 50-70% em água) — aplicado com frequência.
- Microencapsulação — pode melhorar a atividade residual dos hidratantes por permitir a liberação contínua após o banho.
- Emolientes — protegem a pele; suavizam as superfícies ásperas produzidas pela descamação excessiva; em geral, são combinados com agentes oclusivos para estimular a hidratação da epiderme.

Terapia Sistêmica
- As causas específicas necessitam de tratamentos específicos (i. e., reposição da tireoxina em casos de hipotireoidismo; suplementos de zinco em casos de dermatose responsiva a esse elemento).
- Antibióticos sistêmicos — sempre são indicados contra piodermites secundárias.
- Agentes retinoides — sucesso variado em seborreia idiopática ou primária; há relatos de resposta individual a retinoides em casos refratários: isotretinoína (1 mg/kg VO a cada 12-24 h); se for observada uma resposta, reduzir a dose gradativamente (1 mg/kg a cada 48 h ou 0,5 mg/kg a cada 24 h). É difícil aviar os retinoides sintéticos em virtude de procedimentos de prescrição muito rigorosos.
- Ciclosporina — fornecer 5 mg/kg/dia até o controle do quadro, depois diminuir para uma dose mínima e eficaz de manutenção para os casos individuais de distúrbio de queratinização, associados à hipersensibilidade, adenite sebácea, displasia epidérmica, ictiose e/ou dermatite por *Malassezia*.
- Cetoconazol — 10 mg/kg/dia em casos de dermatite grave por *Malassezia*.

PRECAUÇÕES
- Corticosteroides — podem ser utilizados com critério para controlar a inflamação resultante de muitos distúrbios esfoliativos; tais agentes, no entanto, mascaram os sinais de piodermite e impedem o diagnóstico preciso da doença primária.
- Análogos das vitaminas A e D — como os efeitos colaterais podem ser graves, recomenda-se o encaminhamento dos pacientes a um dermatologista antes de tratá-los com esses agentes experimentais.

ACOMPANHAMENTO
MONITORIZAÇÃO DO PACIENTE
- Antibióticos e terapia tópica — monitorizar a resposta terapêutica a cada 3 semanas; os pacientes podem responder de forma diferenciada a várias terapias tópicas.
- Mudanças de estação, desenvolvimento de doenças extras (especialmente hipersensibilidade cutânea) e recidiva da piodermite — podem provocar o agravamento de pacientes previamente controlados; a reavaliação é crítica para determinar o envolvimento de novos fatores de risco e a necessidade de alterações na terapia.
- Endocrinopatias — após a administração de pílulas, é recomendável a monitorização de rotina de função da tireoide por 4-6 h ou a realização dos testes de estimulação com ACTH para a obtenção de tratamento adequado.
- Distúrbios autoimunes seletivos — reavaliar o animal com frequência durante a fase inicial de indução; avaliar com menor frequência após a remissão; nesse caso, há necessidade de avaliações clínicas e dados laboratoriais.
- Terapia imunossupressora — hemogramas, bioquímicas séricas e urinálises frequentes com cultura para monitorizar a ocorrência de complicações.
- Agentes retinoides — bioquímicas séricas, incluindo a mensuração dos triglicerídeos, e testes lacrimais de Schirmer.
- Cetoconazol — bioquímicas séricas.

DIVERSOS
FATORES RELACIONADOS COM A IDADE
O envelhecimento da pele pode estar relacionado com o aumento nos distúrbios esfoliativos ou recidivas.

POTENCIAL ZOONÓTICO
A dermatofitose e diversos ectoparasitas possuem potencial zoonótico ou capacidade de indução de lesões em seres humanos.

GESTAÇÃO/FERTILIDADE/REPRODUÇÃO
Retinoides sistêmicos e vitamina A em doses terapêuticas — extremamente teratogênicos; não usar em fêmeas intactas, em função da teratogenicidade grave e previsível e do período de suspensão extremamente longo; mulheres em idade fértil não devem manipular esses medicamentos.

SINÔNIMO(S)
- Distúrbios de queratinização — seborreia, seborreia idiopática, defeito de queratinização, disqueratinização e termos humanos incorretos (eczema, psoríase, escama, caspa); sebopsoríase: termo correto para descrever as semelhanças entre alguns defeitos de queratinização humanos e caninos.
- Foliculite bacteriana = piodermite.

VER TAMBÉM
- Dermatite atópica (atopia). • Demodicose. • Hiperadrenocorticismo (síndrome de Cushing) — Gatos. • Hiperadrenocorticismo (síndrome de Cushing) — Cães. • Hipotireoidismo. • Dermatite por *Malassezia*. • Piodermite. • Sarna Sarcóptica.

ABREVIATURA(S)
- ACTH = hormônio adrenocorticotrópico.

Sugestões de Leitura
Gross TL, Ihrke PJ, Walder EJ, Affolter V. Skin Diseases of the Dog and Cat: Clinical and Histopathologic Diagnosis. Oxford: Blackwell Science, 2nd ed., 2005.

Autores Guillermina Manigot e Alexander H. Werner
Consultor Editorial Alexander H. Werner

DERMATOSES NASAIS – CÃES

CONSIDERAÇÕES GERAIS

DEFINIÇÃO
Condição patológica da pele nasal, envolvendo tanto a porção que contém pelos (ponte nasal/porção dorsal do focinho) como a porção sem pelos (plano nasal).

FISIOPATOLOGIA
Dependem da causa.

SISTEMA(S) ACOMETIDO(S)
Cutâneo/exócrino.

IDENTIFICAÇÃO
• Dermatofitose, dermatose responsiva ao zinco, dermatomiosite e demodicose — mais provavelmente em cães com <1 ano de idade.
• Dermatose responsiva ao zinco — raças Husky Siberiano, Malamute do Alasca.
• Dermatomiosite — raças Collie, Pastor de Shetland.
• Síndrome uveodermatológica — raças Akita, Samoieda, Husky siberiano.
• LES e LED — raças Collie, Pastor de Shetland, Pastor alemão; o LED pode ocorrer mais frequentemente nas fêmeas.
• Linfoma epiteliotrópico — cães idosos.
• Arterite nasal de cães da raça São Bernardo.
• Dermatose solar nasal — raças de pigmentação clara.
• Paraqueratose nasal de cães da raça Labrador retriever.

SINAIS CLÍNICOS
• Despigmentação.
• Hiperpigmentação.
• Eritema.
• Erosão/ulceração.
• Vesículas/pústulas.
• Crostas.
• Formação cicatricial.
• Alopecia.
• Nódulos/placas.

CAUSAS
• Piodermite/furunculose nasal.
• Demodicose.
• Dermatofitose.
• Outras infecções fúngicas — criptococose, esporotricose, aspergilose.
• LED ou LES.
• Furunculose nasal eosinofílica.
• Dermatite por picada de mosquito.
• Pênfigo foliáceo.
• Pênfigo eritematoso.
• Pênfigo vulgar.
• Dermatite solar nasal.
• Arterite.
• Dermatite solar nasal.
• Dermatomiosite.
• Dermatose responsiva ao zinco.
• Síndrome uveodermatológica.
• Dermatite necrolítica superficial.
• Vitiligo.
• Despigmentação nasal idiopática.
• Hipersensibilidade de contato — dermatite pela tigela de plástico, hipersensibilidade a medicamento tópico (neomicina).
• Tumores — carcinoma de células escamosas, carcinoma de células basais, linfoma epiteliotrópico, fibrossarcoma, histiocitose cutânea.
• Traumatismo.
• Granuloma estéril idiopático.
• Hiperqueratose nasal idiopática.
• Dermatite pelo vírus da cinomose.

FATORES DE RISCO
• Gatos adultos — podem ser portadores inaparentes dos dermatófitos.
• Comportamento de escavar — piodermite, dermatofitose.
• Exposição ao sol — dermatite solar nasal, LED, LES, pênfigo eritematoso.
• Nariz pouco pigmentado — dermatite solar nasal, carcinoma de células escamosas.
• Raças de grande porte e crescimento rápido suplementadas em exagero com cálcio ou dieta rica em cereais — dermatose responsiva ao zinco.
• Imunossupressão — demodicose, piodermite, dermatofitose.
• Exposição a insetos — dermatite por picada de mosquito e, possivelmente, furunculose nasal.

DIAGNÓSTICO

DIAGNÓSTICO DIFERENCIAL

Dermatite Solar Nasal
• Lesões — confinadas ao nariz; desencadeadas por exposição intensa à luz solar.
• Começa na pele pouco pigmentada na junção do plano nasal e ponte do nariz.
• Margens palpebrais levemente pigmentadas também podem ser acometidas.
• Imunofluorescência direta negativa.

LED
• Acomete principalmente a área nasal.
• Pode afetar as margens mucocutâneas dos lábios e das pálpebras.
• Exacerbada pela luz solar.
• Dermatite frequentemente precedida por despigmentação.
• Imunofluorescência direta positiva na zona da membrana basal.
• Biopsia — dermatite de interface com incontinência pigmentar.

LES
• Doença multissistêmica.
• Lesões cutâneas — frequentemente envolvem o nariz, a face, as junções mucocutâneas; multifocal ou generalizada.
• Teste ANA positivo.
• Imunofluorescência direta positiva na zona da membrana basal.

Pênfigo Foliáceo
• Lesões — iniciam, em geral, na face e nas orelhas; costumam envolver os coxins palmoplantares; acabam se generalizando.
• Desenvolvimento progressivo, notado pela primeira vez na junção do plano nasal e da porção dorsal do focinho.
• Biopsia — pústulas subcorneais com acantólise.
• Imunofluorescência direta positiva nos espaços intercelulares da epiderme.

Pênfigo Eritematoso
• Lesões — confinadas principalmente à face e às orelhas; tipicamente mais graves dos que as lesões de LED.
• Com frequência, a despigmentação é uma manifestação inicial.
• Biopsia — pústulas intraepidérmicas com acantólise e incontinência pigmentar.
• Imunofluorescência direta positiva na zona da membrana basal e nos espaços intercelulares.

Demodicose
• Frequentemente começa na face ou nos membros anteriores; não no plano nasal, mas na pele que contém pelos da região nasal.
• A demodicose de início juvenil é frequentemente facial em princípio.
• Pode generalizar.
• Diagnóstico feito mediante raspados cutâneos.

Dermatite pela Tigela de Plástico (ou de Borracha)
• Despigmentação e eritema do plano nasal anterior e da porção anterior dos lábios.
• Sem ulceração ou crostas.
• Histórico de exposição.
• Semelhante à dermatite de contato.
• Incomum; alto índice de suspeita — lesões mais frequentemente atribuídas a traumatismo por tigelas de bordas ásperas.

Dermatomiosite
• Raças de alto risco.
• Idade de início jovem.
• Lesões nasais e faciais, bem como das extremidades — caracterizadas por erosão, alopecia, formação cicatricial e hiperpigmentação.
• As lesões são particularmente notadas nos pontos de traumatismo ou pressão.
• Pode-se observar megaesôfago ou polimiosite.
• Biopsia — dermatite de interface com atrofia folicular.
• Imunofluorescência direta negativa.

Síndrome Uveodermatológica
• Raças de alto risco.
• Os sintomas oculares geralmente antecedem a doença dermatológica.
• Uveíte e despigmentação macular cutânea sem inflamação — nariz, lábios e pálpebras.
• Leucotriquia e leucodermia notáveis.
• Biopsia das lesões precoces — dermatite de interface, incontinência pigmentar.

Dermatose Responsiva ao Zinco
• Raças de alto risco.
• Identificação típica ou dieta (i. e., rica em fibra ou suplementação com cálcio).
• Lesões crostosas — face, junções mucocutâneas, pontos de pressão, coxins palmoplantares.
• Biopsia — hiperqueratose paraqueratótica.

Outros
• Piodermite/furunculose nasal — início agudo de foliculite na porção do nariz que contém pelos.
• Dermatofitose — porção do nariz que contém pelos; diagnosticar por cultura ou biopsia.
• Furunculose nasal eosinofílica — parte dorsal do focinho que contém pelos; diagnosticar por biopsia.
• Vitiligo — despigmentação macular cutânea sem inflamação em regiões como nariz, lábios, pálpebras, coxins palmoplantares e unhas; pode ser observada leucotriquia com leucodermia; diagnosticar por biopsia.
• Hipopigmentação nasal — a coloração negra normal do plano nasal "desbota" e dá lugar a uma cor castanho-claro ou esbranquiçada; pode ser sazonal ou sofrer exacerbação ou remissão; considerado um quadro estético e não patológico.
• Hiperqueratose nasal idiopática — crescimentos córneos e ressecados de queratina localizados no plano nasal; pode ou não estar associada à hiperqueratose digital.

DERMATOSES NASAIS – CÃES

- Outras doenças — diferenciar por meio de anamnese ou biopsia (i. e., infiltrados de células neoplásicas).

HEMOGRAMA/BIOQUÍMICA/URINÁLISE
- Geralmente normais.
- LES — pode haver anemia hemolítica, trombocitopenia, indícios de glomerulonefrite (ureia elevada, proteinúria), artropatia ou outros sintomas baseados no(s) sistema(s) corporal(is) acometido(s).

MÉTODOS DIAGNÓSTICOS
- Raspados cutâneos — para pesquisa de *Demodex*.
- Citologia — para detecção de microrganismos fúngicos, bactérias, eosinófilos ou células acantolíticas (pênfigo).
- Meio para teste de dermatófitos — dermatofitose.
- Cultura em ágar Sabouraud — outras infecções fúngicas.
- Cultura bacteriana e antibiograma ou avaliação citológica — piodermite.
- Punção articular — indícios de poliartrite no LES.
- ANA — positivo na maior parte dos casos de LES.
- Exame oftalmológico — uveíte na síndrome uveodermatológica.
- ECG — indícios de miocardite no LES.
- EMG — indícios de polimiosite no LES e na dermatomiosite.
- Imunofluorescência direta — depósito de imunoglobulinas na zona da membrana basal em casos de LED, LES e pênfigo eritematoso e nos espaços intercelulares da epiderme em casos de pênfigo foliáceo e pênfigo eritematoso.
- Neoplasia — citologia ou biopsia.
- Biopsia cutânea.

ACHADOS PATOLÓGICOS
- Foliculite/furunculose — (± ácaros, bactérias ou elementos fúngicos) — demodicose, dermatofitose, piodermite/furunculose nasal.
- Predominância eosinofílica — dermatite por picada de mosquito, furunculose eosinofílica.
- Atrofia folicular e fibrose perifolicular — dermatomiosite.
- Dermatite de interface — LED, LES, dermatomiosite, síndrome uveodermatológica.
- Pústulas intraepidérmicas com acantólise — pênfigo foliáceo e pênfigo eritematoso.
- Acantólise suprabasilar — pênfigo vulgar.
- Hiperqueratose paraqueratótica — dermatose responsiva ao zinco.
- Hipomelanose — vitiligo, síndrome uveodermatológica.

- Dermatite granulomatosa/piogranulomatosa — piodermite, infecção fúngica, corpo estranho, granuloma estéril idiopático.
- Infiltrado de células neoplásicas — histiocitose cutânea, outras neoplasias.

TRATAMENTO
- Como paciente de ambulatório, exceto em casos de LES com grave falência múltipla de órgãos ou tumores que necessitam de excisão cirúrgica ou radioterapia.
- Reduzir a exposição à luz solar — LED, LES, pênfigo eritematoso, dermatite solar nasal, carcinoma de células escamosas.
- Desestimular o comportamento de escavar — piodermite, dermatofitose.
- Proteção contra insetos.
- Embebições mornas — ajudam a remover os exsudatos e as crostas.
- Substituir a tigela de plástico ou de borracha e evitar o contato com medicamento tópico ou outro agente indutor de reação de hipersensibilidade.

MEDICAÇÕES
MEDICAMENTO(S) DE ESCOLHA
- Infecções fúngicas — antifúngicos sistêmicos: griseofulvina, cetoconazol, itraconazol; enilconazol tópico para aspergilose; excisão cirúrgica de lesões discretas precoces.
- Dermatite solar nasal — corticosteroides tópicos; antibióticos em caso de infecção secundária; filtros solares; pele hipopigmentada com tatuagem (método não utilizado atualmente).
- Granuloma estéril idiopático — excisão cirúrgica quando possível; terapia imunossupressora com glicocorticoides ± azatioprina, ciclosporina, tetraciclina e niacinamida.
- LED — corticosteroides ou tacrolimo tópicos; tetraciclina e niacinamida; terapia oral (igual à do pênfigo foliáceo) se temporariamente necessária em casos graves.
- Pênfigo foliáceo, pênfigo vulgar e LES — terapia imunossupressora com prednisolona ± azatioprina (cães), clorambucila, crisoterapia.
- Vitiligo/despigmentação nasal — sem tratamento.
- Neoplasia — excisão cirúrgica; quimioterapia; radioterapia.

- Hiperqueratose nasal idiopática — creme com antibiótico-corticosteroide para fissuras, umectante tópico (Kerasolv® da DVM Pharmaceuticals), tacrolimo tópico (Protopic®).
- Outras doenças — ver doença específica.

CONTRAINDICAÇÕES
Evitar a crisoterapia em pacientes com nefropatia.

PRECAUÇÕES
- Griseofulvina — pode provocar anorexia, vômito, diarreia e supressão da medula óssea; administrar dieta rica em gordura.
- Cetoconazol — pode provocar anorexia, irritação gástrica, hepatotoxicidade e clareamento da pelagem.

ACOMPANHAMENTO
MONITORIZAÇÃO DO PACIENTE
Varia com a doença específica e com o tratamento prescrito.

COMPLICAÇÕES POSSÍVEIS
Formação cicatricial com infecções profundas ou limpeza excessivamente vigorosa.

DIVERSOS
POTENCIAL ZOONÓTICO
Dermatofitose.

GESTAÇÃO/FERTILIDADE/REPRODUÇÃO
A griseofulvina é teratogênica.

SINÔNIMO(S)
- Dermatite necrolítica superficial = eritema migratório necrolítico superficial e síndrome hepatocutânea.
- Uveodermatológica = síndrome de Vogt-Koyanagi-Harada.

ABREVIATURA(S)
- ANA = anticorpo antinuclear.
- ECG = eletrocardiograma.
- EMG = eletromiografia.
- LED = lúpus eritematoso discoide.
- LES = lúpus eritematoso sistêmico.

Sugestões de Leitura
Muller GH, Kirk RW, Scott DW. Small Animal Dermatology, 4th ed. Philadelphia: Saunders, 1989.

Autor Karen Helton Rhodes
Consultor Editorial Alexander H. Werner

DERMATOSES NEOPLÁSICAS

CONSIDERAÇÕES GERAIS

DEFINIÇÃO
- Proliferação neoplásica de células que se derivam da pele ou migram para a pele.
- Tumores epidérmicos incluem aqueles que se originam de queratinócitos, melanócitos, células de Merkel e de Langerhans, além de linfoma epiteliotrópico.
- Tumores de anexos abrangem aqueles que surgem de folículos pilosos, glândulas sebáceas e glândulas sudoríferas.
- Tumores cutâneos dérmicos e subcutâneos englobam aqueles de origem mesenquimal e outros originários de células redondas.
- Tumores cutâneos secundários ou metastáticos advêm da proliferação, na pele, de células provenientes de neoplasias primárias de outros órgãos.

FISIOPATOLOGIA
- A neoplasia desenvolve-se como resultado de alterações em genes responsáveis pelo controle da proliferação celular e homeostasia.
- Foram identificados mais de 100 genes relacionados com o câncer.
- Oncogenes codificam proteínas que promovem o crescimento celular; genes supressores de tumor codificam proteínas que restringem os processos de proliferação e diferenciação celulares.
- São encontradas mutações no p53, um gene supressor de tumor, em aproximadamente 50% dos cânceres em seres humanos; esse tipo de mutação também é encontrado em muitos tumores que afetam cães e gatos.
- A luz ultravioleta promove o desenvolvimento do tumor por meio de dano ao DNA e supressão do sistema imune.
- Muitos vírus promovem o crescimento do tumor, estimulando a proliferação das células e/ou suprimindo o sistema imune.
- Há relatos de neoplasia cutânea específica associada a medicamentos e/ou vacinações.

SISTEMA(S) ACOMETIDO(S)
Cutâneo/Exócrino.

GENÉTICA
- Foram relatadas predisposições raciais para tumores específicos, embora o modo de herança nessas raças não tenha sido determinado.
- Mutações em oncogenes e/ou genes supressores de tumor (p. ex., p53) estão presentes em muitos tipos de tumores cutâneos.

INCIDÊNCIA/PREVALÊNCIA
- A taxa de incidência combinada para tumores cutâneos foi relatada em 728/100.000 (0,728%) para cães e 84/100.000 (0,084%) para gatos.
- A pele corresponde ao local mais comum de ocorrência de neoplasia no cão (30% dos tumores totais) e o segundo local mais comum no gato (20% dos tumores totais).
- Os tumores de pele no cão são aproximadamente 55% mesenquimais, 40% epiteliais e 5% melanocíticos.
- Os tumores cutâneos mais frequentemente relatados em cães são lipoma, tumores de glândulas sebáceas, mastocitoma, histiocitoma e papilomas.
- Os tumores de pele no gato são cerca de 50% epiteliais, 48% mesenquimais e 2% melanocíticos.
- Os tumores cutâneos relatados com maior frequência em gatos são tumor de células basais (basalioma), carcinoma de células escamosas, mastocitoma, e fibrossarcoma.
- Muitas vezes, os tumores cutâneos em cães e gatos são benignos e malignos, respectivamente.

DISTRIBUIÇÃO GEOGRÁFICA
As regiões geográficas próximas ao Equador, com altas altitudes, ou com areia ou outras superfícies refletoras, têm uma incidência mais alta de dermatoses neoplásicas induzidas pelo sol.

IDENTIFICAÇÃO
Espécies
Cães e gatos.

Raça(s) Predominante(s)
- As raças caninas com a incidência global mais alta de tumores cutâneos incluem Boxer, Terrier escocês, Bullmastiff, Basset hound, Weimaraner, Kerry blue terrier e Elkhound norueguês.
- As raças felinas com a incidência global mais alta de tumores cutâneos englobam Siamês e Persa.
- Certas raças são predispostas a tipos específicos de tumores (ver *Sugestões de Leitura*).
- Cão — raças associadas às neoplasias cutâneas mais comuns:
  - Lipoma — Cocker spaniel, Dachshund, Doberman pinscher, Labrador retriever, Schnauzer miniatura, Weimaraner.
  - Tumor de glândulas sebáceas — Beagle, Cocker spaniel, Dachshund, Setter irlandês, Lhasa apso, Malamute, Schnauzer miniatura, Poodle, Shih tzu, Husky siberiano.
  - Mastocitoma — Staffordshire terrier americano, Beagle, Boston terrier, Boxer, Bull terrier, Dachshund, Buldogue inglês, Fox terrier, Golden retriever, Labrador retriever, Pug, Shar-pei, Weimaraner.
  - Histiocitoma — Staffordshire terrier americano, Boston terrier, Boxer, Cocker spaniel, Dachshund, Doberman pinscher, Springer spaniel inglês, Dinamarquês, Labrador retriever, Schnauzer miniatura, Rottweiler, Terrier escocês, Shar-pei, Pastor de Shetland, West Highland white terrier.
  - Papiloma — Cocker spaniel, Kerry blue terrier.
- Gato — raças associadas às neoplasias cutâneas mais comuns:
  - Tumor de células basais (basalioma) — Persa, Himalaio (carcinoma de células basais — Siamês).
  - Carcinoma de células escamosas — não há relatos de predisposição racial.
  - Mastocitoma — Siamês.
  - Fibrossarcoma — não há relatos de predisposição racial.

Idade Média e Faixa Etária
- A idade média para neoplasia cutânea é de 10 anos e meio em cães e 12 anos em gatos.
- A faixa etária de pico para neoplasia cutânea em cães e gatos é de 6 a 14 anos.

Sexo Predominante
- As fêmeas têm uma incidência maior de tumores em cães (56%).
- Os machos têm uma incidência maior de tumores em gatos (56%).

SINAIS CLÍNICOS
Comentários Gerais
O sinal clínico mais comum consiste em nódulo(s) cutâneo(s) ou subcutâneo(s); alguns tumores apresentam uma superfície ulcerada; outros podem resultar em descamação excessiva ou na formação de placas cutâneas.

Achados Anamnésicos
- Os tumores podem ser de crescimento lento; o proprietário pode encontrá-los durante os atos de acariciar, banhar ou embelezar o animal de estimação.
- Os tumores podem ser de crescimento rápido e aparecer (ou aumentar de tamanho) com rapidez (p. ex., histiocitoma).

Achados do Exame Físico
- Nódulos — cutâneos ou subcutâneos.
- Úlceras cutâneas.
- Descamação excessiva.
- Papilomas cutâneos.
- Placas cutâneas.

CAUSAS
- Genéticas (mutações gênicas).
- Ambientais (p. ex., luz ultravioleta, exposição à radiação).
- Agentes virais (p. ex., papilomavírus, FeLV, FIV).
- Toxinas (p. ex., alcatrão).
- Medicamentos (p. ex., agentes imunossupressores, agentes quimioterápicos).
- Neoplasias epidérmicas:
  - Queratinócitos — papilomas, carcinoma de células escamosas, carcinoma de células basais (basalioma), carcinoma basoscamoso.
  - Melanócitos — melanoma.
  - Células de Merkel — carcinoma de células de Merkel.
  - Células de Langerhans — histiocitoma e histiocitose.
  - Linfoma epiteliotrópico.
- Neoplasias de anexos:
  - Folículos pilosos — tricofoliculoma, tricoepitelioma, acantoma queratinizante infundibular, tricolemoma, pilomatricoma, tricoblastoma.
  - Glândulas sebáceas — adenoma sebáceo, epitelioma sebáceo, adenocarcinoma sebáceo, epitelioma de glândulas perianais, carcinoma de glândulas perianais.
  - Glândulas sudoríferas — cistadenoma apócrino, adenoma/adenocarcinoma secretor apócrino, adenoma/carcinoma ductal apócrino, carcinoma écrino.
- Neoplasia dérmica e subcutânea:
  - Origem mesenquimal — sarcoma de tecidos moles: fibroma/fibrossarcoma, mixoma/mixossarcoma, hemangiopericitoma, linfangioma/linfangiossarcoma, hemangioma/hemangiossarcoma, lipoma/lipossarcoma, neurofibrossarcoma, leiomioma/leiomiossarcoma, sinovioma/sarcoma de células sinoviais, rabdomioma/rabdomiossarcoma.
  - Origem de células redondas — tumor venéreo transmissível, mastocitoma, plasmocitoma, linfoma, histiocitoma e tumores histiocíticos.
- Tumores cutâneos secundários ou metastáticos originam-se de metástases ou neoplasias primárias em outros órgãos para a pele.

FATORES DE RISCO
- Coloração e comprimento da pelagem (p. ex., raças de pele glabra [ou seja, sem pelo], pelagem branca, pele pouco pigmentada — risco elevado de carcinoma de células escamosas).
- Idade (p. ex., os animais jovens apresentam risco mais alto de infecções virais, enquanto os mais velhos, de neoplasia associada ao ambiente).

DERMATOSES NEOPLÁSICAS

- Exposição à luz solar (p. ex., cães e gatos que tomam banho de sol ou gastam horas fora de casa sobre superfícies refletoras têm maior risco de tumores cutâneos induzidos por luz ultravioleta).
- Genética — certas raças exibem maior risco de desenvolver tipos específicos de tumores (ver anteriormente e em *Sugestões de Leitura*).

DIAGNÓSTICO

DIAGNÓSTICO DIFERENCIAL
- Cistos/abscessos.
- Nódulos/granulomas/placas inflamatórios — doença granulomatosa e piogranulomatosa estéril, paniculite estéril, infecções fúngicas, infecções micobacterianas, corpos estranhos.
- Ulceração cutânea autoinduzida ou induzida por traumatismo.
- Hamartoma/nevos.

HEMOGRAMA/BIOQUÍMICA/URINÁLISE
N/D.

OUTROS TESTES LABORATORIAIS
- Citologia (aspirado por agulha fina ou esfregaço por impressão).
- Biopsia.
- Linfonodos regionais (para estadiamento do tumor).

DIAGNÓSTICO POR IMAGEM
Radiografias torácicas e ultrassonografia abdominal são úteis para estadiamento do tumor (avaliar o paciente em busca de doença metastática ou neoplasia primária subjacente).

MÉTODOS DIAGNÓSTICOS
- Citologia.
- Histopatologia.
- Imuno-histoquímica (útil para confirmar certos tipos de tumores).

ACHADOS PATOLÓGICOS
Varia com o tipo de tumor; ver tumores específicos para obtenção de mais informações.

TRATAMENTO

CUIDADO(S) DE SAÚDE ADEQUADO(S)
- Varia com o tipo de tumor.
  - A observação é adequada para alguns tumores benignos.
  - Excisão cirúrgica, criocirurgia, radioterapia, e/ou quimioterapia ou imunoterapia específica para o tumor podem ser curativas ou paliativas.

CUIDADO(S) DE ENFERMAGEM
- Varia com o tipo e o local do tumor.
- Tumores traumatizados podem vir a sofrer infecção secundária.

ATIVIDADE
Varia com o tipo e o local do tumor.

DIETA
Dietas ricas em ácidos graxos ômega-3, arginina e proteína podem ser benéficas para estimulação da resposta imune e prevenção de caquexia associada ao câncer.

ORIENTAÇÃO AO PROPRIETÁRIO
Varia com o tipo e o local do tumor.

CONSIDERAÇÕES CIRÚRGICAS
- Varia com o tipo e o local do tumor — talvez haja necessidade de margens amplas de segurança para evitar a recorrência de tumores infiltrativos.
- O pré-tratamento com anti-histamínicos é adequado na excisão de mastocitomas.

MEDICAÇÕES

MEDICAMENTO(S) DE ESCOLHA
Varia com o tipo de tumor — os protocolos de quimioterapia são úteis em alguns casos.

CONTRAINDICAÇÕES
Varia com o tipo de tumor e a presença de doença concomitante.

PRECAUÇÕES
Varia com o tipo e o local do tumor.

INTERAÇÕES POSSÍVEIS
Varia com o tipo e o local do tumor.

MEDICAMENTO(S) ALTERNATIVO(S)
Varia com o tipo e o local do tumor.

ACOMPANHAMENTO

MONITORIZAÇÃO DO PACIENTE
Varia com o tipo e o local do tumor.

PREVENÇÃO
- Varia com o tipo e o local do tumor.
- Minimizar a exposição à luz ultravioleta pode ajudar a evitar alguns tipos de tumores.

COMPLICAÇÕES POSSÍVEIS
Varia com o tipo e o local do tumor.

EVOLUÇÃO ESPERADA E PROGNÓSTICO
Varia com o tipo e o local do tumor

DIVERSOS

DISTÚRBIOS ASSOCIADOS
Varia com o tipo e o local do tumor.

FATORES RELACIONADOS COM A IDADE
Varia com o tipo e o local do tumor.

POTENCIAL ZOONÓTICO
Nenhum.

GESTAÇÃO/FERTILIDADE/REPRODUÇÃO
Varia com o tipo de tumor; alguns podem ter uma predisposição genética.

SINÔNIMOS
N/D.

VER TAMBÉM
Tipos específicos de tumores.

ABREVIATURAS
- FeLV = vírus da leucemia felina.
- FIV = vírus da imunodeficiência felina.

RECURSOS DA INTERNET
- http://www.oncolink.org/types/section.cfm?c=22&s=69 (OncoLink Vet).
- http://www.vetcancersociety.org/.

Sugestões de Leitura
Campbell KL, ed. Small Animal Dermatology Secrets. Philadelphia: Hanley & Belfus, 2004, pp. 385-458.
Goldschmidt MH, Shofer FS. Skin Tumors of the Dog and Cat. Oxford: Butterworth Heinemann, 1992.
Gross TL, Ihrke PJ, Walder EJ, et al. Skin Diseases of the Dog and Cat: Clinical and Histopathologic Diagnosis, 2nd ed. Oxford: Blackwell, 2005, pp. 561-893.
Scott DW, Miller WH, Griffin CE. Muller & Kirk's Small Animal Dermatology, 6th ed. Philadelphia: Saunders, 2001, pp. 1236-1414.
Shearer D, Dobson J. An approach to nodules and draining sinuses. In: Foster A, Foil C, BSAVA Manual of Small Animal Dermatology, 2nd ed. Gloucestershire, UK: BSAVA, pp. 55-65.

Autor Karen L. Campbell
Consultor Editorial Alexander H. Werner

Dermatoses Nodulares/Granulomatosas Estéreis

CONSIDERAÇÕES GERAIS

DEFINIÇÃO
Doenças cujas lesões primárias consistem em nódulos maciços, elevados e com >1 cm de diâmetro.

FISIOPATOLOGIA
- Nódulos — costumam ser o resultado de infiltração de células inflamatórias na derme ou no tecido subcutâneo; podem ser secundários a estímulos endógenos ou exógenos.
- A inflamação é tipicamente, mas nem sempre, granulomatosa a piogranulomatosa.

SISTEMA(S) ACOMETIDO(S)
Cutâneo/exócrino.

GENÉTICA
Para os casos de sarcoma histiocítico dos cães Montanhês de Berna, é proposta uma transmissão oligogênica.

IDENTIFICAÇÃO
- Pode acometer qualquer idade, raça ou sexo.
- Dermatofibrose nodular — Pastor alemão, 3-5 anos de idade.
- Calcinose circunscrita — Pastor alemão, <2 anos de idade.
- Histiocitose sistêmica e histiocitose maligna — Montanhês de Berna (principalmente) e Rottweiler, além de Golden e Labrador Retrievers.
- Granuloma eosinofílico — cães machos da raça Husky siberiano com <3 anos de idade.

SINAIS CLÍNICOS
- Caracterizados por nódulos isolados ou múltiplos na derme ou no tecido subcutâneo.
- Nódulos firmes a flutuantes.
- Ocasionalmente dolorosos.
- A epiderme sobrejacente pode permanecer normal ou estar ulcerada.

CAUSAS
- Amiloidose.
- Reação a corpos estranhos.
- Esferulocitose.
- Granuloma e piogranuloma estéreis idiopáticos.
- Granuloma eosinofílico canino.
- Calcinose cutânea.
- Calcinose circunscrita.
- Histiocitose maligna (sarcoma histiocítico disseminado).
- Histiocitose reativa (cutânea e sistêmica).
- Paniculite nodular estéril.
- Dermatofibrose nodular.
- Xantoma cutâneo.

FATORES DE RISCO
- Reação a corpos estranhos — induzida por exposição a qualquer material irritante (p. ex., poeira de concreto ou fibra de vidro).
- Corpos estranhos nos pelos — risco elevado em cães de grande porte que repousam em superfícies muito duras.
- Calcinose cutânea — aumento do risco com a exposição a doses altas de glicocorticoides exógenos ou endógenos.
- Paniculite — elevação do risco com dieta deficiente em vitamina E.
- Xantoma cutâneo — petiscos ou dietas ricos em gorduras, diabetes melito, hiperlipidemia.

DIAGNÓSTICO

DIAGNÓSTICO DIFERENCIAL
- Ver a seção "Causas".
- Dermatoses nodulares estéreis — devem ser diferenciadas de infecções bacterianas e fúngicas profundas e de neoplasias dérmicas.
- Todas essas doenças podem ser diagnosticadas por meio de histopatologia e culturas teciduais profundas.
- Imuno-histoquímica — exame útil para diferenciar os distúrbios histiocíticos neoplásicos de outras doenças neoplásicas; também diferencia doenças histiocíticas reativas de malignas.
- A coloração imuno-histoquímica deve ser realizada em tecido fresco congelado e não fixado em formalina.

HEMOGRAMA/BIOQUÍMICA/URINÁLISE
- Amiloidose — possíveis alterações na bioquímica e/ou na urinálise em caso de acometimento de órgãos internos.
- Histiocitose maligna — pancitopenia.
- Calcinose cutânea — alterações características de hiperglicocorticoidismo (p. ex., leucograma de estresse, atividade elevada da fosfatase alcalina, hiperglicemia, densidade urinária baixa).
- Xantomas cutâneos — pode haver glicosúria, hiperglicemia e/ou anormalidades do perfil lipídico.

OUTROS TESTES LABORATORIAIS
Níveis séricos da ferritina — podem ficar elevados em casos de histiocitose maligna, mas não em histiocitose reativa.

DIAGNÓSTICO POR IMAGEM
- Radiologia e ultrassonografia — delineiam o envolvimento de órgãos internos em casos de amiloidose e histiocitose.
- Radiologia — identifica outras áreas de calcificação distrófica em cães com calcinose cutânea.
- Ultrassonografia — permite a identificação de tumores renais ou uterinos em cães com dermatofibrose nodular; em cães com calcinose cutânea, também podem ser observadas alterações hepáticas e tumor ou aumento de volume da adrenal.

MÉTODOS DIAGNÓSTICOS
- Biopsias cutâneas para histopatologia e culturas (fúngicas, aeróbias, anaeróbias e micobacterianas) — são essenciais para o diagnóstico apropriado de dermatoses nodulares.
- As biopsias devem ser excisionais, se possível.
- É recomendável a realização de culturas a partir do tecido nodular e não dos exsudatos; os microrganismos fúngicos e micobacterianos podem passar despercebidos nos exsudatos com facilidade.
- Pode haver a necessidade de colorações histopatológicas especiais para bactérias, micobactérias e fungos a fim de descartar a presença de qualquer agente infeccioso.

ACHADOS PATOLÓGICOS
- Amiloidose — caracterizada pelo acúmulo de depósitos eosinofílicos amorfos, que podem se estender para o tecido subcutâneo; os depósitos coram-se de verde-maçã com o corante vermelho Congo sob luz polarizada.
- Reação a corpos estranhos — caracterizada por inflamação supurativa a piogranulomatosa, que afeta a derme, o tecido subcutâneo e, ocasionalmente, o músculo subjacente. O corpo estranho incitante pode ou não estar presente no tecido amostrado.
- Esferulocitose — caracterizada pela presença de histiócitos que circundam corpúsculos aparentados de parede fina preenchidos com esférulas eosinofílicas homogêneas.
- Granuloma e piogranuloma estéreis idiopáticos — caracterizados por inflamação granulomatosa a piogranulomatosa, que pode se estender da derme para o panículo; a inflamação mimetiza aquela observada em casos de doenças infecciosas nodulares; diferenciados pela obtenção de culturas teciduais aeróbias, anaeróbias, micobacterianas e fúngicas negativas.
- Granuloma eosinofílico canino — caracterizado pelo acúmulo de inúmeros eosinófilos com a formação de edema e possível mucina. É comum a degeneração de colágeno, especialmente em lesões mais agudas.
- Calcinose cutânea — caracterizada pelo depósito difuso de cálcio no colágeno dérmico e nos anexos cutâneos, que pode se estender para as camadas teciduais mais profundas.
- Calcinose circunscrita — caracterizada por depósitos focais a multifocais de minerais, que destroem os tecidos moles.
- Histiocitose reativa (cutânea e sistêmica) — caracterizada por um infiltrado acentuadamente angiocêntrico de histiócitos, que não formam granulomas ou piogranulomas; não é possível diferenciar as doenças cutâneas e sistêmicas por meio de biopsia.
- Histiocitose maligna (sarcoma histiocítico disseminado) — caracterizada por uma proliferação densa de células pleomórficas de células fusiformes ou redondas, que destroem a arquitetura tecidual normal; os tumores provenientes de outros tumores de células fusiformes e redondas são diferenciados por meio da imuno-histoquímica; os sarcomas histiocíticos expressam constantemente os marcadores CD45, CD18, CDI, CD11c e MHC* II.
- Paniculite nodular estéril — caracterizada por inflamação neutrofílica a piogranulomatosa, que afeta predominantemente as camadas profundas da derme e o panículo; os adipócitos podem estar necrosados ou ser infiltrados por macrófagos espumosos.
- Dermatofibrose nodular — caracterizada por espessamento dérmico focal de feixes normais de colágeno; as alterações histopatológicas são muito sutis; é importante fornecer ao patologista a identificação e a anamnese do animal.
- Xantoma cutâneo — caracterizado por uma inflamação granulomatosa difusa composta de grandes macrófagos espumosos; nem sempre há lagos de depósitos lipídicos amorfos extracelulares e fendas de colesterol em todos os casos.

TRATAMENTO

CUIDADO(S) DE SAÚDE ADEQUADO(S)
- Os cães com calcinose cutânea podem necessitar de internação em virtude da ocorrência de sepse e para receber terapia tópica intensiva.

---

* N. T.: Complexo de histocompatibilidade maior.

Dermatoses Nodulares/Granulomatosas Estéreis

- A maior parte desses distúrbios pode ser tratada em um esquema ambulatorial.
- Os distúrbios neoplásicos ou metabólicos podem necessitar de internação e cuidados de suporte.

CUIDADO(S) DE ENFERMAGEM
Os cães acometidos por qualquer uma dessas doenças em que os nódulos sofrem ulceração ou ruptura se beneficiarão da hidroterapia para manter as lesões limpas.

ATIVIDADE
Não há indicação de qualquer restrição da atividade física.

DIETA
Os animais com xantoma devem ser alimentados com uma dieta pobre em gordura.

ORIENTAÇÃO AO PROPRIETÁRIO
- Os quadros de histiocitose maligna, amiloidose, dermatofibrose nodular e histiocitose reativa sistêmica são quase sempre fatais.
- Os prognósticos de doença histiocítica reativa cutânea, paniculite estéril e piogranuloma estéril são reservados, pois essas doenças podem necessitar de terapia imunossupressora a longo prazo; alguns desses casos nem respondem à terapia.

MEDICAÇÕES

MEDICAMENTO(S)
- Amiloidose — não há nenhuma terapia conhecida a menos que a lesão seja solitária e possa ser removida por via cirúrgica.
- Esferulocitose — o único tratamento eficaz é a remoção cirúrgica.
- Granuloma e piogranuloma estéreis idiopáticos:
  - Prednisona (2,2-4,4 mg/kg divididos por VO a cada 12 h) constitui a primeira linha terapêutica; manter os esteroides por 7-14 dias após a remissão completa; depois, reduzir a dose gradativamente.
- Azatioprina (2,2 mg/kg a cada 48 h) pode ser adicionada à terapia como um medicamento que poupa o uso de esteroide.
- Ciclosporina (5-10 mg/kg a cada 24 h) pode ser eficaz em casos irresponsivos a esteroides.
- Reações a corpos estranhos — tratadas de forma mais eficiente por meio da remoção da substância agressora, se possível; no caso de corpos estranhos nos pelos, é recomendável colocar o cão em uma cama mais macia e instituir a terapia tópica com agentes queratolíticos; muitos cães com corpos estranhos nos pelos também apresentam infecções bacterianas profundas secundárias, que precisam ser tratadas com antibióticos tanto tópicos como sistêmicos.
- Granuloma eosinofílico canino — a prednisona (1,1-2,2 mg/kg VO a cada 24 h) costuma ser eficaz.
- Histiocitose maligna — não há nenhuma terapia eficaz a longo prazo; a lomustina foi usada com certo êxito a curto prazo; é rapidamente fatal (o tempo de sobrevida média costuma ser inferior a 3 meses).
- Histiocitose cutânea/sistêmica — altas doses de glicocorticosteroides, ciclosporina, leflunomida e outros agentes citotóxicos podem resultar na remissão, mas as terapias prolongadas costumam ser necessárias e as recidivas são comuns.
- Calcinose cutânea — é imprescindível controlar a doença subjacente, se possível; a maioria dos casos necessita de antibióticos para controlar as infecções bacterianas secundárias; a prática de hidroterapia e a aplicação frequente de banhos com xampus antibacterianos minimizam os problemas secundários; o DMSO tópico é útil (aplicado em não mais do que um terço do corpo, uma vez ao dia, até a resolução das lesões); se as lesões forem amplas, os níveis séricos de cálcio deverão ser monitorizados com rigor enquanto se utiliza o DMSO.
- Calcinose circunscrita — a excisão cirúrgica consiste na terapia de escolha.
- Paniculite nodular estéril — as lesões isoladas e únicas são passíveis de remoção cirúrgica; a prednisona (2,2-4,4 mg/kg VO a cada 24 h ou divididos por VO a cada 12 h) representa o tratamento de escolha e deve ser administrada até a regressão das lesões; em seguida, a dose é reduzida gradativamente; alguns cães permanecem em remissão a longo prazo, mas outros necessitam de terapia prolongada em dias alternados; alguns casos respondem à vitamina E por via oral (400 UI a cada 12 h); os casos refratários podem responder à ciclosporina.
- Dermatofibrose nodular — não há nenhuma terapia para a maioria dos casos, pois os cistoadenocarcinomas costumam ser bilaterais; em caso unilateral raro de cistoadenocarcinoma ou em um cistoadenoma, a remoção do único rim acometido pode ser benéfica.
- Xantoma cutâneo — em geral, a correção do diabetes melito ou da hiperlipoproteinemia subjacentes é curativa.
- Azatioprina (2,2 mg/kg a cada 48 h) pode ser utilizada juntamente com a prednisona como um agente que poupa o uso de corticosteroide.
- Ciclosporina (5-10 mg/kg a cada 24 h) pode ser usada como uma alternativa à terapia com glicocorticoide se o paciente se mostrar intolerante aos esteroides ou se esses agentes não forem suficientemente eficazes.
- Combinação de tetraciclina e niacinamida (250 mg de cada por VO a cada 8 h para cães com <10 kg e 500 mg de cada a cada 8 h para aqueles com >10 kg) também pode ser empregada como uma alternativa à terapia com glicocorticoide; essa combinação é eficaz principalmente em casos leves.

CONTRAINDICAÇÕES
Se possível, deve-se evitar o uso de corticosteroides e de outros agentes imunossupressores em qualquer animal com foliculite secundária.

PRECAUÇÕES
DMSO — manipular com cuidado; monitorizar os níveis séricos de cálcio se esse agente for utilizado para tratar a calcinose cutânea.

ACOMPANHAMENTO

MONITORIZAÇÃO DO PACIENTE
- Em pacientes sob terapia imunossupressora a longo prazo, deve-se monitorizá-los com hemograma, perfil bioquímico, urinálise e urocultura por, no mínimo, a cada 6 meses.
- Em cães submetidos ao DMSO para o tratamento de calcinose cutânea, deve-se checar o nível de cálcio a cada 7-14 dias durante o primeiro mês de terapia se amplas áreas estiverem acometidas.

COMPLICAÇÕES POSSÍVEIS
O uso de terapia imunossupressora a longo prazo (especialmente glicocorticosteroides) pode tornar os pacientes mais suscetíveis a outras dermatoses, como foliculite bacteriana, demodicose e dermatofitose, bem como a efeitos colaterais sistêmicos.

EVOLUÇÃO ESPERADA E PROGNÓSTICO
- Amiloidose sistêmica, histiocitose maligna, histiocitose reativa sistêmica e dermatofibrose nodular — são invariavelmente fatais.
- A maioria dos outros distúrbios exibe prognóstico reservado; muitos deles necessitam de terapia imunossupressora vitalícia para que permaneçam em remissão.

DIVERSOS

DISTÚRBIOS ASSOCIADOS
- Calcinose cutânea — hiperglicocorticoidismo, insuficiência renal crônica e diabetes melito.
- Calcinose circunscrita — (ocasionalmente) osteodistrofia hipertrófica e poliartrite idiopática.
- Dermatofibrose nodular — cistoadenoma/cistoadenocarcinoma, leiomioma/leiomiossarcoma.
- Xantoma cutâneo — diabetes melito e hiperlipoproteinemia.

VER TAMBÉM
- Adenocarcinoma Renal.
- Amiloidose.
- Hiperadrenocorticismo (Síndrome de Cushing) — Cães.

ABREVIATURA(S)
- DMSO = dimetilsulfóxido.

RECURSOS DA INTERNET
http://www.histiocytosis.ucdavis.edu/.

Sugestões de Leitura
Coomer AR, Liptak JM. Canine histiocytic diseases. Compend Contin Educ Pract Vet 2008, 30:202-217.
Griffin CE, Kwochka KW, MacDonald JM, eds. Current Veterinary Dermatology. St. Louis: Mosby, 1993.
Gross TL, Ihrke PJ, Walder EJ. Skin Diseases of the Dog and Cat, 2nd ed. Ames, IA: Blackwell, 2005.
Scott DW, Miller WH, Griffin CE. Muller & Kirk's Small Animal Dermatology, 6th ed. Philadelphia: Saunders, 2001.

Autor Dawn E. Logas
Consultor Editorial Alexander H. Werner

DERMATOSES PAPULONODULARES

CONSIDERAÇÕES GERAIS

DEFINIÇÃO
- Trata-se de doenças cujas lesões primárias se manifestam sob a forma de pápulas e nódulos.
- Pápula: lesões sólidas e elevadas da pele com menos de 1 cm de diâmetro.
- Nódulo: lesões sólidas e elevadas da pele que apresentam mais de 1 cm de diâmetro e se estendem para as camadas cutâneas mais profundas.

FISIOPATOLOGIA
- Pápulas — em geral, resultam de infiltração tecidual por células inflamatórias; concomitantemente, há edema intraepidérmico ou hiperplasia epidérmica e edema dérmico.
- Nódulos — costumam ser o resultado de infiltração maciça de células inflamatórias ou neoplásicas na derme ou no tecido subcutâneo.

SISTEMA(S) ACOMETIDO(S)
Cutâneo/exócrino.

GENÉTICA
Determinada pela causa; doenças específicas podem ser observadas com maior frequência em certas raças.

IDENTIFICAÇÃO
- Cães e gatos.
- Determinada pela causa.

SINAIS CLÍNICOS
- Pápulas e/ou nódulos com distribuição característica da causa.
- Com frequência, observam-se lesões concomitantes de formação de crostas, inflamação, alterações de pigmentação e mudanças na pelagem; também são características da causa.

CAUSAS
- Foliculites bacterianas superficial e profunda.
- Dermatofitose.
- Adenite sebácea.
- Pustulose eosinofílica estéril.
- Acnes canina e felina.
- Quérions.
- Demodicose.
- Dermatite rabdítica.
- Dermatite actínica.
- Dermatite piogranulomatosa idiopática estéril de perianexos.
- Neoplasia.

FATORES DE RISCO
- Foliculite, dermatofitose e demodicose — qualquer doença ou medicamento indutor de comprometimento imunológico.
- Foliculite bacteriana comumente associada à hipersensibilidade cutânea e/ou endocrinopatia.
- Dermatite rabdítica — pode estar associada ao contato com restos orgânicos em decomposição (palha ou feno), que contenham *Pelodera strongyloides*.
- Dermatite actínica — observada com maior frequência em cães errantes de pelo curto e levemente pigmentados, que vivem em áreas com ampla exposição à luz solar; relatada mais comumente em cães das raças Dálmata, Staffordshire terrier americano, Pit Bull terrier, Beagle, Whippet, Galgo italiano, Galgo e Basset hound.

DIAGNÓSTICO

DIAGNÓSTICO DIFERENCIAL
- Determinado pela causa.
- Essas doenças podem ser diferenciadas por meio de testes diagnósticos (ver adiante).

HEMOGRAMA/BIOQUÍMICA/URINÁLISE
- Na maioria dos pacientes, devem permanecer dentro dos limites de normalidade a menos que haja doença subjacente.
- Em casos de pustulose eosinofílica estéril, pode haver uma eosinofilia circulante.

OUTROS TESTES LABORATORIAIS
Determinados pela causa.

DIAGNÓSTICO POR IMAGEM
N/D.

MÉTODOS DIAGNÓSTICOS
- Raspados cutâneos — identificam possíveis ácaros *Demodex* ou larvas rabditiformes.
- Culturas para pesquisa de dermatófitos — identificam possíveis dermatofitoses.
- Preparações de Tzanck para pústulas (se presentes) — determinam a presença de bactérias e neutrófilos degenerados, compatíveis com foliculite bacteriana; os eosinófilos provavelmente são indicativos de pustulose ou furunculose eosinofílicas.
- Aspirado e citologia do nódulo — identificam a existência de infiltrado celular; presença de microrganismos.
- Biopsia cutânea — útil para determinar o diagnóstico definitivo se os procedimentos diagnósticos basais estiverem normais e/ou se o tratamento empírico inicial for ineficaz.

TRATAMENTO

- Em quase todas as causas, o animal pode ser tratado em um esquema ambulatorial (exceto alguns casos de neoplasia).
- A demodicose generalizada com sepse secundária necessita de hospitalização.
- Não é recomendável nenhuma mudança específica da atividade física ou da dieta.

MEDICAÇÕES

MEDICAMENTO(S) DE ESCOLHA

Foliculite Bacteriana
- Piodermite superficial — devem-se administrar antibióticos apropriados por no mínimo 3-4 semanas ou 1 semana após a resolução dos sinais clínicos, escolhidos com base na cultura bacteriana e no antibiograma.
- Piodermite profunda — devem-se administrar antibióticos adequados por no mínimo 6-8 semanas ou 2 semanas após a resolução dos sinais clínicos, selecionados com base na cultura e no antibiograma.
- Identificar e controlar a causa subjacente para evitar recidivas.
- Ver o capítulo específico em busca de recomendações adicionais.

Adenite Sebácea
- A aplicação de uma mistura de propilenoglicol e água (diluição de 50-75%), uma vez ao dia sob a forma de spray sobre as áreas acometidas é uma medida útil em casos leves.
- Suplementos à base de ácidos graxos essenciais na dieta (VO a cada 12 h), além de óleo de prímula (500 mg VO a cada 12 h).
- Terapia tópica: xampus antisseborreicos, enxágues de emolientes (óleo para bebês) e umectantes.
- Ciclosporina (5 mg/kg VO a cada 12-24 h).
- Vitamina A na dose de 8.000-10.000 UI/9 kg a cada 24 h.
- Casos refratários — isotretinoína (1 mg/kg VO a cada 12-24 h); caso se observe uma resposta, reduzir a dose gradativamente (1 mg/kg a cada 48 h ou 0,5 mg/kg a cada 24 h). Não é fácil aviar os retinoides sintéticos em função dos procedimentos de prescrição muito rigorosos.
- A maioria dos casos mostra-se refratária aos corticosteroides.
- Ver capítulo específico em busca de outras recomendações.

Acnes Canina e Felina
- Nos casos leves, podem desaparecer sem terapia.
- Casos mais graves — xampus e/ou géis de peróxido de benzoíla a cada 24 h até a resolução das lesões; depois, conforme a necessidade.
- Pomada de mupirocina a 2% — antibiótico tópico; aplicar a cada 24 h ou alternar com as terapias à base de peróxido de benzoíla; a mupirocina não deve ser utilizada em gatos com lesões profundas.
- Metronidazol a 0,75% sob a forma de gel diariamente ou com menor frequência, conforme a necessidade.
- Infecção recidivante ou muito profunda (furunculose) — antibióticos sistêmicos e impregnação com água tépida.
- Deve-se buscar a causa subjacente e tratá-la de acordo.
- Quando nenhuma causa subjacente é encontrada, deve-se recorrer ao uso de tampões/compressas à base de clorexidina ou tampões/lenços umedecidos de ácido acético/ácido bórico ou géis de peróxido de benzoíla, diariamente ou em dias alternados; o produto Duoxo® spot-on 2 vezes por semana pode ser útil.
- Os gatos podem ser sensíveis aos efeitos irritantes do peróxido de benzoíla.
- Casos bastante refratários — antibióticos sistêmicos; tretinoína tópica (a cada 12 h) ou isotretinoína (1-2 mg/kg VO a cada 24 h). Não é fácil aviar os retinoides sintéticos em função dos procedimentos de prescrição muito rigorosos.
- Ver capítulo específico em busca de mais recomendações.

Dermatite Rabdítica
- Remover e eliminar a cama do animal.
- Lavar canis, camas e gaiolas, bem como tratar com inseticida ou spray antipulga para a dependência.
- Banhar o animal acometido e remover as crostas.
- Aplicar banho de imersão parasiticida — pelo menos 2 vezes em intervalos semanais.
- Utilizar os corticosteroides, conforme a necessidade, para inflamação.
- Infecção grave — pode necessitar do uso de antibióticos.

DERMATOSES PAPULONODULARES

Dermatite Actínica
- Luz solar — evitar a exposição entre 10 h da manhã e 4 h da tarde; aplicar filtro/protetor com fator de proteção solar ≥15, a cada 12 h.
- Inflamação grave — os corticosteroides tópicos ou sistêmicos podem proporcionar conforto ao animal; a hidrocortisona a 1-2,5% tópica costuma ser suficiente; também se faz uso da prednisona sistêmica (inicialmente, 1 mg/kg VO por 3-5 dias); alguns casos podem necessitar de terapia pulsada contínua.
- Infecção secundária — possivelmente requer o uso de antibióticos.
- Neoplasia associada: hemangioma, hemangiossarcoma e carcinoma de células escamosas — hemangiossarcoma induzido pela luz solar raramente sofre metástase e surge como neoplasia primária; carcinoma de células escamosas — o prognóstico é reservado a mau, dependendo do estágio da doença; a terapia inclui retinoides sintéticos, hipertermia, criocirurgia, fotoquimioterapia, radioterapia e excisão cirúrgica.
- O exame de rotina em intervalos regulares (para triagem dos casos de câncer) é recomendado para identificar e remover as lesões neoplásicas à medida que elas se desenvolvem.

Dermatoses Nodulares Estéreis
- Tentar identificar a causa subjacente.
- Ciclosporina 5 mg/kg VO a cada 24 h (sem alimento 2 h antes e depois da dosagem), reduzindo-a gradativamente de acordo com a resposta.
- Combinações de tetraciclina e niacinamida.
- Corticosteroides em doses imunossupressoras, reduzindo-os de forma gradual de acordo com a resposta.
- Medicamentos quimioterápicos (clorambucila ou azatioprina).

Outras
- Dermatofitose — griseofulvina (50-150 mg/kg VO/dia) ou itraconazol (10 mg/kg VO a cada 24 h) por 3 semanas e, depois, terapia pulsada 2 vezes por semana até a resolução das lesões; ver também o capítulo específico.
- Pustulose eosinofílica estéril — prednisolona/prednisona (2,2-4,4 mg/kg a cada 24 h; depois, reduzir gradativamente para uma dosagem inferior em dias alternados).
- Quérion — ver "Dermatofitose".
- Demodicose — ver o capítulo específico.
- Neoplasia — ver o capítulo específico.

CONTRAINDICAÇÕES
Em casos de foliculite, dermatofitose, quérions e demodicose, é recomendável evitar o uso de corticosteroides e outros imunossupressores.

PRECAUÇÕES
- Ácidos graxos — utilizar com cuidado em cães com enteropatia inflamatória ou surtos recidivantes de pancreatite.
- Isotretinoína — pode causar ceratoconjuntivite seca, hiperatividade, prurido otológico, junção mucocutânea eritematosa, letargia com vômito, distensão e eritema abdominais, anorexia com letargia, colapso e língua edemaciada; as anormalidades do hemograma completo e da bioquímica sérica incluem contagem plaquetária alta, hipertrigliceridemia, hipercolesterolemia e atividade elevada da alanina transaminase.
- Ciclosporina — pode causar vômito e diarreia, hiperplasia da gengiva e dos linfócitos B, hirsutismo, lesões cutâneas papilomatosas e alta incidência de infecções; as reações tóxicas potenciais são aparentemente raras e englobam nefro/hepatotoxicidade.

INTERAÇÕES POSSÍVEIS
- Como a ciclosporina e os corticosteroides podem interagir com diversos medicamentos, é aconselhável a consulta de um compêndio ou bulário antes do uso.
- Na prescrição de medicamentos as quais o clínico não está familiarizado, é recomendável a consulta de um compêndio ou bulário.

MEDICAMENTO(S) ALTERNATIVO(S)
N/D.

ACOMPANHAMENTO

MONITORIZAÇÃO DO PACIENTE
- Hemograma completo, perfil bioquímico e urinálise — obter os valores de referência (basais) e, depois, monitorizar a cada 4-6 meses em pacientes submetidos à ciclosporina.
- Hemograma completo, perfil bioquímico e urinálise/urocultura — obter os valores de referência (basais) e, depois, monitorizar a cada 4-6 meses em pacientes submetidos a corticosteroides.
- Hemograma completo, perfil bioquímico e urinálise — monitorizar mensalmente por 4-6 meses em pacientes submetidos à terapia com retinoides sintéticos.
- Produção lacrimal — verificar mensalmente por 4-6 meses e, depois, a cada 6 meses em pacientes submetidos à terapia com retinoides sintéticos.
- Raspados cutâneos — monitorizar a terapia em pacientes com demodicose (ver "Demodicose").
- Repetir as culturas fúngicas — acompanhar a terapia em pacientes com dermatofitose (ver "Dermatofitose").
- Resolução das lesões — analisar a evolução dos quadros de adenite sebácea, distúrbios actínicos e todas as outras doenças.

COMPLICAÇÕES POSSÍVEIS
A dermatite actínica pode evoluir para neoplasia franca, inclusive carcinoma de células escamosas.

DIVERSOS

DISTÚRBIOS ASSOCIADOS
N/D.

FATORES RELACIONADOS COM A IDADE
N/D.

POTENCIAL ZOONÓTICO
Dermatofitose — em seres humanos, relata-se uma incidência de 30-50% dos casos de *Microsporum canis*.

GESTAÇÃO/FERTILIDADE/REPRODUÇÃO
- Retinoides sintéticos — teratogênicos; não usar em animais prenhes, naqueles destinados à reprodução ou em fêmeas intactas; não devem ser manipulados por mulheres em idade fértil.
- Corticosteroides — evitar o uso em animais prenhes.
- Ciclosporina — evitar durante a gestação a menos que seja absolutamente necessária; dosagens de 2 a 5 vezes o normal são feto/embriotóxicas em ratos e coelhos.

VER TAMBÉM
- Acne — Gatos.
- Acne — Cães.
- Demodicose.
- Dermatofitose.
- Piodermite.
- Adenite Sebácea Granulomatosa.

Sugestões de Leitura
Griffin CE, Kwochka KW, MacDonald JM, eds. Current Veterinary Dermatology. St. Louis: Mosby, 1993.
Gross TL, Ihrke PJ, Walder EJ. Veterinary Dermatopathology, 2nd ed. St. Louis: Mosby, 2005.
Medleau LA, Hnilica KA. Small Animal Dermatology: A Color Atlas and Therapeutic Guide. St. Louis: Saunders, 2006.
Scott DW, Miller WH, Griffin CE. Muller & Kirk's Small Animal Dermatology, 6th ed. Philadelphia: Saunders, 2001.

Autor Karen A. Kuhl
Consultor Editorial Alexander H. Werner

DERMATOSES VESICULOPUSTULARES

CONSIDERAÇÕES GERAIS

DEFINIÇÃO
• Pústula — elevação pequena e circunscrita da epiderme, preenchida com pus.
• Vesícula — elevação pequena e circunscrita da epiderme, preenchida com líquido translúcido.

FISIOPATOLOGIA
Pústulas e vesículas — produzidas por edema, acantólise (pênfigo), degeneração balonosa (infecções virais), enzimas proteolíticas liberadas pelos neutrófilos (piodermite), degeneração de células basais (lúpus) ou separação dermoepidérmica (penfigoide bolhoso).

SISTEMA(S) ACOMETIDO(S)
Cutâneo/exócrino.

IDENTIFICAÇÃO
• Lúpus — as raças Collie, Pastor de Shetland e Pastor alemão podem ser predispostas.
• Pênfigo eritematoso — as raças Collie e Pastor alemão podem ser predispostas.
• Pênfigo foliáceo — as raças Akita, Chow chow, Dachshund, Bearded collie, Terra Nova, Doberman pinscher e Schipperkes podem ser predispostas.
• Penfigoide bolhoso — as raças Collie e Doberman pinscher podem ser predispostas
• Dermatomiosite — acomete cães jovens pertencentes às raças Collie e pastor de Shetland.
• Dermatose pustulosa subcórnea — a raça Schnauzer é acometida com maior frequência.
• Dermatose linear por IgA — ocorre exclusivamente em Dachshund.
• Dermatofitose — acomete animais jovens.

SINAIS CLÍNICOS
N/D.

CAUSAS
Pústulas/Vesículas
• Piodermite superficial — impetigo, piodermite disseminada superficial, foliculite bacteriana superficial, acne canina ou felina.
• Complexo pênfigo — pênfigo foliáceo, pênfigo eritematoso, pênfigo pan-epidérmico.
• Dermatose pustulosa subcórnea.
• Dermatofitose.
• Demodicose.
• Pustulose eosinofílica estéril.
• Dermatose linear por IgA.
• LES.
• LED.
• Penfigoide bolhoso.
• Pênfigo vulgar.
• Dermatomiosite.
• Erupção medicamentosa cutânea.
• Epidermólise bolhosa.

FATORES DE RISCO
• Exposição medicamentosa — LES e penfigoide bolhoso.
• A foliculite bacteriana costuma ser secundária a algum fator predisponente (p. ex., demodicose, hipotireoidismo, alergia ou administração de corticosteroide).
• Luz solar (ultravioleta) — pênfigo eritematoso, penfigoide bolhoso, LES, LED e dermatomiosite.

DIAGNÓSTICO

DIAGNÓSTICO DIFERENCIAL
Piodermites Superficiais
• Causa mais comum.
• Caso se trate a causa subjacente de forma eficaz, a resposta à antibioticoterapia apropriada será imediata.
• Pústula intacta — o esfregaço direto revela a fagocitose de bactérias por neutrófilos; a cultura, em geral, recupera o *Staphylococcus pseudintermedius*; a biopsia demonstra pústulas neutrofílicas intraepidérmicas ou foliculite.

Complexo Pênfigo
• Trata-se de um grupo de doenças imunomediadas, caracterizadas por células acantolíticas (falta de adesão dos queratinócitos na epiderme) ao exame histológico.
• Esfregaços diretos — muitas células acantolíticas, neutrófilos não degenerados e nenhuma bactéria.
• Cultura de pústula intacta — negativa.
• Imunofluorescência direta — depósitos nos espaços intercelulares da epiderme em aproximadamente 50% dos casos.
• Tende a aumentar e diminuir, independentemente da antibioticoterapia; responde à terapia imunossupressora.

Dermatose Pustulosa Subcórnea
• Dermatose pustulosa idiopática rara dos cães.
• Tende a aumentar e diminuir.
• Pústulas intactas — os esfregaços diretos revelam inúmeros neutrófilos, nenhuma bactéria e células acantolíticas ocasionais; as culturas permanecem negativas.
• Imunofluorescência direta — negativa.
• Resposta insatisfatória a glicocorticosteroides e antibióticos.

Dermatofitose
• Doença comum tanto de cães como de gatos.
• Cultura positiva para dermatófitos.
• É comum a ocorrência de foliculite bacteriana secundária.
• Biopsia cutânea — foliculite com elementos fúngicos.

Pustulose Eosinofílica Estéril
• Dermatose idiopática rara dos cães.
• Esfregaços diretos — revelam inúmeros eosinófilos, neutrófilos não degenerados, células acantolíticas ocasionais e nenhuma bactéria.
• Biopsia cutânea — pústulas intraepidérmicas eosinofílicas, foliculite e furunculose.
• Imunofluorescência direta negativa.
• Resposta rápida a glicocorticosteroides.

Dermatose Linear por IgA
• Dermatose idiopática rara dos cães da raça Dachshund.
• Tende a aumentar e diminuir.
• Pústulas — estéreis e subcorneais.
• Imunofluorescência direta positiva quanto à presença de IgA na zona da membrana basal.

LES
• Doença multissistêmica com sinais clínicos e manifestações cutâneas variáveis, incluindo ulceração mucocutânea.
• Imunofluorescência direta positiva na zona da membrana basal.
• AAN positivo.

LED
• Acomete apenas a pele; as lesões costumam ficar confinadas à face.
• Despigmentação, eritema e ulceração do plano nasal — são comuns.
• Biopsia cutânea — dermatite de interface.
• Imunofluorescência direta positiva na zona da membrana basal.
• AAN negativo.

Penfigoide Bolhoso
• Distúrbio ulcerativo da pele e/ou das mucosas.
• Biopsia cutânea — formação de fenda subepidérmica.
• Imunofluorescência direta positiva na zona da membrana basal.
• Não se observa acantólise.

Pênfigo Vulgar
• Forma mais grave de pênfigo.
• Caracterizado por ulceração da cavidade bucal, da junção mucocutânea e da pele.
• Biopsia cutânea — presença de acantólise suprabasal e formação de fenda.
• Imunofluorescência direta positiva nos espaços intercelulares da epiderme.

Dermatomiosite
• Doença inflamatória idiopática da pele e dos músculos de cães jovens das raças Collie e Pastor de Shetland.
• As lesões acometem a face, a ponta das orelhas, a extremidade da cauda e os pontos de compressão dos membros.
• Caracterizada por alopecia, formação de crostas e cicatrizes, bem como por distúrbios de pigmentação, além de erosões/ulceração.
• Biopsia cutânea — atrofia folicular, perifoliculite e degeneração hidrópica das células basais.
• Imunofluorescência direta negativa.
• Biopsia muscular e EMG — evidências de inflamação.

HEMOGRAMA/BIOQUÍMICA/URINÁLISE
• Os resultados geralmente não são dignos de nota.
• LES — possível desenvolvimento de anemia, trombocitopenia ou glomerulonefrite.
• Dermatose pustulosa eosinofílica — a maioria dos cães acometidos apresenta eosinofilia periférica.

OUTROS TESTES LABORATORIAIS
N/D.

DIAGNÓSTICO POR IMAGEM
N/D.

MÉTODOS DIAGNÓSTICOS
• Esfregaço direto a partir de pústulas/vesículas intactas.
• Cultura de pústulas/vesículas intactas.
• Biopsia cutânea para exame histopatológico.
• Imunofluorescência direta, incluindo IgA.
• Título do AAN.
• EMG.
• Biopsia muscular.

TRATAMENTO

CUIDADO(S) DE SAÚDE ADEQUADO(S)
• Banhos periódicos com xampus antimicrobianos — ajudam a remover os debris superficiais e a controlar a foliculite bacteriana secundária.

Dermatoses Vesiculopustulares

- Em geral, o tratamento é feito em um esquema ambulatorial.
- LES, pênfigo vulgar e penfigoide bolhoso — podem ser potencialmente letais e necessitar de cuidados terapêuticos intensivos com internação.

MEDICAÇÕES

MEDICAMENTO(S) DE ESCOLHA

Foliculite Bacteriana
- Escolhas empíricas: cefalexina 22 mg/kg a cada 12 h; clindamicina 5,5 mg/kg a cada 12 h; amoxicilina-ácido clavulânico 15 mg/kg a cada 12 h.
- Selecionados com base nos resultados das culturas de pústulas intactas.

Complexo Pênfigo/Penfigoide Bolhoso
- Medicamentos quimioterápicos: azatioprina ou clorambucila.
- Combinação de tetraciclina e niacinamida.
- Ciclosporina.

Dermatose Pustulosa Subcórnea
- Dapsona — 1 mg/kg VO a cada 8 h até a remissão (em geral, 1-4 semanas); depois, reduzir a dose gradativamente para 1 mg/kg a cada 24 h ou 2 vezes por semana.
- Sulfassalazina (Azulfidine®) — 10-20 mg/kg VO a cada 8 h até a remissão; em seguida, conforme a necessidade.

Dermatose Linear por IgA
- Prednisolona — 2,2-4,4 mg/kg VO a cada 24 h até a remissão; depois, diminuir gradativamente para uma terapia em dias alternados.
- Dapsona — 1 mg/kg VO a cada 8 h até a remissão; em seguida, reduzir de modo gradativo e administrar conforme a necessidade; os pacientes podem responder individualmente a um medicamento, mas não a outro.

Pustulose Eosinofílica Estéril
- Prednisolona: 2,2-4,4 mg/kg VO a cada 24 h até a remissão (em geral, 5-10 dias); posteriormente, conforme a necessidade, para evitar recidivas (em geral, exige-se uma terapia a longo prazo em dias alternados).
- Ver doenças específicas.

CONTRAINDICAÇÕES
N/D.

PRECAUÇÕES

Prednisolona
- Infecções secundárias.
- Doença de Cushing iatrogênica.
- Emaciação muscular.
- Hepatopatia por esteroides.
- Mudanças comportamentais.
- Polidipsia, poliúria.
- Polifagia.

Dapsona
- Cães — observam-se quadros leves de anemia, leucopenia e elevação da ALT, não associados aos sinais clínicos; tais alterações costumam retornar ao normal ao se reduzir a dosagem para manutenção.
- Ocasionalmente, verificam-se trombocitopenia fatal ou leucopenia grave.
- Vômito, diarreia ou erupção cutânea pruriginosa ocasionais.
- Gatos — mais suscetíveis à intoxicação por dapsona; há relatos de anemia hemolítica e neurotoxicidade.

Sulfassalazina
- Ceratoconjuntivite seca.

INTERAÇÕES POSSÍVEIS
N/D.

MEDICAMENTO(S) ALTERNATIVO(S)
N/D.

ACOMPANHAMENTO

MONITORIZAÇÃO DO PACIENTE
- Dapsona — monitorizar o hemograma completo, a contagem plaquetária e a ALT a cada 2 semanas inicialmente e caso se desenvolva qualquer efeito colateral clínico.
- Terapia a longo prazo com a sulfassalazina — verificar a produção lacrimal.
- Terapia imunossupressora — acompanhar a cada 1-2 semanas inicialmente; depois, a cada 3-4 meses durante a terapia de manutenção.

COMPLICAÇÕES POSSÍVEIS
N/D.

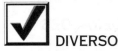

DIVERSOS

DISTÚRBIOS ASSOCIADOS
N/D.

FATORES RELACIONADOS COM A IDADE
N/D.

POTENCIAL ZOONÓTICO
Dermatofitose: as lesões podem se desenvolver em seres humanos que convivem com o animal na mesma casa.

GESTAÇÃO/FERTILIDADE/REPRODUÇÃO
N/D.

VER TAMBÉM
- Acne — Cães.
- Acne — Gatos.
- Dermatomiosite.
- Dermatofitose.
- Lúpus Eritematoso Cutâneo (Discoide).
- Lúpus Eritematoso Sistêmico.
- Pênfigo.
- Piodermite.

ABREVIATURA(S)
- AAN = anticorpo antinuclear.
- ALT = alanina aminotransferase.
- EMG = eletromiografia.
- LED = lúpus eritematoso discoide.
- LES = lúpus eritematoso sistêmico.

Sugestões de Leitura
Muller GH, Kirk RW, Scott DW. Small Animal Dermatology, 4th ed. Philadelphia: Saunders, 1989.

Autor Karen Helton Rhodes
Consultor Editorial Alexander H. Werner

DERMATOSES VIRAIS

CONSIDERAÇÕES GERAIS

REVISÃO
• Dermatoses causadas por infecção viral dentro de estruturas queratinizadas.
• A replicação viral dentro de estruturas queratinizadas pode causar efeitos citossupressores ou suprarregular a queratinização, resultando em problemas hiperplásicos ou crostosos.

IDENTIFICAÇÃO
Cães e gatos
• Dermatoses incomuns.
• Não há relatos de predileções raciais, sexuais ou geográficas.
• Não há base genética para essas doenças.
• De filhotes a cães jovens adultos.
• Gatos de qualquer idade.

SINAIS CLÍNICOS
• É comum o envolvimento da face ou da cabeça.
• Pés e/ou coxins palmoplantares podem ser acometidos.
• Início agudo ou gradual; as lesões podem ser associadas ao histórico de ferida por mordida ou briga.
• Prurido variável.
• Crostas.
• Foliculite bacteriana superficial associada.
• Abscesso.
• Paroníquia.
• Cicatrização deficiente de ferida.
• Seborreia.
• Dermatite esfoliativa.
• Cornos cutâneos.
• Gengivite/estomatite.
• Ulceração cutânea ou bucal.
• Hiperqueratose nasodigital.
• Máculas ou placas pigmentadas.
• Evolução para carcinoma bowenoide *in situ* (papilomavírus).

CAUSAS
• Infecção pelo vírus da leucemia felina.
• Infecção pelo vírus da imunodeficiência felina.
• Infecção pelo vírus cowpox felino.
• Peritonite infecciosa felina.
• Papilomavírus felino.
• Papilomavírus canino.
• Cinomose canina.
• Dermatite pustular viral contagiosa (parapoxvírus).
• Pseudorraiva.
• Infecção por rinotraqueíte felina.
• Infecção por calicivírus felino.
• Comportamento de briga ou caça, exposição a animais infectados e/ou ingestão de material contaminado aumenta o risco de exposição.

DIAGNÓSTICO

DIAGNÓSTICO DIFERENCIAL
• Doenças crostosas — se a formação de crostas anteceder outros sintomas, considerar erupção medicamentosa, pênfigo foliáceo, lúpus eritematoso sistêmico e causas de dermatite esfoliativa.
• Distúrbios alérgicos — se o prurido for o sinal clínico inicial, considerar dermatite alérgica à pulga, reação adversa cutânea aos alimentos, ou dermatite atópica.
• Doenças parasitárias — escabiose, demodicose, queiletielose canina e/ou felina.
• Doenças infecciosas — infecções bacterianas e fúngicas superficiais e profundas, leishmaniose.
• Cães — síndromes de deficiência de zinco, síndrome hepatocutânea, hiperqueratose nasal.
• Neoplasia — em caso de formação extensa de crostas e úlceras, considerar mastocitomas e linfoma epiteliotrópico.

HEMOGRAMA/BIOQUÍMICA/URINÁLISE
Normais.

OUTROS TESTES LABORATORIAIS
• Biopsia cutânea — necessária para demonstrar a origem viral das lesões na pele.
• Isolamento viral.
• Sorologia — confirma a presença de infecção por FeLV, FIV ou outros agentes virais.

DIAGNÓSTICO POR IMAGEM
N/D.

MÉTODOS DIAGNÓSTICOS
• Raspados cutâneos e tricogramas — infestações parasitárias.
• Cultura de dermatófitos — infecções fúngicas.
• Citologia da epiderme — foliculite bacteriana.
• A biopsia cutânea é o teste diagnóstico definitivo.
• Coloração imuno-histoquímica para pesquisa de partículas virais.
• Sorologia viral.

ACHADOS PATOLÓGICOS
• Hiperplasia.
• Degeneração balonosa.
• Dermatite de interface do tipo hidrópica.
• Formação de células gigantes sinciciais dentro da epiderme e/ou da bainha radicular externa do folículo piloso.
• Corpúsculos de inclusão em queratinócitos.

TRATAMENTO

• O tratamento geralmente é ambulatorial, exceto para os pacientes com doença sistêmica.
• Evitar a exposição a outros animais que podem vir a ser infectados.

MEDICAÇÕES

MEDICAMENTO(S) DE ESCOLHA
• Cuidados de suporte e tratamento de infecções secundárias.
• Gatos — herpes-vírus: L-lisina 200-500 mg/gato a cada 12 h; alfainterferona 30 unidades/gato/dia VO.
• Gatos — carcinoma bowenoide *in situ*: imiquimode tópico.
• Cães — papilomavírus; alfainterferona 1,5 MU por via SC 3 vezes por semana.

CONTRAINDICAÇÕES
Corticosteroides ou outras terapias que causam imunossupressão.

ACOMPANHAMENTO

PREVENÇÃO
Evitar não só o comportamento de caça, mas também a exposição a materiais potencialmente infecciosos e animais infectados.

COMPLICAÇÕES POSSÍVEIS
Bacteremia e septicemia.

EVOLUÇÃO ESPERADA E PROGNÓSTICO
• As lesões cutâneas podem não responder à terapia.
• Por fim, pode ocorrer o desenvolvimento de sinais sistêmicos como resultado da infecção viral.
• Dependendo do agente viral causal, os animais podem se curar espontaneamente.
• A infecção pelo papilomavírus pode evoluir para carcinoma bowenoide *in situ*.

DIVERSOS

DISTÚRBIOS ASSOCIADOS
N/D.

POTENCIAL ZOONÓTICO
Considerações zoonóticas — o vírus cowpox felino e a dermatite pustular viral contagiosa (parapoxvírus) podem ser transmitidos não só para seres humanos, mas também para outros cães e gatos.

VER TAMBÉM
• Papilomatose.
• Doenças das vias aéreas superiores — gatos.
• Infecções virais — gatos.
• Infecções virais — cães.

ABREVIATURAS
• FeLV = vírus da leucemia felina.
• FIV = vírus da imunodeficiência felina.

Sugestões de Leitura
Scott DW, Miller WH, Griffin CE. Muller & Kirk's Small Animal Dermatology, 6th ed. Philadelphia: Saunders, 2001.

Autor Elizabeth R. May
Consultor Editorial Alexander H. Werner

Descolamento da Retina

 CONSIDERAÇÕES GERAIS

DEFINIÇÃO
Qualquer separação da retina neural do epitélio pigmentar retiniano.

FISIOPATOLOGIA
• Espaço sub-retiniano — um espaço potencial entre o epitélio pigmentar retiniano e a retina neural, onde se acumulam líquidos ou exsudatos. • Classificada por sua etiopatogenia — um dos mecanismos a seguir ou uma combinação do mecanismo regmatógeno (laceração da retina), exsudação sub-retiniana ou tração.

Regmatógena
• Laceração ou orifício na retina, que pode estar relacionada com fatores como idade, presença de cataratas, tração por debris inflamatórios, traumatismo ou degeneração da retina. O humor vítreo se desloca para o espaço sub-retiniano, o que resulta no descolamento da retina. Provavelmente constitui o tipo predominante que ocorre em associação a cataratas e após cirurgia dessa afecção. Requer alguma anormalidade vítrea (p. ex., liquefação, tração).

Exsudativa
• O líquido se acumula no espaço sub-retiniano por causa da ruptura da barreira hematorretiniana. • Líquido sub-retiniano — pode ser seroso, hemorrágico ou exsudativo (p. ex., granulomatoso nos pacientes com blastomicose). • Fatores patogênicos hematógenos/sistêmicos — comuns. • Vasculite, hipertensão e hiperviscosidade — podem provocar descolamento seroso com ou sem hemorragia.

Tração
• Tração por tecido fibroso ou fibrovascular; descola a retina do epitélio pigmentar retiniano subjacente e/ou pode provocar um orifício ou uma laceração na retina. • Pode ser associada a traumatismo, corpos estranhos intraoculares ou qualquer causa de inflamação vítrea grave.

SISTEMA(S) ACOMETIDO(S)
• Nervoso — cães com meningoencefalomielite granulomatosa frequentemente desenvolverão sintomas neurológicos. • Oftálmico — retina. • Pode ser uma manifestação de alguma doença sistêmica.

GENÉTICA
Depende da causa — cães com cataratas hereditárias ou luxações do cristalino podem desenvolver descolamento regmatógeno. Algumas raças podem apresentar laceração e descolamento da retina por anormalidades vítreas primárias.

INCIDÊNCIA/PREVALÊNCIA
• Exsudativo — mais comum em cães e gatos. • Regmatógeno — mais comum nos cães por causa da prevalência maior de cataratas e de cirurgia dessa afecção.

IDENTIFICAÇÃO

Espécies
Cães e gatos.

Raça(s) Predominante(s)
• Depende da causa. • Raças tipo Terrier — predispostas à luxação primária do cristalino, a qual pode contribuir para a laceração e o descolamento da retina com ou sem cirurgia. • Raças que podem desenvolver cataratas. • Raças Shih tzu, Boston terrier, Galgo italiano — parecem ser predispostas a descolamentos regmatógenos espontâneos atribuídos a vítreo liquefeito anormal. • Cães com coloração merle da pelagem: Pastor australiano, Pastor de Shetland, Dogue alemão arlequim, Collie. • Raças que podem ter displasia grave da retina: Springer spaniel, Labrador, Bedlington terrier. • Raças com retinopatia grave (também conhecida como displasia do epitélio pigmentar retiniano, retinopatia multifocal canina): Grande Pirineu, Mastiff, Coton de Tulear.

Idade Média e Faixa Etária
• Dependem da causa. • Pacientes mais idosos — cataratas e doenças sistêmicas (p. ex., hipertensão, neoplasia e doença imunomediada) estão frequentemente relacionadas com a idade. • Cães jovens: acometidos por displasia grave da retina, retinopatia multifocal canina.

SINAIS CLÍNICOS
• Cegueira ou visão reduzida no olho acometido. • Pupila dilatada com reflexo pupilar à luz lento ou ausente. O reflexo pupilar à luz pode estar quase normal se o descolamento for agudo. • Em geral, podem ser observados vasos sanguíneos com uma "membrana" (que corresponde à retina) com facilidade por meio da pupila, imediatamente atrás do cristalino. • Anormalidades vítreas — moscas volantes*, hemorragia ou sinérese (liquefação); comuns. • Interrupção ou alteração do curso dos vasos sanguíneos em virtude de elevação da retina. • Com líquido sub-retiniano claro — os vasos podem produzir sombras. • Com líquido exsudativo ou sangue, o tapete pode não ser visualizado. • Outros sintomas dependerão de quaisquer doenças sistêmicas subjacentes. • Ver "Coriorretinite" em busca dos sinais de inflamação. Retinopatia multifocal canina: lesões multifocais elevadas de cor cinza a castanha (descolamentos focais) de tamanho variado. Começa em torno de 11 meses de vida, mas evolui com o passar do tempo.

CAUSAS
Bilateral — sugere algum problema sistêmico induzido pela ruptura da barreira hematorretiniana.

Degenerativas
• Degeneração retiniana progressiva em estágio final — pode levar à formação de orifício na retina e descolamento dessa estrutura ocular: ver "Degeneração da Retina".

Anômalas
• Colobomas — anomalia do olho do Collie: retina anormal em torno de nervo óptico colobomatoso ou grandes estafilomas coroidais podem levar a descolamentos regmatógenos; raças Border collie, Pastor australiano e outras raças cujos cães possuem pelagens merles (disgenesia ocular merle). • Anomalias oculares múltiplas — Akita ou em qualquer raça. • Displasia grave da retina — displasia oculosquelética nas raças Labrador retriever e Samoieda; displasia da retina: Springer spaniel inglês e Bedlington terrier. • Retinopatia multifocal canina — suspeitar de displasia do epitélio pigmentar retiniano; Grande Pirineu, Mastiff, Coton de Tulear.

---

* N. T.: As moscas volantes são minúsculos grumos de gel ou células dentro do corpo vítreo, o líquido gelatinoso, que preenche o interior do olho.

Metabólicas
• Hipotireoidismo. • Hiperviscosidade. • Policitemia. • Hipoxia com complicações hemorrágicas. • Cães — hipertensão sistêmica (qualquer causa como insuficiência renal ou feocromocitoma), hipotireoidismo, hipercolesterolemia e hiperproteinemia (p. ex., com mieloma múltiplo). • Gatos — muito frequentemente causado por hipertensão sistêmica como condição primária ou secundária à insuficiência renal ou a hipertireoidismo. Mieloma múltiplo e tumores adrenais também podem causar descolamento da retina em virtude de hiperviscosidade ou hipertensão.

Neoplásicas
• Qualquer neoplasia primária ou metastática. • Comumente associadas a mieloma múltiplo, linfoma, meningoencefalite granulomatosa e massas intraoculares — adenocarcinoma ou melanoma do corpo ciliar. • Hipertensão secundária a tumores adrenais como feocromocitoma; rara.

Infecciosas
• Retinite ou coriorretinite infecciosa — pode provocar descolamento focal ou difuso. • A infecção pode se estender a partir do SNC ou até essa região do corpo. • Ver "Coriorretinite".

Imunomediadas/Inflamatórias
• Doença por imunocomplexo — pode provocar vasculite ou inflamação, que resulta em descolamento exsudativo. • Cães — LES; síndrome uveodermatológica. • Gatos — periarterite nodosa; LES.

Idiopáticas
• Se todas as outras causas forem descartadas, incluindo lacerações da retina. • Descolamento idiopático responsivo a esteroide — relatado em cães pertencentes a raças gigantes, embora possa ocorrer em qualquer raça.

Traumáticas e Tóxicas
• Bilateral — provavelmente nunca ocorre. • Lesão penetrante no corpo estranho que cause lacerações retinianas ou hemorragia intraocular — pode provocar descolamento parcial ou completo. • Traumatismo rombo grave com inflamação ou hemorragia. • Traumatismo cirúrgico — pode contribuir para a laceração da retina. • Tóxica — reações idiossincrásicas a medicamentos (p. ex., trimetoprima-sulfa em cães, griseofulvina em gatos).

FATORES DE RISCO
• Hipertensão sistêmica. • Idade avançada: adelgaçamento da retina, degeneração vítrea grave. • Cataratas hipermaduras. • Cristalinos luxados. • Extração do cristalino. • Hereditários: cães jovens que apresentam displasia mais grave da retina e/ou múltiplas anomalias oculares.

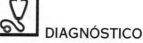 **DIAGNÓSTICO**

DIAGNÓSTICO DIFERENCIAL
• Cegueira ou visão prejudicada — neurite óptica; glaucoma; cataratas; atrofia progressiva da retina; SDSAR (ver "Degeneração da Retina"); doença do SNC.
• Pupila dilatada com reflexos pupilares à luz lentos ou ausentes — glaucoma; lesão do nervo oculomotor; neurite óptica; atrofia progressiva da retina; SDSAR.

Descolamento da Retina

- Membrana ou vasos associados ao cristalino ou atrás dessa estrutura ocular — túnica vascular persistente do cristalino; membranas pupilares persistentes; membrana fibrovascular secundária à neoplasia ou inflamação intraoculares.

HEMOGRAMA/BIOQUÍMICA/URINÁLISE
- Tipicamente normais se o problema estiver confinado ao olho.
- Anormalidades compatíveis com algum processo mórbido sistêmico associado.

OUTROS TESTES LABORATORIAIS
- Dependem do problema sistêmico sob suspeita.
- Eletroforese de proteínas.
- Constatação da proteína de Bence-Jones na urina.
- Perfil de coagulação.
- Cultura bacteriana de líquidos oculares ou corporais.
- Mensuração dos hormônios tireoidianos.
- Teste sorológico para doenças infecciosas — ver "Coriorretinite".

DIAGNÓSTICO POR IMAGEM
- Radiografias toracoabdominais e ultrassonografia abdominal — pesquisa de linfadenopatia, neoplasia primária, doença metastática ou infiltrados compatíveis com agentes infecciosos.
- Radiografias da coluna vertebral — podem revelar alterações ósseas compatíveis com mieloma múltiplo.
- Ultrassom ocular — identifica descolamentos da retina, presença de massas intraoculares e, às vezes, luxações do cristalino; valioso se o meio intraocular não estiver límpido.
- Ultrassom cardíaco — indicado para gatos com retinopatia hipertensiva.

MÉTODOS DIAGNÓSTICOS
- Exame oftalmológico.
- Mensuração isolada ou repetida da pressão arterial — pode revelar hipertensão; em geral, a pressão arterial média em cães e gatos é <160 mmHg.
- Punção do LCS — indicada nos sinais de doença do SNC ou neurite óptica.
- Vitreocentese ou aspirado do líquido sub--retiniano — podem ser realizados quando outros testes diagnósticos falharem na obtenção de uma causa e caso se suspeite de algum agente infeccioso ou neoplasia; podem agravar a inflamação ou induzir à hemorragia.

ACHADOS PATOLÓGICOS
- Retina separada do epitélio pigmentar retiniano e da coroide subjacente.
- Pode-se notar a presença de massas ou exsudato sub-retiniano ou do agente infeccioso etiológico.
- Caso crônico — resulta em atrofia da retina e aparência de lápide ao epitélio pigmentar retiniano.

TRATAMENTO
CUIDADO(S) DE SAÚDE ADEQUADO(S)
- Depende da condição física do paciente.
- O paciente costuma ser tratado em um esquema ambulatorial.
- Cegueira aguda — a visão poderá ser restaurada se a causa subjacente for rapidamente identificada e tratada; fazer todas as tentativas para determinar a causa.
- A degeneração ocorre com rapidez — fornecer o tratamento o mais rápido possível após o diagnóstico.
- Regmatógeno — o oftalmologista está capacitado a fornecer o tratamento cirúrgico.

ORIENTAÇÃO AO PROPRIETÁRIO
- Explicar que o descolamento da retina pode ser um sinal de doença sistêmica e, por essa razão, é importante a realização de testes diagnósticos.
- Informar ao proprietário que o descolamento da retina associado à luxação do cristalino ou cirurgia de catarata é potencialmente bilateral.
- Explicar ao proprietário sobre a possível ocorrência de retorno da visão em casos de descolamento da retina de curta duração se a causa subjacente for tratada.
- Avisar o proprietário que os animais de companhia cegos, sobretudo os gatos, podem se adaptar notavelmente bem e ter boa qualidade de vida (ver "Degeneração da Retina").

CONSIDERAÇÕES CIRÚRGICAS
- Regmatógeno — pode ser submetido a reparo cirúrgico; encaminhar o paciente para um oftalmologista.
- Retinopexia a laser — pode reverter descolamentos associados a colobomas do disco óptico acompanhados de anomalia do olho do Collie; pode estabilizar descolamentos parciais/pequenos.

MEDICAÇÕES
MEDICAMENTO(S) DE ESCOLHA
- Dependem das causas sistêmicas subjacentes, as quais devem ser devidamente identificadas e tratadas.
- Prednisona sistêmica — 2 mg/kg divididos a cada 12 h por 3-10 dias e, em seguida, reduzir de forma gradativa; utilizada caso se descarte uma micose sistêmica e se o descolamento for supostamente imunomediado; pode facilitar a nova fixação da retina; em casos de doença imunomediada, reduzir muito lentamente as medicações, durante meses.
- Doses anti-inflamatórias de prednisona — 0,5 mg/kg e, em seguida, reduzir de forma gradual; podem ser valiosas nos descolamentos exsudativos de natureza infecciosa contanto que a doença subjacente esteja sendo definitivamente tratada.
- Agentes anti-hipertensivos — anlodipino na dose de 0,5-1,0 mg/kg VO a cada 24 h em cães e 0,625-1,25 mg em gatos. Outros agentes como propranolol podem ser usados se o anlodipino falhar no controle da hipertensão. Enalapril (0,25-0,5 mg/kg a cada 12-24 h) ou benazepril (0,25-0,5 mg/kg a cada 24 h) para gatos com hipertensão irresponsiva ao anlodipino isolado; esses agentes também podem ser importantes em gatos com insuficiência renal e proteinúria. Consultar algum especialista em medicina interna. Ver as seções sobre "Insuficiência Renal".

CONTRAINDICAÇÕES
Corticosteroides sistêmicos — não utilizar a menos que a micose sistêmica esteja descartada ou definitivamente tratada.

MEDICAMENTO(S) ALTERNATIVO(S)
- Agentes quimioterápicos — sugeridos para o tratamento de condições neoplásicas.
- Azatioprina — cães, 2 mg/kg VO a cada 24 h inicialmente e, em seguida, 0,5-1,0 mg/kg a cada 48 h; para controlar a inflamação; pode ser necessária em adição aos esteroides na síndrome uveodermatológica ou no descolamento imunomediado idiopático.
- Ciclosporina oral: cães, 5 mg/kg/dia pode ser eficaz em alguns descolamentos imunomediados da retina; i. e., síndrome uveodermatológica.

ACOMPANHAMENTO
MONITORIZAÇÃO DO PACIENTE
- Azatioprina — obter inicialmente o hemograma completo, em seguida a cada 1-2 semanas nos primeiros 1-3 meses; monitorizar a cada 1-2 meses quanto à ocorrência de supressão da medula óssea (se notada, reduzir a dose ou interrompê-la). Obter os perfis bioquímicos logo no início e na fase de acompanhamento para avaliar a presença de toxicidade do fígado ou do pâncreas.
- Monitorizar a pressão arterial nos casos com hipertensão.

COMPLICAÇÕES POSSÍVEIS
- Cegueira permanente. • Cataratas. • Glaucoma.
- Dor ocular crônica. • Morte em caso de descolamento da retina secundário a algum processo mórbido sistêmico/neoplásico.

EVOLUÇÃO ESPERADA E PROGNÓSTICO
- Prognóstico para visão no caso de descolamento completo — reservado. Como exceção, temos a retinopatia hipertensiva, que é diagnosticada e tratada adequadamente.
- Cegueira — pode se desenvolver em dias a semanas, ainda que ocorra nova fixação da retina (mais provável com descolamentos exsudativos do que com os serosos).
- A visão poderá retornar se a causa subjacente for removida e se ocorrer nova fixação da retina.
- Coriorretinite focal ou multifocal — não prejudica acentuadamente a visão; poderá deixar cicatrizes.

DIVERSOS
DISTÚRBIOS ASSOCIADOS
- Exsudativo — doença sistêmica. • Cataratas.
- Traumatismo. • Tração e/ou regmatógeno — hemorragia ou inflamação vítreas. • Sinais do SNC em cães com meningoencefalomielite granulomatosa ou doença sistêmica com envolvimento do SNC.

ABREVIATURA(S)
- LCS = líquido cerebrospinal.
- LES = lúpus eritematoso sistêmico.
- SDSAR = síndrome de degeneração súbita e adquirida da retina.
- SNC = sistema nervoso central.

Sugestões de Leitura
Maggs DJ, Miller PE, Ofri R. Slatter's Fundamentals of Veterinary Ophthalmology, 4th ed. St. Louis: Saunders, 2008.

Autor Patricia J. Smith
Consultor Editorial Paul E. Miller

Desvio Portossistêmico Adquirido

CONSIDERAÇÕES GERAIS

REVISÃO
Desvios portossistêmicos adquiridos desenvolvem-se subsequentemente à hipertensão portal.

IDENTIFICAÇÃO
• Mais comum — cães com hepatopatia crônica, hepatopatia fibrosante juvenil, hipertensão portal não cirrótica e cães com anomalia vascular portossistêmica intolerantes à ligadura cirúrgica, sobretudo aqueles com aplicação de constritor ameroide. • Gatos — em casos avançados e graves de hepatopatia policística (fibrose), síndrome colangite/colangio-hepatite grave ou anomalia vascular portossistêmica intolerante à ligadura cirúrgica. • Cães e gatos — subsequente à obstrução extra-hepática crônica (>6 semanas) do ducto biliar. • Determinados distúrbios — apresentam incidência etária ou racial; a doença policística nos gatos é mais comum nas raças Himalaio e Persa.

SINAIS CLÍNICOS
• Os sinais clínicos representam sequelas de perfusão hepática comprometida e, em caso de hepatopatia crônica, função hepática reduzida; dependem da cronicidade do distúrbio subjacente. • Encefalopatia hepática episódica — principal sinal; podem incluir anormalidades neurocomportamentais, cegueira, poliúria e polidipsia, anorexia, letargia, vômito e sinais neurológicos atribuídos ao cérebro ou tronco cerebral ou sugestivos de mielopatia transversa; os sinais frequentemente melhoram com a fluidoterapia (com glicose e suplementos de potássio), antibióticos de amplo espectro, lactulose e restrição de proteína na dieta (ver "Encefalopatia Hepática"). • Ascite — comum, porém variável; pode regredir e reaparecer. • Vasculopatia esplâncnica hipertensiva — provoca sangramento/ulceração gastroduodenais; pode evoluir para perfuração e peritonite séptica, perda de sangue com risco de morte em caso de coagulopatia coexistente, ou encefalopatia hepática grave por causa do potente efeito encefalogênico do sangue entérico; causa anorexia, vômito, diarreia, dor abdominal e anemia. • Urogenital — uropatia obstrutiva atribuída à urolitíase por biurato de amônio: hematúria macro ou microscópica; polaciúria; disúria.

CAUSAS E FATORES DE RISCO
• Múltiplos vasos tortuosos — representam a formação de ponte vascular entre a circulação esplâncnica e sistêmica. • Falta de válvulas na veia porta — faz com que o sangue siga para "uma via de mínima resistência". • Hipertensão portal — resultante de muitos processos mórbidos: mais importante, fibrose hepática difusa com ou sem cirrose; obstrução extra-hepática crônica do ducto biliar sem resolução (>6 semanas); outras causas, incluindo tromboembolia venosa portal, hipertensão portal idiopática, hipertensão portal não cirrótica (obliteração de vênulas portais terciárias ou delicadas) e obstrução do fluxo de saída dos sinusoides hepáticos (zona 3 ao nível das vênulas hepáticas, veias ou veia cava); menos comumente, distúrbios que prejudicam a perfusão do segmento esplâncnico da veia porta (tromboembolia, estenose, estrangulamento) e, raramente, atresia da veia porta (má-formação congênita de veia porta intra ou extra-hepática) e fístula(s) AV(s) hepática(s) congênita(s) ou adquirida(s) (que arterializam a circulação portal); ver "Hipertensão Portal". • Pode levar ao desenvolvimento de encefalopatia hepática associada à ingestão de alimento rico em proteína, hemorragia entérica (tendências ao sangramento, vasculopatia portal), azotemia, alcalemia, distúrbios eletrolíticos, transfusões sanguíneas ou hemólise, infecções e administração de determinados medicamentos. • Hiperamonemia e metabolismo prejudicado do ácido úrico em alantoína hidrossolúvel provocam urolitíase por urato de amônio.

DIAGNÓSTICO

DIAGNÓSTICO DIFERENCIAL
• Sinais do SNC — distúrbios infecciosos (p. ex., PIF, cinomose, toxoplasmose, infecções relacionadas com FeLV ou FIV); intoxicações (p. ex., chumbo, cogumelos, substâncias psicoativas); hidrocefalia; epilepsia idiopática; distúrbios metabólicos (p. ex., hipoglicemia grave, hipo ou hipercalemia, hipocalcemia, hipofosfatemia grave). • Sinais gastrintestinais — obstrução intestinal; imprudência alimentar; ingestão de corpo estranho; enteropatia inflamatória. • Sinais do trato urinário — infecção bacteriana do trato urinário; urolitíase. • Poliúria e polidipsia — distúrbios da concentração de urina (p. ex., diabetes insípido, função adrenal anormal, hipercalcemia, polidipsia primária, nefropatia congênita ou adquirida). • Causas de efusão abdominal — distúrbios cardiopulmonares indutores de insuficiência cardíaca direita; doença pericárdica; hepatopatias inflamatórias primárias; hepatopatia infiltrativa (p. ex., neoplasia e amiloide); distúrbios abdominais não hepáticos associados a efusões (p. ex., torção esplênica, neoplasia visceral e carcinomatose) ou peritonite: química (p. ex., bile, urina e quilo) ou séptica.

HEMOGRAMA/BIOQUÍMICA/URINÁLISE
• Hemograma completo — a microcitose reflete desvio portossistêmico ou deficiência de ferro; é comum uma leve anemia arregenerativa; pecilocitose (gatos); células-alvo (cães). • Bioquímica — além do baixo nível de ureia, níveis baixos a normais de creatinina, glicose, albumina e colesterol são comuns; atividade enzimática hepática (fosfatase alcalina geralmente elevada nos pacientes jovens [isoenzima óssea]) e bilirrubina variáveis; os achados dependem da causa subjacente. • Urinálise — concentração urinária variável; cristalúria por biurato de amônio, hematúria, piúria e proteinúria refletem urolitíase (traumatismo mecânico, inflamação ou infecção).

OUTROS TESTES LABORATORIAIS
• Ácidos biliares séricos totais — indicadores sensíveis para desvio portossistêmico adquirido ou anomalia vascular portossistêmica; valores em jejum normais a discretamente elevados e pós-prandiais acentuadamente aumentados (em geral, >100 μmol/L) = "padrão de desvio". • Valores da amônia sanguínea — indicadores sensíveis de encefalopatia hepática; as amostras de sangue não podem ser congeladas nem encaminhadas pelo correio para análises subsequentes em virtude da instabilidade da amônia; a presença de cristalúria por biurato de amônio pressupõe níveis sanguíneos elevados de amônia (avaliar três amostras de urina, 4-8 h após a alimentação); teste de tolerância à amônia — método mais confiável de demonstrar a intolerância a essa substância; Cuidado: pode induzir à encefalopatia hepática. • Testes de coagulação — prolongamento do TP e TTPA, além de PIVKA, refletem a gravidade da disfunção hepática, falha na síntese, CID e suficiência da vitamina K_1; as PIVKA são valiosas na tomada de decisão sobre a necessidade de tratamento com suplementação de vitamina K_1. A baixa atividade da proteína C reflete desvio portossistêmico (anomalia vascular portossistêmica, desvio portossistêmico adquirido). • Efusão abdominal — geralmente transudato puro ou modificado; relação elevada da albumina no soro e na efusão (>1,1); corrobora com o papel desempenhado pela hipertensão portal na efusão.

DIAGNÓSTICO POR IMAGEM

Radiografia Abdominal
• O tamanho do fígado depende da causa subjacente; micro-hepatia: comum nos cães com hepatopatia crônica ou variante da anomalia vascular portossistêmica indutora de ascite; variável nos gatos, a doença policística costuma causar hepatomegalia. • Efusão abdominal. • Cálculos de biurato de amônio — radiotransparentes a menos que combinados com minerais radiodensos.

Portovenografia Radiográfica
• Demonstra múltiplos desvios portossistêmicos adquiridos; método não recomendado em virtude dos riscos de complicações iatrogênicas; ver alternativas adiante.

Ultrassonografia Abdominal
• O tamanho do fígado depende da causa subjacente. • Pode revelar alterações do parênquima ou do sistema biliar em virtude de doença. • Desvio portossistêmico adquirido — identificado com o uso do Doppler de fluxo colorido; confirma fluxo portal hepatofugal; desvio portossistêmico adquirido tortuoso geralmente adjacente aos rins ou ao baço. • Efusão abdominal. • Urólitos: pelve renal ou bexiga urinária; raros nos ureteres. • Fístula AV intra-hepática — estrutura vascular pulsante dentro de um lobo hepático aumentado, juntamente com efusão abdominal e desvio portossistêmico adquirido (ver "Má-formação Arteriovenosa do Fígado"). • Doppler de fluxo colorido pode detectar trombos portais.

Cintilografia Colorretal
• Teste sensível e não invasivo, que confirma desvio portossistêmico. • Não é capaz de diferenciar anomalia vascular portossistêmica de desvio portossistêmico adquirido. • Administrar pertecnetato de tecnécio-99m por via retal; a obtenção de imagem em câmara gama determina a taxa de aparecimento do isótopo no fígado e no coração; calcular a fração do desvio a partir de gráficos tempo/atividade (≤15% é normal); não é um método quantitativo.

TC Multissetorial
• Procedimento não invasivo de escolha para obtenção de imagens; define a anatomia vascular com detalhes; identifica anormalidades viscerais; permite a rápida coleta de dados; necessita de anestesia a curto prazo.

Desvio Portossistêmico Adquirido

MÉTODOS DIAGNÓSTICOS
Citologia do Aspirado por Agulha Fina
• Aspirado hepático — aspirados com agulha calibre 22 não são capazes de diferenciar distúrbios indutores de desvio portossistêmico. • Biopsia hepática — biopsia cirúrgica aberta em cunha ou amostragem laparoscópica (pinça para biopsia em cálice); obter tecido de diversos lobos hepáticos; as amostras obtidas com a agulha Tru-Cut® podem não obter tecido adequado para o diagnóstico definitivo; geralmente de um único lobo.

ACHADOS PATOLÓGICOS
• Macroscópicos — fígado pequeno de contorno irregular em casos de hepatopatia crônica (cirrose, fibrose). • Tamanho normal a aumentado no início de obstrução do fluxo de saída venoso (síndrome de Budd-Chiari, lesão veno-oclusiva). • Lobo hepático grande (o restante do fígado encontra-se de tamanho normal a pequeno) em caso de fístula AV hepática. • Normal a pequeno — hipertensão portal idiopática, hipertensão portal não cirrótica, trombos portais. • Fígado pequeno se houver atresia portal congênita. • Fígado normal a grande em gatos com doença policística hepática: pode haver apenas estruturas císticas microscópicas inaparentes ao ultrassom.

TRATAMENTO
CUIDADO(S) DE SAÚDE ADEQUADO(S)
Paciente internado — sinais graves de encefalopatia hepática; para a provisão de cuidados críticos.

CUIDADO(S) DE ENFERMAGEM
Ver "Encefalopatia Hepática".

DIETA
• Suporte nutricional — essencial para manter a condição corporal para o controle ideal da encefalopatia hepática; é importante o fornecimento de dieta balanceada com restrição proteica; otimizar a tolerância de proteína da dieta (ver "Encefalopatia Hepática"); a porção de proteína é titulada de acordo com a resposta do paciente em combinação com tratamentos que melhoram a encefalopatia hepática (ver "Encefalopatia Hepática"); utilizar dietas comerciais formuladas para hepatopatia ou insuficiência renal moderada; cães: proteína do leite e da soja são as melhores fontes; gatos (carnívoros puros): devem receber proteína derivada da carne; proteína titulada com acréscimos de porções de 0,5 g/kg (proteína do leite: queijo, caseinato de cálcio — cães apenas; ou soja), a cada 5-7 dias. • Nutrição parenteral — ver "Encefalopatia Hepática".

ORIENTAÇÃO AO PROPRIETÁRIO
• Depende da causa subjacente. • Orientar o proprietário sobre os sinais de encefalopatia hepática e o potencial para uropatia obstrutiva por biurato de amônio nos machos; cães machos podem necessitar de uretrostomia pré-escrotal permanente. • Esclarecer o proprietário sobre como ajustar os diuréticos (de acordo com a necessidade) para mobilizar o líquido da efusão abdominal. • Instruir o proprietário sobre como ajustar os medicamentos por via oral e enemas (conforme a necessidade) para melhorar a encefalopatia hepática (ver "Encefalopatia Hepática").

MEDICAÇÕES
MEDICAMENTO(S)
• Hemorragia entérica — associada à vasculopatia esplâncnica hipertensiva (diapedese e ulcerações na região gastroduodenal) e coagulopatia; não há provas de que o uso profilático de bloqueadores da acidez e gastroprotetores diminuam o risco; tratar o animal sintomático pelo uso de bloqueador histaminérgico H_2 (prefere-se a famotidina) e sucralfato; talvez haja necessidade de terapia com componente sanguíneo e DDVAP (ver "Coagulopatia por Hepatopatia"). • Efusão abdominal — medir sequencialmente o peso corporal e a circunferência abdominal (cintura); atribuir escores à condição corporal; no início, reforçar a restrição ao exercício (melhora não só a perfusão renal, mas também a eliminação de sódio e água), restrição de sódio na dieta, diuréticos (uso combinado de furosemida e espironolactona); furosemida (0,5-2 mg/kg VO a cada 12-24 h) e espironolactona (0,5-2 mg/kg VO a cada 12 h; utilizar uma única dosagem dobrada como dose de ataque de uma só vez); as titulações da dose são feitas com base na resposta a cada 4 dias, utilizando aumentos de 25-50% na dose; a abdominocentese (terapêutica) de grandes volumes é utilizada em casos de ascite que se mostra refratária à intervenção médica ou compromete o consumo alimentar, a ventilação ou o sono; necessita de técnica asséptica, além da administração concomitante de fluidos poliônicos e coloides, para otimizar a segurança. • Os antagonistas dos receptores V_2 da vasopressina recentemente disponíveis podem ser bem-sucedidos em casos de ascite refratária (no entanto, ainda não há dados disponíveis em cães ou gatos).

PRECAUÇÕES
• Ter consciência do metabolismo alterado dos medicamentos relacionados com a extração reduzida de primeira passagem (desvio portossistêmico), metabolismo/biotransformação hepáticos alterados e ligação proteica diminuída (caso esteja com hipoalbuminemia). • Permanecer vigilante para a desidratação induzida pelo diurético e falta de regulação eletrolítica.

INTERAÇÕES POSSÍVEIS
Evitar a metoclopramida ao utilizar a espironolactona (bloqueia o efeito); evitar medicamentos anti-inflamatórios não esteroides, pois esses agentes podem inibir a diurese induzida pela furosemida e potencializar a lesão renal.

ACOMPANHAMENTO
MONITORIZAÇÃO DO PACIENTE
• Reavaliar o comportamento e o apetite do paciente em casa como reflexo da encefalopatia hepática. • Monitorizar os sinais clínicos, o apetite, a condição e o peso corporais, a circunferência abdominal, o hemograma completo, a bioquímica sérica e a urina (cristalúria por biurato de amônio); os ácidos biliares séricos totais não são válidos para avaliação sequencial, uma vez que se encontram constantemente elevados nos pacientes com desvio portossistêmico adquirido e naqueles tratados com ácido ursodesoxicólico (medicamento medido no ensaio). • Ajustar o tratamento clínico para reduzir a encefalopatia hepática episódica, a cristalúria por biurato de amônio e o potencial de formação do urólito, bem como a ocorrência de efusão abdominal. • Inspecionar cuidadosamente o paciente em busca de indícios de sangramento clínico; determinar a necessidade da administração intermitente crônica da vitamina K_1 pela via parenteral (teste de PIVKA).

PREVENÇÃO
• Efetuar tratamento precoce da hepatopatia adquirida e da obstrução extra-hepática do ducto biliar para minimizar a fibrose hepática. • Considerar a propriedade da ligadura completa da anomalia vascular portossistêmica por técnicas cirúrgicas ou constritor ameroide: com base nos sinais clínicos.

COMPLICAÇÕES POSSÍVEIS
• Tratar o distúrbio subjacente. • Hemorragia entérica associada à vasculopatia hipertensiva; pode necessitar de cuidados intensivos imediatos para tratar a hipovolemia, a coagulopatia e a encefalopatia hepática subsequente; talvez haja necessidade de ressecção cirúrgica do segmento intestinal envolvido (raro). • Desidratação, alcalose por contração, azotemia — complicações dos diuréticos.

EVOLUÇÃO ESPERADA E PROGNÓSTICO
• Variam com a causa subjacente. • O controle da hepatopatia crônica ou da fibrose hepática aparentemente prolonga a vida. • Animais com hipertensão portal não cirrótica e fibrose hepática juvenil poderão viver > 8 anos se forem tratados com sucesso durante a doença sintomática inicial.

DIVERSOS
DISTÚRBIOS ASSOCIADOS
• Urolitíase por urato de amônio. • Ascite. • Coagulopatia. • Encefalopatia hepática. • Sangramento/ulceração intestinais. • Uropatia obstrutiva.

VER TAMBÉM
• Anomalia Vascular Portossistêmica Congênita. • Ascite. • Cirrose e Fibrose do Fígado. • Coagulopatia por Hepatopatia. • Encefalopatia Hepática. • Hepatite Crônica Ativa. • Hepatopatia Fibrosante Juvenil.

ABREVIATURA(S)
• AV = arteriovenoso(a). • CID = coagulação intravascular disseminada. • DDAVP = 1-desamino-8-d-arginina vasopressina (desmopressina). • FeLV = vírus da leucemia felina. • FIV = vírus da imunodeficiência felina. • PIF = peritonite infecciosa felina. • PIVKA = proteínas invocadas pela ausência ou pelo antagonismo da vitamina K. • SNC = sistema nervoso central. • TC = tomografia computadorizada. • TP = tempo de protrombina. • TTPA = tempo de tromboplastina parcial ativada.

Sugestões de Leitura
Bunch SE, Johnson SE, Cullen JM. Idiopathic noncirrhotic portal hypertension in dogs: 33 cases (1982-1998). JAVMA 2001, 218:392-399.

Autor Sharon A. Center
Consultor Editorial Sharon A. Center

Diabetes Insípido

CONSIDERAÇÕES GERAIS

DEFINIÇÃO
O diabetes insípido constitui um distúrbio do metabolismo hídrico, caracterizado por poliúria, densidade ou osmolalidade urinárias baixas (urina denominada insípida ou sem gosto) e polidipsia.

FISIOPATOLOGIA
- Diabetes insípido central — deficiência na secreção do ADH.
- Diabetes insípido nefrogênico — insensibilidade renal ao ADH.

SISTEMA(S) ACOMETIDO(S)
- Endócrino/metabólico.
- Renal/urológico.

INCIDÊNCIA/PREVALÊNCIA
- Diabetes insípido central — rara.
- Diabetes insípido nefrogênico — rara.

IDENTIFICAÇÃO
Espécies
Cães e gatos.

Idade Média e Faixa Etária
- Formas congênitas — <1 ano de idade.
- Formas adquiridas (p. ex., neoplásicas, traumáticas e idiopáticas) — qualquer idade.

SINAIS CLÍNICOS
- Poliúria.
- Polidipsia.
- Incontinência — ocasional.

CAUSAS
Secreção Inadequada do ADH
- Defeito congênito.
- Idiopática.
- Traumatismo.
- Neoplasia.

Insensibilidade Renal ao ADH
- Congênita.
- Secundária a medicamentos (p. ex., lítio, demeclociclina e metoxiflurano).
- Secundária a distúrbios endócrinos e metabólicos (p. ex., hiperadrenocorticismo, hipocalemia, piometra e hipercalcemia).
- Secundária à nefropatia ou infecção (p. ex., pielonefrite, insuficiência renal crônica e piometra).

DIAGNÓSTICO

DIAGNÓSTICO DIFERENCIAL
Distúrbios Poliúricos
- Hiperadrenocorticismo.
- Diabetes melito.
- Hepatopatia — desvio portossistêmico.
- Hiperadrenocorticismo.
- Piometra.
- Pielonefrite.
- Hipertireoidismo — gatos.
- Hipercalcemia.
- Polidipsia psicogênica.
- Insuficiência renal.

HEMOGRAMA/BIOQUÍMICA/URINÁLISE
- Geralmente permanecem normais; em alguns pacientes, observa-se hipernatremia.
- Densidade urinária baixa (em geral, <1,012; com frequência, <1,008).

OUTROS TESTES LABORATORIAIS
Nível plasmático do ADH.

DIAGNÓSTICO POR IMAGEM
RM ou TC — na suspeita de tumor hipofisário.

MÉTODOS DIAGNÓSTICOS
- Teste modificado de privação hídrica (ver o "Apêndice II" em busca do protocolo).
- Tentativa de suplementação do ADH — ensaio terapêutico com o ADH sintético (DDAVP); em caso de resposta positiva, o consumo de água diminui por volta de 50% em 3-5 dias.
- Descartar todas as outras causas de PU/PD antes de se conduzir um ensaio com o ADH.

ACHADOS PATOLÓGICOS
Degeneração e morte de neurônios neurossecretores na neuro-hipófise (diabetes insípido central).

TRATAMENTO

CUIDADO(S) DE SAÚDE ADEQUADO(S)
Para a realização do teste modificado de privação hídrica, deve-se internar o paciente; já o ensaio com o ADH é frequentemente executado como um procedimento ambulatorial.

ATIVIDADE
Sem restrição.

DIETA
Normal, com livre acesso à água.

ORIENTAÇÃO AO PROPRIETÁRIO
- Rever a dose do DDAVP e a técnica de administração.
- Salientar a importância do fornecimento de água *ad libitum*, ou seja, à vontade.

MEDICAÇÕES

MEDICAMENTO(S) DE ESCOLHA
- Diabetes insípido central — DDAVP (1-2 gotas da preparação intranasal no saco conjuntival a cada 12-24 h para controlar a PU/PD); alternativamente, pode-se administrar a preparação intranasal por via SC (2-5 µg a cada 12-24 h). Uma preparação oral de DDAVP está disponível em comprimidos de 0,1-0,2 mg, sendo que cada 0,1 mg é comparável a uma grande gota da preparação intranasal.
- Diabetes insípido nefrogênico — hidroclorotiazida (2-4 mg/kg VO a cada 12 h).

PRECAUÇÕES
A superdosagem do DDAVP pode causar intoxicação hídrica.

MEDICAMENTO(S) ALTERNATIVO(S)
Clorpropamida (Diabinese®; 125-250 mg/dia pode reduzir a PU/PD em casos de diabetes insípido central).

ACOMPANHAMENTO

MONITORIZAÇÃO DO PACIENTE
- Ajustar o tratamento de acordo com os sinais clínicos do paciente; a dosagem e a frequência ideais da administração do DDAVP baseiam-se no consumo de água.
- Os testes laboratoriais (como VG [hematócrito], sólidos totais e concentração sérica de sódio) para detectar desidratação (reposição inadequada do DDAVP) não costumam ser necessários.

PREVENÇÃO
Evitar as circunstâncias que possam aumentar a perda hídrica de forma acentuada.

COMPLICAÇÕES POSSÍVEIS
Prever as complicações de doenças primárias (tumor hipofisário).

EVOLUÇÃO ESPERADA E PROGNÓSTICO
- O distúrbio costuma ser permanente, exceto em raros pacientes nos quais ele foi induzido por traumatismo.
- Em geral, o prognóstico é bom, dependendo do distúrbio subjacente.
- Sem tratamento, a desidratação pode levar a estupor, coma e óbito.

DIVERSOS

FATORES RELACIONADOS COM A IDADE
- Diabetes insípido central e diabetes insípido nefrogênico congênitos — normalmente se manifestam antes dos 6 meses de vida.
- Diabetes insípido central relacionado com tumor hipofisário — observado geralmente em cães com >5 anos de idade.

SINÔNIMO(S)
- Diabetes insípido central.
- Diabetes insípido craniano.
- Diabetes insípido responsivo ao ADH.
- Diabetes insípido nefrogênico.

VER TAMBÉM
Hipostenúria.

ABREVIATURA(S)
- ADH = hormônio antidiurético.
- DDAVP = 1-desamino-8-d-arginina vasopressina (desmopressina).
- PU/PD = poliúria/polidipsia.
- RM = ressonância magnética.
- TC = tomografia computadorizada.
- VG = volume globular.

Sugestões de Leitura
Aroch I, Mazaki-Tovi M, Shemesh O, Sarfaty H, Segev G. Central diabetes insipidus in five cats: Clinical presentation, diagnosis and oral desmopressin therapy. J Feline Med Surg 2005, 7(6):333-339. Epub 2005 May 31.
Campbell FE, Bredhauer B. Trauma-induced central diabetes insipidus in a cat. Australian Vet J 2005, 83(12):732-735.
Feldman EC, Nelson RW. Canine and Feline Endocrinology and Reproduction, 3rd ed. Philadelphia: Saunders, 2006.
Harb MF, Nelson RW, Feldman EC, Scott-Moncrieff JC, Griffey SM. Central diabetes insipidus in dogs: 20 cases (1986-1995). JAVMA 1996, 209(11):1884-1888.

Autor Rhett Nichols
Consultor Editorial Deborah S. Greco

Diabetes Melito com Cetoacidose

CONSIDERAÇÕES GERAIS

DEFINIÇÃO
Trata-se de uma verdadeira emergência médica, secundária à deficiência absoluta ou relativa de insulina, caracterizada por hiperglicemia, cetonemia, acidose metabólica, desidratação e depleção eletrolítica.

FISIOPATOLOGIA
- A deficiência de insulina causa aumento na lipólise, que resulta em produção excessiva de corpos cetônicos e acidose; a incapacidade em manter a homeostasia hidroeletrolítica provoca desidratação, azotemia pré-renal, distúrbios eletrolíticos, obnubilação e óbito.
- Muitos pacientes com cetoacidose diabética apresentam problemas subjacentes (como infecção, inflamação ou cardiopatia) que induzem à secreção de hormônios típicos do estresse (p. ex., glucagon, cortisol, hormônio de crescimento e adrenalina); isso provavelmente contribui para o desenvolvimento de insulinorresistência e cetoacidose diabética, pela promoção dos processos de lipólise, cetogênese, gliconeogênese e glicogenólise.
- A desidratação e as anormalidades eletrolíticas originam-se da diurese osmótica, que promove a perda de água corporal total e eletrólitos.

SISTEMA(S) ACOMETIDO(S)
- Endócrino/metabólico.
- Gastrintestinal.
- Hematológico (gatos).

INCIDÊNCIA/PREVALÊNCIA
Desconhecidas.

IDENTIFICAÇÃO
Espécies
Cães e gatos.

Raça(s) Predominante(s)
- Cães — Poodle miniatura e Dachshund.
- Gatos — nenhuma.

Idade Média e Faixa Etária
- Cães — idade média, 8,4 anos.
- Gatos — idade média, 11 anos (faixa etária, 1-19 anos).

Sexo Predominante
- Caninos — as cadelas são 1,5 vez mais acometidas que os machos.
- Felinos — os machos são 2 vezes mais acometidos que as gatas.

SINAIS CLÍNICOS
- Poliúria.
- Polidipsia ou adipsia.
- Atividade diminuída.
- Anorexia.
- Fraqueza.
- Vômito.
- Letargia e depressão.
- Emaciação muscular e perda de peso.
- Más condições da pelagem.
- Taquipneia.
- Desidratação.
- Condição corporal debilitada (magra).
- Hipotermia.
- Seborreia (caspa).
- Espessamento das alças intestinais.
- Hepatomegalia.
- Hálito de odor cetônico.
- Icterícia.

CAUSAS
- Diabetes melito insulinodependente.
- Infecção (p. ex., cutânea, respiratória, urinária, prostática, além de pielonefrite, piometra e pneumonia).
- Doença concomitante (p. ex., insuficiência cardíaca, pancreatite, insuficiência ou falência renal, asma, neoplasia, acromegalia e estro).
- Idiopático.
- Descumprimento da medicação.
- Estresse.
- Cirurgia.

FATORES DE RISCO
- Qualquer condição indutora de deficiência absoluta ou relativa de insulina.
- Histórico de administração de corticosteroides ou β-bloqueadores.

DIAGNÓSTICO

DIAGNÓSTICO DIFERENCIAL
- Coma hiperosmolar não cetótico.
- Coma hipoglicêmico agudo.
- Uremia.
- Acidose láctica.

HEMOGRAMA/BIOQUÍMICA/URINÁLISE
- Leucocitose com neutrofilia madura.
- Hiperglicemia — glicose sanguínea geralmente >250 mg/dL.
- Atividade elevada das enzimas hepáticas.
- Hipercolesterolemia e lipemia.
- Azotemia.
- Hipocloremia.
- Hipocalemia.
- Hiponatremia.
- Hipofosfatemia.
- Hiato aniônico elevado = (sódio + potássio) — (cloreto + bicarbonato); o normal é de 16 ± 4.
- Glicosúria e cetonúria.
- Densidade urinária variável com sedimento ativo ou inativo.
- Hiperproteinemia.
- Anemia por corpúsculo de Heinz (gatos).

OUTROS TESTES LABORATORIAIS
- Acidose metabólica — CO_2 total venoso <15 mEq/L, causado por cetose.
- Hiperosmolaridade (>330 mOsm/kg).
- Cultura bacteriana de urina e sangue.

MÉTODOS DIAGNÓSTICOS
O ECG pode ajudar a avaliar o *status* do potássio; intervalo QT prolongado em alguns pacientes com hipocalemia; ondas T altas e pontiagudas ("em tenda") em outros pacientes com hipercalemia.

ACHADOS PATOLÓGICOS
Atrofia das células das ilhotas pancreáticas.

TRATAMENTO

CUIDADO(S) DE SAÚDE ADEQUADO(S)
- Se o animal permanecer esperto, alerta e bem hidratado, não haverá necessidade de cuidado intensivo e fluidoterapia intravenosa; iniciar a administração subcutânea de insulina (insulina de ação curta ou intermediária), oferecer alimento e permitir o acesso constante à água; monitorizar o animal de perto quanto ao aparecimento de sinais de doença (p. ex., anorexia, letargia e vômito).
- O tratamento de cães ou gatos cetoacidóticos diabéticos "enfermos" exige a provisão de cuidados intensivos com internação; esse quadro representa uma emergência médica potencialmente letal; os objetivos são corrigir a depleção de água e eletrólitos, reverter a cetonemia e a acidose, além de aumentar a taxa de utilização da glicose pelos tecidos dependentes de insulina.

CUIDADO(S) DE ENFERMAGEM
- Fluidos — necessários para garantir a perfusão tecidual e o débito cardíaco adequados, bem como para manter o volume vascular; também diminuem a concentração sanguínea de glicose.
- O fluido de escolha inicial consiste na administração IV de soro fisiológico a 0,9% suplementada com potássio.
- O volume é determinado pelo déficit de desidratação somado às exigências de manutenção; repor em 24-48 h.

DIETA
Assim que o paciente se encontrar estabilizado, recomenda-se dieta rica em carboidratos complexos e fibras, mas pobre em gorduras.

ORIENTAÇÃO AO PROPRIETÁRIO
Em grande parte dos pacientes, trata-se de uma condição clínica séria que exige a administração de insulina por toda a vida.

MEDICAÇÕES

MEDICAMENTO(S) DE ESCOLHA
Insulina
- Imprescindível para promover a captação periférica de glicose, bem como para inibir a lipólise e a gliconeogênese hepática.
- A insulina regular constitui a insulina de escolha.
- Dosagem inicial — 0,2 U/kg IM (ou SC se a hidratação permanecer normal).
- A dosagem subsequente de 0,1-0,2 U/kg é administrada 3-6 h mais tarde — poderá ser fornecida de hora em hora se o paciente for monitorizado rigorosamente; deve-se considerar a resposta à dosagem prévia de insulina ao se calcular as dosagens subsequentes. Idealmente, a concentração de glicose deve cair para 50-100 mg/dL/h.
- Também é possível administrar a insulina regular sob a forma de infusão contínua por meio de um cateter especialmente destinado para isso. Para os cães, colocar 2,2 unidades/kg em 250 mL de solução de NaCl a 0,9%. Para os gatos, colocar 1,1 unidade/kg em 250 mL de solução de NaCl a 0,9%. Em seguida, permitir o fluxo (i. e., escoamento) de 50 mL de insulina diluída pelo equipo IV e descartar. Se a glicose sanguínea estiver >250 mg/dL, administrar a 10 mL/h. Se a glicose sanguínea estiver entre 200 e 250 mg/dL, administrar a 7 mL/h. Se a glicose sanguínea estiver entre 150 e 200 mg/dL, administrar a 5 mL/h. Se a glicose sanguínea estiver entre 100 e 150 mg/dL, administrar a 5 mL/h e adicionar glicose a 2,5% aos fluidos cristaloides IV. Se a glicose sanguínea estiver <100 mg/dL, interromper a infusão intravenosa de insulina e continuar com glicose a 2,5-5% diluída em infusão cristaloide também por via IV.

Diabetes Melito com Cetoacidose

- Verificar a glicose sanguínea a cada 1-3 h com o uso de fitas reagentes Chemstrip BG® e de um analisador automatizado das fitas de teste (Accu-Chek III®, Boehringer Mannheim; glicosímetro Alpha Trak®, Abbott Laboratories).
- Monitorizar a glicose e as cetonas urinárias diariamente.
- Começar a administrar a insulina de ação mais prolongada quando o paciente já estiver se alimentando e ingerindo líquidos, não estiver mais recebendo os fluidos IV e se a cetose já estiver resolvida ou bastante reduzida; a dosagem baseia-se na insulina de ação curta administrada no hospital.

Suplementação de Potássio
- O potássio corporal total sofre depleção, mas o tratamento (p. ex., fluidos e insulina) reduzirá ainda mais os níveis séricos desse elemento; dessa forma, a suplementação de potássio sempre é imprescindível.
- Se possível, avaliar a concentração de potássio antes de iniciar a insulinoterapia, para orientar a dosagem de suplementação; se essa concentração se encontrar extremamente baixa, poderá ser necessário o adiamento (por horas) da insulinoterapia até que a concentração sérica de potássio aumente.
- A hipocalemia refratária pode indicar depleção de magnésio, exigindo a reposição desse elemento a 0,75-1 mEq/kg/dia sob a forma de cloreto de magnésio ou sulfato de magnésio em velocidade constante de infusão.
- Caso não se conheça a concentração de potássio, adicionar esse elemento (a 40 mEq/L) aos fluidos IV, obter os resultados pré-terapêuticos da análise bioquímica o mais rápido possível e coletar sangue para a análise bioquímica de acompanhamento 24 h após a instituição do tratamento.

Suplementação de Glicose
- Independentemente da concentração sanguínea de glicose, é imprescindível fornecer a insulina para corrigir o estado de cetoacidose.
- Sempre que a glicose sanguínea estiver <200-250 mg/dL, deve-se adicionar glicose a 50% aos fluidos para produzir uma solução de glicose a 2,5% (aumentar para glicose a 5%, se necessário). Suspender a administração de glicose assim que seu nível permanecer acima de 250 mg/dL.
- Não interromper a insulinoterapia.

Suplementação de Bicarbonato
- Controversa; considerar tal suplementação se o pH sanguíneo venoso do paciente for <7,0 ou o CO_2 total estiver <11 mEq/L; o bicarbonato não terá nenhum benefício se o valor do pH for superior a 7,0.
- Dosagem — peso corporal (kg) × 0,3 × déficit de base (déficit de base = bicarbonato sérico normal – bicarbonato sérico do paciente); administrar *lentamente* um quarto à metade da dose IV e o restante diluído em fluidos por 3-6 h.
- Reavaliar a gasometria sanguínea ou o CO_2 total sérico antes da suplementação adicional.

Suplementação de Fósforo
- O nível sérico pré-terapêutico de fósforo costuma permanecer normal; contudo, o tratamento da cetoacidose diminui os níveis desse elemento e as concentrações séricas devem ser avaliadas a cada 12-24 h assim que se iniciar a suplementação.
- Dosagem — 0,01-0,03 mmol/kg/h por 6-12 h em fluidos IV (pode ser preciso aumentar a dose para 0,03-0,06).

CONTRAINDICAÇÕES
Se o paciente estiver anúrico ou oligúrico ou se o nível de potássio ficar >5 mEq/L, não proceder à suplementação de potássio até que se estabeleça o fluxo urinário ou diminua a concentração desse elemento.

PRECAUÇÕES
Utilizar o bicarbonato com cautela em pacientes sem ventilação normal, em virtude de sua incapacidade de excretar o dióxido de carbono gerado durante o tratamento.

ACOMPANHAMENTO

MONITORIZAÇÃO DO PACIENTE
- Monitorizar a postura, a hidratação, o estado cardiopulmonar, o débito urinário e o peso corporal.
- Mensurar a glicose sanguínea a cada 1-3 h em princípio; depois a cada 6 h assim que o paciente se encontrar estabilizado.
- Mensurar os eletrólitos a cada 4-8 h inicialmente; depois a cada 24 h logo que o paciente permanecer estabilizado.
- Mensurar o estado acidobásico a cada 8-12 h também no início; depois a cada 24 h, assim que o paciente ficar estabilizado.

PREVENÇÃO
Administração apropriada da insulina.

COMPLICAÇÕES POSSÍVEIS
- Hipocalemia.
- Hipoglicemia.
- Hipofosfatemia.
- Edema cerebral.
- Edema pulmonar.
- Insuficiência renal.
- Insuficiência cardíaca.

EVOLUÇÃO ESPERADA E PROGNÓSTICO
Reservados.

DIVERSOS

DISTÚRBIOS ASSOCIADOS
- Pancreatite.
- Hiperadrenocorticismo.
- Diestro.
- Infecção bacteriana.
- Depleção de eletrólitos.

GESTAÇÃO/FERTILIDADE/REPRODUÇÃO
- O risco de morte fetal pode ser relativamente alto.
- Com frequência, a regulação da glicose não é uma tarefa fácil.

VER TAMBÉM
- Diabetes Melito sem Complicação — Cães.
- Diabetes Melito sem Complicação — Gatos.

ABREVIATURA(S)
- CO_2 = dióxido de carbono.
- ECG = eletrocardiograma.

Sugestões de Leitura

Brady MA, Dennis JS, Wagner-Mann C. Evaluating the use of plasma hematocrit samples to detect ketones utilizing urine dipstick colorimetric methodology in diabetic cats and dogs. J Vet Emerg Crit Care 2003, 13(1):1-6.

Duarte R, Simoes DMN, Franchini ML, Marquezi ML, Ikesaki JH, Kogika MM, Alves FO. Serum beta-hydroxybutyrate concentrations in the diagnosis of diabetic ketoacidosis in 116 dogs. J Vet Intern Med 2002, 16:411-417.

Durocher LL, Hinchcliff KW, DiBartola SP, Johnson SE. Acid base and hormonal abnormalities in dogs with naturally occurring diabetes mellitus. JAVMA 2008, 232(9):1310-1320.

Hume DZ, Drobatz KJ, Hess RS. Outcome of dogs with diabetic ketoacidosis: 127 dogs (1993-2003). J Vet Intern Med 2006, 20(3):547-555.

Kerl ME. Diabetic ketoacidosis: Pathophysiology and clinical and laboratory presentation. Compend Contin Educ Pract Vet 2001, 23:220-228.

Kerl ME. Diabetic ketoacidosis: Treatment recommendations. Compend Contin Educ Pract Vet 2001, 23:330-339.

Koenig A, Drobatz KJ, Beale AB, King LG. Hyperglycemic, hyperosmolar syndrome in feline diabetics: 17 cases (1995-2001). J Vet Emerg Crit Care 2004, 14(1):30-40.

Parsons SE, Drobatz KJ, Lamb SV, Ward CR, Hess RK. Endogenous serum insulin concentrations in dogs with diabetic ketoacidosis. J Vet Emerg Crit Care 2002, 12:147-152.

Sieber-Ruckstuhl NS, Klev S, Tschuor F, Zini E, Ohlerth S, Boretti FS, Reusch CE. Remission of diabetes mellitus in cats with diabetic ketoacidosis. J Vet Intern Med 2008, 22(6):1326-1332.

Zeugswetter E, Paqitz M. Ketone measurements using dipstick methodology in cats with diabetes mellitus. J Small Anim Pract 2009, 50(1):4-8.

Autor Elisa M. Mazzaferro
Consultor Editorial Deborah S. Greco

Diabetes Melito com Coma Hiperosmolar

CONSIDERAÇÕES GERAIS

DEFINIÇÃO
Doença caracterizada por hiperglicemia grave, hiperosmolaridade, desidratação intensa, falta de cetonas urinárias ou séricas, acidose metabólica nula ou leve a moderada e depressão do SNC.

FISIOPATOLOGIA
- A deficiência de insulina leva à redução no uso de glicose e produção excessiva desse carboidrato.
- A alta concentração sanguínea extracelular resultante de glicose induz a um estado hiperosmolar com declínio no volume do líquido extracelular.
- Ocorre o desenvolvimento de desidratação intracelular, azotemia e uremia, mas a desidratação intracelular torna-se mais pronunciada à medida que a taxa de filtração glomerular diminui; em seguida, ocorre hipoxia tecidual.
- A azotemia, a hiperglicemia e a hiperosmolaridade agravam-se em consequência da retenção de glicose e da diurese osmótica induzida por esse açúcar.
- Embora a cetonemia e a cetonúria não costumem ser características dessa síndrome, a anorexia (especialmente quando prolongada) pode causar cetoacidose leve em alguns pacientes, mas o aumento no ácido láctico representa um colaborador importante para a acidose metabólica que pode se desenvolver nesses pacientes.

SISTEMA(S) ACOMETIDO(S)
- Renal/urológico — desenvolvem-se azotemias renal primária e pré-renal em função da redução no volume do líquido extracelular, do declínio na perfusão tecidual ou de glomerulonefropatia diabética; a densidade urinária fica baixa em decorrência de diurese osmótica, glomerulonefropatia diabética ou insuficiência renal concomitante.
- Cardiovascular — hipotensão decorrente de: baixo volume do líquido extracelular, colapso vascular e depressão na contratilidade miocárdica.
- Nervoso — depressão, desorientação ou confusão mental, crises convulsivas e coma, causados por desidratação intracelular e hiperosmolaridade; a disfunção do SNC piora à medida que a osmolaridade sérica aumenta.

GENÉTICA
N/D.

INCIDÊNCIA/PREVALÊNCIA
Incomum.

DISTRIBUIÇÃO GEOGRÁFICA
N/D.

IDENTIFICAÇÃO
Espécies
Principalmente gatos e, raras vezes, cães.
Raça(s) Predominante(s)
N/D.
Idade Média e Faixa Etária
- Cães — pico de prevalência, 7-9 anos de idade.
- Gatos — qualquer idade; a maioria tem >6 anos de idade.

Sexo Predominante
- Caninos — fêmeas.
- Felinos — machos castrados.

SINAIS CLÍNICOS
Achados Anamnésicos
- Polidipsia/poliúria, polifagia e perda de peso.
- Sinais tardios — fraqueza, vômito, anorexia, depressão, estupor e coma.

Achados do Exame Físico
- Desidratação (grave [10-15%]).
- Hipotermia.
- Prolongamento no tempo de preenchimento capilar.
- Letargia, depressão.
- Crises convulsivas (hiperosmolaridade grave).
- Estupor ou coma (hiperosmolaridade grave).
- Cataratas (cães).

CAUSAS
Diabetes melito associado a hiperosmolaridade, hiperglicemia, azotemia e desidratação graves.

FATORES DE RISCO
- Problemas concomitantes, como cardiopatia, insuficiência renal, pneumonia, pancreatite aguda e outras doenças graves.
- Medicamentos — anticonvulsivantes, glicocorticoides e diuréticos tiazídicos podem precipitar ou agravar essa síndrome.

DIAGNÓSTICO

DIAGNÓSTICO DIFERENCIAL
- Coma mixedematoso — achados clínicos semelhantes, baixo nível de T_4 total, alto nível de TSH.
- Diabetes melito sem complicação — animal alerta mentalmente em casos de hiperglicemia e glicosúria em jejum.
- Diabetes melito cetoacidótico — hiperglicemia em jejum com glicosúria, cetonúria e acidose metabólica.
- Os sinais de letargia e depressão extremas com hiperosmolaridade, hiperglicemia e desidratação graves sem cetonemia e cetonúria costumam diferenciar o diabetes melito com síndrome hiperosmolar não cetótica e o diabetes melito descomplicado e cetoacidótico.

HEMOGRAMA/BIOQUÍMICA/URINÁLISE
- Hiperglicemia grave — geralmente >600 mg/dL.
- Concentrações elevadas de ureia e creatinina.
- Hipernatremia.
- Normocalemia (apesar da depleção do potássio corporal total) ou hipocalemia.
- Em pacientes com insuficiência renal anúrica ou oligúrica, espera-se uma hipercalemia.
- CO_2 total baixo.
- Hiato aniônico elevado.
- Glicosúria.
- Densidade urinária baixa.

OUTROS TESTES LABORATORIAIS
- Hiperosmolaridade grave — geralmente >350 mOsm/L.
- É possível calcular a osmolaridade sérica estimada ou aproximada a partir dos resultados da bioquímica sérica, conforme a fórmula a seguir: 1,86 (Na + K) + ureia/2,8 + glicose/18
- A concentração plasmática elevada do lactato pode ajudar a confirmar acidose láctica metabólica na ausência de cetonemia e cetonúria.

DIAGNÓSTICO POR IMAGEM
N/D.

MÉTODOS DIAGNÓSTICOS
N/D.

ACHADOS PATOLÓGICOS
- Atrofia das células das ilhotas pancreáticas (cães).
- Amiloide pancreático (gatos).
- Necrose cerebral, tromboembolia.

TRATAMENTO

CUIDADO(S) DE SAÚDE ADEQUADO(S)
Corresponde a uma emergência médica potencialmente letal, que requer tratamento com internação.

CUIDADO(S) DE ENFERMAGEM
- A fluidoterapia constitui um componente importante do tratamento clínico. A colocação de sonda nasogástrica possibilita a reposição lenta de água por via oral (cuidado em pacientes com coma).
- Repor metade dos déficits hídricos nas primeiras 12 h e o restante durante as próximas 24 h.
- Administrar soro fisiológico (a 0,9%) por via IV se o animal estiver hipotenso ou hiponatrêmico; utilizar salina a 0,45% se hipernatrêmico (cuidado em reduzir o Na por volta de 2,2 mEq/kg/dia).
- Adicionar potássio (20 mEq/L) aos fluidos iniciais a menos que o paciente tenha hipercalemia.
- Após o restabelecimento da pressão arterial e do débito urinário normais, trocar para a administração IV de solução salina a 0,45%.
- Mudar para glicose a 2,5-5% mais solução salina a 0,45% quando a glicose sanguínea estiver <250 mg/dL e continuar até que o paciente esteja comendo e bebendo por conta própria.

ATIVIDADE
N/D.

DIETA
- Para os cães estabilizados, é recomendável uma dieta pobre em gorduras e rica tanto em fibras como em carboidratos complexos.
- Para os gatos estabilizados, é aconselhável uma dieta pobre em carboidratos e rica em proteínas.

ORIENTAÇÃO AO PROPRIETÁRIO
- Prognóstico mau a reservado.
- Durante a internação, há necessidade de cuidado intensivo e monitorização frequente.

CONSIDERAÇÕES CIRÚRGICAS
N/D.

MEDICAÇÕES

MEDICAMENTO(S) DE ESCOLHA
- Administrar insulina regular 2-4 horas após a instituição da fluidoterapia IV.
- Pode-se usar a insulina regular sob taxa de infusão IV constante na dose de 1,1 U/kg/24 h. Acrescentar 1,1 U/kg da insulina regular em 250 mL de NaCl a 0,9% e administrar a 10 mL/h (0,045 U/kg/h) em equipo separado. Descartar os primeiros 50 mL da solução para compensar a insulina que gruda no tubo plástico.
- Diminuir a dosagem/velocidade constante de infusão quando a glicose sanguínea estiver <250 mg/dL.

Diabetes Melito com Coma Hiperosmolar

- Assim que o paciente se encontrar estabilizado (comendo e bebendo por conta própria, sem vômitos), interromper a administração dos fluidos e da insulina regular; em seguida, pode-se aplicar a insulina glargina, zíncica protamina ou lenta por via SC, como de costume.
- É imprescindível tratar outras doenças concomitantes de forma apropriada.

CONTRAINDICAÇÕES
N/D.

PRECAUÇÕES
Evitar a redução rápida da osmolaridade e da glicose séricas, pois o cérebro ficará hiperosmolar, em comparação ao soro; em seguida, o líquido pode se desviar do espaço extra para o intracelular, resultando em edema cerebral e agravamento do estado neurológico.

INTERAÇÕES POSSÍVEIS
N/D.

MEDICAMENTO(S) ALTERNATIVO(S)
Assim que o quadro estiver estabilizado, podem-se usar agentes hipoglicemiantes orais (p. ex., glipizida) em gatos.

ACOMPANHAMENTO

MONITORIZAÇÃO DO PACIENTE
- Mensurar as concentrações sanguíneas de glicose, com rigor, para evitar hipoglicemia, bem como declínios abruptos e súbitos.
- Idealmente, a glicose sanguínea deve cair 50-100 mg/dL/h até se atingir a concentração de 250 mg/dL.
- Mensurar a glicose sanguínea de hora em hora antes de administrar a próxima dose de insulina regular por via IM durante a estabilização inicial.
- Mensurar o débito urinário para a detecção precoce de insuficiência renal aguda.
- Avaliar estado de hidratação, ECG, pressão venosa central, eletrólitos séricos, ureia e glicose urinária, a cada 2 h durante o período inicial de estabilização.
- Efetuar o controle da glicose a longo prazo, por meio da determinação das concentrações séricas da hemoglobina glicosilada e da frutosamina.
- Ficar atento ao retorno dos sinais clínicos, como polidipsia, poliúria e polifagia.

PREVENÇÃO
- Evitar insulinoterapia inapropriada e insuficiente.
- Evitar hipoglicemia, hipocalemia e hiponatremia.

COMPLICAÇÕES POSSÍVEIS
- São possíveis coma irreversível e óbito, sobretudo em pacientes com insuficiência renal.
- Insuficiência renal aguda.

EVOLUÇÃO ESPERADA E PROGNÓSTICO
Os sinais clínicos e os valores laboratoriais podem melhorar dentro das 24 h iniciais do tratamento, mas esses pacientes apresentam prognóstico reservado.

DIVERSOS

DISTÚRBIOS ASSOCIADOS
Insuficiência cardíaca congestiva, nefropatia, infecção, hemorragia gastrintestinal e outras doenças graves.

FATORES RELACIONADOS COM A IDADE
N/D.

POTENCIAL ZOONÓTICO
N/D.

GESTAÇÃO/FERTILIDADE/REPRODUÇÃO
N/D.

SINÔNIMO(S)
- Coma diabético.
- Coma hiperosmolar.

VER TAMBÉM
- Diabetes Melito com Cetoacidose.
- Diabetes Melito sem Complicação — Cães.
- Diabetes Melito sem Complicação — Gatos.
- Hiperglicemia.
- Hiperosmolaridade.

ABREVIATURA(S)
- CO_2 = dióxido de carbono.
- ECG = eletrocardiograma.
- SNC = sistema nervoso central.
- TSH = hormônio tireostimulante.

Sugestões de Leitura

Brody GM. Diabetic ketoacidosis and hyperosmolar hyperglycemic nonketotic coma. Topics Emerg Med 1992, 14:12-22.

Koenig A, Drobatz KJ, Beale AB, King LG. Hyperglycemic, hyperosmolar syndrome in feline diabetics: 17 cases (1995-2001). J Vet Emerg Crit Care 2004, 14(1):30-40.

MacIntire DK. Emergency therapy of diabetic crises: Insulin overdose, diabetic ketoacidosis, and hyperosmolar coma. Vet Clin North Am 1995, 25:639-650.

Autor Deborah S. Greco
Consultor Editorial Deborah S. Greco
Agradecimento Margaret Kern

Diabetes Melito sem Complicação — Cães

CONSIDERAÇÕES GERAIS

DEFINIÇÃO
• Hiperglicemia de jejum de gravidade suficiente a ponto de resultar em glicosúria concomitante.
• Distúrbio do metabolismo de carboidratos, lipídios e proteínas, causado pela deficiência absoluta ou relativa da insulina. • Em geral, o diabetes melito canino caracteriza-se pela perda da capacidade secretora de insulina por uma suposta destruição imunomediada das células β pancreáticas, resultando em uma dependência de insulina exógena (diabetes melito insulinodependente). • Com uma frequência ainda menor, o diabetes melito canino pode se desenvolver como resultado da combinação de uma deficiência relativa de insulina com insulinorresistência periférica concomitante. Essa combinação de eventos pode culminar em diabetes melito insulinodependente, diabetes melito não insulinodependente ou ambos.

FISIOPATOLOGIA
• A deficiência absoluta ou relativa de insulina resulta em um catabolismo tecidual acelerado, diminuição na capacidade de manutenção da homeostasia de carboidratos, lipídios e proteínas, bem como insulinorresistência. • A hipoinsulinemia, a resistência periférica à insulina e a gliconeogênese hepática contínua culminam em hiperglicemia persistente de gravidade suficiente a ponto de sobrecarregar a reabsorção tubular renal de glicose, levando à glicosúria, consequente diurese osmótica e poliúria/polidipsia compensatórias. • A perda do sinal hipotalâmico de saciedade mediado pela glicose e dependente de insulina culmina em polifagia. • A diminuição na utilização de glicose, dependente de insulina, resulta em catabolismo proteico com perda de peso e aumento na mobilização de lipídios (hiperlipidemia, lipidose hepática, produção de cetonas). • A insulina é muito eficaz para inibir a lipólise periférica e, por essa razão, a produção corporal descontrolada de cetonas ocorre apenas em animais com diabetes melito insulinodependente. • Os acúmulos de grandes quantidades de corpos cetônicos levam ao desenvolvimento de acidose metabólica e à depleção do potássio corporal total.

SISTEMA(S) ACOMETIDO(S)
• Endócrino/metabólico — depleção eletrolítica e acidose metabólica. • Hepatobiliar — lipidose hepática. • Oftálmico — cataratas. • Renal/urológico — glicosúria com consequente diurese osmótica e aumento na probabilidade de infecção bacteriana do trato urinário.

GENÉTICA
Certas raças são drasticamente sub e super-representadas, sugerindo uma suscetibilidade hereditária a insulite (inflamação das ilhotas de Langerhans do pâncreas).

INCIDÊNCIA/PREVALÊNCIA
• A prevalência varia entre 1:400 e 1:500. • Início com incidência sazonal; maior número de animais é diagnosticado no outono e inverno.

IDENTIFICAÇÃO
Espécies
Cães.

Raça(s) Predominante(s)
• As raças super-representadas incluem Samoieda, Terrier tibetano, Cairn terrier e Golden retriever (apenas nos EUA). • Risco possivelmente mais alto que outras raças — Keeshond, Poodle, Dachshund, Schnauzer miniatura, e Beagle. • As raças sub-representadas abrangem Boxer, Pastor alemão e Golden retriever (apenas nos EUA).

Idade Média e Faixa Etária
Média, ~8 anos de idade; faixa etária, 4-14 anos (excluindo a forma juvenil rara).

Sexo Predominante
Fêmeas.

SINAIS CLÍNICOS
• Poliúria e polidipsia (PU/PD), polifagia e perda de peso. • Hepatomegalia. • As cataratas constituem um achado comum em casos crônicos ou em cães com controle insatisfatório de sua doença. • Em animais com cetoacidose acentuada, podem ocorrer letargia, depressão, inapetência, anorexia e vômito.

CAUSAS
• Insulite imunomediada primária. • Distúrbios predisponentes à insulite imunomediada secundária, como pancreatite, diversas doenças virais.

FATORES DE RISCO
• Diestro em cadelas. • Suscetibilidade genética à insulite imunomediada. • Medicamentos como glicocorticoides e progestinas.

DIAGNÓSTICO

DIAGNÓSTICO DIFERENCIAL
Glicosúria renal — não costuma causar hiperglicemia e, geralmente, nenhum sinal de perda de peso com polifagia.

HEMOGRAMA/BIOQUÍMICA/URINÁLISE
• Os resultados do hemograma, em geral, permanecem normais. • Glicose >200 mg/dL. • Atividades elevadas da fosfatase alcalina sérica e da alanina aminotransferase (ALT), em geral com um aumento proporcionalmente maior da primeira enzima, compatível com hepatopatia obstrutiva. • Hipercolesterolemia, lipemia e cetonemia são alterações comuns. • O nível dos eletrólitos varia, mas a hipocalemia e a hipofosfatemia indicam descompensação grave. • O CO_2 total ou o HCO_3 estarão baixos se o paciente apresentar cetoacidose ou desidratação intensa. • A glicosúria é um achado compatível. • A cetonúria é comum. • A densidade urinária pode ser variável, dependendo do nível de glicosúria.

OUTROS TESTES LABORATORIAIS
• Hiato aniônico — alto em pacientes com cetoacidose. • Concentrações plasmáticas de insulina — não são particularmente úteis. Embora uma concentração baixa de insulina sugira uma deficiência absoluta desse hormônio, isso pode ser um reflexo de exaustão reversível das ilhotas pancreáticas, já que a hiperglicemia persistente pode diminuir a atividade secretora desse hormônio, mesmo na presença de células β funcionais.

DIAGNÓSTICO POR IMAGEM
• Radiografia — útil para avaliar doenças concomitantes ou subjacentes (p. ex., cálculos vesicais ou renais, cistite ou colecistite enfisematosas e pancreatite). • Ultrassonografia — indicada em pacientes selecionados, particularmente aqueles com icterícia, para avaliar outras causas possíveis de hepatopatia obstrutiva significativa ou pancreatite concorrente/complicante.

MÉTODOS DIAGNÓSTICOS
Biopsia hepática (percutânea) — indicada em alguns pacientes ictéricos para avaliar outras causas possíveis de hepatopatia obstrutiva.

ACHADOS PATOLÓGICOS
• Achados macroscópicos à necropsia — hepatomegalia com acúmulo significativo de lipídios no fígado. • Os achados histopatológicos revelam, em geral, uma redução drástica no tamanho e no número de ilhotas pancreáticas com arquitetura relativamente normal do tecido exócrino, exceto em cães com doença pancreática exócrina concomitante.

TRATAMENTO

CUIDADO(S) DE SAÚDE ADEQUADO(S)
• Os cães compensados podem ser tratados em um esquema ambulatorial; tais animais encontram-se alertas, bem hidratados e continuam se alimentando e bebendo líquidos, sem vômitos. • Quanto ao tratamento de pacientes descompensados, ver o capítulo sobre "Diabetes Melito com Cetoacidose".

CUIDADO(S) DE ENFERMAGEM
Fluidoterapia — ver "Diabetes Melito com Cetoacidose".

ATIVIDADE
A atividade física vigorosa pode reduzir as necessidades de insulina; um nível constante de atividade diária mostra-se útil.

DIETA
• A dieta deve ser compatível ao quadro — o alimento deve ser controlado e constante em termos calóricos e constitutivos; além disso, o animal deve consumir a mesma ingestão calórica todas as manhãs e todas as noites. • É importante equiparar os efeitos hipoglicêmicos da insulina com os efeitos hiperglicêmicos da refeição. Como a maioria das insulinas atua no máximo 2 a 4 h após a administração de SC e, normalmente, grande parte do alimento está sendo absorvido dentro de 1 h do consumo, o controle glicêmico será quase sempre restabelecido se o cão for alimentado 60-90 minutos APÓS 12 h da dosagem de insulina. Os animais que "beliscam" ao longo do dia podem ser alimentados com ração seca *ad libitum* e duas refeições pequenas de ração enlatada, conforme descrito. Se a insulina não puder ser administrada 1 vez ao dia, fornecer a ingestão calórica diária total em 2 ou 3 refeições dentro das primeiras 6-8 h após a dosagem da insulina. • Fornecer uma quantidade calórica adequada para o peso corporal ideal do animal (~50-70 kcals/kg). O alimento deve ser algo que o cão coma com segurança e dentro de um curto período de tempo. • Cães diabéticos obesos — fornecer uma dieta com restrição calórica para garantir que seu peso corporal ideal seja atingido dentro de 2-4 meses com o uso de alimento rico em fibras e pobre em calorias. Embora uma dieta rica em fibras possa aumentar a saciedade do

Diabetes Melito sem Complicação — Cães

paciente e, possivelmente, a satisfação do proprietário, esse tipo de dieta não desempenha qualquer papel no restabelecimento do controle diabético. • Não é recomendável o fornecimento de petiscos a menos que eles sejam praticamente zero de calorias.

ORIENTAÇÃO AO PROPRIETÁRIO
• Debater sobre os esquemas diários de alimentação e medicamentos, a monitorização domiciliar, os sinais de hipoglicemia, bem como o que fazer diante deles e o momento de se buscar a orientação ou a consulta veterinária. • Os proprietários devem ser incentivados a manter um quadro de informações pertinentes a respeito do animal de estimação, como consumo diário de água, peso corporal semanal, doses atuais de insulina e quantidade de alimento consumido.

CONSIDERAÇÕES CIRÚRGICAS
As fêmeas intactas devem ser submetidas à ovário-histerectomia, quando se encontrarem estabilizadas; a progesterona secretada durante o diestro torna mais imprevisível o tratamento do diabetes melito.

MEDICAÇÕES

MEDICAMENTO(S) DE ESCOLHA
• Insulina — imprescindível para os casos de diabetes melito insulinodependente; utilizada com frequência como parte do tratamento do diabetes melito não insulinodependente. • Vetsulin® (insulina lenta de origem suína) — 0,75 unidades/kg SC a cada 12 h como dose inicial. NOTA: insulina U-40; é imprescindível o uso com seringa de insulina U-40. A disponibilidade pode ser limitada. • Humulin N® — insulina humana de ação intermediária; 0,75 unidades/kg SC a cada 12 h como dose inicial. • Novolin N® — insulina humana de ação intermediária; 0,75 unidades/kg SC a cada 12 h como dose inicial. • PZI Vet® (Idexx Laboratories) raramente é utilizada em cães; insulina humana zíncica protamina de ação intermediária a mais prolongada. NOTA: insulina U-40; é indispensável o uso com seringa de U-40. • Insulinas glargina e detemir: insulinas sintéticas de ação intermediária a mais prolongada, que possuem um nível "sem pico" de atividade e liberação tardia a partir de injeções subcutâneas. Essas insulinas raramente são utilizadas em cães. • As espécies de origem (fonte) da insulina podem influenciar a farmacocinética; as insulinas de origem canina e suína têm sequências idênticas de aminoácidos e, por essa razão, a Vetsulin® não produz uma resposta humoral significativa contra insulina, enquanto grande parte das outras insulinas disponíveis no mercado promove isso. Contudo, não há provas de que o desenvolvimento de anticorpos contra insulina tenha algum significado clínico.

PRECAUÇÕES
• Os glicocorticoides, o acetato de megestrol e a progesterona causam resistência à insulina. • Será preciso ter cuidado com os agentes hiperosmóticos (p. ex., manitol e agentes de contraste radiográfico) se o paciente já estiver hiperosmolar em virtude da hiperglicemia.

MEDICAMENTO(S) ALTERNATIVO(S)
Em geral, o uso de agentes hipoglicemiantes orais não é recomendável. O raro cão com diabetes melito não insulinodependente pode ser responsivo ao tratamento com agentes hipoglicemiantes orais; no entanto, é imprescindível monitorizá-lo com rigor, pois geralmente se trata de uma doença progressiva e o tratamento eficaz pode ter consequências desastrosas.

ACOMPANHAMENTO

MONITORIZAÇÃO DO PACIENTE
• Os cães diabéticos deverão ser tratados por meio de contato regular entre o proprietário e a equipe veterinária. A frequência deverá ser de aproximadamente 3–4 meses se o animal estiver estabilizado e se os sinais clínicos estiverem controlados; ou com maior frequência se o controle se mostrar insatisfatório ou variável. Os critérios eficazes na avaliação de um controle adequado estão listados abaixo. • Sinais clínicos — estimar o grau de PU/PD, o apetite e o peso corporal; se esses itens permanecerem dentro de limites aceitáveis, a doença provavelmente estará bem regulada. • Proteínas glicosiladas — hemoglobina glicosilada ou frutosamina; o grau de glicosilação relaciona-se diretamente com a concentração sanguínea de glicose durante o período de vida das proteínas (normalmente 10-20 dias para a frutosamina, 4-8 semanas para a hemoglobina); dessa forma, essas proteínas não são influenciadas por alterações inexplicáveis no nível isolado de glicose sanguínea nem por efeitos de viagens e/ou internações sobre o esvaziamento gástrico e, consequentemente, a inter-relação entre os efeitos da insulina e a refeição sobre os níveis da glicose sanguínea. • Os níveis das proteínas glicosiladas são modificados por alterações nas concentrações de albumina ou hemoglobina e pela quantidade de tempo gasto na circulação; qualquer coisa que acelere o *turnover* [renovação] da albumina (p. ex., glomerulonefropatia, disfunção hepática, doença GI) reduzirá o nível da frutosamina para uma determinada glicemia média. • Os níveis das proteínas glicosiladas são mais bem utilizados para o tratamento contínuo de paciente diabético relativamente estável; um nível de frutosamina no terço superior da faixa de referência reflete um controle diabético excelente; já um nível de frutosamina no terço inferior é mais sugestivo de um controle diabético demasiadamente zeloso e possível aumento no risco de hipoglicemia clinicamente significativa. • Curva glicêmica — pode fornecer informações sobre a eficácia da insulina, a duração de ação, o nadir (nível sanguíneo mais baixo da glicose, atingido durante o intervalo entre as doses) e o potencial de hiperglicemia de rebote; os resultados estão sujeitos a influências externas; estresse decorrente da internação e coletas múltiplas de sangue; teste utilizado com maior frequência ao se estabilizar o controle inicial, modificar o tipo, a dose ou a frequência de insulina ou se solucionar o quadro em diabéticos problemáticos; idealmente, a duração da curva equipara-se com o intervalo das doses (12 ou 24 h); a identificação do nadir (para evitar hipoglicemia iatrogênica) e o nível de glicose no momento da dosagem constituem os aspectos mais importantes da curva; mimetizar as condições "normais" o mais estritamente possível; antes da internação, pode ser preciso que o proprietário alimente o animal de estimação e aplique a insulina em casa, embora isso não seja ideal, pois introduz fatores adicionais de confusão, relacionados ao esvaziamento gástrico; mensurar a glicose sanguínea a cada 2 ou 4 h; o objetivo é obter uma dose eficaz de insulina (declínio na glicose sanguínea para 100-200 mg/dL) em um intervalo apropriado (a cada 12 ou 24 h, na maioria dos casos) com nadir >80 mg/dL e <150 mg/dL. • Monitorização domiciliar com o uso de estimativas seriadas da glicemia com kits de monitorização da glicose; requer o compromisso, o consentimento e a habilidade do proprietário; essa monitorização é bastante útil como indicador precoce da necessidade de redução na dose em pacientes com sinais clínicos bem controlados; jamais deve ser empregada como critério isolado para o ajuste da insulina pelo proprietário. Os níveis urinários da glicose mensurados pelo proprietário não são particularmente úteis.

PREVENÇÃO
• Castrar as fêmeas; evitar o uso desnecessário do acetato de megestrol. • Não há provas sugestivas de que a obesidade aumente o risco de diabetes melito em cães castrados.

COMPLICAÇÕES POSSÍVEIS
• Pode ocorrer o surgimento de cataratas mesmo com controle glicêmico satisfatório. • Fraqueza, especialmente com exercício; podem ocorrer crises convulsivas ou coma com dosagem excessiva de insulina. • Anemia e hemoglobinemia em caso de hipofosfatemia grave — são complicações extremamente raras e, muito provavelmente, constituem uma consequência do tratamento de cão diabético com cetoacidose.

EVOLUÇÃO ESPERADA E PROGNÓSTICO
• Os cães geralmente apresentam doença permanente a menos que seja influenciada durante um ciclo estral (caso em que a castração pode solucionar o diabetes por um período). • O prognóstico com a aplicação de insulina 2 vezes ao dia e a alimentação alinhada aos efeitos máximos desse hormônio é excelente.

DIVERSOS

DISTÚRBIOS ASSOCIADOS
• Cataratas. • Infecção do trato urinário.

FATORES RELACIONADOS COM A IDADE
O diabetes melito juvenil é raro e seu tratamento pode ser mais difícil.

GESTAÇÃO/FERTILIDADE/REPRODUÇÃO
• O diabetes melito pode se desenvolver durante a prenhez e, nesse caso, é difícil mantê-la. • A administração exógena de insulina pode causar aumento desproporcional do tamanho fetal e distocia. • Também ocorre o desenvolvimento de uma resistência à insulina, o que dificulta o controle da hiperglicemia. • A cadela prenhe é propensa à cetoacidose; dessa forma, poderá ser necessária uma ovário-histerectomia de emergência. • Os cães com diabetes melito não devem se acasalar.

ABREVIATURA(S)
• PU/PD = poliúria e polidipsia.

Autor David Church
Consultor Editorial Deborah S. Greco

Diabetes Melito sem Complicação — Gatos

CONSIDERAÇÕES GERAIS

DEFINIÇÃO
• Distúrbio do metabolismo de carboidratos, lipídios e proteínas, causado pela deficiência absoluta ou relativa da insulina, insulinorresistência e amiloidose insular.
• O tipo II (diabetes melito não insulinodependente) caracteriza-se pela secreção inadequada ou tardia de insulina, em relação às necessidades do paciente; muitos desses pacientes vivem sem a insulina exógena e são menos propensos à cetoacidose; forma mais comum em gatos.

FISIOPATOLOGIA
• A resistência à insulina diminui a capacidade de utilização de carboidratos, lipídios e proteínas pelos tecidos (especialmente da musculatura, do tecido adiposo e do fígado).
• A utilização comprometida da glicose e a gliconeogênese hepática contínua causam hiperglicemia.
• Na sequência, ocorre o desenvolvimento de glicosúria, que leva à diurese osmótica, poliúria e perda de peso compensatória; a mobilização de ácidos graxos livres para o fígado provoca tanto lipidose hepática como cetogênese.

SISTEMA(S) ACOMETIDO(S)
• Endócrino/metabólico — depleção eletrolítica e acidose metabólica.
• Hepatobiliar — lipidose hepática; pode se desenvolver insuficiência hepática.
• Renal/urológico — infecção do trato urinário e diurese osmótica.
• Nervoso — neuropatia periférica.

INCIDÊNCIA/PREVALÊNCIA
A prevalência em gatos é de 1:200.

IDENTIFICAÇÃO
Espécies
Gatos.

Idade Média e Faixa Etária
75% dos casos apresentam-se entre 8-13 anos de idade; faixa etária, 1-19 anos.

Sexo Predominante
Machos.

SINAIS CLÍNICOS
• Sinais precoces — é típica a presença de obesidade.
• É comum a observação de emaciação da musculatura dorsal e oleosidade da pelagem com seborreia (caspas).
• Hepatomegalia, porém a icterícia é mais prevalente em gatos do que em cães.
• Achados menos comuns, postura plantígrada em gatos (neuropatia diabética).
• Sinais tardios — poliúria e polidipsia (PU/PD), polifagia, perda de peso, anorexia, letargia, depressão e vômito.

CAUSAS
• Suscetibilidade genética.
• Amiloide.
• Pancreatite.
• Doenças predisponentes (p. ex., hiperadrenocorticismo e acromegalia).
• Medicamentos (p. ex., glicocorticoides e progestagênios).

FATORES DE RISCO
• Obesidade em caso de diabetes melito do tipo II.
• Ver a seção "Causas".

DIAGNÓSTICO

DIAGNÓSTICO DIFERENCIAL
• Glicosúria renal — geralmente não causa PU/PD, perda de peso ou hiperglicemia.
• Hiperglicemia por estresse em gatos — sem PU/PD ou perda de peso; caso se colete a amostra quando o gato não se encontra estressado, a concentração sanguínea de glicose permanecerá normal. Nível normal de frutosamina.

HEMOGRAMA/BIOQUÍMICA/URINÁLISE
• Os resultados do hemograma, em geral, permanecem normais.
• Glicose >150 mg/dL.
• Atividades elevadas da fosfatase alcalina sérica, alanina aminotransferase (ALT) e aspartato aminotransferase (AST), bem como hipercolesterolemia e lipemia — são comuns.
• O nível dos eletrólitos varia, mas a hipernatremia, a hipocalemia e a hipofosfatemia indicam descompensação grave.
• O CO_2 total ou o HCO_3 estarão baixos se o paciente apresentar cetoacidose ou desidratação intensa.
• A glicosúria é um achado compatível.
• A cetonúria é incomum.
• Com frequência, a densidade urinária encontra-se baixa.

OUTROS TESTES LABORATORIAIS
• Hiato aniônico — alto em pacientes com cetoacidose.
• Frutosamina >350 micromol/L.

DIAGNÓSTICO POR IMAGEM
• Radiografia — útil para avaliar doenças concomitantes ou subjacentes (p. ex., cálculos vesicais ou renais, cistite ou colecistite enfisematosas e pancreatite).
• Ultrassonografia — indicada em pacientes selecionados, particularmente aqueles com icterícia, para pesquisar lipidose hepática, colangio-hepatite e pancreatite.

MÉTODOS DIAGNÓSTICOS
Biopsia hepática (percutânea) — indicada em alguns pacientes ictéricos.

ACHADOS PATOLÓGICOS
• Em geral, não há nenhuma alteração macroscópica à necropsia.
• Os achados histopatológicos podem permanecer normais ou revelar uma degeneração vacuolar das ilhotas de Langerhans ou quantidade pequena de células insulares; em geral, observam-se depósitos de amiloide nas ilhotas.

TRATAMENTO

CUIDADO(S) DE SAÚDE ADEQUADO(S)
• Os gatos compensados podem ser tratados em um esquema ambulatorial; tais animais encontram-se alertas, hidratados e continuam se alimentando e bebendo líquidos, sem vômitos.
• Quanto ao tratamento de pacientes descompensados, ver o capítulo sobre "Diabetes Melito com Cetoacidose".

CUIDADO(S) DE ENFERMAGEM
Fluidoterapia — ver "Diabetes Melito com Cetoacidose".

ATIVIDADE
A atividade física vigorosa pode reduzir as necessidades de insulina; o nível constante de atividade diária mostra-se útil.

DIETA
• Estudos sugerem que dietas enlatadas com teores ultrabaixos de carboidratos podem induzir à remissão do diabetes em 70-95% dos gatos diabéticos recém-diagnosticados; monitorizar de perto em busca de alteração nas necessidades de insulina após qualquer ajuste na dieta.
• Em virtude da indução de hiperglicemia pós-prandial grave, é recomendável evitar os alimentos macios e úmidos.

ORIENTAÇÃO AO PROPRIETÁRIO
• Debater sobre os esquemas diários de alimentação e medicamentos, a monitorização domiciliar, os sinais de hipoglicemia e o que fazer diante deles, bem como sobre o momento de se buscar a orientação ou a consulta veterinária.
• Os proprietários devem ser incentivados a manter um quadro de informações pertinentes a respeito do animal de estimação, como resultados das fitas urinárias reagentes, doses diárias da insulina e pesos corporais semanais.

CONSIDERAÇÕES CIRÚRGICAS
As fêmeas intactas devem ser submetidas à ovário-histerectomia quando se encontrarem estabilizadas; a progesterona secretada durante o diestro dificulta o tratamento do diabetes melito.

MEDICAÇÕES

MEDICAMENTO(S) DE ESCOLHA
• Insulina — tratamento de escolha para a maioria dos gatos.
• Insulina lenta de origem suína (Vetsulin®) — duração intermediária; administrada por via SC; dosagem inicial 2 U a cada 12 h. A disponibilidade pode ser limitada.
• Insulina zíncica protamina (PZI [do inglês *Protamine zinc insulin*], U-40 [concentração]) — insulina de ação prolongada; administrada por via SC, geralmente a cada 24 h; alguns gatos necessitam de injeções a cada 12 h, começando com uma dose de 2 U a cada 12 h.
• Insulina glargina (Lantus®, U-100 [concentração]) — insulina recombinante humana basal sem pico, que confere os melhores resultados quando combinada com uma dieta pobre em carboidrato e rica em proteína. São relatadas taxas de remissão de 70-100% com essa combinação. Dose: 2 U SC a cada 12 h.
• Administração oral de agentes hipoglicemiantes — em gatos com diabetes melito do tipo II, a glipizida mostra-se útil, associada à terapia nutricional; o gato deve apresentar diabetes melito sem complicação e não deve exibir nenhum histórico de cetoacidose; dosagem inicial, 2,5 mg VO a cada 12 h; a monitorização é semelhante àquela realizada em pacientes submetidos à insulina; caso não se controle a hiperglicemia, pode-se tentar a dose de 5 mg VO a cada 12 h; os

Diabetes Melito sem Complicação — Gatos

efeitos colaterais potenciais são: hipoglicemia, alterações das enzimas hepáticas, icterícia e vômito.

PRECAUÇÕES
• Os glicocorticoides, o acetato de megestrol e a progesterona causam insulinorresistência. Se a terapia com esteroides for necessária, utilizar o agente medrol por via oral. Evitar os esteroides injetáveis.
• Utilizar os agentes hiperosmóticos (p. ex., manitol e agentes de contraste radiográfico) se o paciente já estiver hiperosmolar em virtude da hiperglicemia.

INTERAÇÕES POSSÍVEIS
Muitos medicamentos (p. ex., AINEs, sulfonamidas, miconazol, cloranfenicol, inibidores da monoamina oxidase e β-bloqueadores) potencializam o efeito de agentes hipoglicemiantes administrados por via oral; consultar a bula do produto.

MEDICAMENTO(S) ALTERNATIVO(S)
Acarbose —12,5 mg VO a cada 12 h.

ACOMPANHAMENTO

MONITORIZAÇÃO DO PACIENTE
• Curva glicêmica — não é útil em gatos.
• Monitorização da glicose urinária — testa-se a urina quanto à presença de glicose e cetonas, antes das refeições e das injeções de insulina; para utilizar esse procedimento como método regulatório, é imprescindível deixar que o animal mantenha traços (0,25%) de glicosúria para evitar a hipoglicemia.
• Frutosamina — manter <400 micromol/ L. Reavaliar mensalmente durante a regulação inicial, depois a cada 3 meses.
• Sinais clínicos — o proprietário pode estimar o grau de PU/PD, o apetite e o peso corporal; se esses itens permanecerem normais, a doença estará bem regulada.

PREVENÇÃO
Evitar ou corrigir a obesidade; evitar o uso desnecessário de glicocorticoides ou acetato de megestrol.

COMPLICAÇÕES POSSÍVEIS
• Crises convulsivas, cegueira ou coma em caso de superdosagem de insulina.
• Nefropatia diabética.
• Neuropatia diabética.

EVOLUÇÃO ESPERADA E PROGNÓSTICO
• Alguns gatos recuperam-se, mas pode haver recidivas mais tarde.
• O prognóstico com o tratamento é bom; a maioria dos animais apresenta uma expectativa de vida normal.

DIVERSOS

DISTÚRBIOS ASSOCIADOS
Infecção do trato urinário.

FATORES RELACIONADOS COM A IDADE
O diabetes melito juvenil é raro e seu tratamento pode ser mais difícil.

POTENCIAL ZOONÓTICO
Nenhum.

VER TAMBÉM
• Diabetes Melito com Cetoacidose.
• Hiperosmolalidade.

ABREVIATURA(S)
• AINEs = anti-inflamatórios não esteroides.
• ALT = alanina aminotransferase.
• AST = aspartato aminotransferase.
• PU/PD = poliúria e polidipsia.

Sugestões de Leitura
Bennett N, Greco DS, Peterson ME, et al. Comparison of a low carbohydrate-low fiber diet and a moderate carbohydrate-high fiber diet in the management of feline diabetes mellitus. J Feline Med Surg 2006, 8:73-84.
Crenshaw KL, Peterson ME, Heeb LA, et al. Pretreatment clinical and laboratory evaluation of cats with diabetes mellitus: 104 cases (1992-1994). JAVMA 1996, 209:943-949.
Rand JS, Martin GJ. Management of feline diabetes mellitus. Vet Clin North Am Small Anim Pract 2001, 31:881-913.

Autor Deborah S. Greco
Consultor Editorial Deborah S. Greco

Diarreia Aguda

CONSIDERAÇÕES GERAIS

DEFINIÇÃO
Início abrupto ou recente de evacuação com conteúdo anormalmente alto de água e/ou sólido nas fezes.

FISIOPATOLOGIA
• Causada por desequilíbrio nas ações de absorção, secreção e/ou motilidade intestinais.
• Mecanismos da diarreia: (1) Osmótica — quantidade excessiva de moléculas no lúmen intestinal, o que atrai água, sobrepujando a capacidade de absorção do intestino (p. ex., mudanças da dieta, má absorção ou alimentação excessiva). (2) Secretória — estimulação da secreção do intestino delgado que ultrapassa a capacidade de absorção intestinal (p. ex., toxinas, sejam de origem química ou bacteriana [bactérias intestinais]). A estimulação do sistema nervoso parassimpático ou a exposição a uma variedade de secretagogos pode aumentar a secreção intestinal. (3) Exsudativa ou por aumento da permeabilidade — extravasamento de líquido tecidual, proteínas séricas, sangue ou muco a partir de locais de infiltração ou ulceração. (4) Disfunção da motilidade — a hipomotilidade (íleo paralítico) é mais comum que a hipermotilidade. A hipermotilidade pode ser primária (síndrome do intestino irritável) ou secundária (obstrução e/ou má absorção com consequente distensão intestinal). A motilidade intestinal anterógrada (i. e., que se move para a frente) impulsiona o quimo intestinal em direção ao cólon e para fora do corpo; a motilidade segmentar tende a retardar a progressão anterógrada e aumentar o tempo para digestão e absorção do alimento; o aumento na propulsão anterógrada ou a diminuição nas contrações segmentares pode produzir diarreia por alterações na motilidade e declínios secundários na absorção. (5) Mista.

SISTEMA(S) ACOMETIDO(S)
• Cardiovascular — hipovolemia, com indução de taquicardia, mucosas pálidas e pulsos débeis; a hipocalemia pode causar arritmias.
• Endócrino/metabólico — anormalidades eletrolíticas e acidobásicas, desidratação e azotemia pré-renal.
• Gastrintestinal — dor abdominal e possível diminuição da motilidade induzida por hipocalemia.
• Musculosquelético — a hipocalemia pode levar à fraqueza muscular.

IDENTIFICAÇÃO
• Cães e gatos. • Qualquer animal pode sofrer de diarreia aguda; os filhotes caninos e felinos são os mais frequentemente acometidos.

SINAIS CLÍNICOS
Comentários Gerais
• A diarreia aguda costuma ser autolimitante e se apresentar como um episódio isolado, não afetando o animal em termos sistêmicos.
• Outros casos são leves e não sistêmicos, mas desaparecem depois de alguns dias.
• Algumas vezes, trata-se de uma doença grave aguda ou superaguda. Isso é mais comum em cães do que em gatos (p. ex., parvovirose).
• Os sinais de doença mais grave (p. ex., vômitos concomitantes, dor abdominal, hematoquezia, hemoptise, desidratação intensa ou depressão) devem incitar a prática de medidas diagnósticas e terapêuticas mais rigorosas.

Achados Anamnésicos
• Aumento na fluidez e/ou no volume fecais e/ou na frequência de curta duração.
• O proprietário pode relatar a ocorrência de acidentes fecais, alterações na consistência e no volume fecais, presença de sangue ou muco nas fezes ou esforço para defecar.
• Os proprietários ainda podem se mostrar capazes de relatar exposição a toxinas, bem como mudanças da dieta ou indiscrições/imprudências alimentares.

Achados do Exame Físico
• Variam com a gravidade da doença.
• Presença frequente de desidratação, depressão ou letargia em certas intensidades.
• Em indivíduos mais gravemente acometidos, podem ocorrer dor e desconforto abdominais, febre, sinais de hipotensão, náusea e fraqueza.
• O exame retal pode revelar a presença de sangue e/ou muco ou a consistência alterada das fezes.

CAUSAS
• As doenças sistêmicas também podem resultar em diarreia como evento secundário.
• Indiscrição/imprudência alimentar — ingestão de lixo, material não alimentar ou alimento estragado.
• Mudanças da dieta — alterações abruptas na quantidade ou no tipo dos gêneros alimentícios.
• Intolerância alimentar — má digestão ou má assimilação de gêneros alimentícios, hipersensibilidade alimentar.
• Doenças metabólicas — hipoadrenocorticismo (doença de Addison), hepatopatias, nefropatias e pancreatopatias podem causar diarreia aguda ou crônica.
• Obstruções ou corpos estranhos — ingestão de corpos estranhos, intussuscepção, ou vólvulo intestinal.
• Idiopáticas — gastrenterite hemorrágica.
• Virais — parvovírus (parvovírus canino e panleucopenia felina), coronavírus, rotavírus, vírus da cinomose.
• Bacterianas — *Salmonella*, *Campylobacter*, *Clostridium* spp., *Escherichia coli*, etc.
• Parasitárias — verminóticas (anciclóstomos, ascarídeos, tricúris, estrôngilos e cestódeos) ou protozoárias (*Giardia*, coccídios e *Entamoeba*).
• Riquetsianas — intoxicação pelo salmão (*Neorickettsia*).
• Fúngicas — histoplasmose.
• Medicamentos e toxinas — metais pesados (i. e., chumbo), organofosforados, anti-inflamatórios não esteroides, esteroides, antimicrobianos, anti-helmínticos, agentes antineoplásicos, etc.

FATORES DE RISCO
Os cães e gatos jovens apresentam-se com diarreia por exagero/imprudência alimentar, intussuscepção, corpos estranhos e causas infecciosas em frequência maior que os pacientes mais idosos.

DIAGNÓSTICO

DIAGNÓSTICO DIFERENCIAL
• Os pacientes devem ser submetidos aos exames físico completo e fecal (incluindo exame de flutuação e esfregaço direto), coletando-se um banco de dados mínimo para avaliar o estado de hidratação.
• Os testes diagnósticos adicionais dependem da extensão da doença e de outros sinais clínicos.

HEMOGRAMA/BIOQUÍMICA/URINÁLISE
• Em geral, permanecem normais; não são necessários a menos que haja envolvimento sistêmico.
• Em casos de enterite por parvovírus, pode-se observar neutropenia.
• O nível dos eletrólitos comumente se encontra anormal em função das perdas intestinais (hipocalemia, hipocloremia, hiponatremia).

OUTROS TESTES LABORATORIAIS
• Imunorreatividade da lipase pancreática (pancreatite) e imunorreatividade semelhante à da tripsina (insuficiência pancreática exócrina), bem como mensuração dos níveis de cobalamina e folato (absorção alterada) — esses exames são mais comumente realizados em casos de diarreia crônica.
• Exame de fezes com ELISA e IFA — disponível para pesquisa de *Giardia* e *Cryptococcus*.

DIAGNÓSTICO POR IMAGEM
• Radiografias — em geral, não são necessárias em pacientes com doença leve.
• As radiografias abdominais podem ajudar a identificar ou a descartar corpos estranhos ou obstruções intestinais.
• Sinais mais graves (i. e., dor abdominal ou vômitos persistentes) podem aumentar o provável benefício diagnóstico da radiologia.
• A radiografia abdominal contrastada e a ultrassonografia podem ser úteis em alguns pacientes, sobretudo em busca de alguma obstrução.

MÉTODOS DIAGNÓSTICOS
• Efetuar exame de fezes (flutuação e esfregaço) para pesquisa de parasitas em todos os pacientes.
• Como os ovos de helmintos e os oocistos de *Giardia* podem ser eliminados em quantidade pequena ou de forma intermitente, recomendam-se múltiplas análises fecais, embora se possa aconselhar o tratamento empírico. O teste de ELISA para *Giardia* também pode ser benéfico.
• Para a pesquisa dos antígenos parvovirais em cães, podem-se realizar os testes de ELISA nas fezes.
• Endoscopia e biopsia — úteis em casos selecionados; costumam ser mais imprescindíveis em casos de diarreia crônica.

ACHADOS PATOLÓGICOS
Dependem da etiologia.

TRATAMENTO

Depende basicamente da gravidade da doença; quase sempre, os pacientes com doença leve podem ser tratados no ambulatório com terapia sintomática; já aqueles com doença mais grave ou irresponsivos à terapia devem ser submetidos a tratamento mais rigoroso.

CUIDADO(S) DE ENFERMAGEM
• Na maioria dos casos, a fluidoterapia e a correção dos desequilíbrios eletrolíticos constituem a base do tratamento.

Diarreia Aguda

- A fluidoterapia cristaloide pode ser administrada por via oral, subcutânea ou intravenosa, conforme a necessidade; aos pacientes que não estejam vomitando, podem-se fornecer os fluidos por via oral (água ou fluidos que contenham carboidratos e eletrólitos).
- O tratamento visa o retorno do paciente a um estado de hidratação adequado (em 12-24 h) e a reposição de qualquer perda contínua.
- Em casos de diarreia aguda, pode ocorrer depleção volêmica grave; talvez haja necessidade de fluidoterapia rigorosa para evitar o choque.
- Em grande parte dos pacientes, deve-se lançar mão da suplementação de potássio (cloreto de potássio a 20-40 mEq/L), mas não durante a fluidoterapia do choque. A hipocalemia pode agravar o íleo paralítico.

ATIVIDADE
Os animais devem ser submetidos à restrição da atividade física até a interrupção da diarreia.

DIETA
Aos pacientes com doença leve e sem vômitos, um período de jejum (12-24 h) é frequentemente acompanhado por uma dieta branda, como arroz e carne de frango cozidos (na proporção de 4:1), ou uma dieta comercial de prescrição.

ORIENTAÇÃO AO PROPRIETÁRIO
- Também é recomendável restringir a exposição a lixos, outros alimentos não pertencentes à dieta normal do paciente e corpos estranhos em potencial.
- Proceder aos esquemas adequados de vacinação e vermifugação dos filhotes caninos e felinos.

CONSIDERAÇÕES CIRÚRGICAS
Os pacientes com obstruções ou corpos estranhos podem necessitar de cirurgia para avaliação do intestino e remoção desses objetos estranhos.

MEDICAÇÕES

MEDICAMENTO(S) DE ESCOLHA
- Os medicamentos antidiarreicos podem ser classificados como modificadores da motilidade, agentes antissecretores ou protetores intestinais.
- Os modificadores da motilidade atuam geralmente pelo aumento na motilidade segmentar e, consequentemente, incremento no tempo do trânsito intestinal (i. e., antidiarreicos narcóticos, como a loperamida; 0,1 mg/kg VO a cada 8-12 h em cães; 0,08 mg/kg VO a cada 12 h em gatos) ou pela diminuição na motilidade anterógrada (i. e., anticolinérgicos); como as doenças leves costumam ser autolimitantes, esses medicamentos não são necessários. Não utilizá-los por mais de 1-2 dias em função dos efeitos adversos.
- A diarreia aguda que não exibe resolução com os medicamentos antidiarreicos merece pesquisas adicionais.
- Os medicamentos antissecretores (opiáceos, anticolinérgicos, clorpromazina e salicilatos) são utilizados para diminuir o volume de líquido nas fezes.
- Em geral, os protetores intestinais não são úteis em pacientes com diarreia aguda; além disso, não foi demonstrado que esses agentes alterem as perdas hídricas ou eletrolíticas intestinais.
- O subsalicilato de bismuto (0,25 mL/kg VO a cada 4-6 h) pode ter certo benefício em virtude das propriedades antissecretoras do salicilato.
- Em pacientes com diarreia aguda ou naqueles com análises fecais positivas, recomendam-se os anti-helmínticos (i. e., fembendazol, 50 mg/kg VO a cada 24 h por 3-5 dias) e os medicamentos antiprotozoários (i. e., metronidazol, 10-30 mg/kg VO a cada 12 h por 5 dias) como tratamento empírico. Se justificável pela análise fecal, será possível fazer uso de medicamentos coccidiostáticos (i. e., sulfadimetoxina).
- A antibioticoterapia é provavelmente desnecessária em grande parte dos casos de doença leve e, na verdade, pode causar diarreia.
- Os pacientes com enterite bacteriana, doença grave, leucopenia concomitante ou suspeita de descontinuidade da barreira da mucosa gastrintestinal (conforme se evidencia pela presença de sangue nas fezes) devem ser tratados com agentes antimicrobianos.
- Os probióticos (*Lactobacillus*, *Enterococcus*) também podem ser úteis. Sugere-se que os probióticos exerçam efeitos benéficos sobre a saúde dos animais de estimação, por fornecer fontes de enzimas para melhor digestão dos nutrientes da dieta e fatores de estimulação do sistema imunológico.

CONTRAINDICAÇÕES
- Anticolinérgicos em pacientes com suspeita de obstrução intestinal, glaucoma ou íleo paralítico intestinal.
- Analgésicos narcóticos — podem causar depressão do SNC; indesejáveis em pacientes com doença mais grave que já se encontram deprimidos ou letárgicos.
- Analgésicos narcóticos em pacientes com hepatopatias e enterites bacterianas ou tóxicas.

PRECAUÇÕES
- A maioria dos casos de diarreia aguda, porém leve, resolve-se com tratamento mínimo; nesses pacientes, é preciso ter cautela quanto ao exagero tanto nos testes diagnósticos como no tratamento.
- Praticamente qualquer medicamento pode produzir efeitos adversos (que costumam incluir diarreia e vômito); esses efeitos podem ser mais graves do que o problema inicial.
- Os gatos podem ser sensíveis aos subsalicilatos e, portanto, não devem receber doses elevadas ou frequentes.

INTERAÇÕES POSSÍVEIS
Caolina/pectina.

ACOMPANHAMENTO

MONITORIZAÇÃO DO PACIENTE
- A maior parte das diarreias agudas desaparece dentro de alguns dias.
- Se os sinais clínicos persistirem, poderá haver a necessidade de testes diagnósticos e tratamentos adicionais.
- No término da medicação, reavaliar os pacientes que exibiram parasitas por meio do exame de fezes.

PREVENÇÃO
- Os animais devem ser alimentados com uma dieta de alta qualidade e constante.
- É recomendável que os proprietários tentem controlar a alimentação indiscriminada e monitorizem o animal para evitar a ingestão de corpo estranho.

COMPLICAÇÕES POSSÍVEIS
- Acredita-se que a intussuscepção esteja associada ao aumento na motilidade intestinal.
- Monitorizar tal complicação em pacientes com diarreia aguda por outras causas, especialmente cães jovens com enterite parviral e parasitismo.

EVOLUÇÃO ESPERADA E PROGNÓSTICO
A maioria dos casos de diarreia exibe resolução espontânea sem tratamento ou com tratamento mínimo.

DIVERSOS

DISTÚRBIOS ASSOCIADOS
O vômito agudo costuma ocorrer concomitantemente com diarreia aguda.

FATORES RELACIONADOS COM A IDADE
- Os cães e gatos jovens apresentam-se frequentemente com diarreia causada por indiscrição/imprudência alimentar, intussuscepção, corpos estranhos e causas infecciosas, em comparação aos pacientes mais idosos.
- Os animais mais jovens e pertencentes a raças caninas de porte menor também se mostram mais propensos à desidratação e podem necessitar de fluidoterapia mais rigorosa.

POTENCIAL ZOONÓTICO
- A enterite por *Campylobacter* é contagiosa aos seres humanos.
- Algumas cepas de *Giardia* podem ser contagiosas aos seres humanos.
- As larvas parasitárias podem causar *larva migrans visceral* (ascarídeos) e *larva migrans cutânea* (ancilóstomos) em seres humanos, particularmente nas crianças.

GESTAÇÃO/FERTILIDADE/REPRODUÇÃO
Sempre é preciso tomar cuidado ao utilizar medicamentos em animais prenhes.

VER TAMBÉM
- Diarreia Responsiva a Antibióticos.
- Vômito Agudo.

ABREVIATURA(S)
- ELISA = ensaio imunoabsorvente ligado à enzima.
- SNC = sistema nervoso central.

Sugestões de Leitura
Barr SC, Greene CE, Gookin JL. In: Greene CE, ed., Infectious Diseases of the Dog and Cat, 3rd ed. St. Louis: Saunders Elsevier, 2006, pp. 736-750.
Hall EJ, German AJ. Diseases of the small intestine. In: Ettinger SJ, Feldman EC, eds., Textbook of Veterinary Internal Medicine, 6th ed. St. Louis: Elsevier, 2005, pp. 1332-1378.

Autor Erin Portillo
Consultor Editorial Albert E. Jergens

Diarreia Crônica — Cães

CONSIDERAÇÕES GERAIS

DEFINIÇÃO
• Trata-se de uma alteração na frequência, na consistência e no volume das fezes por mais de 3 semanas. • Pode ter origem nos intestinos delgado e/ou grosso (natureza mista ou não).

FISIOPATOLOGIA
• Secreção elevada de solutos e líquidos — diarreia secretória. • Absorção baixa de solutos e líquidos — diarreia osmótica. • Permeabilidade intestinal alta. • Motilidade gastrintestinal anormal. • Muitos casos envolvem várias combinações desses quatro mecanismos fisiopatológicos básicos.

SISTEMA(S) ACOMETIDO(S)
• Endócrino/metabólico. • Exócrino. • Equilíbrio hídrico. • Gastrintestinal. • Linfático.

IDENTIFICAÇÃO
Cães.

SINAIS CLÍNICOS

Comentários Gerais
• O processo patológico subjacente determina a extensão dos sinais clínicos. • As fezes normais são compostas de aproximadamente 68-75% de água. Um aumento de 2-3% no conteúdo de água resulta em uma descrição macroscópica de diarreia. • A classificação dos tipos de diarreia do intestino delgado e/ou grosso (natureza mista ou não) apresenta sobreposição significativa dos achados descritivos.

Achados Anamnésicos
Intestino Delgado
• Volume de fezes maior do que o normal. • Frequência de defecação — normal a moderadamente acima do normal (2-4 vezes por dia). • Perda de peso. • Polifagia. • Pode haver melena. • Sem tenesmo ou disquezia (ou nível mínimo, conforme determinado pelo grau de irritação). • Pode exibir flatulência e borborigmo. • Vômito — variável.

Intestino Grosso
• Volume menor de fezes por defecação, em comparação ao normal. • A frequência de defecação é significativamente mais alta do que o normal (>4 vezes por dia). • Não há perda de peso. • Frequentemente, há hematoquezia e muco. • Tenesmo, urgência, disquezia. • Flatulência e borborigmo — variáveis. • Vômitos — variável.

Achados do Exame Físico
Um exame físico completo, incluindo exame da retina, auscultação e palpação abdominal, é necessário para auxiliar no diagnóstico das possíveis causas de diarreia.

Intestino Delgado
• Má condição corporal associada à má absorção, má digestão e enteropatia com perda de proteína. • Nível variável de desidratação. • A palpação abdominal pode revelar espessamento das alças do intestino delgado, associado a quadros de enteropatia infiltrativa, efusão abdominal, corpo estranho, massa neoplásica, intussuscepção ou linfonodo mesentérico infartado. • Palpação retal normal.

Intestino Grosso
• A condição corporal encontra-se mais tipicamente normal. • Desidratação — incomum. • A palpação abdominal pode revelar espessamento das alças do intestino grosso ou presença de massa abdominal (como corpo estranho, massa neoplásica, intussuscepção ou linfonodo mesentérico infartado). • A palpação retal pode mostrar irregularidade da mucosa retal, massas retais intra ou extraluminais, estenose retal ou linfadenopatia sublombar.

CAUSAS

Intestino Delgado
Doença Primária do Intestino Delgado
• Enteropatia inflamatória (p. ex., enterite linfoplasmocitária, enterite eosinofílica, enterite segmentar granulomatosa, enteropatia imunoproliferativa do Basenji). • Linfangiectasia primária. • Neoplasia. • Infecção bacteriana (*Campylobacter jejuni*, *Salmonella* spp., *Escherichia coli* aderente ou enterotóxica invasiva, outras espécies de enterobactérias, *Yersinia pseudotuberculosis*). • Infecção viral (p. ex., coronavírus, parvovírus, vírus da cinomose, rotavírus). • Infecção fúngica (p. ex., histoplasmose, aspergilose). • Outras infecções (p. ex., prototecose, pitiose). • Parasitas (p. ex., *Giardia*, *Toxocara* spp., *Ancylostoma*, *Toxascaris leonina*, *Cryptosporidium* spp., *Cystoisospora* spp., *Tritrichomonas foetus*, *Strongyloides*). • Obstrução parcial (p. ex., corpo estranho, intussuscepção e neoplasia). • Proliferação bacteriana no intestino delgado. • Síndrome do intestino curto. • Úlceras duodenais.

Má Digestão
• Insuficiência pancreática exócrina. • Doença hepatobiliar — ausência de sais biliares intraluminais necessários para digestão.

Alimentar
• Intolerância alimentar (diarreia responsiva ao alimento). • Alergia alimentar. • Enteropatia sensível ao glúten. • Mudança rápida da dieta.

Distúrbios Metabólicos
• Doença hepatobiliar. • Hipoadrenocorticismo. • Gastrenterite urêmica. • Toxinas — enterotoxinas, aflatoxinas, exotoxinas, intoxicação alimentar. • Reações medicamentosas adversas.

Intestino Grosso
Doença Primária do Intestino Grosso
• Enteropatia inflamatória (p. ex., colite linfoplasmocitária, colite eosinofílica, colite ulcerativa histiocítica). • Neoplasia. • Pólipos retais benignos. • Infecção (p. ex., histoplasmose, *Clostridium perfringens*, *Salmonella* spp., *Campylobacter jejuni*, *Prototheca* e pitiose). • Parasitas (p. ex., *Trichuris vulpis*, *Giardia*, *Ancylostoma caninum*, *Entamoeba histolytica* e *Balantioides coli*). • Intussuscepção ileocólica e inversão cecal.

Alimentar
• Dieta — indiscrição/imprudência alimentares, mudanças na dieta e corpo estranho (p. ex., ossos, plásticos, madeiras, pelos). • Fibra — diarreia responsiva do intestino grosso.

Diversas
Síndrome do intestino irritável.

FATORES DE RISCO

Intestino Delgado
• Mudanças na dieta e oferecimento de dietas com pouca digestibilidade ou ricas em gordura. • As raças caninas de grande porte, especialmente Pastor alemão, apresentam incidência mais alta de insuficiência pancreática exócrina. • Os cães de grande porte também exibem um risco maior de vólvulo/torção intestinais; podem ser observados em associação com insuficiência pancreática exócrina. • A pitiose ocorre com maior frequência em cães jovens de grande porte, residentes em áreas norte-americanas rurais que apresentam uma incidência mais alta e fazem fronteira com o Golfo do México.

Intestino Grosso
• As mudanças na dieta ou a indiscrição/imprudência alimentares, o estresse e os fatores psicológicos podem desempenhar um papel na diarreia. • A colite ulcerativa histiocítica (associada à *Escherichia coli* aderente invasiva) ocorre mais frequentemente em Boxer com <3 anos de idade. • A pitiose é mais comum em cães de grande porte que gastam mais tempo fora de casa com uma vida errante ou hábitos de caça.

DIAGNÓSTICO

DIAGNÓSTICO DIFERENCIAL
Em primeiro lugar, deve-se situar a origem da diarreia aos intestinos delgado ou grosso, ou em ambos.

HEMOGRAMA/BIOQUÍMICA/URINÁLISE
• Eosinofilia — essa anormalidade pode estar associada a parasitismo, enterocolite eosinofílica, hipoadrenocorticismo ou pitiose. • Linfopenia e hipocolesterolemia — podem se relacionar com linfangiectasia. • Anemia e microcitose — sugerem sangramento crônico do trato gastrintestinal e deficiência de ferro. • Pan-hipoproteinemia resultante de enteropatia com perda de proteína — associa-se a distúrbios infiltrativos do intestino delgado e linfangiectasia. • Anormalidades no perfil bioquímico, nos ensaios hormonais, no perfil de ácidos biliares séricos e na urinálise — podem indicar nefropatia, doença hepatobiliar ou endocrinopatia.

OUTROS TESTES LABORATORIAIS

Exame Fecal e/ou Raspado Retal
• Exame fecal direto, flutuação fecal de rotina, teste ELISA nas fezes e centrifugação com sulfato de zinco (em busca de *Giardia*) — podem apontar a presença de parasitas gastrintestinais. Talvez haja necessidade de múltiplas amostras para infestações por tricuris. • Exame citológico de raspados retais — pode revelar microrganismos específicos, como *Histoplasma* ou *Prototheca*. • Exame de fezes com PCR — pode ser útil na triagem de infecções de ocorrência rara ou de diagnóstico difícil (p. ex., enterite viral, criptosporidiose, giardíase, salmonelose, detecção do gene A responsável pela codificação da enterotoxina do *C. perfringens*, infecção por *C. difficile*, infecção por *Campylobacter*). Os resultados do teste de PCR devem ser interpretados diante de dados como identificação, anamnese, manifestação clínica, histórico de vacinação e outros dados laboratoriais do paciente. • Coprocultura na suspeita de *Campylobacter* ou *Salmonella* — são necessários meios de cultura especiais; informar a suspeita ao laboratório antes do envio da amostra.

Provas da Função Pancreática Exócrina
• Imunorreatividade semelhante à da tripsina específica canina — teste de escolha para confirmar os casos de insuficiência pancreática exócrina em cães; imunorreatividade sérica

Diarreia Crônica — Cães

semelhante à da tripsina <2,5 μg/L em jejum é diagnóstica.

Testes quanto à presença de Má Absorção
• Folato sérico — o baixo nível sérico dessa vitamina pode estar associado à má absorção da porção proximal do intestino delgado; podem ocorrer níveis elevados em virtude de proliferação bacteriana no intestino delgado. • Vitamina B_{12} (cobalamina) — o baixo nível sérico dessa vitamina pode estar relacionado com insuficiência pancreática exócrina ou má absorção da porção distal do intestino delgado; as síndromes de deficiência primária da cobalamina são raras.

Testes quanto à presença de Doença Metabólica
• Nível de cortisol em repouso — um valor <1,7 μg/dL é compatível com, mas não diagnóstico de, hipocortisolemia. • Teste de estimulação com ACTH — na suspeita de hipoadrenocorticismo. • Mensuração dos ácidos biliares séricos em jejum e duas horas pós-prandiais — em casos de suspeita de doença hepatobiliar; os valores significativamente elevados sugerem disfunção hepática ou desvio portossistêmico.

DIAGNÓSTICO POR IMAGEM
• As radiografias abdominais simples podem indicar obstrução intestinal, padrão intestinal anormal, organomegalia, massa, corpo estranho, doença pancreática, doença hepatobiliar, doença urinária ou efusão abdominal. • As radiografias contrastadas (estudo sequencial radiográfico da porção anterior do trato gastrintestinal ou enema baritado) podem indicar espessamento da parede intestinal, úlceras intestinais, irregularidades da mucosa, massa, corpo estranho radiotransparente ou estenose. As radiografias contrastadas exigem compromisso com múltiplas radiografias e uso de volume adequado do meio de contraste para ter um valor diagnóstico adequado. • A ultrassonografia abdominal pode demonstrar espessamento da parede intestinal, segmentação anormal da parede intestinal em camadas, massas gastrintestinais ou fora do trato GI, intussuscepção, corpo estranho, íleo paralítico, efusão abdominal, doença hepatobiliar, ou linfadenopatia mesentérica ou mesocólica. • As técnicas avançadas de diagnóstico por imagem (TC, RM) não são efetuadas com rotina como exames de primeira linha.

MÉTODOS DIAGNÓSTICOS
• Caso se excluam as causas metabólicas, parasitárias, alimentares e infecciosas, bem como as de má digestão (insuficiência pancreática exócrina), será aconselhável a realização dos exames de endoscopia e biopsia da mucosa, ultrassonografia e aspirado por agulha fina, biopsia micronuclear ou alguma abordagem cirúrgica para a obtenção do diagnóstico definitivo e a provisão do tratamento.

Endoscopia/Laparoscopia
• A endoscopia flexível do trato gastrintestinal anterior permite o exame e a biopsia das mucosas gástrica e duodenal; sempre se devem obter múltiplas amostras (8-10) da mucosa de cada segmento/área. • A colonoscopia flexível possibilita o exame de todo reto, cólon, ceco e, muitas vezes, da porção distal do íleo; também se recomenda a obtenção de múltiplas amostras da mucosa (8-10) de cada segmento. • As impressões visuais de detalhes da mucosa gastrintestinal podem ser normais ou anormais; sempre há necessidade da obtenção de biopsias. • As biopsias endoscópicas repousam nas doenças infiltrativas e inflamatórias que são representadas nas duas primeiras camadas da parede intestinal e nos segmentos biopsiados que são representativos de outros locais não alcançados. • Biopsias de espessura completa podem ser obtidas via laparoscopia a partir de um ou mais segmentos do intestino delgado (não do intestino grosso) via exteriorização do(s) segmento(s).

Biopsia Cirúrgica
• É possível obter as biopsias de espessura completa a partir de locais/segmentos claramente visualizados do trato intestinal. • Uma abordagem cirúrgica poderá ser a abordagem mais vantajosa/pragmática se biopsias de múltiplos órgãos (intestino delgado, linfonodos, estômago, pâncreas, fígado, etc.) forem desejáveis, ao mesmo tempo em que mantém a capacidade de corrigir os achados anormais se for conveniente.

Biopsia Gastrintestinal Orientada por Ultrassom
• Pode-se realizar o aspirado obtido por agulha fina e guiado por ultrassom em grande parte das lesões gastrintestinais, que se apresentam como alvos razoáveis. • Com essas técnicas, há preocupações quanto ao risco de translocação de células cancerígenas ou microrganismos infecciosos.

TRATAMENTO

CUIDADO(S) DE SAÚDE ADEQUADO(S)
• Tratar a causa subjacente — a terapia sintomática ou empírica raramente soluciona a diarreia crônica. • Informar ao proprietário sobre o fato de que a resolução completa dos sinais clínicos nem sempre é possível, apesar do diagnóstico correto e do tratamento apropriado; isso é particularmente verdadeiro em casos de linfangiectasia, neoplasia intestinal, pitiose e histoplasmose. Algumas causas de diarreia crônica resultam em alterações anatômicas na mucosa intestinal, que podem levar meses para desaparecer ou podem não se resolver (p. ex., fusão das vilosidades, linfangiectasia, fibrose, função alterada do sistema nervoso mioentérico). • O fornecimento de dietas pobres em gordura, constituídas por nova fonte (para o paciente) de proteína e carboidrato, altamente digestíveis ou suplementadas com fibras por 3-4 semanas pode solucionar a diarreia decorrente de intolerância ou alergia alimentares. As mudanças frequentes da dieta para manter uma condição livre de sintomas sugerem a necessidade de outros exames.

CUIDADO(S) DE ENFERMAGEM
• Se o paciente estiver desidratado, administrar fluidoterapia com soluções eletrolíticas balanceadas. • Considerar a administração de coloides em pacientes hipoproteinêmicos que necessitam de fluidoterapia. • Corrigir os desequilíbrios eletrolíticos e acidobásicos.

CONSIDERAÇÕES CIRÚRGICAS
Proceder à laparotomia exploratória e biopsia cirúrgica se houver indícios de obstrução, massa intestinal, comprometimento da porção média do intestino delgado inatingível pelo procedimento guiado por ultrassom ou caso se duvide do diagnóstico, com base na biopsia endoscópica ou no procedimento guiado por ultrassom, em função de uma resposta insatisfatória à terapia.

MEDICAÇÕES

MEDICAMENTO(S) DE ESCOLHA
Específicos à doença.

CONTRAINDICAÇÕES
Os anticolinérgicos podem exacerbar a maioria dos tipos de diarreia crônica; algumas vezes, esses agentes são usados para aliviar as cólicas e os espasmos dolorosos associados à síndrome do intestino irritável.

ACOMPANHAMENTO

MONITORIZAÇÃO DO PACIENTE
• Monitorar o volume e a aparência das fezes, a frequência da defecação e o peso corporal. • Em cães com enteropatia com perda de proteína — mensurar as proteínas séricas e avaliar os sinais clínicos (ascite, edema subcutâneo, efusão pleural). • A resolução da diarreia costuma ser gradativa após o tratamento; se a diarreia não desaparecer com o tratamento, considerar a reavaliação do diagnóstico.

COMPLICAÇÕES POSSÍVEIS
• Desidratação. • Baixa condição corporal. • Efusões abdominais relacionadas com causas específicas de diarreia crônica. • Ascite, edema subcutâneo e/ou efusão pleural em casos de hipoalbuminemia decorrente de enteropatias com perda de proteína.

DIVERSOS

POTENCIAL ZOONÓTICO
• Giardíase. • Salmonelose. • Campilobacteriose. • Ascaridíase.

VER TAMBÉM
Ver a seção "Causas".

ABREVIATURA(S)
• ACTH = hormônio adrenocorticotrópico. • B_{12} = vitamina B_{12}, cobalamina. • ELISA = ensaio imunoabsorvente ligado à enzima. • GI = gastrintestinal. • PCR = reação em cadeia da polimerase. • RM = ressonância magnética. • TC = tomografia computadorizada.

Sugestões de Leitura
Willard MD, Mansell J, Fosgate GT, et al. Effect of sample quality on the sensitivity of endoscopic biopsy for detecting gastric and duodenal lesions in dogs and cats. J Vet Intern Med, 2008, 22(5):1084-1089.

Autor Mark E. Hitt
Consultor Editorial Albert E. Jergens

Diarreia Crônica — Gatos

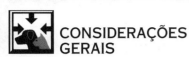

CONSIDERAÇÕES GERAIS

DEFINIÇÃO
- Trata-se de uma alteração na frequência, na consistência e no volume das fezes por mais de 3 semanas ou com padrão de recidiva episódica.
- Pode ter origem nos intestinos delgado e/ou grosso (natureza mista ou não).

FISIOPATOLOGIA
- Secreção elevada de solutos e líquidos — diarreia secretória. • Absorção baixa de solutos e líquidos — diarreia osmótica. • Permeabilidade intestinal alta. • Motilidade gastrintestinal anormal. • Muitos casos envolvem várias combinações desses quatro mecanismos fisiopatológicos básicos para o desenvolvimento da diarreia.

SISTEMA(S) ACOMETIDO(S)
- Gastrintestinal. • Endócrino/metabólico — hídrico, eletrolítico e acidobásico. • Nutricional.
- Linfático. • Exócrino.

IDENTIFICAÇÃO
Gatos.

SINAIS CLÍNICOS
Comentários Gerais
- O processo patológico subjacente determina a extensão dos sinais clínicos. • As fezes normais são compostas de aproximadamente 68-75% de água. Um aumento de 2-3% no conteúdo de água resulta em uma má qualidade das fezes e descrição macroscópica de diarreia. • A classificação dos tipos de diarreia proveniente do intestino delgado e grosso é uma ferramenta clínica conveniente, embora haja sobreposição significativa desses achados descritivos (tipos).

Achados Anamnésicos
Intestino Delgado
- Volume de fezes maior do que o normal.
- A frequência de defecação apresenta-se normal a moderadamente acima do normal (2-4 vezes por dia).
- Perda de peso.
- Polifagia.
- Pode ocorrer melena.
- Sem tenesmo ou disquezia (ou nível mínimo, conforme determinado pelo grau de irritação).
- Pode exibir flatulência e borborigmo.
- Vômito — variável.

Intestino Grosso
- Volume menor de fezes por defecação, em comparação ao normal.
- A frequência de defecação é significativamente mais alta do que o normal (>4 vezes por dia).
- Não há perda de peso.
- Com frequência, há hematoquezia e muco.
- Tenesmo, urgência, disquezia.
- Flatulência e borborigmo — variáveis.
- Vômitos — variável.

Achados do Exame Físico
Um exame físico completo, incluindo exame da retina, ausculação e palpação abdominal, é necessário para auxiliar no diagnóstico das possíveis causas de diarreia.

Intestino Delgado
- Má condição corporal associada à má absorção, má digestão e enteropatia com perda de proteína.
- Nível variável de desidratação.
- A palpação abdominal pode revelar espessamento das alças do intestino delgado, associado a quadros de enteropatia infiltrativa, efusão abdominal, corpo estranho, massa neoplásica, intussuscepção ou linfonodo mesentérico infartado.
- Palpação retal normal.

Intestino Grosso
- A condição corporal encontra-se mais tipicamente normal.
- Desidratação — incomum.
- A palpação abdominal pode revelar espessamento das alças do intestino grosso ou presença de massa abdominal (como corpo estranho, massa neoplásica, intussuscepção ou linfonodo mesentérico infartado).
- A palpação retal pode mostrar irregularidade da mucosa retal, massas retais intra ou extraluminais, estenose retal ou linfadenopatia sublombar.

CAUSAS
Doenças do Intestino Delgado e Grosso
Doença Primária
- Enteropatia inflamatória (p. ex., enterocolite linfoplasmocitária, enterite eosinofílica, enterite segmentar granulomatosa).
- Neoplasia (p. ex., linfoma, adenocarcinoma, mastocitoma).
- Infecção bacteriana (p. ex., *Salmonella* spp., *Escherichia coli* enterotóxica, outras espécies de enterobactérias, *Yersinia pseudotuberculosis*).
- Infecção viral (p. ex., coronavírus intestinal, PIF, infecção associada a FeLV/FIV).
- Infecção fúngica (p. ex., histoplasmose, aspergilose).
- Outras infecções (p. ex., prototecose, pitiose).
- Parasitas (p. ex., *Giardia*, *Toxocara* spp., *Ancylostoma*, *Toxascaris leonina*, *Cryptosporidium* spp., *Cystoisospora* spp., *Tritrichomonas foetus*).
- Obstrução parcial (p. ex., corpo estranho, intussuscepção e neoplasia).
- Linfangiectasia secundária.
- Proliferação bacteriana no intestino delgado.
- Síndrome do intestino curto.
- Atrofia das vilosidades.
- Úlceras duodenais.

Má Digestão
- Doença hepatobiliar — ausência de sais biliares necessários para digestão intraluminal.
- Insuficiência pancreática exócrina.

Alimentar
- Intolerância alimentar (diarreia responsiva ao alimento).
- Alergia alimentar.
- Mudança rápida da dieta.

Distúrbios Metabólicos
- Hipertireoidismo.
- Deficiência da cobalamina (há discussões sobre se isso é causa ou efeito).
- Nefropatia — uremia.
- Doença hepatobiliar — insuficiência hepática.
- Toxinas (p. ex., enterotoxinas, aflatoxinas, exotoxinas, intoxicação alimentar).
- Reações medicamentosas adversas.

Anomalias Congênitas
- Encurtamento do cólon.
- Desvio portossistêmico.
- Ligamento pancreático-mesojejunal persistente.

FATORES DE RISCO
Mudanças na dieta e fornecimento de dieta com pouca digestibilidade ou rica em gorduras; a suprarregulação na produção de enzimas da borda em escova pelas células epiteliais intestinais (transdução do RNAm) necessita de aproximadamente 5 dias da exposição do substrato.

DIAGNÓSTICO

DIAGNÓSTICO DIFERENCIAL
Em primeiro lugar, é recomendável localizar a origem da diarreia aos intestinos delgado ou grosso ou em ambos, com base nos sinais anamnésicos.

HEMOGRAMA/BIOQUÍMICA/URINÁLISE
- Eosinofilia em alguns gatos com parasitismo, enterocolite eosinofílica, síndrome hipereosinofílica ou mastocitoma.
- Macrocitose em certos gatos com hipertireoidismo ou infecção pelo FeLV.
- Anemia (variavelmente regenerativa) e microcitose são sugestivas de sangramento crônico do trato gastrintestinal e deficiência de ferro.
- Leucopenia em determinados gatos com infecção pelos FeLV ou FIV.
- Pan-hipoproteinemia causada por enteropatia com perda proteica é incomum em gatos com comprometimento intestinal, mas pode ocorrer. Hipoalbuminemia também pode ser observada.
- Anormalidades no perfil bioquímico, nos ensaios hormonais, no perfil de ácidos biliares séricos e na urinálise — podem indicar nefropatia, doença hepatobiliar ou endocrinopatia.

OUTROS TESTES LABORATORIAIS
Exame Fecal e/ou Raspado Retal
- Exame fecal direto, flutuação fecal de rotina, teste ELISA nas fezes e centrifugação com sulfato de zinco (em busca de *Giardia*) — podem revelar parasitas gastrintestinais.
- Exame citológico de raspados retais — pode exibir microrganismos específicos, como *Histoplasma* ou *Prototheca*.
- Coloração de Sudan para pesquisa de gorduras fecais — pode indicar esteatorreia, sugestiva de má absorção ou má digestão.
- Exame de fezes com PCR — pode ser útil na triagem de infecções de ocorrência rara ou de diagnóstico difícil (p. ex., enterite viral, criptosporidiose, giardíase, salmonelose, *Tritrichomonas foetus*). Os resultados do teste de PCR devem ser interpretados diante de dados como identificação, anamnese, manifestação clínica, histórico de vacinação e outros dados laboratoriais do paciente.
- Coprocultura na suspeita de *Salmonella* — há necessidade de meios de cultura especiais.

Provas de Função da Tireoide
- Concentração sérica elevada do T_4 total ou T_4 livre — indica hipertireoidismo.
- Na suspeita de hipertireoidismo com T_4 normal, efetuar o teste de supressão com T_3.
- Outras opções de exames: teste de resposta ao TRH, teste de estimulação com TSH (THS recombinante humano) ou cintilografia da tireoide marcada com tecnécio; a mensuração do T_4 livre também pode ser utilizada, embora possam ocorrer alguns resultados falso-positivos com valores elevados.

Teste Sorológico
Teste para detecção de anticorpos contra FeLV e FIV — particularmente na presença de anormalidades hematológicas.

Diarreia Crônica — Gatos

Provas da Função Pancreática Exócrina
- Imunorreatividade semelhante à da tripsina específica felina — teste de escolha para o diagnóstico de insuficiência pancreática exócrina.
- Pode-se mensurar a atividade proteolítica fecal em amostras de fezes obtidas em 3 dias consecutivos com teste de digestão de película/proteína fecal.

DIAGNÓSTICO POR IMAGEM
- As radiografias abdominais simples podem indicar obstrução intestinal, padrão intestinal anormal, organomegalia, massa, corpo estranho, doença pancreática, doença hepatobiliar, doença urinária ou efusão abdominal.
- As radiografias contrastadas (estudo sequencial radiográfico da porção anterior do trato gastrintestinal ou enema baritado) podem indicar espessamento da parede intestinal, úlceras intestinais, irregularidades da mucosa, massa, corpo estranho radiotransparente ou estenose. As radiografias contrastadas exigem compromisso com múltiplas radiografias e uso de volume adequado do meio de contraste para ter um valor diagnóstico adequado.
- A ultrassonografia abdominal pode demonstrar espessamento da parede intestinal, segmentação anormal da parede intestinal em camadas, massas gastrintestinais ou fora do trato GI, intussuscepção, corpo estranho, íleo paralítico, efusão abdominal, doença hepatobiliar, nefropatia, ou linfadenopatia mesentérica ou mesocólica. A ultrassonografia abdominal é utilizada em conjunto com radiografias abdominais.
- As técnicas avançadas de diagnóstico por imagem (TC, RM) não são efetuadas com rotina como exames de primeira linha na avaliação de diarreia crônica.

MÉTODOS DIAGNÓSTICOS
- Caso se excluam as causas metabólicas, parasitárias, alimentares e infecciosas, bem como as de má digestão (insuficiência pancreática exócrina), será aconselhável a realização dos exames de endoscopia e biopsia da mucosa, ultrassonografia e aspirado por agulha fina, biopsia micronuclear ou alguma abordagem cirúrgica para a obtenção do diagnóstico definitivo e a provisão do tratamento.

Endoscopia/Laparoscopia
- A endoscopia flexível do trato gastrintestinal anterior permite o exame e a biopsia das mucosas gástrica e duodenal; sempre se devem obter múltiplas amostras (8-10) da mucosa de cada segmento/área.
- A colonoscopia flexível possibilita o exame de todo reto, cólon e ceco; a coloproctoscopia rígida limita o exame à porção descendente do cólon e ao reto, sendo realizada com menos frequência em virtude de sua limitação; também se recomenda a obtenção de múltiplas amostras da mucosa (8-10) de cada segmento.
- As impressões visuais de detalhes da mucosa gastrintestinal podem ser normais ou anormais; sempre há necessidade da obtenção de biopsias.
- As biopsias endoscópicas repousam nas doenças infiltrativas e inflamatórias que são representadas nas duas primeiras camadas da parede intestinal e nos segmentos biopsiados que são representativos de outros locais não alcançados.
- Biopsias de espessura completa podem ser obtidas via laparoscopia a partir de um ou mais segmentos do intestino delgado (não do intestino grosso) via exteriorização do(s) segmento(s).

Biopsia Cirúrgica
- É possível obter as biopsias de espessura completa a partir de locais/segmentos claramente visualizados do trato intestinal.
- Uma abordagem cirúrgica poderá ser a abordagem mais vantajosa/pragmática se biopsias de múltiplos órgãos (intestino delgado, linfonodos, estômago, pâncreas, fígado, etc.) forem desejáveis, ao mesmo tempo em que mantém a capacidade de corrigir os achados anormais descobertos.

Biopsia Gastrintestinal Orientada por Ultrassom
- Pode-se realizar o aspirado obtido por agulha fina e guiado por ultrassom em grande parte das lesões gastrintestinais, que se apresentam como alvos razoáveis.
- Biopsias micronucleares guiadas por ultrassom com agulha Tru-Cut® em lesões não cavitárias com >2 cm de diâmetro são realizadas com menos frequência.
- É recomendável a técnica de paracentese do líquido peritoneal para análise, cultura e citologia desse líquido.
- Com essas técnicas, há preocupações quanto ao risco de translocação de células cancerígenas ou microrganismos infecciosos.

TRATAMENTO

CUIDADO(S) DE SAÚDE ADEQUADO(S)
- Tratar a causa subjacente — a terapia sintomática ou empírica raramente soluciona a diarreia crônica.
- Informar ao proprietário sobre o fato de que a resolução completa dos sinais clínicos nem sempre é possível, apesar do diagnóstico correto e do tratamento apropriado; isso é particularmente verdadeiro em casos de linfangiectasia, neoplasia intestinal, pitiose e histoplasmose. Algumas causas de diarreia crônica resultam em alterações anatômicas na mucosa intestinal, que podem levar meses para desaparecer ou podem não se resolver (p. ex., fusão das vilosidades, linfangiectasia, fibrose, função alterada do sistema nervoso mioentérico).
- O fornecimento de dietas pobres em gordura, constituídas por nova fonte (para o paciente) de proteína e carboidrato, altamente digestíveis ou suplementadas com fibras por 3-4 semanas pode solucionar a diarreia decorrente de intolerância ou alergia alimentares. As mudanças frequentes da dieta para manter uma condição livre de sintomas sugerem a necessidade de outros exames.

CUIDADO(S) DE ENFERMAGEM
- Administrar fluidoterapia com soluções eletrolíticas balanceadas.
- Corrigir os desequilíbrios eletrolíticos e acidobásicos.

CONSIDERAÇÕES CIRÚRGICAS
Proceder à laparotomia exploratória e biopsia cirúrgica se houver indícios de obstrução, massa intestinal, comprometimento da porção média do intestino delgado inatingível pelo procedimento guiado por ultrassom ou caso se duvide do diagnóstico, com base na biopsia endoscópica ou no procedimento guiado por ultrassom, em função de uma resposta insatisfatória à terapia.

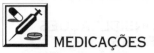

MEDICAÇÕES

MEDICAMENTO(S) DE ESCOLHA
Específicos à doença.

CONTRAINDICAÇÕES
Os anticolinérgicos exacerbam a maior parte dos tipos de diarreia crônica e não devem ser utilizados como tratamentos empíricos.

PRECAUÇÕES
- Os antidiarreicos opiáceos, como o difenoxilato e a loperamida, podem causar hiperatividade e depressão respiratória em gatos e não devem ser usados por mais de 3 dias.

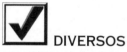

ACOMPANHAMENTO

MONITORIZAÇÃO DO PACIENTE
- Monitorizar o volume e a aparência das fezes, a frequência da defecação e o peso corporal.
- A resolução costuma ocorrer gradativamente com o tratamento; se a diarreia não desaparecer, considerar a reavaliação do diagnóstico.

COMPLICAÇÕES POSSÍVEIS
- Desidratação.
- Baixa condição corporal.
- Efusões abdominais relacionadas com causas específicas de diarreia crônica.

DIVERSOS

POTENCIAL ZOONÓTICO
- Toxoplasmose. • Giardíase. • Criptosporidiose. • Salmonelose. • Campilobacteriose.

VER TAMBÉM
Ver a seção "Causas".

ABREVIATURA(S)
- ELISA = ensaio imunoabsorvente ligado à enzima. • FeLV = vírus da leucemia felina. • FIV = vírus da imunodeficiência felina. • GI = gastrintestinal. • PCR = reação em cadeia da polimerase. • PIF = peritonite infecciosa felina. • RM = ressonância magnética. • TC = tomografia computadorizada. • TRH = hormônio liberador da tireotropina. • TSH = hormônio tireostimulante.

Sugestões de Leitura
Evans SE, Bonczynski JJ, Broussard JD, Han E, Baer KE. Comparison of endoscopic and full-thickness biopsy specimens for diagnosis of inflammatory bowel disease and alimentary tract lymphoma in cats. JAVMA 2006, 229(9):1447-1450.
Tolbert MK, Gookin JL. Tritrichomonas foetus: A new agent of feline diarrhea. Compend Contin Educ Pract Vet 2009, 31(8):374-381.
Willard MD, Mansell J, Fosgate GT, et al. Effect of sample quality on the sensitivity of endoscopic biopsy for detecting gastric and duodenal lesions in dogs and cats. J Vet Intern Med 2008, 22(5):1084-1089.

Autor Mark E. Hitt
Consultor Editorial Albert E. Jergens

Diarreia Responsiva a Antibióticos

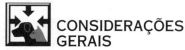

CONSIDERAÇÕES GERAIS

REVISÃO
- Definida como diarreia responsiva a antibióticos, sem uma etiologia subjacente identificável.
- A diarreia responsiva a antibióticos pode ser intercambiável com proliferação bacteriana (primária) idiopática do intestino delgado. A proliferação bacteriana secundária do intestino delgado é o resultado de doenças gastrintestinais concomitantes (p. ex., insuficiência pancreática exócrina).
- As teorias atuais concentram-se na possibilidade de desregulação imune, possivelmente associada à expressão anormal de células-T CD4+, plasmócitos produtores de IgA, e citocinas.

IDENTIFICAÇÃO
Espécies
Cães.
Raça(s) Predominante(s)
A incidência pode ser elevada em Pastor alemão, Boxer e Shar-pei.
Idade Média e Faixa Etária
Desconhecidas, mas pode ser mais comum em filhotes de cães.
Sexo Predominante
N/D.

SINAIS CLÍNICOS
Achados Anamnésicos
- Sinais atribuídos ao intestino delgado — inapetência ou anorexia, vômito, perda de peso, diarreia volumosa.
- Sinais atribuídos ao intestino grosso — tenesmo, hematoquezia, aumento da frequência de defecações.

Achados do Exame Físico
Podem ser detectadas alterações como perda de peso, má condição corporal, borborigmos e flatulência; o sinal de hematoquezia pode estar presente se houver grande envolvimento intestinal.

CAUSAS E FATORES DE RISCO
- Desconhecidos.
- Há suspeita do envolvimento de determinadas bactérias enteropatogênicas (*Clostridium perfringens*, *E. coli* e *Lawsonia intracellularis*), mas tais bactérias não foram confirmadas como agentes etiológicos.

DIAGNÓSTICO

DIAGNÓSTICO DIFERENCIAL
- Proliferação bacteriana secundária do intestino delgado.
- IPE.
- Infecção parasitária.
- Enteropatia inflamatória.
- Neoplasia.

HEMOGRAMA/BIOQUÍMICA/URINÁLISE
- Tipicamente normais.
- Hipoalbuminemia é um achado incomum.

OUTROS TESTES LABORATORIAIS
- É recomendável a realização de exame de fezes para pesquisa de parasitas.
- Os níveis séricos de cobalamina podem estar baixos, enquanto os níveis de folato podem estar aumentados ou diminuídos, compatíveis com a proliferação bacteriana.
- Os ácidos biliares séricos não conjugados não parecem ser úteis no diagnóstico.
- Os níveis séricos de IST (mensurada para descartar IPE) permanecem normais.
- A proteína C-reativa tem tido valor limitado na avaliação.

DIAGNÓSTICO POR IMAGEM
É aconselhável a obtenção de imagens de rotina do abdome (radiografias e ultrassonografia) para descartar outras causas de diarreia. Os resultados desses exames são normais em casos de diarreia responsiva a antibióticos.

MÉTODOS DIAGNÓSTICOS
- Não há um teste definitivo para o diagnóstico de diarreia responsiva a antibióticos além da resolução dos sinais gastrintestinais após a administração desses agentes terapêuticos.
- O diagnóstico depende da exclusão de outras causas de diarreia crônica e da resposta clínica a algum curso adequado de antibioticoterapia.

TRATAMENTO

- A hospitalização geralmente não é indicada e os cães podem ser tratados em um esquema ambulatorial.
- Também não há indicação de restrição da atividade física.
- O papel desempenhado pela dieta em casos de diarreia responsiva a antibióticos não é conhecido. As recomendações atuais envolvem o fornecimento de dieta de alta digestibilidade e baixo teor de gordura. A suplementação de ácidos graxos ou probióticos é controversa.

MEDICAÇÕES

MEDICAMENTO(S)
- Existem várias opções de antibióticos disponíveis:
  ○ Oxitetraciclina (10-20 mg/kg VO a cada 8 h); metronidazol (10-20 mg/kg VO a cada 8 h); tilosina (20 mg/kg VO a cada 8-12 h).
  ○ Em alguns casos, pode haver a necessidade de terapia combinada.
  ○ A antibioticoterapia deve ser administrada por 4-6 semanas.
- Se os níveis séricos de cobalamina estiverem reduzidos, deve-se proceder à suplementação dessa vitamina. Cães com <15 kg de peso corporal: 500 µg de cobalamina parenteral; cães com >15 kg de peso corporal: até 1.000 µg de cobalamina parenteral. As doses são administradas sob a forma de injeções subcutâneas 1 vez por semana por 6 semanas e, depois, em semanas alternadas por 6 semanas. É recomendável a reavaliação dos níveis séricos de cobalamina no final da terapia.

CONTRAINDICAÇÕES/INTERAÇÕES POSSÍVEIS
- A oxitetraciclina pode provocar a formação de manchas no esmalte dos dentes. As doses devem ser diminuídas em animais com insuficiência hepática ou renal.
- O metronidazol sofre metabolismo hepático extenso; as dosagens devem ser reduzidas em animais com insuficiência hepática.

ACOMPANHAMENTO

- A resolução clínica da diarreia é o critério mais importante.
- Também pode ser observado ganho de peso; a hipoalbuminemia (se presente) deve desaparecer.
- Podem ocorrer recidivas em caso de interrupção prematura dos antibióticos.
- Em alguns casos, pode ser necessária a terapia prolongada com baixas doses (1 vez ao dia).

DIVERSOS

ABREVIATURAS
- IPE = insuficiência pancreática exócrina.
- IST = imunorreatividade semelhante à da tripsina.

Sugestões de Leitura
German AJ, Day MJ, Ruaux CG, et al. Comparison of direct and indirect tests for small intestinal bacterial overgrowth and antibiotic-responsive diarrhea in dogs. J Vet Intern Med 2003, 17:33–43.
Hall EJ, German AJ. Diseases of the small intestine. In: Ettinger SJ, Feldman EC, eds., Textbook of Veterinary Internal Medicine, 6th ed. St. Louis: Elsevier, 2005, pp. 1364–1367.
Hostutler RA, Luria BJ, Johnson SE, et al. Antibiotic responsive histiocytic ulcerative colitis in 9 Dogs. J Vet Intern Med 2004, 18:499–504.
Westermarck E, Skrzypczak T, Harmoinen J, et al. Tylosin-responsive chronic diarrhea in dogs. J Vet Intern Med 2005, 19:177–186.

Autor Jo Ann Morrison
Consultor Editorial Albert E. Jergens

DIOCTOPHYMA RENALE (TAMBÉM CONHECIDO COMO VERME RENAL GIGANTE)

CONSIDERAÇÕES GERAIS

REVISÃO
• Em cães, as fêmeas do verme adulto de *D. renale* são significativamente maiores que os machos, atingindo 100 cm de comprimento e 1,2 cm de largura. Em contraste, os machos têm apenas 20-40 cm de comprimento e 6 mm de largura.
• Tanto o macho como a fêmea das formas adultas de *D. renale* são tipicamente de coloração vermelho-viva quando estão vivos, mas ficam preto-acastanhados depois de sua morte e degeneração. A cor vermelha característica pode ser associada a um pigmento sanguíneo semelhante à hemoglobina (eritrocruorina).
• Os ovos são em formato de limão e de tamanho constante. Possuem coloração castanho-clara ou ferrugem com fossas (depressões) profundas em seus envoltórios, exceto nos polos, que contêm opérculos. Foi estimado que uma fêmea típica de *D. renale* produz aproximadamente 18-20 milhões de ovos em seu período de vida. Os ovos podem permanecer viáveis por até 5 anos. As temperaturas de dessecação e congelamento são letais para ovos infecciosos de *D. renale*.
• Os anelídeos de vida livre (*Lumbriculus variegatus*) são hospedeiros intermediários essenciais. As espécies de *Lumbriculus* (também conhecido como verme negro e verme de lama) são filogeneticamente aparentadas com a minhoca. Podem ser facilmente encontrados na Europa, América do Norte e América do Sul. Frequentemente habitam águas superficiais (ou seja, pouco profundas) das margens de lagoas, lagos e pântanos, onde se alimentam de vegetação e microrganismos em decomposição. Qualquer mamífero que beba água contendo anelídeos infectados tem o potencial de ingerir o terceiro estágio infectado do *D. renale*.

EPIDEMIOLOGIA
Foram constatados casos de *D. renale* em praticamente toda parte do mundo com clima temperado. Na América do Norte, os casos foram encontrados com frequência em regiões como Mississippi, Louisiana, Minnesota, Wisconsin e Michigan, bem como em províncias centrais e orientais do Canadá. O verme renal gigante foi relatado em muitas espécies de animais, incluindo cães, martas, coiotes, chacais, guaxinins, raposas, lobos, doninhas, fuinhas, lontras e mustelídeos. Os seres humanos são hospedeiros acidentais; por causa da parte aquática de seu ciclo de vida, a água é um elemento essencial do habitat de *D. renale*. Portanto, não é de se surpreender que os mamíferos semiaquáticos que se alimentam de peixes são os hospedeiros definitivos mais comuns de *D. renale*. Peixes e sapos frequentemente servem como hospedeiros paratênicos para esse parasita. A marta é o mustelídeo mais comumente infectado e constitui o principal hospedeiro definitivo na América do Norte.

CICLO DE VIDA
• Para completar o ciclo de vida, tanto machos como fêmeas devem estar localizados no mesmo rim do hospedeiro; além disso, o trato urinário deve estar patente (desobstruído). Os ovos férteis são eliminados na urina pelo hospedeiro e sofrem processo embrionário na água. Depois de 1-7 meses, eles produzem larvas de primeiro estágio. A velocidade de seu desenvolvimento depende da temperatura da água. A temperatura ideal para o desenvolvimento embrionário dos ovos é de 25-30 °C. Os ovos eclodem somente depois de serem engolidos pelo hospedeiro intermediário, *L. variegatus*. Esse anelídeo é o único hospedeiro intermediário necessário para completar o ciclo de vida. Um período de ≥100 dias no *L. variegatus* é necessário para que o segundo estágio e o terceiro estágio infeccioso do parasita se desenvolvam. O hospedeiro definitivo torna-se infectado por ingerir as larvas infecciosas em anelídeos.
• Os hospedeiros paratênicos também podem fazer parte do ciclo de vida. Nos Estados Unidos, sapos e *northern black bullheads* (peixes de cabeça grande) são hospedeiros paratênicos. As larvas encistam-se no fígado, mesentério, parede gástrica ou músculos abdominais dos hospedeiros paratênicos.
• O hospedeiro definitivo torna-se infectado pela ingestão de peixe cru, sapos, outros hospedeiros paratênicos ou de *L. variegatus*. Depois de serem engolidas pelo hospedeiro definitivo, as larvas infecciosas penetram nas paredes do estômago ou dos intestinos e migram para a submucosa. Depois de aproximadamente 5-7 dias, elas migram para o fígado e permanecem lá por cerca de 50 dias. Na sequência, ocorrem a migração para o rim direito ou esquerdo e a invasão da pelve renal.
• O *D. renale* é encontrado com maior frequência no rim direito do que no esquerdo. A predileção pelo rim direito é atribuída à relação anatômica estreita desse rim com o duodeno. De acordo com alguns pesquisadores, as formas adultas do *D. renale* são encontradas na pelve renal esquerda, onde penetram no estômago na altura da curvatura maior. O encontro de *D. renale* encistado ao redor do fígado é associado à penetração larval na curvatura menor do estômago. Ocasionalmente, o *D. renale* é encontrado na bexiga urinária e/ou no ureter. O número mais alto de adultos encontrados em 1 cão é de 34. O tempo necessário para que as larvas infecciosas se tornem fêmeas grávidas maduras no hospedeiro definitivo é de 3 meses e meio a 6 meses. Todo o ciclo de vida requer aproximadamente 2 anos.

FISIOPATOLOGIA

Rim
Os parasitas adultos atingem um tamanho considerável no momento em que eles penetram no rim. Os mecanismos exatos envolvidos com o acesso à pelve renal não foram relatados. A entrada do *D. renale* no rim provavelmente resulta dos efeitos de enzimas liberadas pelo próprio parasita. Potentes colagenases, hialuronidases e cisteína proteases liberadas pelos nematódeos podem facilmente digerir os tecidos do hospedeiro. As glândulas que contêm essas enzimas podem estar localizadas adjacentes ao esôfago. As evidências disponíveis não apóiam a teoria de que a forma adulta do *D. renale* lentamente devora o tecido renal do hospedeiro, reduzindo-o a um saco oco. A cavidade bucal do parasita não é usada para a ingestão de tecidos renais intactos; não foram detectadas partículas sólidas no esôfago do *D. renale*. Embora o(s) mecanismo(s) exato(s) de destruição seja(m) desconhecido(s), a obstrução causada pelo(s) parasita(s) adulto(s) em crescimento e pela hidronefrose (ou pionefrose) secundária desempenha um papel importante. O exame microscópico óptico de cortes dos rins de cães com infecção renal unilateral revela alterações típicas de hidronefrose avançada (ou seja, obliteração da maioria dos túbulos renais circundados por tecido inflamatório crônico e persistência da arquitetura estrutural de muitos glomérulos). Os ovos de *D. renale* podem ser observados no parênquima renal adjacente à pelve renal. O urotélio que reveste a pelve renal fica frequentemente hiperplásico em algumas áreas e ulcerado em outras áreas. Se apenas um único rim for acometido pelo *D. renale*, o hospedeiro mantém uma função renal adequada em virtude dos processos compensatórios de hipertrofia e hiperplasia do rim remanescente. Se ambos os rins estiverem parasitados, ou se um único rim estiver parasitado e o rim oposto apresentar disfunção comórbida substancial, podem ocorrer estágios variados de insuficiência renal e uremia. Os ovos que são liberados pelos vermes fêmeas passam pelo trato urinário e provocam inflamação na mucosa do ureter e da bexiga urinária.

Cavidade Peritoneal
• Em cães, parasitas viáveis localizados na cavidade abdominal e/ou entre os lobos do fígado frequentemente são relatados como um achado incidental durante ovário-histerectomias. Sob certas condições, é possível que os vermes adultos possam permanecer na cavidade peritoneal por períodos prolongados antes da penetração em um rim.
• Os ovos presentes na cavidade peritoneal podem deflagrar o desenvolvimento de peritonite crônica. O exame das vísceras abdominais de cães com *D. renale* na cavidade peritoneal revelou hemorragia, inflamação granulomatosa e fibrose, envolvendo com maior frequência o omento, a superfície do fígado e, com menor frequência, a superfície do baço. Machos adultos viáveis (mas não fêmeas) foram encontrados na cavidade peritoneal de cães sem uma resposta inflamatória associada, sugerindo que fêmeas e/ou seus ovos estimulem uma resposta inflamatória mais acentuada do hospedeiro que os machos.
• Pode ocorrer ascite em cães com *D. renale* na cavidade peritoneal. O líquido detectado na cavidade abdominal costuma ser hemorrágico. Segundo relatos, a quantidade de líquido ascítico removida de cães infectados por *D. renale* variou de aproximadamente 20 mililitros a 3,2 litros.

IDENTIFICAÇÃO
Espécies
Cães e gatos.

Raça(s) Predominante(s)
N/D.

Idade Média e Faixa Etária
N/D.

Sexo Predominante
N/D.

SINAIS CLÍNICOS
• A ingestão de *L. variegatus* infectado por *D. renale* pelos cães tipicamente induz a vômito em virtude dos efeitos do parasita sobre a mucosa gástrica.
• Se apenas um único rim for invadido pelo *D. renale* e o rim oposto permanecer normal, frequentemente não haverá sinais clínicos.
• Hematúria "silenciosa" pode ser a primeira indicação de alguma anormalidade.
• A palpação do abdome pode revelar um rim hidronefrótico aumentado de volume e/ou deformado.

Dioctophyma Renale (Também Conhecido Como Verme Renal Gigante)

• Se ambos os rins estiverem parasitados, podem ocorrer sinais clínicos atribuíveis à insuficiência renal ou uremia. Contudo, o hospedeiro morrerá antes que a hidronefrose extensa de ambos os rins tenha tempo de se desenvolver. O grau de disfunção renal é influenciado por (1) número de parasitas no rim, (2) duração da infecção, (3) número de rins parasitados e (4) presença e gravidade de doenças renais comórbidas.

CAUSAS E FATORES DE RISCO
Ver as seções *Ciclo de Vida* e *Fisiopatologia*.

DIAGNÓSTICO

DIAGNÓSTICO DIFERENCIAL
Qualquer causa de hidronefrose ou renomegalia.

HEMOGRAMA/BIOQUÍMICA/URINÁLISE
• Na presença de verme fêmea grávida em um ou ambos os rins com trajeto patente (desobstruído) para o exterior, o exame microscópico da urina eliminada pelo hospedeiro geralmente revela os ovos de *D. renale*.
• Hematúria, piúria e proteinúria com ou sem ovos são alterações indicativas de alguma resposta inflamatória.
• Achados típicos de insuficiência renal crônica quando ambos os rins estão parasitados ou quando apenas um único rim contém os parasitas e o rim contralateral está lesado.

OUTROS TESTES LABORATORIAIS
N/D.

DIAGNÓSTICO POR IMAGEM
• A radiografia pode revelar um rim hidronefrótico aumentado de volume. Se a urografia intravenosa for realizada, o exame pode ser caracterizado pela incapacidade do rim parasitado em excretar o agente de contraste.
• A ultrassonografia pode demonstrar que o rim acometido está hidronefrótico e contém quantidade excessiva de líquido. O exame ultrassonográfico também pode revelar alças hipoecoicas características associadas a um ou mais desses parasitas na pelve renal. As ultrassonografias em planos transversais do rim acometido podem mostrar uma borda hiperecoica delgada que contém múltiplas estruturas circulares de diâmetro uniforme. As camadas mais externas dessas estruturas são hiperecoicas, enquanto as mais internas, hipoecoicas. No plano longitudinal, as estruturas aparecem como bandas hiperecoicas alongadas que se alternam com bandas hipoecoicas alongadas. Se houver parasitas viáveis na cavidade peritoneal, a ultrassonografia pode exibir bandas curvilíneas hiperecoicas na região do lobo caudal direito do fígado e/ou do polo cranial do rim direito. A realização seriada de ultrassonografias pode revelar o movimento do(s) parasita(s) de um local para o outro.
• As imagens de TC e RM também podem ser usadas para detectar o *D. renale* na pelve renal de um ou ambos os rins, na cavidade peritoneal, ou em posições variadas entre os lobos do fígado.

MÉTODOS DIAGNÓSTICOS
N/D.

TRATAMENTO

A nefrectomia costuma ser o tratamento de escolha quando apenas um único rim é acometido e o rim oposto ainda se mostra capaz de manter a homeostasia. Em pacientes com parasitas em ambos os rins, o procedimento de nefrotomia e a remoção dos parasitas podem ser indicados se ainda restar uma quantidade suficiente de tecido funcional em ambos os rins para manter uma qualidade de vida razoável. Infelizmente, no momento em que o envolvimento de ambos os rins pelo *D. renal* é identificado, os pacientes com frequência já apresentam insuficiência renal irreversível moderada a grave. Os parasitas encontrados como achados incidentais na cavidade peritoneal durante o procedimento de celiotomia (laparotomia) podem ser removidos sem morbidade adicional.

MEDICAÇÕES

MEDICAMENTO(S)
O tratamento farmacológico de adultos e/ou larvas infecciosas descobertos em qualquer espécie é praticamente inexistente. Há um relato de um homem de 44 anos de idade que exibia dor lombar recorrente atribuída ao *D. renale* e foi curado após dois esquemas terapêuticos de ivermectina.

CONTRAINDICAÇÕES/INTERAÇÕES POSSÍVEIS
N/D.

ACOMPANHAMENTO

PREVENÇÃO
Os cães e gatos não devem ser alimentados com peixe cru ou vísceras de peixe, sobretudo em áreas onde o *D. renale* sabidamente existe. Do mesmo modo, esses animais não devem ter acesso a águas de lagos ou lagoas que provavelmente contenham estágios infecciosos do *D. renale*.

DIVERSOS

ABREVIATURAS
• RM = ressonância magnética
• TC = tomografia computadorizada

RECURSOS DA INTERNET
http://www.capcvet.org.

Sugestões de Leitura
Karmanova EM. Biological peculiarities of nematodes of the order dioctophymidia. In: Dioctophymidia of Animals and Man and Diseases Caused by Them. Fundamentals of Nematology, vol. 20. Moscow: Nauka Publishers, 1968, pp. 24-121.
Osborne CA, Stevens JB, Hanlon GF, et al. Dioctophyma renale in the dog. JAVMA 1969, 155:605-620.

Autores Carl A. Osborne e Hasan Albasan
Consultor Editorial Carl A. Osborne

Dirofilariose — Cães

CONSIDERAÇÕES GERAIS

DEFINIÇÃO
Doença causada pela infecção por *Dirofilaria immitis*.

FISIOPATOLOGIA
• A gravidade da doença está diretamente relacionada com o número de vermes, a duração da infecção e a resposta do hospedeiro.
• O dano endotelial induz à proliferação e inflamação da camada mioíntima, predispondo à formação de edema periarterial.
• Aumento, tortuosidade e obstrução arteriais lobares provocam diminuição da complacência, perda do recrutamento colateral, hipertensão pulmonar e trombose.
• O dano pulmonar é exacerbado após a morte dos vermes adultos e com a prática de atividade física.

SISTEMA(S) ACOMETIDO(S)
• Respiratório — proliferação da camada mioíntima, hipertensão pulmonar (em casos graves), embolização, pneumonite alérgica (algumas infecções ocultas), granulomatose eosinofílica (incomum).
• Cardiovascular — hipertensão pulmonar grave provoca hipertrofia do ventrículo direito e, em alguns animais, insuficiência cardíaca congestiva direita/ascite.
• Hematológico/linfático/imune — o fluxo interno venoso ao coração pode vir a ser obstruído pelos vermes, provocando anemia hemolítica traumática (síndrome da veia cava).
• Renal/urológico — glomerulonefrite/proteinúria por imunocomplexos.

INCIDÊNCIA/PREVALÊNCIA
Praticamente 100% em cães não protegidos que vivem em regiões altamente endêmicas.

DISTRIBUIÇÃO GEOGRÁFICA
• Mais comum em zonas tropicais e subtropicais.
• Comum ao longo da costa do Atlântico e do Golfo do México, bem como nas bacias dos rios Ohio e Mississipi.
• Diagnosticada nos cães em todos os 50 estados dos EUA.
• Ubíquo — por causa do mosquito vetor.

IDENTIFICAÇÃO

Raça(s) Predominante(s)
• Raças de cães de médio a grande porte são mais acometidas que as de pequeno porte.
• É mais comum em cães com acesso a ambientes externos em comparação àqueles que vivem dentro de casa.

Idade Média e Faixa Etária
A infecção pode ocorrer em qualquer idade; a maioria dos animais acometidos tem 3-8 anos de idade.

Sexo Predominante
Os machos são acometidos com maior frequência que as fêmeas.

SINAIS CLÍNICOS

Achados Anamnésicos
• Os animais, em geral, permanecem assintomáticos ou exibem sinais mínimos como tosse ocasional (Classe I).
• Tosse e intolerância ao exercício associados a dano pulmonar moderado (Classe II).
• Caquexia, anemia, intolerância ao exercício, síncope e ascite (ICC direita) em cães gravemente acometidos (Classe III).

Achados do Exame Físico
• Sem anormalidades — animais com infecção leve (Classe I) e alguns com infecção moderadamente grave (Classe II).
• Respiração laboriosa ou crepitações — cães com hipertensão pulmonar grave (Classe III) ou complicações tromboembólicas pulmonares.
• Taquicardia, perda de peso, intolerância ao exercício, síncope, tosse, anemia e dispneia (Classe III).
• Ascite, distensão/pulsação da veia jugular e hepatomegalia indicam ICC direita (Classe III).
• Hemoptise — ocorre ocasionalmente.
• Mucosas pálidas, dispneia, pulsos fracos, hemoglobinemia e hemoglobinúria (síndrome da veia cava).

FATORES DE RISCO
• Residência em regiões endêmicas. • Habitat com acesso a ambientes externos. • Falta de profilaxia.
• Temperatura acima de 17,7°C o dia todo, todos os dias por, no mínimo, 1 mês. • Temperatura superior a 26,6°C todos os dias durante 10-14 dias.

DIAGNÓSTICO

DIAGNÓSTICO DIFERENCIAL
• Outras causas de hipertensão pulmonar e trombose (p. ex., hiperadrenocorticismo, nefro ou enteropatia com perda de proteínas). • Doença pulmonar obstrutiva crônica. • Pneumonia.
• Doença pulmonar alérgica. • Outras causas de ascite (p. ex., miocardiopatia dilatada). • Outras causas de anemia hemolítica (p. ex., imunomediada).

HEMOGRAMA/BIOQUÍMICA/URINÁLISE
• Anemia — ausente, leve ou moderada, dependendo da cronicidade, da gravidade da doença e das complicações tromboembólicas. Anemia associada à infecção de classe III.
• Eosinofilia e basofilia — variam.
• Leucograma inflamatório e trombocitopenia associados à tromboembolia.
• Hiperglobulinemia — achado inconsistente.
• Hemoglobinemia — evidente com síndrome da veia cava e menos frequente com tromboembolia.
• Proteinúria — comum em animais com infecção grave e crônica; causada por glomerulonefrite por imunocomplexo ou amiloidose.
• Hemoglobinúria — síndrome da veia cava ou lise grave com tromboembolia (Classe III).

OUTROS TESTES LABORATORIAIS
• Testes sorológicos altamente específicos e sensíveis que identificam o antígeno da fêmea adulta de *D. immitis*; testar 7 meses após o término da estação prévia de transmissão.
• Antigenemia ausente na ausência de vermes adultos fêmeas.
• Teste positivo fraco é averiguado pela repetição do teste com o uso de algum teste diferente.
• Reação forte indica carga relativa alta de vermes ou morte recente dos vermes.
• Os testes para identificação de microfilárias não são recomendados para a triagem de rotina de dirofilariose; utilizados principalmente para confirmar os testes antigênicos positivos fracos e determinar o estado microfilarêmico antes de os pacientes serem submetidos à dietilcarbamazina ou milbemicina oxima como preventivos de dirofilariose. O esfregaço direto é, no mínimo, 25% menos sensível que os testes de concentração.

DIAGNÓSTICO POR IMAGEM

Achados Radiográficos
• Utilizar projeção dorsoventral.
• O aumento segmentar da artéria pulmonar principal, bem como o aumento e a tortuosidade das artérias lobares, variam de ausentes (Classe I) a graves (Classe III). Ordem de acometimento: artéria caudal direita > artéria caudal esquerda > artérias craniais.
• Infiltrados pulmonares parenquimatosos de gravidade variável — em torno das artérias lobares; podem se estender para a maioria ou todos de um ou múltiplos lobos pulmonares quando ocorre tromboembolia.
• Infiltrados difusos, simétricos, alveolares e intersticiais ocorrem ocasionalmente por causa de reação alérgica às microfilárias (pneumonite alérgica). Cerca de 10% das infecções ocultas.

Achados Ecocardiográficos
• Em geral, não há nada digno de nota; no entanto, podem refletir dilatação do ventrículo direito e hipertrofia da parede, regurgitação da valva atrioventricular direita (tricúspide), hipertensão pulmonar, pequena subcarga do coração esquerdo (obstrução/hipertensão pulmonar).
• Podem-se detectar ecodensidades paralelas lineares produzidas pelas filárias no ventrículo direito, no átrio direito e nas artérias pulmonares.

MÉTODOS DIAGNÓSTICOS

Achados Eletrocardiográficos
• Geralmente normais. • Podem refletir hipertrofia do ventrículo direito em cães com infecção grave.
• Distúrbios do ritmo cardíaco — observados ocasionalmente (é mais comum a ocorrência de contrações atriais prematuras e fibrilação atrial) na infecção grave.

ACHADOS PATOLÓGICOS
• Coração direito grande. • Proliferação da camada mioíntima da artéria pulmonar. • Tromboembolia pulmonar. • Hemorragia pulmonar.
• Hepatomegalia e congestão em animais com ICC direita.

TRATAMENTO

CUIDADO(S) DE SAÚDE ADEQUADO(S)
• A maioria dos pacientes é hospitalizada durante a administração de adulticida.
• Eliminar as microfilárias com profilaxia mensal; o medicamento Interceptor® pode causar um rápido declínio no número de microfilárias, devendo ser utilizado com cuidado nesse quadro.
• A hospitalização é recomendada para cães que sofrem complicações tromboembólicas.

ATIVIDADE
• Há necessidade de restrição intensa por 4-6 semanas após a administração de adulticida.
• O confinamento em gaiola é recomendado por 3-4 semanas após a administração de adulticida para os pacientes de Classe III.
• É aconselhável o confinamento em gaiola por 7 dias para os cães com complicações tromboembólicas pulmonares.

DIROFILARIOSE — CÃES

ORIENTAÇÃO AO PROPRIETÁRIO
• Prognóstico bom para os animais com infecção leve a moderada.
• Complicações pulmonares após a administração de adulticida são prováveis em pacientes com comprometimento moderado a grave da artéria pulmonar e naqueles com alta carga de vermes.
• Pode ocorrer reinfecção a menos que se administre a profilaxia apropriada.

CONSIDERAÇÕES CIRÚRGICAS
• Tratamento de escolha para a síndrome da veia cava. • A remoção de vermes do coração direito e da artéria pulmonar pela veia jugular com o uso de fluoroscopia e uma pinça-jacaré longa flexível ou escova especial confeccionada com a crina de cavalo é altamente eficaz para tratar altas cargas de vermes quando realizada por um profissional experiente.

MEDICAÇÕES
MEDICAMENTO(S) DE ESCOLHA
• Estabilizar os animais acometidos por ICC direita com o uso de diuréticos, inibidor da ECA, repouso em gaiola e restrição moderada de sódio antes do tratamento adulticida.
• Estabilizar o quadro de insuficiência pulmonar com suplementação de oxigênio, agentes antitrombóticos (p. ex., ácido acetilsalicílico ou heparina) ou dosagens anti-inflamatórias de corticosteroides, dependendo dos achados clínicos e radiográficos.
• Medicamento adulticida: dicloridrato de melarsomina (Immiticide®, 2,5 mg/kg IM/dose) — as injeções são aplicadas nos músculos epaxiais com o uso de agulhas calibre 22; aplicar pressão sobre o local da injeção durante e após a retirada da agulha. Um resultado positivo no teste antigênico 6 meses depois pode indicar a necessidade de repetição do tratamento.
• Um protocolo de eliminação gradual é recomendado na maioria dos casos; administrar 1 injeção seguida em 1 mês por 2 injeções (primeira injeção nos músculos epaxiais esquerdo ou direito, seguida pela injeção no lado oposto 24 h depois). Esse protocolo distribui o efeito adulticida e a tromboembolia em 2 tratamentos.
• Para infecção de Classe III em cães de pequeno porte ou infecção grave de Classe III com alta carga de vermes — administrar 1 injeção a cada 4-6 semanas por um total de 3 injeções. Manter o paciente sob confinamento estrito por 4-6 semanas. Realizar o teste antigênico 6 meses após a terceira injeção.
• Pneumonite alérgica — administrar prednisona ou prednisolona (2 mg/kg VO a cada 12-24 h por vários dias) e, em seguida, administrar o Immiticide® imediatamente.
• Não é recomendável a terapia rápida contra microfilárias (p. ex., ivermectina em altas doses ou milbemicina); é aceitável eliminar as microfilárias por meio da profilaxia mensal.

PRECAUÇÕES
• Tratamento adulticida — não indicado em pacientes com insuficiência renal, insuficiência hepática (icterícia) ou síndrome nefrótica.
• Síndrome da veia cava — remover os vermes por meio cirúrgico e estabilizar o paciente com tratamento conservativo por, no mínimo, 1 mês antes da terapia adulticida.

MEDICAMENTO(S) ALTERNATIVO(S)
• Heparina sódica (75 unidades/kg SC a cada 8 h), ácido acetilsalicílico (5-7 mg/kg VO a cada 24 h) ou heparina de baixo peso molecular (dalteparina: 100 unidades/kg SC a cada 12 h) por 1-3 semanas antes, durante e por 3 semanas após a administração do adulticida são recomendações controversas para a maioria dos casos graves da doença de Classe III; a terapia é combinada com confinamento estrito e prolongado em gaiola.
• Heparina sódica (200-500 unidades/kg SC a cada 8 h) é recomendada para cães com tromboembolia pulmonar ou hemoglobinúria com o objetivo de prolongar o TTPA em um valor de 1,5-2 vezes o nível basal.
• Ivermectina administrada mensalmente por, pelo menos, 32 meses mata algumas filárias adultas (em geral, não é recomendada).
• Doxiciclina (5-10 mg/kg VO a cada 12 h) é utilizada por alguns clínicos antes da terapia adulticida para eliminar a *Wolbachia*, uma bactéria intrafilarial Gram-negativa, associada à inflamação pós-adulticida dos pulmões e rins; não há estudos clínicos que demonstrem a utilidade desse medicamento. Não é empregada pelos autores.

ACOMPANHAMENTO
MONITORIZAÇÃO DO PACIENTE
Realizar o teste antigênico 6 meses após o tratamento adulticida. Alguns cães com antigenemia persistente de baixo grau podem não necessitar de tratamento. Antigenemia fraca indica que a maioria dos vermes foi morta; com isso, a doença pulmonar exibirá melhora e a profilaxia com Heartgard® finalmente eliminará os vermes remanescentes.

PREVENÇÃO
• A profilaxia contra dirofilariose deve ser providenciada para todos os cães sob risco. Os autores recomendam a profilaxia durante todo o ano. Caso contrário, essa profilaxia deve ser iniciada na época do mosquito e mantida por 1 mês após a primeira geada (hemisfério Norte).
• Realizar o teste antigênico antes de iniciar o tratamento preventivo.
• Efetuar o teste antigênico 7 meses após o término da estação anterior.
• Dietilcarbamazina (Filarabits®) — não é recomendada pelos autores.
• Ivermectina (Heartgard®) — preventivo mensal altamente eficaz que, quando combinado com o pamoato de pirantel (Heartgard Plus®), também controla as infestações por ancilóstomos e nematódeos; pode ser dada com segurança a cães com microfilaremia.
• Milbemicina oxima (Interceptor®) — profilaxia mensal altamente eficaz, que também controla ancilóstomos, nematódeos e tricúris; a dosagem preventiva é microfilaricida; podem ocorrer reações agudas quando administrada a cães com microfilaremia.
• Moxidectina (Advantage Multi®) — uma solução tópica administrada mensalmente, que também controla pulgas, carrapatos, ancilóstomos, nematódeos, tricúris e ácaros otológicos.
• Selamectina (Revolution®) — uma preparação tópica mensal altamente eficaz.
• Preventivos orais de lactona macrocíclica, como milbemicina oxima, ivermectina, moxidectina e selamectina, possuem eficácia retroativa de 100% por 1 mês e, no mínimo, 75% por 2 meses.
• Administrar a filhotes logo depois de 8 semanas de vida, conforme ditado pelo risco sazonal.
• Todos os medicamentos profiláticos podem ser administrados com segurança a cães da raça Collie nas dosagens apropriadas.
• Para cães que se encontram infectados por vermes adultos e ainda não estão tomando medicamento profilático, qualquer um dos medicamentos supramencionados pode ser iniciado imediatamente, devendo ser instituído dentro de 1 mês do diagnóstico. Os autores não recomendam o uso de Interceptor® em cães com microfilaremia.
• Os autores não costumam iniciar a profilaxia e depois adiar o tratamento adulticida por 1 ou mais meses.
• A ação retroativa do Heartgard® é de quase 100% em 4 meses após a inoculação se administrado por 12 meses consecutivos.
• Todas as lactonas macrocíclicas eliminam as microfilárias em 6-12 meses.

COMPLICAÇÕES POSSÍVEIS
• Complicações tromboembólicas pulmonares após a administração de adulticida — podem ocorrer até 4-6 semanas depois do tratamento; em geral, são mais graves em cães com doença de Classe III e naqueles não submetidos a confinamento adequado.
• Trombocitopenia e coagulação intravascular.
• Efeitos adversos da melarsomina — tromboembolia pulmonar (em geral, 7-30 dias após a terapia); anorexia (incidência de 13%); miosite/reação no local da injeção (incidência de 32%, embora seja leve e só dure 1-2 dias); letargia ou depressão (incidência de 15%); elevação das enzimas hepáticas; paresia/paralisia/atividade mental alterada (raras).

EVOLUÇÃO ESPERADA E PROGNÓSTICO
• Classe I — em geral, sem ocorrências especiais, com prognóstico excelente.
• Classe III — prognóstico reservado com maior risco de complicações.

DIVERSOS
DISTÚRBIOS ASSOCIADOS
Wolbachia.

ANESTESIA
Quando houver necessidade de anestesia/cirurgia, adiar o tratamento de dirofilariose até depois do procedimento.

GESTAÇÃO/FERTILIDADE/REPRODUÇÃO
• O tratamento adulticida deve ser adiado.
• Pode ocorrer infecção transplacentária por microfilárias.

VER TAMBÉM
• Coagulação Intravascular Disseminada.
• Hepatotoxinas. • Hipertensão Pulmonar.
• Insuficiência Cardíaca Congestiva Direita.
• Síndrome Nefrótica. • Tromboembolia Pulmonar.

ABREVIATURA(S)
• ICC = insuficiência cardíaca congestiva.

Autores Justin D. Thomason e Clay A. Calvert

Dirofilariose — Gatos

CONSIDERAÇÕES GERAIS

REVISÃO
- Doença causada pela infecção por *Dirofilaria immitis*.
- A microfilaremia é incomum (menos de 20% dos casos) e, se presente, costuma ser transitória.
- Prevalência de 1/10 daquela observada em cães desprotegidos.
- Carga média de vermes baixa.
- Os vermes são fisicamente menores, mas indícios recentes sugerem que o tempo de vida seja semelhante aos de cães.

IDENTIFICAÇÃO
- Sem predisposição racial ou etária.
- Os machos são mais comumente infectados por via natural e mais fáceis de serem infectados por meio experimental.

SINAIS CLÍNICOS
Achados Anamnésicos
- Tosse (isso é relativamente incomum com insuficiência cardíaca).
- A tosse comumente ocorrerá no início da doença antes de uma infecção estabelecida por vermes adultos.
- Doença respiratória associada à dirofilariose.
- Ocorrência de sinais clínicos e doença pulmonar 2-4 meses depois da infecção mesmo se uma infecção por vermes adultos nunca for estabelecida.
- Dispneia.
- Vômitos (causa indeterminada).
- Tromboembolia pulmonar frequentemente resulta em insuficiência respiratória aguda e morte.
- Vômitos e sinais respiratórios predominam na doença crônica.

Achados do Exame Físico
- Em geral, permanecem normais.
- Aumento dos ruídos broncovesiculares.
- A presença de arritmia, sopro ou ritmo de galope deve aumentar a suspeita de cardiopatia primária.

CAUSAS E FATORES DE RISCO
- Gatos que vivem em ambientes externos correm maior risco (2:1).
- A infecção por FeLV não é um fator predisponente.

DIAGNÓSTICO

DIAGNÓSTICO DIFERENCIAL
- Asma. • Miocardiopatia. • Quilotórax. • Infecção por *Aelurostrongylus abstrusus*. • Infecção por *Paragonimus kellicotti*.

HEMOGRAMA/BIOQUÍMICA/URINÁLISE
- Variam com o estágio da doença.
- Leve anemia arregenerativa.
- Eosinofilia inconsistente.
- Basofilia concomitante deve aumentar a suspeita.
- Hiperglobulinemia.

OUTROS TESTES LABORATORIAIS
Testes de Concentração de Microfilárias Sensibilidade muito baixa, mas especificidade elevada.

Testes para o Antígeno da Dirofilária
- ELISA ou imunocromatografia.
- Os testes que detectam o antígeno circulante da dirofilária são mais específicos que os testes de anticorpo.
- O resultado positivo ao teste de antígeno é fortemente sugestivo de infecção por dirofilárias adultas.
- Cargas baixas de vermes (menos de 5) e infecções por vermes de um único sexo costumam resultar em testes falso-negativos de antígeno.
- O resultado negativo não exclui dirofilariose; mais de 40% dos gatos com infecção por vermes adultos são negativos ao teste de antígeno. Muitos gatos (aqueles acometidos por doença respiratória associada à dirofilariose) ficam sintomáticos bem antes de um teste de antígeno se tornar positivo.

Testes de Anticorpo contra Dirofilária
- ELISA ou imunocromatografia.
- Os testes que detectam anticorpos circulantes contra o antígeno de vermes imaturos e adultos são os mais sensíveis para a dirofilariose felina.
- O resultado positivo não confirma infecção por *vermes adultos*. Em geral, ficam positivos dentro de 4 meses da infecção.
- Quanto mais intensa a resposta de anticorpo, mais provável uma infecção por vermes adultos.
- Podem se tornar negativos em infecções por vermes adultos.

DIAGNÓSTICO POR IMAGEM
Radiografia
- Aumento das artérias pulmonares (>1,6 vez a largura da 9ª costela).
- Artérias pulmonares embotadas e tortuosas.
- Infiltrados pulmonares perivasculares difusos.
- Pode haver efusão pleural.
- Em casos de dirofilariose felina de ocorrência espontânea e de indução experimental, há registro de quilotórax.

Ecocardiografia
- Artéria pulmonar principal dilatada.
- Identificação de vermes no coração ou na artéria pulmonar principal; os vermes são observados mais comumente na artéria pulmonar direita, mas também se encontram no átrio e ventrículo direitos (sinal hiperecoico de "igual").
- Teste sensível nas mãos de um ecocardiografista experiente.
- Exclui ou confirma outras cardiopatias primárias (miocardiopatias).

TRATAMENTO

- Atualmente, não há nenhuma terapia adulticida clínica aprovada ou recomendada.
- A extração por via cirúrgica ou com cateterismo pode ser a opção terapêutica mais razoável.
- Os gatos sintomáticos devem ser estabilizados (ver adiante) antes de se considerar a extração dos vermes.
- A "cura" espontânea é provavelmente mais comum em gatos que em cães.

MEDICAÇÕES

MEDICAMENTO(S)
Estabilização Inicial
- Suplementação de oxigênio.
- Teofilina (formulação de liberação sustentada), 25 mg/kg VO a cada 24 h à noite.
- Prednisolona, 1-2 mg/kg VO a cada 12-24 h por 10-14 dias; em seguida, diminuir gradualmente.
- Doxiciclina, 10 mg/kg VO a cada 24 h durante 30 dias (para eliminar a bactéria endossimbionte *Wolbachia*) pode acelerar a morte dos vermes e diminuir a gravidade da inflamação pulmonar secundária à embolização por vermes.
- Fluidoterapia balanceada deve ser feita cuidado se houver indicação.
- Atualmente, não é recomendada a terapia adulticida clínica.
- Os cuidados de suporte para tromboembolia pulmonar são os mesmos utilizados para estabilização inicial (ver anteriormente).

CONTRAINDICAÇÕES/INTERAÇÕES POSSÍVEIS
- Terapia com ácido acetilsalicílico — nenhum benefício documentado.
- Informações atuais não confirmam o uso de melarsomina (Immiticide®) em gatos.

ACOMPANHAMENTO

MONITORIZAÇÃO DO PACIENTE
A avaliação seriada da resposta clínica, a obtenção de radiografias torácicas, bem como os testes para detecção de antígeno e anticorpo de dirofilárias, são mais informativos.

PREVENÇÃO
- Ivermectina µ24 µg/kg VO a cada 30 dias.
- Milbemicina oxima — 0,5 mg/kg VO a cada 30 dias.
- Selamectina — 6,6–12 mg/kg por via SC a cada 30 dias.
- Moxidectina — 1 mg/kg ou 6,6-20 mg/kg VO a cada 30 dias.
- A administração desses medicamentos em gatos não é impedida por soropositividade de anticorpo ou antígeno.

DIVERSOS

SINÔNIMO(S)
Doença do coração.

ABREVIATURA(S)
- ELISA = ensaio imunoabsorvente ligado à enzima.
- FeLV = vírus da leucemia felina.

RECURSOS DA INTERNET
Diretrizes de 2010 para o Diagnóstico, o Tratamento e a Prevenção de Dirofilariose (*Dirofilaria immitis*) em Gatos. The American Heartworm Society: http://www.heartwormsociety.org/veterinaryresources/feline-guidelines.html.

Sugestões de Leitura
Calvert CA, Thomason JD. Heartworm disease. In: Tilley LP, Smith FWK, Oyama MA, Sleeper MM, eds., Manual of Canine and Feline Cardiology, 4th ed. St. Louis: Saunders Elsevier, 2008, pp. 183-199.

Autor Matthew W. Miller
Consultores Editoriais Larry P. Tilley e Francis W.K. Smith, Jr.

DISAUTONOMIA (SÍNDROME DE KEY-GASKELL)

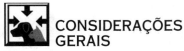

CONSIDERAÇÕES GERAIS

REVISÃO
- Caracterizada por falha da função autonômica em múltiplos órgãos com envolvimento motor ou sensorial mínimo.
- Cães jovens adultos, habitantes de zonas rurais e do Meio-Oeste dos EUA, estão sob maior risco.
- O tratamento é sintomático e o prognóstico, reservado.

IDENTIFICAÇÃO
- Cães e, menos comumente, gatos.
- Não há predileção racial ou sexual.
- A idade média de acometimento é de 18 meses, mas qualquer idade pode ser acometida.

SINAIS CLÍNICOS
- Início agudo a subagudo (5-14 dias).
- Podem estar presentes diversas combinações de sinais clínicos, embora haja necessidade de sinais tanto simpáticos como parassimpáticos em vários órgãos para que a formulação do diagnóstico seja confiável.
- Os déficits sensoriais ou motores são mínimos.

Queixas Apresentadas
- Com maior frequência, observam-se sinais GI de vômito ou regurgitação, diarreia ou, ocasionalmente, constipação.
- Esforço para urinar e gotejamento de urina.
- Fotofobia e protrusão da terceira pálpebra.
- Dispneia, tosse e secreção nasal.
- Depressão, anorexia e perda de peso.

Achados do Exame Físico
- Perda de tônus do esfíncter anal.
- Ressecamento do nariz e das mucosas; ausência de produção lacrimal.
- Bexiga urinária distendida de fácil compressão.
- Aumento de amplitude média até dilatação máxima das pupilas, sem reflexo pupilar à luz, mas visão intacta.
- Protrusão da terceira pálpebra, ptose e enoftalmia.
- Ausência de borborigmos intestinais e, ocasionalmente, dor abdominal.
- Frequência cardíaca e pressão arterial tipicamente no extremo inferior da faixa de normalidade, mas não se elevam em resposta ao estresse.
- Quadros secundários de pneumonia por aspiração ou rinite.
- Caquexia.
- Ocasionalmente, há déficits proprioceptivos leves ou fraqueza.

CAUSAS E FATORES DE RISCO
- A causa é desconhecida.
- Incidência mais alta em Missouri, Oklahoma e Kansas, embora haja relato de casos em toda parte dos EUA.
- Cães errantes (ou seja, de vida livre) e rurais estão sob maior risco.

DIAGNÓSTICO

DIAGNÓSTICO DIFERENCIAL
- Toxicidade anticolinérgica.
- Outros diagnósticos diferenciais dependem, sobretudo, dos sinais clínicos específicos; p. ex., infecção do trato urinário em caso de disúria, úlcera de córnea na presença de fotofobia, desidratação em relação ao ressecamento das mucosas.

HEMOGRAMA/BIOQUÍMICA/URINÁLISE
Não são dignos de nota.

OUTROS TESTES LABORATORIAIS
N/D.

DIAGNÓSTICO POR IMAGEM
- Megaesôfago ± pneumonia por aspiração.
- Distensão das alças intestinais sem peristaltismo.
- Bexiga urinária distendida.

MÉTODOS DIAGNÓSTICOS
- Se as pupilas estiverem acometidas, a instilação de pilocarpina a 0,05% em um único olho produzirá miose dentro de 60 min. Isso descarta toxicidade anticolinérgica.
- A administração de atropina (0,03 mg/kg IV) pode não produzir uma elevação da frequência cardíaca; isso sugere perda do tônus vagal.
- Ecocardiografia pode revelar disfunção sistólica como um encurtamento fracional reduzido.
- A aplicação intradérmica de histamina pode não produzir qualquer resposta ou gerar a formação de pápula, mas sem rubor; isso demonstra a perda de inervação simpática das arteríolas.

TRATAMENTO
- Sintomático.
- Fluidos IV para evitar desidratação.
- Sonda de alimentação para garantir uma nutrição adequada na presença de megaesôfago. Na ausência de motilidade GI, talvez seja necessária a nutrição parenteral.
- Colírios lubrificantes se a produção lacrimal não for suficiente.
- Umidificação do ar pode ser útil em caso de ressecamento das mucosas.
- Compressão manual da bexiga urinária.

MEDICAÇÕES

MEDICAMENTO(S)
- Antibióticos, conforme a necessidade, para tratar as infecções secundárias.
- Betanecol para estimular o lacrimejamento e a micção (iniciar com a dose de 0,05 mg/kg a cada 12-8 h e ajustá-la, com base na resposta).
- Pilocarpina ocular para aliviar a fotofobia.
- Medicamentos procinéticos, como metoclopramida, em caso de acometimento da motilidade GI.

CONTRAINDICAÇÕES/INTERAÇÕES POSSÍVEIS
- Os animais com disautonomia desenvolvem supersensibilidade a agentes colinérgicos ou adrenérgicos de ação direta por causa da denervação.
- É preciso ter muito cuidado no uso desses medicamentos, particularmente dos agentes adrenérgicos que podem precipitar taquiarritmias fatais. É melhor iniciar com < 10% do extremo inferior da faixa de dosagem ao utilizar medicamentos de ação direta e aumentar a dose, conforme a necessidade, para obter o efeito desejado.

ACOMPANHAMENTO
- O prognóstico é reservado. A maioria dos animais vem a óbito em decorrência de pneumonia por aspiração ou é submetida à eutanásia em função da baixa qualidade de vida.
- Os animais que sobrevivem ao quadro frequentemente apresentam certo grau de disfunção autonômica permanente que pode necessitar de cuidados constantes.

DIVERSOS
- A identificação de perda neuronal nos gânglios à necropsia confirma o diagnóstico.
- O diagnóstico clínico baseia-se na insuficiência autonômica em múltiplos órgãos sem causa subjacente ou envolvimento motor ou sensorial significativo e resposta adequada ao teste farmacológico.

ABREVIATURA(S)
- GI = gastrintestinal.

RECURSOS DA INTERNET
http://www.cvm.missouri.edu/neurology/Dysauton/dyshome.htm

Sugestões de Leitura

Berghaus RD, O'Brien DP, Johnson GC, Thorne JG. Risk factors for development of dysautonomia in dogs. JAVMA 2001, 218:1285-1292.

Harkin KR, Andrews GA, Nietfeld JC. Dysautonomia in dogs: 65 cases (1993-2000). JAVMA 2002, 220(5):633-644.

Harkin KR, Bulmer BJ, Biller DS. Echocardiographic evaluation of dogs with dysautonomia. JAVMA 2009, 235(12):1431-1436.

Longshore RC, O'Brien DP, Johnson GC, et al. Dysautonomia in dogs — a retrospective study. J Vet Intern Med 1996, 10(3):103-109.

O'Brien DP, Johnson GC. Dysautonomia and autonomic neuropathies. Vet Clin North Am Small Anim Pract 2002, 32(1):251-265.

Autor Dennis P. O'Brien
Consultor Editorial Joane M. Parent

Disbiose do Intestino Delgado

CONSIDERAÇÕES GERAIS

DEFINIÇÃO
• A disbiose do intestino delgado é uma síndrome clínica provocada por alteração da microbiota do intestino delgado.
• Previamente, diversos termos distintos foram usados para descrever disbiose do intestino delgado:
• A proliferação bacteriana no intestino delgado é definida como >10^4 UFC bacterianas anaeróbias e/ou >10^5 totais/mL no suco duodenal de cães. No entanto, esses critérios são atualmente controversos.
• Diarreia responsiva a antibióticos é usada por vários autores para descrever os pacientes que apresentam diarreia responsiva à antibioticoterapia. Tanto o tipo de bactéria como o tipo de antibiótico eficaz não foram definidos para diarreia responsiva a antibióticos.
• Diarreia responsiva à tilosina foi descrita por um grupo na Finlândia. A expressão surgiu com base no fato de que foram descritos vários cães com diarreia crônica que não respondiam a diversos antibióticos ou corticosteroides, mas respondiam ao tratamento com tilosina.
• Atualmente, não há nenhum consenso sobre a composição quantitativa da microbiota gastrintestinal em cães ou gatos saudáveis.
• A disbiose do intestino delgado difere da colonização do trato alimentar por bactérias patogênicas conhecidas (p. ex., *Salmonella* spp., *Campylobacter jejuni*, *Clostridium perfringens* enterotoxigênica, *E. coli* enterotóxica, ou outras).

FISIOPATOLOGIA
• Bactérias são constantemente ingeridas com alimento e/ou saliva.
• Os mecanismos protetores do hospedeiro evitam a proliferação de bactérias patogênicas ou potencialmente patogênicas por meio de secreção de ácido gástrico, motilidade intestinal (peristaltismo), secreção de substâncias antimicrobianas na bile e no suco pancreático, bem como por produção entérica local de IgA.
• A válvula ileocólica é uma barreira fisiológica entre o intestino grosso, que é povoado por grande número de bactérias, e o intestino delgado menos povoado.
• Quando esses mecanismos de defesa natural falham e um número excessivo de certas espécies de bactérias persiste na parte superior do intestino delgado, elas podem provocar doença, mesmo que não sejam patógenos obrigatórios.
• Bactérias anaeróbias (p. ex., *Bacteroides* spp. e *Clostridium* spp.) foram consideradas como a causa patológica mais provável do que muitas bactérias aeróbias.

SISTEMA(S) ACOMETIDO(S)
• Gastrintestinal — distúrbio na função absortiva normal, resultando em amolecimento das fezes e perda de peso.
• Hepatobiliar — a veia porta conduz toxinas bacterianas e outras substâncias para o fígado, o que pode induzir a alterações hepáticas.

GENÉTICA
• Não foi estabelecida nenhuma base genética para disbiose do intestino delgado. Contudo, estudos recentes sugerem que a colite ulcerativa histiocítica deva ser considerada como um tipo de disbiose do intestino grosso. Como a maioria dos casos foi descrita no Boxer, é provável a existência de fatores genéticos que predisponham os cães dessa raça a esse tipo de disbiose.
• Além disso, algumas raças (Pastor alemão, Shar-pei chinês e Beagle) parecem estar sob risco aumentado de disbiose do intestino delgado.

INCIDÊNCIA/PREVALÊNCIA
Desconhecidas.

IDENTIFICAÇÃO
Espécies
• Cães.
• Gatos — desconhecida; pouco se sabe sobre a microbiota normal do intestino delgado em gatos e, nessa espécie, o efeito de alterações da microbiota é pouco compreendido. Em parte, isso talvez seja atribuído ao fato de que, até há pouco tempo, era usada a expressão proliferação bacteriana do intestino delgado e, como os gatos saudáveis parecem ter contagens bacterianas mais altas do que a de seres humanos ou cães, o conceito de uma proliferação da microbiota não era atrativo. Contudo, certos gatos com diarreia crônica respondem à antibioticoterapia, sugerindo que a disbiose do intestino delgado também possa ocorrer nessa espécie de animais.

Raça(s) Predominante(s)
Subjetivamente, as raças Pastor alemão, Shar-pei chinês e Beagle apresentam uma incidência elevada.

Idade Média e Faixa Etária
• Desconhecidas.
• Pode ser diagnosticada em cães de qualquer idade (faixa etária: <1 ano e >8 anos de idade).

SINAIS CLÍNICOS
Comentários Gerais
Alterações na microbiota intestinal podem causar sinais clínicos de doença do intestino delgado, como fezes moles ou diarreia, perda de peso e outros.

Achados Anamnésicos
• Fezes moles ou diarreia crônicos — comuns.
• Perda de peso, apesar do apetite razoável — habitual.
• Borborimo e flatulência — usuais.
• Vômito — ocasional/variável.
• Podem ser observados sinais clínicos do processo patológico subjacente em casos de disbiose do intestino delgado secundário.
• Os sinais clínicos podem aparecer e desaparecer ou permanecer contínuos.

Achados do Exame Físico
• Perda de peso e má condição corporal.

CAUSAS
• Disbiose do intestino delgado primária é provavelmente incomum; infelizmente, no entanto, uma causa de disbiose do intestino delgado permanece muitas vezes sem diagnóstico e, com isso, muitos cães são diagnosticados com disbiose do intestino delgado idiopática.
• Disbiose do intestino delgado secundária (mais comum):
• Alteração na anatomia do intestino delgado — hereditária ou adquirida (p. ex., alça intestinal cega congênita, obstruções parciais, neoplasia, corpo estranho, intussuscepção, estenose, aderência ou divertículo).
• Modificação na motilidade intestinal — induzida por hipotireoidismo, neuropatias autônomas.
• Insuficiência pancreática exócrina — aproximadamente 70% dos cães com esse tipo de insuficiência apresentam disbiose do intestino delgado concomitante.
• Hipocloridria ou acloridria — espontânea ou iatrogênica (p. ex., bloqueador histaminérgico dos receptores H_2).
• Alteração do sistema imunológico — imunodeficiência, diminuição nas defesas das mucosas e enteropatia preexistente.

FATORES DE RISCO
Doenças intestinais que afetam os mecanismos de defesa local (p. ex., enteropatia inflamatória, reações alimentares adversas, infestação parasitária, outras).

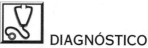

DIAGNÓSTICO

DIAGNÓSTICO DIFERENCIAL
• Doenças gastrintestinais secundárias (i. e., insuficiência hepática, insuficiência renal, insuficiência pancreática exócrina, hipotireoidismo, hipoadrenocorticismo, outras).
• Doenças gastrintestinais primárias (i. e., infecciosas, inflamatórias, neoplásicas, mecânicas, tóxicas ou outras).

HEMOGRAMA/BIOQUÍMICA/URINÁLISE
• Em geral, normais.
• Hipoalbuminemia — rara; quando presente, sugere enteropatia particularmente grave, justificando o diagnóstico e a abordagem terapêutica de forma rigorosa.

DIAGNÓSTICO POR IMAGEM
Não são úteis para o diagnóstico de disbiose do intestino delgado primária. Contudo, podem revelar achados indicativos de alguma causa subjacente.

OUTROS TESTES LABORATORIAIS
Concentrações Séricas de Cobalamina e Folato
• O nível sérico de folato pode estar aumentado, pois muitas espécies de bactérias sintetizam essa vitamina; além disso, a proliferação dessas espécies levarão a uma superabundância de ácido fólico no intestino delgado.
• Já a concentração sérica de cobalamina pode estar diminuída, visto que muitas espécies de bactérias competem com o hospedeiro por essa vitamina.
• O encontro de concentração sérica aumentada de folato e nível sérico diminuído de cobalamina é razoavelmente específico para disbiose do intestino delgado em cães. Contudo, nem todos os pacientes com esse tipo de afecção demonstram esse padrão.
• A concentração sérica de folato e de cobalamina é o único teste para disbiose do intestino delgado disponível atualmente com certa rotina.

Cultura Bacteriana Qualitativa e Quantitativa do Suco do Intestino Delgado
• Culturas quantitativas aeróbicas e anaeróbicas do líquido duodenal são consideradas há muito tempo como o teste com padrão de excelência para o diagnóstico de proliferação bacteriana do intestino delgado em pacientes humanos.
• Método invasivo — necessita de endoscopia ou laparoscopia.
• Trabalho recente sugere que a espécie de bactérias que compõem a microbiota do intestino

delgado pode ser mais importante que o número de bactérias.
• Nenhum protocolo padronizado foi estabelecido para amostragem, manipulação e cultura do suco duodenal, levando à elevada variabilidade nas contagens bacterianas.

Ensaios Terapêuticos
• Tratar os pacientes com suspeita de disbiose do intestino delgado com antibiótico, prebiótico ou probiótico e observar os resultados.
• Talvez seja difícil interpretar os resultados de ensaios terapêuticos, pois pode haver mais de uma doença (p. ex., enteropatia inflamatória mais disbiose do intestino delgado, intolerância alimentar mais disbiose do intestino delgado); a falta de resposta clínica pode levar à conclusão incorreta de que não há disbiose do intestino delgado; a seleção incorreta do tratamento experimentado também pode provocar falha na resposta clínica.

ACHADOS PATOLÓGICOS
• Não há achados macroscópicos à laparotomia exploratória ou endoscopia.
• Histopatologia e citologia da mucosa do intestino delgado tipicamente não exibem nada digno de nota.

TRATAMENTO
CUIDADO(S) DE SAÚDE ADEQUADO(S)
• Tratamento clínico em um esquema ambulatorial.
• A disbiose do intestino delgado pode ser tratada com antibióticos, prebióticos, probióticos ou uma combinação dos mesmos:
• Antibióticos: ver adiante em busca das medicações.
• Prebióticos: consultar o item "Dieta" abaixo.
• Probióticos: há um grande interesse no uso de probióticos para cães e gatos com diarreia crônica, embora pouco se saiba sobre a eficácia desses agentes. Os probióticos devem ser obrigatoriamente seguros, estáveis e eficazes. Com base nesses critérios, atualmente devem ser usados apenas os probióticos planejados para uso em cães e/ou gatos e produzidos por fabricantes importantes.
• A melhora pode levar alguns dias a várias semanas.

CUIDADO(S) DE ENFERMAGEM
• Geralmente nenhum.
• Cuidados de suporte para os pacientes com emaciação ou hipoalbuminemia.

ATIVIDADE
Sem restrição.

DIETA
• Dieta de alta digestibilidade.
• Foi demonstrado que a dieta contendo fruto-oligossacarídeos seja benéfica em cães com proliferação bacteriana do intestino delgado.

ORIENTAÇÃO AO PROPRIETÁRIO
• Alguns pacientes apresentam melhora clínica em dias.
• Certos animais necessitam de semanas de tratamento antes de demonstrarem melhora — tratar por 2-3 semanas antes de tirar conclusões sobre a eficácia da terapia.

• Quaisquer doenças concomitantes ou predisponentes (p. ex., enteropatia inflamatória, insuficiência pancreática exócrina, intolerância/alergia alimentar, neoplasia do trato alimentar e obstrução parcial) também precisam ser tratadas.
• Quase sempre é necessário tratamento contínuo ou repetido.

CONSIDERAÇÕES CIRÚRGICAS
Indicada apenas para algumas causas subjacentes de disbiose do intestino delgado (i. e., obstrução parcial, divertículo ou massa intestinal).

MEDICAÇÕES
MEDICAMENTO(S) DE ESCOLHA
• É preferível o uso de antibióticos de amplo espectro, administrados por via oral, eficazes contra bactérias tanto aeróbias como anaeróbias.
• Tilosina (25 mg/kg VO a cada 12 h por 6 semanas) constitui a principal escolha. Esse agente costuma ser usado sob a forma de pó, comercializado para uso em aves e porcos. É administrado no alimento. Pode ser utilizado a longo prazo, sendo muito seguro e barato. Além disso, não é usado em seres humanos e, portanto, tem pouco risco de promover o surgimento de espécies bacterianas resistentes indutoras de morbidade e mortalidade de pacientes humanos. Para cães de pequeno porte e gatos, o medicamento deve ser manipulado em cápsulas. Para cães de porte maior, a dose pode ser estimada, utilizando-se uma colher das de chá e administrando-se a medicação no alimento.
• Oxitetraciclina (20 mg/kg VO a cada 8 h por 6 semanas) é secretada na bile e sofre circulação entero-hepática. Contudo, a disponibilidade da oxitetraciclina para uso oral é limitada nos Estados Unidos ou na Europa. Não administrar juntamente com o alimento (o cálcio presente na dieta promove a quelação da oxitetraciclina e a torna ineficaz). Não deve ser substituída por tetraciclina ou doxiciclina.
• Metronidazol (10-20 mg/kg VO a cada 8 h por 6 semanas) costuma ser utilizado na clínica geral por causa de sua atividade contra bactérias anaeróbias. Também pode apresentar efeitos imunomoduladores. Entretanto, o metronidazol pode ter efeitos colaterais significativos. Como os cães com disbiose do intestino delgado podem ter deficiência de cobalamina, fica indicada a suplementação parenteral de vitamina B_{12} (cães, 250-1.500 µg dessa vitamina por injeção subcutânea, dependendo do porte do animal; o esquema posológico é tipicamente de 1 dose semanal por 6 semanas e, depois, 1 dose mensal; as concentrações séricas da cobalamina devem ser reavaliadas um mês depois da última dose).

PRECAUÇÕES
• A tetraciclina deve ser usada com cuidado em pacientes com hepatopatia significante.
• Evitar as oxitetraciclinas em pacientes muito jovens.
• Pode ocorrer nefropatia com doses elevadas das oxitetraciclinas.
• A oxitetraciclina pode provocar febre, dor abdominal, perda de pelo e depressão nos gatos.

MEDICAMENTO(S) ALTERNATIVO(S)
Em cães com insuficiência pancreática exócrina e disbiose do intestino delgado, a terapia concomitante para disbiose do intestino delgado só será indicada se a reposição enzimática isolada não resolver a diarreia e/ou induzir ao ganho de peso.

ACOMPANHAMENTO
MONITORIZAÇÃO DO PACIENTE
• Peso corporal e, em pacientes com hipoproteinemia, concentração sérica da albumina são os parâmetros mais importantes; a melhora sugere eficácia do tratamento.
• A diarreia também deve desaparecer.
• Se a diarreia persistir apesar do restabelecimento no peso corporal e/ou aumento na concentração sérica da albumina, ficará indicada a pesquisa em busca de enteropatia concomitante.

EVOLUÇÃO ESPERADA E PROGNÓSTICO
Disbiose do intestino delgado primária sem fatores complicadores (p. ex., enteropatia inflamatória e linfoma) — o prognóstico mediante tratamento adequado costuma ser bom.

DIVERSOS
DISTÚRBIOS ASSOCIADOS
• Há suspeitas de que a disbiose do intestino delgado seja uma causa de enteropatia inflamatória em alguns pacientes.
• Considerar a possibilidade de insuficiência pancreática exócrina concomitante.

GESTAÇÃO/FERTILIDADE/REPRODUÇÃO
Evitar a oxitetraciclina e o metronidazol, sobretudo no início da prenhez.

SINÔNIMO(S)
Proliferação bacteriana do intestino delgado, diarreia responsiva a antibióticos ou diarreia responsiva a tilosina podem ser usados como sinônimos por alguns autores.

VER TAMBÉM
• Diarreia Crônica — Cães.
• Diarreia Crônica — Gatos.
• Enteropatia Inflamatória.
• Insuficiência Pancreática Exócrina.
• Linfoma — Cães.
• Linfoma — Gatos.

ABREVIATURA(S)
• UFC = unidades formadoras de colônias.

RECURSOS DA INTERNET
www.vetmed.tamu.edu/gilab

Sugestões de Leitura
German AJ, Day MJ, Ruaux CG, Steiner JM, Williams DA. Comparison of direct and indirect tests for small intestinal bacterial overgrowth and antibiotic-responsive diarrhea in dogs. J Vet Intern Med 2003, 17(1):33-43.
Johnston KL. Small intestinal bacterial overgrowth. Vet Clin North Am Small Anim Pract 1999, 29(2):523-550.
Westermarck E, Frias R, Skrzypczak T. Effect of diet and tylosin on chronic diarrhea in Beagles. J Vet Intern Med 2005, 19:822-827.

Autores Jan S. Suchodolski e Jörg M. Steiner
Consultor Editorial Albert E. Jergens

Discinesia Ciliar Primária

CONSIDERAÇÕES GERAIS

REVISÃO
- Distúrbio congênito (autossômico recessivo) de disfunção ciliar, envolvendo o trato respiratório, as tubas auditivas, os ventrículos cerebrais, o canal espinal, os ovidutos, os ductos eferentes dos testículos e o flagelo espermático.
- O batimento ciliar é normalmente coordenado, mas tipicamente discinético ou ausente em cães acometidos.
- Hidrocefalia e/ou *situs inversus* [inversão de posição ou de localização; síndrome de Kartagener] podem ser achados concomitantes.
- Os cães com doença crônica do trato respiratório e *situs inversus* provavelmente apresentam discinesia ciliar primária, não justificando uma extensa avaliação diagnóstica.

IDENTIFICAÇÃO
- Geralmente acomete cães jovens (<8 semanas de vida), embora tais cães possam permanecer assintomáticos até uma idade mais avançada (1/2-10 anos).
- Relatada predominantemente em cães de raças puras.

SINAIS CLÍNICOS
Achados Anamnésicos
- Espirro crônico, secreção nasal, tosse, intolerância ao exercício e angústia respiratória. Apesar da drástica resposta inicial a antibióticos, a recidiva após o tratamento é interrompida.
- Histórico familiar — ninhadas grandes podem ter >1 cão acometido.
- Fêmeas férteis; machos caracteristicamente não.

Achados do Exame Físico
- Secreção nasal mucopurulenta bilateral.
- Tosse produtiva.
- Podem ocorrer taquipneia, dispneia e cianose.
- Aumento difuso de intensidade variável nos ruídos pulmonares.
- Sons cardíacos podem ser inaudíveis no caso de broncopneumonia grave ou mais altos no lado direito do tórax com *situs inversus*.

CAUSAS E FATORES DE RISCO
- Genéticos.
- Consanguinidade.

DIAGNÓSTICO

DIAGNÓSTICO DIFERENCIAL
- Doenças congênitas (p. ex., disfunção de neutrófilos e deficiência de imunoglobulina) ou adquiridas (p. ex., cinomose) que produzem rinossinusite e broncopneumonia crônicas.
- Pneumonia por aspiração recidivante.
- Pneumonia bacteriana crônica.
- Fístula broncoesofágica.
- Exposição crônica à fumaça de cigarro — pode retardar a depuração mucociliar.
- Infecção por *Mycoplasma* spp. ou *Bordetella* — pode causar defeitos ciliares adquiridos.

HEMOGRAMA/BIOQUÍMICA/URINÁLISE
- Leucocitose neutrofílica madura — desvio à esquerda e neutrófilos tóxicos em caso de broncopneumonia grave.
- Hiperglobulinemia — cães mais idosos.
- Policitemia — em caso de hipoxemia crônica.

OUTROS TESTES LABORATORIAIS
- Gasometria sanguínea pode revelar hipoxemia com normocapnia ou hipocapnia.
- Lavado broncoalveolar tipicamente recupera material mucoide a mucopurulento caracterizado ao exame citológico como exsudato purulento com uma ou mais espécies de bactérias isoladas na cultura. É recomendável a solicitação de cultura para pesquisa de *Mycoplasma*.

DIAGNÓSTICO POR IMAGEM
Radiografia
- Alterações compatíveis com broncopneumonia crônica.
- Imagem de *situs inversus*.
- Espessamento ou esclerose das bulas timpânicas.

Cintilografia Mucociliar
- Primeiramente, é necessário descartar infecções ou exposição crônica à fumaça de cigarro.
- Estudo de depuração do muco traqueal revela ausência de movimento do radiofármaco a partir da carina traqueal em pacientes acometidos.

MÉTODOS DIAGNÓSTICOS
Microscopia Eletrônica
- Lesões ultraestruturais nos cílios da mucosa nasal ou bronquial são identificadas em grande parte dos pacientes.
- Lesões específicas devem ser encontradas em uma alta porcentagem dos cílios; o mesmo defeito deve ser constatado nos cílios de múltiplas localizações ou dos animais acometidos na mesma ninhada.
- São comuns lesões ultraestruturais adquiridas envolvendo <20% dos cílios em caso de infecção crônica do trato respiratório.
- Foram descritos cães com discinesia ciliar primária, porém sem lesões ciliares ultraestruturais; nesse caso, há necessidade de análise *in vitro* da frequência e sincronia do batimento ciliar para o diagnóstico.

ACHADOS PATOLÓGICOS
Trato Respiratório Superior
- Rinite bacteriana crônica com exsudato mucoide a mucopurulento, além de inflamação da mucosa, hiperplasia da glândula mucosa e, ocasionalmente, hipoplasia dos ossos turbinados nasais, atresia dos seios frontais, sinusite frontal e rinólitos.

Trato Respiratório Inferior
- Material mucoide a mucopurulento dentro das vias aéreas em caso de bronquite, bronquiectasia, atelectasia e enfisema subpleural.

Diversos
- Hidrocefalia.
- *Situs inversus* das vísceras torácicas e/ou abdominais (*situs inversus totalis*).
- Impactação de uma ou de ambas as orelhas médias com material gelatinoso estéril.

TRATAMENTO
- Atividade física de rotina intensifica a depuração de muco pelo aumento da respiração e indução de tosse.
- Suplementação de oxigênio durante os episódios agudos de broncopneumonia grave.
- Terapia das vias aéreas com nebulização de salina e tapotagem são úteis para eliminação das secreções.

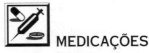

MEDICAÇÕES

MEDICAMENTO(S)
- Os antibióticos são selecionados com base nos testes de cultura e sensibilidade bacterianas; a duração varia com a gravidade da infecção.
- Antibioticoterapia contínua não é aconselhável em virtude da colonização por bactérias resistentes.

CONTRAINDICAÇÕES/INTERAÇÕES POSSÍVEIS
Os supressores da tosse aumentam o encarceramento das secreções e exacerbam a inflamação das vias aéreas.

Anestesia
- Os pacientes apresentam comprometimento da troca gasosa e, portanto, alto risco de complicações.
- Minimizar o quadro de depressão respiratória e o tempo de recuperação.

ACOMPANHAMENTO

COMPLICAÇÕES POSSÍVEIS
- Temperatura ambiente elevada pode produzir hipertermia e possível internação por causa da capacidade reduzida de perda de calor por evaporação pelos pulmões.
- Pneumotórax — cistos subpleurais, cistos bronquiectásicos, cistos intersticiais e bolhas enfisematosas podem se desenvolver a partir do encarceramento prolongado de ar e ruptura.
- Hipertensão da artéria pulmonar, *cor pulmonale* e insuficiência cardíaca direita podem resultar de hipoxemia crônica.
- Amiloidose reativa sistêmica secundária à broncopneumonia bacteriana persistente.

EVOLUÇÃO ESPERADA E PROGNÓSTICO
- A evolução clínica da doença e a longevidade dos pacientes são altamente variáveis.
- Antibioticoterapia adequada e fisioterapia pulmonar podem resultar em prolongamento da sobrevida.

DIVERSOS

VER TAMBÉM
Pneumonia Bacteriana.

Sugestões de Leitura
Daniel GB, Edwards DF, Harvey RC, Kabalka GW. Communicating hydrocephalus in dogs with congenital ciliary dysfunction. Dev Neurosci 1995, 17:230-235.
Edwards DF, Patton CS, Kennedy JR. Primary ciliary dyskinesia in the dog. Probl Vet Med 1992, 4:291-319.
Johnson LR. Diseases of small airways. In: Ettinger SJ, Feldman EC, eds., Textbook of Veterinary Internal Medicine, 6th ed. St. Louis: Elsevier, 2005, pp. 1233-1239.

Autor Ned F. Kuehn
Consultor Editorial Lynelle R. Johnson

Discopatia Intervertebral — Gatos

CONSIDERAÇÕES GERAIS

REVISÃO
- A extrusão ou protrusão de disco com consequente mielopatia é mais comum em cães; as discopatias de Hansen tanto Tipo I como Tipo II são relatadas em gatos.
- A discopatia Tipo I é secundária à metaplasia condroide e mineralização do núcleo pulposo.
- A discopatia tipo II é secundária à degeneração fibroide e protrusão do anel fibroso.

IDENTIFICAÇÃO
- Para todos os gatos relatados com mielopatia secundária à discopatia — a idade média é de 8,4 anos, enquanto a faixa etária, 1,5-17 anos.
- Em gatos com discopatia mineralizada Tipo I — a idade média é de 7,3 anos, enquanto a faixa etária, 2-13 anos.
- Há relatos de envolvimento de raças predominantemente domésticas, além de várias raças puras (Orientais). Também há relatos raros de acometimento de gato exótico de grande porte (tigre).
- Não há predisposição sexual.

SINAIS CLÍNICOS
- A maioria dos gatos sofre de discopatia toracolombar ou lombossacra: os sinais clínicos ficam confinados aos membros pélvicos. Pode ocorrer discopatia cervical; nesse caso, todos os quatro membros podem ser acometidos.
- Os sinais são frequentemente agudos, mas podem ser crônicos.
- Paresia/paralisia.
- Ataxia.
- Anormalidade da marcha, claudicação, relutância em saltar.
- Dor na coluna vertebral e nas costas.
- Incontinência urinária/fecal.
- Anormalidades de postura ou tônus da cauda.
- Perda da percepção à dor (em caso de lesão grave).
- Hipoventilação (na presença de lesão cervical grave).

CAUSAS E FATORES DE RISCO
- Grande parte dos gatos relatados tinha degeneração de disco Tipo I, com extrusão de núcleo pulposo mineralizado em direção ao canal vertebral, resultando em traumatismo e compressão da medula espinal.
- Ao contrário dos cães, cujas raças condrodistróficas (p. ex., Dachshunds) são predispostas à discopatia Tipo I e subsequente extrusão, aparentemente não há nenhum fator de risco óbvio nos gatos.
- Quase todos os gatos relatados apresentavam protrusões ou extrusões de disco clinicamente significativas entre T11 e S1. Semelhantemente aos cães, a presença do ligamento intercapital de T1-T10 pode tornar as protrusões de disco naquela região menos prováveis.

DIAGNÓSTICO

DIAGNÓSTICO DIFERENCIAL
Traumatismo
- Vascular — neuromiopatia isquêmica ("trombo em sela"), isquemia para a medula espinal.
- Neoplasia, especialmente linfoma.
- Infecciosa — PIF, *Cryptococcus*, etc.

HEMOGRAMA/BIOQUÍMICA/URINÁLISE
Geralmente normais.

OUTROS TESTES LABORATORIAIS
N/D.

DIAGNÓSTICO POR IMAGEM
- Radiografias da coluna vertebral — espaço(s) do disco estreitado(s), discos mineralizados *in situ*, material de disco mineralizado dentro do canal vertebral ou sobrejacente aos forames intervertebrais.
- Mielografia — lesão compressiva extradural ao nível do disco acometido.
- TC — compressão extradural; a mineralização do material compressivo pode ser evidenciada.
- RM — hiperintensidade T2 dentro da medula espinal lesionada; o material de disco mineralizado aparece hipointenso em todas as sequências de imagens; a compressão extradural pode estar evidente.

MÉTODOS DIAGNÓSTICOS
- Líquido cerebrospinal — não exibe nada digno de nota ou está contaminado com sangue em grande parte dos gatos; foi observada pleocitose neutrofílica em três gatos.
- Histopatologia de material removido por intervenção cirúrgica — compatível com material de disco degenerativo (Tipo I ou II).

TRATAMENTO

- A descompressão cirúrgica da medula espinal provavelmente é o tratamento mais eficaz para discopatia compressiva.
- Os riscos da cirurgia de coluna vertebral devem ser abordados com o proprietário — hemorragia, lesão iatrogênica da medula espinal, instabilidade.
- As cirurgias de hemilaminectomia, fenda ventral, corpectomia lateral, e laminectomia dorsal lombossacra são descritas no gato.
- No pós-operatório, o fornecimento de cuidados satisfatórios para o paciente em decúbito, o controle da dor, o manejo da bexiga urinária em gatos incontinentes (fixação de sonda urinária de demora ou aplicação de compressão manual) e o uso de fisioterapia adequada ajudam na recuperação neurológica.
- A fenestração de discos mineralizados adjacentes deve ser considerada para evitar recorrência.
- O tratamento médico (repouso em gaiola, controle da dor) pode ser considerado em gatos com deambulação; naqueles sem deambulação e com sinais neurológicos progressivos, é recomendável a aplicação de métodos diagnósticos e terapêuticos mais rigorosos.

MEDICAÇÕES

MEDICAMENTO(S)
- Controle da dor, de preferência opiáceos, se o gato tolerá-los.
- A eficácia de corticosteroides em discopatia felina não foi avaliada.

CONTRAINDICAÇÕES/INTERAÇÕES POSSÍVEIS
N/D.

ACOMPANHAMENTO

- Repetir os exames neurológicos (por, no mínimo, 1-2 vezes ao dia) durante a internação para monitorizar os pacientes pós-operatórios submetidos a tratamento médico quanto à melhora ou queda no estado neurológico.
- Providenciar repouso rigoroso em gaiola aos pacientes pós-operatórios submetidos a tratamento médico por 4-6 semanas e, em seguida, aumentar gradativamente a atividade física e a fisioterapia, conforme a necessidade.
- Não se sabe se a restrição física prolongada seja benéfica.
- Como a discopatia é rara em gatos, a possível taxa de recorrência é desconhecida; entretanto, em um único gato que se recuperou bem após hemilaminectomia, a extrusão de outro disco mineralizado provocou paraplegia e exigiu a realização de nova cirurgia (dados não publicados).
- Alguns gatos exibiram retenção urinária persistente apesar da boa recuperação da deambulação, exigindo a compressão vesical de rotina pelo proprietário.
- A maioria dos gatos tratados por meio cirúrgico (até mesmo dois deles sem percepção de dor) apresentou resultados bons a excelentes.
- Pouquíssimos gatos foram submetidos a tratamento médico a longo prazo e, por essa razão, o prognóstico com esse tipo de tratamento não é conhecido.

DIVERSOS

ABREVIATURAS
- PIF = peritonite infecciosa felina.
- RM = ressonância magnética.
- TC = tomografia computadorizada.

Sugestões de Leitura
Rayward RM. Feline intervertebral disc disease: A review of the literature. Vet Comp Orthop Traumatol 2002, 15:137–144.

Autor Marguerite Knipe
Consultor Editorial Joane M. Parent

Discopatia Intervertebral Cervical

CONSIDERAÇÕES GERAIS

DEFINIÇÃO
Degeneração dos discos intervertebrais cervicais que causa protrusão ou extrusão do material do disco em direção ao canal espinal. O material do disco que sofreu protrusão ou extrusão provoca compressão da medula espinal (mielopatia) e/ou da raiz nervosa (radiculopatia).

FISIOPATOLOGIA
• Classificada como herniação aguda de disco (Hansen tipo I) ou protrusão crônica de disco (Hansen tipo II).
• A degeneração Hansen tipo I caracteriza-se por degeneração condroide do núcleo pulposo e ruptura aguda do anel fibroso com extrusão do núcleo pulposo para dentro do canal espinal.
• A degeneração Hansen tipo II caracteriza-se por degeneração fibrinoide do núcleo pulposo. Isso induz ao abaulamento e à protrusão do anel fibroso dorsal para dentro do canal vertebral.
• A invasão no canal espinal pode provocar compressão focal da medula espinal (mielopatia) e/ou de alguma raiz nervosa (radiculopatia).
• Isquemia e desmielinização são possíveis consequências da compressão da medula espinal.
• A extrusão ou protrusão dorsal de disco é mais comum do que a extrusão ou protrusão lateral de disco.
• Raramente, ocorre extrusão de disco secundária a traumatismo.
• A fusão das vértebras cervicais pode alterar a biomecânica espinal local e, portanto, predispõe o segmento à protrusão (efeito dominó).

SISTEMA(S) ACOMETIDO(S)
Sistema nervoso — mielopatia ou radiculopatia focais.

GENÉTICA
• Desconhecida. • A extrusão de disco Hansen tipo I é mais comum em raças condrodistrofoides (p. ex., Dachshund, Beagle e Cocker spaniel). • A extrusão de disco Hansen tipo II é mais comum em cães de grande porte (p. ex., Doberman pinscher).

INCIDÊNCIA/PREVALÊNCIA
• 15% das discopatias caninas são cervicais. • Nas raças Dachshund, Beagle e Poodle, ocorrem 80% das extrusões de disco. • A incidência global de discopatia em cães é de ± 2%, enquanto a incidência em Dachshund é de ± 25%. • O ponto mais comum da extrusão de disco cervical encontra-se em C3-C4.

IDENTIFICAÇÃO

Espécies
Cães.

Raça(s) Predominante(s)
• Hansen tipo I — Dachshund, Poodle, Beagle, Cocker spaniel.
• Hansen tipo II — Doberman pinscher.

Idade Média e Faixa Etária
• Hansen tipo I — 3-6 anos de idade.
• Hansen tipo II — 8-10 anos de idade.

Sexo Predominante
• Nenhum identificado.

SINAIS CLÍNICOS
A gravidade dos sinais clínicos depende de vários fatores, incluindo a velocidade e o volume da extrusão ou da protrusão de disco, o diâmetro da medula espinal em relação ao diâmetro do canal vertebral e a velocidade da extrusão do material do disco.

Achados Anamnésicos
• Dor cervical (cervicalgia).
• Marcha rígida e descompassada, com relutância ao movimento da cabeça e do pescoço.
• Postura com a cabeça abaixada e espasmos musculares da cabeça, do pescoço e do ombro.
• Relatos sugerem que 10% dos pacientes acometidos são tetraplégicos. Claudicação dos membros torácicos (sinal de raiz ou radiculopatia).

Achados do Exame Físico
• Dor cervical — eliciada à flexão e extensão do pescoço ou rotação do mesmo de um lado para outro. A dor também pode ser eliciada pela palpação profunda dos músculos cervicais.
• Atrofia muscular sobre a escápula.
• Reflexo postural anormal do carrinho de mão.
• Com frequência, observam-se apenas sinais neurológicos mínimos, desde que o amplo canal espinal esteja aliviando o quadro.
• A claudicação dos membros torácicos (curvados ou mantidos em flexão parcial) pode ser o resultado do sinal de raiz/radiculopatia, o que ajuda a localizar a lesão em C4-C7.
• Pode haver paresia com déficits de reação postural, envolvendo tanto os membros torácicos como os pélvicos. Os déficits também podem ser de natureza ipsolateral.
• A paresia do membro pélvico pode ser mais grave que a paresia do membro torácico.
• Os reflexos espinais do membro pélvico podem estar normais ou exagerados.
• Os reflexos espinais do membro torácico podem estar normais a exagerados quando as lesões estão localizadas nos segmentos C1-C6 da medula espinal e podem estar normais a diminuídos quando o segmento C6-T2 da medula espinal estiver acometido.
• A gravidade dos sinais clínicos não se correlaciona com o grau de compressão.
• A função vesical pode ter a natureza de lesão no neurônio motor superior ou permanecer normal.

CAUSAS
• Hansen tipo I — degeneração condroide precoce do disco intervertebral cervical e subsequente mineralização do disco.
• Hansen tipo II — degeneração fibroide gradual do disco intervertebral cervical.

FATORES DE RISCO
Obesidade e eventos traumáticos repetidos naquelas raças predispostas à discopatia intervertebral.

DIAGNÓSTICO

DIAGNÓSTICO DIFERENCIAL
• Discopatia Hansen tipo I. • Discopatia Hansen tipo II. • Neoplasia. • Instabilidade atlantoaxial. • Fratura/luxação espinal. • Discospondilite. • Meningite. • Embolia fibrocartilaginosa. • Instabilidade vertebral cervical. • Endócrina — hipotireoidismo. • Espondilomielopatia. • Osteoartrite. • Doenças do armazenamento de glicogênio.

HEMOGRAMA/BIOQUÍMICA/URINÁLISE
Devem ser realizados em animais idosos antes de anestesia geral e cirurgia.

OUTROS TESTES LABORATORIAIS
• Análise do LCS — coletado sob anestesia geral antes do exame de mielografia, por meio de punção na cisterna e não da punção lombar.
• O LCS pode revelar aumento leve a moderado nos níveis de proteína e pleocitose leve a moderada.
• A herniação aguda de disco costuma exibir mais alterações do LCS do que a herniação crônica.
• EMG poderá ser útil se a compressão causou denervação.

DIAGNÓSTICO POR IMAGEM

Radiografia da Coluna Cervical
• Radiografias simples bem posicionadas da coluna cervical em projeções lateral e ventrodorsal obtidas sob anestesia sempre estão indicadas.
• Os achados clássicos incluem espaço de disco intervertebral estreitado ou encunhamento do espaço do disco, colapso do espaço das facetas articulares, material calcificado do disco no forame intervertebral ou no canal espinal.
• Pode revelar indícios de discospondilite, fratura/luxação, instabilidade atlantoaxial ou vértebras líticas sugestivas de tumor ósseo.

Mielografia
• As radiografias simples podem induzir a erros e equívocos; por essa razão, a mielografia está indicada em 90 a 95% dos pacientes.
• Pode-se optar pela injeção do contraste na cisterna ou na coluna lombar (entre L5 e L6 ou L4 e L5), embora se prefira a injeção lombar.
• Radiografias laterais — revelam desvio dorsal da coluna ventral do contraste sobre o espaço do disco intervertebral, compatível com massa extradural.
• A herniação do disco entre os forames ou dorsolateral é mais bem observada nas radiografias cervicais oblíquas, com toda a coluna cervical posicionada em um ângulo de 45 a 60° em relação à mesa.
• Os casos com tumefação da medula espinal podem causar bloqueio do material de contraste e impedir seu fluxo além da obstrução, limitando o valor diagnóstico da imagem.

Técnicas Avançadas de Diagnóstico por Imagem
• As técnicas de RM e TC também são utilizadas para a localização de protrusão de disco.
• Ambas são úteis para o diagnóstico de extrusões de disco entre os forames ou lateral nos casos em que o exame radiográfico de rotina se mostra normal.
• A RM é o melhor método disponível para a identificação precoce da degeneração de disco em cães. A compressão radicular cervical é identificada por obliteração da gordura epidural no forame neural, deslocamento das raízes nervosas, degeneração ou hipertrofia das facetas articulares e material de disco dentro do forame neural.
• A TC pode fornecer imagens diagnósticas quando houver obstrução do fluxo do meio de contraste.

MÉTODOS DIAGNÓSTICOS
Análise do LCS.

ACHADOS PATOLÓGICOS
Achados Macroscópicos
• Discopatia Hansen tipo I — o material branco do disco em extrusão tem consistência granular e, em geral, é facilmente removido do canal espinal.
• Discopatia Hansen tipo II — protrusão firme do anel fibroso dorsal que se encontra aderido ao

Discopatia Intervertebral Cervical

assoalho do canal espinal e à dura-máter da medula espinal.
• Medula espinal — na extrusão aguda de disco, a medula espinal pode aparecer contusa e tumefata; já na protrusão crônica de disco, a medula espinal pode aparecer atrofiada, mas quase sempre está com aparência normal.

ACHADOS HISTOPATOLÓGICOS
• Discopatia Hansen tipo I — o disco está mais cartilaginoso e sofre calcificação distrófica.
• Discopatia Hansen tipo II — o núcleo não sofre metaplasia cartilaginosa.
• Medula espinal — dependente da gravidade da doença e do tipo de discopatia. Hansen tipo II — observam-se desmielinização e gliose. Hansen tipo I — podem-se observar hemorragia e edema; em casos de doença grave, pode-se observar mielomalacia.

TRATAMENTO

CUIDADO(S) DE SAÚDE ADEQUADO(S)
• Tratamento conservativo — depende da anamnese do paciente e do estado neurológico apresentado. Em geral, o tratamento conservativo fica indicado em casos de início gradual dos sinais clínicos ou em sinais limitados à hiperpatia ou leve ataxia. • Tratamento cirúrgico — indicado em pacientes com episódios repetidos de dor cervical, outros com dor cervical intensa e déficits neurológicos graves ou naqueles irresponsivos ao tratamento conservativo.

CUIDADO(S) DE ENFERMAGEM
• Manejo — proceder à manipulação mínima da coluna cervical e evitar a venopunção jugular.
• Micção — monitorizar os pacientes quanto ao esvaziamento completo da bexiga urinária; os pacientes talvez necessitem de compressão manual ou cateterização intermitente da bexiga urinária. Em alguns casos, pode-se inserir um cateter urinário de demora. A urinálise, incluindo a cultura e o antibiograma, deve ser realizada após a remoção do cateter de demora, para verificar se o paciente não adquiriu cistite bacteriana nosocomial (hospitalar). Estudos recentes sugerem a realização de urocultura e antibiograma em todos os cães submetidos à cirurgia de descompressão espinal.
• Defecação — os pacientes podem necessitar de enemas e receber dieta pobre em resíduos para reduzir o volume das fezes.
• Pacientes em decúbito — devem ser mantidos em colchão bem almofadado e mudados de posição a cada 4 horas. Os animais devem ser examinados quanto à presença de úlceras de decúbito sobre as proeminências ósseas.
• Fisioterapia — os métodos de hidroterapia e amplitude passiva de movimento de todas as articulações devem ser realizados o mais frequentemente possível para evitar atrofia muscular grave.

ATIVIDADE
• Quando os pacientes são levados para passear, é recomendável o uso do peitoral no lugar da coleira cervical; evitar corridas e saltos.
• Os pacientes submetidos ao tratamento conservativo devem ficar estritamente confinados ao repouso em gaiola por 3-4 semanas.
• Após a cirurgia, os pacientes deverão ser confinados e sair para passear na coleira por 4-6 semanas e, só depois disso, ser introduzidos lentamente à atividade plena.

DIETA
Para os pacientes obesos, deve-se instituir dieta de redução do peso.

ORIENTAÇÃO AO PROPRIETÁRIO
• Para o tratamento conservativo, deve-se enfatizar o confinamento estrito em gaiola.
• Perda de peso em animal com obesidade.

CONSIDERAÇÕES CIRÚRGICAS
• Quando indicada, o objetivo da cirurgia é remover o material de disco do canal espinal e, portanto, descomprimir a medula espinal e/ou a raiz nervosa.
• A cirurgia, em geral, confere alívio imediato da dor e consequente função motora normal.
• Uma fenda cervical ventral é a abordagem cirúrgica mais comum para a remoção do material de disco do canal espinal.
• O material de disco que sofreu extrusão dorsolateral para dentro do forame intervertebral é removido por abordagem lateral à coluna cervical ou por meio de laminectomia dorsal.
• O procedimento isolado de fenestração para os cães com dor cervical não costuma solucionar os sinais clínicos e, portanto, não é mais recomendado.

MEDICAÇÕES

MEDICAMENTO(S)
• Glicocorticoterapia em baixas doses pode ser benéfica a fim de reduzir a dor em animais submetidos ao tratamento conservativo.
• Os glicocorticoides administrados a animais sem confinamento simultâneo estrito em gaiola podem exacerbar a extrusão de disco pelo estímulo ao exercício.
• Succinato sódico de metilprednisolona na dose de 30 mg/kg IV nas primeiras 8 h do início dos sinais clínicos pode ser administrado nos casos agudos. Esse tratamento pode ser acompanhado por uma dose de 15 mg/kg 2 h após a dosagem inicial e, em seguida, a cada 6 h por 24 h. Não há provas de que isso exerça algum efeito positivo.
• Se a terapia com esteroides em altas doses for instituída, será recomendável a administração de protetores gastrintestinais. Os medicamentos comumente utilizados são cimetidina, ranitidina, misoprostol e sucralfato.
• Os AINEs podem ser utilizados apenas se o animal não estiver sendo submetido a glicocorticoides ou não recebeu estes medicamentos há pouco tempo.
• Relaxantes musculares podem ser empregados, mas são de valor limitado quando utilizados isoladamente.

CONTRAINDICAÇÕES
Jamais use os glicocorticoides simultaneamente com os AINEs — isso pode provocar irritação gastrintestinal grave e possivelmente perfuração intestinal.

PRECAUÇÕES
Ao se utilizar os corticosteroides em altas doses para discopatia cervical, os pacientes deverão ser submetidos a protetores gástricos para evitar os efeitos colaterais gastrintestinais associados aos corticosteroides. As doses elevadas de glicocorticoides deverão ser usadas apenas em casos agudos se administradas nas primeiras 8 horas da lesão; o valor desses agentes não foi determinado.

INTERAÇÕES POSSÍVEIS
Os AINEs combinados com os glicocorticoides podem provocar perfuração gastrintestinal ou sangramento gastrintestinal grave — ambas as situações levam ao óbito.

ACOMPANHAMENTO

MONITORIZAÇÃO DO PACIENTE
• Devem ser realizadas avaliações semanais até a resolução dos sinais clínicos.
• Todos os pacientes devem ser colocados em coleiras peitorais, evitando-se as do tipo cervical.

PREVENÇÃO
• Inerente a raças específicas.
• A manutenção dos pacientes em um peso ideal pode ajudar.

COMPLICAÇÕES POSSÍVEIS
• As complicações são raras. • Dor cervical contínua. • Deterioração da função motora.
• Subluxação/luxação dos corpos vertebrais.

EVOLUÇÃO ESPERADA E PROGNÓSTICO
• O prognóstico de pacientes submetidos ao tratamento cirúrgico ou conservativo depende dos sinais neurológicos no momento da apresentação.
• O prognóstico, em geral, é favorável para a maior parte dos pacientes.
• A maioria dos pacientes tratados de forma conservativa apresenta recidiva da doença e pode necessitar da intervenção cirúrgica.
• Foi relatada uma taxa de recuperação funcional de 56% nos pacientes com perda de dor profunda que foram submetidos à descompressão cirúrgica bem-sucedida dentro de 12 h do início dos sinais clínicos. Se a cirurgia era adiada por 48 h ou mais, a recuperação caia para menos de 5%.

DIVERSOS

DISTÚRBIOS ASSOCIADOS
Animais predispostos à discopatia cervical também pertencem às mesmas raças predispostas à discopatia toracolombar.

VER TAMBÉM
Discopatia Intervertebral Toracolombar.

ABREVIATURA(S)
• AINE = anti-inflamatório não esteroide.
• EMG = eletromiografia.
• LCS = líquido cerebrospinal.
• RM = ressonância magnética.
• TC = tomografia computadorizada.

Sugestões de Leitura
Toombs JP, Wolf JD. Cervical intervertebral disc disease. In: Textbook of Small Animal Surgery, 3rd ed. Philadelphia: Saunders, 2003, pp. 1196-1201.

Autor Otto I. Lanz
Consultor Editorial Peter K. Shires

Discopatia Intervertebral Toracolombar

CONSIDERAÇÕES GERAIS

DEFINIÇÃO
Alterações degenerativas dentro dos discos intervertebrais caracterizadas por perda de água, necrose celular e calcificação. As propriedades biomecânicas do disco se deterioram, resultando em extrusão ou protrusão do material do disco.

FISIOPATOLOGIA
- A deterioração acelerada dos discos nas raças condrodistróficas recebe o nome de "degeneração condroide".
- Teoria recente relaciona a apoptose induzida por traumatismo como o evento desencadeante na degeneração.
- Hansen tipo I diz respeito à extrusão aguda do núcleo pulposo através do anel fibroso em direção ao canal vertebral; ocorre tipicamente em raças pequenas condrodistróficas, embora também possa ocorrer nos cães maiores não condrodistróficas.
- Lesões Hansen tipo II envolvem protrusão gradual (abaulamento) das fibras anulares dorsais para dentro do canal vertebral; isso é associado à degeneração fibroide do disco.
- A extrusão aguda de disco resulta em lesão direta da medula espinal pelo material do disco e compressão da medula espinal pela massa do disco. A massa do disco (compressão da medula espinal) resulta em isquemia e alterações medulares que variam desde desmielinização leve até necrose de ambas as substâncias, cinzenta e branca; os eventos celulares incluem liberação de substâncias vasoativas, aumento do cálcio intracelular e formação aumentada de radicais livres e peróxidos lipídicos.
- A dor é atribuída à irritação da dura-máter, impingidela da raiz nervosa ou, possivelmente, tem origem discogênica (receptores anulares de dor).
- A herniação de disco é rara entre T3 e T10 em função da presença do ligamento intercapital.

GENÉTICA
Raças condrodistróficas (p. ex., Dachshund, Shih tzu e Pequinês) são predispostas à discopatia Hansen tipo I; raças maiores são mais comumente acometidas por discopatia Hansen tipo II.

INCIDÊNCIA/PREVALÊNCIA
- Disfunção neurológica mais comum em pequenos animais; acomete 2% da população canina.
- Raramente ocorre em gatos.
- A discopatia toracolombar compreende 85% de todas as hérnias de disco.

IDENTIFICAÇÃO
Espécies
Cães e, ocasionalmente, gatos.

Raça(s) Predominante(s)
- Tipo I — Dachshund; Shih tzu, Lhasa apso; Pequinês, Cocker spaniel, Welsh corgi; Poodle miniatura e toy.
- Tipo II — raças maiores, embora possa ocorrer em qualquer raça.

Idade Média e Faixa Etária
- Tipo I — 3 a 6 anos de idade.
- Tipo II — 8-10 anos de idade; gatos, idade média de 10 anos.

SINAIS CLÍNICOS
Comentários Gerais
- Os sinais dependem do tipo de hérnia, da velocidade de contato do disco com a medula espinal, da quantidade e duração da compressão da medula, da localização (neurônio motor superior ou neurônio motor inferior) e da relação entre o diâmetro do canal espinal/medula espinal (cervical *versus* toracolombar).

Achados Anamnésicos
- O início pode ser superagudo ou agudo nos cães condrodistrofoides (doença tipo I) e pode ocorrer durante atividade vigorosa.
- Raças maiores ou cães menores com doença tipo II apresentam início mais insidioso e tendem a piorar com o tempo.

Achados do Exame Físico
- Variam consideravelmente, dependendo do tipo de hérnia e da localização anatômica da lesão.
- Dor toracolombar comum nos cães; relutantes a deambular e postura arqueada; a palpação cuidadosa dos processos espinhosos e da musculatura epaxial produz dor localizada distinta; com frequência, algum grau de paraparesia, com propriocepção diminuída ou ausente ou aptidão motora reduzida nos membros posteriores.
- Os reflexos espinais nos membros posteriores costumam estar exagerados (hiper) quando a lesão se encontra entre T3 e L3; os reflexos estão diminuídos (hipo) quando a lesão é caudal à L3.
- Nos cães, 75% das herniações toracolombares ocorrem entre T11 e L3; aparentemente mais caudal nos gatos (L4-L5).
- A percepção da dor superficial e profunda pode estar diminuída ou ausente nos membros posteriores; a presença da sensação de dor profunda é o único fator prognóstico mais confiável em termos de retorno à função aceitável; a percepção da dor deve ser de natureza cerebral e não confundida com o reflexo de retirada (reflexo espinal local). Nos animais com percepção de dor profunda diminuída, os sinais de midríase ou taquicardia podem ser úteis para confirmar a presença de dor profunda.
- A função do membro anterior permanece normal; ocasionalmente, os fenômenos de Schiff-Sherrington podem provocar aumento do tônus muscular nos membros anteriores.
- Incontinência ou retenção urinárias são comuns quando a lesão acomete a função motora.
- A dor é menos óbvia nos gatos; o local da herniação quase sempre é lombar.

CAUSAS
- Degeneração condroide ou fibroide dos discos intervertebrais toracolombares.
- Há relatos de que 15% dos animais com fraturas espinais tenham extrusões de disco, além da fratura/luxação.

FATORES DE RISCO
A discopatia tipo I acomete raças condrodistróficas com maior frequência.

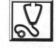

DIAGNÓSTICO

DIAGNÓSTICO DIFERENCIAL
- Tipo I — fratura/luxação induzidas por traumatismo, neoplasia, discospondilite, embolia fibrocartilaginosa; diferenciados por meio do histórico, de radiografia simples e da mielografia.
- Tipo II — mielopatia degenerativa, neoplasia, discospondilite, doença ortopédica; diferenciados por meio do histórico, de radiografia e do exame ortopédico/neurológico minucioso.

HEMOGRAMA/BIOQUÍMICA/URINÁLISE
- Elevação das enzimas hepáticas é comum se o paciente recebeu corticosteroides para dor ou doença neurológica.
- Retenção/incontinência urinárias aumenta o risco de infecção do trato urinário caracterizada por leucócitos, proteína e bacteriúria na urinálise.

OUTROS TESTES LABORATORIAIS
A análise do LCS é realizada rotineiramente em conjunto com a mielografia e se houver altos índices de suspeita de algum outro processo mórbido; pode estar normal, porém mais tipicamente revela aumento leve a moderado na proteína com ou sem pleocitose.

DIAGNÓSTICO POR IMAGEM
- Radiografia da coluna toracolombar.
- Radiografias simples descartam alguns outros processos mórbidos.
- Radiografias diagnósticas obtidas sob anestesia geral podem revelar o espaço do disco estreitado ou em cunha, espaço da faceta articular em colapso e forame intervertebral pequeno, com densidade aumentada ou mineralizada dentro do canal espinal.
- A precisão e a sensibilidade das radiografias simples para determinar o local específico da herniação de disco são baixas.

MÉTODOS DIAGNÓSTICOS
- Mielografia realizada com ioexol é recomendada para todos os pacientes quando houver indicação de cirurgia; o contraste costuma ser aplicado em L5-L6; em geral, esse exame revela compressão da medula espinal por lesão expansiva extradural (tipo massa) adjacente ao disco acometido; a tumefação da medula espinal pode ser evidenciada por adelgaçamento das colunas de contraste sobre diversos espaços intervertebrais.
- A lateralização é mais compatível quando determinada pelas projeções oblíqua e dorsoventral da mielografia.
- TC, RM ou mielografia repetida podem estar indicadas quando os resultados não forem definitivos. A presença de lesão hiperintensa da medula espinal nas imagens ponderadas em T2 tão extensa quanto o corpo da L2 em cães negativos para dor profunda está associada a um prognóstico pior.
- Análise do LCS.

ACHADOS PATOLÓGICOS
Macroscópicos
- Material do disco em extrusão (doença tipo I) — consistência de "pasta dental" branca a amarelada; quando crônico, pode estar endurecido ou aderido a estruturas circunjacentes.
- Material do disco em protrusão (doença tipo II) — consistência geralmente firme e branco-acinzentado, podendo estar aderido às estruturas ao redor.
- A medula espinal pode parecer normal ou estar tumefata e descorada na doença grave aguda.

Histopatológicos
- Discos degenerados apresentam quantidades reduzidas de proteoglicanos, glicosaminoglicanos e água; os discos podem se tornar mineralizados ou cartilaginosos.

DISCOPATIA INTERVERTEBRAL TORACOLOMBAR

- A lesão da medula espinal depende do tipo e da gravidade da extrusão ou da protrusão do disco; doença grave aguda pode causar hemorragia, edema, necrose tecidual; na doença crônica, observa-se desmielinização da substância branca e, em alguns casos, da substância cinzenta.

TRATAMENTO

CUIDADO(S) DE SAÚDE ADEQUADO(S)
- As diretrizes de tratamento são formuladas com base na classificação da condição clínica:
  - Classe 1 — apenas dor nas costas (dorsalgia).
  - Classe 2 — dor nas costas, ataxia, leve paraparesia, boa habilidade motora.
  - Classe 3 — déficits proprioceptivos, habilidade motora comprometida, porém ainda presente.
  - Classe 4 — paraparesia completa (sem habilidade motora), com percepção de dor profunda presente.
  - Classe 5 — paraparesia completa, dor profunda ausente.
- Pacientes da classe 1 são submetidos a tratamento clínico a menos que a dor persista.
- Pacientes da classe 2 são tratados por meio clínico no início com exame neurológico seriado e, depois, com cirurgia se o paciente permanecer estático ou se a condição piorar.
- Classes 3 e 4, tratamento cirúrgico.
- Classe 5, tratamento cirúrgico se estiver dentro das primeiras 12-48 h da ocorrência.
- Exame neurológico seriado é importante para todos os animais acometidos.

CUIDADO(S) DE ENFERMAGEM
- Confinamento restrito absoluto por 2-4 semanas.
- Minimizar a manipulação espinal e sustentar a coluna ao manipular o paciente.
- Garantir a capacidade de micção ou considerar a compressão vesical manual, a cateterização intermitente ou o cateter urinário de demora para os pacientes das classes 3-5.
- Os pacientes em decúbito devem ser mantidos limpos e colocados sobre cama almofadada em gaiolas elevadas e mudados frequentemente de posição para evitar a formação de úlceras de decúbito.
- Talvez haja necessidade de esvaziamento manual do intestino ou aplicação de enemas para promover a defecação.
- Fisioterapia com manipulação passiva dos membros posteriores iniciada logo e seguida por terapia mais intensa (hidroterapia) para os animais com déficits neurológicos.
- Carrinhos ortopédicos são úteis em muitos pacientes para promover o retorno à função; a tolerância do paciente é um fator limitante.

ATIVIDADE
- A restrição do movimento constitui a parte mais importante do tratamento clínico.
- Repouso em gaiola no hospital ou repouso forçado em gaiola como pacientes de ambulatório por 2-4 semanas para aqueles da classe 1 ou animais no pós-operatório.

DIETA
Redução de peso se o paciente estiver obeso.

ORIENTAÇÃO AO PROPRIETÁRIO
- Certo grau de restrição da atividade pode ser um componente importante pelo resto da vida do animal desde que ele tenha discopatia.

- A maior parte dos animais das classes 1-4 apresenta prognóstico bom a excelente em termos de retorno à função, isto é, deambulação com continência intestinal e vesical; os pacientes da classe 5 têm prognóstico pior, mas ainda há esperança; as porcentagens variam, mas até aproximadamente 50% podem recuperar a dor profunda e alguma função.

CONSIDERAÇÕES CIRÚRGICAS
- Fortemente indicada para os animais das classes 3 e 4, bem como dentro das primeiras 12-48 h para os cães da classe 5; igualmente indicada para cães das classes 1 e 2 que se encontrem estáticos ou piorando.
- O principal objetivo cirúrgico é aliviar a compressão da medula espinal pela remoção da massa do disco via hemilaminectomia, laminectomia dorsal ou pediculectomia; embora seja rara a indicação do procedimento isolado de fenestração do disco, esse tipo de intervenção é altamente recomendado como uma terapia adjuvante à descompressão no local primário.
- A recidiva dos sinais clínicos nos animais no período pós-operatório imediato pode ser atribuída à extrusão adicional do disco a partir do local original se não fenestrado. A recidiva mais tardia dos sinais clínicos após a recuperação costuma ser decorrente de protrusão/extrusão nas áreas adjacentes.
- Ainda existem controvérsias cirúrgicas sobre os resultados da fenestração profilática do disco em múltiplos locais realizada durante a cirurgia descompressiva, bem como sobre o prazo e o prognóstico em termos de retorno à função após a cirurgia nos pacientes negativos à dor profunda.

MEDICAÇÕES

MEDICAMENTO(S) DE ESCOLHA
- Succinato sódico de metilprednisolona — usado se o animal apresentar ausência de dor profunda de menos de 12 h de duração e se nenhum outro esteroide foi administrado; aplicado sob a forma de bólus IV de 30 mg/kg. Alguns clínicos recomendam a administração repetida de 15 mg/kg em intervalos de 4 h, sem exceder 4 doses adicionais. O efeito sobre o retorno da sensação de dor não é comprovado.
- AINEs ou narcóticos podem ser mais utilizados como analgésicos nos casos da classe 1.
- Analgésicos narcóticos podem ser necessários no pós-operatório; hidromorfona (0,05-0,2 mg/kg IV ou IM, SC a cada 4 h).
- Metocarbamol (25-45 mg/kg a cada 8 h) pode ser útil nos casos em que o espasmo muscular contribui para a dor; mais aplicável na discopatia cervical.
- Betanecol (5-15 mg/cão VO) e fenoxibenzamina (0,25 mg/kg VO a cada 8-12 h) ou prazosina (1 mg/15 kg VO a cada 8-12 h) são variavelmente úteis no tratamento da disfunção vesical associada à lesão da medula espinal.

PRECAUÇÕES
- O uso dos glicocorticoides sem o confinamento em gaiola pode diminuir a dor, estimulando com isso a atividade excessiva e levando à herniação adicional do disco e deterioração da condição clínica.
- Altas doses de glicocorticoides como a dexametasona, especialmente em combinação com o tratamento cirúrgico, podem resultar em hemorragia gastrintestinal extensa e perfuração intestinal; menos comum com outros glicocorticoides.

MEDICAMENTO(S) E TRATAMENTO(S) ALTERNATIVO(S)
- A acupuntura pode ser eficaz para os animais com dor crônica, em que nenhuma lesão compressiva pode ser demonstrada pela mielografia.
- Apesar de descrita, a discólise por injeção enzimática ou ablação a laser não é uma terapia comprovada nos cães.

ACOMPANHAMENTO

MONITORIZAÇÃO DO PACIENTE
- Os pacientes submetidos ao tratamento clínico devem ser reavaliados 2-3 vezes ao dia quanto à piora dos sinais neurológicos nas primeiras 48 h após o início.
- Se estáveis, reavaliá-los diariamente e, em seguida, semanalmente, até que os sinais clínicos tenham desaparecido.
- Os pacientes tratados por meio cirúrgico são reavaliados duas vezes ao dia até que se observe a melhora; o estado da função vesical ou a espera do desenvolvimento de bexiga autônoma são os fatores limitantes para a hospitalização.

COMPLICAÇÕES POSSÍVEIS
- Recidiva dos sinais associada à herniação do disco no ponto original ou em novo local.
- Deterioração dos sinais clínicos com ou sem cirurgia; é difícil predizer a evolução clínica em muitos casos, especialmente naqueles com lesões graves do tipo 1.
- É raro o desenvolvimento de mielomalacia ascendente ou descendente; ocorre nos cães da classe 4 ou 5, 3-5 dias após a lesão, sendo caracterizada por achados neurológicos variáveis e em processo de mudança, além de possíveis febre e dispneia; eutanásia quando diagnosticada.

EVOLUÇÃO ESPERADA E PROGNÓSTICO
- O prognóstico geral para cães das classes 1-4 é bom a excelente (85-95%); aqueles tratados de modo conservativo podem apresentar recidiva dos sinais clínicos.
- As taxas de recidiva dos cães sem fenestração no momento da laminectomia variam de 5-30%.
- Os cães da classe 5 têm uma chance variável (10-75%) de recuperação; em geral, o prognóstico é reservado, mas aparentemente favorável, se a cirurgia for realizada dentro de 48 h e se o animal tiver tempo suficiente para se recuperar.

DIVERSOS

ABREVIATURA(S)
- AINEs = anti-inflamatórios não esteroides.
- LCS = líquido cerebrospinal.
- RM = ressonância magnética.
- TC = tomografia computadorizada.

Autor Peter K. Shires
Consultor Editorial Peter K. Shires

DISCOSPONDILITE

CONSIDERAÇÕES GERAIS

DEFINIÇÃO
Trata-se de uma infecção bacteriana ou fúngica dos discos intervertebrais e dos corpos vertebrais adjacentes.

FISIOPATOLOGIA
• Disseminação hematógena de microrganismos bacterianos ou fúngicos — causa mais comum.
• Disfunção neurológica — pode ocorrer; em geral, corresponde ao resultado de compressão da medula espinal, causada pela proliferação de tecido ósseo e fibroso; com menor frequência, decorre de luxação ou fratura patológica da coluna vertebral, abscesso epidural ou extensão de infecção às meninges e à medula espinal.

SISTEMA(S) ACOMETIDO(S)
• Musculosquelético — infecção e inflamação da coluna vertebral.
• Nervoso — compressão da medula espinal.

GENÉTICA
• Ainda não se identificou uma predisposição exata.
• Em alguns casos, detectou-se uma imunodeficiência hereditária.

INCIDÊNCIA/PREVALÊNCIA
Aproximadamente 0,1-0,8% das admissões hospitalares de cães.

DISTRIBUIÇÃO GEOGRÁFICA
• Mais comum no sudeste dos EUA.
• Migração de farpas de gramíneas e coccidioidomicose — mais comuns em determinadas regiões.

IDENTIFICAÇÃO
Espécies
Cães; rara em gatos.

Raça(s) Predominante(s)
Raças de porte grande e gigante, especialmente Pastor alemão e Dinamarquês.

Idade Média e Faixa Etária
• Idade média — 4-5 anos.
• Faixa etária — de 5 meses a 12 anos.

Sexo Predominante
Os machos superam as fêmeas em uma proporção de ~2:1.

SINAIS CLÍNICOS
Achados Anamnésicos
• O início costuma ser relativamente agudo; alguns pacientes apresentam sinais leves por vários meses antes do exame.
• Dor — dificuldade de se levantar, relutância em saltar e marcha rígida são os sinais clínicos mais comuns.
• Ataxia ou paresia.
• Perda de peso e anorexia.
• Claudicação.
• Trajetos drenantes.

Achados do Exame Físico
• Áreas focais ou multifocais de dor na coluna vertebral em >80% dos pacientes.
• Pode acometer qualquer espaço discal; o espaço lombossacro é o mais comumente envolvido.
• Paresia ou paralisia, especialmente em casos crônicos sem tratamento.
• Febre em ~30% dos pacientes.
• Claudicação.

CAUSAS
• Bacterianas — *Staphylococcus pseudintermedius* é a mais comum. Outras causas incluem: *Streptococcus*, *Brucella canis* e *E. coli*; no entanto, praticamente qualquer bactéria pode ser o agente causal.
• Fúngicas — *Aspergillus*, *Paecilomyces*, *Scedosporium apiospermum* e *Coccidioides immitis*.
• A migração de farpas de gramíneas associa-se muitas vezes a infecções mistas, especialmente por *Actinomyces*; tende a comprometer os espaços discais e as vértebras entre L2-L4.
• Outras causas — cirurgia; feridas provocadas por mordeduras.

FATORES DE RISCO
• Infecção do trato urinário.
• Doença periodontal.
• Endocardite bacteriana.
• Piodermite.
• Imunodeficiência.

DIAGNÓSTICO

DIAGNÓSTICO DIFERENCIAL
• Protrusão do disco intervertebral — pode causar sinais clínicos semelhantes; diferenciada com base nos exames de radiografia e mielografia.
• Fratura ou luxação vertebrais — detectadas nas radiografias.
• Neoplasias vertebrais — não costumam comprometer as placas terminais vertebrais adjacentes.
• Espondilose deformante — raramente causa sinais clínicos; apresenta características radiográficas semelhantes, incluindo esclerose, formação de esporão ventral e colapso do espaço discal; raras vezes, causa lise das placas terminais vertebrais.
• Meningomielite focal — identificada com frequência por meio da análise do LCS.

HEMOGRAMA/BIOQUÍMICA/URINÁLISE
• Hemograma — frequentemente normal; pode-se observar leucocitose.
• Urinálise — pode revelar piúria e/ou bacteriúria com infecções concomitantes do trato urinário.

OUTROS TESTES LABORATORIAIS
• Hemoculturas aeróbias, anaeróbias e fúngicas identificam o agente causal em cerca de 35% dos casos; obtê-las se estiverem disponíveis.
• Antibiograma — indicado se as culturas forem positivas.
• Uroculturas — indicadas; positivas em aproximadamente 30% dos pacientes.
• Microrganismos que não sejam as espécies de *Staphylococcus* — podem não ser a causa.
• Teste sorológico em busca de *Brucella canis* — indicado.

DIAGNÓSTICO POR IMAGEM
• Radiografias da coluna vertebral — geralmente revelam lise das placas terminais vertebrais adjacentes ao disco acometido, colapso do espaço discal, graus variados de esclerose das placas terminais e formação de esporão ventral; podem não ser observadas lesões até 3-4 semanas após a infecção.
• Mielografia — indicada em casos de déficits neurológicos substanciais; determina a localização e o grau de compressão da medula espinal, particularmente ao se pensar em uma cirurgia descompressiva; a compressão da medula espinal causada por discospondilite tipicamente exibe padrão extradural.
• Tomografia computadorizada ou ressonância magnética — técnicas mais sensíveis do que a radiografia; indicadas quando as radiografias se apresentam normais ou inconclusivas.

MÉTODOS DIAGNÓSTICOS
• Análise do LCS — indicada ocasionalmente para descartar meningomielite; costuma permanecer normal ou revelar conteúdo proteico levemente alto.
• Cintilografia óssea — ocasionalmente útil para detectar lesões precoces; ajuda a esclarecer se as alterações radiográficas são infecciosas ou degenerativas (espondilose deformante).
• Aspiração do disco intervertebral por agulha fina guiada por fluoroscopia — valiosa na obtenção de tecidos para a realização de cultura diante da negatividade das hemo/uroculturas e na ausência de qualquer melhora com a antibioticoterapia empírica.

ACHADOS PATOLÓGICOS
• Macroscópicos — perda do espaço discal normal; proliferação óssea das vértebras adjacentes.
• Microscópicos — destruição piogranulomatosa fibrosante do disco e dos corpos vertebrais.

TRATAMENTO

CUIDADO(S) DE SAÚDE ADEQUADO(S)
• Ambulatorial — os casos de dor leve são tratados com medicação.
• Internação — os casos de dor intensa ou déficits neurológicos progressivos necessitam de cuidados intensivos e monitorização.

CUIDADO(S) DE ENFERMAGEM
Pacientes sem deambulação — mantê-los em superfícies bem acolchoadas, limpas e secas para evitar úlceras de decúbito.

ATIVIDADE
Restrita.

DIETA
Normal.

ORIENTAÇÃO AO PROPRIETÁRIO
• Explicar ao proprietário que a observação da resposta ao tratamento é muito importante para determinar a necessidade de procedimentos diagnósticos ou terapêuticos adicionais.
• Instruir o proprietário a entrar imediatamente em contato com o veterinário em casos de evolução ou recidiva dos sinais clínicos ou do desenvolvimento de déficits neurológicos.

CONSIDERAÇÕES CIRÚRGICAS
• Curetagem de um único espaço discal acometido — ocasionalmente necessária em pacientes refratários à antibioticoterapia.
• Objetivos — remover o tecido acometido; obter tecidos para cultura e avaliação histológica.
• Descompressão da medula espinal por meio de hemilaminectomia ou laminectomia dorsal — indicada em casos de déficits neurológicos substanciais e compressão medular evidente à mielografia, quando não houver nenhuma melhora com a antibioticoterapia; efetuar também a curetagem do espaço discal infectado; pode ser necessário realizar a estabilização cirúrgica caso se remova mais de uma faceta articular.

DISCOSPONDILITE

MEDICAÇÕES

MEDICAMENTO(S) DE ESCOLHA

Antibióticos
- Seleção feita com base nos resultados das hemoculturas e da sorologia.
- Cultura e sorologia negativas — admitir *Staphylococcus* spp. como agente causal; tratar com cefalosporina (p. ex., cefadroxila; cães: 22 mg/kg VO a cada 12 h; gatos: 22 mg/kg VO a cada 24 h) por 8-12 semanas.
- Sinais agudamente progressivos ou déficits neurológicos substanciais — tratados a princípio com antibióticos parenterais (p. ex., cefazolina; cães e gatos: 20-35 mg/kg IV a cada 8 h).
- Brucelose — tratada com tetraciclina (cães: 15 mg/kg VO a cada 8 h) e estreptomicina (cães: 3,4 mg/kg IM a cada 24 h) ou enrofloxacino (cães: 2,5-5 mg/kg VO a cada 12 h).

Analgésicos
- Sinais de dor intensa — tratados com analgésico (p. ex., oximorfona; cães: 0,05-0,2 mg/kg IV, IM, SC a cada 4-6 h).
- Reduzir a dosagem gradativamente após 3-5 dias para estimar a eficácia da antibioticoterapia.

CONTRAINDICAÇÕES
Glicocorticoides.

PRECAUÇÕES
Utilizar os AINEs e outros analgésicos com cuidado — podem causar a resolução temporária dos sinais clínicos mesmo quando a infecção está evoluindo; quando forem usados, suspendê-los após 3-5 dias para avaliar a eficácia da antibioticoterapia.

INTERAÇÕES POSSÍVEIS
Nenhuma.

MEDICAMENTO(S) ALTERNATIVO(S)
- Terapia inicial — cefradina (cães: 20 mg/kg VO a cada 8 h); cloxacilina (cães: 10 mg/kg VO a cada 8 h).
- Pacientes refratários — clindamicina (cães e gatos: 10 mg/kg VO a cada 12 h); enrofloxacino (cães: 5-20 mg/kg VO a cada 24 h; gatos: 5 mg/kg VO a cada 24 h); orbifloxacino (cães e gatos: 2,5-7,5 mg/kg VO a cada 24 h).

ACOMPANHAMENTO

MONITORIZAÇÃO DO PACIENTE
- Reavaliar o animal após 5 dias de terapia.
- Sem melhora na dor, na febre ou no apetite — reavaliar a terapia; considerar a administração de um antibiótico diferente, a aspiração percutânea do espaço discal acometido ou a realização de intervenção cirúrgica.
- Melhora — avaliar o paciente em termos clínicos e radiográficos a cada 4 semanas.

PREVENÇÃO
Identificação precoce das causas predisponentes, aliada ao diagnóstico e tratamento imediatos — ajudam a diminuir a evolução dos sintomas clínicos e a deterioração neurológica.

COMPLICAÇÕES POSSÍVEIS
- Compressão da medula espinal causada por tecidos ósseo e fibroso proliferativos.
- Fratura ou luxação vertebrais.
- Meningite ou meningomielite.
- Abscesso epidural.

EVOLUÇÃO ESPERADA E PROGNÓSTICO
- A recidiva é comum em caso de interrupção prematura da antibioticoterapia (antes de 8-12 semanas de tratamento).
- Alguns pacientes necessitam de terapia prolongada (1 ano ou mais).
- Prognóstico — depende do microrganismo causal e do grau de dano à medula espinal.
- Disfunção neurológica leve ou ausente (cães) — em geral, responde dentro de 5 dias do início da antibioticoterapia.
- Paresia ou paralisia substanciais — prognóstico reservado; pode-se notar a resolução gradativa da disfunção neurológica após várias semanas de terapia; o tratamento é justificável.
- *Brucella canis* — os sinais costumam desaparecer com a terapia; a infecção pode não ser erradicada; a recidiva é comum.

DIVERSOS

DISTÚRBIOS ASSOCIADOS
Ver a seção "Fatores de Risco".

FATORES RELACIONADOS COM A IDADE
N/D.

POTENCIAL ZOONÓTICO
Brucella canis — a infecção humana é incomum, mas pode ocorrer.

GESTAÇÃO/FERTILIDADE/REPRODUÇÃO
N/D.

SINÔNIMO(S)
- Discite.
- Infecção do disco intervertebral.
- Osteomielite intradiscal.
- Osteomielite vertebral.

VER TAMBÉM
Brucelose.

ABREVIATURA(S)
- AINE = anti-inflamatório não esteroide.
- LCS = líquido cerebrospinal.

Sugestões de Leitura

Ameel L, Martlé V, et al. Discospondylitis in the dog: A retrospective study of 18 cases. Vlaams Diergeneeskundig Tijdschrift 2009, 78(5):347-353.

Bagley RS. Diskospondylitis. Fundam Clin Neuro 2005, 172-173(283-285):346.

Braund KG, Sharp NJH. Discospondylitis. In: Clinical Neurology in Small Animals: Localisation, Diagnosis and Treatment. Ithaca, NY: IVIS, 2003.

Burkert BA, Kerwin SC, Hosgood GL, Pechman RD, Ponti Fontenelle J. Signalment and clinical features of diskospondylitis in dogs: 513 cases (1980-2001). JAVMA 2005, 227(2):268-275.

Fischer A, Mahaffey MB, Oliver JE. Fluoroscopically guided percutaneous disk aspiration in 10 dogs with diskospondylitis. J Vet Intern Med 1997, 11:284-287.

Johnson RG, Prata RG. Intradiskal osteomyelitis: A conservative approach. JAAHA 1983, 19:743-750.

Kerwin SC, Lewis DD, Hribernik TN, et al. Diskospondylitis associated with Brucella canis infection in dogs: 14 cases (1989-1991). JAVMA 1992, 201:1253-1257.

Kornegay JN. Diskospondylitis. In: Kirk RW, ed., Current Veterinary Therapy IX. Philadelphia: Saunders, 1986, pp. 810-814.

Thomas WB. Diskospondylitis and other vertebral infections. Vet Clin North Am Small Anim Pract 2000, 30:169-182.

Autor Peter K. Shires
Consultor Editorial Peter K. Shires

DISFAGIA

CONSIDERAÇÕES GERAIS

DEFINIÇÃO
- Deglutição dificultosa ou dolorosa, resultante de dor durante o processo de deglutição ou incapacidade de preensão, formação e deslocamento do bolo alimentar pela orofaringe até o esôfago.
- A discussão a respeito de disfagia esofágica encontra-se nos tópicos sobre "Megaesôfago e Regurgitação".

FISIOPATOLOGIA
- As dificuldades de deglutição podem ser causadas por obstrução mecânica da cavidade bucal ou da faringe, disfunção neuromuscular que resulta em movimentos de deglutição fracos ou incoordenados ou dor associada à preensão, mastigação ou deglutição.
- A disfagia bucal diz respeito à dificuldade com os componentes voluntários da deglutição — preensão e formação do bolo alimentar na base da língua.
- A disfagia faríngea ocorre quando há mau funcionamento dos movimentos involuntários do bolo alimentar pela orofaringe.
- A disfagia cricofaríngea refere-se ao movimento anormal do bolo alimentar desde a faringe, pelo músculo cricofaríngeo, causado por falha no relaxamento desse músculo (acalasia cricofaríngea) ou assincronia entre as contrações faríngeas e a abertura cricofaríngea (assincronia cricofaríngea).
- A deglutição é coordenada pelo centro da deglutição no tronco cerebral; os estímulos aferentes sensoriais são transmitidos ao centro da deglutição pelos V e IX pares de nervos cranianos.
- Os estímulos eferentes motores responsáveis pela deglutição são conduzidos pelos V, VII, XII pares de nervos cranianos (preensão e mastigação), bem como pelos IX e X pares de nervos cranianos (contração faríngea); os distúrbios em qualquer uma dessas áreas podem resultar em disfagia.

SISTEMA(S) ACOMETIDO(S)
- Gastrintestinal.
- Neuromuscular.
- Nervoso.
- Respiratório.

GENÉTICA
- Alguns distúrbios subjacentes têm base genética.
- A disfunção cricofaríngea parece ser hereditária em cães da raça Golden retriever.

INCIDÊNCIA/PREVALÊNCIA
Variáveis, dependendo da etiologia subjacente.

DISTRIBUIÇÃO GEOGRÁFICA
Nenhuma.

IDENTIFICAÇÃO
- Cães e gatos.
- Os distúrbios congênitos indutores de disfagia (p. ex., acalasia cricofaríngea e fenda palatina) costumam ser diagnosticados em animais com <1 ano de idade.
- As disfagias faríngeas adquiridas são mais comuns em pacientes mais idosos.

SINAIS CLÍNICOS
Achados Anamnésicos
- Salivação (em virtude de dor ou incapacidade de engolir a saliva), ânsia de vômito, apetite voraz, tentativas repetidas ou exageradas de deglutição, deglutição com a cabeça em posição anormal, secreção nasal (em função da passagem de alimento e líquidos para a nasofaringe e a cavidade nasal), tosse (causada por aspiração), regurgitação, deglutição dolorosa e, ocasionalmente, anorexia e perda de peso — são todos, sem exceção, possíveis. Se a língua não estiver funcionando normalmente, poderão ser observados problemas com os processos de preensão e mastigação.
- Averiguar o início e a evolução do quadro de disfagia.
- Os corpos estranhos causam disfagia aguda; a disfagia faríngea pode ser crônica e intermitente.

Achados do Exame Físico
- Exame bucal completo, com o paciente sedado ou anestesiado, se necessário, é de suma importância.
- Observar o paciente quanto à presença de assimetria, defeito anatômico, corpo estranho, inflamação, tumor, edema, abscessos dentários ou dentes frouxos.
- É imprescindível observar o paciente se alimentando; isso pode situar a fase anormal da deglutição.
- Realizar exame neurológico completo, com ênfase nos nervos cranianos.

Disfagia Bucal
- A mudança no comportamento alimentar (p. ex., comer com a cabeça inclinada para um lado e jogar a cabeça para trás enquanto come) pode compensar a disfagia bucal.
- Paralisia mandibular, paralisia lingual, odontopatia, tumefação ou atrofia dos músculos mastigatórios, incapacidade de abrir a boca e acúmulo de alimento nas pregas bucais sem retenção de saliva sugerem disfagia bucal.

Disfagia Faríngea
- A preensão de alimentos permanece normal.
- As tentativas repetidas de deglutição enquanto se flexionam e se estendem a cabeça e o pescoço repetidamente, a mastigação excessiva e a ânsia de vômito sugerem disfagia faríngea.
- Também pode haver alimento coberto por saliva retido nas pregas bucais, diminuição no reflexo do vômito e secreção nasal decorrente de aspiração.

Disfagia Cricofaríngea
- Os pacientes fazem esforços repetidos e improdutivos para engolir, apresentam ânsia de vômito e tossem; em seguida, regurgitam com ímpeto imediatamente após a deglutição.
- O reflexo do vômito e a preensão permanecem normais.
- A emaciação é mais comum com essa forma de disfagia, em comparação às outras.

CAUSAS
- As lesões anatômicas ou mecânicas incluem inflamação faríngea (p. ex., abscessos, pólipos inflamatórios e granuloma eosinofílico bucal), linfadenomegalia retrofaríngea, neoplasias, corpos estranhos faríngeos e retrofaríngeos, sialocele, distúrbios da articulação temporomandibular (p. ex., luxação, fratura e osteopatia craniomandibular), fratura mandibular, fenda palatina ou encurtamento congênito do palato, acalasia cricofaríngea (congênita ou adquirida, como raramente se pode observar em associação com hipotireoidismo), distúrbio do frênulo lingual e traumatismo faríngeo.
- A dor decorrente de odontopatias (p. ex., fraturas e abscessos dentários), traumatismo mandibular, estomatite, glossite e inflamação faríngea também pode interromper a preensão normal, a formação do bolo alimentar e a deglutição. Estomatite, glossite e faringite podem ser secundárias a rinotraqueíte viral felina, infecção por FeLV/FIV, pênfigo, LES, uremia e ingestão de substâncias cáusticas ou corpos estranhos.
- Os distúrbios neuromusculares que prejudicam a preensão e a formação do bolo alimentar compreendem os déficits dos nervos cranianos (p. ex., neuropatia idiopática do trigêmeo [V par], paralisia lingual por lesão do XII par dos nervos cranianos) e a miosite dos músculos mastigatórios.
- Fraqueza, paresia ou paralisia faríngeas podem ser causadas por polimiosite infecciosa (p. ex., toxoplasmose e neosporose), polimiosite imunomediada, distrofia muscular, polineuropatias e distúrbios da junção mioneural (p. ex., miastenia grave, paralisia por carrapato e botulismo).
- Outros distúrbios do SNC, especialmente aqueles com envolvimento do tronco cerebral.
- A raiva pode causar disfagia por comprometer tanto o tronco cerebral como os nervos periféricos.
- Outros distúrbios do SNC, especialmente aqueles que envolvem o tronco cerebral.

FATORES DE RISCO
Muitos dos distúrbios neuromusculares causais possuem predisposições raciais.

DIAGNÓSTICO

DIAGNÓSTICO DIFERENCIAL
- É preciso diferenciá-la de vômito e regurgitação decorrentes de doença esofágica.
- Esforços exagerados ou repetidos para engolir — típicos de disfagia; meio mais útil de distingui-la de vômito ou regurgitação.
- Os vômitos associam-se a contrações abdominais; a disfagia, não.

HEMOGRAMA/BIOQUÍMICA/URINÁLISE
- As condições inflamatórias frequentemente geram leucocitose, algumas vezes com desvio à esquerda.
- Em geral, encontra-se uma atividade sérica elevada da creatino fosfocinase em pacientes com distúrbios neuromusculares resultantes em disfagia.
- Em pacientes com úlceras bucais e linguais secundárias à uremia, podem-se encontrar indícios de nefropatias (p. ex., azotemia e concentração urinária baixa).

OUTROS TESTES LABORATORIAIS
- Sorologia para pesquisa de anticorpos musculares do tipo 2M (miosite dos músculos mastigatórios).
- Sorologia para detecção de anticorpos contra os receptores da acetilcolinesterase (miastenia grave adquirida).
- Sorologia em busca de anticorpos antinucleares (doenças imunomediadas).
- Mensuração de T_4, T_4 livre por diálise de equilíbrio, TSH, com ou sem anticorpos antitireoidianos, para descartar hipotireoidismo.
- Teste de supressão com baixas doses de dexametasona ou teste de estimulação com ACTH (hiperadrenocorticismo — pacientes com infecções crônicas ou miopatia).

DIAGNÓSTICO POR IMAGEM
- Obter radiografias simples do crânio e do pescoço, incluindo o aparelho hioide; dar especial atenção às mandíbulas e à articulação

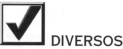

temporomandibular, aos dentes, às regiões faríngea e retrofaríngea, bem como à posição do aparelho hioide.
• A ultrassonografia da faringe pode ser útil em pacientes com lesões expansivas tipo massa e na obtenção de amostras de biopsias guiadas por ultrassom.
• A fluoroscopia, com ou sem contraste positivo, mostra-se útil na avaliação do movimento faríngeo em pacientes com suspeita de disfagia faríngea ou cricofaríngea.
• Exames de TC e/ou RM na suspeita de massa intracraniana.

MÉTODOS DIAGNÓSTICOS
• Biopsias excisionais ou incisionais de lesões expansivas tipo massa.
• Faringoscopia.
• Endoscopia da nasofaringe — retroflexão do endoscópio sobe o palato mole em busca de corpos estranhos.
• Eletromiografia da musculatura faríngea para confirmar a presença de algum distúrbio neuromuscular; avaliar também o paciente quanto à existência de doenças neuromusculares sistêmicas.
• Teste de estimulação repetitiva do nervo e teste de cloreto de edrofônio (0,1-0,2 mg/kg IV) na suspeita de miastenia grave.
• Análise do líquido cerebrospinal em pacientes com distúrbio do SNC.
• Manometria cricofaríngea caso se suspeite de acalasia cricofaríngea.

ACHADOS PATOLÓGICOS
Variáveis, dependendo da etiologia subjacente.

TRATAMENTO
• Determinar a causa subjacente para elaborar o plano terapêutico e estabelecer o prognóstico preciso.
• Direcionar o tratamento primário à causa subjacente.
• A maioria dos pacientes pode ser tratada em um esquema ambulatorial a menos que haja outros fatores de complicação, como pneumonia por aspiração, desidratação causada pela dificuldade de comer e beber, ou fraqueza em virtude da miopatia generalizada.

CUIDADO(S) DE ENFERMAGEM
• Se o animal estiver desidratado, poderá ser necessária a implementação dos cuidados de suporte (fluidos IV).
• Outros cuidados de suporte podem ser necessários no caso de pneumonia por aspiração (oxigênio, etc.).
• Para os pacientes com fraqueza generalizada decorrente de miopatias, há necessidade de bons cuidados de enfermagem, como mudanças de posição, uso de camas satisfatórias e aplicação de fisioterapia.

ATIVIDADE
É recomendável alterações na atividade, com base na etiologia subjacente.

DIETA
• O suporte nutricional é importante em todos os pacientes com disfagia.
• Os pacientes com disfagia bucal poderão se mostrar capazes de deglutir se o bolo alimentar for colocado na porção caudal da faringe; outros podem achar que o ato de lamber um mingau ou uma papa pode facilitar a deglutição; é preciso ter cuidado para evitar a aspiração quando se fornece o alimento por via oral.
• A elevação da cabeça e do pescoço durante a alimentação e por 10-15 minutos após a alimentação pode facilitar a deglutição em pacientes com disfagia faríngea ou cricofaríngea e ajudar a evitar a aspiração de alimento.
• Caso não se consiga suprir as necessidades nutricionais por via oral, poderá ser imprescindível o procedimento de gastrostomia.

ORIENTAÇÃO AO PROPRIETÁRIO
• Variável, dependendo da causa subjacente.
• Orientar o proprietário sobre o fato de que nem todas as doenças subjacentes têm cura, mas sim controle.
• As modificações na alimentação (ver seção acima) podem ser a longo prazo.
• Os proprietários devem ser orientados a monitorar o paciente quanto aos sinais de possível pneumonia por aspiração (secreção nasal mucopurulenta, tosse, dispneia, taquipneia).

CONSIDERAÇÕES CIRÚRGICAS
• A excisão cirúrgica de lesões expansivas tipo massa ou a remoção de corpos estranhos pode ser curativa ou promover a melhora temporária dos sinais clínicos da disfagia.
• O procedimento de miotomia cricofaríngea pode beneficiar os pacientes com disfagia cricofaríngea; o diagnóstico correto é essencial antes da cirurgia, pois a miotomia cricofaríngea exacerbará a dificuldade de deglutição dos animais com disfagia orofaríngea.

MEDICAÇÕES
MEDICAMENTO(S) DE ESCOLHA
A disfagia não representa risco de vida imediato; orientar a terapia medicamentosa à causa subjacente.

PRECAUÇÕES
• Utilizar o sulfato de bário com cautela em pacientes com indícios de aspiração.
• Empregar os corticosteroides com cuidado ou não usá-los, de forma alguma, em pacientes com indícios, ou sob risco, de aspiração.

ACOMPANHAMENTO
MONITORIZAÇÃO DO PACIENTE
• Monitorizar diariamente em busca de sinais de pneumonia por aspiração (p. ex., depressão, febre, secreção nasal mucopurulenta, tosse e dispneia).
• Monitorizar a condição corporal e o estado de hidratação diariamente; se a nutrição oral não suprir as necessidades do paciente, lançar mão da alimentação com sonda aplicada via gastrostomia.

COMPLICAÇÕES POSSÍVEIS
A pneumonia por aspiração representa uma complicação comum em casos de distúrbios de deglutição.

EVOLUÇÃO ESPERADA E PROGNÓSTICO
Variáveis, dependendo da causa.

DIVERSOS
DISTÚRBIOS ASSOCIADOS
• Megaesôfago.
• Pneumonia por aspiração.

FATORES RELACIONADOS COM A IDADE
• Há maior probabilidade de que os animais muito jovens tenham anormalidades congênitas, como acalasia cricofaríngea, observada no momento do desmame e da transição do leite para alimentos sólidos.
• É mais provável que os cães jovens ingiram corpos estranhos e sofram traumatismo facial.
• Os gatos jovens têm maior probabilidade à formação de pólipos inflamatórios.

POTENCIAL ZOONÓTICO
• Considerar a raiva em qualquer paciente com disfagia, especialmente se o estado de vacinação antirrábica do animal for desconhecido ou questionável ou se ele tiver sido exposto a outro animal potencialmente raivoso.
• Caso o animal disfágico morra de neuropatia rapidamente progressiva, enviar a cabeça a um laboratório qualificado e nomeado pelo departamento de saúde local ou estadual para o exame da raiva.

VER TAMBÉM
• Megaesôfago.
• Pneumonia Bacteriana.
• Regurgitação.

ABREVIATURA(S)
• ACTH = hormônio adrenocorticotrópico.
• FeLV = vírus da leucemia felina.
• FIV = vírus da imunodeficiência felina.
• LES = lúpus eritematoso sistêmico.
• SNC = sistema nervoso central.
• RM = ressonância magnética.
• TC = tomografia computadorizada.
• TSH = hormônio tireoestimulante.

Sugestões de Leitura
Woolley CS. Dysphagia and regurgitation. In: Ettinger SJ, Feldman EC, eds., Textbook of Veterinary Internal Medicine, 7th ed. St. Louis: Elsevier, 2010, pp. 191-195.

Autor Krysta Deitz
Consultor Editorial Albert E. Jergens

Displasia Coxofemoral

CONSIDERAÇÕES GERAIS

DEFINIÇÃO
Má-formação e degeneração das articulações coxofemorais.

FISIOPATOLOGIA
• Defeito de desenvolvimento desencadeado por alguma predisposição genética à subluxação da articulação coxofemoral imatura.
• Pouca congruência entre a cabeça femoral e o acetábulo — gera forças anormais entre as articulações; interfere no desenvolvimento normal (levando à irregularidade no formato dos acetábulos e das cabeças femorais); sobrecarrega a cartilagem articular (causando microfraturas e osteoartrite).

SISTEMA(S) ACOMETIDO(S)
Musculosquelético.

GENÉTICA
• Transmissão poligênica complexa.
• Expressão — determinada por uma interação de fatores genéticos e ambientes.
• Índice de hereditariedade — depende da raça.

INCIDÊNCIA/PREVALÊNCIA
• Uma das doenças esqueléticas mais comuns encontradas clinicamente em cães.
• Incidência real — desconhecida; depende da raça.
• A incidência nos gatos é significativamente mais baixa que nos cães.

DISTRIBUIÇÃO GEOGRÁFICA
N/D.

IDENTIFICAÇÃO
Espécies
Cães.

Raça(s) Predominante(s)
• De grande porte — São Bernardo, Pastor alemão, Labrador retriever, Golden retriever, Rottweiler.
• Raças de pequeno porte — podem ser acometidas; menos propensas a demonstrar sinais clínicos.
• Gatos — afeta mais comumente os de raças puras. Segundo relatos, acomete cerca de 18% dos gatos da raça Maine Coon.

Idade Média e Faixa Etária
• Começa no cão imaturo.
• Sinais clínicos — podem se desenvolver depois de 4 meses de vida; podem se desenvolver mais tarde com osteoartrite.

Sexo Predominante
• Nenhum.
• Gatos — mais comum em fêmeas.

SINAIS CLÍNICOS
Comentários Gerais
• Depende do grau de frouxidão articular e de osteoartrite, bem como da cronicidade da doença.
• Precoces — relacionados com a frouxidão articular.
• Tardios — relacionados com a degeneração articular.

Achados Anamnésicos
• Atividade diminuída.
• Dificuldade em se levantar.
• Relutância em correr, saltar ou subir escadas.
• Claudicação intermitente ou persistente nos membros pélvicos — em geral se agrava após o exercício.
• Marcha saltitante tipo coelho ou oscilante.
• Postura estreita nos membros pélvicos.

Achados do Exame Físico
• Dor.
• Articulação frouxa (sinal de Ortolani positivo) — característica de doença precoce; pode não ser observada em casos crônicos em função da fibrose periarticular.
• Crepitação.
• Amplitude de movimento diminuída nas articulações coxofemorais.
• Atrofia dos músculos da coxa.
• Hipertrofia dos músculos do ombro.

CAUSAS
• Predisposição genética para frouxidão coxofemoral.
• Ganho de peso rápido, nível de nutrição e massa muscular pélvica — influenciam a expressão e a evolução.

FATORES DE RISCO
N/D.

DIAGNÓSTICO

DIAGNÓSTICO DIFERENCIAL
• Mielopatia degenerativa.
• Instabilidade lombossacra.
• Doença bilateral da articulação femorotibiopatelar.
• Panosteíte.
• Poliartropatias.

HEMOGRAMA/BIOQUÍMICA/URINÁLISE
N/D.

OUTROS TESTES LABORATORIAIS
N/D.

DIAGNÓSTICO POR IMAGEM
• Radiografias ventrodorsais com a articulação coxofemoral estendida — comumente utilizadas para o diagnóstico; pode ser necessária sedação ou anestesia geral para o posicionamento adequado e preciso do paciente.
• Sinais radiográficos iniciais — subluxação da articulação coxofemoral com má congruência entre a cabeça femoral e o acetábulo; no início, a cabeça do fêmur e o acetábulo encontram-se com formato normal; com a evolução da doença, o acetábulo fica raso e a cabeça do fêmur, achatada.
• Evidência radiográfica de osteoartrite — achatamento da cabeça femoral; acetábulo raso; produção de osteófitos na região periarticular; espessamento da cabeça do fêmur; esclerose do osso subcondral; fibrose do tecido mole periarticular. A remodelagem do colo do fêmur é incomum em gatos.
• Radiografias por distração — quantificam a frouxidão articular; podem acentuar a frouxidão para um diagnóstico mais acurado.
• O registro PennHIP*, desenvolvido na Pensilvânia, faz uso do método radiográfico de distração. A subluxação dorsolateral constitui outro método radiográfico de distração disponível.
• Radiografias de projeção dorsal da margem acetabular — avaliam a margem do acetábulo; avaliam a cobertura dorsal da cabeça femoral.

MÉTODOS DIAGNÓSTICOS
N/D.

ACHADOS PATOLÓGICOS
• Iniciais — cabeça femoral e acetábulo normais; é possível notar frouxidão articular e excesso de líquido sinovial.
• Com a evolução — acetábulo e cabeça do fêmur malformados; degeneração da cartilagem articular.
• Crônicos — pode-se notar erosão de toda a espessura da cartilagem.

TRATAMENTO

CUIDADO(S) DE SAÚDE ADEQUADO(S)
• O tratamento pode ser clínico conservador ou cirúrgico.
• Ambulatorial a menos que seja feita cirurgia.
• Depende(m) do porte e da idade do paciente, da função desejada, da gravidade da frouxidão articular, do grau de osteoartrite, da preferência do clínico e das considerações financeiras do proprietário.

CUIDADO(S) DE ENFERMAGEM
• Fisioterapia (movimento articular passivo) — diminui a rigidez articular; ajuda a manter a integridade muscular.
• Natação (hidroterapia) — excelente forma não concussiva de fisioterapia; estimula a atividade articular e muscular sem exacerbar a lesão articular.

ATIVIDADE
• Conforme a tolerância.
• Natação — recomendada para manter a mobilidade articular ao mesmo tempo em que minimiza as atividades de sustentação do peso.

DIETA
Controle do peso — importante; diminui a carga aplicada à articulação dolorida; minimiza o ganho de peso associado à redução do exercício.

ORIENTAÇÃO AO PROPRIETÁRIO
• Discutir o caráter hereditário da doença.
• Explicar que o tratamento clínico é uma medida paliativa, porque não corrige a instabilidade articular.
• Avisar o proprietário sobre o fato de que a degeneração articular frequentemente evolui a menos que seja feita uma osteotomia corretiva logo no início da doença.
• Esclarecer que os procedimentos cirúrgicos podem recuperar a função articular assim que ocorre degeneração articular grave.

CONSIDERAÇÕES CIRÚRGICAS
Osteotomia Pélvica Tripla ou Dupla
• Procedimento corretivo; destinado a restabelecer a congruência entre a cabeça do fêmur e o acetábulo.
• Paciente imaturo (6-12 meses de vida).
• Rotação do acetábulo — melhora a cobertura dorsal da cabeça do fêmur; corrige as forças que atuam sobre a articulação; minimiza a evolução da osteoartrite; pode permitir o desenvolvimento de uma articulação mais normal se realizada no início (antes que se desenvolva uma degeneração).

---
* N. T.: Mensuração do índice de distração.

DISPLASIA COXOFEMORAL

Sinfisiodese Púbica Juvenil
- A sínfise púbica é fundida em um estágio precoce (com o emprego de eletrocautério).
- Causa ventroversão do acetábulo para cobrir melhor a cabeça do fêmur.
- Melhora a congruência e a estabilidade da articulação — efeitos semelhantes aos da osteotomia pélvica tripla sem implantes cirúrgicos.
- Morbidade mínima; fácil de fazer — precisa ser feita muito cedo (aos 3-4 meses de vida) para ter efeito; obtém-se efeito mínimo se realizada depois de 6 meses de vida.

Substituição Total do Quadril
- Indicada para recuperar a função em cães maduros com doença degenerativa grave irresponsiva ao tratamento clínico.
- Função articular sem dor — relatada em mais de 90% dos casos.
- Substituição unilateral da articulação — proporciona função aceitável em ~80% dos casos.
- Complicações — luxação; neuropraxia ciática; infecção.

Artroplastia por Excisão
- Remoção da cabeça e do colo femorais para eliminar a dor articular (artralgia).
- Trata-se basicamente de um procedimento de recuperação — para osteoartrite significativa; quando a dor não pode ser controlada clinicamente; quando o custo da substituição total do quadril é proibitivo.
- Melhores resultados — cães leves de pequeno porte (menos de 20 kg de peso); pacientes com boa musculatura na região do quadril.
- Com frequência, uma marcha levemente anormal persiste.
- Atrofia muscular pós-operatória — comum, particularmente em cães de grande porte.

Procedimento de Denervação
- Procedimento cirúrgico descrito na literatura especializada para diminuir a dor associada à displasia coxofemoral.
- Não melhora a conformação articular nem a osteoartrite.
- Há poucas provas científicas quanto à eficácia desse procedimento.

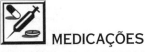

MEDICAÇÕES

MEDICAMENTO(S) DE ESCOLHA
- Analgésicos e anti-inflamatórios — minimizam a dor articular (e, portanto, a rigidez e a atrofia muscular causadas pelo uso restrito); diminuem a sinovite.
- Tratamento clínico — não corrige a anormalidade biomecânica; é provável que o processo degenerativo evolua; em geral, só proporciona alívio temporário dos sinais.
- Agentes — carprofeno (2,2 mg/kg VO a cada 12 h ou 4,4 mg/kg VO a cada 24 h); etodolaco (10-15 mg/kg VO a cada 24 h); deracoxibe (3-4 mg/kg VO a cada 12 h por 1 semana e depois 2 mg/kg VO a cada 12 h).

CONTRAINDICAÇÕES
Evitar o uso de corticosteroides — efeitos colaterais potenciais; dano à cartilagem articular associado ao uso prolongado.

PRECAUÇÕES
- AINEs — desarranjo gastrintestinal pode impedir o uso em alguns pacientes.
- Carprofeno — relatado como causa de hepatotoxicidade aguda em alguns cães.

INTERAÇÕES POSSÍVEIS
N/D.

MEDICAMENTO(S) ALTERNATIVO(S)
Glicosaminoglicanos polissulfatados, glicosamina e sulfato de condroitina — podem exercer efeito condroprotetor em casos de osteoartrite.

ACOMPANHAMENTO

MONITORIZAÇÃO DO PACIENTE
- Monitoração clínica e radiográfica — para avaliar a evolução.
- Tratamento clínico — a deterioração clínica sugere o uso de dosagem ou medicação ou ainda intervenção cirúrgica alternativa.
- Osteotomia pélvica tripla — monitorizada ao exame radiográfico; avalia a consolidação do osso, a estabilidade do implante, a congruência da articulação e a evolução da osteoartrite.
- Substituição do quadril — monitorizada sob avaliação radiográfica; avalia a estabilidade do implante.

PREVENÇÃO
- A melhor forma de prevenir é não acasalar os cães acometidos.
- Radiografias pélvicas — podem ajudar a identificar cães anormais sob o ponto de vista fenotípico; podem não identificar todos os cães portadores da doença.
- Não acasalar novamente machos e fêmeas que tenham tido filhotes acometidos.
- Dietas especiais destinadas às raças caninas de grande porte e crescimento rápido — podem diminuir a gravidade da doença.

COMPLICAÇÕES POSSÍVEIS
N/D.

EVOLUÇÃO ESPERADA E PROGNÓSTICO
A degeneração articular, em geral, evolui — a maioria dos pacientes leva uma vida normal com o tratamento clínico ou cirúrgico apropriado.

DIVERSOS

DISTÚRBIOS ASSOCIADOS
N/D.

FATORES RELACIONADOS COM A IDADE
N/D.

POTENCIAL ZOONÓTICO
N/D.

GESTAÇÃO/FERTILIDADE/REPRODUÇÃO
Não acasalar os cães acometidos; o acréscimo de peso gerado pela prenhez pode exacerbar os sinais clínicos.

ABREVIATURA(S)
- AINEs = anti-inflamatórios não esteroides.

Sugestões de Leitura
Dassler CL. Canine hip dysplasia: Diagnosis and nonsurgical treatment. In: Slatter D, ed., Textbook of Small Animal Surgery, 3rd ed. Philadelphia: Saunders, 2003, pp. 2019-2029.
McLaughlin RM, Tomlinson J. Alternative surgical treatments for canine hip dysplasia. Vet Med 1996, 91:137-143.
McLaughlin RM, Tomlinson J. Radiographic diagnosis of canine hip dysplasia. Vet Med 1996, 91:36-47.
McLaughlin RM, Tomlinson J. Treating canine hip dysplasia with triple pelvic osteotomy. Vet Med 1996, 91:126-136.
Patsikas MN, Papazogoglou LG, Komninou A, et.al. Hip dysplasia in the cat: A report of three cases. J Small Anim Pract 1998, 39:290-294.
Rettenmaier JL, Constantinescu GM. Canine hip dysplasia. Compend Contin Educ Pract Vet 1991, 13:643-653.
Schulz KS, Dejardin LM. Surgical treatment of canine hip dysplasia. In: Slatter D, ed., Textbook of Small Animal Surgery, 3rd ed. Philadelphia: Saunders, 2003, pp. 2029-2059.
Swainson SW, Conzemius MG, Riedesel EA, Smith GK, Riley CB. Effect of pubic symphysiodesis on pelvic development in the skeletally immature greyhound. Vet Surg 2000, 29:178-190.
Todhunter RJ, Lust G. Hip dysplasia: Pathogenesis. In: In: Slatter D, ed., Textbook of Small Animal Surgery, 3rd ed. Philadelphia: Saunders, 2003, pp. 2009-2019.
Tomlinson J, McLaughlin RM. Canine hip dysplasia: Developmental factors, clinical signs and initial examination steps. Vet Med 1996, 91:26-33.
Tomlinson J, McLaughlin RM. Medically managing canine hip dysplasia. Vet Med 1996, 91:48-53.
Tomlinson J, McLaughlin RM. Total hip replacement. Vet Med 1996, 91:118-124.
Wallace LJ. Canine hip dysplasia: Past and present. Semin Vet Med Surg 1987, 2:92-106.

Autor Ron M. McLaughlin
Consultor Editorial Peter K. Shires

Displasia das Valvas Atrioventriculares

CONSIDERAÇÕES GERAIS

DEFINIÇÃO
Má-formação congênita dos aparelhos das valvas atrioventriculares (AV) esquerda (mitral) ou direita (tricúspide).

FISIOPATOLOGIA
• A displasia das valvas AV pode resultar em insuficiência valvar, estenose valvar ou obstrução dinâmica da via de saída, dependendo da anormalidade anatômica. A displasia das valvas AV pode ocorrer de forma isolada ou associada a anormalidades da via ipsilateral de saída, por exemplo, estenose valvular/subvalvular aórtica ou pulmonar. Não é raro que as displasias da mitral e da tricúspide ocorram simultaneamente no mesmo paciente.
• A insuficiência valvar dá origem à dilatação do átrio ipsilateral, hipertrofia excêntrica do ventrículo associado e, se suficientemente grave, sinais de insuficiência cardíaca congestiva (ICC). A miocardiopatia por sobrecarga volêmica crônica e o aumento das pressões atriais representam o resultado final, que culmina em congestão pulmonar em caso de comprometimento da mitral e congestão sistêmica em caso de envolvimento da tricúspide.
• A estenose valvar resulta na dilatação e hipertrofia atriais e, quando grave, hipoplasia do ventrículo receptor. Se as pressões ultrapassarem 15 a 20 mmHg, a estenose da tricúspide ocasionará aumento na pressão do átrio direito e congestão sistêmica. Na presença de defeito do septo atrial ou na persistência do forame oval, poderá ocorrer o desvio sanguíneo da direita para a esquerda. A estenose da mitral, por sua vez, produzirá um aumento na pressão capilar pulmonar e edema pulmonar se as pressões excederem 25 a 30 mmHg. Em animais com estenose da mitral, é comum a ocorrência de hipertensão pulmonar.
• A obstrução da via de saída pode surgir a partir de defeitos que transloquem o folheto anterior para uma posição mais próxima do septo interventricular. Proporcionalmente à gravidade da obstrução, desenvolve-se hipertrofia concêntrica do ventrículo esquerdo.

SISTEMA(S) ACOMETIDO(S)
• Cardiovascular — a obstrução ao fluxo de entrada decorrente de estenose valvar e a sobrecarga volêmica crônica originária de insuficiência valvar resultam em aumento nas pressões venosas pulmonar (valva AV esquerda) ou sistêmica (valva AV direita). Se a lesão for suficientemente grave, surgirão sinais de baixo débito cardíaco. A hipertrofia concêntrica do ventrículo esquerdo desenvolve-se secundariamente à obstrução dinâmica da via de saída.
• Respiratório — subsequente à insuficiência ou estenose da mitral, poderá ocorrer a formação de edema pulmonar. Em animais com estenose da mitral, comumente se observa hipertensão pulmonar como uma complicação.
• Neurológico — durante esforço físico, podem ocorrer com muita frequência sinais de colapso e perda da consciência em casos de doença grave por baixo débito cardíaco e hipotensão. Em animais com obstrução dinâmica da via de saída, o colapso se deve muitas vezes à arritmia ventricular.

GENÉTICA
A displasia da tricúspide é uma condição hereditária, que se expressa como traço autossômico recessivo em cães da raça Labrador retriever. No entanto, ainda não foram estabelecidos os padrões de herança e as questões de hereditariedade em outras raças.

INCIDÊNCIA/PREVALÊNCIA
Uma das anomalias cardíacas congênitas mais comuns em gatos (17% dos defeitos cardíacos congênitos relatados em um único estudo). Diagnosticada com menor frequência em cães.

IDENTIFICAÇÃO
Espécies
Cães e gatos.

Raça(s) Predominante(s)
• Displasia da tricúspide — risco elevado de Labrador retriever, Pastor alemão, Grande Pirineu e, possivelmente, Old English sheepdog. Também é comum em gatos.
• Displasia da mitral — risco elevado em Bull terrier, Terra Nova, Labrador retriever, Dogue alemão, Golden retriever, Dálmata e gato Siamês. Talvez seja o defeito cardíaco congênito mais comum da espécie felina. As más-formações mitrais são frequentemente observadas em gatos com miocardiopatia hipertrófica.

Idade Média e Faixa Etária
Variáveis. Com maior frequência, os sinais manifestam-se dentro dos primeiros anos de vida após o nascimento.

Sexo(s) Predominante(s)
É mais provável a constatação de insuficiência cardíaca em machos.

SINAIS CLÍNICOS
Achados Anamnésicos
• A intolerância ao exercício é o problema mais comum em cães e gatos com displasia das valvas AV.
• Em casos de grave displasia da tricúspide, podem-se observar distensão abdominal, perda de peso e retardo do crescimento.
• Em cães ou gatos com displasia da mitral, é comum a presença de respiração laboriosa.
• Ocorrência de síncope e colapso em casos de estenose crítica da mitral ou tricúspide, obstrução grave da via de saída, arritmia associada ou insuficiência cardíaca por insuficiência das valvas AV.

Achados do Exame Físico
Displasia da Mitral
• Ausculta-se um sopro holossistólico sobre o ápice cardíaco à esquerda. Em casos de doença grave, o sopro é acompanhado por frêmito ou ritmo de galope. Um sopro diastólico tênue pode estar presente na mesma localização em animais com estenose da mitral, mas muitos animais acometidos não apresentam qualquer sopro audível. Em animais com obstruções dinâmicas da via de saída, é audível um sopro de ejeção sistólica que se intensifica durante atividade física ou agitação.
• Indícios de insuficiência cardíaca esquerda — em animais com defeitos graves, observam-se taquipneia, aumento dos esforços respiratórios, crepitações pulmonares e cianose.

Displasia da Tricúspide
• Ausculta-se um sopro holossistólico sobre o ápice cardíaco à direita. Em casos de doença grave, o sopro é acompanhado por frêmito ou ritmo de galope. A regurgitação tricúspide silenciosa está bem descrita em gatos, sendo atribuível a um orifício regurgitante amplo e ao fluxo regurgitante laminar. A distensão e a pulsação das veias jugulares externas podem ser evidentes.
• Indícios de insuficiência cardíaca direita — em casos de más-formações graves, verificam-se ascite e, mais raramente, edema periférico.

DIAGNÓSTICO

DIAGNÓSTICO DIFERENCIAL
• Com a exceção observada da idade de início, a insuficiência congênita das valvas AV assemelha-se à insuficiência degenerativa adquirida dessas valvas no que diz respeito aos achados anamnésicos, às anormalidades do exame físico e às sequelas clínicas.
• Algumas vezes, o sopro do lado direito produzido por insuficiência da tricúspide confunde-se com o sopro do mesmo lado decorrente de um defeito do septo ventricular.
• A ascite causada por regurgitação ou estenose silenciosas da tricúspide é frequentemente atribuída à efusão pericárdica, hepatopatia ou obstrução da veia cava caudal.
• Os cães e gatos com coração triatriado compartilham muitas das características clínicas de estenose das valvas AV.
• Não existe nenhuma forma incontestável para diferenciar a displasia da mitral geradora de obstrução da via de saída e a forma obstrutiva da miocardiopatia. Se a obstrução puder ser abolida com o uso de β-bloqueadores e a hipertrofia do ventrículo esquerdo desaparecer, é provável que a anormalidade primária seja uma displasia da mitral.

HEMOGRAMA/BIOQUÍMICA/URINÁLISE
Geralmente permanecem normais.

DIAGNÓSTICO POR IMAGEM
Achados Radiográficos
Displasia da Mitral
• Na presença de insuficiência valvar, há um aumento de volume do átrio e ventrículo esquerdos. Em caso de estenose valvar, ocorre aumento de volume apenas do átrio esquerdo. Na obstrução dinâmica da via de saída, observa-se um leve aumento de volume do átrio esquerdo.
• Indícios de insuficiência cardíaca esquerda — em casos graves, verificam-se a distensão das veias pulmonares e a formação de edema intersticial ou alveolar.

Displasia da Tricúspide
• Em casos de insuficiência valvar, constata-se um aumento de volume do átrio e ventrículo direitos. A silhueta cardíaca pode parecer globoide em aumentos acentuados de volume. Na estenose valvar, temos um aumento de volume somente do átrio direito.
• Indícios de insuficiência cardíaca direita — em casos graves, observam-se veia cava caudal dilatada, hepatoesplenomegalia ou ascite.

Ecocardiografia
Displasia da Mitral
• A insuficiência valvar resulta na dilatação do átrio esquerdo e na hipertrofia excêntrica do ventrículo esquerdo. Os músculos papilares ficam tipicamente achatados e deslocados no sentido dorsal. As cordas tendíneas encontram-se muitas vezes curtas e espessadas. A ecocardiografia Doppler demonstra um jato transmitral sistólico retrógrado de alta

DISPLASIA DAS VALVAS ATRIOVENTRICULARES

velocidade e velocidades modestamente elevadas do fluxo interno por meio da mitral.
• A estenose da mitral culmina em dilatação do átrio esquerdo, enquanto as dimensões do ventrículo esquerdo permanecem normais ou ficam pequenas. Os folhetos valvares encontram-se com frequência espessados, relativamente imóveis e muitas vezes fundidos. A ecocardiografia Doppler revela um jato transmitral diastólico de alta velocidade, associado a uma fração de ejeção reduzida. Também pode haver indícios de insuficiência mitral e/ou hipertensão pulmonar secundária concomitantes. Descartar a possibilidade de coração triatriado esquerdo.
• A obstrução dinâmica da via de saída do ventrículo esquerdo caracteriza-se por movimento sistólico do folheto anterior da mitral em direção ao septo interventricular, velocidades elevadas da via de saída do ventrículo esquerdo e hipertrofia concêntrica desse ventrículo.

Displasia da Tricúspide
• A insuficiência valvar resulta na dilatação do átrio direito e na hipertrofia excêntrica do ventrículo direito. Os músculos papilares e as cordas tendíneas podem estar fundidos, criando uma aparência de cortina na tricúspide. A ecocardiografia Doppler mostra um jato transtricúspide sistólico retrógrado de alta velocidade e velocidades discretamente elevadas do fluxo interno por meio da tricúspide.
• A estenose da tricúspide culmina na dilatação do átrio direito, associada a dimensões normais ou pequenas do ventrículo direito. Os folhetos valvares não se abrem completamente. A ecocardiografia Doppler exibe um jato transtricúspide diastólico de alta velocidade com fração de ejeção reduzida. Pode haver indícios de insuficiência concomitante da tricúspide e/ou desvio da direita para a esquerda por meio de um forame oval patente ou um defeito do septo atrial associado. Excluir a possibilidade de coração triatriado direito.

Cateterização Cardíaca
• Indicada apenas nos casos em que não foi possível confirmar o diagnóstico pela ecocardiografia ou quando se prevê a correção cirúrgica.
• Displasia da mitral — as mensurações hemodinâmicas devem incluir as pressões do ventrículo esquerdo, a pressão capilar pulmonar em cunha ou a mensuração direta da pressão do átrio esquerdo, além das pressões da artéria pulmonar; e, nos casos de obstrução dinâmica, o registro simultâneo das pressões aórtica e ventricular esquerda com estímulo clínico. Os estudos contrastados são feitos de forma mais eficiente por meio da injeção de contraste no ventrículo esquerdo nos casos de insuficiência valvar e injeção direta no átrio esquerdo via cateterização transeptal nos casos de estenose valvar.
• Displasia da tricúspide — as mensurações hemodinâmicas devem abranger as pressões tanto do átrio como do ventrículo direito. Os estudos contrastados são realizados com maior eficiência por meio da injeção de contraste no ventrículo direito nos casos de insuficiência valvar e injeção no átrio direito nos casos de estenose valvar.

MÉTODOS DIAGNÓSTICOS
Achados Eletrocardiográficos
Em geral, esses achados refletem um padrão de aumento de volume da câmara cardíaca. Os defeitos graves podem ser acompanhados por diversas arritmias, particularmente os batimentos atriais prematuros, taquicardia supraventricular ou fibrilação atrial.

TRATAMENTO
CUIDADO(S) DE SAÚDE ADEQUADO(S)
Em casos de ICC, é necessária a internação do paciente.
ORIENTAÇÃO AO PROPRIETÁRIO
É fundamental informá-lo a respeito da hereditariedade da condição e, consequentemente, aconselhá-lo contra o acasalamento de seus animais.
ATIVIDADE
Restrita, de acordo com a gravidade da doença.
DIETA
Dieta com restrição de sódio se a insuficiência cardíaca for manifesta ou iminente.
CONSIDERAÇÕES CIRÚRGICAS
• O reparo ou a substituição das valvas está disponível em alguns centros cirúrgicos.
• A valvoplastia por balão é, algumas vezes, eficaz para estenose valvar.

MEDICAÇÕES
MEDICAMENTO(S) DE ESCOLHA
• Displasia da mitral ou tricúspide associada à insuficiência — diuréticos, inibidores da ECA e pimobendana (0,3 mg/kg a cada 12 h) para pacientes com ICC manifesta ou iminente. A furosemida (2-4 mg/kg a cada 12-24 h) e o enalapril (0,5 mg/kg a cada 12 h) são utilizados para controlar a congestão. A digoxina (0,002-0,004 mg/kg a cada 12 h) é usada para controlar as taquiarritmias supraventriculares.
• Estenose da mitral ou tricúspide — para controlar o edema, empregam-se os diuréticos. Para solucionar a congestão, ajusta-se a dose da furosemida (2-4 mg/kg a cada 12-24 h). É recomendável manter a frequência cardíaca próxima a 150 bpm, utilizando a digoxina (0,002-0,004 mg/kg a cada 12 h), um bloqueador dos canais de cálcio, como o diltiazem (1,0-1,5 mg/kg a cada 8 h) ou um β-bloqueador, como o atenolol (0,5-1,5 mg/kg a cada 12-24 h).
• Obstrução dinâmica da via de saída — titular um β-bloqueador, como o atenolol (0,5-1,5 mg/kg a cada 12-24 h), para abolir ou diminuir a gravidade da obstrução.
PRECAUÇÕES
Monitorização-padrão do paciente, em busca dos efeitos colaterais provocados pelo medicamento cardíaco (p. ex., intoxicação por digitálicos e azotemia).

ACOMPANHAMENTO
MONITORIZAÇÃO DO PACIENTE
• Na ausência de sinais de insuficiência cardíaca, reavaliar anualmente. Mas, na presença desses sinais, reavaliar o paciente por, no mínimo, a cada 3 meses. É aconselhável a obtenção de radiografias torácicas, ECG e ecocardiografia.
PREVENÇÃO
Não acasalar os animais acometidos.
COMPLICAÇÕES POSSÍVEIS
• ICC: esquerda e direita em casos de displasia da mitral e tricúspide, respectivamente.
• Durante a atividade física, pode ocorrer colapso ou síncope.
• Com uma doença grave, observam-se taquicardia supraventricular paroxística ou fibrilação atrial.
EVOLUÇÃO ESPERADA E PROGNÓSTICO
• A evolução depende da gravidade do defeito subjacente.
• O prognóstico é reservado a mau em defeitos graves.

DIVERSOS
DISTÚRBIOS ASSOCIADOS
• A displasia da mitral costuma acompanhar a estenose aórtica valvular ou subvalvular, enquanto a displasia da tricúspide comumente se associa à estenose pulmonar.
GESTAÇÃO/FERTILIDADE/REPRODUÇÃO
É recomendável evitá-la em função da hereditariedade do defeito e da possível indução de descompensação ou agravamento da insuficiência cardíaca.
VER TAMBÉM
• Insuficiência Cardíaca Congestiva Direita.
• Insuficiência Cardíaca Congestiva Esquerda.
ABREVIATURAS
• AV = atrioventricular.
• ECA = enzima conversora de angiotensina.
• ECG = eletrocardiografia.
• ICC = insuficiência cardíaca congestiva.

Sugestões de Leitura
Bonagura JD, Lehmkuhl LB. Congenital heart disease. In: Fox PR, Sisson D, Moise NS. Textbook of Canine and Feline Cardiology: Principles and Clinical Practice, 2nd ed. Philadelphia: Saunders, 1999, pp. 520-526.
Oyama MA, Sisson DD, Thomas WP, Bonagura JD. Congenital heart disease. In: Ettinger SJ, Feldman EC, eds., Textbook of Veterinary Internal Medicine, 6th ed. St. Louis: Elsevier, 2005.
Strickland KN. Congenital heart disease. In: Tilley LP, Smith FWK, Oyama MA, Sleeper MM, eds., Manual of Canine and Feline Cardiology, 4th ed. St. Louis: Saunders Elsevier, 2008, pp. 215-239.

Autor David Sisson
Consultores Editoriais Larry P. Tilley e Francis W.K. Smith, Jr.

Displasia do Cotovelo

CONSIDERAÇÕES GERAIS

DEFINIÇÃO
Trata-se de um grupo de anormalidades de desenvolvimento que levam à má-formação e degeneração da articulação do cotovelo.

FISIOPATOLOGIA
• Quatro anormalidades — não união do processo ancôneo, osteocondrite dissecante, fragmentação do processo coronoide medial e incongruência; podem ocorrer de forma isolada ou em combinação; podem ser observadas em um ou ambos os cotovelos; a doença bilateral é comum (50% dos casos).
• Não união do processo ancôneo — caracterizada por fechamento tardio da placa de crescimento entre o processo ancôneo e a metáfise ulnar proximal (olécrano) por volta dos 5 meses de vida; pode resultar de um estresse mecânico anormal sobre o processo ancôneo.
• Osteocondrite dissecante — acomete a face medial do côndilo do úmero; um distúrbio na ossificação endocondral provoca retenção da cartilagem articular e o subsequente estresse mecânico leva à formação de lesão de retalho cartilaginoso.
• Fragmentação do processo coronoide medial — fragmentação ou fissura condrais ou osteocondrais do processo coronoide medial da ulna; trata-se de uma manifestação de osteocondrose do processo coronoide; o processo coronoide não possui um centro de ossificação separado; pode resultar de estresse mecânico anormal sobre o processo coronoide medial.
• Incongruência — o crescimento proximal assíncrono entre o rádio e a ulna pode conduzir à carga anormal, ao desgaste e à erosão da cartilagem no compartimento úmero-ulnar; possível má-formação da incisura troclear da ulna; uma incisura troclear levemente elíptica com diminuição no arco da curvatura mostra-se muito pequena para se articular com a tróclea umeral, o que resulta em maior contato em áreas do processo ancôneo, do processo coronoide e do côndilo umeral medial e pouco ou nenhum contato em outras áreas da tróclea.

SISTEMA(S) ACOMETIDO(S)
Musculosquelético.

GENÉTICA
• Doença hereditária.
• Alta hereditariedade — o índice de hereditariedade varia entre 0,25 e 0,45.

INCIDÊNCIA/PREVALÊNCIA
• Causa mais comum de dor e claudicação relacionadas com o cotovelo.
• Representa uma das causas mais comuns de claudicação dos membros torácicos em raças caninas de grande porte.

DISTRIBUIÇÃO GEOGRÁFICA
N/D.

IDENTIFICAÇÃO
Espécies
Cães.
Raça(s) Predominante(s)
Raças grandes e gigantes — Labrador retriever; Rottweiler; Golden retriever; Pastor alemão; cão Montanhês de Berna; Chow Chow; Bearded collie; Terra Nova.
Idade Média e Faixa Etária
• Idade de início dos sinais clínicos — tipicamente 4-10 meses.
• Idade no momento do diagnóstico — geralmente 4-18 meses.
• Idade dos sintomas relacionados com artropatia degenerativa — qualquer idade.
Sexo Predominante
• Fragmentação do processo coronoide medial — predisposição de machos.
• Não união do processo ancôneo, osteocondrite dissecante, incongruência — nenhuma predisposição estabelecida.

SINAIS CLÍNICOS
Comentários Gerais
• Claudicação — caso não se observe nenhuma anormalidade nítida ao exame físico ou nas radiografias, a intervenção inicial poderá exigir o uso de técnicas avançadas de diagnóstico por imagem.
• Nem todos os pacientes se apresentam sintomáticos quando jovens.
• É comum a ocorrência de episódio agudo de claudicação relacionada com o cotovelo decorrente de alterações de artropatia degenerativa avançada em pacientes adultos.
Achados Anamnésicos
Claudicação intermitente ou persistente dos membros torácicos — exacerbada por exercícios; exacerbação progressiva a partir de rigidez observada somente após o repouso.
Achados do Exame Físico
• Dor — eliciada à hiperflexão ou extensão do cotovelo; desencadeada ao se manter o cotovelo e o carpo a 90°, enquanto o carpo é posicionado em pronação e supinação.
• Membro acometido — tendência a ser mantido em abdução e supinação.
• Efusão da articulação e distensão da cápsula articular — observados especialmente entre o epicôndilo lateral e o olécrano.
• Crepitação — pode ser palpada em casos de artropatia degenerativa avançada.
• Diminuição na amplitude dos movimentos.

CAUSAS
• Genéticas.
• Evolutivas (i. e., de desenvolvimento).
• Nutricionais.

FATORES DE RISCO
• Crescimento e ganho de peso rápidos.
• Dieta rica em calorias.

DIAGNÓSTICO

DIAGNÓSTICO DIFERENCIAL
• Traumatismo.
• Artrite séptica.
• Panosteíte.
• Avulsão ou calcificação dos músculos flexores.
• Sarcoma de células sinoviais.

HEMOGRAMA/BIOQUÍMICA/URINÁLISE
N/D.

OUTROS TESTES LABORATORIAIS
N/D.

DIAGNÓSTICO POR IMAGEM
Radiografia
• Obter imagens de ambos os cotovelos — alta incidência de doença bilateral.
• A artropatia degenerativa do cotovelo é identificada pela presença de osteófitos na margem cranial da cabeça do rádio e dos epicôndilos (medial e lateral), bem como no processo coronoide medial; também é comum a constatação de esclerose da ulna caudal ao processo coronoide e à incisura troclear, além de uma inclinação escalonada entre a superfície articular do rádio e o processo coronoide lateral; em casos de não união do processo ancôneo, osteocondrite dissecante, fragmentação do processo coronoide medial e incongruência, essas alterações também podem ser observadas.
• Não união do processo ancôneo — diagnosticada de forma mais eficiente a partir da projeção médio-lateral hiperflexionada; pode-se observar com facilidade a falta de união óssea.
• Osteocondrite dissecante — diagnosticada com maior eficiência a partir das projeções craniocaudal e craniocaudal/látero-medial oblíqua; revela a presença de defeito radiotransparente ou achatamento da face medial do côndilo umeral.
• Fragmentação do processo coronoide medial — pode não ser visualizada em alguns casos; o diagnóstico é, portanto, presuntivo, com base em lesões de artropatia degenerativa e na ausência de lesões típicas da não união do processo ancôneo ou da osteocondrite dissecante; comumente se observa a formação de osteófitos na superfície caudoproximal do processo ancôneo em casos de fragmentação do processo coronoide medial.
Outros
TC, RM e tomografia linear — fornecem provas mais definitivas quanto à presença de fragmentos não deslocados ou fissuras.

MÉTODOS DIAGNÓSTICOS
• Punção da articulação e análise do líquido sinovial — confirmam o envolvimento articular.
• Líquido sinovial — deve ter coloração amarelo-palha, com viscosidade normal a reduzida; a citologia revela <10.000 células nucleadas/μL (>90% são células mononucleares); os resultados normais não descartam necessariamente o diagnóstico. • Artroscopia — pode ajudar no diagnóstico de não união do processo ancôneo, fragmentação do processo coronoide medial e osteocondrite dissecante.

ACHADOS PATOLÓGICOS
• Não união do processo ancôneo — união fibrosa entre o processo ancôneo e a metáfise ulnar proximal; invasão de tecido fibroso e degeneração do processo ancôneo; artropatia degenerativa.
• Osteocondrite dissecante — retalho condral no côndilo umeral medial; esclerose do osso subcondral subjacente com invasão de tecido fibroso; lesão erosiva na cartilagem coronoide justaposta; artropatia degenerativa.
• Fragmentação do processo coronoide medial — fragmentação condral ou osteocondral da extremidade cranial ou da margem lateral do processo coronoide medial; lesão erosiva sobre a cartilagem da face medial justaposta do côndilo umeral; artropatia degenerativa.
• Incongruência — lesões erosivas que envolvem parte ou todo o processo coronoide medial e a cartilagem articular justaposta da face medial do

côndilo umeral; artropatia degenerativa; estriações lineares na cartilagem articular.

TRATAMENTO

CUIDADO(S) DE SAÚDE ADEQUADO(S)
Cirurgia — controversa, mas recomendada na maioria dos pacientes.

CUIDADO(S) DE ENFERMAGEM
• Aplicação de compressas frias sobre a articulação do cotovelo — realizar imediatamente após a cirurgia para ajudar a diminuir a tumefação articular e controlar a dor; aplicar por, no mínimo, 5-10 min a cada 8 h durante 3-5 dias.
• Exercícios com amplitude de movimentos — benéficos até que o paciente consiga sustentar seu peso no(s) membro(s).

ATIVIDADE
Restringir para todos os pacientes no período pós-operatório.

DIETA
• Controle do peso — importante para diminuir a carga e a tensão sobre a(s) articulação(ões) acometida(s).
• Restrição do ganho de peso e do crescimento em cães jovens — pode diminuir a incidência e a gravidade.

ORIENTAÇÃO AO PROPRIETÁRIO
• Discutir sobre a hereditariedade da doença.
• Analisar o potencial de evolução da artropatia degenerativa.
• Examinar a influência do consumo excessivo de nutrientes que promovem o crescimento rápido.

CONSIDERAÇÕES CIRÚRGICAS
• Gravidade da artropatia degenerativa e idade avançada do paciente — influenciam negativamente o resultado.
• Não união do processo ancôneo — há quatro opções: remoção, fixação com parafuso de efeito compressivo, osteotomia ulnar proximal dinâmica e fixação com parafuso de efeito compressivo associada à osteotomia proximal dinâmica; a decisão é tomada com base no grau da artropatia degenerativa, na idade do paciente e na habilidade do cirurgião.
• Osteocondrite dissecante e fragmentação do processo coronoide medial — abordagem medial ao cotovelo (não é necessária a diferenciação diagnóstica); remoção de fragmento(s) solto(s).
• Incongruência — controversa; há quatro opções: tratamento conservativo sem cirurgia, coronoidectomia, osteotomia ulnar proximal dinâmica, osteotomia intra-articular; a decisão baseia-se no tipo de incongruência, no grau da artropatia degenerativa, na idade do paciente e na habilidade do cirurgião.
• Diagnóstico e tratamento artroscópicos — opção excelente em casos de fragmentação do processo coronoide medial, osteocondrite dissecante e incongruência; benefícios: visualização superior e invasividade mínima.

MEDICAÇÕES

MEDICAMENTO(S) DE ESCOLHA
• Nenhum que promova a consolidação dos fragmentos osteocondrais ou condrais.
• AINEs — minimizam a dor, diminuem a inflamação e tratam a artropatia degenerativa associada de forma sintomática.
• Deracoxibe (3-4 mg/kg VO a cada 24 h, mastigável).
• Carprofeno (2,2 mg/kg VO a cada 12 ou 24 h).
• Etodolaco (10-15 mg/kg VO a cada 24 h).
• Meloxicam (dose de ataque 0,2 mg/kg VO, depois 0,1 mg/kg VO a cada 24 h — na forma líquida).
• Tepoxalina (dose de ataque 20 mg/kg, depois 10 mg/kg VO a cada 24 h).

CONTRAINDICAÇÕES
Evitar os corticosteroides — efeitos colaterais em potencial; danos à cartilagem articular associados ao uso a longo prazo.

PRECAUÇÕES
AINEs — a irritação gastrintestinal pode impedir seu emprego em alguns pacientes.

INTERAÇÕES POSSÍVEIS
N/D.

MEDICAMENTO(S) ALTERNATIVO(S)
Medicamentos condroprotetores (p. ex., glicosaminoglicanos polissulfatados, glicosamina e sulfato de condroitina) — podem ajudar a limitar a degeneração e o dano cartilaginosos; também podem ajudar a aliviar a dor e a inflamação.

ACOMPANHAMENTO

MONITORIZAÇÃO DO PACIENTE
• Pós-cirúrgica — limitar a atividade por, no mínimo, 4 semanas; estimular precocemente os movimentos ativos da(s) articulação(ões) acometida(s).
• Exames anuais — recomendados para avaliar a evolução da artropatia degenerativa.

PREVENÇÃO
• Desestimular a reprodução de animais acometidos.
• Não repetir acasalamentos entre reprodutores que resultem em ninhadas comprometidas.

COMPLICAÇÕES POSSÍVEIS
N/D.

EVOLUÇÃO ESPERADA E PROGNÓSTICO
• Evolução da artropatia degenerativa — esperada.
• Prognóstico — de razoável a bom para todas as formas.

DIVERSOS

DISTÚRBIOS ASSOCIADOS
N/D.

FATORES RELACIONADOS COM A IDADE
Os cães de meia-idade a idosos com artropatia degenerativa avançada não são candidatos à intervenção cirúrgica.

POTENCIAL ZOONÓTICO
N/D.

GESTAÇÃO/FERTILIDADE/REPRODUÇÃO
N/D.

SINÔNIMO(S)
Osteocondrose do cotovelo.

VER TAMBÉM
Osteocondrose

ABREVIATURA(S)
• AINEs = anti-inflamatórios não esteroides.
• RM = ressonância magnética.
• TC = tomografia computadorizada.

Sugestões de Leitura
Fujita Y, Schulz KS, Mason DR, Kass PH, Stover SM. Effect of humeral osteotomy on joint surface contact in canine elbow joints. Am J Vet Res 2003, 64(4):506-511.

Haudiquet PR, Marcellin-Little DJ, Stebbins ME. Use of the distomedial-proximolateral oblique radiographic view of the elbow joint for examination of the medial coronoid process in dogs. Am J Vet Res 2002, 63(7):1000-1005.

Hornof WJ, Wind AP, Wallack ST, Schulz KS. Canine elbow dysplasia: The early radiographic detection of fragmentation of the coronoid process. Vet Clin North Am Small Anim Pract 2000, 30(2):257-266.

Janutta V, Hamann H, Klein S, Tellhelm B, Distl O. Genetic analysis of three different classification protocols for the evaluation of elbow dysplasia in German shepherd dogs. J Small Anim Pract 2006, 47(2):75-82.

Janutta V, Hamann H, Klein S, Tellhelm B, Distl O. Genetic evaluation of elbow angles as predictors of elbow dysplasia in German shepherd dogs. J Vet Med A Physiol Pathol Clin Med 2005, 52(5):254-261.

Remy D, Neuhart L, Fau D, Genevois JP. Canine elbow dysplasia and primary lesions in German shepherd dogs in France. J Small Anim Pract 2004, 45(5):244-248.

Sallander MH, Hedhammar A, Trogen ME. Diet, exercise, and weight as risk factors in hip dysplasia and elbow arthrosis in Labrador retrievers. J Nutr 2006, 136 (7 Suppl):2050S-2052S.

Samoy Y, Van Ryssen B, Gielen I, Walschot N, van Bree H. Review of the literature: Elbow incongruity in the dog. Vet Comp Orthop Traumatol 2006, 19(1):1-8.

Snelling SR, Lavelle RB. Radiographic changes in elbow dysplasia following ulnar osteotomy—a case report and review of the literature. Australian Vet J 2004, 82(5):278-281.

Autor Peter K. Shires
Consultor Editorial Peter K. Shires
Agradecimento O autor e os editores agradecem a colaboração de Peter D. Schwarz, que foi o autor deste capítulo em uma edição mais antiga.

Displasia Microvascular Hepatoportal

CONSIDERAÇÕES GERAIS

DEFINIÇÃO
• Anormalidade vascular intra-hepática que causa desvio intra-hepático entre a circulação portal e a sistêmica. • Lesões histológicas: (1) mau desenvolvimento de ramos terciários da veia porta; (2) mau posicionamento das vênulas hepáticas adjacentes às tríades portais ou dentro dessas tríades; (3) músculo liso proeminente (estrangulamento da musculatura das vênulas hepáticas que controla o fluxo sanguíneo por meio do fígado) sugere um efeito fisiológico de fluxo arterializado sinusoidal. • Envolvimento inconsistente de lobos hepáticos: alguns lobos gravemente acometidos (desvio completo), alguns com perfusão portal diminuída, outros normais. • Característica clinicopatológica: aumento dos ácidos biliares séricos totais. • Associada à anomalia vascular portossistêmica em parentescos de cães de pequeno porte; explica a falha de normalização dos ácidos biliares séricos totais após a oclusão completa da anomalia vascular portossistêmica em alguns cães e a incapacidade de atenuação completa dessa anomalia em outros. • O diagnóstico de displasia microvascular é confundido por uma definição histológica inapropriada de hipoplasia portal na literatura veterinária. Qualquer causa adquirida de desvio portal a sistêmico extra-hepático (fluxo sanguíneo hepatofugal) gera características histológicas idênticas, conforme observado em displasia microvascular e anomalia vascular portossistêmica. A hipoplasia indica a falta de desenvolvimento que não pode ser discernida na biopsia do fígado.

FISIOPATOLOGIA
• Más-formações vasculares indutoras de comprometimento na perfusão venosa portal intra-hepática (desvio pelo fígado). • Encefalopatia hepática: rara.

SISTEMA(S) ACOMETIDO(S)
• Gastrintestinal — quando sintomática, muito frequentemente se observam sinais gastrintestinais vagos: vômito, diarreia, inapetência em virtude de enteropatia inflamatória. • Hepatobiliar — encefalopatia hepática: rara a inexistente, altamente sugestiva de anomalia vascular portossistêmica não identificada ou diagnóstico errôneo de encefalopatia hepática. • Renal/urológico — encontro de cristalúria/urolitíase por biurato de amônio; sugere anomalia vascular portossistêmica não identificada.

GENÉTICA
• Hereditária em certas raças de pequeno porte; p. ex., Yorkshire terrier, Maltês, Cairn terrier, Spaniel tibetano, Shih tzu, Havanese, Norfolk terrier, Schnauzer miniatura, Pug, outras. • Herança — complexa; poligênica autossômica dominante de penetrância incompleta. Os ácidos biliares séricos totais são utilizados como marcadores fenotípicos. • Progenitores sem o problema podem ter progênie acometida.

INCIDÊNCIA/PREVALÊNCIA
A prevalência em certas raças caninas de pequeno porte varia de 30 a 80%; ver anteriormente.

DISTRIBUIÇÃO GEOGRÁFICA
Mundial.

IDENTIFICAÇÃO
Espécies
Cães.

Raça(s) Predominante(s)
• Restrita a raças caninas de pequeno porte, especialmente nas raças supramencionadas. • Rara a inexistente em raças caninas de grande porte.

Idade Média e Faixa Etária
Congênita; detectada em animais jovens assintomáticos (por volta de 4-6 meses de idade), já com 6 semanas de vida, utilizando os ácidos biliares séricos totais com teste de amostras pareadas ou relação de ácidos biliares: creatinina na urina (4-8 h após a alimentação).

SINAIS CLÍNICOS
Comentários Gerais
• Embora dois grupos (assintomático e sintomático) tenham sido descritos em termos históricos, é muito provável que os cães sintomáticos apresentem anomalia vascular portossistêmica. • A displasia microvascular é identificada durante avaliações diagnósticas ou triagens de rotina para problemas de saúde não relacionados ou em teste de ácidos biliares séricos totais de rotina em raças e parentescos com alta prevalência conhecida do traço para anomalia vascular portossistêmica/displasia microvascular. • É preciso tomar cuidado para descartar outras causas de aumento dos ácidos biliares séricos totais antes que os sinais clínicos sejam atribuídos à displasia microvascular; doenças concomitantes podem complicar a interpretação dos ácidos biliares séricos totais. • A displasia microvascular sem complicação não é associada à hipertensão portal e ascite.

Achados Anamnésicos
• Cães assintomáticos — apresentam, em geral, nada digno de nota no histórico; ocasionalmente, exibem recuperação anestésica demorada ou intolerância a medicamentos. • Cães sintomáticos — representam aqueles com anomalia vascular portossistêmica erroneamente classificada como displasia microvascular; queixas inespecíficas (anorexia, letargia, vômitos ou diarreia) relacionadas com enteropatia inflamatória concomitante; recuperação lenta de anestesia ou sedação injetável ou oral com certos agentes.

Achados do Exame Físico
Nada digno de nota.

CAUSAS
Distúrbio hereditário congênito.

FATORES DE RISCO
Raças puras de pequeno porte.

DIAGNÓSTICO

DIAGNÓSTICO DIFERENCIAL
• Anomalia vascular portossistêmica — qualquer cão jovem assintomático com aumento nos valores de ácidos biliares séricos totais ou em qualquer cão jovem com encefalopatia hepática; 20% dos cães assintomáticos têm anomalia vascular portossistêmica. • Sintomáticos (com mais de 2 anos de idade) — desvio portossistêmico adquirido atribuído a hepatopatias inflamatórias, infiltrativas, neoplásicas ou tóxicas agudas ou crônicas. • Qualquer distúrbio que diminua a perfusão hepática portal demonstra aspectos histopatológicos idênticos, caracterizados por arterialização, e diminui a visualização da veia porta. Certos distúrbios, como atresia venosa portal (hipoplasia portal intra-hepática verdadeira) e hipertensão portal não cirrótica (hipoperfusão portal adquirida, envolvendo ramos portais terciários), são associados aos quadros de hipertensão portal, ascite e desvio portossistêmico adquirido.

HEMOGRAMA/BIOQUÍMICA/URINÁLISE
• Hemograma completo — geralmente normal. • Bioquímica — em geral, não há nada digno de nota; a atividade das enzimas hepáticas costuma permanecer normal (exceto fosfatase alcalina alta em pacientes jovens em virtude do crescimento ósseo); hipoglobulinemia ou hipoalbuminemia leves observadas em cerca de 50% dos pacientes jovens. Elevação das enzimas ALT e AST em cães com lesão degenerativa/inflamatória adquirida na zona 3; observada em cães com enteropatia inflamatória concomitante. A hiperamonemia não foi documentada em displasia microvascular não complicada. • Urinálise — densidade urinária dentro da faixa de normalidade, mas sem cristalúria por biurato de amônio.

OUTROS TESTES LABORATORIAIS
Ácidos biliares séricos totais
• Estimativas pré e pós-prandiais — teste diagnóstico recomendado; valores >25 μmol/L confirmam função ou perfusão hepáticas anormais. • Padrão de desvio — comum (concentrações pós-prandiais de ácidos biliares séricos totais muito superiores às pré-prandiais); observado também em casos de anomalia vascular portossistêmica e desvio portossistêmico adquirido; 15-20% dos cães apresentam níveis mais altos de ácidos biliares séricos totais em jejum do que pós-prandiais. • Generalização — a magnitude do aumento é menor na displasia microvascular do que na anomalia vascular portossistêmica, mas a sobreposição de valores diminui a capacidade dos ácidos biliares séricos totais em distinguir os distúrbios. • Diferenças quantitativas nos valores anormais de ácidos biliares séricos totais não são capazes de diferenciar a "gravidade" das lesões histológicas da displasia microvascular nem determinar de forma seriada a alteração no estado do paciente.

Estudos de Depuração
• Cães da raça Cairn terrier com displasia microvascular demonstram uma depuração reduzida de ânions orgânicos por meio do corante verde de indocianina, confirmando a perfusão hepática diminuída; o verde de indocianina tem baixa utilidade clínica.

Proteína C
• A maioria dos cães com displasia microvascular apresenta atividade normal da proteína C, em comparação àqueles com anomalia vascular portossistêmica sintomática com baixa atividade dessa proteína (<70%).

DIAGNÓSTICO POR IMAGEM
• Radiografia abdominal — sem micro-hepatia ou renomegalia, conforme observadas na anomalia vascular portossistêmica. • Ultrassonografia abdominal — sem desvio macroscópico de vaso, como constatado na anomalia vascular portossistêmica; fígado geralmente de tamanho normal; um ultrassonografista experiente pode suspeitar de hipoperfusão hepática portal. • Portovenografia mesentérica — falha em demonstrar anomalia vascular portossistêmica e anormalidades sutis da microvasculatura portal. **Cuidado:** na anomalia vascular portossistêmica, o vaso com desvio poderá passar despercebido se a portografia for concluída apenas em um único decúbito. • Cintilografia colorretal — frações de desvio normais ou levemente aumentadas na displasia microvascular; exclui desvio macroscópico (como na anomalia vascular portossistêmica ou no desvio portossistêmico adquirido). A perfusão diferencial de lobo pode ser evidente.

MÉTODOS DIAGNÓSTICOS
• Biopsia do fígado — é importante obter amostras de vários lobos hepáticos, pois a displasia microvascular não afeta os lobos hepáticos uniformemente; evitar a amostragem do lobo caudado, pois ele é o menos acometido. • Exame microscópico do tecido hepático — necessário para obter o diagnóstico definitivo e descartar outros distúrbios que provocam aumento nos valores dos ácidos biliares séricos totais. • Biopsias com agulha — podem não obter tecido suficiente para o diagnóstico definitivo e também limita a amostragem a um ou dois lobos. • Amostras em cunha ou obtidas à laparoscopia — são confiáveis para o diagnóstico. • A biopsia não é capaz de diferenciar entre displasia microvascular e anomalia vascular portossistêmica em grande parte dos casos em virtude dos aspectos histológicos semelhantes. • Também é impossível distinguir a causa da hipoperfusão portal a partir das características presentes em hiperfusão portal não cirrótica ou anomalia vascular portossistêmica atribuída a oclusão/trombo venoso portal extra-hepático.

ACHADOS PATOLÓGICOS
Macroscópicos
• Fígado de aspecto e tamanho normais. • Alguns lobos hepáticos podem parecer pequenos.
Microscópicos
• Displasia microvascular — provoca lesões compatíveis com hipoperfusão portal, conforme observado em anomalia vascular portossistêmica; no entanto, essas lesões costumam ser menos pronunciadas quando todos os outros lobos hepáticos são considerados (alguns lobos não são acometidos ou minimamente afetados); as veias portas são observadas. • Pequenas vênulas portais não perfundidas ou ausentes em algumas tríades portais, enquanto outros exibem vênulas portais de aspecto normal; vasos linfáticos proeminentes; múltiplos cortes transversais de arteríola portal; tríades portais juvenis, atrofia lobular em alguns lobos hepáticos, lipogranulomas dispersos (contêm hemossiderina); musculatura estrangulada proeminente espessa de vênulas hepáticas; alguns cães apresentam vacuolização e inflamação não supurativa na zona 3, que colidem com as vênulas hepáticas (tal lesão costuma estar associada à enteropatia inflamatória). • Nota: a biopsia do fígado em qualquer cão com idade igual ou inferior a 4 meses pode demonstrar tríades portais juvenis.

TRATAMENTO
CUIDADO(S) DE SAÚDE ADEQUADO(S)
• Pacientes assintomáticos — não é recomendado nenhum cuidado médico específico.
• Medicamentos inadequados para prescrição: ácido ursodesoxicólico, S-adenosilmetionina, silibinina (cardo mariano) ou restrição de proteína na dieta se houver apenas displasia microvascular. Sinais gastrintestinais: vômitos ou diarreia prolongados — internar o paciente para o fornecimento de cuidados de suporte e avaliações diagnósticas; esses cães apresentam outros distúrbios ou displasia microvascular complicada (ver "Encefalopatia Hepática"; "Anomalia Vascular Portossistêmica Congênita"; ou "Enteropatia Inflamatória").
• Raramente, os cães com alterações degenerativas na zona 3 desenvolvem uma hepatopatia, que leva à disfunção hepática progressiva, hipertensão portal e ascite; o diagnóstico requer biopsia e imagens do fígado, além do tratamento para insuficiência hepática e ascite. • A displasia microvascular associada à inflamação não supurativa da zona 3 (envolvendo, sobretudo, eosinófilos) e associada à enteropatia inflamatória pode necessitar de dexametasona em baixas doses (0,05 mg/kg VO a cada 48-72 h; a dexametasona é utilizada para evitar os efeitos mineralocorticoides); dieta hipoalergênica; metronidazol em baixas doses (7,5 mg/kg VO a cada 12 h); em caso de atividade baixa da proteína C: adicione uma dose mínima de ácido acetilsalicílico (0,5 mg/kg VO a cada 24-48 h). Lesões na zona 3 podem predispor à oclusão tromboembólica de vênulas hepáticas.

DIETA
• A maioria dos cães com displasia microvascular não necessita de uma dieta com restrição proteica.
• Os cães com encefalopatia hepática provavelmente apresentam doenças adquiridas ou anomalia vascular portossistêmica — ver "Encefalopatia Hepática".

ORIENTAÇÃO AO PROPRIETÁRIO
• Orientar os criadores que, atualmente, a displasia microvascular não pode ser selecionada para o abate a partir de um parentesco com base em testes; progenitores com ácidos biliares séricos totais normais têm gerado progênie acometida; o exame dos ácidos biliares séricos totais em progênie F_1 e F_2 é o único método para definir a melhor estratégia reprodutiva no momento.
• Avisar os proprietários que os valores de ácidos biliares séricos totais não podem ser usados para classificar a gravidade da displasia microvascular.
• O teste de ácidos biliares séricos totais é valioso para identificar a displasia microvascular em cães jovens para evitar confusão diagnóstica no futuro em adultos com doenças não hepáticas.

MEDICAÇÕES
MEDICAMENTO(S) DE ESCOLHA
Para encefalopatia hepática — ver "Encefalopatia Hepática".
PRECAUÇÕES
Cuidado com reações adversas a medicamentos que dependem de remoção ou metabolismo hepáticos de primeira passagem para ser eliminados.

ACOMPANHAMENTO
MONITORIZAÇÃO DO PACIENTE
• Cães assintomáticos — sem recomendações específicas; o acompanhamento a longo prazo de cães sem lesão na zona 3 (descrita anteriormente) não revelou deterioração progressiva na função do fígado nem encurtamento no tempo de vida. • Não é aconselhável a repetição dos testes de ácidos biliares séricos totais, pois os valores permanecem anormais e exibem pequena variação fisiológica.

PREVENÇÃO
• No presente momento, não é possível tecer recomendações para eliminar a displasia microvascular de linhagem genética ou raça em particular. Com base nas informações obtidas de grandes pedigrees de Yorkshire terrier, Cairn terrier, Spaniel tibetano, Maltês, Shih tzu e Havanese, o acasalamento de progenitores não acometidos não elimina a displasia microvascular de uma família.
• Em famílias com alta incidência — permanecer vigilante em relação a cães vagamente enfermos que possam ter anomalia vascular portossistêmica; a anomalia vascular portossistêmica pode passar despercebida pela exploração cirúrgica, assim como pela portovenografia (estudo em um único decúbito); a cintilografia colorretal é capaz de detectar desvio portossistêmico de forma definitiva (fluxo sanguíneo hepatofugal); a atividade da proteína C ajuda a diferenciar cães com anomalia vascular portossistêmica daqueles com displasia microvascular (anomalia vascular portossistêmica: atividade baixa; displasia microvascular: atividade normal).

EVOLUÇÃO ESPERADA E PROGNÓSTICO
• A maioria dos cães acometidos com displasia microvascular permanece assintomática e vive uma vida normal. • Foi documentado um aumento progressivo de valores anormais dos ácidos biliares séricos totais com a idade (juvenil a adulta). • Os cães com a lesão na zona 3 descrita antes podem desenvolver hepatopatia progressiva, que leva a alterações como encefalopatia hepática, hipertensão portal, desvio portossistêmico adquirido, ascite e, raramente, tromboembolia venosa portal.

DIVERSOS
DISTÚRBIOS ASSOCIADOS
As raças caninas de pequeno porte com alta incidência de anomalia vascular portossistêmica são acometidas com maior frequência.

FATORES RELACIONADOS COM A IDADE
Os ácidos biliares séricos totais podem ser usados para fazer a triagem de cães jovens (16 semanas de vida) em raças que sabidamente têm alta prevalência de anomalia vascular portossistêmica e displasia microvascular.

GESTAÇÃO/FERTILIDADE/REPRODUÇÃO
As cadelas assintomáticas acometidas podem levar a gestação a termo.

SINÔNIMO(S)
• Hipoperfusão portal congênita, mas não hipoplasia portal (ver anteriormente). • Displasia microvascular hepática. • Atresia venosa portal intra-hepática. • Displasia portovascular microscópica.

VER TAMBÉM
• Encefalopatia Hepática. • Hepatopatia Fibrosante Juvenil. • Desvio Portossistêmico Adquirido. • Anomalia Vascular Portossistêmica Congênita.

ABREVIATURA(S)
• ALT = alanina aminotransferase. • AST = aspartato aminotransferase. • GI = gastrintestinal.

Sugestões de Leitura
Allen L, Stobie D, Mauldin GN, Baer KE. Clinicopathological features of dogs with hepatic microvascular dysplasia with and without portosystemic shunts: 42 cases (1991-1996). JAVMA 2000, 214(5):218-220.
Schermerhorn T, Center SA, Dykes NL, Rowland PH, et al. Characterization of hepatoportal microvascular dysplasia in a kindred of cairn terriers. J Vet Intern Med 1996, 10:219-230.

Autores Thomas Schermerhorn e Sharon A. Center
Consultor Editorial Sharon A. Center

Dispneia e Angústia Respiratória

CONSIDERAÇÕES GERAIS

DEFINIÇÃO
Dispneia — termo subjetivo que, na medicina humana, significa "uma sensação desconfortável na respiração" ou uma sensação de falta de ar; na medicina veterinária, esse termo descreve uma dificuldade ou angústia respiratória.

FISIOPATOLOGIA
Acredita-se que a dispneia e a angústia respiratória ocorram quando o sistema nervoso central nota uma diferença entre o *feedback* aferente proveniente de um determinado sinal de controle motor eferente (ventilação requerida) e o que o cérebro havia previsto como seria a resposta aferente adequada (ventilação obtida).

SISTEMA(S) ACOMETIDO(S)
Respiratório.

IDENTIFICAÇÃO
Cães e gatos; não há predileção racial, etária nem sexual.

SINAIS CLÍNICOS

Achados Anamnésicos
• Início agudo ou crônico. • Podem ser associados a tosse, taquipneia, intolerância a exercício.

Achados do Exame Físico
• Sinais gerais de angústia respiratória — esforço abdominal aumentado, rubor nasal (especialmente em gatos), respiração de boca aberta, extensão do pescoço, abdução do cotovelo; outros sinais dependem da causa subjacente. • Doença nasal — estertor, ausência de fluxo de ar pelas narinas; a dispneia melhora com a respiração de boca aberta. • Doença das vias aéreas superiores (anteriores)/laringe — estridor, hipertermia, dispneia à inspiração. • Obstrução fixa, como massa ou corpo estranho em alguma via aérea calibrosa — dispneia à inspiração e expiração. • Colapso traqueal — tosse grasnante. • Doença das vias aéreas inferiores (posteriores) — tosse, sibilos expiratórios à auscultação, esforço abdominal. • Pneumopatia parenquimatosa — pode exibir crepitações à auscultação; pode permanecer normal à auscultação. • Pneumonia — febre, sensibilidade da traqueia. • Edema pulmonar cardiogênico — sopro cardíaco, hipotermia, mucosas pálidas, tempo de preenchimento capilar deficiente. • Doença do espaço pleural — ruídos respiratórios diminuídos; porção ventral —líquido; porção dorsal — ar. • Comprometimento da parede torácica — frequentemente padrão respiratório paradoxal, traumatismo visível ou palpável.
• Tromboembolia pulmonar — pode apresentar sinais clínicos da doença subjacente, que predispõe à trombose, p. ex., hiperadrenocorticismo, anemia hemolítica imunomediada, neoplasia. • Outros sinais pertencerão à doença subjacente, p. ex., choque, traumatismo.

CAUSAS E FATORES DE RISCO

Doença das Vias Aéreas Superiores (Anteriores)
• Obstrução nasal — estenose das narinas (pólipos); infecção; inflamação; neoplasia; traumatismo; coagulopatia.
• Faringe — alongamento do palato mole; corpo estranho; neoplasia.
• Laringe — paralisia laríngea; eversão dos sáculos laríngeos; edema; colapso; corpo estranho; neoplasia; traumatismo; formação de malha tecidual.
• Porção cervical da traqueia — colapso; estenose; traumatismo; corpo estranho; neoplasia; parasitas.

Doença das Vias Aéreas Inferiores (Posteriores)
• Porção torácica da traqueia — ver a descrição sobre a porção cervical da traqueia; compressão extraluminal — linfadenopatia; aumento de volume do átrio esquerdo; tumores da base do coração.

Doença das Vias Aéreas de Pequeno Calibre
• Alérgica; inflamatória; infecciosa (*Mycoplasma*); parasitária; neoplásica (carcinoma broncogênico).

Pneumopatia Parenquimatosa
• Edema — edema cardiogênico ou não cardiogênico.
• Pneumonia — infecciosa; parasitária; por aspiração; eosinofílica; intersticial.
• Neoplasia (primária ou metastática).
• Inflamatória — síndrome da angústia respiratória aguda; pneumonite urêmica.
• Hemorragia — traumatismo; coagulopatia.
• Tromboembolia pulmonar — anemia hemolítica imunomediada; nefropatia ou enteropatia com perda de proteínas; dirofilariose; hiperadrenocorticismo; neoplasia.

Doença do Espaço Pleural
• Pneumotórax — traumático; secundário à pneumopatia parenquimatosa; ruptura de bolhas; migração de corpo estranho; espontânea.
• Efusão pleural — observação de transudatos, exsudatos; hemotórax; quilotórax.
• Tecidos moles — neoplasia; hérnia diafragmática.

Comprometimento da Parede Torácica
• Pneumotórax aberto — traumatismo; segmento frouxo — traumatismo; neoplasia; paralisia por botulismo, polirradiculoneurite, paralisia por carrapato, miastenia grave.

Distensão Abdominal
• Organomegalia — hiperplasia; neoplasia; gestação; obesidade; ascite; dilatação/torção gástrica.

DIAGNÓSTICO

DIAGNÓSTICO DIFERENCIAL
• Dispneia inspiratória — indicativa de doença das vias aéreas superiores (anteriores).
• Dispneia expiratória — sugestiva de doença intratorácica das vias aéreas.
• Pode ocorrer dispneia à inspiração e expiração em casos de obstruções fixas das vias aéreas superiores (anteriores) e doença intratorácica grave.
• Insuficiência cardíaca congestiva — sopro, taquicardia, qualidade deficiente do pulso, pulsos jugulares, hipotermia, crepitações à auscultação, secreção nasal líquida.

HEMOGRAMA/BIOQUÍMICA/URINÁLISE
• Anemia — pode causar dispneia não respiratória.
• Policitemia — hipóxia crônica.
• Leucograma inflamatório — pneumonia, piotórax.
• Trombocitose — hiperadrenocorticismo predispõe à tromboembolia pulmonar.
• Relação sódio: potássio <27 — constatação possível em casos de efusões quilosas pleurais ou abdominais.
• Fosfatase alcalina elevada — hiperadrenocorticismo predispõe à tromboembolia pulmonar.
• Azotemia — se grave, poderá levar à pneumonite urêmica.
• Proteinúria — pode predispor à tromboembolia pulmonar.
• Falência múltipla de órgãos — SARA.
• Hipoproteinemia — pode sugerir doença com perda de proteínas, capaz de predispor à tromboembolia pulmonar.

OUTROS TESTES LABORATORIAIS
• Teste de dirofilariose.
• Análise do líquido pleural.
• Gasometria sanguínea — pode ajudar a determinar a gravidade da angústia respiratória do paciente.
• PaO_2 — pressão parcial de oxigênio dissolvido no sangue arterial; normoxemia: PaO_2 de 80-120 mmHg (ar ambiente, nível do mar), hipoxemia: PaO_2 <80 mmHg, hiperoxemia: PaO_2 >120 mmHg; F_IO_2 — a fração de oxigênio inspirado varia de 0,21 (ar ambiente) a 1,0; relação PaO_2/F_IO_2 — mensuração da eficiência pulmonar; $PaO_2/F_IO_2 \geq 500$ — eficiência pulmonar normal; 300-500 — ineficiência leve; 200-300 — ineficiência moderada; <200 — ineficiência grave. A redução da eficiência pulmonar deve-se mais comumente à pneumopatia parenquimatosa.
• P_VO_2 — pressão parcial de oxigênio dissolvido no sangue venoso; é mais confiável uma amostra de sangue central (jugular); a P_VO_2 é determinada pelo consumo e distribuição teciduais de oxigênio; a P_VO_2 normal no ar ambiente = 40-60 mmHg; P_VO_2 <30 mmHg é preocupante do ponto de vista clínico; P_VO_2 <20 mmHg é potencialmente letal.
• $PaCO_2$ — pressão parcial de CO_2 dissolvido no sangue arterial; mensuração da ventilação; $PaCO_2$ normal = 40 mmHg (cães); 31 mmHg (gatos). Hipercapnia = hipoventilação = declínio na ventilação minuto (VM) alveolar.
• Teste de coagulação — na suspeita de hemotórax e/ou hemorragia pulmonar.
• As concentrações plasmáticas de pró-peptídeo natriurético atrial n-terminal, peptídeo natriurético cerebral, endotelina-1, e troponina-I cardíaca podem ajudar na diferenciação de causas cardíacas e não cardíacas de dispneia.

DIAGNÓSTICO POR IMAGEM
• Radiografia cervicotorácica: Doença das vias aéreas superiores (anteriores) — alongamento do palato mole, estreitamento das vias calibrosas, linfadenopatia, anormalidades intraluminais. Pneumonia — infiltrados alveolares; edema pulmonar cardiogênico — sombra cardíaca aumentada, distensão venosa pulmonar, aumento de volume do átrio esquerdo com infiltrados pulmonares peri-hilares em cães; os infiltrados podem ter qualquer distribuição em gatos. Edema pulmonar não cardiogênico — distribuição caudodorsal. SARA — infiltrados alveolares simétricos e difusos. Anormalidades vasculares pulmonares — tromboembolia pulmonar, dirofilariose. Doença do espaço pleural — pneumotórax, efusão pleural, lesões expansivas tipo massa, hérnias diafragmáticas.

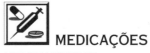
Dispneia e Angústia Respiratória

Comprometimento da parede torácica — fraturas de costela, neoplasia.
• Ultrassonografia torácica: avaliação da distribuição da efusão pleural (excelente como orientação à toracocentese). Identificação de massa pulmonar — orienta o aspirado por agulha fina; avaliação mediastínica. A ausência do "sinal de deslizamento" pode ser utilizada para identificação de pneumotórax.
• Ecocardiografia: avalia a função cardíaca se houver a suspeita de edema pulmonar cardiogênico ou efusão pleural; o aumento na pressão arterial pulmonar e a sobrecarga no ventrículo direito podem apoiar o diagnóstico de tromboembolia pulmonar; permite a observação de massas na base do coração.
• Radiografias ou ultrassonografias abdominais: avaliação da distensão abdominal.
• Fluoroscopia: avalia colapso da traqueia e/ou das vias aéreas calibrosas.
• Tomografia computadorizada: possibilita a avaliação de doença das vias aéreas, do parênquima pulmonar e do espaço pleural; é capaz de detectar lesões não tão claramente definidas nas radiografias, mas exige anestesia geral.
• Angiografia vascular pulmonar: padrão de excelência para o diagnóstico de tromboembolia pulmonar.
• Cintilografia de ventilação-perfusão: o desequilíbrio entre ventilação e perfusão é sugestivo de tromboembolia pulmonar, embora esse exame raramente seja realizado; a perfusão anormal dá suporte ao diagnóstico.

MÉTODOS DIAGNÓSTICOS
• Oximetria de pulso — SpO_2 — porcentagem da hemoglobina saturada com o oxigênio, mensurada por meio de um oxímetro de pulso. A relação entre PaO_2 e SpO_2 é definida pela curva de dissociação de oxigênio-hemoglobina; PaO_2 de 60 mmHg = SpO_2 de 90%; PaO_2 de 80 mmHg = SpO_2 de 95%; PaO_2 > 100 mmHg = SpO_2 de 100%. Abaixo de 95%, pequenas alterações na SpO_2 indicam grandes alterações na PaO_2; as mensurações da SpO_2 em animais sob alto nível de oxigênio inspirado carecem de sensibilidade.
• Toracocentese — análise e cultura do líquido.
• Laringotraqueoscopia — permite a visualização de corpos estranhos e massas.
• Broncoscopia — avalia as vias aéreas de pequeno e grande calibre; permite a obtenção de lavado broncoalveolar para citologia e cultura. Necessita de anestesia e do paciente estabilizado.

TRATAMENTO

CUIDADO(S) DE SAÚDE ADEQUADO(S)
• Prover os cuidados em um esquema de internação até se identificar e tratar a causa ou se determinar a ausência de risco de vida; a terapia depende da causa subjacente.
• SEMPRE administrar oxigênio e manter o paciente em decúbito esternal até se determinar a capacidade de oxigenação do animal.
• Doença das vias aéreas inferiores (posteriores) — broncodilatadores (terbutalina); oxigenoterapia até a estabilização do paciente; os corticosteroides sistêmicos podem ser necessários para estabilizar os gatos com broncoconstrição aguda.
• Pneumopatia parenquimatosa — oxigenoterapia, antibióticos na presença de pneumonia; tratar os distúrbios de coagulação de acordo; o edema cardiogênico requer a administração de furosemida +/– vasodilatadores. O edema não cardiogênico necessita de oxigenoterapia e, possivelmente, de ventilação com pressão positiva.
• Doença do espaço pleural — toracocentese para punção de ar e líquido; remover a maior quantidade possível. Caso haja necessidade de punções torácicas frequentes para manter o paciente estável, proceder à aplicação de sonda torácica.
• Comprometimento da parede torácica — cirurgia, conforme indicação, particularmente na presença de ferida torácica aberta; o tórax frouxo pode necessitar de intervenção cirúrgica, embora ele costume ser o resultado de comprometimento do espaço pleural com risco de vida após traumatismo da parede torácica. Paralisia da parede torácica/fadiga muscular — ventilação com pressão positiva se o animal estiver gravemente hipercapneico.
• Distensão abdominal — drenar a ascite, conforme a necessidade, para manter o paciente confortável; aliviar a distensão gástrica.

CUIDADO(S) DE ENFERMAGEM
• Oxigenoterapia via gaiola, cânula nasal, colar elizabetano coberto com envoltório plástico, máscara facial ou por fluxo. Umidificar a fonte de oxigênio caso se forneça a oxigenoterapia nasal por mais de algumas horas.
• Manter o animal em decúbito esternal e mudar o quarto posterior de posição a cada 3-4 horas, se o paciente não tolerar o decúbito lateral.
Monitorizar a temperatura regularmente, já que o esforço respiratório resulta em hipertermia, o que aumenta a angústia respiratória.

ATIVIDADE
Confinamento rigoroso em gaiola até a dificuldade respiratória desaparecer.

DIETA
Fornecer dieta de redução do peso se a obesidade estiver contribuindo para a causa.

CONSIDERAÇÕES CIRÚRGICAS
• É imprescindível ajustar cuidadosamente a anestesia ao paciente. É essencial assegurar uma via aérea, assim como uma indução intravenosa rápida. É frequentemente necessária a ventilação com pressão positiva nesses pacientes.
• Os animais com obstrução das vias aéreas superiores (anteriores) são frágeis e podem sofrer rápida descompensação. É preciso ter diversas sondas endotraqueais de múltiplos calibres à disposição.
• Dispneia associada a alguma massa laríngea pode responder à cirurgia de debridamento, embora a formação de edema e a ocorrência de hemorragia possam levar ao agravamento da obstrução.
• Evitar a ventilação com pressão positiva em pacientes com pneumotórax fechado. É imprescindível monitorizar o *status* de oxigenação dos pacientes anestesiados com o uso de oximetria de pulso e, sempre que possível, gasometria arterial.

MEDICAÇÕES
MEDICAMENTO(S)
Variam de acordo com a causa subjacente (ver a seção "Cuidado(s) de Saúde Adequado(s)").

ACOMPANHAMENTO
MONITORIZAÇÃO DO PACIENTE
• Os pacientes submetidos à oxigenoterapia podem ser monitorizados por meio da avaliação do grau de esforço respiratório. À medida que o paciente se estabiliza, realizar uma tentativa ao ar ambiente e reavaliar o nível de dificuldade respiratória. A gasometria arterial pode ser uma avaliação útil.
• A oximetria de pulso constitui uma ferramenta eficaz de monitorização dos pacientes sob o ar atmosférico/ambiente e pode descartar hipoxemia.
• Na avaliação dos comprometimentos do parênquima pulmonar e do espaço pleural, frequentemente fica indicada a repetição de radiografias.

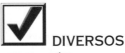
DIVERSOS
VER TAMBÉM
• Asma e Bronquite — Gatos.
• Edema Pulmonar Não Cardiogênico.
• Insuficiência Cardíaca Congestiva Esquerda.
• Insuficiência Cardíaca Congestiva Direita.
• Laringopatias.
• Pneumonia.
• Pneumotórax.
• Síndrome Braquicefálica das Vias Aéreas.
• Síndrome da Angústia Respiratória Aguda (SARA).

ABREVIATURA(S)
• SARA = síndrome da angústia respiratória aguda.

Sugestões de Leitura
Forney S. Dyspnea and tachypnea. In: Ettinger SJ, Feldman EC, eds., Textbook of Veterinary Internal Medicine, 7th ed. St. Louis: Elsevier, 2010, pp. 253-255.
Herndon WE, Rishniw M, et al. Assessment of plasma cardiac troponin I concentration as a means to differentiate cardiac and noncardiac causes of dyspnea in cats. JAVMA 2008, 233:1261-1264.
Mellema MS. The neurophysiology of dsypnea. J Vet Emerg Crit Care 2008, 18:561-571.
Prosek R, Sisson DD, Oyama M, Solter PF. Distinguishing cardiac and noncardiac dypsnea in 48 dogs using plasma atrial natriuretic factor, B-type natriuretic factor, endothelin and cardiac troponin-I. J Vet Intern Med 2007, 21:238-242.

Autor Kate Hopper
Consultor Editorial Lynelle R. Johnson

Disquezia e Hematoquezia

CONSIDERAÇÕES GERAIS

DEFINIÇÃO
- Disquezia — defecação dolorosa ou dificultosa.
- Hematoquezia — sangue vivo nas fezes ou sobre elas.

FISIOPATOLOGIA
- Resulta de diversas causas de inflamação ou irritação do reto ou do ânus.
- A hematoquezia também ocorre em casos de colonopatias.

SISTEMA(S) ACOMETIDO(S)
- Dermatológico.
- Gastrintestinal.

IDENTIFICAÇÃO
- Cães e gatos.
- Não há predileção racial ou sexual.

SINAIS CLÍNICOS
Achados Anamnésicos
- Choro e gemido durante a defecação.
- O tenesmo é comum.
- Se a dor for intensa, poderá ocorrer a ausência de defecação ou obstipação.
- Em pacientes com colonopatia, há diarreia mucoide e sanguinolenta.

Achados do Exame Físico
- O exame retal pode revelar fezes endurecidas (constipação ou obstipação), diarreia (doença colorretal), pólipos, massas, espessamento anorretal, estenose retal ou colônica, aumento de volume/dor das glândulas anais, prostatomegalia ou hérnias perineais.
- Em casos de fístulas perianais, há trajetos fistulosos em torno do ânus.
- Em casos de pseudocoprostase, ocorre oclusão anal com pelos emaranhados e fezes.

CAUSAS
Doença Anorretal
- Estenose ou espasmo.
- Saculite ou abscesso anal.
- Fístulas perianais.
- Corpos estranhos retais ou anais.
- Pseudocoprostase.
- Prolapso retal.
- Traumatismo — feridas ocasionadas por mordeduras, etc.
- Neoplasias — adenocarcinoma, linfoma e tumores dos sacos anais.
- Pólipos retais.
- Lúpus eritematoso mucocutâneo.

Colonopatias
- Neoplasias — adenocarcinoma, linfoma.
- Megacólon idiopático — gatos.
- Inflamação — enteropatia inflamatória, agentes infecciosos ou parasitários, colite alérgica (ver "Colite e Proctite").
- Constipação (ver "Constipação e Obstipação").

Doença Extraintestinal
- Fratura da pelve ou dos membros pélvicos.
- Prostatopatia.
- Hérnia perineal.
- Neoplasias intrapélvicas.

FATORES DE RISCO
- A ingestão de pelos, ossos, corpos estranhos pode contribuir para a constipação e a subsequente disquezia.
- Fatores ambientais, como bandeja sanitária suja e passeios pouco frequentes, podem colaborar para a constipação e a subsequente disquezia.

DIAGNÓSTICO

DIAGNÓSTICO DIFERENCIAL
- Disúria, estrangúria ou hematúria — achados anormais na urinálise, como piúria, cristalúria, bacteriúria.
- Distocia — diferenciar com a anamnese e o diagnóstico por imagem.

HEMOGRAMA/BIOQUÍMICA/URINÁLISE
- Em geral, permanecem normais.
- Neutrofilia em casos de infecção ou inflamação.

OUTROS TESTES LABORATORIAIS
Múltiplos exames de fezes para descartar causas infecciosas/parasitárias de colite.

DIAGNÓSTICO POR IMAGEM
- As radiografias pélvicas podem revelar doença intrapélvica, corpo estranho ou fratura.
- A ultrassonografia pode demonstrar prostatopatias ou massas abdominais caudais.

MÉTODOS DIAGNÓSTICOS
Colonoscopia/proctoscopia para avaliar doença inflamatória ou neoplásica.

TRATAMENTO

- Em geral, é feito em um esquema ambulatorial.
- Considerar o uso de laxantes para facilitar a defecação em caso de doença anorretal.
- Dilatação das estenoses com o uso de cateter com extremidade em balão.
- As doenças anorretais podem necessitar de correção cirúrgica — hérnias perineais, pólipos anorretais.

MEDICAÇÕES

MEDICAMENTO(S) DE ESCOLHA
- Antibióticos — se houver infecção bacteriana (p. ex., abscesso dos sacos anais); amoxicilina/ácido clavulânico 15 mg/kg VO a cada 12 h.
- Medicamentos anti-inflamatórios — sulfassalazina ou prednisona na presença de colite idiopática (ver capítulos sobre "Colite").
- Laxantes — lactulose, 1 mL/4,5 kg VO a cada 8-12 h, até se obter o efeito; docusato de sódio ou docusato de cálcio, cães 50-100 mg VO a cada 12-24 h, gatos 50 mg VO a cada 12-24 h.

CONTRAINDICAÇÕES
Evitar os agentes indutores de aumento no volume fecal (fibras insolúveis), a menos que haja indicação específica (colite).

PRECAUÇÕES
N/D.

INTERAÇÕES POSSÍVEIS
N/D.

MEDICAMENTO(S) ALTERNATIVO(S)
N/D.

ACOMPANHAMENTO

MONITORIZAÇÃO DO PACIENTE
Inicialmente, monitorizar os sinais clínicos a cada 2-3 semanas.

COMPLICAÇÕES POSSÍVEIS
- Se houver a necessidade de terapia cirúrgica rigorosa do ânus, pode-se observar incontinência fecal.
- Poderá ocorrer megacólon secundário se a obstipação for grave e prolongada.

DIVERSOS

DISTÚRBIOS ASSOCIADOS
N/D.

FATORES RELACIONADOS COM A IDADE
N/D.

POTENCIAL ZOONÓTICO
N/D.

GESTAÇÃO/FERTILIDADE/REPRODUÇÃO
É preciso ter cautela com o uso de corticosteroides e antibióticos.

VER TAMBÉM
- Colite e Proctite.
- Constipação e Obstipação.

Sugestões de Leitura
Webb CB. Anal-rectal disease. In: Bonagura JD, Twedt DC, eds., Current Veterinary Therapy XIV. St. Louis: Elsevier, 2009, pp. 527-531.
Zoran DL. Rectoanal disease. In: Ettinger SJ, Feldman EC, eds., Textbook of Veterinary Internal Medicine, 6th ed. St. Louis: Elsevier, 2005, pp. 1408-1420.

Autor Lisa E. Moore
Consultor Editorial Albert E. Jergens

DISRAFISMO ESPINAL

CONSIDERAÇÕES GERAIS

REVISÃO
- Desenvolvimento anormal da medula espinal ao longo do plano mediano, levando a uma variedade de anomalias estruturais (p. ex., hidromielia, canal central duplicado ou ausente, siringomielia e aberrações no septo mediano dorsal e na fissura mediana ventral).
- Segmentos espinais toracolombares são os mais comumente acometidos.
- O termo *disrafismo* sugere uma anormalidade no fechamento do tubo neural; pode ser preferível o uso do termo *mielodisplasia*.

IDENTIFICAÇÃO
Não Progressivo
- Cães e gatos.
- Raça Weimaraner — hereditário.
- Há relatos em cães pertencentes às raças Buldogue inglês, Samoieda, Dálmata, Setter inglês, Golden retriever, Rottweiler e gatos Manx.
- Sem predileção sexual.
- Aparente em torno de 3-6 semanas de vida.

Progressivo
- Animais adultos da raça Cavalier King Charles spaniel com siringomielia resultante de má--formação óssea occipital (má-formação de Chiari I; síndrome de má-formação occipital caudal).
- Cão adulto da raça Pomerânia com siringomielia cervical e hidrocefalia.
- Cão Fox terrier adulto com paresia progressiva no membro pélvico esquerdo.

SINAIS CLÍNICOS
- Variam em termos de gravidade.
- Raça Weimaraner — flexão e extensão simultâneas dos membros pélvicos (marcha saltitante tipo coelho); déficits proprioceptivos, postura em base larga e postura agachada do membro pélvico.
- Raça Cavalier King Charles spaniel — dor no pescoço ou na cabeça; fraqueza progressiva dos membros torácicos, paraparesia; desequilíbrio; arranhadura involuntária paroxística do flanco ou do pescoço.

CAUSAS E FATORES DE RISCO
- Genéticos — raça Weimaraner; condição homozigota letal; heterozigotos clinicamente acometidos.
- Lesão da medula espinal *in utero* provocada por infecção, traumatismo e comprometimento vascular pode causar siringomielia (cavitação da medula espinal).
- Idiopática em pacientes isolados.
- A siringomielia pode ser adquirida como resultado de infecção, traumatismo ou neoplasia.

DIAGNÓSTICO

DIAGNÓSTICO DIFERENCIAL
- Clinicamente diferenciado de mielopatias comuns por estar presente ao nascimento e não ter caráter progressivo.
- Discopatia intervertebral, mielite, cistos aracnoides e neoplasia precisam ser diferenciados de causas progressivas da siringomielia.

HEMOGRAMA/BIOQUÍMICA/URINÁLISE
Geralmente normais.

OUTROS TESTES LABORATORIAIS
N/D.

DIAGNÓSTICO POR IMAGEM
- Radiografias simples e mielografia — anomalias da coluna vertebral e compressão da medula espinal associadas em alguns pacientes.
- Sem técnicas sofisticadas de imagem, pode ser impossível obter o diagnóstico antes da morte em outras raças caninas que não a Weimaraner e nos gatos Manx.
- RM — representa a modalidade definitiva de diagnóstico por imagem para siringomielia, atenuação do quarto ventrículo, compactação do tronco cerebral na fossa caudal e herniação do vermis cerebelar (síndrome de má-formação occipital caudal, má-formação tipo Chiari); hidrocefalia se evidente.
- TC — revela hidrocefalia, se evidente, com síndrome de má-formação occipital caudal.
- Radiografias do crânio — podem demonstrar defeito do osso occipital.

OUTROS MÉTODOS DIAGNÓSTICOS
N/D.

TRATAMENTO

- Pacientes levemente acometidos — podem ser animais de estimação.
- Animais gravemente acometidos podem se beneficiar de um carrinho de rodas ortopédico especial para cães; considerar a eutanásia.
- Considerações cirúrgicas — remodelagem do forame magno (com má-formação occipital caudal) ou colocação de derivação ventriculoperitoneal; laminectomia, ± derivação siringossubaracnoide (pode interromper a evolução do quadro ou melhorar o curso da doença, retardando a progressão dos sinais neurológicos).

MEDICAÇÕES

MEDICAMENTO(S)
- Se houver infecção do trato urinário — tratar com antibióticos, escolhidos com base nos resultados da urocultura e do antibiograma.
- Siringomielia — os corticosteroides podem melhorar os sinais por diminuírem a produção de LCS e a formação de edema na síndrome de má-formação occipital caudal. Reduzir gradativamente para prednisona em dias alternados ou dexametasona duas vezes por semana; inibidores da anidrase carbônica (acetazolamida a 3,5-7,5 mg/kg a cada 8-12 h; metazolamida a 5 mg/kg a cada 8-12 h) ou furosemida (5 mg/kg VO, IM, SC a cada 12 h) ou omeprazol (Prilosec® a 0,5-1 mg/kg VO a cada 24 h; atualmente, não há dados clínicos sobre o uso e a eficácia) também podem aliviar os sinais por reduzirem a produção de LCS e, consequentemente, possibilitam a redução na dose do esteroide.

CONTRAINDICAÇÕES/INTERAÇÕES POSSÍVEIS
N/D.

ACOMPANHAMENTO

- Infecção secundária do trato urinário — observada nos animais gravemente acometidos; atribuída a distúrbios da micção.
- Evitar as úlceras de decúbito, bem como as assaduras por urina e fezes, pelo fornecimento de cuidados adequados aos pacientes nessa posição.

DIVERSOS

DISTÚRBIOS ASSOCIADOS
Arco vertebral congênito (p. ex., espinha-bífida) e má-formação do complexo corpo e disco vertebral (p. ex., hemivértebra e vértebra em bloco) — esses quadros isolados frequentemente não provocam sinais clínicos.

ABREVIATURA(S)
- LCS = líquido cerebrospinal.
- RM = ressonância magnética.
- TC = tomografia computadorizada.

Sugestões de Leitura
Bailey CS, Morgan JP. Congenital malformations. In: Moore MP, ed., Diseases of the Spine. Vet Clin North Am Small Anim Pract 1992, 22:985-1015.
Rusbridge C, Knowler SP. Inheritance of occipital bone hypoplasia (Chiari type I malformation) in Cavalier King Charles spaniels. J Vet Intern Med 2004, 18(5):673-678.
Rusbridge C, MacSweeny JE, Davies JV, et al. Syringohydromyelia in Cavalier King Charles spaniels. JAAHA 2000, 36(1):34-41.
Summers BA, Cummings JH, de Lahunta A. Veterinary Pathology. St. Louis: Mosby, 1995.

Autor Richard J. Joseph
Consultor Editorial Joane M. Parent

DISTOCIA

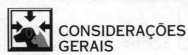

CONSIDERAÇÕES GERAIS

DEFINIÇÃO
Dificuldade de parto.

FISIOPATOLOGIA
• A distocia pode ocorrer como resultado de fatores maternos ou fetais e durante qualquer estágio do parto.
• Anormalidades de apresentação, postura e posição afetam a relação entre a ninhada e o canal de parto materno. Apresentação: relação entre o eixo espinal fetal e o eixo espinal materno — longitudinal anterior ou posterior é normal; transversa é anormal. Posição: relação entre o dorso fetal e os quadrantes pélvicos maternos — dorsossacral é o normal. Postura: relação entre as extremidades ou a cabeça fetais e o corpo fetal — a postura normal consiste em pés e membros estendidos, bem como cabeça estendida.
• A inércia uterina pode ser primária ou secundária. A primária corresponde à falha em iniciar as contrações uterinas sincrônicas, enquanto a secundária se refere à interrupção das contrações uterinas em virtude de fadiga uterina ou hipocalcemia (ver Inércia Uterina).
• Há três estágios do trabalho de parto:

Estágio 1
• Começa com o início das contrações uterinas e relaxamento da cérvix; termina com a ruptura do primeiro saco corioalantoico — duração média de 6-12 h (pode durar até 36 h em cadelas nervosas e primíparas).
• Cadelas — podem ficar inquietas, nervosas e anoréxicas; podem tremer, respirar de forma ofegante, caminhar compassadamente e procurar um lugar para fazer o ninho.
• Gatas — tendem a vocalizar em princípio; ronronam e socializam-se à medida que o estágio 1 do parto se aproxima.

Estágio 2
• Liberação dos fetos.
• Cadelas — contrações abdominais evidentes na tentativa de parir; o período desde o início do estágio 2 até a expulsão do primeiro filhote costuma ser <4 h; o tempo entre a expulsão dos filhotes subsequentes geralmente é de 20-60 min (pode ser de até 2-3 h).
• Gatas — a duração média do parto é de 16 h, com variação de 4-42 h (até 3 dias, em alguns casos, pode ser normal); é importante considerar essa variabilidade ao se intervir no trabalho de parto.
• O número de fetos presentes pode influenciar significativamente a duração dos estágios 2 e 3.

Estágio 3
• Liberação das membranas fetais.
• Cadelas com múltiplos filhotes — podem alternar entre os estágios 2 e 3; pode liberar um ou dois fetos e, depois, uma ou duas membranas fetais ou liberar um feto e, então, sua membrana fetal acompanhante.

INCIDÊNCIA/PREVALÊNCIA
• Cadelas — incidência desconhecida; difícil de estimar, por conta da variabilidade das raças e da intervenção dos criadores.
• Gatas — a média descrita varia de 3,3-5,8%; gatas de raças mestiças, 0,4%; incidência elevada em gatas com *pedigree*, sendo de até 18,2% na raça Devon rex.

IDENTIFICAÇÃO
Raça(s) Predominante(s)
Cadelas
• Incidência mais alta em raças miniaturas e pequenas em virtude do pequeno tamanho da ninhada com tamanho fetal grande concomitantemente; pode ocorrer em raças de grande porte com ninhadas grandes ou singulares (i. e., um único filhote canino grande).
• Raças braquicefálicas — cabeça larga e pelve estreita — Buldogue, Boston terrier, Pug.
• Ampla relação entre cabeça fetal e pelve materna — Sealyham terrier, Scottish terrier.
• Inércia uterina — Scottish terrier, Dachshund, Border terrier, Aberdeen terrier, Labrador retriever (ver "Inércia Uterina").
• Raças mestiças com incidência global elevada de distocia — Chihuahua, Dachshund, Pequinês, Yorkshire terrier, Poodle miniatura, Pomerânia.

Gatas
• Raças braquicefálicas — Persa, Himalaio.
• Raças dolicocefálicas — Devon rex.

SINAIS CLÍNICOS
Achados Anamnésicos
• São indicadores de distocia:
• Mais de 30 min de contrações abdominais vigorosas e persistentes, sem a expulsão dos fetos.
• Mais de 4 h desde o início do estágio 2 até a liberação do primeiro feto (cadelas).
• Mais de 2 h entre o nascimento da ninhada (cadelas).
• Falha em iniciar o trabalho de parto dentro de 24 h depois da queda na temperatura retal (<37,2°C) ou dentro de 36 h do declínio da progesterona sérica <2 ng/mL (cadelas).
• A fêmea chora, exibe sinais de dor e lambe constantemente a região vulvar no momento do parto.
• Prenhez prolongada — >72 dias desde o dia do primeiro cruzamento (cadelas); >59 dias desde o primeiro dia do diestro citológico (cadelas); >66 dias a partir do pico de LH (cadelas); >68 dias a partir do dia do acasalamento (gatas) (ver "Acasalamento, Momento Oportuno").

Achados do Exame Físico
• Presença de corrimento preto-esverdeado (uteroverdina), que antecede o nascimento do primeiro filhote por volta de mais de 2 h.
• Presença de corrimento sanguinolento antes da liberação do primeiro feto ou entre os fetos.
• Ausência ou diminuição do reflexo de Ferguson (a estimulação ou a pressão sobre a parede dorsal da vagina eliciam o esforço abdominal [tato suave]) indica inércia uterina.

CAUSAS
Fetais
• Tamanho fetal exagerado — ninhada de um único filhote canino; monstruosidade fetal, anasarca fetal; hidrocefalia fetal; prenhez prolongada em virtude da incapacidade de um único feto iniciar o trabalho de parto.
• Apresentação, posição ou postura fetais anormais no canal de parto.
• Morte fetal.

Maternas
• Contrações uterinas deficientes — defeito do miométrio; desequilíbrio bioquímico; distúrbio psicogênico; exaustão (ver "Inércia Uterina").
• Compressão abdominal ineficaz — dor; medo; debilidade (exaustão); hérnia diafragmática; idade; perfuração da traqueia.
• Placentite, metrite, endometrite.
• Toxemia da prenhez, diabetes gestacional.
• Canal pélvico anormal decorrente de lesão pélvica prévia, conformação anormal ou imaturidade pélvica.
• Pelve congenitamente pequena — Welsh corgi; raças braquicefálicas.
• Hérnia inguinal.
• Anormalidade do fórnix vaginal — estenose; septos; hiperplasia vaginal; vagina hipoplásica; cisto intra ou extraluminal; neoplasia.
• Anormalidade do orifício vulvar — estenose; vulva invertida; vulva pequena; fibrose por traumatismo; neoplasia.
• Dilatação cervical insuficiente.
• Falta de lubrificação adequada.
• Torção uterina.
• Ruptura uterina.
• Neoplasias, cistos ou aderências uterinos.

FATORES DE RISCO
• Idade.
• Raças braquicefálicas e toys.
• Raças Persa, Himalaio e Devon Rex.
• Obesidade.
• Mudanças ambientais abruptas na proximidade do parto.
• Histórico prévio de distocia.

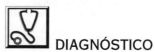

DIAGNÓSTICO

DIAGNÓSTICO DIFERENCIAL
Inércia uterina — hipocalcemia *versus* hipoglicemia.

EXAME FÍSICO
• Exame físico completo — essencial; determinar os problemas concomitantes ou colaboradores (p. ex., hipoglicemia, hipocalcemia, desidratação e febre); realizar palpação abdominal cuidadosa para confirmar a existência de fetos.
• Exame vaginal digital — identifica a presença de feto ou membranas fetais no canal vaginal; revela anormalidades do canal pélvico materno; avalia o reflexo de Ferguson.
• Cadelas que falham em produzir contrações abdominais em resposta ao toque suave ou à ocitocina — é mais provável a presença de inércia uterina do que distocia obstrutiva, a menos que a obstrução tenha várias horas de duração.

HEMOGRAMA/BIOQUÍMICA/URINÁLISE
Banco de dados mínimo — volume globular (hematócrito), proteínas totais, ureia, bem como concentrações séricas de glicose e cálcio (é preferível a mensuração do cálcio ionizado ao cálcio sérico total).

OUTROS TESTES LABORATORIAIS
Concentração de progesterona.

DIAGNÓSTICO POR IMAGEM
• Radiografias (abdome e região pélvica) — determinam a conformação pélvica, o número e o posicionamento dos fetos, a evidência de obstrução fetal; o tamanho fetal exagerado e a morte fetal; pode haver a necessidade de duas projeções.
• Evidência radiográfica de morte fetal — colapso dos esqueletos fetais, associação anormal dos ossos

fetais em relação ao esqueleto axial, presença de ar/gás em torno do feto, formação de bolas no feto.
• Ultrassonografia — recomendada para monitorizar a viabilidade fetal; detecta estresse fetal (p. ex., frequência cardíaca fetal <180 ou >280 bpm — cadelas; <95 ou >260 bpm — gatas) — e para avaliar o descolamento da placenta e a característica dos líquidos fetais (presença de mecônio ou sangue no líquido amniótico indica estresse fetal); a frequência cardíaca fetal é normalmente 2 a 3 vezes à da progenitora em cadelas.
• Evidência ultrassonográfica de morte fetal — falta de batimento cardíaco do feto ou descolamento da placenta.

TRATAMENTO
CUIDADO(S) DE SAÚDE ADEQUADO(S)
• Internação — até o nascimento de toda a ninhada e a estabilização da mãe.
• Inércia uterina — instituir o tratamento se não houver indícios de estresse fetal. Pode ser atribuída à hipoglicemia, hipocalcemia, produção endógena inadequada de ocitocina ou resposta inapropriada à produção normal de ocitocina (ver "Inércia Uterina").
• Agentes ecbólicos não devem ser administrados diante de possível distocia obstrutiva, pois eles podem acelerar o descolamento da placenta e a morte dos fetos ou causar ruptura do útero.
• Hipocalcemia — administração de gliconato de cálcio a 10% a 0,2 mL/kg lentamente por via IV (durante 5-10 min ao mesmo tempo em que se monitoriza a ocorrência de arritmias) ou 1-5 mL/cadela SC; pode ser repetido em intervalos de 4 a 6 h, conforme a necessidade; em gatas, 0,5-1,0 mL de gliconato de cálcio lentamente por via IV — utilizar com cuidado, pois há aumento no risco de ruptura uterina em virtude da força das contrações uterinas após a administração de cálcio em gatas.
• Hipoglicemia — administração de solução eletrolítica balanceada com glicose a 5-10% a uma velocidade de 60-80 mL/kg/dia por via IV.
• Ocitocina — assim que os déficits de cálcio e glicose forem tratados, a administração de microdoses de ocitocina (0,5-4,0 UI por vias IM ou SC, dependendo do porte da cadela e da resposta ao tratamento); pode ser repetida em intervalos de 30 min, contanto que a evolução do parto prossiga. Se houver a necessidade de mais de 3 a 4 doses de ocitocina por feto e a permanência de mais de 4 fetos, deve-se levar o procedimento de cesariana em consideração. Se a cadela não estiver contraindo de forma adequada por conta própria, deve-se esperar um intervalo de no mínimo 30 minutos entre a liberação de um feto e a administração da próxima dose de ocitocina.
• Os sistemas de monitorização WhelpWise® podem ser utilizados para monitorar as frequências cardíacas dos fetos e os padrões das contrações uterinas. Esses sistemas são excelentes para cadelas sem histórico prévio de inércia uterina ou com ninhadas grandes para determinar a necessidade e a resposta ao tratamento médico.

Expulsão Manual
• Para liberar um feto alojado no fórnix vaginal.
• Aplicar lubrificação com liberalidade; posicionar a paciente em estação.
• Uso dos dedos — provoca menor dano ao feto e à mãe.
• Expulsão com o emprego de instrumentos (cadelas) — se o fórnix vaginal for muito pequeno para as manipulações digitais; utilizar com lubrificação adequada; colocar sempre um dedo no fórnix vaginal para direcionar o instrumento; recomendam-se os ganchos de castração ou as pinças sem dentes de trava; aplicar a tração na direção posterior e ventral.
• É preciso ter extrema cautela; as sequelas indesejáveis incluem mutilações do feto e lacerações da mãe.
• Jamais aplique tração às extremidades distais de um feto vivo.
• Gatas — não se recomenda o emprego de instrumentos, em função do tamanho pequeno do fórnix vaginal.
• Falha de expulsão do feto localizado no canal vaginal dentro de 30 min — indica-se a cesariana.

CONSIDERAÇÕES CIRÚRGICAS
• Indicações de cesariana — inércia uterina irresponsiva à ocitocina ou inércia uterina responsiva, mas com mais de 4 fetos remanescentes no útero (para maximizar a sobrevivência fetal); obstrução pélvica ou vaginal; mau posicionamento fetal não passível de correção; tamanho fetal exagerado; estresse fetal; morte fetal intrauterina.
• Cesariana eletiva — raças propensas à distocia; cadelas com histórico de distocia; cadelas com um único feto grande ou ninhadas muito grandes; realizada frequentemente para maximizar a sobrevivência fetal.

Anestesia
Comentários Gerais
• Sempre fornecer fluidoterapia com solução eletrolítica balanceada antes, durante e depois da cirurgia.
• O útero gravídico pode comprimir os grandes vasos e comprometer o retorno venoso ao mesmo tempo em que exerce pressão sobre o diafragma, resultando em um declínio no volume corrente.
• As cadelas prenhes apresentam pressão arterial sistólica, PO_2, volume globular (hematócrito) mais baixos, porém PCO_2, frequências respiratórias e incidência de acidose mais altas do que as não prenhes.
• Os desfechos maternos e neonatais podem melhorar com a pré-oxigenação dos pacientes.

Cadelas
• Pré-medicação com glicopirrolato (0,01 mg/kg IM) se as frequências cardíacas fetais permanecerem normais ou com atropina (0,02-0,04 mg/kg IM) se existir bradicardia fetal; indução com propofol (4-6 mg/kg IV), bem como intubação e manutenção com sevoflurano (ou isoflurano), constitui o protocolo anestésico preferido.
• Se o propofol não estiver disponível, lançar mão da pré-medicação com diazepam (0,1-0,4 mg/kg IV, IM) e butorfanol (0,2-0,4 mg/kg IM), acompanhada por máscara com sevoflurano (ou isoflurano) para indução e manutenção.
• A cetamina não é recomendada na cadela em função de seus efeitos depressores sobre os fetos.
• Também pode ser utilizada anestesia epidural (0,2 mg/kg de bupivacaína a 0,5% e morfina em formulação livre de preservativos a 0,1 mg/kg ou lidocaína a 2% a 0,1-0,3 mL/kg sem adrenalina administrada até o efeito desejado, mas sem exceder 10 mg/kg da dose total de lidocaína) associada à anestesia local. As desvantagens da anestesia local/regional envolvem a incapacidade de oxigenação adequada sem sonda endotraqueal e o aumento do fluxo sanguíneo regional, dificultando ainda mais a hemostasia.
• Butorfanol (0,1-0,4 mg/kg IV, IM) ou buprenorfina (0,005-0,01 mg/kg IV/IM) pode ser utilizado para analgesia pós-operatória se necessário.
• Pré-medicações — caso de faça uso do diazepam, os neonatos deverão ser revertidos com flumazenil (0,01 mg/kg IV); se os opiáceos forem utilizados antes da liberação dos fetos, os neonatos deverão ser revertidos com naloxona (0,04 mg/kg IV, IM, SC); talvez haja necessidade de repetição da dosagem até que os medicamentos sejam completamente metabolizados no neonato.

Gatas
• Gata saudável — pré-medicar com glicopirrolato (0,005-0,01 mg/kg IV, IM) se as frequências cardíacas fetais permanecerem normais ou atropina (0,04 mg/kg IM) se a bradicardia fetal estiver presente.
• Indução com propofol (4-6 mg/kg IV), intubação e manutenção com sevoflurano ou isoflurano, constitui o protocolo anestésico preferido.
• Alternativamente, pode-se usar a pré-medicação com diazepam (0,2-0,4 mg/kg IV, IM) e butorfanol (0,1-0,4 mg/kg IM), acompanhados por máscara com sevoflurano ou isoflurano.
• Se o propofol não estiver disponível, proceder à indução com diazepam (0,2-0,4 mg/kg IV) e cetamina (2,2-4,4 mg/kg IV), acompanhados por manutenção com sevoflurano ou isoflurano. A cetamina afeta o feto de modo dose-dependente, de modo que a dose mínima requerida para indução deva ser utilizada. Com a pré-medicação adequada, uma indução com baixas doses (1 mg/kg IV ou 5 mg/kg IM) pode ser conveniente.
• Anestesia epidural — lidocaína a 2% (0,2 mL/kg) administrada até a obtenção do efeito desejado, associada ao butorfanol (0,2-0,4 mg/kg IV, IM).
• Gata com depressão ou exaustão grave — pré-medicação com diazepam (0,2-0,4 mg/kg IV, IM) ou midazolam (0,066-0,22 mg/kg IV, IM) e butorfanol (0,2-0,4 mg/kg IV, IM) ou oximorfona (0,1-0,4 mg/kg IV, IM); acompanhados por propofol para indução e manutenção com sevoflurano ou isoflurano.

MEDICAÇÕES
MEDICAMENTO(S) DE ESCOLHA
Ocitocina — em casos de inércia uterina (ver "Inércia Uterina").

CONTRAINDICAÇÕES
Ocitocina — contraindicada em casos de distocia obstrutiva de causa fetal ou materna, estresse fetal, morte fetal intrauterina antiga, ruptura uterina, torção uterina.

ACOMPANHAMENTO
PREVENÇÃO
• Cesariana eletiva programada para cadelas com canal pélvico anormal; pelve pequena; anormalidades do fórnix vaginal; raças

DISTOCIA

predispostas à distocia; fêmeas com histórico prévio de inércia uterina.
• Cirurgia marcada — é extremamente importante identificar o primeiro dia do diestro, o pico do LH ou a ovulação durante o cruzamento; isso aumenta significativamente a viabilidade fetal; ver "Acasalamento, Momento Oportuno". Se o momento da ovulação não estiver disponível, haverá necessidade de avaliação da idade e da maturação gestacionais por meio da ultrassonografia.

EVOLUÇÃO ESPERADA E PROGNÓSTICO
• Em caso de identificação imediata da distocia e êxito da intervenção cirúrgica — prognóstico bom a razoável quanto à vida da fêmea; razoável quanto à sobrevida da prole.
• Em caso de não identificação ou na falta de tratamento da distocia por 24-48 h (cadelas) — prognóstico mau a reservado quanto à vida da fêmea; é improvável que algum filhote sobreviva (cadelas).
• Em caso de não identificação ou na falta de tratamento da distocia por 24-48 h (gatas) — prognóstico altamente variável, dependendo da causa.

DIVERSOS

GESTAÇÃO/FERTILIDADE/REPRODUÇÃO
O histórico de distocia pode ou não exercer um impacto sobre a fertilidade da fêmea no futuro, dependendo da causa. A distocia pode predispor o animal a episódios repetidos durante as gestações subsequentes, dependendo da causa (anormalidades anatômicas, inércia uterina primária). O desempenho da cesariana para os casos de distocia durante o parto não exclui a possibilidade de a cadela dar cria naturalmente durante os partos subsequentes e dependerá do motivo pelo qual esse procedimento foi necessário.

ABREVIATURA(S)
• LH = hormônio luteinizante.
• PCO_2 = pressão parcial de dióxido de carbono.
• PO_2 = pressão parcial de oxigênio.

Sugestões de Leitura
Johnston SD, Root Kustritz MV, Olson PNS. Canine parturition; Feline parturition. In: Canine and Feline Theriogenology. Philadelphia: Saunders, 2001, pp. 105-128, 431-437.

Autor Cheryl Lopate
Consultor Editorial Sara K. Lyle
Agradecimento O autor e os editores agradecem a colaboração prévia de Louis F. Archbald.

Distrofia Neuroaxonal

CONSIDERAÇÕES GERAIS

REVISÃO
- Doenças degenerativas hereditárias de neurônios em diversas regiões do SNC, particularmente no cerebelo e nas vias associadas.
- Algumas vezes, os distúrbios primários de distrofia neuroaxonal são classificados como abiotrofias.
- Herança — autossômica recessiva nas raças em que a hereditariedade está comprovada.
- A principal característica patológica da distrofia neuroaxonal, os esferoides axonais, também ocorre no processo de envelhecimento normal, bem como secundariamente a uma série de outras doenças, como doenças metabólicas adquiridas ou hereditárias e toxicidades.

IDENTIFICAÇÃO
- Cães e gatos.
- Raças predispostas — gatos domésticos e Siamês, além de cães das raças Rottweiler, Collie, Papillon, Chihuahua, Pastor alemão, Jack Russell terrier e Boxer.
- Idade de início — específica para a raça, variando de menos de 2 meses de vida em gato, Chihuahua e Papillon até 1-2 anos em Rottweiler.

SINAIS CLÍNICOS
- Ataxia cerebelar — dismetria e hipermetria progressivas dos membros (raramente hipometria) com hiper-reflexia patelar.
- Força e propriocepção normais na maioria dos casos. Os cães da raça Rottweiler podem sofrer extenso envolvimento das colunas dorsais da medula espinal cervical e exibir déficits proprioceptivos.
- Perda das respostas à ameaça apesar da normalidade na visão e nos nervos faciais.
- Sinais progressivos de envolvimento do tronco cerebral podem ser característicos, especialmente em cães da raça Papillon, incluindo perda do reflexo da deglutição e do movimento da língua; nos estágios finais, pode ocorrer o desenvolvimento de tetraplegia.
- Leve tremor intencional ou dismetria da cabeça e do pescoço em alguns pacientes.
- Sinais principalmente cerebelares em cães das raças Rottweiler, Collie e Chihuahua, bem como em gatos domésticos; lesões predominantemente da medula espinal nas raças Pastor alemão e Boxer; presença de tremor e ataxia cerebelar em todos os animais acometidos.

CAUSAS E FATORES DE RISCO
- Desconhecidos.
- Classificada geralmente como abiotrofia neuronal.
- Herança autossômica recessiva comprovada em algumas raças.
- Predisposição racial.

DIAGNÓSTICO
- Suspeita com base nos sinais clínicos em alguma raça predisposta, geralmente em animais jovens.
- O diagnóstico definitivo requer o exame histopatológico do tecido nervoso (SNC), em geral após a morte.

DIAGNÓSTICO DIFERENCIAL
- Outras anomalias cerebelares congênitas, abiotrofias e distúrbios degenerativos. Relatados ocasionalmente em gatos e uma série de raças de cães, tais como Border collie, Brittany, Coton de Tulear, Gordon setter, Jack Russell (Parson Russel) terrier, Labrador retriever, Old English sheepdog e muitas outras.
- Outras anomalias estruturais do tronco cerebral caudal, incluindo síndrome de má-formação occipital caudal e síndrome de Dandy-Walker. Diferenciadas por meio de técnicas de diagnóstico por imagem, particularmente RM. Determinadas raças são predispostas, p. ex., síndrome de má-formação occipital caudal no Cavalier King Charles spaniel.
- Hipoplasia cerebelar causada por infecção de felino *in utero* pelo vírus da panleucopenia felina — aparente por volta de 3-6 semanas de vida; não progressiva.
- Encefalite da cinomose — diferenciada com base nos sinais sistêmicos que antecedem ou acompanham os déficits neurológicos e nos resultados da análise do LCS (normais em casos de distrofia neuroaxonal).
- Encefalites inflamatórias não infecciosas, particularmente meningoencefalomielite granulomatosa. Encefalites específicas da raça (Pug, Maltês, Yorkshire terrier) costumam gerar sinais atribuídos ao prosencéfalo (crises convulsivas), embora possa ocorrer um envolvimento cerebelar. Diferenciadas pela presença de alterações inflamatórias no LCS e, em alguns casos, por lesões cerebrais realçadas pelo contraste na RM.
- Neoplasia com acometimento do cerebelo — primária, metastática ou localmente invasiva. Ocorre em cães e gatos mais idosos, geralmente com mais de 5 anos de idade. Diferenciada com base nas técnicas de diagnóstico por imagem (particularmente RM), análise do LCS em alguns casos e envolvimento sistêmico no caso de neoplasia metastática.
- Mielopatia cervical — déficits proprioceptivos e tetraparesia.
- O diagnóstico de distrofia neuroaxonal é feito por exclusão; pode ser impossível obter o diagnóstico antes da morte.

HEMOGRAMA/BIOQUÍMICA/URINÁLISE
Normais.

OUTROS TESTES LABORATORIAIS
N/D.

DIAGNÓSTICO POR IMAGEM
Atrofia do cerebelo pode ser notável na RM em certos pacientes (p. ex., cães da raça Papillon).

MÉTODOS DIAGNÓSTICOS
Todos os exames diagnósticos antes da morte estão normais.

ACHADOS PATOLÓGICOS
- Esferoides axonais — presentes em toda parte da substância branca ou cinzenta do SNC, dependendo da raça acometida. Os esferoides contêm acúmulos anormais de proteínas intracelulares, particularmente várias associadas ao transporte axonal e à função sináptica.
- Pode ocorrer degeneração da mielina secundariamente ao comprometimento axonal.

TRATAMENTO
- Não existe nenhum tratamento disponível que altere a evolução da doença.
- Atividade — restrita a áreas onde se possam evitar quedas (evitar escadas, piscinas, etc.).

MEDICAÇÕES

MEDICAMENTO(S)
N/D.

CONTRAINDICAÇÕES/INTERAÇÕES POSSÍVEIS
N/D.

ACOMPANHAMENTO
- Rottweiler — piora entre 1-5 anos; os animais dessa raça desenvolvem reflexos patelares e extensores cruzados clônicos.
- Embora não seja fatal, é gravemente incapacitante.

DIVERSOS

ABREVIATURA(S)
- LCS = líquido cerebrospinal.
- RM = ressonância magnética.
- SNC = sistema nervoso central.

Sugestões de Leitura
Diaz JV, Duque C, et al. Neuroaxonal dystrophy in dogs: Case report in 2 litters of papillon puppies. J Vet Intern Med 2007, 21:531-534.
Nibe K, Kita C, et al. Clinicopathological features of canine neuroaxonal dystrophy and cerebellar cortical abiotrophy in papillon and papillon-related dogs. J Vet Med Sci 2007, 69:1047-1052.
Sanders SG, Bagley RS. Cerebellar diseases and tremor syndromes. In: Dewey CW, ed., A Practical Guide to Canine and Feline Neurology, 2nd ed. Ames, IA: Wiley-Blackwell, 2008, pp. 300-301.

Autor Mary O. Smith
Consultor Editorial Joane M. Parent

Distrofias da Córnea

CONSIDERAÇÕES GERAIS

REVISÃO
• Afecção corneana primária, hereditária (ou familiar), bilateral e, muitas vezes, simétrica, não associada a outras doenças oculares ou sistêmicas.
• Há três tipos com base na localização anatômica: epiteliais — associados a células epiteliais disceratóticas e necrosadas, ausência focal de membrana basal epitelial e aumento nas células no estroma corneano anterior; estromais — depósito lipídico no interior do estroma corneano; endoteliais — caracterizadas por células endoteliais distróficas anormais.

IDENTIFICAÇÃO
Geralmente em cães; rara em gatos.

Epiteliais
Pastor de Shetland — idade de início de 6 meses a 6 anos; evolução lenta.

Estromais
• Acometem geralmente cães jovens adultos.
• Raças acometidas — Afghan hound, Airedale terrier, Malamute do Alasca, Cocker spaniel americano, Beagle, Bearded collie, Bichon frisé, Cavalier King Charles spaniel, Pastor alemão, Lhasa apso, Mastife, Pinscher miniatura, Rough collie (Collie de pelo áspero), Samoieda, Husky siberiano, Weimaraner, Whippet e outras; somente em algumas raças, já se identificou o padrão de herança.

Endoteliais
• Cães — acometem principalmente as raças Boston terrier, Chihuahua e Dachshund; podem comprometer outras raças; tipicamente, os animais são de meia-idade ou mais idosos no início dos sinais clínicos; sugere-se a predileção por cadelas.
• Gatos — acometem os animais jovens; descrição mais frequente em gatos domésticos de pelo curto; um problema semelhante que ocorre sem comprometimento endotelial é hereditário na raça Manx como um distúrbio autossômico recessivo.

SINAIS CLÍNICOS
Todos causam certo grau de opacidade na córnea.

Epiteliais
• Podem ser assintomáticas ou apresentar blefarospasmo; opacidades em anéis circulares a irregulares, brancos ou cinzas, multifocais; associados algumas vezes a erosões corneanas multifocais.
• Visão — costuma não ser acometida.

Estromais
• Geralmente assintomáticas, sem inflamação associada.
• Centrais — mais comuns; opacidade oval a circular, de coloração cinza, branca ou prateada, na córnea central ou paracentral; sob aumento, podem-se notar múltiplas opacidades fibrilares a coalescentes, que conferem uma aparência de cristal ou de vidro fosco (distrofia corneana cristalina).
• Difusas — acomete a raça Airedale; opacidade densa mais difusa do que nos casos de distrofia central.
• Anulares — acomete mais comumente a raça Husky siberiano; opacidade em formato de rosquinha na córnea paracentral ou periférica.

• Visão — costuma não ser acometida; em casos de doença avançada ou difusa, é possível o surgimento de déficit visual.

Endoteliais
• Assintomáticas nas fases iniciais.
• Edema da córnea temporal ou inferotemporal, que geralmente evolui até envolver toda a córnea depois de meses a anos.
• Possível desenvolvimento de bolhas epiteliais corneanas (ceratopatia bolhosa) e ulceração/erosão corneanas subsequentes; a erosão ou a ulceração pode causar blefarospasmo em virtude da dor.
• Visão — pode exibir diminuição na acuidade visual em casos de doença avançada.

CAUSAS E FATORES DE RISCO
• Epiteliais — resultado de anormalidades degenerativas ou inatas do epitélio e/ou da membrana basal corneanos.
• Estromais — resultado de anormalidade inata ou erro localizado no metabolismo lipídico corneano; podem ser influenciadas por hiperlipoproteinemia (possivelmente aumenta a opacidade).
• Endoteliais — resultado de degeneração da camada endotelial; a perda subsequente da função de bombeamento do endotélio resulta em edema da córnea.

DIAGNÓSTICO

DIAGNÓSTICO DIFERENCIAL
• Epiteliais, estromais — outras causas de opacidade corneana: degenerações, úlceras, cicatrizes, infiltrados inflamatórios corneanos.
• Endoteliais — outras causas de edema difuso da córnea: uveíte e glaucoma.

HEMOGRAMA/BIOQUÍMICA/URINÁLISE
Epiteliais, estromais — concentrações elevadas nos níveis de colesterol e triglicerídeos podem modificar a evolução da doença, mas não constituem a causa.

MÉTODOS DIAGNÓSTICOS
• Estromais — costumam não reter o corante de fluoresceína.
• Epiteliais ou endoteliais — podem reter o corante de fluoresceína, muitas vezes em áreas puntiformes multifocais, particularmente em casos de doença avançada.
• Tonometria — para eliminar o glaucoma como causa do edema da córnea.

TRATAMENTO

• Doença epitelial ou endotelial avançada com ulceração — podem necessitar de tratamento contra ceratite ulcerativa.
• Estromais — em geral, não necessitam de tratamento; pode-se efetuar a ceratectomia superficial para remover os depósitos lipídicos (se forem graves), mas isso não costuma ser necessário e os depósitos podem recidivar após a cirurgia.
• Informar ao proprietário sobre a natureza hereditária de algumas distrofias da córnea.
• Distrofia endotelial avançada — pode-se fazer uso de lentes de contato terapêuticas flexíveis, com ou sem debridamento do excesso de epitélio corneano; cirurgia com a criação de retalhos (*flaps*) conjuntivais; termoceratoplastia (cauterização térmica da córnea); ceratoplastia penetrante (transplante de córnea) pode ser benéfica, mas os índices de sucesso variam (de razoável a bom em gatos, porém ruim em cães).

MEDICAÇÕES

MEDICAMENTO(S)
• Ulceração da córnea — antibióticos e, possivelmente, atropina tópicos (ver "Ceratite Ulcerativa").
• Epiteliais — ciclosporina a 1-2% em veículo oleoso ou pomada oftalmológica desse agente a 0,2% a cada 8-24 h, conforme a necessidade, para alívio dos sinais clínicos.
• Endoteliais — pomada tópica de cloreto de sódio a 5%; tratamento paliativo; não promove a remoção acentuada de debris da córnea, mas pode evitar a evolução e a ruptura de bolhas epiteliais corneanas.

CONTRAINDICAÇÕES/INTERAÇÕES POSSÍVEIS
Corticosteroides tópicos — não demonstram qualquer benefício em casos de distrofia lipídica (estromal); além disso, apresentam benefício questionável em outras formas de distrofia.

ACOMPANHAMENTO

• Reavaliação — necessária apenas diante do desenvolvimento de dor ocular (oftalmalgia) ou ulceração corneana.
• Opacidade da córnea — pode aumentar e diminuir em casos de distrofia lipídica; sua resolução é improvável.
• Ulceração da córnea — pode acompanhar a evolução de distrofia epitelial ou endotelial.
• Visão — não é acometida de forma considerável, exceto em casos avançados.

DIVERSOS

VER TAMBÉM
• Ceratite Ulcerativa.
• Degenerações e Infiltrações da Córnea.

RECURSOS DA INTERNET
www.eyevet.info/corneal_dystrophy.html.

Sugestões de Leitura
Crispin SM, Barnett KC. Dystrophy, degeneration and infiltration of the canine cornea. J Small Anim Pract 1983;24:63-83.

Autor Ellison Bentley
Consultor Editorial Paul E. Miller
Agradecimentos O autor gostaria de agradecer as contribuições feitas por B. Keith Collins na preparação deste capítulo.

Distúrbios da Articulação Temporomandibular

CONSIDERAÇÕES GERAIS

REVISÃO
• Distúrbios da ATM levam à alteração da função normal do sistema mastigador*, uma vez que a mobilidade e a função da articulação ficam comprometidas.
• Causas genéticas, traumáticas, degenerativas ou idiopáticas podem resultar em dor, disfunção oclusal, frouxidão articular, artrite crônica ou travamento com a boca aberta.

IDENTIFICAÇÃO
• Cães e gatos.
• Nenhuma predisposição racial, sexual nem etária na maior parte dos distúrbios da ATM.
• Travamento mandibular com a boca aberta — raças Basset hound e Setter irlandês.
• Pode haver predisposição genética em determinadas raças (p. ex. Basset hound) para o desenvolvimento de distúrbios da ATM.

SINAIS CLÍNICOS
Gerais
• Dificuldade de abertura da boca.
• Dificuldade de fechamento da boca.
• Frouxidão ou movimento lateral excessivo da mandíbula.
• Dor e/ou crepitação à mastigação, ao bocejo e/ou à vocalização.

Específicos
• Luxação/subluxação da ATM — histórico de traumatismo ou travamento com a boca aberta; evidência radiográfica de luxação.
• Travamento mandibular com a boca aberta — o processo coronoide da mandíbula "desliza" lateralmente à superfície ventral do arco zigomático e fica travado naquela posição; grande saliência palpada no lado acometido da face.
• Lesão traumática — indícios do traumatismo; boca aberta caída; mobilidade da mandíbula (pode apresentar fraturas múltiplas); radiografias indicam fratura.
• Osteoartrite/alterações pós-traumáticas crônicas — crepitação e dor ao comer ou se a mandíbula for forçada a se mover; radiografias podem demonstrar reação óssea indicativa de alterações artríticas.

CAUSAS E FATORES DE RISCO
• Pacientes sob maior risco de sofrer lesões — jovens; animais de vida livre.
• Traumatismo pode provocar fraturas ou luxação, resultando em problemas imediatos, bem como problemas degenerativos futuros.
• Neurapraxia mandibular — carregar objetos pesados na boca.
• Miosite dos músculos da mastigação — adulto; raça de grande porte (p. ex., Pastor alemão).

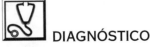

DIAGNÓSTICO

DIAGNÓSTICO DIFERENCIAL
• Osteopatia craniomandibular.
• Hiperparatireoidismo primário ou secundário.

---
* N. T.: Estrutura osteoarticular e muscular que constitui o aparelho da mastigação.

• Neurapraxia mandibular — estiramento dos ramos nervosos (motores) dos músculos da mastigação; em geral, causado por se transportar objetos pesados com a boca; a mandíbula pende aberta, porém pode ser fechada manualmente com facilidade.
• Miosite dos músculos da mastigação — doença autoimune de miofibras tipo 2M dos músculos em questão, inervadas pelo nervo trigêmeo, com necrose, fagocitose e fibrose; o trismo evolui para a incapacidade total de abertura dos maxilares.

HEMOGRAMA/BIOQUÍMICA/URINÁLISE
Espera-se que os achados se encontrem dentro dos limites de normalidade.

OUTROS TESTES LABORATORIAIS
• Autoanticorpos séricos contra a miosina tipo 2M — para descartar miosite dos músculos da mastigação.
• Citologia do líquido aspirado da ATM — pode ser benéfica no diagnóstico de uma poliartropatia caracterizada por inflamação das superfícies articulares.

DIAGNÓSTICO POR IMAGEM
• Radiografia do crânio — é essencial efetuar uma técnica radiográfica adequada para visualização da ATM.
• RM — exame com padrão de excelência pela formação de imagens da ATM.

MÉTODOS DIAGNÓSTICOS
• Geralmente nenhum.
• Biopsia muscular — para descartar miosite dos músculos da mastigação.

TRATAMENTO

• O tratamento definitivo é direcionado à eliminação ou alteração do fator etiológico responsável pelo distúrbio, bem como à correção do problema.
• Luxação da ATM — traumática: a luxação frequentemente ocorre no sentido rostral; em casos agudos, colocar um "pino" (um lápis) atravessando a boca entre os dentes carniceiros (4º pré-molar superior); fechar delicadamente a porção rostral da boca com uma "tração" suave para reduzir a luxação (empurrar no sentido caudal em caso de luxação rostral); pode não ser possível a redução de luxações crônicas, o que talvez exija a realização de cirurgia.
• Travamento mandibular com a boca aberta — exige atendimento imediato; sedar o animal, abrir mais a boca e aplicar delicada pressão sobre a saliência do processo coronoide para permitir seu deslizamento para trás, sob o arco zigomático; tratamento cirúrgico: excisar a porção ventral do arco zigomático e/ou a porção dorsal do processo coronoide para aliviar futuros travamentos.
• Lesão ou fratura na ATM — dependem da extensão do dano; a fixação não é uma tarefa fácil; às vezes, há necessidade de condilectomia.
• Osteoartrite ou anquilose crônicas — quando graves, a condilectomia pode ser necessária.
• "Mandíbula caída" (neurapraxia [mandibular] do trigêmeo) — tratamento conservador: repouso, medicamentos anti-inflamatórios.
• Miosite dos músculos da mastigação — medicações imunossupressoras; abertura da boca forçada gradual dentro do possível.

MEDICAÇÕES

MEDICAMENTO(S) DE ESCOLHA
• Analgésicos — nos distúrbios dolorosos.
• Medicamentos anti-inflamatórios — na dor pós-operatória e na inflamação crônica.
• Relaxantes musculares — ajudam a evitar atividade muscular acentuada em virtude da resposta à dor crônica.

ACOMPANHAMENTO

MONITORIZAÇÃO DO PACIENTE
Cada caso deve ser acompanhado com cuidado por causa das alterações progressivas que podem ocorrer na ATM, especialmente após lesão traumática.

PREVENÇÃO
Evitar situações que permitam o traumatismo (animais correndo soltos).

COMPLICAÇÕES POSSÍVEIS
Em muitos casos após o tratamento cirúrgico envolvendo distúrbios da ATM, pode ocorrer o subsequente desenvolvimento de artrite.

EVOLUÇÃO ESPERADA E PROGNÓSTICO
Dependem do distúrbio que acomete a ATM e do grau desse acometimento.

DIVERSOS

GESTAÇÃO/FERTILIDADE/REPRODUÇÃO
A condição tipicamente não é afetada pela prenhez. Todavia, se o tratamento clínico for considerado, agentes como os corticosteroides não devem ser usados nas pacientes prenhes.

VER TAMBÉM
Fraturas Maxilares e Mandibulares.

ABREVIATURA(S)
• ATM = articulação temporomandibular.
• RM = ressonância magnética.

RECURSOS DA INTERNET
http://www.avdc.org/Nomenclature.html.

Sugestões de Leitura
Harvey CE, Emily PP. Oral lesions of soft tissues and bone: Differential diagnosis. In: Harvey CE, Emily PP, eds., Small Animal Dentistry. St. Louis: Mosby, 1993, pp. 85-88.
Lobprise HB. Blackwell's Five-Minute Veterinary Consult Clinical Companion—Small Animal Dentistry. Ames, IA: Blackwell, 2007 (for additional topics, including diagnostics and techniques).
Okeson JP. Management of Temporomandibular Disorders and Occlusion. St. Louis: Mosby, 1998.
Wiggs, RB, Lobprise, HB. Clinical oral pathology. In: Wiggs RB, Lobprise HB, Veterinary Dentistry: Principles and Practice. Philadelphia: Lippincott-Raven, 1997, pp. 127-130.

Autores Heidi B. Lobprise e Bonnie C. Bloom
Consultor Editorial Heidi B. Lobprise

Distúrbios da Imunodeficiência Primária

CONSIDERAÇÕES GERAIS

DEFINIÇÃO
Baixa capacidade de elaborar uma resposta imune eficaz em virtude de defeitos hereditários no sistema imunológico.

FISIOPATOLOGIA
• Na literatura especializada veterinária, foram descritos defeitos nos sistemas mediado por células e do complemento, bem como nos sistemas humorais e fagocitários. • Defeitos que envolvem a resposta imune humoral — associados a maior suscetibilidade à infecção bacteriana. • Defeitos que envolvem a resposta imune mediada por células — associados a maior suscetibilidade a infecções virais, fúngicas e protozoárias. • Defeitos no sistema fagocitário ou do complemento — associados à infecção disseminada.

SISTEMA(S) ACOMETIDO(S)
• Hematológico/linfático/imune — defeito em uma população celular específica no tecido linfoide. • Cutâneo/exócrino/respiratório/gastrintestinal — infecções crônicas ou recidivantes. • Outros sistemas orgânicos — disseminação de infecção, falha de desenvolvimento.

GENÉTICA
Tipicamente específicos da raça com modos de herança variáveis.

INCIDÊNCIA/PREVALÊNCIA
Raros.

IDENTIFICAÇÃO

Espécies
Cães e gatos.

Raça(s) Predominante(s)
• Imunodeficiência combinada grave ligada ao cromossomo X — Basset hound, Cardigan Welsh corgi. • Imunodeficiência combinada grave — Jack Russel terrier. • Deficiência de IgA — Beagle, Pastor alemão e Shar-pei chinês. • Deficiência de IgM — Doberman pinscher. • Hipoplasia do timo — Weimaraner anão. • Hematopoiese cíclica — Collie cinza. • Síndrome de Chediak-Higashi — gato Persa. • Deficiência de adesão leucocitária — Setter irlandês. • Deficiência de complemento — Spaniel britânico. • Defeito bactericida — Doberman pinscher. • Hipogamaglobulinemia transitória — Samoieda.

Idade Média e Faixa Etária
As imunodeficiências primárias tipicamente se manifestam no primeiro ano de vida.

Sexo Predominante
Imunodeficiência combinada grave recessiva ligada ao cromossomo X de Basset hound — machos acometidos e fêmeas portadoras do defeito.

SINAIS CLÍNICOS

Comentários Gerais
Dependem do nível de defeito da resposta imune; variam desde sinais respiratórios e gastrintestinais crônicos e infecções cutâneas até condições potencialmente letais.

Achados Anamnésicos
• Alta suscetibilidade a infecções e falha em responder à antibioticoterapia convencional apropriada. • Letargia. • Anorexia. • Infecção cutânea. • Desenvolvimento insuficiente. • Os sinais frequentemente aparecem quando a concentração de anticorpos maternos declina. • Doença induzida por vacina com vírus vivo modificado.

Achados do Exame Físico
• Característicos — desenvolvimento insuficiente. • Sinais clínicos atribuíveis a infecções.

CAUSAS
Congênitas.

DIAGNÓSTICO

DIAGNÓSTICO DIFERENCIAL
• Os pacientes precisam ser rigorosamente examinados em busca do processo mórbido subjacente capaz de causar um estado de imunodeficiência secundário (adquirido) (p. ex., hiperadrenocorticismo, FeLV e FIV). • Os pacientes são tipicamente jovens com infecção recidivante que não respondem ao tratamento convencional.

HEMOGRAMA/BIOQUÍMICA/URINÁLISE
O hemograma completo pode indicar deficiências em linhagens celulares afetadas de forma específica ou algum processo inflamatório crônico.

OUTROS TESTES LABORATORIAIS
• Eletroforese de proteínas séricas — demonstra deficiência visível na concentração de imunoglobulina. • Quantificação de imunoglobulina sérica — avalia o sistema imune humoral, identifica a deficiência seletiva de imunoglobulina e confirma o diagnóstico de agamaglobulinemia. • Teste da transformação de linfócitos — avalia o sistema imune mediado por células e identifica os animais com deficiência de linfócitos T. • Ensaios bactericidas — avaliam a função dos neutrófilos. • Concentração sérica de componentes do complemento — diagnostica a deficiência de complemento. • Enumeração de subgrupos de linfócitos por imunofluorescência com anticorpos monoclonais — identifica a deficiência de linhagens celulares específicas.
• Existem outros testes mais específicos disponíveis para avaliar a função imunológica em espécies veterinárias; no entanto, para a obtenção de resultados confiáveis, há necessidade do acesso a laboratórios de pesquisa que realizem esses testes.

MÉTODOS DIAGNÓSTICOS
Em alguns pacientes, a biopsia de medula óssea e linfonodos ajuda a classificar o tipo de imunodeficiência.

ACHADOS PATOLÓGICOS
• As lesões variam, pois dependem do defeito específico. A maioria resulta de infecção recidivante ou oportunista envolvendo a pele, o canal auditivo e os sistemas respiratório e gastrintestinal. • Lesões de septicemia são comuns em animais com defeitos graves. • Defeitos dos linfócitos T — lesões hipoplásicas ou displásicas do timo e de áreas de tecidos linfoides secundários dependentes dessas células. • Defeitos dos linfócitos B — lesões hipoplásicas ou displásicas da medula óssea ou de áreas de tecidos linfoides secundários dependentes dessas células. • Pode-se detectar hipoplasia ou hiperplasia linfoide, dependendo do defeito geral e da ocorrência de infecção.

TRATAMENTO

CUIDADO(S) DE SAÚDE ADEQUADO(S)
• Talvez haja necessidade de internação para controlar as infecções potencialmente letais. • O tratamento ambulatorial é possível para alguns pacientes.

CUIDADO(S) DE ENFERMAGEM
Cuidados de suporte adequados à natureza da infecção.

ATIVIDADE
Determinada basicamente pela gravidade do defeito e pela ocorrência de infecção.

DIETA
• Pode ser necessário o manejo nutricional para garantir que o paciente seja mantido em um nível adequado de nutrição. • É imprescindível evitar o consumo de fontes potenciais de agentes infecciosos, como carne crua.

ORIENTAÇÃO AO PROPRIETÁRIO
• Informar ao proprietário que não há cura para o animal. • Explicar porque o paciente tem alta suscetibilidade à infecção. • Abordar o caráter hereditário da doença. • Discutir a possibilidade de outros indivíduos da ninhada estarem acometidos. • Evitar a exposição a animais doentes.

MEDICAÇÕES

MEDICAMENTO(S) DE ESCOLHA
• Antibióticos para controlar as infecções.
• Gamaglobulina ou preparações de plasma podem ser usadas em conjunto com antibióticos para controlar as infecções em pacientes com defeito humoral. • Tratamento sintomático de estados mórbidos secundários.

CONTRAINDICAÇÕES
Não é recomendável a administração de gamaglobulina ou preparações de plasma a pacientes com deficiência seletiva de IgA, porque muitos pacientes acometidos têm altas concentrações de anticorpos anti-IgA e podem desenvolver uma reação anafilática.

PRECAUÇÕES
Vacinas de vírus vivos modificados não devem ser administradas a pacientes com suspeita de deficiências de linfócitos T, pois podem induzir à doença.

ACOMPANHAMENTO

MONITORIZAÇÃO DO PACIENTE
• Monitorizar o paciente em busca de sinais clínicos de infecções secundárias. • Efetuar exame físico de rotina para avaliar a eficácia da antibioticoterapia.

PREVENÇÃO
• Não acasalar os animais acometidos. • Realizar a análise do *pedigree* para determinar o modo de herança e evitar a propagação do defeito.

COMPLICAÇÕES POSSÍVEIS
Infecções.

EVOLUÇÃO ESPERADA E PROGNÓSTICO
• A gravidade do defeito determina a evolução da doença e seu prognóstico. • Os pacientes com defeitos mínimos podem ser tratados com sucesso.

DIVERSOS

ABREVIATURA(S)
• FeLV = vírus da leucemia felina. • FIV = vírus da imunodeficiência felina.

Autor Paul W. Snyder
Consultor Editorial A.H. Rebar

Distúrbios da Motilidade Gástrica

CONSIDERAÇÕES GERAIS

DEFINIÇÃO
Os distúrbios da motilidade gástrica resultam de condições que interrompem direta ou indiretamente o esvaziamento gástrico normal, o que, por sua vez, pode causar retenção gástrica anormal, distensão gástrica e sinais gástricos subsequentes associados a anorexia, náuseas e vômitos.

FISIOPATOLOGIA
O estômago possui duas regiões motoras distintas. A região proximal relaxa para acomodar o alimento e regular a expulsão dos líquidos. Contrações lentas intrínsecas dessa região empurram os líquidos pelo piloro. A porção distal do estômago fragmenta mecanicamente os sólidos, expelindo-os por meio de fortes contrações peristálticas. A motilidade e o esvaziamento gástricos distais são regulados por um marca-passo gástrico, uma área de atividade elétrica intrínseca encontrada na curvatura maior. A atividade elétrica gástrica, a composição alimentar e os fatores extrínsecos, sem exceção, influenciam o esvaziamento. Durante o jejum, sólidos indigeríveis são expelidos do estômago por complexos mioelétricos migratórios que produzem fortes contrações em todo o estômago e nos intestinos a cada 2 h no estado de jejum. Essa motilidade está sob a regulação do hormônio motilina. Disritmias na atividade elétrica gástrica normal podem ser fundamentais na fisiopatologia dos distúrbios que afetam a motilidade gástrica.

SISTEMA(S) ACOMETIDO(S)
Gastrintestinal.

INCIDÊNCIA/PREVALÊNCIA
Desconhecidas. Muitos fatores podem alterar o esvaziamento gástrico, embora possam não resultar em doença clínica.

IDENTIFICAÇÃO
Espécies
Cães e gatos.

Raça(s) Predominante(s)
Desconhecidas.

Idade Média e Faixa Etária
Os sintomas ocorrem em qualquer idade, embora seja incomum observar distúrbios primários da motilidade em animais jovens.

SINAIS CLÍNICOS
Comentários Gerais
Os sinais clínicos são frequentemente secundários à etiologia primária do distúrbio da motilidade gástrica.

Achados Anamnésicos
• O principal sinal clínico consiste em vômitos pós-prandiais crônicos de alimento. O estômago deve ser esvaziado após uma refeição média em aproximadamente 6-8 h em cães e 4-6 h em gatos (nota: os tempos normais de esvaziamento variam muito entre os animais, sendo influenciados pelo volume da refeição, densidade de calorias e conteúdo de fibras). O vômito de alimento não digerido mais de 12 h após uma refeição sugere algum distúrbio da motilidade gástrica ou, possivelmente, obstrução do fluxo de saída. No entanto, pode ocorrer vômito a qualquer momento após uma refeição.
• Outros sinais incluem distensão gástrica, náuseas, anorexia, eructação, pica e perda de peso.
• O esfíncter esofágico distal também pode estar incompetente com hipomotilidade gástrica, podendo haver sinais associados a esofagite por refluxo.

Achados do Exame Físico
• Normais ou associados à causa subjacente do distúrbio.
• Palpação de estômago grande e distendido.
• Ruídos gástricos diminuídos à auscultação abdominal.

CAUSAS
• Os distúrbios idiopáticos primários da motilidade gástrica podem surgir de defeitos na atividade mioelétrica normal. A maioria dos distúrbios da motilidade ocorre secundariamente a outras condições primárias.
• Distúrbios metabólicos incluem hipocalemia, uremia, encefalopatia hepática e hipotireoidismo.
• Inibição nervosa como resultado de estresse, medo, dor ou traumatismo.
• Medicamentos como anticolinérgicos, agonistas β-adrenérgicos e narcóticos.
• Doença gástrica primária como obstruções do fluxo de saída, gastrite, úlceras gástricas, parvovirose e cirurgia gástrica.
• Há suspeitas de que a síndrome de dilatação e vólvulo gástricos resulte de algum distúrbio primário da motilidade associado à atividade mioelétrica e mecânica anormal. Os cães podem continuar tendo sinais de hipomotilidade gástrica após gastropexia cirúrgica.
• Os refluxos gastresofágicos e enterogástricos (ver "Síndrome do Vômito Bilioso") podem resultar de hipomotilidade gástrica.
• As síndromes de disautonomia apresentam a hipomotilidade gástrica como parte de uma doença generalizada.

FATORES DE RISCO
Qualquer doença gástrica potencial pode resultar em hipomotilidade secundária.

DIAGNÓSTICO

DIAGNÓSTICO DIFERENCIAL
Além de ser amplo, o diagnóstico diferencial deve incluir qualquer condição que cause vômito. Sempre é preciso excluir obstruções do fluxo de saída gástrico.

HEMOGRAMA/BIOQUÍMICA/URINÁLISE
O hemograma de rotina, o perfil bioquímico sérico, a urinálise e o teste de flutuação fecal precisam ser realizados para descartar a causa potencial de hipomotilidade gástrica. Vômitos contínuos podem resultar em desidratação, anormalidades eletrolíticas ou desequilíbrio acidobásico. Hipocalemia é uma anormalidade eletrolítica comum associada à motilidade gastrintestinal anormal.

OUTROS TESTES LABORATORIAIS
Talvez haja necessidade de exames especiais para determinar a causa específica da hipomotilidade gástrica, sendo individualizados para cada paciente.

DIAGNÓSTICO POR IMAGEM
Radiografias Simples
Radiografias abdominais podem revelar estômago distendido com gás, líquido ou ingesta.

Radiografia Contrastada com Bário Líquido
Pode exibir indícios de atraso do esvaziamento gástrico e contrações gástricas diminuídas à fluoroscopia. Alguns casos podem apresentar esvaziamento normal de líquidos, mas anormal de sólidos (nota: o estresse das radiografias pode diminuir o esvaziamento gástrico mesmo no animal normal).

Radiografia Contrastada com Bário Ingerido
O bário misturado a uma refeição normal pode demonstrar o atraso do esvaziamento gástrico de sólidos. Os cães normais esvaziam o estômago em aproximadamente 6-8 h. A retenção gástrica anormal está associada a tempos mais prolongados de esvaziamento gástrico.

Radiografia Contrastada com Marcador Ingerido
Pequenos marcadores impregnados com bário ou outros marcadores radiopacos misturados com uma refeição normal provocam atraso na passagem semelhantemente àquele observado na radiografia contrastada com bário ingerido com alimento.

Emissão de Radionuclídeo
Marcadores radionuclídeos misturados com uma refeição fornecem a medida mais precisa do esvaziamento em termos clínicos. O tempo de esvaziamento gástrico (tempo que uma refeição normal leva para deixar o estômago) varia de 4-8 h.

Ultrassonografia
Pode-se usar o ultrassom para avaliar a motilidade antral e pilórica.

Smartpill (dispositivo médico)
Trata-se de uma cápsula sensora sem fio não invasiva, que é administrada por via oral e transmite dados sobre pressão, tempo de trânsito, pH do lúmen e temperatura à medida que passa pelo estômago e pelos intestinos (delgado e grosso). É um teste utilizado em seres humanos para estudar a motilidade GI que vem sendo aplicado no cão.

MÉTODOS DIAGNÓSTICOS
Endoscopia
Os achados endoscópicos frequentemente permanecem normais em condições idiopáticas. É possível encontrar alimento no estômago quando ele deveria estar vazio após um período de jejum pré-endoscópico de 12 h. A endoscopia detecta doenças obstrutivas ou inflamatórias do estômago.

ACHADOS PATOLÓGICOS
• Em condições idiopáticas, a mucosa gástrica encontra-se normal.
• A histologia do estômago pode identificar causas inflamatórias ou neoplásicas que expliquem a hipomotilidade gástrica.

TRATAMENTO

CUIDADO(S) DE SAÚDE ADEQUADO(S)
• A maioria dos pacientes é tratada em um esquema ambulatorial.
• Nos casos de vômitos ou desidratação graves e desequilíbrio eletrolítico, há necessidade de hospitalização e terapia específica.

CUIDADO(S) DE ENFERMAGEM
Desidratação com desequilíbrio hidreletrolítico requer reposição apropriada de líquidos.

Distúrbios da Motilidade Gástrica

ATIVIDADE
As restrições baseiam-se na doença subjacente.

DIETA
- A manipulação da dieta é importante no tratamento dos distúrbios primários da motilidade gástrica.
- Devem ser formuladas dietas de consistência líquida ou semilíquida, com baixo teor de gorduras e fibras.
- É recomendável o fornecimento de refeições em pequenas quantidades várias vezes ao dia.
- Em geral, a mera manipulação da dieta é bem-sucedida no tratamento de pacientes com esvaziamento gástrico tardio causado por algum distúrbio da motilidade.

ORIENTAÇÃO AO PROPRIETÁRIO
Discutir as possíveis etiologias subjacentes de alteração da motilidade gástrica e a variação da resposta à terapia para cada indivíduo.

CONSIDERAÇÕES CIRÚRGICAS
- Os cães acometidos pela síndrome crônica de dilatação-vólvulo gástricos e retenção gástrica devem ser submetidos à gastropexia cirúrgica.
- Após qualquer cirurgia gástrica, podem levar até 14 dias para que a motilidade volte ao normal.
- Pacientes com obstruções do fluxo de saída necessitam de correção cirúrgica.

MEDICAÇÕES

MEDICAMENTO(S)
Agentes Procinéticos Gástricos
- A metoclopramida (Reglan®) aumenta a amplitude das contrações do antro e inibe o relaxamento receptivo do fundo, além de coordenar a motilidade duodenal e gástrica. É um antagonista dos receptores dopaminérgicos no trato GI proximal, resultando em aumento na liberação de acetilcolina pelos neurônios entéricos. Também tem efeitos antieméticos, bloqueando a zona de deflagração dos quimiorreceptores no tronco cerebral em cães, mas não em gatos. A dosagem oral é de 0,2-0,4 mg/kg a cada 6-8 h, administrados 30 min antes das refeições (usar uma dose menor em gatos). A metoclopramida é considerada um procinético fraco.
- A cisaprida atua diretamente por neurotransmissão colinérgica da musculatura lisa gastrintestinal, estimulando a motilidade. O mecanismo de ação proposto é que ela acentua a liberação de acetilcolina no plexo mioentérico, mas não induz à estimulação dos receptores nicotínicos ou muscarínicos. Esse agente também aumenta a pressão no esfíncter esofágico inferior, melhora o esvaziamento gástrico e promove maior motilidade dos intestinos delgado e grosso. A dose sugerida é de 0,1 mg/kg VO a cada 8-12 h antes das refeições. Atualmente, a cisaprida está disponível em farmácias de manipulação, pois o produto humano foi retirado do mercado em função dos efeitos de arritmias cardíacas.
- Antibióticos macrolídeos, incluindo eritromicina e claritromicina, são agonistas dos receptores da motilina e aumentam a motilidade gastrintestinal. A eritromicina em doses baixas (submicrobiológicas) atua como agonista dos receptores da motilina, promovendo a liberação de acetilcolina que, por sua vez, promove o esvaziamento gástrico. A dose sugerida de eritromicina para a obtenção de efeitos específicos sobre a motilidade é de 0,5-1 mg/kg VO a cada 8-12 h, administrados 30 min antes das refeições. A eritromicina parece ser mais eficaz que a metoclopramida como agente procinético.
- Domperidona é um antagonista dos receptores dopaminérgicos periféricos que é comercializado fora dos EUA. Esse agente regula a motilidade da musculatura lisa do estômago e do intestino delgado do mesmo modo que a metoclopramida.
- Os antagonistas dos receptores H_2 — ranitidina (2 mg/kg VO a cada 8 h) e nizatidina (5 mg/kg VO a cada 24 h) — têm efeitos procinéticos significativos sobre a motilidade gástrica em virtude da inibição da acetilcolinesterase. Nem a cimetidina nem a famotidina afetam o esvaziamento gástrico.

CONTRAINDICAÇÕES
- Os procinéticos gástricos não devem ser administrados a pacientes com obstrução do fluxo de saída gástrico.
- A metoclopramida está contraindicada com a administração concomitante de fenotiazina e narcóticos ou em animais com epilepsia.

PRECAUÇÕES
- A metoclopramida pode causar nervosismo, ansiedade ou depressão.
- A cisaprida pode provocar depressão, vômitos, diarreia ou cólica abdominal.
- A eritromicina pode induzir a vômitos.

ACOMPANHAMENTO

MONITORIZAÇÃO DO PACIENTE
- A resposta ao tratamento varia de acordo com a causa subjacente.
- A falha em responder ao tratamento clínico requer pesquisa adicional em busca de obstrução mecânica.

EVOLUÇÃO ESPERADA E PROGNÓSTICO
- A duração do tratamento depende da capacidade de resolução do distúrbio subjacente ou da resposta à terapia.
- Nos casos de cirurgia gástrica ou parvovirose, a função gástrica pode levar 10-14 dias para voltar ao normal.
- A disautonomia generalizada tem prognóstico grave.

DIVERSOS

DISTÚRBIOS ASSOCIADOS
A hipomotilidade gástrica pode estar associada à esofagite por refluxo e gastrite por refluxo (síndrome do vômito bilioso).

GESTAÇÃO/FERTILIDADE/REPRODUÇÃO
Evitar os procinéticos gástricos em animais prenhes.

SINÔNIMO(S)
- Hipomotilidade gástrica.
- Atonia gástrica.

VER TAMBÉM
- Gastrite Atrófica.
- Gastrite Crônica.
- Refluxo Gastresofágico.
- Síndrome da Dilatação e Vólvulo Gástricos.
- Síndrome do Vômito Bilioso.

ABREVIATURA(S)
- GI = gastrintestinal.

Sugestões de Leitura
Hall, J.A. Diseases of the stomach. In: Ettinger, S.J., Feldman, E.C., eds. Textbook of veterinary internal medicine, 5th ed. Philadelphia: Saunders, 2000;1154-1181.
Hall, J.A., Washabau, F Diagnosis and treatment of gastric motility disorders. Vet Clin North Am Small Anim Pract 1999; 29:377-395.
Harkin, K.R., Andrews, G.A., Nietfeld, J.C. Dysautonomia in dogs: 65 cases (1993-2000). J Am Vet Med Assoc. 2002, 220(5):633-639.
Washabau, R.J. Gastrointestinal motility disorders and gastrointestinal prokinetic therapy.Vet Clin North Am Small Anim Pract. 2003, 33(5):1007-2.

Autor David C. Twedt
Consultor Editorial Albert E. Jergens

DISTÚRBIOS DA UNHA E DO LEITO UNGUEAL

CONSIDERAÇÕES GERAIS

DEFINIÇÃO
• Paroníquia — inflamação do tecido mole ao redor da unha. • Dobra ungueal — tecido em formato de lua crescente que circunda a porção proximal da unha. • Banda coronária e crista dorsal — produz grande parte da unha.
• Onicomicose — infecção fúngica da unha.
• Onicorrexe — unhas quebradiças que tendem a fender ou quebrar. • Onicomadese — esfacelamento da unha. • Distrofia ungueal — deformidade provocada por crescimento anormal; frequentemente uma sequela de algum distúrbio.
• Onicomalacia — amolecimento das unhas.

FISIOPATOLOGIA
• Unhas e dobras ungueais — sujeitas a traumatismo, infecção, insuficiência vascular, doença imunomediada, neoplasia, defeitos de queratinização e anormalidades congênitas.

SISTEMA(S) ACOMETIDO(S)
Cutâneo/exócrino.

IDENTIFICAÇÃO
• Cães e gatos. • Dachshund — onicorrexe. • Pastor alemão, Rottweiler, possivelmente Schnauzer gigante e Doberman pinscher — onicodistrofia lupoide simétrica. • Husky siberiano, Dachshund, Rhodesian ridgeback, Rottweiler, Cocker spaniel — onicodistrofia idiopática. • Pastor alemão, Whippet, Springer spaniel inglês — onicomadese idiopática. • Faixa etária média — 3-8 anos para onicodistrofia lupoide simétrica. • Não há relatos de predominância sexual.

SINAIS CLÍNICOS
• Lambedura dos pés e/ou das unhas/dobras ungueais. • Claudicação. • Dor. • Eritema, tumefação e exsudato das unhas/dobras ungueais.
• Deformidade ou esfacelamento da unha.
• Alteração de cor da unha. • Hemorragia proveniente da unha ou na perda de alguma unha.
• Descrição prévia de "pés sensíveis".

CAUSAS
Paroníquia
• Infecção — bactérias, dermatófito, levedura (*Candida*, *Malassezia*), demodicose, leishmaniose.
• Imunomediada — pênfigo, penfigoide bolhoso, LES, erupção medicamentosa, onicodistrofia lupoide simétrica. • Neoplasia — carcinoma subungueal de células escamosas, melanoma, carcinoma écrino, osteossarcoma, queratoacantoma subungueal, papiloma escamoso invertido. • Fístula arteriovenosa.

Onicomicose
• Cães — *Trichophyton mentagrophytes* — geralmente generalizado. • Gatos — *Microsporum canis*.

Onicorrexe
• Idiopática — especialmente no Dachshund; múltiplas unhas. • Traumatismo. • Infecção — dermatofitose, leishmaniose.

Onicomadese
• Traumatismo. • Infecção. • Imunomediada — pênfigo, penfigoide bolhoso, LES, erupção medicamentosa, onicodistrofia lupoide simétrica.
• Insuficiência vascular — vasculite, doença da aglutinina fria. • Neoplasia — ver anteriormente.
• Idiopática.

Distrofia Ungueal
• Acromegalia. • Hipertireoidismo felino.
• Dermatose responsiva ao zinco. • Más-formações congênitas.

DIAGNÓSTICO

DIAGNÓSTICO DIFERENCIAL
• Traumatismo ou neoplasia frequentemente acomete uma única unha. • Envolvimento de várias unhas sugere doença sistêmica. • Doenças imunomediadas (exceto onicodistrofia lupoide simétrica) apresentam, em geral, outras lesões cutâneas além das lesões das unhas/dobras ungueais.

HEMOGRAMA/BIOQUÍMICA/URINÁLISE
Podem revelar indícios de LES, diabetes melito, hipertireoidismo ou outra doença sistêmica.

OUTROS TESTES LABORATORIAIS
• FeLV. • Tiroxina sérica. • Título de ANA.

DIAGNÓSTICO POR IMAGEM
Radiografias — osteomielite da terceira falange, alteração neoplásica.

OUTROS MÉTODOS DIAGNÓSTICOS
• Biopsia — frequentemente envolve a amputação da terceira falange; a inclusão da banda coronária é necessária para o diagnóstico de grande parte dos casos. • Citologia do exsudato obtido da unha e/ou da dobra ungueal. • Raspado cutâneo.
• Cultura bacteriana e fúngica.

TRATAMENTO

Paroníquia
• Remoção cirúrgica da placa ungueal (cobertura externa). • Embebições antimicrobianas.
• Identificação da causa subjacente e tratamento específico.

Onicomicose
• Embebições antifúngicas — clorexidina, iodopovidona, solução de enxofre. • Remoção cirúrgica da placa ungueal — pode melhorar a resposta à medicação sistêmica. • Amputação da terceira falange.

Onicorrexe
• Reparo com cola ungueal (tipo utilizado para colar unhas falsas nas pessoas). • Remoção de pedaços lascados. • Amputação da terceira falange.
• Tratamento da causa subjacente.

Onicomadese
• Embebições antimicrobianas. • Tratamento da causa subjacente.

Neoplasia
• Determinado pelo comportamento biológico do tumor específico. • Excisão cirúrgica. • Amputação do dedo ou do membro. • Quimioterapia e/ou radioterapia.

Distrofia Ungueal
• Tratamento da causa subjacente.

MEDICAÇÕES

MEDICAMENTO(S) DE ESCOLHA
• Paroníquia por bactérias — antibióticos sistêmicos selecionados com base na cultura e no antibiograma. • Paroníquia por leveduras — por *Candida* ou *Malassezia* — cetoconazol (10 mg/kg VO a cada 12-24 h); nistatina ou miconazol tópicos. • Onicomicose — griseofulvina (50-150 mg/kg VO por dia) ou cetoconazol (10 mg/kg VO a cada 12 h) durante 6-12 meses até a obtenção de resultados negativos à cultura; itraconazol (10 mg/kg VO a cada 24 h) durante 3 semanas e, em seguida, pulsoterapia 2 vezes por semana até a resolução do quadro. • Onicomadese — o tratamento é determinado pela causa; terapia imunomoduladora para doenças imunomediadas; os medicamentos incluem ciclosporina, tetraciclina com niacinamida, pentoxifilina, vitamina E, suplementações com ácidos graxos essenciais e agentes quimioterápicos (azatioprina, clorambucila, etc.).

CONTRAINDICAÇÕES
Griseofulvina — não utilizar em fêmeas prenhes.

PRECAUÇÕES
• Griseofulvina — pode provocar mielossupressão, anorexia, vômito e diarreia; a absorção é intensificada se administrada com refeição rica em gordura. • Cetoconazol — pode provocar anorexia, irritação gástrica, hepatotoxicidade e clareamento da pelagem.

ACOMPANHAMENTO

EVOLUÇÃO ESPERADA E PROGNÓSTICO
• Paroníquia por bactérias ou leveduras e onicomicose — o tratamento pode ser prolongado e a resposta, influenciada por fatores subjacentes.
• Onicorrexe — talvez haja necessidade de amputação da terceira falange para a resolução.
• Onicomadese — o prognóstico é determinado pela causa subjacente; doenças imunomediadas e problemas vasculares carreiam um prognóstico mais reservado do que causas traumáticas ou infecciosas. • Distrofia ungueal — o prognóstico é bom quando se consegue tratar a causa subjacente.
• Neoplasia — excisadas por amputação do dedo; tumores malignos já sofreram metástase no momento do diagnóstico.

DIVERSOS

POTENCIAL ZOONÓTICO
Dermatofitose.

SINÔNIMO(S)
• Unha/dobra ungueal = leito ungueal. • Oniquite lupoide = onicodistrofia lupoide simétrica.

ABREVIATURA(S)
• ANA = anticorpo antinuclear. • FeLV = vírus da leucemia felina. • LES = lúpus eritematoso sistêmico.

Sugestões de Leitura
Muller GH, Kirk RW, Scott DW. Small Animal Dermatology, 4th ed. Philadelphia: Saunders, 1989.

Autor Karen Helton Rhodes
Consultor Editorial Alexander H. Werner

Distúrbios do Desenvolvimento Sexual

CONSIDERAÇÕES GERAIS

DEFINIÇÃO
• Erros no estabelecimento do sexo cromossômico, gonadal ou fenotípico que causam diferenciação sexual anormal.
• Variedade de padrões desde genitália ambígua até genitália aparentemente normal com esterilidade.

FISIOPATOLOGIA
Diferenciação sexual normal é um processo sequencial — estabelecimento do sexo cromossômico na fertilização (cão: 78, XX ou 78, XY; gato: 38, XX ou 38, XY), desenvolvimento do sexo gonadal e, finalmente, desenvolvimento do sexo fenotípico.

Distúrbios do Sexo Cromossômico
• Defeitos no número ou na estrutura dos cromossomos sexuais — não disjunção cromossômica durante a meiose leva à trissomia, monossomia; não disjunção mitótica de um único zigoto conduz ao mosaicismo; fusão de zigotos induz ao quimerismo.
• Síndrome XXY (Klinefelter) — 79, XXY (cão); 39, XXY (gato); testículos hipoplásicos; macho fenotípico (genitália normal a hipoplásica); estéril; alguns machos felinos com pelagem casco de tartaruga.
• Síndrome XO (Turner) — 77, XO (cão); 37, XO (gato); ovários disgênicos; fêmea fenotípica; genitália infantil; estéril.
• Síndrome XXX — 79, XXX; ovários sem folículos; fenótipo feminino; FSH e LH elevados; cães.
• Quimera hermafrodita verdadeira — XX/XY ou XX/XXY; tecido ovariano e testicular; o sexo fenotípico depende da quantidade de tecido testicular; cães e gatos.
• Quimera XX/XY com testículos e quimera XY/XY com testículos — variam de fêmea fenotípica com genitália anormal até macho com possível fertilidade; cães e gatos (alguns machos com pelagem casco de tartaruga).

Distúrbios do Sexo Gonadal
• Diferenciação testicular — determinada normalmente pela constituição cromossômica sexual; o gene *SRY* (localizado no cromossoma Y) codifica uma proteína que inicia a diferenciação testicular; o gene *SOX9* (relacionado com o gene *SRY* [Grupo de Alta Mobilidade] box 9) é um gene autossômico expresso em todas as células de Sertoli, crítico também para a diferenciação testicular.
• Diferenciação ovariana — antigamente se acreditava que fosse um processo passivo (falha na diferenciação testicular); atualmente, sabe-se que é um processo ativo, envolvendo os genes *WNT4/RSPO1* e β-catenina.
• Sexo invertido — os indivíduos acometidos possuem gônadas que não estão de acordo com o sexo cromossômico; apenas a inversão do sexo XX negativo para o gene *SRY* foi relatada no cão; o sexo invertido XX não foi descrito em gatos; relatado em 18 raças de cães; no momento, não se conhece o gene autossômico responsável pela indução testicular; o sexo invertido XX canino não se deve à mutação do gene *PIRST1* (um gene afetado por inversão do sexo em cabras tosquiadas); a análise de *linkage* (ligação genética) em Cocker spaniel americano acometido indica que os genes *SOX9* e *RSPO1* são candidatos improváveis (genes envolvidos na inversão de sexo no homem); são observados dois fenótipos; ambos os fenótipos podem ser vistos na mesma família de cães:
• Sexo XX invertido, hermafrodita verdadeiro XX — ovários e testículos [ovotestículo] (pelo menos um); fenótipo feminino masculinizado; varia desde vulva normal a anormal, clitóris de tamanho normal a grande (ou clitóris semelhante a um possível pênis), útero, oviductos, epidídimos e ductos espermáticos; raramente fértil; apenas cães.
• Sexo XX invertido, machos XX — testículos (geralmente criptorquídicos); epidídimos, ductos espermáticos, próstata; útero bicórneo, porém oviductos ausentes; pênis e prepúcio hipoplásicos; hipospadias são comuns; apenas cães.

Distúrbios do Sexo Fenotípico
• Diferenciação sexual fenotípica (trato reprodutivo e genitália externa tubulares) — depende do sexo gonadal; o plano embrionário básico ("padrão") é feminino; o fenótipo masculino culminará apenas se os testículos forem capazes de secretar a substância inibidora mulleriana e a testosterona, mas também se os receptores androgênicos funcionais (gene ligado ao cromossomo X) estiverem presentes; sexo gonadal e cromossômico são concordantes; genitália interna ou externa ambígua; o trato tubular do macho provém de derivados do ducto wolffiano (mesonéfrico), enquanto o trato tubular da fêmea surge de derivados do ducto mülleriano (paramesonéfrico).
• Pseudo-hermafrodita feminino — XX; ovários; genitália masculinizada (leve aumento do clitóris até genitália masculina quase normal); oviductos, útero, parte cranial da vagina; próstata variavelmente presente; provocado por administração de esteroide sexual durante a prenhez; raro em cães e gatos; único relato de hiperplasia adrenal congênita (síndrome adrenogenital) em um gato macho fenotípico, 38, XX, com ovários, oviductos, epidídimos, ductos espermáticos, útero bicórneo em virtude da 11 β-hidroxilase responsável pelo aumento nas concentrações de testosterona.
• Síndrome do ducto mülleriano persistente (pseudo-hermafrodita masculino) — XY; testículos (50% são criptorquídicos uni ou bilaterais); todos os derivados dos ductos wolffianos e müllerianos estão presentes (sistema masculino normal com oviductos, útero e parte cranial da vagina); pênis, prepúcio e escroto geralmente normais; cães e gatos.
• Hipospadias (defeito na masculinização dependente de androgênio) — XY; localização anormal do orifício urinário (desde a glande peniana até o períneo); genitália externa sem ambiguidade; testículos (podem ser criptorquídicos); falha de masculinização completa do trajeto urogenital durante o desenvolvimento da uretra; cães.
• Feminização testicular completa (defeito na masculinização dependente de androgênio) — XY; testículos (quase sempre abdominais); sem derivados dos ductos wolffianos ou müllerianos; vulva externamente; gatos.
• Feminização testicular incompleta — XY; grau variável de masculinização (machos inférteis ambíguos a fenotípicos); testículos escrotais ou dentro do escroto bífido; genitália externa semelhante à vulva até hipospadias perineais a macho um tanto normal; vagina de fundo cego com orifício uretral feminino em algumas; sem derivados dos ductos müllerianos; gatos (um único relato em cão).

SISTEMA(S) ACOMETIDO(S)
• Reprodutivo — anomalias das gônadas, do trato tubular e da genitália externa.
• Renal/urológico — ocasionalmente acometidos (p. ex., incontinência, hematúria e cistite).
• Cutâneo/exócrino — dermatite perivulvar (vulva hipoplásica); dermatite perineal ou periprepucial (hipospadias); hiperpigmentação (neoplasia testicular).

GENÉTICA
• Anormalidades do sexo cromossômico — causadas geralmente por eventos ao acaso durante a formação do gameta ou desenvolvimento embrionário precoce.
• Anormalidades do sexo gonadal — sexo XX invertido no Cocker spaniel americano herdado como traço autossômico recessivo; sexo XX invertido no Beagle, Pointer alemão de pelo curto, herança compatível com traço autossômico recessivo; sexo XX invertido considerado de caráter familiar no Cocker spaniel inglês, Pug, Kerry blue terrier, Elkhound norueguês, Weimaraner; outras raças relatadas incluem Wheaten terrier de pelo macio, Vizla, Walker hound, Doberman pinscher, Basset hound, Pit bull terrier americano, Border collie, Afghan hound.
• Anormalidades do sexo fenotípico — síndrome do ducto mülleriano persistente nos cães das raças Schnauzer miniatura nos EUA e Basset hound na Holanda e, possivelmente, nos gatos da raça Persa, herdada como traço autossômico recessivo com expressão limitada aos indivíduos XY; hipospadias são consideradas hereditárias no Boston terrier; feminização testicular (sobretudo em gatos) provavelmente ligada ao cromossomo X.

INCIDÊNCIA/PREVALÊNCIA
• Em geral, raros.
• Nas raças acometidas — podem ser comuns dentro de famílias ou mesmo dentro da raça como um todo.

IDENTIFICAÇÃO

Espécies
Cães e gatos.

Raça(s) Predominante(s)
Cães (ver as seções "Genética" e "Sugestões de Leitura").

Idade Média e Faixa Etária
• Distúrbios congênitos; defeitos presentes ao nascimento.
• Indivíduos acometidos com genitália externa normal podem não ser identificados até a idade do acasalamento ou na gonadectomia de rotina.

Sexo Predominante
Encontrados tanto nas fêmeas fenotípicas como nos machos fenotípicos.

SINAIS CLÍNICOS

Comentários Gerais
• Dependem do tipo de distúrbio.
• Aqui se encontram relacionados os possíveis achados para qualquer uma das condições; nem todos ocorrem em cada distúrbio específico.

Achados Anamnésicos
• Falha para entrar no cio.
• Infertilidade e esterilidade (macho ou fêmea).
• Vulva, clitóris, prepúcio ou pênis — tamanho, formato ou localização anormais.
• Jato de urina — localização anormal.

DISTÚRBIOS DO DESENVOLVIMENTO SEXUAL

- Machos fenotípicos acometidos são atraentes para outros machos.
- Incontinência urinária.
- Corrimento vulvar.
- PD/PU.

Achados do Exame Físico
- Vulva normal ou hipoplásica.
- Clitóris normal ou aumentado; osso no clitóris.
- Dermatite perivulvar e corrimento vulvar.
- Testículos escrotais, unilaterais, ou criptorquídicos bilaterais; escroto bífido.
- Pênis e prepúcio normais ou hipoplásicos.
- Meato uretral normal ou anormalmente localizado.
- Sinais dermatológicos de hiperestrogenismo nos machos.
- Massa abdominal.

CAUSAS
- Congênitas — hereditárias ou não.
- Administração de hormônio esteroide exógeno durante a prenhez.

FATORES DE RISCO
Administração de androgênio ou progestagênio durante a prenhez (fêmea canina pseudo-hermafrodita).

DIAGNÓSTICO

DIAGNÓSTICO DIFERENCIAL
Indivíduos com Genitália sem Ambiguidade
- Infertilidade (feminina) — infertilidade do macho; acasalamento não sincronizado; hiperplasia endometrial cística subclínica; hipotireoidismo.
- Falha para entrar no ciclo estral (fêmea) — cio silencioso; hipotireoidismo; hipercorticismo; gonadectomia anterior.
- Infertilidade (masculina) — infertilidade da fêmea; acasalamento sem sincronização; utilização de medicamento exógeno com influência sobre a fertilidade; orquite ou epididimite; degeneração ou hipoplasia testiculares; prostatite.

HEMOGRAMA/BIOQUÍMICA/URINÁLISE
- Geralmente normais.
- Neutrofilia; anemia normocítica normocrômica; hiperglobulinemia, hiperproteinemia; azotemia; níveis elevados de ALT e fosfatase alcalina com piometra (síndrome do ducto mülleriano persistente).
- Urinálise — pode revelar indícios de cistite com anormalidades anatômicas que afetam a localização do meato uretral.

OUTROS TESTES LABORATORIAIS
- Hormônios esteroides sexuais (progesterona, testosterona e estradiol) — geralmente abaixo da faixa normal; podem estar normais em alguns distúrbios brandos (paciente não estéril); elevação da testosterona em resposta ao GnRH ou hCG sugere produção testicular de androgênio (ver "Criptorquidismo").
- Cariotipagem — necessária para definir o sexo cromossômico (Molecular Cytogenetics Laboratory, Texas A&M University; 10 mL de sangue heparinizado com sódio, 5 mL de EDTA; amostra enviada no gelo, de um dia para o outro).
- Teste da reação em cadeia de polimerase para o gene *SRY* — sexo XX invertido (não está disponível comercialmente).
- Estudos de ligação do androgênio em fibroblastos genitais — feminização testicular (não está disponível no mercado).

DIAGNÓSTICO POR IMAGEM
- Radiografia e ultrassonografia de rotina — podem ser de valor diagnóstico na suspeita de massa abdominal (p. ex., neoplasia testicular na síndrome do ducto mülleriano persistente, feminização testicular ou sexo XX invertido); machos com sinais atribuíveis à piometra (útero presente com pseudo-hermafrodita feminino ou síndrome do ducto mülleriano persistente).
- Estudos contrastados do trato urogenital inferior — podem ser valiosos no diagnóstico de pseudo-hermafroditas femininos.

ACHADOS PATOLÓGICOS
Macroscópicos
- Todos os pacientes — descrição exata da genitália externa: particular atenção conferida ao tamanho e à localização da vulva ou do prepúcio; presença e aspecto de estruturas como clitóris, pênis, escroto, próstata, parte caudal da vagina ou osso no clitóris; posição do orifício urinário (necessária para denominar a estrutura fálica como pênis ou clitóris).
- Na maior parte dos pacientes sem anormalidades cromossômicas identificadas — efetuar laparotomia exploratória para determinar a localização e a morfologia das gônadas e da genitália interna.

Histopatológicos
- Exame de todos os tecidos removidos — fundamental para definir o tipo de distúrbio.
- Gônadas — variam desde arquitetura quase normal à disgênica ou combinação de ovário e testículo (ovotestículo).
- Essencial para descrever os componentes do sistema de ductos müllerianos e/ou wolffianos, se encontrados.

TRATAMENTO

CUIDADO(S) DE SAÚDE ADEQUADO(S)
- Geralmente como paciente de ambulatório.
- Internação — para laparotomia exploratória.

CUIDADO(S) DE ENFERMAGEM
Fêmeas fenotípicas com dermatite perivulvar secundária à vulva hipoplásica e machos fenotípicos com hipospadias — terapia local para melhorar as sequelas dermatológicas, conforme a necessidade (ver "Dermatoses Erosivas ou Ulcerativas").

ORIENTAÇÃO AO PROPRIETÁRIO
- Aconselhar o proprietário a castrar os animais acometidos.
- Orientar o proprietário a remover os portadores de distúrbios hereditários conhecidos ou sob suspeita do programa de reprodução.

CONSIDERAÇÕES CIRÚRGICAS
- Gonadectomia e histerectomia (caso se encontre o útero) — procedimentos recomendados.
- Amputação de clitóris aumentado — recomendado quando a superfície mucosa sofre repetidos traumatismos.
- Cirurgia reconstrutora do prepúcio e de má-formação peniana — cães; pode ser necessária na síndrome do macho XX ou em casos de hipospadias.

MEDICAÇÕES

CONTRAINDICAÇÕES
Evitar a utilização de androgênio ou progesterona durante a prenhez.

ACOMPANHAMENTO

PREVENÇÃO
- Castrar os animais com distúrbios hereditários.
- Remover os portadores de distúrbios hereditários do programa de reprodução.

COMPLICAÇÕES POSSÍVEIS
- Infertilidade.
- Esterilidade.
- Problemas do trato urinário — incontinência; cistite.
- Neoplasia testicular.
- Piometra.

DIVERSOS

FATORES RELACIONADOS COM A IDADE
Pacientes não diagnosticados em idade precoce — piometra (p. ex., síndrome do ducto mülleriano persistente; fêmea pseudo-hermafrodita); neoplasia testicular (p. ex., síndrome do ducto mülleriano persistente; feminização testicular; sexo XX invertido).

SINÔNIMO(S)
- Hermafroditas. • Pseudo-hermafroditas.
- Intersexos. • Síndrome de Klinefelter.
- Síndrome de Turner.

ABREVIATURA(S)
- ALT = alanina aminotransferase.
- FSH = hormônio foliculoestimulante.
- GnRH = hormônio liberador da gonadotropina.
- hCG = gonadotropina coriônica humana.
- LH = hormônio luteinizante.
- PD/PU = polidipsia/poliúria.

RECURSOS DA INTERNET
Meyers-Wallen VN. Inherited abnormalities of sexual development in dogs and cats. In: Concannon PW, England G, Verstegen III J, Linde-Forsberg C, eds., Recent Advances in Small Animal Reproduction. International Veterinary Information Service, Ithaca NY, www.ivis.org, 2001; A1217.0901.

Sugestões de Leitura
Johnston SD, Root Kustritz MV, Olson PN. Disorders of the canine ovary. In: Johnston SD, Root Kustritz MV, Olson PN, Canine and Feline Theriogenology. Philadelphia: Saunders, 2001, pp. 193-205.
Lyle SK. Disorders of sexual development in the dog and cat. Theriogenology 2007, 68(3):338-343.

Autor Sara K. Lyle
Consultor Editorial Sara K. Lyle
Agradecimento O autor e os editores agradecem a colaboração prévia de Vicki N. Meyers-Wallen.

Distúrbios dos Cílios (Triquíase/Distiquíase/Cílios Ectópicos)

CONSIDERAÇÕES GERAIS

REVISÃO
• Triquíase — quando o pelo originário de locais normais entra em contato com as superfícies da córnea ou da conjuntiva.
• Distiquíase — quando os cílios emergem dos orifícios da glândula meibomiana ou próximos a eles na margem palpebral e podem ou não entrar em contato com a córnea.
• Cílios ectópicos — pelos isolados ou múltiplos que surgem da superfície conjuntival palpebral, a vários milímetros da margem palpebral, mais comumente perto da porção média da pálpebra superior.

IDENTIFICAÇÃO
• Comuns em cães; raros em gatos.
• Mais comuns em cães jovens.
• Qualquer raça pode ser acometida.
• Triquíase: (a) triquíase da prega facial — raças com pregas faciais proeminentes (p. ex., Pequinês, Pug e Buldogue), (b) agenesia palpebral — comumente bilateral na face lateral das pálpebras superiores em gatos jovens, (c) entrópio — comum em cães jovens em raças predispostas (Shar-pei, Retrievers e muitas outras raças) e, ocasionalmente, em gatos.
• Distiquíase — encontrada até certo ponto na maioria dos cães da raça Cocker spaniel.
• Cílios ectópicos — mais comuns que a média nas raças Dachshund, Lhasa apso e Pastor de Shetland.

SINAIS CLÍNICOS
Triquíase da Prega Facial
• Vascularização corneana e pigmentação nasal.
• Blefarospasmo.
• Epífora.

Agenesia Palpebral
• Ceratite.
• Lagoftalmia.

Entrópio
• Blefarospasmo.
• Epífora.
• Ceratite, inclusive do tipo ulcerativa.

Distiquíase
• Em geral, assintomática.
• Cílios rígidos e retos em contato com a córnea — é possível notar blefarospasmo, epífora, vascularização da córnea, pigmentação e ulceração.

Cílios Ectópicos
• Dor ocular (oftalmalgia).
• Blefarospasmo intenso.
• Epífora.

• Úlceras de córnea superficiais com aspecto linear (correspondentes ao movimento da pálpebra) na córnea superior — comum; resistentes à cicatrização ou recidivantes até que o problema subjacente seja diagnosticado e corrigido.

CAUSAS E FATORES DE RISCO
Em geral, estão relacionados com a conformação facial ou a predisposição racial ou, então, são idiopáticos.

DIAGNÓSTICO

DIAGNÓSTICO DIFERENCIAL
• Secundários a outras anormalidades de anexos — i.e., entrópio, agenesia palpebral.
• Ceratoconjuntivite seca.
• Corpo estranho conjuntival.
• Conjuntivite infecciosa.
• Diagnóstico formulado com base na observação direta de cílios anormais.

HEMOGRAMA/BIOQUÍMICA/URINÁLISE
N/D.

OUTROS TESTES LABORATORIAIS
N/D.

DIAGNÓSTICO POR IMAGEM
N/D.

MÉTODOS DIAGNÓSTICOS
N/D.

TRATAMENTO

TRIQUÍASE
• Pode ser submetida a tratamento conservativo em alguns pacientes.
• Pode ajudar o ato de manter os pelos perioculares curtos; contudo, a depilação dos pelos das pregas faciais pode torná-los mais rígidos e irritantes.
• Correção cirúrgica de anormalidades dos anexos — indicada.
• É possível a ressecção das pregas faciais.
• Fechamento do canto medial dos olhos — em geral, constitui um procedimento mais eficiente; também elimina a lagoftalmia e o entrópio medial.
• Reparo do entrópio.
• Reparo de agenesia palpebral ou tratamento de distiquíase, conforme exposto a seguir.

DISTIQUÍASE
• Costuma ser assintomática e não necessitar de tratamento.
• Sintomática — pode ser submetida a tratamento cirúrgico por crioterapia, eletrocautério, eletroepilação, ablação a laser ou ressecção da superfície conjuntival.
• Técnicas cirúrgicas de divisão palpebral — evitar; a cicatrização pós-operatória pode predispor o paciente a entrópio cicatricial e prejudicar a função palpebral.

CÍLIOS ECTÓPICOS
• Podem ser tratados por meio cirúrgico — ressecção em bloco dos cílios e da glândula meibomiana associada.
• Crioterapia — pode ser usada como tratamento isolado ou adjuvante após a ressecção cirúrgica.
• Alertar o proprietário sobre o fato de que o paciente corre risco de desenvolver cílios ectópicos em outros locais.
• Avisar o proprietário para levar o paciente a uma nova consulta em caso de recidiva dos sinais clínicos.

MEDICAÇÕES

MEDICAMENTO(S)
• Raramente indicados.
• Pomadas lubrificantes — às vezes, são valiosas para amolecer os cílios e diminuir a irritação antes da correção cirúrgica.
• Antibióticos tópicos — perioperatórios; recomendados em pacientes submetidos à cirurgia para minimizar a flora conjuntival nos locais cirúrgicos.

CONTRAINDICAÇÕES/INTERAÇÕES POSSÍVEIS
N/D.

ACOMPANHAMENTO

Distiquíase — é comum a ocorrência de novo crescimento, pois os procedimentos destrutivos (crioterapia, eletroepilação, ablação a laser) devem ser realizados de forma conservadora para minimizar o dano palpebral.

DIVERSOS

Sugestões de Leitura
Maggs DJ, Miller PE, Ofri R. Slatter's Fundamentals of Veterinary Ophthalmology, 4th ed. St. Louis: Saunders, 2008, pp. 107-119.

Autor Erin S. Champagne
Consultor Editorial Paul E. Miller

DISTÚRBIOS DOS SACOS ANAIS

CONSIDERAÇÕES GERAIS

REVISÃO
- Os sacos anais são reservatórios para as secreções normalmente evacuadas durante a defecação.
- Os distúrbios incluem impactação, infecção (saculite) e neoplasia.
- As opções terapêuticas envolvem a compressão manual, a irrigação, o uso de antibióticos e a excisão cirúrgica.

IDENTIFICAÇÃO
- Cães e, raramente, gatos.
  - Impactação — Poodle miniatura e toy, Cocker americano e Springer spaniel inglês, Chihuahua.
  - Neoplasia (adenocarcinoma) — Pastor alemão, Golden retriever, Cocker americano e Springer spaniel inglês.
- Raças predispostas:
- Sem predileção etária ou sexual.

SINAIS CLÍNICOS
- Prurido anal, que se manifesta frequentemente por arrastamento da região perineal no chão ("*scooting*").
- Prurido perianal.
- Hesitação para defecar.
- Tenesmo.
- Perseguição da cauda.
- Secreção anal de matéria não fecal e de odor fétido.
- Recusa a se sentar e/ou elevar a cauda.

CAUSAS E FATORES DE RISCO
- Possíveis fatores predisponentes — fezes moles ou diarreia, secreções glandulares excessivas e distúrbios dermatológicos que alteram as características (celularidade e colonização de microrganismos) de secreções dos sacos anais.
- A retenção das secreções pode levar à infecção e à formação de abscesso.

DIAGNÓSTICO

DIAGNÓSTICO DIFERENCIAL
- Reação alimentar adversa ou hipersensibilidade alimentar.
- Hipersensibilidade à picada de pulgas.
- Dermatite atópica.
- Infestação por tênias.
- Foliculite bacteriana das pregas da cauda.
- Dermatite por *Malassezia*.
- Transtorno compulsivo (lambedura anal).
- Colite ou outro distúrbio intestinal.
- Distúrbio de queratinização.
- Neoplasia dos sacos anais (incluindo adenocarcinoma, carcinoma de células escamosas).
- Adenoma perianal.
- Adenocarcinoma perianal.
- Fístulas perianais.

HEMOGRAMA/BIOQUÍMICA/URINÁLISE
- Costumam permanecer normais.
- Hipercalcemia — adenocarcinoma dos sacos anais.

OUTROS TESTES LABORATORIAIS
Nenhum a menos que indicados por alguma causa subjacente.

DIAGNÓSTICO POR IMAGEM
Nenhum a menos que indicado por alguma causa subjacente.

MÉTODOS DIAGNÓSTICOS
- Palpação digital dos sacos anais — os sacos anais normais não são palpáveis externamente.
- O conteúdo dos sacos anais normais varia amplamente em termos de aspecto macroscópico e características microscópicas; em geral, o conteúdo é fino ou aquoso, com celularidade mínima ou microrganismos principalmente extracelulares.
- Impactação — secreção pastosa geralmente mais espessa de coloração castanha; número mais elevado de *Malassezia* e bactérias intracelulares.
- Saculite anal e abscedação — secreção purulenta de odor fétido, frequentemente manchada de sangue.
- Citologia de secreções dos sacos anais — o aumento na quantidade de neutrófilos, *Malassezia* e bactérias intracelulares indica infecção; embora os relatos variem, a presença de cocos gram-positivos é mais comum nas secreções normais.
- Cultura bacteriana e antibiograma — as secreções normais podem conter *Proteus mirabilis*, *Streptococcus* spp., *Escherichia coli*, *Bacillus* spp., *Clostridium perfringens* e *Pseudomonas aeruginosa*.

TRATAMENTO

- Em casos de impactação e saculite, espremer o conteúdo com delicada compressão manual.
- Talvez haja necessidade de sedação para irrigar os sacos anais gravemente impactados ou doloridos.
- Infusão de antibióticos e/ou corticosteroides diretamente nos sacos anais.
- Drenagem de abscessos.
- Uso de antibióticos orais adequados e/ou medicamentos contra leveduras.
- Excisão dos sacos anais em caso de doença crônica.
- Excisão cirúrgica e estadiamento de neoplasia dos sacos anais; combinar com quimioterapia.
- Identificação das causas subjacentes de doença predisponente.
- O fornecimento de dietas ricas em fibras pode ajudar na compressão manual dos sacos anais.

MEDICAÇÕES

MEDICAMENTO(S)
- Infecção — uso de antibióticos adequados: cefalexina (22 mg/kg a cada 12 h), amoxicilina tri-hidratada e clavulanato de potássio (10-15 mg/kg a cada 12 h), clindamicina (11 mg/kg a cada 12-24 h), trimetoprima-sulfametoxazol (15 mg/kg a cada 12 h); metronidazol (15 mg/kg a cada 12 h); enrofloxacino (10-20 mg/kg a cada 12 h [cães], 5 mg/kg/dia [gatos]) e orbifloxacino (5 mg/kg a cada 24 h).
- Doença crônica associada a fístulas perianais; ciclosporina (5 mg/kg a cada 24 h) e/ou tacrolimo tópico.

CONTRAINDICAÇÕES/INTERAÇÕES POSSÍVEIS
N/D.

ACOMPANHAMENTO

- Reavaliar os pacientes semanalmente no início e, depois, conforme a necessidade, para monitorizar a cicatrização.
- Espremer manualmente o conteúdo dos sacos anais e/ou irrigar o conteúdo até que esses sacos se esvaziem sem intervenção.

DIVERSOS

VER TAMBÉM
- Adenocarcinoma dos Sacos Anais.
- Fístula Perianal.

Sugestões de Leitura

Muse R. Diseases of the anal sac. In: Bonagura JD, Twedt DC, eds., Kirk's Current Veterinary Therapy, 14th ed. St. Louis: Saunders, 2009, pp. 465-468.

Zoran DL. Rectoanal disease. In: Ettinger SJ, ed., Textbook of Veterinary Internal Medicine, 6th ed. Philadelphia: Saunders, 2005, pp. 1408-1420.

Autor Alexander H. Werner
Consultor Editorial Alexander H. Werner

Distúrbios Mieloproliferativos

CONSIDERAÇÕES GERAIS

REVISÃO
- Proliferação neoplásica de linhagens celulares não linfoides que se originam na medula óssea (células granulocíticas, monocíticas, eritrocíticas e megacariocíticas), resultando em leucemia.
- Acredita-se que os distúrbios mieloproliferativos representem um espectro de distúrbios em que a célula-tronco envolvida é um precursor hematopoiético capaz de se diferenciar em todos os tipos celulares sanguíneos, exceto os linfócitos.

IDENTIFICAÇÃO
- Cães e gatos — mais comum em gatos.
- Podem ser mais comuns em cães de grande porte do que nos de pequeno porte.

SINAIS CLÍNICOS
- Mucosas pálidas.
- Letargia.
- Inapetência.
- Perda de peso.
- Hepatosplenomegalia.
- Linfadenomegalia periférica — ocasionalmente.

CAUSAS E FATORES DE RISCO
- Gatos — mais comumente associados à infecção pelo FeLV; ao se recuperar de panleucopenia ou hemobartonelose, pode haver um risco relativamente mais alto de desenvolver uma linhagem celular mutante induzida pelo FeLV.
- Cães — foram experimentalmente induzidos com exposição crônica à radiação em baixas doses.

DIAGNÓSTICO

DIAGNÓSTICO DIFERENCIAL
- Leucemia linfocítica aguda — costuma ser diferenciada por técnicas especiais de coloração (imuno-histoquímica ou imunocitoquímica para marcadores linfoides) ou PCR para rearranjo de receptores antigênicos.
- Resposta leucemoide secundária à inflamação.
- Outras causas de eosinofilia — parasitose; doença alérgica; gastrenterite eosinofílica; mastocitomas; diferenciar de leucemia eosinofílica.
- Anemia hemolítica grave deve ser diferenciada de eritroleucemia aguda.

HEMOGRAMA/BIOQUÍMICA/URINÁLISE
- Anemia grave arregenerativa.
- Hemácias nucleadas circulantes.
- Eritrócitos megaloblásticos.
- Leucocitose ou leucopenia
- Trombocitopenia com morfologia plaquetária anormal.
- Circulação de células mieloides imaturas.

OUTROS TESTES LABORATORIAIS
- Exame de aspirado ou biopsia nuclear da medula óssea — revela uma medula óssea hipercelular com morfologia anormal em todas as linhagens celulares; proliferação neoplásica ou ausência de alguma linhagem celular.
- Coloração imuno-histoquímica ou outra coloração especial — pode ser necessária para determinar a linhagem celular.

DIAGNÓSTICO POR IMAGEM
Radiografia simples e ultrassonografia abdominais — é comum a constatação de hepatosplenomegalia.

MÉTODOS DIAGNÓSTICOS
Exame de aspirado ou biopsia nuclear da medula óssea.

TRATAMENTO

- Internação ou tratamento ambulatorial.
- Cuidado de suporte — transfusões de sangue e administração de fluido para corrigir a desidratação.
- Procurar veterinário especialista em oncologia para consulta e tratamento.

MEDICAÇÕES

MEDICAMENTO(S)
- Pouca informação disponível na literatura especializada sobre o tratamento.
- Citosina arabinosídeo — pode ser utilizada; 100 mg/m² SC divididos a cada 12 h em 4 dias por semana ou velocidade de infusão constante em 6-8 h a uma dose de 400 mg/m².
- Hidroxiureia — 30-45 mg/kg a cada 24 h por 7-10 dias; em seguida, 30-45 mg/kg a cada 48 h; titular a dosagem basicamente em relação à resposta do paciente.
- Antibióticos — podem ser indicados para combater infecção secundária.

CONTRAINDICAÇÕES/INTERAÇÕES POSSÍVEIS
A quimioterapia pode ser tóxica; procurar orientação antes do tratamento se não estiver familiarizado com medicamentos citotóxicos.

ACOMPANHAMENTO

- Hemograma completo e exame do aspirado da medula óssea — para determinar a resposta ao tratamento e a evolução da doença.
- Prognóstico — grave; em geral, apresentam evolução clínica rápida e fatal.

DIVERSOS

GESTAÇÃO/FERTILIDADE/REPRODUÇÃO
- Medicamentos quimioterápicos estão contraindicados em fêmeas prenhes.
- Não é recomendável o acasalamento de animais com neoplasia.

ABREVIATURA(S)
- FeLV = vírus da leucemia felina.
- PCR = reação em cadeia da polimerase.

Sugestões de Leitura
Reagan WJ, DeNicola DB. Myeloproliferative and lymphoproliferative disorders. In: Morrison WB, ed., Cancer in Dogs and Cats: Medical and Surgical Management. Jackson, WY: Teton NewMedia, 2002, pp. 89-114.

Autor Rebecca G. Newman
Consultor Editorial Timothy M. Fan
Agradecimento O autor e os editores agradecem a colaboração prévia de Linda S. Fineman.

DISÚRIA E POLACIÚRIA

CONSIDERAÇÕES GERAIS

DEFINIÇÃO
- Disúria — dificuldade ou dor à micção.
- Polaciúria — eliminação de pequenas quantidades de urina com aumento na frequência.

FISIOPATOLOGIA
A bexiga urinária e a uretra servem normalmente como reservatórios de armazenamento e liberação periódica de urina. Os distúrbios inflamatórios e não inflamatórios do trato urinário inferior podem diminuir a complacência e a capacidade de armazenamento vesicais por dano aos componentes estruturais da parede vesical ou por estímulo às terminações nervosas sensoriais localizadas na bexiga ou na uretra. As sensações de repleção, urgência e dor vesicais estimulam a micção prematura e reduzem a capacidade funcional da bexiga urinária. A disúria e a polaciúria são causadas por lesões na bexiga urinária e/ou na uretra e fornecem indícios claros de doença do trato urinário inferior; esses sinais clínicos não excluem o envolvimento concomitante do trato urinário superior ou de distúrbios em outros sistemas corporais.

SISTEMA(S) ACOMETIDO(S)
Renal/urológico — bexiga, uretra e próstata.

IDENTIFICAÇÃO
Cães e gatos.

SINAIS CLÍNICOS
N/D.

CAUSAS

Bexiga Urinária
- Infecção do trato urinário — bacteriana, viral, fúngica, parasitária ou micoplásmica.
- Urocistolitíase.
- Neoplasias — por exemplo, carcinoma das células de transição.
- Traumatismo.
- Anormalidades anatômicas — por exemplo, ureterocele, persistência de útero masculino, hérnias perineais incluindo a bexiga urinária em seu conteúdo, e granulomas por castração.
- Atonia do músculo detrusor — por exemplo, obstrução parcial crônica e disautonomia.
- Substâncias químicas/medicamentos — por exemplo, ciclofosfamida.
- Iatrogênicas — por exemplo, cateterização, palpação, fluxo reverso, distensão vesical excessiva durante radiografia contrastada, uro-hidropropulsão, uretrocistoscopia e cirurgia.
- Idiopáticas — por exemplo, doença idiopática do trato urinário inferior felino.

Uretra
- Infecção do trato urinário — ver seção anterior.
- Uretrolitíase — ver seção anterior.
- Tampões uretrais — por exemplo, compostos de matriz e matriz-cristalina.
- Neoplasias — ver seção anterior; invasão local por neoplasias malignas de estruturas adjacentes.
- Traumatismos.
- Anomalias anatômicas — por exemplo, estenoses congênitas ou adquiridas, fístulas uretrorretais e pseudo-hermafroditas.
- Hipertonicidade do esfíncter uretral — por exemplo, lesões medulares do neurônio motor superior, dissinergia reflexa e espasmo uretral.
- Iatrogênicas — ver seção anterior.
- Idiopáticas — ver seção anterior.

Próstata
- Prostatite ou abscesso prostático.
- Neoplasias — adenocarcinoma e carcinoma das células de transição.
- Hiperplasia cística.
- Cistos paraprostáticos.

FATORES DE RISCO
- Doenças, métodos diagnósticos ou tratamentos que (1) alteram as defesas normais do trato urinário do hospedeiro e predispõem o animal à infecção, (2) predispõem à formação de urólitos ou (3) causam dano ao urotélio ou outros tecidos do trato urinário inferior.
- Doenças murais ou extramurais que comprimem a bexiga urinária ou o lúmen uretral.

DIAGNÓSTICO

DIAGNÓSTICO DIFERENCIAL

Diferenciar de Outros Padrões Anormais de Micção
- Descartar poliúria — aumento na frequência e no volume urinários >50 mL/kg/dia.
- Descartar obstrução uretral — estrangúria, anúria, distensão vesical excessiva, sinais de uremia pós-renal.
- Descartar incontinência urinária — micção involuntária, gotejamento urinário, enurese, esvaziamento vesical incompleto.
- Descartar borrifamento de urina ou marcação territorial com urina — eliminação de pequenas quantidades de urina em superfícies verticais ou outros locais socialmente significativos.

Diferenciar as Causas de Disúria e Polaciúria
- Descartar infecção do trato urinário — hematúria; urina fétida ou turva; bexiga urinária pequena, dolorosa, espessada.
- Descartar urolitíase — hematúria; urólitos palpáveis na uretra ou na bexiga urinária.
- Descartar neoplasias — hematúria; massas palpáveis na uretra ou na bexiga urinária.
- Descartar distúrbios neurogênicos — parede vesical flácida; urina residual no lúmen vesical após micção; outros déficits neurológicos em estruturas como membros pélvicos, cauda, períneo e esfíncter anal.
- Descartar prostatopatias — secreção uretral, prostatomegalia, pirexia, depressão, tenesmo, dor abdominal caudal, marcha rígida.
- Descartar cistite por ciclofosfamida — por meio da anamnese.
- Descartar distúrbios iatrogênicos — histórico de cateterização, fluxo reverso, radiografia contrastada, uro-hidropropulsão, uretrocistoscopia ou cirurgia.

HEMOGRAMA/BIOQUÍMICA/URINÁLISE
- Os resultados do hemograma completo e da bioquímica sérica frequentemente permanecem normais. Uma doença do trato urinário inferior complicada por obstrução uretral pode estar associada a azotemia, hiperfosfatemia, acidose e hipercalemia. Os pacientes com pielonefrite concomitante podem exibir diminuição na capacidade de concentração urinária, leucocitose e azotemia. Os animais com prostatite aguda ou abscessos prostáticos podem apresentar leucocitose, enquanto os pacientes desidratados podem ter elevação nas proteínas plasmáticas totais.
- É melhor avaliar os distúrbios vesicais em amostras urinárias coletadas por cistocentese. Já os distúrbios uretrais são mais bem avaliados, coletando-se as amostras por micção espontânea ou comparando-se os resultados de análise das amostras obtidas por micção espontânea e por cistocentese. (**Cuidado:** o procedimento de cistocentese pode induzir à hematúria.)
- Piúria, hematúria e proteinúria indicam inflamação do trato urinário; entretanto, tais anormalidades constituem achados inespecíficos, que podem resultar de causas infecciosas e não infecciosas de doença do trato urinário inferior.
- A identificação de bactérias, fungos ou ovos de parasitas no sedimento urinário sugere, mas não prova, que uma infecção do trato urinário esteja causando ou complicando uma doença do trato urinário inferior. Ao se interpretar os resultados da urinálise, deve-se considerar a possibilidade de contaminação da urina durante a coleta e o armazenamento.
- A identificação de células neoplásicas no sedimento urinário indica neoplasia do trato urinário. É preciso ter cautela na formulação do diagnóstico de neoplasia, com base no exame do sedimento urinário. Uma inflamação do trato urinário ou os extremos no pH ou na osmolalidade urinários podem causar atipia epitelial de difícil diferenciação com neoplasias.
- A cristalúria ocorre em pacientes normais, em outros com urolitíase ou naqueles com doença do trato urinário inferior não associada a urólitos. É fundamental interpretar o significado da cristalúria com cuidado.
- Em gatos com doença idiopática não obstrutiva do trato urinário inferior, ocorrem hematúria, proteinúria e cristalúria variável. Nesses pacientes, é rara a piúria significativa.

OUTROS TESTES LABORATORIAIS
- Urocultura quantitativa — representa o meio mais definitivo de identificar e caracterizar as infecções bacterianas do trato urinário; os resultados negativos da urocultura sugerem uma causa não infecciosa (p. ex., urólitos e neoplasias) ou inflamação associada à infecção do trato urinário causada por microrganismos fastidiosos (p. ex., micoplasmas ou agentes virais).
- Avaliação citológica de sedimento urinário, líquido prostático, secreções uretrais ou corrimentos vaginais ou amostras de biopsia, obtidos por meio de sonda ou aspirado por agulha — pode ajudar na avaliação de pacientes com doença localizada do trato urinário; pode estabelecer o diagnóstico definitivo de neoplasia do trato urinário, mas não é capaz de descartá-la.

DIAGNÓSTICO POR IMAGEM
Radiografias abdominais simples, uretrocistografia e cistografia contrastadas, ultrassonografia do trato urinário e urografia excretora são importantes meios de identificação e localização das causas de disúria e polaciúria.

MÉTODOS DIAGNÓSTICOS
- Utilizar a uretrocistografia em pacientes com lesões persistentes do trato urinário inferior para as quais ainda não se estabeleceu nenhum diagnóstico definitivo por outros meios menos invasivos.
- Utilizar a avaliação sob microscopia óptica de amostras teciduais obtidas por biopsia de pacientes com lesões persistentes do trato urinário para as

DISÚRIA E POLACIÚRIA

quais ainda não se estabeleceu nenhum diagnóstico definitivo por outros meios menos invasivos. As amostras teciduais podem ser adquiridas por meio de biopsia com cateter, uretrocistoscopia e biopsia com pinça ou cirurgia.

TRATAMENTO

- Os animais com doenças não obstrutivas do trato urinário inferior são tipicamente tratados como pacientes de ambulatório; a avaliação diagnóstica pode exigir uma internação breve.
- A disúria e a polaciúria associadas a sinais sistêmicos de doença (p. ex., pirexia, depressão, anorexia, vômito e desidratação) ou a achados laboratoriais de azotemia ou leucocitose justificam não só a avaliação diagnóstica rigorosa, mas também a instituição dos tratamentos de suporte e sintomático.
- O tratamento depende da causa subjacente e dos locais envolvidos. Ver os capítulos específicos que descrevem as doenças listadas na seção sobre causas.
- Com frequência, os sinais clínicos de disúria e polaciúria apresentam rápida resolução após o tratamento específico da(s) causa(s) subjacente(s).

MEDICAÇÕES

MEDICAMENTO(S) DE ESCOLHA

- Os pacientes com incontinência por urgência miccional, sinais clínicos graves ou persistentes ou doença intratável do trato urinário inferior podem se beneficiar da terapia sintomática com propantelina, oxibutinina, ou tolterodina, agentes anticolinérgicos que podem diminuir a força e a frequência de contrações descontroladas do músculo detrusor.
- Os pacientes com carcinoma das células de transição vesicais ou uretrais podem ser tratados de forma sintomática com o piroxicam (anti-inflamatório não esteroide), que diminui a gravidade dos sinais clínicos, melhora a qualidade de vida e, em alguns casos, induz à remissão do tumor.

CONTRAINDICAÇÕES

- Glicocorticoides ou outros agentes imunossupressores em pacientes com suspeita de infecção dos tratos urinário ou genital.
- Medicamentos potencialmente nefrotóxicos (p. ex., gentamicina) em pacientes febris, desidratados ou azotêmicos ou sob suspeita de pielonefrite, septicemia ou nefropatia preexistente.

PRECAUÇÕES
N/D.

INTERAÇÕES POSSÍVEIS
N/D.

MEDICAMENTO(S) ALTERNATIVO(S)
N/D.

ACOMPANHAMENTO

MONITORIZAÇÃO DO PACIENTE

- Monitorar a resposta ao tratamento por meio dos sinais clínicos, exames físicos seriados, testes laboratoriais, bem como pelas avaliações radiográficas e ultrassonográficas apropriadas para cada causa específica.
- Consultar os capítulos específicos que descrevem as doenças listadas na seção "Causas".

COMPLICAÇÕES POSSÍVEIS

- A disúria e a polaciúria podem estar associadas à formação de divertículos vesicouracais macroscópicos.
- Consultar os capítulos específicos que descrevem as doenças listadas na seção "Causas".

DIVERSOS

DISTÚRBIOS ASSOCIADOS

- Hematúria, piúria e proteinúria.
- Distúrbios predisponentes à infecção do trato urinário.
- Distúrbios predisponentes à formação de urólitos.
- Divertículos vesicouracais macroscópicos.

FATORES RELACIONADOS COM A IDADE
N/D.

POTENCIAL ZOONÓTICO
Nenhum.

GESTAÇÃO/FERTILIDADE/REPRODUÇÃO
N/D.

SINÔNIMO(S)

- Síndrome urológica felina*.
- Doença do trato urinário inferior.

VER TAMBÉM

- Capítulos sobre Urolitíase.
- Divertículos Vesicouracais.
- Doença Idiopática do Trato Urinário Inferior Felino.
- Infecção Bacteriana do Trato Urinário Inferior.
- Infecção Fúngica do Trato Urinário Inferior.
- Obstrução do Trato Urinário.
- Retenção Urinária Funcional.

Sugestões de Leitura

Adams LG, Syme HM. Canine lower urinary tract disease. In: Ettinger SJ, Feldman EC, eds., Textbook of Veterinary Internal Medicine, 6th ed. St. Louis: Elsevier, 2005, pp. 1850-1874.

Bartges JW. Urinary tract infections. In: Ettinger SJ, Feldman EC, eds., Textbook of Veterinary Internal Medicine, 6th ed. St. Louis: Elsevier, 2005, pp. 1800-1808.

Chun R, Garrett L. Urogenital and mammary gland tumors. In: Ettinger SJ, Feldman EC, eds., Textbook of Veterinary Internal Medicine, 6th ed. St. Louis: Elsevier, 2005, pp. 784-789.

Lane IF. Use of anticholinergic agents in lower urinary tract disease. In: Bonagura JD, ed., Kirk's Current Veterinary Therapy XIII: Small Animal Practice. Philadelphia: Saunders, 2000, pp. 899-902.

Westropp JL, Buffington CAT, Chew D. Feline lower urinary tract diseases. In: Ettinger SJ, Feldman EC, eds., Textbook of Veterinary Internal Medicine, 6th ed. St. Louis: Elsevier, 2005, pp. 1828-1850.

Autores John M. Kruger and Carl A. Osborne
Consultor Editorial Carl A. Osborne

---

* N. T.: Termo obsoleto.

DIVERTÍCULOS ESOFÁGICOS

CONSIDERAÇÕES GERAIS

REVISÃO
- Saculações em forma de bolsa da parede esofágica que promovem o acúmulo de líquidos e ingesta.
- Os divertículos podem ser congênitos ou adquiridos, mas são raros.
- Ocorrem divertículos por pulsão como consequência do aumento da pressão intraluminal, conforme é observado em casos de distúrbios obstrutivos esofágicos como corpo estranho.
- Ocorrem divertículos por tração secundários à inflamação periesofágica, em que os processos de fibrose e contração empurram a parede do esôfago, formando uma bolsa.
- Os divertículos ocorrem mais comumente na entrada torácica ou perto do hiato.
- Os sistemas orgânicos acometidos incluem o gastrintestinal (regurgitação), o musculosquelético (perda de peso) e o respiratório (pneumonia por aspiração).

IDENTIFICAÇÃO
- Raros; mais comuns em cães do que em gatos.
- Congênitos ou adquiridos (sem base genética comprovada).
- Sem predileção importante por sexo ou raça.

SINAIS CLÍNICOS
- Regurgitação pós-prandial, disfagia, anorexia, tosse.
- Perda de peso, angústia respiratória.

CAUSAS E FATORES DE RISCO

Divertículo por Pulsão
- Distúrbios do desenvolvimento embrionário da parede esofágica.
- Corpo estranho esofágico ou distúrbio focal da motilidade (incomum).

Divertículo por Tração
- Processo inflamatório associado à traqueia, aos pulmões, aos linfonodos hilares ou ao pericárdio; a consequente formação de tecido conjuntivo fibroso adere-se à parede esofágica.

DIAGNÓSTICO

DIAGNÓSTICO DIFERENCIAL

Esôfago redundante (comprimento excessivo do esôfago)
O acúmulo do contraste de bário na região da entrada torácica pode ocorrer normalmente em cães jovens (especialmente em raças braquicefálicas).

Massa Periesofágica
O esofagograma ou a esofagoscopia devem diferenciar a presença de massa.

HEMOGRAMA/BIOQUÍMICA/URINÁLISE
Em geral, permanecem dentro dos limites de normalidade.

OUTROS TESTES LABORATORIAIS
N/D.

DIAGNÓSTICO POR IMAGEM
- Radiografia torácica — pode exibir a presença de ar ou a opacidade de tecido mole cranial ao diafragma ou à entrada torácica.
- Esofagograma contrastado — revela o acúmulo de contraste no divertículo.
- Fluoroscopia — útil para avaliar a motilidade esofágica.

MÉTODOS DIAGNÓSTICOS
A esofagoscopia confirma a existência de bolsas com ingesta/restos de alimento no esôfago.

TRATAMENTO
- Se o divertículo for pequeno e não estiver causando sinais clínicos significativos, proceder ao tratamento conservativo com dieta pastosa e leve, administrada com o animal com a cabeça elevada e acompanhada por bastante líquido.
- Se o divertículo for grande ou estiver associado a sinais clínicos expressivos, recomenda-se a ressecção cirúrgica.
- A orientação do proprietário deve incluir a importância do manejo nutricional e o potencial de pneumonia por aspiração.
- Fornecer fluidoterapia, antibióticos e enfermagem rigorosa na presença concomitante de pneumonia por aspiração; a nutrição enteral alternativa via gastrostomia ou jejunostomia endoscópicas percutâneas pode ser necessária em pacientes com pneumonia por aspiração.
- Tratar a esofagite se estiver presente.

MEDICAÇÕES

MEDICAMENTO(S)
- Terapia medicamentosa para esofagite, se presente.
- Fornecer antagonistas histaminérgicos dos receptores H_2 (p. ex., ranitidina 2 mg/kg VO a cada 12 h ou famotidina) se o paciente tiver esofagite concomitante.
- Administrar antibióticos de amplo espectro se o paciente tiver pneumonia por aspiração concomitante; em caso de pneumonia grave, selecionar o antibiótico específico com base na cultura e no antibiograma de amostras obtidas por lavagem transtraqueal ou broncoalveolar.

CONTRAINDICAÇÕES/INTERAÇÕES POSSÍVEIS
N/D.

ACOMPANHAMENTO

MONITORIZAÇÃO DO PACIENTE
- Avaliar o paciente em busca de evidência de infecção ou pneumonia por aspiração.
- Manter um equilíbrio nutricional positivo durante todo o processo patológico.

COMPLICAÇÕES POSSÍVEIS
Pacientes com divertículos e impactação ficam predispostos à perfuração, fístula e estenose, bem como à deiscência pós-operatória da incisão.

EVOLUÇÃO ESPERADA E PROGNÓSTICO
O prognóstico é reservado em pacientes com grandes divertículos e sinais clínicos francos.

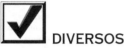

DIVERSOS

RECURSOS DA INTERNET
Rede de Informações Veterinárias: www.vin.com/VIN.plx.

Sugestões de Leitura
Jergens AE. Diseases of the esophagus. In: Ettinger SJ, Feldman EC, eds., Textbook of Veterinary Internal Medicine, 7th ed. Philadelphia: Saunders, 2009.

Autor Albert E. Jergens
Consultor Editorial Albert E. Jergens

Divertículos Vesicouracais

CONSIDERAÇÕES GERAIS

REVISÃO
• Trata-se de uma anomalia congênita comum da bexiga urinária, que ocorre quando a porção do úraco (i. e., um conduto fetal que permite a passagem de urina da bexiga para a placenta) localizada no vértice vesical falha em se fechar; o resultado é um divertículo cego de tamanho variável que se projeta a partir do vértice vesical.
• Outras características incluem divertículos microscópicos congênitos (lúmens microscópicos que podem persistir no vértice vesical).
• Os divertículos macroscópicos adquiridos desenvolvem-se após o início de doenças do trato urinário inferior, adquiridas e concomitantes, mas não relacionadas; presumivelmente, a obstrução da uretra ou a hiperatividade do detrusor induzidas por inflamação gera elevação da pressão intraluminal e subsequente aumento dos divertículos microscópicos.
• Os divertículos macroscópicos congênitos, causados mais provavelmente por diminuição do fluxo urinário, desenvolvem-se antes ou logo depois do nascimento e persistem por tempo indefinido.

IDENTIFICAÇÃO
• Cães e gatos.
• Os divertículos vesicouracais são encontrados com frequência em gatos com doenças adquiridas do trato urinário inferior; são duas vezes mais comuns em felinos machos do que em fêmeas.
• Não há predisposição racial ou etária.

SINAIS CLÍNICOS
• Dependem da presença de distúrbios concomitantes, que predispõem à formação de divertículos vesicouracais macroscópicos.
• Hematúria, disúria, polaciúria ou sinais de obstrução uretral em alguns pacientes com doenças concomitantes e adquiridas do trato urinário inferior.

CAUSAS E FATORES DE RISCO
• Divertículos microscópicos congênitos persistentes — causa desconhecida.
• Divertículos microscópicos congênitos — fatores de risco para divertículos macroscópicos adquiridos.
• Doenças associadas ao aumento da pressão vesical intraluminal (p. ex., infecção bacteriana do trato urinário, urólitos, tampões uretrais e doença idiopática) — fatores de risco para divertículos macroscópicos adquiridos.

DIAGNÓSTICO

DIAGNÓSTICO DIFERENCIAL
• Úraco persistente (ou patente); muito raro — caracterizado por perda inapropriada de urina pelo umbigo.
• Os ligamentos uracais persistentes são resquícios fibrosos não patentes do úraco, que conectam o vértice vesical ao umbigo.
• Os cistos uracais são acúmulos focais de líquido em segmentos isolados do úraco persistente e podem ser assépticos ou sépticos.

HEMOGRAMA/BIOQUÍMICA/URINÁLISE
• Achados anormais relacionados com o distúrbio subjacente indutor dos divertículos vesicouracais a menos que sejam complicados por doenças adquiridas e concomitantes do trato urinário inferior.
• Achados anormais relacionados com a infecção secundária do trato urinário.

OUTROS TESTES LABORATORIAIS
N/D.

DIAGNÓSTICO POR IMAGEM
• Divertículos macroscópicos congênitos e adquiridos — mais bem identificados por meio de uretrocistografia com contraste positivo.
• As radiografias obtidas com a bexiga completamente cheia e depois parcialmente distendida com meio de contraste podem facilitar a detecção de divertículos pequenos.

MÉTODOS DIAGNÓSTICOS
N/D.

ACHADOS PATOLÓGICOS
• Os divertículos macroscópicos extramurais aparecem como projeções luminais cônicas ou convexas a partir do vértice vesical.
• Os divertículos microscópicos intramurais aparecem como lúmens revestidos pelo epitélio de transição, que persistem no vértice vesical desde a camada da submucosa até a subserosa.

TRATAMENTO

• Muitos divertículos macroscópicos em gatos (e, provavelmente, em cães) serão adquiridos e autolimitantes se a doença subjacente for removida.
• Os esforços terapêuticos diretos visam a eliminação da(s) causa(s) subjacente(s) da doença do trato urinário inferior.
• Considerar a realização de diverticulectomia se algum divertículo macroscópico persistir no paciente com infecção bacteriana persistente ou recidivante do trato urinário, apesar do fornecimento de antibioticoterapia apropriada.

MEDICAÇÕES

MEDICAMENTO(S) DE ESCOLHA
N/D.

CONTRAINDICAÇÕES/INTERAÇÕES POSSÍVEIS
N/D.

ACOMPANHAMENTO

MONITORIZAÇÃO DO PACIENTE
Se a infecção bacteriana do trato urinário persistir ou recidivar independentemente da administração de antibioticoterapia adequada, o estado do divertículo deverá ser reavaliado por meio de radiografia contrastada.

PREVENÇÃO
Evitar os procedimentos diagnósticos ou os tratamentos que alteram as defesas normais do trato urinário do hospedeiro e predispõem o animal à infecção do trato urinário.

COMPLICAÇÕES POSSÍVEIS
Os divertículos macroscópicos congênitos persistentes são fatores de risco para infecção bacteriana recidivante do trato urinário.

EVOLUÇÃO ESPERADA E PROGNÓSTICO
• Os divertículos microscópicos congênitos costumam ser clinicamente silenciosos a menos que complicados por doença concomitante do trato urinário inferior.
• Os divertículos macroscópicos adquiridos tipicamente cicatrizam em 2-3 semanas após a melhora dos sinais clínicos de doença do trato urinário inferior.
• Em geral, o procedimento de diverticulectomia e o fornecimento de antibioticoterapia adequada estão associados à resolução de infecções recidivantes do trato urinário em pacientes com divertículos macroscópicos congênitos persistentes.

DIVERSOS

DISTÚRBIOS ASSOCIADOS
• Os divertículos macroscópicos congênitos persistentes são fatores de risco potenciais para infecções bacterianas recidivantes do trato urinário.
• Os divertículos macroscópicos adquiridos são tipicamente encontrados em pacientes com doenças concomitantes do trato urinário inferior.

VER TAMBÉM
• Doença Idiopática do Trato Urinário Inferior Felino.
• Infecção do Trato Urinário Inferior.

Sugestões de Leitura
Osborne CA, Johnston GR, Kruger JM, et al. Etiopathogenesis and biological behavior of feline vesicourachal diverticula. Vet Clin North Am 1987, 17:697.

Autores John M. Kruger e Carl A. Osborne
Consultor Editorial Carl A. Osborne

Doença da Aglutinina Fria

CONSIDERAÇÕES GERAIS

REVISÃO
• Distúrbio autoimune raro do tipo II, no qual os anticorpos antieritrocitários apresentam atividade acentuada a temperaturas <37,2°C e geralmente a <31,1°C.
• Tipicamente, as aglutininas frias correspondem à IgM, embora já haja descrição de IgG e IgG-IgM mistas.
• As aglutininas frias com amplitude térmica inferior costumam estar associadas com aglutinação eritrocitária direta a temperaturas corporais baixas na microvasculatura periférica e com uma doença acrocianótica ou outros fenômenos vasoclusivos periféricos, todos desencadeados ou intensificados pela exposição ao frio.
• A fixação de complemento e o fenômeno de hemólise constituem um processo reativo morno, que ocorre a temperaturas corporais elevadas; por essa razão, os pacientes podem apresentar títulos altíssimos de aglutininas frias, embora esses anticorpos possam se mostrar incapazes de promover a hemólise de eritrócitos nas temperaturas atingidas na corrente sanguínea.
• Grande parte das aglutininas frias causa encurtamento pequeno ou nulo no tempo de vida do eritrócito.
• Aglutininas frias de amplitude térmica elevada (raras) — podem causar hemólise contínua; com frequência, a anemia resultante apresenta-se branda e estável, mas a exposição ao frio pode aumentar enormemente a ligação das aglutininas frias e a hemólise intravascular mediada pelo complemento.

IDENTIFICAÇÃO
• Distúrbio raro em cães e gatos.
• Em cães e gatos saudáveis, pode-se encontrar um título baixo das aglutininas frias de ocorrência natural (em geral, na proporção de 1:32 ou menor); no entanto, isso não tem importância clínica.
• Não se conhecem a base genética, a idade média e a faixa etária de acometimento, bem como as predileções raciais e sexuais.
• Ocorrência mais provável em climas mais frios.

SINAIS CLÍNICOS
• Com frequência, há histórico de exposição ao frio.
• Acrocianose associada à sedimentação de aglutinados eritrocitários na microvasculatura cutânea.
• Eritema.
• Ulceração cutânea com formação secundária de crostas.
• Necrose gangrenosa e seca da extremidade da orelha, da ponta da cauda, do nariz e dos pés.
• As áreas acometidas podem estar doloridas.
• A anemia pode ou não representar uma característica importante; os sinais clínicos incluem palidez, fraqueza, taquicardia, taquipneia, icterícia, pigmentúria, esplenomegalia leve e sopro cardíaco tênue.

CAUSAS E FATORES DE RISCO
• Doença primária — idiopática.
• Doença secundária — associada à infecção respiratória superior (gatos), isoeritrólise neonatal, intoxicação pelo chumbo (cães) e neoplasia.
• Exposição ao frio como fator de risco.
• Em seres humanos, a doença da aglutinina fria foi descrita em pacientes pós-transplante de fígado e pode ser deflagrada pela administração de tacrolimo.

DIAGNÓSTICO

DIAGNÓSTICO DIFERENCIAL
• Diagnóstico estabelecido por meio de achados anamnésicos (exposição ao frio), resultados do exame físico, demonstração da aglutinação fria *in vitro*.
• Lesões cutâneas — vasculite cutânea, síndrome hepatocutânea, eritema multiforme, necrólise epidérmica tóxica, dermatomiosite, CID, LES, neoplasias linforreticulares, crioulcerações, intoxicação pelo chumbo e pênfigo.
• Anemia — anemia hemolítica por anticorpos mornos; outras causas de anemia.
• Hemaglutinação macroscópica *in vitro* — as disproteinemias podem levar à formação de *rouleaux**, mimetizando a aglutinação eritrocitária em lâmina de vidro.

HEMOGRAMA/BIOQUÍMICA/URINÁLISE
• Autoaglutinação à temperatura ambiente.
• Anormalidades laboratoriais secundárias à hemólise.

OUTROS TESTES LABORATORIAIS
• Quando uma amostra de sangue em heparina ou EDTA em lâmina de vidro sofrer aglutinação espontânea à temperatura ambiente, com intensificação a 3,9°C, e os eritrócitos voltarem a se dispersar após aquecimento a 37,2°C, deve-se suspeitar de aglutininas frias.
• Caso não se consiga induzir à aglutinação *in vitro*, será inconcebível sua ocorrência *in vivo* nas extremidades.
• Os casos duvidosos podem ser confirmados por meio do teste de Coombs a 3,9°C e 37,2°C.
• Teste de Coombs a 37,2°C — em geral, as aglutininas frias não são detectadas, pois elas podem ser extraídas dos eritrócitos durante a lavagem; dessa forma, o teste requer o uso de soro anticomplemento.
• Teste de Coombs a 3,9°C — em cães saudáveis, relata-se incidência >50% de resultados positivos, o que pode ser causado por ligação inespecífica do próprio reagente ou por ligação de aglutininas frias não patogênicas de título baixo e ocorrência natural.
• A classe das globulinas pode ser estabelecida por meio de imunoeletroforese do eluato** concentrado (i. e., do material obtido por lavagem) de eritrócitos do paciente, o que é importante para o prognóstico e o tratamento.

ACHADOS PATOLÓGICOS
• Necrose dérmica.
• Ulceração com características secundárias de infecções oportunistas.
• Trombose vascular com indícios de necrose isquêmica.

---

* N. T.: Fenômeno de Rouleaux corresponde ao empilhamento de eritrócitos observado nas distensões sanguíneas, decorrentes da concentração elevada de fibrinogênio ou globulinas. A formação de rouleaux é especialmente marcante na paraproteinemia (gamopatia monoclonal).
** N. T: produto advindo da eluição (separação).

TRATAMENTO

• O paciente deve ficar internado em ambiente aquecido até que a doença pare de evoluir.
• O cuidado de suporte e o tratamento da ferida dependem dos sinais clínicos; se a necrose na ponta da cauda ou nos pés for grave, poderá haver a necessidade de amputação.
• A esplenectomia é de pouco auxílio em pacientes com distúrbios hemolíticos mediados pela IgM, mas pode ser útil naqueles com anemia hemolítica mediada pela IgG resistentes à terapia.
• Orientar o proprietário a sempre manter o paciente em ambiente aquecido para evitar recidivas.
• Em seres humanos, a terapia é frequentemente ineficaz. Plasmaférese, gamaglobulinas intravenosas e rituximabe já se mostraram benéficos em alguns pacientes.

MEDICAÇÕES

MEDICAMENTO(S)

Aglutininas Frias IgM
• A terapia imunossupressora não é muito eficaz contra os distúrbios mediados pela IgM, mas deve ser tentada (i. e., corticosteroides, azatioprina, leflunomida). • Plasmaférese.

Aglutininas Frias IgG
• Terapia imunossupressora.

CONTRAINDICAÇÕES/INTERAÇÕES POSSÍVEIS
• Monitorizar o paciente quanto à presença de sinais de infecção secundária à terapia imunossupressora.
• Não utilizar fluidos IV frios.

ACOMPANHAMENTO

• Um paciente com a doença da aglutinina fria conhecida deve ser mantido constantemente em ambientes aquecidos.
• Em geral, a doença da aglutinina fria caracteriza-se por início agudo e evolução rápida.
• O prognóstico é reservado a razoável.
• A recuperação pode levar semanas.

DIVERSOS

VER TAMBÉM
Anemia Imunomediada.

ABREVIATURA(S)
• CID = coagulação intravascular disseminada.
• EDTA = ácido etilenodiaminotetracético.
• LES = lúpus eritematoso sistêmico.

Sugestões de Leitura
Dickson NJ. Cold agglutinin disease in a puppy associated with lead intoxication. J Small Anim Pract 1990;31:105-108.

Autor Jörg Bücheler
Consultor Editorial A. H. Rebar.

Doença de Chagas (Tripanossomíase Americana)

CONSIDERAÇÕES GERAIS

REVISÃO
- Causada pelo parasita protozoário hemoflagelado zoonótico *Trypanosoma cruzi*. • Infecção — as fezes infectadas de um vetor (Triatominae, denominado comumente de barbeiro) são depositadas em uma ferida (local de picada do vetor) ou em uma mucosa; o cão alimenta-se do vetor infectado; a transmissão ocorre por meio da transfusão de sangue contaminado. • Após a multiplicação no local de ingresso (5 dias após a infecção), ocorre a disseminação hematógena à maioria dos órgãos, mas principalmente ao coração e ao cérebro. • Os microrganismos tornam-se intracelulares, multiplicam-se e depois se irrompem na circulação, de modo a gerar parasitemias maciças, associadas particularmente à miocardite aguda e, menos comumente, à encefalite difusa (14 dias após a infecção).
- Ocorre o declínio das parasitemias (subpatentes 30 dias após a infecção). • Há uma ascensão dos títulos de anticorpos (detectáveis por volta de 26 dias após a infecção). • Se sobreviver à miocardite aguda, o cão entrará em um período assintomático prolongado (pode durar de meses a anos); desenvolvimento progressivo e insidioso de degeneração miocárdica; miocardiopatia dilatada final. • Américas do Sul e Central — doença endêmica (tanto em seres humanos como nos animais de estimação). • Estados Unidos — principalmente no Texas; além de Louisiana, Oklahoma, Carolina do Sul e Virgínia; há relatos de vetores e hospedeiros reservatórios infectados em regiões como Califórnia, Novo México, Flórida, Geórgia, Carolina do Norte e Maryland.

IDENTIFICAÇÃO
- Cães jovens — mais comum. • Doença aguda — cães geralmente com menos de 2 anos de idade. • Doença crônica — cães idosos. • Raças de caça — probabilidade de contato com vetores ou hospedeiros reservatórios. • Mais frequentemente nos machos. • Gatos — não há casos relatados na América do Norte.

SINAIS CLÍNICOS
Comentários Gerais
Duas síndromes — aguda (miocardite ou encefalite em cães jovens) e crônica (miocardiopatia dilatada em cães idosos).

Achados Anamnésicos
Aguda
- Morte súbita. • Letargia. • Depressão. • Anorexia. • Diarreia. • Fraqueza. • Intolerância a exercícios. • Disfunção leve a grave do SNC (semelhante à da cinomose). • Ataxia, crises convulsivas.

Crônica
- Fraqueza. • Intolerância a exercícios. • Síncope. • Morte súbita.

Achados do Exame Físico
Aguda
- Linfadenopatia generalizada. • Insuficiência cardíaca. • Taquicardia e arritmias. • Sinais neurológicos — fraqueza; ataxia, coreia; crises convulsivas (indistinguíveis da cinomose).

Crônica
Taquicardia — sustentada ou paroxística.

CAUSAS E FATORES DE RISCO
T. cruzi.

DIAGNÓSTICO

DIAGNÓSTICO DIFERENCIAL
- Miocardiopatia. • Defeitos cardíacos congênitos. • Miocardite traumática. • Cinomose. • Toxoplasmose. • Neosporose.

HEMOGRAMA/BIOQUÍMICA/URINÁLISE
Em geral, normais.

OUTROS TESTES LABORATORIAIS
- Sorologia — o título positivo confirma o diagnóstico; exame disponível na unidade de parasitologia dos CDCs, Centers for Disease Control and Prevention, nos EUA. • Testes sorológicos imunocromatográficos *in situ* (desenvolvidos para o diagnóstico em ser humano na América do Sul) possuem alta sensibilidade e especificidade quando utilizados em cães — excelente ferramenta para estudo não somente em cães, mas também em animais selvagens. • Os títulos de anticorpos são muito sensíveis e específicos; se descartarem *Leishmania*: proceder à reação cruzada com essa espécie de parasita. • Isolamento do microrganismo — cultura em infusão de fígado e triptose; coletar 50 mL de sangue heparinizado. • Examinar a camada leucocitária em um tubo de micro-hematócrito (centrifugado para a leitura do VG), utilizando a objetiva de 40° do microscópio — observam-se microrganismos durante o período de alta parasitemia. • PCR — exame muito útil durante os estágios indeterminados e crônicos quando os tripomastigotas sanguíneos são muito difíceis de demonstrar. Possui alta especificidade, porém baixa sensibilidade, a menos que se examinem amostras obtidas de múltiplos tecidos. • Troponina I elevada — doença aguda.

DIAGNÓSTICO POR IMAGEM
- Radiografia — aguda: cardiomegalia, edema pulmonar e, raramente, leve efusão pleural; crônica: cardiomegalia. • Ecocardiografia — aguda: raras vezes revela anormalidades da câmara ou da parede cardíaca; crônica: fração de ejeção reduzida, encurtamento fracional e adelgaçamento das paredes livres dos ventrículos direito e esquerdo.

MÉTODOS DIAGNÓSTICOS
Eletrocardiografia
- Aguda — bloqueio atrioventricular; depressão na amplitude do complexo QRS; bloqueio do ramo direito do feixe de His. • Crônica — amplitude baixa do QRS; bloqueio do ramo direito do feixe de His; arritmias ventriculares (em princípio, observam-se CVPs unifocais, que se tornam multiformes e depois se degeneram em diversas formas de taquicardia ventricular).

TRATAMENTO

- A terapia clínica não produz cura clínica. • Em casos de prognóstico mau e potencial zoonótico, a eutanásia representa uma opção.

ORIENTAÇÃO AO PROPRIETÁRIO
- Alertar o proprietário sobre o possível risco zoonótico e o potencial de morte súbita. • Aguda — em geral, evolui para a forma crônica, o que é muitas vezes fatal. • Fêmea intacta infectada — pode transmitir a infecção à prole.

MEDICAÇÕES

MEDICAMENTO(S)
- Diversos medicamentos possuem eficácia limitada durante o estágio agudo da doença; nenhum deles produz a cura clínica; até mesmo os animais tratados podem evoluir para doença crônica. • Benzimidazol (Ragonil®) — 5 mg/kg VO a cada 12 h por 60 dias; medicamento preferido para uso em cães; melhora acentuada da doença aguda em seres humanos e, provavelmente, em cães. Disponível no Communicable Disease Center. • Nifurtimox (Lampit®) — 30 mg/kg VO a cada 12 h por 90-120 dias; medicamento sob pesquisa que, quando combinado com corticosteroides, pode melhorar as taxas de mortalidade e morbidade em cães. Disponível no Communicable Disease Center. • Alopurinol — exibe certa eficácia em seres humanos, mas provavelmente não em cães. Tentar 30 mg/kg VO a cada 12 h por 100 dias. • Cetoconazol — eficácia baixa. • Verapamil (bloqueador dos canais de cálcio) — melhora a cardiopatia aguda e aumenta a sobrevida de camundongos infectados pelo *T. cruzi*; o emprego desse medicamento em cães não teve o mesmo êxito. • Citioato (Proban®) — 3,3 mg/kg VO a cada 48 h; eficaz na redução das populações do vetor. Foi demonstrado que o fipronil sob a forma de *spot-on* (Frontline® Top Spot, Merial) é ineficaz em impedir o repasto sanguíneo de vetores da família Reduviidae nos cães. • Tratamento de suporte da miocardiopatia dilatada (insuficiência cardíaca direita e esquerda) e das arritmias ventriculares.

ACOMPANHAMENTO

- Cardiopatia — prognóstico sempre reservado.
- Crônica — prognóstico de reservado a ruim.

DIVERSOS

POTENCIAL ZOONÓTICO
Existente; por ser basicamente incurável em seres humanos, a eutanásia de cães infectados constitui uma opção.

ABREVIATURA(S)
- CVP = complexo ventricular prematuro.
- PCR = reação em cadeia da polimerase. • VG = volume globular (hematócrito). • SNC = sistema nervoso central.

Sugestões de Leitura
Barr SC. American trypanosomiasis. In: Greene CE, ed., Infectious Diseases of the Dog and Cat, 3rd ed. St. Louis: Saunders Elsevier, 2006, pp. 676-681.
Nieto PD, Boughton R, Dorn PL, et al. Comparison of two immunochromatographic assays and the indirect immunofluorescence antibody test for diagnosis of Trypanosoma cruzi infection in dogs in south central Louisiana. Vet Parasitol 2009, 165:241-247.

Autor Stephen C. Barr
Consultor Editorial Stephen C. Barr

DOENÇA DE LEGG-CALVÉ-PERTHES

CONSIDERAÇÕES GERAIS

DEFINIÇÃO
Degeneração espontânea da cabeça e do colo femorais, levando a colapso da articulação coxofemoral e osteoartrite.

FISIOPATOLOGIA
- Causa exata desconhecida; não foi identificada uma lesão vascular específica.
- Evidência histológica — pontos de infarto dos vasos que nutrem o fêmur proximal.
- Necrose do osso subcondral — levando a colapso e deformação da cabeça femoral durante aplicação de carga normal.
- Cartilagem articular — torna-se espessada; desenvolvimento de fenda; desgaste das camadas superficiais.
- Degeneração e reparo ósseos simultâneos — característica da isquemia e da revascularização do osso.
- Nenhuma evidência de hipercoagulabilidade ou de outras anormalidades da coagulação sanguínea.

SISTEMA(S) ACOMETIDO(S)
Musculosquelético — provoca a claudicação do membro posterior; início insidioso.

GENÉTICA
- Manchester terrier — padrão de herança multifatorial com alto grau de hereditariedade.
- Provável predisposição hereditária.

INCIDÊNCIA/PREVALÊNCIA
- Comum entre raças caninas miniatura, toy e pequena.
- Não há nenhuma estimativa precisa disponível.

DISTRIBUIÇÃO GEOGRÁFICA
N/D.

IDENTIFICAÇÃO
Espécies
Cães.

Raça(s) Predominante(s)
- Raças Toy e Terrier — mais suscetíveis.
- Manchester terrier, Pinscher miniatura, Poodle toy, Lakeland terrier, West Highland white terrier e Cairn terrier — maiores do que a incidência esperada.

Idade Média e Faixa Etária
- Maior parte dos pacientes tem 5-8 meses de vida.
- Variação — 3-13 meses.

Sexo Predominante
Nenhum.

SINAIS CLÍNICOS
Comentários Gerais
Geralmente, unilateral; apenas 12-16% dos casos são bilaterais.

Achados Anamnésicos
Claudicação — em geral, exibe início gradual em 2-3 meses; sustenta o peso; ocasionalmente, o membro é conduzido.

Achados do Exame Físico
- Dor à manipulação do quadril — muito comum.
- Crepitação da articulação — inconsistente.
- Atrofia dos músculos da coxa — quase sempre observada.
- Paciente normal sob outros aspectos.

CAUSAS
- Desconhecidas.
- Tamponamento dos vasos subsinoviais intracapsulares que nutrem a cabeça femoral — causa sugerida de isquemia, levando a alterações patológicas.

FATORES DE RISCO
- Raças pequenas, toy e miniatura — risco aumentado.
- Traumatismo na região do quadril.

DIAGNÓSTICO

DIAGNÓSTICO DIFERENCIAL
- Luxação patelar medial — pode ocorrer independentemente; principal diagnóstico diferencial em cães jovens.
- Ruptura do ligamento cruzado cranial — principal diagnóstico diferencial em cães idosos.
- Displasia coxofemoral — sinais radiográficos semelhantes.

HEMOGRAMA/BIOQUÍMICA/URINÁLISE
N/D.

OUTROS TESTES LABORATORIAIS
N/D.

DIAGNÓSTICO POR IMAGEM
- Alterações radiográficas precoces — alargamento do espaço articular; diminuição da densidade óssea da epífise; esclerose e espessamento do colo femoral.
- Alterações radiográficas tardias — áreas transparentes dentro da cabeça femoral.
- Alterações radiográficas do estágio terminal da doença — achatamento e deformação extrema da cabeça femoral; osteoartrose grave — fratura do colo femoral.

MÉTODOS DIAGNÓSTICOS
N/D.

ACHADOS PATOLÓGICOS
- Cabeça femoral — removida durante o procedimento de excisão da cabeça e do colo femoral; geralmente deformada com superfície articular irregular espessada.
- Doença precoce — caracterizada ao exame histológico por perda dos osteócitos lacunares e necrose dos elementos medulares; trabéculas circundadas por tecido de granulação.
- Doença tardia — trabéculas metafisárias espessadas; mistura de necrose e reparo tecidual típicos de revascularização óssea.
- Doença avançada — atividade osteoclástica; neoformação óssea.

TRATAMENTO

CUIDADO(S) DE SAÚDE ADEQUADO(S)
- Repouso e analgésicos — sucesso relatado no alívio da claudicação em poucos pacientes.
- Tipoia de Ehmer — êxito descrito em um único paciente; mantida por 10 semanas; aumenta o risco de anquilose.
- O início insidioso quase sempre impede a identificação precoce e a possibilidade de tratamento conservativo bem-sucedido.
- Excisão da cabeça e do colo femoral com exercício precoce e vigoroso após a cirurgia — constitui o tratamento de escolha.

CUIDADO(S) DE ENFERMAGEM
Pós-Cirúrgicos
- Fisioterapia — extremamente importante para a reabilitação do membro acometido.
- Analgésicos, medicamentos anti-inflamatórios e compressas com gelo — 3-5 dias; são relevantes.
- Exercícios de amplitude de movimento — extensão e flexão; devem ser instituídos imediatamente.
- Pequenos pesos de chumbo — presos como braceletes no boleto, acima da articulação do jarrete; estimula a utilização precoce do membro tratado.

ATIVIDADE
- Pós-cirúrgica — a atividade precoce é estimulada para melhorar a utilização do membro.
- Tratamento conservativo — nesse caso, é recomendável a restrição da atividade.

DIETA
Evitar a obesidade.

ORIENTAÇÃO AO PROPRIETÁRIO
- Alertar os proprietários sobre a base genética da doença em cães da raça Manchester terrier; desestimular o cruzamento dos cães acometidos.
- Avisar o proprietário sobre o fato de que a recuperação após a excisão da cabeça e do colo femoral pode levar de 3-6 meses.

CONSIDERAÇÕES CIRÚRGICAS
Excisão da cabeça e do colo femoral — tratamento de escolha.

MEDICAÇÕES

MEDICAMENTO(S) DE ESCOLHA
AINEs — antes ou depois da cirurgia; minimizam a dor articular (artralgia); diminuem a sinovite; carprofeno (2,2 mg/kg VO a cada 12 h), etodolaco (10-15 mg/kg VO a cada 24 h), meloxicam (0,2 mg/kg VO, IV ou SC no primeiro dia, depois 0,1 mg/kg 1 vez ao dia), deracoxibe (1-2 mg/kg VO 1 vez ao dia para osteoartrite, 3-4 mg/kg para dor pós-operatória VO 1 vez ao dia; não exceder 7 dias), firocoxibe (5 mg/kg VO 1 vez ao dia), ácido acetilsalicílico tamponado ou com revestimento entérico (10-25 mg/kg VO a cada 8 ou 12 h).

CONTRAINDICAÇÕES
AINEs — o desconforto gastrintestinal pode impedir o uso em alguns pacientes.

PRECAUÇÕES
- AINEs — a inibição da atividade plaquetária pode aumentar a hemorragia durante o procedimento cirúrgico; se possível, interromper o ácido acetilsalicílico por, no mínimo, 1 semana antes da cirurgia; costuma provocar algum grau de ulceração gástrica.

INTERAÇÕES POSSÍVEIS
AINEs — não utilizar em conjunto com os glicocorticoides; risco de ulceração gastrintestinal; considerar tempos de intervalo adequados ao se trocar de um AINE para outro.

MEDICAMENTO(S) ALTERNATIVO(S)
Medicamentos condroprotetores (p. ex., glicosaminoglicanos polissulfatados, glicosamina e sulfato de condroitina) — pouca utilidade em

Doença de Legg-Calvé-Perthes

casos de doença avançada; nenhuma prova sugere que esses medicamentos evitem ou revertam o processo mórbido.

ACOMPANHAMENTO

MONITORIZAÇÃO DO PACIENTE
• Monitorizar a evolução do quadro após a cirurgia — intervalos de 2 semanas; necessária para garantir a complacência com as recomendações de exercícios.
• Reavaliar o tratamento conservativo com exame físico e radiografias para determinar a necessidade de cirurgia.

PREVENÇÃO
• Não incentivar o cruzamento dos animais acometidos.
• Não repetir cruzamentos entre machos e fêmeas que deram origem a filhotes acometidos.

COMPLICAÇÕES POSSÍVEIS
Limitar o exercício pós-operatório pode resultar em uma função do membro abaixo do ideal.

EVOLUÇÃO ESPERADA E PROGNÓSTICO
• Excisão da cabeça e do colo femoral — prognóstico bom a excelente quanto à recuperação completa (taxas de sucesso de 84-100%).
• Tratamento conservativo — há relatos de alívio da claudicação depois de 2-3 meses em cerca de 25% dos pacientes.

DIVERSOS

DISTÚRBIOS ASSOCIADOS
N/D.

FATORES RELACIONADOS COM A IDADE
Em geral, acomete cães jovens pertencentes a raças de pequeno porte, embora cães maduros também possam ser acometidos por doença crônica.

POTENCIAL ZOONÓTICO
N/D.

GESTAÇÃO/FERTILIDADE/REPRODUÇÃO
N/D.

SINÔNIMO(S)
• Doença de Perthes.
• Coxa plana.
• Coxa magna.
• Necrose avascular da cabeça femoral.
• Necrose asséptica da cabeça femoral.
• Osteocondrite juvenil.

VER TAMBÉM
• Displasia Coxofemoral — Cães.
• Doença do Ligamento Cruzado Cranial.
• Luxação Patelar.

ABREVIATURA(S)
• AINEs = anti-inflamatórios não esteroides.

Sugestões de Leitura
Brenig B, Leeb T, Jansen S, Kopp T. Analysis of blood clotting factor activities in canine Legg-Calvé-Perthes disease. J Vet Intern Med 1999, 13:570-573.
Gambardella PC. Legg-Calvé-Perthes disease in dogs. In: Bojrab MJ, ed., Disease Mechanisms in Small Animal Surgery, 2nd ed. Philadelphia: Saunders, 1993, pp. 804-807.
Gibson KL, Lewis DD, Perchman RD. Use of external coaptation for the treatment of avascular necrosis of the femoral head in a dog. JAVMA 1990, 197:868-869.
LaFond E, Breur GJ, Austin CC. Breed susceptibility for developmental orthopedic diseases in dogs. JAAHA 2002, 38:467-477.
Peycke L. Femoral head and neck ostectomy. NAVC Clinician's Brief 2011, 9(2):55-59.
Piek CJ, Hazewinkel HAW, Wolvekamp WTC, et al. Long term follow-up of avascular necrosis of the femoral head in the dog. J Small Anim Pract 1996, 37:12-18.
Piermattei DL, Flo GL, DeCamp CE. Hip joint. In: Handbook of Small Animal Orthopedics and Fracture Repair, 4th ed. Philadelphia: Saunders, 2006, pp. 507-508.
Trostel CT, Pool RR, McLaughlin RM. Canine lameness caused by developmental orthopedic diseases: Panosteitis, Legg-Calvé-Perthes disease, and hypertophic osteodystrophy. Compend Contin Educ Pract Vet 2003, 25(4):282-292.

Autor Larry Carpenter
Consultor Editorial Peter K. Shires

Doença de Tyzzer

CONSIDERAÇÕES GERAIS

REVISÃO
- *Clostridium piliformis* (antigamente conhecido como *Bacillus piliformis*) — bactéria Gram-negativa de 0,5 × 10-40 µm; patógeno intracelular obrigatório.
- Infecção — acredita-se que o microrganismo se prolifere inicialmente nas células epiteliais do intestino; dissemina-se ao fígado pela veia porta hepática; a colonização hepática é associada à necrose hepática periportal multifocal.

IDENTIFICAÇÃO
- Cães e gatos.
- Qualquer idade; os jovens apresentam um risco mais elevado.
- Roedores — são clinicamente acometidos.

SINAIS CLÍNICOS
- Início rápido de letargia, depressão, anorexia, desconforto e distensão abdominais, hepatomegalia; seguidos por hipotermia.
- Óbito — ocorre em 24-48 h.
- Material fecal — a diarreia é pouco frequente; é mais comum encontrar pequenas quantidades de fezes pastosas.

CAUSAS E FATORES DE RISCO
- *C. piliformis*.
- Contato com roedores — pode representar um fator de risco.
- Neonatos e animais imunocomprometidos (p. ex., cinomose, FeLV, panleucopenia felina e hiperlipoproteinemia familiar) — parecem ter maior risco.

DIAGNÓSTICO

DIAGNÓSTICO DIFERENCIAL
- O diagnóstico costuma ser feito à necropsia — diagnóstico de doença aguda e altamente fatal.
- Distinguida de outras causas de morte súbita e hepatite aguda.
- Outras causas de enterocolite aguda em filhotes de gatos.

HEMOGRAMA/BIOQUÍMICA/URINÁLISE
ALT — elevações acentuadas em amostras sanguíneas coletadas pouco antes do óbito.

OUTROS TESTES LABORATORIAIS
- Sorologia — para identificar infecções latentes em colônias de roedores; pode ser utilizada para pesquisar a doença em cães e gatos.
- Isolamento do microrganismo — requer a inoculação em camundongos, ovos embrionados ou cultura celular.
- Imunocitoquímica e PCR de tecidos acometidos.

DIAGNÓSTICO POR IMAGEM
N/D.

MÉTODOS DIAGNÓSTICOS
N/D.

ACHADOS PATOLÓGICOS
Macroscópicos
- Focos cinza-esbranquiçados a hemorrágicos multifocais em todo o fígado; também podem ocorrer em outras vísceras.
- Já foram relatadas alterações como miocardite focal, espessamento e congestão intestinais, linfadenopatia mesentérica.
- Na espécie canina, há relatos de lesões amplamente disseminadas, incluindo miocardite grave, hepatite, enterocolite, leiomiosite intestinal e adenite cortical adrenal.

Histológicos
- Necrose hepática multifocal.
- Ileíte ou colite necrótica.
- Microrganismos filamentosos intracelulares — costumam ser numerosos; a observação com o corante de H&E não é fácil; exige corantes argênticos (p. ex., Steiner ou Warthin-Starry modificados).

TRATAMENTO

Não há nenhum tratamento eficaz.

MEDICAÇÕES

MEDICAMENTO(S)
Nenhum.

CONTRAINDICAÇÕES/INTERAÇÕES POSSÍVEIS
Nenhuma.

ACOMPANHAMENTO

PREVENÇÃO
Evitar os fatores predisponentes — isso pode limitar a doença.

DIVERSOS

ABREVIATURA(S)
- ALT = alanina aminotransferase.
- FeLV = vírus da leucemia felina.
- H&E = hematoxilina e eosina.
- PCR = reação em cadeia da polimerase.

Sugestões de Leitura
Barr SC, Bowman DD. Tyzzer's disease. In: Canine and Feline Infectious Diseases and Parasitology. Ames, IA: Blackwell, 2006, pp. 535-537.
Jones BR, Greene CE. Tyzzer's disease. In: Greene CE, ed., Infectious Diseases of the Dog and Cat, 3rd ed. St. Louis: Saunders Elsevier, 2006, pp. 362-363.
Young JK, Baker DC, Burney DP. Naturally occurring Tyzzer's disease in a puppy. Vet Pathol 1995, 32:63-65.

Autor Stephen C. Barr
Consultor Editorial Stephen C. Barr

Doença de von Willebrand

CONSIDERAÇÕES GERAIS

DEFINIÇÃO
- Defeito hemostático primário causado por alguma deficiência quantitativa ou funcional do vWF.
- A manifestação clínica varia desde diátese hemorrágica leve a grave.

FISIOPATOLOGIA
- vWF consiste em uma proteína plasmática adesiva necessária para a ligação normal das plaquetas nos locais de lesão de pequenos vasos. Além disso, o vWF plasmático é uma proteína carreadora do fator VIII de coagulação.
- A falta do vWF prejudica a adesão e agregação plaquetárias. As formas de maior peso molecular do vWF demonstram uma reatividade mais elevada em manter as interações plaqueta-colágeno.

SISTEMA(S) ACOMETIDO(S)
- A deficiência do vWF pode causar hemorragia espontânea, hemorragia pós-traumática prolongada e, por fim, anemia por perda de sangue.
- Hemorragia espontânea tipicamente se manifesta como sangramento proveniente das superfícies de mucosas.

GENÉTICA
- Traço autossômico; tanto os machos como as fêmeas expressam e transmitem o defeito em uma frequência equivalente.
- O padrão de expressão das formas graves (doença de von Willebrand tipos 2 e 3) é recessivo; já o padrão das formas mais brandas (doença de von Willebrand tipo 1) parece recessivo ou dominante incompleto.

INCIDÊNCIA/PREVALÊNCIA
- O defeito hemostático hereditário é mais comum em cães.
- Raramente relatado em gatos.

DISTRIBUIÇÃO GEOGRÁFICA
Nenhuma.

IDENTIFICAÇÃO
Raça(s) Predominante(s)
- Três classificações de tipo são encontradas em cães; um único tipo predomina dentro de cada raça acometida:
- Doença de von Willebrand tipo 1 (sinais leves a moderados): deficiência quantitativa da proteína. Baixos níveis do antígeno do vWF com diminuição proporcional na função do vWF. O tipo 1 é a classificação mais comum.
- Raças: Airedale, Akita, Basset hound, Montanhês de Berna, Dachshund, Doberman pinscher, Pastor alemão, Golden retriever, Galgo, Wolfhound irlandês, Manchester terrier, Pinscher miniatura, Pembroke Welsh corgi e Poodle, além de casos esporádicos em qualquer raça e cães mestiços.
- Doença de von Willebrand tipo 2 (sinais graves): defeito quantitativo e funcional da proteína; baixos níveis do antígeno do vWF com deficiência desproporcional de atividade em virtude da ausência de multímeros de alto peso molecular.
- Raças: Pointer alemão de pelo duro e o de pelo curto.
- Doença de von Willebrand tipo 3 (sinais graves): ausência completa do vWF plasmático.
- Raças: Chesapeake Bay retriever, Kooiker holandês, Terrier escocês, Pastor de Shetland e casos esporádicos em qualquer raça.

Idade Média e Faixa Etária
- As formas graves (doença de von Willebrand tipos 2 e 3) tipicamente se manifestam por volta de 3-6 meses de vida.
- As formas mais brandas tipicamente demonstram sangramento anormal após cirurgia ou traumatismo ou em associação com algum outro distúrbio que comprometa a hemostasia.

SINAIS CLÍNICOS
Achados do Exame Físico
- Hemorragia proveniente das superfícies de mucosas: epistaxe, hemorragia gastrintestinal, hematúria, hemorragia vaginal e/ou gengival.
- Sangramento prolongado após cirurgia ou traumatismo.
- Anemia por perda sanguínea em caso de hemorragia prolongada.

CAUSAS
A doença de von Willebrand hereditária é causada por mutações que afetam a síntese, a liberação ou a estabilidade do vWF.

FATORES DE RISCO
Condições patológicas adquiridas ou terapias medicamentosas que diminuem a função das plaquetas podem exacerbar os sinais clínicos da doença de von Willebrand.

DIAGNÓSTICO

DIAGNÓSTICO DIFERENCIAL
- Trombocitopenia (a primeira causa a ser excluída em qualquer paciente com hemorragia anormal).
- Deficiência adquirida de fator de coagulação (frequentemente associada à hepatopatia, deficiência de vitamina K ou CID).
- Defeitos adquiridos da função plaquetária (vinculada muitas vezes à terapia medicamentosa, uremia, hiperproteinemia).
- Deficiências hereditárias de fator de coagulação.
- Defeitos hereditários na função das plaquetas.

HEMOGRAMA/BIOQUÍMICA/URINÁLISE
- Desenvolvimento de anemia regenerativa após perda sanguínea.
- A contagem das plaquetas permanece normal a menos que o paciente tenha sofrido sangramento agudo e maciço.

OUTROS TESTES LABORATORIAIS
- Testes de triagem do perfil de coagulação (TCA, TTPA, TP, TCT, fibrinogênio) — normais.
- Diagnóstico clínico formulado com base na mensuração específica da concentração plasmática do vWF (antígeno do vWF).
- Níveis do antígeno do vWF <50% indicam deficiência do vWF, embora os sinais clínicos de sangramento anormal tipicamente se desenvolvam em animais com níveis <25%.
- As doenças de von Willebrand tipos 1 e 2 são caracterizadas por baixos níveis do antígeno do vWF, enquanto a doença de von Willebrand tipo 3 é definida como a ausência completa de proteína detectável (antígeno do vWF <0,1%).
- As doenças de von Willebrand tipos 1 e 2 são diferenciadas com base nas análises funcionais e/ou estruturais do vWF.
- O ensaio de ligação do vWF ao colágeno é uma medida funcional de afinidade do vWF pelo colágeno. Os cães com a doença de von Willebrand tipo 2 apresentam uma deficiência relativa do ensaio de ligação do vWF ao colágeno em comparação ao antígeno do vWF, resultando em uma relação de concentração:função proteicas >2:1. Os cães acometidos pela doença de von Willebrand tipo 1 possuem concentração e função proteicas proporcionais.
- A estrutura dos multímeros do vWF é visualizada em exames de *western blot* (também conhecido como mancha ocidental). Os cães com a doença de von Willebrand tipo 2 carecem das formas de maior peso molecular.

DIAGNÓSTICO POR IMAGEM
N/D.

MÉTODOS DIAGNÓSTICOS
- Tempo de sangramento da mucosa bucal e função das plaquetas mensurados com o analisador PFA-100® são testes de triagem na fase de cuidados, cujos pontos finais se encontram prolongados em pacientes com defeitos da agregação plaquetária e deficiência do vWF. O prolongamento é inespecífico e pode acompanhar trombocitopenia grave, anemia ou alterações na viscosidade sanguínea.
- Tempo de sangramento da mucosa bucal (valores esperados de 2-4 min): valores típicos para doença de von Willebrand tipo 1 = 5-10 min; doença de von Willebrand tipos 2 e 3 >12 min.
- Tempos de oclusão* do PFA-100® (tempo esperado de oclusão de ADP/colágeno <120 s): valores típicos para doença de von Willebrand tipo 1 = 150-300 s; doença de von Willebrand tipos 2 e 3 >300 s.

ACHADOS PATOLÓGICOS
A hemorragia é a única anormalidade associada. A morbidade e a mortalidade são causadas por perda sanguínea ou hemorragia para locais críticos (i. e., SNC, trato respiratório).

TRATAMENTO

- Transfusão de sangue total fresco, plasma fresco, plasma fresco congelado e crioprecipitado fornecerá o vWF.
- Terapia com algum componente (plasma fresco congelado a 10-12 mL/kg) ou crioprecipitado (a definição de unidade e a dosagem variam de acordo com a fonte) é mais eficiente para profilaxia cirúrgica e pacientes não anêmicos, para evitar a sensibilização das hemácias e a sobrecarga de volume.
- Os pacientes com doença de von Willebrand grave talvez necessitem de transfusões repetidas (a cada 6-12 h) para controlar ou evitar hemorragia.

CONSIDERAÇÕES CIRÚRGICAS
- A transfusão pré-operatória deve ser administrada imediatamente antes do procedimento. O vWF de pico é obtido logo após a transfusão, sendo que os valores declinam até o nível basal em 24 h depois de uma única dose.
- O repouso em gaiola e a monitorização rigorosa do paciente (hematócrito e avaliação seriados da

---

* N. T.: Tempo requerido para o agregado plaquetário obstruir a abertura e cessar o fluxo de sangue.

DOENÇA DE VON WILLEBRAND

ferida cirúrgica) por 24 h após a cirurgia são ideais para confirmar a hemostasia adequada. O tratamento da doença de von Willebrand grave tipicamente requer pelo menos uma transfusão pós-operatória.

MEDICAÇÕES

MEDICAMENTO(S) DE ESCOLHA
- Acetato de desmopressina (DDAVP) é um análogo da vasopressina que pode ser administrado no período pré-operatório a cães com a doença de von Willebrand tipo 1 leve a moderada para intensificar a hemostasia cirúrgica. A dosagem é de 1 μg/kg SC; aplicado 30 min antes da cirurgia.
- A resposta é variável; a transfusão deve estar disponível se o DDAVP sozinho não evitar o sangramento.

CONTRAINDICAÇÕES
Evitar medicamentos com efeitos anticoagulantes ou antiplaquetários: AINEs, antibióticos de sulfonamida, heparina, varfarina sódica (Coumadin®), expansores plasmáticos, estrogênios, agentes citotóxicos.

ACOMPANHAMENTO

MONITORIZAÇÃO DO PACIENTE
Observar rigorosamente o animal em busca de hemorragias associadas a traumatismo ou procedimentos cirúrgicos.

PREVENÇÃO
- Fazer a triagem dos cães no período pré-operatório para determinar o nível basal do antígeno do vWF em raças ou linhagens com alta prevalência da doença de von Willebrand. O risco de sangramento anormal é maior para níveis de antígeno do vWF <25%.
- Os cães clinicamente acometidos não devem ser acasalados. Os portadores da doença de von Willebrand podem ser identificados com base no baixo nível de antígeno do vWF (<50%); no entanto, os valores de cães portadores e negativos (livres) podem se sobrepor no extremo inferior da faixa normal (nível do antígeno do vWF de 50-70%). Atualmente, testes comerciais (VetGen®) para detectar mutações específicas do vWF no DNA estão disponíveis para variantes da doença de von Willebrand em diversas raças. Os cães heterozigotos para uma mutação específica são considerados "portadores" da doença de von Willebrand, enquanto os homozigotos são tidos como "acometidos" para essa doença.
- As práticas de reprodução seletiva podem reduzir ou eliminar a doença de von Willebrand de algum pedigree acometido. O ideal é acasalar dois progenitores livres da doença, pois com isso se espera que toda a ninhada também seja livre. O acasalamento de um progenitor livre com outro portador pode ser aceitável; nesse caso, os filhotes negativos gerados a partir desses cruzamentos são utilizados para futuros fins reprodutivos. Os acasalamentos entre portadores não são aconselháveis em função da alta probabilidade de se gerar uma ninhada clinicamente acometida.

EVOLUÇÃO ESPERADA E PROGNÓSTICO
- A maioria dos cães com doença de von Willebrand leve a moderada tem uma boa qualidade de vida e necessita de um tratamento específico mínimo ou nulo.
- Os cães com as formas mais graves necessitam de transfusão para cirurgia e devem ser transfundidos se os cuidados de suporte falharem no controle do sangramento espontâneo. Grande parte desses cães pode ser mantida de forma confortável em seus lares.

DIVERSOS

DISTÚRBIOS ASSOCIADOS
- O desenvolvimento de qualquer condição patológica que prejudique a função plaquetária pode exacerbar a tendência hemorrágica da doença de von Willebrand. As condições comuns incluem trombocitopenia, endocrinopatia (hipotireoidismo, hipocortisolismo), hiperproteinemia e uremia.
- A doença de von Willebrand adquirida ocorre em seres humanos com estenose aórtica; além disso, traços da doença de von Willebrand tipo 2 foram relatados em cães da raça Cavalier King Charles spaniel com valvulopatia mitral.

GESTAÇÃO/FERTILIDADE/REPRODUÇÃO
Ver a seção "Prevenção" em busca das recomendações em termos de reprodução.

SINÔNIMO(S)
Antigamente, a proteína do vWF era referida como antígeno relacionado com o fator VIII.

ABREVIATURA(S)
- ADP = adenosina 5'difosfato.
- AINE = anti-inflamatório não esteroide.
- CID = coagulação intravascular disseminada.
- DDAVP = 1-desamino-8-D-arginina vasopressina.
- TCA = tempo de coagulação ativada.
- TCT = tempo de coagulação da trombina.
- TP = tempo de protrombina.
- TTPA = tempo de tromboplastina parcial ativada.
- vWF = fator de von Willebrand.

Sugestões de Leitura
Brooks MB, Catalfamo JL. Platelet disorders and von Willebrand disease. In: Ettinger S, Feldman E. eds. Textbook of Veterinary Internal Medicine, 6th ed. St. Louis: Elsevier, 2004, pp. 1918-1929.
Johnson GS. Canine von Willebrand's disease. In: Feldman BF, ed., Hemostasis. Vet Clin North Am Small Anim Pract 1988, 18:195-229.
Stokol T, Parry BW. Canine von Willebrand disease; a review. Aust Vet Pract 1993, 23:94-103.
Venta PJ, Li J, Yuzbasiyan-Gurkan V, Brewer GJ, Schall W. Mutation causing vWDin Scottish terriers. J Vet Intern Med 2000, 14:10-19.

Autor Marjory Brooks
Consultor Editorial A.H. Rebar

Doença do Armazenamento de Glicogênio

CONSIDERAÇÕES GERAIS

REVISÃO
- Também conhecida como glicogenoses. Trata-se de distúrbios hereditários raros que se caracterizam pela atividade enzimática defeituosa ou deficiente no controle do metabolismo do glicogênio.
- Acúmulo tecidual de glicogênio — acarreta aumento de volume e disfunção de órgãos; pode acometer o fígado, o coração, a musculatura esquelética, os rins e o SNC.
- Glicogenólise hepática comprometida — produz hipoglicemia sintomática.
- Classificação — de acordo com o tipo de defeito enzimático e do(s) órgão(s) primário(s) acometido(s): mais de 12 tipos em seres humanos, 4 tipos em cães (Ia, II, III e VII), 1 tipo em gatos (IV).

IDENTIFICAÇÃO
- Os sinais clínicos manifestam-se em animais jovens — dias a vários meses após o nascimento na maioria dos distúrbios.
- Tipo Ia (doença de von Gierke) — filhotes de cães da raça Maltês; subunidade catalítica do gene da glicose-6-fosfatase.
- Tipo II (doença de Pompe) — cães da raça Lapland; início aos 6 meses de vida.
- Tipo III (doença de Cori) — cadelas jovens da raça Pastor alemão e cães da raça Retriever de pelo ondulado. Mutação do gene AGL (amilo-1-6 glicosidase).
- Tipo IV (doença de Andersen) — gatos dos Bosques da Noruega; pode haver natimortos; podem diminuir logo após o nascimento; os sinais podem se manifestar aos 5-7 meses de declínio neurológico progressivo. Mutação do gene GBE1(enzima de ramificação do glicogênio).
- Tipo VII (doença de Tarui) — cães da raça Springer Spaniel inglês com 2-9 anos de idade. Mutação do gene M-PFK (fosfofrutoquinase do músculo).
- Sem predominância sexual conhecida.
- Herança autossômica recessiva — gatos dos Bosques da Noruega, além de cães das raças Springer Spaniel inglês, Lapland e Maltês; suspeita no Pastor alemão.

SINAIS CLÍNICOS
- Dependem do defeito enzimático.
- Tipo Ia (filhotes de Maltês) — desenvolvimento deficiente; depressão mental; hipoglicemia; distensão abdominal; hepatomegalia; morte ou eutanásia aos 60 dias de vida.
- Tipo II (cães da raça Lapland) — vômitos e regurgitação relacionados com megaesôfago; fraqueza muscular progressiva; alterações cardíacas; morte antes dos 2 anos de idade.
- Tipo III (cães da raça Pastor alemão e Retriever de pelo ondulado) — depressão; fraqueza; falha de crescimento; distensão abdominal decorrente da hepatomegalia; hipoglicemia leve; atividade elevada das enzimas hepáticas e da creatinoquinase.
- Tipo IV (gatos dos Bosques da Noruega) — a morte costuma ocorrer no período perinatal; febre intermitente; tremores musculares generalizados; atrofia e fraqueza muscular que evoluem para tetraplegia; morte súbita causada por degeneração miocárdica e disritmia terminal. A administração de glicose pode manter os gatos até a fase adulta.
- Tipo VII (Springer Spaniel inglês) — anemia hemolítica compensada; hemólise intravascular episódica; hemoglobinúria; um único paciente desenvolveu miopatia progressiva aos 11 anos de idade.

CAUSAS E FATORES DE RISCO
Deficiências
- Tipo Ia — glicose-6-fosfatase.
- Tipo II — α-glicosidase ácida.
- Tipo III — amilo-1,6-glicosidase.
- Tipo IV — enzima de ramificação do glicogênio (α-1,4-D-glucano).
- Tipo VII — fosfofrutoquinase.

DIAGNÓSTICO

DIAGNÓSTICO DIFERENCIAL
- Alto índice de suspeita diagnóstica.
- Afiliação racial.
- Diferenciar outras causas de hipoglicemia juvenil — desnutrição; endoparasitismo; hipoglicemia transitória de jejum; anomalia vascular portossistêmica.
- Outras causas de fraqueza muscular — doenças infecciosas; endocrinopatia; causas imunomediadas; hipocalemia; outras neuromiopatias.

HEMOGRAMA/BIOQUÍMICA/URINÁLISE
- Tipos I e II — hipoglicemia; tipo I: um trabalho recente demonstrou hiperlactacidemia, hipercolesterolemia, hipertrigliceridemia e hiperuricemia.
- Tipo VII — anemia; reticulocitose; pigmentúria.

OUTROS TESTES LABORATORIAIS
- Teste genético: tipo I em cães da raça Maltês; tipo III em cães da raça Retriever de pelo ondulado; tipo IV em gatos dos Bosques da Noruega; tipo VII em cães da raça Springer Spaniel inglês.
- Tipo VII — teste com eritrócitos *in vitro*.

DIAGNÓSTICO POR IMAGEM
- Tipo II — radiografia torácica; pode revelar cardiomegalia e megaesôfago.
- Tipos Ia e III — radiografia abdominal; pode demonstrar hepatomegalia.
- Ultrassonografia abdominal — pode exibir parênquima hiperecoico e hepatomegalia compatíveis com acúmulo hepático de glicogênio.
- Tipos II e IV — ecocardiografia; pode mostrar alterações cardíacas.

MÉTODOS DIAGNÓSTICOS
- Análise de enzima tecidual e determinação do glicogênio.
- Eletromiografia.
- Eletrocardiografia.
- Teste genético.

ACHADOS PATOLÓGICOS
- Tipo Ia — emaciação; hepatomegalia maciça; acúmulo de glicogênio e lipídio (vacuolização) em hepatócitos e células epiteliais tubulares renais.
- Tipo II — acúmulo de glicogênio nos músculos esqueléticos, liso e cardíaco.
- Tipo III — hepatomegalia provocada pelo acúmulo hepático de glicogênio; também nos músculos esqueléticos.
- Tipo IV — atrofia muscular generalizada; acúmulo de glicogênio: músculos esqueléticos, SNC e sistema nervoso periférico.
- Tipo VII — depósitos de polissacarídeos na musculatura esquelética.

TRATAMENTO

CUIDADO(S) DE ENFERMAGEM
- De suporte.
- Tipos I e III — podem necessitar da administração intravenosa de glicose para tratar a crise hipoglicêmica; o tratamento a longo prazo costuma não ter utilidade.
- Terapia genética experimental com vetor associado ao adenovírus induziu à sobrevida de cães acometidos pelo tipo Ia.

DIETA
- Controlar a hipoglicemia (tipos I e III) com refeições frequentes de uma dieta rica em carboidrato até que o diagnóstico seja confirmado.

ORIENTAÇÃO AO PROPRIETÁRIO
- Avisar o proprietário sobre o fato de que as amostras serão enviadas a laboratórios especializados em caracterização genética/enzimática.
- Discutir os mecanismos conhecidos de hereditariedade para modificar os programas de reprodução.

ACOMPANHAMENTO
- Monitorizar a possível ocorrência de hipoglicemia.
- Excluir os pais de programas reprodutivos.
- Prognóstico — mau; a maioria dos pacientes vem a óbito ou é submetida à eutanásia em virtude da deterioração progressiva; exceção para a raça Springer Spaniel com manifestações hematológicas.

DIVERSOS

VER TAMBÉM
- Anomalia Vascular Portossistêmica Congênita.
- Doenças do Armazenamento Lisossomal.
- Mucopolissacaridoses.

ABREVIATURA(S)
- SNC = sistema nervoso central.

Sugestões de Leitura
Brix AE, Howerth EW, et al. Glycogen storage disease type Ia in two littermate maltese puppies. Vet Pathol 1995, 32:460-465.
Harvey JW, Calderwood MB. Polysaccharide storage myopathy in canine phosphofructokinase deficiency (type VII glycogen storage disease). Vet Pathol 1990, 27:1-8.
Koeberl DD, Pinto C, Brown T, et al. Gene therapy for inherited metabolic disorders in companion animals. ILAR J 2009, 50:122-127.
Walvoort HC. Glycogen storage disease type II in the lapland dog. Vet Q 1985, 7:187-190.

Autor Sharon A. Center
Consultor Editorial Sharon A. Center

Doença do Ligamento Cruzado Cranial

CONSIDERAÇÕES GERAIS

DEFINIÇÃO
Corresponde à lesão aguda ou progressiva do ligamento cruzado cranial, que resulta em instabilidade parcial a completa da articulação femorotibial (soldra).

FISIOPATOLOGIA
- Função do ligamento cruzado cranial — contenção passiva da articulação femorotibial, limitando a rotação medial (interna) e o deslocamento cranial da tíbia em relação ao fêmur; também limita a hiperextensão da articulação mencionada.
- Sem o ligamento cruzado cranial, as contenções ativas (músculos) em torno da articulação femorotibial constituem as principais limitações para o deslizamento da tíbia no sentido cranial.
- Lesão do ligamento cruzado cranial — por traumatismo (agudo) ou lesão repetitiva (crônica).
- Ruptura aguda — <20% dos casos são causados pela superação na resistência do ligamento em cães por meio de ações traumáticas; ocasionada geralmente por hiperextensão ou rotação medial (interna) excessiva, com a articulação femorotibial em flexão parcial (20-50°); o traumatismo agudo constitui a causa mais comum em gatos.
- Lesão subclínica repetitiva — incoordenação neuromuscular, envelhecimento, anormalidades conformacionais, tônus muscular deficiente relacionado com hábitos sedentários ou imobilização de membro e, possivelmente, dano imunomediado.
- Microrrupturas de feixes de fibras individuais do ligamento mantêm a principal estrutura intacta, mas comprometida em termos funcionais; o reparo deixa o local enfraquecido; consequentemente, o enfraquecimento cumulativo acaba levando à ruptura por um insulto secundário.
- Lesão subclínica — relacionada com o porte do animal; cães >15 kg exibem mais alterações significativas na resistência do ligamento cruzado cranial; a constatação de alterações histológicas e a diminuição das propriedades teciduais são mais comuns em cães com >5 anos de idade.
- Anormalidades conformacionais — soldra e jarrete retilíneos, inclinação caudal do platô tibial, luxação patelar e estreitamento da incisura intercondilar — podem predispor o paciente à lesão repetitiva.
- Ruptura parcial — responde por 25-30% dos casos de claudicação da articulação femorotibial.
- Instabilidade não tratada — alterações degenerativas dentro de algumas semanas; alterações graves dentro de alguns meses.
- Dano ao menisco medial (corno caudal) — ocorre em >50% dos casos.

SISTEMA(S) ACOMETIDO(S)
Musculosquelético e, possivelmente, neurológico.

GENÉTICA
- Desconhecida.
- Pode ser importante em pacientes predispostos a déficits de contenção ativa da articulação femorotibial e/ou anormalidades conformacionais.

INCIDÊNCIA/PREVALÊNCIA
Ruptura do ligamento cruzado cranial — a causa mais comum de claudicação dos membros pélvicos em cães; principal causa de artropatia degenerativa na articulação femorotibial.

DISTRIBUIÇÃO GEOGRÁFICA
N/D.

IDENTIFICAÇÃO
Espécies
- Cães.
- Incomum em gatos.

Raça(s) Predominante(s)
- Todas são suscetíveis.
- Rottweiler e Labrador retriever — incidência elevada de ruptura do ligamento cruzado cranial quando apresentam <4 anos de idade.

Idade Média e Faixa Etária
- Cães com >5 anos de idade.
- Cães de grande porte — entre 1-2 anos de idade.

Sexo Predominante
Fêmeas — castradas.

SINAIS CLÍNICOS
Comentários Gerais
Relacionados com o grau de ruptura (parcial *versus* completo), o modo de ruptura (agudo *versus* crônico) e a ocorrência de lesão meniscal, bem como a gravidade da inflamação e da artropatia degenerativa.

Achados Anamnésicos
- Eventos atléticos ou traumáticos — geralmente antecedem as lesões agudas.
- Atividade normal com consequente claudicação aguda — sugere ruptura degenerativa.
- Claudicação intermitente sutil a acentuada (por semanas a meses) — compatível com lacerações parciais, que estão evoluindo para a ruptura completa.

Achados do Exame Físico
- A ruptura aguda resulta em claudicação sem sustentação do peso e aparecimento de efusão articular, com o membro acometido mantido em flexão parcial enquanto o animal se encontra em estação.
- Teste de gaveta cranial — método diagnóstico em casos de ruptura; testado em flexão, ângulo normal em estação, e extensão; não é uma tarefa fácil apreciar esse movimento de gaveta em casos de ruptura parcial com a articulação femorotibial em extensão ou ângulo normal em estação.
- Teste de compressão tibial — movimento cranial da tíbia em relação ao fêmur ao se contrair o gastrocnêmio por meio da flexão do jarrete.
- Efusão articular evidente no início, com subsequente achado radiográfico.
- Espessamento palpável da face medial da articulação femorotibial (suporte medial).
- Atrofia da musculatura dos membros pélvicos — particularmente o grupo do músculo quadríceps.
- Resultados falso-negativos dos testes de gaveta cranial e de compressão tibial em casos de lacerações crônicas ou parciais ou em pacientes sensíveis (por dor) ou inquietos, que não são submetidos à sedação nem anestesia.

CAUSAS
- Traumatismo.
- Microlesão repetitiva.
- Anormalidades conformacionais.

FATORES DE RISCO
- Obesidade.
- Luxação patelar.
- Conformação deficiente.
- Inclinação caudal excessiva do platô tibial.
- Estreitamento da incisura intercondilar.

DIAGNÓSTICO

DIAGNÓSTICO DIFERENCIAL
- Movimento de gaveta positivo, que é interrompido abruptamente à medida que o ligamento cruzado cranial sofre estiramento, é comum em filhotes caninos.
- Ruptura do ligamento cruzado caudal — incomum como uma ocorrência isolada.
- Luxação patelar (medial ou lateral) — isolada ou associada com ruptura do ligamento cruzado cranial.
- Lesão do(s) ligamento(s) colateral(is), lesão do tendão extensor longo dos dedos.
- Osteocondrite dissecante do côndilo femoral.
- Neoplasias (p. ex., sarcoma das células sinoviais).

HEMOGRAMA/BIOQUÍMICA/URINÁLISE
N/D.

OUTROS TESTES LABORATORIAIS
N/D.

DIAGNÓSTICO POR IMAGEM
Radiografias
- Úteis na avaliação de doença degenerativa e outras doenças intra-articulares.
- Achados comuns — efusão articular com distensão da cápsula e compressão do coxim gorduroso infrapatelar; osteófitos periarticulares; entesiófitos*; fraturas por avulsão do ligamento cruzado cranial; calcificação do ligamento cruzado cranial.

Ressonância Magnética
Demonstra por meio gráfico os processos patológicos do ligamento cruzado e dos meniscos.

MÉTODOS DIAGNÓSTICOS
- Artrocentese — citologia articular para classificar as alterações sinoviais e descartar sepse ou doença imunomediada.
- Artroscopia — permite a inspeção direta dos ligamentos cruzados, dos meniscos e de outras estruturas intra-articulares.

ACHADOS PATOLÓGICOS
- Graus variados de fibrilação e erosão cartilaginosas.
- Formação de osteófitos periarticulares.
- Danos meniscais.
- Sinovite.
- Fibras rompidas do ligamento cruzado cranial — hialinização; invasão tecidual fibrosa; necrose; perda da orientação paralela dos feixes ligamentares.

TRATAMENTO

CUIDADO(S) DE SAÚDE ADEQUADO(S)
- Cães <15 kg — há possibilidade de tratamento conservativo em um esquema ambulatorial; 65% apresentam melhora ou ficam normais por volta de 6 meses.
- Cães >15 kg — tratamento por meio de estabilização cirúrgica; apenas 20% exibem

---

* N. T.: Proliferações ósseas no local de inserção de tecidos moles em uma superfície óssea.

DOENÇA DO LIGAMENTO CRUZADO CRANIAL

melhora ou ficam normais em torno de 6 meses com o tratamento conservativo.
• Cirurgia de estabilização — recomendada em todos os cães; acelera a taxa de recuperação; diminui as alterações degenerativas; intensifica a função do membro.

CUIDADO(S) DE ENFERMAGEM
Pós-cirúrgico(s) — fisioterapia (i. e., compressas com gelo, exercícios com amplitude de movimentos, massagens e estimulação mioelétrica); importantes para restabelecer a mobilidade e a força.

ATIVIDADE
Restrita — em casos de tratamento conservativo e imediatamente após estabilização cirúrgica; a duração depende do método de tratamento e do progresso do paciente.

DIETA
Controle do peso — importante para diminuir a carga e, com isso, o estresse (tensão) sobre a articulação femorotibial.

ORIENTAÇÃO AO PROPRIETÁRIO
• Alertar o proprietário que, independentemente do método terapêutico utilizado, um pouco de artropatia degenerativa é comum.
• Informar o proprietário que o retorno à função atlética plena é possível, mas exige considerável reabilitação.
• Avisar o proprietário que 20-40% dos cães com ruptura unilateral do ligamento cruzado cranial sofrerão ruptura do ligamento contralateral.

CONSIDERAÇÕES CIRÚRGICAS
• Nenhuma técnica tem se mostrado superior às outras em termos clínicos ou radiográficos.
• Estudos recentes de placa de força revelam diferenças mínimas entre as técnicas comuns.

Métodos Extra-articulares
• Diversas técnicas utilizam um implante de calibre robusto para imbricar a tíbia ao fêmur e restabelecer a estabilidade.
• Material implantado — aplicado no plano aproximado da origem e da inserção do ligamento cruzado cranial.

Métodos Intra-articulares
• Planejados para substituir o ligamento cruzado cranial do ponto de vista anatômico.
• Autoenxertos (ligamento patelar, fáscia), aloenxertos (osso-tendão-osso) e materiais sintéticos — comumente utilizados.
• Incisuroplastia intercondilar femoral — recomendada para minimizar a lesão do enxerto.
• Substituição artroscópica — recém-descrita, mas com sucesso desconhecido.

Métodos Extra-articulares Modificados
• Transposição da cabeça fibular ou transposição do tendão poplíteo.
• Realinhamento e tensão do ligamento colateral lateral ou do tendão poplíteo para limitar a rotação medial (interna) e o movimento de gaveta cranial.

Osteotomia de Nivelamento do Platô Tibial
• Osteotomia rotacional da porção proximal da tíbia.
• Mantida no local com placas e parafusos especiais.
• Nivelar o platô tibial e neutralizar a propulsão tibial cranial.
• O controle ativo do deslocamento tibial cranial é restabelecido, o que ajuda a estabilizar a articulação femorotibial.

MEDICAÇÕES

MEDICAMENTO(S) DE ESCOLHA
• AINEs — minimizam a dor; diminuem a inflamação.
• Meloxicam (dose de ataque de 0,2 mg/kg VO, depois 0,1 mg/kg diariamente VO na forma líquida).
• Carprofeno (2,2 mg/kg VO a cada 12 h).
• Etodolaco (10-15 mg/kg VO 1 vez ao dia).
• Deracoxibe (3-4 mg/kg VO 1 vez ao dia — mastigável) por 7 dias para dor pós-operatória).

CONTRAINDICAÇÕES
Evitar os corticosteroides — efeitos colaterais potenciais; danos à cartilagem articular associados ao uso prolongado.

PRECAUÇÕES
• AINEs — podem causar irritação gastrintestinal, o que pode impedir o uso em alguns pacientes.
• Ceratite seca observada com o uso do etodolaco por mais de 6 meses.

INTERAÇÕES POSSÍVEIS
N/D.

MEDICAMENTO(S) ALTERNATIVO(S)
Agentes condroprotetores (glicosaminoglicanos polissulfatados, glicosamina e sulfato de condroitina) — podem ajudar a limitar o dano e melhorar a regeneração das cartilagens.

ACOMPANHAMENTO

MONITORIZAÇÃO DO PACIENTE
• Depende do método terapêutico.
• A maior parte das técnicas exige 2-4 meses de reabilitação.

PREVENÇÃO
Evitar o acasalamento de animais com anormalidades conformacionais.

COMPLICAÇÕES POSSÍVEIS
Segunda intervenção cirúrgica — necessária em 10-15% dos casos, em função dos danos meniscais subsequentes.

EVOLUÇÃO ESPERADA E PROGNÓSTICO
Independentemente da técnica cirúrgica, o índice de sucesso gira em torno de 85%.

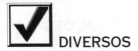

DIVERSOS

DISTÚRBIOS ASSOCIADOS
Danos meniscais.

FATORES RELACIONADOS COM A IDADE
Ver a seção "Fisiopatologia".

POTENCIAL ZOONÓTICO
N/D.

GESTAÇÃO/FERTILIDADE/REPRODUÇÃO
N/D.

VER TAMBÉM
• Artrite (Osteoartrite).
• Luxação Patelar.

ABREVIATURA(S)
• AINEs = anti-inflamatórios não esteroides.

Sugestões de Leitura
Aragon CL, Budsberg SC. Applications of evidence-based medicine: Cranial cruciate ligament injury repair in the dog. Vet Surg 2005, 34:93-98.
Brinker WO, Piermattei DL, Flo GL. Rupture of the cranial cruciate ligament. In: Brinker WO, Piermattei DL, Flo GL, eds., Handbook of Small Animal Orthopedics and Fracture Repair, 3rd ed. Philadelphia: Saunders, 1997, pp. 534-563.
Hoffmann DE, Miller J, Ober C, Shires PK. Tibial tuberosity advancement in 65 canine stifles. Vet Comp Orthop Traumatol 2007, 19:219-227.
Johnson JM, Johnson AL. Cranial cruciate ligament rupture: Pathogenesis, diagnosis, and postoperative rehabilitation. Vet Clin North Am 1993, 23:717-733.
Lampman T, Lund E, Lipowitz A. Cranial cruciate disease: Current status of diagnosis, surgery, and risk of disease. Vet Comp Orthop Traumatol 2003, 16:122-126.
Miller J, Shires PK. Effect of 9mm tibial tuberosity advancement on cranial tibial translation in the canine cranial cruciate ligament deficient stifle. Vet Surg 2007, 36:335-340.
Slocum B, Slocum TD. Treatment of the stifle for cranial cruciate ligament rupture. In: Bojrab MJ, ed., Current Techniques in Small Animal Surgery, 4th ed. Philadelphia: Lea & Febiger, 1998, pp. 1187-1215.

Autor Peter K. Shires
Consultor Editorial Peter K. Shires
Agradecimento O autor e o editor agradecem as contribuições feitas por Peter D. Schwarz, que foi o autor deste capítulo em uma edição anterior.

Doença Idiopática do Trato Urinário Inferior dos Felinos

CONSIDERAÇÕES GERAIS

DEFINIÇÃO
As expressões *síndrome urológica felina* e *SUF* eram utilizadas indevidamente pelos veterinários como diagnósticos para descrever distúrbios de gatos domésticos, caracterizados por hematúria, disúria, polaciúria, periúria e obstrução uretral parcial ou completa, porque várias combinações desses sinais podem estar associadas a qualquer causa de doença do trato urinário inferior felino. A similaridade dos sinais clínicos com diversas causas não surpreende, pois o trato urinário felino responde a várias doenças de forma limitada e previsível. Felizmente, com a maior compreensão das causas e consequências dos distúrbios no trato urinário inferior felino, essas expressões foram abandonadas. No momento de redigir este capítulo, as expressões *doença idiopática do trato urinário inferior* e *cistite idiopática felina* estão em uso comum. No entanto, essas expressões representam diagnósticos de exclusão estabelecidos somente depois da eliminação de causas conhecidas.

FISIOPATOLOGIA
- Ver capítulos específicos que descrevam as doenças listadas na seção "Diagnóstico Diferencial".
- Episódios iniciais de doenças idiopáticas do trato urinário inferior costumam ocorrer na ausência de números significativos de bactérias detectáveis e piúria. Estudos diagnósticos prospectivos de machos e fêmeas com e sem obstrução identificaram infecções bacterianas do trato urinário em menos de 3% dos gatos adultos jovens e de meia-idade e em aproximadamente 10% dos gatos idosos.
- A etiopatogênese da doença idiopática do trato urinário inferior é incerta. Os mecanismos propostos incluem disfunção da barreira urotelial, cistite neurogênica, doença neuroimune induzida por mastócitos e disfunção psiconeuroendócrina sistêmica.
- Estudos experimentais e clínicos têm implicado a atuação de agentes virais, especialmente calicivírus, como agentes etiológicos potenciais em alguns gatos.
- Alguns gatos com doenças do trato urinário inferior exibem achados semelhantes aqueles observados em pessoas com cistite intersticial, um distúrbio neuroinflamatório não maligno caracterizado por concentrações urinárias diminuídas de glicosaminoglicanos e aumento da permeabilidade urinária, o que é associado ao dano à camada de glicosaminoglicanos que reveste a superfície luminal do trato urinário. Tais similaridades incitam a hipótese de que algumas doenças do trato urinário inferior são análogas à cistite intersticial humana.
- As observações clínicas sugerem que o estresse possa desempenhar um papel na precipitação ou exacerbação dos sinais associados à cistite idiopática.

SISTEMA(S) ACOMETIDO(S)
- Renal/urológico — trato urinário inferior.
- A obstrução persistente ao fluxo de saída uretral resulta em azotemia pós-renal.

INCIDÊNCIA/PREVALÊNCIA
- A incidência de hematúria, disúria e/ou obstrução uretral em gatos domésticos nos EUA e na Grã-Bretanha foi relatada antes como sendo de aproximadamente 0,5-1% ao ano.
- O índice de morbidade hospitalar proporcional para doença idiopática do trato urinário inferior felino em gatos internados com sinais do trato urinário inferior gira em torno de 65%.

IDENTIFICAÇÃO
Espécie
Felina, tanto machos como fêmeas.

Idade Média e Faixa Etária
- Pode ocorrer em qualquer idade, embora seja mais comum em adultos jovens a de meia-idade (média etária de 3 anos e meio).
- Incomum em gatos com <1 ano de idade e >10.

SINAIS CLÍNICOS
Achados Anamnésicos
- Disúria.
- Hematúria.
- Polaciúria.
- Periúria — micção em locais impróprios.
- Obstrução ao fluxo de saída.

Achados do Exame Físico
Parede vesical espessada, firme e contraída.

CAUSAS
- Ver a seção "Fisiopatologia".
- Doenças não infecciosas, inclusive cistite idiopática.
- É implicado o envolvimento de agentes virais.

FATORES DE RISCO
Estresse — pode desempenhar um papel na precipitação ou exacerbação dos sinais; é improvável que haja alguma causa primária.

DIAGNÓSTICO

DIAGNÓSTICO DIFERENCIAL
- Distúrbios metabólicos, inclusive vários tipos de urólitos e tampões uretrais.
- Agentes infecciosos, inclusive bactérias, micoplasma/ureaplasma, agentes fúngicos e parasitas.
- Traumatismo.
- Distúrbios neurogênicos, inclusive dissinergia reflexa, espasmo uretral e hipotonia ou atonia vesical (primária ou secundária).
- Doença iatrogênica, inclusive soluções de fluxo reverso, cateteres uretrais, cateteres uretrais permanentes* (em especial sistemas abertos), cateteres uretrais pós-cirúrgicos e complicações de uretrostomia.
- Anormalidades anatômicas, inclusive anomalias do úraco e estenoses adquiridas da uretra.
- Neoplasia (benigna ou maligna).
- Os sinais clínicos podem ser confundidos com constipação, que pode ser descartada à palpação abdominal.

HEMOGRAMA/BIOQUÍMICA/URINÁLISE
- Hematúria e proteinúria sem piúria ou bacteriúria significativa — em geral, presentes.
- Se a obstrução uretral persistir, os perfis bioquímicos séricos revelarão azotemia, hiperfosfatemia, hipercalemia e conteúdo total de CO_2 diminuído.

OUTROS TESTES LABORATORIAIS
- Ausência de bacteriúria — verificar por urocultura quantitativa; coletar amostras de urina por cistocentese para evitar contaminação com microrganismos (bacteriúria) que normalmente inibem o trato urinário distal.
- A microscopia eletrônica de transmissão pode revelar partículas semelhantes ao calicivírus em alguns tampões uretrais.

DIAGNÓSTICO POR IMAGEM
- Radiografias simples — podem excluir urólitos radiopacos ou tampões uretrais.
- Uretrocistografia retrógrada com contraste positivo ou cistografia anterógrada — podem descartar estenoses uretrais, divertículos vesicouracais e neoplasia.
- Cistografia com duplo contraste — pode excluir urólitos pequenos ou radiolúcidos, coágulos de sangue e espessamento da parede vesical atribuído à inflamação ou neoplasia.
- Ultrassonografia — pode descartar urólitos.

MÉTODOS DIAGNÓSTICOS
- Cistoscopia — pode excluir urólitos e divertículos.
- Biopsias obtidas com cateteres urinários, cistoscópios ou via cirurgia — podem permitir a caracterização morfológica de lesões inflamatórias ou neoplásicas; não são necessárias com rotina.

ACHADOS PATOLÓGICOS
- A cistoscopia pode revelar hemorragias petequiais (também chamadas glomerulações) da superfície mucosa da bexiga urinária.
- Ulceração da mucosa, congestão, edema da submucosa, hemorragia e fibrose; células inflamatórias podem não ser proeminentes a menos que infecções bacterianas secundárias do trato urinário tenham se originado do cateterismo ou de uretrostomia perineal.

TRATAMENTO

CUIDADO(S) DE SAÚDE ADEQUADO(S)
- Pacientes com doenças não obstrutivas do trato urinário inferior — são tratados tipicamente em um esquema ambulatorial; a avaliação diagnóstica pode exigir breve hospitalização.
- Pacientes com doenças obstrutivas do trato urinário inferior — em geral, são hospitalizados para diagnóstico e tratamento.

DIETA
- É recomendável um manejo nutricional apropriado para cristalúria persistente associada a tampões uretrais de matriz cristalina.
- Observações empíricas sugerem que a recidiva dos sinais pode ser minimizada com alimentos úmidos ao invés de secos. O objetivo é promover a ação de irrigação exercido pelo aumento do volume urinário e diluir mais as toxinas, os irritantes químicos, os mediadores inflamatórios e os constituintes que promovem a formação de urólitos.

ORIENTAÇÕES AO PROPRIETÁRIO
- Hematúria, disúria e polaciúria — em geral autolimitantes; diminuem em 4-7 dias, mas geralmente recidivam de forma imprevisível.

---

* N. T.: Também conhecidos como cateteres de demora.

Doença Idiopática do Trato Urinário Inferior dos Felinos

- Faltam estudos controlados que demonstrem a eficácia da maioria dos medicamentos usados para tratar o distúrbio de modo sintomático.
- Os machos devem ser monitorizados quanto à presença de sinais de obstrução uretral.
- Reduzir o estresse ambiental, minimizando o impacto exercido por mudanças de casa e mantendo uma dieta constante. O enriquecimento ambiental de gatos que vivem dentro de casa consiste na provisão de recursos necessários (água, alimento, bandejas sanitárias, espaço, brinquedos), fornecendo um local seguro para o gato se esconder, além de permitir o aperfeiçoamento das interações entre o gato e o proprietário e o controle de conflitos.
- Proporcionar a higiene com bandejas sanitárias apropriadas.

CONSIDERAÇÕES CIRÚRGICAS
- Não recomendamos a cistotomia para lavagem e debridamento da mucosa da bexiga urinária como uma modalidade terapêutica.
- Não fazer uretrostomias perineais para minimizar a obstrução uretral recidivante sem localizar a doença obstrutiva na uretra peniana por uretrografia contrastada.

MEDICAÇÕES

MEDICAMENTO(S) DE ESCOLHA
- Tolterodina pode ser considerada como um agente anticolinérgico e antiespasmódico para minimizar a hiperatividade do músculo detrusor da bexiga e a incontinência de urgência; a dose empírica sugerida é de 0,05 mg/kg VO a cada 12 h. No entanto, não há relatos de estudos controlados que avaliem a segurança ou a eficácia desse medicamento.
- Amitriptilina, um antidepressivo tricíclico e ansiolítico (com propriedades anticolinérgicas, anti-histamínicas, anti-α-adrenérgicas, anti-inflamatórias e analgésicas) — defendida empiricamente para tratar gatos com sinais persistentes ou recidivantes graves; a dose empírica sugerida é de 5-10 mg/gato a cada 24 h, à noite. Não recomendamos a amitriptilina para o tratamento de episódios agudos e autolimitantes de doença idiopática do trato urinário inferior dos felinos.
- Butorfanol, buprenorfina e fentanila — recomendados empiricamente para analgesia a curto prazo em gatos com cistite idiopática. No entanto, não há relatos de estudos controlados que avaliem a segurança ou a eficácia desses medicamentos.
- Fenoxibenzamina — pode ser usada para minimizar a dissinergia reflexa e a obstrução funcional do fluxo de saída uretral; a dose empírica sugerida é de 0,5 mg/kg VO a cada 12 h.
- Prazosina — pode ser utilizada para minimizar a dissinergia reflexa e a obstrução funcional ao fluxo de saída; a dose empírica sugerida é de 0,25 a 0,5 mg/gato VO a cada 12-24 h.
- Polissulfato sódico de pentosana, um glicosaminoglicano semissintético — recomendado empiricamente para ajudar a reparar o revestimento de glicosaminoglicano da mucosa do trato urinário. Os resultados de estudos clínicos controlados não demonstraram quaisquer efeitos benéficos do polissulfato de pentosana sobre a redução da gravidade ou frequência dos sinais clínicos em gatos com doença idiopática do trato urinário inferior dos felinos.
- Glicosamina oral isolada ou em combinação com sulfato de condroitina oral é recomendada empiricamente para ajudar a reparar a camada lesionada de glicosaminoglicano que reveste o urotélio. Os resultados de estudos clínicos controlados não demonstraram quaisquer efeitos benéficos da glicosamina sobre a redução da gravidade ou frequência dos sinais clínicos em gatos com doença idiopática do trato urinário inferior dos felinos.
- Corticosteroides — nenhum efeito detectável sobre a remissão de sinais clínicos agudos demonstrados; predispõem a infecções bacterianas do trato urinário, especialmente em gatos com cateteres transuretrais permanentes.
- Anti-inflamatórios não esteroides — recomendados empiricamente para alguns por conta de suas propriedades anti-inflamatórias e analgésicas. Contudo, a segurança dos AINEs no tratamento de cistite idiopática não foi avaliada por ensaios clínicos controlados.
- Dimetilsulfóxido (DMSO) — nenhum efeito detectável sobre a remissão dos sinais clínicos foi demonstrado.
- Antibióticos e metenamina — nenhum efeito detectável sobre a remissão dos sinais clínicos foi demonstrado em gatos.

CONTRAINDICAÇÕES
- Fenazopiridina — analgésico do trato urinário utilizado isoladamente ou em combinação com medicamentos à base de sulfa; pode resultar em metemoglobinemia e alterações oxidativas irreversíveis na hemoglobina, resultando na formação de corpúsculos de Heinz e anemia.
- Azul de metileno — antisséptico fraco; pode causar a formação de corpúsculos de Heinz e o surgimento de anemia grave.
- Betanecol — colinérgico usado para tratar hipotonia vesical; não usar em pacientes com obstrução uretral.

PRECAUÇÕES
- Gatos com obstrução uretral e azotemia pós-renal correm maior risco de eventos medicamentosos adversos, especialmente no caso de medicamentos e anestésicos que dependem da eliminação ou do metabolismo renal.
- Cateteres urinários permanentes, sobretudo quando associados à diurese induzida por fluidos, predispõem os pacientes a infecções bacterianas do trato urinário.

ACOMPANHAMENTO

MONITORIZAÇÃO DO PACIENTE
Monitorizar a hematúria por urinálise; a cistocentese pode causar hematúria iatrogênica e, por essa razão, preferem-se amostras eliminadas naturalmente, ou seja, por micção espontânea.

PREVENÇÃO
- Observações empíricas sugerem que a recidiva dos sinais clínicos pode ser minimizada pelo fornecimento de alimentos úmidos ao invés de secos.
- Reduzir o estresse ambiental.

COMPLICAÇÕES POSSÍVEIS
- Cateteres transuretrais permanentes — em geral, causam traumatismo; predispõem a infecções bacterianas ascendentes do trato urinário.
- Uretrostomias perineais — podem predispor a infecções bacterianas do trato urinário e estenoses da uretra.

EVOLUÇÃO ESPERADA E PROGNÓSTICO
Hematúria, disúria e polaciúria são, em geral, autolimitantes em pacientes com grande parte das doenças idiopáticas do trato urinário inferior e desaparecem em 4-7 dias. Esses sinais frequentemente recidivam de forma imprevisível; a frequência de recidiva parece declinar com o avanço da idade.

DIVERSOS

FATORES RELACIONADOS COM A IDADE
A frequência de recidiva parece diminuir com a idade.

SINÔNIMO(S)
- Cistite idiopática felina.
- Cistite intersticial felina.
- Doença urológica felina.
- Inflamação do trato urinário felino.
- SUF (ver a seção "Definição").

VER TAMBÉM
- Disúria e Polaciúria.
- Hematúria.
- Infecção Bacteriana do Trato Urinário Inferior.
- Infecção Fúngica do Trato Urinário Inferior.
- Urolitíase por Estruvita — Gatos.

ABREVIATURA(S)
- AINE = anti-inflamatório não esteroide.

Sugestões de Leitura
Kruger JM, Osborne CA, Lulich JP. Changing paradigms of feline idiopathic cystitis. Vet Clin North Am Small Anim Pract 2009, 31:15-40.
Lekcharoensuk C, Osborne CA, Lulich JP. Epidemiologic study of risk factors for lower urinary tract diseases in cats. JAVMA 2001, 218:1429-1435.
Osborne CA, Kruger JM, Lulich JP, et al. Feline lower urinary tract diseases. In: Ettinger SJ, Feldman EC, eds., Textbook of Veterinary Internal Medicine, 5th ed. Philadelphia: Saunders, 2000, pp. 1710-1747.
Westropp JL, Buffington CAT, Chew D. Feline lower urinary tract diseases. In: Ettinger SJ, Feldman EC, eds., Textbook of Veterinary Internal Medicine, 6th ed. St. Louis: Elsevier, 2005, pp. 1828-1850.

Autores Carl A. Osborne, John M. Kruger e Jody P. Lulich
Consultor Editorial Carl A. Osborne

DOENÇA PERIODONTAL

CONSIDERAÇÕES GERAIS

DEFINIÇÃO
Inflamação de algumas ou de todas as estruturas de sustentação dos dentes (gengiva, cemento, ligamento periodontal e osso alveolar); comparada com a gengivite (inflamação da gengiva marginal), a periodontite indica algum grau de perda do tecido de inserção periodontal.

FISIOPATOLOGIA
• A barreira epitelial intacta, a alta taxa de renovação epitelial e a descamação superficial impedem o acesso direto das bactérias ao tecido.
• Alguns produtos bacterianos podem se difundir pelo epitélio da junção até atingir o tecido conjuntivo gengival subjacente; os mecanismos normais de defesa do hospedeiro limitam a penetração desses produtos e seus efeitos nocivos.
• Oscilações no equilíbrio hospedeiro-parasita podem resultar em ciclos de intensidade diminuída ou aumentada da resposta inflamatória; pode-se pensar na periodontite como o resultado de uma interação hospedeiro-parasita imperfeitamente equilibrada.
• Causada pelas bactérias localizadas na fenda gengival; inicialmente se forma uma película na superfície do esmalte de um dente sadio; a película é composta de proteínas e glicoproteínas depositadas a partir da saliva e do líquido da fenda gengival; a película atrai bactérias aeróbias Gram-positivas (predominantemente actinomicetos e estreptococos); imediatamente, ocorre a adesão de mais bactérias, formando a placa; em alguns dias, a placa se espessa, torna-se mineralizada e transforma-se no cálculo, que é rugoso e irritante para a gengiva. Com o tempo, cria-se um ambiente anaeróbico na região subgengival, fazendo com que espiroquetas e bastonetes móveis anaeróbios povoem essa região; maior quantidade de placa acumula-se na parte superior do cálculo; as endotoxinas liberadas pelas bactérias anaeróbias provocam destruição tecidual e perda óssea (periodontite).

SISTEMA(S) ACOMETIDO(S)
• Gastrintestinal — cavidade bucal.
• Lesões hepáticas, renais e neurológicas (SNC) microscópicas são encontradas em alguns animais.

GENÉTICA
N/D.

INCIDÊNCIA/PREVALÊNCIA
Comum.

DISTRIBUIÇÃO GEOGRÁFICA
Nenhuma.

IDENTIFICAÇÃO
Espécies
Cães e gatos (menos comum).

Raça(s) Predominante(s)
Nenhuma.

Idade Média e Faixa Etária
Mais comum em animais mais idosos.

Sexo Predominante
Nenhum.

SINAIS CLÍNICOS
Nenhum.

Achados do Exame Físico
• O nível de gravidade da doença periodontal relaciona-se com o dente isolado; um paciente pode ter os dentes em diferentes estágios de doença periodontal:
  ◦ Normal (nível 0 da doença periodontal): clinicamente normal — sem inflamação gengival ou periodontite evidente do ponto de vista clínico.
  ◦ Estágio 1 (nível 1 da doença periodontal): gengivite apenas sem perda da inserção. A altura e a arquitetura da margem alveolar encontram-se normais.
  ◦ Estágio 2 (nível 2 da doença periodontal): periodontite precoce — menos de 25% de perda da inserção ou, no máximo, há um envolvimento da furcação do estágio 1 em dentes com múltiplas raízes. Há sinais radiológicos precoces de periodontite. A perda da inserção periodontal é inferior a 25%, conforme mensurada pela sondagem do nível de inserção clínica ou pela determinação radiográfica da distância da margem alveolar a partir da junção cemento-esmalte em relação ao comprimento da raiz.
  ◦ Estágio 3 (nível 3 da doença periodontal): periodontite moderada — perda de 25-50% da inserção, conforme mensurada pela sondagem do nível de inserção clínica, pela determinação radiográfica da distância da margem alveolar a partir da junção cemento-esmalte em relação ao comprimento da raiz, ou pela existência de envolvimento da furcação do estágio 2 em dentes com múltiplas raízes.
  ◦ Estágio 4 (nível 4 da doença periodontal): periodontite avançada — perda de mais de 50% da inserção, conforme mensurada pela sondagem do nível de inserção clínica, pela determinação radiográfica da distância da margem alveolar a partir da junção cemento-esmalte em relação ao comprimento da raiz ou pela existência de envolvimento da furcação do estágio 3 em dentes com múltiplas raízes.
• A perda da inserção pode envolver a perda da gengiva inserida e/ou do osso alveolar (bem como do ligamento periodontal). Pode ocorrer a formação de bolsas periodontais ou a retração do tecido com exposição das raízes e/ou da área de furcação.

CAUSAS
• Gengivite — cães; *Streptococcus* e *Actinomyces* spp.
• Periodontite — cães; bacteroides pigmentados ou não, *Porphyromonas denticanis*, *Porphyromonas salivosa*, *Porphyromonas gulae*, *Prevotella* spp., *Fusobacterium* spp.
• Gatos — *Peptostreptococcus*, *Actinomyces* e *Porphyromonas* spp.

FATORES DE RISCO
• Raças toy com dentes encavalados.
• Cães que se lambem — isso faz com que os pelos fiquem incrustados no sulco gengival.
• Outras doenças debilitantes.
• Mau estado de nutrição.

DIAGNÓSTICO

DIAGNÓSTICO DIFERENCIAL
• Pênfigo.
• Lúpus.
• Neoplasia bucal.
• Estomatite.

HEMOGRAMA/BIOQUÍMICA/URINÁLISE
N/D.

OUTROS TESTES LABORATORIAIS
N/D.

DIAGNÓSTICO POR IMAGEM
• Radiografia — ferramenta diagnóstica importante; até 60% da doença fica escondida abaixo da linha gengival.
• Nenhuma alteração radiográfica na doença de estágio 1 (gengivite).
• Sinais radiográficos precoces da doença de estágio 2/3 incluem perda da densidade e da nitidez da margem alveolar; à medida que a doença periodontal evolui, há perda apical de mineralização da lâmina dura e envolvimento da furcação nos dentes com múltiplas raízes.
• A doença periodontal grave aparece ao exame radiográfico como perda da sustentação óssea ao redor de uma ou mais raízes; a perda óssea pode ser horizontal (diminuição na altura do osso em torno de um ou mais dentes), vertical (defeito infraósseo) ou oblíqua (combinação de ambas).

MÉTODOS DIAGNÓSTICOS
• Sondagem periodontal — "profundidade da sondagem": distância entre a margem livre da gengiva e a extensão apical da bolsa; profundidades >2 mm no cão e 1 mm no gato são anormais.
• A "perda da inserção" mede o espaço entre a junção cemento-esmalte e a extensão apical da bolsa; normalmente, o sulco gengival fica localizado nessa junção; qualquer perda de inserção é anormal.

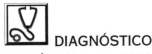

TRATAMENTO

• O objetivo final da terapia periodontal é controlar a placa e evitar a perda de inserção; um paciente disposto e um proprietário capaz de fornecer os cuidados em casa são considerações importantes na criação de um plano terapêutico.
• Foi concedida uma licença condicional para a Bacterina Porphyromonas Denticanis-Gulae-Salivosa®, como um auxílio na prevenção de periodontite, evidenciada pela redução nos processos de osteólise e osteosclerose (Pfizer Animal Health, Exton PA).
• Estágio 1 ou 2 — limpeza profissional, raspagem manual, polimento, irrigação, aplicação de flúor.
• Estágio 3 — profundidades da bolsa: 3-5 mm nos cães, 2-3 mm nos gatos; acima disso, acrescentar aplainamento radicular fechado e curetagem subgengival.
• Após a limpeza minuciosa de bolsa de profundidade moderada, a aplicação de gel antibiótico local (Doxirobe® gel, Pfizer Animal Health, Exton PA) pode ajudar a rejuvenescer os tecidos periodontais e reduzir a profundidade da bolsa.
• Estágio 4 — há necessidade de cirurgia para exposição da raiz para o tratamento (curetagem com retalho aberto) ou extração.
• Se houver 2-3 mm de gengiva sadia inserida — aplicar retalho de reposição apical para reduzir a profundidade da bolsa nas áreas de perda óssea alveolar; se não houver resquícios de gengiva sadia suficiente para o retalho de reposição apical, usar

DOENÇA PERIODONTAL

retalho rotacionado (a partir da gengiva adjacente), retalho gengival livre ou extração.
• Procedimentos de substituição óssea — com bolsas infraósseas de duas, três ou quatro paredes.
• Regeneração tecidual guiada — utilizar barreiras teciduais para separar o tecido gengival e a superfície radicular.

MEDICAÇÕES

MEDICAMENTO(S) DE ESCOLHA
A clindamicina e a amoxicilina/ácido clavulânico são antimicrobianos aprovados para doença periodontal; podem ser utilizados por uma semana antes do tratamento periodontal, antes da anestesia, 7-10 dias no pós-operatório e/ou sob a forma de terapia intermitente em pacientes seletos cujos proprietários fornecem cuidados de higiene bucodentária em casa.

Cuidados em Casa
• Flúor — preparações com fluoreto estanhoso (Omni Gel® e Gel Kam®) ajudam a controlar a doença periodontal, reduzindo a deposição da placa na superfície do esmalte, e também diminuem a dor nos dentes (odontalgia); usar uma potência de 0,4% em pacientes com a doença periodontal nos estágios 3 e 4, especialmente naqueles com as superfícies radiculares expostas.
• Clorexidina — o produto mais eficaz para inibir a formação da placa nos seres humanos; bacteriostática e bactericida contra bactérias, fungos e alguns vírus; uma vez absorvida, essa substância continua sendo eficaz por até 24 h; nos humanos, para obtenção do máximo efeito, ela é bochechada por 1 min duas vezes ao dia; o tempo de contato da aplicação é importante para que o produto se una ao dente e ao sulco gengival; no entanto, não é fácil conseguir 1 min de irrigação (enxágue) bucal nos animais; dessa forma, a clorexidina pode ser aplicada com chumaço de gaze ou aplicadores com ponta de algodão, sob a forma de *spray* ou com dedais próprios para escovação. A clorexidina encontra-se incorporada no produto mastigável CHEXTRA® (Virbac).
• CHX Guard solution® [solução protetora de clorexidina] (VRx Products, Harbor City, CA) contém gliconato de clorexidina a 0,12% mais gliconato de zinco, o qual promove a cicatrização do tecido ulcerado; CHX gel clorhexidine gluconate 0,12%® [gliconato de clorexidina a 0,12% sob a forma de gel]; o gel permite maior tempo de contato e possui sabor agradável.

• Hexarinse® contém clorexidina a 0,12%, cetilpiridínio, cloreto e zinco.
• Novaldent® — acetato de clorexidina a 0,1%.
• Lenços umedecidos DentAcetic® (Dermapet) são utilizados diariamente para remover as placas.
• OraVet® (Merial) sob a forma de gel para prevenção de placa, aplicado semanalmente.
• Dieta — alimentos tipo biscoitos de textura dura são preferíveis a barrinhas de textura macia.
• Dieta t/d para controle de tártaro (Hill) — especificamente indicado para controlar o tártaro (cálculo dentário) em cães e gatos.
• A quantidade e o tipo de produtos receitados para a dispensação de cuidados bucodentários em casa dependem da doença periodontal.
 ◦ Estágios 1 e 2 — escovação diária com dentifrício (no caso, uma pasta própria para pacientes veterinários).
 ◦ Estágio 3, doença periodontal estabelecida — escovação diária com pasta de dentes contendo flúor mais aplicação de gel com fluoreto estanhoso duas vezes por semana.
 ◦ Estágio 4, doença periodontal avançada — gel de ascorbato de zinco (Maxi/Guard®, Addison Biological) 3-4 vezes ao dia para ajudar a regenerar o colágeno celular mais *spray* de clorexidina a 0,2% duas vezes ao dia; ou CHX-Guard® (VRx Products), gliconato de clorexidina e zinco, depois de 2 semanas, podem substituir o gel com fluoreto estanhoso duas vezes por semana pelo *spray* de clorexidina.

CONTRAINDICAÇÕES
N/D.

PRECAUÇÕES
N/D.

INTERAÇÕES POSSÍVEIS
Não utilizar produtos com clorexidina e flúor concomitantemente; o contato de ambos os produtos pode inativá-los; melhor esperar 30 min a 1 h entre o uso de dentifrício contendo flúor e colutório ou gel contendo clorexidina.

MEDICAMENTO(S) ALTERNATIVO(S)
• Tetraciclina.
• Metronidazol (Flagyl®).

ACOMPANHAMENTO

MONITORIZAÇÃO DO PACIENTE
O grau da doença periodontal determina o intervalo de retorno à consulta; alguns pacientes são reavaliados mensalmente, enquanto outros podem ser reavaliados a cada 3-6 meses.

PREVENÇÃO
Cuidados satisfatórios de higiene bucodentária em casa.

COMPLICAÇÕES POSSÍVEIS
N/D.

EVOLUÇÃO ESPERADA E PROGNÓSTICO
Em virtude do aspecto multifatorial da doença periodontal e da resposta de cada animal, a evolução esperada e o prognóstico podem ser altamente variáveis, mas a avaliação precoce do paciente, o estabelecimento do diagnóstico e a formulação de tratamento adequado podem minimizar os efeitos destrutivos dessa doença.

DIVERSOS

DISTÚRBIOS ASSOCIADOS
N/D.

FATORES RELACIONADOS COM A IDADE
N/D.

POTENCIAL ZOONÓTICO
N/D.

GESTAÇÃO/FERTILIDADE/REPRODUÇÃO
N/D.

ABREVIATURA(S)
• SNC = sistema nervoso central.

RECURSOS DA INTERNET
http://www.avdc.org/Nomenclature.html.

Sugestões de Leitura
Harvey CE. Periodontal disease in dogs. Vet Clin North Am 1998, 28:1111-1128.
Wiggs RB, Lobprise HB. Veterinary Dentistry: Principles and Practice. Philadelphia: Lippincott-Raven, 1997.

Autor Jan Bellows
Consultor Editorial Heidi B. Lobprise

Doença Renal Policística

CONSIDERAÇÕES GERAIS

REVISÃO
Distúrbio no qual grandes porções do parênquima renal normalmente diferenciado são deslocadas por múltiplos cistos; os cistos renais se desenvolvem nos néfrons preexistentes e nos ductos coletores; ambos os rins são invariavelmente envolvidos, porque a doença é hereditária na maioria dos casos.

IDENTIFICAÇÃO
• Gato Persa e relacionados com essa raça (p. ex., Exótico de pelo curto, Himalaio, Fold escocês) são mais comumente acometidos que outras raças.
• As raças caninas acometidas incluem Cairn terrier e Beagle.

SINAIS CLÍNICOS
• Os cistos frequentemente permanecem silenciosos em termos clínicos até se tornarem grandes e numerosos o suficiente a ponto de contribuir para a insuficiência renal ou o aumento abdominal; desse modo, os pacientes tipicamente se encontram normais do ponto de vista clínico durante as fases iniciais da formação e crescimento do cisto.
• Podem-se detectar rins protuberantes ("encaroçados") por palpação abdominal.
• Em sua maioria, os cistos renais não são dolorosos quando palpados, mas a infecção secundária aguda dos cistos pode estar associada à rápida distensão da cápsula renal e consequente dor.

CAUSAS E FATORES DE RISCO
• Herança autossômica dominante no gato Persa. Uma transversão de nucleotídeos (citosina para adenina) que gera um códon de interrupção prematura é fortemente associada ao fenótipo.
• Os estímulos para a formação de cisto renal permanecem obscuros; fatores genéticos, endógenos e ambientais parecem influenciar o processo.
• As substâncias químicas cistogênicas incluem difeniltiazol, ácido nordi-hidroguaiarético, difenilamina, ácido triclorofenoxiacético e corticosteroides de longa ação.

DIAGNÓSTICO

DIAGNÓSTICO DIFERENCIAL
• Outras doenças multicísticas dos rins.
• Doença glomerulocística do Collie.
• Cistadenocarcinoma renal associado à fibrose nodular nos cães da raça Pastor alemão.
• Cistos renais associados à insuficiência renal crônica ou à displasia renal.
• Causas não císticas de renomegalia.
• Neoplasia renal.
• Hidronefrose.
• Pseudocistos perirrenais.
• Peritonite infecciosa felina.
• Nefrite micótica ou bacteriana.

HEMOGRAMA/BIOQUÍMICA/URINÁLISE
• Os resultados não costumam ser dignos de nota a menos que o paciente tenha insuficiência renal.
• Hematúria é rara.

OUTROS TESTES LABORATORIAIS
• Existem testes genéticos disponíveis para identificar a mutação da doença renal policística autossômica dominante tipo 1 em gatos. Esse teste é particularmente útil para fazer a triagem de filhotes felinos com menos de 3-4 meses de vida, momento em que a ultrassonografia pode ser menos sensível. O teste também é proveitoso para confirmar a presença de doença renal policística autossômica dominante tipo 1 hereditária em gatos reprodutivos com cistos detectados ao exame ultrassonográfico. Outras mutações também podem gerar cistos renais hereditários.
• O líquido do cisto pode ser claro, turvo ou hemorrágico; além disso, o líquido de cistos diferentes no mesmo rim pode diferir.
• A cultura bacteriana do líquido do cisto ajuda a diagnosticar infecção concomitante.
• É incomum a ocorrência de hipertensão sem insuficiência renal.

DIAGNÓSTICO POR IMAGEM
Radiografia
Radiografia simples e urografia contrastada intravenosa não são métodos sensíveis para confirmar doença cística.

Ultrassonografia
• Revela lesões cavitárias anecoicas caracterizadas por paredes lisas de margens nítidas e aumento distal, que são diagnósticas.
• Como já foi detectada a presença de cistos em gatos com até 7 semanas de vida, a triagem de gatos com menos de 6 meses de vida está associada a maiores taxas de resultados falso-negativos.
• Revela cavidades císticas hipoecoicas em alguns pacientes com cistos infectados por bactérias.
• Utilizada para detectar cistos em outros órgãos (p. ex., fígado, pâncreas), o que ajuda a diferenciar entre doença renal policística autossômica dominante e distúrbios renais multicísticos adquiridos.

MÉTODOS DIAGNÓSTICOS
A avaliação de aspirados do rim por agulha fina pode permitir a diferenciação entre doença cística e outras doenças indutoras de renomegalia.

TRATAMENTO
• Embora não costume ser imediatamente letal, o processo de nefrite bacteriana e o envolvimento do cisto justificam a tomada de medidas imediatas para evitar sepse e mortalidade. Em nossa experiência, a ocorrência de infecção bacteriana de cistos é rara.
• A resolução espontânea dos cistos não foi relatada em cães nem em gatos; com o tempo, a maioria dos cistos aumenta de tamanho e em número, comprometendo muitas vezes o parênquima renal adjacente de funcionamento normal.
• A eliminação dos cistos renais e das lesões parenquimatosas renais associadas ainda não é praticável; o tratamento frequentemente é limitado a minimizar as consequências fisiopatológicas da formação do cisto renal (i. e., insuficiência renal, infecção renal, hematúria e dor).
• Pode-se utilizar a aspiração percutânea do líquido de cistos renais grandes para minimizar a dor e a compressão do parênquima renal adjacente normal. No entanto, esse procedimento é impraticável para rins com centenas de cistos. É necessária a aspiração periódica de líquido (a cada 7-15 dias) para manter o volume reduzido do cisto.
• Alguns pacientes podem necessitar de tratamento para insuficiência renal concomitante.
• Considerar a realização de nefrectomia se houver uma sepse incontrolável associada a cistos infectados.
• A erradicação da doença por meio de cruzamento seletivo de gatos não acometidos pode ser impossível, já que quase 40% dos Persas são afetados. O acasalamento seletivo pode diminuir a diversidade genética, aumentando a frequência de outros traços hereditários indesejáveis.

MEDICAÇÕES

MEDICAMENTO(S)
• Apesar de rara, a infecção bacteriana dos cistos foi observada em gatos. A menos que a infecção seja acompanhada por pielonefrite, as bactérias podem não ser observadas na urina. Considerar a presença de infecção parenquimatosa quando os cistos renais estiverem associados à dor renal e febre, mesmo na ausência de bacteriúria.
• O tratamento de cistos infectados requer uma consideração especial. A natureza ácida do líquido cístico e sua contenção pela barreira epitelial podem inibir o estabelecimento de concentrações bactericidas dos antibióticos ácidos comumente utilizados (p. ex., cefalosporinas e penicilinas) dentro dos lúmens císticos. Antibióticos lipossolúveis e alcalinos (p. ex., combinações de trimetoprima-sulfonamida, fluoroquinolonas, cloranfenicol, tetraciclina e clindamicina), que penetram nas barreiras epiteliais e ficam ionizados e presos nos lúmens do cisto, são recomendados para seres humanos com cistos infectados e devem ser considerados para o tratamento de cães e gatos.

ACOMPANHAMENTO
• Monitorizar os pacientes a cada 2-6 meses quanto à existência de doença associada (p. ex., insuficiência renal, infecção renal e dor).
• Na ausência de sepse, o prognóstico a curto prazo parece ser favorável sem tratamento.
• O prognóstico a longo prazo para pacientes com doença do rim policístico frequentemente depende da gravidade e da evolução da insuficiência renal.

DIVERSOS

Sugestões de Leitura
Bonazzi M, Volta A, Gnudi G, et al. Comparison between ultrasound and genetic testing for early diagnosis of polycystic kidney disease in Persian and Exotic Shorthair cats. J Feline Med Surg 2009, 11:430-434.

Autores Jody P. Lulich e Carl A. Osborne
Consultor Editorial Carl A. Osborne

Doenças do Armazenamento Lisossomal

CONSIDERAÇÕES GERAIS

REVISÃO
• Distúrbios hereditários raros, causados pela deficiência parcial ou completa de alguma enzima lisossomal ou proteína ativadora da enzima, a qual leva ao acúmulo intracitoplasmático (armazenamento) do substrato daquela enzima.
• Produtos de armazenamento — proteínas, carboidratos, lipídios ou uma combinação deles.
• Principais classes de doença — proteinoses, glicoproteinoses, oligossacaridoses, esfingolipidoses, mucopolissacaridoses.
• Muitos tipos diferentes são relatados tanto em cães como em gatos.
• A herança é autossômica recessiva.

IDENTIFICAÇÃO
• Cães — raças Pastor alemão, Pointer alemão de pelo curto, Setter inglês, Beagle, Cairn terrier, Bluetick hound, West Highland terrier, Sidney silky terrier, Springer spaniel inglês, Cão d'água português, Spaniel japonês, Labrador retriever, Buldogue americano, Setter irlandês, cães de raças mistas e muitas outras.
• Gatos — raças Persa, Siamês, Korat, Balinês, Doméstico de pelo curto.
• A maior parte dos animais acometidos tem <1 ano de idade, porém foram descritas algumas doenças de início no adulto.

SINAIS CLÍNICOS
Comentários Gerais
• Variam com a gravidade da deficiência enzimática.
• Em certas doenças, os animais portadores podem ser acometidos com a forma mais leve da doença.
• Muitos sistemas orgânicos são acometidos, mas os sinais neurológicos tendem a predominar.

Achados Anamnésicos
• Os animais acometidos geralmente são normais ao nascimento.
• Além da falha no desenvolvimento, os animais acometidos podem manifestar más-formações esqueléticas, particularmente nas mucopolissacaridoses.
• Manifestação de diversos sinais neurológicos dentro dos primeiros meses de vida, sugestivos de doença neurológica multifocal.

Achados do Exame Físico/Neurológico
• É comum a disfunção cerebelar — tremor intencional, nistagmo, dismetria.
• Ocorre neuropatia periférica em algumas doenças — fraqueza, hiporreflexia ou arreflexia, emaciação.
• Outros sinais neurológicos — ataxia, intolerância ao exercício, crises convulsivas, mudanças comportamentais, déficits visuais, surdez, comportamentos estereotipados, déficits proprioceptivos, tremores.
• Sinais não neurológicos — podem ser observadas organomegalia ou más-formações esqueléticas.
• Oftalmopatia presente em algumas doenças — opacificação da córnea, formação de catarata.

CAUSAS E FATORES DE RISCO
• Genéticos — deleção ou mutação envolvendo um único gene que causa deficiência parcial ou absoluta de alguma enzima lisossomal ou proteína ativadora; produção deficiente de enzimas que não apresentam atividade biológica normal.
• Raça suscetível.

DIAGNÓSTICO

DIAGNÓSTICO DIFERENCIAL
• Encefalopatia metabólica — costuma exibir sinais clínicos episódicos; os resultados do hemograma completo, da análise bioquímica e da urinálise quase sempre são diagnósticos.
• Intoxicações — início agudo de sinais clínicos; histórico de exposição.
• Hipoplasia cerebelar — início com 3-6 semanas de vida; não progressiva.
• Abiotrofia cerebelar — déficits limitados ao cerebelo; pode ser difícil diferenciar nos estágios iniciais sem testes específicos.
• Infecções pré-natais ou neonatais (sobretudo virais), resultando em meningoencefalomielite — diferenciadas pelo exame do LCS; pode haver outros sinais, como coriorretinite.
• Doenças metabólicas — especialmente orgânicas e aminoacidúrias.

HEMOGRAMA/BIOQUÍMICA/URINÁLISE
• Esfregaços regulares de sangue e exame do LCS — vacuolização citoplasmática dos leucócitos, provocada pelo acúmulo dos produtos de armazenamento, está presente em alguns casos.
• Urina — pode-se constatar o acúmulo anormal de substâncias (p. ex., oligossacarídeo na α-manosidose).

OUTROS TESTES LABORATORIAIS
N/D.

DIAGNÓSTICO POR IMAGEM
• Radiografia — má-formação óssea pode estar presente em doenças caracterizadas por processo patológico esquelético (p. ex., mucopolissacaridoses).
• Imagem por ressonância magnética — foi utilizada em um único caso para revelar o envolvimento difuso da substância branca no cérebro de cão com leucodistrofia de células globoides; pode estar anormal em outras doenças.

MÉTODOS DIAGNÓSTICOS
• Teste genético molecular — disponível para o diagnóstico específico de um número cada vez maior de doenças do armazenamento lisossomal; pode ser utilizado para identificar potenciais portadores.
• Aspirados ou biopsias de órgãos parenquimatosos, particularmente do fígado e baço, podem revelar material de armazenamento intracelular.
• Testes bioquímicos — o diagnóstico pode ser feito pela demonstração da baixa atividade enzimática ou presença de substratos ou intermediários metabólicos acumulados nas preparações de soro, cérebro, vísceras, leucócitos ou fibroblastos cutâneos.
• Eletromiografia e estudos da condução nervosa — anormais em doenças caracterizadas por neuropatia ou miopatia periférica.
• Biopsia de nervo periférico ou músculo esquelético — pode demonstrar o processo patológico específico.

TRATAMENTO
• Paciente de ambulatório — a menos que déficits graves impeçam o cuidado de enfermagem em casa.
• Atividade — restrita a áreas seguras; evitar escadas.
• Dieta e líquidos — garantir a ingestão apropriada (os pacientes quase sempre estão debilitados); fluidoterapia parenteral e suporte nutricional (enteral ou parenteral) podem ser necessários em casos de doença grave.
• Transplante de medula óssea — utilizado experimentalmente com algum sucesso.
• Terapia genética — área de pesquisa intensa que pode trazer esperança para o tratamento específico.
• Terapia de reposição enzimática — a reposição enzimática intratecal direta demonstrou certa eficácia em um quadro experimental.
• Tratamento primário — preventivo; controle da reprodução; aconselhamento genético.
• Os pacientes podem estar sob alto risco de desenvolvimento de infecção secundária; monitorizar rigorosamente; iniciar o tratamento adequado se a infecção se desenvolver.

MEDICAÇÕES

MEDICAMENTO(S)
N/D.

CONTRAINDICAÇÕES/INTERAÇÕES POSSÍVEIS
N/D.

ACOMPANHAMENTO
• Progressivas e basicamente fatais.
• Análise do *pedigree* — pode ser valioso no diagnóstico; importante para a identificação de animais portadores potenciais.

DIVERSOS

ABREVIATURA(S)
• LCS = líquido cerebrospinal.

Sugestões de Leitura
Bannasch D. Canine genetic disease testing: Methods and availability. In: Proceedings, American College of Veterinary Internal Medicine, Charlotte, NC, June 4-8, 2003.
Dewey CW. Lysosomal storage disease. In: Dewey CW, ed., A Practical Guide to Canine and Feline Neurology, 2nd ed. Ames, IA: Wiley-Blackwell, 2008, pp. 115-121.
Skelly BJ, Franklin RJM. Recognition and diagnosis of lysosomal storage diseases in the cat and dog. J Vet Intern Med 2002, 16:133-141.

Autor Mary O. Smith
Consultor Editorial Joane M. Parent

Doenças Endomiocárdicas — Gatos

CONSIDERAÇÕES GERAIS

REVISÃO
- Endomiocardite — doença cardiopulmonar aguda que tipicamente se desenvolve após algum evento estressante; caracterizado por pneumonia intersticial e inflamação endomiocárdica; a pneumonia em geral é grave e costuma levar ao óbito; um único relato registrou a incidência de endomiocardite à necropsia como equivalente à da miocardiopatia hipertrófica.
- Fibroelastose endocárdica — cardiopatia congênita em que o espessamento endocárdico fibroso grave acarreta insuficiência cardíaca secundária à insuficiência diastólica e sistólica.
- Faixas moderadoras excessivas — trata-se de uma entidade patológica rara e única. As faixas moderadoras são bandas musculares normais no ventrículo direito, mas às vezes podem ocorrer no ventrículo esquerdo.

IDENTIFICAÇÃO
- Gatos.
- Endomiocardite — predominantemente machos (62%) com 1-4 anos de idade.
- Fibroelastose endocárdica — desenvolvimento precoce de insuficiência biventricular ou cardíaca esquerda, em geral antes dos 6 meses de vida.
- Faixas moderadoras excessivas — podem ser vistas em gatos de qualquer idade.

SINAIS CLÍNICOS

Achados Anamnésicos

Endomiocardite
- Dispneia após algum evento estressante em gato jovem e saudável.
- Os sinais respiratórios, em geral, ocorrem 5-21 dias após o evento estressante.
- Em um único relato, 73% dos casos foram levados à consulta entre agosto e setembro (EUA).

Fibroelastose Endocárdica e Faixas Moderadoras Excessivas
- Letargia, fraqueza, colapso, síncope.
- Hiporexia e perda de peso.
- Dispneia.
- Taquipneia.
- Cianose.
- Distensão abdominal.
- Paresia ou paralisia; sinais de doença tromboembólica.

Achados do Exame Físico

Endomiocardite
- Dispneia grave.
- Crepitações ocasionais.
- Pode haver sopro ou ritmo de galope; a intensidade do sopro pode variar.
- Pode haver indícios de doença tromboembólica.
- Tipicamente, não há anormalidades significativas antes do evento estressante.

Fibroelastose Endocárdica e Faixas Moderadoras Excessivas
- Ritmo de galope.
- Sopro sistólico, possível regurgitação mitral.
- Dispneia e aumento dos ruídos pulmonares ou crepitações.
- Paresia ou paralisia com pulsos femorais fracos ou ausentes.
- Possíveis arritmias.

CAUSAS E FATORES DE RISCO
- A causa de todas as três doenças é desconhecida.
- Os fatores de risco para endomiocardite incluem incidentes estressantes como anestesia (comumente associada à castração ou remoção das garras), vacinação, novo lar ou banho.
- A fibroelastose endocárdica pode ser familiar em gatos das raças Sagrado da Birmânia e Siamês.
- O aparecimento de faixas moderadoras excessivas em gato jovem é sugestivo de má-formação congênita.

DIAGNÓSTICO

DIAGNÓSTICO DIFERENCIAL

Outras Causas de Doença Cardíaca
Miocardiopatia hipertrófica, miocardiopatia não classificada, miocardiopatia restritiva, miocardiopatia dilatada, más-formações cardíacas congênitas.

Outras Causas de Dispneia
- Outras formas de doença cardíaca, miocardiopatia hipertrófica, miocardiopatia não classificada, miocardiopatia restritiva, miocardiopatia dilatada, más-formações congênitas.
- Doença respiratória primária.
- Doença do espaço pleural.
- Distúrbios mediastínicos, infecção, traumatismo, neoplasia.
- Distúrbios da hemoglobina, anemia, metemoglobinemia, causas de cianose central.

Outras Causas de Colapso, Fraqueza ou Síncope
- Arritmias.
- Doença neurológica ou musculosquelética.
- Doença metabólica ou distúrbios eletrolíticos.
- Outras formas de paresia ou paralisia.
- Tromboembolia arterial secundária a qualquer forma de cardiopatia ou neoplasia.
- Doença neurológica ou musculoesquelética.
- Neoplasia.

HEMOGRAMA/BIOQUÍMICA/URINÁLISE
Não são diagnósticos.

OUTROS TESTES LABORATORIAIS
N/D.

DIAGNÓSTICO POR IMAGEM

Achados Radiográficos Torácicos em Todas as Três Doenças
- Cardiomegalia.
- Infiltrados intersticiais ou alveolares ou efusão pleural mediante o desenvolvimento de congestão.

Achados Ecocardiográficos

Endomiocardite
- Átrio esquerdo normal a levemente aumentado.
- A espessura da parede ventricular esquerda pode estar normal ou discretamente aumentada (0,6-0,7 cm).
- Relato de endomiocárdio hiperecoico — a incidência parece variar, além de ser subjetiva; em um único relato, chegou a 86%.

Fibroelastose Endocárdica
- Os dados disponíveis são limitados.
- Função ventricular esquerda reduzida e átrio esquerdo aumentado.

Faixas Moderadoras Excessivas
Muitos achados podem se sobrepor ao quadro de miocardiopatia restritiva. Às vezes, pode-se observar uma rede de falsos tendões nas imagens da ecocardiografia bidimensional.

MÉTODOS DIAGNÓSTICOS

Achados Eletrocardiográficos
- Endomiocardite — é comum a constatação de taquicardia sinusal; há relatos de complexos ventriculares e atriais prematuros, bloqueio de ramo do feixe de His e bloqueio AV completo.
- Fibroelastose endocárdica — indícios de aumento do lado esquerdo do coração; ritmo sinusal tipicamente está presente, embora sejam possíveis várias arritmias.
- Faixas moderadoras excessivas — vários achados eletrocardiográficos foram relatados: bloqueio AV, bradicardia sinusal, bloqueio do ramo direito do feixe de His e desvio do eixo para a esquerda.

ACHADOS PATOLÓGICOS

Endomiocardite
- Pneumonia intersticial.
- Aumento do lado esquerdo do coração e opacidade do endomiocárdio ventricular esquerdo com focos de hemorragia; é notável a fibroplasia do endocárdio.
- Vários graus de inflamação endomiocárdica com infiltrados de neutrófilos, linfócitos, plasmócitos, histiócitos e macrófagos ao exame histológico.

Fibroelastose Endocárdica
- Dilatação do ventrículo e do átrio esquerdos com espessamento grave, difuso, opaco e branco do endocárdio.
- Espessamento hipocelular fibroelástico difuso do endomiocárdio; edema endomiocárdico proeminente com dilatação dos vasos linfáticos.

Faixas Moderadoras Excessivas
- As alterações tipicamente incluem contorno irregular do endocárdio ventricular esquerdo com ápice arredondado e numerosos tendões falsos irregulares no ventrículo esquerdo. O peso do coração pode ser maior do que o normal. As faixas moderadoras são compostas de fibras de Purkinje centrais e colágeno.

TRATAMENTO

ENDOMIOCARDITE
- Não há nenhum protocolo terapêutico até o momento.
- Uma pequena porcentagem de gatos sobrevive e fica sob terapia a longo prazo.
- Cuidados de suporte com oxigênio e possivelmente ventilação.

FIBROELASTOSE ENDOCÁRDICA E FAIXAS MODERADORAS EXCESSIVAS
- A oxigenoterapia em gaiola é menos estressante.
- Toracocentese se houver efusão pleural.

MEDICAÇÕES

MEDICAMENTO(S) DE ESCOLHA

Endomiocardite
Esteroides, furosemida e vasodilatadores já foram tentados, mas a eficácia desses agentes ainda é desconhecida.

Fibroelastose Endocárdica e Faixas Moderadoras Excessivas
ICC aguda
- Administração parenteral de furosemida na dose de 0,5-1 mg/kg IV ou IM a cada 1-6 h.

Doenças Endomiocárdicas — Gatos

- Aplicação tópica de pomada de nitroglicerina a 2%, 3-6 mm a cada 4-6 h.
- As arritmias podem desaparecer com a estabilização do paciente. Na presença de fibrilação atrial (frequência cardíaca >200), pode-se administrar algum bloqueador dos canais de cálcio ou β-bloqueador para ajudar a controlar a resposta ventricular. Se houver miocardiopatia dilatada, a digoxina poderá ser uma escolha mais eficiente para controlar a frequência cardíaca da fibrilação atrial. Para outras arritmias supraventriculares e ventriculares, pode ser preferível aguardar uma resposta à terapia de insuficiência cardíaca antes de se iniciar a terapia antiarrítmica.
- Edema intratável — nitroprusseto, 1-5 μg/kg/min, pode ser útil.

ICC crônica
- Tratar como outra ICC, com furosemida e enalapril.
- Pode-se acrescentar digoxina quando o paciente se encontrar estabilizado e estiver comendo.

CONTRAINDICAÇÕES/INTERAÇÕES POSSÍVEIS
N/D.

ACOMPANHAMENTO
EVOLUÇÃO ESPERADA E PROGNÓSTICO
- Endomiocardite — prognóstico mau, embora alguns animais sobrevivam; os animais que sobrevivem à fase respiratória podem evoluir para fibrose endocárdica ventricular esquerda.
- Fibroelastose endocárdica e faixas moderadoras excessivas — o tratamento clínico da ICC pode prolongar a vida, mas a recuperação é improvável.

DIVERSOS
DISTÚRBIOS ASSOCIADOS
- Tromboembolia aórtica.
- Pode haver uma relação entre a endomiocardite e a fibrose endocárdica ventricular esquerda.

VER TAMBÉM
- Insuficiência Cardíaca Congestiva Direita.
- Insuficiência Cardíaca Congestiva Esquerda.
- Miocardite.
- Tromboembolia Aórtica.

ABREVIATURA(S)
- AV = atrioventricular.
- ICC = insuficiência cardíaca congestiva.

Sugestões de Leitura
Bossbaly MB, Stalis I, Knight D, Van Winkle T. Feline endomyocarditis: A clinical/pathological study of 44 cases. Proceedings of the 12th ACVIM Forum, 1994, p. 975.
Liu S, Tilley LP. Excessive moderator bands in the left ventricle of 21 cats. JAVMA 1982, 180:1215-1219.
Stalis IH, Bossbaly MJ, Van Winkle TJ. Feline endomyocarditis and left ventricular endocardial fibrosis. Vet Pathol 1995, 32(2):122-126.
Wray JD, Gajanayake I, Smith SH. Congestive heart failure associated with a large transverse left ventricular moderator band in a cat. J Feline Med Surg 2007, 9:56-60.

Autor Carl D. Sammarco
Consultores Editoriais Larry P. Tilley e Francis W.K. Smith, Jr.

Doenças Orbitais (Exoftalmia, Enoftalmia, Estrabismo)

CONSIDERAÇÕES GERAIS

DEFINIÇÃO
- Posição anormal do bulbo ocular.
- Exoftalmia — deslocamento anterior do bulbo ocular.
- Enoftalmia — deslocamento posterior do bulbo ocular.
- Estrabismo — desvio do bulbo ocular da posição correta de fixação, a qual o paciente não consegue corrigir.

FISIOPATOLOGIA
- Não é possível examinar a órbita diretamente; dessa forma, as doenças orbitais manifestam-se apenas por sinais que alteram a posição, o aspecto ou a função do bulbo e dos anexos.
- Bulbo ocular malposicionado — causado por alterações no volume (perda ou ganho) do conteúdo orbital ou função anormal dos músculos extraoculares.
- Exoftalmia — causada por lesões expansivas em posição posterior ao equador do bulbo ocular.
- Enoftalmia — gerada pela perda de volume orbital ou por lesões expansivas em posição anterior ao equador do bulbo ocular.
- Estrabismo — provocado geralmente por desequilíbrio do tônus dos músculos extraoculares ou lesões que restrinjam a mobilidade desses músculos.

SISTEMA(S) ACOMETIDO(S)
- Oftálmico.
- Respiratório — por causa da estreita proximidade, as doenças orbitais podem envolver não só a cavidade nasal, mas também os seios frontais e maxilares.

IDENTIFICAÇÃO
- Cães e gatos.
- Abscesso ou celulite orbitais e miosite — mais comuns nos cães jovens adultos.
- Miosite — raças predispostas: Pastor alemão, Golden retriever, Weimaraner.
- Neoplasia orbital — mais comum nos cães de meia-idade a idosos.

SINAIS CLÍNICOS

Exoftalmia
- Sinais secundários de doença orbital expansiva.
- Dificuldade de retropulsão do bulbo ocular.
- Secreção ocular serosa a mucopurulenta.
- Quemose.
- Tumefação palpebral.
- Lagoftalmia — incapacidade de fechar as pálpebras sobre a córnea adequadamente durante o ato de piscar.
- Ceratite por exposição — com ou sem ulceração.
- Dor à abertura da boca.
- Protrusão da terceira pálpebra atribuída à massa extraconal ou mais tarde durante a evolução de massa intraconal.
- Comprometimento visual provocado por neuropatia óptica.
- Anormalidades do fundo ocular, incluindo o descolamento da retina.
- Congestão dos vasos retinianos.
- Desvio focal para dentro da parte posterior do bulbo ocular.
- Tumefação do disco óptico.
- Ceratite neurotrópica após lesão do ramo oftálmico do V par de nervo craniano.
- Febre e mal-estar — em caso de abscesso ou celulite orbitais.
- PIO — raramente elevada.

Enoftalmia
- Ptose.
- Protrusão da terceira pálpebra.
- Atrofia dos músculos extraoculares.
- Entrópio — com doença grave.

Estrabismo
- Desvio de um ou de ambos os olhos da posição normal.
- Pode-se notar exoftalmia ou enoftalmia.

CAUSAS

Exoftalmia
- Neoplasia — primária ou secundária.
- Abscesso ou celulite — bacteriana ou fúngica; a fúngica é mais provável nos gatos; procurar por corpos estranhos.
- Mucocele zigomática — não descrita nos gatos.
- Miosite — músculos mastigatórios ou extraoculares (polimiosite eosinofílica ou extraocular).
- Hemorragia orbital secundária a traumatismo.
- Fístulas ou varizes arteriovenosas — raras.

Enoftalmia
- Dor ocular.
- Microftalmia.
- Encolhimento do bulbo ocular.
- Bulbo ocular colapsado.
- Síndrome de Horner.
- Desidratação.
- Perda de gordura ou músculo orbitais.
- Enoftalmia conformacional nas raças dolicocefálicas.
- Neoplasia — especialmente aquelas que se originam da parte rostral da órbita.

Estrabismo
- Inervação anormal dos músculos extraoculares.
- Restrição da mobilidade dos músculos extraoculares por tecido cicatricial formado por traumatismo ou inflamação anteriores.
- Destruição das inserções dos músculos extraoculares após proptose.
- Estrabismo convergente — congênito; resulta do cruzamento anormal de fibras visuais no SNC (gato Siamês).
- Estrabismo do Shar-pei.

FATORES DE RISCO
Proptose — ocorre mais facilmente nos cães braquicefálicos com órbitas rasas.

DIAGNÓSTICO

DIAGNÓSTICO DIFERENCIAL

Sinais Semelhantes
- Bulbo ocular buftálmico — pode simular a presença de massa expansiva e provocar o deslocamento anterior do olho em virtude de seu tamanho em relação ao volume orbital; PIO geralmente elevada; diâmetro da córnea é maior do que o normal, edema corneano, pupila em midríase, ↓ da visão (i. e., sinais de glaucoma).
- Episclerite — pode provocar espessamento difuso ou focal grave da túnica fibrosa, mimetizando muitas vezes um bulbo buftálmico; edema corneano; PIO normal ou baixa; rubor aquoso.

Causas
- Início agudo de exoftalmia — frequentemente uma doença orbital inflamatória. É mais provável que a dor, eliciada sobretudo à abertura da boca, seja atribuída à doença orbital inflamatória do que à neoplasia orbital.
- Mucoceles — mais variáveis na velocidade de início e no grau de desconforto do paciente.
- Miosite extraocular ou eosinofílica — doenças bilaterais; o microrganismo *Neospora caninum* causou polimiosite extraocular em uma ninhada de Pointer alemão de pelo curto.
- Neoplasia — costuma ser lentamente progressiva, mas indolor; provoca exoftalmia unilateral.

HEMOGRAMA/BIOQUÍMICA/URINÁLISE
- Geralmente normais.
- Leucograma — pode revelar inflamação em caso de abscesso, celulite ou miosite.
- Eosinofilia periférica — ocasionalmente observada em cães com miosite eosinofílica dos músculos da mastigação.

DIAGNÓSTICO POR IMAGEM
- Radiografias do crânio (sobretudo dos seios frontais e da cavidade nasal).
- Ultrassonografia, TC e RM da órbita — são extremamente valiosas para definir a extensão da(s) lesão(ões) e diferenciar entre os tipos de miosite.
- Radiografias torácicas — podem ajudar a identificar doença metastática.

MÉTODOS DIAGNÓSTICOS
- Falta de retropulsão do bulbo — confirma a presença de massa expansiva.
- Exame da boca, radiografias do crânio e aspirado por agulha fina da órbita — podem ser concluídos após a anestesia do paciente.
- Aspirado por agulha fina (calibre 18-20) — enviar amostras para culturas aeróbia, anaeróbia e fúngica; coloração de Gram; e exame citológico.
- Citologia — frequentemente diagnóstica para abscesso ou celulite, mucocele da glândula salivar zigomática e neoplasia.
- Biopsia — indicada se o aspirado por agulha não for diagnóstico. Biopsia dos músculos masseter, temporal ou extraocular na suspeita de miosite; as análises em busca de fibras do tipo 2M podem ser úteis.
- Teste de ducção* forçada do bulbo ocular (estrabismo) — apanhar a conjuntiva com um par de pinças finas após anestesia tópica; diferencia doença neurológica (na qual o bulbo ocular se move livremente) de condição restritiva (na qual o bulbo ocular não pode ser movimentado manualmente).

TRATAMENTO

PROPTOSE
Ver "Proptose".

---

* N. T.: Trata-se de um movimento monocular, ou seja, um movimento executado só por um olho. A ducção forçada é utilizada para avaliar se um determinado desvio ocular é secundário ou não à obstrução mecânica. O olho é movimentado por meio da aplicação de uma pinça na conjuntiva e episclera junto ao limbo esclerocorneano.

Doenças Orbitais (Exoftalmia, Enoftalmia, Estrabismo)

ABSCESSO OU CELULITE ORBITAIS
• Observa-se a drenagem em menos da metade dos pacientes, em geral porque a lesão se encontra no estágio de celulite e um abscesso verdadeiro ainda não se formou.
• Se não houver tumefação evidente da mucosa bucal atrás do último dente molar e o ultrassom não revelar a presença de abscesso, é melhor evitar a incisão da mucosa bucal e tratar com antibióticos sistêmicos e medicamentos anti-inflamatórios; deve-se manter o bulbo ocular acometido úmido com lubrificantes tópicos a cada 6 h.
• Os casos graves podem necessitar de fluidos intravenosos para manter a hidratação e repor os déficits hídricos até que o paciente consiga se alimentar.
• Se houver uma tumefação evidente da mucosa bucal atrás do último dente molar, estabelecer uma drenagem ventral da órbita enquanto o paciente estiver anestesiado.
• Incisar a mucosa preparada por meio cirúrgico a cerca de 1 cm atrás do último molar.
• Impulsionar uma pinça de ponta romba (p. ex., Kelly ou Carmalt) no espaço orbital e abri-lo; em geral, avançar a pinça até o abscesso drenar, na altura da trava, ou até que o movimento do olho ocorra com a pinça aberta.
• Tomar cuidado para minimizar o traumatismo retrobulbar e a lesão ao nervo óptico; utilizar apenas dissecção romba; jamais cortar ou esmagar o tecido.
• As complicações que podem ocorrer com dissecção agressiva incluem dano ao nervo óptico e aos nervos ciliares.
• Coletar amostras para cultura bacteriana e exame citológico por essa via.
• Fornecer alimento pastoso até que o bulbo ocular esteja de volta à posição normal e a dor aparentemente tenha desaparecido.
• Compressa quente — a cada 6 h; ajuda a diminuir a tumefação e limpa a secreção.

NEOPLASIAS ORBITAIS
• Geralmente primárias e malignas.
• Exenteração precoce ou cirurgia exploratória orbital e debridamento da massa por abordagem lateral à órbita para recuperar o bulbo ocular são escolhas terapêuticas racionais.
• Quimio ou radioterapia adjuvantes — dependendo do tipo da neoplasia e da extensão da lesão.
• Sem terapia adjuvante — a sobrevida será de semanas a meses se a neoplasia for maligna, porque o paciente costuma ser examinado tardiamente na evolução da doença.
• Assim que o diagnóstico for estabelecido, recomenda-se a consulta com algum oncologista.

MUCOCELE ZIGOMÁTICA
Pode se resolver com a administração de antibiótico e corticosteroide; caso contrário, a excisão cirúrgica do cisto e da glândula associada geralmente é curativa.

ESTRABISMO
• Neurológico — mais bem tratado pela identificação e tratamento da causa subjacente, se possível.
• Restritivo ou pós-traumático — pode ser tratado de modo cirúrgico; reposicionar ou excisar as inserções dos músculos extraoculares; aliviar a tensão excessiva sobre esses músculos; geralmente é método muito difícil.

MEDICAÇÕES
MEDICAMENTO(S) DE ESCOLHA
• Exoftalmia (todos os pacientes) — lubrificar a córnea (p. ex., pomada ou gel de lágrima artificial a cada 6 h) para evitar dessecação e ulceração.
• Ulceração — antibiótico tópico (p. ex., bacitracina, neomicina, polimixina a cada 8 h) e cicloplégico (p. ex., atropina a 1% a cada 12-24 h), para evitar a infecção e reduzir o espasmo ciliar, respectivamente.

Abscesso ou Celulite Orbitais
• Antibióticos por via intravenosa — ampicilina sódica (20 mg/kg a cada 6-8 h) ou cloranfenicol (25 mg/kg a cada 8 h); enquanto se aguardam os resultados do exame de cultura bacteriana e citologia se os proprietários desistirem dos testes diagnósticos. Em alguns pacientes com abscessos profundos e bem-selados, deve-se considerar o uso de medicamentos com espectro anaeróbio (amoxicilina com ácido clavulânico ou metronidazol).
• Infecções orbitais bacterianas — podem ser mistas; é comum o envolvimento de *Pasteurella multocida* e *Enterobacteriaceae*.
• Antibióticos por via oral — prescritos depois que o paciente começa a comer; escolhidos com base na cultura e no antibiograma.
• A maior parte dos pacientes se recupera dentro de aproximadamente duas semanas de tratamento.
• Fluconazol (2,5 mg/kg a cada 12 h ou 5 mg/kg a cada 24 h) ou posaconazol (5 mg/kg a cada 12 h) pode ser considerado em casos de aspergilose orbital.
• Prednisona —1 mg/kg SC ou IM a cada 24 h, uma ou duas vezes; não só minimiza a neurite óptica, mas também diminui a tumefação orbital e a exposição do bulbo ocular.
• Alternativamente, os AINE sistêmicos (p. ex., carprofeno ou meloxicam) podem ser utilizados no lugar da prednisona.

Miosite Aguda
• Dificuldade de preensão — corticosteroides sistêmicos (prednisona, 2 mg/kg SC ou IM); depois, corticosteroides por via oral nas 4-6 semanas seguintes (prednisona, 2 mg/kg a cada 24 h) até que a tumefação desapareça; em seguida, reduzir de forma gradativa.
• Azatioprina — 1-2 mg/kg VO a cada 24 h por 3-7 dias; em seguida, a cada 48 h e subsequente redução gradual; com ou sem corticosteroides, pode ser utilizada de forma crônica para tratar doença recidivante.

PRECAUÇÕES
• Corticosteroides sistêmicos — usar com extremo cuidado em caso de doença orbital fúngica profunda.
• Azatioprina — pode ser hepatotóxica e provocar mielossupressão.
• Acompanhar o paciente com a contagem de plaquetas e a mensuração das enzimas hepáticas a cada 1-2 semanas por 8 semanas e, depois, periodicamente.

ACOMPANHAMENTO
MONITORIZAÇÃO DO PACIENTE
• Doença orbital inflamatória — examinar no mínimo semanalmente até que os sinais clínicos desapareçam.
• Aconselhar o proprietário a esperar pela recidiva dos sinais clínicos, especialmente se um corpo estranho orbital for provável.
• Tratar as infecções fúngicas por 60 dias após os sinais clínicos cessarem.

COMPLICAÇÕES POSSÍVEIS
• Perda da visão.
• Perda do olho.
• Malposicionamento permanente do bulbo ocular.
• Morte.

DIVERSOS
FATORES RELACIONADOS COM A IDADE
Administrar a antibioticoterapia primeiro antes de tentar a drenagem ventral da órbita.

GESTAÇÃO/FERTILIDADE/REPRODUÇÃO
Evitar o uso de corticosteroides sistêmicos, medicações antifúngicas e azatioprina em fêmeas prenhes.

VER TAMBÉM
• Olho Vermelho.
• Proptose.

ABREVIATURA(S)
• AINE = anti-inflamatório não esteroide.
• PIO = pressão intraocular.
• RM = ressonância magnética.
• SNC = sistema nervoso central.
• TC = tomografia computadorizada.

Sugestões de Leitura
Dubey JP, Oestner A, Piper RC. Repeated transplacental transmission of Neospora caninum in dogs. JAVMA 1990, 197:857-860.
Lindley DM. Disorders of the orbit. In: Kirk RW, Bonagura JD, eds., Current Veterinary Therapy XI. Philadelphia: Saunders, 1992, pp. 1081-1085.
Speiss BM. Diseases and surgery of the canine orbit. In: Gelatt KN, ed., Veterinary Ophthalmology, 4th ed. Ames, IA: Blackwell, 2007, pp. 539-562.

Autor Carmen M.H. Colitz
Consultor Editorial Paul E. Miller

Doenças Renais de Natureza Congênita e de Desenvolvimento

CONSIDERAÇÕES GERAIS

DEFINIÇÕES
- Anormalidades funcionais ou morfológicas, resultantes de processos mórbidos hereditários (genéticos) ou adquiridos, que comprometem a diferenciação e o crescimento dos rins em desenvolvimento antes ou logo depois do nascimento.
- Agenesia renal — ausência completa de um ou ambos os rins.
- Displasia renal — desenvolvimento desorganizado do parênquima renal.
- Ectopia renal — mau posicionamento congênito de um ou ambos os rins; os rins ectópicos podem estar fundidos.
- Glomerulopatia — doença glomerular de qualquer tipo.
- Nefropatia tubulointersticial — distúrbio não inflamatório dos túbulos renais e do interstício.
- Doença renal policística — caracterizada pela formação de múltiplos cistos de tamanho variável em toda parte do córtex e da medula renal.
- Telangiectasia renal — caracterizada por más-formações vasculares multifocais, envolvendo os rins e outros órgãos.
- Amiloidose renal — consiste no depósito extracelular de amiloide em capilares glomerulares, glomérulos e interstício.
- Nefroblastoma — neoplasia renal congênita, originária do blastema* metanéfrico pluripotente.
- Cistadenocarcinoma renal multifocal — neoplasia renal hereditária em cães.
- Síndrome de Fanconi — anomalia funcional tubular renal generalizada, que se caracteriza pela diminuição na reabsorção de glicose, fosfato, eletrólitos, aminoácidos e ácido úrico.
- Glicosúria renal primária — defeito funcional isolado na reabsorção tubular renal de glicose.
- Cistinúria — excreção urinária excessiva de cistina, em função de um defeito funcional isolado na reabsorção tubular renal desse aminoácido e de outros aminoácidos dibásicos.
- Xantinúria — excreção urinária exagerada de xantina causada por uma deficiência na xantina oxidase e conversão reduzida da hipoxantina em xantina e da xantina em ácido úrico.
- Hiperuricúria — excreção urinária demasiada de ácido úrico, urato de sódio ou urato de amônio, causada pelo dano na conversão hepática do ácido úrico em alantoína e pela intensificação na secreção tubular renal de ácido úrico.
- Hiperoxalúria primária — distúrbio caracterizado por hiperoxalúria intermitente, acidúria L-glicérica, nefropatia por oxalato e insuficiência renal aguda.
- Diabetes insípido nefrogênico congênito — distúrbio na capacidade de concentração renal, causado pela diminuição na responsividade renal ao hormônio antidiurético.

FISIOPATOLOGIA
- Muitos distúrbios renais congênitos e evolutivos são causados por anormalidades genéticas que interrompem o desenvolvimento normal sequencial e coordenado, bem como a interação de múltiplos tecidos embrionários envolvidos na formação dos rins maduros. • Os distúrbios renais congênitos e evolutivos também podem ser gerados por fatores não genéticos que comprometam os rins em desenvolvimento antes ou logo depois do nascimento.

___
*N. T.: Conjunto de células embrionárias em estágio indiferenciado, do qual vai se originar futuro órgão ou estrutura.

SISTEMA(S) ACOMETIDO(S)
Renal/urológico.

GENÉTICA
Os distúrbios renais familiares foram descritos nas seguintes raças de cães e gatos:
- Agenesia renal em cães das raças Beagle e Doberman pinscher.
- Displasia renal em cães das raças Malamute do Alasca, Boxer, Chow chow, Golden retriever, Keeshond, Lhasa apso, Schnauzer miniatura, Shih tzu, Wheaten terrier de pelo macio e Poodle standard (padrão).
- Glomerulopatia em cães Beagle, Montanhês de Berna, Spaniel britânico, Bull terrier, Doberman pinscher, Cocker spaniel inglês, Terra nova, Rottweiler, Samoieda e Wheaten terrier de pelo macio.
- Nefropatia tubulointersticial em cães da raça Elkhound norueguês.
- Doença renal policística em cães das raças Beagle, Bull terrier, Cairn terrier e West highland white terrier, bem como em gatos das raças Persa, exótico do pelo curto e Himalaio.
- Telangiectasia renal em cães Pembroke Welsh Corgi.
- Amiloidose renal em gatos das raças Abissínio, Oriental de pelo curto e Siamês, bem como em cães das raças Beagle, Foxhound inglês e Shar-pei.
- Cistadenocarcinoma renal em cães da raça Pastor alemão.
- Síndrome de Fanconi em cães das raças Basenji e Border terrier.
- Glicosúria renal primária em cães das raças Elkhound norueguês, Scottish terrier e Basenji.
- Cistinúria em cães das raças Basset hound, Buldogue inglês, Dachshund, Buldogue francês, Terrier irlandês, Mastife, Terra nova, Scottish deer hound, Staffordshire bull terrier e Boiadeiro australiano, além de gatos domésticos.
- Xantinúria em cães da raça Cavalier King Charles spaniel e gatos domésticos de pelo curto.
- Hiperuricúria em cães das raças Dálmata, Terrier preto russo e Buldogue inglês.
- Hiperoxalúria primária em gatos domésticos de pelo curto e no cão Spaniel tibetano.

INCIDÊNCIA/PREVALÊNCIA
Raramente identificadas; no entanto, os distúrbios causados por fatores genéticos ocorrem com maior frequência em animais aparentados em mais de uma geração do que na população em geral.

IDENTIFICAÇÃO
Espécies
Cães e gatos.

Raça(s) Predominante(s)
A ocorrência de casos esporádicos de doença renal de natureza congênita e de desenvolvimento é possível, sem uma predisposição familiar aparente em qualquer raça canina ou felina.

Idade Média e Faixa Etária
A maioria dos pacientes tem menos de 5 anos de idade no momento do diagnóstico.

Sexo Predominante
- A cistinúria familiar ocorre principalmente em cães machos.
- A glomerulopatia hereditária da raça Samoieda é mais comum em machos do que em fêmeas; na raça Terra nova, ambos os sexos são acometidos.
- A glomerulonefropatia familiar dos cães da raça Montanhês de Berna é mais comum em fêmeas do que em machos.

SINAIS CLÍNICOS
Comentários Gerais
Não se consegue distinguir grande parte dos distúrbios de natureza congênita e de desenvolvimento das doenças renais não congênitas/evolutivas, com base na anamnese ou no exame físico.

Achados Anamnésicos
- Indicam insuficiência renal crônica.
- Algumas glomerulopatias associadas a distensão abdominal, edema e outros sinais da síndrome nefrótica.
- Distensão abdominal em certos pacientes com rins policísticos ou neoplasias renais.
- Hematúria em determinados pacientes com telangiectasia renal ou neoplasias renais.
- Dor abdominal aparente em alguns animais com telangiectasia renal.
- Com frequência, os pacientes com agenesia renal unilateral, rins ectópicos e defeitos isolados de transporte tubular renal permanecem assintomáticos.

Achados do Exame Físico
- Sinais clínicos associados à insuficiência renal crônica.
- Ascite ou edema depressível (i. e., que cede à pressão digital) em alguns pacientes acometidos por glomerulopatias com perda de proteínas ou amiloidose.
- Renomegalia ou lesões expansivas abdominais em determinados pacientes com rins policísticos, neoplasias renais ou rins ectópicos fundidos.
- Dor renal em certos pacientes com telangiectasia renal.

CAUSAS
Não Hereditárias
- Agentes infecciosos — infecção pelo vírus da panleucopenia felina e pelo herpes-vírus canino, associada à displasia renal. • Medicamentos — corticosteroides, difenilamina e bifenilas, associados a rins policísticos; clorambucila e arseniato de sódio, associados à agenesia renal.
- Fatores nutricionais — hipo ou hipervitaminose A, associados à ectopia renal.

DIAGNÓSTICO

DIAGNÓSTICO DIFERENCIAL
- Descartar as causas adquiridas e não evolutivas de doença renal primária. • Excluir as causas não renais de hematúria, proteinúria, glicosúria, distensão abdominal ou ascite.

HEMOGRAMA/BIOQUÍMICA/URINÁLISE
- Anemia arregenerativa em pacientes com insuficiência renal crônica.
- Azotemia e densidade urinária <1,030 em cães e <1,035 em gatos caso se desenvolva uma insuficiência renal.
- Proteinúria, hipoalbuminemia e hipercolesterolemia em pacientes com síndrome nefrótica.
- Glicosúria normoglicêmica em animais com síndrome de Fanconi ou glicosúria renal primária.

Doenças Renais de Natureza Congênita e de Desenvolvimento

- Hematúria em pacientes com neoplasia renal congênita ou telangiectasia renal.
- Cristalúria por cistina em pacientes com cistinúria.
- Cristalúria por xantina em pacientes com xantinúria.
- Cristalúria por urato em pacientes com hiperuricúria.

OUTROS TESTES LABORATORIAIS
Existem testes genéticos diretos disponíveis para a detecção de mutações genéticas específicas associadas aos quadros de nefropatia familiar em Cocker spaniel inglês, cistinúria familiar em Terra nova e doença renal policística familiar em gatos Persa e mestiços dessa raça.

DIAGNÓSTICO POR IMAGEM
A radiografia abdominal simples, a ultrassonografia renal e a urografia excretora são métodos diagnósticos importantes para a identificação e a caracterização dos distúrbios renais de natureza congênita e de desenvolvimento, bem como de suas sequelas associadas.

MÉTODOS DIAGNÓSTICOS
Considerar a avaliação sob microscopia óptica de amostras obtidas por biopsia renal de pacientes com anormalidades morfológicas ou funcionais dos rins para as quais ainda não se estabeleceu um diagnóstico definitivo por outros meios menos invasivos.

ACHADOS PATOLÓGICOS
- Os distúrbios renais de natureza congênita e de desenvolvimento podem estar associados a diversas combinações de lesões primárias, compensatórias e degenerativas. De modo inverso, alguns distúrbios funcionais podem não estar ligados com alterações na morfologia renal.
- Displasia renal — rins em fase terminal; as lesões primárias incluem glomérulos imaturos ("fetais"), persistência do mesênquima e dos ductos metanéfricos, epitélio tubular atípico e metaplasia disontogênica; as lesões primárias costumam estar relacionadas com lesões degenerativas, inflamatórias e compensatórias secundárias e podem estar mascaradas por tais danos.
- Glomerulopatias — rins geralmente normais a pequenos; a maioria das glomerulopatias hereditárias caracteriza-se por uma glomerulonefrite membranoproliferativa primária com graus variados de doença tubulointersticial, mas uma glomerulopatia membranosa atrófica cística corresponde à lesão característica em Rottweiler acometido.
- Nefropatia tubulointersticial — rins em fase terminal; as lesões renais incluem fibrose periglomerular e intersticial, hiperplasia e hipertrofia epiteliais parietais e infiltrado mononuclear intersticial.
- Doença renal policística — ver o capítulo específico.
- Amiloidose renal — ver o capítulo específico.
- Telangiectasia renal — as lesões englobam múltiplos nódulos e coágulos de tamanho variável e de cor vermelho-escuro, repletos de sangue no córtex e na medula renais, além de fibrose intersticial, infiltrado mononuclear intersticial e hidronefrose.
- Nefroblastoma — massa renal unilateral; do ponto de vista microscópico, caracteriza-se pela presença de componentes teciduais epiteliais e mesenquimatosos embrionários.
- Cistadenocarcinoma renal multifocal — aumento de volume bilateral dos rins, com estruturas císticas protrusas irregulares ou proliferações epiteliais tubulares renais neoplásicas multifocais; frequentemente associado a dermatofibrose nodular cutânea e leiomiomas uterinos múltiplos.
- Ectopia renal — os rins podem estar situados no espaço retroperitoneal do canal pélvico, na fossa ilíaca ou no abdome; os rins fundidos assumem diversos formatos; os rins com aspecto de ferradura exibem uma fusão simétrica ao longo da borda medial de cada polo.
- Síndrome de Fanconi — achados microscópicos incompatíveis de atrofia tubular, fibrose intersticial, cariomegalia tubular e necrose papilar aguda.
- Hiperoxalúria primária — rins aumentados de volume e de formato irregular; as lesões microscópicas incluem depósito de cristais de oxalato de cálcio nos túbulos renais, bem como fibrose intersticial e periglomerular variável.

TRATAMENTO
- A característica dos distúrbios renais de natureza congênita e de desenvolvimento frequentemente dificulta o tratamento específico.
- O tratamento de suporte ou de acordo com os sintomas (i. e., sintomático) pode melhorar a qualidade de vida e minimizar a evolução da doença em pacientes com disfunção renal.
- As opções terapêuticas são escolhidas com base nos sinais clínicos e nas avaliações laboratoriais apropriadas.
- Consultar outros capítulos que descrevem doenças renais ou síndromes clínicas específicas.

MEDICAÇÕES
MEDICAMENTO(S) DE ESCOLHA
Recorrer aos capítulos que falam sobre doenças renais ou síndromes clínicas específicas.

CONTRAINDICAÇÕES
Sempre que possível, evitar os medicamentos potencialmente nefrotóxicos (p. ex., gentamicina, anti-inflamatórios não esteroides) ou os agentes anestésicos que diminuem a função renal (p. ex., metoxiflurano).

PRECAUÇÕES
Em pacientes com insuficiência renal, evitar os medicamentos que exigem a excreção renal; se necessário, modificar os esquemas posológicos para compensar a depuração renal reduzida dos medicamentos e de outros metabólitos.

ACOMPANHAMENTO
MONITORIZAÇÃO DO PACIENTE
Dirigir-se também aos capítulos que abordam doenças renais ou síndromes clínicas específicas.

PREVENÇÃO
Os distúrbios renais de natureza congênita e de desenvolvimento são irreversíveis; dessa forma, o controle repousa no não acasalamento de animais acometidos. Sempre considerar a identificação e a correção precoces dos fatores predisponentes (genéticos ou não), que possam comprometer uma descendência futura.

COMPLICAÇÕES POSSÍVEIS
- Insuficiência renal aguda ou crônica.
- Síndrome nefrótica.
- Urolitíase.
- Hidronefrose.
- Infecção do trato urinário.

EVOLUÇÃO ESPERADA E PROGNÓSTICO
- Altamente variável; depende do distúrbio específico, do grau das lesões primárias e da gravidade da disfunção renal.
- A maioria dos distúrbios de natureza congênita e de desenvolvimento é irreversível e pode resultar em insuficiência renal crônica avançada, mas alguns pacientes com disfunção renal leve a moderada podem permanecer estáveis por períodos prolongados.
- Os pacientes com alguns distúrbios (p. ex., agenesia renal unilateral, ectopia renal, cistinúria, hiperuricúria e glicosúria renal primária) podem permanecer assintomáticos a menos que o distúrbio seja complicado por urolitíase, infecção do trato urinário ou outros processos mórbidos promotores de uma disfunção renal progressiva.

DIVERSOS
DISTÚRBIOS ASSOCIADOS
- Doença renal policística, associada a cistos hepatobiliares.
- Cistinúria, xantinuria e hiperuricúria, associadas à formação de urólitos.
- Amiloidose em cães da raça Shar-pei, associada à pirexia ou tumefação intermitentes dos jarretes.
- Neoplasias renais, associadas à osteoartropatia hipertrófica, policitemia ou outras síndromes paraneoplásicas.

SINÔNIMO(S)
Doença renal familiar, doença renal juvenil.

VER TAMBÉM
- Acidose Tubular Renal.
- Amiloidose.
- Anemia de Nefropatia Crônica.
- Doença Renal Policística.
- Hematúria.
- Hiperparatireoidismo Renal Secundário.
- Insuficiência Renal Aguda.
- Insuficiência Renal Crônica.
- Oligúria e Anúria.
- Poliúria e Polidipsia.
- Renomegalia.
- Síndrome de Fanconi.
- Síndrome Nefrótica.
- Urolitíase por Cistina.

Sugestões de Leitura
DiBartola SP. Familial renal disease in dogs and cats. In: Ettinger SJ, Feldman EC, eds., Textbook of Veterinary Internal Medicine, 6th ed. St. Louis: Elsevier, 2005, pp. 1819–1824.
Patterson EE. Methods and availability of tests for hereditary disorders of dogs. In: Bonagura JD, Twedt DC, eds., Kirk's Current Veterinary Therapy XIV. St. Louis: Elsevier Saunders, 2009, pp. 1054–1059.

Autores John M. Kruger, Carl A. Osborne, e Scott D. Fitzgerald
Consultor Editorial Carl A. Osborne

Dor Aguda, Crônica e Pós-operatória

CONSIDERAÇÕES GERAIS

DEFINIÇÃO
• Dor é uma sensação desagradável ou experiência emocional associada à lesão tecidual real ou potencial.
• A incapacidade do animal em se comunicar não anula a presença de dor e a necessidade de tratamento apropriado para o alívio desse sintoma.

FISIOPATOLOGIA
• A aplicação de algum estímulo nocivo ativa terminações nervosas especializadas denominadas nociceptores; os nociceptores fazem a transdução dos estímulos químicos, mecânicos ou térmicos nocivos para potenciais eletroquímicos que são transmitidos via nervos sensoriais desde o tecido acometido até a medula espinal.
• No corno dorsal da medula espinal, o nervo periférico aferente de primeira ordem faz sinapse com neurônios espinais ascendentes, os quais terminam no tronco cerebral. As informações nocivas aferentes podem ser moduladas na altura do corno dorsal por outras informações aferentes, impulsos nervosos descendentes inibitórios, ou inibição farmacológica por várias classes de medicamentos. Os neurônios ascendentes fazem sinapse no tronco cerebral para formar tratos ascendentes que terminam no córtex, onde ocorre a percepção da sensação de dor. Respostas neuroendócrinas e fisiológicas (p. ex., taquicardia e cortisol elevado) a estímulos nocivos podem se originar na altura do tronco cerebral e não se correlacionar necessariamente à intensidade percebida da dor.
• Processos nociceptivos (i. e., transdução, transmissão e modulação) parecem ser semelhantes em termos anatômicos e fisiológicos na maioria dos mamíferos e em muitas espécies não mamíferas. A percepção da dor pode variar entre as espécies e nos indivíduos da mesma espécie, pois existem diferenças anatômicas no desenvolvimento cortical; além disso, a integração de experiências passadas e comportamentos aprendidos varia.
• A atividade prolongada nas vias nociceptivas (p. ex., dias, semanas ou meses) decorrente de lesão ou doença crônica ou de dano tecidual ao sistema nervoso pode provocar uma alteração no processamento neurológico, resultando em sensibilização dessas vias e hiper-responsividade. Isso pode causar uma resposta acentuada a algum estímulo não considerado normalmente como nocivo (alodinia*).

SISTEMA(S) ACOMETIDO(S)
• A dor pode se originar de qualquer tecido, incluindo aqueles dentro do próprio sistema nervoso. Em seres humanos, a dor pode ser associada ao medo, à ansiedade ou à depressão na ausência de qualquer lesão observável.
• A resposta fisiológica à dor pode incluir função imune diminuída, catabolismo aumentado e marcadores neuroendócrinos elevados de estresse. A dor pode resultar em perda da função dos tecidos acometidos.

GENÉTICA
Fatores como idade, sexo, estirpe reprodutiva e espécie podem alterar as respostas a estímulos nocivos. Recentemente, foram descritos genes que modificam as respostas comportamentais de camundongos individualmente aos estímulos nocivos.

INCIDÊNCIA/PREVALÊNCIA
• Do ponto de vista evolutivo, a aversão aos estímulos nocivos era uma reação protetora para os organismos, mantendo-os fora do perigo. Semelhanças na anatomia e nas respostas aos estímulos nocivos sugerem que os mamíferos humanos e não humanos possam sentir dor de maneiras semelhantes.
• Embora a dor aguda seja benéfica para alertar ou ensinar um animal sobre a presença de objetos perigosos em potencial em seu ambiente, esse tipo de dor associada à cirurgia ou lesão não beneficia o paciente e deve ser tratado de forma adequada.

DISTRIBUIÇÃO GEOGRÁFICA
N/D.

IDENTIFICAÇÃO
N/D.

SINAIS CLÍNICOS
• Sinais comportamentais de dor e de sofrimento variam de forma considerável entre os animais individualmente.
• Experiência, ambiente, idade, espécie e outros fatores podem modificar a intensidade da reação aos estímulos nocivos.
• Os sinais clínicos mais evidentes de sofrimento no cão e no gato incluem vocalização, agitação, postura ou marcha anormais, solavancos, hiperestesia ou hiperalgesia, e alodinia.
• Os sinais mais sutis compartilhados por muitas condições incluem tremores, depressão, apetite diminuído, estupor e mordidas.
• Taquipneia, taquicardia, midríase e hipertensão são sinais observados na resposta ao estresse, que também podem acompanhar a dor; entretanto, esses sinais são inespecíficos e estão presentes em muitas condições não dolorosas.
• Sinais clínicos associados a condições cronicamente dolorosas podem ser muito sutis ou difíceis de avaliar, já que os mecanismos homeostáticos tendem a ajudar o animal a compensar. Com frequência, condições cronicamente dolorosas estão associadas à atividade reduzida, claudicação ou depressão.

CAUSAS
• A dor pode ser provocada não só por dano tecidual associado a traumatismo ou cirurgia, mas também por alterações degenerativas crônicas, como a osteoartrite.
• A dor que sobrevive à lesão tecidual inicial é patológica e pode indicar processamento alterado do sistema nervoso.

FATORES DE RISCO
• Todos os animais que sofrem lesão tecidual cirúrgica ou traumática devem ser avaliados quanto à presença da dor.

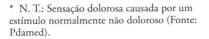

* N. T.: Sensação dolorosa causada por um estímulo normalmente não doloroso (Fonte: Pdamed).

DOR AGUDA, CRÔNICA E PÓS-OPERATÓRIA

• A intensidade da dor nem sempre pode se correlacionar com o grau de dano tecidual. Contudo, métodos mais invasivos em tecidos moles e procedimentos ortopédicos provavelmente estão associados a maior intensidade da dor.

DIAGNÓSTICO
DIAGNÓSTICO DIFERENCIAL
• A identificação da dor em pacientes veterinários é um diagnóstico, mas o prontuário clínico deve refletir o plano diagnóstico e terapêutico do veterinário.
• A dor aguda é quase sempre acompanhada por lesão tecidual ou doença, mas o diagnóstico e o tratamento do distúrbio primário devem ser realizados antes ou concomitantemente com o tratamento da dor. A presença ou a ausência de dor, às vezes, é utilizada como forma de monitoramento e diagnóstico de algumas condições, mas o tratamento deve estar de acordo com o correto exercício clínico. A dor deve ser diferenciada do sofrimento associado a outros fatores, como a contenção, a bandagem restritiva e a separação dos proprietários. Os medicamentos usados para tratamento da dor, sobretudo os opioides e os anestésicos dissociativos, podem provocar disforia, que frequentemente lembra os sinais de dor e sofrimento.

HEMOGRAMA/BIOQUÍMICA/URINÁLISE
• Aumentos no cortisol associados à dor aguda podem aparecer sob a forma de leucograma de estresse.
• A hiperglicemia também pode ser observada em alguns pacientes.
• Resultados normais dos testes laboratoriais não devem descartar a presença de dor.

OUTROS TESTES LABORATORIAIS
N/D.

DIAGNÓSTICO POR IMAGEM
• Muitas condições que podem ser dolorosas são associadas a alterações nos exames de ultrassonografia, radiografia, TC ou RM.
• Alterações crônicas como o grau de formação de osteófitos em casos de osteoartrite não se correlacionam necessariamente com o grau de dor e disfunção sofridas pelo paciente.

MÉTODOS DIAGNÓSTICOS
• Realizar uma avaliação diagnóstica completa em busca de algum distúrbio subjacente (p. ex., ruptura do ligamento cruzado cranial) quando o animal aparece com dor. No caso do diagnóstico de alguma condição subjacente, haverá necessidade de tratamento adequado. A dor em pacientes veterinários é mais comumente causada por alguma condição clínica ou cirúrgica subjacente, passível de tratamento.
• Iniciar a avaliação da dor pela identificação, anamnese e exame físico do animal. Em seguida, o comportamento do animal é observado a distância e, depois, avaliado durante a interação humana. Por fim, efetua-se uma palpação delicada da região de interesse do corpo, se necessária, para determinar a resposta do animal.
• Ao se administrar analgésicos, o processo deve ser repetido periodicamente para avaliar a eficácia. Não se deve assumir que a administração de um analgésico resulte no alívio aceitável da dor.
• A supressão completa da dor pode não ser possível nem desejável se a administração do analgésico resultar em efeitos adversos excessivos. A terapia deve ter como objetivo tornar a dor tolerável.

TRATAMENTO
CUIDADO(S) DE SAÚDE ADEQUADO(S)
• A seleção de analgésico e anestésico depende da espécie, da intensidade da dor e da causa subjacente.
• Tratar a causa subjacente ao mesmo tempo, se possível.
• Acupuntura e manipulação física (massagem, manipulação dos pontos deflagradores, quiroprática) podem ser modalidades terapêuticas adjuvantes para certos tipos de condições.
• Se a qualidade de vida do paciente não for aceitável, a realização de eutanásia poderá ser a opção mais humanitária.

CUIDADO(S) DE ENFERMAGEM
• Boas práticas gerais de enfermagem.
• Tratamentos não farmacológicos, incluindo bandagem e hidroterapia, podem ser apropriados.

ATIVIDADE
• A medicina de reabilitação é um adjuvante útil para algumas condições dolorosas.
• Repouso em gaiola ou restrição da atividade podem ser valiosos para alguns tipos de problemas.

DIETA
• Mudanças na dieta para ajudar no tratamento da condição subjacente (p. ex., redução do peso na displasia coxofemoral) podem ser benéficas.
• Muitos suplementos e nutracêuticos são comercializados, pois há alegações de que esses agentes exercem efeitos benéficos sobre a cartilagem articular.
• Muitas rações veterinárias comerciais estão disponíveis no mercado para cães com osteoartrite.

ORIENTAÇÃO AO PROPRIETÁRIO
• Quando a medicação para a dor é prescrita, instruir o proprietário sobre os pontos aos quais ele deverá prestar atenção para um tratamento eficaz, bem como os efeitos adversos.
• Informar ao proprietário que a eficiência analgésica varia, podendo haver a necessidade de experimentar diversos medicamentos antes de se encontrar o tratamento eficaz.
• O proprietário também deve participar da avaliação da dor, especialmente a dor crônica. O uso de escalas simplificadas de classificação, como a Oxford Pain Chart [Tabela de Dor da Universidade de Oxford], pode auxiliar na comprovação da eficácia do tratamento.

DOR AGUDA, CRÔNICA E PÓS-OPERATÓRIA

CONSIDERAÇÕES CIRÚRGICAS
• O tratamento cirúrgico da condição subjacente indutora da dor pode ser a melhor modalidade terapêutica.
• Ruptura cirúrgica de nervos (neurectomia) para interromper a transmissão da dor nem sempre é associada a resultados positivos e pode resultar em piora da condição dolorosa.

MEDICAÇÕES

MEDICAMENTO(S) DE ESCOLHA (VER APÊNDICE VIII)
• Opioides, isolados ou combinados com outras classes de medicamentos, como sedativos/tranquilizantes ou AINE, são amplamente utilizados para o tratamento da dor pós-operatória aguda. Agonistas totais do receptor opioide µ, como a morfina, a hidromorfona e a fentanila, costumam ser eficazes para dor moderada a grave. Medicamentos agonistas parciais ou agonistas-antagonistas, como a buprenorfina e o butorfanol, ficam, em geral, reservados para dor leve a moderada. Os opioides geralmente apresentam baixa biodisponibilidade por via oral e, por essa razão, as doses orais devem ser ajustadas de acordo. Agonistas totais do receptor opioide µ podem ser utilizados com segurança nos gatos. Entretanto, as doses são normalmente reduzidas com relação às doses para os cães. Caso ocorra o aparecimento de disforia, a tranquilização com α_2-agonista ou acepromazina pode ser eficaz.
• AINE são usados mais comumente no tratamento crônico de condições dolorosas nos cães. Em geral, os AINE mais recentes são mais seguros quando administrados de forma crônica, porém os efeitos colaterais gastrintestinais e renais ainda são possíveis. A melhor estratégia parece ser reduzir a dose para a dosagem mais baixa, porém eficaz, em cada animal. Se a administração crônica for prevista, os exames de bioquímica sérica deverão ser considerados para monitorizar a ocorrência de efeitos adversos hepáticos e renais.
• A segurança e a eficácia da maior parte dos AINE não foram bem demonstradas nos gatos e, por isso, o uso desses agentes a longo prazo pode ser limitado nessa espécie.
• O tratamento de dor neuropática (dor originária de dentro do sistema nervoso) é uma subcategoria da dor patológica. A dor neuropática pode se originar de massas cerebrais ou espinais, lesões (como em casos de discopatia intervertebral), processos inflamatórios ou estímulo repetitivo do sistema de transmissão da dor por lesão crônica fora do sistema nervoso. Os sinais clássicos que acompanham a dor neuropática são a alodinia e a hiperalgesia. A dor neuropática nem sempre responde de forma satisfatória aos analgésicos tradicionais, como AINE e opioides, embora esses medicamentos geralmente sejam tentados no início (exceto para os AINE quando a intervenção neurocirúrgica é iminente). Os antidepressivos tricíclicos, os anticonvulsivantes, os antagonistas dos receptores NMDA e outras terapias alternativas (complementares) podem ser eficazes. A maior parte desses tratamentos requer o uso de medicações da medicina humana fora da indicação da bula.

CONTRAINDICAÇÕES
• Os opioides podem estar associados à depressão respiratória grave em pacientes humanos, mas a grande maioria dos cães e gatos apresenta apenas uma depressão respiratória mínima. Nos pacientes com comprometimento respiratório grave ou hipertensão intracraniana, os opioides podem estar contraindicados. A maioria dos agonistas dos receptores opioides µ também pode alterar a motilidade dos tratos gastrintestinal e urinário, resultando em constipação, retenção urinária e vômito.
• Os AINE podem provocar ulceração gastrintestinal, hepatopatias e comprometimento da função renal. Doença gastrintestinal, hepática ou renal preexistente pode ser contraindicação para o uso desses agentes. Terapia concomitante com glicocorticoide, estresse grave ou anorexia podem predispor muitos animais a efeitos colaterais. Os AINE que inibem de modo significativo a ciclo-oxigenase (COX-1) também podem alterar a função plaquetária e resultar em hemorragia ou tempos de sangramento prolongados. O paracetamol ou analgésicos que o contenham não devem ser utilizados nos gatos.

PRECAUÇÕES
• Monitorizar cuidadosamente os pacientes quanto aos efeitos adversos e à eficácia clínica após a administração de medicamentos analgésicos.
• Há relatos de hipertermia induzida por opioides em pacientes felinos, mais comumente após a aplicação de emplastros de fentanila ou a administração de hidromorfona.
• A administração de opioides pode resultar em alteração da motilidade gastrintestinal (constipação), inapetência e retenção urinária. Esses sinais costumam aparecer logo após o início da terapia com opioide e devem desaparecer dentro de 12-36 h do término da administração desses agentes. Nesse ínterim, pode haver a necessidade de cuidados de suporte, como a passagem de cateter urinário.

INTERAÇÕES POSSÍVEIS
• Os opioides podem reduzir as necessidades anestésicas da maior parte das espécies, sobretudo quando combinados com α_2-agonistas ou acepromazina como pré-medicação antes da anestesia. Em seres humanos, a combinação de certos opioides com antidepressivos pode resultar em toxicidade serotoninérgica; os antidepressivos (p. ex., L-deprenil, amitriptilina, trazodona) são ocasionalmente receitados aos pacientes veterinários e, nesse caso, a interação com opioides é possível.

DOR AGUDA, CRÔNICA E PÓS-OPERATÓRIA

- A terapia concomitante com glicocorticoide pode aumentar a toxicidade dos AINE.
- Outros medicamentos que predispõem os animais a comprometimento gastrintestinal ou renal, como os antimicrobianos aminoglicosídeos, devem ser utilizados com cautela quando os AINE também estão sendo administrados.

MEDICAMENTO(S) ALTERNATIVO(S)
- Medicamentos analgésicos adjuvantes (p. ex., gabapentina, amantadina, amitriptilina) podem ser benéficos para os pacientes com alterações do processamento neurológico após doença crônica ou lesão do sistema nervoso. Para selecionar e administrar algum analgésico adjuvante de forma adequada, o veterinário deverá ter conhecimento sobre a farmacologia clínica do medicamento. Portanto, são necessárias as informações a seguir a respeito do agente terapêutico: (1) indicação aprovada, (2) indicação não aprovada (p. ex., como analgésico) amplamente aceita na prática médica veterinária, (3) efeitos colaterais comuns e efeitos adversos potencialmente graves, (4) características farmacocinéticas e (5) diretrizes posológicas específicas para dor (ver Apêndice VIII).
- Tratamentos clínicos não tradicionais são comuns, porém devem ser avaliados em termos de segurança e eficácia antes da recomendação e do uso.
- Há pouco tempo, a medicina regenerativa (i. e., terapia de células-tronco) se tornou mais comum. Dois tipos são populares: células-tronco mesenquimais derivadas do tecido adiposo e células-tronco derivadas da medula óssea. Ambos são usados para o tratamento de osteoartrite crônica em cães e cavalos. Outros usos também estão sendo investigados. A eficácia com muitas terapias para condições crônicas parece ser imprevisível, mas os resultados podem mudar a vida em um pequeno número de pacientes.

ACOMPANHAMENTO
MONITORIZAÇÃO DO PACIENTE
- Deve ser realizada uma avaliação frequente da eficácia dos medicamentos analgésicos.
- Os pacientes submetidos à medicação analgésica de forma crônica, sobretudo os AINE, devem ser periodicamente avaliados para monitorizar as funções gastrintestinal, hepática e renal.
- É da responsabilidade do veterinário garantir que as informações sobre os efeitos das medicações prescritas sejam divulgadas aos proprietários.

PREVENÇÃO
Embora algum grau de dor geralmente seja uma consequência inevitável de cirurgia ou traumatismo, a administração preemptiva** (prévia) dos medicamentos analgésicos pode conferir um melhor controle da dor e diminuir a potencialização da dor pelo sistema nervoso central, sempre que possível. A utilização de técnicas anestésicas adequadas, incorporando pré-medicações analgésicas, e técnicas analgésicas locais e regionais quando apropriadas, é a forma mais eficaz de praticar a analgesia preemptiva.

EVOLUÇÃO ESPERADA E PROGNÓSTICO
A dor aguda associada a cirurgia ou traumatismo costuma desaparecer com a cicatrização do tecido. Os opioides podem ser mais eficazes nas 12-24 h após a cirurgia, enquanto os AINE podem ser mais eficientes após esse período. Alguns AINE são analgésicos eficazes quando administrados imediatamente após a cirurgia. Quando os sinais de dor persistem além da evolução normal de alguns dias a semanas, suspeitar de doença persistente, lesão ou alterações no sistema nervoso central e consultar um anestesiologista ou especialista com experiência no controle da dor em busca de sugestões acerca do tratamento apropriado.

DIVERSOS
GESTAÇÃO/FERTILIDADE/REPRODUÇÃO
- Os opioides podem provocar depressão respiratória fetal após o parto. Os AINE podem

---

** N. T.: O termo "preemptiva" implica uma forma de analgesia que, iniciada antes de o estímulo doloroso ser gerado, previne ou diminui a dor subsequente (Fonte: Revista Brasileira de Anestesiologia).

alterar a produção materna ou fetal de prostaglandina, resultando em complicações na gestação.
- Os efeitos de muitos dos medicamentos analgésicos aprovados para uso em cães e gatos sobre o feto não estão amplamente relatados.

ABREVIATURA(S)
- AINE = anti-inflamatórios não esteroides.
- NMDA = N-metil-D-aspartato.
- RM = ressonância magnética.
- TC = tomografia computadorizada.

RECURSOS DA INTERNET
- Trabalho sobre a posição dos anestesiologistas do American College of Veterinary sobre o controle da dor: http://www.acva.org/professional/Position/pain.htm.
- International Veterinary Academy of Pain Management: http://www.ivapm.org.

Sugestões de Leitura
AAHA/AAFP Pain Management Guidelines Task Force Members, Peter Hellyer, Ilona Rodan, Jane Brunt, Robin Downing, James E. Hagedorn, and Sheilah Ann Robertson. AAHA/AAFP Pain Management Guidelines for Dogs & Cats. JAAHA 2007, 43:235-248.
Gaynor JS, Muir III, WW, eds. Veterinary Pain Management, 2nd ed. St. Louis: Mosby, 2009.
Mathews K. Pain assessment and management in dogs and cats. In: Mathews K, ed., Veterinary Emergency and Critical Care, 2nd ed. Guelph, Ontario: Lifelearn, 2006, pp. 117-123.
Mathews KA, ed. Update on management of pain. Vet Clin North Am Small Anim Pract 2008.
Tranquilli WJ, Thurmon JC, Grimm KA, eds. Lumb and Jones Veterinary Anesthesia and Analgesia, 4th ed. Ames, IA: Blackwell, 2007.

Autores Leigh A. Lamont, Kurt A. Grimm e William J. Tranquilli
Consultor Editorial Joane M. Parent

DOR NO PESCOÇO E NO DORSO

CONSIDERAÇÕES GERAIS

DEFINIÇÃO
Desconforto ao longo da coluna vertebral.

FISIOPATOLOGIA
Causada por inúmeras doenças neurológicas ou não neurológicas (p. ex., poliartrite). Secundária à estimulação de nociceptores localizados nas meninges, nas raízes nervosas, nos nervos espinais, nas vértebras e estruturas associadas (p. ex., periósteo, cápsulas articulares), bem como na musculatura epaxial. Uma doença intracraniana pode desenvolver dor cervical referida quando a pressão intracraniana estiver elevada.

SISTEMA(S) ACOMETIDO(S)
• Nervoso. • Neuromuscular. • Musculosquelético.

IDENTIFICAÇÃO
Espécies
• Cães e gatos.

Raça(s) Predominante(s)
• Discopatia intervertebral — cães; tipo 1 em raças condrodistróficas e tipo 2 em raças de grande porte. Incomum nos gatos. • Espondilomielopatia cervical — Doberman, Dinamarquês, Rottweiler, Dálmata. • Subluxação atlantoaxial — raças caninas pequenas e miniaturas (p. ex., Yorkshire terrier). • Meningite-arterite responsivas a esteroides — Montanhês de Berna, Boxer, Beagle. • Síndrome de má-formação occipital caudal — Cavalier King Charles spaniel. • Polimiosite imunomediada — Terra Nova, Boxer.

Idade Média e Faixa Etária
• Discopatia intervertebral tipo 1 — incomum com menos de 2 anos de idade, pico entre 3 e 8 anos de idade. • Discopatia intervertebral tipo 2 — >5 anos. • Espondilomielopatia cervical (síndrome de Wobbler) — cães de meia-idade a idosos da raça Doberman (média: 6 anos), cães jovens da raça Dinamarquês (<3 anos). • Subluxação atlantoaxial — cães jovens aos de meia-idade. • Meningite-arterite responsivas a esteroides — <2 anos (8-18 meses).

SINAIS CLÍNICOS
Achados Anamnésicos
Queixa principal — relaciona-se com o desconforto percebido; p. ex., vocalização, atividade diminuída, relutância em se levantar ou deitar, relutância em descer ou subir escadas, incapacidade de beber ou comer nas tigelas colocadas no chão (por conta da dor cervical). Além disso, a dor no pescoço pode ser intermitente.

Achados do Exame Físico
• Condução anormal do pescoço, relutância em movimentar a cabeça, postura cervical rígida.
• Dorso arqueado (cifose).
• Dor à palpação da coluna vertebral e/ou manipulação do pescoço.
• Rigidez abdominal (referida a partir da dor no dorso).
• Aumento no tônus da musculatura epaxial.
• Espasmos intermitentes dos músculos do pescoço.
• Relutância em caminhar, marcha afetada e forçada, rigidez dos membros, passos curtos e cautelosos.
• Claudicação sem sustentação do peso (sinal de compressão de raiz nervosa).
• Sinais autonômicos (p. ex., taquicardia, dilatação pupilar).
• Possíveis déficits neurológicos (p. ex., paresia, ataxia).
• Pirexia (meningite-arterite responsivas a esteroides, doenças infecciosas).

CAUSAS
Degenerativas
• Discopatia intervertebral — causa mais comum de dor espinal em cães.
• Espondilomielopatia cervical (síndrome de Wobbler).
• Cistos sinoviais espinais.
• Hipertrofia de faceta vertebral.
• Calcinose circunscrita.
• Espondilose deformante, ossificação dural (geralmente assintomática).

Anômalas/Evolutivas (desenvolvimento)
• Subluxação atlantoaxial.
• Síndrome de má-formação occipital caudal e siringomielia.
• Más-formações vertebrais: p. ex., hemivértebra (geralmente assintomática).
• Osteocondromatose.
• Seio dermoide.

Neoplásicas
• Neoplasia da coluna vertebral (o tipo intramedular é raramente doloroso), de raiz nervosa-nervo periférico (p. ex., tumor da bainha de nervos periféricos) e de músculo.
• Tumores intracranianos com PIC elevada secundária (dor cervical referida).

Nutricionais
• Hipervitaminose A felina.

Inflamatórias
• Discospondilite, osteomielite vertebral, fisite.
• Meningite-meningomielite infecciosa — viral (p. ex., PIF), bacteriana, riquetsial, fúngica, protozoária, parasitária ou por algas.
• Meningite-meningomielite não infecciosa — p. ex., meningite-arterite responsivas a esteroides, meningoencefalomielite granulomatosa.
• Empiema epidural espinal.
• Abscesso paraspinal.
• Poliartrite — imunomediada, infecciosa.
• Polimiosite — polimiosite imunomediada, infecciosa, rabdomiólise por exercício.

Idiopáticas
• Cisto subaracnoide (raramente doloroso).

Traumáticas
• Fratura e/ou luxação da coluna vertebral.
• Hérnia de disco traumática.

Vasculares
• Hemorragia espinal (extramedular).

FATORES DE RISCO
• Raças — condrodistróficas (discopatia intervertebral).
• Traumatismo.
• Procedimento cirúrgico prévio (discospondilite, subluxação).
• Neoplasia maligna.
• Ferida por mordedura, corpo estranho, infecção do trato urinário, endocardite.
• Coagulopatia.
• Dieta hepática (hipervitaminose A).
• Infecção por FeLV (linfoma espinal).

DIAGNÓSTICO

DIAGNÓSTICO DIFERENCIAL
• Doença ortopédica.
• Dor abdominal (dorso).
• Mudança comportamental ou atividade mental anormal (delírio).
• PIC elevada (dor cervical referida).
• Mielopatia não dolorosa — p. ex., mielopatia degenerativa, mielopatia fibrocartilaginosa.
• Distúrbios paroxísticos.
• Síndrome de hiperestesia felina.

HEMOGRAMA/BIOQUÍMICA/URINÁLISE
• Hemograma completo geralmente normal. Podem-se observar neutrofilia (meningite-arterite responsivas a esteroides, discospondilite), trombocitopenia (riquetsiose, neoplasia maligna).
• Elevação da CK e AST — miosite, decúbito, traumatismo, anorexia (gato).
• Hiperproteinemia — neoplásica, infecciosa.
• Infecção do trato urinário — foco de discospondilite, com retenção de urina.
• Mioglobinúria — miosite.

OUTROS TESTES LABORATORIAIS
• Títulos sorológicos e PCR (sangue, LCS) para pesquisa de doenças infecciosas.
• Hemo/uroculturas — discospondilite.
• Níveis de IgA e de proteínas de fase aguda (sangue, LCS) em meningite-arterite responsivas a esteroides.
• Eletroforese de proteínas séricas.
• Perfil de coagulação.

DIAGNÓSTICO POR IMAGEM
Radiografias Simples da Coluna Vertebral
• Não são capazes de identificar compressão da medula espinal.
• Discopatia intervertebral — podem detectar espaço intervertebral estreitado e disco calcificado.
• Detectam discospondilite (radiografias normais nas primeiras 2-3 semanas).
• Neoplasias espinais — osteólise, proliferação óssea, canal vertebral mais amplo.
• Detectam fraturas, luxações (atlantoaxiais), hipertrofia de faceta articular, más-formações, calcinose circunscrita, espondilose, osteocondromatose.

Radiografia Torácica e Ultrassonografia
• Detectam neoplasias (primárias ou metastáticas), infecções disseminadas, endocardite, lesões relacionadas com traumatismo.

Mielografia
• Detecta e delineia lesões da medula espinal como extradurais, intradurais-extramedulares e intramedulares. Baixa sensibilidade na detecção de lesões paranquimatosas.

TC
• Mais sensível que as radiografias para detectar discospondilite, fraturas vertebrais, tumores ósseos. Delimita claramente as lesões ósseas, porém exibe menos contraste para tecidos moles em comparação à RM. Pode ser útil para diagnosticar discopatia intervertebral tipo 1 se o material estiver calcificado.
• Mielograma por TC — mais sensível para avaliar lesões compressivas da medula espinal.

RM
• Mais sensível que a TC para os tecidos moles. Modalidade de diagnóstico por imagem mais

Dor no Pescoço e no Dorso

recompensadora para identificar o local e a extensão de lesões parenquimatosas da medula espinal, raízes nervosas, nervos e músculos.

MÉTODOS DIAGNÓSTICOS

LCS
- Análise útil em caso de meningite/meningomielite, mas normal ou inespecífica em muitas outras situações. É rara, porém possível a detecção de células neoplásicas.
- Considerar a mensuração dos níveis de IgA, proteínas de fase aguda e títulos sorológicos, bem como a realização de PCR e cultura.

Artrocentese e Análise do Líquido Sinovial
- Poliartrite.

Eletrodiagnóstico
- EMG, estudos de condução nervosa — detectam e localizam doença neuromuscular (p. ex., polimiosite).

Aspirado Percutâneo por Agulha Fina Guiada por Fluoroscopia ou TC
- Discospondilite, neoplasias.

Biopsia
- Óssea (p. ex., neoplasia, osteomielite), muscular (p. ex., polimiosite).

TRATAMENTO

CUIDADO(S) DE SAÚDE ADEQUADO(S)
- Internação — em casos de sinais clínicos graves, exigência do tratamento ou impossibilidade de repouso em gaiola. Fornecer cuidados intensivos de emergência em casos de dor intensa ou déficit neurológico grave.
- Ambulatorial — quando se busca o tratamento conservador (nesse caso, pode ser justificável a restrição do exercício).
- Cirurgia de emergência — em caso de instabilidade espinal traumática ou déficit neurológico grave (paraparesia não deambulatória, tetraplegia) em virtude de compressão aguda da medula espinal.

CUIDADO(S) DE ENFERMAGEM
- Pacientes não deambulatórios — fornecer cama macia e alternar o lado de decúbito.
- Instabilidade vertebral — ter extremo cuidado à manipulação para evitar exacerbação da lesão.

ATIVIDADE
Restringir o exercício por, no mínimo, 3-4 semanas em pacientes submetidos a tratamento clínico.

DIETA
Modificar a dieta em caso de hipervitaminose A.

ORIENTAÇÃO AO PROPRIETÁRIO
- Monitorizar a dor, a resposta ao tratamento e possíveis anormalidades da marcha. É comum a ocorrência de recidiva em muitas doenças.
- A causa mais comum de dor espinal em cães é a discopatia intervertebral. Esclarecer a necessidade de restrição da atividade física e de confinamento em gaiola por 3-4 semanas quando se buscar por tratamento clínico; é frequente a recidiva. Se a dor persistir ou o estado neurológico se deteriorar, o tratamento cirúrgico será recomendado, até mesmo como um procedimento de emergência.

CONSIDERAÇÕES CIRÚRGICAS
Variam de acordo com a doença. Em geral, a percepção de dor profunda é considerada o indicador prognóstico mais importante quanto à recuperação funcional em doença neurológica. A correção de subluxação atlantoaxial é associada a altos índices de morbidade e mortalidade perioperatórias.

MEDICAÇÕES

MEDICAMENTO(S) DE ESCOLHA
- Opioides — tramadol (1-5 mg/kg a cada 6-12 h VO, cão), morfina (0,1-1,0 mg/kg a cada 4 h, cão), hidromorfona (0,05-0,2 mg/kg a cada 4 h, cão), fentanila (emplastro transdérmico). • Glicocorticoides — prednisona a 0,5-1 mg/kg a cada 24 h (cão) em doses decrescentes. O uso de glicocorticoides em traumatismo agudo da medula espinal é controverso. O tratamento clínico de discopatia intervertebral aguda deve se concentrar no confinamento em gaiola. Há necessidade de doses mais altas (2-4 mg/kg a cada 24 h) em casos de doença imunomediada. • AINEs — potencialmente mais eficazes em discopatia intervertebral cervical aguda. Meloxicam (0,1 mg/kg a cada 24 h, cão), carprofeno (2,2 mg/kg a cada 12 h, cão). • Gabapentina a 10-15 mg/kg a cada 8 h VO, cão; dor neuropática crônica (siringomielia, doença radicular nervosa). • De acordo com a doença — antimicrobianos (p. ex., discospondilite), medicamentos imunossupressores, quimioterapia (neoplasias).

CONTRAINDICAÇÕES
- Glicocorticoides, agentes imunossupressores — contraindicados em infecções. • Opioides — contraindicados em diarreia causada por ingestão de substâncias tóxicas e nos casos de obstrução gastrintestinal.

PRECAUÇÕES
- A administração concomitante de AINEs e glicocorticoides é fortemente contraindicada. • Glicocorticoides e AINEs — podem causar ulceração/hemorragia gastrintestinais. • Glicocorticoides — podem causar infecção do trato urinário. • Instabilidade vertebral ou discopatia intervertebral — é obrigatório o repouso estrito em gaiola enquanto o paciente está sendo submetido a agentes anti-inflamatórios e analgésicos; o aumento da atividade física pode exacerbar o problema. • Opioides — tomar cuidado na presença de disfunção respiratória, PIC elevada, depressão do SNC e bradiarritmias. • Gabapentina — ter cautela se houver insuficiência renal.

INTERAÇÕES POSSÍVEIS
- Opioides — aumento na depressão neurológica (SNC) e respiratória quando combinados com outros depressores do SNC. • Gabapentina — antiácidos orais podem diminuir 20% da biodisponibilidade oral.

MEDICAMENTO(S) ALTERNATIVO(S)
- Antagonistas dos receptores NMDA (p. ex., cetamina) — analgésicos. • Pregabalina, antidepressivos tricíclicos — dor neuropática crônica. • Furosemida — para síndrome de má-formação occipital caudal/siringomielia. • Azatioprina, ciclosporina — para frear doenças imunomediadas. • Relaxantes musculares — benzodiazepínicos, metocarbamol (podem ser prejudiciais se houver instabilidade da coluna vertebral).

ACOMPANHAMENTO

MONITORIZAÇÃO DO PACIENTE
- A monitorização é feita principalmente com base nos sinais clínicos e na resposta terapêutica. Em princípio, deve-se monitorizar o animal, pelo menos, uma vez por semana. Na presença de dor intensa aguda e/ou déficit neurológico, é recomendável a internação ou a monitorização diária. Fazer ajustes ou considerar a realização de cirurgia quando o tratamento clínico não for eficaz.
- Análise do LCS (p. ex., meningite-arterite responsivas a esteroides), radiografias da coluna vertebral (p. ex., discospondilite), níveis de proteínas de fase aguda, exame de sangue/radiografias torácicas/ultrassonografia (p. ex., neoplasias, doenças infecciosas).

PREVENÇÃO
Evitar atividade excessiva, saltos/pulos, subida e descida de escadas, bem como excesso de peso. Evitar também o uso de coleiras cervicais.

COMPLICAÇÕES POSSÍVEIS
- Recidivas ou deterioração. O tratamento cirúrgico pode ser recomendado em um esquema de emergência de acordo com a doença.
- Dor irresponsiva crônica.
- Disfunção neurológica permanente.
- Disseminação para outros locais, fratura/luxação vertebrais patológicas (discospondilite, neoplasias).
- Artropatia degenerativa (poliartrite).

EVOLUÇÃO ESPERADA E PROGNÓSTICO
- Varia com a doença, a gravidade dos sinais clínicos e o déficit neurológico.
- Discopatia intervertebral tipo 1 — o êxito com o tratamento clínico em cães que apresentam dor ou déficits brandos apenas gira em torno de 50%.

DIVERSOS

DISTÚRBIOS ASSOCIADOS
- Poliartrite imunomediada não erosiva e meningite-arterite responsivas a esteroides.
- Discospondilite e infecção do trato urinário.
- FeLV e linfoma espinal felino. • Polimiosite e linfoma. • Polimiopatias/miosite — megaesôfago/disfagia e pneumonia por aspiração.

ABREVIATURA(S)
- AINEs = anti-inflamatórios não esteroides.
- AST = aspartato aminotransferase. • CK = creatina quinase. • EMG = eletromiografia. • FeLV = vírus da leucemia felina. • LCS = líquido cerebrospinal. • NMDA = N-metil-D-aspartato. • PCR = reação em cadeia da polimerase. • PIC = pressão intracraniana. • PIF = peritonite infecciosa felina. • RM = ressonância magnética. • SNC = sistema nervoso central. • TC = tomografia computadorizada.

Sugestões de Leitura
Dewey CW. A Practical Guide to Canine and Feline Neurology, 2nd ed. Ames, IA: Wiley-Blackwell, 2008.

Autor Luis Gaitero
Consultor Editorial Joane M. Parent

ECLÂMPSIA

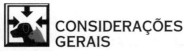

CONSIDERAÇÕES GERAIS

REVISÃO
- Hipocalcemia pós-parto.
- Costuma se desenvolver 1-4 semanas após o parto; pode ocorrer na gestação a termo, no pré-parto ou no final da lactação.
- Altera os potenciais de membrana celular, gerando uma descarga espontânea das fibras nervosas e uma contração tônico-clônica da musculatura esquelética.
- Exibe tetania e convulsões potencialmente letais, que levam a hipertermia.
- É possível o desenvolvimento de edema cerebral.

IDENTIFICAÇÃO
- Cães — cadela no pós-parto; mais comum em raças toy; incidência mais alta com a primeira ninhada.
- Mais comum antes do dia 40 pós-parto; ocasionalmente, ocorre antes do parto.
- Raças sob alto risco: Chihuahua, Pinscher miniatura, Shih tzu, Poodle miniatura, Pelado mexicano, Pomerânia.
- Gatos — rara.

SINAIS CLÍNICOS
Achados Anamnésicos
- Cuidado materno deficiente.
- Inquietação, nervosismo.
- Respiração ofegante, choro.
- Vômito, diarreia.
- Ataxia, marcha rígida.
- Prurido facial.
- Tremores musculares, tetania, convulsões.
- Decúbito, rigidez extensora — observados geralmente 8-12 h após o início dos sinais clínicos.

Achados do Exame Físico
- Hipertermia.
- Frequência respiratória acelerada.
- Pupilas dilatadas, respostas pupilares luminosas lentas.
- Tremores musculares, rigidez muscular, convulsões.

CAUSAS E FATORES DE RISCO
- Suplementação de cálcio durante a prenhez.
- Relação inadequada de Ca:P na dieta gestacional.
- Proporção baixa entre peso corporal: tamanho da ninhada.
- Nutrição pré-natal deficiente.
- Primeira ninhada.

DIAGNÓSTICO

DIAGNÓSTICO DIFERENCIAL
- Hipoglicemia — pode ser um achado concomitante; não ocorre rigidez muscular somente com a hipoglicemia.
- Toxicose — distinguida por meio da identificação e da anamnese.
- Epilepsia ou outro distúrbio neurológico — diferenciados por meio da identificação; a concentração de cálcio é diagnóstica.

HEMOGRAMA/BIOQUÍMICA/URINÁLISE
- Cálcio sérico total <7 mg/dL.
- Embora o cálcio ionizado (<2,4-3,2 mg/dL) seja a forma relevante da função neuromuscular normal, a mensuração do cálcio sérico total é suficiente para o diagnóstico.
- Hipoglicemia — pode ser um achado concomitante.
- Relata-se hipomagnesemia em 44% das cadelas acometidas; essa anormalidade pode promover tetania.
- Nível sérico elevado de potássio em 56% dos casos, em virtude de acidose metabólica ou alcalose respiratória.

DIAGNÓSTICO POR IMAGEM
N/D.

OUTROS TESTES LABORATORIAIS
N/D.

MÉTODOS DIAGNÓSTICOS
O ECG revela intervalo QT prolongado, bradicardia, taquicardia ou contrações ventriculares prematuras.

TRATAMENTO
- Internação de emergência.
- Hipertermia — resfriar o animal com embebição em água fresca e ventiladores; é preciso ter cautela com enemas de água fresca.
- Filhotes caninos — afastá-los da mãe e criá-los manualmente; se isso for impossível ou indesejável em função da necessidade comportamental de contato com a mãe, afastá-los por 24 h ou até a estabilização do cálcio sérico e fornecer a suplementação pelo resto da lactação; continuar a monitorização do nível sérico de cálcio.

MEDICAÇÕES

MEDICAMENTO(S)
- Gliconato de cálcio — administração IV lenta de 0,5-1,50 mL/kg de solução a 10% até se obter o efeito por 5 min; monitorizar a frequência cardíaca ou o ECG durante a aplicação; pode-se fornecer um medicamento extra por via intramuscular ou subcutânea.
- Corrigir a hipoglicemia.
- Diazepam — 5 mg IV; em casos de crises convulsivas irresponsivas.
- Edema cerebral — tratar, se for indicado.
- Lactato, carbonato ou gliconato de cálcio — 30-100 mg/kg/dia VO até o término da lactação.
- A suplementação com magnésio pode ser útil em cadelas hipomagnesêmicas.

CONTRAINDICAÇÕES/INTERAÇÕES POSSÍVEIS
Corticosteroides — evitar, pois causam diminuição na absorção intestinal e aumento na excreção renal de cálcio.

ACOMPANHAMENTO

MONITORIZAÇÃO DO PACIENTE
- Concentração sérica de cálcio — monitorizar até a estabilização dentro dos limites de normalidade.
- Evitar a suplementação de cálcio durante a prenhez.
- Dieta — materna: garantir a relação cálcio:fósforo de 1:1 ou 1,2:1; evitar os alimentos ricos em fitatos (p. ex., soja); filhotes caninos: suplementar a alimentação em ninhadas grandes.

COMPLICAÇÕES POSSÍVEIS
- Edema cerebral.
- Óbito.
- Criação manual dos filhotes caninos.

EVOLUÇÃO ESPERADA E PROGNÓSTICO
- É provável a recidiva em ninhadas subsequentes.
- Prognóstico — bom em casos de tratamento imediato; mau em casos de tratamento tardio.

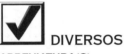

DIVERSOS

ABREVIATURA(S)
- ECG = eletrocardiograma.

Sugestões de Leitura
Aroch I, Srebro H, Shpigel NY. Serum electrolyte concentration in bitches with eclampsia. Vet Record 1999, 145:318-320.
Drobatz KJ, Casey KK. Eclampsia in dogs: 31 cases (1995-1998). JAVMA 2000, 217(2):216-219.
Johnston SD, Kustritz MVR, Olson PN. Periparturient disorders in the bitch. In: Johnston SD, Kustritz MVR, Olson PN, eds., Canine and Feline Theriogenology. Philadelphia: Saunders, 2001, pp. 129-145.

Autor Joni L. Freshman
Consultor Editorial Sara K. Lyle

ECTRÓPIO

CONSIDERAÇÕES GERAIS

REVISÃO
- Eversão ou movimento para fora da margem da pálpebra, resultando em exposição da conjuntiva palpebral.
- Exposição e distribuição lacrimal deficiente — podem predispor o paciente à doença de córnea com risco de perda da visão.

IDENTIFICAÇÃO
- Cães e, raramente, gatos.
- Raças com prevalência mais alta do que a média — raças esportivas (p. ex., Spaniel, Hound e Retriever); raças gigantes (p. ex., São Bernardo e Mastife); qualquer raça com pele facial frouxa (especialmente o Bloodhound).
- Evolutivo — predisposição genética nas raças listadas; pode ocorrer em cães com <1 ano de idade.
- Adquirido — observado em outras raças; ocorre em uma fase tardia da vida, secundariamente à perda da musculatura facial e ao desenvolvimento de frouxidão cutânea relacionados com a idade.
- Intermitente — causado por fadiga; pode ser observado após exercício vigoroso ou quando o animal se encontra sonolento ou inativo.

SINAIS CLÍNICOS
- Eversão da pálpebra inferior com falta de contato dessa pálpebra com o bulbo ocular e exposição da conjuntiva palpebral e da terceira pálpebra — costumam ser evidentes.
- Mancha facial causada por drenagem lacrimal deficiente — as lágrimas rolam pela face em vez de passarem do olho para o nariz via ductos nasolacrimais.
- Histórico de secreção mucoide a mucopurulenta decorrente da exposição conjuntival.
- Irritação recidivante por corpo estranho.
- Histórico de conjuntivite bacteriana.

CAUSAS E FATORES DE RISCO
- Geralmente secundário a alterações associadas às raças na conformação facial e na sustentação palpebral.
- Perda de peso acentuada ou perda de massa muscular na cabeça e em torno da órbita — podem resultar em doença adquirida.
- Expressão facial trágica (do latim *facies tragica*) em cães hipotireóideos.
- Formação de cicatriz nas pálpebras, secundária à lesão ou à correção excessiva de entrópio — podem resultar em doença cicatricial.

DIAGNÓSTICO

DIAGNÓSTICO DIFERENCIAL
- Em geral, é evidente do ponto de vista clínico.
- Procurar por qualquer distúrbio subjacente em raças não predispostas e pacientes em idade de início tardia.
- Perda de massa orbital ou periorbital — pode causar a condição em pacientes com miosite dos músculos da mastigação.
- Paralisia do nervo palpebral — distúrbio associado à falta de tônus muscular nos músculos orbiculares do olho.

HEMOGRAMA/BIOQUÍMICA/URINÁLISE
N/D.

OUTROS TESTES LABORATORIAIS
- Possível miosite dos músculos da mastigação — teste em busca de autoanticorpos contra as fibras musculares do tipo 2M.
- Paralisia do nervo palpebral ou expressão facial trágica — considerar a realização de testes quanto à presença de hipotireoidismo.

DIAGNÓSTICO POR IMAGEM
N/D.

MÉTODOS DIAGNÓSTICOS
- Paralisia do nervo palpebral — avaliação neurológica completa; potencial em casos de hipotireoidismo.
- Conjuntivite secundária — considerar os exames de cultura bacteriana ou citologia para ajudar a selecionar o antibiótico tópico apropriado.
- Coloração da córnea e da conjuntiva com o uso de fluoresceína ou rosa-bengala — pode registrar ulcerações de córneas; pode revelar a gravidade do problema de exposição.

TRATAMENTO

- Cuidados de suporte (pomadas antibióticas ou lubrificantes tópicas) e boa higiene oculofacial — são suficientes em grande parte das doenças leves.
- Tratamento cirúrgico — encurtamento palpebral ou cirurgia plástica facial radical para a remoção de dobras ou pregas cutâneas; necessário para os pacientes gravemente acometidos que tenham irritação ocular crônica.
- Condição intermitente induzida por fadiga — não tratar por meio cirúrgico.

MEDICAÇÕES

MEDICAMENTO(S)
- Antibióticos oftálmicos tópicos de amplo espectro — conjuntivite bacteriana ou ulceração corneana. Neomicina/polimixina B/bacitracina (ou outros selecionados com base nos resultados de cultura e antibiograma) a cada 6-8 h.
- Colírios ou pomadas lubrificantes — diminuem os ressecamentos conjuntival e corneano, secundários à exposição.
- Condições induzidas por hipotireoidismo e miosite dos músculos da mastigação — podem responder de forma satisfatória ao tratamento clínico adequado da doença subjacente.

CONTRAINDICAÇÕES/INTERAÇÕES POSSÍVEIS
N/D.

ACOMPANHAMENTO

- Pode ficar mais grave à medida que o paciente envelhece.
- Paciente tratado sem cirurgia — monitorizar quanto à presença de sinais de conjuntivite infecciosa, ceratopatia por exposição, ulceração de córnea e dermatite facial.

DIVERSOS

DISTÚRBIOS ASSOCIADOS
- Hipotireoidismo.
- Miosite Inflamatória Focal — Miosite dos Músculos da Mastigação e Miosite dos Músculos Extraoculares.

FATORES RELACIONADOS COM A IDADE
É mais provável que os animais idosos sofram ectrópio secundariamente à perda do tônus muscular facial.

VER TAMBÉM
- Hipotireoidismo.
- Miopatia Inflamatória Focal — Miosite dos Músculos da Mastigação e Miosite dos Músculos Extraoculares.

Sugestões de Leitura
Stades FC, Gelatt KN. Diseases and surgery of the canine eyelid. In: Gelatt KN, ed., Veterinary Ophthalmology, 4th ed. Ames, IA: Blackwell, 2007, pp. 583-594.

Autor J. Phillip Pickett
Consultor Editorial Paul E. Miller

EDEMA PERIFÉRICO

CONSIDERAÇÕES GERAIS

DEFINIÇÃO
Edema consiste no acúmulo focal ou difuso excessivo de líquido tecidual dentro do interstício; frequente em superfícies gravitacionais, se localizado ou generalizado.

FISIOPATOLOGIA
- Pressão hidrostática capilar elevada.
- Permeabilidade capilar aumentada.
- Anormalidade da drenagem linfática.
- Baixa pressão coloidosmótica plasmática.

SISTEMA(S) ACOMETIDO(S)
- Pele/exócrino.
- Musculosquelético.

GENÉTICA
- Linfedema primário predominantemente hereditário foi descrito em cães da raça Poodle.
- Edema congênito letal foi comprovado em cães de raça Buldogue.

INCIDÊNCIA/PREVALÊNCIA
Variáveis.

DISTRIBUIÇÃO GEOGRÁFICA
Pertinente ao se considerar os mecanismos de doenças infecciosas.

IDENTIFICAÇÃO
Espécies
Cães e gatos.

Raça(s) Predominante(s)
Linfedema primário ou congênito foi relatado em cães das raças Buldogue, Poodle, Old English sheepdog e Labrador.

SINAIS CLÍNICOS
Achados Anamnésicos
- Doença alérgica ou outra imune, cardíaca, hepática ou outra orgânica.
- Traumatismo.
- Exposição a agentes tóxicos (venenosos) ou infecciosos como os carrapatos ou outros aracnídeos.

Achados do Exame Físico
- Inicialmente, pode-se notar um ganho de peso inexplicável; por outro lado, a detecção precoce é improvável.
- Com frequência, identifica-se um edema subcutâneo não inflamatório primeiro nas regiões pendentes do tórax ou do abdome ou na parte distal dos membros.
- Edema inflamatório pode ser notado em focos não pendentes do interstício.

CAUSAS
Edema Localizado ou em um Único Membro
- Pressão hidrostática capilar elevada.
- Obstrução venosa ou arterial, por exemplo, trombose ou síndrome pós-caval.
- Fístula arteriovenosa.
- Permeabilidade capilar aumentada.
- Agressões (p. ex., mordida de cobra ou picada de abelha) focais ou multifocais imunes, infecciosas ou tóxicas (químicas ou biológicas).
- Traumatismo.
- Queimaduras.
- Obstrução linfática.
- Linfangite estéril (piodermite juvenil) ou infecciosa.
- Invasão neoplásica primária ou metastática do tecido linfático.
- Aplasia ou disgenesia congênita do sistema linfático.

Edema Regional ou Generalizado
- Pressão hidrostática capilar elevada.
- Insuficiência cardíaca congestiva (ICC).
- Tamponamento cardíaco.
- Trombose da veia cava cranial ou caudal.
- Insuficiência renal e hipernatremia (retenção de sal).
- Paralisia ou decúbito prolongado com subsequente falha da bomba venosa.
- Efeito de torniquete exercido por alguma bandagem.
- Permeabilidade capilar aumentada.
- Insultos (p. ex., sepse ou vasculite) sistêmicos imunes, infecciosos ou tóxicos.
- Anormalidades linfáticas.
- Processos regionais adquiridos traumáticos, imunes, infecciosos ou neoplásicos.
- Aplasia congênita ou outra disgenesia linfática.
- Pressão coloidosmótica plasmática baixa.
- Doença indutora de perda de proteínas (p. ex., síndrome nefrótica ou linfangiectasia intestinal).
- Falha na produção de proteínas (p. ex., cirrose).
- Perda exsudativa de proteínas (p. ex., queimadura grave).

FATORES DE RISCO
Variáveis.

DIAGNÓSTICO

DIAGNÓSTICO DIFERENCIAL
- Edema periférico secundário a mixedema ou inflamação é tipicamente não depressível.
- Edema bilateral dos membros torácicos com distensão venosa jugular implica síndrome da veia cava cranial.
- Edema bilateral dos membros pélvicos com ou sem ascite denota hipoalbuminemia ou obstrução da veia cava caudal.
- Edema dos membros torácicos e/ou pélvicos com distensão venosa jugular, hidrotórax e/ou ascite pressupõe cardiopatia.
- Edema focal com ruído e frêmito indica fístula arteriovenosa.
- Edema focal com eritema pode ser secundário à mordida de inseto ou de outra natureza.
- Edema multifocal ou difuso com formação de petéquias e/ou equimose pode estar associado à coagulopatia ou vasculite.

HEMOGRAMA/BIOQUÍMICA/URINÁLISE
- Leucocitose sugere doença inflamatória ou infecciosa.
- Trombocitopenia pode ser secundária à vasculite (p. ex., febre maculosa das Montanhas Rochosas), lúpus eritematoso sistêmico (LES) ou coagulopatia (p. ex., CID).
- Pan-hipoproteinemia é compatível com gastrenteropatia, porém a diarreia não constitui um sinal clínico obrigatório.
- Pan-hipoproteinemia e hipocolesterolemia são observadas em caso de linfangiectasia intestinal.
- Pode ocorrer hipoalbuminemia na insuficiência hepática.
- Hipoalbuminemia com proteinúria sugere glomerulopatia.
- Hipoalbuminemia com proteinúria e hipercolesterolemia em paciente edematoso define a síndrome nefrótica.

OUTROS TESTES LABORATORIAIS
- Teste da antitrombina III é indicado em condições com perda de albumina.
- Delinear ainda mais a trombocitopenia com biopsia da medula óssea, anticorpo antinuclear (ANA), títulos para *Ehrlichia* e febre maculosa das Montanhas Rochosas, além do perfil da coagulação.
- Pan-hipoproteinemia pode determinar a necessidade de biopsia intestinal.
- Hipoalbuminemia pode justificar as provas de função hepática (p. ex., teste do ácido biliar e biopsia do fígado).
- Confirmar a presença de proteinúria com a relação de proteína:creatinina urinárias.
- Culturas bacteriana e fúngica de fístulas cegas podem ser valiosas.
- Títulos fúngicos ou outros ensaios de doenças infecciosas podem ser justificáveis; a residência primária e o histórico de viagens do paciente devem ser considerados.
- Análise do líquido pleural ou peritoneal é sugerida se houver efusão.
- Hormônio da tireoide (T_4) baixo em repouso deve ser elaborado com o teste de estimulação com o hormônio liberador da tireotropina (TRH), T_4 livre por diálise de equilíbrio, ou concentração do hormônio tireostimulante (TSH).

DIAGNÓSTICO POR IMAGEM
- A suspeita de cardiopatia necessita de radiografias torácicas e ecocardiograma.
- Angiografia (p. ex., venocavografia) pode ajudar a definir obstrução vascular.
- Ultrassom diagnóstico pode ajudar a delinear oclusão vascular.
- Termografia e varreduras de perfusão (p. ex., cintilografia) são compreensíveis apenas para poucos, porém foram utilizadas para diagnosticar vasculopatia oclusiva.

MÉTODOS DIAGNÓSTICOS
- Aspirado por agulha fina de alguma área acometida para a realização de citologia e cultura pode ser útil.
- Biopsia e cultura profunda podem ajudar a definir uma causa subjacente para o edema.

ACHADOS PATOLÓGICOS
Dependem da causa do edema.

TRATAMENTO

CUIDADO(S) DE SAÚDE ADEQUADO(S)
Dependem da causa do edema.

CUIDADO(S) DE ENFERMAGEM
- É recomendável a aplicação de compressas mornas para os pacientes com edema secundário à infecção.
- Há necessidade de bons cuidados de enfermagem para evitar a formação de úlceras de decúbito nos pacientes nessa condição.

ATIVIDADE
Depende da causa do edema — por exemplo, recomenda-se a restrição ao exercício em pacientes com insuficiência cardíaca congestiva.

DIETA
Depende da causa do edema — por exemplo, os pacientes acometidos por nefropatia com perda de

EDEMA PERIFÉRICO

proteínas necessitam de dieta com restrição proteica.

ORIENTAÇÃO AO PROPRIETÁRIO
Depende da causa do edema.

CONSIDERAÇÕES CIRÚRGICAS
• Cirurgias como linfangioplastia, trombectomia ou desvio linfaticovenoso podem ser paliativas.
• A amputação do membro edematoso, às vezes, é indicada.
• Fístulas arteriovenosas podem ser tratadas por vários métodos cirúrgicos.

MEDICAÇÕES

MEDICAMENTO(S)
• Anafilaxia — adrenalina (1 mg/mL) na dose de 0,01 mL/kg IM ou SC até, no máximo, 0,02-0,05 mL; succinato sódico de prednisona na dose de 10-30 mg/kg IV; os anti-histamínicos possuem benefício duvidoso se já houver anafilaxia.
• Linfedema — o uso da benzopirona fornece resultados variáveis na medicina veterinária; rutina, 50 mg/kg VO a cada 8 h, foi misturada ao alimento para gatos com quilotórax.
• Edema cardiogênico — combinações de agentes inotrópicos positivos ou negativos, vasodilatadores e diuréticos são comumente usadas em pacientes com ICC.
• Edema imunomediado requer terapia imunossupressora (p. ex., prednisona e ciclofosfamida).
• Vasculite e edema secundários à doença riquetsiana tipicamente respondem à tetraciclina (22 mg/kg VO a cada 8 h) ou doxiciclina (5 mg/kg VO a cada 12 h).
• Edema associado a outros agentes infecciosos necessita de terapia antifúngica ou antibioticoterapia (determinada idealmente pelos resultados da cultura e do antibiograma).
• Mixedema secundário ao hipotireoidismo deve responder de modo gradual à suplementação com T_4.
• Edema associado a insultos tóxicos pode ser retardado com antídotos (p. ex., antiveneno).
• Terapia anticoagulante (p. ex., heparina e varfarina) pode beneficiar os pacientes com CID ou depleção de antitrombina III, respectivamente.
• Expansores volêmicos vasculares, como hidroxietilamido ou plasma, frequentemente beneficiam os pacientes com baixa pressão oncótica plasmática; furosemida em doses muitos baixas sob taxa de infusão constante de 0,1 mg/kg/h é eficaz em conjunto com algum expansor volêmico.

CONTRAINDICAÇÕES
• Diuréticos — geralmente agravam o edema de origem não cardiogênica.
• Esteroides — podem piorar o edema secundário à doença infecciosa.
• Adrenalina — contraindicada, em geral, no choque, exceto em casos de anafilaxia.
• Propranolol (β-bloqueador) — contraindicado em pacientes predispostos a broncospasmo.

PRECAUÇÕES
• Evitar injeções IM em pacientes com trombocitopenia.
• Reduzir gradativamente a terapia com esteroide a longo prazo, de forma que a produção endógena de esteroides seja retomada.
• Utilizar a adrenalina com cuidado em pacientes predispostos à fibrilação ventricular.
• Usar o enalapril de forma cautelosa em animais com nefropatia.
• Antibioticoterapia a longo prazo pode facilitar a ocorrência de superinfecção por fungo (p. ex., *Candida*) ou bactéria resistente.
• Monitorizar rigorosamente os anticoagulantes para evitar hemorragia fatal.

ACOMPANHAMENTO

MONITORIZAÇÃO DO PACIENTE
• Repetição dos exames de hemograma completo, bioquímica sanguínea e relações de proteína:creatinina urinárias para pesquisa de discrasias sanguíneas e avaliação das concentrações séricas e urinárias de proteína, respectivamente.
• Avaliação semanal do tempo de protrombina ou do tempo de tromboplastina parcial para os pacientes sob varfarina ou heparina, respectivamente.
• Biopsias seriadas do tecido acometido, como de rim na glomerulonefrite, podem ajudar a fornecer o prognóstico.
• Repetição das culturas ou dos títulos agudos e convalescentes para os pacientes que sofrem de doença infecciosa.
• Análise periódica de T_4 para os pacientes que recebem suplementação de hormônio da tireoide.

PREVENÇÃO
Depende da causa do edema.

COMPLICAÇÕES POSSÍVEIS
• Úlcera de decúbito.
• Hemorragia fatal.
• Trombose fatal.
• Insuficiências cardíaca, gastrintestinal, hepática ou renal refratárias.
• Desnutrição.
• Edema e herniação cerebrais.
• Infecção e sepse resistentes.

EVOLUÇÃO ESPERADA E PROGNÓSTICO
Dependem da causa do edema.

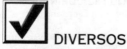

DIVERSOS

DISTÚRBIOS ASSOCIADOS
Efusão pericárdica, pleural ou peritoneal.

FATORES RELACIONADOS COM A IDADE
Anomalias vasculares ou linfedema primário geralmente são comprovados nos pacientes jovens (p. ex., anasarca).

POTENCIAL ZOONÓTICO
• Exposição recente a carrapatos é um elemento comum nos animais de estimação e em seus proprietários, que podem sofrer simultaneamente de doença riquetsiana.
• Certos microrganismos protozoários (*Leishmania*), fúngicos (*Sporothrix*) e bacterianos (*Brucella*) podem ser transmitidos para as pessoas por contato direto.

GESTAÇÃO/FERTILIDADE/REPRODUÇÃO
A brucelose foi associada a edema vulvar, vasculite necrosante e morte embrionária ou abortamento fetal.

SINÔNIMO(S)
Anasarca.

VER TAMBÉM
• Ascite.
• Cirrose e Fibrose do Fígado.
• Hiperlipidemia.
• Hipoalbuminemia.
• Linfedema.
• Proteinúria.
• Quilotórax.
• Trombocitopenia.
• Vasculite Cutânea — Cães.
• Vasculite Sistêmica.

ABREVIATURA(S)
• CID = coagulação intravascular disseminada.
• ICC = insuficiência cardíaca congestiva.
• T_4 = tiroxina.
• TRH = hormônio liberador da tireotropina.
• TSH = hormônio tireostimulante.

Sugestões de Leitura
Fossum TW, King LA, Miller MW, et al. Lymphedema: Clinical signs, diagnosis and treatment. J Vet Intern Med 1992, 6:312-319.
Fossum TW, Miller MW. Lymphedema: Etiopathogenesis. J Vet Intern Med 1992, 6:283-293.
Fox PR, Petrie JP, Hohenhaus AE. Peripheral vascular disease. In: Ettinger SJ, Feldman EC, eds., Textbook of Veterinary Internal Medicine, 6th ed. St. Louis: Elsevier, 2005.
Raffe MR, Roberts J. Edema. In: Ettinger SJ, Feldman EC, eds., Textbook of Veterinary Internal Medicine, 6th ed. St. Louis: Elsevier, 2005.

Autor Marc Elie
Consultores Editoriais Larry P. Tilley e Francis W.K. Smith, Jr.

Edema Pulmonar Não Cardiogênico

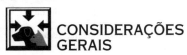

CONSIDERAÇÕES GERAIS

DEFINIÇÃO
Acúmulo de líquido de edema no interstício e nos alvéolos pulmonares, na ausência de cardiopatia.

FISIOPATOLOGIA
- Associado ao aumento da permeabilidade vascular pulmonar e ao extravasamento de líquido para o interstício e os alvéolos; se grave, pode ser acompanhado por resposta inflamatória e acúmulo de neutrófilos e macrófagos no interstício e nos alvéolos.
- Diversos mecanismos podem contribuir para alterações na permeabilidade vascular pulmonar.
- Liberação sistêmica de catecolaminas — pode levar à vasoconstrição sistêmica, desviando temporariamente o sangue para a circulação pulmonar e levando à sobrecarga circulatória pulmonar transitória e lesão endotelial; provavelmente ocorre nos pacientes com edema neurogênico, mordedura de fio elétrico e obstrução das vias aéreas superiores.
- Em pacientes com obstrução das vias aéreas superiores, a pressão intratorácica negativa gerada por tentativas inspiratórias diante de uma obstrução aérea contribui para a formação de edema.
- O aumento da permeabilidade vascular pode fazer parte de uma resposta inflamatória generalizada que se desenvolve em pacientes com síndrome da resposta inflamatória sistêmica, sepse ou pancreatite.
- Para todas as formas, o insulto incitante pode deflagrar uma resposta da cascata inflamatória que frequentemente piora nas 24 h seguintes após o episódio inicial.
- Gravidade da manifestação clínica — varia, desde leve até grave; os pacientes mais gravemente acometidos podem evoluir de normais até a morte em algumas horas após o incidente.

SISTEMA(S) ACOMETIDO(S)
- Respiratório.
- Hemático/linfático/imune — se for grave e induzir à insuficiência respiratória, pode estar associado à CID.
- Cardiovascular — hipotensão, taquicardia e choque.
- Renal/urológico — insuficiência renal aguda.

GENÉTICA
Desconhecida.

INCIDÊNCIA/PREVALÊNCIA
Raro.

IDENTIFICAÇÃO
Espécies
Principalmente cães, ocasionalmente gatos. Não há predileção racial ou sexual, exceto no que diz respeito à obstrução das vias aéreas.

Raça(s) Predominante(s)
Nenhuma específica; os cães braquicefálicos são mais propensos à obstrução das vias aéreas.

Idade Média e Faixa Etária
- Incidência mais alta nos filhotes caninos com <1 ano de idade.
- Jovem — associado a estrangulamento, traumatismo cefálico e mordeduras de fio elétrico.
- Idoso — associado a obstrução laríngea e neoplasia.

SINAIS CLÍNICOS
Comentários Gerais
Variam, dependendo da causa subjacente e da gravidade.

Achados Anamnésicos
- Causa predisponente — obstrução das vias aéreas; mordedura de fio elétrico; crises convulsivas; traumatismo cefálico.
- Início agudo de dispneia.

Achados do Exame Físico
- Dispneia leve a grave.
- Frequência e esforço respiratórios aumentados; respiração com a boca aberta.
- Adaptações posturais à angústia respiratória (se grave).
- Indisposição para se deitar.
- Mucosas pálidas ou cianóticas (grave).
- Ruídos ásperos (leves no início) ou crepitações generalizadas (graves no final) à auscultação.
- Expectoração de espuma ou bolhas rosadas; no paciente entubado gravemente acometido, podem-se notar grandes volumes de líquido sanguinolento fluindo para fora da sonda endotraqueal.
- Auscultação cardíaca normal; podem-se notar arritmias; é comum a presença de taquicardia.

CAUSAS
- Obstrução das vias aéreas superiores — paralisia laríngea; lesão por corrente asfixiante; massa; abscesso.
- Mordedura de fio elétrico.
- Doença neurológica aguda — traumatismo cefálico; crises convulsivas prolongadas.
- Inalação de fumaça.
- Pneumonia por aspiração.
- Síndrome da resposta inflamatória sistêmica — sepse; endotoxemia; pancreatite.
- Anafilaxia (gatos).

FATORES DE RISCO
- Hipoproteinemia.
- Reanimação com fluido cristaloide.

DIAGNÓSTICO

DIAGNÓSTICO DIFERENCIAL
- Edema pulmonar cardiogênico.
- Infecção pulmonar — pneumonia bacteriana, viral ou fúngica.
- Neoplasia pulmonar.
- Hemorragia pulmonar.
- Tromboembolia pulmonar.

HEMOGRAMA/BIOQUÍMICA/URINÁLISE
- Embora seja comum a constatação de leucocitose, as anormalidades de leucopenia e trombocitopenia são possíveis — em virtude de sequestro neutrofílico no pulmão e consumo de plaquetas.
- Exames bioquímicos — geralmente normais; pode-se notar hipoalbuminemia atribuída à perda proteica pulmonar; há relatos de hiperglicemia leve.
- Urinálise — usualmente normal.

OUTROS TESTES LABORATORIAIS
- Oximetria de pulso e gasometria sanguínea arterial — costumam demonstrar hipoxemia e hipocapnia leves a graves; os resultados não são específicos, mas indicam a gravidade da disfunção pulmonar.
- Teste de coagulação (pacientes gravemente acometidos) — pode revelar prolongamento leve a moderado do TP e do TTP por causa do consumo e de CID.

DIAGNÓSTICO POR IMAGEM
- Radiografias torácicas — vitais; podem simplesmente revelar um padrão intersticial proeminente em casos de doença leve ou precoce; podem-se notar infiltrados alveolares em casos de doença moderada ou grave; infiltrados alveolares são comuns nos campos pulmonares dorsocaudais; tais infiltrados também podem ser observados em outros campos pulmonares e, às vezes, são assimétricos e predominantemente do lado direito. A silhueta cardíaca geralmente se encontra normal.
- Ecocardiografia — descarta edema pulmonar cardiogênico.

MÉTODOS DIAGNÓSTICOS
- Citologia de líquido das vias aéreas — inflamatório com neutrófilos e alguns macrófagos alveolares. O líquido tende a ter altos valores de proteína (>3 g/dL). A cultura pode ser negativa inicialmente, mas ficar positiva se houver pneumonia bacteriana sobreposta.
- Oximetria de pulso — método não invasivo; monitorização contínua da saturação da hemoglobina arterial; fornece informações sobre a gravidade e a evolução da disfunção pulmonar.
- Pressão arterial pulmonar em cunha — valores normais confirmam a origem não cardiogênica; a medição não é comumente realizada.

ACHADOS PATOLÓGICOS
- Macroscópicos — os pulmões geralmente se encontram pesados, vermelhos ou congestos; podem não estar colabados; podem apresentar superfície de corte úmida; é possível notar a presença de espuma nas vias aéreas principais.
- Histopatológicos — dependem da gravidade do insulto; leve no início: pode-se notar material amorfo eosinofílico preenchendo os alvéolos ou pode estar próximo do normal, porque o líquido foi removido no processamento da lâmina; grave: membranas hialinas alveolares, alveolite e infiltrados inflamatórios intersticiais com neutrófilos e macrófagos evidentes e acompanhados por atelectasia, congestão vascular e hemorragia; podem ser encontrados dentro de horas de um grave insulto.

TRATAMENTO

CUIDADO(S) DE SAÚDE ADEQUADO(S)
- Tratamento hospitalar *vs* ambulatorial — depende da gravidade da manifestação clínica da disfunção respiratória; depende da causa subjacente da doença (p. ex., cães com obstrução das vias aéreas superiores ou crises convulsivas graves podem necessitar de hospitalização).
- Empreender todos os esforços para resolver e tratar a causa subjacente (p. ex., aliviar a obstrução das vias aéreas ou tratar as crises convulsivas).
- Leve a moderado — os pacientes geralmente melhoram sozinhos dentro de 24-48 h com a resolução completa; oferecer suporte da função pulmonar e cardiovascular durante o reparo pulmonar.
- Grave — difícil de tratar; pode necessitar de ventilação com pressão positiva por causa da

Edema Pulmonar Não Cardiogênico

insuficiência respiratória; muitos pacientes morrem apesar dos extensos cuidados de suporte.

CUIDADO(S) DE ENFERMAGEM
• Minimizar o estresse nos animais dispneicos.
• Oxigenoterapia — vital em doença moderada a grave; administrar via máscara ou capuz, cateter nasal ou gaiola de oxigênio; a concentração do oxigênio inspirado depende da gravidade da doença; a maior parte dos pacientes passa bem com oxigênio a 40-50%, porém a doença grave pode necessitar de 80-100% para manter a vida.
• Grave — pode necessitar de ventilação com pressão positiva e pressão expiratória final positiva.
• Fluidoterapia com solução eletrolítica balanceada — administrar como solução de reposição em casos de desidratação ou choque; ter cuidado com os fluidos se o animal estiver dispneico.
• Plasma ou coloides sintéticos — considerar na hipoproteinemia; melhora a pressão oncótica, minimizando o deslocamento de líquido para os pulmões.

ATIVIDADE
Cães com hipoxia moderada a grave e angústia respiratória — repouso e mínimo estresse são vitais para minimizar as necessidades de oxigênio.

ORIENTAÇÃO AO PROPRIETÁRIO
• Avisar o proprietário que a condição pode piorar antes da melhora.
• Informar o proprietário que a doença grave que evolui rapidamente para edema pulmonar fulminante e insuficiência respiratória está associada a um prognóstico muito mau.

CONSIDERAÇÕES CIRÚRGICAS
Relevantes apenas para o tratamento da causa subjacente.

MEDICAÇÕES

MEDICAMENTO(S) DE ESCOLHA
• Endotélio lesado na vasculatura pulmonar — não há nenhum tratamento específico disponível.
• Resposta inflamatória — gerada por uma variedade de mediadores e cascatas; não pode ser bloqueada por um único medicamento anti-inflamatório específico que leve à resolução do edema.
• Diuréticos — são, em geral, minimamente ineficazes; o edema é provocado por alterações na permeabilidade, não pela pressão hidrostática elevada; pode-se usar a furosemida com cuidado em bólus de 0,5-2 mg/kg IV, IM ou na dose de 0,1-1 mg/kg/hora IV sob infusão contínua.
• Corticosteroides — usados para reduzir a tumefação nos pacientes com obstrução das vias aéreas superiores; geralmente ineficazes para resposta inflamatória pulmonar; podem predispor os pacientes a complicações infecciosas (p. ex., pneumonia bacteriana); no caso de sua utilização, recomenda-se a dosagem anti-inflamatória (p. ex., fosfato sódico de dexametasona na dose de 0,05-0,1 mg/kg IV).

PRECAUÇÕES
Diuréticos (p. ex., furosemida) — utilização excessiva pode provocar desidratação e redução acentuada no volume intravascular com resolução mínima do edema; o volume intravascular baixo pode exacerbar o colapso cardiovascular ou o choque.

ACOMPANHAMENTO

MONITORIZAÇÃO DO PACIENTE
• Observar a frequência e o padrão respiratórios e auscultar frequentemente (a cada 2-4 h) nas primeiras 24-48 h, dependendo da gravidade da doença.
• Avaliar a função pulmonar por meio da oximetria de pulso ou gasometria do sangue arterial (inicialmente a cada 2-4 h).
• Determinar o hematócrito e os sólidos totais e examinar as mucosas, a qualidade do pulso, a frequência cardíaca, a pressão arterial e o débito urinário a cada 2-4 h para avaliar o estado cardiovascular e possível evolução para o choque.

PREVENÇÃO
• Evitar o contato com fio elétrico.
• Corrigir a obstrução das vias aéreas.
• Tratar as crises convulsivas e a pressão intracraniana elevada.

COMPLICAÇÕES POSSÍVEIS
Geralmente nenhuma caso o paciente se recupere da crise aguda.

EVOLUÇÃO ESPERADA E PROGNÓSTICO
• Leve a moderado — resolução habitual dos sinais clínicos em 24-72 horas; não há necessidade de tratamento específico, exceto para o oxigênio e cuidadosa suplementação com fluido.
• Grave — difícil de tratar; pode necessitar de ventilação com pressão positiva em função de insuficiência respiratória.
• Taxas gerais de sobrevida — 80-90%.
• Prognóstico a longo prazo — excelente para os pacientes recuperados.

DIVERSOS

DISTÚRBIOS ASSOCIADOS
Síndrome da angústia respiratória aguda.

SINÔNIMO(S)
• Choque pulmonar.
• Pulmão úmido traumático.
• Insuficiência alveolar aguda.
• Lesão pulmonar aguda.
• Síndrome do extravasamento capilar.
• Angústia respiratória positiva.
• Atelectasia congestiva.
• Síndrome do pulmão hemorrágico.

VER TAMBÉM
Síndrome da Angústia Respiratória Aguda (SARA).

ABREVIATURA(S)
• CID = coagulação intravascular disseminada.
• TP = tempo de protrombina.
• TTP = tempo de tromboplastina parcial.

Sugestões de Leitura
Drobatz KJ, Saunders HM. Noncardiogenic pulmonary edema. In: Kirk's Current Veterinary Therapy XIII: Small Animal Practice. Philadelphia: Saunders, 2000, pp. 800-812.
Drobatz KJ, Saunders HM, Pugh C, Hendricks JC. Noncardiogenic pulmonary edema: 26 cases (1987-1993). JAVMA 1995, 206:1732-1736.
Kerr LY. Pulmonary edema secondary to upper airway obstruction in the dog: A review of nine cases. JAAHA 1989, 25:207-212.
Kolata RJ, Burrows CF. The clinical features of injury by chewing electrical cords in dogs and cats. JAAHA 1981, 17:219-222.

Autor Lesley G. King
Consultor Editorial Lynelle R. Johnson

EFUSÃO PERICÁRDICA

CONSIDERAÇÕES GERAIS

DEFINIÇÃO
Volume anormalmente elevado de líquido dentro do saco pericárdico; o tamponamento cardíaco refere-se à síndrome clínica que resulta do baixo débito cardíaco ocasionado por compressão mecânica do coração.

FISIOPATOLOGIA
O acúmulo de líquido excede as capacidades elástica ou de estiramento do saco pericárdico; o acúmulo adicional leva ao aumento da pressão intrapericárdica. Ocorrerá tamponamento cardíaco quando a pressão intrapericárdica exceder a pressão de enchimento diastólico cardíaco. O átrio direito e o ventrículo direito normalmente possuem a pressão de enchimento cardíaco mais baixa e, por essa razão, são predominantemente acometidos. O declínio resultante no retorno venoso diminui o débito cardíaco. Em animais com doença pericárdica crônica, o baixo débito cardíaco ativa mecanismos compensatórios que levam ao acúmulo de líquido. Essa queda no débito cardíaco tipicamente se manifesta como ICC do lado direito. Animais com o desenvolvimento agudo de efusões tipicamente apresentam sinais de fraqueza ou de colapso.

SISTEMA(S) ACOMETIDO(S)
- Cardiovascular — sinais de baixo débito cardíaco e ICC.
- Hepatobiliar — congestão passiva crônica e enzimas hepáticas leve a moderadamente elevadas.
- Renal/urológico — azotemia pré-renal.
- Respiratório — taquipneia ou efusão pleural.

INCIDÊNCIA/PREVALÊNCIA
Os distúrbios pericárdicos compreendem cerca de 8% dos casos de cardiologia canina encaminhados a instituições de referência.

IDENTIFICAÇÃO
Espécies
Cães; rara nos gatos.

Raça(s) Predominante(s)
- As raças Golden retriever e Pastor alemão são predispostas tanto a hemangiossarcoma atrial direito como à efusão idiopática.
- As raças braquicefálicas são predispostas a tumores do corpo aórtico.

Idade Média e Faixa Etária
Cães de meia-idade a idosos estão predispostos.

Sexo Predominante
Cães machos podem ser predispostos à efusão idiopática.

SINAIS CLÍNICOS
Comentários Gerais
Efusão pericárdica crônica frequentemente provoca distensão jugular e ascite sem sopro cardíaco.

Achados Anamnésicos
- Letargia.
- Anorexia.
- Fraqueza.
- Intolerância ao exercício.
- Distensão abdominal.
- Angústia respiratória.
- Síncope ou colapso.
- Vômito.

Achados do Exame Físico
- Distensão da veia jugular.
- Ascite (especialmente com efusão crônica).
- Sons cardíacos abafados.
- Pulsos arteriais fracos.
- Pulso paradoxal.
- Palidez ou tempo de preenchimento capilar lento.
- Taquipneia e/ou taquicardia.

CAUSAS
- Neoplasia — hemangiossarcoma, tumor da base do coração, adenoma ou adenocarcinoma da tireoide, mesotelioma, neoplasia metastática e linfoma (especialmente em gatos).
- Idiopática — benigna ou hemorrágica.
- Coagulopatia — intoxicação por rodenticida antagonista da vitamina K, outras coagulopatias.
- Infecção — peritonite infecciosa felina, coccidioidomicose, pericardite bacteriana.
- Distúrbios congênitos — hérnia diafragmática peritoneopericárdica, cistos intrapericárdicos.
- Laceração atrial esquerda ou traumatismo cardíaco.
- ICC (sobretudo nos gatos).
- Corpo estranho.
- Pericardite constritiva com fibrose.

DIAGNÓSTICO

DIAGNÓSTICO DIFERENCIAL
- ICC secundária a outras causas (p. ex., valvulopatia e miocardiopatia), insuficiência hepática, neoplasia abdominal com hemorragia, nefropatia ou enteropatia com perda de proteína.
- Outras causas de ascite (p. ex., insuficiência hepática, hipoproteinemia, neoplasia intra-abdominal e hemorragia) — caracteristicamente resultam em anormalidades notáveis no hemograma completo e no perfil bioquímico, com a falta de distensão venosa jugular. O exame da veia jugular pode ser útil na diferenciação entre essas condições e insuficiência cardíaca.

HEMOGRAMA/BIOQUÍMICA/URINÁLISE
- Hemograma completo — em geral, normal; possível anemia em animais com hemangiossarcoma, linfoma ou coagulopatia; morfologia das hemácias pode estar anormal; pode haver trombocitopenia em animais com neoplasia ou CID.
- Perfil bioquímico — frequentemente normal; pode haver enzimas hepáticas leve a moderadamente elevadas (nos animais com congestão hepática passiva crônica), azotemia branda (tipicamente pré-renal), hipoproteinemia e anormalidades eletrolíticas leves (p. ex., hiponatremia, hipocloremia e hipercalemia).
- Urinálise — geralmente normal com capacidade normal de concentração renal a menos que algum diurético tenha sido administrado.

OUTROS TESTES LABORATORIAIS
- Altas concentrações séricas de troponina I cardíaca foram demonstradas em cães com efusão pericárdica, especialmente naqueles com hemangiossarcoma.
- Tempos de coagulação (p. ex., tempo de tromboplastina parcial ativada e tempo de protrombina de único estágio) — prolongados nos animais com intoxicação por rodenticida antagonista da vitamina K ou CID.
- Apesar de limitada em termos de sensibilidade e especificidade diagnósticas, a análise do líquido pericárdico pode ser útil na identificação de etiologias neoplásicas (p. ex., linfoma) ou causas infecciosas.
- Os testes para a peritonite infecciosa felina ou para o vírus da leucemia felina podem ter utilidade em gatos.

DIAGNÓSTICO POR IMAGEM
Achados da Radiografia Torácica
- Aumento de volume cardíaco de leve a grave; silhueta cardíaca frequentemente globoide com bordas muito nítidas evidenciadas, quase sempre, na projeção dorsoventral por causa da ausência de artefatos produzidos pelo movimento cardíaco.
- Efusão pleural em alguns pacientes.
- Ascite em muitos pacientes.
- Veia cava caudal grande em alguns pacientes.
- Em pacientes com neoplasia metastática, pode-se observar a presença de infiltrados pulmonares nodulares.

Ecocardiografia
- Teste diagnóstico superior para confirmar o diagnóstico.
- Espaço livre de eco claramente identificado entre o pericárdio parietal e a superfície epicárdica do coração.
- Com frequência, esse exame demonstra a causa da efusão pericárdica em pacientes com neoplasia (p. ex., hemangiossarcoma atrial direito ou tumor da base do coração) ou hérnia diafragmática peritoneopericárdica; raramente demonstra ruptura do átrio direito.
- A efusão pericárdica facilita a detecção de massas intrapericárdicas; a ecocardiografia é idealmente realizada antes da pericardiocentese se o paciente estiver estabilizado.
- O colapso diastólico do átrio ou ventrículo direitos é indicativo de tamponamento cardíaco.

MÉTODOS DIAGNÓSTICOS
Achados Eletrocardiográficos
- Taquicardia sinusal em muitos pacientes; ocasionalmente, detectam-se arritmias ventriculares ou supraventriculares.
- Complexos QRS de baixa voltagem (<1 mV nas derivações I, II, III, aVR, aVL e aVF) em alguns animais.
- Elevação do segmento ST em alguns pacientes.
- Alternância elétrica, uma variação regular (1:1 ou 2:1) na altura ou na morfologia da onda QRS-T, resulta da oscilação do coração para frente e para trás dentro do saco pericárdico em alguns pacientes.

TRATAMENTO

CUIDADO(S) DE SAÚDE ADEQUADO(S)
O tamponamento cardíaco justifica a realização de pericardiocentese imediata; caso o clínico não se sinta confortável para executar a pericardiocentese, é fortemente aconselhável o encaminhamento do animal a indivíduos com habilidade nessa técnica. Talvez haja necessidade de pericardiocenteses repetidas; a cirurgia pode ser indicada em cães selecionados. Raramente, a pericardiocentese é necessária em gatos.

Pericardiocentese
- Colocar o paciente em decúbito esternal. Fazer a tricotomia no lado direito do tórax, entre o 3º e o

EFUSÃO PERICÁRDICA

8º espaço intercostal, desde uma área acima da junção costocondral ventralmente até o esterno. O lado direito do tórax é preferido em relação ao esquerdo em virtude da menor probabilidade de laceração da artéria coronária. É aconselhado o monitoramento simultâneo com ECG para detectar arritmias. A ecocardiografia é valiosa para identificar o melhor espaço intercostal; todavia, se esse exame não estiver disponível, deve-se realizar a pericardiocentese no 5º espaço intercostal, logo abaixo da junção costocondral. Após a preparação asséptica da pele e a realização do bloqueio anestésico local com lidocaína, avançar um cateter longo (~2 cm) e calibroso (calibre ~18) no saco pericárdico; pode-se obter uma pequena quantidade de líquido pleural claro antes de avançar o cateter dentro do saco pericárdico. Nos cães, a efusão pericárdica costuma ser hemorrágica, embora alguns pacientes tenham efusão serosa ou serossanguinolenta. Remover o máximo possível da efusão (a menos que se suspeite de laceração atrial esquerda). Caso ocorra o desenvolvimento de arritmias, reposicionar a agulha ou o cateter e ficar preparado para administrar lidocaína IV.
• A menos que o paciente tenha hemorragia ativa dentro do saco pericárdico, a efusão obtida pela pericardiocentese não deve coagular, mas deve apresentar um volume globular diferente daquele do sangue periférico. O sobrenadante da efusão crônica quase sempre é xantocrômico.

CUIDADO(S) DE ENFERMAGEM
A menos que o paciente exiba uma desidratação acentuada, os fluidos, em geral, não são necessários nem recomendados em casos de efusão pericárdica crônica. A leve expansão volêmica pode ser valiosa em determinados animais com efusão pericárdica aguda. Administrar oxigênio aos cães com taquipneia ou sinais de instabilidade hemodinâmica.

ATIVIDADE
Repouso em gaiola, acompanhada por restrição de exercícios.

ORIENTAÇÃO AO PROPRIETÁRIO
Os proprietários devem ser informados sobre a natureza tipicamente recidivante das efusões pericárdicas, embora o prognóstico possa ser muito variável, dependendo da causa subjacente. Também é recomendável orientar e alertar os proprietários sobre a importância da monitorização rigorosa quanto à ocorrência de recidiva da efusão e ao potencial de morte súbita.

CONSIDERAÇÕES CIRÚRGICAS
• Além de prolongar a sobrevida, a pericardiectomia pode ter utilidade no tratamento de efusão pericárdica resultante de tumores da base do coração.
• Os casos de efusão pericárdica idiopática podem responder à pericardiocentese; a pericardiectomia fica indicada em efusão recidivante.
• Massas do apêndice auricular direito podem ser tratadas por meio cirúrgico; no entanto, é improvável que a ressecção isolada sem quimioterapia adjuvante prolongue a vida de forma significativa.
• A toracoscopia permite a pericardiectomia parcial com diminuição do risco e da dor no pós-operatório.

MEDICAÇÕES

MEDICAMENTO(S) DE ESCOLHA
• Os medicamentos não devem ser utilizados no lugar da pericardiocentese.
• Diuréticos — podem ajudar a reduzir a ascite, embora possam levar à azotemia progressiva e à fraqueza do paciente; geralmente, não são aconselháveis.
• Vitamina K — indicada para os pacientes com intoxicação por rodenticida anticoagulante.
• Antibióticos apropriados — indicados em animais com pericardite infecciosa.
• Quimioterapia — pode ser útil para o tratamento de efusão causada por linfoma; parcialmente eficaz no tratamento de hemangiossarcoma atrial e, em geral, ineficaz nos casos de tumor da base do coração; foi demonstrado que a quimioterapia adjuvante à base de doxorrubicina após ressecção de massa atrial direita aumente os tempos de sobrevida, embora os cães raramente sobrevivam por mais de 6 meses após a cirurgia.

CONTRAINDICAÇÕES
Digitálicos, vasodilatadores e inibidores da enzima conversora de angiotensina — descritos por serem relativa ou absolutamente contraindicados.

PRECAUÇÕES
A administração de diuréticos frequentemente leva à exacerbação de fraqueza e azotemia.

MEDICAMENTO(S) ALTERNATIVO(S)
• Para o tratamento de mesotelioma, pode-se tentar a aplicação de quimioterapia intracavitária.
• Os corticosteroides podem ser valiosos em cães selecionados com efusão pericárdica idiopática.
• Imunossupressores adicionais ou quimioterapia intracavitária podem ser considerados em efusões recidivantes, especialmente nos casos com efusão pleural recidivante após pericardiectomia.

ACOMPANHAMENTO

MONITORIZAÇÃO DO PACIENTE
• ECG — aconselhado durante as primeiras 24 h, já que a pericardiocentese quase sempre leva a arritmias ventriculares.
• A efusão pericárdica pode recidivar em qualquer estágio; o exame do paciente e a realização de ecocardiografia em 10-14 dias e a cada 2-4 meses são recomendados para detectar a efusão pericárdica idiopática.

COMPLICAÇÕES POSSÍVEIS
• Hipotensão ou choque.
• Pneumotórax, arritmias e perfuração miocárdica ou laceração coronária secundárias à pericardiocentese.

EVOLUÇÃO ESPERADA E PROGNÓSTICO
• Hemangiossarcoma atrial direito — mau; o tumor é altamente maligno e minimamente responsivo à quimioterapia; em geral, não é passível de ressecção no momento do diagnóstico; a realização de pericardiectomia é controversa.
• Quimiodectoma — razoável; tumor de crescimento lento; tardio para sofrer metástase; a pericardiectomia frequentemente resolve os sinais clínicos; foi relatada sobrevida de até 3 anos após a pericardiectomia.
• O prognóstico é bom na efusão pericárdica idiopática; cerca de 50% dos casos se resolvem depois de 1 ou 2 pericardiocenteses; a pericardiectomia, em geral, é curativa nos casos persistentes.

DIVERSOS

DISTÚRBIOS ASSOCIADOS
Hemangiossarcoma do baço.

FATORES RELACIONADOS COM A IDADE
• Efusão pericárdica idiopática pode ser mais comum nos cães de meia-idade a idosos.
• Hemangiossarcoma e tumores da base do coração são mais comuns nos animais idosos.

POTENCIAL ZOONÓTICO
Coccidioidomicose.

SINÔNIMO(S)
• Tamponamento cardíaco.
• Tamponamento pericárdico.
• Pericardite.

VER TAMBÉM
• Coccidioidomicose.
• Envenenamento por Rodenticidas Anticoagulantes.
• Hemangiossarcoma Cardíaco.
• Laceração da Parede Atrial.
• Peritonite Infecciosa Felina (PIF).
• Quimiodectoma.
• Tumores Miocárdicos.

ABREVIATURA(S)
• CID = coagulação intravascular disseminada.
• ECG = eletrocardiograma.
• ICC = insuficiência cardíaca congestiva.

Sugestões de Leitura
Chun R, Kellihan HB, Henik RA, et al. Comparison of plasma cardiac troponin I concentrations among dogs with cardiac hemangiosarcoma, noncardiac hemangiosarcoma, other neoplasms, and pericardial effusion of nonhemangiosarcoma origin. JAVMA 2010, 237(7):806-811.
Nelson OL, Ware WA. Pericardial effusion. In: Bonagura JD, Twedt DC, eds., Kirk's Current Veterinary Therapy XIV. St. Louis: Saunders Elsevier, 2009, pp. 825-831.
Shaw SP, Rush JE. Canine pericardial effusion: Diagnosis, treatment and prognosis. Compend Contin Educ Pract Vet 2007, 29:405-411.
Vicari ED, Brown DC, Holt DE, et al. Survival times of and prognostic indicators for dogs with heart base masses: 25 cases (1986-1999) JAVMA 2001, 219:485-487.
Weisse C, Soares N, Beal MW, et al. Survival times in dogs treated with right atrial hemangiossarcoma treated by means of surgical resection with or without adjuvant chemotherapy: 23 cases (1986-2000). JAVMA 2005, 226:575-579.

Autores Suzanne M. Cunningham e John E. Rush
Consultores Editoriais Larry P. Tilley e Francis W.K. Smith, Jr.

EFUSÃO PLEURAL

CONSIDERAÇÕES GERAIS

DEFINIÇÃO
Acúmulo anormal de líquido dentro da cavidade pleural.

FISIOPATOLOGIA
- Produção maior que a normal ou reabsorção menor que a normal de líquido pleural.
- Alterações nas pressões hidrostática e oncótica ou na permeabilidade vascular e na função linfática podem contribuir para o acúmulo de líquido pleural.

SISTEMA(S) ACOMETIDO(S)
- Respiratório.
- Cardiovascular.

IDENTIFICAÇÃO
Espécies
Cães e gatos.

Raça(s) Predominante(s)
Varia com a causa subjacente.

Idade Média e Faixa Etária
Varia com a causa subjacente.

Sexo Predominante
Varia com a causa subjacente.

SINAIS CLÍNICOS
Comentários Gerais
- Depende do volume de líquido, da rapidez de acúmulo desse líquido e da causa subjacente.

Achados Anamnésicos
- Dispneia.
- Taquipneia.
- Ortopneia.
- Respiração com a boca aberta.
- Cianose.
- Intolerância ao exercício.
- Letargia.
- Inapetência.
- Tosse.

Achados do Exame Físico
- Dispneia — respirações frequentemente superficiais e rápidas.
- Sons cardíacos e ruídos pulmonares abafados ou inaudíveis ventralmente.
- Preservação dos ruídos respiratórios dorsalmente.
- Macicez ventralmente à percussão torácica.

CAUSAS
Pressão Hidrostática Alta
- ICC.
- Super-hidratação.
- Neoplasia intratorácica.

Pressão Oncótica Baixa
- Hipoalbuminemia — ocorre na enteropatia com perda de proteínas, nefropatia com perda de proteínas e na hepatopatia.

Anormalidade Vascular ou Linfática
- Infecciosa — bacteriana, viral ou fúngica.
- Neoplasia (p. ex., linfoma mediastínico, timoma, mesotelioma, tumor pulmonar primário e doença metastática).
- Quilotórax (p. ex., gerado por linfangiectasia, ICC, obstrução da veia cava cranial [associada algumas vezes a implante de marca-passo transvenoso], neoplasia, infecções fúngicas, dirofilárias, hérnia diafragmática, torção de lobo pulmonar e traumatismo).
- Hérnia diafragmática.
- Hemotórax (p. ex., causado por traumatismo, neoplasia, coagulopatia, *Angiostrongylus vasorum*).
- Torção de lobo pulmonar.
- Tromboembolia pulmonar.
- Pancreatite.

DIAGNÓSTICO

DIAGNÓSTICO DIFERENCIAL
- Indícios físicos ou anamnésicos de traumatismo externo — considerar hemotórax ou hérnia diafragmática.
- A febre sugere alguma causa inflamatória, infecciosa ou neoplásica.
- Sopros, ritmos de galope ou arritmias combinadas com distensão ou pulsação da veia jugular sugerem alguma causa cardíaca subjacente.
- A ascite concomitante sugere PIF, ICC (principalmente cães), hipoalbuminemia grave, hérnia diafragmática, neoplasia disseminada ou pancreatite.
- Nos gatos, a compressibilidade diminuída da porção cranial do tórax sugere a presença de massa mediastínica cranial.
- Alterações oculares concomitantes (p. ex., coriorretinite e uveíte) sugerem PIF ou doença fúngica.

HEMOGRAMA/BIOQUÍMICA/URINÁLISE
- Os resultados do hemograma podem estar anormais nos pacientes com piotórax, PIF, neoplasia ou torção de lobo pulmonar.
- A hipoalbuminemia grave (em geral, <1 g/dL para causar efusão) sugere enteropatia com perda de proteínas, nefropatia com perda de proteínas ou hepatopatia.
- A hiperglobulinemia (policlonal) sugere PIF.

OUTROS TESTES LABORATORIAIS
- A análise do líquido deve incluir as características físicas (i. e., cor, claridade, odor e coágulos), o pH, o nível de glicose, o teor de proteína total, a contagem de células nucleadas totais e o exame citológico; a Tabela 1 fornece as características de vários tipos de líquidos pleurais e suas associações patológicas.
- Nos gatos, a concentração de LDH nos transudatos é de <200 UI/L, enquanto nos exsudatos, >200 UI/L.
- O pH do líquido pleural <6,9 sugere piotórax nos gatos.
- A concentração de glicose no líquido pleural geralmente se iguala aos níveis no soro. Nos gatos, o piotórax e os processos malignos diminuem a concentração de glicose no líquido pleural em relação à concentração desse açúcar no soro; por isso, o líquido pleural com pH normal e a baixa concentração de glicose sugerem malignidade nos gatos.
- Os testes sorológicos para detecção do vírus da leucemia felina (se o paciente tiver linfoma mediastínico), do vírus da imunodeficiência felina (se o paciente tiver piotórax) e do coronavírus (na suspeita de PIF) estão disponíveis.
- Suspeita de cardiopatia — considerar o teste para dirofilariose em cães e gatos, bem como a avaliação da tireoide nos gatos.
- Suspeita de infecção — fazer cultura bacteriana aeróbica e anaeróbica, além dos testes de sensibilidade e considerar o uso de corantes especiais (p. ex., colorações de Gram e acidorresistentes) do líquido.
- Suspeita de PIF — considerar a eletroforese proteica do líquido; nível de γ-globulina >32% da proteína total é fortemente sugestivo do diagnóstico de PIF.
- Suspeita de quilo — fazer o teste de depuração com éter ou realizar coloração de Sudan no líquido pleural, além de avaliações de triglicerídeos e colesterol do líquido e do soro.

DIAGNÓSTICO POR IMAGEM
Achados Radiográficos
- Utilizados para confirmar a efusão pleural; não deve ser realizado até depois da toracocentese em pacientes dispneicos com indícios de efusão pleural ao exame físico.
- Os indícios radiográficos de efusão pleural incluem o afastamento das margens pulmonares da parede torácica e do esterno por densidade líquida no espaço pleural, linhas de fissura interlobar preenchida com líquido, perda ou mancha nas bordas cardíaca e diafragmática, embotamento das margens pulmonares nos ângulos costofrênicos (projeção ventrodorsal) e ampliação do mediastino (projeção ventrodorsal).
- Arredondamento das margens do lobo pulmonar caudal (projeção lateral) — mais comum em pacientes com pleurite fibrosante causada por quilotórax, piotórax ou PIF.
- Efusão unilateral — mais comum em pacientes com quilotórax e piotórax; hemotórax, neoplasia pulmonar, hérnia diafragmática e torção de lobo pulmonar.
- Avaliar as radiografias pós-toracocentese de forma meticulosa em busca de cardiomegalia, lesões intrapulmonares, massas mediastínicas, hérnia diafragmática, torção de lobo pulmonar e indícios de traumatismo (p. ex., fraturas de costelas).
- O diagnóstico de hérnia diafragmática é possível com peritoneografia de contraste positivo.
- O ducto torácico pode ser avaliado por linfangiografia de contraste positivo.

Achados Ecocardiográficos
- A avaliação ultrassonográfica do tórax será recomendada se houver suspeita de cardiopatia, hérnia diafragmática ou massa mediastínica cranial.
- É mais fácil realizar a ecocardiografia antes da toracocentese, desde que o paciente esteja estável.

MÉTODOS DIAGNÓSTICOS
- Toracocentese — permite a caracterização do tipo de líquido e a determinação da causa subjacente potencial.
- Toracotomia ou toracoscopia exploratória — para obter amostras de biopsia de órgãos como pulmão, linfonodos ou pleura, se houver indicação.

TRATAMENTO

- Primeiro, efetuar a toracocentese para aliviar a angústia respiratória; se o paciente se estabilizar após a toracocentese, o tratamento ambulatorial será possível para algumas doenças. Na grande maioria das vezes, os pacientes são hospitalizados, porque necessitam de tratamento intensivo como sondas torácicas de retenção (p. ex., pacientes com piotórax) ou cirurgia torácica.
- A prevenção de novo acúmulo de líquido requer tratamento com base no diagnóstico definitivo.
- A cirurgia fica indicada para tratamento de algumas neoplasias, reparo de hérnia diafragmática, linfangiectasia (i. e., ligadura do

EFUSÃO PLEURAL

Tabela 1

	\multicolumn{6}{c}{Caracterização do fluido pleural}
	Transudato	Transudato Modificado	Exsudato Asséptico	Exsudato Séptico	Quilo	Hemorragia
Cor	Incolor a amarelo pálido	Amarelo ou rosa	Amarelo ou rosa	Amarelo a vermelho-acastanhado	Branco leitoso	Vermelho
Turbidez	Claro	Claro a turvo	Claro a turvo; fibrina	Turvo a opaco; fibrina	Opaco	Opaco
Proteína (g/dL)	<1,5	2,5-5,0	3,0-8,0	3,0-7,0	2,5-6,0	3,0
Células nucleadas/μL	<1.000	1.000-7.000 (até 100.000 em casos de linfoma)	5.000-20.000 (até 100.000 em casos de linfoma)	5.000-300.000	1.000-20.000	Semelhante ao sangue periférico
Citologia	Predominantemente células mesoteliais e macrófagos	Principalmente macrófagos e células mesoteliais; poucos PMN não degenerados; células neoplásicas em alguns casos	Maioria PMN não degenerados e macrófagos; células neoplásicas em alguns casos	Grande parte de PMN degenerados; também há macrófagos; bactérias	Pequenos linfócitos, PMN e macrófagos	Maioria hemácias; macrófagos com eritrofagocitose
Associações mórbidas	Hipoalbuminemia (nefropatia com perda de proteínas, enteropatia com perda de proteínas ou hepatopatia); ICC precoce	ICC; neoplasia; hérnia diafragmática; pancreatite	PIF; neoplasia; hérnia diafragmática; torção de lobo pulmonar	Piotórax	Linfangiectasia; ICC; obstrução da veia cava cranial; neoplasia; infecção fúngica; dirofilariose; hérnia diafragmática; torção de lobo pulmonar; traumatismo	Traumatismo; coagulopatia; neoplasia; torção de lobo pulmonar

Modificado de Sherding RG. Diseases of the pleural cavity, In: Sherding RG, ed. The cat: diseases and clinical management. 2. ed. New York: Churchill Livingstone, 1994, p. 1061.

ducto torácico), remoção de corpo estranho e torção de lobo pulmonar (lobectomia pulmonar).
• Desvios pleuroperitoneais podem aliviar os sinais clínicos em animais com efusão pleural intratável.

MEDICAÇÕES

MEDICAMENTO(S) DE ESCOLHA
• O tratamento varia de acordo com a doença específica.
• Os diuréticos geralmente ficam reservados para os pacientes com doenças indutoras de retenção de líquido e sobrecarga de volume (p. ex., ICC).

PRECAUÇÕES
• Evitar medicamentos que deprimem as respirações ou diminuem a pressão arterial.
• A utilização inadequada de diuréticos predispõe o paciente à desidratação e a distúrbios eletrolíticos sem a eliminação da efusão.

ACOMPANHAMENTO

MONITORIZAÇÃO DO PACIENTE
A avaliação radiográfica é fundamental para avaliar o tratamento em grande parte dos pacientes.

COMPLICAÇÕES POSSÍVEIS
• Morte atribuída ao comprometimento respiratório.
• Pode ocorrer o desenvolvimento de nova expansão do edema pulmonar depois de a efusão pleural ser manualmente removida.

EVOLUÇÃO ESPERADA E PROGNÓSTICO
Varia com a causa subjacente, mas costuma ser de reservado a mau. Em um estudo de 81 casos de efusão pleural em cães, 25% se recuperaram completamente e 33% vieram a óbito durante o tratamento ou foram submetidos à eutanásia imediatamente após o término da avaliação diagnóstica.

DIVERSOS

SINÔNIMO(S)
• Hidrotórax = transudatos e transudatos modificados.
• Piotórax = empiema, pleurite séptica.

VER TAMBÉM
Ver "Causas".

ABREVIATURA(S)
• ICC = insuficiência cardíaca congestiva.
• LDH = lactato desidrogenase.
• PIF = peritonite infecciosa felina.
• PMN = neutrófilos polimorfonucleares.

Sugestões de Leitura
Mellanby RJ, Villiers E, Herrtage ME. Canine pleural effusions: A retrospective study of 81 cases. J Small Anim Pract 2002, 43(10):447-451.
Sherding RG, Birchard SJ. Pleural effusion. In: Birchard SJ, Sherding RG, eds., Saunders Manual of Small Animal Practice, 3rd ed. St. Louis: Saunders Elsevier, 2006, pp. 1696-1707.
Smeak DD, Birchard SJ, McLoughlin MA, et al. Treatment of chronic pleural effusion with pleuroperitoneal shunts in dogs: 14 cases (1985-1999). JAVMA 2001, 219(11):1590-1597.

Autor Francis W.K. Smith, Jr.
Consultores Editoriais Larry P. Tilley e Francis W.K. Smith, Jr.

ENCEFALITE

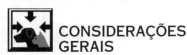

CONSIDERAÇÕES GERAIS

DEFINIÇÃO
Inflamação encefálica que pode ser acompanhada por envolvimento da medula espinal e/ou das meninges.

FISIOPATOLOGIA
• Inflamação — causada por algum agente infeccioso ou pelo próprio sistema imune do paciente. • Imunomediada — geralmente não se conhece a causa do distúrbio no sistema imune.

SISTEMA(S) ACOMETIDO(S)
• Nervoso. • Sinais multissistêmicos — podem ser observados em pacientes com doenças infecciosas.

INCIDÊNCIA/PREVALÊNCIA
Desconhecidas.

DISTRIBUIÇÃO GEOGRÁFICA
Varia com a causa ou o agente implicados.

IDENTIFICAÇÃO
Espécies
Cães e gatos.

Raça(s) Predominante(s)
• Meningoencefalite granulomatosa — acomete principalmente raças caninas de pequeno porte, sobretudo Terrier e Poodle miniatura; os cães de grande porte também são acometidos. • Encefalite do Pug — Pug. • Meningoencefalite piogranulomatosa — Pointer alemão de pelo curto. • Encefalite do Maltês — Maltês.
• Encefalite necrosante do Yorkshire terrier — Yorkshire terrier.

SINAIS CLÍNICOS
Achados Anamnésicos
• Início agudo de sinais clínicos, que evoluem com rapidez.

Achados do Exame Físico
• Em casos de microrganismos micóticos, riquetsiais, virais e prototecais — frequentemente se observam lesões no fundo ocular.

Achados do Exame Neurológico
• Determinados pela porção cerebral mais acometida.
• Fossa rostral — crises convulsivas; andar em círculos e a passos compassados; mudança de personalidade; diminuição no nível de responsividade.
• Fossa caudal — anormalidades relacionadas com o tronco cerebral (p. ex., sonolência, inclinação da cabeça, paresia/paralisia facial e incoordenação).
• Evolução (p. ex., anisocoria, pupilas puntiformes, redução no nível de consciência e nistagmo fisiológico deficiente) — sugere herniação tentorial.

CAUSAS
Cães
• Idiopáticas, imunomediadas — meningoencefalite granulomatosa; encefalite do Pug; encefalite do Maltês; encefalite necrosante do Yorkshire terrier; meningoencefalite eosinofílica.
• Virais — cinomose; raiva; herpes; parvovírus; adenovírus; pseudorraiva; vírus das encefalomielites equinas oriental e venezuelana.
• Encefalomielite pós-vacinal — cinomose; raiva; corona/parvovírus caninos.
• Riquetsiais — febre maculosa das Montanhas Rochosas; erliquiose.

• Micóticas — criptococose; blastomicose; histoplasmose; coccidioidomicose; aspergilose; feoifomicose.
• Bacterianas — anaeróbias e aeróbias.
• Protozoárias — toxoplasmose; neosporose; encefalitozoonose.
• Espiroquetas — borreliose.
• Migração parasitária — *Dirofilaria immitis*; *Toxocara canis*; *Ancylostoma caninum*; *Cuterebra*; cisticercose.
• Migração de corpo estranho — farpas de plantas; outros.
• Prototecose.
• Meningoencefalite piogranulomatosa.

Gatos
• Idiopáticas, imunomediadas — meningoencefalite granulomatosa; meningoencefalite eosinofílica.
• Polioencefalomielite idiopática.
• Virais — PIF; raiva; FIV; pseudorraiva; panleucopenia; rinotraqueíte.
• Micóticas — criptococose; blastomicose; feoifomicose.
• Bacterianas — anaeróbias e aeróbias.
• Protozoárias — toxoplasmose.
• Migração parasitária — *Dirofilaria immitis*; *Cuterebra*.

FATORES DE RISCO
• Medicamentos imunossupressores e infecções pelo FIV ou FeLV — encefalites infecciosas.
• Áreas infectadas por carrapatos — infecções por riquétsias e *Borrelia*.
• Histórico de viagem — infecções micóticas.

DIAGNÓSTICO

DIAGNÓSTICO DIFERENCIAL
• Encefalites fúngicas — frequentemente acompanhadas por sinais sistêmicos.
• Doenças protozoárias — sistêmicas; podem apresentar um histórico crônico.
• Riquetioses — é comum a constatação de anormalidades no hemograma.
• PIF — os pacientes costumam ter <3 anos de idade; curso prolongado; resultados característicos da análise do LCS.
• Cinomose — observada comumente na forma de encefalite aguda com sinais sistêmicos em pacientes com <1 ano de idade; pode ser difícil confirmá-la no período *antemortem*.
• Neoplasia primária do SNC — os sinais podem ser semelhantes aos da encefalite.
• Distúrbios degenerativos — em geral, de início lento e evolução insidiosa.
• Encefalopatia metabólica ou tóxica — anormalidades neurológicas simétricas e bilaterais, que se relacionam com o cérebro; confirmar as toxinas por meio de testes laboratoriais ou ensaios sorológicos.

HEMOGRAMA/BIOQUÍMICA/URINÁLISE
• Hemograma — frequentemente permanece normal; pode-se observar leucocitose em doenças produtoras de sinais sistêmicos; pode haver linfopenia nos estágios precoces das infecções pelo vírus da cinomose e por riquétsias; a encefalite riquetsial pode ser acompanhada por trombocitopenia e anemia.
• Bioquímica sérica — também permanece frequentemente normal; com frequência, observa-se hiperproteinemia juntamente com

gamopatia policlonal em casos de PIF e infecções sistêmicas crônicas; pode ocorrer elevação moderada da creatina cinase em casos de infecção por *Neospora*.

OUTROS TESTES LABORATORIAIS
• Sorologia — disponível em casos de doenças fúngicas, protozoárias, riquetsiais e virais; embora seja útil, esse exame deve ser interpretado com cautela, pois um título positivo nem sempre indica doença ativa (p. ex., toxoplasmose em gatos) e um título negativo nem sempre descarta doença ativa (p. ex., PIF).
• Anticorpos fluorescentes indiretos — um único título positivo de 1:10 ou superior confirma erliquiose.
• ELISA — uma elevação de quatro vezes entre os títulos de IgG nas fases aguda e convalescente quando o primeiro título se encontra >1:128 confirma febre maculosa das Montanhas Rochosas; um título de IgM >1:256 sugere infecção nas 16 semanas prévias por *Toxoplasma gondii* e pode indicar exacerbação de infecção crônica.
• Teste de aglutinação em látex — um único título positivo a partir do soro ou do LCS confirma a presença de antígenos criptocócicos.
• Imunodifusão em ágar gel — diagnostica blastomicose com alto grau de precisão.
• Produção local de anticorpos (IgG e IgM) específicos contra o vírus da cinomose —no LCS após a infecção viral do SNC.
• Título positivo quanto à presença de *Neospora caninum* — correlaciona-se satisfatoriamente com doença ativa.
• Título positivo em relação à PIF — indica apenas infecção por um coronavírus; pode não ser patogênico.
• Título positivo para *Borrelia burgdorferi* — indica exposição ao microrganismo, mas não necessariamente uma doença ativa.

DIAGNÓSTICO POR IMAGEM
• Radiografias torácicas — podem confirmar anormalidades pulmonares.
• Radiografias cranianas — podem confirmar sinusite/rinite em alguns gatos com criptococose.
• TC ou RM encefálicas — podem detectar lesões expansivas (tipo massa) multifocais ou isoladas.

MÉTODOS DIAGNÓSTICOS
• Análise do LCS — realizar em todos os animais com sinais clínicos sugestivos de encefalite; os resultados quase sempre são anormais; no entanto, resultados normais não descartam os casos de encefalite viral aguda, limitados ao parênquima; em casos de pleocitose, efetuar culturas bacterianas (aeróbias e anaeróbias).
• Resultados do LCS — a presença de neutrófilos indica processo inflamatório ativo agudo; linfócitos pequenos são indicativos de resposta antigênica; eosinófilos sugerem resposta alérgica ou reação a corpo estranho (tumores, parasitas).

ACHADOS PATOLÓGICOS
As lesões dependem da resposta encefálica ao agente infeccioso ou a outras causas.

TRATAMENTO

CUIDADO(S) DE SAÚDE ADEQUADO(S)
Internação — para o diagnóstico e a terapia inicial.

ENCEFALITE

CUIDADO(S) DE ENFERMAGEM
• Tratamento sintomático — controlar o edema cerebral e a atividade convulsiva, conforme a necessidade.
• Edema cerebral — administrar manitol a 20% (2,2 g/kg IV durante 30-45 min); essa administração pode ser repetida dentro de 1-2 h para se obter uma resposta máxima; limitar o uso de fluidos parenterais para evitar edema cerebral de rebote; com o emprego do manitol, fica indicado o tratamento com corticosteroides a curto prazo (72 h) para a obtenção de controle adicional (fosfato sódico de dexametasona a 0,5 mg/kg IV a cada 12 h por 24 h; reduzir em seguida para 0,25 mg/kg a cada 12 h por 48 h).
• Crises convulsivas — tratar com medicamentos anticonvulsivantes; administração sob a forma de bólus ou infusão em velocidade constante.

ATIVIDADE
Conforme a tolerância.

DIETA
Em casos de depressão grave ou vômito — não fornecer nada por via oral até que a condição melhore, para evitar aspiração.

ORIENTAÇÃO AO PROPRIETÁRIO
• Notificar o proprietário sobre a possível recidiva em casos de encefalite idiopática ou imunomediada quando se interrompe a terapia.

CONSIDERAÇÕES CIRÚRGICAS
Biopsia cerebral — pode ser necessária para o diagnóstico específico.

MEDICAÇÕES

MEDICAMENTO(S) DE ESCOLHA
• Aplicar terapia específica assim que o diagnóstico for obtido ou caso haja alto índice de suspeita.
• Idiopática e imunomediada — prednisona a 2 mg/kg a cada 12 h inicialmente; reduzida de forma gradual em 6 meses.
• Riquetsial e borreliose — doxiciclina.
• Protozoária — clindamicina.
• Micótica — exige tratamento por 1-2 anos; utilizar itraconazol (5 mg/kg VO a cada 12 h com alimento) ou fluconazol (6,25-12,5 mg/kg VO ou IV a cada 12 h); os corticosteroides são frequentemente necessários durante as primeiras 4-6 semanas para controlar o edema cerebral.
• Viral e pós-vacinal — não há nenhum tratamento definitivo; tratar de forma sintomática.
• Bacteriana — antibióticos de amplo espectro que penetram na barreira hematoencefálica; caso não se conheça o agente infeccioso, tentar uma combinação de enrofloxacino (5-10 mg/kg VO ou IV a cada 12 h) e ticarcilina-clavulanato (50 mg/kg IV a cada 8 h) ou amoxicilina-clavulanato (13,75 mg/kg VO a cada 8 h).

CONTRAINDICAÇÕES
• Encefalite bacteriana e febre maculosa das Montanhas Rochosas — os corticosteroides são contraindicados.
• Filhotes caninos com <6 meses de vida acometidos por doença riquetsial — utilizar o cloranfenicol (em virtude das manchas nos dentes induzidas pela doxiciclina).
• Filhotes caninos com <8 meses de vida — o enrofloxacino é contraindicado, em função dos danos cartilaginosos; utilizar amoxicilina-clavulanato ou ticarcilina-clavulanato isoladamente.
• Infecções do SNC — não empregar aminoglicosídeos e cefalosporinas de primeira geração, pois a penetração no SNC não é satisfatória.

PRECAUÇÕES
• Para diminuir a pressão intracraniana, administrar manitol por via intravenosa 10 min antes de se administrar a anestesia para a coleta do LCS.
• Corticosteroides — observar o paciente de perto quanto ao agravamento dos sinais clínicos, sugestivos de causa infecciosa.

INTERAÇÕES POSSÍVEIS
• Cloranfenicol e cimetidina — não usar concomitantemente com fenobarbital para evitar níveis séricos tóxicos desse anticonvulsivante, secundários à interferência no metabolismo hepático.
• Os corticosteroides alteram a análise do LCS se utilizados por 12 h ou mais.

MEDICAMENTO(S) ALTERNATIVO(S)
• Leflunomida — 1,5-4 mg/kg a cada 24 h individualizada com base no nível sanguíneo de seu metabólito ativo, teriflunomida, mensurado 24 h após a medicação 4 semanas depois da instituição da terapia em virtude da meia-vida prolongada de 2 semanas. A faixa terapêutica de segurança é de 20-40 mcg/mL. Com frequência, esse agente é eficaz em casos de encefalite imunomediada irresponsiva à terapia convencional. Leucopenia, trombocitopenia e colite hemorrágica são possíveis efeitos adversos. Obtenção mensal do hemograma completo; o tratamento dura 1 ano.
• Citarabina — 100 mg/m² SC a cada 12 h por 4 doses no total a cada 4 semanas pode ser utilizada em acréscimo à leflunomida e prednisona em cães com encefalite imunomediada para se obter imunossupressão adicional. Os efeitos adversos são semelhantes aos da leflunomida. O *nadir* (nível mais baixo) ocorre por volta de 1-2 semanas. É recomendável a realização do hemograma 2 semanas após a terapia.

ACOMPANHAMENTO

MONITORIZAÇÃO DO PACIENTE
• Avaliações neurológicas frequentes nas primeiras 48-72 h para monitorizar a evolução do quadro.
• Recidiva conforme a medicação é retirada — repetir a análise do LCS.
• Mensuração do título sérico para o antígeno capsular criptocócico a cada 3 meses até sua negatividade.

PREVENÇÃO
• Em animais que residem em áreas endêmicas, deve-se empregar um método eficaz de controle de carrapatos.
• Evitar a vacinação de cães que já tiveram meningoencefalite granulomatosa.

COMPLICAÇÕES POSSÍVEIS
• Corticoterapia a longo prazo — sinais de hiperadrenocorticismo iatrogênico.
• Coleta do LCS e evolução natural da doença — herniação tentorial e óbito.

EVOLUÇÃO ESPERADA E PROGNÓSTICO
• Resolução dos sinais — geralmente gradativa (2-8 semanas).
• Prototecal — quase sempre evolui para o óbito.
• Imunomediada — prognóstico razoável a bom quanto à remissão completa em casos de imunossupressão rigorosa.
• Infecções riquetsiais, micóticas, bacterianas, protozoárias e espiroquetais — possibilidade razoável de sobrevida.
• Migração parasitária, corpos estranhos migratórios, meningoencefalite piogranulomatosa, encefalite necrosante do Yorkshire terrier e polioencefalomielite — costumam ser fatais.
• Encefalite do Pug e do Maltês — podem ser fatais; a evolução é bastante variável; alguns pacientes respondem ao tratamento com esteroides por períodos prolongados.
• Encefalomielite pós-vacinal — pode exibir resolução espontânea; muitas vezes, causa danos permanentes e leva ao óbito.

✓ DIVERSOS

FATORES RELACIONADOS COM A IDADE
• Animais jovens (<2 anos) e idosos (>8 anos) — maior risco de doenças infecciosas.
• Cães com <6 anos de idade — encefalites imunomediadas e idiopáticas.

POTENCIAL ZOONÓTICO
• Raiva — considerar em áreas endêmicas se o paciente for um animal de rua que apresenta encefalite de evolução rápida.
• Os seres humanos podem ser infectados pelo mesmo carrapato-vetor que afetou o paciente.
• Os exsudatos obtidos de animais com micose podem se reverter ao estágio micelial infeccioso formador de esporos.
• As culturas são altamente contagiosas e devem ser manipuladas com extrema cautela.

VER TAMBÉM
• "Causas".
• Crises Convulsivas (Convulsões, Estado Epiléptico) — Cães.
• Crises Convulsivas (Convulsões, Estado Epiléptico) — Gatos.
• Estupor e Coma.

ABREVIATURA(S)
• ELISA = ensaio imunoabsorvente ligado à enzima.
• LCS = líquido cerebrospinal.
• PIF = peritonite infecciosa felina.
• RM = ressonância magnética.
• TC = tomografia computadorizada.
• FIV = vírus da imunodeficiência felina.
• FeLV = vírus da leucemia felina.
• SNC = sistema nervoso central.

RECURSOS DA INTERNET
http://www.ivis.org/advances/Vite/toc.asp.

Sugestões de Leitura
Greene CE, ed. Infectious Diseases of the Dog and Cat, rev. reprint, 3rd ed. Philadelphia: Saunders, 2006.
Schatzberg S. Idiopathic granulomatous and necrotizing inflammatory disorders of the canine central nervous system. Vet Clin North Am Small Anim Pract 2010, 40(1):101-120.

Autor Allen Sisson
Consultor Editorial Joane M. Parent

ENCEFALITE NECROSANTE

CONSIDERAÇÕES GERAIS

DEFINIÇÃO
Encefalite necrosante, restrita em termos históricos a algumas raças como Pug, Yorkshire terrier e Maltês, também é descrita hoje em dia em outras raças, como Chihuahua, Shih tzu e outras. Por essa razão, o termo "encefalite necrosante específica à raça" não é mais utilizado.

SISTEMA(S) ACOMETIDO(S)
SNC.

GENÉTICA
Provável base genética; suspeita de distúrbio multifatorial.

INCIDÊNCIA/PREVALÊNCIA
Embora a incidência e a prevalência sejam indeterminadas, essa doença ocorre regularmente.

DISTRIBUIÇÃO GEOGRÁFICA
Ocorre em todo o mundo, sendo observada principalmente em raças *toys*.

IDENTIFICAÇÃO
Raça(s) Predominante(s)
Maltês, Pug, Yorkshire terrier, Buldogue francês, Chihuahua, Shih tzu e outras raças *toys*.
Idade Média e Faixa Etária
Acomete, sobretudo, cães jovens adultos (faixa etária de 4 meses a 10 anos).
Sexo Predominante
Não há predileção sexual.

SINAIS CLÍNICOS
Sinais progressivos relacionados com uma lesão do prosencéfalo (comportamento anormal, crises convulsivas, andar em círculo, cegueira), lesões do tronco encefálico com sinais vestibulares centrais, ou uma lesão multifocal.

CAUSAS E FATORES DE RISCO
• Desconhecidos.
• Talvez haja suspeita de algum agente infeccioso.

DIAGNÓSTICO

DIAGNÓSTICO DIFERENCIAL
• Outras doenças inflamatórias/infecciosas do SNC — diferenciadas nos resultados dos exames de sorologia, LCS e RM.
• Neoplasia — diferenciada nos achados da RM.

HEMOGRAMA/BIOQUÍMICA/URINÁLISE
Os resultados costumam ser normais.

OUTROS TESTES LABORATORIAIS
N/D.

DIAGNÓSTICO POR IMAGEM
TC/RM — os resultados ajudam a apoiar o diagnóstico clínico, considerando-se a raça, a idade, os sinais clínicos e a evolução da doença. As lesões podem ser prosencefálicas multifocais assimétricas com realce de contraste variável e incluir múltiplas áreas císticas de necrose.

MÉTODOS DIAGNÓSTICOS
• LCS — pleocitose com células predominantemente mononucleares; elevação leve a acentuada de proteínas.
• Biopsia cerebral — para confirmar o diagnóstico.

ACHADOS PATOLÓGICOS
• Necrose e inflamação não supurativa das substâncias branca e cinzenta do cérebro; lesões multifocais; as lesões ativas consistem em um grande centro gliótico malácico circundado por uma parede de inflamação mononuclear grave.
• As lesões antigas consistem em áreas rarefeitas ou císticas circundadas por esclerose astroglial intensa.

TRATAMENTO

CUIDADO(S) DE SAÚDE ADEQUADO(S)
• Tratamento hospitalar ou ambulatorial com base no estado neurológico do paciente.
• Não há tratamento específico conhecido.

CUIDADO(S) DE ENFERMAGEM
N/D.

ATIVIDADE
N/D.

DIETA
N/D.

ORIENTAÇÃO AO PROPRIETÁRIO
• Não é possível o tratamento específico da doença; com o uso de agentes anti-inflamatórios ou imunossupressores, pode haver melhora, mas não cura.
• As crises convulsivas podem ser o único sinal clínico no início da doença em cães da raça Pug — é recomendada a avaliação diagnóstica de cães dessa raça que se apresentam com crises convulsivas.

CONSIDERAÇÕES CIRÚRGICAS
N/D.

MEDICAÇÕES

MEDICAMENTO(S) DE ESCOLHA
• Tratamento sintomático.
• Para controle das crises convulsivas, usar fenobarbital (2-8 mg/kg VO a cada 12 h).
• Os corticosteroides podem reduzir a resposta inflamatória e melhorar os sinais clínicos (p. ex., prednisolona ou prednisona 1-2 mg/kg VO a cada 24 h nas primeiras 1-2 semanas; em seguida, a dose pode ser reduzida de forma lenta e gradual).

CONTRAINDICAÇÕES/INTERAÇÕES POSSÍVEIS
N/D.

PRECAUÇÕES
N/D.

MEDICAMENTO(S) ALTERNATIVO(S)
Citosina-arabinosídeo, procarbazina, azatioprina, ciclosporina, leflunomida, lomustina, micofenolato de mofetila, principalmente em uma terapia combinada com corticosteroides.

ACOMPANHAMENTO

MONITORIZAÇÃO DO PACIENTE
• Exames clínicos e neurológicos regulares para monitorizar a resposta ao tratamento sintomático.
• Monitorização dos níveis séricos de fenobarbital.

PREVENÇÃO
N/D.

COMPLICAÇÕES POSSÍVEIS
N/D.

EVOLUÇÃO ESPERADA E PROGNÓSTICO
• A evolução da doença é crônica por meses ou até mesmo anos; em todo caso confirmado, os sinais neurológicos foram progressivos.
• O prognóstico é reservado.

DIVERSOS

DISTÚRBIOS ASSOCIADOS
Em um único cão da raça Pug, foi observada necrose do miocárdio além das lesões encefálicas.

FATORES RELACIONADOS COM A IDADE
N/D.

POTENCIAL ZOONÓTICO
N/D.

GESTAÇÃO/FERTILIDADE/REPRODUÇÃO
Três cães da raça Pug descritas no Japão tiveram um histórico de gestação antes do início dos sinais clínicos.

ABREVIATURAS
• LCS = líquido cerebrospinal.
• RM = ressonância magnética.
• SNC = sistema nervoso central.
• TC = tomografia computadorizada.

Sugestões de Leitura
Cordy DR, Holliday TA. A necrotizing meningoencephalitis of pug dogs. Vet Pathol 1989, 26:191-194.
Stalis IH, Chadwick B, Dayrell-Hart B, Summers BA, VanWinkle TJ. Necrotizing meningoencephalitis of Maltese dogs. Vet Pathol 1995, 32:230-235.
Talarico LR, Schatzberg SJ. Idiopathic granulomatous and necrotising inflammatory disorders of the canine central nervous system: A review and future perspectives. J Small Anim Pract 2010, 51:150-154.
Tipold A, Fatzer R, Jaggy A, Zurbriggen A, Vandevelde M. Necrotizing encephalitis in Yorkshire terriers. J Small Anim Pract 1993, 34:623-628.

Autor Andrea Tipold
Consultor Editorial Joane M. Parent

Encefalite Secundária à Migração Parasitária

CONSIDERAÇÕES GERAIS

REVISÃO
- Migração parasitária aberrante para o SNC.
- Os parasitas normalmente podem comprometer um outro sistema orgânico do mesmo hospedeiro (p. ex., *Dirofilaria immitis*, *Taenia*, *Ancylostoma caninum*, *Angiostrongylus* ou *Toxocara canis*) ou uma espécie diferente de hospedeiro (p. ex., nematódeo dos guaxinins [*Baylisascaris procyonis*]; nematódeo dos cangambás [*B. columnaris*]; *Coenurus* spp. ou *Cysticercus cellulosae*).
- Acesso ao SNC — em geral por via hematógena (dirofilariose) ou por meio dos tecidos adjacentes, incluindo a orelha média, os forames cranianos, as cavidades nasais, a placa cribriforme e as fontanelas abertas (cuterebrose).

IDENTIFICAÇÃO
- Dirofilariose — apenas animais adultos.
- Outros parasitas — animais jovens com acesso a ambientes externos — ocorrência rara e esporádica.

SINAIS CLÍNICOS
- Variam de acordo com a porção acometida do SNC.
- Provavelmente assimétricos.
- Podem sugerir a presença de lesão expansiva focal tipo massa ou o processo patológico multifocal.
- Cuterebrose — sazonal (Julho-Outubro), com início agudo ou superagudo de mudanças comportamentais, crises convulsivas, déficits visuais, etc. É comum a constatação de histórico prévio de doença respiratória.
- Parasita murino, *Angiostrongylus cantonensis* (Austrália) — síndrome lombossacra (paralisia/paresia dos membros pélvicos, da cauda e da bexiga) que pode ascender aos membros torácicos e nervos cranianos em filhotes caninos.

CAUSAS E FATORES DE RISCO
Abrigo em gaiola previamente ocupada por animais silvestres (guaxinins, cangambás).

DIAGNÓSTICO

DIAGNÓSTICO DIFERENCIAL
- Descartar outras causas de encefalopatia focal — doenças infecciosas (virais, bacterianas, protozoárias ou fúngicas); meningoencefalomielite granulomatosa; tumor cerebral.
- O diagnóstico costuma ser feito à necropsia.

HEMOGRAMA/BIOQUÍMICA/URINÁLISE
Normais a menos que o parasita também comprometa os tecidos não neurais.

OUTROS TESTES LABORATORIAIS
LCS — pode revelar pleocitose eosinofílica, neutrofílica ou mononuclear (encontrada também em casos de encefalites protozoárias, fúngicas e prototecais); pode permanecer normal em lesões estritamente parenquimatosas.

DIAGNÓSTICO POR IMAGEM
TC e RM — cerebrais; lesão focal e/ou infarto cerebral em virtude da oclusão de vasos cerebrais. Esses exames são inespecíficos e frequentemente inconclusivos, mas podem conduzir à exploração cirúrgica e remoção do parasita migratório.

ACHADOS PATOLÓGICOS
- O parasita ou seus trajetos podem ou não ser identificados.
- Infarto, ruptura vascular e hemorragia ou êmbolos vasculares podem causar necrose e malácia locais a extensas. Pode haver proliferação granulomatosa e/ou hidrocefalia obstrutiva.
- *Dirofilaria immitis* — intra ou extravascular.
- Os vermes adultos produzem inflamação focal.
- Suspeita-se da cuterebrose como causa de encefalopatia isquêmica felina.

TRATAMENTO

- Remoção cirúrgica de *Cuterebra* intracraniana.
- Medicamentos (ver adiante) podem potencializar a doença.
- Cuidados de suporte e enfermagem.

MEDICAÇÕES

MEDICAMENTO(S)
- Dirofilariose e angiostrongilose neural — os tratamentos anti-helmínticos podem levar ao agravamento dos sinais clínicos e, algumas vezes, ao óbito.
- Angiostrongilose neural branda — os filhotes caninos podem se recuperar com os cuidados de suporte e a corticoterapia.
- Uma única dose de ivermectina (400 mg/kg SC) pode matar as larvas de *Cuterebra* em gatos com suspeita de cuterebrose. O pré-tratamento com difenidramina (4 mg/kg) e dexametasona intravenosa (0,1 mg/kg) pode amenizar as reações alérgicas/anafiláticas às larvas mortas ou agonizantes.

CONTRAINDICAÇÕES/INTERAÇÕES POSSÍVEIS
N/D.

ACOMPANHAMENTO

MONITORIZAÇÃO DO PACIENTE
Conforme a necessidade.

PREVENÇÃO
- Manter os animais domésticos dentro de casa e/ou afastados de animais silvestres.
- Utilizar anti-helmínticos e preventivos contra dirofilariose.

COMPLICAÇÕES POSSÍVEIS
N/D.

EVOLUÇÃO ESPERADA E PROGNÓSTICO
Geralmente progressivos após o início agudo ou insidioso.

DIVERSOS

VER TAMBÉM
- Dirofilariose — Cães.
- Dirofilariose — Gatos.
- Encefalite.
- Encefalitozoonoses.
- Encefalopatia Isquêmica Felina.

ABREVIATURA(S)
- LCS = líquido cerebrospinal.
- RM = ressonância magnética.
- SNC = sistema nervoso central.
- TC = tomografia computadorizada.

RECURSOS DA INTERNET
- Braund KG. Neurovascular disorders (atualizado em 2003). In: Clinical Neurology in Small Animals — Localization, Diagnosis and Treatment. www.ivis.org.
- Vite CH. Inflammatory diseases of the central nervous system (updated 2005). In: Clinical Neurology in Small Animals — Localization, Diagnosis and Treatment. www.ivis.org.

Sugestões de Leitura
Dewey CW. Verminous encephalitis. In: A Practical Guide to Canine and Feline Neurology, 2nd ed. Ames, IA: Wiley-Blackwell, 2008, pp. 184-185.
Glass EN, et al. Clinical and clinicopathologic features in 11 cats with Cuterebra Larvae myasis of the central nervous system. J Vet Intern Med 1998, 12:365-368.
Williams KJ, Summers BA, de Lahunta A. Cerebrospinal cuterebriasis in cats and its association with feline ischemic encephalopathy. Vet Pathol 1998, 35:330-343.

Autor Christine Berthelin-Baker
Consultor Editorial Joane M. Parent

ENCEFALITOZOONOSE

CONSIDERAÇÕES GERAIS

REVISÃO
- A encefalotozoonose é conhecida atualmente como microsporidiose.
- Infecção causada pelos parasitas *Encephalitozoon cuniculi* e outras espécies.
- Acomete os pulmões, o coração, os rins e o cérebro.
- Incomum nos EUA.

IDENTIFICAÇÃO
- Cães e gatos.
- Não há predileção etária, sexual ou racial.

SINAIS CLÍNICOS

Neonatos
- Surge algumas semanas após o parto.
- Retardo do crescimento.
- Falta de desenvolvimento.
- Evolui para insuficiência renal.
- Anormalidades neurológicas.

Adultos
- Os mesmos sinais apresentados pelos neonatos.
- Pode exibir comportamento agressivo, crises convulsivas ou cegueira.

CAUSAS E FATORES DE RISCO
- A via mais provável é a oronasal, a partir de urina contaminada com esporos.
- Os canis constituem um fator de risco.

DIAGNÓSTICO

DIAGNÓSTICO DIFERENCIAL
- Raiva.
- Cinomose.
- Neosporose.
- Toxoplasmose.

HEMOGRAMA/BIOQUÍMICA/URINÁLISE
- Anemia normocítica normocrômica.
- Linfocitose e monocitose.
- Espera-se uma elevação dos níveis séricos da ALT e da fosfatase alcalina.

OUTROS TESTES LABORATORIAIS
Sorologia — sangue e LCS.

DIAGNÓSTICO POR IMAGEM
Pode contribuir, mas não é diagnóstico.

MÉTODOS DIAGNÓSTICOS
- Urinálise — sedimento corado pelo corante de Gram ou Ziehl-Neelsen; esporos Gram-positivos; birrefringente.
- A identificação positiva requer procedimentos imunológicos.

ACHADOS PATOLÓGICOS
- Nefrite intersticial não supurativa — achado compatível.
- Hepatomegalia e petéquias em toda a superfície de vários órgãos.
- Rins intumescidos, cistite hemorrágica, cistos corticais renais ou infartos.
- Cérebro — na presença de lesões, observam-se trombose e encefalomalacia, espaços císticos no parênquima.

TRATAMENTO

- Internação com terapia de suporte.
- Eutanásia — quando há sinais neurológicos graves.

MEDICAÇÕES

MEDICAMENTO(S)
Quimioterapia — desconhecida para cães e gatos; tentar os benzimidazóis, em particular albendazol (50 mg/kg a cada 8 h por 7 dias), porque funcionam em camundongos e seres humanos.

CONTRAINDICAÇÕES/INTERAÇÕES POSSÍVEIS
N/D.

ACOMPANHAMENTO

PREVENÇÃO
Higienização — importante; conseguida com etanol a 70%.

EVOLUÇÃO ESPERADA E PROGNÓSTICO
Vários pacientes se recuperarão sem outros sinais clínicos se as manifestações renais ou cerebrais não se agravarem.

DIVERSOS

POTENCIAL ZOONÓTICO
Riscos potenciais para seres humanos, sobretudo os imunossuprimidos.

ABREVIATURA(S)
- ALT = alanina aminotransferase.
- LCS = líquido cerebrospinal.

RECURSOS DA INTERNET
www.dpd.cdc.gov/DPDx/HTML/Microsporidiosis.htm.

Sugestões de Leitura
Didier PJ, Snowden K, Alvarez X, Didier ES. Microsporidiosis. In: Greene CE, ed., Infectious Diseases of the Dog and Cat, 3rd ed. St. Louis: Saunders Elsevier, 2006, pp. 711-716.

Autor Johnny D. Hoskins
Consultor Editorial Stephen C. Barr

ENCEFALOPATIA HEPÁTICA

CONSIDERAÇÕES GERAIS

DEFINIÇÃO
Amplo espectro de sinais neuropsiquiátricos associados à insuficiência hepática aguda, desvio portossistêmico sem hepatopatia intrínseca ou fibrose/cirrose hepáticas com hipertensão portal.

FISIOPATOLOGIA
• A maioria dos sinais neurocomportamentais é atribuída a substâncias derivadas do intestino (metabolismo bacteriano e proteico), particularmente amônia. A amônia e o glutamato são neurotoxinas. • Os fatores fisiopatológicos incluem: falha de energia (neuroglicopenia), alteração do pH cerebral e do fluxo iônico de cálcio, anormalidades que envolvem neurotransmissores como glutamato, GABA e catecolaminas, distúrbio do metabolismo de aminoácidos aromáticos, níveis cerebrais elevados de substâncias endógenas semelhantes a benzodiazepinas, citocinas inflamatórias, lesão oxidativa, sendo que cada um deles contribui para desarranjos eletrofisiológicos.

SISTEMA(S) ACOMETIDO(S)
• Nervoso — há um predomínio de função cerebral anormal; consciência e função diminuídas que evoluem para sonolência ou coma ou, então, agitação que evolui para atividade convulsiva; agressividade e crises convulsivas são mais prováveis em gatos com anomalia vascular portossistêmica. • GI — vômitos, diarreia e anorexia. • Renal/urológico — cristalúria por biurato de amônio; cálculos renais pélvicos e císticos.

GENÉTICA
• Anomalia vascular portossistêmica congênita — hereditária em algumas raças (ver "Anomalia Vascular Portossistêmica Congênita").

INCIDÊNCIA/PREVALÊNCIA
Distúrbio incomum.

IDENTIFICAÇÃO
Espécies
Cães e gatos.

Raça(s) Predominante(s)
• Anomalia vascular portossistêmica — em geral, ocorre em raças puras de cães; ocorrência elevada em algumas raças (ver "Anomalia Vascular Portossistêmica Congênita"). • Hepatite crônica e hepatopatia por armazenamento de cobre são mais comuns em determinadas raças (ver capítulos).

Idade Média e Faixa Etária
• Anomalia vascular portossistêmica — em geral, afeta animais jovens. • Hepatopatia adquirida com desvio portossistêmico adquirido — qualquer idade.

SINAIS CLÍNICOS
Comentários Gerais
• Neurológicos — costumam ter relação com o consumo de refeições, particularmente aquelas ricas em proteína, ou infecção sistêmica; hemorragia GI; desidratação; azotemia; constipação; catabolismo. • Pode ocorrer resolução temporária com restrição de proteína na dieta ± tratamento com antibiótico ou lactulose ± resolução das condições associadas. • Recuperação prolongada da sedação ou anestesia.

Achados Anamnésicos
• Anormalidades episódicas. • Dificuldades de aprendizado (adestramento, no caso). • Letargia, sonolência, coma. • Anorexia, vômitos, ptialismo.
• Poliúria e polidipsia. • Desorientação — vagar sem rumo; marcha compulsiva; compressão da cabeça contra objetos. • Cegueira amaurótica.
• Crises convulsivas. • Mais frequente em gatos do que em cães — ptialismo; crises convulsivas; agressividade; desorientação; estupor atáxico.
• Mais frequente em cães do que em gatos — comportamento compulsivo (compressão da cabeça contra objetos, andar em círculo, vagar sem rumo, vocalização); vômitos; diarreia; poliúria e polidipsia; hematúria; polaciúria e disúria associada a urólitos de biurato de amônio.

Achados do Exame Físico
• Anomalia vascular portossistêmica — os gatos podem parecer de porte normal, embora a maioria tenha baixa estatura; micro-hepatia; e íris de cor dourada/acobreada (gatos sem olhos azuis e não pertencentes à raça Persa). • Anomalia vascular portossistêmica — os cães podem parecer de porte normal, mas costumam exibir retardo do crescimento; micro-hepatia; incidência elevada de criptorquidismo em um único estudo.
• Hepatopatia adquirida — depende da cronicidade do distúrbio subjacente e da formação de desvio portossistêmico adquirido; a formação de ascite é comum em cães com encefalopatia hepática causada por hepatopatia adquirida e frequentemente sofre exacerbação e remissão em termos de gravidade; nesses animais, podem ocorrer coagulopatias incomuns/variáveis. • Sinais atribuídos ao trato urinário inferior; uropatia obstrutiva em função de urolitíase por biurato de amônio; coloração laranja ou castanha à urina pela presença de cristais.

CAUSAS
• Anomalia vascular portossistêmica — más-formações congênitas. • Desvio portossistêmico adquirido — ocorre com doenças que induzem à hipertensão portal (cirrose, fístula AV intra-hepática, fibrose); ver "Hipertensão Portal"; "Desvio Portossistêmico Adquirido".
• Insuficiência hepática aguda — induzida por medicamentos, toxinas ou infecção (ver "Insuficiência Hepática Aguda"; "Hepatotoxinas").

FATORES DE RISCO
• Alcalose, hipocalemia, hipoglicemia. • Certos anestésicos e sedativos. • Determinados medicamentos (p. ex., metionina, tetraciclina e anti-histamínicos). • Sangramento entérico — causa precipitante aguda mais comum de encefalopatia hepática. • Transfusão — hemoderivados armazenados podem conter altas concentrações de amônia; transfusões de sangue incompatível. • Infecções. • Constipação.
• Catabolismo — distúrbios que causam emaciação muscular; grandes quantidades de amônia normalmente sofrem destoxificação transitória por armazenamento no tecido muscular.

DIAGNÓSTICO

DIAGNÓSTICO DIFERENCIAL
• Toxicidade pelo chumbo. • Infecção do trato urinário — outra urolitíase. • Parasitismo intestinal. • Doença gastrintestinal primária. • Hipoglicemia: muitas causas. • Toxoplasmose. • Doença congênita ou má-formação do SNC — hidrocefalia; doenças de armazenamento; tumor cerebral. • Intoxicação aguda por etilenoglicol ou xilitol. • Doenças infecciosas — raiva; cinomose. • Neoplasia do SNC. • Deficiência de tiamina — encefalopatia de Wernicke (especialmente em gatos). • Intoxicação por medicamentos; drogas recreacionais para seres humanos.

HEMOGRAMA/BIOQUÍMICA/URINÁLISE
Hemograma Completo
• Anomalia vascular portossistêmica e desvio portossistêmico adquirido — microcitose eritrocitária; leve anemia arregenerativa; pecilocitose (gatos); células em alvo (cães); o desvio portossistêmico adquirido pode se apresentar com ou sem plasma ictérico.

Bioquímica
• Níveis baixos de ureia e creatinina — os valores refletem poliúria e polidipsia, TFG alta e síntese hepática reduzida em anomalia vascular portossistêmica e hepatopatia grave adquirida.
• Hipoglicemia — cães jovens de raças toy com anomalia vascular portossistêmica; insuficiência hepática fulminante; cirrose. • Colesterol baixo — comum; anomalia vascular portossistêmica e desvio portossistêmico adquirido; insuficiência hepática fulminante. • Enzimas hepáticas — atividade variável com desvio portossistêmico adquirido; a fosfatase alcalina, em geral, apresenta-se elevada em pacientes jovens com anomalia vascular portossistêmica em virtude da isoenzima óssea. • Bilirrubina — normal com anomalia vascular portossistêmica, mas pode estar alta com desvio portossistêmico adquirido.
• Hipoalbuminemia — comum com desvio portossistêmico adquirido, mas inconsistente e discreta com anomalia vascular portossistêmica.

Urinálise
• Baixa concentração — comum com anomalia vascular portossistêmica. • Cristalúria por urato de amônio — causa hematúria, piúria e proteinúria por inflamação mecânica e infecção secundária a cálculos metabólicos.

OUTROS TESTES LABORATORIAIS
• Amônia sanguínea — indicador sensível de encefalopatia hepática, mas inconsistente; hiperamonemia de jejum não é confiável, porque a encefalopatia hepática pode ocorrer sem hiperamonemia em função de sua patogenia multifatorial; os valores de amônia no sangue são menos confiáveis que os ácidos biliares séricos totais em virtude de problemas analíticos/metodológicos e pelo fato de as amostras não poderem ser enviadas para análise; teste de tolerância à amônia — método mais confiável para detectar intolerância a essa substância; **Cuidado:** pode induzir à encefalopatia hepática. • Ácidos biliares séricos totais — confirmam insuficiência hepática ou desvio associado à encefalopatia hepática. • Provas de coagulação — anomalia vascular portossistêmica: as anormalidades, em geral, não estão associadas a sangramento; desvio portossistêmico adquirido: aumentos do TP, do TTPA, da PIVKA, mas diminuição do fibrinogênio, refletem a gravidade da disfunção hepática, a falha na síntese, a presença de CID e a suficiência da vitamina K. • Proteína C — baixa em cães com desvio considerável, insuficiência hepática, enteropatia com perda de proteínas, CID.
• Efusão abdominal — hepatopatia adquirida; fístula AV hepatoportal; transudato puro ou modificado. • Valores hepáticos de zinco — em geral, baixos (<120 µg/g de tecido hepático).

DIAGNÓSTICO POR IMAGEM
Ver "Anomalia Vascular Portossistêmica Congênita" e "Desvio Portossistêmico Adquirido".

ENCEFALOPATIA HEPÁTICA

MÉTODOS DIAGNÓSTICOS
• Aspiração hepática — não é capaz de diferenciar os distúrbios que causam desvio portossistêmico. • Biopsia hepática — amostra, obtida por biopsia em cunha durante cirurgia aberta ou laparoscopia (com pinças de biopsia dotadas de ventosas), de tecido de vários lobos hepáticos. • Biopsia realizada com agulha (Tru-Cut®) — pode coletar amostras teciduais de forma inadequada.

ACHADOS PATOLÓGICOS
• Macroscópicos — as alterações hepáticas refletem o distúrbio subjacente; herniação cerebral em casos de encefalopatia hepática aguda. • Microscópicos — lesões do SNC: polimicrocavitação e astrocitose tipo II de Alzheimer.

TRATAMENTO

CUIDADO(S) DE SAÚDE ADEQUADO(S)
• Depende(m) da condição subjacente. • Anomalia vascular portossistêmica — é preferível a correção cirúrgica, mas pode-se optar pelo tratamento clínico prolongado.

CUIDADO(S) DE ENFERMAGEM
• Depende(m) da condição subjacente; eliminar os fatores que promovem a encefalopatia hepática. • Aumentar a tolerância à proteína da dieta com o uso de enemas, tratamentos orais (ver "Medicações") e alteração do consumo proteico. • Se houver coma hepático — interromper as medicações orais. • Fluidos — usar cristaloides balanceados, mas evitar o uso de lactato em caso de insuficiência hepática fulminante; se o paciente estiver hipoglicêmico, suplementar os fluidos com glicose a 2,5-5,0%; fornecer cloreto de potássio a 20-30 mEq/L (não exceder 0,5 mEq/kg/h) e titular de acordo com as necessidades; fluidos com restrição de sódio na presença de ascite e/ou hipalbuminemia acentuada. • Vitaminas solúveis do complexo B (2 mL/L de fluidos).

ATIVIDADE
Manter o paciente aquecido, inativo e hidratado.

DIETA
• Nível adequado de calorias — evitar o catabolismo e manter a massa muscular (local para destoxificação/armazenamento temporários da amônia). • Restrição de proteína na dieta — base do tratamento clínico; usar dieta específica para hepatopatia ou insuficiência renal moderada; cães: as melhores fontes de proteína são os laticínios e a soja; 2,5 g de proteína/kg; gatos: precisam de proteína derivada da carne; 3,5 g de proteína/kg. • S-adenosilmetionina — é preferível para a suplementação de metionina: 20 mg/kg VO/d. • Tiamina — para evitar encefalopatia de Wernicke; 50-100 mg diários por 3 dias, em seguida com vitaminas hidrossolúveis nos fluidos. **Cuidado:** podem ocorrer reações anafilactoides com a tiamina injetável. • Nutrição parenteral parcial — recomendada no caso de inapetência a curto prazo a fim de minimizar a mobilização catabólica de músculo; usar a nutrição parenteral total se a inapetência durar mais de 5 dias e se a via enteral não estiver disponível; o uso de soluções de aminoácidos de cadeia ramificada é controverso.

ORIENTAÇÃO AO PROPRIETÁRIO
• Encefalopatia hepática — frequentemente episódica e recidivante caso não se consiga curar o distúrbio subjacente. • Ensinar o proprietário a aplicar enemas e ajustar a dose das medicações com critério. • Anomalia vascular portossistêmica — a ligadura cirúrgica pode ser curativa, embora possa causar complicações adversas em alguns cães; os sinais clínicos pós-operatórios podem persistir, exigindo tratamento nutricional crônico e clínico. • Desvio portossistêmico adquirido — depende da causa subjacente.

CONSIDERAÇÕES CIRÚRGICAS
• Ver "Anomalia Vascular Portossistêmica Congênita". • Desvio portossistêmico adquirido — não fazer ligadura.

MEDICAÇÕES

MEDICAMENTO(S)
• Os agentes terapêuticos que aumentam a tolerância à proteína da dieta alteram a microbiota ou as condições entéricas, reduzindo a produção ou a disponibilidade de substâncias indutoras de encefalopatia hepática. • Antibióticos — de um espectro que altere a microbiota intestinal (aeróbica e anaeróbica) ou seus produtos; escolhas antibióticas de primeira escolha: sistêmicos (metronidazol 7,5 mg/kg VO a cada 12 h ou amoxicilina, especialmente em gatos, 12,5-25 mg/kg VO a cada 8-12 h), combinados com lactulose e neomicina (10-22 mg/kg VO a cada 12 h [o tratamento crônico com neomicina pode resultar em nefro ou ototoxicidade]); antimicrobianos locais sob a forma de enema: usar as mesmas doses que as orais; não administrar tanto pela via oral como retal.
• Carboidratos fermentados inabsorvíveis — lactulose, lactitol ou lactose (se houver deficiência de lactase); diminuem a produção ou a absorção de amônia; efeito catártico; aprisiona o nitrogênio em bactérias; a lactulose é mais comumente utilizada (iniciar com 0,5-1,0 mL/kg a cada 8-12 h); a meta terapêutica são 2-3 evacuações de fezes moles por dia; também pode ser administrada como enema na encefalopatia hepática aguda e no coma *após* a remoção de debris pelos enemas de limpeza.
• Probióticos com carboidratos fermentados inabsorvíveis podem alterar favoravelmente a flora intestinal de forma a diminuir a produção de toxina da encefalopatia hepática. • Enemas — *enemas de limpeza* (fluidos poliônicos aquecidos) promovem a limpeza mecânica do cólon (10-15 mL/kg); *enemas de retenção* liberam diretamente substratos fermentáveis ou alteram diretamente o pH e os microrganismos do cólon; lactulose, lactitol ou lactose diluídos (1:2 em água); neomicina em água (não exceder a dose oral, não administrar por via oral e retal); Betadine® diluída (1:10 em água, enxaguar bem em 15 min); vinagre diluído (1:10 em água). • Suplementação com zinco — 2 enzimas do ciclo da ureia necessitam de zinco; medir o nível plasmático basal desse elemento, dose de 1-3 mg/kg VO de zinco elementar (acetato de zinco); titular a dose com base nas mensurações de zinco plasmático; evitar valores > 800 μg/dL. • Edema cerebral — complica a encefalopatia hepática aguda; manitol (1 g/kg diluído em solução fisiológica, durante 30 min); oxigênio nasal; *N*-acetilcisteína (140 mg/kg IV diluídos a 1:2 em solução fisiológica e administrados por meio de filtro não pirogênico; em seguida, 70 mg/kg a cada 8 h); o uso de glicocorticoides é controverso, pois esses agentes podem promover sangramento entérico. • Terapia de salvamento para encefalopatia hepática intratável (experimental) — L-ornitina/L-aspartato (humanos, ratos: 180-300 mg/kg/dia fracionados em 3 doses); L-carnitina (100 mg/kg VO ou IV) pode atenuar a hiperamonemia. • Na presença de atividade convulsiva — o levetiracetam é o anticonvulsivante preferido; os anticonvulsivantes secundários incluem zonisamida (cuidado: medicamento à base de sulfa) e, por último, brometo de potássio (complicado pela fluidoterapia) como agentes preferidos em relação ao fenobarbital.

CONTRAINDICAÇÕES
Se possível, evitar os medicamentos que dependem do metabolismo, da biotransformação ou da excreção hepática.

PRECAUÇÕES
Usar com cautela anestésicos, sedativos, tranquilizantes, diuréticos poupadores de potássio, analgésicos e medicamentos que ficam altamente ligados a proteínas (o baixo nível de albumina diminui a ligação proteica).

INTERAÇÕES POSSÍVEIS
Medicamentos que afetam o metabolismo hepático ou dependem dele — por exemplo, cimetidina, cloranfenicol, barbitúricos, cetoconazol.

ACOMPANHAMENTO

MONITORIZAÇÃO DO PACIENTE
• Reavaliar o comportamento do paciente em casa, bem como sua condição corporal e seu peso. • Monitorizar a albumina e a glicose — em pacientes com distúrbios que não são passíveis de correção; ajustar a nutrição. • Monitorizar os eletrólitos — especialmente potássio, porque a hipocalemia agrava a hiperamonemia.

PREVENÇÃO
Evitar desidratação, azotemia, hemólise, constipação, sangramento entérico, endoparasitismo, infusão de sangue armazenado, desafio com amônio, infecções do trato urinário (em especial por microrganismos produtores de urease, p. ex., *Staphylococcus*), hipocalemia, hipomagnesemia e alcalemia.

COMPLICAÇÕES POSSÍVEIS
Dano neurológico permanente (raro).

EVOLUÇÃO ESPERADA E PROGNÓSTICO
Dependem do distúrbio subjacente.

DIVERSOS

SINÔNIMO(S)
• Coma hepático.

VER TAMBÉM
• Anomalia Vascular Portossistêmica Congênita.
• Desvio Portossistêmico Adquirido.
• Insuficiência Hepática Aguda. • Má-formação Arteriovenosa do Fígado.

ABREVIATURA(S)
• AV = arteriovenosa(o)(s). • CID = coagulação intravascular disseminada. • GABA = ácido γ-aminobutírico. • PIVKA = proteínas invocadas pela ausência ou antagonismo da vitamina K. • SNC = sistema nervoso central. • TFG = taxa de filtração glomerular. • TP = tempo de protrombina. • TTPA = tempo de tromboplastina parcial ativada.

Autor Sharon A. Center

Encefalopatia Isquêmica Felina

CONSIDERAÇÕES GERAIS

DEFINIÇÃO
- Doença neurológica sazonal que ocorre em gatos de vida livre ou naqueles com acesso a ambientes externos na América do Norte durante os meses de verão; geralmente resulta em início súbito de crises convulsivas, andar em círculo, alteração da atividade mental e/ou cegueira.
- Migração aberrante de larvas de *Cuterebra* no cérebro de gato; tal migração frequentemente provoca trombose ou vasospasmo da artéria cerebral média com consequente necrose isquêmica; degeneração das camadas superficiais do córtex cerebral e destruição do parênquima associadas à migração física da larva no parênquima cerebral.
- É preciso diferenciá-la de outras causas de doenças vasculares que envolvem os cérebros de gatos, bem como de outras doenças neurológicas felinas.

FISIOPATOLOGIA
- Na encefalopatia isquêmica felina, as larvas de *Cuterebra* ingressam no gato pelas vias nasais, migram por meio da placa cribriforme para o bulbo olfatório do cérebro e, em seguida, ao longo do pedúnculo olfatório e, algumas vezes, prosseguem no parênquima cerebral ou, alternativamente, no espaço subaracnóideo; se ainda estiverem vivos, os parasitas migram no sentido caudal, onde podem comprometer a artéria cerebral média; o comprometimento dessa artéria pode ser físico por meio das espinhas existentes no corpo das larvas ou, possivelmente, por meio de substâncias químicas secretadas pelo parasita, responsáveis pela produção de vasospasmo; ou esse vasospasmo pode ser secundário à hemorragia causada pelos parasitas; os parasitas podem, então, morrer no espaço subaracnóideo ou dentro do parênquima.
- A mosca adulta do cavalo deposita os ovos pela entrada na toca de roedores. Os ovos eclodem e liberam as larvas de 1º estágio ou L1, que se aderem ao pelo do rato ou coelho, ingressam no corpo por meio de algum orifício natural (boca, nariz, olho ou ânus) e migram para os tecidos associados (nasofaringe, traqueia, cavidade torácica, diafragma, cavidade abdominal). Em seguida, as larvas continuam sua migração até atingirem um local subcutâneo na região inguinal ou torácica, onde sofrem maturação primeiro para o 2º estágio ou L2 e depois dentro da hipoderme para o 3º estágio ou L3, emergem através da pele, deixam o hospedeiro, passam para a fase de pupa no solo durante o inverno e, então, surgem na primavera como a mosca adulta do cavalo; quando o gato caça próximo da toca de roedores, a larva L1 adere-se ao pelo do gato e ganha acesso às vias nasais deste animal, dando início ao trajeto catastrófico de encefalopatia isquêmica felina.
- Ocasionalmente, as larvas não migram por meio da placa cribriforme, mas ficam incrustadas nas vias nasais ou no trato respiratório do gato, provocando sinais respiratórios focais.

SISTEMA(S) ACOMETIDO(S)
- Cérebro e, menos comumente, medula espinal.
- As larvas podem ser encontradas em regiões como pele, vias nasais, faringe, laringe, olhos, traqueia e tórax de gatos.

GENÉTICA
Nenhuma base genética.

INCIDÊNCIA/PREVALÊNCIA
Desconhecidas.

DISTRIBUIÇÃO GEOGRÁFICA
- Apenas na América do Norte.
- Mesma distribuição que a mosca de cavalo do gênero *Cuterebra*.
- A doença não é identificada em locais que não possuem a mosca de cavalo do gênero *Cuterebra*, como Austrália e Japão.

IDENTIFICAÇÃO
Raça(s) Predominante(s)
Nenhuma.

Idade Média e Faixa Etária
- Média — 2 anos.
- Variação — 1-7 anos.

Sexo Predominante
Nenhum.

SINAIS CLÍNICOS
- Início súbito de sinais neurológicos.
- Frequentemente precedidos por sinais respiratórios superiores 1-3 semanas antes dos sinais neurológicos (em virtude da migração do parasita pelas vias nasais).
- Com frequência, há sinais prosencefálicos.
- Muito comumente, observam-se crises convulsivas, andar em círculo, atividade mental alterada, cegueira.
- Algumas vezes, ocorrem sinais neurológicos multifocais.
- Raramente, há sinais atribuídos à medula espinal.

CAUSAS
Larvas de *Cuterebra*.

FATORES DE RISCO
- Gatos de vida livre; acesso a ambientes externos.
- Meses de julho, agosto e setembro na região nordeste dos Estados Unidos e sudeste do Canadá.
- Gatos com hábitos de caça.

DIAGNÓSTICO

DIAGNÓSTICO DIFERENCIAL
- Outras causas de acidentes vasculares no cérebro, como doença renal em caso de hipertensão.
- Traumatismo externo.
- Tumores — de início progressivo e não súbito.
- Doenças infecciosas/inflamatórias — como aquelas causadas por *Cryptococcus* sp., *Toxoplasma gondii*, vírus da peritonite infecciosa felina e vírus da imunodeficiência felina.

HEMOGRAMA/BIOQUÍMICA/URINÁLISE
- Costumam permanecer normais.
- Hemograma completo — ocasionalmente, há neutrofilia, leucocitose ou eosinofilia.
- Bioquímica — de vez em quando, observam-se globulinas elevadas ou hiperglicemia.

OUTROS TESTES LABORATORIAIS
- Sorologia para FeLV, FIV, PIF — negativa.
- Títulos para detecção do antígeno criptocócico — negativos.
- IgG e IgM contra *Toxoplasma* — negativos.

DIAGNÓSTICO POR IMAGEM
- RM — modalidade diagnóstica de escolha; detecta a lesão em trilha que se estende da placa cribriforme para o bulbo olfatório e os lobos frontais, parietais e temporais, sendo mais bem identificadas nas sequências dorsais; também se pode observar a área de infarto isquêmico; se realizada logo após o início dos sinais, observa-se o aumento na intensidade dos sinais nas imagens ponderadas em T2, naquelas ponderadas em densidade de prótons e em outras obtidas pela técnica de recuperação de imagem por inversão de atenuação líquida, associado à isquemia das camadas superficiais do córtex cerebral ou da área irrigada pela artéria cerebral média; realce parenquimatoso escasso na área de infarto após a administração de contraste. Se a RM for realizada em mais de 2-3 semanas após o início dos sinais, pode-se constatar a perda da substância cinzenta sobrejacente na região irrigada pela artéria cerebral média e hidrocefalia ex-vácuo associada. A angiografia por RM (tempo de voo ou pós-contraste) pode ter certa utilidade em alguns casos.
- TC — valor limitado.

MÉTODOS DIAGNÓSTICOS
Líquido cerebrospinal — normal ou inflamação não supurativa com macrófagos, linfócitos ou eosinófilos.

ACHADOS PATOLÓGICOS
- Áreas locais de malacia e hemorragia, envolvendo os bulbos e pedúnculos olfatórios, além de cortes transversais do cérebro. Por meio do exame da placa cribriforme, os bulbos e pedúnculos olfatórios, bem como o parênquima remanescente, as meninges e a calvária sobrejacente, podem revelar as larvas, que têm aproximadamente 5-10 mm de comprimento (larvas de 2º estágio), coloração castanha e anéis concêntricos de espinhas ao longo do corpo.
- As características histopatológicas podem incluir necrose e hemorragia do trajeto de migração do parasita ou achados menos específicos, como necrose cerebrocortical laminar superficial, infarto cerebral, rarefação e astrogliose subependimárias, além de astrogliose subpial.

TRATAMENTO

CUIDADO(S) DE SAÚDE ADEQUADO(S)
N/D.

CUIDADO(S) DE ENFERMAGEM
- Se o gato estiver exibindo muitas crises convulsivas, talvez haja necessidade de gaiola almofadada.
- Pode-se lançar mão de cateter IV articulado se o paciente exibir o andar em círculo propulsivo ou perda do equilíbrio.

ATIVIDADE
N/D.

DIETA
N/D.

ORIENTAÇÃO AO PROPRIETÁRIO
- Ocorre apenas em gatos de vida livre e naqueles com acesso a ambientes externos; os gatos que vivem estritamente dentro de casa não desenvolvem encefalopatia isquêmica felina.
- Sua ocorrência se dá somente nos meses de verão na maioria dos pacientes examinados durante os meses de julho, agosto e setembro na região nordeste dos Estados Unidos e sudeste do Canadá.

ENCEFALOPATIA ISQUÊMICA FELINA

• Pode não ocorrer em grandes áreas metropolitanas que não possuem os hospedeiros apropriados habituais, como o coelho-de--rabo-de-algodão.

CONSIDERAÇÕES CIRÚRGICAS
A remoção do parasita do cérebro e/ou da medula espinal não foi relatada em gatos, mas será possível se a neuroimagem estiver disponível logo após o início dos sinais clínicos.

MEDICAÇÕES
MEDICAMENTO(S) DE ESCOLHA
• Cuidados de suporte, incluindo medicamentos anticonvulsivantes e suplementação hídrica adequada, o que pode envolver a administração de tiamina e a adição de potássio por via IV, dependendo do estado nutricional do paciente; tipicamente, o fenobarbital é utilizado a uma dose de manutenção de 7,5-15 mg VO, IM ou IV a cada 12 h/gato; além disso, o fenobarbital pode ser administrado a uma dose total de ataque de 16 mg/kg IV, VO ou IM; essa dose costuma ser dividida em 24-48 h (p. ex., 4 mg/kg a cada 12 h por 2 dias); em seguida, inicia-se a dose de manutenção; o diazepam pode ser utilizado a uma dose de 2,5-5 mg IV para interromper as crises convulsivas aglomeradas ou o estado epiléptico.
• Foi proposto o uso de um coquetel de medicamentos para os gatos recém-acometidos — difenidramina IM a 4 mg/kg, 1-2 h antes de administrar a ivermectina SC a 200-500 µg/kg e o succinato sódico de prednisolona a 30 mg/kg IV; o tratamento é repetido 24 e 48 h após a primeira injeção da ivermectina; além disso, os pacientes recebem a prednisona a 5 mg/gato a cada 12 h VO por 14 dias e o enrofloxacino a 22,7 mg VO a cada 12 h por 14 dias; como a ivermectina não é aprovada para uso contra larvas de *Cuterebra*, é imprescindível a obtenção de autorização pelo proprietário antes da administração; o coquetel terapêutico supramencionado não é indicado para os pacientes com sinais clínicos há >1 semana, pois é provável que o parasita já esteja morto.

CONTRAINDICAÇÕES
Não utilizar a ivermectina em gatos com sensibilidade conhecida.

PRECAUÇÕES
Não foram observados quaisquer efeitos adversos advindos da ivermectina; no entanto, pode ocorrer uma reação anafiláctica ou alérgica em caso de morte súbita das larvas de *Cuterebra* e subsequente liberação de possíveis antígenos estranhos.

INTERAÇÕES POSSÍVEIS
N/D.

MEDICAMENTO(S) ALTERNATIVO(S)
Pode-se usar a dexametasona no lugar da prednisona.

ACOMPANHAMENTO
MONITORIZAÇÃO DO PACIENTE
Avaliações neurológicas sequenciais.

PREVENÇÃO
• Manter os gatos dentro de casa.
• Foi sugerida a aplicação mensal de fipronil, imidacloprida, selamectina ou ivermectina para prevenir infecções pelo parasita.

COMPLICAÇÕES POSSÍVEIS
• Pode continuar tendo crises convulsivas não controladas.
• Ainda pode exibir o andar em círculo compulsivo.
• Pode apresentar mudanças comportamentais, como agressividade.

EVOLUÇÃO ESPERADA E PROGNÓSTICO
Após o ataque inicial, muitos pacientes melhoram e se tornam animais de estimação aceitáveis; pode haver déficits persistentes, crises convulsivas, andar em círculo e comportamento indesejável, como agressividade; os sinais clínicos persistentes dependem do dano causado pelo infarto e pela migração parasitária.

DIVERSOS
DISTÚRBIOS ASSOCIADOS
Nenhum.

FATORES RELACIONADOS COM A IDADE
N/D.

POTENCIAL ZOONÓTICO
Nenhum; no entanto, há relatos de migração aberrante de larvas de *Cuterebra* em seres humanos, mais comumente como uma forma ocular em crianças.

GESTAÇÃO/FERTILIDADE/REPRODUÇÃO
N/D.

SINÔNIMO(S)
Cuterebríase do SNC.

ABREVIATURA(S)
• RM = ressonância magnética.
• TC = tomografia computadorizada.
• FIV = vírus da imunodeficiência felina.
• FeLV = vírus da leucemia felina.
• PIF = peritonite infecciosa felina.

RECURSOS DA INTERNET
• http://Botfly.ifas.ufl.edu/links1.htm.
• http://Cal.vet.upenn.edu/dxendopar/parasitepages/unknown/cutebra.html.
• http://web.vet.cornell.edu/public/oed/neuropathology.

Sugestões de Leitura
Bowman DD, Hendrix CM, Lindsay DS, et. al. Feline Clinical Parasitology. Ames: Iowa State University Press, 2002, pp. 430-439.
De Lahunta A, Glass EN. Veterinary Neuroanatomy and Clinical Neurology, 3rd ed. St. Louis: Saunders/Elsevier, 2009, pp. 413-418.
Glass EN, Cornetta AM, de Lahunta A, et. al. Clinical and clinicopathologic features in 11 cats with Cuterebra larvae myiasis of the central nervous system. J Vet Intern Med 1998, 12:365-368.
Williams KJ, Summers BA, de Lahunta A. Cerebrospinal cuterebriasis in cats and its association with feline ischemic encephalopathy. Vet Pathol 1998, 35:330-343.

Autores Eric Glass e Alexander de Lahunta
Consultor Editorial Joane M. Parent

Endocardiose das Valvas Atrioventriculares

CONSIDERAÇÕES GERAIS

DEFINIÇÃO
Doença degenerativa crônica que compromete as valvas atrioventriculares (AV) esquerda (mitral) e direita (tricúspide), levando às insuficiências cardíaca e valvar.

FISIOPATOLOGIA
• A proliferação e o depósito de mucopolissacarídeos dentro da camada esponjosa subendotelial leva ao espessamento, à distorção e ao enrijecimento das valvas AV; a princípio, as tumefações apresentam-se nodulares, mas ocorre uma coalescência até envolver toda a valva e muitas vezes as cordas tendíneas unidas a ela.
• A incompetência das valvas AV provoca regurgitação, pressão atrial alta, débito cardíaco reduzido, ativação de mecanismos compensatórios (sistema nervoso simpático, sistema renina-angiotensina-aldosterona e peptídeos natriuréticos) e ICC.
• A sobrecarga por volume induz à dilatação ventricular progressiva, rigidez ventricular avançada e função ventricular prejudicada; isso resulta em insuficiência congestiva e de baixo débito (fluxo anterógrado).
• Em casos de laceração atrial, pode ocorrer tamponamento cardíaco agudo.
• As alterações degenerativas nas cordas tendíneas levam à distorção, ao enfraquecimento e à ruptura dessas estruturas, gerando instabilidade nas valvas e aumento na regurgitação.

SISTEMA(S) ACOMETIDO(S)
• Cardiovascular — ambas as valvas AV são acometidas, mas um único estudo em amostras de necropsia constatou uma distribuição de 62% somente para a mitral, 1% apenas para a tricúspide e 33% para ambas.
• Respiratório — caso ocorra o desenvolvimento de edema.
• Renal/urológico — azotemia pré-renal.
• Hepatobiliar — congestão passiva.

GENÉTICA
Algumas raças (Cavalier King Charles spaniel, Dachshund) parecem ter um componente hereditário a essa doença.

INCIDÊNCIA/PREVALÊNCIA
A doença valvar crônica aumenta de aproximadamente 5% em cães de meia-idade (5-7 anos) para >35% em cães idosos (12 anos).

IDENTIFICAÇÃO
Espécies
Acomete principalmente os cães, mas pode ser observado em gatos idosos.

Raça(s) Predominante(s)
• Tipicamente, acomete raças de pequeno porte (<20 kg, embora possa ser observado com menor frequência em cães de porte maior).
• Prevalência mais elevada — Cavalier King Charles spaniel, Chihuahua, Schnauzer miniatura, Maltês, Lulu da Pomerânia, Cocker spaniel, Pequinês, Fox terrier, Boston terrier, Poodle miniatura e toy, Pinscher miniatura e Whippet.

Idade Média e Faixa Etária
Início da insuficiência cardíaca aos 10-12 anos de idade, embora se possa detectar um sopro alguns anos mais cedo; a raça Cavalier King Charles spaniel é caracteristicamente acometida em uma idade muito mais precoce (6-8 anos).

Sexo(s) Predominante(s)
Machos — proporção de machos:fêmeas de 1,5:1.

SINAIS CLÍNICOS
Os sinais dependem do estágio da doença. Foram desenvolvidos vários esquemas de classificação para categorizar os pacientes, com base na gravidade da doença e nos sinais exibidos. Esses graus são usados para facilitar a tomada de decisões terapêuticas. As descrições feitas aqui se alinham com o sistema de classificação descrito na declaração de consenso do American College of Veterinary Internal Medicine (ACVIM) sobre doença valvar e o esquema de classificação modificado do New York Heart Association (NYHA).

Doença Valvar Assintomática
• É melhor auscultar o sopro sistólico no quinto espaço intercostal esquerdo (mitral) ou no quarto espaço intercostal direito (tricúspide).
• Os sopros podem variar desde um sopro holossistólico em faixa de baixa frequência até um sopro mesossistólico mais breve de alta frequência; ocasionalmente, detecta-se apenas um estalido mesossistólico.
• À medida que a doença evolui, o sopro tipicamente se torna mais sonoro e se propaga de forma mais ampla; em casos de doença grave, o volume da regurgitação fica tão amplo que tanto a frequência como a sonoridade do sopro podem diminuir.
• Inicialmente, os pacientes não exibem evidência radiográfica ou ecocardiográfica óbvia de "remodelagem" (alterações nas câmaras cardíacas ou nos componentes musculares) (estágio 2a do ACVIM). Conforme a doença evolui, será observada evidência de cardiomegalia, muitas vezes antes de os sinais clínicos evidentes de insuficiência cardíaca serem identificados (estágio 2b do ACVIM). Qualquer animal com sinais de insuficiência cardíaca (independentemente da gravidade) está no estágio C do ACVIM, mas varia em sua classe do NYHA, dependendo da gravidade.

Insuficiência Cardíaca Leve (Classe II do NYHA)
• Tosse, intolerância ao exercício e dispneia durante atividade física extenuante; ocasionalmente, a síncope pode ser a única queixa do proprietário.

Insuficiência Cardíaca Moderada (Classe III do NYHA)
• Tosse, intolerância ao exercício e dispneia em grande parte do tempo.

Insuficiência Cardíaca Grave (Requer Internação — Classe IV do NYHA)
• Dispneia grave, fraqueza profunda, distensão abdominal, tosse produtiva (i. e., líquido espumoso e róseo), ortopneia, cianose e síncope.

Insuficiência Cardíaca Refratária
• Os sinais clínicos persistem apesar da conduta terapêutica convencional.

CAUSAS
Idiopáticas, embora o papel de uma série de moduladores inflamatórios esteja sendo investigado no início ou na propagação da doença.

FATORES DE RISCO
N/D.

DIAGNÓSTICO

DIAGNÓSTICO DIFERENCIAL
• Miocardiopatia dilatada.
• Cardiopatia congênita.
• Doença crônica das vias aéreas ou do interstício pulmonar.
• Pneumonia.
• Embolia pulmonar.
• Neoplasia pulmonar.
• Dirofilariose.

HEMOGRAMA/BIOQUÍMICA/URINÁLISE
• Azotemia pré-renal secundária a um dano à perfusão renal; a densidade urinária encontra-se alta a menos que seja complicada por nefropatia subjacente ou administração diurética prévia.
• Em muitos pacientes com congestão passiva, observa-se atividade elevada das enzimas hepáticas.
• Pode ser observado um "leucograma de estresse".

OUTROS TESTES LABORATORIAIS
Em pacientes com doença e insuficiência das valvas atrioventriculares, foi registrada uma elevação da porção N-terminal do pró-peptídeo natriurético cerebral. Estudos demonstraram que os níveis se correlacionam com a gravidade da doença, a presença de insuficiência cardíaca como causa de sinais clínicos e possível redução na resposta à terapia. As elevações na porção N-terminal do pró-peptídeo natriurético cerebral também podem ajudar não só a predizer quais pacientes assintomáticos provavelmente evoluem para insuficiência cardíaca, mas também a determinar o prognóstico naqueles que sofrem essa evolução.

DIAGNÓSTICO POR IMAGEM
Achados Radiográficos
• O tamanho do coração varia de normal à cardiomegalia esquerda ou generalizada.
• O aumento de volume do átrio esquerdo na projeção lateral exibe deslocamento dorsal da quarta parte distal da traqueia e fragmentação dos brônquios do tronco principal; a projeção dorsoventral revela acentuação do ângulo entre os brônquios do tronco principal, sombreamento duplo na posição de seis horas, local onde a margem caudal do átrio se estende além do ventrículo esquerdo, e abaulamento do apêndice atrial esquerdo na posição de uma a três horas.
• Insuficiência cardíaca esquerda — a veia pulmonar fica maior do que a artéria pulmonar associada; o padrão intersticial aumentado ± os broncogramas aéreos são típicos de edema pulmonar cardiogênico, mas não patognomônicos; inicialmente, a congestão e o edema são peri-hilares; em seguida, todos os campos pulmonares acabam exibindo alterações. O pulmão direito pode ser acometido antes do esquerdo.

Achados Ecocardiográficos
• Espessamento e distorção da mitral; o folheto septal é o mais gravemente acometido.
• Alongamento e ruptura das cordas tendíneas, ocasionando o prolapso da mitral.
• Aumento de volume do átrio esquerdo.
• O ventrículo esquerdo poderá estar distendido e ficará hiperdinâmico se o fluxo regurgitante estiver elevado e a função miocárdica permanecer intacta; o ventrículo pode ficar hipodinâmico por insuficiência do miocárdio à medida que essa

ENDOCARDIOSE DAS VALVAS ATRIOVENTRICULARES

câmara cardíaca se torna mais distendida do ponto de vista macroscópico.
- Efusão pericárdica em alguns pacientes.
- Os estudos com Doppler registram um jato de regurgitação em direção ao átrio esquerdo e a área do jato regurgitante no fluxo colorido.
- Os índices do Doppler, incluindo a fração regurgitante, são utilizados para avaliar a gravidade do quadro.
- A avaliação com Doppler quanto à presença de hipertensão pulmonar deve ser um componente de rotina de qualquer avaliação ecocardiográfica em pacientes com doença valvar crônica.

MÉTODOS DIAGNÓSTICOS
- Abdominocentese/pleurocentese — um transudato modificado é característico de ICC.
- Para quantificar a hipoxemia e monitorar a resposta terapêutica, emprega-se a gasometria sanguínea arterial/venosa.
- Em todos os pacientes com doença valvar crônica, é recomendável a avaliação da pressão sanguínea sistêmica para averiguar a existência de hipertensão sistêmica concomitante.

Achados Eletrocardiográficos
- Em animais com ICC, é comum a constatação de taquicardia sinusal.
- O ECG pode revelar indícios de aumento de volume do átrio esquerdo (onda P *mitrale*) ou do ventrículo esquerdo (ondas R altas e largas).
- Também podem se desenvolver arritmias atrioventriculares.

ACHADOS PATOLÓGICOS
- As alterações valvares macroscópicas dividem-se em quatro tipos — o tipo I demonstra apenas alguns nódulos discretos na linha de oclusão/fechamento valvar; já o tipo IV exibe uma distorção macroscópica da valva por placas e nódulos cinza-esbranquiçados indutores de contração das cúspides e rolamento da margem livre; as cordas encontram-se irregularmente espessadas, com regiões de adelgaçamento e ruptura.
- Lesões provocadas pelo jato — espessamento e opacidade irregulares do endocárdio atrial.
- Em alguns pacientes, observam-se fissuras ou lacerações recentes e cicatrizadas no átrio esquerdo; as lacerações de espessura completa levam à formação de hemopericárdio (parede livre) ou ao surgimento de defeito do septo atrial adquirido (septo).
- Em muitos pacientes, verifica-se a dilatação do átrio e do ventrículo esquerdo.
- O grau de hipertrofia do ventrículo esquerdo pode ficar claro somente após a pesagem do coração.
- Pequenos trombos no átrio esquerdo — são raros nos cães, porém mais comuns e extensos nos gatos.

TRATAMENTO

CUIDADO(S) DE SAÚDE ADEQUADO(S)
Internação para os pacientes que necessitam de suporte de oxigênio; se estáveis, esses pacientes poderão ficar menos estressados em casa.

CUIDADO(S) DE ENFERMAGEM
Oxigenoterapia em casos de hipoxemia, conforme a necessidade.

ATIVIDADE
- Recomenda-se a restrição absoluta de exercícios para pacientes sintomáticos.
- Pacientes estáveis submetidos ao tratamento clínico — limitar a atividade física a caminhadas com guia/coleira; evitar exercícios explosivos e súbitos.

DIETA
- A prevenção de caquexia cardíaca por meio da ingestão calórica adequada deve ser o principal objetivo do manejo nutricional de pacientes com doença valvar crônica.
- Se tolerável, indica-se uma dieta com restrição de sal ao paciente em insuficiência cardíaca; é aconselhável a monitorização rigorosa da concentração de sódio.
- Pode ocorrer o desenvolvimento de hiponatremia à medida que a ICC evolui e nos pacientes alimentados com dietas intensamente restritas em sódio associado ao emprego de diuréticos de alça e dos inibidores da enzima conversora da angiotensina (ECA).
- Caso se desenvolva a hiponatremia, efetuar a troca do tipo de alimentação para uma dieta com menor restrição de sódio (p. ex., dieta própria para pacientes nefropatas ou geriátricos).

ORIENTAÇÃO AO PROPRIETÁRIO
- Discutir a natureza progressiva da doença.
- Enfatizar a importância da dosagem constante e compatível de todos os medicamentos, bem como do controle de exercícios.
- Destacar a relevância de evitar a caquexia cardíaca, prestando especial atenção ao apetite e utilizando a dieta apropriada.
- Ressaltar os sinais de intoxicação pela digoxina e aconselhar o proprietário a interromper o tratamento e notificar imediatamente o veterinário mediante o aparecimento de qualquer um deles.
- A orientação dos proprietários sobre técnicas simples, como monitorização da frequência respiratória ou cardíaca do paciente em repouso, ajuda a envolvê-los nos cuidados de seus animais de estimação e pode detectar aumentos sugestivos de insuficiência congestiva em desenvolvimento ou recidivante.

CONSIDERAÇÕES CIRÚRGICAS
São utilizadas técnicas cirúrgicas de substituição valvar e de sutura em bolsa de tabaco para reduzir a área do orifício da mitral; embora a experiência com essas técnicas seja limitada, o reparo cirúrgico pode representar uma opção quando se tiver acesso a um cirurgião cardiovascular e a um desvio cardiopulmonar.

MEDICAÇÕES

MEDICAMENTO(S) DE ESCOLHA
O tratamento recomendado depende do estágio da doença; essas recomendações seguem as diretrizes estabelecidas pela declaração de consenso desenvolvida pelo ACVIM.

Pacientes Assintomáticos
- Na ausência de aumento de volume cardíaco, não se recomenda qualquer tratamento.
- A administração dos inibidores da ECA a pacientes assintomáticos que exibem cardiomegalia progressiva é defendida naqueles com cardiomegalia esquerda significativa por alguns cardiologistas. Atualmente, a administração de pimobendana a pacientes assintomáticos é de valor desconhecido, mas estudos estão em andamento para avaliar esse agente terapêutico.

ICC Crônica (Tipicamente Tratado em um Esquema Ambulatorial)
- Diuréticos — furosemida (1-2 mg/kg a cada 8-12 h).
- Inibidores da ECA: enalapril (0,5 mg/kg a cada 12-24 h), benazepril (0,25-0,5 mg/kg a cada 24 h).
- Pimobendana, um inodilatador, tem um início de ação rápido (30-60 min), sendo recomendada para o tratamento de insuficiência cardíaca.
- Embora a espironolactona tipicamente seja utilizada por seu efeito diurético em combinação com outros diuréticos, demonstrou-se que esse agente exerce uma influência positiva sobre a remodelagem deletéria que ocorre à medida que a cardiopatia evolui. Inicialmente, esse medicamento é usado a uma dose de 0,5-1 mg/kg VO a cada 24 h. A dose pode ser aumentada para 1-2 mg/kg VO a cada 12 h em casos de insuficiência cardíaca refratária.
- Nitroglicerina — pomada percutânea a 2% (~0,3-2,5 cm a cada 6 h até que o paciente se estabilize).
- Digoxina — especialmente em casos de arritmias supraventriculares, inclusive fibrilação atrial (0,005 mg/kg ou 0,22 mg/m² VO a cada 12 h).
- Se tolerável, implementar a restrição de sódio.
- Antiarrítmicos — conforme a necessidade.
- Bloqueadores dos canais de cálcio — para tratar as arritmias atriais.
- β-bloqueadores — para tratar as arritmias atriais e ventriculares. Alguns cardiologistas defendem o uso de β-bloqueadores em pacientes com função intacta do miocárdio para anular os efeitos negativos da estimulação excessiva dos receptores β.
- Antiarrítmicos da classe I — procainamida, mexiletina e tocainida; para tratar as arritmias ventriculares de importância clínica.
- Antiarrítmicos da classe III — sotalol e amiodarona para arritmias intratáveis.
- Inibidores da fosfodiesterase tipo 5 (sildenafila) devem ser considerados na presença de hipertensão pulmonar.

Insuficiência Cardíaca Congestiva Aguda (Frequentemente Tratada com Internação)
- Oxigênio — a 40% em gaiola de O_2 (podendo chegar até 100%) por até 24 horas; utilizar O_2 nasal em cães de grande porte, 50-100 mL/kg/min por meio de um umidificador.
- Diuréticos — furosemida (2-4 mg/kg IV a cada 4-8 h).

Vasodilatadores
- Benazepril (0,25-0,5 mg/kg a cada 24 h).
- Enalapril (0,5 mg/kg a cada 12-24 h).
- Pimobendana (0,25 mg/kg VO a cada 12 h) é usado isoladamente ou em combinação com outros vasodilatadores e/ou digoxina.
- Hidralazina (0,5 mg/kg a cada 12 h, titulados em até 2 mg/kg, se necessário) — utilizada nos estágios agudos para diminuir a pós-carga com rapidez; pode causar hipotensão.
- Nitroglicerina — pomada (~0,6 cm/5 kg até 5,0 cm por via percutânea) ou injetável (1-5 μg/kg/min sob infusão em velocidade constante).
- Nitroprusseto de sódio (1-10 μg/kg/min) — monitorizar a pressão sanguínea.
- Vasodilatadores arteriais pulmonares, como sildenafila (inibidores da fosfodiesterase tipo 5), devem ser considerados em pacientes com hipertensão pulmonar.

Inotrópicos Positivos
- Pimobendana (0,25 mg/kg VO a cada 12 h).

ENDOCARDIOSE DAS VALVAS ATRIOVENTRICULARES

- Digoxina (0,005 mg/kg ou 0,22 mg/m² VO a cada 12 h).
- Dobutamina (cães, 1-10 μg/kg/min; gatos, 1-5 μg/kg/min) — pode ocasionar crises convulsivas.
- Dopamina (1-10 μg/kg/min).
- Os agentes com propriedades β-bloqueadoras (p. ex., carvedilol) estão sendo pesquisados por sua capacidade de suprarregular os receptores beta em pacientes com disfunção grave do miocárdio. O carvedilol (0,1-0,4 mg/kg VO a cada 12 h) é um α e β-bloqueador com atividade antioxidante. Iniciar com a dose mais baixa e aumentá-la gradativamente se tolerável.

PRECAUÇÕES
- Utilizar a digoxina, os diuréticos e os inibidores da ECA com cautela em pacientes nefropatas.
- Se intervalos apropriados isentos de nitrato (de 12 h) forem negligenciados da posologia, é possível que se desenvolva tolerância a esse sal.
- Os β-bloqueadores são inotrópicos negativos e podem ter um efeito adverso agudo sobre a função do miocárdio, embora o uso desses agentes a longo prazo possa restabelecer o papel desse músculo.

INTERAÇÕES POSSÍVEIS
Em pacientes submetidos à administração concomitante de bloqueadores dos canais de cálcio ou quinidina, é recomendável monitorizar a concentração da digoxina.

MEDICAMENTO(S) ALTERNATIVO(S)
- Diuréticos — adicionar os diuréticos tiazídicos e os poupadores de potássio (p. ex., espironolactona) em animais refratários.
- A bumetanida representa uma alternativa à furosemida.
- Vasodilatadores — outros inibidores da ECA incluem o lisinopril; pode-se utilizar o dinitrato de isossorbida no lugar da pomada de nitroglicerina em pacientes que necessitam da administração de nitrato a longo prazo.

 ACOMPANHAMENTO

MONITORIZAÇÃO DO PACIENTE
- Para registrar uma cardiomegalia progressiva, é recomendável obter radiografias basais ao se detectar um sopro pela primeira vez e depois a cada 6-12 meses.
- Evidências sugerem que a porção N-terminal do pró-peptídeo natriurético cerebral pode ser utilizada de forma semelhante. Uma referência basal é obtida quando se ausculta o sopro pela primeira vez e, em seguida, o teste é feito de forma seriada para avaliar uma alteração significativa.
- Após um episódio de ICC, avaliar os pacientes semanalmente durante o primeiro mês de tratamento; caso se observem quaisquer alterações ao exame físico, será possível repetir as radiografias torácicas e o ECG na primeira avaliação semanal e nas consultas subsequentes.
- Monitorizar os níveis de ureia e creatinina ao se utilizar os diuréticos e os inibidores da ECA em combinação. Na administração concomitante da espironolactona e dos inibidores da ECA (especialmente quando combinados com digoxina), devem-se monitorizar os níveis séricos do potássio.

COMPLICAÇÕES POSSÍVEIS
Embora as provas permaneçam controversas, foi sugerido endocardite, em virtude da colonização bacteriana da mitral comprometida.

EVOLUÇÃO ESPERADA E PROGNÓSTICO
Ocorre degeneração progressiva tanto das valvas como da função do miocárdio, o que exige dosagens crescentes dos agentes terapêuticos; o prognóstico a longo prazo depende da resposta ao tratamento e do estágio da insuficiência cardíaca.

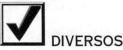 DIVERSOS

SINÔNIMO(S)
- Doença Valvar Degenerativa.
- Doença Valvar Crônica.
- Insuficiência Valvar Adquirida.
- Fibrose Valvar.

VER TAMBÉM
- Insuficiência Cardíaca Congestiva Direita.
- Insuficiência Cardíaca Congestiva Esquerda.
- Laceração da Parede Atrial.

ABREVIATURA(S)
- AV = atrioventricular.
- ECA = enzima conversora da angiotensina.
- ICC = insuficiência cardíaca congestiva.

Sugestões de Leitura
Abbott JA. Acquired valvular disease. In:Tilley LP, Smith FWK, Oyama MA, Sleeper MM, eds., Manual of Canine and Feline Cardiology, 4th ed. St. Louis: Saunders Elsevier, 2008, pp. 2110-2138.
Atkins C, et al. Guidelines for the diagnosis and treatment of canine chronic valvular heart disease. J Vet Intern Med 2009, 23:1142-1150.
Kvart C, Haggstrom J, Pedersen HD, et al. Efficacy of enalapril for prevention of congestive heart failure in dogs with myxomatous valve disease and asymptomatic mitral regurgitation. J Vet Intern Med 2002, 16(1):80-88.

Autor Andrew Beardow
Consultores Editoriais Larry P. Tilley e Francis W.K. Smith, Jr.

ENDOCARDITE INFECCIOSA

CONSIDERAÇÕES GERAIS

DEFINIÇÃO
Invasão do endocárdio cardíaco, em geral das valvas, por agentes infecciosos. Em geral, bactérias Gram-positivas, especialmente estafilococos ou estreptococos. Ocasionalmente, *Rickettsia* ou *Bartonella* em cães. Raras vezes, envolve a participação de fungos em cães. Os casos com culturas negativas podem ser atribuídos a *Bartonella* ou fungos (i. e., *Aspergillus*). Menos provavelmente decorrente de *Brucella*, *Coxiella* e *Chlamydia*.

FISIOPATOLOGIA
• Desenvolve-se bacteremia a partir de várias portas de entrada; as bactérias invadem e colonizam as valvas e válvulas cardíacas — em geral a aórtica, em alguns casos a mitral (valva atrioventricular esquerda) e, raramente, a tricúspide (valva atrioventricular direita) e a pulmonar.
• A ulceração endocárdica expõe o colágeno, causando agregação de plaquetas, ativação da cascata de coagulação e formação de vegetações.
• As vegetações nas valvas/válvulas cardíacas são compostas por uma camada interna de plaquetas, fibrina, hemácias e bactérias, mais uma camada média de bactérias e outra externa de fibrina.
• Ocorre o desenvolvimento de insuficiência valvar/valvular em particularmente todos os pacientes; a insuficiência aórtica quase invariavelmente acarreta ICC esquerda intratável em questão de semanas a vários meses.
• A ICC é menos frequente e latente quando apenas a mitral está acometida.
• As lesões vegetativas podem desalojar, provocando infarto ou infecção metastática em qualquer órgão; os órgãos comumente infectados incluem o baço, os rins, o cérebro e os músculos esqueléticos.

SISTEMA(S) ACOMETIDO(S)
• Cardiovascular — insuficiência valvar/valvular; arritmias; miocardite.
• Musculosquelético — poliartropatia séptica ou imunomediada; osteopatia hipertrófica; discospondilite.
• Respiratório — edema pulmonar e/ou êmbolos.
• Renal/urológico — infarto renal; glomerulonefrite imunomediada; infecções do trato urinário.
• Sanguíneo/linfático/imune — hipercoagulação.
• SNC — para/tetraparesia; déficits dos nervos cranianos; atividade mental anormal.

IDENTIFICAÇÃO
Espécies
Cães e, raramente, gatos.
Raça(s) Predominante(s)
• Raças caninas de porte médio a grande.
• Aquelas predispostas à estenose subaórtica.
Idade Média e Faixa Etária
A maioria dos cães acometidos tem 4-8 anos de idade; no entanto, a infecção pode ocorrer em qualquer idade.
Sexo Predominante
A maioria dos estudos revela predominância em machos — pode ser até de 2:1.

SINAIS CLÍNICOS
Comentários Gerais
• A bacteremia Gram-negativa resulta em sinais clínicos superagudos ou agudos, enquanto a bacteremia Gram-positiva, em sinais clínicos subagudos ou crônicos.
• Os sinais sistêmicos são secundários a quadros de infarto, infecção (inflamação), toxemia ou dano imunomediado; em geral, os sinais clínicos se sobrepõem (ICC e/ou arritmias).

Achados Anamnésicos
• Doença infecciosa nas últimas semanas a vários meses em alguns pacientes, envolvendo a pele e a boca, bem como os tratos GI e genital (i. e., prostatite).
• Histórico de fatores predisponentes — terapia imunossupressora, estenose aórtica, cirurgia recente, feridas infectadas, abscessos ou piodermite.
• Os motivos comuns para a consulta incluem letargia, paresia, febre, anorexia, distúrbios GI e claudicação.

Achados do Exame Físico
• Em geral, diversos e confusos — quadro conhecido como o "grande imitador".
• Febre e mal-estar generalizado.
• Dispneia causada por ICC.
• Arritmias (geralmente ventriculares, embora também ocorram bloqueio cardíaco e taquiarritmias supraventriculares).
• Claudicação ou desvio de um ou ambos os membros.
• Sopro sistólico.
• Sopro "vai e vem" — associado à vegetação na válvula aórtica, causando turbulência sistólica e regurgitação diastólica — difícil detecção sem auscultação cuidadosa do precórdio cranioventral direito.
• Sopro diastólico com pulsos femorais hiperdinâmicos constitui uma forte indicação de endocardite aórtica avançada.

CAUSAS
• Infecção bacteriana associada à cavidade bucal, ao osso, à próstata, à pele e a outros locais.
• Procedimentos diagnósticos ou cirúrgicos invasivos que forçam a entrada de bactérias na corrente sanguínea.

FATORES DE RISCO
• Estenose subaórtica congênita.
• Imunossupressão causada por uso prolongado ou altas doses de corticosteroides, neoplasia ou administração de medicamentos citotóxicos.

DIAGNÓSTICO

DIAGNÓSTICO DIFERENCIAL
• A bacteremia por qualquer causa provoca anormalidades hematológicas idênticas e sinais clínicos semelhantes.
• Distúrbios polissistêmicos imunomediados.
• ICC esquerda causada por miocardiopatia dilatada ou estenose subaórtica congênita.

HEMOGRAMA/BIOQUÍMICA/URINÁLISE
• Infecção ativa grave associada a um leucograma inflamatório (i. e., neutrofilia, desvio para a esquerda e monocitose) — pacientes com infecção crônica relativamente inativa ou encapsulada podem ter leucogramas normais ou quase normais; aqueles com infecção crônica podem ter neutrofilia madura com monocitose.
• Anemia arregenerativa.
• Trombocitopenia — gravidade variável.
• Albumina baixa-normal ou baixa, glicose baixa-normal ou baixa e atividade elevada da fosfatase alcalina sérica estão associadas de forma inconsistente à sepse.
• Azotemia renal — secundária à embolização renal, pielonefrite e/ou insuficiência renal induzida por hipovolemia.
• Proteinúria causada por embolização séptica, glomerulonefrite imunomediada ou infarto dos rins; hematúria, piúria e cilindros granulosos associados à pielonefrite.

OUTROS TESTES LABORATORIAIS
• Hemocultura — três amostras obtidas em intervalos de pelo menos 1 hora durante 24 h; pelo menos duas devem recuperar o mesmo microrganismo; são recomendadas culturas aeróbias e anaeróbias; existem sistemas de remoção de antibióticos disponíveis para o diagnóstico de pacientes submetidos a esses agentes.
• Bacteremia com cultura negativa é frequentemente atribuída à administração prévia de antibióticos ou microrganismos fastidiosos, especialmente *Bartonella*.
• Pontas de cateter — cultura.
• Uroculturas (não substituem as hemoculturas) — fáceis; em geral, dão resultados positivos; não incriminam necessariamente o trato urinário como a fonte de infecção.
• Exames para detectar infecção de próstata, rins e ossos podem ser justificáveis.
• Ocasionalmente, verificam-se resultados positivos para anticorpo antinuclear, lúpus eritematoso, fator reumatoide e teste de Coombs — inespecíficos; tendem a confundir o diagnóstico.
• Meio de cultura para crescimento de *Bartonella* antiproteobactéria e PCR — para detecção de *Bartonella* na suspeita de endocardite infecciosa.

DIAGNÓSTICO POR IMAGEM
Achados Radiográficos
Aumento de volume do lado esquerdo do coração; raramente, observam-se calcificações de uma ou mais valvas/válvulas cardíacas.

Ecocardiografia
Melhor exame — a endocardite vegetativa da válvula aórtica é distinguida com facilidade; é difícil diferenciar infecção da mitral de degeneração mixomatosa. Pesquisar por massa volumosa e oscilante que se move para frente e para trás entre o ventrículo esquerdo e a aorta ou o átrio esquerdo. Imagem hiperecoica com a cronicidade.

MÉTODOS DIAGNÓSTICOS
Amostras de líquido articular obtidas por meio de punção das articulações para exame citológico e cultura — o exame citológico geralmente não diferencia a artrite séptica da imunomediada; em geral, asséptica ou pode coexistir com endocardite infecciosa. Em geral, os neutrófilos não estão degenerados, independentemente da causa.

Achados Eletrocardiográficos
• ECG — pode estar normal; em alguns casos, reflete aumento de volume do lado esquerdo do coração; em geral, detecta taquiarritmias ventriculares; ocasionalmente, revela bloqueio cardíaco de gravidade variável ou taquiarritmias supraventriculares.
• Bloqueio cardíaco sugere acometimento da válvula aórtica com infecção ou infarto do septo adjacente.

ACHADOS PATOLÓGICOS
• Cardiomegalia, quase sempre do lado esquerdo, quando presente.
• Lesões vegetativas e coágulos sanguíneos em uma ou mais valvas/válvulas.

Endocardite Infecciosa

- Infecção, hemorragia e infarto do miocárdio adjacente.
- Infartos renais sempre estão presentes e levam à proteinúria e, possivelmente, insuficiência renal.
- Locais de infecção primária ou secundária, sobretudo rins e baço.
- Hemorragia ou edema pulmonar.

TRATAMENTO

O alto índice de suspeita no início do quadro com testes diagnósticos rigorosos e rápidos, acompanhados por tratamento adequado, é imperativo para a cura. A cura será uma expectativa razoável quando a endocardite infecciosa (isolada) da mitral for identificada no início de sua evolução e se o tratamento for rigoroso.

CUIDADO(S) DE ENFERMAGEM
- Fluidoterapia rigorosa — pelo menos o dobro do nível de manutenção para pacientes com insuficiência renal.
- ICC franca ou iminente limita os volumes de líquido que podem ser administrados, problema praticamente insuperável em pacientes com insuficiência renal concomitante.
- ICC iminente — fornecer não mais do que os volumes de manutenção de líquido; alternar glicose a 5% com solução de Ringer lactato (ou glicose a 2,5% em solução de Ringer lactato diluído à metade); em geral, é necessária a suplementação de potássio.

ORIENTAÇÃO AO PROPRIETÁRIO
Prognóstico reservado se apenas a mitral estiver acometida. Contudo, com o diagnóstico relativamente precoce e o tratamento adequado, a sobrevida será provável; prognóstico grave se a válvula aórtica estiver acometida.

MEDICAÇÕES

MEDICAMENTO(S) DE ESCOLHA
Tratamento variável — depende da gravidade da sepse e da presença ou ausência de ICC.

Antibióticos
- Constituem a base do tratamento, mas em geral não erradicam a infecção antes que ocorra dano irreversível da válvula aórtica (quando infectada); o dano maior do que o mínimo dessa válvula acarreta risco de vida, porque a insuficiência aórtica tende a ser uma complicação letal.
- A administração IV de altas doses de antibióticos bactericidas é indispensável e recomendada pelo maior tempo possível (pelo menos, 1 semana), seguida pela administração SC por uma ou mais semanas.
- Administração oral — recomendada somente depois de pelo menos 4 semanas de terapia injetável e pelo menos 1 semana a partir do desaparecimento dos sinais hematológicos e clínicos de infecção e inflamação; o tratamento prolongado (>4 meses) é necessário para erradicar a infecção das vegetações.
- A seleção do antibiótico é determinada tanto pela urgência das complicações sépticas como pelos resultados da cultura bacteriana; estafilococos coagulase-positivos e estreptococos são os microrganismos mais frequentemente incriminados e, por essa razão, as escolhas podem ser feitas antes dos resultados das culturas.
- Estafilococos coagulase-positivos — em geral, são resistentes aos antibióticos penicilina, hetacilina, amoxicilina e ampicilina.
- Estreptococos — costumam ser resistentes aos aminoglicosídeos e às fluoroquinolonas.
- Bactérias Gram-negativas — frequentemente sensíveis às cefalosporinas de terceira geração, às fluoroquinolonas e aos aminoglicosídeos.
- *Bartonella* — apenas os aminoglicosídeos parecem ser eficientes; pode-se tentar o uso de doxiciclina, fluoroquinolona, rifampicina ou azitromicina.
- Cefalosporinas de primeira geração — escolha razoável para pacientes estáveis até que se obtenham os resultados da cultura.
- Tratar a sepse potencialmente letal de imediato com combinações medicamentosas. Na espera dos resultados da cultura, recomenda-se um dos três esquemas: (1) penicilina, ampicilina, ticarcilina ou alguma cefalosporina de primeira geração combinada com algum aminoglicosídeo. Os aminoglicosídeos não constituem uma boa escolha para animais com ICC franca ou iminente ou aqueles com azotemia renal. A gentamicina (2 mg/kg a cada 8 h) é recomendada por apenas 5-10 dias em função da toxicidade renal. Uma fluoroquinolona pode substituir um aminoglicosídeo. (2) Clindamicina (2-10 mg/kg IV a cada 8 h) mais enrofloxacino (10 mg/kg a cada 24 h diluídos em água estéril 1:1 e injetados lentamente durante 15-20 minutos). (3) Cefalosporinas de geração avançada ou ticarcilina-ácido clavulânico (Timentin®) — altas dosagens, mas apenas as doses normais se o paciente tiver insuficiência renal.

Tratamento da ICC
- Pimobendana, inibidor da ECA, espironolactona, anlodipino e furosemida indicados para pacientes com ICC franca ou iminente.
- Oxigênio, nitroglicerina, furosemida em altas doses (2-8 mg/kg IV) e hidralazina (1-2 mg/kg a cada 12 h) para pacientes com edema pulmonar grave e agudo.

CONTRAINDICAÇÕES
- Evitar antibióticos que não conseguem penetrar na fibrina (p. ex., sulfonamidas).
- Corticosteroides.

MEDICAMENTOS ALTERNATIVOS
- Terapia anticoagulante — controversa na prevenção de embolização. A heparina não é recomendada na medicina humana, pois aumenta o risco de hemorragia.
- Ácido acetilsalicílico (5-7 mg/kg VO a cada 24 h) e/ou dalteparina (100 U/kg SC a cada 8 h) e/ou clopidogrel (2-4 mg/kg VO a cada 24 h) — podem reduzir a disseminação bacteriana e a embolização. O último medicamento é dispendioso.
- Heparina sódica (200-500 U/kg SC a cada 8 h) — pode ser utilizada no ambiente hospitalar com objetivo de prolongar o TTPA em 1,5-2 vezes o valor basal.

ACOMPANHAMENTO

MONITORIZAÇÃO DO PACIENTE
- Surgimento de resistência a antibiótico — febre recidivante e leucograma inflamatório; é indispensável ajustar o tratamento com base nos resultados da cultura.
- Exame frequente e hemograma após a alta hospitalar.
- Repetir as hemoculturas 1 semana após suspender a administração dos antibióticos ou se a febre voltar.

PREVENÇÃO
- Cateteres permanentes (também conhecidos como cateteres de demora) — restringir às indicações apropriadas; colocação asséptica; trocar em 3-5 dias.
- Administrar antibióticos a cães com estenose subaórtica, submetidos a procedimentos odontológicos.
- Evitar o uso de corticosteroides sem critério.

COMPLICAÇÕES POSSÍVEIS
- ICC.
- Insuficiência renal.
- Embolização séptica de muitos tecidos e órgãos.
- Poliartropatia imunomediada persistente ou latente.

EVOLUÇÃO ESPERADA E PROGNÓSTICO
- Prognóstico melhor associado ao breve histórico de bacteremia, diagnóstico rápido e tratamento rigoroso.
- Mortalidade relativamente mais alta em animais que tenham recebido corticosteroides há pouco tempo.
- Prognóstico grave para os pacientes com endocardite da válvula aórtica.
- Os pacientes com endocardite na mitral podem ser salvos com tratamento adequado.
- Pode ocorrer ICC latente com o avanço, o diagnóstico tardio ou o tratamento inadequado para endocardite na mitral.

DIVERSOS

DISTÚRBIOS ASSOCIADOS
Defeitos cardíacos congênitos (em geral, estenose subaórtica) em alguns animais.

SINÔNIMO(S)
- Endocardite bacteriana.
- Endocardite vegetativa.

VER TAMBÉM
- Bartonelose.
- Discospondilite.
- Insuficiência Cardíaca Congestiva Esquerda.
- Insuficiência Renal Aguda.
- Prostatite e Abscesso Prostático.
- Sepse e Bacteremia.

ABREVIATURA(S)
- ICC = insuficiência cardíaca congestiva.
- TTPA = tempo de tromboplastina parcial ativada.
- ECG = eletrocardiograma.
- ECA = enzima conversora de angiotensina.
- GI = gastrintestinal.
- SNC = sistema nervoso central.

Sugestões de Leitura
Calvert, C, Wall, M. Cardiovascular Infections In: Greene, CE, ed. Infectious diseases of the dog and cat. St. Louis: Saunders Elsevier, 2006; 841-865.

Autores Justin D. Thomason e Clay A. Calvert
Consultores Editoriais Larry P. Tilley e Francis W.K. Smith, Jr.

Enteropatia Causada pelo Glúten no Setter Irlandês

CONSIDERAÇÕES GERAIS

REVISÃO
Doença hereditária rara em que há uma predisposição ao desenvolvimento de sensibilidade ao glúten da dieta presente no trigo e em outros grãos.

IDENTIFICAÇÃO
• Acomete a raça Setter irlandês.
• Os sinais se desenvolvem em cães jovens a de meia-idade.
• A transmissão genética de enteropatia sensível ao glúten está provavelmente sob o controle de um único lócus recessivo autossômico importante.

SINAIS CLÍNICOS
• Baixo ganho de peso (ou perda de peso).
• Baixa condição corporal.
• Diarreia leve que pode ser intermitente.

CAUSAS E FATORES DE RISCO
A enteropatia e os sinais clínicos são exacerbados pela dieta com glúten em sua composição.

DIAGNÓSTICO

DIAGNÓSTICO DIFERENCIAL
• Enteropatia inflamatória.
• Doenças infecciosas como *Giardia*, ancilóstomos e nematódeos.
• Anormalidades metabólicas.
• Insuficiência pancreática exócrina.

HEMOGRAMA/BIOQUÍMICA/URINÁLISE
• Geralmente permanecem normais.
• O hemograma completo pode revelar eosinofilia.

OUTROS TESTES LABORATORIAIS
• As concentrações séricas de folato encontram-se abaixo do normal em alguns pacientes, refletindo má absorção crônica.
• Para a exclusão de outros diagnósticos diferenciais, é recomendável a realização de outros testes, tais como flutuação fecal para excluir parasitas intestinais e imunorreatividade sérica semelhante à da tripsina para descartar insuficiência pancreática exócrina.
• A imunorreatividade semelhante à da tripsina e as concentrações de cobalamina costumam permanecer normais.

DIAGNÓSTICO POR IMAGEM
Sem utilidade.

MÉTODOS DIAGNÓSTICOS
Amostras de biopsia intestinal (do jejuno) obtidas via endoscopia ou laparotomia.

ACHADOS PATOLÓGICOS
• O exame histológico de amostras de biopsia do jejuno dos cães acometidos criados com dieta contendo trigo revela atrofia parcial das vilosidades e acúmulo de linfócitos intraepiteliais.
• As anormalidades jejunais melhoram após a retirada do glúten, mas retornam em caso de desafio com esse ingrediente.

TRATAMENTO

O tratamento é feito em um esquema ambulatorial. Evitar dietas contendo glúten pelo resto da vida.

MEDICAÇÕES

MEDICAMENTO(S)
Fornecimento de folato (0,5-2 mg VO a cada 24 h por 2-4 semanas) se a concentração sérica dessa vitamina estiver acentuadamente abaixo do normal (<4 µg/L).

CONTRAINDICAÇÕES/INTERAÇÕES POSSÍVEIS
N/D.

ACOMPANHAMENTO

Considerar a avaliação periódica do folato sérico (a cada 6-12 meses).

DIVERSOS

Sugestões de Leitura
Hall EJ, German AJ. Diseases of the small intestine. In: Ettinger SJ, Feldman EC, eds., Textbook of Veterinary Internal Medicine, 7th ed. St. Louis: Elsevier, 2010, p. 1557.

Autor Krysta Deitz
Consultor Editorial Albert E. Jergens

Enteropatia com Perda de Proteínas

CONSIDERAÇÕES GERAIS

DEFINIÇÃO
• Qualquer processo patológico caracterizado por perda excessiva de proteínas para o lúmen gastrintestinal.
• As doenças associadas à enteropatia com perda de proteínas incluem gastrenteropatias primárias e distúrbios sistêmicos, como linfangiectasia ou insuficiência cardíaca congestiva.

FISIOPATOLOGIA
• Sob condições fisiológicas, dois terços da perda proteica normal nos cães ocorre pelo intestino delgado.
• As proteínas plasmáticas que extravasam para o lúmen gastrintestinal são rapidamente digeridas em aminoácidos constituintes, que podem ser reabsorvidos e utilizados para a síntese de novas proteínas.
• Essa perda normal de proteínas plasmáticas pode ser acelerada por doença da mucosa gastrintestinal ou por extravasamento elevado de linfa para o lúmen gastrintestinal.
• A perda gastrintestinal de proteína está associada à perda tanto de albumina como de globulina.
• Em resposta à perda proteica gastrintestinal aumentada, o fígado aumenta a síntese de albumina. Entretanto, esse órgão não consegue aumentar a síntese de albumina além de duas vezes o débito normal.
• Quando a perda de proteína excede sua síntese, o resultado será a hipoproteinemia.
• A hipoproteinemia grave provoca declínio na pressão oncótica plasmática, o qual pode estar associado a alterações hemodinâmicas e pode levar à efusão nas cavidades corporais ou, menos comumente, à formação de edema periférico.

SISTEMA(S) ACOMETIDO(S)
• Coagulação — pacientes acometidos por enteropatia com perda de proteínas também perdem a antitrombina III e podem estar hipercoaguláveis.
• Gastrintestinal — gastrenteropatia primária que pode estar associada a diarreia, vômito ou outros sinais clínicos de doença GI.
• Linfático — linfangiectasia.
• Hemodinâmico — ascite ou efusão pleural atribuídas a queda da pressão oncótica, levando a desconforto abdominal ou até à dispneia.
• Respiratório — dispneia causada por efusão pleural.
• Pele — edema subcutâneo.

GENÉTICA
Há suspeitas de uma natureza hereditária da enteropatia com perda de proteínas atribuída a causas subjacentes específicas, com base em uma alta prevalência de tais condições em raças caninas específicas (Lundehund norueguês, Wheaten terrier de pelo macio, Yorkshire terrier e outras). Contudo, nada foi comprovado até o momento.

INCIDÊNCIA/PREVALÊNCIA
• A incidência e a prevalência reais da enteropatia com perda de proteínas são desconhecidas.
• Muitos cães com gastrenterite subaguda ou aguda apresentam enteropatia com perda de proteínas transitória.

IDENTIFICAÇÃO
Espécies
Cães e gatos.

Raça(s) Predominante(s)
Raças de cães com prevalência aumentada de enteropatia com perda de proteínas incluem as seguintes: Wheaten terrier de pelo macio, Basenji, Yorkshire terrier e Lundehund norueguês.

Idade Média e Faixa Etária
Qualquer idade.

SINAIS CLÍNICOS
Comentários Gerais
Os sinais clínicos são variáveis.

Achados Anamnésicos
• Diarreia (crônica, contínua ou intermitente, aquosa a semissólida), perda de peso e letargia são os achados mais frequentemente relatados. Entretanto, um número significativo de cães acometidos por enteropatia com perda de proteínas apresenta fezes normais.
• Raramente se relata a ocorrência de vômito.

Achados do Exame Físico
• Ascite, edema em regiões pendentes e dispneia gerada pela efusão pleural podem ser detectados em casos de hipoproteinemia acentuada.
• A palpação abdominal pode revelar alças intestinais espessadas.

CAUSAS
Distúrbios dos Linfáticos
• Linfangiectasia intestinal.
• Linfoma gastrintestinal.
• Infiltração granulomatosa do intestino delgado.
• Insuficiência cardíaca congestiva que leva à hipertensão linfática.

Doenças Associadas à Permeabilidade Aumentada da Mucosa ou Ulceração da Mucosa
• Gastrenterite viral — parvovírus e outros.
• Gastrenterite bacteriana — salmonelose e outras.
• Gastrenterite fúngica — histoplasmose e outras.
• Enterite parasitária — ancilóstomos, tricúris e outros.
• Enteropatia inflamatória — gastrenterites linfocítica, linfocítico-plasmocitária, eosinofílica.
• Reações adversas a alimentos — alergia alimentar, intolerância alimentar e outras.
• Enteropatias mecânicas — intussuscepção crônica, corpo estranho crônico e outras.
• Neoplasia intestinal — linfoma, adenocarcinoma.
• Úlceras gástricas ou intestinais.

FATORES DE RISCO
• Gastrenteropatia.
• Distúrbios linfáticos.
• Cardiopatia.

DIAGNÓSTICO

DIAGNÓSTICO DIFERENCIAL
• Hipoalbuminemia atribuída à enteropatia com perda de proteínas deve ser diferenciada de outras causas de redução dos níveis de albumina.
• Hipoalbuminemia causada por insuficiência hepática está mais frequentemente associada à concentração normal ou até aumentada da globulina sérica. Também pode haver elevação na atividade das enzimas hepáticas, diminuição nos níveis séricos de ureia, colesterol e até mesmo da glicose, além de possível aumento nas concentrações pré e pós-prandiais séricas de ácidos biliares.
• Hipoalbuminemia gerada por nefropatia com perda de proteínas: leve nos pacientes com febre ou hiperadrenocorticismo, mas moderada a grave naqueles com glomerulonefrite ou amiloidose; comumente associada à concentração normal ou até aumentada da globulina sérica — descartar pela relação normal de proteína:creatinina urinárias.
• Hipoalbuminemia provocada por perda sanguínea grave está associada à hipoglobulinemia — a perda sanguínea pode ser excluída por meio da medição do hematócrito e do exame físico completo do paciente; em alguns casos, pode ser necessário o teste para pesquisa de sangue oculto.
• Ingestão inadequada de proteína (i. e., inanição) é uma causa rara de hipoalbuminemia.
• Hipoalbuminemia ocasionada por enteropatia com perda de proteínas quase sempre está associada à hipoglobulinemia — confirmação pelo aumento fecal na concentração de inibidor da α_1-proteinase (deve ser avaliada em amostras fecais obtidas por três dias consecutivos, de fezes eliminadas de forma natural e recém-congeladas).

HEMOGRAMA/BIOQUÍMICA/URINÁLISE
• Hipoalbuminemia e frequentemente hipoglobulinemia (pan-hipoproteinemia).
• Em alguns casos, pode-se observar uma concentração normal ou até aumentada da globulina sérica, quando o processo patológico subjacente está associado à estimulação antigênica crônica (p. ex., enteropatia imunoproliferativa de Basenjis).
• Hipocalcemia — secundária à hipoalbuminemia.
• Pode ser observada hipocolesterolemia.
• Na linfangiectasia, pode-se constatar linfopenia.

OUTROS TESTES LABORATORIAIS
• Concentração fecal aumentada do inibidor da α_1-proteinase.
• Uma vez identificada a enteropatia com perda de proteínas como a causa da hipoalbuminemia, a realização de testes específicos pode ser valiosa para determinar a causa específica desse tipo de enteropatia — múltiplos exames de fezes (esfregaços e flutuações) para descartar parasitose intestinal como causa da enteropatia com perda de proteínas; concentrações séricas de cobalamina e folato para diagnosticar disbiose do intestino delgado (também chamada de proliferação bacteriana no intestino delgado) ou deficiência de cobalamina.
• Outros, conforme a necessidade.

DIAGNÓSTICO POR IMAGEM
• Radiografias torácicas podem revelar indícios de doença cardíaca ou fúngica.
• Radiografias abdominais podem demonstrar indícios de enteropatia mecânica ou outras causas de enteropatia com perda de proteínas.
• Ultrassonografia abdominal também pode exibir indícios de enteropatia mecânica ou outras causas de enteropatia com perda de proteínas.
• Ecocardiografia pode mostrar indícios de cardiopatia.

MÉTODOS DIAGNÓSTICOS
• Agente anti-helmíntico de amplo espectro — para tratar parasitose potencial por uma variedade de endoparasitas gastrintestinais.

ENTEROPATIA COM PERDA DE PROTEÍNAS

- Ensaio alimentar — para descartar reações adversas a alimentos.
- Raspado da mucosa retal — para excluir histoplasmose.
- Gastroduodenoscopia e colonoscopia — para visualizar a mucosa gastrintestinal e coletar biopsias endoscópicas para avaliação histopatológica. O responsável técnico pela endoscopia pode fazer um diagnóstico presuntivo de linfangiectasia pela visualização de "placas" brancas (p. ex., vasos lácteos* distendidos por quilomícron) ao longo da mucosa. As biopsias endoscópicas devem conter toda a espessura da mucosa para maximizar a recuperação diagnóstica das amostras teciduais.
- Laparotomia exploratória abdominal não só pode demonstrar os vasos linfáticos intestinais dilatados, mas também permite a realização de biopsias de espessura total dos intestinos e dos linfonodos.
- Concentração fecal de inibidor da α_1-proteinase — para documentar a perda gastrintestinal excessiva de proteína (essa análise é espécie-específica para cães e gatos, mas está disponível apenas no Gastrointestinal Laboratory na Universidade A&M do Texas).

ACHADOS PATOLÓGICOS

Enteropatia com perda de proteínas
- A enteropatia com perda de proteínas não está associada a nenhuma lesão macroscópica ou histopatológica específica. Em vez disso, as lesões identificadas são aquelas da causa específica de enteropatia com perda de proteínas.

Linfangiectasia Intestinal
- Patologia macroscópica — observação dos vasos linfáticos dilatados no mesentério e na superfície serosa dos intestinos; podem ser observados nódulos amarelo-esbranquiçados e depósitos granulares espumosos adjacentes aos vasos linfáticos.
- Histopatologia — distorção balonosa das vilosidades provocada pelos vasos lácteos acentuadamente dilatados; as vilosidades podem ser edematosas e alguns apresentam aspecto rombo; geralmente, há edema de mucosa; além disso, acúmulos difusos ou multifocais de linfócitos e de plasmócitos podem ser identificados na lâmina própria.
- Outras causas de enteropatia com perda de proteínas também podem levar a alterações macroscópicas ou histológicas específicas. Ver os capítulos que tratam dessas condições.

TRATAMENTO

CUIDADO(S) DE ENFERMAGEM
- Nos casos de hipoalbuminemia grave e complicações decorrentes da hipoalbuminemia, transfusões de plasma ou coloides (hetamido ou dextrana) devem ser consideradas a fim de aumentar a pressão oncótica plasmática quando os sinais clínicos de edema ou de efusão forem graves.
- Abdominocentese para drenar ascite ou pleurocentese para remover efusão pleural nos casos com comprometimento por grave efusão.

---

* N. T.: Os vasos linfáticos do intestino delgado recebem a denominação especial de vasos quilíferos ou lácteos de um modo geral.

ATIVIDADE
Normal.

DIETA
- Modificada, dependendo da causa subjacente da enteropatia com perda de proteínas.
- Se a linfangiectasia for diagnosticada ou altamente suspeita, deve-se usar uma dieta com baixo teor de gordura. Uma dieta elementar também pode ser utilizada em pacientes com doença grave.

ORIENTAÇÃO AO PROPRIETÁRIO
Preparar os proprietários para o tratamento a longo prazo; as curas espontâneas são raras.

CONSIDERAÇÕES CIRÚRGICAS
- A hipoalbuminemia aumenta a morbidade pós-operatória por causa da lenta cicatrização de feridas.
- Algumas causas de enteropatia com perda de proteínas (p. ex., intussuscepção, corpo estranho crônico e algumas neoplasias intestinais) necessitam de intervenção cirúrgica.

MEDICAÇÕES

MEDICAMENTO(S) DE ESCOLHA
- Não existe tratamento farmacológico para a própria enteropatia com perda de proteínas. Por outro lado, a causa subjacente da enteropatia com perda de proteínas precisa ser tratada. Ver "Tratamento" para essas condições.
- Contudo, os pacientes acometidos por enteropatia com perda de proteínas também perdem a antitrombina III e podem ser hipercoaguláveis. Assim, os pacientes devem ser tratados com algum inibidor da agregação plaquetária:
- Em cães: ácido acetilsalicílico em baixas doses (0,5 mg/kg a cada 12 h VO; utilizar um comprimido de 81 mg e colocar no interior de uma seringa de 10 mL, adicionar 8,1 mL de água, misturar até dissolver completamente e perfazer uma solução de 10 mg/mL; descartar a porção não utilizada imediatamente); ou
- Em cães ou gatos: bissulfato de clopidogrel (3-5 mg/kg a cada 24 h VO em cães; 18,75 mg/gato a cada 24 h VO, o que equivale a um quarto de um comprimido de 75 mg).

CONTRAINDICAÇÕES
- Não é recomendável o uso concomitante de ácido acetilsalicílico e clopidogrel.
- O clopidogrel também não deve ser utilizado com outros AINE, fenitoína, torsemida e varfarina.

PRECAUÇÕES
O sangramento pode ser intensificado em pacientes que são submetidos a inibidores da agregação plaquetária e precisam passar por cirurgia.

MEDICAMENTO(S) ALTERNATIVO(S)
Diuréticos como a furosemida foram utilizados por alguns clínicos para controlar o edema e a efusão pleural. Entretanto, tais agentes não funcionaram bem em pacientes acometidos por enteropatia com perda de proteínas por causa da pressão oncótica plasmática reduzida e ainda podem estar associados a efeitos colaterais.

ACOMPANHAMENTO

MONITORIZAÇÃO DO PACIENTE
Verificar o peso corporal, a concentração da albumina sérica e os indícios de sinais clínicos recidivantes (efusão pleural, ascite e/ou edema). A frequência depende da gravidade da condição.

COMPLICAÇÕES POSSÍVEIS
- Dificuldade respiratória gerada pela efusão pleural.
- Desnutrição proteico-calórica grave.
- Diarreia intratável.

EVOLUÇÃO ESPERADA E PROGNÓSTICO
- O prognóstico é reservado. Cães pertencentes a raças de porte menor carreiam um prognóstico mais favorável, pois é mais fácil realizar o suporte nutricional nesses animais.
- Em muitos casos, é impossível tratar a doença primária.

DIVERSOS

DISTÚRBIOS ASSOCIADOS
Animais da raça Wheaten terrier de pelo macio podem apresentar nefropatia com perda de proteínas em conjunto com a enteropatia com perda de proteínas.

POTENCIAL ZOONÓTICO
Histoplasmose, anciióstomos e coccídeos apresentam potencial zoonótico para os seres humanos.

ABREVIATURA(S)
- AINE = anti-inflamatório não esteroide.
- GI = gastrintestinal.

RECURSOS DA INTERNET
http://vetmed.tamu.edu/gilab/.

Sugestões de Leitura
Littman MP, Dambach DM, Vaden SL, et al. Familial protein-losing enteropathy and protein-losing nephropathy in soft coated Wheaten terriers: 222 cases (1983-1997). J Vet Intern Med 2000, 14:68-80.
Peterson PB, Willard MD. Protein-losing enteropathies. Vet Clin North Am Small Anim Pract 2003, 33:1061-1082.
Vaden SL. Protein-losing enteropathies. In: Steiner JM, ed., Small Animal Gastroenterology. Hannover: Schlütersche-Verlagsgesellschaft mbH, 2008, pp. 207-210.

Autor Jörg M. Steiner
Consultor Editorial Albert E. Jergens

Enteropatia Imunoproliferativa de Basenjis

CONSIDERAÇÕES GERAIS

REVISÃO
- Doença imunologicamente mediada que se caracteriza por diarreia crônica intermitente, anorexia e perda de peso progressivas, com tais sinais associados à gastrenterite ou enterite linfoplasmocitária intensa infiltrativa e indícios concomitantes de enteropatia com perda proteica, má absorção e má digestão.
- Presença de hipergamaglobulinemia em virtude do aumento nas concentrações de IgA sérica.
- Os sistemas acometidos incluem o gastrintestinal, o imunológico, o cutâneo, o renal, o endócrino e o hepatobiliar.

IDENTIFICAÇÃO
- Basenjis jovens a de meia-idade — em geral, com menos de 3 anos de idade.
- Cães aparentados são frequentemente acometidos.

SINAIS CLÍNICOS
- Diarreia crônica intermitente.
- Perda de peso progressiva grave.
- Anorexia que, muitas vezes, antecede a diarreia.
- Alopecia bilateral simétrica.
- Escore diminuído da condição corporal.
- Atitude — em geral vivaz e alerta.
- Apesar de comuns, os vômitos são variáveis em termos de gravidade.

CAUSAS E FATORES DE RISCO
- Embora a patogênese seja incerta, há hipóteses de uma interação entre respostas imunológicas anormais, genótipo e possivelmente uma contribuição de fatores ambientais.
- O modo de herança não é conhecido.
- O agravamento episódico dos sintomas foi associado a eventos estressantes — embarque, estro, transporte, vacinação etc.

DIAGNÓSTICO

DIAGNÓSTICO DIFERENCIAL
Linfangiectasia, enterite linfoplasmocitária, enterite eosinofílica, histoplasmose, insuficiência pancreática exócrina, linfoma intestinal, proliferação bacteriana no intestino delgado, giardíase, distúrbios metabólicos, parasitismo intestinal.

HEMOGRAMA/BIOQUÍMICA/URINÁLISE
- Hipoproteinemia.
- Hipoalbuminemia grave.
- Hiperglobulinemia.
- Em geral, há neutrofilia madura.
- Anemia pouco regenerativa associada à doença inflamatória crônica.
- Aumento moderado das enzimas hepáticas — observado em casos de doença avançada.

OUTROS TESTES LABORATORIAIS
- Hipergamaglobulinemia decorrente do aumento da IgA sérica.
- Depressão da curva de absorção da xilose correlaciona-se com a gravidade da doença clínica.
- Pode haver hipergastrinemia e hipercloridria.
- Nenhum teste ou achado histológico é definitivo ou patognomônico.

DIAGNÓSTICO POR IMAGEM
A ultrassonografia abdominal pode demonstrar espessamento difuso do intestino delgado (4-6 mm), camadas normais da parede gastrintestinal e ausência de outras anormalidades viscerais.

OUTROS MÉTODOS DIAGNÓSTICOS
- O aspecto endoscópico da parede do intestino delgado costuma aparecer anormal, mas pode estar normal. Sempre há necessidade de biopsias para a obtenção do diagnóstico preciso.
- O teste genético (DNA) não está disponível no momento.

ACHADOS PATOLÓGICOS
- Lesões patológicas compatíveis incluem espessamento uniforme do intestino delgado, infiltração generalizada da lâmina própria intestinal por linfócitos e plasmócitos, bem como enfraquecimento e fusão das extremidades vilosas.
- Pode ocorrer hipertrofia das pregas gástricas, gastrite linfocitária e/ou atrofia da mucosa gástrica, enfraquecimento e alargamento das vilosidades intestinais e leve dilatação dos vasos linfáticos.
- A presença e a gravidade das lesões gástricas não se correlacionam com a gravidade das lesões intestinais.
- Outras lesões associadas incluem atrofia das células parafoliculares da tireoide, ulceração da pina, atrofia acinar gástrica e glomerulonefrite.

TRATAMENTO
- Tratamento clínico ambulatorial a menos que existam desidratação ou outras complicações graves.
- Recomendar aos proprietários que não acasalem os cães acometidos nem suas ninhadas.
- Minimizar os episódios estressantes.
- Utilizar dietas de eliminação, frequentemente com teor reduzido de triglicerídeos de cadeia longa, para determinar qual dieta é mais bem tolerada.

MEDICAÇÕES

MEDICAMENTO(S)
Imunossupressores/Anti-inflamatórios
- Embora haja relatos de sucesso variável, esses medicamentos são considerados como a base do tratamento.
- Prednisona (1 mg/kg VO a cada 12 h por 2-4 semanas, depois reduzir de forma lenta e gradual em 4-6 meses até atingir 0,5-1 mg/kg VO a cada 48 h).
- Pode-se tentar o uso da clorambucila (0,25 mg/kg VO a cada 72 h com monitorização dos efeitos adversos) ou de outros medicamentos imunossupressores.

Antibióticos
- Tentativas de antibióticos são variavelmente úteis para indivíduos acometidos que possam ter proliferação bacteriana no intestino delgado.
- Metronidazol (10-20 mg/kg VO a cada 12-24 h).
- Tilosina (10 mg/kg VO a cada 12 h).
- Oxitetraciclina (10-20 mg/kg VO a cada 8 h).

Suplementos Nutricionais/Tratamento Adjuvante
- Acredita-se que o emprego de dietas ou suplementos ricos em ácidos graxos ômega-3 possa favorecer a estabilidade da membrana e diminuir as respostas inflamatórias no intestino acometido, embora existam poucos dados específicos disponíveis para apoiar essa hipótese.
- O uso de probióticos pode reduzir o risco de proliferação bacteriana e diminuir o estado de respostas inflamatórias pelo intestino associado aos tecidos linfoides, mas não há dados específicos disponíveis para apoiar essa hipótese.

CONTRAINDICAÇÕES/INTERAÇÕES POSSÍVEIS
Os anticolinérgicos são contraindicados.

ACOMPANHAMENTO
- Os sinais de diarreia e perda de peso geralmente apresentam uma melhora inicial com o tratamento.
- É comum a recidiva dos sinais.
- Ao longo de meses a alguns anos, o prognóstico é mau a longo prazo.

DIVERSOS

Sugestões de Leitura
Breitschwerdt EB. Immuno-proliferative enteropathy of Basenjis. Semin Vet Med Surg Small Anim 1992, 7:153-161.
MacLachian NJ, Breitschwerdt EB, Chambers JM, et al. Gastroenteritis of Basenji dogs. Vet Pathol 1988, 25(1):36-41.
Spohr A, Koch J, Jensen AL. Ultrasonographic findings in a Basenji with immuno-proliferative enteropathy. J Small Anim Pract 1995, 36:79-82.

Autor Mark E. Hitt
Consultor Editorial Albert E. Jergens

Enteropatia Inflamatória

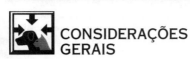

CONSIDERAÇÕES GERAIS

DEFINIÇÃO
Grupo de enteropatias crônicas, caracterizado por sinais gastrintestinais persistentes e indícios histopatológicos de inflamação intestinal.

FISIOPATOLOGIA
• Respostas imunes aberrantes do hospedeiro provavelmente são deflagradas pela microbiota intestinal.
• O dano resulta da elaboração de citocinas, liberação de enzimas proteolíticas e lisossomais, ativação do complemento secundária ao depósito de imunocomplexos e geração de radicais livres de oxigênio.
• Há suspeitas de suscetibilidade genética do hospedeiro envolvendo defeitos na imunidade inata em cães, embora isso seja possível em gatos.

SISTEMA(S) ACOMETIDO(S)
• Gastrintestinal.
• Hepatobiliar.
• Hemático/linfático/imune — raramente.
• Musculosquelético — raramente.
• Oftálmico — raramente.
• Respiratório — raramente.
• Cutâneo/exócrino — raramente.

GENÉTICA
Ainda não foram identificados os genes de suscetibilidade semelhantes àqueles observados em enteropatia inflamatória em seres humanos.

INCIDÊNCIA/PREVALÊNCIA
O diagnóstico histopatológico mais comum em cães e gatos com sinais gastrintestinais crônicos.

DISTRIBUIÇÃO GEOGRÁFICA
N/D.

IDENTIFICAÇÃO
Espécies
Cães e gatos.

Raça(s) Predominante(s)
• Algumas raças caninas são predispostas (p. ex., enteropatia imunoproliferativa do Basenji e Lundehund, colite histiocítica de Buldogue francês e Boxer, além de enteropatia sensível ao glúten em Setter irlandês); também se observa uma incidência elevada em Pastor alemão.
• Os gatos da raça Siamês podem ser predispostos.
• Comum em cães e gatos sem raça definida.

Idade Média e Faixa Etária
Mais comum em animais de meia-idade, embora os mais jovens (com menos de 2 anos de idade) possam ser acometidos.

Sexo Predominante
N/D.

SINAIS CLÍNICOS
Achados Anamnésicos
• Cães — vômito intermitente crônico, diarreia do intestino grosso e/ou delgado e perda de peso são comuns.
• Gatos — anorexia é o sinal mais comum, seguida por perda de peso, vômito e diarreia.
• Borborigmo, flatulência, hematoquezia, dor abdominal e fezes mucoides são menos comumente relatados.

Achados do Exame Físico
• Variam de um animal aparentemente saudável a magro e deprimido.
• Com frequência, observa-se o mau aspecto da pelagem.
• A palpação abdominal pode revelar dor, alças intestinais espessadas e linfadenopatia mesentérica (especialmente nos gatos). Pode ocorrer ascite em cães acometidos por enteropatia com perda de proteínas.

CAUSAS
• É muito provável que a etiologia seja multifatorial.
• A etiologia provavelmente envolve interações complexas entre a genética do hospedeiro, a imunidade da mucosa e os fatores relacionados com o ambiente (microbiota).

Agentes Infecciosos
• A *E. coli* aderente e evasiva foi associada a lesões granulomatosas da mucosa em cães com colite ulcerativa histiocítica.
• *Giardia*, *Salmonella*, *Campylobacter* e flora gastrintestinal residente normal são envolvidas no quadro de enteropatia inflamatória.

Agentes Nutricionais
• Proteínas da carne, aditivos alimentares, corantes artificiais, conservantes, proteínas do leite e glúten (trigo) são, sem exceção, agentes causais sugeridos.
• Os fatores nutricionais parecem importantes na patogenia da inflamação crônica em enteropatia inflamatória canina e felina.

Fatores Genéticos
• Determinadas formas de enteropatia inflamatória são mais comuns em algumas raças de cães e gatos.
• Defeitos na imunidade inativa (p. ex., mutações no gene TLR5, conforme observado em cães da raça Pastor alemão) que afetam a homeostasia da mucosa podem predispor um animal suscetível ao desenvolvimento de enteropatia inflamatória.

FATORES DE RISCO
As hipóteses atuais sugerem que a enteropatia inflamatória seja um distúrbio multifatorial condicionado por fatores genéticos, imunológicos e ambientais.

DIAGNÓSTICO

DIAGNÓSTICO DIFERENCIAL
• Gatos — hipertireoidismo, neoplasia intestinal (especialmente linfossarcoma bem diferenciado), reações alimentares adversas, PIF granulomatosa e outras infecções virais (p. ex., FeLV e FIV), insuficiência renal e hepática, insuficiência pancreática exócrina, parasitismo intestinal e enteropatia responsiva a antibióticos são os principais diferenciais.
• Cães — neoplasia intestinal, distúrbios da motilidade, reações alimentares adversas, linfangiectasia, insuficiência pancreática exócrina, parasitismo intestinal e diarreia responsiva a antibióticos são os principais diferenciais.

HEMOGRAMA/BIOQUÍMICA/URINÁLISE
• Os resultados podem permanecer normais; esses testes servem mais frequentemente para eliminar outros diagnósticos diferenciais.
• Leve anemia arregenerativa de doença crônica. Algumas vezes, observa-se leve leucocitose com ou sem desvio à esquerda em casos de solução de continuidade na mucosa (p. ex., erosões).
• Os gatos com enteropatia inflamatória podem revelar alterações nas concentrações séricas de proteína total (i. e., hiperproteinemia) e albumina, além de aumento na atividade das enzimas hepáticas (p. ex., ALT e/ou fosfatase alcalina).
• Hipoproteinemia é mais comum nos cães com enteropatia inflamatória do que nos gatos.
• A deficiência de cobalamina é relatada tanto em cães como em gatos com doença significativa do intestino delgado.

OUTROS TESTES LABORATORIAIS
• Valiosos para eliminar outros diagnósticos diferenciais.
• Cães — os testes incluem avaliação da função pancreática exócrina (imunorreatividade sérica canina semelhante à da tripsina), sorologia para pancreatite (imunorreatividade sérica canina da lipase pancreática) e ensaios de cobalamina e folato séricos para situar a doença do intestino delgado.
• Gatos — mensuração de T_4 e sorologia para FeLV/FIV são recomendadas; imunorreatividade sérica semelhante à da tripsina em jejum (na suspeita de insuficiência pancreática exócrina); ensaios de cobalamina e folato séricos para localizar a doença do intestino delgado.

DIAGNÓSTICO POR IMAGEM
• Radiografias abdominais simples — geralmente normais.
• Estudos contrastados com bário — podem revelar anormalidades da mucosa e alças intestinais espessadas. Entretanto, achados normais não eliminam a possibilidade de enteropatia inflamatória.
• Ultrassonografia — pode indicar o aumento na espessura da parede intestinal e a presença de linfadenopatia mesentérica. No entanto, essas anormalidades, mesmo se presentes, não são específicas de enteropatia inflamatória.

MÉTODOS DIAGNÓSTICOS
• Realizar um ensaio com dieta hipoalergênica (teste de eliminação) para descartar reações alimentares adversas. Se os sinais gastrintestinais desaparecerem, o diagnóstico será de alergia ou intolerância alimentar, não havendo mais necessidade de outras avaliações diagnósticas.
• Sempre fazer exame de fezes para pesquisa de parasitas nematódeos e protozoários.
• O diagnóstico definitivo requer os exames de biopsia e histopatologia de amostra do intestino, obtida geralmente por endoscopia.
• A laparotomia exploratória pode ser indicada na indisponibilidade do exame de endoscopia ou para a coleta de amostras de mucosa de espessura completa.
• Utilizar índices de escore clínico (p. ex., índice de atividade da enteropatia inflamatória canina) para definir a carga patológica inicial e avaliar a resposta à terapia. A avaliação concomitante da proteína-C reativa serve como um biomarcador útil de inflamação ativa em cães.

ACHADOS PATOLÓGICOS
Indícios morfológicos de inflamação da mucosa, incluindo alterações epiteliais, distorção estrutural (p. ex., hiperplasia das criptas, processo de fibrose) e celularidade aumentada da lâmina própria. Recentemente, foram descritas novas diretrizes histopatológicas para definir a gravidade da inflamação gastrintestinal.

Enteropatia Inflamatória

TRATAMENTO

CUIDADO(S) DE SAÚDE ADEQUADO(S)
O tratamento é feito em um esquema ambulatorial a menos que o paciente esteja debilitado por desidratação, hipoproteinemia ou caquexia.

CUIDADO(S) DE ENFERMAGEM
• Se o paciente estiver desidratado ou precisar passar por um esquema de nada por via oral por causa do vômito, qualquer fluido balanceado como a solução de Ringer lactato é adequado (para o paciente sem outra doença concomitante); por outro lado, é recomendável selecionar os fluidos com base nas doenças secundárias.
• Se houver hipoalbuminemia grave gerada pela enteropatia com perda de proteínas, considerar os coloides como dextranas ou hetamido.

ATIVIDADE
Sem restrições.

DIETA
• Fornecer dieta de eliminação com proteína intacta ou hidrolisado para ajudar a diminuir a inflamação intestinal.
• Corrigir a hipocobalaminemia por meio de injeções parenterais semanais de cobalamina.
• Em cães e gatos com colite, sugere-se a suplementação com fibras.
• Óleo de peixe (ácidos graxos ômega-3) como uma espécie de varredor de radicais livres é utilizado para reduzir a inflamação intestinal.
• Probióticos podem ser benéficos em alguns animais, mas até o momento não são clinicamente comprovados.

ORIENTAÇÃO AO PROPRIETÁRIO
• Enfatizar ao proprietário o fato de que a enteropatia inflamatória não tem cura, mas sim controle na maioria dos casos.
• As recidivas são comuns; o proprietário deve ter paciência durante os vários ensaios com alimentos e medicação, frequentemente necessários para manter a doença sob controle.

CONSIDERAÇÕES CIRÚRGICAS
Não existe nenhum procedimento cirúrgico disponível para o alívio da enteropatia inflamatória em pacientes veterinários.

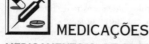

MEDICAÇÕES

MEDICAMENTO(S) DE ESCOLHA
• Ver a discussão nas doenças específicas.

• Os animais acometidos devem ser tratados com esquemas terapêuticos imunossupressores.

CONTRAINDICAÇÕES
Caso haja problemas secundários, evitar o uso de agentes terapêuticos que possam estar contraindicados para essas condições.

PRECAUÇÕES
Ver a discussão nas doenças específicas.

INTERAÇÕES POSSÍVEIS
Ver a discussão nas doenças específicas.

MEDICAMENTO(S) ALTERNATIVO(S)
Ver a discussão nas doenças específicas.

ACOMPANHAMENTO

MONITORIZAÇÃO DO PACIENTE
• Talvez haja necessidade de reavaliação periódica (a cada 2-4 semanas) até que a condição do paciente se estabilize.
• Nenhum outro acompanhamento é necessário, exceto exames físicos anuais e avaliação durante a recidiva.

PREVENÇÃO
N/D.

COMPLICAÇÕES POSSÍVEIS
Desidratação, desnutrição, reações adversas a medicamentos, hipoproteinemia, hipocobalaminemia, anemia e doenças secundárias ao tratamento ou resultantes dos problemas supramencionados.

EVOLUÇÃO ESPERADA E PROGNÓSTICO
• Em geral, o prognóstico é bom a excelente a curto prazo.
• O prognóstico mau a longo prazo em cães com enteropatia inflamatória foi associado com doença clínica grave, anormalidades acentuadas à endoscopia, ascite e hipoalbuminemia.

DIVERSOS

DISTÚRBIOS ASSOCIADOS
• Ver a discussão nas doenças específicas.
• Os gatos podem demonstrar lesões inflamatórias concomitantes no fígado e/ou no pâncreas (a chamada "triadite").

FATORES RELACIONADOS COM A IDADE
• Ver a discussão nas doenças específicas.
• A avaliação diagnóstica e os diferenciais são basicamente os mesmos, independentemente da idade.

• Alguns diferenciais são mais prováveis nos animais mais jovens (i. e., parasitismo intestinal *versus* neoplasia).
• Orientar os proprietários sobre acasalamento e monitorização quanto ao aparecimento de outras doenças.

POTENCIAL ZOONÓTICO
N/D.

GESTAÇÃO/FERTILIDADE/REPRODUÇÃO
Ver a discussão nas doenças específicas.

VER TAMBÉM
• Gastrenterite Eosinofílica.
• Gastrenterite Linfocítica-plasmocitária.
• Colite Granulomatosa.

ABREVIATURA(S)
• ALT = alanina aminotransferase.
• PIF = peritonite infecciosa felina.
• T_4 = tiroxina.
• FIV = vírus da imunodeficiência felina.
• FeLV = vírus da leucemia felina.

RECURSOS DA INTERNET
Rede de Informações Veterinárias: www.vin.com/VIN.plx.

Sugestões de Leitura
Allenspach K, Wieland B, Grone A. et al. Chronic enteropathies in dogs: Evaluation of risk factors for negative outcome. J Vet Intern Med 2007, 21:700-708.
Day MJ, Bilzer T, Mansell J, et al. International standards for the histopathological diagnosis of gastrointestinal inflammation in the dog and cat: A report from the World Small Animal Veterinary Association Gastrointestinal Standardization Group. J Comp Pathol 2008, Suppl 1:S1-S43.
Jergens AE, Schreiner CA, Frank DE, et al. A scoring index for disease activity in canine inflammatory bowel disease. J Vet Intern Med 2003, 17:291-297.

Autor Albert E. Jergens
Consultor Editorial Albert E. Jergens

ENTEROTOXICOSE CLOSTRÍDICA

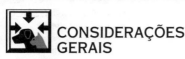

CONSIDERAÇÕES GERAIS

DEFINIÇÃO
- Síndrome complexa e pouco compreendida, que se caracteriza por diarreia em cães e gatos e se associa ao *Clostridium perfringens*.
- A presença da enterotoxina desse microrganismo e de isolamentos fecais enterotoxigênicos parece fornecer os melhores indícios de diarreia associada ao *Clostridium perfringens*.
- É considerado que o *Clostridium perfringens* seja uma das etiologias de distúrbios associados à diarreia responsiva a antibióticos.

FISIOPATOLOGIA
- O *Clostridium perfringens* é um microrganismo residente intestinal comum, encontrado geralmente na forma vegetativa, que vive em uma relação simbiótica com o hospedeiro.
- Parecem existir determinadas cepas de *Clostridium perfringens* (usualmente do tipo A, com base na análise da PCR), capazes de produzir enterotoxinas, que se ligam à mucosa intestinal, alteram a permeabilidade celular e resultam em dano celular e/ou subsequente morte celular.
- Acredita-se que a produção de enterotoxinas do *Clostridium perfringens* esteja associada à esporulação intestinal do microrganismo; essa enterotoxina, no entanto, não causa doença sistêmica. Isso contrasta com as endotoxinas associadas ao *Clostridium perfringens*, vinculadas a sinais sistêmicos.
- Parece haver uma série de fatores intrínsecos relacionados com o hospedeiro, que influenciam a produção de enterotoxinas e a patogenicidade do *Clostridium perfringens*.

SISTEMA(S) ACOMETIDO(S)
Gastrintestinal.

INCIDÊNCIA/PREVALÊNCIA
- Não se conhece a incidência; entretanto, suspeita-se que até 15-20% dos casos de diarreia em cães estejam relacionados com o *Clostridium perfringens*. Menos comum em gatos.
- Também pode estar associada a uma diarreia nosocomial.

IDENTIFICAÇÃO
Espécies
Cães e gatos.
Idade Média e Faixa Etária
- A doença pode ocorrer em animais de qualquer idade.
- A maioria dos pacientes que desenvolvem sinais clínicos crônicos tende a ser de meia-idade ou mais idosa.

SINAIS CLÍNICOS
Comentários Gerais
- As síndromes clínicas associam-se à diarreia autolimitante aguda e adquirida, com duração de 5-7 dias, à diarreia intermitente crônica ou a sinais relacionados com outras gastrenteropatias ou doenças não gastrintestinais.
- Os sinais crônicos caracterizam-se muitas vezes por episódios intermitentes, que recorrem a cada 4-6 semanas e podem persistir por meses a anos. A síndrome pode ser consequência de uma doença nosocomial (adquirida em hospital), com sinais precipitados durante ou logo após a internação ou a hospedagem em um canil.
- O *Clostridium perfringens* também está associado a gastrenterite hemorrágica aguda e, com frequência, é observado concomitantemente com casos de parvovirose.

Achados Anamnésicos
- O sinal mais comum consiste em diarreia do intestino grosso, com muco fecal, pequenas quantidades de sangue fresco, fezes escassas e tenesmo com aumento na frequência de defecação.
- Os cães também podem apresentar sinais de diarreia do intestino delgado, caracterizada por volume abundante de fezes aquosas.
- Outros sinais incluem vômito, flatulência, hematoquezia, desconforto abdominal ou emaciação generalizada em casos crônicos.

Achados do Exame Físico
- Raramente se evidenciam doença sistêmica ou debilidade.
- O desconforto abdominal pode ser detectado à palpação.
- Pode haver evidências de sangue ou muco nas fezes.
- A febre é incomum.

CAUSAS
- Não se sabe se o *Clostridium perfringens* enterotoxigênico é uma infecção adquirida verdadeira ou um patógeno oportunista. Há apenas algumas cepas do *Clostridium perfringens* geneticamente capazes de produzir enterotoxinas, mas somente determinados animais são acometidos do ponto de vista clínico. A doença pode estar associada à proliferação bacteriana no intestino delgado.
- A diarreia pode estar vinculada a imprudências alimentares ou mudanças na dieta.

FATORES DE RISCO
- Fatores indutores de estresse ao trato gastrintestinal, mudança da dieta, doença concomitante ou internação podem precipitar os sinais clínicos.
- A patogenicidade do *Clostridium perfringens* pode depender da integridade metabólica e imunológica do trato gastrintestinal, bem como da integridade de sua mucosa.
- Possivelmente deficiência da IgA.
- O ambiente alcalino no lúmen intestinal promove a esporulação do *Clostridium perfringens* e a produção da enterotoxina.
- Proliferação bacteriana intestinal primária.

DIAGNÓSTICO

- Deve-se suspeitar do *Clostridium perfringens* como agente etiológico em casos com sinais clínicos intermitentes agudos ou crônicos.
- Os testes diagnósticos sempre devem ser avaliados durante o início dos episódios clínicos.
- No final da evolução da doença, a evidência do *Clostridium perfringens* ou da enterotoxina pode estar ausente.
- O quadro provocado pelo *Clostridium perfringens* consiste em uma diarreia responsiva a antibióticos; sendo assim, a resposta ao uso de antibióticos adequados ajudaria a apoiar um diagnóstico presuntivo de diarreia associada a esse microrganismo.

DIAGNÓSTICO DIFERENCIAL
- É aconselhável considerar todas as causas de diarreia, incluindo doenças sistêmicas ou metabólicas, bem como distúrbios intestinais específicos.
- Os parasitas gastrintestinais, a enteropatia inflamatória, a colite idiopática crônica e a síndrome do intestino irritável (acometimento do sistema nervoso entérico) podem se assemelhar à enterotoxicose produzida pelo *Clostridium perfringens*.

HEMOGRAMA/BIOQUÍMICA/URINÁLISE
Em geral, permanecem normais.

OUTROS TESTES LABORATORIAIS
A confirmação diagnóstica da enterotoxicose por *Clostridium perfringens* ainda é controversa e nenhum teste parece ser completamente exato.

Microbiologia
- As culturas fecais anaeróbias costumam identificar concentrações altas dos microrganismos *Clostridium perfringens*, mas ocasionalmente são negativas.
- Os cães normais frequentemente exibem cultura positiva para o *Clostridium perfringens*.
- As culturas específicas de esporos fecais detectam concentrações elevadas de esporos clostrídicos (>10^6 esporos por grama de fezes) em animais acometidos e correlacionam-se bem com a doença clínica, mas raramente são realizadas.

Análise da Enterotoxina
- A identificação da enterotoxina produzida pelo *Clostridium perfringens* (positiva nas fezes), associada a sinais clínicos, coprocultura e resposta à antibioticoterapia, apoia o *Clostridium perfringens* como um patógeno coparticipante.
- Essa análise da enterotoxina é efetuada, lançando-se mão do teste de ELISA nas fezes. O ensaio de aglutinação passiva reversa em látex é considerado impreciso. A análise necessita de 1 grama (amostra do tamanho de uma ervilha) de fezes. Como a enterotoxina do *Clostridium perfringens* é bastante estável, as fezes podem ser refrigeradas ou congeladas antes da análise.
- Os achados da análise nem sempre se correlacionam com a doença clínica. Em muitos cães assintomáticos, já se observaram resultados falso-positivos, o que sugere uma resistência inerente à patogenicidade da enterotoxina. A interferência de certas substâncias nas fezes ou de amostras obtidas durante o período de convalescença pode gerar resultados falso-negativos.
- A identificação do gene da enterotoxina do *Clostridium perfringens* por meio da técnica de PCR tende a se correlacionar com a diarreia em cães acometidos.

Citologia Fecal
- A identificação de grande quantidade de endósporos do *Clostridium perfringens* nas fezes nem sempre se correlaciona com a doença clínica ou com a análise da enterotoxina fecal. A presença ou a falta de endósporos é variável; alguns endósporos do *Clostridium perfringens* não são patogênicos, enquanto outros endósporos são provenientes de outras bactérias formadoras de esporos. A presença de endósporos patogênicos do *Clostridium perfringens* ocorre no início da doença e pode não ser observada caso se avaliem as fezes em uma fase mais tardia da doença. Uma quantia superior a 5 esporos por campo óptico sob imersão em óleo é considerada anormal.
- A citologia envolve o preparo de esfregaço fecal delgado em lâmina de microscópio, a secagem ao ar ou a fixação pelo calor e a coloração com os

Enterotoxicose Clostrídica

corantes de Diff-Quick ou panótico ou de Wright. Para a identificação dos esporos, também se pode utilizar o corante verde malaquita específico para tais estruturas.
- Os esporos do *Clostridium perfringens* exibem uma aparência de "alfinete de segurança", com estrutura oval e corpo denso em uma das extremidades da parede do esporo.
- A detecção dos esporos deve ser feita logo após o início dos sinais clínicos.
- É recomendável avaliar a presença de esporos, juntamente com outros achados laboratoriais e clínicos.

MÉTODOS DIAGNÓSTICOS
A colonoscopia ajuda a descartar enteropatias concomitantes.

ACHADOS PATOLÓGICOS
- As amostras colônicas obtidas por biopsias em períodos assintomáticos costumam permanecer normais.
- Os pacientes com enterotoxicose por *Clostridium perfringens* podem exibir evidências colonoscópicas de hiperemia ou ulceração na mucosa.
- A histologia pode revelar colite catarral ou supurativa.
- Ocasionalmente, verifica-se uma leve enteropatia inflamatória.

TRATAMENTO

CUIDADO(S) DE SAÚDE ADEQUADO(S)
- A maior parte dos casos é tratada em um esquema ambulatorial.
- Em casos de vômito ou diarreia grave com consequente desidratação e desequilíbrio eletrolítico, poderá haver a necessidade de internação.

CUIDADO(S) DE ENFERMAGEM
Para a reposição das perdas decorrentes da diarreia (incomum), poderá ser imprescindível a terapia hidroeletrolítica.

ATIVIDADE
Restrita durante a doença aguda.

DIETA
- A manipulação da dieta desempenha um papel importante no tratamento e no controle dos casos de doença recidivante crônica. As dietas formuladas com alto teor de fibras solúveis (fermentáveis) ou insolúveis frequentemente resultam na melhora clínica, pela redução na quantidade de clostrídios entéricos. Isso pode ser atribuído à acidificação na porção distal do intestino, limitando dessa forma a esporulação do *Clostridium perfringens* e a produção da enterotoxina.
- As rações comerciais ricas em fibras podem ser suplementadas com psílio (1/2-2 colheres das de chá/dia) como fonte de fibras solúveis.
- As dietas pobres em fibras devem ser suplementadas com farelo bruto (1-3 colheres das de sopa/dia) como fonte de fibras insolúveis ou com psílio como fonte de fibras solúveis.
- As dietas à base de prebióticos contendo substâncias fermentáveis (como fruto-oligossacárideos) podem ser benéficas pela modificação da flora GI.

ORIENTAÇÃO AO PROPRIETÁRIO
A doença aguda é muitas vezes autolimitante, enquanto os casos crônicos podem necessitar de terapia prolongada.

MEDICAÇÕES

MEDICAMENTO(S) DE ESCOLHA
Antibióticos
- A doença aguda autolimitante costuma exigir um curso antibiótico de 5-7 dias. A maioria dos pacientes responde de forma satisfatória à antibioticoterapia adequada (p. ex., ampicilina ou amoxicilina, clindamicina, metronidazol ou tilosina orais). As tetraciclinas não constituem uma boa escolha ao se tratar os casos de *Clostridium perfringes*, pois muitos são resistentes.
- Os casos recidivantes crônicos frequentemente necessitam de antibioticoterapia prolongada. Para um tratamento a longo prazo, sugere-se a administração de tilosina (Tylan® solúvel) a uma dose de 7-15 mg/kg a cada 12-24 h, misturada com alimento ou formulada em cápsulas. A tilosina também pode ter outros efeitos gastrintestinais além de sua ação antimicrobiana.
- O fornecimento de altas doses de antibióticos parece não ser necessário para evitar a recidiva em casos crônicos. A administração de antibióticos por via oral em concentrações inibitórias submicrobianas pode ser eficaz em casos crônicos. De fato, níveis baixos de antibióticos podem não reduzir a quantidade do *Clostridium perfringens* entéricos, mas podem alterar o microambiente ecológico, impedindo a esporulação do microrganismo e a produção das enterotoxinas.

MEDICAMENTO(S) ALTERNATIVO(S)
- Probióticos (como lactobacilo ou outros) podem ter efeitos antibacterianos sobre o microrganismo *Clostridium* e relatos não publicados sugerem certo benefício em casos crônicos.
- Os casos crônicos podem exibir uma resposta favorável a dietas ricas em fibras (ver "Dieta"); assim, pode-se tentar a manipulação na dieta como uma terapia isolada após a resolução dos sinais clínicos.

ACOMPANHAMENTO

MONITORIZAÇÃO DO PACIENTE
A resposta do paciente à terapia apoia o diagnóstico e, raramente, a repetição dos testes diagnósticos é necessária.

PREVENÇÃO
- A infecção é associada à contaminação do ambiente, mas a desinfecção não é uma tarefa fácil.
- O fornecimento de dietas ricas em fibras pode diminuir a incidência de diarreia nosocomial adquirida.

EVOLUÇÃO ESPERADA E PROGNÓSTICO
- Grande parte dos animais responde bem à terapia. Os casos crônicos podem necessitar de terapia vitalícia para o controle dos sinais clínicos.
- Uma falha na resposta sugere a presença de doença concomitante; assim, fica indicada avaliação diagnóstica adicional.

DIVERSOS

DISTÚRBIOS ASSOCIADOS
A enterotoxicose por *Clostridium perfringens* associa-se com frequência a outras enteropatias, como parvovirose, gastrenterite hemorrágica aguda ou enteropatia inflamatória.

POTENCIAL ZOONÓTICO
Desconhecido.

GESTAÇÃO/FERTILIDADE/REPRODUÇÃO
A antibioticoterapia pode ser contraindicada.

SINÔNIMO(S)
Colite crônica idiopática.

VER TAMBÉM
- Colite e Proctite.
- Disbiose do Intestino Delgado.

ABREVIATURA(S)
- ELISA = ensaio imunoabsorvente ligado à enzima.
- GI = gastrintestinal.
- PCR = reação em cadeia da polimerase.

Sugestões de Leitura
Albini S, Brodard I, Jaussi A. Real-time multiplex PCR assays for reliable detection of Clostridium perfringens toxin genes in animal isolates. Vet Microbiology 2008,127;179-185.
Cave NJ, Marks SL, Kass PH, et al. Evaluation of a routine diagnostic fecal panel for dogs with diarrhea, JAVMA 2002, 221(1):52-59.
Kirth SA, Prescott JF, Welch MK, et al. Nosocomial diarrhea associated with enterotoxigenic Clostridium perfringens infection in dogs. JAVMA 1989, 195:331-334.
Marks SL, Kather EJ. Antimicrobial susceptibilities of canine Clostridium difficile and Clostridium perfringens isolates to commonly utilized antimicrobial drugs. Vet Microbiology 2003, 94(1):39-45.
Marks SL, Kather EJ. Bacterial-associated diarrhea in the dog: A critical appraisal. Vet Clin North Am Small Anim Pract 2003, 33(5):1029-1060.
Marks SL, Kather EJ, Kass PH, Melli AC. Genotypic and phenotypic characterization of Clostridium perfringens and Clostridium difficile in diarrheic and healthy dogs. J Vet Intern Med 2002, 16:533-540.
Weese JS, Staempfli HR, Prescott JF, et al. The roles of Clostridium difficile and enterotoxigenic Clostridium perfringens in diarrhea in dog. J Vet Intern Med 2001, 15:374-378.

Autor David C. Twedt
Consultor Editorial Albert E. Jergens

ENTRÓPIO

CONSIDERAÇÕES GERAIS

REVISÃO
- Inversão de parte ou de toda a margem palpebral.
- Irritação da córnea por atrito — por causa do contato com os cílios ou as sobrancelhas; pode resultar em ulceração ou perfuração da córnea ou ceratite pigmentar.
- A visão pode ficar ameaçada.

IDENTIFICAÇÃO
- Comum em cães; ocasional em gatos.
- Gatos — costuma ser constatado em raças braquicefálicas (p. ex., Persa e Himalaio).
- Cães — observado em Chow Chow, Shar pei, Elkhound norueguês, raças desportivas (p. ex., Spaniel e Retriever), braquicefálicas (p. ex., Buldogue inglês, Pug e Pequinês), toys (p. ex., Poodle e Yorkshire terrier) e gigantes (p. ex., Mastife, São Bernardo e Terra Nova).
- Idade — observado em filhotes caninos com 2-6 semanas de vida (especialmente Chow Chow e Shar pei); geralmente identificado em cães com menos de 1 ano de idade; em gatos, pode acometer qualquer idade.

SINAIS CLÍNICOS
- Dependem do tipo e do grau do problema.
- Discreto, medial — epífora crônica e ceratite pigmentar medial (raças toys e braquicefálicas de cães e gatos).
- Discreto, lateral — secreção ocular mucoide a mucopurulenta crônica (cães de raças gigantes).
- Pálpebra superior, pálpebra inferior ou canto lateral — blefarospasmo grave, secreção purulenta, ceratite pigmentar ou ulcerativa e potencial ruptura da córnea (Chow Chow, Shar pei e raças desportivas).

CAUSAS E FATORES DE RISCO
- Há principalmente uma predisposição genética na conformação facial e na sustentação palpebral.
- Raças braquicefálicas (de cães e gatos) — tensão excessiva sobre as estruturas ligamentares do canto medial acopladas às pregas nasais e defeitos na conformação facial resultam em interiorização das faces mediais das pálpebras superiores e inferiores no canto medial.
- Raças gigantes e aquelas com muita pele na face (Bloodhound) ou excesso de pregas faciais (Chow Chow e Shar pei) — a frouxidão das estruturas ligamentares do canto lateral permite o entrópio das pálpebras superiores e inferiores e do canto lateral.
- Conjuntivite ou ceratite infecciosa crônica (gatos) — podem ocasionar entrópio funcional por blefarospasmo crônico (entrópio espástico).
- Raças predispostas (cães) — entrópio espástico se a irritação ocular (p. ex., distiquíase, cílios ectópicos, triquíase, corpo estranho e conjuntivite irritante) acarretarem blefarospasmo excessivo.
- Raças não predispostas — pode ser o resultado de algum irritante primário indutor de entrópio espástico secundário.
- Perda de peso grave ou atrofia da musculatura, causada por miosite dos músculos da mastigação (cães) — a perda da gordura orbital ou da musculatura periorbital pode levar a enoftalmia e entrópio.

DIAGNÓSTICO

DIAGNÓSTICO DIFERENCIAL
- Em geral, óbvio ao exame clínico — as causas subjacentes de entrópio espástico devem ser excluídas e corrigidas, se possível, antes de se tentar a correção cirúrgica.
- Filhotes caninos — comum em criadores novatos de Chow Chow e Shar pei que acreditam erroneamente que seja normal o fato de as pálpebras não estarem abertas com 4-5 semanas de vida, quando na verdade os filhotes sofrem de blefarospasmo grave e entrópio espástico.

HEMOGRAMA/BIOQUÍMICA/URINÁLISE
N/D.

OUTROS TESTES LABORATORIAIS
N/D.

DIAGNÓSTICO POR IMAGEM
N/D.

MÉTODOS DIAGNÓSTICOS
A aplicação de algum anestésico tópico pode reduzir o componente espástico e permitir a diferenciação entre entrópio espástico e fisiológico.

TRATAMENTO

FILHOTES CANINOS
- Jovens (em especial Shar pei e Chow Chow) — NÃO fazer a ressecção cirúrgica cutânea logo de início.
- Em casos de úlcera de córnea — aplicar pomadas antibióticas tópicas (p. ex., neomicina/polimixina B/bacitracina) a cada 6-8 h.
- Em casos de entrópio discreto sem ulceração da córnea — lubrificar com pomada de lágrima artificial a cada 8-12 h.
- Em casos de entrópio moderado a grave — everter temporariamente as margens palpebrais com suturas para tentar interromper o ciclo de espasmo-irritação-espasmo; se isso for bem-sucedido, não será necessário o procedimento permanente. Talvez haja necessidade de repetição do procedimento a cada 2-4 semanas até que a conformação facial adulta esteja concluída.
- Técnica de ressecção cutânea permanente — adiada até que a conformação da face do paciente se desenvolva (geralmente aos 6 meses de vida na maioria das raças), pois isso aumenta as taxas de êxito.

ENTRÓPIO MEDIAL
- A eversão temporária do canto medial com o uso de suturas pode ajudar a determinar a contribuição do entrópio medial para o sinal de epífora observado em raças caninas *toys* e braquicefálicas de cães e gatos.
- A reconstrução do canto medial deverá ser realizada se o entrópio resultar em ceratite pigmentar, epífora crônica ou formação cicatricial corneana.

CÃES E GATOS ADULTOS
- Entrópio crônico — requer algum tipo de cirurgia para eversão da margem palpebral; procedimento simples de Hotz-Celsus ou cantoplastia lateral mais radical.
- Nenhum histórico de entrópio prévio e sinais clínicos de problema agudo — examinar meticulosamente em busca da causa do problema espástico e corrigi-la; pode-se tentar uma técnica de sutura para eversão temporária antes da ressecção cutânea permanente, se necessário.

MEDICAÇÕES

MEDICAMENTO(S)
- Pomada oftálmica tópica — com 3 antibióticos ou com base nos resultados da cultura e do antibiograma; a cada 6-12 h; pode ser utilizada em caso de úlcera de córnea, no pós-operatório ou como lubrificante pré-cirúrgico.
- Pomadas de lágrima artificial à base de vaselina tópica (Duratears®, Puralube® ou Labrilube®) a cada 8-12 h podem ser usadas temporariamente em casos leves sem ulceração de córnea.

CONTRAINDICAÇÕES/INTERAÇÕES POSSÍVEIS
N/D.

ACOMPANHAMENTO

Técnica de sutura para eversão temporária — poderá reverter o entrópio quando as suturas forem removidas ou tracionadas espontaneamente através da pele; repetida se necessário até que o paciente esteja adulto o bastante para ser submetido a uma forma de reparo por ressecção cutânea mais permanente (aproximadamente aos 6 meses de vida).

DIVERSOS

Sugestões de Leitura
Stades FC, Gelatt KN. Diseases and surgery of the canine eyelid. In: Gelatt KN, ed., Veterinary Ophthalmology, 4th ed. Ames, IA: Blackwell, 2007, pp. 574-583.
Williams DL, Kim JY. Feline entropion: A case series of 50 affected animals (2003-2008). Vet Ophthalmology 2009, 12(4):221-226.

Autor J. Phillip Pickett
Consultor Editorial Paul E. Miller

Envenenamento (Intoxicação)

CONSIDERAÇÕES GERAIS

DEFINIÇÃO
- Com frequência, os pacientes agudamente doentes recebem diagnóstico de envenenamento quando não há nenhum outro diagnóstico óbvio.
- Os esforços devem ser direcionados para a estabilização do paciente.
- O diagnóstico será formulado após a determinação das condições preexistentes e do controle inicial dos sinais clínicos.
- Objetivos do tratamento — efetuar intervenção de emergência; evitar exposição adicional; impedir absorção extra; aplicar antídotos específicos; acelerar a eliminação; fornecer medidas de suporte; oferecer orientação ao proprietário.
- Suspeita de intoxicação — amostras e materiais tóxicos suspeitos podem ser valiosos do ponto de vista médico-legal; sustentam uma cadeia adequada de provas físicas; permitem guardar prontuários médicos completos.
- Pode-se poupar um tempo valioso, aplicando o tratamento adequado para a substância tóxica conhecida ou sob suspeita.

Instruções Iniciais ao Proprietário
- Podem ser benéficas para o tratamento subsequente.
- Levar o paciente ao veterinário o mais rápido possível.
- Em caso de atraso no transporte — manter o paciente aquecido; evitar qualquer outro tipo de estresse.
- Advertir os espectadores sobre a condição do paciente.
- Talvez seja necessário amordaçar o paciente.
- Encaminhar o vômito não contaminado e os materiais tóxicos suspeitos e seus recipientes ao hospital.
- Se o paciente urinar, coletar qualquer urina e enviá-la ao hospital.
- Utilizar recipientes limpos de plástico ou de vidro para o envio das amostras.

DIAGNÓSTICO

DIAGNÓSTICO DIFERENCIAL
- Diagnóstico definitivo — difícil; os animais entram em contato com um amplo arsenal de substâncias tóxicas; ver "Apêndice V: Toxicoses Clínicas — Sistemas Acometidos e Efeitos Clínicos".
- Locais onde recorrer em casos de emergências — National Animal Poison Control Center [Centro Norte-americano de Controle Toxicológico Animal]; laboratórios diagnósticos estaduais; centros locais de controle toxicológico; grande valor para casos sob suspeita de intoxicação, especialmente quando rótulos ou recipientes estão disponíveis.
- Quando o composto suspeito e os sinais clínicos não coincidem — tratar os sinais, desconsiderando o rótulo.
- Confirmação do diagnóstico — por meio de análise química (pode ocorrer após o fato); o diagnóstico preciso e os prontuários detalhados podem ajudar futuros pacientes acometidos pela mesma substância tóxica, mas são valiosos nos processos médico-legais.

TRATAMENTO

CUIDADOS DE SUPORTE
- Controle da temperatura corporal.
- Manutenção da função respiratória e cardiovascular.
- Controle do equilíbrio acidobásico.
- Alívio da dor.
- Controle dos distúrbios do SNC — ver tópicos específicos.

TRATAMENTO DE EMERGÊNCIA
- Estabelecimento de via aérea patente (desobstruída).
- Respiração artificial.
- Massagem cardíaca — externa ou interna.
- Aplicação de técnicas de desfibrilação.
- Após a estabilização — pode-se prosseguir com medidas terapêuticas mais específicas.

EVITAR A ABSORÇÃO
- Principal fator terapêutico.
- Em primeiro lugar, é necessário remover o paciente do ambiente contaminado.
- Medidas disponíveis — lavagem; utilização criteriosa de eméticos; técnicas de lavagem gástrica; uso de adsorventes e catárticos.

Lavagem da Pele
- Indicada para substâncias tóxicas externas.
- Lavar a pele do paciente para remover o agente nocivo.
- **CUIDADO:** evitar a contaminação das pessoas que manipulam o paciente.

Eméticos
- De pouco valor além de 4 h após a ingestão; depois desse período, a maior parte do material já terá passado para o duodeno.
- Não induzir a êmese em pacientes inconscientes ou gravemente deprimidos ou após a ingestão de ácidos fortes, álcalis, destilados de petróleo, tranquilizantes ou outros antieméticos.
- Apomorfina — mais eficaz e mais segura para uso em cães e gatos; disponibilidade desconhecida em qualquer época determinada; pequenos animais, 0,04 mg/kg IV ou 0,08 mg/kg IM, SC; controlar os sinais clínicos adversos causados pela apomorfina com algum antagonista narcótico intravenoso apropriado (p. ex., naloxona na dose de 0,04 mg/kg).
- Ipeca — pouca eficácia; nunca utilizar quando o carvão ativado fizer parte do esquema terapêutico.
- Xilazina — administração intravenosa; usada com algum sucesso em cães e gatos.
- Peróxido de hidrogênio (água oxigenada) — nem sempre é eficaz.

Carvão Ativado
- Não desintoxica, mas evita a absorção se utilizado adequadamente.
- Altamente absortivo de muitas substâncias tóxicas — inseticidas organofosforados; outros inseticidas; rodenticidas; cloreto de mercúrio; estricnina; outros alcaloides (p. ex., morfina e atropina); barbitúricos; etilenoglicol.
- Ineficaz contra cianeto, etanol, metanol, destilados de petróleo, cloreto de sódio e clorato.
- Administrado em combinação com eméticos — aumenta a eficácia da eliminação da substância tóxica por êmese.
- Usar banheira ou alguma outra área de fácil limpeza quando se administra carvão ativado a pequenos animais.
- Dosagem — 1-5 g/kg de peso corporal na concentração de 1g de carvão/5-10 mL de água 3-4 vezes ao dia por 2-3 dias.
- Um pouco de carvão deve permanecer no estômago e ser acompanhado por catártico para evitar a dessorção* da substância tóxica.
- Catártico — sulfato de sódio; administrado 30 min após a administração do carvão.

Lavagem Gástrica
- Meio eficaz de esvaziar o estômago.
- Tamanho da sonda gástrica — utilizar a maior possível; uma boa regra nesse caso é usar o mesmo tamanho da sonda endotraqueal com manguito (1 mm = 3 Fr**).
- Volume de água ou solução de lavagem para cada irrigação — 5-10 mL/kg de peso corporal.
- Ciclo de infusão e aspiração — repetido 10-15 vezes.
- O carvão ativado na solução aumenta a eficácia.
- Uso de carvão ativado a uma taxa de 1-3 g/kg de peso corporal.
- Acompanhar a administração do carvão ativado com catártico salino, como sulfato de sódio a 250 mg/kg.
- Precauções — (1) utilizar baixa pressão para não forçar a substância tóxica para o duodeno; (2) reduzir o volume infundido em estômagos obviamente enfraquecidos (p. ex., no paciente que ingeriu alguma substância tóxica cáustica ou corrosiva); (3) não forçar a sonda gástrica pelo esôfago ou pela parede do estômago.
- O carvão ativado tem uma eficácia maior contra muitas toxinas em comparação a outros adsorventes como terra de Fuller* e/ou bentonita.
- As combinações de sorbitol e carvão ativado podem produzir desidratação hipernatrêmica, sobretudo em pacientes que já se encontram fisiologicamente estressados.

Óleos
- Óleo mineral ou vegetal — valioso para substâncias tóxicas lipossolúveis.
- Óleo mineral (petrolato líquido) — inerte; é menos provável que seja absorvido.
- Utilizar com catártico.
- Sulfato de sódio — 1 g/kg por via oral; agente mais eficaz para evacuação do intestino do que o sulfato de magnésio; preferido com carvão ativado e óleo mineral.

Enemas
- Lavagem colônica ou enema superior — podem acelerar a eliminação das substâncias tóxicas a partir do trato gastrintestinal.
- Água morna com sabão Castile* — solução excelente.
- Preparações disponíveis no mercado atuam como agentes osmóticos.
- Cuidado para evitar a indução de desidratação e desequilíbrios eletrolíticos em tratamento com excesso de zelo.
- Evitar sabões com hexaclorofeno em gatos.

ACELERAR A ELIMINAÇÃO
- Substâncias tóxicas absorvidas — geralmente excretadas pelos rins; podem ser excretadas por outras vias (p. ex., bile, fezes, pulmões e outras secreções corporais).

---

* N. T.: Entende-se por dessorção a transferência de átomos, moléculas ou agregados de um sólido para a fase gasosa (Fonte: Laboratório Van de Graaf).

** N. T.: Fr corresponde a French (unidade de medida).

ENVENENAMENTO (INTOXICAÇÃO)

- Excreção renal — pode ser manipulada em muitos animais.
- Excreção urinária — pode ser intensificada pela utilização de diuréticos ou pela modificação do pH da urina.

Diuréticos
- Para intensificar a excreção urinária de substâncias tóxicas — requer a manutenção de função renal adequada.
- Quando não se consegue estabelecer um fluxo urinário mínimo — é obrigatório o uso de diálise peritoneal.
- Agentes de escolha — manitol (1-2 g/kg IV a cada 6 h) e furosemida (5 mg/kg a cada 6-8 h).

Manipulando o pH da Urina
- Técnica farmacológica clássica.
- Os compostos ácidos permanecem ionizados na urina alcalina, enquanto os compostos alcalinos ficam ionizados na urina ácida.
- Cloreto de amônio (200 mg/kg por via oral diariamente em doses divididas) e cloridrato de etilenodiamina (1-2 comprimidos a cada 8 h para cães de porte médio) — acidificação urinária a longo prazo.
- Solução fisiológica — acidificante urinário bom e rápido.
- Bicarbonato de sódio (5 mEq/kg/h) — pode ser utilizado como agente alcalinizante.

Diálise Peritoneal
- Indicada para oligúria ou anúria.
- Apontada para a simples remoção de substâncias tóxicas absorvidas no paciente com função renal normal.
- pH da solução — pode ser alterado para manter o estado ionizado do composto nocivo.

FLUIDOTERAPIA
Considerar a reposição volêmica com cristaloides e coloides se necessário.

Terapia por Infusão de Emulsão Lipídica
- Se a intoxicação for atribuída a complicações anestésicas locais, considerar a terapia com a infusão IV de lipídios.
- A terapia com lipídios IV pode ser útil em casos de colapso cardíaco relacionado não só com anestésicos locais em particular, mas também com clomipramina e verapamil.
- Há relatos de caso do uso bem-sucedido em intoxicação por moxidectina em filhote de cão.
- Potencialmente útil para o tratamento de intoxicações causadas por toxinas lipossolúveis, embora haja poucos indícios clínicos da eficácia de antídoto lipídico sobre a intoxicação causada por medicamentos ingeridos.

MEDICAÇÕES
Antídotos ou procedimentos específicos estão disponíveis para as substâncias tóxicas mais comuns; ver o tópico específico.

ACOMPANHAMENTO
A monitorização específica depende da substância tóxica e dos sinais clínicos do paciente, além das anormalidades laboratoriais.

DIVERSOS
ABREVIATURA(S)
- SNC = sistema nervoso central.

RECURSOS DA INTERNET
- ASPCA Poison Control Center: http://www.aspca.org/pet-care/poison-control/.
- Toxiban: http://www.lloydinc.com/pdfs/ToxiBan.pdf.

Sugestões de Leitura
Peterson ME, Talcott PA, eds. Small Animal Toxicology. Philadelphia: Saunders, 2006.
Plumlee KH, ed. Clinical Veterinary Toxicology. St. Louis: Mosby, 2004.

Autores Tam Garland e E. Murl Bailey
Consultor Editorial Gary D. Osweiler

ENVENENAMENTO POR ARSÊNICO

CONSIDERAÇÕES GERAIS

REVISÃO
- Causado por herbicidas, inseticidas, conservantes de madeira e tratamentos contra hemoparasitas.
- Leva à interrupção de muitas reações metabólicas importantes.
- Exposição — oral é a mais comum; a percutânea pode causar toxicose sistêmica.

IDENTIFICAÇÃO
- Cães e gatos.
- Qualquer raça, idade ou sexo pode ser acometido.

SINAIS CLÍNICOS
Exposição Aguda
- Dor abdominal.
- Vômito.
- Fraqueza.
- Diarreia.
- Hematoquezia.
- Pulso débil e rápido.
- Prostração.
- Temperatura abaixo do normal.
- Colapso.
- Óbito.

Exposição Oral Subcrônica a Crônica
- Anorexia.
- Perda de peso.

CAUSAS E FATORES DE RISCO
- Exposição oral, percutânea ou terapêutica a compostos que contenham arsênico.
- A toxicidade é amplamente variável.
- Os animais fracos e debilitados são mais suscetíveis.

DIAGNÓSTICO

DIAGNÓSTICO DIFERENCIAL
- Toxicose por metais pesados.
- Ingestão de agentes cáusticos.
- Ingestão de plantas irritantes.
- Parvovírus canino ou felino.

HEMOGRAMA/BIOQUÍMICA/URINÁLISE
Análise bioquímica sérica — para pesquisar indícios de danos hepáticos e renais.

OUTROS TESTES LABORATORIAIS
Concentração de arsênico — testar urina, vômito ou conteúdo gástrico (envenenamento agudo), rins ou fígado (subagudo) e pelos (crônico); diminui drasticamente na urina, nos rins e no fígado 1-2 dias após a exposição; não confiável no sangue.

DIAGNÓSTICO POR IMAGEM
N/D.

MÉTODOS DIAGNÓSTICOS
N/D.

ACHADOS PATOLÓGICOS
- Envenenamento superagudo — leva ao óbito sem lesões.
- Lesões no trato gastrintestinal — comuns e graves; hiperemia da mucosa gástrica e porção proximal do intestino delgado; conteúdo gastrintestinal aquoso; presença de sangue e mucosa esfacelada nas fezes.
- Fígado — ictérico e friável.
- Pulmões — congestos; edematosos.
- Lesões cutâneas (exposição da pele) — formação de vesículas/bolhas; edema; rachaduras/fissuras; sangramento; infecções secundárias.

TRATAMENTO

- Remover a fonte de arsênico.
- Eméticos seguidos por lavagem gástrica — caso não tenha ocorrido vômito.
- Estimular a excreção.
- Diálise em casos de insuficiência renal.
- Fluidoterapia apropriada.
- Caulim-pectina — alivia o trato gastrintestinal.
- Manter o paciente aquecido e confortável.

DIETA
Nos casos em que o paciente mantém o alimento no trato digestório, fornecer quantidades pequenas de alimento de alta qualidade; aumentar essa quantidade conforme a tolerância.

MEDICAÇÕES

MEDICAMENTO(S)
Dimercaprol (BAL)
- Administrar 2,5-5 mg/kg em veículo oleoso por via IM profunda a cada 4 h por 2 dias; a cada 8 h no 3º dia; a cada 12 h por até 10 dias; 5 mg/kg apenas no 1º dia em pacientes acometidos de forma aguda.
- Os sinais de toxicose (dor no local da injeção, vômito, tremores, convulsões) desaparecem à medida que a BAL é excretada em 3-4 h.
- Esse medicamento libera o arsênico, o que pode agravar os sinais; fornecer, então, uma dose extra.

Outros Medicamentos
DMSA (succímer) — menos tóxico que a BAL; tratamento oral eficaz para intoxicação pelo chumbo em pequenos animais. Potencialmente útil para envenenamento por arsênico, embora não haja estudos controlados sobre o tratamento de cães e gatos envenenados por essa substância na literatura especializada.

ACOMPANHAMENTO

- O prognóstico será grave em casos de exposição a altas doses a menos que se formule o diagnóstico e se institua o tratamento precocemente.
- Monitorizar o paciente de perto quanto à presença de sinais de toxicose por BAL.

DIVERSOS

VER TAMBÉM
Envenenamento (Intoxicação).

ABREVIATURA(S)
- BAL = British anti-Lewisite*.
- DMSA = ácido 2,3-dimercaptossuccínico.

Sugestões de Leitura
Garland T. Arsenic. In: Gupta RC, ed., Veterinary Toxicology: Basic and Clinical Principles. New York: Academic Press, 2007, pp. 418-421.
National Research Council. Arsenic. In: Mineral Tolerance of Animals, 2nd ed. Washington, DC: National Academies Press, 2005, pp. 31-45.
Neiger RD. Arsenic. In: Peterson ME, Talcott PA, eds., Small Animal Toxicology, 2nd ed. Philadelphia: Saunders, 2006, pp. 592-602.

Autor Regg D. Neiger
Consultor Editorial Gary D. Osweiler

ENVENENAMENTO POR COGUMELO

CONSIDERAÇÕES GERAIS

REVISÃO
- Existem oito categorias classificadas com base na toxina e no toxidromo* (sete delas têm relevância veterinária; Tab. 1).
- Podem ocorrer toxidromos mistos (espécies em >1 categoria ou mistura de espécies consumidas).

FISIOPATOLOGIA
SISTEMA(S) ACOMETIDO(S)
INCIDÊNCIA/PREVALÊNCIA
- Ciclopeptídeo e grupos gastrintestinais — comuns.
- Outros — ocasionais.

DISTRIBUIÇÃO GEOGRÁFICA
Grupo de insuficiência renal aguda — principalmente na Europa, não registrado na América do Norte.

IDENTIFICAÇÃO
Espécies
Cães.

Idade Média e Faixa Etária
Todas as idades.

SINAIS CLÍNICOS
Comentários Gerais
- Espécies psicoativas são frequentemente desidratadas para transporte e venda; o produto desidratado permanece tóxico por no mínimo 6 meses.
- Muitas vezes, as espécies psicoativas são preparadas como extratos aquosos para consumo ou armazenamento sob refrigeração.
- Com frequência, as espécies psicoativas são cobertas com chocolate para facilitar a ingestão e o contrabando; pode ocorrer toxicidade do cogumelo e chocolate combinados.
- As espécies psicoativas são geralmente oferecidas como presentes de Natal.

Achados Anamnésicos
- Os proprietários frequentemente se mostram relutantes em fornecer detalhes, já que muitos casos envolvem tentativas do uso abusivo de substâncias ilícitas.

Achados do Exame Físico
Ciclopeptídeo
- Geralmente, envolve três fases sequenciais — GI, latente e hepatorrenal.
- O início tardio da fase GI e a recidiva da doença hepatorrenal após um período latente são características diagnósticas-chave. Com a exceção do MMA, todos os outros tipos de envenenamento por cogumelo ocorrem com relativa rapidez e em geral se resolvem de forma relativamente rápida. A recidiva caracterizada por doença hepatorrenal não ocorre no envenenamento por MMA.
- Fase de gastrenterite (início >6 h; dura cerca de 24 h) — vômitos intensos, diarreia sanguinolenta, dor abdominal, febre, desidratação, distúrbio eletrolítico, hipoglicemia.
- Fase latente (dura de 12-24 h) — aparente remissão.
- Fase hepatorrenal (começa 3-4 d após a ingestão) — insuficiência hepática e renal, icterícia, depressão, sinais de encefalopatia hepática e edema cerebral, hipoglicemia, crises convulsivas, coagulopatias, acidose metabólica, insuficiência renal, íleo paralítico grave, anormalidades de condução cardíaca, coma.
- Altos índices de morbidade e mortalidade; o óbito ocorre durante a fase hepatorrenal (3-7 dias após a ingestão).

Monometil-hidrazina
- Gastrenterite (início >6 h) — vômitos, diarreia sanguinolenta, dor abdominal, febre, desidratação, distúrbio eletrolítico, hipoglicemia.
- Ataxia.
- Ansiedade, hiperatividade, tremor, crise convulsiva.
- Tipicamente autolimitante, desaparecendo em alguns dias.
- Em casos graves raros, pode ocorrer o desenvolvimento de insuficiência hepática.

Muscarina
- Início rápido (15-60 min).
- Geralmente se resolve em 2-6 h (24 h no máximo).
- Sintomas do envenenamento — diarreia, micção, miose, broncorreia, broncoconstrição, êmese, lacrimejamento, salivação.
- Ocasionalmente, ocorre dano hepático.

Ácido Ibotênico/Muscimol
- Início rápido (30-60 min).
- Estimulação inicial do SNC, ataxia, hiperatividade, corrida sem sentido, excitação maníaca, crise convulsiva, alucinações visuais ("morder moscas imaginárias").
- Subsequente depressão do SNC — sonolência, estupor, sono e coma.
- Períodos de excitação do SNC alternados com depressão do SNC.
- A morte é muito rara.
- Distúrbio GI NÃO é uma característica.

Alucinógenos
- Início em até 4 h.
- Sinais simpaticomiméticos.
- Disforia, agitação, ansiedade, agressão.
- Hipertermia.
- Raramente — convulsões, coma, morte.
- Distúrbio GI NÃO é uma característica.

Irritantes GI
- Início em até 2 h.
- Mal-estar, fraqueza, êmese, diarreia.
- Distúrbios hidreletrolíticos.
- Geralmente autolimitante; desaparece em 24 h.

CAUSAS
Ver Tabelas 2 e 3.

FATORES DE RISCO
- Inexperiência na colheita de cogumelos silvestres.
- Abuso de substâncias pelo proprietário.
- Cultivo/tráfico de espécies alucinógenas.
- Época de colheita de cogumelo.

DIAGNÓSTICO

DIAGNÓSTICO DIFERENCIAL
HEMOGRAMA/BIOQUÍMICA/URINÁLISE
OUTROS TESTES LABORATORIAIS
MÉTODOS DIAGNÓSTICOS
Biopsia do fígado.

TRATAMENTO

CUIDADO(S) DE SAÚDE ADEQUADO(S)
- Tratamento médico de paciente internado.
- Cuidados intensivos para ciclopeptídeos.
- Não dar alta até que o envenenamento por ciclopeptídeo tenha sido refutado.

Tabela 1

Grupo	Espécies-chave
Ciclopeptídeo	*Amanita phalloides*, muitas espécies de *Amanita*, *Galerina* sp.
Monometil-hidrazina (MMA)	*A. muscaria* (cogumelo agário-das-moscas), *A. pantherina* (cogumelo amanita-pantera), *Gyromitra* sp., *Lycoperdon* sp.
Muscarina	*Clitocybe* sp., *Inocybe* sp., *A. pantherina*
Ácido ibotênico/muscimol	*Coprinus atramentarius*, *A. pantherina*, *A. muscaria*
Alucinógenos	*Psilocybe* sp., *Panaeolus* sp., *Gymnopilus* sp., *Stropharia* sp., *Conocybe* sp.
Irritantes GI	*Chlorophyllum* sp. e muitos outros
Insuficiência renal aguda	*Cortinarius* sp.

---

* N. T.: Conjunto de sinais e sintomas observados depois da exposição a alguma substância.

ENVENENAMENTO POR COGUMELO

Tabela 2

Grupo	Mecanismo
Ciclopeptídeo	Amatoxinas inibem a RNA polimerase II, bloqueando a transcrição de RNA e DNA. Os alvos são expostos rapidamente, dividindo as células (epitélio da cripta intestinal, hepatócitos e epitélio tubular renal) A falotoxina polimeriza irreversivelmente os filamentos de actina no árvore hepatobiliar, resultando em colestase
MMA	A giromitrina hidrolisa-se em MMA, o que provoca diminuição do GABA no SNC
Muscarina	Agonista colinérgico pós-ganglionar M_1 e M_2.
Ácido ibotênico/muscimol	Ácido ibotênico, um agonista do glutamato, é rapidamente metabolizado em muscimol, um agonista GABA-B
Alucinógenos	A psilocibina é metabolizada em psilocina, um agonista serotoninérgico $5\text{-}HT_{1A}$ e $5\text{-}HT_{2A/2C}$
Desarranjo GI	Irritantes, alérgenos
Insuficiência renal aguda	As toxinas são 2,2-bipiridina e compostos que se assemelham a paraquat e diquat — o ciclo redox é o mecanismo provável

Tabela 3

Grupo	Alvo
Ciclopeptídeo	Gastrintestinal — gastrenterite grave 6-24 h após a ingestão Hepatobiliar — necrose hepática centrolobular de início tardio (3-4 dias) Renal — nefrose tubular renal aguda de início tardio (3-4 dias) Metabólico — hipoglicemia Hematológico — coagulopatia Imune — propensão à sepse Nervoso — edema cerebral, encefalopatia hepatorrenal, coma
MMA	Gastrintestinal — vômito/diarreia 6-8 h após a ingestão Nervoso — excitação do SNC, crise convulsiva Neuromuscular — ataxia, tremor Hepatobiliar — necrose e insuficiência (rara) hepáticas
Muscarina	Gastrintestinal — diarreia, êmese, lacrimejamento excessivo Urinário — micção frequente Oftálmico — miose, cicloplegia Respiratório — broncorreia, broncoconstrição Cardiovascular — bradicardia, hipotensão
Ácido ibotênico/muscimol	Nervoso — ciclos de estimulação do SNC, seguidos por depressão, alucinações visuais, confusão mental, agitação, agressividade, atividade motora inútil ou sem sentido, crise convulsiva, coma, sinais simpaticomiméticos Oftálmico — midríase Metabólico — hipertermia
Alucinógenos	Nervoso — disforia, ansiedade, confusão mental, agitação, agressividade, atividade motora inútil ou sem sentido, crise convulsiva, coma, sinais simpaticomiméticos Neuromuscular — ataxia, hiper-reflexia
Desarranjo GI	Gastrintestinal — êmese, diarreia
Insuficiência renal aguda	Renal — nefrose tubulointersticial de início tardio (até 20 dias).

Tabela 4

Grupo	Diagnósticos Diferenciais Comuns
Ciclopeptídeo	Fase GI — gastrenterite infecciosa, irritantes GI e corrosivos Fase hepatorrenal — fósforo branco, micotoxinas hepatotóxicas e toxinas hepatotóxicas de algas, plantas hepatotóxicas
MMA	Antagonistas do GABA, estimulantes do SNC, agentes convulsivantes, isoniazida
Muscarina	Pesticidas anticolinesterásicos, medicamentos colinérgicos e toxinas
Ácido ibotênico/muscimol	Outros alucinógenos, estimulantes, lesão cerebral, infecção do SNC
Alucinógenos	LSD e outros alucinógenos, lesão cerebral, infecção do SNC
Desarranjo GI	Gastrenterite infecciosa, irritantes GI e corrosivos
Insuficiência renal aguda	Etilenoglicol, diquat, plantas que afetam os rins

CUIDADO(S) DE ENFERMAGEM

• Descontaminação do trato GI superior (de preferência, indução de êmese com o uso de apomorfina a 0,04 mg/kg IV ou no saco conjuntival; ou lavagem gástrica) é justificável no caso de envenenamento confirmado por ciclopeptídeos desde que: (1) o paciente seja levado à consulta em até 2 h após a ingestão; (2) a êmese ainda não tenha ocorrido; (3) não haja contraindicações (excitação do SNC, doença cardiovascular preexistente).

ENVENENAMENTO POR COGUMELO

Tabela 5

Grupo	Efeitos
Ciclopeptídeo	Fase GI — hemoconcentração, distúrbios eletrolíticos, perda de sangue GI Insuficiência hepatorrenal — evidência enzimática de necrose e colestase hepatocelulares, níveis séricos e urinários elevados de bilirrubina, ácidos biliares séricos aumentados, uremia, distúrbios eletrolíticos, poliúria inicial seguida por isostenúria ou anúria, hipoglicemia, coagulopatias, cilindros urinários, evidência de sepse
MMA	Inespecíficos; evidência de lesão oxidativa aos eritrócitos (metemoglobinemia, ↑ hemoglobina livre, ↑ sulfa-hemoglobina) pode estar presente nos estágios iniciais
Muscarina	Inespecíficos; raramente, há evidência enzimática de lesão hepatocelular
Ácido ibotênico/muscimol	Inespecíficos
Alucinógenos	Inespecíficos
Desarranjo GI	Hemoconcentração, distúrbios eletrolíticos
Insuficiência renal aguda	Poliúria inicial seguida por isostenúria ou anúria, distúrbios eletrolíticos (notavelmente hipercalemia), uremia

Tabela 6

Grupo	Outros Testes
Ciclopeptídeo	Identificação da espécie de cogumelo por especialista; teste de Meixner para detectar amatoxinas (podem ocorrer falso-negativos); mensuração de amanitina nos líquidos corporais
MMA	Identificação da espécie de cogumelo por especialista; o nível sanguíneo não se correlaciona bem com a gravidade; detecção da substância no conteúdo gástrico e/ou nos cogumelos
Muscarina	Identificação da espécie de cogumelo por especialista; detecção da substância nos líquidos corporais, no conteúdo gástrico e/ou nos cogumelos
Ácido ibotênico/muscimol	Identificação da espécie de cogumelo por especialista; detecção da substância nos líquidos corporais, no conteúdo gástrico e/ou nos cogumelos
Alucinógenos	Identificação da espécie de cogumelo por especialista; detecção da substância nos líquidos corporais, no conteúdo gástrico e/ou nos cogumelos
Desarranjo GI	Identificação da espécie de cogumelo por especialista
Insuficiência renal aguda	Identificação da espécie de cogumelo por especialista; detecção de oralanina nos líquidos corporais, nas fezes, no conteúdo gástrico e/ou nos cogumelos

- A administração de carvão ativado em dose repetida (1-4 g/kg a cada 3-6 h por 24-36 h; mistura em água 1 g/5-10 mL de água) visando diminuir o ciclo entero-hepático da toxina é de potencial benefício, apesar de não ser comprovado, no envenenamento por ciclopeptídeos.
- A administração de carvão ativado em dose única em até 2 h após a ingestão é possivelmente benéfica, mas não comprovada, em envenenamento por outros tipos de cogumelo na ausência de contraindicações.
- Ressuscitação hídrica (cristaloides IV) conforme houver necessidade.

ATIVIDADE
Evitar infortúnios.

DIETA
Nada por via oral se houver desarranjo GI.

ORIENTAÇÃO AO PROPRIETÁRIO
Segundo um velho ditado de Klingensmith, "Os caçadores de cogumelos sempre consomem o que encontram" (tradução nossa). Quanto mais informações se têm sobre a identificação de cogumelos silvestres, maiores serão as chances de consumi-los, pois sempre existirão aqueles que fogem da regra. Portanto, é melhor evitar a exposição dos animais a qualquer tipo de cogumelo.

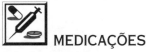

MEDICAÇÕES

MEDICAMENTO(S)
- Antídotos (Tab. 7).
- Cuidados de suporte (Tab. 8).

CONTRAINDICAÇÕES
- Envenenamento por MMA — hipnóticos de ação curta.
- Ácido ibotênico/muscimol — atropina, propofol.

MEDICAMENTO(S) ALTERNATIVO(S)
Metocarbamol 55-220 mg/kg IV, sem exceder 330 mg/kg/dia; administrar metade da dose rapidamente e, depois, o restante até fazer efeito; para controle das crises convulsivas.

ACOMPANHAMENTO

MONITORIZAÇÃO DO PACIENTE
- Ciclopeptídeos — enzimas hepáticas séricas, bilirrubina sérica, ácidos biliares séricos.
- Nível sérico de eletrólitos.
- Estado do SNC.

EVOLUÇÃO ESPERADA E PROGNÓSTICO
- Ciclopeptídeos — reservado.
- Outros — geralmente bom a menos que haja dano a órgãos.

DIVERSOS

VER TAMBÉM
- Insuficiência Hepática Aguda.
- Insuficiência Renal Aguda.
- Crises Convulsivas (Convulsões, Estado Epiléptico) — Gatos.
- Crises Convulsivas (Convulsões, Estado Epiléptico) — Cães.

ABREVIATURA(S)
- GABA = ácido gama-aminobutírico.
- GI = gastrintestinal.
- MMA = monometil-hidrazina.
- SNC = sistema nervoso central.

Sugestões de Leitura
Rumack BH, Spoerke DG. Handbook of Mushroom Poisoning: Diagnosis and Treatment. New York: CRC Press, 1994.
Schonwald S. Mycotoxins and toxigenic fungi. In: Dart RC, ed., Medical Toxicology, 3rd ed. Baltimore: Lippincott, Williams & Wilkins, 2004, pp. 1719-1735.

Autor Rhian Cope
Consultor Editorial Gary D. Osweiler

ENVENENAMENTO POR COGUMELO

Tabela 7

Grupo	Antídoto
Ciclopeptídeo	Não há nenhum tratamento comprovadamente eficaz Ácido tióctico (1-2 mg/kg a cada 6 h) creditado com ↓ mortalidade humana Silibinina (50 mg/kg/dia a cada 6 h); combinar com N-acetilcisteína A penicilina é teoricamente benéfica, embora a eficácia seja limitada na prática clínica
MMA	Piridoxina 25 mg/kg
Muscarina	Atropina até fazer efeito (o ponto extremo é o ressecamento das secreções)
Ácido ibotênico/muscimol	N/D
Alucinógenos	N/D
Desarranjo GI	N/D
Insuficiência renal aguda	N/D

Tabela 8

Grupo	Cuidados de Suporte
Ciclopeptídeo	Glicose ou dextrose IV se necessário Plasma fresco congelado Transfusão sanguínea Vitamina K (K_1 — 0,5-1,5 mg/kg IM ou SC a cada 12 h por até 3 doses em intervalo de 24 h 1 vez; vitamina K_1 oral — 1 mg/kg VO a cada 24 h se os ácidos biliares entéricos e sua absorção estiverem adequados Potássio na presença de hipocalemia de insuficiência hepática Furosemida 2-4 mg/kg IV a cada 8-12 h; para insuficiência renal oligúrica ou anúrica em pacientes com estado de hidratação normal; combinar com dopamina Dopamina 0,5-3 mcg/kg para insuficiência renal oligúrica ou anúrica; combinar com furosemida
MMA	Diazepam 0,25-0,5 mg/kg IV ou IM; para crises convulsivas
Muscarina	Atropina até fazer efeito (ressecamento das secreções; 0,02-0,04 mg/kg com metade da dose por via IV e a outra metade por via IM; titular até fazer efeito)
Ácido ibotênico/muscimol	Diazepam 0,25-0,5 mg/kg IV ou IM; para crises convulsivas
Alucinógenos	Diazepam 0,25-0,5 mg/kg IV ou IM; para crises convulsivas
Desarranjo GI	N/D
Insuficiência renal aguda	Furosemida 2-4 mg/kg IV a cada 8-12 h; para insuficiência renal oligúrica ou anúrica em pacientes com estado de hidratação normal; combinar com dopamina Dopamina 0,5-3 mcg/kg para insuficiência renal oligúrica ou anúrica; combinar com furosemida

Envenenamento por Rodenticidas Anticoagulantes

CONSIDERAÇÕES GERAIS

DEFINIÇÃO
Coagulopatia causada por declínio dos fatores de coagulação (dependentes da vitamina K_1) na circulação, após exposição a rodenticidas anticoagulantes.

FISIOPATOLOGIA
• Inibição da vitamina K_1 epóxido redutase, da DT-diaforase e possivelmente de outras enzimas envolvidas na redução da vitamina K_1 epóxido em vitamina K_1. • Vitamina K_1 — necessária para a carboxilação dos fatores II, VI, IX e X de coagulação; os fatores de coagulação não carboxilados não se ligam ao cálcio o suficiente a ponto de participarem da formação de coágulos.

SISTEMA(S) ACOMETIDO(S)
Hematológico/linfático/imune.

INCIDÊNCIA/PREVALÊNCIA
Comum — muitas iscas de ratos são vendidas sem prescrição médica (ou seja, constituem produtos de venda livre) e são amplamente utilizadas nos ambientes domésticos.

IDENTIFICAÇÃO
• Cães e gatos. • Não há predisposição racial ou sexual; os animais mais jovens podem ingerir as iscas com maior facilidade.

SINAIS CLÍNICOS

Comentários Gerais
Pode ser levemente mais prevalente na primavera e no outono, época em que os produtos rodenticidas são mais utilizados.

Achados Anamnésicos
• Uso de rodenticidas anticoagulantes. • Dispneia — intolerância a exercício. • Sangramento.

Achados do Exame Físico
• Hematomas — frequentemente situados na região ventral e nos locais de venopunção.
• Abafamento dos sons cardíacos ou dos ruídos respiratórios. • Mucosas pálidas. • Letargia.

CAUSAS
• Exposição a produtos rodenticidas anticoagulantes. • Anticoagulantes cumarínicos de primeira geração (p. ex., varfarina e pindona) — basicamente foram substituídos por anticoagulantes mais potentes de segunda geração.
• Anticoagulantes de segunda geração (p. ex., brodifacum, bromadiolona, difacinona e clorofacinona) — em geral, são mais tóxicos do que os agentes de primeira geração e alguns persistem por mais tempo antes de serem excretados. • Difentialona (D-Cease®) — menos tóxico aos cães (DL50* de 4 mg/kg) do que o brodifacum (DL50 de 0,25-2,5 mg/kg), a bromadiolona (DL50 de 11-20 mg/kg), a clorofacinona (DL50 de 50-100 mg/kg) e a varfarina (DL50 de 20-50 mg/kg); semelhante à difacinona (DL50 de 3-7,5 mg/kg); em gatos, a DL50 é >16 mg/kg; a concentração nas iscas é mais baixa (0,0025%; 25 ppm) do que em outras iscas de rodenticidas de segunda geração (0,005%;

---
* N. T.: DL50 é a dose de uma substância química que provoca a morte de 50% de um grupo de animais da mesma espécie, quando administrada pela mesma via.

50 ppm); dessa forma, cães e gatos podem tolerar a ingestão de quantidades maiores.

FATORES DE RISCO
• Doses pequenas durante alguns dias são mais perigosas do que uma única dose ampla; qualquer tipo de exposição pode causar toxicose.
• Toxicidade secundária ao consumo de roedores envenenados — improvável.

DIAGNÓSTICO

DIAGNÓSTICO DIFERENCIAL
• CID. • Deficiências congênitas dos fatores de coagulação.

HEMOGRAMA/BIOQUÍMICA/URINÁLISE
Anemia — em casos de hemorragia acentuada.

OUTROS TESTES LABORATORIAIS
• TCA >150 segundos — indicativo de coagulopatia. • TP e TTP prolongados — sugestivos de exposição a rodenticidas; o TP é acometido antes do TTP. • Análises sanguínea ou hepática — confirmatórios da exposição a algum produto específico.

DIAGNÓSTICO POR IMAGEM
Radiografia torácica — pode detectar hemotórax ou hemopericárdio.

MÉTODOS DIAGNÓSTICOS
Toracocentese — pode confirmar a presença de hemotórax.

ACHADOS PATOLÓGICOS
• Sangue livre tanto nas cavidades torácica e abdominal como nos pulmões — comum.
• Hemorragia na abóbada craniana e nos tratos gastrintestinal e urinário — menos comum; pode ocorrer tanto por via subcutânea como intramuscular.

TRATAMENTO

CUIDADO(S) DE SAÚDE ADEQUADO(S)
• Internação — em casos de crise aguda. • Esquema ambulatorial — hipótese a ser considerada assim que a coagulopatia estiver estabilizada.

CUIDADO(S) DE ENFERMAGEM
Transfusão de sangue total ou plasma frescos — pode ser necessária em casos de hemorragia; promove o acesso imediato dos fatores de coagulação dependentes da vitamina K; o sangue total pode representar a escolha mais adequada em casos de anemia grave.

ATIVIDADE
Confinar o paciente durante os estágios precoces do envenenamento, uma vez que a atividade física intensifica a perda sanguínea.

DIETA
Não há nenhum efeito identificável.

ORIENTAÇÃO AO PROPRIETÁRIO
Alertar o proprietário a respeito das sérias consequências de uma nova exposição.

CONSIDERAÇÕES CIRÚRGICAS
• Toracocentese — pode ser importante para a remoção de sangue livre no tórax, responsável pela dispneia e insuficiência respiratória. • Antes da cirurgia, é fundamental corrigir a coagulopatia.

MEDICAÇÕES

MEDICAMENTO(S) DE ESCOLHA
• Vitamina K_1 — 2,5-5,0 mg/kg VO a cada 24 horas durante 5 dias a 6 semanas (dependendo do produto específico); a biodisponibilidade é acentuada pelo fornecimento concomitante de pequenas quantidades de gordura, como as rações enlatadas para cães. • Administração da vitamina K_1 — mantida por 3-4 semanas na suspeita de toxicose por anticoagulantes de segunda geração.

CONTRAINDICAÇÕES
• Vitamina K_3 — não tem eficácia no tratamento de toxicose causada por rodenticidas anticoagulantes; portanto, é contraindicada.
• Vitamina K_1 intravenosa — há relatos de reações anafiláticas; evitar essa via de administração.

PRECAUÇÕES
• Evitar as injeções parenterais e os procedimentos cirúrgicos desnecessários. • Utilizar a menor agulha possível na aplicação de injeções ou na coleta de amostras.

INTERAÇÕES POSSÍVEIS
Sulfonamidas e fenilbutazona — podem deslocar os rodenticidas anticoagulantes dos locais de ligação do plasma, levando à toxicose e aumentando a quantidade de agentes tóxicos livres.

ACOMPANHAMENTO

MONITORIZAÇÃO DO PACIENTE
TCA e TP — para avaliar a eficácia da terapia; monitorização contínua por 3-5 dias após a interrupção do tratamento.

PREVENÇÃO
Não permitir o acesso dos animais aos rodenticidas anticoagulantes.

COMPLICAÇÕES POSSÍVEIS
• Subsequentemente à hemorragia intrapulmonar, pode-se observar uma pneumonia bacteriana secundária. • Hemorragia intracraniana e/ou intra-articular.

EVOLUÇÃO ESPERADA E PROGNÓSTICO
Se o paciente sobreviver nas primeiras 48 horas da coagulopatia aguda, há uma melhora no prognóstico.

DIVERSOS

GESTAÇÃO/FERTILIDADE/REPRODUÇÃO
Varfarina e difacinona, talvez outros — podem passar para o líquido amniótico e para os fetos quando uma cadela prenhe é exposta; há preocupações semelhantes quanto ao fornecimento de leite contaminado a filhotes caninos.

ABREVIATURA(S)
• CID = coagulação intravascular disseminada.
• TCA = tempo de coagulação ativada. • TP = tempo de protrombina. • TTP = tempo de tromboplastina parcial.

RECURSOS DA INTERNET
http://www.aspcapro.org/animal-poison-control-center-articles.php.

Autor Michael J. Murphy
Consultor Editorial Gary D. Osweiler

Epididimite/Orquite

CONSIDERAÇÕES GERAIS

REVISÃO
- Epididimite — inflamação do epidídimo; sinal clínico mais significativo e grave de brucelose.
- Orquite — inflamação dos testículos.
- Podem ser agudas ou crônicas.
- Traumatismo direto ao escroto — causa mais comum da forma aguda.
- Podem ocorrer separadamente ou em combinação (orquiepididimite); também é possível a propagação para as túnicas vaginais (periorquiepididimite).

IDENTIFICAÇÃO
- Não são incomuns em cães; raras em gatos.
- Sem base genética nem predileção racial.
- Idade média de 3,7 anos; faixa etária de 11 meses a 10 anos.

SINAIS CLÍNICOS
- Testículos intumescidos.
- Dor (aguda).
- Lambedura do escroto — pode acarretar dermatite.
- Inquietação.
- Anorexia.
- Relutância em andar e acasalar.
- Ferida aberta ou abscesso.
- Infertilidade.
- Pirexia.

CAUSAS E FATORES DE RISCO
- *Brucella canis* — predileção por infectar a cauda do epidídimo.
- Cinomose.
- Febre maculosa das Montanhas Rochosas.
- Infecção ascendente — associada à prostatite (especialmente em casos de brucelose) e cistite.
- Contaminação urinária retrógrada do ducto deferente — sequela de pressão intra-abdominal alta, como aquela causada por traumatismo em acidente automobilístico.
- Feridas por mordedura e outros ferimentos penetrantes — microrganismos isolados de testículos infectados: *Staphylococcus*, *Streptococcus*, *Escherichia coli*, *Proteus* e *Mycoplasma*.
- Resposta autoimune a antígenos de espermatozoides — secundária a traumatismo ou inflamação.
- Tireoidite linfocítica autoimune — familiar na raça Beagle.

DIAGNÓSTICO

DIAGNÓSTICO DIFERENCIAL
- Hérnia inguinoscrotal.
- Dermatite escrotal.
- Torção do cordão espermático.
- Hidrocele.
- Granuloma espermático.
- Neoplasia testicular.
- Prostatite.
- Cistite.

HEMOGRAMA/BIOQUÍMICA/URINÁLISE
- Leucocitose — pode ser encontrada em casos de orquite aguda ou infecciosa.
- Piúria, hematúria, proteinúria — poderão ser constatadas se a epididimite/orquite for secundária à prostatite ou cistite.

OUTROS TESTES LABORATORIAIS
- Anticorpos contra *B. canis* — fazer testes imediatamente em qualquer cão com aumento de volume do escroto (ver "Brucelose").
- Teste de aglutinação rápida em lâmina — utilizado como triagem; sensível, mas inespecífico (D-Tec CB, Synbiotics Corp.).
- Se os resultados forem positivos — será recomendável a reavaliação por meio do teste de imunodifusão em ágar gel (Cornell University Diagnostic Laboratory) ou da cultura bacteriana de sangue total ou aspirado de linfonodo.

DIAGNÓSTICO POR IMAGEM
- Avaliação ultrassonográfica da próstata — aspiração orientada por ultrassom para exame citológico e cultura bacteriana.
- Avaliação ultrassonográfica dos testículos e epidídimos — os testículos inflamados exibem áreas hipoecoicas irregulares; já os epidídimos inflamados apresentam contornos irregulares e áreas hipo ou hiperecoicas; obter medidas para comparações futuras.

MÉTODOS DIAGNÓSTICOS
- Sêmen — coletar se possível; avaliação citológica; cultura bacteriana.
- Citologia (sêmen) — leucócitos; bactérias; espermatozoides com caudas espiraladas, cabeças destacadas (separadas) e gotículas citoplasmáticas proximais e distais retidas; aglutinação de cabeça com cabeça (*B. canis*).
- Massagem da próstata — exame citológico; cultura bacteriana; amostra coletada de forma asséptica por cateter uretral.
- Feridas abertas — culturas bacterianas.
- Aspirado por agulha fina — amostra dos testículos/epidídimos aumentados de volume para citologia e cultura; os leucócitos variam desde inúmeros neutrófilos (supurativas) até quantidade mínima de células inflamatórias (granulomatosas).

TRATAMENTO

- Se não houver interesse em preservar a fertilidade — coletar uma quantidade adequada de amostra para realização de cultura; estabilizar o paciente por meio clínico; administrar os antibióticos necessários no período pré-operatório para evitar a formação de cordão cirroso; e, por fim, castrar.
- Se houver interesse em preservar a fertilidade (orquite unilateral) — proceder à castração unilateral se a manutenção do futuro do animal como reprodutor for imprescindível; administrar os antibióticos adequados no pré-operatório.

MEDICAÇÕES

MEDICAMENTOS(S)
Antibióticos — continuar por pelo menos 3 semanas; utilizar inicialmente oxacilina, trimetoprima-sulfonamida, aminoglicosídeo ou enrofloxacino; trocar mediante a disponibilidade dos resultados da cultura e do antibiograma; é improvável que a antibioticoterapia sem castração uni ou bilateral seja bem-sucedida.

CONTRAINDICAÇÕES/INTERAÇÕES POSSÍVEIS
N/D.

ACOMPANHAMENTO

- Prognóstico em termos de fertilidade — reservado a mau, especialmente em casos de orquite bilateral.
- O aquecimento dos testículos provoca degeneração desse órgão — a degeneração no testículo contralateral pode ser resultante de doença primária ou de temperatura intraescrotal elevada após castração unilateral.
- Traumatismo ou inflamação pode causar obstrução de túbulos eferentes ou do ducto epididimário, acarretando a formação de espermatoceles ou granuloma espermático.
- Sêmen (cães) — avaliar as características 3 meses após o término do tratamento da orquite.

DIVERSOS

VER TAMBÉM
Brucelose.

Sugestões de Leitura
Feldman EC, Nelson RW. Canine and Feline Endocrinology and Reproduction. Philadelphia: Saunders, 1987, pp. 705-709.
Johnston SD, Root Kustritz MV, Olson PNS. Disorders of the canine testis and epididymes. In: Johnston SD, Kustritz MVR, Olson PN, eds., Canine and Feline Theriogenology. Philadelphia: Saunders, 2001, pp. 313-317.

Autor Carlos R.F. Pinto
Consultor Editorial Sara K. Lyle

EPÍFORA

CONSIDERAÇÕES GERAIS

DEFINIÇÃO
Fluxo anormal excessivo da porção aquosa do filme lacrimal pré-corneano.

FISIOPATOLOGIA
Causada por um de três problemas comuns: (1) produção excessiva da porção aquosa das lágrimas (geralmente em resposta à irritação ocular); (2) disfunção da pálpebra secundária à má-formação ou deformidade; ou (3) obstrução do sistema de drenagem nasolacrimal.

SISTEMA(S) ACOMETIDO(S)
Oftálmico e pele periocular.

IDENTIFICAÇÃO
Ver a seção "Causas".

SINAIS CLÍNICOS
N/D.

CAUSAS

Produção Excessiva de Lágrimas Secundária a Irritantes Oculares

Congênitas
- Distiquíase ou triquíase — comum em animais jovens das raças Sheltie, Shih tzu, Lhasa apso, Cocker spaniel, Poodle miniatura.
- Entrópio — Shar pei, Chow Chow, Labrador retriever.
- Agenesia palpebral — gatos domésticos de pelo curto.

Adquiridas
- Corpos estranhos na córnea ou na conjuntiva — em geral, cães ativos jovens pertencentes às raças de grande porte.
- Neoplasias palpebrais — cães idosos (todas as raças).
- Blefarite — infecciosa ou imunomediada.
- Conjuntivite — infecciosa ou imunomediada.
- Ceratite ulcerativa.
- Uveíte anterior.
- Glaucoma.

Anormalidades Palpebrais ou Disfunção Palpebral
- As lágrimas nunca alcançam os pontos nasolacrimais, mas sim escorrem pela margem palpebral.
- A função normal das pálpebras não direciona as lágrimas para o canto medial e os pontos nasolacrimais.

Congênitas
- Fissuras macropalpebrais — raças braquicefálicas.
- Ectrópio — Dinamarquês, Bloodhound, Spaniel.
- Entrópio — raças braquicefálicas — face medial da pálpebra inferior; Labrador retriever — face lateral da pálpebra inferior.

Adquiridas
- Formação cicatricial palpebral pós-traumática.
- Paralisia do nervo facial.

Obstrução do Sistema de Drenagem Nasolacrimal

Congênita
- Pontos nasolacrimais imperfurados — Cocker spaniel, Buldogue, Poodle.
- Orifícios nasolacrimais ectópicos — aberturas extras ao longo do lado da face ventral para o canto medial.
- Atresia nasolacrimal — ausência das aberturas distais para o nariz.

Adquirida
- Rinite ou sinusite — causa tumefação adjacente ao ducto nasolacrimal.
- Traumatismo ou fraturas dos ossos lacrimais ou maxilares.
- Corpos estranhos — farpas de gramíneas, sementes, areia, parasitas.
- Neoplasia — de estruturas como terceira pálpebra, conjuntivas, pálpebras mediais, cavidade nasal, osso maxilar ou seios perioculares.
- Dacriocistite — inflamação dos canalículos, saco lacrimal ou ductos nasolacrimais.

FATORES DE RISCO
- Raças propensas a anormalidades palpebrais congênitas (ver a seção "Causas").
- Cães ativos com acesso à rua — sob risco de corpos estranhos.

DIAGNÓSTICO

DIAGNÓSTICO DIFERENCIAL
- Outras secreções oculares (p. ex., mucosas ou purulentas) — a epífora é uma secreção aquosa e serosa.
- Olho — geralmente vermelho quando causada por produção excessiva de lágrimas; "silencioso" quando secundária a comprometimento do fluxo de saída.
- Causas irritantes e algumas congênitas de obstrução — exame ocular completo.
- Condição de início agudo, unilateral, com dor ocular (blefarospasmo) — costuma indicar a presença de corpo estranho ou lesão da córnea.
- Condição bilateral crônica — geralmente indica um problema congênito.
- Dor facial, tumefação, secreção nasal ou espirros — podem indicar infecção nasal ou sinusal; pode ser indício de obstrução por neoplasia.
- Com secreção mucosa ou purulenta no canto medial — pode ser indício de dacriocistite.

HEMOGRAMA/BIOQUÍMICA/URINÁLISE
N/D.

OUTROS TESTES LABORATORIAIS
N/D.

DIAGNÓSTICO POR IMAGEM
- Radiografias de crânio — podem revelar lesão nasal, sinusal ou maxilar.
- Dacriocistorrinografia — material de contraste radiopaco para ajudar a localizar a obstrução.
- RM ou TC — podem ajudar a localizar a obstrução (geralmente com meio de contraste) e caracterizar as lesões associadas.

MÉTODOS DIAGNÓSTICOS
- Cultura bacteriana, antibiograma e exame citológico do material — em casos de material purulento no canto medial (p. ex., dacriocistite); realizados antes de se instilar qualquer substância no olho.
- Aplicação tópica do corante fluoresceína no olho — teste mais fisiológico para função nasolacrimal; deve ser efetuado em primeiro lugar; o corante flui através do sistema nasolacrimal e alcança as narinas externas em aproximadamente 10 segundos em cães normais.
- Irrigação nasolacrimal — ver informações adiante.
- Rinoscopia — com ou sem biopsia ou cultura bacteriana; poderá ser indicada se os exames anteriores sugerirem a existência de lesão nasal ou sinusal.
- Cirurgia exploradora — pode ser a única forma de se obter o diagnóstico definitivo.
- Fechamento temporário da pálpebra medial inferior com sutura — poderá ajudar a determinar se o reparo do entrópio medial inferior ou o reposicionamento da pálpebra reduziria a epífora secundária a anormalidades da conformação palpebral.

Irrigação Nasolacrimal
- Confirma a obstrução.
- Pode deslocar algum material estranho.
- O procedimento consiste na inserção de cânula nasolacrimal no ponto nasolacrimal superior.
- Por meio da cânula, instila-se colírio — se o líquido não sair no ponto nasolacrimal inferior, a obstrução estará localizada nos canalículos superiores ou inferiores, no saco nasolacrimal ou no ponto inferior (imperfurado).
- Obstrução manual do ponto inferior — se o líquido irrigado não sair pelas narinas externas, a obstrução estará situada no ducto nasolacrimal ou em sua abertura distal (atresia ou bloqueio por lesão em seio nasal).

TRATAMENTO

- Eliminar a causa de irritação ocular — remoção de corpo estranho na conjuntiva ou na córnea; tratamento da doença ocular primária (p. ex., conjuntivite, ceratite ulcerativa e uveíte); criocirurgia ou eletroepilação para distiquíase; correção de entrópio; cantoplastia medial ou lateral (para triquíase medial e fissuras macropalpebrais); correção de anormalidades palpebrais cicatriciais.
- Tratar a lesão obstrutiva primária (p. ex., massa na terceira pálpebra, massa nasal ou sinusal, e infecção) — fazer logo de início; o sucesso do tratamento pode permitir o restabelecimento do fluxo nasolacrimal normal.
- Avisar o proprietário que o animal fica predisposto à obstrução nasolacrimal e que a recidiva é comum.
- Informar ao proprietário que a detecção e a intervenção precoces resultam em um prognóstico melhor a longo prazo.

CONSIDERAÇÕES CIRÚRGICAS

Pontos Imperfurados
- Fica indicada a abertura cirúrgica dos pontos.
- Se um dos pontos estiver patente/desobstruído (em geral, o superior), a irrigação com colírio por meio da abertura superior fará com que a conjuntiva "forme uma tenda" no local do ponto inferior. Submeter o paciente à anestesia tópica ou geral. Pinçar a conjuntiva sobrejacente aos canalículos inferiores com pinça e cortar com tesoura para deixar um ponto patente. Para os pontos fechados por formaçã`o cicatricial conjuntival (simbléfaro) causada por conjuntivite grave (p. ex., conjuntivite por herpes-vírus em gatos), usar o mesmo procedimento. Em caso de doença recidivante, talvez haja necessidade da sutura de tubo de Silastic® no local para evitar a formação de estenose.

EPÍFORA

Ducto Nasolacrimal Distal Obstruído ou Obliterado
• Dacriocistorrinostomia ou conjuntivorrinostomia — criar uma abertura para drenar as lágrimas à cavidade nasal.
• Ver técnicas cirúrgicas na seção "Sugestões de Leitura".

MEDICAÇÕES

MEDICAMENTO(S) DE ESCOLHA
• Soluções oftálmicas tópicas de antibiótico de amplo espectro — enquanto se aguardam os resultados dos exames diagnósticos (p. ex., cultura bacteriana e antibiograma; radiografias diagnósticas); a cada 4-6 h; pode-se tentar o uso de soluções oftálmicas tópicas com 3 antibióticos (neomicina, gramicidina e polimixina B) ou solução oftálmica de ciprofloxacino.
• Dacriocistite — com base nos resultados da cultura bacteriana e do antibiograma; continuar por pelo menos 21 dias.

CONTRAINDICAÇÕES
• Corticosteroides tópicos ou combinações tópicas deles com antibiótico — evitar a menos que tenha sido estabelecido o diagnóstico definitivo.
• Corticosteroides tópicos — nunca usar se a córnea ainda reter o corante fluoresceína.

PRECAUÇÕES
N/D.

INTERAÇÕES POSSÍVEIS
N/D.

MEDICAMENTO(S) ALTERNATIVO(S)
Tetraciclina — 5 mg/kg VO a cada 24 h; pode ajudar a reduzir a mancha idiopática dos pelos faciais perioculares por lágrimas; a mancha volta quando se interrompe a administração do medicamento.

ACOMPANHAMENTO

MONITORIZAÇÃO DO PACIENTE
Dacriocistite
• Reavaliar a cada 7 dias até a resolução do problema.
• Continuar o tratamento por pelo menos 7 dias após o desaparecimento dos sinais clínicos para ajudar a evitar a recidiva.
• Se o problema persistir por mais de 7-10 dias com o tratamento ou se houver recidiva logo após o término do tratamento — isso indica a presença de corpo estranho ou foco de infecção persistente, o que exige a realização de outros exames diagnósticos (p. ex., dacriocistorrinografia).

Cateter Nasolacrimal
• Costuma ser necessário para a dacriocistite persistente.
• Mantém a patência do ducto e evita a ocorrência de estenose.
• Cateter — tubo de Silastic® ou polietileno (PE90); deixar no lugar por 2-4 semanas.
• Procedimento — introduzir um fio de sutura de náilon 2-0 pelo ponto superior e através do ducto nasolacrimal até sair nas narinas externas; passar o tubo de forma retrógrada sobre a sutura; suturar as partes superior e inferior do tubo à face.
• A maioria dos cães é bem tolerante ao tubo.
• Prosseguir com os antibióticos tópicos como antes.

Dacriocistorrinotomia/Conjuntivorrinostomia
• Tubo — reavaliar a cada 7 dias para garantir a manutenção da integridade desse dispositivo; poderá ser necessária uma nova aplicação de sutura se o tubo ficar frouxo ou sair do lugar.
• Após a retirada do tubo — reavaliar 14 dias depois; nesse exame e em exames futuros, instilar fluoresceína no olho e verificar a patência nasolacrimal, examinando as narinas externas para ver se o corante passa por elas; pode-se avaliar o sistema nasolacrimal de forma mais minuciosa por meio de canulação e irrigação com colírio.
• Dacriocistorrinografia contrastada — repetida 3-4 meses após a cirurgia para avaliar o tamanho da abertura nasal; repetida em caso de recidiva ou na ausência de drenagem nasolacrimal da fluoresceína.

COMPLICAÇÕES POSSÍVEIS
Recidiva — complicação mais comum; causada pela recidiva de irritação ocular (p. ex., ulceração da córnea, distiquíase e entrópio), recidiva de dacriocistite ou fechamento das aberturas da dacriocistorrinotomia ou conjuntivorrinostomia na cavidade nasal.

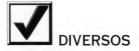

DIVERSOS

DISTÚRBIOS ASSOCIADOS
• Conjuntivite crônica — gatos.
• Conjuntivite crônica — cães.
• "Infecções" oculares recidivantes.
• Dermatite úmida ("manchas quentes") ventral ao canto medial.
• Secreção nasal.

FATORES RELACIONADOS COM A IDADE
N/D.

POTENCIAL ZOONÓTICO
N/D.

GESTAÇÃO/FERTILIDADE/REPRODUÇÃO
N/D.

VER TAMBÉM
• Ceratite Ulcerativa.
• Conjuntivite — Cães.
• Conjuntivite — Gatos.
• Distúrbios dos Cílios (Triquíase, Distiquíase/Cílios Ectópicos).
• Protrusão da Terceira Pálpebra.

ABREVIATURA(S)
• RM = ressonância magnética.
• TC = tomografia computadorizada.

Sugestões de Leitura
Grahn BH, Sandmeyer LS. Diseases and surgery of the canine nasolacrimal system. In: Gelatt KN, ed., Veterinary Ophthalmology, 4th ed. Ames, IA: Blackwell, 2007, pp. 618-632.
Miller PE. Lacrimal system. In: Maggs DJ, Miller PE, Ofri R, Slatter's Fundamentals of Veterinary Ophthalmology, 4th ed. St. Louis: Saunders, 2008, pp. 157-174.

Autor Brian C. Gilger
Consultor Editorial Paul E. Miller

Epilepsia Idiopática (Genética)

CONSIDERAÇÕES GERAIS

DEFINIÇÃO
Síndrome caracterizada apenas por epilepsia, na ausência de lesão cerebral subjacente demonstrável ou outros sinais ou sintomas neurológicos; relacionada com a idade; supostamente genética.

FISIOPATOLOGIA
• Mecanismo exato desconhecido. • A disfunção pode ser bioquímica ou o animal pode ter uma propensão intrínseca a ter crises convulsivas.
• Mecanismos provavelmente diferentes entre as raças.

SISTEMA(S) ACOMETIDO(S)
Nervoso.

GENÉTICA
Com base na análise do pedigree, suspeita-se de base genética em raças como Beagle, Pastor belga (Groenendael e Tervuren), Montanhês de Berna, Alsatian britânico, Dachshund, Springer spaniel inglês, Finnish spitz, Golden retriever, Keeshond, Wolfhound irlandês, Spinone italiano, Labrador retriever, Pastor de Shetland, Poode standard, Vizla.

INCIDÊNCIA/PREVALÊNCIA
• Entre 0,5 e 2,3% de todos os cães, maior naqueles em colônias de pesquisa. • Gatos — rara; pouco documentada.

DISTRIBUIÇÃO GEOGRÁFICA
Disseminada.

IDENTIFICAÇÃO
Espécies
Cães.

Raça(s) Predominante(s)
Beagle; todos os pastores (alemão, australiano e belga); Montanhês de Berna; Boxer; Cocker spaniel; Collie e Border collie; Dachshund; Golden retriever; Setter irlandês; Wolfhound irlandês, Keeshond; Labrador retriever; Poodle (todos os portes); São Bernardo; Pastor de Shetland; Husky siberiano; Springer spaniel; Welsh corgi; Fox terrier de pelo duro.

Idade Média e Faixa Etária
• Idade média — 10 meses a 3 anos. • Faixa etária — 6 meses a 5 anos.

Sexo Predominante
Predisposição do sexo masculino em cães da raça Montanhês de Berna.

SINAIS CLÍNICOS
Comentários Gerais
• As crises convulsivas podem ser generalizadas desde o início ou exibir uma breve aura (início focal) com rápida generalização secundária. • A presença de aura é frequente (o animal parece assustado, atordoado, busca por atenção ou se esconde, etc.) antes das crises convulsivas generalizadas. • Podem ocorrer crises convulsivas focais nas raças Finnish spitz, Springer spaniel inglês, Labrador retriever, Viszla, Pastor belga, Poodle standard.

Achados Anamnésicos
• Crises convulsivas — a maioria ocorre enquanto o paciente está em repouso ou dormindo; geralmente à noite ou no início da manhã; a frequência tenderá a aumentar se não for tratada; o animal acometido cai de um lado, fica rígido, movimenta a mandíbula, saliva bastante, urina, defeca, vocaliza e patinha com os 4 membros em combinações variáveis. Duração breve (30-90 segundos). • Comportamento pós-ictal (i. e., após a convulsão) — períodos de confusão mental e desorientação; marcha a esmo, compulsiva e às cegas; polidipsia e polifagia frequentes; recuperação imediata ou até em 24 h. • Cães com epilepsia estabelecida apresentam crises convulsivas generalizadas e agrupadas em intervalos regulares de 1-4 semanas. • Durante as crises convulsivas, não se deve observar assimetria, como espasmo mais pronunciado em um dos lados, contrações dos membros em um dos lados, andar em círculo imediatamente antes ou depois das crises.

Achados do Exame Físico
• Com frequência, o paciente já se recuperou no momento da consulta. • Os pacientes podem exibir comportamento pós-ictal.

CAUSAS
Genéticas em algumas raças; idiopáticas em outras.

FATORES DE RISCO
Epilepsia conhecida nos progenitores.

DIAGNÓSTICO

DIAGNÓSTICO DIFERENCIAL
• Padrão das crises convulsivas (idade de início, tipo e frequência das crises) — fator mais importante no diagnóstico de epilepsia idiopática.
• Primeira crise convulsiva — entre 6 meses e 5 anos de idade; quanto mais jovem for o animal, mais grave será a epilepsia; se início ocorrer antes dos 2 anos de idade, o problema frequentemente se torna intratável (i. e., refratário à medicação).
• Início agudo de uma série de crises convulsivas ou estado epiléptico — excluir intoxicação ou doença cerebral estrutural. • Mais de 2 crises convulsivas na primeira semana no início — considerar outro diagnóstico que não a epilepsia idiopática. • Crises convulsivas antes dos 6 meses de vida ou depois dos 5 anos de idade — origem metabólica ou intracraniana e estrutural; descartar hipoglicemia em cães mais idosos. • Crises convulsivas focais ou presença de déficits neurológicos — excluir doença intracraniana estrutural.

HEMOGRAMA/BIOQUÍMICA/URINÁLISE
• Geralmente normais. • Realizar antes do início da medicação antiepiléptica para obter os dados basais.

OUTROS TESTES LABORATORIAIS
A mensuração dos ácidos biliares para descartar encefalopatia hepática é desnecessária em cães com crises convulsivas sem comportamento anormal episódico concomitante.

DIAGNÓSTICO POR IMAGEM
RM — exame indicado apenas se o padrão das crises convulsivas não se enquadrar em um quadro de epilepsia idiopática, se houver déficits neurológicos ou na suspeita de doença intracraniana estrutural.

MÉTODOS DIAGNÓSTICOS
• Análise do LCS — na suspeita de doenças intracranianas estruturais. • Eletroencefalografia — podem ser observadas alterações como espículas interictais, poliespículas e complexos espícula-onda lenta.

ACHADOS PATOLÓGICOS
• Ausência de lesão primária. • Perda neuronal secundária e gliose, causadas pelas crises convulsivas prolongadas ou repetidas.

TRATAMENTO

CUIDADO(S) DE SAÚDE ADEQUADO(S)
• Paciente ambulatorial — recidiva de crises convulsivas isoladas. • Paciente internado — em casos de crises convulsivas seguidas (mais de 1 a cada 24 h) ou estado epiléptico.

CUIDADO(S) DE ENFERMAGEM
Pacientes internados com distúrbio convulsivo necessitam de monitorização constante.

ATIVIDADE
Evitar a prática de natação para prevenir afogamento.

DIETA
• As mudanças na dieta alteram a farmacocinética do fenobarbital. • Os cães sob medicação antiepiléptica crônica ficam acima do peso ideal; nesse caso, deve-se adicionar um programa de redução do peso, conforme a necessidade. • Tratamento com brometo de potássio — os pacientes devem ter níveis constantes de sal em suas dietas; um aumento no teor de sal provoca um incremento na excreção de brometo, de preferência em detrimento ao cloreto, com subsequente redução nos níveis séricos do brometo de potássio. Por outro lado, uma diminuição no conteúdo de sal leva ao aumento no nível sérico de brometo de potássio. • Tentativa com dieta rica em gordura e pobre em carboidrato — sem melhora no controle das crises convulsivas.

ORIENTAÇÃO AO PROPRIETÁRIO
• Informar ao proprietário que as crises convulsivas seguidas graves e o estado epiléptico são emergências médicas potencialmente letais, que necessitam de atendimento médico imediato.
• Incentivar o proprietário a manter uma espécie de calendário com anotações sobre a data, o horário, a duração e a gravidade das crises convulsivas para avaliar a resposta ao tratamento. • Informar ao proprietário que, uma vez instituído o tratamento, o paciente necessitará de medicação pelo resto da vida na maioria dos casos. • Orientar o proprietário sobre o fato de que a retirada abrupta da medicação pode causar crises convulsivas.

MEDICAÇÕES

MEDICAMENTO(S) DE ESCOLHA
• Iniciar o tratamento em casos de crises convulsivas generalizadas secundárias, se houver crises agrupadas agudas ou estado epiléptico agudo. • Tratamento antiepiléptico — visa diminuir a frequência, a gravidade e a duração das crises convulsivas; o controle ideal raramente é atingido. • Pode ocorrer o desenvolvimento de tolerância e refratariedade ao tratamento.

Fenobarbital
• Medicamento tradicional de primeira linha; dosagem inicial: 3-5 mg/kg VO a cada 12 h; os níveis estacionários e constantes são atingidos em 12-15 dias, mas diminuem significativamente nos primeiros 6 meses, devido à ativação das enzimas lisossomais. • Níveis séricos terapêuticos ideais:

Epilepsia Idiopática (Genética)

100-120 μmol/L ou 23-28 μg/mL; reavaliar os níveis a cada 2 semanas até que a faixa terapêutica ideal seja atingida. • Dose de ataque por via oral (se necessária) — 5-10 mg/kg a cada 12 h por 2 dias para atingir a faixa terapêutica com rapidez.

Brometo de Potássio
• Medicamento tradicional de primeira linha; dosagem inicial: 30 mg/kg VO a cada 24 h ou fracionados a cada 12 h; o estado estacionário e constante é atingido em 3-4 semanas, mas varia com a concentração de sal na dieta. • Níveis séricos terapêuticos ideais: 20-25 mmol/L ou 1,6-2 mg/mL; se o brometo de potássio for utilizado como o único antiepiléptico, o nível sérico de 25-32 mmol/L ou 2-2,25 mmol/L poderá ser usado com segurança. • Poderá ser combinado com o fenobarbital se as crises convulsivas não forem controladas com o nível sérico ideal desse último medicamento — essa combinação pode produzir um efeito benéfico e sinérgico. • Dose de ataque — não recomendada, pois pode causar vômito, diarreia, sedação duradoura e profunda; se necessária, dobrar as doses diárias (30-60 mg/kg a cada 12 h). • A insuficiência renal diminui a eliminação de brometo; nesse caso, a dosagem inicial deve ser reduzida pela metade.

Diazepam (Uso Domiciliar)
• Para abortar crises convulsivas em andamento — cães com crises convulsivas seguidas ou estado epiléptico. • Inserir 0,5-1 mg/kg do medicamento injetável no reto por uma espécie de dreno (cânula de teto, por exemplo) assim que ocorrer a crise convulsiva; repetir 20 e 40 min mais tarde até um total de 3 inserções em 40 min; procedimento realizado no início das crises convulsivas em andamento, aumenta a possibilidade de abortar crises subsequentes.

CONTRAINDICAÇÕES
Aminofilina, teofilina — podem causar atividade convulsiva.

PRECAUÇÕES
Agonistas α-adrenérgicos (p. ex., fenilpropanolamina) — excitação do sistema nervoso central.

INTERAÇÕES POSSÍVEIS
• Cimetidina e cloranfenicol — interferem no metabolismo do fenobarbital; podem gerar níveis tóxicos desse anticonvulsivante. • Sempre que os medicamentos tiverem de ser administrados aos animais pelo resto da vida, o clínico e/ou o proprietário deverá recorrer à bula do produto ou ao farmacêutico para obter informações sobre as interações medicamentosas.

MEDICAMENTO(S) ALTERNATIVO(S)
• No caso de polifarmácia (i. e., administração concomitante de diversos medicamentos), iniciar a adição de forma gradativa para evitar sedação. • Zonisamida — possível medicamento de primeira linha; 5 mg/kg a cada 12 h VO; 10 mg/kg a cada 12 h VO se adicionada ao fenobarbital; meia-vida de 15 h em cães; faixa terapêutica em seres humanos (10-40 μg/mL); segura e bem-tolerada; não disponível no Canadá. • Levetiracetam — 20 mg/kg a cada 12-8 h VO; pode-se observar uma melhora e, depois, um aumento na frequência das crises convulsivas (efeito "lua de mel"); sem metabolismo hepático; seguro e bem-tolerado; preferido em crises convulsivas de início focal. • Gabapentina — 25-50 mg/kg/24 h VO divididos em 3 ou 4 doses; eficácia moderada sob a forma de adição. O análogo mais recente, a pregabalina, pode ser mais eficaz (2-4 mg/kg a cada 8 h VO). • Clorazepato — 0,5-1 mg/kg VO a cada 8 h. • Felbamato — 30-70 mg/kg a cada 12-8 h; não disponível no Canadá. • Fenitoína, ácido valproico e carbamazepina e etossuximida — farmacocinética inadequada em cães. • Outros tratamentos — acupuntura, estimulação do nervo vago, estimulação motora magnética transcraniana, implantes de fios de ouro.

ACOMPANHAMENTO
MONITORIZAÇÃO DO PACIENTE
• Níveis séricos dos medicamentos — mensurados preferencialmente nos níveis de vale (contrário ao pico) e, ao mesmo tempo, para cada amostragem. • Fenobarbital — mensurar o nível 4 semanas após o início do tratamento; ajustar a dose oral conforme a necessidade; repetir a cada 2 semanas até que os níveis séricos ideais sejam alcançados; com o uso prolongado, obter os exames de hemograma e bioquímica sérica e, ainda, mensurar os níveis do fenobarbital a cada 6-12 meses; medir também os níveis de albumina, enzimas hepáticas e níveis medicamentosos séricos para monitorizar as tendências; por ser um medicamento essencialmente hepatotóxico, a maioria dos cães acaba desenvolvendo hepatotoxicidade se os níveis séricos estiverem acima de 140 μmol/L (>33 μg/mL) por um longo período de tempo (>1 ano). Na suspeita de hepatotoxicidade, mensurar os ácidos biliares. • Brometo de potássio — medir os níveis séricos (juntamente com os do fenobarbital) 4-6 semanas após o início do tratamento (devem girar em torno de 8-12 mmol/L ou 0,5-1 mg/mL) e depois em 3-4 meses; o brometo de potássio pode fazer com que os níveis do fenobarbital declinem. • Monitorizar atentamente os níveis do brometo de potássio na presença de insuficiência renal (isostenúria ou azotemia). • Mensurar os níveis séricos de triglicerídeos a cada 6-12 meses em caso de tratamento crônico com fenobarbital e fenobarbital/brometo de potássio — o aumento é um fator de risco para pancreatite. • Se o cão submetido ao brometo de potássio necessitar de mudança da dieta, considerar o teor de sal da nova dieta; monitorizar o nível de forma adequada.

PREVENÇÃO
• A suspensão abrupta da medicação pode precipitar crises convulsivas. • Evitar o fornecimento de petiscos salgados aos cães tratados com brometo de potássio.

COMPLICAÇÕES POSSÍVEIS
• Episódios recorrentes de crises convulsivas agrupadas e estado epiléptico. • Fenobarbital e brometo de potássio — poliúria, polidipsia, polifagia e ganho de peso. • Fosfatase alcalina sérica alta induzida pelo fenobarbital (isoenzima esteroide) — ocorre frequentemente; pode ser um sinal precoce de hepatotoxicidade, mas será menos preocupante se a ALT estiver dentro dos valores de referência. • Hepatotoxicidade induzida pelo fenobarbital — ocorre após tratamento crônico com níveis séricos elevados (>140 μmol/L ou >33 μg/mL); muitas vezes, pode ter início insidioso; a única anormalidade bioquímica pode ser uma queda na albumina. • Incidência mais alta de pancreatite em pacientes tratados com fenobarbital e/ou brometo de potássio; assim que a pancreatite se desenvolve, a recidiva é frequente. • Fenobarbital — pode ocorrer o desenvolvimento de rara supressão da medula óssea com neutropenia grave e sepse no início do tratamento; suspender a administração. • O tratamento com fenobarbital pode resultar em hiperexcitabilidade paradoxal; interromper a medicação. • Brometo de potássio — quando os níveis se encontram >22 mmol/L ou >1,8 mg/mL, os proprietários podem se queixar de que o animal tem instabilidade ao subir ou descer escadas. • Zonisamida, levetiracetam, gabapentina sob a forma de adição — sedação passageira.

EVOLUÇÃO ESPERADA E PROGNÓSTICO
• Tratamento pelo resto da vida. • Alguns cães são satisfatoriamente controlados com o mesmo medicamento e a mesma dosagem durante anos; outros permanecem sob controle insatisfatório apesar da polifarmácia. • O paciente pode desenvolver estado epiléptico e vir a óbito. • Os episódios de estado epiléptico são mais frequentes em cães de grande porte; entretanto, o tratamento precoce não diminui a ocorrência desse estado. • A expectativa de vida é geralmente normal; no entanto, o tempo de sobrevida será mais curto em casos de estado epiléptico. • Aumento no risco de morte prematura. • O prognóstico dependerá da habilidade do veterinário, do sucesso terapêutico e da motivação do proprietário.

DIVERSOS
DISTÚRBIOS ASSOCIADOS
• A epilepsia idiopática pode ser a causa de síndrome do eutireóideo doente em cães. • A fenobarbital pode reduzir os níveis de T_4 e causar uma tendência crescente (i. e., para cima) no TSH sem hipotireoidismo.

FATORES RELACIONADOS COM A IDADE
• Se o início for antes dos 2 anos de idade, provavelmente será mais difícil o controle da epilepsia. • Se o início for depois dos 3 anos de idade, haverá maior probabilidade de controle adequado da epilepsia.

GESTAÇÃO/FERTILIDADE/REPRODUÇÃO
• Evitar que os animais acometidos se acasalem. • A relação entre os hormônios sexuais e a ocorrência de crises convulsivas em cães epilépticos não foi pesquisada.

SINÔNIMO(S)
Epilepsia.

VER TAMBÉM
• Crises Convulsivas (Convulsões, Estado Epiléptico) — Cães. • Crises Convulsivas (Convulsões, Estado Epiléptico) — Gatos.

ABREVIATURA(S)
• ALT = alanina aminotransferase. • LCS = líquido cerebrospinal. • RM = ressonância magnética. • TSH = hormônio tireostimulante.

RECURSOS DA INTERNET
http://www.ivis.org/advances/Vite/berendt/chapter_frm.asp?LA=1.

Sugestões de Leitura
Thomas WB. Idiopathic epilepsy in dogs and cats. Vet Clin North Am Small Anim Pract 2010, 40:161-179.

Autor Joane M. Parent
Consultor Editorial Joane M. Parent

EPISCLERITE

CONSIDERAÇÕES GERAIS
REVISÃO
- Infiltração focal ou difusa da episclera* e/ou do estroma escleral por uma mistura variável de células inflamatórias e fibroblastos.
- Primária — acomete apenas o olho; provavelmente imunomediada; surge como um nódulo episcleral/escleral perilímbico (episclerite nodular) ou como um espessamento difuso da episclera (episclerite difusa); a forma nodular pode acometer a córnea e a terceira pálpebra com nódulos de aspecto similar.
- Secundária — em geral difusa; decorre do derramamento de células inflamatórias na episclera por causa de outros distúrbios oculares (p. ex., endoftalmite e panoftalmite); pode acometer particularmente qualquer outro sistema orgânico.

IDENTIFICAÇÃO
- Cães.
- Collie e Pastor de Shetland jovens aos de meia-idade.

SINAIS CLÍNICOS
- Nodulares — aparecem tipicamente sob a forma de massa episcleral/escleral lisa, indolor, localizada, elevada, róseo-acastanhada e de consistência firme.
- Difusos — menos comuns; surgem como eritema e espessamento difusos de toda a episclera/esclera; acompanhados por dor ocular (oftalmalgia) de intensidade variável.
- Secundários — uveíte frequentemente pronunciada.
- Conjuntiva — em geral, move-se livremente sobre a superfície da lesão.
- Nódulos — tendem a ser lentamente progressivos, bilaterais e propensos à recidiva.

CAUSAS E FATORES DE RISCO
- Nodular e primária difusa — idiopática; acredita-se que seja imunomediada.
- Secundária — pode resultar de infecção ocular fúngica ou bacteriana profunda, linfoma, histiocitose sistêmica na raça Montanhês de Berna, glaucoma crônico e traumatismo ocular.

DIAGNÓSTICO
DIAGNÓSTICO DIFERENCIAL
- Outras causas de congestão ocular ("olho vermelho") — diferenciadas por exame oftalmológico minucioso e pela tonometria.
- Outras lesões semelhantes a massas — diferenciadas por biopsia ou exame citológico.
- Neoplasia — linfoma; carcinoma de células escamosas; disseminação de massa intraocular; outros tumores.
- Granuloma — infecção fúngica profunda; corpo estranho retido.
- Tecido de granulação — traumatismo; úlcera de córnea cicatrizada ou em processo de cicatrização; perfuração do bulbo ocular com prolapso da úvea.

HEMOGRAMA/BIOQUÍMICA/URINÁLISE
- Em geral, permanecerão normais se a lesão estiver confinada ao olho ou aos anexos.

---
* N. T.: Estrutura mais externa da esclera.

- Secundária — é possível a observação de anormalidades compatíveis com outras doenças sistêmicas (p. ex., infecção fúngica profunda ou histiocitose sistêmica).

OUTROS TESTES LABORATORIAIS
- Fator reumatoide, anticorpo antinuclear e preparações para pesquisa de células do lúpus eritematoso — geralmente não são úteis.
- Sorologia — pode ajudar a descartar infecções fúngicas profundas.

DIAGNÓSTICO POR IMAGEM
- Radiografias toracoabdominais ou ultrassonografia abdominal — podem ajudar a excluir infecção fúngica profunda ou neoplasia disseminada.
- Ultrassonografia ocular — poderá ajudar a revelar outras anormalidades oculares se opacidades dos meios oculares impedirem o exame ocular completo.

MÉTODOS DIAGNÓSTICOS
- Biopsia incisional e exame histopatológico do tecido acometido.
- Nodular — caracterizada por números variáveis de histiócitos, linfócitos, plasmócitos e fibroblastos.
- Se houver uveíte proeminente — fazer uma pesquisa de uveíte (ver "Uveíte Anterior — Cães").

TRATAMENTO
- Tentar a confirmação histológica ou citológica do diagnóstico antes do tratamento.
- Nodular primária — tende a ter evolução benigna; em casos de doença leve, a mera observação pode ser suficiente.
- Paciente ambulatorial — se houver dor ocular, acometimento escleral difuso, alteração da função palpebral, envolvimento da córnea ou ameaça à visão.

MEDICAÇÕES
MEDICAMENTO(S)
- Prosseguir na lista citada abaixo apenas se a modalidade prévia for ineficaz.
- Acetato de prednisolona tópico a 1% — a cada 4 h por 1 semana; em seguida, a cada 6 h por 2 semanas; depois, diminuir gradativamente.
- Prednisolona sistêmica — 1-2 mg/kg/dia; reduzir de forma gradual com a melhora.
- Azatioprina sistêmica — 1-2 mg/kg/dia por 3-7 dias; em seguida, proceder à redução gradual da dose para a mais baixa possível.
- Criocirurgia ou tentativa de excisão.
- Alternativa aos medicamentos listados ou à cirurgia — pode-se tentar uma combinação de tetraciclina e niacinamida (a cada 8 h VO); 250 mg de cada para cães com menos de 10 kg; 500 mg de cada para cães com mais de 10 kg; pode-se não observar uma boa resposta clínica por pelo menos 8 semanas; efeitos colaterais incomuns e resultantes principalmente do efeito de desarranjo gastrintestinal causado pela niacinamida.

CONTRAINDICAÇÕES/INTERAÇÕES POSSÍVEIS
- Evitar medicamentos imunossupressores sistêmicos com infecções fúngicas profundas.

- Prednisolona ou azatioprina sistêmicas — podem precipitar pancreatite potencialmente hepatotóxicas.
- Azatioprina — pode induzir à mielossupressão potencialmente fatal.
- Niacina — não substitui a niacinamida.

ACOMPANHAMENTO
MONITORIZAÇÃO DO PACIENTE
- Primária — monitorizar a regressão de nódulo(s) ou a redução do espessamento episcleral ou da congestão a cada 2-3 semanas por 6-9 semanas e depois conforme a necessidade; prognóstico geralmente bom; pode necessitar de terapia por meses ou pelo resto da vida.
- Secundária — o acompanhamento, o prognóstico e as complicações geralmente dependem da doença primária.
- Azatioprina — repetir o hemograma completo, a contagem de plaquetas e a mensuração das enzimas hepáticas a cada 1-2 semanas nas primeiras 8 semanas e, em seguida, periodicamente.

COMPLICAÇÕES POSSÍVEIS
- Perda da visão.
- Dor ocular crônica.
- Uveíte.
- Glaucoma secundário.

DIVERSOS
SINÔNIMO(S)
- Granuloma do Collie.
- Histiocitoma fibroso.
- Granuloma do limbo.
- Esclerouveíte necrogranulomatosa.
- Fasciite nodular.
- Episclerite nodular granulomatosa.
- Ceratoconjuntivite proliferativa.

Sugestões de Leitura
Maggs DJ. Cornea and sclera. In: Maggs DJ, Miller PE, Ofri R, Slatter's Fundamentals of Veterinary Ophthalmology, 4th ed. St. Louis: Saunders, 2008, pp. 175-202.
Rothstein E, Scott DW, Riis RC. Tetracycline and niacinamide for the treatment of sterile pyogranuloma/granuloma syndrome in a dog. JAAHA 1997, 33:540-543.

Autor Paul E. Miller
Consultor Editorial Paul E. Miller

EPISTAXE

CONSIDERAÇÕES GERAIS

DEFINIÇÃO
Sangramento pelo nariz.

FISIOPATOLOGIA
Resulta de uma dentre três anormalidades — coagulopatia; doença local ou expansiva; e doença vascular ou sistêmica.

SISTEMA(S) ACOMETIDO(S)
- Respiratório — hemorragia; espirros.
- Hematológico/linfático/imune — anemia.
- Gastrintestinal — melena.

GENÉTICA
Varia, dependendo da causa subjacente.

INCIDÊNCIA/PREVALÊNCIA
Variam, dependendo da causa subjacente.

IDENTIFICAÇÃO
Espécies
Cães e gatos.

Raça(s) Predominante(s)
Variam, dependendo da causa subjacente.

Idade Média e Faixa Etária
Variam, dependendo da causa subjacente.

Sexo Predominante
Varia, dependendo da causa subjacente.

SINAIS CLÍNICOS
Achados Anamnésicos
- Hemorragia nasal.
- Espirros e/ou respiração estertorosa.
- Melena.
- Com coagulopatia — hematoquezia, melena, hematúria ou hemorragia advinda de outras áreas do corpo.

Achados do Exame Físico
- Hemorragia nasal.
- Melena — pode ser de sangue deglutido.
- Estridor nasal — pode estar presente em caso de neoplasia, corpo estranho ou doença inflamatória avançada.
- Com coagulopatia — possivelmente petéquias, equimoses, hematomas, sangramentos intracavitários, hematoquezia, melena e hematúria.
- Com coagulopatia ou hipertensão — possivelmente hemorragias retinianas.

CAUSAS
Coagulopatia

Trombocitopenia
- Doença imunomediada — doença idiopática; LES; reação medicamentosa; reação à vacina de vírus vivo modificado.
- Doença infecciosa — erliquiose; neorriquetsiose; febre maculosa das Montanhas Rochosas; babesiose; doença relacionada com FeLV ou FIV.
- Doença da medula óssea — neoplasia; anemia aplásica; infecciosa (fúngica, riquetsiana ou viral).
- Distúrbio paraneoplásico.
- CID.

Trombopatia
- Congênita — doença de von Willebrand; trombastenia; trombopatia.
- Adquirida — AINE; clopidogrel; hiperglobulinemia (*Ehrlichia*, mieloma múltiplo); uremia; CID.

Defeitos dos fatores de coagulação
- Congênitos: hemofilia A (deficiência do fator VIIIc) e hemofilia B (deficiência do fator IX).
- Adquiridos: intoxicação pelo rodenticida anticoagulante (varfarina), doença hepatobiliar e CID.

Lesão Local
- Corpo estranho.
- Traumatismo.
- Infecção — fúngica (*Aspergillus, Cryptococcus* e *Rhinosporidium*); viral ou bacteriana. Em geral, produz um exsudato mucopurulento manchado de sangue em vez de hemorragia franca.
- Neoplasia — adenocarcinoma; carcinoma; condrossarcoma; carcinoma de células escamosas; fibrossarcoma; linfoma; tumor venéreo transmissível.
- Odontopatia — fístula oronasal; abscesso da raiz dentária.
- Rinite linfoplasmocítica.

Doença Vascular ou Sistêmica
- Hipertensão — nefropatia; hipertireoidismo; hiperadrenocorticismo; doença idiopática.
- Hiperviscosidade — hiperglobulinemia (mieloma múltiplo, *Ehrlichia*); policitemia.
- Vasculite — doenças imunomediadas e riquetsioses.

FATORES DE RISCO
Coagulopatia
- Doença imunomediada — cadelas jovens a de meia-idade, de porte pequeno a médio.
- Doença infecciosa — cães que vivem ou viajam para áreas endêmicas; exposição a carrapatos.
- Trombastenia — cães caçadores de lontra.
- Trombopatia — Basset hound, Spitz.
- Doença de von Willebrand — raças Doberman pinscher, Airedale, Pastor alemão, Scottish terrier, Chesapeake Bay retriever e muitas outras; gatos.
- Hemofilia A — Pastor alemão e muitas outras raças; gatos.
- Hemofilia B — Cairn terrier, Coonhound, São Bernardo e outras raças; gatos.

Lesões Expansivas
- Aspergilose — Pastor alemão, Rottweiler.
- Neoplasia — raças dolicocefálicas.

DIAGNÓSTICO

DIAGNÓSTICO DIFERENCIAL
Ver a seção "Causas".

HEMOGRAMA/BIOQUÍMICA/URINÁLISE
- Anemia — se tiver ocorrido hemorragia suficiente.
- Trombocitopenia — possível.
- Neutrofilia — infecção; neoplasia.
- Pancitopenia — em caso de doença da medula óssea.
- Hipoproteinemia — se tiver ocorrido hemorragia suficiente.
- BUN alto com creatinina normal — possível, em virtude da ingestão de sangue.
- Hiperglobulinemia — possível em casos de erliquiose, mieloma múltiplo.
- Azotemia — hipertensão induzida por insuficiência renal.
- ALT, AST e bilirrubina total elevadas — com coagulopatia por hepatopatia grave.
- Urinálise — geralmente normal; é possível a observação de hematúria (se houver coagulopatia), isostenúria (em caso de hipertensão induzida por insuficiência renal) e proteinúria (na presença de LES ou doença glomerulotubular e hipertensão).

OUTROS TESTES LABORATORIAIS
- Perfil de coagulação — tempos prolongados com defeitos dos fatores de coagulação; normal com trombocitopenia e trombopatia.
- Teste do anticorpo antinuclear — positivo em alguns casos de LES.
- Provas de função plaquetária (p. ex., tempo de sangramento da mucosa bucal, análise do fator de von Willebrand) — podem ser anormais em caso de disfunção plaquetária (a contagem das plaquetas e o perfil de coagulação podem permanecer normais).
- Títulos de *Ehrlichia*, *Neorickettsia*, febre maculosa das Montanhas Rochosas ou *Babesia* — podem ser positivos em epistaxe induzida por trombocitopenia ou trombopatia.
- Sorologia fúngica — pode ajudar a estabelecer um diagnóstico de rinite fúngica; é possível a obtenção de resultados falso-positivos e falso-negativos e, por essa razão, é imprescindível interpretá-los diante de outros achados clínicos e diagnósticos.
- Análise dos hormônios tireoidianos — elevados em gatos com epistaxe em virtude de hipertensão induzida pelo estado hipertireóideo.

DIAGNÓSTICO POR IMAGEM
- Radiografia torácica — triagem para pesquisa de metástase.
- Série radiográfica nasal — realizada sob anestesia, incluindo projeções ventrodorsal com a boca aberta e tangencial (*skyline*) dos seios nasais quando se suspeita de lesão expansiva ou local; observa-se osteólise em caso de neoplasia e sinusite fúngica; corpos estranhos não costumam ser observados; pode-se identificar a presença de odontopatia.
- TC ou RM — técnica mais sensível que as radiografias.

MÉTODOS DIAGNÓSTICOS
- Avaliação da pressão sanguínea — quando tiverem sido excluídas coagulopatias e lesões expansivas e for observada azotemia.
- Rinoscopia, lavagem nasal, biopsia nasal (cega ou guiada por rinoscopia ou TC) — indicada para doença expansiva; serve não só para remover corpos estranhos, mas também para avaliar e obter amostras de tecido nasal para o diagnóstico etiológico (p. ex., examinar amostras de tecido nasal quanto à presença de neoplasia e infecção por meio de citologia e/ou histopatologia e cultura bacteriana/fúngica e antibiograma).
- Biopsia por aspiração da medula óssea — indicada caso se identifique pancitopenia.

TRATAMENTO

CUIDADO(S) DE SAÚDE ADEQUADO(S)
- Coagulopatia — o paciente costuma ser internado.
- Lesão expansiva ou doença vascular ou sistêmica — paciente ambulatorial ou internado, dependendo da doença e de sua gravidade.
- Radioterapia — tumores nasais; várias taxas de resposta.

EPISTAXE

CUIDADO(S) DE ENFERMAGEM
• Fornecer cuidados de suporte básicos se houver necessidade (fluidos, nutrição).

ATIVIDADE
• Minimizar a atividade ou os estímulos que precipitem episódios hemorrágicos.

ORIENTAÇÃO AO PROPRIETÁRIO
• Informar o proprietário a respeito da doença.
• Ensinar o proprietário a reconhecer uma hemorragia grave (p. ex., fraqueza, colapso, palidez e perda sanguínea >30 mL/kg de peso corporal).

CONSIDERAÇÕES CIRÚRGICAS
• A cirurgia ficará indicada se a remoção do corpo estranho por rinoscopia ou às cegas for impossível.
• Rinite fúngica (p. ex., *Aspergillus* e *Rhinosporidium*) pode necessitar de debridamento (ver também a seção sobre "Medicações" adiante).

MEDICAÇÕES
MEDICAMENTO(S) DE ESCOLHA
Considerações Gerais
• Transfusão de sangue total, papa de hemácias ou solução de hemoglobina — pode ser necessária na presença de anemia grave.
• Acepromazina (0,05-0,1 mg/kg SC, IV em caso de animal normotérmico e na ausência de distúrbio plaquetário) para reduzir a pressão arterial e promover a coagulação; pode ajudar a controlar hemorragia séria.
• Interromper todos os AINEs.

Coagulopatia
• Doença imunomediada — prednisona (1,1 mg/kg a cada 12 h; reduzir gradativamente em 4-6 meses); outros medicamentos podem ser utilizados, além da prednisona, para casos refratários: azatioprina (cães, 2,2 mg/kg VO a cada 24 h por 14 dias, depois a cada 48 h; gatos, 0,3 mg/kg VO a cada 48 h), ciclosporina (5-10 mg/kg VO a cada 12 h); imunoglobulina humana (0,5-1 g/kg IV de uma solução a 6% por 6-12 h) é útil para o controle imediato.
• Doença infecciosa — riquetsiose (doxiciclina, 5 mg/kg VO a cada 12 h por 3-6 semanas); *Babesia* (imidocarbe, 6,6 mg/kg SC, 2 doses em intervalo de 2 semanas, aceturato de diminazeno 5 mg/kg IM uma vez, ou 10 dias de atovaquona 13,3 mg/kg VO a cada 8 h com azitromicina 10 mg/kg VO a cada 24 h).
• Neoplasia da medula óssea — ver Distúrbios Mieloproliferativos.
• Trombopatia e trombastenia — não há nenhum tratamento a menos que haja doença linfoproliferativa.
• Doença de von Willebrand — plasma ou crioprecipitado para sangramento agudo; DDVAP 1 μg/kg SC ou IV diluído em 20 mL de NaCl a 0,9% e administrado durante 10 minutos pode ajudar a controlar ou evitar a ocorrência de hemorragia antes de procedimentos invasivos (a formulação intranasal [mais barata] pode ser usada após a passagem de filtro bacteriostático).
• Hemofilia A — plasma ou crioprecipitado para sangramento agudo; não há tratamento a longo prazo.
• Hemofilia B — plasma para sangramento agudo; não há tratamento a longo prazo.

• Intoxicação por rodenticida anticoagulante — plasma para sangramento agudo; vitamina K em uma dose de ataque de 5 mg/kg, seguida por 1,25 mg/kg a cada 12 h por 1 semana (em caso de formulação com varfarina) a 4 semanas (em caso de formulação de ação mais prolongada).
• Hiperglobulinemia — plasmaférese.
• Policitemia — flebotomia.
• Hepatopatia e CID — tratar e dar suporte à causa subjacente; o plasma pode ser benéfico.

Lesão Expansiva
• Infecção bacteriana secundária — antibióticos escolhidos com base na cultura e no antibiograma.
• Infecção fúngica — tratamento tópico da cavidade nasal e dos seios frontais com clotrimazol a 1% em polietilenoglicol (ver a seção "Precauções") ou enilconazol a 1-5% (ver protocolo para Aspergilose Nasal); dapsona (1 mg/kg VO a cada 8 h por 2 semanas e, em seguida, 1 mg/kg VO a cada 12 h por 4 meses) após a cirurgia para rinosporidiose.

Doença Vascular ou Sistêmica
• Hiperviscosidade — tratar a doença subjacente (p. ex., erliquiose e mieloma múltiplo); plasmaférese.
• Vasculite — doxiciclina para riquetsiose (5 mg/kg a cada 12 h por 3-6 semanas); prednisona para doença imunomediada (1,1 mg/kg a cada 12 h; diminuir gradativamente por 4-6 meses).

Hipertensão
• Tratar a doença subjacente — nefropatia, hipertireoidismo, hiperadrenocorticismo.
• Reduzir o peso.
• Restringir o sódio.
• Bloqueadores dos canais de cálcio — anlodipino (cães: 0,1 mg/kg VO a cada 12-24 h; gatos: 0,625-1,25 mg/gato VO a cada 12-24 h) — tratamento de escolha; diltiazem (cães: 0,5-1,5 mg/kg a cada 8 h; gatos: 1,75-2,5 mg/kg a cada 8 h).
• Inibidores da ECA — benazepril (0,5 mg/kg a cada 24 h); enalapril (0,25-0,5 mg/kg a cada 12-24 h).
• β-Bloqueadores — propranolol (0,5-1 mg/kg a cada 8 h); atenolol (2 mg/kg a cada 24 h).
• Diuréticos — hidroclorotiazida (2-4 mg/kg a cada 12 h); furosemida (0,5-2 mg/kg a cada 8-12 h).

CONTRAINDICAÇÕES
• Evitar medicamentos que possam predispor o paciente à hemorragia — AINEs; heparina; clopidogrel; tranquilizantes fenotiazínicos.
• Antifúngicos tópicos — não usar em pacientes com ruptura da placa cribriforme.

PRECAUÇÕES
• Quimioterápicos (p. ex., azatioprina) — monitorizar as contagens de neutrófilos semanalmente até que se tenha estabelecido um padrão demonstrando que o paciente tolera o medicamento.
• Enalapril e/ou diuréticos — monitorizar atentamente o paciente com insuficiência renal; evitar restrição intensa de sal ao usar os inibidores da ECA.
• Evitar preparações tópicas de clotrimazol com propilenoglicol, pois podem ocorrer irritação e ulceração potencialmente letais da mucosa, além de tumefação nasofaríngea.

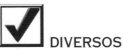
ACOMPANHAMENTO
MONITORIZAÇÃO DO PACIENTE
• Contagem de plaquetas em caso de trombocitopenia.
• Perfil de coagulação em defeitos dos fatores de coagulação.
• Pressão arterial na presença de hipertensão.
• Monitorizar os sinais clínicos.

PREVENÇÃO
• Restringir o acesso a áreas que possam ter rodenticidas anticoagulantes.
• Fornecer cuidados odontológicos preventivos.

COMPLICAÇÕES POSSÍVEIS
Anemia e colapso (raros).

EVOLUÇÃO ESPERADA E PROGNÓSTICO
Variam, dependendo da causa subjacente.

DIVERSOS
GESTAÇÃO/FERTILIDADE/REPRODUÇÃO
Evitar medicamentos teratogênicos (p. ex., itraconazol).

VER TAMBÉM
Ver a seção "Causas".

ABREVIATURA(S)
• AINE = anti-inflamatório não esteroide.
• ALT = alanina aminotransferase.
• AST = aspartato aminotransferase.
• CID = coagulação intravascular disseminada.
• DDAVP = 1-desamino-8-D-arginina vasopressina.
• ECA = enzima conversora da angiotensina.
• FeLV = vírus da leucemia felina.
• FIV = vírus da imunodeficiência felina.
• LES = lúpus eritematoso sistêmico.
• RM = ressonância magnética.
• TC = tomografia computadorizada.

Sugestões de Leitura
Brooks M. Coagulopathies and thrombosis. In: Ettinger SJ, Feldman EC, eds., Textbook of Veterinary Internal Medicine, 5th ed. Philadelphia: Saunders, 2000, pp. 1829-1841.
Brooks MB, Catalfamo JL. Platelet disorders and von Willebrand disease. In: Ettinger SJ, Feldman EC, eds., Textbook of Veterinary Internal Medicine, 6th ed. St. Louis: Elsevier, 2005, pp. 1918-1937.
Stepien RL, Henik RA. Systemic hypertension. In: Bonagura JD, Twedt DC, eds., Kirk's Current Veterinary Therapy XIV. St. Louis: Saunders Elsevier, 2009, pp. 713-717.
Venker-van Haagen AJ. Diseases of the nose and nasal sinuses. In: Ettinger SJ, Feldman EC, eds., Textbook of Veterinary Internal Medicine, 6th ed. St. Louis: Elsevier, 2005, pp. 1186-1196.

Autor Mitchell A. Crystal
Consultor Editorial Lynelle R. Johnson

Epúlide

CONSIDERAÇÕES GERAIS

REVISÃO
- As categorias das epúlides são fibromatosa, ossificante e acantomatosa.
- Classicamente, são considerados tumores de origem não odontogênica que surgem do estroma do tecido conjuntivo periodontal e não sofrem metástase.
- A maioria dos tumores adere-se ao osso e não é encapsulada, exibindo superfície lisa a levemente nodular.
- As classificações recentes listam as epúlides fibromatosas e ossificantes como fibromas odontogênicos periféricos e as epúlides acantomatosas como ameloblastoma periférico ou ameloblastoma acantomatoso periférico.

IDENTIFICAÇÃO
- Cães — quarta malignidade bucal mais comum.
- Gatos — rara.
- Mais comum em raças braquicefálicas.
- A raça Boxer tem maior incidência de epúlides fibromatosas.
- Idade média de 7 anos.
- Não há predileção sexual.

SINAIS CLÍNICOS
Achados Anamnésicos
- Em geral nenhum — achado incidental, detectado ao exame físico de rotina.
- Salivação excessiva.
- Halitose.
- Disfagia.
- Secreção bucal sanguinolenta.
- Perda de peso.

Achados do Exame Físico
- Massa bucal — nos estágios iniciais, pode surgir como pequenas massas pedunculadas.
- Os ameloblastomas acantomatosos periféricos são mais comumente encontrados na parte rostral da mandíbula.
- Observa-se o deslocamento de estruturas dentárias em virtude da natureza expansiva da massa.
- Possível deformidade facial em função de assimetria do maxilar ou da mandíbula.
- Ocasionalmente, há linfadenopatia cervical.

CAUSAS E FATORES DE RISCO
Nada foi identificado.

DIAGNÓSTICO

DIAGNÓSTICO DIFERENCIAL
- Fibroma.
- Pólipo benigno.
- Ameloblastoma.
- Tumor bucal maligno.
- Hiperplasia gengival.
- Abscesso.
- Diferenciada de outros tipos de massas por biopsia excisional aliada ao aspecto radiográfico.

HEMOGRAMA/BIOQUÍMICA/URINÁLISE
Os resultados costumam permanecer normais.

OUTROS TESTES LABORATORIAIS
Raras vezes, as preparações citológicas são diagnósticas.

DIAGNÓSTICO POR IMAGEM
- Determinar as margens do tumor por meio de radiografias intrabucais.
- As radiografias de ameloblastoma acantomatoso periférico demonstram tipicamente alterações ósseas significativas com expansão para os tecidos adjacentes; os fibromas odontogênicos periféricos não possuem margens bem-definidas ao exame radiográfico; as estruturas dentárias costumam ser deslocadas, podendo ocorrer reabsorção unidirecional ao longo da borda da lesão em qualquer epúlide; as epúlides ossificantes podem apresentar margens ósseas por causa de seu componente osteoide.
- A TC pode ser necessária para obter imagens detalhadas da invasividade de um ameloblastoma acantomatoso periférico.

MÉTODOS DIAGNÓSTICOS
É necessária a realização de biopsia tecidual ampla e profunda (abaixo do osso) para diferenciar de outras malignidades bucais — fibroma, fibrossarcoma ou fibrossarcoma de baixo grau.

TRATAMENTO

DIETA
Alimentos pastosos podem ser recomendados para evitar ulceração do tumor ou após a excisão conservadora ou radical.

CONSIDERAÇÕES CIRÚRGICAS
- Fibroma odontogênico periférico — a excisão cirúrgica com pelo menos 1 cm de margem de segurança costuma ser curativa; esses tumores têm origem no estroma do ligamento periodontal, de modo que a extração dos dentes acometidos e a curetagem da cavidade alveolar estão indicadas; os casos mais avançados podem exigir a excisão dentária e óssea em bloco; a criocirurgia pode estar indicada para pequenas lesões minimamente aderentes ao osso.
- Epúlide ossificante — caracteristicamente possui uma matriz óssea e, por esse motivo, a excisão costuma ser mais difícil; as técnicas são semelhantes àquelas empregadas no fibroma odontogênico periférico.
- Ameloblastoma acantomatoso periférico — em virtude da agressividade desse tumor, são recomendadas margens de segurança de pelo menos 2 cm; os procedimentos de mandibulectomia ou maxilectomia parciais são frequentemente indicados, por causa da localização do tumor.
- A radioterapia proporciona um controle a longo prazo em cães com ameloblastoma acantomatoso periférico considerado inoperável; a maioria dos esquemas de radioterapia tenta a aplicação de 40-60 Gy por 3-6 semanas.

MEDICAÇÕES

MEDICAMENTO(S)
- Não há relatos de eficácia da quimioterapia ambulatorial; a maioria dos tumores de origem mesenquimatosa não responde satisfatoriamente.
- Há relatos de controle local (paliativo) com administração intralesional de cisplatina.
- A injeção local de bleomicina foi bem-sucedida no tratamento de epúlide acantomatosa.

CONTRAINDICAÇÕES/INTERAÇÕES POSSÍVEIS
A quimioterapia pode ser tóxica; o clínico deve buscar por orientação antes de iniciar o tratamento se ele não estiver familiarizado com agentes citotóxicos.

ACOMPANHAMENTO

MONITORIZAÇÃO DO PACIENTE
- Exames completos da boca, da cabeça e do pescoço em 1, 2, 3, 6, 9, 12, 15, 18 e 24 meses após o tratamento.
- Radiografias intrabucais periódicas, sobretudo em casos de ameloblastoma acantomatoso periférico.

EVOLUÇÃO ESPERADA E PROGNÓSTICO
- As epúlides não sofrem metástase.
- A maioria das epúlides é curada quando as margens excisionais estão isentas de células neoplásicas; a recidiva será provável se as margens cirúrgicas não incluírem estruturas periodontais (i. e., a excisão inclui osso normal).
- O tempo médio de sobrevida após a cirurgia de ameloblastoma acantomatoso periférico é de 43 meses (faixa etária de 6-134 meses); os tempos médios de sobrevida em pacientes com ameloblastoma acantomatoso periférico, epúlide ossificante e fibroma odontogênico periférico são de 52, 29 e 47 meses, respectivamente. Os tempos de sobrevida acima são de fontes diferentes.
- A sobrevida média após a aplicação de radioterapia em cães com ameloblastoma acantomatoso periférico varia de 1-102 meses (média de 37 meses); a taxa de sobrevida em um período de 1 ano é de 85% e, em 2 anos, de 67%.
- Há relatos de transformação maligna de epúlide acantomatosa (ameloblastoma acantomatoso periférico) em até 20% dos pacientes submetidos à irradiação anos após o tratamento, sugerindo que esse quadro possa ser uma lesão pré-cancerosa.
- Os ameloblastomas acantomatosos periféricos são altamente invasivos em ossos.

DIVERSOS

SINÔNIMOS
- Epúlide. • Ameloblastoma Periférico.
- Ameloblastoma Acantomatoso Periférico.
- Fibroma Odontogênico Periférico.

VER TAMBÉM
Massas Bucais.

ABREVIATURA(S)
- TC = tomografia computadorizada.

RECURSOS DA INTERNET
http://www.avdc.org/Nomenclature.html.

Sugestões de Leitura
Bjorling DE, Chambers JN, Mahaffey EA. Surgical treatment of epulides in dogs: 25 cases (1974-1984). JAVMA 1987, 190:1315-1318.
Thrall DE. Orthovoltage radiotherapy of acanthomatous epulides in 39 dogs. JAVMA 1984, 184:826-829.

Autores Thomas Klein e Heidi B. Lobprise
Consultor Editorial Heidi B. Lobprise

ERLIQUIOSE

CONSIDERAÇÕES GERAIS

DEFINIÇÃO
Causadas por *Ehrlichia* spp. — causam riquetsiose transmitida por carrapato.

Cães
• Dentro da família Anaplasmataceae — existem três gêneros patogênicos: *Ehrlichia*, *Anaplasma*, e *Neorickettsia*. • *Ehrlichia* spp. — divididas em três grupos: (1) *E. canis*: erliquiose encontrada no meio intracitoplasmático de leucócitos circulantes; (2) *E. ewingii*: erliquiose granulocítica canina; semelhantemente a *A. phagocytophilum*, infecta as células granulocíticas em cães, mas difere em termos de distribuição geográfica (encontrado principalmente nas regiões sudeste e centro-sul dos Estados Unidos); (3) *E. chaffeensis*: semelhante à *E. canis*, com tropismo por células mononucleares; trata-se principalmente de um patógeno humano, mas provoca doença em cães; a distribuição da doença baseia-se na faixa de ocorrência do vetor (principalmente *Amblyomma americanum*).
• *Anaplasma* spp. — existem dois microrganismos importantes: (1) *A. phagocytophilum*: infecta principalmente cavalos, mas também as células granulocíticas de cães; encontrado, sobretudo, nos estados do nordeste e meio-oeste superior dos EUA e na Califórnia, com base na distribuição dos vetores (carrapatos *Ixodes* spp.); (2) *A. platys*: tropismo por plaquetas; compartilha reatividade cruzada sorológica com o *A. phagocytophilum*.
• Apesar da constatação habitual em regiões definidas, os indícios sorológicos sugerem que a *E. canis* e o *A. phagocytophilum* ocorram em todos os 48 estados contíguos. • *Neorickettsia* spp. — existem dois microrganismos relevantes: (1) *N. risticii*: causa febre do cavalo de Potomac, mas também infecta cães e gatos; infecções adquiridas pela ingestão de caracóis infectados, estágios de vida livre de nematódeos ou insetos aquáticos com metacercárias encistadas; o pastoreio ou o consumo de água estagnada explica o motivo pelo qual os equinos são infectados com maior frequência que os cães; os cães infectados apresentam títulos negativos para *E. canis*; (2) *N. helminthoeca*: provoca intoxicação pelo salmão em cães.

Gatos
• Erliquiose mononuclear felina. • Extremamente rara. • *E. risticii* e *A. phagocytophilum*. • Evidência sorológica — sugere uma espécie que tenha reatividade cruzada com a *E. canis* possa causar a doença.

FISIOPATOLOGIA
• *E. canis*. • *Rhipicephalus sanguineus* — carrapato marrom do cão; transmite a doença aos cães pela saliva; período de incubação de 1-3 semanas; 3 estágios da doença:
  ◦ Forma aguda — dissemina-se do local da picada até o baço, o fígado e os linfonodos (causa organomegalia); depois, torna-se subclínica com trombocitopenia leve; acomete principalmente o endotélio; vasculite; anticorpos antiplaquetários podem exacerbar a trombocitopenia; leucopenia variável; anemia leve; a gravidade depende do microrganismo.
  ◦ Forma subclínica — o microrganismo persiste; a resposta humoral aumenta (hiperglobulinemia); também ocorre a persistência da trombocitopenia.
  ◦ Forma crônica — diminuição na produção da medula óssea (plaquetas, supressão eritroide); hipercelularidade da medula com plasmócitos.

SISTEMA(S) ACOMETIDO(S)
• Tendências hemorrágicas — trombocitopenia e vasculite. • SNC, olhos (uveíte anterior) e pulmões — raramente acometidos por vasculite.
• Linfadenopatia. • Multissistêmico.
• Esplenomegalia.

INCIDÊNCIA/PREVALÊNCIA
• Ocorre em todo o ano; insidiosa. • Duração média desde o início até a manifestação — geralmente >2 meses. • A prevalência varia, dependendo da localização geográfica.

DISTRIBUIÇÃO GEOGRÁFICA
• Mundial. • América do Norte — principalmente na Costa do Golfo do México e no litoral oriental; também no Meio-Oeste e na Califórnia.

IDENTIFICAÇÃO
Espécies
• Cães — podem ser infectados por diversas espécies; *E. canis*, *A. platys*, *A. phagocytophilum*, *E. ewingii* e *E. chaffeensis* produzem as principais entidades patológicas. • Gatos — *E. risticii*; a sorologia sugere uma espécie semelhante à *E. canis*.

Raça(s) Predominante(s)
Crônica (*E. canis*) — parece mais grave em Doberman pinscher e Pastor alemão.

Idade Média e Faixa Etária
• Idade média — 5,22 anos. • Faixa etária — 2 meses até 14 anos.

SINAIS CLÍNICOS
Comentários Gerais
Duração dos sinais clínicos desde a doença aguda inicial até a manifestação — geralmente >2 meses.

Achados Anamnésicos
• Letargia, depressão, anorexia e perda de peso.
• Febre. • Sangramento espontâneo — espirro, epistaxe. • Angústia respiratória. • Ataxia, inclinação da cabeça. • Dor ocular (uveíte).

Achados do Exame Físico
Aguda
• Diátese hemorrágica (formação de petéquias nas mucosas, em consequência da trombocitopenia) associada à febre (com depressão, anorexia, perda de peso) e linfadenopatia generalizada devem levantar a suspeita de erliquiose. • Carrapatos — encontrados em 40% dos casos. • Respiratória — dispneia (até mesmo cianose); aumento nos ruídos broncovesiculares. • Doença difusa no SNC (meningite). • Ataxia com disfunção do neurônio motor superior. • Disfunção vestibular.
• Hiperestesia generalizada ou local. • A maioria dos cães recupera-se sem tratamento e entra em um estado subclínico.

Crônica
• Em áreas não endêmicas. • Sangramento espontâneo. • Anemia. • Linfadenopatia generalizada. • Edema do escroto e dos membros.
• Esplenomegalia. • Hepatomegalia. • Uveíte, geralmente bilateral (75%), embora possa ser o único sinal apresentado. • Hifema. • Hemorragia e descolamento da retina com cegueira. • Edema de córnea. • Artrite (rara). • Crises convulsivas (raras).

FATORES DE RISCO
Infecção concomitante por *Babesia*, *Haemobartonella*, *A. platys* e *Hepatozoon canis* — agrava a síndrome clínica.

DIAGNÓSTICO

DIAGNÓSTICO DIFERENCIAL
• Febre maculosa das Montanhas Rochosas (*Rickettsia rickettsii*) — geralmente sazonal entre os meses de março e outubro (nos EUA); testes sorológicos para o diagnóstico; responde ao mesmo tratamento da erliquiose.
• Trombocitopenia imunomediada — não costuma estar associada com febre ou linfadenopatia; os testes sorológicos são os mais eficientes para a distinção; é possível tratar ambos os quadros até que se conheçam os resultados.
• Lúpus eritematoso sistêmico — teste do AAN geralmente negativo em casos de erliquiose; testes sorológicos para o diagnóstico.
• Mieloma múltiplo — testes sorológicos para diferenciar e determinar a causa da hiperglobulinemia.
• Leucemia linfocítica crônica — diferenciar por meio da linfocitose e da citologia medular óssea.
• Brucelose — testes sorológicos para o diagnóstico.

HEMOGRAMA/BIOQUÍMICA/URINÁLISE
Aguda
• Trombocitopenia — antes do início dos sinais clínicos.
• Anemia.
• Leucopenia — por linfopenia e eosinopenia.
• Leucocitose e monocitose — à medida que a doença se torna mais crônica.
• Mórulas — são raros os corpúsculos de inclusão intracitoplasmáticos nos leucócitos. • Alterações inespecíficas — aumentos leves na ALT, fosfatase alcalina, ureia, creatinina e bilirrubina total (rara).
• Hiperglobulinemia — aumenta progressivamente 1-3 semanas após a infecção.
• Hipoalbuminemia — decorre, em geral, da perda renal.
• Proteinúria — com ou sem azotemia; cerca de metade dos pacientes.

Crônica
• Pancitopenia — típica; pode haver monocitose e linfocitose.
• Hiperglobulinemia — a magnitude do aumento da globulina correlaciona-se com a duração da infecção; em geral, há uma gamopatia policlonal, mas também ocorrem gamopatias monoclonais (IgG).
• Hipoalbuminemia.
• Níveis elevados de ureia e creatinina — decorrentes de doença renal primária.

OUTROS TESTES LABORATORIAIS
Teste Sorológico
• Constitui o método diagnóstico mais útil e confiável do ponto de vista clínico.
• O IFA é altamente sensível; especificidade baixa com reatividade cruzada entre *E. canis* e *A. phagocytophila*, mas não entre *E. canis* e *A. platys*.
• Há testes mais específicos em desenvolvimento.
• Títulos — confiáveis 3 semanas após a infecção; títulos >1:10 são diagnósticos.
• Anemia positiva ao teste de Coombs — pode ser observada; pode confundir o diagnóstico.
• Teste em busca de outros patógenos associados — *Babesia*, *Mycoplasma haemofelis*, *A. platys* e *Hepatozoon canis*.
• Teste sorológico de triagem no local de atendimento — Snap 3Dx (inclui *E. canis*) e 4Dx

ERLIQUIOSE

(inclui *E. canis* e *A. phagocytophilum*, que também sofre reação cruzada com *A. platys*) estão disponíveis (IDEXX Labs, Westbrook, ME). Os testes positivos devem ser confirmados com IFA e outros exames (como hemograma completo) antes de se instituir o tratamento.
- PCR — mais confiável do que o encontro de mórulas circulantes.
- PCR do sangue para pesquisa de *E. canis* fornece um diagnóstico espécie-específico, sendo positivo por volta do dia 7 após a infecção, em geral antes do desenvolvimento de doença clínica (9-12 dias pós-infecção). O exame de PCR fica negativo 9 dias após o tratamento. A técnica de PCR realizada em amostras sanguíneas é muito mais sensível que aquela feita em amostras conjuntivais.

MÉTODOS DIAGNÓSTICOS
Aspirado da Medula Óssea
- Aguda — hipercelularidade das séries megacariocítica e mieloide.
- Crônica — frequentemente há hipoplasia eritroide com aumento nas proporções M:E e plasmocitose.
- Além disso, observa-se aumento no número de mastócitos em esfregaços da medula óssea.

ACHADOS PATOLÓGICOS
- Aguda — hemorragias petequiais nas superfícies serosas e mucosas da maioria dos órgãos; linfadenopatia generalizada (mancha acastanhada), hepatosplenomegalia e medula óssea vermelha (hipercelularidade).
- Crônica — medula pálida (hipoplásica); edema subcutâneo; ao exame histológico, é mais característico um infiltrado perivascular de plasmócitos em inúmeros órgãos; é comum uma meningoencefalite não supurativa multifocal com infiltrado celular linfoplasmocitário nas meninges.

TRATAMENTO
CUIDADO(S) DE SAÚDE ADEQUADO(S)
- Internação — estabilização clínica inicial em casos de anemia e/ou tendência hemorrágica resultante de trombocitopenia.
- Ambulatório — pacientes estabilizados; monitorizar frequentemente o sangue e a resposta aos medicamentos.

CUIDADO(S) DE ENFERMAGEM
- Soluções eletrolíticas balanceadas — indicadas em casos de desidratação.
- Transfusão sanguínea — recomendada em casos de anemia.
- Transfusão de plasma rico em plaquetas ou de sangue — aconselhável em casos de hemorragia decorrente de trombocitopenia.

ORIENTAÇÃO AO PROPRIETÁRIO
- Aguda — prognóstico excelente com a terapia apropriada.
- Crônica — a resposta à terapia pode levar 1 mês; prognóstico mau se a medula óssea estiver gravemente hipoplásica.
- A evolução de aguda para crônica pode ser facilmente evitada por meio de tratamento eficaz e precoce; entretanto, muitos cães permanecem soropositivos e podem apresentar recidivas (mesmo anos mais tarde).
- Pastor alemão e Doberman pinscher — forma mais crônica e grave da doença.

MEDICAÇÕES
MEDICAMENTO(S) DE ESCOLHA
- Doxiciclina (tratamento de escolha) — 5 mg/kg VO a cada 12 h por 3-4 semanas; administrar por via intravenosa por 5 dias se o cão estiver vomitando.
- Dipropionato de imidocarbe — 2 doses de 6,6 mg/kg IM em intervalo de 14 dias; supostamente eficaz contra *E. canis*, embora tenha falhado em remover a infecção experimental de cães com a doença.
- Glicocorticoides — prednisolona ou prednisona; 1-2 mg/kg VO a cada 12 h por 5 dias; podem ser indicados quando a *trombocitopenia* representar um risco de vida (acredita-se que ela resulte de mecanismos imunomediados); como a trombocitopenia imunomediada constitui o principal diagnóstico diferencial, esses agentes poderão ser indicados até que os resultados dos testes sorológicos estejam disponíveis.
- Esteroides androgênicos — utilizados para estimular a produção da medula óssea em cães cronicamente acometidos com medulas hipoplásicas; oximetolona (2 mg/kg a cada 24 h VO até se obter a resposta) ou decanoato de nandrolona (1,5 mg/kg IM semanalmente).

CONTRAINDICAÇÕES
- Tetraciclinas (e derivados) — não usar em cães com <6 meses de vida (produz manchas amareladas permanentes nos dentes); não utilizar em casos de insuficiência renal (tentar a doxiciclina, pois ela pode ser excretada pelo trato gastrintestinal).
- O enrofloxacino não se mostra eficaz contra *Erhlichia* spp., mas sim contra *Anaplasma* spp.

PRECAUÇÕES
Glicocorticoides — o uso prolongado em níveis imunossupressores pode interferir na depuração e eliminação da *E. canis* após o emprego das tetraciclinas.

MEDICAMENTO(S) ALTERNATIVO(S)
- Oxitetraciclina e tetraciclina — 22 mg/kg VO a cada 8 h por 21 dias; eficazes e mais baratas.
- Cloranfenicol — 20 mg/kg VO a cada 8 h por 14 dias; para filhotes caninos com <6 meses de vida; evita as manchas amareladas dos dentes em fase de erupção, causadas pelas tetraciclinas; alertar o proprietário quanto aos riscos à saúde pública; evitar em cães com trombocitopenia, pancitopenia ou anemia.

ACOMPANHAMENTO
MONITORIZAÇÃO DO PACIENTE
- Contagem plaquetária — a cada 3 dias após a instituição do agente antirriquetsiano até voltar aos níveis normais; a melhora é rápida em casos agudos.
- Testes sorológicos — repetir em 9 meses; a maioria dos cães ficará soronegativa; títulos positivos sugerem reinfecção ou tratamento ineficaz (reinstituir o esquema terapêutico).

PREVENÇÃO
- Controle da infestação por carrapatos — banhos de imersão ou *sprays* que contenham diclorvós, clorfenvinfós, dioxationa, propoxur ou carbarila; as coleiras contra pulgas e carrapatos podem diminuir a reinfestação, mas ainda não se comprovou a confiabilidade dessas coleiras; evitar as áreas infestadas por carrapatos.
- Remoção manual dos carrapatos — utilizar luvas (ver a seção "Potencial Zoonótico"); certificar-se de que as partes bucais do parasita foram removidas para evitar reação ao corpo estranho.

EVOLUÇÃO ESPERADA E PROGNÓSTICO
- Aguda — prognóstico excelente com o tratamento apropriado.
- Crônica — pode levar 4 semanas para obtenção da resposta clínica; prognóstico mau em casos de hipoplasia medular.

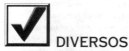

DIVERSOS
DISTÚRBIOS ASSOCIADOS
- *Babesia*.
- *Haemobartonella*.
- *A. platys*.

POTENCIAL ZOONÓTICO
- Os indícios sorológicos mostram a ocorrência da *E. canis* (ou, possivelmente, uma espécie relacionada) em pessoas; provavelmente não há infecção direta a partir dos cães; acredita-se que a exposição a carrapatos seja necessária; o *R. sanguineus* provavelmente não constitui o vetor em seres humanos.
- A maioria dos casos ocorre no sul e no centro-sul dos EUA.
- Sinais clínicos relevantes em seres humanos — febre, cefaleia, mialgia, dor ocular e desarranjo gastrintestinal.

SINÔNIMO(S)
- Febre hemorrágica canina.
- Riquetsiose canina.
- Tifo canino.
- Febre canina de Lahore.
- Doença hemorrágica de Nairobi.
- Doença dos cães rastreadores.
- Pancitopenia tropical canina.

ABREVIATURA(S)
- AAN = anticorpo antinuclear.
- ALT = alanina aminotransferase.
- IFA = anticorpo fluorescente indireto.
- M:E = proporção mieloide:eritroide.
- PCR = reação em cadeia da polimerase.
- SNC = sistema nervoso central.

Sugestões de Leitura
Eddlestone SM, Diniz PP, Neer TM, et al. Doxycycline clearance of experimentally induced chronic Ehrlichia canis infection in dogs. J Vet Intern Med 2007, 21:1237-1242.
Hegarty BC, de Paiva Diniz PP, Bradley JM, et al. Clinical relevance of annual screening using a commercial enzyme-linked immunosorbent assay (SNAP 3Dx) for canine ehrlichiosis. JAAHA 2009, 45:118-124.

Autor Stephen C. Barr
Consultor Editorial Stephen C. Barr

Erupções Medicamentosas Cutâneas

CONSIDERAÇÕES GERAIS

REVISÃO
- Corresponde a um amplo espectro de doenças e sinais clínicos que variam acentuadamente em termos de aparência clínica.
- É provável que muitas reações medicamentosas leves passem despercebidas ou não sejam descritas; assim, não se conhecem as taxas de incidência para medicamentos específicos.

IDENTIFICAÇÃO
- Cães e gatos.
- Predisposições etária, racial e sexual — basicamente desconhecidas.
- Certos tipos de erupções medicamentosas parecem ter base familiar (p. ex., reações à vacina antirrábica em ninhadas de cães).

SINAIS CLÍNICOS
- Prurido — pode ser ativado por uma ampla variedade de compostos; sintoma mais comum de erupção medicamentosa em seres humanos.
- Exantemas maculopapulares — comumente acompanham o prurido como sinal inespecífico de inflamação.
- Eritrodermia esfoliativa — resposta eritematosa difusa causada por vasodilatação; frequentemente leva à esfoliação (descamação difusa).
- Urticária/angioedema — origina-se de uma reação de hipersensibilidade imediata (tipo I); exige sensibilização prévia; o aumento na permeabilidade vascular leva ao extravasamento de líquido para o interstício.
- Vasculite por hipersensibilidade — inflamação da vasculatura cutânea; resulta em fluxo sanguíneo deficiente e lesão anóxica ao tecido receptor; na maioria dos casos, acredita-se que essa vasculite represente uma reação de hipersensibilidade do tipo III.
- Dermatite eosinofílica com edema (síndrome semelhante à de Wells) de cães — placas ou máculas intensamente eritematosas (possivelmente semelhantes a alvos), que podem ser acompanhadas por edema acentuado; distribuição localizada, regional ou generalizada; o aspecto clínico das lesões pode ser indistinguível de vasculite e eritema multiforme.
- Eritema multiforme — máculas ou placas eritematosas, que se expandem no sentido periférico e podem clarear no centro, produzindo uma aparência de "olho de boi" (semelhante a um alvo); podem-se observar múltiplas configurações/formas.
- Síndrome de Stevens-Johnson — semelhante à necrólise epidérmica tóxica com descolamento epidérmico menos extenso (<30%) e, muitas vezes, envolvimento da mucosa bucal.
- Necrólise epidérmica tóxica — necrose e esfacelamento extensos (>30%) da epiderme em camadas; resulta em uma superfície cutânea úmida e intensamente inflamada.
- Pênfigo/penfigoide induzidos por medicamentos — reação medicamentosa menos comum em animais; podem mimetizar estreitamente as formas autoimunes (espontâneas) dessas doenças; os sintomas podem persistir após a suspensão do medicamento.

CAUSAS E FATORES DE RISCO
- Medicamentos de qualquer tipo.
- Podem ocorrer após a primeira dose ou semanas a meses depois da administração do mesmo medicamento.
- Eritrodermia esfoliativa — associada mais frequentemente ao uso de xampus e banhos de imersão; também costuma ser observada com reações a medicamentos otológicos tópicos (nos canais auditivos e nos pavilhões auriculares côncavos).
- Dermatite eosinofílica com edema — forte associação com gastrenteropatia aguda concomitante e uso de medicamentos antidiarreicos e/ou antieméticos.
- Associação temporal em cães entre a aplicação de metaflumizona (Promeris®) e o início de pênfigo foliáceo.

DIAGNÓSTICO

DIAGNÓSTICO DIFERENCIAL
- Prurido, exantemas maculopapulares e urticária/angioedema — doenças alérgicas (atopia, reações adversas a alimentos, hipersensibilidade de contato) e reações a ectoparasitas (escabiose, dermatite à picada de pulga, hipersensibilidade à picada de pulga, ferroadas de insetos).
- Eritrodermia esfoliativa — descartar linfoma epiteliotrópico em cães e gatos idosos.
- Vasculite — confirmada por meio de biopsia; descartar doenças infecciosas, neoplásicas e autoimunes como a causa; muitos casos de vasculite são idiopáticos.
- Eritema multiforme — descartar infecções respiratórias e neoplasias internas; em cães adultos mais idosos, ocorre uma forma idiopática/crônica.
- Pênfigo/penfigoide — considerar reações medicamentosas sempre que essas doenças forem diagnosticadas; entretanto, a doença autoimune de ocorrência espontânea é muito mais comum.

HEMOGRAMA/BIOQUÍMICA/URINÁLISE
Em casos de vasculite, existe o potencial de doenças hepáticas, renais e gastrintestinais concomitantes.

OUTROS TESTES LABORATORIAIS
- Cães com vasculite — sorologia em busca de riquétsias, AAN.
- Gatos com vasculite — sorologia quanto à presença de FeLV e FIV, além de testes para descartar PIF.
- Tanto em cães como em gatos — culturas bacterianas e fúngicas em casos de vasculite com inflamação piogranulomatosa.

MÉTODOS DIAGNÓSTICOS
Biopsia cutânea para exame histopatológico — obrigatória para o diagnóstico de grande parte das doenças induzidas por medicamentos (vasculite, eritema multiforme, necrólise epidérmica tóxica, pênfigo/penfigoide).

ACHADOS PATOLÓGICOS
Variam de acordo com o processo patológico específico.

TRATAMENTO

- Interromper o uso do medicamento agressor ou sob suspeita.
- Síndrome de Stevens Johnson/necrólise epidérmica tóxica — cuidado de suporte intensivo e suporte hídrico/nutricional, em virtude das exsudações líquida e proteica e do risco de sepse.
- Alívio da dor quando houver indicação; no entanto, é recomendável o uso de quantidade mínima de medicamentos na suspeita de erupção medicamentosa.
- Para eritema multiforme idiopático crônico/persistente, os agentes azatioprina ou ciclosporina podem ser eficazes.

MEDICAÇÕES

MEDICAMENTO(S)
- A maioria dos problemas responde à terapia imunossupressora se apenas a suspensão do medicamento agressor for insuficiente (controverso no caso de síndrome de Stevens Johnson/necrólise epidérmica tóxica por causa do risco de sepse).

CONTRAINDICAÇÕES/INTERAÇÕES POSSÍVEIS
Evitar o medicamento agressor ou qualquer outro agente terapêutico da mesma classe ou família.

ACOMPANHAMENTO

MONITORIZAÇÃO DO PACIENTE
- Internação — se o paciente estiver debilitado.
- Esquema ambulatorial — reavaliações regulares, dependendo da condição física do animal.

PREVENÇÃO
Ver "Contraindicações/Interações Possíveis".

COMPLICAÇÕES POSSÍVEIS
- Infecções secundárias. • Depleção de eletrólitos e proteínas plasmáticas (síndrome de Stevens Johnson/necrólise epidérmica tóxica).

EVOLUÇÃO ESPERADA E PROGNÓSTICO
- Algumas reações parecem ativar respostas imunes autoperpetuantes.
- Determinados metabólitos medicamentosos podem persistir por dias a semanas e provocar uma resposta contínua.
- Necrólise epidérmica tóxica — prognóstico mau.
- Vasculite — prognóstico reservado quando houver complicações sistêmicas.

DIVERSOS

DISTÚRBIOS ASSOCIADOS
Vasculite cutânea — artropatia, hepatite, glomerulonefrite e distúrbios neuromusculares, entre outros.

VER TAMBÉM
- Pênfigo. • Vasculite Cutânea — Cães.

ABREVIATURA(S)
- AAN = anticorpo antinuclear. • FeLV = vírus da leucemia felina. • FIV = vírus da imunodeficiência felina. • PIF = peritonite infecciosa felina.

Sugestões de Leitura
Scott DW, Miller WH, Griffin GE, eds. Adverse cutaneous drug reactions. In: Muller & Kirk's Small Animal Dermatology, 6th ed. Philadelphia: Saunders, 2001, pp. 720-756.

Autor Daniel O. Morris
Consultor Editorial Alexander H. Werner

ESOFAGITE

CONSIDERAÇÕES GERAIS

DEFINIÇÃO
• Inflamação do esôfago — tipicamente do corpo esofágico e do esfíncter gastresofágico; ocasionalmente do esfíncter cricofaríngeo.
• Varia desde uma leve inflamação da superfície mucosa até ulceração grave, envolvendo as camadas submucosa e muscular.

FISIOPATOLOGIA
• A mucosa esofágica possui vários mecanismos importantes de barreira para resistir a substâncias cáusticas, incluindo epitélio escamoso estratificado com junções intracelulares estreitas, gel mucoso e íons bicarbonato de superfície.
• Depuração esofágica rápida por peristaltismo e neutralização do ácido pela saliva rica em bicarbonato são mecanismos de defesa importantes para evitar esofagite por refluxo.
• O rompimento dessas barreiras e mecanismos de defesa causa inflamação, erosão e/ou ulceração de estruturas subjacentes.
• A inflamação contínua provoca diminuição da motilidade do esôfago e do tônus do esfíncter esofágico inferior, o que faz com que ocorra maior refluxo e perpetua a inflamação.

SISTEMA(S) ACOMETIDO(S)
• Gastrintestinal — corpo esofágico (muito comum); esfíncter gastresofágico; ocasionalmente, o esfíncter cricofaríngeo.
• Respiratório — se a regurgitação for grave, poderá surgir pneumonia por aspiração com laringite e faringite concomitantes.

INCIDÊNCIA/PREVALÊNCIA
Desconhecida; acredita-se que seja baixa.

DISTRIBUIÇÃO GEOGRÁFICA
Esofagite causada por *Pythium* spp. — em geral, distribuído regionalmente nos estados dos EUA que fazem fronteira com o Golfo do México.

IDENTIFICAÇÃO
Espécies
Cães e gatos.
Raça(s) Predominante(s)
Nenhuma relatada.
Idade Média e Faixa Etária
• Qualquer idade; os animais jovens com hérnia de hiato esofágica congênita podem correr maior risco de esofagite por refluxo.
• Animais idosos correm maior risco de desenvolver refluxo e possivelmente esofagite durante anestesia.
Sexo Predominante
Nenhum.

SINAIS CLÍNICOS
Achados Anamnésicos
• Regurgitação.
• Hipersalivação.
• Uivo, choro ou ganido durante a deglutição (odinofagia).
• Extensão da cabeça e do pescoço durante a deglutição (odinofagia).
• Disfagia.
• Apetite diminuído (hiporexia).
• Perda de peso.
• Tosse e/ou secreção nasal em animais com pneumonia por aspiração concomitante.

Achados do Exame Físico
• Em geral, não são dignos de nota.
• Debilidade generalizada em caso de esofagite grave.
• Inflamação bucal e faríngea e/ou ulceração se tiverem sido ingeridas substâncias cáusticas ou irritantes.
• Febre e hipersalivação em alguns pacientes com esofagite ulcerativa grave.
• Dor à palpação do pescoço e do esôfago.
• Caquexia e perda de peso com doença prolongada.
• Sibilos pulmonares e tosse em pacientes com pneumonia por aspiração.
• Secreção nasal causada por inflamação nasal com aspiração.

CAUSAS
• Anestesia que resulta em refluxo gastresofágico.
• Doença do refluxo gastresofágico.
• Vômito crônico.
• Retenção esofágica de comprimidos ou cápsulas (doxiciclina, clindamicina, AINEs — muito comum em gatos).
• Corpo estranho esofágico.
• Agentes infecciosos — calicivírus, pitiose, *Candida*.
• Sondas de alimentação nasogástrica ou aquelas inseridas por esofagostomia ou faringostomia.
• Cirurgia esofágica e/ou torácica.
• Esofagite eosinofílica — rara.

FATORES DE RISCO
• Hérnia de hiato — aumenta o risco de refluxo gastresofágico.
• Anestesia — o uso de certos medicamentos, como diazepam, atropina, pentobarbital e tranquilizantes derivados de fenotiazina, antes da anestesia diminui a pressão do esfíncter gastresofágico e pode resultar em refluxo gastresofágico.
• O jejum por períodos prolongados ou a falta de jejum coloca os pacientes sob maior risco de refluxo gastresofágico durante a anestesia e possível esofagite.

DIAGNÓSTICO

DIAGNÓSTICO DIFERENCIAL
• Corpo estranho esofágico — geralmente detectado em radiografias simples ou esofagoscopia.
• Estenose esofágica — estreitamento segmentar revelado pela radiografia contrastada com bário ou esofagoscopia.
• Disfagia orofaríngea — diagnosticada ao se avaliar a deglutição de bário à fluoroscopia.
• Hérnia de hiato — a forma congênita costuma ser reconhecida como uma opacidade caudodorsal repleta de gás na cavidade torácica; podem ser necessários exames contrastados para documentar hérnia de hiato adquirida.
• Megaesôfago — a radiografia simples, em geral, revela dilatação difusa do corpo esofágico.
• Divertículos esofágicos — bolsas focais detectadas por meio de radiografias simples ou contrastadas ou esofagoscopia.
• Anomalia do anel vascular — geralmente revelada pela radiografia contrastada com bário como uma dilatação focal do corpo esofágico proximal.

HEMOGRAMA/BIOQUÍMICA/URINÁLISE
Costumam permanecer normais; os pacientes com esofagite ulcerativa ou pneumonia por aspiração podem ter leucocitose e neutrofilia.

DIAGNÓSTICO POR IMAGEM
• Radiografia torácica simples — em geral, não há alteração digna de nota; pneumonia por aspiração pode ser evidente nas partes pendentes do pulmão; raramente, demonstra dilatação do esôfago cranial à estenose (pode-se observar alimento retido na parte dilatada do esôfago) ou massa intra ou extraluminal.
• Radiografia contrastada com bário — pode revelar retenção do contraste no esôfago em caso de doença do refluxo gastresofágico, estreitamento segmentar, dilatação esofágica ou hipomotilidade esofágica difusa; a formação de estenose pode ser aparente em pacientes gravemente acometidos; é capaz de identificar o número, a localização e o comprimento das estenoses.

MÉTODOS DIAGNÓSTICOS
• Endoscopia e biopsia — meios mais confiáveis de diagnóstico; em pacientes com esofagite grave, a mucosa parece hiperêmica e edematosa, com áreas de ulceração e sangramento ativo; pode haver crescimentos polipoides.
• Casos discretos de esofagite podem parecer normais à endoscopia, como gatos com esofagite crônica por refluxo gastresofágico, e necessitar de biopsia da mucosa para confirmar o diagnóstico.
• Aspiração transtraqueal e/ou broncoscopia para citologia, cultura e antibiograma se houver suspeita de pneumonia por aspiração.

ACHADOS PATOLÓGICOS
• Inflamação linfoplasmocitária esofágica com componente neutrofílico na fase aguda e/ou ulcerações e erosões.
• Hiperplasia ou displasia de células escamosas.

TRATAMENTO

CUIDADO(S) DE SAÚDE ADEQUADO(S)
Os animais com acometimento leve podem ser tratados em um esquema ambulatorial; aqueles com esofagite mais grave (p. ex., anorexia total, desidratação e pneumonia por aspiração) precisam ser hospitalizados.

CUIDADO(S) DE ENFERMAGEM
• Fluidos intravenosos para manter a hidratação — casos mais graves.
• Medicações — talvez tenham de ser administradas por via parenteral durante a hospitalização.
• Oxigenoterapia — pode ser necessária em pacientes com pneumonia por aspiração grave.

DIETA
• Esofagite grave — suspender o alimento e a água por, no mínimo, 3-5 dias; manter a dieta com sondas de alimentação por gastrostomia (de preferência) ou nutrição parenteral total.
• Aos pacientes aptos a se alimentar por via oral:
  ○ Ao se retomar a alimentação, fornecer várias refeições em pequenas quantidades.
  ○ É recomendável uma dieta de alta digestibilidade (os valores de digestibilidade da matéria seca devem ultrapassar 85-88% e da proteína, 92%) com níveis baixos a moderados de gordura (o alto teor de gordura na dieta atrasa o esvaziamento gástrico) e conteúdos

baixos de fibras de consistência líquida ou pastosa.

ORIENTAÇÃO AO PROPRIETÁRIO
- Discutir a necessidade de restringir o consumo de alimentos no caso de pacientes com esofagite grave.
- Abordar as complicações potenciais, inclusive pneumonia por aspiração, estenose esofágica, perfuração esofágica e/ou anormalidades da motilidade esofágica.

CONSIDERAÇÕES CIRÚRGICAS
Nos casos graves, fica indicada a gastrostomia endoscópica percutânea ou a colocação cirúrgica de sonda de gastrostomia.

MEDICAÇÕES
MEDICAMENTO(S) DE ESCOLHA
- Geralmente, são administrados por via parenteral (exceto o sucralfato) nos casos graves; quando administrados por via enteral, dissolver em água e administrar por via oral (p. ex., com uma seringa ou conta-gotas) ou sonda de gastrostomia.
- Suspensão de sucralfato (0,5-1 g VO a cada 8 h) — mais terapêutica que os comprimidos inteiros de sucralfato.
- Antibióticos — indicados em caso de pneumonia por aspiração concomitante ou ulceração esofágica grave ou perfuração esofágica.
- Agente antissecretor de ácido gástrico (p. ex., famotidina, 0,5 mg/kg VO, SC, IV a cada 12-24 h; ranitidina, 1-2 mg/kg VO, SC, IV a cada 8-12 h; cimetidina, 5-10 mg/kg VO, SC, IV a cada 8 h; omeprazol, 0,7 mg/kg VO a cada 24 h) — para evitar a ocorrência de irritação adicional por refluxo gastresofágico.
- Solução de lidocaína (0,5 mg/kg VO a cada 4-6 h) — para tratar a dor esofágica intensa.
- Dosagem anti-inflamatória de corticosteroides (p. ex., prednisona, 0,5-1 mg/kg VO a cada 12 h) — para diminuir a possibilidade da formação de estenose esofágica nos casos graves.
- Agentes procinéticos gastrintestinais (cisaprida, 0,1-0,5 mg/kg VO a cada 8-12 h; metoclopramida, 0,2-0,5 mg/kg VO, SC a cada 8 h) — podem ajudar a diminuir o refluxo gastresofágico; podem estimular a motilidade esofágica distal em gatos.

CONTRAINDICAÇÕES
Nenhuma.

PRECAUÇÕES
Nenhuma.

INTERAÇÕES POSSÍVEIS
- A cimetidina e a ranitidina ligam-se à enzima do citocromo hepático P-450 e podem interferir no metabolismo de outros medicamentos.
- Os antagonistas do receptor H_2 impedem a captação do omeprazol pelas células oxínticas.
- O sucralfato pode interferir na absorção gastrintestinal de outros medicamentos (p. ex., cimetidina, ranitidina e omeprazol); isso, no entanto, pode não ter importância clínica.

MEDICAMENTO(S) ALTERNATIVO(S)
- Emplastros analgésicos à base de fentanila — podem ser úteis nos casos graves de esofagite dolorosa.
- Análogos da eritromicina — podem ser proveitosos para tratar gatos com esofagite secundária à doença do refluxo gastresofágico.

ACOMPANHAMENTO
MONITORIZAÇÃO DO PACIENTE
- Pacientes com esofagite leve não requerem necessariamente acompanhamento com endoscopia; o rastreamento dos sinais clínicos pode ser suficiente.
- Considerar a endoscopia de acompanhamento em pacientes com esofagite ulcerativa e naqueles sob risco de estenose esofágica.

PREVENÇÃO
- Omeprazol — 1 mg/kg VO 4 h antes da anestesia ou bólus de metoclopramida, seguido por infusão em velocidade constante durante a cirurgia, diminuem o risco do desenvolvimento de refluxo gastresofágico.
- Se o refluxo gastresofágico for a causa da esofagite, o proprietário deverá evitar o fornecimento de refeições ao animal tarde da noite, pois isso tende a diminuir a pressão do esfíncter gastresofágico durante o sono.
- A preparação adequada do paciente antes de anestesia (jejum) diminui o risco de refluxo gastresofágico.
- Após a administração oral de cápsulas e comprimidos, fornecer bólus de água (5 mL) em cães e gatos; acelerar o tempo de trânsito dos comprimidos para o estômago em gatos, revestindo os comprimidos com manteiga ou aplicando o suprimento Nutrical no nariz dos gatos para estimular a lambedura após a administração de comprimidos; incentivar o animal de estimação a comer depois da administração oral para estimular a deglutição.

COMPLICAÇÕES POSSÍVEIS
- Formação de estenose.
- Perfuração esofágica.
- Pneumonia por aspiração.
- Disfunção permanente da motilidade esofágica.
- Esofagite por refluxo crônico.
- Esôfago de Barrett (complicação rara de esofagite por refluxo crônico em gatos).

EVOLUÇÃO ESPERADA E PROGNÓSTICO
- Obtenção dos melhores resultados quando os pacientes são tratados com uma barreira à difusão (p. ex., sucralfato) e inibidor da secreção de ácido gástrico (p. ex., famotidina, ranitidina, cimetidina e omeprazol).
- Esofagite leve — em geral, o prognóstico é favorável.
- Esofagite grave ou ulcerativa — prognóstico reservado.
- A recuperação completa será possível se o distúrbio for reconhecido e tratado antes do desenvolvimento de complicações sérias.

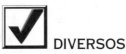
DIVERSOS
POTENCIAL ZOONÓTICO
Nenhum.

GESTAÇÃO/FERTILIDADE/REPRODUÇÃO
Antagonistas do receptor H_2 (p. ex., cimetidina, ranitidina e famotidina), inibidores da bomba de prótons (p. ex., omeprazol) e glicocorticoides devem ser usados com cautela durante a gestação.

SINÔNIMO(S)
Inflamação esofágica.

VER TAMBÉM
- Corpos Estranhos Esofágicos.
- Disfagia.
- Divertículos Esofágicos.
- Estenose Esofágica.
- Hérnia de Hiato.
- Megaesôfago.
- Refluxo Gastresofágico.
- Regurgitação.

ABREVIATURA(S)
- AINE = anti-inflamatório não esteroide.

Sugestões de Leitura
Glazer A, Walters PC. Esophagitis and esophageal strictures. Compend Contin Educ Pract Vet 2008, 30(5):281-292.
Jergens AE. Diseases of the esophagus. In: Ettinger SJ, Feldman EC, eds., Textbook of Veterinary Internal Medicine, 6th ed. St. Louis: Elsevier, 2005, pp. 1298-1310.
Sellon RK, Willard MD. Esophagitis and esophageal strictures. Vet Clin North Am Small Anim Pract 2003, 33(5):945-967.

Autor Jocelyn Mott
Consultor Editorial Albert E. Jergens

Espermatocele/Granuloma Espermático

CONSIDERAÇÕES GERAIS

REVISÃO
- Espermatocele — distensão cística dos dúctulos eferentes ou do epidídimo contendo espermatozoides, geralmente associada à perda de patência do ducto.
- Granuloma espermático — reação inflamatória crônica granulomatosa que se desenvolve quando os espermatozoides escapam dos dúctulos eferentes ou do ducto epididimário para o tecido circundante; clinicamente importante quando a obstrução bilateral do sistema de ductos leva à azoospermia.

IDENTIFICAÇÃO
Cães e gatos.

SINAIS CLÍNICOS
- Suspeita em cão azoospérmico que possui testículos de tamanho normal.
- Raramente associada à dor ou a lesões visíveis ou palpáveis.

CAUSAS E FATORES DE RISCO
- Traumatismo indutor de ruptura do ducto epididimário — libera antígenos espermáticos para o tecido circundante.
- Adenomiose — invasão das células de revestimento epitelial do epidídimo nas camadas musculares; pode ser um fator; associada a excesso de estímulo estrogênico.
- Hiperplasia epitelial do epidídimo — pode ser um precursor da adenomiose; não é frequentemente observada nos cães com <2,5 anos de idade; notada em certo grau em 75% dos cães com >7,75 anos de idade; o risco aumenta com a idade.
- Complicação da vasectomia — especialmente quando a técnica cirúrgica não foi meticulosa.
- Oclusão congênita do ducto epididimário.

DIAGNÓSTICO

DIAGNÓSTICO DIFERENCIAL
- Azoospermia (cães) — degeneração testicular; hipoplasia; ejaculação retrógrada; ejaculação incompleta.
- Sinais escrotais (p. ex., dor e lesões palpáveis; cães) — epididimite; orquite; dermatite escrotal.

HEMOGRAMA/BIOQUÍMICA/URINÁLISE
- Urinálise (por cistocentese) após a ejaculação — descartar ejaculação retrógrada.
- Hemograma completo e perfil bioquímico — geralmente normais.

OUTROS TESTES LABORATORIAIS
- Análise do FSH canino — alta concentração associada à degeneração e hipoplasia; concentração normal nos cães com azoospermia e com os testículos de tamanho normal associados à obstrução bilateral do epidídimo ou ejaculação retrógrada.
- Concentração da fosfatase alcalina do plasma seminal — amostras azoospérmicas com fosfatase alcalina <5.000 U/L são compatíveis com obstrução bilateral do epidídimo ou ejaculação incompleta; ver "Infertilidade do Macho — Cães".

DIAGNÓSTICO POR IMAGEM
A ultrassonografia é útil para diferenciar espermatocele/granuloma espermático de outras condições que provocam aumento de volume do escroto.

MÉTODOS DIAGNÓSTICOS
Biopsia cirúrgica do testículo e biopsia excisional do tecido epididimário acometido — permitem a identificação do epidídimo; possibilitam a avaliação da espermatogênese; as espermatoceles aparecem como cistos amarelados dentro do epidídimo.

ACHADOS PATOLÓGICOS
Exame histológico de amostra testicular — espermatogênese completa em cão com azoospermia indica obstrução.

TRATAMENTO

- Cão azoospérmico — raramente exibem recuperação espontânea.
- Obstrução bilateral do epidídimo — provavelmente não é passível de tratamento, exceto por meio de anastomose microcirúrgica do ducto deferente com a estrutura cística ou o segmento patente do epidídimo; poucas tentativas foram feitas para realizar esse procedimento nos cães.

MEDICAÇÕES

MEDICAMENTO(S)
Nenhum medicamento foi descrito na literatura especializada para desobstruir o sistema de ductos.

ACOMPANHAMENTO

EVOLUÇÃO ESPERADA E PROGNÓSTICO
- Granuloma espermático unilateral — razoável a reservado quanto à fertilidade; o manejo reprodutivo irá melhorar a fertilidade; ver "Acasalamento, Momento Oportuno".
- Granuloma espermático bilateral — prognóstico mau em termos de fertilidade.

DIVERSOS

VER TAMBÉM
- Acasalamento, Momento Oportuno.
- Infertilidade do Macho — Cães.

ABREVIATURA(S)
- FSH = hormônio foliculoestimulante.

Sugestões de Leitura
Althouse GC, Evans LE, Hopkins SM. Episodic scrotal mutilation with concurrent bilateral sperm granuloma in a dog. JAVMA 1993, 202:776-778.
Mayenco Aguirre AM, Garcia Fernandez P, Sanchez Muela M. Sperm granuloma in the dog: Complication of vasectomy. J Small Anim Pract 1996, 37:392-393.
Perez-Marin CC, Lopez R, Dominguez KM, Zafra R. Clinical and pathological findings in testis, epididymis, deferens duct and prostate following vasectomy in a dog. Reprod Dom Anim 2006, 41:169-174.

Autor Carlos R. F. Pinto
Consultor Editorial Sara K. Lyle

ESPIRRO, ESPIRRO REVERSO, ÂNSIA DE VÔMITO

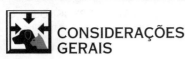

CONSIDERAÇÕES GERAIS

DEFINIÇÃO
- Espirro — um reflexo expiratório protetor normal que serve para expelir ar e material através da cavidade nasal; comumente associado à secreção nasal.
- Espirro reverso — um reflexo inspiratório repetitivo protetor normal que serve para remover irritantes da nasofaringe (também conhecido como o reflexo da aspiração).
- Ânsia de vômito (também conhecida como vômito seco ou esforço para vomitar) — um reflexo protetor normal para remover secreções da laringe, traqueia proximal, faringe ou esôfago; frequentemente mal-interpretada como vômito pelos proprietários.

FISIOPATOLOGIA
- Irritação de receptores irritantes da submucosa; vários estímulos (infecciosos, parasitários, irritantes, mecânicos — especialmente secreções acumuladas) eliciarão esses reflexos, dependendo do local onde a irritação é aplicada.
- Espirro — irritação da mucosa nasal; a frequência muitas vezes diminui em caso de doença crônica.
- Espirro reverso — irritação da mucosa nasofaríngea caudodorsal.
- Ânsia de vômito — irritação da mucosa da traqueia cervical (ou laringe); a irritação da mucosa orofaríngea e esofágica também pode estar envolvida. Pode acompanhar um episódio de tosse à medida que as secreções são conduzidas por meio da laringe ou anteceder a tosse por aspiração para a traqueia.

SISTEMA(S) ACOMETIDO(S)
- Respiratório — frequentemente associados a distúrbios infecciosos ou inflamatórios envolvendo o trato respiratório superior.
- Gastrintestinal — a ânsia de vômito também pode ser causada por distúrbios de deglutição, esôfago ou estômago.

GENÉTICA
N/D

INCIDÊNCIA/PREVALÊNCIA
Esses reflexos normais são comuns tanto no cão como no gato em resposta à irritação da mucosa.

DISTRIBUIÇÃO GEOGRÁFICA
Mundial

IDENTIFICAÇÃO
- Qualquer raça de cão ou gato pode ser acometida.
- Esses reflexos por si só não são associados a qualquer idade específica, mas sim a problemas que os causam; os exemplos incluem:
  ○ Animais jovens — infecção, fenda palatina, discinesia ciliar primária
  ○ Animais mais idosos — tumores nasais, doença odontológica.
- Espirro agudo em cães é mais frequentemente causado por corpo estranho nasal, enquanto em gatos é associado com maior frequência à rinite viral aguda.

SINAIS CLÍNICOS
- A posição da cabeça e da boca do animal pode ajudar os proprietários a determinar quais desses reflexos estão presentes.
- O espirro tipicamente resulta em esforço(s) expiratório(s) explosivo(s) súbito(s) com a boca fechada e a cabeça lançada para baixo; pode fazer com que o nariz do cão bata contra o chão.
- O espirro reverso é um esforço inspiratório, ruidoso, súbito, frequentemente paroxístico, com a cabeça tracionada para trás, boca fechada e lábios para dentro.
- A ânsia de vômito é um esforço expiratório; tipicamente com a cabeça e o pescoço estendidos e a boca mantida aberta; em geral, termina com a deglutição do animal (com pouco ou nada expelido).

CAUSAS
- Qualquer irritação ou inflamação da mucosa pode eliciar esses reflexos. O mesmo agente na cavidade nasal pode eliciar um espirro, mas, quando aplicado na nasofaringe, resultaria em um espirro reverso. O reflexo, portanto, situa o local da irritação para avaliações futuras.
- As causas nasais comuns de espirro e espirro reverso incluem secreções nasais excessivas (ver capítulo sobre Secreção Nasal), corpo estranho (especialmente se os sinais forem de início agudo e violento), alergia, neoplasia, e parasitas; cães — *Pneumonyssoides*; cães e gatos — *Cuterebra*, *Eucoleus* (*Capillaria*), *Linguatula*.
- Doenças extranasais que resultam em espirro reverso, espirro (e secreção nasal), já que as secreções podem ser forçadas para a nasofaringe e as cavidades nasais — pneumonia, megaesôfago, vômito crônico, disfagia cricofaríngea, ou acalasia.
- O espirro reverso pode ser idiopático, sobretudo em raças caninas de pequeno porte. Nesse caso, não há outros sinais clínicos associados.
- As causas de ânsia de vômito incluem:
  ○ Secreções expelidas das vias aéreas inferiores e para a traqueia cervical ou laringe.
  ○ Disfunção da faringe/laringe com consequente aspiração das vias aéreas em virtude da perda de função motora e/ou sensorial que normalmente protege as vias aéreas.
  ○ Vômito por doença esofágica ou gastrintestinal.

FATORES DE RISCO
- Os animais com vacinação deficiente podem desenvolver infecção/inflamação nasal e espirro (filhotes felinos com infecções do trato respiratório superior, filhotes caninos com tosse dos canis).
- Tosse produtiva pode produzir secreções excessivas que podem ser impulsionadas para a nasofaringe e induzir a espirro reverso.
- As doenças odontológicas crônicas podem causar rinite e espirro ou espirro reverso.
- Os ácaros nasais podem causar tanto espirro reverso como espirro em cães (mas não em gatos); nos Estados Unidos, a incidência é inversamente proporcional ao uso de preventivo contra dirofilariose.
- Corpos estranhos nasais eliciam espirro e/ou espirro reverso, dependendo de sua localização; animais de rua, especialmente aqueles de caça, talvez exibam maior risco.
- O espirro reverso é frequentemente associado à agitação.

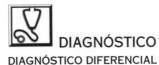

DIAGNÓSTICO

DIAGNÓSTICO DIFERENCIAL
Sinais Similares
- Diferenciar espirro regular (ocorre à expiração) de espirro reverso (ocorre à inspiração e situa o local da irritação à nasofaringe).
- A ânsia de vômito é frequentemente mal-interpretada como vômito.

HEMOGRAMA/BIOQUÍMICA/URINÁLISE
Os resultados não são específicos de qualquer causa de espirro, espirro reverso ou ânsia de vômito em particular.

OUTROS TESTES LABORATORIAIS
Esses reflexos são secundários a outro processo que tenha irritado e estimulado as superfícies da mucosa em uma ou mais áreas. O teste diagnóstico visa à determinação dessa causa específica.

DIAGNÓSTICO POR IMAGEM
- Espirro e espirro reverso — radiografias ou TC do crânio.
- Ânsia de vômito — radiografias torácicas e broncoscopia podem ser necessárias para pesquisa de secreções excessivas nas vias aéreas inferiores e pneumonia.

MÉTODOS DIAGNÓSTICOS
- Espirro e espirro reverso — rinoscopia ântero-posterior, sonda periodontal.
- Ânsia de vômito — determinar a presença ou ausência de reflexo do vômito, laringoscopia para determinar a função intrínseca (utilizar doxapram para estimular a respiração).

ACHADOS PATOLÓGICOS
Pode ser encontrada uma inflamação inespecífica na cavidade nasal ou nasofaringe.

TRATAMENTO

CUIDADO(S) DE SAÚDE ADEQUADO(S)
A remoção da irritação incitante da mucosa, sempre que possível, resultará no alívio desses reflexos.

CUIDADO(S) DE ENFERMAGEM
A terapia ambulatorial é geralmente indicada, exceto talvez após biopsia rinoscópica.

ATIVIDADE
É recomendável a restrição da prática de exercício e atividade física após biopsias rinoscópicas para evitar sangramento excessivo.

DIETA
N/D

ORIENTAÇÃO AO PROPRIETÁRIO
- Orientar os proprietários para que eles compreendam que esses reflexos são normais. O teste diagnóstico é necessário para determinar a causa subjacente e permitir o tratamento adequado.
- O contato direto com outros animais deve ser limitado até que o tratamento da causa subjacente (se infecciosa) seja concluído.
- Os episódios de espirro reverso paroxístico podem ser reduzidos, induzindo à deglutição (fricção da garganta com ingestão de água) ou apneia (tampar o nariz e a boca).

CONSIDERAÇÕES CIRÚRGICAS
- Dependendo da causa subjacente, pode haver a necessidade de anestesia para a realização de cirurgia ou endoscopia direcionada à remoção de abscesso dentário ou corpo estranho responsável pelo espirro ou espirro reverso.
- Fazer cirurgia em caso de laringopatia com cautela nos casos em que a ânsia de vômito é proeminente em virtude do aumento no risco de

Espirro, Espirro Reverso, Ânsia de Vômito

pneumonia por aspiração na presença de disfunção esofágica concomitante.

MEDICAÇÕES

MEDICAMENTO(S) DE ESCOLHA
• Não há medicamento que suprima especificamente esses reflexos; o tratamento é direcionado ao irritante subjacente.
• As infecções bacterianas nasais (secundárias a corpo estranho, doença odontológica, tumor, etc.) são mais bem tratadas com antibióticos direcionados contra bactérias gram-positivas (mais comuns).
• Os ácaros nasais são tratados com ivermectina (200-300 µg/kg VO ou SC semanalmente por 3 semanas) ou milbemicina (em Collies e raças similares na dose de 0,5-1 mg/kg VO semanalmente por 3 semanas). É recomendável que todos os cães da casa sejam tratados para evitar nova infecção.
• Quando não se encontra nenhum problema nasal subjacente para explicar o espirro, é aconselhável o tratamento contra ácaros nasais. Se nenhuma melhora for observada, pode-se tentar o tratamento inespecífico e prolongado com doxiciclina e piroxicam (0,3 mg/kg VO diariamente).
• Doenças das vias aéreas inferiores com excesso de secreções são tratadas com antibióticos se houver confirmação de infecção bacteriana; é mais comum o envolvimento de bactérias gram-negativas.
• Para inflamação inespecífica das vias aéreas, utilizar algum anti-inflamatório, como prednisolona (1-2 mg/kg a cada 12-24 h) ou piroxicam (0,3 mg/kg VO a cada 24-48 h) se nenhuma infecção for confirmada.

• Não há tratamento para ânsia de vômito secundária à perda sensorial na laringe com aspiração recorrente; é recomendada a elevação das tigelas de água e ração. A modificação da consistência do alimento oferecido também pode ser útil.

CONTRAINDICAÇÕES
• Ivermectina em Collies e raças semelhantes.
• Uso de piroxicam concomitantemente com outros AINEs ou corticosteroides, bem como em pacientes com insuficiência renal.

PRECAUÇÕES
A segurança dos medicamentos mais recomendados não foi estabelecida em animais gestantes.

INTERAÇÕES POSSÍVEIS
N/D

MEDICAMENTO(S) ALTERNATIVO(S)
Descongestionantes (efedrina, vasoconstritores tópicos) ou anti-histamínicos podem reduzir as secreções e o espirro em alguns casos.

ACOMPANHAMENTO

MONITORIZAÇÃO DO PACIENTE
Esperar a redução do espirro ou espirro reverso com o uso de terapia adequada.

PREVENÇÃO
Limitar o acesso a corpos estranhos e fornecer cuidados odontológicos adequados.

COMPLICAÇÕES POSSÍVEIS
Se a ânsia de vômito for secundária à perda sensorial da laringe, pode ocorrer o desenvolvimento de grave pneumonia por aspiração.

EVOLUÇÃO ESPERADA E PROGNÓSTICO
• Os ácaros nasais devem responder ao tratamento em até 3 semanas.
• Os espirros ou espirros reversos secundários a corpo estranho desaparecem rapidamente após a remoção do mesmo.

DIVERSOS

DISTÚRBIOS ASSOCIADOS
N/D

FATORES RELACIONADOS COM A IDADE
N/D

POTENCIAL ZOONÓTICO
N/D

GESTAÇÃO/FERTILIDADE/REPRODUÇÃO
N/D

VER TAMBÉM
• Secreção Nasal
• Rinite e Sinusite

ABREVIATURA(S)
• AINE = anti-inflamatório não esteroide
• TC = tomografia computadorizada

Sugestões de Leitura
Doust R, Sullivan M. Nasal discharge, sneezing and reverse sneezing. In: King LG, ed., Textbook of Respiratory Disease in Dogs and Cats. Philadelphia: Saunders, 2004, pp. 17-29.
McKiernan BC. Sneezing and nasal discharge. In: Ettinger SJ, Feldman EC, eds., Textbook of Veterinary Internal Medicine, 4th ed. Philadelphia: Saunders, 1994, pp. 79-85.

Autores Dominique Peeters e Brendan C. McKiernan
Consultor Editorial Lynelle R. Johnson

ESPLENOMEGALIA

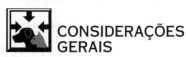

CONSIDERAÇÕES GERAIS

DEFINIÇÃO
Aumento de volume do baço; caracterizado como difuso ou nodular.

FISIOPATOLOGIA
• Funções do baço — remoção de eritrócitos senis e anormais; filtração e fagocitose de partículas antigênicas como microrganismos, material celular degradado, macromoléculas; produção de linfócitos e plasmócitos; produção de anticorpos; reservatório de eritrócitos e de plaquetas; metabolismo e armazenamento do ferro; hematopoiese, conforme a necessidade.
• Muitos distúrbios afetam a função do baço.

Difusa
Quatro Mecanismos Patológicos Gerais
• Inflamação (esplenite) — associada a agentes infecciosos; classificada de acordo com o tipo celular (p. ex., supurativa, necrosante, eosinofílica, linfoplasmocitária e granulomatosa-piogranulomatosa).
• Hiperplasia linforreticular — hiperplasia de fagócitos mononucleares e elementos linfoides (em resposta aos antígenos); destruição eritrocitária acelerada.
• Congestão — associada à drenagem venosa prejudicada.
• Infiltração — envolve a invasão celular do baço ou o depósito de substâncias anormais.

Nodular
• Associada a distúrbios neoplásicos (tumor) ou não neoplásicos (infecção, hiperplasia/regeneração, ou inflamação).

SISTEMA(S) ACOMETIDO(S)
Os distúrbios do baço também podem ser associados a alterações no fígado.

IDENTIFICAÇÃO
• Cães e gatos.
• Torção esplênica — super-representada nas raças caninas de grande porte e tórax profundo (p. ex., Pastor alemão e Dinamarquês).
• Hemangiossarcoma — cães de meia-idade; raças de grande porte; possivelmente mais comum nos machos do que nas fêmeas; predileção pelas raças Pastor alemão, Golden retriever e Labrador retriever.
• Baço proeminente — pode ser normal em determinadas raças (Pastor alemão, Terrier escocês).

SINAIS CLÍNICOS

Comentários Gerais
• Aumento de volume do baço — com frequência inespecífico.
• Frequentemente reflete mais algum distúrbio subjacente do que doença primária do baço.

Achados Anamnésicos
• Diarreia, vômito, anorexia — secundários a linfoma, mastocitoma, PIF e enterite linfoplasmocitária (gatos).
• Dor abdominal vaga; distensão leve a modesta.
• Sinais vagos/letargia, desconforto abdominal, anorexia, vômito, perda de peso — torção esplênica (cães).
• Fraqueza e colapso — secundários a hemoabdome decorrente de ruptura esplênica e hematoma associado ou hemangiossarcoma (cães); ou raramente outra neoplasia.

Achados do Exame Físico
• Baço proeminente à palpação abdominal; o baço não palpável não exclui esplenomegalia.
• Cães — superfície lisa ou irregular.
• Gatos — aumento uniforme, geralmente difuso.
• Palidez, tempo de preenchimento capilar lento, pulsos periféricos fracos e taquicardia em caso de hemorragia ou torção esplênicas.
• Distensão abdominal em caso de esplenomegalia maciça ou ruptura esplênica.
• Petéquias e equimoses em caso de coagulopatia secundária a distúrbio esplênico primário ou doença subjacente.
• Hematomegalia concomitante, intestinos espessados e/ou linfadenopatia mesentérica implica doença infiltrativa ou inflamatória.
• Linfadenomegalia periférica — sugere linfoma/leucemia.
• Arritmias cardíacas — podem indicar anormalidade cardíaca clinicamente significativa com envolvimento do baço (congestão), embora as arritmias ventriculares também estejam associadas a distúrbios esplênicos primários.

CAUSAS

Cães

Inflamação (Esplenite)
• Supurativa — ferida abdominal penetrante; corpo estranho migratório; endocardite; sepse; complicação infecciosa de torção esplênica.
• Necrosante — geralmente secundária à torção ou neoplasia; anaeróbios; *Salmonella*; hepatite infecciosa canina aguda.
• Eosinofílica — gastrenterite eosinofílica.
• Linfoplasmocitária — distúrbios infecciosos subagudos ou crônicos; hepatite infecciosa canina; erliquiose; piometra; *Brucella*; *Leishmania*; enteropatia inflamatória concomitante.
• Granulomatosa — histoplasmose; *Leishmania*.
• Piogranulomatosa — blastomicose; *Mycobacterium*; esporotricose.

Hiperplasia
• Infecção — bacteremia crônica (endocardite bacteriana; discospondilite; *Brucella*).
• Doença imunomediada — LES; anemia hemolítica ou trombocitopenia.

Congestão
• Tranquilizantes; barbitúricos; hipertensão portal; insuficiência cardíaca direita; torção esplênica.

Infiltração
• Neoplasia — linfoma; leucemia aguda e crônica; sarcoma histiocítico; mieloma múltiplo; mastocitose sistêmica.
• Hematopoiese extramedular — anemia hemolítica imunomediada ou trombocitopenia; anemia crônica; doença infecciosa; malignidade; LES.
• Amiloidose.

Gatos

Inflamação
• Supurativa — ferida penetrante ou corpo estranho migratório; septicemia; salmonelose.
• Necrosante — salmonelose.
• Eosinofílica — síndrome hipereosinofílica.
• Linfoplasmocitária — enterite linfoplasmocitária; micoplasmas hemotrópicos; piometra.
• Granulomatosa — histoplasmose; micobacteriose.
• Piogranulomatosa — PIF, *Mycobacterium*.

Hiperplasia
• Infecção — micoplasmose hemotrópica.
• Imunomediada — hemólise crônica, LES.

Congestão
• Hipertensão portal, insuficiência cardíaca congestiva.

Infiltração
• Neoplásica — mastocitoma (mais comum); linfoma; doença mieloproliferativa; doença linfoproliferativa; sarcoma histiocítico; mieloma múltiplo; hemangiossarcoma (raro).
• Não neoplásica — amiloidose, hematopoiese extramedular.

FATORES DE RISCO
Gatos — FeLV, PIF.

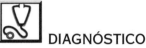

DIAGNÓSTICO

DIAGNÓSTICO DIFERENCIAL
Outra organomegalia ou massas craniais.

HEMOGRAMA/BIOQUÍMICA/URINÁLISE

Cães
• Anemia regenerativa secundária a sangramento esplênico ou doença hemolítica.
• Hemácias nucleadas — podem acompanhar hematopoiese extramedular e indicar disfunção esplênica.
• Esferócitos — hemólise, cisalhamento microangiopático (também se observam esquizócitos).
• Leucocitose com desvio à esquerda — pode indicar condições infecciosas ou inflamatórias, resposta regenerativa acentuada ou hematopoiese extramedular.
• Trombocitopenia — por aumento de consumo (CID ou sangramento) secundário à hemangiossarcoma, destruição elevada (imunomediada), sequestro ou produção diminuída na medula óssea.
• Hipercalcemia pode estar associada à neoplasia, especialmente linfoma.
• Hiperglobulinemia pode estar associada à neoplasia ou infecção por *Ehrlichia*.
• Hemoglobinemia e hiperbilirrubinemia — podem ocorrer em caso de anemia microangiopática, torção esplênica, hemangiossarcoma e anemia imunomediada com o baço como o local de remoção de hemácias extravasculares.

Gatos
• Exame direto das hemácias para pesquisa de hemoparasitas.
• Anemia regenerativa e esplenomegalia — podem indicar micoplasmose hemotrópica.
• Macrocitose e anemia arregenerativa — sugerem infecção por retrovírus ou doença mieloproliferativa.
• Eosinofilia — sugere síndrome hipereosinofílica, mastocitose sistêmica ou linfoma.
• Blastos circulantes — indicam distúrbio mieloproliferativo ou linfoproliferativo.
• Hemácias nucleadas — podem acompanhar hematopoiese extramedular e disfunção esplênica.
• Trombocitopenia — por aumento do consumo (CID), destruição aumentada (imunomediada), sequestro ou produção diminuída na medula óssea.

OUTROS TESTES LABORATORIAIS
• Teste de FeLV e FIV.
• Esfregaços da camada leucocitária — mastócitos circulantes (podem ocorrer com doença inflamatória e neoplasia); blastos.

ESPLENOMEGALIA

- Perfil de coagulação — CID comumente observada com hemangiossarcoma (inclui tempos de coagulação prolongados, hipofibrinogenemia e PDFs aumentados; dímeros D não são específicos para aplicação clínica nos diagnósticos diferenciais).

DIAGNÓSTICO POR IMAGEM
Radiografia Abdominal
- Confirma ou detecta a esplenomegalia.
- Pode aparecer um efeito expansivo (tipo massa) na porção mesoabdominal cranial esquerda.
- Pode fornecer indícios de alguma causa subjacente — hepatomegalia concomitante pode indicar doença infiltrativa ou cardiopatia direita; a torção esplênica pode ocorrer secundariamente à dilatação e vólvulo gástricos.
- Efusão — pode indicar hemorragia por ruptura esplênica (hemangiossarcoma, hematoma) ou hipertensão portal que exerce influência sobre a perfusão esplênica. A visualização da cauda esplênica ao longo da parede corporal ventral em radiografias laterais de gatos apoia o diagnóstico de esplenomegalia.

Radiografia Torácica
- Três projeções (lateral esquerda e direita, além de dorsoventral) — triagem para pesquisa de metástases e doença subjacente na cavidade torácica, além de efusão.
- Avaliação dos linfonodos esternais, sobretudo nos gatos — esses linfonodos realizam a drenagem da cavidade abdominal, refletindo distúrbios indutores de linfadenomegalia.

Ultrassonografia Abdominal
- Diferencia entre padrões parenquimatosos difusos e nodulares; as anormalidades nodulares são facilmente identificadas.
- Aumento difuso com parênquima normal — pode ocorrer em caso de congestão ou infiltração celular.
- Ecogenicidade reduzida — pode ser observada em casos de torção esplênica, trombose da veia esplênica, linfoma ou leucemia.
- Padrão ecogênico misto e complexo — hemangiossarcoma ou hematoma.
- Hematomas — ecogenicidade variável; podem apresentar septação interna e encapsulação, bem como passar por um estágio em que se assemelham a lesões em alvo sugestivas de neoplasia.
- Pode identificar doenças abdominais concomitantes em órgãos como fígado, rins, intestinos e linfonodos.
- Não é capaz de diferenciar entre distúrbios esplênicos benignos e malignos.
- O sinal de interrogação no Doppler de fluxo colorido pode detectar trombos da veia esplênica ou torção do baço.

Ecocardiografia
- Avaliação do átrio direito em busca de lesões expansivas tipo massa — indicada quando se suspeita de hemangiossarcoma (com base no aspecto ultrassonográfico e nos achados hematológicos).

MÉTODOS DIAGNÓSTICOS
Aspirado por Agulha Fina
- Método — colocar o paciente em decúbito lateral direito ou dorsal; utilizar agulha calibre 23 ou 25, com 2,5-3,75 cm de comprimento; para distúrbios difusos: pode-se aspirar sem o auxílio da ultrassonografia; para distúrbios nodulares: necessita da orientação ultrassonográfica.
- Método sem aspiração (em que NÃO se aplica uma pressão negativa à seringa) — resulta em uma recuperação maior de células nucleadas em relação à quantidade de sangue do que o método com aspiração.
- Amostras — submeter à avaliação citológica para a pesquisa de agentes infecciosos (encontrados com maior frequência nos macrófagos); identificar o tipo celular inflamatório ou infiltrativo predominante.
- Infiltrados neoplásicos — classificados como epiteliais, mesenquimais ou discretos (células redondas).
- Aspiração do baço — pode romper hemangiossarcoma.

Aspirado da Medula Óssea
- Indicado na presença de citopenias antes da esplenectomia (o baço pode ser a única fonte hematopoiética).
- Pode fornecer o diagnóstico de distúrbio infeccioso (p. ex., erliquiose, micose, toxoplasmose, leishmaniose) ou neoplasia hematopoiética.

TRATAMENTO
- Depende da causa subjacente; fornecer cuidados de enfermagem de suporte de acordo com a necessidade.
- É importante determinar se a esplenomegalia é pertinente de condições sistêmicas.
- Tratamento e prognóstico após a esplenectomia — baseiam-se nos aspectos histopatológicos: o hemangiossarcoma pode passar despercebido em alguns tumores em virtude de necrose regional, fazendo-se o diagnóstico de hematoma.

CONSIDERAÇÕES CIRÚRGICAS
Esplenectomia
- Na presença de anemia ou leucopenia — descartar aplasia/hipoplasia da medula óssea antes da cirurgia; o baço pode ser a fonte da hematopoiese.
- Indicada em casos de torção esplênica, ruptura esplênica, massas esplênicas isoladas provavelmente consideradas como neoplásicas e infiltração de mastócitos (gatos).
- Laparotomia exploratória — permite a avaliação direta de todos os órgãos abdominais.

MEDICAÇÕES
MEDICAMENTO(S)
Depende(m) da causa subjacente.

ACOMPANHAMENTO
MONITORIZAÇÃO DO PACIENTE
Arritmias ventriculares (cães) — associadas a lesões expansivas esplênicas ou torção esplênica; podem ocorrer antes, durante e até 3 dias depois da esplenectomia; avaliar (por meio de auscultação e eletrocardiograma) os candidatos cirúrgicos antes da anestesia; monitorização cardíaca contínua durante a cirurgia e no pós-operatório.

COMPLICAÇÕES POSSÍVEIS
- Paciente sem baço — risco elevado de infecção e hemoparasitismo.
- Sepse pós-operatória — complicação rara.
- Antibióticos — indicados nos pacientes sem o baço submetidos à terapia imunossupressora caso se observe algum sinal de infecção.
- Esplenectomia — pode comprometer a adaptação do cão à atividade física (por comprometimento nas adaptações de transporte do oxigênio).

DIVERSOS
FATORES RELACIONADOS COM A IDADE
As causas neoplásicas são mais prováveis em animais idosos.

POTENCIAL ZOONÓTICO
Uma variedade de doenças infecciosas pode envolver o baço.

VER TAMBÉM
Ver a seção "Causas".

ABREVIATURA(S)
- CID = coagulação intravascular disseminada.
- LES = lúpus eritematoso sistêmico.
- PDF = produtos de degradação da fibrina.
- PIF = peritonite infecciosa felina.
- FeLV = vírus da leucemia felina.
- FIV = vírus da imunodeficiência felina.

Sugestões de Leitura
Christensen NI, Canfield PJ, Martin PA, et al. Cytopathological and histopathological diagnosis of canine splenic disorders. Australian Vet J 2009, 87:175-181.
Hammer AS, Couto CG. Disorders of the lymph nodes and spleen. In: Scherding RG, ed., The Cat: Diseases and Clinical Management, 2nd ed. New York: Churchill Livingstone, 1994, pp. 671-689.
Neer MT. Clinical approach to splenomegaly in dogs and cats. Compend Contin Educ Pract Vet 1996, 18:35-48.
Spangler WL, Culbertson MR. Prevalence and type of splenic diseases in cats: 455 cases (1985-1991). JAVMA 1992, 201:773-776.
Spangler WL, Culbertson MR. Prevalence and type of splenic diseases in dogs: 1,480 cases (1985-1989). JAVMA 1992, 200:829-834.
Spangler WL, Kass PH. Pathologic factors affecting postsplenectomy survival in dogs. J Vet Intern Med 1997, 11:166-171.

Autor Cheryl E. Balkman
Consultor Editorial Sharon A. Center

ESPONDILOMIELOPATIA CERVICAL (SÍNDROME DE WOBBLER)

CONSIDERAÇÕES GERAIS

DEFINIÇÃO
• Espondilomielopatia cervical (EMC) ou síndrome de Wobbler é uma doença da coluna cervical de raças caninas de porte grande e gigante.
• EMC é caracterizada por compressão da medula espinal e/ou das raízes nervosas, o que leva a déficits neurológicos e/ou cervicalgia (dor no pescoço).

FISIOPATOLOGIA
• A fisiopatologia envolve uma lesão compressiva causada por herniação de disco intervertebral, má-formação óssea, ou ambas, em um canal vertebral estenótico.
• Compressão associada ao disco — cães >3 anos. A degeneração do disco intervertebral e a subsequente protrusão podem ser secundárias à articulação de faceta articular anormal em Doberman pinschers, o que predispõe ao aumento do esforço rotacional nos discos intervertebrais.
• Má-formação vertebral (compressão óssea associada) — observada mais comumente em raças gigantes de cães, em geral naqueles jovens adultos (<3 anos). A má-formação óssea pode comprimir a medula espinal nos sentidos dorsoventral (má-formação do arco vertebral), dorsolateral (má-formação do processo articular) ou lateral (má-formação pedicular).
• Compressão dinâmica da medula espinal (aquela que se altera com os movimentos da coluna cervical) sempre é um componente da fisiopatologia em qualquer tipo de compressão.
• As evidências atuais não sugerem que a instabilidade desempenhe um papel primário na patogênese da EMC.

SISTEMA(S) ACOMETIDO(S)
Nervoso.

GENÉTICA
• Base hereditária proposta para as raças Borzoi e Basset hound.
• Não há dados definitivos sobre a hereditariedade da ECM em Doberman pinschers.

INCIDÊNCIA/PREVALÊNCIA
A ECM é provavelmente o distúrbio neurológico mais comum da coluna cervical de raças caninas de porte grande e gigante.

DISTRIBUIÇÃO GEOGRÁFICA
N/D.

IDENTIFICAÇÃO
Raça(s) Predominante(s)
• Os cães da raça Doberman pinscher são os mais comumente acometidos, com cerca de 50% dos casos observados nessa raça.
• Outras raças com uma alta incidência incluem Dinamarquês, Rottweiler, Weimaraner, e Dálmata. A ECM pode ser observada em qualquer raça, inclusive naquelas de pequeno porte.

Idade Média e Faixa Etária
• Nos cães Doberman pinschers e outras raças de grande porte, o problema costuma se apresentar com >3 anos de idade, com uma idade média de 6 anos.
• Os cães de raças gigantes geralmente apresentam o problema com <3 anos de idade, embora as manifestações tardias possam ser observadas.

Sexo Predominante
Os machos são levemente super-representados.

SINAIS CLÍNICOS
Comentários Gerais
• A apresentação clínica clássica corresponde a uma ataxia lentamente progressiva dos membros pélvicos com envolvimento menos grave dos membros torácicos.

Achados Anamnésicos
• Uma disfunção crônica lentamente progressiva da marcha é característica. As apresentações agudas costumam ser associadas à dor no pescoço. Ocasionalmente, observa-se o agravamento agudo de um cão com histórico crônico.
• A dor no pescoço ou hiperestesia cervical é um achado anamnésico comum, que ocorre em aproximadamente 65-70% dos Dobermans e 40-50% de outras raças.

Achados do Exame Neurológico
• A dor no pescoço constitui a principal queixa em 5-10% dos pacientes.
• A marcha é caracterizada por ataxia proprioceptiva e paresia (fraqueza). A ataxia e a paresia são mais evidentes nos membros pélvicos com lesões na porção caudal da coluna cervical (C5-6, C6-7). Lesões compressivas na coluna cervical média tendem a causar ataxia em todos os quatro membros.
• A marcha dos membros torácicos pode parecer de passos curtos, espástica com aparência oscilante, ou muito fraca.
• Os déficits proprioceptivos costumam estar presentes, mas os cães com ataxia crônica podem não exibi-los. A análise da marcha (ataxia) fornece uma indicação mais sensível de mielopatia do que os déficits proprioceptivos.
• Os cães podem se apresentar sem deambulação.
• Em alguns casos, podem ser observadas as alterações de atrofia do músculo supraespinal e desgaste das unhas dos dedos.
• O tônus dos músculos extensores costuma estar aumentado em todos os quatro membros.
• Os reflexos patelares permanecem normais ou aumentados. Pode ser difícil eliciar o reflexo flexor nos membros torácicos em virtude do aumento do tônus extensor.

CAUSAS
• Internação hospitalar caso se eleja o tratamento cirúrgico.
• Nutrição — foi proposto o consumo excessivo de proteína, cálcio e calorias em Dinamarquês. A nutrição não parece desempenhar um papel no desenvolvimento de EMC em raças caninas de grande porte.
• A causa da EMC é provavelmente multifatorial.

FATORES DE RISCO
• Conformação corporal — foram propostos cabeça grande e pescoço longo, mas estudos mais recentes não descobriram qualquer correlação entre as dimensões do corpo e a incidência de EMC.
• Também foi proposta uma rápida taxa de crescimento, mas isso não foi confirmado por outros estudos.

DIAGNÓSTICO

DIAGNÓSTICO DIFERENCIAL
• Distúrbios ortopédicos, como displasia coxofemoral e ruptura do ligamento cruzado. Diferenciados pelo exame neurológico (ausência de ataxia).
• Neoplasia espinal, cistos subaracnoides espinais, cistos sinoviais espinais, discospondilite, osteomielite, meningomielite, traumatismo. Diferenciados pelos resultados dos exames de radiografias simples, análise do LCS, mielografia, TC ou RM.

HEMOGRAMA/BIOQUÍMICA/URINÁLISE
N/D.

OUTROS TESTES LABORATORIAIS
N/D.

DIAGNÓSTICO POR IMAGEM
Radiografias Cervicais Simples
• As radiografias simples servem como uma ferramenta de triagem para descartar distúrbios ósseos. Embora possa ser visto estreitamento do disco intervertebral ou ponto de inflexão vertebral, esses achados não são específicos para EMC, pois podem ser observados em raças caninas de grande porte clinicamente normais.
• Alterações osteoartríticas dos processos articulares podem ser observadas em raças gigantes.

Mielografia
• A mielografia pode definir a(s) localização(ões) e a direção (ventral, dorsal, lateral) da compressão da medula espinal. Projeções obtidas sob estresse (flexão ou extensão) podem causar um risco significativo de deterioração neurológica. A mielografia por tração linear é um procedimento mais seguro, capaz de distinguir lesões estáticas e dinâmicas.

Técnicas Avançadas de Diagnóstico por Imagem
• Mielografia por TC — visualização transversal da compressão da medula espinal e determinação dos locais com atrofia da medula espinal.
• RM — visualização de estruturas como parênquima da medula espinal, disco intervertebral, tecidos moles e raízes nervosas; as imagens podem ser obtidas nos planos sagitais, transversais e dorsais. Alterações de sinal da medula espinal permitem uma identificação mais precisa do principal local de compressão em comparação aos exames de TC e mielografia.

MÉTODOS DIAGNÓSTICOS
Análise do LCS — geralmente normal; pode ser observada leve pleocitose mista ou neutrofílica em cães com apresentações agudas; é possível a observação de concentrações proteicas elevadas nas apresentações crônicas.

ACHADOS PATOLÓGICOS
• Desmielinização do trato da substância branca da medula espinal no local de compressão medular. A ocorrência de dano axonal pode levar à degeneração walleriana nos tratos ascendente e descendente da substância branca.
• Alterações como perda neuronal, gliose e necrose podem ser observadas na substância cinzenta.
• Compressão crônica, grave e focal da medula espinal pode levar à mielomalacia focal.

TRATAMENTO

CUIDADO(S) DE SAÚDE ADEQUADO(S)
• Internação hospitalar caso se eleja o tratamento cirúrgico.

Espondilomielopatia Cervical (Síndrome de Wobbler)

- Tratamento ambulatorial caso se escolha a terapia médica.

CUIDADO(S) DE ENFERMAGEM
- Cães sem deambulação — manter os pacientes em camas macias e alternar o lado de decúbito a cada 4 horas para evitar a formação de úlceras.
- Cateterização vesical.
- A fisioterapia é essencial não só para evitar atrofia muscular e ancilose, mas também para acelerar a recuperação.

ATIVIDADE
- É recomendável a restrição da atividade física por pelo menos 2 meses para os cães submetidos a tratamento médico.
- A restrição da atividade também é importante nos 2 ou 3 primeiros meses do pós-operatório para permitir a fusão do osso e evitar o deslocamento do implante.

DIETA
- Evitar a ingestão excessiva de proteína, cálcio ou calorias em raças caninas de porte gigante com compressão óssea.

ORIENTAÇÃO AO PROPRIETÁRIO
- Informar ao proprietário que a cirurgia oferece as melhores chances de restabelecimento do animal (cerca de 80%), mas há um risco de 1-5% de complicações significativas associadas aos procedimentos cirúrgicos cervicais.

CONSIDERAÇÕES CIRÚRGICAS
- Fenda ventral — técnica comumente utilizada e recomendada para compressões ventrais isoladas. Também pode ser usada para compressões ventrais múltiplas.
- Laminectomia dorsal — principal indicação para compressões dorsais ou dorsolaterais. Também pode ser usada para compressões ventrais múltiplas.
- Técnicas de distração/estabilização/fusão são recomendadas para compressões ventrais dinâmicas únicas ou múltiplas. Artroplastia de disco cervical — permite o restabelecimento da largura normal do disco com preservação do movimento do segmento acometido. Também permite a descompressão direta da medula espinal, porque a técnica de fenda ventral é realizada antes da inserção do disco de titânio. A artroplastia de disco é amplamente utilizada no tratamento de EMC em seres humanos.
- A taxa de recorrência gira em torno de 20% com qualquer técnica cirúrgica.
- A fenestração fornece uma taxa de sucesso muito baixa e não é recomendada.

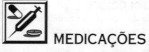

MEDICAÇÕES

MEDICAMENTO(S) DE ESCOLHA
- Corticosteroides — dexametasona 0,1-0,25 mg/kg a cada 24 h. Os cães com EMC parecem responder melhor à dexametasona do que à prednisona em princípio. O uso de prednisona na dose de 1 mg/kg a cada 24 h, com redução progressiva da dosagem e da frequência, é a abordagem mais comum para uso moderado a prolongado. Na maioria dos cães, pode-se interromper a prednisona depois de 4-8 semanas de tratamento.

CONTRAINDICAÇÕES
N/D.

PRECAUÇÕES
Monitorizar o paciente quanto à ocorrência de sinais de gastrenterite, hemorragia gástrica e cistite.

INTERAÇÕES POSSÍVEIS
Não usar corticosteroides em combinação com AINEs.

MEDICAMENTO(S) ALTERNATIVO(S)
AINEs como meloxicam na dose de 0,1 mg/kg a cada 24 h podem ser utilizados em cães com hiperestesia cervical ou leve ataxia apenas.

ACOMPANHAMENTO

MONITORIZAÇÃO DO PACIENTE
Repetir a avaliação neurológica, quantas vezes for necessária, para monitorizar a resposta ao tratamento.

PREVENÇÃO
- É recomendável evitar atividade excessiva, bem como pulos, saltos e corridas.
- Evitar o uso de coleiras cervicais; optar pelos modelos peitorais.

COMPLICAÇÕES POSSÍVEIS
- Podem ocorrer crises convulsivas e deterioração neurológica transitória após o exame de mielografia.
- Também pode ocorrer recorrência dos sinais clínicos em cães tratados por meios médicos ou cirúrgicos.

EVOLUÇÃO ESPERADA E PROGNÓSTICO
- Cerca de 80% dos pacientes melhoram com a cirurgia.
- Aproximadamente 50% dos pacientes melhoram com o tratamento médico (restrição da atividade física ± corticosteroides) e 25% permanecem estáveis.

DIVERSOS

DISTÚRBIOS ASSOCIADOS
Miocardiopatia dilatada, hipotireoidismo e doença de von Willebrand são comuns em cães da raça Doberman pinscher. Essas doenças podem influenciar as opções diagnósticas e terapêuticas. Os Doberman pinschers com suspeita de EMC devem ser submetidos à avaliação de rotina para pesquisa desses distúrbios.

FATORES RELACIONADOS COM A IDADE
- Cães jovens de porte gigante ou grande — má-formação vertebral e compressão medular.
- Cães mais idosos — compressão associada ao disco.

POTENCIAL ZOONÓTICO
N/D.

GESTAÇÃO/FERTILIDADE/REPRODUÇÃO
N/D.

SINÔNIMOS
- Má-formação/Má-articulação cervical.
- Espondilopatia cervical.
- Instabilidade vertebral cervical.

VER TAMBÉM
Discopatia Intervertebral — Gatos.

ABREVIATURA(S)
- AINE = anti-inflamatórios não esteroides.
- EMC = espondilomielopatia cervical.
- LCS = líquido cerebrospinal.
- RM = ressonância magnética.
- TC = tomografia computadorizada.

Sugestões de Leitura
Burbidge HM. A review of wobbler syndrome in the Doberman pinscher. Aust Vet Pract 1995, 25:147-156.
da Costa RC. Cervical spondylomyelopathy (wobbler syndrome). Vet Clin North Am Small Anim Pract 2010, 40:881-913.
da Costa RC, Parent JM. Outcome of medical and surgical treatment in dogs with cervical spondylomyelopathy: 104 cases. JAVMA 2008, 233:1284-1290.
da Costa RC, Parent JP, Dobson H, et al. Comparison of magnetic resonance imaging and myelography in 18 Doberman pinscher dogs with cervical spondylomyelopathy. Vet Radiol Ultrasound 2006, 47:523-531.
da Costa RC, Parent JM, Partlow G, et al. Morphologic and morphometric magnetic resonance imaging features of Doberman pinscher dogs with and without clinical signs of cervical spondylomyelopathy. Am J Vet Res 2006, 67:1601-1612.
Jeffery ND, McKee WM. Surgery for disc-associated wobbler syndrome in the dog – an examination of the controversy. J Small Anim Pract 2001, 42:574-581.

Autor Ronaldo Casimiro da Costa
Consultor Editorial Joane M. Parent

ESPONDILOSE DEFORMANTE

CONSIDERAÇÕES GERAIS

REVISÃO
- Distúrbio degenerativo não inflamatório da coluna vertebral, caracterizado pela produção de osteófitos ao longo das faces ventral, lateral e dorsolateral das placas terminais vertebrais.
- Localização mais comum — cães: coluna toracolombar na área da vértebra anticlinal* e das vértebras lombares superiores; gatos: vértebras torácicas relatadas em 68% dos gatos domésticos assintomáticos.

IDENTIFICAÇÃO
- Cães e gatos.
- Cães — comumente observada nas raças de grande porte, particularmente Pastor alemão; também afeta animais das raças Boxer, Airedale terrier e Cocker spaniel.
- A ocorrência aumenta com a idade; 50% dos cães têm em torno de 6 anos e 75%, por volta de 9 anos; pode ser evidenciada nos cães jovens com predisposição hereditária.
- As fêmeas são mais acometidas que os machos.

SINAIS CLÍNICOS
Comentários Gerais
- Os pacientes tipicamente se encontram assintomáticos; as lesões são de menor importância clínica.
- A dor pode acompanhar a fratura de esporões ou pontes ósseas.

Achados Anamnésicos
- Rigidez.
- Movimento restrito.
- Dor.

Achados do Exame Físico
- Déficits neurológicos atribuídos à compressão da medula espinal ou de raiz nervosa são raros.

CAUSAS E FATORES DE RISCO
- Microtraumatismo repetido.
- Traumatismos maiores.
- Predisposição hereditária.

DIAGNÓSTICO

DIAGNÓSTICO DIFERENCIAL
- Discospondilite — diferenciada por evidência radiográfica de lise da placa terminal.
- Osteoartrite espinal — degeneração das facetas articulares das articulações.

HEMOGRAMA/BIOQUÍMICA/URINÁLISE
Normais.

OUTROS TESTES LABORATORIAIS
N/D.

DIAGNÓSTICO POR IMAGEM
Radiografia da coluna vertebral — inicialmente revela osteófitos sob a forma de projeções triangulares a alguns milímetros da margem do corpo vertebral; com a evolução, parecem unir o espaço intervertebral; é rara a constatação de anquilose verdadeira.

MÉTODOS DIAGNÓSTICOS
Mielografia e TC ou RM — para casos raros; demonstram a presença de osteófito dorsal atípico, comprimindo a medula espinal ou as raízes nervosas ou invadindo estruturas críticas de tecido mole.

TRATAMENTO

- Informar ao proprietário que o distúrbio costuma ser um achado assintomático e acidental, além de possivelmente não ser responsável pelos sinais clínicos.
- Dorsalgia ou déficits neurológicos — fazer avaliação diagnóstica da coluna vertebral.
- Espondilose — tratar como paciente de ambulatório com repouso estrito e administração de analgésico ou, possivelmente, acupuntura.
- Obesidade — é recomendável a implementação de programa de redução do peso.

MEDICAÇÕES

MEDICAMENTO(S)
Utilizar apenas quando o paciente estiver apresentando os sinais.

AINEs
- Preferíveis em relação aos esteroides nos cães a menos que o paciente apresente déficits neurológicos por provocarem menos efeitos colaterais; administrar após as refeições.
- Carprofeno (Rimadyl®) — 2,2 mg/kg VO a cada 12 h nos cães.
- Etodolaco (Etogesic®) — 5-15 mg/kg uma vez ao dia nos cães.
- Deracoxibe (Deramaxx®) — 1-2 mg/kg uma vez ao dia nos cães.
- Meloxicam (Metacam®) — 0,2 mg/kg uma única vez e, depois, 0,1 mg/kg a cada 24 h nos cães; 0,2 mg/kg uma única vez, seguido por 0,1 mg/kg a cada 24 h por 2 dias e, então, 0,025 mg/kg 2-3 vezes/semana nos gatos.
- Tepoxalina (Zubrin®) — 20 mg/kg no primeiro dia e, depois, 10 mg/kg a cada 24 h nos cães.
- Paracetamol (Tylenol®) — 5 mg/kg a cada 12 h VO apenas nos cães; analgésico sem ação de AINE.
- Em caso de sensibilidade GI, utilizar em combinação com algum antiácido (cimetidina a 6-10 mg/kg VO a cada 8 h ou ranitidina a 1-2 mg/kg VO a cada 12 h ou famotidina a 0,5-1 mg/kg a cada 24 h ou omeprazol a 0,5-1 mg/kg a cada 24 h) ou algum protetor gastrintestinal (misoprostol a 3-5 μg/kg VO a cada 6-8 h ou sucralfato a 0,5-1 g a cada 8 h) para diminuir a possibilidade de ulceração gastrintestinal.

Corticosteroides
- Prednisona — 0,5-1 mg/kg dividido a cada 12 h; reduzir gradativamente para dias alternados ou menos, se possível.
- Usar apenas em pacientes com déficits neurológicos.
- Acupuntura — a aplicação de agulha seca ou eletroacupuntura em intervalos semanais ou quinzenais e reduzidos conforme a necessidade pode ser muito eficaz no alívio da dor; valiosa nos animais intolerantes à medicação ou quando os proprietários preferem a "medicina alternativa natural".

CONTRAINDICAÇÕES/INTERAÇÕES POSSÍVEIS
- Paracetamol (Tylenol®) — não utilizar nos gatos.
- Evitar a administração prolongada dos AINEs ou a combinação de AINEs e esteroides por causa do risco de ulceração gastrintestinal.

ACOMPANHAMENTO

- Retornar o animal gradativamente à atividade normal após o desaparecimento dos sinais há várias semanas.
- Podem ocorrer recidivas com atividade extenuante.

DIVERSOS

ABREVIATURA(S)
- AINEs = anti-inflamatórios não esteroides.
- GI = gastrintestinal.
- RM = ressonância magnética.
- TC = tomografia computadorizada.

Sugestões de Leitura
Morgan JP, Hansson K, Miyabayashi T. Spondylosis deformans in the female beagle dog: A radiographic study. J Small Anim Pract 1989, 30(8):457-460.
Romatowski J. Spondylosis deformans in the dog. Compend Contin Educ Pract Vet 1986, 8:531-536.

Autor Richard J. Joseph
Consultor Editorial Joane M. Parent

---

* N.T.: Diz-se de vértebra torácica que tem espinha neural situada em sentido contrário à da espinha neural adjacente.

ESPOROTRICOSE

CONSIDERAÇÕES GERAIS

REVISÃO
- Doença fúngica zoonótica que pode acometer o tegumento, os vasos linfáticos ou ser generalizada.
- Provocada pelo fungo dimórfico ubíquo *Sporothrix schenkii*, via inoculação direta.

IDENTIFICAÇÃO
- Cães e gatos. • Raça Doberman pinscher — pode ser predisposta à doença multicêntrica.

SINAIS CLÍNICOS
- Cães — forma cutânea: inúmeros nódulos, que podem drenar ou formar crostas, acometendo tipicamente a cabeça ou o tronco. • Gatos — forma cutânea: as lesões quase sempre aparecem, no início, como feridas ou abscessos que mimetizam ferimentos associados a brigas, encontrados na cabeça, na região lombar ou na parte distal dos membros. • Forma cutaneolinfática — corresponde, em geral, à extensão da forma cutânea através dos vasos linfáticos, resultando na formação de novos nódulos e trajetos drenantes ou crostas; a linfadenopatia é comum. • Forma disseminada — sinais sistêmicos de mal-estar e febre.

CAUSAS E FATORES DE RISCO
- Cães — animais de caça em função de feridas penetrantes associadas a espinhos ou farpas.
- Gatos — machos intactos de vida livre em virtude de brigas.
- Animais expostos a solo rico em material orgânico em decomposição são predispostos.
- Exposição a animais infectados ou gatos clinicamente saudáveis que compartilham o mesmo ambiente com algum gato acometido é um fator de risco.
- Doença imunossupressora também constitui um fator de risco.
- Prevalência elevada em regiões tropicais e subtropicais.

DIAGNÓSTICO

ATENÇÃO: A esporotricose é uma doença zoonótica e, por essa razão, devem ser tomadas medidas de precaução adequadas para evitar a infecção. A ausência de solução de continuidade na pele não protege o animal contra a doença.

DIAGNÓSTICO DIFERENCIAL
- Processos infecciosos — doenças bacterianas e fúngicas que se apresentam com nódulos e trajetos drenantes (p. ex., criptococose, blastomicose, lepra felina, histoplasmose). • Neoplasia. • Infecção bacteriana profunda. • Parasitas — *Demodex* ou *Pelodera*.

HEMOGRAMA/BIOQUÍMICA/URINÁLISE
Nenhuma alteração a menos que esteja associada à doença generalizada.

OUTROS TESTES LABORATORIAIS
- Culturas do tecido profundamente acometido.
- ATENÇÃO: a esporotricose trata-se de uma doença zoonótica; os funcionários do laboratório devem ser alertados sobre o possível diagnóstico diferencial; as culturas não devem ser tentadas até que outros diagnósticos diferenciais tenham sido eliminados.

MÉTODOS DIAGNÓSTICOS
- Citologia de exsudatos — pode-se encontrar a levedura arredondada em forma de charuto no meio intracelular ou livre no exsudato.
- Biopsia — microrganismos geralmente numerosos, sobretudo nos gatos; colorações fúngicas especiais (PAS ou metenamina argêntica de Gomori) podem auxiliar no diagnóstico; a ausência de microrganismos demonstráveis nos tecidos de cães não exclui o diagnóstico.

TRATAMENTO

- A natureza zoonótica da esporotricose deve ser considerada ao se tratar um animal acometido por essa doença. • A terapia ambulatorial pode ser uma consideração, embora aumente o potencial de exposição humana.

MEDICAÇÕES

MEDICAMENTO(S)

Solução Supersaturada de Iodeto de Potássio
- Tratamento de escolha do ponto de vista histórico — cães: 40 mg/kg VO a cada 8 h juntamente com o alimento; gatos: 10-20 mg/kg VO a cada 12 h juntamente com o alimento.
- Tratar por, no mínimo, 2 meses e continuar por 30 dias após a resolução das lesões clínicas.
- Cães — se os sinais de iodismo forem notados (pelagem ressecada, escamas em excesso, secreção oculonasal, vômito, depressão ou colapso), interromper a solução por 1 semana; em caso de sintomas leves, reiniciar com a mesma dose; se os sintomas forem graves ou recidivantes, deve-se considerar o uso de outros medicamentos.
- Gatos — sinais de iodismo (depressão, vômito, anorexia, fasciculação, hipotermia e colapso cardiovascular) são mais comuns; se observados, é recomendável a interrupção do medicamento.

Cetoconazol e Itraconazol
- Apresentam resultados animadores no tratamento de doenças fúngicas em cães e gatos.
- Cães:
  - Cetoconazol: 5-15 mg/kg VO a cada 12 h até 1 mês após a resolução clínica ou por, no mínimo, 2 meses; a resolução deve ocorrer dentro de aproximadamente 3 meses; os efeitos colaterais são relativamente brandos, sendo a anorexia o mais comum.
  - Itraconazol: sob a formulação de cápsulas na dose de 5-10 mg/kg a cada 12-24 h por, no mínimo, 2 meses; menos efeitos colaterais são observados com a dose mais baixa de 5 mg/kg a cada 24 h; com frequência, é mais bem tolerado do que o cetoconazol; há relatos de hepatopatia e vasculite agudas (ver "Dermatofitose").
- Gatos:
  - Cetoconazol: 5-10 mg/kg VO a cada 12-24 h por 1-2 meses além da cura clínica; os distúrbios gastrintestinais são mais comumente observados nos gatos do que outros efeitos colaterais como depressão, febre, icterícia e sinais neurológicos.
  - Itraconazol: 15 mg/kg VO a cada 24 h por, no mínimo, 1 mês após a cura clínica; tratamento de escolha para os gatos (mais eficaz e menos efeitos colaterais); a dosagem da suspensão oral (contendo ciclodextrina) é de 1,25-1,5 mg/kg a cada 24 h.
- Não é recomendável a formulação manipulada de itraconazol em virtude da absorção potencialmente inconstante; a suspensão oral é mais eficiente se administrada com o estômago vazio para melhorar a absorção.

ACOMPANHAMENTO

MONITORIZAÇÃO DO PACIENTE
É recomendada a reavaliação do animal a cada 2-4 semanas, incluindo a mensuração das enzimas hepáticas.

PREVENÇÃO
Determinar a fonte da infecção original, se possível, para evitar infecções repetidas.

EVOLUÇÃO ESPERADA E PROGNÓSTICO
- Não se deve esperar falha na resposta terapêutica.
- Nesse caso, deve-se considerar o uso de tratamento alternativo ou esquema terapêutico combinado (solução supersaturada de iodeto de potássio e cetoconazol).
- Os agentes fluconazol e terbinafina continuam relativamente sem teste, mas podem se mostrar promissores para o tratamento.

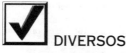

DIVERSOS

POTENCIAL ZOONÓTICO
- ATENÇÃO: doença zoonótica que exige a tomada de medidas de precaução adequadas para evitar a infecção.
- A orientação do proprietário é de suma importância.
- A ausência de solução de continuidade na pele não protege o animal contra a doença.
- Há relatos de transmissão zoonótica a partir de mordidas e arranhões de roedores, papagaios, gatos, cães, cavalos e tatus.
- Os gatos clinicamente saudáveis que compartilham o mesmo ambiente com algum gato infectado podem ser uma fonte de infecção.

ABREVIATURA(S)
- PAS = ácido periódico de Schiff.

Sugestões de Leitura
Hirano M, Watanabe K, Murakami M, Kano R, Yanai T, Yamazoe K, Fukata T, Kudo T. A case of feline sporotrichosis. J Vet Med Sci 2006, 68:283-284.
Lima Barros MB, Oliveira Schubach A, Valle ACF, Galhardo MCG, et al. Cat-transmitted sporotrichosis epidemic in Rio de Janeiro, Brazil: Description of a series of cases. Clin Infect Dis 2004, 38:529-535.
Rosser EJ, Dunstan RW. Sporotrichosis. In: Greene CE, ed., Infectious Diseases of the Dog and Cat, 3rd ed. St. Louis: Saunders Elsevier, 2006, pp. 550-569.
Scott DW, Miller WH, Griffin CE. Muller & Kirk's Small Animal Dermatology, 6th ed. Philadelphia: Saunders, 2001, pp. 386-390, 410-415.

Autores W. Dunbar Gram e Marlene Pariser
Consultor Editorial Alexander H. Werner

Esquistossomíase Canina (Heterobilharzíase)

CONSIDERAÇÕES GERAIS

REVISÃO
- *Heterobilharzia americanum* — parasita esquistossomatídeo de guaxinins.
- Os ovos eliminados nas fezes dos guaxinins eclodem para liberar miracídios que penetram nos caramujos hospedeiros de água doce. Após um período de desenvolvimento e multiplicação assexuada, os caramujos liberam cercárias que infectam o hospedeiro seguinte (podem ser os cães) por penetração cutânea. Depois de penetrarem na pele, as larvas sofrem migração para o pulmão e, em seguida, prosseguem sua trajetória para as veias mesentéricas, onde machos e fêmeas separados formam pares. Os ovos postos pelas fêmeas dos vermes são conduzidos até a parede intestinal, onde promovem erosão em seu trajeto pelo lúmen para serem eliminados nas fezes. Outros ovos são transportados para o fígado ou para outros órgãos pela corrente sanguínea, onde se alojam e provocam doença granulomatosa.
- Os cães são infectados quando entram em contato com água doce contendo cercárias.
- Restrita aos guaxinins no sudoeste dos Estados Unidos. Casos caninos relatados em regiões como Texas, Flórida, Louisiana e Carolina do Norte.

IDENTIFICAÇÃO
Cães, tipicamente adultos, que têm acesso a áreas pantanosas ou alagadiças.

SINAIS CLÍNICOS
- Letargia (sinal clínico mais comum), perda de peso e diminuição do apetite constituem os sinais mais comumente apresentados.
- Outros sinais incluem vômito, diarreia, anorexia e poliúria/polidipsia; mais raramente se observam melena e borborigmo.

CAUSAS E FATORES DE RISCO
Nadar em água doce em áreas contaminadas com cercárias provenientes de miracídios.

DIAGNÓSTICO

DIAGNÓSTICO DIFERENCIAL
- Coccidiose.
- Diarreia bacteriana.
- Enterite viral.

HEMOGRAMA/BIOQUÍMICA/URINÁLISE
- Anemia e eosinofilia leves.
- Proteinúria.
- Possível hipercalemia.

OUTROS TESTES LABORATORIAIS
Teste ELISA — realizado por laboratório particular, College of Veterinary Medicine (Faculdade de Medicina Veterinária), North Carolina State University (Universidade do Estado da Carolina do Norte).

DIAGNÓSTICO POR IMAGEM
Radiografias contrastadas e ultrassom podem revelar o espessamento das paredes intestinais.

MÉTODOS DIAGNÓSTICOS
- Os ovos com miracídios podem ser identificados nas fezes, porém as fezes devem ser mantidas em solução salina — não na água — ou os miracídios eclodirão espontaneamente, tornando impossível o diagnóstico.
- Identificação dos ovos por meio de flutuação fecal com o uso de solução de açúcar com densidade 1,3 ou sedimentação fecal. A flutuação fecal de rotina não detectará esses ovos pesados.
- Diversos casos anteriores foram diagnosticados após laparotomia.

TRATAMENTO

Os cuidados fornecidos ao paciente internado durante os primeiros dias do tratamento provavelmente são justificáveis, já que a resposta à morte do verme poderá necessitar de cuidados de suporte.

MEDICAÇÕES

MEDICAMENTO(S)
- Praziquantel (50 mg/kg, VO, uma vez).
- Fembendazol (50 mg/kg, VO, a cada 24 h, durante 10 dias).

ACOMPANHAMENTO

Verificar as fezes depois de 12 meses para garantir que não contenham ovos.

DIVERSOS

No Japão e em outros países com *Schistosoma japonicum* endêmico, os cães podem ser infectados com essa espécie humana e zoonótica.

POTENCIAL ZOONÓTICO
Os estágios no cão não representam qualquer risco para as pessoas que os manipulam nem para os proprietários. As pessoas que entram nas mesmas águas podem desenvolver lesões.

SINÔNIMO(S)
Esquistossomose.

ABREVIATURA(S)
- ELISA = ensaio imunoabsorvente ligado à enzima.

Sugestões de Leitura
Fabrick C, Bugbee A, Fosgate, G. Clinical features and outcome of Heterobilharzia americana infection in dogs. J Vet Intern Med 2010, 24:140-144.
Flowers JR, Hammerberg B, Wood SL, et al. *Heterobilharzia americana* infection in a dog. JAVMA 2002, 220:193-196.

Autor Dwight D. Bowman
Consultor Editorial Stephen C. Barr

ESTEATITE

CONSIDERAÇÕES GERAIS

REVISÃO
- Esteatite consiste na inflamação do tecido adiposo (gorduroso); pode ser chamada de "doença da gordura amarela".
- A nutrição está envolvida na patologia da condição. A ingestão de grandes quantidades de gorduras insaturadas na dieta sem atividade antioxidante suficiente (na maioria dos casos, é comum a deficiência de vitamina E) pode resultar na peroxidação com subsequente necrose da gordura e esteatite. A esteatite também pode ocorrer secundariamente a infecção, distúrbio inflamatório, vasculopatia, neoplasia e doença imunomediada. Alguns casos são associados a dietas à base de peixe ou derivados de peixe, enquanto outros são idiopáticos.
- Doença rara, que se torna menos prevalente com a adição de antioxidantes às rações comerciais padrão.

IDENTIFICAÇÃO
Espécies
- Predominantemente gatos.
- Relatada em cães com doenças concomitantes (p. ex., carcinoma pancreático).

Idade Média e Faixa Etária
- Gatos jovens a meia-idade (4 meses-7 anos).
- Cães mais idosos.

SINAIS CLÍNICOS
- Apetite reduzido (hiporexia).
- Letargia, fadiga, dor generalizada.
- Relutância a se mover, saltar, brincar.
- Dor à manipulação ou palpação abdominal.
- Febre.
- Tecido subcutâneo nodular (gordura) e pelagem opaca, além de pele oleosa e escamosa.

CAUSAS E FATORES DE RISCO
- Deficiência da vitamina E.
- Capacidade antioxidante diminuída, com subsequente peroxidação lipídica mediada pelos radicais livres.
- Dieta à base de óleo de peixe (atum vermelho, peixe branco, sardinhas, cavala, arenque, bacalhau); raramente, dieta à base de fígado.
- Dieta caseira com grande quantidade de peixe ou cérebro de porco.
- Grandes quantidades de ácidos graxos insaturados na dieta.
- Pancreatite ou carcinoma pancreático.
- Infecção (viral, fúngica, bacteriana).
- Doença imunomediada, neoplasia.
- Traumatismo, pressão, frio, corpo estranho.
- Radioterapia, irradiação.
- Idiopática.

DIAGNÓSTICO

DIAGNÓSTICO DIFERENCIAL
- Osteodistrofia nutricional.
- Peritonite (qualquer causa).
- Abscesso subcutâneo, infecção.
- Meningite espinal, hiperestesia (qualquer causa).
- PIF.
- Miosite (qualquer causa).
- Doença pancreática.

HEMOGRAMA/BIOQUÍMICA/URINÁLISE
- Leucocitose neutrofílica grave +/– desvio à esquerda.
- Leve anemia normocítica normocrômica.
- Possível hipocalcemia.
- Eosinofilia ocasional.
- Alterações inespecíficas atribuídas à inflamação/febre (atividade enzimática hepática levemente elevada, elevação da creatina quinase, azotemia).
- Resultados do teste sanguíneo indicativos de distúrbio concomitante.

OUTROS TESTES LABORATORIAIS
- Citologia de aspirado por agulha fina (neutrófilos e macrófagos, ± bactérias).
- Cultura fúngica/bacteriana.
- Teste para detecção de FeLV/FIV.

DIAGNÓSTICO POR IMAGEM
- Gordura subcutânea, inguinal ou falciforme mosqueada.
- Perda de contraste na cavidade abdominal.

MÉTODOS DIAGNÓSTICOS
- Biopsia.
- Histologia (H&E, PAS, Ziehl-Neelsen).

ACHADOS PATOLÓGICOS
- Gordura subcutânea granulosa protuberante.
- Coloração da gordura corporal normal a amarelo-alaranjado.
- Edema gorduroso, mineralização, necrose com infiltrado inflamatório.
- Predominantemente neutrófilos, inflamação mista, incluindo linfócitos, plasmócitos e macrófagos, além de adipócitos necróticos.
- Paniculite piogranulomatosa lobular e septal.
- Pigmento ceroide intra/extracelular (produto inerte da peroxidação de ácidos graxos insaturados).

TRATAMENTO

CUIDADO(S) DE ENFERMAGEM
- Atenção ao nível de conforto do paciente.
- Medidas para estimular o apetite.
- Tratamento dos distúrbios concomitantes.

ATIVIDADE
Limitada em função do desconforto.

DIETA
- Remover os produtos à base de peixe da dieta.
- Fornecer ração comercial balanceada e completa para gatos.
- Talvez haja necessidade de nutrição enteral (p. ex., sonda de gastrostomia endoscópica percutânea e sonda de alimentação inserida via esofagostomia).

ORIENTAÇÃO AO PROPRIETÁRIO
- Importância da dieta balanceada.
- Quaisquer alterações na dieta felina devem ser feitas de forma gradativa.

MEDICAÇÕES

MEDICAMENTO(S)
- Vitamina E (acetato de α-tocoferol, 10-25 UI VO a cada 12 h).
- Corticosteroides na dose anti-inflamatória.
- S-adenosilmetionina (SAMe) como antioxidante na dose de 18 mg/kg/dia VO, administrada com o estômago vazio.
- Ciclosporina, 5 mg/kg/dia VO.

CONTRAINDICAÇÕES/INTERAÇÕES POSSÍVEIS
Corticosteroides são contraindicados diante de infecção ativa.

ACOMPANHAMENTO

MONITORIZAÇÃO DO PACIENTE
Pode demorar semanas a meses para a resolução.

PREVENÇÃO
Fornecer ração comercial balanceada para gatos.

COMPLICAÇÕES POSSÍVEIS
- Anorexia.
- Lipidose hepática.

EVOLUÇÃO ESPERADA E PROGNÓSTICO
- Recuperação demorada.
- Prognóstico bom uma vez estabelecida a ingestão da dieta apropriada.

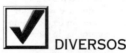

DIVERSOS

DISTÚRBIOS ASSOCIADOS
- Carcinoma pancreático.
- Ascite quilosa.
- Peritonite.

SINÔNIMO(S)
- Doença da gordura amarela.
- Pansteatite.
- Paniculite.

VER TAMBÉM
- Adenocarcinoma Pancreático.
- Peritonite.

ABREVIATURA(S)
- FeLV = vírus da leucemia felina.
- FIV = vírus da imunodeficiência felina.
- H&E = hematoxilina e eosina.
- PAS = ácido periódico de Schiff.
- PIF = peritonite infecciosa felina.

RECURSOS DA INTERNET
Alimentando seu gato: www.vet.cornell.edu/FHC/brochures/.

Sugestões de Leitura
Hoskins JD. Nutrition and nutritional problems. In: Hoskins JD, ed., Veterinary Pediatrics, 3rd ed. Philadelphia: Saunders, 2001, pp. 487-488.

Autor Craig B. Webb
Consultor Editorial Deborah S. Greco

ESTENOSE AÓRTICA

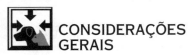

CONSIDERAÇÕES GERAIS

DEFINIÇÃO
Estreitamento do trajeto do fluxo de saída do ventrículo esquerdo, observado mais comumente como uma doença congênita ou perinatal, que se agrava no primeiro ano de vida. O defeito pode ser valvular, subvalvular (mais comum em cães) ou supravalvular (mais comum em gatos). Como uma anomalia congênita em cães, a obstrução costuma ser causada pela formação de tecido fibroso proximal à válvula; nesse caso, a doença recebe o nome de estenose subaórtica. Menos comumente, a displasia da valva atrioventricular esquerda (mitral) pode causar estenose subaórtica, ligando essa valva ao septo interventricular.

FISIOPATOLOGIA
A obstrução aórtica acentuada requer um aumento na pressão intraventricular para manter o fluxo sanguíneo anterógrado e a pressão sanguínea sistêmica. A sobrecarga pressórica leva à hipertrofia dos miócitos e ao subsequente espessamento das paredes cardíacas. Isso pode resultar em doença arterial coronariana, isquemia cardíaca relativa, arritmias, regurgitação aórtica ou mitral, insuficiência cardíaca congestiva esquerda e fluxo sanguíneo sistêmico diminuído. O mecanismo de morte súbita é pouco compreendido.

SISTEMA(S) ACOMETIDO(S)
• Cardiovascular — sobrecarga (por pressão) do ventrículo esquerdo. • Pulmonar — caso ocorra o desenvolvimento de edema pulmonar.
• Possibilidade do aparecimento de sinais multissistêmicos, secundariamente à ICC ou ao baixo débito cardíaco. Múltiplos sinais sistêmicos na presença de endocardite bacteriana.

GENÉTICA
Traço hereditário em cães da raça Terra Nova. A transmissão poligênica exibe uma pseudodominância; um gene dominante maior associado a modificadores pode estar envolvido. Outras raças podem exibir características hereditárias semelhantes.

INCIDÊNCIA/PREVALÊNCIA
Acomete cerca de 1,5 a 2,0 dentre 1.000 cães e 0,2 dentre 1.000 gatos atendidos nas instituições veterinárias de ensino; a estenose subaórtica provavelmente representa o segundo defeito cardíaco congênito mais comum em cães e o mais comum em raças de grande porte. Em um único estudo, a estenose aórtica foi responsável por 6% dos defeitos cardíacos congênitos em gatos.

IDENTIFICAÇÃO

Espécies
Cães e gatos.

Raça(s) Predominante(s)
A estenose subaórtica é mais comum em cães das raças Terra Nova, Pastor alemão, Golden retriever, Bouvier des Flandres, Rottweiler e Boxer. As raças Samoieda, Buldogue inglês e Dogue alemão também exibem risco mais elevado do que outras raças; os cães da raça Bull terrier são predispostos à estenose da válvula aórtica, tipicamente associada à displasia concomitante da valva atrioventricular esquerda (mitral). Os cães da raça Boxer exibem um maior estreitamento do trajeto do fluxo de saída em comparação com outras raças de porte semelhante; a diferenciação de estenose subaórtica leve por essa variação racial é problemática.

Idade Média e Faixa Etária
A estenose subaórtica desenvolve-se no período pós-natal, nas primeiras semanas ou nos primeiros meses de vida; o desenvolvimento fenotípico é concluído por volta de 1 ano de idade. O início dos sinais clínicos pode ocorrer em qualquer idade, dependendo da gravidade da obstrução. Os sinais podem ser observados no exame físico, sem qualquer indício anamnésico de doença.

SINAIS CLÍNICOS

Achados Anamnésicos
• Relacionados com a gravidade da obstrução; variam desde a ausência de achados até ICC, síncope e morte súbita. • Histórico genético de ninhadas acometidas do mesmo pai ou mãe.

Achados do Exame Físico
• Sopro sistólico de ejeção, mais audível próximo ao quarto espaço intercostal esquerdo, desde a base do coração até a junção costocondral; esse sopro pode se propagar à entrada torácica, às artérias carótidas e, se muito sonoro, até mesmo ao crânio. A propagação à porção esquerda do ápice e à porção cranial direita do tórax é comum. A intensidade do sopro é mais ou menos correlacionada com a gravidade da doença. Em filhotes caninos com menos de 2 meses de vida, pode não haver sopro, embora possa se tornar mais proeminente durante os 6 primeiros meses de vida. • Em alguns animais, é palpável um frêmito ao nível da base cardíaca esquerda até a junção costocondral. • No desenvolvimento de regurgitação aórtica, pode-se auscultar um sopro diastólico no ápice esquerdo. • Em caso de regurgitação mitral, pode haver um sopro holossistólico no ápice esquerdo. • Associados ao início de ICC esquerda, observam-se dispneia, taquipneia e crepitações. • Em animais com doença suficientemente grave a ponto de comprometer a hemodinâmica, verificam-se pulsos femorais tipicamente débeis (fracos) e tardios. • Em animais com hipertrofia do ventrículo esquerdo, constata-se uma espécie de "asma" ventricular esquerda (i. e., impulso cardíaco prolongado e pronunciado palpável no tórax). • Arritmias.

CAUSAS
• Doença congênita ou perinatal. • Em alguns cães, é secundária à endocardite bacteriana da válvula aórtica. • Em gatos com miocardiopatia hipertrófica, é comum uma estenose funcional (p. ex., muscular ou subvalvular), mas seu significado é desconhecido. • Em cães com estreitamento do trajeto do fluxo de saída aórtico associado à hipertrofia muscular, relata-se uma estenose subaórtica "dinâmica". • Uma complicação ou variante de displasia da valva atrioventricular esquerda (mitral).

FATORES DE RISCO
• Histórico familiar de estenose subaórtica. • A endocardite aórtica é predisposta por imunossupressão, infecção sistêmica, bacteremia e fluxo sanguíneo intracardíaco anormal, incluindo estenose subaórtica.

DIAGNÓSTICO

DIAGNÓSTICO DIFERENCIAL
• Um sopro sistólico de ejeção pode representar um sopro inocente/fisiológico no animal jovem, causado por anemia, dor, febre e agitação. Os sopros sistólicos no tórax esquerdo são comumente causados por persistência do ducto arterioso (em geral, é um sopro contínuo, mas o componente diastólico pode ser localizado), estenose pulmonar, regurgitação mitral, defeito do septo ventricular, defeito do septo atrial ou tetralogia de Fallot em cães. Algumas dessas condições podem coexistir com a estenose subaórtica. • Os pulsos podem estar débeis (fracos) em animais com outras cardiopatias em que o volume sistólico esteja reduzido (p. ex., estenose pulmonar e miocardiopatia) ou naqueles com obstrução aórtica distal ao trajeto do fluxo de saída (p. ex., coarctação aórtica, interrupção aórtica e tromboembolia aórtica).

HEMOGRAMA/BIOQUÍMICA/URINÁLISE
Tipicamente normais.

DIAGNÓSTICO POR IMAGEM

Achados Radiográficos Torácicos
• Podem ser sutis, já que a hipertrofia do miocárdio decorrente da sobrecarga por pressão pode não aumentar o tamanho da silhueta cardíaca (hipertrofia concêntrica). • Aumento de volume do lado esquerdo do coração. • Os campos pulmonares apresentam-se normais a menos que se desenvolva uma ICC indutora de distensão venosa pulmonar e de infiltrados pulmonares intersticiais ou alveolares. • O mediastino pode estar alargado e a cintura cranial da silhueta cardíaca preenchida, em consequência da dilatação pós-estenótica da aorta.

Achados Ecocardiográficos
• O espectro de achados depende da gravidade da doença; as anormalidades podem ser sutis.
• Espessamento da parede ventricular esquerda e do septo interventricular. • Na estenose subaórtica, podem ser visíveis uma crista ecogênica e/ou um estreitamento macroscópico do trajeto de fluxo de saída do ventrículo esquerdo proximalmente à válvula aórtica. • Em caso de estenose subaórtica valvular, nota-se o espessamento e o aumento na ecogenicidade da válvula; na presença de endocardite, há lesões vegetativas. • O folheto anterior da valva atrioventricular esquerda (mitral) também pode se apresentar espesso e ecogênico.
• Em alguns animais, constata-se uma dilatação pós-estenótica da aorta. • Em outros animais, verifica-se o aumento na ecogenicidade do miocárdio, particularmente da zona subendocardial e dos músculos papilares.
• Muitas vezes, observa-se um "fechamento prematuro" da válvula aórtica na ecocardiografia em modo M.

Achados Ecocardiográficos de Doppler
• A estenose produz um alto pico na velocidade de ejeção (>2,25 m/s), que pode ser adiado para uma fase mais tardia na ejeção; observam-se uma aceleração do fluxo proximalmente à obstrução e um jato de fluxo sanguíneo turbulento distalmente à válvula. • O gradiente pressórico transvalvular pode ser estimado a partir da velocidade de fluxo (gradiente de pressão = $4 \times [\text{velocidade de fluxo}]^2$) com uma precisão variável. A ecocardiografia Doppler de fluxo colorido permite a observação direta do jato turbulento distalmente à obstrução e a "convergência do fluxo" proximalmente. • A área efetiva do orifício diminui.

Achados Angiocardiográficos/ Cateterização Cardíaca
• A radiografia contrastada pode revelar o espessamento da parede ventricular esquerda e do

Estenose Aórtica

septo, o estreitamento do trajeto do fluxo de saída do ventrículo esquerdo e do orifício valvular, bem como a dilatação pós-estenótica da aorta. • A cateterização cardíaca possibilita a determinação do gradiente pressórico transvalvular. Os gradientes de pressão indicam a gravidade da doença: <50 mmHg (doença leve), 50-75 mmHg (moderada), 75-100 mmHg (grave) e >100 mmHg (muito grave). Tais categorias, no entanto, são um tanto arbitrárias e grosseiramente relacionadas com a evolução clínica. Os gradientes de pressão (obtidos por cateterização ou ecocardiografia Doppler) ficam maiores com o aumento no volume de ejeção e, por essa razão, devem ser interpretados levando-se em consideração outros aspectos da função cardíaca. A anestesia realizada durante a cateterização cardíaca pode afetar os gradientes. • A elevação na pressão diastólica do ventrículo esquerdo pode acompanhar a perda da complacência ventricular, bem como uma ICC iminente ou manifesta. • A angiografia e a cateterização cardíacas permitem a caracterização de tipos incomuns de estenose (incluindo as estenoses valvulares, as supravalvulares e as de "canalização do fluxo de saída"), bem como a avaliação de defeitos concomitantes.

MÉTODOS DIAGNÓSTICOS

Achados Eletrocardiográficos
• O ECG pode exibir sinais de hipertrofia do ventrículo esquerdo, como ondas R altas, complexos QRS amplos e desvio do eixo elétrico médio para a esquerda. • Um ponto de inclinação (*slurring*) do segmento ST é compatível com hipertrofia ou isquemia do ventrículo esquerdo; o desvio do segmento ST após exercícios leves sugere fortemente a presença de insuficiência coronariana. • Nos casos gravemente acometidos, podem ocorrer taquiarritmias ventriculares, que constituem uma causa potencial dos sinais clínicos e de morte súbita. A monitorização eletrocardiográfica com Holter em um período de 24 horas é apropriada em animais sintomáticos ou significativamente acometidos.

TRATAMENTO

CUIDADO(S) DE SAÚDE ADEQUADO(S)
As recomendações terapêuticas para pequenos animais são controversas e variam entre os especialistas. A internação é conveniente para as complicações, como arritmias, episódios de síncope e ICC.

ATIVIDADE
Restrita em animais acometidos por mais do que uma doença branda. Em animais gravemente acometidos, um esforço físico poderá levar à ocorrência de síncope, colapso e morte súbita.

ORIENTAÇÃO AO PROPRIETÁRIO
• Os animais acometidos devem ser castrados ou, caso contrário, vetados para a reprodução. • É preciso avaliar rigorosamente os cães aparentados, em busca de indícios de doença clínica. • Alertar os proprietários quanto às complicações potenciais (p. ex., morte súbita e ICC) em animais gravemente acometidos e em relação ao aumento no risco de endocardite e complicações anestésicas.

CONSIDERAÇÕES CIRÚRGICAS
• O tratamento definitivo exige uma cirurgia cardíaca aberta com desvio cardiopulmonar, para a ressecção, o reparo (valvuloplastia) ou a substituição (reposição valvular) da lesão obstrutiva. Infelizmente, a relação risco-benefício para a ressecção aberta da estenose subaórtica em cães não apoia a recomendação; além disso, essa espécie ainda pode sofrer morte súbita após o procedimento. • Em alguns cães sintomáticos, a dilatação da via de saída com o auxílio de um balão durante a cateterização cardíaca resulta na redução aguda dos gradientes transvalvulares e na melhora dos sinais clínicos. Contudo, apesar da diminuição no gradiente valvular, um pequeno ensaio clínico falhou em demonstrar uma vantagem desse procedimento em termos de sobrevida para cães gravemente acometidos, em comparação à terapia isolada com β-bloqueador (atenolol).

MEDICAÇÕES

MEDICAMENTO(S) DE ESCOLHA
• O tratamento clínico é paliativo e empírico; não foram publicados ensaios clínicos placebo-controlados que apoiem um tratamento específico.
• O uso de bloqueadores β-adrenérgicos é defendido para os cães acometidos por estenose subaórtica com histórico de síncope ou colapso, gradiente pressórico transvalvular >75 mmHg ou na evidência de arritmias ventriculares ou de alterações do segmento ST em um ECG obtido após atividade física. Os benefícios potenciais incluem a limitação das exigências de oxigênio pelo miocárdio, a proteção contra arritmias ventriculares e a lentificação da frequência cardíaca. Os β-bloqueadores devem ser administrados até se obter o efeito desejado. É recomendável instituir a terapia com cautela em dosagens baixas, titulando-as para cima em um período de dias a semanas. Atenolol (cães, 0,5-1,5 mg/kg VO a cada 12 h; gatos, 6,25 mg/gato VO a cada 12-24 h).
• Também pode haver a necessidade de tratamento específico para arritmias ventriculares, fibrilação atrial ou ICC esquerda.
• Os animais acometidos estão sob risco de desenvolver endocardite bacteriana. Recomenda-se o tratamento meticuloso das infecções, assim como uma quimioprofilaxia para os procedimentos odontológicos ou geniturinários.
• O tratamento de estenose dinâmica em gatos com miocardiopatia hipertrófica é controverso.

CONTRAINDICAÇÕES
Os β-bloqueadores são contraindicados em animais com distúrbios broncoconstritivos. O uso contínuo em pacientes com ICC manifesta é controverso.

PRECAUÇÕES
• Os β-bloqueadores limitam a capacidade de aumento do débito cardíaco por disfunção cardíaca. Esses medicamentos devem ser iniciados com uma dose baixa e gradativamente titulados para cima a fim de evitar complicações iatrogênicas.
• O uso abusivo de diuréticos ou venodilatadores pode provocar uma queda súbita no débito cardíaco.
• Uma redução acentuada da pressão sanguínea sistêmica por inibidores da ECA, bloqueadores dos canais de cálcio ou dilatadores arteriolares pode agravar a obstrução ao fluxo de saída ou a insuficiência coronariana.
• Os glicosídeos digitálicos e os agentes inotrópicos positivos, como a pimobendana, podem exacerbar a obstrução ao fluxo de saída ou as arritmias ventriculares.
• É recomendável evitar o uso dos agentes anestésicos e sedativos com efeitos colaterais hipotensores, arritmogênicos ou cardiodepressores notáveis. Se necessário, um agente narcótico (p. ex., butorfanol ou oximorfona) poderá ser combinado com diazepam para sedação e com baixas concentrações inspiradas de isofluorano para anestesia.

MEDICAMENTO(S) ALTERNATIVO(S)
• O tartarato de metoprolol (0,5-1,0 mg/kg VO a cada 8-12 h para cães; 2-15 mg/gato VO a cada 8 h) e carvedilol (0,5-1,5 mg/kg VO a cada 12 h para cães) estão entre os β-bloqueadores alternativos.
• O diltiazem (0,5-2,0 mg/kg VO a cada 8 h para cães; 7,5-15,0 mg/gato VO a cada 8 h) pode teoricamente ter efeitos semelhantes nessa doença.

ACOMPANHAMENTO

MONITORIZAÇÃO DO PACIENTE
Monitorizar por meio de ECG, radiografias torácicas, ecocardiografias bidimensional e Doppler. O tratamento das complicações (p. ex., ICC e arritmias) exige a monitorização rigorosa para detectar os efeitos colaterais renais/eletrolíticos, pró-arrítmicos, inotrópicos negativos e hipotensores dos medicamentos.

COMPLICAÇÕES POSSÍVEIS
ICC, arritmias, infarto miocárdico, regurgitação aórtica, regurgitação mitral, morte súbita e endocardite bacteriana.

EVOLUÇÃO ESPERADA E PROGNÓSTICO
• Os cães levemente acometidos podem ter uma expectativa de vida normal sem tratamento.
• Uma doença grave tipicamente limita a longevidade por ICC ou morte súbita.
• Os quadros de ICC, colapso ou síncope sugerem doença grave e prognóstico assustador.

DIVERSOS

FATORES RELACIONADOS COM A IDADE
Na estenose subaórtica, um sopro não se encontra tipicamente presente ao nascimento; ele se desenvolve nas primeiras semanas a meses no período pós-natal, juntamente com o desenvolvimento da lesão estenótica.

GESTAÇÃO/FERTILIDADE/REPRODUÇÃO
Contraindicada.

VER TAMBÉM
• Endocardite Infecciosa.
• Insuficiência Cardíaca Congestiva Esquerda.
• Miocardiopatia Hipertrófica — Cães.
• Miocardiopatia Hipertrófica — Gatos.

ABREVIATURA(S)
• ECG = eletrocardiografia.
• ICC = insuficiência cardíaca congestiva.

Autor Donald J. Brown
Consultores Editoriais Larry P. Tilley e Francis W.K. Smith, Jr.

Estenose das Valvas Atrioventriculares

CONSIDERAÇÕES GERAIS

DEFINIÇÃO
A estenose das valvas atrioventriculares (AV) é um estreitamento patológico do orifício da mitral (esquerda) ou da tricúspide (direita).

FISIOPATOLOGIA
- O enchimento ventricular em doença clinicamente significativa requer um gradiente de pressão diastólica persistente entre o átrio e o ventrículo.
- É comum a ocorrência de regurgitação valvar concomitante.
- O aumento na pressão atrial pode levar à dilatação atrial, congestão venosa e ICC. Em casos de estenose da mitral, ocorre a formação de edema pulmonar; em casos de estenose grave da tricúspide, podem se desenvolver ascite, efusão pleural e quilotórax.
- Em pacientes com estenose da tricúspide, o forame oval pode permanecer patente, permitindo o desvio sanguíneo da direita para a esquerda com sinais de cardiopatia cianótica.
- O débito cardíaco e a capacidade física ficam limitados em casos de estenose das valvas AV.
- A estenose da mitral pode levar à dispneia por esforço por edema pulmonar transitório.
- Pode ocorrer o desenvolvimento de hipertensão pulmonar como resultado de estenose da mitral, levando à intolerância ao exercício e hipertrofia do ventrículo direito. Isso pode ser grave, sobretudo em gatos com estenose da mitral.

SISTEMA(S) ACOMETIDO(S)
- Respiratório — em casos de estenose da mitral — compressão dos brônquios por aumento de volume do átrio esquerdo, além de edema pulmonar; efusão pleural com atelectasia na estenose da tricúspide.
- Hepatobiliar — em casos de estenose da tricúspide — congestão hepática e ascite.

GENÉTICA
Incerta.

INCIDÊNCIA/PREVALÊNCIA
Rara.

DISTRIBUIÇÃO GEOGRÁFICA
Mundial.

IDENTIFICAÇÃO
Espécies
Cães e gatos.

Raça(s) Predominante(s)
- A estenose da mitral é super-representada nos cães das raças Bull terrier e Terra Nova e, possivelmente, nos gatos Siameses.
- A estenose da tricúspide é descrita com maior frequência em cães Old English sheepdog e Labrador retriever.

Idade Média e Faixa Etária
A maioria dos pacientes apresenta-se em uma idade jovem, embora ocorram exceções, especialmente nos gatos.

SINAIS CLÍNICOS
Achados Anamnésicos
- Intolerância ao exercício.
- Síncope.
- Dispneia ou taquipneia por esforço.
- Tosse — estenose da mitral.
- Cianose.
- Distensão abdominal — estenose da tricúspide.
- Paresia posterior aguda — gatos com estenose da mitral.
- Retardo do crescimento.
- Hemoptise por ruptura de vasos intrapulmonares — estenose da mitral.

Achados do Exame Físico
- Sopro diastólico tênue com seu ponto de intensidade máxima sobre o ápice esquerdo (estenose da mitral) ou no hemitórax direito (estenose da tricúspide).
- É comum um sopro holossistólico decorrente da regurgitação mitral ou tricúspide.
- Na estenose da mitral, ainda se observam crepitações, taquipneia e dispneia.
- Na estenose da tricúspide, há distensão jugular, pulsos jugulares, ascite e hepatomegalia.
- Ocorre cianose pelo desvio sanguíneo da direita para a esquerda na presença de estenose da tricúspide.

CAUSAS
- Atribuída, em geral, à displasia congênita das valvas AV esquerda (mitral) ou direita (tricúspide).
- Anéis teciduais responsáveis por obstrução supravalvar são associados à estenose AV.
- Endocardite infecciosa, neoplasia intracardíaca, miocardiopatia hipertrófica em gatos são possíveis causas de estenose adquirida.
- Estenose da tricúspide foi observada em casos de formação de fibrose cicatricial da tricúspide em cães com derivações de marca-passo transvenoso.

FATORES
Ver a seção "Fatores de Risco" para Endocardite Infecciosa; marca-passo transvenoso permanente.

DIAGNÓSTICO

DIAGNÓSTICO DIFERENCIAL
Na ausência de estenose, é imprescindível diferenciar a estenose das valvas AV das causas mais comuns de regurgitação mitral e tricúspide. Tais causas incluem lesões congênitas e adquiridas das valvas AV e do aparelho de sustentação.

HEMOGRAMA/BIOQUÍMICA/URINÁLISE
Podem permanecer normais ou refletir as alterações relacionadas com ICC ou terapia medicamentosa para insuficiência cardíaca.

DIAGNÓSTICO POR IMAGEM
Radiografia Torácica
- O aumento de volume atrial representa o achado mais compatível e proeminente; pode-se observar uma cardiomegalia generalizada.
- Estenose da mitral — é possível verificar congestão venosa pulmonar e edema pulmonar; a hemorragia intrapulmonar pode ser erroneamente interpretada como pneumonia ou alguma outra doença parenquimatosa.
- Estenose da tricúspide — pode haver hepatomegalia; o diâmetro da veia cava caudal possivelmente se encontra ampliado.

Ecocardiografia
- Constitui o teste diagnóstico de escolha.
- A ecocardiografia bidimensional revela um átrio acentuadamente dilatado com excursão valvar atenuada durante a diástole, muitas vezes com evidência de folhetos valvares AV irregulares e espessados; os folhetos valvares aparentemente podem se elevar como uma "cúpula" no decorrer da diástole. Também pode ser evidenciada a presença de anel responsável por obstrução supravalvar, bem como outras lesões (ver a seção "Causas" anteriormente).
- Os estudos em modo M exibem um aumento de volume atrial com movimento harmonioso dos folhetos valvares AV, indicando uma fusão comissural; a inclinação EF sofre uma diminuição.
- A obtenção de imagens de fluxo colorido demonstra um jato diastólico turbulento, que se origina na valva estenosada e se projeta em direção ao ápice do ventrículo; com frequência, também há um jato turbulento decorrente da regurgitação das valvas AV.
- Os estudos de Doppler espectral demonstram um aumento nas velocidades do fluxo transvalvar diastólico; o prolongamento no tempo médio da pressão calculada constitui uma característica típica e referencial; também se pode observar uma reversão na amplitude das ondas E e A em casos que ainda se encontram em ritmo sinusal (fisiológico).
- Na estenose da mitral com hipertensão pulmonar, observa-se o aumento de volume das câmaras cardíacas do lado direito.

Angiografia
- Átrio direito: a injeção de contraste demonstra dilatação acentuada dessa câmara cardíaca; ocorre em casos de estenose da tricúspide e, em geral, persistência do forame oval ou desvio do septo atrial; a opacificação do átrio esquerdo pode ser observada após a injeção do contraste no átrio direito.
- Podem-se visualizar os folhetos valvares irregulares e espessados ou as valvas estenosas.
- Tipicamente, a injeção ventricular de contraste revela a regurgitação valvar.
- Pode haver opacificação tardia do ventrículo e dos grandes vasos.

Cateterização Cardíaca
- Entre o átrio e o ventrículo, identifica-se um gradiente de pressão diastólica. Uma ampla onda "A" será comum se a função atrial for preservada.
- Em casos de estenose da mitral, ocorre elevação das pressões atrial esquerda, capilar pulmonar em cunha e arterial pulmonar.
- Na estenose da tricúspide, temos um aumento nas pressões atrial direita e venosa central.
- A pressão ventricular pode permanecer normal na ausência de defeitos concomitantes.

MÉTODOS DIAGNÓSTICOS
Eletrocardiografia
- Pode haver padrões variáveis de aumento de volume.
- Com frequência, observam-se ritmos ectópicos, especialmente de origem atrial. A fibrilação atrial é o distúrbio de ritmo mais importante, pois se perde a contribuição atrial para o enchimento da câmara cardíaca.

ACHADOS PATOLÓGICOS
- A valva AV acometida encontra-se anormal, com folhetos espessados e comissuras fundidas. Podem ser identificadas outras lesões, como anel supramitral (ver a seção "Causas").
- Muitos casos também exibem anormalidades nas cordas tendíneas e nos músculos papilares.
- É comum a constatação de dilatação e hipertrofia atriais.

Estenose das Valvas Atrioventriculares

TRATAMENTO

CUIDADO(S) DE SAÚDE ADEQUADO(S)
Os pacientes em ICC manifesta devem ser tratados com internação. As intervenções cirúrgicas ou efetuadas à base de cateter podem ser consideradas assim que a insuficiência cardíaca se encontrar estabilizada. O controle dos distúrbios do ritmo cardíaco, sobretudo fibrilação atrial, também é importante. Como esses pacientes tipicamente constituem um caso complexo, é recomendável a consulta com algum cardiologista.

CUIDADO(S) DE ENFERMAGEM
A oxigenoterapia deve ser administrada ao paciente com dispneia ou hipoxemia por insuficiência cardíaca congestiva esquerda. Tipicamente, a fluidoterapia é contraindicada no paciente com ICC manifesta, exceto em casos de azotemia moderada a grave, comprometimento renal ou desidratação grave concomitantes. O procedimento de paracentese terapêutica pode ser considerado no paciente com efusões pleurais ou ascite timpânica. A sedação com butorfanol é adequada para os pacientes dispneicos.

ATIVIDADE
É recomendável a restrição de exercícios para qualquer animal acometido por essa condição. O repouso em gaiola é ideal em pacientes com ICC.

DIETA
Fornecer uma dieta hipossódica (ou seja, com baixo teor de sódio) em pacientes com ICC.

ORIENTAÇÃO AO PROPRIETÁRIO
O proprietário precisa ser orientado sobre os sintomas associados à ICC e a urgência do tratamento, particularmente em casos de ICC esquerda. A probabilidade de ataques recidivantes de ICC também deve ser abordada.

CONSIDERAÇÕES CIRÚRGICAS
• A reposição ou o reparo cirúrgicos da valva acometida requer desvio cardiopulmonar ou hipotermia; o custo e a viabilidade desses procedimentos são fatores altamente limitantes.
• A valvoplastia por balão é um tratamento alternativo e já foi usado com sucesso para o tratamento de estenose das valvas AV.

MEDICAÇÕES

MEDICAMENTO(S)

ICC
• Furosemida — cães, 2-6 mg/kg IV, IM, SC, VO a cada 8-24 h; gatos, 1-4 mg/kg IV, IM, SC, VO a cada 8-24 h.
• Enalapril — cães, 0,25-0,5 mg/kg VO a cada 12 h; gatos, 0,25-0,5 mg/kg VO a cada 12-24 h; ver a seção "Acompanhamento" para a monitorização do paciente.
• Pasta de nitroglicerina (~0,6-2,5 cm por via tópica a cada 12 h) para diminuir as pressões venosas pulmonares; entretanto, isso não foi avaliado de forma criteriosa.

Taquiarritmias Atriais
• Digoxina — cães, 0,003-0,005 mg/kg VO a cada 12 h; gatos, ¼ de um comprimido de 0,125 mg VO a cada 24-48 h; ajustar a dose, com base nas concentrações séricas.
• β-bloqueadores, como o atenolol, ou bloqueadores dos canais de cálcio, como o diltiazem, para a supressão de complexos atriais prematuros frequentes e para o controle da frequência cardíaca em taquiarritmias atriais, como taquicardia/flutter/fibrilação atriais. Cuidado ao utilizar esses medicamentos em ICC não controlada.
• Dosagens típicas de atenolol: cães, 0,25-1,0 mg/kg a cada 12 h; gatos, 6,25-12,5 mg/gato a cada 12-24 h; iniciar com a dose baixa e titular até fazer efeito.
• Dosagens de diltiazem: cães, 2-6 mg/kg diariamente em duas (diltiazem de ação prolongada) ou três doses divididas; iniciar com a dose baixa e titular até fazer efeito); gatos, cloridrato de diltiazem de 7,5 mg VO a cada 8 h, Dilacor XR® de 15-30 mg a cada 12-24 h ou Cardizem CD® a 10 mg/kg a cada 24 h.
• Sotalol para arritmias intratáveis — cães, 1-2 mg/kg VO a cada 12 h; gatos, 10-20 mg/gato a cada 12 h.
• Os cães podem ser encaminhados para eletrocardioversão, visando converter a fibrilação atrial em ritmo sinusal (com terapia de acompanhamento com sotalol ou amiodarona); no entanto, é comum a reversão de volta à fibrilação atrial em virtude da dilatação atrial acentuada.

Hipertensão Pulmonar
• Sildenafila — cães, 0,5-3 mg/kg VO a cada 8-12 h.

PRECAUÇÕES
• Como regra geral, a pimobendana não deve ser utilizada em casos de estenose valvar pura; entretanto, alguns cães e gatos com ICC avançada foram submetidos a esse medicamento com aparente sucesso, sobretudo quando havia estenose/regurgitação valvar combinada.
• Utilizar inibidores da ECA ou outros vasodilatadores com bom senso em pacientes com ICC; o débito cardíaco fica limitado e a vasodilatação pode induzir à hipotensão. Monitorizar a pressão sanguínea arterial e a função renal.

INTERAÇÕES POSSÍVEIS
• A furosemida e os inibidores da ECA podem afetar a função renal, alterar os eletrólitos sanguíneos e reduzir a pressão sanguínea; esses parâmetros devem ser monitorizados.
• A sildenafila também pode diminuir a pressão sanguínea sistêmica e, por essa razão, não deve ser usada com pasta de nitroglicerina ou algum outro nitrato.

MEDICAMENTO(S) ALTERNATIVO(S)
A espironolactona (2 mg/kg VO a cada 12-24 h) pode ser considerada como diurético complementar e por seu efeito antifibrótico (como um antagonista da aldosterona).

ACOMPANHAMENTO

MONITORIZAÇÃO DO PACIENTE
• Radiografias torácicas — para avaliar a presença de edema pulmonar ou efusão pleural.
• Ecocardiografia aliada a estudos com Doppler — para estimar as pressões pulmonares e avaliar subjetivamente a função cardíaca direita se o animal estiver sob a sildenafila.
• Nível da digoxina — avaliar 7-10 dias após a instituição da terapia; em 8-12 h, esse nível deverá estar em 0,8-1,5 ng/mL.
• Quando submetido à administração de diurético e/ou de algum inibidor da ECA, o paciente deverá ser monitorizado quanto à função renal, ao nível eletrolítico e à pressão sanguínea arterial.
• Avaliação-padrão do ritmo cardíaco com ECG ou Holter (ECG ambulatorial) na presença de arritmias.

COMPLICAÇÕES POSSÍVEIS
• ICC.
• Fibrilação atrial.
• Síncope.
• Tromboembolia arterial — gatos.
• Hemorragia pulmonar em casos de estenose da mitral.

EVOLUÇÃO ESPERADA E PROGNÓSTICO
• A morbidade é alta; exceto em casos brandos, o prognóstico é geralmente mau. Contudo, alguns animais vivem por 6-8 anos, mesmo com estenose relativamente grave da mitral.
• A intervenção cirúrgica ou a valvoplastia por balão pode alterar a evolução da doença, mas os dados são limitados.

DIVERSOS

DISTÚRBIOS ASSOCIADOS
Os defeitos congênitos concomitantes são comuns (p. ex., estenose subaórtica em casos de estenose da mitral e persistência do forame oval em casos de estenose da tricúspide).

GESTAÇÃO/FERTILIDADE/REPRODUÇÃO
A possibilidade de que esse quadro seja um defeito hereditário precisa ser considerada ao se avaliar a adequação do animal para fins reprodutivos, particularmente nas raças com predileção por esse defeito. A carga hemodinâmica extra da gestação pode ser pouco tolerada por um coração já comprometido.

SINÔNIMOS
Displasia atrioventricular com estenose

VER TAMBÉM
• Displasia das Valvas Atrioventriculares.
• Endocardite Infecciosa.

ABREVIATURA(S)
• AV = atrioventricular.
• ECA = enzima conversora da angiotensina.
• ECG = eletrocardiografia.
• ICC = insuficiência cardíaca congestiva.

Sugestões de Leitura
Brown WA, Thomas WP. Balloon valvuloplasty of tricuspid stenosis in a Labrador Retriever. J Vet Intern Med 1995, 9:419-424.
Lehmkuhl LB, Ware WA, Bonagura JD. Mitral stenosis in 15 dogs. J Vet Intern Med 1994, 8:2-17.
Stamoulis ME, Fox PR. Mitral valve stenosis in three cats. J Small Anim Pract 1993, 34:452-456.

Autores Lora S. Hitchcock e John D. Bonagura
Consultores Editoriais Larry P. Tilley e Francis W.K. Smith, Jr.

Estenose Esofágica

CONSIDERAÇÕES GERAIS

DEFINIÇÃO
Estreitamento circunferencial anormal do lúmen esofágico.

FISIOPATOLOGIA
• Pode ocorrer secundariamente à lesão esofágica grave da mucosa quando a inflamação se estende além da mucosa e para as camadas submucosa e muscular, o que resulta em fibrose.
• As principais causas de estenose incluem esofagite e corpos estranhos esofágicos.

SISTEMA(S) ACOMETIDO(S)
• Gastrintestinal — acometimento segmentar ou difuso do esôfago.
• Respiratório — pode ocorrer pneumonia por aspiração secundária à regurgitação.

GENÉTICA
Não há base genética aparente.

INCIDÊNCIA/PREVALÊNCIA
Desconhecida; acredita-se que seja baixa.

DISTRIBUIÇÃO GEOGRÁFICA
Estenoses granulomatosas por *Spirocerca lupi* — observadas ocasionalmente no sudeste dos EUA.

IDENTIFICAÇÃO
Espécies
Cães e gatos.

Raça(s) Predominante(s)
Nenhuma relatada.

Idade Média e Faixa Etária
Qualquer idade; estenoses neoplásicas tendem a ocorrer em animais de meia-idade a idosos.

SINAIS CLÍNICOS
Comentários Gerais
• Em geral, acomete toda a circunferência do esôfago; pode ocorrer em qualquer localização ou segmento do esôfago.
• Os sinais clínicos estão relacionados com a gravidade e a extensão da estenose.

Achados Anamnésicos
• Regurgitação.
• Refeições líquidas em geral são mais bem toleradas do que as sólidas.
• Disfagia — em caso de estenoses esofágicas proximais.
• Salivação.
• Uivo, choro ou ganido durante a deglutição (odinofagia) na presença de esofagite ativa.
• Apetite satisfatório inicialmente; por fim, anorexia com o estreitamento esofágico progressivo e a inflamação.
• Perda de peso e desnutrição à medida que a doença evolui.
• Tosse e/ou secreção nasal em caso de aspiração.

Achados do Exame Físico
• Em geral, não são dignos de nota.
• Perda de peso e caquexia — em animais com estenose crônica ou avançada.
• Hipersalivação e/ou dor à palpação do pescoço e do esôfago — possivelmente observadas em animais com esofagite concomitante.
• Sibilos pulmonares e tosse — podem ser detectadas em animais com pneumonia por aspiração.

CAUSAS
• Refluxo gastresofágico durante a anestesia — mais comum.
• Ingestão de irritantes químicos.
• Vômito persistente.
• Retenção esofágica de comprimidos e cápsulas (doxiciclina, clindamicina e AINEs — muito comum em gatos).
• Doença do refluxo gastresofágico.
• Corpo estranho esofágico.
• Cirurgia esofágica.
• Processos neoplásicos — intra ou extramurais.
• Estenoses congênitas — raras.
• Esofagite eosinofílica — rara.
• Granuloma por *Spirocerca lupi*.

FATORES DE RISCO
• A preparação inadequada (sem jejum ou jejum prolongado) antes da cirurgia colocam alguns pacientes sob risco de refluxo gastresofágico, esofagite e subsequente formação de estenose.
• O uso de certos medicamentos durante a anestesia (p. ex., diazepam, atropina, pentobarbital, tranquilizantes derivados da fenotiazina, opioides, propofol, inalantes) diminui a pressão do esfíncter gastresofágico e pode resultar em refluxo gastresofágico.
• Administração de comprimidos em gatos.
• Obstrução por corpo estranho esofágico.

DIAGNÓSTICO

DIAGNÓSTICO DIFERENCIAL
• Anomalia do anel vascular — diagnóstico diferencial importante em animal jovem com estenose mesoesofágica e dilatação esofágica proximal; em geral, esses animais apresentam problemas logo após o desmame.
• Esofagite — o paciente pode ter sinais clínicos idênticos aos de estenose esofágica; a diferenciação requer radiografia contrastada com bário e endoscopia.
• Corpo estranho esofágico — os sinais clínicos podem ser idênticos aos de estenose esofágica; radiografias simples podem identificar a presença de corpo estranho esofágico, embora o contraste com bário ou a endoscopia possam ser necessários.
• Massa intraluminal — rara; pode ser detectada em radiografias, mas muitas requerem endoscopia; leiomioma, carcinoma de células escamosas, fibrossarcoma e osteossarcoma são as malignidades esofágicas mais comuns.
• Massa periesofágica extraluminal — frequentemente detectada em radiografias, mas pode requerer ultrassonografia torácica; linfoma, tumores da base do coração e abscesso mediastínico são as causas mais comuns de compressão esofágica extraluminal.

HEMOGRAMA/BIOQUÍMICA/URINÁLISE
• Costumam permanecer normais.
• Pacientes com esofagite ulcerativa ou pneumonia por aspiração podem ter leucocitose e neutrofilia.

DIAGNÓSTICO POR IMAGEM
• Radiografia torácica simples; geralmente normal; raras vezes, demonstra a dilatação do esôfago cranial à estenose (pode-se observar alimento retido na parte dilatada do esôfago) ou massa intra ou extraluminal; pneumonia por aspiração pode ser evidente em pacientes com regurgitação frequente.
• Radiografia contrastada com bário — frequentemente diagnóstica; dependendo da gravidade da estenose, o bário líquido pode passar sem impedimentos; para identificar a estenose, costuma ser necessário o uso de bário em pasta ou misturado com alimento; é possível observar o estreitamento segmentar ou difuso do esôfago com alguma dilatação proximal à estenose; esse tipo de radiografia identifica o número, a localização e o comprimento da(s) estenose(s).

MÉTODOS DIAGNÓSTICOS
• Endoscopia — realizar em todos os pacientes para confirmar o local e a gravidade da estenose e excluir a presença de processo maligno intraluminal.
• Histopatologia — é algumas vezes necessária para diferenciar neoplasia de estenose não neoplásica (p. ex., fibrótica). É recomendável a realização de citologia esfoliativa juntamente com biopsia da mucosa.

ACHADOS PATOLÓGICOS
• Estenose esofágica.
• Esofagite em alguns pacientes.
• Dilatação e hipertrofia muscular proximal à estenose.

TRATAMENTO

CUIDADO(S) DE SAÚDE ADEQUADO(S)
• Inicialmente tratamento hospitalar.
• Pode-se dar alta aos pacientes depois de satisfazer as necessidades de hidratação, conseguir a dilatação (pelo menos, parcial) do segmento acometido e iniciar qualquer tratamento necessário de pneumonia por aspiração e esofagite.

CUIDADO(S) DE ENFERMAGEM
• Fluidos intravenosos — podem ser necessários para corrigir o estado de hidratação.
• Medicações — talvez tenham de ser administradas por via parenteral após os procedimentos de dilatação para facilitar a cicatrização.
• Oxigênio — pode ser necessário em pacientes com pneumonia por aspiração grave concomitante.

ATIVIDADE
Irrestrita.

DIETA
• Suspender a alimentação por via oral em pacientes com esofagite grave e após os procedimentos de dilatação.
• Pode-se inserir uma sonda de gastrostomia temporária no momento da dilatação esofágica como meio de fornecer suporte nutricional contínuo.
• Oferecer refeições líquidas ao reinstituir a alimentação por via oral.

ORIENTAÇÃO AO PROPRIETÁRIO
• Os animais, em geral, não se recuperam de uma estenose esofágica não tratada.
• O melhor tratamento para estenoses benignas é a dilatação esofágica.
• Pacientes com estenoses malignas têm prognóstico mau.
• Discutir a alta probabilidade de recidiva e a necessidade habitual de múltiplos procedimentos de dilatação.

Estenose Esofágica

- Abordar a possibilidade de melhora (p. ex., diminuir ou acabar com a regurgitação, capacidade de comer alimentos enlatados macios, mas não os secos), mas não de cura.

CONSIDERAÇÕES CIRÚRGICAS
- Dilatação com vela ou cânula — relato recente revela desfechos semelhantes aos obtidos pela dilatação com balão.
- Dilatação mecânica via cateter com balão à endoscopia ou fluoroscopia — melhor opção terapêutica; acredita-se que seja superior à vela ou cânula, pois a aplicação de forças radiais, em vez de cisalhamento, resulta em menos possibilidade de perfuração esofágica; realizar endoscopia após a dilatação para verificar se houve dano à mucosa esofágica; podem ser necessárias novas dilatações em intervalos de 1-2 semanas até que a estenose se resolva; alguns clínicos combinam esse procedimento com injeções intralesionais de corticosteroides para ajudar a evitar a recidiva da estenose.
- Ressecção da estenose esofágica — segundo relatos, a taxa comprovada de sucesso é <50% e, em geral, está associada a complicações pós-operatórias substanciais.
- Outros métodos cirúrgicos — esofagotomia, esofagectomia com anastomose; interposição jejunal e criação de um divertículo por tração.
- A colocação de *stent** esofágico autoexpansivo por fluoroscopia ou endoscopia também pode ser uma opção adequada.

MEDICAÇÕES

MEDICAMENTO(S) DE ESCOLHA
- Administrar medicações por via parenteral após os procedimentos de dilatação e se houver esofagite grave.
- Ao retomar a terapia por via oral, dissolver os medicamentos em água e administrar com seringa ou diretamente via tubo de gastrostomia para garantir que eles alcancem o estômago.
- Dosagem anti-inflamatória de corticosteroides (p. ex., prednisona, 0,5-1 mg/kg VO a cada 12 h) — pode ajudar a evitar o processo de fibrose e a formação de nova estenose durante a fase de cicatrização.
- Injeções intralesionais de triancinolona após a dilatação de estenose esofágica podem ser úteis para diminuir a fibrose do esôfago.
- Suspensão de sucralfato — 0,5-1 g VO a cada 8 h.
- Agentes antissecretores de ácido gástrico — famotidina, 0,5 mg/kg VO, IV a cada 12-24 h; ranitidina, 1-2 mg/kg VO, IV, SC a cada 8-12 h; cimetidina, 5-10 mg/kg VO, SC, IV a cada 8 h; omeprazol, 0,7 mg/kg VO a cada 24 h.
- Agente procinético (i. e., cisaprida 0,1-0,5 mg/kg VO a cada 8-12 h; metoclopramida 0,2-0,5 mg/kg VO, SC a cada 8 h) — para aumentar o tônus do esfíncter gastresofágico após a resolução da estenose.
- Solução de lidocaína — 0,5 mg/kg VO a cada 4-6 h; para tratar a dor esofágica intensa.

CONTRAINDICAÇÕES
Eméticos.

INTERAÇÕES POSSÍVEIS
- A cimetidina e a ranitidina ligam-se à enzima do citocromo hepático P-450 e podem interferir no metabolismo de outros medicamentos.
- Os antagonistas do receptor H_2 impedem a captação do omeprazol pelas células oxínticas.
- O sucralfato pode inibir a absorção gastrintestinal de outros medicamentos (p. ex., cimetidina, ranitidina e omeprazol); isso, no entanto, pode não ter importância clínica.

ACOMPANHAMENTO

MONITORIZAÇÃO DO PACIENTE
Repetir a radiografia contrastada com bário ou a endoscopia e o procedimento de dilatação com balão/vela ou cânula a cada 2-4 semanas até que os sinais clínicos tenham se resolvido e o lúmen esofágico tenha alcançado o diâmetro adequado.

PREVENÇÃO
- Preparação adequada do paciente antes da anestesia (8 a 12 h de jejum pré-operatório).
- Evitar certos medicamentos (p. ex., atropina, diazepam, pentobarbital, morfina e tranquilizantes derivados da fenotiazina) antes da anestesia.
- Se houver refluxo gastresofágico, aconselhar o proprietário a evitar o fornecimento de refeições para o animal tarde da noite, pois elas tendem a diminuir a pressão do esfíncter gastresofágico durante o sono.
- Omeprazol — 1 mg/kg VO 4 h antes da anestesia e o bólus de metoclopramida, seguido por infusão em velocidade constante durante a cirurgia, diminuem o risco do desenvolvimento de refluxo gastresofágico.
- Após a administração oral de cápsulas e comprimidos, fornecer bólus de água (5 mL) em cães e gatos; acelerar o tempo de trânsito dos comprimidos para o estômago em gatos, revestindo os comprimidos com manteiga ou aplicando o suprimento Nutrical® no nariz dos gatos para estimular a lambedura após a administração de comprimidos; incentivar o animal de estimação a comer depois da administração oral para estimular a deglutição.

COMPLICAÇÕES POSSÍVEIS
- Perfuração esofágica — complicação potencialmente letal da dilatação de estenose esofágica; em geral, ocorre no momento da dilatação, embora tenha sido observada vários dias a semanas depois.
- Os pacientes correm risco de pneumonia por aspiração.
- Podem ocorrer sangramento esofágico excessivo e/ou bacteremia, secundariamente à dilatação do esôfago.
- Recidiva de estenose.

EVOLUÇÃO ESPERADA E PROGNÓSTICO
- Geralmente, quanto maior a estenose, mais reservado será o prognóstico.
- Estenoses esofágicas fibrosantes — em geral, o prognóstico é bom a reservado; pode recidivar apesar de dilatações esofágicas repetidas; melhora sem a cura é uma meta mais realista (ver a seção "Orientação ao Proprietário").
- Estenose maligna — prognóstico mau.

DIVERSOS

GESTAÇÃO/FERTILIDADE/REPRODUÇÃO
Estenose esofágica e desnutrição — a gestação pode ser difícil.

SINÔNIMO(S)
- Estreitamento esofágico.
- Obstrução esofágica.

VER TAMBÉM
- Corpos Estranhos Esofágicos.
- Disfagia.
- Esofagite.
- Megaesôfago.
- Refluxo Gastresofágico.
- Regurgitação.

ABREVIATURA(S)
- AINE = anti-inflamatório não esteroide.

Sugestões de Leitura
Bissett SA, Davis J, Subler K, et al. Risk factors and outcome of bougienage for treatment of benign esophageal strictures in dogs and cats: 28 cases (1995-2004). JAVMA 2009, 235:844-850.
Glazer A, Walters PC. Esophagitis and esophageal strictures. Compend Contin Educ Pract Vet 2008, 30(5):281-292.
Jergens AE. Diseases of the esophagus. In: Ettinger SJ, Feldman EC, eds., Textbook of Veterinary Internal Medicine, 6th ed. St. Louis: Elsevier, 2005, pp. 1298-1310.

Autor Jocelyn Mott
Consultor Editorial Albert E. Jergens

---

* N. T.: Dispositivo metálico, utilizado com a finalidade de manter o lúmen de uma artéria permeável, com seu calibre próximo do normal, formando uma nova "parede" para o vaso.

Estenose Lombossacra e Síndrome da Cauda Equina

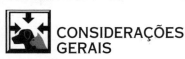

CONSIDERAÇÕES GERAIS

DEFINIÇÃO
- Causada pelo estreitamento dorsoventral do canal vertebral lombossacro, acompanhado pela compressão das raízes nervosas lombares (a partir de L7), sacrais ou caudais.
- A síndrome diz respeito aos sinais clínicos relacionados com a lesão dessas raízes nervosas.

FISIOPATOLOGIA
- Congênita — o desenvolvimento anormal do arco dorsal das vértebras L7-S1 provoca estreitamento do canal vertebral lombossacro; o estresse biomecânico crônico pode contribuir para as alterações degenerativas que diminuem o diâmetro do canal e provocam a compressão das raízes nervosas espinais; quanto menor o canal, menos estenose será necessária antes que os sinais clínicos apareçam.
- Adquirida — provocada por alterações degenerativas nos tecidos ósseos e moles, que levam à redução gradual no canal espinal lombossacro.

SISTEMA(S) ACOMETIDO(S)
Nervoso — especificamente as raízes nervosas, a partir de L7 no sentido caudal.

GENÉTICA
Não há nenhuma base genética conhecida.

INCIDÊNCIA/PREVALÊNCIA
Desconhecida.

DISTRIBUIÇÃO GEOGRÁFICA
N/D.

IDENTIFICAÇÃO
Espécies
- Comum nos cães.
- Rara nos gatos.

Raça(s) Predominante(s)
- Congênita — cães de porte pequeno a médio; raça Border collie.
- Adquirida — cães pertencentes a raças de grande porte; raças Pastor alemão, Boxer, Rottweiler.

Idade Média e Faixa Etária
- Congênita — 3-8 anos.
- Adquirida — idade média de início 6-7 anos.

Sexo Predominante
- Congênita — nenhum.
- Adquirida — machos.

SINAIS CLÍNICOS
- Relacionam-se com graus variados de compressão das raízes nervosas L7, sacrais e caudais.
- Dor lombossacra — característica clínica proeminente; pode ser o único sinal.
- Disfunção do nervo ciático — pode inicialmente se manifestar como claudicação; pode evoluir para fraqueza do membro pélvico, emaciação muscular e déficits de reação postural.
- Envolvimento da raiz do nervo pudendo — incontinência urinária e/ou fecal.
- Envolvimento da raiz nervosa caudal — condução anormal da cauda; fraqueza a paralisia da cauda.
- Compressão tanto das meninges como das raízes nervosas — distúrbios sensoriais que variam desde sensações desagradáveis até dor lombar baixa óbvia.
- Congênita — lesões autoinfligidas são comuns.
- Pacientes com ambas as formas — extensão dos membros pélvicos ou flexão da cauda sobre o dorso diminui o diâmetro do canal lombossacro e costuma eliciar uma resposta dolorosa.

CAUSAS
- Má-formação vertebral congênita, inclusive da vértebra de transição ou osteocondrose das placas terminais sacrais.
- Protrusão de disco tipo II.
- Hipertrofia ou hiperplasia do ligamento interarqueado.
- Proliferação das facetas articulares.
- Subluxação ou instabilidade da junção lombossacra.

FATORES DE RISCO
Cães, particularmente os da raça Pastor alemão, com vértebra de transição lombossacra apresentam um risco elevado de desenvolvimento da síndrome. Não foi identificada nenhuma característica radiografia capaz de predizer o desenvolvimento da doença em animais normais do ponto de vista clínico.

DIAGNÓSTICO

DIAGNÓSTICO DIFERENCIAL
- Displasia coxofemoral ou outra lesão ortopédica — dor lombar baixa; distinguir por meio de exame ortopédico completo.
- Discospondilite crônica, osteomielite e tumores vertebrais primários ou metastáticos — não podem ser diferenciados apenas pelos sinais clínicos.
- Fraturas e subluxações vertebrais — agudas; caracterizam-se por sinais mais bilaterais.
- Meningomielite ou radiculoneurite localizada — geralmente dor mais difusa.

HEMOGRAMA/BIOQUÍMICA/URINÁLISE
- Em geral, normais.
- Urinálise — pode revelar infecção do trato urinário inferior secundária à incontinência urinária.

OUTROS TESTES LABORATORIAIS
N/D.

DIAGNÓSTICO POR IMAGEM
- Radiologia — espondilose na junção lombossacra; estreitamento do espaço entre os discos em L7-S1; deslocamento ventral do sacro em relação às vértebras lombares; interpretar com cuidado, porque todas essas alterações podem ser observadas nos animais clinicamente normais.
- Mielografia — raramente benéfica, uma vez que o espaço subaracnóideo raras vezes se estende além da vértebra L6 em cães pertencentes a raças de grande porte; indicada para descartar lesões rostrais à junção lombossacra.
- Epidurografia — pode delinear massa expansiva sobre o espaço do disco lombossacro.
- Discografia do espaço L7-S1 — pode ajudar a destacar a elevação da fibrose do anel dorsal.
- TC e RM — modalidades diagnósticas de escolha.

MÉTODOS DIAGNÓSTICOS
- Eletromiografia — diagnóstica e prognóstica; denervação pode ser detectada nos músculos inervados pelas raízes nervosas lombares (a partir de L7) a caudais; a denervação confirma a localização da lesão e implica déficits permanentes.
- As latências de potenciais evocados espinais lombares induzidos por estimulação do nervo tibial podem ser prolongadas.

ACHADOS PATOLÓGICOS
- Podem ser uma ou mais das características a seguir:
  - Discopatia tipo II com abaulamento do anel dorsal.
  - Hipertrofia do ligamento interarqueado.
  - Espondilose indutora de estenose do forame intervertebral, com consequente compressão das raízes nervosas.
  - Deslocamento ventral do sacro em relação às vértebras lombares.
  - Proliferação das facetas articulares e hipertrofia da cápsula articular.
  - Má-formação congênita, consistindo em pedículos encurtados.
  - Lâmina e processos articulares esclerosados e espessados.
  - Presença de vértebra de transição lombossacra.

TRATAMENTO

CUIDADO(S) DE SAÚDE ADEQUADO(S)
- Continência urinária — paciente de ambulatório aguardando cirurgia.
- Incontinência urinária — paciente internado para tratamento clínico inicial.

CUIDADO(S) DE ENFERMAGEM
Incontinência urinária — cateterizar a bexiga até o retorno do controle voluntário adequado; monitorar rigorosamente quanto à presença de infecção do trato urinário e administrar antibióticos apropriados se houver necessidade.

ATIVIDADE
- Após a descompressão cirúrgica — restringir por 4 semanas; em seguida, retornar gradualmente à função atlética.
- Tratamento não cirúrgico — confinamento e caminhadas restritas a correias, isoladamente ou em combinação com corticosteroides, aliviam com frequência a dor; os sinais clínicos frequentemente retornam com o aumento no nível dos exercícios.

DIETA
Evitar a obesidade; o excesso de peso aumenta o estresse biomecânico sobre a coluna.

ORIENTAÇÃO AO PROPRIETÁRIO
- Informar ao proprietário que, sem o tratamento, haverá comprometimento neurológico progressivo dos membros pélvicos, incontinência urinária e fecal, além de paralisia da cauda.
- Esclarecer o proprietário sobre o fato de que a claudicação do membro pélvico e as lesões autoinfligidas resultam da dor associada à irritação e compressão da raiz nervosa.
- Discutir o tratamento cirúrgico, mencionando os seguintes pontos: (1) esse tipo de tratamento interrompe a evolução e remove a origem da dor, (2) alguns déficits neurológicos podem permanecer e (3) o tratamento clínico isolado não costuma ser insatisfatório.

CONSIDERAÇÕES CIRÚRGICAS
- Descompressão cirúrgica — tratamento preferido.

Estenose Lombossacra e Síndrome da Cauda Equina

- Laminectomia dorsal das vértebras L7-S1 — alivia a compressão com eficiência em grande parte dos pacientes sem gerar instabilidade; poderá ser combinada com a facetectomia ou com a foraminotomia se as raízes nervosas estiverem comprimidas.
- As técnicas de distração e fusão das vértebras com ou sem laminectomia devem ser consideradas se a junção lombossacra parecer instável (nas radiografias ou durante a cirurgia).

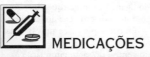

MEDICAÇÕES

MEDICAMENTO(S) DE ESCOLHA
AINEs ou corticosteroides — geralmente insatisfatórios.

CONTRAINDICAÇÕES
N/D.

PRECAUÇÕES
N/D.

INTERAÇÕES POSSÍVEIS
N/D.

MEDICAMENTO(S) ALTERNATIVO(S)
N/D.

ACOMPANHAMENTO

MONITORIZAÇÃO DO PACIENTE
N/D.

PREVENÇÃO
N/D.

COMPLICAÇÕES POSSÍVEIS
- Formação de seroma — sequela frequente da cirurgia; pode ser tratado de forma eficaz pelo repouso em gaiola e drenagem cirúrgica.
- Formação de tecido fibroso excessivo (membrana de laminectomia) na área cirúrgica — causa rara de recidiva dos sinais clínicos; minimizar por meio de técnica cirúrgica apropriada; além de difícil, a remoção cirúrgica apresenta uma taxa de sucesso mais baixa do que a laminectomia dorsal inicial.
- Recidiva dos sinais >6 meses após a cirurgia.

EVOLUÇÃO ESPERADA E PROGNÓSTICO
- Variam com o grau de lesão neurológica.
- Em caso de dor lombar baixa e déficits neurológicos leves (cães) — prognóstico bom após a cirurgia; 70-80% exibem desfechos excelentes ou bons.
- Na presença de incontinência fecal e urinária — prognóstico reservado.

DIVERSOS

DISTÚRBIOS ASSOCIADOS
Infecções do trato urinário inferior frequentemente acompanham a incontinência urinária.

FATORES RELACIONADOS COM A IDADE
- Pastor alemão — osteoartrite coxofemoral e/ou mielopatia degenerativa concomitante.
- Na existência de vértebra de transição lombossacra, a síndrome poderá se desenvolver 1-2 anos antes do que a média (cães).

POTENCIAL ZOONÓTICO
N/D.

GESTAÇÃO/FERTILIDADE/REPRODUÇÃO
N/D.

SINÔNIMO(S)
- Má articulação ou má-formação lombossacra.
- Instabilidade lombossacra.
- Espondilopatia lombossacra.
- Espondilolistese lombossacra.

VER TAMBÉM
- Discospondilite.
- Discopatia Intervertebral — Toracolombar.

ABREVIATURA(S)
- AINEs = anti-inflamatórios não esteroides.
- RM = ressonância magnética.
- TC = tomografia computadorizada.

RECURSOS DA INTERNET
http://veterinarymedicine.dvm360.com/vetmed/Medicine/Degenerative-lumbosacral-stenosis-in-dogs/ArticleStandard/Article/detail/169902.

Sugestões de Leitura
De Risio L, Sharp NJ, Olby NJ, Munan KR, Thomas WB. Predictors of outcome after dorsal decompressive laminectomy for degenerative lumbosacral stenosis in dogs: 69 cases (1987-1997). JAVMA 2001, 219(5):624-628.
Jones JC, Banfield CM, Ward DL. Association between postoperative outcome and results of magnetic resonance imaging and computed tomography in working dogs with degenerative lumbosacral stenosis. JAVMA 2000, 216(11):1769-1774.
Jones JC, Shires PK, Inzana KD, Sponenberg DP, Massicotte C, Renberg W, Giroux A. Evaluation of canine lumbosacral stenosis using intravenous contrast-enhanced computed tomography. Vet Radiol Ultrasound 1999, 40(2):108-114.
Linn L, Bartels K, Rochat M, Payton M, Moore G. Lumbosacral stenosis in 29 military working dogs: Epidemiologic findings and outcome after surgical intervention (1990-1999). Vet Surg 2003, 32:21-29.
Suwankong N, Voorhout G, Hazewinkle HA, Meij BP. Agreement between computed tomography, magnetic resonance imaging, and surgical findings in dogs with degenerative lumbosacral stenosis. JAVMA 2006, 229(12):1924-1929.

Autor Karen Dyer Inzana
Consultor Editorial Joane M. Parent

Estenose Nasofaríngea

CONSIDERAÇÕES GERAIS

REVISÃO
• Formação de membrana fina, porém resistente, no meato nasal interno, resultando na oclusão da abertura nasofaríngea caudal ou no estreitamento do orifício de uma abertura oval de >1 cm para uma abertura de 1 a 2 mm ou menos.
• Inflamação e fibrose crônicas ao exame histológico sugerem alguma causa infecciosa.
• Inflamação secundária à regurgitação ou vômito crônico de material ácido em direção à nasofaringe deve ser considerada como uma possível causa.
• Também há suspeitas de estreitamento ou disgenesia congênita da região; há relatos de músculos palatofaríngeos espessados como uma causa de estenose nasofaríngea no Dachshund.

IDENTIFICAÇÃO
• Gatos de qualquer raça ou sexo.
• Observada menos comumente em cães.
• Idade — qualquer idade contanto que tenha transcorrido muito tempo desde a exposição até a causa incitante; os casos congênitos podem se manifestar no início ou final da vida.

SINAIS CLÍNICOS
• Indícios de obstrução do trato respiratório superior.
• Ruído de assobio ou de ronco durante a respiração.
• Respiração de boca aberta.
• Secreção nasal mínima em muitos casos.
• Duração dos sinais de, no mínimo, alguns meses.
• Agravamento dos sinais clínicos durante a alimentação.
• Falha em responder a antibióticos ou corticosteroides.
• Ausência de fluxo aéreo nasal de uma ou ambas as narinas.

CAUSAS E FATORES DE RISCO
• Doença respiratória superior, potencialmente desencadeada por causas virais ou bacterianas.
• Corpo estranho ou área acometida por irritante de contato (regurgitação perianestésica, refluxo de conteúdo gástrico secundário à doença esofágica ou gástrica).

DIAGNÓSTICO

DIAGNÓSTICO DIFERENCIAL
• Pólipos nasofaríngeos — observados durante o exame bucal ou por radiografia ou endoscopia.
• Rinite ou sinusite crônicas — secreção nasal moderada a grave e espirros; alterações radiográficas óbvias costumam ser observadas.
• Corpo estranho — secreção nasal mucopurulenta unilateral; anormalidades radiográficas.
• Neoplasia intranasal — obstrução unilateral; secreção nasal frequentemente sanguinolenta; alterações radiográficas.
• Rinite micótica — secreção nasal moderada a grave, quase sempre hemorrágica; alterações radiográficas.
• Laringopatia — sem melhora com a respiração de boca aberta; ausência de ronco e de secreção nasal; anormalidades ao exame bucal.

HEMOGRAMA/BIOQUÍMICA/URINÁLISE
N/D.

OUTROS TESTES LABORATORIAIS
N/D.

DIAGNÓSTICO POR IMAGEM
• Achados radiográficos quase normais.
• Pode-se visualizar a estenose nasofaríngea ao exame de TC. Talvez haja necessidade de reconstrução sagital das imagens.

MÉTODOS DIAGNÓSTICOS
• Impossibilidade de atravessar um cateter de 3,5 French pelo meato ventral em direção à faringe.
• Visualização da estenose pelo uso de broncoscópio pediátrico retrofletido em direção à nasofaringe ou uso de espelho odontológico iluminado.

TRATAMENTO

• Cirurgia — sob anestesia geral; paciente posicionado em decúbito dorsal com a boca amplamente aberta; incisar o palato mole; ressecar a membrana; suturar o palato mole.
• Dilatação com balão — método não invasivo; a fluoroscopia simplifica o procedimento; a aplicação intralesional de triancinolona pode evitar recidivas.

MEDICAÇÕES

MEDICAMENTO(S)
Antibióticos após a cirurgia.

CONTRAINDICAÇÕES/INTERAÇÕES POSSÍVEIS
N/D.

ACOMPANHAMENTO

• Avisar o proprietário sobre a possibilidade de recidiva.
• Considerar o uso de corticosteroides intralesionais ou inalados se houver a necessidade de um segundo procedimento.

DIVERSOS

ABREVIATURA(S)
• TC = tomografia computadorizada.

Sugestões de Leitura
Berent AC, Kinns J, Weisse C. Balloon dilatation of nasopharyngeal stenosis in a dog. JAVMA 2006, 229:385-388.
Glaus TM, Gerber B, Tomsa K, Keiser M. Reproducible and long-lasting success of balloon dilation of nasopharyngeal stenosis in cats. Vet Record 2005, 157:257-259.
Unterer S, Kirberger RM, Steenkamp G, Spotswood TC, Boy SC, Miller DB, van Zyl M. Stenotic nasopharyngeal dysgenesis in the dachshund: Seven cases (2002-2004). JAAHA 2006, 42:290-297.

Autor Lynelle R. Johnson
Consultor Editorial Lynelle R. Johnson
Agradecimento a Justin H. Straus por ter escrito este capítulo nas edições anteriores.

Estenose Pulmonar

CONSIDERAÇÕES GERAIS

DEFINIÇÃO
Estreitamento congênito do trato do fluxo de saída do ventrículo direito, obstruindo a passagem do fluxo deste ventrículo para a artéria pulmonar; geralmente é valvular, embora possa ser subvalvular ou supravalvular.

FISIOPATOLOGIA
A estenose provoca uma sobrecarga de pressão do ventrículo direito, resultando em hipertrofia concêntrica. O ventrículo direito desenvolve pressões sistólicas elevadas para superar a estenose, cuja magnitude se correlaciona com a gravidade da estenose. A diferença entre a pressão ventricular direita elevada e a pressão arterial pulmonar normal (i. e., o gradiente de pressão) é frequentemente utilizada para descrever a gravidade da estenose. A hipertrofia do ventrículo direito aumenta o risco de isquemia e de arritmias. As alterações geométricas no formato do ventrículo direito podem resultar em insuficiência tricúspide secundária, embora a insuficiência tricúspide também possa estar associada à displasia concomitante dessa valva atrioventricular direita. Com o exercício, o ventrículo direito pode ficar incapaz de aumentar o volume sistólico de forma adequada. A insuficiência tricúspide com ou sem insuficiência miocárdica do ventrículo direito pode levar a pressões atriais direitas elevadas e ICC direita. Um quadro concomitante de defeito do septo atrial ou persistência do forame oval pode causar desvio da direita para a esquerda, especialmente com o exercício, o que pode resultar em cianose de esforço. Em geral, uma leve estenose pulmonar não produz efeitos hemodinâmicos significativos além do sopro de ejeção.

SISTEMA(S) ACOMETIDO(S)
• Cardiovascular — ICC direita, arritmias.
• Hepatobiliar — hepatomegalia com ICC direita.
• Nervoso — hipoperfusão cerebral durante o exercício.

GENÉTICA
Defeito hereditário nos cães da raça Beagle; sugere-se um modo poligênico de transmissão.

INCIDÊNCIA/PREVALÊNCIA
• A maior parte das pesquisas revela a estenose pulmonar como o terceiro defeito cardíaco congênito mais comum nos cães, compreendendo 21% dos defeitos cardíacos congênitos em um único estudo.
• Rara nos gatos, especialmente como defeito isolado, abrangendo 3% dos defeitos cardíacos congênitos em um único estudo.

IDENTIFICAÇÃO
Espécies
Cães e gatos.

Raça(s) Predominante(s)
Buldogue inglês, Terrier escocês, Fox terrier de pelo duro, Schnauzer miniatura, West Highland white terrier, Chihuahua, Samoieda, Mastife, Cocker spaniel, Beagle, Boxer.

Idade Média e Faixa Etária
Presente desde o nascimento e pode ser detectada sob a forma de sopro em filhotes de cão; caso não se detecte qualquer sopro, os animais acometidos podem não ser identificados até o subsequente desenvolvimento dos sinais clínicos.

Sexo Predominante
Predileção para os machos na raça Buldogue inglês e possivelmente em outras raças.

SINAIS CLÍNICOS
Comentários Gerais
• Estenose leve — geralmente sem sinais clínicos.
• Pacientes gravemente acometidos — podem desenvolver ICC, síncope por esforço ou morte súbita.

Achados Anamnésicos
• Distensão abdominal.
• Dispneia.
• Síncope por esforço, intolerância ao exercício ou morte súbita.
• Assintomática.

Achados do Exame Físico
• Sopro sistólico mais alto sobre a base do coração do lado esquerdo; pode se propagar amplamente, porém mais no sentido dorsal à esquerda em particular.
• Sopro — mesossistólico ou holossistólico e crescendo-decrescendo.
• Sopros mais sonoros com frêmito precordial — geralmente associados à estenose mais grave.
• Podem ocorrer arritmias; a frequência cardíaca pode estar alta na ICC.
• Outros sinais de ICC incluem ascite, distensão venosa jugular e taquipneia.

CAUSAS
Congênitas.

DIAGNÓSTICO

DIAGNÓSTICO DIFERENCIAL
• Sopros Semelhantes Podem Ser Encontrados em Casos de:
  ◦ Estenose aórtica.
  ◦ Defeitos dos septos atriais ou ventriculares com desvio acentuado da esquerda para a direita.
  ◦ Tetralogia de Fallot.
• ICC Direita Associada a Sopro Pode Ser Observada em Casos de:
  ◦ Valvulopatia adquirida (endocardiose).
  ◦ Miocardiopatia dilatada.

HEMOGRAMA/BIOQUÍMICA/URINÁLISE
• Geralmente, não há alterações dignas de nota.
• Pode haver policitemia com desvio da direita para a esquerda.

DIAGNÓSTICO POR IMAGEM
Achados Radiográficos
• Radiografias torácicas costumam revelar aumento cardíaco do lado direito, com abaulamento pós-estenótico da artéria pulmonar visível na projeção dorsoventral na posição de 1-2 h.
• A veia cava caudal pode estar ampla, podendo haver ascite com ou sem efusão pleural na insuficiência congestiva.

Achados Ecocardiográficos
• Hipertrofia do ventrículo direito, com achatamento do septo interventricular e aparência de "figura em oito" nas projeções de eixo curto nos casos graves.
• Em geral, é possível obter imagem do local da estenose, embora isso possa ser mais difícil quando a válvula está hipoplásica; válvulas pulmonares displásicas aparecem como folhetos ecodensos espessados; folhetos fundidos apresentam movimento anormal com cúpula sistólica; estenoses subvalvulares ou supravalvulares discretas podem aparecer como estreitamento hiperecoico localizado.
• "Ventrículo direito com dupla câmara" é uma variante da estenose pulmonar subvalvular, caracterizada por estenose muscular ou fibromuscular focal na porção média do ventrículo direito. Pode ser difícil obter a imagem dessa alteração nas projeções convencionais.
• Hipertrofia localizada pode ser vista na região infundibular do ventrículo direito.
• Pode-se observar dilatação pós-estenótica da artéria pulmonar.

Ecocardiografia com Doppler
• Pode-se usar o Doppler espectral para medir a velocidade elevada do fluxo da artéria pulmonar a fim de calcular o gradiente de pressão por meio da estenose. Gradientes de pressão abaixo de 50 mmHg geralmente representam estenose leve; aqueles acima de 100 mmHg indicam estenose grave.
• Doppler de fluxo colorido pode revelar regurgitação tricúspide.

Angiografia
• Angiografia cardíaca seletiva pode ajudar a identificar as anormalidades morfológicas exatas antes de cirurgia; podem-se obter imagens de válvulas displásicas e hipertrofia infundibular com mais clareza.
• Valiosa na identificação da estenose pulmonar causada por artéria coronária anômala circundando o trato do fluxo de saída ventricular direito, a qual pode afetar a escolha do tratamento; recomendada para o Buldogue inglês, já que essa anomalia é relatada com frequência.

MÉTODOS DIAGNÓSTICOS
Eletrocardiografia
• Alterações na forma da onda do complexo QRS incluem ondas S profundas nas derivações I, II, III e aVF, além de desvio do eixo para a direita.
• Pode ocorrer fibrilação atrial com aumento grave do átrio direito.

Cateterismo Cardíaco
A mensuração da pressão por essa técnica raramente é necessária para o diagnóstico; os gradientes de pressão podem ser avaliados de forma não invasiva por meio da ecocardiografia com Doppler.

ACHADOS PATOLÓGICOS
• Existem várias formas; a maior parte delas resulta em hipertrofia do ventrículo direito e dilatação pós-estenótica da artéria pulmonar; pode ocorrer hipertrofia infundibular em local proximal à obstrução.
• Válvula pulmonar hipoplásica com folhetos espessados ("válvula pulmonar displásica").
• Anel da válvula pulmonar normal com as comissuras fundidas.
• Artérias coronárias anômalas.
• Estenose supravalvular ou subvalvular discreta, com possível displasia tricúspide concomitante.
• Bandas fibromusculares que dividem os tratos do fluxo de entrada e de saída ventriculares direitos ("ventrículo direito com dupla câmara").

ESTENOSE PULMONAR

TRATAMENTO

CUIDADO(S) DE SAÚDE ADEQUADO(S)
A maioria dos casos é tratada em um esquema ambulatorial; a hospitalização inicial daqueles com ICC grave pode ser a melhor opção.

CUIDADO(S) DE ENFERMAGEM
Raramente, efusões pleurais podem necessitar de drenagem; em geral, a ascite é tratada de modo clínico.

ATIVIDADE
O exercício deve ficar restrito nos casos com síncope ou insuficiência congestiva; entretanto, é recomendável evitar a atividade física nos casos assintomáticos com estenose grave.

DIETA
Dietas pobres em sal (hipossódicas) podem beneficiar aqueles com ascite refratária.

ORIENTAÇÃO AO PROPRIETÁRIO
- Animais levemente acometidos podem levar vida normal.
- Pacientes moderada a gravemente acometidos podem se beneficiar de intervenções como dilatação com cateter em balão ou cirurgia; a melhora dos sinais clínicos e o aumento da sobrevida são associados a procedimentos bem-sucedidos com dilatação por balão.
- O prognóstico será reservado assim que os sinais congestivos se desenvolverem.
- Não acasalar os animais acometidos.

CONSIDERAÇÕES CIRÚRGICAS
- Dilatação com cateter em balão — método raramente seguro que envolve a passagem de cateter através da estenose e a insuflação de balão para dilatar a obstrução; em muitos casos, o gradiente de pressão fica significativamente reduzido, sobretudo quando a lesão é provocada pelas comissuras fundidas; menor êxito com válvulas displásicas ou hipoplásicas e contraindicada com artérias coronárias anômalas.
- Em geral, a cirurgia não é bem-sucedida em ventrículo direito com dupla câmara.
- Técnicas cirúrgicas alternativas incluem valvulotomia ou métodos de enxerto tipo remendo; os índices de mortalidade tendem a ser mais elevados do que com a valvuloplastia com balão.

MEDICAÇÕES

MEDICAMENTO(S) DE ESCOLHA
Se houver sinais de ICC, tratar a ascite com furosemida (2-4 mg/kg VO a cada 8-12 h); na insuficiência refratária, pode ser válido adicionar espironolactona (1-2 mg/kg VO a cada 12 h); tratar a fibrilação atrial com digoxina (0,22 mg/m^2 VO a cada 12 h).

CONTRAINDICAÇÕES
Vasodilatadores (p. ex., hidralazina) podem provocar hipotensão sem aliviar a estenose, mas o melhor é evitá-los.

PRECAUÇÕES
Evitar o uso exagerado de diuréticos; administrar fluidos intravenosos (quando necessários) com cuidado para evitar a exacerbação dos sinais congestivos. Inibidores da ECA podem ser valiosos com sinais congestivos, embora possam provocar hipotensão. Iniciar com baixas doses e monitorizar a pressão arterial.

ACOMPANHAMENTO

MONITORIZAÇÃO DO PACIENTE
Utilizar ecocardiogramas seriados para acompanhar o gradiente de pressão e o tamanho da câmara cardíaca.

PREVENÇÃO
Não acasalar os animais acometidos.

COMPLICAÇÕES POSSÍVEIS
- ICC direita.
- Arritmias.
- Intolerância ao exercício.
- Síncope por esforço.
- Morte súbita.

EVOLUÇÃO ESPERADA E PROGNÓSTICO
- Animais levemente acometidos podem permanecer assintomáticos com tempo de vida normal.
- Animais gravemente acometidos apresentam prognóstico reservado, pois podem desenvolver ICC ou sofrer morte súbita; os sinais clínicos geralmente são mais comuns nos animais com mais de 1 ano de idade.

DIVERSOS

DISTÚRBIOS ASSOCIADOS
- Defeitos dos septos atriais ou ventriculares e persistência do forame oval.
- A raça Buldogue inglês é descrita com artéria coronária direita única de onde surge uma artéria coronária principal esquerda anômala que circunda e faz constrição na base da válvula pulmonar.

FATORES RELACIONADOS COM A IDADE
Defeito e sopro estão presentes desde o nascimento.

GESTAÇÃO/FERTILIDADE/REPRODUÇÃO
Não acasalar os animais acometidos.

SINÔNIMO(S)
Estenose pulmônica.

VER TAMBÉM
- Insuficiência Cardíaca Congestiva Direita.
- Sopros Cardíacos.

ABREVIATURA(S)
- ECA = enzima conversora de angiotensina.
- ICC = insuficiência cardíaca congestiva.

Sugestões de Leitura
Buchanan JW. Pathogenesis of single right coronary artery and pulmonic stenosis in English Bulldogs. J Vet Intern Med 2001, 15:101-104.
Bussadori C, DeMadron E, Santilli RA, Borgarelli M. Balloon valvuloplasty in 30 dogs with pulmonic stenosis: Effect of valve morphology and annular size on initial and 1-year outcome. J Vet Intern Med 2001, 15:553-558.
Fingland RB, Bonagura JD, Myer CW. Pulmonic stenosis in the dog: 29 cases (1975-1984). JAVMA 1986, 189:218-226.
Johnson MS, Martin M, Edwards D, et al. Pulmonic stenosis in dogs: Balloon dilation improves clinical outcome. J Vet Intern Med 2004, 18:656-662.
Koffas H, Luis Fuentes V, Boswood A, et al. Double chambered right ventricle in 9 cats. J Vet Intern Med 2007, 21:76-80.

Autor Virginia Luis Fuentes
Consultores Editoriais Larry P. Tilley e Francis W.K. Smith, Jr.

Estenose Retal

CONSIDERAÇÕES GERAIS

REVISÃO
- Diminuição do tamanho do lúmen retal ou anal causada por contratura ou formação cicatriciais como resultado de cicatrização de ferida ou processo de inflamação crônica ou por doença neoplásica proliferativa.
- A função gastrintestinal fica comprometida por causa da obstrução ao fluxo de saída.
- Não há relatos de base genética.

IDENTIFICAÇÃO
- Cães e gatos.
- Também não há relatos de predileção etária, racial ou sexual.

SINAIS CLÍNICOS
- Variam com a gravidade da lesão.
- Tenesmo.
- Disquezia e constipação.
- Hematoquezia.
- Fezes mucoides.
- Diarreia do intestino grosso.
- Pode ocorrer o desenvolvimento de megacólon secundário.

CAUSAS E FATORES DE RISCO
- Inflamatórias — abscesso retoanal, saculite anal, fístulas perianais, proctite, corpo estranho, infecção fúngica (p. ex., histoplasmose e pitiose).
- Traumáticas — lacerações.
- Neoplásicas — adenocarcinoma retal, leiomioma, pólipos retais.
- Iatrogênicas — anastomose retal, excisão de massa retal, biopsia retal.
- Congênitas — atresia anal.

DIAGNÓSTICO

DIAGNÓSTICO DIFERENCIAL
- Processos expansivos que levem à diminuição da capacidade retal (compressão retal extraluminal [p. ex., prostatopatias e fraturas pélvicas], obstrução retal intraluminal [p. ex., pseudocopróstase e corpo estranho]) e constrição funcional (espasmos musculares do reto).
- Diferenciar por palpação retal e diagnóstico por imagem.

HEMOGRAMA/BIOQUÍMICA/URINÁLISE
- Geralmente normais.
- Pacientes com infecção ou inflamação podem apresentar leucograma inflamatório.

OUTROS TESTES LABORATORIAIS
N/D

DIAGNÓSTICO POR IMAGEM
- Radiografias abdominais simples e estudos contrastados (p. ex., enema baritado, com ar ou de duplo contraste e séries gastrintestinais com bário) podem revelar estreitamento consistente no diâmetro do lúmen retal.
- Radiografias contrastadas necessitam de preparo adequado do paciente (enemas de água morna ± polietilenoglicol 30-50 mL/kg VO 12 e 6 h antes do procedimento) seguido pela instilação de 10 mL de bário/kg por meio de cateter-balão.
- A combinação de ar e bário permite melhor observação da mucosa colônica e ajuda a determinar a extensão da lesão; pode ser difícil delinear as lesões muito próximas do ânus.
- Ultrassonografia abdominal poderá revelar espessamento e arquitetura alterada se houver doença retocolônica infiltrativa (p. ex., pitiose ou neoplasia).

MÉTODOS DIAGNÓSTICOS
- Palpação retal digital para caracterizar e determinar a extensão e a localização da estenose.
- Proctoscopia/colonoscopia pode ser valiosa para observar a estenose, determinar a extensão da lesão e obter amostra de biopsia.
- Raspados colônicos podem auxiliar no diagnóstico citológico de doenças fúngicas (histoplasmose) e neoplásicas.
- Realizar biopsia e avaliar a lesão ao exame histopatológico para classificar o processo mórbido e estabelecer o prognóstico.

TRATAMENTO

- Resolver a causa subjacente antes de tratar especificamente a estenose sempre que possível.
- Efetuar tratamento clínico paliativo com a utilização de amolecedores fecais e enemas ou a eliminação dos agentes infectantes ou das condições inflamatórias.
- Administrar fluidoterapia para otimizar a hidratação antes de aplicar o enema para pacientes constipados ou obstipados.
- Talvez haja necessidade de anestesia para a administração do enema.
- Proceder à dilatação de estenoses não neoplásicas e pós-operatórias com balão — pode ser necessário mais de um procedimento com base na resposta do paciente.
- Realizar reconstrução cirúrgica de estenoses focais (procedimentos de plástica) (ver a seção "Sugestões de Leitura" em busca de mais detalhes).
- Pode haver a necessidade de anastomose com ressecção completa para lesões extensas e estenoses recidivantes.
- Radio e/ou quimioterapia podem beneficiar o tratamento de algumas neoplasias.

MEDICAÇÕES

MEDICAMENTO(S)
- Amolecedores de fezes — docusato de sódio (cães, 50-200 mg VO a cada 8-12 h; gatos, 50 mg VO a cada 12-24 h); lactulose (solução a 10 g/15 mL, na dose de 1 mL/4,5 kg a cada 8-12 h até fazer efeito). A injeção intralesional de corticosteroides, como triancinolona antes da dilatação, pode melhorar os resultados. A injeção pode ser repetida mais uma vez se houver necessidade de mais dilatações.
- Corticosteroides — pode-se usar a prednisona para tratar condições inflamatórias não infecciosas (0,5-1 mg/kg VO a cada 24 h ou dividido a cada 12 h) e após a dilatação com balão ou a passagem de vela ou de cânula para evitar a recidiva da estenose.
- A quimioterapia pode ser indicada para diversas neoplasias.
- Terapia antifúngica na presença de infecção por fungos.
- Terapia antimicrobiana perioperatória apropriada é defendida em conjunto com dilatação por balão ou terapia cirúrgica; escolher um agente com amplo espectro de atividade contra anaeróbios e coliformes (p. ex., cefoxitina sódica [30 mg/kg IV]).
- Os antibióticos podem ser administrados após dilatação caso ocorra laceração da mucosa (p. ex., amoxicilina ou metronidazol).

CONTRAINDICAÇÕES/INTERAÇÕES POSSÍVEIS
- Corticosteroides quando houver possibilidade de infecção.
- Os corticosteroides podem afetar de modo adverso a cicatrização após correção cirúrgica da estenose.

ACOMPANHAMENTO

MONITORIZAÇÃO DO PACIENTE
- Resolução ou recidiva dos sinais clínicos.
- Pacientes com lesões neoplásicas — recidiva e doença metastática.

COMPLICAÇÕES POSSÍVEIS
- Tratamento clínico — podem incluir ineficácia, diarreia e efeitos adversos das medicações.
- A dilatação com balão pode resultar em lacerações retais profundas, hemorragia ou, possivelmente, perfuração de toda a espessura.
- Tratamento cirúrgico — incontinência fecal, formação de estenose secundária e deiscência da ferida.

EVOLUÇÃO ESPERADA E PROGNÓSTICO
- Varia com a gravidade da estenose.
- Pacientes com estenoses benignas que são facilmente submetidos à terapia clínica ou a procedimentos cirúrgicos como dilatação com balão ou passagem de vela ou de cânula podem apresentar resultados bons a longo prazo.
- A ressecção cirúrgica possui prognóstico mais reservado por causa da frequência de complicações.
- A maior parte dos pacientes com sinais clínicos identificáveis em virtude de neoplasia apresenta prognóstico reservado a mau quanto à resolução completa.

DIVERSOS

FATORES RELACIONADOS COM A IDADE
Observa-se atresia anal depois de semanas do nascimento.

VER TAMBÉM
- Colite e Proctite.
- Constipação e Obstipação.
- Disquezia e Hematoquezia.
- Fístula Perianal.
- Histoplasmose.
- Pitiose.
- Pólipos Retoanais.

Sugestões de Leitura
Webb CB, McCord KW, Twedt DC. Rectal strictures in 19 dogs: 1997-2005. JAAHA 2007, 43:332-336.
Zoran DL. Rectoanal disease. In: Ettinger SJ, Feldman EC, eds., Textbook of Veterinary Internal Medicine, 6th ed. St. Louis: Elsevier, 2005, pp. 1408-1420.

Autor Eric R. Pope
Consultor Editorial Albert E. Jergens

ESTERTOR E ESTRIDOR

CONSIDERAÇÕES GERAIS

DEFINIÇÃO
• Ruídos anormalmente elevados que resultam da passagem de ar pela nasofaringe, faringe, laringe ou traqueia estreitadas.
• Ruídos descontínuos audíveis sem o estetoscópio.
• Estertor — ruído de ronco de baixa intensidade que, em geral, surge da vibração de tecido flácido ou de líquido; geralmente se origina de obstrução das vias aéreas nasais e faríngeas.
• Estridor — ruídos de intensidade mais elevada que ocorrem quando tecidos relativamente rígidos são vibrados pela passagem do ar; resultado da obstrução parcial ou completa da laringe ou da porção cervical da traqueia.

FISIOPATOLOGIA
• A obstrução das vias aéreas provoca turbulência à medida que o ar passa por uma via estreitada; com a piora da obstrução ou com o aumento da velocidade do fluxo de ar, a amplitude do ruído aumenta à medida que o tecido, a secreção ou o corpo estranho responsável pela obstrução vibra.
• Uma obstrução suficiente a ponto de aumentar a atividade respiratória promove o aumento do esforço muscular respiratório e exacerba a turbulência; podem ocorrer o desenvolvimento de inflamação e a formação de edema dos tecidos na região da obstrução, diminuindo ainda mais o lúmen das vias aéreas e aumentando ainda mais a atividade respiratória, criando um círculo vicioso.
• A obesidade potencializa o esforço respiratório acentuado, exacerbando com isso a obstrução das vias aéreas.

SISTEMA(S) ACOMETIDO(S)
Respiratório.

GENÉTICA
• A síndrome braquicefálica das vias aéreas é hereditária em muitas raças.
• A paralisia hereditária da laringe é identificada nas raças Bouvier des Flandres, Rottweiler, Husky siberiano e Dálmata.

INCIDÊNCIA/PREVALÊNCIA
Comuns.

DISTRIBUIÇÃO GEOGRÁFICA
Mundial.

IDENTIFICAÇÃO
Espécies
Cães e gatos.

Raça(s) Predominante(s)
• Comuns em cães ou gatos braquicefálicos.
• Paralisia adquirida da laringe — super-representada em determinadas raças gigantes (p. ex., São Bernardo e Terra Nova) e em raças de grande porte (p. ex., Setter irlandês, Labrador e Golden retriever).

Idade Média e Faixa Etária
• Animais braquicefálicos acometidos e cães ou gatos com paralisia hereditária da laringe tipicamente têm menos de 1 ano de idade quando o proprietário detecta o problema.
• Paralisia adquirida da laringe ocorre tipicamente em cães e gatos mais idosos.
• Gatos — diagnosticados menos comumente do que nos cães; sem padrão etário óbvio.

Sexo Predominante
Sem predileção sexual para qualquer causa embora a paralisia hereditária da laringe apresente predominância masculina da ordem de 3:1.

SINAIS CLÍNICOS
• Alteração ou perda da vocalização.
• Obstrução parcial — produz aumento nos ruídos das vias aéreas antes de produzir alteração evidente no padrão respiratório ou na troca gasosa.
• Os proprietários podem indicar que o ruído existe há muitos anos.
• Ruídos respiratórios audíveis a certa distância sem o estetoscópio — suspeita de estreitamento das vias aéreas.
• Natureza do ruído — varia desde anormalmente alto a tremor evidente até chiado de alta intensidade, dependendo do grau de estreitamento das vias aéreas.
• Podem-se notar esforço respiratório aumentado e movimentos respiratórios paradoxais (colapsos da parede torácica para dentro durante a inspiração e saltos para fora durante a expiração) quando o esforço é extremo; os movimentos respiratórios quase sempre são acompanhados por alterações posturais evidentes (p. ex., membros anteriores abduzidos, cabeça e pescoço estendidos e respiração com a boca aberta).

CAUSAS
• Síndrome braquicefálica das vias aéreas (estenose das narinas, alongamento do palato mole, eversão dos sáculos laríngeos, colapso da laringe).
• Paralisia da laringe — herdada ou adquirida.
• Neoplasia da laringe — benigna ou maligna.
• Laringite granulomatosa/inflamatória.
• Colapso, estenose, obstrução, neoplasia ou corpo estranho traqueais.
• Pólipo, estenose, corpo estranho nasofaríngeos.
• Acromegalia.
• Disfunção neuromuscular ou traumatismo.
• Anestesia ou sedação — apenas se existir anatomia predisponente.
• Cisto da fenda de Rathke.
• Palato mole fendido.
• Aplasia do palato mole.
• Pregas excessivas da mucosa faríngea.
• Massa no palato mole.
• Edema ou inflamação do palato, da faringe e da laringe (incluindo o revestimento mucoso evertido dos ventrículos laríngeos) — secundários à tosse, ao vômito ou à regurgitação, fluxo aéreo turbulento, infecção respiratória superior e hemorragia.
• Secreções (p. ex., pus, muco e sangue) no lúmen das vias aéreas — de forma aguda depois de cirurgia; o animal consciente normal as expectoraria ou engoliria.

FATORES DE RISCO
• Temperatura ambiente elevada.
• Febre.
• Taxa metabólica elevada — como ocorre nos quadros de hipertireoidismo ou sepse.
• Exercício.
• Ansiedade ou agitação.
• Qualquer doença cardiovascular ou respiratória que aumente a ventilação.
• A turbulência provocada pelo aumento do fluxo de ar pode levar à tumefação e piorar a obstrução das vias aéreas.

DIAGNÓSTICO

DIAGNÓSTICO DIFERENCIAL
• Sem indicadores valiosos, deve-se auscultar o animal sistematicamente sobre o nariz, a faringe, a laringe e a traqueia para identificar não só o ponto de máxima intensidade de qualquer ruído anormal, mas também a fase da respiração em que ele seja mais evidente.
• É importante identificar a localização anatômica de onde surge o ruído anormal, para procurar as causas exacerbantes (ver a seção "Fatores de Risco"; p. ex., uma obstrução crônica das vias aéreas pode se tornar manifesta quando o paciente fica exposto a temperaturas ambientes extremamente elevadas).
• É imprescindível diferenciar os ruídos de estreitamento faríngeo, laríngeo e traqueal daqueles que surgem em qualquer outro local do sistema respiratório.
• Estreitamento das vias nasais e da traqueia, além de estreitamento grave ou extenso dos brônquios — podem provocar o aumento dos ruídos respiratórios.
• Se o ruído persistir quando o paciente abrir a boca, praticamente é possível descartar uma causa nasal.
• Se o proprietário descrever uma mudança na vocalização do animal, a laringe provavelmente será o local da anormalidade.

OUTROS TESTES LABORATORIAIS
Ocasionalmente, fica indicado o exame de gasometria arterial; em casos de obstrução grave e prolongada das vias aéreas, ocorrem hipoxia e hipoventilação.

DIAGNÓSTICO POR IMAGEM
• Radiografias laterais da cabeça e do pescoço — podem ajudar a identificar tecidos moles anormais das vias aéreas (p. ex., palato mole alongado ou pólipo nasal); utilização limitada para identificar paralisia da laringe embora radiologistas experientes consigam identificar sáculos laríngeos anormalmente dilatados ou tumefatos; a destruição cartilaginosa sugere neoplasia ou laringite granulomatosa; pode permitir a avaliação adicional de massas externas que comprimem as vias aéreas superiores.
• Radiografia e fluoroscopia — exames importantes para avaliar o sistema cardiorrespiratório; descartar outras causas ou causas adicionais de dificuldade respiratória; tais condições podem contribuir para uma obstrução subjacente das vias aéreas superiores, fazendo com que a condição subclínica se torne clínica (sintomática).
• A técnica de radiologia digital é a preferida para obtenção de imagens com mais detalhes.
• O ultrassom pode ser utilizado para avaliar a estrutura e a função da laringe, embora também possa ser usado para registrar algum colapso da porção cervical da traqueia; no entanto, o ar não é uma boa janela acústica.
• A tomografia computadorizada pode ser empregada para fornecer detalhes anatômicos adicionais.

MÉTODOS DIAGNÓSTICOS
Faringoscopia e Laringoscopia
• Testes diagnósticos definitivos para inspeção direta de alterações faríngeas ou laríngeas.

ESTERTOR E ESTRIDOR

- Necessitam de sedação intensa que preserve a função da laringe.
- Lembrar que a capacidade do paciente em utilizar os músculos para abrir as vias aéreas fica comprometida pela anestesia; o veterinário e os proprietários devem determinar se eles estão preparados para efetuar correções cirúrgicas se indicadas.
- Caso não se identifiquem nem se corrijam os problemas passíveis de correção — a recuperação do paciente da anestesia pode ficar complicada pela obstrução grave das vias aéreas; é preciso ficar preparado para realizar uma traqueostomia se a via aérea estiver obstruída e caso não se consiga efetuar a correção cirúrgica definitiva imediatamente.
- Determinar a sincronização e o grau de movimento das pregas vocais durante leve anestesia — avaliar a presença de paralisia da laringe. Utilizar o doxapram (1 mg/kg IV) para estimular a respiração, se houver necessidade.
- Palato normal — delgado; ele mal se sobrepõe às pontas da epiglote; deslocado facilmente no sentido dorsal, utilizando-se a lâmina do laringoscópio.
- Palato mole superalongado — espesso; em geral, inflamado; pode repousar 1 cm ou mais além da ponta da epiglote.
- O paciente deve estar o mais estabilizado possível antes de ser submetido à anestesia geral, mas não se deve adiar o procedimento de forma desmedida; o tratamento cirúrgico apropriado geralmente constitui o único meio de reduzir a obstrução das vias aéreas.

TRATAMENTO
CUIDADO(S) DE SAÚDE ADEQUADO(S)
- Para o tratamento cirúrgico, há necessidade de internação.
- Monitorizar com rigor os efeitos dos sedativos; tais agentes podem relaxar os músculos das vias aéreas superiores e piorar a obstrução; por essa razão, é preciso ficar preparado com recursos de emergência para manter as vias aéreas caso ocorra obstrução completa dessas vias. O diazepam é o sedativo preferido.
- Obstrução extrema das vias aéreas — tentar uma entubação de emergência; se a obstrução impedir a entubação, a traqueostomia de emergência ou a passagem de cateter traqueal para administrar oxigênio poderá ser o único meio disponível para manter a vida; um cateter traqueal pode manter a oxigenação apenas por um breve período enquanto se busca uma solução mais permanente.

CUIDADO(S) DE ENFERMAGEM
- O tratamento requer a remoção da obstrução, embora a suplementação de oxigênio seja variavelmente útil.
- Talvez haja necessidade de fluidoterapia intravenosa, particularmente se ocorrer o desenvolvimento de hipertermia por causa do aumento na atividade respiratória.
- Medidas ativas de resfriamento (bolsas de gelo nas regiões axilares e inguinais, aplicação de álcool nos coxins palmoplantares, fluidos IV resfriados) são úteis para aliviar a hipertermia, mas não são indicadas em casos de febre.

ATIVIDADE
Manter o paciente em ambiente fresco, quieto e calmo — ansiedade, esforço e dor levam ao aumento da ventilação, agravando potencialmente a obstrução.

DIETA
- Nada por via oral caso se planeje a realização de anestesia.
- Evitar a obesidade que piora o esforço respiratório.

ORIENTAÇÃO AO PROPRIETÁRIO
Informar o proprietário sobre o fato de que o paciente pode passar de uma respiração ruidosa para uma via aérea obstruída em alguns minutos ou até mesmo segundos.

CONSIDERAÇÕES CIRÚRGICAS
- Laringoscopia e broncoscopia são utilizadas não só para a recuperação de corpo estranho, mas também para a realização de biopsia de região da laringe e do lúmen da traqueia. O uso de pequenos cateteres tipo balão que passam pelo corpo estranho antes da expansão pode ser útil na remoção de alguns objetos.
- Tomar um cuidado especial na indução da anestesia geral ou no emprego de sedativos em qualquer paciente com obstrução das vias aéreas superiores.
- Cirurgia — indicada para obter o diagnóstico por meio de biopsia com exame histopatológico, tratar a obstrução enquanto se aguardam os resultados desse exame ou a resolução da inflamação/infecção (p. ex., traqueotomia) ou solucionar a doença por excisão, correção da lesão obstrutiva e remoção de corpos estranhos.

MEDICAÇÕES
MEDICAMENTO(S)
- Abordagens clínicas — serão apropriadas apenas se a causa subjacente for algum quadro de infecção, edema, inflamação ou hemorragia; causas anatômicas ou neurológicas não são responsivas ao tratamento clínico sintomático.
- Esteroides — poderão ser indicados se o edema ou a inflamação forem supostamente um fator que contribui para o quadro; o efeito obtido com a administração intravenosa deve ser evidenciado em aproximadamente 1 hora. Uma única dose pode ser suficiente ou talvez haja necessidade de uma redução gradativa da dosagem. A presença de laringite inflamatória quase sempre requer a administração de doses mais elevadas por um esquema posológico mais longo, com diminuição gradual da dose de acordo com a resolução dos sinais clínicos.

PRECAUÇÕES
Sedativos, analgésicos e anestésicos — evitar a supressão excessiva dos movimentos laríngeos e a supressão respiratória para prevenir a aspiração nos animais com laringopatia.

ACOMPANHAMENTO
MONITORIZAÇÃO DO PACIENTE
É necessário que a frequência e o esforço respiratórios sejam rigorosamente monitorizados. Quando o proprietário opta pelo tratamento de paciente aparentemente estável em casa ou caso a observação contínua não seja possível, informá-lo sobre a possibilidade de obstrução completa.

PREVENÇÃO
Aconselhar o proprietário a evitar exercícios, temperaturas ambientes elevadas e agitação extrema.

COMPLICAÇÕES POSSÍVEIS
Podem ocorrer sérias complicações sem o tratamento para aliviar a obstrução; essas complicações incluem edema das vias aéreas, edema pulmonar (pode evoluir para lesão pulmonar aguda com risco de morte) e hipoventilação; pode necessitar de traqueotomia e/ou ventilação artificial.

EVOLUÇÃO ESPERADA E PROGNÓSTICO
- Variam com a causa subjacente.
- Mesmo com o tratamento cirúrgico, algum grau de obstrução pode permanecer por 7-10 dias em virtude da tumefação.

DIVERSOS
DISTÚRBIOS ASSOCIADOS
Neuropatia periférica frequentemente associada à paralisia da laringe.

SINÔNIMO(S)
Ronco.

VER TAMBÉM
- Acromegalia — Gatos.
- Colapso Traqueal.
- Hipotireoidismo.
- Laringopatias.
- Miastenia Grave.
- Pólipos Nasais e Nasofaríngeos.
- Síndrome Braquicefálica das Vias Aéreas.

Sugestões de Leitura
Hendricks JC. Respiratory condition in critical patients. Vet Clin North Am Small Anim Pract 1989, 19:1167-1188.

Autor James C. Prueter
Consultor Editorial Lynelle R. Johnson

ESTOMATITE

CONSIDERAÇÕES GERAIS

DEFINIÇÃO
Inflamação do revestimento mucoso de qualquer uma das estruturas da cavidade bucal; no âmbito clínico, o termo deve ficar reservado para descrever inflamação bucal disseminada (além de gengivite e periodontite), que também pode se estender para os tecidos da submucosa (p. ex., a mucosite caudal acentuada que se estende para os tecidos da submucosa pode ser denominada "estomatite caudal".)

FISIOPATOLOGIA
- Processo inflamatório e outras alterações podem se desenvolver na mucosa bucal normal por causa da enorme quantidade de vasculatura na área e de sua proximidade com o ambiente externo.
- Também pode afetar o comportamento em função do desconforto e das dificuldades de alimentação; problemas oftalmológicos em virtude da proximidade de algumas estruturas bucais com as estruturas oculares; e pele se a inflamação se estender para a região peribucal.

GENÉTICA
N/D.

INCIDÊNCIA/PREVALÊNCIA
N/D.

DISTRIBUIÇÃO GEOGRÁFICA
Nenhuma.

IDENTIFICAÇÃO
Espécies
Cães e gatos.

Raça(s) Predominante(s)
- Estomatite ulcerativa na raça Maltês — incidência maior nos machos.
- Granuloma eosinofílico bucal — mais comumente na raça Husky siberiano (pode ser hereditário).
- Hiperplasia gengival em raças de grande porte (ver "Hiperplasia Gengival").
- Periodontite de rápida evolução, observada principalmente em animais jovens adultos como os das raças Galgo e Shih tzu.
- Periodontite juvenil localizada na região dos incisivos maxilares ou mandibulares — particularmente comum na raça Schnauzer miniatura.

Idade Média e Faixa Etária
- Periodontite de início juvenil em gatos jovens.
- Doença periodontal associada à formação de cálculo dentário é observada com maior frequência em cães e gatos idosos, bem como em raças suscetíveis.

Sexo Predominante
Nenhum.

SINAIS CLÍNICOS
Comentários Gerais
Com frequência, não se consegue fazer um diagnóstico definitivo de inflamação com base apenas nos achados do exame físico.

Achados do Exame Físico
- Halitose.
- Dor.
- Lesões ulceradas.
- Ptialismo.
- Edema.
- Possível inflamação periocular em virtude da proximidade com a cavidade bucal.
- Placa e cálculo dentários extensos. Procurar por lesões na cavidade bucal e nas superfícies labiais adjacentes aos dentes com grande quantidade de cálculo.

CAUSAS
Anatômicas
- Doença periodontal causada por apinhamento dos dentes.
- Inserção do frênulo labial.
- Síndrome dos lábios apertados* na raça Shar-pei.

Metabólicas
- Uremia e altos níveis de amônia na saliva.
- Vasculite e xerostomia são observadas em casos de diabetes melito.
- Macroglossia** e lábios tumefatos conforme vistos no hipoparatireoidismo.
- Possível envolvimento do palato e/ou da língua por linfoma.

Imunomediadas
- Pênfigo foliáceo.
- Pênfigo vulgar.
- Penfigoide bolhoso.
- Lúpus eritematoso sistêmico e lúpus eritematoso discoide no cão.
- Hipersensibilidade aguda a medicamentos.

Infecciosas
- Flora bucal oportunista secundária a lesões bucais.
- Estomatite micótica.
- Infecções sistêmicas.
- Leptospirose: petéquias.
- Lepra felina (micobactéria): placas elevadas (ou seja, em relevo).
- Infecções por calicivírus ou herpes-vírus — gatos.
- Cinomose.
- Papilomatose viral — cães.

Traumáticas
- Irritação por cálculo e placa dentárias.
- Corpos estranhos — síndrome dos mastigadores de chiclete.
- Choque por fio elétrico.
- Queimaduras químicas.
- Lacerações.
- Picadas de cobras.
- Pancadas.
- Traumatismo do palato pelos dentes caninos mandibulares de base estreita.

Tóxicas
- Determinadas plantas.
- Quimioterapia.
- Radioterapia.
- Irritantes químicos.

FATORES DE RISCO
Saúde bucal insatisfatória.

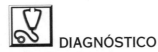

DIAGNÓSTICO

DIAGNÓSTICO DIFERENCIAL
- Úlceras bucais.

---

* N.T.: É uma doença em cães na ração Shar-pei, na qual o lábio inferior se dobra e cobre os dentes mandibulares.
** N.T.: Aumento extraordinário do volume da língua.

- Estomatite periodontal ulcerativa crônica.
- Osteomielite idiopática.
- Linfoma.

HEMOGRAMA/BIOQUÍMICA/URINÁLISE
Exames bioquímicos para detectar outras doenças.

OUTROS TESTES LABORATORIAIS
- Teste imunológico.
- Culturas micóticas.
- Isolamento viral.
- Estudos toxicológicos.
- Eletroforese de proteínas séricas.
- Testes endócrinos.

DIAGNÓSTICO POR IMAGEM
Radiografia para identificar anormalidades ósseas ou dentárias.

MÉTODOS DIAGNÓSTICOS
Biopsia.

TRATAMENTO

CUIDADO(S) DE SAÚDE ADEQUADO(S)
- Corrigir as deficiências nutricionais ou hídricas, conforme a necessidade, em um esquema ambulatorial ou internação.
- Doenças dentária ou periodontal presentes devem ser tratadas.

CUIDADO(S) DE ENFERMAGEM
Pode-se colocar sonda alimentar, se for preciso.

ATIVIDADE
N/D.

DIETA
Considerar o uso de dieta hipoalergênica para diminuir a carga antigênica que se acumula nas superfícies dentárias em casos de placas. Talvez haja necessidade de ajustes na dieta, dependendo da capacidade de alimentação do paciente na presença de dor.
O proprietário deve estar ciente de que esta é uma condição crônica e multifatorial que requer atenção constante, com respostas variáveis dos pacientes.

CONSIDERAÇÕES CIRÚRGICAS
Às vezes, a maior parte dos dentes, ou todos os dentes, precisam ser extraídos para resolver a estomatite.

MEDICAÇÕES

MEDICAMENTO(S) DE ESCOLHA
- Antimicrobianos — antibióticos de amplo espectro; amoxicilina-clavulanato; clindamicina; metronidazol (10 mg/kg VO a cada 12 h ou 40-50 mg/kg como dose de ataque no primeiro dia, seguida por 20-25 mg/kg a cada 8 h por 7 dias ou menos); doxiciclina (5 mg/kg VO como dose de ataque, 2,5 mg/kg VO 12 h depois e 2,5 mg/kg VO 1 vez ao dia daí em diante); solução ou gel de clorexidina (CHX®, VRx Products, Harbor City, CA) — retardante da placa; e Maxi-Guard® (Addison Biological Laboratory, Fayette, MO) — soluções e géis de zinco-ácido orgânico para promover a cicatrização tecidual e retardar o acúmulo de placa.
- Agentes anti-inflamatórios — prednisolona ou prednisona; para úlcera eosinofílica (2-4,4 mg/kg

ESTOMATITE

VO 1 vez ao dia; para os casos crônicos, utilizar 0,5-1 mg/kg VO em dias alternados); como terapia adjuvante de gengivite-faringite plasmocitária felina — pode melhorar a inflamação e o apetite.
• Medicamentos imunossupressores em caso de estomatite secundária à doença autoimune.
• Quimioterapia em caso de estomatite secundária a linfoma.
• Omegainterferona (interferona recombinante felina) — infiltrações da submucosa: 1-2 MU/cavidade bucal, repetidas 3 vezes em intervalos de 2 semanas se necessárias ou 1 MU/kg SC a cada 48 h por 5 injeções.

CONTRAINDICAÇÕES
Terapia imunossupressora em caso de estomatite secundária à doença infecciosa.

PRECAUÇÕES
N/D.

INTERAÇÕES POSSÍVEIS
N/D.

MEDICAMENTO(S) ALTERNATIVO(S)
N/D.

 ACOMPANHAMENTO

MONITORIZAÇÃO DO PACIENTE
Avaliar a cavidade bucal periodicamente para monitorizar a resolução ou a recidiva das lesões bucais.

PREVENÇÃO
• A aplicação semanal de OraVet® (Merial, Atlanta, GA) aos dentes sem cálculo pode ser útil para prevenir inflamação adicional aos tecidos bucais.
• Colutórios bucais e escovação dentária com medicamentos bucais podem ser valiosos, especialmente no caso de doença periodontal.
• Foi desenvolvida uma vacina periodontal (Pfizer, New York, NY), que está sendo comercializada para auxiliar na prevenção de perda óssea causada por periodontite em cães.

COMPLICAÇÕES POSSÍVEIS
A bacteremia gerada pela doença periodontal pode provocar doença renal, cardíaca, hepática e pulmonar.

EVOLUÇÃO ESPERADA E PROGNÓSTICO
Varia de acordo com a causa subjacente

 DIVERSOS

DISTÚRBIOS ASSOCIADOS
• Periodontite.
• Inflamação orofaríngea.
• Gengivite.
• Mucosite alveolar.
• Mucosite sublingual.
• Mucosite labial/bucal.
• Mucosite caudal.
• Palatite.
• Glossite.
• Queilite.
• Osteomielite.
• Tonsilite.
• Faringite.

FATORES RELACIONADOS COM A IDADE
N/D.

POTENCIAL ZOONÓTICO
Procedimentos de profilaxia dentária em pequenos animais têm causado infecções em seres humanos por bactérias aerossolizadas. Por isso, é recomendável o uso de óculos de segurança e máscara de proteção ao se efetuar tais procedimentos.

GESTAÇÃO/FERTILIDADE/REPRODUÇÃO
N/D.

SINÔNIMO(S)
• Estomatite de São Vicente, uma estomatite ulceromembranosa causada por *Fusobacterium* spp. e espiroquetas.
• Boca de trincheira.

VER TAMBÉM
• Inflamação Orofaríngea Felina.
• Hiperplasia Gengival.
• Ulceração Bucal.
• Doença Periodontal.

RECURSOS DA INTERNET
http://www.avdc.org/Nomenclature.html.

Sugestões de Leitura
Harvey CE, Emily PP. Oral lesions of soft tissues and bone: Differential diagnosis. In: Harvey CE, Emily PP, eds., Small Animal Dentistry. St. Louis: Mosby, 1993, pp. 42-88.
Wiggs RB, Lobprise HB. Veterinary Dentistry: Principles and Practice. Philadelphia: Lippincott-Raven, 1997, pp. 104-139.

Autor Larry Baker
Consultor Editorial Heidi B. Lobprise

ESTRONGILOIDÍASE

CONSIDERAÇÕES GERAIS

REVISÃO
- Cães — infecção da paramucosa do intestino delgado por *Strongyloides stercoralis* (*S. canis*); presença apenas de nematódeos fêmeas; pode causar diarreia.
- Gatos — não há relatos da infecção natural por *S. stercoralis* nos EUA; é rara a infecção do intestino grosso por *S. tumefaciens*, causando nódulos macroscopicamente visíveis.
- Múltiplas vias de transmissão de larvas infectantes, incluindo penetração cutânea, ingestão e via transmamária (neonatos); as larvas infectantes podem se desenvolver a partir dos ovos no trato GI e autoinfectar o hospedeiro, resultando em infecção persistente.
- Parasita com relativa especificidade para o hospedeiro; potencial de transmissão para os seres humanos.

IDENTIFICAÇÃO
- Cães e gatos.
- Filhotes caninos (e, possivelmente, filhotes felinos) em virtude da transmissão transmamária de larvas pela progenitora.

SINAIS CLÍNICOS
- *S. stercoralis* — geralmente assintomática, podendo ser grave, sobretudo em animais jovens.
- O desenvolvimento dos sinais clínicos acompanha a via de migração das larvas desde a penetração cutânea até os pulmões e, depois, para o intestino delgado.
- Filhotes caninos e felinos debilitados.
- Dermatite.
- Tosse, broncopneumonia.
- Diarreia (especialmente em neonatos) de consistência variável (fezes aquosas a mucoides ou moles e não formadas); pode conter sangue, muco; constipação.
- Os gatos (*S. tumefaciens*) costumam permanecer assintomáticos; cólon firme palpável.

CAUSAS E FATORES DE RISCO
- Transmissão transmamária se a cadela for infectada durante a fase final da gestação ou na lactação; não ocorrem larvas latentes (dormentes) nos tecidos da cadela.
- As larvas infectantes no ambiente contaminado por fezes penetram na pele, particularmente sob condições de saneamento insatisfatório, bem como de temperatura e umidade elevadas.
- Alta prevalência em canis.
- Possível autoinfecção atribuída ao rápido desenvolvimento de larvas para o estágio infectante dentro do trato GI do hospedeiro.

DIAGNÓSTICO

DIAGNÓSTICO DIFERENCIAL
Diversas outras infecções entéricas parasitárias, virais ou bacterianas e causas não infecciosas de diarreia.

HEMOGRAMA/BIOQUÍMICA/URINÁLISE
Pode ocorrer eosinofilia.

OUTROS TESTES LABORATORIAIS
N/D.

DIAGNÓSTICO POR IMAGEM
Nódulos de *S. tumefaciens* podem ser visíveis por colonoscopia.

MÉTODOS DIAGNÓSTICOS
- Detecção de larvas rabditiformes de primeiro estágio com esôfago de três partes em fezes recém-coletadas (frescas) ou larvas filariformes de terceiro estágio com esôfago cilíndrico reto e cauda bifurcada nas fezes incubadas; pode haver a necessidade de exames fecais repetidos por causa da liberação irregular e em baixa quantidade das larvas.
- Técnica de Baermann é a mais sensível, embora existam outros métodos (formalina-acetato de etila).
- *S. tumefaciens* — examinar também a presença de nódulos sob microscopia em busca de fêmeas adultas, ovos e larvas.
- Necropsia — exame microscópico de raspados da mucosa do intestino delgado em busca de fêmeas adultas (2-2,5 mm × 35 μm) com esôfago cilíndrico longo ocupando um terço do comprimento do corpo e larvas de primeiro estágio (200-250 μm de comprimento) com esôfago rabditiforme.

TRATAMENTO

Geralmente, o tratamento consiste no uso de agentes anti-helmínticos em um esquema ambulatorial a menos que seja necessária a suplementação com fluido intravenoso para a desidratação.

MEDICAÇÕES

MEDICAMENTO(S)
- Uso de anti-helmínticos fora da indicação da bula.
- Fembendazol 50 mg/kg VO a cada 24 h por 5 dias; talvez haja necessidade de repetição.
- Ivermectina 0,2 mg/kg SC ou VO como dose única; pode ser necessário repetir o tratamento; a dose é estabelecida fora da indicação da bula.
- É recomendado algum agente adulticidade/larvicida (fembendazol) para infecção em neonatos a fim de eliminar as larvas que sofrem migração pulmonar.

CONTRAINDICAÇÕES/INTERAÇÕES POSSÍVEIS
Não administrar a ivermectina na dose de 0,2 mg/kg a pacientes positivos para dirofilária ou a raças caninas sensíveis a esse medicamento (p. ex., Collies).

ACOMPANHAMENTO

MONITORIZAÇÃO DO PACIENTE
Repetir o exame de fezes mensalmente por 6 meses após o tratamento para garantir a eliminação da infecção; a liberação das larvas é intermitente.

PREVENÇÃO
Canis — instituir limpeza diária minuciosa e completa, além de desinfecção com água sanitária a 1% e tratamento anti-helmíntico mensal, para eliminar ou minimizar o número de larvas infectantes presentes no ambiente.

COMPLICAÇÕES POSSÍVEIS
Há relatos de migração aberrante das larvas para a medula espinal em filhotes caninos.

DIVERSOS

POTENCIAL ZOONÓTICO
Os seres humanos podem desenvolver dermatite (erupção cutânea), desconforto abdominal grave e diarreia.

ABREVIATURA(S)
- GI = gastrintestinal.

RECURSOS DA INTERNET
www.cdc.gov.

Sugestões de Leitura
Bowman D.D. Georgis' Parasitology for Veterinarians, 9th ed. St. Louis: Saunders, 2009, pp. 191-193.

Autor Julie Ann Jarvinen
Consultor Editorial Stephen C. Barr

ESTUPOR E COMA

CONSIDERAÇÕES GERAIS

DEFINIÇÃO
• Estupor — inconsciência, embora possa acordar com estímulos nocivos. • Coma — inconsciência e sem possibilidade de acordar com estímulos nocivos.

FISIOPATOLOGIA
Sistema ativador reticular ascendente — rede de neurônios situados no núcleo do tronco cerebral; funciona como sistema de despertamento para o córtex cerebral; qualquer alteração patológica grave (anatômica ou metabólica) que provoque interrupção pode levar a depressão, estupor ou coma.

SISTEMA(S) ACOMETIDO(S)
• Cardiovascular. • Nervoso. • Neuromuscular. • Respiratório. • Oftálmico.

IDENTIFICAÇÃO
• Cães e gatos. • Sem predileção racial, etária ou sexual.

SINAIS CLÍNICOS

Achados Anamnésicos
• Possibilidade de traumatismo ou perambulação sem supervisão. • Problemas prévios de importância clínica — diabetes melito e insulinoterapia; hipoglicemia; problemas cardiovasculares; episódios hipóxicos; insuficiência renal; insuficiência hepática; neoplasia. • Ambiente do paciente — possível intermação; hipotermia; afogamento por um triz; exposição a medicamentos, narcóticos e toxinas (p. ex., etilenoglicol, chumbo e anticoagulantes), incluindo as medicações do proprietário. • O início pode ser agudo ou lentamente progressivo, dependendo da causa subjacente.

Achados do Exame Físico
• Buscar por indícios de traumatismo externo ou interno. • Examinar quanto à presença de hipotermia ou hipertermia graves. • Indícios de hipoxia ou cianose, equimoses ou formação de petéquias, ou ainda insuficiência cardíaca ou respiratória — justifica a pesquisa por causas metabólicas. • Palpar com cuidado em busca de indícios de neoplasia. • Hemorragias retinianas ou vasos distendidos — hipertensão. • Papiledema — edema cerebral. • Descolamento da retina — causas infecciosas, neoplásicas ou hipertensivas. • Coriorretinite — causas infecciosas (cinomose, doenças relacionadas com o FeLV, toxoplasmose, criptococose ou PIF). • Bradicardia contínua (com potássio sérico normal) — lesão no mesencéfalo, na ponte ou na medula oblonga.

Achados do Exame Neurológico
• Determinar o nível de consciência e se o paciente pode ser despertado. • Reflexos pupilares à luz — pupilas responsivas pequenas: lesão cerebral ou diencefálica; pupilas irresponsivas dilatadas (uni ou bilaterais) ou fixas na posição central: lesões mesencefálicas ou medulares graves. • Reflexo oculocefálico (quando a manipulação cervical for possível) — perda do nistagmo vestibular fisiológico: envolvimento do tronco cerebral. • Padrões respiratórios — respiração de Cheyne-Stokes: lesão cerebral difusa ou diencefálica grave; hiperventilação: lesão no mesencéfalo; respiração atáxica ou apnêustica: lesão na ponte ou na medula oblonga. • Nervos cranianos — sem déficits com lesão do cérebro-diencéfalo; déficits do III par de nervos cranianos: lesão do mesencéfalo; déficits dos V-XII pares de nervos cranianos: lesões da medula oblonga e da ponte. • Alterações posturais — rigidez descerebrada: lesão no mesencéfalo.

CAUSAS
• Farmacológicas — narcóticos; depressores; ivermectina. • Anatômicas — hidrocefalia. • Metabólicas — hipoglicemia grave; hiperglicemia; síndromes hiperosmolares; hipernatremia; hiponatremia; encefalopatia hepática; hipoxemia; hipercarbia; hipotermia; hipertermia; hipotensão; coagulopatias; insuficiência renal; doença de armazenamento lisossomal. • Nutricionais — hipoglicemia; deficiência de tiamina. • Neoplásicas (primárias) — meningioma; astrocitoma; gliomas; papiloma do plexo coroide; adenoma hipofisário; outras. • Metastáticas — hemangiossarcoma; linfoma; carcinoma mamário; outros. • Inflamatórias não infecciosas — meningoencefalomielite granulomatosa. • Infecciosas — bacteriana; viral (cinomose, PIF); parasitária (larva migrans aberrante); protozoária (neosporose, toxoplasmose); fúngica (criptococose, blastomicose, histoplasmose, coccidioidomicose, actinomicose); doenças originárias de carrapatos. • Idiopáticas — epilepsia (pós-estado epiléptico). • Imunomediadas — vasculite e trombocitopenia com consequente hemorragia. • Traumáticas. • Tóxicas — etilenoglicol; chumbo; rodenticida anticoagulante; outras toxinas. • Vasculares — hemorragia (distúrbios de sangramento, hipertensão); infarto (encefalopatia isquêmica felina, microfilária ou larvas adultas migratórias de dirofilária).

FATORES DE RISCO
• Diabetes melito — insulinoterapia.
• Insulinomas.
• Exposição a calor ou frio intensos sem proteção.
• Animal de vida livre — traumatismo.
• Animais jovens e não vacinados.

DIAGNÓSTICO

DIAGNÓSTICO DIFERENCIAL
• Início agudo — causados mais comumente por toxinas, medicamentos, traumatismo ou acidentes vasculares.
• Evolução lenta dos sinais neurológicos sem anormalidades sistêmicas — sugere distúrbios neurológicos primários de causas inflamatórias, neoplásicas ou anatômicas. • Sinais corticais difusos bilaterais — doenças metabólicas, toxinas, infecção sistêmica, medicamentos e causas nutricionais.
• Sinais do tronco cerebral — traumatismo, inflamação, neoplasia, acidentes vasculares ou comumente por evolução de doença cerebral com consequente herniação tentorial.

HEMOGRAMA/BIOQUÍMICA/URINÁLISE

Hemograma Completo
• Intoxicação pelo chumbo — pode revelar hemácias nucleadas ou pontilhado basófilo.
• Infecção grave — hemograma inflamatório.
• Anemia grave — sugere hipoxemia.

Bioquímica Sérica
• Podem-se observar hipoglicemia, hiperglicemia, hipernatremia, azotemia, hiperosmolaridade e outros desarranjos metabólicos.

Urinálise
• Diabetes melito — glicosúria.
• Insuficiência renal — isostenúria, cilindros granulosos.
• Doença imunomediada ou infecção grave — proteinúria.
• Encefalopatia hepática — cristais de biurato de amônio.
• Intoxicação pelo etilenoglicol — cristais de oxalato de cálcio ou de hipurato.

OUTROS TESTES LABORATORIAIS
• Teste do etilenoglicol sérico e mensuração do hiato osmolar — início agudo.
• Concentrações da amônia sérica e dos ácidos biliares pré e pós-prandiais — níveis elevados indicam encefalopatia hepática.
• Títulos no soro e no LCS — na suspeita de doença infecciosa.
• Gasometria arterial — indícios de hipoxemia; alterações graves do pH; hipercarbia.
• Coagulograma — incluindo TP, TTP, fibrinogênio, PDF, contagem plaquetária, antitrombina III e tempo de sangramento bucal; suspeita de sangramento ou trombose intracraniana.
• Teste sorológico — FeLV, FIV e dirofilariose.
• Níveis séricos de chumbo.

DIAGNÓSTICO POR IMAGEM
• Radiografias simples (tórax e abdome) — indícios de comprometimento orgânico, infiltração ou neoplasia.
• Radiografias do crânio — fraturas nos casos traumáticos, pesquisa de massas.
• TC — método excelente para detectar hemorragia aguda dentro da calvária*; fraturas deprimidas; corpos estranhos penetrantes.
• RM com contraste — revela edema cerebral, hemorragia, massa, doenças infiltrativas.

MÉTODOS DIAGNÓSTICOS
• Análise do LCS — envolve o exame de citologia, as concentrações de imunoglobulinas e proteínas, bem como os títulos para doenças infecciosas; efetuar apenas quando não houver indícios de traumatismo, PIC aumentada, coagulopatias ou doença metabólica.
• RAETC — determina a função do tronco cerebral.
• ECG — determina disfunção cardíaca; as anormalidades podem contribuir para o desenvolvimento de estupor ou coma ou podem ser provocadas por doença cerebral.
• EEG — detecta atividade convulsiva não clínica capaz de prolongar os quadros de estupor e coma.

ACHADOS PATOLÓGICOS
Podem-se detectar alterações como edema cerebral, hemorragia, infarto, isquemia, inflamação, neoplasia, herniação, laceração, contusão, hematomas, fratura de crânio, necrose e apoptose.

TRATAMENTO

---

* N.T.: Parte superior do crânio em forma de cúpula ou calota.

ESTUPOR E COMA

EM CASO DE MÁ PERFUSÃO
- Utilizar uma quantidade mínima de cristaloides, porque esses fluidos contribuirão para a formação de edema cerebral se a barreira hematencefálica estiver rompida; uma combinação de coloides de alto peso molecular (p. ex., hetamido) com cristaloides possibilita a ressuscitação volêmica com pequenos volumes de fluido.
- Manter a pressão sanguínea arterial sistólica >90 mmHg com cristaloides e/ou coloides; evitar a ocorrência de hipertensão.
- Hidratação — manter com uma solução cristaloide eletrolítica balanceada.
- A cabeça do paciente deve ser nivelada com o corpo ou elevada a um ângulo de 20°; a cabeça nunca deve ficar em um nível mais baixo que o corpo para evitar o aumento da PIC.
- Evitar o reflexo da tosse ou espirro durante a entubação ou a suplementação de oxigênio por meio de cânula nasal; pode elevar gravemente a PIC; a lidocaína (cães, 0,75 mg/kg IV) administrada antes da entubação pode atenuar a reação de engasgo e o reflexo da tosse.
- $PaCO_2$ — manter entre 35 e 45 mmHg; hiperventilar pode reduzir o fluxo sanguíneo cerebral e a PIC; a PaO_2 precisa estar >50 mmHg para manter a autorregulação do fluxo sanguíneo cerebral.
- Utilizar as veias periféricas, deixando o fluxo sanguíneo da veia jugular desobstruído; o desvio do volume de sangue para as veias jugulares é um mecanismo compensatório importante durante PIC elevada.
- Evitar agitação violenta, crises convulsivas ou qualquer outra forma de atividade motora descontrolada; podem elevar a PIC; a infusão de diazepam (0,5-1 mg/kg/h), midazolam (0,2-0,4 mg/kg) ou propofol (3-6 mg/kg IV titulado até fazer efeito; em seguida, 0,1-0,6 mg/kg/min em velocidade constante) pode ser necessária para as crises convulsivas.
- Evitar as complicações secundárias do decúbito — lubrificação dos olhos; técnica asséptica com o uso de cateteres; mudança de posição do animal.
- Ventriculostomia para drenagem do LCS se a elevação crítica da PIC não for responsiva ao tratamento clínico.
- Considerar a descompressão e a exploração cirúrgicas — se a disfunção cerebral estiver evoluindo para sinais no mesencéfalo com histórico de traumatismo ou sangramento (herniação tentorial); PIC elevada não responsiva à terapia clínica (se os instrumentos de monitorização estiverem disponíveis); fragmentos de fraturas deprimidas do crânio; corpo estranho penetrante.
- Nutrição — técnicas com sonda de fluxo de gotejamento para manter a nutrição durante o período inconsciente; ajustar as necessidades nutricionais para compensar as demandas metabólicas.
- Cisaprida (modificador da motilidade) na dose de 0,5 mg/kg a cada 12-8 h pode ser necessária.

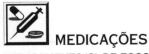

MEDICAÇÕES
MEDICAMENTO(S) DE ESCOLHA
PIC Elevada
- Hiperventilação ou terapia com diurético.
- Furosemida — 0,75 mg/kg IV; diminui a produção do LCS e o nível da PIC.
- Manitol — 0,1-0,5 g/kg em bólus IV a cada 2 h por 3-4 doses em cães e 2-3 doses em gatos; restabelece o fluxo sanguíneo cerebral e reduz a PIC; administrar após a furosemida.
- Não usar agentes osmóticos na presença de hemorragia intracraniana.
- Considerar a dose de ataque do fenobarbital (4 mg/kg/h por 3 doses) em casos de atividade convulsiva contínua.

Doença Subjacente
- Glicocorticosteroides — para anormalidades intracranianas inflamatórias e expansivas.
- Enemas com lactulose, flumazenil (0,02 mg/kg IV) e suporte hídrico — encefalopatia hepática.
- Diurese hídrica — insuficiência renal.
- Reidratação e insulina — para diabetes melito com hiperosmolalidade; reduzem a glicose lentamente.
- Suplementação com glicose — hipoglicemia.
- Manter o volume intravascular; resfriar — na hipertermia.
- Manter o volume intravascular; aquecer para 36,6°C — na hipotermia.
- Lavagem gástrica e instilação de carvão ativado com catártico — na ingestão de toxina.
- Toxinas específicas podem necessitar de agentes terapêuticos específicos (p. ex., etilenoglicol tratado com etanol e diálise peritoneal).
- Antibióticos — utilizar agentes que atravessem a barreira hematencefálica na suspeita de infecções bacterianas (p. ex., trimetoprima-sulfa, doxiciclina e metronidazol); usar agentes de amplo espectro se a barreira hematencefálica estiver rompida (p. ex., cefalosporinas de primeira geração).
- Ajustar a seleção de fluido cristaloide para corrigir distúrbios eletrolíticos.
- Tiamina (100 mg IM) — possível deficiência de tiamina.

CONTRAINDICAÇÕES
- Coloides — utilizar quantidades mínimas de coloides de alto peso molecular para corrigir a hipotensão na presença de hemorragia intracraniana.

PRECAUÇÕES
- Evitar a ocorrência de hipertensão.
- Evitar a sobrecarga de volume intravascular.
- Manitol e solução salina hipertônica — podem agravar o estado neurológico se houver hemorragia intracraniana.
- Hiperventilar — manter a $PaCO_2$ >30 mmHg; não fazer por períodos prolongados (>48 h).

ACOMPANHAMENTO
MONITORAÇÃO DO PACIENTE
- Exames neurológicos seriados — detectam a deterioração da função que justifica uma intervenção terapêutica rigorosa.
- Pressão sanguínea — manter a fluidoterapia adequada para perfusão ao mesmo tempo em que se evita a hipertensão.
- Gasometria sanguínea — avaliar a necessidade de suplementação com oxigênio ou de ventilação; monitorizar a PCO_2 ao hiperventilar.
- Glicose sanguínea — garantir um nível sanguíneo para manter as funções cerebrais ao mesmo tempo em que se evita a hiperosmolalidade.
- ECG — detecta arritmias que possam afetar a perfusão, a oxigenação e o fluxo sanguíneo cerebral.
- PIC — detecta elevações acentuadas; revela o sucesso do tratamento.
- Eletrólitos — detectam hipernatremia e hipocalemia.

PREVENÇÃO
- Manter os animais de estimação confinados ou acorrentados.
- Evitar a exposição a toxinas ou medicamentos existentes dentro de casa.
- Estabelecer um programa de cuidados de saúde de rotina para minimizar as complicações infecciosas e metabólicas.

COMPLICAÇÕES POSSÍVEIS
- Déficits neurológicos residuais como crises convulsivas. • Complicações compatíveis com doença subjacente.

EVOLUÇÃO ESPERADA E PROGNÓSTICO
- A doença do tronco cerebral é pior que a doença do córtex cerebral.
- O Escore de Coma de Glasgow pode fornecer informações prognósticas.

DIVERSOS
ABREVIATURA(S)
- ECG = eletrocardiograma.
- EEC = eletroencefalograma.
- LCS = líquido cerebrospinal.
- $PaCO_2$ = pressão parcial de dióxido de carbono no sangue arterial.
- PaO_2 = pressão parcial de oxigênio arterial.
- PDF = produtos de degradação da fibrina.
- PIC = pressão intracraniana.
- PIF = peritonite infecciosa felina.
- RAETC = resposta auditiva evocada do tronco cerebral.
- RM = ressonância magnética.
- TC = tomografia computadorizada.
- TP = tempo de protrombina.
- TTP = tempo de tromboplastina parcial.
- FIV = vírus da imunodeficiência felina.
- FeLV = vírus da leucemia felina.

RECURSOS DA INTERNET
- www.accessmedicine.com.
- www.cvmbs.colostate.edu/clinsci/wing/comascor.html.

Sugestões de Leitura
Chrisman CL, Mariani C, Platt S. Dementia, stupor and coma. In: Neurology for the Small Animal Practitioner. Jackson, WY: Teton NewMedia, 2003, pp. 41-84.
Mathews K. Stupor/coma. In: Mathews KA, ed., Veterinary Emergency and Critical Care Manual, 2nd ed. Guelph, Ontario: Lifelearn, 2006, pp. 478-482.
Mathews K, Parent J. Head trauma. In: Mathews KA, ed., Veterinary Emergency and Critical Care Manual, 2nd ed. Guelph, Ontario: Lifelearn, 2006, pp. 691-701.

Autor Rebecca Kirby
Consultor Editorial Joane M. Parent

Evacuação e Micção Domiciliares pelos Cães

CONSIDERAÇÕES GERAIS

DEFINIÇÃO
Micção e/ou defecação, por necessidade de eliminação ou para marcação territorial, em local considerado impróprio pelo proprietário.

FISIOPATOLOGIA
• Adestramento doméstico inadequado ou incompleto. • Micção por submissão ou agitação. • Testosterona, que leva ao comportamento de marcação. • Comportamento de marcação por territorialidade, ansiedade. • Ansiedade (ansiedade da separação, fobia de ruídos). • Disfunção cognitiva.

SISTEMA(S) ACOMETIDO(S)
Comportamental — abandono em abrigos, levando à eutanásia ou troca de proprietário.

GENÉTICA
Algumas raças de cães parecem ser mais fáceis de adestrar que outras.

INCIDÊNCIA/PREVALÊNCIA
• Em pesquisas com proprietários de cães, entre 6,4 e 7,4% mencionaram alguma forma desse problema. • 37% dos proprietários que relataram ter procurado um veterinário por causa de algum problema comportamental declararam que seu cão sujava a casa indevidamente. • A incidência de eliminação imprópria, incluindo o comportamento de marcação territorial, em machos intactos é quase 60% maior do que aquela observada em machos castrados e cadelas intactas ou castradas.

DISTRIBUIÇÃO GEOGRÁFICA
Nenhuma foi descrita.

IDENTIFICAÇÃO
Espécie
Cães.

Raça(s) Predominante(s)
Segundo relatos breves, é descrito um potencial genético de predisposição racial quanto à facilidade de adestramento doméstico e em termos de micção por submissão ou agitação.

Idade Média e Faixa Etária
• Eliminação imprópria atribuída a adestramento doméstico inadequado ou incompleto vista em idade precoce. • Micção por submissão ou agitação observada principalmente em cães mais jovens. • A marcação territorial com urina começa a ser exibida à medida que o cão atinge a maturidade sexual. • A evacuação domiciliar é uma queixa comum de donos de cães idosos.

Sexo Predominante
• Em geral, é mais fácil adestrar as cadelas que os machos. • É mais provável que os machos intactos marquem o território com urina do que os castrados e as cadelas intactas ou castradas.

SINAIS CLÍNICOS
Comentários Gerais
• A eliminação imprópria é o motivo pessoal mais comum para o abandono de um animal em um abrigo. • É imprescindível abordar o adestramento adequado com os proprietários desde muito cedo. • A evacuação domiciliar pode ser associada a problemas clínicos, como distúrbios endócrinos, distúrbios do trato urinário e doença metabólica.

Achados Anamnésicos
• Histórico de micção e/ou defecação em áreas impróprias. • Pode estar associada a sinais de outros distúrbios comportamentais (como ansiedade da separação). • Pode estar vinculada à falta de tempo gasto pelo proprietário em adestrar o animal de forma adequada. • Pode estar ligada à punição de um cão que urina em sinal de submissão. • A obtenção de histórico médico e comportamental completo ajudará a determinar os possíveis deflagradores, incluindo o momento, o local e a frequência em que ocorre a eliminação, além da viabilidade de o animal fazer suas necessidades fora de casa.

Achados do Exame Físico
• Se não houver achados anormais ao exame físico, é provável que a evacuação domiciliar seja atribuída a alguma causa comportamental. • Talvez tenha havido alguma causa médica incitante que se resolveu há muito tempo em relação ao problema comportamental e o animal tenha aprendido a fazer suas necessidades dentro de casa. • Achados anormais ao exame físico precisam ser investigados e podem estar relacionados com alguma causa clínica subjacente de eliminação imprópria.

CAUSAS
As causas de eliminação imprópria em cães podem ser atribuídas principalmente a algum problema comportamental ou ser secundárias ou simultâneas a algum distúrbio clínico.

Causas Comportamentais
• Falta de adestramento domiciliar adequado ou adestramento incompleto.
• Comportamento de marcação.
• Micção por submissão.
• Micção por agitação.
• Ansiedade da separação.
• Síndrome de disfunção cognitiva.
• Fobia a ruídos.
• Induzida por medo.
• Polidipsia/poliúria psicogênicas.

Causas Clínicas
Degenerativas
• Displasia do quadril/osteoartrite/artropatia degenerativa. • Insuficiência renal.

Anatômicas
• Ureteres ectópicos.

Metabólicas
• Incontinência.
• Diabetes melito.
• Diabetes insípido
• Insuficiência hepática.
• Hiperadrenocorticismo.
• Hipoadrenocorticismo.
• Crises convulsivas.

Neoplásicas
• Neoplasia renal. • Neoplasia vesical. • Outras doenças neoplásicas que causem fraqueza.

Infecciosas/Inflamatórias
• Infecção ou inflamação do trato urinário. • Cristalúria com cistite. • Distúrbio intestinal inflamatório. • Doença pancreática. • Parasitas intestinais.

FATORES DE RISCO
• Macho intacto (i. e., não castrado).
• Problema comportamental concomitante, como ansiedade da separação.
• Proprietários desinformados ou desmotivados quanto ao adestramento de seu cão.

DIAGNÓSTICO

DIAGNÓSTICO DIFERENCIAL
Diferenciar causas comportamentais de eliminação imprópria das causas clínicas por meio de avaliação médica adequada.

HEMOGRAMA/BIOQUÍMICA/URINÁLISE
• Indicados para excluir causas clínicas.
• Normais se a eliminação imprópria for atribuída a causas comportamentais.

DIAGNÓSTICO POR IMAGEM
Não indicado, a não ser para descartar causas clínicas, principalmente urolitíase ou ureteres ectópicos.

MÉTODOS DIAGNÓSTICOS
• Filmar o cão quando o proprietário estiver presente para ver suas interações em casa com esse animal de estimação.
• Fazer um relatório para monitorar os fatores causais potenciais de eliminação imprópria, bem como para monitorar a melhora do problema.
• Filmar o cão quando o proprietário estiver saindo de casa para verificar se há ansiedade da separação ou outros distúrbios de ansiedade.

ACHADOS PATOLÓGICOS
Nenhum no caso de causas comportamentais.

TRATAMENTO

CUIDADO(S) DE SAÚDE ADEQUADO(S)
Qualquer medida apropriada que garanta a manutenção de uma saúde satisfatória do animal.

ATIVIDADE
• Manter o cão do lado de fora a fim de garantir que ele tenha acesso suficiente para suas necessidades fisiológicas; ou proporcionar um acesso aceitável a algum ambiente externo por meio de uma portinhola, por exemplo, se o cão for adestrado para isso.
• Aumentar o nível de atividade para ajudar no tratamento de outros problemas comportamentais, bem como para melhorar a saúde do cão.

DIETA
• Se o cão apresentar eliminação imprópria, fornecer refeições em horários predeterminados (em vez de comida à vontade) que possam ajudar a manter um cronograma de eliminação das necessidades fisiológicas.
• Fornecer dieta de alta densidade calórica pode ajudar a diminuir a urgência de defecar com tanta frequência.
• Em geral, a água não deve ser retirada do cão.

ORIENTAÇÃO AO PROPRIETÁRIO
Comentários Gerais
• Orientar o proprietário sobre a(s) causa(s) da eliminação imprópria, bem como o potencial de tratamento prolongado do problema.
• Tratar os problemas clínicos subjacentes/contribuintes.
• Tratar outros problemas comportamentais subjacentes/contribuintes.
• Limpar as áreas sujas com um produto à base de enzimas, para ajudar a eliminar qualquer odor que possa atrair o cão para fazer as necessidades no mesmo local. Se o objeto sujo for um pedaço de

ESPÉCIES CANINA E FELINA

EVACUAÇÃO E MICÇÃO DOMICILIARES PELOS CÃES

pano ou qualquer outro pano menor, como um tapete destruído, lave-o em máquina.
• A punição não é apropriada, especialmente se o ato de eliminação não for testemunhado pelo proprietário, pois isso pode gerar ansiedade, medo e agressividade defensiva.

Adestramento Incompleto
• Manter o cão completamente supervisionado todo o tempo. Se ele não for supervisionado, mantê-lo confinado a menos que o confinamento provoque pânico, destruição e/ou lesão no cão.
• Em alguns casos, amarrar o cão junto aos donos ou próximo a eles permite uma melhor supervisão. Os cães nunca devem ser amarrados sem supervisão.
• Levar o cão para fora de casa com frequência para ele fazer suas necessidades.
• Recompensá-lo quando a eliminação ocorrer nas horas e nos locais apropriados; isso requer que o proprietário saia com o cão.
• Limpar as áreas sujas total e minuciosamente.
• Usar uma "expressão-chave" regularmente para ajudar a associar o ato com o local e o horário da eliminação.
• Alimentar o animal em horários predeterminados, com água sempre à disposição.

Micção por Submissão ou por Agitação
• Não punir o comportamento, pois isso pode agravar o problema.
• Fazer com que os proprietários ignorem o cão quando ele entrar em casa (sem interações verbais ou físicas ou contato visual).
• O cão deve sair para fazer suas necessidades antes de ser recepcionado.
• É recomendável que o cão seja abordado sem confronto e com calma; não se inclinar na direção dele nem brincar de forma interativa ao abordá-lo.
• Atividades alternadas ao retorno para casa, como perguntar por um brinquedo ou mandá-lo "sentar", podem ajudar nos casos leves.

Comportamento de Marcação com Urina
• Orientar os proprietários sobre a eficácia de castrar o animal para diminuir o comportamento de marcação com urina.
• Determinar pelo histórico a presença de quaisquer deflagradores possíveis do comportamento, inclusive estímulos indutores de ansiedade.
• Combater os deflagradores com dessensibilização e contracondicionamento e/ou evitá-los, conforme o caso.
• Tornar as áreas marcadas com urina aversivas para o cão, usando "armadilhas", como tapetes ou folhas de plástico que deslizam. Pode-se usar punição à distância bem no início de todo e qualquer episódio de marcação com urina, mas somente se o proprietário conseguir pegar o animal no ato.
• Evitar o acesso aos locais de marcação preferidos.
• Como alternativa, o proprietário pode transformar a área em um local positivo, passando a alimentar o cão nela.

CONSIDERAÇÕES CIRÚRGICAS
A castração de cão intacto diminui rapidamente a marcação com urina em 30% dos casos, com declínio gradual em 20% e nenhuma alteração em 50%. Os resultados são os mesmos, independentemente da idade do animal no momento da castração.

 MEDICAÇÕES

MEDICAMENTO(S) DE ESCOLHA
• A modificação do comportamento deve ser usada em conjunto com medicações psicotrópicas.
• Raramente, esse tipo de tratamento é eficaz quando a ansiedade não faz parte do problema comportamental. Efeito desprezível em animais que não são adestrados ou exibem micção por submissão. • Se a marcação com urina ou a eliminação imprópria for induzida por ansiedade, as medicações podem ser úteis, mas apenas em conjunto com a mudança comportamental.
• Inibidores seletivos de recaptação da serotonina (ISRSs) ou antidepressivos tricíclicos/ansiolíticos (ATCs) podem ser úteis. Um exemplo de ISRSs é a fluoxetina, na dose de 1 mg/kg VO a cada 24 h. Um exemplo de ATC é a clomipramina, na dose de 1-2 mg/kg VO a cada 12 h. • O início completo de ação dessas medicações pode ser 4-6 semanas após a instituição do tratamento e os proprietários devem estar cientes disso. • Os efeitos colaterais dos ISRSs podem incluir náuseas, vômitos, diarreia e letargia. • Os efeitos colaterais dos ATCs podem compreender náuseas, vômitos, diarreia, letargia, arritmias cardíacas e potencialização de atividade convulsiva.

CONTRAINDICAÇÕES
• Uso de medicamentos sem modificação comportamental concomitante. • Agentes ansiolíticos tricíclicos são contraindicados em crises convulsivas e cardiopatia; além disso, podem interferir nas medicações antitireóideas.

PRECAUÇÕES
Tomadas com base na escolha de cada medicamento.

INTERAÇÕES POSSÍVEIS
Não usar ISRSs e ATCs juntos ou em conjunto com algum inibidor da MAO como o L-deprenil ou amitraz.

MEDICAMENTO(S) ALTERNATIVO(S)
• Os produtos à base de feromônios têm o potencial de ajudar a diminuir a ansiedade.
• Raramente se recomenda o uso de progestinas para o controle da marcação com urina, por conta dos efeitos colaterais graves e potenciais.

 ACOMPANHAMENTO

MONITORIZAÇÃO DO PACIENTE
Os pacientes devem ser monitorizados junto ao proprietário em consultas de acompanhamento ou por telefone. O proprietário deve manter um relatório de incidentes, fatores desencadeantes e tratamentos instituídos para fornecer uma avaliação objetiva da melhora.

PREVENÇÃO
• Realizar adestramento adequado do cão em casa.
• Castrar cães e cadelas.
• Tratar qualquer condição clínica subjacente.
• Tratar qualquer problema comportamental subjacente.

COMPLICAÇÕES POSSÍVEIS
A recidiva é possível se o proprietário negligenciar o tratamento, abandonando o animal de estimação.

EVOLUÇÃO ESPERADA E PROGNÓSTICO
• O prognóstico de qualquer problema comportamental é altamente dependente da capacidade do proprietário em seguir as instruções. As estimativas de prognóstico a seguir baseiam-se nas instruções seguidas pelo proprietário para a modificação do comportamento.
• O prognóstico quanto ao declínio da micção por submissão e agitação é bom.
• O prognóstico em relação à conduta no caso de adestramento incompleto é bom.
• Prognóstico da marcação em machos previamente intactos: 50% de melhora (30% rapidamente, 20% mais devagar) com a castração, mesmo sem modificação complementar do comportamento.
• O prognóstico quanto ao controle da marcação com urina em cães castrados será bom se os fatores desencadeantes forem identificados e controlados com evasão (ou seja, evitando-os) ou outras formas de modificação do comportamento.
• Alguns animais com histórico de alguma causa clínica de eliminação imprópria ainda podem manter o comportamento após a causa clínica ter sido tratada da devida forma.

 DIVERSOS

FATORES RELACIONADOS COM A IDADE
• É mais provável que os filhotes não recebam adestramento ou sejam adestrados de forma incompleta e exibam micção por submissão e agitação.
• A disfunção cognitiva torna-se mais provável à medida que o cão envelhece.

POTENCIAL ZOONÓTICO
Baixo potencial zoonótico.

SINÔNIMO(S)
• Marcação com urina. • Micção imprópria.
• Defecação imprópria. • Eliminação imprópria.

VER TAMBÉM
• Síndrome de Ansiedade da Separação.
• Síndrome de Disfunção Cognitiva.

ABREVIATURA(S)
• MAO = monoamina oxidase. • ISRS = inibidor seletivo de recaptação da serotonina. • ATC = antidepressivo tricíclico.

RECURSOS DA INTERNET
• American College of Veterinary Behaviorists: www.dacvb.org.
• American Veterinary Society of Animal Behavior: www.avsabonline.org.

Sugestões de Leitura
Hart BL, Hart LA. The Perfect Puppy: How to Choose Your Dog by Its Behavior. New York: Freeman, 1988.
Landsberg G, Hunthausen W, Ackerman L. Handbook of Behavior Problems of the Dog and Cat, 2nd ed. Philadelphia: Elsevier Saunders, 2003.
Yeon SC, Erb HN, Houpt KA. A retrospective study of canine house soiling: Diagnosis and treatment. JAAHA 1999, 35(2):101-106.

Autor Melissa Bain
Consultor Editorial Debra F. Horwitz

Evacuação e Micção Domiciliares pelos Gatos

CONSIDERAÇÕES GERAIS

DEFINIÇÃO
Eliminação de urina fora da bandeja sanitária (também chamada periúria), o que inclui micção inadequada, comportamento de toalete, micção (agachada) em superfícies horizontais fora da bandeja sanitária e marcação territorial com a função normal de comunicação, além de jatos de urina em superfícies verticais como parte de um ritual de exibição da cauda ereta. Do mesmo modo, a defecação imprópria é um comportamento de toalete, caracterizado pelo depósito de fezes fora da bandeja sanitária*; nesse caso, a marcação com fezes, conhecida como *middening*, caracteriza-se pelo depósito de fezes em locais proeminentes, sem cobri-las. Em todos os casos, causas clínicas potenciais devem ser investigadas antes de se assumir um diagnóstico de problema comportamental. De qualquer forma, a evacuação domiciliar exerce um impacto negativo sobre a relação homem-animal.

FISIOPATOLOGIA
• Micção/defecação inadequadas — pode ser uma resposta normal à insatisfação com o ambiente da bandeja sanitária ou preferência específica por um local ou substrato alternativo ou, então, refletir um estado fisiopatológico subjacente, como associação negativa (dor) à bandeja sanitária secundariamente à presença de urólitos ou constipação.
• Marcação com urina — um comportamento normal observado em gatos de vida livre e nos confinados; diferenças individuais significativas na tendência à marcação com urina em um dado ambiente; alguns gatos nunca parecem exibir o comportamento e outros gatos exibem o comportamento regularmente. Os gatos que fazem marcação com urina também utilizam a bandeja sanitária para toalete.
• Marcação com fezes (*middening*) — deve ser um diagnóstico de exclusão.

SISTEMA(S) ACOMETIDO(S)
• Comportamental.
• Endócrino.
• Gastrintestinal.
• Renal/urológico.
• Outros.

GENÉTICA
• Embora não tenha sido especificamente identificado, pode haver um componente hereditário para a marcação com urina; relatos breves envolvem os progenitores de indivíduos acometidos que exibem o comportamento.
• As raças Persa e Himalaio que exibem micção imprópria devem ser submetidas ao teste de DNA quanto à presença de distúrbio genético (no caso, doença renal policística).

INCIDÊNCIA/PREVALÊNCIA
• Em um único levantamento, 11% dos proprietários de gatos relataram a eliminação imprópria como um problema.
• Foi estimado que 10% dos gatos machos castrados e 5% das fêmeas castradas praticam a marcação com urina.
• A evacuação domiciliar é o problema comportamental mais comum que levam os proprietários de gatos a buscar orientação veterinária e a segunda razão mais comum de abandono de gatos em abrigos de animais.

DISTRIBUIÇÃO GEOGRÁFICA
A evacuação domiciliar é mais problemática em países, onde os gatos costumam ficar presos dentro de casa.

IDENTIFICAÇÃO
Espécies
Gatos.
Raça(s) Predominante(s)
A evacuação domiciliar pode ocorrer em qualquer raça, embora os Persas, Himalaios e parentescos sejam super-representados em alguns estudos.
Idade Média e Faixa Etária
A micção imprópria pode ocorrer em qualquer idade.
Sexo Predominante
• A evacuação domiciliar pode ocorrer em qualquer sexo, intacto ou castrado.
• A micção em jato é mais comum em machos (intactos e castrados) do que em fêmeas (intactas e castradas).

SINAIS CLÍNICOS
Comentários Gerais
Identificar o Gato Acometido em um Ambiente com Inúmeros Gatos
• Observação direta, embora os gatos possam se tornar reservados se forem punidos.
• Isolar todo gato, um de cada vez, em um pequeno cômodo ou sala para identificar o culpado pelo processo de eliminação; esse protocolo, no entanto, pode alterar o meio social o suficiente a ponto de inibir a eliminação inadequada durante o confinamento seriado.
• Se a urina estiver alcalina, administrar o corante fluoresceína (6 fitas reagentes de fluoresceína em uma cápsula gelatinosa VO ou 10 mg/gato) sequencialmente a cada gato. A urina eliminada fora da bandeja sanitária emite fluorescência sob iluminação com a lâmpada de Wood por aproximadamente 24 h; se negativa após 36 h, o teste poderá ser repetido em outro gato. Resultados negativos são comuns em ambientes onde a frequência de micção em jato é baixa. Cuidado: a fluoresceína pode manchar tecidos.

Identificar os Locais de Evacuação Domiciliar dentro da Casa
• O proprietário deve fazer um mapa da casa, indicando os locais de eliminação de urina e fezes, bem como os locais das bandejas sanitárias.

Achados Anamnésicos
Micção Imprópria
• A micção nos arredores da bandeja sanitária pode sugerir insatisfação com a qualidade das caixas de areia ou granulado.
• Padrão anormal de micção (incontinência, poliúria, hematúria, disúria) é sugestivo de algum problema congênito ou clínico subjacente.
• Histórico de polidipsia, anorexia, vômito e diarreia sugere alguma etiologia clínica subjacente.

Marcação com Urina
• A marcação pode ser uma resposta a uma desorganização da casa ou à presença de outro(s) gato(s) dentro ou fora dela.
• Histórico de desalojamento, agressividade ou comportamento de evasão entre os gatos em uma casa com inúmeros felinos.
• Observação da postura do jato de urina: o gato orienta-se no sentido caudal para uma superfície vertical, enrijece sua postura, eleva e estremece sua cauda e direciona um pequeno jato de urina caudalmente.
• Observação das marcações com urina em superfícies verticais.
• As marcações com urina em volta de janelas e portas do lado de fora sugere uma resposta à presença de algum gato fora de casa.
• Marcações com urina em mobílias ou outros objetos proeminentes ou jatos de urina em objetos novos trazidos para casa. O jato de urina em sacolas de mercado ou móveis novos sugere marcação olfativa associada à excitação em reposta a novos estímulos.
• As marcações com urina em superfícies horizontais podem ser encontradas em vestimentas ou camas associadas a uma pessoa em particular ou em resposta a visitantes ou objetos novos.

Defecação Imprópria
• Histórico de esforço para defecar (tenesmo); vocalização ao defecar; fezes duras, ressecadas ou volumosas sugerem defecações dolorosas que podem levar a uma fuga condicionada da bandeja sanitária para a defecação.

Marcação com Fezes
• Depósito de fezes em locais proeminentes e visíveis.

Achados do Exame Físico
• A presença de achados físicos anormais depende da natureza do problema, seja fisiopatológica ou comportamental.
• Se o problema for estritamente comportamental, o exame físico será normal.

CAUSAS
Causas Clínicas
• Doença do trato urinário inferior, inclusive cistite intersticial idiopática.
• Urolitíase.
• Diabetes melito.
• Hipertireoidismo.
• FeLV.
• FIV.
• Hepatopatia.
• Disfunção cognitiva (senilidade).
• Iatrogênicas — administração de fluidos, corticosteroides, diuréticos.

Causas Comportamentais
• Bandeja sanitária suja.
• Número inadequado de bandejas ou locais (é recomendável ter uma bandeja por gato mais uma).
• Bandeja sanitária posicionada em local afastado ou desagradável para o gato ou sujeita à interferência por cães ou crianças.
• Tipo de bandeja sanitária imprópria — uma bandeja coberta capaz de reter um odor aversivo ou muito pequena para que os gatos grandes se movimentem de forma confortável; ou uma bandeja que faz com que outros gatos, cães e crianças pequenas sejam o alvo do gato quando ele sair.
• Fatores relativos ao tempo — padrões diários ou semanais de micção imprópria sugerem uma causa ambiental; início agudo em gato que antes usava a bandeja sanitária de forma adequada sugere algum problema clínico.
• Substrato — tipo inaceitável; os testes de preferência indicam que a maioria dos gatos prefere um substrato de granulado fino e inodoro;

---

* N.T.: Também conhecida como caixa de areia ou granulado.

Evacuação e Micção Domiciliares pelos Gatos

uma mudança nos hábitos de uso da bandeja que coincida com um novo tipo de bandeja sugere uma associação; mudança súbita da preferência de um substrato (p. ex., bandeja de plástico) por outro não habitual (p. ex., pia ou lavatório) sugere algum distúrbio do trato urinário inferior.
- Localização — a micção fora da bandeja sanitária pode ser sugestiva de preferência por determinado local ou influência de fatores sociais.
- Dinâmica social — considerar os conflitos sociais entre os gatos e quaisquer modificações concomitantes no mundo social do gato na época em que o problema começou (p. ex., chegada de um novo gato).
- Probabilidade de jato de urina — diretamente proporcional ao número de gatos na casa.
- Presença de gatos no ambiente externo — pode eliciar a micção em jato em portas e janelas.

FATORES DE RISCO
Micção/Defecação Impróprias
- Higiene inadequada da bandeja sanitária.
- Características das bandejas sanitárias (tipo, odor, tamanho ou estilo da bandeja).

Marcação com Urina
- Macho.
- Sexualmente intacto.
- Casa com inúmeros gatos.
- Histórico de marcação com urina por algum progenitor.

DIAGNÓSTICO
DIAGNÓSTICO DIFERENCIAL
- É imprescindível identificar se há algum problema clínico subjacente ao problema comportamental.
- Se o problema for comportamental, será preciso diferenciar micção imprópria de marcação com urina.

HEMOGRAMA/BIOQUÍMICA/URINÁLISE
Em geral, permanecem normais nos casos em que a marcação com urina e a micção imprópria são problemas estritamente comportamentais; a urinálise constitui o banco de dados mínimo em qualquer gato examinado por conta de micção imprópria; coletar amostras seriadas de gatos, cujos sinais comportamentais apresentem remissão e exacerbação; o hemograma completo e a bioquímica sérica são recomendados antes da administração de qualquer medicação e para avaliar o estado clínico.

OUTROS TESTES LABORATORIAIS
Gatos com micção imprópria refratária ou sinais progressivos devem ser submetidos a testes para hipertireoidismo, FeLV e FIV.

DIAGNÓSTICO POR IMAGEM
Ultrassonografia ou radiografias abdominais para descartar a urolitíase como causa subjacente de micção imprópria; estudos contrastados adicionais.

MÉTODOS DIAGNÓSTICOS
Informações anamnésicas úteis: mapeamento da casa, com as bandejas sanitárias e as marcações com urina; diário comportamental com a frequência diária calculada de micções em cada bandeja sanitária e fora das bandejas.

ACHADOS PATOLÓGICOS
Nenhum a menos que haja alguma etiologia clínica subjacente.

TRATAMENTO
CUIDADO(S) DE SAÚDE ADEQUADO(S)
- Tratar qualquer condição clínica subjacente.
- Usar terapias ambientais e comportamentais antes do tratamento farmacológico ou juntamente com ele. Ver http://indoorpet.osu.edu.
- Restringir o acesso do gato a ambientes onde ocorre a eliminação domiciliar de urina.
- Se o proprietário quiser a interrupção imediata do problema, será proveitoso confinar o gato a um ambiente na ausência do proprietário. Providenciar bandeja sanitária, água, comida e local para repouso. O gato pode ser deixado no ambiente quando o proprietário retornar e estiver disponível para a supervisão estrita do animal. Iniciar outros tratamentos mais permanentes.
- Limpar os "acidentes" fisiológicos de micção com removedores à base de enzimas, específicos para essa finalidade.

Micção Imprópria
- Remover o conteúdo das bandejas sanitárias diariamente e substituí-lo por completo uma vez por semana.
- Evitar o uso de desodorizantes, bandejas sanitárias perfumadas ou outros odores fortes nos arredores da bandeja.
- Afastar as tigelas de comida para longe da bandeja sanitária.
- Providenciar pelo menos uma bandeja sanitária para cada gato, distribuídas em mais de um local, e evitar áreas de fluxo intenso de pessoas ou muito ruído.
- Se a bandeja sanitária for coberta, providenciar outra maior, plana e sem tampa, preenchida com substrato granulado fino inodoro, sem forro. Podem ser fornecidas bandejas adicionais (um "buffet de bandejas sanitárias") para avaliar a preferência do gato quanto ao tipo e substrato.
- Se o gato tiver preferência por um lugar da casa para micção imprópria, colocar outra bandeja sanitária nesse local. Depois do uso regular, afastá-la 2,5 cm por dia para um local mais aceitável pelo proprietário.
- Talvez seja necessário o confinamento do gato em uma "sala segura" nos momentos em que o proprietário não estiver disponível para supervisionar.

Marcação com Urina
- Se houver sinais de que o gato está emitindo jatos de urina em resposta à presença de gatos da rua, evite que ele tenha acesso visual ou olfativo a esses gatos. Um produto destinado ao ambiente (Feliway*, Ceva Animal Health), um concentrado de ferormônio facial felino sintético, está disponível no mercado como tratamento para a marcação com urina. O produto é aspergido regularmente ou difundido no ambiente e pode melhorar o comportamento de eliminação de jatos de urina.
- Impedir que o gato da casa veja os de fora.
- Para distrair seu gato e evitar que ele volte sua atenção para outros gatos, o proprietário deve ter tempo para interagir com seu animal diariamente.
- A farmacoterapia desempenha um papel importante no controle do problema.

CUIDADO(S) DE ENFERMAGEM
N/D.

ATIVIDADE
N/D.

DIETA
Nenhuma dieta específica é necessária a menos que sugerida por alguma etiologia clínica subjacente, como urolitíase.

ORIENTAÇÃO AO PROPRIETÁRIO
- Os gatos não sujam a casa por maldade ou vingança.
- A repressão e a punição são contraindicadas e farão com que o gato evite seu próprio dono.
- É importantíssimo compreender a motivação de base para o comportamento de evacuação domiciliar para o sucesso do tratamento.
- A criação de um ambiente harmonioso e previsível diminuirá a ansiedade e a excitação que podem contribuir para a evacuação domiciliar.

CONSIDERAÇÕES CIRÚRGICAS
Os gatos que usam a urina para marcar o território devem ser castrados. Nos casos de marcação com urina, a castração diminui o comportamento de eliminação de jatos em até 90% dos machos e 95% das fêmeas.

MEDICAÇÕES
MEDICAMENTO(S) DE ESCOLHA
Micção Imprópria
- Em geral, não se indica o uso de medicação, exceto nos casos refratários ao tratamento ou quando associados à ansiedade generalizada ou excitação acentuada.
- Podem ser utilizados os agentes farmacológicos pertencentes a uma série de classes medicamentosas. Todos eles possuem o efeito genérico de diminuir a excitação e a ansiedade. Os efeitos colaterais podem ser a sedação e/ou a mudança do comportamento social (ver Apêndice IX: Bulário). Os medicamentos mais comumente utilizados incluem fluoxetina, clomipramina, amitriptilina, buspirona.

Marcação com Urina
Para diminuir a frequência de jatos de urina, talvez haja necessidade de medicação com o objetivo de reduzir a excitação.

Defecação Imprópria
Em geral, não é indicado o uso de medicação.

Marcação com Fezes
Talvez seja necessária a utilização de medicamentos para diminuir a excitação que impulsiona e move esse comportamento.

CONTRAINDICAÇÕES
- Benzodiazepínicos — contraindicados em gatos, em virtude do potencial de necrose hepática idiopática fatal.
- Antidepressivos tricíclicos — contraindicados em gatos com antecedentes de distúrbios da condução cardíaca, retenção urinária ou fecal, megacólon, obstruções do trato urinário inferior e glaucoma.
- A via transdérmica não parece produzir níveis medicamentosos satisfatórios e constantes.

PRECAUÇÕES
- Todos os medicamentos relacionados são usados fora da indicação da bula. Explicar ao proprietário a natureza experimental desses tratamentos e os efeitos colaterais comuns; documentar a discussão mediante anotação no prontuário médico ou utilizar um termo de liberação. Começar com o

Evacuação e Micção Domiciliares pelos Gatos

Tabela 1.

Medicamentos e Dosagens Utilizados para Controlar o Hábito de Marcação Territorial com Urina pelos Gatos				
Medicamento	Classe Medicamentosa	Dosagem Oral em Gatos	Frequência	Efeitos Colaterais
Fluoxetina	ISRS	0,5-1,0 mg/kg	a cada 24 h	Diminuição do apetite, sonolência
Paroxetina	ISRS	0,25-0,50 mg/kg	a cada 24 h	Constipação
Clomipramina	ATC	0,2-0,50 mg/kg	a cada 24 h	Sonolência
Amitriptilina	ATC	0,25-1,0 mg/kg	a cada 24 h	Sonolência
Buspirona	Azapirona	0,5-1,0 mg/kg	a cada 12 h	Efeitos colaterais GI (raros)

uso de psicotrópicos quando o proprietário estiver presente para monitorizar o paciente.
- Os benzodiazepínicos podem causar necrose hepática idiopática (uma condição potencialmente fatal) em gatos aparentemente saudáveis; portanto, esses agentes raramente são utilizados para o tratamento.
- Efeito colateral comum da paroxetina: constipação.
- Efeito colateral comum da fluoxetina: diminuição do apetite; para evitar anorexia em gatos obesos, inicie com baixas doses e aumente aos poucos.

INTERAÇÕES POSSÍVEIS
Não usar inibidores da MAO (inclusive amitraz e L-deprenil) simultaneamente com ATCs ou ISRSs.

MEDICAMENTO(S) ALTERNATIVO(S)
- Progestinas sintéticas — o risco de efeitos colaterais graves, inclusive discrasias sanguíneas, piometra, hiperplasia mamária, carcinoma de mama, diabetes melito e obesidade, diminuiu seu uso, outrora comum.
- Terapia com ferormônios (Feliway®) — pode diminuir os jatos de urina.

ACOMPANHAMENTO

MONITORIZAÇÃO DO PACIENTE
- É essencial o acompanhamento regular do animal.
- O proprietário deve manter um registro diário dos padrões de eliminação, para que o sucesso do tratamento possa ser avaliado, permitindo os subsequentes ajustes na terapia. Numere as bandejas sanitárias e peça para o proprietário contar e registrar o número de micções em cada bandeja e fora das bandejas todos os dias.
- Para o comportamento de marcação, a medicação poderá ser retirada de forma gradativa ao longo de 2 semanas como um teste, após 2 meses de controle terapêutico bem-sucedido. No entanto, se os aspectos sociais ainda estiverem presentes como a base do comportamento, a medicação talvez tenha de ser mantida para o êxito da terapia. Para a monitorização do paciente, é recomendável a obtenção de hemograma completo, perfil bioquímico, urinálise e exame físico anualmente.

PREVENÇÃO
- Proceder à castração dos gatos.
- Restringir o número de gatos para diminuir a probabilidade de marcação com urina.
- Orientar os proprietários sobre a higiene, a seleção e o local adequados das bandejas sanitárias para evitar problemas de evacuação domiciliar.
- Os clínicos veterinários devem questionar os donos de gatos sobre evacuação domiciliar em cada consulta de rotina, pois a identificação e o tratamento precoces otimizam o sucesso terapêutico.

COMPLICAÇÕES POSSÍVEIS
- As expectativas do proprietário precisam ser realistas. O controle imediato de um problema de longa data como este é improvável; o objetivo, portanto, é a melhora gradual com o passar do tempo.
- A falha no tratamento pode resultar na eutanásia do gato, sua entrega a um abrigo de animais ou abandono.

EVOLUÇÃO ESPERADA E PROGNÓSTICO
- O prognóstico quanto à melhora do quadro será bom se a etiologia subjacente for identificada e tratada.
- Se o comportamento de marcação com urina não for tratado, ele destruirá os pertences da casa e abalará a relação homem-animal, levando ao desamparo do animal, à desistência da posse, ao abandono para algum abrigo de animais e até à eutanásia.

DIVERSOS

DISTÚRBIOS ASSOCIADOS
A agressividade entre os gatos pode estar associada à marcação territorial com jatos de urina.

FATORES RELACIONADOS COM A IDADE
- Os gatos mais idosos podem considerar o acesso às bandejas sanitárias difícil e procurar locais alternativos.
- A não utilização da bandeja sanitária pode ser associada ao declínio cognitivo relacionado com a idade.

POTENCIAL ZOONÓTICO
Mulheres grávidas não devem limpar as bandejas sanitárias de gatos em virtude do risco de transmissão de toxoplasmose.

GESTAÇÃO/FERTILIDADE/REPRODUÇÃO
Os antidepressivos tricíclicos estão contraindicados em animais utilizados para fins reprodutivos.

SINÔNIMO(S)
- Geral: evacuação domiciliar felina.
- Urina: eliminação imprópria felina, micção agachada fora da bandeja sanitária, marcação com urina, jato de urina.
- Fezes: defecação imprópria felina, defecação fora da bandeja sanitária, marcação com fezes, *middening*.

ABREVIATURA(S)
- ATC = antidepressivo tricíclico.
- FeLV = vírus da leucemia felina.
- FIV = vírus da imunodeficiência felina.
- GI = gastrintestinal.
- ISRS = inibidor seletivo de recaptação da serotonina.

RECURSOS DA INTERNET
- Cornell University Feline Health Center, "Housesoiling": http://www.vet.cornell.edu/fhc/brochures/Housesoiling.html.
- Ohio State University Indoor Cat Initiative: http://indoorpet.osu.edu/cats/, http://indoorpet.osu.edu.

Sugestões de Leitura
King JN, Steffan J, Heath SE, et al. Determination of the dosage of clomipramine for the treatment of urine spraying in cats. JAVMA 2004, 225:881-887.
Neilson JC. House soiling by cats. In: Horwitz DF, Mills D, eds., BSAVA Manual of Canine and Feline Behavioural Medicine, 2nd ed. Gloucestershire, UK: BSAVA, 2009, pp. 117-126.
Pryor PA, Hart BL, Bain MJ, Cliff CK. Causes of urine marking in cats and the effects of environmental management on the frequency of marking. JAVMA 2001, 219:1709-1713.
Pryor PA, Hart BL, Cliff KD, Bain MJ. Effects of a selective serotonin reuptake inhibitor on urine spraying behavior in cats. JAVMA 2001, 219:1557-1561.
Tynes VV, Hart BL, Pryor PA, et al. Evaluation of the role of lower urinary tract disease in cats with urine-marking behavior. JAVMA 2003, 223:457-461.

Autor Barbara L. Sherman
Consultor Editorial Debra F. Horwitz

FALHA OVULATÓRIA

CONSIDERAÇÕES GERAIS

REVISÃO
- A falha ovulatória é uma interrupção do processo de liberação dos oócitos pelos folículos com consequente formação de corpo lúteo e produção de progesterona. • Embora possa ocorrer em cadelas ou gatas de qualquer idade, há um aumento da frequência com o avanço da idade.
- A falha ovulatória pode se manifestar com sintomas de ninfomania ou anestro prolongado.
- As cadelas com ninfomania apresentam produção elevada de estrogênios e podem exibir sinais de toxicidade causada por esses hormônios, incluindo anormalidades dermatológicas ou hematológicas.

IDENTIFICAÇÃO
- Pode acometer cadelas ou gatas intactas de qualquer idade, embora haja uma predisposição maior em fêmeas mais idosas. • A falha ovulatória é relatada em 1,2% das cadelas que se apresentam para manejo reprodutivo; não há relato de prevalência nas gatas. • Não há predisposição racial relatada para anovulação; os cistos foliculares são mais comumente relatados em Malamute, Pastor alemão, Golden retriever, Bouvier des Flandres, e Labrador retriever. • Hereditariedade desconhecida.

SINAIS CLÍNICOS
- Proestro ou estro prolongado. • Vulva edematosa.
- Corrimento vulvar sanguinolento (cadela).
- Ninfomania. • Anestro. • Alopecia bilateral simétrica (progressiva, não pruriginosa). • Em caso de neoplasia: ○ Abdome aumentado de volume.
- Massa craniomesoabdominal palpável. ○ ± Ascite.
- Em caso de anormalidade cromossômica: ○ A genitália varia de normal a infantil ou ambígua.
- Aumento de volume do clitóris ou do osso clitoriano. ○ Baixa estatura. ○ Anestro.

CAUSAS E FATORES DE RISCO
- Falha de liberação do hormônio liberador de gonadotropina ou do hormônio luteinizante do hipotálamo ou da hipófise, respectivamente.
- Falha de resposta ao LH pelos receptores presentes na parede folicular. • Falha na produção de quantidade adequada de estrogênios pelos folículos para eliciar uma onda no GnRH. • Cistos foliculares funcionais: ○ Podem mimetizar um ciclo estral normal em princípio, mas o estro persiste e a ovulação não ocorre. • Ooforite imunomediada. • Caquexia ou obesidade.
- Estresse (desempenho, viagem, canil). • Doença de Addison. • Síndrome de Cushing.

DIAGNÓSTICO

DIAGNÓSTICO DIFERENCIAL
- Prolongamento de proestro (até 30 dias) ou estro (até 30 dias). • Cio dividido: ○ Nesse caso, o ciclo anovulatório será acompanhado por um ciclo normal, fértil e ovulatório em 1-8 semanas.
- Tumor de células da granulosa ou cistadenoma seroso: ○ massa abdominal ± palpável. ○ ovário aumentado de volume ao exame ultrassonográfico, muitas vezes com um aspecto de favo de mel. – ± ascite. ○ ± alopecia bilateral simétrica, hiperpigmentação, liquenificação em caso de neoplasia funcional em termos endócrinos.
- Senescência ovariana. • Ooforite imunomediada.
- Anormalidade cromossômica: ○ Intersexos, hermafroditas, pseudo-hermafroditas, quimeras*, mosaicos** podem desenvolver folículos que acabam ovulando ou simplesmente regridem.
- Administração exógena de estrogênios ou exposição a esses hormônios.

HEMOGRAMA/BIOQUÍMICA/URINÁLISE
- Na presença de toxicidade dos estrogênios:
  ○ Anemia normocítica normocrômica.
  ○ Trombocitopenia. ○ Leucocitose inicial seguida por leucopenia.

OUTROS TESTES LABORATORIAIS
- Níveis de progesterona <4-10 ng/mL em múltiplas amostras uma vez que a citologia vaginal tenha excedido 70% de células superficiais anucleadas. Frequentemente oscilam em torno de 3-5 ng/mL por um período de tempo prolongado e nunca ultrapassam 10 ng/mL. • A cariotipagem é indicada nos casos com suspeita de anormalidade cromossômica.

DIAGNÓSTICO POR IMAGEM
- A radiologia pode ser benéfica na existência de massa ovariana. Pode ser observada uma hiperdensidade de tecido mole na porção mesoabdominal. Na presença de ascite, pode haver uma perda dos detalhes abdominais gerais ou um aspecto em vidro fosco. • A ultrassonografia é extremamente útil para avaliar as estruturas ovarianas. ○ Múltiplas estruturas anecoicas no ovário podem ser consideradas folículos.
○ Estruturas de origem folicular com mais de 1 cm são consideradas císticas. ○ Ovários aumentados de volume podem ser neoplásicos. ○ Estruturas anecoicas com paredes espessas podem indicar luteinização (parcial ou completa) de estruturas foliculares. ○ Há necessidade de ultrassonografia seriada (diária) para registrar a ovulação.

MÉTODOS DIAGNÓSTICOS
- Laparotomia exploratória para examinar os ovários ou obter biopsias ovarianas. • A bolsa ovariana deve ser obrigatoriamente aberta para visualizar o ovário.

TRATAMENTO

Manter a cadela separada de machos intactos para evitar acasalamento acidental.

MEDICAÇÕES

MEDICAMENTO(S)
- Agentes indutores de ovulação: ○ Uma vez que a citologia tenha atingido >70% de células anucleadas e os folículos tenham >4-5 mm (raças caninas *toys* a pequeno porte); 5-7 mm (raças caninas de médio a grande porte); 7-10 mm (raças caninas de porte gigante); 2-3 mm (espécie felina) — pode-se tentar a indução da ovulação. ○ GnRH

---

* N.T.: Animal no qual foi introduzido, natural ou artificialmente, células alogênicas com sucesso (Fonte: Pdamed).

** N.T.: Estrutura que, em genética, corresponde a um organismo produzido por uma mistura de células com genótipos diferentes (Fonte: Pdamed).

---

na dose de 1,1-2,2 μg/kg IM ou IV ou 25 μg/gato IM. A administração pode ser repetida diariamente por 1-3 dias em cadelas; dose única para gatas.
○ hCG na dose de 500-1.000 UI/cadela IM ou 500 UI/gata IM. A administração pode ser repetida em 2-3 dias se a ovulação não ocorrer. ○ Os hormônios GnRH e hCG podem ser administrados concomitantemente. ○ Deslorrelina (implante de 2,1 mg; Ovuplant®). ○ O implante deve ser removido assim que a ovulação for registrada (progesterona >10 ng/mL). ○ O implante é aplicado na mucosa dos lábios vulvares utilizando o bloqueio anestésico com lidocaína e, depois, removido com bloqueio semelhante e dissecção cortante. ○ Em gatas, a estimulação mecânica da cérvix uterina pode ser realizada começando no momento da medicação inicial de indução, mas repetida várias vezes ao dia por 24-48 horas.

ACOMPANHAMENTO

- É aconselhável a monitorização das concentrações de progesterona durante a gestação, pois a falha luteal ou o hipoluteoidismo são comuns com a ovulação induzida. • É recomendável a monitorização dos níveis de progesterona após o uso dos medicamentos de indução para confirmar uma elevação normal desse hormônio. • Os exames ultrassonográficos seriados podem ser úteis para registrar a ovulação.

DIVERSOS

DISTÚRBIOS ASSOCIADOS
Alopecia bilateral simétrica não pruriginosa com estro significativamente prolongado.

GESTAÇÃO/FERTILIDADE/REPRODUÇÃO
- Dependendo da etiologia, a anovulação pode ser hereditária; portanto, isso deve ser levado em consideração antes do acasalamento. • Com frequência, o ciclo estral após um ciclo anovulatório é normal, não exigindo qualquer medicamento para indução da ovulação.

VER TAMBÉM
- Infertilidade, fêmea — Cães. • Distúrbios do Desenvolvimento Sexual.

ABREVIATURAS
- GnRH = hormônio liberador de gonadotropina.
- hCG = gonadotropina coriônica humana.
- LH = hormônio luteinizante.

RECURSOS DA INTERNET
Concannon PW, England G, Verstegen III J, Linde-Forsberg C, eds. Recent Advances in Small Animal Reproduction. International Veterinary Information Service, Ithaca NY, www.ivis.org.

Sugestões de Leitura
Johnston SD, Root Kustritz MV, Olson PNS. Disorders of the feline ovary. In: Canine and Feline Theriogenology. Philadelphia: Saunders, 2001, pp. 453-462.
Meyers-Wallen VN. Unusual and abnormal canine estrous cycles. Theriogenology 2007, 68:1205-1210.

Autor Cheryl Lopate
Consultor Editorial Sara K. Lyle

FEBRE

CONSIDERAÇÕES GERAIS

DEFINIÇÃO
Temperatura corporal acima do normal por causa de alteração no ponto de ajuste do centro termorregulador no hipotálamo; a temperatura corporal normal em cães e gatos é de 37,8-39,3°C. Febre de origem indeterminada — pelo menos 39,7°C em, no mínimo, quatro ocasiões em um período de 14 dias e doença de 14 dias de duração sem causa óbvia.

FISIOPATOLOGIA
Pirogênios endógenos ou exógenos provocam liberação de substâncias endógenas, que reajustam o centro termorregulador hipotalâmico para uma temperatura mais alta, ativando respostas fisiológicas apropriadas para elevar a temperatura corporal até o novo ponto de ajuste. As consequências fisiológicas incluem aumento das demandas metabólicas, catabolismo muscular, supressão da medula óssea, maiores necessidades hídricas e calóricas e, possivelmente, CID e choque.

SISTEMA(S) ACOMETIDO(S)
- Cardiovascular — taquicardia.
- Hematológico/linfático/imune — depressão da medula óssea e CID.
- Nervoso — edema cerebral, depressão.

DISTRIBUIÇÃO GEOGRÁFICA
A incidência de infecções fúngicas e algumas infecções riquetsiais e bacterianas varia de forma bastante expressiva.

IDENTIFICAÇÃO
Espécies
- Cães e gatos.

Raça(s) Predominante(s)
Alguns distúrbios associados à raça podem resultar em febre de origem indeterminada (p. ex., febre do Shar-pei, meningite/arterite).

Idade Média e Faixa Etária
Qualquer idade.

SINAIS CLÍNICOS
Comentários Gerais
- A febre em si é benéfica — o aumento da temperatura corporal diminui a divisão bacteriana e aumenta a imunocompetência.
- Febre prolongada >40,5°C acarreta desidratação e anorexia.
- Febres >41,1°C podem levar a edema cerebral, depressão da medula óssea e CID.

Achados Anamnésicos
- Histórico clínico (p. ex., contato com agentes infecciosos, estilo de vida, viagem, vacinação recente, administração de medicamentos, picadas de insetos, doença prévia, alergias) e exame físico (incluindo o exame da retina) podem ajudar a identificar alguma condição patológica subjacente.
- A elucidação dos padrões de febre (p. ex., contínua, intermitente) raramente é proveitosa.

Achados do Exame Físico
- Hipertermia.
- Letargia.
- Inapetência.
- Taquicardia.
- Hiperpneia.
- Mucosas hiperêmicas.
- Desidratação.
- Choque.

CAUSAS
Agentes Infecciosos (Mais Comuns)
- Agentes virais — FeLV, FIV, parvovírus, cinomose, herpes-vírus e calicivírus.
- Bactérias — endotoxinas Gram-positivas e Gram-negativas, *Mycoplasma*, *Bartonella*.
- Fungos sistêmicos — *Histoplasma*, *Blastomyces*, *Coccidioidomyces* e *Cryptococcus*.
- Rickettsiaceae — *Rickettsia rickettsii* (febre maculosa das Montanhas Rochosas).
- Anaplasmataceae — *Ehrlichia canis*, *Anaplasma phagocytophila*, *Neorickettsia helminthoeca*.
- Parasitas e protozoários — *Babesia*, *Toxoplasma*, *larva migrans aberrante*, *Dirofilaria thromboemboli*, *Leishmania*, *Cytauxzoon*, *Hepatozoon*, *Neospora*.
- *Leptospira* spp.
- *Borrelia burgdorferi* (doença de Lyme).

Processos Imunomediados
Lúpus eritematoso sistêmico, anemia hemolítica imunomediada, trombocitopenia imunomediada, pênfigo, poliartrite, polimiosite, artrite reumatoide, vasculite, reações de hipersensibilidade, reação à transfusão e infecção secundária a defeitos imunes hereditários ou adquiridos.

Endócrinos e Metabólicos
Hipertireoidismo, hipoadrenocorticismo (raro), feocromocitoma, hiperlipidemia e hipernatremia.

Neoplasia
Linfoma, doença mieloproliferativa, plasmocitoma, mastocitoma, histiocitose maligna, doença metastática, tumor necrótico e tumor sólido, particularmente em órgãos como fígado, rins, ossos, pulmões e linfonodos.

Outros Distúrbios Inflamatórios
Colangio-hepatite, lipidose hepática, hepatopatia tóxica, cirrose, enteropatia inflamatória, pancreatite, peritonite, pleurite, doenças granulomatosas, desvio portossistêmico, tromboflebite, infartos, pan-esteatite, paniculite, osteodistrofia hipertrófica, traumatismo contuso (rombo), neutropenia cíclica, lesões intracranianas (encefalite, traumatismo) e tromboembolia pulmonar.

Medicamentos e Toxinas
Tetraciclina, sulfonamida, penicilinas, nitrofurantoína, anfotericina B, barbitúricos, iodo, atropina, cimetidina, salicilatos (altas dosagens), anti-histamínicos, procainamida e metais pesados.

Febre de Origem Indeterminada — Cães
- Infecção (28%) — discospondilite, blastomicose e outras infecções fúngicas, endocardite valvular, abscessos de tecidos moles ou parênquima, bacteremia, artrite séptica, meningite séptica, piotórax, corpo estranho/abscesso pulmonar, piometra de coto uterino, broncopneumonia, osteomielite, peritonite, prostatite, pancreatite, pielonefrite, osteomielite, sepse secundária à imunodeficiência, leptospirose, leishmaniose, toxoplasmose, doença de Lyme, infecção por *Ehrlichia*, *Anaplasma*, *Bartonella*.
- Doença imunomediada (27%) poliartrite, meningite ou vasculite imunomediadas, dentre outras.
- Doença da medula óssea, incluindo neoplasia (16%).
- Neoplasia (7%).
- Diversos (10%) osteodistrofia hipertrófica, meningite, linfadenite, panosteíte, desvio portossistêmico, reação medicamentosa, toxina, febre do Shar-pei.
- Não diagnosticada (12%).

Febre de Origem Indeterminada — Gatos
- A maioria é mediada por vírus (p. ex., FeLV, FIV, PIF, menos comumente parvovírus, herpes-vírus e calicivírus).
- Infecção bacteriana oculta persistente por bactérias atípicas, às vezes secundária a feridas por mordedura (p. ex., *Yersinia*, *Mycobacteria*, *Nocardia*, *Actinomyces* e *Brucella*).
- O piotórax é comum.
- Outras causas — pielonefrite, traumatismo contuso (rombo), lesão intestinal penetrante, abscesso dentário, micoses sistêmicas (p. ex., *Histoplasma*, *Blastomyces* e *Coccidioides*), linfoma e tumores sólidos.
- Os distúrbios imunes são raros, assim como prostatite, endometrite, discospondilite, pneumonia e endocardite.

FATORES DE RISCO
- Viagem recente.
- Exposição a agentes biológicos.
- Imunossupressão.
- Animais muito jovens ou idosos.

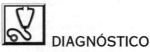

DIAGNÓSTICO

DIAGNÓSTICO DIFERENCIAL
É preciso diferenciar a febre verdadeira de hipertermia. O estresse e a ansiedade gerados no hospital podem causar um aumento discreto da temperatura. Temperaturas de até 39,4°C podem ser causadas por estresse ou doença. Temperaturas >40°C quase sempre são relevantes. Temperaturas >41,7°C não costumam ser febre; é mais provável que sejam hipertermia primária.

HEMOGRAMA/BIOQUÍMICA/URINÁLISE
- Hemograma completo e esfregaço sanguíneo — leucopenia ou leucocitose, desvio à esquerda, monocitose, linfocitose, trombocitopenia ou trombocitose, esferócitos, microrganismos.
- O perfil bioquímico e a urinálise variam com o sistema orgânico envolvido.

OUTROS TESTES LABORATORIAIS
- Se houver suspeita de doença infecciosa, tentar a cultura do microrganismo — urocultura, hemoculturas (i. e., 3 anaeróbias e 3 aeróbias, obtidas durante uma elevação da temperatura ou em intervalos de 20 minutos; tentar o uso do maior volume possível para aumentar a recuperação diagnóstica; considerar o emprego de frascos de resina que se ligam a antibióticos), cultura de fungos e do LCS, cultura dos líquidos sinovial e prostático, bem como de amostras de biopsia, se houver indicação clínica.
- Testes para FeLV e FIV, teste Snap 4DX®, sorologia ou PCR para *Toxoplasma*, *Borrelia*, *Mycoplasma*, *Bartonella*, *Anaplasma*, *Ehrlichia*, *Rickettsia*, PIF, micoses sistêmicas.
- Exame fecal na presença de sinais gastrintestinais.
- Lavado traqueal ou broncoalveolar se houver comprometimento respiratório.
- Teste para dirofilariose oculta diante da suspeita de embolia pulmonar.
- Na suspeita de distúrbios imunes — exame citológico do líquido sinovial; testes de Coombs, fator reumatoide (o título do anticorpo antinuclear

e o teste do fator reumatoide frequentemente não são recompensadores).
• Teste de imunorreatividade da lipase pancreática.
• T_4 para descartar hipertireoidismo em gatos.

DIAGNÓSTICO POR IMAGEM
Radiografia
• Radiografias abdominais para fazer a varredura de tumores e efusão.
• Radiografias torácicas para excluir pneumonia, neoplasia e piotórax.
• Radiografias simples do esqueleto para detectar tumores ósseos, mieloma múltiplo, osteomielite, discospondilite, panosteíte, osteopatia hipertrófica e osteodistrofia hipertrófica.
• Radiografias dos dentes e do crânio para pesquisar abscessos das raízes dentárias, infecções dos seios nasais, corpos estranhos e neoplasia.
• Radiografia contrastada (p. ex., gastrintestinal e urografia excretora) para buscar por indícios de neoplasia ou infecção.

Ultrassonografia
• Abdominal (mais biopsia ou aspirado orientado pelo ultrassom, se indicado) à procura de neoplasia abdominal e abscesso ou outro local de infecção (p. ex., pielonefrite, pancreatite, piometra).
• Ecocardiografia se houver suspeita de endocardite.

Imagens Nucleares
• Procedimentos de varredura com radionuclídeos para avaliar o paciente em busca de tumores ósseos, osteomielite e embolia pulmonar.
• TC ou RM, se indicados por outros achados.
• Fusão de imagem (combinação de tomografia por emissão de pósitrons com o uso de fluordesoxiglicose marcada radioativamente e TC).

MÉTODOS DIAGNÓSTICOS
• Artrocentese (cultura e citologia).
• Aspirado e biopsia da medula óssea diante da suspeita de malignidade ou mielodisplasia.
• Biopsia de linfonodo, pele ou músculo se houver indicação clínica.
• Exame do aspirado obtido por agulha fina ou biopsia de qualquer massa ou órgão anormal.
• Punção do LCS se os sinais neurológicos sugerirem tumor cerebral ou meningite.
• Endoscopia e biopsia na presença de sinais gastrintestinais.
• Laparotomia exploratória — último recurso se todos os outros exames diagnósticos falharem na determinação da causa e se o paciente não estiver melhorando.

TRATAMENTO
CUIDADO(S) DE SAÚDE ADEQUADO(S)
• Objetivos do tratamento:
  ○ Reajustar o ponto de ajuste do centro termorregulador do hipotálamo para um nível mais baixo.
  ○ Remover a causa subjacente.

CUIDADO(S) DE ENFERMAGEM
• A administração de fluidos (IV) frequentemente reduz a temperatura corporal.
• Se o paciente estiver desidratado, iniciar o fornecimento de cristaloides isotônicos.
• Resfriamento tópico em caso de febre intensa (resfriamento por convecção com ventiladores, resfriamento por evaporação com álcool isopropílico nos coxins palmoplantares, nas axilas e nas virilhas).
• Utilizar o tratamento antipirético apenas em casos de febre prolongada e potencialmente fatal (>41,1ºC), além de insucesso no resfriamento tópico. Os pacientes comprometidos (p. ex., aqueles com insuficiência cardíaca, crises convulsivas ou doença respiratória) necessitam de tratamento antipirético mais cedo. O tratamento antipirético pode dificultar a elucidação da causa, atrasar a terapia correta e complicar a monitorização do paciente (p. ex., a redução da febre é uma indicação importante de resposta ao tratamento).

ATIVIDADE
Restrita.

DIETA
Os pacientes febris encontram-se em um estado hipercatabólico e necessitam de alta ingestão calórica.

ORIENTAÇÃO AO PROPRIETÁRIO
Explicar ao proprietário que a avaliação diagnóstica de pacientes com febre de origem indeterminada é, muitas vezes, vasta, cara e invasiva, e nem sempre fornece o diagnóstico definitivo.

CONSIDERAÇÕES CIRÚRGICAS
Talvez haja necessidade de cirurgia em alguns animais com causa infecciosa (p. ex., piometra, peritonite, piotórax, e abscesso hepático) ou neoplásica localizada subjacente de febre.

MEDICAÇÕES
MEDICAMENTO(S) DE ESCOLHA
• A seleção depende do diagnóstico.
• Não usar antibióticos de amplo espectro (ou seja, "de ataque") sem antes fazer uma avaliação diagnóstica completa a menos que o estado do paciente seja crítico e esteja deteriorando rapidamente.

Antibióticos
• Selecionados com base nos resultados da cultura bacteriana ou da sorologia.
• Em situações de emergência, a terapia com antibióticos combinados pode ser iniciada após a obtenção de amostras para cultura (p. ex., cefalotina, 20 mg/kg IV a cada 6-8 h; combinada com enrofloxacino a 2,5-5 mg/kg IV a cada 12 h). A escolha de outros antimicrobianos depende da suspeita clínica principal, com base nos achados clínicos e laboratoriais preliminares.
• Não administrar antibióticos por mais de 1-2 semanas se a resposta não for favorável.

Antipiréticos
• Ácido acetilsalicílico — cães, 10 mg/kg VO a cada 12 h; gatos, 6 mg/kg VO a cada 48 h.
• Deracoxibe — cães, 1-2 mg/kg/dia.
• Flunixino meglumina — cães, 0,5-1 mg/kg IV ou IM uma única vez (administrar fluidos IV).

Glicocorticoides
• Não usar a menos que as causas infecciosas tenham sido excluídas.
• Podem mascarar os sinais clínicos e acarretar imunossupressão, além de não serem recomendados para uso como antipiréticos; a administração de corticosteroides a gatos com febre de origem indeterminada intratável após a exclusão de doenças infecciosas pode promover uma resposta favorável.
• Indicados principalmente para a febre associada à doença imunomediada e certos tumores responsivos aos esteroides (p. ex., linfoma).

PRECAUÇÕES
Os efeitos colaterais dos antipiréticos incluem êmese, diarreia, ulceração gastrintestinal, dano renal, hemólise, hepatotoxicidade (paracetamol, particularmente perigoso em gatos) e rigidez muscular (flunixino meglumina).

INTERAÇÕES POSSÍVEIS
A combinação de anti-inflamatórios não esteroides (AINE) e esteroides aumenta o risco de hemorragia gastrintestinal.

ACOMPANHAMENTO
MONITORIZAÇÃO DO PACIENTE
• Monitorizar a temperatura corporal do paciente pelo menos a cada 12 h.
• Se a causa da febre permanecer desconhecida para o clínico, repetir a anamnese e o exame físico juntamente com os exames laboratoriais de triagem.
• Caso a febre se desenvolva ou se agrave durante a hospitalização, considerar a ocorrência de infecção nosocomial ou superinfecção.

EVOLUÇÃO ESPERADA E PROGNÓSTICO
Variam com a causa; em alguns pacientes (mais comumente em gatos), não se consegue determinar a causa subjacente.

DIVERSOS
FATORES RELACIONADOS COM A IDADE
• Animais jovens — é mais provável que eles tenham doença infecciosa do que outras causas; o prognóstico é melhor do que nos animais idosos.
• Animais idosos — as causas comuns incluem infecção intra-abdominal e neoplasia; os sinais tendem a ser mais inespecíficos; prognóstico frequentemente reservado.

SINÔNIMO(S)
Pirexia.

VER TAMBÉM
Intermação e Hipertermia.

ABREVIATURA(S)
• AINE = anti-inflamatório não esteroide.
• CID = coagulação intravascular disseminada.
• FIV = vírus da imunodeficiência felina.
• FeLV = vírus da leucemia felina.
• LCS = líquido cerebrospinal.
• PCR = reação em cadeia da polimerase.
• PIF = peritonite infecciosa felina.
• RM = ressonância magnética.
• TC = tomografia computadorizada.

Autores Maria Vianna e Jörg Bucheler
Consultores Editoriais Larry P. Tilley e Francis W.K. Smith, Jr.

Febre Familiar do Shar-Pei

CONSIDERAÇÕES GERAIS

DEFINIÇÃO
Distúrbio familiar imunorreativo na raça chinesa Shar-pei, caracterizado por febre episódica e jarretes tumefatos, com amiloidose sistêmica progressiva associada.

FISIOPATOLOGIA
- A raça em questão tem predisposição ao depósito sistêmico reativo de amiloide. O mecanismo exato é desconhecido; no entanto, sugere-se que ela seja secundária a níveis elevados de IL-6, possivelmente com outros mediadores inflamatórios.
- A IL-6 pode induzir ao aumento dos níveis séricos de amiloide A (um reagente de fase aguda). A produção excessiva de amiloide A sérico resulta no depósito extracelular de amiloide, que acarreta insuficiência de órgãos, dependendo do local do depósito.
- O amiloide é depositado em todos os tecidos, porém os locais mais importantes em termos clínicos são os rins e o fígado.
- A amiloidose hepática pode tornar o fígado friável e suscetível à ruptura e ao hemoabdome secundário.
- A amiloidose renal e a síndrome nefrótica secundária predispõem os cães dessa raça a estados de hipercoagulabilidade.
- Do mesmo modo que a febre familiar do Mediterrâneo em pessoas, esses mediadores inflamatórios causam febre e inflamação serosa, acometendo a pleura, o peritônio e as membranas sinoviais.

SISTEMA(S) ACOMETIDO(S)
- Cardiovascular — trombose venosa (p. ex., tromboembolia pulmonar); hipertensão sistêmica.
- Gastrintestinal — dor abdominal; vômito; diarreia; hemoabdome; ascite.
- Hematológico/linfático/imune — anemia; leucocitose, com ou sem desvio à esquerda; defeitos de coagulação; estados hipercoaguláveis; queda nos níveis de imunoglobulina.
- Hepatobiliar — hepatomegalia; ruptura hepática; elevação das enzimas hepáticas; comprometimento da função hepática.
- Musculosquelético — efusão articular, especialmente da articulação tibiotarsal; claudicação; rigidez; marcha cautelosa como se estivesse "pisando em ovos"; dorso arqueado ("dorso de carpa"); indisposição em se locomover.
- Nervoso — acidente vascular; sinais neurológicos de início agudo (p. ex., inclinação da cabeça, ataxia vestibular e crises convulsivas).
- Oftálmico — descolamento da retina.
- Renal/urológico — proteinúria; baixa densidade urinária; poliúria; polidipsia.
- Respiratório — taquipneia ou dispneia.
- Pele — tumefação periarticular edematosa do tecido mole, especialmente na região da articulação tibiotarsal; focinho tumefato; icterícia; esfacelamento da pele.

GENÉTICA
Existe a hipótese de que seja um distúrbio hereditário autossômico recessivo.

INCIDÊNCIA/PREVALÊNCIA
- Estima-se que 23-28% dos cães da raça Shar-pei sejam acometidos pelo distúrbio.
- Estima-se que 53% dos cães da raça Shar-pei com febre tenham a febre do Shar-pei.

IDENTIFICAÇÃO
- Idade média — 4 anos.
- Faixa etária — 19 semanas a 9 anos.
- Predisposição sexual — nenhuma.

SINAIS CLÍNICOS

Comentários Gerais
- Os achados da anamnese e do exame físico podem variar, dependendo do órgão acometido e da gravidade da amiloidose.
- Alguns casos podem exibir apenas alguns dos achados expostos a seguir.

Achados Anamnésicos
- Anorexia episódica, letargia, rigidez, jarretes e/ou focinho tumefatos —autolimitantes (24-36 h) ou responsivos a AINEs.
- Surtos intermitentes de dor abdominal, vômitos e/ou diarreia.
- Poliúria e polidipsia.
- Perda de peso.

Achados do Exame Físico
- Febre acentuada (39,4-41,7°C) que dura 24-36 h.
- Letargia e desidratação.
- Tumefações periarticulares edematosas do tecido mole em uma ou mais articulações.
- Efusão articular.
- Focinho tumefato.
- Dor abdominal.
- Relutância ao movimento e postura arqueada.
- Taquipneia.
- Hepatomegalia, ascite e icterícia.
- Mucosas pálidas, secundariamente à anemia induzida por insuficiência renal crônica ou, em casos raros, ao hemoabdome.

CAUSAS
- Acredita-se que a falta de regulação de processos imunes e inflamatórios nos cães da raça Shar-pei predisponha a raça ao desenvolvimento de amiloidose secundária ou reativa.
- Qualquer infecção crônica, inflamação, doença imunomediada ou neoplasia pode causar amiloidose reativa ou secundária.

FATORES DE RISCO
O estresse pode deflagrar um episódio de febre.

DIAGNÓSTICO

DIAGNÓSTICO DIFERENCIAL
- Causas infecciosas ou imunomediadas de poliartrite — p. ex., *Ehrlichia*, doença de Lyme, lúpus eritematoso sistêmico, poliartrite idiopática.
- Icterícia (ver capítulo sobre o assunto).
- Insuficiência renal crônica (*idem*).
- Poliúria e polidipsia (*idem*).
- Febre de origem indeterminada.

HEMOGRAMA/BIOQUÍMICA/URINÁLISE
- Anemia arregenerativa — secundária à insuficiência renal crônica ou ao hemoabdome agudo.
- Leucocitose com ou sem desvio à esquerda.
- Alterações compatíveis com insuficiência renal — por exemplo, elevações dos níveis de ureia, creatinina e fósforo, além de aumento do hiato aniônico.
- Hipoalbuminemia — secundária à proteinúria ou insuficiência hepática.
- Hipercolesterolemia — compatível com a síndrome nefrótica (hipoalbuminemia, proteinúria, ascite e colesterol elevado).
- Elevações na atividade da fosfatase alcalina e da ALT; nível de bilirrubina elevado.
- Proteinúria — nos casos em que o amiloide se deposita no córtex renal. **Nota:** na maioria dos cães, há depósito medular de amiloide; desse modo, a proteinúria pode estar ausente.
- Isostenúria — em casos de acometimento renal ou insuficiência hepática.
- Bilirrubinúria — secundária à colestase.

OUTROS TESTES LABORATORIAIS
- Sorologia para pesquisa de *Ehrlichia*, *Anaplasma* e *Borrelia*/Snap 4Dx/ou PCR.
- Testes para detecção de dirofilária — excluir glomerulonefrite secundária ao depósito de imunocomplexos induzidos por dirofilariose.
- Teste de Coombs, AAN e fator reumatoide — para identificar doença imunomediada subjacente concomitante.
- TP e TTP — os fatores IX e X podem ser perdidos por meio dos glomérulos e prolongar o TTP; a insuficiência hepática pode causar prolongamento do TP e do TTP; a trombose de órgãos pode provocar CID e prolongamento concomitante do TP e do TTP, além de aumento dos D-dímeros.
- Nível de antitrombina III — pode estar baixo por causa da perda através dos glomérulos; acredita-se que esse nível decline em relação direta com o grau de hipoalbuminemia; é possível que a mensuração da antitrombina III seja preditiva quanto ao risco de formação de trombo.
- Níveis de IgA ou IgG — podem estar baixos em alguns casos; acredita-se que níveis baixos aumentem o risco de inflamação ou infecção.
- Relação de proteína:creatinina urinárias — elevada com o depósito de amiloide nos glomérulos; tipicamente >13 com amiloidose (normal: <1).

DIAGNÓSTICO POR IMAGEM
- Radiografia abdominal — as anormalidades podem incluir hepatomegalia ou imagens com detalhes reduzidos por causa de efusão peritoneal secundária; a efusão abdominal pode ser secundária à hipoalbuminemia, hipertensão portal ou hemorragia.
- Radiografia torácica — as anormalidades podem incluir efusão pleural secundária à hipoalbuminemia grave ou inflamação pleural.
- Radiografia articular — mostra tipicamente a tumefação periarticular dos tecidos moles, sem acometimento ósseo.
- Ultrassonografia abdominal — pode revelar um aspecto hipoecoico homogêneo difuso do parênquima hepático; os rins podem aparecer hiperecoicos.

MÉTODOS DIAGNÓSTICOS
- Análise do líquido sinovial — pode ou não revelar indícios de sinovite aguda (i. e., presença de PMN e viscosidade reduzida do líquido sinovial); a inflamação pode estar limitada às estruturas de sustentação inferiores da sinóvia.
- Biopsia ou aspiração renal e/ou hepática por agulha fina (desde que o TP, o TTP, o número de plaquetas e o tempo de sangramento na mucosa bucal estejam normais) — depósito de amiloide. A biopsia é o método preferido; no entanto, o corante vermelho Congo e a luz polarizada são utilizados para confirmar a presença de amiloide em amostras citológicas.

Febre Familiar do Shar-Pei

ACHADOS PATOLÓGICOS
- Depósito sistêmico de amiloide em vários órgãos (p. ex., rins, fígado, trato gastrintestinal, baço, linfonodos, glândulas adrenais, coração, pulmões, tireoide, próstata e pâncreas).
- O depósito de amiloide pode estar associado primariamente a vasos ou dentro do parênquima (p. ex., o espaço de Disse no fígado).

TRATAMENTO
CUIDADO(S) DE SAÚDE ADEQUADO(S)
- Paciente ambulatorial — durante episódios mínimos de dor e febre, responsivos aos AINEs.
- Paciente hospitalizado — a hospitalização é necessária durante períodos de anorexia, febre, claudicação acentuada ou dor inespecífica, vômitos ou diarreia, ascite ou episódios de colestase.
- Unidade de terapia intensiva — necessária durante a falência de órgãos ou a ocorrência de eventos tromboembólicos.
- Cirurgia de emergência — indicada para hemoabdome ou na suspeita de trombose venosa esplênica, porta ou renal.

CUIDADO(S) DE ENFERMAGEM
- Líquidos poliônicos balanceados — se o paciente estiver desidratado ou com anorexia, vômitos e/ou diarreia.
- Oxigênio — nos casos em que se suspeita de tromboembolia pulmonar.
- Abdominocentese — poderá ser necessária se a ascite estiver causando um comprometimento respiratório.
- Transfusões de sangue — poderão ser indicadas se a anemia for grave.
- Plasma fresco congelado — pode ser considerado para CID ou outras coagulopatias.
- Antibióticos — se houver suspeita de sepse ou diagnóstico de infecção concomitante; diante da suspeita de sepse, devem ser usados os agentes de amplo espectro; do contrário, a escolha do antibiótico deve ser orientada pelo teste de sensibilidade (antibiograma). **Nota:** o enrofloxacino é geralmente contraindicado em casos de síndrome de choque tóxico estreptocócico.
- AINE ou outros analgésicos (p. ex., opioides) — podem ser necessários para a febre e a dor; os AINE estão contraindicados em casos com doença renal concomitante ou sinais gastrintestinais.
- Protetores da mucosa gástrica — se houver suspeita de úlcera gástrica secundária à doença renal ou hepática.

ATIVIDADE
Limitar a atividade durante os episódios febris; em outras circunstâncias, depende da gravidade e da extensão do distúrbio sistêmico subjacente.

DIETA
- Com restrição de proteína — pode estar indicada na insuficiência renal para diminuir os sinais clínicos de uremia ou se a relação de proteína:creatinina urinárias estiver elevada; cães com evidência de encefalopatia hepática deverão ser submetidos à dieta com restrição proteica assim que estiverem estabilizados.
- Ácidos graxos ômega-3 — podem ser benéficos para a glomerulopatia.

ORIENTAÇÃO AO PROPRIETÁRIO
- Não existe cura para a amiloidose familiar do Shar-pei; portanto, a terapia é paliativa.
- A terapia pode diminuir o depósito de amiloide, mas a condição geralmente já terá evoluído além do estágio em que a medicação se mostra benéfica.
- O diagnóstico deve ser estabelecido para garantir que não haja um problema subjacente ou concomitante passível de tratamento.
- Os cães acometidos não devem ser usados como reprodutores.

MEDICAÇÕES
MEDICAMENTO(S)
- Colchicina — 0,03 mg/kg VO a cada 12-24 h; para retardar o depósito de amiloide; não se sabe se a colchicina terá algum efeito benéfico se já tiver ocorrido o depósito de amiloide. Considerar o uso da colchicina assim que o diagnóstico de febre familiar do Shar-pei for confirmado.
- DMSO — 80 mg/kg SC 3 vezes por semana ou 125 mg/kg VO a cada 12 h; o uso é controverso, pois geralmente há dúvidas quanto à ocorrência de algum efeito clínico significativo.
- Esteroides — apenas se houver uma doença imunomediada concomitante.
- Ácido acetilsalicílico em dose baixa — 0,5-1 mg/kg VO a cada 12-24 h; se houver preocupação com hipercoagulabilidade.
- Inibidores da ECA (0,25-0,5 mg/kg a cada 12-24 h VO) e/ou bloqueadores dos receptores de angiotensina para proteinúria significativa.

CONTRAINDICAÇÕES
Os AINEs estão contraindicados na presença de doença renal e úlceras gastrintestinais.

PRECAUÇÕES
- O uso de esteroides pode acelerar o depósito de amiloide.
- A colchicina pode causar desconforto gastrintestinal; o uso crônico pode estar associado à supressão da medula óssea.
- O DMSO tem odor muito forte.

ACOMPANHAMENTO
MONITORIZAÇÃO DO PACIENTE
- Densidade urinária — monitorizar em busca de isostenúria.
- Relações de proteína:creatinina urinárias — monitorizar quanto à presença de glomerulopatia.
- Perfil bioquímico — monitorizar os parâmetros renais e hepáticos, inclusive hipoalbuminemia.
- Monitorizar o hematócrito — para detectar anemia.
- Monitorizar a pressão arterial e o exame do fundo de olho — em pacientes hipertensos.

PREVENÇÃO
Evitar filhotes de linhagens com histórico de febre do Shar-pei.

COMPLICAÇÕES POSSÍVEIS
- Morte — causada por ruptura hepática ou tromboembolia pulmonar.
- Vasculite imunomediada secundária indutora de esfacelamento intenso da pele, síndrome de choque tóxico estreptocócico causadora de fasciíte necrosante localizada e/ou choque ou falência múltipla de órgãos concomitante.

EVOLUÇÃO ESPERADA E PROGNÓSTICO
- Distúrbio progressivo que apresenta exacerbações e remissões, com prognóstico reservado a mau, dependendo do momento do diagnóstico.
- Inevitavelmente fatal em virtude de insuficiência renal ou hepática crônica.
- A evolução pode levar de semanas a anos.

DIVERSOS
FATORES RELACIONADOS COM A IDADE
Tende a ser mais grave nos casos diagnosticados em uma idade precoce.

GESTAÇÃO/FERTILIDADE/REPRODUÇÃO
Não deixar que cães acometidos se acasalem.

SINÔNIMO(S)
Síndrome do jarrete inchado.

ABREVIATURA(S)
- AAN = anticorpo antinuclear.
- AINEs = anti-inflamatórios não esteroides.
- ALT = alanina aminotransferase.
- CID = coagulação intravascular disseminada.
- ECA = enzima conversora de angiotensina.
- DMSO = dimetilsulfóxido.
- IL-6 = interleucina 6.
- PCR = reação em cadeia da polimerase.
- PMN = neutrófilo polimorfonuclear.
- TP = tempo de protrombina.
- TTP = tempo de tromboplastina parcial.

RECURSOS DA INTERNET
- www.drjwv.com
- www.wvc.vetsuite.com

Sugestões de Leitura
DiBartola SP, Tarr MJ, Webb DM, Giger U. Familial renal amyloidosis in Chinese Shar Pei dogs. JAVMA 1990, 197:483-487.
May C, Hammill J, Bennett D. Chinese shar pei fever: A preliminary report. Vet Record 1992, 26:586-587.
Rivas AL, Tintle L, Kimball ES, et al. A canine febrile disorder associated with elevated interleukin-6. Clin Immunol Immunopathol 1992, 64:36-45.

Autor Julie Armstrong
Consultor Editorial A.H. Rebar

Febre Maculosa das Montanhas Rochosas

CONSIDERAÇÕES GERAIS

DEFINIÇÃO
- Riquetsiose originária do carrapato, causada por *Rickettsia rickettsii*, que acomete os cães, além de ser considerada a riquetsiose mais importante nos seres humanos.
- Anticorpos contra *R. akari* (agente causal da varíola por riquétsia nos seres humanos) foram encontrados nos cães de Nova York, NY, nos EUA. Não se sabe se essa riquétsia provoca doença nos cães.
- Outros microrganismos riquetsiais ainda não definidos também podem provocar sinais clínicos nos cães.

FISIOPATOLOGIA
- Vetor — carrapato (*Dermacentor variabilis*) do cão americano, encontrado a leste da Grande Planície [vasta região central de pastagens dos EUA]; carrapato da madeira (*D. andersoni*), encontrado desde as Cascatas até as Montanhas Rochosas.
- Transmissão — via saliva do vetor ou transfusão de sangue; o carrapato deve ficar aderido por 5-20 h para infectar o hospedeiro (seres humanos, cães e gatos) ou o hospedeiro reservatório (roedores e cães).
- Período de incubação — 2 dias a 2 semanas.
- Infecção — o microrganismo invade o endotélio vascular e nele se multiplica; provoca hemorragia microvascular; agregação plaquetária e anticorpos antiplaquetários causam trombocitopenia, vasoconstrição, aumento da permeabilidade vascular, perda elevada de plasma para o espaço intersticial (tumefação orgânica), hipotensão e, por fim, CID e choque; leva à vasculite disseminada nos órgãos com circulação endarterial (causa dos sinais clínicos).

SISTEMA(S) ACOMETIDO(S)
- Envolvimento multissistêmico.
- Cardiovascular — vasculite, hipotensão, choque.
- Hemático/linfático/imune — tendência ao sangramento gerada por trombocitopenia, vasculite, linfadenopatia, esplenomegalia.
- Musculosquelético — dor articular (artralgia).
- Nervoso — estupor, crises convulsivas, déficits vestibulares, coma, dor cervical (cervicalgia).
- Oftálmico — conjuntivite, congestão escleral.
- Respiratório — dispneia, tosse.
- Pele/exócrino — edema das extremidades e/ou da face.

GENÉTICA
N/D.

INCIDÊNCIA/PREVALÊNCIA
- Época dos carrapatos — final de março ao final de setembro [no hemisfério norte].
- Prevalência — infecções gerais nos carrapatos <2%; varia com a localização geográfica.

DISTRIBUIÇÃO GEOGRÁFICA
- Américas do Norte e do Sul.
- EUA — não há dados exatos para os cães; distribuição semelhante à dos seres humanos: estados costeiros do leste (especialmente os estados da Carolina do Norte e do Sul), vale do Rio Mississipi e estados do centrossul; pesquisa sorológica de cães de abrigos de Rhode Island: 21%.

IDENTIFICAÇÃO
Espécies
Cães.

Raça(s) Predominante(s)
- Cães de raça pura parecem mais propensos ao desenvolvimento da doença clínica do que os de raças mistas.
- Cães da raça Pastor alemão — mais comum.

Idade Média e Faixa Etária
Qualquer idade.

Sexo Predominante
Nenhum.

SINAIS CLÍNICOS
Achados Anamnésicos
- Febre — dentro de 2-3 dias da aderência do carrapato.
- Letargia.
- Depressão.
- Anorexia.
- Tumefação (edema) — lábios, escroto, prepúcio, orelhas, extremidades.
- Marcha rígida — especialmente com tumefação escrotal ou prepucial.
- Sangramento espontâneo — espirro, epistaxe.
- Angústia respiratória.
- Neurológicos — ataxia, inclinação da cabeça.
- Dor ocular (oftalmalgia).

Achados do Exame Físico
- Ocorre doença tanto clínica como subclínica.
- Clínica — variável em termos de gravidade; dura 2-4 semanas sem tratamento.
- Os carrapatos ainda podem estar presentes nos casos agudos.
- Pirexia.
- Lesões cutâneas — edema da face, dos membros, do prepúcio e do escroto.
- Extremidades — necrose.
- Conjuntivite.
- Congestão escleral.
- Respiratórios — dispneia, intolerância ao exercício resultante de pneumonite, ruídos broncovesiculares aumentados.
- Linfadenopatia generalizada.
- Neurológicos — disfunção vestibular, estado mental alterado, crises convulsivas.
- Mialgia/artralgia.
- Petéquias.
- Equimoses — regiões ocular, bucal, genital; 20% dos pacientes.
- Diáteses hemorrágicas — epistaxe, melena, hematúria; nos casos graves.
- Arritmias cardíacas — morte súbita.
- CID e morte por choque — nos casos agudos graves.

CAUSAS
R. rickettsii.

FATORES DE RISCO
- Exposição aos carrapatos.
- Coinfecção com outros patógenos (originários do carrapato).

DIAGNÓSTICO

DIAGNÓSTICO DIFERENCIAL
- Erliquiose canina — *Ehrlichia canis*; não sazonal; pode ser clinicamente indistinguível da febre maculosa das Montanhas Rochosas (sobretudo, os casos agudos); diferenciar por meio de teste sorológico; ambas respondem ao mesmo tratamento.
- Trombocitopenia imunomediada — não costuma estar associada à febre ou linfadenopatia; diferenciar pelo teste sorológico; podem-se tratar ambas até que os resultados sejam conhecidos.
- Lúpus eritematoso sistêmico — o título do anticorpo antinuclear, em geral, apresenta-se negativo em caso da febre maculosa das Montanhas Rochosas; o teste sorológico é diagnóstico.
- Brucelose — edema escrotal; o teste sorológico é diagnóstico.

HEMOGRAMA/BIOQUÍMICA/URINÁLISE
Hemograma completo
- Trombocitopenia (~40% dos casos) — parcialmente atribuída ao anticorpo antiplaquetário.
- Megatrombocitose, leve anemia (normocrômica, normocítica), leucopenia branda (no início da infecção), leucocitose (e monocitose) — à medida que a doença se torna mais crônica.

Bioquímica
- Geralmente inespecífica.
- Leves aumentos em ALT, fosfatase alcalina, ureia, creatinina e bilirrubina total (raros).
- Hipercolesterolemia — constantemente encontrada; causa desconhecida.
- Hipoalbuminemia — causada por dano ao endotélio vascular.
- Foram relatadas, sem exceção, alterações como azotemia, hiponatremia, hipocloremia e acidose metabólica.

Urinálise
- Proteinúria — com ou sem azotemia; gerada por lesão glomerular/tubular.
- Hematúria — defeitos da coagulação.

OUTROS TESTES LABORATORIAIS
- Existem diversos testes sorológicos disponíveis, incluindo imunofluorescência microscópica, ELISA e teste de aglutinação em látex. O teste de imunofluorescência microscópica é mais comumente utilizado em laboratórios diagnósticos; mede a IgG; os títulos séricos levam 2 a 3 semanas para subir; podem ser negativos nos casos muito agudos; títulos pareados — fazer com 3 semanas de intervalo; aumento de quatro vezes entre os títulos agudo e convalescente; evitar erros no diagnóstico por conta da considerável reatividade cruzada com outros microrganismos riquetsiais; títulos elevados podem ser detectados até 1 ano após o tratamento.
- ELISA — alta sensibilidade, pois essa técnica é capaz de mensurar tanto a IgG como a IgM; detecta infecção mais cedo do que os testes que só medem a IgG.
- Teste de aglutinação em látex — especificidade mais alta e sensibilidade mais baixa do que o teste de imunofluorescência microscópica (ocorrem resultados falso-negativos); um único título elevado é diagnóstico.
- PCR no sangue total ou em amostras teciduais — técnica mais sensível do que a cultura, embora possa detectar DNA não viável. Também pode detectar o DNA antes da soroconversão em alguns cães. Disponível no estado da Carolina do Norte (EUA).

DIAGNÓSTICO POR IMAGEM
N/D.

MÉTODOS DIAGNÓSTICOS
- Imunofluorescência direta — biopsias de pele obtidas com anestesia local e saca-bocado (também conhecido como *punch*) das áreas acometidas;

FEBRE MACULOSA DAS MONTANHAS ROCHOSAS

detecta os antígenos riquetsiais já com 3-4 dias após a infecção.
• LCS — frequentemente normal; pode revelar aumento no conteúdo de proteínas e células nucleadas.

ACHADOS PATOLÓGICOS
• Petéquias disseminadas, esplenomegalia e linfadenopatia hemorrágica generalizada.
• Vasculite necrosante com infiltração celular (mononuclear e neutrofílica) perivascular.
• Lesões vasculares — mais proeminentes na pele, nos rins, no miocárdio, nas meninges, na retina, no pâncreas, no trato gastrintestinal e na bexiga urinária.
• Necrose hepática e miocárdica focal, gliose nodular no cérebro e pneumonia intersticial são comuns.
• Colorações especiais — para identificar os microrganismos.

TRATAMENTO

CUIDADO(S) DE SAÚDE ADEQUADO(S)
Proceder à internação até a estabilização do paciente e a constatação de resposta ao tratamento.

CUIDADO(S) DE ENFERMAGEM
• Desidratação — solução eletrolítica balanceada; utilizar com cuidado por causa do aumento da permeabilidade vascular e do volume expandido do líquido extracelular (que exacerbam os edemas cerebral e pulmonar).
• Anemia — transfusão sanguínea.
• Hemorragia por trombocitopenia — transfusão de plasma rico em plaquetas ou de sangue total.

ATIVIDADE
Restrita.

DIETA
N/D.

ORIENTAÇÃO AO PROPRIETÁRIO
• Prognóstico — bom nos casos agudos com tratamento apropriado e imediato.
• A resposta ocorre dentro de horas do tratamento.
• Se o tratamento não for instituído até que ocorram os sinais do SNC ou mais tarde no processo mórbido, a mortalidade será elevada; o paciente com sinais do SNC pode morrer dentro de horas.

CONSIDERAÇÕES CIRÚRGICAS
Se houver necessidade de cirurgia por outras razões, poderá ser necessária a realização de transfusão sanguínea para corrigir a anemia e/ou a trombocitopenia.

MEDICAÇÕES

MEDICAMENTO(S) DE ESCOLHA
• Doxiciclina — derivado sintético da tetraciclina, 10 mg/kg VO a cada 12 h durante 10 dias; ou IV por 5 dias se o paciente estiver vomitando.
• Prednisona — utilização concomitante; dose anti-inflamatória ou imunossupressora; se administrada logo no início da doença, não parece ser nociva para a recuperação clínica.

CONTRAINDICAÇÕES
• Tetraciclinas (ou derivados) — não usar nos pacientes com <6 meses de vida por causa do surgimento de manchas amareladas permanentes nos dentes.
• Insuficiência renal — não utilizar a tetraciclina; pode-se usar a doxiciclina (excretada também pelo trato gastrintestinal).
• Enrofloxacino — evitar em cães jovens, pois pode ocorrer lesão da cartilagem articular (precedida por claudicação); desarranjo gastrintestinal (vômito, anorexia).

PRECAUÇÕES
Cloranfenicol
• Evitar se a confirmação sorológica for realizada após o início do tratamento; diminui os títulos em um maior grau em comparação às tetraciclinas.
• Informar o proprietário sobre os riscos à saúde pública; interfere diretamente na síntese da molécula heme e da medula óssea.
• Evitar sua utilização em cães com trombocitopenia, pancitopenia ou anemia.

INTERAÇÕES POSSÍVEIS
Nenhuma.

MEDICAMENTO(S) ALTERNATIVO(S)
• Tetraciclinas, cloranfenicol e enrofloxacino — igualmente eficazes se utilizados no início da doença.
• Oxitetraciclina e tetraciclina — 22 mg/kg VO a cada 8 h por 14 dias; eficazes e menos dispendiosas.
• Cloranfenicol — para filhotes caninos com <6 meses de vida; 20 mg/kg VO a cada 8 h por 14 dias; é recomendado para evitar a coloração amarelada dos dentes em erupção.
• Enrofloxacino — 3 mg/kg VO a cada 12 h por 7 dias.

ACOMPANHAMENTO

MONITORIZAÇÃO DO PACIENTE
Monitorizar a contagem de plaquetas a cada 3 dias até a normalidade.

PREVENÇÃO
• Controlar a infestação por carrapatos nos cães — utilizar banhos de imersão ou *sprays* contendo diclorvós, clorfenvinfós, dioxation, propoxur ou carbaril.
• Coleiras contra pulgas e carrapatos — podem reduzir a reinfestação; não está comprovada a confiabilidade.
• Evitar as áreas infestadas por carrapatos.
• Ambiente — é impossível a erradicação dos carrapatos; o microrganismo é preservado nos roedores e em outros hospedeiros reservatórios.
• Remoção manual dos carrapatos* — usar luvas (ver a seção "Potencial Zoonótico");
ter a certeza de que as peças bucais foram removidas, pois tais estruturas podem gerar reação por corpo estranho se deixadas no local.

COMPLICAÇÕES
N/D.

EVOLUÇÃO ESPERADA E PROGNÓSTICO
• Tratamento precoce com antibiótico — não só diminui a febre e o extravasamento de albumina, mas também melhora a condição do paciente dentro de 24-48 h.

---

* N. T.: Para a remoção manual dos carrapatos, utilize um algodão embebido em álcool.

• Contagens de plaquetas — repetir a cada 3 dias após o início do tratamento até que estejam dentro dos limites de normalidade; devem retornar ao normal dentro de 2-4 dias depois do início do tratamento.
• Títulos sorológicos — mais baixos nos cães tratados do que naqueles não submetidos a tratamento; os títulos permanecem positivos durante o período de convalescença.
• Cães naturalmente infectados parecem nunca sofrerem reinfecção.
• Casos agudos — prognóstico excelente com o tratamento adequado.
• Com doença do SNC — prognóstico pior.

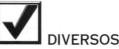

DISTÚRBIOS ASSOCIADOS
Nenhum.

FATORES RELACIONADOS COM A IDADE
Nenhum.

POTENCIAL ZOONÓTICO
• Incidência (em seres humanos) — está declinando nos EUA; da metade de 1992 à metade de 1993: 300 casos; incidência anterior: até 1.000 casos/ano.
• Acomete principalmente os jovens adultos e as crianças.
• Fonte de infecção (seres humanos) — originária dos carrapatos transmitidos a partir dos cães; não diretamente dos cães; quando se removem os carrapatos infectados dos cães.
• Principais sinais clínicos (seres humanos) — mimetizam aqueles nos cães; sobretudo febre e dor de cabeça (cefaleia); os sinais neurológicos ocorrem mais tarde; erupções cutâneas observadas em apenas 50% dos pacientes.
• O tratamento com tetraciclinas resulta na rápida recuperação.

GESTAÇÃO/FERTILIDADE/REPRODUÇÃO
N/D.

ABREVIATURA(S)
• ALT = alanina aminotransferase.
• CID = coagulação intravascular disseminada.
• ELISA = ensaio imunoabsorvente ligado à enzima.
• LCS = líquido cerebrospinal.
• SNC = sistema nervoso central.
• PCR = reação em cadeia da polimerase.

Sugestões de Leitura
Greene CE, Breitschwerdt EB. Rocky Mountain spotted fever, murine tryphuslike disease, rickettsialpox, typhus, and Q fever. In: Greene CE, ed., Infectious Diseases of the Dog and Cat, 3rd ed. St. Louis: Saunders Elsevier, 2006, pp. 232-245.
Kidd L, Maggi R, Diniz PP, et al. Evaluation of conventional and real-time PCR assays for detection and differentiation of spotted fever group rickettsia in dog blood. Vet Microbiology 2008, 129:294-303.
Mikszewski JS, Vite CH. Central nervous system dysfunction associated with Rocky Mountain spotted fever infection in five dogs. JAAHA 2005, 41:259-266.

Autor Stephen C. Barr
Consultor Editorial Stephen C. Barr

Febre Q

CONSIDERAÇÕES GERAIS

REVISÃO
- Causada pela riquétsia zoonótica *Coxiella burnetii*.
- Infecção — mais comumente por inalação ou ingestão de microrganismos enquanto se alimentam nos líquidos corporais infectados (urina, fezes, leite ou corrimentos da parturiente), tecidos (especialmente placenta) ou carcaças de hospedeiros reservatórios animais infectados (bovinos, ovinos, caprinos); pode ocorrer após exposição ao carrapato (há muitas espécies de carrapatos implicadas).
- Pulmões — acredita-se que sejam a principal porta de entrada para a circulação sistêmica.
- O microrganismo se replica no endotélio vascular; provoca vasculite disseminada; a gravidade depende da patogenicidade da cepa do microrganismo; a vasculite resulta em necrose e hemorragia nos pulmões, no fígado e no SNC.
- Existe um extenso período latente após a recuperação até que se desenvolva o fenômeno crônico de formação de imunocomplexos; o microrganismo é reativado do estado latente durante o parto, resultando no ingresso de grande quantidade na placenta, nos líquidos da parturiente, na urina, nas fezes e no leite.
- Mundialmente endêmica. A maioria dos casos nos Estados Unidos ocorre nos estados ocidentais.

IDENTIFICAÇÃO
Cães e gatos de qualquer idade, sexo ou raça.

SINAIS CLÍNICOS
Achados Anamnésicos
- Frequentemente há um histórico de contato com animais de criação ou carrapatos.
- Febre.
- Letargia.
- Depressão.
- Anorexia.
- Abortamento — especialmente gatas.
- Ataxia e crises convulsivas — sobretudo cães.

Achados do Exame Físico
- Geralmente assintomática.
- A esplenomegalia é frequentemente o único achado clínico.
- Sinais neurológicos multifocais — cães.

CAUSAS E FATORES DE RISCO
- *C. burnetii*.
- Exposição a animais infectados (especialmente após o parto) e a carrapatos.

DIAGNÓSTICO

DIAGNÓSTICO DIFERENCIAL
- Gatos — outras causas de abortamento: infecções (rinotraqueíte viral, panleucopenia, FeLV, toxoplasmose, bactérias, incluindo coliformes, *Streptococcus* spp., *Staphylococcus* spp., *Salmonella*); defeitos fetais; problemas maternos (nutrição, anormalidades do trato genital); estresse ambiental; distúrbios endócrinos (hipoluteidismo).
- Cães — outras causas de encefalite.

HEMOGRAMA/BIOQUÍMICA/URINÁLISE
Inespecíficos.

OUTROS TESTES LABORATORIAIS
Sorologia
- Sorologia — existem os métodos de IF e ELISA disponíveis; um aumento de quatro vezes no título de IgG em um período de 4 semanas é diagnóstico; o uso de técnicas sorológicas mais recentes que mensuram a IgM em uma única amostra não foi bem documentado em pequenos animais.
- Coletar 2-3 mL de soro e refrigerar, para identificação do microrganismo.
- Coletar amostra tecidual (p. ex., placenta) e refrigerar, para inoculação em animal.
- PCR — técnica também realizada no laboratório mencionado acima; utilizada para detectar os microrganismos em culturas ou amostras teciduais obtidas do paciente.

DIAGNÓSTICO POR IMAGEM
N/D.

MÉTODOS DIAGNÓSTICOS
N/D.

TRATAMENTO
- Alertar o proprietário quanto ao possível risco zoonótico.
- Internação — evita o risco zoonótico para o proprietário.
- Utilizar luvas e máscaras ao se tratar um animal infectado ou ao atender um caso de abortamento em gata.

MEDICAÇÕES

MEDICAMENTO(S)
- Tetraciclina — 22 mg/kg VO a cada 8 h por 2 semanas.
- Doxiciclina — 20 mg/kg VO a cada 12 h por 1 semana.
- Enrofloxacino — 10 mg/kg VO a cada 12 h por 1 semana; deve ser eficaz, embora não haja relatos clínicos; eficaz *in vitro*.

CONTRAINDICAÇÕES/INTERAÇÕES POSSÍVEIS
- Os medicamentos à base de tetraciclina são associados a amarelamento dos dentes em animais jovens; não utilizar em animais com insuficiência renal.
- A doxiciclina pode causar esofagite e estenose.
- O enrofloxacino pode gerar defeitos nas cartilagens em animais jovens.
- Além disso, o enrofloxacino pode causar degeneração da retina quando utilizado em gatos com doença renal ou hepática concomitante ou sob altas doses.

ACOMPANHAMENTO
- Não é fácil determinar o sucesso do tratamento, porque muitos animais melhoram espontaneamente.
- Até mesmo os casos assintomáticos devem ser submetidos a tratamento rigoroso por causa do potencial zoonótico.
- Não se conhece a utilidade de previsão do sucesso do tratamento com base na melhora sorológica.

DIVERSOS

POTENCIAL ZOONÓTICO
- Potencial zoonótico importante.
- No momento em que o diagnóstico é formulado em gato ou cão, já ocorreram exposição humana e infecção.
- Instruir os proprietários e as pessoas contactantes (ou seja, aquelas que estão em contato com o animal) a procurar atendimento médico imediato.
- Os seres humanos contraem a doença por inalação de aerossóis infectados (p. ex., após o parto); as crianças costumam ser infectadas pela ingestão de leite cru, embora geralmente permaneçam assintomáticas.
- Há relatos de surtos urbanos prévios pela exposição a gatos infectados.
- Período de incubação desde o tempo de contato até os primeiros sinais da doença — 5-32 dias.
- Possível transmissão de pessoa a pessoa.

ABREVIATURA(S)
- ELISA = ensaio imunoabsorvente ligado à enzima.
- FeLV = vírus da leucemia felina.
- IF = imunofluorescência.
- PCR = reação em cadeia da polimerase.
- SNC = sistema nervoso central.

Sugestões de Leitura
Brouqui P, Badiaga S, Raoult D. Q fever outbreak in homeless shelter. Emer Infect Dis 2004, 10:1297-1299.
Greene CE, Breitschwerdt EB. Q-Fever. In: Greene CE, ed., Infectious Diseases of the Dog and Cat, 3rd ed. St. Louis: Saunders Elsevier, 2006, pp. 242-245.
Komiya T, Sadamasu K, Kang MI, et al. Seroprevalence of Coxiella burnetii infections among cats in different living environments. J Vet Med Sci 2003, 65:1047-1048.

Autor Stephen C. Barr
Consultor Editorial Stephen C. Barr

FENÔMENO DE SCHIFF-SHERRINGTON

CONSIDERAÇÕES GERAIS

REVISÃO
• Extensão do membro torácico associada à paralisia ou paresia do membro pélvico depois de lesão da medula espinal aguda e, em geral, grave, caudalmente à intumescência cervical; fenômeno mais bem observado quando o paciente está em decúbito lateral.
• Postura — provocada por dano às células limítrofes ou a seus processos ascendentes, que são interneurônios localizados na medula espinal lombar (sobretudo, L2-4) e normalmente inibem os neurônios motores extensores da intumescência cervical.

IDENTIFICAÇÃO
Qualquer cão que sofra de lesão grave da medula espinal toracolombar.

SINAIS CLÍNICOS
• Membros torácicos — rigidamente estendidos; marcha e reações posturais normais (porque a lesão é caudal à intumescência cervical).
• Membros pélvicos — dependem da gravidade e da localização da lesão; os sinais costumam ser atribuídos ao neurônio motor superior, embora possam ser decorrentes do neurônio motor inferior.
• Em mielopatias toracolombares agudas graves, pode haver choque espinal, além do fenômeno de Schiff-Sherrington: há uma paralisia flácida inicial caudal ao nível da lesão, com perda dos reflexos miotáticos e flexores. Em cães e gatos, o choque espinal é incomum e costuma desaparecer dentro de uma hora, com subsequente desenvolvimento de sinais mais típicos de doença do neurônio motor superior caudal à lesão da medula espinal.

CAUSAS E FATORES DE RISCO
• Traumatismo (especialmente acidentes em vias de trânsito) e discopatia intervertebral — mais comuns.
• Mielopatias vasculares (p. ex., embolia fibrocartilaginosa, coagulopatias, etc.).

DIAGNÓSTICO

DIAGNÓSTICO DIFERENCIAL
• Rigidez descerebrada — observada com doença do tronco cerebral, em que todos os membros estão rígidos e apresentam disfunção do neurônio motor superior; presença de opistótono; o paciente está inconsciente.
• Rigidez descerebelada — observada com doença cerebelar, em que os membros torácicos se encontram rígidos, enquanto os membros pélvicos se apresentam flexionados; a consciência costuma estar alterada.
• Lesão da medula espinal cervical — pode apresentar hipertonia extensora nos membros torácicos; também se observam déficits do neurônio motor superior e de propriocepção de todos os membros.
• O aspecto-chave no diagnóstico diferencial é que, no fenômeno de Schiff-Sherrington, a função e as reações posturais nos membros torácicos permanecem normais apesar da rigidez extensora, embora tais quesitos estejam anormais nos membros pélvicos.

HEMOGRAMA/BIOQUÍMICA/URINÁLISE
N/D.

OUTROS TESTES LABORATORIAIS
N/D.

DIAGNÓSTICO POR IMAGEM
Radiologia (radiografia, mielografia, TC, RM) — demonstram a lesão espinal toracolombar.

MÉTODOS DIAGNÓSTICOS
N/D.

TRATAMENTO

• Direcionado à lesão toracolombar subjacente.
• Não há nenhum tratamento específico disponível.
• O problema desaparecerá se a função adequada da medula espinal for restabelecida.
• O fenômeno de Schiff-Sherrington não é um indicador prognóstico: o prognóstico, então, é determinado pela gravidade dos sinais caudais à lesão da medula espinal.

MEDICAÇÕES

MEDICAMENTO(S)
Conforme indicados pela mielopatia subjacente.

CONTRAINDICAÇÕES/INTERAÇÕES POSSÍVEIS
N/D.

ACOMPANHAMENTO

• A postura pode persistir por dias a semanas; no entanto, isso não é indicação de um prognóstico sem esperanças.
• Com o tratamento rápido e rigoroso, o paciente poderá se recuperar, sobretudo se houver percepção de dor caudal à lesão.

DIVERSOS

ABREVIATURA(S)
• RM = ressonância magnética.
• TC = tomografia computadorizada.

Sugestões de Leitura
Dewey CW. Functional and dysfunctional neuroanatomy: The key to lesion localization. In: Dewey CW, ed., A Practical Guide to Canine and Feline Neurology, 2nd ed. Ames, IA: Wiley-Blackwell, 2008, p. 41.

Autor Mary O. Smith
Consultor Editorial Joane M. Parent

Feocromocitoma

CONSIDERAÇÕES GERAIS

DEFINIÇÃO
APUDomas são tumores das células conhecidas como células de captação e descarboxilação de aminas precursoras (APUD, em inglês). Os APUDomas são células secretoras de peptídeos que sintetizam e metabolizam aminas biogênicas; tais células são encontradas em todo o corpo (tireoide, medula adrenal) e trato gastrintestinal. Os feocromocitomas consistem em células cromafins que se originam de células da crista neural dentro da medula adrenal ou dos gânglios simpáticos (paragangliomas).

FISIOPATOLOGIA
Os sinais clínicos desenvolvem-se como resultado da natureza invasiva do tumor e suas metástases ou da secreção excessiva de catecolaminas (p. ex., hipertensão, taquicardia). Os sinais de hipertensão e taquicardia podem ser constantes ou paroxísticos.

SISTEMA(S) ACOMETIDO(S)
- Cardiovascular.
- Neurológico.
- Renal.
- Respiratório.

INCIDÊNCIA/PREVALÊNCIA
Doença incomum em cães; rara em gatos.

IDENTIFICAÇÃO
Espécies
Cães e, raramente, gatos.

Raça(s) Predominante(s)
Boxer, Poodle miniatura e Pastor alemão.

Idade Média e Faixa Etária
- A idade média em cães é de 11 anos; a faixa etária é de 1-16 anos de idade.
- Gatos mais idosos.

SINAIS CLÍNICOS
Comentários Gerais
- Os sinais predominantes originam-se de vasoconstrição mediada por receptores alfa e efeitos cardíacos mediados por receptores beta que causam hipertensão sistêmica ou taquiarritmias.
- Os sinais de hipertensão podem ser constantes ou paroxísticos. Os sinais podem estar presentes há mais de um ano ou se desenvolver subitamente, culminando no óbito.
- Trinta por cento dos casos permanecem assintomáticos e são identificados apenas à necropsia.

Achados Anamnésicos
- Os sinais clínicos são frequentemente episódicos ou agudos.
- São comuns os achados de fraqueza generalizada e letargia.
- Anorexia.
- Vômito.
- Perda de peso.
- Respiração ofegante, dispneia.
- Diarreia.
- Gemido, andar compassado.
- Ascite, edema.
- Poliúria/polidipsia.
- Tremores/calafrios.
- Epistaxe.
- Adipsia.

Achados do Exame Físico
- Podem permanecer normais.
- Letargia, depressão.
- Taquipneia, dispneia.
- Magro, emaciado.
- Fraqueza.
- Edema periférico.
- Ascite.
- Arritmias cardíacas.
- Sopro sistólico.
- Estertores.
- Mucosas pálidas ou hiperêmicas.
- Massa abdominal.
- Desidratação.
- Cegueira.
- Dor abdominal.

CAUSAS
Os feocromocitomas são tumores das células cromafins.

DIAGNÓSTICO

DIAGNÓSTICO DIFERENCIAL
- Hiperadrenocorticismo.
- Hiperaldosteronismo.
- Hipertensão essencial (gatos).
- Doença renal com hipertensão secundária.

HEMOGRAMA/BIOQUÍMICA/URINÁLISE
- Anemia arregenerativa.
- Hemoconcentração.
- Leucocitose.
- Hiperglicemia leve.
- Uremia branda.
- Aumento das enzimas hepáticas.
- Hipoalbuminemia.
- Hipocalcemia.
- Proteinúria.

OUTROS TESTES LABORATORIAIS
Pressão Arterial
Pressão sistólica >180 ou diastólica >95 mmHg é diagnóstica para hipertensão. Apenas 50% dos animais com feocromocitoma encontram-se hipertensos quando a pressão arterial é mensurada por causa da natureza episódica da secreção de alguns tumores.

Eletrocardiografia
Taquicardia sinusal é a arritmia mais comum; contrações ventriculares prematuras são menos comuns.

DIAGNÓSTICO POR IMAGEM
Radiografia Abdominal
- Massa abdominal (30%).
- Calcificação da massa adrenal (10%).
- Hepatomegalia.
- Deslocamento renal.
- Contorno renal anormal.
- Ascite.
- Aumento de volume da veia cava caudal.

Radiografia Torácica
- Cardiomegalia generalizada.
- Congestão ou edema pulmonar.

Ultrassonografia Abdominal
- Massa adrenal unilateral.
- Invasão da veia cava caudal e de outras estruturas adjacentes pelo tumor.
- Metástase intra-abdominal e hepática.

OUTRAS MODALIDADES DE IMAGEM
- TC e RM.
- Cintilografia com o uso de iodo 123 — varredura com metaiodobenzilguanidina.

MÉTODOS DIAGNÓSTICOS
- Catecolaminas plasmáticas:
  - >2.000 pg/mL apoia o diagnóstico de feocromocitoma.
- Catecolaminas e metabólitos de catecolaminas urinários:
  - É necessária a excreção total durante o período de 24 h.
  - Sem ingestão de baunilha, medicamentos ou agentes de contraste radiográfico antes de obter a amostra urinária.
  - 10-15% de falso-positivos.
  - A urina deve ser acidificada (pH <3).
  - Baixa sensibilidade (0,42) em comparação com as catecolaminas plasmáticas (0,97).
  - Ácido vanilmandélico — normal <7,0 µg/dia.
  - Metanefrina/normetanefrina — normais <1,3 µg/dia.
  - Catecolaminas urinárias totais — normais <250 µg/dia.
- Teste da fentolamina:
  - Usada em pacientes hipertensos para avaliar a dependência de catecolaminas na manutenção da hipertensão.
  - Após a obtenção de uma pressão arterial estável, administra-se um bólus IV de fentolamina (0,5-1,5 mg).
  - A pressão arterial é registrada a cada 30 segundos nos primeiros 3 minutos e depois a cada minuto por mais 7 minutos.
  - O teste será positivo se a queda na pressão arterial for superior a 35 mmHg (sistólica) ou 25 mmHg (diastólica) e o declínio durar no mínimo 5 minutos.
  - Alta incidência de falso-positivos e hipotensão.
  - Testes provocativos:
  - Histamina, tiramina, glucagon podem causar crise hipertensiva.

ACHADOS PATOLÓGICOS
A coloração imuno-histoquímica dos tecidos tumorais com cromogranina A ou sinaptofisina permite a diferenciação de feocromocitomas de outros tipos tumorais.

TRATAMENTO

CUIDADO(S) DE SAÚDE ADEQUADO(S)
- A remoção cirúrgica do tumor constitui o tratamento de escolha.
- A terapia clínica é mais comumente utilizada para estabilizar os pacientes antes da cirurgia.

ORIENTAÇÃO AO PROPRIETÁRIO
Os tempos de sobrevida podem ser de até 3 anos após a ressecção cirúrgica bem-sucedida do tumor. Em gatos, a remoção do tumor é frequentemente curativa; tais tumores são muitas vezes benignos, exatamente o oposto dos tumores malignos observados em cães.

CONSIDERAÇÕES CIRÚRGICAS
Cuidado Pré-operatório
- Fenoxibenzamina (0,2-1,5 mg/kg VO a cada 12 h) 1-2 semanas antes da cirurgia.
- Atenolol, um antagonista β-1 seletivo (0,2-1 mg/kg VO a cada 12-24 h), pode ser utilizado para

FEOCROMOCITOMA

controlar taquicardia supraventricular clinicamente significativa.

Complicações e Monitorização do Paciente
• Complicações comuns — hipertensão, taquicardia grave, outras arritmias cardíacas e hipovolemia/hipotensão.

Anestesia
• Induzir à anestesia com algum agente narcótico ou propofol.
• Manter a anestesia com isoflurano.

Cirurgia
Adrenalectomia unilateral e frequentemente trombectomia. A manipulação do tumor pode causar hipertensão grave se o paciente não for pré-medicado de forma adequada.

MEDICAÇÕES

MEDICAMENTO(S) DE ESCOLHA
• A hipertensão pré-operatória e intraoperatória pode ser tratada com fentolamina (0,02-0,1 mg/kg IV até fazer efeito).
• Arritmias cardíacas e taquicardia grave — problemas comuns; geralmente respondem aos agentes β-bloqueadores como o esmolol (0,5 mg/kg em bólus IV lento, seguido por 0,05-0,2 mg/kg/min em infusão IV).

CONTRAINDICAÇÕES
• Agentes anestésicos — morfina, meperidina, xilazina e cetamina.

• Poderá ocorrer o desenvolvimento de hipertensão grave se um β-bloqueador não seletivo (p. ex., propranolol) for utilizado sem bloqueio alfa-adrenérgico prévio (p. ex., fentolamina, fenoxibenzamina).

PRECAUÇÕES
O beta-bloqueio não seletivo pode levar à hipertensão fatal.

MEDICAMENTO(S) ALTERNATIVO(S)
N/D.

ACOMPANHAMENTO

MONITORIZAÇÃO DO PACIENTE
Pressão arterial, pressão venosa central e ECG são rigorosamente monitorizados no período pós-operatório imediato (24-72 h).

COMPLICAÇÕES POSSÍVEIS
Pós-operatórias — hemorragia intra-abdominal, hemorragia, hipotensão, peritonite, sepse.

EVOLUÇÃO ESPERADA E PROGNÓSTICO
O prognóstico é reservado a razoável.

DIVERSOS

DISTÚRBIOS ASSOCIADOS
Neoplasias endócrinas múltiplas tipos II e III.

FATORES RELACIONADOS COM A IDADE
Nenhum.

POTENCIAL ZOONÓTICO
Nenhum.

GESTAÇÃO/FERTILIDADE/REPRODUÇÃO
N/D.

VER TAMBÉM
Hipertensão Sistêmica.

ABREVIATURA(S)
• ECG = eletrocardiograma.
• RM = ressonância magnética.
• TC = tomografia computadorizada.

Sugestões de Leitura
Greco DS. APUDomas and other emerging feline endocrinopathies. In: August JR, ed., Consultations in Feline Internal Medicine IV. Philadelphia: Saunders, 2001, pp. 181-185.
Kyles AE, Feldman EC, De Cock HEV, et al. Surgical management of adrenal gland tumors with and without associated tumor thrombi in dogs: 40 cases (1994-2001). JAVMA 2003, 223:654-662.

Autor Deborah S. Greco
Consultor Editorial Deborah S. Greco

Fibrilação e Flutter Atriais

CONSIDERAÇÕES GERAIS

DEFINIÇÃO
- Fibrilação atrial — ritmo supraventricular rápido e variavelmente irregular. Há duas formas identificadas: primária (uma doença rara que ocorre principalmente em cães de grande porte com ou sem uma leve cardiopatia subjacente) e secundária (que ocorre em cães e gatos, secundariamente a uma cardiopatia subjacente).
- O flutter atrial é similar à fibrilação atrial; no flutter, entretanto, a frequência atrial apresenta-se de modo geral mais lenta e caracteriza-se por ondas serrilhadas na linha basal do ECG. Via de regra, a resposta ventricular é rápida, mas pode ser regular ou irregular.

CARACTERÍSTICAS DO ECG
Flutter Atrial
- O ritmo atrial costuma ser regular; a frequência é de aproximadamente 300-400 bpm.
- Em geral, as ondas P distinguem-se como ondas P discretas ou como linhas basais "serrilhadas".
- O ritmo e a frequência ventriculares dependem geralmente da frequência atrial e da condução nodal AV, mas costumam ser regulares ou variavelmente irregulares e rápidos.
- O padrão de condução rumo aos ventrículos é variável — em alguns casos, despolarizações atriais alternadas produzem uma despolarização ventricular (proporção de condução de 2:1), conferindo um ritmo ventricular regular; outras vezes, o padrão de condução parece aleatório, estabelecendo um ritmo ventricular irregular capaz de mimetizar a fibrilação atrial.

Fibrilação Atrial Secundária
- Ausência de ondas P — a linha basal pode ficar achatada ou exibir pequenas ondulações irregulares (ondas "f"); algumas ondulações podem se assemelhar às ondas P.
- Frequência ventricular elevada — geralmente 180-240 bpm em cães e >220 bpm em gatos.
- O intervalo entre os complexos QRS é variavelmente irregular; em geral, esses complexos parecem normais.

Fibrilação Atrial Primária
Similar à fibrilação atrial secundária, exceto por apresentar uma frequência ventricular dentro dos limites de normalidade.

FISIOPATOLOGIA
- Fibrilação atrial — causada por inúmeras e pequenas vias de reentrada, que geram um padrão de despolarização rápido (>500 despolarizações/minuto) e desorganizado nos átrios, resultando na interrupção da contração atrial. As despolarizações bombardeiam continuamente o tecido nodal AV, que atua como um filtro e não permite a condução de todas as despolarizações até os ventrículos. Muitas despolarizações atriais ativam apenas uma parte dos átrios, pois a frequência cardíaca elevada torna porções dos átrios refratárias; dessa forma, tais despolarizações não conseguem chegar à junção AV. Outros impulsos atriais penetram no tecido juncional AV, mas não são intensos o suficiente a ponto de penetrar em toda a sua extensão. Os impulsos bloqueados comprometem as propriedades de condução do tecido juncional AV e alteram a condução dos impulsos elétricos subsequentes; os impulsos elétricos são conduzidos irregularmente por meio da junção AV, produzindo um ritmo ventricular irregular.
- Flutter atrial — provavelmente se origina de um único local de reentrada que se desloca de forma contínua por todo o miocárdio atrial e estimula o nodo AV de modo frequente e regular. Quando a frequência atrial se torna suficientemente rápida, o período refratário do nodo AV excede a duração do ciclo (intervalo entre as ondas P) da taquicardia supraventricular e algumas despolarizações atriais são impedidas de atravessar o nodo AV (bloqueio AV de segundo grau funcional).

SISTEMA(S) ACOMETIDO(S)
Cardiovascular
A perda da contração atrial pode resultar na redução do volume sistólico e do débito cardíaco, dependendo da frequência cardíaca; uma frequência cardíaca elevada pode culminar na deterioração da função do miocárdio (insuficiência miocárdica induzida por taquicardia).

GENÉTICA
Não há estudos reprodutivos disponíveis.

INCIDÊNCIA E PREVALÊNCIA
N/D.

DISTRIBUIÇÃO GEOGRÁFICA
N/D.

IDENTIFICAÇÃO
Espécies
Cães e gatos.
Raça(s) Predominante(s)
Os cães de raças grandes e gigantes são mais propensos à fibrilação atrial primária.
Idade Média e Faixa Etária
N/D.
Sexo(s) Predominante(s)
N/D.

SINAIS CLÍNICOS
Comentários Gerais
- Em geral, relacionam-se mais com o processo patológico subjacente e/ou a ICC do que com a arritmia propriamente dita; no entanto, os animais previamente estáveis podem sofrer descompensação.
- Os pacientes com fibrilação atrial primária costumam permanecer assintomáticos, mas podem exibir uma leve intolerância ao exercício.

Achados Anamnésicos
- Tosse/dispneia/taquipneia.
- Intolerância ao exercício.
- Raramente, ocorre síncope.
- Tipicamente, os cães com fibrilação atrial primária apresentam-se assintomáticos.

Achados do Exame Físico
- À auscultação, os pacientes com fibrilação atrial exibem um ritmo cardíaco errático que se assemelha a um "par de tênis em uma secadora".
- Na fibrilação atrial, a intensidade da primeira bulha cardíaca é variável; a segunda bulha cardíaca, por sua vez, é auscultada apenas nos batimentos com ejeção efetiva, não em todos os batimentos.
- A terceira bulha cardíaca (som de galope) pode estar presente.
- Os pacientes com fibrilação atrial apresentam déficits de pulso e uma qualidade variável do pulso.
- Com frequência, constatam-se sinais de ICC (p. ex., tosse, dispneia e cianose).

CAUSAS
- Valvulopatia crônica.
- Miocardiopatia.
- Cardiopatia congênita.
- Toxicidade da digoxina.
- Idiopáticas.
- Pré-excitação ventricular (flutter atrial).

DIAGNÓSTICO

DIAGNÓSTICO DIFERENCIAL
- Despolarizações atriais (supraventriculares) prematuras frequentes.
- Taquicardia supraventricular com bloqueio AV.

HEMOGRAMA/BIOQUÍMICA/URINÁLISE
N/D.

OUTROS TESTES LABORATORIAIS
N/D.

DIAGNÓSTICO POR IMAGEM
- A ecocardiografia e a radiografia podem caracterizar o tipo e a gravidade da cardiopatia subjacente; é comum um aumento de volume (moderado a grave) do átrio esquerdo.
- O diagnóstico por imagem é tipicamente normal em pacientes com fibrilação atrial primária, embora um aumento de volume (leve) do átrio esquerdo possa acompanhar as alterações hemodinâmicas impostas pela arritmia.

MÉTODOS DIAGNÓSTICOS
N/D.

ACHADOS PATOLÓGICOS
N/D.

TRATAMENTO

CUIDADO(S) DE SAÚDE ADEQUADO(S)
- Os pacientes com fibrilação atrial (secundária) rápida são submetidos à terapia clínica para retardar a frequência ventricular. A conversão da fibrilação atrial em ritmo sinusal seria ideal, mas tais tentativas em pacientes com cardiopatia subjacente ou aumento de volume graves do átrio esquerdo são fúteis, em virtude do baixo índice de sucesso e da alta taxa de recidiva. Em cães com fibrilação atrial primária, considerar o emprego da quinidina ou da cardioversão elétrica ao ritmo sinusal.
- Os pacientes com fibrilação atrial primária podem ser convertidos de volta ao ritmo sinusal (fisiológico). A taxa de sucesso depende da cronicidade do quadro. Em geral, os pacientes que se encontram em fibrilação atrial por >4 meses apresentam uma taxa de sucesso mais baixa e uma frequência de recidiva mais alta. Nesses pacientes, o controle da frequência, se necessário, é o tratamento recomendado.
- Cardioversão elétrica com corrente direta — consiste na aplicação de choque elétrico transtorácico em um momento específico do ciclo cardíaco; necessita de equipamentos especiais, pessoal treinado e anestesia geral. Um pequeno choque elétrico (10 joules) pode ser suficiente, porém a maioria dos casos exige uma potência mais alta (50-150 joules). A cardioversão bifásica com corrente direta consistentemente promove a

Fibrilação e Flutter Atriais

conversão do ritmo cardíaco, utilizando uma potência mais baixa (<50 joules).

CUIDADO(S) DE ENFERMAGEM
Conforme indicado para ICC.

ATIVIDADE
Restringir a atividade física até que se controle a taquicardia.

DIETA
Em casos de ICC, restrição de sódio leve a moderada.

ORIENTAÇÃO AO PROPRIETÁRIO
• A fibrilação atrial secundária costuma estar associada a uma grave cardiopatia subjacente; o objetivo terapêutico consiste na redução da frequência cardíaca e no controle dos sinais clínicos.
• Em casos de fibrilação atrial secundária, é improvável uma cardioversão contínua ao ritmo sinusal.

CONSIDERAÇÕES CIRÚRGICAS
N/D.

MEDICAÇÕES

MEDICAMENTO(S) DE ESCOLHA
Para retardar a condução por meio do nodo AV, frequentemente se empregam a digoxina, os bloqueadores β-adrenérgicos, o esmolol e os bloqueadores dos canais de cálcio (diltiazem); a definição de uma resposta adequada da frequência cardíaca varia entre os clínicos, mas em geral é de 140-160 bpm nos cães.

Cães
• Digoxina — a dose oral de manutenção é de 0,005-0,01 mg/kg VO a cada 12 h; para atingir uma concentração sérica terapêutica com maior rapidez, pode-se duplicar a dose de manutenção no primeiro dia. Se a digoxina for administrada isoladamente e a frequência cardíaca permanecer elevada, avaliar o nível desse antiarrítmico e ajustar a dose para nivelá-la ao limite terapêutico. Caso a frequência cardíaca permaneça alta, considerar a adição de um bloqueador dos canais de cálcio ou um bloqueador β-adrenérgico.
• Diltiazem — administrado inicialmente a uma dose de 0,5 mg/kg VO a cada 8 h, com subsequente titulação até a dose máxima de 1,5 mg/kg VO a cada 8 h ou até que se alcance uma resposta conveniente.
• Para converter a fibrilação atrial primária em ritmo sinusal, pode-se utilizar a quinidina oral em altas doses ou a cardioversão elétrica. A quinidina pode ser usada com segurança em doses de até 20 mg/kg VO a cada 2 h se rigorosamente monitorizada; doses abaixo de 12,5 mg/kg a cada 6 h não costumam ser eficazes.
• A terapia para fibrilação atrial visa suprimir o circuito de reentrada atrial com o uso de sotalol, amiodarona ou procainamida. A conversão ao ritmo sinusal não costuma ser bem-sucedida.

Gatos
• Na maioria dos gatos, o diltiazem (1-2,5 mg/kg VO a cada 8 h) ou o atenolol (6,25-12,5 mg/gato VO a cada 12-24 h) constituem os medicamentos de escolha.
• Se a frequência cardíaca não for suficientemente reduzida com o uso desses medicamentos ou se insuficiência do miocárdio estiver presente, será possível a adição da digoxina (0,005 mg/kg VO a cada 24-48 h).

CONTRAINDICAÇÕES
• Em pacientes com bloqueio AV preexistente, não se recomenda o uso da digoxina, do diltiazem, do propranolol e do atenolol.
• Pela possibilidade do desenvolvimento de bradiarritmias e/ou bloqueio AV significativos do ponto de vista clínico, deve-se evitar a combinação de bloqueadores dos canais de cálcio e β-bloqueadores.

PRECAUÇÕES
• Em animais com insuficiência do miocárdio, é preciso ter cautela ao utilizar os bloqueadores dos canais de cálcio e os β-bloqueadores, pois ambos são inotrópicos negativos.
• O emprego da quinidina oral em altas doses para a conversão ao ritmo sinusal implica o risco de intoxicação por esse medicamento (p. ex., hipotensão, fraqueza, ataxia e crises convulsivas) — a administração de diazepam por via intravenosa controla as crises; os outros sinais diminuem dentro de algumas horas da interrupção da quinidina.

INTERAÇÕES POSSÍVEIS
A quinidina eleva o nível da digoxina, o que geralmente exige uma redução na dose desse último antiarrítmico.

MEDICAMENTO(S) ALTERNATIVO(S)
Propranolol — administrado inicialmente a uma dose de 0,1-0,2 mg/kg VO a cada 8 h e, depois, titulada para cima até que se obtenha uma resposta adequada. Não ultrapassamos a dose de 0,5 mg/kg VO a cada 8 h. Além de ser pouco tolerado quando utilizado de forma crônica, o propranolol também afeta os receptores-β2; por essa razão, raramente se emprega esse medicamento.

ACOMPANHAMENTO

MONITORIZAÇÃO DO PACIENTE
• Monitorizar rigorosamente a frequência cardíaca e o ECG.
• Como as frequências cardíacas obtidas no hospital e aquelas mensuradas em ECGs de superfície podem não ser exatas (em virtude da ansiedade do paciente e de outros fatores ambientais), a monitorização com o Holter representa um meio mais preciso de avaliar a necessidade de controle da frequência cardíaca e/ou a eficácia da terapia clínica.

COMPLICAÇÕES POSSÍVEIS
Agravamento da função cardíaca com início de arritmia.

EVOLUÇÃO ESPERADA E PROGNÓSTICO
• Fibrilação atrial secundária — associada à cardiopatia grave; portanto, tem um prognóstico reservado a mau.
• Fibrilação atrial primária com achados ultrassonográficos normais — em geral, apresenta um prognóstico bom.

DIVERSOS

FATORES RELACIONADOS COM A IDADE
N/D.

GESTAÇÃO/FERTILIDADE/REPRODUÇÃO
N/D.

ABREVIATURA(S)
• AV = atrioventricular.
• bpm= batimentos por minuto.
• ECG = eletrocardiografia.
• ICC = insuficiência cardíaca congestiva.

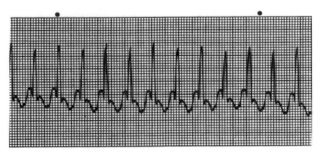

Figura 1. Flutter atrial com condução AV 2:1 a uma frequência ventricular de 330 bpm em cão com defeito do septo atrial. Essa taquicardia supraventricular foi associada a um padrão de Wolff-Parkinson-White. (De: Tilley LP. *Essentials of canine and feline electrocardiography*, 3.ed. Baltimore: Williams & Wilkins, 1992, com permissão.)

Fibrilação e Flutter Atriais

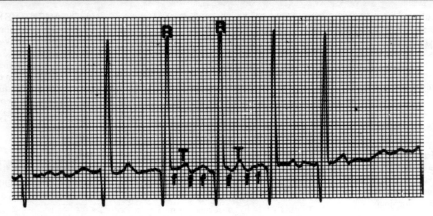

Figura 2. Fibrilação atrial "grosseira" em cão com persistência do ducto arterioso. As ondas f apresentam-se proeminentes. (De: Tilley LP. *Essentials of canine and feline electrocardiography*, 3.ed. Baltimore: Williams & Wilkins, 1992, com permissão.)

Sugestões de Leitura

Kittleson MD. Electrocardiography. In: Kittleson MD, Kienle RD, eds., Small Animal Cardiovascular Medicine. St Louis: Mosby, 1998, pp. 72-94.

Kraus MS, Gelzer ARM, Moise S. Treatment of cardiac arrhythmias and conduction disturbances. In: Tilley LP, Smith FWK, Oyama MA, Sleeper MM, eds., Manual of Canine and Feline Cardiology, 4th ed. St. Louis: Saunders Elsevier, 2008, pp. 315-332.

Tilley LP, Smith FWK Jr. Electrocardiography. In: Tilley LP, Smith FWK, Oyama MA, Sleeper MM, eds., Manual of Canine and Feline Cardiology, 4th ed. St. Louis: Saunders Elsevier, 2008, pp. 49-77.

Autor Richard D. Kienle
Consultores Editoriais Larry P. Tilley e Francis W.K. Smith, Jr.

Fibrilação Ventricular

CONSIDERAÇÕES GERAIS

DEFINIÇÃO
Ritmo ventricular associado à perda de atividade ventricular organizada, resultando em fibrilação do músculo cardíaco.

Características do ECG
- Ritmo rápido, caótico e irregular, com ondas bizarras ou oscilações. As oscilações podem ser amplas (fibrilação grosseira) ou pequenas (fibrilação fina).
- Sem ondas P.
- Sem complexos QRS.

FISIOPATOLOGIA
A perda da atividade ventricular organizada resulta em declínio agudo e intenso no débito cardíaco, usualmente seguido por óbito.

SISTEMA(S) ACOMETIDO(S)
- Cardiovascular.
- Todos os sistemas orgânicos são acometidos pela perda da perfusão.

GENÉTICA
N/D.

INCIDÊNCIA/PREVALÊNCIA
Desconhecidas.

DISTRIBUIÇÃO GEOGRÁFICA
Nenhuma.

IDENTIFICAÇÃO

Espécies
Cães e gatos.

Raça(s) Predominante(s)
Nenhuma.

Idade Média e Faixa Etária
Desconhecidas, mas provavelmente é mais comum em animais idosos.

SINAIS CLÍNICOS

Achados Anamnésicos
- Em muitos pacientes, há doença sistêmica ou cardíaca graves.
- Em alguns pacientes, há arritmias cardíacas prévias.

Achados do Exame Físico
- Parada cardíaca.
- Colapso.
- Óbito.

CAUSAS
- Anoxia.
- Estenose aórtica.
- Desequilíbrios autônomos, especialmente aumento do tônus simpático ou administração de catecolaminas.
- Cirurgia cardíaca.
- Reações medicamentosas — por exemplo, agentes anestésicos, particularmente halotano e barbitúricos de ação ultracurta, digoxina.
- Choque elétrico.
- Desequilíbrios eletrolíticos e acidobásicos.
- Hipotermia.
- Lesão do miocárdio.
- Miocardite.
- Choque.

FATORES DE RISCO
Qualquer doença sistêmica ou cardiopatia graves.

DIAGNÓSTICO

DIAGNÓSTICO DIFERENCIAL
Descartar os artefatos eletrocardiográficos. Reaplicar os eletrodos do ECG, assegurando o contato satisfatório com a pele e a aplicação de quantidade adequada de álcool sobre eles. Verificar o pulso.

HEMOGRAMA/BIOQUÍMICA/URINÁLISE
Em geral, as anormalidades relacionam-se com o problema metabólico subjacente, indutor da fibrilação ventricular.

OUTROS TESTES LABORATORIAIS
N/D.

DIAGNÓSTICO POR IMAGEM
N/D.

MÉTODOS DIAGNÓSTICOS
N/D.

ACHADOS PATOLÓGICOS
N/D.

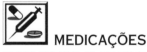

TRATAMENTO

CUIDADO(S) DE SAÚDE ADEQUADO(S)
- Ritmo rapidamente fatal, que requer tratamento imediato e rigoroso.
- O paciente provavelmente virá a óbito, sem a realização de cardioversão elétrica.

Desfibrilação com Corrente Direta
- Contrachoque externo — 50-100 watts/s (pacientes de pequeno porte); 100-360 watts/s (pacientes de grande porte).
- Contrachoque interno —10-25 watts/s (pacientes de pequeno porte); 25-100 watts/s (pacientes de grande porte).
- Se a primeira tentativa falhar, deve-se repeti-la duas vezes.
- Iniciar com a potência mais baixa, aumentando-a a cada choque.
- Caso não se tenha acesso ao desfibrilador elétrico, administrar um golpe pré-cordial. Aplicar um golpe pronunciado, com o pulso aberto na parede torácica sobre o coração. Esse procedimento raramente é bem-sucedido, mas não há nada a perder.

CUIDADO(S) DE ENFERMAGEM
Tratar o surgimento de quaisquer problemas, como hipotermia, hipercalemia e distúrbios acidobásicos.

ATIVIDADE
N/D.

DIETA
N/D.

ORIENTAÇÃO AO PROPRIETÁRIO
Se o paciente for convertido de volta ao ritmo sinusal, avisar o proprietário sobre o alto risco de recidiva da arritmia no período imediatamente após a reanimação.

CONSIDERAÇÕES CIRÚRGICAS
N/D.

MEDICAÇÕES

MEDICAMENTO(S) DE ESCOLHA
- Instituir a RCPC.
- Adrenalina (0,2 mg/kg IV, intratraqueal, intralingual; dobrar a dose e diluir com volume equivalente de soro fisiológico para administração intratraqueal) — pode converter a fibrilação fina em fibrilação grosseira e aumentar as possibilidades de cardioversão elétrica.
- Assim que o animal for submetido a uma cardioversão bem-sucedida, deve-se administrar

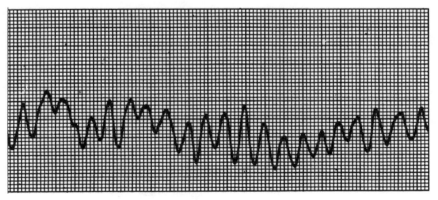

Figura 1 Fibrilação ventricular grosseira. (De: Tilley LP: *Essentials of canine and feline electrocardiography*. 3. ed., Baltimore: Williams & Wilkins, 1992, com permissão.)

FIBRILAÇÃO VENTRICULAR

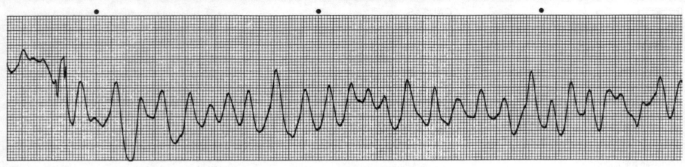

Figura 2 Flutter-fibrilação ventricular em gato com danos miocárdicos graves decorrentes de uma queda do 11° andar. Os complexos apresentam-se bastante largos, bizarros, altos e rápidos. (De: Tilley LP: *Essentials of canine and feline electrocardiography*. 3. ed., Baltimore: Williams & Wilkins, 1992, com permissão.)

lidocaína ou amiodarona intravenosa para diminuir o risco de nova fibrilação ou do desenvolvimento de taquicardia ventricular.

CONTRAINDICAÇÕES
Nenhuma.

PRECAUÇÕES
A lidocaína aumenta o limiar de fibrilação, mas dificulta ainda mais a desfibrilação.

INTERAÇÕES POSSÍVEIS
Em seres humanos, emprega-se o bretílio para tratar a fibrilação ventricular recorrente; em cães e gatos, no entanto, esse medicamento pode precipitar arritmias ventriculares, incluindo a fibrilação ventricular.

MEDICAMENTO(S) ALTERNATIVO(S)
Se não houver acesso ao desfibrilador elétrico, pode-se tentar a cardioversão química. Administrar 1,0 mEq de potássio/kg e 6,0 mg de acetilcolina/kg por via intracardíaca; entretanto, raramente se tem sucesso com tal conduta.

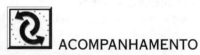
ACOMPANHAMENTO

MONITORIZAÇÃO DO PACIENTE
• Hemograma completo, urinálise, perfil bioquímico, gasometria arterial e estado acidobásico.

• Na suspeita de cardiopatia primária — efetuar ecocardiograma e obter radiografias torácicas.
• Monitorizar o ECG de perto e com frequência.

PREVENÇÃO
Monitorização cuidadosa de pacientes criticamente enfermos para evitar e corrigir desequilíbrios acidobásicos, hipotensão e hipoxemia.

COMPLICAÇÕES POSSÍVEIS
• Óbito.
• CID e falência múltipla de órgãos.

EVOLUÇÃO ESPERADA E PROGNÓSTICO
A maioria dos pacientes vem a óbito, em função da arritmia ou da doença subjacente.

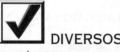
DIVERSOS

DISTÚRBIOS ASSOCIADOS
Nenhum.

FATORES RELACIONADOS COM A IDADE
Nenhum.

POTENCIAL ZOONÓTICO
Nenhum.

GESTAÇÃO/FERTILIDADE/REPRODUÇÃO
N/D.

VER TAMBÉM
Parada Cardiopulmonar.

ABREVIATURA(S)
• CID = coagulação intravascular disseminada.
• ECG = eletrocardiograma.
• RCPC = ressuscitação cardiopulmonar e cerebral.

Sugestões de Leitura

Crowe DT, Fox PR, Devey JJ, Spreng D. Cardiopulmonary and cerebral resuscitation. In: Fox PR, Sisson D, Moise NS, eds., Textbook of Canine and Feline Cardiology, 2nd ed. Philadelphia: Saunders, 1999, pp. 427-454.

Kraus MS, Gelzer ARM, Moise S. Treatment of cardiac arrhythmias and conduction disturbances. In: Tilley LP, Smith FWK, Oyama MA, Sleeper MM, eds., Manual of Canine and Feline Cardiology, 4th Ed. St. Louis: Saunders Elsevier, 2008, pp. 315-332.

Tilley LP, Smith FWK, Jr. Electrocardiography. In: Tilley LP, Smith FWK, Oyama MA, Sleeper MM, eds., Manual of Canine and Feline Cardiology, 4th Ed. St. Louis: Saunders Elsevier, 2008, pp. 49-77.

Autor Francis W.K. Smith, Jr.
Consultores Editoriais Larry P. Tilley e Francis W.K. Smith, Jr.

FIBROSSARCOMA DA GENGIVA

CONSIDERAÇÕES GERAIS

REVISÃO
• O fibrossarcoma é um tumor mesenquimal caracterizado por células fusiformes malignas que produzem quantidades variadas de colágeno. • O fibrossarcoma bucal origina-se mais comumente na gengiva. O palato pode ser afetado, mas geralmente isso se deve à extensão de algum tumor gengival maxilar. Ocasionalmente, o fibrossarcoma surge dos lábios ou da bochecha, mas raras vezes da língua. • Em cães, o fibrossarcoma constitui a terceira malignidade bucal mais comum (20% de todos os tumores bucais). • Em gatos, o fibrossarcoma representa a segunda malignidade bucal mais comum (5-15% de todos os tumores bucais).

IDENTIFICAÇÃO
• Cães e gatos. • Em geral, raças caninas de grande porte são predispostas. Os cães da raça Golden retriever são super-representados, sobretudo para a variante de fibrossarcoma de baixo e alto grau em termos histológico e biológico, respectivamente (ver a seção de "Achados Patológicos"). Não há relatos de predileção racial em gatos. • Uma leve predisposição dos machos foi inconsistentemente relatada em cães. • A idade média é de 7 anos (faixa, 1-16 anos) em cães e 10 anos (faixa, 1-21 anos) em gatos.

SINAIS CLÍNICOS
Achados Anamnésicos
• Massa visível. • Halitose. • Hipersalivação. • Secreção bucal sanguinolenta. • Disfagia. • Dor bucal — comportamento avesso a toques ou afagos e/ou consumo alimentar reduzido apesar de demonstrar interesse pela comida. • Perda de peso.

Achados do Exame Físico
• A realização de exame oral sob sedação ou anestesia é frequentemente útil. • É muito comum a constatação de massa firme e lisa. • A mucosa sobrejacente costuma permanecer intacta, embora o traumatismo e a ulceração ocasionados pela oclusão dos dentes sejam comuns em casos de tumores volumosos. • Halitose, hipersalivação e/ou sangramento bucal. • Dentes frouxos ou ausentes. • Dificuldade ou dor à abertura da boca (especialmente em tumores caudais). • Deformidade facial. • Linfadenomegalia mandibular ipsolateral (hiperplasia reativa ou metástase). • Secreção nasal, epistaxe ou fluxo de ar diminuído por meio das narinas (tumores maxilares).

CAUSAS E FATORES DE RISCO
Nenhum identificado.

DIAGNÓSTICO

DIAGNÓSTICO DIFERENCIAL
• Melanoma amelanótico.
• Carcinoma de células escamosas.
• Ameloblastoma (epúlide acantomatoso).
• Periodontoma fibromatoso ou ossificante (epúlide).
• Osteossarcoma.
• Abscesso da raiz dentária.
• Osteomielite.
• Cisto dentígero.
• Osteopatia craniomandibular (cães, especialmente das raças West Highland White terrier, Cairn terrier e Scottish terrier).

HEMOGRAMA/BIOQUÍMICA/URINÁLISE
Geralmente normais.

DIAGNÓSTICO POR IMAGEM
• Radiografias do crânio ou dos dentes são recomendadas para avaliar o envolvimento ósseo (presente em 60-70% dos casos).
• A imagem obtida por TC pode permitir o estadiamento mais preciso da doença, além de ser útil para o planejamento da cirurgia e/ou radioterapia. É particularmente útil para tumores maxilares e tumores mandibulares volumosos ou caudais.
• É recomendável a obtenção de radiografias torácicas para fazer a triagem quanto à presença de metástase.
• Se o paciente for submetido à TC, será aconselhável a obtenção de imagem concomitante do tórax como um meio mais sensível de pesquisar metástase pulmonar.

MÉTODOS DIAGNÓSTICOS
• A histopatologia é necessária para obtenção do diagnóstico definitivo. Todo tecido removido deve ser enviado ao patologista. Isso possibilita a formulação de um diagnóstico mais preciso e permite a avaliação das margens para estimar a eficácia da excisão.
• Os exames de citologia ou histopatologia do linfonodo mandibular ipsolateral são recomendados para fazer a triagem de metástase.

ACHADOS PATOLÓGICOS
Foram descritos tumores de baixo grau ao exame histológico, mas de alto grau em termos biológicos, particularmente em Golden retriever e outras raças caninas de grande porte. Em princípio, esses tumores foram classificados como lesões benignas (fascíite nodular, nódulos inflamatórios crônicos, tecido de granulação) ou fibrossarcoma de baixo grau ao exame histopatológico. Contudo, um comportamento biológico agressivo, incluindo destruição do tecido ósseo (75%), metástase para linfonodos (20%) e metástase pulmonar (12%), está presente nos cães acometidos.

TRATAMENTO

• Excisão cirúrgica — recomenda-se a remoção da massa e do osso adjacente (maxilectomia ou mandibulectomia) com margem de segurança de, no mínimo, 2-3 cm, sempre que possível.
• Se a excisão for incompleta, será aconselhável a aplicação de radioterapia adjuvante para melhorar o controle local.
• A radioterapia pode ser considerada como uma modalidade terapêutica local isolada quando a cirurgia não for possível ou em caso de desistência por parte do proprietário.
• A quimioterapia adjuvante é razoável dado o potencial metastático moderado do fibrossarcoma bucal, embora haja relativamente pouca informação a respeito da eficácia.
• Os cuidados paliativos concentram-se no controle da dor. Os analgésicos orais estão abordados adiante. O bloqueio nervoso regional também pode conferir analgesia por até algumas semanas. Também é recomendável o fornecimento de alimentos pastosos.

MEDICAÇÕES

MEDICAMENTO(S)
• Agentes anti-inflamatórios não esteroides:
  ○ Ácido acetilsalicílico (10-25 mg/kg VO a cada 8-24 h).
  ○ Carprofeno (2 mg/kg VO a cada 12 h).
  ○ Deracoxibe (1-2 mg/kg VO a cada 24 h).
  ○ Meloxicam (0,1 mg/kg VO a cada 24 h).
  ○ Firocoxibe (5 mg/kg VO a cada 24 h).
  ○ Tramadol (2-5 mg/kg VO a cada 6-12 h).
  ○ Gabapentina (10-15 mg/kg VO a cada 8-12 h).
• Antibioticoterapia empírica pode ser considerada em infecções bacterianas secundárias.
• Quimioterapia adjuvante — podem ser instituídos protocolos à base de doxorrubicina; consultar um oncologista veterinário em busca das recomendações atuais.

CONTRAINDICAÇÕES/INTERAÇÕES POSSÍVEIS
Não utilizar a doxorrubicina em cães com arritmias ou função miocárdica diminuída; utilizar com cuidado em gatos com insuficiência renal.

ACOMPANHAMENTO

MONITORIZAÇÃO DO PACIENTE
Realização de exame físico e obtenção de radiografias torácicas a cada 2-3 meses.

EVOLUÇÃO ESPERADA E PROGNÓSTICO
• A maioria dos pacientes vem a óbito ou é submetida à eutanásia em virtude da doença local.
• A taxa metastática global é de 20-30% (linfonodos regionais e pulmões).
• Apenas com a cirurgia, o prognóstico individual depende da agressividade da cirurgia, bem como do tamanho e da localização do tumor. A sobrevida média é de 9-12 meses, embora seja possível o controle a longo prazo com a excisão completa.
• Com a associação de cirurgia (excisão parcial) e radioterapia, a sobrevida média é de 18 meses.
• Com a radioterapia isolada, a sobrevida média livre de progressão é de 45 meses para tumores com <2 cm, 31 meses para aqueles de 2-4 cm e 7 meses para outros com >4 cm.
• Embora haja poucas informações a respeito dos gatos, o prognóstico provavelmente é mais reservado em função da dificuldade de excisão cirúrgica completa.

DIVERSOS

ABREVIATURA(S)
• TC = tomografia computadorizada.

Sugestões de Leitura
Coyle VJ, Garrett LD. Finding and treating oral melanoma, squamous cell carcinoma, and fibrosarcoma in dogs. Vet Med 2009, 104:292-305.

Autor Dennis B. Bailey
Consultor Editorial Timothy M. Fan

Fibrossarcoma de Osso

CONSIDERAÇÕES GERAIS

REVISÃO
- O fibrossarcoma ósseo primário origina-se de elementos estromais dentro da cavidade medular. Caracteriza-se por células fusiformes malignas que produzem quantidades variadas de colágeno, mas não qualquer osteoide ou cartilagem.
- Em cães, o fibrossarcoma responde por <5% de todos os tumores ósseos primários. A metáfise ou diáfise de ossos longos parece ser afetada com maior frequência. Também há relatos de tumores das costelas ou vértebras.
- Em gatos, os tumores ósseos primários são incomuns. Há relatos de que o fibrossarcoma seja o segundo tumor ósseo mais comum em gatos, mas nem todos os estudos diferenciam os tumores ósseos primários daqueles que envolvem o tecido ósseo secundariamente por invasão local. Os locais relatados incluem o maxilar, a mandíbula, o úmero, a escápula, o carpo, os dedos, as costelas e o osso sacro.

IDENTIFICAÇÃO
- Cães e gatos.
- Não há predileção racial ou sexual evidente em cães ou gatos.
- As idades relatadas variam de 1,5 a 12 anos em cães e 9 a 13 anos em gatos.

SINAIS CLÍNICOS
Achados Anamnésicos
Fibrossarcoma Apendicular
- Claudicação progressiva.
- Pode haver tumefação palpável.

Fibrossarcoma Axial
- É comum a presença de tumefação localizada com ou sem dor.
- Tumores que se originam da mandíbula ou do maxilar podem ser associados a sinais de halitose, disfagia, dor à abertura da boca ou secreção nasal.
- Tumores vertebrais podem induzir a déficits neurológicos.
- Tumores das costelas são associados raramente a sinais respiratórios.

Achados do Exame Físico
Fibrossarcoma Apendicular
- Claudicação de gravidade variável, desde mínima até sem sustentação do peso.
- Pode haver tumefação palpável.

Fibrossarcoma Axial
- Achados variáveis do exame físico (ver a seção sobre "Achados Anamnésicos" anteriormente).
- Os sinais de dor ou desconforto não são tão compatíveis quanto em tumores apendiculares.
- Dependendo do tamanho e da localização do tumor, a presença de massa pode ser visível ou palpável.

CAUSAS E FATORES DE RISCO
Desconhecidas.

DIAGNÓSTICO

DIAGNÓSTICO DIFERENCIAL
- Outros tumores ósseos primários (osteossarcoma, condrossarcoma, hemangiossarcoma).
- Tumores ósseos metastáticos (carcinomas de células de transição, próstata, glândulas mamárias, tireoide, glândulas apócrinas dos sacos anais).
- Tumores com invasão local de ossos adjacentes (carcinoma nasal; carcinoma bucal de células escamosas, melanoma, fibrossarcoma, ameloblastoma; sarcoma de células sinoviais; sarcoma histiocítico; carcinoma de células escamosas dos dedos, melanoma).
- Tumores hematopoiéticos (mieloma, linfoma).
- Osteomielite bacteriana ou fúngica.

HEMOGRAMA/BIOQUÍMICA/URINÁLISE
Geralmente normais.

DIAGNÓSTICO POR IMAGEM
- Radiografias da lesão primária revelam características de uma lesão óssea agressiva (osteólise, destruição cortical, formação óssea não homogênea, zona de transição maldefinida).
- Radiografias torácicas são recomendadas para fazer a triagem de metástase pulmonar.
- TC é recomendável em casos de tumores axiais para o estadiamento mais preciso de doença local e o planejamento de cirurgia e/ou radioterapia.
- Se o paciente for submetido à TC, será aconselhável a obtenção de imagens concomitantes do tórax como um meio mais sensível para fazer a triagem de metástase pulmonar.

MÉTODOS DIAGNÓSTICOS
- Os exames de biopsia e histopatologia são necessários para a formulação do diagnóstico definitivo. É recomendável o exame cuidadoso do *tumor inteiro* por algum patologista experiente; até metade dos tumores identificados inicialmente como fibrossarcoma é reclassificada no final das contas como osteossarcoma.
- Há relatos de que o fibrossarcoma ósseo primário sofra metástase para diversos locais, tais como: pulmões, linfonodos regionais, outros ossos, pele, pericárdio e miocárdio. Considerar a avaliação diagnóstica adicional, conforme indicado, para descartar metástase para estes ou outros locais.

TRATAMENTO
- O procedimento de amputação é recomendado para tumores apendiculares.
- Para tumores axiais, recomenda-se uma ampla excisão cirúrgica sempre que possível. Se a excisão cirúrgica for incompleta, a radioterapia adjuvante poderá ajudar a melhorar o controle local, embora haja pouca informação a respeito da eficácia.
- A terapia paliativa é aconselhável em pacientes com doença local ou metástase macroscópica não ressecável ou em caso de desistência da terapia definitiva. Os cuidados paliativos concentram-se no alívio da dor.

MEDICAÇÕES

MEDICAMENTO(S)
- Analgésicos anti-inflamatórios não esteroides:
  - Ácido acetilsalicílico (10-25 mg/kg VO a cada 8-24 h).
  - Carprofeno (2 mg/kg VO a cada 12 h).
  - Deracoxibe (1-2 mg/kg VO a cada 24 h).
  - Meloxicam (0,1 mg/kg VO a cada 24 h).
  - Firocoxibe (5 mg/kg VO a cada 24 h).
- Tramadol (2-5 mg/kg VO a cada 6-12 h).
- Gabapentina (10-15 mg/kg VO a cada 8-12 h).
- Pamidronato (1-2 mg/kg IV a cada 3-4 semanas) diminui a reabsorção óssea, aumenta a densidade mineral óssea e pode reduzir a dor associada a tumores ósseos.
- Prednisona (0,5-1 mg/kg VO a cada 24 h) pode ser útil em pacientes com metástase pulmonar.
- Quimioterapia adjuvante — a doxorrubicina como agente isolado ou alternado com cisplatina ou carboplatina pode retardar a evolução do tumor; consultar um veterinário oncologista em busca das recomendações atuais.

CONTRAINDICAÇÕES/INTERAÇÕES POSSÍVEIS
- Não combinar os AINEs com prednisona ou cisplatina.
- Não fazer uso da cisplatina em cães com insuficiência renal nem em gatos.
- Não utilizar a doxorrubicina em cães com arritmias ou função miocárdica reduzida; usar com cuidado em gatos com insuficiência renal.

ACOMPANHAMENTO

MONITORIZAÇÃO DO PACIENTE
Realização de exames físicos e obtenção de radiografias torácicas a cada 2-3 meses.

EVOLUÇÃO ESPERADA E PROGNÓSTICO
- Há informações limitadas a respeito do prognóstico a longo prazo.
- A excisão completa do tumor primário pode conferir um controle potencial a longo prazo.
- Até metade dos pacientes desenvolverá metástase. A metástase foi identificada em até 19 meses após a amputação.

DIVERSOS

VER TAMBÉM
- Condrossarcoma Ósseo.
- Osteossarcoma.

ABREVIATURA(S)
- AINEs = anti-inflamatórios não esteroides.
- TC = tomografia computadorizada.

Sugestões de Leitura
Albin LW, Berg J, Schelling SH. Fibrosarcoma of the canine appendicular skeleton. JAAHA 1991, 27:303-309.

Autor Dennis B. Bailey
Consultor Editorial Timothy M. Fan

Fibrossarcoma dos Seios Nasais e Paranasais

CONSIDERAÇÕES GERAIS

REVISÃO
- Fibrossarcoma é um tumor maligno de células fusiformes que produzem uma quantidade variada de estroma (fibroso) colagenoso.
- Em cães, o fibrossarcoma responde por até 15% de todos os tumores caninos dos seios nasais, sendo o segundo tumor nasal não epitelial mais comum.
- O fibrossarcoma nasal é raro em gatos.

IDENTIFICAÇÃO
- Em cães, nenhuma predileção racial ou sexual foi identificada.
- A idade média é de 9 anos (faixa etária, 1-16 anos).
- Raro em gatos — não há predileção evidente.

SINAIS CLÍNICOS
Achados Anamnésicos
- Epistaxe e/ou secreção mucopurulenta uni ou bilateral.
- Espirros.
- Respiração estertorosa.
- Deformidade facial.
- Apetite diminuído e/ou halitose, secundários à invasão da cavidade bucal.
- Crises convulsivas, mudanças comportamentais e/ou obnubilação, secundárias à invasão craniana.

Achados do Exame Físico
- Epistaxe e/ou secreção nasal (uni ou bilateral).
- Diminuição do fluxo de ar nasal (uni ou bilateral).
- Dor à palpação ou percussão dos seios nasais ou paranasais.
- Deformidade facial.
- Retropulsão diminuída dos olhos ou exoftalmia.
- Epífora e/ou secreção ocular.
- Efeito expansivo visível com massa que se projeta por meio do palato em direção à cavidade bucal.

DIAGNÓSTICO

DIAGNÓSTICO DIFERENCIAL
- Outros tumores nasais — adenocarcinoma, carcinoma de células escamosas, condrossarcoma, osteossarcoma, linfoma, tumor venéreo transmissível (cães), pólipo nasofaríngeo (gatos).
- Rinite fúngica — aspergilose e penicilose (cães), criptococose (gatos), esporotricose (ambos).
- Rinosporidiose (cães).
- Rinite viral — herpes-vírus e calicivírus (gatos).
- Corpo estranho.
- Trombocitopenia ou outra coagulopatia.
- Hipertensão.
- Abscesso da raiz dentária.
- Rinite alérgica.
- Sinusite bacteriana — incomum.
- Fístula oronasal.

HEMOGRAMA/BIOQUÍMICA/URINÁLISE
- Geralmente normais.
- Relatos raros de eritrocitose paraneoplásica.

OUTROS TESTES LABORATORIAIS
- Irrigação nasal para realização de citologia e cultura — raramente útil.
- Perfil de coagulação.
- Tempo de sangramento da mucosa bucal.

DIAGNÓSTICO POR IMAGEM
- Radiografias do crânio — revelam opacidade dos tecidos moles na cavidade nasal e/ou nos seios frontais, bem como destruição de estruturas como ossos turbinados, septo nasal, vômer ou ossos palatinos, maxilares e/ou frontais circunjacentes.
- Radiografias torácicas — para fazer a triagem de metástases pulmonares.
- TC — é superior às radiografias para detectar a opacidade dos tecidos moles dentro da cavidade nasal e dos seios circunjacentes, além de destruição óssea e extensão por meio da placa cribriforme em direção ao cérebro. A TC também é utilizada para fins de planejamento da radioterapia (ver a seção sobre "Tratamento" adiante).
- Se o paciente for submetido à TC, será recomendável a obtenção de imagens concomitantes do tórax como um meio mais sensível para fazer a triagem de metástase pulmonar.

MÉTODOS DIAGNÓSTICOS
- Medição da pressão arterial e exame do fundo ocular.
- Citologia dos linfonodos mandibulares para triagem de possível metástase.
- Às vezes, o exame de rinoscopia pode ser útil para visualizar a presença de massa ou placa fúngica e orientar a realização de subsequente biopsia.
- Os exames de biopsia tecidual e histopatologia são necessários para a formulação do diagnóstico definitivo. O instrumento de biopsia não deve passar na altura do canto medial do olho para evitar a penetração da placa cribriforme.

TRATAMENTO

- A radioterapia constitui o tratamento de escolha.
- Protocolos definitivos comuns:
  - Aplicação de 57 Gy em 19 frações de 3,0 Gy cada de segunda a sexta-feira.
  - Aplicação de 42 Gy em 10 frações de 4,2 Gy cada de segunda a sexta-feira.
- Protocolos paliativos (menor número de tratamentos e menor dose de radiação total) podem ser preferíveis para cães com doença muito avançada.
- A cirurgia sozinha é ineficaz, embora haja alguns indícios de que a exenteração da cavidade nasal após a radioterapia aumente o tempo de sobrevida em cães com vários tumores nasais.
- A quimioterapia não foi avaliada especificamente para casos de fibrossarcoma nasal, mas protocolos à base de doxorrubicina são utilizados com sucesso modesto para fibrossarcomas originários de outros locais.
- Consultar um veterinário oncologista e/ou um oncologista especialista em radiação em busca das recomendações atuais.

MEDICAÇÕES

MEDICAMENTO(S)
- Fenilefrina sob a forma de spray nasal pode ser utilizada de forma intermitente para interromper a epistaxe.
- Pode ser considerado o uso de antibioticoterapia empírica para infecções bacterianas secundárias.
- Quimioterapia (doxorrubicina isolada ou em combinação com ifosfamida, cisplatina ou carboplatina) pode ser levada em consideração. Consultar um veterinário oncologista em busca das recomendações atuais.

CONTRAINDICAÇÕES/INTERAÇÕES POSSÍVEIS
- Não utilizar a doxorrubicina em cães com arritmias ou função miocárdica reduzida; usar com cuidado em gatos com insuficiência renal.
- Não usar a cisplatina em cães com insuficiência renal nem em gatos.
- Não fazer uso da ifosfamida em cães ou gatos com insuficiência renal.

ACOMPANHAMENTO

MONITORIZAÇÃO DO PACIENTE
- São recomendáveis a realização de exames físicos e a obtenção de radiografias torácicas a cada 2-3 meses.
- TC da cavidade nasal pode ser considerada para monitorizar a involução ou evolução da doença.

EVOLUÇÃO ESPERADA E PROGNÓSTICO
- A taxa metastática global é <20% (geralmente envolve os linfonodos regionais e/ou os pulmões).
- A sobrevida média apenas com cuidados paliativos é de 3 meses.
- Com a aplicação de radioterapia definitiva, as taxas de sobrevida livre de recidiva em um período de 1 e 2 anos giram em torno de 50% e 30%, respectivamente.
- Para os pacientes com tumores nasais em geral, a extensão para os seios frontais e/ou a erosão através dos ossos das vias nasais é associada a um aumento de três vezes no risco de recidiva local.
- O envolvimento cerebral é um sinal prognóstico mau.
- O envolvimento uni *versus* bilateral não é um fator prognóstico significativo.

DIVERSOS

VER TAMBÉM
- Adenocarcinoma Nasal.
- Condrossarcoma dos Seios Nasais e Paranasais.
- Epistaxe.

ABREVIATURA(S)
- TC = tomografia computadorizada.

Sugestões de Leitura
Theon AP, Madewell BR, Harb MF, Dungworth DL. Megavoltage irradiation of neoplasms of the nasal and paranasal cavities in 77 dogs. JAVMA 1993, 202:1469-1475.

Autor Dennis B. Bailey
Consultor Editorial Timothy M. Fan

FISALOPTEROSE

CONSIDERAÇÕES GERAIS

REVISÃO
- *Physaloptera* spp., ocorrem em cães e gatos; os adultos aderem-se à mucosa gástrica; não há migração de larvas para fora do trato gastrintestinal.
- A infecção pode ser assintomática ou causar gastrite e, consequentemente, vômito.
- Tipicamente, há poucos vermes; é comum a ocorrência de infecções por um único verme.
- Transmitida pela ingestão de larvas infectantes em hospedeiros intermediários (p. ex., larvas de insetos, besouros, baratas, grilos coprófagos) ou em hospedeiros de transporte (p. ex., pássaros, roedores, sapos, cobras, lacertílios).

IDENTIFICAÇÃO
Cães e gatos; qualquer raça, idade ou sexo.

SINAIS CLÍNICOS
- Vômito, muitas vezes crônico e intermitente; ocasionalmente, os vermes são encontrados no vômito.
- Melena.
- Pode ocorrer perda de peso, sobretudo com infecção crônica.
- Podem ocorrer sinais clínicos sem a produção de ovos durante o período pré-patente ou infecção por um único verme.

CAUSAS E FATORES DE RISCO
- Exposição a ambientes externos; acesso a hospedeiros intermediários (insetos) ou hospedeiros de transporte (pequenos vertebrados).
- Acesso ao habitat ocupado por espécies de vida selvagem (guaxinim, raposa, coiote, lince, puma, texugo, gambá) infectadas por *Physaloptera*.

DIAGNÓSTICO

DIAGNÓSTICO DIFERENCIAL
- Outras causas infecciosas de vômito, incluindo infecções parasitárias, virais ou bacterianas.
- *Spirocerca*, o verme do esôfago, produz ovos menores semelhantes (11-15 × 30-37 μm); pode causar vômito em jatos; os vermes não costumam estar no vômito; infecção relativamente rara nos Estados Unidos.
- *Ollulanus*, um nematódeo tricostrongilídeo, pode causar vômito crônico; observado principalmente em gatos de colônias e em outros selvagens; as larvas e os adultos (<1 mm de comprimento), mas não os ovos, estão presentes no vômito ou nas fezes.
- Nematódeos (ascarídeos) em filhotes caninos e felinos; os vermes podem estar presentes nas fezes e no vômito; um pouco maiores que o *Physaloptera*; caracterizados por três lábios e asas cervicais.
- Outras causas não infecciosas de vômito, incluindo imprudência alimentar, corpos estranhos no estômago, ingestão acidental de substâncias nocivas, neoplasia gastrintestinal, doenças metabólicas.

HEMOGRAMA/BIOQUÍMICA/URINÁLISE
Podem ocorrer anemia leve e eosinofilia.

OUTROS TESTES LABORATORIAIS
N/D.

DIAGNÓSTICO POR IMAGEM
Radiografia abdominal, incluindo estudos contrastados, para eliminar outras causas de vômito.

MÉTODOS DIAGNÓSTICOS
- Endoscopia (gastroscopia) para visualizar e remover os vermes, geralmente aderidos à mucosa gástrica ou duodenal; é necessária a realização de exame meticuloso e completo para detectar todos os vermes; tipicamente, poucos vermes estão presentes; além disso, eles podem estar escondidos por muco, ingesta, pregas gástricas; podem ser observadas hemorragias puntiformes a partir dos locais prévios de fixação.
- *Physaloptera* spp. são pequenos (2,5-5 cm de comprimento), robustos, brancos ou rosados, com colar cuticular anterior; os *P. praeputialis* machos e fêmeas possuem uma bainha cuticular posterior semelhante a prepúcio.
- Esfregaço direto, câmara úmida ou flutuação fecal para detectar os ovos no vômito ou nas fezes; os ovos são densos e podem ser de difícil detecção via flutuação fecal com o uso de soluções de baixa densidade; utilizar solução de flutuação com densidade >1,25.
- Os ovos são pequenos (42-58 × 29-42 μm), larvados, ovoides a elipsoidais, incolores e de parede espessa.

TRATAMENTO
- O tratamento é feito em um esquema ambulatorial; uso de anti-helmíntico com ou sem remoção endoscópica dos vermes.
- O uso de anti-helmíntico é fora da indicação da bula e casual.

MEDICAÇÕES

MEDICAMENTO(S)
- Na ausência de migração além da parede gástrica, utilizar anti-helmínticos adulticidas com liberação no estômago.
- Fembendazol (cães), 50 mg/kg VO a cada 24 h por 3-5 dias; repetir mediante a persistência dos sinais.
- Pamoato de pirantel (cães/gatos), 5 mg/kg duas vezes em intervalo de 3 semanas ou 15-20 mg/kg uma única vez; repetir mediante a persistência dos sinais.
- Ivermectina (gatos), 0,2 mg/kg VO ou SC uma única vez.
- Medicação para reduzir a gastrite — antagonistas histaminérgicos H_2 (p. ex., famotidina 0,5 mg/kg VO a cada 24 h); sucralfato 0,25-1 g VO a cada 8-12 h no cão; 0,25 g VO a cada 8-12 h no gato.

CONTRAINDICAÇÕES/INTERAÇÕES POSSÍVEIS
Não administrar ivermectina a 0,2 mg/kg a cães ou gatos positivos para dirofilárias.

ACOMPANHAMENTO

MONITORIZAÇÃO DO PACIENTE
Reavaliar 1-2 semanas após o tratamento e repetir a terapia anti-helmíntica se os ovos ainda estiverem presentes no exame de fezes e/ou se o vômito persistir.

PREVENÇÃO
- Remover e descartar as fezes imediatamente para evitar infecção de hospedeiros intermediários artrópodes.
- Impedir hábitos errantes (ou seja, de vida livre) para os animais de estimação; evitar práticas de caça e canibalismo.

EVOLUÇÃO ESPERADA E PROGNÓSTICO
Os sinais clínicos e/ou a eliminação de ovos nas fezes devem desaparecer dentro de 2 semanas do tratamento.

Sugestões de Leitura
Campbell KL, Graham JC. Physaloptera infection in dogs and cats. Compend Contin Educ Pract Vet 1999, 21:299-314.

Autor Julie Ann Jarvinen
Consultor Editorial Stephen C. Barr

Fístula Arteriovenosa

CONSIDERAÇÕES GERAIS

REVISÃO
Corresponde a uma conexão (comunicação) anormal de baixa resistência entre uma artéria e uma veia. A presença de ampla fístula arteriovenosa faz com que uma fração significativa do débito cardíaco total se desvie do leito capilar. O aumento resultante no débito cardíaco pode levar à insuficiência cardíaca congestiva (ICC) de "alto débito". A localização da fístula arteriovenosa é variável. Os locais relatados incluem: cabeça, pescoço, orelha, língua, membros, flanco, medula espinal, cérebro, pulmões, fígado, veia cava e trato gastrintestinal. Em geral, é observada como uma lesão adquirida.

IDENTIFICAÇÃO
- Cães e gatos (rara em ambos).
- Não há predisposição etária, racial ou sexual específica conhecida.

SINAIS CLÍNICOS
Achados Anamnésicos
- Os animais com doença adquirida frequentemente apresentam histórico de traumatismo sobre a área acometida.
- O proprietário pode notar uma tumefação (inchaço) quente e indolor no local da lesão.
- É possível um histórico compatível com ICC iminente ou manifesta, dependendo do tamanho e da duração do desvio.
- Outros achados históricos dependem da localização da lesão.
- O desvio pode causar disfunção orgânica local.

Achados do Exame Físico
- Variam e dependem da localização da fístula arteriovenosa.
- Em animais com doença prolongada e fluxo sanguíneo elevado, podem se desenvolver sinais de ICC (p. ex., tosse, dispneia, taquipneia e intolerância ao exercício).
- Alguns animais exibem pulsos saltitantes, em decorrência do alto volume de ejeção e do rápido escoamento através da fístula arteriovenosa.
- No local, verifica-se um sopro contínuo (ruído) causado pelo fluxo sanguíneo através da lesão.
- A compressão cuidadosa da artéria em posição proximal à lesão suprime o ruído. Quando o fluxo sanguíneo se encontra alto, essa compressão também poderá eliciar um declínio reflexo imediato na frequência cardíaca (sinal de Branham).
- Além disso, observam-se edema, isquemia e congestão de órgãos e tecidos causados pela pressão venosa elevada nas proximidades da lesão.
- Se a lesão ocorrer em um membro, isso resultará em edema depressível, claudicação, ulceração, formação de crostas e gangrena.
- Uma lesão próxima a órgãos vitais pode causar sinais associados à insuficiência do órgão envolvido, como ascite (fígado), crises convulsivas (cérebro), paresia (medula espinal) e dispneia (pulmões).

CAUSAS E FATORES DE RISCO
- Raramente se trata de uma lesão congênita.
- Uma fístula arteriovenosa adquirida tipicamente se origina de danos locais à vasculatura, secundariamente a traumatismo, cirurgia, venopunção, injeção perivascular (p. ex., barbitúricos) ou tumor.

DIAGNÓSTICO

DIAGNÓSTICO DIFERENCIAL
- A lesão pode se assemelhar a um aneurisma ou um pseudoaneurisma.
- Achados clínicos bizarros, dependendo da localização da fístula arteriovenosa, podem sugerir outros processos mórbidos; uma fístula arteriovenosa pode representar uma consideração diagnóstica tardia.

HEMOGRAMA/BIOQUÍMICA/URINÁLISE
Podem refletir danos aos sistemas adjacentes à lesão, ou seja, é possível a constatação de anormalidades bioquímicas sugestivas de disfunções hepáticas, renais ou em outros órgãos.

OUTROS TESTES LABORATORIAIS
N/D.

DIAGNÓSTICO POR IMAGEM
Achados Radiográficos Torácicos
- Em alguns animais com fístula arteriovenosa significativa em termos hemodinâmicos, observam-se aumento do volume cardíaco e hipercirculação pulmonar.

Achados Ecocardiográficos
- Pode permitir o diagnóstico por imagem da fístula arteriovenosa, retratando sua natureza cavernosa.
- O ultrassom Doppler pode demonstrar o fluxo turbulento de alta velocidade dentro da lesão.

Achados Angiográficos
- A angiografia seletiva delineia a lesão, pode ser necessária para o diagnóstico definitivo e ainda é altamente desejável para uma avaliação pré-cirúrgica. São imprescindíveis a colocação do cateter próximo à lesão e a injeção rápida do contraste; um fluxo sanguíneo de alto volume dilui o meio de contraste com rapidez.

MÉTODOS DIAGNÓSTICOS
N/D.

TRATAMENTO
- Do ponto de vista histórico, o tratamento definitivo exigia a realização de cirurgia para romper e remover as conexões vasculares anormais. Em animais com sinais clínicos relacionados com a fístula arteriovenosa, é recomendável o tratamento definitivo, uma vez que as lesões podem aumentar de tamanho.
- Além de necessitar de possível transfusão sanguínea, a cirurgia pode ser difícil e trabalhosa; é aconselhável a delimitação da lesão antes do procedimento cirúrgico por meio da angiografia.
- Embora a intervenção cirúrgica seja muitas vezes bem-sucedida, a fístula arteriovenosa poderá sofrer recidiva. Em alguns animais, pode ser necessária a amputação da parte acometida.
- A embolização transcateter com espirais vaso-oclusivos constitui uma opção terapêutica mais recente. As vantagens potenciais incluem tratamento relativamente não invasivo e acesso intravascular para remover as lesões.

MEDICAÇÕES

MEDICAMENTO(S)
- O tratamento clínico concomitante depende do local da fístula arteriovenosa e dos aspectos clínicos secundários.
- Antes da cirurgia, pode ser indispensável o tratamento clínico da ICC.

CONTRAINDICAÇÕES/INTERAÇÕES POSSÍVEIS
Evitar a administração excessiva de fluido, pois os animais com fístula arteriovenosa apresentam sobrecarga por volume.

ACOMPANHAMENTO
Haverá necessidade de reavaliação pós-operatória para determinar a ocorrência ou não de recidivas da fístula arteriovenosa.

DIVERSOS

VER TAMBÉM
Insuficiência Cardíaca Congestiva Esquerda

ABREVIATURA(S)
- ICC = insuficiência cardíaca congestiva.

Sugestões de Leitura
Fox PR, Petrie J-P, Hohenhaus AE. Peripheral vascular disease. In: Ettinger SJ, Feldman EC, eds., Textbook of Veterinary Internal Medicine, 6th ed. St. Louis: Elsevier, 2005.

Autor Donald J. Brown
Consultores Editoriais Larry P. Tilley e Francis W.K. Smith, Jr.

Fístula Oronasal

CONSIDERAÇÕES GERAIS

REVISÃO
- Defeito entre as cavidades bucal e nasal.
- Pode ocorrer uma comunicação entre a boca e a cavidade nasal por doença em qualquer um dos tecidos que envolvem os dentes maxilares e o palato duro.
- Os caninos maxilares são os mais comumente envolvidos.
- A raiz palatina do quarto pré-molar maxilar é a próxima área mais comumente envolvida.

IDENTIFICAÇÃO
- Cão — tipos dolicocéfalos de cabeça são acometidos com maior frequência, sobretudo da raça Dachshund.
- Gatos — rara.

SINAIS CLÍNICOS
- Rinite crônica — com ou sem sangue.
- Espirros — também são comuns, especialmente quando os caninos maxilares são palpados com o dedo.

CAUSAS E FATORES DE RISCO
- Geralmente associada ao estágio final de periodontite do dente canino maxilar, levando à lise (destruição) do osso que separa as cavidades nasal e bucal.
- Outras causas incluem traumatismo, penetração de corpo estranho, ferimentos por mordedura, extração traumática de dente, choque elétrico ou câncer bucal.
- A largura da fístula está relacionada com o tamanho do dente acometido, enquanto a profundidade da fístula, com a cronicidade da infecção periodontal.
- Cães com caninos mandibulares de base estreita e deslocamento lingual não corrigido e aqueles com maloclusões mandibulares acentuadas (sobremordida) que fazem com que os caninos mandibulares penetrem no palato duro são predispostos.
- Os cães da raça Dachshund são predispostos.

DIAGNÓSTICO

DIAGNÓSTICO DIFERENCIAL
- Doença periodontal.
- Neoplasia bucal.
- Traumatismo.
- Penetração de corpo estranho.

HEMOGRAMA/BIOQUÍMICA/URINÁLISE
N/D.

OUTROS TESTES LABORATORIAIS
N/D.

DIAGNÓSTICO POR IMAGEM
- As radiografias do crânio raramente são úteis para o diagnóstico de fístula oronasal, porque as lesões em geral são isoladas à superfície medial.
- As radiografias intrabucais são altamente recomendadas para avaliar o estado periodontal dos dentes do paciente.
- As radiografias podem demonstrar o encarceramento de corpo estranho ou lise compatível com neoplasia.

MÉTODOS DIAGNÓSTICOS
Sondagem periodontal — se a sondagem resultar em extensão direta para a cavidade nasal ou levar à epistaxe, existe fístula oronasal.

TRATAMENTO

- Extração do dente e oclusão do defeito; após a extração, o objetivo da oclusão cirúrgica é colocar uma camada epitelial nas cavidades bucal e nasal.
- Aplicação de retalho (*flap*) de espessura completa — após a extração do dente, um retalho pediculado de mucoperiósteo pode ser suspenso a partir da face dorsal da fístula, liberado, avançado até recobrir o defeito e suturado no local; a aplicação bem-sucedida de retalho de espessura completa necessita de pelo menos 2 mm de gengiva aderida acima do defeito, suturas na borda do defeito (não sobre o vazio) e ausência de tensão na linha de sutura.
- Retalho duplo de reposição — usado nas grandes fístulas ou nas falhas de reparo, onde não há nenhuma gengiva aderida ou onde não se consegue incluir o tecido periosteal; após a extração, o primeiro retalho é coletado a partir do palato duro e invertido, de forma que o epitélio bucal fique na direção da passagem nasal; o segundo retalho é mucobucal e coletado a partir da mucosa alveolar e da face inferior do lábio rostral à fístula; esse retalho é suturado sobre o primeiro retalho e o local doador.
- Regeneração tecidual guiada do dente canino maxilar — pode ser utilizada para o reparo de bolsa palatina profunda se ainda não estiver fistulada; um retalho palatino é elevado até se aproximar do defeito infraósseo; os tecidos moles e os cálculos dentários são removidos do defeito com o uso de cureta.
- Em bolsas infraósseas profundas antes da fistulação, enxertos ósseos, como PerioGlas®, Consil® (Nutramax Laboratories, Edgewood, MD), hidroxiapatita natural e sintética, osso autógeno e heterólogo, ácido poliláctico e molde de gesso foram usados para excluir o novo crescimento de tecido conjuntivo e epitélio gengivais, promovendo a regeneração do osso e do ligamento periodontal. Não é recomendável o uso de materiais de implante na presença de fístula oronasal.
- Fístulas oronasais localizadas na porção central do palato duro podem ser submetidas a reparo com o uso de retalho de transposição do mucoperiósteo do palato duro coletado a partir do tecido adjacente ao defeito.

MEDICAÇÕES

MEDICAMENTO(S)
N/D.

CONTRAINDICAÇÕES/INTERAÇÕES POSSÍVEIS
N/D.

ACOMPANHAMENTO

MONITORIZAÇÃO DO PACIENTE
Monitorização pós-operatória normal.

EVOLUÇÃO ESPERADA E PROGNÓSTICO
Mesmo com o uso de tecido suficiente, a liberação excelente de tensão exercida sobre o retalho e a aplicação de técnica satisfatória, pode ocorrer a formação de uma abertura persistente em virtude da constante tensão sobre o local durante cada respiração. Com o uso de tecido insuficiente ou técnica inadequada, o prognóstico declina, havendo a necessidade de outras intervenções cirúrgicas com o avanço de retalhos.

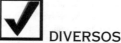

DIVERSOS

RECURSOS DA INTERNET
http://www.avdc.org/Nomenclature.html.

Sugestões de Leitura
Bellows JE. Small Animal Dental Equipment, Materials and Techniques. Ames, IA: Blackwell, 2004.
Wiggs RB, Lobprise HB. Veterinary Dentistry: Principles and Practice. Philadelphia: Lippincott-Raven, 1997.

Autor Jan Bellows
Consultor Editorial Heidi B. Lobprise

FÍSTULA PERIANAL

CONSIDERAÇÕES GERAIS

REVISÃO
• Distúrbio inflamatório crônico caracterizado por múltiplos seios ulcerados, dolorosos e progressivos ou, com frequência muito menor, por verdadeiros trajetos fistulosos envolvendo a região perianal.
• Sinônimos: furunculose anal, seio perianal, fístulas pararretais, fístulas no ânus.

IDENTIFICAÇÃO
• Cães. • Acomete principalmente cães da raça Pastor alemão; também afeta cães da Setter irlandês. • Cães de meia-idade, com idade média de 5-7 anos; faixa etária, 7 meses a 14 anos. • Na maioria dos estudos, os machos são mais comumente acometidos.

SINAIS CLÍNICOS
• Disquezia. • Tenesmo. • Hematoquezia.
• Constipação. • Diarreia. • Corrimento anal mucopurulento fétido. • Ulceração da pele perianal, com formação de trajeto sinuoso.
• Lambedura e automutilação. • Relutância em sentar; dificuldades de postura; mudanças comportamentais de personalidade. • Dor à manipulação da cauda e ao exame da área perianal.
• Incontinência fecal. • Anorexia. • Perda de peso.

CAUSAS E FATORES DE RISCO
• A causa não está claramente definida, embora haja fortes suspeitas de algum mecanismo imunomediado multifatorial. • Parece ser uma resposta inapropriada mediada por células-T.
• Também foi proposta uma associação com colite, particularmente nos cães da raça Pastor alemão.
• Foi sugerida, mas não comprovada, uma predisposição genética, com base na incidência racial. • Foram implicados alguns fatores anatômicos, em particular nos cães da raça Pastor alemão. • O animal conduz a cauda abaixada, além de ter uma cauda ampla; apenas uma pequena porcentagem de cães com essa conformação vem a ser acometida. • Densidade elevada de glândulas sudoríferas apócrinas na zona cutânea do canal anal dos cães da raça Pastor alemão.

DIAGNÓSTICO

DIAGNÓSTICO DIFERENCIAL
• Outros processos inflamatórios — por exemplo, anusite e hidradenite supurativa. • Abscesso crônico do saco anal. • Adenoma ou adenocarcinoma perianal, com ulceração e drenagem. • Carcinoma de células escamosas.
• Infecção bacteriana atípica. • Oomicose. • Fístula retal.

HEMOGRAMA/BIOQUÍMICA/URINÁLISE
• Geralmente normais.
• Pacientes com inflamação podem apresentar leucograma inflamatório.

MÉTODOS DIAGNÓSTICOS
• Diagnóstico presuntivo — com base nos sinais clínicos do animal e resultados do exame físico.
• Diagnóstico definitivo — estabelecido por meio de biopsia da área acometida.
• Colonoscopia com biopsia — pode revelar colite associada.

TRATAMENTO

CUIDADO(S) DE SAÚDE ADEQUADO(S)
• Inicialmente, é recomendável a terapia médica em um esquema ambulatorial em todos os casos.
• A tricotomia e a limpeza da região perianal facilitam a terapia local. • A aplicação de banho com xampu antimicrobiano pode ser útil.

DIETA
• Modificação da dieta — uso de nova fonte proteica, como carne de veado ou peixe e batata.
• Amolecedores fecais — com dor ou tenesmo.

CONSIDERAÇÕES CIRÚRGICAS
• Do ponto de vista histórico, a cirurgia era considerada como o principal tratamento; no entanto, com uma melhor compressão da fisiopatologia, a cirurgia fica indicada principalmente para os pacientes com resolução incompleta ou pseudocicatrização dos trajetos sinuosos. • Saculectomia anal — realizar em caso de envolvimento confirmado dos sacos anais.
• Opções cirúrgicas — é preferível a ressecção do tecido inflamatório e/ou a ablação dos seios remanescentes com laser de dióxido de carbono.
• Debridamento cirúrgico (remoção da pele que reveste cada trajeto) com fulguração (destruição de tecido vivo) por meio de cautério químico ou eletrocautério; a ressecção cirúrgica acompanhada por fechamento primário ou a cicatrização por segunda intenção são outras opções se o laser não estiver disponível. • A excisão radical do anel retal com abaixamento retrorretal modificado não costuma ser necessária e está associada a um maior risco de incontinência fecal.

MEDICAÇÕES

MEDICAMENTO(S) DE ESCOLHA
• Prednisona oral, tacrolimo tópico, metronidazol e uma nova fonte proteica parecem ser eficazes e econômicos. ○ Prednisona — administrar por via oral na dose de 2 mg/kg a cada 24 h por 2 semanas, diminuir para 1 mg/kg a cada 24 h por 4 semanas e, depois, 1 mg/kg a cada 48 h por 10 semanas. ○ Pomada de tacrolimo a 0,1% — aplicar por via tópica 2 vezes ao dia com mão enluvada inicialmente e, depois, reduzir de forma gradativa para a cada 24-72 h conforme as lesões desaparecem. ○ É provável que a terapia de manutenção crônica com tacrolimo e, possivelmente, prednisona em uma frequência reduzida de aplicação e dose seja necessária para o controle a longo prazo, respectivamente.
○ Metronidazol — 10 mg/kg a cada 12 h por 2 semanas. ○ Nova fonte proteica — deve ser estritamente forçada. ○ Amolecedor fecal se houver necessidade. ○ Esse protocolo terapêutico é consideravelmente mais barato do que o protocolo imunossupressor oral descrito adiante. ○ Admita que o paciente colabore o suficiente para permitir a aplicação de 2 vezes ao dia do tacrolimo OU ciclosporina ± cetoconazol. • Microemulsão de ciclosporina A como agente único — administrar 4-8 mg/kg VO por dia como dose de indução e, depois, reduzir a dose gradativamente com base na resposta clínica. • Ciclosporina A e cetoconazol — administrar a ciclosporina por via oral a 2-5 mg/kg/dia VO e o cetoconazol a 5-10 mg/kg/dia VO como dose de indução e, depois, reduzir a ciclosporina gradativamente à medida que os sinais clínicos desaparecerem. • O cetoconazol diminui a dose necessária da ciclosporina, inibindo as enzimas responsáveis pela metabolização deste último medicamento; no entanto, a inibição pode ser muito variável entre os pacientes, dificultando a predição da concentração sanguínea da ciclosporina. • Manter o tratamento por, no mínimo, 4 semanas após a resolução completa da(s) fístula(s), embora muitos pacientes necessitem de tratamento crônico com uma frequência reduzida para evitar recidivas.
• Tacrolimo (pomada a 0,1%) aplicado por via tópica como terapia de manutenção pode ser suficiente para controlar as lesões; iniciar a aplicação conforme a dose dos medicamentos orais for reduzida. • Aplicar por via tópica a cada 12 h com mão enluvada e, depois, reduzir gradativamente para a cada 24-72 h.

MEDICAMENTO(S) ALTERNATIVO(S)
• Azatioprina — é usada para diminuir a gravidade das lesões antes da cirurgia; é improvável que esse medicamento resulte em resolução completa por si só. • Talvez haja necessidade de analgésicos, especialmente durante a fase de indução, para facilitar a terapia local.

ACOMPANHAMENTO

MONITORIZAÇÃO DO PACIENTE
• Avaliar os níveis mínimos (também conhecidos como níveis terapêuticos de vale) da ciclosporina, sobretudo quando o cetoconazol for utilizado na suspeita de toxicidade.
• Examinar novamente para avaliar a cicatrização, os sinais de recidiva e as complicações associadas.

COMPLICAÇÕES POSSÍVEIS
• Alopecia reversível. • Vômito, diarreia, anorexia.
• Perda de peso. • Recidiva. • Falha de cicatrização.
• Deiscência da ferida cirúrgica. • Tenesmo.
• Incontinência fecal. • Estenose anal.
• Flatulência. • Síndrome de Cushing iatrogênica por corticosteroides.

EVOLUÇÃO ESPERADA E PROGNÓSTICO
• Reservado quanto à resolução completa, exceto em pacientes levemente acometidos.
• Talvez haja necessidade de tratamento crônico.
• Se todo o tratamento for interrompido, o paciente deverá ser monitorizado de perto quanto à ocorrência de recidiva.

DIVERSOS

DISTÚRBIOS ASSOCIADOS
• Colite. • Pode ocorrer o desenvolvimento de constipação e/ou obstipação.

Sugestões de Leitura
Stanley BJ, Hauptman JG. Long-term prospective evaluation of topically applied 0.1% tacrolimus ointment for treatment of perianal sinuses in dogs. JAVMA 2009, 235:397-404.

Autor Eric R. Pope
Consultor Editorial Albert E. Jergens

FLATULÊNCIA

CONSIDERAÇÕES GERAIS

DEFINIÇÃO
Formação excessiva de gases no estômago ou no trato intestinal. A eructação consiste na passagem de gás do estômago para a boca, enquanto o flato se refere ao gás liberado pelo ânus.

FISIOPATOLOGIA
• Em geral, resulta de alguma mudança na dieta ou imprudência alimentar, mas pode ser o prenúncio de uma doença gastrintestinal mais séria, especialmente em gatos.
• A deglutição de ar (aerofagia) e a fermentação bacteriana de nutrientes são as principais fontes de gás gastrintestinal; fontes menos significativas incluem a interação do ácido gástrico e do bicarbonato pancreático/salivar e a difusão de gases pelo sangue.
• Dietas pouco digeríveis que escapam da assimilação intestinal e, portanto, ficam disponíveis para a fermentação colônica e dietas que liberam gases odoríferos estão associadas à flatulência; elas incluem oligossacarídeos não absorvíveis (soja, feijão e ervilha), alimento deteriorado, dietas ricas em gordura, laticínios e condimentos.
• Alimentos com fibras contribuem indiretamente para a formação de flatos ao reduzirem a digestibilidade da matéria seca e diretamente pela fermentação da fibra no cólon.
• Os cães e gatos são intolerantes à lactose; a concentração de 1,5 g/kg/dia na dieta (11 g de lactose em 1 xícara de leite) pode produzir flatos e diarreia.
• A rápida troca na dieta ou o aumento na concentração de algum componente alimentar, sobretudo carboidrato ou fibra, pode causar flatos durante um período de adaptação intestinal.
• Até 99% dos flatos são compostos de nitrogênio, oxigênio, hidrogênio, dióxido de carbono e metano, dos quais todos são inodoros.
• Gases fétidos, incluindo amônia, sulfeto de hidrogênio, indol, escatol, aminas voláteis, ácidos graxos de cadeia curta, compõem o 1% restante. A má digestão de proteínas é frequentemente responsável pela produção de gases fétidos.
• Estados mórbidos que prejudicam a assimilação de nutrientes, tornando-os disponíveis para a fermentação no cólon, podem causar flatos.

SISTEMA(S) ACOMETIDO(S)
Gastrintestinal.

GENÉTICA
Não há nenhuma base genética conhecida, embora as raças braquicefálicas sejam super-representadas.

INCIDÊNCIA/PREVALÊNCIA
Desconhecidas.

DISTRIBUIÇÃO GEOGRÁFICA
N/D.

IDENTIFICAÇÃO
Espécies
Queixa comum em cães; rara em gatos.
Raça(s) Predominante(s)
Observa-se aerofagia excessiva em raças braquicefálicas, cães desportistas e aqueles com comportamento alimentar glutão/competitivo.
Idade Média e Faixa Etária
Qualquer idade.
Sexo Predominante
Nenhum.

SINAIS CLÍNICOS
Achados Anamnésicos
Aumento da frequência e, possivelmente, do volume de flatos detectados pelo proprietário.
Achados do Exame Físico
• Leve desconforto abdominal causado por possível distensão gastrintestinal — embora possa ser difícil identificar um leve desconforto, esse sinal pode ser relatado pelo proprietário como um animal de estimação que exibe esforços repetidos de deglutição, inquietação ou letargia.
• Quando o flato se deve à doença gastrintestinal, pode haver sinais gastrintestinais concomitantes, como diarreia, vômito, borborigmo, alterações no apetite e perda de peso.

CAUSAS
Aumento da Aerofagia
• Comportamento alimentar glutão ou competitivo.
• Doença respiratória ou qualquer causa de aumento da frequência respiratória.
• Alimentação logo após o exercício.
• Raças braquicefálicas.

Relacionadas com a Dieta
• Dietas ricas em oligossacarídeos não absorvíveis — soja, ervilha, feijão.
• Dietas ricas em fibras fermentáveis — lactose, pectina, inulina, psílio, farelo de aveia.
• Alimentos deteriorados.
• Laticínios.
• Modificações abruptas na dieta.
• Condimentos e aditivos alimentares/suplementos.

Condições Mórbidas
• Doença intestinal aguda e crônica — enteropatia inflamatória; enteropatias responsivas a antibióticos ou proliferação bacteriana excessiva no intestino delgado; neoplasia; síndrome do intestino irritável; parasitismo; enterite bacteriana, protozoária ou viral; e alergia ou intolerância alimentares.
• Insuficiência pancreática exócrina.

FATORES DE RISCO
• Comportamento nervoso, glutão ou competitivo.
• Alimentação logo após o exercício.
• Raças braquicefálicas.
• Modificações abruptas na dieta.
• Alimentos impróprios (fornecimento de restos de comida da mesa, provavelmente fermentados) ou deteriorados.
• Estilo de vida sedentário. Um estudo feito em 1998 relatou que 43% dos proprietários de cães escolhidos aleatoriamente detectaram flatulência, mais comumente em cães sedentários, sem associação a uma dieta específica.

DIAGNÓSTICO

DIAGNÓSTICO DIFERENCIAL
• Diferenciar causas nutricionais e comportamentais de flatos de doença gastrintestinal por meio da avaliação completa dos antecedentes do paciente; isso permite que o clínico se certifique do tipo de dieta, da quantidade ingerida, da frequência das refeições e das modificações ou acréscimos na dieta, bem como do ambiente onde o paciente é alimentado.
• Pesquisar o método de alimentação — frequência, quantidade, relação com o exercício, a maneira como é oferecida e a incidência de comportamento alimentar competitivo. Talvez seja necessário observar o paciente enquanto ele come para verificar se existe algum comportamento glutão.
• Realizar um exame físico completo com foco na avaliação gastrintestinal. Palpar o abdome à procura de alças intestinais cheias de gás, dor e distensão e ainda auscultar o abdome em busca de ruídos intestinais, cuja ausência indica íleo paralítico. Exame retal para a avaliação da anatomia pélvica e retal.
• Avaliar o escore da condição corporal; se baixo, isso pode indicar doença gastrintestinal concomitante ou consumo alimentar inadequado. A obesidade pode ser associada a um estilo de vida sedentário, que pode ser um fator de risco.

HEMOGRAMA/BIOQUÍMICA/URINÁLISE
Geralmente normais a menos que haja doença intestinal significativa (p. ex., hipoalbuminemia em enteropatia com perda de proteínas).

OUTROS TESTES LABORATORIAIS
• Citologia retal para avaliar a presença de neoplasia, parasitas, neutrófilos.
• Cultura para clostrídios e análise de toxinas.
• Testes de flutuação em sulfato de zinco ou ELISA fecal para verificar se há giardíase.
• PCR fecal para pesquisar *Tritrichomonas* em gatos jovens ou filhotes felinos.
• Coproculturas para averiguar a existência de salmonelose ou campilobacteriose.
• Imunorreatividade semelhante à da tripsina para examinar se há insuficiência pancreática exócrina.
• Concentrações séricas de cobalamina e folato para saber se há doença grave da mucosa.

DIAGNÓSTICO POR IMAGEM
• Ultrassonografia abdominal para diagnosticar massas gastrintestinais ou espessamento mural.
• Em alguns casos, pode ser necessária a realização de estudos contrastados para detectar algum padrão obstrutivo.
• Na melhor das hipóteses, a avaliação da motilidade intestinal não é uma tarefa fácil; no entanto, pode-se fazer uso de marcadores cintilográficos em algumas instituições de referência.

MÉTODOS DIAGNÓSTICOS
Amostras de biopsia gastrintestinal obtidas à cirurgia ou via endoscopia para detectar doença gastrintestinal infiltrativa.

TRATAMENTO

CUIDADO(S) DE SAÚDE ADEQUADO(S)
Ambulatoriais — tratar qualquer doença gastrintestinal subjacente.

CUIDADO(S) DE ENFERMAGEM
Nenhum.

ATIVIDADE
Incentivar um estilo de vida ativo — o exercício aumenta a motilidade GI, o que ajudará a expelir os flatos e aumentará a regularidade da defecação.

FLATULÊNCIA

DIETA
- Fornecer refeições em pequenas quantidades várias vezes ao dia em um ambiente isolado e tranquilo.
- Mudar a alimentação para uma de alta digestibilidade, com baixas concentrações de fibras e gordura (p. ex., Eukanuba Low Residue Formula, Hill's i/d Diet, Purina EN Formula, Royal Canin Low Fat Formula), ou refeições preparadas em casa contendo arroz branco cozido (cães) com frango sem pele ou queijo *cottage* (balanceadas com vitaminas e minerais) (nota: os gatos não precisam ser alimentados com carboidrato para um ensaio alimentar).
- Uma troca na fonte de proteína ou carboidrato ou a remoção dos aditivos beneficia alguns animais.
- Nos gatos, dietas ricas em proteínas ou pobres em carboidratos poderão ser benéficas se houver intolerância a carboidrato.

ORIENTAÇÃO AO PROPRIETÁRIO
Desestimular as imprudências na dieta (p. ex., ingestão de lixo ou coprofagia).

CONSIDERAÇÕES CIRÚRGICAS
Nenhuma.

MEDICAÇÕES

MEDICAMENTO(S) DE ESCOLHA
- Carminativos são medicações que aliviam a flatulência — não há estudos que demonstrem a segurança ou o benefício desses agentes em cães ou gatos.
- O acetato de zinco liga-se a compostos sulfidrílicos.
- *Yucca schidigera* liga-se à amônia e, por essa razão, é adicionada a rações como flavorizante.
- O carvão ativado seco absorve praticamente todos os gases odoríferos quando misturado diretamente com fezes e flatos humanos; no entanto, o número de eventos com flatos, o volume ou o odor do gás não diminuem nas pessoas.
- A inclusão de carvão ativado, *Y. schidigera* e acetato de zinco em um petisco reduziu a frequência de episódios altamente odoríferos em cães.
- O subsalicilato de bismuto (cães, 1 mL/kg VO inicialmente e, em seguida, 0,25 mL/kg a cada 6 h) adsorve sulfeto de hidrogênio e tem propriedades antibacterianas; contudo, múltiplas doses diárias a longo prazo dificultam sua praticidade. Não recomendado para uso em gatos em função do potencial de toxicidade pelo salicilato.
- A simeticona é um agente antiespumante que diminui a tensão superficial das bolhas de gás, conferindo a coalescência com maior facilidade e a liberação dos gases intestinais; entretanto, não há alteração na produção de gás.
- Suplementos de enzimas pancreáticas podem reduzir a flatulência em alguns pacientes com produção diminuída dessas enzimas.

CONTRAINDICAÇÕES
Evitar o subsalicilato de bismuto em gatos e em cães com ulceração gastroduodenal e distúrbios hemorrágicos.

PRECAUÇÕES
N/D.

INTERAÇÕES POSSÍVEIS
N/D.

MEDICAMENTO(S) ALTERNATIVO(S)
- Mais de 30 preparações à base de ervas e plantas estão disponíveis, mas a dosagem, a segurança e a eficácia são desconhecidas.
- Recentemente, o uso de probióticos para normalizar ou estabilizar o microambiente intestinal é defendido e, portanto, pode ser uma tentativa segura; entretanto, não foi conduzido nenhum estudo sobre a eficácia dessa abordagem.

ACOMPANHAMENTO

MONITORIZAÇÃO DO PACIENTE
Resposta à terapia.

PREVENÇÃO
- Evitar dietas ricas em oligossacarídeos não absorvíveis e fibras fermentáveis ou não fermentáveis.
- Evitar laticínios, alimentos deteriorados e modificações súbitas na alimentação.
- Não alimentar o animal logo após o exercício.
- O uso de probióticos para melhorar a flora bacteriana comensal pode ser benéfico se o desarranjo da flora for a principal causa da flatulência.

COMPLICAÇÕES POSSÍVEIS
Nenhuma.

EVOLUÇÃO ESPERADA E PROGNÓSTICO
N/D.

DIVERSOS

DISTÚRBIOS ASSOCIADOS
Doença gastrintestinal.

FATORES RELACIONADOS COM A IDADE
N/D.

POTENCIAL ZOONÓTICO
N/D.

GESTAÇÃO/FERTILIDADE/REPRODUÇÃO
N/D.

SINÔNIMO(S)
N/D.

VER TAMBÉM
- Campilobacteriose.
- Enteropatia Inflamatória.
- Insuficiência Pancreática Exócrina.
- Proliferação Bacteriana no Intestino Delgado.
- Salmonelose.
- Síndrome do Intestino Irritável.

ABREVIATURA(S)
- ELISA = ensaio imunoabsorvente ligado à enzima.
- GI = gastrintestinal.
- PCR = reação em cadeia da polimerase.

RECURSOS DA INTERNET
Rede de Informações Veterinárias: www.vin.com/VIN.plx.

Sugestões de Leitura
Davenport DJ, Remillard RL, Simpson KW, et al. Gastrointestinal and exocrine pancreatic disease. In: Hand MS, Thatcher CD, Remillard RL, et al., eds. Small Animal Clinical Nutrition, 4th ed. Topeka, KS: Mark Morris Institute, 2000, pp. 725-810.

Giffard CJ, Collins SB, Stoodley N, et al. Ability of an antiflatulence treat to reduce the hydrogen sulfide content of canine flatulence. Proceedings 18th ACVIM, 2000, p. 726.

Guilford WG. New ideas for management of gastrointestinal tract disease. J Small Anim Pract 1994, 35:620-624.

Matz ME. Flatulence. In: Ettinger SJ, Feldman EC, eds., Textbook of Veterinary Internal Medicine, 6th ed. St. Louis: Elsevier, 2005, pp. 148-149.

Roudebush P. Flatulence: What do we know about intestinal gas? Proceedings 19th ACVIM, 2001, pp. 592-594.

Autor Debra L. Zoran
Consultor Editorial Albert E. Jergens
Agradecimento O autor e os editores agradecem a colaboração prévia de Marc C. Walker e Randall C. Longshore, que foram os autores deste capítulo na edição anterior.

FLEBITE

CONSIDERAÇÕES GERAIS

DEFINIÇÃO
- Um processo inflamatório que envolve a túnica íntima da parede do endotélio vascular, geralmente associado a, e considerado como, uma complicação de terapia IV periférica.
- A tromboflebite implica a formação de coágulo de fibrina, podendo envolver a vasculatura superficial ou tecidos profundos.

FISIOPATOLOGIA
- A sensibilização do endotélio vascular provoca a liberação de substâncias vasoativas que causam vasoconstrição, aumentam a permeabilidade vascular, ativam os sistemas de coagulação e promovem a quimiotaxia de leucócitos.
- O extravasamento de proteínas e do plasma leva à formação de inchaço e edema.
- A formação trombótica obstrui o fluxo sanguíneo e pode causar espessamento palpável ou cordão vascular, o que pode evoluir para esclerose vascular irreversível.
- Os pirogênios liberados pelos leucócitos podem causar inflamação sistêmica e febre. Os exsudatos podem estar presentes no local de venopunção, especialmente em caso de colonização bacteriana.

SISTEMA(S) ACOMETIDO(S)
- Cutâneo — inflamação/infecção locais.
- Cardiovascular — alteração da permeabilidade vascular e do fluxo sanguíneo.
- Hematológico/Linfático/Imunológico — bactérias, mediadores inflamatórios e êmbolos podem provocar resposta inflamatória sistêmica e disfunção orgânica.
- Respiratório — tromboflebite venosa profunda pode causar embolia pulmonar.

INCIDÊNCIA/PREVALÊNCIA
- 20-80% dos pacientes hospitalizados que recebem terapia IV periférica.
- É mais comum uma tromboflebite superficial, mas 10-12% podem evoluir para trombose venosa profunda.

IDENTIFICAÇÃO
- Cães e gatos.
- Não há predisposição etária, racial ou sexual específica em medicina veterinária.
- Os pacientes neonatais e geriátricos podem ser predispostos em virtude da baixa função imunológica.

SINAIS CLÍNICOS
- No mínimo, há dois dos indicadores de inflamação local mencionados a seguir — eritema, dor, calor, inchaço e enrijecimento dos vasos.
- Pode haver drenagem ou exsudação em caso de infecção ou abscesso concomitante.
- O sinal de febre pode estar presente com infecção ou inflamação sistêmica associada.

CAUSAS
- Lesão mecânica — calibre/rigidez/integridade/duração do cateter IV, colocação traumática, venopunção prévia, altas velocidades de infusão de fluido.
- Lesão química — material do cateter IV, medicamentos, fluidos de extrema osmolalidade ou pH, nutrição parenteral, outras soluções vesicantes.
- Colonização bacteriana — técnica asséptica inadequada durante a colocação, cuidados insatisfatórios do cateter pós-colocação, sepse ou imunossupressão. São fontes comuns de bactérias: pontos de ruptura no sistema de infusão, micróbios da pele e microrganismos circulantes.
- Fluxo sanguíneo obstruído — cateter de amplo calibre, vasoconstrição, hipotensão, formação de trombo.

FATORES DE RISCO
- Duração da cateterização — incidência mais alta com cateteres que permanecem no local por mais de 72 horas.
- Tipos de infusado — cáustico, hiperosmolar, imunogênico e/ou bólus de grande volume.
- Tríade de Virchow — estado hipercoagulável, anormalidades do fluxo sanguíneo e dano à parede dos vasos predispõem o paciente à trombose.
- Características do paciente — obesidade, imobilidade, má qualidade das veias, imunodeficiência, trombofilia, policitemia ou hemoconcentração, doença cardíaca ou renal crônica, gestação.
- Características da doença — processo maligno, infecção, traumatismo, insuficiência respiratória ou circulatória.

DIAGNÓSTICO

DIAGNÓSTICO DIFERENCIAL
- Hipersensibilidade cutânea, vasculite, ou outra reação imunomediada.
- Infecção ou inflamação tecidual subcutânea ou intersticial.
- Lesão ou infecção prévia não relacionada no vaso ou no local de colocação do cateter IV.

HEMOGRAMA/BIOQUÍMICA/URINÁLISE
- As alterações do hemograma completo são compatíveis com o grau de resposta inflamatória sistêmica e o consumo de plaquetas.
- As alterações dos exames de bioquímica e urinálise podem ser aplicáveis em caso de dano a órgãos secundário à embolia (p. ex., lesão hepática, renal, portal, caval, cerebral, cardíaca, pulmonar).

OUTROS TESTES LABORATORIAIS
Testes de coagulação — podem ser observadas alterações nas mensurações de TP, TTP, D-dímero, antitrombina, proteína-C, tromboelastografia.

DIAGNÓSTICO POR IMAGEM
- Angiografia/flebografia — técnicas com padrão de excelência para o diagnóstico de embolia, apesar de invasivas; necessitam do uso de contraste e podem aumentar os fatores de risco do paciente.
- TC ou RM — permitem o diagnóstico de embolia tecidual profunda mediante suspeita com base no dano ou disfunção de órgãos.
- Ultrassonografia em modo-B, ultrassonografia duplex ou pletismografia — métodos mais recentes e menos invasivos de avaliação da patência (desobstrução) venosa, da característica dos vasos e do fluxo sanguíneo, mas com disponibilidade limitada.

MÉTODOS DIAGNÓSTICOS
- Doppler — exame barato para avaliação da patência venosa e do fluxo sanguíneo.
- Cultura da cânula intravenosa e drenagem do local (se presente) — as hemoculturas também podem ser indicadas com sinais de inflamação sistêmica.

ACHADOS PATOLÓGICOS
- Achados macroscópicos — estreitamento e espessamento vasculares, focais ou localmente extensos com inchaço e alteração de cor do tecido circunjacente. Pode haver a presença de trombos.
- Histopatologia — inchaço das células endoteliais, infiltração leucocítica da parede vascular com depósito de fibrina e formação de trombo.

TRATAMENTO

CUIDADO(S) DE SAÚDE ADEQUADO(S)
- Remover o(s) cateter(es) IV(s) dos locais acometidos o mais rápido possível. Iniciar antibioticoterapia adequada, terapia tópica e cuidados das feridas.
- Monitorizar o paciente quanto à ocorrência de reações anafiláticas e outras reações durante a infusão de produtos sanguíneos ou quaisquer medicamentos novos. Dor no local da inserção é frequentemente o primeiro indicador de flebite, infiltração ou extravasamento.
- Evitar a infusão de medicamentos ou soluções hiperosmolares com pH abaixo de 5 ou acima de 9 através de cânulas periféricas. Em caso de acesso venoso central, sempre se deve avaliar o retorno venoso antes de iniciar a infusão.
- Na suspeita de infiltração cáustica, interromper a infusão e deixar a cânula no local temporariamente para aspirar qualquer fluido remanescente no cateter e para instilar um antídoto específico no tecido acometido quando aplicável.
- Aplicar compressas úmidas e quentes intermitentes ou hidroterapia; algumas substâncias extravasadas podem necessitar de crioterapia.
- Para evitar estagnação do fluxo sanguíneo e ocorrência de tromboembolia, é fundamental garantir a ressuscitação volêmica sanguínea adequada e promover a mobilidade do paciente; considerar o uso de fisioterapia e/ou terapia compressiva.

CUIDADO(S) DE ENFERMAGEM
- Colocação de cateter IV — utilizar técnica asséptica rigorosa e curativo estéril. Com curativo de gazes, verificar o local a cada 48 horas para minimizar a manipulação durante a troca de bandagem; curativos semipermeáveis transparentes são os preferidos para permitir uma avaliação mais frequente dos locais de inserção do cateter. Pomadas ou géis antimicrobianos tópicos não diminuem a incidência de infecções relacionadas com o cateter, mas podem promover o desenvolvimento de microrganismos resistentes a antibióticos; portanto, não são recomendados. Evitar extremidades inferiores, articulações e nervos na escolha dos locais de inserção dos cateteres. Utilizar cateteres mais longos e de calibre menor sempre que possível; o material de poliuretano é preferível ao Teflon.
- Manutenção de cateter IV — as cânulas IV devem ser examinadas em termos de patência, integridade e inchaço associado a cada 1-2 horas com infusões contínuas. A incidência de flebite aumenta significativamente com cateteres periféricos que são mantidos no local por mais de 72 horas, mas não se altera de 72 a 96 horas. Trocar os cateteres periféricos a cada 3-4 dias ou em até 24 horas se colocados em uma situação de

FLEBITE

emergência. Não é recomendada a substituição de rotina de cateteres venosos centrais.

ATIVIDADE
- É recomendável a prática de atividade regular moderada para diminuir o risco de trombose.
- Realizar fisioterapia regularmente com foco sobre o membro acometido, sobretudo nos pacientes sem deambulação.

DIETA
- Suporte nutricional adequado ao tratamento de doença(s) subjacente(s).
- Considerar o uso de dieta não glicêmica e/ou controle glicêmico se houver sepse ou risco dessa infecção.

ORIENTAÇÃO AO PROPRIETÁRIO
- Orientar os proprietários sobre os riscos e as complicações de cateter IV, especialmente em pacientes com fatores predisponentes.
- Os proprietários devem ser treinados e manter a fisioterapia e os cuidados básicos de enfermagem em casa.

CONSIDERAÇÕES CIRÚRGICAS
- Os locais infectados e/ou o amplo dano tecidual advindos da colocação de cateter podem necessitar de debridamento cirúrgico e sutura tardia.
- Os procedimentos de ligadura cirúrgica ou denudação dos vasos cordados podem ser indicados para evitar trombose venosa profunda.

MEDICAÇÕES

MEDICAMENTO(S) DE ESCOLHA
- Antibióticos (na suspeita de infecção) — utilizar terapia empírica, com base no local da infecção (p. ex., cefalexina 20 mg/kg VO ou IV a cada 8 horas para pele) e nos potenciais contaminantes se os exames de cultura e antibiograma não estiverem disponíveis.
- AINE — p. ex., meloxicam na dose de 0,1-0,2 mg/kg VO ou SC pode melhorar significativamente a morbidade e o conforto do paciente.
- Heparina — considerar a terapia com heparina de baixo peso molecular para evitar o desenvolvimento de embolia. A heparinização do cateter intravenoso (100 U/mL) pode diminuir a incidência de embolia e prolongar o uso desse cateter.
- Terapia tópica — substâncias heparinoides, como polissulfato de mucopolissacarídeo (p. ex., Hirudoid®), têm ação anticoagulante, inibem a formação de trombo, estimulam a fibrinólise e podem ativar o fluxo sanguíneo local. Os heparinoides podem ser mais eficazes para o tratamento de flebite preexistente do que para a prevenção. Foi demonstrado que o creme de notoginseng, derivado da raiz de ginseng, seja eficaz na redução dos sinais de dor e eritema, bem como da formação de edema e cordão fibroso. Emplastros, cremes ou géis de nitroglicerina (os sprays não são eficazes) promovem vasodilatação local em até 10 minutos, duram 3-6 horas e são eficientes para prevenção e tratamento dos primeiros estágios de flebite. Os AINE tópicos, como gel de piroxicam ou diclofenaco, podem ajudar a aliviar os sinais clínicos e acelerar a resolução.

CONTRAINDICAÇÕES/INTERAÇÕES POSSÍVEIS
- Infusões ou agentes tópicos cáusticos, irritantes, ou imunogênicos.
- Uso de AINE com doses anti-inflamatórias ou imunossupressoras de corticoterapia concomitante.

PRECAUÇÕES
- Evitar o uso de AINE sistêmicos em caso de disfunção renal, hepática ou gastrintestinal.
- A menos que utilizados como um pré-tratamento adequado para quimioterapia, os corticosteroides são associados à cicatrização tardia da ferida e podem predispor à infecção.

INTERAÇÕES POSSÍVEIS
- AINE sistêmicos com inibição significativa de tromboxano (p. ex., salicilato) utilizados em combinação com heparina podem predispor à coagulopatia.
- Terapia vasopressora concomitante pode predispor à tromboflebite; é recomendável o uso de algum vasodilatador tópico.

MEDICAMENTO(S) ALTERNATIVO(S)
- Cremes tópicos para dermatite, como cremes à base de sulfadiazina de prata e calamina (p. ex., Calmoseptine®), podem ajudar a diminuir a irritação e evitar a infecção.
- Em caso de umidade excessiva ou extravasamento transdérmico de líquido, pode ser útil manter a pele seca com o uso de medicamento sob a forma de pó (p. ex., Gold Bond®). Não usar sobre solução de continuidade na pele.

ACOMPANHAMENTO

MONITORIZAÇÃO DO PACIENTE
- Vermelhidão, inchaço, dor ou calor persistentes ou progressivos — ajustar a antibioticoterapia com base nos resultados mais atuais da cultura e do antibiograma.
- Em caso de necrose tecidual, ocorrem enrijecimento, palidez, coloração negra ou formação de escara na pele.

PREVENÇÃO
- Evitar o uso de veias flebóticas para terapia IV ou coleta de sangue até que os vasos estejam completamente cicatrizados.
- Considerar o uso de filtros submícrons de cateter IV, que podem reduzir a incidência de flebite pela remoção de particulados, endotoxinas e outros mediadores solúveis de morbidade.

COMPLICAÇÕES POSSÍVEIS
- Necrose tecidual.
- Neurite ou perda de função.
- Linfangite.
- Septicemia.
- Extensão para o sistema venoso profundo.

EVOLUÇÃO ESPERADA E PROGNÓSTICO
- A maioria dos casos é leve e autolimitante depois de 1-3 dias com a remoção do cateter. O prognóstico é bom, embora a patência vascular comumente seja comprometida.
- As lesões locais graves podem levar 3-4 semanas para desaparecer, podendo resultar em perda de função ou dano tecidual permanente.
- O prognóstico é reservado em caso de flebite associada à tromboembolia pulmonar e/ou sepse.

DIVERSOS

DISTÚRBIOS ASSOCIADOS
- Tromboembolia pulmonar.
- Infecção/celulite/sepse.

FATORES RELACIONADOS COM A IDADE
- Pacientes neonatais e geriátricos podem ser predispostos à infecção.
- Pacientes geriátricos podem apresentar má cicatrização de feridas.

GESTAÇÃO/FERTILIDADE/REPRODUÇÃO
- A gestação pode predispor à tromboembolia.
- A incidência de complicações fetais com flebite é desconhecida.

SINÔNIMOS
- Tromboflebite.
- Extravasamento/infiltração.
- Vasculite.

VER TAMBÉM
- Tromboembolia Pulmonar.
- Sepse e Bacteremia.

ABREVIATURAS
- AINE = anti-inflamatório não esteroide.
- RM = ressonância magnética.
- TC = tomografia computadorizada.
- TP = tempo de protrombina.
- TTP = tempo de tromboplastina parcial.

RECURSOS DA INTERNET
- http://emedicine.medscape.com/article/463256-overview.
- www.emedicinehealth.com/phlebitis/article_em.htm.
- www.patient.co.uk/health/Phlebitis.htm.

Sugestões de Leitura
Cesarone MR, et al. Management of superficial vein thrombosis and thrombophlebitis: Status and expert opinion. Angiology 2007, 58 Suppl 1:7S-15S.
Diniz dos Reis PE, et al. Pharmacological interventions to treat phlebitis, systematic review. J Infus Nurs 2009, 32(2):74-79.
Marino PL. The ICU Book, 3rd ed. Baltimore: Williams & Wilkins, 2007, pp. 130-145.
Webster J, et al. Routine care of peripheral intravenous catheters versus clinically indicated replacement: Randomised controlled trial. BMJ 2008, 337:a339.

Autor Kathryn M. Long
Consultor Editorial Larry P. Tilley e Francis W.K. Smith, Jr.

Fobias a Trovões e Relâmpagos

CONSIDERAÇÕES GERAIS

REVISÃO
A fobia a trovões e relâmpagos é um distúrbio caracterizado por medo persistente e exagerado a tempestades ou aos estímulos associados a elas. A fisiopatologia envolve componentes fisiológicos, emocionais e comportamentais.

SISTEMA(S) ACOMETIDO(S)
• Comportamental — tentativas de fuga ou escape. • Cardiovascular — taquicardia. • Endócrino/metabólico — aumento nos níveis de cortisol, hiperglicemia induzida por estresse. • Gastrintestinal — inapetência, desarranjo gastrintestinal. • Musculosquelético — traumatismo autoinduzido resultante das tentativas de escape. • Nervoso — estimulação adrenérgica/noradrenérgica excessiva. • Respiratório — taquipneia. • Cutâneo/exócrino — dermatite acral por lambedura.

IDENTIFICAÇÃO
• Ocorre tanto em cães como em gatos, mas a primeira espécie aparece com maior frequência nas consultas. • A distribuição quanto ao sexo e ao estado de castração é uniforme nos cães acometidos. • Pode acometer qualquer raça. Em um estudo, as fobias a trovões e relâmpagos eram mais prevalentes entre as raças de pastoreio. • Há suspeitas de predisposição genética. • Os cães podem começar a exibir os sinais ainda quando filhotes, mas podem não ser levados à consulta até a idade adulta.

SINAIS CLÍNICOS
Achados Anamnésicos
• Durante as tempestades, observa-se a ocorrência de um ou mais dos sinais clínicos expostos a seguir: respiração ofegante, marcha estereotipada, tremores, permanência próxima ao proprietário, busca de esconderijos, salivação, comportamento destrutivo, vocalização excessiva, traumatismo autoinfligido e evacuação/micção inapropriadas.
• Os estímulos indutores do medo incluem chuva, relâmpago, trovão, temporais fortes e, possivelmente, mudanças na pressão barométrica e na eletricidade estática.

Achados do Exame Físico
Não são dignos de nota exceto em casos de lesões autoinfligidas.

CAUSAS E FATORES DE RISCO
A causa exata não é conhecida, mas pode envolver combinações dos fatores expostos a seguir: • Falta de exposição a tempestades na fase precoce do desenvolvimento. • Reforço não intencional de resposta ao medo por parte do proprietário. • Experiência altamente aversiva, como exposição a temporais violentos. • Predisposição genética a reações emocionais.

DIAGNÓSTICO

DIAGNÓSTICO DIFERENCIAL
• As condições indutoras de respostas comportamentais semelhantes incluem ansiedade causada por separação, frustração gerada por obstáculos e fobias a ruídos. • As afecções clínicas indutoras de sinais clínicos similares compreendem distúrbios metabólicos, cardíacos, neurológicos, dermatológicos e gastrintestinais ou qualquer condição desencadeadora de dor ou desconforto.

HEMOGRAMA/BIOQUÍMICA/URINÁLISE
Os resultados devem permanecer dentro dos limites de normalidade.

OUTROS TESTES LABORATORIAIS
Podem ser indicados os testes das funções tireóidea ou adrenal.

DIAGNÓSTICO POR IMAGEM
Radiografias para ajudar a identificar as fontes de dor.

MÉTODOS DIAGNÓSTICOS
• Eletrocardiograma para detectar anormalidades de condução cardíaca. • Biopsias cutâneas na suspeita de dermatopatias primárias.

TRATAMENTO

AMBIENTE
Evitar o confinamento em engradados se houver risco de lesão.

MUDANÇA COMPORTAMENTAL
• Não se deve punir nem tentar confortar o animal durante as tempestades. • Com frequência, empregam-se a dessensibilização e o contracondicionamento associados. • A dessensibilização envolve a exposição ao estímulo gravado em um volume que não induza ao medo. O volume será gradativamente aumentado apenas se o animal permanecer tranquilo. • O contracondicionamento envolve o adestramento de uma resposta (sentar, relaxar) incompatível com a reação de medo. As recompensas alimentares são frequentemente utilizadas para facilitar o aprendizado. • As gravações de tempestades em áudio estão disponíveis no mercado. Com exceção dos ruídos de tempestades, a reprodução dos estímulos naturais que ocorrem durante os temporais não é uma tarefa fácil. • O emprego inapropriado desses adestramentos pode agravar a condição. • Tais adestramentos serão ineficazes em animais irresponsivos aos ruídos gravados de tempestades.

MEDICAÇÕES

MEDICAMENTO(S) DE ESCOLHA
• O uso de medicamentos nessa condição está fora da indicação recomendada no rótulo. • As azapironas, os antidepressivos tricíclicos (ATC) e os inibidores seletivos de recaptação da serotonina (ISRS) necessitam de 2-4 semanas para fazer efeito e devem ser administrados diariamente durante a estação chuvosa para controlar a ansiedade. Tais agentes terapêuticos podem ser utilizados em combinação com os benzodiazepínicos de ação rápida.

Benzodiazepínicos
• Medicamentos de eleição. • Empregados para o controle imediato (a curto prazo) da ansiedade. • Alprazolam — cães: 0,02-0,1 mg/kg VO a cada 4-12 h. • Clonazepam — cães: 0,1-0,5 mg/kg a cada 12 h. • Diazepam — cães: 0,5-1 mg/kg VO a cada 4-12 h.

Azapironas
• Buspirona — cães: 0,5-2,0 mg/kg VO a cada 8-12 h; gatos: 2,5-7,5 mg/gato VO a cada 12 h.

Inibidores Seletivos de Recaptação da Serotonina
• Fluoxetina — cães: 1 mg/kg VO a cada 24 h; gatos: 0,5-1 mg/kg VO a cada 24 h. • Paroxetina — cães: 1 mg/kg VO a cada 24 h; gatos: 0,5-1 mg/kg VO a cada 24 h. • Efeitos colaterais: inapetência e irritabilidade.

Antidepressivos Tricíclicos (ATCs)
• Amitriptilina — cães: 1-3 mg/kg VO a cada 12 h; gatos: 0,5-2 mg/kg VO a cada 24 h.
• Clomipramina — cães: 2 mg/kg VO a cada 12 h; gatos: 2,5-5 mg/gato VO a cada 24 h. • Efeitos colaterais: sedação, efeitos GI e anticolinérgicos, além de distúrbios da condução cardíaca.

Tranquilizantes Fenotiazínicos
• Acepromazina — cães: 0,1-1 mg/kg VO a cada 6-8 h. • Propriedades ansiolíticas insatisfatórias.
• Utilizar **apenas** quando houver a necessidade de contenção química para evitar lesões.

CONTRAINDICAÇÕES/INTERAÇÕES POSSÍVEIS
• É preciso ter cautela com o uso de benzodiazepínicos em cães agressivos e gatos — em virtude da possibilidade de desinibição da agressão. • Evitar o emprego de ATC e fenotiazínicos em machos reprodutores e pacientes com distúrbios convulsivos, cardiopatia, diabetes melito, glaucoma ou doença da tireoide.
• Diminuir a dose ou evitar o uso desses medicamentos em pacientes geriátricos e animais hepatopatas ou nefropatas. • Jamais se deve associar o uso de ATC, ISRS e fenotiazínicos com os inibidores da monoamina oxidase.

ACOMPANHAMENTO

MONITORIZAÇÃO DO PACIENTE
Com o uso de medicamentos, é aconselhável a monitorização periódica do paciente com hemogramas completos e perfis bioquímicos.

PREVENÇÃO
• Os filhotes de cães e de gatos devem ser expostos a diversos estímulos sob condições favoráveis.
• Ignorar os sinais leves de ansiedade durante as tempestades para evitar o reforço desses comportamentos.

COMPLICAÇÕES POSSÍVEIS
Lesões graves e danos a propriedades.

EVOLUÇÃO ESPERADA E PROGNÓSTICO
O prognóstico depende da gravidade, da duração e da possibilidade de prevenção das lesões. Se a condição não for tratada, sua evolução será provável.

DIVERSOS

GESTAÇÃO/FERTILIDADE/REPRODUÇÃO
N/D.

ABREVIATURA(S)
• ATC = antidepressivo tricíclico. • GI = gastrintestinal. • ISRS = inibidor seletivo de recaptação da serotonina.

Autor Lynne M. Seibert
Consultor Editorial Debra F. Horwitz

FOBIAS, MEDO E ANSIEDADE — CÃES

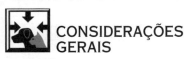

CONSIDERAÇÕES GERAIS

DEFINIÇÃO

Medo
Uma emoção que consiste em uma resposta psicológica e fisiológica (i. e., resposta ao estresse) à presença de algum estímulo perigoso (p. ex., pessoa, animal, situação, som, objeto), induzindo a uma reação de adaptação e esquivamento.

Fobias
- Um medo acentuado, irracional e excessivo de algum estímulo (p. ex., animal, situação, pessoa, som, objeto). Tal medo consiste em uma resposta fisiológica e psicológica, que resulta em uma reação mal-adaptativa.
- Muito comum — ruídos (p. ex., trovões, relâmpagos ou fogos de artifício).

Ansiedade
Reação que consiste em uma resposta fisiológica e psicológica, deflagrada pela antecipação de perigo futuro ou memória de perigos passados. Não há necessidade que o estímulo esteja presente para provocar a resposta.

FISIOPATOLOGIA
- As informações sobre um estímulo indutor de medo são conduzidas dos órgãos sensoriais até o núcleo central (NC) da amígdala. O NC envia estímulos para a substância cinzenta central (resposta musculoesquelética), o hipotálamo lateral (resposta do SNA) e a estria terminal (resposta hormonal), montando uma resposta de estresse fisiológico.
- A resposta de estresse fisiológico é graduada com base no nível percebido de controle pelo animal e no nível percebido de dificuldade.
- Qualquer estímulo neutro no ambiente pode ser pareado com a resposta de estresse fisiológico até que o estímulo cause uma resposta fisiológica.
- Certos hormônios do estresse aumentam o aprendizado, a consolidação da memória e a recuperação.
- Há provas de que, embora as memórias de pavor e espanto possam ser significativamente reduzidas, elas não podem ser "apagadas".

SISTEMA(S) ACOMETIDO(S)
- Comportamental — imobilidade, inquietação, marcha compassada, andar em círculo, fixação/afeição excessiva, escape, esquivamento, postura defensiva, comportamento destrutivo, vocalização, agressividade.
- Cardiovascular — taquicardia.
- Endócrino/metabólico — alterações no eixo HPA, aumento da glicose sanguínea.
- Gastrintestinal — inapetência, hipersalivação, vômito, diarreia, defecação.
- Hematológico/linfático/imune — leucograma de estresse.
- Musculoesquelético — lesões autoinfligidas.
- Neuromuscular — aumento da atividade motora, tremores, percepção diminuída à dor, catatonia.
- Oftálmico — congestão episcleral, midríase.
- Renal/urológico — micção.
- Respiratório — taquipneia.
- Pele/exócrino — lesão traumática, granuloma acral por lambedura.

GENÉTICA
A hereditariedade influencia o desenvolvimento de medos e fobias, embora não esteja claro até que ponto os medos específicos (p. ex., ruídos) sejam hereditários.

INCIDÊNCIA/PREVALÊNCIA
Desconhecidas para medos, ansiedades e fobias como um grupo.

IDENTIFICAÇÃO
Nenhuma idade, raça ou sexo é super-representada. Medos/ansiedades/fobias podem se desenvolver em qualquer idade.

SINAIS CLÍNICOS

Comentários Gerais
Vigilância demasiada, despertar do SNA, catatonia, aumento da atividade motora, eliminação, destruição, vocalização excessiva, hipersalivação, respiração ofegante, busca por esconderijos, tremores, comportamentos de escape, linguagem corporal de medo.

Achados Anamnésicos
Experiência traumática, socialização inadequada, mãe medrosa/ansiosa, histórico de impossibilidade de escape a algum estímulo (p. ex., preso em uma caixa ou engradado) ou exposição enquanto se encontra sozinho.

Achados do Exame Físico
Geralmente não são dignos de nota; é possível a observação de lesões autoinfligidas.

CAUSAS
- Socialização inadequada, evento traumático, hereditariedade, síndrome de disfunção cognitiva, aprendizado prévio.
- Doenças ou condições físicas dolorosas podem aumentar a ansiedade e contribuir para o desenvolvimento de medos, fobias e ansiedades.

FATORES DE RISCO
Gerais — medos, ansiedades e fobias existentes; socialização inadequada, realojamento, mãe ansiosa/medrosa/fisicamente doente, evento traumático — especialmente quando o animal está sozinho.

DIAGNÓSTICO

DIAGNÓSTICO DIFERENCIAL
- Transtornos comportamentais — síndrome de disfunção cognitiva, comportamento indisciplinado, adestramento domiciliar incompleto, marcação com urina/fezes, comportamento de busca por atenção, falta de estimulação, comportamento territorial.
- Distúrbios médicos — neoplasia (p. ex., massa intracraniana), endocrinopatia (p. ex., encefalopatia hepática, diabetes, hipotireoidismo), cistite, pielonefrite, diabetes, doença gastrintestinal (p. ex., colite, parasitas, alergias alimentares, enteropatia inflamatória, síndrome do intestino irritável), doença neurológica (p. ex., crises convulsivas, neurite), problemas de pele (p. ex., dermatite acral por lambedura, atopia, dermatite alérgica à pulga, alergias alimentares), toxicidade (p. ex., chumbo, medicamentos recreativos).

HEMOGRAMA/BIOQUÍMICA/URINÁLISE
- Devem permanecer normais.
- Fazer antes de iniciar o tratamento medicamentoso.

OUTROS TESTES LABORATORIAIS
- T_4, T_4 livre — realizar antes de iniciar o tratamento medicamentoso.
- Provas de função da adrenal.

DIAGNÓSTICO POR IMAGEM
TC ou RM para descartar distúrbios cerebrais estruturais. Lançar mão de outras técnicas de diagnóstico por imagem, conforme a necessidade, para diagnosticar e tratar distúrbios médicos subjacentes.

MÉTODOS DIAGNÓSTICOS
- Anamnese e observação minuciosas do paciente (é útil filmar o comportamento).
- Fazer a triagem de pacientes quanto à presença de agressividade.
- Exposição ao estímulo se essa medida for segura.
- Procedimentos diagnósticos adequados para avaliar qualquer problema médico concomitante.

TRATAMENTO

CUIDADO(S) DE SAÚDE ADEQUADO(S)
- Tipicamente ambulatorial.
- Internação (pensões ou estabelecimentos de cuidados diários) — quando não se consegue evitar o estímulo indutor de medo/ansiedade/fobia e se o paciente estiver causando lesões autoinfligidas ou ainda se os medicamentos ansiolíticos não se mostrarem eficazes.
- O tratamento deve incluir orientação do proprietário, medidas de segurança, modificação do comportamento, alteração do ambiente e diminuição da ansiedade.
- Diagnosticar e tratar qualquer problema médico que possa causar dor, desconforto ou alterações de humor, bem como quaisquer lesões.

Segurança
- Proprietários — não devem manipular fisicamente o paciente quando ele estiver assustado ou buscando se esconder, pois isso pode resultar em agressividade. Em vez disso, tente distrair o cão com alimento ou brinquedo.
- Paciente — se houver tentativas intensas de escape ou lesões autoinfligidas, evite colocar o animal em engradados e limite o acesso do cão a janelas, portas, fios de eletricidade e canos de água. Considerar a acomodação do animal em pensões de cuidados diários.
- Público — se o cão tiver exibido um comportamento agressivo em casos de medo e ansiedade, o proprietário deverá evitar situações provocativas e utilizar dispositivos de controle adequados (p. ex., coleiras do tipo Gentle Leader ou Halti, focinheira em cesta).

Modificação do Comportamento
- Evitar o estímulo por 2-8 semanas, dependendo da gravidade da reação, ao mesmo tempo em que se ensinam habilidades de enfrentamento ao paciente (p. ex., sentar, observar, olhar, relaxar) e se estabelece uma zona de segurança.
- Interações estruturadas com o proprietário (p. ex., sentar para todas as interações).
- Exercícios de independência — sentar ou permanecer em estação com um brinquedo comestível.
- A punição (p. ex., correção com coleira de choque, grito, pancada) é contraindicada.
- Os proprietários devem evitar mimar o cão, mas sim distraí-lo e redirecioná-lo a brincadeiras ou

Fobias, Medo e Ansiedade — Cães

brinquedos comestíveis em situações de medo ou ansiedade.
- Dessensibilização e contracondicionamento — iniciar depois de ensinar as ferramentas de enfrentamento. A dessensibilização e o contracondicionamento devem ser tentados com supervisão, pois tais medidas podem sensibilizar o animal ao estímulo, fazendo com que o comportamento piore.

Modificação do Ambiente
- Criar um local seguro onde a exposição ao estímulo indutor do medo possa ser limitada.
- Considerar o estabelecimento em pensões de cuidados diários.
- Limitar o uso de caixas ou engradados a menos que o cão seja adestrado para isso, saia facilmente deles e não entre em pânico quando confinado.
- Aumentar a atividade física.
- Alternar os brinquedos.

ORIENTAÇÃO AO PROPRIETÁRIO
- Orientar os proprietários sobre o fato de que o paciente não é rancoroso/vingativo nem culpado; as fobias podem exigir um curso terapêutico prolongado; muito provavelmente, elas serão controladas, mas não curadas.
- Ajudar o proprietário a compreender a sutileza dos sinais envolvidos e aprender a reconhecer os sinais físicos associados à resposta de estresse fisiológico.

MEDICAÇÕES

MEDICAMENTO(S) DE ESCOLHA
- Sempre devem ser prescritos com um plano terapêutico completo, compatível com o padrão de cuidado.
- Grande parte dos tratamentos será a longo prazo, possivelmente por anos; o tratamento mínimo é, em geral, de 6 meses, com modificação comportamental concomitante. Se o cão tiver melhorado significativamente em 6 meses, tentar retardar o desmame, reduzindo a dose em 25-50% a cada 14 dias.
- Se o estímulo for previsível, fica indicado um medicamento leve (p. ex., benzodiazepínico, inibidor/antagonista da recaptação de serotonina), dependendo da situação e conforme a necessidade.
  - O medicamento será mais eficiente se administrado antes de quaisquer sinais de ansiedade, medo ou pânico; deve ser administrado por no mínimo 30-90 min antes do estímulo provocativo previsto.
  - Benzodiazepínicos:
    - Diazepam 0,50-2,2 mg/kg VO até a cada 4 h.
    - Clorazepato 0,50-2,2 mg/kg VO até a cada 4 h.
    - Alprazolam 0,01-0,1 mg/kg VO até a cada 4 h.
  - Inibidor/antagonista da recaptação de serotonina:
    - Trazodona 2,0-8,0 mg/kg VO até a cada 8 h.
  - Para estímulo generalizado inevitável ou grave — fica indicada a administração diária do medicamento.
  - Inibidores seletivos de recpatação da serotonina e antidepressivos tricíclicos. Ambas as classes de medicamentos podem levar até 6 semanas para fazer efeito. Para ambas, os pacientes devem ser iniciados com a dose baixa da faixa posológica e, depois, lentamente submetidos a incrementos em 2 a 4 semanas, com base na resposta para evitar os efeitos colaterais.
    - ATC:
      - Clomipramina 1,0-3,0 mg/kg VO a cada 12 h.
    - ISRS:
      - Sertralina 1,0-3,0 mg/kg VO a cada 24 h.
      - Fluoxetina 0,5-2,0 mg/kg VO a cada 24 h.

PRECAUÇÕES
- Todos os medicamentos listados são usados fora da indicação da bula, exceto a clomipramina (Clomicalm®) e fluoxetina (Reconcile®) para o tratamento de ansiedade da separação em cães nos Estados Unidos — seguir as recomendações do Health and Human Services.
- Anomalias da condução cardíaca — ter cuidado e monitorizar o paciente durante a administração de ATCs.
- Tomar cuidado ao prescrever medicamentos a pacientes geriátricos ou àqueles com comprometimento hepático ou renal — rever o metabolismo e a eliminação do medicamento em compêndios antes de prescrevê-lo.
- Os proprietários devem receber informações sobre os medicamentos, incluindo os efeitos colaterais potenciais.
- A maioria dos medicamentos modificadores do humor tem o potencial de aumentar a agitação, o medo e a agressividade.

INTERAÇÕES POSSÍVEIS
- Ter cuidado ao prescrever diversos medicamentos ao mesmo tempo com o mesmo modo de ação. Rever a bula de cada medicamento antes de prescrevê-lo.
- Não utilizar IARS, ISRS ou ATC com inibidores da MAO, incluindo, mas não se limitando a, selegilina, coleiras preventivas e imersões de amitraz.
- Não usar ISRS e ATC em combinação — possível risco de síndrome serotoninérgica, o que pode ser fatal.

MEDICAMENTO(S) ALTERNATIVO(S)
- Suplementos:
  - Anxitane® — conforme instrução da bula.
  - Novifit® — conforme instrução da bula.
  - Melatonina — <5 kg → 1,0 mg; 5-12 kg → 1,5 mg; >12 kg → 3,0-6,0 mg.

ACOMPANHAMENTO

MONITORIZAÇÃO DO PACIENTE
- Os proprietários deverão entrar em contato com o veterinário em intervalos de 2 semanas nas primeiras 6-8 semanas de tratamento. Tipicamente, o plano terapêutico terá de ser alterado.
- Hemograma completo, bioquímica, urinálise, T_4 e T_4 livre — a cada 12 meses para animais com <8 anos de idade sob medicamentos administrados diariamente; a cada 6 meses para cães com >8 anos de idade.

COMPLICAÇÕES POSSÍVEIS
Se o animal não for deixado sem tratamento ou tratado apenas com medicações, será provável a evolução desses distúrbios.

EVOLUÇÃO ESPERADA E PROGNÓSTICO
- O curso terapêutico dependerá da resposta à medicação, da adequação do ambiente e da capacidade do proprietário em efetuar a modificação comportamental.
- A duração do tratamento varia de 2 a 12 meses, dependendo da gravidade e do número de problemas. Pode-se esperar a possibilidade de desmame (retirada) da medicação apenas nos cães responsivos às modificações comportamental e ambiental.
- Tipicamente, o tratamento prosseguirá até certo ponto durante a vida do animal.

DIVERSOS

FATORES RELACIONADOS COM A IDADE
A disfunção cognitiva precoce pode se apresentar como um medo inespecífico.

GESTAÇÃO/FERTILIDADE/REPRODUÇÃO
A maioria dos medicamentos citados não foi avaliada ou está contraindicada em animais prenhes.

SINÔNIMO(S)
- Ansiedade generalizada.
- Neofobia.
- Ansiedade específica.

ABREVIATURA(S)
- ATC = antidepressivo tricíclico.
- HHA = eixo hipotálamo-hipófise-adrenal.
- ISRS = inibidor seletivo da recaptação de serotonina.
- IARS = inibidor/antagonista da recaptação de serotonina.
- MAO = monoamina oxidase.
- NC = núcleo central.
- RM = ressonância magnética.
- SNA = sistema nervoso autônomo.
- TC = tomografia computadorizada.
- T_4 = tiroxina.

RECURSOS DA INTERNET
- American College of Veterinary Behaviorists: www.dacvb.org.
- American Veterinary Society of Animal Behavior: www.avsabonline.org.

Sugestões de Leitura
Horwitz D, Mills D, Heath S, eds. BSAVA Manual of Canine and Feline Behavioural Medicine. Gloucestershire, UK: BSAVA, 2002.
King J, Simpson B, Overall KL, et al. Treatment of separation anxiety in dogs with clomipramine: Results from a prospective, randomized, double-blinded, placebo-controlled clinical trial. Appl Anim Beh Sci 2000, 67:255-275.
Landsberg G, Hunthausen W, Ackerman L. Handbook of Behavior Problems of the Dog and Cat, 2nd ed. Philadelphia: Elsevier Saunders, 2003.
Sherman BL, Mills DS. Canine anxieties and phobias: An update on separation anxiety and noise aversions. Vet Clin North Am Small Anim Pract 2008, 38:1081-1106.
Sherman B, Landsberg GM, Reisner I, et al. Effects of Reconcile (fluoxetine) chewable tablets plus behavior management for canine separation anxiety. Vet Therapeutics 2007, 8:18-31.

Autor Lisa Radosta
Consultor Editorial Debra F. Horwitz

Fobias, Medo e Ansiedade — Gatos

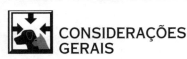

CONSIDERAÇÕES GERAIS

DEFINIÇÃO
• Medo é a sensação de apreensão que resulta da proximidade de alguma situação ou objeto que represente uma ameaça externa. A resposta do sistema nervoso autônomo prepara o corpo para "se eriçar, lutar ou fugir". Como tal, trata-se de um comportamento normal, essencial para a adaptação e sobrevida. • Ansiedade é a antecipação de perigos de origem desconhecida ou imaginária que culmina em reações fisiológicas associadas ao medo. Pode ocorrer ansiedade diante de algum evento amedrontador ou como resultado de modificações que não estejam não relacionadas com o ambiente e sejam imprevisíveis. • Fobia é um medo persistente e demasiado de algum estímulo específico, como uma tempestade ou a separação de alguém ou algo querido.

FISIOPATOLOGIA
• As respostas ao estresse tornam-se problemáticas quando o indivíduo não é capaz de controlar a situação estressante por suas próprias ações ou escapar dela por meio de respostas comportamentais adequadas.
• A ansiedade ou o medo crônicos podem gerar problemas secundários de comportamento, como se lamber demais, urinar em jato ou agredir outros gatos ou, então, predispor o gato a problemas de saúde em função de um sistema imune comprometido.

SISTEMA(S) ACOMETIDO(S)
• Comportamental — excesso de vigilância, evita comportamentos, possível agressão quando se tenta manusear ou conter o animal.
• Cardiovascular — aumento da frequência cardíaca e do fluxo sanguíneo para órgãos internos durante incidentes que causem medo.
• Endócrino/metabólico — liberação de glicose na corrente sanguínea, liberação de glicocorticoides.
• Gastrintestinal — queda do apetite.
• Hematológico/linfático/imune — efeitos do estresse crônico sobre a função imunológica.
• Musculosquelético — perda de peso com o tempo como resposta aos efeitos do estresse crônico sobre o apetite, além de consumo alimentar reduzido devido ao comportamento de se esconder.
• Neuromuscular — pode-se observar uma redução na atividade, porque o animal evita contato e se esconde. Reações de medo e ansiedade também podem incluir andar compassado, tremores e atividade repetitiva.
• Oftálmico — pupilas dilatadas (midríase) em resposta à estimulação do sistema nervoso autônomo.
• Respiratório — aumento da frequência respiratória quando o animal está ansioso ou disposto a lutar.
• Pele/exócrino — pode mostrar sinais de problemas secundários de comportamento, como se lamber excessivamente.

GENÉTICA
Componente genético desconhecido, mas possível. A raça, a coloração da pelagem e a personalidade paterna estão ligadas a traços individuais de personalidade nos gatos.

IDENTIFICAÇÃO
Qualquer idade, sexo ou raça.

SINAIS CLÍNICOS
Comentários Gerais
• Os sinais de medo ou ansiedade podem variar entre os indivíduos e de acordo com diferentes estímulos.
• Nos casos leves de ansiedade ou medo, o gato pode ficar tenso e mais reativo aos estímulos do ambiente. Alguns animais podem se retirar para lugares de esconderijo considerados seguros. No outro extremo, os gatos em pânico podem ficar muito agressivos ou destrutivos em suas tentativas de fugir daquilo que temem.
• Os estímulos que deflagram respostas ansiosas ou medrosas podem ser muito específicos (um indivíduo, situação ou ruído específico) ou mais generalizados.

Achados Anamnésicos
• Obter uma descrição clara da linguagem corporal e do comportamento do gato, bem como de quaisquer eventos ou situações que sempre desencadeiam ansiedade ou medo. As informações acerca de fatores desencadeantes específicos associados ao comportamento ansioso ou medroso podem ser úteis para estabelecer um programa de modificação comportamental e ambiental.
• Posturas corporais associadas ao comportamento medroso incluem orelhas para trás ou para o lado da cabeça, corpo abaixado em repouso ou movimento, cabeça baixa, cauda dobrada ao longo do corpo ou abaixada, piloereção, silhueta de "gato de Halloween".
• As pupilas costumam estar dilatadas; além disso, o gato pode estar ofegante, sacudindo-se, babando ou trocando os pelos.
• Se estiver com muito medo, o gato pode perder o controle vesicointestinal e espremer as glândulas adanais.
• As vocalizações costumam ser mínimas a menos que o gato mostre comportamento defensivo em resposta a uma ameaça percebida.
• O gato pode caminhar compassado, vocalizar e solicitar atenção do proprietário.
• Micção em jato e comportamento destrutivo de arranhadura podem ser observados em gatos ansiosos.
• Os detalhes da vida pregressa do gato, se conhecidos, podem indicar antecedentes de pouca socialização e exposição ao ambiente ou apontar possíveis influências genéticas, como pais ariscos ou ancestrais ferozes.

Achados do Exame Físico
Em geral, não são dignos de nota a menos que o gato se machuque tentando escapar ou procurando um abrigo ao fugir.

CAUSAS E FATORES DE RISCO
O comportamento medroso em gatos pode estar relacionado com os seguintes fatores:
• Influências genéticas sobre o temperamento.
• Experiência prévia e socialização, além de aprendizado por observação de mãe medrosa e outros gatos adultos.
• Aprendizado tardio por meio de experiências negativas.
• Estresse social, pressão populacional.

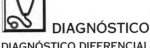

DIAGNÓSTICO

DIAGNÓSTICO DIFERENCIAL
Nos casos em que os gatos mostram um afastamento social súbito ou uma resistência mais generalizada a serem manuseados, a anamnese e o exame físico completos ajudam a delinear as causas físicas de um problema de comportamento.

HEMOGRAMA/BIOQUÍMICA/URINÁLISE
Os exames laboratoriais podem ser indicados pela informação obtida à anamnese e ao exame físico ou como uma triagem pré-medicação.

OUTROS TESTES LABORATORIAIS
Conforme indicação na suspeita de causas físicas.

DIAGNÓSTICO POR IMAGEM
As técnicas de diagnóstico por imagem poderão ser indicadas se a anamnese, o exame físico e os exames laboratoriais forem fortemente sugestivos de alguma causa orgânica para o comportamento do gato.

TRATAMENTO

ATIVIDADE
Estimular interações normais com os proprietários, embora o contato/comportamento contínuo não devam ser forçados.

DIETA
• Rotina alimentar normal.
• Talvez haja necessidade de mudar o local dos comedouros/bebedouros e das bandejas sanitárias (caixas de areia) se o comportamento ansioso ou medroso estiver restringindo o acesso.

ORIENTAÇÃO AO PROPRIETÁRIO
Comentários Gerais
• Discutir as expectativas de comportamento. As expectativas do proprietário em relação às interações sociais com ele(a) ou com outros gatos podem estar contribuindo para o problema e influenciar o prognóstico.
• Um plano terapêutico razoável envolvendo modificações comportamentais adaptadas ao caso e ajustes ambientais, bem como informações complementares como apostilas, folhetos ou artigos, ajudarão o proprietário a compreender melhor a situação e implementar o tratamento.

Terapia Comportamental
• Identificar o estímulo específico que provoca o comportamento de medo ou ansiedade.
• Evitar a exposição a estímulos que causam medo, se possível. Dar oportunidades para o próprio gato contornar a situação, observando as preferências dele por "esconderijos" e fornecendo-lhe um "lugar seguro" para se esconder, caso não consiga evitar a situação.
• Se o gato tiver de ser manipulado enquanto está com medo, é preciso ter cuidado e utilizar contenções físicas (mordaças, sacolas) para evitar lesões tanto no gato como na equipe veterinária.
• Dessensibilização e contracondicionamento para ajudar a diminuir a reatividade ao estímulo indutor do medo. A dessensibilização sistemática é um programa de exposição lentamente progressiva ao objeto ou situação que o gato teme. O contracondicionamento consiste em melhorar um ambiente interno e externo para se contrapor ao que causa medo, o que, em geral, é conseguido por meio de recompensas alimentares ou outros estímulos prazerosos, como brinquedos. Ver a lista de "Sugestões de Leitura" em busca de referências que forneçam mais detalhes a respeito do assunto.
• Resolver problemas secundários como interações sociais forçadas subsequentes à agressão defensiva

FOBIAS, MEDO E ANSIEDADE — GATOS

voltada para pessoas ou outros gatos ou eliminar problemas que possam resultar de medo ou ansiedade.

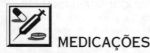
MEDICAÇÕES

MEDICAMENTO(S)
• Os medicamentos poderão constituir um adjuvante útil à modificação comportamental se o comportamento de medo ou ansiedade do animal for tão intenso a ponto de interferir no aprendizado ou em outras atividades comportamentais normais.
• Nenhum medicamento está aprovado pela FDA para uso em gatos com comportamento medroso; por essa razão, os proprietários têm de ser alertados sobre o fato de que as informações sobre a eficácia, as contraindicações e os efeitos colaterais são limitadas e, em geral, extrapoladas da literatura humana.
• Se houver dúvidas ou preocupações sobre um paciente ou medicamento específico, a consulta ao veterinário especialista em comportamento poderá ser proveitosa.

Inibidores Seletivos de Recaptação da Serotonina (ISRSs)
• Fluoxetina (Prozac®) — 0,5-1 mg/kg VO a cada 24 h. Efeitos colaterais: diminuição do apetite e irritabilidade.
• Paroxetina (Paxil®) — 0,5-1 mg/kg VO a cada 24 h. Efeitos colaterais: diminuição do apetite, irritabilidade, constipação.

Antidepressivos Tricíclicos (ATCs)
• Clomipramina — 0,5 mg/kg a cada 24 h, 2,5-5 mg/gato VO a cada 24 h. Efeitos colaterais: sedação, anticolinérgicos, possíveis distúrbios da condução cardíaca em animais predispostos.
• Amitriptilina — 0,5-1,0 mg/kg VO a cada 12-24 h. Efeitos colaterais: sedação, anticolinérgicos, possíveis distúrbios da condução cardíaca em animais predispostos.

Azapirona
• Buspirona — 0,5-1,0 mg/kg VO a cada 12 h, 2,5-7,5 mg/gato VO a cada 12 h. Efeitos colaterais: desarranjo GI, sedação leve, desinibição do comportamento agressivo.

Benzodiazepínicos
• Alprazolam — 0,125-0,25 mg/gato VO a cada 12 h. Efeitos colaterais: sedação, desinibição da agressão, aumento do apetite.

CONTRAINDICAÇÕES
• O uso de buspirona, ATC e ISRS não é recomendado em animais que sofram de crises convulsivas. Os ISRS e ATC não devem ser utilizados em conjunto com inibidores da MAO, como amitraz ou selegilina.
• Em virtude dos casos relatados de necrose hepática idiopática fatal, o uso do diazepam (Valium®) não é recomendado atualmente para uso em gatos.

PRECAUÇÕES
• Exames laboratoriais básicos são fortemente sugeridos antes do uso de medicação psicotrópica em algum animal, para ter certeza de que as funções hepática e renal são suficientes para metabolizar a medicação, e verificar se alguma condição física poderia contraindicar os medicamentos específicos.
• O ato de medicar os gatos pode vir a ser estressante, sobretudo quando a medicação não é palatável, como muitos dos medicamentos mencionados anteriormente. A manipulação de medicamentos em uma formulação mais palatável pode facilitar a administração, aumentando o consumo e a eficácia do agente terapêutico.

INTERAÇÕES POSSÍVEIS
O leitor deve abordar quaisquer dúvidas sobre possíveis interações medicamentosas com um veterinário especialista em comportamento ou um farmacêutico.

MEDICAMENTO(S) ALTERNATIVO(S)
A terapia com feromônio (Feliway®, ComfortZone®), desenvolvida inicialmente para casos de marcação territorial com urina, é utilizada sob a forma de spray aerossol e/ou difusor de ambiente para tranquilizar gatos ansiosos e medrosos em casa, durante viagens e durante internação ou consultas clínicas. Embora medicamentos alternativos como preparações à base de ervas tenham sido sugeridas para comportamentos ansiosos e medrosos em animais, nenhum estudo científico demonstrou a eficácia desses agentes para tais distúrbios em gatos. O uso desses compostos deve ser supervisionado por um veterinário conhecedor de métodos diagnósticos e terapêuticos complementares e alternativos. A utilização concomitante de algumas ervas medicinais e medicamentos psicotrópicos pode induzir a interações medicamentosas graves; por essa razão, os proprietários devem ser questionados sobre o emprego atual de medicamentos de venda livre aos gatos.

ACOMPANHAMENTO

MONITORIZAÇÃO DO PACIENTE
É necessário o acompanhamento frequente, pessoal ou telefônico, especialmente durante os primeiros meses de tratamento, para motivar o proprietário e monitorizar a eficácia de qualquer tratamento medicamentoso adjuvante.

PREVENÇÃO
• Interações pacíficas e calmas, bem como associações positivas com estímulos indutores de medo, podem manter as reações relacionadas a essa sensação em um nível muito baixo.
• A exposição precoce positiva a pessoas, lugares e coisas durante os 3-9 primeiros meses de vida e durante o primeiro ano pode ser útil para evitar alguns problemas tardios com o comportamento do medo.

COMPLICAÇÕES POSSÍVEIS
Problemas comportamentais secundários poderão surgir ou persistir depois que o comportamento de medo ou ansiedade tiver diminuído e, portanto, necessitarão de tratamento específico.

EVOLUÇÃO ESPERADA E PROGNÓSTICO
• Animais com personalidade tímida ou pouco sociáveis podem mostrar uma resposta mínima ao tratamento.
• Uma "meta" realista depende dos antecedentes do animal (histórico de socialização, genética e diferenças individuais na personalidade), da situação em casa e de outros fatores que geram confusão, como a frequência de exposição natural a estímulos indutores de medo.
• A medicação pode ajudar a melhorar a resposta à modificação de comportamento, mas não elimina completamente os sinais.

DIVERSOS

DISTÚRBIOS ASSOCIADOS
• Transtornos estereotípicos ou compulsivos.
• Marcação territorial com urina, eliminação inadequada.
• Agressividade defensiva em direção a pessoas e outros animais: também pode tornar o gato um alvo de agressividade por outros gatos.

POTENCIAL ZOONÓTICO
A agressividade relacionada ao medo pode levar a mordeduras ou arranhões defensivos e subsequente infecções.

GESTAÇÃO/FERTILIDADE/REPRODUÇÃO
Deve-se evitar o uso de medicamentos em animais prenhes.

VER TAMBÉM
• Agressividade, Revisão — Gatos.
• Transtornos Compulsivos — Gatos.
• Evacuação Domiciliar — Gatos.
• Marcação Territorial e Comportamento Errante — Gatos.

ABREVIATURA(S)
• FDA = U.S. Food and Drug Administration (departamento do governo norte-americano responsável pelo controle de alimentos e medicações).
• GI = gastrintestinal.
• MAO = monoamina oxidase.
• ISRS = inibidor seletivo de recaptação da serotonina.
• ATC = antidepressivo tricíclico.

RECURSOS DA INTERNET
Para mais informações sobre a terapia com feromônios (Feliway® e ComfortZone®): acesse www.feliway.com.

Sugestões de Leitura
Levine ED. Feline fear and anxiety. Vet Clin North Am Small Anim Pract 2008, 38(5):1065-1079.
Mendl M, Harcourt R. Individuality in the domestic cat: Origins, development and stability. In: Turner DC, Bateson P, eds., The Domestic Cat, the Biology of Its Behaviour, 2nd ed. Cambridge: Cambridge University Press, 2000, pp. 48-64.
Mills DS, Simpson BS. Psychotropic agents. In: Horwitz D, Mills D, Heath F, eds., BSAVA Manual of Canine and Feline Behavioural Medicine. Gloucestershire, UK: BSAVA, 2002, pp. 237-238.

Autor Leslie Larson Cooper
Consultor Editorial Debra F. Horwitz

Formação e Estrutura Anormais do Dente

CONSIDERAÇÕES GERAIS

DEFINIÇÃO

Variação no Tamanho do Dente
- Macrodontia — tamanho demasiadamente grande da coroa, raiz normal.
- Microdontia — formato normal da coroa, mas pequeno.
- Dente assimétrico — dente pequeno em formato de cone com uma única cúspide.

Variação na Estrutura/Formato do Dente
- Fusão — dois botões dentários separados, que são unidos para formar um único dente inteiro ou unidos nas raízes por cimento e dentina.
- Geminação — o botão dentário em desenvolvimento sofre separação incompleta, resultando em duas coroas com um canal radicular comum.
- Dilaceração — dente distorcido ou malformado (coroa ou raiz) — um termo geral que pode ser usado para muitas apresentações diferentes.
- Invaginação (dente invaginado, ou seja, um dentro do outro) — as camadas externas invaginam-se nas estruturas internas com gravidade variada.
- Dentes em concha — presença de coroa, mas pouco a nenhum desenvolvimento radicular.
- Amelogênese imperfeita — redução hereditária na quantidade de matriz do esmalte desenvolvida.

FISIOPATOLOGIA
- Estresse ou estímulo (traumatismo) no momento do desenvolvimento pode alterar a formação do dente.
- Infecção, traumatismo aos botões dentários, ou extração traumática de dentes decíduos durante a formação do dente permanente pode alterar significativamente a estrutura dentária.
- Tendências genéticas ou familiares não conhecidas para a maioria dos problemas.
- Cão/gato.

IDENTIFICAÇÃO

Aspectos Clínicos
Ver Definição.
- Fusão (dentes fundidos) — a coroa fundida será maior que um único dente. Haverá um número reduzido de dentes (dois são contados como um).
- Geminação (dentes geminados) — o número real dos dentes permanecerá inalterado, mas um dente será maior, com duplicação de parte da coroa (e, possivelmente, das raízes ao exame radiográfico). Dentes conhecidos como *gêmeos siameses*.
- Dilaceração (dentes dilacerados)
  ○ Qualquer variação na estrutura ou na forma — raiz extra, raiz curva.
  ○ Todo dente deve ser avaliado quanto à integridade do sistema pulpar, pois qualquer ruptura na continuidade da coroa e das raízes pode resultar em exposição da polpa ao ambiente externo.

DIAGNÓSTICO

DIAGNÓSTICO DIFERENCIAL
- Traumatismo às estruturas dentárias.
- Anormalidades de desenvolvimento.

MÉTODOS DIAGNÓSTICOS
- Exame bucal completo.
- Radiografias intrabucais.
- Na presença de qualquer estrutura anormal (dilaceração, p. ex.), é imprescindível a avaliação da integridade do sistema pulpar e do potencial de compressão.
- Métodos diagnósticos pré-operatórios adequados, quando indicados, antes de qualquer procedimento.

TRATAMENTO
- Desenvolvimento anormal dos primeiros molares mandibulares em raças caninas de pequeno porte.
- A dilaceração é mais comum, descrita algumas vezes como dente invaginado.
- Como um dos primeiros dentes permanentes a se formar, pode haver um desafio mecânico (falta de espaço) em cães de pequeno porte — desafio este que impede o desenvolvimento adequado da coroa e da raiz.
- Invaginação do esmalte e/ou cimento no colo do dente, muitas vezes com certo grau de retração gengival.

SINAIS RADIOGRÁFICOS
- Descontinuidade entre as coroas e as raízes.
- Possível exposição da polpa e cálculos dentários na polpa.
- Raízes convergentes com amplos canais (polpa não vital).
- Abscedação periapical/radicular com extensa perda óssea.

MEDICAÇÕES

MEDICAMENTO(S)
Procedimentos
- Terapias antimicrobiana e analgésica adequadas, quando indicadas.
- Monitorização e suporte adequados do paciente durante procedimentos anestésicos.
- Fusão dentária — não há necessidade de nenhum tratamento a menos que o sulco entre os dois dentes e/ou as coroas se estenda para a margem gengival ou abaixo dela (ninho para doença periodontal).
- Geminação dentária — se isso resultar em compressão do dente, pode haver a necessidade de extração.
- Dilaceração dentária — se houver exposição ou comprometimento da polpa, a extração geralmente é necessária.
  ○ Em alguns casos, a terapia endodôntica e restauradora pode permitir a conservação do dente.

ACOMPANHAMENTO

EVOLUÇÃO ESPERADA E PROGNÓSTICO
- Prognóstico bom em dentes com alterações moderadas (dentes assimétricos, dentes fundidos, dentes geminados).
- Prognóstico reservado em dentes dilacerados com comprometimento da polpa, embora a extração tipicamente seja bem-sucedida.

DIVERSOS

RECURSOS DA INTERNET
http://www.avdc.org/Nomenclature.html.

Sugestões de Leitura
Lobprise HB. Blackwell's Five-Minute Veterinary Consult Clinical Companion—Small Animal Dentistry. Ames, IA: Blackwell, 2007(for additional topics, including diagnostics and techniques).
Regezi JA, Sciubba JJ, Jordan RCK. Oral Pathology Clinical Pathologic Correlations, 4th ed. St. Louis: Saunders, 1999, pp. 367-370.
Wiggs RB, Lobprise HB. Veterinary Dentistry: Principles and Practice. Philadelphia: Lippincott-Raven, 1997, pp. 105-107.

Autor Heidi B. Lobprise
Consultor Editorial Heidi B. Lobprise

Fraqueza e Colapso Induzidos por Exercício em Labradores Retrievers

CONSIDERAÇÕES GERAIS

REVISÃO
Distúrbio hereditário que causa fraqueza e colapso durante exercício intensivo em Labradores retrievers normais sob outros aspectos.

IDENTIFICAÇÃO
• Labradores retrievers — quase 10% de todos os animais de estimação, cães de exposição e Labradores retrievers de campo são acometidos.
• Raro em Chesapeake Bay retrievers e retrievers de pelo ondulado.
• Os sinais tipicamente se tornam aparentes entre 5 meses e 3 anos de idade (idade média de 12 meses).
• Não há predileção por sexo ou cor da pelagem.

SINAIS CLÍNICOS
Comentários Gerais
• Ausência de sinais sistêmicos.
• Tipicamente, os episódios de colapso são pouco frequentes e ocorrem apenas com extremos de exercício e agitação.
• Os cães podem se engajar normalmente em exercícios de caminhada, natação, corrida e outras atividades que não são associadas a um alto nível de agitação ou estresse.
• É comum o relato de que os cães sintomáticos tenham um temperamento agitado.

Achados do Exame Físico
• Além de estarem em boa forma, os cães acometidos são saudáveis e musculosos.
• Entre os episódios de fraqueza e colapso, os exames físicos e neurológicos são normais.

Características dos Episódios de Fraqueza e Colapso
• A fraqueza ocorre 5-20 minutos depois de exercício intenso com agitação ou estresse.
• A primeira anormalidade observada é uma marcha oscilante ou forçada.
• Os membros posteriores ficam fracos e incapazes de suportar o peso.
• Muitos cães continuarão correndo, arrastando seus membros posteriores em uma postura agachada.
• Alguns cães exibem incoordenação com postura em base larga, hipermetria e queda durante o episódio e durante a recuperação.
• Durante um episódio grave, todos os quatro membros podem ser acometidos e o cão pode ficar em decúbito e incapaz de mover seus membros ou levantar sua cabeça.
• A maioria dos cães permanece consciente e alerta durante os episódios — 10-25% parecem desorientados ou confusos.
• Os músculos dos membros posteriores apresentam-se flácidos durante o colapso e há uma perda dos reflexos patelares.
• Pode haver um aumento no tônus extensor nos membros anteriores de alguns cães com colapso quando eles se encontram em decúbito lateral.
• Não há dor ou desconforto aparente à palpação ou manipulação dos músculos, das articulações ou da coluna vertebral durante ou após o colapso.
• A recuperação completa do animal ocorre em até 5-30 minutos.
• Apesar de elevada (média >41,6°C), a temperatura retal não é diferente de Labradores que praticam exercícios semelhantes, mas não sofrem colapso induzido por exercício.
• Alguns cães com colapso induzido por exercício vêm a óbito durante o colapso — a morte costuma ser precedida por uma breve crise convulsiva generalizada.

CAUSAS
• Distúrbio genético — hereditário como um traço autossômico recessivo.
• Cães sintomáticos — homozigotos para uma mutação no gene dinamina 1. A dinamina 1 (DNM1) é uma proteína importante nos processos de neurotransmissão no cérebro e na medula espinal durante atividade neuronal de alto nível. Há evidências de que a mutação do DNM1 associada ao colapso induzido por exercício exerça seu efeito mais acentuado sobre a função desse gene quando a temperatura corporal está elevada, como normalmente ocorre com o exercício.

FATORES DE RISCO
• Os cães geneticamente acometidos estão sob alto risco de colapso ao participarem de exercícios de alta intensidade com agitação ou estresse concomitante.
• Os cães acometidos com estilo de vida sedentário ou temperamento dócil (calmo) podem nunca exibir fraqueza ou colapso, mas a maioria daqueles geneticamente afetados (>80%) terá pelo menos 1 episódio de colapso antes de atingirem 3 anos de idade.
• O colapso ocorre somente durante atividades deflagradoras específicas associadas a um alto nível de agitação ou ansiedade.
• As atividades deflagradoras que mais provavelmente induzem ao colapso incluem retomadas repetitivas de atividades divertidas ou adestramentos, caça de aves não aquáticas, atividades lúdicas intensas com outros cães e corridas ao lado de veículos 4X4 (ou seja, de todo tipo de terreno).
• A elevação na temperatura ambiente e na umidade parece aumentar o risco de colapso em cães acometidos.

DIAGNÓSTICO

DIAGNÓSTICO DIFERENCIAL
• A natureza episódica do colapso, a associação com exercício e agitação, a evolução típica de fraqueza durante um episódio e a rápida recuperação completa devem levar a um diagnóstico presuntivo de colapso induzido por exercício em Labrador retriever jovem. Embora os exames físicos e neurológicos permaneçam normais, há necessidade de avaliações mais detalhadas não só para eliminar outras causas de fraqueza e colapso, mas também para confirmar a suscetibilidade genética ao colapso induzido por exercício.
• Os cães com miopatias metabólicas, polimiosite e miastenia grave são tipicamente muito mais intolerantes ao exercício que aqueles com colapso induzido por exercício e sofrerão colapso com exercício leve de curta duração.
• Miopatia centronuclear (conhecida previamente como miopatia hereditária do Labrador retriever ou deficiência de miofibras do tipo II) — distúrbio muscular hereditário em Labradores retrievers que causa atrofia muscular generalizada, fraqueza constante que piora com o exercício, e reflexos patelares ausentes em repouso. O diagnóstico desse distúrbio é feito por biopsia do músculo ou teste de DNA (www.labradorcnm.com).
• Arritmia cardíaca como causa de intolerância ao exercício pode ser descartada por meio de auscultação do coração, palpação dos pulsos femorais e realização de ECG em repouso e durante o colapso. Talvez haja necessidade de um monitor tipo Holter ou de um traçado eletrocardiográfico para registro de eventos com o objetivo de descartar arritmia cardíaca intermitente como causa de colapso.
• Hipoglicemia — excluída pela mensuração da glicemia durante algum episódio.
• Hipo ou hipercalemia — descartada pela mensuração dos níveis de potássio durante algum episódio.
• Hipoadrenocorticismo (doença de Addison) — excluída pelo teste de estimulação com ACTH.
• Crises convulsivas — de início abrupto e associadas à perda de consciência, atividade convulsiva, recuperação rápida e sinais pós-ictais.
• Epilepsia atípica/discinesia paroxística — episódios breves de marcha agachada anormal, desequilíbrio, balançar da cabeça ou incoordenação podem ser observados em Labradores retrievers como um distúrbio convulsivo ou locomotor. Os episódios podem ser induzidos por exercício/agitação em alguns cães, confundindo-se com o colapso induzido por exercício. O início dos sinais é superagudo, os episódios são breves (em geral, menos de 5 minutos) e a recuperação é imediata, ajudando na distinção entre esse problema e o distúrbio mais progressivo de marcha causado pelo colapso induzido por exercício. O diagnóstico pode ser feito apenas por meio da exclusão de outros distúrbios (inclusive do colapso induzido por exercício) com teste.
• Cataplexia — episódios breves, superagudos e não progressivos de paralisia flácida completa.
• Intermação — o colapso atribuído à intermação costuma ser associado a sangramento, choque e atividade mental anormal. Insuficiência renal aguda, CID e morte são comuns. A recuperação, se ocorrer, é prolongada.
• Hipertermia maligna (também conhecida como síndrome do estresse canino) — estado hipermetabólico deflagrado por certos anestésicos, calor extremo, atividade intensa ou estresse psicológico em cães geneticamente suscetíveis. Ocorrem hipertermia, contração generalizada dos músculos esqueléticos, rabdomiólise e CID, e muitos cães acabam morrendo. A recuperação, se ocorrer, é prolongada. Testes de contratura *in vitro* nas biopsias de músculo ou identificação da mutação genética causal do receptor de rianodina (RYR1) são necessários para a obtenção do diagnóstico.

HEMOGRAMA/BIOQUÍMICA/URINÁLISE
Normais em repouso e durante o colapso.

OUTROS TESTES LABORATORIAIS
• Gasometria arterial — normal em repouso; durante o colapso, no entanto, observam-se alcalose respiratória extrema e acidose metabólica leve idênticas àquelas constatadas em Labradores sob atividade física intensa sem colapso induzido por exercício.
• Mensuração dos níveis de lactato e piruvato — normais em repouso, mas iguais durante o colapso de Labradores que se exercitam sem colapso induzido por exercício.
• Avaliação da tireoide — normal.

- Teste de estimulação com ACTH — normal.
- Análise de mutação no receptor de rianodina (RYR1) responsável por hipertermia maligna — negativa.
- Teste para detecção de anticorpos antirreceptores de acetilcolina responsáveis por miastenia grave adquirida — negativo.

DIAGNÓSTICO POR IMAGEM
Radiografias toracoabdominais, ultrassonografia abdominal, ecocardiografia — normais.

MÉTODOS DIAGNÓSTICOS
Achados eletrocardiográficos (ECG) em repouso e durante o colapso — normais.

Teste de DNA
- O diagnóstico definitivo requer a demonstração de que um cão tem duas cópias da mutação do gene DNM1.
- O teste pode ser realizado no sangue, em *swabs* de células da bochecha, em unhas removidas de filhotes de cães ou no sêmen.
- Aproximadamente 10% de todos os Labradores retrievers testados possuem duas cópias da mutação do gene DNM1 (acometidos); >30% de todos os Labradores retrievers testados apresentam apenas uma única cópia da mutação desse gene (portadores).
- O encontro de duas cópias da mutação do gene DNM1 confirma que o cão sofre de colapso induzido por exercício, mas não descarta necessariamente outras causas de intolerância ao exercício ou colapso por exercício. É importante realizar os testes necessários para descartar outras causas de colapso que podem ser potencialmente mais tratáveis.

ACHADOS PATOLÓGICOS
- Histologia do músculo — normal.
- Exames completos *post-mortem* (à necropsia) de cães que morrem durante o colapso induzido por exercício — normais.

TRATAMENTO

ATIVIDADE
A maioria dos cães acometidos pode ter vidas ativas normais se as atividades deflagradoras específicas forem evitadas ou feitas com moderação.

ORIENTAÇÃO AO PROPRIETÁRIO
- Os sinais costumam piorar nos 3-5 minutos após o término do exercício; alguns cães acometidos (<5%) morrem durante o colapso.
- Toda atividade deve ser interrompida ao primeiro sinal de fraqueza ou incoordenação.
- Considerar o fornecimento de água fresca por via oral, a aspersão com água ou a imersão em água para reduzir a temperatura corporal.

CONSIDERAÇÕES CIRÚRGICAS
Alguns cães machos têm sofrido menos episódios de colapso após a castração.

MEDICAÇÕES

MEDICAMENTO(S)
- Quando a mudança de atividade não for eficaz, pode-se tentar o tratamento médico.
- Fenobarbital 2 mg/kg a cada 12 h VO — pode diminuir o número e a gravidade dos episódios associados a atividades deflagradoras. O fenobarbital pode simplesmente diminuir o nível de agitação em cães acometidos, reduzindo a probabilidade de colapso. O leve efeito sedativo pode afetar adversamente o desempenho em atividades de adestramento e competição. Pode ser desnecessário atingir níveis séricos terapêuticos adequados como em caso de epilepsia. Os efeitos adversos incluem polifagia, polidipsia e poliúria. Há necessidade de monitorização vitalícia para pesquisa de hepatotoxicidade.

CONTRAINDICAÇÕES/INTERAÇÕES POSSÍVEIS
Cimetidina e cloranfenicol — interferem no metabolismo de fenobarbital; podem levar a níveis sanguíneos tóxicos.

ACOMPANHAMENTO

- A maioria dos cães acometidos pode ser tratada de forma eficaz, evitando as atividades deflagradoras e observando esses animais rigorosamente quanto ao aparecimento dos primeiros sinais de fraqueza.
- O tratamento médico pode permitir que alguns cães gravemente acometidos participem de atividades deflagradoras sem sofrer colapso.
- À medida que os cães acometidos envelhecem, os episódios de colapso tornam-se menos frequentes, mas ainda podem ser fatais.

DIVERSOS

DISTÚRBIOS ASSOCIADOS
Os cães com colapso induzido por exercício não desenvolvem outros problemas médicos associados conforme envelhecem.

FATORES RELACIONADOS COM A IDADE
Os episódios de colapso podem se tornar menos frequentes com o avanço da idade dos cães, possivelmente por causa da agitação menos intensa associada às atividades deflagradoras.

POTENCIAL ZOONÓTICO
N/D.

GESTAÇÃO/FERTILIDADE/REPRODUÇÃO
- Os animais devem ser submetidos a exames para estabelecer seu *status* de colapso induzido por exercício antes de cruzar.
- Os cães acometidos (com duas cópias da mutação do gene DNM1) não devem ser reproduzidos ou, então, devem ser acasalados apenas com animais que sabidamente não são portadores para evitar a geração de prole acometida.
- Os cães portadores (com uma única cópia da mutação do gene DNM1) devem ser acasalados apenas com animais que sabidamente não são portadores para evitar a geração de prole acometida.

ABREVIATURAS
- ACTH = hormônio adrenocorticotrófico.
- CID = coagulação intravascular disseminada.
- DNM1 = dinamina 1.
- ECG = eletrocardiograma.
- RYR1 = receptor de rianodina.

RECURSOS DA INTERNET
Respostas a perguntas frequentes e instruções para envio de amostras para o teste de DNA — acessar o website do Laboratório Diagnóstico Veterinário da Universidade de Minnesota: http://www.cvm.umn.edu/vdl/ourservices/canineneuromuscular/home.html.

Sugestões de Leitura
Paterson EE, Minor KM, Tchernatynskaia AV, et al. A canine DNM1 mutation is highly associated with the syndrome of exercise-induced collapse. Nature Genetics 2008, 40(10):1235-1239.
Taylor SM, Shmon CL, Shelton GD, et al. Exercise induced collapse of Labrador retrievers: Survey results and preliminary investigation of heritability. JAAHA 2008, 44:295-301.
Taylor SM, Shmon CL, Adams VJ, et al. Evaluations of Labrador retrievers with exercise-induced collapse, including response to a standardized strenuous exercise protocol. JAAHA 2009, 45:3-13.

Autor Susan M. Taylor
Consultor Editorial Joane M. Parent

Fratura Dentária

CONSIDERAÇÕES GERAIS

DEFINIÇÃO
- As lesões traumáticas dos dentes podem envolver fraturas do esmalte, da dentina, do cemento ou danos ao periodonto.
- Pode envolver a coroa e a raiz do dente acometido.
- As fraturas serão classificadas como não complicadas (simples) se não envolverem a exposição da polpa, e complicadas se a polpa for exposta pela linha de fratura.

FISIOPATOLOGIA
- A polpa exposta não tratada invariavelmente leva à pulpite e, por fim, à necrose pulpar e ao comprometimento periapical.
- A pulpite e a necrose pulpar também poderão ocorrer em casos de fraturas não complicadas, particularmente se a linha de fratura estiver próxima à câmara pulpar, o que expõe um grande número de túbulos dentinários calibrosos e permite a comunicação entre a polpa e o ambiente externo.

SISTEMA(S) ACOMETIDO(S)
- Gastrintestinal — cavidade bucal.
- A infecção na cavidade bucal pode causar complicações sistêmicas.

GENÉTICA
N/D.

INCIDÊNCIA/PREVALÊNCIA
N/D.

DISTRIBUIÇÃO GEOGRÁFICA
Nenhuma.

IDENTIFICAÇÃO
Espécies
Cães e gatos.
Raça(s) Predominante(s)
Nenhuma.
Idade Média e Faixa Etária
Qualquer idade.
Sexo Predominante
Nenhum.

SINAIS CLÍNICOS
Fraturas Coronárias
- Perda clínica de substância da coroa dentária; pode afetar apenas o esmalte ou o esmalte e a dentina; a linha de fratura pode ser transversa ou oblíqua.
- Fraturas não complicadas com a linha de fratura próxima à câmara pulpar — a polpa de coloração rosa-pálida fica visível por meio da dentina; a exploração delicada não possibilita a penetração da sonda na cavidade pulpar.
- Em fraturas coronárias complicadas, a câmara pulpar encontra-se aberta e, portanto, facilmente acessível à sonda.
- As fraturas complicadas recentes estão associadas a hemorragias provenientes da polpa.
- As fraturas mais antigas podem exibir necrose pulpar; do ponto de vista clínico, a câmara pulpar apresenta-se preenchida por material necrótico escuro e, muitas vezes, o dente mostra-se manchado.

Fraturas Radiculares
- Podem ocorrer em qualquer ponto ao longo da superfície radicular; embora possam ocorrer de forma isolada, tais fraturas frequentemente ocorrem em combinação com as fraturas coronárias.
- A linha de fratura pode ser transversa ou oblíqua; os segmentos podem permanecer alinhados ou sofrer deslocamentos.
- Os sinais clínicos indicativos de possível fratura radicular incluem dor à oclusão da boca ou durante a respiração de boca aberta.
- A mobilidade anormal horizontal ou vertical de dente com periodonto sadio pode levantar a suspeita de fratura radicular.

CAUSAS
Em geral, as fraturas dentárias resultam de algum incidente traumático (p. ex., acidente automobilístico, pancada contundente na face e mastigação de objetos duros).

FATORES DE RISCO
O comportamento errante aumenta o risco de traumatismo.

DIAGNÓSTICO

DIAGNÓSTICO DIFERENCIAL
- Fratura coronária — atrito, formação dentária anormal.
- Fratura radicular — luxação; o diagnóstico definitivo de fraturas radiculares é feito por meio de radiografias.

HEMOGRAMA/BIOQUÍMICA/URINÁLISE
Exames inalterados por fratura dentária.

OUTROS TESTES LABORATORIAIS
Nenhum.

DIAGNÓSTICO POR IMAGEM
- As radiografias são obrigatórias.
- É imprescindível o uso de técnicas radiográficas intrabucais e de filmes radiográficos intrabucais dentários.
- As radiografias revelam a extensão completa da lesão e permitem o planejamento terapêutico.
- Além disso, as radiografias são indispensáveis para o desempenho adequado dos procedimentos endodônticos e a monitorização dos resultados terapêuticos.

MÉTODOS DIAGNÓSTICOS
Transiluminação — para ajudar a determinar a vitalidade do dente: incidir um foco luminoso por meio do dente (luz do otoscópio); um dente viável deverá transiluminar de forma satisfatória.

ACHADOS PATOLÓGICOS
A polpa exposta não tratada invariavelmente leva à pulpite e, por fim, à necrose pulpar e ao comprometimento periapical.

TRATAMENTO

CUIDADO(S) DE SAÚDE ADEQUADO(S)
Depende(m) da extensão e da gravidade do traumatismo ao paciente.

CUIDADO(S) DE ENFERMAGEM
Depende(m) da extensão e da gravidade do traumatismo ao paciente.

ATIVIDADE
Restringir, conforme indicado pela natureza do traumatismo.

DIETA
No período pós-operatório imediato (24-72 h), o ato de umedecer a ração seca do paciente pode ajudar a diminuir as chances de traumatismos na linha de sutura. Continue a monitorização do local.

ORIENTAÇÃO AO PROPRIETÁRIO
Pode haver a necessidade de uma série de tratamentos.

CONSIDERAÇÕES CIRÚRGICAS
Fraturas Coronárias Não Complicadas
Remover as margens pontiagudas com broca e selar os túbulos dentinários expostos com material de restauração adequado.

Fraturas Coronárias Complicadas
Todas as fraturas desse tipo necessitarão de terapia endodôntica se o dente for mantido; a extração é preferível a nenhum tratamento.

Dentes Maduros
- Fratura recente de dente maduro com a polpa ainda viável — existem duas opções terapêuticas: (1) procedimento de pulpectomia parcial e capeamento direto da polpa (pulpotomia vital), seguida por restauração ou (2) terapia convencional do canal radicular e restauração.
- Para que a pulpectomia parcial e o capeamento pulpar direto sejam bem-sucedidos, os procedimentos devem ser realizados poucas horas após a lesão.
- Logo no início, informar ao proprietário que o procedimento pode não ser o tratamento final — o dente poderá necessitar do tratamento convencional de canal se a polpa vier a sofrer necrose.
- Quando a polpa já se encontra cronicamente inflamada ou necrótica, o tratamento convencional de canal e a restauração constituirão as terapias de escolha se o periodonto estiver sadio.

Dentes Imaturos
- Para o desenvolvimento radicular contínuo, é imprescindível uma polpa viável; assim, contanto que a polpa esteja viável, o tratamento de escolha consistirá na pulpectomia parcial e no capeamento pulpar direto, seguidos por restauração.
- Se a polpa estiver necrótica, não ocorrerá nenhum desenvolvimento subsequente da raiz; os dentes imaturos necrosados necessitam de tratamento endodôntico para serem mantidos; remover o tecido necrótico e obliterar o canal radicular com pasta de hidróxido de cálcio; certo grau de apexogênese (evento fisiológico, desenvolvimento radicular contínuo) e de apexificação (fechamento apical, induzido pelo tratamento) pode ser estimulado caso se efetue tal procedimento; trocar o hidróxido de cálcio a cada 6 meses até o ápice se fechar ao se realizar o tratamento convencional de canal.
- Os dentes imaturos poderão estar presentes no animal maduro se o traumatismo aos dentes em desenvolvimento causar necrose pulpar; tratar tais dentes da mesma forma que qualquer outro dente imaturo.

Fraturas Radiculares
- O tratamento de fraturas coronárias e radiculares depende da extensão da linha de fratura abaixo da margem gengival.
- Se a linha de fratura não envolver a polpa e não se estender mais de 4-5 mm abaixo da margem gengival, pode-se executar o tratamento odontológico de restauração; se a fratura se estender mais de 5 mm abaixo da margem

Fratura Dentária

gengival e envolver a polpa, costuma-se recomendar a extração do dente.
• O nível da fratura determina a escolha do tratamento para as fraturas radiculares horizontais; fraturas na região apical apresentam prognóstico melhor do que aquelas próximas à margem gengival.
• Uma fratura horizontal da porção coronária da raiz geralmente obriga à extração do dente; a principal exceção é o canino inferior, já que a estabilidade e a resistência mandibulares dependem das raízes dos dentes caninos. Se a raiz tiver o periodonto sadio, ela deverá ser submetida a tratamento endodôntico após a remoção da porção coronária.
• As fraturas mesorradiculares e apicais horizontais consolidarão se o dente for imobilizado; as fraturas radiculares horizontais podem se consolidar por meio de calos dentinocementários, uniões fibrosas ou uniões osteofibrosas.
• Se a polpa do fragmento coronário se tornar necrótica, a fratura não se consolidará; nesse caso, fica indicado o tratamento endodôntico do segmento coronário; o segmento apical poderá ser deixado *in situ* (i. e., no local) se não houver nenhum indício radiográfico de comprometimento periapical; na presença de indícios radiográficos de tal acometimento, deve-se remover o segmento apical.

MEDICAÇÕES
MEDICAMENTO(S) DE ESCOLHA
Pode ser indicado o uso de antibiótico bactericida de amplo espectro por 5 a 7 dias (p. ex., na presença de infecção antiga).
CONTRAINDICAÇÕES
Nenhuma.
PRECAUÇÕES
Nenhuma.

INTERAÇÕES POSSÍVEIS
Nenhuma.
MEDICAMENTO(S) ALTERNATIVO(S)
Nenhum.

ACOMPANHAMENTO
MONITORIZAÇÃO DO PACIENTE
• Avaliar os procedimentos de pulpectomia parcial e capeamento pulpar direto com a obtenção de radiografias pós-operatórias após 6 e 12 meses ou em intervalos determinados pelos sinais clínicos, para detectar necrose pulpar e alterações periapicais consequentes, indicativos da necessidade do tratamento de canal.
• Verificar o resultado do tratamento convencional de canal por meio radiográfico 6-12 meses do pós-operatório; a presença de indícios de comprometimento periapical nesse período indica a necessidade de novo tratamento endodôntico ou da extração do dente; a terapia endodôntica extra deverá refazer o tratamento de canal, muitas vezes junto da cirurgia endodôntica.
• Examinar as fraturas radiculares por meio radiográfico 6-12 meses do pós-operatório.
• Checar as fraturas não complicadas também por meio radiográfico 4-6 meses do pós-operatório para avaliar o estado periapical.

PREVENÇÃO
• Evitar as situações de provável dano aos dentes; impedir a mastigação de objetos duros (como pedras) pelos animais.
• Para evitar complicações, instituir o tratamento em poucas horas após a lesão.

COMPLICAÇÕES POSSÍVEIS
• A polpa exposta não tratada invariavelmente leva à pulpite e, por fim, à necrose pulpar e ao comprometimento periapical.
• Interrupção no desenvolvimento de dentes imaturos.

EVOLUÇÃO ESPERADA E PROGNÓSTICO
Variam de acordo com a vitalidade da polpa, o local da fratura e o estágio de desenvolvimento do dente (maduro ou imaturo); ver a seção "Tratamento" em busca de discussões mais detalhadas.

DIVERSOS
DISTÚRBIOS ASSOCIADOS
Nenhum.
FATORES RELACIONADOS COM A IDADE
O tratamento de dentes maduros e imaturos difere; ver a seção "Tratamento".
POTENCIAL ZOONÓTICO
Nenhum.
GESTAÇÃO/FERTILIDADE/REPRODUÇÃO
N/D.
RECURSOS DA INTERNET
Classificação de fraturas dentárias: http://avdc.org/Nomeclature.pdf.

Sugestões de Leitura
Gorrel C. Emergencies. In: Veterinary Dentistry for the General Practitioner. Philadelphia: Saunders, 2004, pp. 131-155.
Gorrel C, Robinson J. Endodontic therapy. In: Crossley DA, Penman S, eds., Manual of Small Animal Dentistry. Gloucestershire, UK: BSAVA, 1995, pp. 168-181.

Autor Cecilia Gorrel
Consultor Editorial Heidi B. Lobprise

Fraturas Maxilares e Mandibulares

CONSIDERAÇÕES GERAIS

REVISÃO
Fraturas das mandíbulas, dos maxilares e das estruturas associadas são classificadas segundo a localização, a gravidade (i. e., envolvimento dos dentes, lacerações do tecido mole e tipo de fratura óssea) e os efeitos dos músculos da mastigação exercidos sobre a redução.

FISIOPATOLOGIA
Efeitos dos Músculos da Mastigação
- Os músculos responsáveis pela abertura da boca (p. ex., o músculo digástrico) podem ajudar a reduzir ou deslocar a fratura.
- Favoráveis — fratura reduzida pelos músculos da mastigação.
- Desfavoráveis — fratura deslocada pelos músculos da mastigação.

Classificação de Lesão da Sínfise
- Tipo I — separação; sem solução de continuidade no tecido mole.
- Tipo II — separação; com solução de continuidade no tecido mole.
- Tipo III — separação; com solução de continuidade no tecido mole e cominuição do osso; não é incomum a presença de dentes fraturados.
- Os dentes envolvidos podem ser mantidos durante o processo ósseo (i. e., com tratamento endodôntico ou restauração). Se necessário, esses dentes poderão ser extraídos após a consolidação óssea.

NOTA: a frouxidão da sínfise é um achado clínico comum em gatos geriátricos e cães de raças toy.

Classificação de Fratura da Mandíbula pela Localização
- A — dos incisivos centrais (linha média) aos dentes caninos (a sínfise é um local comum de fratura da mandíbula no gato).
- B — do canino ao segundo pré-molar.
- C — do segundo pré-molar ao primeiro molar (dente carniceiro).
- D — do primeiro molar ao ângulo da mandíbula.
- E — ângulo da mandíbula.
- F — processo coronoide.
- G — processo condilar.
- H — linha média do palato.
- I — palato fora da linha média.
- J — maciça ou combinação de fraturas.

IDENTIFICAÇÃO
Espécies
- Cães e gatos.

SINAIS CLÍNICOS
- Variam muito de acordo com a localização, o tipo, a extensão, a causa e os fatores de risco subjacentes que resultam na lesão.
- Deformidade facial, maloclusão, dentes fraturados, sangramento bucal ou nasal e incapacidade de fechar a mandíbula de forma adequada são sinais comuns.

CAUSAS
Lesão, traumatismo e fatores predisponentes.

FATORES DE RISCO
- Ambiente ou temperamento de alto risco.
- Infecções bucais (p. ex., doença periodontal e osteomielite), neoplasia ou determinadas doenças metabólicas (p. ex., hipoparatireoidismo) — podem resultar em mandíbulas mais fracas que ficam mais propensas à lesão.
- Lesão traumática com envolvimento das mandíbulas ou dos dentes.
- Fatores congênitos ou hereditários, resultando no osso da mandíbula enfraquecido ou deformado.

DIAGNÓSTICO

DIAGNÓSTICO DIFERENCIAL
- Formulado com base na inspeção, na palpação e nos achados radiográficos.
- Condições da ATM — ver "Distúrbios da Articulação Temporomandibular".
- Subluxação ou luxação dentária (i. e., interferência no fechamento da mandíbula).
- Doença endodôntica (p. ex., abscesso dentário).
- Corpo estranho alojado na cavidade bucal ou próximo a ela.
- Lesão ou doença do nervo maxilar ou mandibular.
- Miosite eosinofílica.
- Osteopatia craniomandibular.
- Neoplasia.

HEMOGRAMA/BIOQUÍMICA/URINÁLISE
Conforme a necessidade — para avaliar e testar o impacto da lesão inicial; para avaliar o animal antes da cirurgia.

DIAGNÓSTICO POR IMAGEM
Radiografia — TC e RM intra e extrabucal.

MÉTODOS DIAGNÓSTICOS
- Exame bucal.
- Exame neurológico.
- Biopsia para exame histopatológico se houver indicação.

ACHADOS PATOLÓGICOS
- Não união.
- Neoplasia.
- Osteomielite.
- Doença periodontal e/ou endodôntica.

TRATAMENTO

CONSIDERAÇÕES CIRÚRGICAS
- Tecidas com base no tipo de fratura, nos equipamentos disponíveis e nos materiais utilizados, bem como no conhecimento, na experiência e no nível de conforto do profissional.
- A seleção do tratamento baseia-se em quatro pontos importantes: (1) redução da fratura e contato razoável das extremidades da fratura, se possível; (2) restabelecimento da oclusão natural, se possível; (3) estabilização suficiente para consolidação adequada; (4) condição de recuperação (condição não passível de reparo nem de estabilização).

TIPOS CARACTERÍSTICOS DE TRATAMENTOS PARA AS CLASSES DE FRATURAS

Estabilização Interarco (tipicamente para as classes D, E, F, G e J)
- Focinheira.
- Fio de arco cruzado (do maxilar à mandíbula).
- Fixação dos dentes em arco cruzado com resina composta; utilizada, algumas vezes, em combinação com pinos dentários (i. e., TMS; Whaledent, New York, NY).

Estabilização Intra-arco (tipicamente para as classes H e I)
- Combinação de pino e fio.
- Fio dental.
- Imobilização com resina acrílica ou composta.

Estabilização Intrabucal com Imobilização (tipicamente para as classes A, B, C, H, I e J)
- Imobilização com resina acrílica ou composta.

Estabilização Intrabucal com Fio (tipicamente para as classes A, B, C, H, I e J)
- Fio interdental — amarrilho de Ivy, amarrilho múltiplo de Stout, técnicas cirúrgicas de Essig e Risdon para aplicação de fio.
- Conexão dental com fio metálico ortodôntico — fio circundental utilizado para a ancoragem das imobilizações com resina composta e acrílica (fios flexíveis, torcidos ou de cerclagem).
- Conexão óssea com fio metálico ortodôntico — fio circunferencial; transósseo; transcircunferencial.

Fixação Interna (para a maior parte das classes de fraturas, embora deva ser usada seletivamente, considerando os dentes e as raízes)
- Fio ortopédico; pinos intramedulares; placas; parafusos.
- NOTA: NÃO introduza um pino intramedular dentro do canal mandibular.

Fixação Externa (para a maior parte das classes de fraturas, embora deva ser usada seletivamente, considerando os dentes e as raízes)
- Pinos intramedulares com barras (de aço inoxidável ou carbono) ou tubos (p. ex., Penrose) reforçados com resina composta ou acrílica.

Cirurgia de Recuperação (tipicamente para as fraturas da classe J)
- Condilectomia — fraturas da ATM não passíveis de reparo.
- Queiloplastia — procedimento de recuperação para manter um suporte mandibular razoável em determinadas condições de não união.
- Mandibulectomia rostral (ou outra) — utilizada em certos casos de não união ou com lesão maciça.

TÉCNICAS
A seguir estão descritas as técnicas mais comumente empregadas; opções mais avançadas estão além do escopo deste capítulo (ver a seção "Sugestões de Leitura").

Tratamento Inicial
- O conhecimento de oclusão, das raízes dentárias e da anatomia durante o tratamento é crítico.
- O paciente deve ser entubado e, nesse caso, um tubo de faringostomia ajuda nos testes de oclusão no período intraoperatório.
- Os dentes na linha de fratura devem ser avaliados e mantidos por meio de tratamento apropriado até que a fratura se consolide, se possível, pois a remoção pode resultar em instabilidade.
- Lacunas ou defeitos ósseos devem ser preenchidos com material de enxerto autógeno de osso esponjoso, material ósseo condutivo (Consil, Nutramax Labs Inc., Edgewood, MD), material ósseo indutivo (PepGen P-15, Cerimed Corp) ou material de enxerto ósseo.
- O tratamento com imobilizações de resina composta/acrílica em associação com aplicação de fio (amarrilho de Ivy, amarrilho múltiplo de Stout

FRATURAS MAXILARES E MANDIBULARES

costuma ser muito eficaz; pode conferir um melhor restabelecimento da oclusão e menos traumatismo aos dentes.
• Avaliar o dano aos tecidos moles, promover o debridamento e aplicar sutura quando apropriado.

Procedimento
• Desinfetar com clorexidina e, em seguida, limpar e polir os dentes (pedra-pomes sem flúor).
• Reduzir a fratura em oclusão adequada.
• Cobrir os dentes adjacentes e os tecidos moles com vaselina.
• Realizar ataque ácido sobre os dentes com gel de ácido fosfórico a 37%; deixar por 30-60 s; enxaguar completamente e secar os dentes com jato de ar.
• Aplicar a imobilização.

Materiais
Resina Acrílica
• Apesar de barato, esse material produz calor quando misturado e vapores perigosos necessitam de ventilação.
• Assim que os dentes forem preparados e submetidos à aplicação de fio, moldar a imobilização, colocando o pó e o líquido no estilo sal e pimenta em pequenos incrementos (para evitar reação hipertérmica) até a densidade e o formato desejados da imobilização obtida.
• Finalizar e polir com broca de acrílico em peça manual de alta velocidade.

Resina Composta (ProtempGarant – ESPE)
• Menos reação exotérmica e vapores; mais cara.
• Após o ataque ácido, utilizar um adesivo para dentina e aplicar um agente isolante à arcada oposta para evitar que a resina composta se una a esses dentes durante o teste de oclusão.
• Com a extremidade de um instrumental (espátula, no caso), aplicar o produto à área da imobilização, moldando-o à medida que ele endurece.
• Finalizar e polir com broca em pedra branca e colocar uma camada final de adesivo.

Conexão ou Sutura Óssea Circunferencial com Fio Metálico Ortodôntico
• Passar o fio ao redor do osso — técnica utilizada mais comumente para separações da sínfise.
• Agulha calibre 20 ou 18 — para passar o fio.
• Fio calibre 24 a 28 — em neonatos, cães de pequeno porte ou gatos, um material de sutura absorvível (de longa duração — p. ex., PDS) ou não absorvível 1 a 2-0 pode algumas vezes ser substituído pelo fio.
• Introduzir o fio pela incisão perfurante (espaço intermandibular ventral) até o vestíbulo; passar por trás dos caninos, descer pelo vestíbulo no lado oposto e voltar para trás pela incisão ventral.
• Apertar o fio para reduzir a fratura, mas sem apertar muito as extremidades do fio ou, então, os dentes poderão ser tracionados em uma direção muito mais medial (base estreita, deslocados no sentido lingual) e ferir o palato.
• Se os dentes tiverem base estreita, afrouxar as extremidades do fio ou inserir um fio em formato de 8 ao redor dos dentes caninos e sob a mandíbula.

CUIDADOS DOMÉSTICOS
• Cera ortodôntica — cera mole, flexível, deixada com o proprietário para cobrir periodicamente os fios irritantes.
• Produtos de irrigação bucal — utilizar duas vezes ao dia para promover a higiene bucal e reduzir as bactérias; soluções de clorexidina ajudam a diminuir as bactérias; soluções de zinco e de ácido ascórbico (Maxi-Guard Gel, Addison Biological) ajudam a reduzir as bactérias e estimular a cicatrização dos tecidos moles.
• Dieta — talvez haja necessidade de alimentos pastosos ou papas durante a consolidação da fratura.
• Também é necessário o suporte nutricional, além de fluidos de manutenção.
• Exercício de mastigação — evitar a mastigação de itens muito duros durante o processo de consolidação da fratura.

MEDICAÇÕES
MEDICAMENTO(S)
Controle da Dor
• Anestesia local — bloqueios anestésicos locais intrabucais; bloqueios de nervos regionais: n. mentoniano, n. mandibular, n. infraorbital, n. palatino e n. maxilar.
• Injetáveis — tartarato de butorfanol; buprenorfina; nalbufina.
• Emplastros transdérmicos — fentanila.
• Orais — carprofeno; tartarato de butorfanol; hidrocodona.

Antibióticos
• De amplo espectro, selecionados com base na anamnese, no estado de saúde e no perfil bioquímico.

ACOMPANHAMENTO
MONITORIZAÇÃO DO PACIENTE
• Física — reavaliar 2 semanas do pós-operatório.
• Radiográfica — reavaliar 4-6 semanas do pós-operatório e, em seguida, a cada 2 semanas até que a fratura se consolide e/ou a imobilização seja removida.
• O local da fratura pode ficar temporariamente (1-2 semanas) sob maior risco de novas fraturas após o suporte da imobilização ser removido.
• Assim que a linha de fratura estiver estabilizada, os dentes comprometidos poderão necessitar de tratamento endodôntico adicional (p. ex., tratamento de canal radicular) ou cuidadosa extração.
• Se o processo de consolidação resultar em maloclusão — poderá haver a necessidade de tratamento ortodôntico, endodôntico e/ou exodôntico seletivo (extração).
• Outras considerações — estabilidade da fratura e aplicação da imobilização; higiene bucal; ingestão oral de água e alimento; manutenção do peso; micção e defecação apropriadas; indicações de dor ou tumefação (inchaço).

PREVENÇÃO
Tentar minimizar o risco de traumatismo.

COMPLICAÇÕES POSSÍVEIS
• Maloclusão. • Doença endodôntica. • Osteomielite. • Não união. • Sequestro. • Deiscência. • Defeitos neurológicos. • Síndrome da dor facial. • Mastigação prejudicada. • Perda de peso temporária. • Traumatismo do tecido mole atribuído à aplicação da imobilização ou dos fios.

POSSÍVEIS SEQUELAS
Mastigação Prejudicada
• Artrite da ATM — dor crônica ou intermitente dessa articulação; pode necessitar do procedimento de condilectomia.
• Maloclusão — atrito dentário; pode requerer extrações.
• Não união — pode exigir mandibulectomia ou maxilectomia parcial ou completa.
• Anquilose da mandíbula na ATM ou na área do arco zigomático.

Síndrome da Dor Facial
• Aguda ou crônica.
• Atribuída a traumatismo de nervo por lesão ou como complicação da cirurgia.

Lesão de Nervo
• Envolvimento da função motora.

EVOLUÇÃO ESPERADA E PROGNÓSTICO
• Geralmente bons; entretanto, fatores predisponentes, força desencadeante, localização, tipo de fratura, qualidade dos cuidados domésticos e seleção da modalidade terapêutica podem afetar o resultado da consolidação da fratura.
• 4-12 semanas para união óssea.

DIVERSOS
DISTÚRBIOS ASSOCIADOS
• Maloclusão.
• Dificuldade de mastigação.
• Falta de simetria na cabeça.
• Traumatismo do tecido mole.
• Doença periodontal.
• Dentes lascados, fraturados, luxados ou avulsionados.

FATORES RELACIONADOS COM A IDADE
A consolidação de fratura pode ser mais rápida em animais mais jovens.

VER TAMBÉM
Articulação Temporomandibular — Deslocamento/Luxação/Travamento Intermitente da Boca.

ABREVIATURA(S)
• ATM = articulação temporomandibular.
• TC = tomografia computadorizada.
• RM = ressonância magnética.

RECURSOS DA INTERNET
http://www.avdc.org/Nomenclature.html.

Sugestões de Leitura
Fossum TW. Small Animal Surgery, 2nd ed. St. Louis: Mosby, 2002, pp. 901-913.
Legendre L. Maxillofacial fracture repairs. Vet Clin North Am Small Anim Pract 2005, 35:1009-1040.
Lobprise HB. Blackwell's Five-Minute Veterinary Consult Clinical Companion — Small Animal Dentistry. Ames, IA: Blackwell, 2007 (for additional topics, including diagnostics and techniques).
Marretta SM. Maxillofacial surgery. Vet Clin North Am Small Anim Pract 1998, 28:1285-1296.
Wiggs RB, Lobprise HB. Veterinary Dentistry: Principles and Practice. Philadelphia: Lippincott-Raven, 1997, pp. 259-279.

Autores Robert B. Wiggs e Barron P. Hall
Consultor Editorial Heidi B. Lobprise

Gastrenterite Eosinofílica

CONSIDERAÇÕES GERAIS

DEFINIÇÃO
Doença inflamatória do estômago e do intestino, caracterizada por infiltração de eosinófilos, em geral na lâmina própria, embora ocasionalmente envolva as camadas submucosa e muscular.

FISIOPATOLOGIA
• Os antígenos ligam-se à IgE na superfície de mastócitos, resultando em degranulação dessas células.
• Alguns dos produtos liberados são potentes quimiotáticos de eosinófilos.
• Os eosinófilos contêm grânulos com substâncias que lesam diretamente os tecidos circundantes.
• Os eosinófilos também podem ativar diretamente os mastócitos, desencadeando um ciclo vicioso de degranulação e destruição tecidual.

SISTEMA(S) ACOMETIDO(S)
• Gastrintestinal — geralmente acomete o estômago e o intestino delgado, mas o intestino grosso também pode ser acometido.
• Em gatos, a síndrome hipereosinofílica pode envolver o trato gastrintestinal, o fígado, o baço, os rins, as adrenais e o coração. Também há relatos raros em cães, particularmente na raça Rottweiler.

GENÉTICA
N/D.

INCIDÊNCIA/PREVALÊNCIA
• Segundo relatos, a gastrenterite eosinofílica é mais comum em cães do que em gatos.
• Menos comum que a gastrenterite linfocítica-plasmocitária.
• Ocasionalmente, pode haver um infiltrado celular misto composto de eosinófilos, linfócitos e plasmócitos.

DISTRIBUIÇÃO GEOGRÁFICA
N/D.

IDENTIFICAÇÃO
Espécies
Cães e gatos.

Raça(s) Predominante(s)
Pastor alemão, Rottweiler, Weathen terrier de pelo macio e Shar-pei podem ser predispostos.

Idade Média e Faixa Etária
• Cães — mais comum naqueles com menos de 5 anos de idade, embora os animais de qualquer idade possam ser acometidos.
• Gatos — idade média, 8 anos; variação relatada de 1,5-11 anos.

Sexo Predominante
Nenhum relatado.

SINAIS CLÍNICOS
Achados Anamnésicos
• Vômitos intermitentes, diarreia do intestino delgado, anorexia e/ou perda de peso são as queixas mais comuns do proprietário, semelhantemente a outras causas de gastrenterite.
• Um único relato afirma que 50% dos gatos com gastrite/enterite eosinofílica tinham hematoquezia ou melena.

Achados do Exame Físico
• Gatos — podem-se palpar alças intestinais espessadas.
• Pode haver evidência de perda de peso.
• Se a síndrome hipereosinofílica for a causa da doença gastrintestinal, será possível observar linfonodos periféricos aumentados, linfadenopatia mesentérica e hepatosplenomegalia.

CAUSAS
• Gastrenterite eosinofílica idiopática.
• Parasitária.
• Imunomediada — alergia alimentar; reação medicamentosa adversa; associada a outras formas de enteropatia inflamatória.
• Mastocitose sistêmica.
• Síndrome hipereosinofílica.
• Leucemia eosinofílica.
• Granuloma eosinofílico.

FATORES DE RISCO
N/D.

DIAGNÓSTICO

DIAGNÓSTICO DIFERENCIAL
• Todas as causas supramencionadas estão incluídas no diagnóstico diferencial de infiltrados eosinofílicos no estômago e no intestino delgado.
• A gastrenterite eosinofílica idiopática é um diagnóstico de exclusão.
• É imperativa a realização de múltiplos exames de flutuação fecal e esfregaços diretos para excluir parasitismo intestinal. A vermifugação de rotina com algum produto de amplo espectro costuma ser indicada, mesmo quando todos os exames de fezes forem negativos.
• A biopsia intestinal diferencia as outras causas de enteropatia inflamatória da gastrenterite eosinofílica.
• Ensaios alimentares devem descartar alergia ou hipersensibilidade alimentar.

HEMOGRAMA/BIOQUÍMICA/URINÁLISE
• O hemograma pode revelar eosinofilia periférica — mais comum em gatos do que em cães, particularmente comum e pronunciada em casos de síndrome hipereosinofílica.
• Pode haver pan-hipoproteinemia ou hipoalbuminemia se também houver enteropatia com perda de proteínas.
• Na síndrome hipereosinofílica, pode-se observar o aumento das enzimas hepáticas e/ou a presença de azotemia.
• A urinálise costuma permanecer normal.

OUTROS TESTES LABORATORIAIS
O esfregaço da camada leucocitária exclui mastocitose sistêmica, quando houver suspeita.

DIAGNÓSTICO POR IMAGEM
• Radiografias abdominais simples fornecem poucas informações, mas são úteis para descartar outras doenças que podem se manifestar com sinais clínicos semelhantes.
• Radiografias contrastadas com bário podem demonstrar o espessamento das paredes intestinais e as irregularidades da mucosa, mas não fornecem nenhuma informação sobre a etiologia ou a natureza do espessamento.
• Ultrassonografia — pode ser usada para medir o estômago e a espessura da parede intestinal, bem como para excluir outras doenças e examinar órgãos como fígado, baço e linfonodos mesentéricos em gatos com síndrome hipereosinofílica. Com frequência, fica indicada a obtenção de aspirados desses órgãos quando visualizados.

MÉTODOS DIAGNÓSTICOS
• O diagnóstico definitivo frequentemente requer o exame histopatológico de amostras de biopsia obtidas por endoscopia ou cirurgia exploratória.
• Aspirados de medula óssea serão recomendados se houver mastocitose sistêmica ou eosinofilia periférica significativa aparente.
• A laparotomia exploratória pode ficar indicada quando partes do trato gastrintestinal, inacessíveis à endoscopia, estiverem acometidas ou na presença de organomegalia abdominal.

ACHADOS PATOLÓGICOS
• Pode haver pregas rugosas espessadas, erosões, úlceras e aumento da friabilidade da mucosa do estômago, embora esse órgão possa parecer normal ao exame macroscópico.
• Ulcerações e erosões também podem ser observadas no intestino.
• Infiltrados eosinofílicos podem estar dispersos pelo intestino; pode ser necessária a realização de múltiplas biopsias para se obter uma amostra diagnóstica.
• A histopatologia revela a presença de infiltrado difuso de eosinófilos na lâmina própria; as camadas submucosa e muscular também podem estar envolvidas (o que é mais comum em gatos com essa doença, segundo relatos).

TRATAMENTO

CUIDADO(S) DE SAÚDE ADEQUADO(S)
• A maioria dos pacientes pode ser tratada com sucesso em um esquema ambulatorial.
• Os pacientes com mastocitose sistêmica, enteropatias com perda de proteínas ou outras doenças concomitantes podem precisar de hospitalização até que estejam estabilizados.

CUIDADO(S) DE ENFERMAGEM
• Se o paciente estiver desidratado ou tiver de ficar em jejum (i. e., nada por via oral) por causa de vômitos, qualquer fluido balanceado como Ringer lactato será adequado (caso o paciente não tenha outra condição concomitante); do contrário, escolher os fluidos com base nas doenças secundárias.
• Se o paciente tiver hipoalbuminemia grave em decorrência de enteropatia com perda de proteínas, considerar o uso de coloides como hetamido. Infelizmente, a maioria dos casos necessita de quantidades proibitivas de plasma em termos de custo para serem benéficas.

ATIVIDADE
Não há necessidade de restrição a menos que o animal esteja gravemente debilitado.

DIETA
• Manipulação da dieta — representa, em geral, um componente crítico da terapia; pode ser feita de várias formas.
• Dietas altamente digeríveis com fontes limitadas de nutrientes (dietas hipoalergênicas) — são extremamente úteis para estimular a remissão; podem ser usadas como dietas de manutenção assim que o paciente estiver estabilizado. A maior parte dos casos é tratada com êxito dessa forma.
• Cães — os exemplos incluem as rações comerciais vendidas com prescrição Hill's d/d, z/d e i/d, Purina EN, HA e LA, Royal Canin com restrição proteica, Eukanuba Low Residue Diet e

Gastrenterite Eosinofílica

Canine Response Formula FP ou KO; também se pode fazer uso de dietas caseiras balanceadas.
- Gatos — os exemplos incluem as rações comerciais vendidas com prescrição Hill's i/d, z/d, m/d e d/d; Purina DM e EN; Royal Canin com restrição proteica; Eukanuba Low Residue Diet.
- Dietas monoméricas (p. ex., elementar) — têm componentes não alergênicos; podem ser usadas em pacientes que não estejam vomitando, mas tenham inflamação gastrintestinal moderada a grave; úteis quando se suspeita de alergia alimentar. Em geral, o tratamento com dietas monoméricas não é necessário.
- Em pacientes com acometimento intestinal grave e enteropatia significativa com perda de proteínas, pode ser indicado o uso de nutrição parenteral total (NPT) até que a remissão seja obtida. No entanto, é raro haver necessidade de NPT.
- Assim que o paciente estiver estabilizado, poderá ser instituído um ensaio alimentar com dieta de eliminação se a causa sob suspeita for alergia ou intolerância alimentar para determinar o nutriente agressor. Isso, entretanto, não costuma ser feito.

ORIENTAÇÃO AO PROPRIETÁRIO
Explicar a natureza flutuante da doença, com exacerbações e remissões, a necessidade de vigilância pelo resto da vida do animal em relação aos fatores desencadeantes e o potencial de terapia prolongada.

CONSIDERAÇÕES CIRÚRGICAS
N/D.

MEDICAÇÕES

MEDICAMENTO(S) DE ESCOLHA
- Corticosteroides — prednisona a 2-4 mg/kg VO a cada 24 h (raramente requer o extremo superior da dose para começar).
- Diminuir os corticosteroides gradativamente em cerca de 25% a cada 2-3 semanas até 25% da dose original e, em seguida, estender para intervalos de 4 a 8 semanas antes de interromper; as recidivas são mais comuns nos pacientes em que os corticosteroides são retirados com muita rapidez.
- Ocasionalmente, outros imunossupressores podem ser usados para permitir uma redução na dose do corticosteroide e evitar alguns dos efeitos adversos da terapia esteroide. Essas medicações também são adicionadas em casos refratários.
- Imunossupressores como azatioprina (2,2 mg/kg a cada 24 h VO, reduzindo para um esquema em dias alternados depois de 2-3 semanas) na suspeita de algum mecanismo imunomediado e se a resposta à dieta e à administração de glicocorticoide for inadequada. Espera-se que ocorra uma resposta em 2-3 semanas.
- Para imunossupressão adicional nos casos em que há necessidade de uma resposta imediata, adicionar a clorambucila (0,1-0,2 mg/kg a cada 24 h por 7 dias e, em seguida, em dias alternados). Com frequência, a clorambucila é utilizada no lugar da azatioprina, embora possa ser usada em adição a este medicamento.
- A budenosida, um novo glicocorticoide oral, foi utilizada com sucesso para tratar cães e gatos com enteropatia inflamatória; parece ter mais que um efeito tópico sobre o trato intestinal. Os relatos demonstraram a ocorrência de certa absorção e efeitos secundários sobre o eixo hipófise-adrenal. As recomendações atuais de dose são de 2-3 mg/m² (não formuladas com base em pesquisas científicas), mas frequentemente exigem a manipulação para qualquer cão, exceto os de grande porte.

CONTRAINDICAÇÕES
Se houver problemas secundários, evitar o uso de agentes terapêuticos possivelmente contraindicados para tais condições.

PRECAUÇÕES
- Prednisona e budenosida (menos comumente) podem causar ulcerações gastrintestinais. Se houver indícios de ulcerações, fica indicada a adição de protetores gástricos. Não foi demonstrado que o uso de protetores gástricos evite o dano, mas é tão eficaz quanto um tratamento.
- A azatioprina e a clorambucila raramente provocam supressão da medula óssea; em geral, causam mais de um problema em gatos do que em cães. Em todos os pacientes submetidos à azatioprina ou clorambucila, deve-se realizar um hemograma completo 10-14 dias após o início do tratamento, com reavaliações mensais e depois bimestrais durante todo o período terapêutico; a supressão da medula óssea pode ser observada em qualquer momento durante a terapia, mas costuma ser reversível com a interrupção do medicamento. Também é recomendável a avaliação regular do perfil bioquímico.
- Pancreatite, lesão hepática e anorexia constituem outros efeitos colaterais potenciais desses medicamentos.

INTERAÇÕES POSSÍVEIS
N/D.

MEDICAMENTO(S) ALTERNATIVO(S)
N/D.

ACOMPANHAMENTO

MONITORIZAÇÃO DO PACIENTE
- Em princípio, a monitorização é frequente em alguns pacientes mais gravemente acometidos; as contagens dos eosinófilos periféricos podem ser úteis; a dosagem de corticosteroide costuma ser ajustada durante essas consultas.
- Pacientes com doença menos grave — podem ser examinados 2-5 semanas após a avaliação inicial; mensalmente ou, depois, a cada 2 meses, até que a terapia com corticosteroide seja concluída.
- Pacientes submetidos à azatioprina — monitorizar conforme mencionado anteriormente.
- Em geral, os pacientes não precisam de acompanhamento a longo prazo a menos que o problema recidive.

PREVENÇÃO
Em caso de suspeita ou confirmação de intolerância ou alergia alimentar, evitar o nutriente em questão e seguir estritamente as modificações da dieta.

COMPLICAÇÕES POSSÍVEIS
- Perda de peso e debilidade nos casos refratários.
- Efeitos adversos da terapia com corticosteroide.
- Supressão da medula óssea, pancreatite, hepatite ou anorexia causada pela azatioprina e/ou clorambucila.

EVOLUÇÃO ESPERADA E PROGNÓSTICO
- A grande maioria dos cães com gastrenterite eosinofílica responde a uma combinação de manipulação da dieta e terapia com esteroide.
- Os gatos, em geral, apresentam uma forma mais grave da doença, com prognóstico pior do que os cães.
- Com frequência, os gatos necessitam de doses maiores de corticosteroides por períodos mais longos para que ocorra remissão.

DIVERSOS

DISTÚRBIOS ASSOCIADOS
Nenhum.

FATORES RELACIONADOS COM A IDADE
Nenhum.

POTENCIAL ZOONÓTICO
Esse potencial só é levado em consideração quando os infiltrados eosinofílicos são secundários a parasitas (p. ex., *Ancylostoma*, *Giardia* e ascarídeos).

GESTAÇÃO/FERTILIDADE/REPRODUÇÃO
- A prednisona foi utilizada com segurança em gestantes; no entanto, os corticosteroides foram associados à maior incidência de defeitos congênitos, abortamentos e morte fetal.
- A azatioprina já foi usada em mulheres grávidas de forma segura e pode ser uma boa substituta para os corticosteroides em animais prenhes.

VER TAMBÉM
- Enteropatia Inflamatória.
- Gastrenterite Linfocítica-plasmocitária.
- Mastocitomas.

ABREVIATURA(S)
- IgE = imunoglobulina E.

Sugestões de Leitura
Strombeck DR, Guilford WG. Idiopathic inflammatory bowel diseases. In: Guilford WG, Center SA, Strombeck DR, et al., eds., Strombeck's Small Animal Gastroenterology, 3rd ed. Philadelphia: Saunders, 1996.
Tarris TR. Feline inflammatory bowel disease. Vet Clin North Am 1993, 23:569-586.

Autor Michelle Pressel
Consultor Editorial Albert E. Jergens

Gastrenterite Hemorrágica

CONSIDERAÇÕES GERAIS

DEFINIÇÃO
Trata-se de uma enterite hemorrágica superaguda de cães, caracterizada por início súbito de diarreia sanguinolenta grave que, em geral, é explosiva, com vômitos, hipovolemia e hemoconcentração acentuada em virtude da perda notável de água e eletrólitos para o lúmen intestinal.

FISIOPATOLOGIA
Muitas condições resultam em diarreia hemorrágica, mas a síndrome de gastrenterite hemorrágica aguda em cães parece ter aspectos clínicos únicos que a diferenciam como uma entidade clínica distinta de outras causas. A gastrenterite hemorrágica caracteriza-se por perda superaguda de integridade da mucosa intestinal, com deslocamento rápido de sangue, líquido e eletrólitos para o lúmen intestinal. Ocorrem desidratação e choque hipovolêmico rapidamente. A translocação de bactérias ou toxinas por meio da mucosa intestinal lesada pode resultar em choque séptico ou endotóxico. Raramente se observam inflamação e necrose. O aumento na permeabilidade intestinal pode representar uma reação de hipersensibilidade do tipo I.

SISTEMA(S) ACOMETIDO(S)
- Gastrintestinal.
- Cardiovascular.

GENÉTICA
Desconhecida; no entanto, parece haver raças pequenas específicas em que a síndrome é super-representada.

INCIDÊNCIA/PREVALÊNCIA
Condição clínica comum.

DISTRIBUIÇÃO GEOGRÁFICA
N/D.

IDENTIFICAÇÃO
Espécies
Cães.

Raça(s) Predominante(s)
- Todas as raças podem ser acometidas, mas a incidência é maior nas de pequeno porte.
- As raças mais representadas incluem Schnauzer miniatura, Dachshund, Yorkshire terrier e Poodle miniatura.

Idade Média e Faixa Etária
Em geral, ocorre em cães adultos com idade média de 5 anos.

Sexo Predominante
N/D.

SINAIS CLÍNICOS
Comentários Gerais
- Os achados clínicos são variáveis tanto em termos de evolução como de gravidade da doença que, em geral, é superaguda e associada a choque hipovolêmico concomitante.
- A maioria dos animais acometidos encontrava-se saudável, sem histórico de mudanças ambientais ou doença gastrintestinal concomitante.

Achados Anamnésicos
- Os sinais costumam ser benignos com vômitos agudos, anorexia e depressão, seguidos por diarreia aquosa que, rapidamente, se transforma em diarreia sanguinolenta.
- Os sinais evoluem com rapidez e se agravam em questão de horas (em geral, 8-12 h), sendo o resultado do choque hipovolêmico e da hemoconcentração.

Achados do Exame Físico
- O paciente geralmente se encontra deprimido e fraco, com tempo de preenchimento capilar prolongado e pressão de pulso fraca.
- O turgor cutâneo como um reflexo de desidratação pode estar aparentemente normal em virtude da natureza superaguda da doença e do lapso de tempo transcorrido nos desvios de líquido entre os compartimentos.
- A palpação abdominal pode ser dolorosa e detectar as alças intestinais repletas de líquido.
- O exame retal identifica diarreia sanguinolenta e, mais tarde durante a evolução da doença, surgem fezes características com aspecto de "geleia de framboesa".
- Embora ocasionalmente haja febre, a temperatura costuma permanecer normal ou até mesmo abaixo do normal.

CAUSAS
- A etiologia é desconhecida.
- Reação de hipersensibilidade do tipo I direcionada contra a mucosa entérica do hospedeiro.
- Culturas de alguns cães com gastrenterite hemorrágica resultam principalmente em culturas puras de *Clostridium perfringens* e enterotoxina, mas o significado é desconhecido.
- As pesquisas em busca de cepas toxigênicas de *E. coli* não são recompensadoras, embora sejam possíveis.

FATORES DE RISCO
- Desconhecidos.
- A maioria dos cães encontra-se previamente sadia, sem doença concomitante importante.

DIAGNÓSTICO

DIAGNÓSTICO DIFERENCIAL
- Parvovírus.
- Enterite bacteriana como salmonelose ou campilobacteriose.
- Condições que resultam em choque endotóxico ou hipovolêmico.
- Obstrução ou intussuscepção intestinal.
- Hipoadrenocorticismo.
- Pancreatite.
- Coagulopatia.

HEMOGRAMA/BIOQUÍMICA/URINÁLISE
- Hemoconcentração com hematócrito em geral >60% e às vezes até 75%. Geralmente, observa-se leucograma de estresse.
- O perfil bioquímico pode revelar elevações secundárias das enzimas hepáticas e aumento da ureia em função de causas pré-renais. A proteína total pode estar normal ou baixa por causa da perda de proteína no trato GI.

OUTROS TESTES LABORATORIAIS
Exames de Fezes
- Negativos para parasitas.
- ELISA negativo para parvovírus.
- A citologia fecal revela muitos eritrócitos e alguns leucócitos.
- É possível cultivar clostrídios em alta concentração, embora as culturas sejam negativas para outros patógenos entéricos.

Coagulograma
Geralmente se apresenta normal; ocasionalmente, entretanto, a ocorrência de CID secundária é uma complicação.

DIAGNÓSTICO POR IMAGEM
As radiografias abdominais revelam os intestinos delgado e grosso repletos de líquido e gás.

MÉTODOS DIAGNÓSTICOS
Eletrocardiograma
Podem ser observadas arritmias cardíacas como contrações ventriculares prematuras e taquicardia ventricular.

Endoscopia
- O exame de colonoscopia não está indicado nem é útil para o diagnóstico.
- Pode revelar hemorragia, ulceração e hiperemia difusas da mucosa.

ACHADOS PATOLÓGICOS
As alterações no intestino incluem congestão macroscópica e indícios microscópicos de autólise sem inflamação acentuada.

TRATAMENTO

CUIDADO(S) DE SAÚDE ADEQUADO(S)
Os pacientes sob suspeita de gastrenterite hemorrágica aguda devem ser hospitalizados e submetidos a tratamento rigoroso, porque a deterioração clínica costuma ser rápida e pode ser fatal.

CUIDADO(S) DE ENFERMAGEM
- Em todos os casos, é imprescindível a rápida reposição volêmica.
- Administram-se soluções eletrolíticas balanceadas a uma velocidade de 40-60 mL/kg/h IV até que o hematócrito decline para menos de 50%.
- Fluidos de manutenção são administrados a uma velocidade moderada para manter a função circulatória e corrigir quaisquer déficits de potássio ou outros eletrólitos durante o período de recuperação.
- Perdas GI contínuas de líquido devem ser estimadas e o volume encontrado acrescentado às necessidades hídricas.
- Animais com hipoproteinemia podem necessitar de coloides ou plasma.

ATIVIDADE
Restrita.

DIETA
- Nada por via oral durante a doença aguda.
- Durante o período de recuperação, é recomendável o fornecimento de dieta branda, com baixo teor de fibras e pobre em gorduras, por vários dias antes de voltar à alimentação normal.

ORIENTAÇÃO AO PROPRIETÁRIO
- Discutir a necessidade de tratamento clínico imediato e rigoroso. Com a terapia apropriada, a mortalidade costuma ser baixa.
- Há relatos de recidiva em cerca de 10% dos casos.

CONSIDERAÇÕES CIRÚRGICAS
N/D.

GASTRENTERITE HEMORRÁGICA

MEDICAÇÕES

MEDICAMENTO(S) DE ESCOLHA
• Antibióticos parenterais são administrados em função do potencial de septicemia e das possíveis implicações de infecção por *Clostridium perfringens*. Recomenda-se o uso da ampicilina.
• As escolhas alternativas incluem trimetoprima-sulfa ou cefalosporinas. Nos casos em que se suspeita de septicemia, sugere-se o emprego de ampicilina combinada com alguma fluoroquinolona (enrofloxacino).
• Glicocorticoides de ação curta são sugeridos (fosfato sódico de dexametasona na dose de 0,5-1,0 mg/kg IV) por conta da possível reação de hipersensibilidade.
• Talvez haja necessidade de transfusão de sangue (raramente) em caso de perda sanguínea excessiva.

CONTRAINDICAÇÕES
N/D.

PRECAUÇÕES
Como pode ocorrer o rápido desenvolvimento de choque séptico e/ou hipovolêmico, é recomendável a monitorização rigorosa do animal.

INTERAÇÕES POSSÍVEIS
N/D.

MEDICAMENTO(S) ALTERNATIVO(S)
• Antibióticos orais e protetores intestinais são de pouco benefício e, em geral, não são administrados.
• A administração retal de protetores da mucosa tem valor questionável.
• Antieméticos podem ser administrados para controlar vômitos graves. Modificadores da motilidade intestinal não são considerados necessários nem são recomendados.

ACOMPANHAMENTO

MONITORIZAÇÃO DO PACIENTE
• Monitorizar o hematócrito e os sólidos totais com frequência (pelo menos a cada 4-6 h).
• Modificar a reposição hídrica com base no hematócrito, nas perdas contínuas de líquidos GI e na função circulatória.
• Se não houver melhora clínica em 24-48 h, reavaliar o paciente, pois é provável que haja outras causas de diarreia hemorrágica.

PREVENÇÃO
N/D.

COMPLICAÇÕES POSSÍVEIS
• Ocasionalmente, pode haver o desenvolvimento de CID. Podem ocorrer sinais neurológicos ou até mesmo crises convulsivas secundárias à hemoconcentração.
• Ocorrem arritmias cardíacas em decorrência da lesão miocárdica sob suspeita por reperfusão.
• Pode ocorrer síndrome hemolítico-urêmica (raramente).
• A maioria dos cães se recupera. A taxa de mortalidade pode ser alta em cães não submetidos a tratamento. Menos de 10% dos cães tratados morrem, enquanto 10-15% apresentam ocorrências repetidas.

EVOLUÇÃO ESPERADA E PROGNÓSTICO
• A evolução da doença, em geral, é curta, durando de 24-72 h.
• O prognóstico é bom, pois a maioria dos pacientes se recupera sem complicações.
• É incomum a ocorrência de morte súbita.

DIVERSOS

DISTÚRBIOS ASSOCIADOS
N/D.

FATORES RELACIONADOS COM A IDADE
N/D.

POTENCIAL ZOONÓTICO
Desconhecido.

GESTAÇÃO/FERTILIDADE/REPRODUÇÃO
N/D.

SINÔNIMO(S)
Enterocolite hemorrágica aguda.

VER TAMBÉM
• Diarreia Aguda.
• Vômito Agudo.

ABREVIATURA(S)
• CID = coagulação intravascular disseminada.
• ELISA = ensaio imunoabsorvente ligado à enzima.
• GI = gastrintestinal.

Sugestões de Leitura
Hall JH, German AJ. Diseases of the small intestine. In: Ettinger SJ, Feldman EC, eds., Textbook of Veterinary Internal Medicine, 6th ed. St. Louis: Elsevier, 2005, pp. 1332-1378.
Sasaki J, Goryo M, Asahina M, et al. Hemorrhagic enteritis associated with *Clostridium perfringens* type A in a dog. J Vet Med Sci 1999, 61:175-177.
Spielman BL, Garvey MS. Hemorrhagic gastroenteritis in dogs. JAAHA 1993, 29:341-344.
Strombeck DR, Guilford WG. In: Guilford WG, Center SA, et al., eds., Strombeck's Small Animal Gastroenterology. Philadelphia: Saunders, 1996, pp. 433-435.

Autor David C. Twedt
Consultor Editorial Albert E. Jergens

Gastrenterite Linfoplasmocitária

CONSIDERAÇÕES GERAIS

DEFINIÇÃO
• A forma mais comum de enteropatia inflamatória que se caracteriza por infiltração de linfócitos e plasmócitos na lâmina própria do estômago e do intestino; geralmente acompanhada por outros critérios de inflamação da mucosa.
• Menos comumente, os infiltrados podem se estender para a submucosa e a muscular da mucosa.

FISIOPATOLOGIA
• Trata-se de uma resposta imune aberrante a estímulos ambientais que provavelmente resultam em perda de hemostasia da mucosa; alterações na microbiota intestinal (ou seja, proliferação bacteriana no intestino delgado) podem ser um deflagrador.
• Exposição contínua a antígeno, aliada à inflamação desregulada, resulta na doença, embora os mecanismos exatos e os fatores relacionados com o paciente continuem desconhecidos.

SISTEMA(S) ACOMETIDO(S)
• Gastrintestinal — tipicamente acomete o intestino delgado e, às vezes, o estômago; o cólon pode ser independente ou simultaneamente acometido.
• Ocasionalmente, observam-se manifestações extraintestinais de inflamação (p. ex., trombocitopenia leve) apesar de não serem bem caracterizados.

GENÉTICA
As raças Basenji, Lundehund e Wheaten terrier de pelo macio apresentam formas familiares de enteropatia inflamatória.

INCIDÊNCIA/PREVALÊNCIA
A forma mais comum de enteropatia inflamatória que afeta cães e gatos.

IDENTIFICAÇÃO
Raça(s) Predominante(s)
• Lundehunde e Basenji exibem formas peculiares de enteropatia inflamatória; a enteropatia causada pelo glúten acomete cães da raça Setter irlandês; os quadros de enteropatia e nefropatia com perda proteica afetam a raça Wheaten terrier de pelo macio.
• Segundo relatos, o Pastor alemão e o Shar-pei chinês são predispostos à gastrenterite linfoplasmocitária.
• Os gatos de raça pura (raças asiáticas) podem ter uma incidência maior.

Idade Média e Faixa Etária
• Mais comum em animais de meia-idade a mais idosos.
• Há relatos de cães com apenas 8 meses e gatos com 5 meses de vida.

Sexo Predominante
Nenhum relatado.

SINAIS CLÍNICOS
Achados Anamnésicos
• Os sinais associados à gastrite linfoplasmocitária com ou sem enterite podem variar em termos de tipo, gravidade e frequência.
• Em geral, a evolução é crônica e intermitente ou cíclica, mas a frequência aumenta com o tempo. Os surtos são caracterizados por exacerbações e remissões espontâneas.
• Gatos — vômitos crônicos intermitentes constituem o sinal mais comum; diarreia crônica do intestino delgado é o segundo.
• Cães — diarreia crônica do intestino delgado é o mais comum; se apenas o estômago estiver envolvido, vômitos serão o sinal mais comum.
• Cães e gatos — anorexia e perda de peso crônica são comuns; ocasionalmente, observam-se hematoquezia, hematêmese e melena.

Achados do Exame Físico
Variam de animais perfeitamente normais a pacientes desidratados, caquéticos e deprimidos, dependendo da gravidade da doença e do órgão acometido.

CAUSAS
A patogênese é provavelmente multifatorial e envolve interações complexas entre fatores genéticos, imunológicos e ambientais (p. ex., microbiota).

Agentes Infecciosos
• Microrganismos como *Giardia*, *Salmonella*, *Campylobacter* e microbiota gastrintestinal normal são implicados na patogênese. Foi constatado um aumento de bactérias associadas à mucosa em cães e gatos com enteropatia inflamatória em comparação a animais saudáveis.

Agentes Nutricionais
• Proteínas da carne e do leite, aditivos alimentares, corantes artificiais, conservantes e glúten (trigo) podem contribuir para a patogênese da inflamação crônica da mucosa.

Fatores Genéticos
• Certas formas de enteropatia inflamatória são mais comuns em algumas raças de cães (ver anteriormente).
• Certos genes do complexo de histocompatibilidade maior podem tornar um indivíduo suscetível ao desenvolvimento de enteropatia inflamatória.

FATORES DE RISCO
Ver a seção "Causas".

DIAGNÓSTICO

DIAGNÓSTICO DIFERENCIAL
• Outros distúrbios intestinais inflamatórios infiltrativos (p. ex., gastrenterite eosinofílica e enteropatia inflamatória granulomatosa).
• Hipersensibilidade alimentar e outras causas de reações alimentares adversas.
• Distúrbios metabólicos.
• Neoplasia.
• Doenças infecciosas (p. ex., histoplasmose, toxoplasmose, giardíase, salmonelose, enterite por *Campilobacter* e proliferação bacteriana excessiva).
• Outras doenças (p. ex., linfangiectasia, distúrbios da motilidade gastrintestinal e insuficiência pancreática exócrina).
• Em gatos, considerar hipertireoidismo, infecções virais sistêmicas (p. ex., FeLV, FIV e PIF) e pancreatite crônica.

HEMOGRAMA/BIOQUÍMICA/URINÁLISE
• Geralmente normais.
• Anemia arregenerativa e leucocitose discretas com ou sem um leve desvio à esquerda.
• Hipoproteinemia é mais comum em cães do que em gatos com enteropatia inflamatória.

OUTROS TESTES LABORATORIAIS
• Alterações nos níveis séricos de cobalamina e folato podem servir para localizar as regiões acometidas por inflamação do intestino delgado.
• Mensuração do nível sérico da lipase pancreática para fazer a triagem de inflamação do pâncreas.
• Inibidor da alfa 1-proteinase fecal para avaliar a presença de enteropatia com perda de proteínas.
• Imunorreatividade semelhante à da tripsina deve ser realizada para avaliar a existência de insuficiência pancreática exócrina.
• Gatos — é recomendável a sorologia de T_4 e FeLV/FIV/toxoplasmose para fazer a triagem de causas infecciosas para sinais gastrintestinais.

DIAGNÓSTICO POR IMAGEM
• Radiografias simples do abdome são geralmente normais.
• Radiografias contrastadas com bário ocasionalmente revelam anormalidades da mucosa e espessamento das alças intestinais; tipicamente, no entanto, não são úteis para estabelecer o diagnóstico definitivo.

MÉTODOS DIAGNÓSTICOS
• Em primeiro lugar, pode-se tentar uma dieta hipoalergênica para descartar reações alimentares adversas; se os sinais desaparecerem, não haverá necessidade de testes diagnósticos adicionais.
• Sempre realizar exame coprológico direto e indireto em busca de parasitas.
• O diagnóstico definitivo requer biopsia e histopatologia da mucosa, obtidas em geral por endoscopia. Obter biopsias do íleo em função do desempenho de ileoscopia retrógrada se possível.
• A laparotomia ou laparoscopia exploratória poderá ser indicada em caso de envolvimento de partes do trato gastrintestinal inacessíveis à endoscopia ou na presença de organomegalia abdominal.
• A avaliação clínica da gravidade da doença com o uso de um índice de atividade da enteropatia inflamatória canina é uma ferramenta útil.

ACHADOS PATOLÓGICOS
• Ao exame macroscópico, o aspecto do estômago e dos intestinos pode variar de normal a edematoso, espessado e ulcerado.
• O aspecto histopatológico típico consiste em um infiltrado de linfócitos e plasmócitos na lâmina própria; pode haver alterações estruturais, incluindo atrofia das vilosidades, fusão, fibrose, abscedação das criptas e linfangiectasia, em graus variados.
• A distribuição pode ser irregular, exigindo a realização de várias biopsias para formular o diagnóstico.

TRATAMENTO

CUIDADO(S) DE SAÚDE ADEQUADO(S)
• Ambulatoriais a menos que o paciente esteja debilitado por desidratação, hipoproteinemia ou caquexia.
• Monitorizar as respostas terapêuticas com o uso dos escores do índice de atividade da enteropatia inflamatória canina.

CUIDADO(S) DE ENFERMAGEM
• Se o paciente estiver desidratado ou precisar de nada por via oral em virtude de vômitos intensos, um cristaloide balanceado, como Ringer lactato, será adequado; suplementação eletrolítica adicional

Gastrenterite Linfoplasmocitária

poderá ser necessária na presença de alterações (p. ex., cloreto de potássio, sulfato de magnésio).
- Se houver hipoalbuminemia grave causada por enteropatia com perda de proteína, será recomendável a administração de coloides (p. ex., dextranas ou hetamido).

ATIVIDADE
Sem restrições.

DIETA
- A terapia nutricional com dieta de eliminação é um componente essencial do tratamento.
- Pacientes com acometimento intestinal grave e enteropatia com perda de proteína talvez necessitem de nutrição parenteral total até a estabilidade.
- É recomendável o uso de dietas de alta digestibilidade e com restrição antigênica (ou seja, com uma única fonte proteica) para minimizar as contribuições potenciais de reações alimentares adversas.
- Dietas altamente digeríveis diminuem a carga antigênica intestinal, ajudando com isso a diminuir a inflamação da mucosa; a terapia nutricional adequada pode contribuir para a remissão clínica e ser usada como uma dieta de manutenção.
- A modificação da relação de ácidos graxos ômega 3:6 também pode ajudar a modular a resposta inflamatória.
- A suplementação parenteral de cobalamina será essencial se os níveis séricos dessa vitamina estiverem abaixo do normal. As deficiências da cobalamina podem não só contribuir para os sinais clínicos, mas também limitar a eficácia da terapia nutricional e clínica.
- Inúmeras dietas comerciais de eliminação que atendem aos critérios supramencionados estão disponíveis para cães e gatos; as dietas caseiras também constituem uma excelente opção, porém consomem mais tempo dos proprietários.
- Utilizar suplementação de fibras em cães e gatos com colite.

ORIENTAÇÃO AO PROPRIETÁRIO
- É mais provável que a enteropatia inflamatória seja controlada e não curada, pois as recidivas são comuns.
- É preciso ter paciência durante as várias tentativas com alimentos e medicações que costumam ser necessárias.

MEDICAÇÕES

MEDICAMENTO(S) DE ESCOLHA
- Corticosteroides — a base do tratamento da enterite linfoplasmocitária idiopática; a prednisona ou a prednisolona é usada com maior frequência (1-2 mg/kg VO a cada 12 h) em cães e gatos; os gatos podem necessitar de uma dose maior para controlar sua doença. Quando os sinais clínicos desaparecerem, diminuir gradualmente a dose do corticosteroide após 2-4 semanas da terapia de indução; as recidivas serão comuns se a dose for reduzida muito rapidamente. Talvez haja necessidade de doses de manutenção a cada 48-72 h em alguns pacientes. Os gatos podem responder melhor à prednisolona do que à prednisona. Budesonida, um esteroide localmente ativo, pode ser usada em pacientes intolerantes aos efeitos colaterais sistêmicos da prednisona. Os esteroides parenterais podem ser necessários em casos graves em que a absorção oral pode ser limitada.
- Azatioprina (2 mg/kg a cada 24-48 h VO em cães; não recomendada em gatos) — imunossupressor que pode ser usado para permitir a redução na dose do corticosteroide; o início tardio de ação (até 3 semanas) limita a eficácia em casos agudos.
- Clorambucila (2 mg/kg a cada 48-72 h VO em gatos) é uma alternativa eficaz ao uso da azatioprina.
- Metronidazol — tem propriedades antibacterianas e antiprotozoárias; há alguns indícios de que esse agente também tenha efeitos imunomoduladores; a dose para enteropatia inflamatória em cães e gatos é de 10 mg/kg VO a cada 12 h.

MEDICAMENTO(S) ALTERNATIVO(S)
- Ciclosporina — pode ser útil na terapia de casos refratários de gastrenterite linfoplasmocitária; utilizar Atopica® na dose de 2-5 mg/kg VO a cada 12 h para cães e 1-4 mg/kg a cada 12-24 h para gatos; como a dosagem é bastante individualizada, é recomendável a monitorização dos níveis de vale (contrário aos níveis de pico); seu custo proíbe o uso de rotina desse medicamento.
- Sulfassalazina — um análogo da sulfa que é degradado pelas bactérias do lúmen em sulfapiridina e ácido 5-aminossalicílico; este último composto exerce efeitos anti-inflamatórios no cólon; a dosagem para cães com enteropatia inflamatória colônica é de 10-30 mg/kg VO a cada 8-12 h. Utilizar com cuidado em gatos e sob dosagem reduzida em função do potencial de toxicidade do salicilato.

PRECAUÇÕES
- Azatioprina — provoca mielossupressão, sobretudo em gatos; os hemogramas completos de rotina são recomendados em 2 semanas, 1 mês e, depois, a cada 2 meses; a mielossupressão será tipicamente reversível se o medicamento for interrompido assim que se constatar a supressão.
- Metronidazol — pode causar neurotoxicidade reversível com dosagens elevadas; a interrupção desse medicamento costuma reverter os sinais neurológicos.
- Ciclosporina — pode causar irritação gastrintestinal, hiperplasia gengival e papilomatose; associada ao desenvolvimento de linfoma em seres humanos.

INTERAÇÕES POSSÍVEIS
- A ciclosporina pode interferir no metabolismo do fenobarbital e da fenitoína.
- O cetoconazol, a eritromicina e a cimetidina podem diminuir o metabolismo hepático da ciclosporina.
- Quaisquer medicamentos potencialmente nefrotóxicos devem ser usados com cautela em conjunto com a ciclosporina.

ACOMPANHAMENTO

MONITORIZAÇÃO DO PACIENTE
- Os pacientes gravemente acometidos sob medicamentos supressores da medula óssea necessitam de monitorização frequente (ver acima); ajustar os medicamentos durante as consultas, com base nos exames de sangue e nos sinais clínicos.
- Reavaliar os pacientes com doença menos grave 2-3 semanas depois da avaliação inicial e, depois, mensalmente ou a cada 2 meses até que os medicamentos sejam reduzidos e os sinais clínicos desapareçam.

PREVENÇÃO
Na suspeita ou confirmação de alergia ou intolerância alimentar, evitar o item em questão e seguir estritamente as modificações da dieta.

COMPLICAÇÕES POSSÍVEIS
- Perda de peso e debilidade em casos refratários.
- Hiperadrenocorticismo iatrogênico e efeitos colaterais da terapia com esteroides.
- Mielossupressão, pancreatite, hepatopatia ou anorexia podem ser causadas pela azatioprina.
- Vômito, diarreia e anorexia com ciclosporina; tipicamente, a redução temporária da dose resultará em resolução dos sinais gastrintestinais.
- Ceratoconjuntivite seca com sulfassalazina.

EVOLUÇÃO ESPERADA E PROGNÓSTICO
- Cães e gatos com inflamação leve a moderada exibem prognóstico bom a excelente quanto à recuperação completa.
- Pacientes com infiltrados graves, em particular se outras partes do trato GI estiverem acometidas, apresentam um prognóstico mais reservado.
- Outros índices prognósticos associados a desfechos negativos a longo prazo incluem lesões graves da mucosa à endoscopia, hipocobalaminemia e hipoalbuminemia.
- Em geral, a resposta inicial à terapia ocorre de acordo com a capacidade de recuperação do indivíduo.

DIVERSOS

GESTAÇÃO/FERTILIDADE/REPRODUÇÃO
- Os corticosteroides são associados à maior incidência de defeitos congênitos, abortamento e morte fetal.
- A azatioprina é usada com segurança em mulheres grávidas e pode ser uma boa substituta para os corticosteroides em animais prenhes.
- A sulfassalazina deve ser utilizada com extrema cautela durante a gestação.

VER TAMBÉM
- Enteropatia Inflamatória.
- Gastrenterite Eosinofílica.

ABREVIATURA(S)
- FeLV = vírus da leucemia felina.
- FIV = vírus da imunodeficiência felina.
- GI = gastrintestinal.
- PIF = peritonite infecciosa felina.

Sugestões de Leitura
Hall EJ, German AJ. Diseases of the small intestine. In: Ettinger SJ, Feldman EC, eds., Textbook of Veterinary Internal Medicine, 6th ed. St. Louis: Elsevier, 2005, pp. 1332-1378.
Jergens AE, Schreiner CA, Frank DE, et al. A scoring index for disease activity in canine inflammatory bowel disease. J Vet Intern Med 2003, 17:291-297.

Autor John M. Crandell
Consultor Editorial Albert E. Jergens

Gastrite Atrófica

CONSIDERAÇÕES GERAIS

REVISÃO
Um tipo de gastrite crônica que se caracteriza histologicamente por redução focal ou difusa no tamanho e na profundidade das glândulas gástricas com células inflamatórias associadas.

IDENTIFICAÇÃO
- Variável, mas incomum em pacientes jovens.
- Alta prevalência no Lundehund norueguês (faixa etária de 4-13 anos), mas os machos são super-representados.
- Incomum em outras raças.

SINAIS CLÍNICOS
- Vômitos crônicos, muitas vezes intermitentes, de alimento ou bile.
- Anorexia, letargia, perda de peso.

CAUSAS E FATORES DE RISCO
- Gastrenterite inflamatória idiopática constitui um fator de risco potencial.
- Podem refletir gastrite crônica de qualquer causa.
- Há suspeita de predisposição genética no Lundehund norueguês.

DIAGNÓSTICO

DIAGNÓSTICO DIFERENCIAL
Outras formas de gastrite e enterite crônicas.

HEMOGRAMA/BIOQUÍMICA/URINÁLISE
- Na presença de ulceração gástrica, pode haver anemia com trombocitopenia ou trombocitose.
- Na raça Lundehund, pode-se observar pan-hipoproteinemia sem proteinúria, bem como em outras acometidas por enteropatia com perda proteica.

OUTROS TESTES LABORATORIAIS
- O aumento na concentração sérica de folato pode sugerir proliferação bacteriana, embora o folato não seja um biomarcador confiável.
- Foi relatada acloridria em cães; pode levar à proliferação bacteriana ou enterite por aderência íntima da bactéria e destruição das microvilosidades.
- Considerar o exame diagnóstico para doença hepatobiliar e pancreática, bem como para concentração de cobalamina abaixo do normal, em gatos.
- É recomendável a realização de biopsias endoscópicas dos intestinos delgados para descartar inflamação da mucosa em cães e gatos.

DIAGNÓSTICO POR IMAGEM
- As radiografias simples podem revelar metástase pulmonar ou linfadenopatia na presença de processo maligno concomitante, enquanto as radiografias contrastadas podem exibir esvaziamento gástrico tardio. A ultrassonografia pode mostrar a parede gástrica espessada e uma linfadenopatia mesentérica.
- Com neoplasia gástrica, pode haver linfadenopatia.

MÉTODOS DIAGNÓSTICOS
O diagnóstico definitivo é obtido via gastroscopia com biopsia e avaliação histopatológica.

ACHADOS PATOLÓGICOS
- O exame histopatológico de amostras de biopsia gástrica revela atrofia glandular e infiltrados inflamatórios (neutrófilos ou células mononucleares). A maioria das lesões é observada no fundo gástrico. Em cães de outras raças que não o Lundehund, foi constatada gastrite linfoplasmocitária com atrofia.
- A coloração de mucina em cães da raça Lundehund exibe células mucosas anormais do colo e presença de metaplasia pseudopilórica. A transformação neoplásica pode ser associada à hiperplasia linear de células neuroendócrinas (requer coloração especial em casos sob suspeita: cromogranina A, sinaptofisina, método de Sevier-Munger).
- O papel da infecção pelo *Helicobacter* é controverso. Foi constatado que os gatos que desenvolvem gastrite atrófica tenham infecções pelo *H. pylori*, mas infecções ativas pelo *Helicobacter* não foram documentadas em casos caninos. A atividade da urease em biopsias gástricas não é diagnóstica e está pouco correlacionada com infecção real. A infecção clínica é confirmada pela documentação histológica de bactérias espirais na mucosa gástrica e depressões com inflamação associada.

TRATAMENTO

- A terapia ideal é desconhecida. Pode-se tentar a terapia utilizada em casos de gastrenterite responsiva a alimentos e a antibióticos. Tratar qualquer etiologia subjacente identificada.
- As sondas de alimentação podem ser indicadas em pacientes com caquexia.
- Em caso de lentidão no esvaziamento gástrico, as dietas pobres em gordura com restrição proteica moderada (cuidado com a restrição excessiva em gatos) podem ajudar no esvaziamento; uma nova fonte proteica também pode ser útil.

MEDICAÇÕES

MEDICAMENTO(S)
- Antagonistas dos receptores de histamina do tipo 2 (p. ex., famotidina, 0,5 mg/kg VO a cada 12-24 h) ou inibidores da bomba de prótons (p. ex., omeprazol, 0,7 mg/kg VO a cada 24 h) para inibir a secreção de ácido gástrico. Não é recomendável o uso do omeprazol a longo prazo.
- Se os vômitos persistirem, agentes procinéticos como metoclopramida (0,2-0,5 mg/kg VO a cada 8 h) ou cisaprida (0,1-0,5 mg/kg VO a cada 8-12 h) podem ser indicados.
- Tratamento triplo (p. ex., amoxicilina, 11-22 mg/kg VO a cada 12 h; metronidazol, 33 mg/kg VO a cada 24 h; e sucralfato, 0,5-1 g VO a cada 8 h, ou omeprazol, 0,66 mg/kg VO a cada 24 h; todos por 3 semanas) se a infecção por *Helicobacter* spp. for confirmada. Essas infecções frequentemente persistem apesar da terapia.

CONTRAINDICAÇÕES/INTERAÇÕES POSSÍVEIS
Cuidado com medicações que sabidamente exacerbam a gastrite, como corticosteroides e anti-inflamatórios não esteroides.

ACOMPANHAMENTO

- Pode ser necessária terapia prolongada intermitente com antiácido — não se incentiva o uso do omeprazol a longo prazo, pois esse agente pode estar associado ao desenvolvimento de desequilíbrios bacterianos intestinais.
- Monitorizar o paciente quanto ao desenvolvimento de megaesôfago secundário a vômitos crônicos.
- Há suspeitas de correlação com a evolução para câncer gástrico na raça Lundehund norueguês, embora isso não tenha sido comprovado. Tumores como adenocarcinoma e carcinoma neuroendócrino são associados. Monitorizar o animal em busca do desenvolvimento de tumores gástricos (radiografias torácicas, ultrassonografia abdominal).

DIVERSOS

Nesses pacientes, há suspeita, mas sem comprovação, de hipergastrinemia e hipoacidez.

DISTÚRBIOS ASSOCIADOS
- Enterite crônica de causas inflamatórias, autoimunes ou infecciosas.
- Enteropatia com perda proteica no Lundehund.

VER TAMBÉM
- Gastrite Crônica.
- Vômito Crônico.

Sugestões de Leitura
Berghoff N, Ruaux CG, Steiner JM, et al. Gastroenteropathy in Norwegian Lundehunds. Compend Contin Educ Pract Vet 2007, 29(8):456-465, 468-470.

Qvigstad G, Kolbjornsen O, Skancke E, et al. Gastric neuroendocrine carcinoma associated with atrophic gastritis in the Norwegian Lundehund. J Comp Pathol 2008, 139:194-201.

Simpson KW. Diseases of the stomach. In: Ettinger SJ, Feldman EC, eds., Textbook of Veterinary Internal Medicine, 6th ed. St. Louis: Elsevier, 2005, pp. 1321-1326.

Autor Jessica M. Clemans
Consultor Editorial Albert E. Jergens

GASTRITE CRÔNICA

CONSIDERAÇÕES GERAIS

DEFINIÇÃO
- Vômitos intermitentes com mais de 1-2 semanas de duração, secundários à inflamação gástrica.
- Presença de erosões ou úlceras gástricas, dependendo da causa desencadeante e da duração.

FISIOPATOLOGIA
- Irritação crônica da mucosa gástrica por irritantes químicos, medicamentos, corpos estranhos, agentes infecciosos ou síndromes de hiperacidez que resultam em resposta inflamatória na superfície mucosa passível de se estender até acometer as camadas submucosas.
- Exposição crônica a alérgenos ou doença imunomediada também podem ocasionar inflamação crônica.

SISTEMA(S) ACOMETIDO(S)
- Gastrintestinal — esofagite pode resultar de vômitos crônicos ou refluxo gastroesofágico.
- Respiratório — pneumonia por aspiração é observada com pouca frequência, secundariamente a vômitos crônicos; será mais provável se houver doença esofágica concomitante ou se o paciente estiver debilitado.

INCIDÊNCIA/PREVALÊNCIA
Relativamente comum.

IDENTIFICAÇÃO
Espécies
Cães e gatos.

Raça(s) Predominante(s)
- Cães idosos de pequeno porte (p. ex., Lhasa apso, Shih tzu e Poodle miniatura) são mais comumente acometidos por hiperplasia e hipertrofia da mucosa do antro.
- Basenji e Drentse patrijshond podem desenvolver gastrite hipertrófica crônica.

Idade Média e Faixa Etária
Varia com a causa subjacente.

Sexo Predominante
Varia com a causa subjacente.

SINAIS CLÍNICOS
Achados Anamnésicos
- O vômito costuma estar manchado de bile e pode conter alimento não digerido, manchas de sangue ou sangue digerido ("borra de café").
- A frequência varia de dias a poucas semanas e aumenta à medida que a gastrite evolui.
- O vômito pode ser estimulado quando o animal come ou bebe.
- A ocorrência de vômito logo pela manhã antes de comer pode indicar síndrome do vômito bilioso.
- Pode haver perda de peso com anorexia crônica.
- Pode-se observar melena com ulceração (incomum).
- Diarreia se houver enteropatia concomitante.

Achados do Exame Físico
- Em geral, permanecem dentro dos limites de normalidade.
- O animal pode estar magro e com anorexia persistente.
- As mucosas podem estar pálidas na presença de anemia causada pela perda sanguínea crônica.
- Pode haver dor abdominal cranial (raramente observada).

CAUSAS
- Inflamatórias — imunomediadas, alergia ou intolerância alimentar, idiopáticas.
- Imprudência alimentar — plantas, corpos estranhos, irritantes químicos.
- Toxinas — fertilizantes, herbicidas, agentes de limpeza, metais pesados.
- Doenças metabólicas/endócrinas — azotemia, hepatopatia crônica, hipoadrenocorticismo, pancreatite.
- Neoplásicas — comuns: linfoma gastrintestinal, adenocarcinoma gástrico, linfoma de células pequenas (especialmente gatos, aumento recente em cães); pouco frequentes: pólipos gástricos, gastrinoma, leiomiossarcoma, plasmocitoma, mastocitoma.
- Parasitismo — *Physaloptera* spp. (cães, gatos), *Ollulanus tricuspis* e *Gnathostoma* spp. (gatos).
- Medicamentos — AINE, glicocorticoides.
- Infecciosas — *Helicobacter* spp., pitiose, virais (cinomose em cães, FeLV em gatos).
- Outras — refluxo duodenogástrico (síndrome do vômito bilioso), estresse, acloridria.

FATORES DE RISCO
- Medicações — AINE, glicocorticoides.
- Ambientais — animais que vivem soltos e vagam pelas ruas sem supervisão são mais propensos a ingerir alimentos ou materiais inadequados.
- Ingestão de antígeno alimentar ao qual o animal adquiriu alergia ou intolerância.

DIAGNÓSTICO

DIAGNÓSTICO DIFERENCIAL
- Embora as causas supramencionadas estejam incluídas no diagnóstico diferencial de gastrite crônica, é comum a existência de causa não identificável para a inflamação gástrica.
- É preciso diferenciar vômitos crônicos de regurgitação crônica (vômito ativo versus passivo).
- Inflamação do intestino delgado e neoplasia do estômago ou do intestino delgado frequentemente se apresentam com sinais e achados do exame físico semelhantes aos de inflamação gástrica.
- Gastrite idiopática — diagnóstico de exclusão; costuma ser caracterizada por infiltrado predominantemente linfoplasmocitário (superficial ou difuso).
- Gastrite eosinofílica, gastrite hipertrófica, gastrite granulomatosa/histiocítica e gastrite atrófica são menos comuns; em geral, há sobreposição de alterações histológicas nos tipos de infiltrados inflamatórios.
- A gastrite atrófica difere ao exame endoscópico — visualização dos vasos da submucosa secundariamente ao adelgaçamento da mucosa gástrica.
- Gastrite hipertrófica — pregas mucosas proeminentes que não ficam achatadas com a insuflação gástrica.

HEMOGRAMA/BIOQUÍMICA/URINÁLISE
- O hemograma completo não costuma revelar nada digno de nota a menos que haja doença sistêmica.
- Hemoconcentração em casos de desidratação grave.
- Pode-se observar anemia arregenerativa (anemia de doença crônica) ou regenerativa (por perda de sangue).
- Com ulceração — anemia microcítica hipocrômica associada à deficiência de ferro se houver perda sanguínea grave e prolongada.
- Pode-se verificar eosinofilia com gastrenterite eosinofílica.
- Azotemia com densidade urinária baixa na gastrite urêmica.
- Aumento da atividade das enzimas hepáticas séricas e das bilirrubinas totais ou hipoalbuminemia com hepatopatia crônica.
- Hipercalemia e hiponatremia sugerem doença de Addison.
- Hiponatremia, hipocalemia, hipocloremia e nível elevado de bicarbonato com urina acidótica sugerem obstrução ao fluxo de saída gástrico (alcalose metabólica hipoclorêmica).

OUTROS TESTES LABORATORIAIS
O nível sérico elevado de gastrina sem azotemia sugere gastrinoma.

DIAGNÓSTICO POR IMAGEM
- Radiografias abdominais simples — geralmente permanecem normais, embora possam revelar corpos estranhos radiodensos, parede gástrica espessada ou obstrução ao fluxo de saída gástrico com distensão persistente do estômago.
- Radiografias contrastadas — podem detectar corpos estranhos, obstrução ao fluxo de saída gástrico, esvaziamento gástrico tardio, defeitos ou espessamentos da parede gástrica.
- Ultrassonografia — pode detectar espessamento da parede gástrica, presença de ulcerações e existência de corpos estranhos no estômago.

MÉTODOS DIAGNÓSTICOS
- Gastroscopia — técnica, em geral, adequada para inspeção da mucosa gástrica e realização de biopsia; na maioria dos casos, no entanto, também se devem avaliar e fazer biopsia do duodeno.
- A biopsia gástrica e o exame histopatológico são necessários para o diagnóstico, mesmo se a mucosa gástrica estiver aparentemente normal.
- Corpos estranhos podem ser identificados e recuperados via endoscopia.
- A laparotomia exploratória fica indicada na suspeita de úlcera perfurada ou lesão de submucosa da parede gástrica e quando há necessidade de gastrectomia parcial ou biopsia de espessura completa.
- A flutuação fecal pode revelar a presença de parasitas intestinais.

ACHADOS PATOLÓGICOS
- Gastrite idiopática — os infiltrados inflamatórios variam; podem ser compostos de linfócitos, plasmócitos, neutrófilos, eosinófilos e/ou histiócitos.
- As alterações da mucosa podem ser degenerativas, hiperplásicas ou atróficas.
- Pode haver níveis variáveis de edema e tecido fibroso; podem-se observar *Helicobacter* spp. Precisam ser observados dentro das glândulas gástricas como significativos; podem ser solicitadas colorações especiais para hifas de fungos e *Helicobacter*.
- Pode-se constatar inflamação linfoplasmocitária juntamente com *Helicobacter* spp. O tratamento para *Helicobacter* pode resultar na resolução de sinais clínicos sem terapia imunossupressora.
- Se forem observadas alterações hiperplásicas, deve-se obter o nível de gastrina antes de instituir ou depois de interromper a administração de antiácidos, bloqueadores dos receptores

GASTRITE CRÔNICA

histaminérgicos H₂ ou bloqueadores da bomba de prótons.

TRATAMENTO

CUIDADO(S) DE SAÚDE ADEQUADO(S)
• A maioria dos pacientes encontra-se estável à apresentação a menos que os vômitos sejam graves o suficiente a ponto de provocar desidratação.
• Tipicamente, o paciente pode ser tratado em um esquema ambulatorial, dependendo dos exames diagnósticos ou dos ensaios clínicos em andamento com dietas especiais ou medicações.
• Se o paciente estiver desidratado ou se houver agravamento dos vômitos, hospitalizar e instituir a terapia IV apropriada com fluidos cristaloides (ver "Vômito Agudo").

DIETA
• Ração de consistência macia e baixo teor de gordura, formulada a partir de uma única fonte de carboidrato e proteína.
• Queijo *cottage* sem gordura, carne branca de frango sem pele, hambúrguer cozido ou tofu como fonte de proteína, além de arroz, massa ou batata como fonte de carboidrato, na proporção de 1:3.
• Refeições em pequenas quantidades várias vezes ao dia (a cada 4-6 h ou mais frequentes).
• Pode-se usar uma nova fonte de proteína ou dieta proteica hidrolisada caso se suspeite de alergia alimentar.
• As dietas devem ser consumidas por, no mínimo, 3 semanas para se avaliar a adequação da resposta. Com frequência, há necessidade de períodos mais prolongados de teste (6-8 semanas).
• O fornecimento de refeição no final do período da noite pode ajudar a evitar a síndrome do vômito bilioso logo pela manhã.

ORIENTAÇÃO AO PROPRIETÁRIO
• A gastrite tem inúmeras causas.
• Avaliação diagnóstica — pode ser extensa; em geral, o diagnóstico definitivo requer a realização de biopsia.

CONSIDERAÇÕES CIRÚRGICAS
• Tratamento cirúrgico se alguma massa granulomatosa ou hipertrofia estiver causando obstrução ao fluxo de saída gástrico.
• Gastrotomia para remoção de corpos estranhos se a recuperação endoscópica não for bem-sucedida ou não estiver disponível.

MEDICAÇÕES

MEDICAMENTO(S) DE ESCOLHA
• Tratar quaisquer erosões e úlceras gástricas (ver "Úlcera Gastroduodenal").
• Administrar glicocorticoides (prednisona, 2-4 mg/kg VO a cada 24 h [raramente requer o extremo superior da dose para iniciar]; diminuir a dose por volta de 25% a cada 2-3 semanas por 2-3 meses) em caso de gastrite crônica secundária a mecanismos imunomediados sob suspeita se não houver resposta clínica ao tratamento nutricional.
• Tratamento para gastrite por *Helicobacter* — amoxicilina (22 mg/kg VO a cada 12 h), pepto-bismol (15 mg/kg VO a cada 6-8 h) e metronidazol (10 mg/kg VO a cada 12 h) por 3 semanas (ver "Infecção por *Helicobacter*").
• Antieméticos para distúrbios hidreletrolíticos causados por vômitos frequentes ou profusos (ver "Vômito Agudo").
• Metoclopramida (0,2-0,4 mg/kg VO a cada 6-8 h), cisaprida (0,5-1 mg/kg VO a cada 8 h) ou eritromicina em baixas doses (0,5-1 mg/kg VO a cada 8 h) para aumentar o esvaziamento gástrico e normalizar a motilidade intestinal se o esvaziamento gástrico estiver lento ou se houver refluxo gastroduodenal.

CONTRAINDICAÇÕES
• Não usar procinéticos, metoclopramida ou cisaprida se houver obstrução ao fluxo de saída gástrico.
• Antiácidos não estão indicados na gastrite atrófica e na acloridria.

PRECAUÇÕES
• Os esteroides são imunossupressores, o que torna importante a monitorização rigorosa quanto à ocorrência de infecções secundárias.
• Tais agentes também podem inibir a barreira da mucosa gástrica normal, ocasionando ulceração.

MEDICAMENTO(S) ALTERNATIVO(S)
• Prostaglandina E sintética (misoprostol, 1-3 μg/kg VO a cada 6-8 h) para evitar úlceras na mucosa gástrica em casos de toxicidade dos AINE.
• Imunossupressores como a azatioprina (2,2 mg/kg VO a cada 24 h, reduzindo gradativamente para um esquema em dias alternados depois de 2-3 semanas) na suspeita de mecanismo imunomediado e se a resposta à dieta e à administração de glicocorticoides não for adequada. Espera-se que a resposta ocorra em 2-3 semanas.
• Para imunossupressão adicional caso haja necessidade de uma resposta imediata, adicionar a clorambucila (0,1-0,2 mg/kg a cada 24 h por 7 dias e, depois, em dias alternados). Frequentemente utilizada no lugar da azatioprina, embora possa ser usada em adição a este medicamento.

ACOMPANHAMENTO

MONITORIZAÇÃO DO PACIENTE
• A resolução dos sinais clínicos indica uma resposta positiva.
• Mensuração dos eletrólitos e do estado acidobásico se estiverem inicialmente anormais.
• Hemogramas completos devem ser solicitados semanalmente e, depois, reduzidos para cada 4-6 semanas em pacientes submetidos à medicação mielossupressora (i. e., azatioprina, clorambucila). Também é necessária a monitorização bioquímica adicional a cada 2-3 meses.
• Repetir a avaliação diagnóstica e considerar a possível repetição da biopsia se os sinais diminuírem mas não desaparecerem.

PREVENÇÃO
• Evitar medicações (p. ex., corticosteroides e AINE) e alimentos que causem irritação gástrica ou resposta alérgica no paciente.
• Impedir o comportamento errante do animal e o potencial de imprudência alimentar.

COMPLICAÇÕES POSSÍVEIS
• Evolução da gastrite de superficial para atrófica.
• Erosões e úlceras gástricas com dano progressivo à mucosa.
• Pneumonia por aspiração.
• Desequilíbrios eletrolíticos ou acidobásicos.

EVOLUÇÃO ESPERADA E PROGNÓSTICO
Varia com a causa subjacente.

DIVERSOS

FATORES RELACIONADOS COM A IDADE
Animais jovens são mais propensos a ingerir corpos estranhos.

GESTAÇÃO/FERTILIDADE/REPRODUÇÃO
• A prednisona foi utilizada com segurança em gestantes; no entanto, os corticosteroides são associados a um aumento na incidência de defeitos congênitos, abortamento e morte fetal.
• A azatioprina também foi usada com segurança em gestantes e pode ser um bom substituto de corticosteroides em animais prenhes.
• Não administrar o misoprostol a animais prenhes.

VER TAMBÉM
• Fisalopterose.
• Gastrite Atrófica.
• Gastrenterite Eosinofílica.
• Gastrenterite Linfoplasmocitária.
• Gastropatia Pilórica Hipertrófica Crônica.
• Infecção por *Helicobacter*.
• Úlcera Gastroduodenal.

ABREVIATURA(S)
• AINE = anti-inflamatórios não esteroides.
• FeLV = vírus da leucemia felina.

Sugestões de Leitura
Neiger R. Diseases of the stomach: Chronic gastritis. In: Steiner JM, ed., Small Animal Gastroenterology. Hannover, Germany: Schlutersche Verlagsgesellschaft mbH & Co., 2008, pp. 161-165.
Simpson KW. Diseases of the stomach. In: Ettinger SJ, Feldman EC, eds., Textbook of Veterinary Internal Medicine, 6th ed. St. Louis: Elsevier, 2005, pp. 1321-1331.

Autor Michelle Pressel
Consultor Editorial Albert E. Jergens

Gastropatia Pilórica Hipertrófica Crônica

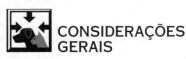

CONSIDERAÇÕES GERAIS

DEFINIÇÃO
Estenose pilórica ou gastropatia pilórica hipertrófica crônica é um estreitamento obstrutivo do canal pilórico, resultante de graus variados de hipertrofia da camada muscular ou hiperplasia da mucosa.

FISIOPATOLOGIA
• Pode resultar de alguma lesão congênita composta principalmente de hipertrofia do músculo liso ou corresponder a um dos três tipos da forma adquirida — basicamente hipertrofia do músculo circular (tipo 1), uma combinação de hipertrofia da camada muscular e hiperplasia da mucosa (tipo 2) ou essencialmente hiperplasia da mucosa (tipo 3).
• A causa é desconhecida; os fatores propostos incluem aumento dos níveis de gastrina (que exerce efeito trófico sobre o músculo e a mucosa) ou alterações no plexo mioentérico que acarretam distensão crônica do antro e seus efeitos associados.

SISTEMA(S) ACOMETIDO(S)
• Gastrintestinal — vômito intermitente crônica; também há relatos de regurgitação.
• Musculosquelético — perda de peso.
• Respiratório — possível pneumonia por aspiração.

GENÉTICA
Padrão de herança desconhecido.

INCIDÊNCIA/PREVALÊNCIA
Desconhecidas.

DISTRIBUIÇÃO GEOGRÁFICA
N/D.

IDENTIFICAÇÃO
Espécies
• Mais comum em cães.
• Rara em gatos.

Raça(s) Predominante(s)
• Congênita — raças braquicefálicas (Boxer, Boston terrier, Buldogue); gatos da raça Siamês.
• Adquirida — Lhasa apso, Shih tzu, Pequinês, Poodle.

Idade Média e Faixa Etária
• Congênita — logo após o desmame (introdução de alimento sólido) e até 1 ano de idade.
• Adquirida — 9,8 anos de idade.

Sexo Predominante
Duas vezes mais comum em machos do que em fêmeas.

SINAIS CLÍNICOS
Comentários Gerais
• Sinais clínicos relacionados com o grau de estreitamento pilórico.
• Vômitos em jato geralmente não constituem uma queixa à apresentação. Em geral, os animais encontram-se em boa condição corporal.

Achados Anamnésicos
• Vômitos crônicos intermitentes de alimento não digerido ou parcialmente digerido (raras vezes contendo bile) em geral várias horas depois de uma refeição.
• Lesões congênitas começam a provocar sinais clínicos logo após o desmame.
• A frequência dos vômitos aumenta com o tempo.
• Ausência de resposta a agentes antieméticos ou procinéticos (modificadores da motilidade gástrica).
• Anorexia ocasional com perda de peso.
• Regurgitação.

Achados do Exame Físico
A maioria dos cães, em geral, está em boa condição física.

CAUSAS
• Congênitas ou adquiridas.
• Podem ser influenciadas por doenças murais infiltrativas.
• Elevações crônicas nos níveis de gastrina.
• Fatores neuroendócrinos podem desempenhar algum papel.

FATORES DE RISCO
Estresse crônico, distúrbios inflamatórios, gastrite crônica, úlceras gástricas e predisposições genéticas influenciam o processo mórbido em humanos e podem exercer algum papel em pequenos animais.

DIAGNÓSTICO

DIAGNÓSTICO DIFERENCIAL
• Neoplasia gástrica.
• Corpo estranho gástrico.
• Doença fúngica granulomatosa (p. ex., pitiose).
• Granuloma eosinofílico.
• Distúrbios da motilidade.
• Massa abdominal cranial — pancreática ou duodenal.

HEMOGRAMA/BIOQUÍMICA/URINÁLISE
• Os achados variam, dependendo do grau e da cronicidade da obstrução.
• Alcalose metabólica hipoclorêmica (característica de obstrução ao fluxo de saída pilórico) ou acidose metabólica (ou desequilíbrio acidobásico misto).
• Hipocalemia.
• Anemia — se houver ulceração gastrintestinal (GI) concomitante.
• Azotemia pré-renal — se houver desidratação.

OUTROS TESTES LABORATORIAIS
N/D.

DIAGNÓSTICO POR IMAGEM
Radiografias Abdominais
• Estômago normal a acentuadamente distendido.

Radiografia do Trato GI Superior Contrastada com Bário
• Pode exibir um sinal de "bico" criado pelo estreitamento pilórico, fazendo com que uma quantidade mínima de bário passe para o antro pilórico.
• Retenção de grande parte do bário no estômago 6 h depois indica esvaziamento gástrico tardio.
• Defeitos do enchimento intraluminal ou espessamento da parede pilórica.

Fluoroscopia
• Contratilidade gástrica normal.
• Passagem tardia do bário por meio do piloro.

Ultrassonografia Abdominal
• Espessamento mensurável da parede do piloro e do antro.

MÉTODOS DIAGNÓSTICOS
Endoscopia — permite avaliar a mucosa quanto à presença de ulceração, hiperplasia e lesões expansivas; possibilita a obtenção de amostras para exame histopatológico.

ACHADOS PATOLÓGICOS
• Incluem pólipos focais a multifocais na mucosa, espessamento difuso da mucosa e da parede pilórica, com grau variável de estreitamento pilórico.
• As alterações variam desde hipertrofia do músculo liso circular até hiperplasia da mucosa e estruturas glandulares associadas; há um amplo espectro de infiltração por células inflamatórias.

TRATAMENTO

CUIDADO(S) DE SAÚDE ADEQUADO(S)
• Dependem da gravidade dos sinais clínicos.
• Os pacientes devem ser examinados e a cirurgia marcada o mais rapidamente possível.

CUIDADO(S) DE ENFERMAGEM
• Fluidos parenterais apropriados para corrigir quaisquer desequilíbrios eletrolíticos e alcalose ou acidose metabólica.
• Solução fisiológica isotônica (com suplementação de potássio) é o fluido de escolha para a alcalose metabólica hipoclorêmica.
• É importante considerar o suporte nutricional pós-operatório.
• Nos casos graves tratados com gastroduodenostomia ou gastrojejunostomia, a colocação cirúrgica de tubo de jejunostomia para nutrição enteral pode ser vantajosa.

ATIVIDADE
Restrita.

DIETA
Alta digestibilidade e pobre em gordura — até que a intervenção cirúrgica seja viável.

ORIENTAÇÃO AO PROPRIETÁRIO
• O tratamento cirúrgico é altamente bem-sucedido.
• Se houver recidiva dos sinais clínicos no pós-operatório, talvez haja indicação de procedimentos cirúrgicos mais rigorosos.

CONSIDERAÇÕES CIRÚRGICAS
• A intervenção cirúrgica é o tratamento de escolha.
• Os objetivos envolvem o estabelecimento do diagnóstico com amostras histopatológicas, a excisão de tecido anormal e o restabelecimento da função GI com o procedimento minimamente invasivo.
• Os procedimentos cirúrgicos dependem do grau de obstrução — piloromiotomia (Fredet-Ramstedt), piloroplastia (Heineke-Mikulicz ou retalho com avanço antral), gastroduodenostomia (Billroth 1), gastrojejunostomia (Billroth 2).

MEDICAÇÕES

MEDICAMENTO(S) DE ESCOLHA
• Antieméticos e modificadores da motilidade, em geral, não são eficazes.
• Antagonistas dos receptores H_2 e inibidores da bomba de prótons podem conferir alívio sintomático.

CONTRAINDICAÇÕES
• Indícios de obstrução pilórica completa impedem o uso de medicamentos pró-motilidade.

Gastropatia Pilórica Hipertrófica Crônica

• Evitar agentes anticolinérgicos em virtude de seus efeitos inibitórios sobre a motilidade GI.

PRECAUÇÕES
N/D.

INTERAÇÕES POSSÍVEIS
N/D.

MEDICAMENTO(S) ALTERNATIVO(S)
N/D.

 ACOMPANHAMENTO

MONITORIZAÇÃO DO PACIENTE
Pós-operatória para detectar recidiva dos sinais clínicos por causa da má escolha do procedimento cirúrgico.

PREVENÇÃO
N/D.

COMPLICAÇÕES POSSÍVEIS
As complicações cirúrgicas no pós-operatório incluem recidiva dos sinais clínicos, ulceração gástrica, pancreatite, obstrução do ducto biliar e deiscência da ferida cirúrgica com peritonite.

EVOLUÇÃO ESPERADA E PROGNÓSTICO
• 85% dos cães revelam resultados bons a excelentes, com resolução dos sinais clínicos após a intervenção cirúrgica apropriada.
• Prognóstico mau se a causa subjacente for neoplasia gástrica (em especial adenocarcinoma).

 DIVERSOS

DISTÚRBIOS ASSOCIADOS
Ulceração gástrica.

FATORES RELACIONADOS COM A IDADE
• Vômitos intermitentes em cães jovens braquicefálicos ao desmame indicam estenose congênita.
• Vômitos crônicos intermitentes em cães adultos de pequeno porte (8-10 anos de idade) confirmam o diagnóstico de hipertrofia pilórica adquirida.

POTENCIAL ZOONÓTICO
Nenhum.

GESTAÇÃO/FERTILIDADE/REPRODUÇÃO
Altos níveis de gastrina em fêmeas prenhes podem predispor ao desenvolvimento da síndrome.

SINÔNIMO(S)
• Gastropatia antral hipertrófica crônica.
• Gastrite hipertrófica.
• Hipertrofia pilórica antral adquirida.
• Estenose pilórica congênita.

ABREVIATURA(S)
• GI = gastrintestinal.

Sugestões de Leitura
Bellenger, C.R.; Maddison, J.E.; Macpherson, G.C.; Ilkiw, J.E.: Chronic hypertrophic pyloric gastropathy in 14 dogs. Aust Vet J 67:317-320, 1990.
Fossum, T.W.: Surgery of the digestive system. In: Fossum, T.W., ed., Small Animal Surgery. St. Louis: Mosby, 2007, pp. 433-436.

Autor Steven L. Marks
Consultor Editorial Albert E. Jergens

GIARDÍASE

CONSIDERAÇÕES GERAIS

REVISÃO
- Infecção intestinal de cães e gatos por um protozoário que habita no lúmen, a *Giardia*.
- Transmissão direta ou indireta pela ingestão de cistos que se tornam imediatamente infectantes quando eliminados nas fezes.
- Trofozoítos, microrganismos móveis (flagelados) liberados a partir dos cistos ingeridos, aderem-se à superfície dos enterócitos no intestino delgado por meio de disco de sucção ventral; movem-se de um local para outro.
- Pode causar diarreia do intestino delgado, embora a infecção frequentemente permaneça assintomática.

IDENTIFICAÇÃO
- Cães — até 50% em filhotes de cães e até 100% em canis.
- Gatos — até 11%.

SINAIS CLÍNICOS
- Os sinais clínicos são mais comuns em hospedeiros jovens; cães mais idosos e gatos costumam permanecer assintomáticos.
- Podem ser agudos, transitórios, intermitentes ou crônicos.
- Síndrome de má absorção com fezes moles, espumosas, gordurosas e volumosas (diarreia), geralmente com odor rançoso.
- A infecção crônica pode levar à debilidade.

CAUSAS E FATORES DE RISCO
- Transmitida pela ingestão de cistos provenientes de fezes em alimentos, água, ambiente ou pelo.
- É mais comum a transmissão indireta pela água; condições úmidas e frias favorecem a sobrevivência do cisto.
- Risco mais alto de infecção em filhotes caninos e felinos, populações de alta densidade (canis, gatis, abrigos de animais) e cães/gatos imunocomprometidos.

DIAGNÓSTICO

DIAGNÓSTICO DIFERENCIAL
- Outras causas infecciosas e não infecciosas de diarreia do intestino delgado, má digestão e síndromes de má absorção, sobretudo insuficiência pancreática exócrina, enteropatia inflamatória.
- Em gatos, deve-se diferenciar de infecção por *Tritrichomonas fetus*, uma causa de diarreia do intestino grosso.

HEMOGRAMA/BIOQUÍMICA/URINÁLISE
Geralmente normais.

OUTROS TESTES LABORATORIAIS
N/D.

DIAGNÓSTICO POR IMAGEM
N/D.

MÉTODOS DIAGNÓSTICOS
- Detecção de trofozoítos, cistos ou antígenos de *Giardia* nas fezes.
- Trofozoítos (15 × 8 μm) são detectáveis em fezes frescas, especialmente diarreia, e em aspirados duodenais obtidos por endoscopia; identificá-los em esfregaço corado por Diff-Quick ou lugol (uma solução com iodo) pelo formato de gota de lágrima, com dois núcleos proeminentes, e em câmara úmida de aspirado ou pequena quantidade de fezes em salina pelo aspecto de "folha caída"; os meios de flutuação lisam os trofozoítos.
- Cistos, com aproximadamente 12 μm de comprimento, são ovais com 2-4 núcleos e eliminados de forma intermitente; a flutuação centrífuga de fezes frescas em sulfato de zinco (densidade igual a 1,18) constitui o método de escolha; o exame de três amostras coletadas em intervalos de 2 a 3 dias detecta >70% das infecções; cistos distorcidos (em formato de lua crescente) em flutuação com açúcar ou outra solução de flutuação com densidade >1,25; a sedimentação com formalina e acetato de etila é útil em casos de esteatorreia.
- Existem *kits* disponíveis no mercado à base de ELISA para detecção do antígeno de *Giardia* nas fezes dentro do ambiente da clínica; esses *kits* têm sensibilidade variável em comparação à flutuação centrífuga com sulfato de zinco; são capazes de detectar infecção assintomática. Podem ocorrer resultados falso-negativos ou positivos com todos os métodos.

TRATAMENTO
- Tratar como pacientes ambulatoriais, a menos que estejam debilitados ou desidratados.
- A terapia medicamentosa deve ser combinada com limpeza e desinfecção do ambiente, além de banho do paciente para evitar infecção.
- Existem vacinas contra *Giardia* disponíveis no mercado; foram constatados resultados variáveis em estudos de eficácia; podem constituir um adjuvante útil à terapia medicamentosa em alguns casos.

MEDICAÇÕES

MEDICAMENTO(S)
- Todos os medicamentos utilizados estão fora da indicação da bula.
- Fembendazol, 50 mg/kg VO a cada 24 h por 3 dias (cães) ou 5 dias (gatos); pode ser necessário um segundo curso terapêutico.
- Febantel/praziquantel/pirantel, dose da bula por 3 dias (cães) ou 5 dias (gatos).
- Metronidazol, 20-22 mg/kg a cada 12 h por 5 dias em cães.
- Benzoato de metronidazol, 22-25 mg/kg VO a cada 12 h por 5-7 dias em gatos.

CONTRAINDICAÇÕES/INTERAÇÕES POSSÍVEIS
- O metronidazol só tem 67% de eficácia em cães; sabor amargo; pode causar anorexia, vômitos, sinais neurológicos (SNC).
- Embora seja eficaz, o albendazol (25 mg/kg VO a cada 12 h por 2 dias em cães ou 5 dias em gatos) não é recomendado, pois pode ser teratogênico e/ou causar anorexia, depressão, vômito, ataxia, diarreia, abortamento ou mielossupressão.

ACOMPANHAMENTO
- Repetir os exames fecais para confirmar a eficácia do tratamento e detectar nova infecção.
- A infecção crônica pode levar à debilidade.

DIVERSOS

POTENCIAL ZOONÓTICO
- A *Giardia* constitui o parasita intestinal mais comum em pessoas que residem na América do Norte.
- Embora existam genótipos hospedeiro-específicos muito comuns em cães (*G. canis*) e gatos (*G. felis*), ambas as espécies (canina e felina) podem ser infectadas por genótipos zoonóticos de *G. lamblia*.
- A importância de animais domésticos como reservatórios da infecção humana e a frequência da transmissão zoonótica são desconhecidas, mas parecem ser mínimas.
- O risco de transmissão zoonótica dos animais domésticos para seres humanos imunocompetentes parece ser baixo, mas provavelmente é elevado em pessoas com imunidade comprometida.

GESTAÇÃO/FERTILIDADE/REPRODUÇÃO
Não utilizar o albendazol em cadelas ou gatas prenhes, pois esse agente pode ser teratogênico.

ABREVIATURA(S)
- SNC = sistema nervoso central.
- ELISA = ensaio imunoabsorvente ligado à enzima.

RECURSOS DA INTERNET
- www.capcvet.org.
- www.cdc.gov.

Sugestões de Leitura
Bowman DD. Georgis' Parasitology for Veterinarians, 9th ed. St. Louis: (Saunders) Elsevier Science, 2009, pp. 89-91.

Autor Julie Ann Jarvinen
Consultor Editorial Stephen C. Barr

GLAUCOMA

CONSIDERAÇÕES GERAIS

DEFINIÇÃO
- Corresponde à PIO elevada, que causa alterações degenerativas características no nervo óptico e na retina, com subsequente perda da visão.
- Diagnóstico — PIO >25-30 mmHg (cães) ou >31 mmHg (gatos) conforme determinada via tonometria de aplanação, tonometria de rebote ou tonometria de Schiotz (com o uso da tabela de conversão humana de Friedenwald de 1955 que acompanha o instrumento Schiotz) com alterações na visão ou no aspecto do nervo óptico ou da retina.

FISIOPATOLOGIA
- Desenvolve-se quando o fluxo de saída normal do humor aquoso fica prejudicado.
- Pode resultar de doença ocular primária (ângulos de filtração estreitados ou fechados e goniodisgenesia, que têm predisposição genética).
- Pode ser secundário a outras doenças oculares (luxação primária do cristalino, uveíte anterior, tumor intraocular ou hifema).

SISTEMA(S) ACOMETIDO(S)
Oftálmico.

GENÉTICA
Cães — acredita-se que a configuração anômala predisponente dos ângulos de filtração seja hereditária; o modo de herança é incerto.

INCIDÊNCIA/PREVALÊNCIA
Cães — mais comum em algumas raças; a incidência global é maior que 0,8% de todas as admissões hospitalares listadas no banco de dados das faculdades de medicina veterinária da América do Norte.

IDENTIFICAÇÃO
Espécies
- Cães — primário e secundário.
- Gatos — o primário é raro; o secundário é observado em pacientes com sinais de uveíte de longa data ou luxação do cristalino.

Raça(s) Predominante(s)
- Goniodisgenesia — raças do círculo ártico (p. ex., Elkhound norueguês, Husky siberiano, Malamute, Akita e Samoieda); Bouvier des flandres; Basset hound; Chow chow; Shar-pei; Spaniel (p. ex., Cocker americano e inglês, Springer inglês e galês).
- Ângulos de filtração estreitos — Spaniel; Chow chow; Shar-pei; raças toy (p. ex., Poodle, Maltês e Shih tzu).
- Secundário a luxações do cristalino — Terrier (p. ex., Boston, Cairn, Manchester, Dandie dinmont, Norfolk, Norwich, Scottish, Sealyham, West Highland white, Parson Jack Russell e Fox) e Shar-pei.

Idade Média e Faixa Etária
- Primário (cães) — qualquer idade; acomete predominantemente os de meia-idade (4-9 anos de idade).
- Secundário à luxação do cristalino (cães) — acomete, em geral, animais jovens (2-6 anos de idade).
- Secundário à uveíte crônica (gatos) — costuma afetar gatos idosos (com mais de 6 anos).

SINAIS CLÍNICOS
Comentários Gerais
- Não pode ser diagnosticado com acurácia sem a tonometria instrumental.
- Todos os hospitais veterinários bem equipados devem ter um tonômetro.

Achados Anamnésicos
- Glaucoma de ângulo agudo — dor aparente (blefaroespasmo, sensibilidade em torno da cabeça, secreção serosa ou seromucoide); o olho pode estar visivelmente turvo ou vermelho; a menos que o glaucoma seja bilateral, geralmente não se nota a perda da visão.
- Secundário — depende da doença primária.
- Uveíte — podem-se notar dor (por muitos dias), congestão na esclera e edema de córnea.
- Luxação anterior do cristalino — podem-se notar dor aguda, congestão na esclera e edema de córnea; pode-se ver o cristalino na câmara anterior (se o edema de córnea não for grave).
- Uveíte crônica (gatos) — os sinais de dor podem não ser notados; é comum verificar o olho aumentado e aparentemente indolor ou a pupila dilatada.
- Aumento do globo ocular — pode ser notado primeiro pelos proprietários.

Achados do Exame Físico
Primário Agudo
- PIO alta.
- Blefaroespasmo.
- Enoftalmia.
- Congestão da esclera.
- Edema de córnea.
- Pupila dilatada.
- Perda da visão — pode ser detectada pela ausência do reflexo de ameaça ou resposta de ofuscamento e/ou ausência de reflexo pupilar à luz direto ou consensual.
- O nervo óptico pode estar com depressão ou em forma de cálice.

Crônico (Estágio Terminal)
- Aumento do globo ocular (buftalmia).
- Estrias de Descemet ("estrias de Haab").
- Subluxação do cristalino com crescente afáquico.
- Atrofia da cabeça do nervo óptico.
- Necrose da retina — detectada por hiper-refletividade peripapilar ou generalizada do tapete.

Induzido por Uveíte
- PIO elevada.
- Congestão da esclera.
- Edema de córnea.
- Debris inflamatórios na câmara anterior.
- Pupila miótica (±).
- Sinéquia posterior (±).
- *Íris bombé* (seclusão pupilar, abaulamento da íris pelo acúmulo de humor aquoso) (±).

CAUSAS
- Primário — anomalias do ângulo de filtração.
- Secundário — impedimento do fluxo de saída do humor aquoso (p. ex., uveíte: células inflamatórias ou debris celulares; luxação do cristalino: cristalino ou vítreo aderido; hifema; eritrócitos; tumores oculares; células neoplásicas).

FATORES DE RISCO
- Uveíte anterior.
- Luxação do cristalino.
- Hifema.
- Neoplasia intraocular.
- Aplicação de midriáticos tópicos — pode precipitar glaucoma agudo em animais predispostos.
- Primário (cães) — considerar todos os casos como bilaterais, mesmo que um olho esteja normotenso; fica indicada a avaliação do olho ileso (i. e., não acometido) por oftalmologista veterinário em busca de anomalias do ângulo de filtração para determinar o risco de glaucoma futuro naquele olho.

DIAGNÓSTICO

DIAGNÓSTICO DIFERENCIAL
- Ver "Olho Vermelho".
- Conjuntivite — PIO não elevada; pupila não dilatada; hiperemia conjuntival mais difusa e avermelhada, em vez de congestão dos vasos da esclera.
- Uveíte — inicialmente PIO abaixo do normal ou hipotenso; resulta, em geral, em pupila miótica.
- Tonometria — em geral, diferencia o glaucoma de outras causas de olho vermelho.

HEMOGRAMA/BIOQUÍMICA/URINÁLISE
- Primário — tipicamente normais.
- Secundário — anormalidades compatíveis com a doença sistêmica primária (p. ex., trombocitopenia com hifema).

OUTROS TESTES LABORATORIAIS
Sorologia para doenças infecciosas — pode ajudar a diagnosticar a causa da uveíte.

DIAGNÓSTICO POR IMAGEM
- Radiografia ou ultrassonografia (doença secundária) — pode demonstrar lesões compatíveis com disseminação fúngica ou neoplásica para o olho como uma causa de uveíte ou hifema.
- Ultrassom ocular (doença secundária) — poderá facilitar a avaliação do olho se os meios oculares estiverem opacos.

MÉTODOS DIAGNÓSTICOS
- Tonometria instrumental — essencial.
- Doença aguda — encaminhar a um oftalmologista veterinário para o exame ocular detalhado de ambos os olhos, inclusive a avaliação dos ângulos de filtração (gonioscopia).
- ERG — pode ajudar a determinar se o olho acometido é capaz de recuperar a visão com o tratamento clínico e/ou cirúrgico; o traçado normal não indica necessariamente que a visão no olho esteja normal; amplitude diminuída ou traçado plano é garantia de que a visão não será recuperada apesar do tratamento.

ACHADOS PATOLÓGICOS
- Colapso do ângulo de filtração.
- Perda de células ganglionares da retina.
- Alteração de fotorreceptor.
- Gliose e "escavação" da cabeça do nervo óptico.

TRATAMENTO

CUIDADO(S) DE SAÚDE ADEQUADO(S)
- Agudo (cães) — tratamento médico com internação.

- Depois da alta — reavaliar a cada 1-2 dias durante 1 semana para monitorizar o retorno ao aumento da PIO.

ORIENTAÇÃO AO PROPRIETÁRIO
- Avisar o proprietário que o glaucoma primário é uma doença bilateral; sem a terapia profilática, mais de 50% dos casos desenvolvem glaucoma no outro olho em 8 meses.
- Alertar o proprietário que 40% ou mais dos cães ficarão cegos do olho acometido no primeiro ano, independentemente do tratamento clínico ou cirúrgico.

CONSIDERAÇÕES CIRÚRGICAS
- Os casos induzidos de glaucoma primário e luxação do cristalino são tratados de forma mais eficiente por meio cirúrgico.
- Primário (cães) — menos de 10% dos pacientes submetidos apenas a tratamento clínico recuperam a visão no fim do primeiro ano.
- Procedimentos — intensificam o fluxo de saída do humor aquoso (dispositivos de filtração); diminuem a produção do humor aquoso (p. ex., ciclofotocoagulação com laser de Nd:YAG ou diodo; ciclofotocoagulação endoscópica com laser de diodo; ou ciclocriocirurgia transescleral para ablação do corpo ciliar); possivelmente a ciclofotocoagulação endoscópica com laser de diodo é mais eficaz na manutenção da PIO normal e da visão. A remoção do cristalino luxado anteriormente pode resultar no retorno da visão do olho acometido, além de ajudar a reduzir a PIO.
- Olhos cegos e dolorosos — enucleação; evisceração e implantação de prótese intraocular (se não houver infecção ou neoplasia intraocular); injeção de gentamicina dentro da câmara vítrea; tudo para minimizar o tratamento clínico a longo prazo.

MEDICAÇÕES
MEDICAMENTO(S) DE ESCOLHA
Uso de múltiplos agentes para diminuir a PIO até os valores normais o mais rápido possível na tentativa de recuperar a visão.

Primário Agudo (Cães)
O tratamento clínico de emergência pode incluir um ou mais dos medicamentos a seguir:
- Se disponíveis, tentar primeiro os agentes mióticos análogos de prostaglandina, como latanoprosta a 0,005% (Xalatan®; a cada 12 h), travoprosta a 0,004% (Travatan®; a cada 12 h) ou bimatoprosta a 0,03% (Lumigan®; a cada 12 h).
- Se a PIO não se normalizar em 2 h (ou se os agentes mióticos análogos de prostaglandina não estiverem disponíveis), usar:
- Agentes hiperosmóticos — manitol (1-2 g/kg IV por 20 min) ou glicerina (1-2 mL/kg VO a cada 8-12 h); desidratam o humor vítreo.
- Agentes mióticos — solução de pilocarpina a 2% (a cada 6-12 h); brometo de demecário a 0,25% (a cada 12 h); intensificam o fluxo de saída do humor aquoso.
- Inibidora da anidrase carbônica oral — metazolamida (2-4 mg/kg a cada 8-12 h); diminui a produção do humor aquoso.
- Inibidores da anidrase carbônica tópicos (±) — dorzolamida a 2% (Trusopt®; a cada 8 h), brinzolamida a 1% (Azopt®; a cada 8 h); reduzem a produção do humor aquoso.
- Antagonistas beta-adrenérgicos tópicos (±) — maleato de timolol a 0,5% (a cada 12 h), levobunalol a 0,5% (a cada 12 h), betaxolol a 0,5% (a cada 12 h); diminuem a produção do humor aquoso.

Induzido por Luxação Anterior do Cristalino ou Uveíte (Cães)
- Tratar como doença primária.
- Agentes mióticos — não usar.
- Corticosteroides tópicos — utilizados para diminuir a inflamação se não houver ceratite ulcerativa.

Uveíte Crônica Escaldante (Gatos)
- Corticosteroides tópicos.
- β-bloqueadores tópicos.
- Inibidores da anidrase carbônica tópicos ou, possivelmente, sistêmicos.

CONTRAINDICAÇÕES
- Atropina tópica — não usar.
- Agentes mióticos — não utilizar com luxação anterior primária do cristalino ou uveíte.
- Utilizar apenas um agente miótico.
- Usar somente um beta-agonista.
- Só usar um inibidor da anidrase carbônica (tópico ou sistêmico).

PRECAUÇÕES
- Pilocarpina tópica — irritante; pode causar conjuntivite e dor na área da sobrancelha; pode agravar a uveíte.
- Absorção sistêmica de antagonistas β-adrenérgicos tópicos — pode causar broncoconstrição e bradicardia em cães de pequeno porte e gatos.
- Inibidores da anidrase carbônica sistêmicos — provocam acidose metabólica e desequilíbrios eletrolíticos observados sob a forma de respiração ofegante, fraqueza, desorientação e/ou mudança comportamental.
- Diuréticos osmóticos — podem desencadear edema pulmonar agudo em pacientes com doença indutora de comprometimento cardiovascular-pulmonar.
- Glicerina — não usar com diabetes melito; causa hiperglicemia.

INTERAÇÕES POSSÍVEIS
Brometo de demecário — inibidor da colinesterase; pode causar envenenamento por organofosforado se usado em conjunto com produtos à base desse tipo de parasiticida.

MEDICAMENTO(S) ALTERNATIVO(S)
Outros diuréticos (furosemida, tiazidas, etc.) — não reduzem a PIO.

ACOMPANHAMENTO
MONITORIZAÇÃO DO PACIENTE
- PIO — monitorizada com frequência e regularidade após a instituição da terapia inicial; se o nível hipotenso for mantido por muitas semanas, diminuir a terapia medicamentosa de forma lenta e gradual.
- Monitorizar as reações medicamentosas.

PREVENÇÃO
- Primário — doença bilateral; recomendar o exame do olho ileso (i. e., não acometido) por oftalmologista veterinário para determinar o risco de desenvolvimento de glaucoma.
- Terapia profilática para o olho ileso predisposto — brometo de demecário a 0,25% (a cada 24 h antes de dormir) ou latanoprosta a 0,005% (a cada 24 h antes de dormir) ou maleato de timolol a 0,5% (a cada 12 h) ou dorzolamida a 2% (a cada 8-12 h); retarda o início de glaucoma no segundo olho predisposto.

COMPLICAÇÕES POSSÍVEIS
- Cegueira.
- Dor ocular crônica.

EVOLUÇÃO ESPERADA E PROGNÓSTICO
- Doença crônica que requer tratamento clínico constante (mesmo com intervenção cirúrgica).
- Apenas com tratamento clínico — a maioria dos pacientes acaba ficando cega.
- Tratamento cirúrgico — maiores chances de preservar a visão por mais tempo; grande parte dos pacientes não conserva a visão por mais de 2 anos após o diagnóstico inicial.
- Secundário à luxação do cristalino — pode ter prognóstico razoável com a remoção bem-sucedida do cristalino luxado.
- Secundário à uveíte anterior — pode carrear prognóstico razoável com o controle da uveíte.

DIVERSOS
GESTAÇÃO/FERTILIDADE/REPRODUÇÃO
- Todos os medicamentos mencionados podem afetar a prenhez.
- Casos de glaucoma primário e luxação do cristalino — hereditários; não acasalar os animais acometidos.

VER TAMBÉM
- Olho Vermelho.
- Uveíte Anterior — Cães.
- Uveíte Anterior — Gatos.

ABREVIATURA(S)
- ERG = eletrorretinograma.
- Nd:YAG = neodímio, ítrio, alumínio e granada.
- PIO = pressão intraocular.

Sugestões de Leitura
Gaarder J. Canine glaucoma. In: Bonagura JD, ed. Kirk's Current Veterinary Therapy XIII. Philadelphia: Saunders, 2000, pp. 1075-1081.
Gelatt KN, Brooks DE, Kallberg ME. The canine glaucomas. In: Gelatt KN, ed., Veterinary Ophthalmology, 4th ed. Ames, IA: Blackwell, 2007, pp. 753-811.
Stiles J, Townsend WM. Feline ophthalmology. In: Gelatt KN, ed., Veterinary Ophthalmology, 4th ed. Ames, IA: Blackwell, 2007, pp. 1127-1130.
Miller PE, Schmidt GM, Vainisi SJ, et al. The efficacy of topical prophylactic antiglaucoma therapy in primary closed angle glaucoma in dogs: A multicenter clinical trial. JAAHA 2000, 36:431-438.

Autor J. Phillip Pickett
Consultor Editorial Paul E. Miller

GLICOSÚRIA

CONSIDERAÇÕES GERAIS

DEFINIÇÃO
Concentração urinária semiquantitativa positiva de glicose detectável pelos exames laboratoriais de rotina (p. ex., fitas reagentes). Concentrações baixas normalmente presentes (2-10 mg/dL em seres humanos) não são detectáveis com o uso dos testes habituais de triagem. Glicosúria persistente (detectada com os testes de triagem) é um achado anormal (patológico).

FISIOPATOLOGIA
• A glicose é livremente filtrada por meio dos capilares glomerulares; portanto, o nível sanguíneo e o filtrado glomerular possuem concentrações equivalentes de glicose.
• A glicose é ativamente reabsorvida pelo lúmen dos túbulos renais proximais por cotransporte com o sódio, utilizando uma proteína de transporte existente na borda em escova das células epiteliais. Os níveis fisiológicos de glicose filtrada são removidos basicamente dessa maneira durante o estado de saúde (os níveis excretados são muito baixos para serem detectados com o uso dos testes de triagem de rotina).

Glicosúria Hiperglicêmica
• Haverá glicosúria quando a concentração plasmática de glicose exceder a capacidade máxima de transporte renal das células epiteliais tubulares (aproximadamente 170-180 mg/dL para cães e 260-310 mg/dL para gatos). Quando há hiperglicemia, a próxima etapa é determinar se a glicosúria é transitória ou persistente.

Transitória
• Fisiológica — geralmente transitória e associada à liberação dos hormônios endógenos do "estresse" (glucagon, catecolaminas, glicocorticoides), particularmente comum nos gatos. O soro pode estar normoglicêmico ou hiperglicêmico no momento em que a urina é coletada, porque concentrações diferentes de glicose excretada na urina se acumulam na bexiga urinária com o passar do tempo.
• Farmacológica — pode ocorrer após a administração de soluções (p. ex., glicose e soluções de nutrição parenteral total) que contenham glicose. Alguns hormônios (hormônio adrenocorticotrópico, glicocorticoides, glucagon, adrenalina, progesterona) e medicamentos (adrenalina, morfina, fenotiazinas, xilazina em gatos, diazóxido, l-asparaginase) podem causar glicosúria.
• Tóxica — etilenoglicol.
• Patológica — possível em casos de pancreatite aguda.

Persistente
• Patológica — diabetes melito, hiperadrenocorticismo (±), feocromocitoma, glucagonoma, acromegalia, progesterona (endógena ou exógena), estresse extremo, hepatopatia crônica, lesões do SNC (±).

Glicosúria Normoglicêmica
• Capacidade reabsortiva prejudicada das células epiteliais dos túbulos renais proximais.

Congênita
• Glicosúria primária, após jejum durante a noite (Terrier escocês).
• Síndrome de Fanconi (cães da raça Basenji; esporádica também em Elkhound norueguês, Pastor de Shetland, Schnauzer miniatura, Labrador retriever, Border terrier, Whippet, Yorkshire terrier e raças caninas mistas); reabsorção diminuída de glicose, aminoácidos e fósforo, bem como secreção reduzida de íons de hidrogênio.

Adquirida
• Síndrome de Fanconi atribuída à toxicidade, como intoxicação por metais pesados (chumbo, mercúrio, cádmio, urânio), medicamentos (gentamicina, cefalosporinas, tetraciclina vencida, cisplatina, estreptozotocina, amoxicilina), substâncias químicas (Lysol®, ácido maleico).
• Insuficiência renal aguda com lesões tubulares significativas (±).
• Toxicidade — intoxicação por metais pesados (p. ex., chumbo, mercúrio), medicamentos (p. ex., gentamicina, cisplatina) e substâncias químicas (p. ex., Lysol®, ácido maleico).

SISTEMA(S) ACOMETIDO(S)
• Renal/urológico — pacientes normoglicêmicos apresentam função anormal das células epiteliais dos túbulos renais. Os cães com síndrome de Fanconi podem desenvolver acidose metabólica e doença renal crônica com envolvimento secundário de múltiplos sistemas. A glicosúria predispõe o paciente à infecção bacteriana do trato urinário.
• Endócrino — pacientes hiperglicêmicos podem ter diabetes melito e/ou hiperadrenocorticismo.

IDENTIFICAÇÃO
• Com frequência, cães e gatos adultos desenvolvem glicosúria hiperglicêmica persistente causada por diabetes melito de início no adulto.
• Os cães com síndrome de Fanconi congênita tipicamente desenvolvem doença clínica em virtude da reabsorção defeituosa de glicose e aminoácidos aos 4-5 anos de idade; machos e fêmeas são igualmente acometidos.
• Há relatos de distúrbios tubulares renais familiares (ver a seção "Fisiopatologia").
• Glicosúria renal primária (Terrier escocês) pode ser identificada em uma idade precoce como um achado incidental.

SINAIS CLÍNICOS

Comentários Gerais
Os sinais clínicos são variáveis, dependendo da causa primária.

Achados Anamnésicos
• Glicosúria persistente resulta em poliúria (diurese osmótica), levando à polidipsia compensatória.
• A glicosúria predispõe o animal a infecções do trato urinário; os sinais resultantes são associados à infecção do trato urinário superior e/ou inferior.
• A raça (ver a seção "Fisiopatologia") e o histórico terapêutico (ver a seção "Fisiopatologia") são importantes.

Achados do Exame Físico
• Os pacientes com glicosúria hiperglicêmica podem exibir sinais sistêmicos; ver os capítulos sobre diabetes melito.
• Os pacientes com glicosúria normoglicêmica podem apresentar funções corporais normais.
• Os cães com síndrome de Fanconi podem desenvolver sinais de acidose metabólica, anormalidades eletrolíticas e doença renal crônica.

CAUSAS

Glicosúria Hiperglicêmica

Transitória
• Fisiológica — hiperglicemia por estresse; comum nos gatos.
• Farmacológica — ver a seção "Fisiopatologia".

Persistente
• Diabetes melito (100% dos pacientes); deficiência de insulina ou resistência a esse hormônio.
• Hiperadrenocorticismo (5-10% dos pacientes); insulinorresistência.
• Pancreatite aguda (±); deficiência de insulina.
• Outras causas menos comuns — lesões do SNC, feocromocitoma, concentração elevada do hormônio de crescimento em função do aumento da progesterona (endógena ou exógena) ou acromegalia, glucagonoma, insuficiência hepática crônica (atribuída à falha em metabolizar o glucagon).

Glicosúria Normoglicêmica

Congênita
• Glicosúria renal primária (Terrier escocês).
• Síndrome de Fanconi (ver a seção "Fisiopatologia").
• Doenças congênitas podem ser associadas à disfunção renal (Elkhound norueguês).

Adquirida
• Insuficiência renal aguda associada a lesões tubulares proximais significativas.
• Síndrome de Fanconi (ver a seção "Fisiopatologia").
• Doença renal crônica (rara).

FATORES DE RISCO
Variam com as causas subjacentes.

DIAGNÓSTICO

DIAGNÓSTICO DIFERENCIAL
• Glicosúria hiperglicêmica persistente nos pacientes em jejum é frequentemente associada a endocrinopatias (p. ex., diabetes melito e hiperadrenocorticismo).
• Pancreatite aguda.
• Disfunções reabsortivas tubulares renais provocam glicosúria normoglicêmica.
• Com frequência, os pacientes sob estresse exibem hiperglicemia e glicosúria transitórias leves.

ACHADOS LABORATORIAIS

Testes de Triagem
• Normalmente negativos (a concentração urinária de glicose é muito baixa para ser detectada).

Testes de Glicose Oxidase
• Específicos para glicose; mais sensíveis (~40-100 mg/dL) do que os métodos de redução do cobre.

$$\text{Glicose} + O_2 \text{ (ar)} + H_2O \xrightarrow{\text{oxidase}} \text{ácido glicurônico} + H_2O$$

$$H_2O \xrightarrow{\text{peroxidase do rábano silvestre}} H_2O + O \text{ (oxigênio nascente)}$$

$$O + \text{indicador colorido} \longrightarrow \text{complexo oxidado de mudança da coloração}$$

• Glicose oxidase, peroxidase e indicador colorido são impregnados nas fitas reagentes; tais fitas reagem especificamente com a glicose à temperatura ambiente dentro de um intervalo de tempo curto e definido após a imersão na urina. A mudança de cor é comparada com uma cartela de cores; no entanto, a pigmentúria pode prejudicar a interpretação da cor.

- Resultados falso-positivos — contaminação com peróxido de hidrogênio, hidrocloreto, cloro ou outros agentes oxidantes fortes.
- Resultados falso-negativos — (1) Ácido ascórbico é supostamente sintetizado e excretado em baixas concentrações nos cães (até 90 mg/dL) e gatos (até 50 mg/dL). Baixas concentrações de ácido ascórbico podem inibir a detecção de concentrações urinárias baixas de glicose ou subestimar concentrações urinárias mais altas de glicose por meio de fitas reagentes com o método da glicose oxidase de alguns fabricantes. O iodato foi incorporado na Chemstrip® (fita reagente da Boehringer Mannheim) para diminuir a interferência do ácido ascórbico, eliminando praticamente os resultados falso-negativos sob concentrações urinárias baixas, mas significativas em termos patológicos, de glicose, segundo relatos. Além disso, a ingestão de grandes quantidades de ácido ascórbico (suplementos de vitamina C, medicamentos de tetraciclina com formulação de ácido ascórbico) pode resultar em leituras falsamente diminuídas. (2) Ingestão de salicilato. (3) Amostras refrigeradas que não foram aquecidas à temperatura ambiente antes do teste (reação dependente da temperatura). (4) Cetonúria (moderadamente aumentada, 40 mg/dL) em amostras com baixas concentrações de glicose. (5) Densidade elevada pode resultar em redução na sensibilidade de glicose com o uso de Multistix® (fita reagente da Bayer). (6) Reagentes vencidos (as enzimas glicose oxidase e peroxidase são lábeis) ou reagentes expostos à luz solar.

Testes de Redução do Cobre
- Inespecíficos para a glicose; menos sensíveis (250 mg/dL) e limite de detecção mais alto do que os métodos da glicose oxidase.

Íons cúpricos + glicose $\xrightarrow{\text{álcali}}$ + íons cuprosos + glicose oxidada
(azul)   (laranja-vermelho)

- Clinitest® é adicionado a 5 (ou 2 para diminuir a sensibilidade) gotas de urina e 10 gotas de água em um tubo-teste e a cor da reação final é comparada a uma escala de cor após o término da ebulição (cerca de 15 segundos).
- Resultados falso-positivos — (1) Substâncias redutoras (glicose, frutose, lactose, galactose, maltose, pentose). (2) Ácido ascórbico. (3) Glicuronatos conjugados (p. ex., bilirrubina conjugada). (4) Determinados medicamentos (salicilatos, penicilina, sulfonamidas, hidrato de cloral). (5) Formaldeído.

Exames Confirmatórios
- Testes baseados nas enzimas hexoquinase ou glicoquinase desidrogenase com o uso de analisador químico automatizado podem ser utilizados para confirmar a presença ou a ausência de glicose quando se encontram resultados inesperados ou urina pigmentada.

Medicamentos Capazes de Alterar os Resultados Laboratoriais
Ver a seção "Achados Laboratoriais — Testes de Triagem".

Distúrbios Capazes de Alterar os Resultados Laboratoriais
Ver a seção "Achados Laboratoriais — Testes de Triagem".

Os Resultados Serão Válidos se os Exames Forem Realizados em Laboratório Humano?
Sim.

HEMOGRAMA/BIOQUÍMICA/URINÁLISE
Glicosúria Hiperglicêmica
- Detecção de cetonúria, hiperglicemia e glicosúria indica cetoacidose diabética.
- A presença de leucograma inflamatório com atividades elevadas da lipase e/ou amilase séricas apoia o diagnóstico de pancreatite em cães não azotêmicos ou levemente azotêmicos.
- Os cães com atividade acentuadamente aumentada da fosfatase alcalina sérica, hiperglicemia, glicosúria (bem como hipercolesterolemia, hipertrigliceridemia) devem ser avaliados em busca de hiperadrenocorticismo.
- É provável que a glicosúria leve com hiperglicemia transitória seja fisiológica em pacientes sob estresse.

OUTROS TESTES LABORATORIAIS
- Glicosúria hiperglicêmica — conduzir o teste de supressão com dexametasona em baixas doses ou teste de estimulação com ACTH na suspeita de hiperadrenocorticismo.
- Glicosúria normoglicêmica — a mensuração das concentrações de fósforo, glicose e aminoácidos em amostras sincronizadas de urina pode ajudar a diferenciar síndrome de Fanconi e glicosúria renal primária.
- Ver capítulos relacionados com causas específicas.

DIAGNÓSTICO POR IMAGEM
Ultrassonografia pode ser útil no diagnóstico de hiperadrenocorticismo e pancreatite.

TRATAMENTO
- Suspender a administração de quaisquer medicamentos associados a defeitos adquiridos do transporte tubular renal.
- O tratamento varia com a causa; ver capítulos relacionados com causas específicas.

MEDICAÇÕES
MEDICAMENTO(S) DE ESCOLHA
- Glicosúria hiperglicêmica — tratar os pacientes com diabetes melito por conta da hiperglicemia.
- Glicosúria normoglicêmica — não há necessidade de tratamento para distúrbios de transporte tubular a menos que haja acidose metabólica e anormalidades eletrolíticas (p. ex., síndrome de Fanconi).

CONTRAINDICAÇÕES
Os pacientes com diabetes melito não devem ser submetidos a medicamentos diabetogênicos, como corticosteroides ou fluidos contendo glicose.

ACOMPANHAMENTO
MONITORIZAÇÃO DO PACIENTE
Variável, dependendo da condição subjacente.

COMPLICAÇÕES POSSÍVEIS
- A glicosúria persistente predispõe o paciente ao desenvolvimento de infecções bacterianas do trato urinário (cistite, pielonefrite ascendente e possível sepse).
- Diurese osmótica com poliúria obrigatória resulta em polidipsia, exigindo o acesso à água para evitar desidratação.

DIVERSOS
DISTÚRBIOS ASSOCIADOS
Infecções do trato urinário, doença renal crônica, retinopatia diabética ou cataratas.

GESTAÇÃO/FERTILIDADE/REPRODUÇÃO
A secreção de progesterona em excesso em cadelas intactas pode induzir a diabetes melito por causa da insulinorresistência.

OUTROS
Tumores hipofisários secretores do hormônio de crescimento em gatos mais idosos (sobretudo machos) podem induzir a diabetes melito (insulinorresistência).

VER TAMBÉM
- Diabetes Melito sem Complicação — Cães.
- Diabetes Melito sem Complicação — Gatos.
- Doenças Renais de Natureza Congênita e de Desenvolvimento.
- Hiperadrenocorticismo (Síndrome de Cushing) — Gatos.
- Hiperadrenocorticismo (Síndrome de Cushing) — Cães.
- Síndrome de Fanconi.
- Pancreatite.

ABREVIATURA(S)
- ACTH = hormônio adrenocorticotrópico.
- SNC = sistema nervoso central.

Sugestões de Leitura
Finco DR. Congenital, inherited, and familial renal diseases. In: Osborne CA, Finco DR, eds., Canine and Feline Nephrology and Urology. Philadelphia: Williams & Wilkins, 1995, pp. 136-205, 471-483.
Nagel D, Seiler D, Hohenberger EF, Ziegler M. Investigations of ascorbic acid interference in urine test strips. Clin Lab 2006, 52:149-153.
Osborne CA, Lees GE. A clinician's analysis of urinalysis. In: Osborne CA, Finco DR, eds., Canine and Feline Nephrology and Urology. Philadelphia: Williams & Wilkins, 1995, pp. 136-205.
Osborne CA, Stevens JB. Handbook of Canine and Feline Urinalysis. St. Louis: Ralston Purina, 1981.
Osborne CA, Stevens, JB eds. In: Urinalysis: A Compassionate Guide to Patient Care. Shawnee, KS: Bayer, 1999.

Autores Cheryl L. Swenson e Carl A. Osborne
Consultor Editorial Carl A. Osborne

Glomerulonefrite

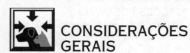

CONSIDERAÇÕES GERAIS

DEFINIÇÃO
- Inflamação e disfunção concomitante dos glomérulos. A glomerulonefrite costuma ser atribuída ao depósito de imunocomplexos intraglomerulares (nem sempre há células inflamatórias).
- "Glomerulonefrite" é um termo utilizado de forma imprecisa como uma espécie de guarda-chuva para cobrir todas as glomerulopatias, mas muitas doenças glomerulares não são "glomerulonefrite" de fato, porque a lesão primária não se deve à inflamação dos glomérulos.

FISIOPATOLOGIA
- Complexos antígeno-anticorpo circulantes solúveis podem sofrer deposição ou ficar aprisionados nos glomérulos. Alternativamente, os imunocomplexos também podem se formar *in situ* dentro da parede do capilar glomerular quando os anticorpos circulantes reagem com os antígenos "depositados" nesse local. Após a formação ou o depósito de imunocomplexos glomerulares, determinados fatores, incluindo a ativação da cascata do complemento, a infiltração de neutrófilos e macrófagos, a agregação de plaquetas, a ativação do sistema de coagulação e a deposição de fibrina, contribuem para a lesão glomerular.
- O glomérulo responde com proliferação celular (glomerulonefrite proliferativa), espessamento da membrana basal glomerular (glomerulopatia membranosa) ou ambos (glomerulonefrite membranoproliferativa). Se a inflamação e a lesão persistirem, os processos de hialinização e esclerose dos glomérulos acarretarão a perda dos néfrons e, por fim, insuficiência e falência renais crônicas.
- A perda de proteína e outros componentes do soro para os lumens dos túbulos renais também contribui para a falência renal progressiva por meio de inúmeros mecanismos.

SISTEMA(S) ACOMETIDO(S)
- Renal/urológico — proteinúria inicialmente, com poucos ou nenhum leucócitos e hemácias. Em caso de doença progressiva e perda dos néfrons, ocorrem azotemia e falência renal crônica.
- Cardiovascular — proteinúria grave pode resultar em edema e ascite secundários à hipoalbuminemia e retenção de sódio. É comum a ocorrência de hipertensão. Também ocorrem hipercolesterolemia e hipercoagulabilidade com doença tromboembólica secundária em associação com proteinúria moderada a grave.

GENÉTICA
- Há relatos de doença glomerular familiar nas raças Montanhês de Berna, Spaniel britânico, Bull terrier, Bullmastiff, Mastiff francês, Dálmata, Samoieda, Doberman pinscher, Cocker spaniel, Terra Nova, Rottweiler, Pembroke Welsh corgi, Beagle, e Wheaten terrier de pelo macio.
- Ocorre amiloidose familiar em cães da raça Shar-pei; foram relatados casos esporádicos de ninhadas acometidas em outras raças. A amiloidose familiar ocorre em gatos Abissínios. Contudo, tanto nos cães Shar-peis como nos gatos Abissínios, os depósitos de amiloide renal são encontrados principalmente no interstício medular; a amiloidose glomerular ocorre em alguns animais acometidos.

INCIDÊNCIA/PREVALÊNCIA
- A doença glomerular subclínica é comum. Em alguns estudos, 90% dos cães de fontes aleatórias tinham lesões glomerulares.
- Pode ser a principal causa de doença renal progressiva crônica que leva à falência renal em cães; no entanto, a glomerulonefrite possivelmente é subdiagnosticada, porque a glomerulosclerose progressiva faz com que a magnitude da proteinúria diminua no momento em que se desenvolve a azotemia.

IDENTIFICAÇÃO
Espécies
Cães; menos comumente, gatos.
Raça(s) Predominante(s)
- Ver a seção "Genética".
- Labrador e Golden retriever parecem ser predispostos ao desenvolvimento de glomerulonefrite, necrose tubular aguda e inflamação intersticial associada à infecção por *Borrelia burgdorferi*.
Idade Média e Faixa Etária
- Cães — idade média, 6,5-8,5 anos; faixa etária, 0,8-17 anos. Os cães com nefrite hereditária podem desenvolver proteinúria antes dos 6 meses de vida.
- Gatos — idade média, 4 anos.
Sexo Predominante
- Cães — sem predileção sexual.
- Gatos —75% são machos.

SINAIS CLÍNICOS
Comentários Gerais
- Em geral, descobre-se proteinúria significativa à triagem anual de animais saudáveis ou durante a avaliação de outros problemas.
- Ocasionalmente, sinais associados a alguma doença infecciosa, inflamatória ou neoplásica subjacente constituem a razão da ida ao veterinário.
Achados do Histórico e do Exame Físico
- Perda leve a moderada de proteína — a proteinúria permanece assintomática. Contudo, sinais inespecíficos podem incluir letargia e/ou perda de peso.
- Perda grave de proteína (concentração sérica de albumina <1-1,5 g/dL) — frequentemente ocorrem edema transudativo e/ou ascite.
- Se a doença evoluiu para falência renal, podem ocorrer os sinais de poliúria/polidipsia, anorexia, náusea e vômito.
- Dispneia aguda ou respiração ofegante grave em cães podem ser causadas por tromboembolia pulmonar (incomum), que ocorre em associação com hipoalbuminemia moderada a grave (concentração sérica de albumina <2-2,5 g/dL).
- Cegueira aguda atribuída a hemorragia ou descolamento da retina pode ser associada à hipertensão sistêmica (incomum).

CAUSAS
- Glomerulonefrite autoimune verdadeira (i. e., glomerulonefropatia antimembrana basal), em que os anticorpos são direcionados contra antígenos renais endógenos, é muito rara em cães e gatos.
- Várias doenças infecciosas e inflamatórias são associadas à deposição glomerular ou formação *in situ* de imunocomplexos (ver adiante). Em muitos casos, não se identifica qualquer fonte antigênica ou processo mórbido subjacente; nesse caso, a doença é considerada idiopática. As doenças a seguir são associadas à glomerulonefrite:
  ◦ Cães — infecciosas (p. ex., hepatite infecciosa canina, endocardite bacteriana, brucelose, dirofilariose, erliquiose, hepatozoonose, leishmaniose, piometra, borreliose, qualquer infecção bacteriana crônica, tripanossomíase); neoplásicas; inflamatórias (p. ex., lúpus eritematoso sistêmico); endócrinas (p. ex., hiperadrenocorticismo, diabetes melito, administração prolongada de corticosteroides); nefrites hereditárias; causas diversas (sulfonamidas).
  ◦ Gatos — infecciosas (p. ex., FeLV, PIF, FIV, e poliartrite por micoplasma); neoplásicas; familiares (amiloidose); e idiopáticas (especialmente glomerulopatia membranosa).

DIAGNÓSTICO

DIAGNÓSTICO DIFERENCIAL
- Proteinúria — comumente associada à inflamação e/ou hemorragia do trato urinário pós-glomerular (p. ex., cistite/pielonefrite bacteriana, urolitíase, falência renal tubular, ou neoplasia); inflamação do trato urinário geralmente (mas nem sempre) é associada a sedimento urinário ativo (i. ex., aumento no número de hemácias, leucócitos, células epiteliais, cilindros e bactérias por campo óptico). Hiperglobulinemia secundária a gamopatias monoclonais ou policlonais pode causar proteinúria, particularmente quando analisada pelo método turbidimétrico com ácido sulfossalicílico. Semelhantemente à glomerulonefrite, a amiloidose renal muitas vezes provoca proteinúria grave com sedimento urinário inativo (pode haver cilindros hialinos). A biopsia renal constitui o único método preciso para distinguir amiloidose de outras formas de doença glomerular.
- Hipoalbuminemia — pode estar associada à baixa produção de albumina (hepatopatia grave) ou ao aumento da perda de albumina (enteropatias e nefropatias com perda de proteína).

HEMOGRAMA/BIOQUÍMICA/URINÁLISE
- O hemograma completo geralmente não apresenta alterações dignas de nota.
- Nos casos graves, ocorrem hipoalbuminemia e hipercolesterolemia.
- Proteinúria significativa persistente com sedimento urinário inativo (podem ser observados cilindros hialinos).
- A microalbuminúria frequentemente precede a proteinúria franca e pode ajudar na detecção precoce de dano glomerular.
- Em caso de doença avançada, há alterações compatíveis com falência renal. Azotemia leve pode preceder a perda completa da capacidade de concentração da urina.

OUTROS TESTES LABORATORIAIS
Relação de Ureia:Creatinina Urinárias
- Usada para confirmar e quantificar a proteinúria anormal.
- A magnitude da proteinúria tem certa correlação com a gravidade das lesões glomerulares, o que torna a relação de ureia:creatinina urinárias um parâmetro útil para avaliar a resposta à terapia e a evolução ou remissão da doença glomerular.
- Assim que a falência renal se desenvolve em virtude de esclerose progressiva dos glomérulos, a

GLOMERULONEFRITE

relação de proteína:creatinina urinárias pode diminuir.

Eletroforese de Proteína
- A eletroforese de proteína sérica e urinária pode ajudar a identificar a origem da proteinúria.
- Imunoglobulinas de cadeia leve (proteínas de Bence Jones) podem estar presentes na urina em casos de malignidade linfoide.

DIAGNÓSTICO POR IMAGEM
Esses procedimentos são úteis para descartar condições concomitantes. Pode ser observada uma leve renomegalia.

MÉTODOS DIAGNÓSTICOS
- Biopsia renal — se houver proteinúria significativa e persistente associada a sedimento urinário inativo, a avaliação histopatológica do tecido renal geralmente permitirá a diferenciação entre glomerulonefrite e amiloidose. Os resultados da biopsia também podem ajudar a formular o prognóstico e o plano terapêutico. Considerar a realização de biopsia somente depois de efetuar exames menos invasivos (p. ex., hemograma completo, perfil bioquímico sérico, urinálise e quantificação de proteinúria) e avaliar a capacidade de coagulação do sangue.
- Contraindicações relativas à biopsia renal — um rim solitário, trombocitopenia ou outra coagulopatia, e lesões renais associadas a acúmulo de líquido (p. ex., hidronefrose e cistos/abscessos renais).
- As complicações relacionadas com a biopsia são mais comuns em pacientes com < 5 kg e gravemente azotêmicos.

ACHADOS PATOLÓGICOS
- Várias combinações de espessamento da membrana (forma membranosa) e aumento da celularidade (forma proliferativa); também se pode notar a formação de cicatriz glomerular (glomerulosclerose).
- Usar coloração imunofluorescente e/ou imuno-histoquímica e microscopia eletrônica para maximizar as informações obtidas com a amostra de biopsia. Esses exames necessitam da colocação do tecido de biopsia em fixadores e preservativos especiais, e não em formalina.
- Solicitar uma coloração com vermelho Congo para detectar a presença de amiloide, além dos corantes de tecido.

TRATAMENTO

DIETA
Dietas hipossódicas e hipoproteicas de alta qualidade. Muitas rações disponíveis no mercado para problemas renais atendem a esses critérios.

ORIENTAÇÃO AO PROPRIETÁRIO
Assim que ocorrer o desenvolvimento de azotemia e falência renal, o prognóstico será em geral mau em função do caráter rapidamente progressivo da doença.

MEDICAÇÕES

MEDICAMENTO(S) DE ESCOLHA
- Como a maioria das doenças glomerulares é mediada por mecanismos imunopatogênicos, a terapia mais específica e eficaz consiste na eliminação da fonte de estimulação antigênica. Com frequência, isso não é uma tarefa fácil, porque o processo mórbido ou a fonte antigênica não é identificada ou é impossível eliminá-la (p. ex., neoplasia).
- Inibidores da ECA diminuem a proteinúria por meio de alterações na pressão da filtração glomerular. Em um único estudo prospectivo, o enalapril (0,5 mg/kg a cada 12-24 h) exerceu efeitos anti-hipertensivos e antiproteinúricos, além de diminuir a evolução da doença renal, em cães com glomerulonefrite idiopática. Como a proteinúria pode ser diretamente tóxica aos túbulos renais, a terapia com inibidores da ECA deve ser iniciada no momento do diagnóstico a menos que haja azotemia grave.
- Embora a glomerulonefrite frequentemente tenha uma base autoimune, nenhum ensaio clínico controlado em medicina veterinária demonstrou qualquer benefício advindo da terapia imunossupressora. Pelo contrário, foi demonstrado que os glicocorticoides e a ciclosporina independentemente agravem o prognóstico em muitos pacientes.
- O ácido acetilsalicílico diminui a produção de tromboxano, uma causa importante de inflamação glomerular, e reduz a agregação plaquetária e a consequente doença tromboembólica. O ácido acetilsalicílico em baixas doses (0,5 mg/kg VO a cada 12-24 h) pode reduzir a agregação plaquetária e evitar declínios nas prostaglandinas benéficas ao mesmo tempo em que diminui as concentrações de tromboxano. A terapia com ácido acetilsalicílico costuma ser iniciada assim que a albumina sérica estiver abaixo de 2,2-2,5 g/dL.

CONTRAINDICAÇÕES
Medicamentos imunossupressores (sobretudo corticosteroides quando utilizados isoladamente). Contudo, a glomerulopatia membranosa (antes do início da azotemia) possivelmente é uma doença glomerular que pode ser tratada de forma eficaz com agentes imunossupressores; há necessidade de confirmação por biopsia antes de instituir a terapia.

PRECAUÇÕES
- As dosagens de medicamentos altamente ligados a proteínas e/ou eliminados pelos rins (p. ex., ácido acetilsalicílico) talvez tenham de ser ajustadas; as concentrações séricas de albumina mudam com o tratamento ou a evolução da doença.
- Utilizar os inibidores da ECA com cuidado em pacientes azotêmicos. Assim que a creatinina sérica estiver maior do que aproximadamente 3,5 g/dL, deve-se considerar a redução das doses; além disso, a creatinina deverá ser reavaliada após cerca de 4-7 dias.

ACOMPANHAMENTO

MONITORIZAÇÃO DO PACIENTE
- Relação de proteína:creatinina urinárias — método menos invasivo para avaliar a evolução ou remissão das glomerulopatias.
- A magnitude da proteinúria diminuirá à medida que ocorrer a perda de mais néfrons com a evolução da doença; portanto, sempre é preciso interpretar as alterações na relação de proteína:creatinina urinárias diante de alterações na concentração sérica de creatinina.
- Acompanhar as concentrações séricas de ureia, creatinina, albumina e eletrólitos, bem como a pressão arterial e o peso corporal.
- O ideal é reavaliar o paciente 1, 3, 6, 9 e 12 meses depois do início do tratamento.

PREVENÇÃO
Não acasalar os animais com suspeita de doença glomerular familiar.

COMPLICAÇÕES POSSÍVEIS
- Distúrbios tromboembólicos.
- Hipertensão.
- Síndrome nefrótica.
- Insuficiência ou falência renais crônicas.

EVOLUÇÃO ESPERADA E PROGNÓSTICO
- O prognóstico a longo prazo é reservado a mau.
- O quadro frequentemente evolui apesar do tratamento.

DIVERSOS

SINÔNIMO(S)
- Doença glomerular.
- Glomerulonefropatia.
- Nefropatia com perda de proteína.

VER TAMBÉM
- Amiloidose.
- Borreliose de Lyme.
- Proteinúria.
- Síndrome Nefrótica.

ABREVIATURA(S)
- ECA = enzima conversora de angiotensina.
- FeLV = vírus da leucemia felina.
- FIV = vírus da imunodeficiência felina.
- PIF = peritonite infecciosa felina.

Sugestões de Leitura
Vaden, S.L. Glomerular diseases. In: Ettinger, S.J., Feldman, E.C., eds. Textbook of veterinary internal medicine. 7th ed. Philadelphia: Saunders, 2010:2021-2036.

Autores George E. Lees, Gregory F. Grauer, e Barrak M. Pressler
Consultor Editorial Carl A. Osborne

Glucagonoma

CONSIDERAÇÕES GERAIS

REVISÃO
- Trata-se de um tumor pancreático raro, que se origina das células alfa das ilhotas pancreáticas, responsáveis pela secreção do glucagon. Os glucagonomas também podem secretar outros hormônios, como gastrina, polipeptídeo pancreático e, em casos raros, insulina.
- O excesso de glucagon circulante resulta em aumento do catabolismo proteico, lipólise, gliconeogênese e glicogenólise. O ápice dessas alterações bioquímicas resulta em hiperglicemia, hipoaminoacidemia, anemia e perda de peso. O glucagon também pode exercer um efeito secretor sobre o intestino delgado, levando à diarreia.
- Os glucagonomas podem afetar inúmeros sistemas orgânicos, incluindo musculosquelético, tegumentar, endócrino, gastrintestinal, nervoso/comportamental e hepatobiliar.

IDENTIFICAÇÃO
- Cães — raro; animais mais idosos.
- Gatos — não há relatos até o momento.

SINAIS CLÍNICOS
- O principal sinal é uma dermatopatia característica conhecida mais comumente como eritema migratório necrolítico. Isso também foi relatado na literatura veterinária como necrose epidérmica metabólica, dermatite necrolítica superficial, síndrome hepatocutânea e dermatopatia diabética.
- As lesões cutâneas incluem eritema, crostas e erosões, localizadas geralmente em torno de junções mucocutâneas na face, no períneo e na genitália, bem como ao longo da parte distal dos membros e nos coxins palmoplantares. As lesões são frequentemente pruriginosas, exibindo coxins palmoplantares hiperqueratóticos e dolorosos. Em muitos casos, os coxins são a única área acometida.
- Outros sinais sistêmicos podem incluir letargia, poliúria/polidipsia, diarreia, piodermites e/ou infecções leveduriformes secundárias, além de perda de peso.

CAUSAS E FATORES DE RISCO
A etiologia do glucagonoma é desconhecida; no entanto, os glucagonomas são comumente representados na síndrome de neoplasia endócrina múltipla.

DIAGNÓSTICO

DIAGNÓSTICO DIFERENCIAL
- O glucagonoma sempre deve ser adicionado à lista de diagnóstico diferencial ao se constatar a presença de lesões cutâneas compatíveis com eritema migratório necrolítico; entretanto, outros diferenciais mais comuns devem incluir hepatopatia inespecífica e hipoaminoacidemia.
- A necrose epidérmica metabólica foi associada a diabetes, tumores pancreáticos e hepatopatia. Outras dermatopatias que devem ser diferenciadas incluem o pênfigo foliáceo, o lúpus eritematoso sistêmico, a vasculite, as dermatoses alimentares, a dermatose responsiva à vitamina A e a dermatopatia causada por deficiência de zinco.
- É importante notar que a hiperglucagonemia leve a moderada pode ser vista secundariamente a doenças não relacionadas com o glucagonoma, como hepatopatia, doença pancreática, insuficiência renal crônica, inanição, bacteremia, cetoacidose diabética e hiperadrenocorticismo.

HEMOGRAMA/BIOQUÍMICA/URINÁLISE
- Hemograma completo — pode permanecer normal; no entanto, é comum a constatação de anemia normocítica normocrômica e/ou neutrofilia madura.
- Bioquímica sanguínea — também pode estar normal; todavia, podem ser observadas elevações discretas das enzimas hepáticas e/ou da bilirrubina total, além de leve hiperglicemia e/ou hipoalbuminemia.
- Mensuração dos ácidos biliares e provas da função hepática costumam estar dentro dos limites de normalidade.
- Urinálise — é comum um declínio na densidade urinária. Pode haver glicosúria na presença de diabetes melito secundário.

OUTROS TESTES LABORATORIAIS
- Os níveis plasmáticos de glucagon encontram-se, em geral, extremamente elevados (i. e., >1.000 pg/mL); contudo, os níveis de glucagon normais a levemente elevados não descartam o glucagonoma.
- Em geral, os níveis plasmáticos de aminoácidos apresentam-se gravemente diminuídos; além disso, acredita-se que a hipoaminoacidemia esteja associada ao desenvolvimento de eritema migratório necrolítico.
- Além de os níveis de zinco estarem geralmente reduzidos, também se acredita que esses níveis estejam associados ao desenvolvimento de eritema migratório necrolítico.
- A frutosamina pode estar elevada em pacientes com diabetes melito secundário.

DIAGNÓSTICO POR IMAGEM
- Ultrassonografia é útil para detectar glucagonomas pancreáticos, metástases peripancreáticas e metástases hepáticas.
- TC, RM, tomografia por emissão de pósitrons, angiografia visceral seletiva e cintilografia para receptores de somatostatina (com octreotida e meta-iodo-benzil-guanida marcado com iodo radioativo) são utilizados para aumentar a sensibilidade de detecção de glucagonoma em seres humanos.

MÉTODOS DIAGNÓSTICOS
O aumento nos níveis séricos de glucagon e a presença de sinais clínicos compatíveis com eritema migratório necrolítico são indicativos de glucagonoma, embora o diagnóstico definitivo só possa ser feito por meio de biopsia, exame histopatológico e documentação da expressão imuno-histoquímica do glucagon. Os ensaios imuno-histoquímicos para outros hormônios pancreáticos e gastrintestinais são comumente realizados.

ACHADOS PATOLÓGICOS
- Ao exame histopatológico, as biopsias cutâneas obtidas de lesões de eritema migratório necrolítico associadas ao glucagon tipicamente exibem edema superficial a mesoepidérmico grave, hiperqueratose paraqueratótica difusa e hiperplasia epidérmica irregular. Essa tríade de achados histopatológicos costuma ser mencionada como um padrão "vermelho, branco e azul".
- Em termos histopatológicos, as biopsias coletadas do glucagonoma primário (e/ou de metástases) tipicamente revelam células pleomórficas das ilhotas com grânulos citoplasmáticos finos e mitoses ocasionais com expressão imuno-histoquímica do glucagon (e, muitas vezes, outros hormônios secretores).

TRATAMENTO

- A excisão cirúrgica de glucagonoma pancreático primário não metastático representa a melhor chance de cura. Infelizmente, é relatada uma alta taxa de morbidade e mortalidade no pós-operatório. Além disso, a síndrome do glucagonoma relatada em seres humanos está associada à doença tromboembólica, o que pode exacerbar ainda mais os índices de morbidade e mortalidade.
- A combinação de debridamento (tumor primário e/ou metástases) e da terapia médica com octreotida pode solucionar temporariamente as lesões cutâneas e conferir alívio ao animal.
- Se a cirurgia e/ou a terapia com octreotida não forem possíveis, as terapias paliativas sintomáticas poderão ser benéficas, incluindo dieta rica em proteína com claras de ovo (aproximadamente 2 a 4 claras/dia para um cão de 25 kg), suplementação de zinco (pode ser benéfica diante de níveis séricos normais desse elemento), conforme esboçado adiante, e suplementação de ácidos graxos.
- Infecções cutâneas secundárias por bactérias e/ou leveduras são comuns e devem ser tratadas de acordo.

MEDICAÇÕES

MEDICAMENTO(S)
- Octreotida é um análogo da somatostatina, que inibe a conversão de pré-pró-glucagon em glucagon, podendo ser benéfico em pacientes com glucagonoma metastático e/ou não ressecável. Os efeitos colaterais relatados no uso humano incluem dor no local da injeção, vômito, diarreia e colestase. A dosagem segura e eficaz de octreotida (ou lanreotida de ação prolongada) não foi relatada em cães; todavia, há relatos de uma dose de 10-20 μg/cão por via SC a cada 8-12 h; também foi relatada uma dose única e segura de 50 μg/cão SC em cães saudáveis.
- Vários quimioterápicos já foram usados na síndrome humana do glucagonoma. A doxorrubicina e a estreptozotocina parecem ter a melhor atividade, apesar de limitada. O uso de estreptozotocina como um agente lítico para as células das ilhotas pancreáticas foi relatado previamente em um pequeno número de cães com insulinoma, mas não foi descrito em cães com glucagonoma.
- Os glicocorticoides podem melhorar o prurido secundário das lesões cutâneas no eritema migratório necrolítico, mas não são recomendados para uso em glucagonomas, pois esses agentes provavelmente exacerbam a hiperglicemia (considerando-se que muitos pacientes com glucagonoma têm diabetes melito secundário).
- Aminoácidos intravenosos (500 mL de aminoácidos essenciais acrescentados à solução fisiológica ou de Ringer lactato durante 12 h ou solução de aminoácidos a 10% a 24 mL/kg administrada em 8-12 h em uma veia central calibrosa) demonstraram uma melhora variável nas lesões cutâneas em cães. Se eficazes, os tratamentos

GLUCAGONOMA

podem ser repetidos a cada 1-2 semanas até que os sinais clínicos diminuam ou desapareçam.
• Xampus à base de enxofre/ácido salicílico ou bem suaves podem ajudar a remover as crostas, amaciar a pele e melhorar a dor e/ou o prurido associado(s) às lesões da pele e/ou dos coxins palmoplantares.
• Pode ser considerado o uso de sulfato de zinco oral a 10 mg/kg/dia ou metionina zíncica a 2 mg/kg/dia ou gliconato de zinco a 3 mg/kg/dia.

CONTRAINDICAÇÕES/INTERAÇÕES POSSÍVEIS
Os glicocorticoides podem exacerbar a hiperglicemia na presença de diabetes melito secundário.

ACOMPANHAMENTO
MONITORIZAÇÃO DO PACIENTE
• A monitorização hematológica seriada deve ser feita no pós-operatório para se certificar de que a hiperglucagonemia prévia (e quaisquer outras anormalidades) esteja se resolvendo e continue dentro dos limites de normalidade.
• É fortemente sugerida a realização de ultrassonografias seriadas de acompanhamento e radiografias torácicas em três projeções para monitorizar a ocorrência de metástase.

DIVERSOS
VER TAMBÉM
• Hepatopatia Diabética.
• Dermatite Necrolítica Superficial.

ABREVIATURA(S)
• TC = tomografia computadorizada.
• RM = ressonância magnética.

Sugestões de Leitura
Allenspach K, et al. Glucagon-producing neuroendocrine tumour associated with hypoaminoacidemia and skin lesions. J Small Anim Pract 2000, 41:402-406.
Chastain MA. The glucagonoma syndrome: A review of its features and discussion of new perspectives. Am J Med Sci 2001, 321(5):306-320.
Kasper CS, McMurry K. Necrolytic migratory erythema without glucagonoma versus canine superficial necrolytic dermatitis: Is hepatic impairment a clue to pathogenesis? J Am Acad Dermatol 1991, 25(3):534-541.
Langer NB, Jergens AE, Miles KG. Canine glucagonoma. Compend Contin Educ Pract Vet 2003, 25(1):56-63.
Mizuno T, Hiraoka H, Yoshioka C, Takeda Y, Matsukane Y, Shimoyama N, Morimoto M, Hayashi T, Okuda M. Superficial necrolytic dermatitis associated with extrapancreatic glucagonoma in a dog. Vet Dermatol 2009, 20(1):72-79.

Autor Phil Bergman
Consultor Editorial Deborah S. Greco

Granulomatose Linfomatoide

CONSIDERAÇÕES GERAIS

REVISÃO
- Doença pulmonar rara de cães e gatos, caracterizada por proliferação angiocêntrica e angiodestrutiva, além de infiltração por células linfoides atípicas.
- Não se trata de uma doença granulomatosa, como foi anteriormente relatada.

IDENTIFICAÇÃO
- Cães e gatos.
- Idade média — 5,75 anos (faixa etária de 1,5-14 anos) em cães.
- Embora não haja qualquer predileção racial, é mais comum em raças de grande porte e raças puras.
- Não há predileção sexual.

SINAIS CLÍNICOS
- Sinais respiratórios progressivos, incluindo tosse e dispneia.
- Secreção nasal serosa.
- Intolerância ao exercício.
- Perda de peso.
- Anorexia.
- Febre em 50% dos pacientes.
- Duração — dias a semanas.

CAUSAS E FATORES DE RISCO
Desconhecidos.

DIAGNÓSTICO

DIAGNÓSTICO DIFERENCIAL
- Pneumonia micótica, bacteriana ou por aspiração.
- Neoplasia pulmonar primária ou metastática.

HEMOGRAMA/BIOQUÍMICA/URINÁLISE
- Nada consistente.
- Leucocitose neutrofílica é comum.
- Eosinofilia comum.
- Basofilia comum.

OUTROS TESTES LABORATORIAIS
Alguns cães apresentam dirofilariose concomitante e resultado positivo no teste para pesquisa de dirofilárias.

DIAGNÓSTICO POR IMAGEM
- Radiografia — revela consolidação pulmonar lobar (p. ex., lesões expansivas tipo massa), linfadenomegalia hilar e efusão pleural.
- Lesões — uni ou bilaterais.

MÉTODOS DIAGNÓSTICOS
- Biopsia — para o diagnóstico definitivo.
- Aspirado com citologia — para diagnóstico presuntivo.

ACHADOS PATOLÓGICOS
- Macroscópicos — múltiplos nódulos pulmonares com predileção pelos lobos caudais dos pulmões com metástase ou envolvimento de linfonodos hilares.
- Histológicos — caracterizados por lâminas de células linfoides e plasmoides atípicas misturadas com poucos eosinófilos e linfócitos pequenos nos vasos sanguíneos pulmonares. Os linfócitos podem ser compostos por linhagens das células B e T.
- Citológicos — podem aparecer como inflamação eosinofílica e neutrofílica estéril com macrófagos reativos.
- É possível a ocorrência de metástase para fígado, coração, rins, baço, pâncreas, glândula adrenal e outros órgãos.

TRATAMENTO

- Medicamentos citotóxicos com a excisão cirúrgica quando apropriada.
- Sempre consulte um veterinário especialista em oncologia.

MEDICAÇÕES

MEDICAMENTO(S)
Protocolo quimioterápico combinado — CHOP ou outro protocolo combinado adequado para linfoma.

CONTRAINDICAÇÕES/INTERAÇÕES POSSÍVEIS
- Mielossupressão — causada por medicamentos citotóxicos.
- Cistite hemorrágica — causada pela ciclofosfamida.

ACOMPANHAMENTO

MONITORIZAÇÃO DO PACIENTE
Mesmo que aquele realizado para linfoma tratado por quimioterapia.

COMPLICAÇÕES POSSÍVEIS
- Dispneia à medida que a doença evolui.
- Depressão.
- Anorexia.
- Mielossupressão provocada pela quimioterapia.

EVOLUÇÃO ESPERADA E PROGNÓSTICO
A sobrevida média em cães submetidos à quimioterapia sistêmica é de 12 meses e meio; no entanto, a faixa etária quanto à sobrevida pode ser muito ampla com base na resposta inicial à terapia.

DIVERSOS

DISTÚRBIOS ASSOCIADOS
Pode evoluir para linfoma.

SINÔNIMO(S)
- Granulomatose Pulmonar Eosinofílica.
- Granulomatose.
- Granulomatose Linfoide.
- Angiite Linfoproliferativa.

ABREVIATURA(S)
- CHOP = ciclofosfamida, hidroxidaunorrubicina, vincristina (Oncovin®) e prednisona.

Sugestões de Leitura

Baez J, Sorenmo KU. Pulmonary and bronchial neoplasia. In: King LG, ed., Textbook of Respiratory Disease in Dogs and Cats. St. Louis: Saunders, 2004, pp. 508-516.

Berry CR, Moore PF, Thomas WP, et al. Pulmonary lymphomatoid granulomatosis in seven dogs (1976-1987). J Vet Intern Med 1990, 4:157-166.

Bounous DI, Bienzle D, Miller-Liebl D. Pleural effusion in a dog. Vet Clin Path 2000, 29:55-58.

Morrison WB. Tumors of uncertain origin. In: Morrison WB, ed., Cancer in Dogs and Cats: Medical and Surgical Management. Jackson, WY: Teton NewMedia, 2002, pp. 745-750.

Park HM, Hwang DN, Kang BT, et al. Pulmonary lymphomatoid granulomatosis in a dog: Evidence of immunophenotypic diversity and relationship to human pulmonary lymphomatoid granulomatosis and pulmonary Hodgkin's disease. Vet Pathol 2007, 44:921-923.

Autor Wallace B. Morrison
Consultor Editorial Timothy M. Fan

HALITOSE

CONSIDERAÇÕES GERAIS

DEFINIÇÃO
Odor desagradável que emana da cavidade bucal.

FISIOPATOLOGIA
- O cheiro de leite azedo que acompanha a doença periodontal pode resultar de populações bacterianas associadas a placas, cálculos, tecidos não sadios da cavidade bucal, partículas de alimento em decomposição retidas na cavidade bucal e necrose tecidual.
- Ao contrário do que comumente se acredita, o ar do pulmão normal ou o aroma do estômago não contribuem para a halitose.
- A causa mais comum é a doença periodontal causada por placa bacteriana.
- Uma biopelícula de bactérias se forma sobre um dente recentemente limpo e polido assim que o paciente começa a salivar; as bactérias aderem-se à película em 6-8 h; em questão de dias, a placa torna-se mineralizada, produzindo o cálculo dentário; à medida que a placa envelhece e a gengivite evolui para periodontite (perda óssea), a flora bacteriana muda de predominantemente cocos aeróbios Gram-positivos imóveis para uma população anaeróbia Gram-negativa móvel que inclui *Prophyromonas*, Bacteroides, *Fusobacterium* e *Actinomyces* spp.
- A superfície áspera do cálculo dentário atrai mais bactérias, irritando a margem gengival livre; à medida que a inflamação prossegue, o sulco gengival transforma-se em uma bolsa periodontal, onde se acumulam restos de alimentos e produtos de degradação bacteriana, gerando a halitose.
- A principal causa do mau cheiro é a putrefação promovida pelas bactérias anaeróbias Gram-negativas, que geram compostos sulfurados voláteis, como sulfeto de hidrogênio, metilmercaptano, sulfeto de dimetila e ácidos graxos voláteis.
- Os compostos sulfurados voláteis também podem desempenhar um papel na doença periodontal, pois afetam a integridade da barreira tecidual, fazendo com que as endotoxinas acarretem destruição periodontal, endotoxemia e bacteremia.

SISTEMA(S) ACOMETIDO(S)
Gastrintestinal — cavidade bucal.

IDENTIFICAÇÃO
Espécies
Cães e gatos.

Raça(s) Predominante(s)
Raças de pequeno porte e braquicefálicas são mais propensas à doença bucal, porque os dentes estão mais unidos, os animais pequenos vivem por mais tempo e seus proprietários tendem a lhes oferecer alimentos mais pastosos.

Idade Média e Faixa Etária
Os animais mais idosos são predispostos.

SINAIS CLÍNICOS
- Se a halitose for atribuída à doença bucal, podem ocorrer ptialismo (com ou sem alimento), patadas na boca, anorexia.
- Na maioria dos casos, nenhum sinal clínico é observado, além do odor.

CAUSAS
- Ingestão de alimentos com mau cheiro.
- Metabólicas — diabetes, uremia.
- Respiratórias — rinite, sinusite, neoplasia.
- Gastrintestinais — megaesôfago, neoplasia, corpo estranho.
- Dermatológicas — piodermite das pregas labiais.
- Nutricionais — gêneros alimentícios fétidos, coprofagia.
- Doença bucal — doença periodontal e ulceração, ortodônticas, faringite, tonsilite, neoplasia, corpos estranhos.
- Traumatismo — lesão por fio de eletricidade, fraturas abertas, agentes cáusticos indutores de dano à cavidade bucal.
- Infecciosas — infecções bacterianas, fúngicas, virais da cavidade bucal.
- Doenças autoimunes da cavidade bucal.
- Complexo granuloma eosinofílico.

DIAGNÓSTICO

HEMOGRAMA/BIOQUÍMICA/URINÁLISE
Geralmente, permanecem normais. Podem ser observadas alterações compatíveis com diabetes melito ou nefropatia.

DIAGNÓSTICO POR IMAGEM
Radiografias intrabucais são adequadas para ajudar no diagnóstico das causas de halitose.

MÉTODOS DIAGNÓSTICOS
- Sulfeto de hidrogênio, mercaptanos e ácidos graxos voláteis constituem os principais componentes da halitose; pode-se usar um monitor industrial de sulfeto para medir a concentração desse elemento em partes por milhão de pico.
- Outros métodos diagnósticos para avaliação de doença periodontal incluem radiografia intrabucal, sondagem da profundidade da bolsa, níveis de aderência e mobilidade do dente.

TRATAMENTO

CUIDADO(S) DE SAÚDE ADEQUADO(S)
- O tratamento é ambulatorial.
- Assim que a causa específica da halitose for descoberta, direcionar a terapia para a correção da doença existente. • Com frequência, múltiplos dentes são extraídos em caso de doença periodontal avançada como causa da halitose.

ORIENTAÇÃO AO PROPRIETÁRIO
- A halitose geralmente é um sinal de cavidade bucal não saudável e deve incitar ao exame imediato da boca.
- Tomar medidas preventivas para garantir a boa saúde bucal (p. ex., escovação dos dentes).

CONSIDERAÇÕES CIRÚRGICAS
A avaliação bucal é realizada sob anestesia geral por meio de radiografias intrabucais. O tratamento envolve a extração de dentes com perda de sustentação superior a 50%.

MEDICAÇÕES

MEDICAMENTO(S) DE ESCOLHA
- Os antibióticos não são indicados para o tratamento de halitose.
- O controle dos patógenos periodontais ajuda a controlar as infecções dentárias e acompanhar o mau cheiro. Doxirobe® Gel (Pfizer) é indicado na doença periodontal em estágio 2, caracterizada pela existência de bolsas. Quando acompanhadas por cuidados domésticos, essas bolsas têm demonstrado uma redução em sua profundidade.
- Foi demonstrado que a aplicação semanal de OraVet®, um gel para prevenção de placas, diminui a formação dessas placas bacterianas.
- O uso de produtos para cuidados bucais que contenham íons metálicos, especialmente zinco, inibe a produção de odor por causa da afinidade dos íons metálicos pelo enxofre; o zinco forma complexos com o sulfeto de hidrogênio até formar sulfeto de zinco insolúvel; o zinco interfere na proliferação microbiana e na calcificação de depósitos microbianos (por interferir no desenvolvimento de cálculo de cristais). O tratamento tópico com gel de cisteína e ascorbato de zinco costuma diminuir a halitose em 30 minutos. Nos EUA, há um produto de ascorbato de zinco associado a aminoácido (Maxi/Guard Oral Cleansing Gel, Addison Biological).
- A clorexidina utilizada como colutório bucal ou como pasta também ajuda a controlar a placa, diminuindo o odor; nos EUA, ela é comercializada como CHX Guard®, CHX Guard LA® (VRx Products, Harbor City, CA); CET Oral Hygiene Spray, pasta de dentes DentiVet® e Hexarinse® (Virbac, Fort Worth, TX).

ACOMPANHAMENTO

MONITORIZAÇÃO DO PACIENTE
Avaliar o paciente quanto à recidiva dos sinais.

PREVENÇÃO
A escovação ou fricção diária ajuda não só a remover a placa, mas também a controlar a doença dentária e o odor bucal; realizar exames periódicos para monitorizar os cuidados.

EVOLUÇÃO ESPERADA E PROGNÓSTICO
Variam com a causa subjacente.

DIVERSOS

SINÔNIMO(S)
- Respiração fétida.
- Hálito pútrido.
- Mau cheiro.
- *Fetor ex ore.*
- *Fetor oris.*

VER TAMBÉM
Doença periodontal.

Sugestões de Leitura
Harvey CE, Emily PP. Small Animal Dentistry. Philadelphia: Mosby, 1993.
Wiggs RB, Lobprise HB. Veterinary Dentistry: Principles and Practice. Philadelphia: Lippincott-Raven, 1997.

Autor Jan Bellows
Consultor Editorial Heidi B. Lobprise

Hemangiopericitoma

CONSIDERAÇÕES GERAIS

REVISÃO
- Um sarcoma de tecido mole que surge em torno dos vasos sanguíneos no tecido subcutâneo.
- Frequentemente referido como tumor da bainha dos nervos periféricos.
- Localmente invasivo, que muitas vezes se estende além das margens visíveis.
- Sofre metástase em menos de 15% dos pacientes.
- Pode exibir um crescimento lento.
- O crescimento local pode interferir na função dos membros.

IDENTIFICAÇÃO
- Comum em cães, mas raro em gatos.
- Mais comum em raças caninas de grande porte do que naquelas de pequeno porte.
- Cães e gatos de meia-idade a mais idosos.

SINAIS CLÍNICOS

Achados Anamnésicos
- Tipicamente, massa flutuante a firme, indolor e de crescimento lento (semanas a meses).
- É incomum o crescimento rápido a menos que seja uma variante de alto grau.

Achados do Exame Físico
- Massa de tecido mole no subcutâneo, mais frequentemente localizada em um membro do que no tronco.
- Mole, flutuante ou firme.
- Indolor a menos que esteja ulcerada ou promova a invasão de tecidos musculares ou nervosos.
- Geralmente aderida ao tecido subjacente.
- É rara a ocorrência de metástase para linfonodos regionais.

CAUSAS E FATORES DE RISCO
Cães de grande porte estão sob alto risco.

DIAGNÓSTICO

DIAGNÓSTICO DIFERENCIAL
- Outros sarcomas de tecido mole, incluindo tumor da bainha dos nervos periféricos, fibrossarcoma, rabdomiossarcoma, sarcoma de tecido mole indiferenciado, mixossarcoma, histiocitoma fibroso maligno, sarcoma histiocítico.
- Lipoma e outros tumores subcutâneos — benignos e malignos.

HEMOGRAMA/BIOQUÍMICA/URINÁLISE
Geralmente normais.

DIAGNÓSTICO POR IMAGEM
- Radiografias torácicas são recomendadas antes do tratamento, embora a ocorrência de metástase seja identificada em menos de 10-15% dos casos.
- Exames de TC ou RM contrastadas são recomendados não só para determinar a extensão da doença, mas também para otimizar o tratamento cirúrgico e a radioterapia.

MÉTODOS DIAGNÓSTICOS
- Aspirado por agulha fina e citologia podem fornecer o diagnóstico presuntivo, mas as células nem sempre esfoliam de forma satisfatória.
- É essencial a realização de biopsia incisional e histopatologia para confirmar o diagnóstico, determinar o grau do tumor e planejar a abordagem cirúrgica.
- A avaliação imuno-histoquímica da biopsia pode ajudar na diferenciação de outros tumores mesenquimais.
- A avaliação dos linfonodos regionais (citologia ou histopatologia) é adequada em tumores de alto grau para confirmar ou negar a presença de metástases regionais.

TRATAMENTO

CONSIDERAÇÕES CIRÚRGICAS
- Excisão cirúrgica em bloco rigorosa e precoce constitui o tratamento de escolha.
- À microscopia, as células cancerosas estendem-se bem além das bordas macroscópicas do tumor.
- É comum haver a formação de pseudocápsula composta de células cancerosas comprimidas.
- Excisão do tumor em bloco; se for "esfoliado", um leito sadio de células cancerosas será deixado para trás.
- Enviar toda a amostra a um patologista para avaliação da margem cirúrgica; é aconselhável a aplicação de tinta apropriada às bordas cirúrgicas para avaliar as margens por completo.
- Talvez haja necessidade da amputação de membro ou dedo acometido por tumores volumosos que podem não ser passíveis de ressecção.
- A ressecção de costela ou parede abdominal pode ser necessária para tumores do tronco.
- A radioterapia deve ser considerada como uma opção terapêutica quando a excisão cirúrgica completa não for possível, podendo ser aplicada à doença microscópica (fracionada no pós-operatório) ou macroscópica (hipofracionada).

MEDICAÇÕES

MEDICAMENTO(S)
- A quimioterapia à base de doxorrubicina não é consistentemente relatada como benéfica, mas continua sendo recomendada após a excisão de tumor de alto grau (grau III).
- A quimioterapia em baixas doses com piroxicam e ciclofosfamida pode ajudar a retardar a recidiva local em caso de ressecção incompleta do sarcoma.
- Pode haver novas opções terapêuticas para doença metastática. Portanto, o proprietário deve entrar em contato com o oncologista veterinário para atualização dos tratamentos que podem estar disponíveis.
- É recomendável a administração de terapia analgésica, conforme a necessidade, na presença de dor ou desconforto.

ACOMPANHAMENTO

MONITORIZAÇÃO DO PACIENTE
- Se a ressecção cirúrgica completa for acessível e o tumor categorizado como de baixo grau, será improvável o novo crescimento do tumor ou a ocorrência de metástases; com isso, a monitorização contínua do paciente pode ser dispensada.
- Se a ressecção cirúrgica for parcial ou o tumor categorizado como de alto grau, o paciente deverá ser monitorizado quanto à presença de novo crescimento local e metástases à distância com exame físico repetido e radiografias torácicas a cada 3 meses.

EVOLUÇÃO ESPERADA E PROGNÓSTICO
- A recidiva local, a metástase e o tempo de sobrevida global são muito influenciados pela largura da margem cirúrgica e pelo grau histológico, conforme for determinado pelo médico-anatomista patológico.
- A cura da doença será possível quando a cirurgia for rigorosa e as margens cirúrgicas estiverem livres do tumor, especialmente em tumores de grau I e II. Em um único estudo, a sobrevida média chegou a 2 anos com sarcomas de tecido mole de grau baixo (I) dos membros tratados apenas com cirurgia.
- A recidiva será inevitável se o tratamento não for rigoroso; maior risco de doença metastática, sobretudo em tumores de grau elevado (III).
- O controle do tumor a longo prazo com radioterapia após debridamento cirúrgico do tumor confere taxas de controle de 60-85% por 1 a 5 anos.
- É recomendável o controle de excisão cirúrgica parcial com uma segunda cirurgia rigorosa ou radioterapia o mais rápido possível. A quimioterapia em baixas doses também constitui uma opção terapêutica.

DIVERSOS

ABREVIATURA(S)
- RM = ressonância magnética.
- TC = tomografia computadorizada.

Sugestões de Leitura

Ehrhart N. Soft-tissue sarcomas in dogs: A review. JAAHA 2005, 41:241-246.

Elmslie RE, Glawe P, Dow SW. Metronomic therapy with cyclophosphamide and piroxicam effectively delays tumor recurrence in dogs with incompletely resected soft tissue sarcomas. J Vet Intern Med 2008, 22:1373-1379.

Kuntz CA, Dernell WS, Powers BE, et al. Prognostic factors for surgical treatment of soft tissue sarcomas in dogs: 75 cases (1986-1996). JAVMA 1997, 211:1147-1151.

Mazzei M, Millante F, Ati S, et al. Haemangiopericytoma: Histological spectrum, immunohistochemical characterization and prognosis. Vet Dermatol 2002, 13:15-21.

Stefanello D, Morello E, Roccabianca P, et al. Marginal excision of low-grade spindle cell sarcoma of canine extremities: 35 dogs (1996-2006). Vet Surg 2008, 37:461-465.

Autor Louis-Philippe de Lorimier
Consultor Editorial Timothy M. Fan
Agradecimento O autor e os editores agradecem a colaboração prévia de Phyllis Glawe.

Hemangiossarcoma Cutâneo

CONSIDERAÇÕES GERAIS

REVISÃO
- Tumor maligno que surge de células endoteliais.
- O tumor primário desenvolve-se dentro da derme ou de tecidos subcutâneos.
- Responsável por 14% de todos os hemangiossarcomas em cães.
- Prevalência (cães e gatos) — 0,3-2%.

IDENTIFICAÇÃO
- Cães e gatos.
- Pit bull, Boxer e Pastor alemão — acometidos mais comumente que outras raças.
- Hemangiossarcoma dérmico — cães das raças Whippet, Galgo e aparentadas.
- Idade média, 9 anos; faixa etária, 4,5-15,6 anos.

SINAIS CLÍNICOS
Dérmicos
- Em geral, massa solitária (especialmente gatos), embora possam ocorrer múltiplas massas.
- Nódulos firmes, elevados, escuros são comuns em regiões como membros, cabeça, face, orelhas, prepúcio, plano nasal e abdome ventral.
- As lesões não costumam ser ulcerativas.

Subcutâneos
- Em geral, massa solitária (especialmente gatos), embora possam ocorrer múltiplas massas.
- Massas firmes ou moles, flutuantes, com ou sem contusões associadas.
- É comum o sangramento intratumoral.
- As massas são tipicamente maiores do que os tumores dérmicos.
- Os membros pélvicos costumam ser acometidos (cães e gatos), mas podem surgir em qualquer local.
- Em gatos, os locais mais comumente envolvidos são o flanco e o abdome ventral, bem como as regiões inguinal e cervical.

CAUSAS E FATORES DE RISCO
- Hemangiossarcoma dérmico associado à radiação ultravioleta (indução actínica).
- Hemangiossarcoma subcutâneo pode ser secundário à radioterapia ionizante prévia.

DIAGNÓSTICO

DIAGNÓSTICO DIFERENCIAL
- Hematoma subcutâneo induzido por traumatismo.
- Hamartoma ou mastocitoma.

HEMOGRAMA/BIOQUÍMICA/URINÁLISE
Geralmente normais.

OUTROS TESTES LABORATORIAIS
Perfil de coagulação — pode haver anormalidades laboratoriais compatíveis com CID (tempos de sangramento prolongados, trombocitopenia, fibrinogênio baixo e produtos de degradação da fibrina altos), resultantes de uma coagulopatia de consumo em cães com lesões subcutâneas amplas de hemangiossarcoma com sangramento ativo.

DIAGNÓSTICO POR IMAGEM
- Radiografias torácicas são recomendadas para a detecção de metástase pulmonar (rara em gatos).
- Ultrassonografia abdominal para detectar metástase intra-abdominal (rara em gatos).
- TC ou RM para determinar a extensão da doença e o planejamento cirúrgico.

MÉTODOS DIAGNÓSTICOS
Citologia
- Com frequência, esse exame não é recompensador em virtude do número insuficiente de células e da contaminação sanguínea da amostra.
- As células neoplásicas são em formato de fuso, círculo oval, chama ou estrela com anisocitose e anisocariose, núcleos únicos arredondados, ovais ou pleomórficos, nucléolos proeminentes, baixa relação núcleo/citoplasma e citoplasma basofílico moderado a abundante e geralmente vacuolizado.

Histopatologia
- Necessária para confirmar o diagnóstico; permite a diferenciação entre hemangioma e hemangiossarcoma e origem dérmica *versus* subcutânea.
- Revela células endoteliais neoplásicas que formam canais vasculares irregulares com áreas sólidas compostas de células estromais intensamente anaplásicas.

ACHADOS PATOLÓGICOS
- Dérmicos — bem circunscritos, limitados à derme.
- Subcutâneos — pouco circunscritos; muito invasivos.

TRATAMENTO

CONSIDERAÇÕES CIRÚRGICAS
- A excisão cirúrgica rigorosa constitui o tratamento de escolha.
- Cães — a excisão completa de hemangiossarcoma dérmico (estágio I) é associada a um tempo médio de sobrevida de 780 dias *versus* hemangiossarcoma subcutâneo (estágio II) com tempo médio de sobrevida de 172 dias.
- Gatos — a excisão completa é mais comum em casos de tumores dérmicos e controle local satisfatório (intervalo livre de doença >450 dias). A excisão parcial é mais comum em casos de tumores subcutâneos e tem alta probabilidade de recidiva local (<300 dias).

RADIOTERAPIA
- Protocolo definitivo como parte de múltiplas modalidades terapêuticas (cirurgia, quimioterapia, radioterapia) — indicado para o controle de carga tumoral residual microscópica.
- Protocolo paliativo (hipofracionado) para o tratamento de carga tumoral macroscópica não ressecável — produz taxas de resposta de ~70% e tempos de sobrevida de <100 dias.

MEDICAÇÕES

MEDICAMENTO(S)
- Quimioterapia é recomendada para hemangiossarcoma subcutâneo.
- Quimioterapia neoadjuvante é indicada para diminuir o tamanho dos tumores antes de cirurgia; observa-se taxa de resposta de ~35% em cães submetidos à doxorrubicina.
- Quimioterapia adjuvante com doxorrubicina prolonga significativamente os tempos de sobrevida em casos de hemangiossarcoma subcutâneo.
- Quimioterapia contínua em baixas doses — protocolos terapêuticos metronômicos que consistem em piroxicam diário e ciclofosfamida em baixas doses (10 mg/m^2 VO a cada 24 h) podem ter supostas capacidades antiangiogênicas e retardar a evolução da doença.

ACOMPANHAMENTO

EVOLUÇÃO ESPERADA E PROGNÓSTICO
- Dérmico — tempo médio de sobrevida em cães de 780 dias apenas com a cirurgia; intervalo livre de doença em gatos >450 dias somente com a intervenção cirúrgica.
- Subcutâneo — tempo médio de sobrevida em cães de 172 dias com cirurgia isolada *versus* >1.100 dias em caso de cirurgia e quimioterapia adjuvante com doxorrubicina; intervalo livre de doença em gatos <300 dias com a cirurgia.
- Nos casos de hemangiossarcomas em estágios II e III, espera-se a ocorrência de metástase à distância para os pulmões.

DIVERSOS

ABREVIATURA(S)
- CID = coagulação intravascular disseminada.
- RM = ressonância magnética.
- TC = tomografia computadorizada.

Sugestões de Leitura
Bulakowski EJ, Philibert JC, Siegel S, et al. Evaluation of outcome associated with subcutaneous and intramuscular hemangiosarcoma treated with adjuvant doxorubicin in dogs: 21 cases (2001-2006). JAVMA 2008, 233:122-128.
Johannes CM, Henry CJ, Turnquist SE, et al. Hemangiosarcoma in cats: 53 cases (1992-2002). JAVMA 2007, 231:1851-1856.
McAbee KP, Ludwig LL, Bergman PJ, et al. Feline cutaneous hemagiosarcoma: A retrospective study of 18 cases. JAAHA 2005, 41:110-116.
Ward H, Fox LE, Calderwood-Mays MB, et al. Cutaneous hemangiosarcoma in 25 dogs: A retrospective study. J Vet Intern Med 1994, 8:345-348.

Autor Craig Clifford
Consultor Editorial Timothy M. Fan
Agradecimento O autor e os editores agradecem a colaboração prévia de Phyllis Glawe.

Hemangiossarcoma do Baço e do Fígado

CONSIDERAÇÕES GERAIS

DEFINIÇÃO
Neoplasia altamente maligna que surge de células endoteliais vasculares e/ou células-tronco hemangioblásticas transformadas.

FISIOPATOLOGIA
• A ruptura do tumor primário leva a hemorragia aguda, colapso e, frequentemente, morte súbita.
• Tumor altamente metastático que se dissemina no início do curso da doença por via hematógena ou implantação intra-abdominal.

SISTEMA(S) ACOMETIDO(S)
• Hematológico/linfático/imune — baço.
• Podem ocorrer metástases em qualquer órgão, incluindo pulmões, rins, músculos, peritônio, omento, linfonodos, mesentério, adrenais, medula espinal, cérebro, tecido subcutâneo e diafragma.

GENÉTICA
Nenhuma relação identificada.

INCIDÊNCIA/PREVALÊNCIA
• Cães — 0,3-2% dos tumores registrados em necropsias, representando 7% de todas as malignidades.
• Gatos — raro.

DISTRIBUIÇÃO GEOGRÁFICA
N/D.

IDENTIFICAÇÃO

Espécies
Cães e gatos.

Raça(s) Predominante(s)
• Cães — as raças Pastor alemão, Golden retriever, Boxer, Dinamarquês, Setter inglês e Pointer costumam ser mais acometidas.
• Gatos — os domésticos de pelo curto são super-representados.

Idade Média e Faixa Etária
• Cães — idade média, 8-10 anos; raramente documentado em animais muito jovens com menos de 1 ano de idade.
• Gatos — idade média, 10 anos.

Sexo Predominante
Não há predileção sexual.

SINAIS CLÍNICOS

Comentários Gerais
• A queixa mais comumente apresentada é o colapso agudo como resultado de ruptura tumoral e subsequente hemorragia.
• Outros sinais são especificamente relacionados com os órgãos envolvidos.

Achados Anamnésicos
• Colapso agudo devido à ruptura tumoral/perda sanguínea aguda.
• Fraqueza.
• Colapso intermitente.
• Perda de peso.
• Claudicação.
• Sinais neurológicos: ataxia, paresia, crises convulsivas.

Achados do Exame Físico
• Mucosas pálidas.
• Taquicardia.
• Líquido peritoneal.
• Massa abdominal cranial palpável.

CAUSAS
• Cães — as anormalidades genéticas incluem superexpressão da oncoproteína STAT3, mutações dentro dos genes supressores tumorais $p53$ e PTEN, bem como superexpressão de fatores angiogênicos, como fator de crescimento do endotélio vascular e angioproteínas.
• Gatos — nenhuma identificada.

FATORES DE RISCO
N/D.

DIAGNÓSTICO

DIAGNÓSTICO DIFERENCIAL
• Outras causas de massas esplênicas e hepáticas — linfoma; leiomiossarcoma; lipossarcoma; hematoma; hemangioma; cisto esplênico; hepatoma; carcinoma hepatocelular; cisto hepático.
• Na presença de hemoabdome, o hemangiossarcoma constitui o diagnóstico mais comum (variando de 63 a 92,6%).

HEMOGRAMA/BIOQUÍMICA/URINÁLISE
• Anemia regenerativa com policromasia, reticulocitose, anisocitose e eritrócitos nucleados.
• Leucocitose caracterizada por neutrofilia madura.
• Trombocitopenia.
• Atividade elevada das enzimas hepáticas em casos de envolvimento hepático.

OUTROS TESTES LABORATORIAIS
Prolongamento de TP e TPP, além de aumento nos produtos de degradação da fibrina.

DIAGNÓSTICO POR IMAGEM

Radiografia
• Radiografias abdominais para identificar a presença de massa abdominal cranial e indícios de líquido abdominal (perda de detalhes da serosa).
• Radiografias torácicas para identificar doença metastática pulmonar, caracterizada por padrão miliar coalescente ou padrão intersticial miliar nodular/generalizado.

Ultrassonografia
• Ultrassonografia abdominal para detectar lesões esplênicas ou hepáticas, nódulos omentais e líquido abdominal livre (hemoabdome).
• Ecocardiografia para identificar massas no átrio direito (mais bem identificadas na presença de, pelo menos, algum grau de efusão pericárdica).

RM/TC
Os exames de RM/TC possuem alta sensibilidade e especificidade na determinação de processos benignos e malignos do fígado e do baço.

MÉTODOS DIAGNÓSTICOS
• Abdominocentese para caracterizar o acúmulo de líquido — geralmente um líquido serossanguinolento ou efusão hemorrágica não coagulada.
• Citologia — relata-se que a recuperação diagnóstica de hemangiossarcoma com esse exame seja baixa (25%).

ESTÁGIOS DA DOENÇA
• Estágio I — tumor confinado ao órgão, sem ruptura.
• Estágio II — tumor rompido.
• Estágio III — doença metastática evidente.

ACHADOS PATOLÓGICOS
• Hemangiossarcoma esplênico — massa friável hemorrágica.
• Hemangiossarcoma hepático — nódulos hemorrágicos solitários ou múltiplos de tamanho variável.
• Exame histopatológico — necessário para o diagnóstico definitivo; caracterizado geralmente por grandes espaços sanguíneos revestidos por células mesenquimais anaplásicas, numerosas estruturas capilares pequenas e áreas sólidas de células endoteliais neoplásicas sem estrutura vascular aparente.

TRATAMENTO

CUIDADO(S) DE SAÚDE ADEQUADO(S)
Paciente hospitalizado — tratamento inicial clínico e cirúrgico.

CUIDADO(S) DE ENFERMAGEM
• Soluções eletrolíticas isotônicas balanceadas para corrigir choque hipovolêmico e débito cardíaco diminuído.
• Transfusão de sangue total fresco para repor a perda sanguínea e a capacidade carreadora de oxigênio decorrentes do sangramento agudo.
• Tratar a CID conforme a necessidade.

ATIVIDADE
Restrita até a recuperação cirúrgica inicial.

DIETA
Sem alteração.

ORIENTAÇÃO AO PROPRIETÁRIO
• Informar ao proprietário sobre a possível indicação de cirurgia de emergência.
• Avisar o proprietário sobre a possibilidade de morte súbita caso não se procure por qualquer outra terapia.
• Discutir a importância do acompanhamento da terapia (quimioterapia ou terapia metronômica).

CONSIDERAÇÕES CIRÚRGICAS
• O procedimento de esplenectomia constitui o padrão de cuidado e o tratamento inicial de escolha. Remove a carga tumoral macroscópica e diminui a probabilidade de morte aguda por hemorragia. A cirurgia sozinha é um tratamento paliativo, com tempos médios de sobrevida de 1-3 meses.
• Avaliar o perfil de coagulação antes da cirurgia.

MEDICAÇÕES

MEDICAMENTO(S) DE ESCOLHA

Quimioterapia Adjuvante
• Doxorrubicina é o medicamento mais eficaz e, por essa razão, é incluída em todos os protocolos citotóxicos convencionais:
  ○ 30 mg/m^2 IV para cães com >10 kg; 1 mg/kg IV para cães e gatos com <10 kg.
  ○ Intervalo a cada 2 semanas em cães e a cada 3 semanas em gatos por 5 ciclos terapêuticos.
• Consultar um oncologista veterinário em busca de qualquer tratamento atualizado disponível.

CONTRAINDICAÇÕES
• Doxorrubicina — não usar na presença de arritmias ou fração de encurtamento do coração reduzida.

HEMANGIOSSARCOMA DO BAÇO E DO FÍGADO

- A quimioterapia pode causar efeitos tóxicos no trato gastrintestinal, na medula óssea e no coração; buscar orientação antes do tratamento se não estiver familiarizado com agentes citotóxicos.

PRECAUÇÕES
- Monitorizar o leucograma — adiar a quimioterapia se a contagem de neutrófilos estiver <2.000/µL.
- Monitorizar as plaquetas — adiar a quimioterapia se a contagem de plaquetas estiver <50.000/µL.

INTERAÇÕES POSSÍVEIS
Nenhuma.

MEDICAMENTO(S) ALTERNATIVO(S)
- Imunoterapia:
  - Muramil tripeptídeo-fosfatidiletanolamida lipossomal, um ativador sintético de macrófagos derivado da parede celular de micobactérias, associado ao protocolo de doxorrubicina/ciclofosfamida (tempo médio de sobrevida de 273 dias).
  - Vacina alogênica contra hemangiossarcoma + doxorrubicina (tempo médio de sobrevida de 182 dias).
- Terapia metronômica (quimioterapia em baixas doses):
  - Administração oral diária de ciclofosfamida (10 mg/m^2) e piroxicam (0,3 mg/kg).

 ACOMPANHAMENTO

MONITORIZAÇÃO DO PACIENTE
- Radiografias torácicas a cada 2 meses para monitorizar metástases à distância.
- Ultrassonografia abdominal a cada 2 meses para monitorizar metástases regionais.

PREVENÇÃO
Nenhuma.

COMPLICAÇÕES POSSÍVEIS
- Sepse secundária à neutropenia induzida pela quimioterapia.
- Toxicidade gastrintestinal (vômito e diarreia) secundária à administração quimioterápica.
- Miocardiopatia induzida pela doxorrubicina.
- Descamação ou esfacelamento cutâneo secundário ao extravasamento de doxorrubicina.

EVOLUÇÃO ESPERADA E PROGNÓSTICO
- Tempo médio de recidiva (gatos) — 4-5 meses.
- Tempo médio de sobrevida apenas com a cirurgia (cães) — 19-65 dias.
- Tempo médio de sobrevida com cirurgia associada à quimioterapia (cães) — 145-179 dias.

 DIVERSOS

DISTÚRBIOS ASSOCIADOS
CID.

FATORES RELACIONADOS COM A IDADE
Nenhum.

POTENCIAL ZOONÓTICO
Nenhum.

GESTAÇÃO/FERTILIDADE/REPRODUÇÃO
Não usar quimioterapia em animais prenhes.

SINÔNIMO(S)
- Angiossarcoma.
- Hemangioendotelioma maligno.

VER TAMBÉM
- Hemangiossarcoma do Coração.
- Hemangiossarcoma do Osso.
- Hemangiossarcoma da Pele.

ABREVIATURA(S)
- CID = coagulação intravascular disseminada.
- RM = ressonância magnética.
- TC= tomografia computadorizada.
- TP = tempo de protrombina.
- TTP = tempo de tromboplastina parcial.

Sugestões de Leitura
Brown NO, Patnaik AK, MacEwen EG. Canine hemangiosarcoma: Retrospective analysis of 104 cases. JAVMA 1985, 186:56-58.
Clifford CA, Mackin AJ, Henry CJ. Treatment of canine hemangiosarcoma: 2000 and beyond. J Vet Intern Med 2000, 14:479-485.
de Lorimier LP, Kitchell BE. How to manage patients with hemangiosarcoma. Vet Med 2002, 97:46-57.
Fosmire SP, Dickerson EB, Scott AM, et al. Canine malignant hemangiosarcoma as a model of primitive angiogenic endothelium. Lab Invest 2004, 84:562-572.
Prymak C, McKee LJ, Goldschmidt MH, et al. Epidemiologic, clinical, pathologic, and prognostic characteristics of splenic hemangiosarcoma and splenic hematoma in dogs: 217 cases (1985). JAVMA 1988, 193:706-712.
Scavelli TD, Patnaik AK, Melhaff CJ, et al. Hemangiosarcoma in the cat: Retrospective evaluation of 31 surgical cases. JAVMA 1985, 187:817-819.
Soremno KU, Baez JL, Clifford CA, et al. Efficacy and toxicity of a dose-intensified doxorubicin protocol in canine hemangiosarcoma. J Vet Intern Med 2004, 18:209-213.

Autor Craig Clifford
Consultor Editorial Timothy M. Fan

Hemangiossarcoma do Coração

CONSIDERAÇÕES GERAIS

REVISÃO
- O tumor cardíaco mais comum em cães.
- O coração pode ser um local primário ou de metástase em cães e gatos.
- A maioria dos tumores acomete o átrio direito e/ou o apêndice auricular direito.
- Raramente, envolve a parede ventricular direita ou valva/válvula cardíaca.

IDENTIFICAÇÃO
- Cães e, raramente, gatos.
- Relatado mais comumente em Pastor alemão e Golden retriever.

SINAIS CLÍNICOS
Comentários Gerais
Os sinais clínicos são mais comumente causados pelo desenvolvimento de efusão pericárdica e insuficiência cardíaca congestiva direita.

Achados do Exame Físico
- Efusão abdominal.
- Ruídos pulmonares ventrais baixos ou ausentes — secundários à efusão pleural.
- Dispneia.
- Perda de peso.
- Bulhas cardíacas abafadas com efusão pericárdica ou pleural.
- Síncope.
- Arritmia.
- Déficits de pulso.
- Pulso paradoxal.
- Intolerância ao exercício.
- Hepatomegalia.
- Distensão jugular.

CAUSAS E FATORES DE RISCO
Desconhecidos.

DIAGNÓSTICO

DIAGNÓSTICO DIFERENCIAL
- Outras causas de insuficiência cardíaca direita — p. ex., dirofilariose.
- Outras causas de arritmia.
- Outra neoplasia cardíaca.
- Efusão pericárdica hemorrágica idiopática.
- Outras causas de efusão pericárdica, especialmente linfoma.

HEMOGRAMA/BIOQUÍMICA/URINÁLISE
- Pode haver anemia e hemácias nucleadas.
- Hemácias fragmentadas (esquizócitos) e trombocitopenia.

OUTROS TESTES LABORATORIAIS
N/D.

DIAGNÓSTICO POR IMAGEM
- Radiografias frequentemente revelam a presença de efusão pericárdica e/ou pleural; raramente detectam o efeito expansivo gerado por massa cardíaca.
- Ecocardiografia é útil para identificar a localização e a extensão do envolvimento tumoral.

MÉTODOS DIAGNÓSTICOS
- O diagnóstico definitivo requer a realização de biopsia tecidual.
- A avaliação citológica de líquido pericárdico pode fornecer um diagnóstico de apoio, especialmente se as células mesenquimais malignas esfoliarem para a efusão pericárdica.
- Eletrocardiografia pode revelar a presença de arritmia; alternância elétrica ou complexos de baixa voltagem são possíveis na presença de efusão pericárdica.

TRATAMENTO

- Cirurgia e quimioterapia devem ser consideradas como opções terapêuticas de primeira linha.
- A utilidade da radioterapia é basicamente inexplorada para o tratamento dessa doença.
- Centese periódica da efusão pericárdica e pleural pode proporcionar alívio sintomático.
- Sempre consultar um oncologista veterinário em busca de qualquer avanço nas opções terapêuticas.

MEDICAÇÕES

MEDICAMENTO(S)
Quimioterapia, especialmente doxorrubicina intravenosa, pode ser eficaz em adiar o início e a evolução do tumor primário e do crescimento de metástases.

CONTRAINDICAÇÕES/INTERAÇÕES POSSÍVEIS
N/D.

ACOMPANHAMENTO

MONITORIZAÇÃO DO PACIENTE
Os pacientes devem ser monitorados mensalmente por meio de exames físicos seriados, radiografias torácicas e ecocardiografias.

PREVENÇÃO
Nenhuma.

COMPLICAÇÕES POSSÍVEIS
As complicações podem ser associadas a centese repetida dos espaços pericárdico e pleural, resultando no desenvolvimento de arritmias, pneumotórax e infecção.

EVOLUÇÃO ESPERADA E PROGNÓSTICO
Prognóstico — reservado a mau.

DIVERSOS

DISTÚRBIOS ASSOCIADOS
- Hemangiossarcoma concomitante em outros locais (p. ex., fígado e baço).
- Sinais clínicos de insuficiência cardíaca congestiva secundária à efusão pericárdica.

Sugestões de Leitura
Aronsohn M. Cardiac hemangiosarcoma in the dog: A review of 38 cases. JAVMA 1985, 187:922-926.
Morrison WB. Nonpulmonary intrathoracic cancer. In: Morrison WB, ed., Cancer in Dogs and Cats: Medical and Surgical Management. Jackson, WY: Teton NewMedia, 2002, pp. 513-526.
Weisse C, Soares N, Beal MW, et al. Survival times in dogs with right atrial hemangiosarcoma treated by means of surgical resection with or without adjuvant chemotherapy: 23 cases (1986-2000). JAVMA 2005, 226(4):575-579.

Autor Wallace B. Morrison
Consultor Editorial Timothy M. Fan

Hemangiossarcoma do Osso

CONSIDERAÇÕES GERAIS

REVISÃO
- Tumor maligno altamente metastático de células endoteliais vasculares.
- Doença primária rara.
- Responde por <5% de todos os tumores ósseos (o acometimento apendicular varia; em caso de envolvimento axial, a costela é o local mais comumente afetado).
- Pode ser difícil distinguir lesões primárias de metastáticas.
- Há necessidade do exame de imuno-histoquímica para diferenciar de osteossarcoma telangiectásico.

IDENTIFICAÇÃO
- Cães e gatos.
- As raças Golden retriever, Boxer, Dinamarquês e Pastor alemão são predispostas.
- Idade média — cães, 6 anos; gatos, 17-18 anos.

SINAIS CLÍNICOS
Achados Anamnésicos
- Apendicular — claudicação; tumefação/massa de tecido mole no local; fratura patológica.
- Axial — tumefação da parede torácica em caso de hemangiossarcoma de costela; dispneia na presença de efusão pleural hemorrágica.

Achados do Exame Físico
- Tumefação de tecido mole no local do tumor.
- Fratura palpável.
- Ruídos pulmonares ventrais baixos ou ausentes (se houver efusão pleural).
- Taquicardia/mucosas pálidas em caso de anemia induzida pela hemorragia.

CAUSAS E FATORES DE RISCO
Desconhecidos.

DIAGNÓSTICO

DIAGNÓSTICO DIFERENCIAL
- Outros tumores ósseos primários ou metastáticos (osteossarcoma, osteossarcoma telangiectásico, fibrossarcoma e condrossarcoma).
- Osteomielite (bacteriana ou fúngica).

HEMOGRAMA/BIOQUÍMICA/URINÁLISE
- Embora sejam menos comuns do que aquelas observadas em casos de hemangiossarcoma esplênico, as anormalidades podem incluir:
  - Anemia regenerativa.
  - Eritrócitos nucleados.
  - Pecilocitose — acantócitos; esquistócitos; esferócitos.
  - Trombocitopenia.
  - Leucocitose.

OUTROS TESTES LABORATORIAIS
Perfil de coagulação — pode indicar CID.

DIAGNÓSTICO POR IMAGEM
- Radiologia óssea pode revelar lesão osteolítica sem margens definidas e reação perióstea mínima; possíveis fraturas patológicas.
- Radiografia torácica para identificar metástase pulmonar.
- Ultrassonografia abdominal e ecocardiografia — para pesquisar por tumor visceral primário (baço, fígado, ou coração) ou metástase.
- TC pode determinar a extensão do tumor ósseo para excisão cirúrgica (especialmente de costela) e fornecer uma avaliação mais sensível de metástase pulmonar.

MÉTODOS DIAGNÓSTICOS
- A realização de biopsia incisional pode ser útil em termos diagnósticos, mas, em virtude da natureza vascular do tumor, a contaminação sanguínea da amostra pode invalidar o diagnóstico ou impedir a diferenciação entre hemangiossarcoma e osteossarcoma telangiectásico.
- A biopsia excisional constitui o método preferido para o diagnóstico.

ACHADOS PATOLÓGICOS
- A avaliação macroscópica revela a existência de massa escura e friável frequentemente dentro da cavidade medular do osso.
- A histopatologia caracteriza-se por células mesenquimais anaplásicas dispostas em cordões separados por uma base colagenosa para canais e espaços vasculares preenchidos com hemácias, trombos e debris necróticos.

TRATAMENTO

- Excisão cirúrgica rigorosa de locais com tumor.
  - A amputação é necessária em caso de envolvimento apendicular.
  - Pode ser mais difícil remover tumores axiais.
- Quimioterapia adjuvante é indicada em função do alto potencial metastático.
  - Protocolos à base de doxorrubicina (isolada ou em combinação com vincristina e/ou ciclofosfamida).
- A radioterapia pode ser usada como tratamento paliativo de dor relacionada com o osso.

MEDICAÇÕES

MEDICAMENTO(S)
- Doxorrubicina isolada: 30 mg/m^2 IV para cães com mais de 10 kg; 1 mg/kg IV para cães com menos de 10 kg a cada 2 semanas por 5 ciclos; e gatos 1 mg/kg IV a cada 3 semanas.
- A adição de ciclofosfamida e vincristina pode ser considerada para dosar a intensidade da terapia sistêmica.

CONTRAINDICAÇÕES/INTERAÇÕES POSSÍVEIS
- Em cães, a doxorrubicina tem um efeito cardiotóxico cumulativo, não sendo recomendada em animais com miocardiopatia. Avaliar a função cardíaca por meio de ecocardiografia antes da terapia em raças predispostas à miocardiopatia dilatada.
- Para gatos, a doxorrubicina pode causar nefrotoxicidade; por essa razão, os valores da função renal (densidade urinária, ureia, creatinina) devem ser avaliados antes da terapia e a cada 2 a 3 ciclos.

ACOMPANHAMENTO

MONITORIZAÇÃO DO PACIENTE
Radiografia torácica, ecocardiografia, ultrassonografia abdominal e exame físico — 1, 4, 7, 10, 13, 18 e 24 meses após o tratamento.

COMPLICAÇÕES POSSÍVEIS
- Fraturas patológicas.
- Tumores (costela) e lesões metastáticas podem se romper, resultando em sinais clínicos relacionados com efusão ou anemia.

EVOLUÇÃO ESPERADA E PROGNÓSTICO
- O tempo médio de sobrevida global é desconhecido em virtude da raridade dos casos.
- Menos de 10% dos pacientes sobrevivem 1 ano após a cirurgia isolada.
- A sobrevida média (todas as localizações) após cirurgia e quimioterapia é desconhecida, mas provavelmente semelhante àquela observada em casos de hemangiossarcoma do baço.

DIVERSOS

ABREVIATURA(S)
- CID = coagulação intravascular disseminada.
- TC = tomografia computadorizada.

Sugestões de Leitura
Dernell WS, Ehrhart NP, Straw RC, Vail DM. Tumors of the skeletal system. In: Withrow SJ, Vail DM, eds., Small Animal Clinical Oncology, 4th ed. Philadelphia: Saunders, 2007, pp. 540-582.
Waters DJ, Cooley DM. Skeletal neoplasms. In: Morrison WB, ed., Cancer in Dogs and Cats: Medical and Surgical Management. Jackson, WY: Teton NewMedia, 2002, pp. 610-625.

Autor Craig Clifford
Consultor Editorial Timothy M. Fan
Agradecimento O autor e os editores agradecem a colaboração prévia de Joanne C. Graham.

HEMATÊMESE

CONSIDERAÇÕES GERAIS

DEFINIÇÃO
Vômito de sangue.

FISIOPATOLOGIA
Ruptura na barreira da mucosa do esôfago, estômago ou intestino delgado superior, acarretando inflamação e sangramento. Coagulopatias também podem se manifestar com hematêmese. Um animal também pode vomitar sangue originário da cavidade bucal ou do sistema respiratório (superior ou inferior) e que foi engolido.

SISTEMA(S) ACOMETIDO(S)
• Gastrintestinal — inflamação, traumatismo, ulceração, neoplasia e/ou corpo estranho na cavidade bucal, na região da faringe, no esôfago, no estômago e/ou no duodeno.
• Cardiovascular — hemorragia aguda grave pode resultar em taquicardia, sopro cardíaco sistólico e/ou hipotensão.
• Respiratório — hemorragia respiratória com ingestão pode levar à hematêmese.
• Hematológico — coagulopatia com hemorragia gastrintestinal pode ocasionar hematêmese.

INCIDÊNCIA/PREVALÊNCIA
A incidência real é desconhecida.

IDENTIFICAÇÃO
Espécies
Cães e, menos comumente, gatos.

Raça(s) Predominante(s)
Parece haver uma super-representação dos cães da raça Chow chow e dos gatos da raça Siamês com adenocarcinoma gástrico.

Idade Média e Faixa Etária
Todas as idades.

Sexo Predominante
Machos caninos apresentam maior incidência de carcinoma gástrico.

SINAIS CLÍNICOS
Achados Anamnésicos
• Vômitos com sangue — pode aparecer sangue no vômito na forma de flocos frescos, coágulos ou sangue digerido, parecido com borra de café.
• Pode ou não haver melena. • Anorexia. • Dor abdominal (o animal pode adotar a postura de oração).

Achados do Exame Físico
• Dor abdominal. • Melena. • Se o paciente estiver anêmico — haverá taquicardia, sopro cardíaco, palidez, fraqueza e/ou colapso.

CAUSAS
Coagulopatias
• Trombocitopenia. • Trombocitopatia — doença de von Willebrand, AINE, medicamentos, uremia.
• Síndrome de hiperviscosidade. • Coagulopatia intravascular disseminada. • Intoxicação por rodenticida anticoagulante. • Deficiência de fator de coagulação. • Insuficiência hepática.
• Policitemia.

Medicamentos
• AINE, glicocorticoides.

Doenças Gastrintestinais
• Enteropatia inflamatória. • Neoplasia bucal, esofágica, gástrica ou duodenal. • Corpo estranho bucal, esofágico, gástrico ou duodenal. • Torção ou vólvulo mesentéricos, intestinais, cecocólicos ou colônicos. • Gastrenterite hemorrágica.
• Esofagite. • Úlceras gastroduodenais. • Hérnia de hiato. • Intussuscepção gastresofágica.

Intoxicação
• Intoxicação por metais pesados (arsênico, zinco, tálio, ferro ou chumbo). • Envenenamento por plantas (diefenbáquia, sagueiro, cogumelo, mamona). • Intoxicação por substâncias químicas (fenol, etilenoglicol, agentes corrosivos, cremes para psoríase — análogos da vitamina D).
• Toxicidade de pesticidas/rodenticidas (colecalciferol). • Picada de cobra. • Aflatoxinas.

Doenças Infecciosas
• Parasitismo gastrintestinal. • Pitiose.
• Gastrenterite viral, fúngica ou bacteriana.
• Infecção por riquétsia.

Doenças Metabólicas
• Insuficiência renal. • Hepatopatia.
• Hipoadrenocorticismo. • Pancreatite.

Neoplasias
• Mastocitose. • Gastrinoma. • Tumores bucais, nasais, respiratórios ou gastrintestinais.
• APUDomas.

Doenças Neurológicas
• Traumatismo craniano. • Mielopatia.

Doenças Respiratórias
• Doença nasal — neoplasia, infecção fúngica, corpo estranho. • Doença dos pulmões e das vias aéreas — neoplasia, pneumonia grave, infecção fúngica, corpo estranho, dirofilariose.

Estresse/Doença Clínica Grave
• Choque séptico ou hipovolêmico. • Doença grave. • Queimaduras. • Intermação. • Cirurgia de grande porte. • Traumatismo. • Hipertensão sistêmica. • Hipotensão.

FATORES DE RISCO
• Administração de medicamentos ulcerogênicos — AINE ou glicocorticoides. • Pacientes criticamente enfermos. • Choque hipovolêmico ou séptico. • Trombocitopenia. • Administração concomitante de AINE e glicocorticoides.

DIAGNÓSTICO

DIAGNÓSTICO DIFERENCIAL
• Hemoptise — as radiografias torácicas podem revelar a presença de doença nos pulmões ou nas vias aéreas.
• Regurgitação ou vômito de sangue engolido por causa de doenças extragastrintestinais (p. ex., orofaríngea, nasofaríngea ou cutânea, bem como do trato urogenital e dos sacos anais).
• Ingestão e vômito de corpos estranhos ou alimentos que se pareçam com sangue fresco ou digerido (p. ex., ferro por VO).

HEMOGRAMA/BIOQUÍMICA/URINÁLISE
• Em caso de perda sanguínea aguda (3-5 dias) — anemia arregenerativa (normocítica e normocrômica, com reticulocitose mínima).
• Na perda sanguínea com >7 dias de duração — anemia regenerativa (macrocítica, com reticulocitose).
• Em caso de perda sanguínea crônica — anemia ferropriva (microcítica e hipocrômica, além de reticulocitose variável, com ou sem trombocitose).
• Pode ou não exibir trombocitopenia.
• Pode ou não ter pan-hipoproteinemia com hemorragia digestiva.
• Pode apresentar neutrofilia madura ou neutrofilia com desvio à esquerda com sepse e/ou perfuração de úlcera gastroduodenal.
• A relação de ureia:creatinina pode estar elevada com hemorragia gastrintestinal

OUTROS TESTES LABORATORIAIS
• Teste de sangue oculto nas fezes pode ser positivo — o cão não deve ter se alimentado de carne por 3 dias antes do teste.
• Flutuação fecal — triagem em busca de parasitismo gastrintestinal.
• Perfil de coagulação — na suspeita de distúrbio hemorrágico.
• Ácidos biliares — se houver suspeita de hepatopatia.
• Teste de estimulação com ACTH — na suspeita de hipoadrenocorticismo.

DIAGNÓSTICO POR IMAGEM
• Radiografias abdominais podem identificar corpo estranho ou massa no estômago ou no duodeno, pancreatite, pneumoperitônio, efusão ou alterações compatíveis com doença renal, pancreática ou hepática.
• Radiografias torácicas podem revelar corpo estranho ou massa no esôfago, intussuscepção gastresofágica, doença nos pulmões ou nas vias aéreas e/ou metástase pulmonar.
• Ultrassonografia abdominal pode identificar massa gástrica ou duodenal, espessamento da parede gástrica ou duodenal ou estratificação alterada, úlcera gástrica e/ou linfadenopatia abdominal.
• O ultrassom abdominal também pode fazer a triagem de anormalidades no pâncreas, no fígado, nos rins e em outros órgãos abdominais como fonte de hematêmese.
• Cintilografia gastrintestinal, se disponível, pode ser utilizada para localizar perda sanguínea gastrintestinal.

MÉTODOS DIAGNÓSTICOS
• Endoscopia para avaliar o aspecto da mucosa do esôfago, estômago e trato intestinal delgado superior se as causas extragastrintestinais tiverem sido excluídas.
• Biopsia de lesões da mucosa e envio para exame histopatológico a fim de determinar a natureza da doença gastrintestinal subjacente.
• Abdominocentese pode identificar peritonite séptica.
• Obtenção de aspirados por agulha fina ou amostras de biopsia de massas cutâneas ou intra-abdominais para identificar neoplasia/doença.

ACHADOS PATOLÓGICOS
• Inflamação e hemorragia gastroduodenais.
• As úlceras podem exibir mais necrose, microtrombos e hemorragia, além de uma penetração mais profunda que as erosões.

TRATAMENTO

CUIDADO(S) DE SAÚDE ADEQUADO(S)
• Tratar qualquer causa subjacente.
• Tratar em um esquema ambulatorial se a causa for identificada e eliminada, os vômitos não forem excessivos e o sangramento gastroduodenal for mínimo.

HEMATÊMESE

- Pacientes hospitalizados — aqueles com hemorragia gastroduodenal grave, úlcera perfurada, vômitos excessivos e/ou peritonite séptica.

CUIDADO(S) DE ENFERMAGEM
- Fluidos intravenosos para manter a hidratação.
- Pode ser necessária a implementação de tratamento rigoroso com fluido intravenoso para o choque — cristaloides e/ou coloides.
- Pacientes com hipoproteinemia grave podem precisar de coloides e/ou plasma para aumentar a pressão oncótica vascular.
- Pacientes com hemorragia gastroduodenal grave podem necessitar de transfusões (de sangue total ou papa de hemácias).
- Pacientes com coagulopatias subjacentes podem precisar de sangue total, plasma fresco ou plasma fresco congelado para reposição dos fatores de coagulação.
- Nos casos graves de hematêmese — para interromper o sangramento gastrintestinal, pode-se tentar a lavagem com água gelada (10-20 mL/kg, deixando no estômago por 15-30 min) ou a lavagem com noradrenalina (8 mg/500 mL) diluída em água gelada.

ATIVIDADE
Restrita.

DIETA
- Interromper o consumo oral na presença de vômito.
- Quando a alimentação for retomada, fornecer refeições em pequenas quantidades várias vezes ao dia.

ORIENTAÇÃO AO PROPRIETÁRIO
- AINE só devem ser administrados com a orientação do veterinário.
- A administração de AINE pode resultar em ulcerações e perfurações gastroduodenais.
- Os efeitos adversos dos AINE podem ser minimizados, administrando-os com alimento e mediante a administração concomitante de algum análogo sintético da prostaglandina (p. ex., misoprostol).

CONSIDERAÇÕES CIRÚRGICAS
O tratamento cirúrgico ficará indicado em casos de falha do tratamento clínico depois de 5-7 dias, hemorragia incontrolável, perfuração de úlcera gastroduodenal e/ou identificação de tumor potencialmente ressecável.

MEDICAÇÕES

MEDICAMENTO(S) DE ESCOLHA
- Antagonistas dos receptores histaminérgicos (H_2) inibem competitivamente a secreção de ácido gástrico e representam os medicamentos de escolha inicial (cimetidina, 5-10 mg/kg VO, SC, IV a cada 8 h para cão e gato; ranitidina, 0,5-2 mg/kg SC, VO, IV a cada 8-12 h para cão e gato; famotidina, 0,5 mg/kg VO, IV a cada 12-24 h para cão e gato; nizatidina 5 mg/kg VO a cada 24 h para cão). Os antagonistas dos receptores H_2 diferem em termos de potência e duração de ação. A famotidina é o agente mais potente seguido pela ranitidina, depois, pela cimetidina. Tratar por, no mínimo, 6-8 semanas. Pode ocorrer o efeito rebote ácido de hipersecreção gástrica quando os bloqueadores dos receptores H_2 são interrompidos; no entanto, esse efeito pode ser minimizado, reduzindo-se a dose gradativamente conforme o medicamento é interrompido.
- Antiácidos neutralizam a acidez gástrica e alguns induzem à síntese local de protetores da mucosa, mas devem ser administrados por no mínimo 4 a 6 vezes ao dia para serem eficazes. A obediência do proprietário a esse esquema terapêutico é muitas vezes insatisfatória.
- Suspensão de sucralfato (0,5-1 g VO a cada 6-8 h) protege o tecido ulcerado (citoproteção) não só por se ligar aos locais ulcerados, à pepsina e aos sais biliares, mas também por estimular a síntese de prostaglandina. A ligação é maior em úlceras duodenais do que nas gástricas.
- Antibiótico(s) com atividade contra bactérias gram-negativas entéricas e anaeróbias devem ser administrados por via parenteral na suspeita de solução de continuidade na barreira da mucosa gastrintestinal ou na presença de pneumonia por aspiração.
- Antieméticos (clorpromazina 0,5 mg/kg a cada 6-8 h SC, IM, IV para cão e gato; proclorperazina 0,1-0,5 mg/kg a cada 6-8 h SC, IM para cão e gato; ondansetrona 0,5 mg/kg IV a cada 12 h para cão; 0,2 mg/kg IV a cada 12 h para gato; metoclopramida 1 mg/kg a cada 24 h sob infusão em velocidade constante para cão e gato; maropitanto 1 mg/kg SC a cada 24 h por 5 dias para cão; 2 mg/kg VO a cada 24 h por 5 dias para cão) serão administrados se os vômitos forem frequentes ou resultarem em perdas significativas de líquido.
- Omeprazol (0,7 mg/kg VO a cada 24 h para cão) — inibidor mais potente da secreção de ácido gástrico; tratamento de escolha para gastrinoma com evidência de metástase ou doença não passível de ressecção e doença gastroduodenal irresponsiva à terapia com bloqueadores dos receptores H_2.

CONTRAINDICAÇÕES
- Evitar os medicamentos que possam lesar a barreira da mucosa gastroduodenal (p. ex., AINE e corticosteroides).

INTERAÇÕES POSSÍVEIS
- Bloqueadores dos receptores H_2 impedem a captação do omeprazol pelas células oxínticas.
- O sucralfato pode alterar a absorção de outros medicamentos. Por essa razão, esse agente deve ser administrado com o estômago vazio 2 horas antes ou depois de outros medicamentos por via oral.
- Os antiácidos podem alterar a absorção oral e a eliminação renal de outros medicamentos.

MEDICAMENTO(S) ALTERNATIVO(S)
O misoprostol, um análogo sintético da prostaglandina (3 µg/kg VO a cada 8-12 h), com ações antissecretoras e citoprotetoras, ajuda a prevenir e tratar as úlceras induzidas por AINE. Pode haver alguma eficácia no tratamento de ulcerações gastroduodenais de outras etiologias.

ACOMPANHAMENTO

MONITORIZAÇÃO DO PACIENTE
- A melhora em alguns casos pode ser avaliada pela resolução dos sinais clínicos; exames como hematócrito, proteína total, sangue oculto nas fezes e ureia podem ajudar a detectar perda sanguínea contínua.
- Dependendo da causa subjacente da hematêmese, podem ser necessários exames laboratoriais ou técnicas de diagnóstico por imagem específicos para monitorizar a resposta à terapia.

COMPLICAÇÕES POSSÍVEIS
- Perda sanguínea intensa. • Sepse. • Perfuração de úlcera.

EVOLUÇÃO ESPERADA E PROGNÓSTICO
- Variam com as causas subjacentes.
- Pacientes com neoplasia gástrica maligna, insuficiência renal, insuficiência hepática, pitiose, mastocitose sistêmica, sepse e/ou perfuração gástrica — prognóstico reservado a mau.
- Hematêmese secundária à administração de AINE ou a quadros de coagulopatia, enteropatia inflamatória ou hipoadrenocorticismo — o prognóstico pode ser bom a excelente, dependendo da gravidade da doença.
- Hematêmese secundária à intermação, toxicidades e mordidas de cobra pode ter prognóstico variável.

DIVERSOS

DISTÚRBIOS ASSOCIADOS
Anemia.

FATORES RELACIONADOS COM A IDADE
Neoplasia é mais comum em animais mais idosos.

POTENCIAL ZOONÓTICO
O potencial zoonótico do *Helicobacter* spp. é controverso.

GESTAÇÃO/FERTILIDADE/REPRODUÇÃO
Prostaglandinas sintéticas (p. ex., misoprostol) causam abortamento.

VER TAMBÉM
- Úlcera Gastroduodenal. • Melena.

ABREVIATURA(S)
- ACTH = hormônio adrenocorticotrópico.
- AINE = anti-inflamatórios não esteroides.

Sugestões de Leitura
Liptak JM, Hunt GB, Barrs VRD, et al. Gastroduodenal ulceration in cats: Eight cases and a review of the literature. J Feline Med Surg 2002, 4:27-42.
Simpson KW. Diseases of stomach. In: Ettinger SJ, Feldman EC, eds., Textbook of Veterinary Internal Medicine, 6th ed. St. Louis: Elsevier, 2005, pp. 1310-1331.

Autor Jocelyn Mott
Consultor Editorial Albert E. Jergens

HEMATOPOIESE CÍCLICA

CONSIDERAÇÕES GERAIS

REVISÃO
• A hematopoiese cíclica em filhotes da raça Collie de pelagem de coloração cinza diluída caracteriza-se por episódios frequentes de infecção com falha no desenvolvimento e morte precoce. Os sistemas acometidos são o hematopoiético e a pele, bem como os tratos respiratório e gastrintestinal. Do ponto de vista clínico, os filhotes podem parecer normais nas primeiras 4-6 semanas e, depois, desenvolver diarreia, conjuntivite, gengivite, pneumonia, infecções cutâneas, artralgia cárpica e febre. A intussuscepção do intestino delgado constitui uma causa frequente de óbito.
• Episódios mórbidos, que variam desde inatividade acompanhada por febre até infecções potencialmente letais, repetem-se em intervalos de 11-14 dias.
• Os filhotes de pelagem cinza costumam ser menores que seus companheiros de ninhada ao nascimento, mostram-se fracos e, frequentemente, são abandonados pela cadela.
• A afecção foi observada em muitas linhagens sanguíneas de Collie nos EUA e em outros países; entretanto, os criadores experientes dessa raça não tentam criar os filhotes acometidos e, muitas vezes, não têm conhecimento da presença do gene responsável em sua linhagem sanguínea. Em consequência disso, raramente se observam filhotes de Collie cinza.
• Também foram relatados casos de hematopoiese cíclica em dois gatos com infecção pelo FeLV.

IDENTIFICAÇÃO
• A hematopoiese cíclica em Collie está presente apenas em filhotes de pelagem diluída. A diluição da cor e o distúrbio da medula óssea correspondem a uma condição hereditária, que se perpetua como traço autossômico recessivo (presumivelmente o mesmo gene). O distúrbio da medula óssea e a diluição da cor estariam presentes em filhotes mestiços de Collie/Beagle e poderiam ocorrer em qualquer cão com raça definida com linhagens sanguíneas de Collie em ambos os progenitores se tais progenitores tivessem o gene recessivo.
• Os sinais clínicos ocorrem precocemente em até 1-2 semanas de vida e sempre são evidenciados em torno de 4-6 semanas de vida.
• No Reino Unido, já foi relatada uma doença aparentemente semelhante em filhotes de coloração normal em duas ninhadas da raça Border collie. Foram descritos casos isolados de hematopoiese cíclica em cães das raças Pomerânia e Cocker spaniel; nessas raças, a doença ainda não está bem caracterizada.
• A agregação plaquetária *in vitro* apresenta-se reduzida em Collies de pelagem cinza acometidos. As alterações relatadas nas populações de linfócitos incluem um número elevado de linfócitos T gama e uma quantidade reduzida de linfócitos T mu no timo, nos linfonodos e no sangue. Ambas as populações de células-T ciclaram com as alterações nos neutrófilos e monócitos no sangue.
• A hematopoiese cíclica observada nos dois gatos parece ser outra manifestação não neoplásica possível de infecção por FeLV.

SINAIS CLÍNICOS
Achados Anamnésicos
• Fraqueza. • Falha no desenvolvimento.
• Conjuntivite. • Gengivite. • Diarreia.
• Pneumonia. • Infecções cutâneas. • Artralgia cárpica.

Achados do Exame Físico
• Coloração diluída da pelagem com diluição na cor do epitélio nasal. • Filhotes menores e mais fracos, quando comparados aos companheiros de ninhada com coloração normal. • Febre. • Olhos lacrimejantes, gengivas avermelhadas, tonsilite e diarreia — quase sempre estão presentes durante a fase do ciclo hematopoiético quando os sinais clínicos ficam evidentes; outros sinais variam, dependendo do local de sepse. • Articulações cárpicas doloridas observadas durante a fase de recuperação inicial do ciclo patológico. • Sinais e sintomas de FeLV em gatos.

CAUSAS E FATORES DE RISCO
• Doença hereditária em cães puros ou mestiços da raça Collie.
• Infecção pelo vírus da FeLV em gatos.

DIAGNÓSTICO

DIAGNÓSTICO DIFERENCIAL
• A diluição na coloração da pelagem é patognomônica para a doença em Collie ou raças mestiças de Collie.
• Em filhotes de Collie, também se observa a diluição na coloração não associada à hematopoiese cíclica. Contudo, os filhotes são de porte normal, não desenvolvem episódios frequentes de infecção, podem atingir a intensidade normal na cor da pelagem por volta dos 6 meses de vida e apresentam intensidade normal na cor do nariz.
• Os filhotes de Collie com hematopoiese cíclica sempre exibem diluição na coloração do epitélio nasal.
• Gatos com sinais e sintomas compatíveis com infecção pelo FeLV.

HEMOGRAMA/BIOQUÍMICA/URINÁLISE
• Neutropenia grave, que dura 2-5 dias e ocorre em intervalos de 11-14 dias com anemia marginal normocítica a microcítica em cães; anemia normocítica ou macrocítica leve a moderada em gatos.
• É importante saber que os sinais clínicos de infecção são frequentemente mínimos durante os episódios neutropênicos.
• Sinais locais de tumefação e rubor, juntamente com sinais sistêmicos de infecção, costumam ocorrer durante os primeiros dias da fase neutrofílica do ciclo patológico; por essa razão, observa-se neutrofilia com monocitose moderada ao exame inicial do hemograma completo.
• O hemograma deve ser repetido em intervalos de 1-2 dias para confirmar o diagnóstico.

TRATAMENTO

• Aconselhar os proprietários a não tentar a criação do(s) filhote(s).
• A administração de antibióticos e a terapia de suporte podem prolongar a vida dos filhotes por alguns anos, mas sob considerável custo.
• O ciclo mórbido já foi interrompido no campo experimental por meio de transplante da medula óssea e do tratamento diário com endotoxina, carbonato de lítio (10 mg/kg VO a cada 12 h) ou fator recombinante humano ou estimulante de colônia canino.

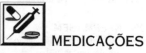

MEDICAÇÕES

MEDICAMENTO(S)
Antibióticos e fluidos, conforme a necessidade, contra infecções.

ACOMPANHAMENTO

MONITORIZAÇÃO DO PACIENTE
É aconselhável que os proprietários fiquem atentos aos sinais de infecção.

PREVENÇÃO
Os cães não devem ficar alojados em pensões.

COMPLICAÇÕES POSSÍVEIS
A infecção respiratória pode ser potencialmente letal se não for tratada.

EVOLUÇÃO ESPERADA E PROGNÓSTICO
São esperadas infecções intermitentes. O prognóstico é reservado.

DIVERSOS

GESTAÇÃO/FERTILIDADE/REPRODUÇÃO
Os cães portadores ou acometidos da raça Collie não devem ser acasalados.

VER TAMBÉM
Neutropenia.

ABREVIATURAS
• FeLV = vírus da leucemia felina.

Sugestões de Leitura
Dale DC, Rodger E, Cebon J, Ramiesh N, Hammond WP, Zsebo KM. Long-term treatment of canine cyclic hematopoiesis with recombinant canine stem cell factor. Blood 1995, 85:74-79.
DiGiacomo RF, Hammond WP, Kunz LL, Cox PA. Clinical and pathologic features of cyclic hematopoiesis in grey collie dogs. Am J Pathol 1983, 111:224-233.
Hammond WP, Boone TC, Donahue RE, et al. A comparison of treatment of canine cyclic hematopoiesis with recombinant human granulocyte-macrophage colony-stimulating factor (GM-CSF), G-CSF interleukin-3, and canine G-CSF. Blood 1990, 76:523-532.
Swenson CL, Kociba GJ, O'Keefe DA, Crisp MS, Jacobs RM, Rojko JL. Cyclic hematopoiesis associated with feline leukemia virus infection in two cats. JAVMA 1987, 191:93-96.
Yang TJ. Recovery of hair coat color in gray collie (cyclic neutropenia)—normal bone marrow transplant chimeras. Am J Pathol 1978, 91:149-154.

Autor Peter MacWilliams
Consultor Editorial A. H. Rebar
Agradecimento Dr. John E. Lund é o autor original deste capítulo. Seu conhecimento e experiência representam as maiores contribuições.

Hematúria

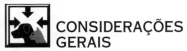

CONSIDERAÇÕES GERAIS

DEFINIÇÃO
Presença de sangue na urina.

FISIOPATOLOGIA
Secundária à perda da integridade do endotélio no trato urinário, deficiência de fator da coagulação ou trombocitopenia.

SISTEMAS ACOMETIDOS
• Renal/urológico. • Reprodutivo.

IDENTIFICAÇÃO
• Cães e gatos.
• Hematúria familiar em animais jovens, neoplasia em animais mais idosos.
• Fêmeas sob maior risco de infecção do trato urinário.

SINAIS CLÍNICOS
Achados Anamnésicos
Urina manchada de sangue com ou sem polaciúria.

Achados do Exame Físico
• Massa palpável em pacientes com neoplasia.
• Dor abdominal em alguns pacientes.
• Próstata aumentada de volume e/ou dolorida em machos.
• Petéquias ou equimoses em pacientes com coagulopatia.

CAUSAS
Sistêmicas
• Coagulopatia. • Trombocitopenia. • Vasculite.

Trato Urinário Superior
• Anatômicas — por exemplo, doença renal cística e má-formação familiar.
• Metabólicas — por exemplo, nefrolitíase.
• Neoplásicas — por exemplo, linfoma renal, adenocarcinoma e hemangiossarcoma.
• Infecciosas — por exemplo, leptospirose, PIF e bactérias.
• Inflamatórias — por exemplo, glomerulonefrite.
• Idiopáticas.
• Traumatismo.

Trato Urinário Inferior
• Anatômicas — por exemplo, más-formações da bexiga.
• Metabólicas — por exemplo, urólitos.
• Neoplásicas — por exemplo, carcinoma de células de transição e linfossarcoma.
• Infecciosas — por exemplo, doenças bacterianas, fúngicas e virais.
• Idiopáticas — gatos (cistite idiopática).
• Traumatismo.
• Cistite hemorrágica induzida por ciclofosfamida.

Genitália
• Metabólicas — por exemplo, estro.
• Neoplásicas — por exemplo, tumor venéreo transmissível, leiomioma e adenocarcinoma da próstata.
• Infecciosas — por exemplo, doenças bacterianas e fúngicas.
• Inflamatórias — por exemplo, hiperplasia prostática benigna.
• Traumatismo.

FATORES DE RISCO
Raça predisposta à urolitíase (p. ex., Dálmata e a urolitíase por urato), coagulopatia (p. ex., Doberman e a doença de von Willebrand) ou neoplasia (p. ex., Pastor alemão e o cistadenocarcinoma renal).

DIAGNÓSTICO

Ver Figura 1.

DIAGNÓSTICO DIFERENCIAL
Outras causas de alteração da cor da urina (p. ex., mioglobinúria, hemoglobinúria e bilirrubinúria).

ACHADOS LABORATORIAIS
Medicamentos Capazes de Alterar os Resultados Laboratoriais
• Doses substanciais de vitamina C (ácido ascórbico) podem causar resultados falso-negativos ao teste com tira reagente; gerações mais novas de tiras reagentes são mais resistentes à interferência ao reduzir substâncias como o ácido ascórbico.

Distúrbios Capazes de Alterar os Resultados Laboratoriais
• Testes urinários comuns com tira reagente para detectar hemácias, hemoglobina ou mioglobina.
• Densidade urinária baixa (síndromes poliúricas) lisa os eritrócitos.
• Bacteriúria (peroxidase bacteriana) provoca resultados falso-positivos com as tiras reagentes.
• Conservantes à base de formalina geram resultados falso-negativos com as tiras reagentes.

Os Resultados Serão Válidos se os Exames Forem Realizados em Laboratório Humano?
• Sim.

HEMOGRAMA/BIOQUÍMICA/URINÁLISE
• Trombocitopenia e anemia grave em alguns pacientes.
• Azotemia em alguns pacientes com doença renal bilateral.
• Eritrócitos (>5-10 células/campo óptico) e, possivelmente, agentes infecciosos podem ser observados no sedimento urinário.
• Cristalúria em alguns pacientes com urolitíase.

OUTROS TESTES LABORATORIAIS
• TCA ou perfil da coagulação para excluir coagulopatia.
• Cultura bacteriana da urina para identificar infecção do trato urinário.
• Exame de ejaculado para identificar doença da próstata.

DIAGNÓSTICO POR IMAGEM
Ultrassonografia, radiografia e, possivelmente, radiografia contrastada são frequentemente úteis para localizar a causa subjacente.

MÉTODOS DIAGNÓSTICOS
• Biopsia de lesão expansiva tipo massa.
• Vaginoscopia em fêmeas ou uretrocistoscopia em machos e fêmeas.

TRATAMENTO

• Hematúria pode indicar a presença de processo patológico grave.
• Urolitíase e insuficiência renal podem necessitar de modificação da dieta.
• Infecção do trato urinário pode ser causada por outra doença, local (p. ex., neoplasia e urolitíase) ou sistêmica (p. ex., hiperadrenocorticismo e diabetes melito), que também requer tratamento.

MEDICAÇÕES

MEDICAMENTO(S) DE ESCOLHA
• Talvez haja necessidade de transfusão de sangue se o paciente estiver gravemente anêmico.
• Cristaloides para tratar a desidratação.
• Antibióticos para tratar infecção do trato urinário e septicemia.
• Heparina para CID.

CONTRAINDICAÇÕES
Medicamentos imunossupressores, exceto para tratar doença imunomediada.

INTERAÇÕES POSSÍVEIS
Meios de contraste intravenosos podem causar insuficiência renal aguda.

ACOMPANHAMENTO

MONITORIZAÇÃO DO PACIENTE
Depende das doenças primárias ou associadas.

COMPLICAÇÕES POSSÍVEIS
• Anemia.
• Hipovolemia se a hemorragia for grave.
• Obstrução ureteral ou uretral causada por coágulos sanguíneos.

DIVERSOS

FATORES RELACIONADOS COM A IDADE
• Tende a ocorrer neoplasia em animais mais idosos. • Tendem a ocorrer doenças imunomediadas em animais jovens adultos.

POTENCIAL ZOONÓTICO
Leptospirose.

VER TAMBÉM
• Cilindrúria.
• Cristalúria.
• Deficiência dos Fatores de Coagulação.
• Disúria e Polaciúria.
• Doença Idiopática do Trato Urinário Inferior Felino.
• Glomerulonefrite.
• Hemoglobinúria e Mioglobinúria.
• Infecção do Trato Urinário Inferior.
• Nefrolitíase.
• Pielonefrite.
• Prostatite e Abscesso Prostático.
• Prostatomegalia.
• Proteinúria.
• Trombocitopenia.
• Urolitíase.

ABREVIATURA(S)
• CID = coagulação intravascular disseminada.
• PIF = peritonite infecciosa felina.
• TCA = tempo de coagulação ativada.

Sugestões de Leitura
Bartges JW. Discolored urine. In: Ettinger SJ, Feldman EC, eds., Textbook of Veterinary Internal Medicine, 6th ed. St. Louis: Elsevier, 2005, pp. 112–114.

Autor Joseph W. Bartges
Consultor Editorial Carl A. Osborne

HEMATÚRIA

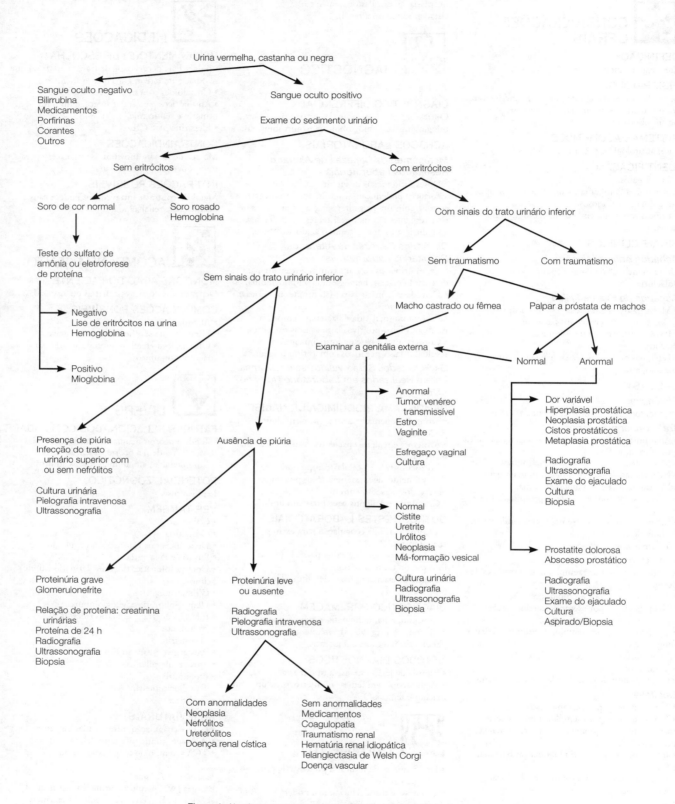

Figura 1. Algoritmo para o diagnóstico de urina vermelha, castanha ou negra.

HEMOGLOBINÚRIA E MIOGLOBINÚRIA

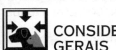

CONSIDERAÇÕES GERAIS

DEFINIÇÃO
Concentração semiquantitativa positiva de heme na urina (também relatada como sangue oculto), detectada por meio de exames laboratoriais de rotina (p. ex., fita reagente).

FISIOPATOLOGIA
• A hemoglobina liberada pelas hemácias durante hemólise intravascular (hemoglobinemia) fica ligada (alta afinidade) à haptoglobina, inibindo com isso a destruição tecidual oxidativa. Os complexos hemoglobina-haptoglobina são muito grandes para atravessar os capilares glomerulares normais, sendo removidos pelo sistema reticuloendotelial, principalmente no baço. A haptoglobina fica saturada quando a concentração de hemoglobina se encontra elevada; a hemoglobina livre (cadeias contendo 4 moléculas hemes, 64.000 daltons) rapidamente se dissocia em dímeros instáveis (32.000 daltons) pequenos o suficiente para atravessar os capilares glomerulares, resultando em hemoglobinúria (coloração vermelha na urina). A hemoglobina livre sofre endocitose de fase líquida (via receptores de megalina e tubulina expressos na membrana apical) nas células epiteliais tubulares renais. A globina sofre degradação, enquanto a molécula heme livre é catabolizada pela heme oxigenase, resultando em peroxidação lipídica e depósito de Fe. Além disso, um ambiente intratubular ácido favorece a precipitação da hemoglobina, a formação de cilindros e a obstrução dos túbulos. A metemoglobinemia provoca um processo patológico análogo.
• Em contraste, a mioglobina, cadeia contendo uma única molécula heme (aproximadamente 17.500 daltons), é liberada pelo músculo após diminuição do aporte energético ou ocorrência de lesão. A interação da molécula heme com a porção proteica (globina) faz com que a mioglobina transporte o oxigênio sem oxidação do ferro ferroso (Fe^{2+}) em ferro férrico (Fe^{3+}). A mioglobina é livre e rapidamente removida, atravessando a barreira glomerular (tamanho pequeno, sem proteína de transporte) e o plasma permanece incolor. Contudo, o acúmulo de mioglobina na urina provoca alteração da cor para castanho, enquanto um ambiente ácido favorece a precipitação da mioglobina, a formação de cilindros e a obstrução dos túbulos. Além disso, a mioglobina penetra nas células epiteliais tubulares renais proximais via receptores de megalina e tubulina, causando peroxidação lipídica sem a liberação de ferro livre (via ciclo de oxirredução do centro da molécula heme). Condições alcalinas evitam a peroxidação lipídica induzida pela mioglobina por (1) estabilizar o complexo ferril-mioglobina reativo e (2) reduzir a precipitação de mioglobina nos túbulos renais.

SISTEMA(S) ACOMETIDO(S)
Renal/urológico — a hemoglobina, a metemoglobina e a mioglobina são nefrotóxicas, especialmente na presença de perfusão renal diminuída e condições ácidas.

IDENTIFICAÇÃO
• Bedlington terrier — toxicose hereditária por cobre pode causar hemólise em virtude da liberação desse elemento químico do fígado para o sangue. Embora haja relatos de hepatopatia associada ao cobre em outras raças de cães, foi relatado que apenas o Bedlington terrier tenha um desfecho hemolítico.
• Springer spaniel inglês, Cocker spaniel americano, Cocker spaniel inglês, Cocker spaniel — deficiência hereditária de fosfofrutoquinase (PFK) pode provocar hemólise intravascular com hemoglobinúria e miopatia.
• Cães de corrida de trenó e galgos — miopatia por exercício pode resultar em mioglobinúria.
• Old English sheepdog — acidose láctica por exercício com hemoglobinúria.
• Isoeritrólise neonatal em gatos — (gata com tipo sanguíneo B e filhotes com os tipos A ou AB) nas raças Britânico de pelo curto, Cornish rex, Devon rex, Abissínio, Birmanês, Himalaio, Persa, Fold escocês e Somali; os neonatos morrem em até 2 dias.

SINAIS CLÍNICOS
Comentários Gerais
Uma diversidade de sinais clínicos pode estar associada a causas específicas; ver a seção "Causas".
Achados Anamnésicos
A raça do animal e os antecedentes de tratamento medicamentoso são particularmente importantes; ver a seção "Causas".
Achados do Exame Físico
• Sinais associados à anemia (mucosas pálidas, taquicardia, letargia, icterícia).
• Sinais associados a dano muscular (sensibilidade, contusão).

CAUSAS
Hemoglobinúria
• Dano oxidativo — medicamentos (paracetamol, benzocaína, vitamina K_3, novo azul de metileno, fenacetina, fenazopiridina, monensina sódica); alimentos (cebolas, alho); metais pesados (cobre, zinco).
• Agentes físicos — queimaduras, intermação/insolação, lesões por esmagamento, choque elétrico, administração IV de fluido hipotônico, microangiopatia (p. ex., coagulopatia intravascular disseminada, síndrome da veia cava por *D. immitis*).
• Toxinas (perda da integridade da membrana) — veneno de cobra (p. ex., coral) ou de aranha (p. ex., reclusa-castanha).
• Agentes infecciosos — babesiose (p. ex., *B. canis*), leptospirose (p. ex., *L. icterohemorrhagica*), citauxzoonose (p. ex., *C. felis*), micoplasmose (p. ex., *M. hemofelis*).
• Imunomediadas — anemia hemolítica imunomediada idiopática, transfusão de sangue incompatível, isoeritrólise (p. ex., em gata com tipo sanguíneo B e filhotes com os tipos A ou AB).
• Deficiências — hipofosfatemia (p. ex., após tratamento com insulina em pacientes com diabetes melito).
• Associada à genética — deficiência da PFK, toxicidade do cobre.
• Outras causas — hemorragia retroperitoneal.

Mioglobinúria
• Miosite — infecciosa (p. ex., toxoplasmose, neosporose), eosinofílica (Pastor alemão, outras raças), imunomediada.
• Associada à genética — distrofia muscular ligada ao cromossomo X (p. ex., Golden retriever, Weimaraner, Rottweiler, Samoieda, Pastor de Groenendael, Schnauzer miniatura); glicogenoses (doenças de armazenamento) — Tipo II (Spitz), Tipo III (Pastor alemão), Tipo VII (colônia de Springer spaniel, um único Cocker spaniel americano); anormalidades mitocondriais (Clumber spaniel, Sussex spaniel, possivelmente Old English sheepdog).
• Toxinas (perda da integridade da membrana) — veneno de cobra (p. ex., coral) ou de aranha (p. ex., reclusa-castanha).
• Físicas — isquemia, lesão por esmagamento, síndrome de compartimentalização.
• Temperatura corporal excessiva (p. ex., intermação/insolação, crises convulsivas prolongadas).
• Exercício extremo.

FATORES DE RISCO
• Predisposição genética (ver a seção "Identificação").
• Exposição a toxinas ou medicamentos específicos.
• Certos agentes infecciosos.
• Esforço físico extremo.
• Intermação/insolação.
• Veneno de cobra ou de aranha.

DIAGNÓSTICO

DIAGNÓSTICO DIFERENCIAL
• Pesquisa de sangue oculto (molécula heme) com fita reagente na urina detecta hemácias, hemoglobina (ou metemoglobina) e mioglobina; os itens a seguir ajudam na diferenciação:
• Plasma/soro límpido (claro) com hemácias ou hemácias fantasmas no sedimento urinário sugere hematúria.
  ○ Plasma/soro hemolisado (não relacionado com a coleta) sugere hemoglobinúria.
  ○ Sangue total cor de chocolate sugere metemoglobinúria.
  ○ Plasma/soro límpido (claro) com concentração elevada de CK e indícios clínicos de dano muscular sugere mioglobinúria.
  ○ Resultados falso-positivos (ver a seção "Achados Laboratoriais").

ACHADOS LABORATORIAIS
Medicamentos Capazes de Alterar os Resultados Laboratoriais
• Administração de vitamina C (ácido ascórbico) pode causar resultados falso-negativos nos testes com fitas reagentes.
• Administração de transportadores de oxigênio (Oxyglobin) à base de hemoglobina gera resultados positivos nos testes com fitas reagentes.

Distúrbios Capazes de Alterar os Resultados Laboratoriais
• Hipostenúria (densidade urinária baixa) pode causar hemólise *in vitro* (sem hemácias intactas no sedimento) com uma reação positiva.
• Bacteriúria pode gerar resultados falso-positivos nos testes (peroxidase bacteriana).
• Reagentes oxidantes (p. ex., de desinfetantes) podem provocar resultados falso-positivos.
• Hemoglobina livre de sangue ou produtos sanguíneos transfundidos pode induzir a uma reação positiva.
• A formalina ocasiona resultados falso-negativos.

Os Resultados Serão Válidos se os Exames Forem Realizados em Laboratório Humano?
• Sim.

Hemoglobinúria e Mioglobinúria

HEMOGRAMA/BIOQUÍMICA/URINÁLISE
- Proteinúria.
- Hemólise intravascular — hematócrito decrescente (pode ser acompanhado por leucocitose), anormalidades no esfregaço sanguíneo (hemoparasitas, corpúsculos de Heinz, hemácias fantasmas [mediadas pelo complemento]), bilirrubinemia, atividade elevada da ALT, bilirrubinúria.
- Rabdomiólise — atividades aumentadas da CK e AST.

OUTROS TESTES LABORATORIAIS
- Teste de precipitação com sulfato de amônio — misturar 5 mL de urina com 2,8 g de sulfato de amônio e centrifugar; a hemoglobina sofre precipitação, mas a mioglobina permanece na solução. Precipitado escuro é sugestivo de hemoglobinúria, enquanto sobrenadante escuro é indicativo de mioglobinúria; se ambos forem escuros, haverá hemoglobina e mioglobina.
- Esfregaço sanguíneo corado pelo novo azul de metileno para detectar corpúsculos de Heinz.
- Detecção de metemoglobina confirma a presença de toxina como oxidante.
- A concentração de haptoglobina está diminuída em caso de hemólise intravascular.
- Concentração sérica elevada de cobre ou zinco.
- Teste de DNA para deficiência de PFK.

DIAGNÓSTICO POR IMAGEM
Radiografia ou ultrassonografia abdominal — pode revelar moedas, dispositivos de hardware ou outros objetos metálicos no trato gastrintestinal; tamanho anormal do fígado em pacientes com hepatopatia associada ao cobre.

MÉTODOS DIAGNÓSTICOS
- Biopsia do fígado para mensurar a concentração de cobre.
- Exercício forçado (p. ex., Old English sheepdog).

TRATAMENTO
- Quantidades abundantes de fluido para manter a função renal (50% de sódio sob a forma de bicarbonato de sódio na presença de acidose para evitar precipitação e peroxidação).
- Evitar estresse em pacientes anêmicos.
- Evitar hiperventilação se o paciente tiver deficiência de PFK.
- Hematúria induzida por exercício tem uma evolução benigna autolimitante.
- Ver causas suspeitas para instituir o tratamento específico.

MEDICAÇÕES

MEDICAMENTO(S) DE ESCOLHA
Variam de acordo com a causa subjacente.

CONTRAINDICAÇÕES
Ver a lista de causas dos medicamentos contraindicados.

PRECAUÇÕES
N/D.

INTERAÇÕES POSSÍVEIS
N/D.

MEDICAMENTO(S) ALTERNATIVO(S)
N/D.

ACOMPANHAMENTO

MONITORIZAÇÃO DO PACIENTE
Hematócrito, PO_2, urinálise, creatinina sérica, ALT (hepatopatia associada ao cobre), CK (associada à miopatia).

COMPLICAÇÕES POSSÍVEIS
Pode ocorrer o desenvolvimento de dano renal (insuficiência).

DIVERSOS

DISTÚRBIOS ASSOCIADOS
N/D.

FATORES RELACIONADOS COM A IDADE
Isoeritrólise neonatal.

POTENCIAL ZOONÓTICO
- Leptospirose.
- Toxoplasmose.

GESTAÇÃO/FERTILIDADE/REPRODUÇÃO
N/D.

SINÔNIMO(S)
Pigmentúria.

VER TAMBÉM
Ver a seção "Causas".

ABREVIATURA(S)
- ALT = alanina aminotransferase.
- AST = aspartato aminotransferase.
- CK = creatina quinase.
- PFK = fosfofrutoquinase.

Sugestões de Leitura
Giger U. Regenerative anemias caused by blood loss or hemolysis. In: Ettinger SJ, Feldman EC, eds., Textbook of Veterinary Internal Medicine, 6th ed. St. Louis: Elsevier, 2005, pp. 1886-1907.
Harvey JW. Pathogenesis, laboratory diagnosis, and clinical implications of erythrocyte enzyme deficiencies in dogs, cats, and horses. Vet Clin Pathol 2006, 35:144-156.
Osborne CA, Stevens JB. Biochemical analysis of urine: Indications, methods, interpretation. In: Urinalysis: A Compassionate Guide to Patient Care. Shawnee, KS: Bayer, 1999, pp. 86-124.
Shelton DG. Rhabdomyolysis, myoglobinuria, and necrotizing myopathies. Vet Clin Small Anim 2004, 34:1469-1482.
Singh D, Chander V, Chopra K. Rhabdomyolysis. Methods Find Exp Clin Pharmacol 2005, 27:39-48.

Autores Cheryl L. Swenson e Carl A. Osborne
Consultor Editorial Carl A. Osborne
Agradecimento Frederic Jacob e Leslie Sharkey.

HEMORRAGIA DA RETINA

CONSIDERAÇÕES GERAIS

DEFINIÇÃO
- Áreas focais ou generalizadas de sangramento em parte ou em todas as camadas da retina.
- Pode ser aguda ou crônica.

FISIOPATOLOGIA
- Depende da causa. • Pode ser o resultado de diversas causas. • Descolamentos da retina induzidos por traumatismo — podem lacerar vasos sanguíneos da retina. • Frequentemente envolvida em más-formações congênitas, anormalidades vasculares concomitantes e síndromes de neovascularização. • Pode-se notar retinopatia em conjunto com diabetes melito — envolve a formação de microaneurismas vasculares com hemorragia ou exsudação concomitante.
- Intoxicações, coagulação sistêmica, distúrbios neoplásicos, doença fúngica sistêmica — podem provocar hemorragia focal ou mais disseminada.
- Hipertensão sistêmica e doenças imunomediadas (p. ex., aquelas indutoras de anemia) — podem provocar hemorragia local em conjunto com anormalidades vasculares e/ou descolamentos completos ou parciais da retina.

SISTEMA(S) ACOMETIDO(S)
Oftalmológico.

GENÉTICA
- Anomalia do olho do Collie — traço autossômico recessivo.
- Displasia da retina — há suspeitas de que seja transmitida por herança autossômica recessiva.
- Descolamento da retina — depende do fator causal; tipo hereditário quando observado em conjunto com a anomalia do olho do Collie ou com a displasia da retina.

INCIDÊNCIA/PREVALÊNCIA
- Baixa incidência na anomalia do olho do Collie.
- Relativamente comum em retinopatia hipertensiva de gatos idosos.

IDENTIFICAÇÃO
Espécies
Cães e gatos: qualquer raça, idade ou sexo.

Raça(s) Predominante(s)
- A causa pode ter base genética e ser altamente específica para a raça e para a idade — cães jovens da raça Collie com anomalia do olho do Collie; cães da raça Labrador retriever com displasia vitreorretiniana congênita.
- Defeitos hereditários congênitos específicos para a raça capazes de provocar descolamento ou displasia grave da retina — cães das raças Collie e Sheltie com anomalia do olho do Collie; cães da raça Pastor australiano com disgenesia ocular merle; cães das raças Labrador, Sealyham, Bedlington terrier e Springer spaniel com displasia da retina; e cães da raça Schnauzer miniatura com displasia da retina e vítreo primário hiperplásico persistente.

Idade Média e Faixa Etária
- Gatos idosos de ambos os sexos — frequentemente acometidos por hipertensão sistêmica.
- Anomalia do olho do Collie e displasia da retina — são defeitos congênitos que podem ser observados em cães com 5 a 7 semanas de vida.

Sexo Predominante
Não há predileção sexual.

SINAIS CLÍNICOS
Comentários Gerais
Os sinais dependem das causas subjacentes, como doença inflamatória no segmento posterior, doença sistêmica ou más-formações oculares.

Achados Anamnésicos
- Frequentemente nenhum. • Perda da visão.
- Colisão contra objetos.

Achados do Exame Físico
- Dependem da causa subjacente. • Aspecto vermelho-claro ou escuro do segmento posterior.
- Câmara anterior preenchida de sangue (hifema).
- Indícios de sangramento em outros locais — petéquias, equimoses, melena, hematúria.
- Leucocoria (pupila de aspecto esbranquiçado) com ou sem coloração avermelhada atrás do cristalino. • Ausência de resposta à ameaça.
- Respostas pupilares anormais.

CAUSAS
Congênitas
- Descolamento da retina secundário a más-formações congênitas graves no olho. • Defeitos vitreorretinianos; p. ex., em TVCHP/VPHP.
- Defeitos retinianos em displasia geográfica ou completa da retina ou em descolamento parcial ou completo dessa estrutura ocular.

Adquiridas
Traumatismo
- Hipertensão sistêmica (especialmente gatos idosos) — nefropatia; cardiopatia; hipertireoidismo; hiperadrenocorticismo; idiopática.
- Intoxicação — dicumarol; paracetamol; sulfonamida; estradurina.
- Riquétsia — *Rickettsia rickettsia*, *Ehrlichia* spp. associadas.
- Micose sistêmica — criptococose.
- Neoplasia — linfossarcoma.
- Mieloma de plasmócitos.
- Distúrbios hematológicos — distúrbio da coagulação sanguínea (doença de von Willebrand); anemia grave; trombocitopenia; gamopatia monoclonal e síndrome de hiperviscosidade.
- Retinopatia diabética.
- Descolamento da retina.
- Vasculite imunomediada.

FATORES DE RISCO
- Hipertensão sistêmica ou distúrbios de coagulação.
- Hematológicos como anemia e policitemia.
- Membranas vasculares.

DIAGNÓSTICO

DIAGNÓSTICO DIFERENCIAL
- Padrão normal dos vasos da coroide em um fundo subalbinótico. Olhos pouco pigmentados. O sangue fica contido nos canais vasculares e não fora do lúmen do vaso.
- Hemorragia vítrea — coloração avermelhada da pupila, sendo impossível descartar hemorragia concomitante da retina.
- As causas de hemorragia vítrea incluem persistência anormal de sistema vascular hialoide (TVCHP/VPHP hereditários e certas outras formas de múltiplas anomalias oculares de desenvolvimento) observada em cães jovens; neoplasia — especialmente linfossarcoma ou tumores do corpo ciliar; uveíte; glaucoma; luxação do cristalino; e alterações inflamatórias graves no vítreo associadas a traumatismo rombo ou penetrante, corpos estranhos e disseminadas a partir de doenças locais ou sistêmicas (p.ex., riquetsiose ou micose sistêmica).
- Turvamento generalizado ou local ou ausência de detalhes do fundo ocular — em geral, não se observa qualquer coloração avermelhada, sem hemorragia vítrea ou retiniana.

HEMOGRAMA/BIOQUÍMICA/URINÁLISE
- Geralmente normais a menos que secundários a alguma doença sistêmica.
- Hiperglicemia e/ou glicosúria — anormalidades possivelmente observadas em casos de retinopatia diabética.
- Níveis séricos aumentados de ureia ou creatinina e proteinúria — comuns em gatos com descolamento e hemorragia da retina secundários à hipertensão sistêmica.
- Trombocitopenia ou outras alterações compatíveis com distúrbios hematológicos sistêmicos.

OUTROS TESTES LABORATORIAIS
Avaliação diagnóstica completa e minuciosa — suspeita de doença sistêmica; inclui testes endócrinos da tireoide e adrenal, testes sorológicos para agentes infecciosos e estudos imunológicos.

DIAGNÓSTICO POR IMAGEM
- Oftalmoscopia com laser de varredura com angiografia por fluoresceína e verde de indocianina (ver adiante) é uma técnica vantajosa para diferenciar hemorragia superficial ou profunda da retina.
- Ultrassonografia para avaliar a posição do cristalino e o estado da retina em casos com segmento posterior preenchido de sangue.
- Se a presença de neoplasia for possível, considerar a obtenção de radiografias torácicas.
- Ultrassonografia abdominal poderá ser considerada na suspeita de doença sistêmica.

MÉTODOS DIAGNÓSTICOS
- Exame oftalmológico com foco de luz — permite, em geral, o diagnóstico de descolamento completo da retina com hemorragia parcial dessa estrutura ocular; com frequência, pode-se visualizar a neurorretina descolada através da pupila como um véu esbranquiçado de tecido.
- Oftalmoscopia indireta — diagnóstico de alterações fundoscópicas e vítreas; pode-se avaliar a profundidade da hemorragia por seu formato e coloração; pré-retiniana (entre a membrana limitante interna e o corpo vítreo): frequentemente tem a forma de quilha de barco e cor vermelho-clara; intrarretiniana: mais arredondada e mais escura.
- Paracentese vítrea e exame citológico — ajuda no diagnóstico em casos de suspeita de neoplasia ou doença micótica.
- Mensuração da pressão arterial — indicada em todos os pacientes com hemorragia retiniana e vítrea grave.
- Angiografia — para o diagnóstico de anomalias vasculares, descolamento da retina e outros distúrbios do segmento posterior. A fluoresceína é utilizada por via IV para obtenção de imagens detalhadas da vasculatura da retina, enquanto o verde de indocianina acrescenta informações sobre os vasos da coroide.

ACHADOS PATOLÓGICOS
- Dependem da causa.

HEMORRAGIA DA RETINA

- Os achados incluem hemorragia pré-retiniana, intrarretiniana ou sub-retiniana que pode ser focal ou envolver grandes áreas.
- Alterações morfológicas secundárias incluem áreas fibróticas com proliferação de extensões celulares para o espaço sub-retiniano, intrarretiniano e espessamento da membrana limitante externa.

TRATAMENTO

CUIDADO(S) DE SAÚDE ADEQUADO(S)
- Inicialmente, os animais costumam ser internados — às vezes, nos setores de cuidados intensivos para o máximo acompanhamento.
- Intoxicações — quase sempre necessitam de tratamento específico.
- Considerar o encaminhamento para exame oftalmológico mais detalhado, incluindo o ultrassom, antes de tentar a terapia empírica.

CUIDADO(S) DE ENFERMAGEM
- Depende(m) da causa.
- Com frequência, há necessidade de cuidados de suporte com técnicos veterinários bem-habilitados para monitorar a evolução do quadro várias vezes ao dia.

ATIVIDADE
Descolamento da retina — repouso em gaiola até que a retina se fixe novamente em casos traumáticos.

DIETA
Depende da causa subjacente; poderá haver restrições na dieta se o distúrbio primário for atribuído à hepato ou nefropatia.

ORIENTAÇÃO AO PROPRIETÁRIO
- Discutir o convívio com animais cegos ou a eutanásia de filhotes caninos com hemorragia bilateral grave atribuída a anormalidades congênitas (das raças listadas na seção "Identificação").
- Avisar o proprietário que os cães unilateralmente acometidos podem servir como animais de estimação, mas não devem ser utilizados no acasalamento, fato nem sempre óbvio para o proprietário.

CONSIDERAÇÕES CIRÚRGICAS
Cirurgia — encaminhar o paciente a algum oftalmologista para a realização de vitrectomia e/ou cirurgia de fixação da retina.

MEDICAÇÕES

MEDICAMENTO(S) DE ESCOLHA
- Dependem da causa subjacente.
- Corticosteroides sistêmicos — caso se desista da avaliação diagnóstica minuciosa e seja improvável a presença de doença infecciosa; prednisolona (1-2 mg/kg/dia por 7-14 dias e, em seguida, diminuir de forma gradativa; tratamento a longo prazo por até 4-6 semanas); especialmente no descolamento da retina como sequela de traumatismo em cães e gatos.
- Cloranfenicol ou outro antibiótico sistêmico de amplo espectro — na suspeita de doença infecciosa bacteriana; pode ser administrado concomitantemente com os corticosteroides.
- Hipertensão sistêmica primária — tratar conforme a necessidade; frequentemente se emprega tratamento combinado com corticosteroides (conforme descrição prévia), diuréticos (p. ex., furosemida, 3-4 mg/kg/dia por 5-7 dias) e bloqueadores dos canais de cálcio.
- Azatioprina oral — 1-2 mg/kg/dia por até uma semana e, em seguida, reduzir de forma gradual; para os descolamentos da retina imunomediados; combinar com corticosteroides sistêmicos; fazer hemograma completo, contagem plaquetária e análise das enzimas hepáticas a cada 2 semanas nos primeiros dois meses e, depois, periodicamente.
- Itraconazol — para criptococose ou outra infecção fúngica profunda; ver "Criptococose" ou a micose sistêmica apropriada.

CONTRAINDICAÇÕES
- Corticosteroides sistêmicos e outros medicamentos imunossupressores — não utilizar em processos infecciosos manifestos no segmento posterior do olho.
- AINE sistêmicos — contraindicados em distúrbios hemorrágicos, função renal prejudicada ou hipersensibilidades preexistentes; predispõem o paciente (especialmente gatos) à ulceração gastrintestinal.

PRECAUÇÕES
AINE — flunixino meglumina e ácido acetilsalicílico são comumente utilizados, mas podem exacerbar o sangramento; qualquer um desses agentes pode ser usado para controlar a inflamação intraocular nos cães. Utilizar com cautela nos gatos.

MEDICAMENTO(S) ALTERNATIVO(S)
- Flunixino meglumina — 0,5 mg/kg IV; dose única; pode ser utilizado em cães se o olho estiver inflamado e se as causas infecciosas não foram descartadas.
- Azatioprina oral — pode ser usada em doença imunomediada do fundo ocular; ver a seção "Medicamento(s) de Escolha".

ACOMPANHAMENTO

MONITORIZAÇÃO DO PACIENTE
- Monitoramento repetido — necessário para garantir o desaparecimento da condição e a normalização da morfologia da retina.
- Hemorragias pré-retinianas — absorvidas, em geral, dentro de algumas semanas a vários meses caso sejam localizadas.
- Hemorragias maiores ou repetidas — podem ser acompanhadas por processos fibroblásticos; podem levar à formação de membranas pré-retinianas fibrosas e aderências vitreorretinianas, as quais podem provocar tração vitreorretiniana e descolamento da retina.
- Hemorragia intrarretiniana — reabsorvida dentro de algumas semanas a meses; pode produzir cicatrização da retina.

COMPLICAÇÕES POSSÍVEIS
- Descolamento da retina. • Cegueira. • Visão prejudicada. • Uveíte crônica. • Glaucoma.

EVOLUÇÃO ESPERADA E PROGNÓSTICO
- Dependem da causa subjacente.
- Além de pequenas, praticamente todas as lesões hemorrágicas da retina são observadas durante o exame oftalmoscópico de rotina, costumam cicatrizar rápido e não geram problemas de visão.
- Hemorragias da retina atribuídas a doenças sistêmicas ou más-formações retinianas geralmente são mais graves, mas a maioria delas tem prognóstico incerto.

DIVERSOS

DISTÚRBIOS ASSOCIADOS
- Traumatismo — com frequência, podem-se notar lesões concomitantes em outras partes do olho ou do corpo.
- Hipertensão — cardíaca, nefropatia, hipertireoidismo ou hiperadrenocorticismo — comuns; podem provocar problemas clínicos sistêmicos, que precisam ser monitorizados.
- Intoxicação — com frequência, trata-se de um distúrbio hemorrágico generalizado que envolve outros órgãos.
- Infecção por *Cryptococcus* — quase sempre provoca leptomeningite e pneumonite concomitantes.
- Linfoma — pode acometer diversas partes do organismo; doença fatal.
- Distúrbios hematológicos — provocam doença sistêmica; os sintomas dependem da fisiopatologia; são comuns as alterações de anemia e sangramento recidivante.
- Cataratas secundárias — podem se desenvolver dentro de semanas após o início de diabetes melito nos cães.

FATORES RELACIONADOS COM A IDADE
- Pode ocorrer em qualquer idade.
- Frequentemente se deve a doenças congênitas (em geral, possuem base hereditária) ou a processos mórbidos de desenvolvimento (ver a seção "Causas").

GESTAÇÃO/FERTILIDADE/REPRODUÇÃO
- Os cães acometidos por doença hereditária da retina indutora de hemorragia nessa estrutura ocular não devem ser utilizados no programa reprodutivo.
- Corticosteroides e medicamentos imunossupressores podem provocar complicações no que diz respeito à prenhez.

VER TAMBÉM
- Coriorretinite. • Descolamento da Retina.
- Hifema. • Hipertensão Sistêmica.

ABREVIATURA(S)
- AINE = anti-inflamatórios não esteroides.
- TVCHP = túnica vascular do cristalino hiperplásica persistente.
- VPHP = vítreo primário hiperplásico persistente.

Sugestões de Leitura

Bjerkas E, Ekesten B, Narfström K, Grahn B. Visual impairment. In: Peiffer RL, Petersen-Jones SM, eds., Small Animal Ophthalmology: A Problem-Oriented Approach, 4th ed. London: Saunders, 2008, pp. 116-202.

Narfström K, Petersen-Jones S. Diseases of the canine ocular fundus. In: Gelatt KN, ed., Veterinary Ophthalmology, 4th ed. Ames, IA: Blackwell, 2007.

Petersen-Jones SM, Crispin SM. Manual of Small Animal Ophthalmology. Gloucestershire, UK: BSAVA, 1993.

Autor Kristina Narfström
Consultor Editorial Paul E. Miller

HEMOTÓRAX

CONSIDERAÇÕES GERAIS

REVISÃO
- Acúmulo de sangue no espaço pleural.
- Pode-se desenvolver de forma aguda (por traumatismo ou coagulopatia) ou crônica com o passar do tempo.
- Os sistemas cardiovascular e respiratório são comumente acometidos.

IDENTIFICAÇÃO
Qualquer idade, raça ou sexo de cães e gatos.

SINAIS CLÍNICOS
- Início superagudo a agudo — em geral, ocorrem sinais de hipovolemia antes que um volume suficiente de sangue se acumule no espaço pleural a ponto de prejudicar a respiração. • Angústia respiratória, taquipneia. • Mucosas pálidas.
- Fraqueza e colapso. • Pulso rápido e fraco.
- Macicez torácica ventral; hiper-ressonância dorsal se houver pneumotórax concomitante em associação com alguma causa traumática.

CAUSAS E FATORES DE RISCO
- Traumatismo — sangramento proveniente de qualquer artéria ou veia da parede torácica, do mediastino ou da coluna torácica; lesão ao coração, aos pulmões, ao timo e ao diafragma; víscera abdominal herniada (fígado ou baço).
- Neoplasia — em qualquer estrutura adjacente à cavidade pleural.
- Coagulopatias — podem ser congênitas ou adquiridas; é comum a ingestão de rodenticida; insuficiência hepática; colangio-hepatite com doença concomitante do intestino delgado.
- Torção de lobo pulmonar.
- Hemorragia tímica aguda em animais jovens.
- *Dirofilaria immitis*, *Spirocerca lupi*, *Angiostrongylus vasorum*.

DIAGNÓSTICO

DIAGNÓSTICO DIFERENCIAL
- Contusão pulmonar. • Pneumotórax. • Hérnia diafragmática. • Tórax frouxo. • Efusões pleurais não hemorrágicas — quilotórax; piotórax; transudatos modificados; transudatos.
- Insuficiência cardíaca congestiva.

HEMOGRAMA/BIOQUÍMICA/URINÁLISE
- Hematócrito e hemoglobina — refletem perda sanguínea após a ocorrência de desvios iniciais do compartimento líquido.
- A contagem plaquetária pode estar baixa (~ 100.000) com perda sanguínea aguda.
- A contagem plaquetária muito baixa (<20.000) é compatível com sangramento espontâneo.
- Avaliação de esfregaço periférico — menos de 3-5 plaquetas/campo óptico indica trombocitopenia.
- O perfil bioquímico pode revelar níveis baixos de glicose, ureia, albumina e colesterol em casos com insuficiência hepática.

OUTROS TESTES LABORATORIAIS

Análise do Líquido
- Efusão causada por hemorragia — hematócrito e nível de proteína semelhantes aos do sangue periférico; é comum observar plaquetas ao exame citológico.
- Efusão causada por inflamação ou congestão vascular — hematócrito <8%.
- Exame citológico — em geral, não identifica causas malignas.

Provas da Coagulação
- TCA ou TP/TTP prolongados — sugestivos de coagulopatia.
- PIVKA (uma forma modificada de TTPA) — aumentadas em caso de envenenamento por rodenticida.
- TP/TTPA prolongados e contagem plaquetária baixa — indicativos de CID.
- D-dímeros positivos auxiliam na detecção de CID.
- Análise de fatores específicos — pode diagnosticar defeito congênito ou coagulopatia adquirida.
- Tempo de sangramento da mucosa bucal — identifica a presença de defeito na função plaquetária.

DIAGNÓSTICO POR IMAGEM
- Radiologia — revela efusão pleural que varia desde um aumento difuso na radiopacidade até a formação de folhetos ventrais, fissuras interlobares e densidades pleurais localizadas.
- É possível observar lesões associadas (p. ex., fraturas de costelas, pneumotórax, contusões pulmonares, lesões diafragmáticas e massas).
- Padrão gasoso vesicular — sugestivo de torção do lobo pulmonar.
- Ultrassonografia — confirma a efusão pleural; pesquisar por massas, torção de lobo pulmonar e herniação do fígado, da vesícula biliar, do baço ou do intestino.
- Em pacientes estáveis sem coagulopatia — a avaliação do espaço pleural pode permitir uma melhor visualização radiográfica de massas ou de outra doença.

MÉTODOS DIAGNÓSTICOS
- Toracocentese.
- Exploração cirúrgica — pode ser necessária para estabelecer o diagnóstico; se a imagem não sugerir o lado apropriado para acessar, recomenda-se o lado esquerdo. A tomografia computadorizada pré-operatória pode ser útil.

TRATAMENTO

- Agudo — uso criterioso de fluidos IV. Tentar atingir uma pressão arterial sistólica acima de 90 mmHg, mas não necessariamente acima de 110 mmHg, com o uso de hetamido; utilizar salina hipertônica para corrigir a hipovolemia.
- Pneumotórax coexistente — em geral, requer toracocentese com agulha ou toracostomia com sonda.
- Plasma, fatores de coagulação específicos e/ou transfusão sanguínea podem ser necessários para restabelecer os fatores de coagulação ou fornecer hemácias para transporte de oxigênio.
- Contusão pulmonar — pode necessitar de suporte ventilatório.
- Hemorragia torácica grave ou recidivante — pode exigir a exploração cirúrgica.
- Oxigenoterapia.
- Manutenção do calor corporal.
- A maioria dos casos de coagulopatia exibe dificuldade respiratória associada a sangramento do parênquima e não a hemorragia pleural e, portanto, raramente necessita de remoção do líquido pleural para solucionar a taquipneia.
- Autotransfusão.

MEDICAÇÕES

MEDICAMENTO(S)
- Hipovolemia — ver "Choque Hemorrágico".
- Vitamina K_1 — 5 mg/kg SC como dose de ataque (utilizando uma agulha de pequeno calibre), seguida por 1,5-2,5 mg/kg VO a cada 12 h por 21-30 dias. Levam 12 h ou mais para carboxilação dos fatores de coagulação e restauração da atividade. • Analgésicos — sistêmicos ou sob a forma de bloqueios nervosos.
- Antibióticos de amplo espectro — quando indicados.

CONTRAINDICAÇÕES/INTERAÇÕES POSSÍVEIS
Evitar o ácido acetilsalicílico e outros AINE.

ACOMPANHAMENTO

MONITORIZAÇÃO DO PACIENTE
- Sinais clínicos, frequência e esforço respiratórios, frequência cardíaca. • Temperatura. • Produção de urina. • Alívio da dor. • Radiografias de acompanhamento em intervalos de 48 h até a estabilização do paciente. • Perfil de coagulação em 48 h se a coagulopatia for diagnosticada e 48 h depois da interrupção do suplemento de vitamina K.

COMPLICAÇÕES POSSÍVEIS
- Piotórax. • Sepse. • Encarceramento e constrição dos pulmões por tecido cicatricial e fibrose.

DIVERSOS

DISTÚRBIOS ASSOCIADOS
- Peritonite — com feridas penetrantes (p. ex., por arma de fogo) no abdome. • Perfuração esofágica.

VER TAMBÉM
- Coagulação Intravascular Disseminada.
- Contusões Pulmonares. • Efusão Pleural.
- Envenenamento por Rodenticidas Anticoagulantes. • Torção de Lobo Pulmonar.

ABREVIATURA(S)
- AINE = anti-inflamatório não esteroide.
- CID = coagulação intravascular disseminada.
- PIAVK = proteínas invocadas pela ausência ou antagonismo da vitamina K.
- TCA = tempo de coagulação ativada.
- TP = tempo de protrombina.
- TTP = tempo de tromboplastina parcial.
- TTPA = tempo de tromboplastina parcial ativada.

Sugestões de Leitura
Berry CR, Gallaway A, Thrall DE, Carlisle, C. Thoracic radiographic features of anticoagulant rodenticide toxicity in fourteen dogs. Vet Radiol Ultrasound 1993, 34:391–396.

Autor Bradley L. Moses
Consultor Editorial Lynelle R. Johnson

Hepatite Crônica Ativa

CONSIDERAÇÕES GERAIS

DEFINIÇÃO
Lesão hepática associada à lesão necroinflamatória não supurativa ativa. Quando crônica, ocorre o desenvolvimento de fibrose progressiva, que acaba culminando em cirrose.

FISIOPATOLOGIA
• Uma grande variedade de eventos desencadeantes provoca lesão hepática: tais eventos alteram a arquitetura do fígado, danificam as membranas ou organelas e ativam as citocinas e respostas imunes mediadas por células; os componentes hepáticos tornam-se focos de alvo; a lesão inicial pode envolver agentes infecciosos, toxinas ou agentes terapêuticos, mas a causa frequentemente permanece indeterminada.
• Células inflamatórias, predominantemente linfócitos, células de Kupffer e neutrófilos são células efetoras iniciais; citocinas, quimiocinas e radicais livres oxidativos são moléculas comuns.
• A zona inicial da lesão delimita a área de resposta necroinflamatória. A zona 1 (periportal) é comum em muitas formas de hepatite idiopática, enquanto a zona 3 incrimina lesão primária associada a cobre, certas toxinas e insultos isquêmicos ou hipóxicos repetidos.
• A inflamação crônica resulta em fibrose progressiva com formação de ponte entre as zonas envolvidas. A fibrose em ponte distorce a arquitetura lobular, levando a cirrose e insuficiência hepática com a cronicidade.
• Desenvolvimento progressivo de colestase.

SISTEMA(S) ACOMETIDO(S)
• Gastrintestinal — êmese; diarreia; anorexia; vasculopatia gastrentérica hipertensiva portal.
• Hematológico/linfático/imune — coagulopatia (estágio avançado da doença).
• Hepatobiliar.
• Nervoso — encefalopatia hepática (estágio avançado da doença).
• Urinário — poliúria e polidipsia; cristalúria por urato de amônio (estágio avançado da doença).

GENÉTICA
Hepatotoxicidade hereditária do cobre — ver "Hepatopatia por Armazenamento de Cobre".

INCIDÊNCIA/PREVALÊNCIA
N/D.

IDENTIFICAÇÃO

Espécies
Cães.

Raça(s) Predominante(s)
Bedlington terrier, Doberman pinscher, Cocker spaniel, Labrador retriever, talvez Skye terrier, Poodle standard, West Highland white terrier.

Idade Média e Faixa Etária
Média — 6-8 anos (variação de 2-10 anos).

Sexo Predominante
Cocker spaniel — os machos podem exibir maior risco.

SINAIS CLÍNICOS

Achados Anamnésicos
• Pode permanecer assintomático no início da doença.
• Letargia.
• Anorexia, perda de peso, vômito.
• Poliúria e polidipsia.
• Icterícia (estágio tardio da doença).
• Ascite (estágio tardio da doença, indicando início de hipertensão portal e desenvolvimento de desvio portossistêmico adquirido, fibrose, cirrose).

Achados do Exame Físico
• Pode permanecer assintomático no início da doença.
• Letargia, mau aspecto da pelagem e má condição corporal.
• Icterícia.
• Ascite.
• Encefalopatia hepática — estágio tardio da doença.

CAUSAS
• Infecciosas — vírus da hepatite canina; leptospirose; bacteremia ou endotoxemia portal entérica associada à enteropatia inflamatória; administração parenteral acidental de vacina intranasal contra *Bordettella*.
• Imunomediadas — autoimune com título de ANA positivo; sensibilização imune adquirida; inflamação não supurativa.
• Tóxicas — doença do armazenamento de cobre; exposição aguda ou crônica a medicamentos (p. ex., trimetoprima-sulfa, zonisamida, fenobarbital, fenitoína, CCNU, amiodarona, carprofeno) e exposição repetida a toxinas de origem ambiental ou alimentar (p. ex., dimetilnitrosamina, aflatoxina, cicadácea, cianobactéria).

FATORES DE RISCO
• Imunoestimulantes (vacinações?) e mimetismo molecular de epítopos celulares por agentes infecciosos ou infecção do endotélio sinusoidal.
• Medicamentos — indutores ou inibidores de enzimas microssomais ou condições que diminuem o estado antioxidante hepático podem aumentar o dano ao fígado por certas toxinas.

DIAGNÓSTICO

DIAGNÓSTICO DIFERENCIAL
• Hepatite aguda — histórico; biopsia hepática.
• Desvio portossistêmico congênito (anomalia vascular portossistêmica) — ultrassonografia abdominal; venografia contrastada por radiografia ou TC multissetorial; cintilografia colorretal; biopsia hepática.
• Neoplasia hepática — radiografia ou ultrassonografia; citologia; biopsia.
• Causas de efusão abdominal — hipoalbuminemia; insuficiência cardíaca direita; carcinomatose; peritonite biliar.
• Outras causas de hipertensão portal — ver "Hipertensão Portal".
• Icterícia — obstrução extra-hepática do ducto biliar; peritonite biliar; hemólise.

HEMOGRAMA/BIOQUÍMICA/URINÁLISE
• Hemograma completo — anemia arregenerativa; microcitose eritrocitária com desvio portossistêmico adquirido; leucograma e trombocitopenia variáveis; proteína total baixa em caso de doença crônica.
• Bioquímica — enzimas hepáticas elevadas; bilirrubina total, albumina, ureia, glicose e colesterol variáveis; insuficiência hepática sugerida por níveis baixos de albumina, ureia, glicose e colesterol, na ausência de outras explicações.
• Urinálise — concentração urinária variável; bilirrubinúria; cristalúria por biurato de amônio em caso de desvio portossistêmico adquirido.

OUTROS TESTES LABORATORIAIS
• Ácidos biliares séricos totais — valores normais em jejum, mas elevados após as refeições.
• Intolerância à amônia — reflete desvio portossistêmico adquirido; insensível a alterações colestáticas.
• Provas de coagulação — podem revelar TP, TTPA e PIAVK prolongados, fibrinogênio baixo e aumento de PDF ou D-dímeros; baixa atividade da proteína C sugere desvio portossistêmico adquirido ou insuficiência hepática.
• Efusão abdominal — hepatopatia crônica ou hipertensão portal: transudato puro ou modificado.
• Valores do zinco hepático — baixos com doença crônica e, particularmente, com desvio portossistêmico adquirido.
• Sorologia — p. ex., leptospirose, riquetsioses, borreliose, bartonelose, agentes fúngicos endêmicos.
• Título de ANA — níveis baixos com títulos positivos são inespecíficos.
• Coloração imuno-histoquímica de amostra hepática — para confirmar a atuação de agente infeccioso ou a origem das células infiltrativas.

DIAGNÓSTICO POR IMAGEM

Radiografia Abdominal
• Micro-hepatia — sugere doença em estágio terminal.
• Efusão abdominal — imagem obscura.
• Cálculos de urato de amônio — radiolucentes a menos que combinados com minerais radiodensos.

Ultrassonografia Abdominal
• O tamanho do fígado depende do estágio da doença; micro-hepatia no estágio tardio da doença.
• Ecogenicidade normal a variavelmente alterada do parênquima e do trato biliar; pode-se notar nodularidade, além de bordas hepáticas irregulares.
• Desvio portossistêmico adquirido — vasos tortuosos caudais ao rim esquerdo ou próximos à veia esplênica; fluxo de Doppler colorido.
• Efusão abdominal.
• Urólitos (muito pequenos ou grandes) podem ser observados na pelve renal ou na bexiga urinária, podendo indicar biuratos de amônio.
• Excluir obstrução extra-hepática do ducto biliar (icterícia, enzimas hepáticas elevadas); identificar lesões expansivas tipo massa e colelitíase; mucocele da vesícula biliar; colecistite; coledoquite; lesões císticas (abscesso). Possibilita a obtenção de aspirado por agulha fina — citologia e colecistocentese para coleta de bile.

Cintigrafia Colorretal
• Sensível e não invasiva — detecta desvio portossistêmico adquirido.

MÉTODOS DIAGNÓSTICOS

Citologia de Aspirado por Agulha Fina
• Aspiração hepática — não é capaz de diagnosticar hepatite crônica, fibrose hepática ou hepatopatia por armazenamento de cobre de forma definitiva com o exame citológico.

Biopsia Hepática
• Laparotomia para obtenção de amostras cuneiformes ou laparoscópicas para biopsia em cálice — preferidas às amostras obtidas com o uso da agulha Tru-Cut® (calibre 18), que pode obter

HEPATITE CRÔNICA ATIVA

tecido inadequado. Obter amostras de biopsia de vários lobos hepáticos.
• Cultura bacteriana — aeróbia e anaeróbia do fígado e da bile com antibiograma.
• Análise de metal — determina as concentrações de cobre, ferro e zinco (com base na matéria seca). Níveis baixos de zinco são comuns em distúrbios associados a desvio portossistêmico; níveis altos de ferro são usuais em distúrbios necroinflamatórios; níveis elevados de cobre podem representar uma causa primária de hepatite ou refletir secundariamente dano hepático.

ACHADOS PATOLÓGICOS
• Macroscópicos — iniciais: nenhuma alteração macroscópica; estágio tardio: micro-hepatia com bordas ou superfícies irregulares (nódulos finos ou grosseiros) ou desvio portossistêmico adquirido tortuoso.
• Microscópicos — inflamação não supurativa, envolvendo a zona de lesão; colestase e hiperplasia biliar variáveis; necrose por etapas e/ou em ponte; hepatite de interface; ruptura da placa limitante em lesões da zona 1; na doença em estágio tardio: ponte entre as zonas ou dentro delas; nódulos regenerativos e transição para cirrose.

TRATAMENTO

CUIDADO(S) DE SAÚDE ADEQUADO(S)
• Paciente internado — para a realização de exames diagnósticos e o início da terapia clínica em cães muito doentes.
• Ambulatoriais — se a condição estiver estabilizada para o diagnóstico; titular lentamente para a terapia clínica.

CUIDADO(S) DE ENFERMAGEM
• Depende(m) da condição subjacente.
• Fluidoterapia — fluidos poliônicos balanceados e suplementados para corrigir as anormalidades eletrolíticas ou a hipoglicemia; restringir o sódio na presença de ascite.
• Vitaminas hidrossolúveis (2 mL/L de fluidos).
• Ascite — tratada com dieta restrita em sódio, repouso forçado, diuréticos (furosemida combinada com espironolactona); ver "Cirrose e Fibrose do Fígado".
• Abdominocentese terapêutica — procedimento asséptico para remover grande volume de ascite sintomática, que comprometa a ingestão alimentar, a ventilação e o sono; a abdominocentese será realizada se os diuréticos e a restrição de sódio forem ineficazes.

ATIVIDADE
Manter o paciente aquecido, inativo e hidratado; a inatividade pode promover a regeneração hepática, a normoglicemia e a mobilização da ascite.

DIETA
• Níveis adequados de calorias e proteínas — evitar o catabolismo e manter a massa muscular (atenua a hiperamonemia); monitorizar a condição corporal.
• Proteína da dieta — restringir apenas se houver sinais de encefalopatia hepática (ver "Encefalopatia Hepática").
• Frequência das refeições — refeições em pequenas quantidades várias vezes ao dia otimizam a assimilação de nutrientes.

• Restrição de sódio — com ascite ou hipoalbuminemia grave: <100 mg/100 kcal ou <0,2% com base na matéria seca.
• Suplemento vitamínico de boa qualidade — ocorre comprometimento no metabolismo de vitaminas em casos de hepatopatia e perdas urinárias; evitar suplementos de cobre em casos de hepatopatia por armazenamento desse mineral.
• Tiamina — assegurar a reposição para evitar encefalopatia de Wernicke; 50-100 mg VO diários; **Cuidado:** podem ocorrer reações anafilactoides com a tiamina injetável.
• Nutrição parenteral parcial — recomendada para inapetência a curto prazo a fim de minimizar o catabolismo.
• Nutrição parenteral total — se a inapetência durar mais de 7 dias; o uso de soluções de aminoácidos de cadeia ramificada continua controverso em cães e gatos com disfunção hepática.

ORIENTAÇÃO AO PROPRIETÁRIO
• Espera-se mais o controle do que a cura; as medicações são necessárias pelo resto da vida; a doença é cíclica; por essa razão, há necessidade de avaliações trimestrais ou semestrais.
• As recomendações originam-se de experiências clínicas, estudos em seres humanos e modelos animais da doença em virtude da falta de estudos veterinários a longo prazo que comprovem a eficácia dos tratamentos.

CONSIDERAÇÕES CIRÚRGICAS
Desvio portossistêmico adquirido — não fazer ligadura nem bandagem na veia cava.

MEDICAÇÕES

MEDICAMENTO(S)

Diuréticos
• Para ascite — combinação de furosemida (0,5-2 mg/kg IV, SC, VO a cada 12 h) e espironolactona (0,5-2 mg/kg VO a cada 12 h; e espironolactona é a dose de ataque da espironolactona; usar o dobro da dose uma única vez); reavaliar e ajustar a dose para 25-50% em intervalos de 4-7 dias. Titular a dose de acordo com a resposta.

Para Encefalopatia Hepática
• Ver "Encefalopatia Hepática".

Antioxidantes
• Vitamina E — α-tocoferol, 10 UI/kg VO diariamente.
• S-adenosilmetionina — (utilizar o doador de metila, comprovadamente biodisponível, para a formação de glutationa reduzida) — 20 mg/kg de comprimido com revestimento entérico VO a cada 24 h com o estômago vazio para melhor absorção.
• Evitar a vitamina C em caso de alta concentração tecidual de cobre ou ferro — aumenta a lesão oxidativa associada a metais de transição.

Zinco (Acetato de Zinco)
• Antioxidante; antifibrótico; bloqueia a captação intestinal de cobre, necessário para as enzimas do ciclo da ureia.
• Zinco elementar, 1,5-3 mg/dia VO; ajustar a dose, utilizando as concentrações plasmáticas sequenciais de zinco (evitar valores plasmáticos >800 μg/dL).

Quelação do Cobre
• Ver "Hepatopatia por Armazenamento de Cobre".

Imunomodulação
• Prednisolona ou prednisona — 2-4 mg/kg/dia VO; com ascite: usar dexametasona para evitar o efeito mineralocorticoide (dividir a dose de prednisona por 8-10), administrar a cada 2-4 dias.
• Azatioprina — terapia adjuvante para inflamação imunomediada; 0,5-2 mg/kg VO a cada 24 h por 3-5 dias e, em seguida, em dias alternados; titular para uma redução de 25-50% da dose após 2-6 meses, com base em perfis bioquímicos sequenciais que demonstrem melhora (p. ex., declínio nos níveis da bilirrubina total e na atividade das enzimas hepáticas); monitorizar o hemograma completo e o perfil bioquímico a cada 7-10 dias no primeiro mês para assegurar a ausência de toxicidade hematopoiética, hepática e pancreática; em caso de toxicidade hematopoiética aguda, interromper a terapia, aguardar a recuperação do animal e, depois, retomar o tratamento com redução de 25% da dose; em caso de toxicidade hematopoiética crônica insidiosa (após meses) ou lesão hepática colestática ou pancreática aguda, interromper a terapia permanentemente.
• Micofenolato de mofetila — para pacientes intolerantes à azatioprina; 5-10 mg/kg VO a cada 24-48 h; monitorizar o animal quanto à ocorrência de toxicidade hematopoiética (rara).
• Ciclosporina microemulsificada — embora seja uma opção, a experiência com esse medicamento a longo prazo é limitada.
• Outros imunomoduladores estão relacionados a seguir.

Ácido Ursodesoxicólico
• Efeito imunomodulador, hepatoprotetor, antifibrótico, colerético, antiendotóxico, antioxidante.
• 7,5 mg/kg VO a cada 12 h; administrado com alimento para melhor assimilação; os comprimidos têm melhor biodisponibilidade; pode ser preparado sob a forma de solução aquosa; seguro; manter o tratamento por tempo indefinido.

Antifibróticos
• Polienilfosfatidilcolina poli-insaturada (fosfatidilcolina poli-insaturada) — 25-100 mg/kg VO diários com o alimento; tão potente quanto a colchicina em alguns modelos testados de hepatopatia; o efeito poupador de corticosteroide permite a titulação para baixo da prednisolona para controlar a doença; outros efeitos: imunomoduladores, antioxidantes e hepatoprotetores; a prescrição é rotineira.
• Colchicina — inibe a produção de colágeno, além de ter efeito anti-inflamatório; 0,03 mg/kg VO diários; os efeitos tóxicos incluem diarreia hemorrágica e mielossupressão; evitar a formulação unida com a probenecida sob a forma de complexos; selecionada como terapia quando a fibroplasia for o aspecto histológico mais importante; papel controverso; não combinar com a azatioprina.
• Silibinina com fosfatidilcolina poli-insaturada — efeitos hepatoprotetores (numerosas toxinas), antifibróticos e antioxidantes; promove a regeneração hepatocelular; 2-5 mg/kg VO diários (apenas a formulação unida à fosfatidilcolina poli-insaturada sob a forma de complexos); desempenha papel no controle de hepatite crônica não resolvida.

CONTRAINDICAÇÕES
Sempre que possível, evitar medicamentos que exijam metabolismo hepático.

Hepatite Crônica Ativa

PRECAUÇÕES
- Glicocorticoides — podem precipitar encefalopatia hepática, sangramento entérico, vômitos e/ou ascite.
- Dose excessiva de zinco — pode causar hemólise.

INTERAÇÕES POSSÍVEIS
- Evitar medicações que alteram a biotransformação hepática ou as vias de excreção (p. ex., cimetidina, quinidina e cetoconazol).
- A metoclopramida diminui a eficácia da espironolactona.

ACOMPANHAMENTO

MONITORIZAÇÃO DO PACIENTE
- Comportamento, condição corporal e peso — ajustar a ingestão proteica e calórica à tolerância ao nitrogênio e às necessidades aparentes de energia.
- Hemograma completo, bioquímica e urinálise — procurar por sinais de toxicidade medicamentosa, remissão da doença, capacidade de síntese, urolitíase por biurato de amônio e infecção do trato urinário.

PREVENÇÃO
Manter um alto nível de vigilância para detectar sinais precoces de hepatite em raças predispostas (p. ex., atividade elevada das enzimas hepáticas); apurar o diagnóstico e iniciar a terapia precocemente.

COMPLICAÇÕES POSSÍVEIS
- Sepse secundária à imunossupressão.
- Encefalopatia hepática.
- CID.
- Ulceração entérica.
- Insuficiência hepática e morte.

EVOLUÇÃO ESPERADA E PROGNÓSTICO
- Variam com a causa.
- Doença crônica, icterícia e ascite — apresenta prognóstico pior, embora possa sobreviver por anos com o fornecimento de cuidado conscencioso.
- Polifarmácia (administração concomitante de diversos medicamentos) e suporte nutricional prolongam a sobrevida de qualidade quando comparado com os casos não tratados.
- O diagnóstico e o tratamento precoces em Doberman pinscher, Bedlington terrier e Cocker spaniel, bem como nos casos de hepatopatias por armazenamento de cobre, parecem suspender a evolução da doença durante anos em alguns cães.

DIVERSOS

POTENCIAL ZOONÓTICO
Leptospirose; *Bartonella*; riquétsias (vetores endêmicos).

SINÔNIMO(S)
- Hepatite do Doberman.
- Hepatite do Cocker spaniel.
- Hepatopatia por armazenamento de cobre.
- Hepatite ativa crônica.

VER TAMBÉM
- Ascite.
- Desvio Portossistêmico Adquirido.
- Insuficiência Hepática Aguda.

ABREVIATURA(S)
- ANA = anticorpo antinuclear.
- CID = coagulação intravascular disseminada.
- CCNU = 1-(2-cloroetil)-3-ciclohexil-1-nitroso-ureia (lomustina).
- PDF = produtos de degradação da fibrina.
- PIAVK = proteínas invocadas pela ausência ou antagonismo da vitamina K.
- TC = tomografia computadorizada.
- TP = tempo de protrombina.
- TTPA = tempo de tromboplastina parcial ativada.

Autor Sharon A. Center
Consultor Editorial Sharon A. Center
Agradecimento a Dr. Robert M. Hardy, autor deste capítulo na edição anterior.

HEPATITE GRANULOMATOSA

CONSIDERAÇÕES GERAIS

REVISÃO
- Diagnóstico histopatológico incomum.
- Ocorre secundariamente à infecção por bactérias, vírus, parasitas, protozoários ou fungos específicos, resultando na formação de granuloma ou infiltração de fagócitos mononucleares e inflamação do fígado.
- Pode refletir algum distúrbio imunomediado ou imunorregulador.
- Pode refletir neoplasias histiocíticas.
- Pode estar localizada no fígado ou envolver esse órgão como parte de uma doença multissistêmica (baço, linfonodos), o que pode mascarar a hepatopatia subjacente.
- A toxicidade hepática por cobre é associada a pequenos focos granulomatosos multifocais, envolvendo a fagocitose de hepatócitos necróticos carregados de cobre por macrófagos e neutrófilos.

IDENTIFICAÇÃO
- Cães e gatos.
- Não há predileção por raça, sexo ou idade.

SINAIS CLÍNICOS
Achados Anamnésicos
- Anorexia, vômito, diarreia, perda de peso.
- Letargia.
- Poliúria ou polidipsia.

Achados do Exame Físico
- Hepatomegalia grave.
- Dor abdominal: vaga, em virtude da distensão da cápsula hepática.
- Icterícia.
- Distensão abdominal — ascite, hepatomegalia.
- Esplenomegalia — reação granulomatosa coexistente ou hiperplasia reticuloendotelial.
- Linfadenopatia.
- Febre.
- Taquipneia: por distensão abdominal, envolvimento de doença pulmonar.

CAUSAS E FATORES DE RISCO
- Infecção fúngica sistêmica — mais comum; histoplasmose; blastomicose; coccidioidomicose; pitiose.
- Infecção bacteriana — por *Brucella*; *Nocardia*, *Borrelia*, *Propionibacterium acnes*, doença micobacteriana; *Bartonella*.
- Infecção por riquétsia.
- Parasitismo — larva migrans visceral; trematódeos hepáticos; esquistossomíase; dirofilariose.
- Vírus — PIF.
- Doenças causadas por protozoários — toxoplasmose; leishmaniose visceral.
- Outros — linfangiectasia intestinal; neoplasia (histiocitose maligna, linfoma, reação reticuloendotelial associada a carcinoma hepatocelular); distúrbios imunomediados (síndrome hemofagocítica); reações medicamentosas; idiopáticos.

DIAGNÓSTICO

DIAGNÓSTICO DIFERENCIAL
Características muito distintas iniciam a busca por considerações diagnósticas; o histórico medicamentoso precisa ser cuidadosamente revisto.

HEMOGRAMA/BIOQUÍMICA/URINÁLISE
- Hemograma completo — leucograma inflamatório ou de estresse; anemia arregenerativa (inflamação crônica); esferócitos com anemia microangiopática ou imunomediada ou síndrome hemofagocítica; monocitose em caso de inflamação/infecção crônicas.
- Bioquímica — enzimas hepáticas elevadas; hiperbilirrubinemia; achado variável: hipoglicemia; hipoalbuminemia; nível baixo de ureia; proteínas séricas totais altas ou baixas; hipergamaglobulinemia; é possível notar anormalidades eletrolíticas com distúrbios hídricos e acidobásicos.
- Urinálise — pode permanecer normal, embora seja possível o encontro de proteinúria, eritrócitos, leucócitos, cilindros celulares e outros, além de bilirrubinúria.

OUTROS TESTES LABORATORIAIS
- Concentrações dos ácidos biliares séricos — frequentemente elevadas com envolvimento hepático maciço.
- Provas de coagulação — normais, exceto em casos de insuficiência hepática em estágio terminal.
- Exames sorológicos — os títulos para agentes infecciosos precisam ser avaliados com cuidado; considerar os títulos convalescentes; títulos elevados de IgM para toxoplasmose confirmam infecção ativa; a sorologia para *Bartonella* deve ser considerada.
- Testes diagnósticos moleculares: PCR ou hibridização *in situ* fluorescente (para bactérias ou outros microrganismos) no tecido hepático podem confirmar certos agentes infecciosos não visualizados ao exame histopatológico.
- Título do anticorpo antinuclear — positivo no caso de LES, mas títulos positivos baixos são inespecíficos.
- Culturas bacterianas — em tecido hepático, bile ou sangue; as culturas para micobactérias crescem lentamente (meses); a detecção das micobactérias pode ser mais eficiente com o uso de PCR; coloração tecidual (Ziehl-Neelsen; a coloração em seres humanos com infecção micobacteriana granulomatosa costuma ser negativa).

DIAGNÓSTICO POR IMAGEM
- Radiografia abdominal — hepatomegalia; massa abdominal; perda de detalhes da imagem em função da ascite.
- Ultrassonografia abdominal — avalia o tamanho do fígado e o padrão de alteração do parênquima hepático (difuso *versus* focal); delimita lesões expansivas tipo massa; outras lesões viscerais; linfadenopatia; possibilita a obtenção de amostras para o diagnóstico.

MÉTODOS DIAGNÓSTICOS
- Aspirado para obtenção de amostras — parênquima hepático; outras lesões viscerais; efusão abdominal.
- Biopsia do fígado — para obtenção do diagnóstico definitivo da reação granulomatosa, embora não costume definir a causa. Aplicar corantes específicos para cobre e quantificar esse elemento no tecido hepático (com base no peso seco).
- Aspirados e biopsia do fígado — corantes fúngicos; coloração de Gram; culturas e sensibilidades bacterianas e fúngicas — importantes do ponto de vista diagnóstico.

ACHADOS PATOLÓGICOS
- Macroscópicos — hepatomegalia; superfície normal ou finamente irregular; textura firme; bordas arredondadas.
- Microscópicos — reação piogranulomatosa com orientação zonal variável.

TRATAMENTO
- Internação *vs* tratamento ambulatorial — determinado pela gravidade dos sinais clínicos.
- Fluidoterapia — com solução poliônica balanceada para desidratação; pode requerer glicose (a 2,5-5%); suplementação criteriosa com potássio.
- É essencial o fornecimento de suporte nutricional; proporcionar um balanço nitrogenado positivo; não restringir a proteína na ausência de sinais de encefalopatia hepática.
- Informar ao proprietário que as causas dessa síndrome (p. ex., PIF, neoplasia) são frequentemente difíceis de confirmar e tratar.
- Se a resposta granulomatosa estiver associada à hepatotoxicidade por cobre, ver "Hepatopatia por Armazenamento de Cobre".

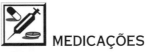

MEDICAÇÕES

MEDICAMENTO(S)
- Remover as terapias medicamentosas consideradas como possível causa de reação hepática granulomatosa.
- Depende(m) da causa; ver capítulos específicos.
- Imunomodulação — na suspeita de mecanismos imunomediados e resultados negativos para etiologia infecciosa.
- Doença idiopática (sem causa subjacente ou possíveis marcadores de processo imunomediado) — os glicocorticoides combinados com azatioprina demonstraram sucesso comprovado em um pequeno número de casos; podem exacerbar condições infecciosas não detectadas.
- Vômitos — antieméticos (p. ex., metoclopramida, 0,2-0,5 mg/kg VO ou SC a cada 6-8 h; ondansetrona, 0,5-1,0 mg/kg 30 min antes das refeições, a cada 12-24 h); maropitant (1,0 mg/kg SC, VO por, no máximo, 5 dias).
- Sangramento gastrintestinal — antagonistas dos receptores H_2 (p. ex., famotidina, 0,5 mg/kg VO, IM, SC a cada 12-24 h) e gastroproteção com sucralfato.

INTERAÇÕES POSSÍVEIS
- Considerar as interações medicamentosas potenciais por conta do amplo espectro de possíveis causas.
- Ponderar o ajuste das medicações que necessitem de ativação, biotransformação ou eliminação hepáticas.
- Imunossupressão — pode agravar os sinais clínicos de distúrbios infecciosos primários.

ACOMPANHAMENTO

MONITORIZAÇÃO DO PACIENTE
- Monitoramento de rotina do estado hídrico, equilíbrio acidobásico, eletrólitos e resposta geral ao tratamento.
- Avaliações hematológicas, bioquímicas e sorológicas sequenciais, além das técnicas de diagnóstico por imagem — podem ser úteis.

Hepatite Granulomatosa

COMPLICAÇÕES POSSÍVEIS
- Hepatite crônica.
- Fibrose ou cirrose hepáticas.
- Insuficiência hepática.
- Coagulopatia.

EVOLUÇÃO ESPERADA E PROGNÓSTICO
- Dependem da causa primária.
- Na melhor das hipóteses, o prognóstico costuma ser reservado, em virtude da natureza multissistêmica dessa síndrome.

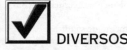

DIVERSOS
POTENCIAL ZOONÓTICO
- Brucelose — principal agente causal de caráter preocupante.
- Blastomicose, coccidioidomicose, bartonelose, leishmaniose — não são contagiosas; o animal de estimação pode servir como sentinela de exposição ambiental ou vetor de transmissão.

VER TAMBÉM
- Bartonelose.
- Blastomicose.
- Coccidioidomicose.
- Histoplasmose.
- Leishmaniose.
- Lúpus Eritematoso Sistêmico.
- Peritonite Infecciosa Felina (PIF).
- Pitiose.

ABREVIATURA(S)
- PCR = reação em cadeia da polimerase.
- PIF = peritonite infecciosa felina.

Sugestões de Leitura
Chapman BL, et al. Granulomatous hepatitis in dogs: Nine cases (1987-1990). JAVMA 1993, 203:680.
Rallis T, Day MJ, Saridomichelikis MN, et al. Chronic hepatitis associated with canine leishmaniosis (Leishmania infantum): A clinicopathological study of 26 cases. J Comp Pathol 2005, 132:145-152.
Ramachandran R, Kakar S. Histological patterns in drug-induced liver disease. J Clin Pathol 2009, 62:481-492.
Wainwright H. Hepatic granulomas. Eur J Gastroenterol Hepatol 2007, 93-95.

Autor Sharon A. Center
Consultor Editorial Sharon A. Center
Agradecimento a Dr. Robert M. Hardy, autor deste capítulo na edição anterior.

HEPATITE INFECCIOSA CANINA

CONSIDERAÇÕES GERAIS

REVISÃO
- Doença viral de cães (família Canidae) causada por CAV-1 sorologicamente homogêneo e antigenicamente distinto de CAV-2 respiratório.
- Infecção — afeta órgãos parenquimatosos (especialmente o fígado), olhos e endotélio.
- Exposição oronasal — acarreta viremia (4-8 dias); o vírus é disseminado pela saliva e nas fezes; dispersão inicial para macrófagos hepáticos (células de Kupffer) e endotélio; replica-se nas células de Kupffer; provoca dano a hepatócitos adjacentes com subsequente viremia maciça quando liberado.
- A resposta humoral adequada depura os órgãos em 10-14 dias; no entanto, o vírus persiste nos túbulos renais e pode ser eliminado na urina por 6-9 meses.
- Hepatite crônica — ocorre após a infecção em cães, com resposta de anticorpo neutralizante apenas parcial.
- Lesão ocular citotóxica — uveíte anterior; acarreta o clássico "olho azul da hepatite".

IDENTIFICAÇÃO
- Cães e outros animais da família Canidae.
- Sem predileção racial ou sexual.
- Mais comum em cães com menos de 1 ano de idade.

SINAIS CLÍNICOS
- Dependem do estado imunológico do hospedeiro e do grau de lesão citotóxica inicial.
- Superagudos — febre; sinais do SNC; colapso vascular; CID; morte em questão de horas.
- Agudos — febre; anorexia; letargia; vômitos; diarreia; hepatomegalia; dor abdominal; efusão abdominal; vasculite (petéquias, equimoses); CID; linfadenopatia; raramente, encefalite não supurativa.
- Sem complicações — letargia; anorexia; febre transitória; tonsilite; vômitos; diarreia; linfadenopatia; hepatomegalia; dor abdominal.
- Tardios — 20% dos casos desenvolvem uveíte anterior e edema corneano 4-6 dias após a infecção; recuperação em 21 dias; pode evoluir para glaucoma e ulceração da córnea.

CAUSAS E FATORES DE RISCO
- CAV-1.
- Cães não vacinados são suscetíveis.

DIAGNÓSTICO

DIAGNÓSTICO DIFERENCIAL
- Herpes-vírus canino (neonatal).
- Outras hepatopatias infecciosas.
- Leptospirose.
- Hepatite granulomatosa.
- Hepatite tóxica.
- Doença infecciosa fulminante — p. ex., parvovírus e cinomose.

HEMOGRAMA/BIOQUÍMICA/URINÁLISE
- Hemograma completo — esquistócitos; leucopenia durante a viremia aguda, seguida por leucocitose com linfocitose reativa e eritrócitos nucleados.
- Bioquímica — atividade inicialmente elevada das enzimas hepáticas; essa atividade começa a declinar em 14 dias; níveis baixos de glicose e albumina refletem insuficiência hepática fulminante, vasculite e endotoxemia; níveis baixos de sódio e potássio refletem perdas GI; hiperbilirrubinemia se o animal sobreviver vários dias.
- Urinálise — proteinúria reflete lesão glomerular; cilindros granulosos refletem dano tubular renal; bilirrubinúria é compatível com icterícia.

OUTROS TESTES LABORATORIAIS
- Provas de coagulação — refletem a gravidade da lesão hepática e CID.
- Sorologia para anticorpos contra o CAV-1— aumento de 4 vezes nos títulos de IgM e IgG; anticorpos induzidos por vacinação recente confundem a interpretação.
- Isolamento viral — segmento anterior do olho, rim, tonsila e urina; difícil em órgãos parenquimatosos (especialmente o fígado), exceto na primeira semana de infecção.

DIAGNÓSTICO POR IMAGEM
- Radiografia abdominal — fígado normal ou grande; perda de detalhes da imagem causada por efusão.
- Ultrassonografia abdominal — é possível observar hepatomegalia, parênquima hipoecoico (padrão multifocal ou difuso) e efusão.

MÉTODOS DIAGNÓSTICOS
- Biopsia hepática.
- Cultura viral.
- Sorologia aguda e convalescente.

ACHADOS PATOLÓGICOS
- Agudos — edema e hemorragia de linfonodos; hemorragias de serosas viscerais; fígado grande, escuro e mosqueado; vesícula biliar edematosa; exsudato fibrinoso no fígado, na vesícula biliar e em outras vísceras; esplenomegalia; infartos renais; efusão abdominal. Em casos de infecção por herpes-vírus canino em neonatos, também se observam necrose perivascular no fígado e em outros órgãos, alteração na coloração hepática e efusão abdominal.
- Crônicos — fígado pequeno, fibrótico ou cirrótico.

TRATAMENTO

- Em geral, o tratamento é feito com o paciente internado.
- Fluidoterapia — fluidos poliônicos balanceados; evitar o uso de lactato em caso de insuficiência hepática fulminante; monitorizar com cuidado os líquidos para evitar super-hidratação diante do aumento da permeabilidade vascular.
- Suplementação criteriosa de potássio (e outro eletrólito), pois a depleção de eletrólitos pode acentuar a encefalopatia hepática.
- Evitar neuroglicopenia — suplementar os fluidos com glicose (a 2,5-5%) conforme a necessidade.
- Terapia de componentes sanguíneos para coagulopatia; os componentes sanguíneos são preferidos aos coloides sintéticos para manter a pressão osmótica coloidal.
- Com CID franca — produtos sanguíneos (hemoderivados) frescos e heparina de baixo peso molecular (p. ex., enoxaparina, 100 U/kg [1 mg/kg] a cada 24 h).
- Suporte nutricional — refeições em pequenas quantidades várias vezes ao dia conforme a tolerância; otimizar o consumo de nitrogênio pelo paciente; a restrição inadequada de proteína pode prejudicar o reparo e a regeneração teciduais; a restrição de nitrogênio é aconselhada apenas se houver sinais evidentes de encefalopatia hepática.
- Se a alimentação oral não for tolerada, fornecer nutrição parenteral parcial (por, no máximo, 5 dias) ou, de preferência, nutrição parenteral total.

MEDICAÇÕES

MEDICAMENTO(S)
- Antimicrobianos profiláticos — para a migração transmural prevista de microbiota entérica e endotoxemia na ocorrência de insuficiência hepática; por exemplo, ticarcilina (33-50 mg/kg a cada 6-8 h) combinada com metronidazol (reduzir a dose convencional para 7,5 mg/kg IV a cada 8-12 h) e alguma fluoroquinolona.
- Antieméticos — para os vômitos; por exemplo, metoclopramida (0,2-0,5 mg/kg VO ou SC a cada 6-8 h ou em velocidade de infusão constante); ondansetrona (0,5-1,0 mg/kg VO a cada 12 h); maropitanto (1 mg/kg/dia SC por, no máximo, 5 dias).
- Antagonistas dos receptores histaminérgicos H_2 — para gastroproteção; por exemplo, famotidina (0,5 mg/kg VO, IV, SC a cada 12-24 h) e sucralfato (0,25-1,0 g VO a cada 8-12 h).
- Medicamentos para a encefalopatia hepática (ver "Encefalopatia Hepática").
- Ácido ursodesoxicólico — colerético e hepatoprotetor (10-15 mg/kg/dia em duas doses divididas com o alimento); administrar por tempo indefinido em caso de hepatite crônica.
- Antioxidantes — vitamina E (10 UI/kg/dia VO), N-acetilcisteína IV (dose de ataque de 140 mg/kg, seguida por 70 mg/kg a cada 8 h) até a via oral ser possível; depois, mudar para S-adenosilmetionina (20 mg/kg/dia VO com o estômago vazio); utilizar até a normalização das enzimas hepáticas ou por tempo indefinido em hepatite crônica.

CONTRAINDICAÇÕES
Considerar a gravidade da lesão hepática, depleção proteica e idade ao calcular as doses dos medicamentos.

ACOMPANHAMENTO

MONITORIZAÇÃO DO PACIENTE
- Monitorizar o estado hidreletrolítico e acidobásico, bem como o perfil de coagulação, para ajustar as medidas de suporte.
- Monitorizar o animal quanto à ocorrência de insuficiência renal aguda.

PREVENÇÃO
Vacinação com vírus vivo modificado — com 6-8 semanas de vida; 2 reforços em intervalos de 3-4 semanas até a 16ª semana de vida; reforço em 1 ano; vacina altamente eficaz; pode não haver necessidade de mais reforços.

COMPLICAÇÕES POSSÍVEIS
- Insuficiência hepática fulminante.
- Insuficiência renal aguda.
- CID.
- Glaucoma.
- Hepatite crônica.
- Septicemia.
- Encefalopatia hepática.

Hepatite Infecciosa Canina

EVOLUÇÃO ESPERADA E PROGNÓSTICO
• Superaguda — prognóstico mau; morte em horas.
• Aguda — variável: prognóstico reservado a bom.
• Resposta humoral deficiente (título 1:16-1:50) — pode ocorrer o desenvolvimento de hepatite crônica.
• Resposta humoral satisfatória (título >1:500 de IgG) — é possível a recuperação completa em 5-7 dias.
• Pacientes recuperados — podem desenvolver doença hepática ou renal crônica.

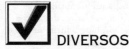

DIVERSOS

FATORES RELACIONADOS COM A IDADE
• Anticorpos maternos — podem proteger alguns filhotes de cães nas primeiras 8 semanas; depende da concentração de anticorpos na cadela e da transferência passiva eficaz.
• Vacinação de filhotes com altos níveis de anticorpos adquiridos passivamente — bem-sucedida com 14-16 semanas de vida.

VER TAMBÉM
• Coagulação Intravascular Disseminada.
• Encefalopatia Hepática.
• Infecção por Herpes-vírus — Cães.
• Insuficiência Hepática Aguda.
• Insuficiência Renal Aguda.
• Uveíte Anterior — Cães.
• Hepatite Crônica Ativa.

ABREVIATURA(S)
• CAV-1 = adenovírus canino 1.
• CID = coagulação intravascular disseminada.
• GI = gastrintestinal.
• SNC = sistema nervoso central.

Sugestões de Leitura
Greene CE. Infectious canine hepatitis and canine acidophil cell hepatitis. In: Greene CE, ed., Infectious Diseases of the Dog and Cat, 3rd ed. St. Louis: Saunders Elsevier, 2006, pp. 41-53.

Autor Sharon A. Center
Consultor Editorial Sharon A. Center

HEPATITE SUPURATIVA E ABSCESSO HEPÁTICO

CONSIDERAÇÕES GERAIS

REVISÃO
- Infecções bacterianas restritas ao sistema hepatobiliar — incomuns; consistem em microabscedação multifocal, colangite ou colangio-hepatite difusas, colecistite, coledoquite ou lesões necróticas supurativas unifocais discretas; associadas a microrganismos piogênicos.
- Grandes abscessos isolados em neoplasia hepática primária que infecta secundariamente o núcleo tumoral isquêmico.

IDENTIFICAÇÃO
- Cães e gatos.
- Sem predominância racial.
- Abscesso hepático — mais comum em cães idosos, associado à neoplasia hepática primária (adenoma, adenocarcinoma) com focos necróticos onde o tumor excedeu seu aporte sanguíneo, ou secundário à imunossupressão ou diabetes melito; em neonatos, pode-se desenvolver subsequentemente à onfalite.
- Colangite ou colangio-hepatite sépticas supurativas — mais comum em felinos machos jovens aos de meia-idade; infecção entérica ductal retrógrada ou translocação bacteriana entérica.
- Distúrbios colestáticos (p. ex., obstrução extra-hepática do ducto biliar, mucocele da vesícula biliar).

SINAIS CLÍNICOS
Achados Anamnésicos
- Letargia.
- Sinais gastrintestinais: vômito, diarreia.
- Perda de peso.
- Poliúria e polidipsia.
- Tremores.
- Febre.

Achados do Exame Físico
- Febre.
- Dor na porção epigástrica do abdome.
- Desidratação.
- Hepatomegalia: focal com abscesso volumoso.
- Coagulopatia.
- Distensão abdominal ou onda líquida.
- Icterícia.
- Sinais de endotoxemia: taquicardia, taquipneia, hipotensão, colapso hipoglicêmico.

CAUSAS E FATORES DE RISCO
- Infecção hematógena pela veia porta, artéria hepática ou veia umbilical.
- Obstruções da árvore biliar ou doença hepatobiliar ou pancreática preexistente com predisposição à translocação de bactérias intestinais.
- Infecção ascendente do trato biliar.
- Neoplasia hepática primária: adenoma ou adenocarcinoma com focos necróticos.
- Respostas imunes comprometidas: diabetes melito, administração de glicocorticoides, hiperadrenocorticismo, quimioterapia, distúrbios imunomediados sob imunossupressores.
- Feridas penetrantes.
- Complicação de biopsia hepática.

DIAGNÓSTICO

DIAGNÓSTICO DIFERENCIAL
- Doença infecciosa ou necroinflamatória — a maioria dos pacientes apresenta-se febril.
- Abscesso hepático — febre, dor abdominal e/ou hepatomegalia (especialmente se houver fatores de risco).
- Pancreatite ou abscesso pancreático.
- Neoplasia hepatobiliar.
- Obstrução ou perfuração gastrintestinal.
- Peritonite ou outro abscesso intra-abdominal.
- Colecistite, coledoquite, colelitíase.

HEMOGRAMA/BIOQUÍMICA/URINÁLISE
- Hemograma completo — leucocitose neutrofílica com desvio à esquerda; alterações tóxicas nos leucócitos; monocitose; trombocitopenia; anemia arregenerativa.
- Bioquímica — atividade elevada variável da fosfatase alcalina, com maior atividade da ALT e AST; hipoalbuminemia, hiperglobulinemia, hiperbilirrubinemia inconsistente e hipoglicemia; características que refletem endotoxemia (por bactérias Gram-negativas).
- Urinálise — geralmente normal; bilirrubinúria; a cultura pode ou não revelar microrganismos disseminados por via hematógena.

OUTROS TESTES LABORATORIAIS
- Ácidos biliares séricos — podem estar altos; dependem do grau de acometimento hepático ou da colestase ou podem refletir colestase associada à sepse.
- Testes de coagulação e morfologia dos eritrócitos (esquistócitos) — compatíveis com CID.

DIAGNÓSTICO POR IMAGEM
Radiografia Abdominal
- Hepatomegalia.
- Efeito expansivo hepático na presença de abscesso volumoso.
- Perda (focal ou difusa) de detalhes abdominais reflete efusão.
- Presença de gás dentro do parênquima hepático ou da árvore biliar (bactérias produtoras de gás; rara).

Ultrassonografia
- Abscesso — principal método não invasivo de detecção (>0,5 cm); lesões solitárias, variavelmente ecogênicas, cavitárias, com margem hiperecoica.
- Mineralização de tecido distrófico ou aprisionamento de gás — aparecem hiperecoicos.
- Múltiplas massas — algumas parecem complexas.
- Interface altamente ecogênica em massa cavitária — pode ser gás; a combinação com efusão abdominal e efeito perilesional hiperecoico confirma a presença de abscesso.
- Abscesso miliar — é impossível discernir de outros distúrbios hepáticos parenquimatosos.
- Síndrome colangite/colangio-hepatite séptica supurativa — a imagem não é exclusiva.

MÉTODOS DIAGNÓSTICOS
Citologia
- As avaliações citológicas são essenciais; as amostras histológicas raramente revelam microrganismos bacterianos.
- Amostras — efusão; aspirado do parênquima hemático e de lesões discretas, obtido por meio de orientação ultrassonográfica; colecistocentese para coleta de líquido e debris biliares.
- Corantes — Wright-Giemsa para detecção citológica de bactérias; corante de Gram para avaliação da morfologia.
- Procurar por bactérias dentro de leucócitos e sinais de processo patológico predisponente primário (p. ex., neoplasia).

Cultura e Antibiograma
- Em caso de reação supurativa ou piogranulomatosa (citologia) — efetuar cultura para bactérias aeróbias e anaeróbias, bem como para fungos.
- Sangue (culturas aeróbias e anaeróbias) — é mais provável que sejam positivas se houver múltiplos abscessos.
- Infecções polimicrobianas — ~30%.
- Bactérias Gram-negativas — comuns; *E. coli* (mais comum); *Klebsiella* spp.; *Pseudomonas* spp.; *Enterobacter* spp.; *Proteus* spp.; *Serratia marcescens*; *Citrobacter* spp.
- Bactérias Gram-positivas — *Enterococcus* spp. (mais comum); *Staphylococcus* spp.; *Streptococcus* spp.
- Microrganismos anaeróbios — menos comuns; *Clostridium* spp. (mais comum); *Propionibacterium acnes*; *Bacteroides* spp. sugere infecção polimicrobiana e facilita o crescimento de outras bactérias.

TRATAMENTO

- Paciente internado — se houver sinais de sepse.
- Fluidos e antibióticos intravenosos — são essenciais.
- Suporte hídrico — corrige déficits de desidratação; retifica distúrbios acidobásicos e eletrolíticos.
- Abscesso — drenar via lobectomia hepática durante laparotomia ou sob orientação ultrassonográfica; em alguns casos (choque endotóxico), a drenagem facilitada pelo ultrassom é o melhor método; após a drenagem, monitorizar a temperatura corporal, as enzimas hepáticas, o leucograma e, de forma sequencial, as imagens com ultrassom (monitorizar o tamanho do abscesso, a presença de peritonite focal ou difusa); repetir a drenagem com prudência (talvez haja necessidade da inserção de cateter de demora na área de supuração para drenagem contínua).
- Obstrução extra-hepática do ducto biliar — a descompressão biliar é essencial; é preciso administrar antimicrobianos intravenosos antes de manipulações cirúrgicas da árvore biliar para evitar septicemia.

MEDICAÇÕES

MEDICAMENTO(S)
- Antibióticos — escolhidos inicialmente com base na citologia e na coloração de Gram, mas ajustados com base nos resultados da cultura e do antibiograma; continuar por 3-4 meses.
- Tratamento inicial — antibióticos combinados para eliminar uma possível infecção polimicrobiana (patógenos aeróbios e anaeróbios comuns); uma combinação empírica eficaz comum inclui ticarcilina (25-50 mg/kg por 15 min em

Hepatite Supurativa e Abscesso Hepático

velocidade de infusão constante) ou amoxicilina clavulanato (10-20 mg/kg VO a cada 12 h), enrofloxacino (2,5 mg/kg VO ou SC a cada 12 h para cães ou gatos; pode-se usar a dose de 5 mg/kg VO ou SC a cada 12 h em cães) e metronidazol (15 mg/kg IV a cada 12 h; reduzir a dose pela metade se houver disfunção hepática ou colestase grave) ou clindamicina (10-16 mg/kg SC por dia; diminuir a dose em caso de disfunção hepática ou colestase grave para 5 mg/kg SC por dia).
• Coleréticos — são aconselhados se houver envolvimento da árvore biliar (ver obstrução extra-hepática do ducto biliar ou síndrome colangite/colangio-hepatite).
• Antioxidantes — são recomendados (ver "Hepatite Crônica Ativa").

CONTRAINDICAÇÕES
• Aminoglicosídeos — não administrar até que o estado de hidratação esteja normalizado; podem não penetrar na cápsula do abscesso.
• Evitar medicamentos metabolizados ou excretados pelo fígado ou aqueles reconhecidamente hepatotóxicos se houver comprometimento da função hepática; ajustar as doses ou a frequência dos medicamentos quando a eliminação estiver reduzida por colestase ou disfunção hepática.

ACOMPANHAMENTO

MONITORIZAÇÃO DO PACIENTE
• Avaliar os sinais vitais e a condição física.
• Exames sequenciais por ultrassom — monitorizar o paciente quanto à recidiva de abscesso.

COMPLICAÇÕES POSSÍVEIS
• CID.
• Septicemia/endotoxemia.
• Insuficiência hepática fulminante.
• Peritonite séptica.

EVOLUÇÃO ESPERADA E PROGNÓSTICO
• Prognóstico favorável — detecção e tratamento rigoroso precoces.
• Prognóstico pior — distúrbios concomitantes, especialmente neoplasia hepática primária não passível de ressecção.

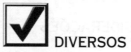

DIVERSOS

ABREVIATURA(S)
• ALT = alanina aminotransferase.
• AST = aspartato aminotransferase.
• CID = coagulação intravascular disseminada.

Sugestões de Leitura

Center SA. Hepatobiliary infections. In: Greene CE, ed., Infectious Diseases of the Dog and Cat, 4th ed. St. Louis: Saunders Elsevier (in press).

Schwarz LA, Penninck DG, Leveille-Webster C. Hepatic abscesses in 13 dogs: A review of the ultrasonographic findings, clinical data, and therapeutic options. Vet Radiol Ultrasound 1998, 39:357-365.

Zatelli A, Bonfanti U, Zini E, et al. Percutaneous drainage and alcoholization of hepatic abscesses in five dogs and a cat. JAAHA 2005, 41:34-38.

Autor Sharon A. Center
Consultor Editorial Sharon A. Center
Agradecimento a C. R. L. Webster, autor deste capítulo na edição anterior.

HEPATOMEGALIA

CONSIDERAÇÕES GERAIS

DEFINIÇÃO
Fígado grande detectado ao exame físico, em radiografias abdominais, ultrassonografia ou à inspeção direta do órgão; normalmente, o fígado corresponde a 1,3-5% do peso corporal; filhotes de cães e de gatos geralmente possuem uma relação de fígado:massa corporal maior que a de adultos.

FISIOPATOLOGIA
• O tamanho normal do fígado é determinado por fatores hepatotrópicos (produzidos no intestino e no pâncreas, mas liberados no sangue portal).
• O aumento é atribuído a (1) capacitância dos sinusoides (represamento de sangue) ou (2) acúmulo parenquimatoso ou sinusoidal de células, substratos ou produtos de armazenamento.

Difusa ou Generalizada
• Inflamatória — hepatite imunomediada ou infecciosa; classificada de acordo com o tipo de célula. • Hiperplasia linforreticular — resposta a antígenos ou destruição acelerada de eritrócitos. • Congestão — comprometimento da drenagem venosa. • Infiltração — invasão de células (em geral, neoplásicas) ou acúmulo excessivo de glicogênio ou lipídios, amiloides ou outros produtos metabólicos. • Lesões císticas. • Colestase — obstrução extra-hepática do ducto biliar, colestase intra-hepática. • Hematopoiese extramedular.

Nodular, Focal ou Assimétrica
• Neoplasia. • Hemorragia. • Infecção ou inflamação. • Hiperplasia nodular hepática.
• Regeneração nodular. • Fístula arteriovenosa — envolve um lobo maior do que outros lobos.
• Regeneração assimétrica após ressecção hepática volumosa. • Lesões císticas. • Torção de lobo hepático.

SISTEMA(S) ACOMETIDO(S)
• Gastrintestinal — compressão ou deslocamento gástricos; efusão decorrente de hipertensão portal hepática. • Pulmonar — diminuição do espaço ventilatório (rara).

IDENTIFICAÇÃO
• Cães e gatos. • Animais idosos costumam ser mais acometidos.

SINAIS CLÍNICOS

Achados Anamnésicos
• Distensão abdominal ou massa palpável.
• Desconforto abdominal — localização vaga.
• Dependem da causa subjacente.

Achados do Exame Físico
• Cães — fígado palpável além da margem costal (o fígado normal é palpado em algumas raças).
• Gatos — fígado palpável em mais de 1,5 cm além da margem costal (em alguns gatos, o fígado normal é palpável). • Pode não ser detectado em animais obesos.

CAUSAS

Inflamação
• Hepatite infecciosa ou crônica (no início).
• Necrose hepática aguda — muitas causas.
• Síndrome colangite/colangio-hepatite felina.
• Obstrução extra-hepática do ducto biliar.
• Hiperplasia linforreticular — doença imunomediada (anemia hemolítica, lúpus eritematoso sistêmico, idiopática), distúrbios infecciosos (p. ex., por riquétsias, *Babesia*).

Oclusão do Fluxo Venoso
• Pressão venosa central elevada — insuficiência cardíaca congestiva direita secundária à doença da valva atrioventricular direita (tricúspide); miocardiopatia; anomalia congênita (coração triatriado direito); neoplasia; doença pericárdica; dirofilariose; hipertensão pulmonar; arritmia grave. • Oclusão elevada nas veias cava e hepática — secundária à trombose; invasão tumoral ou oclusão extramural; síndrome da veia cava por dirofilariose; estenose ou dobra congênita da veia cava; hérnia diafragmática; oclusão intra-hepática da veia hepática (síndrome de Budd-Chiari; doença venoclusiva, zona 3); torção de lobo hepático.

Infiltração
• Neoplasia. • Anormalidades metabólicas — cães: glicogênio (ver "Hepatopatia Vacuolar"); gatos: lipídios (ver "Lipidose Hepática"): cães e gatos: recém-nascidos; secundariamente a diabetes melito ou síndromes hiperlipidêmicas; doença metabólica de armazenamento; amiloide. • Hiperplasia linforreticular — doença infecciosa, resposta imune, estimulação antigênica.

Hematopoiese Extramedular
• Anemias regenerativas — hemolíticas (imunomediadas, congênitas, metabólicas, infecciosas); lesão oxidativa; eritroparasitemia; insuficiência da medula óssea.

Neoplasia
• Tumores infiltrativos, difusos ou focais grandes.
• Hepática primária — linfoma; adenoma ou carcinoma hepatocelular; colangiocarcinoma (carcinoma do ducto biliar). • Linfoma.
• Hemangioma ou hemangiossarcoma. • Fibroma ou fibrossarcoma. • Leiomioma ou leiomiossarcoma. • Osteossarcoma. • Vários tumores metastáticos.

Obstrução Biliar (Obstrução Extra-Hepática do Ducto Biliar)
• Pancreatite; neoplasia pancreática. • Neoplasias na porta hepática (p. ex., carcinoma do ducto biliar). • Granuloma/fibrose do ducto biliar comum. • Síndrome da bile espessa, mucocele do colédoco ou da vesícula biliar. • Colelitíase.
• Duodenite proximal; corpo estranho duodenal.
• Migração de trematódeos (gatos).

Lesões Císticas
• Cistos hepáticos ou biliares. • Cistadenoma (gatos). • Doenças policísticas — podem estar associadas a cistos renais (comuns em gatos da raça Persa). • Cistos adquiridos — tumores. • Abscessos hepáticos (cavitações císticas).

Outras
• Medicamentos — corticosteroides (ver "Hepatopatia Vacuolar"), fenobarbital (cães).
• Hiperplasia nodular hepática (associada à hepatopatia vacuolar), hiperplasia adenomatosa hepática.

FATORES DE RISCO
• Cardiopatia. • Dirofilariose. • Neoplasia.
• Hepatopatia primária — inflamatória, neoplásica ou cística. • Corticosteroides — exógenos ou endógenos. • Tratamento com fenobarbital.
• Diabetes melito mal controlado. • Anorexia em gatos obesos — lipidose hepática. • Obstrução extra-hepática do ducto biliar. • Certas anemias — hematopoiese extramedular hepática difusa.

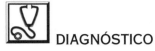

DIAGNÓSTICO

DIAGNÓSTICO DIFERENCIAL

Sinais Semelhantes
• Distinguir de outros distúrbios indutores de aumento das vísceras (estômago, baço), massas abdominais craniais ou efusões via radiografia e ultrassonografia.

Causas Diferenciais
• Distúrbios cardíacos (p. ex., sopro cardíaco, pulsos femorais fracos, reflexo hepatojugular, distensão e pulsos jugulares, além de bulhas cardíacas abafadas). • Anemia sintomática (palidez com ou sem icterícia; taquicardia; taquipneia; intolerância ao exercício; pulsos saltitantes).
• Hepatopatia parenquimatosa — caracteriza-se por letargia, anorexia, vômitos, diarreia, perda de peso, icterícia, coagulopatias, encefalopatia hepática, poliúria/polidipsia e ascite.
• Hepatopatia vacuolar (cães) — sinais de hiperadrenocorticismo ou hiperplasia adrenal ou outra doença crônica. • Lipidose hepática — icterícia em gatos obesos anoréxicos ou diabetes melito mal controlado (cães ou gatos); filhotes caninos ou felinos.

HEMOGRAMA/BIOQUÍMICA/URINÁLISE

Hemograma Completo
• Identificar a presença de anemia e a causa; esferócitos (anemia hemolítica imunomediada, anemia microangiopática); esquistócitos (anemia microangiopática por cisalhamento vascular, síndrome da veia cava, hemangiossarcoma, CID), corpúsculos de Heinz (lesão oxidativa); hemoparasitas (*Mycoplasma hemofelis*, *Babesia*).
• Células blásticas circulantes — doença mieloproliferativa ou linfoproliferativa.
• Hemácias nucleadas — hematopoiese extramedular, doença esplênica. • Macrocitose e anemia arregenerativa — FIV, FeLV.
• Trombocitopenia — aumento do consumo ou da destruição; produção reduzida. • Trombocitose — neoplasia; inflamação; hiperadrenocorticismo; doença esplênica.

Bioquímica
• Distúrbios hepáticos inflamatórios — em geral, apresentam atividade elevada das enzimas hepáticas; hiperglobulinemia variável; concentrações variáveis de bilirrubina e albumina.
• Hiperplasia linforreticular — enzimas hepáticas leve a moderadamente elevadas. • Neoplasia hepática primária — enzimas hepáticas moderada a acentuadamente elevadas (ALT, fosfatase alcalina, GGT). • Neoplasia metastática — níveis variáveis das enzimas hepáticas; ocasionalmente, há hipercalcemia ou hiperglobulinemia. • Distúrbios infiltrativos — alterações mínimas nas enzimas hepáticas; hiperbilirrubinemia variável.
• Hepatopatia vacuolar (cães) — fosfatase alcalina acentuadamente elevada; colesterol alto com glicocorticoides ou esteroides sexuais. • Lipidose hepática (gatos) — fosfatase alcalina, AST e ALT acentuadamente elevadas; aumento mínimo na GGT a menos que haja pancreatite, síndrome colangite/colangio-hepatite ou obstrução extra-hepática do ducto biliar concomitante.
• Doenças de armazenamento — poucas anormalidades. • Obstrução extra-hepática do ducto biliar — fosfatase alcalina, GGT e outras enzimas acentuadamente elevadas;

HEPATOMEGALIA

hiperbilirrubinemia e hipercolesterolemia. • Lesões císticas — resultados normais, exceto com abscessos hepáticos (ALT e AST acentuadamente elevadas). • Associada a tratamento com fenobarbital — enzimas hepáticas altas (especialmente fosfatase alcalina em cães).
• Hiperplasia nodular — fosfatase alcalina normal ou moderadamente elevada, associada muitas vezes à hepatopatia vacuolar.

OUTROS TESTES LABORATORIAIS
• Testes para pesquisa de FIV e FeLV — gatos.
• Esfregaços da camada leucocitária — para detecção de blastos circulantes (neoplasia). • Perfil de coagulação — a ocorrência de CID é comum com hemangiossarcoma ou linfoma difuso; tempos de coagulação prolongados são comuns com obstrução extra-hepática do ducto biliar (em especial no teste de PIAVK). • Ácidos biliares séricos totais — altos com distúrbios difusos e obstrução extra-hepática do ducto biliar; *excessivos em caso de* icterícia *não hemolítica*. • Teste do eixo hipofisário-adrenal (cães) — ver "Hepatopatia Vacuolar". • Teste para dirofilariose — em áreas endêmicas. • Sorologia para fungos — em áreas endêmicas. • Outras sorologias — p. ex., riquétsias, *Bartonella*.

DIAGNÓSTICO POR IMAGEM
Radiografia Abdominal
• Hepatomegalia — extensão de margens hepáticas arredondadas além do arco costal; deslocamento caudodorsal do estômago; deslocamento caudal da flexura duodenal cranial, do rim direito e do cólon transverso. • Pode sugerir a causa.

Radiografia Torácica
• Três projeções (laterais direita e esquerda, dorsoventral) — para pesquisa de metástases e outros distúrbios. • Distúrbios do coração, dos pulmões, do pericárdio e da veia cava.
• Linfadenopatia esternal — reflete inflamação ou neoplasia abdominais. • Filhotes (de cães e de gatos) e obtenção de imagens à inspiração profunda — hepatomegalia falsa.

Ultrassonografia Abdominal
• Tamanho do fígado e contorno da superfície.
• Aumento difuso com ecogenicidade normal — congestão; infiltração celular (linfoma); inflamação; hematopoiese extramedular; hiperplasia reticuloendotelial. • Aumento difuso com parênquima hipoecoico — variação normal; congestão, linfoma e sarcoma difuso; amiloidose.
• Aumento difuso com parênquima hiperecoico (nodularidade mínima) — acúmulo de lipídio ou glicogênio; inflamação; fibrose; linfoma.
• Aumento difuso com nódulos hipoecoicos — neoplasia; abscessos; hepatopatia vacuolar (cães) e glicogênio; lesões císticas. • Identifica obstrução extra-hepática do ducto biliar. • Identifica doenças abdominais concomitantes — dos rins; intestinos; linfonodos; efusão; sinal de interrogação da porta hepática. • Não é capaz de diferenciar doença benigna de maligna. • Identifica efusão abdominal — padrões de distribuição e de ecogenicidade.

OUTROS MÉTODOS DIAGNÓSTICOS
Eletrocardiografia e Ecocardiografia
• Caracterizam a condução e a estrutura cardíacas.

Aspirado por Agulha Fina
• Procedimento — agulha de calibre 22, com 2,5-3,75 cm de comprimento; aspirar diretamente o fígado com aumento difuso sem o auxílio da ultrassonografia; lesões focais aspiradas com orientação do ultrassom. • Citologia — pode revelar agentes infecciosos, alteração vacuolar, neoplasia, inflamação ou hematopoiese extramedular; raras vezes, o diagnóstico definitivo é confirmado de forma confiável, pois podem ocorrer resultados falso-positivos e falso-negativos.
• Biopsia hepática — realizada se a ultrassonografia excluir obstrução extra-hepática do ducto biliar, a citologia não indicar inflamação séptica ou neoplasia e se não houver outros diagnósticos óbvios; realizar biopsia aspirativa percutânea com agulha (Tru-Cut®) guiada por ultrassom na suspeita de neoplasia ou amiloide (evitar na presença de abscesso ou obstrução extra-hepática do ducto biliar); caso contrário, é melhor obter amostras com abordagens exploratórias laparoscópica ou cirúrgica. • Cultura microbiana — bacteriana aeróbia e anaeróbia; fúngica se for o caso. • Colorações — hematoxilina e eosina (corante de rotina); tricromo de Masson (fibrose); rodanina (cobre); PAS (glicogênio); corante acidorresistente (para pesquisa de micobactérias se houver inflamação granulomatosa); vermelho Congo (amiloide); óleo vermelho O (lipídio, corte congelado), reticulina (para avaliação de desarranjo na arquitetura do órgão). • Provas de coagulação — antes de obter amostras do fígado, considerar a mensuração de TP, TTPA ou TCA, fibrinogênio, PIAVK e tempo de sangramento da mucosa bucal; é amplamente reconhecida a falta de predição segura e confiável de hemorragia iatrogênica. • Efusão abdominal — citologia; teor de proteína; culturas; avaliar antes de obter amostras de tecidos.
• Pericardiocentese — em caso de tamponamento pericárdico.

TRATAMENTO

CUIDADO(S) DE SAÚDE ADEQUADO(S)
• Ambulatoriais — exceto na insuficiência cardíaca ou hepática. • Metas gerais de suporte — eliminar ou tratar a causa desencadeante; prevenir complicações; limitar os desarranjos associados à insuficiência hepática. • Desarranjos importantes — desidratação e hipovolemia; encefalopatia hepática; hipoglicemia; anormalidades acidobásicas e eletrolíticas; coagulopatias; hemorragia entérica; sepse; endotoxemia.

CUIDADO(S) DE ENFERMAGEM
• Suplemento de cloreto de potássio caso se faça uso de fluidos IV — escala móvel (manutenção = 20 mEq/L de fluido). • Suplementação de vitaminas solúveis do complexo B.

ATIVIDADE
Restrita; repouso inicial em gaiola em alguns distúrbios.

DIETA
• Proteína da dieta — restringir apenas em caso de encefalopatia hepática. • Bem balanceada com quantidade adequada de energia; é essencial um balanço nitrogenado positivo; teores adequados de vitaminas e micronutrientes. • Sódio — restringir na presença de insuficiência cardíaca ou ascite.

ORIENTAÇÃO AO PROPRIETÁRIO
• O tratamento e o prognóstico dependem da causa subjacente. • Muitas causas são potencialmente letais.

CONSIDERAÇÕES CIRÚRGICAS
• Ressecção de lesões hepáticas primárias ou focais em forma de massas — será indicada a descompressão biliar se houver obstrução extra-hepática do ducto biliar. • Pericardiectomia — se a efusão voltar após pericardiocentese inicial.

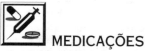

MEDICAÇÕES

MEDICAMENTO(S)
Varia(m) com a causa subjacente.

CONTRAINDICAÇÕES
• Evitar medicamentos hepatotóxicos.
• Hepatopatia vacuolar (cães) — evitar glicocorticoides. • Lipidose hepática (gatos) — evitar medicamentos que promovam catabolismo; evitar jejum.

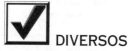

ACOMPANHAMENTO

MONITORIZAÇÃO DO PACIENTE
• Avaliação física e imagens hepáticas — reavaliar o tamanho do fígado. • Hemograma completo, bioquímica, ácidos biliares séricos totais — avaliação seriada de anormalidades e da função hepática; contagem de reticulócitos com anemia.
• Radiografia torácica, eletrocardiografia e ecocardiografia — reavaliar o estado do paciente.
• Eixo hipofisário-adrenal — com distúrbios adrenais. • Frutosamina — com diabetes melito.
• Ajustar as dosagens dos medicamentos de acordo com a função hepática, a condição e o peso corporais.

COMPLICAÇÕES POSSÍVEIS
Muitas causas são potencialmente letais.

DIVERSOS

POTENCIAL ZOONÓTICO
Certos agentes infecciosos são preocupantes.

VER TAMBÉM
• Adenoma Hepatocelular. • Amiloidose. • Anemia Imunomediada. • Carcinoma Hepatocelular.
• Hepatite Granulomatosa. • Hepatite Supurativa e Abscesso Hepático. • Hepatopatia Vacuolar.
• Insuficiência Cardíaca Congestiva Direita.
• Obstrução do Ducto Biliar. • Síndrome Colangite/Colangio-hepatite.

ABREVIATURA(S)
• FeLV = vírus da leucemia felina. • FIV = vírus da imunodeficiência felina. • PAS = ácido periódico de Schiff. • PIAVK = proteínas invocadas pela ausência ou antagonismo da vitamina K. • TCA = tempo de coagulação ativada. • TP = tempo de protrombina. • TTPA = tempo de tromboplastina parcial ativada.

Autor Sharon A. Center
Agradecimento Keith P. Richter

Hepatopatia Diabética

CONSIDERAÇÕES GERAIS

REVISÃO
• Lesão hepática caracterizada por hepatopatia degenerativa vacuolar e colapso parenquimatoso, que resultam em formação acentuada de nódulos hepáticos; associada a dermatose rara nos pontos de pressão e diabetes melito. • As lesões hepáticas podem anteceder o desenvolvimento das lesões cutâneas e do diabetes melito; tais lesões podem se desenvolver em alguns cães submetidos a tratamento crônico com fenobarbital.

IDENTIFICAÇÃO
• Cães de idade média a mais idosos. • Os machos podem apresentar uma predisposição mais notável. • Não há raça predominante.

SINAIS CLÍNICOS
Achados Anamnésicos
• Início agudo; podem manifestar poucos sinais clínicos. • Sinais comuns — perda de peso; letargia; poliúria e polidipsia; icterícia; anorexia; diarreia; vômito; algumas vezes, claudicação.

Achados do Exame Físico
• Letargia, má condição corporal e lesões dolorosas no cotovelo e nos pés que comprometem as posturas em estação e em decúbito. • Lesões cutâneas — ver "Dermatite Necrolítica Superficial". • Volume hepático — variável (pequeno a grande); raramente se mostra possível a palpação das bordas hepáticas irregulares.

CAUSAS E FATORES DE RISCO
• Etiologia — associada a hipoaminoacidemia; papel etiológico nas lesões cutâneas. • Papel etiopatogênico secundário — sugerido nas deficiências pouco definidas de zinco, ácidos graxos ou niacina. • Hiperglucagonemia — proposta originalmente como o mecanismo causal; incompatível (apenas 30-40% dos cães submetidos a exames demonstram níveis plasmáticos elevados do glucagon); a correlação deficiente pode refletir a especificidade dos ensaios ou a extração hepática reforçada do glucagon; em <25% dos cães, foi demonstrada a presença de tumor pancreático produtor de glucagon. • Demonstração de insulinorresistência. • Lesões cutâneas semelhantes descritas em associação com hepatopatias primárias, causadas por fenobarbital ou micotoxicose crônica.

DIAGNÓSTICO

DIAGNÓSTICO DIFERENCIAL
• Cirrose — hiperplasia nodular regenerativa, com deposição extensa de tecido conjuntivo e perda da organização arquitetural. • Hepatite crônica — infiltrados de células inflamatórias; necrose periportal gradativa. • Hepatopatia por armazenamento de cobre — nível tecidual elevado desse elemento, associado inicialmente à lesão necroinflamatória da zona 3. • Hiperplasia nodular difusa. • Hepatopatia vacuolar.

HEMOGRAMA/BIOQUÍMICA/URINÁLISE
• Hemograma completo — desde anemia arregenerativa leve a moderada até anemia levemente regenerativa; em casos de lesão hepática avançada, há microcitose (hemácias de tamanho pequeno); a leucocitose neutrofílica reflete as infecções cutâneas. • Bioquímica — enzimas hepáticas elevadas (especialmente a fosfatase alcalina e a alanina aminotransferase); hipoproteinemia; hipoalbuminemia; hiperglicemia de jejum; níveis variáveis de colesterol e ureia. • Urinálise — cristalúria por biurato de amônio pode refletir insuficiência hepática.

OUTROS TESTES LABORATORIAIS
• Ácidos biliares séricos totais — anormalmente aumentados. • Glucagon plasmático — contraditoriamente alto. • Aminoácidos plasmáticos — 30-50% das concentrações normais em relação à maior parte dos aminoácidos em cães com lesões cutâneas; declínios intermediários em cães com lesões hepáticas que precedem as lesões cutâneas.

DIAGNÓSTICO POR IMAGEM
• Radiografia abdominal — tamanho variável do fígado (frequentemente normal a aumentado de volume); é rara a presença de efusão. • Ultrassonografia abdominal — pode-se observar irregularidade nas bordas hepáticas; padrão nodular característico: focos hipoecoicos no parênquima hiperecoico, conhecido como "padrão em queijo suíço"; embora seja sugerido como um aspecto patognomônico, outras hepatopatias vacuolares graves também podem demonstrar esse padrão; não se conseguem obter imagens de nodularidades difusas ocasionais; observa-se massa pancreática em <20% dos cães.

MÉTODOS DIAGNÓSTICOS
• Amostragem por aspiração — os hepatócitos exibem vacuolização associada à presença de glicogênio e lipídio. • Biopsia hepática — a biopsia aspirativa com agulha pode comprometer o diagnóstico definitivo por limitar a detecção de nódulos regenerativos e fibroplasias; pode ser mais eficiente para cães com lesões cutâneas extensas; prefere-se a coleta de amostras laparoscópicas mais volumosas; como os cães acometidos por lesões cutâneas não apresentam boa cicatrização, deve-se evitar a laparotomia se possível. • Caso se encontre a presença de massa(s) pancreática(s), proceder à ressecção para o exame histológico e a coloração imuno-histoquímica para a detecção de glucagon e outros produtos. • Biopsia cutânea — ver "Dermatite Necrolítica Superficial".

TRATAMENTO

• Tratar o diabetes e, se associado ao fenobarbital, interromper a medicação. • Dieta — rica em proteínas de alta qualidade; pode ser necessária a alimentação por via enteral ou parenteral; aumentar a tolerância ao nitrogênio com o emprego de lactulose e metronidazol (ver "Encefalopatia Hepática"). • Suplementação de aminoácidos — gemas de ovo (3-6 gemas por dia); produto anabólico a base de proteína do soro do leite em pó (1 porção tipicamente contém 7 g de proteína, 25-35 kcal; 1 porção/5-7 kg de peso corporal; misturada com a dieta; em caso de encefalopatia hepática, utilizar uma dieta formulada para insuficiência hepática); infusão IV de solução de aminoácidos cristalinos a 10% (Aminosyn®, Abbott Laboratories; 100 mL fornecem 10 g de aminoácidos, 25 mL/kg de peso corporal durante 8-12 h pela veia jugular a menos que haja coagulopatia; em seguida, fazer uso de cateter jugular longo inserido profundamente até uma veia periférica; é rara a indução de encefalopatia hepática. As lesões cutâneas podem desaparecer somente depois do tratamento com um único aminoácido; em caso de resposta tênue, repetir a cada 7-10 dias por 4 tratamentos; na ausência de resposta, o prognóstico será grave. • Suplementação de ácidos graxos ômega-3 — duplicar a dose normal de um suplemento de alta potência.

MEDICAÇÕES

MEDICAMENTO(S)
• Infecções da pele ou do leito ungueal — antimicrobianos ou antifúngicos sistêmicos; banhos antissépticos. • Suplementação de zinco — 2 mg/kg a cada 24 h com metionina de zinco (ou acetato de zinco em casos de encefalopatia hepática). • Niacinamida — relatos não publicados; 250-500 mg/cão a cada 12 h (500 mg para os cães com >10 kg); ficar atento aos efeitos tóxicos; evitar a formulação de liberação estendida. • Glicocorticoides tópicos — em casos de lesões cutâneas inflamatórias não responsivas, após o tratamento da infecção (**Cuidado:** os glicocorticoides sistêmicos podem promover encefalopatia hepática, ulceração entérica e infecção). • Cetoconazol — para eliminar as infecções secundárias por leveduras. • Análogo da somatostatina (octreotídeo: 2-3,7 μg/kg a cada 6-12 h) — há teorias quanto ao uso dessa medicação como possível tratamento, com base em causas endocrinológicas especulativas; pode controlar tumores pancreáticos metastáticos secretores de glucagon. • Ácido ursodesoxicólico — 10-15 mg/kg VO diariamente, sendo a dose dividida e administrada com alimento. • Antioxidantes — vitamina E (10 UI/kg diariamente VO); S-adenosilmetionina (20 mg/kg VO diariamente).

INTERAÇÕES POSSÍVEIS
• Indução de encefalopatia hepática em casos de consumo de suplementos ricos em proteínas e infusões de aminoácidos. • Efeitos tóxicos do cetoconazol e sua interferência no metabolismo de medicamentos, bem como efeitos tóxicos da niacinamida e do zinco.

ACOMPANHAMENTO

MONITORIZAÇÃO DO PACIENTE
• Exame físico mensal para avaliar a necessidade da infusão de aminoácidos e do tratamento de infecções secundárias. • Hemograma completo, bioquímica e urinálise em intervalos trimestrais. • Tratamento meticuloso do diabetes melito.

COMPLICAÇÕES POSSÍVEIS
• Cetoacidose — incomum. • Encefalopatia hepática. • Sepse — em virtude do diabetes e das lesões cutâneas. • Dor — decorrente das lesões cutâneas.

EVOLUÇÃO ESPERADA E PROGNÓSTICO
• Alguns cães alcançam a remissão cutânea em >2 anos com as terapias descritas; outros apresentam evolução ininterrupta, necessitando de eutanásia; há relatos não publicados de melhora das lesões hepáticas com o tratamento.

Autor Sharon A. Center
Consultor Editorial Sharon A. Center

Hepatopatia Fibrosante Juvenil

CONSIDERAÇÕES GERAIS

DEFINIÇÃO
- Hepatopatia não inflamatória de cães jovens adultos, associada à fibrose hepática.
- Fibrose progressiva provoca hipertensão portal, desvios portossistêmicos adquiridos, ascite e encefalopatia hepática.
- Alguns casos são associados a más-formações da placa ductal (conforme descrito em fibrose hepática juvenil em seres humanos); essas más-formações desenvolvem fibrose portal em ponte e dúctulos/ductos biliares malformados.
- Hipoperfusão da veia porta é associada a cada síndrome.

FISIOPATOLOGIA
- Fibrose hepática — gravidade variável.
- A gênese de fibrose hepatoportal ou centrolobular permanece incerta; as possibilidades incluem (1) más-formações embriológicas; (2) exposição crônica a ácidos biliares tóxicos; (3) exposição a toxinas entéricas (componentes bacterianos Gram-negativos); ou (4) resposta "juvenil" contínua à lesão hepática.
- O processo de fibrose é mais grave quando a síndrome é diagnosticada em animais mais idosos (condição crônica).
- A relação com hipertensão portal não cirrótica não está clara.
- Também se sugere que a fibrose hepatoportal represente um espectro de hipoplasia primária ou congênita da veia porta. No entanto, qualquer causa de hipoperfusão da veia porta gera características histológicas idênticas (ver "Displasia Microvascular Hepatoportal"; "Anomalia Vascular Portossistêmica Congênita").

SISTEMA(S) ACOMETIDO(S)
- Fígado — micro-hepatia.
- Gastrintestinal — anorexia; vômito ou diarreia intermitentes que refletem vasculopatia intestinal hipertensiva ou enteropatia inflamatória.
- Hematológico/linfático/imune — microcitose das hemácias em função de desvio portossistêmico adquirido.
- Musculoesquelético — retardo do crescimento e má condição corporal: doença crônica, inapetência, má assimilação intestinal.
- Nervoso — encefalopatia hepática episódica.
- Urogenital — poliúria e polidipsia; se associada à má-formação da placa ductal, pode haver cistos renais; urolitíase por biurato de amônio reflete desvio portossistêmico adquirido.

IDENTIFICAÇÃO
- Apenas cães.
- Jovens adultos; idade média — 2 anos (faixa etária de 0,2-8 anos) (em um único estudo).
- Não há predileção sexual.
- Pode acometer ninhadas, embora não se conheça uma base genética.

SINAIS CLÍNICOS
- Sinais episódicos do SNC atribuídos à encefalopatia hepática.
- Distensão abdominal: ascite.
- Retardo do crescimento, má-formação corporal.
- Sinais GI: inapetência, êmese, diarreia, hemorragia intestinal.
- Poliúria e polidipsia.
- Urolitíase por uratos de amônio.

CAUSAS E FATORES DE RISCO
- Exposição crônica a toxinas entéricas.
- Pode refletir doenças GI hemorrágicas em cães jovens (endotoxemia portal) como a lesão desencadeante.

DIAGNÓSTICO

DIAGNÓSTICO DIFERENCIAL
- Sinais do SNC — distúrbios infecciosos (p. ex., cinomose); intoxicações (p. ex., chumbo); hidrocefalia; epilepsia; distúrbios metabólicos (p. ex., hipoglicemia, hipocalemia e hipercalemia).
- Encefalopatia hepática — desvio portossistêmico adquirido ou anomalia vascular portossistêmica.
- Ascite — transudato puro (ver "Hipertensão Portal").

HEMOGRAMA/BIOQUÍMICA/URINÁLISE
- Hemograma completo — microcitose eritrocitária; células-alvo.
- Bioquímica — hipoalbuminemia e hipocolesterolemia; globulina e ureia normais a baixas; atividade normal a aumento modesto na fosfatase alcalina e ALT.
- Urinálise — cristalúria por biurato de amônio.

OUTROS TESTES LABORATORIAIS
- Testes de coagulação de rotina — anormalidades variáveis (ver "Coagulopatia por Hepatopatia"). Baixa atividade da proteína C (desvio portossistêmico adquirido).
- Ácidos biliares séricos totais — aumentados: padrão em casos de desvio.
- Análise do líquido peritoneal — transudato puro (proteína total, em geral, <2,5 g/dL); transudato modificado em casos crônicos.

DIAGNÓSTICO POR IMAGEM
Radiografias
- Abdominais — efusão, micro-hepatia.
- Torácicas — normais (para descartar cardiopatia do lado direito).

Ultrassonografia Abdominal
- Efusão abdominal, fígado normal a pequeno.
- Textura hepática variável; vasculatura sem alterações dignas de nota até hipoperfusão portal; pode detectar desvio portossistêmico adquirido.
- Doppler de fluxo colorido — fluxo hepatofugal; desvio portossistêmico adquirido atrás de um único rim; descartar trombose portal e fístula(s) AV hepática(s).

Outras Técnicas de Diagnóstico por Imagem
- Portografia venosa — não recomendada, mas pode confirmar a presença de desvio portossistêmico adquirido.
- Cintilografia colorretal — confirma o desvio.
- TC multissetorial com contraste vascular — pode fornecer detalhes sobre a anatomia vascular.

Ecocardiografia
- Descarta cardiopatia do lado direito e oclusão da veia cava (ver "Hipertensão Portal").

MÉTODOS DIAGNÓSTICOS
- Biopsia hepática.
- Hipertensão portal — >13 cmH$_2$O; atenuada por desvio portossistêmico adquirido; a mensuração não é útil em termos clínicos.

ACHADOS PATOLÓGICOS
- Macroscópicos — fígado pequeno; aspecto nodular fino.
- Microscópicos — gravidade variável e padrão da fibrose em zonas; pequenas vênulas portais refletem a hipoperfusão portal, mas não definem hipoplasia; múltiplos cortes transversais de arteríolas portais refletem o fluxo arterial aumentado em resposta à hipoperfusão portal.
- Más-formações da placa ductal — fibrose associada a dúctulos/ductos biliares malformados.
- Atrofia dos lóbulos e hepatócitos — reflete desvio portossistêmico adquirido.

TRATAMENTO

CUIDADO(S) DE SAÚDE ADEQUADO(S)
- Internação — para encefalopatia hepática grave (ver "Encefalopatia Hepática").
- Tratamento ambulatorial — para pacientes estáveis.
- Eliminar endoparasitas.
- Evitar o uso de AINE: aumentam a ascite (retenção de sódio e água) e o sangramento gastrintestinal.
- Tratar as infecções imediatamente — em pacientes imunocomprometidos: vigilância reduzida das células de Kupffer, opsonização bacteriana prejudicada.
- Permanecer vigilante para as uropatias obstrutivas por biurato de amônio (todos os níveis do sistema urinário); a obstrução uretral (machos) pode exigir a realização de uretrostomia permanente.

CUIDADO(S) DE ENFERMAGEM
Encefalopatia Hepática
- Eliminar os fatores causais; individualizar a dieta; suplementar com vitaminas hidrossolúveis, vitamina K (dependendo do teste de PIVKA) e vitamina E; otimizar o tratamento de encefalopatia hepática de acordo com a resposta individual (ver "Encefalopatia Hepática"). Esforçar-se para manter a condição corporal — a massa muscular atenua a toxicidade da amônia; fornecer múltiplas refeições diárias em pequenas quantidades.
- Ascite (ver "Hipertensão Portal").

MEDICAÇÕES

MEDICAMENTO(S) DE ESCOLHA
Encefalopatia Hepática
- Lactulose (0,5-1,0 mL/kg VO a cada 8-12 h) — dose ajustada com o objetivo de manter as fezes amolecidas; pode ser retirada com modificações ideais da dieta.
- Antibióticos por via oral — as primeiras escolhas são metronidazol (8 mg/kg VO a cada 12 h) ou amoxicilina (22 mg/kg VO a cada 12 h). A última escolha é representada pela neomicina (20 mg/kg VO a cada 8-12 h): tome cuidado com a absorção intestinal aumentada em casos de enteropatia inflamatória, além de possível nefro e ototoxicidade (administração crônica de neomicina: absorção de 3% por dose pode levar à toxicidade).

Ascite
- Restrição de sódio na dieta.
- Furosemida (1-4 mg/kg VO, IM ou IV a cada 12-24 h) — o efeito de depleção do potássio é modulado pela combinação terapêutica com espironolactona.

HEPATOPATIA FIBROSANTE JUVENIL

- Espironolactona (1-4 mg/kg VO a cada 12 h como dose de ataque e, depois, dose de manutenção de 2-4 mg/kg) — poupadora de potássio; menos potente do que a furosemida.
- Reduzir a dose do diurético após obtenção de resposta positiva inicial; individualizar o tratamento crônico em relação à resposta; os diuréticos podem ser utilizados de forma intermitente para mobilizar a ascite recidivante.
- Ascite refratária a diuréticos — considerar a realização de abdominocentese terapêutica ou o uso de antagonistas dos receptores V_2.

Medicamentos Antifibróticos e Antioxidantes
- Ver "Cirrose e Fibrose do Fígado".

Tendências Hemorrágicas
- Ver "Coagulopatia por Hepatopatia".

Hemorragia Gastrintestinal
- Ver "Cirrose e Fibrose do Fígado"; "Hipertensão Portal".

CONTRAINDICAÇÕES/INTERAÇÕES POSSÍVEIS
- Evitar ou diminuir a dose de medicamentos que dependem de biotransformação hepática ou do metabolismo hepático de primeira passagem; evitar os medicamentos que reagem com receptores GABA-benzodiazepínicos; evitar os medicamentos que inibem a biotransformação e o metabolismo de outros agentes terapêuticos (p. ex., cimetidina, cloranfenicol, quinidina, alguns bloqueadores dos canais de cálcio).
- Evitar a metoclopramida se a espironolactona for utilizada como diurético (aumenta os níveis da aldosterona).

ACOMPANHAMENTO

MONITORIZAÇÃO DO PACIENTE
- Bioquímica — monitorizar inicialmente a cada 2-4 semanas até a estabilização e depois a cada 4-6 meses; monitorizar quanto à ocorrência de intoxicação medicamentosa iatrogênica, descompensação, lesão hepática progressiva ou ativa.
- Caso se faça uso da colchicina, monitorizar o hemograma completo quanto à mielossupressão e observar toxicidade intestinal e neurotoxicidade.

COMPLICAÇÕES POSSÍVEIS
Encefalopatia hepática — necessita de tratamento nutricional e clínico por tempo indefinido.

EVOLUÇÃO ESPERADA E PROGNÓSTICO
- Informar o proprietário sobre a inexistência de base de dados que fundamentam o tratamento e o prognóstico.
- É possível a sobrevida a longo prazo (anos).
- Pode haver a necessidade de tratamentos a curto prazo ou por toda a vida — antifibróticos, modificações nutricionais, tratamentos complementares para encefalopatia hepática e vasculopatia portal hipertensiva (hemorragia intestinal, inapetência) e ascite.
- Exacerbações ocasionais de encefalopatia hepática e ascite podem necessitar de internações para o ajuste das intervenções nutricional e clínica. Pode ser necessária a titulação da restrição de sódio e do uso de diuréticos para se obter o controle ideal da ascite.

DIVERSOS

DISTÚRBIOS ASSOCIADOS
- Encefalopatia hepática.
- Ascite.
- Sangramento gastrintestinal.
- Desvio portossistêmico adquirido.

FATORES RELACIONADOS COM A IDADE
- O prognóstico depende do grau de fibrose e de insuficiência hepática no momento do diagnóstico inicial.
- A fibrose pode evoluir com a idade; pouco fundamentada em função da escassez de biopsias hepáticas de acompanhamento.

POTENCIAL ZOONÓTICO
Nenhum.

VER TAMBÉM
- Ascite.
- Desvio Portossistêmico Adquirido.
- Encefalopatia Hepática.
- Hipertensão Portal.

ABREVIATURA(S)
- AINE = anti-inflamatório não esteroide.
- ALT = alanina aminotransferase.
- AV = arteriovenoso.
- GABA = ácido gama-aminobutírico.
- GI = gastrintestinal.
- PIAVK = proteínas invocadas pela ausência ou antagonismo da vitamina K.
- SNC = sistema nervoso central.
- TC = tomografia computadorizada.

Sugestões de Leitura
Brown DL, Van Winkle T, Cecere T, et al. Congenital hepatic fibrosis in 5 dogs. Vet Pathol 2010, 47:102-107.
Bunch SE, Johnson SE, Cullen JM. Idiopathic noncirrhotic portal hypertension in dogs: 33 cases (1982-1998). JAVMA 2000, 218:392-399.
Rutgers HC, Haywood S, Kelly DF. Idiopathic hepatic fibrosis in 15 dogs. Vet Record 1993, 133:115-118.

Autor Sharon A. Center
Consultor Editorial Sharon A. Center

Hepatopatia por Armazenamento de Cobre

CONSIDERAÇÕES GERAIS

DEFINIÇÃO
Corresponde ao acúmulo hepático anormal de cobre, que causa hepatite aguda ou crônica e finalmente cirrose. Acredita-se que a doença primária reflita uma anormalidade de base genética no metabolismo do cobre.

FISIOPATOLOGIA
• A anormalidade nas concentrações hepáticas de cobre origina-se tanto de um defeito metabólico hepático primário como de um evento secundário ao equilíbrio anormal de cobre por colestase ou ingestão excessiva desse elemento.
• O cobre é normalmente absorvido a partir do intestino delgado, armazenado no fígado, e o excesso é excretado pelo sistema biliar. O acúmulo primário de cobre (defeito genético ou consumo demasiado) aparece primeiramente na zona 3 (centrolobular) no lóbulo hepático; o acúmulo secundário de cobre associado à lesão hepática ou colestase frequentemente ocorre na zona 1 (periportal) ou adjacente às regiões lesadas.
• O acúmulo colestástico secundário de cobre raramente excede 1.000 μg/g de tecido hepático seco, enquanto os distúrbios hereditários no metabolismo desse elemento muitas vezes ultrapassam 1.000 μg/g de tecido hepático seco. O cobre resulta em dano hepatocelular, que ocorre em parte como resultado do dano oxidativo às membranas e mitocôndrias.
• A hepatite focal evolui para hepatite crônica e finalmente para cirrose.
• A necrose hepática aguda grave pode liberar o cobre armazenado no fígado para a corrente sanguínea, provocando hemólise (raro).

SISTEMA(S) ACOMETIDO(S)
• Hepatobiliar.
• Sanguíneo/linfático — a anemia hemolítica constitui uma sequela rara em casos de necrose hepática aguda que libera o cobre do fígado, gerando níveis séricos elevados desse elemento.

GENÉTICA
• Um traço autossômico recessivo em Bedlington terrier em virtude de mutação do gene COMMD1 está envolvido na excreção biliar de cobre.
• Uma relação causal com algum distúrbio genético permanece sem comprovação em cães das raças West Highland white terrier, Skye terrier, Dálmata, Doberman pinscher e Labrador retriever, embora tenha se demonstrado que parentes dessas raças tenham indivíduos com hepatopatia e valores teciduais elevados de cobre; alguns indivíduos apresentam níveis hepáticos elevados de cobre sem evidência histológica de hepatopatia.

INCIDÊNCIA/PREVALÊNCIA
• Bedlington terrier — em uma época, possivelmente, o equivalente a dois terços dos animais dessa raça nos Estados Unidos era composta de portadores ou acometidos; a incidência tem declinado significativamente por meio de triagem genética.
• West Highland white terrier — a prevalência em certas linhagens parece alta, mas a incidência global nessa raça é baixa. O cobre hepático elevado nem sempre pode estar associado à hepatite crônica.
• Doberman pinscher — 4-6% dos animais dessa raça podem ter hepatite crônica e concentrações hepáticas anormais de cobre. Suspeita-se de excreção biliar anormal de cobre em alguns cães acometidos; no entanto, os defeitos de excreção desse elemento podem apenas fazer parte da doença global.
• Labrador retriever — super-representados em casos de hepatite e concentração hepática anormal de cobre; a incidência é desconhecida, mas pode ser alta em comparação a outras raças listadas adiante.

IDENTIFICAÇÃO
Espécies
Cães e, raramente, gatos.

Raça(s) Predominante(s)
Há relatos de que as raças Bedlington terrier, West Highland white terrier, Skye terrier, Doberman pinscher, Dálmata e Labrador retriever tenham concentrações hepáticas elevadas de cobre.

Idade Média e Faixa Etária
• Bedlington terrier — o cobre acumula-se com o passar do tempo, atingindo o máximo aos 6 anos de idade; os cães podem ser clinicamente acometidos em qualquer idade, embora a maioria se apresente como animais de meia-idade a idosos com hepatite crônica.
• West Highland white terrier — observa-se o acúmulo máximo do cobre por volta de 1 ano de idade; no entanto, a doença clínica pode ocorrer em qualquer momento.
• Skye terrier — pode acometer todas as idades.
• Doberman pinscher — podem começar a desenvolver hepatite com aumentos da ALT e acúmulo de cobre em 1-3 anos de idade; os sinais de hepatopatia frequentemente ocorrem após os 7 anos de idade.
• Labrador retriever e Dálmata — idade média no momento do diagnóstico de hepatite crônica.

Sexo Predominante
Doberman pinscher — fêmeas.

SINAIS CLÍNICOS
Comentários Gerais
• As hepatopatias primárias por armazenamento de cobre geralmente se enquadram em uma de três categorias: doença subclínica; doença aguda (incomum) observada em cães jovens com necrose hepática aguda; ou doença progressiva crônica em cães de meia-idade a idosos com hepatite crônica que frequentemente evolui para cirrose.
• O acúmulo hepático secundário de cobre pode ocorrer em casos de hepatopatia necroinflamatória progressiva crônica e colestase hepática.

Achados Anamnésicos
• Sinais agudos — início súbito de letargia, anorexia e vômito.
• Sinais crônicos — histórico variável de letargia intermitente, anorexia, perda de peso, vômito, diarreia, polidipsia e poliúria. Os sinais mais tardios podem incluir distensão abdominal (ascite), icterícia, sangramento espontâneo e encefalopatia hepática.

Achados do Exame Físico
• Sinais agudos — letargia, fraqueza, icterícia, mucosas pálidas (anemia) e urina escura (bilirrubinúria e rara hemoglobinúria).
• Sinais crônicos — perda de peso, ascite, icterícia e micro-hepatia são comuns. Em alguns cães, observam-se melena e hemorragias petequiais.

CAUSAS
• Primárias — comprovadas em cães da raça Bedlington terrier, mas suspeitas em alguns parentes de Dálmata, Labrador retriever e West Highland white terrier.
• Secundárias — a hepatopatia colestática resulta em retenção secundária de cobre em alguns cães; frequentemente culmina em confusão diagnóstica quanto à relação causal de cobre com lesões patológicas.

FATORES DE RISCO
Primários — o fornecimento de dietas ricas em cobre ou água com alto teor desse elemento; o estresse também pode precipitar a doença aguda.

DIAGNÓSTICO

DIAGNÓSTICO DIFERENCIAL
• Doenças agudas — doenças infecciosas (p. ex., hepatite infecciosa canina, leptospirose e septicemia), necrose hepática aguda, abscedação hepática, lesão hepática induzida por medicamentos ou toxinas, pancreatite aguda, linfoma hepático, anemia hemolítica autoimune ou intoxicação pelo zinco.
• Doenças crônicas — hepatite crônica, fibrose hepática idiopática, colangio-hepatite de origem inflamatória ou imunomediada, lesão hepática induzida por medicamentos ou toxinas, hepatite infecciosa, doença biliar obstrutiva crônica, pancreatite fibrosante crônica, desvio portossistêmico congênito, neoplasia hepática ou neoplasia metastática.

HEMOGRAMA/BIOQUÍMICA/URINÁLISE
• Hemograma — os resultados podem permanecer normais. Em alguns animais com hemólise aguda associada ao cobre, observam-se anemia regenerativa, leucocitose e neutrofilia. Em certos cães com doença progressiva crônica, verifica-se anemia arregenerativa normocrômica microcítica ou normocítica.
• Bioquímica — nível elevado na atividade das enzimas hepáticas (aumento proeminente das transaminases) e hiperbilirrubinemia em alguns animais. O nível anormal das enzimas hepáticas sem sinais clínicos em raças predispostas deve levantar um alto índice de suspeita de hepatopatia por acúmulo de cobre. À medida que a função hepática se deteriora, podem ocorrer hipoalbuminemia, hiperglobulinemia, baixo nível de ureia, hipoglicemia ou hipocalcemia.
• Urinálise — os resultados costumam permanecer normais ou positivos quanto à presença de bilirrubinúria; mais tarde, observam-se urina diluída, cristalúria por biurato de amônio; a rara síndrome de Fanconi reflete toxicidade dos túbulos renais proximais pelo cobre.

OUTROS TESTES LABORATORIAIS
• Concentração elevada de ácidos biliares séricos totais em jejum ou pós-prandiais.
• Em casos avançados, há um prolongamento nos tempos de coagulação (i. e., TP, TTPA e TCA) e no tempo de sangramento da mucosa bucal.
• Em cães com necrose hepática aguda resultante de hepatotoxicose por cobre, as concentrações séricas desse elemento podem estar aumentadas; caso contrário, as concentrações séricas de cobre não refletem as concentrações teciduais desse elemento.
• As mensurações hepáticas de cobre devem ser conciliadas com os achados histopatológicos hepáticos.

HEPATOPATIA POR ARMAZENAMENTO DE COBRE

• Marcador genético de DNA para detecção de cães acometidos e portadores da raça Bedlington terrier: relata-se uma precisão de 95%. O teste específico para pesquisa da mutação do gene COMMD1 é mais preciso; no entanto, há relatos de que alguns cães acometidos da raça mencionada exibam resultados negativos para esse teste da mutação genética.

DIAGNÓSTICO POR IMAGEM
• Radiografias — na maioria dos cães, as radiografias abdominais não são dignas de nota; micro-hepatia (fígado diminuído de volume) em alguns cães cronicamente acometidos; detalhes abdominais insatisfatórios em casos de ascite.
• Ultrassonografia — ecogenicidade hepática normal no início; mais tarde, ecogenicidade nodular hiperecoica a mista.

MÉTODOS DIAGNÓSTICOS
Biopsia hepática — necessária para confirmar o tipo de lesão hepática e determinar as concentrações de cobre por meio de coloração (retenção qualitativa desse elemento) e quantificação. As concentrações hepáticas normais desse elemento são <400 µg/g de tecido hepático seco. As concentrações relatadas de cobre em cães com suspeita de hepatopatia primária por armazenamento desse elemento, de acordo com as raças, são as seguintes: Bedlington terrier: 850-12.000 µg/g de tecido hepático seco; West Highland white terrier: até 3.500 µg/g de tecido hepático seco; Doberman pinscher: 1.000-2.000 µg/g de tecido hepático seco; Dálmata: 750-8.400 µg/g de tecido hepático seco; Labrador retriever: 400-2.575 µg/g de tecido hepático seco. As concentrações de cobre por retenção secundária desse elemento costumam ser <1.000 µg/g de tecido hepático seco. A determinação hepática do cobre deve ser realizada no tecido hepático recém-coletado por biopsia.

ACHADOS PATOLÓGICOS
• Em casos de hepatopatia em fase terminal, o fígado encontra-se pequeno, nodular e cirrótico.
• O cobre acumula-se em lisossomos hepáticos na zona 3 (centrolobular) em casos de armazenamento primário desse elemento. A coloração histoquímica do cobre é semiquantitativa; ao exame histológico, a lesão envolve primeiramente necrose hepática focal, além de lesões piogranulomatosas, mas evolui para hepatite crônica e, finalmente, cirrose.

TRATAMENTO

CUIDADO(S) DE SAÚDE ADEQUADO(S)
• Tratamento feito em um esquema ambulatorial para a maioria dos cães.
• Avaliação e tratamento hospitalares para os cães com sinais de insuficiência hepática. Ver "Hepatite Crônica Ativa" e "Cirrose e Fibrose do Fígado" em busca de mais detalhes sobre o tratamento de hepatopatia.

CUIDADO(S) DE ENFERMAGEM
Os animais em insuficiência hepática necessitam de correção hidroeletrolítica adequada; tratamento de encefalopatia hepática; talvez haja necessidade de tratamento para coagulopatia.

ATIVIDADE
Normal.

DIETA
• É recomendável o fornecimento de dietas pobres em cobre aos animais acometidos; pode-se lançar mão das dietas caseiras balanceadas, evitando-se os alimentos ricos em cobre (p. ex., vísceras); no entanto, preferem-se as rações comerciais. Fornecer uma dieta hepática de prescrição que contenha o conteúdo mais baixo de cobre (aproximadamente 4 mg/kg). A administração de quelantes, em conjunto com as rações comerciais, pode ser bem-sucedida no tratamento do Bedlington terrier. Alguns cães da raça Labrador retriever submetidos a uma terapia de quelação bem-sucedida foram mantidos apenas sob dieta com baixo teor de cobre. Fornecer uma dieta de alta qualidade com níveis suficientes de proteínas e níveis moderados de gordura para atender às necessidades de energia. O conteúdo proteico deve ser reduzido apenas quando o paciente exibir encefalopatia hepática.
• Suplementar a dieta com vitaminas hidrossolúveis e evitar os suplementos minerais com cobre em sua composição.
• Medir o nível de cobre da água e restringir o acesso à água com níveis >0,2 ppm desse elemento.

ORIENTAÇÃO AO PROPRIETÁRIO
• Deve-se fazer a triagem de todos os cães da raça Bedlington terrier por meio do teste de mutação do gene COMMD1.
• Outras raças devem ser monitorizadas quanto à atividade anormal das enzimas hepáticas pelo exame de sangue ou à retenção de cobre por meio de biopsia do fígado.
• A terapia é necessária pelo resto da vida.
• Existem dúvidas quanto ao grau de predisposição genética em várias raças; no entanto, não se devem acasalar os animais acometidos a menos que o alto consumo de cobre na dieta seja considerado como a causa da doença.

CONSIDERAÇÕES CIRÚRGICAS
Os animais com insuficiência hepática apresentam riscos cirúrgicos e anestésicos.

MEDICAÇÕES

MEDICAMENTO(S) DE ESCOLHA
Ver as demais seções em busca de outros tratamentos específicos de hepatite e cirrose crônicas.

Terapia de Quelação
• D-Penicilamina (10-15 mg/kg VO a cada 12 h) — promove a quelação e a excreção urinária do cobre; supostamente, possui outros efeitos protetores. Deve-se instituir o tratamento em cães acometidos com concentrações hepáticas do cobre >1.000-2.000 µg/g de tecido hepático seco. Podem-se esperar quedas de aproximadamente 1.000 µg/g de tecido hepático seco por ano de tratamento em Bedlington terrier com concentrações de cobre >2.000 µg/g de tecido hepático seco. Outras raças, que possuem concentrações de cobre <2.000 µg/g de tecido hepático seco, podem chegar a níveis normais em 3 a 6 meses. Administrar 1 h antes das refeições. Pode-se associar esse medicamento com a ocorrência de vômitos; nesse caso, deve-se fornecê-lo com pequenas quantidades de alimento, embora o efeito desse medicamento diminua quando administrado com alimento. Após um curso terapêutico (6-12 meses), é recomendável repetir a biopsia para monitorizar a resposta. A quelação bem-sucedida em cães acometidos resulta em uma melhora histológica da hepatite (normalização da atividade da ALT).
• Cloridrato de trientina (5-15 mg/kg VO a cada 12 h) — constitui um quelante alternativo do cobre, que parece ser tão eficaz quanto à penicilamina com diretrizes semelhantes. Administrar 1 h antes das refeições. Em alguns cães submetidos a altas doses de trientina, foi observada insuficiência renal aguda.

Bloqueio da Captação Entérica de Cobre
• Zinco (100 mg de zinco elementar VO a cada 12 h, como dose de ataque por 2 meses, depois 25-50 mg VO a cada 12 h para cães do porte da raça Bedlington terrier); administrar sob a forma de acetato de zinco, 1 h antes das refeições. O zinco diminui a absorção intestinal de cobre; estudos demonstraram concentrações hepáticas reduzidas desse elemento com 2 anos de terapia em alguns cães das raças Bedlington terrier e West Highland white terrier. Pode ser benéfico em cães nos estágios precoces da doença ou com concentrações hepáticas mais baixas de cobre (geralmente <1.000 µg/g de tecido hepático seco). O zinco pode não ser eficaz em cães com concentrações elevadas de cobre (>1.000 µg/g de tecido hepático seco) e hepatite; nesse caso, é preferível a terapia de quelação. O vômito é um efeito colateral frequente da administração de zinco. Baixas doses de zinco administradas com uma dieta pobre nesse elemento em cães da raça Labrador retriever submetidos previamente à quelação não se mostraram mais eficazes do que apenas o uso da dieta com baixo teor de cobre.

Antioxidantes
• Dextroalfatocoferol (vitamina E na dose de 10 U/kg a cada 24 h VO); utilizar como terapia adjuvante.
• SAMe: utilizar também como terapia adjuvante.

Hepatoprotetores
• Silibinina (extrato de cardo mariano [*Silybum marianum*]) — utilidade indeterminada em casos de hepatopatia por armazenamento de cobre.
• Ácido ursodesoxicólico — recomendado em casos de hepatite crônica (ver "Hepatite Crônica Ativa") e altos níveis de ácidos biliares séricos totais.

CONTRAINDICAÇÕES
Ácido ascórbico (vitamina C) — não recomendado, pois pode aumentar a hepatotoxicidade do cobre.

INTERAÇÕES POSSÍVEIS
A penicilamina ou a trientina podem não ser eficazes quando administradas por via oral juntamente com o zinco.

ACOMPANHAMENTO

MONITORIZAÇÃO DO PACIENTE
• Nível das enzimas hepáticas a cada 3-6 meses; avaliar o peso e a condição corporais.
• Mensuração da concentração hepática do cobre dentro de 1 ano após o início do tratamento.
• Avaliação da concentração sérica do zinco em caso de terapia com esse elemento nas primeiras 2-3 semanas até a estabilização e em uma faixa não

Hepatopatia por Armazenamento de Cobre

tóxica (200-500 µg/dL) e, em seguida, a cada 4-6 meses.

PREVENÇÃO
• Acasalar apenas os cães da raça Bedlington terrier que não sejam portadores do defeito genético. Com base na concentração hepática de cobre <400 µg/g de tecido hepático seco com 1 ano de idade ou no teste genético, há um registro hepático disponível para os cães da raça Bedlington terrier comprovadamente não acometidos.
• A determinação das concentrações hepáticas de cobre depois de 1 ano de idade ajuda no diagnóstico dos animais acometidos.
• A mensuração periódica da ALT em raças de risco auxilia na identificação de cães acometidos para uma intervenção precoce.

COMPLICAÇÕES POSSÍVEIS
• Em casos raros, a D-Penicilamina pode causar glomerulonefrite, poliartrite ou doença vesicular semelhante a distúrbio autoimune das junções mucocutâneas que desaparece com a suspensão do medicamento.
• O excesso de zinco (dose oral >200 mg/dia ou concentração sanguínea >800 µg/dL) pode causar anemia hemolítica.

EVOLUÇÃO ESPERADA E PROGNÓSTICO
• Cães jovens agudamente acometidos por insuficiência hepática fulminante ou cães mais idosos com cirrose apresentam prognóstico mau.
• Cães jovens com lesão hepática aguda leve a moderada costumam responder à terapia com quelantes e apresentam prognóstico razoável.
• Em caso de detecção da doença (realização de biopsia hepática com base na atividade elevada da ALT e no alto índice de suspeita de hepatotoxicidade do cobre) antes do desenvolvimento de hepatite em cães submetidos à terapia apropriada, o prognóstico é bom.

DIVERSOS

GESTAÇÃO/FERTILIDADE/REPRODUÇÃO
Não acasalar os cães acometidos da raça Bedlington terrier nem os portadores.

SINÔNIMO(S)
• Hepatite do Bedlington terrier.
• Hepatite crônica ativa.
• Toxicidade crônica do cobre.
• Toxicose pelo cobre.

VER TAMBÉM
• Cirrose e Fibrose do Fígado.

• Hepatite Crônica Ativa.

ABREVIATURA(S)
• ALT = alanina aminotransferase.
• SAMe = dissulfato tosilato de S-adenosil-L--metionina.
• TCA = tempo de coagulação ativada.
• TP = tempo de protrombina.
• TTPA = tempo de tromboplastina parcial ativada.

RECURSOS DA INTERNET
www.vetgen.com em busca da triagem genética em cães da raça Bedlington terrier.

Sugestões de Leitura
Hoffmann G, van den Ingh TS, Bode P, et al. Cu-associated chronic hepatitis in Labrador Retrievers. J Vet Intern Med 2006, 20(4):856-861.
Mandigers PJ, van den Ingh TS, Bode P, et al. Association between liver Cu concentration and subclinical hepatitis in Doberman Pinschers. J Vet Intern Med 2004, 18(5):647-650.
Rolfe DS, Twedt DC. Cu-associated hepatopathies in dogs. Vet Clin North Am Small Anim Pract 1995, 25(2):399-417.

Autor David C. Twedt
Consultor Editorial Sharon A. Center

HEPATOPATIA VACUOLAR

CONSIDERAÇÕES GERAIS

DEFINIÇÃO
• Hepatopatia vacuolar — alteração vacuolar citosólica reversível dos hepatócitos em cães, associada, em geral, à vacuolização por acúmulo de glicogênio e, raramente, de lipídios. • Hepatopatia vacuolar por armazenamento de glicogênio — secundária a muitos distúrbios primários, incluindo tratamento com glicocorticoide, hiperadrenocorticismo, hiperplasia adrenal atípica (hormônios sexuais, especialmente 17-hidroxiprogesterona), doenças crônicas (inflamatórias, neoplásicas) em outros sistemas. • Caracteriza-se por atividade elevada da fosfatase alcalina, geralmente sem sinais de insuficiência hepática. • Aspecto histológico semelhante, mas notavelmente grave, à doença hepatocutânea (ver "Hepatopatia Diabética"); pode se desenvolver em cães sob terapia crônica com fenobarbital.
• Hepatopatia vacuolar com inclusões lipídicas discretas — hiperlipidemia idiopática; acúmulo de lipídio e glicogênio em casos de diabetes melito e hipotireoidismo.

FISIOPATOLOGIA
• Glicocorticoides — induzem ao aumento reversível do glicogênio nos hepatócitos dentro de 2-3 dias do tratamento; as formas injetáveis e as de depósito induzem à hepatopatia vacuolar mais grave em comparação às vias orais ou tópicas.
• Expansão celular — associada à hepatomegalia e degeneração dos hepatócitos, levando ao colapso e à nodularidade do parênquima, confundidos macroscopicamente com cirrose. • A resposta variável aos glicocorticoides entre os cães relaciona-se com (1) o tipo de medicamento, (2) a via, (3) a dose, (4) a duração do tratamento e (5) a sensibilidade de cada animal; a hepatopatia vacuolar pode ocorrer até depois da administração de glicocorticoides orais em baixas doses e a curto prazo. • A hepatopatia vacuolar pode refletir: reação ao estresse, citocinas ou resposta de fase aguda desencadeadas por distúrbios sistêmicos não hepáticos ou neoplasia (especialmente linfoma) na ausência de exposição a glicocorticoides ou doença adrenal. • A ocorrência de hepatopatia vacuolar é comum em casos de mucocele da vesícula biliar.

SISTEMA(S) ACOMETIDO(S)
Hepatobiliar — em geral, a função hepática permanece normal; hepatopatia vacuolar grave pode levar à insuficiência hepática.

INCIDÊNCIA/PREVALÊNCIA
• Cães — comum. • Gatos — rara; vacuolização hepática por acúmulo de triglicerídeos (ver "Lipidose Hepática").

IDENTIFICAÇÃO
Espécies
Cães; raramente, gatos.

Raça(s) Predominante(s)
Raças predispostas ao hiperadrenocorticismo (p. ex., Poodle miniatura, Dachshund, Boxer e Boston terrier), Terrier escocês (distúrbio dos hormônios sexuais por hiperplasia adrenal; hiperlipidemia) e outras com hiperlipidemia (Schnauzer miniatura, Pastor de Shetland, Beagle).

Idade Média e Faixa Etária
• Cães de meia-idade a idosos — quando causada por hiperadrenocorticismo espontâneo (>75% encontram-se acima de 9 anos de idade); quando associada à inflamação sistêmica crônica ou neoplasia. • Cães de qualquer idade — hepatopatia vacuolar iatrogênica subsequente à administração de glicocorticoides. • Cães ou gatos jovens — hiperlipidemia genética; filhotes caninos ou felinos — lipidose hepática juvenil.

SINAIS CLÍNICOS
Comentários Gerais
• Com frequência, os sinais clínicos refletem os glicocorticoides ou outra doença sistêmica subjacente. • Raramente, observam-se sinais clínicos de hepatopatia ou insuficiência hepática; em casos crônicos e graves de hepatopatia vacuolar e encefalopatia hepática, pode-se desenvolver insuficiência hepática, além de esses sinais serem observados em muitos cães com doença hepatocutânea (ver "Hepatopatia Diabética").

Achados Anamnésicos
• Excesso de glicocorticoides — poliúria e polidipsia; polifagia; alopecia endócrina; distensão abdominal; fraqueza muscular; respiração ofegante; letargia; pele friável; contusões.
• Hiperplasia adrenal produtora de hormônios sexuais — sinais semelhantes ao excesso de glicocorticoides, embora possam ser mais raros e menos graves; alopecia endócrina pode ser o único sinal apresentado; alguns cães permanecem assintomáticos, exceto pela atividade progressiva e crônica da fosfatase alcalina.

Achados do Exame Físico
• Hepatomegalia. • Relacionam-se com o excesso de hormônios esteroides ou com a doença subjacente; dependem da gravidade e da duração da doença.

CAUSAS
• Administração de glicocorticoides.
• Hiperadrenocorticismo típico. • Hiperplasia adrenal atípica — produção demasiada de múltiplos hormônios esteroides (especialmente 17-hidroxiprogesterona). • Administração crônica de fenobarbital — pode causar degeneração vacuolar grave. • Doenças sistêmicas associadas à resposta de fase aguda ou estresse — por exemplo, odontopatia grave, enteropatia inflamatória, pancreatite crônica, neoplasia sistêmica (especialmente linfoma), infecções crônicas (trato urinário, pele), hipotireoidismo, erros inatos do metabolismo lipídico (acúmulo de lipídio ou glicogênio).

FATORES DE RISCO
• Doses farmacológicas de fenobarbital.
• Raças sob risco de hiperadrenocorticismo.
• Raças sob risco de hiperlipidemia.

DIAGNÓSTICO

DIAGNÓSTICO DIFERENCIAL
• Outras hepatopatias difusas (especialmente aquelas indutoras de hepatomegalia e aumento na atividade sérica das enzimas hepáticas) — congestão passiva; neoplasia (primária ou metastática ao fígado); doença inflamatória; hepatopatia por anticonvulsivantes; distensão hepática por acúmulo de amiloide (raro).
• Características de distinção da hepatopatia vacuolar — a maioria dos cães apresenta aumentos mais acentuados nas atividades séricas da fosfatase alcalina em relação a ALT e AST; concentração sérica normal de bilirrubina; níveis normais a leves aumentos na concentração dos ácidos biliares séricos totais; parênquima hepático hiperecoico heterogêneo ou homogêneo à ultrassonografia (podem-se observar nódulos ou padrão semelhante a "queijo suíço"); aspecto citológico característico de hepatócitos.

HEMOGRAMA/BIOQUÍMICA/URINÁLISE
Hemograma Completo
• Depende da doença subjacente. • Anemia arregenerativa — anemia de doença crônica ou hipotireoidismo. • Policitemia relativa — excesso de esteroide. • Leucograma de estresse — hiperadrenocorticismo; exposição a glicocorticoides; estresse por doença.
• Trombocitose — neoplasia; hiperadrenocorticismo; doença esplênica.

Bioquímica
• Fosfatase alcalina e GGT — atividades acentuadamente elevadas; a isoenzima da fosfatase alcalina induzida por glicocorticoides não é capaz de diferenciar a causa de hepatopatia vacuolar, já que outros distúrbios hepáticos também induzem à formação dessa isoenzima; atividade variável das enzimas ALT e AST. • Albumina sérica e bilirrubina total — costumam permanecer normais; em geral, os níveis elevados de bilirrubina implicam algum outro processo hepatobiliar ou hemolítico. • Hipercolesterolemia — hiperadrenocorticismo, hiperplasia adrenal produtora de hormônios sexuais; certos erros inatos do metabolismo lipídico (hiperlipidemias); hipotireoidismo; pancreatite; síndrome nefrótica.

OUTROS TESTES LABORATORIAIS
• Ácidos biliares séricos totais — podem exibir modesta elevação. • Teste de tolerância à amônia — geralmente normal. • Isoenzima da fosfatase alcalina induzida por glicocorticoides — não tem utilidade clínica (ver anteriormente). • Eixo hipofisário-adrenal — o teste de resposta ao ACTH ou o teste de supressão com a dexametasona em altas e baixas doses, bem como o ACTH endógeno, podem ajudar a diferenciar distúrbio adrenal *versus* distúrbio hipofisário primário. • Relação de cortisol:creatinina urinários — a urina coletada em casa ajuda a descartar hiperadrenocorticismo; a alta relação pode refletir estresse hospitalar ou doença não adrenal. • Em casos de hepatopatia vacuolar confirmada por biopsia do fígado, causa subjacente não evidenciada, paciente assintomático ou presença de sintomas de doença adrenal — avaliar o perfil do cortisol e dos hormônios sexuais com o teste de resposta ao ACTH e usar o ultrassom para visualizar as adrenais. • Teste de função da tireoide — descarta hipotireoidismo. • Determinações dos triglicerídeos (em jejum) — quantificam o grau da hiperlipidemia. • Imunorreatividade da lipase pancreática canina — pode indicar inflamação pancreática ou enteropatia inflamatória "subclínica".

DIAGNÓSTICO POR IMAGEM
• Radiografia abdominal — revela hepatomegalia ou outras condições subjacentes. • Radiografia torácica — pode demonstrar linfadenopatia, doença metastática, distúrbios cardíacos ou pulmonares.
• Ultrassonografia abdominal — detecta hepatomegalia, parênquima hepático hiperecoico difuso ou imagem "mosqueada" nodular multifocal; as lesões multifocais são sugestivas de nódulos ("padrão de queijo suíço"); além disso, pode revelar comprometimento primário subjacente das vísceras (p. ex., linfadenopatia mesentérica) ou distúrbios da

Hepatopatia Vacuolar

adrenal (tamanho/formato; as adrenais podem estar aumentadas de volume em casos de hiperadrenocorticismo ou estresse crônico) ou neoplasia.

MÉTODOS DIAGNÓSTICOS
• Citologia hepática a partir de aspirado por agulha fina — agulha de calibre 22 com 2,5-3,75 cm de comprimento; pode-se aspirar o fígado difusamente aumentado de volume, sem a orientação por ultrassom; no caso de fígado com lesões multifocais, direcionar a agulha para os nódulos e o parênquima normal com a orientação ultrassonográfica. • Citologia — a vacuolização por acúmulo de glicogênio é comum em muitos distúrbios hepáticos primários. Exame utilizado para descartar alteração vacuolar; não é capaz de confirmar a hepatopatia vacuolar de forma definitiva. • Biopsia hepática — comprova a hepatopatia vacuolar e exclui outras hepatopatias primárias; prosseguir caso não se encontre outro distúrbio sistêmico que poderia explicar a atividade elevada da fosfatase alcalina e a hepatopatia vacuolar de origem hepática; para confirmar a hepatopatia vacuolar, pode-se usar a agulha de biopsia Tru-Cut® guiada por ultrassom; no entanto, o quadro de hepatopatia primária pode passar despercebido nesse tipo de exame; nesse caso, é recomendável a realização de laparoscopia ou laparotomia (se houver indicação de inspeções e biopsias viscerais). • Características citológicas — distensão citosólica vacuolar dos hepatócitos, causadora de "rarefação" ou aspecto granular do citosol dessas células. • Cultura tecidual e antibiograma — se houver suspeita de inflamação supurativa, enviar amostra para culturas bacterianas e fúngicas aeróbias e anaeróbias. • Avaliações dos perfis de coagulação — TP, TTPA, TCA, fibrinogênio, PIAVK e tempo de sangramento das mucosas; baixo valor preditivo para hemorragia iatrogênica.

ACHADOS PATOLÓGICOS
• Macroscópicos — variáveis; desde fígado normal até hepatomegalia moderada; irregularidade inconsistente da superfície; perda do padrão lobular normal; confundida com cirrose em caso de hepatopatia vacuolar avançada com colapso do parênquima. • Microscópicos — vacuolização e balonamento acentuados dos hepatócitos em padrões zonais, difusos ou focais; focos de degeneração/necrose hepáticas e macrófagos; agregados focais de neutrófilos associados à hematopoiese extramedular.

TRATAMENTO

DIETA
• Hiperlipidemia ou pancreatite — restrição de gordura na dieta; restrição de suplementos com alto teor de gordura. • Obesidade — restrição cautelosa de calorias; tratar quaisquer distúrbios predisponentes.

CONSIDERAÇÕES CIRÚRGICAS
• Dependem das condições subjacentes. • As massas adrenocorticais podem ser submetidas à ressecção. • Massas hipofisárias — a ressecção deve ser realizada apenas por cirurgiões experientes; se a experiência cirúrgica for limitada, a aplicação de radioterapia constituirá a melhor opção terapêutica das lesões expansivas hipofisárias.

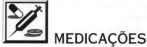

MEDICAÇÕES

MEDICAMENTO(S) DE ESCOLHA
• Dependem da doença subjacente. • Hiperadrenocorticismo dependente da hipófise ou síndrome de hiperplasia adrenal (anormalidade nos níveis dos hormônios sexuais) — costumam ser tratados por meio clínico: op'-DDD, trilostano ou cetoconazol (as duas últimas medicações diminuem as enzimas necessárias para a síntese de esteroides pela adrenal); o op'-DDD é o agente preferido para hiperplasia adrenal produtora de hormônios sexuais; o L-deprenil e a melatonina são ineficazes. • Tratamento de distúrbios inflamatórios primários que necessitam de medicamentos imunossupressores ou anti-inflamatórios — utilizar diversos medicamentos para minimizar a exposição aos glicocorticoides [ver "Medicamento(s) Alternativo(s)"] em casos de hepatopatia vacuolar sintomática. • Neoplasias — ressecção tumoral, quimio ou radioterapia, conforme for pertinente. • Odontopatias — antibioticoterapia e procedimentos odontológicos apropriados. • Enteropatia inflamatória — dietas proteicas hidrolisadas hipoalergênicas e imunomodulação (evitar o uso de glicocorticoides). • Pielonefrite, dermatite crônica ou outros distúrbios infecciosos — antibioticoterapia a longo prazo, selecionada com base nos resultados da cultura microbiana e do antibiograma; outros medicamentos adequados. • Hipotireoidismo — suplementação da tiroxina.

CONTRAINDICAÇÕES
• Evitar os medicamentos hepatotóxicos em caso de hepatopatia vacuolar sintomática. • Ao utilizar o cetoconazol (agente que prejudica o metabolismo de certos agentes terapêuticos), deve-se ter cuidado com as interações medicamentosas. • Evitar os medicamentos com efeitos de indução das enzimas hepáticas.

PRECAUÇÕES
Glicocorticoides — é preciso ter cautela com o uso desses medicamentos em pacientes com hepatopatia vacuolar; utilizar a dose mais baixa, porém eficaz, do esquema posológico (p. ex., empregar um protocolo em dias alternados caso se faça uso da prednisona ou prednisolona); tomar cuidado especial se o paciente estiver hiperlipidêmico: os glicocorticoides podem agravar os sinais clínicos de dor abdominal, vômito, pancreatite; aumentam as necessidades de insulina em animais com diabetes melito; podem aumentar a formação de mucocele da vesícula biliar; podem provocar lipidose hepática em gatos.

MEDICAMENTO(S) ALTERNATIVO(S)
Componentes de diversos agentes que podem ajudar no tratamento de distúrbios imunomediados ou inflamatórios; p. ex., metronidazol, azatioprina, clorambucila, ciclofosfamida, micofenolato ou ciclosporina.

ACOMPANHAMENTO

MONITORIZAÇÃO DO PACIENTE
• Hepatomegalia — palpação abdominal; inspeção com técnicas de diagnóstico por imagem.

• Normalização enzimática — bioquímica. • Função da adrenal — testes de estimulação com o ACTH. • Neoplasia — exame físico e diagnóstico por imagem. • Controle da infecção — repetição das culturas. • Hiperlipidemia — avaliação das concentrações plasmáticas de lipidemia; mensuração dos níveis de triglicerídeos e colesterol.

PREVENÇÃO
• Limitar a exposição a glicocorticoides. • Utilizar a terapia em dias alternados (se possível) com a prednisona; titular para a dose mais baixa, porém eficaz.

COMPLICAÇÕES POSSÍVEIS
Inúmeras — relacionadas com os efeitos multissistêmicos de glicocorticoides e distúrbios associados.

EVOLUÇÃO ESPERADA E PROGNÓSTICO
• A maioria dos pacientes permanece assintomática para hepatopatia vacuolar apesar da elevação da fosfatase alcalina; entretanto, em casos de hepatopatia vacuolar crônica em cães com aumento crônico na atividade da fosfatase alcalina, pode se desenvolver uma hepatopatia degenerativa progressiva que leva à formação de nódulos difusos e ao desenvolvimento de insuficiência hepática. • As anormalidades laboratoriais e os aspectos patológicos são reversíveis antes do colapso degenerativo do parênquima.

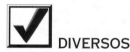

DIVERSOS

DISTÚRBIOS ASSOCIADOS
• Tromboembolia pulmonar e miopatia em virtude de hiperadrenocorticismo. • Pancreatite atribuível à hiperlipidemia. • Mucocele da vesícula biliar.

GESTAÇÃO/FERTILIDADE/REPRODUÇÃO
Falhas reprodutivas com o excesso de glicocorticoides — atrofia testicular; estro anormal.

SINÔNIMO(S)
• Hepatopatia por glicocorticoides. • Hepatopatia por esteroides. • Hepatopatia por corticosteroides. • Alteração vacuolar.

VER TAMBÉM
• Hepatopatia Diabética. • Hiperadrenocorticismo (Síndrome de Cushing). • Hiperplasia Nodular Hepática. • Mucocele da Vesícula Biliar.

ABREVIATURA(S)
• ACTH = hormônio adrenocorticotrópico. • ALT = alanina aminotransferase. • AST = aspartato aminotransferase. • GGT = gama-glutamiltransferase. • PIAVK = proteínas invocadas pela ausência ou pelo antagonismo da vitamina K. • TCA = tempo de coagulação ativada. • TP = tempo de protrombina. • TTPA = tempo de tromboplastina parcial ativada.

Sugestões de Leitura
Sepesy LM, Center SA, Randolph JF, et al. Vacuolar hepatopathy in dogs: 336 cases (1993-2005). JAVMA 2006, 229:246-252.

Autor Sharon A. Center
Consultor Editorial Sharon A. Center
Agradecimento Reconhecimento pela autoria prévia de Keith P. Richter

HEPATOTOXINAS

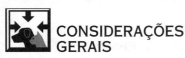

CONSIDERAÇÕES GERAIS

DEFINIÇÃO
- Substâncias endógenas ou exógenas (medicamentos, xenobióticos, toxinas) que causam lesão hepática.
- Direta — causa previsível de lesão.
- Idiossincrásica — imprevisível, não relacionada com a dose, apresentando hipersensibilidade imunomediada ou lesão metabólica.

FISIOPATOLOGIA
- O fígado tem alta suscetibilidade por causa de sua localização e de seu papel central em vias metabólicas e de destoxificação. A hepatotoxicidade é a intoxicação de órgão mais comumente relatada com reações adversas reais a medicamentos.
- Os mecanismos de dano podem ser diretos, decorrentes de subprodutos metabólicos ativos e/ou causados por processos oxidativos gerados por metabólitos de radicais livres.
- Pode causar lesão hepatocelular ou citolítica (necrose e apoptose), colestase, reação imunológica (espectador inocente ou mediada por hapteno) ou padrões histopatológicos mistos de lesão.
- Suscetibilidade e gravidade da lesão — influenciados por idade, espécie, estado nutricional, administração concomitante de medicamentos, doença anterior, estado antioxidante, fatores hereditários e exposição atual ou prévia aos mesmos compostos ou a similares.

SISTEMA(S) ACOMETIDO(S)
- Hepatobiliar. • Nervoso — encefalopatia hepática. • Renal — necrose tubular proximal; síndrome hepatorrenal (rara).

GENÉTICA
Algumas raças de cães podem ter predisposição à hepatotoxicidade associada a determinados medicamentos.

INCIDÊNCIA/PREVALÊNCIA
Não é incomum.

IDENTIFICAÇÃO
Espécies
- Cães e gatos. • Os gatos apresentam maior risco que os cães a algumas toxinas, em virtude de sua menor capacidade de destoxificação endógena e suscetibilidade à depleção de glutationa.

Raça(s) Predominante(s)
- Gatos da raça Siamês — algumas famílias exibem alto risco por causa da formação diminuída de glicuronídeos.
- Algumas raças de cães têm maior risco de certas intoxicações medicamentosas — Doberman, Dálmata e Samoieda por sulfato de trimetoprima; Doberman por oxibendazol; Labrador retriever por AINE (possivelmente); Cocker spaniel e Pastor alemão por fenobarbital; raças de pastoreio por polimorfismos do gene MDR1 (desarranjo na produção da glicoproteína P), com envolvimento de várias medicações e outros fatores farmacogenéticos.

Idade Média e Faixa Etária
- Qualquer idade.
- Animais jovens (menos de 16 semanas de vida) — vias metabólicas e excretoras hepáticas imaturas; discriminam menos as toxinas ingeridas.

SINAIS CLÍNICOS
Comentários Gerais
- Os sintomas podem refletir exposição crônica prolongada ou uma única exposição aguda a alguma toxina. • Anamnese detalhada — importante: incluir ambiente, medicamentos e histórico médico prévio.

Achados Anamnésicos
- Mal-estar a estado moribundo.
- Desenvolvimento de anorexia, vômito, diarreia, icterícia.

Achados do Exame Físico
- Temperatura corporal variável (hipotérmico a febre), vômito, diarreia, fraqueza. • Icterícia — manifesta ou progressiva (p. ex., 48-96 h após a exposição). • Ascite — rara (sinal grave).
- Encefalopatia hepática ou coma. • CID secundária à necrose hepática — hemorragia; petéquias; equimose.

CAUSAS
Qualquer medicamento, toxina ou xenobiótico pode causar hepatotoxicidade; são de gravidade variável; e ocorrem em qualquer indivíduo.

Medicamentos Comumente Relatados
- Paracetamol (cães e gatos). • Antifúngicos azólicos (cães e gatos). • Amiodarona.
- Amoxicilina. • Azatioprina. • Carprofeno — qualquer AINE (cães). • CCNU (cães).
- Ciclosporina. • Diazepam (gatos). • Doxiciclina (gatos, cães). • Glicocorticoides (cães).
- Griseofulvina (gatos). • Halotano (cães).
- Mebendazol (cães). • Metimazol (gatos).
- Metoxiflurano (cães). • Mitotano (Lysodren®, op'-DDD) (cães). • Fenitoína (cães). • Primidona (cães). • Fenobarbital (cães). • Estanozolol (gatos).
- Antibióticos tipo sulfa (cães). • Tetraciclina (gatos, cães). • Tiacetarsamida (cães, gatos).
- Trimetoprima-sulfadiazina (cães).

Toxinas Ambientais Comuns
- Cogumelos do gênero *Amanita* (cogumelos que contêm amanitina). • Aflatoxinas/micotoxinas.
- Algas cianofíceas (Cyanobacteria). • Compostos clorados. • Cicadáceas (castanha da palmeira do sagu). • Metais pesados (Pb, Zn, Mn, Ar, Fe, Cu).
- Substâncias químicas fenólicas (especialmente gatos). • Gossipol da semente de algodão.

Endotoxinas
- Microrganismos entéricos — *Clostridium perfringens*; *Clostridium difficile*; microrganismos Gram-negativos. • Intoxicação alimentar — *Staphylococcus*; *E. coli*; *Salmonella*.

Fatores Nutricionais/Herbários
- *Atractylis gummifera*. • Cimicífuga. • *Callilepis laureola*. • Chaparral. • Extratos de confrei (alcaloides pirrolizidínicos). • Ervas medicinais chinesas (certos constituintes, embora seja difícil caracterizar o conteúdo). • Germândrea (erva-carvalhinha). • Quelidônia-maior (erva-andorinha). • Extrato de chá verde. • Ácido lipoico (gatos). • Kava-kava (cães). • Alcaçus.
- Visco. • Poejo. • Sene. • Ácido úsnico.
- Valeriana. • Xilitol (adoçante; cães).

FATORES DE RISCO
- Medicações que influenciam o metabolismo hepático (indutores e inibidores enzimáticos).
- Hepatopatia prévia.
- Paciente submetido à exposição anterior, exposto atualmente (administração atual do medicamento) ou exposição recente não elimina sua consideração como uma causa de hepatotoxicidade.

DIAGNÓSTICO

DIAGNÓSTICO DIFERENCIAL
- Outros distúrbios hepáticos.
- Distúrbios infecciosos que acometem o fígado: leptospirose, hepatite infecciosa canina, PIF, toxoplasmose, riquetsioses (febre maculosa das Montanhas Rochosas, Erliquiose).
- Pancreatite necrosante hemorrágica aguda.
- Lesão hepática traumática ou hipóxica.
- O diagnóstico de evento hepatotóxico envolve a integração de fatores como histórico do paciente, ambiente, alimento, medicações e relação temporal.

HEMOGRAMA/BIOQUÍMICA/URINÁLISE
- Hematócrito e sólidos totais — frequentemente normais ou altos em hepatotoxicoses agudas (choque ou desidratação).
- ALT e AST séricas — podem estar extremamente altas; proporcionalmente mais altas que a atividade sérica da fosfatase alcalina; monitorizar o paciente de forma sequencial em busca dos valores máximos (pode ser de 10 a 100 vezes o normal) e o subsequente declínio na ALT e AST em 3-28 dias; sem importância prognóstica para um valor enzimático elevado inicialmente. Em casos de lesão citolítica, a atividade das aminotransferases pode preceder os aumentos na bilirrubina e na fosfatase alcalina.
- Fosfatase alcalina — em geral, continua subindo por vários dias a semanas à medida que a ALT declina.
- Creatino quinase — é preciso determinar seus níveis; alta atividade associada a mionecrose; algumas hepatotoxinas também lesam os músculos (p. ex., intoxicação por diazepam em gatos); atividade elevada da AST com níveis normais da creatino quinase implica lesão de origem hepática.
- Hiperbilirrubinemia — pode ser mínima ou se tornar progressivamente elevada.
- Albumina, ureia e glicose — variáveis.
- Glicosúria e cilindros granulares em caso de lesão dos túbulos renais proximais (p. ex., carprofeno). Algumas toxinas suprimem a síntese de enzimas hepáticas, dificultando o reconhecimento clínico da lesão hepática (p. ex., algas cianofíceas, aflatoxina).

OUTROS TESTES LABORATORIAIS
- Perfil de coagulação — TP, TTPA, PDF e plaquetas; antitrombina variável; monitorizar o paciente quanto à ocorrência de CID.
- Baixa atividade da proteína C — biomarcador para transcrição proteica bloqueada em aflatoxicose.
- Animal não ictérico — ácidos biliares séricos totais pareados para ajudar a avaliar função hepática ou níveis basais de referência.
- Ensaios para pesquisa de medicamentos ou toxinas — onerosos; resultados demorados.

DIAGNÓSTICO POR IMAGEM
- Radiografia abdominal — toxicidade aguda: fígado normal a aumentado de tamanho; lesão crônica: fígado de tamanho variável.
- Ultrassonografia abdominal — ecogenicidade, tamanho e margens hepáticas variáveis.

MÉTODOS DIAGNÓSTICOS
- Biopsia com agulha (do fígado) — pode confirmar ou apoiar o diagnóstico de lesão hepática; avaliará a gravidade se a lesão demonstrar

HEPATOTOXINAS

um padrão acinar ou zonal; se forem coletadas biopsias com agulha, serão necessárias múltiplas amostras (de preferência, com agulha de calibre 14 a 16); as amostras obtidas por laparoscopia são mais confiáveis.
• Aspiração com agulha: hepatócitos necróticos, inclusão lipídica citosólica; morfologia variável de células displásicas em toxicidade por aflatoxinas e cicadáceas.

ACHADOS PATOLÓGICOS
Variáveis, dependendo da toxina, do mecanismo de lesão celular, da zona acinar de metabolismo ou acúmulo de produto ou lesão vascular.

TRATAMENTO
CUIDADO(S) DE SAÚDE ADEQUADO(S)
Paciente hospitalizado — ambiente de cuidados críticos.

CUIDADO(S) DE ENFERMAGEM
• É imperativa a prevenção ou a correção do choque. • Fluidoterapia — manter a perfusão hepática para melhorar a oxigenação e a remoção de toxina; administrar uma vez e meia a necessidade de manutenção com atenção à pressão oncótica e ao estado de hidratação; administrar coloide se o nível de albumina estiver em 1,5 g/dL; fluidoterapia — evitar fluidos que contenham lactato em insuficiência hepática fulminante.
• Administração de coloide — é preferível o plasma inicialmente para o fornecimento de proteínas precursoras coagulantes e anticoagulantes, acompanhado pelo uso cauteloso de hetamido se justificável. • Tendências hemorrágicas — fornecer vitamina K1 (0,5-1,5 mg/kg SC ou IM, a cada 12-24 h); administrar sangue total ou plasma fresco congelado conforme a necessidade. (**Cuidado:** os produtos sanguíneos armazenados podem ter altas concentrações de amônia, causando encefalopatia hepática.)
• Oxigênio nasal — em caso de perfusão periférica comprometida (hipotensão) ou edema pulmonar; pode melhorar a distribuição de oxigênio ao tecido hepático. • Suspeitar de dano oxidativo como um componente da maioria dos eventos hepatotóxicos — administrar doadores de tiol ou de glutationa (ver adiante); a glutationa é importante para a conjugação direta de certas toxinas, pode facilitar a destoxificação de alguns metabólitos, aumentar a proteção antioxidante, ajudar a corrigir o estado de redox das células, conferindo resistência à apoptose e promovendo o reparo da membrana celular e a regeneração das células. • Monitorizar o débito urinário — diuréticos e dopamina (dose baixa sob infusão em velocidade constante) conforme o caso; ver "Insuficiência Renal Aguda". • Hipoglicemia — administrar glicose para manter a normoglicemia.

ATIVIDADE
Manter o animal quieto e em repouso.

DIETA
• Proteína — normal a menos que haja encefalopatia hepática franca.
• Suporte nutricional — NPP; mudar para NPT se houver inapetência por mais de 5 dias; considerar a colocação de cateter venoso central para NPT se as tendências hemorrágicas estiverem controladas; mais tarde, passar para suporte nutricional enteral com sonda nasoesofágica.

• Energia — estimada em 99 × (peso corporal em kg)^{0,67} para cães, 60 × (peso corporal ideal em kg) para gatos.
• Vitamina K1 — 0,5-1,5 mg/kg a cada 12 h por 3 doses e, em seguida, conforme a necessidade, com base no PIVKA ou TP.

ORIENTAÇÃO AO PROPRIETÁRIO
• Discutir o potencial de 3-10 dias da unidade de cuidados intensivos.
• Muitos se recuperam por completo; cirrose pós-necrótica e hepatite crônica podem se desenvolver após lesões hepáticas difusas.

MEDICAÇÕES
MEDICAMENTO(S) DE ESCOLHA
• Suplementação de eletrólitos — uso criterioso de cloreto de potássio e fosfato de potássio.
• Glicocorticoides de ação curta — para choque endotóxico (succinato sódico de prednisolona); o uso permanece controverso.
• Ampicilina, metronidazol, imipeném ou ticarcilina (intravenosos) concomitantemente com aminoglicosídeo ou enrofloxacina parenteral — aconselhados para proteger o animal contra infecções derivadas de migração transmural de microbiota entérica.
• Terapia antioxidante — para intervenção em crise: N-acetilcisteína para necrose hepática aguda ou fulminante (dose de ataque de 140 mg/kg IV, seguida por 70 mg/kg IV a cada 6-8 h; administrar durante 20 min e não por infusão em velocidade constante), diluir em solução fisiológica e administrar por meio de filtro não pirogênico de 0,25 μm; quando o paciente aceitar medicamentos por via oral e a condição se estabilizar, trocar para a S-adenosilmetionina oral (20 mg/kg, comprimidos com revestimento entérico VO a cada 24 h e com o estômago vazio); vitamina E sob a forma de acetato de d-α-tocoferol (10 UI/kg VO a cada 24 h).
• Vitaminas do complexo B — parenterais; cofatores essenciais para o metabolismo hepático.
• Silibinina (componente ativo da silimarina [extrato de cardo mariano]; utilizar a formulação complexada com a fosfatidilcolina (2-5 mg/kg a cada 24 h VO); benefícios mais bem caracterizados para toxicidade por *Amanita*; pode aumentar a regeneração hepática e conferir propriedades antioxidantes, hepatoprotetoras e antifibróticas.
• Ácido ursodesoxicólico — não é justificável a menos que haja hepatopatia crônica (10-15 mg/kg VO divididos a cada 12 h); administrar juntamente com alimento para melhor absorção. Em gatos anoréxicos, é prudente fornecer a suplementação de taurina (conjugação obrigatória de ácidos biliares com esse aminoácido).

CONTRAINDICAÇÕES
Evitar ou avaliar o risco de usar medicamentos que sabidamente provocam hepatotoxicose ou que necessitam ou inibem o metabolismo hepático.

PRECAUÇÕES
• Medicamentos relacionados como hepatotoxinas — usar com cautela.
• Cateterismo de grandes vasos e aspirados ou biopsias diagnósticos com agulha — ter cuidado na presença de testes de coagulação prolongados ou sangramento/contusão espontâneo.

ACOMPANHAMENTO
MONITORIZAÇÃO DO PACIENTE
• Evitar hipotermia. • Glicemia, eletrólitos e hematócrito — monitorizar diariamente; podem ocorrer oscilações rapidamente. • Hemograma completo, análise bioquímica sérica, TTPA, TP ou PIVKA — repetir a cada 48 h, conforme for justificável. • Monitorizar o débito urinário.

PREVENÇÃO
Verificar com detalhes o ambiente e as medicações futuras.

COMPLICAÇÕES POSSÍVEIS
• CID ou hemorragia. • Encefalopatia hepática.
• Insuficiência hepática progressiva. • Cirrose pós-necrótica.

EVOLUÇÃO ESPERADA E PROGNÓSTICO
• São necessários 3-5 dias para estimar o prognóstico.
• Agravamento progressivo do estado: êmese e hematêmese intratáveis, intolerância aos tratamentos de suporte, oligúria, CID e encefalopatia hepática — indicadores negativos.
• Declínio da ALT em 30% ou mais a cada 48 h com outros indícios de melhora é um indicador positivo; o declínio da ALT em insuficiência hepática fulminante pode indicar perda da massa hepática, evidenciada por sinais contínuos de função hepática reduzida ou progressiva.
• Cirrose pós-necrótica — possível em 3-6 meses.

DIVERSOS
DISTÚRBIOS ASSOCIADOS
• Hepatite. • Fibrose. • Encefalopatia hepática.
• Lipidose hepática (gatos). • Icterícia. • Ascite.
• Hipoglicemia. • Sepse.

FATORES RELACIONADOS COM A IDADE
• Animais jovens — podem estar sob maior risco de exposição e ingestão de toxina.
• Animais mais idosos — podem ter doenças que necessitam de medicamentos responsáveis pelo aumento do risco (p. ex., cimetidina, fenobarbital, AINE).

VER TAMBÉM
• Cirrose e Fibrose do Fígado. • Encefalopatia Hepática. • Envenenamento (Intoxicação).
• Insuficiência Hepática Aguda. • Toxicidade do Paracetamol.

ABREVIATURA(S)
• AINE = anti-inflamatório não esteroide. • ALT = alanina aminotransferase. • AST = aspartato aminotransferase. • CCNU = cloroetil-ciclo-hexil--nitrosureia. • CID = coagulação intravascular disseminada. • MDR1 = gene 1 de resistência a múltiplos medicamentos. • NPP = nutrição parenteral parcial. • NPT = nutrição parenteral total. • PDF = produtos de degradação da fibrina.
• PIF = peritonite infecciosa felina. • PIVKA = proteínas invocadas pela ausência ou antagonismo da vitamina K. • TP = tempo de protrombina.
• TTPA = tempo de tromboplastina parcial ativada.

Autor Mark E. Hitt
Consultor Editorial Sharon A. Center

HEPATOZOONOSE

CONSIDERAÇÕES GERAIS

REVISÃO
• Infecção sistêmica pelo protozoário *Hepatozoon americanum*.
• Pode envolver ossos, fígado, baço, músculos, capilares do miocárdio e epitélio do intestino delgado.
• Cães — mais comum no sul e no sudeste dos EUA.
• Gatos — incomum nos EUA; foi relatado um único caso no Havaí.

IDENTIFICAÇÃO
• Cães e, raramente, gatos.
• Sem predominância etária, racial ou sexual.

SINAIS CLÍNICOS
• Em geral, trata-se de uma infecção subclínica.
• Podem ser intermitentes e recidivantes.
• Doença clínica grave — febre; inapetência; perda de peso; diarreia sanguinolenta; sinais neurológicos (hiperestesia sobre as regiões paralombares).

CAUSAS E FATORES DE RISCO
Amblyomma maculatum — carrapato; picada ou ingestão.

DIAGNÓSTICO

DIAGNÓSTICO DIFERENCIAL
• Neoplasia.
• Endocardite.
• Poliartrite ou polimiosite imunomediadas.
• Doença de Chagas.
• Leishmaniose.
• Babesiose.
• Erliquiose.
• Discospondilite.

HEMOGRAMA/BIOQUÍMICA/URINÁLISE
• Leucocitose neutrofílica, algumas vezes com desvio à esquerda.
• Anemia — leve a moderada.
• Atividade sérica elevada da fosfatase alcalina.

OUTROS TESTES LABORATORIAIS
Esfregaços sanguíneos — identificam os microrganismos nos neutrófilos e monócitos circulantes.

DIAGNÓSTICO POR IMAGEM
Radiografias — da pelve, das vértebras lombares e dos ossos longos; revelam proliferação periosteal.

MÉTODOS DIAGNÓSTICOS
Biopsia muscular.

ACHADOS PATOLÓGICOS
• Caquexia.
• Atrofia muscular.
• Aumento de volume do fígado e do baço — podem conter estágios de esquizonte ao exame histopatológico.
• Proliferação periosteal do osso.

TRATAMENTO

• Paciente hospitalizado — para dor intensa; providenciar alívio sintomático.
• Controle da dor — como aquele efetuado para qualquer doença musculosquelética.
• Nível geral de atividade e apetite — dependem da magnitude da dor.
• Não é possível prever a responsividade à terapia medicamentosa (exceto o controle da dor), pois os dados são limitados.

MEDICAÇÕES

MEDICAMENTO(S)
• Principalmente paliativos.
• Glicocorticoides — podem conferir um alívio temporário.
• AINE.
• Terapia combinada inicial:
• Trimetoprima-sulfadiazina — 15 mg/kg VO a cada 12 h por 14 dias.
• Clindamicina — 10 mg/kg VO a cada 8 h por 14 dias.
• Pirimetamina — 0,25 mg/kg VO a cada 24 h por 14 dias.
• Seguidos por terapia prolongada:
• Decoquinato — 10-20 mg/kg VO a cada 12 h por até 33 meses.

CONTRAINDICAÇÕES/INTERAÇÕES POSSÍVEIS
Nenhuma.

ACOMPANHAMENTO

MONITORIZAÇÃO DO PACIENTE
• É difícil monitorizar os microrganismos em cães com infecção crônica.
• É melhor monitorizar a melhora.

PREVENÇÃO
Controle dos carrapatos dentro de casa ou no canil.

COMPLICAÇÕES POSSÍVEIS
• Glicocorticoides — podem exacerbar a doença clínica.
• É possível que nunca ocorram alterações radiográficas.

EVOLUÇÃO ESPERADA E PROGNÓSTICO
• A infecção frequentemente permanece assintomática.
• A qualidade de vida a longo prazo pode não ser satisfatória, mesmo com bons resultados terapêuticos.

DIVERSOS

POTENCIAL ZOONÓTICO
Não há risco relatado para seres humanos.

ABREVIATURA(S)
• AINE = anti-inflamatórios não esteroides.

RECURSOS DA INTERNET
www.vet.uga.edu/vpp/clerk/ludlow/index.htm

Sugestões de Leitura
Macintire DK, Vincent-Johnson NA, Craig TM. Hepatozoon americanum infection. In: Greene CE, ed., Infectious Diseases of the Dog and Cat, 3rd ed. St. Louis: Saunders Elsevier, 2006, pp. 705-711.
Macintire DK, Vincent-Johnson NA, Kane CW, et al. Treatment of dogs infected with Hepatozoon americanum: 53 cases (1989-1998). JAVMA 2001, 218:77-82.

Autor Johnny D. Hoskins
Consultor Editorial Stephen C. Barr

Hérnia de Hiato

CONSIDERAÇÕES GERAIS

REVISÃO
- Definida como a protrusão de qualquer conteúdo abdominal através do hiato esofágico do diafragma. Os órgãos mais comumente herniados incluem partes do esôfago abdominal e o fundo do estômago.
- Foram descritos vários tipos distintos de hérnias de hiato. A forma mais comum é a deslizante ou axial, em que ocorre um deslocamento simples do esôfago terminal, da junção gastresofágica e de parte do estômago em direção cranial através do hiato. Quando uma parte do estômago se desloca através do hiato paralelamente ao esôfago e à junção gastresofágica em posições normais, ocorre uma hérnia de hiato paraesofágica ou rolante.
- A doença pode ser congênita ou adquirida.

IDENTIFICAÇÃO
- Cães e gatos.
- A forma congênita é mais comum e os sinais tipicamente surgem em animais com menos de 1 ano de idade.
- A forma adquirida pode ocorrer em qualquer idade.
- Os machos são possivelmente super-representados.
- Os cães Shar-pei e Buldogue inglês são as raças mais comumente acometidas.

SINAIS CLÍNICOS
- O sinal clínico mais comum é a regurgitação, embora os pacientes também possam sofrer de outros sinais gastrintestinais, como diarreia, vômito, perda de peso e anorexia. Os sintomas podem ser episódicos em função da natureza dinâmica da doença.
- Também é possível a observação de sinais respiratórios. Esses sinais incluem tosse, dispneia e intolerância a exercícios. Os sinais respiratórios podem ser secundários ao deslocamento físico de órgãos respiratórios ou à pneumonia por aspiração.

CAUSAS E FATORES DE RISCO
- Congênita — as raças Shar-pei e Buldogue inglês são predispostas.
- Adquirida — pode ser decorrente de algum evento traumático ou atribuída a um aumento do esforço inspiratório. Também foi relatada como uma possível sequela do tétano.

DIAGNÓSTICO

DIAGNÓSTICO DIFERENCIAL
- Hérnia diafragmática peritoneopericárdica.
- Hérnia diafragmática traumática.
- Corpo estranho esofágico.
- Neoplasia esofágica.
- Esofagite.
- Megaesôfago.
- Anomalia do anel vascular.
- Intussuscepção gastresofágica.

HEMOGRAMA/BIOQUÍMICA/URINÁLISE
Em geral, permanecem dentro dos limites normais, embora seja possível a constatação de leucograma inflamatório, especialmente em animais com quadro subjacente de pneumonia por aspiração.

OUTROS TESTES LABORATORIAIS
N/D.

DIAGNÓSTICO POR IMAGEM
Radiografia Torácica
Classicamente, observa-se uma densidade de tecido mole na região do hiato esofágico. Em virtude da natureza dinâmica da doença, esse aspecto nem sempre pode estar presente em radiografias estáticas; nesse caso, a obtenção de radiografias seriadas pode ser útil para detectar a doença. As radiografias torácicas também podem detectar megaesôfago e/ou pneumonia por aspiração concomitante se presentes.

Esofagograma Contrastado e Fluoroscopia
Os estudos contrastados podem ter utilidade para confirmar o diagnóstico, bem como para descartar outras causas potenciais dos sinais clínicos e/ou das alterações radiográficas. O agente de contraste deve delinear as estruturas gastrintestinais responsáveis pela anormalidade e pode ajudar a excluir outros diagnósticos diferenciais. A confirmação do diagnóstico de hérnia de hiato é obtida quando se detectam a junção gastresofágica e/ou as pregas rugais em posição cranial ao hiato esofágico.

MÉTODOS DIAGNÓSTICOS
A esofagoscopia pode ser útil para confirmar o diagnóstico e traçar a gravidade da esofagite subjacente que costuma ser observada nesses pacientes.

TRATAMENTO

- Como muitos cães com hérnia de hiato permanecem assintomáticos, o diagnóstico pode ser um achado incidental.
- Nesses pacientes, não se justifica uma terapia rigorosa.
- O tratamento médico é tipicamente instituído em primeiro lugar nos cães mais idosos ou naqueles com sinais clínicos leves a moderados.
- Com frequência, há necessidade de terapia clínica para pneumonia por aspiração.
- A modificação da dieta é frequentemente uma medida adjuvante útil à intervenção médica. Os pacientes devem receber refeições frequentes em pequenas quantidades de uma dieta com baixo teor de gordura.
- Fica indicado o tratamento cirúrgico em casos irresponsivos a mais de 30 dias da terapia médica adequada, bem como em pacientes gravemente acometidos e naqueles com hérnias muito amplas.
- A correção cirúrgica é complexa e, portanto, deve ser realizada por um cirurgião experiente. Para a correção cirúrgica, é necessário que o cirurgião esteja bastante familiarizado com as técnicas de modificação de hérnia diafragmática e cirurgia gastresofágica. A intervenção cirúrgica envolve uma combinação de hiatoplastia diafragmática, esofagopexia e gastropexia. Foram descritos procedimentos de reforço do esfíncter, como vários procedimentos de fundoplicatura; tais procedimentos, no entanto, são relacionados com altas taxas de complicação e mortalidade perioperatória. As decisões quanto ao procedimento costumam ser tomadas durante a cirurgia pelo cirurgião e são ditadas pelos achados intraoperatórios, bem como pela experiência do cirurgião.

MEDICAÇÕES

MEDICAMENTO(S)
- Em geral, são prescritos medicamentos procinéticos para facilitar o esvaziamento gástrico e aumentar o tônus do esfíncter esofágico inferior.
- Gastroprotetores (como sucralfato) podem ajudar no tratamento de esofagite e gastrite concomitantes.
- Antagonistas dos receptores H2 (ranitidina ou famotidina) diminuem a acidez do refluxo gástrico.
- Omeprazol e outros inibidores da bomba de prótons podem ser administrados para reduzir a secreção ácida pelo estômago.
- Os antibióticos são adequados na presença de pneumonia por aspiração.

ACOMPANHAMENTO

- Os proprietários devem compreender que a terapia médica a longo prazo é frequentemente indicada em pacientes com hérnias de hiato submetidas a tratamento médico ou cirúrgico.
- O prognóstico varia de reservado a razoável.
- Os pacientes submetidos a tratamento clínico ou cirúrgico bem-sucedido poderão exibir uma persistência dos sinais clínicos se houver disfunção esofágica subjacente.

DIVERSOS

Sugestões de Leitura
Adamantos S, Boag A. Thirteen cases of tetanus in dogs. Vet Record 2007, 161:298-302.
Callan MB, Washabau RJ, Saunders HM, Kerr L, Prymak C, Holt D. Congenital esophageal hiatal hernia in the Chinese Shar-Pei dog. J Vet Intern Med 1993, 7:210-215.
Lorinson D, Bright RM. Long-term outcome of medical and surgical treatment of hiatal hernias in dogs and cats: 27 cases (1978-1996). JAVMA 1998, 213:381-384.

Autor S. Brent Reimer
Consultor Editorial Albert E. Jergens
Agradecimento O autor e os editores agradecem a colaboração de Margo L. Mehl, que foi o autor deste capítulo em edições anteriores.

HÉRNIA DIAFRAGMÁTICA

CONSIDERAÇÕES GERAIS

REVISÃO
- Protrusão de algum órgão abdominal através de abertura anormal no diafragma, na forma de lesão adquirida ou defeito congênito.
- Traumática — causa adquirida mais comum; costuma ser o resultado de traumatismo automobilístico, mas também pode resultar de qualquer pancada ou golpe violento; o aumento súbito na pressão culmina em um gradiente de pressão toracoabdominal, provocando laceração no diafragma, geralmente em uma porção muscular.
- Congênita — pleuroperitoneal ou peritoneopericárdica; podem-se mencionar outros defeitos congênitos (p. ex., defeito do septo ventricular, estenose aórtica, desvio portocaval e defeitos da parede abdominal cranioventral).
- Diminuição na expansão pulmonar normal — em função da falta de contato pulmonar com a pleura parietal.
- Alterações intrapulmonares (p. ex., contusão pulmonar, atelectasia e mudanças na permeabilidade capilar indutoras da formação de edema) — contribuem para uma troca gasosa deficiente.
- Fraturas de costelas causadas por traumatismo — podem contribuir para a hipoventilação, em virtude da dor ou de fatores mecânicos (tórax frouxo).
- O traumatismo miocárdico pode resultar em diversas disritmias — taquiarritmias ventriculares: mais comuns; observadas dentro de 24-72 h após o traumatismo; o controle não é uma tarefa fácil com o tratamento convencional; costumam desaparecer dentro de 5 dias.
- Vários estágios de choque — podem levar à falência múltipla dos órgãos.

IDENTIFICAÇÃO
- Cães e gatos.
- Adquirida — não há raça predominante.
- Congênita — as raças Weimaraner e Cocker spaniel podem ser predispostas; os gatos da raça Himalaio pode ser super-representados; pode ser diagnosticada em qualquer idade, pois os sinais clínicos são variáveis e intermitentes.
- Os animais jovens estão sob maior risco de hérnias diafragmáticas, tanto por causas congênitas como pelas traumáticas.

SINAIS CLÍNICOS
Traumática
- Pode ser aguda, subaguda ou crônica (sem histórico de traumatismo).
- É possível a constatação de sinais respiratórios de baixa intensidade ou histórico vago de problemas gastrintestinais.
- Os sinais clínicos podem ser progressivos.
- Taquipneia e angústia respiratória — sinais clínicos mais comuns; com frequência, os pacientes acometidos de forma aguda apresentam-se em choque.
- Arritmias — podem ser detectadas.
- Abafamento das bulhas cardíacas e dos ruídos respiratórios, juntamente com borborigmos intestinais — podem ser auscultados no tórax.
- Abdome — pode parecer vazio à palpação.
- Encarceramento agudo do intestino ou do estômago — pode causar vômito, diarreia, ânsia de vômito, timpanismo, dor e colapso agudo.

Congênita
- Pode ser assintomática, mas possivelmente se torna sintomática em uma fase posterior.
- Os sinais clínicos são atribuíveis aos sistemas respiratório, cardíaco ou gastrintestinal.
- Dispneia, abafamento das bulhas cardíacas, sopros e defeitos concomitantes da parede abdominal ventral — sinais mais comuns.
- Pode ser aguda, decorrente do estrangulamento de intestino, fígado ou baço encarcerados ou consequente à rápida formação de efusões pericárdicas.

CAUSAS E FATORES DE RISCO
Traumática — falta de confinamento e exposição a automóveis; qualquer traumatismo rombo; os animais errantes e os machos caninos estão sob risco mais elevado, em comparação a outros.

DIAGNÓSTICO

DIAGNÓSTICO DIFERENCIAL
- Ver "Dispneia e Angústia Respiratória".
- Ver "Respiração Ofegante e Taquipneia".
- Ver "Efusão Pleural".

HEMOGRAMA/BIOQUÍMICA/URINÁLISE
Podem-se observar alterações inespecíficas decorrentes de isquemia ou choque.

OUTROS TESTES LABORATORIAIS
N/D.

DIAGNÓSTICO POR IMAGEM
- Radiografia toracoabdominal padrão em duas projeções.
- Radiografia com feixe horizontal.
- Ultrassonografia.
- Radiografia contrastada — série gastrintestinal superior ou peritoneografia.

MÉTODOS DIAGNÓSTICOS
Indicação de toracocentese na presença de efusão pleural.

TRATAMENTO

Traumática
- Internação — tratar o choque; restabelecer a ventilação e o débito cardíaco; tratar a lesão concomitante; estabilizar o paciente antes da cirurgia.
- Cirurgia — fica indicada a intervenção precoce em casos de hipotensão persistente apesar da fluidoterapia adequada (incluindo transfusão, quando necessária), insuficiência respiratória grave por compressão pulmonar excessiva, insuficiência hepática grave secundária ao encarceramento de órgãos, ruptura intestinal ou intestino preenchido com gás e aumentado de volume, observado em radiografias; caso não se consiga estabilizar o paciente, o reparo cirúrgico não restabelecerá necessariamente os estados cardiovascular e respiratório.
- Dilatação gástrica intratorácica — exige a descompressão imediata.

Congênita
- Reparo cirúrgico — realizar o mais cedo possível para evitar a formação de aderências e o encarceramento de órgãos.
- Estabilizar os pacientes antes da cirurgia.

MEDICAÇÕES

MEDICAMENTO(S)
Agentes antiarrítmicos — conforme indicação; muitas vezes, o controle das arritmias cardíacas não se mostra uma tarefa fácil.

CONTRAINDICAÇÕES/INTERAÇÕES POSSÍVEIS
É preciso ter cuidado ao se tratar o animal em choque com contusão pulmonar grave concomitante; produtos como o hetamido podem ser benéficos.

ACOMPANHAMENTO

MONITORIZAÇÃO DO PACIENTE
Monitorização eletrocardiográfica frequente ou contínua — aconselhada; avaliar o paciente em busca de arritmias pós-operatórias.

COMPLICAÇÕES POSSÍVEIS
- Pneumotórax — pode se desenvolver a partir de uma pressão excessiva exercida sobre o tecido pulmonar lesionado durante a insuflação anestésica ou por falha na remoção de ar da cavidade torácica após o fechamento do diafragma.
- Hipertermia pós-operatória é comum em gatos.
- Edema pulmonar — pode se desenvolver a partir da administração demasiada de fluidos diante de pressão oncótica baixa decorrente de perda sanguínea, alterações na permeabilidade capilar secundárias à inflamação em resposta à contusão pulmonar, ou reexpansão.

EVOLUÇÃO ESPERADA E PROGNÓSTICO
Prognóstico — sempre é reservado no início; torna-se razoável, subsequentemente ao controle bem-sucedido do choque, à eliminação de qualquer arritmia cardíaca e ao sucesso da cirurgia, bem como na ausência de edema pulmonar de reexpansão. É pouco provável que os gatos mais idosos com hérnia diafragmática traumática sobrevivam ao reparo cirúrgico.

DIVERSOS

DISTÚRBIOS ASSOCIADOS
As hérnias diafragmáticas peritoneopericárdicas congênitas podem estar associadas a outros defeitos congênitos da linha média, como defeitos septais, fendas palatinas e defeitos da parede abdominal.

Sugestões de Leitura

Gibson TW, Brisson BA, Sears W. Perioperative survival rates after surgery for diaphragmatic hernia in dogs and cats: 92 cases (1990-2002). JAVMA 2005, 227:105-109.

Reimer SB, Kyles AE, Filipowicz DE, Gregory CR. Long-term outcome of cats treated conservatively or surgically for peritoneopericardial diaphragmatic hernia: 66 cases (1987-2002). JAVMA 2004, 224:728-732.

Schmiedt CW, Tobias KM, Stevenson MA. Traumatic diaphragmatic hernia in cats: 34 cases (1991-2001). JAVMA 2003, 222:1237-1240.

Autor Catriona MacPhail
Consultor Editorial Lynelle R. Johnson

HÉRNIA DIAFRAGMÁTICA PERITONEOPERICÁRDICA

CONSIDERAÇÕES GERAIS

REVISÃO
• Má-formação embriológica da linha média ventral, permitindo a comunicação entre as cavidades pericárdica e peritoneal.
• Pode estar associada a outras más-formações congênitas, incluindo deformidades do esterno (especialmente nos gatos), presença de hérnia abdominal cranial e defeitos do septo ventricular.
• Os sinais podem ser atribuídos à compressão do coração ou dos pulmões por grandes quantidades de vísceras abdominais e ao encarceramento dos órgãos abdominais (p. ex., fígado e intestino delgado).

IDENTIFICAÇÃO
• Cães e gatos.
• A idade em que ocorrem os primeiros sinais clínicos varia; mais de um terço dos pacientes tem 4 anos de idade ou mais.
• Weimaraner e Persa podem estar predispostos.
• Não há provas de que as lesões sejam hereditárias, embora haja relatos em ninhadas.

SINAIS CLÍNICOS
Comentários Gerais
• Depende da natureza e da quantidade de conteúdo abdominal que sofreu herniação.

Achados Anamnésicos
• Vômito.
• Diarreia.
• Perda de peso.
• Dor abdominal.
• Tosse.
• Dispneia.

Achados do Exame Físico
• Sons cardíacos abafados.
• Impulso cardíaco apical deslocado ou atenuado.
• Deformidade esternal palpável ou hérnia abdominal cranial.
• Tamponamento cardíaco e sinais de insuficiência cardíaca congestiva do lado direito (raros).

CAUSAS E FATORES DE RISCO
• Má-formação embriológica.
• Lesão pré-natal do septo transverso e das dobras pleuroperitoneais.

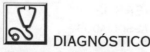

DIAGNÓSTICO

DIAGNÓSTICO DIFERENCIAL
• Nunca se trata de um defeito traumático adquirido, porque não há comunicação direta natural existente entre as cavidades peritoneal e pericárdica após o nascimento.
• Efusão pericárdica.

HEMOGRAMA/BIOQUÍMICA/URINÁLISE
Nenhuma alteração hematológica ou bioquímica associada.

OUTROS TESTES LABORATORIAIS
N/D.

DIAGNÓSTICO POR IMAGEM
• Os achados radiográficos dependem do tamanho do defeito e da quantidade de conteúdo abdominal herniado; a margem cardíaca caudal e o diafragma podem se sobrepor; as radiografias torácicas podem mostrar o abdome "vazio" e possíveis densidades radiográficas múltiplas.
• A peritoneografia com contraste positivo e negativo é utilizada para avaliar o diafragma. A injeção de 1-2 mL/kg de peso corporal de material de contraste positivo hidrossolúvel dentro da cavidade peritoneal, seguida por radiografias em decúbito lateral direito e esquerdo, esternal e dorsal, permitem a avaliação completa do diafragma. A identificação do contraste dentro do espaço pleural confirma o diagnóstico de ruptura diafragmática. Materiais como ar, dióxido de carbono ou óxido nitroso também podem ser usados.
• A sequência radiográfica com bário pode demonstrar as alças intestinais, atravessando o diafragma e dentro do saco pericárdico.
• A angiografia não seletiva delineia as câmaras cardíacas dentro da grande silhueta cardíaca.
• A ecocardiografia fornece o diagnóstico definitivo.

MÉTODOS DIAGNÓSTICOS
O ECG poderá revelar complexos pequenos em caso de herniação do conteúdo abdominal ou na presença de efusão acentuada.

TRATAMENTO

A oclusão cirúrgica da hérnia após o retorno dos órgãos viáveis a seus locais normais geralmente é curativa. Nos pacientes adultos assintomáticos com pequenas hérnias, o tratamento pode ser dispensável.

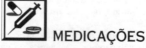

MEDICAÇÕES

MEDICAMENTO(S)
• A contratilidade miocárdica não é acometida na maioria dos pacientes; não é indicado o uso de medicamentos para aumentar o débito cardíaco.
• Pode-se administrar um tratamento sintomático com base na natureza e na quantidade de conteúdo abdominal herniado.

CONTRAINDICAÇÕES/INTERAÇÕES POSSÍVEIS
Os medicamentos que diminuem a pós-carga (p. ex., vasodilatadores arteriolares) ou a pré-carga (p. ex., dilatadores venosos e diuréticos) ventricular não são úteis e podem causar redução de enchimento ventricular, hipotensão e baixo débito cardíaco.

ACOMPANHAMENTO

O prognóstico após a cirurgia é excelente nos animais sem anomalias congênitas significativas ou fatores indutores de complicação.

DIVERSOS

RECURSOS DA INTERNET
www.vetgo.com/cardio.

Sugestões de Leitura
Kienle RD. Pericardial disease and cardiac neoplasia. In: Kittleson MD, Kienle RD, eds., Small Animal Cardiovascular Medicine. St. Louis: Mosby, 1999, pp. 413-432.
Neiger R. Peritoneopericardial diaphragmatic hernia in cats. Compend Contin Educ Pract Vet 1996, 461-479.
Reimer SB, Kyles AE, Filipowicz DE, et al. Long-term outcome of cats treated conservatively or surgically for peritoneopericardial diaphragmatic hernia: 66 cases (1987-2002). JAVMA 2004, 224:728-732.
Tobias AH, McNiel EA. Pericardial disorders and cardiac tumors. In: Tilley LP, Smith FWK, Oyama MA, Sleeper MM, eds., Manual of Canine and Feline Cardiology, 4th ed. St. Louis: Saunders Elsevier, 2008, pp. 200-214.

Autor Larry P. Tilley
Consultores Editoriais Larry P. Tilley e Francis W. K. Smith, Jr.

HÉRNIA PERINEAL

CONSIDERAÇÕES GERAIS

REVISÃO
Resulta da falha dos músculos do diafragma pélvico em conferir sustentação adequada, fazendo com que as estruturas pélvicas e/ou abdominais sofram herniação para a região perineal.

FISIOPATOLOGIA
- A herniação ocorre mais comumente entre o músculo levantador do ânus e o esfíncter externo do ânus. Também pode ocorrer entre os músculos levantador do ânus e coccígeo.
- É amplamente defendida a ideia de que os músculos do diafragma pélvico sofrem um enfraquecimento progressivo. Esforço crônico, atrofia neurogênica ou influência hormonal de androgênios são hipóteses que conquistaram considerável apoio como causa do enfraquecimento.
- A prostatopatia é um fator potencial que contribui para a hérnia perineal.

IDENTIFICAÇÃO
- É mais comumente diagnosticada em cães do que em gatos.
- Machos intactos são acometidos com uma frequência muito maior do que machos castrados ou quaisquer fêmeas.
- Existem predileções raciais por Pequinês, Boston terrier, Welsh corgi, Dachshund, Collie e Old English sheepdog.
- Costuma ser diagnosticada em cães com mais de 5 anos de idade.

SINAIS CLÍNICOS
Achados Anamnésicos
- Tenesmo.
- Disquezia.
- Estrangúria/anúria em caso de encarceramento da bexiga urinária.
- Incontinência (urinária e fecal).
- O proprietário pode ter observado uma tumefação (inchaço) não clínico na região perineal.

Achados do Exame Físico
- Tumefação perineal — tipicamente visualizada/palpada na região entre o túber isquiático e o ânus. Pode ser uni (59%) ou bilateral (41%).
- Pode estar sistemicamente enfermo em casos de estrangulamento de vísceras ou encarceramento do trato urinário.
- Tipicamente, o diagnóstico é feito por uma combinação do histórico do paciente e dos achados do exame físico, bem como pela detecção de defeito no diafragma pélvico durante o exame retal.

CAUSAS E FATORES DE RISCO
- Desconhecidos.
- As causas sugeridas incluem influência crônica de androgênios, prostatopatia, tenesmo crônico, doença colorretal, atrofia neurogênica dos músculos do diafragma pélvico.

DIAGNÓSTICO

DIAGNÓSTICO DIFERENCIAL
- Neoplasia perianal.
- Doença do saco anal (inflamação ou neoplasia).
- Neoplasia do trato genital ou urinário.

HEMOGRAMA/BIOQUÍMICA/URINÁLISE
- Sem alterações previsíveis.
- Azotemia pós-renal secundária à obstrução urinária se presente.

DIAGNÓSTICO POR IMAGEM
- Radiografias — podem registrar as vísceras envolvidas na hérnia. Também podem confirmar a localização da bexiga urinária dentro da hérnia ou da cavidade abdominal.
- Radiografia contrastada — cistogramas ou uretrogramas podem ser utilizados para ajudar na localização do trato urinário inferior. Os colonogramas raramente são usados para confirmar envolvimento colônico, bem como para comprovar qualquer saculação ou dilatação retal.
- Ultrassonografia — raras vezes empregada para confirmar o encarceramento de estruturas dentro da hérnia, como bexiga urinária, próstata, gordura retroperitoneal.

MÉTODOS DIAGNÓSTICOS
Exame retal — revela enfraquecimento palpável do diafragma pélvico. Também pode revelar saculação ou desvio retal.

TRATAMENTO

- Em virtude das sequelas potencialmente letais de encarceramento vesical ou estrangulamento visceral, não é recomendável a protelação da intervenção cirúrgica.
- O aumento do conteúdo de fibra na dieta e a administração de amolecedores fecais, laxantes e enemas, conforme a necessidade, podem ajudar a manter a consistência das fezes, o que minimiza os sinais clínicos até a instituição da correção cirúrgica.

CONSIDERAÇÕES CIRÚRGICAS
- A cirurgia deve ser realizada no paciente estável. Os pacientes com obstrução urinária podem necessitar de cateterização uretral e estabilização no período pré-operatório para estabelecer a eliminação de urina, bem como para corrigir a azotemia ou as anormalidades eletrolíticas. A intervenção cirúrgica não deve ser adiada em pacientes com obstrução urinária ou gastrintestinal.
- Foram descritos muitos procedimentos cirúrgicos distintos. Herniorrafia com o uso de retalho (*flap*) do músculo obturador interno constitui a técnica de escolha para muitos.
- Outras técnicas incluem transposição do músculo glúteo superficial, transposição do músculo semitendíneo e janela anal, bem como reposição anatômica tradicional.
- Caso haja escassez de tecido, poderá ser empregada uma combinação de técnicas ou implantes cirúrgicos biocompatíveis como uso de submucosa de intestino delgado de suíno ou malha de polipropileno.
- Procedimentos como colopexia, cistopexia e vasopexia também podem ser utilizados na tentativa de manter seus respectivos órgãos abdominais dentro da cavidade abdominal de forma permanente.
- A castração de cães machos intactos também é necessária, pois os cães não castrados têm uma taxa de recidiva 2,7 vezes maior que os castrados.

MEDICAÇÕES

MEDICAMENTO(S)
- Em virtude da proximidade anatômica da incisão cirúrgica ao ânus, sugere-se o uso perioperatório de antibióticos.
- Alguns cirurgiões preferem utilizar amolecedores fecais no período pós-operatório para minimizar o tenesmo, enquanto outros preferem aumentar o volume das fezes pelo uso de um teor elevado de fibras na dieta.

ACOMPANHAMENTO

PREVENÇÃO
É recomendável a castração de cães para prevenção dessa doença.

COMPLICAÇÕES POSSÍVEIS
As complicações cirúrgicas são frequentes e incluem infecção, incontinência fecal, prolapso retal, recidiva e paralisia do nervo ciático, bem como tenesmo contínuo.

EVOLUÇÃO ESPERADA E PROGNÓSTICO
Há relatos de que as taxas de recidiva estejam entre 0 e 50%.

DIVERSOS

DISTÚRBIOS ASSOCIADOS
- Prostatopatias (hipertrofia prostática benigna, prostatite, cistos prostáticos etc.).
- Megacólon.
- Tenesmo.
- Saculação, divertículo, desvio retais.

Sugestões de Leitura
Bellenger CR, Canfield RB. Perineal hernia. In: Slatter D, ed., Textbook of Small Animal Surgery, 3rd ed. Philadelphia: Saunders, 2003, pp. 487-498.
Stoll MR, Cook JL, Pope ER, et al. The use of porcine small intestinal submucosa as a biomaterial for perineal herniorrhaphy in the dog. Vet Surg 2002, 31:379-390.
Szabo S, Wilkens B, Radasch RM. Use of polypropylene mesh in addition to internal obturator transposition: A review of 59 cases (2000-2004). JAAHA 2007, 43:136-142.

Autor S. Brent Reimer
Consultor Editorial Albert E. Jergens

HIDROCEFALIA

CONSIDERAÇÕES GERAIS

DEFINIÇÃO
- Dilatação anormal do sistema ventricular atribuída ao aumento de volume do LCS.
- Pode ser simétrica ou assimétrica.
- Pode envolver todo o sistema ventricular ou apenas elementos proximais ao local de obstrução do sistema ventricular.

FISIOPATOLOGIA
- A hidrocefalia consiste em uma distensão ativa do sistema ventricular — mais comumente obstrutiva, mas muito raramente por produção excessiva do LCS.
- Obstrutiva — o LCS acumula-se antes da obstrução, com um padrão circulatório normal do LCS (não comunicante) ou em seu local de reabsorção pelas vilosidades aracnoides meníngeas (comunicante); dependendo do equilíbrio entre a produção de LCS (que é constante e independente da PIC) e da capacidade de absorção desse líquido, a PIC pode estar normal ou elevada; podem ser observados sinais clínicos em qualquer um dos casos.
- Obstrução congênita — hidrocefalia obstrutiva primária; o local mais comum é na altura do aqueduto mesencefálico em virtude da fusão dos colículos rostrais; infecções pré-natais (sobretudo pelo vírus da parainfluenza) podem causar estenose do aqueduto com subsequente hidrocefalia; pode resultar em alteração considerável da arquitetura do cérebro.
- Obstrução adquirida — hidrocefalia obstrutiva secundária; os locais incluem os forames interventriculares, o aqueduto mesencefálico ou as aberturas laterais do quarto ventrículo.
- Produção excessiva de LCS (comunicante) — rara; causada, por exemplo, por algum tumor do plexo coroide.
- "Hidrocefalia compensatória" é um termo utilizado antigamente para descrever uma condição em que o LCS ocupa o espaço onde o parênquima neural foi destruído; essa condição não é uma hidrocefalia verdadeira; tal terminologia, portanto, é obsoleta.
- Os sinais clínicos de disfunção neurológica resultam de dano ao parênquima neural, o que possui etiologia multifatorial.

SISTEMA(S) ACOMETIDO(S)
Nervoso.

GENÉTICA
Gatos da raça Siamês — autossômica recessiva.

INCIDÊNCIA/PREVALÊNCIA
Desconhecidas.

IDENTIFICAÇÃO
Espécies
Cães e gatos.

Raça(s) Predominante(s)
- Congênita — cães de pequeno porte e braquicefálicos: Buldogue, Chihuahua, Maltês, Pomerânia, Poodle toy, Yorkshire terrier, Lhasa apso, Cairn terrier, Boston terrier, Pug e Pequinês.
- Hereditária — gatos da raça Siamês e cães da raça Yorkshire terrier. Alta incidência de ventriculomegalia clinicamente assintomática em Beagles adultos normais.
- Adquirida — qualquer raça de cão ou gato.

Idade Média e Faixa Etária
- Congênita — em geral se torna aparente em algumas semanas de vida a 1 ano de idade. Pode ocorrer início agudo dos sinais em cães com hidrocefalia congênita não diagnosticada antes. A causa exata dessa descompensação é incerta.
- Adquirida — qualquer idade.

Sexo Predominante
Nenhum.

SINAIS CLÍNICOS
Comentários Gerais
- Congênita — pode ocorrer sem sinais clínicos, especialmente em cães de raças toy; é possível notar outras más-formações ou anomalias do SNC (p. ex., más-formações do cerebelo ou siringomielia), o que pode contribuir ainda mais para a miríade de sinais.
- Adquirida — os sinais atribuíveis à doença subjacente podem ser tão ou mais proeminentes que os atribuíveis à hidrocefalia.
- A gravidade dos sinais clínicos pode não corresponder ao grau de aumento ventricular.

Achados Anamnésicos
- Comportamentais — diminuição da consciência; falta ou perda da capacidade de ser adestrado (inclusive em casa); sonolência excessiva; vocalização; às vezes, hiperexcitabilidade.
- Déficits visuais, incluindo cegueira.
- Crises convulsivas — podem ser observadas.

Achados do Exame Físico
- Cabeça — pode parecer grande e em forma de abóbada, com um "topo" exagerado; com frequência, existem suturas abertas e/ou fontanelas persistentes; esses achados, no entanto, podem estar presentes sem hidrocefalia e vice-versa. Alguns cães com hidrocefalia congênita grave apresentam estrabismo bilateral divergente — em virtude de má-formação da órbita ou disfunção do tronco cerebral.

Achados do Exame Neurológico
- Os sinais podem ser de início agudo ou gradativo, embora possam ser estáticos ou progressivos.
- Pode ocorrer uma ampla variedade de sinais de disfunção cerebral.
- Doença cerebral — comportamento anormal (entorpecimento e sonolência), cegueira cortical (perda da visão com olhos e reflexos pupilares à luz normais), vocalização imprópria, às vezes hiperexcitável; pode haver o andar em círculos na doença lateralizada.
- Anormalidades da marcha — incoordenação, ataxia e reações posturais diminuídas.
- Crises convulsivas — podem ocorrer.
- Forma congênita — a má-formação da órbita durante o crescimento pode resultar em estrabismo ventrolateral com movimentos oculocefálicos normais; os movimentos oculocefálicos podem estar anormais se a disfunção do tronco cerebral for a causa do estrabismo.
- Aumento acentuado da PIC — estupor ou coma, pupilas extremamente mióticas (puntiformes) ou fixas dilatadas, perda dos movimentos oculocefálicos normais (nistagmo fisiológico), padrões respiratórios anormais e postura descerebrada; pode levar à herniação tentorial fatal.
- A gravidade dos sinais clínicos pode não se correlacionar com o tamanho do ventrículo, embora haja uma tendência de agravamento dos sinais clínicos com o maior aumento dos ventrículos.

CAUSAS
- Congênita — inúmeras más-formações congênitas provocam obstrução do sistema ventricular e resultam em hidrocefalia; má-formação hereditária, infecção pré-natal (p. ex., cães: vírus da parainfluenza, gatos: coronavírus), exposição aos teratógenos, hemorragia cerebral secundária à distocia, deficiência nutricional (vitamina A) e outras.
- Adquirida — tumores, abscessos e doenças inflamatórias (incluindo inflamação resultante de hemorragia causada por lesões traumáticas ou outras causas de sangramento).

FATORES DE RISCO
Os animais com hidrocefalia compensada podem descompensar diante de algum insulto como infecção ou traumatismo, resultando no desenvolvimento de sinais clínicos.

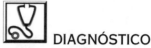

DIAGNÓSTICO

DIAGNÓSTICO DIFERENCIAL
- Outras anomalias cerebrais congênitas.
- Doenças tóxicas ou metabólicas que resultam em disfunção cerebral.
- Lesões cerebrais expansivas ou doenças infecciosas que resultam em elevação da PIC (podem coexistir com hidrocefalia).
- Lesão cerebral traumática (pode haver hidrocefalia coexistente).

HEMOGRAMA/BIOQUÍMICA/URINÁLISE
Geralmente normais.

DIAGNÓSTICO POR IMAGEM
- Radiografia do crânio (congênita) — revela aumento do crânio em forma de abóbada com suturas abertas e fontanelas persistentes; a abóbada craniana pode ter um aspecto em vidro fosco. As radiografias do crânio também podem revelar adelgaçamento da calvária.
- TC e RM — fornecem o diagnóstico definitivo.
- Ultrassom realizado através das fontanelas abertas — pode revelar aumento dos ventrículos.

MÉTODOS DIAGNÓSTICOS
- Análise do LCS — ter extremo cuidado ao coletar a amostra se o paciente estiver com a PIC elevada (isso pode ocasionar herniação cerebral fatal através do forame magno e/ou abaixo do tentório do cerebelo); a composição permanecerá normal se não houver outra doença intracraniana (p. ex., neoplasia e inflamação); no entanto, essa composição estará frequentemente anormal na presença de doença subjacente adquirida.
- EEG — congênita: em geral característico, incluindo hipersincronia, alta amplitude (25-300 μV) e baixa frequência (1-7 Hz); adquirida: os achados variam.

ACHADOS PATOLÓGICOS
- Cérebro — pode estar aumentado com perda do padrão normal de sulcos e giros; é possível observar distorção do parênquima, inclusive adelgaçamento do córtex cerebral, ruptura do septo pelúcido e atrofia de outras estruturas adjacentes; com doença grave, pode ocorrer herniação cerebral, seja do cérebro e do mesencéfalo sob o tentório cerebelar ou do

cerebelo e da medula oblonga caudal através do forame magno.
• Sistema ventricular — distensão leve a grave (de todo o sistema ou apenas da parte rostral à lesão obstrutiva); com a forma não comunicante, observa-se estreitamento ou obstrução do sistema ventricular em virtude de inflamação ou lesões expansivas.

TRATAMENTO

CUIDADO(S) DE SAÚDE ADEQUADO(S)
• Paciente hospitalizado — cuidados intensivos para aqueles com sinais graves ou quando submetidos a tratamento cirúrgico.
• Paciente de ambulatório — aqueles com sinais leves a moderados que podem receber tratamento clínico.

CUIDADO(S) DE ENFERMAGEM
Evitar as complicações secundárias do decúbito nos pacientes em estado de estupor ou coma — evitar úlceras de pressão; ressecamento ocular; e congestão pulmonar hipostática.

ORIENTAÇÃO AO PROPRIETÁRIO
Alertar o proprietário a observar sinais de deterioração no estado de alerta mental, na visão e no comportamento, o que pode sinalizar agravamento do problema.

CONSIDERAÇÕES CIRÚRGICAS
• Desvio cirúrgico do LCS dos ventrículos para a cavidade peritoneal ou o átrio direito — tratamento definitivo.
• A cirurgia deve ser considerada apenas quando o tratamento clínico for ineficaz ou resultar em efeitos colaterais adversos.
• Complicações — ocorre obstrução do desvio em até 50% dos pacientes; a ocorrência de infecção é menos comum; comumente há necessidade de revisão do desvio; o desvio exagerado pode resultar em complicações graves e potencialmente fatais (colapso do manto cerebral).
• Os sinais clínicos podem não se resolver por completo; sinais residuais, em geral, indicam dano cerebral irreversível.
• Cirurgia de tumor cerebral ou outra lesão expansiva — considerar se for a causa subjacente.

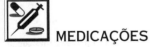

MEDICAÇÕES

MEDICAMENTO(S) DE ESCOLHA
• Reduzir a produção de LCS. Os dados sobre a eficácia de corticosteroides em diminuir a produção do LCS são conflitantes, mas é comum a observação de efeitos clínicos benéficos (prednisona a 0,25-0,5 mg/kg VO a cada 12 h ou dexametasona a 0,25 mg/kg VO a cada 12 h); devem ser reduzidos de forma gradativa para um esquema em dias alternados e a dose reduzida ao máximo possível. Inibidores da anidrase carbônica: acetazolamida (10 mg/kg VO a cada 8 h) com ou sem furosemida (1 mg/kg a cada 24 h); os eletrólitos precisam ser monitorizados com frequência; é improvável que o uso a longo prazo seja benéfico, podendo levar a consequências adversas. Foi relatado que o omeprazol reduza a produção do LCS em cães normais em um modelo experimental, mas não há dados disponíveis sobre a utilidade desse medicamento no quadro clínico; além disso, os relatos de estudos sem comprovação científica ou verificação experimental são desapontadores.
• Diminuir a PIC — diuréticos osmóticos: manitol (1 g/kg sob infusão IV lenta durante 20 min; pode ser repetido 2 vezes em intervalos de 6 h); e/ou diuréticos de alça: furosemida (cães, 2-8 mg/kg IV, IM, SC a cada 12 h; gatos, 1-2 mg/kg IV, IM, SC a cada 12 h). Esses tratamentos são apenas a curto prazo, sendo úteis para o tratamento agudo de casos graves.
• Tratar a causa subjacente — administrar medicamentos específicos sempre que possível (p. ex., antibióticos para infecção bacteriana, radiação ou cirurgia para neoplasia).

CONTRAINDICAÇÕES
Fluidoterapia — usar com cautela no caso de doença grave; não super-hidratar.

PRECAUÇÕES
• Corticosteroides — o tratamento prolongado poderá causar hiperadrenocorticismo ou hipoadrenocorticismo iatrogênicos se a administração do medicamento for subitamente interrompida.
• Diuréticos — podem causar choque ou desequilíbrios eletrolíticos, em especial hipocalemia com a administração de furosemida.

ACOMPANHAMENTO

MONITORIZAÇÃO DO PACIENTE
• Monitorizar a exacerbação da hidrocefalia e sinais atribuíveis a alguma causa subjacente (p. ex., neoplasia intracraniana).

COMPLICAÇÕES POSSÍVEIS
• Herniação cerebral e morte.
• Infecção e obstrução quando se efetua o desvio ventriculoperitoneal; por essa razão, ficam indicados a revisão do desvio e o tratamento específico de infecção bacteriana.

EVOLUÇÃO ESPERADA E PROGNÓSTICO
• Bom a mau — depende da causa e da gravidade.
• Forma congênita discreta — prognóstico bom; pode necessitar apenas de tratamento clínico ocasional.

DIVERSOS

DISTÚRBIOS ASSOCIADOS
Hipoplasia cerebelar em filhotes de gatos com infecção congênita pelo vírus da panleucopenia felina.

FATORES RELACIONADOS COM A IDADE
Congênita — observada, em geral, em animais com menos de 1 ano de idade.

VER TAMBÉM
Estupor e Coma.

ABREVIATURA(S)
• EEG = eletroencefalograma.
• LCS = líquido cerebrospinal.
• PIC = pressão intracraniana.
• RM = ressonância magnética.
• SNC = sistema nervoso central.
• TC = tomografia computadorizada.

Sugestões de Leitura
Coates JR, Sullivan SA. Congenital cranial and intracranial malformations. In: August J, ed., Consultations in Feline Internal Medicine, 4th ed. Philadelphia: Saunders, 2001, pp. 413-423.
Dewey CW. Encephalopathies: Disorders of the brain. In: Dewey CW, ed., A Practical Guide to Canine and Feline Neurology, 2nd ed. Ames, IA: Wiley-Blackwell, 2008, pp. 126-129, 193.
Kawasaki Y, Tsuruta T, et al. Hydrocephalus with visual deficits in a cat. J Vet Med Sci 2006, 65:1361-1364.
Saito M, Olby N, et al. Relationship among basilar artery resistance index, degree of ventriculomegaly, and clinical signs in hydrocephalic dogs. Vet Radiol Ultrasound 2003, 44:687-694.
Summers BA, Cummings JF, de Lahunta A. Veterinary Neuropathology. St. Louis: Mosby, 1995, pp. 75-77.
Thomas WB. Hydrocephalus in dogs and cats. Vet Clin North Am Small Anim Pract 2010, 40:143-159.

Autor Mary O. Smith
Consultor Editorial Joane M. Parent

HIDRONEFROSE

CONSIDERAÇÕES GERAIS

REVISÃO
• A hidronefrose provoca distensão progressiva da pelve renal e dos divertículos renais, com atrofia do parênquima renal secundária à obstrução.
• A doença costuma ser unilateral e ocorre secundariamente à obstrução parcial ou completa do rim ou ureter por urólitos, neoplasia, doença retroperitoneal, traumatismo, radioterapia e ligadura acidental do ureter durante a ovário--histerectomia e após a cirurgia para ureter ectópico.
• Hidronefrose bilateral é rara e geralmente resulta de doença do trígono vesical, da próstata ou da uretra. Em cães, podem ocorrer graus variados de hidronefrose como resultado de prolapso da bexiga urinária em direção a alguma hérnia perineal.

IDENTIFICAÇÃO
Cães e gatos.

SINAIS CLÍNICOS
Achados Anamnésicos
• Subclínicos em alguns cães e gatos.
• Inapetência.
• Polidipsia e poliúria.
• Hematúria.
• Depressão, diarreia e vômitos associados à uremia em pacientes com hidronefrose bilateral ou em caso de comprometimento na função do rim contralateral.
• Podem ser atribuíveis à causa da obstrução (p. ex., dor abdominal).

Achados do Exame Físico
• Normais em alguns pacientes.
• Renomegalia.
• Dor renal, abdominal ou lombar.
• Massa abdominal — bexiga ou próstata.
• Massa no trígono vesical, na próstata, na vagina ou na uretra (incluindo ureterólitos), palpável ao exame retal.

CAUSAS E FATORES DE RISCO
Doenças Ureterais
• Ureterólitos.
• Neoplasia.
• Estenose, atresia e fibrose ureterais.
• Ligadura acidental do ureter durante o procedimento de ovário-histerectomia.
• Secundárias a ureter ectópico congênito.
• Complicação da cirurgia de ureter ectópico.

Doenças do Trato Urogenital Inferior
• Massas vesicais (p. ex., carcinoma de células de transição).
• Prostatopatia (p. ex., neoplasia da próstata).
• Massa vaginal.

Doença Retroperitoneal
• Massas — granuloma, neoplasia, cisto, abscesso, hematoma. • Hérnia perineal.

DIAGNÓSTICO

DIAGNÓSTICO DIFERENCIAL
• Outras causas de renomegalia — p. ex., amiloidose, neoplasia, granuloma, cistos e pseudocistos perinéfricos (gatos).
• Outras causas de dor abdominal — p. ex., pancreatite e peritonite.
• Discopatia intervertebral indutora de dor lombar.
• Pielonefrite sem obstrução.

HEMOGRAMA/BIOQUÍMICA/URINÁLISE
• Normais em alguns pacientes.
• Perda da capacidade de concentração urinária (primeira anormalidade detectada), hematúria, piúria.
• Azotemia, hiperfosfatemia, hipercalcemia e acidemia em pacientes com hidronefrose bilateral grave que resulta em doença renal avançada e uremia.

DIAGNÓSTICO POR IMAGEM
• Radiografias abdominais podem permanecer normais ou revelar renomegalia, prostatomegalia, urólitos, contraste retroperitoneal reduzido ou distensão vesical.
• A realização de urografia excretora ou cistografia ou a injeção de contraste radiográfico por nefropielocentese pode ser necessária para determinar a localização e a causa da obstrução.
• A ultrassonografia revela dilatação da pelve renal e dos divertículos renais, com adelgaçamento do parênquima renal; em alguns cães e gatos, detecta-se dilatação de um ou ambos os ureteres.
• Em caso de obstrução bilateral, a morte por insuficiência renal sobrevirá antes de ambos os rins serem extensivamente acometidos.

MÉTODOS DIAGNÓSTICOS
A uretrocistoscopia ou a vaginoscopia podem ajudar a determinar a causa e a localização de obstrução do trato urinário inferior.

TRATAMENTO

• Internar o paciente e iniciar os cuidados de suporte (p. ex., fluidos ± antibióticos) enquanto se realizam os exames diagnósticos.
• Corrigir os déficits hidroeletrolíticos com fluidoterapia intravenosa (NaCl a 0,9% ou solução de Ringer lactato) durante 4-6 h, seguida por fluidos de manutenção conforme a necessidade. Os pacientes com poliúria extrema talvez necessitem de taxas mais elevadas de fluido de manutenção para manter a hidratação.
• Restabelecer a patência (desobstrução) urinária, aliviar a obstrução do trato urinário inferior por cateterização, realizar cistocentese seriada ou inserir tubo de cistostomia o mais rápido possível.
• O tratamento específico (p. ex., cirúrgico) depende da causa e da presença ou não de insuficiência renal concomitante ou outro processo patológico (p. ex., urólitos bilaterais com envolvimento do rim e/ou ureter contralaterais, neoplasia metastática).
• Raramente, há necessidade de cirurgia de emergência; as anormalidades metabólicas e eletrolíticas devem ser corrigidas antes da cirurgia.
• Em alguns pacientes, pode ser indicado o procedimento de nefrectomia (p. ex., para abscessos renais, neoplasias).

MEDICAÇÕES

MEDICAMENTO(S)
• Administrar bicarbonato de sódio para tratar a acidemia metabólica grave. Para um déficit de ácido mensurado, fornecer 1/4 da dose calculada (peso em kg × 0,3 × déficit de base) de bicarbonato sob a forma de bólus intravenoso lento e o restante com fluidos intravenosos. Se o déficit de base não for conhecido, administrar o bicarbonato na dose de 2-4 mEq/kg/dose, dependendo da gravidade dos sinais.
• A hipercalcemia (leve a moderada) costuma desaparecer com a reposição de fluido e/ou a administração de bicarbonato. A hipercalcemia sintomática grave requer um tratamento clínico mais rigoroso.
• Ver outros princípios sobre o tratamento de pacientes com insuficiência renal atribuída à hidronefrose bilateral nos capítulos sobre doença renal aguda ou crônica.

CONTRAINDICAÇÕES/INTERAÇÕES POSSÍVEIS
• Não acrescentar nem misturar o bicarbonato de sódio com fluidos que contenham cálcio.
• Não administrar material de contraste radiográfico por via IV até que o paciente esteja reidratado.

ACOMPANHAMENTO

MONITORIZAÇÃO DO PACIENTE
• Ultrassonografia — pode ser repetida em intervalos de 2-4 semanas após o alívio da obstrução, para avaliar a melhora do paciente; alguns sinais de resolução costumam aparecer por volta de 3 meses depois do alívio da obstrução.
• Monitorização seriada da bioquímica sérica e dos eletrólitos em pacientes com achados iniciais anormais.
• Após o alívio da obstrução — a ocorrência de poliúria e diurese pós-obstrutiva pode levar a hipocalemia, perda de peso, desidratação e, possivelmente, lesão renal permanente.

COMPLICAÇÕES POSSÍVEIS
Ruptura do sistema excretor e dano renal irreversível.

EVOLUÇÃO ESPERADA E PROGNÓSTICO
• Variáveis, dependendo da causa, do tempo de duração da obstrução e da presença ou ausência de infecção concomitante.
• O dano renal irreversível geralmente tem início 15-45 dias após a obstrução.
• Se a obstrução for aliviada em 1 semana, o dano renal será reversível.
• Alguma função pode ser recuperada com o alívio da obstrução por até 4 semanas.
• Infecção concomitante acelera a gravidade do dano renal.

DIVERSOS

VER TAMBÉM
• Acidose Metabólica.
• Hipercalcemia.
• Insuficiência Renal Aguda.
• Insuficiência Renal Crônica.

Autor S. Dru Forrester
Consultor Editorial Carl A. Osborne
Agradecimento O autor e o consultor editorial agradecem as colaborações do antigo autor deste capítulo, Marc G. Bercovitch.

HIFEMA

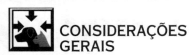

CONSIDERAÇÕES GERAIS

DEFINIÇÃO
Sangue dentro da câmara anterior na forma de coágulo, sangue sedimentado na câmara anterior ventral ou hemácias suspensas por todo o humor aquoso, conferindo o aspecto de "cereja" a esse humor.

FISIOPATOLOGIA
• Desintegração da barreira hematoaquosa e/ou lesão direta aos vasos sanguíneos da íris e do corpo ciliar. As causas incluem traumatismo tecidual direto à córnea ou à úvea anterior (íris e corpo ciliar); liberação de prostaglandina por traumatismo tecidual ou mediadores inflamatórios, como agentes infecciosos; e dano direto às paredes dos vasos sanguíneos, como ocorre com hipertensão sistêmica, complexos antígeno-anticorpo ou microrganismos infecciosos ou células neoplásicas circulantes.
• Hemostasia anormal por deficiência de coagulação ou trombocitopenia.
• Sangramento proveniente de vasos anormais dentro do olho. Isso se deve mais comumente às membranas fibrovasculares pré-iridianas, que se formam em resposta à doença intraocular crônica (uveíte, descolamento da retina, neoplasia); tal doença, por sua vez, gera hipoxia intraocular. Raramente, os vasos sanguíneos congênitos anormais no olho, como membranas pupilares persistentes, túnica vascular do cristalino ou artéria hialoide, podem sangrar, causando hifema.

SISTEMA(S) ACOMETIDO(S)
Oftálmico.

INCIDÊNCIA/PREVALÊNCIA
Não é um achado oftalmológico incomum e nem um achado que seja importante identificar, pois pode ser o sinal clínico apresentado de alguma doença sistêmica subjacente grave.

IDENTIFICAÇÃO
Espécies
Cães e gatos.

Raça(s) Predominante(s)
Collie com anomalia ocular específica dessa raça.

SINAIS CLÍNICOS
Achados Anamnésicos – Causas Oftalmológicas Primárias
• Em geral, apresenta manifestação unilateral em paciente normal sob outros aspectos sistêmicos.
• Traumatismo rombo no globo ocular frequentemente apresentará um histórico de colisão por carro ou exposição a grandes animais, como bovinos ou equinos.
• Perfuração da córnea pode ter histórico de úlcera nessa estrutura ocular com subsequente perfuração; ou encontro prévio com gato, que resulta em laceração pelas garras deste animal, especialmente em filhotes de cães.

Achados Anamnésicos – Causas Sistêmicas
• Manifestação uni ou bilateral; a apresentação bilateral é fortemente sugestiva de etiologia sistêmica.
• Perda de peso, anorexia, letargia e diminuição ou perda da visão podem acompanhar algumas causas sistêmicas.
• Dor ocular geralmente acompanha causas infecciosas atribuídas à uveíte concomitante.

Achados do Exame Físico – Causas Oftalmológicas Primárias
• Exceto em casos de traumatismo generalizado (colisão por carro), o exame físico não exibirá nada digno de nota, com anormalidades restritas ao globo ocular e aos tecidos moles periorbitais.
• Traumatismo rombo apresentará tumefação dolorosa dos tecidos moles periorbitais e, raramente, fraturas da rima orbital; com frequência, há hifema total obscurecendo outras estruturas intraoculares.
• Traumatismo perfurante é associado a sinais de dor intensa, secreção ocular sanguinolenta ou límpida (aquosa), graus variados de hifema, miose e sinequia anterior, além de câmara anterior rasa (superficial); o edema de córnea circundará o local da perfuração, podendo haver prolapso da íris através da perfuração.
• Os hifemas atribuídos a membranas fibrovasculares pré-iridianas, descolamento da retina, neoplasia ou vasculatura congênita costumam ser indolores com pouquíssima inflamação intraocular (rubor aquoso, miose).
• Catarata hipermadura apoia o desenvolvimento de membrana fibrovascular pré-iridiana ou descolamento da retina como causa do hifema.

Achados do Exame Físico – Causas Sistêmicas
• Na suspeita de alguma doença sistêmica subjacente, é justificável a realização de exame físico completo; dependendo da doença sistêmica, o exame físico pode não revelar nada digno de nota ou apresentar achados significativos, como linfadenopatia.
• Os achados do exame oftalmológico serão variáveis, dependendo da etiologia do hifema.
• Etiologias não inflamatórias, como hipertensão e distúrbios de coagulação, geralmente exibirão desconforto mínimo e uveíte (traços ou ausência de rubor aquoso, sem miose e sem hiperemia conjuntival). A hipertensão quase sempre está associada ao envolvimento da retina, como hemorragias e/ou descolamento dessa estrutura ocular.
• Deficiências de coagulação podem exibir sangramento em qualquer lugar, incluindo o tecido subconjuntival e o espaço retrobulbar; em casos de trombocitopenia, pode haver petéquias na conjuntiva palpebral ou membrana nictitante. Etiologias infecciosas e neoplásicas frequentemente apresentarão dor significativa, uveíte anterior (miose, rubor aquoso e fibrina, além de hiperemia e tumefação iridianas), coriorretinite com descolamento da retina e possível glaucoma secundário.

CAUSAS
Ver Tabela 1.

FATORES DE RISCO
• Oftalmológicos: catarata hipermadura, descolamento da retina, uveíte anterior crônica.
• Sistêmicos: qualquer doença, distúrbio ou localização geográfica que predisponha o animal a doenças sistêmicas que, sabidamente, provocam uveíte (p. ex., doença renal crônica ou hipertireoidismo com predisposição à hipertensão sistêmica).

DIAGNÓSTICO

DIAGNÓSTICO DIFERENCIAL
Vascularização profunda da córnea, ao longo do limbo ventral, pode ser confundida com hifema.

HEMOGRAMA/BIOQUÍMICA/URINÁLISE
Achados anormais podem apoiar a presença de doença sistêmica.

OUTROS TESTES LABORATORIAIS
Com base nos achados do histórico e do exame físico, poderão ser indicados o perfil de coagulação e a sorologia (para riquétsias e fungos) na suspeita de doença sistêmica.

DIAGNÓSTICO POR IMAGEM
• Ultrassonografia ocular é indicada para avaliar descolamento da retina ou tumores da úvea quando não estiverem visíveis ao exame oftalmológico.
• Com base nos achados do histórico e do exame físico, poderão ser indicadas tanto a obtenção de radiografias toracoabdominais como a realização de ultrassonografia abdominal se houver suspeita de doença sistêmica.

MÉTODOS DIAGNÓSTICOS
• Mensuração da pressão arterial com Doppler na suspeita de hipertensão.
• Obtenção de aspirados de linfonodos na presença de linfadenopatia ou caso se suspeite de neoplasia ou doença fúngica.

ACHADOS PATOLÓGICOS
Hemorragia macroscópica na câmara anterior.

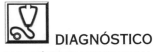

TRATAMENTO

CUIDADO(S) DE SAÚDE ADEQUADO(S)
O tratamento clínico ambulatorial é apropriado a menos que se identifique alguma doença sistêmica subjacente que necessite de hospitalização.

ATIVIDADE
Não há necessidade de restrição da atividade física a menos que o paciente esteja cego (ambiente restrito a jardins com cercas, sem piscinas, com passeios de coleira etc.) ou se o hifema for atribuído à trombocitopenia ou a algum distúrbio de coagulação (evitar brincadeiras bruscas, corrida sem restrição etc.).

ORIENTAÇÃO AO PROPRIETÁRIO
• O hifema, por si só, não é doloroso, embora pareça um quadro drástico.
• É muito importante identificar a causa subjacente do hifema, pois algumas etiologias representam um sério risco à saúde.
• É importante iniciar o tratamento oftalmológico imediatamente para tentar evitar sequelas dolorosas e, algumas vezes, irreversíveis e indutoras de cegueira, como glaucoma.

CONSIDERAÇÕES CIRÚRGICAS
• O hifema secundário à ulceração ou laceração perfurante da córnea deve ser submetido a reparo cirúrgico pela aplicação direta de sutura (laceração) ou enxerto (úlcera perfurada) nessa estrutura ocular quando se espera um resultado visual. Em casos de perfuração grave com prolapso extenso da íris e perda da pupila, é recomendável o procedimento de enucleação.
• Olhos permanentemente cegos e dolorosos devem ser enucleados (com exame histopatológico) para obtenção de conforto permanente.
• O procedimento de irrigação/remoção cirúrgicas do hifema não é bem-sucedido, pois o traumatismo da cirurgia resulta em exacerbação do hifema e inflamação intraocular.

HIFEMA

Tabela 1

Causas de hifema	
Etiologias Oftalmológicas Primárias	*Etiologias Sistêmicas*
Traumatismo: Lesão perfurante ao globo ocular Traumatismo rombo ao globo ocular Compressão vascular extraocular grave (asfixia, compressão torácica)	Hipertensão
Membrana fibrovascular pré-iridiana: Uveíte crônica (induzida pelo cristalino a partir de catarata hipermadura, pós-cirurgia intraocular) Descolamento crônico da retina (catarata hipermadura, displasia da retina, anomalia do olho do Collie, traumatismo)	Riquetsiose: Ehrlichia Febre maculosa das Montanhas Rochosas
Descolamento da retina (sangramento proveniente dos vasos retinianos): Anomalia do olho do Collie Displasia grave da retina Catarata hipermadura Pós-cirurgia de catarata	Neoplasia metastática: Linfoma (mais comum) Carcinomas, sarcomas, melanoma, tumor venéreo transmissível Mieloma múltiplo, leucemias, policitemia vera
Neoplasia intraocular primária (avançada) — é menos provável que provoque hifema em comparação à neoplasia metastática: Melanoma da íris Adenoma/adenocarcinoma do corpo ciliar	Distúrbios de coagulação: Intoxicação por rodenticidas Doença de von Willebrand
Uveíte pigmentar do Golden retriever com ruptura de cisto uveal preenchido de sangue	Doença fúngica: Blastomicose (Criptococose, histoplasmose e coccidioidomicose são menos prováveis)
Sangramento proveniente de vasos sanguíneos intraoculares congênitos anômalos: Membranas pupilares persistentes patentes Persistência da túnica vascular do cristalino Artéria hialoide persistente	PIF Protótheca Parasitárias — migração intraocular aberrante de larvas

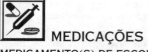

MEDICAÇÕES

MEDICAMENTO(S) DE ESCOLHA
• Instilação tópica de acetato de prednisolona a 1% ou dexametasona a 0,1% a cada 4-8 h para ajudar a estabilizar a barreira hematoaquosa; *não utilizar se houver úlcera ou perfuração de córnea.*
• Atropina a 1% a cada 6-24 h para ajudar a evitar a formação de sinequia posterior; *a atropina é contraindicada na presença de glaucoma secundário.*
• AINE sistêmicos (tepoxalina, carprofeno, meloxicam) em casos de traumatismo perfurante para obter analgesia e ajudar na estabilização da barreira hematoaquosa.
• Prednisona sistêmica em casos de envolvimento conhecido ou sob suspeita da coroide e/ou da retina, *dependendo da causa subjacente*; pode ser utilizada a dose anti-inflamatória (0,5-1,0 mg/kg VO a cada 24 h) para traumatismo rombo, PIF e doença riquetsiana ou fúngica com terapia antimicrobiana adequada.
• Pode-se fazer uso da aplicação tópica de inibidores da anidrase carbônica (dorzolamida a 2%, brinzolamida a 1%) a cada 8 h, β-bloqueador (timolol a 0,5%) a cada 8-12h e/ou agente simpaticomimético (dipivefrina a 0,1%) a cada 8-12 h na presença de glaucoma secundário.

CONTRAINDICAÇÕES
• AINE tópicos (flurbiprofeno, diclofenaco etc.) costumam ser contraindicados em casos de hifema.
• Análogos da prostaglandina (latanoprosta, travoprosta, bimatoprosta) tópicos são contraindicados se houver glaucomas secundários.

ACOMPANHAMENTO

MONITORIZAÇÃO DO PACIENTE
• O exame de tonometria deve ser utilizado para monitorizar o paciente quanto ao desenvolvimento de glaucoma secundário, o que diminui o prognóstico em termos de recuperação da visão.
• Efetuar a tonometria a cada 1-2 dias se a PIO estiver normal a elevada ou mais acentuada ou se houver fatores de risco, como fibrina e/ou sinequia posterior.
• Realizar a tonometria semanalmente em caso de PIO baixa ou se o hifema e a uveíte anterior forem leves a moderadas em termos de gravidade.
• *A tonometria é contraindicada em casos de perfuração da córnea.*

COMPLICAÇÕES POSSÍVEIS
Glaucoma secundário, sinequia/discoria posterior, formação de catarata, perda da visão, possível perda do olho em casos de cegueira permanente e dor ocular.

EVOLUÇÃO ESPERADA E PROGNÓSTICO
• Caso se consiga tratar a causa subjacente do hifema de forma bem-sucedida, como o reparo de laceração da córnea ou o controle de hipertensão, e ainda se o dano intraocular não for extenso, o prognóstico será bom quanto à resolução completa do hifema.
• Se o traumatismo ocular for grave ou se a doença subjacente não for controlada, o hifema persistirá, podendo culminar em cegueira; a ausência de melhora do hifema 2 semanas após o traumatismo rombo tem prognóstico mau.
• O hifema causado por sangramento proveniente de membranas fibrovasculares pré-iridianas geralmente não exibe resolução ou, então, desaparece e recidiva.
• Em caso de dor ocular gerada por globo perfurado ou glaucoma secundário, sem qualquer esperança razoável de recuperação da visão, será recomendado o procedimento de enucleação.

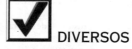

DIVERSOS

ABREVIATURA(S)
• AINE = anti-inflamatório não esteroide.
• PIF = peritonite infecciosa felina.
• PIO = pressão intraocular.

Autor Margi A. Gilmour
Consultor Editorial Paul E. Miller

HIPERADRENOCORTICISMO (SÍNDROME DE CUSHING) — CÃES

CONSIDERAÇÕES GERAIS

DEFINIÇÃO
- Hiperadrenocorticismo espontâneo é um distúrbio causado pela produção excessiva de cortisol pelo córtex adrenal.
- Hiperadrenocorticismo iatrogênico resulta da administração exógena excessiva de glicocorticoides de qualquer forma ou por qualquer via.
- Qualquer que seja o caso, os sinais clínicos são atribuídos aos efeitos deletérios das concentrações circulantes elevadas de glicocorticoide, exercidos sobre múltiplos sistemas orgânicos.

FISIOPATOLOGIA
- Aproximadamente 80-85% dos casos de hiperadrenocorticismo de ocorrência natural se devem à hiperplasia adrenocortical bilateral resultante de tumores corticotróficos hipofisários ou hiperplasia com hipersecreção de ACTH.
- Nos outros 15-20% dos casos, há neoplasia adrenocortical secretora de cortisol; cerca da metade desses é maligna.
- Raramente causado pela secreção ectópica de ACTH por tumor não hipofisário.
- O hiperadrenocorticismo iatrogênico resulta da administração exógena excessiva de glicocorticoides.

SISTEMA(S) ACOMETIDO(S)
- O grau de acometimento de cada sistema varia de forma considerável; em alguns pacientes, podem predominar sinais atribuíveis a um único sistema; outros, por sua vez, sofrem envolvimento de vários sistemas em um grau comparável.
- Os sinais atribuíveis ao trato urinário ou à pele costumam predominar.
- Endócrino/metabólico — hiperglicemia; ocorre diabetes melito em 10% dos casos.
- Cardiovascular — hipertensão (em geral, leve).
- Gastrintestinal — polifagia.
- Hematológico/linfático/imune — leucograma de estresse; imunossupressão; eritrocitose e trombocitose leves.
- Hepatobiliar — hepatopatia atribuída ao depósito de glicogênio; aumento na atividade sérica da fosfatase alcalina em virtude da produção de isoenzima induzida por corticosteroide.
- Neuromuscular — fraqueza muscular; sinais do SNC, incluindo anorexia, ataxia, desorientação e, raramente, crises convulsivas na presença de macroadenoma hipofisário.
- Renal/urológico — poliúria/polidipsia em 90% dos casos; proteinúria; é comum a ocorrência de infecção do trato urinário.
- Reprodutor — atrofia testicular e anestro.
- Respiratório — respiração ofegante; possível tromboembolia pulmonar em função de um estado hipercoagulável.
- Cutâneo — é comum o surgimento de alopecia bilateral simétrica; comedões; hiperpigmentação; piodermite recidivante.

GENÉTICA
Não há base genética conhecida.

INCIDÊNCIA/PREVALÊNCIA
- Não se dispõe dos números exatos.
- Considerado um dos distúrbios endócrinos mais comuns em cães.

DISTRIBUIÇÃO GEOGRÁFICA
N/D.

IDENTIFICAÇÃO
Espécies
Cães.

Raça(s) Predominante(s)
Poodle, Dachshund, Boston terrier, Pastor alemão e Beagle.

Idade Média e Faixa Etária
Em geral, trata-se de um distúrbio de animais de meia-idade a idosos; muito raramente, pode-se observar hiperadrenocorticismo dependente da hipófise em cães com até 1 ano de idade.

Sexo Predominante
Sem predominância de hiperadrenocorticismo dependente da hipófise em cães; possível predominância de tumores adrenais em cadelas.

SINAIS CLÍNICOS
Comentários Gerais
- A gravidade é bastante variável, dependendo da duração e da gravidade do excesso de cortisol.
- Em alguns casos, a presença física do processo neoplásico (hipofisário ou adrenal) contribui para os sinais clínicos.

Achados do Histórico e do Exame Físico
Poliúria e polidipsia, polifagia, abdome penduloso, respiração mais ofegante, hepatomegalia, perda de pelos, hiperpigmentação cutânea, adelgaçamento da pele, fraqueza muscular, obesidade, letargia, atrofia muscular, comedões, equimose, atrofia testicular, anestro, calcinose cutânea, paralisia do nervo facial.

CAUSAS
- Dependente da hipófise — o adenoma é mais comum; os adenocarcinomas são raros; hipófise anterior acometida em aproximadamente 80% dos casos; envolvimento do lobo intermediário da hipófise no restante dos casos; a incidência exata de macroadenomas hipofisários (i. e., >1 cm de diâmetro) é desconhecida, mas pode ser de 10-25%.
- Tumor adrenal — adenoma ou carcinoma (50/50).
- Secreção ectópica de ACTH — rara.
- Iatrogênico — atribuído à administração de glicocorticoide.

FATORES DE RISCO
- Nenhum conhecido para a doença espontânea.
- A presença de qualquer condição que leve à administração exógena de glicocorticoide é um fator de risco para hiperadrenocorticismo iatrogênico.

DIAGNÓSTICO

DIAGNÓSTICO DIFERENCIAL
- Depende das anormalidades clínicas e laboratoriais exibidas.
- Inclui hipotireoidismo, dermatoses por hormônios sexuais, alopecia X, tumores secretores de hormônios sexuais, acromegalia, diabetes melito, hepatopatias, doença renal e outras causas de poliúria/polidipsia.

HEMOGRAMA/BIOQUÍMICA/URINÁLISE
- O hemograma pode revelar eosinopenia, linfopenia, leucocitose, neutrofilia, eritrocitose e/ou trombocitose.
- A bioquímica sérica pode mostrar elevação das enzimas hepáticas, do colesterol e do CO_2 total; a atividade da fosfatase alcalina encontra-se alta em aproximadamente 90% dos cães com hiperadrenocorticismo; além disso, as elevações da fosfatase alcalina são proporcionalmente maiores que as de ALT; é comum a constatação de hiperglicemia, embora apenas cerca de 10% dos cães com hiperadrenocorticismo tenham diabetes melito concomitante.
- A urinálise pode revelar densidade baixa, proteinúria, hematúria, piúria e/ou bacteriúria.

OUTROS TESTES LABORATORIAIS
- Testes endócrinos são necessários em cães com histórico, sinais clínicos e anormalidades laboratoriais sugestivos de hiperadrenocorticismo.
- Não efetuar os testes para hiperadrenocorticismo em cães doentes a menos que haja sinais clínicos compatíveis com essa endocrinopatia.
- Testes de triagem são destinados a determinar se o hiperadrenocorticismo está presente ou não.
- Assim que o diagnóstico definitivo de hiperadrenocorticismo for feito, deve-se proceder a um teste de diferenciação para determinar se há hiperadrenocorticismo dependente da hipófise ou tumor adrenal; a diferenciação fornece informações cruciais para a tomada de decisões terapêuticas e a formulação de prognóstico preciso.
- Testes de diferenciação nunca devem ser feitos antes do diagnóstico de hiperadrenocorticismo por meio de testes de triagem.
- Ver no Apêndice II tabela de protocolos de testes endócrinos.
- Para converter a concentração de cortisol em nmol/L para μg/dL, dividir por 27,6.
- Todas as concentrações de cortisol utilizadas abaixo são para fins ilustrativos; verificar junto ao laboratório em busca das faixas normais de referência e dos valores de corte.

Testes de Triagem
Relação de Cortisol:Creatinina Urinários
- A excreção urinária de cortisol aumenta como reflexo do aumento na secreção adrenal do hormônio, independentemente da presença de hiperadrenocorticismo dependente da hipófise ou de tumor adrenal.
- A relação de cortisol:creatinina urinários elevada é um marcador sensível de hiperadrenocorticismo, estando presente em 90-100% dos cães acometidos.
- Essa relação deve ser mensurada em amostra coletada em casa quando o animal não estiver estressado.
- Resultados falso-positivos são comuns; apenas cerca de 20% dos cães com relação de cortisol:creatinina urinários elevada têm hiperadrenocorticismo.
- Uma relação normal torna muito improvável o diagnóstico de hiperadrenocorticismo (possibilidade ≤10%).
- A relação elevada é compatível com o diagnóstico de hiperadrenocorticismo; no entanto, como as chances de resultado falso-positivo são grandes, sempre se deve fazer um teste de estimulação com ACTH ou um teste de supressão com dexametasona em baixas doses para confirmar a presença de hiperadrenocorticismo.

Teste de Supressão com Dexametasona em Baixas Doses (TSDBD)
- A ausência de supressão 8 h após a injeção de dexametasona em baixas doses é compatível com o diagnóstico de hiperadrenocorticismo.

Hiperadrenocorticismo (Síndrome de Cushing) — Cães

- A sensibilidade do TSDBD é de aproximadamente 95% em cães.
- Em cães, há uma possibilidade relativamente alta de resultado falso-positivo, de até 50%, se houver doença não adrenal.
- A ausência de supressão em 4 h, mas com supressão completa em 8 h, tecnicamente não é compatível com hiperadrenocorticismo, embora se suspeite de sua presença; é justificável a realização de mais testes.
- Com certos resultados, o TSDBD também pode servir como teste diferencial ou de triagem; se a amostra de 8 h tiver >30 nmol/dL, o resultado será compatível com hiperadrenocorticismo; se, além disso, houver supressão para <30 nmol/L em 4 h após a administração de dexametasona (i. e., um "escape" em 8 h após a aplicação de dexametasona) ou as amostras coletadas em 4 e/ou 8 h após a dexametasona estiverem com <50% do valor basal, os resultados serão compatíveis com hiperadrenocorticismo dependente da hipófise; se os critérios de hiperadrenocorticismo dependente da hipófise não forem atendidos, as chances ainda serão de aproximadamente 50% para esse tipo de hiperadrenocorticismo *versus* 50% para tumor adrenal.
- Se os valores basais se aproximarem de 30 nmol/L ou ocorrer supressão apenas em 50%, a presença de hiperadrenocorticismo dependente da hipófise deverá ser confirmada por outros meios.

Teste de Estimulação com ACTH
- Uma resposta maior do que a normal é compatível com o diagnóstico de hiperadrenocorticismo espontâneo.
- A sensibilidade global desse teste é de aproximadamente 80%. Para hiperadrenocorticismo dependente da hipófise, a sensibilidade gira em torno de 87%, enquanto para o hiperadrenocorticismo atribuído a algum tumor adrenal é de cerca de 61%.
- Esse teste é mais específico em cães que o TSDBD (há uma chance de apenas 15% de resultado falso-positivo com doença não adrenal).
- O teste de estimulação com ACTH jamais pode diferenciar entre hiperadrenocorticismo dependente da hipófise e tumor adrenal.
- Único teste capaz de diagnosticar hiperadrenocorticismo iatrogênico; o diagnóstico é feito com histórico de exposição a glicocorticoide por qualquer via, presença de sinais clínicos compatíveis e concentração de cortisol pós-ACTH abaixo da faixa de referência.
- A formulação recomendada de ACTH é o Cortrosyn®; caso se faça uso de ACTH manipulado, devem-se coletar amostras antes, bem como 1 e 2 h depois, da administração de ACTH, para que a resposta de pico não passe despercebida.

Testes Diferenciais
Teste de Supressão com Dexametasona em Altas Doses (TSDAD)
- Duas respostas são compatíveis com hiperadrenocorticismo dependente da hipófise; se houver supressão para <30 nmol/L em 4 e/ou 8 h após a administração de dexametasona ou as amostras estiverem com <50% do valor basal 4 e/ou 8 h depois da dexametasona, haverá hiperadrecorticismo dependente da hipófise.
- Se os valores basais se aproximarem de 30 nmol/L ou ocorrer supressão em apenas 50% do valor, a presença de hiperadrenocorticismo dependente da hipófise deverá ser confirmada por outros meios.

- O TSDAD *jamais* consegue confirmar a presença de tumor adrenal; se os critérios para o diagnóstico de hiperadrenocorticismo dependente da hipófise não forem atendidos, haverá a possibilidade de 50% de que o paciente tenha hiperadrenocorticismo dependente da hipófise ou tumor adrenal.

Concentração de ACTH Endógeno
- Requer apenas uma única amostra de sangue, embora haja necessidade de manipulação especial.
- Em pacientes com hiperadrenocorticismo dependente da hipófise, a concentração de ACTH endógeno deve estar normal a aumentada; em casos de tumor adrenal, a concentração de ACTH endógeno deve estar abaixo do normal.
- Esse teste pode ser usado para confirmar a presença de tumor adrenal.
- Existe uma zona obscura nos resultados; se a concentração de ACTH endógeno do paciente cair nessa zona, os resultados não serão diagnósticos.
- Com a repetição do teste nos momentos em que a concentração original mensurada cair nessa zona duvidosa (chance em torno de 15%), cerca de 96% dos casos serão definitivamente diferenciados.
- Não há como prever quando a concentração de ACTH endógeno cairá nessa zona obscura.

DIAGNÓSTICO POR IMAGEM
- Radiografias abdominais podem diferenciar hiperadrenocorticismo dependente da hipófise de tumor adrenal; aproximadamente 40-50% dos tumores adrenais caninos são observados; a mineralização da adrenal é altamente suspeita da presença de tumor nessa glândula.
- Radiografias torácicas ficam indicadas em pacientes com tumor adrenal para verificar se há metástases.
- Ultrassonografia, TC e RM — úteis não só para diferenciar hiperadrenocorticismo dependente da hipófise de tumor adrenal, mas também para realizar o estadiamento de tumor adrenal; a ultrassonografia abdominal nunca pode ser usada como teste de triagem, pois o aumento de volume bilateral da adrenal também pode ser observado em doença crônica não relacionada a essa glândula; o tumor adrenal pode ser pequeno e de difícil visualização à ultrassonografia; a invasão da veia cava, do fígado ou dos rins é um indicador de malignidade; pode não ser uma tarefa fácil determinar a presença de atrofia adrenal com o exame de ultrassom.
- TC e RM — em geral, são úteis para demonstrar macroadenomas hipofisários.
- Como a radioterapia, uma modalidade terapêutica necessária para macroadenoma hipofisário, é mais eficaz para tumores menores, alguns autores defendem a obtenção de imagens da hipófise com certa rotina em todos os cães diagnosticados com hiperadrenocorticismo dependente da hipófise; as recomendações de acompanhamento e tratamento variam, dependendo do tamanho do tumor.

MÉTODOS DIAGNÓSTICOS
Biopsia adrenal (realizada, em geral, em amostra de tumor adrenal obtida via adrenalectomia) é frequentemente necessária para diferenciar tumor benigno *versus* maligno.

ACHADOS PATOLÓGICOS
- Hiperadrenocorticismo dependente da hipófise — o exame macroscópico revela hipófise de tamanho normal a aumentado e aumento adrenocortical bilateral.

- Ao exame microscópico, podem ser observados adenoma, adenocarcinoma ou hiperplasia corticotrófica da parte distal ou da intermediária da hipófise e hiperplasia adrenocortical.
- Tumor adrenal — o exame macroscópico revela massa adrenal de tamanho variável, atrofia da glândula contralateral (raramente os tumores são bilaterais) e metástase em alguns pacientes com carcinoma adrenal; é possível ver invasão ou trombose na veia cava com tumores malignos.
- À microscopia, observa-se adenoma ou carcinoma adrenocortical.
- Com qualquer forma de hiperadrenocorticismo, podem ser observadas alterações generalizadas do cortisol em excesso, como atrofia cutânea e glomerulopatia.

TRATAMENTO
CUIDADO(S) DE SAÚDE ADEQUADO(S)
Determinados pela gravidade dos sinais clínicos, pela condição geral do paciente e por quaisquer fatores complicantes (p. ex., diabetes melito e tromboembolia pulmonar).

CUIDADO(S) DE ENFERMAGEM
Variáveis, conforme exposto anteriormente.

ATIVIDADE
Não há necessidade de alteração da atividade física.

DIETA
Em geral, não é necessária a modificação; usar dieta apropriada se houver diabetes melito concomitante.

ORIENTAÇÃO AO PROPRIETÁRIO
- Se o tratamento clínico for utilizado, ele deverá ser feito pelo resto da vida do animal.
- Em caso de reação adversa ao mitotano ou trilostano — interromper a administração do medicamento, administrar prednisona e fazer uma reavaliação veterinária no dia seguinte; caso não se observe resposta à prednisona em algumas horas, o animal deverá ser submetido a um exame veterinário imediatamente.

CONSIDERAÇÕES CIRÚRGICAS
- Hipofisectomia — embora seja descrita, em geral não está disponível nos EUA.
- A adrenalectomia bilateral não é usada para o tratamento de hiperadrenocorticismo dependente da hipófise em cães.
- A cirurgia é o tratamento de escolha em cães com adenomas adrenocorticais e carcinomas pequenos a menos que o paciente seja de alto risco cirúrgico; no entanto, há necessidade de uma equipe especializada, além de estabelecimentos apropriados, pois esse tipo de intervenção é tecnicamente exigente, necessitando de cuidados pós-operatórios intensivos.
- Dependendo da condição do paciente, o controle clínico do hiperadrenocorticismo pode ser desejável antes da cirurgia, se possível.

MEDICAÇÕES
MEDICAMENTO(S) DE ESCOLHA
Mitotano
- O mitotano (o,p'-DDD, Lysodren®) é um dos dois principais agentes utilizados para o

HIPERADRENOCORTICISMO (SÍNDROME DE CUSHING) — CÃES

tratamento clínico do hiperadrenocorticismo dependente da hipófise em cães; ele destrói seletivamente as células secretoras de glicocorticoide do córtex adrenal; talvez seja o medicamento de escolha para o tratamento clínico de tumor adrenal, pois pode destruir as células tumorais e controlar a secreção de cortisol.

• Hiperadrenocorticismo dependente da hipófise — administrar uma dose inicial de ataque de 40-50 mg/kg fracionados 2 vezes ao dia; avaliar a eficácia por meio do teste de estimulação com ACTH após 8 dias ou antes disso se o animal exibir diminuição do apetite, vômitos, diarreia, inquietação ou baixo consumo de água (<60 mL/kg/dia); o objetivo é que a concentração de cortisol basal e pós-ACTH fique na faixa ideal de 30-150 nmol/L; continuar a indução com repetição do teste, conforme a necessidade, até se observar uma resposta adequada; em seguida, iniciar a terapia de manutenção com 50 mg/kg/semana divididos em 2 a 3 doses; realizar ajustes da dose com base no teste de estimulação com ACTH (manter os níveis de cortisol basal e pós-ACTH dentro da faixa ideal); se a concentração sérica de cortisol antes ou depois do ACTH estiver <30 nmol/L, interromper a administração do mitotano e administrar doses fisiológicas de prednisona (0,1 mg/kg a cada 12 h); não se pode administrar a prednisona em até 12 h antes do teste de estimulação com ACTH; efetuar esse teste a cada 7-14 dias inicialmente; a secreção de cortisol costuma se recuperar em semanas a alguns meses, mas pode levar mais tempo; assim que a concentração de cortisol estiver na faixa ideal, interromper a prednisona e iniciar a terapia de manutenção; se foi na terapia de manutenção que o cortisol se tornou deficiente, reiniciar a manutenção com uma dose 25% mais baixa; se ocorrer recidiva em qualquer momento durante a terapia de manutenção, conforme indicado pelos níveis de cortisol acima da faixa ideal, haverá necessidade de ajuste da dose; se a concentração sérica de cortisol pós-ACTH for de 150-300 nmol/L, aumentar a dose de manutenção em 25% e reavaliar em 4 semanas; se a concentração sérica de cortisol pós-ACTH estiver >300 nmol/L, repetir a dose de ataque por 5-7 dias e realizar um teste de estimulação com ACTH; continuar a dose de ataque até que a concentração de cortisol esteja na faixa ideal e, depois, reiniciar a dose de manutenção semanal com uma dose aproximadamente 50% mais alta.

• Tumor adrenal — o objetivo de uso do mitotano é atingir níveis de cortisol basal e pós-ACTH baixos a indetectáveis (i. e., <30 nmol/L); a dose inicial é de 50-75 mg/kg fracionados diariamente; efetuar o teste de estimulação com ACTH após 10-14 dias para avaliar a eficácia ou antes disso caso se observem os sinais de diminuição do apetite, vômitos, diarreia, inquietação ou baixo consumo de água (<60 mL/kg/dia); a indução tipicamente requer doses maiores e por mais tempo do que para o tratamento do hiperadrenocorticismo dependente da hipófise; a dose deve ser aumentada em 50 mg/kg/dia a cada 10-14 dias se o controle não tiver sido alcançado, conforme estabelecido pelo teste de estimulação com ACTH; se surgirem efeitos adversos atribuídos ao mitotano, a administração deverá continuar com a dose mais alta tolerável; assim que o controle for obtido, a terapia de manutenção deverá começar com a dose de 75-100 mg/kg/semana divididos em 2-3 doses; se os níveis de cortisol pré e pós-ACTH subirem para a faixa

normal em repouso (i. e., 10-160 nmol/L), aumentar a dose de manutenção em 50%; se os níveis de cortisol subirem acima dos parâmetros normais em repouso pré e pós-ACTH, repetir a dose de ataque até atingir o controle e aumentar semanalmente a dose de manutenção em cerca de 50%; durante a indução e a manutenção, visto que a meta é criar uma insuficiência de glicocorticoide, deve-se administrar a prednisona na dose de 0,2 mg/kg/dia.

• É possível a deficiência de aldosterona, secundariamente à terapia com mitotano; se isso ocorrer, provavelmente o paciente apresentará insuficiência adrenocortical completa permanente; nesse caso, deve-se iniciar o tratamento para hipoadrenocorticismo.

Trilostano

• O trilostano (Vetoryl®) é aprovado para uso na Europa e nos EUA; a eficácia para o tratamento de hiperadrenocorticismo dependente da hipófise é alta, em comparação ao mitotano; a sobrevida de cães com hiperadrenocorticismo dependente da hipófise é a mesma para aqueles tratados com mitotano ou trilostano; inibe a enzima adrenocortical 11-β-hidroxiesteroide desidrogenase e talvez outras, suprimindo com isso a produção de progesterona e seus produtos finais, incluindo cortisol e aldosterona.

• A dose inicial é de 2,2-6,7 mg/kg VO a cada 24 h ou divididos a cada 12 h; caso se observem efeitos colaterais secundários (i. e., anorexia, vômitos, diarreia), interromper o medicamento por 3-5 dias e, depois, reinstituir a cada 48 h por 1 semana antes de prosseguir com o esquema posológico inicial; deve ser realizado um teste de estimulação com ACTH, começando 4-6 h após a ingestão do comprimido em 10-14 dias, 30 dias e 90 dias depois de estar sob a dose plena; se, na reavaliação em 10-14 dias, for observada qualquer melhora, não aumentar a dose mesmo se as concentrações de cortisol estiverem acima do ideal, mas esperar até a reavaliação em 30 dias e modificar a dose se houver necessidade. Se a concentração de cortisol pós-ACTH for <40 nmol/L e o paciente estiver aparentemente bem, interromper o trilostano por 48-72 h e, em seguida, reiniciar com uma dose mais baixa, ou, idealmente, deve-se fazer um teste de estimulação com ACTH sem reinstituir o trilostano até que a secreção de cortisol tenha se recuperado; se a concentração de cortisol pós-ACTH for de 40-150 nmol/L e os sinais clínicos tiverem desaparecido, a dose deverá continuar como está; se a concentração de cortisol pós-ACTH estiver em 150-250 nmol/L, aumentar a dose do trilostano na presença de sinais clínicos ou, se esses sinais tiverem desaparecido, deixar como está, mas monitorizar o paciente com cuidado quanto à recidiva dos sinais; se a concentração sérica de cortisol pós-ACTH estiver >250 nmol/L, aumentar a dose diária ou usar o esquema posológico de 2 vezes ao dia; a mesma dose administrada 1 vez ao dia deve ser dividida e fornecida 2 vezes ao dia (p. ex., se for administrada a dose de 60 mg 1 vez ao dia, então a dose será de 30 mg a cada 12 h); se a concentração sérica de cortisol pós-ACTH for de 40-150 nmol/L e os sinais clínicos persistirem, utilizar o esquema posológico de 2 vezes ao dia; assim que a condição clínica do cão e a dose do medicamento tiverem sido estabilizadas, um teste de estimulação com ACTH deverá ser efetuado a cada 3-6 meses e a

concentração sérica de potássio mensurada para verificar se há hipercalemia.

• Como o trilostano é capaz de suprimir a secreção de aldosterona, poderá ocorrer uma crise addisoniana; a ocorrência de necrose adrenocortical secundária à administração de trilostano pode ser mais comum do que se acreditava; a hipocortisolemia secundária à administração de trilostano costuma se resolver em até 48-72 h da interrupção do medicamento, embora possa ocorrer a supressão temporária de semanas a meses e até mesmo a supressão permanente.

• O trilostano pode ser usado para tratar o tumor adrenal e controlar os sinais clínicos (pelo menos transitoriamente), mas não constitui o medicamento de escolha; para os casos de tumor adrenal, o mitotano é o agente terapêutico de escolha, pois verdadeiramente se trata de um quimioterápico e pode matar as células tumorais.

L-Deprenil

• O L-deprenil (cloridrato de selegilina; Anipryl®) é aprovado pela FDA para o tratamento de hiperadrenocorticismo dependente da hipófise; diminui a secreção de ACTH pela hipófise por aumentar o tônus dopaminérgico no eixo hipotalâmico-hipofisário, reduzindo com isso as concentrações séricas de cortisol; indicado apenas para o tratamento do hiperadrenocorticismo dependente da hipófise sem complicações; não recomendado para os cães com doenças concomitantes, como diabetes melito; não pode ser usado para tratar tumor adrenal; iniciar a terapia com a dose de 1 mg/kg diariamente e aumentar para 2 mg/kg/dia depois de 2 meses se a resposta for inadequada; se essa dose mais alta também não for eficaz, fornecer terapia alternativa; não há monitorização objetiva; a avaliação da eficácia é feita com base na avaliação subjetiva de remissão dos sinais clínicos.

• Eficácia questionável; um único estudo constatou eficácia de 20%, enquanto outro julgou o L-deprenil como um agente ineficaz.

• Efeitos adversos como anorexia, letargia, vômitos e diarreia são incomuns (menos de 5% dos cães) e costumam ser leves; as desvantagens incluem a necessidade de administração diária pelo resto da vida do animal e o custo da medicação.

Cetoconazol

• O cetoconazol (10 mg/kg VO a cada 12 h inicialmente; até 20 mg/kg VO a cada 12 h em alguns cães) inibe as enzimas responsáveis pela síntese de cortisol; indicado para os cães que não toleram o mitotano nas doses necessárias para controlar o hiperadrenocorticismo; pode ser útil para o alívio dos sinais clínicos de hiperadrenocorticismo em cães com tumor adrenal; a monitorização é feita pelo desempenho nos testes de estimulação com ACTH com os mesmos objetivos que os do mitotano; a eficácia é de aproximadamente 50% ou menos; os efeitos adversos incluem anorexia, vômitos, diarreia, letargia, trombocitopenia e hepatopatia idiossincrática.

CONTRAINDICAÇÕES

• Não usar agentes anti-inflamatórios não esteroides em cães com hiperadrenocorticismo não controlado.

• Os medicamentos que aumentam a pressão arterial ou a coagulação devem ser utilizados com cuidado.

Hiperadrenocorticismo (Síndrome de Cushing) — Cães

PRECAUÇÕES
- Os efeitos colaterais do mitotano não são raros; leves na maioria dos cães; incluem letargia, fraqueza, anorexia, vômitos, diarreia, ataxia e hipoadrenocorticismo iatrogênico.
- Os efeitos colaterais são mais comuns em cães com tumor adrenal submetidos a altas doses de mitotano.
- Em relação ao mitotano, utilizá-lo com cautela em pacientes com insuficiência renal e hepatopatia primária.
- Os efeitos colaterais do cetoconazol parecem ser menos comuns; incluem anorexia, vômitos, diarreia, trombocitopenia e hepatopatia.
- No que diz respeito ao cetoconazol, também é preciso ter cuidado quanto ao uso em pacientes com hepatopatia primária ou trombocitopenia; o efeito sobre a capacidade reprodutiva é desconhecido.
- Os efeitos colaterais do L-deprenil são incomuns.
- Os efeitos colaterais do trilostano incluem anorexia, letargia, vômitos e diarreia; podem ocorrer em aproximadamente 60% dos pacientes; também há relatos de crise addisoniana e necrose adrenocortical.
- O uso do trilostano também deve ser cauteloso em pacientes com insuficiência renal e hepatopatia primária; contraindicado na prenhez.
- Para todos os medicamentos, haverá necessidade de monitorização rigorosa se forem utilizados em pacientes diabéticos; as necessidades de insulina podem diminuir rapidamente com o controle do hiperadrenocorticismo.

MEDICAMENTO(S) ALTERNATIVO(S)
A radioterapia é necessária para os animais com macroadenomas hipofisários; os níveis de ACTH podem levar vários meses para diminuir; nesse ínterim, controlar o hiperadrenocorticismo com os medicamentos supracitados.

ACOMPANHAMENTO

MONITORIZAÇÃO DO PACIENTE
Resposta à terapia — usar testes de estimulação com ACTH periódicos para avaliar a eficácia do mitotano, do cetoconazol ou do trilostano (ver anteriormente em busca de mais detalhes); se o animal estiver sob terapia de manutenção com o mitotano, testar em 1, 3 e 6 meses e, em seguida, a cada 3-6 meses ou em caso de recidiva dos sinais clínicos de hiperadrenocorticismo; a suficiência de qualquer período de repetição da dose de ataque necessária do mitotano é checada pelo teste de estimulação com ACTH antes de se iniciar uma dose maior de manutenção desse medicamento; a suficiência da dose de cetoconazol ou trilostano é averiguada pelo teste de estimulação com ACTH após qualquer alteração da dose; com o trilostano, deve-se realizar o teste de estimulação com ACTH, começando 4-6 h após a ingestão do comprimido, embora com o mitotano e o cetoconazol a realização do teste depois da ingestão do comprimido não faça diferença; os sinais clínicos do hiperadrenocorticismo desaparecem alguns dias a meses após o controle ter sido atingido; avaliar a eficácia da terapia com L-deprenil exclusivamente com base na resolução dos sinais clínicos do hiperadrenocorticismo.

PREVENÇÃO
Para a prevenção de recidiva, é necessária a administração regular das medicações com acompanhamento adequado.

COMPLICAÇÕES POSSÍVEIS
- Hipertensão.
- Proteinúria.
- Infecção recidivante.
- Cálculos urinários (oxalato de cálcio).
- Diabetes melito.
- Tromboembolia pulmonar.
- Sinais neurológicos secundários a algum macroadenoma hipofisário.

EVOLUÇÃO ESPERADA E PROGNÓSTICO
- Hiperadrenocorticismo não tratado — geralmente um distúrbio progressivo com prognóstico mau.
- Hiperadrenocorticismo dependente da hipófise tratado — em geral, apresenta prognóstico bom; o tempo médio de sobrevida para cão submetido ao mitotano ou ao trilostano é de aproximadamente 2 anos; pelo menos, 10% sobrevivem 4 anos; os cães que vivem mais de 6 meses tendem a vir a óbito por causas não relacionadas com o hiperadrenocorticismo.
- Macroadenomas e sinais neurológicos — prognóstico mau a grave; macroadenomas sem sinais neurológicos ou com sinais discretos — prognóstico razoável a bom com radioterapia e tratamento clínico.
- Adenomas adrenais — costumam exibir prognóstico bom a excelente; carcinomas pequenos (sem metástases) têm prognóstico razoável a bom em termos gerais, porém bom a excelente com ressecção cirúrgica.
- Carcinomas grandes e tumor adrenal com metástases disseminadas — demonstram, em geral, prognóstico mau a razoável, embora ocasionalmente se observem respostas impressionantes a altas doses de mitotano.

DIVERSOS

DISTÚRBIOS ASSOCIADOS
Sinais neurológicos em cães com grandes tumores hipofisários; intolerância à glicose ou diabetes melito concomitante; tromboembolia pulmonar; aumento na incidência de infecções, especialmente do trato urinário e da pele; hipertensão; proteinúria/glomerulopatia.

FATORES RELACIONADOS COM A IDADE
N/D.

POTENCIAL ZOONÓTICO
N/D.

GESTAÇÃO/FERTILIDADE/REPRODUÇÃO
N/D.

SINÔNIMO(S)
Doença de Cushing; síndrome de Cushing.

VER TAMBÉM
Hiperadrenocorticismo (Síndrome de Cushing) — Gatos.

ABREVIATURA(S)
- ACTH = hormônio adrenocorticotrópico.
- ALT = alanina aminotransferase.
- RM = ressonância magnética.
- SNC = sistema nervoso central.
- TC = tomografia computadorizada.
- TSDAD = teste de supressão com dexametasona em altas doses.
- TSDBD = teste de supressão com dexametasona em baixas doses.

RECURSOS DA INTERNET
www.dechra.com: informações úteis sobre o uso de trilostano.

Sugestões de Leitura
Behrend EN, Kemppainen RJ. Diagnosis of canine hyperadrenocorticism. Vet Clin North Am 2001, 31:985-1003.
Braddock JA, Church DB, Robertson ID, et al. Inefficacy of selegiline in treatment of canine pituitary-dependent hyperadrenocorticism. Australian Vet J 2004, 82:272-277.
Braddock JA, Church DB, Robertson ID, et al. Trilostane treatment in dogs with pituitary-dependent hyperadrenocorticism. Australian Vet J 2003, 81:600-607.
Feldman EC, Nelson RW. Canine hyperadrenocorticism (Cushing's syndrome). In: Feldman EC, Nelson RW, eds., Feline and Canine Endocrinology and Reproduction, 3rd ed. Philadelphia: Saunders, 2004, pp. 252-357.
Kintzer PP, Peterson ME. Mitotane treatment of cortisol secreting adrenocortical neoplasia: 32 cases (1980-1992). JAVMA 1994, 205:54-61.
Kintzer PP, Peterson ME. Mitotane (o, p'-ddd) treatment of 200 dogs with pituitary-dependent hyperadenocorticism. J Vet Intern Med 1991, 5:182-190.
Vaughn MA, Feldman EC, Hoar BR, Nelson RW. Evaluation of twice-daily, low-dose trilostane treatment administered orally in dogs with naturally occurring hyperadrenocorticism. JAVMA 2008, 232:1321-1328.

Autor Ellen N. Behrend
Consultor Editorial Deborah S. Greco

HIPERADRENOCORTICISMO (SÍNDROME DE CUSHING) — GATOS

CONSIDERAÇÕES GERAIS

DEFINIÇÃO
A síndrome de Cushing (hiperadrenocorticismo) felina é um distúrbio causado pela secreção excessiva de cortisol pelas glândulas adrenais.

FISIOPATOLOGIA
• Síndrome de Cushing felina espontânea — causada pela hiperprodução de cortisol pelas glândulas adrenais. • Aproximadamente 85% dos gatos com síndrome de Cushing apresentam hiperplasia adrenocortical bilateral resultante de hiperplasia ou tumor hipofisário. Os outros 15% possuem tumor adrenal, cuja metade é benigna e a outra metade, maligna. Independentemente da causa, a síndrome de Cushing felina costuma ser acompanhada por diabetes melito (80% dos casos).

IDENTIFICAÇÃO
• Gatos. • Nenhuma predisposição racial ou sexual conhecida. • Gatos de meia-idade a mais idosos.

SINAIS CLÍNICOS
• Poliúria, polidipsia, polifagia, fragilidade cutânea (contusão, laceração, adelgaçamento), perda de peso e fraqueza muscular são os sinais mais comuns. • Também se observam obesidade, hepatomegalia, alopecia, diarreia, vômito, aumento de volume abdominal, pontas das orelhas dobradas e aspecto descuidado. • Há relatos de letargia (embotamento) atribuída à fraqueza muscular ou aos efeitos de massa hipofisária. • Os hormônios sexuais em excesso podem causar sinais como barbas penianas e mudanças comportamentais (comportamento sexual).

CAUSAS E FATORES DE RISCO
• Adenoma hipofisário com subsequente hiperplasia corticotrófica e secreção adrenocortical excessiva de cortisol. • Adenoma benigno (50%) ou adenocarcinoma maligno (50%) funcionais autônomos. • É rara a forma iatrogênica causada pela administração de glicocorticoides.

DIAGNÓSTICO

DIAGNÓSTICO DIFERENCIAL
• Diabetes melito. • Insulinorresistência.
• Acromegalia. • Hepatopatia. • Doença renal.
• Tumores adrenais secretores de hormônios sexuais. • Hipotireoidismo.

HEMOGRAMA/BIOQUÍMICA/URINÁLISE
• Leucograma de estresse. • Hiperglicemia, hipercolesterolemia, ALT levemente elevada em virtude de diabetes melito concomitante desregulada. • Não é comum a elevação da fosfatase alcalina sérica, porque os gatos não possuem a isoenzima induzida por corticoide. • É comum uma relação elevada de cortisol:creatinina urinários. • Anormalidades menos comuns — azotemia, proteinúria e hiperglobulinemia.

OUTROS TESTES LABORATORIAIS
Testes de Triagem
• Relação de cortisol:creatinina urinários — exame sensível (útil por seu valor preditivo negativo, ou seja, caso se obtenha uma relação normal de creatinina:cortisol urinários, a síndrome de Cushing felina será improvável) e barato, além de ser fácil de realizar e interpretar. É preferível a coleta de urina em casa sem estresse. • Teste de supressão com dexametasona em baixas doses (TSDBD) — extremamente sensível. Exige 10 vezes a mais que a dose utilizada em cães: 0,1 mg/kg IV. O plasma é obtido para mensuração do cortisol antes e ainda 4 e 8 horas depois da administração de dexametasona. A falha na supressão é compatível com a síndrome de Cushing felina. • Teste de estimulação com ACTH constitui principalmente um teste de reserva adrenal. Esse teste requer menos tempo, além de ser fácil de interpretar, relativamente barato e específico para síndrome de Cushing felina quando os resultados estiverem anormais.

Testes Diferenciais
• Teste de supressão com dexametasona em altas doses (TSDAD) — dose de 1 mg/kg, seguindo o mesmo protocolo do teste de supressão com dexametasona em baixas doses. É mais fácil realizar e interpretar uma versão "caseira" utilizando múltiplas relações de creatinina:cortisol urinários e dexametasona oral do que o protocolo hospitalar.
• A mensuração endógena plasmática de ACTH é alta a normal ou superior em casos de hiperadrenocorticismo dependente da hipófise em comparação a níveis plasmáticos baixos desse hormônio em casos de tumor adrenal (<10 pg/mL). A faixa normal para gatos é de 0-60 pg/mL. O sangue é coletado em frasco de EDTA, centrifugado imediatamente, e o plasma é transferido para um frasco plástico e congelado.
• No protocolo de supressão com a dexametasona "em casa", os proprietários devem coletar amostras de urina pela manhã nos dias 1, 2 e 3. Administrar doses orais de dexametasona (TSDBD [0,1 mg/kg] ou TSDAD [1 mg/kg]) em intervalos de 6 h por 2 dias. Enviar as três amostras de urina ao laboratório para medir a relação de creatinina:cortisol urinários. Nos dias 1 e 2, os valores são basais. A supressão no dia 3 abaixo de 50% não é observada em gatos com tumor adrenal, mas pode ser vista em casos de hiperadrenocorticismo dependente da hipófise.

DIAGNÓSTICO POR IMAGEM
• A ultrassonografia abdominal é o exame preferido para visualizar as glândulas adrenais. Apesar de subjetiva, a ultrassonografia pode ser uma excelente ferramenta para discernir entre hiperadrenocorticismo dependente da hipófise e tumor adrenal. As glândulas adrenais simétricas de tamanho normal ou aumentado são sugestivas de hiperadrenocorticismo dependente da hipófise, enquanto o aumento unilateral apoia a presença de tumor adrenal. • Os exames de TC e RM permitem a visualização de macroadenomas hipofisários.

MÉTODOS DIAGNÓSTICOS
Os perfis dos hormônios sexuais ou a mensuração do fator de crescimento insulinossímile-1 (IGF-1) são obtidos para descartar os diagnósticos diferenciais.

TRATAMENTO

• A síndrome de Cushing felina é uma doença debilitante. Em comparação aos cães, as opções para gatos são mais limitadas e não tão bem-sucedidas. • O tratamento médico antes da cirurgia é benéfico para evitar complicações decorrentes de fragilidade cutânea, infecções e contusões. • A radiação da hipófise com cobalto em casos de hiperadrenocorticismo dependente da hipófise pode se tornar parte integrante do tratamento da síndrome de Cushing felina. • Os procedimentos de adrenalectomia unilateral para tumor adrenal e adrenalectomia bilateral para hiperadrenocorticismo dependente da hipófise (com tratamento médico para hipoadrenocorticismo) parecem ser as opções terapêuticas mais bem-sucedidas. • Talvez haja necessidade de pivalato de desoxicortisona e Depo-medrol®. • A hipofisectomia (transesfenoidal com microcirurgia) está disponível em algumas instituições.

MEDICAÇÕES

MEDICAMENTO(S)
• Mitotano (o,p'-DDD, Lysodren®) provoca destruição seletiva das células adrenocorticais secretoras de cortisol. Já foram utilizadas doses de 50 mg/kg/dia divididas; no entanto, até mesmo o dobro da dose algumas vezes não demonstrou melhora. • Trilostano inibe a 3 xyxyβ-17-hidroxiesteroide desidrogenase de forma reversível, o que bloqueia a síntese de esteroide. Em um pequeno número de casos de síndrome de Cushing felina com hiperadrenocorticismo dependente da hipófise, o trilostano diminuiu os sinais clínicos e melhorou os resultados dos testes endócrinos. Já foram utilizadas doses de até 60 mg/gato VO a cada 12 h. • Outros medicamentos são usados com sucesso limitado (cetoconazol, metirapona e aminoglutetimida).

ACOMPANHAMENTO

• A melhora clínica com diminuição dos sinais de síndrome de Cushing felina é indicativa do benefício da terapia medicamentosa. • Testes repetidos da relação de creatinina:cortisol urinários e da estimulação com ACTH podem ser benéficos.

DIVERSOS

ABREVIATURA(S)
• ACTH = hormônio adrenocorticotrópico. • RM = ressonância magnética. • TC = tomografia computadorizada. • TSDAD = teste de supressão com dexametasona em altas doses. • TSDBD = teste de supressão com dexametasona em baixas doses.

Sugestões de Leitura
Feldman EC, Nelson RW. Hyperadrenocorticism in cats (Cushing's syndrome). In: Canine and Feline Endocrinology and Reproduction, 3rd ed. Philadelphia: Saunders, 2004, pp. 358-393.
Neiger R, Witt AL, et al. Trilostane therapy for treatment of pituitary-dependent hyperadrenocorticism in 5 cats. J Vet Intern Med 2004, 18:160-165.

Autor Deirdre Chiaramonte
Consultor Editorial Deborah S. Greco

Hiperandrogenismo

CONSIDERAÇÕES GERAIS

REVISÃO
- Síndrome rara em cães, caracterizada por elevações absolutas ou relativas nas concentrações séricas de hormônios sexuais masculinizantes, como a testosterona e seus derivados. É mais frequentemente documentada em cães machos intactos.
- Não há relatos de hiperandrogenismo em gatos.
- Em machos, os androgênios (testosterona e di-hidrotestosterona) são produzidos pelas células intersticiais dos testículos, sendo responsáveis pelo desenvolvimento sexual fenotípico normal, pelo comportamento e pela espermatogênese. Esses hormônios também são produzidos pelo córtex adrenal e pelos ovários nas fêmeas.
- Pode ocorrer como resultado da produção excessiva pelos testículos, ovários ou córtex adrenal. Este último pode ocorrer secundariamente à alteração na atividade enzimática da via esteroidogênica, resultando em desvio do substrato (i. e., a deficiência da 21-hidroxilase resultará em aumento na disponibilidade do substrato para produção de androstenediona).
- Também pode ocorrer de forma iatrogênica em associação à administração de androgênios sintéticos exógenos.
- O hiperandrogenismo pode resultar em alterações comportamentais, anormalidades do trato reprodutivo e problemas dermatológicos.

Hiperandrogenismo e Alopecia
- As causas endócrinas e metabólicas de alopecia no tronco têm nomenclatura confusa. Há muitos nomes diferentes usados para descrever a alopecia do tronco que, supostamente, está relacionada com um desequilíbrio relativo nos hormônios sexuais ou concentrações séricas circulantes elevadas de hormônios sexuais como a testosterona.
- Pode ocorrer desequilíbrio nos hormônios sexuais, secundário à produção excessiva, conforme observado em associação à hiperplasia adrenal ou a tumores adrenais. Pode ser visto associado a tumores testiculares ou cães com hiperandrogenismo verdadeiro; ou pode ser constatado com esteroidogênese adrenal alterada, como ocorre com a síndrome semelhante à hiperplasia adrenal (também conhecida como síndrome semelhante à hiperplasia adrenal congênita, alopecia responsiva ao hormônio do crescimento, desequilíbrio de hormônio sexual adrenal, alopecia ligada a hormônio sexual). A terminologia mais recente menciona essas condições como alopecia X de raças nórdicas. Os termos são usados para a síndrome nas raças Pomerânia, Chow chow, Keeshond e Samoieda; acredita-se que o problema resulte da deficiência de 21-hidroxilase cortical adrenal, ocasionando hiperandrogenismo e uma queda secundária no hormônio do crescimento.
- Em virtude das etiologias diferentes do estado hiperandrogênico, o sucesso do tratamento com castração, administração de mitotano ou hormônio do crescimento varia de acordo com a condição. Para aqueles animais com anormalidades clínicas limitadas à alopecia, deve-se dar uma atenção especial aos benefícios (principalmente estéticos) *versus* os riscos terapêuticos antes de se instituir o tratamento. Em relação aos animais com esteroidogênese adrenal alterada, não se sabe ao certo por que os cães apresentam respostas variáveis à mesma terapia.

IDENTIFICAÇÃO
Cães — raças Pomerânia, Chow chow, Poodle, Keeshond e Samoieda.

SINAIS CLÍNICOS

Achados Anamnésicos
- Agressividade.
- Parada do crescimento (secundária ao fechamento prematuro das placas de crescimento epifisárias).
- Ciclos estrais irregulares.
- Anestro.
- Síndromes de virilização.

Achados do Exame Físico
Gerais
- Alopecia endócrina (bilateralmente simétrica, envolvendo o pescoço, o tronco, a parte caudal das coxas, o pavilhão auricular e a cauda).
- Pelagem ressecada e quebradiça.
- Hiperpigmentação da pele.
- Epífora.
- Seborreia oleosa.

Fêmeas
- Hipertrofia do clitóris.
- Epífora.
- Seborreia oleosa.
- Vaginite (associada à exposição anormal do clitóris).
- Virilização.
- Diferenciação sexual anormal (com a exposição *in utero*).

Machos
- Prostatomegalia secundária à hiperplasia.
- Anormalidades da morfologia espermática.
- Hiperplasia das glândulas adanais.
- Puberdade prematura.
- Fechamento prematuro das placas de crescimento epifisárias.

CAUSAS E FATORES DE RISCO
- Administração exógena de androgênios.
- Aumento da secreção endógena de androgênios.
- Tumor testicular (mais comumente secundário a tumores testiculares intersticiais).
- Exposição *in utero* de feto do sexo feminino a androgênios.

DIAGNÓSTICO

DIAGNÓSTICO DIFERENCIAL
Alopecia Simétrica Não Pruriginosa ("Alopecia Endócrina")
- Hipotireoidismo.
- Hiperadrenocorticismo.
- Hiperestrogenismo.

Hipertrofia do Clitóris
- Anormalidades das gônadas sexuais (pseudo--hermafroditismo, hermafroditismo verdadeiro).
- Hiperadrenocorticismo.

Agressividade
- Doença neurológica.
- Distúrbios comportamentais.

HEMOGRAMA/BIOQUÍMICA/URINÁLISE
Geralmente normais; pode ocorrer elevação das enzimas hepatocelulares.

OUTROS TESTES LABORATORIAIS
- Cariótipo — para detectar intersexo/anormalidades das gônadas.
- Teste de estimulação com hormônio do crescimento — esse teste é concluído com o uso de xilazina ou clonidina; pode ser empregado para demonstrar a falta de aumento nas concentrações séricas de hormônio do crescimento após a administração. O teste não é confiável para documentar hiperandrogenismo; alguns cães apresentam resposta normal ao hormônio do crescimento, mas respondem bem à suplementação desse hormônio. Concentrações séricas de testosterona — concentrações séricas isoladas podem estar dentro dos limites de normalidade. Mensurações repetidas podem ser mais indicativas de concentrações séricas verdadeiras de testosterona; no entanto, em virtude dos níveis séricos flutuantes, tanto as mensurações isoladas como as repetidas não são confiáveis para a documentação do estado hiperandrogênico. O método mais confiável para mensurar a testosterona é o teste de estimulação com o uso de GnRH (25-50 mcg/cão ou 2,0 mcg/kg, IM) ou hCG (44 UI/kg). Devem ser obtidas amostras sanguíneas basais e 1 h (GnRH) ou 4 h (hCG) após a estimulação. O nível sérico normal de testosterona é de 0,1-4,0 ng/mL antes da estimulação, mas de 3,0-7,0 ng/mL após a estimulação.
- Teste de estimulação com ACTH — enviar amostras de soro para avaliação de hormônios sexuais. Os resultados podem ser variáveis.
- Relação de cortisol:creatinina urinários — muitos cães com alopecia X exibem elevação na relação de cortisol:creatinina urinários, apoiando o estado hipercortisolêmico, independentemente do teste dos hormônios sexuais estimulados com o ACTH.

DIAGNÓSTICO POR IMAGEM
Radiografia e ultrassonografia testicular para avaliação do parênquima adrenal e testicular, triagem em busca de massas intra-abdominais ou exame do tecido gonadal como fonte dos androgênios.

MÉTODOS DIAGNÓSTICOS
A biopsia de pele pode revelar alterações inespecíficas associadas à alopecia endócrina; entretanto, esse exame de biopsia de pele não permitirá a diferenciação entre as diferentes causas endócrinas de alopecia (p. ex., hipotireoidismo, hiperandrogenismo).

TRATAMENTO

- Castração cirúrgica de animais intactos.
- Excisão cirúrgica de massas secretoras de testosterona, tecido neoplásico.

MEDICAÇÕES

MEDICAMENTO(S)
- Progestágenos — como acetato de megestrol são antiandrogênicos e podem ser usados para diminuir as concentrações séricas de testosterona; no entanto, seu uso pode estar associado a efeitos colaterais sérios (ver "Contraindicações/Interações Possíveis"); além disso, é preciso considerar os

riscos e os benefícios antes do uso em cães. É aconselhável a obtenção de um termo de consentimento informado assinado pelo proprietário.
• Inibidores da esteroidogênese — como o cetoconazol, a cimetidina ou o trilostano (não aprovado pela FDA).
• Destruição controlada do córtex adrenal (zona reticulada) — via administração de mitotano.
• Melatonina — experimental até o momento.
• Administração de hormônio do crescimento — 0,1 UI (0,05 mg/kg) SC 3 vezes por semana durante 4-6 semanas.

CONTRAINDICAÇÕES/INTERAÇÕES POSSÍVEIS
• Progestágenos — seu uso pode estar associado a níveis elevados de hormônio do crescimento, diabetes melito e supressão adrenocortical.
• Melatonina — regula os eventos reprodutivos mediados pela luz e seu uso deve ser evitado em animais reprodutores.
• Hormônio do crescimento e acetato de megestrol — são potencialmente diabetogênicos e aumentam o risco de câncer de mama. A glicemia ou as fitas reagentes de imersão urinária devem ser monitorizadas durante a terapia. O diabetes pode não ser reversível na interrupção da terapia.
• Inibidores da 5-α-redutase — como a finasterida, inibem a conversão de testosterona em di-hidrotestosterona apenas na próstata e não induzirá a uma diminuição sistêmica nas concentrações circulantes de testosterona.

ACOMPANHAMENTO
• Repetir o teste de estimulação com ACTH conforme for pertinente quando se fizer uso de mitotano ou trilostano.
• Repetir o teste de estimulação com ACTH para avaliação dos hormônios sexuais após a terapia; todavia, as anormalidades dos hormônios sexuais podem persistir apesar da resposta clínica ao tratamento.
• Exame físico para avaliação da resposta à terapia.
• Reavaliar as concentrações séricas estimuladas de testosterona após a terapia se estiverem inicialmente excessivas.

DIVERSOS
DISTÚRBIOS ASSOCIADOS
• Tumores de células intersticiais.
• Síndrome semelhante à hiperplasia adrenal.
• Hiperadrenocorticismo.
• Hiperplasia prostática benigna.
• Hipertrofia do clitóris, vaginite.

ABREVIATURA(S)
• ACTH = hormônio adrenocorticotrófico.
• GnRH = hormônio liberador de gonadotropina.
• hCG = gonadotropina coriônica humana.

Sugestões de Leitura
Scott DW, Miller WH, Griffin CE. Endocrine and metabolic diseases. In: Muller & Kirk's Small Animal Dermatology, 6th ed. Philadelphia: Saunders, 2001, pp. 780–885.

Autores Autumn P. Davidson e Sophie A. Grundy
Consultor Editorial Deborah S. Greco

HIPERCALCEMIA

CONSIDERAÇÕES GERAIS

DEFINIÇÃO
- Cálcio sérico total >11,5 mg/dL (cães).
- Cálcio sérico total >10,5 mg/dL (gatos).
- Cálcio sérico ionizado >1,45 mmol/L (cães).
- Cálcio sérico ionizado >1,4 mmol/L (gatos).
- A hipercalcemia deve ser confirmada pela demonstração de concentrações elevadas de cálcio ionizado.
- As concentrações de cálcio total e as fórmulas de correção não predizem o cálcio ionizado com precisão.

FISIOPATOLOGIA
- O controle do cálcio é complexo, sendo influenciado pelas ações do PTH e da vitamina D e pela interação desses hormônios com os intestinos, os ossos, os rins e os paratireoides.
- O desarranjo funcional desses fatores pode acarretar hipercalcemia.
- A produção secretora de algumas células neoplásicas também pode alterar a homeostasia do cálcio.

SISTEMA(S) ACOMETIDO(S)
- Cardiovascular — hipertensão e alteração da contratilidade cardíaca.
- Gastrintestinal — diminui a excitabilidade da musculatura lisa e pode alterar a função gastrintestinal.
- Neuromuscular — a contratilidade deprimida da musculatura esquelética provoca fraqueza.
- Renal/urológico — altos níveis de cálcio são tóxicos para os túbulos renais e podem causar poliúria e polidipsia (PU/PD) e insuficiência renal; também podem induzir à urolitíase e doença associada do trato urinário inferior.

IDENTIFICAÇÃO
- Cães e gatos.
- Hiperparatireoidismo primário em cães da raça Keeshond e gatos da raça Siamês.

SINAIS CLÍNICOS
Comentários Gerais
- Dependem da causa de hipercalcemia.
- Pacientes com neoplasia, insuficiência renal ou hipoadrenocorticismo subjacentes, em geral, parecem doentes.
- Animais com hiperparatireoidismo primário apresentam sinais clínicos discretos, se presentes, atribuídos apenas aos efeitos da hipercalcemia.
- Os sinais tornam-se evidentes quando a hipercalcemia é grave e crônica.

Achados Anamnésicos
- Muitos animais permanecem assintomáticos.
- PU/PD — mais comum em cães.
- Anorexia.
- Letargia — mais comum em gatos.
- Vômitos.
- Constipação.
- Fraqueza.
- Estupor e coma — casos graves.
- Sinais do trato urinário inferior em animais que apresentam urólitos secundários com cálcio em sua composição.

Achados do Exame Físico
- Linfadenomegalia ou organomegalia abdominal em pacientes com linfoma.
- Em geral, não são dignos de nota em cães com hiperparatireoidismo primário.
- Adenoma da paratireoide — raramente palpável em cães; com frequência palpável em gatos com hiperparatireoidismo primário, embora possa ser confundido com a tireoide.

CAUSAS
- Neoplasia — linfoma (mais comum em cães, menos comum em gatos) e adenocarcinoma das glândulas apócrinas dos sacos anais (cães), mieloma múltiplo, leucemia linfocítica, tumor ósseo metastático, fibrossarcoma (gatos), vários tipos de carcinoma.
- Hiperparatireoidismo primário.
- Insuficiência renal — aguda ou crônica.
- Doenças granulomatosas.
- Hipoadrenocorticismo.
- Intoxicação por rodenticidas análogos à vitamina D — não são mais comercializados nos EUA.
- Intoxicação por vitamina D a partir de plantas ou dietas.
- Doenças osteolíticas.
- Intoxicação por alumínio.
- Hipercalcemia idiopática em gatos.

FATORES DE RISCO
- Raça Keeshond — hiperparatireoidismo.
- Insuficiência renal.
- Neoplasia.
- Uso de suplementos de cálcio ou quelantes de fosfato intestinal que contenham cálcio.
- Uso de calcitriol ou outras preparações à base de vitamina D.

DIAGNÓSTICO

DIAGNÓSTICO DIFERENCIAL
- A anamnese deve incluir a exposição a fontes exógenas de vitamina D e qualquer resposta prévia a esteroides.
- Histórico de doença que se exacerba e diminui sugere hipoadrenocorticismo.
- A palpação completa de linfonodos, bem como do reto e do abdome, pode levantar a suspeita de linfoma e outra neoplasia.
- Avaliação do estado de hidratação, palpação renal e antecedentes urinários apontam para doença do trato urinário inferior ou insuficiência renal.

ACHADOS LABORATORIAIS
Medicamentos Capazes de Alterar os Resultados Laboratoriais
- Os anticoagulantes oxalato, citrato e EDTA ligam-se ao cálcio e reduzem falsamente sua estimativa.
- Preparações à base de vitamina D e diuréticos tiazídicos podem elevar as concentrações séricas de cálcio.

Distúrbios Capazes de Alterar os Resultados Laboratoriais
- Hemólise e lipidemia podem elevar falsamente as concentrações de cálcio.
- Hipoalbuminemia pode reduzir falsamente a concentração de cálcio total.

Os Resultados Serão Válidos se os Exames Forem Realizados em Laboratório Humano?
Sim.

HEMOGRAMA/BIOQUÍMICA/URINÁLISE
- Cálcio sérico — as concentrações de cálcio total dependem das proteínas de ligação; o cálcio ajustado (corrigido) pode ser estimado pelas fórmulas expostas a seguir:

$$\text{Ca corrigido} = \text{Ca (mg/dL)} - \text{albumina (g/dL)} + 3,5$$

ou

$$\text{Ca corrigido} = \text{Ca (mg/dL)} - [0,4 \times \text{proteína total (g/dL)}] + 3,3$$

- Essas fórmulas nem sempre indicam o nível real do cálcio ionizado no cão e não foram bem avaliadas no gato.
- Azotemia e isostenúria ajudam a definir o grau de comprometimento renal.
- O fósforo sérico costuma estar baixo ou nos limites inferiores da normalidade em pacientes com hiperparatireoidismo primário ou hipercalcemia associada à malignidade.
- Hiperfosfatemia na ausência de azotemia sugere alguma causa não paratireóidea de hipercalcemia.
- É difícil interpretar a combinação de hiperfosfatemia e azotemia, pois a insuficiência renal pode ser a causa ou o efeito da hipercalcemia.
- Hipercalcemia e hiponatremia sugerem hipoadrenocorticismo.
- Hiperglobulinemia está associada a mieloma múltiplo.
- Em pacientes com doença mieloftísica, observam-se citopenias.

OUTROS TESTES LABORATORIAIS
- O cálcio sérico ionizado encontra-se elevado em pacientes com hiperparatireoidismo primário ou hipercalcemia associada à malignidade; geralmente normal em pacientes com hipercalcemia associada à insuficiência renal.
- Estimativa do PTH sérico — os métodos para mensuração da molécula intacta e ensaio em dois locais possuem a maior especificidade; concentração alta-normal ou alta sugere hiperparatireoidismo primário; pode estar elevado em pacientes com insuficiência renal crônica; concentração baixa torna mais provável a presença de neoplasia.
- O nível de PTH-rp sérico geralmente se apresenta alto em pacientes com hipercalcemia associada à malignidade.
- Ensaios para a vitamina D não estão amplamente disponíveis.

DIAGNÓSTICO POR IMAGEM
- A radiografia é útil para avaliar o tamanho e a forma dos rins, bem como a presença de urolitíase, lise óssea e neoplasia oculta.
- A ultrassonografia é valiosa para examinar a arquitetura renal e ainda verificar se há linfadenomegalia abdominal, tumores da paratireoide e urolitíase.

MÉTODOS DIAGNÓSTICOS
- Citologia de aspirado de linfonodos obtido por agulha fina para confirmar linfoma.
- Exame do aspirado de medula óssea para confirmar neoplasia hematopoiética oculta. • Teste de estimulação com ACTH para confirmar hipoadrenocorticismo.

TRATAMENTO

- Internar por causa dos efeitos deletérios da hipercalcemia e da necessidade de fluidoterapia.
- Considerar a hipercalcemia grave como uma emergência médica.

HIPERCALCEMIA

MEDICAÇÕES

MEDICAMENTO(S) DE ESCOLHA
• Soro fisiológico — fluido de escolha.
• Evitar fluidos que contenham cálcio.
• Diuréticos (furosemida) e corticosteroides podem ser úteis.

CONTRAINDICAÇÕES
• Não usar glicocorticoides até que o diagnóstico de linfoma seja excluído, pois esses agentes podem mascarar o diagnóstico; caso haja suspeita de hipoadrenocorticismo, não administrar os glicocorticoides até se efetuar um teste de estimulação com ACTH.
• Diuréticos tiazídicos podem causar retenção de cálcio.

PRECAUÇÕES
N/D.

INTERAÇÕES POSSÍVEIS
Evitar o uso de compostos que contenham cálcio ou fósforo, pois podem causar mineralização de tecidos moles em pacientes gravemente hipercalcêmicos ou hiperfosfatêmicos.

MEDICAMENTO(S) ALTERNATIVO(S)
• Bicarbonato de sódio (1-4 mEq/kg) pode ser útil em combinação com outros tratamentos.
• A mitramicina já foi utilizada em crises hipercalcêmicas graves; se possível, evitar seu uso por causa da nefro e hepatotoxicidade associadas.
• A calcitonina pode ser útil no tratamento da hipervitaminose D.
• O pamidronato também foi utilizado com êxito no tratamento de hipercalcemia atribuída a várias causas em cães e gatos.

ACOMPANHAMENTO

MONITORIZAÇÃO DO PACIENTE
• Cálcio sérico a cada 12 h (mensurar o cálcio ionizado, se possível).
• Provas de função renal — a presença de cilindros no sedimento urinário pode ser o primeiro sinal de dano tubular renal.
• É preciso monitorizar o débito urinário, em particular quando se suspeita de insuficiência renal oligúrica, caso em que o débito urinário deve ser medido com cuidado; não é possível determinar se há oligúria a menos que o paciente esteja plenamente hidratado.
• É indispensável monitorizar o estado de hidratação; os indicadores de super-hidratação incluem o aumento do peso corporal e da pressão venosa central, bem como a formação de edema (pulmonar ou subcutâneo).

COMPLICAÇÕES POSSÍVEIS
• Insuficiência renal irreversível.
• Mineralização de tecidos moles.

DIVERSOS

DISTÚRBIOS ASSOCIADOS
Urolitíase contendo cálcio.

FATORES RELACIONADOS COM A IDADE
• Elevações discretas nos níveis de cálcio e fósforo podem ser normais nos animais em fase de crescimento.
• Cães e gatos de meia-idade e idosos com hipercalcemia correm maior risco de ter câncer.

POTENCIAL ZOONÓTICO
Nenhum.

GESTAÇÃO/FERTILIDADE/REPRODUÇÃO
Os fetos correm o mesmo risco que as mães; não modificar o tratamento por causa de prenhez.

VER TAMBÉM
• Hiperparatireoidismo.
• Insuficiência Renal Aguda.
• Insuficiência Renal Crônica.
• Linfoma — Cães.
• Síndromes Paraneoplásicas.
• Toxicidade da Vitamina D.

ABREVIATURA(S)
• ACTH = hormônio adrenocorticotrópico.
• Ca = cálcio.
• EDTA = ácido etilenodiaminotetracético.
• PTH = paratormônio.
• PTH-rp = peptídeo relacionado com o paratormônio.
• PU/PD = poliúria e polidipsia.

Sugestões de Leitura
Messinger JS, Windham WR, Ward CR. Ionized hypercalcemia in dogs: A retrospective study of 109 cases (1998-2003). J Vet Intern Med 2009, 23(3):514-519.
Midkiff AM, Chew DJ, Randolph JF, Center SA, DiBartola SP. Idiopathic hipercalcemia in cats. J Vet Intern Med 2000, 14(6):619-626.
Savary KC, Price GS, Vaden SL. Hypercalcemia in cats: A retrospective study of 71 cases (1991-1997). J Vet Intern Med 2000, 14(2):184-189.
Schenck PA, Chew DJ. Hypercalcemia: A quick reference. Vet Clin North Am Small Anim Pract 2008, 38(3):449-453.
Schenck PA, Chew DJ. Prediction of serum ionized calcium concentration by use of serum total calcium concentrations in dogs. Am J Vet Res 2005, 66(8):1330-1336.

Autor Thomas K. Graves
Consultor Editorial Deborah S. Greco

HIPERCALEMIA

CONSIDERAÇÕES GERAIS

DEFINIÇÃO
Concentração sérica de potássio acima do limite superior de normalidade do laboratório de teste, em geral >5,7 mEq/L (mmol/L).

FISIOPATOLOGIA
• O potássio é principalmente intracelular; suas concentrações séricas não refletem as concentrações teciduais com precisão. • A hipercalemia costuma estar associada à lesão celular (p. ex., traumatismo e isquemia) e outras causas de translocação do potássio para fora do espaço intracelular (p. ex., acidose). • O potássio é eliminado pelos rins e sua eliminação é facilitada pela aldosterona; condições que inibem a eliminação renal de potássio causam hipercalemia.

SISTEMA(S) ACOMETIDO(S)
• Cardiovascular — como o potássio afeta a condução cardíaca, as alterações refletem-se no ECG; à medida que o nível de potássio sobe, as ondas T tornam-se altas e espiculadas com base estreita, os complexos QRS alargam-se e os intervalos P-R ficam mais longos; as ondas P tornam-se menores e mais largas e, em animais com hipercalemia grave, desaparecem (parada atrial); concentrações mais altas de potássio provocam fusão de QRS-T, o que acarreta um ritmo idioventricular complexo largo, seguido por fibrilação ventricular ou assistolia; as alterações no ECG em animais com hipercalemia variam e diminuem com a hipernatremia, a hipercalcemia e a alcalose. • Nervoso — a função neuromuscular é acometida.

IDENTIFICAÇÃO
• Cães e gatos. • Pseudo-hipercalemia em certas raças de cães da Ásia Oriental (p. ex., Akita, Shiba, Jindo e Shar-pei chinês).

SINAIS CLÍNICOS
Achados Anamnésicos
• Fraqueza. • Colapso. • Paralisia flácida. • Morte.
Achados do Exame Físico
Além dos achados anamnésicos, observam-se arritmias, especialmente bradiarritmias, em alguns animais.

CAUSAS
• Pseudo-hipercalemia — algumas células sanguíneas (i. e., hemácias [relatos em raças caninas da Ásia Oriental, incluindo Akita, Shiba, Jindo e Shar-pei chinês], plaquetas, leucócitos) contêm altas concentrações de potássio; se a amostra de sangue não for analisada ou separada imediatamente, o potássio intracelular será liberado no soro, fazendo com que a concentração desse elemento sofra um aumento artificial (pseudo-hipercalemia). • Baixa eliminação de potássio — insuficiência renal anúrica ou oligúrica; ruptura do trato urinário ou obstrução da uretra; administração de diuréticos poupadores de potássio, inibidores da ECA, trimetoprima, anti-inflamatórios não esteroides ou heparina (causando hipoaldosteronismo); algumas doenças gastrintestinais (p. ex., salmonelose, tricuríase e perfuração duodenal). • Translocação de potássio — acidose, síndrome de reperfusão, síndrome da lise tumoral, lesão muscular (traumatismo, deficiência de fosfofrutoquinase), superdosagem grave de digitálicos, infusão de manitol e hiperosmolalidade induzida por hiperglicemia.
• Consumo elevado de potássio — suplementos orais ou parenterais desse elemento.
• Outras — efusões pleurais e ascite.

FATORES DE RISCO
• Fluidoterapia com suplementação de potássio.
• Administração de diuréticos poupadores de potássio e inibidores da ECA, principalmente em pacientes com doença renal. • Condições associadas a acidose. • Traumatismo. • Doença renal. • Doença do trato urinário inferior em gatos machos. • Cálculos císticos em cães machos.
• Trombocitose e leucemia. • Akita, Shiba, Jindo e Shar-pei chinês — pseudo-hipercalemia.
• Deficiência de fosfofrutoquinase.

DIAGNÓSTICO

DIAGNÓSTICO DIFERENCIAL
• Histórico de queixas gastrintestinais que se exacerbam e diminuem, fraqueza, colapso — considerar hipoadrenocorticismo. • Esforço para urinar ou débito urinário baixo — considerar obstrução urinária ou insuficiência renal anúrica/oligúrica.

ACHADOS LABORATORIAIS
Distúrbios Capazes de Alterar os Resultados Laboratoriais
• Trombocitose (>1.000.000 células/mm^3), leucocitose (>200.000 células/mm^3) e leucócitos anormais (leucêmicos) podem causar a liberação de grandes quantidades de potássio no soro se este não for separado rapidamente.

Os Resultados Serão Válidos se os Exames Forem Realizados em Laboratório Humano?
Sim.

HEMOGRAMA/BIOQUÍMICA/URINÁLISE
• Em pacientes com relação de Na:K <27, considerar hipoadrenocorticismo; em alguns pacientes com diarreia e acidose metabólica, ascite, quilotórax ou prenhez, a relação de Na:K também pode ser baixa. • Em pacientes com azotemia, considerar hipoadrenocorticismo, insuficiência renal anúrica ou oligúrica e ruptura ou obstrução do trato urinário. • Em pacientes com elevação das enzimas creatina quinase, aspartato aminotransferase e desidrogenase láctica, considerar lesão muscular. • Em pacientes com trombocitose ou leucocitose graves ou se o paciente pertencer à raça de cão da Ásia Oriental, considerar pseudo-hipercalemia.

OUTROS TESTES LABORATORIAIS
Teste de resposta ao ACTH para excluir hipoadrenocorticismo.

DIAGNÓSTICO POR IMAGEM
Radiografias contrastadas ou ultrassonografia para descartar ruptura ou obstrução do trato urinário.

TRATAMENTO

• Varia, dependendo da causa subjacente de hipercalemia. • A natureza agressiva do quadro é determinada pelo aspecto do paciente e pela gravidade das anormalidades no ECG. • Iniciar as medidas de suporte para diminuir o potássio enquanto se busca pelo diagnóstico definitivo.
• Solução fisiológica (a 0,9%) é o fluido de escolha para diminuir as concentrações de potássio e neutralizar os efeitos da hipercalemia sobre a condução cardíaca; se o paciente estiver desidratado ou hipotenso, os fluidos poderão ser administrados rapidamente (cães, até 90 mL/kg/h; gatos, 60 mL/kg/h ou mais rápido com monitorização da pressão venosa central).

MEDICAÇÕES

MEDICAMENTO(S) DE ESCOLHA
• Pode-se administrar o bicarbonato de sódio a pacientes com hipercalemia grave para induzir à translocação do potássio para as células; se o pH do sangue e o déficit de base não puderem ser determinados, administrar 1-2 mEq/kg lentamente por via IV; para calcular a dose do bicarbonato com maior precisão: cães, 0,3 × peso corporal (kg) × (21 − HCO$_3^-$ do paciente) e gatos, 0,3 × peso corporal (kg) × (19 − HCO$_3^-$ do paciente). • Administrar metade da dose e reavaliar. • Pode-se optar pela administração de glicose e insulina regular a pacientes com hipercalemia grave para induzir à translocação do potássio para as células (insulina regular, 0,5 U/kg IV com glicose a 50%, 1 g/kg IV); a glicose também pode ser usada sem insulina.
• No caso de pacientes com hipercalemia potencialmente letal, administrar o gliconato de cálcio a 10% (0,5-1 mL/kg lentamente por via IV durante 10 min) enquanto se monitoriza o ECG; o cálcio antagoniza o efeito do potássio sobre o sistema de condução cardíaca sem diminuir a concentração desse elemento.

CONTRAINDICAÇÕES
• Evitar os fluidos que contenham potássio e aqueles que causam hiponatremia, acidose ou hipocalcemia. • Evitar os medicamentos que contenham potássio ou interfiram na eliminação desse elemento (p. ex., inibidores da ECA, antibióticos à base de trimetoprima e diuréticos poupadores de potássio).

PRECAUÇÕES
• Kayexalate® e bicarbonato de sódio provocam uma carga de sódio que pode levar à retenção de líquido em pacientes com insuficiência cardíaca ou renal. • O bicarbonato de sódio baixa os níveis de cálcio ionizado. Usar com cautela em pacientes com hipocalcemia.

MEDICAMENTO(S) ALTERNATIVO(S)
O poliestirenossulfonato de sódio (Kayexalate®) por via oral ou retal liga-se ao potássio no trato intestinal, limitando a absorção e a reabsorção; raramente usado na clínica veterinária.

ACOMPANHAMENTO

MONITORIZAÇÃO DO PACIENTE
• Verificar novamente o potássio em uma frequência determinada pela doença subjacente.
• Verificar o ECG frequentemente até que os distúrbios do ritmo se resolvam.

PREVENÇÃO
• Monitorizar o potássio em pacientes submetidos a medicamentos que alteram a eliminação desse elemento. • Administrar o potássio por via IV em uma taxa <0,5 mEq/kg/h.

HIPERCALEMIA

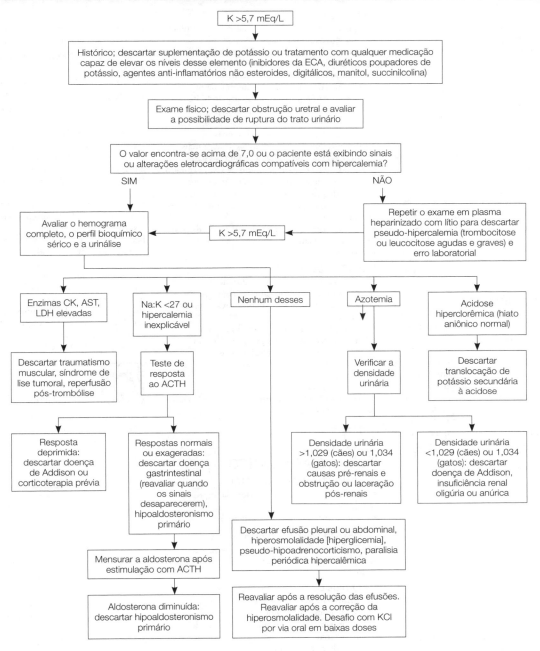

Figura 1. Algoritmo para o diagnóstico de hipercalemia.

COMPLICAÇÕES POSSÍVEIS
Morte de animais com hipercalemia grave.

EVOLUÇÃO ESPERADA E PROGNÓSTICO
Variam com a gravidade da hipercalemia e a causa subjacente.

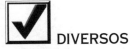

DIVERSOS

GESTAÇÃO/FERTILIDADE/REPRODUÇÃO
Há relatos de hipercalemia e hiponatremia combinadas em várias cadelas prenhes.

VER TAMBÉM
• Acidose Metabólica. • Deficiência da Fosfofrutoquinase. • Hipoadrenocorticismo (Doença de Addison). • Insuficiência Renal Aguda. • Obstrução do Trato Urinário. • Parada Atrial.

ABREVIATURA(S)
• AST = aspartato aminotransferase. • ACTH = hormônio adrenocorticotrópico. • CK = creatina quinase. • ECA = enzima conversora de angiotensina. • ECG = eletrocardiograma. • KCl = cloreto de potássio. • LDH = desidrogenase láctica.

Sugestões de Leitura
DiBartola SP. Fluid, Electrolyte and Acid-Base Disorders in Small Animal Practice, 3rd ed. Philadelphia: Saunders, 2005.
Schaer M. Therapeutic approach to chronic electrolyte emergencies. Vet Clin North Am Small Anim Pract 2008, 38(3):513-533.
Willard M. Therapeutic approach to chronic electrolyte disorders. Vet Clin North Am Small Anim Pract 2008, 38(3):535-541.

Autor Francis W.K. Smith, Jr.
Consultor Editorial Deborah S. Greco

HIPERCAPNIA

CONSIDERAÇÕES GERAIS

DEFINIÇÃO
- Aumento na pressão parcial de dióxido de carbono no sangue arterial.
- Valores normais da $PaCO_2$ — 35-45 mmHg.
- A hipercapnia é sinônimo de hipoventilação.

FISIOPATOLOGIA
- CO_2 — produto final do metabolismo celular aeróbio; considerado a principal força-motriz para a ventilação por meio de estimulação dos quimiorreceptores centrais na medula oblonga; esse gás é transportado no sangue em três formas: bicarbonato (65%), ligado à hemoglobina (30%) e dissolvido no plasma (5%; a fonte dos valores da $PaCO_2$); acrescentado constantemente ao gás alveolar da circulação pulmonar e removido pela ventilação alveolar.
- Raramente encontrada no paciente não anestesiado, clinicamente normal; resulta de hipoventilação alveolar.

SISTEMA(S) ACOMETIDO(S)
- Cardiovascular — pode resultar em liberação de catecolaminas endógenas, o que pode induzir a arritmias cardíacas; pode causar vasodilatação, levando à hipotensão.
- Hematológico/linfático/imune — pode alterar o equilíbrio acidobásico; o aumento agudo resulta na produção excessiva de íons hidrogênio e queda no pH (acidose respiratória).
- Nervoso — o cérebro é o principal órgão acometido; o fluxo sanguíneo cerebral tem uma relação linear com a $PaCO_2$; a hipercapnia resulta em aumento do fluxo sanguíneo cerebral e da pressão intracraniana; uma $PaCO_2$ >90 mmHg pode ocasionar narcose por CO_2 e perda da consciência.

IDENTIFICAÇÃO
Qualquer raça, idade e sexo de cães e gatos.

SINAIS CLÍNICOS
Achados Anamnésicos
- Padrão respiratório anormal.
- Fraqueza — secundária à hipoxemia concomitante ou doença neuromuscular primária.

Achados do Exame Físico
- Pacientes anestesiados — em geral, não exibem sinais óbvios; condição grave pode causar taquipneia e taquicardia.
- Hipoventilação atribuída à fraqueza muscular ou neuropatia — esforços respiratórios fracos; movimentos torácicos diminuídos; esforço abdominal excessivo; movimento exagerado dos músculos faciais durante a inspiração; fraqueza possivelmente generalizada em decorrência de distúrbio neuromuscular primário (miastenia grave, polirradiculoneuropatia).
- Obstrução de vias aéreas superiores — esforços inspiratórios acentuados e prolongados, com expirações variáveis, dependendo da natureza da obstrução, seja ela fixa (p. ex., massa) ou não (p. ex., paralisia laríngea); é comum a constatação de estertor ou estridor.
- Efusão pleural — pode haver respiração rápida superficial; pode-se notar um componente abdominal acentuado; ruídos pulmonares diminuídos na porção ventral do tórax.
- Doença do parênquima pulmonar — aumento dos ruídos broncovesiculares; crepitações (edema, infecção, contusões).

CAUSAS
- Hipoventilação — aumento na $PaCO_2$ resultante de uma queda na ventilação alveolar; pode ser decorrente de anestesia, paralisia muscular, obstrução de vias aéreas superiores, presença de ar ou líquido no espaço pleural, restrição no movimento da caixa torácica, hérnia diafragmática, doença do parênquima pulmonar e do SNC.
- Pode ocorrer em pacientes que estejam respirando espontaneamente durante a anestesia inalatória (isoflurano ou sevoflurano).
- Aumento do CO_2 inspirado — a causa mais comum é o paciente voltar a respirar os gases expirados por causa do acúmulo de CO_2 expirado no aparelho de anestesia; também ocorre com o fluxo inadequado de gás fresco em um circuito de anestesia não respiratório (p. ex., circuito de Bain e circuito T de Ayres).
- Administração exógena de bicarbonato de sódio, que se dissocia em CO_2, com ventilação inadequada.

FATORES DE RISCO
- Uso de agente inalatório (isoflurano ou sevoflurano) como único anestésico, já que os anestésicos inalatórios são depressores respiratórios potentes.
- Planos profundos de anestesia inalatória.
- Fluxo inadequado de oxigênio fresco com circuitos anestésicos não respiratórios.
- Doença brônquica ou alveolar.
- Obstrução de vias aéreas superiores.
- Doença pleural.
- Ventilação inadequada durante a administração de bicarbonato de sódio.

DIAGNÓSTICO

DIAGNÓSTICO DIFERENCIAL
- Paciente consciente — hipertermia; hipoxemia; traumatismo craniano.
- Paciente anestesiado — hipoxemia.

ACHADOS LABORATORIAIS
Medicamentos Capazes de Alterar os Resultados Laboratoriais
N/D.

Distúrbios Capazes de Alterar os Resultados Laboratoriais
Bolhas de ar na amostra de sangue arterial e/ou acondicionamento impróprio da amostra de sangue arterial — valores de $PaCO_2$ falsamente baixos após cerca de 30 min.

Os Resultados Serão Válidos se os Exames Forem Realizados em Laboratório Humano?
Sim.

OUTROS TESTES LABORATORIAIS
- Hemogasometria arterial — diagnóstico determinado a partir de uma amostra de sangue coletada em condições anaeróbias, como se segue: usar heparina suficiente para cobrir a agulha e o interior da seringa; obter amostra da artéria femoral ou podal dorsal; colocar uma tampa de borracha na agulha ou cobrir o canhão da seringa para evitar a entrada de ar do ambiente na amostra.
- Analisar a amostra em até 15 min se deixada à temperatura ambiente; colocar a amostra em gelo para aumentar o tempo de segurança e a precisão da análise para 2-4 h.
- Analisadores dos gases sanguíneos portáteis ou à beira do leito — existem vários modelos disponíveis; tornam a análise mais conveniente.

DIAGNÓSTICO POR IMAGEM
Radiografia torácica — pode revelar doença dos brônquios, dos alvéolos ou do espaço pleural.

OUTROS MÉTODOS DIAGNÓSTICOS
- Endoscopia das vias aéreas superiores — utilizada para descartar massa ou paralisia laríngea.
- Método alternativo de análise — capnômetro (ver Figs. 1 e 2).
- O gás corrente final é quase inteiramente alveolar e tem quase o mesmo valor de CO_2 em relação à $PaCO_2$, muito próximo do valor médio de alvéolos perfundidos.
- Vantagem da capnometria — é capaz de monitorizar a $PaCO_2$ com base em cada respiração, enquanto uma amostra para hemogasometria tem um valor finito em um período de tempo limitado.
- Desvantagens — taquipneia e volume corrente insuficiente resultarão em valores falsamente baixos do CO_2 corrente final; a $PaCO_2$ encontra-se muito mais alta do que o CO_2 corrente final em caso de tromboembolia pulmonar; a cavidade torácica aberta (em caso de cirurgia) relata valores falsamente baixos do CO_2 corrente final em função do excesso de espaço morto.

TRATAMENTO
- Providenciar ventilação alveolar adequada.
- Anestesia — proporcionar ventilação manual ou mecânica com o ventilador do aparelho anestésico.

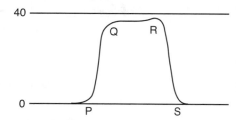

Figura 1 Capnograma normal. O segmento de P a Q da onda corresponde à exalação; o trecho Q a R representa o platô após a exalação, enquanto o ponto R se refere ao CO_2 corrente final; R a S equivale à inalação.

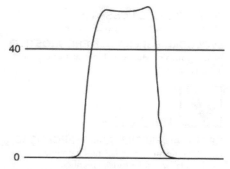

Figura 2 Capnograma com hipercapnia. O platô e o CO_2 corrente final encontram-se acima do normal.

HIPERCAPNIA

- Paciente não anestesiado com doença pulmonar ou neurológica (SNC) grave — conferir ventilação mecânica com ventilador de cuidado intensivo; geralmente requer sedação intensa.
- Suplementação de oxigênio — necessidade determinada pela doença primária; o fornecimento desse gás sem ventilação provavelmente não corrigirá a hipercapnia.
- Tratamento definitivo — tratar a causa primária; interromper a anestesia inalatória ou fornecer ventilação durante a anestesia; efetuar diagnóstico de doença neuromuscular.

MEDICAÇÕES

MEDICAMENTO(S) DE ESCOLHA
Estimulantes respiratórios não são indicados e raramente produzem hipoventilação reversível.

CONTRAINDICAÇÕES
Anestésicos ou outros depressores respiratórios — contraindicados em doença do SNC caso não se consiga fornecer o suporte ventilatório adequado; o aumento da $PaCO_2$ pode resultar em elevações perigosas da pressão intracraniana e predispor o paciente à herniação do tronco cerebral.

PRECAUÇÕES
N/D.

INTERAÇÕES POSSÍVEIS
N/D.

MEDICAMENTO(S) ALTERNATIVO(S)
N/D.

ACOMPANHAMENTO

MONITORIZAÇÃO DO PACIENTE
- Avaliar a eficácia dos cuidados de suporte (ventilação) e do tratamento definitivo — devem resultar em diminuição do esforço respiratório.
- Reavaliar a hemogasometria arterial ou a capnometria — determinam a melhora; avaliar a adequação da ventilação.

COMPLICAÇÕES POSSÍVEIS
Doença concomitante do SNC pode não só causar aumento da pressão intracraniana, mas também predispor o paciente à herniação do tronco cerebral e à morte.

DIVERSOS

DISTÚRBIOS ASSOCIADOS
N/D.

FATORES RELACIONADOS COM A IDADE
N/D.

POTENCIAL ZOONÓTICO
Nenhum.

GESTAÇÃO/FERTILIDADE/REPRODUÇÃO
N/D.

SINÔNIMO(S)
- Hipercarbia.
- Hipoventilação.

VER TAMBÉM
- Dispneia e Angústia Respiratória.
- Respiração Ofegante e Taquipneia.

ABREVIATURA(S)
- $PaCO_2$ = pressão parcial de dióxido de carbono no sangue arterial.
- SNC = sistema nervoso central.

Sugestões de Leitura
Martin L. All You Really Need to Know to Interpret Arterial Blood Gases. Philadelphia: Lippincott Williams & Wilkins, 1999, pp. 27-47.
West JB. Pulmonary Physiology and Pathophysiology. Philadelphia: Lippincott Williams & Wilkins, 2001, pp. 84-111, 125-144.
West JB. Respiratory Physiology: The Essentials, 6th ed. Philadelphia: Lippincott Williams & Wilkins, 2000, pp. 11-21, 103-115.

Autor Thomas Kevin Day
Consultor Editorial Lynelle R. Johnson

HIPERCLOREMIA

CONSIDERAÇÕES GERAIS

DEFINIÇÃO
Concentração sérica de cloreto >122 mEq/L em cães e >129 mEq/L em gatos.

FISIOPATOLOGIA
• O cloreto é o ânion mais abundante no líquido extracelular.
• A hipercloremia está associada a condições semelhantes àquelas indutoras de hipernatremia — perda de água superior à de sódio e cloreto ou consumo excessivo de NaCl.
• A concentração de cloreto é inversamente proporcional à de bicarbonato; a perda elevada de bicarbonato (i. e., GI ou por desgaste renal), acompanhada por baixa reabsorção renal de cloreto superior a de bicarbonato, pode causar hipercloremia.

SISTEMA(S) ACOMETIDO(S)
Relacionados com a causa subjacente.

DISTRIBUIÇÃO GEOGRÁFICA
Mundial.

IDENTIFICAÇÃO
Espécies
Cães e gatos.

SINAIS CLÍNICOS
Comentários Gerais
• Relacionados com hipernatremia concomitante e/ou doença subjacente.
• A gravidade dos sinais neurológicos possui relação com o grau de hipernatremia e a velocidade com que se desenvolve.
Achados do Histórico e do Exame Físico
• Polidipsia. • Desorientação. • Coma. • Crises convulsivas.

CAUSAS
Cloreto Corporal Total Elevado
• Ingestão oral — rara.
• NaCl administrado por via IV durante a reanimação cardiovascular.
Cloreto Corporal Total Normal com Déficit de Água
• Baixo consumo (p. ex., sem acesso à água).
• Grande perda urinária de água (p. ex., diabetes insípido).
• Alta perda insensível de água (p. ex., respiração ofegante).
Cloreto Corporal Total Baixo com Perda de Líquido Hipotônico
• Perda urinária — diabetes melito, diurese osmótica e após obstrução urinária.
Acidose Metabólica Hiperclorêmica
• Acidose tubular renal — distúrbios tubulares renais que causam depleção renal de bicarbonato ou baixa secreção de íon hidrogênio.
• Diarreia associada à perda gastrintestinal de bicarbonato e reabsorção renal de cloreto.

DIAGNÓSTICO

DIAGNÓSTICO DIFERENCIAL
• Acidose metabólica com hiato aniônico normal (p. ex., acidose tubular renal e perda gastrintestinal de bicarbonato).
• Diabetes insípido.
• Desidratação hipertônica.
• Formas graves de diabetes melito (p. ex., cetoacidose diabética e síndrome hiperosmolar não cetótica).
• Ingestão de sal — rara.

ACHADOS LABORATORIAIS
Medicamentos Capazes de Alterar os Resultados Laboratoriais
• Uma ampla variedade de medicamentos pode interferir na capacidade renal de concentrar a urina, causando perda de água superior à de sódio, bem como altas concentrações de sódio e cloreto; tais medicamentos incluem o lítio, a demeclociclina e a anfotericina.
• Outros medicamentos que podem aumentar a concentração de cloreto incluem a acetazolamida, o cloreto de amônio, os androgênios e a colestiramina.
• Pode ocorrer uma concentração de cloreto falsamente alta com uma concentração sérica elevada de iodeto ou brometo — observada mais comumente em pacientes com epilepsia tratada com brometo de potássio.

Distúrbios Capazes de Alterar os Resultados Laboratoriais
• Hemoglobina e bilirrubina causarão leituras falsamente elevadas de cloreto caso se faça uso de testes colorimétricos.

Os Resultados Serão Válidos se os Exames Forem Realizados em Laboratório Humano?
Sim.

HEMOGRAMA/BIOQUÍMICA/URINÁLISE
• Cloreto elevado, frequentemente associado a altos níveis de sódio.
• Diabetes insípido — densidade urinária baixa, poliúria e sódio urinário reduzido.
• Cetoacidose diabética e síndrome hiperosmolar não cetótica — glicose sanguínea elevada.
• Desidratação hipertônica — sódio urinário baixo e densidade urinária alta (em geral, >1,030).
• Acidose tubular renal — acidose hiperclorêmica, pH urinário >5,3, potássio sérico frequentemente baixo e outras causas de acidose metabólica são excluídas.

OUTROS TESTES LABORATORIAIS
Acidose tubular renal — resposta ao $NaHCO_3$ ou NH_4Cl.

DIAGNÓSTICO POR IMAGEM
TC ou RM em pacientes com diabetes insípido para descartar tumor hipofisário.

TRATAMENTO

CUIDADO(S) DE SAÚDE ADEQUADO(S)
Hipercloremia com hipernatremia — fluidos hipotônicos (glicose a 5% em água); diminuir o sódio por volta de 0,5 mEq/h ou não mais de 20 mEq/L/dia.

MEDICAÇÕES

MEDICAMENTO(S) DE ESCOLHA
• Hipovolemia — solução fisiológica isotônica (solução fisiológica ou de Ringer lactato) ou fluido isotônico (glicose a 5% com metade de solução fisiológica).
• Diabetes insípido central — DDAVP (1-2 gotas no saco conjuntival a cada 12-24 h). • Diabetes insípido nefrogênico — clorotiazida (10-40 mg/kg VO a cada 12 h).
• Acidose metabólica hiperclorêmica — tratar a causa subjacente; considerar a reposição de bicarbonato e potássio, se necessário.

PRECAUÇÕES
• A correção rápida da hipercloremia com hipernatremia pode causar edema pulmonar.
• Durante a correção da hipercloremia, pode surgir hipocalcemia.

ACOMPANHAMENTO

MONITORIZAÇÃO DO PACIENTE
Eletrólitos, peso corporal e estado de hidratação.

PREVENÇÃO
É preciso ter a certeza de que os animais sempre têm acesso à água.

COMPLICAÇÕES POSSÍVEIS
• Relacionadas com a hipernatremia associada ou com o distúrbio subjacente.
• As complicações neurológicas incluem trombose ou hemorragias no SNC, crises convulsivas e hiperatividade.

EVOLUÇÃO ESPERADA E PROGNÓSTICO
Varia com a causa subjacente.

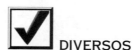

VER TAMBÉM
Hipernatremia.

ABREVIATURA(S)
• DDAVP = nome comercial da desmopressina, uma preparação sintética do hormônio antidiurético.
• GI = gastrintestinal.
• SNC = sistema nervoso central.

Sugestões de Leitura
DiBartola SP. Fluid, Electrolyte and Acid-Base Disorders in Small Animal Practice, 3rd ed. Philadelphia: Saunders, 2005.
Rose DB, Post T. Clinical Physiology of Acid-Base and Electrolyte Disorders, 5th ed. New York: McGraw-Hill, 2000.

Autor Rhett Nichols
Consultor Editorial Deborah S. Greco

HIPERCOAGULABILIDADE

CONSIDERAÇÕES GERAIS

REVISÃO
• Trata-se de um desequilíbrio entre pró-coagulantes e anticoagulantes que alteram a formação do coágulo, resultando em predisposição à trombose.
• A hipercoagulabilidade pode resultar de hiperagregabilidade plaquetária; quantidades elevadas, ativação excessiva ou remoção diminuída dos fatores de coagulação; quantidades diminuídas ou inibição acentuada de anticoagulantes (p. ex., antitrombina III, proteína C); ou fibrinólise defeituosa. • De fato, a trombose é frequentemente considerada como uma prova de que ocorreu a hipercoagulabilidade. Contudo, é improvável que a trombose ocorra exclusivamente por um desequilíbrio da hipercoagulabilidade. • A formação de trombo depende de três grandes influências (tríade de Virchow): lesão endotelial, fluxo sanguíneo alterado (estase ou turbulência) e hipercoagulabilidade. É provável que apenas a lesão endotelial cause trombose de forma independente.
• Os locais comuns de trombose são: artérias pulmonares, aorta distal, veia cava, vasos intestinais/mesentéricos, veia porta, artérias periféricas.

SINAIS CLÍNICOS
• A hipercoagulabilidade é um quadro assintomático. A evolução para trombose pode gerar sinais dependentes do local de acometimento. • Tromboembolia pulmonar — dispneia e taquipneia agudas e graves ou respiração laboriosa crônica. Pode-se constatar a presença de distensão jugular, sopro cardíaco, hepatosplenomegalia. • Tromboembolia aórtica — paresia/paralisia agudas, dor nas extremidades, pulso femoral diminuído e extremidades frias. O início pode ser gradativo em cães, mas muito agudo em gatos. • CID — tromboembolia inicial, seguida por sangramento (ver "Coagulação Intravascular Disseminada").

CAUSAS E FATORES DE RISCO
• CID. • Hiperadrenocorticismo. • Anemia hemolítica imunomediada. • Neoplasia. • Infecção por parvovírus. • Ativação plaquetária. • Nefropatia (ou enteropatia) com perda de proteínas. • Sepse.
• Trombocitose. • Considerar também as causas de dano endotelial e fluxo sanguíneo alterado que podem fazer parte de todo o processo patológico.

DIAGNÓSTICO

DIAGNÓSTICO DIFERENCIAL
• A tromboembolia pulmonar pode mimetizar pneumopatias como pneumonia bacteriana ou fúngica, edema pulmonar e dirofilariose. • A tromboembolia aórtica distal requer a diferenciação de outras causas de paraparesia e paraplegia; ausência de pulsos femorais e extremidades frias confirmam a presença de tromboembolia aórtica distal.

HEMOGRAMA/BIOQUÍMICA/URINÁLISE
Tipicamente refletem a existência de doença subjacente ou os efeitos da trombose sobre órgãos específicos.

OUTROS TESTES LABORATORIAIS
• As elevações do D-dímero confirmam a ocorrência de fibrinólise dos coágulos, mas são inespecíficas quanto ao tipo e mecanismo. • Os declínios da antitrombina III (60-75% como taxa de referência) aumentam o risco de trombose.
• TP, TTPA — tempos de coagulação encurtados constituem um marcador não confiável de hipercoagulabilidade. • Tromboelastografia — há relatos de que esse exame identifique os estados de hipercoagulabilidade em casos de CID, infecção por parvovírus, anemia hemolítica imunomediada e nefropatia com perda de proteínas. • Gasometria arterial — observa-se hipoxemia em casos de tromboembolia pulmonar.

DIAGNÓSTICO POR IMAGEM
• Radiografia torácica — pode revelar poucas anormalidades apesar da dispneia grave em alguns casos de tromboembolia pulmonar; as anormalidades mais comuns incluem oligoemia regional, infiltrados pulmonares alveolares, alterações vasculares pulmonares e efusão pleural.
• Ultrassonografia abdominal — pode confirmar a oclusão aórtica distal em muitos pacientes com tromboembolia aórtica. • Ecocardiografia — para identificar trombos intracardíacos e obter indícios de hipertensão pulmonar associada à tromboembolia pulmonar (dilatação ou hipertrofia do ventrículo direito, aumento da artéria pulmonar principal e regurgitação da valva atrioventricular direita [tricúspide]).

MÉTODOS DIAGNÓSTICOS
• Angiografia — para localizar e confirmar a existência de tromboembolia. • Cintilografia nuclear por perfusão — estudo não invasivo usado para confirmar o diagnóstico de tromboembolia pulmonar.

TRATAMENTO

• Internação — necessária para o tratamento inicial de trombose e o início da terapia anticoagulante. • Cuidados de suporte — garantir um nível de hidratação adequado, manter a perfusão, minimizar a estase vascular, corrigir e monitorizar as anormalidades acidobásicas e eletrolíticas, bem como utilizar e manipular os cateteres intravenosos de forma apropriada.
• Restrição acentuada da atividade.
• Oxigenoterapia — indicada em muitos casos de tromboembolia pulmonar. • Administração de analgésicos para dor aguda. • Informar os proprietários sobre a existência de risco de futuros eventos tromboembólicos, especialmente se a doença subjacente persistir.

MEDICAÇÕES

MEDICAMENTO(S)

Anticoagulantes
• Heparina não fracionada — (para terapia inicial — escolha mais comum), iniciando com doses de 150-200 UI/kg SC a cada 6 h (cães) e 200 UI/kg a cada 8 h (gatos); titular até atingir um aumento de 1,5-2 vezes no TTPA; verificar o TTPA uma vez ao dia (2 horas após a administração de heparina).
• Heparina de baixo peso molecular (p. ex., enoxaparina, dalteparina); (alternada para terapia inicial — mais segura, porém cara); o TTPA tipicamente permanece inalterado (a atividade antiXa é utilizada para avaliação do efeito anticoagulante); dose inicial apropriada: 1 mg/kg (1.000 U/kg) a cada 12 h. • Varfarina — (para terapia crônica) antagonista da vitamina K; a terapia é ajustada para prolongar o TP em aproximadamente o dobro do nível basal; doses iniciais apropriadas: 0,1-0,2 mg/kg VO a cada 24 h.

Inibição Plaquetária
• Ácido acetilsalicílico — como medida profilática para lidar com condições predisponentes ou evitar nova trombose; 0,5-5,0 mg/kg a cada 24 h ou a cada 12 h (cães); 5 mg/gato a cada 72 h.

Trombólise
• Estreptoquinase, ativador do plasminogênio tecidual, uroquinase — a terapia fibrinolítica é um ramo lógico para os casos de tromboembolia aguda. No entanto, o emprego seguro e eficaz desses medicamentos potentes não está bem estabelecido.

CONTRAINDICAÇÕES/INTERAÇÕES POSSÍVEIS
• Não tratar com varfarina de início ou exclusivamente; possível estado inicial de hipercoagulabilidade; sobrepor com anticoagulação adequada com heparina por 4 dias.
• Alta taxa de interação entre a varfarina e outros medicamentos; reavaliar o TP com quaisquer alterações na medicação. • A ocorrência de sangramento representa o maior risco com a anticoagulação; interromper a administração do anticoagulante e administrar a protamina (para casos de superdosagem de heparina) ou a vitamina K (para casos de uso de varfarina) e plasma, conforme a necessidade, para tratar a hemorragia.

ACOMPANHAMENTO

TP — monitorizar diariamente por 4-5 dias (8 h depois da dose) e interromper a administração de heparina ao se atingir o TP apropriado; verificar o TP 6-8 h após a última dose de heparina, pois ele pode diminuir; após a alta hospitalar, verificar o TP 2 vezes por semana, depois 1 vez por semana durante várias semanas e, em seguida, a cada 2 meses.

DIVERSOS

VER TAMBÉM
• Amiloidose. • Coagulação Intravascular Disseminada. • Glomerulonefrite. • Síndrome Nefrótica. • Tromboembolia Aórtica.
• Tromboembolia Pulmonar.

ABREVIATURA(S)
• CID = coagulação intravascular disseminada.
• TP = tempo de protrombina.
• TTPA = tempo de tromboplastina parcial ativada.

Sugestões de Leitura
Thromboembolic therapies in dogs and cats: An evidence-based approach. Vet Clin Small Anim 2007, 37:579-609.

Autor John A. Christian
Consultor Editorial A. H. Rebar
Agradecimento Agradecemos as colaborações de Mary F. Thompson feitas na edição anterior.

Hiperestrogenismo (Toxicidade do Estrogênio)

CONSIDERAÇÕES GERAIS

REVISÃO
• Síndrome que se caracteriza por alta concentração sérica de estrogênios (estradiol, estriol e estrona).
• Pode ocorrer como resultado da secreção excessiva de estrogênio ou da administração exógena de estrogênios, como o dietilestilbestrol.
• Os locais de produção endógena de estrogênio incluem os folículos ovarianos, os cistos ovarianos foliculares, as células de Leydig e o córtex da adrenal (zonas glomerular e fascicular); também pode ocorrer como resultado da conversão periférica de androgênios em excesso.
• Os estrogênios endógenos na fêmea são responsáveis pelo comportamento sexual normal, bem como pelo desenvolvimento e pela função do trato reprodutivo feminino; no macho, os estrogênios são responsáveis pela função das células de Leydig.
• Os estrogênios potencializam o efeito estimulante da progesterona no endométrio e permitem o relaxamento da cérvix — ambos os efeitos aumentam o risco de hiperplasia endometrial cística e piometra. No macho, os estrogênios potencializam a ação de androgênios na próstata. Os estrogênios também aumentam a atividade osteoblástica, a retenção de cálcio e fósforo, bem como a proteína total do corpo e a taxa metabólica.
• Altas concentrações séricas de estrogênio — representam uma fonte de retroalimentação (*feedback*) negativa no eixo hipotalâmico-hipofisário e resultam em supressão da secreção de gonadotropina; interferem na diferenciação das células-tronco na medula óssea e no metabolismo do ferro nas hemácias.

IDENTIFICAÇÃO
Hiperestrogenismo Endógeno
• Caninos machos mais idosos (secundário a tumores testiculares).
• Cadelas mais idosas (secundário a tumores de células da granulosa e outros tipos de tumores ovarianos, além de cistos ovarianos foliculares).
• Cadelas jovens (cistos ovarianos foliculares).

Hiperestrogenismo Exógeno
• Todas as espécies e idades em associação à administração de estrogênio ou exposição a esse hormônio.
• As raças caninas *toys* expostas à terapia de reposição hormonal transdérmica pelo proprietário.

SINAIS CLÍNICOS
Achados Anamnésicos
• Atraente para caninos machos.
• Infertilidade.
• Proestro e estro prolongados (fêmeas).
• Libido diminuída (machos).
• Ninfomania.
• Sangramento e aumento de volume vulvar.
• Hematúria (em associação com hiperplasia prostática benigna ou trombocitopenia).

Achados do Exame Físico
• Cutâneos/endócrinos — alopecia simétrica não pruriginosa (alopecia endócrina); hiperplasia de glândula sebácea da cauda; hiperpigmentação.
• Reprodutivos (em machos) — massa testicular; assimetria testicular (em associação com massa tumoral ou atrofia testicular); atrofia testicular: pode ser unilateral no testículo sem tumor, como observada em associação com tumor testicular funcional produtor de estrogênio, ou bilateral, como constatada em associação com hiperestrogenismo exógeno; criptorquidismo; prostatomegalia (secundária à metaplasia escamosa); ginecomastia.
• Reprodutivos (em fêmeas) — edema e aumento de volume vulvar; corrimento vulvar; ginecomastia.
• Hematológico/linfático/imune — mucosas pálidas; hemorragia trombocitopênica; petéquias; febre (por infecção bacteriana secundária associada à neutropenia); depressão.

CAUSAS E FATORES DE RISCO
• Cistos ovarianos foliculares.
• Tumor ovariano funcional (tumor de células da granulosa e outros tumores ovarianos).
• Tumor testicular (em particular sertolinoma, embora também possa ocorrer secundariamente a tumores de células de Leydig e intersticiais).
• Administração exógena de estrogênio ou exposição a esse hormônio — forma iatrogênica.

DIAGNÓSTICO

DIAGNÓSTICO DIFERENCIAL
Alopecia Simétrica Não Pruriginosa (Alopecia Endócrina)
• Hipotireoidismo — o diagnóstico baseia-se nos sinais clínicos apropriados em conjunto com anormalidades hematológicas e bioquímicas típicas (anemia arregenerativa normocítica normocrômica, hipercolesterolemia) e provas de função da tireoide (T_4 total, T_4 livre, TSH).
• Hiperadrenocorticismo — os sinais clínicos costumam incluir poliúria, polidipsia e intolerância ao exercício; o hemograma completo pode revelar leucocitose e eritrocitose; as anormalidades bioquímicas séricas abrangem elevação da fosfatase alcalina, da ALT e do colesterol, além de queda da ureia; outros exames compreendem relação de cortisol:creatinina urinárias, estimulação com ACTH, teste com dexametasona em baixas doses, ACTH endógeno, ultrassonografia abdominal.
• Dermatose responsiva ao GH — ver "Hiperandrogenismo".
• Dermatose por hormônio sexual adrenal — ver "Hiperandrogenismo".

Atraente para Machos
• Vaginite — pode ser diferenciada de hiperestrogenismo pela citologia vaginal (ausência de cornificação de células epiteliais vaginais), ausência de indícios de anormalidades ovarianas ou histórico de ovário-histerectomia.
• Anormalidade do comportamento — diagnóstico de exclusão.
• Infecção, inflamação (corpo estranho) ou neoplasia do trato geniturinário.

Infertilidade
• Degeneração/atrofia/orquite testiculares imunomediadas — diagnóstico formulado com base no exame físico, na ausência de massas testiculares ou intra-abdominais, na avaliação do sêmen (azoospermia) e no aspirado testicular por agulha fina para os exames de citologia ou biopsia.
• Anormalidades intersexuais — incomuns; o diagnóstico é confirmado pelos achados do exame físico (genitália externa anormal), pelo cariótipo anormal e pelo exame histológico do trato reprodutor, quando viáveis.

HEMOGRAMA/BIOQUÍMICA/URINÁLISE
Hemograma completo — as alterações são extremamente variáveis; se presentes, caracterizam-se por trombocitopenia ou trombocitose, anemia progressiva e leucocitose (as contagens de leucócito podem ultrapassar 100.000 leucócitos/μL nas 2-3 primeiras semanas; depois de 3 semanas, é possível observar pancitopenia e anemia aplásica; hematúria (secundária à trombocitopenia).

OUTROS TESTES LABORATORIAIS
• Concentrações séricas de estrogênio (estradiol) — podem ser avaliadas por meio de radioimunoensaio; no entanto, concentrações séricas fisiológicas podem estar dentro dos limites de normalidade em virtude da precisão do ensaio. A elevação prolongada de estradiol em níveis esperados para o proestro ou estro é responsável pelos sinais clínicos.
• Citologia vaginal/prepucial — extremamente confiável como bioensaio para estrogênio; sob a influência do estrogênio, revela predominância de células epiteliais cornificadas anucleares ou com núcleos picnóticos.
• GnRH — pode ser administrado na tentativa de induzir à luteinização em casos sob suspeita da síndrome dos ovários remanescentes ou de cistos foliculares; administram-se 50 μg de hCG por via intramuscular e verifica-se a progesterona sérica 7-10 dias depois para verificar se ocorreu a luteinização; os resultados são variáveis; além disso, cistos foliculares patológicos costumam ser irresponsivos. A citologia vaginal refletirá níveis de estradiol mais baixos por um retorno às células parabasais.

DIAGNÓSTICO POR IMAGEM
• Ultrassonografia do abdome e dos testículos — para verificar se há massas testiculares, estruturas císticas ou aumento de volume de estruturas ovarianas e massas intra-abdominais, bem como para avaliar o tamanho e a ecogenicidade dos linfonodos locais.
• Vaginoscopia — pode ser feita para avaliar a mucosa vaginal; sob a influência do estrogênio, a mucosa vaginal deve parecer edematosa e rosada ou crenulada.

MÉTODOS DIAGNÓSTICOS
• Citologia de aspirado de massas testiculares obtido por agulha fina — pode fornecer o diagnóstico citológico antes de se prosseguir com a cirurgia.
• Aspirado percutâneo de grandes cistos foliculares ovarianos guiado por ultrassom — raramente resulta em resolução clínica, pois a estrutura cística persiste. O líquido cístico obtido pode ser avaliado em termos de concentração hormonal.
• Avaliação radiográfica de metástases da cavidade torácica em três projeções — fazer antes de qualquer intervenção cirúrgica na suspeita de neoplasia.
• Hemograma completo, bioquímica sérica e urinálise — efetuar sempre no pré-operatório.
• Exame e biopsia de linfonodos locais — para verificar se há doença metastática; podem ser feitos, se indicados, no momento da exploração cirúrgica ou da ultrassonografia.
• Biopsia da parte central da medula óssea — pode confirmar a presença de mielossupressão.

HIPERESTROGENISMO (TOXICIDADE DO ESTROGÊNIO)

- Laparoscopia ou laparotomia — podem ser usadas para identificar e retirar massas intra-abdominais, tecido ovariano ou tecido testicular.
- Biopsia cutânea — pode revelar alterações inespecíficas associadas à alopecia endócrina, como hiperqueratose ortoqueratótica, atrofia e melanose epidérmicas, queratose folicular, folículos pilosos telogênicos e atrofia de glândulas sebáceas.

TRATAMENTO

- O tratamento de escolha do hiperestrogenismo endógeno na fêmea e no macho intactos é a castração cirúrgica.
- Pode-se considerar a orquiectomia ou ovariectomia unilateral do testículo ou ovário neoplásico acometido em animais reprodutores valiosos. O uso de próteses testiculares não é aconselhável e nem ético. Podem ocorrer alterações endometriais secundárias à exposição prolongada a estrogênios; tais alterações, por sua vez, podem contribuir para uma fertilidade abaixo do ideal mesmo se o ovário anormal tiver sido removido, tornando reservado o prognóstico quanto à fertilidade. O exame histopatológico sempre deve ser feito para avaliar as alterações neoplásicas e as metástases locais.
- Interromper a administração ou exposição exógena de estrogênio em casos de hiperestrogenismo exógeno. Cães de pequeno porte estão sob alto risco de exposição à terapia de reposição hormonal transdérmica (frequentemente aplicada nos antebraços) em consequência de sua frequente manutenção.

MEDICAÇÕES

MEDICAMENTO(S)
- Cuidados de suporte — envolvem a administração de terapia antimicrobiana adequada e derivados do sangue.
- Eritropoietina sintética, darbopoietina, G-CSF, GM-CSF — podem ser considerados como estimulantes da produção da série eritroide e de granulócitos no nível da medula óssea; segundo relatos, o lítio mostrou-se benéfico em casos de aplasia da medula óssea induzida por estrogênio.
- GnRH — é improvável que esse hormônio induza à ovulação em casos de cistos foliculares.

CONTRAINDICAÇÕES/INTERAÇÕES POSSÍVEIS
A administração de agentes quimioterápicos para o tratamento de metástases testiculares ou neoplasias ovarianas deve ser feita com cuidado em virtude do alto risco de mielossupressão secundária ao hiperestrogenismo.

ACOMPANHAMENTO

- Repetir hemogramas completos seriados — para avaliar a resposta à terapia e a evolução da doença.
- Repetir citologia de aspirados da medula óssea seriados — para avaliar a resposta da medula óssea e a regeneração eritroide, mieloide e megacariocítica quando há mielossupressão. Pode não haver sinais periféricos de regeneração durante semanas a meses após o insulto inicial.
- Administração concomitante de ferrodextrana por via IM ou múltiplas doses diárias de ferro por via oral — fundamental para manter a regeneração de eritrócitos.
- Uso de eritropoietina, darbopoietina, G-CSF, GM-CSF — monitorizar atentamente a regeneração de eritrócitos e leucócitos.
- Avaliação da concentração sérica de progesterona — pode ser usada para avaliar a ovulação; a concentração sérica de progesterona >2 ng/dL (em geral, >5) confirma a ocorrência de ovulação e luteinização, mas não descarta neoplasia ovariana concomitante.
- Os sinais clínicos da síndrome de feminização do macho devem desaparecer em 2-6 semanas após a remoção do tumor testicular.
- Não resolução da pancitopenia e manutenção da hipoplasia da medula óssea 3 semanas após a remoção cirúrgica de neoplasia ovariana ou testicular ou de cistos foliculares — associadas a prognóstico grave.

DIVERSOS

DISTÚRBIOS ASSOCIADOS
- Prostatomegalia secundária à hiperplasia.
- Hiperplasia endometrial cística e fertilidade abaixo do ideal.
- Hepatotoxicidade (secundária à administração exógena de estrogênio).
- Infertilidade.
- Aplasia da medula óssea, pancitopenia.
- Sepse.

ABREVIATURA(S)
- ACTH = hormônio adrenocorticotrópico.
- ALT = alanina aminotransferase.
- G-CSF = fator estimulante das colônias de granulócitos.
- GM-CSF = fator estimulante das colônias de granulócitos e macrófagos.
- hCG = gonadotropina coriônica humana.
- GH = hormônio do crescimento.
- GnRH = hormônio liberador da gonadotropina.
- TSDBD = teste de supressão com dexametasona em baixas doses.
- T_4 = tiroxina.
- TSH = hormônio tireostimulante.

Sugestões de Leitura
Johnston SD, Root Kustritz MV, Olson PNS, eds. Disorders of the canine ovary. In: Canine and Feline Theriogenology. Philadelphia: Saunders, 2001, pp. 193-205.
Johnston SD, Root Kustritz MV, Olson PNS, eds. Disorders of the canine testes and epididymis. In: Canine and Feline Theriogenology. Philadelphia: Saunders, 2001, pp. 312-332.

Autores Autumn P. Davidson e Sophie A. Grundy
Consultor Editorial Deborah S. Greco

HIPERFOSFATEMIA

CONSIDERAÇÕES GERAIS

DEFINIÇÃO
- Fósforo sérico total >5,5 mg/dL (cães).
- Fósforo sérico total >6 mg/dL (gatos).

FISIOPATOLOGIA
- O controle do fósforo é complexo, sendo influenciado pelas ações do PTH e da vitamina D e pela interação desses hormônios com órgãos como intestinos, ossos, rins e paratireoides.
- O aumento do fósforo sérico origina-se da absorção gastrintestinal excessiva de fósforo, de sua reabsorção óssea também excessiva e de sua excreção renal reduzida.

SISTEMA(S) ACOMETIDO(S)
- Renal.
- Endócrino.
- Metabólico.

IDENTIFICAÇÃO
- Cães e gatos.
- Qualquer idade, embora seja mais comum em animais jovens em fase de crescimento ou idosos com insuficiência renal.

SINAIS CLÍNICOS
Achados Anamnésicos
- Dependem da causa subjacente de hiperfosfatemia.
- Não há sinais específicos atribuíveis diretamente à hiperfosfatemia.
- A hiperfosfatemia aguda provoca tetania hipocalcêmica e/ou colapso vascular.

Achados do Exame Físico
A hiperfosfatemia crônica gera calcificação de tecidos moles, resultando em insuficiência renal crônica e calcinose tumoral.

CAUSAS
- Taxa de filtração glomerular reduzida.
- Azotemia pré-renal.
- Azotemia renal.
- Azotemia pós-renal.
- Hiperfosfatemia secundária à reabsorção óssea excessiva ou degradação muscular.
- Cães jovens em crescimento.
- Hipoparatireoidismo.
- Hipersomatotropismo.
- Hiperfosfatemia causada por absorção gastrintestinal excessiva de fósforo.
- Osteólise.
- Osteoporose por desuso.
- Neoplasia óssea.
- Hipertireoidismo.
- Enemas contendo fósforo.
- Toxicose por vitamina D.
- Suplementação de fósforo na dieta.
- Hiperparatireoidismo secundário nutricional.

FATORES DE RISCO
- Doença renal.
- Uso de enemas contendo fósforo em pequenos animais, como gatos.

DIAGNÓSTICO

DIAGNÓSTICO DIFERENCIAL
- Hipoparatireoidismo — também se caracteriza por sinais clínicos de hipocalcemia, como crises convulsivas e tetania.
- Azotemia pré-renal como causa de hiperfosfatemia — associada a estados patológicos que resultam em baixo débito cardíaco, como insuficiência cardíaca congestiva, desidratação, hipoadrenocorticismo e choque.
- Insuficiência renal aguda ou crônica — considerada pela presença de sinais de azotemia e achados anormais na urinálise (densidade urinária baixa).
- Animais jovens em crescimento — podem ter o dobro das concentrações séricas de fósforo encontradas em animais adultos.
- Intoxicação por vitamina D — histórico de suplementação dessa vitamina ou ingestão de rodenticidas análogos a essa vitamina (p. ex., Rampage®).
- Hiperparatireoidismo secundário nutricional — histórico de desequilíbrio entre o cálcio e o fósforo da dieta.
- Hipertireoidismo em gatos — sinais clínicos de perda de peso, polifagia e polidipsia/poliúria.
- Hipersomatotropismo — cogitado pelo histórico de administração de progesterona em cães e diabetes melito resistente à insulina em gatos.
- Calcinose tumoral sem azotemia — observada em seres humanos como um distúrbio autossômico dominante; causa rara de hiperfosfatemia associada a grandes lesões ósseas.
- Intoxicação por jasmim — histórico de ingestão da planta.
- Factícia (artificial).

ACHADOS LABORATORIAIS
Medicamentos Capazes de Alterar os Resultados Laboratoriais
- Enemas contendo fósforo.
- Fosfato de potássio intravenoso.
- Esteroides anabolizantes.
- Furosemida.
- Hidroclorotiazida.
- Minociclina.

Distúrbios Capazes de Alterar os Resultados Laboratoriais
- Hemólise e lipidemia podem causar um aumento falso das concentrações de fósforo.
- Coleta de sangue com determinados anticoagulantes, como citrato, oxalato ou EDTA.

Os Resultados Serão Válidos se os Exames Forem Realizados em Laboratório Humano?
Sim.

HEMOGRAMA/BIOQUÍMICA/URINÁLISE
- Fósforo sérico >6 mg/dL.
- Cálcio sérico baixo em pacientes com hipoparatireoidismo primário.
- Cálcio sérico elevado em animais com intoxicação pela vitamina D.
- Azotemia e isostenúria ajudam a definir o grau de comprometimento renal.
- Hipercalemia e hiponatremia sugerem hipoadrenocorticismo.

OUTROS TESTES LABORATORIAIS
- Estimativa do PTH sérico — os métodos de ensaio da molécula intacta e em dois locais apresentam a maior especificidade; concentrações altas a normais ou elevadas sugerem hiperparatireoidismo primário; concentrações baixas sugerem neoplasia.
- Concentrações de tiroxina — indicadas em gatos com hiperfosfatemia e sinais clínicos compatíveis com hipertireoidismo.
- Concentrações do fator de crescimento insulinossímile 1 (IGF-1) — indicadas em cães ou gatos com hiperfosfatemia inexplicável e sinais clínicos compatíveis com acromegalia; as concentrações de IGF-1 estão elevadas em animais com hipersomatotropismo.
- Ensaios para a vitamina D não se encontram facilmente disponíveis.
- Teste de estimulação com ACTH para confirmar hipoadrenocorticismo.

DIAGNÓSTICO POR IMAGEM
- Radiografia abdominal para avaliar o tamanho e a simetria dos rins.
- Ultrassonografia renal para detectar mineralização de tecido mole.
- Cintilografia da tireoide para excluir hipertireoidismo.
- Radiografia de ossos longos para detectar osteoporose ou neoplasia.

MÉTODOS DIAGNÓSTICOS
Biopsia renal.

TRATAMENTO
- Internação, por causa dos efeitos deletérios da hiperfosfatemia e da necessidade de fluidoterapia; considerar hiperfosfatemia grave como uma emergência clínica.
- Restrição de fósforo na dieta.
- Soro fisiológico é o fluido de escolha.

MEDICAÇÕES

MEDICAMENTO(S) DE ESCOLHA
Hiperfosfatemia Aguda
- Glicose (1 g/kg IV) e insulina (0,5 U/kg IV).
- Evitar os fluidos que contenham fósforo.

Hiperfosfatemia Crônica
- Administração de quelantes de fósforo (p. ex., hidróxido de alumínio ou carbonato de alumínio, 30-100 mg/kg/dia VO juntamente com as refeições).

CONTRAINDICAÇÕES
N/D.

PRECAUÇÕES
N/D.

INTERAÇÕES POSSÍVEIS
N/D.

MEDICAMENTO(S) ALTERNATIVO(S)
N/D.

ACOMPANHAMENTO

MONITORIZAÇÃO DO PACIENTE
- Cálcio sérico a cada 12 h.
- Provas de função renal — é preciso monitorar o débito urinário, particularmente se houver suspeita de insuficiência renal oligúrica, caso em que o débito urinário deve ser medido com cuidado; não é possível determinar a oligúria a menos que o paciente esteja completamente hidratado.
- Estado de hidratação — os indicadores de super-hidratação incluem aumento do peso

corporal e da pressão venosa central, bem como a formação de edema (pulmonar ou subcutâneo).

COMPLICAÇÕES POSSÍVEIS
- Hipofosfatemia que resulta em hemólise.
- Mineralização de tecido mole.

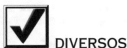
DIVERSOS
DISTÚRBIOS ASSOCIADOS
Hipocalcemia.

FATORES RELACIONADOS COM A IDADE
Elevações discretas no fósforo podem ser normais nos animais em crescimento.

POTENCIAL ZOONÓTICO
Nenhum.

GESTAÇÃO/FERTILIDADE/REPRODUÇÃO
N/D.

VER TAMBÉM
- Hipoparatireoidismo.
- Insuficiência Renal Aguda.
- Insuficiência Renal Crônica.

ABREVIATURA(S)
- ACTH = hormônio adrenocorticotrópico.
- EDTA = ácido etilenodiaminotetracético.
- IGF-1 = fator de crescimento insulinossímile 1.
- PTH = paratormônio.

Sugestões de Leitura
Aurbach GD, Marx SJ, Spiegel AM. Parathyroid hormone, calcitonin, and the calciferols. In: Wilson JD, Foster DW, eds., Williams Textbook of Endocrinology, 7th ed. Philadelphia: Saunders, 1985, pp. 1208-1209.

Willard MD, Tvedten H, Turnwald GH. Clinical Diagnosis by Laboratory Methods. Philadelphia: Saunders, 1989.

Autor Deborah S. Greco
Consultor Editorial Deborah S. Greco

HIPERGLICEMIA

CONSIDERAÇÕES GERAIS

DEFINIÇÃO
Aumento transitório ou persistente das concentrações séricas de glicose.

FISIOPATOLOGIA
- Insulinorresistência e amiloidose pancreática (diabetes melito tipo 2 em gatos).
- Insulinorresistência gerada por hormônios endógenos (hormônio do crescimento) ou medicamentos (corticosteroides).
- Deficiência absoluta ou relativa de insulina (diabetes melito tipo 1 em cães).
- Aumento da gliconeogênese e da glicogenólise (liberação de adrenalina por estresse, diabetes melito tipo 2).

SISTEMA(S) ACOMETIDO(S)
- Endócrino/metabólico — insulinorresistência, glicogenólise hepática.
- Nervoso — hiperglicemia grave pode causar desidratação do SNC por aumentar a osmolalidade sérica. Fraqueza dos membros pélvicos e postura plantígrada causadas por neuropatia diabética em gatos.
- Oftálmico — hiperglicemia persistente pode causar cataratas em cães.
- Renal/urológico — diurese osmótica causada por glicemia que exceda o limiar renal (maior no gato que no cão) provoca poliúria com polidipsia secundária.

IDENTIFICAÇÃO
Cães e gatos de qualquer idade ou raça.

SINAIS CLÍNICOS

Comentários Gerais
- Os sinais clínicos variam e, em geral, refletem a doença subjacente.
- Alguns pacientes permanecem assintomáticos, sobretudo aqueles com hiperglicemia induzida por medicamentos, estresse e pós-prandial.

Achados Anamnésicos
- Variáveis, de acordo com a espécie do animal e a duração da hiperglicemia.
- Podem permanecer normais.
- Cães com diabetes: polidipsia, poliúria, depressão, perda de peso, obesidade, polifagia.
- Gatos com diabetes: obesidade, postura plantígrada, anorexia, vômitos, diarreia, polidipsia/poliúria.
- Depressão do SNC, coma — hiperglicemia grave com hiperosmolalidade.

Achados do Exame Físico
- Podem permanecer normais.
- Obesidade em gatos com diabetes melito tipo 2.
- Postura plantígrada em gatos.
- Cataratas em cães.
- Emaciação em cães com diabetes melito tipo 1.
- Hepatomegalia resultante de hepatopatia diabética.
- Infecções crônicas: respiratórias, cutâneas.
- Má condição da pelagem.

CAUSAS CLÍNICAS
- Deficiência relativa ou absoluta de insulina — diabetes melito tipo 1 e tipo 2.
- Insulinorresistência — diabetes melito tipo 2 em gatos, hiperadrenocorticismo, feocromocitoma, glucagonoma, hipersomatotropismo, hipertireoidismo, níveis elevados de progesterona durante o diestro (cães), insuficiência renal, infecção do trato urinário.
- Fisiológica — flutuação pós-prandial e estresse (hiperglicemia induzida pela adrenalina) em gatos.
- Medicamentos — diuréticos tiazídicos, morfina, fluidos contendo glicose, progestinas (p. ex., acetato de megestrol), hormônio do crescimento, glicocorticoides e ACTH.
- Problemas de regulação em diabéticos submetidos a tratamento — dietas ricas em carboidratos (gatos), problemas com a administração de insulina, hiperglicemia hipoglicêmica induzida pela insulina (rara).
- Administração parenteral de soluções nutricionais.
- Erro laboratorial.

FATORES DE RISCO
- Estresse em gatos.
- Doenças concomitantes — hiperadrenocorticismo, acromegalia e pancreatite aguda.
- Medicamentos diabetogênicos — esteroides, progestágenos.
- Fluidos contendo glicose.

DIAGNÓSTICO

DIAGNÓSTICO DIFERENCIAL
- Uma elevação leve e transitória da glicemia pode estar associada a estresse.
- Em pacientes com hiperglicemia discreta e sem histórico de polidipsia/poliúria, repetir a determinação da glicemia depois de 12 h de jejum e mensurar a frutosamina sérica.

ACHADOS LABORATORIAIS

Medicamentos Capazes de Alterar os Resultados Laboratoriais
- Glicemia elevada — glicocorticoides, ACTH, fluidos contendo glicose, adrenalina, asparaginase, agonistas β-adrenérgicos e diazóxido.

Distúrbios Capazes de Alterar os Resultados Laboratoriais
- Lipidemia, hemólise e icterícia podem interferir nos ensaios espectrofotométricos.
- O atraso na separação artificial do soro diminui as concentrações de glicose; é preciso separar o soro até 1 h depois da coleta para evitar a utilização de glicose pelas células.
- Uso de glicosímetros humanos — pode fazer uma leitura 25% abaixo do valor glicêmico real; repetir com monitor validado para sangue total de cães ou gatos.
- Tiras reagentes para glicemia precisam de sangue total.
- Medir a concentração de glicose no sangue total até 30 min depois da coleta.

Os Resultados Serão Válidos se os Exames Forem Realizados em Laboratório Humano?
Sim.

HEMOGRAMA/BIOQUÍMICA/URINÁLISE
- A hiperglicemia pode ser o único achado anormal.
- Hemograma completo — pode estar normal; possível leucograma inflamatório em pacientes com sepse.
- Urinálise — pode estar normal; as possíveis anormalidades incluem glicosúria, piúria, bacteriúria e cetonúria.
- Hiperglicemia em jejum mais glicosúria sugerem diabetes melito.
- Lipidemia em pacientes com baixos níveis de lipoproteína lipase (Schnauzer miniatura), hiperadrenocorticismo, pancreatite aguda e amostra de sangue pós-prandial.
- Atividade elevada das enzimas lipase e amilase sugere pancreatite aguda, especialmente em animais não azotêmicos.
- Imunorreatividade aumentada da lipase plasmática em pacientes com pancreatite aguda.
- Atividade elevada das enzimas hepáticas pode acompanhar infiltração gordurosa com diabetes.

OUTROS TESTES LABORATORIAIS
- Frutosamina — valores normais descartam diabetes como a causa de hiperglicemia.
- Estimulação com ACTH ou teste de supressão com dexametasona em baixas doses para excluir hiperadrenocorticismo.

DIAGNÓSTICO POR IMAGEM
N/D.

MÉTODOS DIAGNÓSTICOS
N/D.

TRATAMENTO
- Insulinoterapia (cães e alguns gatos) e agentes hipoglicemiantes orais (gatos). • Interromper a administração de medicamentos diabetogênicos.
- Fluidos sem glicose.

DIETA
- Dieta rica em proteína e pobre em carboidrato em gatos com diabetes melito.
- Dieta com alto teor de fibras solúveis e baixo conteúdo de gordura em cães com diabetes melito.

MEDICAÇÕES

MEDICAMENTO(S) DE ESCOLHA
- Insulina — a regular (cristalina) para cetoacidose diabética, insulina Lente® (cães).
- Insulina glargina ou insulina zíncica protamina em gatos com diabetes melito.
- Hipoglicemiantes orais, como glipizida (gatos com diabetes melito tipo 2).

CONTRAINDICAÇÕES
- Medicamentos diabetogênicos (p. ex., glicocorticoides). • Fluidos contendo glicose.

PRECAUÇÕES
Evitar a insulinoterapia rápida e rigorosa que diminua a glicemia de forma abrupta e provoque hipoglicemia ou edema cerebral.

INTERAÇÕES POSSÍVEIS
N/D.

MEDICAMENTO(S) ALTERNATIVO(S)
Acarbose a 12,5 mg VO a cada 12 h; bloqueador de amido intestinal.

ACOMPANHAMENTO

MONITORIZAÇÃO DO PACIENTE
- Monitorizar o animal quanto ao retorno dos sinais clínicos de diabetes, como poliúria, polidipsia e polifagia.

HIPERGLICEMIA

- Mensurar a glicemia após a suspensão dos medicamentos diabetogênicos.
- Medir a hemoglobina glicosilada e a frutosamina em um esquema ambulatorial para monitorizar o controle glicêmico a longo prazo.

COMPLICAÇÕES POSSÍVEIS
- Alta incidência de sepse (e infecção).
- Hiperglicemia grave pode estar associada à depressão do SNC e coma em função da hiperosmolaridade.

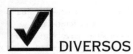

DIVERSOS

DISTÚRBIOS ASSOCIADOS
- Hiperosmolaridade.
- Uremia pode estar associada à hiperglicemia.

FATORES RELACIONADOS COM A IDADE
Nenhum.

POTENCIAL ZOONÓTICO
Nenhum.

GESTAÇÃO/FERTILIDADE/REPRODUÇÃO
N/D.

SINÔNIMO(S)
Alto nível de açúcar no sangue.

VER TAMBÉM
- Diabetes Melito sem Complicação — Cães.
- Diabetes Melito sem Complicação — Gatos.
- Hiperosmolaridade.

ABREVIATURA(S)
- ACTH = hormônio adrenocorticotrópico.
- SNC = sistema nervoso central.

Sugestões de Leitura
Kaneko JJ. Carbohydrate metabolism and its diseases. In: Kaneko JJ, ed., Clinical Biochemistry of Domestic Animals, 4th ed. San Diego: Academic, 1989, pp. 44–85.

Autor Deborah S. Greco
Consultor Editorial Deborah S. Greco
Agradecimento Margaret Kern

HIPERLIPIDEMIA

CONSIDERAÇÕES GERAIS

DEFINIÇÕES
- Concentração sanguínea elevada de lipídios de paciente em jejum (há mais de 12 h); inclui tanto a hipercolesterolemia como a hipertrigliceridemia.
- Lipêmica — soro ou plasma separado do sangue que contenha uma concentração excessiva de triglicerídios (>200 mg/dL).
- Lactescência — aspecto leitoso opaco do soro ou plasma que contenha uma concentração ainda maior de triglicerídios (>1.000 mg/dL) do que o soro lipêmico.

FISIOPATOLOGIA
Hiperlipidemia Primária
- Hiperlipidemia (idiopática) primária — defeito no metabolismo de lipídios que causa hipertrigliceridemia com ou sem hiperquilomicronemia; provavelmente hereditária em cães da raça Schnauzer miniatura, embora o defeito genético ainda deva ser determinado.
- Hiperquilomicronemia em gatos — defeito familiar autossômico recessivo na atividade da lipase lipoproteica.
- Hipercolesterolemia primária — ocorre em algumas famílias de Briard, Collie de pelagem áspera, Pastor de Shetland, Doberman pinscher e Rottweiler; o colesterol LDL encontra-se elevado.

Hiperlipidemia Secundária
- Pós-prandial — ocorre absorção de quilomícrons no trato gastrintestinal 30-60 min após a ingestão de uma refeição contendo gordura; pode aumentar os triglicerídios séricos por até 12 h.
- Diabetes melito — baixa atividade da lipase lipoproteica; síntese elevada de lipoproteína de densidade muito baixa (VLDL) pelo fígado.
- Hipotireoidismo — baixa atividade da lipase lipoproteica e atividade lipolítica por outros hormônios (p. ex., catecolaminas); degradação hepática reduzida de colesterol em ácidos biliares.
- Hiperadrenocorticismo — síntese aumentada de VLDL pelo fígado e baixa atividade da lipase lipoproteica causam hipercolesterolemia e hipertrigliceridemia.
- Hepatopatia — hipercolesterolemia causada pela excreção reduzida de colesterol na bile.
- Síndrome nefrótica — a via sintética comum para albumina e colesterol e, possivelmente, a baixa pressão oncótica acarretam aumento da síntese de colesterol.
- Pancreatite — associada à hipertrigliceridemia em cães, embora a relação causal não tenha sido estabelecida.
- Obesidade — síntese hepática excessiva de VLDL.

SISTEMA(S) ACOMETIDO(S)
- Endócrino/metabolismo.
- Gastrintestinal.
- Hepatobiliar.
- Nervoso.
- Oftálmico.

IDENTIFICAÇÃO
- Cães e gatos.
- Variáveis, dependendo da causa.
- Hiperlipidemias hereditárias — idade de início >8 meses em gatos e >4 anos em raças predispostas de cães como Schnauzer miniatura.

SINAIS CLÍNICOS
Achados Anamnésicos
- Pode permanecer assintomático.
- Ingestão recente de algum metal.
- Crises convulsivas, sinais neurológicos.
- Dor e desconforto abdominais.
- Neuropatias.

Achados do Exame Físico
- Lipidemia da retina.
- Lipidemia do humor aquoso.
- Neuropatia.
- Xantomas cutâneos.
- Granulomas lipídicos em órgãos abdominais.

CAUSAS
Aumento da Absorção de Triglicerídios ou Colesterol
- Pós-prandial.

Aumento da Produção de Triglicerídios ou Colesterol
- Idiopático.
- Síndrome nefrótica.
- Prenhez.
- Defeitos nas enzimas responsáveis pela depuração de lipídios ou nas proteínas carreadoras de lipídios.
- Hiperquilomicronemia idiopática.
- Hiperquilomicronemia em gatos.

Diminuição na Depuração de Triglicerídios ou Colesterol
- Hipotireoidismo.
- Hiperadrenocorticismo.
- Diabetes melito.
- Pancreatite.
- Colestase.

FATORES DE RISCO
- Obesidade.
- Alto consumo de gordura na dieta.
- Predisposição genética em cães da raça Schnauzer miniatura e gatos da raça Himalaio.
- Hipercolesterolemia idiopática observada em famílias de Briard, Collie de pelagem áspera, Pastor de Shetland, Doberman pinscher e Rottweiler.

DIAGNÓSTICO

DIAGNÓSTICO DIFERENCIAL
Hiperlipidemia de Jejum
- Excluir lipidemia pós-prandial com 12 h de jejum.

Hiperlipoproteinemia Primária
- Observa-se hiperlipidemia idiopática mais comumente em cães da raça Schnauzer miniatura.
- Hiperquilomicronemia em gatos manifesta-se, em geral, sob a forma de polineuropatias e lipogranulomas.
- Nota-se hipercolesterolemia idiopática em uma variedade de raças; os animais costumam permanecer assintomáticos.

Hiperlipidemia Secundária
- Diabetes melito — os sinais incluem polifagia, perda de peso, polidipsia e poliúria; os achados de glicosúria e hiperglicemia em jejum confirmam o diagnóstico.
- Hipotireoidismo — os sinais compreendem letargia, hipotermia, busca por calor e alterações dermatológicas (p. ex., alopecia e hiperpigmentação).
- Pancreatite — os sinais englobam dor abdominal, vômitos, diarreia e anorexia; muitas vezes, a hiperlipidemia é acompanhada por atividade alta das enzimas hepáticas, bem como da amilase e lipase.
- Hiperadrenocorticismo — os sinais abrangem polidipsia, poliúria, polifagia, alterações dermatológicas (p. ex., alopecia e pele fina) e hepatomegalia; a hipercolesterolemia frequentemente é acompanhada por aumento na atividade da fosfatase alcalina.
- Hepatopatia e distúrbios colestáticos — os sinais abarcam anorexia, perda de peso e icterícia.
- Síndrome nefrótica — os sinais envolvem ascite e edema periférico; observa-se hipercolesterolemia em conjunto com hipoproteinemia e proteinúria.

ACHADOS LABORATORIAIS
Manipulação das Amostras
- Enviar o soro para exame.
- A lipidemia provocará hemólise se o soro permanecer com as hemácias por muito tempo; questionar sobre o método laboratorial de depuração das amostras lipidêmicas antes de enviá-las para análise.
- Podem ser enviadas duas amostras: uma para análise bioquímica, que pode ser depurada, e outra para verificação das concentrações de triglicerídios e colesterol.

Medicamentos Capazes de Alterar os Resultados Laboratoriais
- Corticosteroides.
- Fenitoína.
- Proclorperazina.
- Tiazidas.
- Fenotiazinas.

Distúrbios Capazes de Alterar os Resultados Laboratoriais
- Colesterol falsamente elevado.
- Amostras obtidas sem jejum (com menos de 12 h).
- Icterícia — técnicas espectrofotométricas.
- Anticoagulantes à base de fluoreto e oxalato — técnicas enzimáticas.
- Lipidemia.

Os Resultados Serão Válidos se os Exames Forem Realizados em Laboratório Humano?
Sim.

HEMOGRAMA/BIOQUÍMICA/URINÁLISE
- Os resultados do hemograma costumam permanecer normais.
- Hiperadrenocorticismo — policitemia, hemácias nucleadas, atividade elevada da fosfatase alcalina.
- Hipotireoidismo — leve anemia normocítica normocrômica.
- Triglicerídios altos — cães, >150 mg/dL; gatos, >100 mg/dL.
- Colesterol alto — cães, >300 mg/dL; gatos, >200 mg/dL.
- Síndrome nefrótica — albumina baixa; proteinúria.
- Diabetes melito — glicose sérica alta, glicosúria.
- Pancreatite — imunorreatividade elevada da lipase pancreática (espécie-específica); hipocalcemia.
- Os resultados da urinálise frequentemente se encontram normais.

OUTROS TESTES LABORATORIAIS
- Determinações de HDL e LDL — usadas na medicina humana; não se pode assumir que os

HIPERLIPIDEMIA

valores relatados de HDL e LDL em cães e gatos sejam confiáveis.
• Teste para quilomícrons — obter amostra de soro após 12 h de jejum e refrigerar por 12-14 h; não congelar; os quilomícrons sobem para a superfície e formam uma camada leitosa.
• Eletroforese de lipoproteínas — separa LDL, VLDL, HDL1 e HDL2.
• Atividade de lipase lipoproteica — coletar soro para determinar as concentrações de triglicerídios e colesterol e realizar eletroforese de lipoproteínas antes e 15 min depois da administração IV de heparina (90 UI/kg); se não houver alteração nos valores antes e depois da administração de heparina, deve-se suspeitar de um sistema enzimático defeituoso da lipase lipoproteica.
• Determinações de T_4, T_4 livre e TSH são indicadas na suspeita de hipotireoidismo.
• Teste de estimulação com hormônio adrenocorticotrópico (ACTH) ou teste de supressão com baixas doses de dexametasona são indicados se houver suspeita de hiperadrenocorticismo.

DIAGNÓSTICO POR IMAGEM
N/D.

MÉTODOS DIAGNÓSTICOS
N/D.

TRATAMENTO
A dieta deve conter menos de 10% de gordura (p. ex., Royal Canin com baixo teor de gordura, Hill's Prescription Diet r/d ou w/d, Iams com restrição de calorias, Purina OM).

MEDICAÇÕES
MEDICAMENTO(S) DE ESCOLHA
• O tratamento inicial é direcionado à modificação da dieta.

• Ver "Medicamento(s) Alternativo(s)" se a dieta falhar no controle da hiperlipidemia.

CONTRAINDICAÇÕES
N/D.

PRECAUÇÕES
N/D.

INTERAÇÕES POSSÍVEIS
N/D.

MEDICAMENTO(S) ALTERNATIVO(S)
• Genfibrozila — 7,5 mg/kg VO a cada 12 h; 200 mg/cão/dia.
• Óleos de peixe — gordura poli-insaturada ômega-3, 50-300 mg/kg VO a cada 24 h.
• Niacina — 25-100 mg/cão/dia (liberação lenta).

ACOMPANHAMENTO
MONITORIZAÇÃO DO PACIENTE
• Manter as concentrações de triglicerídios <500 mg/dL para evitar episódios possivelmente fatais de pancreatite aguda.
• Não é necessário verificar o colesterol com frequência, porque a hipercolesterolemia não está associada a sinais clínicos.

COMPLICAÇÕES POSSÍVEIS
• Pancreatite e crises convulsivas são complicações comuns da hiperlipidemia em cães da raça Schnauzer miniatura.
• Em gatos com quilomicronemia hereditária, foram relatadas alterações como formação de xantoma, lipidemia da retina e desenvolvimento de neuropatias; as neuropatias periféricas costumam desaparecer 2-3 meses após a instituição de dieta com pouco teor de gordura.

DIVERSOS
DISTÚRBIOS ASSOCIADOS
• Pancreatite.

• Crises convulsivas.
• Neuropatias.

FATORES RELACIONADOS COM A IDADE
Nenhum.

POTENCIAL ZOONÓTICO
Nenhum.

GESTAÇÃO/FERTILIDADE/REPRODUÇÃO
Causa potencial de aumento do colesterol.

SINÔNIMO(S)
• Lipidemia — soro ou plasma turvo secundário à hipertrigliceridemia significativa.
• Hiperlipoproteinemia — concentração sanguínea elevada de lipoproteínas.

VER TAMBÉM
Ver "Causas".

ABREVIATURA(S)
• HDL = lipoproteína de alta densidade.
• LDL = lipoproteína de baixa densidade.
• T_4 = tiroxina.
• TSH = hormônio tireostimulante.
• VLDL = lipoproteína de densidade muito baixa.

Sugestões de Leitura
Barrie J, Watson TOG. Hyperlipidemia. In: Bonagura JD, ed., Kirk's Current Veterinary Therapy XII. Philadelphia: Saunders, 1995, pp. 430-434.
Ford R. Canine hyperlipidemias. In: Ettinger SJ, Feldman EC, eds., Textbook of Veterinary Internal Medicine, 4th ed. Philadelphia: Saunders, 1994, pp. 1414-1418.
Jones B. Feline hyperlipidemias. In: Ettinger SJ, Feldman EC, eds., Textbook of Veterinary Internal Medicine, 4th ed. Philadelphia: Saunders, 1994, pp. 1410-1413.
Xenoulis PG, Steiner JM. Lipid metabolism and hyperlipidemia in dogs. Vet J 183(1):12-21.

Autor Craig B. Webb
Consultor Editorial Deborah S. Greco

HIPERMAGNESEMIA

CONSIDERAÇÕES GERAIS

DEFINIÇÃO
- Cães — magnésio sérico >2,5 mg/dL.
- Gatos — magnésio sérico >2,3 mg/dL.

FISIOPATOLOGIA
- A hipermagnesemia é muito menos significativa do ponto de vista clínico do que o baixo nível de magnésio corporal total nos pacientes veterinários.
- Magnésio — perde apenas para o potássio como o cátion intracelular mais abundante; a maior parte é encontrada em ossos e músculos; necessário para muitas funções metabólicas.
- O magnésio no soro ocorre em três formas: uma forma não ultrafiltrável, ligada à proteína (cerca de 25-30%) e duas formas ultrafiltráveis, as formas quelada e ionizada, que juntas respondem por 70-75% do magnésio sérico.
- A forma quelada é unida ao fosfato, citrato e a outros compostos sob a forma de complexos e constitui uma pequena porcentagem do magnésio ultrafiltrável.
- A absorção do magnésio ocorre principalmente no íleo, embora também ocorra no jejuno e cólon.
- O magnésio é um cofator importante na bomba ATPase de sódio e potássio que mantém um gradiente elétrico através das membranas e, portanto, desempenha um papel importante na atividade de tecidos eletricamente excitáveis.
- A interferência no gradiente elétrico pode alterar os potenciais de repouso da membrana; distúrbios da repolarização resultam em anormalidades neuromusculares e cardíacas.
- Os rins mantêm o equilíbrio de magnésio com reabsorção de 10-15% nos túbulos proximais, 60-70% no ramo ascendente espesso da alça de Henle e 10-15% nos túbulos contorcidos distais. Os túbulos contorcidos distais não só estão sob controle hormonal e neuro-hormonal, mas também determinam a concentração urinária final de magnésio.
- Como a homeostasia do magnésio é basicamente controlada por eliminação renal, qualquer condição que provoque um declínio intenso na taxa de filtração glomerular pode eliciar a hipermagnesemia.
- A alta concentração de magnésio prejudica a transmissão de impulsos nervosos e diminui a resposta pós-sináptica na junção neuromuscular. Quando o magnésio foi administrado a cães anestesiados na dose de 0,12 mEq/kg/min, os efeitos cardiovasculares não eram observados até que os níveis plasmáticos excedessem 12,2 mEq/L. A dose total do magnésio necessária para atingir esse nível era de 1-2 mEq/kg. Para causar arritmias cardíacas fatais (fibrilação ventricular), eram necessárias doses cumulativas de 5,9-10,9 mEq/kg.
- O magnésio é conhecido como o bloqueador de cálcio na natureza; as complicações mais graves da hipermagnesemia originam-se do antagonismo do cálcio no sistema de condução cardíaca.

SISTEMA(S) ACOMETIDO(S)
- Cardiovascular. • Musculosquelético. • Nervoso.

GENÉTICA
N/D.

INCIDÊNCIA/PREVALÊNCIA
A hipermagnesemia foi constatada em 18% e 13% dos gatos e cães (ambos hospitalizados), respectivamente. A maioria desses pacientes também tinha insuficiência renal ou azotemia pós-renal.

DISTRIBUIÇÃO GEOGRÁFICA
N/D.

IDENTIFICAÇÃO
Espécies
Cães e gatos.

Raça(s) Predominante(s)
N/D.

Idade Média e Faixa Etária
N/D.

Sexo Predominante
N/D.

SINAIS CLÍNICOS
Comentários Gerais
- Causada, em geral, por insuficiência renal; os sinais clínicos podem ser atribuídos à azotemia e insuficiência renal. A hipermagnesemia clínica é relatada com maior frequência quando os pacientes com doença renal preexistente são suplementados de forma exagerada com sais de magnésio por via parenteral.
- Caracterizada por perda progressiva da função neuromuscular, respiratória e cardiovascular.

Achados do Histórico e do Exame Físico
- Náusea, vômito, fraqueza, bradicardia, paralisia flácida, depressão mental e hiporreflexia.
- Observam-se hipotensão e alterações do ECG, inclusive condução intraventricular tardia e intervalo QT prolongado, à medida que os níveis séricos de magnésio sobem.
- Foram detectados bloqueio atrioventricular, depressão respiratória, coma e parada cardíaca em pessoas com concentrações séricas de magnésio >16 mg/dL.

CAUSAS
- Insuficiência renal.
- Distúrbios de hipomotilidade intestinal e constipação.
- Distúrbios endócrinos, inclusive hipoadrenocorticismo, hipotireoidismo e hiperparatireoidismo.
- Administração excessiva de magnésio em soluções catárticas que contêm esse elemento em sua composição em conjunto com carvão ativado, laxantes contendo magnésio e excesso de magnésio em soluções de diálise peritoneal.
- Suplementação iatrogênica demasiada em pacientes com doença renal concomitante.

FATORES DE RISCO
- Doença renal.
- Hemólise maciça.
- Hipoadrenocorticismo.
- Hiperparatireoidismo.
- Uso excessivo de soluções catárticas que contêm magnésio, sobretudo em pacientes com insuficiência renal.
- Hipomotilidade intestinal.

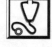

DIAGNÓSTICO

DIAGNÓSTICO DIFERENCIAL
- Os sinais são muito parecidos com os de hipocalcemia que, em geral, ocorre simultaneamente.
- A bradicardia pode ser causada por doença neurológica, hipercalemia, hipertensão, hipotireoidismo, síndrome do nó sinusal doente e vários medicamentos.

ACHADOS LABORATORIAIS
Nota: 12 mg de magnésio = 1 mEq de magnésio; para converter de mg/dL para mEq/L, dividir por 1,2.

Medicamentos Capazes de Alterar os Resultados Laboratoriais
- O soro é preferível ao plasma, porque o anticoagulante usado em amostras de plasma pode conter citrato ou outros íons capazes de se ligar ao magnésio.
- EDTA, oxalato com fluoreto de sódio, citrato de sódio e gliconato de cálcio IV podem resultar em valores séricos falsamente baixos de magnésio.

Distúrbios Capazes de Alterar os Resultados Laboratoriais
- Hemólise pode causar falsos aumentos no magnésio sérico; a concentração de magnésio nos eritrócitos corresponde a aproximadamente o triplo da sérica.
- A conservação de soro ou urina em recipientes de metal pode elevar falsamente os valores de magnésio.
- A hiperbilirrubinemia pode causar quedas falsas no magnésio sérico.

Os Resultados Serão Válidos se os Exames Forem Realizados em Laboratório Humano?
Sim.

HEMOGRAMA/BIOQUÍMICA/URINÁLISE
- Magnésio sérico — cães, >2,5 mg/dL; gatos, >2,3 mg/dL.
- É comum o encontro de hipocalcemia.
- Azotemia em alguns pacientes.

OUTROS TESTES LABORATORIAIS
O magnésio ionizado pode ser medido com algum eletrodo íon-seletivo ou por ultrafiltração do plasma; os métodos alternativos de avaliação do nível de magnésio incluem a medição dos níveis desse elemento nas células sanguíneas mononucleares ou a quantificação da retenção de alguma dose de ataque.

DIAGNÓSTICO POR IMAGEM
N/D.

MÉTODOS DIAGNÓSTICOS
Recursos eletrodiagnósticos (p. ex., EMG e ECG) revelam os efeitos da hipermagnesemia, mas não ajudam a diferenciar a causa.

TRATAMENTO

- O tratamento envolve medidas para intensificar a eliminação do magnésio do corpo e o uso de terapia sintomática.
- Interromper a administração de todas as medicações e suplementos nutricionais que contenham magnésio.
- Diurese salina e diuréticos de alça aumentam a depuração renal do magnésio.
- Fluidoterapia com NaCl a 0,9% confere volume hídrico para combater os quadros de hipovolemia, hipotensão e azotemia.
- Pacientes com oligúria podem necessitar de diálise peritoneal para tratar a hipermagnesemia grave.
- A administração parenteral de cálcio antagoniza diretamente o efeito do magnésio, revertendo a

HIPERMAGNESEMIA

depressão respiratória, as arritmias cardíacas e a hipotensão; o cálcio também favorece a excreção de magnésio.

CUIDADO(S) DE ENFERMAGEM
Os pacientes com manifestações neurológicas de hipermagnesemia podem necessitar de cuidados intensivos de enfermagem para evitar pneumonia por aspiração, atelectasia pulmonar, necrose por compressão (úlceras de decúbito), além de assaduras por urina e fezes.

DIETA
É recomendável a interrupção de qualquer suplemento de magnésio.

ORIENTAÇÃO AO PROPRIETÁRIO
Os proprietários devem entender as condições preexistentes que induziram à hipermagnesemia.

ATIVIDADE
O nível de atividade do paciente depende das condições subjacentes e da resposta à terapia.

MEDICAÇÕES
MEDICAMENTO(S) DE ESCOLHA
• A furosemida promove a excreção renal de magnésio por diminuir sua absorção na alça de Henle.
• A administração enteral e parenteral de cálcio ajuda a reverter as manifestações clínicas de hipermagnesemia e a corrigir a hipocalcemia concomitante; a suplementação oral com qualquer preparação pode ser administrada na dosagem de 25-50 mg/kg/dia; a hipermagnesemia grave pode ser tratada com gliconato de cálcio a 10%: 1-2 mL/kg (diluído a 1:1 com solução fisiológica) IV ou SC a cada 8 h, administrado muito lentamente.

CONTRAINDICAÇÕES
Compostos e fluidos que contenham magnésio.

PRECAUÇÕES
Monitorizar o ECG durante as infusões de cálcio.

INTERAÇÕES POSSÍVEIS
N/D.

MEDICAMENTO(S) ALTERNATIVO(S)
N/D.

ACOMPANHAMENTO
MONITORIZAÇÃO DO PACIENTE
• Concentrações séricas de magnésio e cálcio.
• Função renal — azotemia e débito urinário.
• Eletrocardiograma contínuo, se possível.

PREVENÇÃO
A suplementação de magnésio deve ser abordada com cautela em pacientes com insuficiência renal.

COMPLICAÇÕES POSSÍVEIS
• Hipermagnesemia e hipocalcemia graves podem ser fatais.
• É 2,6 vezes menos provável que os cães com hipermagnesemia sobrevivam à doença do que os pacientes com níveis séricos normais de magnésio.

EVOLUÇÃO ESPERADA E PROGNÓSTICO
Os pacientes veterinários submetidos à administração iatrogênica de doses excessivas podem ter bons desfechos com a identificação imediata do quadro e o fornecimento de cuidados de suporte.

DIVERSOS
DISTÚRBIOS ASSOCIADOS
• Hipocalcemia.
• Hiperfosfatemia.
• Azotemia.

FATORES RELACIONADOS COM A IDADE
Nenhum.

POTENCIAL ZOONÓTICO
Nenhum.

GESTAÇÃO/FERTILIDADE/REPRODUÇÃO
Os efeitos sobre o feto são idênticos aos observados na mãe.

VER TAMBÉM
Hipocalcemia.

ABREVIATURA(S)
• ECG = eletrocardiografia.
• EMG = eletromiografia.

Sugestões de Leitura
Bateman SW. Disorders of magnesium: Magnesium deficit and excess. In: DiBartola SP, ed., Fluid, Electrolyte and Acid-Base Disorders in Small Animal Practice, 3rd ed. Philadelphia: Elsevier, 2006, pp. 210-226.
Jackson CB, Drobatz KJ. Iatrogenic magnesium overdose: 2 case reports. J Vet Emerg Crit Care 2004, 14(2):115-123.
Martin LG. Hypercalcemia and hypermagnesemia. Vet Clin North Am Small Anim Pract 1998, 28(3):565-585.
Nakayama T, Nakayama H, Hiyamoto M, Hamlin RL. Hemodynamic and electrocardiographic effects of magnesium sulfate in healthy dogs. J Vet Intern Med 1999, 13:485-490.
Toll J, Erb H, Brinbaum N, Schermerhorn T. Prevalence and incidence of serum magnesium abnormalities in hospitalized cats. J Vet Intern Med 2002, 16(3):217-221.

Autor Tim B. Hackett
Consultor Editorial Deborah S. Greco

HIPERMETRIA E DISMETRIA

CONSIDERAÇÕES GERAIS

DEFINIÇÃO
• Dismetria descreve a incoordenação dos membros durante o movimento voluntário, caracterizada pela incapacidade de julgar a velocidade, a amplitude e a força dos movimentos. • Hipermetria descreve os movimentos de alcance excessivo com os membros, conferindo um tipo de marcha característico, semelhante à de ganso. O termo dismetria inclui tanto hipo como hipermetria. • O cerebelo desempenha um papel central não só na geração de movimentos habilidosos, mas também na manutenção do tônus muscular e da postura corporal. Ele não inicia, mas coordena e suaviza os movimentos. • O dano ao cerebelo resulta em graduação e calibração imprecisas dos movimentos voluntários e, portanto, marcha dismétrica ou hipermétrica. A força motora é preservada; a propriocepção consciente não é acometida.
• Raramente, a compressão dos tratos espinocerebelares em distúrbios da medula espinal pode provocar dismetria. É mais provável que isso ocorra com lesões de localização dorsal, além de estar associada geralmente à paresia. • Em certas raças de cães e gatos, ocorrem abiotrofias cerebelares autossômicas recessivas.

IDENTIFICAÇÃO
Cães e gatos de qualquer idade, quaisquer raças e ambos os sexos.

SINAIS CLÍNICOS
Outros sinais de doença cerebelar que podem estar presentes incluem oscilação do tronco, tremor intencional, postura em base larga, inclinação da cabeça, perda da resposta a ameaças e anisocoria.

CAUSAS
Cerebelares
• Cães — hipoplasia (hereditária ou secundária à infecção por herpes-vírus canino no período perinatal); abiotrofia; doenças do armazenamento lisossomal; vírus da cinomose; infecções por protozoários (*Toxoplasma gondii* e *Neospora caninum*); infecções por riquétsias (*Ehrlichia canis* e febre maculosa das Montanhas Rochosas); criptococose e outras infecções fúngicas; meningoencefalite granulomatosa; síndrome do tremor responsiva a esteroides (tremor idiopático ou síndrome de tremor do cão branco*); neoplasia; traumatismo; infarto; hemorragia e intoxicação por metronidazol. • Gatos — hipoplasia mais comumente secundária à infecção *in utero* pelo vírus da panleucopenia felina; doenças do armazenamento lisossomal; peritonite infecciosa felina; vírus da leucemia felina e vírus da imunodeficiência felina (a imunossupressão associada predispõe o animal a outras encefalites e a neoplasia); toxoplasmose; criptococose e outras infecções fúngicas; neoplasia; hemorragia e traumatismo.

Espinais
• Cães — cistos subaracnoides; neoplasia; má-formação vertebral e calcinose circunscrita.

FATORES DE RISCO
Cerebelares
• Há relatos de abiotrofia cerebelar em cães das raças Setter gordon e irlandês, Kerry blue terrier, Airedale terrier, Finnish harrier, Samoieda, cães de corrida de Berna, Cocker spaniel, Cairn terrier, Kelpy australiano, Bulmastife, Spinone italiano, Old English sheepdog, Rhodesian ridgeback, Collie border e de pelo duro, Staffordshire terrier americano, Spaniel britânico e Terriers escocês.
• Há relatos de hipoplasia cerebelar nas raças Chow chow, Setter irlandês e Fox terrier de pelo duro. • Doenças de armazenamento lisossomal indutoras de dismetria foram relatadas em gatos das raças Siamês, Balinês, Persa e domésticos de pelo curto, bem como nos cães de raças Springer Spaniel inglês, Cão d'água português, Pointer alemão de pelo curto, Silky terrier australiano, Schipperkes, Setter inglês, Border collie, Saluki, Chihuahua, Queensland blue heeler, Dachshund, Pastor iugoslavo e Terrier tibetano. • Cães brancos de pequeno porte, como os das raças Maltês e West highland white terrier, são predispostos à síndrome do tremor responsiva a esteroides (idiopática). • Metronidazol em dosagens acima de 60 mg/kg/dia pode induzir a sinais vestibulocerebelares em cães. Os sinais são induzidos em alguns cães com doses mais baixas.
• Eventos vasculares, tanto tromboembólicos como hemorrágicos, podem causar sinais cerebelares. Em cães mais idosos, ocorre trombose da artéria cerebelar rostral.

Espinais
• Cães de raças gigantes são predispostos à má-formação e instabilidade vertebral.
• Cães jovens pertencentes a raças de grande porte são predispostos a cistos subaracnoides e calcinose circunscrita.

DIAGNÓSTICO

DIAGNÓSTICO DIFERENCIAL
• Alguns cães, em especial os de pequeno porte, têm marcha de passadas altas em seus membros torácicos como um achado normal. Se não houver outros sinais de doença cerebelar, será importante informar ao proprietário que esse tipo de marcha é normal no animal em questão.

HEMOGRAMA/BIOQUÍMICA/URINÁLISE
• O hemograma completo pode refletir doença infecciosa/inflamatória.
• Em algumas doenças de armazenamento lisossomal, pode haver produtos do armazenamento nos leucócitos.

OUTROS TESTES LABORATORIAIS
• Mensuração dos títulos sorológicos nas fases aguda e convalescente — para diagnosticar doenças causadas por riquétsias, protozoários, fungos e vírus.
• Mensuração dos títulos de anticorpos ou antígeno no LCS (criptococos) — no caso de algumas infecções (p. ex., toxoplasmose e criptococose), além dos títulos sorológicos.
• Análise de PCR no LCS e no soro — para diagnosticar doenças causadas por riquétsias, bactérias, protozoários, fungos e vírus; exame sensível e específico se o agente infeccioso estiver presente no LCS ou no soro.

DIAGNÓSTICO POR IMAGEM
• Radiografia torácica — para identificar doença metastática em paciente idoso.
• Ultrassonografia abdominal — na suspeita de neoplasia intra-abdominal.
• TC ou RM do cérebro — para diagnosticar neoplasia, atrofia cerebelar por hipoplasia ou abiotrofia; a RM é modalidade preferida para avaliar a fossa caudal.
• Radiografia simples da coluna vertebral — se houver suspeita de mielopatia; pode ser útil para identificar más-formações vertebrais e calcinose circunscrita.
• RM espinal — método não invasivo que fornece informações sobre o parênquima da medula espinal.

MÉTODOS DIAGNÓSTICOS
• Exame de fundo de olho — para identificar coriorretinite (indícios de doença infecciosa/inflamatória) e lesões vasculares.
• Análise do LCS — para diagnosticar encefalite; produtos do armazenamento podem estar presentes nos leucócitos em algumas doenças de armazenamento lisossomal.
• Biopsia hepática — pode ser útil para diagnosticar certas doenças do armazenamento lisossomal em animais com hepatomegalia.

TRATAMENTO

CUIDADO(S) DE SAÚDE ADEQUADO(S)
• Sinais clínicos graves e/ou rapidamente progressivos — hospitalização para avaliação diagnóstica e tratamento imediatos.
• Sinais clínicos leves e lentamente progressivos — tratamento ambulatorial, embora os exames diagnósticos que exigem anestesia necessitem de hospitalização.
• Os pacientes devem ter as atividades limitadas e ficar em áreas restritas, onde não haja probabilidade de quedas e lesões autoinfligidas.

MEDICAÇÕES

MEDICAMENTO(S) DE ESCOLHA
Interromper a administração de metronidazol, independentemente da dose, para verificar se os sinais clínicos melhoram.

ACOMPANHAMENTO

MONITORIZAÇÃO DO PACIENTE
Exames neurológicos repetidos periódicos.

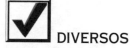

DIVERSOS

POTENCIAL ZOONÓTICO
As infecções fúngicas podem ser zoonóticas.

ABREVIATURA(S)
• LCS = líquido cerebrospinal.
• PCR = reação em cadeia da polimerase.

Autor Natasha J. Olby
Consultor Editorial Joane M. Parent

---

* N. T.: Também conhecida como "síndrome do cão branco sacudidor".

HIPERNATREMIA

CONSIDERAÇÕES GERAIS

DEFINIÇÃO
Concentração sérica de sódio >158 mEq/L em cães ou >165 mEq/L em gatos.

FISIOPATOLOGIA
- Como o sódio representa o cátion mais abundante no líquido extracelular, a hipernatremia costuma refletir um estado de hiperosmolalidade.
- As causas comuns de hipernatremia incluem perda renal ou gastrintestinal de água superior à perda de sódio e baixo consumo de água.

SISTEMA(S) ACOMETIDO(S)
- Endócrino/metabólico.
- Nervoso.

IDENTIFICAÇÃO
Cães e gatos.

SINAIS CLÍNICOS
- Polidipsia.
- Desorientação.
- Coma.
- Crises convulsivas.
- Outros achados dependem da causa subjacente.
- A gravidade dos sinais costuma estar correlacionada com o grau de hipernatremia.

CAUSAS
- Sódio corporal total elevado — ingestão oral (rara); administração IV de NaCl durante a reanimação cardiovascular; hiperaldosteronismo (raro).
- Sódio corporal total normal mais déficit de água — baixo consumo de água (p. ex., falta de acesso à água e adipsia ou hipodipsia); alta perda urinária de água (p. ex., diabetes insípido); grande perda insensível de água (p. ex., respiração ofegante e hipertermia).
- Sódio corporal total baixo e perda de líquido hipotônico (i. e., perda de líquido contendo sódio, sem reposição adequada de água) — perda urinária (p. ex., diabetes melito, diurese osmótica e diurese após obstrução urinária aguda); perda gastrintestinal de sódio (p. ex., administração de catárticos osmóticos, vômitos e diarreia).

DIAGNÓSTICO

DIAGNÓSTICO DIFERENCIAL
- Diabetes insípido.
- Síndrome hiperosmolar não cetótica.
- Desidratação hipertônica.
- Ingestão de sal — rara.

ACHADOS LABORATORIAIS

Medicamentos Capazes de Alterar os Resultados Laboratoriais
Uma ampla variedade de medicamentos interfere na capacidade renal de concentrar a urina, ocasionando perda de água superior à de sódio e alta concentração sérica de sódio; tais medicamentos incluem o lítio, a demeclociclina e a anfotericina.

Distúrbios Capazes de Alterar os Resultados Laboratoriais
Lipidemia ou hiperproteinemia (>11 g/dL) pode elevar a concentração de sódio como artefato quando se utiliza o método da fotometria de chama.

Os Resultados Serão Válidos se os Exames Forem Realizados em Laboratório Humano?
Sim.

HEMOGRAMA/BIOQUÍMICA/URINÁLISE
- Concentração sérica elevada de sódio.
- Diabetes insípido — poliúria, densidade urinária baixa e concentração urinária reduzida de sódio.
- Síndrome hiperosmolar não cetótica — hiperglicemia, débito urinário baixo e densidade urinária elevada (em geral, >1,025).
- Desidratação hipertônica — concentração urinária reduzida de sódio e densidade urinária alta (em geral, >1,030).

OUTROS TESTES LABORATORIAIS
- Teste modificado de privação de água (ver protocolo do teste no Apêndice II) para diferenciar diabetes insípido de outras causas de poliúria e polidipsia; feito após os resultados do hemograma completo, da análise bioquímica, da urinálise e da avaliação dos testes endócrinos, para descartar hiperadrenocorticismo.
- Após a restrição de água, os pacientes com diabetes insípido apresentam pouco ou nenhum aumento na densidade ou osmolalidade urinárias.
- Após administração de ADH ou DDAVP, os pacientes com diabetes insípido nefrogênico sofrem aumento <10% na densidade urinária; aqueles com diabetes insípido central exibem aumento de 10-800%.

DIAGNÓSTICO POR IMAGEM
TC ou RM em pacientes com diabetes insípido para excluir tumor hipofisário.

TRATAMENTO
- Após a resolução da hipernatremia, considerar o uso de dieta hipossódica (especialmente em pacientes com diabetes insípido nefrogênico).
- A água tem de estar disponível o tempo todo para os pacientes com diabetes insípido.

MEDICAÇÕES

MEDICAMENTO(S) DE ESCOLHA
- Em caso de hipovolemia grave — repor o volume com solução fisiológica isotônica (i. e., solução de Ringer lactato ou solução fisiológica) ou fluidos isotônicos (p. ex., glicose a 5% com metade de solução fisiológica).
- Hipernatremia — administrar fluidos hipotônicos (p. ex., glicose a 5% em água) para reduzir o sódio sérico em 0,5 mEq/h ou não mais que 20 mEq/L/dia; suplementar com potássio e fosfato se necessário.
- Diabetes insípido central — DDAVP (1-2 gotas no saco subconjuntival a cada 12-24 h).
- Diabetes insípido nefrogênico — hidroclorotiazida (2-4 mg/kg VO a cada 12 h).

CONTRAINDICAÇÕES
Consultar a literatura especializada do fabricante.

PRECAUÇÕES
- A correção rápida da hipernatremia pode causar edema pulmonar.
- Durante a correção da hipernatremia, pode surgir hipocalcemia.

ACOMPANHAMENTO

MONITORIZAÇÃO DO PACIENTE
- Quadro agudo — eletrólitos, débito urinário e peso corporal.
- Diabetes insípido — consumo de água.

COMPLICAÇÕES POSSÍVEIS
- Trombose ou hemorragia do SNC.
- Hiperatividade.
- Crises convulsivas.
- Sódio sérico >180 mEq/L frequentemente associado a dano residual do SNC.
- Embora muitos pacientes se recuperem, a possibilidade de dano neurológico é maior.

DIVERSOS

FATORES RELACIONADOS COM A IDADE
N/D.

POTENCIAL ZOONÓTICO
Nenhum.

SINÔNIMO(S)
Nenhum.

VER TAMBÉM
- Diabetes Insípido.
- Hipostenúria.

ABREVIATURA(S)
- ADH = hormônio antidiurético.
- DDAVP = nome comercial da desmopressina, uma preparação sintética do ADH.
- RM = ressonância magnética.
- SNC = sistema nervoso central.
- TC = tomografia computadorizada.

Sugestões de Leitura
DiBartola SP. Fluid, Electrolyte, and Acid-Base Disorders in Small Animal Practice, 3rd ed. Philadelphia: Saunders, 2005.
Marks SL, Taboada J. Hypernatremia and hypertonic syndromes. Vet Clin North Am Small Anim Pract 1998, 28(3):533-543.
Ross DB. Clinical Physiology of Acid-Base and Electrolyte Disorders, 3rd ed. New York: McGraw-Hill, 1989.

Autor Rhett Nichols
Consultor Editorial Deborah S. Greco

HIPEROSMOLARIDADE

CONSIDERAÇÕES GERAIS

DEFINIÇÃO
- Osmolaridade — expressa em mOsm/L; representa o número de partículas de soluto por litro de solução.
- Osmolalidade — expressa em mOsm/kg; representa o número de partículas de soluto por quilograma de solução.
- Hiperosmolaridade — alta concentração de partículas de soluto por litro de solução.
- Concentrações séricas >310 mOsm/L em cães e >330 mOsm/L em gatos, em geral, são consideradas hiperosmolares.

FISIOPATOLOGIA
- O sódio sérico é responsável pela maioria das partículas osmoticamente ativas que contribuem para a osmolaridade sérica; a glicose sérica e a ureia também contribuem para a osmolaridade sérica.
- Qualquer coisa que gere a perda de água aumenta as concentrações de solutos no plasma ou no soro, elevando com isso a osmolaridade sérica.
- O volume de sangue, o estado de hidratação e o nível do ADH estão intimamente envolvidos no controle de volume do líquido extracelular.
- O baixo volume de sangue circulante estimula os barorreceptores carotídeos e aórticos a responderem às alterações na pressão arterial, provocando a secreção de ADH.
- A hiperosmolaridade acomete os osmorreceptores no hipotálamo e estimula a secreção de ADH pela neuro-hipófise; o centro hipotalâmico da sede também é estimulado e provoca o aumento do consumo de água para neutralizar a hiperosmolaridade sérica por diluição dos solutos.
- Aumentos rápidos na osmolaridade sérica geram deslocamento da água ao longo de seu gradiente de concentração do espaço intracelular para o extracelular, resultando em desidratação neuronal, encolhimento e morte celular; os vasos cerebrais podem enfraquecer e gerar hemorragia.

SISTEMA(S) ACOMETIDO(S)
- Cardiovascular — hipotensão e contratilidade ventricular diminuída.
- Nervoso — a sede excessiva pode ser o primeiro sinal de hiperosmolaridade. A depressão do SNC pode levar ao coma.
- Renal/urológico — baixo débito urinário.

IDENTIFICAÇÃO
- Cães e gatos.
- Hipodipsia e hiperosmolaridade foram relatadas em cadelas jovens da raça Schnauzer miniatura.

SINAIS CLÍNICOS
Comentários Gerais
- Principalmente neurológicos ou comportamentais.
- A gravidade está mais relacionada com a rapidez com que ocorre a hiperosmolaridade do que com a magnitude absoluta da alteração.
- É mais provável que os sinais clínicos ocorram se a osmolaridade sérica estiver > 350 mOsm/L e, em geral, eles serão graves a níveis >375 mOsm/L.

Achados Anamnésicos
- Anorexia, letargia, vômitos, fraqueza, desorientação, ataxia, crises convulsivas e coma; polidipsia seguida por hipodipsia.

Achados do Exame Físico
- O animal pode permanecer assintomático ou exibir anormalidades que podem refletir a doença subjacente.
- Além dos achados anamnésicos, podem ser detectados os sinais de desidratação, taquicardia, hipotensão, pulsos fracos e febre.

CAUSAS
Aumento de Solutos
Hipernatremia, hiperglicemia, azotemia grave, intoxicação por etilenoglicol, envenenamento por sal, enemas de fosfato de sódio em cães de pequeno porte e gatos, manitol, solução de contraste radiográfico, administração de etanol, intoxicação por ácido acetilsalicílico, choque, lactato em pacientes com acidose láctica, acetoacetato e β-hidroxibutirato em pacientes com cetoacidose, nutrição enteral líquida e soluções de nutrição parenteral.

Diminuição de Volume do Líquido Extracelular
Desidratação — perda gastrintestinal, perda cutânea, perda para o terceiro espaço, baixo consumo de água e poliúria sem polidipsia compensatória adequada.

FATORES DE RISCO
- Condições clínicas predisponentes — insuficiência renal, diabetes insípido, diabetes melito, hiperadrenocorticismo, hiperaldosteronismo e intermação/insolação.
- Soluções hiperosmolares terapêuticas — fisiológica hipertônica, bicarbonato de sódio, enemas de fosfato de sódio em cães de pequeno porte e gatos, manitol e soluções de nutrição parenteral.
- Temperaturas ambientais elevadas.
- Febre.

DIAGNÓSTICO

DIAGNÓSTICO DIFERENCIAL
- Doença e neoplasia primárias do SNC podem ser caracterizadas por alteração da atividade mental, mas a osmolaridade sérica costuma permanecer normal.
- Em geral, os indícios físicos ou o histórico de lesão ajudam a excluir depressão do SNC causada por traumatismo craniano.
- Realizar um exame físico completo para avaliar o estado de hidratação e obter informações a respeito de terapia prévia que possa ter incluído fluidos contendo sódio ou soluções hiperosmolares.

ACHADOS LABORATORIAIS
Medicamentos Capazes de Alterar os Resultados Laboratoriais
A administração excessiva de fluidos contendo sódio ou soluções hiperosmolares aumenta a osmolaridade sérica.

Distúrbios Capazes de Alterar os Resultados Laboratoriais
N/D.

Os Resultados Serão Válidos se os Exames Forem Realizados em Laboratório Humano?
Sim.

HEMOGRAMA/BIOQUÍMICA/URINÁLISE
- Aumento do hematócrito, da hemoglobina e das proteínas plasmáticas em pacientes desidratados; também pode haver aumento dos eletrólitos séricos.
- Hiperosmolaridade é uma indicação para se avaliar as concentrações séricas de sódio e glicose.
- Sem a presença de osmoles excessivos não mensurados, a estimativa da osmolaridade sérica pode ser calculada a partir do perfil bioquímico sérico da seguinte maneira:

$$2(Na^+ + K^+) + glicose/18 + ureia/2,8 = mOsm/L$$

- Normalmente, a osmolaridade calculada não deve exceder a mensurada; se isso acontecer, considerar erro do laboratório.
- Se a osmolaridade mensurada exceder a calculada, determinar o hiato osmolar.
- Hiato osmolar = osmolaridade mensurada — osmolaridade calculada.
- Osmolaridade mensurada alta e osmolaridade calculada normal com hiato osmolar elevado indicam a presença de solutos não mensurados (exceto Na, K, glicose e ureia).
- Osmolaridade mensurada alta com hiato osmolar normal, em geral, indicam que a hiperosmolaridade é causada por hiperglicemia ou hipernatremia.
- A concentração sérica de sódio pode estar artificialmente baixa em pacientes com hiperglicemia grave e hiperosmolaridade.
- Hiperglicemia em jejum e glicosúria confirmam o diagnóstico de diabetes melito.
- Inúmeros cristais de oxalato de cálcio na urina sugerem intoxicação por etilenoglicol.
- Densidade urinária elevada exclui diabetes insípido.
- Densidade urinária baixa, em especial hipostenúria, sugere diabetes insípido.

OUTROS TESTES LABORATORIAIS
Osmolaridade urinária inferior à sérica sugere diabetes insípido; urina concentrada descarta diabetes insípido.

DIAGNÓSTICO POR IMAGEM
A ultrassonografia renal pode revelar rins hiperecoicos brilhantes em pacientes com intoxicação por etilenoglicol.

MÉTODOS DIAGNÓSTICOS
N/D.

TRATAMENTO

- Uma leve hiperosmolaridade sem sinais clínicos pode não justificar um tratamento específico, mas é preciso diagnosticar e tratar as doenças subjacentes.
- Internar os pacientes com osmolaridade moderada a alta (>350 mOsm/L) e aqueles com sinais clínicos e, gradativamente, diminuir a osmolaridade sérica com fluidos IV enquanto se busca o diagnóstico definitivo.
- Administrar glicose a 5% em água ou solução fisiológica a 0,45% IV lentamente.
- O déficit de água livre deve ser calculado pela seguinte fórmula:

$$\text{Déficit de água livre} = 0,4 \times \text{peso corporal magro em kg} \times [(Na\ \text{plasmático}/140) - 1]$$

- O objetivo é não diminuir o sódio em mais de 15 mEq/L no período de 8 h; ou seja, o objetivo

definitivo é não diminuir o sódio mais de 2 mEq/L por hora.
• Inicialmente, pode-se usar solução fisiológica a 0,9% para restaurar a hemodinâmica normal e repor os déficits causados pela desidratação; repor metade dos déficits gerados pela desidratação no decorrer de 12 h e o restante nas 24 h subsequentes; em seguida, passar a usar a glicose a 5% em água ou solução fisiológica a 0,45%.

MEDICAÇÕES
MEDICAMENTO(S) DE ESCOLHA
As crises convulsivas podem ser controladas com diazepam, fenobarbital, propofol ou pentobarbital.
CONTRAINDICAÇÕES
Soluções fisiológica hipertônica e hiperosmolar.
PRECAUÇÕES
• Inicialmente, pode-se usar solução fisiológica, mas sua administração rápida pode agravar os sinais neurológicos.
• A administração rápida de fluidos hipotônicos (p. ex., glicose a 5% em água e solução fisiológica a 0,45%) também pode causar edema cerebral e agravar os sinais neurológicos.
INTERAÇÕES POSSÍVEIS
N/D.
MEDICAMENTO(S) ALTERNATIVO(S)
Pode-se administrar a insulina regular, 0,1 unidade/kg IM ou IV, se ocorrer uma crise hiperglicêmica secundária à administração de nutrição parenteral.

ACOMPANHAMENTO
MONITORIZAÇÃO DO PACIENTE
• Estado de hidratação; evitar super-hidratação.
• Tamanho da bexiga, débito urinário e padrões respiratórios durante a administração IV de fluidos.
• Anúria, padrões respiratórios irregulares, agravamento da depressão, coma ou crises convulsivas podem ser sinais de deterioração.
COMPLICAÇÕES POSSÍVEIS
Alteração da consciência e comportamento anormal.

DIVERSOS
DISTÚRBIOS ASSOCIADOS
Hipernatremia e hiperglicemia.
FATORES RELACIONADOS COM A IDADE
Nenhum.
POTENCIAL ZOONÓTICO
Nenhum.
GESTAÇÃO/FERTILIDADE/REPRODUÇÃO
N/D.
VER TAMBÉM
• Diabetes Melito com Coma Hiperosmolar.
• Hiperglicemia.
• Hipernatremia.

ABREVIATURA(S)
• ADH = hormônio antidiurético.
• SNC = sistema nervoso central.

Sugestões de Leitura
DiBartola SP, ed. Fluid Therapy in Small Animal Practice. Philadelphia: Saunders, 1992.
DiBartola SP, Green RA, Autran de Morais HS. Osmolality and osmolal gap. In: Willard MD, Tvedten H, Turnwald GH, eds., Small Animal Clinical Diagnosis by Laboratory Methods, 2nd ed. Philadelphia: Saunders, 1994, pp. 106-107.
Goldcamp C, Schaer M. Hypernatremia in dogs. Compend Contin Educ Pract Vet 2007, 29(3):148-152.
Koenig A, Drobatz KJ, Beale AB, King LG. Hyperglycemic, hyperosmolar syndrome in feline diabetics: 17 cases (1995-2001). J Vet Emerg Crit Care 2004, 14:30-40.
Moens NMM, Remedios AM. Hyperosmolar hyperglycemic syndrome in a dog resulting from parenteral nutrition overload. J Small Anim Pract 1997, 38:417-420.
Riley JH, Cornelius LM. Osmolality. In: Loeb WF, Quimby FW, eds., The Clinical Chemistry of Laboratory Animals. New York: Pergamon Press, 1989, pp. 395-397.
Schermerhorn T, Barr SC. Relationships between glucose, sodium, and effective osmolality in dogs and cats. J Vet Emerg Crit Care 2006, 16:19-24.

Autor Elisa M. Mazzaferro
Consultor Editorial Deborah S. Greco

Hiperparatireoidismo

CONSIDERAÇÕES GERAIS

DEFINIÇÃO
Concentração circulante alta, patológica e contínua de PTH.

FISIOPATOLOGIA
• PTH — secretado pelas paratireoides em resposta a alterações na concentração de cálcio ionizado no soro; a concentração sérica de cálcio sobe por seus efeitos sobre a reabsorção óssea e tubular renal de cálcio e a absorção intestinal de cálcio dependente da vitamina D.
• Pode se desenvolver como uma condição primária ou ser secundária a algum distúrbio da homeostase do cálcio; o hiperparatireoidismo primário está associado a adenomas benignos (em geral) da(s) paratireoide(s); o hiperparatireoidismo secundário pode ser causado por deficiência de cálcio e vitamina D associada à desnutrição ou doença renal crônica.

SISTEMA(S) ACOMETIDO(S)
• Gastrintestinal.
• Neuromuscular.
• Cardiovascular.
• Renal/urológico.

GENÉTICA
• Não há nenhuma base genética conhecida para o hiperparatireoidismo primário, mas sua associação a certas raças sugere uma possível base hereditária em alguns casos.
• Pode ocorrer o desenvolvimento de hiperparatireoidismo secundário associado à nefropatia hereditária, embora não seja um distúrbio herdado em si.

INCIDÊNCIA/PREVALÊNCIA
• A prevalência da forma primária não é conhecida.
• Diagnosticado mais comumente em cães do que em gatos.
• Razoavelmente comum entre as causas de hipercalcemia, porém muito menos comum que a hipercalcemia por malignidade em cães.
• A prevalência do hiperparatireoidismo secundário nutricional está diminuindo à medida que o público se torna mais instruído sobre a nutrição dos animais de estimação.
• Insuficiência renal crônica com hiperparatireoidismo secundário é extremamente comum, mais ainda em gatos do que em cães.

DISTRIBUIÇÃO GEOGRÁFICA
N/D.

IDENTIFICAÇÃO
Espécies
Cães e gatos.

Raça(s) Predominante(s)
• Cães da raça Keeshond.
• Gatos da raça Siamês.

Idade Média e Faixa Etária
• Gatos — idade média, 13 anos; faixa, 8-15 anos.
• Cães — idade média, 10 anos; faixa, 5-15 anos.

Sexo Predominante
Nenhum.

SINAIS CLÍNICOS
Comentários Gerais
• A maioria dos cães e gatos com hiperparatireoidismo primário não parece doente.
• Os sinais costumam ser leves e atribuídos exclusivamente aos efeitos da hipercalcemia.
• Os sinais tornam-se evidentes quando a hipercalcemia é grave e crônica.

Achados Anamnésicos
• Poliúria.
• Polidipsia.
• Anorexia.
• Letargia.
• Vômitos.
• Fraqueza.
• Urolitíase.
• Estupor e coma.

Achados do Exame Físico
• Em geral, não exibem nada digno de nota.
• O adenoma da paratireoide não é palpável em cães, mas costuma ser em gatos.
• A doença secundária nutricional, às vezes, está associada a fraturas ósseas patológicas e má condição corporal geral.

CAUSAS
• Hiperparatireoidismo primário — adenoma da paratireoide secretor de PTH. Na maioria dos casos, apenas uma única glândula paratireoide encontra-se adenomatosa. Os tumores malignos das paratireoides são raros e geralmente não invasivos.
• Hiperparatireoidismo secundário renal — perda renal de cálcio e absorção intestinal reduzida de cálcio em virtude de deficiência na produção de calcitriol pelas células tubulares renais.
• Hiperparatireoidismo secundário nutricional — deficiência nutricional de cálcio e vitamina D.

FATORES DE RISCO
• Hiperparatireoidismo primário — desconhecidos.
• Hiperparatireoidismo secundário — doença tubular renal coexistente ou nutrição deficiente em cálcio/vitamina D.

DIAGNÓSTICO

DIAGNÓSTICO DIFERENCIAL
A lista de diagnóstico diferencial inclui causas de hipercalcemia.
• Linfoma — comum em cães, raro em gatos.
• Adenocarcinoma das glândulas apócrinas dos sacos anais — cães.
• Outros carcinomas — cães e gatos.
• Doença mieloproliferativa — gatos.
• Fibrossarcoma — gatos.
• Insuficiência renal crônica.
• Hipoadrenocorticismo.
• Intoxicação por rodenticidas análogos à vitamina D — tais produtos não são mais comercializados nos EUA, mas a exposição pode vir de fontes vegetais e suplementos vitamínicos.
• Doenças granulomatosas.
• Hipercalcemia idiopática em gatos.

HEMOGRAMA/BIOQUÍMICA/URINÁLISE
• Alta concentração sérica de cálcio.
• Concentração sérica de fósforo baixa ou normal a baixa no hiperparatireoidismo primário.
• Hiperfosfatemia no hiperparatireoidismo secundário ou hipervitaminose D.
• Concentrações séricas de ureia e creatinina costumam permanecer normais em pacientes com hiperparatireoidismo primário, exceto naqueles com insuficiência renal induzida por hipercalcemia.

OUTROS TESTES LABORATORIAIS
• O cálcio sérico ionizado encontra-se frequentemente normal em pacientes com insuficiência renal crônica e alto naqueles com hiperparatireoidismo primário ou hipercalcemia associada à malignidade.
• A alta concentração sérica de PTH é diagnóstica de hiperparatireoidismo primário na ausência de azotemia; os ensaios que medem a molécula intacta de PTH são mais úteis. A concentração sérica normal de PTH em animal com hipercalcemia pode ser considerada como um achado anormal e sinalizar hipercalcemia dependente da paratireoide.

DIAGNÓSTICO POR IMAGEM
• As radiografias podem ser úteis para verificar se há urolitíase, avaliar a morfologia renal e a densidade óssea e ainda identificar neoplasia oculta.
• A ultrassonografia da região ventral do pescoço, às vezes, revela a presença de adenoma da paratireoide.
• O ultrassom do abdome pode revelar linfadenomegalia, urolitíase ou anormalidades morfológicas renais.

MÉTODOS DIAGNÓSTICOS
Exploração cirúrgica da região ventral do pescoço.

ACHADOS PATOLÓGICOS
• O adenoma da paratireoide costuma ser uma massa solitária, pequena (= 1 cm), redonda, castanho-clara ou avermelhada, localizada na proximidade da tireoide.
• Ocasionalmente se encontram múltiplos adenomas.
• As distinções histológicas entre adenomas, hiperplasia e carcinomas da paratireoide geralmente são obscuras.

TRATAMENTO

CUIDADO(S) DE SAÚDE ADEQUADO(S)
• O hiperparatireoidismo primário, em geral, requer cuidados hospitalares e cirurgia.
• O hiperparatireoidismo secundário nutricional ou renal em pacientes que não estejam em estado crítico pode ser tratado em um esquema ambulatorial.

CUIDADO(S) DE ENFERMAGEM
N/D.

ATIVIDADE
Nenhuma modificação é recomendada.

DIETA
Suplementação de cálcio para as formas secundárias.

ORIENTAÇÃO AO PROPRIETÁRIO
Explicar os sinais atribuíveis às alterações no nível de cálcio, pois a hipocalcemia é uma complicação potencial da paratireoidectomia.

CONSIDERAÇÕES CIRÚRGICAS
• A cirurgia é o tratamento de escolha para o hiperparatireoidismo primário e, em geral, é importante para o estabelecimento do diagnóstico.
• Ablação térmica (i. e., por emissão de calor) percutânea guiada por ultrassom foi utilizada com

êxito para o tratamento de adenoma da paratireoide e pode ser recomendada se disponível.
• Há relatos de que a ablação por injeção percutânea de etanol guiada por ultrassom tenha menos sucesso do que a cirurgia ou a ablação térmica.

MEDICAÇÕES
MEDICAMENTO(S) DE ESCOLHA
• Soro fisiológico é o fluido escolha para o tratamento da hipercalcemia.
• Diuréticos (furosemida) e corticosteroides podem ser úteis no tratamento da hipercalcemia.
• Não há tratamento clínico para o hiperparatireoidismo primário em si.
• Hiperparatireoidismo secundário renal é, algumas vezes, tratado com calcitriol, mas o uso dessa medicação não ganhou ampla aceitação.
• Uma nova classe de medicamentos calcimiméticos está sendo utilizada para tratar hiperparatireoidismo secundário renal em pacientes humanos, mas não há relatos de estudos sobre o uso desses agentes em cães e gatos.

CONTRAINDICAÇÕES
• Não usar glicocorticoides até que o diagnóstico de linfoma tenha sido excluído, pois tais agentes podem dificultar o diagnóstico.
• Evitar o uso de fluidos que contenham cálcio.

PRECAUÇÕES
Usar a furosemida apenas em pacientes com hidratação adequada.

INTERAÇÕES POSSÍVEIS
N/D.

MEDICAMENTO(S) ALTERNATIVO(S)
O pamidronato é usado para tratar hipercalcemia por várias causas em cães e gatos.

ACOMPANHAMENTO
MONITORIZAÇÃO DO PACIENTE
• Hipocalcemia pós-operatória é relativamente comum após o tratamento do hiperparatireoidismo primário, sobretudo em pacientes com concentração sérica pré-cirúrgica de cálcio >14 mg/dL; verificar o cálcio sérico 1-2 vezes ao dia por 1 semana após a cirurgia.
• Hipocalcemia pós-operatória requer o tratamento com vitamina D (é recomendável o calcitriol) e suplementos de cálcio (ver "Tratamento do Hipoparatireoidismo"), devendo-se monitorizar o cálcio ionizado para orientar os ajustes da dosagem.
• Em pacientes com comprometimento renal, verificar a concentração sérica de ureia e creatinina.

PREVENÇÃO
• Não há estratégias para a prevenção do hiperparatireoidismo primário.
• O fornecimento de nutrição adequada previne o hiperparatireoidismo secundário nutricional.

COMPLICAÇÕES POSSÍVEIS
Insuficiência renal irreversível secundária à hipercalcemia.

EVOLUÇÃO ESPERADA E PROGNÓSTICO
• A doença não tratada costuma evoluir para doença renal ou neurológica em estágio terminal.
• O prognóstico em relação ao tratamento de adenoma da paratireoide é excelente.
• Observa-se recidiva em pequena porcentagem de casos.
• Em animais que desenvolvem hipoparatireoidismo pós-operatório, o retorno de função da paratireoide ao normal é imprevisível e pode levar semanas a meses.

DIVERSOS
DISTÚRBIOS ASSOCIADOS
Urolitíase contendo cálcio.

FATORES RELACIONADOS COM A IDADE
N/D.

POTENCIAL ZOONÓTICO
N/D.

GESTAÇÃO/FERTILIDADE/REPRODUÇÃO
N/D.

VER TAMBÉM
• Hipercalcemia.
• Hiperparatireoidismo Secundário Renal.
• Insuficiência Renal Crônica.

ABREVIATURA(S)
• PTH = paratormônio.

Sugestões de Leitura
Feldman EC, Hoar B, Pollard R, Nelson RW. Pretreatment clinical and laboratory findings in dogs with primary hyperparathyroidism: 210 cases (1987-2004). JAVMA 2005, 227(5):756-761.
Feldman EC, Nelson RW. Hypercalcemia and primary hyperparathyroidism. In: Canine and Feline Endocrinology and Reproduction, 3rd ed. St. Louis: Saunders, 2004, pp. 660-715.
Gear RN, Skelly BJ, Herrtage ME. Primary hyperparathyroidism in 29 dogs: Diagnosis, treatment, outcome and associated renal failure. J Small Anim Pract 2005, 46(1):10-16.
Rasor L, Pollard R, Feldman EC. Retrospective evaluation of three treatment methods for primary hyperparathyroidism in dogs. JAAHA 2007, 43(2):70-77.
Richter KP, Kallet AJ, Feldman EC, Brum DE. Primary hyperparathyroidism in cats: Seven cases (1984-1989). JAVMA 1991, 199(12):1767-1771.

Autor Thomas K. Graves
Consultor Editorial Deborah S. Greco

Hiperparatireoidismo Secundário Renal

CONSIDERAÇÕES GERAIS

REVISÃO
- Síndrome clínica caracterizada por alta concentração de PTH biologicamente ativo secundária à doença renal crônica; a principal causa é a ausência absoluta ou relativa na síntese de calcitriol, embora baixas concentrações de cálcio ionizado e hiperfosfatemia também contribuam para o quadro.
- A hiperfosfatemia secundária ao declínio da função renal diminui a atividade da 1-α-hidroxilase nos rins que, por sua vez, reduz a produção de calcitriol (1,25-di-hidroxicolecalciferol). A massa tubular renal diminuída também contribui para a síntese reduzida de calcitriol. Concentrações normais de calcitriol exercem um efeito negativo sobre a síntese de PTH no núcleo da paratireoide. Concentrações baixas de calcitriol e cálcio sérico ionizado resultam em aumento da produção de PTH e hiperplasia da paratireoide. A alta produção de PTH aumenta as baixas concentrações séricas de calcitriol e cálcio, à custa da concentração contínua elevada de PTH.
- A síntese de calcitriol fica comprometida em pacientes com doença renal crônica grave e números baixos de túbulos renais, qualquer que seja o nível de compensação do PTH. O PTH pode não só atuar como uma toxina urêmica, mas também promover nefrocalcinose e evolução de insuficiência renal crônica.

IDENTIFICAÇÃO
Cães e gatos — ver "Insuficiência Renal Crônica" em busca das predileções etárias e raciais.

SINAIS CLÍNICOS
- Aqueles associados à doença renal crônica subjacente constituem o motivo habitual para o exame.
- Ocorre osteodistrofia renal grave ou "mandíbula de borracha" em alguns pacientes, mais comumente nos cães jovens com hiperparatireoidismo secundário renal grave.
- Dor em torno da cabeça ou nos ossos — algumas vezes, muito acentuada.

CAUSAS E FATORES DE RISCO
- Qualquer doença que provoque doença renal crônica.
- Consumo excessivo de fósforo na dieta.

DIAGNÓSTICO

DIAGNÓSTICO DIFERENCIAL
- Nefropatia hipercalcêmica — doença (ou insuficiência) renal causada por hipercalcemia ionizada; pode ser difícil diferenciar de hiperparatireoidismo secundário renal de longa duração, em que a hiperplasia das paratireoides limita sua capacidade de interromper a liberação de PTH diante de altas concentrações de cálcio ionizado (hiperparatireoidismo terciário).
- A concentração sérica de cálcio total costuma ser mais alta em pacientes com nefropatia hipercalcêmica do que naqueles com hiperparatireoidismo secundário renal; a concentração sérica de cálcio ionizado, em geral, é baixa ou normal no hiperparatireoidismo secundário renal, mas alta na nefropatia hipercalcêmica.
- A concentração sérica de PTH é baixa em animais com hipercalcemia decorrente de malignidade; é possível detectar causas subjacentes de hipercalcemia como linfoma ou adenocarcinoma das glândulas apócrinas dos sacos anais.
- Hiperparatireoidismo primário — caracterizado inicialmente por hipercalcemia (ionizada e total), concentração sérica normal ou baixa de fósforo e alta de PTH; no início, a função renal encontra-se normal, mas pode vir a ser comprometida com a evolução da doença.

HEMOGRAMA/BIOQUÍMICA/URINÁLISE
- Azotemia.
- Hiperfosfatemia.
- Densidade urinária <1,030 em cães e <1,035 em gatos.
- A concentração sérica de cálcio total pode estar baixa, normal ou levemente alta; ver "Insuficiência Renal Crônica".

OUTROS TESTES LABORATORIAIS
- O diagnóstico definitivo e a monitorização terapêutica do hiperparatireoidismo secundário renal exigem a mensuração de alta concentração sérica de PTH; é necessário um imunoensaio para o PTH direcionado contra a parte aminoterminal ou a molécula intacta desse hormônio e validado em cães ou gatos para a obtenção de resultados passíveis de reprodução e significativos.
- A concentração sérica de cálcio ionizado baixa a normal é útil para diferenciar o hiperparatireoidismo secundário renal de outras causas de hipercalcemia.

DIAGNÓSTICO POR IMAGEM
As radiografias podem revelar baixa densidade óssea, perda da lâmina dura em torno dos dentes e mineralização de tecido mole da mucosa gástrica ou de outros tecidos.

TRATAMENTO

- Ver princípios terapêuticos gerais em "Insuficiência Renal Crônica".
- Fornecer dieta com baixo teor de fósforo (formulada, de preferência, para cães ou gatos com doença renal crônica) para minimizar a retenção desse elemento químico.
- Proporcionar livre acesso à água fresca para manter a hidratação do animal.

MEDICAÇÕES

MEDICAMENTO(S)

Quelantes Intestinais de Fosfato
- Prescrever se o tratamento nutricional não fizer com que a concentração de fósforo volte ao normal.
- Hidróxido de alumínio (30-90 mg/kg/dia VO juntamente com as refeições), carbonato de cálcio (90-150 mg/kg/dia VO juntamente com as refeições), acetato de cálcio (60-90 mg/kg/dia VO juntamente com as refeições) ou carbonato de lantânio (mesma dose do hidróxido de alumínio).
- Em casos raros, pode ocorrer o aparecimento de hipercalcemia quando um quelante de fosfato contendo cálcio é combinado com calcitriol. Quelantes de fosfato quimicamente distintos podem ser usados em combinação para reduzir a dosagem de cada um e, assim, minimizar o risco de hipercalcemia ou intoxicação pelo alumínio.

Calcitriol
- Em dose baixa (2,0-3,5 ng/kg VO a cada 24 h) — pode-se usar após o início da restrição de fósforo na dieta e quelantes orais de fosfato; note que a dose é em ng/kg, e não em mg/kg; é preciso contar com uma farmácia especializada na reformulação de doses baixas dessa prescrição.
- Manter a concentração sérica de fósforo dentro dos parâmetros normais antes e durante a terapia com calcitriol; fósforo sérico <4,5 mg/dL no estágio 2 da doença renal crônica; <5,0 no estágio 3 da doença renal crônica; e <6,0 mg/dL no estágio 4 da doença renal crônica.

CONTRAINDICAÇÕES/INTERAÇÕES POSSÍVEIS
- A administração de calcitriol pode resultar em hipercalcemia, especialmente se combinada com algum quelante intestinal de fosfato contendo cálcio. Às vezes, ocorre o aumento na concentração de cálcio total em pacientes com doença renal crônica de longa data, mas não relacionado com o tratamento à base de calcitriol. Em tais casos, a concentração de cálcio ionizado é normal ou baixa, mas a hipercalcemia não desaparece quando se interrompe o tratamento com calcitriol.
- Não usar quelantes intestinais de fosfato contendo cálcio em pacientes com o produto cálcio × fósforo >70. Usar quelantes intestinais de fosfato contendo alumínio inicialmente, para corrigir a hiperfosfatemia, seguidos por quelantes intestinais de fosfato contendo cálcio assim que a concentração sérica de fósforo estiver normal.

ACOMPANHAMENTO

MONITORIZAÇÃO DO PACIENTE
- Concentrações séricas de cálcio, fósforo, creatinina e ureia — monitorizar semanal a mensalmente, dependendo da terapia e da gravidade da doença renal crônica.
- Pacientes submetidos ao calcitriol devem ser monitorizados quanto ao aparecimento de hipercalcemia e/ou hiperfosfatemia semanalmente durante 4 semanas, em seguida mensalmente se estiverem estabilizados e depois a cada 3-4 meses.
- Avaliações seriadas da concentração de PTH — a maioria dos cães e gatos tratados com baixas doses de calcitriol atinge níveis de PTH próximos do normal em 3 meses; pode ser necessário aumentar a dose naqueles com hiperplasia grave da paratireoide.
- Caso surja hipercalcemia, suspender o uso do calcitriol. A estimativa do cálcio ionizado é recomendável, pois alguns animais com doença renal crônica desenvolvem hipercalcemia não ionizada sem relação com o tratamento à base de calcitriol. Se a hipercalcemia for atribuída ao tratamento com calcitriol (cálcio ionizado alto), ela deverá diminuir em 5 dias. O tratamento intermitente com calcitriol com o dobro da dose em dias alternados pode aliviar uma hipercalcemia discreta. Pacientes com hipercalcemia mais grave podem se beneficiar do uso de 3,5 vezes a dose normal, administrada a cada 3 dias e meio. Tais efeitos sobre a redução da hipercalcemia se devem

HIPERPARATIREOIDISMO SECUNDÁRIO RENAL

à menor programação das células epiteliais intestinais para a absorção do cálcio.

PREVENÇÃO
A restrição de fósforo na dieta de pacientes com doença renal crônica pode adiar o início de hiperparatireoidismo secundário renal.

COMPLICAÇÕES POSSÍVEIS
Osteodistrofia renal e fraturas patológicas (raras).

EVOLUÇÃO ESPERADA E PROGNÓSTICO
• A evolução da doença renal crônica subjacente pode ser mais lenta com o tratamento do hiperparatireoidismo secundário renal em cães; não se sabe se isso também se aplica aos gatos.

• O prognóstico a longo prazo é reservado a mau em pacientes com doença renal crônica e hiperparatireoidismo secundário renal.

DIVERSOS

FATORES RELACIONADOS COM A IDADE
Animais jovens podem desenvolver osteodistrofia renal grave e se beneficiar do tratamento à base de calcitriol e carbonato de cálcio.

ABREVIATURA(S)
• PTH = paratormônio.

Sugestões de Leitura

Polzin D. Chronic kidney disease. In: Ettinger SJ, Feldman EC, eds., Textbook of Veterinary Internal Medicine, 7th ed. St. Louis: Elsevier, 2009, pp. 2036-2067.

Polzin DJ, Ross SJ, Osborne CA. Calcitriol therapy in chronic kidney disease. In: Bonagura J, ed., Current Veterinary Therapy XIV. Philadelphia: Saunders, 2008, pp. 892-895.

Autor David J. Polzin
Consultor Editorial Carl A. Osborne

Hiperplasia das Glândulas Mamárias – Gatas

CONSIDERAÇÕES GERAIS

REVISÃO
Aumento de volume de uma ou mais glândulas mamárias.

IDENTIFICAÇÃO
• Gatas jovens, intactas, em ciclo estral ou prenhes.
• Gatos de qualquer sexo após gonadectomia (raro em gato).
• Gatos de qualquer sexo submetidos a progestogênio exógeno (p. ex., acetato de megestrol).

SINAIS CLÍNICOS
• Aumento de volume localizado ou difuso de uma ou mais glândulas mamárias.
• Massas firmes e indolores em casos não complicados.
• Sem sinais concomitantes de doença sistêmica; possível leucocitose com mastite secundária.

CAUSAS E FATORES DE RISCO
• Secundária à influência da progesterona.
• Pode surgir após gonadectomia; a patogênese pode envolver hormônios como progesterona, hormônio de crescimento, prolactina, fator de crescimento insulinossímile.
• Aumento dos níveis da progesterona — pseudociese na gata induzida a ovular, porém não prenhe por 40-50 dias após a indução da ovulação; observado por toda a gestação; também ocorre com progestogênios exógenos.

DIAGNÓSTICO

DIAGNÓSTICO DIFERENCIAL
• Mastite — gata lactante; glândulas mamárias eritematosas e dolorosas; doença sistêmica com febre e neutrofilia imatura; células inflamatórias e bactérias no líquido espremido da(s) glândula(s) acometida(s).
• Neoplasia mamária — gatas idosas (>6 anos de idade); aparência macroscópica pode ser indistinguível; diferenciada por meio de biopsia do tecido acometido.

HEMOGRAMA/BIOQUÍMICA/URINÁLISE
Normais.

OUTROS TESTES LABORATORIAIS
N/D.

DIAGNÓSTICO POR IMAGEM
N/D.

MÉTODOS DIAGNÓSTICOS
• Exame citológico do líquido espremido das glândulas acometidas — não inflamatório.
• Biopsia excisional — proliferação fibroglandular benigna sem inflamação nem necrose.

TRATAMENTO
• Hipertrofia causada pela elevação da progesterona endógena — regride quando a progesterona declina no final da pseudociese ou da gestação; considerar o procedimento de ovário-histerectomia se a fertilidade não for uma preocupação.
• Hipertrofia atribuída a progestogênios exógenos — regride quando a medicação é interrompida.
• Hipertrofia após gonadectomia — ocorrerá a resolução espontânea; em animais que manifestam certo incômodo, pode-se tentar o uso de bloqueadores dos receptores de progesterona (aglepristona), inibidores da prolactina (bromocriptina) ou testosterona.

MEDICAÇÕES

MEDICAMENTO(S)
• Mesilato de bromocriptina — 0,25 mg (por gato) VO a cada 24 h por 5-7 dias; no entanto, não é aprovado para utilização nos felinos; pode provocar náusea.
• Náusea — metoclopramida (0,2 mg/kg VO a cada 6-8 h) ou dose da bromocriptina dividida (administrar 2 vezes ao dia).
• Acetato de megestrol (Ovaban®) — o sucesso relatado é duvidoso; o uso a longo prazo pode aumentar o risco de neoplasia mamária.
• Aglepristona (15 mg/kg SC em 2 dias consecutivos ou 20 mg/kg SC uma única vez); não aprovado para uso nos felinos; não é encontrado facilmente disponível nos Estados Unidos (mifepristona, um composto aparentado, está disponível nesse país como um produto para seres humanos; a dose para gatos não está definida).
• Cipionato de testosterona ou enantato de testosterona (2 mg/kg IM uma única vez); não aprovado para uso nos felinos.

CONTRAINDICAÇÕES/INTERAÇÕES POSSÍVEIS
Aglepristona — provoca abortamento em gatas prenhes. Pode-se observar uma dermatite no local da injeção.

ACOMPANHAMENTO
• Probabilidade de recidiva nas gatas deixadas intactas — desconhecida.
• Correlação com outras condições anormais do trato reprodutivo — desconhecida.

DIVERSOS

SINÔNIMO(S)
• Fibroadenomatose mamária.
• Hipertrofia mamária benigna.
• Hipertrofia mamária fibroglandular.

Sugestões de Leitura
Burstyn U. Management of mastitis and abscessation of mammary glands secondary to fibroadenomatous hyperplasia in a primiparturient cat. JAVMA 2010, 236:326-329.
Gimenz F, Hecht S, Craig LE, et al. Early detection, aggressive therapy: Optimizing the management of feline mammary masses. J Feline Med Surg 2010, 12:214-224.
Hayden DW, Johnston SD, Krang DT, et al. Feline mammary hypertrophy/fibroadenoma complex: Clinical and hormonal aspects. Am J Vet Res 1981, 42:1699-1703.
Johnston SD, Root Kustritz MV, Olson PN. Disorders of the mammary glands of the queen. In: Canine and Feline Theriogenology. Philadelphia: Saunders, 2001, pp. 474-485.

Autor Margaret V. Root Kustritz
Consultor Editorial Sara K. Lyle

HIPERPLASIA E PROLAPSO VAGINAIS

CONSIDERAÇÕES GERAIS

REVISÃO
• Protrusão de massa esférica ou em formato de rosquinha a partir da vulva durante o proestro ou o estro, raramente durante o parto ou após a administração de medicamentos estrogênicos para indução do estro.
• Tipo I — eversão leve do assoalho vaginal, mas sem protrusão através da vulva.
• Tipo II — prolapso do tecido vaginal através do orifício vulvar (massa em formato de língua).
• Tipo III — eversão em formato de rosquinha de toda a circunferência da parede vaginal, incluindo o orifício uretral, o qual pode ser observado ventralmente no tecido prolapsado.
• Resposta exagerada da mucosa vaginal aos estrogênios; alguns animais acometidos possuem cistos foliculares.
• Apesar do nome, as alterações observadas ao exame histopatológico são mais compatíveis com edema do que com hiperplasia ou hipertrofia se ocorrerem durante o proestro ou o estro.
• Prolapso grave — pode obstruir a uretra e impedir a micção normal.

IDENTIFICAÇÃO
• Cadelas jovens (maioria entre 18-22 meses, faixa de 6 meses a 4,6 anos) de grande porte.
• Raças predispostas — raças grandes e braquicefálicas (Boxer, Mastiff, Buldogue inglês e São Bernardo); Labrador e Chesapeake Bay retriever; Pastor alemão; Springer spaniel; Walker hound; Airedale terrier; Pit bull terrier americano.
• É provável um componente hereditário — incidência elevada em algumas linhagens familiares.

SINAIS CLÍNICOS
Achados Anamnésicos
• Início do proestro ou do estro.
• Apesar de serem raros, esses achados podem ser constatados durante o diestro ou no momento do parto (8-12% dos casos ocorrem na hora do parto) ou após a administração de medicamentos estrogênicos para a indução do estro.
• Lambedura da região vulvar.
• A cadela não permite a cópula.
• Disúria.
• Ocorrência prévia.

Achados do Exame Físico
• Protrusão de massa tecidual em formatos de círculo (ou seja, arredondado), de língua ou de rosquinha através da vulva.
• Exame vaginal — localizar o lúmen e o orifício uretral; tipos I e II: o lúmen vaginal encontra-se em posição dorsal ao prolapso; tipo III: o lúmen situa-se em um ponto central ao prolapso; nos três tipos, o orifício uretral apresenta-se ventralmente ao prolapso.
• O tecido pode estar seco ou necrosado.

CAUSAS E FATORES DE RISCO
• Estimulação estrogênica.
• Predisposição genética.
• Distocia.
• Pressão abdominal elevada.

DIAGNÓSTICO

DIAGNÓSTICO DIFERENCIAL
• Pólipo vaginal — diferenciado por meio do exame vaginal.
• Neoplasia vaginal — tumor venéreo transmissível e leiomioma; diferenciada por meio da identificação do animal, da fase do ciclo e do exame da vagina.
• Hipertrofia do clitóris — diferenciada por meio de exame físico meticuloso.

HEMOGRAMA/BIOQUÍMICA/URINÁLISE
N/D.

OUTROS TESTES LABORATORIAIS
N/D.

DIAGNÓSTICO POR IMAGEM
N/D.

MÉTODOS DIAGNÓSTICOS
Biopsia (cadela idosa) — diferenciar de neoplasia.

TRATAMENTO

• O tratamento é feito em um esquema ambulatorial a menos que ocorra obstrução da uretra.
• Reprodução — possível por meio de inseminação artificial (discutir possível hereditariedade).
• Tecido prolapsado — manter limpo e lubrificado com lubrificante hidrossolúvel estéril.
• Colar elizabetano e ambiente limpo — minimizam o traumatismo tecidual.
• Instruir o proprietário a monitorizar a capacidade miccional do paciente.
• Na presença de obstrução uretral, inserir cateter urinário de demora.
• Regressão — começa geralmente no final do estro; deve estar resolvida durante o início do diestro.
• Taxa de recidiva — 66-100% no próximo ciclo estral.
• Ovário-histerectomia — impede a recidiva; pode acelerar a resolução.
• Condição grave — exige a redução ou a ressecção cirúrgicas; se possível, a intervenção cirúrgica deverá ser realizada quando a massa estiver começando a regredir; identificar e sondar a uretra, pois a taxa de recidiva no próximo ciclo é de 25% após a cirurgia.
• Em caso de distocia, há necessidade de cesariana e, possivelmente, ovário-histerectomia.

MEDICAÇÕES

MEDICAMENTO(S)
GnRH (2,2 μg/kg IM) ou hCG (1.000 UI IM) — caso não se tenha intenção reprodutiva nesse ciclo; pode acelerar a ovulação e a resolução em alguns dias; não são eficazes se administrados após a ovulação (níveis de progesterona >8-10 ng/mL).

CONTRAINDICAÇÕES/INTERAÇÕES POSSÍVEIS
Evitar os medicamentos progestacionais, pois podem induzir à piometra.

ACOMPANHAMENTO

MONITORIZAÇÃO DO PACIENTE
Monitorizar a integridade do tecido prolapsado e a capacidade de micção.

PREVENÇÃO
Ovário-histerectomia — recomendada em função do componente genético e da probabilidade de recidiva.

COMPLICAÇÕES POSSÍVEIS
Tipo III — pode comprometer a uretra e impedir a micção normal.

EVOLUÇÃO ESPERADA E PROGNÓSTICO
• Tratamento clínico — o prognóstico quanto à recuperação é bom, exceto em casos de envolvimento da uretra.
• Intervenção cirúrgica em casos do tipo III — o prognóstico é bom.

DIVERSOS

ABREVIATURA(S)
• GnRH = hormônio liberador da gonadotropina.
• hCG = gonadotropina coriônica humana.

RECURSOS DA INTERNET
Schaeferes-Okkens AC. Vaginal Edema and Vaginal Fold Prolapse in the Bitch, Including Surgical Management, 2001. http://www.ivis.org/advances/Concannon/schaeferes/IVIS.pdf.

Sugestões de Leitura
Feldman EC, Nelson RW. Vaginal defects, vaginitis, and vaginal infections. In: Feldman EC, Nelson RW, eds., Canine and Feline Endocrinology and Reproduction. Philadelphia: Saunders, 2004, pp. 901-928.
Johnston SD, Root Kustritz MV, Olson PNS. Disorders of the canine vagina, vestibule, and vulva. In: Johnston SD, Root Kustritz MV, Olson PNS, eds., Canine and Feline Theriogenology. Philadelphia: Saunders, 2001, pp. 225-242.
Post K, Van Haaften BV, Okkens AC. Vaginal hyperplasia in the bitch: Literature review and commentary. Can Vet J 1991, 32:35-37.

Autor Joni L. Freshman
Consultor Editorial Sara K. Lyle

Hiperplasia Gengival

CONSIDERAÇÕES GERAIS

DEFINIÇÃO
• Aumento do tecido gengival causado pela proliferação de seus elementos (multiplicação anormal ou aumento do número normal de células em arranjo normal).
• Provável tendência familiar — Boxer.

IDENTIFICAÇÃO
• Cães e, raramente, gatos.
• Raças predominantes — Boxer, Dinamarquês, Collie, Doberman pinscher, Dálmata.

SINAIS CLÍNICOS
• Espessamento e aumento na altura da inserção gengival e na margem gengival — às vezes, cobre completamente a superfície do dente.
• Formação resultante de "pseudobolsas" — aumento na profundidade da bolsa em virtude do aumento na altura da gengiva; não se deve à perda da inserção a menos que não haja tratamento e o quadro evolua para doença periodontal concomitante.
• O aumento da margem gengival pode ser simétrico, especialmente nos incisivos.
• É possível o acometimento local de áreas (Sheltie), embora o padrão mais generalizado seja típico.
• O envolvimento focal, além da margem gengival, pode originar áreas hiperplásicas em função da irritação crônica, como a lesão típica de "mastigador de goma". Essas áreas devem ser avaliadas quanto à necessidade terapêutica (excisão).
• Pode formar massas protuberantes (semelhantes a cachos de uvas) nas margens gengivais — há necessidade de biopsia para descartar neoplasia.

CAUSAS
Resposta inflamatória crônica à presença de bactérias na placa associada à doença periodontal.

FATORES DE RISCO
• Predominância racial (ver a seção "Identificação").
• Administração crônica de medicamentos — difenil-hidantoína; ciclosporina; nitrendipino; nifedipino.

DIAGNÓSTICO

DIAGNÓSTICO DIFERENCIAL
• Presuntivo, com base no aspecto clínico, especialmente se generalizada e encontrada na raça predominante.
• Neoplasia bucal — por exemplo, fibromas odontogênicos periféricos; não costumam ser generalizadas; às vezes, há alterações ósseas.
• Papilomatose oral — papilomas formados, em geral, nas superfícies mucosas.
• Opérculo — observado em animais jovens durante a fase de erupção dos dentes; perda incompleta e/ou persistência do tecido gengival que cobre o dente em erupção.

HEMOGRAMA/BIOQUÍMICA/URINÁLISE
N/D.

OUTROS TESTES LABORATORIAIS
N/D.

DIAGNÓSTICO POR IMAGEM
Radiografia intrabucal — para descartar quaisquer alterações ósseas subjacentes (mais comuns em casos de epúlides ou tumores).

MÉTODOS DIAGNÓSTICOS
• Biopsia — área(s) focal(is) irresponsiva(s) à terapia padrão.
• Histopatologia — para excluir neoplasia e outras causas; a avaliação histológica é o único método de confirmação.

TRATAMENTO

CUIDADO(S) DE SAÚDE ADEQUADO(S)
Limpeza dentária regular e cuidados domésticos — para minimizar os efeitos da placa e do acúmulo de bactérias.

ORIENTAÇÃO AO PROPRIETÁRIO
• Problema crônico recidivante que, em geral, exige a repetição da terapia.
• Incentivar o nível mais alto de cuidados em casa e a limpeza profissional regular.

CONSIDERAÇÕES CIRÚRGICAS
Gengivoplastia (Novo Contorno)
• Para remover o excesso de tecido gengival e restabelecer a profundidade normal da bolsa.
• Fornecer monitorização e suporte adequados para o paciente durante os procedimentos anestésicos.
• Injeções de anestésico local ou géis tópicos.
• Sonda periodontal — para determinar a profundidade da pseudobolsa; pode-se marcar a profundidade da bolsa do lado de fora dela com a extremidade da sonda ("pontos").
• Excisar o excesso de tecido e formar uma nova margem gengival.
• Aço frio — tesoura ou lâmina de bisturi resistente e afiada.
• Unir os pontos feitos pela sonda com a lâmina para aproximar a margem gengival normal ou usar tesoura, acompanhando a profundidade da bolsa para remover o excesso de tecido.
• Broca 12 de alta velocidade — para contornar a margem fazendo ângulo; ajudar na hemostasia.
• Eletrocautério ou radiocirurgia — usar corrente retificada completa ou parcialmente; evitar dano ao osso ou tecido subjacente.
• Laser — utilizar de forma adequada e evitar dano a dentes e ossos.
• Espessura excessiva (região dos incisivos e caninos) — técnica de Widman modificada; envolver um retalho (*flap*) para levantar a gengiva das superfícies dentárias; excisar uma cunha de tecido para remover a gengiva na parte interna da bolsa, de modo a diminuir a largura da inserção gengival; suturar de forma interdental para firmar a gengiva; usar pressão digital para reposicionar.
• Tintura de mirra e benzoína — usar gotejamento; cobrir as margens seccionadas e secar; 4-5 camadas.
• Soluções hemostáticas — ajudam a controlar a hemorragia se houver necessidade.

MEDICAÇÕES

MEDICAMENTO(S)
• Antimicrobianos orais — clorexidina; gel de ascorbato de zinco.
• Para controle da dor pós-operatória.

CONTRAINDICAÇÕES/INTERAÇÕES POSSÍVEIS
Pacientes sob medicação crônica com difenil-hidantoína ou ciclosporina — podem ficar predispostos a alterações hiperplásicas.

ACOMPANHAMENTO

MONITORIZAÇÃO DO PACIENTE
• Conforto pós-operatório — administrar medicação para dor conforme a necessidade.
• Exames regulares, além de limpeza e tratamento profissionais — para evitar recidiva, que é comum.

PREVENÇÃO
Limpeza profissional regular e cuidados domésticos meticulosos.

COMPLICAÇÕES POSSÍVEIS
• Possível exacerbação da doença periodontal em pseudobolsas se não for tratada; bolsas mais profundas são mais suscetíveis a infecções bacterianas anaeróbias.
• A aplicação de calor excessivo com tratamento eletrocirúrgico pode lesionar os dentes (pulpite, morte da polpa) e o osso alveolar.

EVOLUÇÃO ESPERADA E PROGNÓSTICO
• Prognóstico bom com cuidados regulares.
• A recidiva é comum.

DIVERSOS

VER TAMBÉM
Massas Bucais.

RECURSOS DA INTERNET
http://www.avdc.org/Nomenclature.html.

Sugestões de Leitura
Lobprise HB. Blackwell's Five-Minute Veterinary Consult Clinical Companion — Small Animal Dentistry. Ames, IA: Blackwell, 2007 (for additional topics, including diagnostics and techniques).
Wiggs RB, Lobrise HB. Veterinary Dentistry: Principles and Practice. Philadelphia: Lippincott-Raven, 1997.

Autora Heidi B. Lobprise
Consultora Editorial Heidi B. Lobprise

HIPERPLASIA HEPÁTICA NODULAR

CONSIDERAÇÕES GERAIS

REVISÃO
• Hiperplasia hepática nodular — lesão aparentemente benigna, observada no fígado de cães de meia-idade a idosos, que consiste em acúmulo discreto de hepatócitos hiperplásicos misturados com hepatócitos vacuolizados contendo glicogênio. • Quadro associado ao aumento na atividade das enzimas hepáticas em cães idosos, especialmente fosfatase alcalina. • A suspeita clínica provém de alta atividade enzimática hepática e da detecção ultrassonográfica de nódulos hepáticos ou nodularidade ou "massa" hepática observada durante cirurgia exploratória. • Aspecto ultrassonográfico variável. • As amostras de biopsia devem incluir fígado acometido e normal para interpretação apropriada. • A hiperplasia nodular pode ser confundida com regeneração secundária à hepatite crônica ou neoplasia hepatocelular (adenoma) com biopsias centrais com agulha ou quando apenas o tecido nodular sem tecido hepático normal é amostrado. • Aparentemente é mais comum em cães com hepatopatia vacuolar e naqueles com hiperplasia adrenal (atípica) dos hormônios sexuais; pode representar uma resposta ao colapso lobular secundário à degeneração vacuolar. • Diagnóstico controverso; não está claro que isso seja uma "síndrome" verdadeira.

IDENTIFICAÇÃO
• Cães. • Lesão relacionada com a idade; os nódulos desenvolvem-se por volta de 6-8 anos de idade; um único estudo documentou a presença de lesões em todos os cães com mais de 14 anos de idade. • Pode ser mais comum em Terrier escocês.

SINAIS CLÍNICOS
Comentários Gerais
Achados do Exame Físico
• A hiperplasia nodular não causa doença clínica a menos que nódulos amplos sofram ruptura e sangramento (raro) ou se os nódulos diminuírem a perfusão hepática sinusoidal; pode ser confundida com hiperplasia adenomatosa e adenoma hepático. • Hepatomegalia; é possível palpar a margem hepática irregular (raramente). • É comum a descoberta casual da hiperplasia hepática difusa durante as avaliações de outras doenças.

CAUSAS E FATORES DE RISCO
• Etiologia — desconhecida; fatores metabólicos (causas de hepatopatia vacuolar) e eventos lesivos prévios.

DIAGNÓSTICO

DIAGNÓSTICO DIFERENCIAL
• Cirrose — a hiperplasia nodular regenerativa envolve todo o fígado; formação de nódulos irregulares de tamanho variável, separados por tecido fibroso; perda da arquitetura acinar e processo de fibrose. • Neoplasia — grandes nódulos isolados ou multifocais de hiperplasia nodular podem ser confundidos com neoplasia hepática primária ou secundária; maior confusão com neoplasia hepatocelular primária (adenoma ou carcinoma hepatocelular), diferenciados com base na (1) displasia de hepatócitos, (2) atipia nuclear, (3) formação pseudoglandular, (4) perda ou redução de fibras de reticulina e (5) integração arquitetural com o tecido hepático circundante normal. • Hepatopatia vacuolar — vacuolização de hepatócitos nas lesões de hiperplasia nodular ou adjacentes a elas; considerar a adequação da amostra de tecido antes de prosseguir com os testes para hepatopatia vacuolar (ver "Hepatopatia Vacuolar").

HEMOGRAMA/BIOQUÍMICA/URINÁLISE
• Hemograma completo — sem características compatíveis. • Perfil bioquímico — é comum o aumento na atividade da fosfatase alcalina sérica (variação de 2,5-16 vezes o normal); pode estar associado a aumentos em outras enzimas hepáticas; supõe-se que a atividade da fosfatase alcalina reflita colestase intralesional ou compressão mecânica de tecido hepático normal adjacente, mas pode refletir um fenômeno de indução associado à hepatopatia vacuolar; atividade elevada da ALT pode refletir compressão e hipoxia de hepatócitos normais adjacentes ou aumento da replicação celular dentro das lesões; em geral, não há alterações nos níveis de proteína total, albumina, bilirrubina total e colesterol. • Urinálise — sem achados compatíveis.

OUTROS TESTES LABORATORIAIS
Ácidos biliares séricos totais — geralmente normais a menos que a hiperplasia seja difusa e grave.

DIAGNÓSTICO POR IMAGEM
• Radiografia abdominal — em geral, sem anormalidades; raramente, observam-se margens hepáticas irregulares na projeção lateral. • Ultrassonografia abdominal — ecogenicidade variável relacionada com as alterações do exame histológico e o tamanho do nódulo; a ecogenicidade pode ser hipoecoica, hiperecoica ou mista; nódulos com ecogenicidade idêntica ao parênquima adjacente normal passam despercebidos.

MÉTODOS DIAGNÓSTICOS
• Aspiração de amostras — pode recuperar hepatócitos normais, hepatócitos com rarefação citosólica e fragilidade compatíveis com hepatopatia vacuolar (retenção de glicogênio) ou algumas células com vacúolos lipídicos discretos (triglicerídeos); hepatócitos binucleados ocasionais; os hepatócitos podem ser pequenos com variação acentuada em termos de tamanho e demonstrar características "displásicas" (células de divisão rápida). • Biopsia hepática — a biopsia coletada por agulha pode não diferenciar a lesão com clareza, por causa do pequeno tamanho da amostra; o diagnóstico definitivo requer amostras de tecido grandes o bastante para incluir a lesão e o parênquima hepático normal adjacente. • Métodos de biopsia recomendados — laparoscópico, biopsia aberta em cunha durante a laparotomia ou múltiplas amostras obtidas com agulha de calibre 14.

ACHADOS PATOLÓGICOS
• Macroscópicos — lesões expansivas tipo massa isoladas ou múltiplas, raramente, apresentam >3 cm de diâmetro; cor semelhante à do tecido hepático normal adjacente; há relatos de que lesões extensas mimetizem cirrose macronodular (esse quadro pode representar lesões em hepatopatia vacuolar grave com colapso do parênquima). • Microscópicos — lesão expansiva bem-delimitada em que os hepatócitos hiperplásicos comprimem o parênquima adjacente; aspecto hepatocelular variável; o diagnóstico definitivo fica comprometido por amostras teciduais inadequadas (p. ex., técnica de biopsia por agulha Tru-Cut®). • A diferenciação de neoplasia hepática primária (adenoma) pode ser ambígua.

TRATAMENTO

Geralmente, não há necessidade de qualquer tratamento; a ruptura de grandes nódulos pode necessitar de transfusão sanguínea e excisão de emergência da lesão expansiva tipo massa. Efetuar tratamento paliativo ou proporcionar alívio da causa subjacente de hepatopatia vacuolar se presente.

MEDICAÇÕES

MEDICAMENTO(S)
Embora haja relatos de que a hiperplasia nodular tenha uma evolução benigna, é preciso ter cuidado para determinar sua associação com hepatopatia vacuolar e distúrbios relacionados, especialmente hiperplasia adrenal atípica (ver "Hepatopatia Vacuolar").

ACOMPANHAMENTO

MONITORIZAÇÃO DO PACIENTE
• Perfis bioquímicos trimestrais.
• Ultrassonografias abdominais sequenciais para avaliar a evolução dos nódulos hepáticos.
• Ver "Hepatopatia Vacuolar" em busca dos distúrbios relacionados.

COMPLICAÇÕES POSSÍVEIS
• Lesões de hiperplasia nodular — podem incitar a avaliações hepáticas macro e microscópicas, bem como a exames laboratoriais e técnicas de diagnóstico por imagem, que distraem a atenção clínica dos problemas médicos sintomáticos.
• Não é possível a distinção de neoplasia com base apenas nos dados obtidos nos exames laboratoriais ou nas técnicas de diagnóstico por imagem.

EVOLUÇÃO ESPERADA E PROGNÓSTICO
Podem se desenvolver nódulos mais extensos; raramente, ocorrem focos necróticos ou hemorragia grave com lesões que se comportam do mesmo modo que grandes hepatomas (necrose central).

DIVERSOS

VER TAMBÉM
• Adenoma Hepatocelular. • Carcinoma Hepatocelular. • Cirrose e Fibrose Hepáticas.
• Hepatite Crônica Ativa. • Hepatopatia Vacuolar.

ABREVIATURA(S)
• ALT = alanina aminotransferase.

Autor Sharon A. Center

Hiperplasia Prostática Benigna

CONSIDERAÇÕES GERAIS

REVISÃO
- Alteração patológica na próstata, relacionada com a idade, que a torna aumentada de volume e indolor.
- Ocorre em duas fases: glandular e complexa.
- A fase glandular caracteriza-se por uma quantidade alta de células prostáticas grandes e próstata simetricamente aumentada.
- A fase complexa caracteriza-se por hiperplasia glandular, atrofia glandular, formações císticas pequenas, inflamação crônica e metaplasia escamosa epitelial.

IDENTIFICAÇÃO
- Observada inicialmente em machos caninos intactos com 1-2 anos de idade.
- A prevalência aumenta com a idade; 60 e 95% dos machos caninos são acometidos, respectivamente, por volta dos 6 e 9 anos de idade.

SINAIS CLÍNICOS
Achados Anamnésicos
- Ausentes na maioria dos cães.
- Secreção uretral sanguinolenta.
- Hematúria.
- Presença de sangue no ejaculado.
- Tenesmo (esforço durante a defecação).
- Fezes semelhantes a tiras.
- Disúria.

Achados do Exame Físico
- Próstata aumentada de volume, simétrica e indolor.
- Dor prostática em cães com complicações de infecção bacteriana ou carcinoma prostático.

CAUSAS E FATORES DE RISCO
- Testosterona e 5-α-di-hidrotestosterona.
- Estrogênios.
- Envelhecimento.
- Eliminação do risco por meio da castração.

DIAGNÓSTICO

DIAGNÓSTICO DIFERENCIAL
- Prostatite bacteriana aguda — associada tipicamente à febre, depressão, dor à palpação retal, neutrofilia, piúria e bacteriúria; pode ocorrer de forma concomitante com a hiperplasia prostática benigna em cães.
- Prostatite bacteriana crônica — relacionada tipicamente com infecções recidivantes do trato urinário inferior e subfertilidade; também pode acompanhar a hiperplasia prostática benigna em cães.
- Adenocarcinoma prostático — ligado normalmente à hiporexia, perda de peso, fraqueza dos membros pélvicos, disúria, hematúria e disquezia; no sedimento urinário, podem-se observar células neoplásicas.
- Cistos prostáticos e paraprostáticos — podem gerar massas císticas abdominais palpáveis, preenchidas por líquido de coloração amarela a laranja.

HEMOGRAMA/BIOQUÍMICA/URINÁLISE
- Hemograma completo e perfil bioquímico — normais.
- Urinálise — pode permanecer normal ou revelar hematúria; ausência de piúria e bacteriúria a menos que o cão tenha infecção bacteriana concomitante.

OUTROS TESTES LABORATORIAIS
- O líquido prostático obtido por meio da ejaculação ou massagem prostática apresenta-se límpido ou hemorrágico; contagem eritrocitária elevada; contagem leucocitária normal; a cultura revela <100.000 unidades formadoras de colônias de bactérias/mL, exceto se o cão apresentar infecção bacteriana concomitante.
- Em alguns cães, a concentração sérica da esterase prostática encontra-se elevada.

DIAGNÓSTICO POR IMAGEM
Radiografia
- As radiografias abdominais revelam a prostatomegalia.
- A uretrocistografia retrógrada pode se mostrar normal ou exibir estreitamento da uretra prostática e/ou refluxo do meio de contraste para o interior da próstata.

Ultrassonografia
- Mostra o aumento de volume prostático com o parênquima de ecogenicidade uniforme; em alguns cães, observam-se pequenos cistos preenchidos por líquido.
- O aspirado com agulha fina guiada por ultrassom pode ser utilizado para o diagnóstico correto de prostatopatia em 80% dos casos.

MÉTODOS DIAGNÓSTICOS
N/D.

TRATAMENTO

- Frequentemente, não é necessário.
- Castração — método mais eficaz, que evita a recidiva; em casos de hiperplasia prostática benigna complicada por prostatite bacteriana aguda, é recomendável o adiamento da cirurgia até a resolução da infecção.

MEDICAÇÕES

MEDICAMENTO(S)
- Se a castração não for aceitável, os medicamentos expostos a seguir podem reduzir temporariamente o volume da próstata:
  - Finasterida (0,1-0,5 mg/kg/dia por até 4 meses).
  - Acetato de megestrol (0,11 mg/kg VO diariamente por 3 semanas).
  - Medroxiprogesterona (3 mg/kg SC).

CONTRAINDICAÇÕES/INTERAÇÕES POSSÍVEIS
- Evitar os estrogênios, em função da possível toxicidade hematológica e do desenvolvimento de metaplasia escamosa prostática.
- A administração a longo prazo do acetato de megestrol ou da medroxiprogesterona pode resultar no desenvolvimento de diabetes melito.

ACOMPANHAMENTO

- A castração culminará na rápida involução do volume prostático aumentado.
- O tratamento com a finasterida não é associado a declínio na libido, diminuição na qualidade do sêmen ou indução de defeitos congênitos. A hiperplasia prostática benigna apresentará recidiva após a suspensão da finasterida; o período de tempo até a recorrência dos sinais clínicos é variável.

DIVERSOS

DISTÚRBIOS ASSOCIADOS
- Prostatite bacteriana e carcinoma bacteriano.
- Prostatomegalia em cães castrados é fortemente sugestiva de carcinoma prostático.

VER TAMBÉM
- Cistos Prostáticos
- Prostatite e Abscesso Prostático
- Prostatomegalia

Sugestões de Leitura
Johnston SD, Root Kustritz MV, Olson PN. Disorders of the canine prostate. In: Canine and Feline Theriogenology. Philadelphia: Saunders, 2001, pp. 337-355.
Smith J. Canine prostatic disease: A review of anatomy, pathology, diagnosis, and treatment. Theriogenology 2008, 70:375-383.

Autores Margaret V. Root Kustritz e Jeffrey S. Klausner
Consultor Editorial Carl A. Osborne

HIPERSENSIBILIDADE À PICADA DE PULGA E CONTROLE DE PULGAS

CONSIDERAÇÕES GERAIS

DEFINIÇÃO
- Hipersensibilidade à picada de pulga — reação alérgica aos antígenos existentes na saliva das pulgas, com ou sem evidência desses ectoparasitas ou de seus dejetos.
- Infestação por pulgas — grande número de pulgas e grande quantidade de seus dejetos com ou sem dermatite por hipersensibilidade à picada de pulga.
- Dermatite à picada de pulga — reação irritante (sem hipersensibilidade) às picadas de pulga.

FISIOPATOLOGIA
- Hipersensibilidade à picada de pulgas — causada por um hapteno de baixo peso molecular e dois alérgenos de alto peso molecular que ajudam a iniciar a reação alérgica.
- Alérgenos de alto peso molecular — aumentam a ligação ao colágeno dérmico; quando ligados, formam um antígeno completo necessário para desencadear a hipersensibilidade à picada de pulgas.
- Saliva da pulga — contém compostos semelhantes à histamina que irritam a pele.
- A exposição intermitente favorece a hipersensibilidade à picada de pulgas; é menos provável que a exposição contínua resulte em hipersensibilidade.
- Relata-se o encontro de anticorpos IgE e IgG contra as pulgas.
- Há relatos de reações de hipersensibilidade imediata e tardia.
- Resposta de fase tardia mediada por IgE — parte da reação de hipersensibilidade à picada de pulgas; ocorre 3-6 h após a exposição.
- Hipersensibilidade de basófilos cutâneos — parte da reação de hipersensibilidade à picada de pulgas; infiltração de basófilos na derme; mediada por IgE ou IgG; exposições subsequentes provocam a degranulação dos basófilos; manifesta-se sob a forma de hipersensibilidade imediata e tardia.

SISTEMA(S) ACOMETIDO(S)
Cutâneo/exócrino.

GENÉTICA
Hipersensibilidade à picada de pulgas — padrão de herança desconhecido; mais comum em raças atópicas.

INCIDÊNCIA/PREVALÊNCIA
Varia com as condições do clima e a população de pulgas.

DISTRIBUIÇÃO GEOGRÁFICA
Hipersensibilidade à picada de pulgas — pode ocorrer em qualquer lugar; não sazonal apenas nos climas quentes e úmidos durante o ano todo, bem como nos animais que vivem dentro de casa.

IDENTIFICAÇÃO
Espécies
Cães e gatos.

Raça(s) Predominante(s)
Hipersensibilidade à picada de pulgas — qualquer raça; mais comum em raças atópicas.

Idade Média e Faixa Etária
Hipersensibilidade à picada de pulgas — rara antes dos 6 meses de vida; a idade média varia de 3-6 anos, embora possa ser observada em qualquer idade.

Sexo Predominante
N/D.

SINAIS CLÍNICOS
Achados Anamnésicos
- Prurido.
- Mastigação em regiões do corpo ("bater de dentes" como se estivesse roendo uma espiga de milho).
- Lambedura, principalmente na metade dorsal do corpo, mas pode incluir as regiões do antebraço.
- Histórico de pulgas e dejetos.
- Exposição a outros animais.
- Controle prévio de pulgas/falta de controle desses ectoparasitas.
- Casa com animais de estimação.

Achados do Exame Físico
- Determinados pela gravidade da reação e pelo grau de exposição a pulgas (i. e., sazonal *versus* anual).
- O encontro de pulgas e de seus dejetos é útil, embora não seja fundamental, para o diagnóstico de hipersensibilidade à picada desses ectoparasitas.
- Animais sensíveis necessitam de baixa exposição e tendem a se auto-higienizar, o que remove indícios da infestação e dificulta a identificação do parasita.
- Cães — lesões concentradas em uma área triangular da região lombossacra caudodorsal; envolvimento de regiões como face caudal das coxas, parte inferior do abdome, região inguinal e face cranial dos antebraços; as lesões primárias consistem em pápulas; lesões secundárias (p. ex., hiperpigmentação, liquenificação, alopecia e descamação) e dermatite piotraumática (conhecida como *hotspots* ou manchas quentes) são comuns na hipersensibilidade à picada de pulgas sem controle; podem ser observadas foliculite e furunculose secundárias; é rara a presença de nódulos fibropruriginosos.
- Gatos — nessa espécie, são constatados diversos padrões; o mais comum é uma dermatite crostosa miliar com padrão em forma de cunha sobre a região lombossacra caudodorsal e, em geral, ao redor da cabeça e do pescoço; outras apresentações ocorrem sob a forma de alopecia da região inguinal com ou sem inflamação ou placas eosinofílicas e outras formas do complexo granuloma eosinofílico.

CAUSAS
Ver a seção "Fisiopatologia".

FATORES DE RISCO
Hipersensibilidade à picada de pulgas — a exposição intermitente a pulgas aumenta a probabilidade de desenvolvimento; costuma ser observada em conjunto com atopia.

DIAGNÓSTICO

DIAGNÓSTICO DIFERENCIAL
- Alergia alimentar.
- Atopia.
- Sarna sarcóptica/notoédrica.
- Queiletielose.
- Qualquer dermatopatia pruriginosa.

HEMOGRAMA/BIOQUÍMICA/URINÁLISE
- Geralmente normais.
- Gatos — é possível detectar hipereosinofilia.

OUTROS TESTES LABORATORIAIS
- Raspados cutâneos — negativos.
- Uso de pentes antipulgas — para o encontro de pulgas ou seus dejetos.
- RAST e ELISA — acurácia variável; há relatos de ambos com resultados falso-positivos e falso-negativos.

DIAGNÓSTICO POR IMAGEM
N/D.

MÉTODOS DIAGNÓSTICOS
- O diagnóstico, em geral, baseia-se nas informações obtidas à anamnese e na distribuição das lesões e/ou na resposta ao controle adequado das pulgas.
- O encontro de pulgas ou seus dejetos confirma o diagnóstico, embora seja muito difícil encontrá-los, especialmente nos gatos.
- A identificação de segmentos de *Dipylidium caninum* também confirma a presença de pulgas.
- Teste alérgico intradérmico com antígeno de pulga — revela reações positivas imediatas em grande número de animais alérgicos a pulgas; às vezes, podem ser observadas reações tardias (24-48 h) em animais alérgicos que não demonstram reação imediata.
- O teste mais preciso pode ser a resposta ao tratamento adequado.

ACHADOS PATOLÓGICOS
- Dermatite perivascular superficial.
- Microabscessos eosinofílicos intraepidérmicos — fortemente sugestivos de hipersensibilidade à picada de pulgas.
- Eosinófilos como o principal componente celular da derme — confirma a hipersensibilidade à picada de pulgas.
- Avaliação histopatológica — não é capaz de diferenciar a hipersensibilidade à picada de pulgas dos quadros de atopia, alergia alimentar ou outras hipersensibilidades com precisão.

TRATAMENTO

CUIDADO(S) DE SAÚDE ADEQUADO(S)
Terapia ambulatorial.

CUIDADO(S) DE ENFERMAGEM
N/D.

ATIVIDADE
N/D.

DIETA
N/D.

ORIENTAÇÃO AO PROPRIETÁRIO
- Informar os proprietários que não há cura para a hipersensibilidade à picada de pulgas.
- Avisar os proprietários que os animais alérgicos a pulgas geralmente ficam mais sensíveis a picadas desses ectoparasitas à medida que envelhecem.
- Esclarecer os proprietários que o controle da exposição a pulgas constitui atualmente a única forma de tratamento; a hipossensibilização não é um método eficaz.

CONSIDERAÇÕES CIRÚRGICAS
N/D.

MEDICAÇÕES

MEDICAMENTO(S) DE ESCOLHA
- Corticosteroides — dosagens anti-inflamatórias para alívio sintomático ao mesmo tempo em que se institui o controle adequado das pulgas.

HIPERSENSIBILIDADE À PICADA DE PULGA E CONTROLE DE PULGAS

- Anti-histamínicos — alívio sintomático.
- Dinotefurano/piriproxifeno — produto tópico de ação rápida para gatos; o produto para cães contém permetrina em altas doses e não deve ser utilizado em gatos.
- Fipronil (antagonista do GABA) — tratamento tópico mensal para cães e gatos (sob a forma de *spray* para cães); atividade contra pulgas e carrapatos; resistente à remoção com água; perfil excelente de segurança e eficácia.
- Imidacloprida — tratamento tópico mensal (*spot*) para cães e gatos; perfil excelente de segurança e eficácia.
- Metaflumizona — interrompe o influxo de sódio necessário para a propagação dos impulsos nervosos; resulta em diminuição do repasto sanguíneo, perda da coordenação, paralisia e morte da pulga; estudos demonstraram uma excelente redução das pulgas e dos ovos desses ectoparasitas até 7 semanas com uma alta margem de segurança; o produto para cães contém amitraz e não deve ser usado em gatos.
- Nitenpiram — adulticida neonicotinoide contra pulgas; administrado por via oral; início de ação rápido, mas atuação breve; remove mais de 95% das pulgas adultas de cães e gatos dentro de 4-6 h da administração oral, embora tenha atividade residual por 48-72 h.
- Spinosad — tratamento oral mensal aprovado para uso apenas em cães; o modo de ação envolve receptores alfa D nicotínicos de acetilcolina com alguns efeitos sobre o GABA, resultando em paralisia por excitação nervosa e morte da pulga; considera-se que o spinosad seja seguro em conjunto com todos os outros produtos de controle de pulgas e preventivos de dirofilariose.
- *Sprays*/outros tratamentos tópicos — contêm, em geral, piretrinas e piretroides (piretrinas sintéticas) com algum regulador do crescimento de insetos ou sinergista; geralmente eficazes em menos de 48-72 h; as vantagens abrangem a baixa toxicidade e a atividade repelente; as desvantagens incluem as aplicações frequentes e o custo.
- Tratamento do interior da casa — nebulizadores e *sprays*; em geral, contêm organofosforados, piretrinas e/ou reguladores do crescimento de insetos; aplicar de acordo com as instruções do fabricante; tratar todos os cômodos da casa; podem ser aplicados pelo proprietário; as vantagens envolvem o fato de serem substâncias químicas fracas e geralmente de baixo custo; a desvantagem está na aplicação trabalhosa; esses *sprays* concentram as substâncias químicas nas áreas que mais necessitam de tratamento.
- Exterminadores profissionais — entre as vantagens, destaca-se o fato de dar menos trabalho para o proprietário do animal; exigem relativamente poucas aplicações; às vezes, têm garantia; as desvantagens compreendem a potência das substâncias químicas e o custo; recomendações específicas e orientações têm de ser seguidas.
- Substâncias inertes — ácido bórico, terra diatomácea e aerogel de sílica; tratar a cada 6-12 meses; seguir as recomendações do fabricante; muito seguras e eficazes se aplicadas corretamente.
- Tratamento da parte externa da casa — concentrado nas áreas sombreadas; os *sprays*, em geral, contêm piretroides ou organofosforados e algum regulador do crescimento do inseto; os pós costumam ser compostos por organofosforados; o produto que contém nematoides (*Steinerma carpocapsae*) é muito seguro e isento de substâncias químicas.

CONTRAINDICAÇÕES
N/D.

PRECAUÇÕES
- As instruções do rótulo a respeito da idade mínima de aplicação e da espécie devem ser rigorosamente seguidas.
- Spinosad pode potencializar os efeitos neurológicos de ivermectina em altas doses (utilizada para o tratamento de demodicose generalizada).
- Produtos antipulgas tipo piretrina/piretroide — as reações adversas incluem depressão, hipersalivação, tremores musculares, vômitos, ataxia, dispneia e anorexia.
- Organofosforados — as reações adversas incluem hipersalivação, lacrimejamento, micção, defecação, vômitos, diarreia, miose, febre, tremores musculares, crises convulsivas, coma e morte; a toxicidade torna seu uso inadequado considerando-se as alternativas atuais.
- Toxicidade — se qualquer um desses sinais for observado, o animal deverá ser totalmente banhado para remover toda a substância química remanescente e tratado de forma adequada; entrar em contato com algum centro toxicológico local em busca de sugestões terapêuticas adicionais.
- Roedores e peixes são muito sensíveis às piretrinas.

INTERAÇÕES POSSÍVEIS
Spinosad não deve ser utilizado com ivermectina em altas doses (usada em sarna demodécica generalizada); seguro quando combinado com preventivos contra dirofilariose.

MEDICAMENTO(S) ALTERNATIVO(S)
- Talcos — contêm, em geral, organofosforados ou carbamatos; a vantagem está na alta eficácia residual; as desvantagens incluem o ressecamento da pele e a toxicidade; organofosforados e carbamatos devem ser evitados em gatos.
- Banhos de imersão, *sprays*, talcos e espumas — os banhos de imersão contêm, em geral, organofosforados e piretrinas sintéticas e não devem ser usados mais de uma vez por semana; seguir as instruções do fabricante por questões de segurança e para obter os melhores resultados; após o uso repetido, esses agentes podem causar ressecamento ou ser irritantes; tratamentos mais seguros e mais modernos sob a forma de *spots* basicamente substituíram esses produtos.

ACOMPANHAMENTO

MONITORIZAÇÃO DO PACIENTE
- Prurido — a diminuição significa que a hipersensibilidade à picada de pulgas está sendo controlada.
- Pulgas e seus dejetos — a ausência nem sempre é um indicador confiável de sucesso do tratamento em animais muito sensíveis.

PREVENÇÃO
- Ver a seção "Medicações".
- Climas quentes o ano todo exigem o controle de pulgas durante todo o ano.
- Climas quentes em termos sazonais — começar o controle de pulgas nos meses de maio ou junho no Hemisfério Norte.

COMPLICAÇÕES POSSÍVEIS
- Foliculite bacteriana secundária.
- Dermatite úmida aguda.
- Dermatite acral por lambedura.

EVOLUÇÃO ESPERADA E PROGNÓSTICO
O prognóstico será bom se o controle estrito das pulgas for instituído.

DIVERSOS

DISTÚRBIOS ASSOCIADOS
Aproximadamente 80% dos cães atópicos também são alérgicos à picada de pulgas.

FATORES RELACIONADOS COM A IDADE
A embalagem dos produtos deverá ser consultada quanto à idade mínima aprovada para a aplicação.

POTENCIAL ZOONÓTICO
Em áreas de infestação moderada a grave por pulgas, as pessoas podem ser picadas por elas; as lesões papulares costumam ficar localizadas nos pulsos e tornozelos.

GESTAÇÃO/FERTILIDADE/REPRODUÇÃO
- Corticosteroides e organofosforados — não usar em cadelas e gatas prenhes.
- Seguir cuidadosamente as instruções do rótulo de cada produto para determinar sua segurança.

SINÔNIMO(S)
Alergia a picadas de pulgas.

ABREVIATURA(S)
- ELISA = ensaio imunoabsorvente ligado à enzima.
- GABA = ácido γ-aminobutírico.
- RAST = teste radioalergossorvente.

RECURSOS DA INTERNET
http://capcvet.org/. The Companion Animal Parasite Council, um conselho independente de veterinários e outros profissionais da área de saúde animal, firmado com o objetivo de criar diretrizes para o controle ideal de endo e ectoparasitas.

Sugestões de Leitura
Sousa CA, Halliwell RE. The ACVD task force on canine atopic dermatitis (XI): The relationship between arthropod hypersensitivity and atopic dermatitis in the dog. Vet Immunol Immunopathol 2001, 81(3-4):233-237.

Autores Jean S. Greek e Karen A. Kuhl
Consultor Editorial Alexander H. Werner

HIPERTENSÃO PORTAL

CONSIDERAÇÕES GERAIS

DEFINIÇÃO
Pressão portal >13 cmH$_2$O ou 10 mmHg.

FISIOPATOLOGIA
• Causas — aumento do fluxo sanguíneo portal; resistência elevada ao fluxo sanguíneo portal ou uma combinação de ambos. • Aumento do fluxo portal — arterialização da circulação portal como ocorre em casos de fístula arteriovenosa ou subsequente à resistência hepática elevada (desvio intra-hepático arteriovenoso) e circulação portal hepatofugal. • Resistência elevada — geralmente adquirida; a região anatômica é utilizada para classificar os mecanismos: pré-hepático (parte abdominal da veia porta), hepático (dentro do fígado) ou pós-hepático (estruturas craniais ao fígado: veias hepáticas, veia cava, coração, pericárdio). • Consequências — desenvolvimento de múltiplos desvios portossistêmicos adquiridos, efusão abdominal em virtude do aumento na produção de linfa, predisposição à encefalopatia hepática. • Desvio portossistêmico adquirido leva à formação de ascite: causas hepáticas — transudato puro reflete hipertensão portal e hipoalbuminemia concomitantes (proteína <1,5 g/dL); causas pós-hepáticas — transudato modificado (proteína >2,5 g/dL); causas pré-hepáticas — transudato puro ou modificado; a baixa celularidade reflete linfa esplâncnica.

SISTEMA(S) ACOMETIDO(S)
• Distúrbios hepatobiliares — distensão e hipertensão da vasculatura portal; esplenomegalia: distúrbios pós-hepáticos — congestão passiva do fígado, congestão venosa intra-hepática, hepatomegalia e hipertensão venosa portal variável. • Distúrbios pré-hepáticos — hipertensão portal esplâncnica, esplenomegalia e desvio portossistêmico adquirido. • Nervoso — encefalopatia hepática atribuída a desvio portossistêmico adquirido. • Cardiovascular — pode ocorrer o desenvolvimento de múltiplos desvios portossistêmicos e ascite em casos de obstrução da veia cava/hepática (ao nível do diafragma), mas não com insuficiência cardíaca congestiva ou tamponamento pericárdico, pois ambos provocam aumento da pressão hidrostática nos sistemas das veias hepática e cava.
• Gastrintestinal — edema entérico, aumento na permeabilidade da parede intestinal com predisposição à translocação transmural de bactérias (endotoxemia, bacteremia), vasculopatia entérica hipertensiva (sangramento entérico, ulceração) e má assimilação.

GENÉTICA
Ocorrência elevada em algumas raças e afins — certas anomalias vasculares hepáticas; fibrose hepática idiopática; hipertensão portal não cirrótica; hepatopatia causada pelo cobre.

IDENTIFICAÇÃO
Espécies
Cães e, raramente, gatos.

Raça(s) Predominante(s)
Distúrbios vasculares hepáticos familiares — Doberman pinscher (hipertensão portal não cirrótica); São Bernardo (fístula arteriovenosa); Poodle standard de pelagem preta, Pastor alemão (fibrose hepática idiopática ou juvenil); doença hepatobiliar adquirida: Cocker spaniel, Doberman pinscher, Labrador retriever; as raças Yorkshire terrier, Maltês e Pug, bem como os gatos, são menos tolerantes à ligadura cirúrgica de anomalia venosa portossistêmica (especialmente a constritores ameroides).

Idade Média e Faixa Etária
• Juvenis — distúrbios hereditários ou congênitos; más-formações da veia cava e do coração. • Cães jovens (com <2 anos de idade) — fibrose hepática idiopática ou juvenil ou, então, más-formações envolvendo a placa ductal; p. ex., hepatopatia policística (afeta gatos, mas é rara nos cães). • Cães jovens com início dos sinais antes de 1 ano e meio de idade — más-formações vasculares hepáticas congênitas em casos de agenesia portal com fístula arteriovenosa hepática (rara). • Animais de meia-idade e idosos — distúrbios hepatobiliares adquiridos.

SINAIS CLÍNICOS
Comentários Gerais
Dependem da localização, do grau e da velocidade de início da hipertensão portal e dos fatores causais.

Achados Anamnésicos
• Distensão abdominal — ascite. • Encefalopatia hepática — secundária a desvio portossistêmico adquirido. • Distúrbios cardíacos ou restrição pericárdica — tosse; intolerância ao exercício; dispneia; pulso jugular; pulsos femorais fracos ou pulso alternante. • Tromboembolia portal — diarreia sanguinolenta; íleo paralítico; dor abdominal; letargia; inapetência.

Achados do Exame Físico
• Efusão abdominal. • Hepatomegalia — apenas causas pós-hepáticas. • Esplenomegalia — congestão esplâncnica ou trombos venosos.
• Distensão da veia jugular — causas cardíacas ou pericárdicas pós-hepáticas. • Bulhas cardíacas abafadas — efusão pericárdica ou pleural.
• Arritmias ou sopros cardíacos — cardiopatia.
• "Crepitações" pulmonares (edema) — causas cardíacas ou pericárdicas. • Confusão mental, estupor, coma, cegueira, outras anormalidades comportamentais neurológicas — encefalopatia hepática. • Icterícia — causas hepáticas. • Ruído hepático (fístula arteriovenosa).

CAUSAS
Pré-hepáticas
• Trombose da veia porta, estenose ou neoplasia.
• Compressão da veia porta — linfonodos grandes; neoplasia, granuloma; abscesso.
• Complicação pós-operatória de ligadura de desvio portossistêmico adquirido: especialmente por constritores ameroides. • Atresia congênita da veia porta — hipertensão portal amenizada por desvio portossistêmico adquirido.

Intra-hepáticas
• Fibrose/cirrose do fígado. • Hepatopatia inflamatória crônica. • Obstrução extra-hepática crônica do ducto biliar (mais de 6 semanas).
• Fibrose hepática juvenil ou idiopática. • Neoplasia hepática — localização no sistema porta hepático.
• Encarceramento do fígado — em hérnia diafragmática. • Doença venoclusiva. • Hipertensão portal não cirrótica. • Atresia da veia porta (intra ou extra-hepática). • Fístula arteriovenosa hepática.

Pós-hepáticas
• Insuficiência cardíaca congestiva direita.
• Dirofilariose. • Tamponamento pericárdico.
• Pericardite — restritiva ou constritiva.
• Neoplasia cardíaca. • Coração triatriado direito.
• Tromboembolia pulmonar grave — distúrbios que afetam a veia cava caudal supradiafragmática — trombose; ocorrência de torção ou formação de membrana congênitos; síndrome da veia cava por dirofilariose; oclusão por neoplasia; encarceramento em hérnia diafragmática.

DIAGNÓSTICO

DIAGNÓSTICO DIFERENCIAL
• Análise físico-química de efusão abdominal — ajuda a estreitar o diagnóstico. • Transudato puro — hipoalbuminemia secundária à enteropatia com perda de proteínas, nefropatia com perda de proteínas, insuficiência hepática. • Transudato modificado com albumina normal ou baixa — enteropatia com perda de proteínas, nefropatia com perda de proteínas, insuficiência hepática (efusão crônica), neoplasia, tromboembolia abdominal, encarceramento hepático (visceral) em hérnia diafragmática. • Transudato modificado com fígado grande e distensão jugular — anormalidades cardíacas ou pericárdicas; dirofilariose; tumor do átrio direito. • Transudato modificado com fígado grande, sem distensão jugular, bulha cardíaca abafada ou edema pulmonar — veia cava dobrada; síndrome semelhante à de Budd-Chiari (efeito venoclusivo sobre a veia hepática). • Encefalopatia hepática — fibrose hepática; cirrose; hepatopatia fibrosante juvenil; fístula arteriovenosa hepática; qualquer causa de desvio portossistêmico adquirido.
• Icterícia — hepatite ou colangite crônicas; obstrução extra-hepática crônica do ducto biliar; neoplasia hepática infiltrativa. • Diarreia sanguinolenta, dor abdominal, íleo paralítico, sinais de endotoxemia —tromboembolia portal extra-hepática aguda.

HEMOGRAMA/BIOQUÍMICA/URINÁLISE
• Hemograma completo — esquistócitos ou esquizócitos em casos de tromboembolia; microcitose eritrocitária em casos de desvio portossistêmico adquirido ou anomalia venosa portossistêmica; plasma ictérico em casos de hepatopatia ou anemia microangiopática por cisalhamento (também revelam a presença de esquistócitos). • Bioquímica — hepatopatia: enzimas hepáticas elevadas variáveis, baixa concentração de ureia, creatinina, colesterol e glicose, hiperbilirrubinemia e anormalidades da coagulação; distúrbios pós-hepáticos: atividade elevada das enzimas hepáticas, às vezes com azotemia. • Urinálise — cristalúria por biurato de amônio na presença de desvio portossistêmico adquirido; é possível observar cilindros granulares em casos de tromboembolia; pode-se notar proteinúria em casos de dirofilariose.

OUTROS TESTES LABORATORIAIS
• Ácidos biliares séricos totais — concentrações normais a altas em jejum e elevadas 2 h após as refeições em casos de desvio portossistêmico adquirido ou doença hepatobiliar; padrão de desvio: valores normais em jejum e acentuadamente elevados após as refeições.
• Amônia sanguínea — hiperamonemia em casos de desvio portossistêmico adquirido; é preferível a mensuração dos ácidos biliares séricos totais.
• Caracterização físico-química de efusão

HIPERTENSÃO PORTAL

abdominal — relação elevada de albumina no soro:efusão (>1,1) compatível com hipertensão portal; uma relação alta pode predizer uma resposta positiva à diureticoterapia.

DIAGNÓSTICO POR IMAGEM

Radiografias
• Radiografia torácica — pode revelar a causa de hipertensão portal pós-hepática (p. ex., veia cava dobrada, efusão pericárdica, doença pulmonar, efusão pleural e hérnia diafragmática). • Radiografia abdominal — pode revelar efusão, esplenomegalia ou fígado grande (p. ex., com congestão, neoplasia difusa ou fístula arteriovenosa hepática); fígado pequeno na maioria dos distúrbios hepáticos que causam desvio portossistêmico adquirido e anomalia venosa portossistêmica.

Ultrassonografia Abdominal
• Inspeciona a dinâmica circulatória com o uso do Doppler de fluxo colorido para identificar perfusão hepatofugal (fluxo retrógrado da veia porta), procurar por trombos e detectar desvio portossistêmico adquirido ou anomalia venosa portossistêmica (caudal ao rim esquerdo). • Identifica anormalidades que envolvem a veia porta abdominal ou extra-hepática: atresia, estenose, trombos, lesões oclusivas no sistema porta hepático. • Identifica lobo(s) contendo fístula(s) arteriovenosa(s). • Avalia o parênquima visceral, além de identificar linfadenomegalia e lesões expansivas (neoplasia). • Estima a distensão venosa hepática.

Ecocardiografia
• Detecta distúrbios cardíacos e pericárdicos, além de neoplasias, trombos, dirofilárias, efusões pleurais, más-formações ou trombos na veia cava, hérnia diafragmática.

Angiografia e Imagens Nucleares
• Cintilografia colorretal — confirma o desvio portossistêmico. • Angiografia radiográfica — demonstra o tronco celíaco e a artéria hepática para confirmar a presença de fístula arteriovenosa hepática; estudos não seletivos ou seletivos — cardiopatia congênita; tromboêmbolos; distúrbios da veia hepática. • Portovenografia — confirma a existência de desvio portossistêmico adquirido. • TC multissetorial — caracterização de alta qualidade da vasculatura regional na área de interesse; método não invasivo; exame preferido atualmente em detrimento de outros.

MÉTODOS DIAGNÓSTICOS
• Eletrocardiografia e pressão venosa central — em casos de cardiopatia. • Biopsia hepática — necessária para o diagnóstico de distúrbios hepáticos parenquimatosos ou vasculares. • Pressão portal — mensuração não recomendada; não é confiável para deduzir as causas subjacentes; a hipertensão portal é confirmada de forma adequada pelas técnicas de diagnóstico por imagem.

TRATAMENTO

CUIDADO(S) DE SAÚDE ADEQUADO(S)
Internação — na presença de sinais de encefalopatia hepática; amenização da ascite tensa por abdominocentese terapêutica.

CUIDADO(S) DE ENFERMAGEM
• Fluidoterapia — em todas as causas, deve-se restringir a concentração de sódio (evitar NaCl a 0,9%) em função da alta probabilidade de sobrecarga de sódio corporal total. Ter cuidado para evitar edema pulmonar iatrogênico, sobretudo em animal com hipoalbuminemia. • Monitorizar o peso e a condição corporais, a circunferência abdominal, as proteínas plasmáticas e o hematócrito. • Pressão oncótica baixa — fica indicado o uso de coloides ou albumina; evitar a utilização de dextrana em casos de disfunção hepática; prefere-se a administração de plasma para pacientes hepatopatas (ou hetamido na dose de 20 mL/kg/dia administrada em velocidade de infusão constante). • Suplementação de glicose — em casos de disfunção hepática e hipoglicemia; glicose a 2,5-5% com fluidos poliônicos com metade da potência inicialmente; titular a concentração de glicose até atingir a normoglicemia e evitar a hiperglicemia. • Abdominocentese terapêutica — realizada se a distensão abdominal estiver causando desconforto, comprometimento ventilatório, privação do sono, restrição do consumo alimentar ou se essa distensão for refratária ao tratamento clínico; a remoção repetida de grandes volumes de líquido pode resultar em hipovolemia, hipoproteinemia e depleção eletrolítica, além de introduzir infecções; administrar concomitantemente fluidos poliônicos com coloides com moderação. Fornecer 4-8 g de albumina/L de ascite removida.

ATIVIDADE
Depende da causa; restringir a atividade na presença de ascite.

DIETA
• Ascite — restrição de sódio na dieta para <100 mg/100 kcal. • Restrição de proteína apenas se houver encefalopatia hepática.

ORIENTAÇÃO AO PROPRIETÁRIO
Pode não haver como prever a cura ou a melhora crônica até que se determine o diagnóstico definitivo.

CONSIDERAÇÕES CIRÚRGICAS
• A realização de ligadura de desvio portossistêmico adquirido ou a aplicação de bandagem na veia cava é fortemente contraindicada. • Se ocorrer o desenvolvimento de hipertensão portal sintomática aguda após a ligadura cirúrgica de desvio portossistêmico adquirido — a remoção da ligadura será obrigatória. • A embolectomia de trombos não é recomendada; tais trombos podem ser recanalizados com cuidados de suporte; a dissolução do coágulo (estreptoquinase, ativador de plasminogênio tecidual) é uma medida complicada e cara, além de ter um prognóstico mau (ver "Coagulopatia por Hepatopatia"). • Correção de hérnia diafragmática crônica; a liberação de vísceras encarceradas pode causar endotoxemia perioperatória/pós-operatória. • É possível realizar a correção cirúrgica e obter a cura de coração triatriado e veia cava dobrada. • Pericardiectomia — restrição ou tamponamento pericárdicos; o procedimento toracoscópico é menos invasivo, exibe menor índice de mortalidade e apresenta os melhores resultados. • Remoção de tumor ou aderências fibrosas que causam oclusão venosa. • Remoção (lobectomia) ou embolização (acrilamida) de fístula arteriovenosa hepática; o desvio intra-hepático microscópico geralmente mantém a hipertensão portal e o desvio portossistêmico adquirido.

MEDICAÇÕES

MEDICAMENTO(S) DE ESCOLHA
• Tratamento da efusão abdominal — restrição de sódio (ver anteriormente a seção "Dieta"); diureticoterapia combinada. • Furosemida (1-4 mg/kg VO, IM ou IV a cada 12-24 h) e espironolactona (1-4 mg/kg VO a cada 12 h, iniciada com dose de ataque; dose de manutenção de no mínimo 2-4 mg/kg). • Reduzir gradativamente a dose do diurético após resposta positiva inicial; individualizar o tratamento crônico até obtenção da resposta; os diuréticos são utilizados de forma intermitente para mobilizar as ascites recidivantes. • Furosemida e enalapril ou outros medicamentos, conforme indicados por distúrbios cardíacos específicos. • Tratamento de encefalopatia hepática (ver "Encefalopatia Hepática").

INTERAÇÕES POSSÍVEIS
• Evitar medicamentos que sofrem extração hepática de primeira passagem, biotransformação ou eliminação hepática, se possível; se isso não for possível, ajustar a dose dos medicamentos. • Reduzir a dose de medicamentos que ficam altamente ligados a proteínas na presença de hipoalbuminemia.

ACOMPANHAMENTO

MONITORIZAÇÃO DO PACIENTE
• Registrar sequencialmente o peso e a condição corporais, além de medir a circunferência abdominal. • De forma sequencial também, avaliar a hidratação do paciente, o nível de eletrólitos, o estado acidobásico e a pressão arterial, conforme a necessidade. • Monitorizar os níveis de albumina em casos de hipoalbuminemia e as concentrações de glicose na presença de hepatopatia ou desvio portossistêmico adquirido. • Monitorizar os ruídos pulmonares, a oximetria de pulso e o esforço ventilatório — em distúrbios cardiovasculares.

COMPLICAÇÕES POSSÍVEIS
• Trombose. • Endotoxemia. • Hipotensão. • Encefalopatia hepática.

EVOLUÇÃO ESPERADA E PROGNÓSTICO
Dependem da causa.

DIVERSOS

DISTÚRBIOS ASSOCIADOS
• Hepatopatia crônica. • Distúrbios indutores de oclusão venosa pré ou pós-hepática.

GESTAÇÃO/FERTILIDADE/REPRODUÇÃO
Afeta a perfusão uterina e provavelmente causa abortamento ou gera natimortos.

VER TAMBÉM
• Anomalia Vascular Portossistêmica Congênita. • Ascite. • Cirrose e Fibrose do Fígado. • Desvio Portossistêmico Adquirido. • Encefalopatia Hepática. • Insuficiência Cardíaca Congestiva Direita. • Pericardite.

Autor Sharon A. Center

HIPERTENSÃO PULMONAR

CONSIDERAÇÕES GERAIS

DEFINIÇÃO
Pressão sistólica de pico da artéria pulmonar >30 mmHg e/ou pressão diastólica de pico da artéria pulmonar >15 mmHg.

FISIOPATOLOGIA
• Várias anormalidades podem ocasionar elevações na pressão da artéria pulmonar: (1) vasoconstrição arterial pulmonar (primária ou secundária à hipoxemia e acidemia), (2) obstrução da artéria pulmonar, (3) pressão atrial esquerda elevada com consequente elevação da pressão arterial e venosa pulmonar, ou (4) fluxo sanguíneo pulmonar excessivo.
 • À medida que as pressões nas veias, capilares e/ou artérias pulmonares sobem, as pressões do lado direito do coração aumentam para manter o fluxo sanguíneo pulmonar. Isso pode resultar em hipertrofia excêntrica e/ou concêntrica do ventrículo direito, depressão da função cardíaca direita, queda do fluxo sanguíneo pulmonar e diminuição do enchimento do lado esquerdo do coração com consequente desenvolvimento de sinais clínicos. As pressões elevadas no coração direito podem causar congestão venosa sistêmica, regurgitação tricúspide e consequente insuficiência cardíaca congestiva direita.

SISTEMA(S) ACOMETIDO(S)
• Cardiovascular — ver a seção "Fisiopatologia".
• Hepatobiliar — ICC direita pode causar congestão hepática e ascite.
• Respiratório — pode haver doença pulmonar. ICC direita pode causar efusão pleural.

GENÉTICA
• Não foi encontrada nenhuma base genética específica.
• A hipertensão pulmonar pode ser secundária a vários defeitos cardíacos congênitos que podem ter uma base genética.
• Os pacientes com predisposição genética à cardiopatia esquerda provavelmente têm uma alta prevalência de hipertensão pulmonar.

INCIDÊNCIA/PREVALÊNCIA
Desconhecidas.

DISTRIBUIÇÃO GEOGRÁFICA
Desconhecida; pode ser que haja uma prevalência relativamente alta em áreas onde a dirofilariose é endêmica e em altitudes elevadas.

IDENTIFICAÇÃO
Espécies
Cães e gatos.

Raça(s) Predominante(s)
Possível com base na causa subjacente de hipertensão pulmonar (p. ex., cardiopatia congênita, fibrose pulmonar). Foi sugerida uma alta incidência nas raças terriers.

Sexo Predominante
Há relatos de incidência elevada em fêmeas.

Idade Média e Faixa Etária
Geralmente cães idosos.

SINAIS CLÍNICOS
Comentários Gerais
Os sinais podem ser atribuídos à hipertensão pulmonar e/ou à doença primária subjacente.

Achados Anamnésicos
• Intolerância ao exercício/dispneia por esforço.
• Dispneia/taquipneia.
• Tosse/hemoptise.
• Síncope.
• Distensão abdominal.
• Perda de peso.
• Letargia.
• Morte súbita.

Achados do Exame Físico
• Dispneia/taquipneia.
• Tosse.
• Hemoptise.
• Segunda bulha cardíaca sonora e/ou desdobrada.
• Estertores pulmonares e/ou ruídos broncovesiculares ásperos.
• Cianose.
• Sopro cardíaco.
• Distensão abdominal.
• Distensão jugular.
• Edema subcutâneo.
• Perda de peso.

CAUSAS
Hipertensão Pulmonar Primária
• Em seres humanos, foi identificado um distúrbio congênito da vasculatura pulmonar.
• Anormalidades em substâncias vasodilatadoras e vasoconstritoras derivadas do endotélio resultam em obstrução vascular e vasoconstrição.
• Não identificada em animais de companhia.

Doença do Parênquima Pulmonar
• *Obstrução vascular* — resultante de lesões pulmonares (p. ex., fibrose, neoplasia), hipertrofia vascular e inflamação vascular pulmonar.
• *Vasoconstrição* — constrição vascular reativa secundária à hipoxia e acidemia.
• *Causas específicas*:
  ○ Pneumonia (bacteriana, viral, fúngica, parasitária).
  ○ Bronquite crônica.
  ○ Doença pulmonar obstrutiva crônica.
  ○ Fibrose pulmonar.
  ○ Bronquite eosinofílica.
  ○ Neoplasia pulmonar.
  ○ Síndrome da angústia respiratória do adulto.

Tromboembolia Pulmonar
• *Obstrução vascular* — por trombo.
• *Vasoconstrição* — constrição vascular reativa secundária à hipoxia e/ou no local do trombo.
• *Causas*:
  ○ Hiperadrenocorticismo.
  ○ Nefropatia com perda de proteínas.
  ○ Enteropatia com perda de proteínas.
  ○ Sepse.
  ○ Anemia hemolítica imunomediada.
  ○ Neoplasia.
  ○ Pancreatite.
  ○ Endocardite.
  ○ Coagulação intravascular disseminada.
  ○ Cardiopatia primária (tipicamente do lado direito).

Dirofilariose
• *Obstrução vascular* — secundária à hipertrofia vascular, inflamação, tromboembolia e presença de dirofilárias.
• *Vasoconstrição* — no local de estabelecimento de dirofilárias e trombos e/ou secundária à hipoxia.

Cardiopatia Congênita com Desvio da Esquerda para a Direita
• *Fluxo sanguíneo pulmonar excessivo* em virtude de desvio da esquerda para a direita através de vários defeitos congênitos resulta em dano à vasculatura pulmonar, causando *vasoconstrição* e *obstrução vascular* atribuídas à hipertrofia vascular.
• *Causas*:
  ○ Persistência do ducto arterioso.
  ○ Defeito do septo ventricular.
  ○ Defeito do septo atrial.

Cardiopatia Esquerda
• *Pressão atrial esquerda elevada* reflui para as veias pulmonares, resultando em hipertensão pulmonar.
• *Causas*:
  ○ Regurgitação mitral.
  ○ Miocardiopatia (dilatada, hipertrófica, restritiva, não classificada).
  ○ Estenose mitral.
  ○ Obstrução venosa pulmonar congênita (coração triatriado esquerdo).
  ○ Tumores atriais esquerdos.

Causas Extrapulmonares de Hipoxia Crônica
• *Vasoconstrição* — alguns fatores ambientais podem resultar em hipoxia e acidemia, levando à vasoconstrição pulmonar.
• *Causas*:
  ○ Hipoventilação (síndrome de Pickwick, distúrbios neuromusculares).
  ○ Doença de altitude elevada.

FATORES DE RISCO
• Doença cardíaca e pulmonar.
• Dirofilariose.
• Doenças associadas à tromboembolia pulmonar.
• Obesidade.
• Altitudes elevadas.

DIAGNÓSTICO

DIAGNÓSTICO DIFERENCIAL
• ICC esquerda sem hipertensão pulmonar.
• Colapso da traqueia.
• ICC direita.
• Doença pulmonar significativa sem hipertensão pulmonar.
• Dirofilariose sem hipertensão pulmonar.
• Pneumotórax.
• Efusão pleural (piotórax, quilotórax, hemotórax, hidrotórax).
• Paralisia/doença da laringe.

HEMOGRAMA/BIOQUÍMICA/URINÁLISE
• Não há anormalidades compatíveis.
• Pode-se observar policitemia em caso de hipoxia crônica acentuada.

OUTROS TESTES LABORATORIAIS
• Gasometria arterial (hipoxemia).
• Teste para dirofilariose oculta.
• Pesquisa de causas de tromboembolia pulmonar (relação de proteína:creatinina urinárias, nível de antitrombina III, D-dímero, perfil de coagulação, teste de estimulação com ACTH, teste de supressão com dexametasona).
• Análise de efusões pleurais ou abdominais.

DIAGNÓSTICO POR IMAGEM
Radiografia
• Artéria pulmonar dilatada e/ou vasos pulmonares tortuosos.
• Aumento de volume do átrio e ventrículo direitos.
• Veia cava caudal dilatada.
• Efusão pleural.

Hipertensão Pulmonar

- Hepatomegalia.
- Ascite.
- Possíveis indícios de doença pulmonar primária, embolia pulmonar ou dirofilariose.

Ecocardiografia
- Hipertrofia concêntrica/excêntrica do ventrículo direito.
- Movimento paradoxal de septo.
- Dilatação do átrio direito.
- Dilatação da artéria pulmonar.
- Efusão pleural/pericárdica.
- Regurgitação tricúspide: se houver regurgitação dessa valva atrioventricular direita sem estenose pulmonar ou estenose da artéria pulmonar, o gradiente de pressão *sistólica* entre o ventrículo direito e o átrio direito poderá ser estimado com o uso de Doppler espectral, utilizando a equação de Bernoulli modificada: $4 \times$ (velocidade de regurgitação tricúspide de pico)^2.
- Gradiente pressórico >30 mmHg (velocidade de regurgitação tricúspide >2,8 m/s) é compatível com hipertensão pulmonar.
- Gradiente entre 30 e 50 mmHg é compatível com hipertensão pulmonar leve, 51-80 mmHg com hipertensão pulmonar moderada e >80 mmHg com hipertensão pulmonar grave.
- Insuficiência da válvula pulmonar: se houver insuficiência dessa válvula sem estenose pulmonar ou estenose da artéria pulmonar, o gradiente de pressão *diastólica* entre a artéria pulmonar e o ventrículo direito poderá ser estimado com o uso de Doppler espectral, utilizando a equação de Bernoulli modificada.
- Gradiente pressórico >15 mmHg (velocidade de insuficiência da válvula pulmonar >2,0 m/s) é compatível com hipertensão pulmonar.
- Indícios de cardiopatia esquerda, dirofilariose, cardiopatia congênita ou tromboembolia pulmonar, dependendo da causa de hipertensão pulmonar.

TC/RM
- Podem ter valor diagnóstico ao se considerar o diagnóstico de neoplasia pulmonar ou outras doenças infiltrativas; considerar os riscos da anestesia.

MÉTODOS DIAGNÓSTICOS
Lavado transtraqueal, lavado broncoalveolar ou aspirado/biopsia pulmonar podem ser valiosos se houver indícios de doença pulmonar primária; considerar os riscos da anestesia.

Eletrocardiografia
- Desvio do eixo elétrico médio para a direita.
- Ondas S profundas nas derivações I, II, III e aVF.
- Alargamento do complexo QRS.
- Ondas P altas (i. e., P *pulmonale*).
- Pode ocorrer depressão/elevação do segmento ST com hipoxia significativa.
- Arritmias induzidas por hipoxia, como complexos ventriculares prematuros.

Cateterismo Cardíaco e Angiografia Pulmonar
- Raramente necessários para confirmar hipertensão pulmonar.
- Podem demonstrar anormalidades como dirofilárias, tromboembolia pulmonar, alterações vasculares ou cardiopatia congênita que confirmam a causa subjacente de hipertensão pulmonar.
- Considerar os riscos da anestesia.

ACHADOS PATOLÓGICOS
- Dependem da doença subjacente e da gravidade:
  - Lesões pulmonares primárias.
  - Trombo na artéria pulmonar.
  - Artéria pulmonar dilatada.
  - Aumento de volume do lado direito do coração.
  - Dilatação da veia cava.
  - Dirofilárias.
  - Efusão pleural/pericárdica.
  - Ascite.
  - Hipertrofia da camada média da vasculatura pulmonar.
  - Proliferação da camada íntima e esclerose da vasculatura pulmonar.
  - Arterite necrosante.

TRATAMENTO

CUIDADO(S) DE SAÚDE ADEQUADO(S)
- Internar os pacientes em angústia respiratória grave até que estejam estabilizados.
- Administrar oxigenoterapia, broncodilatadores, diuréticos e antibióticos em um esquema emergencial de acordo com a doença subjacente.
- Se o paciente estiver em um estado crítico, talvez seja preciso adiar alguns procedimentos diagnósticos até sua estabilização.

CUIDADO(S) DE ENFERMAGEM
- Monitorizar o estado de hidratação e a temperatura do corpo com rigor.
- A fluidoterapia criteriosa pode ser benéfica, embora seja imprescindível considerar o estado cardíaco do paciente e o possível desenvolvimento de ICC.
- Manter o ambiente com o mínimo de estresse.

ATIVIDADE
Restrita.

DIETA
Diretrizes específicas com base na doença subjacente; se houver insuficiência cardíaca, pode ser benéfico restringir o sódio na dieta.

ORIENTAÇÃO AO PROPRIETÁRIO
- O diagnóstico, em geral, é presuntivo sem a realização de cateterismo e/ou ecocardiografia Doppler.
- O prognóstico varia com a reversibilidade da doença subjacente, mas é bastante reservado na maioria dos casos.
- Evitar ambientes que possam predispor à angústia respiratória — frio excessivo ou ar seco, calor demasiado, tabagismo passivo, altitudes elevadas.

CONSIDERAÇÕES CIRÚRGICAS
A extração cirúrgica de dirofilárias é uma consideração em pacientes com infestação grave.

MEDICAÇÕES

MEDICAMENTO(S) DE ESCOLHA
- Tratar o processo patológico subjacente primário sempre que possível.
- O agente terapêutico ideal deve reduzir a resistência vascular pulmonar e a hipertensão pulmonar sem provocar hipotensão sistêmica significativa; o oxigênio pode conseguir isso, mas a administração prolongada desse gás não costuma ser viável nesses pacientes; o uso a curto prazo ou intermitente de oxigênio pode ser benéfico.

Inibidores da Fosfodiesterase Tipo V
- Inibem a degradação do GMPc, provocando o aumento do óxido nítrico com consequente vasodilatação pulmonar; também podem causar uma leve vasodilatação sistêmica, ocasionando o declínio na pressão sanguínea sistêmica.
- Não administrar com outros medicamentos que possam ter efeitos semelhantes, como os nitratos.
- Sildenafila: inúmeros estudos demonstram melhora clínica e ecocardiográfica em cães com hipertensão pulmonar.
- Tadalafila: benefício sugerido por um único estudo publicado.
- Vardenafila: ainda não foi avaliado nos animais de companhia; *não* demonstra efeitos vasodilatadores sobre a vasculatura pulmonar em seres humanos.

Outros Vasodilatadores
- Benefício limitado como vasodilatadores pulmonares diretos em virtude da hipotensão sistêmica concomitante que ocorre com a administração.
- Muito importantes no tratamento de hipertensão pulmonar decorrente de cardiopatia esquerda; a vasodilatação sistêmica aumentará o fluxo anterógrado que pode resultar em diminuição na pressão do átrio esquerdo.
- As opções incluem inibidores da ECA (p. ex., enalapril e benazepril), hidralazina e bloqueadores dos canais de cálcio (diltiazem ou anlodipino).
- A pimobendana é um inibidor da fosfodiesterase tipo III (vasodilatação sistêmica), mas também pode provocar uma leve inibição da fosfodiesterase tipo V conforme discussão prévia.

Broncodilatadores
- Podem ser benéficos em pacientes com doença pulmonar.
- As metilxantinas podem ocasionar uma leve vasodilatação arterial pulmonar.
- Podem ter efeitos inotrópicos positivos possivelmente benéficos em alguns tipos de disfunção cardíaca.
- As opções incluem simpaticomiméticos (p. ex., terbutalina) e metilxantinas (p. ex., teofilina).

Inotrópicos Positivos (Digoxina, Dobutamina)
- Não constituem o principal tratamento de hipertensão pulmonar.
- Podem ser benéficos em casos de ICC.
- Monitorizar o paciente com rigor quanto à ocorrência de arritmias.

Terapia Anticoagulante
- Indicada para doença tromboembólica.
- As opções incluem heparina, varfarina e ácido acetilsalicílico.
- Atualmente, os medicamentos clopidogrel e heparinas de baixo peso molecular estão sob investigação em animais.
- O ácido acetilsalicílico e o clopidogrel podem ser administrados simultaneamente, já que esses agentes possuem mecanismos de ação distintos.
- Todos os anticoagulantes têm sucesso variável na prevenção de tromboembolia nos animais de companhia.

Terapia Trombolítica
- As indicações e a eficácia são questionáveis.
- Estreptoquinase e ativador de plasminogênio tecidual são os principais agentes trombolíticos.

HIPERTENSÃO PULMONAR

• Provavelmente indicada apenas se houver tromboembolia pulmonar aguda com comprometimento cardíaco significativo.

Terapia Anti-inflamatória e Antibiótica
• Doses anti-inflamatórias de esteroides podem ser benéficas quando a causa subjacente da hipertensão pulmonar tiver um componente inflamatório (p. ex., dirofilariose, alguns casos de doença pulmonar primária).
• Os antibióticos são indicados se houver algum componente infeccioso bacteriano (pneumonia).

CONTRAINDICAÇÕES
• Medicamentos ou situações que possam agravar a hipoxia pulmonar (p. ex., depressores respiratórios).
• Medicamentos que deprimem a função cardíaca (p. ex., β-bloqueadores).
• Medicamentos que possam gerar broncoconstrição (p. ex., β-bloqueadores inespecíficos).
• Medicamentos que possam causar vasoconstrição.

PRECAUÇÕES
• Os vasodilatadores podem causar hipotensão sistêmica.
• Raramente, os broncodilatadores podem levar à taquicardia e hiperexcitabilidade.
• Monitorizar os perfis de coagulação de perto durante a terapia anticoagulante.
• A hipovolemia pode interferir no enchimento do lado direito do coração e, portanto, deprimir a função cardíaca e o fluxo sanguíneo pulmonar; monitorizar os pacientes sob diureticoterapia com rigor.

MEDICAMENTO(S) ALTERNATIVO(S)
N/D.

ACOMPANHAMENTO

MONITORIZAÇÃO DO PACIENTE
• Exame físico com auscultação cardiopulmonar meticulosa.
• Monitorizar o animal quanto ao agravamento dos sinais clínicos.
• Ecocardiografia seriada para avaliar a melhora ou a piora da hipertensão pulmonar.
• Monitorização seriada da pressão arterial se o paciente estiver sendo submetido a vasodilatadores.
• Possível repetição de radiografias torácicas, ECG e hemogasometrias arteriais.

PREVENÇÃO
Avaliação e prevenção precoces de condições que predisponham à hipertensão pulmonar.

COMPLICAÇÕES POSSÍVEIS
• Insuficiência cardíaca direita.
• Síncope.
• Sinais debilitantes progressivos (p. ex., dispneia por esforço, letargia, fraqueza, anorexia).
• Arritmias cardíacas.
• Morte súbita.
• Caquexia cardíaca.

EVOLUÇÃO ESPERADA E PROGNÓSTICO
• Determinados com base na capacidade de reversão da doença subjacente.
• Quando as alterações forem irreversíveis, o tratamento será paliativo.
• Em geral, o prognóstico é bastante reservado.

DIVERSOS

DISTÚRBIOS ASSOCIADOS
Ver a seção "Causas".

FATORES RELACIONADOS COM A IDADE
N/D.

GESTAÇÃO/FERTILIDADE/REPRODUÇÃO
Alto risco.

VER TAMBÉM
Capítulos sobre doenças que causam hipertensão pulmonar.

ABREVIATURA(S)
• ACTH = hormônio adrenocorticotrópico.
• ECA = enzima conversora de angiotensina.
• ECG = eletrocardiograma.
• ICC = insuficiência cardíaca congestiva.
• RM = ressonância magnética.
• TC = tomografia computadorizada.

Sugestões de Leitura
Bach JF, Rozanski EA, MacGregor J, Betkowski JM, Rush JE. Restrospective evaluation of Sildenafil Citrate as a therapy for pulmonary hypertension. J Vet Intern Med 2006, 20:1132-1135.
Henik RA. Pulmonary hypertension. In: Bonagura JD, Twedt DC, eds., Current Veterinary Therapy XIV. St. Louis: Saunders Elsevier, 2009, pp. 697-702.
Kellum HB, Stepien RL. Sildenafil citrate therapy in 22 dogs with pulmonary hypertension. J Vet Intern Med 2007, 21:1258-1264.

Autor Donald P. Schrope
Consultores Editoriais Larry P. Tilley e Francis W.K. Smith, Jr.

Hipertensão Sistêmica

CONSIDERAÇÕES GERAIS

DEFINIÇÃO
Elevação contínua da pressão arterial sistólica ou diastólica (ou ambas). Em cães e gatos, a pressão arterial sistólica ≥140 mmHg ou a pressão arterial diastólica ≥90 mmHg obtida por qualquer método é considerada anormal. O aumento na pressão arterial pode ser transitório e relacionado com artefato de medição (induzido por estresse ou efeito do avental branco) ou contínuo e patológico. Em pacientes veterinários, a hipertensão costuma ser atribuída a algum outro processo patológico e, nesse caso, recebe o nome de hipertensão secundária. Caso não haja uma doença subjacente ou não se consiga determiná-la, empregam-se os termos hipertensão primária, essencial ou idiopática.

FISIOPATOLOGIA
- A pressão arterial é o produto do débito cardíaco e da resistência vascular sistêmica; o débito cardíaco é determinado pela frequência cardíaca e pelo volume sistólico.
- A regulação da pressão arterial depende da integração de mecanismos complexos nos sistemas nervosos central e periférico, tecidos renal e cardíaco, além de fatores humorais, que afetam de forma sinérgica o débito cardíaco e a resistência vascular.
- Os barorreceptores existentes no seio carotídeo e no arco aórtico respondem a alterações na pressão arterial; uma queda na pressão arterial aumenta a descarga simpática, causando vasoconstrição e aumento da contratilidade/frequência cardíacas. As substâncias humorais que modulam a pressão arterial incluem catecolaminas, vasopressina, cininas, renina, angiotensina, aldosterona, prostaglandinas e peptídeo natriurético atrial.
- A hipertensão primária não é totalmente compreendida em pacientes veterinários, mas alguns casos têm um componente hereditário. A hipertensão secundária é mais comumente associada à doença renal crônica e a endocrinopatias em cães e gatos.
- A hipertensão também pode ocorrer secundariamente à fluidoterapia, ao uso de medicamentos vasoconstritores, à administração de esteroides ou à terapia com eritropoietina.

SISTEMA(S) ACOMETIDO(S)
- Cardiovascular.
- Renal/urológico.
- Ocular.
- Nervoso.

GENÉTICA
Colônias de cães hipertensos foram reproduzidas pelo cruzamento de cães com hipertensão essencial; o modo de herança, no entanto, é desconhecido.

INCIDÊNCIA/PREVALÊNCIA
- Cães: Prevalência de hipertensão causada por doença — doença renal crônica (9-93%; a maioria dos estudos apoia uma taxa de 60-80%), hiperadrenocorticismo (73-80%), diabetes melito (24-46%).
- Gatos: Prevalência de hipertensão em doença renal crônica (19-65%).

IDENTIFICAÇÃO
Espécies
Cães e gatos.

Raça(s) Predominante(s)
Nenhuma.

Idade Média e Faixa Etária
- Em geral, ocorre em cães e gatos mais idosos.
- Os animais mais jovens podem ser acometidos em caso de doença renal causada por infecção (p. ex., leptospirose) ou doença hereditária (p. ex., doença renal policística, displasia).

SINAIS E ACHADOS CLÍNICOS
- Oculares: cegueira aguda, hemorragia intraocular, pupilas dilatadas, descolamento exsudativo da retina, tortuosidade dos vasos retinianos, edema perivascular da retina, papiledema, degeneração da retina (sinal tardio).
- Neurológicos: depressão, inclinação da cabeça, crises convulsivas, nistagmo, paresia, ataxia, andar em círculo, desorientação.
- Renais: poliúria/polidipsia associada à evolução de doença renal crônica, hematúria, proteinúria.
- Cardíacos: sopro, ritmo de galope, raramente ICC.
- Epistaxe.

CAUSAS
Primária ou Essencial
- Desconhecidas; familiar em alguns cães.

Secundária
- Responde pela maioria dos casos em cães e gatos.
- Doença renal — doença renal em estágio terminal, glomerulonefrite, amiloidose.
- Hiperadrenocorticismo.
- Hipertireoidismo.
- Diabetes melito — menos comum.
- Feocromocitoma — condição mais rara.
- Hiperaldosteronismo — incomum.
- Doença do sistema nervoso central — causa rara.

DIAGNÓSTICO

DIAGNÓSTICO DIFERENCIAL
- Cardiovascular — miocardiopatia hipertrófica, cardiopatia tireotóxica, estenose aórtica, doença tromboembólica arterial.
- Oftálmico — traumatismo ocular, infecções sistêmicas (bacterianas, fúngicas, virais), coagulopatias, vasculopatia.
- Neurológico — doença primária do cérebro, da medula espinal ou de nervo periférico.

HEMOGRAMA/BIOQUÍMICA/URINÁLISE
- Hemograma completo: costuma permanecer normal; observam-se queda e aumento do hematócrito em casos de doença renal crônica grave e hiperadrenocorticismo, respectivamente.
- Perfil bioquímico: azotemia, hiperfosfatemia, hipocalemia (insuficiência renal); hiperglicemia (diabetes melito); fosfatase alcalina sérica elevada (hiperadrenocorticismo); aumento da ALT (hipertireoidismo); hipocalemia (hiperaldosteronismo).
- Urinálise: proteinúria (glomerulonefrite, amiloidose, hiperadrenocorticismo); hematúria; baixa capacidade de concentração urinária (insuficiência renal, hiperadrenocorticismo); glicosúria (diabetes melito).

OUTROS TESTES LABORATORIAIS
- Glomerulonefropatia — alta relação de proteína:creatinina urinárias, baixa depuração da creatinina.
- Disfunção renal — baixa depuração da creatinina.
- Hiperadrenocorticismo — resposta exagerada ao teste de estimulação com ACTH, falha na supressão com dexametasona, alta relação de cortisol:creatinina urinárias.
- Hipertireoidismo (gatos) — T_4 alto, supressão inadequada no teste de supressão com T_3.
- Hipotireoidismo (cães) — níveis baixos de T_3, T_4, T_3 livre, T_4 livre; possivelmente, nível elevado de autoanticorpos contra T_3 e T_4; TSH endógeno alto.
- Feocromocitoma — aumento de metabólitos urinários das catecolaminas.
- Hiperaldosteronismo — elevação dos níveis plasmáticos de aldosterona.

DIAGNÓSTICO POR IMAGEM
- Ecocardiografia para avaliar a presença de cardiopatia hipertensiva (os achados incluem hipertrofia da parede livre do ventrículo esquerdo e/ou do septo interventricular, disfunção diastólica ou estrutura e função normais).
- Radiografias torácicas para avaliar a existência de alterações cardíacas secundárias (tipicamente uma leve cardiomegalia sem ICC).
- Radiografias abdominais para avaliar o fígado, as adrenais e os rins.
- Ultrassonografia abdominal para avaliar os rins, o fígado, as adrenais e a bexiga urinária.
- TC ou RM se houver suspeita de tumor cerebral, hemorragia ou hiperadrenocorticismo.
- TC, RM ou mielograma para determinar a causa da paresia.
- Cintilografia da tireoide para avaliar hipertireoidismo.

MÉTODOS DIAGNÓSTICOS
O diagnóstico definitivo de hipertensão requer o registro de pressão arterial alta por métodos diretos ou indiretos.

Diretos (Invasivos)
Considerados como métodos com padrão de excelência, mas raramente realizados em um esquema ambulatorial nos animais alertas; procedimentos reservados para monitorização intraoperatória ou tratamento emergencial de hipertensão grave.

Indiretos (Não Invasivos)
- Quando efetuadas de forma correta, as mensurações indiretas da pressão arterial correlacionam-se bem com as mensurações diretas, além de serem facilmente realizadas no ambiente clínico. Medidas indiretas da pressão arterial costumam ser obtidas com técnicas oscilométricas ou Doppler, dependendo do porte do animal.
- Emprega-se um manguito inflável em torno da extremidade; a largura do manguito deve ser de aproximadamente 30-40% (gatos) ou 40% (cães) da circunferência do membro ou da cauda no local de aplicação. O manguito deve ser posicionado na altura do coração ou próximo a ele ao se mensurar a pressão arterial.
- Um manguito muito pequeno resultará em uma mensuração falsamente elevada da pressão arterial, enquanto um manguito muito grande resultará em uma medição falsamente baixa.
- Deve ser obtida uma média de 5 a 7 mensurações da pressão arterial; descartar a primeira medida.
- Um registro permanente de mensuração da pressão arterial deve incluir a técnica utilizada, o tamanho do manguito, o membro usado, a hora

do dia, o horário da medicação, a disposição do animal e o nome do operador.
• Técnicas constantes produzem resultados mais confiáveis. Interpretar os resultados levando em conta o nível de agitação do animal durante o procedimento e repetir se os resultados forem questionáveis.

Técnica Oscilométrica
• A técnica oscilométrica (Cardell, Memoprint, PetMap) detecta oscilações na pressão do pulso abaixo do manguito, resultantes de alterações no diâmetro arterial.
• Colocar o animal em decúbito lateral ou esternal e deixá-lo em ambiente calmo. Posicionar o marcador arterial (seta) do manguito na face palmar da região do metacarpo (ou proximal ao carpo com a seta apontada no sentido medial), sobre a região craniomedial do metatarso (ou proximal ao tarso) ou na face ventral da cauda em uma posição cômoda e justa. O aparelho pode insuflar o manguito automaticamente com exibição da pressão arterial (sistólica, diastólica e média) e da frequência cardíaca.
• A técnica oscilométrica não é tão confiável quanto o método Doppler para animais com frequências cardíacas rápidas, artérias muito pequenas ou tremores musculares.

Técnica Doppler
• Fluxômetros por Doppler (Parks, Vet-Dop, Jorgensen) detectam o fluxo sanguíneo como uma alteração na frequência do som refletido (desvio do Doppler) em virtude do movimento das hemácias subjacentes. Para as mensurações obtidas do membro torácico, um manguito pneumático é confortavelmente envolto em torno do antebraço acima do carpo. Um manômetro aneroide conecta-se ao manguito oclusivo. O transdutor Doppler é colocado sobre a artéria mediana na face ventral da pata dianteira, entre os coxins do metacarpo e do carpo (distalmente ao manguito). O pelo entre os coxins deve ser umedecido para remover as bolsas de ar antes de aplicar o transdutor com gel. Não há necessidade de se fazer tricotomia da região.
• Depois de insuflar o manguito em 30-40 mmHg a mais do que a pressão sistólica esperada, o manguito é desinsuflado em aproximadamente 3-4 mmHg/segundo. Um sinal audível do fluxo sanguíneo é ouvido pelo operador, indicando a pressão arterial sistólica.
• A principal limitação da técnica Doppler é a discriminação imprecisa dos sons que designam a pressão diastólica e, portanto, média.
• A técnica Doppler é o método preferido de mensuração da pressão arterial em gatos.

Categorias de Pressão Arterial e Diretrizes Terapêuticas para Cães e Gatos
• Para diminuir o risco de dano a órgãos-alvo, a pressão arterial deve ser idealmente reduzida para uma pressão arterial sistólica <140 mmHg e uma pressão diastólica <90 mmHg. Isso pode não ser uma tarefa fácil em muitos pacientes com doença refratária; por essa razão, a ACVIM tem classificado as faixas de pressão arterial com base na probabilidade de dano a órgãos-alvo.
• A presença de dano a órgãos-alvo, independentemente da pressão arterial, dita o tratamento. Se não houver dano a órgãos-alvo, deve-se repetir uma mensuração variável ou questionável da pressão arterial.
• Hipertensão em estágio I ou leve é definida como uma pressão arterial sistólica entre 140 e 159 mmHg e uma pressão arterial diastólica entre 90 e 99. Uma pressão arterial nessa faixa representa um risco mínimo de dano a órgãos-alvo e, nesse caso, o tratamento não é recomendado.
• Hipertensão em estágio II ou moderada é definida como uma pressão arterial sistólica entre 160 e 179 mmHg e uma pressão arterial diastólica entre 100 e 109.
• Hipertensão em estágio III ou grave é definida como uma pressão arterial sistólica ≥180 mmHg e uma pressão arterial diastólica ≥110 mmHg. O tratamento é recomendado para os pacientes tanto em estágio II como em estágio III para limitar o dano a órgãos-alvo.

ACHADOS PATOLÓGICOS
• Hipertrofia das arteríolas, hiperplasia da túnica média dos vasos e destruição da camada interna da lâmina elástica; o dano vascular nos olhos e nos rins, bem como nos tecidos do sistema cardiovascular e nervoso, acarreta hemorragia, trombose, edema e necrose.
• Desenvolve-se hipertrofia ventricular em resposta ao aumento da sobrecarga.

TRATAMENTO
CUIDADO(S) DE SAÚDE ADEQUADO(S)
Em geral, o tratamento é feito em um esquema ambulatorial. Talvez haja necessidade de cuidados hospitalares, dependendo da condição subjacente (p. ex., fluidoterapia em casos de insuficiência renal) ou complicações graves relacionadas com a hipertensão (p. ex., sinais neurológicos ou hemorragia retiniana aguda).

DIETA
• Influenciada pela causa subjacente; a restrição de sódio é controversa, pois ela ativará o eixo renina-angiotensina-aldosterona. É improvável que só a restrição de sódio reduza a pressão arterial.
• Evitar o alto consumo de sal.

ORIENTAÇÃO AO PROPRIETÁRIO
• A menos que a causa subjacente seja passível de cura (p. ex., hipertireoidismo) ou de controle (p. ex., hiperadrenocorticismo), é provável que o paciente tenha de tomar medicação anti-hipertensiva pelo resto da vida.
• Alertar os proprietários a respeito do dano a órgãos-alvos decorrente de hipertensão não controlada (p. ex., hemorragia da retina, descolamento da retina, comprometimento renal progressivo, cardiopatia e sinais neurológicos).

CONSIDERAÇÕES CIRÚRGICAS
Podem ser indicadas em casos de hipertireoidismo, feocromocitoma, hiperaldosteronismo e algumas formas de hiperadrenocorticismo.

MEDICAÇÕES
MEDICAMENTO(S) DE ESCOLHA
Terapia de Escolha
• Tratar a causa subjacente se possível.
• Gatos — anlodipino constitui o medicamento oral de primeira linha, com adição de algum inibidor da ECA na presença de proteinúria.
• Cães — inibidor da ECA (p. ex., enalapril, benazepril) representa o agente terapêutico de primeira linha (em função da frequência de proteinúria subjacente), com adição de anlodipino como o segundo medicamento, se houver necessidade.
• Espironolactona e hidralazina podem ser adicionados ao esquema anti-hipertensivo se os inibidores da ECA e o anlodipino forem ineficazes em reduzir a pressão arterial para <160 mmHg.
• Em uma emergência hipertensiva, pode-se lançar mão da administração parenteral de hidralazina, nitroprusseto de sódio ou labetolol. Há necessidade da monitorização direta contínua da pressão arterial.

Bloqueadores dos Canais de Cálcio Di-hidropiridínicos
• Diminuem a resistência vascular periférica por meio de vasodilatação.
• Anlodipino — cães, 0,1-0,5 mg/kg VO a cada 24 h; gatos, 0,625-1,25 mg/gato VO a cada 24 h.

Inibidores da ECA
• Diminuem a resistência vascular periférica e o volume sistólico ao bloquearem a conversão de angiotensina I em angiotensina II; promovem renoproteção; reduzem a remodelagem vascular.
• Enalapril — cães, 0,5 mg/kg VO a cada 12 h; gatos, 0,25-0,5 mg/kg VO a cada 12 h.
• Benazepril — cães e gatos, 0,5 mg/kg VO a cada 12 h.

Vasodilatadores de Ação Direta
• Diminuem a resistência vascular periférica.
• Hidralazina — cães e gatos, 0,25-0,5 mg/kg VO a cada 12 h, com aumento gradual para 3 mg/kg VO a cada 12 h se necessário.

Antagonistas dos Receptores Alfa
• Utilizados mais comumente com antagonistas dos receptores beta em casos de feocromocitoma.
• Fenoxibenzamina — cães, 0,25 mg/kg VO a cada 12 h; gatos, 2,5 mg/gato VO a cada 12 h.

Diuréticos
• Espironolactona — cães e gatos, 1-2 mg/kg VO a cada 12 h; utilizada principalmente em virtude dos efeitos antialdosterona para limitar o processo de fibrose; diurético fraco.
• Furosemida — cães, 2-4 mg/kg VO a cada 12 h; gatos, 1-2 mg/kg VO a cada 12 h; não é usada com rotina em terapia anti-hipertensiva.

Antagonistas dos Receptores Beta
• Diminuem a frequência cardíaca e o débito cardíaco, além de suprimirem a secreção de renina.
• Bloqueiam os efeitos exercidos pelo excesso dos hormônios tireoidianos, embora haja necessidade de outros medicamentos para controlar a pressão arterial.
• Raramente utilizados em cães a menos que haja feocromocitoma.
• Propranolol — cães, 0,2-1 mg/kg VO a cada 8 h; gatos, 2,5-5 mg/gato VO a cada 8-12 h.
• Atenolol — cães, 0,25-1 mg/kg VO a cada 12-24 h; gatos, 6,25-12,5 mg/gato VO a cada 12-24 h.

CONTRAINDICAÇÕES
Reduzir ou suspender o uso de esteroides e vasoconstritores.

PRECAUÇÕES
• Os vasodilatadores arteriais podem provocar taquicardia reflexa; os medicamentos de ação rápida aumentam o risco de hipotensão e insuficiência renal aguda.
• Os β-bloqueadores podem agravar os quadros de doença bronquiolar, ICC e distúrbios de condução (p. ex., bloqueio AV de segundo e terceiro graus).

Hipertensão Sistêmica

INTERAÇÕES POSSÍVEIS
- As combinações de medicamentos aumentam o risco de hipotensão.
- O emprego de inibidores da ECA e espironolactona pode resultar em hipercalemia, especialmente com doença renal subjacente.

MEDICAMENTO(S) ALTERNATIVO(S)
Em uma emergência hipertensiva, pode-se usar hidralazina (0,2 mg/kg SC ou IM), nitroprusseto de sódio (1-5 µg/kg/min até 10 µg/kg/min em velocidade de infusão constante) ou labetolol (0,25 µg/kg a cada 10 min; 20-30 µg/kg/min em velocidade de infusão constante). É necessária a monitorização direta contínua da pressão arterial.

ACOMPANHAMENTO

MONITORIZAÇÃO DO PACIENTE
- Mensurações da pressão arterial <140/90 constituem o objetivo do tratamento, embora a pressão arterial sistólica <160 mmHg seja razoável e minimizará o risco de dano a órgãos-alvo.
- A pressão arterial e as complicações hipertensivas (sobretudo retinopatia) devem ser checadas semanalmente até o controle da pressão arterial.
- Exames laboratoriais para medir os efeitos colaterais de medicações e a resposta da doença clínica (p. ex., proteinúria, hematúria, anemia, trombocitopenia, equilíbrio do sódio e potássio, azotemia e albumina).

COMPLICAÇÕES POSSÍVEIS
- ICC.
- Glomerulonefropatia (proteinúria, hematúria).
- Insuficiência renal.
- Retinopatia (hemorragia, descolamento da retina).
- Acidente vascular cerebral (vários sinais do sistema nervoso central).

EVOLUÇÃO ESPERADA E PROGNÓSTICO
- Ditados pela causa subjacente da hipertensão.
- A pressão arterial pode ser controlada com terapia adequada/combinada em grande parte dos pacientes, mas a terapia anti-hipertensiva não melhora necessariamente o tempo de sobrevida.

DIVERSOS

FATORES RELACIONADOS COM A IDADE
Doença renal crônica, hipertireoidismo e hiperadrenocorticismo — mais comum em animais mais idosos.

SINÔNIMO(S)
- Pressão arterial elevada.
- Hipertensão arterial sistêmica.

VER TAMBÉM
- Diabetes Melito sem Complicação — Cães.
- Diabetes Melito sem Complicação — Gatos.
- Feocromocitoma.
- Glomerulonefrite.
- Hiperadrenocorticismo (Síndrome de Cushing) — Gatos.
- Hiperadrenocorticismo (Síndrome de Cushing) — Cães.
- Hipertireoidismo.
- Insuficiência Renal Aguda.
- Insuficiência Renal Crônica.

ABREVIATURA(S)
- ACVIM = American College of Veterinary Internal Medicine.
- ACTH = hormônio adrenocorticotrópico.
- AV = atrioventricular.
- ALT = alanina aminotransferase.
- ECA = enzima conversora da angiotensina.
- ICC = insuficiência cardíaca congestiva.
- RM = ressonância magnética.
- TC = tomografia computadorizada.
- T_3 = tri-iodotironina.
- T_4 = tiroxina.
- TSH = hormônio tireostimulante.

RECURSOS DA INTERNET
http://www.vin.com/proceedings/Proceedings.plx?CID=WALTHAMOSU2002&PID=2989http://www3.interscience.wiley.com/cgi-bin/fulltext/120715479/PDFSTART?CRETRY=1&SRETRY=0.

Sugestões de Leitura
Brown S, Atkins C, Bagley R, Carr A, et al. ACVIM consensus statement: Guidelines for the identification, evaluation, and management of systemic hypertension in dogs and cats. J Vet Intern Med 2007, 21:542-558.
Henik RA, Brown SA. Systemic hypertension. In: Tilley LP, Smith FWK, Oyama MA, Sleeper MM, eds., Manual of Canine and Feline Cardiology, 4th ed. St. Louis: Saunders Elsevier, 2008, pp. 277-286.

Autor Rosie Henik
Consultores Editoriais Larry P. Tilley e Francis W.K. Smith, Jr.

HIPERTIREOIDISMO

CONSIDERAÇÕES GERAIS

DEFINIÇÃO
Metabolismo geral patológico, contínuo e acentuado, causado por altas concentrações circulantes de hormônios tireoidianos.

FISIOPATOLOGIA
• Em gatos, é causado mais frequentemente por nódulos hiperfuncionais autônomos da glândula tireoide que secretam T_4 e T_3, sem o controle de influências fisiológicas (p. ex., secreção de TSH); um ou ambos os lobos da tireoide podem ser acometidos.
• Casos raros de hipertireoidismo felino (1-2%) são causados por carcinoma hiperfuncional da tireoide.
• Extremamente incomum em cães, foi observado em alguns com carcinoma da tireoide (a maioria dos cães com neoplasia da tireoide é eutireóidea) e naqueles que recebem suplementação excessiva de hormônio tireoidiano exógeno.

SISTEMA(S) ACOMETIDO(S)
• Comportamental.
• Cardiovascular — hipertrofia do miocárdio e hipertensão.
• Gastrintestinal — desnutrição celular crônica, tempo de trânsito gastrintestinal diminuído, má absorção e dano hepatocelular.
• Musculoesquelético — caquexia.
• Nervoso.
• Renal/urológico — TFG alta pode mascarar insuficiência renal crônica subjacente, possível lesão por hiperfiltração e baixa capacidade de concentrar a urina.

GENÉTICA
Não há predisposição genética conhecida.

INCIDÊNCIA/PREVALÊNCIA
• Endocrinopatia mais comum em gatos; uma das doenças mais comuns em gatos no final da meia-idade e idosos; a incidência verdadeira é desconhecida, mas o diagnóstico da doença está aumentando.
• Raro em cães.

IDENTIFICAÇÃO

Espécies
Gatos e (raramente) cães.

Idade Média e Faixa Etária
A idade média em gatos é de aproximadamente 13 anos; variação de 4-22 anos. Incomum em gatos com menos de 6 anos de idade.

SINAIS CLÍNICOS

Comentários Gerais
• Polissistêmicos; refletem o aumento global no metabolismo.
• Menos de 10% dos pacientes são mencionados como "apáticos"; tais pacientes exibem sinais atípicos (p. ex., apetite deficiente, anorexia, depressão e fraqueza).

Achados Anamnésicos
• Perda de peso.
• Polifagia.
• Vômitos.
• Diarreia.
• Polidipsia.
• Taquipneia.
• Hiperatividade.
• Dispneia.
• Agressividade.

Achados do Exame Físico
• Aumento de volume da tireoide — 70% dos pacientes apresentam acometimento bilateral.
• Má condição corporal.
• Sopro cardíaco.
• Taquicardia.
• Ritmo de galope.
• Aspecto desleixado.
• Unhas engrossadas.

CAUSAS
• Gatos — nódulos hiperfuncionais autônomos; raramente, carcinoma da tireoide.
• Cães — secreção de T_4 ou T_3 por algum carcinoma da tireoide ou iatrogênica pela suplementação excessiva de tiroxina.

FATORES DE RISCO
• Alguns relatos relacionaram o hipertireoidismo felino com algumas rações enlatadas.
• Estudos recentes implicaram toxinas de disfunção endócrina (p. ex., PBDE) como possíveis causas de hipertireoidismo felino, mas não há provas disso.
• A idade avançada aumenta o risco.

DIAGNÓSTICO

DIAGNÓSTICO DIFERENCIAL
Os sinais clínicos de hipertireoidismo felino podem se sobrepor àqueles de insuficiência renal crônica, hepatopatia crônica e neoplasia (especialmente linfoma intestinal); eles podem ser excluídos com base nos achados laboratoriais de rotina e nas provas de função da tireoide.

HEMOGRAMA/BIOQUÍMICA/URINÁLISE
• Eritrocitose (leve) e, menos comumente, leucocitose, linfopenia e eosinopenia — resposta ao estresse associada a altos níveis de T_3 e T_4.
• Atividade elevada da ALT — comum.
• Elevação de fosfatase alcalina, LDH, AST, ureia, creatinina, glicose, fósforo e bilirrubina — menos comum; causada por complicações mais graves do hipertireoidismo.

OUTROS TESTES LABORATORIAIS
• Concentrações séricas de T_4 total — mede a T_4 ligada à proteína e a forma livre (não ligada); a alta concentração em repouso confirma o diagnóstico de hipertireoidismo.
• Concentração sérica de T_3 total — a concentração elevada é menos confiável que a T_4 total sérica.
• T_4 livre por diálise de equilíbrio — útil para diagnosticar hipertireoidismo leve ou precoce em gatos, que podem ter concentrações séricas em repouso normais de T_4 total.
• Na teoria, a T_4 livre reflete com maior precisão o verdadeiro estado secretor da tireoide, mas alguns gatos com doença não relacionada com a tireoide exibem elevações inexplicáveis de T_4 livre; portanto, não se deve usar apenas a T_4 livre como teste de triagem de primeira linha.
• Teste de supressão com T_3 — útil para diagnosticar hipertireoidismo leve (ver protocolo e interpretação no Apêndice II).
• Teste de estimulação com TRH — proveitoso para diagnosticar hipertireoidismo leve (ver protocolo e interpretação no Apêndice II).

DIAGNÓSTICO POR IMAGEM
• A radiografia torácica e a ecocardiografia podem ser úteis para avaliar a gravidade da miocardiopatia.
• Cães — obter radiografias torácicas para detectar metástase pulmonar.
• Gatos — o ultrassom abdominal pode ser útil para explorar doença renal subjacente.
• Cintilografia da tireoide pode ser usada para diagnosticar hipertireoidismo e determinar a localização de tecido tireóideo anormal.

MÉTODOS DIAGNÓSTICOS
• O tratamento do hipertireoidismo pode diminuir significativamente a função renal; procurar qualquer valor anormal revelado pelo hemograma completo, pelo perfil bioquímico sérico ou pela urinálise por meio de cultura bacteriana da urina, além de radiografia e ultrassonografia abdominais do trato urinário.
• Pode-se medir a TFG pelo desaparecimento de io-hexol do plasma ou radiofármacos apropriados (se disponíveis) em gatos com suspeita de doença renal subjacente. Ao contrário de alguns relatos, a urina concentrada (densidade >1,035) não diminui o risco de insuficiência renal pós-tratamento.
• A mensuração não invasiva da pressão arterial pode ser útil na avaliação completa antes do tratamento e na monitorização da terapia.

ACHADOS PATOLÓGICOS
• Hiperplasia adenomatosa de um ou ambos os lobos da tireoide.
• Carcinoma em cães e 1-2% dos gatos.

TRATAMENTO

CUIDADO(S) DE SAÚDE ADEQUADO(S)
• O tratamento ambulatorial, em geral, é suficiente para gatos caso se faça uso de medicações antitireóideas.
• O tratamento com iodo radioativo e a tireoidectomia cirúrgica necessitam de hospitalização e monitoramento.
• Casos raros de insuficiência cardíaca congestiva franca requerem cuidados intensivos de emergência em hospital.

ATIVIDADE
Não é recomendável qualquer modificação.

DIETA
• A resolução da tireotoxicose dispensa a necessidade de modificações.
• A má absorção de muitos nutrientes e o metabolismo aumentado sugerem a necessidade de dieta altamente digerível com boa biodisponibilidade de proteína no hipertireoidismo não submetido a tratamento.

ORIENTAÇÃO AO PROPRIETÁRIO
• Informar os proprietários sobre os efeitos adversos das medicações antitireóideas (ver adiante) e as complicações cirúrgicas.
• Os proprietários devem estar cientes da possibilidade de recidiva (rara) após o tratamento.

CONSIDERAÇÕES CIRÚRGICAS
• A tireoidectomia cirúrgica é um tratamento recomendado para o hipertireoidismo em gatos.
• O tratamento cirúrgico do carcinoma da tireoide (cães e gatos), em geral, não leva à cura, mas pode ser paliativo.

HIPERTIREOIDISMO

MEDICAÇÕES

MEDICAMENTO(S) DE ESCOLHA
• A terapia com iodo radioativo é indiscutivelmente o tratamento mais seguro e mais eficaz. A disponibilidade de estabelecimentos veterinários que oferecem esse tipo de tratamento é limitada, mas está crescendo.
• O metimazol (Tapazole®) é o medicamento recomendado com maior frequência (5-15 mg/dia fracionados a cada 8-12 h).
• A aplicação do metimazol pode ser por via transdérmica (formulado por meio de farmácias de manipulação em gel PLO [sigla em inglês para Organogel Lecitina Plurônica]). A resolução da tireotoxicose leva mais tempo com o metimazol transdérmico do que com aquele administrado por via oral.
• Bloqueadores β-adrenérgicos — ocasionalmente utilizados para tratar alguns dos efeitos cardiovasculares e neurológicos do excesso de hormônio tireoidiano; podem ser usados em combinação com o metimazol; usados principalmente no preparo do paciente para a tireoidectomia cirúrgica ou a terapia com iodo radioativo. O atenolol é útil para o controle de taquicardia, embora seja necessária a adição de algum inibidor da ECA para controlar a hipertensão em gatos com hipertireoidismo.

PRECAUÇÕES
• Os medicamentos antitireóideos têm vários efeitos colaterais.
• Anorexia e vômitos são efeitos colaterais comuns do metimazol; os efeitos colaterais raros incluem escoriação autoinduzida da face, trombocitopenia, diátese hemorrágica, agranulocitose, anticorpos antinucleares séricos e hepatopatia.
• Os efeitos colaterais geralmente se desenvolvem nos três primeiros meses de tratamento e podem ou não exigir a interrupção do medicamento e o uso de terapia alternativa (dependendo da gravidade).
• Efeitos como sangramento, icterícia e agranulocitose requerem a suspensão imediata do medicamento.
• Com a exceção dos vômitos, também podem ocorrer efeitos colaterais com o metimazol transdérmico.

MEDICAMENTO(S) ALTERNATIVO(S)
• Carbimazol — outro antitireóideo útil; não está disponível nos EUA.
• Propiltiouracila — pode ser útil se o metimazol não estiver disponível; os efeitos adversos podem ser mais comuns e mais graves que os do metimazol.
• Ipodato — um agente de contraste radiográfico; pode ser usado na dose de 15 mg/kg VO a cada 12 h para tratar alguns casos de hipertireoidismo leve, mas não é eficaz em grande parte dos pacientes hipertireóideos; não foi estabelecida a eficácia a longo prazo.

ACOMPANHAMENTO

MONITORIZAÇÃO DO PACIENTE
• Metimazol — exame físico, hemograma completo (com contagem de plaquetas), perfil bioquímico sérico e determinação da T_4 sérica a cada 2-3 semanas nos três primeiros meses de tratamento; ajustar a dosagem para manter a concentração sérica de T_4 nos parâmetros normais a baixos.
• Tireoidectomia cirúrgica — ficar atento para o desenvolvimento de hipocalcemia e/ou paralisia laríngea durante o período pós-operatório inicial; medir as concentrações séricas de T_4 na primeira semana da cirurgia e depois a cada 3-6 meses para verificar a ocorrência de recidiva.
• Iodo radioativo — medir as concentrações séricas de T_4 2 semanas após o tratamento e subsequentemente a cada 3-6 meses.
• Função renal — a TFG declina após o tratamento na maioria dos pacientes; portanto, é preciso realizar o exame físico, a bioquímica sérica e a urinálise 1 mês depois do tratamento e, em seguida, conforme indicado pelo histórico clínico.

COMPLICAÇÕES POSSÍVEIS
• A doença não tratada pode ocasionar insuficiência cardíaca congestiva, diarreia intratável, dano renal, descolamento da retina (como resultado de hipertensão) e morte.
• As complicações do tratamento cirúrgico incluem hipoparatireoidismo, hipotireoidismo e paralisia laríngea.
• O surgimento de hipotireoidismo é raro após a terapia com iodo radioativo.

EVOLUÇÃO ESPERADA E PROGNÓSTICO
• Doença sem complicações — prognóstico excelente; a recidiva é possível e mais comumente associada à negligência do proprietário com relação ao tratamento clínico; o novo crescimento de tecido hipertireóideo é possível, mas incomum após tireoidectomia cirúrgica ou tratamento com iodo radioativo.
• O tempo médio de sobrevida relatado em gatos submetidos a tratamento com iodo radioativo é de 4 anos; o tempo médio de sobrevida com metimazol é de 2 anos; o tempo médio de sobrevida de gatos tratados com iodo radioativo e metimazol é de 5,3 anos.
• Gatos com doença renal preexistente apresentam um prognóstico pior. A insuficiência renal é a causa mais comum de morte em gatos hipertireóideos.
• Cães ou gatos com carcinoma da tireoide — prognóstico mau; o tratamento com iodo radioativo, cirúrgico ou ambos, em geral, é acompanhado por recidiva da doença; a quimioterapia adjuvante é de benefício questionável.

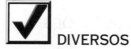

DIVERSOS

DISTÚRBIOS ASSOCIADOS
• Em gatos com doença renal subjacente (secundária à hipertensão crônica ou sem relação com doença da tireoide), o prognóstico é menos favorável.
• Insuficiência renal pode não se tornar evidente até que o eutireoidismo se estabeleça; por essa razão, uma forma reversível de tratamento (i. e., medicamentos antitireóideos) será recomendada se houver suspeita de doença renal em gato com hipertireoidismo. Estudos recentes revelam que o declínio pós-tratamento mais significativo na TFG ocorre durante o primeiro mês depois do tratamento e, por esse motivo, um período de 30 dias deve ser suficiente para a realização de uma tentativa com medicamentos antitireóideos antes do uso de um tratamento mais permanente para hipertireoidismo.
• Em alguns pacientes, pode ser melhor deixar o hipertireoidismo sem tratamento.

SINÔNIMO(S)
• Tireotoxicose.
• Bócio tóxico multinodular.
• Doença de Plummer.

VER TAMBÉM
• Hipertensão Sistêmica.
• Hipoparatireoidismo.
• Insuficiência Cardíaca Congestiva Esquerda.
• Miocardiopatia Hipertrófica — Gatos.

ABREVIATURA(S)
• AST = aspartato aminotransferase.
• ALT = alanina aminotransferase.
• ECA = enzima conversora de angiotensina.
• LDH = desidrogenase láctica (lactato desidrogenase).
• T_3 = tri-iodotironina.
• T_4 = tiroxina.
• TFG = taxa de filtração glomerular.
• TRH = hormônio liberador de tireotropina.
• TSH = hormônio tireostimulante.

Sugestões de Leitura
Graves TK. Hyperthyroidism and the kidneys. In: August JR, ed. Consultations in Feline Internal Medicine. Philadelphia: Saunders, 1997.
Henik RA, Stepien RL, Wenholz LJ, Dolson MK. Efficacy of atenolol as a single antihypertensive agent in hyperthyroid cats. J Feline Med Surg 2008, 10(6):577-582.
Milner RJ, Channell CD, Levy JK, Schaer M. Survival times for cats with hyperthyroidism treated with iodine 131, methimazole, or both: 167 cases (1996-2003). JAVMA 2006, 228(4):559-563.
Trepanier LA. Medical management of hyperthyroidism. Clin Tech Small Anim Pract 2006, 21(1):22-28.

Autor Thomas K. Graves
Consultor Editorial Deborah S. Greco

HIPOADRENOCORTICISMO (DOENÇA DE ADDISON)

CONSIDERAÇÕES GERAIS

DEFINIÇÃO
- Distúrbio endócrino que resulta da produção deficiente de glicocorticoides e/ou mineralocorticoides.
- A doença de Addison refere-se a uma deficiência tanto de glicocorticoides como de mineralocorticoides.

FISIOPATOLOGIA
- A deficiência de mineralocorticoides (aldosterona) resulta na incapacidade de excretar potássio e reter sódio; a deficiência de sódio acarreta diminuição do volume circulante efetivo que, por sua vez, contribui para azotemia pré-renal, hipotensão, desidratação, fraqueza e depressão.
- A hipercalemia (juntamente com outros desarranjos metabólicos) pode resultar em toxicidade miocárdica.
- A deficiência de glicocorticoide (cortisol) contribui para os sinais de anorexia, vômitos, melena, letargia e perda de peso; predispõe o animal à hipoglicemia e resulta em comprometimento na excreção de água.

SISTEMA(S) ACOMETIDO(S)
- Cardiovascular.
- Gastrintestinal.
- Musculosquelético.
- Renal/Urológico.
- Cutâneo.

GENÉTICA
Foi determinada uma base genética em cães das raças Poodle standard, Bearded collie e Leonberger.

INCIDÊNCIA/PREVALÊNCIA
Não se dispõe de números exatos; considerado incomum a raro em cães e muito raro em gatos.

DISTRIBUIÇÃO GEOGRÁFICA
N/D.

IDENTIFICAÇÃO
Espécies
Cães e gatos.

Raça(s) Predominante(s)
- Dinamarquês, Rottweiler, Cão d'água português, Poodle standard, Bearded collie, Leonberger, West Highland white terrier e Wheaten terrier apresentam risco relativo elevado.
- Sem predominância em gatos.

Idade Média e Faixa Etária
- Cães — variação, <1 a >12 anos de idade; média, 4 anos.
- Gatos — variação, 1-9 anos; a maioria é de meia-idade.

Sexo Predominante
As cadelas estão sob maior risco relativo; não há predileção em gatos.

SINAIS CLÍNICOS
Comentários Gerais
Os sinais variam de leves e raros em alguns pacientes com hipoadrenocorticismo crônico a graves e potencialmente letais em uma crise addisoniana aguda. Múltiplos sistemas orgânicos podem ser envolvidos; o tipo e a extensão de acometimento variam de caso a caso.

Achados Anamnésicos
- Cães — letargia, anorexia, vômitos, perda de peso, exacerbação/remissão, diarreia, resposta prévia à terapia, tremores, PU/PD.
- Gatos — letargia, anorexia, vômitos, PU/PD, perda de peso.

Achados do Exame Físico
- Cães — depressão, fraqueza, desidratação, colapso, hipotermia, tempo de preenchimento capilar lento, melena, pulso fraco, bradicardia, abdome doloroso, perda de pelos.
- Gatos — desidratação, fraqueza, tempo de preenchimento capilar lento, pulso fraco, bradicardia.

CAUSAS
- Hipoadrenocorticismo primário — idiopáticas (imunomediadas), dosagem excessiva de mitotano e/ou trilostano, doença granulomatosa, tumores metastáticos, doença fúngica, coagulopatia.
- Hipoadrenocorticismo secundário — iatrogênicas após suspensão da administração prolongada de glicocorticoides, deficiência isolada de ACTH, pan-hipopituitarismo, tumor hipofisário não funcional.

FATORES DE RISCO
N/D.

DIAGNÓSTICO

DIAGNÓSTICO DIFERENCIAL
- Os sinais são inespecíficos e observados em outros distúrbios clínicos mais comuns, em particular doenças gastrintestinais e renais.
- Embora não haja sinais patognomônicos, uma evolução inconstante (com exacerbação e remissão) e uma resposta prévia à intervenção clínica inespecífica ("fluidos e esteroides") devem alertar o clínico a considerar o diagnóstico.

HEMOGRAMA/BIOQUÍMICA/URINÁLISE
- As anormalidades hematológicas podem incluir anemia, eosinofilia e linfocitose.
- Os achados bioquímicos séricos podem incluir hipercalemia, azotemia, hiponatremia, hipocloremia, CO_2 total diminuído, hipercalcemia, aumento das enzimas hepáticas, elevação da fosfatase alcalina sérica e hipoglicemia.
- A urinálise, em geral, revela comprometimento na capacidade de concentração urinária.
- Alguns pacientes com hipoadrenocorticismo exibem níveis normais de eletrólitos (hipoadrenocorticismo atípico).

OUTROS TESTES LABORATORIAIS
- O diagnóstico definitivo é feito pela demonstração de concentrações séricas basais não detectáveis a baixas de cortisol, que não aumentam 1 h depois da administração IV de ACTH sintético (5 µg/kg em cães, 0,125 mg em gatos). Alternativamente, o ACTH em forma de gel pode ser aplicado por via IM (2 U/kg em cães, 10 U em gatos), com a coleta da amostra de cortisol sérico feita dentro de 2 h após a administração do ACTH.
- Em animais desidratados hipovolêmicos, usar o ACTH sintético por via IV ou adiar o teste até depois da administração inicial de fluidos ter sido concluída.
- Determinar a concentração plasmática de ACTH em pacientes com níveis normais de eletrólitos para diferenciar hipoadrenocorticismo primário do secundário; é preciso coletar a amostra antes de administrar os glicocorticoides.

DIAGNÓSTICO POR IMAGEM
- As radiografias podem revelar microcardia, estreitamento da veia cava ou da aorta descendente, campos pulmonares hipoperfundidos, micro-hepatia com menor frequência e, muito raramente, megaesôfago.
- A ultrassonografia abdominal pode revelar glândulas adrenais pequenas.

MÉTODOS DIAGNÓSTICOS
N/D.

ACHADOS PATOLÓGICOS
- Exame macroscópico — atrofia das adrenais.
- Microscópicos — adrenalite linfocítica-plasmocitária e/ou atrofia adrenocortical.

TRATAMENTO

CUIDADO(S) DE SAÚDE ADEQUADO(S)
- Uma crise addisoniana aguda é uma emergência médica que requer terapia intensiva.
- O tratamento do hipoadrenocorticismo crônico depende da gravidade dos sinais clínicos; geralmente, a estabilização e a terapia iniciais são conduzidas em um esquema ambulatorial.

CUIDADO(S) DE ENFERMAGEM
- Tratar a crise addisoniana aguda com correção rápida da hipovolemia, utilizando fluidos isotônicos (de preferência, NaCl a 0,9%).
- Monitorizar a pressão arterial e o débito urinário, bem como a frequência e o ritmo cardíacos.

ATIVIDADE
Evitar estresse e esforço desnecessários durante uma crise addisoniana.

DIETA
Sem necessidade de alteração.

ORIENTAÇÃO AO PROPRIETÁRIO
- É necessária a terapia de reposição com glicocorticoide e/ou mineralocorticoide pelo resto da vida.
- São necessárias doses maiores de glicocorticoide (acima das necessidades de manutenção) durante períodos de estresse como viagens, internações e cirurgias.

CONSIDERAÇÕES CIRÚRGICAS
N/D.

MEDICAÇÕES

MEDICAMENTO(S) DE ESCOLHA
- Hipoadrenocorticismo primário crônico — a maioria dos pacientes necessitará da reposição diária de glicocorticoide (prednisona, 0,2 mg/kg/dia), bem como da reposição de mineralocorticoide (pivalato de desoxicorticosterona, 2 mg/kg IM ou SC a cada 21-30 dias, ajustados, conforme a necessidade, com base nas determinações dos eletrólitos séricos). Alternativamente, pode-se utilizar uma reposição de mineralocorticoide por via oral (acetato de fludrocortisona, 10-20 µg/kg/dia divididos, ajustados em incrementos de 0,05 a 0,1 mg com base nas determinações seriadas de eletrólitos séricos).

HIPOADRENOCORTICISMO (DOENÇA DE ADDISON)

- Em uma crise addisoniana, fica indicada a administração parenteral de algum glicocorticoide de ação rápida como fosfato sódico de dexametasona ou succinato sódico de prednisolona; o fosfato sódico de dexametasona é preferível, porque a prednisolona sofre reação cruzada com os ensaios de cortisol. O fosfato sódico de dexametasona é administrado a uma dose de 2-4 mg/kg IV; essa dose pode ser repetida em 2-6 h, se necessário. A dose do glicocorticoide é gradativamente reduzida à medida que a condição melhora.
- Fluidoterapia com NaCl a 0,9%, conforme a necessidade, com base na hidratação, no estado volêmico e na pressão arterial do paciente. Em uma crise addisoniana, os fluidos são instituídos a uma velocidade de 60-80 mL/kg/h nas primeiras 1-2 h e, em seguida, reduzidos gradativamente com base no estado clínico do animal.
- Tratar a hipoglicemia, se presente, com glicose IV.
- Raramente, há necessidade de terapia com bicarbonato de sódio; fica reservado para os casos com acidose grave.
- Pacientes com hipoadrenocorticismo secundário confirmado só precisam da suplementação de glicocorticoide (prednisona, 0,2 mg/kg/dia).

CONTRAINDICAÇÕES
N/D.

PRECAUÇÕES
N/D.

INTERAÇÕES POSSÍVEIS
N/D.

MEDICAMENTO(S) ALTERNATIVO(S)
Ver "Hipercalemia" em busca do tratamento de emergência dos casos de hipercalemia grave.

ACOMPANHAMENTO

MONITORIZAÇÃO DO PACIENTE
- Após as 2 primeiras injeções de pivalato de desoxicorticosterona, o ideal é medir os níveis de eletrólitos séricos em 2, 3 e 4 semanas para determinar a duração do efeito; em seguida, verificar os níveis de eletrólitos no momento da injeção nos próximos 3-6 meses (e ajustar a dose do pivalato de desoxicorticosterona, se houver necessidade) e, depois, a cada 6 meses.
- O pivalato de desoxicorticosterona costuma ser necessário em intervalos mensais; alguns pacientes necessitam de injeções a cada 3 semanas, mas raros pacientes precisam de injeções a cada 2 semanas; alternativamente, para manter as injeções mensais, a dosagem do pivalato de desoxicorticosterona pode ser aumentada de forma gradual.
- A grande maioria dos cães com hipoadrenocorticismo será bem controlada com uma dose de manutenção do pivalato de desoxicorticosterona de 2 mg/kg/injeção todo mês. Se necessário, a dose do pivalato de desoxicorticosterona pode ser sequencialmente reduzida, com base nas determinações de eletrólitos séricos, pois alguns cães podem ser controlados com uma dosagem mensal abaixo de 2 mg/kg. Alternativamente, o intervalo entre as injeções pode ser aumentado ao mesmo tempo em que se monitorizam as concentrações de eletrólitos séricos.
- Ajustar a dose diária de fludrocortisona em incrementos de 0,05-0,1 mg, conforme a necessidade, com base nas determinações seriadas dos eletrólitos séricos; após o início da terapia, verificar os níveis séricos de eletrólitos semanalmente até que os valores se estabilizem na faixa normal; daí em diante, averiguar as concentrações de eletrólitos séricos, bem como a ureia ou a creatinina, mensalmente nos primeiros 3-6 meses e, depois, a cada 3-12 meses.
- Em muitos cães submetidos à fludrocortisona, a dose diária necessária para controlar o distúrbio é aumentada de forma gradativa, em geral nos primeiros 6-24 meses de tratamento; para a maioria dos cães, a dosagem final necessária da fludrocortisona é de 20-30 µg/kg/dia; a dose de 10 µg/kg/dia ou menos é capaz de controlar pouquíssimos cães.

PREVENÇÃO
- Continuar a terapia de reposição hormonal pelo resto da vida do paciente.
- Aumentar a dosagem de reposição do glicocorticoide durante períodos de estresse como viagens, internações e cirurgias.

COMPLICAÇÕES POSSÍVEIS
- Podem ocorrer os efeitos de PU/PD em virtude da administração de prednisona, exigindo a redução da dose ou a interrupção do medicamento.
- Também é possível a ocorrência de PU/PD após a administração de fludrocortisona, exigindo uma troca para a terapia com pivalato de desoxicorticosterona.

EVOLUÇÃO ESPERADA E PROGNÓSTICO
Exceto nos casos de pacientes com hipoadrenocorticismo primário causado por doença granulomatosa ou metastática e hipoadrenocorticismo secundário provocado por massa hipofisária, o prognóstico para a grande maioria de pacientes é bom a excelente após a estabilização e o tratamento adequados.

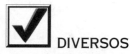

DIVERSOS

DISTÚRBIOS ASSOCIADOS
Ocorre insuficiência concomitante de glândula endócrina em até 5% dos cães —hipotireoidismo, diabetes melito e/ou hipoparatireoidismo.

FATORES RELACIONADOS COM A IDADE
N/D.

POTENCIAL ZOONÓTICO
Nenhum.

GESTAÇÃO/FERTILIDADE/REPRODUÇÃO
N/D.

SINÔNIMO(S)
Doença de Addison (hipoadrenocorticismo primário).

VER TAMBÉM
- Hipercalemia.
- Hiponatremia.

ABREVIATURA(S)
- ACTH = hormônio adrenocorticotrópico.
- PU/PD = poliúria e polidipsia.

Sugestões de Leitura
Greco DS, Peterson ME. Feline hypoadrenocorticism. In: Kirk RW, ed., Current Veterinary Therapy X. Philadelphia: Saunders, 1989, pp. 1042-1045.
Kintzer PP, Peterson, ME. Canine hypoadrenocorticism. In: Kirk RW, Bonagura JD, Twedt DC, eds., Current Veterinary Therapy XIV. Philadelphia: Saunders Elsevier, 2009, pp. 231-235.
Peterson ME, Kintzer PP, Kass PH. Pretreatment clinical and laboratory findings in dogs with hypoadrenocorticism: 225 cases (1979-1993). JAVMA 1996, 208:85-91.

Autor Peter P. Kintzer
Consultor Editorial Deborah S. Greco

HIPOALBUMINEMIA

CONSIDERAÇÕES GERAIS

DEFINIÇÃO
• A concentração sérica baixa de albumina é identificada na maioria dos ensaios se estiver <2 g/dL.

FISIOPATOLOGIA
• Albumina — uma proteína constitutiva sintetizada exclusivamente no fígado. • Representa 75-80% da pressão coloidoncótica plasmática. • Uma pressão oncótica baixa permite o extravasamento de líquido para o espaço intersticial e os compartimentos potenciais do terceiro espaço, provocando a formação de edema e o surgimento de efusão nas cavidades corporais. • Valores <1,5 g/dL levam ao desenvolvimento de edema e efusão. • Valores de 1,5-2,5 g/dL não geram edema nem efusão a menos que outros fatores desregulem as forças de Starling: p. ex., aumento da pressão hidrostática (oclusão venosa, hipertensão do leito vascular, retenção renal de sódio e água, sobrecarga hídrica) e aumento da permeabilidade vascular. • Concentrações relativas de albumina e globulina — ajudam a diferenciar os fatores causais; declínios equivalentes se desenvolvem em casos de enteropatia com perda de proteínas, perda de sangue e hemodiluição.

SISTEMA(S) ACOMETIDO(S)
• Cardiovascular e respiratório — efusão transudativa em cavidades corporais (p. ex., efusão pleural e ascite); edema periférico; edema pulmonar. • Endócrino e metabólico — ligação proteica alterada confere o aumento dos efeitos de hormônios e medicamentos livres não ligados. • Cutâneo e musculosquelético — cicatrização tardia de feridas (controverso); alteração do turgor cutâneo.

IDENTIFICAÇÃO
Espécies
Cães e gatos.

SINAIS CLÍNICOS
Achados Anamnésicos
• Distensão abdominal — ascite. • Diarreia e/ou vômitos — enteropatia com perda de proteínas. • Dispneia — causada por edema pulmonar ou efusão pleural. • Membros tumefatos — por edema gravitacional. • Anasarca.

Achados do Exame Físico
• Distensão abdominal — efusão. • Bulhas cardíacas abafadas — efusão pleural. • Dispneia ou crepitações pulmonares — edema. • Edema periférico. • Alças intestinais espessadas — enteropatia com perda de proteínas.

CAUSAS
Produção Diminuída de Albumina
• Hepatopatia crônica — hepatite crônica; cirrose; fibrose hepática idiopática; variável em desvio portossistêmico congênito (cães). • Consumo inadequado — desnutrição/má assimilação.

Perda Extracorporal de Albumina
• Nefropatia com perda de proteínas — amiloidose; glomerulonefrite. • Enteropatia com perda de proteínas — linfangiectasia; linfoma; enteropatia inflamatória grave; histoplasmose. • Lesões cutâneas gravemente exsudativas. • Perda sanguínea crônica grave — intestinal.

• Paracentese repetida de grandes volumes — efusão abdominal ou pleural.

Sequestro para Cavidades Corporais e Tecidos
• Efusões inflamatórias — pancreatite; peritonite séptica ou asséptica ou efusões pleurais; efusões quilosas. • Vasculopatias — imunomediadas (LES); infecciosas (*Ehrlichia*, febre maculosa das Montanhas Rochosas); síndrome de sepse; hepatite infecciosa canina; outras.

Outras
• Síntese sub-regulada de albumina — hiperglobulinemia, resposta de fase aguda negativa; balanço nitrogenado negativo, catabolismo. • Diluição — expansão vascular iatrogênica; síndrome de liberação inadequada do ADH. • Hipoadrenocorticismo.

FATORES DE RISCO
• Doenças em órgãos como fígado, rins, intestinos e vasos sanguíneos. • Balanço nitrogenado negativo; nutrição deficiente.

DIAGNÓSTICO

DIAGNÓSTICO DIFERENCIAL
• Hepatopatia grave — o paciente pode estar ictérico; pode desenvolver encefalopatia hepática ou poliúria e polidipsia; predispõe à formação de ascite. • Enteropatia com perda de proteínas — é comum a presença de diarreia; em geral, há segmentos intestinais espessados, podendo ser segmentares ou difusos. • Lesões cutâneas — precisam ser graves e exsudativas (p. ex., queimaduras, necrólise epidérmica tóxica, vasculite). • Perda sanguínea externa — associada à palidez; os sinais vitais indicam anemia; indícios extracorporais de perda sanguínea (intestinal; urinária; outras). • Desnutrição — hipoalbuminemia leve. • Fluidoterapia rigorosa — pode exacerbar a hipoalbuminemia ou gerar anormalidades transitórias.

ACHADOS LABORATORIAIS
Medicamentos Capazes de Alterar os Resultados Laboratoriais
A ampicilina pode causar valores falsamente altos (dependendo do sistema de ensaio).

Distúrbios Capazes de Alterar os Resultados Laboratoriais
Lipidemia extrema ou hemólise excessiva — podem gerar valores falsamente elevados com o método do verde de bromocresol.

Os Resultados Serão Válidos se os Exames Forem Realizados em Laboratório Humano?
Sim.

HEMOGRAMA/BIOQUÍMICA/URINÁLISE
Hemograma Completo
• Depende da causa subjacente. • Hepatopatia grave — hemácias com microcitose (comum) indicam desvio portossistêmico. • Perda sanguínea grave — anemia regenerativa. • Enteropatia com perda de proteínas — linfopenia na linfangiectasia.

Bioquímica
• Fracionamento da proteína total — pode revelar indícios do distúrbio subjacente; os padrões são influenciados pela resposta de fase aguda; a hiperglobulinemia confere *feedback* negativo sobre a síntese de albumina. • Hepatopatia crônica — albumina baixa; globulina normal a alta.

• Enteropatia com perda de proteínas — albumina baixa; globulina baixa. • Nefropatia com perda de proteínas — albumina baixa; a globulina costuma permanecer normal, mas pode ser variável a baixa com proteinúria não seletiva (nefropatia grave com perda de proteínas). • Perdas exsudativas — albumina baixa; globulina variável. • Desnutrição — albumina baixa; globulina normal. • Perda sanguínea grave — albumina baixa; globulina baixa a normal. • Colesterol — baixo em casos de hepatopatia crônica, enteropatia grave com perda de proteínas, doença de Addison e desnutrição grave; alto em casos de nefropatia com perda de proteínas e pancreatite. • Enzimas hepáticas — podem estar elevadas em casos de hepatite crônica, enteropatia inflamatória indutora da perda de proteínas, além de fosfatase alcalina alta (indução) como uma resposta generalizada à inflamação sistêmica. • Bilirrubina — pode estar alta com hepatopatia crônica. • Ureia — pode estar baixa com hepatopatia crônica ou em pacientes sob diurese; alta com função renal reduzida ou desidratação. • Hipercalemia e hiponatremia — indicam doença de Addison ou pseudo-hipoadrenocorticismo associado ao intestino. • Hipocalcemia falsa — atribuída à proteína baixa.

Urinálise
• Descartar nefropatia com perda de proteínas e perda urológica de sangue. • Obter a amostra de urina por cistocentese para evitar contaminação do trato urinário inferior. **Cuidado:** evitar micro-hematúria induzida por cistocentese. • Proteinúria — confirmar a detecção com fita de imersão mediante determinação bioquímica. • Relação de proteína:creatinina urinárias — essencial; o valor >3,0 é compatível com proteinúria de faixa nefrótica; é imprescindível interpretar os resultados juntamente com o sedimento urinário; valores positivos falsos com sedimento ativo (leucócitos, eritrócitos) indicando piúria substancial ou hematúria macroscópica; nota: muitos cães com glomerulonefrite possuem cilindros hialinos, céreos ou granulares na urina.
• Microalbuminúria: não acrescenta informações adjuvantes importantes em comparação à relação de proteína:creatinina urinárias. • Cristalúria por biurato de amônio — em insuficiência hepática, desvio portossistêmico adquirido.

OUTROS TESTES LABORATORIAIS
• Ácidos biliares séricos totais — altos com hepatopatia grave; é possível notar valores baixos falsos em enteropatia com perda de proteínas (má absorção de gordura). • Avaliação físico-química da efusão — transudato (puro ou modificado) se a hipoalbuminemia representar um fator causal. • Antitrombina — proteína anticoagulante com peso molecular semelhante ao da albumina e sintetizada basicamente no fígado; pode estar baixa em casos de enteropatia/nefropatia com perda de proteínas e falha de síntese hepática. • Proteína C — proteína anticoagulante com peso molecular semelhante ao da albumina e sintetizada basicamente no fígado; pode estar baixa em casos de doença/insuficiência hepática grave, desvio portossistêmico, sepse.

DIAGNÓSTICO POR IMAGEM
• Radiografia torácica — efusão pleural; edema pulmonar. • Radiografias abdominais — efusão; alteração de tamanho do fígado; lesões expansivas; sinais quadrantes de doença pancreática.
• Ultrassonografia abdominal — ajuda a identificar anormalidades viscerais (p. ex., fígado

HIPOALBUMINEMIA

pequeno e parede intestinal espessada), lesões expansivas, bolsas de líquido, alteração do fluxo sanguíneo portal, linfadenopatia mesentérica e anormalidades da árvore biliar.

MÉTODOS DIAGNÓSTICOS
• Biopsia hepática — após avaliar o estado de coagulação (tempo de sangramento de mucosa, PIAVK, TP, TTPA, contagem de plaquetas); solicitar coloração especial para o fígado (H&E, Rodanina, Azul da Prússia, Reticulina, PAS).
• Biopsia renal — diferencia amiloidose de glomerulonefrite; enviar amostras para coloração especial dos rins e estudos ultraestruturais; do contrário, é improvável que as características da biopsia influenciem as opções terapêuticas.
• Biopsia intestinal — via endoscopia (pequeno pedaço) ou cirurgia (espessura total); podem ocorrer cicatrização tardia de feridas cirúrgicas e formação de seroma após laparotomia em pacientes com hipoalbuminemia grave.

TRATAMENTO
CUIDADO(S) DE SAÚDE ADEQUADO(S)
• Depende(m) da causa definitiva. • Efusão pleural que restringe a ventilação — realizar o procedimento de toracocentese com ou sem tubo torácico.

CUIDADO(S) DE ENFERMAGEM
Aplicar fisioterapia e fazer o paciente caminhar para aumentar a mobilização do edema periférico.

Fluidoterapia
• Evitar carga de sódio. • Coloides — utilizados para aumentar a pressão oncótica e reduzir a quantidade de cristaloides necessária para a expansão volêmica; prever a administração intravenosa contínua em velocidade de infusão constante; as proteínas não são retidas pelos pacientes com perdas extracorporais (enteropatia com perda de proteínas, nefropatia com perda de proteínas, exsudação em superfície), administrar para expansão volêmica aguda; note que os coloides se equilibram com o interstício. • Plasma — melhor coloide, particularmente nos casos de coagulopatia ou alto risco de trombose (baixo nível de antitrombina e proteína C); fornece antitrombina e albumina; efeito oncótico e retenção sistêmica mais prolongados em comparação com os coloides sintéticos.
• Hetamido — polímero sintético; aumenta a pressão oncótica; solução a 6% em NaCl a 0,9% (10-20 mL/kg IV durante 6-8 h ou em velocidade lenta sob infusão contínua por 24 h); em geral, há necessidade de múltiplas doses ao longo dos dias; pode exacerbar ou gerar tendências hemorrágicas; não fornece a albumina (importante proteína de transporte e ligação). • Dextrana 70 — polissacarídeo; aumenta a pressão oncótica; considerado o último recurso como coloide alternativo; solução a 6% em NaCl a 0,9% (1 mL/kg/h IV); não fornece a albumina (importante proteína de transporte e ligação); pode exacerbar ou gerar tendências hemorrágicas por interferir na função plaquetária; evitar seu uso em pacientes com problemas hepáticos, pois pode provocar sangramento. • Albumina humana — terapia controversa na medicina veterinária e nos cães; além de ser antigênica nos cães, pode provocar resposta de hipersensibilidade imediata (anafilática) ou tardia; a reação adversa pode culminar no óbito;

dose máxima de 6,25 g/kg (25 mL/kg) IV administrada durante 4-72 h (infusão em velocidade constante que varia de 0,1-1,7 mL/kg/h [0,025-0,425 g/kg] durante 4-72 h); a albumina rapidamente se equilibra com o interstício; a albumina humana é modificada em termos moleculares durante a produção e tem propriedades reduzidas de ligação proteica; a administração não deve ser repetida em cães.

DIETA
• Obter um balanço energético e nitrogenado positivo. • Encefalopatia hepática — restringir o consumo de proteína (ver "Encefalopatia Hepática"). • Efusões ou edema atribuídos à hipoalbuminemia — restringir o sódio.
• Enteropatia com perda de proteínas associada à linfangiectasia — triglicerídeos de cadeia média (apenas cães; controversos) combinados com restrição de gordura na dieta.

MEDICAÇÕES
MEDICAMENTO(S)
• Glicocorticoides — usados para alguns tipos de hepatite crônica e enteropatia inflamatória; selecionar os agentes que carecem de efeitos mineralocorticoides (p. ex., dexametasona) para evitar retenção de sódio e água. • Diuréticos — ajudam a mobilizar e excretar o excesso de água e sódio do corpo; furosemida (1-4 mg/kg IV, IM ou VO a cada 4-12 h): utilizada com critério para evitar contração do volume intravascular e combinada com espironolactona (1-4 mg/kg a cada 12 h) nos casos de hepato ou cardiopatia.
• Tratamento antitrombótico (baixos níveis de antitrombina e proteína C, além de indícios de trombos) — ácido acetilsalicílico (0,5 mg/kg VO ou por via retal a cada 24 h), especialmente nos casos de nefropatia com perda de proteínas.
• Enalapril (0,5 mg/kg VO a cada 12-24 h) — para cães com nefropatia com perda de proteínas; o benazepril é uma alternativa de uso.

CONTRAINDICAÇÕES
Coloides sintéticos — evitar na presença de anúria, insuficiência renal, insuficiência cardíaca congestiva, coagulopatia grave ou doença de von Willebrand.

PRECAUÇÕES
• Fluidoterapia — grandes doses de coloides sintéticos podem causar sobrecarga volêmica e coagulopatia; evitar a dosagem excessiva de fluidos cristaloides quando administrados com coloides sintéticos, pois estes se distribuem rapidamente para os espaços intersticiais (70% do volume em 1 h), agravando o edema prévio dos pulmões ou dos membros e as efusões em cavidades corporais; restringir o volume de cristaloides como fluido de manutenção para um terço do normal, dependendo das perdas atuais, se usados com coloides. • Transfusão de plasma canino ou albumina humana — pode ser complicada por reações transfusionais ou alérgicas; a transfusão de plasma é de valor dúbio se houver perda extracorporal atual grave de albumina (p. ex., nefropatia/enteropatia com perda de proteínas, vasculite). • Terapia diurética — pode causar contração volêmica grave, predispondo os pacientes à azotemia e hipotensão, bem como a distúrbios eletrolíticos e acidobásicos. • Efeitos

colaterais imprevistos dos medicamentos — atribuídos à ligação reduzida da albumina com o medicamento. • Uso de DDAVP para sangramento — pode agravar a retenção de líquido e as complicações associadas.

INTERAÇÕES POSSÍVEIS
Dosagem excessiva inadvertida de medicamentos com alta ligação proteica.

ACOMPANHAMENTO
MONITORIZAÇÃO DO PACIENTE
• Peso corporal — especialmente durante a fluidoterapia; monitorizar a retenção de líquido.
• Sinais vitais, auscultação torácica à procura de crepitações — monitorizar a ocorrência de edema pulmonar. • Concentrações séricas seriadas de albumina. • Pressão arterial — monitorizar para detectar expansão vascular. • Circunferência abdominal — monitorizar quanto à formação de ascite. • Oximetria de pulso — para detectar hipoxemia secundária a edema pulmonar.
• Pressão venosa central — não é confiável; monitoriza o equilíbrio hídrico; evitar o uso de cateteres venosos centrais em pacientes com tendências hemorrágicas ou trombóticas.

COMPLICAÇÕES POSSÍVEIS
• Nefropatia com perda de proteínas — pode ser complicada por tromboembolia; minimizar o procedimento de cateterismo intravenoso e a indução de traumatismo iatrogênico. • Hipovolemia — em animais com desidratação, crise addisoniana, perda sanguínea ou sob doses excessivas de diuréticos; pode predispor o animal à insuficiência renal aguda, CID ou encefalopatia hepática.

EVOLUÇÃO ESPERADA E PROGNÓSTICO
Dependem da causa subjacente.

DIVERSOS
GESTAÇÃO/FERTILIDADE/REPRODUÇÃO
A condição complica a prenhez.

VER TAMBÉM
• Amiloidose.
• Anomalia Vascular Portossistêmica Congênita.
• Cirrose e Fibrose do Fígado.
• Desvio Portossistêmico Adquirido.
• Enteropatia com Perda de Proteínas.
• Glomerulonefrite.
• Hepatopatia Fibrosante Juvenil.

ABREVIATURA(S)
• ADH = hormônio antidiurético.
• CID = coagulação intravascular disseminada.
• DDAVP = 1-desamino-8-D-arginina (vasopressina).
• H&E = hematoxilina e eosina.
• LES = lúpus eritematoso sistêmico.
• NaCl = cloreto de sódio.
• PAS = ácido periódico de Schiff.
• PIAVK = proteínas invocadas pela ausência ou antagonismo da vitamina K.
• TP = tempo de protrombina.
• TTPA = tempo de tromboplastina parcial ativada.

Autor Sharon A. Center

HIPOANDROGENISMO

CONSIDERAÇÕES GERAIS

REVISÃO
- Hipoandrogenismo refere-se à deficiência relativa ou absoluta de hormônios sexuais masculinizantes, como a testosterona e seus derivados. Os androgênios são produzidos pelo córtex da adrenal, pelo ovário na fêmea e pelas células de Leydig (intersticiais) dos testículos no macho.
- Machos — o hipoandrogenismo clínico primário no macho é uma condição rara associada à alopecia bilateral simétrica (alopecia endócrina) em cães castrados idosos. Também pode ser visto em associação à degeneração testicular resultante de doença testicular inflamatória (orquite); no entanto, a última não costuma estar associada a outros sinais clínicos, além da ausência de espermatogênese, já que as células produtoras de testosterona frequentemente são poupadas. O distúrbio pode ser iatrogênico após a administração prolongada de certos medicamentos (ver adiante) que interferem na produção de testosterona.
- Fêmeas — o hipoandrogenismo primário é documentado em cadelas, embora o secundário (relativo) seja muito mais comum em virtude de condições como hiperadrenocorticismo e hipotireoidismo.

IDENTIFICAÇÃO
- Cães e gatos.
- Mais comum em animais idosos, embora exista a forma congênita.
- O hipoandrogenismo primário é raro em fêmeas, porém mais comum em machos caninos castrados (especialmente da raça Afghan hound).

SINAIS CLÍNICOS
Achados Anamnésicos
- Falha dos ciclos estrais.
- Diminuição da libido, falha de fecundação da fêmea.

Achados do Exame Físico
- Pelagem seca e opaca, além de alopecia simétrica.
- Alteração de cor da pelagem.
- Testículos pequenos e macios.
- Sêmen de baixa qualidade (oligospermia, azoospermia).
- Ausência de espículas penianas em gatos.

CAUSAS E FATORES DE RISCO
- Castração.
- Cães da raça Boston terrier — baixa produção de androgênio fetal associada à ocorrência de hipospadias.
- Gatos com pelagem calico e semelhante a casco de tartaruga — associado à síndrome de Klinefelter (39 XXY).
- Administração de medicamentos antiandrogênicos — mitotano, cetoconazol, cimetidina, acetato de megestrol.
- Degeneração testicular (avançada).

DIAGNÓSTICO

DIAGNÓSTICO DIFERENCIAL
- Hipotireoidismo — diagnóstico formulado com base nos sinais clínicos apropriados, em conjunto com anormalidades hematológicas e bioquímicas típicas (anemia arregenerativa normocítica normocrômica, além de hipercolesterolemia) e provas de função da tireoide (T_4 total, T_4 livre, TSH canino).
- Hiperadrenocorticismo — os sinais clínicos incluem, em geral, poliúria/polidipsia e intolerância ao exercício; o hemograma completo pode revelar leucocitose, eritrocitose; as anormalidades bioquímicas séricas englobam elevação de fosfatase alcalina, ALT e colesterol, mas nível baixo de ureia; outros exames incluem relação de creatinina:cortisol urinários, estimulação com ACTH, TSDBD, ACTH endógeno, ultrassonografia abdominal.
- Hipossomatotropismo — também conhecido como dermatose responsiva ao GH. Acredita-se que essa síndrome seja um problema secundário que ocorre em associação com alopecia X (ver "Hiperandrogenismo"). O diagnóstico definitivo é estabelecido mediante a consideração cuidadosa da raça, da anamnese, do exame físico, dos resultados laboratoriais, excluindo outras causas endócrinas de alopecia, bem como de biopsia cutânea e da resposta à terapia.
- O diagnóstico baseia-se na avaliação do histórico, no exame físico, nos testes laboratoriais para descartar outros diagnósticos diferenciais e na resposta à terapia.

HEMOGRAMA/BIOQUÍMICA/URINÁLISE
Em geral, não há nada digno de nota.

OUTROS TESTES LABORATORIAIS
- A biopsia cutânea pode revelar alterações inespecíficas associadas à alopecia endócrina, como hiperqueratose ortoqueratótica, atrofia epidérmica e melanose, queratose folicular, folículos pilosos telogênicos (ou seja, inativos) e atrofia das glândulas sebáceas.
- Cariótipo — para detectar anormalidades de intersexo.
- Concentrações séricas de testosterona — os valores isolados são de pouco significado clínico em virtude da oscilação diária na concentração sérica em animais normais. O método mais confiável para mensurar a testosterona é um teste de estimulação com GnRH (25-50 mcg/cão, ou 2,0 mcg/kg, IM) ou hCG (44 UI/kg). Devem ser obtidas amostras sanguíneas basais e 1 (GnRH) ou 4 h (hCG) após a estimulação. A testosterona sérica normal é de 0,1-4,0 ng/mL antes da estimulação, mas 3,0-7,0 ng/mL após a estimulação.
- Aspirado testicular por agulha fina para exame citológico, ou biopsia testicular — para documentar doença testicular inflamatória prévia ou atual.
- Análise do sêmen.
- Concentração sérica de LH — para avaliar a função das células de Leydig.

DIAGNÓSTICO POR IMAGEM
Ultrassonografia testicular e abdominal para avaliar o parênquima dos testículos e as glândulas adrenais.

TRATAMENTO

Terapia de reposição hormonal com assinatura do termo de consentimento informado pelo proprietário do animal em virtude dos efeitos colaterais potenciais.

MEDICAÇÕES

MEDICAMENTO(S) DE ESCOLHA
Metiltestosterona
- Cães: 5-25 mg/cão VO a cada 24-48 h.
- Gatos: 1-2,5 mg/gato VO a cada 48 h.

CONTRAINDICAÇÕES/INTERAÇÕES POSSÍVEIS
- O uso de metiltestosterona pode resultar em hepatopatia colestática, epífora, seborreia e alterações do comportamento, como agressividade.
- É recomendável evitar os medicamentos que interferem na síntese de esteroide.

ACOMPANHAMENTO

MONITORIZAÇÃO DO PACIENTE
Monitorizar a resposta à terapia.

PREVENÇÃO
Evitar fármacos que sabidamente causam hipoandrogenismo em animais reprodutores.

COMPLICAÇÕES POSSÍVEIS
Hipogonadismo permanente e infertilidade são possíveis como uma consequência de *feedback* negativo.

EVOLUÇÃO ESPERADA E PROGNÓSTICO
Varia com a causa; pode ser permanente, temporário ou intermitente.

DIVERSOS

DISTÚRBIOS ASSOCIADOS
- Dermatose responsiva à testosterona em machos.
- Hipogonadismo.
- Anormalidades de intersexo.

ABREVIATURA(S)
- ACTH = hormônio adrenocorticotrópico.
- ALT = alanina aminotransferase.
- GH = hormônio de crescimento.
- GnRH = hormônio liberador de gonadotropina.
- hCG = gonadotropina coriônica humana.
- LH = hormônio luteinizante.
- TSDBD = teste de supressão com dexametasona em baixas doses.
- T_4 = tiroxina.
- TSH = hormônio tireostimulante.

Sugestões de Leitura
Griffin CE, Scott DW, Miller WH. Endocrine and metabolic diseases. In: Scott DW, Miller WH, Griffin CE, eds., Muller and Kirk's small animal dermatology. Philadelphia: Saunders, 2001, 780-885.

Autores Autumn P. Davidson e Sophie A. Grundy
Consultor Editorial Deborah S. Greco

Hipocalcemia

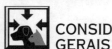

CONSIDERAÇÕES GERAIS

DEFINIÇÃO
Baixa concentração sérica total de cálcio.

FISIOPATOLOGIA
Do cálcio sérico circulante total, 40-50% apresentam-se ligados à proteína, 40-50% mostram-se ionizados e 10% encontram-se unidos sob a forma de complexos com outras substâncias. O cálcio ligado à proteína e aquele unido sob a forma de complexos não estão disponíveis para uso por tecidos. Apenas a forma ionizada fica disponível para os tecidos, sendo responsável pelos problemas clínicos (hipo e hipercalcemia). A mensuração de rotina do cálcio ionizado não é um procedimento fácil; os perfis bioquímicos registram apenas o cálcio sérico total. Os mecanismos envolvidos na hipocalcemia incluem:
• Baixa concentração de proteínas de ligação — hipoalbuminemia. • Absorção intestinal diminuída — deficiência de vitamina D (doença renal, enteropatia grave, raquitismo). • Reabsorção óssea e renal reduzida — hipoparatireoidismo.
• Ingestão inadequada na dieta. • Perda excessiva — lactação (eclâmpsia). • Sequestro — saponificação (pancreatite aguda). • Ligação/formação de complexo com substâncias químicas administradas, ingeridas ou endógenas — enemas contendo fosfato, toxicidade por citrato (múltiplas transfusões de anticoagulantes contendo essa substância), intoxicação por etilenoglicol, toxicidade por oxalato, dieta com baixos níveis de cálcio e altos teores de fósforo (hiperparatireoidismo secundário nutricional), síndrome de lise tumoral aguda (hiperfosfatemia decorrente da rápida destruição das células tumorais induzida por terapia antineoplásica).
• Síntese comprometida ou refratariedade ao PTH — hipomagnesemia. • Resistência de órgão-alvo ao calcitriol (vitamina D) (raquitismo tipo 2 dependente dessa vitamina).

SISTEMA(S) ACOMETIDO(S)
• Nervoso/neuromuscular — crises convulsivas, tetania, ataxia e fraqueza.
• Cardiovascular — alterações no ECG e bradicardia.
• Gastrintestinal — anorexia e vômitos (especialmente em gatos).
• Oftálmico — cataratas lenticulares posteriores.
• Respiratório — respiração ofegante.

GENÉTICA
Ver doenças/causas específicas.

INCIDÊNCIA/PREVALÊNCIA
Ver doenças/causas específicas.

IDENTIFICAÇÃO

Espécies
Cães e gatos.

Raça(s) Predominante(s)
Varia dependendo da causa subjacente.

Idade Média e Faixa Etária
Varia dependendo da causa subjacente.

Sexo Predominante
Varia dependendo da causa subjacente.

SINAIS CLÍNICOS

Comentários Gerais
Podem ser observados sinais da doença subjacente sem sinais clínicos de hipocalcemia, porque os últimos não ocorrem até que o cálcio sérico total decline abaixo de 6,7 mg/dL.

Achados Anamnésicos
• Crises convulsivas. • Tremores, contrações ou fasciculações musculares. • Ataxia ou marcha rígida. • Fraqueza. • Respiração ofegante. • Fricção facial. • Vômitos. • Anorexia.

Achados do Exame Físico
• Ataxia, marcha rígida, fraqueza, fasciculação muscular, tremor, contração espasmódica. • Febre.
• Cataratas lenticulares posteriores em pacientes com hipoparatireoidismo primário.

CAUSAS

Hipocalcemia Não Patológica
• Erro laboratorial — é recomendável repetir a determinação do cálcio sérico para confirmar hipocalcemia verdadeira, especialmente se os resultados indicarem hipocalcemia significativa apesar da ausência de sinais clínicos.
• Hipoalbuminemia — causa mais comum; responsável por mais de 50% dos pacientes; acarreta redução do cálcio ligado à proteína sem afetar o cálcio ionizado; não está associada a sinais clínicos; corrigir a hipoalbuminemia, utilizando uma das seguintes fórmulas:

$$Ca\ corrigido = [Ca\ (mg/dL) - albumina\ (g/dL)] + 3{,}5$$

ou

$$Ca\ corrigido = [Ca\ (mg/dL) - \{0{,}4 \times proteína\ total\ (g/dL)\}] + 3{,}3$$

Nota: Fórmulas inválidas em gatos, embora a hipoalbuminemia provoque uma queda na concentração de cálcio.
• Alcalose — provoca redução no cálcio mensurado total e ionizado; não associada a sinais clínicos.

Hipocalcemia Patológica
• Hipoparatireoidismo primário.
• Hipoparatireoidismo secundário à tireoidectomia (ou outras terapias corretivas para hipertireoidismo, como injeção de etanol na tireoide guiada por ultrassom ou ablação da tireoide por emissão de calor [radiofrequência]) e dano à paratireoide.
• Hipoparatireoidismo secundário à ablação da paratireoide por emissão de calor [frequência] guiada por ultrassom (para hiperparatireoidismo/massas paratireoides) e dano à paratireoide.
• Insuficiência renal — aguda ou crônica.
• Intoxicação por etilenoglicol.
• Toxicidade por oxalato (lírio, filodendro, etc.).
• Pancreatite aguda.
• Tetania puerperal — eclâmpsia.
• Enemas contendo fosfato.
• Hiperparatireoidismo secundário nutricional.
• Hipomagnesemia.
• Má absorção intestinal.
• Intoxicação por citrato — múltiplas transfusões de sangue ou desproporção entre o sangue e o citrato.
• Pós-correção de hiperparatireoidismo em virtude de hipofunção das paratireoides normais induzida por *feedback* negativo prolongado.
• Raquitismo (hipovitaminose D, calcitriol plasmático reduzido) ou raquitismo tipo 2 dependente da vitamina D (resistência de receptores do órgão-alvo ao calcitriol).
• Síndrome de lise tumoral aguda.

FATORES DE RISCO
• Tetania puerperal (eclâmpsia) — em cadelas pertencentes a raças de pequeno porte durante os primeiros 21 dias de amamentação de uma ninhada.
• Pós-procedimentos de correção para hipertireoidismo e hiperparatireoidismo (dano à paratireoide ou hipofunção da paratireoide normal induzida por *feedback* negativo prolongado).

DIAGNÓSTICO

DIAGNÓSTICO DIFERENCIAL
• Sinais clínicos de hipocalcemia — descartar hipoparatireoidismo primário, hipoparatireoidismo secundário à terapia corretiva de hipertireoidismo e hiperparatireoidismo e dano à paratireoide, tetania puerperal (eclâmpsia) e intoxicação indutora de rápida ligação/formação de complexos com o cálcio (p. ex., enemas contendo fosfato, intoxicação por etilenoglicol); outras causas raramente diminuem os níveis séricos de cálcio o bastante a ponto de causar sinais clínicos.
• Poliúria e polidipsia — excluir insuficiência renal.
• Sinais neurológicos — descartar intoxicação por etilenoglicol.
• Vômitos e diarreia — excluir pancreatite aguda, má absorção intestinal, insuficiência renal e intoxicação por etilenoglicol.
• Ostealgia (dor nos ossos) ou fraturas ósseas — descartar hiperparatireoidismo secundário nutricional.

ACHADOS LABORATORIAIS

Medicamentos Capazes de Alterar os Resultados Laboratoriais
• O bicarbonato de sódio pode causar alcalose e diminuir a concentração sérica de cálcio.
• Amostras coletadas em tubos com EDTA podem resultar na concentração sérica de cálcio falsamente baixa por causa da quelação desse mineral.

Distúrbios Capazes de Alterar os Resultados Laboratoriais
• A lipidemia pode aumentar significativamente o cálcio sérico.
• Hipoalbuminemia pode diminuir falsamente o cálcio sérico (ver causas de hipocalcemia não patogênica).

Os Resultados Serão Válidos se os Exames Forem Realizados em Laboratório Humano?
Sim.

HEMOGRAMA/BIOQUÍMICA/URINÁLISE
• Cálcio baixo.
• Possível anemia leve a moderada em pacientes com insuficiência renal crônica, hiperparatireoidismo secundário nutricional ou má absorção intestinal.
• Possível leucocitose em animais com pancreatite aguda.
• Hipoalbuminemia em pacientes com hipocalcemia induzida por hipoproteinemia — má absorção intestinal, nefropatia com perda de proteína, outras causas.
• CO_2 total elevado em casos de hipocalcemia induzida por alcalose.
• Altos níveis de ureia e creatinina em pacientes com insuficiência renal aguda e crônica, intoxicação por etilenoglicol ou toxicidade por oxalato.

HIPOCALCEMIA

- Níveis elevados de fósforo em pacientes com insuficiência renal aguda e crônica, intoxicação por etilenoglicol, toxicidade por oxalato, hipoparatireoidismo primário, hipoparatireoidismo secundário a procedimentos corretivos de hipertireoidismo ou hiperparatireoidismo e dano à paratireoide, síndrome de lise tumoral aguda, ou em pacientes submetidos a enemas contendo fosfato.
- Atividades aumentadas das enzimas amilase e lipase em muitos dos pacientes, mas não em todos, com pancreatite aguda.
- Isostenúria em pacientes com insuficiência renal crônica, insuficiência renal aguda moderada a avançada, intoxicação por etilenoglicol ou toxicidade por oxalato.
- Glicosúria em alguns animais com insuficiência renal aguda, intoxicação por etilenoglicol ou toxicidade por oxalato.

OUTROS TESTES LABORATORIAIS
- Cálcio ionizado — ajuda a determinar se os sinais clínicos são atribuídos à hipocalcemia, pois esta é a forma ativa do cálcio.
- Teste do etilenoglicol — indicado nos pacientes com suspeita da ingestão de etilenoglicol nas 12-16 horas prévias.
- Imunorreatividade da lipase pancreática — indicada em animais com suspeita de pancreatite aguda.
- Ensaio com PTH — indicado na suspeita de hipoparatireoidismo primário.
- Concentração sérica de magnésio — a hipomagnesemia é uma causa rara de hipocalcemia.
- Calcitriol plasmático (vitamina D, 1,25-di--hidroxicolecalciferol) — indicado para fazer a triagem de raquitismo ou raquitismo tipo 2 dependente da vitamina D (raro).

DIAGNÓSTICO POR IMAGEM
- As radiografias, em geral, permanecem normais.
- Possivelmente, rins pequenos em pacientes com insuficiência renal crônica e rins grandes naqueles com insuficiência renal aguda, intoxicação por etilenoglicol ou toxicidade por oxalato.
- Possivelmente, baixa densidade óssea em animais com hiperparatireoidismo secundário nutricional.
- Possivelmente, efusão pleural discreta e poucos detalhes abdominais em virtude da efusão nos casos de pancreatite.

MÉTODOS DIAGNÓSTICOS
As alterações no ECG incluem prolongamento dos segmentos ST e QT; bradicardia sinusal e ondas T largas ou alternantes em alguns pacientes.

ACHADOS PATOLÓGICOS
Variam, dependendo da causa subjacente.

TRATAMENTO

CUIDADO(S) DE SAÚDE ADEQUADO(S)
- Internação para hipocalcemia clínica.
- Em geral, há necessidade de tratamento de emergência apenas para os pacientes com hipoparatireoidismo primário, hipoparatireoidismo secundário a procedimentos corretivos de hipertireoidismo ou hiperparatireoidismo e dano à paratireoide, tetania puerperal (eclâmpsia), administração recente de enema contendo fosfato, toxicidade por citrato (rara) e intoxicação por etilenoglicol.
- O tratamento a curto e longo prazos costuma ser necessário apenas para o hipoparatireoidismo primário e a tetania puerperal (eclâmpsia).
- Para a tetania puerperal (eclâmpsia), é preciso retirar os filhotes da cadela e efetuar o aleitamento manual até o desmame.

CUIDADO(S) DE ENFERMAGEM
Varia(m), dependendo da causa subjacente.

ATIVIDADE
Varia, dependendo da causa subjacente.

DIETA
É recomendável a modificação da dieta em casos de hiperparatireoidismo secundário nutricional (para uma dieta balanceada) e insuficiência renal (ver "Insuficiência Renal Crônica").

ORIENTAÇÃO AO PROPRIETÁRIO
Varia, dependendo da causa subjacente.

CONSIDERAÇÕES CIRÚRGICAS
Variam, dependendo da causa subjacente.

MEDICAÇÕES

MEDICAMENTO(S) DE ESCOLHA
Tratamento de Emergência
- Solução de gliconato de cálcio a 10% — 5-15 mg/kg (0,5-1,5 mL/kg) lentamente até fazer efeito em um período de 10 minutos; monitorizar a frequência cardíaca e interromper a administração temporariamente caso ocorra bradicardia; se a monitorização ECG for possível, o encurtamento do intervalo QT será uma indicação para interromper temporariamente a administração.
- Solução de cloreto de cálcio a 10% — também é eficaz; extremamente cáustica se administrada por via extravascular e três vezes mais potente que o gliconato de cálcio; a dose em mg/kg é a mesma do gliconato de cálcio (5-15 mg/kg), mas é necessário apenas um terço do volume (0,15-0,5 mL/kg).

Tratamento a Curto Prazo Imediatamente após a Correção da Tetania
É possível evitar a recidiva dos sinais clínicos após o tratamento de emergência com solução de gliconato de cálcio a 10%, fazendo uso de uma das medidas a seguir:
- Infusão IV em velocidade constante de 60-90 mg/kg/dia (6,5-9,75 mL/kg/dia) acrescentados aos fluidos.
- Administração subcutânea 3-4 vezes ao dia da dosagem necessária para o controle inicial da tetania; diluir essa dose em um volume equivalente de solução fisiológica.

Tratamento a Longo Prazo
- Ver "Hipoparatireoidismo".

CONTRAINDICAÇÕES
Evitar o uso de bicarbonato, já que a alcalinização pode reduzir ainda mais os níveis séricos de cálcio.

PRECAUÇÕES
Ver "Hipoparatireoidismo".

INTERAÇÕES POSSÍVEIS
- Os sais de cálcio podem precipitar se adicionados às soluções que contenham bicarbonato, lactato, acetato ou fosfatos.
- Ver "Hipoparatireoidismo".

ACOMPANHAMENTO

MONITORIZAÇÃO DO PACIENTE
- Para os pacientes que necessitam de terapia para hipocalcemia a longo prazo, o cálcio sérico deverá ser avaliado 4-7 dias depois do tratamento inicial, depois (se normocalcêmico) mensalmente nos primeiros 6 meses e, em seguida, a cada 2-4 meses.
- O objetivo é manter a concentração sérica de cálcio entre 8-10 mg/dL.

PREVENÇÃO
Varia, dependendo da causa subjacente.

COMPLICAÇÕES POSSÍVEIS
Hipocalcemia e hipercalcemia (que podem levar à insuficiência renal) são preocupações em pacientes sob tratamento prolongado.

EVOLUÇÃO ESPERADA E PROGNÓSTICO
- Varia, dependendo da causa subjacente.
- É comum a recidiva da hipocalcemia após a administração de cálcio até que a causa subjacente seja tratada; fica indicada a monitorização dos sinais clínicos e do cálcio sérico.

DIVERSOS

GESTAÇÃO/FERTILIDADE/REPRODUÇÃO
- A hipocalcemia pode levar à fraqueza e distocia.
- Em geral, observa-se tetania puerperal (eclâmpsia) em cadelas pertencentes a raças de pequeno porte durante os primeiros 21 dias de amamentação da ninhada.

VER TAMBÉM
- Eclâmpsia. • Hipoalbuminemia.
- Hipomagnesemia. • Hipoparatireoidismo.
- Pancreatite. • Insuficiência Renal Aguda.
- Insuficiência Renal Crônica. • Intoxicação por Etilenoglicol. • Intoxicação por Lírio.

ABREVIATURA(S)
- Ca = cálcio. • ECG = eletrocardiograma.
- EDTA = ácido etilenodiaminotetracético.
- PTH = paratormônio.

RECURSOS DA INTERNET
- http://www.vet.uga.edu/VPP/CLERK/mcfarland/index.php
- http://www.clevelandclinicmeded.com/medicalpubs/diseasemanagement/endocrinology/hypocalcemia/

Sugestões de Leitura
Feldman EC, Nelson RW. Hypocalcemia and primary hypoparathyroidism. In: Feldman EC, Nelson RW, eds., Canine and Feline Endocrinology and Reproduction, 3rd ed. St. Louis: Saunders, 2004, pp. 716-742.
Nelson EC. Hypoparathyroidism and hypocalcemia calcium. In: Ettinger SJ, Feldman EC, eds., Textbook of Veterinary Internal Medicine, 6th ed. St. Louis: Elsevier, 2005, pp. 1529-1535.
Waters CB, Scott-Moncrieff JCR. Hypocalcemia in cats. Compend Contin Educ Pract Vet 1992, 14:497-507.

Autor Mitchell A. Crystal
Consultor Editorial Deborah S. Greco

HIPOCALEMIA

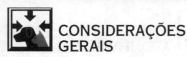

CONSIDERAÇÕES GERAIS

DEFINIÇÃO
Concentração sérica de potássio <3,5 mEq/L (faixa normal: 3,5-5,5 mEq/L).

FISIOPATOLOGIA
• O potássio é principalmente um eletrólito intracelular; os níveis séricos, no entanto, podem não refletir com precisão as concentrações corporais totais.
• Esse íon é predominantemente responsável pela manutenção do volume do líquido intracelular, além de ser necessário para a função normal de muitas enzimas.
• O potencial de membrana celular em repouso é determinado pela relação da concentração de potássio intra e extracelular, sendo mantido pela bomba de Na$^+$,K$^+$-ATPase. Os distúrbios de condução em tecidos suscetíveis (cardíaco, nervoso e muscular) são causados por rápidos desvios nessa relação.
• A hipocalemia pode ser causada por ingestão diminuída, perda (pelo trato gastrintestinal ou pelos rins) ou translocação de potássio para o líquido extracelular.

SISTEMA(S) ACOMETIDO(S)
• Neuromuscular — fraqueza muscular, incluindo músculos esqueléticos e ventilatórios.
• Cardíaco — alterações eletrocardíacas e arritmias.
• Renal — hipostenúria, nefropatia e insuficiência renal.
• Metabólico — afeta o equilíbrio acidobásico.

IDENTIFICAÇÃO
• Cães e gatos com predisposições à perda elevada de potássio, translocação de potássio ou ingestão reduzida desse elemento.
• Gatos jovens da raça Birmanês com episódios recidivantes de paralisia periódica hipocalêmica.

SINAIS CLÍNICOS
• Fraqueza muscular generalizada ou paralisia.
• Cãibras musculares.
• Letargia e confusão mental.
• Vômito.
• Anorexia.
• Intolerância a carboidrato e perda de peso.
• Poliúria.
• Polidipsia.
• Motilidade intestinal reduzida.
• Hipostenúria.
• Ventroflexão do pescoço (gatos).
• Falência dos músculos respiratórios.

CAUSAS

Ingestão Diminuída
• Anorexia ou inanição.
• Administração de fluidos intravenosos deficientes ou isentos de potássio.
• Ingestão de argila bentonita (p. ex., aglomerado de bandeja sanitária para gatos).

Perda Gastrintestinal
• Vômito.
• Diarreia.
• Obstrução gastrintestinal.

Perda Urinária
• Doença renal crônica.
• Acidose tubular renal.
• Nefropatia hipocalêmica.
• Diurese pós-obstrutiva.

• Diálise (hemodiálise ou peritoneal).
• Diurese com fluido intravenoso.
• Excesso de mineralocorticoide (hiperadrenocorticismo e hiperaldosteronismo primário).
• Alcalose metabólica.
• Hipocloremia.
• Medicamentos (diuréticos de alça, anfotericina B, penicilinas, envenenamento por cascavel).

Translocação (do Líquido Extracelular para o Intracelular)
• Administração de insulina e glicose.
• Administração de bicarbonato de sódio.
• Catecolaminas.
• Alcalemia.
• Dosagem excessiva de agonista β_2-adrenérgico (p. ex., albuterol).
• Paralisia periódica hipocalêmica (gatos da raça Birmanês).
• Envenenamento por cascavel.

FATORES DE RISCO
• Dietas acidificantes com quantidade desprezível de potássio.
• Diurese ou diálise com fluidos deficientes em potássio.
• Doença crônica (anorexia e emaciação muscular prolongadas).

DIAGNÓSTICO

DIAGNÓSTICO DIFERENCIAL
• PU/PD, hiperglicemia e glicosúria — descartar diabetes melito.
• PU/PD, azotemia e isostenúria — excluir insuficiência renal crônica e nefropatia.
• Vômito, alcalose metabólica e hipocloremia — descartar obstrução do trato gastrintestinal superior.
• Acidose metabólica com pH urinário >6,5 — excluir acidose tubular renal.
• Obstrução uretral — descartar diurese pós-obstrutiva.
• Gato jovem da raça Birmanês com fraqueza muscular episódica — excluir paralisia periódica hipocalêmica.

ACHADOS LABORATORIAIS

Medicamentos Capazes de Alterar os Resultados Laboratoriais
A mensuração falsamente elevada de potássio pode ser causada por quantidade excessiva de K$_3$EDTA em relação à amostra de sangue.

Distúrbios Capazes de Alterar os Resultados Laboratoriais
Nenhum.

Os Resultados Serão Válidos se os Exames Forem Realizados em Laboratório Humano?
Sim.

HEMOGRAMA/BIOQUÍMICA/URINÁLISE
• Hiperglicemia, glicosúria, ± cetonúria, ± cetoacidose em pacientes com diabetes melito.
• Anemia arregenerativa normocítica normocrômica em pacientes com insuficiência renal crônica.
• Ureia e creatinina elevados com isostenúria em pacientes com insuficiência renal crônica ou nefropatia hipocalêmica.
• CO$_2$ total ou HCO$_3^-$ baixos em pacientes com acidose tubular renal ou insuficiência renal.

• pH urinário >6,5 em pacientes com acidose tubular distal.
• CO$_2$ total ou HCO$_3^-$ altos em pacientes com alcalose metabólica.

OUTROS TESTES LABORATORIAIS
• Aldosterona aumentada e renina diminuída em pacientes com hiperaldosteronismo primário.
• Excreção fracional urinária elevada de potássio em pacientes com insuficiência renal crônica ou nefropatia hipocalêmica.
• Testes de estimulação com ACTH são utilizados para diagnosticar distúrbios das glândulas adrenais.

DIAGNÓSTICO POR IMAGEM
• As radiografias e ultrassonografias são úteis no diagnóstico de obstruções do trato gastrintestinal (massas ou corpos estranhos), pancreatite e doenças das glândulas adrenais (hiperadrenocorticismo, hiperaldosteronismo e tumores adrenais), bem como na avaliação de insuficiência renal crônica.
• Estudo do trato gastrintestinal superior com bário para o diagnóstico adicional de obstruções gastrintestinais (anatômicas ou funcionais).
• Tomografia computadorizada ou ressonância magnética para o diagnóstico mais detalhado de doenças das glândulas adrenais.

OUTROS MÉTODOS DIAGNÓSTICOS
Endoscopia gastrintestinal superior para diagnosticar distúrbios dessa porção do trato GI.

TRATAMENTO
• Hipocalemia branda (3,0-3,5 mEq/L) pode ser tratada por meio de suplementação oral com potássio.
• Hipocalemia moderada (2,5-3,0 mEq/L) é mais bem tratada pela administração de suplementos orais ± intravenosos e monitorização rigorosa sob internação.
• Hipocalemia grave (<2,5 mEq/L) também deve ser submetida à hospitalização para suplementação intravenosa intensiva de potássio. Os pacientes devem ser cuidadosamente monitorados quanto à ocorrência de arritmias cardíacas e insuficiência respiratória.

MEDICAÇÕES

MEDICAMENTO(S) DE ESCOLHA
• A suplementação oral com gliconato de potássio (p. ex., Tumil-K®) é um tratamento eficaz em pacientes levemente acometidos. A dosagem inicial é ¼ de colher das de chá (2 mEq) por 4,5 kg de peso corporal no alimento 2 vezes ao dia.

Tabela 1

Concentração de K$^+$ do Paciente	KCl/L (mEq)
3,5-4,5	20
3,0-3,5	30
2,5-3,0	40
2,0-2,5	60
<2,0	80

Nota: não exceder uma velocidade de suplementação intravenosa de 0,5 mEq/kg/h a menos que o animal seja submetido à monitorização contínua e esteja à beira de falência dos músculos ventilatórios.

HIPOCALEMIA

• A suplementação parenteral é necessária em pacientes com anorexia ou vômito ou naqueles com hipocalemia moderada a grave. O cloreto de potássio é adicionado aos fluidos intravenosos de acordo com a tabela, sendo mais bem distribuído via bomba de infusão. Monitorizar e reduzir a dose de acordo.

CONTRAINDICAÇÕES
• Suplementação de glicose.
• Administração de insulina.
• Administração de bicarbonato de sódio.
• Hipoadrenocorticismo não tratado.
• Hipercalemia.
• Insuficiência renal ou comprometimento renal grave.
• Desidratação aguda.
• Reações hemolíticas graves.
• Motilidade gastrintestinal diminuída.

PRECAUÇÕES
Administrar com cautela, evitar a suplementação excessiva e monitorizar com frequência.

INTERAÇÕES POSSÍVEIS
A suplementação concomitante de potássio com inibidores da ECA (p. ex., enalapril), diuréticos poupadores de potássio (p. ex., espironolactona), inibidores da prostaglandina (p. ex., agentes anti-inflamatórios não esteroides), β-bloqueadores (p. ex., atenolol) ou glicosídeos cardíacos (p. ex., digoxina) pode causar efeitos adversos.

MEDICAMENTO(S) ALTERNATIVO(S)
Em pacientes com hipofosfatemia concomitante, pode-se usar o fosfato de potássio.

ACOMPANHAMENTO

MONITORIZAÇÃO DO PACIENTE
Verificar o potássio sérico a cada 6-24 h com base na gravidade da hipocalemia.

COMPLICAÇÕES POSSÍVEIS
Distúrbios eletrolíticos e arritmias.

DIVERSOS

DISTÚRBIOS ASSOCIADOS
• Nefropatia hipocalêmica.
• Hipofosfatemia.
• Hipomagnesemia.
• Alcalose metabólica.

FATORES RELACIONADOS COM A IDADE
Nenhum.

POTENCIAL ZOONÓTICO
Nenhum.

GESTAÇÃO/FERTILIDADE/REPRODUÇÃO
N/D.

VER TAMBÉM
• Alcalose Metabólica.
• Capítulos sobre Diarreia.
• Hiperadrenocorticismo (Síndrome de Cushing) — Cães.
• Hipocloremia.
• Insuficiência Renal Crônica.
• Acidose Tubular Renal.
• Vômito Crônico.

ABREVIATURA(S)
• ACTH = hormônio adrenocorticotrópico.
• ATPase = trifosfato de adenosina.
• CO_2 = dióxido de carbono.
• ECA = enzima conversora de angiotensina.
• HCO_3^- = bicarbonato.
• K^+ = potássio.
• K_3EDTA = sal tripotássico do ácido etilenodiaminotetracético.
• Na^+ = sódio.
• PU/PD = poliúria/polidipsia.

Sugestões de Leitura
DiBartola SP, Autran de Morais H. Disorders of potassium: Hypokalemia and hyperkalemia. In: DiBartola SP, ed., Fluid Therapy in Small Animal Practice, 3rd ed. Philadelphia: Saunders, 2006, pp. 101-107.

Autor Deirdre Chiaramonte
Consultor Editorial Deborah S. Greco

HIPOCLOREMIA

CONSIDERAÇÕES GERAIS

DEFINIÇÃO
Concentração sérica de cloreto abaixo do limite inferior da normalidade — cães, <105 mEq/L; gatos, <117 mEq/L (os valores podem variar entre os laboratórios).

FISIOPATOLOGIA
- O cloreto é o ânion mais abundante no líquido extracelular.
- A concentração de cloreto é controlada pelos gradientes eletroquímicos resultantes do transporte ativo de sódio.
- Em geral, a concentração de cloreto varia diretamente com a de sódio e inversamente com a de bicarbonato.

SISTEMA(S) ACOMETIDO(S)
Dependem do distúrbio subjacente.

GENÉTICA
N/D.

INCIDÊNCIA/PREVALÊNCIA
N/D.

DISTRIBUIÇÃO GEOGRÁFICA
N/D.

IDENTIFICAÇÃO
Espécies
Cães e gatos.
Raça(s) Predominante(s)
N/D.
Idade Média e Faixa Etária
N/D.
Sexo Predominante
N/D.

SINAIS CLÍNICOS
Dependem do distúrbio subjacente.

CAUSAS
- Vômitos gástricos.
- Hipoadrenocorticismo.
- Alcalose metabólica.
- Nefropatia com perda de sal.
- Terapia diurética.

FATORES DE RISCO
N/D.

DIAGNÓSTICO

DIAGNÓSTICO DIFERENCIAL
Se a magnitude da hipocloremia ultrapassar a da hiponatremia, sugere-se a perda seletiva de cloreto, conforme observada em pacientes com vômitos gástricos.

ACHADOS LABORATORIAIS
Medicamentos Capazes de Alterar os Resultados Laboratoriais
Furosemida, tiazidas, bicarbonato e laxantes diminuem a concentração sérica.
Distúrbios Capazes de Alterar os Resultados Laboratoriais
Lipidemia e hiperproteinemia podem diminuir falsamente a concentração de cloreto caso não se faça uso de eletrodos íon-específicos.
Os Resultados Serão Válidos se os Exames Forem Realizados em Laboratório Humano?
Sim.

HEMOGRAMA/BIOQUÍMICA/URINÁLISE
- Baixo nível de cloreto.
- Outras anormalidades dependem do distúrbio subjacente; possivelmente, hiponatremia, hipercalemia e alta concentração de bicarbonato.

OUTROS TESTES LABORATORIAIS
- A estimativa da excreção urinária fracionada de cloreto pode demonstrar a excreção excessiva.
- A gasometria sanguínea pode revelar alcalose metabólica.

DIAGNÓSTICO POR IMAGEM
N/D.

MÉTODOS DIAGNÓSTICOS
N/D.

ACHADOS PATOLÓGICOS
N/D.

TRATAMENTO

CUIDADO(S) DE SAÚDE ADEQUADO(S)
- Depende do distúrbio subjacente.
- Usar NaCl a 0,9% se houver indicação de fluidoterapia.

CUIDADO(S) DE ENFERMAGEM
N/D.

ATIVIDADE
N/D.

DIETA
Não há necessidade de alteração.

ORIENTAÇÃO AO PROPRIETÁRIO
Depende do distúrbio subjacente.

CONSIDERAÇÕES CIRÚRGICAS
N/D.

MEDICAÇÕES

MEDICAMENTO(S) DE ESCOLHA
Outra fluidoterapia e medicação conforme determinado pela causa subjacente.

CONTRAINDICAÇÕES
N/D.

PRECAUÇÕES
N/D.

INTERAÇÕES POSSÍVEIS
N/D.

MEDICAMENTO(S) ALTERNATIVO(S)
N/D.

ACOMPANHAMENTO

MONITORIZAÇÃO DO PACIENTE
Mensuração das concentrações séricas de eletrólitos, conforme a necessidade, para assegurar a resposta adequada.

COMPLICAÇÕES POSSÍVEIS
Dependem do distúrbio subjacente.

PREVENÇÃO
Depende do distúrbio subjacente.

EVOLUÇÃO ESPERADA E PROGNÓSTICO
Depende da causa subjacente.

DIVERSOS

DISTÚRBIOS ASSOCIADOS
Em geral, acompanhada por hiponatremia.

FATORES RELACIONADOS COM A IDADE
N/D.

POTENCIAL ZOONÓTICO
Nenhum.

GESTAÇÃO/FERTILIDADE/REPRODUÇÃO
N/D.

VER TAMBÉM
Hiponatremia.

Sugestões de Leitura
DiBartola SP. Fluid, Electrolyte and Acid-Base Disorders in Small Animal Practice, 3rd ed. Philadelphia: Saunders, 2005.
Rose DB, Post T. Clinical Physiology of Acid-Base and Electrolyte Disorders, 5th ed. New York: McGraw-Hill, 2000.

Autor Peter P. Kintzer
Consultor Editorial Deborah S. Greco

HIPOFOSFATEMIA

CONSIDERAÇÕES GERAIS

DEFINIÇÃO
Concentração sérica de fósforo <2,5 mg/dL.

FISIOPATOLOGIA
- O controle do fósforo é influenciado pelas ações e interações do PTH e da vitamina D em órgãos como trato gastrintestinal, osso, rins e glândulas paratireoides.
- Um declínio na concentração sérica de fósforo pode ser causado por translocação desse elemento a partir do líquido extracelular nas células, bem como por reabsorção renal diminuída ou absorção intestinal reduzida de fósforo.
- O baixo nível sérico de fósforo pode levar à depleção de ATP, o que afeta as células com altas demandas energéticas (músculo esquelético, miocárdio, músculo neurológico e hemácias).
- Os pacientes diabéticos (cetóticos e não cetóticos) estão sob alto risco de hipofosfatemia em virtude da depleção das reservas de fósforo, perda de massa muscular e perdas urinárias. A administração de insulina gera ATP por glicólise, provocando translocação do fósforo.
- A hipofosfatemia diminui as concentrações da eritrócito 2,3-difosfoglicerato, levando à distribuição tecidual comprometida de oxigênio.

SISTEMA(S) ACOMETIDO(S)
- Hematológico/linfático/imune — hemólise, distribuição tecidual prejudicada de oxigênio, comprometimento da função de leucócitos e plaquetas.
- Musculosquelético — fraqueza, dor, insuficiência ventilatória e íleo gastrintestinal.
- Neurológico — a captação prejudicada de glicose leva a encefalopatia, crises convulsivas e coma.
- Cardíaco — diminuição na contratilidade.

IDENTIFICAÇÃO
- Cães e gatos mais idosos.
- Pacientes diabéticos.

SINAIS CLÍNICOS
Achados Anamnésicos
- Geralmente compatíveis com a doença primária responsável pela hipofosfatemia; no entanto, indícios de hipofosfatemia grave (p. ex., hemólise) não costumam ser observados até que as concentrações séricas declinem para 1,0 mg/dL ou menos.

Achados do Exame Físico
- Anemia hemolítica provoca palidez, taquipneia, dispneia e/ou urina manchada de vermelho.
- Fraqueza da musculatura esquelética e respiratória.
- Embotamento mental.

CAUSAS
- Má distribuição (translocação) — tratamento de cetoacidose diabética, administração de insulina ou carga de carboidrato, nutrição parenteral total ou recuperação nutricional, hiperventilação ou alcalose respiratória.
- Reabsorção renal reduzida (aumento da perda renal) — hiperparatireoidismo primário, distúrbios tubulares renais (p. ex., síndrome de Fanconi), diuréticos dos túbulos proximais (p. ex., inibidores da anidrase carbônica), eclâmpsia (tetania hipocalcêmica), hiperadrenocorticismo, administração de bicarbonato de sódio.
- Absorção intestinal diminuída (redução da ingestão) — dietas deficientes em fósforo, deficiência da vitamina D, distúrbios de má absorção, quelantes de fosfato.
- Erro laboratorial — hemólise, icterícia, administração de diurético osmótico (p. ex., manitol).

FATORES DE RISCO
- Dietas deficientes em fósforo ou nutrição parenteral.
- Diabetes melito.
- Anorexia prolongada, desnutrição ou inanição.

DIAGNÓSTICO

DIAGNÓSTICO DIFERENCIAL
- Hiperglicemia, glicosúria, cetonúria e acidose metabólica com hiato aniônico elevado concomitantes — descartar cetoacidose diabética.
- Glicosúria, normoglicemia, isostenúria ± azotemia concomitantes — excluir defeitos tubulares renais.
- Hipercalcemia e proteinúria concomitantes — descartar hiperparatireoidismo primário.
- Hipocalcemia concomitante — excluir tetania hipocalcêmica.
- Fosfatase alcalina sérica elevada concomitante — descartar hiperadrenocorticismo.
- Pan-hipoproteinemia concomitante — excluir má absorção intestinal.

ACHADOS LABORATORIAIS
Medicamentos Capazes de Alterar os Resultados Laboratoriais
Os diuréticos osmóticos (p. ex., manitol) podem reduzir falsamente as concentrações séricas de fósforo.

Distúrbios Capazes de Alterar os Resultados Laboratoriais
Hemólise e icterícia podem diminuir falsamente as concentrações séricas de fósforo.

Os Resultados Serão Válidos se os Exames Forem Realizados em Laboratório Humano?
Sim.

HEMOGRAMA/BIOQUÍMICA/URINÁLISE
- Fósforo sérico abaixo de 2,5 mg/dL.
- Hiperglicemia, glicosúria, cetonúria e acidose metabólica com hiato aniônico elevado em caso de cetoacidose diabética.
- Glicosúria, normoglicemia, isostenúria ou azotemia em caso de defeito tubular renal.
- Hipercalcemia em caso de hiperparatireoidismo primário.
- Hipocalcemia em caso de tetania hipocalcêmica.
- Fosfatase alcalina sérica elevada e proteinúria em caso de hiperadrenocorticismo.
- Pan-hipoproteinemia em caso de má absorção intestinal.

OUTROS TESTES LABORATORIAIS
- Frutosamina sérica — para diagnosticar ou descartar diabetes melito.
- Ensaio com PTH — para diagnosticar ou excluir hiperparatireoidismo.
- Medida dos metabólitos da vitamina D — para diagnosticar ou descartar deficiência dessa vitamina.

DIAGNÓSTICO POR IMAGEM
- A radiografia pode revelar urolitíase em casos de hiperparatireoidismo primário ou baixa qualidade do osso/fraturas patológicas em casos de distúrbios do metabolismo da vitamina D.
- Ultrassonografia (cervical) pode revelar a presença de massa na paratireoide.

OUTROS MÉTODOS DIAGNÓSTICOS
A cirurgia exploratória da região cervical pode revelar a existência de massa na paratireoide.

TRATAMENTO
- É preferível a prevenção.
- Os pacientes assintomáticos com concentrações baixas (1,5-2,5 mg/dL), mas não depletadas, de fósforo podem não necessitar de tratamento com fosfato.
- Se a hipofosfatemia for causada pela administração de insulina ou superalimentação, realizar a suplementação de fósforo.
- Os pacientes com hipofosfatemia grave (<1,5 mg/dL) necessitam de internação e monitoramento quanto à ocorrência de hemólise ou crise hemolítica. Administrar solução eletrolítica isotônica sem cálcio por via IV, suplementada com fosfato de potássio.
- Transfusão de sangue total fresco para crise hemolítica grave.

MEDICAÇÕES

MEDICAMENTO(S) DE ESCOLHA
- Fosfato potássico (3 mMol de fosfato/mL e 4,4 mEq de potássio/mL) administrado por via IV.
- Fosfato sódico (3 mMol de fosfato/mL e 4 mEq de sódio/mL) por via IV.
- Dosagem — 0,01-0,03 mMol/kg/h sob infusão em velocidade constante. Monitorizar o fósforo sérico a cada 6-8 h.
- Interromper a terapia quando a concentração sérica de fósforo atingir 2 mg/dL.

CONTRAINDICAÇÕES
- Hiperfosfatemia.
- Hipocalcemia.
- Hipercalcemia.
- Insuficiência renal.
- Dextrose a 2,5% e dextrose a 5% concomitantes na administração de Ringer lactato e dobutamina.

PRECAUÇÕES
- Administração concomitante de diurético, sobretudo dos inibidores da anidrase carbônica.
- Doença renal.

INTERAÇÕES POSSÍVEIS
- Administração de inibidores da ECA (p. ex., enalapril).
- Administração de glicosídeo cardíaco (p. ex., digoxina).
- Diuréticos poupadores de potássio (p. ex., espironolactona).

MEDICAMENTO(S) ALTERNATIVO(S)
- Suplemento oral de fosfato (p. ex., fosfato sódico) se o paciente não estiver vomitando.
- Leite (desnatado ou pobre em gordura) pode ser suplementado.

HIPOFOSFATEMIA

 ACOMPANHAMENTO

MONITORIZAÇÃO DO PACIENTE
• Medir os níveis séricos de fósforo a cada 6-8 h até a concentração retornar dentro dos limites de normalidade.
• Monitorizar os animais com hiperfosfatemia e interromper o tratamento imediatamente.
• Verificar o nível sérico de potássio diariamente até a estabilização.

COMPLICAÇÕES POSSÍVEIS
• Hemólise.
• Depressão e insuficiência respiratórias.
• Parada cardíaca.

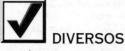 DIVERSOS

DISTÚRBIOS ASSOCIADOS
• Hipocalemia concomitante é comum em pacientes com cetoacidose diabética.
• Hipercalcemia concomitante em cães da raça Keeshond.

FATORES RELACIONADOS COM A IDADE
Presentes, em geral, em cães mais idosos.

POTENCIAL ZOONÓTICO
Nenhum.

GESTAÇÃO/FERTILIDADE/REPRODUÇÃO
Hipocalcemia concomitante no animal periparto é causada por excreção renal de fósforo promovida por PTH, causando hipofosfatemia.

VER TAMBÉM
• Diabetes Melito com Cetoacidose.
• Hiperparatireoidismo.

ABREVIATURA(S)
• ATP = trifosfato de adenosina.
• ECA = enzima conversora de angiotensina.
• PTH = paratormônio.

Sugestões de Leitura
DiBartola SP, Autran de Morais H. Disorders of phosphorous: Hypophosphatemia and hyperphosphatemia. In: DiBartola SP, ed., Fluid Therapy in Small Animal Practice, 3rd ed. Philadelphia: Saunders, 2006, pp. 197-200.

Autor Deirdre Chiaramonte
Consultor Editorial Deborah S. Greco

HIPOGLICEMIA

CONSIDERAÇÕES GERAIS

DEFINIÇÃO
Concentração anormalmente baixa de glicose no sangue.

FISIOPATOLOGIA
Mecanismos responsáveis pela hipoglicemia:
- Excesso de insulina ou fatores semelhantes a ela (p. ex., insulinoma, paraneoplasia extrapancreática, toxicidade do xilitol e dose excessiva iatrogênica de insulina).
- Redução dos hormônios necessários para manter a glicemia normal (p. ex., hipoadrenocorticismo).
- Gliconeogênese hepática diminuída (p. ex., hepatopatia, doenças do armazenamento de glicogênio e sepse).
- Uso metabólico excessivo de glicose (p. ex., em cães de caça, na prenhez, em casos de neoplasia, policitemia e sepse).
- Consumo reduzido ou produção de glicose abaixo do normal (p. ex., em filhotes de cães e gatos, raças toy e em casos de desnutrição ou inanição graves).

SISTEMA(S) ACOMETIDO(S)
- Nervoso.
- Musculosquelético.

IDENTIFICAÇÃO
- Cães e gatos.
- Variável, dependendo da causa subjacente.

SINAIS CLÍNICOS
- Crises convulsivas.
- Paresia posterior.
- Fraqueza.
- Colapso.
- Fasciculações musculares.
- Comportamento anormal.
- Letargia e depressão.
- Ataxia.
- Polifagia.
- Ganho de peso.
- PU/PD.
- Intolerância ao exercício.
- Alguns animais parecem normais, exceto pelos achados associados à doença subjacente.
- Muitos animais apresentam sinais episódicos.

CAUSAS
Endócrinas
- Insulinoma.
- Paraneoplasia extrapancreática (p. ex., carcinoma hepatocelular, adenoma hepatocelular, leiomioma intestinal, leiomiossarcoma intestinal).
- Dose excessiva iatrogênica de insulina.
- Hipoadrenocorticismo.

Hepatopatia
- Desvio portossistêmico.
- Cirrose.
- Hepatite grave (p. ex., tóxica e inflamatória).
- Doenças do armazenamento de glicogênio.

Uso Excessivo
- Hipoglicemia do cão de caça.
- Prenhez.
- Policitemia.
- Neoplasia.
- Sepse.

Consumo Reduzido/Produção Abaixo do Normal
- Filhotes jovens de cães e gatos.
- Cães de raças toy.
- Desnutrição ou inanição grave.

Toxicidade
- Dose excessiva iatrogênica de insulina.
- Toxicidade do xilitol.
- Intoxicação por agentes hipoglicemiantes (p. ex., sulfonilureias).

FATORES DE RISCO
- O baixo consumo calórico predispõe ao surgimento de hipoglicemia em pacientes com condições indutoras de uso excessivo ou produção abaixo do normal.
- Jejum, agitação, exercício e alimentação podem ou não aumentar o risco de episódios hipoglicêmicos em pacientes com insulinoma.

DIAGNÓSTICO

DIAGNÓSTICO DIFERENCIAL
- Pacientes com hiperinsulinismo — sinais de hipoglicemia ou exame físico normal.
- Pacientes com hipoadrenocorticismo — exacerbação, alívio, sinais inespecíficos (p. ex., vômitos, diarreia, melena e fraqueza); os pacientes com a doença de Addison que se apresentam em crise costumam exibir hipovolemia e hipercalemia, em vez de hipoglicemia (p. ex., choque, bradicardia e desidratação).
- Pacientes com desvios portossistêmicos — em geral, são jovens aos de meia-idade; frequentemente magros ou parecem ter crescimento estacionado; raras vezes, apresentam ascite ou edema.
- Pacientes com cirrose e hepatite grave, em geral, têm outros sinais de sua doença (p. ex., sinais gastrintestinais, icterícia e ascite ou edema).
- Pacientes com sepse — críticos; geralmente em choque; pirexia ou hipotermia ao exame; podem ter sinais gastrintestinais.
- Doenças do armazenamento de glicogênio — raras; observadas, em geral, em animais com menos de 1 ano de idade.
- Paraneoplasia extrapancreática e grandes processos neoplásicos indutores de hipoglicemia podem ser detectados com frequência ao exame físico.

ACHADOS LABORATORIAIS
Medicamentos Capazes de Alterar os Resultados Laboratoriais
Nenhum.

Distúrbios Capazes de Alterar os Resultados Laboratoriais
A separação tardia do soro produz valores séricos falsamente baixos de glicose; se o sangue não puder ser centrifugado e o soro separado dentro de 30 minutos após sua coleta, ele deverá ser coletado em frasco contendo fluoreto de sódio.

Os Resultados Serão Válidos se os Exames Forem Realizados em Laboratório Humano?
Sim.

HEMOGRAMA/BIOQUÍMICA/URINÁLISE
- Pacientes com hiperinsulinismo podem apresentar resultados normais.
- Pacientes com hipoadrenocorticismo podem ter linfocitose, eosinofilia, hipercalemia, hiponatremia, azotemia ou hipercalcemia.
- Pacientes com desvios portossistêmicos podem exibir microcitose, hipoalbuminemia, nível baixo da ureia, atividade levemente elevada das enzimas hepáticas, cristais de urato e baixa densidade urinária.
- Pacientes com cirrose, hepatite grave e neoplasia hepática podem ter anemia associada à doença crônica, atividade elevada das enzimas hepáticas, hiperbilirrubinemia, hipoalbuminemia, bilirrubinúria e baixa densidade urinária.
- Pacientes com policitemia têm o hematócrito >65.
- Pacientes com intoxicação pelo xilitol podem revelar hipocalemia, atividade elevada das enzimas hepáticas e hiperbilirrubinemia.

OUTROS TESTES LABORATORIAIS
- Determinação simultânea de glicose e insulina em jejum — indicada diante da suspeita de insulinoma; insulina plasmática elevada na presença de hipoglicemia sugere insulinoma.
- Relação de insulina:glicose corrigida — indicada quando se suspeita de insulinoma:

Relação de insulina:glicose corrigida =
$$\frac{\text{insulina plasmática [µU/mL]} \times 100}{\text{glicose plasmática [mg/dL]} - 30}$$

- Usar o número 1 como denominador se a glicose for <30; relação de insulina:glicose corrigida >30 sugere insulinoma; relação de insulina:glicose corrigida = 19-30 é uma zona obscura — repetir o teste; relação de insulina:glicose corrigida <19 indica que insulinoma é improvável. (**Nota:** resultados falso-positivos serão possíveis, especialmente quando a concentração sanguínea de glicose estiver <40 mg/dL).
- Teste de estimulação com ACTH — indicado na suspeita de hipoadrenocorticismo.
- Ácidos biliares séricos em jejum e pós-prandiais — indicados quando se suspeita de desvio portossistêmico ou hepatopatia funcional.
- Cultura bacteriana de sangue — indicada mediante a suspeita de sepse.
- Frutosamina — a hipoglicemia crônica resultará em baixas concentrações de frutosamina.

DIAGNÓSTICO POR IMAGEM
- Radiografia e ultrassonografia abdominais — úteis em pacientes com paraneoplasia extrapancreática e grandes processos neoplásicos (podem revelar organomegalia ou massas), bem como desvio portossistêmico (micro-hepatia), cirrose (micro-hepatia, hiperecogenicidade) e hepatite grave (hepatomegalia).
- Biopsia hepática guiada por ultrassom, laparoscópica ou cirúrgica — proveitosa para avaliar a existência de cirrose, hepatite e doenças do armazenamento de glicogênio.
- Cintilografia hepática quantitativa por via retal com tecnécio 99m — útil para detectar desvio portossistêmico.
- Portografia mesentérica — vantajosa para detectar desvio portossistêmico (requer cirurgia).

MÉTODOS DIAGNÓSTICOS
- ECG — útil para avaliar bradicardia em pacientes com hipoadrenocorticismo.
- Biopsia hepática guiada por ultrassom ou cirúrgica — proveitosa para verificar se há cirrose, hepatite e doença do armazenamento de glicogênio.

HIPOGLICEMIA

TRATAMENTO

- Tratar os animais com hipoglicemia clínica, cuja doença subjacente precisa de tratamento hospitalar.
- Se o animal conseguir comer (i. e., caso ele se mostre responsivo e não esteja vomitando), a alimentação deverá fazer parte ou compor todo o tratamento inicial.
- Caso o animal não consiga se alimentar, começar a fluidoterapia contínua com glicose a 2,5%; se os sinais clínicos persistirem, usar uma solução de glicose a 5%.
- A cirurgia ficará indicada se a causa da hipoglicemia for algum desvio portossistêmico ou neoplasia secretora de insulina (i. e., insulinoma).

MEDICAÇÕES

MEDICAMENTO(S) DE ESCOLHA

Tratamento de Emergência/Agudo
- No hospital — administrar glicose a 50%, na dose de 1 mL/kg sob a forma de bólus IV lento (1-3 min).
- Em casa — não tentar fazer com que o proprietário administre a medicação por via oral durante uma crise convulsiva; as convulsões hipoglicêmicas costumam desaparecer dentro de 1-2 min; em caso de crise convulsiva prolongada, recomendar o encaminhamento para o hospital; se uma crise convulsiva breve tiver chegado ao fim ou se houver outros sinais de crise hipoglicêmica, é recomendável passar xarope de milho ou glicose a 50% na mucosa bucal, seguido por 2 mL/kg da mesma solução por via oral assim que o paciente conseguir engolir; em seguida, levá-lo para atendimento veterinário imediato.
- Iniciar uma alimentação frequente com dieta pobre em açúcares simples ou, se o paciente não conseguir comer, continuar a fluidoterapia com glicose a 2,5%.

Tratamento a Longo Prazo
- Ver em "Insulinoma" o tratamento desse tumor e da paraneoplasia extrapancreática.
- Hipoglicemia do cão de caça — fornecer refeição com quantidade moderada de gordura, proteína e carboidratos complexos algumas horas antes da caçada; o animal pode comer petiscos (p. ex., biscoitos caninos) a cada 3-5 h durante a caçada.
- Hipoglicemia de raças toy — aumentar a frequência das refeições.

- Hipoglicemia de filhotes de cães e gatos — aumentar a frequência das refeições (colocando-os para mamar nas mães ou fornecendo-lhes mamadeiras).
- Outras causas de hipoglicemia exigem o tratamento da doença subjacente e em geral não requerem tratamento a longo prazo.

CONTRAINDICAÇÕES
- Insulina.
- Barbitúricos e diazepam em pacientes com convulsões hipoglicêmicas — tais agentes não tratam a causa da crise convulsiva e podem agravar a encefalopatia hepática em pacientes com desvio portossistêmico, cirrose ou insuficiência hepática induzida por intoxicação pelo xilitol.

PRECAUÇÕES
- A glicose a 50% provocará necrose e esfacelamento teciduais se for administrada por via extravascular; nunca administrar a glicose em concentrações acima de 5% sem confirmar o acesso venoso.
- Administrar a glicose sob a forma de bólus sem o acompanhamento de refeições frequentes ou fluidos IV contínuos com glicose pode predispor o paciente a episódios hipoglicêmicos subsequentes.

INTERAÇÕES POSSÍVEIS
N/D.

MEDICAMENTO(S) ALTERNATIVO(S)
N/D.

ACOMPANHAMENTO

MONITORIZAÇÃO DO PACIENTE
- Em casa — em caso de retorno ou evolução dos sinais clínicos de hipoglicemia; avaliar a glicose sérica se os sinais retornarem.
- Determinações isoladas intermitentes da glicose sérica podem não refletir verdadeiramente o estado glicêmico do paciente por causa da produção normal de hormônios contrarreguladores.
- Qualquer outra monitorização baseia-se na doença subjacente.

COMPLICAÇÕES POSSÍVEIS
Episódios progressivos recidivantes de hipoglicemia.

DIVERSOS

DISTÚRBIOS ASSOCIADOS
A hipoglicemia prolongada pode causar cegueira transitória (horas a dias) ou permanente em decorrência de necrose laminar do córtex cerebral occipital.

FATORES RELACIONADOS COM A IDADE
Os animais recém-nascidos têm pouca capacidade de armazenamento de glicogênio e capacidade reduzida de realizar a gliconeogênese; assim, períodos curtos de jejum (6-12 h) podem causar hipoglicemia.

POTENCIAL ZOONÓTICO
Nenhum.

GESTAÇÃO/FERTILIDADE/REPRODUÇÃO
- A hipoglicemia pode acarretar fraqueza e distocia.
- A prenhez juntamente com jejum provoca hipoglicemia em raras circunstâncias.

VER TAMBÉM
- Cirrose e Fibrose do Fígado.
- Doença do Armazenamento de Glicogênio.
- Adenoma Hepatocelular.
- Carcinoma Hepatocelular.
- Hipoadrenocorticismo (Doença de Addison).
- Insulinoma.
- Leiomioma do Estômago e dos Intestinos Delgado e Grosso.
- Leiomiossarcoma do Estômago e dos Intestinos Delgado e Grosso.
- Síndrome Paraneoplásica.
- Policitemia.
- Desvio Portossistêmico Adquirido.
- Anomalia Vascular Portossistêmica Congênita.
- Sepse e Bacteremia.
- Toxicidade do Xilitol.

ABREVIATURA(S)
- ACTH = hormônio adrenocorticotrófico.
- ECG = eletrocardiograma.
- PU/PD = poliúria e polidipsia.

Sugestões de Leitura
Feldman EC, Nelson RW. Beta-cell neoplasia: Insulinoma. In: Canine and Feline Endocrinology and Reproduction. St. Louis: Saunders, 2004, pp. 616-644.
Leifer CE. Hypoglycemia. In: Kirk RW, ed., Current Veterinary Therapy IX. Philadelphia: Saunders, 1986, pp. 982-987.
Meleo KA, Caplan ER. Treatment of insulinoma in the dog, cat and ferret. In: Bonagura JD, ed., Current Veterinary Therapy XIII. Philadelphia: Saunders, 2000, pp. 357-361.

Autor Mitchell A. Crystal
Consultor Editorial Deborah S. Greco

HIPOMAGNESEMIA

CONSIDERAÇÕES GERAIS

DEFINIÇÃO
- Cães — magnésio sérico <1,89 mg/dL.
- Gatos — magnésio sérico <1,8 mg/dL.

FISIOPATOLOGIA
- Magnésio — segundo cátion intracelular mais abundante, perdendo apenas para o potássio; a maior parte é encontrada nos ossos (60%) e tecidos moles (38%); grande parte do magnésio de tecidos moles fica na musculatura esquelética e no fígado; necessário para muitas funções metabólicas; um ativador ou catalisador para mais de 300 sistemas enzimáticos, inclusive fosfatases e enzimas que envolvem o ATP.
- O magnésio no soro coexiste de três formas: uma ligada à proteína, outra forma não ultrafiltrável (aproximadamente 25-30%) e duas formas ultrafiltráveis, a forma quelada e ionizada que, juntas, respondem por 70-75% do Mg sérico.
- A forma quelada encontra-se unida sob a forma de complexos com fosfato, citrato e outros compostos, constituindo uma pequena porcentagem de Mg ultrafiltrável.
- Como apenas 1-2% do total de magnésio fica no compartimento extracelular, a concentração sérica de magnésio nem sempre reflete o estado do elemento em todo o corpo.
- A absorção de magnésio ocorre principalmente no íleo, embora também ocorra no jejuno e no cólon.
- Os rins mantêm o equilíbrio de magnésio com reabsorção de 10-15% nos túbulos proximais, 60-70% no ramo ascendente espesso da alça de Henle e 10-15% nos túbulos contorcidos distais. Esses túbulos contorcidos distais estão sob controle hormonal e neuro-hormonal, determinando a concentração urinária final de magnésio.
- Hipomagnesemia — muitas causas; relatam-se taxas de incidência >50% em pacientes humanos criticamente enfermos.
- O magnésio é um cofator importante na bomba ATPase de sódio e potássio, que mantém um gradiente elétrico através das membranas; em consequência disso, o magnésio desempenha um papel importante na atividade de tecidos eletricamente excitáveis. O magnésio também é importante na produção e na eliminação de acetilcolina; uma concentração baixa de magnésio no líquido extracelular pode aumentar as concentrações de acetilcolina nas placas motoras terminais e causar tetania.
- A interferência no gradiente elétrico pode alterar os potenciais de repouso das membranas e provocar distúrbios de repolarização, resultando em anormalidades neuromusculares e cardíacas.
- O magnésio regula o deslocamento de cálcio para as células da musculatura lisa, elementos importantes para a força contrátil e o tônus vascular periférico.
- A hipomagnesemia pode alterar as funções dos músculos esqueléticos, resultando em tetania e uma variedade de miopatias observadas em pacientes submetidos à cisplatina e a outros medicamentos nefrotóxicos.
- As concentrações de magnésio são importantes na condução, excitabilidade e contração cardíacas por regular o deslocamento de cálcio.
- A depleção de magnésio pode afetar a bomba existente nas membranas das células cardíacas, resultando na despolarização dessas células e no desenvolvimento de taquiarritmias; as arritmias cardíacas associadas à hipomagnesemia incluem arritmias ventriculares, *torsades de pointes*, prolongamento do QT, encurtamento do segmento ST e alargamento das ondas T; a hipomagnesemia aumenta o risco de intoxicação por digoxina, porque ambos inibem a bomba da membrana.
- A hipomagnesemia causa resistência aos efeitos do PTH e pode aumentar a captação de cálcio no osso.

SISTEMA(S) ACOMETIDO(S)
- Múltiplos sistemas orgânicos.
- Cardiovascular.
- Gastrintestinal.
- Renal.
- Endócrino.
- Neuromuscular.

IDENTIFICAÇÃO
Cães e gatos.

INCIDÊNCIA/PREVALÊNCIA
Relata-se que 28-54% dos cães e gatos criticamente enfermos tinham hipomagnesemia.

SINAIS CLÍNICOS
Ocorre hipomagnesemia em uma variedade de doenças, com diversos sinais:
- Fraqueza.
- Fibrilação muscular.
- Ataxia e depressão.
- Hiper-reflexia.
- Tetania.
- Mudanças comportamentais.
- Arritmias.

CAUSAS
- Quatro categorias gerais — gastrintestinais, renais, endócrinas e outras.
- Desnutrição grave ou enteropatias indutoras de má absorção significativa podem ocasionar hipomagnesemia, que também pode ocorrer após perda excessiva de líquidos corporais (p. ex., diarreia prolongada grave); o magnésio é encontrado em alta concentração no trato gastrintestinal inferior, razão pela qual a diarreia secretora em humanos é associada à hipomagnesemia profunda; isso foi relatado em cão com enteropatia com perda de proteínas. A homeostasia do magnésio é regulada pelos rins; o controle renal da reabsorção tubular ocorre principalmente no ramo ascendente da alça de Henle; a perda renal de magnésio pode ser decorrente da administração de medicamentos nefrotóxicos, inclusive cisplatina, aminoglicosídeos e anfotericina B; a reabsorção de magnésio também pode ser prejudicada por diurese osmótica (diabetes melito), diuréticos de alça, hipercalciúria e acidose tubular. A hipomagnesemia associada à administração de diurético é um problema significativo em pacientes humanos com insuficiência cardíaca e foi observada experimentalmente em camundongos.
- A hipomagnesemia se desenvolve durante a terapia crônica com diurético tiazídico pela sub-regulação do receptor transitório epitelial dos canais de Mg^{2+} e inibição ou inativação concomitante do cotransportador de Na^+-Cl^-. Os problemas endócrinos associados à hipomagnesemia incluem hipercalcemia, hipertireoidismo e hiperparatireoidismo.
- A lactação pode causar perda excessiva de magnésio.
- O magnésio pode ser redistribuído com o retorno da alimentação após inanição, terapia com insulina em pacientes diabéticos, após paratireoidectomia, com o uso de formulação para nutrição parenteral com conteúdo inadequado de magnésio e em pacientes com pancreatite aguda ou condições indutoras de excesso de catecolaminas. As causas de hipomagnesemia em pacientes criticamente enfermos incluem baixo consumo, ausência de magnésio em fluidos parenterais em pacientes sob fluidoterapia prolongada ou diálise, perda gastrintestinal excessiva, redistribuição e sequestro.
- A hipomagnesemia está associada ao diabetes melito em seres humanos, sendo que quase 25% dos pacientes humanos diabéticos ambulatoriais apresentam níveis séricos baixos de magnésio.
- Embora um único estudo não tenha demonstrado qualquer diferença na apresentação dos níveis de magnésio ionizado em cães com diabetes em comparação aos controles, a hipomagnesemia ainda deve ser considerada em pacientes diabéticos após insulinoterapia rigorosa para cetoacidose diabética.

FATORES DE RISCO
- Nutrição parenteral total.
- Doença renal poliúrica.
- Administração de diurético.
- Diálise peritoneal.
- Diabetes melito e cetoacidose diabética.
- Lactação.
- Síndromes de má absorção gastrintestinal.

DIAGNÓSTICO

DIAGNÓSTICO DIFERENCIAL
- Os sinais de hipomagnesemia são vagos e polissistêmicos, mas outras causas de anormalidades neuromusculares, especialmente outras anormalidades eletrolíticas, precisam ser investigadas.
- Considerar anormalidades cardíacas, intoxicações e doenças renais.

ACHADOS LABORATORIAIS
Nota: 12 mg de magnésio = 1 mEq de magnésio; para converter de mg/dL em mEq/L, dividir por 1,2.

Medicamentos Capazes de Alterar os Resultados Laboratoriais
- O soro é melhor do que o plasma, porque o anticoagulante usado para obter amostras de plasma pode conter citrato ou outros íons que se ligam ao magnésio.
- EDTA, oxalato-fluoreto de sódio, citrato de sódio e gliconato de cálcio intravenoso podem gerar valores séricos de magnésio falsamente baixos.

Distúrbios Capazes de Alterar os Resultados Laboratoriais
- Hemólise pode elevar falsamente o magnésio sérico.
- Hipercalcemia (>16 mg/dL) e hiperproteinemia (>10 g/dL) também podem elevar falsamente o magnésio sérico.
- Hiperbilirrubinemia e lipidemia podem causar quedas falsas no magnésio sérico.

Os Resultados Serão Válidos se os Exames Forem Realizados em Laboratório Humano?
Sim.

HIPOMAGNESEMIA

HEMOGRAMA/BIOQUÍMICA/URINÁLISE
- Baixo nível sérico de magnésio.
- Se o paciente tiver azotemia, considerar o envolvimento de causas renais.
- Cilindros tubulares no sedimento urinário podem ser indício de nefrotoxicidade.
- Hipocalemia, hiponatremia e hipocalcemia são achados comuns em casos de hipomagnesemia.
- Hipocalemia ou hiponatremia deve alertar o clínico para a possibilidade de hipomagnesemia.

OUTROS TESTES LABORATORIAIS
- O diagnóstico de depleção de magnésio pode não ser uma tarefa fácil, pois menos de 1% do magnésio corporal total se encontra no soro; apenas 55% do magnésio no plasma estão na forma ativa (ionizada); 33% estão ligados a proteínas plasmáticas e 12% estão quelados com ânions divalentes como fosfato e sulfato; ensaios com magnésio (espectrofotometria) medem todas as três frações.
- O magnésio ionizado pode ser medido com o uso de eletrodo íon-seletivo ou por ultrafiltração do plasma; métodos alternativos de avaliar o estado do magnésio incluem os níveis desse elemento nas células sanguíneas mononucleares ou a quantificação da retenção a partir de uma dose de ataque.
- A determinação do magnésio urinário pode ajudar a diferenciar entre condições associadas à perda urinária elevada de magnésio e condições de baixo consumo ou pouca absorção.
- Estudos em humanos sugerem que a retenção de mais de 40-50% de uma dose de ataque de magnésio administrada indica depleção de magnésio, enquanto a retenção de menos de 20% indica reservas adequadas desse elemento.

MÉTODOS DIAGNÓSTICOS
Eletrodiagnósticos (p. ex., eletromielografia e eletrocardiografia) podem revelar os efeitos da hipomagnesemia, mas não ajudam a diferenciar a causa.

TRATAMENTO

CUIDADO(S) DE SAÚDE ADEQUADO(S)
- O tratamento depende da causa subjacente da anormalidade e da gravidade da hipomagnesemia.
- A experiência no tratamento de pacientes veterinários com hipomagnesemia é limitada ao tratamento da(s) condição(ões) subjacente(s) e à reposição de magnésio.
- A hipomagnesemia discreta pode se resolver com o tratamento do distúrbio subjacente; no entanto, se a hipomagnesemia for grave, haverá necessidade do fornecimento de cuidados intensivos e da reposição de magnésio.

CUIDADO(S) DE ENFERMAGEM
A hipomagnesemia é um achado comum em pacientes veterinários hospitalizados criticamente enfermos. Os cuidados de enfermagem devem se concentrar no(s) distúrbio(s) subjacente(s).

ATIVIDADE
As restrições da atividade física devem ser feitas com base nas condições concomitantes.

DIETA
Não há recomendações nutricionais para hipomagnesemia a não ser a de suprir as necessidades calóricas dos pacientes com uma dieta balanceada e apropriada, que leve em consideração todos os problemas concomitantes.

MEDICAÇÕES

MEDICAMENTO(S) DE ESCOLHA
- O sulfato de magnésio pode ser diluído em glicose a 5% em água.
- A dose de ataque de emergência é feita com 0,15-0,3 mEq/kg de sulfato de magnésio ou cloreto de magnésio em 5-60 minutos.
- A rápida reposição pode ser concluída pela administração de 0,75-1 mEq/kg/dia (0,03 mEq/kg/h) de sulfato de magnésio ou cloreto de magnésio sob infusão intravenosa em velocidade constante; a solução de sais de magnésio deve ter uma concentração <20%; a infusão de magnésio deve utilizar um equipo intravenoso separado para minimizar as interações com outros minerais.
- Administrar 0,3-0,5 mEq/kg/dia (0,013-0,02 mEq/kg/h) de sulfato de magnésio ou cloreto de magnésio para reposição lenta.

CONTRAINDICAÇÕES
- Não usar aminoglicosídeos, pois a hipomagnesemia potencializa sua nefrotoxicidade.
- Não usar quimioterapia com cisplatina.

PRECAUÇÕES
- Interromper o uso de digoxina, se possível.
- Usar diuréticos com cautela.
- É possível ocorrer hipermagnesemia com o tratamento excessivo.
- Pacientes com azotemia que necessitam de terapia com magnésio devem receber uma dose mais baixa desse elemento e ser submetidos à monitorização mais frequente que aqueles com função renal normal, para evitar hipermagnesemia iatrogênica.

INTERAÇÕES POSSÍVEIS
- O sulfato de magnésio é incompatível com bicarbonato de sódio, hidrocortisona e cloridrato de dobutamina; evitar a mistura de outros fármacos com solução de sulfato de magnésio.
- Evitar compostos que contenham cálcio, pois eles diminuem a concentração sérica de magnésio.
- Pode ocorrer depressão adicional do SNC ao se utilizar sulfato de magnésio parenteral com sedativos depressores do SNC, bloqueadores neuromusculares e anestésicos.
- O sulfato de magnésio parenteral usado com bloqueadores neuromusculares não despolarizantes causou bloqueio neuromuscular excessivo.
- Ter cautela ao usar suplementação de magnésio com compostos digitálicos para evitar distúrbios sérios da condução cardíaca.
- Os suplementos de cálcio podem anular os efeitos do magnésio parenteral.

ACOMPANHAMENTO

MONITORIZAÇÃO DO PACIENTE
- Concentrações séricas diárias de magnésio e cálcio.
- ECG contínuo, especialmente durante a infusão de magnésio.

COMPLICAÇÕES POSSÍVEIS
A hipomagnesemia grave pode ser fatal.

EVOLUÇÃO ESPERADA E PROGNÓSTICO
Os resultados dependem da resolução da(s) doença(s) subjacente(s).

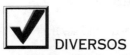

DIVERSOS

DISTÚRBIOS ASSOCIADOS
- Hipertireoidismo.
- Hipocalemia.
- Hiponatremia.
- Hipocalcemia.
- Hipoparatireoidismo.
- Hipofosfatemia.

GESTAÇÃO/FERTILIDADE/REPRODUÇÃO
Os efeitos sobre o feto são idênticos aos observados sobre a mãe.

VER TAMBÉM
Ver a seção "Causas".

ABREVIATURA(S)
- ATP = trifosfato de adenosina.
- Cl⁻ = cloreto.
- EDTA = ácido etilenodiaminotetracético.
- Mg = magnésio.
- Na = sódio.
- PTH = paratormônio.
- SNC = sistema nervoso central.

RECURSOS DA INTERNET
http://www.merck.com/mmpe/sec12/ch156/ch156i.html.

Sugestões de Leitura
Bateman SW. Disorders of magnesium: Magnesium deficit and excess. In: DiBartola SP, ed., Fluid, Electrolyte and Acid-Base Disorders in Small Animal Practice, 3rd ed. Philadelphia: Elsevier, 2006, pp. 210-226.
Fincham SC, Drobatz KJ, Gillespie TN, Hess RS. Evaluation of plasma-ionized magnesium concentration in 122 dogs with diabetes mellitus: A retrospective study. J Vet Intern Med 2004, 18(5):612-617.
Khanna C, Lund EM, Raffe M, et al. Hypomagnesemia in 188 dogs: A hospital population-based prevalence study. J Vet Intern Med 1998, 12(4):304-309.
Martin LG, Matteson VL, Wingfield WE, et al. Abnormalities of serum magnesium in critically ill dogs: Incidence and implications. J Vet Emerg Crit Care 1994, 4:15-20.
Schenck PA, Chew DJ. Understanding recent developments in hypocalcemia and hypomagnesemia. In: Proceedings of the American College of Veterinary Internal Medicine, Baltimore, 2005, pp. 666-668.

Autor Tim B. Hackett
Consultor Editorial Deborah S. Greco

HIPOMIELINIZAÇÃO

CONSIDERAÇÕES GERAIS

DEFINIÇÃO
• Distúrbio causado pela produção insuficiente de mielina durante a gestação.
• Os axônios com mais de 1-2 mm de diâmetro têm um revestimento de mielina originária de oligodendrócitos no SNC e células de Schwann no SNP.
• A mielina isola os axônios e facilita a propagação dos potenciais de ação.

IDENTIFICAÇÃO
SNC
• Cães e gatos.
• Relatada nas raças de cães Welsh Springer spaniel, Samoieda, Chow chow, Weimaraner, Montanhês de Berna, Dálmata e Lurcher (mestiços ingleses).
• Gato Siamês.
• Predominância sexual — os filhotes machos de Springer spaniel e Samoieda são acometidos em termos clínicos, enquanto as fêmeas permanecem basicamente como portadoras assintomáticas; não há relatos de diferenças sexuais em outras raças.
SNP
• Cães.
• Golden retriever — relatada em ambos os sexos.

SINAIS CLÍNICOS
SNC
• Os sinais clínicos aparecem dentro de dias após o nascimento.
• Tremores corporais generalizados que se agravam com o exercício e diminuem em repouso.
• Melhoram por volta de 1 ano de idade, exceto em Springer spaniel e Samoieda, que são acometidos pelo resto da vida.
SNP
• Os sinais clínicos aparecem com 5-7 semanas de vida.
• Fraqueza generalizada, ataxia dos membros pélvicos, emaciação muscular e hiporreflexia.
• Melhoram com a idade.

CAUSAS E FATORES DE RISCO
• Genéticos — distúrbio recessivo ligado ao cromossomo X comprovado para doença do SNC em cães da raça Springer spaniel; especulativos em outras raças.
• Virais ou tóxicos — possíveis nas raças Chow chow, Weimaraner, Montanhês de Berna, Dálmata e Lurcher, porque os sinais clínicos de doença do SNC melhoram ou desaparecem.
• SNP — indeterminados; possivelmente genéticos.

DIAGNÓSTICO

DIAGNÓSTICO DIFERENCIAL
SNC
• Hipoplasia ou abiotrofia cerebelar — tremores em neonatos; no entanto, os sinais de ataxia e tremores intencionais são mais proeminentes.
• Doenças do armazenamento — associadas a tremores; os neonatos permanecem normais.
• Tremores idiopáticos em cães brancos não se desenvolvem antes dos 8 meses de vida.
SNP
• Distrofia muscular.
• Miastenia grave congênita.
• Outras polineuropatias ou miopatias.

HEMOGRAMA/BIOQUÍMICA/URINÁLISE
Geralmente normais.

OUTROS TESTES LABORATORIAIS
N/D.

DIAGNÓSTICO POR IMAGEM
RM — detecta a forma da doença no SNC.

MÉTODOS DIAGNÓSTICOS
SNC
• O diagnóstico baseia-se nos sinais clínicos.
• Biopsia cerebral.
• Necropsia.
SNP
• Eletromiografia — geralmente exibe uma atividade espontânea difusa normal a leve.
• Velocidade da condução nervosa motora — potenciais evocados pequenos ou ausentes e condução lenta.
• Biopsia de nervo — mielina insuficiente em torno de axônios periféricos.

TRATAMENTO
Não há tratamento eficaz para ambas as formas.

MEDICAÇÕES

MEDICAMENTO(S)
N/D.

CONTRAINDICAÇÕES/INTERAÇÕES POSSÍVEIS
N/D.

ACOMPANHAMENTO

PREVENÇÃO
Evitar o acasalamento de animais em que se suspeita de alguma causa genética.

EVOLUÇÃO ESPERADA E PROGNÓSTICO
• SNC — cães das raças Springer spaniel e Samoieda são acometidos por toda a vida; outras raças melhoram por volta de 1 ano de idade.
• SNP — cães com expectativa de vida normal.

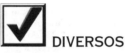

DIVERSOS

ABREVIATURA(S)
• RM = ressonância magnética.
• SNC = sistema nervoso central.
• SNP = sistema nervoso periférico.

Sugestões de Leitura
Braund KG, Mehta JR, Toivio-Kinnucan M, Amling KA, Shell LG, Matz ME. Congenital hypomyelinating polyneuropathy in two golden retriever littermates. Vet Pathol 1989, 26:202-208.
Duncan ID. Abnormalities of myelination of the central nervous system associated with congenital tremor. J Vet Intern Med 1987, 1:10-23.
Matz ME, Shell L, Braund K. Peripheral hypomyelinization in two golden retriever litter mates. JAVMA 1990, 197:228-230.
Stoffregen DA, Huxtable CR, Cummings JF, et al. Hypomyelination of the central nervous system of two Siamese kitten littermates. Vet Pathol 1993, 30:388-391.

Autor Karen Dyer Inzana
Consultor Editorial Joane M. Parent

Hiponatremia

CONSIDERAÇÕES GERAIS

DEFINIÇÃO
Concentração sérica de sódio abaixo do limite inferior da faixa de referência.

FISIOPATOLOGIA
O sódio é o cátion mais abundante presente no líquido extracelular. A hiponatremia em geral, mas nem sempre, reflete hiposmolalidade e tipicamente está associada ao conteúdo corporal total diminuído desse cátion. Teoricamente, a perda de soluto ou a retenção de água podem causar hiponatremia. A maior parte da perda de soluto ocorre em soluções isosmóticas (p. ex., vômitos e diarreia) e, em consequência disso, a retenção de água em relação ao soluto constitui a causa subjacente em quase todos os pacientes com hiponatremia. Em geral, ocorre hiponatremia somente quando há um defeito na excreção renal de água.

SISTEMA(S) ACOMETIDO(S)
• Nervoso — em geral, não se observa disfunção neurológica grave até que a concentração sérica de sódio caia abaixo de 110-115 mEq/L. Os sinais clínicos podem estar mais relacionados com a velocidade de declínio na concentração sérica de sódio do que com o nadir (nível mais baixo) atual. Os cães com hiponatremia crônica frequentemente apresentam sinais clínicos leves ou ausentes.
• A correção muito rápida da hiponatremia também pode causar dano neurológico.

IDENTIFICAÇÃO
Espécies
Cães e gatos.

SINAIS CLÍNICOS
• Letargia. • Fraqueza. • Confusão mental.
• Náusea e vômitos. • Crises convulsivas.
• Obnubilação. • Coma. • Outros achados dependem da causa subjacente.

CAUSAS
Hiponatremia Osmolar Normal
• Hiperlipidemia. • Hiperproteinemia.
Hiponatremia Hiperosmolar
• Hiperglicemia. • Infusão de manitol.
Hiponatremia Hiposmolar
Normovolêmica
• Polidipsia primária. • Coma mixedematoso do hipotireoidismo. • Infusão de fluido hipotônico.
• Síndrome da secreção inadequada de ADH.
Hipervolêmica
• Insuficiência cardíaca congestiva. • Cirrose hepática. • Síndrome nefrótica. • Insuficiência renal grave.
Hipovolêmica
• Perdas gastrintestinais. • Insuficiência renal.
• Perdas para o terceiro espaço. • Perdas cutâneas.
• Diurese. • Hipoadrenocorticismo.

DIAGNÓSTICO

ACHADOS LABORATORIAIS
Medicamentos Capazes de Alterar os Resultados Laboratoriais
• O manitol pode causar pseudo-hiponatremia.
• A administração de diuréticos pode causar hiponatremia.
Distúrbios Capazes de Alterar os Resultados Laboratoriais
• Hiperlipidemia, hiperglicemia e hiperproteinemia podem causar pseudo-hiponatremia.
Os Resultados Serão Válidos se os Exames Forem Realizados em Laboratório Humano?
Sim.

HEMOGRAMA/BIOQUÍMICA/URINÁLISE
• Baixa concentração sérica de sódio.
• Outras anormalidades podem apontar a causa subjacente.

OUTROS TESTES LABORATORIAIS
• A osmolalidade plasmática costuma estar baixa; se ela estiver normal ou alta, descartar hiperlipidemia, hiperglicemia, hiperproteinemia e administração de manitol.
• Osmolalidade urinária <100-150 mOsmol/kg indica polidipsia primária ou reajuste do osmostato. Osmolalidade urinária >150-200 mOsmol/kg indica comprometimento da excreção renal de água.
• A concentração urinária de sódio <15-20 mEq/L indica baixo volume efetivo circulante, deficiência pura de cortisol, polidipsia primária com débito urinário alto, enquanto a concentração urinária de sódio >20-25 mEq/L indica síndrome da secreção inadequada de ADH, insuficiência adrenal, insuficiência renal, reajuste do osmostato, administração de diurético ou vômitos com perda acentuada de bicarbonato.

TRATAMENTO

O tratamento hospitalar *versus* ambulatorial depende da gravidade da hiponatremia, da existência de disfunção neurológica associada e do distúrbio subjacente.

ORIENTAÇÃO AO PROPRIETÁRIO
Depende do distúrbio subjacente.

MEDICAÇÕES

MEDICAMENTO(S) DE ESCOLHA
• O tratamento consiste em aumentar a concentração sérica de sódio e tratar a causa subjacente, se necessário. A normalização muito rápida da hiponatremia pode dar origem a sequelas neurológicas potencialmente graves e ser mais prejudicial que a hiponatremia em si. Portanto, a salina isotônica constitui o fluido de escolha na grande maioria dos casos. Raramente, há necessidade de uma correção mais rigorosa da concentração sérica de sódio com salina hipertônica.
• Os pacientes (edematosos) hipervolêmicos são tipicamente tratados com diuréticos e restrição de sal. A salina isotônica e a furosemida podem ser úteis em pacientes mais acometidos.
• Os pacientes hipovolêmicos são tratados por meio da reposição do déficit volêmico com o uso de salina isotônica.
• O emprego de salina hipertônica pode ser considerado em pacientes selecionados com hiponatremia sintomática grave. O déficit de sódio é estimado em 0,5 × peso corporal magro (kg) × (120 – concentração sérica de sódio). A concentração sérica de sódio é corrigida em uma velocidade de 10-12 mEq/L/dia (0,5 mEq/L/h) ou menos. Assim que a concentração sérica de sódio atingir 120-150 mEq/L, é preciso interromper a salina hipertônica e prosseguir com o uso da salina isotônica ou a restrição de sódio até normalizar lentamente a concentração sérica desse cátion, conforme ditado pela causa subjacente da hiponatremia.
• Outras intervenções terapêuticas são determinadas pela causa subjacente da hiponatremia.

PRECAUÇÕES
A rápida correção da hiponatremia pode resultar em dano neurológico (desmielinização); evitar o aumento na concentração sérica de sódio em mais de 10-12 mEq/L/dia (0,5 mEq/L/h).

ACOMPANHAMENTO

MONITORIZAÇÃO DO PACIENTE
• Efetuar determinações seriadas do sódio sérico para evitar a correção muito rápida da concentração sérica desse cátion e para garantir a resposta adequada ao NaCL e a outras terapias indicadas.
• Monitorizar o estado de hidratação.
• Monitorizar as concentrações de outros eletrólitos séricos, conforme indicado pela condição clínica do paciente e pelo distúrbio subjacente.

PREVENÇÃO
Depende do distúrbio subjacente.

COMPLICAÇÕES POSSÍVEIS
Depende do distúrbio subjacente.

EVOLUÇÃO ESPERADA E PROGNÓSTICO
Depende do distúrbio subjacente.

DIVERSOS

DISTÚRBIOS ASSOCIADOS
Outras anormalidades eletrolíticas e acidobásicas são frequentemente associadas aos distúrbios clínicos que causam hiponatremia.

VER TAMBÉM
• Cirrose e Fibrose do Fígado.
• Insuficiência Cardíaca Congestiva Esquerda.
• Hiperglicemia.
• Hiperlipidemia.
• Hipoadrenocorticismo (doença de Addison).
• Mixedema e Coma Mixedematoso.
• Síndrome Nefrótica.
• Poliúria e Polidipsia.
• Insuficiência Renal Crônica.

ABREVIATURA(S)
• ADH = hormônio antidiurético.

Autor Peter P. Kintzer
Consultor Editorial Deborah S. Greco

HIPOPARATIREOIDISMO

CONSIDERAÇÕES GERAIS

DEFINIÇÃO
Deficiência absoluta ou relativa da secreção de paratormônio que acarreta hipocalcemia.

FISIOPATOLOGIA
• Cães — é mais comum uma paratireoidite imunomediada idiopática.
• Gatos — mais comumente iatrogênico secundário a paratireoides lesionadas ou removidas durante tireoidectomia por causa de hipertireoidismo; atrofia idiopática e paratireoidite imunomediada também são observadas (incomuns).

SISTEMA(S) ACOMETIDO(S)
• Nervoso/neuromuscular — crises convulsivas, tetania, ataxia e fraqueza causadas por aumento da atividade neuromuscular resultante da diminuição na estabilidade da membrana neuronal.
• Cardiovascular — alterações no ECG e bradicardia causadas por modificação na atividade neuromuscular.
• Gastrintestinal — anorexia e vômitos (sobretudo em gatos) de causa desconhecida, possivelmente alterações na atividade muscular gastrintestinal.
• Oftálmico — cataratas lenticulares posteriores de causa desconhecida.
• Respiratório — respiração ofegante causada por fraqueza neuromuscular e ansiedade associada a alterações neurológicas e neuromusculares.
• Renal/urológico — poliúria e polidipsia (PU/PD) de causa desconhecida.

GENÉTICA
Desconhecida.

INCIDÊNCIA/PREVALÊNCIA
• Cães — incomum; a prevalência exata não é relatada.
• Gatos — comum naqueles submetidos à tireoidectomia (10-82% dos pacientes, dependendo da técnica cirúrgica e da habilidade do cirurgião); ocorrência espontânea rara (9 casos relatados na literatura especializada, mais 5 casos de gatos discutidos no livro *Canine and Feline Endocrinology and Reproduction* — ver a seção de "Sugestões de Leitura").

IDENTIFICAÇÃO
Espécies
Cães e gatos.

Raças Predominantes
Poodle toy, Schnauzer miniatura, Pastor alemão, Labrador retriever e raças terrier; gatos mestiços.

Idade Média e Faixa Etária
• Cães — idade média, 4,8 anos; variação, 6 semanas a 13 anos.
• Gatos — secundário à tireoidectomia: idade média 12-13 anos, com variação de 4-22 anos; espontâneo: idade média 2,25 anos, com variação de 6 meses a 7 anos.

Sexo Predominante
• Caninos — fêmeas (60%).
• Felinos — machos (64%).

SINAIS CLÍNICOS
Achados Anamnésicos
Cães
• Crises convulsivas (49-86%).
• Ataxia/marcha rígida (43-62%).
• Fricção facial (62%).
• Tremores, torções e fasciculações musculares (57%).
• Rugido (57%).
• Respiração ofegante (35%).
• Fraqueza.
• PU/PD.
• Vômitos.
• Anorexia.
Gatos
• Letargia, anorexia e depressão (100%).
• Crises convulsivas (50%).
• Tremores, torções e fasciculações musculares (83%).
• Respiração ofegante (33%).
• Bradicardia (17%).

Achados do Exame Físico
Cães
• Abdome tenso, dividido (50-65%).
• Ataxia/marcha rígida (43-62%).
• Febre (30-70%).
• Tremores, torções e fasciculações musculares (57%).
• Respiração ofegante (35%).
• Cataratas lenticulares posteriores (15-32%).
• Fraqueza.
• Até 20% podem exibir resultados normais ao exame físico.
Gatos
• Tremores, torções e fasciculações musculares (83%).
• Respiração ofegante (33%).
• Cataratas lenticulares posteriores (33%).
• Bradicardia (17%).
• Febre (17%).
• Hipotermia (17%).

CAUSAS
Ver a seção "Fisiopatologia".

FATORES DE RISCO
• Cães — N/D.
• Gatos — tireoidectomia para hipertireoidismo.

DIAGNÓSTICO

DIAGNÓSTICO DIFERENCIAL
Os principais problemas associados ao hipoparatireoidismo, que precisam ser diferenciados de outros processos mórbidos, são crises convulsivas, fraqueza e tremores, torções e fasciculações musculares.

Crises Convulsivas
• Cardiovasculares — síncope.
• Metabólicas — encefalopatia hepática e hipoglicemia.
• Neurológicas — epilepsia, neoplasia, toxinas e doença inflamatória.

Fraqueza
• Cardiovasculares — defeitos anatômicos congênitos, arritmias, insuficiência cardíaca e efusão pericárdica.
• Metabólicas — hipoadrenocorticismo, hipoglicemia, anemia, hipocalcemia (especialmente em gatos) e hipotireoidismo.
• Neurológicas/neuromusculares — miastenia grave, polimiosite, polirradiculoneuropatia e mielopatia.
• Tóxicas — paralisia causada por carrapatos, botulismo, exposição crônica a organofosforados e intoxicação pelo chumbo.

Tremores, Torções e Fasciculações Musculares
• Metabólicas — hipercalcemia, hiperadrenocorticismo e tetania puerperal (i. e., eclâmpsia).
• Tóxicas — tétano e envenenamento pela estricnina.

HEMOGRAMA/BIOQUÍMICA/URINÁLISE
• Os resultados do hemograma e da urinálise costumam permanecer normais; esses exames são feitos para excluir outros diagnósticos diferenciais.
• Hipocalcemia (em geral, <6,5 mg/dL) e níveis normais de fosfato ou hiperfosfatemia leve a moderada.
• Avaliar a albumina sérica com cuidado em todos os pacientes com hipocalcemia; hipoalbuminemia é a causa mais comum de hipocalcemia; em cães com hipoalbuminemia, deve-se usar uma das seguintes fórmulas para corrigir o cálcio sérico:

$$\text{Ca corrigido} = [\text{Ca (mg/dL)} - \text{albumina (g/dL)}] + 3,5$$

ou

$$\text{Ca corrigido} = [\text{Ca (mg/dL)} - \{0,4 \times \text{proteína total (g/dL)}\}] + 3,3$$

• A hipocalcemia causada por hipoalbuminemia em gatos não pode ser corrigida por essas fórmulas, embora a última diminua o cálcio sérico nesses animais.
• O outro único processo mórbido que reduz o cálcio sérico e aumenta o fósforo sérico é a insuficiência renal, fácil de distinguir do hipoparatireoidismo pela presença de azotemia.

OUTROS TESTES LABORATORIAIS
Determinação do PTH sérico — demonstra uma concentração não detectável ou muito baixa desse hormônio; os pacientes com outros processos indutores de hipocalcemia (p. ex., insuficiência renal) têm uma concentração de PTH normal a alta.

DIAGNÓSTICO POR IMAGEM
Radiografia e ultrassonografia normais.

MÉTODOS DIAGNÓSTICOS
• As alterações no ECG observadas em pacientes com hipocalcemia incluem prolongamento dos segmentos ST e QT; ocasionalmente, observam-se bradicardia sinusal e ondas T largas ou alternantes.
• A exploração cervical revela ausência ou atrofia das paratireoides.

ACHADOS PATOLÓGICOS
• Cães — tecido normal com linfócitos maduros, plasmócitos e tecido conjuntivo fibroso juntamente com degeneração de células principais.
• Gatos — a atrofia da paratireoide é mais comum, embora os achados histopatológicos semelhantes àqueles observados em cães tenham sido encontrados em gatos.

TRATAMENTO

CUIDADO(S) DE SAÚDE ADEQUADO(S)
• Internar para o tratamento clínico da hipocalcemia até que os sinais clínicos de hipocalcemia sejam controlados e a concentração sérica de cálcio esteja >7 mg/dL.

HIPOPARATIREOIDISMO

- Ver em "Hipocalcemia" o tratamento hospitalar de emergência e a fluidoterapia apropriada.

CUIDADO(S) DE ENFERMAGEM
Em geral, não há necessidade; fornecer hidratação e suporte nutricional em animal anoréxico.

ATIVIDADE
Normal.

DIETA
Evitar dietas pobres em cálcio.

ORIENTAÇÃO AO PROPRIETÁRIO
- Hipoparatireoidismo primário de ocorrência natural necessitará de tratamento e monitorização pelo resto da vida.
- A maioria dos casos de hipoparatireoidismo iatrogênico (p. ex., após tireoidectomia) apresentará recuperação espontânea, necessitando apenas de tratamento e monitorização transitórios.

CONSIDERAÇÕES CIRÚRGICAS
Nenhuma.

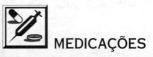

MEDICAÇÕES
MEDICAMENTO(S) DE ESCOLHA
Terapia de Emergência/Aguda
- Ver "Hipocalcemia".

Terapia a Curto Prazo após Tetania
- Ver "Hipocalcemia".

Terapia a Longo Prazo
- A administração de vitamina D é necessária por tempo indefinido; a dose deve ser aumentada ou ajustada de acordo com a concentração sérica de cálcio.
- Preparações de ação mais curta de vitamina D são preferíveis, para que a dosagem excessiva (hipercalcemia) possa ser rapidamente corrigida (ver Tab. 1).
- Uma abordagem mais econômica ao tratamento consiste em maximizar a administração oral de cálcio e reduzir a de vitamina D; o cálcio em geral é menos oneroso que a vitamina D (ver Tab. 2).

CONTRAINDICAÇÕES
Ver "Hipocalcemia".

PRECAUÇÕES
Todas as preparações de cálcio administradas por via oral podem causar distúrbios gastrintestinais; o carbonato de cálcio pode ser menos irritante por causa de sua alta disponibilidade de cálcio e necessidade de menor dosagem.

INTERAÇÕES POSSÍVEIS
- Segundo relatos, soluções injetáveis de cálcio são incompatíveis com tetraciclina, cefalotina, succinato sódico de metilprednisolona, dobutamina, metoclopramida e anfotericina B.
- Diuréticos tiazídicos usados em conjunto com grandes doses de cálcio podem causar hipercalcemia.
- Pacientes que estejam tomando digitálicos serão mais propensos ao desenvolvimento de arritmias se o cálcio for administrado por via intravenosa.
- A administração de cálcio pode antagonizar os efeitos dos agentes bloqueadores dos canais de cálcio (p. ex., diltiazem, verapamil, nifedipino e anlodipino).

MEDICAMENTO(S) ALTERNATIVO(S)
Nenhum.

ACOMPANHAMENTO
MONITORAÇÃO DO PACIENTE
- Hipocalcemia e hipercalcemia são preocupações no tratamento a longo prazo.
- Assim que o cálcio sérico estiver estabilizado e normal, verificar a concentração sérica desse elemento mensalmente nos primeiros 6 meses e, em seguida, a cada 2-4 meses; o objetivo é manter o cálcio sérico entre 8 e 10 mg/dL.
- Informar os proprietários sobre os sinais clínicos de hipo e hipercalcemia.

Tabela 1.

	Preparações de Vitamina D		
Preparação	Dose	Efeito Máximo	Tamanho
1,25 Di-hidroxicolecalciferol (vitamina D$_3$ ativa, calcitriol)	0,03-0,06 mcg/kg/dia	1-4 dias	Cápsulas de 0,25 e 0,5 µg, solução oral de 1,0 µg/mL e injetável de 1 e 2 mcg/mL
Di-hidrotaquisterol	Inicial: 0,02-0,03 mg/kg/dia Manutenção: 0,01-0,02 mg/kg/24-48 h	1-7 dias	Atualmente indisponível; disponível antigamente sob a forma de comprimidos de 0,125 mg, 0,2 mg e 0,4 mg e xarope de 0,2 mg/mL.
Ergocalciferol (vitamina D$_2$)	Inicial: 4.000-6.000 U/kg/dia Manutenção: 1.000-2.000 U/kg/dia-semana	5-21 dias	Cápsulas de 25.000 e 50.000 U e xarope de 8.000 U/mL

Tabela 2.

	Preparações de Cálcio		
Preparação	Dose de Cálcio Elementar	Cálcio Disponível	Tamanho Disponível (Necessidades a serem convertidas em Cálcio Elementar)
Carbonato de cálcio	Cães: 1-4 g/dia Gatos: 0,5-1 g/dia	40%	Comprimidos — 500, 600, 650, 1.250, 1.500 mg Comprimidos mastigáveis — 400, 420, 500, 750, 850, 1.000, 1.250 mg Cápsulas — 1.250 mg Suspensão oral — 250 mg/mL
Gliconato de cálcio	Cães: 1-4 g/dia Gatos: 0,5-1 g/dia	10%	Comprimidos — 500, 650, 975 mg Comprimidos mastigáveis — 500 mg Cápsulas — 500, 700 mg Pó para suspensão — 70 mg/mL
Lactato de cálcio	Cães: 1-4 g/dia Gatos: 0,5-1 g/dia	13%	Comprimidos — 650, 770 mg Cápsulas — 500 mg
Acetato de cálcio	Cães: 1-4 g/dia Gatos: 0,5-1 g/dia	25%	Comprimidos, cápsulas gelatinosas e cápsulas — 667 mg
Citrato de cálcio	Cães: 1-4 g/dia Gatos: 0,5-1 g/dia	21%	Comprimidos — 950, 1.150 mg Comprimidos efervescentes — 2.380 mg Cápsulas — 850, 1.070 mg Pó para suspensão oral — 725 mg/mL
Glibionato de cálcio	Cães: 1-4 g/dia Gatos: 0,5-1 g/dia	30%	Xarope — 360 mg/mL

HIPOPARATIREOIDISMO

PREVENÇÃO
N/D.

COMPLICAÇÕES POSSÍVEIS
• Hipocalcemia.
• Hipercalcemia, que pode levar à insuficiência renal (ver "Hipercalcemia").

EVOLUÇÃO ESPERADA E PROGNÓSTICO
• Com a monitorização estrita do cálcio sérico e a dedicação do proprietário, o prognóstico em termos de sobrevida a longo prazo é excelente.
• Ajustes na administração de vitamina D e cálcio oral podem ser esperados durante o curso terapêutico, especialmente nos 2-6 primeiros meses.
• Gatos com hipoparatireoidismo secundário à tireoidectomia, em geral, necessitam apenas de tratamento transitório, porque costumam recuperar a função paratireóidea normal em 4-6 meses, muitas vezes em 2-3 semanas.

DIVERSOS

DISTÚRBIOS ASSOCIADOS
O excesso de atividade muscular pode acarretar hipertermia, o que pode necessitar de tratamento.

FATORES RELACIONADOS COM A IDADE
N/D.

POTENCIAL ZOONÓTICO
Nenhum.

GESTAÇÃO/FERTILIDADE/REPRODUÇÃO
A hipocalcemia pode acarretar fraqueza e distocia.

VER TAMBÉM
• Hipercalcemia.
• Hipertireoidismo.
• Hipocalcemia.

ABREVIATURA(S)
• Ca = cálcio.
• ECG = eletrocardiograma.
• PTH = paratormônio.
• PU/PD = poliúria e polidipsia.

RECURSOS DA INTERNET
http://www.vet.uga.edu/VPP/CLERK/mcfarland/index.php.

Sugestões de Leitura
Bruyette DS, Feldman EC. Primary hypoparathyroidism in the dog: Report of 15 cases and review of 13 previously reported cases. J Vet Intern Med 1988, 2:7-14.
Feldman EC, Nelson RW. Hypocalcemia and primary hypoparathyroidism. In: Feldman EC, Nelson RW, eds., Canine and Feline Endocrinology and Reproduction, 3rd ed. St. Louis: Saunders, 2004, pp. 716-742.
Henderson AK, Mahony O. Hypoparathyroidism: Pathophysiology and diagnosis. Compend Contin Educ Pract Vet 2005, 27(4):270-279.
Henderson AK, Mahony O. Hypoparathyroidism: Treatment. Compend Contin Educ Pract Vet 2005, 27(4):280-287.
Peterson ME, James KM, Wallace M, et al. Idiopathic hypoparathyroidism in five cats. J Vet Intern Med 1991, 5:47-51.
Waters CB, Scott-Moncrieff JCR. Hypocalcemia in cats. Compend Contin Educ Pract Vet 1992, 14:497-507.

Autor Mitchell A. Crystal
Consultor Editorial Deborah S. Greco

Hipópio e Depósito Lipídico

CONSIDERAÇÕES GERAIS

REVISÃO
• Hipópio — acúmulo de leucócitos na câmara anterior do olho. A ruptura inflamatória da barreira hematoaquosa permite a entrada de células sanguíneas na câmara anterior; o influxo é mediado por fatores quimiotáticos. As células frequentemente se depositam por causa da gravidade.
• Depósito lipídico — embora se assemelhe ao hipópio, a turbidez da câmara anterior é causada pela alta concentração de lipídios no humor aquoso. A ocorrência depende da ruptura da barreira hematoaquosa e da presença de hiperlipidemia concomitante.

IDENTIFICAÇÃO
Acomete tanto cães como gatos, sem predominância etária ou sexual.

SINAIS CLÍNICOS
• Hipópio — opacidade branca a amarelada dentro da câmara anterior; pode ser um acúmulo ventral de células ou preencher completamente a câmara anterior. O acúmulo de fibrina na câmara anterior pode impedir o depósito discreto de leucócitos, resultando em células suspensas dentro da matriz de fibrina. Os sinais oftálmicos concomitantes incluem blefarospasmo, epífora, edema difuso da córnea, rubor aquoso, miose, tumefação da íris e perda da visão.
• Depósito lipídico — aspecto leitoso difuso da câmara anterior. Os sinais oftálmicos concomitantes podem incluir perda da visão, blefarospasmo discreto e edema difuso da córnea leve a moderado.

CAUSAS E FATORES DE RISCO
Hipópio
Qualquer causa de uveíte pode resultar em hipópio. Mais comumente, ele está associado à uveíte grave. Também pode resultar do acúmulo de células neoplásicas em caso de linfoma ocular.

Depósito Lipídico
Resulta de hiperlipidemia e uveíte concomitante. A hiperlipidemia também pode desestabilizar a barreira hematoaquosa por via direta. Ocasionalmente, a lipidemia pós-prandial pode resultar em humor aquoso lipidêmico na presença de uveíte.

DIAGNÓSTICO

DIAGNÓSTICO DIFERENCIAL
Hipópio
Fibrina na câmara anterior — em geral, forma um coágulo irregular, não uma linha horizontal localizada ventralmente.

Depósito Lipídico
• Rubor aquoso intenso — não tem o aspecto leitoso/esbranquiçado do depósito lipídico. Os animais com rubor aquoso intenso costumam exibir muito mais dor ocular do que aqueles com depósito lipídico.
• Edema difuso da córnea — o edema grave dessa estrutura ocular pode ser confundido com opacidade da câmara anterior, mas no primeiro há espessamento do estroma da córnea, ceratocone* e bolhas na córnea.

HEMOGRAMA/BIOQUÍMICA/URINÁLISE
Hipópio
Geralmente normais; pode haver anormalidades relacionadas com a causa subjacente da uveíte.

Depósito Lipídico
Níveis séricos elevados de triglicerídeos e colesterol; pode haver outras anormalidades relacionadas com o(s) distúrbio(s) metabólico(s) subjacente(s).

OUTROS TESTES LABORATORIAIS
Hipópio
Nenhum se o hipópio estiver relacionado com doença de córnea óbvia; se relacionado com uveíte, procurar a causa subjacente dessa condição (ver "Uveíte Anterior — Cães"; "Uveíte Anterior — Gatos").

Depósito Lipídico
Ver "Hiperlipidemia".

MÉTODOS DIAGNÓSTICOS
A centese (punção) da câmara anterior fica indicada na suspeita de hipópio de origem neoplásica (p. ex., linfoma); esse procedimento não é recompensador em outras circunstâncias.

TRATAMENTO

• O hipópio requer o tratamento rigoroso da uveíte e da causa subjacente. O tratamento ambulatorial é adequado.
• O depósito lipídico necessita do tratamento da uveíte e do distúrbio metabólico subjacente. O tratamento ambulatorial também é adequado.

MEDICAÇÕES

MEDICAMENTO(S)
Hipópio

Corticosteroides
Tópicos
• Acetato de prednisolona a 1% — aplicar 2-6 vezes ao dia, dependendo da gravidade da doença.
• Dexametasona a 0,1% — aplicar 2-6 vezes ao dia, dependendo da gravidade da doença.
• Diminuir a frequência da medicação à medida que a condição desaparece.

Subconjuntivais
• Acetonida de triancinolona — 4-6 mg (cães); 4 mg (gatos) por injeção subconjuntival.
• Metilprednisolona — 3-10 mg (cães); 4 mg (gatos) por injeção subconjuntival.
• Indicados sob a forma de dose única, seguidos por anti-inflamatórios tópicos e/ou sistêmicos.

Sistêmicos
• Prednisona — 0,5-2,2 mg/kg/dia (cães); 1-3 mg/kg/dia (gatos); diminuir a dose depois de 7-10 dias.
• Utilizar apenas se as causas infecciosas sistêmicas de uveíte tiverem sido descartadas.

---

* N. T.: Doença degenerativa, progressiva e não inflamatória da córnea, que provoca a percepção de imagens distorcidas ao deformar essa membrana.

Anti-inflamatórios Não Esteroides
Tópicos
• Flurbiprofeno — aplicar 2-4 vezes ao dia, dependendo da gravidade da doença.
• Diclofenaco — aplicar 2-4 vezes ao dia, dependendo da gravidade da doença.
• Muito menos eficazes que os corticosteroides.

Sistêmicos
• Carprofeno — 2,2 mg/kg VO a cada 12 h ou 4,4 mg/kg VO a cada 24 h (cães).
• Ácido acetilsalicílico — 10-25 mg/kg VO a cada 12 h (cães); 10 mg/kg VO a cada 48 h (gatos; apenas para uso a curto prazo).
• Tepoxalina — 10 mg/kg VO a cada 24 h (cães).
• Meloxicam — 0,2 mg/kg VO a cada 24 h (cães).
• Não usar simultaneamente com corticosteroides sistêmicos.

Midriáticos/Cicloplégicos Tópicos
• Sulfato de atropina a 1% — aplicar 1-4 vezes ao dia, dependendo da gravidade da doença. Usar a frequência mais baixa e adequada para manter a pupila dilatada e o conforto ocular. Em gatos, utilizar pomada em vez de solução para minimizar a salivação.

Depósito Lipídico

Corticosteroides Tópicos
• Acetato de prednisolona a 1% — aplicar 2-4 vezes ao dia, dependendo da gravidade da doença.
• Dexametasona a 0,1% — aplicar 2-4 vezes ao dia, dependendo da gravidade da doença.
• Diminuir a frequência da medicação à medida que a condição desaparece.

Midriáticos/Cicloplégicos Tópicos
• Sulfato de atropina a 1% — aplicar 1-2 vezes ao dia, se necessário, caso se note um desconforto ocular.

CONTRAINDICAÇÕES/INTERAÇÕES POSSÍVEIS
• Evitar o uso de agentes mióticos tópicos.
• Corticosteroides tópicos e subconjuntivais estão contraindicados na presença de ceratite ulcerativa concomitante.
• Além da preocupação com glaucoma secundário, a atropina tópica deve ser usada com critério e a pressão intraocular monitorizada.

ACOMPANHAMENTO

MONITORIZAÇÃO DO PACIENTE
Reavaliar em 2-3 dias. A pressão intraocular deve ser monitorizada para se detectar glaucoma secundário. A frequência dos exames subsequentes é determinada pela resposta ao tratamento.

EVOLUÇÃO ESPERADA E PROGNÓSTICO
• Hipópio — prognóstico reservado; depende da doença subjacente e da resposta ao tratamento.
• Depósito lipídico — prognóstico bom; em geral, responde rapidamente (em 24-72 h) à terapia moderada com anti-inflamatórios; é possível a ocorrência de recidiva.

Autor Ian P. Herring
Consultor Editorial Paul E. Miller

HIPOPITUITARISMO

CONSIDERAÇÕES GERAIS

REVISÃO
- Distúrbio resultante da destruição da hipófise por algum processo neoplásico, degenerativo ou anômalo.
- Associado à baixa produção de hormônios hipofisários, incluindo os hormônios tireostimulante (TSH), adrenocorticotrópico (ACTH), luteinizante (LH) e foliculoestimulante (FSH), bem como o hormônio de crescimento (GH).

IDENTIFICAÇÃO
- Cães.
- Idade: 2-6 meses.
- Raças — Pastor alemão, Carnelian bear, Spitz, Pinscher toy e Weimaraner.
- Distúrbio autossômico recessivo simples no Pastor alemão e no Carnelian bear.

SINAIS CLÍNICOS

Achados Anamnésicos
- Retardo mental que se manifesta como dificuldade em domesticar os animais para fazer as necessidades fora de casa.
- Crescimento lento notado nos primeiros 2-3 meses de vida.
- Nanismo proporcional.

Achados do Exame Físico
- Pelagem de filhote retida.
- Pele fina e hipotônica.
- Latido estridente.
- Alopecia no tronco.
- Hiperpigmentação cutânea.
- Genitália infantil.
- Erupção tardia dos dentes.

CAUSAS E FATORES DE RISCO

Congênitas
- Bolsa de Rathke cística.
- Deficiência isolada de GH.

Adquiridas
- Tumor hipofisário.
- Traumatismo.
- Radioterapia.

DIAGNÓSTICO

DIAGNÓSTICO DIFERENCIAL
- Nanismo hipotireóideo; predominância racial e nanismo desproporcional observados em pacientes com hipotireoidismo.
- Outras causas de atrasos do crescimento — desvio portossistêmico, diabetes melito, hiperadrenocorticismo, desnutrição, parasitismo.

HEMOGRAMA/BIOQUÍMICA/URINÁLISE
- Eosinofilia.
- Linfocitose.
- Hipofosfatemia.
- Hipoglicemia.

OUTROS TESTES LABORATORIAIS
- Testes de resposta à corticotropina e ao TSH; resposta abaixo do normal ao TSH e ACTH.
- Análises do hormônio de crescimento e fator de crescimento insulinossímile (IGF-1); a análise do hormônio de crescimento não se encontra disponível atualmente nos EUA; recomenda-se a mensuração do IGF-1, que se encontra baixa.
- Teste de estimulação com grelina — monitoriza as alterações nos níveis de GH em resposta à grelina; exige a análise do GH.

DIAGNÓSTICO POR IMAGEM
A radiografia pode revelar disgenesia epifisária e retenção anormal das placas de crescimento fisárias.

MÉTODOS DIAGNÓSTICOS
N/D.

TRATAMENTO

Tratamento clínico em um esquema ambulatorial.

MEDICAÇÕES

MEDICAMENTO(S)
- Hormônio de crescimento — humano, suíno ou bovino, se disponível; 0,1 UI/kg SC 3 vezes por semana durante 4-6 semanas; repetir se necessário.
- Tratar o hipotireoidismo com levotiroxina (22 µg/kg VO a cada 24 h).
- Glicocorticoides (p. ex., prednisona, 0,2 mg/kg VO a cada 24 h) se o resultado do teste de resposta ao ACTH estiver abaixo do normal; é necessária uma dosagem maior de esteroides durante períodos de estresse.

CONTRAINDICAÇÕES/INTERAÇÕES POSSÍVEIS
Podem ocorrer reações de hipersensibilidade e intolerância aos carboidratos na suplementação com o hormônio de crescimento.

ACOMPANHAMENTO

MONITORIZAÇÃO DO PACIENTE
- Mensurar as concentrações sanguíneas e urinárias de glicose.
- Interromper a suplementação com hormônio de crescimento caso se desenvolva glicosúria ou se a glicemia estiver > 150 mg/dL.

COMPLICAÇÕES POSSÍVEIS
Complicações neurológicas causadas pela expansão da bolsa de Rathke.

EVOLUÇÃO ESPERADA E PROGNÓSTICO
- A pele e a pelagem melhoram em 6-8 semanas do início da suplementação com hormônio de crescimento e tireoidiano.
- Em geral, não há aumento da estatura, porque as placas de crescimento já se fecharam no momento do diagnóstico.
- Os cães frequentemente vêm a óbito ainda jovens (3-4 anos) por causa das complicações neurológicas.
- Prognóstico mau a longo prazo.

DIVERSOS

VER TAMBÉM
- Hipoadrenocorticismo (Doença de Addison).
- Hipotireoidismo.

ABREVIATURA(S)
- ACTH = hormônio adrenocorticotrópico.
- GH = hormônio de crescimento.
- IGF-1 = fator de crescimento insulinossímile-1.
- TSH = hormônio tireostimulante.

Sugestões de Leitura
Bhatti SF, De Vliegher SP, Mol JA, Van Ham LM, Kooistra HS. Ghrelin-stimulation test in the diagnosis of canine pituitary dwarfism. Res Vet Sci 2006, 81(1):24-30.
Campbell KL. Growth hormone-related disorders in dogs. Compend Cont Educ Pract Vet 1988, 10:477-482.

Autor Deborah S. Greco
Consultor Editorial Deborah S. Greco

Hipoplasia Cerebelar

CONSIDERAÇÕES GERAIS

REVISÃO
Causada pelo desenvolvimento parcial de partes do cerebelo, decorrente de fatores intrínsecos (hereditários) ou extrínsecos (infecciosos, tóxicos ou nutricionais).

IDENTIFICAÇÃO
• Os sinais clínicos são evidenciados quando os filhotes caninos e felinos começam a se manter em estação e caminhar (por volta de 6 semanas de vida).
• Hereditária em Airedale, Chow chow, Boston terrier e Bull terrier.

SINAIS CLÍNICOS
• Distúrbio cerebelar simétrico não progressivo — oscilações da cabeça; tremores dos membros; agravados pelo movimento ou pela alimentação (tremores intencionais); desaparecem durante o sono.
• Ataxia cerebelar com postura em base larga.
• Dismetria e desequilíbrio — quedas e movimentos bruscos.

CAUSAS E FATORES DE RISCO
• Gatos — em geral ocorre uma infecção transplacentária ou perinatal pelo vírus da panleucopenia (vírus selvagem ou vírus vivo modificado utilizado em algumas vacinas), que ataca de forma seletiva as células de divisão rápida (p. ex., camada germinativa externa do cerebelo ao nascimento e por 2 semanas do pós-natal).
• Cães — distúrbio hereditário em algumas raças.

DIAGNÓSTICO

DIAGNÓSTICO DIFERENCIAL
• Idade, raça, anamnese e sinais simétricos não progressivos típicos — costumam ser suficientes para o diagnóstico presuntivo.
• Abiotrofia cerebelar precoce — degeneração pós-natal após o desenvolvimento normal; evolução lenta dos sinais em semanas a meses; início na idade neonatal (Beagle, Samoieda, Rhodesian ridgeback, Setter irlandês, Jack Russell terrier, Poodle miniatura) ou pós-natal (Kelpie australiano entre 5-6 semanas de vida; Kerry blue terrier entre 8-16 semanas; Collie de pelo áspero entre 4-8 semanas; Bulmastife entre 4-9 semanas).
• Distrofia neuroaxonal — sinais cerebelares lentamente progressivos, que iniciam em torno de 5 semanas de vida em gatos e 7 semanas em Chihuahua.
• Sequelas cerebelares decorrentes de infecção sistêmica por herpes-vírus canino — seguem a doença sistêmica.
• Crises convulsivas ou outros sinais cerebrais concomitantes — sugerem outras más-formações, como lissencefalia (Fox terrier de pelo duro e Setter irlandês) ou hidrocefalia.
• O diagnóstico final é possível apenas à necropsia.

HEMOGRAMA/BIOQUÍMICA/URINÁLISE
Em geral, permanecem normais.

OUTROS TESTES LABORATORIAIS
N/D.

DIAGNÓSTICO POR IMAGEM
Varredura por RM — atrofia ou má-formação cerebelar (preenchimento incompleto ou assimétrico da fossa craniana posterior pelo cerebelo); descartar outras más-formações.

ACHADOS PATOLÓGICOS
• Cerebelo — normalmente se apresenta bem pequeno nos filhotes caninos ou felinos recém-nascidos (o desenvolvimento cerebelar continua por até 10 semanas do pós-natal); observa-se atrofia sutil a acentuada; como a necropsia é realizada entre semanas a meses após o nascimento, não há qualquer sinal de inflamação ativa.
• Fibras transversais da ponte — diminuição de tamanho, associada à atrofia cerebelar cortical acentuada.
• Hidrocefalia — pode ser um achado concomitante; origina-se de inflamação multifocal ou de más-formações múltiplas (p. ex., síndrome de Dandy-Walker).
• Achados microscópicos — depleção de camadas celulares do córtex cerebelar.

TRATAMENTO
Nenhum.

MEDICAÇÕES

MEDICAMENTO(S)
N/D.

CONTRAINDICAÇÕES/INTERAÇÕES POSSÍVEIS
N/D.

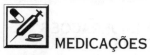

ACOMPANHAMENTO

MONITORIZAÇÃO DO PACIENTE
Ajuda a confirmar o diagnóstico (conforme a necessidade).

PREVENÇÃO
N/D.

COMPLICAÇÕES POSSÍVEIS
N/D.

EVOLUÇÃO ESPERADA E PROGNÓSTICO
• Pode ocorrer uma leve melhora, pois os pacientes compensam seus déficits.
• Déficits — permanentes; sem evolução; compatíveis com a expectativa de vida normal.
• Alguns pacientes podem ser animais de estimação aceitáveis.

CUIDADO(S)
• Limitar o ambiente físico para evitar lesões e acidentes automobilísticos — não permitir que o animal suba em objetos, sofra quedas ou fuja.
• Eutanásia — para os animais gravemente acometidos, incapazes de se alimentar ou se auto-higienizar ou de serem adestrados para defecar ou urinar.

DIVERSOS

Sugestões de Leitura
De Lahunta A, Glass E. Veterinary Neuroanatomy and Clinical Neurology, 3rd ed. St Louis: Saunders Elsevier, 2009, pp. 360-370.

Autor Christine Berthelin-Baker
Consultor Editorial Joane M. Parent

Hipoplasia/Hipocalcificação do Esmalte

CONSIDERAÇÕES GERAIS

REVISÃO
- Defeito aparente nas superfícies do esmalte, frequentemente erodido e manchado; focal ou generalizado.
- Defeitos decorrentes da interrupção na formação do esmalte normal.
- As influências sistêmicas durante a formação do esmalte (cinomose, febre, etc.) por um período de tempo prolongado podem causar alterações generalizadas; em um período de tempo curto, as influências locais ou focais (p. ex., traumatismo, até mesmo oriundo da extração de dentes decíduos) podem causar bandas ou padrões específicos.
- A maior parte dos casos é principalmente estética; alguns pacientes podem apresentar danos estruturais extensos e até mesmo envolvimentos radiculares.
- A descrição mais correta seria hipocalcificação do esmalte, já que a quantidade dessa estrutura dentária permanece adequada (não hipoplásico); no entanto, os defeitos na calcificação levam a defeitos no esmalte.
- Os dentes podem ficar mais sensíveis em caso de exposição da dentina e, ocasionalmente, ocorrem fraturas de dentes gravemente acometidos; em geral, os dentes continuam plenamente funcionais.

IDENTIFICAÇÃO
- Cães e, menos comumente, gatos.
- Com frequência, a hipoplasia/hipocalcificação do esmalte fica evidente no momento da erupção dentária (após 6 meses de vida) ou logo depois disso (com sinais de desgaste).

SINAIS CLÍNICOS

Achados Anamnésicos
Mancha nos dentes.

Achados do Exame Físico
- Superfície do esmalte erodida e irregular, com mancha do esmalte comprometido e possibilidade de exposição da dentina subjacente (castanho-clara).
- Acúmulo precoce ou rápido de placa e cálculo bacterianos na superfície dentária rugosa; possível presença de gengivite e/ou doença periodontal acelerada.

CAUSAS E FATORES DE RISCO
- Lesão durante a formação do esmalte.
- Vírus da cinomose, febre, traumatismo (p. ex., acidentes e aplicação de força excessiva durante a extração de dentes decíduos).

DIAGNÓSTICO

DIAGNÓSTICO DIFERENCIAL
- Pigmentação do esmalte — superfície manchada, porém lisa (uso de tetraciclinas).
- Lesões cariadas — cavidades com cáries.
- Amelogênese imperfeita — distúrbio genético do esmalte.
- Reabsorção dentária — semelhantes àquelas encontradas em gatos.

HEMOGRAMA/BIOQUÍMICA/URINÁLISE
- Costumam permanecer normais.
- Métodos diagnósticos pré-anestésicos adequados, quando houver indicação.

OUTROS TESTES LABORATORIAIS
N/D.

DIAGNÓSTICO POR IMAGEM
- As radiografias intrabucais são necessárias para avaliar a estrutura e a viabilidade das raízes.
- Há casos relatados de formação anormal da raiz, ausência de formação radicular ou separação de coroa e raiz.

MÉTODOS DIAGNÓSTICOS
Nenhum.

TRATAMENTO

- O tratamento depende, sobretudo, da extensão das lesões, bem como dos equipamentos e materiais disponíveis.
- O objetivo terapêutico consiste em tornar a superfície o mais lisa possível.
- Terapia analgésica e antimicrobiana pré-operatórias adequadas, quando houver indicação.

Tratamento Ideal
- O tratamento ideal baseia-se na remoção delicada do esmalte comprometido (escarificação do esmalte) com brocas de pedra branca ou discos de acabamento montados em peças manuais de alta velocidade (com irrigação adequada de resfriamento); as brocas rotativas podem causar dano e calor excessivos — manipular com cuidado!
- É preciso ter cuidado para não lesar os dentes — remoção demasiada de esmalte/dentina; dano hipertérmico à polpa.
- Os defeitos focais podem ser submetidos à restauração com cimento de ionômero de vidro ou compósito de resina, mas o sucesso a longo prazo não é satisfatório; é preferível o uso de restaurações com coroas metálicas; muitos materiais de restauração (agentes ligantes, compostos) exigem o uso de unidades de fotopolimerização e certa dose de habilidade.
- É recomendável o emprego de selantes para vedar os túbulos dentinários expostos e proteger a superfície dentária.

Tratamento Alternativo
- Na falta de equipamentos manuais de alta rotação e fixadores apropriados, o tratamento poderá ser um grande desafio.
- Algumas vezes, é possível remover o esmalte mole e comprometido com o auxílio de ultrassom para raspagem; entretanto, é preciso ter cuidado para evitar danos e hipertermia.
- Para diminuir a sensibilidade do dente e aumentar a resistência do esmalte, pode-se lançar mão do tratamento hospitalar efetuado com base na aplicação de verniz com flúor ou de pasta à base de fluoreto de sódio na superfície dentária seca.

MEDICAÇÕES

MEDICAMENTO(S)
N/D.

CONTRAINDICAÇÕES/INTERAÇÕES POSSÍVEIS
N/D.

ACOMPANHAMENTO

MONITORIZAÇÃO DO PACIENTE
Informar ao proprietário sobre a possibilidade de ocorrência de degeneração do esmalte remanescente, que futuramente necessitará de terapia adicional.

PREVENÇÃO
- Recomendar a limpeza regular dos dentes com profissional especializado e programa de escovação diária em casa; além disso, pode-se incluir a aplicação doméstica semanal de fluoreto estanoso (minimizar a ingestão, em virtude da toxicidade).
- Evitar a mastigação excessiva de objetos duros.

DIVERSOS

RECURSOS DA INTERNET
http://www.avdc.org/Nomenclature.html.

Sugestões de Leitura
Lobprise HB. Blackwell's Five-Minute Veterinary Consult Clinical Companion—Small Animal Dentistry. Ames, IA: Blackwell, 2007 (em busca de outros assuntos, técnicas e métodos diagnósticos).
Wiggs RB, Lobprise HB. Veterinary Dentistry: Principles and Practice. Philadelphia: Lippincott-Raven, 1997.

Autor Heidi B. Lobprise
Consultor Editorial Heidi B. Lobprise

HIPOSTENÚRIA

CONSIDERAÇÕES GERAIS

DEFINIÇÃO
Densidade urinária entre 1,000 e 1,006.

FISIOPATOLOGIA
A capacidade de concentrar a urina normalmente (cães, >1,030; gatos, >1,035) depende da interação complexa entre o ADH, o receptor proteico para ADH no túbulo renal e o interstício medular renal hipertônico; a interferência na síntese, na liberação ou nas ações do ADH, o dano ao túbulo renal e a alteração na tonicidade do interstício medular (falência medular) podem causar hipostenúria.

SISTEMA(S) ACOMETIDO(S)
Depende do distúrbio subjacente.

IDENTIFICAÇÃO
Espécies
Cães e gatos.

Raça(s) Predominante(s)
Nenhuma.

Idade Média e Faixa Etária
Nenhuma.

Sexo Predominante
Nenhum.

SINAIS CLÍNICOS
- Poliúria e polidipsia.
- Incontinência urinária — ocasional.
- Outros sinais dependem do distúrbio subjacente.

CAUSAS
Qualquer distúrbio ou medicamento que interfira na liberação ou nas ações do ADH, provoque danos ao túbulo renal, cause falência medular ou acarrete distúrbio primário da sede (ver "Diagnóstico Diferencial").

DIAGNÓSTICO

DIAGNÓSTICO DIFERENCIAL
- Piometra.
- Síndrome de Cushing.
- Diabetes insípido.
- Pielonefrite.
- Hipercalcemia.
- Insuficiência renal precoce.
- Hepatopatia primária.
- Hipocalemia.
- Hipoadrenocorticismo.
- Polidipsia primária — ingestão compulsiva de água.

ACHADOS LABORATORIAIS
Medicamentos Capazes de Alterar os Resultados Laboratoriais
Cortisona, lítio, demeclociclina, metoxiflurano, diuréticos tiazídicos e administração intravenosa de líquidos, sem exceção, podem diminuir a densidade urinária para a faixa hipostenúrica.

Os Resultados Serão Válidos se os Exames Forem Realizados em Laboratório Humano?
Sim.

HEMOGRAMA/BIOQUÍMICA/URINÁLISE
- Baixa densidade urinária (1,000 a 1,006) e outras anormalidades podem indicar a causa subjacente.
- Alta atividade sérica da fosfatase alcalina sugere hiperadrenocorticismo ou hepatopatia primária.
- Colesterol alto é comum em pacientes com hiperadrenocorticismo.
- Leucocitose com desvio à esquerda em alguns pacientes com piometra ou pielonefrite.
- Hipercalemia e hiponatremia sugerem hipoadrenocorticismo.
- Nível sérico baixo de potássio confirma hipocalemia.
- Sedimento inflamatório ou bacteriúria são compatíveis com pielonefrite.
- Proteinúria é comum em pacientes com pielonefrite, piometra e hiperadrenocorticismo.

OUTROS TESTES LABORATORIAIS
Verificar os níveis de ACTH para determinar a causa do hiperadrenocorticismo (i. e., dependente da hipófise *versus* tumor adrenal).

DIAGNÓSTICO POR IMAGEM
- Radiografia para avaliar o tamanho e a forma dos rins e também para detectar a presença de tumor adrenal calcificado ou útero aumentado de volume.
- Pielograma intravenoso para ajudar a diagnosticar pielonefrite.
- Ultrassonografia para avaliar o tamanho e a arquitetura das adrenais, dos rins e do fígado, além do tamanho do útero.
- RM ou TC para avaliar a existência de massa hipofisária ou hipotalâmica que pode ser a causa de diabetes insípido central ou hiperadrenocorticismo.

MÉTODOS DIAGNÓSTICOS
- Teste de estimulação com ACTH para triagem de hiperadrenocorticismo e hipoadrenocorticismo.
- Teste de supressão com dexametasona em baixas doses e teste da relação de creatinina:cortisol urinários para triagem de hiperadrenocorticismo.
- Mensuração dos ácidos biliares séricos para avaliar a função hepática.
- **Nota:** os cães com hiperadrenocorticismo frequentemente apresentam um leve aumento dos ácidos biliares.
- Teste modificado da privação de água para diferenciar entre diabetes insípido e polidipsia psicogênica; ver o protocolo do teste no Apêndice II.

TRATAMENTO

- Depende do distúrbio subjacente.
- Não restringir o consumo de água pelo paciente a menos que seja conveniente para o diagnóstico definitivo.
- Depende do distúrbio subjacente.

MEDICAÇÕES

MEDICAMENTO(S) DE ESCOLHA
Depende(m) do distúrbio subjacente.

ACOMPANHAMENTO

MONITORIZAÇÃO DO PACIENTE
Densidade urinária, estado de hidratação, função renal e nível de eletrólitos.

COMPLICAÇÕES POSSÍVEIS
Desidratação.

DIVERSOS

DISTÚRBIOS ASSOCIADOS
Ver a lista de "Diagnóstico Diferencial".

POTENCIAL ZOONÓTICO
Nenhum.

VER TAMBÉM
- Diabetes Insípido.
- Hiperadrenocorticismo (Síndrome de Cushing) — Gatos.
- Hiperadrenocorticismo (Síndrome de Cushing) — Cães.

ABREVIATURA(S)
- ACTH = hormônio adrenocorticotrópico.
- ADH = hormônio antidiurético.
- RM = ressonância magnética.
- TC = tomografia computadorizada.

Sugestões de Leitura
DiBartola SP. Fluid, Electrolyte and Acid-Base Disorders in Small Animal Practice, 3rd ed. Philadelphia: Saunders, 2005.
Rose DB, Post T. Clinical Physiology of Acid-Base and Electrolyte Disorders, 5th ed. New York: McGraw-Hill, 2000.

Autor Rhett Nichols
Consultor Editorial Deborah S. Greco

HIPOTERMIA

CONSIDERAÇÕES GERAIS

Em virtude da literatura clínica limitada na medicina veterinária, grande parte das informações a seguir foi extrapolada da literatura médica humana e de estudos experimentais em animais.

DEFINIÇÃO
• Hipotermia é uma condição em que a temperatura corporal central declina abaixo daquela necessária para o metabolismo normal. Em casos de hipotermia primária, as respostas compensatórias de indivíduo saudável à perda de calor são subjugadas por exposição, enquanto a hipotermia secundária complica muitas doenças sistêmicas. • Hipotermia leve — 32-37,2°C.
• Hipotermia moderada — 28-32°C.
• Hipotermia grave — qualquer temperatura abaixo de 28°C.

FISIOPATOLOGIA
• A termorregulação normal equilibra o controle do calor adquirido ou perdido para o ambiente com o calor produzido via termogênese central. A temperatura é controlada pelo hipotálamo com impulsos vindos dos termorreceptores. O calor pode ser adquirido ou perdido para o ambiente por meio de quatro mecanismos, incluindo evaporação, radiação, convecção e condução. A termogênese central gera calor via metabolismo basal, atividade muscular e desacoplamento da gordura marrom (neonatos).
• A produção de calor pode ser aumentada por meio de tremor e aumento da taxa metabólica basal. A ativação tanto do sistema nervoso simpático como do sistema endócrino resulta em níveis circulantes elevados de hormônio liberador dos hormônios tireoidianos, catecolaminas, hormônio do crescimento e glicocorticoides que, juntos, contribuem para o aumento na utilização da glicose e na taxa metabólica basal.
• As adaptações para minimizar a perda de calor incluem vasoconstrição cutânea, piloereção e respostas comportamentais como se encolher, compartilhar o calor do corpo e buscar por abrigo.

SISTEMA(S) ACOMETIDO(S)
• Cardiovascular — nos casos de hipotermia leve, a estimulação simpática induz inicialmente à taquicardia e vasoconstrição periférica com débito cardíaco e pressão arterial normais ou elevados. À medida que o paciente se esfria, a despolarização das células do marca-passo cardíaco fica mais lenta, resultando em bradicardia resistente ao tratamento com atropina; a consequente queda no débito cardíaco é equilibrada por um aumento na resistência vascular sistêmica. Sob temperaturas mais baixas, a bradicardia torna-se progressivamente extrema e a resistência vascular sistêmica declina conforme a liberação de catecolaminas e a responsividade dos receptores adrenérgicos são enfraquecidas. Os achados eletrocardiográficos clássicos incluem a presença da onda de Osborn ou J, disritmias atriais e ventriculares, além de prolongamento dos intervalos PR, QRS e QT. A sequência típica é uma evolução de bradicardia sinusal, passando por fibrilação atrial até fibrilação ventricular e, por fim, assistolia.
• Endócrino — a ativação do sistema simpático e a liberação de hormônios contrarreguladores deflagram o aumento dos processos de glicogenólise, gliconeogênese e lipólise, bem como inibem a liberação e a captação de insulina, resultando em hiperglicemia. Quando a hipotermia se desenvolve lentamente ou é de longa duração, as reservas de glicogênio sofrem depleção, ocorrendo o desenvolvimento de hipoglicemia.
• Gastrintestinal — o aumento na produção de ácido gástrico e o declínio na secreção de bicarbonato duodenal podem predispor os pacientes à ulceração gastrintestinal. É comum a ocorrência de íleo paralítico.
• Hematológico — ocorre desvio de plasma para o espaço extravascular e, consequentemente, a hemoconcentração pode levar a CID hiper e hipocoagulável. A atividade enzimática deprimida dos fatores de coagulação e a hiporreatividade das plaquetas exacerbam a hipocoagulabilidade.
• Hepatobiliar/pancreático — hipoxia tecidual leva a dano hepatocelular e pancreatite.
• Musculosquelético — aumento na viscosidade do líquido articular e rigidez muscular.
• Nervoso — o metabolismo do SNC e o nível de consciência diminuem de forma linear à medida que a temperatura central declina. Incoordenação leve é acompanhada por letargia, obnubilação e coma. Redução progressiva na velocidade de condução dos nervos periféricos conforme a temperatura abaixa.
• Renal — a vasoconstrição periférica aumenta o fluxo sanguíneo dos rins e a taxa de filtração glomerular, resultando em aumento na produção de urina. Conforme a temperatura corporal central declina, a disfunção progressiva dos túbulos renais e a resistência ao hormônio antidiurético contribuem ainda mais para a diurese por frio. Mais tarde, a produção de urina diminui como resultado da queda do débito cardíaco. Consequentemente, pode ocorrer insuficiência renal aguda.
• Respiratório — em casos de hipotermia leve, a taquipneia inicial é substituída por diminuição na frequência respiratória e no volume corrente, mas aumento na produção de secreção das vias aéreas. À medida que a temperatura declina, os reflexos protetores das vias aéreas sofrem diminuição. Em temperaturas abaixo de 34°C, o controle ventilatório é atenuado e, com isso, o aumento na resistência vascular pulmonar leva a desequilíbrio entre os processos de ventilação e perfusão. Em casos de hipotermia grave, desenvolvem-se hipoventilação progressiva e apneia e (mais raramente) edema pulmonar. A hipotermia também faz com que a curva de dissociação da oxiemoglobina se desvie para a esquerda. Esse efeito pode ser mascarado por acidose láctica e respiratória concomitante, que pode se tornar tão profunda a ponto de resultar em um desvio global para a direita.
• Cutâneo — ocorre o desenvolvimento de edema, secundariamente ao aumento na permeabilidade vascular.

INCIDÊNCIA/PREVALÊNCIA
Varia com a localização geográfica.

DISTRIBUIÇÃO GEOGRÁFICA
Mais comum em climas frios.

IDENTIFICAÇÃO
Espécies
Cães e gatos.

Raça(s) Predominante(s)
Raças menores com área de superfície corporal aumentada.

Idade Média e Faixa Etária
Mais comum em neonatos e idosos.

SINAIS CLÍNICOS
Comentários Gerais
• Uma avaliação completa deve ser feita para encontrar as condições comórbidas precipitantes.

Achados Anamnésicos
• Exposição prolongada conhecida a temperaturas ambientes frias. • Possivelmente, fuga de casa ou histórico de traumatismo.

Achados do Exame Físico

Hipotermia leve (32-37,2°C)
Gerais
• Letargia. • Fraqueza. • Tremores vigorosos (variáveis).
Cardiovasculares
• Frequência e ritmo cardíacos, bem como pressão arterial, variáveis. • Mucosas róseas claras a pálidas.
Neurológicos
• Confusão mental, agitação ou obnubilação.
Respiratórios
• Frequência respiratória variável.

Hipotermia moderada (28-32°C)
Gerais
• Colapso. • Tremores reduzidos (variáveis).
Cardiovasculares
• Bradiarritmia com hipotensão. • Mucosas pálidas.
Musculosqueléticos
• Rigidez muscular e articular.
Neurológicos
• Obnubilação, estupor ou coma. • Ataxia e hiporreflexia.
Respiratórios
• Diminuição na profundidade e na frequência da respiração.

Hipotermia grave (<28°C)
Gerais
• Animal moribundo (agonizante) com pele fria e edematosa. • Perda dos tremores (variável).
Cardiovasculares
• Bradiarritmia com hipotensão ou parada cardíaca. • Mucosas pálidas.
Musculosqueléticos
• Rigidez muscular e articular.
Neurológicos
• Coma com pupilas fixas e dilatadas. • Arreflexia.
Respiratórios
• Diminuição na profundidade e na frequência da respiração ou parada respiratória. • Edema pulmonar.

CAUSAS
Termogênese inadequada
• A termogênese normal é subjugada. • Doença grave.

Perda extrema de calor
• Evaporação, condução, convecção e radiação excessivas. • Incapacidade de vasoconstrição ou piloereção. • Perda das adaptações comportamentais.

Falha do centro termorregulador
• Lesão ou doença hipotalâmica.

FATORES DE RISCO
• Idade muito jovem ou avançada. • Reservas corporais baixas de gordura e glicogênio. • Lesão por queimadura. • Lesão ou doença intracraniana.

HIPOTERMIA

- Hipotireoidismo. • Cetoacidose diabética.
- Sepse. • Traumatismo. • Anestesia geral. • Uso de medicamentos, incluindo mas não limitados a, β-bloqueadores, barbitúricos, narcóticos, fenotiazinas.

DIAGNÓSTICO

DIAGNÓSTICO DIFERENCIAL
- Doença primária do SNC, hipoglicemia, anemia, encefalopatia hepática, coma mixedematoso, distúrbios eletrolíticos, sepse, intoxicação, neoplasia e morte. • Bradiarritmia — cardiopatia, efeitos colaterais de medicamentos e intoxicação.

HEMOGRAMA/BIOQUÍMICA/URINÁLISE
- Os resultados são variáveis, dependendo do grau de hipotermia e da presença de condições comórbidas. • Hemograma completo — hemoconcentração e trombocitopenia.
- Bioquímica — azotemia, hiper e hipoglicemia, atividade elevada das enzimas hepáticas, hiperbilirrubinemia. • Urinálise — isostenúria, glicosúria.

OUTROS TESTES LABORATORIAIS
- Gasometria arterial — variável, embora o quadro de acidose metabólica e respiratória seja comum.
- Eletrólitos — não há valores preditivos ou tendências. • Coagulação — hiperfibrinogenemia, CID. O prolongamento *in vivo* nos tempos de coagulação sanguínea pode não refletir os ensaios *in vitro*, devendo ser corrigido com reaquecimento.
- Avaliação dos hormônios tireoidianos — pode confirmar hipotireoidismo subjacente.

DIAGNÓSTICO POR IMAGEM
Para investigar as complicações da recuperação ou a presença de condições comórbidas.

MÉTODOS DIAGNÓSTICOS
- Termômetros de registro baixo podem ser úteis para monitorizar temperaturas corporais abaixo de 34°C. As sondas devem ser inseridas profundamente e não nas fezes. • ECG para avaliar o ritmo cardíaco e os complexos QRS.

ACHADOS PATOLÓGICOS
- Os achados em pacientes que sucumbem à hipotermia acidental primária são variáveis e inespecíficos. Se o resfriamento do corpo e o óbito ocorrerem rapidamente, os achados da necropsia serão mínimos, mas poderão incluir coloração avermelhada da pele, erosões gástricas hemorrágicas e depósitos lipídicos em células epiteliais dos túbulos renais proximais e de outros órgãos. • Os pacientes que morrem de hipotermia secundária agravada por exposição podem exibir achados semelhantes; no entanto, eles também terão evidência de algum processo patológico isolado e significativo.

TRATAMENTO

CUIDADO(S) DE SAÚDE ADEQUADO(S)
Fornecer cuidados intensivos emergenciais para o paciente internado até que ele esteja normotérmico e estável.

CUIDADO(S) DE ENFERMAGEM
- O reaquecimento externo ativo com o uso de cobertores aquecidos, colchões térmicos, calor irradiante, banhos mornos ou ar quente forçado é utilizado em pacientes com hipotermia leve a moderada. As complicações incluem pós-queda da temperatura central por meio do qual o retorno de sangue frio da periferia para a circulação central provoca maior resfriamento central. O reaquecimento do tronco deve ser realizado antes das extremidades para minimizar esse risco. Outra complicação potencial envolve queimaduras iatrogênicas. • As técnicas para aquecer os pacientes com hipotermia grave abrangem a inalação de oxigênio umidificado aquecido, a administração de fluidos intravenosos aquecidos e a lavagem vesical ou gástrica com soro fisiológico morno. Os métodos mais invasivos e mais exigentes do ponto de vista técnico compreendem a lavagem torácica e peritoneal fechada, a hemodiálise, o reaquecimento arteriovenoso ou venovenoso contínuo e o desvio cardiopulmonar.
- A imersão de todo o corpo em água quente é contraindicada, pois isso causará vasodilatação e hipotensão acentuadas, sendo provável a indução de disritmias e colapso cardiovascular.
- Fluidoterapia — a maioria dos pacientes encontra-se inicialmente com depleção volêmica; no entanto, eles precisam ser monitorizados de perto durante a ressuscitação para evitar sobrecarga por volume. Os fluidos cristaloides administrados por via intravenosa devem ser aquecidos até 40°C.
- A hipotensão é tratada com ressuscitação volêmica. O uso de agentes inotrópicos como dopamina em baixas doses é considerado apenas em casos irresponsivos à ressuscitação volêmica.
- Os pacientes com insuficiência respiratória precisam ser submetidos à ventilação mecânica.

ATIVIDADE
Os pacientes minimamente acometidos devem ser incentivados à prática de exercícios, já que a atividade muscular promoverá a geração endógena de mais calor corporal.

DIETA
A nutrição enteral ou parenteral é escolhida com base nas necessidades e nas aptidões de cada paciente.

ORIENTAÇÃO AO PROPRIETÁRIO
É imperativa a prevenção de exposição a temperaturas baixas para evitar hipotermia primária. Os proprietários de pacientes muito jovens e muito idosos, bem como aqueles de animais acometidos por problemas clínicos graves ou submetidos a medicações que inibem a capacidade termorreguladora, devem ser aconselhados a manter seus animais de estimação dentro de casa e tomar as medidas protetoras cabíveis se tiverem de ser expostos a temperaturas baixas.

MEDICAÇÕES

MEDICAMENTO(S) DE ESCOLHA
- Oxigênio. • A suplementação de glicose (a 2,5-5%) via infusão em velocidade constante no fluido cristaloide é indicada em pacientes hipoglicêmicos.

CONTRAINDICAÇÕES
- Hipotermia grave — evitar fluidos que contenham lactato, já que a depuração hepática desse componente pode estar prejudicada.
- Não há provas para apoiar o uso de rotina de esteroides ou antibióticos.

ACOMPANHAMENTO

MONITORIZAÇÃO DO PACIENTE
- Mensuração contínua da temperatura corporal central durante o reaquecimento. • Registro contínuo do ECG e medição frequente da pressão arterial (a cada 1 h) durante o reaquecimento.
- Estimativa frequente (a cada 6-12 h) dos eletrólitos (sódio, potássio, cloreto, cálcio ionizado, magnésio e fósforo), estado acidobásico, hematócrito, proteína total e glicemia.
- Monitorização diária de ureia, densidade urinária, índices de coagulação e enzimas hepáticas em pacientes gravemente acometidos. • Observação do paciente quanto ao desenvolvimento de crioulceração (feridas causadas pelo frio).

PREVENÇÃO
- Evitar a exposição prolongada ao frio, especialmente no caso de animais de alto risco.
- Aquecer os pacientes e monitorizar a temperatura corporal em animais anestesiados.

COMPLICAÇÕES POSSÍVEIS
- A vasodilatação periférica durante o reaquecimento pode fazer com que a temperatura corporal caia ainda mais. • O retorno do sangue periférico frio ao coração pode precipitar arritmias cardíacas. • A hipotermia grave pode causar parada cardíaca.

EVOLUÇÃO ESPERADA E PROGNÓSTICO
Variam com a gravidade da hipotermia, a causa subjacente e o estado de saúde geral do paciente.

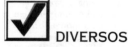

DIVERSOS

FATORES RELACIONADOS COM A IDADE
Neonatos doentes ou hipoglicêmicos podem sofrer hipotermia acentuada em ambientes normais.

VER TAMBÉM
Choque Cardiogênico.

ABREVIATURA(S)
- ECG = eletrocardiograma.
- CID = coagulação intravascular disseminada.
- SNC = sistema nervoso central.

Sugestões de Leitura
Ao H, et al. Delayed platelet dysfunction in prolonged induced canine hypothermia. Resuscitation 2001, 51:83-90.
Armstrong SR, et al. Perioperative hypothermia. J Vet Emerg Crit Care 2005, 15:32-37.
Aslam AF, et al. Hypothermia: Evaluation, electrocardiographic manifestations, and management. Am J Med 2006, 119:297-301.
Danzl D. Hypothermia. Semin Resp Crit Care Med 2002, 23:57-68.
Dhupa N. Hypothermia in dogs and cats. Compend Contin Educ Pract Vet 1995, 17:61-69.
Yoshihara H, Yamamoto T, Mihara H. Changes in coagulation and fibrinolysis occurring in dogs during hypothermia. Thrombosis Res 1985, 37:503-512.

Autores Gretchen Lee Schoeffler e Nishi Dhupa
Consultores Editoriais Larry P. Tilley e Francis W. K. Smith, Jr.

HIPOTIREOIDISMO

CONSIDERAÇÕES GERAIS

DEFINIÇÃO
Manifestações clínicas que resultam da produção inadequada de tiroxina (T_4) e 3,5,3'-tri-iodotironina (T_3) pela glândula tireoide. Quadro caracterizado por diminuição generalizada na atividade metabólica celular.

FISIOPATOLOGIA

Hipotireoidismo Adquirido
• Em cães, o hipotireoidismo adquirido pode ser primário, secundário ou terciário.
• O hipotireoidismo primário é associado a algum defeito localizado na glândula tireoide. O tecido tireóideo sofre destruição ou substituição e, consequentemente, fica menos responsivo ao TSH; com isso, os níveis de T_3 e T_4 declinam de forma gradual, com aumento compensatório no TSH.
• Existem duas formas comuns de hipotireoidismo primário. Tireoidite linfocítica é um processo imunomediado caracterizado por infiltração crônica e progressiva de linfócitos, bem como por destruição da glândula tireoide. Esse processo é gradativo e responde pelo início lento de sinais clínicos associados ao hipotireoidismo. O processo imunomediado é associado à produção de autoanticorpos, predominantemente contra a tireoglobulina; no entanto, há relatos de autoanticorpos contra T_3 e T_4.
• A atrofia idiopática da tireoide é uma forma isolada de destruição dessa glândula que não demonstra um componente inflamatório e é causada pela substituição do tecido tireóideo normal por tecido adiposo.
• Juntos, esses processos respondem por 95% dos casos clínicos de hipotireoidismo nos cães, sendo cada um deles responsável por 50% dos casos relatados. As causas raras de hipotireoidismo primário incluem destruição neoplásica do tecido tireóideo, deficiência de iodo, infecção e destruição iatrogênica secundária a medicamentos, cirurgia e tratamento com iodo radioativo.
• O hipotireoidismo adquirido secundário é raro. O defeito está localizado na hipófise, onde a capacidade de sintetizar e secretar o TSH se encontra prejudicada. O hipotireoidismo secundário pode ser causado por tumores hipofisários, má-formação congênita da hipófise, infecção, ou supressão do TSH. Medicamentos, hormônios ou doenças concomitantes podem causar supressão do TSH.
• O hipotireoidismo terciário (não relatado na literatura veterinária) é de origem hipotalâmica, mas a produção de TRH está diminuída ou é inexistente.

Hipotireoidismo Congênito
• O hipotireoidismo congênito é uma doença rara, caracterizada pela presença ou não de bócio. O *bócio* (aumento de volume da glândula tireoide) desenvolve-se quando há uma liberação aumentada de TSH, juntamente com receptores intactos desse hormônio na tireoide.
• Uma forma autossômica recessiva de hipotireoidismo congênito foi relatada em cães das raças Fox terrier toy e Schnauzer gigante, bem como em gatos da raça Abissínio. Os animais acometidos apresentam uma deficiência da tireoperoxidase.
• O hipotireoidismo congênito também é observado como um componente do pan-hipopituitarismo.

SISTEMA(S) ACOMETIDO(S)
• Comportamental.
• Cardiovascular.
• Endócrino/metabólico.
• Gastrintestinal.
• Nervoso.
• Neuromuscular.
• Oftálmico.
• Reprodutor.
• Cutâneo/exócrino.

GENÉTICA
• Não há base genética conhecida para a herança associada ao hipotireoidismo primário em cães.
• Foi relatada uma forma autossômica recessiva de hipotireoidismo congênito em cães das raças Fox terrier toy e Schnauzer gigante, bem como em gatos da raça Abissínio.

INCIDÊNCIA/PREVALÊNCIA
• O hipotireoidismo primário é a endocrinopatia mais comum em cães. A prevalência parece girar em torno de 1:250.
• O hipotireoidismo é raro em gatos.

DISTRIBUIÇÃO GEOGRÁFICA
Mundial.

IDENTIFICAÇÃO

Espécies
Cães e, raramente, gatos.

Raça(s) Predominante(s)
É mais provável que as raças caninas de porte maior desenvolvam hipotireoidismo (Golden retriever, Doberman pinscher, Dinamarquês, Setter irlandês), embora várias raças de porte menor também pareçam ser predispostas (Schnauzer miniatura, Cocker spaniel, Poodle, Dachshund).

Idade Média e Faixa Etária
Mais comumente observado em cães de meia-idade, com a idade média de início aos 7 anos.

Sexo Predominante
Nenhum.

SINAIS CLÍNICOS

Comentários Gerais
• Os sinais clínicos associados ao hipotireoidismo são vagos e envolvem muitos sistemas diferentes.

Achados Anamnésicos
• Letargia, ganho de peso e perda de pelo são os sinais mais comuns relatados pelos proprietários (40-50% de todos os casos).
• Piodermite (frequentemente recidivante), hiperpigmentação da pele, pelagem seca e quebradiça (10% dos casos).
• Raramente (<5% dos casos), há paralisia facial, fraqueza ou conjuntivite.

Achados do Exame Físico
• Os achados mais comuns incluem anormalidades dermatológicas, ganho de peso, letargia e fraqueza. Muitas alterações parecem ser secundárias à diminuição no metabolismo em virtude da falta de hormônios tireoidianos circulantes.
• Apesar de comuns, as alterações dermatológicas não são observadas em todos os pacientes.
• Pode ser observada uma pelagem seca e opaca. Alopecia bilateral simétrica não pruriginosa do tronco é relatada em 88% dos cães com hipotireoidismo. A perda de pelo é constatada em áreas de atrito intenso e costuma envolver a porção toracoabdominal e cervical ventral, bem como os cotovelos e a cauda. A perda de pelo primário é mais comum, com retenção dos pelos de proteção, resultando em uma pelagem curta e fina.
• A seborreia é comum e pode ser localizada ou ter um padrão de distribuição mais generalizado.
• A piodermite é observada em 14% dos cães com hipotireoidismo e pode ser de natureza recidivante. A falta de hormônios tireoidianos diminuirá a função das células-T e a imunidade humoral, fazendo com que a pele fique mais suscetível a infecções. Demodicose generalizada e infecções por *Malassezia* spp. são comuns. Embora as condições dermatológicas primárias não sejam pruriginosas, o prurido pode acompanhar infecções parasitárias, leveduriformes ou bacterianas secundárias. Alterações crônicas na pele podem resultar em espessamento e hiperpigmentação.
• Otite externa.
• Ganho de peso.
• Nível reduzido de atividade.
• A maioria dos sinais neurológicos é associada à polineuropatia e inclui fraqueza, paralisia do nervo facial, sinais vestibulares (em geral, periféricos) e hiporreflexia. Não há dados que apoiem uma associação entre megaesôfago ou paralisia da laringe e hipotireoidismo.
• Os sinais atribuídos ao sistema nervoso central, incluindo crises convulsivas, ataxia e coma (coma mixedematoso), são raros.
• Nos machos, foram relatadas alterações como diminuição da fertilidade, atrofia dos testículos, motilidade deficiente do sêmen e redução da libido em cães com hipotireoidismo. Nas fêmeas, foi sugerido que o hipotireoidismo esteja associado a períodos interestro prolongados, falha no ciclo, diminuição da libido e desenvolvimento inadequado da glândula mamária. Contudo, não há dados para apoiar uma associação entre níveis reduzidos dos hormônios tireoidianos e falha reprodutiva nos machos ou nas fêmeas.
• As anormalidades cardiovasculares são raras. Há relatos de bradicardia, arritmias, condução cardíaca diminuída, contratilidade reduzida e disfunção diastólica.
• Alterações oculares, incluindo depósitos de colesterol na córnea, ceratoconjuntivite seca e conjuntivite, são observadas em menos de 1% dos cães com hipotireoidismo.

Hipotireoidismo Congênito
• Letargia e inatividade geral.
• Dwarfismo.
• Alopecia.
• Constipação (mais comum em gatos).

CAUSAS
• Tireoidite linfocítica.
• Atrofia idiopática da tireoide.
• Neoplasia.
• Doença hipofisária.
• Anormalidades congênitas.
• Deficiência de iodo na dieta.
• Iatrogênica (secundária à cirurgia ou radiação).

FATORES DE RISCO
Remoção cirúrgica (bilateral) da glândula tireoide.

DIAGNÓSTICO

DIAGNÓSTICO DIFERENCIAL
• Doença dermatológica primária.
• Outras endocrinopatias (hiperadrenocorticismo, diabetes melito, deficiência do hormônio de crescimento).

Hipotireoidismo

- Pancreatite.
- Síndrome nefrótica.
- Doença hepatobiliar.

HEMOGRAMA/BIOQUÍMICA/URINÁLISE
- Úteis para descartar doença não tireóidea.
- Anemia normocítica, normocrômica e arregenerativa é um achado comum. Vinte e oito a 32% dos cães com hipotireoidismo demonstram anemia. O estado hipotireóideo não influencia o tempo de vida da hemácia.
- Hiponatremia.
- Hipercolesterolemia está presente em mais de 75% dos cães com hipotireoidismo.
- Hipertrigliceridemia.
- Altos níveis de colesterol e triglicerídeos foram associados a aterosclerose em cães, embora isso seja raro.
- Nenhuma alteração específica observada na urinálise.

OUTROS TESTES LABORATORIAIS
- O diagnóstico de hipotireoidismo é complexo. O teste de estimulação com TSH é o único teste confiável utilizado para diagnosticar o hipotireoidismo, sendo considerado o método com padrão de excelência. Contudo, existe um acesso limitado aos reagentes do teste, além de ser de alto custo.
- Vários testes estão disponíveis para avaliar a função da tireoide, os níveis dos hormônios tireoidianos e os níveis do anticorpo antitireoglobulina. Esses testes incluem a T_4 total, a T_4 livre, o TSH endógeno, os anticorpos antitireoglobulina, os anticorpos contra T_3 e T_4, a T_3 total, a T_3 reversa e a T_3 livre.
- A combinação dos testes produzirá um resultado altamente confiável.

T_4 Total
- Teste de triagem inicial (alta sensibilidade) de função da tireoide.
- Esse teste mensura os níveis de T_4 ligada à proteína e livre.
- O teste é uma avaliação direta da capacidade da glândula tireoide em produzir hormônio.
- Um nível reduzido de T_4 total é um achado comum nos animais com hipotireoidismo, mas não é diagnóstico dessa endocrinopatia, já que doenças concomitantes podem gerar uma diminuição artificial no nível de T_4 total.
- O nível de T_4 total pode ser mensurado por meios dos testes de ELISA, quimioluminescência ou radioimunoensaio. Há indícios de que o ELISA feito na clínica seja menos confiável do que o radioimunoensaio.

T_4 Livre
- Mais valioso como teste de triagem (alta sensibilidade).
- Mensura a porção metabolicamente ativa do nível de T_4 total.
- Seria de se esperar que os animais com hipotireoidismo tenham um nível baixo de T_4 livre.
- Doenças concomitantes exercem menos efeito sobre o nível de T_4 livre, em comparação ao nível de T_4 total.
- Foi demonstrado que a mensuração por diálise de equilíbrio seja mais confiável do que o radioimunoensaio, pois ela atenua a influência dos anticorpos antitireoglobulina.

Nível de TSH Endógeno
- A mensuração do TSH endógeno está disponível com o uso de ensaio para cães.
- A reatividade cruzada permite que esse ensaio seja utilizado em gatos; no entanto, ele pode ter exatidão apenas 50% das vezes na espécie felina.
- Esse teste tem alta especificidade e baixa sensibilidade, sendo mais bem utilizado como teste confirmatório e não como teste de triagem.
- Espera-se que o nível de TSH esteja elevado em animais hipotireóideos primários em virtude da perda de *feedback* negativo.
- A interpretação do nível de TSH requer o conhecimento do nível de T_4 total ou livre.
- Os métodos de avaliação dos níveis de TSH não são sensíveis em baixos níveis e a avaliação do TSH endógeno não pode ser usada para diagnosticar hipotireoidismo secundário.

Anticorpos Antitireoglobulina
- Anticorpos antitireoglobulina incluem aqueles contra a tireoglobulina, a T_3 e a T_4.
- Um título positivo é preditivo de tireoidite imunomediada, mas sugestivo de hipotireoidismo.
- Anticorpos contra T_3 e T_4 são semelhantes aos hormônios T_3 e T_4, podendo reagir de forma cruzada de modo a elevar falsamente os níveis desses ensaios. Nos animais levemente hipotireóideos (conforme mensurados pelo nível de T_4 total), a presença de anticorpos contra T_4 fará com que pareça que eles sejam eutireóideos, levando a um atraso no diagnóstico e no tratamento do hipotireoidismo.

Teste de Estimulação com TSH
- Do ponto de vista histórico, esse teste é considerado como a técnica com padrão de excelência para o diagnóstico de hipotireoidismo.
- Para a condução desse teste, era utilizado o TSH bovino de classificação farmacêutica; no entanto, a produção desse TSH foi interrompida.
- O TSH humano recombinante pode ser usado com segurança tanto em cães como em gatos para a condução eficiente desse teste embora seja caro. Portanto, é improvável que esse teste se torne uma rotina e substitua os testes de T_4 livre e total e o ensaio de TSH como os métodos diagnósticos de escolha.

T_3 Total, T_3 Reversa e T_3 Livre
- A mensuração de T_3 total não é um indicador confiável de função da tireoide.
- Foi demonstrado que o nível de T_3 permanece normal em até 90% dos cães com hipotireoidismo.
- O nível de T_3 reversa não foi validado nos animais de companhia.
- Por todas essas razões, não é recomendada a avaliação de T_3 total, T_3 reversa e T_3 livre para avaliar a função da tireoide.

Fatores Não Tireóideos que Alteram os Testes de Função da Tireoide
- Além da síndrome do eutireoideo doente, outros fatores alteram os resultados dos testes de função da tireoide, o que pode resultar no erro de diagnóstico.
- Muitos fatores não tireóideos provocam uma *diminuição* artificial nos níveis dos hormônios tireoidianos.
- Alguns medicamentos podem diminuir os níveis dos hormônios tireoidianos e resultar em um animal que desenvolve sinais clínicos de hipotireoidismo. Sulfonamidas, glicocorticoides, fenobarbital, AINE e clomipramina podem reduzir os níveis dos hormônios tireoidianos circulantes.
- Com as sulfonamidas, observa-se que esse efeito ocorre dentro de semanas do início da terapia e desaparece 2 semanas após a interrupção do medicamento.
- Os glicocorticoides inibem todo o eixo hipotálamo-hipófise-adrenal e exercem um efeito direto contra os hormônios tireoidianos.
- O fenobarbital provoca um declínio nos níveis dos hormônios tireoidianos apenas nos animais submetidos ao tratamento a longo prazo. Esse anticonvulsivante não deve ser administrado por 4 semanas antes dos testes de função da tireoide.
- A influência do AINE é variável e, por isso, a avaliação de função da tireoide deve ser feita com cautela e, de preferência, depois de interromper esses agentes bem antes do teste.
- Cães bem condicionados e atléticos possuem níveis constantemente mais baixos de T_4 total e livre.
- A vacinação recente gera um aumento transitório nos níveis de autoanticorpos circulantes, o que pode fazer com que um animal verdadeiramente hipotireóideo se pareça eutireóideo. Portanto, os testes de função da tireoide não deverão ser conduzidos se o paciente tiver sido vacinado nas 2 últimas semanas.

DIAGNÓSTICO POR IMAGEM

Achados Radiográficos
- Problemas ósseos de desenvolvimento (ossificação ou disgenesia epifisária tardia) costumam ser observados nos casos de hipotireoidismo congênito.

Achados Ultrassonográficos
- Existem diferenças significativas no volume e na ecogenicidade da glândula tireoide entre os pacientes hipotireóideos e eutireóideos.
- Nenhuma diferença significativa é observada entre os animais eutireóideos e os eutireóideos doentes.
- A ultrassonografia pode ser uma ferramenta diagnóstica adjuvante para ajudar no diagnóstico de hipotireoidismo canino.

ACHADOS PATOLÓGICOS
- A tireoidite linfocítica caracteriza-se por infiltração crônica e progressiva de linfócitos, além de destruição da glândula tireoide. As células-T citotóxicas desencadeiam um processo inflamatório, levando à destruição de células da tireoide (tirócitos) e fibrose do parênquima.
- A atrofia idiopática da tireoide caracteriza-se pela substituição do parênquima tireóideo normal por tecido adiposo e conjuntivo.
- Muitas alterações cutâneas são inespecíficas. Contudo, certos achados, incluindo espessamento da derme, mixedema e vacuolização dos músculos eretores do pelo, são mais característicos.

TRATAMENTO

CUIDADO(S) DE SAÚDE ADEQUADO(S)
Tratamento médico ambulatorial.

ORIENTAÇÃO AO PROPRIETÁRIO
- É necessária a terapia vitalícia (i. e., pelo resto da vida).
- O quadro é facilmente controlado com a suplementação oral de hormônios tireoidianos.
- Os ajustes da dose são comuns nos estágios iniciais do tratamento.
- A maioria dos sinais clínicos desaparece com o passar do tempo com a suplementação adequada de hormônios tireoidianos.

HIPOTIREOIDISMO

MEDICAÇÕES

MEDICAMENTO(S) DE ESCOLHA
- A suplementação de hormônios tireoidianos sintéticos facilmente trata o hipotireoidismo.
- A levotiroxina sódica está disponível sob a forma de produtos tanto humanos como veterinários.
- É recomendável evitar as formulações genéricas, pois os estudos em seres humanos demonstraram uma grande variabilidade na biodisponibilidade dessas formulações. Caso se faça uso de alguma formulação genérica, sempre se deve prescrever a mesma formulação.
- A suplementação de hormônios é iniciada a uma dose de 0,02 mg/kg VO a cada 12 h. Os níveis de suplementação podem ser aumentados até, no máximo, 0,8 mg por cão por tratamento.
- Por fim, a suplementação pode ser frequentemente reduzida para 1 vez ao dia assim que se obter o controle adequado.
- As doses de levotiroxina para cães excedem aquelas de seres humanos e podem confundir os farmacêuticos e endocrinologistas da medicina humana.

PRECAUÇÕES
Os pacientes com distúrbios metabólicos concomitantes (hepatopatia, endocrinopatias, doença renal, cardiopatia) devem ser submetidos à suplementação (cerca de 25% da dose recomendada) com aumento lento e gradual com o passar do tempo (3 meses) até o nível de manutenção recomendado.

INTERAÇÕES POSSÍVEIS
- Glicocorticoides, AINE e furosemida podem aumentar o metabolismo da levotiroxina.
- Protetores GI podem diminuir a absorção e, por esse motivo, a administração deve ser separada da suplementação dos hormônios tireoidianos em 2 h.

MEDICAMENTO(S) ALTERNATIVO(S)
- Se os níveis de T_4 não se normalizarem após tentativas de monitorização e tratamento com várias marcas distintas de levotiroxina, pode-se tentar o tratamento com liotironina (4-6 mg/kg VO a cada 8-12 h).
- A monitorização baseia-se nos níveis de T_3. No entanto, não há nenhum método confiável de mensuração desse hormônio.

ACOMPANHAMENTO

MONITORIZAÇÃO DO PACIENTE
- O teste de função da tireoide é recomendado 6 semanas após o início da terapia e, em seguida, a cada 6-8 semanas nos primeiros 6-8 meses e, depois, 1 a 2 vezes ao ano.
- O nível de T_4 total deve ser monitorizado e cronometrado, para que o sangue seja coletado 6 h após a administração do medicamento.
- Assim que o paciente estiver estabilizado e bem controlado, a dose terapêutica total poderá ser administrada 1 vez ao dia com resultados clínicos excelentes.
- Para os animais submetidos à suplementação diária, o sangue deverá ser coletado imediatamente antes da administração do medicamento e, outra vez, depois de 6 h.
- Quando a terapia de suplementação é adequada, o nível de T_4 total pós-dose deve estar normal a levemente acima do normal.
- Se o nível de T_4 total estiver significativamente aumentado acima da faixa normal, a dose da medicação ou a frequência da administração deverá ser reduzida.
- Se o nível de T_4 total estiver baixo, talvez haja necessidade de aumento na dose.
- Antes de aumentar a dose, é preciso avaliar a obediência do proprietário em relação ao tratamento, examinar o estado gastrintestinal para garantir a ausência de impacto sobre a absorção e confirmar se não houve alteração na formulação da levotiroxina.

PREVENÇÃO
A suplementação hormonal adequada com monitorização de rotina deve evitar a recidiva do problema.

COMPLICAÇÕES POSSÍVEIS
- Se não forem tratados, os animais hipotireóideos estão sob alto risco de desenvolver mixedema, coma mixedematoso e aterosclerose.
- A suplementação excessiva de hormônios tireoidianos pode resultar em hipertireoidismo iatrogênico.

EVOLUÇÃO ESPERADA E PROGNÓSTICO
- O hipotireoidismo primário pode ser controlado com facilidade e de forma bem-sucedida. O prognóstico para os animais acometidos que recebem tratamento adequado é excelente. A resolução dos sinais clínicos é um indicador importante da suplementação terapêutica adequada.
- Dentro de 1 semana do início da terapia, deve ocorrer uma melhora significativa na postura, no nível de atividade e no estado de alerta do animal.
- As anormalidades dermatológicas melhoram lentamente, com resolução completa em até 3 meses.
- Em geral, as polineuropatias começam a melhorar com rapidez; a resolução completa pode levar alguns meses.
- O quadro de anemia e os níveis séricos de colesterol gradativamente se resolvem nas primeiras semanas de terapia.
- Espera-se que a expectativa de vida seja normal.
- O hipotireoidismo congênito tem um prognóstico reservado a mau.

DIVERSOS

DISTÚRBIOS ASSOCIADOS
Raramente, o hipotireoidismo pode estar associado a outras endocrinopatias.

FATORES RELACIONADOS COM A IDADE
Nenhum.

POTENCIAL ZOONÓTICO
Nenhum.

GESTAÇÃO/FERTILIDADE/REPRODUÇÃO
- Não há problemas relativos à prenhez.
- Não há nenhuma prova definitiva que sugere uma associação com alteração na fertilidade.

VER TAMBÉM
Mixedema e Coma Mixedematoso.

ABREVIATURA(S)
- AINE = anti-inflamatório não esteroide.
- ELISA = ensaio imunoabsorvente ligado à enzima.
- GI = gastrintestinal.
- T_3 = liotironina, 3,5,3′-tri-iodotironina.
- T_4 = tiroxina, tetraiodotironina.
- TRH = hormônio liberador da tirotropina.
- TSH = hormônio tireostimulante.

Sugestões de Leitura
Feldman ED, Nelson RW, eds. Hypothyroidism. In: Canine and Feline Endocrinology and Reproduction, 3rd ed. St. Louis: Elsevier Saunders, 2004, pp. 86-151.
Finora K, Greco DS. Hypothyroidism and myxedema coma in veterinary medicine — physiology, diagnosis and treatment. Compend Contin Educ Pract Vet 2007, 29;19-32.
Meeking SA. Thyroid disorders in the geriatric patient. Vet Clin North Am Small Anim Pract 2005, 35:635-653.
Scott-Moncrieff JCR, Guptill-Yoran L. Hypothyroidism. In: Ettinger SJ, Feldman EC, eds., Textbook of Veterinary Internal Medicine, 6th ed. St. Louis: Elsevier, 2005, pp. 1535-1544.

Autor Kevin Finora
Consultor Editorial Deborah S. Greco

HIPOXEMIA

CONSIDERAÇÕES GERAIS

DEFINIÇÃO
• Queda na PaO_2, resultando em dessaturação acentuada da hemoglobina.
• A PaO_2 ao nível do mar varia de 80 a 100 mmHg.

FISIOPATOLOGIA
Há seis causas fisiológicas — (1) PIO_2 baixa; (2) hipoventilação (aumento na $PaCO_2$); (3) desequilíbrio entre ventilação-perfusão alveolar, de modo que as áreas do pulmão não ventiladas de forma conveniente também não são perfundidas adequadamente; (4) defeito de difusão através da membrana alveolocapilar; (5) desvio cardíaco da direita para a esquerda ou pulmonar; (6) baixo débito cardíaco.

SISTEMA(S) ACOMETIDO(S)
• Todos os órgãos — o oxigênio é essencial para a função celular normal; a necessidade individual de oxigênio para os tecidos varia de acordo com o órgão.
• Cardiovascular — a hipoxemia pode resultar em isquemia focal ou global; se prolongada, podem se desenvolver arritmias e insuficiência cardíaca.
• Nervoso — o cérebro e o SNC são os órgãos mais importantes; a hipoxemia nesses órgãos pode resultar em lesão cerebral irreversível, pois não há grandes reservas de oxigênio no tecido cerebral.

IDENTIFICAÇÃO
Qualquer raça, idade e sexo de cães e gatos.

SINAIS CLÍNICOS

Achados Anamnésicos
• Episódios de tosse.
• Problemas respiratórios — especialmente respiração com a boca aberta.
• Traumatismo.
• Engasgo.
• Intolerância ao exercício.
• Cianose.
• Colapso.

Achados do Exame Físico
• Taquipneia.
• Dispneia.
• Ortopneia.
• Mucosas pálidas.
• Cianose.
• Tosse.
• Respiração com a boca aberta.
• Taquicardia.
• Pulso periférico fraco.
• Auscultação torácica anormal.

CAUSAS
• PIO_2 baixa — altitude elevada (quanto maior a elevação, menor será a pressão barométrica, o que resulta em uma queda da PIO_2; a FIO_2 é fixada em 0,21); sufocação; confinamento em áreas pequenas com ventilação imprópria.
• Hipoventilação — resulta de ventilação alveolar inadequada; paralisia muscular; obstrução de vias aéreas superiores; presença de ar ou líquido no espaço pleural; restrição da caixa torácica, hérnia diafragmática; doença do SNC.
• Desequilíbrio entre ventilação-perfusão alveolar — além de ser a causa mais comum de hipoxemia, esse desequilíbrio ocorre em praticamente qualquer doença pulmonar: tromboembolia pulmonar; doença do parênquima pulmonar (infecciosa ou neoplásica); doença de vias aéreas inferiores; pneumonia; contusões pulmonares; edema pulmonar; ocorre também durante anestesia ou decúbito prolongado em que uma grande área do pulmão se torna atelectásica.
• Defeito de difusão através da membrana alveolocapilar — raramente tem importância clínica.
• Desvio cardíaco da direita para a esquerda ou pulmonar — tetralogia de Fallot; defeito do septo ventricular; ducto arterioso patente invertido; desvio arteriovenoso intrapulmonar.
• Baixo débito cardíaco — insuficiência cardíaca por qualquer causa; choque por qualquer causa.

FATORES DE RISCO
• Ida súbita para altitudes elevadas.
• Traumatismo.
• Broncopneumonia.
• Doença pleural.
• Anestesia.
• Cardiopatia.
• Doença brônquica — doença pulmonar obstrutiva crônica; asma felina.
• Alterações pulmonares ou cardíacas geriátricas.
• Doenças associadas ao risco de embolização, p. ex., anemia hemolítica imunomediada, hiperadrenocorticismo, neoplasia, pancreatite, sepse.

DIAGNÓSTICO

DIAGNÓSTICO DIFERENCIAL
• Sinais de taquipneia e/ou dispneia.
• Agitação ou ansiedade.
• Hipertermia.
• Pirexia.
• Traumatismo craniano.
• Dor.

ACHADOS LABORATORIAIS

Medicamentos Capazes de Alterar os Resultados Laboratoriais
N/D.

Distúrbios Capazes de Alterar os Resultados Laboratoriais
• Bolhas de ar na amostra de sangue arterial — valores falsamente altos da PaO_2.
• Acondicionamento inadequado da amostra de sangue arterial — valores falsamente altos da PaO_2 após cerca de 30 min à temperatura ambiente.

Os Resultados Serão Válidos se os Exames Forem Realizados em Laboratório Humano?
Sim.

HEMOGRAMA/BIOQUÍMICA/URINÁLISE
Hematócrito — pode estar alto em casos de condição crônica; pode estar baixo se a causa for inflamatória ou neoplásica.

OUTROS TESTES LABORATORIAIS

Hemogasometria Arterial
Coletar amostra de sangue arterial de maneira anaeróbia, como se segue:
• Usar heparina suficiente para cobrir a agulha e a parte interna da seringa.
• Coletar amostra de artéria femoral ou podal dorsal.
• Colocar uma tampa de borracha na agulha ou cobrir o canhão da seringa para evitar entrada de ar do ambiente na amostra.
• Analisar a amostra nos primeiros 15 min se ela ficar à temperatura ambiente; colocar a amostra em gelo, para que a análise possa ser feita em 2-4 h.
• Utilizar analisadores dos gases sanguíneos à beira do leito ou portáteis — existem vários modelos disponíveis; tornam a análise mais conveniente.

DIAGNÓSTICO POR IMAGEM
Radiografias torácicas e ecocardiografia — avaliam doença intratorácica; diferenciam doença pulmonar de cardíaca.

MÉTODOS DIAGNÓSTICOS

Oximetria de Pulso
• Determina indiretamente a SaO_2; a relação entre a PaO_2 e a SaO_2 baseia-se na curva de dissociação da oxiemoglobina: SaO_2 >90% quando a PaO_2 >60 mmHg.
• SaO_2 <95% — além de ser considerada normal, indica PaO_2 <80 mmHg.
• Os melhores resultados são obtidos quando se usa sonda na língua dos animais; por essa razão, o uso de sonda pode ser limitado a pacientes anestesiados, intensamente sedados ou gravemente doentes com baixo nível de consciência; manter a língua umedecida para obtenção de leituras mais precisas.
• Outros locais bons para usar a sonda — lábios; orelhas; vulva (fêmea) e prepúcio (macho); pele interdigital (i. e., entre os dedos); pele fina na área do flanco.
• Resultados ruins — menos precisos em estados de baixo fluxo como hipotensão (fluxo global baixo) ou hipotermia (baixo fluxo em direção à pele); valores falsamente baixos (em geral, <85%) durante carboxiemoglobinemia (inalação de fumaça).
• Sondas retais — devem estar disponíveis; permitem leituras em pacientes acordados.

Endoscopia ou Biopsia Pulmonar
É frequente a necessidade de amostragem das vias aéreas para determinar a anormalidade primária que resulta em hipoxemia.

TRATAMENTO

É imprescindível identificar e corrigir a causa primária.

Oxigenoterapia
• Tratamento de suporte mais comum.
• Corrige o baixo nível de oxigênio inspirado, a hipoventilação e os defeitos de difusão através da membrana alveolocapilar; pode não corrigir totalmente o desequilíbrio entre ventilação--perfusão; não corrige desvios cardíacos da direita para a esquerda ou pulmonares e baixo débito cardíaco.
• Pode não ser completamente benéfica até que se restabeleça o volume sanguíneo adequado.
• Distribuído diretamente a partir de uma fonte de oxigênio do aparelho de anestesia via máscara facial fixada em torno do focinho ou de E-tank (tanque de energia) adaptado a regulador de oxigênio através de máscara facial, cateter intranasal ou gaiola de oxigênio.
• Aumento na FIO_2 — determinado pelo fluxo de oxigênio e pela quantidade de oxigênio misturado com o ar ambiente.
• Ventilação com pressão positiva — pode ser necessária para SARA ou hipoventilação grave.

HIPOXEMIA

Fluidoterapia
- Baixo débito cardíaco — a administração de fluido e o uso de suporte inotrópico (p. ex., dobutamina ou dopamina) são importantes.
- Insuficiência cardíaca — requer tratamento clínico rigoroso; diuréticos; redução da pré e pós-carga; suporte inotrópico; administração de oxigênio; fluidos indicados após a instituição do tratamento primário; ter cuidado com o tipo e a velocidade de fluidos após a estabilização inicial.
- Choque hipovolêmico, hemorrágico, traumático ou séptico — requer a administração intensa de fluidos; cristaloides (90 mL/kg o mais rapidamente possível), soluções hipertônicas (NaCl a 7%, 4 mL/kg), coloides (hetamido, 20 mL/kg), soluções carreadoras de oxigênio à base de hemoglobina, ou combinação.
- Contusão pulmonar grave — fluidos hipertônicos ou coloides, ou uma combinação preferida.

MEDICAÇÕES
MEDICAMENTO(S) DE ESCOLHA
Para broncospasmo — broncodilatadores; terbutalina (0,01 mg/kg SC, IM ou IV a cada 8 h).

CONTRAINDICAÇÕES
- Administração intensa de fluidos — não indicada na presença de insuficiência cardíaca e edema pulmonar.
- Diuréticos — não indicados em casos de choque, baixa PIO_2, defeitos de difusão através da membrana alveolocapilar, desequilíbrio entre ventilação-perfusão alveolar e desvios da direita para a esquerda.

PRECAUÇÕES
- Medicamentos inotrópicos — podem se desenvolver arritmias.

- Toxicidade do oxigênio — decorrente da exposição prolongada (> 12 h) a alta concentração (> 70%) desse gás; edema pulmonar, crises convulsivas e morte.

INTERAÇÕES POSSÍVEIS
N/D.

MEDICAMENTO(S) ALTERNATIVO(S)
N/D.

ACOMPANHAMENTO
MONITORIZAÇÃO DO PACIENTE
- Diminuição no esforço respiratório e na cianose (se observada inicialmente) — verificar a eficácia do tratamento e do suporte.
- Hemogasometria arterial — determina a resolução.
- Oximetria de pulso — técnica alternativa; interpretar os resultados com cautela diante de hipotensão, hipotermia, inalação de fumaça e sonda em outro local que não a língua.

COMPLICAÇÕES POSSÍVEIS
- Lesão cerebral — depende da gravidade e da duração da hipoxemia; perda parcial ou completa da função neuronal; demência; crises convulsivas; perda da consciência.
- Arritmias — podem se desenvolver secundariamente à hipoxia miocárdica; pode ser muito difícil tratá-las de modo eficaz.

DIVERSOS
DISTÚRBIOS ASSOCIADOS
N/D.

FATORES RELACIONADOS COM A IDADE
N/D.

POTENCIAL ZOONÓTICO
Nenhum.

GESTAÇÃO/FERTILIDADE/REPRODUÇÃO
Pode afetar adversamente os fetos, sobretudo durante o primeiro trimestre de gravidez.

VER TAMBÉM
- Cianose.
- Dispneia e Angústia Respiratória.
- Respiração Ofegante e Taquipneia.

ABREVIATURA(S)
- FIO_2 = fração de oxigênio no ar inspirado.
- $PaCO_2$ = pressão parcial de dióxido de carbono no sangue arterial.
- PaO_2 = pressão parcial de oxigênio arterial.
- PIO_2 = pressão parcial de oxigênio inspirado.
- SaO_2 = saturação de oxigênio no sangue arterial.
- SARA = síndrome da angústia respiratória aguda.
- SNC = sistema nervoso central.

Sugestões de Leitura
Haskin SC. Interpretation of blood gas measurement. In: King LG, ed., Textbook of Respiratory Disease in Dogs and Cats. Philadelphia: Elsevier, 2004, pp. 181-193.
Hendricks JC. Pulse oximetry. In: King LG, ed., Textbook of Respiratory Disease in Dogs and Cats. Philadelphia: Elsevier, 2004, pp. 194-197.

Autor Thomas Kevin Day
Consultor Editorial Lynelle R. Johnson

Histiocitoma

CONSIDERAÇÕES GERAIS

REVISÃO
Tumor cutâneo benigno que surge de células de Langerhans (p. ex., histiócitos) da pele.

IDENTIFICAÇÃO
- Comum em cães, mas extremamente raro em gatos.
- Mais de 50% dos pacientes caninos têm menos de 2 anos de idade.
- As raças comumente acometidas incluem Boxer, Dachshund, Cocker spaniel, Staffordshire terrier americano, Dinamarquês, Boston terrier, Doberman pinscher, Schnauzer miniatura, Pastor de Shetland, Labrador retriever, West Highland white terrier e Bull terrier.
- Sem predominância racial em gatos.
- Sem predominância sexual em cães ou gatos.

SINAIS CLÍNICOS
- Lesão dérmica solitária, elevada, bem-circunscrita, sem pelo e em forma de botão, que pode estar ulcerada.
- Frequentemente exibe crescimento rápido nas primeiras 1-4 semanas.
- Considerada indolor.
- Locais comuns — cabeça, pavilhão auricular (pina) e membros.
- Há relatos de múltiplos tumores e histiocitomas metastáticos (raros).

CAUSAS E FATORES DE RISCO
Há hipóteses de que a população celular representa uma proliferação atípica ou hiperplasia reativa e não um câncer verdadeiro.

DIAGNÓSTICO

DIAGNÓSTICO DIFERENCIAL
Exame histopatológico e colorações imuno-histoquímicas são necessários para distinguir de inflamação granulomatosa focal e outros tumores de células redondas (tumor venéreo transmissível, linfoma, sarcoma histiocítico e mastocitoma).

HEMOGRAMA/BIOQUÍMICA/URINÁLISE
Geralmente normais.

OUTROS TESTES LABORATORIAIS
N/D.

DIAGNÓSTICO POR IMAGEM
N/D.

OUTROS MÉTODOS DIAGNÓSTICOS
- Exame citológico:
  - Caracterizado por lâminas de células redondas pleomórficas com citoplasma cinza/azul pálido abundante, núcleos arredondados a levemente denteados (recortados) localizados no centro e nucléolos imperceptíveis.
  - Pode haver a presença de infiltrado de células inflamatórias (linfócitos) que, frequentemente, precederá a regressão espontânea da lesão.

ACHADOS PATOLÓGICOS
- Caracterizados por lâminas de histiócitos que se infiltram na derme e no subcutâneo, seguem o rastro de folículos pilosos e elevam o epitélio hiperplásico sobrejacente e muitas vezes ulcerado.
- Nas lesões em remissão, frequentemente se identifica a presença de infiltração linfocítica e necrose.
- Alto índice mitótico compatível com a rápida taxa de crescimento é uma característica desse tumor.

TRATAMENTO

- Pode regredir espontaneamente em 2-3 meses.
- Excisão cirúrgica ou criocirurgia — geralmente são medidas curativas.
- Será importante diferenciar histiocitoma de tumor maligno se o proprietário preferir uma abordagem expectante.
- Os casos com múltiplos histiocitomas podem ter uma evolução clínica mais prolongada, embora a resolução espontânea ainda seja possível.

MEDICAÇÕES

MEDICAMENTO(S)
N/D.

CONTRAINDICAÇÕES/INTERAÇÕES POSSÍVEIS
N/D.

ACOMPANHAMENTO

MONITORIZAÇÃO DO PACIENTE
Excisão cirúrgica é recomendada se a massa não tiver regredido espontaneamente em 2-3 meses.

EVOLUÇÃO ESPERADA E PROGNÓSTICO
- Prognóstico é considerado excelente com a remoção cirúrgica.
- A regressão espontânea é provável em 2-3 meses.

DIVERSOS

Sugestões de Leitura

Clifford CA, Skorupski KS. Tumors of the skin, subcutis and soft tissue; histiocytic diseases. In: Henry CJ, Higginbotham ML, eds., Cancer Management in Small Animal Practice. St Louis: Saunders Elsevier, 2010, pp. 326-330.

Moore PF, Affolter V, Olivry T, et al. The use of immunological reagents in defining the pathogenesis of canine skin disease involving proliferation of leukocytes. In: Kwochka KW, Wilemse T, von Tscharner C, eds., Advances in Veterinary Dermatology. Oxford: Butterworth-Heinemann, 1998, pp. 77-94.

Moore PF, Schrenzel MD, Affolter VK, et al. Canine cutaneous histiocytoma is an epidermotropic Langerhans cell histiocytosis that expresses CD1 and specific beta 2-integrin molecules. Am J Pathol 1996, 148:1699-1708.

Autor Craig Clifford
Consultor Editorial Timothy M. Fan

Histiocitoma Fibroso Maligno (Tumor de Células Gigantes)

CONSIDERAÇÕES GERAIS

REVISÃO
• O nome baseia-se nas características histológicas de células semelhantes a fibroblastos e histiócitos.
• Neoplasia mesenquimal primitiva, embora a origem celular definitiva seja desconhecida; as possibilidades prováveis incluem fibroblastos, histiócitos e células mesenquimais indiferenciadas.
• Diversas variantes histológicas.
• Tipo estoriforme-pleomórfico e célula gigante — duas variantes principais; ambas são localmente invasivas; massas subcutâneas ou viscerais firmes ao exame.
• A despeito dos relatos anteriores em contrário, o potencial metastático nos cães parece ser moderado a alto.
• Foi relatado sob a forma de sarcomas relacionados com o local de injeção dos gatos.

IDENTIFICAÇÃO
• Mais comumente relatado nos gatos do que nos cães.
• Comportamento biológico semelhante em ambas as espécies.
• Idade média — gatos: 9 anos (faixa etária, 2-12 anos); cães: 8 anos (faixa etária, <1-10 anos).
• Sem predileção racial ou sexual comprovada, embora os cães da raça Retriever de pelo liso possam ser predispostos.

SINAIS CLÍNICOS
Achados Anamnésicos
• Podem ocorrer anorexia, perda de peso e letargia.
• Dependem do local de envolvimento.

Achados do Exame Físico
• Tumor invasivo e firme, que surge no tecido subcutâneo.
• Pode apresentar uma extensão profunda para o músculo esquelético subjacente.
• Pode se desenvolver em local adjacente ao osso e induzir a destruição e proliferação ósseas.
• Locais mais comuns — região torácica dorsal e escapular, membros e região pélvica.
• Também pode ser um tumor esplênico primário; pode-se constatar uma esplenomegalia palpável.
• Metástase à distância — é comum.

CAUSAS E FATORES DE RISCO
• Desconhecidos.
• Pode ser induzido por carcinógenos em espécies de animais de laboratório.
• Locais de injeção nos gatos.

DIAGNÓSTICO

DIAGNÓSTICO DIFERENCIAL
• Fibrossarcoma.
• Condrossarcoma.
• Osteossarcoma (extraesquelético).
• Neoplasia de mastócitos.
• Rabdomioma ou rabdomiossarcoma.
• Lipossarcoma.
• Tumores da bainha de nervos periféricos.
• Doenças histiocíticas, como histiocitose maligna ou sistêmica.
• Sarcoma histiocítico.

HEMOGRAMA/BIOQUÍMICA/URINÁLISE
• Hemograma completo — pode variar entre resultados normais e constatação de anemia regenerativa ou arregenerativa.
• Bioquímica — variavelmente anormal.
• Urinálise — em geral, normal.

OUTROS TESTES LABORATORIAIS
Exame citológico de aspirado — pode revelar células semelhantes a histiócitos e fibroblastos.

DIAGNÓSTICO POR IMAGEM
• Radiografia — revela massa densa de tecido mole; pode-se notar proliferação ou destruição óssea.
• Radiografia torácica em três projeções — para verificar a presença de metástase pulmonar.
• RM ou TC — esses exames podem ser superiores para delinear o grau de invasão tumoral para os tecidos circunjacentes.
• Ultrassonografia — pode detectar anormalidades compatíveis com metástase abdominal (mais comum nos linfonodos e no fígado).

MÉTODOS DIAGNÓSTICOS
Exame histológico de amostra obtida por biopsia — necessário para o diagnóstico definitivo.

ACHADOS PATOLÓGICOS
• Classificação — existe considerável debate entre os patologistas, o que pode ter ocasionado as aparentes diferenças no comportamento relatadas na literatura especializada.
• Tipo estoriforme-pleomórfico (também conhecido como inflamatório) e células gigantes (também conhecido como tipo semelhante a osteoclastos) constituem as duas principais variantes relatadas.
• Muitos são histologicamente de alto grau.
• Corantes imuno-histológicos especializados, como vimentina, desmina, alfa-actina de músculo liso, extradomínio 1 (ED1) e/ou azana (para colágeno) podem ajudar na classificação.
• Relato recente de características histológicas sobrepostas consideráveis com doenças histiocíticas na forma esplênica.

TRATAMENTO

• Excisão cirúrgica — difícil em virtude da natureza invasiva local; a taxa de recidiva é elevada.
• Amputação do membro acometido — pode ser apropriada; radiografias toracoabdominais e ultrassonografias abdominais são exames críticos para avaliar a presença de metástase detectável antes da amputação.
• Radioterapia — pode ser útil como tratamento adjuvante para tumor localizado não acessível à ressecção cirúrgica completa. As taxas esperadas de controle tumoral local podem ser semelhantes a outros sarcomas de tecido mole de alto grau.

MEDICAÇÕES

MEDICAMENTO(S)
Quimioterapia — pode ser valiosa em casos de tumor residual de grau elevado ou doença metastática estabelecida; os protocolos à base de doxorrubicina são mais populares (paciente >10 kg, 30 mg/m² IV a cada 3 semanas; pacientes <10 kg, 1 mg/kg IV a cada 3 semanas).

CONTRAINDICAÇÕES/INTERAÇÕES POSSÍVEIS
N/D.

ACOMPANHAMENTO

MONITORIZAÇÃO DO PACIENTE
Reavaliação — o potencial metastático sugeriria exame físico e possível diagnóstico por imagem — mensalmente durante 3 meses e, em seguida, a cada 3 meses.

COMPLICAÇÕES POSSÍVEIS
Efeitos colaterais agudos temporários (p. ex., dermatite úmida e alopecia) podem ser esperados com a radioterapia; por essa razão, é recomendável a consulta com algum oncologista especialista em radiação sobre os efeitos colaterais específicos relacionados com a região anatômica.

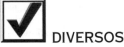

DIVERSOS

ABREVIATURA(S)
• RM = ressonância magnética.
• TC = tomografia computadorizada.

Sugestões de Leitura
Do SH, Hong IH, Park JK, et al. Two different types of malignant fibrous histiocytomas from pet dogs. J Vet Sci 2009, 10:169-171.

Autor Anthony J. Mutsaers
Consultor Editorial Timothy M. Fan

HISTIOCITOSE — CÃES

CONSIDERAÇÕES GERAIS

REVISÃO
- Distúrbio incomum que resulta da proliferação de células das linhagens de monócitos/macrófagos (células fagocitárias) e Langerhans/dendríticas (células apresentadoras de antígenos).
- Sistemas orgânicos acometidos — cutâneo; linfático; hematológico; nervoso; oftálmico; musculoesquelético; gastrintestinal; respiratório.
- Condições não neoplásicas reativas caninas ocorrem sob a forma de histiocitose cutânea e sistêmica de aspecto semelhante, mas diferem em seu aspecto clínico, histológico e fenotípico das doenças histiocíticas neoplásicas.
- As condições histiocíticas neoplásicas em cães incluem histiocitoma cutâneo, sarcoma histiocítico e leucemia de células dendríticas; em gatos, ocorrem histiocitose progressiva e sarcoma histiocítico.
- O sarcoma histiocítico que surge de células dendríticas da derme pode ser localizado ou disseminado (denominado antigamente como "histiocitose maligna").
- O sarcoma histiocítico hemofagocítico é uma variante derivada de macrófagos CD11d-positivos.
- Talvez haja necessidade dos perfis de marcadores imunoquímicos para confirmar a origem histiocítica e diferenciar essas doenças entre si.

IDENTIFICAÇÃO
Histiocitose Reativa
- Uma doença rara em cães que variam de 2 a 11 anos (idade média de 5 anos).
- Não há predileção sexual aparente na forma cutânea, mas uma predominância de machos na doença sistêmica em cães da raça Montanhês de Berna.
- Há uma grande variedade de raças descritas para a histiocitose cutânea, embora as raças Montanhês de Berna, Rottweiler, Golden retriever e Labrador retriever sejam mais predispostas à histiocitose sistêmica.

Histiocitoma Cutâneo Canino
- Doença muito comum de cães jovens com menos de 3 anos de idade, embora tenha sido observada em cães mais idosos.
- Não há predileção sexual.
- A raça Shar-pei é predisposta a histiocitomas múltiplos.

Sarcoma Histiocítico (Localizado/Disseminado/Hemofagocítico)
- Doença incomum de cães entre 2 e 14 anos de idade (idade média de 8 anos).
- Relatada em diversas raças, porém mais comumente em Rottweiler, Montanhês de Berna, Golden retriever, Labrador retriever ou retrievers de pelagem lisa.
- Raras vezes, é documentada como lesões localizadas, disseminadas ou hemofagocíticas em gatos.

SINAIS CLÍNICOS
Comentários Gerais
- Histiocitose cutânea — apresenta, em geral, evolução crônica flutuante; é possível a regressão espontânea das lesões.
- Histiocitose sistêmica — doença debilitante crônica e flutuante; podem ocorrer episódios clínicos múltiplos e períodos assintomáticos.
- Histiocitoma cutâneo canino — frequentemente regride dentro de 3 meses.
- Sarcoma histiocítico — rapidamente progressivo e fatal.
- Leucemia de células dendríticas — pode se originar da medula óssea; rapidamente progressiva e fatal.

Achados Anamnésicos
- Letargia, anorexia, perda de peso.
- Presença de massa(s).
- Claudicação.
- Respirações ruidosas, tosse, dispneia.
- Pode não haver sinais de doença sistêmica em cães com histiocitose cutânea e em alguns com histiocitose sistêmica.

Achados do Exame Físico
Histiocitose Cutânea
- Múltiplos nódulos ou placas intradérmicos não pruriginosos e não dolorosos de regiões como cabeça, pescoço, extremidades, escroto e, menos frequentemente, tronco ou abdome.
- Não há relatos de casos de envolvimento ocular.
- Não há acometimento sistêmico de órgãos.

Histiocitose Sistêmica
- Predileção acentuada por regiões de pele, cavidade nasal, olhos e linfonodos.
- Massas cutâneas — múltiplas; nodulares; bem-circunscritas e em geral ulceradas, com crostas ou alopécicas; costumam ocorrer no focinho, no plano nasal, nas pálpebras, no flanco e no escroto, com aspecto semelhante à histiocitose cutânea.
- Com frequência, há linfadenomegalia periférica moderada a grave.
- Manifestações oculares — conjuntivite; quemose; esclerite; episclerite; nódulos episclerais; edema de córnea; uveíte anterior e posterior; descolamento da retina; glaucoma e exoftalmia.
- Ruídos respiratórios anormais ou ruidosos e/ou infiltração da mucosa nasal.
- Pode ocorrer organomegalia.

Histiocitoma Cutâneo Canino
- Geralmente, um nódulo solitário eritematoso ou ulcerado, não pruriginoso, sem pelo e em relevo.
- Predileção por regiões de cabeça, pescoço, orelhas ou membros.

Sarcoma Histiocítico
- Palidez, fraqueza, dispneia com ruídos pulmonares anormais e sinais neurológicos (p. ex., crises convulsivas, distúrbios centrais, paresia posterior) — comuns.
- Linfadenomegalia e hepatosplenomegalia moderadas a graves.
- Massas — lesões localizadas dentro dos pulmões, medula óssea, pele, cérebro e região periarticular de extremidades.

CAUSAS E FATORES DE RISCO
- Histiocitose cutânea e sistêmica — doenças reativas (inflamatórias) não neoplásicas que surgem da expansão de células dendríticas dérmicas ativadas; a ausência de agentes infecciosos e respostas a medicamentos imunomoduladores sugere o possível envolvimento de mecanismos de falta de regulação imunológica.
- Sarcoma histiocítico disseminado — doença histiocítica neoplásica; origem desconhecida de células dendríticas em processo de proliferação.
- Doença familiar de cães da raça Montanhês de Berna — modo de herança poligênico; responsável por até 25% de todos os tumores nessa raça.
- Cães das raças Retriever de pelo liso, Golden retriever e Rottweiler parecem predispostos, sugerindo fatores genéticos.

DIAGNÓSTICO

DIAGNÓSTICO DIFERENCIAL
- Doença inflamatória — pode ser semelhante à histiocitose reativa com um misto de histiócitos, linfócitos e neutrófilos; no entanto, espera-se maior variação nos tipos celulares.
- Linfoma ou leucemia linfoide — o diagnóstico definitivo frequentemente requer citoquímica e/ou imunoquímica especial.
- Sarcoma anaplásico com células gigantes, conhecido antigamente como histiocitoma fibroso maligno — sarcoma de tecidos moles, localmente agressivo e composto de histiócitos e fibroblastos; coloração imuno-histoquímica positiva para actina e vimentina; a falta de expressão da molécula CD18 indica origem mesenquimal.
- Nódulos esplênicos fibro-histiocíticos — esplenomegalia nodular resultante da proliferação de células fibro-histiocíticas dentro de nódulos linfoides esplênicos; as raças Retriever, Pastor alemão e Cocker spaniel parecem super-representadas; espectro de lesões esplênicas.
- Histiocitose esplênica — esplenomegalia com alterações microscópicas distintivas, incluindo metaplasia mieloide (hematopoiese difusa), histiocitose, eritrofagocitose e trombose com infarto; o acometimento multicêntrico de órgãos é comum; o prognóstico é grave e a presença de células gigantes pode ser preditiva de um desfecho fatal; pode representar parte do espectro de doenças histiocíticas; doenças imunomediadas e infecções sistêmicas podem ser causas subjacentes.
- Dermatite granulomatosa multinodular perianexial — nódulos cutâneos bem-delimitados; comumente no focinho, mas pode acometer os olhos; ao exame histológico, há granulomas distintos e números variáveis de células inflamatórias; a não ser pela associação perianexial, pode não ser uma tarefa fácil diferenciá-la de histiocitose cutânea.
- Granulomatose linfomatoide — infiltrado pulmonar composto de linfócitos, plasmócitos, histiócitos e células linforreticulares atípicas; acomete cães jovens a de meia-idade; ausência de acometimento de linfonodos, outros órgãos ou da medula óssea.
- Doenças granulomatosas — cães com doenças infecciosas como nocardiose, actinomicose e doenças micóticas podem ter opacidades pulmonares nodulares; a citologia e a histopatologia de macrófagos associados podem parecer atípicas e bizarras.
- Síndrome hemofagocítica (histiocitose) — proliferação histiocítica benigna secundária a doenças infecciosas, neoplásicas ou metabólicas; histiócitos são bem diferenciados e podem envolver a medula óssea, os linfonodos, o fígado e o baço; provoca citopenias de pelo menos 2 linhagens celulares.
- Carcinomas ou sarcomas anaplásicos — os achados histopatológicos em cães com histiocitose podem se assemelhar a um tumor pouco diferenciado; marcadores teciduais específicos possibilitam a diferenciação.

HISTIOCITOSE — CÃES

HEMOGRAMA/BIOQUÍMICA/URINÁLISE
• Cães com histiocitose cutânea não têm anormalidades sistêmicas.
• Anemia (regenerativa ou arregenerativa) e trombocitopenia leves a graves são comuns em cães com sarcoma histiocítico sistêmico e disseminado ou sarcoma histiocítico hemofagocítico; em princípio, as citopenias se devem à fagocitose por histiócitos e, mais tarde, ao declínio na produção pelo envolvimento da medula óssea.
• Raramente se observam células de sarcoma histiocítico disseminado na circulação.
• Os resultados bioquímicos variam e podem refletir o grau do acometimento orgânico. É comum a constatação de hipoalbuminemia em cães com sarcoma histiocítico.

OUTROS TESTES LABORATORIAIS
Ferritina sérica — pode ser um marcador tumoral para sarcoma histiocítico; um cão acometido apresentou concentração sérica muito alta de ferritina, sugerindo secreção por fagócitos mononucleares neoplásicos.

DIAGNÓSTICO POR IMAGEM
• Radiografia torácica — opacidades pulmonares nodulares bem-definidas (isoladas ou múltiplas); efusão pleural; consolidação de lobo pulmonar; infiltrados intersticiais difusos; massas mediastínicas; linfadenomegalia esternal e traqueobrônquica.
• Radiografia e ultrassonografia abdominais — hepatomegalia; esplenomegalia; efusão abdominal.
• Outras modalidades de diagnóstico por imagem, como radiografia da coluna vertebral e ressonância magnética dos membros para avaliar a presença de massas periarticulares.

MÉTODOS DIAGNÓSTICOS
• Histopatologia ou citologia de órgãos e/ou linfonodos acometidos.
• Biopsia, tanto para exame histológico como citológico da medula óssea — pode revelar infiltração histiocítica.
• Análise do líquido cerebrospinal — pode ser útil para avaliação de sinais neurológicos.
• Imunoquímica — o diagnóstico de vários distúrbios histiocíticos exige perfis que avaliem a presença de células linfoides, células dendríticas, células de Langerhans e macrófagos, mas eliminem células epiteliais ou mesenquimais.
• Falta de expressão de marcadores linfoides como CD3 (células-T), CD79a (células-B) com CD18-positivo apoia a origem histiocítica.
• Histiocitose cutânea/sistêmica, sarcoma histiocítico localizado/disseminado e leucemia de células dendríticas — coram-se positivamente com o uso de marcadores para células de origem dendrítica mieloide, como CD1, classe II do complexo de histocompatibilidade maior, molécula de adesão CD11c e molécula de adesão intercelular ICAM-1, bem como marcadores de superfície expressos por leucócitos como CD45 e CD18.
• A histiocitose reativa é positiva para Thy-1 e CD4, enquanto o sarcoma histiocítico é negativo para CD4 e, ocasionalmente, Thy-1.
• Histiocitoma cutâneo canino expressa a E-caderina, além de CD1, CD11c e MHCII, mas carece de CD4 e Thy-1.
• Macrófagos neoplásicos de sarcoma histiocítico hemofagocítico expressam CD11b e CD11d (encontrados em macrófagos da polpa vermelha esplênica e da medula óssea), mas possuem baixa expressão dos marcadores dendríticos, CD1 e CD11c.

ACHADOS PATOLÓGICOS
Macroscópicos
• Massas cutâneas.
• Aumento discreto dos linfonodos.
• Focos brancos pouco definidos no baço, nos pulmões, nos rins, nos testículos, nos músculos esqueléticos da cabeça, no fígado e no pâncreas.
• Esplenomegalia e/ou hepatomegalia com possíveis lesões expansivas tipo massa.

Histopatológicos
Histiocitose Cutânea/Sistêmica
• Os infiltrados histiocíticos não revelam as características citológicas bizarras das células da histiocitose maligna.
• Os histiócitos parecem ter como alvo os pequenos vasos sanguíneos (angiocêntricos).
• Raramente se observam células gigantes multinucleadas.
• Números variáveis de outras células inflamatórias ficam entremeados.
• Na pele, a ausência de acometimento epitelial diferencia a doença dos histiocitomas cutâneos benignos.

Sarcoma Histiocítico
• Atipia citológica é a principal característica; os histiócitos são grandes e pleomórficos, com citoplasma espumoso.
• O índice mitótico, em geral, é alto, podendo haver figuras mitóticas anormais.
• Com frequência, observam-se células gigantes multinucleadas.
• Em alguns casos, a eritrofagocitose por histiócitos neoplásicos é evidente.
• Ocasionalmente, podem ser demonstradas leucofagocitose e trombofagocitose.
• A histopatologia da histiocitose pode lembrar sarcoma ou linfoma anaplásicos.
• Talvez haja necessidade de estudos imunoquímicos para confirmar a origem dendrítica mieloide.

TRATAMENTO
• Fluidoterapia ou transfusões de sangue podem ser necessárias, dependendo dos achados clínicos.
• É recomendável a remoção cirúrgica rigorosa de sarcoma histiocítico localizado cutâneo ou a amputação de membro para sarcoma histiocítico localizado periarticular não metastático.

MEDICAÇÕES
MEDICAMENTO(S)
Histiocitose Reativa
• Os cães apresentam episódios de doença clínica seguidos por períodos assintomáticos, sem nenhuma terapia.
• Responsiva a corticosteroides, inclusive com remissão completa e parcial, relatada em até 50% dos casos, principalmente em cães com histiocitose cutânea.
• Em casos de histiocitose sistêmica, foi observado sucesso terapêutico com o uso de medicamentos imunossupressores, como ciclosporina A ou leflunomida.
• Frequentemente ocorrem recidivas, podendo exigir terapia contínua.

Sarcoma Histiocítico
• Há relatos de respostas a protocolos à base de corticosteroides, lomustina, ciclofosfamida, vincristina e doxorrubicina.
• É mais provável que os cães sem hipoalbuminemia, trombocitopenia, anemia e envolvimento esplênico atinjam a remissão parcial ou completa com a lomustina.

ACOMPANHAMENTO
• A eficácia do tratamento é determinada por exames físicos repetidos, hemogramas completos e perfis bioquímicos, bem como por imagens diagnósticas.
• O prognóstico para cães com histiocitose maligna é extremamente mau; a morte em geral ocorre dentro de alguns meses após o diagnóstico.

DIVERSOS
Sugestões de Leitura
Moore PF, Affolter VK. Canine and feline histiocytic diseases. In: Ettinger SJ, Feldman EC, eds., Textbook of Veterinary Internal Medicine: Diseases of the Dog and Cat, 6th ed. St. Louis: Elsevier, 2005, pp. 779-783.

Autor Rose E. Raskin
Consultor Editorial A.H. Rebar
Agradecimento a Kenneth M. Rasnick

HISTOPLASMOSE

CONSIDERAÇÕES GERAIS

DEFINIÇÃO
Infecção fúngica sistêmica causada por *Histoplasma capsulatum*.

FISIOPATOLOGIA
- A forma de micélio cresce melhor em esterco de aves ou no solo enriquecido com matéria orgânica.
- Micélio no solo — produz esporos infecciosos (microconídios); inalado para as vias aéreas terminais.
- Esporos — germinam nos pulmões; desenvolvem-se em leveduras, que são fagocitadas por fagócitos mononucleares.
- Fagócitos mononucleares — distribuem os microrganismos pelo corpo.
- Os microrganismos ingeridos podem infectar diretamente o trato intestinal.
- Resposta imune — determina o desenvolvimento ou não da doença; os animais acometidos costumam desenvolver infecção assintomática transitória.

SISTEMA(S) ACOMETIDO(S)
- Gatos — o trato respiratório é o principal local de infecção; ossos, medula óssea, fígado, baço, pele e linfonodos também são acometidos; o trato intestinal, os olhos, os rins, as adrenais e o cérebro são afetados com menor frequência.
- Cães — o trato intestinal é o local mais frequentemente envolvido; fígado, pulmões, baço e linfonodos são afetados com frequência; ossos, medula óssea, rins, adrenais, cavidade bucal, língua, olhos e testículos são menos frequentemente acometidos.

GENÉTICA
N/D.

INCIDÊNCIA/PREVALÊNCIA
A prevalência da histoplasmose de relevância clínica é relativamente baixa em cães e gatos; na prática ativa, mesmo em áreas endêmicas, observam-se 3-4 casos por ano.

DISTRIBUIÇÃO GEOGRÁFICA
- Áreas endêmicas nos EUA — bacias dos rios Ohio, Missouri, Mississippi, Tennessee e St. Lawrence.
- Observada também no Texas, no sudeste dos EUA, na região dos Grandes Lagos e na Califórnia.

IDENTIFICAÇÃO
Espécies
Cães e gatos.

Raça(s) Predominante(s)
N/D.

Idade Média e Faixa Etária
- Gatos — predominantemente jovens; muitos com menos de 1 ano de idade; todas as idades podem ser infectadas.
- Cães — mais frequente nos animais jovens aos de meia-idade; no entanto, todas as idades podem ser acometidas pela infecção.

Sexo Predominante
N/D.

SINAIS CLÍNICOS
Achados Anamnésicos
Gatos
- Início insidioso em questão de dias a semanas.
- Anorexia, perda de peso e dispneia — mais comuns.
- Ocasionalmente há tosse.
- Claudicação.
- Secreção ocular.
- Diarreia.

Cães
- Perda de peso, depressão e diarreia com tenesmo — mais comuns.
- Tosse.
- Dispneia.
- Intolerância ao exercício.
- Linfadenopatia.
- Claudicação e alterações oculocutâneas — menos comuns.

Achados do Exame Físico
Gatos
- Febre de até 40°C.
- Esforço respiratório aumentado e ruídos pulmonares ásperos.
- Mucosas pálidas.
- Aumento dos linfonodos.
- Claudicação e secreção ocular podem ser encontradas.

Cães
- Magros a emaciados.
- Febre de até 40°C.
- Hepatosplenomegalia.
- Mucosas, em geral, pálidas.
- Ocasionalmente se observa icterícia.
- Tosse e dispneia associadas a ruídos pulmonares ásperos.

CAUSAS
H. capsulatum.

FATORES DE RISCO
- Poleiros de aves onde o solo seja enriquecido com dejetos de aves e de morcegos são ambientes de alto risco; gaiolas, comedouros e bebedouros antigos de frangos também são implicados como fatores de risco.
- Exposição à poeira contaminada com esporos fúngicos provenientes de locais de crescimento de fungos (especialmente no caso de gatos domésticos).
- Amostras de tecidos obtidas de quase metade dos cães e gatos errantes de uma área endêmica foram positivas para *Histoplasma*, apoiando a teoria de que muitas pessoas e animais se encontram infectados, mas poucos desenvolvem doença significativa do ponto de vista clínico.

DIAGNÓSTICO

DIAGNÓSTICO DIFERENCIAL
Gatos
- Dispneia decorrente de pneumonia fúngica — diferenciar de insuficiência cardíaca, asma felina, linfoma, pneumonia, piotórax e outras pneumonias fúngicas.
- Claudicação — diferenciar de traumatismo.
- Alterações oculares — diferenciar de linfoma, toxoplasmose e peritonite infecciosa felina.

Cães
- Diarreia crônica grave e perda de peso — considerar enterite linfocítica plasmocitária, enterite eosinofílica, linfoma, parasitismo crônico e insuficiência pancreática exócrina.
- Diarreia e anemia — considerar infecção grave por ancilóstomos.
- Hepatosplenomegalia e linfadenopatia periférica — compatíveis com linfoma.
- Sinais respiratórios — cinomose, pneumonia bacteriana e cardiopatia.

HEMOGRAMA/BIOQUÍMICA/URINÁLISE
- É comum o desenvolvimento de anemia arregenerativa moderada a grave.
- Contagens de leucócitos — geralmente normais; alguns pacientes apresentam leucocitose; os pacientes com acometimento da medula óssea podem estar leucopênicos.
- Microrganismos de *Histoplasma* — podem ser encontrados nos neutrófilos e monócitos circulantes.
- Acometimento hepático grave — é possível observar hiperbilirrubinemia e atividade elevada da ALT.
- Cães com histoplasmose intestinal grave frequentemente exibem níveis baixos das proteínas totais.

OUTROS TESTES LABORATORIAIS
- Teste de imunodifusão em ágar gel — para detecção de anticorpos; confirma o diagnóstico; resultados positivos indicam doença ativa; infecções prévias podem gerar resultados falso-positivos; muitos animais com doença ativa são negativos à sorologia.
- Teste antigênico — a excreção de antígeno na urina pode representar um método mais preciso de identificação dos animais infectados, embora existam poucos dados disponíveis a respeito disso. Recurso da internet: www.miravistalabs.com.
- Teste de Coombs — pode ser positivo, já que os anticorpos contra *Histoplasma* podem exibir reação cruzada com os eritrócitos; a terapia com esteroides está contraindicada.

DIAGNÓSTICO POR IMAGEM
Radiografia Torácica
- Cães — pneumonia intersticial a nodular difusa; aumento dos linfonodos traqueobrônquicos, comprimindo a bifurcação da traqueia; lesões pulmonares antigas podem ser opacidades calcificadas em forma de moeda, sugestivas de tumores metastáticos.
- Gatos — em geral, padrão intersticial difuso de acometimento pulmonar; calcificação e linfadenopatia traqueobrônquica são incomuns.

Radiografia Abdominal e Óssea
- Cães — aumento de linfonodos esplênicos e mesentéricos, bem como do fígado.
- Gatos e, com menor frequência, cães — lesões ósseas predominantemente osteolíticas que, em geral, ocorrem distalmente aos cotovelos e joelhos.

MÉTODOS DIAGNÓSTICOS
- Identificação de microrganismos à citologia, histopatologia ou cultura — diagnóstico definitivo.
- Amostras de tecidos — órgãos aumentados como fígado, baço e linfonodos são os melhores locais de coleta; raspados retais podem ser ricos em microrganismos; medula óssea; aspirados pulmonares (quando procedimentos menos invasivos não são diagnósticos); lavados traqueais são inconsistentes.

ACHADOS PATOLÓGICOS
- Lesões granulomatosas multifocais em órgãos ricos em células reticuloendoteliais (p. ex., baço, fígado, linfonodos, pulmões e medula óssea).

- Cães — o intestino é o primeiro local a ser acometido; o aumento de linfonodos traqueobrônquicos é comum.
- Gatos — acometimento predominantemente respiratório.

TRATAMENTO

CUIDADO(S) DE SAÚDE ADEQUADO(S)
- O tratamento costuma ser feito em um esquema ambulatorial com itraconazol por via oral.
- Paciente internado para receber anfotericina B por via IV — cães com enteropatia grave e má absorção.

CUIDADO(S) DE ENFERMAGEM
- Cães sob terapia com anfotericina B — mantê-los bem hidratados com solução eletrolítica balanceada para diminuir o potencial de toxicidade renal.
- Animais emaciados com má absorção — fornecer nutrição parenteral total para reverter a emaciação até que a enteropatia tenha se resolvido o suficiente a ponto de promover uma absorção adequada.
- Animais com dispneia grave — suplementação de oxigênio.

ATIVIDADE
Cães com dispneia — reduzir.

DIETA
É indispensável uma alimentação de boa qualidade, de fácil absorção e de sabor agradável (i. e., palatável).

ORIENTAÇÃO AO PROPRIETÁRIO
- Abordar as possíveis áreas de exposição no ambiente doméstico.
- Informar ao proprietário que tanto os animais de estimação como os membros da família podem ter sido expostos à mesma fonte e que o animal não representa um risco para a família.

MEDICAÇÕES

MEDICAMENTO(S) DE ESCOLHA

Itraconazol
- Medicamento de escolha se houver uma função intestinal adequada para absorção de agentes terapêuticos.
- Cães e gatos — 5 mg/kg VO a cada 12 h; administrar com uma refeição rica em gordura.
- Ter cuidado com o itraconazol manipulado, porque a absorção pode não ser boa.
- A duração depende da resposta clínica; o tratamento dura no mínimo 90 dias.

Anfotericina B Intravenosa

Cães
- Com enteropatia inflamatória grave e má absorção — usar até que o paciente comece a ganhar peso; em seguida, iniciar o itraconazol.
- O paciente precisa estar bem hidratado antes de se iniciar o tratamento; não administrar a anfotericina B em soluções eletrolíticas que possam precipitar o medicamento.
- Ureia — verificar antes da administração de cada dose; interromper se o nível se aproximar de 50 mg/dL e manter a hidratação; voltar a administrar quando o nível estiver <30 mg/dL.
- Dose habitual — 0,5 mg/kg IV a cada 48 h.
- Reconstituir em glicose a 5% e diluir para administração.
- Função renal normal — diluir em 60-120 mL de glicose a 5% e administrar durante 15 min.
- Algum comprometimento renal — diluir em 0,5-1 L de glicose a 5% e fornecer durante 3-4 h para reduzir a toxicidade renal.

Gatos
- Usar com cautela.
- Dose habitual — 0,25 mg/kg IV em glicose a 5% durante 3-4 h a cada 48 h.
- Mais sensíveis ao medicamento em comparação aos cães.

Fluconazol
- O envolvimento dos olhos e do cérebro pode ser mais bem tratado com fluconazol, pois esse agente penetra na barreira hematencefálica.
- Usar em cães que não possam receber a anfotericina B.
- Dose habitual (forma intravenosa) — 5 mg/kg IV a cada 12 h até que a absorção intestinal permita o tratamento com o itraconazol por via oral.

CONTRAINDICAÇÕES
Anfotericina B — insuficiência renal impede seu uso.

PRECAUÇÕES
- Esteroides — utilizar com cuidado; permitem a proliferação de *Histoplasma*; angústia respiratória potencialmente letal atribuída à doença pulmonar infiltrativa ou linfadenopatia hilar justifica o uso de dexametasona (0,2 mg/kg IV diariamente por 2-3 dias), mas é provável que o tempo de tratamento com antifúngicos aumente.
- Itraconazol e fluconazol — toxicidade hepática; interromper temporariamente se o paciente estiver com anorexia ou se a atividade sérica da ALT for >300 U/L; reiniciar com metade da dose após o restabelecimento do apetite.

INTERAÇÕES POSSÍVEIS
Itraconazol — contraindicado com terfenadina e cisaprida em seres humanos.

MEDICAMENTO(S) ALTERNATIVO(S)
Nenhum.

ACOMPANHAMENTO

MONITORIZAÇÃO DO PACIENTE
- ALT sérica — mensurar no tratamento com itraconazol; verificar mensalmente ou se o paciente exibir anorexia.
- Radiografias torácicas — em casos de envolvimento pulmonar; avaliar após 60 dias de tratamento para determinar a melhora; repetir em intervalos de 30 dias e interromper o tratamento quando os infiltrados tiverem desaparecido ou as lesões pulmonares remanescentes não melhorarem, indicando fibrose residual; pode não ser fácil diferenciar entre lesões fibróticas residuais e doença ativa; continuar o tratamento por pelo menos 1 mês após todos os sinais de doença ativa terem se resolvido. A monitorização dos níveis de antígenos urinários pode ser útil.

PREVENÇÃO
- Evitar áreas suspeitas de exposição (p. ex., poleiros/hábitats de aves).
- É provável que os cães recuperados fiquem imunes à doença.

COMPLICAÇÕES POSSÍVEIS
A recidiva é possível; nesse caso, há necessidade de um segundo curso terapêutico.

EVOLUÇÃO ESPERADA E PROGNÓSTICO
- Tratamento — a duração, em geral, gira em torno de 4 meses; os medicamentos são caros, especialmente para cães de grande porte.
- Prognóstico — bom para os pacientes estáveis sem dispneia grave; influenciado pela gravidade do acometimento pulmonar e pela debilidade do paciente.

DIVERSOS

DISTÚRBIOS ASSOCIADOS
Sem condições predisponentes aparentes.

FATORES RELACIONADOS COM A IDADE
N/D.

POTENCIAL ZOONÓTICO
- Não se dissemina dos animais para as pessoas.
- É preciso ter cuidado para evitar picadas de agulha durante a coleta de aspirados.
- Pode ocorrer infecção em decorrência de cortes gerados durante as necropsias de animais infectados.

GESTAÇÃO/FERTILIDADE/REPRODUÇÃO
Itraconazol — não tem efeitos teratogênicos em ratos e camundongos nas doses terapêuticas; foi detectada embriotoxicidade sob altas doses; não há estudos em cães e gatos; uma única cadela submetida à medicação no meio da gestação teve uma ninhada normal.

ABREVIATURA(S)
- ALT = alanina aminotransferase.

Sugestões de Leitura
Bromel C, Sukes JE. Histoplasmosis in dogs and cats. Clin Tech Small Anim Pract 2005: 20;227-232.
Greene CE. Histoplasmosis. In: Greene CE, ed., Infectious Diseases of the Dog and Cat, 3rd ed. St. Louis: Saunders Elsevier, 2006, pp. 577-584.
Hodges RD, Legendre AM, Adams LG, et al. Itraconazole for the treatment of histoplasmosis in cats. J Vet Intern Med 1994, 8:409-413.
Schulman RL, McKiernan BC, Schaeffer DJ. Use of corticosteroids for treating dogs with airway obstruction secondary to hilar lymphadenopathy caused by chronic histoplasmosis: 16 cases (1979-1997). JAVMA 1999, 214:1345-1448.

Autor Alfred M. Legendre
Consultor Editorial Stephen C. Barr

Icterícia

CONSIDERAÇÕES GERAIS

DEFINIÇÃO
Concentração sérica de bilirrubina total maior do que a faixa de referência, o que provoca amarelamento dos tecidos.

FISIOPATOLOGIA
• Bilirrubina — derivada da degradação de proteínas com a molécula heme em seu conteúdo; a maioria (80%) provém de eritrócitos senis; o restante de outras proteínas que contêm a molécula heme. • Bilirrubina não conjugada — transportada no plasma ligada à albumina; diglicuronídeo conjugado após captação hepatocelular.
• Bilirrubina conjugada — transportada (com outros componentes da bile) para o sistema biliar; excretada nos intestinos, onde grande parte dela é convertida em outros produtos (o urobilinogênio pode sofrer circulação enterepática); as estercobilinas conferem a cor castanha às fezes.
• Hiperbilirrubinemia — causada pela produção elevada (destruição eritrocitária; icterícia hemolítica) da molécula heme acima da capacidade de captação, conjugação ou depuração biliar do fígado (icterícia hepática) ou da eliminação biliar entérica (icterícia pós-hepática). • A icterícia não hemolítica é causada por doença hepatobiliar ou peritonite biliar.

SISTEMA(S) ACOMETIDO(S)
• Hepatobiliar — a retenção de ácidos biliares e, possivelmente, a bilirrubina podem contribuir para a lesão hepatocelular. • Nervoso — a extrema hiperbilirrubinemia não conjugada pode causar lesões cerebrais degenerativas (raras). • Renal/Urológico — a hiperbilirrubinemia extrema pode provocar lesão tubular renal. • Cutâneo/Exócrino — o amarelamento da pele (icterícia) reflete níveis séricos de bilirrubina >2,5 mg/dL.

IDENTIFICAÇÃO

Espécies
Cães e gatos.

Raça(s) Predominante(s)
• Nenhuma. • Hepatopatias familiares — ver *Fatores de Risco*.

Idade Média e Faixa Etária
• Maioria das causas — doenças de animais adultos. • Cães jovens e não vacinados — sob risco de hepatite infecciosa canina.

Sexo Predominante
Cadelas adultas de raça pura — sob risco de anemia hemolítica imunomediada.

SINAIS CLÍNICOS

Achados Anamnésicos

Formação Elevada de Bilirrubina — Hemólise
• Sinais vagos: letargia, fraqueza. • Sinais gastrintestinais: anorexia, constipação, vômito, perda de peso. • Icterícia. • Transfusão sanguínea recente. • Traumatismo grave: sangramento muscular e/ou abdominal, ou formação de hematoma.

Eliminação Reduzida de Bilirrubina — Colestase
• Sinais GI vagos: anorexia, vômito, diarreia, alteração na cor das fezes (verde ou laranja em caso de icterícia não obstrutiva; acólica em caso de icterícia obstrutiva). • Icterícia. • Mudança na cor da urina: laranja. • Aumento de volume abdominal: na presença de ascite. • Poliúria e polidipsia. • Alteração do estado mental: na presença de encefalopatia hepática.

Achados do Exame Físico

Formação Elevada de Bilirrubina — Hemólise
• Palidez, taquicardia, taquipneia, fraqueza, pulsos femorais saltitantes, sopro cardíaco anêmico.
• Icterícia. • Hepato/esplenomegalia.
• Linfadenopatia. • Tendências hemorrágicas — em animal trombocitopênico. • Fezes laranja.
• Febre. • Sensação "gelatinosa" à palpação da pele (vasculopatia).

Eliminação Reduzida de Bilirrubina — Colestase
• Perda de peso. • Icterícia. • Hepato/esplenomegalia. • Efusão/massa/dor abdominais.
• Fezes melênicas, laranja, verdes ou acólicas.
• Febre.

CAUSAS

Icterícia Pré-hepática
• Distúrbios hemolíticos: hemólise imunomediada; certos medicamentos (portadores de propileno glicol em gatos, trimetoprima-sulfa); LES; distúrbios infecciosos: toxinas (p. ex., lesão oxidativa: zinco, cebolas, fenóis), hipofosfatemia grave. • Transfusão sanguínea incompatível.
• Infecções — FeLV; *Mycoplasma haemofelis*; dirofilariose; *Babesia*; *Ehrlichia*; *Cytauxzoon*.
• Reabsorção de grande volume de sangue — hematomas, cavidades corporais (p. ex., hemangiossarcoma, varfarina).

Icterícia Hepática
• Hepatite idiopática ou familiar crônica.
• Reações medicamentosas adversas — p. ex., anticonvulsivantes; paracetamol; trimetoprima-sulfato; carprofeno; estanozolol (gatos); benzodiazepínicos (gatos); ver "Hepatotoxinas".
• Colangite/colangioepatite.
• Neoplasia infiltrativa — linfoma.
• Cirrose (cães).
• Lipidose hepática (gatos).
• Necrose hepática maciça: p. ex., aflatoxina, cicadácea.
• Doenças sistêmicas com envolvimento hepático — leptospirose (cães); histoplasmose; PIF; hipertireoidismo (gatos); toxoplasmose (gatos).
• Sepse bacteriana — originária em qualquer lugar no corpo; pode elaborar produtos bacterianos que comprometem o processamento hepático da bilirrubina.

Icterícia Pós-hepática
Obstrução mecânica transitória ou persistente dos ductos biliares: (1) pancreatite (obstrução transitória); (2) neoplasia — ducto biliar, pâncreas, duodeno; (3) oclusão do ducto intraluminal — colelitíase, bile lodosa, fascíola hepática (gatos), destruição imunomediada do ducto (colangite esclerosante em gatos); (4) ruptura da árvore biliar com consequente peritonite biliar.

FATORES DE RISCO
• Cães jovens não vacinados — doença infecciosa.
• Predisposição racial para hepatopatia familiar — Doberman pinschers, Bedlington terriers, Cocker spaniels, Dálmatas, Labradores retrievers.
• Cães obesos de meia-idade — pancreatite.
• Gatos obesos anoréxicos — lipidose hepática.
• Medicamentos hepatotóxicos.
• Traumatismo abdominal rombo, doença crônica do trato biliar, mucocele da vesícula biliar — peritonite biliar.
• Anemia hemolítica.

DIAGNÓSTICO

DIAGNÓSTICO DIFERENCIAL
• Icterícia pré-hepática — geralmente de início abrupto; palidez das mucosas; icterícia leve a moderada; fraqueza; taquipneia; sopro cardíaco com anemia grave.
• Icterícia hepática — risco reprodutivo para hepatite familiar; icterícia variável; alteração no tamanho do fígado (grande ou pequeno); efusão abdominal (transudato puro ou modificado); poliúria e polidipsia; mudanças comportamentais de encefalopatia hepática; sangramento.
• Icterícia pós-hepática — ataques crônicos e/ou recorrentes de sinais GI evidentes ou pancreatite com colelitíase; icterícia moderada ou acentuada; mucosas normais sob outros aspectos; dor abdominal difusa ou cranial; massa abdominal cranial; efusão abdominal (séptica ou não séptica, ou peritonite biliar); tendências hemorrágicas; fezes acólicas.

ACHADOS LABORATORIAIS

Medicamentos Capazes de Alterar os Resultados Laboratoriais
Hemoglobina derivada bovina polimerizada para anemia agrava os quadros de icterícia e bilirrubinemia.

Distúrbios Capazes de Alterar os Resultados Laboratoriais
• Ensaio de bilirrubina — com base na reação diazo; estimativas de bilirrubinas séricas totais e diretas; a maioria gera resultados razoáveis de bilirrubina total; os valores de bilirrubina direta variam.
• Leituras superiores em plasma heparinizado.
• Manejo da amostra — importante; a bilirrubina total pode diminuir em 50% por hora com exposição direta à luz solar ou iluminação artificial.
Hemólise — efeitos variáveis sobre a bilirrubina total mensurada por meio de espectrofotometria. Lipemia — aumenta falsamente os valores da bilirrubina total mensurada pelos testes finais. Fracionamento em bilirrubinas conjugadas e não conjugadas — *incapaz de definir as causas de icterícia*, contrário aos dogmas.

Válidos em Laboratórios de Medicina Humana?
Sim.

HEMOGRAMA/BIOQUÍMICA/URINÁLISE

Icterícia Pré-hepática
• Hemograma completo — anemia grave (geralmente regenerativa); o esfregaço sanguíneo pode revelar autoaglutinação, esferócitos, corpúsculos de Heinz, ou parasitas; hemoglobinemia com hemólise intravascular, plaquetas normais a baixas e leucócitos normais a altos, com desvio à esquerda.
• Bioquímica — nível de ALT, atividade da fosfatase alcalina e concentração de nitrogênio ureico sanguíneo normais a altos; albumina normal a baixa; globulina normal a alta; glicose e colesterol normais; bilirrubina elevada.

ICTERÍCIA

Icterícia Hepática
• Hemograma completo — anemia arregenerativa leve; VCM baixo com hepatopatia crônica e desvio portossistêmico.
• Bioquímica — níveis de ALT e/ou fosfatase alcalina leve a acentuadamente elevados; albumina, nitrogênio ureico sanguíneo, glicose e colesterol normais a baixos.
• Urinálise — urina normal a diluída; a bilirrubinúria antecede a hiperbilirrubinemia.

Icterícia Pós-hepática
Hemograma completo — anemia arregenerativa leve ou hematócrito normal.
Bioquímica — ALT aumentada e fosfatase alcalina moderada a acentuadamente elevada; concentrações geralmente normais de albumina, nitrogênio ureico sanguíneo e glicose; colesterol normal a alto.

OUTROS TESTES LABORATORIAIS
• Teste de autoaglutinação em salina ou lâmina de dispersão — na suspeita de aglutinação eritrocitária; VCM alto em analisadores automatizados.
• Teste de Coombs direto — realizar esse exame se não houver evidência de autoaglutinação.
• Teste de fragilidade osmótica — detecta a hemólise.
• Esfregaços sanguíneos — para pesquisa de hemoparasitas.
• Mensuração do zinco plasmático — se houver anemia hemolítica.
• Título de AAN — em caso de anemia hemolítica.
• Ácidos biliares séricos — redundantes se já houver suspeita de icterícia não hemolítica.
• Sorologia — para doenças infecciosas (p. ex., FeLV, leptospirose, micoses) com sinais de doença multissistêmica e icterícia hepática.
• Efusão abdominal — caracterizar as células e o conteúdo proteico.
• Testes de coagulação — valores prolongados, especialmente PIAVK e TP, com oclusão dos ductos biliares; responsiva à vitamina K_1.
• Cultura microbiana e antibiograma — sangue e/ou outras amostras; com leucograma inflamatório e possível foco de infecção bacteriana (p. ex., trato urinário, trato biliar).

DIAGNÓSTICO POR IMAGEM
• Radiografia abdominal — detalhes mascarados e obscurecidos pela efusão; pode revelar hepatomegalia, efeito expansivo ou de massa, ou interfaces minerais ou gasosas no fígado; esplenomegalia (anemia hemolítica, hipertensão portal, neoplasia abdominal); corpo estranho metálico com hemólise induzida pelo zinco.
• Radiografia torácica — pode revelar doença metastática; linfadenopatia esternal (reflete doença abdominal); linfadenopatia geral (linfoma).
• Ultrassonografia abdominal — pode distinguir entre hepatopatia parenquimatosa e obstrução biliar extra-hepática; caracteriza lesões parenquimatosas hepáticas; pode revelar neoplasia abdominal; pode determinar a causa de efusão abdominal; utilizada para direcionar a amostragem da lesão (biopsia aspirativa por agulha).

OUTROS MÉTODOS DIAGNÓSTICOS
• Aspiração com agulha fina — citologia de massa, linfonodo ou lesões teciduais parenquimatosas.
• Biopsia do fígado — cultura bacteriana de tecido hepático, bile e amostras obtidas via celiotomia (laparotomia), percutânea cega, por orifício, laparoscópica ou guiada por ultrassom.
• Intervenção cirúrgica — necessária para o diagnóstico e tratamento de distúrbios pós-hepáticos.

TRATAMENTO
• Depende da causa subjacente.
• Tratamento hospitalar — para cuidados médicos iniciais.
• Repouso em gaiola — para facilitar a regeneração do fígado.
• Dieta — importante em icterícia hepática e pós-hepática; nutricionalmente balanceada com nível proteico máximo tolerado pelo paciente; à base de carboidrato (cães) com restrição proteica para encefalopatia hepática; restrição de sódio na presença de ascite.
• Suplementação de vitamina — vitaminas hidrossolúveis em todos os pacientes; administração parenteral de vitamina K_1 para obstrução do ducto biliar ou colestase grave.

MEDICAÇÕES
MEDICAMENTO(S)
• Icterícia pré-hepática — eliminar a causa incitante; ver "Anemia, Imunomediada; transfusão de sangue total para anemia potencialmente letal".
• Icterícia hepática/pós-hepática — tratar os distúrbios específicos com base nos resultados do diagnóstico por imagem e nos exames de biopsia e cultura.

CONTRAINDICAÇÕES
• Evitar os medicamentos hepatotóxicos conhecidos.
• Evitar as tetraciclinas a menos que claramente indicadas — suprimem a síntese de proteínas pelo fígado, promovendo lipidose hepática.
• Evitar analgésicos, anestésicos, barbitúricos — em caso de insuficiência hepática.

PRECAUÇÕES
• Sedativos — podem precipitar encefalopatia hepática.
• Corticosteroides — utilizá-los com cuidado para inflamação não séptica; aumentam o risco de infecção intercorrente; agravam a ascite (retenção de água e sódio), promovem hepatopatia vacuolar em cães, lipidose hepática em gatos.

INTERAÇÕES POSSÍVEIS
Utilizar qualquer medicamento com cuidado em pacientes ictéricos, pois o metabolismo hepático pode se alterar drasticamente, tornando a farmacocinética imprevisível; na presença de hipoalbuminemia, os medicamentos ligados à proteína apresentam efeitos acentuados, podendo levar à toxicidade.

ACOMPANHAMENTO
MONITORIZAÇÃO DO PACIENTE
• Icterícia pré-hepática — reavaliar o volume globular e os esfregaços sanguíneos, conforme a necessidade; pode necessitar de transfusões repetidas; reduzir gradativamente os agentes imunossupressores.
• Icterícia hepática e pós-hepática — reavaliar o perfil bioquímico sérico conforme ditado pela doença subjacente; manter os tratamentos sintomáticos e específicos.

COMPLICAÇÕES POSSÍVEIS
As doenças que provocam icterícia podem causar morte.

DIVERSOS
DISTÚRBIOS ASSOCIADOS
• Pacientes acometidos por hemólise imunomediada e tratados com doses imunossupressoras de corticosteroides são predispostos a tromboembolia, úlceras gastrintestinais e infecção.
• Pacientes com insuficiência hepática são suscetíveis a infecção e sangramento entéricos.
• Pacientes submetidos à cirurgia biliar reconstrutiva exibem alto risco de colangite bacteriana.

POTENCIAL ZOONÓTICO
Certos sorotipos de leptospirose.

VER TAMBÉM
• Anemia, por Corpúsculo de Heinz.
• Anemia, Imunomediada.
• Anemia, Regenerativa.
• Babesiose.
• Reações à Transfusão Sanguínea.
• Síndrome Colangite/Colangioepatite.
• Colelitíase.
• Cirrose e Fibrose do Fígado.
• Hepatopatia por Armazenamento de Cobre.
• Mucocele da Vesícula Biliar.
• Micoplasmose Hemotrópica (Hemoplasmose).
• Insuficiência Hepática, Aguda.
• Lipidose Hepática.
• Hepatite, Crônica Ativa.
• Hepatite, Infecciosa Canina.
• Hepatite, Supurativa, e Abscesso Hepático.
• Hepatotoxinas.
• Infestação por Fascíola Hepática.
• Lúpus Eritematoso, Sistêmico.
• Pancreatite.
• Toxicidade do Zinco.

ABREVIATURAS
• AAN = anticorpo antinuclear.
• ALT = alanina aminotransferase.
• FeLV = vírus da leucemia felina.
• GI = gastrintestinal.
• LES = lúpus eritematoso sistêmico.
• PIAVK = proteínas invocadas pela ausência ou antagonismo da vitamina K.
• PIF = peritonite infecciosa felina.
• TP = tempo de protrombina.
• VCM = volume corpuscular médio.

Sugestões de Leitura
Willard MD, Twedt DC. Gastrointestinal, pancreatic, and hepatic disorders. In: Clinical Diagnosis By Laboratory Methods, 4th ed, St. Louis: Saunders, 2004, pp. 208-247.

Autor Sharon A. Center
Consultor Editorial Sharon A. Center

ÍLEO PARALÍTICO

CONSIDERAÇÕES GERAIS

REVISÃO
- Define-se como íleo adinâmico (paralítico, funcional) uma obstrução intestinal transitória e reversível resultante da inibição da motilidade intestinal. • A ausência de peristalse no estômago, no intestino delgado ou no intestino grosso provoca obstrução funcional, pois o conteúdo intestinal se acumula nas áreas pendentes do trato gastrintestinal em vez de ser impulsionado em uma direção aboral. • O íleo paralítico não é uma doença primária, mas uma complicação secundária de diversos distúrbios. • Acredita-se que o íleo adinâmico ocorra secundariamente à dissociação eletromecânica da musculatura intestinal em razão de aumento do tônus simpático, liberação de fatores inibidores humorais (catecolaminas, vasopressina, opiáceos endógenos), liberação diminuída de hormônios procinéticos (neurotensina, motilina) ou hipocalemia.

SISTEMA(S) ACOMETIDO(S)
Gastrintestinal.

IDENTIFICAÇÃO
Cães e gatos.

SINAIS CLÍNICOS
- Anorexia. • Vômitos. • Depressão. • Leve distensão ou desconforto abdominal secundário ao acúmulo de gás no intestino com baixa motilidade. • A falha na auscultação de borborigmos intestinais após 2-3 min é sugestiva de íleo paralítico. • Durante o estado inicial (perda parcial da motilidade), os borborigmos intestinais podem estar aumentados.

CAUSAS E FATORES DE RISCO
- Operações cirúrgicas (especialmente cirurgia gastrintestinal). • Desequilíbrio eletrolítico (hipocalemia, hipomagnesemia, hipocalcemia). • Lesões inflamatórias agudas do intestino, da cavidade peritoneal ou de outros órgãos abdominais (particularmente associadas à enterite canina por parvovírus, pancreatite aguda). • Obstrução mecânica não aliviada. • Isquemia intestinal. • Sepse por Gram-negativos. • Endotoxemia. • Choque. • Lesão retroperitoneal. • Uremia. • Neuropatias autônomas (disautonomia, lesão da medula espinal). • Miopatias viscerais. • Uso de anticolinérgicos. • Hiperdistensão intestinal (aerofagia). • Intoxicação por chumbo. • Estresse (por frio e ruído).

DIAGNÓSTICO

DIAGNÓSTICO DIFERENCIAL
É preciso diferenciar o íleo paralítico (adinâmico) de obstruções mecânicas por:
- Corpos estranhos intestinais. • Intussuscepção. • Abscesso intramural. • Hérnia encarcerada ou estrangulada. • Vólvulo. • Infarto mesentérico. • Parasitas. • Aderências. • Estenose pós-operatória. • Impactação. • Má-formação congênita. • Lesões inflamatórias ou traumáticas. • Neoplasia.

HEMOGRAMA/BIOQUÍMICA/URINÁLISE
- As alterações no hemograma dependem da causa primária do íleo paralítico.
- Os perfis bioquímicos séricos e a urinálise ajudam a avaliar a existência de distúrbios eletrolíticos (especialmente hipocalemia) e a presença de azotemia.

OUTROS TESTES LABORATORIAIS
- Mensuração da concentração de lipase pancreática (lipase pancreática específica canina, imunorreatividade da lipase pancreática felina, teste SNAP para lipase pancreática canina).
- Teste ELISA para o parvovírus fecal em filhotes caninos com íleo paralítico e diarreia.

DIAGNÓSTICO POR IMAGEM
Achados Radiográficos Abdominais
- As alças intestinais encontram-se distendidas com gás e líquido. Os padrões radiográficos comuns incluem:
- Íleo paralítico generalizado gasoso — considerar aerofagia, medicamentos paralisantes da musculatura lisa, peritonite generalizada ou enterite.
- Íleo paralítico generalizado líquido — considerar enterite, neoplasia intestinal difusa.
- Íleo paralítico localizado gasoso — considerar peritonite localizada (pancreatite), obstrução intestinal em estágio inicial, ruptura do suprimento arterial.
- Íleo paralítico localizado líquido — considerar corpo estranho, obstrução neoplásica, intussuscepção.

Ultrassonografia
- Diferencia íleo paralítico (adinâmico) de obstruções intestinais mecânicas.
- Identifica pancreatite ou peritonite.

MÉTODOS DIAGNÓSTICOS
EPIB (Esferas de Polietileno Impregnadas com Bário)
- Confirma o íleo paralítico (adinâmico).
- Trânsito gastrintestinal tardio com retenção das EPIB no estômago.
- Dispersão das EPIB por todo o trato gastrintestinal superior.

Outros Procedimentos a Serem Considerados
- Eletrogastrografia não invasiva é utilizada de forma experimental para avaliar a atividade mioelétrica gástrica em cães.
- Abdominocentese com efusão peritoneal para confirmar peritonite.
- Endoscopia gastrintestinal ou laparotomia exploratória para excluir obstrução mecânica.
- Radiografias da coluna vertebral, mielograma, RM da coluna vertebral, TC, análise do LCS para identificar lesão da medula espinal.
- Teste de resposta ocular com pilocarpina a 0,1% e fisostigmina a 0,25% para disautonomia.

TRATAMENTO
- Identificar e tratar a causa primária subjacente.
- Corrigir as anormalidades eletrolíticas (sobretudo hipocalemia), se presentes.
- Acredita-se que o uso de medicamentos procinéticos seja útil.
- Descompressão gastrintestinal via sonda nasogástrica raramente é necessária.

MEDICAÇÕES

MEDICAMENTO(S)
Metoclopramida (0,4 mg/kg IV a cada 6 h).

CONTRAINDICAÇÕES/INTERAÇÕES POSSÍVEIS
- Anticolinérgicos (p. ex., atropina, glicopirrolato).
- Opiáceos (p. ex., morfina, hidromorfona, oximorfona, butorfanol).
- Antidiarreicos opiáceos (p. ex., elixir paregórico, cloridrato de difenoxilato/sulfato de atropina, cloridrato de loperamida).

ACOMPANHAMENTO

MONITORIZAÇÃO DO PACIENTE
- Monitorizar a correção do desequilíbrio eletrolítico, se presente.
- Auscultação abdominal para avaliar a motilidade intestinal.

PREVENÇÃO
Se não houver indicação, evitar anticolinérgicos e opiáceos.

COMPLICAÇÕES POSSÍVEIS
Os animais com íleo paralítico (adinâmico) ficam predispostos ao desenvolvimento de proliferação bacteriana no intestino delgado, translocação bacteriana e sepse.

EVOLUÇÃO ESPERADA E PROGNÓSTICO
O prognóstico depende da resolução bem-sucedida do processo mórbido primário.

DIVERSOS

DISTÚRBIOS ASSOCIADOS
Ver na seção "Causas e Fatores de Risco".

GESTAÇÃO/FERTILIDADE/REPRODUÇÃO
Há relatos de íleo paralítico em cadelas lactantes com hipomagnesemia e hipocalcemia.

SINÔNIMO(S)
- Íleo adinâmico — íleo funcional, íleo paralítico.
- Pseudo-obstrução — íleo adinâmico crônico, mais segmentar.
- Íleo mecânico — costuma ser mencionado na literatura especializada atual como obstrução mecânica.

ABREVIATURA(S)
- ELISA = ensaio imunoabsorvente ligado à enzima.
- LCS = líquido cerebrospinal.
- RM = ressonância magnética.
- TC = tomografia computadorizada.

Sugestões de Leitura
Guilford WG. Motility disorders of the bowel. In: Guilford WG, Center SA, Strombeck DR, Williams DA, Meyer DJ. Strombeck's Small Animal Gastroenterology, 3rd ed. Philadelphia: Saunders, 1996, pp. 335-336.

Autor Susanne K. Lauer
Consultor Editorial Albert E. Jergens

INALAÇÃO DE FUMAÇA

CONSIDERAÇÕES GERAIS

REVISÃO
- O dano ocorre como resultado de lesão direta gerada pelo calor nas vias aéreas superiores e na mucosa nasal. Além disso, a inalação do monóxido de carbono diminui a distribuição tecidual de oxigênio, por se ligar preferencialmente à hemoglobina; a inalação de outras toxinas irrita diretamente as vias aéreas, enquanto a inalação de material particulado se adere às vias aéreas e aos alvéolos.
- A extensão do dano depende do grau e da duração de exposição, bem como do material em combustão.
- Cães e gatos podem apresentar lesão pulmonar grave com pouca evidência cutânea ou bucal da queimadura.
- Reação pulmonar — inicialmente broncoconstrição, edema das vias aéreas e produção de muco; em seguida, resposta inflamatória, traqueobronquite necrosante e acúmulo de líquido pulmonar em virtude do aumento na permeabilidade capilar.
- A maioria dos pacientes exibe progressão da disfunção pulmonar nos 2-3 primeiros dias da exposição.
- Infecções bacterianas sobrepostas — causa comum de morbidade tardia na evolução da doença.

IDENTIFICAÇÃO
Cães e gatos.

SINAIS CLÍNICOS
- Achados anamnésicos compatíveis com a exposição.
- O paciente pode apresentar odor de fumaça.
- Taquipneia e profundidade aumentada da respiração.
- Esforço inspiratório sugestivo de obstrução das vias aéreas superiores pelo edema.
- Adaptações posturais à angústia respiratória.
- As mucosas podem estar de coloração vermelho-cereja (em função da monoxiemoglobina carbônica), pálidas ou cianóticas.
- Auscultação de sibilos, ruídos broncovesiculares ásperos ou crepitações.
- Tosse.
- Bigodes queimados ou enrugados, edema da conjuntiva, úlceras de córnea.

CAUSAS E FATORES DE RISCO
Exposição à fumaça, geralmente por terem ficado presos em edifício em chamas.

DIAGNÓSTICO

HEMOGRAMA/BIOQUÍMICA/URINÁLISE
- Neutropenia — sinal prognóstico mau; indica sequestro de neutrófilos nos pulmões.
- Trombocitopenia — pode sugerir sequestro ou consumo de plaquetas.
- Perfil bioquímico sérico — pode revelar dano hipóxico a outros sistemas orgânicos.
- Urinálise — geralmente normal.

DIAGNÓSTICO POR IMAGEM
Radiografias torácicas — sempre radiografar para estabelecer uma base de referência; os achados variam desde padrão normal até broncointersticial ou alveolar.

MÉTODOS DIAGNÓSTICOS
- Exame citológico e cultura de amostra do lavado transtraqueal — realizar diante da suspeita de traqueobronquite ou pneumonia bacterianas sobrepostas; em geral, os resultados revelam reação supurativa aguda com muco excessivo, neutrófilos e macrófagos alveolares; podem ser observadas bactérias, embora a ausência desses microrganismos não descarte uma infecção bacteriana.
- Oximetria de pulso ou obtenção de gasometria arterial — podem confirmar a hipoxemia; de menor valor para determinar a distribuição tecidual de oxigênio em caso de exposição ao monóxido de carbono.
- Broncoscopia — pode demonstrar a gravidade do dano às vias aéreas; o lavado broncoalveolar permite a coleta de amostras adequadas para exame citológico ou cultura.

TRATAMENTO

- Tratamento inicial — estabilização da função respiratória; estabelecimento de via aérea patente (desobstruída); edema ou obstrução graves das vias aéreas superiores podem necessitar de entubação ou traqueostomia.
- Oxigênio — administrar imediatamente para deslocar o monóxido de carbono da hemoglobina; utilizar a concentração disponível mais elevada por, no mínimo, 2-4 h (ou por mais tempo); após a eliminação da monoxiemoglobina carbônica, continuar a suplementação com 40-60% de FiO_2, conforme a necessidade.
- Administração de fluido — pode ser necessária para manter a função cardiovascular, embora deva ser realizada de forma prudente, se possível, para minimizar a formação de edema pulmonar; usar coloides sintéticos (p. ex., hetamido) nos animais com hipoproteinemia; necessidades elevadas de fluidos nas queimaduras dérmicas extensas em função da considerável perda de líquido e proteína pela superfície cutânea.
- Transfusões de sangue ou de plasma — podem ser necessárias.
- Nebulização de solução salina — facilita a depuração das secreções respiratórias.
- Tapotagem e fisioterapia — facilitam a depuração das secreções respiratórias.
- Suporte nutricional — se necessário para manter a condição corporal e o estado imunológico.

MEDICAÇÕES

MEDICAMENTO(S)
- Suspeita de infecção bacteriana — considerar o uso de antibióticos de amplo espectro após a obtenção de amostras adequadas para cultura bacteriana.
- Broncodilatadores — podem melhorar a função respiratória em caso de broncoconstrição grave gerada pela inflamação, especialmente nos gatos (p. ex., terbutalina a 0,01 mg/kg IV ou IM). Evitar medicamentos por via oral durante crises agudas.
- Edema grave — pode-se tentar o emprego de diuréticos (p. ex., furosemida na dose de 0,5-2 mg/kg IV ou IM), embora costumem ser de pouco benefício.
- Dose anti-inflamatória inicial e única de corticosteroides pode reduzir o edema das vias aéreas.

CONTRAINDICAÇÕES/INTERAÇÕES POSSÍVEIS
- Diuréticos — podem diminuir o volume intravascular sem um efeito benéfico importante sobre a função das vias aéreas ou a formação de edema pulmonar.
- Corticosteroides — utilizar apenas uma vez e se forem absolutamente necessários; podem predispor o paciente à infecção bacteriana.

ACOMPANHAMENTO

MONITORIZAÇÃO DO PACIENTE
- Monitorizar de forma rigorosa a frequência e o esforço respiratórios, a coloração das mucosas, a frequência cardíaca e a qualidade do pulso e a auscultação dos pulmões, bem como o hematócrito e os sólidos totais por 24-72 h.
- Repetir as radiografias em 48 h — para ter certeza da resolução do problema; monitorizar quanto à presença de pneumonia bacteriana.
- Oximetria de pulso e obtenção de gasometria arterial — conforme a necessidade para monitorizar o grau de hipoxemia e a resposta ao tratamento.

COMPLICAÇÕES POSSÍVEIS
- Traqueobronquite ou pneumonia bacterianas — atribuídas à imunossupressão sistêmica e a defesas pulmonares reduzidas, incluindo depuração mucociliar deficiente.
- Resposta inflamatória pulmonar generalizada profunda ou síndrome de resposta inflamatória sistêmica grave — podem desenvolver SARA.
- Pacientes gravemente acometidos podem desenvolver sequelas neurológicas tardias (3-10 dias após a exposição), incluindo crises convulsivas ou edema cerebral.

EVOLUÇÃO ESPERADA E PROGNÓSTICO
- A maior parte dos pacientes deteriora-se durante as 24-48 h iniciais após a exposição à fumaça e, em seguida, melhoram gradativamente, a menos que desenvolvam pneumonia bacteriana ou SARA.
- Queimaduras graves ou lesão orgânica — associadas a um prognóstico mau.

DIVERSOS

ABREVIATURA(S)
- FiO_2 = fração inspirada de oxigênio.
- SARA = síndrome da angústia respiratória aguda.

Sugestões de Leitura
Berent AC, Todd J, Sergeeff J, Powell LL. Carbon monoxide toxicity: A case series. J Vet Emerg Crit Care 2005, 15(2):128-135.
Fitzgerald KT, Flood AA. Smoke inhalation. Clin Tech Small Anim Pract 2006, 21(4):205-214.
Mariani CL. Full recovery following delayed neurologic signs after smoke inhalation in a dog. J Vet Emerg Crit Care 2003, 13(4):235-239.

Autor Lesley G. King
Consultor Editorial Lynelle R. Johnson

INCLINAÇÃO DA CABEÇA

CONSIDERAÇÕES GERAIS

DEFINIÇÃO
Inclinação da cabeça distante de sua orientação normal em relação ao tronco e aos membros, associada em geral a distúrbios do sistema vestibular.

FISIOPATOLOGIA
• Sistema vestibular — coordena a posição e o movimento da cabeça com os dos olhos, do tronco e dos membros ao detectar a aceleração linear e os movimentos de rotação da cabeça; inclui os núcleos vestibulares na medula rostral do tronco cerebral, a porção vestibular do nervo vestibulococlear (VIII par de nervos cranianos) e os receptores nos canais semicirculares da orelha interna.
• Inclinação da cabeça — sinal mais compatível de doenças que acometem o sistema vestibular e suas projeções para o cerebelo, a medula espinal, o córtex cerebral, a formação reticular e os músculos extraoculares (via fascículo longitudinal medial); geralmente ipsolateral à lesão.

SISTEMA(S) ACOMETIDO(S)
Nervoso — periférico ou central.

SINAIS CLÍNICOS
• Certificar-se de que a postura anormal da cabeça é uma inclinação verdadeira e não o ato de virar a cabeça (i. e., a cabeça e o pescoço virados para o lado como se fizessem um círculo).
• Se a doença for bilateral, pode não haver inclinação da cabeça.

CAUSAS

Doença Periférica
• Anatômicas — inclinação congênita da cabeça.
• Metabólicas — hipotireoidismo; adenoma hipofisário cromófobo; doença paraneoplásica.
• Neoplásicas — tumor da bainha nervosa do VIII par de nervos cranianos; neoplasia do osso e do tecido circundante (p. ex., osteossarcoma, fibrossarcoma, condrossarcoma e carcinoma de células escamosas).
• Inflamatórias — otite média e interna; principalmente bacteriana, mas também de origem parasitária (p. ex., *Otodectes*) e fúngica; corpo estranho; pólipo(s) nasofaríngeo(s).
• Idiopáticas — vestibulopatia geriátrica canina; vestibulopatia idiopática felina.
• Imunomediadas — neuropatia de nervos cranianos.
• Tóxicas — aminoglicosídeos, chumbo, hexaclorofeno.
• Traumáticas — ruptura da bula timpânica ou fratura da porção petrosa do osso temporal; rubor da orelha.

Doença Central
• Degenerativas — doença de armazenamento; doença desmielinizante; evento vascular.
• Anatômicas — hidrocefalia.
• Neoplásicas — glioma, papiloma do plexo coroide, meningioma, linfoma, tumor da bainha nervosa, meduloblastoma, tumor do crânio (p. ex., osteossarcoma); metástase (p. ex., hemangiossarcoma e melanoma).
• Nutricionais — deficiência de tiamina.
• Inflamatórias, infecciosas — virais (p. ex., vírus da PIF e da cinomose); por protozoários (p. ex., toxoplasmose e neosporose); fúngicas (p. ex., criptococose, blastomicose, histoplasmose, coccidioidomicose e nocardiose); bacterianas (p. ex., extensão de otite média e interna); parasitárias (p. ex., larvas de *Cuterebra*); por riquétsias (p. ex., erliquiose); por algas (p. ex., prototecose).
• Inflamatórias, não infecciosas — meningoencefalomielite granulomatosa, meningoencefalite específica à raça (p. ex., encefalite necrosante).
• Traumatismo — fratura da porção petrosa do osso temporal com lesão do tronco cerebral.
• Tóxicas — metronidazol.

FATORES DE RISCO
• Hipotireoidismo.
• Administração de medicamentos ototóxicos.
• Tratamento com metronidazol.
• Dieta deficiente em tiamina.
• Otite externa, média e interna.

DIAGNÓSTICO

DIAGNÓSTICO DIFERENCIAL

Vestibulopatia
• Doença unilateral — inclinação da cabeça, em geral, para o lado da lesão; costuma ser acompanhada por outros sinais vestibulares, p. ex., nistagmo anormal (em repouso, postural) com a fase rápida geralmente na direção oposta à inclinação; desvio ventral do olho (estrabismo vestibular) ipsolateral à inclinação observada com a elevação da cabeça; ataxia e desequilíbrio com tendência a cair, apoiar-se e/ou andar em círculo para o lado da inclinação.
• Doença bilateral — a inclinação da cabeça pode não estar presente ou ser discreta do lado mais gravemente acometido; pode haver nistagmo anormal; o nistagmo fisiológico (p. ex., nistagmo vestibular normal) pode estar deprimido ou ausente; também pode exibir amplos movimentos oscilantes da cabeça de um lado para o outro (evidentes, sobretudo, em gatos); pode-se observar uma postura em base larga ou postura agachada com relutância para se mover.
• Inclinação da cabeça — situa a lesão no sistema nervoso periférico (p. ex., porção vestibular do VIII par de nervos cranianos ou receptores na orelha interna) ou central (p. ex., núcleos vestibulares e suas vias neuronais).
• Déficits periféricos — nistagmo horizontal ou rotatório com a fase rápida na direção oposta à inclinação da cabeça; o paciente pode ter paresia ou paralisia concomitante do nervo facial ipsolateral e/ou síndrome de Horner e/ou produção lacrimal diminuída, por causa da estreita associação do VIII par de nervos cranianos com o VII par de nervos cranianos e o sistema nervoso simpático na porção petrosa do osso temporal e na bula timpânica.
• Déficits centrais — nistagmo vertical, horizontal ou rotatório que pode mudar de direção com a posição da cabeça; alteração da atividade mental; paresia ipsolateral e/ou déficits proprioceptivos; sinais centrais relacionados com o cerebelo, a medula rostral e a ponte; em alguns pacientes, há o envolvimento de múltiplos nervos cranianos.
• Síndrome vestibular paradoxal — causada por lesões nos pedúnculos cerebelares caudais ou nos lóbulos floculonodulares do cerebelo; os sinais vestibulares (p. ex., inclinação da cabeça e nistagmo) são opostos ao lado da lesão, enquanto os sinais cerebelares e os déficits proprioceptivos são ipsolaterais à lesão.

Inclinação e Postura da Cabeça de Origem Não Vestibular
• Incomuns.
• Precisam ser diferenciadas de inclinação verdadeira da cabeça de origem vestibular.
• Lesões unilaterais do mesencéfalo podem causar rotação grave da cabeça (>90°) para o lado oposto da lesão; não há outros sinais vestibulares; a inclinação é corrigida quando se põe uma venda nos olhos do paciente.
• Síndrome adversiva — observada em casos de lesões dos lobos talâmico rostral ou frontoparietal; o ato de virar a cabeça, a curvatura do pescoço e/ou o andar em círculo compulsivo podem ser erroneamente interpretados como déficits vestibulares; pode haver reação postural, resposta à ameaça e/ou déficits sensoriais contralaterais à lesão; a virada compulsiva ocorre geralmente em grandes círculos e sem o desequilíbrio e a inclinação verdadeira da cabeça de origem vestibular.

HEMOGRAMA/BIOQUÍMICA/URINÁLISE
• Geralmente normais.
• Leve anemia — hipotireoidismo.
• Leucocitose com neutrofilia — otite média e interna.
• Trombocitopenia — erliquiose.
• Hipercolesterolemia — hipotireoidismo.
• Alta concentração sérica de globulina — PIF.

OUTROS TESTES LABORATORIAIS
• T_4, T_4 livre, T_4 livre por diálise de equilíbrio e níveis de TSH endógeno — quando se suspeita de hipotireoidismo com base nos achados do exame físico e no acometimento uni ou bilateral associado do VIII par de nervos cranianos e, possivelmente, do VII.
• Cultura bacteriana e antibiograma — amostra obtida por miringotomia ou drenagem cirúrgica da bula timpânica caso se suspeite de otite média ou interna.
• Exame microscópico de *swab* da orelha — parasitas (p. ex., *Otodectes*).
• Sorologia — causas infecciosas (p. ex., cinomose; PIF; doenças causadas por protozoários, fungos e riquétsias).

DIAGNÓSTICO POR IMAGEM
• Radiografias da bula timpânica e do crânio — radiografias normais não descartam o comprometimento da bula.
• TC e RM — valiosas para confirmar a presença de lesões da bula timpânica e a extensão de doença periférica para o SNC, localizar tumores e/ou granulomas e documentar a extensão da inflamação.

MÉTODOS DIAGNÓSTICOS
• Análise do LCS — amostra coletada da cisterna cerebelomedular; valiosa para avaliar vestibulopatia central; detectar processo inflamatório; eletroforese de proteína e títulos para comparar com a sorologia se houver indicação, a coleta de amostra poderá colocar o paciente sob risco de herniação se houver pressão intracraniana elevada.
• RAETC — avalia a porção coclear do VIII par de nervos cranianos e as vias auditivas do tronco cerebral; particularmente valiosa para avaliar vestibulopatia periférica, porque algumas doenças podem causar surdez ipsolateral (p. ex., otite média e interna), enquanto outras doenças (p. ex., vestibulopatia geriátrica canina e idiopática felina)

afetam apenas a porção vestibular do VIII par de nervos cranianos.
• Biopsia — de osso e/ou tecido da bula timpânica quando se suspeita de tumor, pólipo ou osteomielite; massas do tronco cerebral (p. ex., ângulo cerebelomedular) são de difícil abordagem e remoção cirúrgica.

TRATAMENTO

• Hospitalar *versus* ambulatorial — depende da gravidade dos sinais (especialmente ataxia vestibular), do porte e da idade do paciente, bem como da necessidade de cuidados de suporte.
• Fluidos de suporte — fluidos intravenosos de reposição ou manutenção podem ser necessários na fase aguda nos casos em que os sinais de desorientação, náuseas e vômitos impedem o consumo oral; isso é particularmente importante em pacientes geriátricos.
• Atividade — restrita, de acordo com o grau de desequilíbrio.
• Dieta — como de costume, a menos que haja deficiência de tiamina (p. ex., dieta exclusivamente à base de peixe sem suplementação vitamínica); restringir o consumo oral na presença de náuseas e vômitos; **CUIDADO:** com aspiração secundária à postura anormal do corpo em pacientes com inclinação grave da cabeça e desequilíbrio ou disfunção do tronco cerebral.
• Interromper a medicação caso se suspeite de toxicidade.
• Tratamento cirúrgico — para drenar a bula timpânica em casos de otite média, remover pólipo(s) nasofaríngeo(s) em gatos e efetuar a ressecção de tumor, se acessível.

MEDICAÇÕES

MEDICAMENTO(S) DE ESCOLHA
• Otite média e interna — antibiótico de amplo espectro (parenteral ou oral) que penetra no osso enquanto se aguardam os resultados da cultura; trimetoprima-sulfa (15 mg/kg VO a cada 12 h ou 30 mg/kg VO a cada 12-24 h); cefalosporinas de primeira geração, como cefalexina (10-30 mg/kg VO a cada 6-8 h) ou amoxicilina/ácido clavulânico (Clavamox®, 12,5 mg/kg VO a cada 12 h para cães e 62,5 mg/gato VO a cada 12 h; Claviseptin®, 12,5 mg/kg VO a cada 12 h); o tratamento dura 4-6 semanas.
• Hipotireoidismo — a reposição de T_4 (cães: levotiroxina, 22 μg/kg VO a cada 12 h) deve ser instituída gradualmente em pacientes geriátricos, sobretudo naqueles com cardiopatia; a resposta varia, dependendo em parte da duração dos sinais (p. ex., em alguns pacientes, a neuropatia não é reversível).
• Infecções no SNC — tratamento específico se houver indicação; para doenças bacterianas, utilizar algum antibiótico que penetre na barreira hematencefálica (p. ex., trimetoprima-sulfa, 15 mg/kg VO a cada 12 h; metronidazol, 15 mg/kg a cada 12 h ou 10 mg/kg a cada 8 h VO ou lentamente por via IV; cefalosporina de terceira geração, p. ex., cefotaxima 25-50 mg/kg IV a cada 8 h); para doenças causadas por protozoários, usar clindamicina (12,5-25 mg/kg VO a cada 12 h); para doenças fúngicas, lançar mão de itraconazol (cães: 2,5 mg/kg VO a cada 12 h ou 5 mg/kg VO a cada 24 h; gatos: 5 mg/kg VO a cada 12 h), fluconazol (cães: 5-8 mg/kg VO a cada 12 h, 10-12 mg/kg VO a cada 24 h; gatos: 50 mg/gato VO a cada 12-24 h); o prognóstico de doenças causadas por protozoários, fungos e vírus (p. ex., PIF) costuma ser mau.
• Meningoencefalomielite granulomatosa — inicialmente, costuma ser tratada com esteroides: dexametasona (0,25 mg/kg VO, IM a cada 12 h por 3 dias; seguida por prednisona (2 mg/kg VO a cada 24 h por 1-2 semanas; em seguida, diminuir lentamente); dependendo da evolução, pode ser necessária uma imunossupressão mais forte — p. ex., citosina arabinosídeo a 50 mg/m² a cada 12 h por 4 tratamentos repetidos a cada 3 semanas (há necessidade de monitorização do hemograma completo); radioterapia.
• Traumatismo — cuidados de suporte (p. ex., anti-inflamatórios, antibióticos e administração intravenosa de fluidos); o reparo específico de fraturas ou a remoção de hematomas é potencialmente difícil, considerando-se a localização.
• Vestibulopatia geriátrica canina e idiopática felina — apenas cuidados de suporte.
• Polineuropatia de nervos cranianos — a resposta à prednisona será boa se o paciente tiver algum distúrbio imune primário.
• Deficiência de tiamina — modificação da dieta e reposição de tiamina.

CONTRAINDICAÇÕES
Medicamentos potencialmente tóxicos para o sistema vestibular — antibióticos aminoglicosídeos; administração prolongada de metronidazol em altas doses.

PRECAUÇÕES
• Administração de trimetoprima-sulfa — ceratoconjuntivite seca (ressecamento ocular).
• Evitar a administração de medicamentos no canal auditivo externo (especialmente à base de óleos) em caso de ruptura da membrana timpânica.

ACOMPANHAMENTO

MONITORIZAÇÃO DO PACIENTE
• Repetir o exame neurológico conforme ditado pela causa subjacente.
• A inclinação da cabeça pode persistir.
• Hipotireoidismo — medir a concentração de T_4 4-6 h após o tratamento, 3-4 semanas depois do início da terapia de reposição hormonal ou da mudança da dosagem.
• Repetir a análise do LCS e as imagens do cérebro — no caso de alguns distúrbios vestibulares centrais.
• Monitorizar a produção de lágrimas (teste lacrimal de Schirmer) com a administração de trimetoprima-sulfa.

COMPLICAÇÕES POSSÍVEIS
• Evolução da doença.
• Herniação cerebral.

EVOLUÇÃO ESPERADA E PROGNÓSTICO
• O prognóstico para distúrbios vestibulares centrais costuma ser pior em comparação aos periféricos.
• O prognóstico para vestibulopatia geriátrica canina e idiopática felina é excelente.

DIVERSOS

DISTÚRBIOS ASSOCIADOS
• Paresia ou paralisia do nervo facial.
• Síndrome de Horner.

FATORES RELACIONADOS COM A IDADE
A síndrome vestibular geriátrica canina acomete cães mais idosos.

VER TAMBÉM
• Vestibulopatia Geriátrica — Cães.
• Vestibulopatia Idiopática — Gatos.
• Encefalite.
• Meningoencefalomielite Granulomatosa.
• Otite Média e Interna.
• Pólipos Nasais e Nasofaríngeos.

ABREVIATURA(S)
• LCS = líquido cerebrospinal.
• PIF = peritonite infecciosa felina.
• RAETC = resposta auditiva evocada do tronco cerebral.
• RM = ressonância magnética.
• SNC = sistema nervoso central.
• TC = tomografia computadorizada.
• TSH = hormônio tireostimulante.

Sugestões de Leitura
Chrisman C, Mariani C, Platt S, Clemmons R. Neurology for the Small Animal Practitioner. Jackson, WY: Teton NewMedia, 2003, pp. 126-143.
De Lahunta A, Glass E. Veterinary Neuroanatomy and Clinical Neurology, 3rd ed. St. Louis: Saunders/Elsevier, 2009, pp. 72, 319-347.
Dewey CW. A Practical Guide to Canine and Feline Neurology, 2nd ed. Ames, IA:Wiley-Blackwell, 2008, pp. 265-285.
Lorenz MD, Kornegay JN. Handbook of Veterinary Neurology, 4th ed. St. Louis: Saunders/Elsevier, 2004, pp. 219-245.
Munana KR. Head tilt and nystagmus. In: Platt SR, Olby NJ, eds. BSAVA Manual of Canine and Feline Neurology, 3rd ed. Gloucester: BSAVA, 2004, pp. 155-171.

Autor Susan M. Cochrane
Consultor Editorial Joane M. Parent

Incontinência Fecal

CONSIDERAÇÕES GERAIS

DEFINIÇÃO
Incapacidade de retenção das fezes, que resulta na passagem involuntária de material fecal.

FISIOPATOLOGIA
• A incontinência do reservatório fecal desenvolve-se quando o processo mórbido diminui a capacidade ou a complacência do reto.
• Ocorre o desenvolvimento de incontinência do esfíncter quando o esfíncter anal externo é anatomicamente rompido (i. e., incontinência não neurogênica do esfíncter) ou desnervado (i. e., incontinência neurogênica do esfíncter).
• A incontinência neurogênica do esfíncter pode ser causada por lesão do nervo pudendo, doença da medula espinal sacral, disfunção autônoma e neuropatia ou miopatia periféricas generalizadas.
• A lesão ou a degeneração dos músculos levantadores do ânus e coccígeo também podem contribuir para a incontinência fecal.

SISTEMA(S) ACOMETIDO(S)
• Gastrintestinal. • Nervoso.

GENÉTICA
Não há nenhuma base genética conhecida para o desenvolvimento de qualquer tipo de incontinência — do reservatório, do esfíncter ou neurogênica.

INCIDÊNCIA/PREVALÊNCIA
Desconhecidas.

DISTRIBUIÇÃO GEOGRÁFICA
Nenhuma.

IDENTIFICAÇÃO
• Cães e gatos. • Embora animais de qualquer idade possam ser acometidos, a incidência aumenta nos pacientes mais idosos.

SINAIS CLÍNICOS

Achados Anamnésicos
• Incontinência do reservatório — promove a urgência na defecação; os sinais incluem defecação frequente e consciente, sem gotejamento das fezes; a defecação pode estar associada a sinais de tenesmo, disquezia ou hematoquezia.
• Incontinência do esfíncter — associada à expulsão involuntária ou gotejamento de material fecal, especialmente durante agitação ou com latidos e tosse.
• Perguntar aos clientes sobre doença neurológica prévia, cirurgia anorretal e/ou traumatismo, adestramento doméstico, vermifugação e se o animal parece defecar de forma voluntária ou involuntária; obter ainda informações sobre a dieta do animal, as medicações atuais e os sinais clínicos sistêmicos concomitantes, especialmente sinais neurológicos.
• Incontinência urinária concomitante sugere incontinência neurogênica do esfíncter.

Achados do Exame Físico
• Incontinência do reservatório — pode incluir sensibilidade anorretal ou dor à palpação digital, massa retal ou espessamento da mucosa retal; o tônus do esfíncter anal externo e o reflexo anal da incontinência não neurogênica do esfíncter permanecem normais.
• Incontinência não neurogênica do esfíncter — pode incluir evidência de traumatismo perineal ou fístulas perianais; embora o reflexo anal esteja presente, o esfíncter anal externo poderá não se fechar completamente se o esfíncter for rompido em termos anatômicos.
• Incontinência neurogênica do esfíncter — pode incluir perda do tônus do esfíncter anal externo, apesar de o tônus anal ser um mau indicador da função do esfíncter anal; o reflexo anal fica ausente ou diminuído.
• Fazer o exame neurológico completo em todos os animais com incontinência do esfíncter; achados adicionais sugestivos de doença da medula espinal lombossacra incluem perda do movimento voluntário e do tônus da cauda, dor lombossacra, paresia ou paralisia flácida posterior e reflexos miotáticos hiporreflexivos para os membros pélvicos.
• Sinais difusos atribuídos à lesão no neurônio motor inferior sugerem neuropatia ou miopatia periféricas generalizadas; sinais relativos à lesão do neurônio motor superior para os membros pélvicos sugerem doença do SNC cranial ao plexo lombossacro.

CAUSAS

Incontinência do Reservatório
• Doença colorretal — colite, síndrome do intestino irritável e neoplasia.
• Diarreia — grandes volumes de fezes por qualquer causa podem sobrecarregar a capacidade de absorção e armazenamento do cólon.

Incontinência Não Neurogênica do Esfíncter
• Lesões anais traumáticas — feridas por mordedura, abscedação grave dos sacos anais, laceração ou ferimento por arma de fogo.
• Iatrogênica — o esfíncter anal externo e os músculos levantadores do ânus podem ser anatomicamente rompidos durante a cirurgia anorretal. • Fístulas perianais.

Incontinência Neurogênica do Esfíncter
• SNC — mielopatia degenerativa, disrafismo espinal, espinha bífida, traumatismo, extrusão do disco intervertebral, neoplasia, meningomielite (várias causas), embolia fibrocartilaginosa, outros comprometimentos vasculares.
• Síndrome da cauda equina — extrusão do disco intervertebral em L6-L7 ou L7-S1, espondilose deformante, estenose congênita do canal espinal, instabilidade lombossacra, discospondilite e neoplasia.
• Neuropatia periférica — infecciosa, imunomediada, induzida por medicamento (p. ex., sulfato de vincristina), disautonomia e idiopática.
• Miopatia/distúrbio neuromuscular.
• Degeneração (envelhecimento) — é provável que múltiplos fatores estejam envolvidos, incluindo-se atrofia dos músculos envolvidos na continência fecal, fraqueza, neuropatia degenerativa e senilidade.

FATORES DE RISCO
• Doença colônica. • Doença e cirurgia anorretal.
• Doença do SNC e neuropatia periférica.

DIAGNÓSTICO

DIAGNÓSTICO DIFERENCIAL
• Doença gastrintestinal por qualquer causa pode aumentar a urgência de defecação sem alterar diretamente a capacidade de reservatório do cólon.
• Ao contrário da incontinência do esfíncter, a doença gastrintestinal quase sempre está associada a sinais de perda de peso, vômito, tenesmo, disquezia e hematoquezia.
• Distúrbios do comportamento (p. ex., ansiedade pela separação), diferentemente da incontinência fecal, estão muitas vezes associados a atividades destrutivas ou vocalização excessiva.
• Em geral, ocorre adestramento doméstico inadequado em cães jovens ou naqueles recentemente introduzidos em algum ambiente interno ou em gatos com aversão à bandeja sanitária (número insuficiente de bandejas, bandejas sujas, localização desfavorável, ninhada nova, etc.).

HEMOGRAMA/BIOQUÍMICA/URINÁLISE
• Os resultados costumam permanecer normais.
• A urinálise pode revelar indícios de infecção do trato urinário inferior (p. ex., piúria e hematúria), especialmente com incontinência urinária concomitante.

OUTROS TESTES LABORATORIAIS
• Realizar o exame de flutuação fecal para ajudar a descartar o parasitismo como causa de diarreia.
• É indicada a realização de raspado retal em regiões onde a histoplasmose ou a pitiose são endêmicas.

DIAGNÓSTICO POR IMAGEM
• Radiografias simples lateral e ventrodorsal da coluna lombossacra podem apresentar evidência de extrusão do disco intervertebral, discospondilite, neoplasia vertebral, espinha bífida, traumatismo lombossacro ou má-formação vertebral.
• Mielografia e epidurografia também são valiosas para demonstrar lesões compressivas dentro do canal espinal.
• TC e RM podem ser necessárias para demonstrar algumas lesões compressivas e lesões intraparenquimatosas da medula espinal.

OUTROS MÉTODOS DIAGNÓSTICOS
• Realizar eletromiografia (EMG) para avaliar o esfíncter anal externo, bem como os músculos levantadores do ânus e coccígeo, em busca de indícios de desnervação ou miopatia.
• Também é recomendada a avaliação de outros músculos para ajudar a localizar a lesão neurológica — desnervação difusa *versus* lesão focal da medula espinal.
• Podem avaliar o reflexo pudendo-anal do ponto de vista eletrofisiológico.
• Efetuar biopsias do músculo e do nervo para pesquisa de miopatia e neuropatia periférica.
• A análise do LCS coletado por punção lombar pode revelar indícios de processo infeccioso ou inflamatório, neoplasia ou traumatismo do SNC.
• Fazer colonoscopia e biopsia da mucosa colorretal caso se suspeite de incontinência do reservatório.

TRATAMENTO

• Se possível, identificar a causa subjacente; a incontinência fecal poderá se resolver se a causa básica for tratada com sucesso (p. ex., descompressão da medula espinal, colite, etc.).
• Dieta — o volume fecal pode ser reduzido, administrando-se rações comerciais pobres em resíduos ou alimentos como queijo cottage e arroz

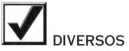

e/ou tofu. Alimentar os animais em horários estabelecidos para melhorar os tempos de controle necessários para defecação. É contraindicado o aumento do volume fecal com dietas ricas em fibras insolúveis.
- Enemas frequentes com água tépida (morna) diminuirão o volume das fezes no cólon e, portanto, reduzirão a incidência de defecação inadequada.
- Mudanças ambientais (p. ex., mudar o animal para algum ambiente externo) podem aumentar a satisfação do proprietário e, dessa forma, evitar a eutanásia de um animal sadio sob outros aspectos.
- Algumas vezes, o reflexo de defecação pode ser induzido nos animais com paralisia posterior (p. ex., pinçamento leve do dedo no membro pélvico ou da cauda); da mesma forma, a aplicação de toalha aquecida na região do ânus ou do períneo pode estimular a defecação.
- A reconstrução cirúrgica de lesões anorretais pode melhorar acentuadamente a continência fecal nos pacientes com incontinência não neurogênica do esfíncter.
- Tipoias fasciais e tipoias de elastômero de silicone obtiveram sucesso variável no tratamento da incontinência neurogênica do esfíncter nos cães.
- O prognóstico será mau se a causa subjacente não puder ser identificada e corrigida com êxito; discutir o prognóstico com o proprietário logo no início da avaliação para evitar expectativas não realistas.

MEDICAÇÕES

MEDICAMENTO(S) DE ESCOLHA
- Medicamentos opiáceos modificadores da motilidade (p. ex., cloridrato de difenoxilato e cloridrato de loperamida) aumentam a contração segmentar do intestino e lentificam a passagem de material fecal, aumentando com isso a quantidade de água absorvida a partir das fezes.
- Agentes anti-inflamatórios, como os glicocorticoides e a sulfassalazina, podem trazer benefício aos pacientes com suspeita de incontinência do reservatório atribuída à enteropatia inflamatória ou colite.
- A melhora nos sinais poderá ser obtida caso se administrem terapias específicas para fístula perianal, enteropatia inflamatória ou outras causas de incontinência relacionadas com o reservatório ou de origem não neurogênica; no entanto, não existem medicamentos específicos eficazes em pacientes com incontinência neurogênica.

CONTRAINDICAÇÕES
- Não utilizar medicamentos modificadores da motilidade em pacientes com diarreia na suspeita de causa infecciosa ou tóxica.
- Não usar opiáceos modificadores da motilidade em pacientes com doença respiratória; ter cuidado quanto ao uso em pacientes com hepatopatia.
- O uso de opiáceos em felinos geralmente não é recomendado.
- Não fornecer dietas que contenham altas concentrações de fibras insolúveis, pois isso produzirá grande quantidade de fezes volumosas, que, por sua vez, são difíceis de serem eliminadas ou podem causar obstipação (sobretudo em gatos).

PRECAUÇÕES
- Medicamentos modificadores da motilidade podem provocar constipação e timpanismo.
- Medicamentos opiáceos modificadores da motilidade podem causar sedação.

INTERAÇÕES POSSÍVEIS
É possível a ocorrência de sedação intensa e depressão respiratória quando os opiáceos são utilizados concomitantemente com outros depressores do SNC (p. ex., barbitúricos, anestésicos gerais e tranquilizantes).

MEDICAMENTO(S) ALTERNATIVO(S)
N/D.

ACOMPANHAMENTO

MONITORIZAÇÃO DO PACIENTE
- Se a incontinência fecal for atribuída a alguma causa neurológica subjacente, utilizar exames neurológicos seriados para monitorizar o progresso do paciente.
- Métodos radiográficos, EMG, análise do LCS e estudos eletrodiagnósticos também podem ser utilizados para acompanhar a evolução do quadro.
- Verificar a consistência e o volume das fezes e ainda certificar-se de que o animal de estimação não se tornou constipado.
- Ajustar a dieta e as dosagens de medicamentos modificadores da motilidade para encontrar a terapia apropriada para cada paciente.

COMPLICAÇÕES POSSÍVEIS
- A incontinência neurogênica do esfíncter frequentemente não é responsiva a despeito de tratamento nutricional, clínico e cirúrgico apropriado.
- Em um estudo recente, 50% dos animais com incontinência fecal foram sacrificados.

DIVERSOS

DISTÚRBIOS ASSOCIADOS
N/D.

FATORES RELACIONADOS COM A IDADE
N/D.

POTENCIAL ZOONÓTICO
- A exposição às fezes do animal aumenta o risco de exposição a parasitas zoonóticos.
- Orientar os proprietários sobre doenças zoonóticas (p. ex., larva migrans cutânea e visceral, bem como toxoplasmose).

GESTAÇÃO/FERTILIDADE/REPRODUÇÃO
N/D.

VER TAMBÉM
- Discopatia Intervertebral Toracolombar.
- Incontinência Urinária.

ABREVIATURA(S)
- EMG = eletromiografia.
- LCS = líquido cerebrospinal.
- RM = ressonância magnética.
- SNC = sistema nervoso central.
- TC = tomografia computadorizada.

RECURSOS DA INTERNET
Rede de Informações Veterinárias: www.vin.com/VIN.plx.

Sugestões de Leitura

Guilford WG. Fecal incontinence in dogs and cats. Compend Contin Educ Pract Vet 1990, 12:313-326.

Richter KP. Diseases of the rectum and anus. In: Kirk's Current Veterinary Therapy XI. Philadelphia: Saunders, 1992, pp. 615-616.

Zoran DL. Recto-anal disease. In: Ettinger SJ, Feldman EC, eds., Textbook of Veterinary Internal Medicine, 6th ed. St. Louis: Elsevier, 2005, pp. 1419-1420.

Autor Debra L. Zoran
Consultor Editorial Albert E. Jergens
Agradecimento O autor e os editores agradecem a colaboração prévia de Marc C. Walker e Randall C. Longshore, que foram os autores deste capítulo na edição anterior.

Incontinência Urinária

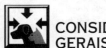

CONSIDERAÇÕES GERAIS

DEFINIÇÃO
Perda do controle voluntário da micção, observada geralmente como extravasamento involuntário da urina.

FISIOPATOLOGIA
Em geral, trata-se de um distúrbio da fase de armazenamento da micção. A falha no armazenamento de urina é provocada pela acomodação comprometida da bexiga urinária, pelo comprometimento dos mecanismos de continência uretral ou pelo desvio anatômico das estruturas de armazenamento urinário. A obstrução parcial ao fluxo de saída e outras causas de hiperdistensão vesical podem resultar na incontinência urinária paradoxal ou por fluxo exagerado.

SISTEMA(S) ACOMETIDO(S)
- Renal/urológico.
- Nervoso.
- Cutâneo/exócrino — assadura pela urina com consequente dermatite perineal e ventral, recesso vulvar.

INCIDÊNCIA/PREVALÊNCIA
A incontinência urinária pode acometer mais de 20% das cadelas castradas, especialmente as raças de grande porte.

IDENTIFICAÇÃO
- Cães e (raramente) gatos.
- Mais comum nas cadelas castradas de meia-idade a idosas; observada também em fêmeas jovens e (raramente) nos machos castrados.
- Cães de raças médias a grandes são mais frequentemente acometidos.

CAUSAS

Neurológicas
- Desorganização de neurorreceptores locais, nervos periféricos, trajetos espinais ou centros superiores envolvidos no controle da micção pode comprometer o armazenamento de urina. Distúrbios periféricos generalizados atribuídos à lesão de neurônio motor inferior ou distúrbios autônomos também podem causar incontinência urinária.
- Lesões da medula espinal sacral, como má-formação congênita, compressão da cauda equina, discopatia lombossacra ou ainda fraturas ou deslocamentos traumáticos, podem resultar em bexiga urinária superdistendida e flácida, com fraca resistência à saída. Com isso, ocorrem retenção de urina e incontinência por fluxo exagerado.
- Lesões do cerebelo ou do centro cerebral da micção afetam a inibição e o controle voluntário do esvaziamento, resultando geralmente em micção frequente e involuntária ou extravasamento de pequenas quantidades de urina.

Disfunção de Armazenamento da Bexiga Urinária
- Acomodação deficiente da urina durante a estocagem ou hiperatividade vesical (instabilidade do detrusor) levam ao extravasamento frequente de pequenas quantidades de urina.
- Infecções do trato urinário, distúrbios inflamatórios crônicos, lesões neoplásicas infiltrativas, compressão externa e obstrução parcial crônica da saída são causas potenciais.
- Hipoplasia congênita da bexiga urinária pode acompanhar ureteres ectópicos ou outros distúrbios de desenvolvimento do trato urogenital.
- Instabilidade idiopática do detrusor foi associada à infecção pelo FeLV nos gatos e a causas desconhecidas nos cães.

Distúrbios Uretrais
- Se o fechamento da uretra conferido pelo músculo liso uretral, músculo estriado e tecido conjuntivo não evitar o extravasamento da urina durante o armazenamento, será observada incontinência urinária intermitente.
- Exemplos — hipoplasia ou incompetência uretral congênita, incompetência uretral adquirida (i. e., incontinência urinária responsiva a hormônio sexual), infecção ou inflamação do trato urinário, prostatopatia ou cirurgia prostática.

Anatômicas
- Anormalidades anatômicas evolutivas (i. e., de desenvolvimento) ou adquiridas desviam a urina dos mecanismos normais de armazenamento ou interferem na função vesical ou uretral.
- Ureteres ectópicos podem desembocar na uretra distal, no útero ou na vagina.
- Resquícios do úraco persistente desviam o fluxo urinário para o umbigo.
- Anomalias vestibulovaginais, hipoplasia urocística congênita ou hipoplasia uretral.
- Localização intrapélvica do colo vesical pode contribuir para o extravasamento da urina em função de incompetência uretral.
- Anormalidades de conformação vulvar e perivulvar podem contribuir para o acúmulo e o extravasamento intermitente de urina.

Retenção de Urina
- Fluxo exagerado é observado quando a pressão intravesicular excede a resistência à saída.

Incontinência Urinária Mista
- Causas mistas ou múltiplas são observadas em humanos e provavelmente ocorrem em cães e gatos. São mais prováveis as combinações de disfunção da uretra e de armazenamento vesical e as combinações de distúrbios anatômicos e funcionais.

FATORES DE RISCO
- A castração aumenta o risco do desenvolvimento de incompetência uretral, especialmente em cães de grande porte (>20 kg).
- Não foi demonstrado que a castração precoce (<3 meses) aumente o risco de incontinência urinária nas cadelas.
- Características de conformação, como a posição do colo vesical, o comprimento da uretra e as anomalias concomitantes da vagina, podem aumentar o risco de incontinência urinária nas cadelas.
- A obesidade pode aumentar o risco de incontinência urinária nas cadelas castradas.
- Outros possíveis fatores de risco para a incompetência uretral incluem a raça, o grande porte corporal, o sinal de poliúria e a caudectomia precoce.

DIAGNÓSTICO

DIAGNÓSTICO DIFERENCIAL

Sinais Semelhantes de Diferenciação
- Micção voluntária, porém inadequada (geralmente comportamental).
- Secreções uretrais frequentemente associadas a prostatopatias nos machos e a distúrbios vaginais nas fêmeas.
- Jato de urina ou micção inadequada nos gatos podem ser confundidos com incontinência urinária; é mais provável que o jato seja emitido pelos gatos na posição ereta (i. e., em estação), com marcação de urina encontrada nas superfícies verticais de móveis, paredes e cortinas.
- Poliúria — pode precipitar ou exacerbar a incontinência urinária ou levar à noctúria e micção inadequada; medir a densidade urinária em amostra aleatória de urina para excluir ou não o sinal de poliúria relevante do ponto de vista clínico.

Causas Diferenciais
- Causas neurogênicas de incontinência urinária — geralmente induzem a uma bexiga urinária grande e distendida, além de outros déficits neurológicos como tônus fraco do ânus ou da cauda, sensibilidade perineal deprimida e déficits proprioceptivos.
- Cães com incompetência uretral tipicamente apresentam ocorrências intermitentes de incontinência urinária, observada com maior frequência à noite ou enquanto o animal está dormindo. O exame físico revela uma bexiga urinária pequena e nenhum outro defeito.
- Acúmulo (represamento) de urina — os cães acometidos podem extravasar pequenas quantidades de urina após a micção.
- Os achados da anamnese e do exame físico nos pacientes com disfunção de armazenamento vesical assemelham-se àqueles observados nos pacientes com incompetência uretral, embora a frequência aumentada de micção ou a urgência aparente possam ser sinais clínicos adicionais.
- Anisocoria é frequentemente encontrada nos gatos com incontinência urinária associada à infecção pelo FeLV.
- Os sinais da anamnese nos cães com prostatopatia incluem tenesmo, fraqueza dos membros posteriores, disúria e polaciúria. Os achados físicos incluem prostatomegalia, dor lombossacra, dor à palpação prostática e tremor ou fraqueza dos membros posteriores.
- Conformação vulvar em recesso ou juvenil pode contribuir para o acúmulo (represamento) de urina.

HEMOGRAMA/BIOQUÍMICA/URINÁLISE
- As análises hematológicas e bioquímicas podem estar indicadas nos pacientes com distúrbios poliúricos (ver "Poliúria e Polidipsia").
- A urinálise pode revelar indícios de infecção do trato urinário (p. ex., piúria, hematúria e bactérias) ou poliúria (p. ex., densidade urinária baixa).

OUTROS TESTES LABORATORIAIS
- Testar os gatos para o FeLV.
- Urocultura em cães com incompetência uretral.

DIAGNÓSTICO POR IMAGEM

Achados Radiográficos
- A radiografia contrastada está indicada nos animais jovens e naqueles que apresentam incontinência urinária logo após procedimentos cirúrgicos ou incidentes traumáticos.
- Os exames de urografia excretora ou tomografia contrastada permitem a inspeção dos rins, das terminações ureterais e da bexiga urinária.
- A vaginouretrografia retrógrada possibilita a visualização da abóbada vaginal, da uretra e da bexiga urinária. Em geral, os ureteres ectópicos são

preenchidos pelo meio de contraste nesses estudos retrógrados.
- A cistografia com duplo contraste pode ser necessária para a visão completa da estrutura vesical e a identificação de lesões vesicais.

Achados Ultrassonográficos
- Possível uso para avaliação dos rins, dos ureteres e da bexiga urinária para identificar urólitos, massas, hidronefrose ou hidroureter ou, ainda, indícios de pielonefrite.

MÉTODOS DIAGNÓSTICOS
- Exame neurológico — o exame da sensibilidade perineal e dos reflexos bulboesponjosos, bem como do tônus do ânus e da cauda, proporciona uma avaliação breve da função nervosa espinal caudal e periférica.
- Cateterização uretral — pode ser necessária para avaliar a patência (desobstrução) da uretra caso se observe retenção urinária.
- Métodos urodinâmicos — considerar os procedimentos de cistometrografia, medida do perfil da pressão uretral e eletromiografia para avaliar a função vesical, uretral e neurológica de forma mais objetiva.
- Cistoscopia — permite a visualização da bexiga urinária, da uretra e das terminações ureterais ectópicas.

TRATAMENTO
CUIDADO(S) DE SAÚDE ADEQUADO(S)
- Geralmente como paciente ambulatorial.
- Tratar os distúrbios obstrutivos parciais e os distúrbios neurológicos primários de forma específica, se possível.
- Identificar a presença de infecção do trato urinário e tratar adequadamente.
- Ureteres ectópicos e hipoplasia uretral congênita frequentemente podem ser submetidos à correção cirúrgica; a ablação a laser guiada por endoscopia já foi utilizada para ureteres ectópicos. Anormalidades funcionais da competência uretral ou do armazenamento vesical podem acompanhar o distúrbio anatômico e necessitar de tratamento clínico auxiliar.
- Agentes formadores de volume de teflon ou colágeno podem ser injetados na submucosa uretral para controlar a incontinência.
- Métodos cirúrgicos, como a colpossuspensão, a cistouretropexia e o implante de prótese para esfíncter, foram descritos para o tratamento de incontinência refratária; no entanto, são constatadas baixas taxas de continência no acompanhamento a longo prazo.

MEDICAÇÕES
MEDICAMENTO(S) DE ESCOLHA
Incompetência Uretral
- Tratar com hormônios sexuais (p. ex., estilbestrol, dietilestilbestrol [0,1-1,0 mg/cão VO a cada 24 h durante 5-7 dias e, em seguida, 0,1-1,0 mg/cão VO a cada 4-7 dias conforme a necessidade], estrogênios conjugados, estriol [1-2 mg/cão VO a cada 24 h por 7 dias e, em seguida, 0,5-1 mg/cão a cada 24-48 h se necessário] e testosterona) ou agonistas α-adrenérgicos (p. ex.,

fenilpropanolamina [1,5 mg/kg VO a cada 8-12 h], fenilefrina, pseudoefedrina [1,1 mg/kg VO a cada 12 h]).
- Os agentes α-adrenérgicos e os hormônios sexuais podem ser administrados em combinação para obtenção de efeito terapêutico sinérgico.
- Imipramina (5-15 mg/cão VO a cada 12 h), um antidepressivo tricíclico com ações anticolinérgicas e α-agonistas, representa um método alternativo de tratamento.
- Deslorrelina, um análogo do GnRH, também já foi usada em casos refratários.

Instabilidade do Detrusor
- Tratar com agentes anticolinérgicos ou antiespasmódicos (p. ex., oxibutinina [aproximadamente 0,2 mg/kg VO a cada 8-12 h, até a dose total de 5 mg], propantelina, imipramina, flavoxato e diciclomina).
- A tolterodina não é amplamente usada em cães.

Prostatopatia
- Ver "Prostatomegalia", além de "Prostatite e Abscesso Prostático".

CONTRAINDICAÇÕES
- Agonistas adrenérgicos em pacientes com cardiopatia, nefropatia e distúrbios hipertensivos.
- Agentes anticolinérgicos em pacientes com glaucoma ou cardiopatia.

PRECAUÇÕES
- Compostos estrogênicos raramente provocam sinais de estro e supressão da medula óssea, mas exacerbam doença imunomediada. Contudo, a supressão da medula óssea atribuída à terapia com estrogênios costuma ser fatal. Portanto, utilizar a dose mínima, porém eficaz, no menor tempo possível.
- A administração de testosterona pode causar sinais de agressividade ou libido, exacerbar a prostatopatia e contribuir para o desenvolvimento de hérnia perineal ou de adenoma perianal.
- Agonistas adrenérgicos podem produzir inquietação, taquicardia e hipertensão.
- Agentes anticolinérgicos podem provocar náusea, vômito e constipação.

INTERAÇÕES POSSÍVEIS
- Antidepressivos tricíclicos não devem ser administrados concomitantemente com inibidores da monoamina oxidase (p. ex., Anipryl®).
- O risco de hipertensão aumentará se os agonistas α-adrenérgicos forem administrados concomitantemente com os antidepressivos tricíclicos.

ACOMPANHAMENTO
MONITORIZAÇÃO DO PACIENTE
- Pacientes submetidos a agentes α-adrenérgicos — observar durante o período terapêutico inicial quanto ao surgimento de efeitos adversos da medicação, incluindo-se taquicardia, ansiedade e hipertensão.
- Pacientes submetidos a estrogênios a longo prazo — inicialmente, monitorizar em 1 mês e fazer hemogramas periódicos.
- Urinálise e urocultura periódicas.
- Esperar uma resposta excelente ao tratamento clínico em 60-90% dos pacientes tratados.
- Uma vez observado o efeito terapêutico, reduzir lentamente a dosagem e a frequência de

administração dos agentes farmacológicos ao mínimo necessário.
- Considerar o uso de combinações terapêuticas (agonista α-adrenérgico com hormônios sexuais ou agentes anticolinérgicos), deslorrelina ou opções cirúrgicas em caso de resposta deficiente à monoterapia (i. e., medicação com um único agente).

COMPLICAÇÕES POSSÍVEIS
- Infecção recidivante e ascendente do trato urinário.
- Assadura pela urina com consequente dermatite perineal e ventral.
- Incontinência refratária e intratável.

DIVERSOS
DISTÚRBIOS ASSOCIADOS
- Infecção do trato urinário.
- Vaginite.

GESTAÇÃO/FERTILIDADE/REPRODUÇÃO
Apesar de a incontinência urinária ser rara nas fêmeas prenhes, não é aconselhável a utilização de estrogênios ou agentes anticolinérgicos.

SINÔNIMO(S)
Enurese.

VER TAMBÉM
- Obstrução do Trato Urinário.
- Poliúria e Polidipsia.
- Prostatite e Abscesso Prostático.
- Retenção Urinária Funcional.

ABREVIATURA(S)
- FeLV = vírus da leucemia felina.
- GnRH = hormônio liberador da gonadotropina.

Sugestões de Leitura
Barth A, Reichler IM, Hubler M, et al. Evaluation of long-term effects of endoscopic injection of collagen into the urethral submucosal for treatment of urethral sphincter incompetence in female dogs: 40 cases. JAVMA 2005, 226:73-76.
Berent AC, Mayhew PD, Porat-Mosenco Y. Use of cystoscopic-guided laser ablation for treatment of intramural ureteral ectopia in male dogs: Four cases (2006-2007). JAVMA 2008, 232:1026-1034.
Lane IF, Westropp JL. Urinary incontinence and micturition disorders: Pharmacologic management. In Bonagura JD, Twedt DC, eds., Kirk's Current Veterinary Therapy XIV. St. Louis: Saunders Elsevier, 2009, pp. 955-959.
McLoughlin MA, Chew DJ. Surgical treatment of urethral sphincter mechanism incompetence in female dogs. Compend Contin Educ Pract Vet 2009, 31:360-373.
Spain CV, Scarlett JM, Houpt K. Long-term risks and benefits of early-age gonadectomy in dogs. JAVMA 2004, 224:380-387.

Autor Jo Smith
Consultor Editorial Carl A. Osborne
Agradecimento O autor e o consultor editorial gostariam de agradecer as colaborações de Dr. Jeanne Barsanti e Dr. India Lane.

Inércia Uterina

CONSIDERAÇÕES GERAIS

REVISÃO
Falha na expulsão de fetos de tamanho normal com apresentação e posturas normais através do canal normal de parto ao término de uma gestação normal.

Primária
- Falha em iniciar o parto ao término da gestação.
- Observada em cadelas de grande porte com um a dois filhotes na ninhada — falha em iniciar o parto.
- Ocorre com ninhadas de tamanho grande — estiramento excessivo do útero.

Secundária
- Ocorre após contrações uterinas prolongadas, em que alguns filhotes ou toda a ninhada não são expelidos.
- Pode ser secundária à distocia ou a ninhadas grandes.

IDENTIFICAÇÃO
Cadelas e gatas de qualquer idade.

SINAIS CLÍNICOS
- Primária — falha em iniciar o parto ao término da gestação; a paciente tipicamente permanece assintomática, exceto por possível corrimento vaginal após separação da placenta; as frequências cardíacas fetais declinam.
- Secundária — as contrações cessam apesar das contrações normais no início; pode expulsar parte da ninhada e, depois, parar; também há declínio nas frequências cardíacas fetais.

CAUSAS E FATORES DE RISCO
- Primária — estimulação inadequada dos fetos para desencadear a cascata de eventos que induzem ao parto (ninhadas pequenas); hormônios ou receptores anormais ou inadequados; doença sistêmica; obesidade; administração de tocolíticos; hipocalcemia; infecção uterina; torção uterina; nutrição inadequada; traumatismo.
- Secundária — acompanha exaustão da musculatura uterina durante o parto normal de ninhadas grandes; ocorre durante distocia após períodos prolongados de contração uterina e consequente fadiga uterina.

DIAGNÓSTICO

DIAGNÓSTICO DIFERENCIAL
- Primária — data prevista imprecisa do parto; pseudociese; gestação inviável.
- Secundária — parto normal; parto já concluído.

HEMOGRAMA/BIOQUÍMICA/URINÁLISE
- Anemia normocítica normocrômica (normal na gestação).
- Hipercolesterolemia (normal na gestação).
- Pode exibir baixos níveis de cálcio total ou ionizado.
- Hipoglicemia.

OUTROS TESTES LABORATORIAIS
Níveis séricos da progesterona <2 ng/mL por 48 h antes do parto em grande parte dos casos.

DIAGNÓSTICO POR IMAGEM
- Achados ultrassonográficos — frequências cardíacas fetais mantidas a <160-170 bpm indicam a presença de estresse e a necessidade de intervenção; separação da placenta do útero — necessidade de intervenção imediata para otimizar a sobrevida da ninhada.
- Achados radiográficos — avaliação da paciente quanto à presença de feto(s), bem como quanto ao tamanho, à posição e à apresentação desse(s) feto(s).

MÉTODOS DIAGNÓSTICOS
Exame da vagina por palpação digital para avaliar a presença de feto dentro do canal de parto caudal e a existência de anormalidade na anatomia causadora de estreitamento do canal do parto.

TRATAMENTO

- Internação — na presença de feto(s) vivo(s) e na documentação de estresse fetal, a melhor opção terapêutica para a sobrevida é a cesariana imediata; a cirurgia constitui a única opção para inércia uterina primária quando se deseja a sobrevivência dos fetos.
- Clínico — para inércia uterina secundária com distocia não obstrutiva.

MEDICAÇÕES

MEDICAMENTO(S)
- Gliconato de cálcio a 5% (0,5-1 mL/5 kg SC ou IV ou 0,2 mL/kg IV) — em caso de hipocalcemia.
- Fluidos contendo glicose a 2,5-5% na presença de hipoglicemia.
- A ocitocina não é tipicamente eficaz para os casos de inércia uterina verdadeira; utilizar após o tratamento com cálcio; 0,5-4 UI/cão SC ou IM; 1-2 UI/gata SC ou IM; não administrar em casos de distocia obstrutiva.

CONTRAINDICAÇÕES/INTERAÇÕES POSSÍVEIS
- Surgimento de arritmias cardíacas no tratamento com o cálcio; monitorizar o eletrocardiograma e interromper o tratamento caso se constate a presença de arritmias.
- As contrações podem ser retomadas apenas com a administração de cálcio e a reidratação da paciente.
- O adiamento da cirurgia enquanto se prossegue o tratamento clínico pode diminuir a taxa de sobrevida dos fetos.
- Ruptura uterina (rara).

ACOMPANHAMENTO

MONITORIZAÇÃO DA PACIENTE
- Acompanhar os níveis de cálcio ionizado em casos de hipocalcemia; a suplementação de cálcio fica indicada durante a lactação nos casos com eclâmpsia.
- Monitorizar a temperatura da fêmea e a natureza do corrimento vaginal diariamente por 5-7 dias após distocia ou cesariana — preocupação quanto à ocorrência de metrite.
- Tocodinamometria para monitorizar as contrações (WhelpWise, Veterinary Perinatal Specialties, Wheatridge, CO, 303-423-3429).

PREVENÇÃO
- Otimizar o manejo reprodutivo para ajudar a aumentar o tamanho da ninhada em casos de inércia primária causada por ninhada pequena.
- É aconselhável reproduzir apenas as cadelas em boa condição corporal e monitorizar a nutrição durante a prenhez.
- Utilizar a tocodinamometria para identificar inércia uterina secundária precocemente permite o reforço imediato das contrações.
- Remover os animais com inércia uterina primária repetida da reprodução.

COMPLICAÇÕES POSSÍVEIS
- Óbito de fetos viáveis caso transcorra muito tempo antes da intervenção.
- Acredita-se que a inércia primária seja hereditária em algumas raças de cães e gatos.

EVOLUÇÃO ESPERADA E PROGNÓSTICO
- Primária — pode apresentar recidiva em gestações subsequentes; a cesariana eletiva pode otimizar a taxa de sobrevida dos fetos.
- Secundária — não apresenta necessariamente recidiva se for atribuída a fatores relacionados com o feto, como tamanho grande da ninhada ou distocia por má apresentação.

DIVERSOS

VER TAMBÉM
Distocia.

ABREVIATURA(S)
- bpm = batimentos por minuto.

Sugestões de Leitura
Bergstrüm A, Fransson B, Lagerstedt AS, Olsson K. Primary uterine inertia in 27 bitches: Aetiology and treatment. J Small Anim Pract 2006, 47(8):456-460.
Johnston SD, Root Kustritz MV, Olson PN. Canine parturition — eutocia and dystocia. In: Canine and Feline Theriogenology. Philadelphia: Saunders, 2001, pp. 105-128.
Pretzer SD. Medical management of canine and feline dystocia. Theriogenology 2008, 70:332-336.

Autor Milan Hess
Consultor Editorial Sara K. Lyle

INFARTO DO MIOCÁRDIO

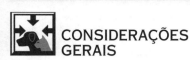

CONSIDERAÇÕES GERAIS

REVISÃO
- Desenvolvimento rápido de necrose miocárdica, resultante da redução completa e mantida do fluxo sanguíneo para uma parte do miocárdio, provocada pela formação de trombo.
- Rara como doença de ocorrência natural nos cães.
- Infartos intramurais microscópicos do miocárdio e áreas focais de fibrose miocárdica são comuns em cães com doença cardiovascular adquirida.
- Características do ECG compatíveis com infarto espontâneo do miocárdio não são bem caracterizadas em cães e gatos.

IDENTIFICAÇÃO
Raro em cães e gatos.

SINAIS CLÍNICOS

Achados Anamnésicos
- Letargia.
- Anorexia.
- Fraqueza.
- Dispneia.
- Colapso.
- Vômito.
- Obesidade.
- Morte inesperada.

Achados do Exame Físico
- Claudicação.
- Taquicardia.
- Sopro cardíaco.
- Distúrbios do ritmo cardíaco.
- Febre de baixo grau.

CAUSAS E FATORES DE RISCO

Cães
- Aterosclerose e doença da artéria coronária.
- Síndrome nefrótica.
- Vasculite.
- Hipotireoidismo.
- Endocardite bacteriana.
- Neoplasia.
- Septicemia.
- Arteriosclerose coronária intramural em cães idosos.
- Estenose aórtica subvalvular.

Gatos
- Miocardiopatia.
- Tromboembolia.

DIAGNÓSTICO
Geralmente presuntivo, com base no início agudo dos sinais em paciente com fatores predisponentes e alterações eletrocardiográficas compatíveis (alterações no segmento ST).

DIAGNÓSTICO DIFERENCIAL

Outras Causas de Alterações no Segmento ST
- Variação normal.
- Isquemia/hipoxia do miocárdio.
- Hiper ou hipocalemia.
- Intoxicação por digitálicos.
- Traumatismo ao coração.
- Pericardite.
- Artefato — linha basal migratória.

Outras Causas de Fraqueza e Colapso
- Traumatismo.
- Doença neurológica.
- Tromboembolia.
- Efusão pericárdica.
- Arritmia.

HEMOGRAMA/BIOQUÍMICA/URINÁLISE
- Leucocitose branda.
- Enzimas hepáticas elevadas.
- Hiperlipidemia — se o animal estiver com hipotireoidismo.
- Aumento da amilase.
- Atividade elevada da creatina quinase e das isoenzimas cardíacas.

OUTROS TESTES LABORATORIAIS
T_4 e T_3 baixas.

DIAGNÓSTICO POR IMAGEM
- Ecocardiografia — as modalidades bidimensional e modo M são úteis para avaliar as anormalidades de movimento da parede e a função global do ventrículo esquerdo.
- Angiocardiografia — raramente, ou quase nunca, utilizada na cardiologia clínica veterinária.

MÉTODOS DIAGNÓSTICOS

Achados Eletrocardiográficos
- Desvio repentino do segmento ST.
- Ondas T altas em pico — nas primeiras horas.
- Desenvolvimento súbito de ondas Q ou mudança na direção da onda T.
- Desvio de eixo do plano frontal.
- Complexos QRS de baixa voltagem.
- Desenvolvimento súbito de bloqueio de ramo do feixe de His ou bloqueio cardíaco.
- Início repentino de arritmias ventriculares por causa de isquemia do miocárdio.
- O declive da onda "R" pode estar associado a infarto miocárdico intramural.

TRATAMENTO
- Tratar o distúrbio subjacente; da mesma forma, efetuar o tratamento sintomático (p. ex., ICC).
- Arritmias com risco de vida precisam ser identificadas e tratadas imediatamente.
- Restringir a atividade física.

MEDICAÇÕES

MEDICAMENTO(S)
- Agentes trombolíticos IV — (p. ex., estreptoquinase); uso proibido em função do custo e da falta de experiência em casos de infarto do miocárdio na medicina veterinária com a dosagem e a própria utilização.
- Lidocaína para as arritmias ventriculares.
- β-bloqueadores — utilizar com cuidado na miocardiopatia dilatada por causa do possível desenvolvimento de ICC de baixo débito.
- Atenolol — cães, 0,25-1 mg/kg VO a cada 12-24 h; gatos, 6,25-12,5 mg VO a cada 24 h.

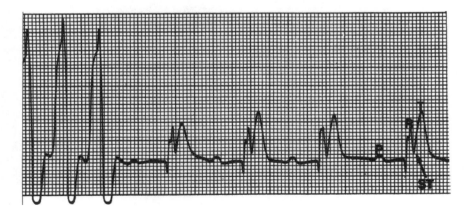

Figura 1. Infarto transmural do ventrículo esquerdo em cão com arteriosclerose e hipotireoidismo. Os três primeiros complexos sucessivos rápidos representam taquicardia ventricular. O ritmo sinusal subsequente ilustra complexos pequenos, elevação acentuada do segmento ST e bloqueio AV de primeiro grau (intervalo P-R prolongado). (De: Tilley LP. *Essentials of canine and feline electrocardiography*. 3. ed. Baltimore: Williams & Wilkins, 1992, com permissão).

INFARTO DO MIOCÁRDIO

• Agentes antitrombóticos (p. ex., dalteparina; heparina de baixo peso molecular, heparina e ácido acetilsalicílico).

ACOMPANHAMENTO
• Determinado pelo estado clínico do paciente e pelo diagnóstico do distúrbio subjacente.
• Monitorizar o paciente submetido a anticoagulante; hemograma e perfis de sangramento, incluindo-se o fibrinogênio.

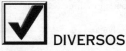

DIVERSOS
ABREVIATURA(S)
• ICC = insuficiência cardíaca congestiva.
• T_3 = tri-iodotironina.
• T_4 = tiroxina.

Sugestões de Leitura
Driehuys E, Van Winkle TJ, Sammarco CD, Drobatz KJ. Myocardial infarction in dogs and cats: 37 cases (1985-1994). JAVMA 1998, 213:1444-1448.

Falk T, Jonsson L. Ischaemic heart disease in the dog: A review of 65 cases. J Small Anim Pract 2000, 3:97-103.

Kidd L, Stepien RL, Amoheim DP. Clinical findings and coronary artery disease in dogs and cats with acute & subacute myocardial necrosis: 28 cases. JAAHA 2000, 36:199-208.

Smith FWK, Jr., Schrope DP, Sammarco CD. Cardiovascular effects of systemic diseases. In: Tilley LP, Smith FWK, Oyama MA, Sleeper MM, eds., Manual of Canine and Feline Cardiology, 4th ed. St. Louis: Saunders Elsevier, 2008, pp. 243-246.

Autor Larry P. Tilley
Consultores Editoriais Larry P. Tilley e Francis W.K. Smith, Jr.

INFECÇÃO BACTERIANA DO TRATO URINÁRIO INFERIOR

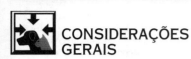

CONSIDERAÇÕES GERAIS

DEFINIÇÃO
Resultado da colonização bacteriana da bexiga urinária e/ou da porção proximal da uretra.

FISIOPATOLOGIA
Micróbios, geralmente bactérias aeróbias, ascendem o trato urinário sob condições que lhes permitem persistir na urina ou aderir ao epitélio e subsequentemente se multiplicar. A colonização do trato urinário requer, no mínimo, um comprometimento transitório dos mecanismos que normalmente o defendem contra a infecção. A inflamação dos tecidos infectados resulta nos sinais clínicos e nas anormalidades dos exames de laboratório apresentados pelo paciente.

SISTEMA(S) ACOMETIDO(S)
Renal/urológico — trato urinário inferior.

GENÉTICA
N/D.

INCIDÊNCIA/PREVALÊNCIA
Comum nas cadelas; menos comum nos cães machos; rara nos gatos com idade igual ou inferior a 6 anos; comum nos gatos com idade igual ou superior a 10 anos.

DISTRIBUIÇÃO GEOGRÁFICA
N/D.

IDENTIFICAÇÃO
Espécies
Mais comum nos cães do que nos gatos.
Raça(s) Predominante(s)
Nenhuma.
Idade Média e Faixa Etária
Todas as idades podem ser acometidas; entretanto, a ocorrência aumenta com a idade em virtude da maior frequência de outras lesões urinárias (p. ex., urólitos, prostatopatia e tumores), que predispõem à infecção secundária do trato urinário.
Sexo Predominante
Mais comum nas fêmeas do que nos machos caninos; ocorrência em machos e fêmeas de felinos é semelhante.

SINAIS CLÍNICOS
Achados Anamnésicos
• Nenhum em alguns pacientes.
• Polaciúria — eliminação frequente de pequenos volumes de urina.
• Disúria.
• Urgência miccional (ou perda aparente da capacidade de controle da micção durante períodos de confinamento).
• Urinar em lugares que não são costumeiros.
• Hematúria e urina turva ou fétida em alguns pacientes.
Achados do Exame Físico
• Nenhuma anormalidade em alguns pacientes.
• Infecção aguda — a bexiga urinária ou a uretra podem parecer sensíveis à palpação.
• A palpação da bexiga urinária pode estimular a micção.
• Infecção crônica — a parede da bexiga urinária ou da uretra pode estar espessada ou anormalmente firme à palpação.
• Infecção secundária — achados atribuíveis ao problema subjacente.

CAUSAS
• Bactérias aeróbias — mais comuns.
• Mais comuns — *Escherichia*, *Staphylococcus* e *Proteus* spp. (mais da metade de todos os casos).
• Comuns — *Streptococcus*, *Klebsiella*, *Enterobacter*, *Pseudomonas* e *Corynebacterium* spp.
• Raras — alguns outros agentes bacterianos e fúngicos.

FATORES DE RISCO
• Condições que causam estase urinária ou esvaziamento incompleto da bexiga urinária.
• Condições que abalam as propriedades de defesa da mucosa.
• Condições que diminuem ou desviam as barreiras anatômicas e funcionais à ascensão microbiana do trato urinário (p. ex., perda do tônus muscular ou comprimento da uretra e das junções vesicoureterais).
• Condições que comprometem as propriedades antibacterianas da urina (p. ex., alterações no pH ou na osmolalidade urinários e baixas concentrações de ureia e de determinados ácidos orgânicos).

DIAGNÓSTICO

DIAGNÓSTICO DIFERENCIAL
• Qualquer outra doença da bexiga urinária ou da uretra.
• Condições comumente confundidas com infecção do trato urinário ou complicadas por esta infecção incluem urolitíase e neoplasia. Nos gatos, a cistite hemorrágica idiopática também é problema comum que deve ser diferenciado de infecção do trato urinário.
• Doença do trato urinário inferior pode vir a ser complicada por infecção secundária do trato urinário; isso recebe o nome de *infecção complicada do trato urinário* e exige estratégias terapêuticas diferentes daquelas utilizadas para episódios não complicados (i. e., simples) de infecção do trato urinário.
• A reinfecção frequente (mais de um episódio de infecção recém-adquirida do trato urinário dentro de um ano) geralmente indica o comprometimento nos mecanismos de defesa do hospedeiro. Procurar alguma causa subjacente. Caso não se consiga identificar nem corrigir nenhuma causa subjacente, considerar o tratamento profilático com medicamento antibacteriano.

HEMOGRAMA/BIOQUÍMICA/URINÁLISE
• Resultados normais do hemograma completo e da bioquímica sérica.
• A piúria está mais comumente associada à infecção do trato urinário, embora lesões urinárias não infecciosas também possam provocar piúria. Hematúria e proteinúria também são comuns. As bactérias podem ou não ser detectadas pelo exame microscópico do sedimento urinário. Às vezes, relata-se bacteriúria em animais sem infecção do trato urinário.

OUTROS TESTES LABORATORIAIS
Cultura e Teste de Sensibilidade Urinários
• A urocultura é necessária para o diagnóstico definitivo.
• A interpretação correta dos resultados da urocultura requer: (1) a obtenção de amostra de uma forma que minimize a contaminação, (2) a manipulação e o armazenamento da amostra, de modo que o número de bactérias viáveis não se altere *in vitro* e (3) o uso de método quantitativo de cultura. Manter a amostra em frasco estéril selado; se a cultura não for processada imediatamente, a urina poderá ser refrigerada por até 8 h sem alterações importantes nos resultados.
• A cistocentese é a técnica preferida na coleta de urina para cultura.
• Os valores de corte para bacteriúria significativa na urina dos cães dependem da forma de coleta — por cistocentese, >1.000/mL; por cateterização, >10.000/mL; por micção espontânea, >100.000/mL.
• Os valores de corte para bacteriúria expressiva na urina dos gatos também dependem da forma de coleta — por cistocentese ou por cateterização, >1.000/mL; por micção espontânea, >10.000/mL.
• Os valores que se aproximam, mas não excedem esses valores de corte (i. e., menos de uma ordem de grandeza), são suspeitos, havendo indicação de novos exames. As culturas de urina que produzem valores com mais de uma ordem de grandeza abaixo desses valores de corte são negativas.
• Teste de suscetibilidade *in vitro* que determina a concentração inibitória mínima (CIM) de cada medicamento contra o microrganismo isolado é preferido para os patógenos urinários. Os agentes que costumam ser utilizados para o tratamento de infecção do trato urinário ficam altamente concentrados na urina; no entanto, é provável que qualquer medicamento com valor de CIM igual ou inferior a ¼ da concentração urinária média da medicação durante o tratamento seja eficaz.

DIAGNÓSTICO POR IMAGEM
Estudos radiográficos simples e contrastados, bem como ultrassonografia da bexiga urinária ou da uretra, podem detectar lesão subjacente do trato urinário (i. e., infecção complicada do trato urinário).

TRATAMENTO

CUIDADO(S) DE SAÚDE ADEQUADO(S)
Tratar como paciente de ambulatório a menos que alguma outra anormalidade urinária (p. ex., obstrução) necessite de internação.

ATIVIDADE
• Sem restrição.
• Regular a micção do paciente de forma a coordená-la com os tratamentos antibacterianos pode melhorar a eficiência terapêutica.

DIETA
As restrições são necessárias, mas podem ser indicadas para outras doenças urinárias concomitantes (p. ex., urolitíase).

ORIENTAÇÃO AO PROPRIETÁRIO
O prognóstico quanto à cura de infecção simples do trato urinário é excelente; já o prognóstico para a infecção complicada do trato urinário depende da anormalidade subjacente. A obediência às recomendações terapêuticas e as avaliações subsequentes de acompanhamento são decisivas para a obtenção dos resultados desejados.

CONSIDERAÇÕES CIRÚRGICAS
Exceto quando um distúrbio concomitante necessita de intervenção cirúrgica, o tratamento não envolve a cirurgia.

Infecção Bacteriana do Trato Urinário Inferior

MEDICAÇÕES

MEDICAMENTO(S) DE ESCOLHA
- Um antibiótico adequado frequentemente pode ser selecionado com base no gênero das bactérias infectantes — penicilina (p. ex., ampicilina, 25 mg/kg VO a cada 8 h) para *Staphylococcus*, *Streptococcus* ou *Proteus* spp.; trimetoprima-sulfadiazina (15 mg/kg combinados VO a cada 12 h) para *Escherichia coli*; cefalexina (30 mg/kg VO a cada 8 h) para *Klebsiella* spp.; tetraciclina (20 mg/kg VO a cada 8 h) para *Pseudomonas* spp.
- Para microrganismo cuja suscetibilidade previsível a algum medicamento específico não é conhecida ou que não responda conforme o esperado ao primeiro medicamento, basear a escolha do medicamento nos resultados do teste de sensibilidade.
- Medicamentos antibacterianos geralmente são mais eficazes quando administrados a cada 8 h; entretanto, as fluoroquinolonas e os produtos à base de trimetoprima-sulfa são eficazes quando administrados a cada 12 h.
- Para infecção aguda não complicada, tratar com medicamentos antimicrobianos por 7-10 dias. Cistite bacteriana crônica pode necessitar de tratamento por até 4-6 semanas. A duração apropriada do tratamento para a infecção complicada do trato urinário inferior depende do problema subjacente.
- Tratamento antibacteriano à noite em baixas doses pode ser empregado para evitar infecções nos animais que apresentam reinfecções frequentes. Iniciar tal tratamento profilático imediatamente após a cura do episódio mais recente de infecção do trato urinário pelo tratamento convencional. Administrar um medicamento antibacteriano adequado, em geral ampicilina ou nitrofurantoína, uma vez ao dia por 4-6 meses ou mais. A dosagem deve ser cerca de um terço da dose diária convencional para o medicamento escolhido, mas o medicamento deve ser administrado após o animal ter urinado pela última vez à tarde.

CONTRAINDICAÇÕES
Reação alérgica ao medicamento.

PRECAUÇÕES
- O uso a longo prazo ou repetido dos medicamentos antibacterianos é associado a efeitos adversos (p. ex., reação alérgica) em alguns animais.
- Ceratoconjuntivite seca está associada à administração de produtos à base de trimetoprima-sulfa.
- Em função da nefrotoxicidade potencial com a administração a prazo longo, usar os aminoglicosídeos apenas quando não houver alternativas.

INTERAÇÕES POSSÍVEIS
Pacientes com a função renal comprometida podem apresentar excreção urinária reduzida dos medicamentos utilizados para tratar a infecção do trato urinário. Além de induzir ao acúmulo não intencional do medicamento em tais pacientes, a excreção urinária prejudicada pode reduzir a eficácia do medicamento.

MEDICAMENTO(S) ALTERNATIVO(S)
- Enrofloxacino e nitrofurantoína.
- Ceftiofur, gentamicina ou amicacina, os quais devem ser administrados por injeção.

ACOMPANHAMENTO

MONITORIZAÇÃO DO PACIENTE
- Quando a eficácia do medicamento antibacteriano for questionável, submeter a urina à cultura 2-3 dias após iniciar o tratamento. Se o medicamento for eficaz, a cultura será negativa.
- Prosseguir o tratamento por, no mínimo, 1 semana após a resolução dos sinais de hematúria, piúria e proteinúria. A falha nos achados da urinálise em retornar ao normal enquanto um episódio de infecção do trato urinário está sendo tratado com antibiótico eficiente (i. e., indicado pela cultura de urina negativa) geralmente indica alguma outra anormalidade do trato urinário (p. ex., urólito e/ou tumor). A rápida recidiva dos sinais quando o tratamento é interrompido quase sempre indica a presença de anormalidade concomitante do trato urinário inferior ou a extensão da infecção para alguma área de localização profunda (p. ex., parênquima prostático ou renal).
- A cura com sucesso de um episódio de infecção do trato urinário é mais bem demonstrada pela realização da urocultura 7-10 dias após o término da terapia antimicrobiana.
- Os animais que estiverem recebendo tratamento profilático antibacteriano à noite em baixas doses para reinfecção frequente devem ser submetidos à urocultura via cistocentese a cada 1-2 meses.

PREVENÇÃO
- Evitar o uso indiscriminado de cateteres urinários.
- Os animais com reinfecção frequente podem receber tratamento à noite para aumentar as defesas do hospedeiro e evitar a ocorrência de novas infecções.

COMPLICAÇÕES POSSÍVEIS
A falha em detectar ou tratar uma infecção bacteriana do trato urinário com eficiência pode levar ao surgimento de pielonefrite ou à formação de urólitos de estruvita.

EVOLUÇÃO ESPERADA E PROGNÓSTICO
- Se não for tratada, espera-se que a infecção persista por tempo indefinido. Os riscos de saúde associados incluem o desenvolvimento da urolitíase e a extensão da infecção para outros locais do trato urinário (p. ex., os rins) ou além (p. ex., septicemia, discospondilite e endocardite bacteriana).
- Em geral, o prognóstico para os animais com infecção não complicada do trato urinário inferior é bom a excelente. Os pacientes que apresentam reinfecção frequente são candidatos a tratamento profilático à noite em baixas doses, como já foi descrito, mas até esses pacientes costumam ficar bem. O prognóstico para os animais com infecção complicada fica determinado pelo prognóstico da outra anormalidade urinária.

DIVERSOS

DISTÚRBIOS ASSOCIADOS
- Urolitíase por estruvita.
- Diabetes melito ou hiperadrenocorticismo.

FATORES RELACIONADOS COM A IDADE
A infecção complicada é mais comum nos animais de meia-idade a idosos do que nos jovens.

GESTAÇÃO/FERTILIDADE/REPRODUÇÃO
Dependendo do estágio da prenhez, da intensidade dos sinais e da presença ou ausência de anormalidades concomitantes, considerar o adiamento da terapia. Evitar o uso de tetraciclina, nitrofurantoína ou enrofloxacino.

SINÔNIMO(S)
- Cistite bacteriana.
- Uretrocistite.
- Uretrite.

VER TAMBÉM
- Pielonefrite.
- Urolitíase por Estruvita — Cães.
- Urolitíase por Estruvita — Gatos.

ABREVIATURA(S)
- CIM = concentração inibitória mínima.

Sugestões de Leitura
Barsanti JA. Multidrug resistant urinary tract infection. In: Bonagura JD, Twedt DC, eds., Kirk's Current Veterinary Therapy. Philadelphia: Saunders, 2009, pp. 921-925.
Labato MA. Uncomplicated urinary tract infection. In: Bonagura JD, Twedt DC, eds., Kirk's Current Veterinary Therapy. Philadelphia: Saunders, 2009, pp. 918-921.
Pressler B, Bartges JW. Urinary tract infections. In: Ettinger SJ, Feldman EC, eds., Textbook of Veterinary Internal Medicine, 7th ed. St. Louis: Elsevier, 2010, pp. 2036-2047.

Autor George E. Lees
Consultor Editorial Carl A. Osborne

Infecção Fúngica do Trato Urinário Inferior

CONSIDERAÇÕES GERAIS

DEFINIÇÃO
- Fungos/leveduras infectantes costumam fazer parte da flora comensal normal da pele e das mucosas ou são ubíquos no ambiente.
- *Candida albicans* é o microrganismo fúngico mais comumente isolado; outras espécies de *Candida* são menos comuns, mas os fungos não pertencentes à espécie *Candida* são menos comuns ainda.
- Infecções fúngicas sistêmicas podem ser associadas ao aparecimento de fungos na urina após a disseminação para os rins. Deve-se suspeitar disso, particularmente em caso de infecção por *Aspergillus* spp. em cães e *Cryptococcus neoformans* em gatos.
- Sistema orgânico acometido: renal/urológico.
- Incomum em cães e gatos.

IDENTIFICAÇÃO
- Cães e gatos.
- Sem predileção racial, etária ou sexual.

SINAIS CLÍNICOS
- Sinais típicos de doença do trato urinário inferior: disúria e polaciúria; é rara a ocorrência de hematúria.
- Muitos animais permanecem assintomáticos.

CAUSAS E FATORES DE RISCO
- Fatores de risco conhecidos: diabetes melito, estomas do trato urinário (p. ex., uretrostomia perineal, tubos de cistotomia, sondas urinárias de demora), doença do trato urinário inferior (p. ex., carcinoma de células de transição da bexiga, infecção bacteriana crônica do trato urinário).
- Fatores de risco sob suspeita: administração recente ou crônica de antibióticos ou glicocorticoides.

DIAGNÓSTICO

DIAGNÓSTICO DIFERENCIAL
- Infecções fúngicas isoladas do trato urinário inferior precisam ser diferenciadas de infecções fúngicas sistêmicas com aparecimento secundário de fungos na urina.
- Infecções do trato urinário inferior podem evoluir para pielonefrite.
- Pode ocorrer a contaminação de amostras de urina durante a coleta em animais com proliferação cutânea ou mucocutânea de leveduras (i. e., dermatite abdominal ventral ou perivulvar ou balanopostite), levando a um diagnóstico falso de infecção fúngica do trato urinário.

HEMOGRAMA/BIOQUÍMICA/URINÁLISE
- Os exames de hemograma completo e bioquímica sérica não são geralmente dignos de nota. Se a infecção ascendeu para o trato urinário superior ou se disseminou para outros locais além do trato urinário, as anormalidades refletirão os órgãos envolvidos.
- Leveduras/fungos podem ser visíveis no sedimento urinário. Contudo, os microrganismos podem ser tão raros a ponto de exigir o uso de preparações de sedimento concentrado para visualizá-los.
- As espécies de fungo, em geral, não podem ser determinadas com base no aspecto citológico.

DIAGNÓSTICO POR IMAGEM
N/D.

MÉTODOS DIAGNÓSTICOS

Cultura Urinária
- As espécies de *Candida* crescerão geralmente dentro de 3 dias em ágar-sangue padrão.
- Outros fungos podem crescer mais lentamente e, com isso, podem não ser detectados por meio dos protocolos padrão de urocultura.
- Na suspeita ou mediante a confirmação de infecção fúngica do trato urinário, é recomendável a solicitação de cultura da urina para pesquisa de fungos. A identificação dos fungos é feita com base nas características de crescimento e nos aspectos morfológicos em ágar dextrose Sabouraud.

Teste de Sensibilidade Antifúngica
- O *C. albicans* é geralmente sensível ao fluconazol; portanto, não há necessidade do teste de sensibilidade de rotina no momento do diagnóstico inicial.
- As outras espécies de *Candida* são mais comumente resistentes ao fluconazol e, nesse caso, o teste de sensibilidade deve ser realizado.
- Os testes de suscetibilidade também devem ser efetuados em princípio nos microrganismos não pertencentes às espécies de *Candida* e em quaisquer infecções por *Candida* sp. irresponsivas à terapia adequada dentro de 4-6 semanas.

TRATAMENTO
- Identificar e corrigir quaisquer fatores de risco concomitantes.
- Era recomendada a alcalinização urinária, mas essa medida é de valor questionável.

MEDICAÇÕES

MEDICAMENTO(S)
- Fluconazol por via oral (5-10 mg/kg VO a cada 12 h) constitui o tratamento inicial de escolha.
- Itraconazol ou cetoconazol são eficazes em alguns casos, mas não representam os tratamentos de escolha por causa da excreção insatisfatória desses medicamentos pela urina.
- Nos casos em que um período de 4-8 semanas de fluconazol se mostra ineficaz para eliminar a infecção, pode-se considerar a infusão intravesicular (bexiga) de clotrimazol a 1% (solução a 1% em polietilenoglicol 400).
- Protocolo para infusão intravesicular de clotrimazol a 1%: sondar e esvaziar a bexiga urinária. Infundir 7,5-10 mL/kg de solução de clotrimazol a 1% (o volume deve ser determinado por meio de palpação vesical durante a infusão). O líquido infundido deve ficar retido por, no mínimo, 15-30 min; a maioria dos gatos conservará o medicamento infundido se não tiver acesso à bandeja sanitária ou área de micção; já nos cães, poderá haver a necessidade de cateteres-balão para evitar a micção prematura. Repetir a infusão a cada 7 dias por, no mínimo, três tratamentos. Repetir a cultura urinária fúngica em aproximadamente 1 semana após o terceiro tratamento para determinar a necessidade ou não de mais infusões. A terapia com fluconazol por via oral deve ser mantida durante todo o protocolo de infusão.
- O tratamento com anfotericina B (intravenosa ou intravesicular) foi tentado em casos esporádicos, mas a eficácia é desconhecida.
- Uma negligência benigna e um monitoramento regular podem ser considerados em pacientes assintomáticos com infecções persistentes apesar de tentativas terapêuticas repetidas. Contudo podem ocorrer infecção ascendente (i. e., pielonefrite fúngica) e disseminação sistêmica.

CONTRAINDICAÇÕES/INTERAÇÕES POSSÍVEIS
- A administração intravesicular de clotrimazol parece ser segura até o momento, mas não foi completamente investigada.
- É recomendável evitar a aplicação intravesicular de clotrimazol em pacientes submetidos a cirurgia vesical ou traumatismo uretral recente.

ACOMPANHAMENTO

MONITORIZAÇÃO DO PACIENTE
- O tratamento deve ser mantido até a ausência de qualquer crescimento fúngico em duas culturas urinárias sucessivas com 14-21 dias de intervalo.
- A cultura urinária fúngica deve ser repetida cerca de 60 dias após a interrupção da terapia e, depois, em intervalos regulares.

DIVERSOS

DISTÚRBIOS ASSOCIADOS
- Diabetes melito.
- Carcinoma de células de transição.

VER TAMBÉM
- Capítulos sobre Aspergilose.
- Criptococose.

Sugestões de Leitura
Jin Y, Lin D. Fungal urinary tract infections in the dog and cat: A retrospective study (2001-2004). JAAHA 2005, 41:373-381.
Pressler B, Vaden SL, Lane IF, et al. Candida spp. urinary tract infections in 13 dogs and seven cats: Predisposing factors, treatment, and outcome. JAAHA 2003, 39:263-270.
Toll J, Ashe CM, Trepanier LA. Intravesicular administration of clotrimazole for treatment of candiduria in a cat with diabetes mellitus. JAVMA 2003, 223:1156-1158.

Autor Barrak M. Pressler
Consultor Editorial Carl A. Osborne

Infecção pelo Calicivírus Felino

CONSIDERAÇÕES GERAIS

DEFINIÇÃO
Doença respiratória viral comum de gatos domésticos e exóticos, caracterizada por sinais respiratórios superiores, ulceração bucal, pneumonia e, ocasionalmente, artrite ou uma doença hemorrágica sistêmica altamente fatal.

FISIOPATOLOGIA
Citólise rápida de células infectadas com comprometimento tecidual e doença clínica resultantes.

SISTEMA(S) ACOMETIDO(S)
- Gastrintestinal — ulceração da língua é comum; ulceração ocasional do palato duro e dos lábios; ocorre infecção dos intestinos; em geral, não há doença clínica.
- Hematológico/linfático/imune — hemorragia.
- Musculosquelético — artrite aguda.
- Oftálmico — conjuntivite serosa aguda sem ceratite ou úlceras de córnea.
- Respiratório — rinite; pneumonia intersticial; ulceração da ponta do nariz.

GENÉTICA
Nenhuma.

INCIDÊNCIA/PREVALÊNCIA
- É comum uma infecção persistente.
- Doença clínica — comum em locais com muitos gatos, abrigos de animais e gatis de reprodução.
- Vacinação de rotina — a incidência da doença clínica diminuiu, embora não tenha reduzido a prevalência do vírus.

DISTRIBUIÇÃO GEOGRÁFICA
Mundial.

IDENTIFICAÇÃO
Espécie
Felina.

Raça(s) Predominante(s)
Nenhuma.

Idade Média e Faixa Etária
- Filhotes jovens com mais de 6 semanas de vida — mais comum.
- Gatos de qualquer idade podem exibir a doença clínica.

Sexo Predominante
Nenhum.

SINAIS CLÍNICOS
Comentários Gerais
Pode se manifestar sob a forma de (a) infecção respiratória superior com acometimento ocular e nasal, (b) doença ulcerativa inicialmente da boca, (c) pneumonia, (d) artrite aguda, (e) doença hemorrágica sistêmica ou (f) qualquer combinação dessas.

Achados Anamnésicos
- Início súbito.
- Anorexia.
- Secreção ocular ou nasal, geralmente com pouco ou nenhum espirro.
- Úlceras na língua, no palato duro, nos lábios, na ponta do nariz ou em torno das garras.
- Dispneia por causa da pneumonia.
- Claudicação dolorosa aguda.

Achados do Exame Físico
- Geralmente alerta e em boas condições.
- Febre.
- As úlceras podem ocorrer sem outros sinais.
- Hemorragia sistêmica.

CAUSAS
- Um pequeno RNA vírus de fita simples e não envelopado (calicivírus felino).
- Existem inúmeras cepas na natureza, com graus variáveis de reatividade antigênica cruzada.
- Mais de um sorotipo.
- Relativamente estável e resistente a muitos desinfetantes.

FATORES DE RISCO
- Falta de vacinação ou vacinação inadequada.
- Instituições com muitos gatos.
- Infecções concomitantes por outros patógenos (p. ex., FHV-1 ou FVP).
- Má ventilação.

DIAGNÓSTICO

DIAGNÓSTICO DIFERENCIAL
- Rinotraqueíte viral felina.
- Clamidiose.
- *Bordetella bronchiseptica*.

HEMOGRAMA/BIOQUÍMICA/URINÁLISE
Nenhum achado característico ou compatível.

OUTROS TESTES LABORATORIAIS
Sorologia em amostras pareadas — detecta a elevação dos títulos de anticorpos neutralizantes contra o vírus.

DIAGNÓSTICO POR IMAGEM
Radiografias dos pulmões — consolidação do tecido pulmonar em gatos com pneumonia.

MÉTODOS DIAGNÓSTICOS
- Culturas celulares para isolamento do vírus — faringe bucal; tecido pulmonar; fezes; sangue; secreções do nariz e da conjuntiva.
- PCR.
- Imunofluorescência do tecido pulmonar — para detecção do antígeno viral.

ACHADOS PATOLÓGICOS
- Macroscópicos — infecção respiratória superior; secreção ocular e nasal; pneumonia com consolidação de grandes partes de lobos pulmonares individuais; possíveis ulcerações na língua, nos lábios e no palato duro; hemorragias sistêmicas.
- Histopatológicos — pneumonia intersticial de grandes partes de lobos pulmonares individuais; ulcerações no epitélio da língua, nos lábios e no palato duro; reações inflamatórias discretas no nariz e nas conjuntivas; hemorragias sistêmicas.

TRATAMENTO

CUIDADO(S) DE SAÚDE ADEQUADO(S)
Ambulatoriais a menos que ocorram pneumonia grave ou hemorragias.

CUIDADO(S) DE ENFERMAGEM
- Limpar os olhos e o nariz conforme indicado.
- Fornecer alimentos pastosos.
- Oxigênio — em caso de pneumonia grave.

ATIVIDADE
Os pacientes não devem ter contato com outros gatos, para evitar a transmissão do agente viral causador da doença.

DIETA
- Sem restrições.
- Dietas especiais — possivelmente para atrair os gatos com anorexia, para que eles voltem a se alimentar.
- Alimentos pastosos — se as ulcerações impedirem que o animal coma.

ORIENTAÇÃO AO PROPRIETÁRIO
Abordar a necessidade do uso de vacinas adequadas e da modificação do protocolo de vacinação em gatis de reprodução de modo a incluir filhotes antes que eles venham a ser infectados (em geral, com 6-8 semanas de vida) pela mãe portadora.

CONSIDERAÇÕES CIRÚRGICAS
Nenhuma.

MEDICAÇÕES

MEDICAMENTO(S) DE ESCOLHA
- Nenhum antiviral específico é eficaz.
- Antibióticos de amplo espectro — costumam ser indicados (p. ex., amoxicilina, 22 mg/kg VO a cada 12 h).
- Infecções bacterianas secundárias em gatos acometidos não são tão importantes quanto aquelas pelo FHV-1.
- Pomadas oftálmicas de antibiótico — para diminuir as infecções bacterianas secundárias da conjuntiva.
- Analgésicos adequados — para a artrite dolorosa transitória.

CONTRAINDICAÇÕES
Nenhuma.

PRECAUÇÕES
Nenhuma.

INTERAÇÕES POSSÍVEIS
Nenhuma.

MEDICAMENTO(S) ALTERNATIVO(S)
Nenhum.

ACOMPANHAMENTO

MONITORIZAÇÃO DO PACIENTE
- Monitorizar o paciente quanto ao desenvolvimento súbito de dispneia associada à pneumonia.
- Não há exames laboratoriais específicos.

PREVENÇÃO
- Todos os gatos deverão receber a vacina ao mesmo tempo em que forem vacinados contra o FHV-1 e o FPV; a vacinação de rotina com vacinas vivas modificadas ou inativadas deve ser feita até 6 semanas de vida e repetida a cada 3-4 semanas até, pelo menos, 16 semanas.
- Gatis de reprodução — a doença respiratória é um problema; vacinar os filhotes em idade precoce com uma vacinação adicional quando tiverem 4-5 semanas de vida ou com uma vacina intranasal aos 10-14 dias de vida; realizar vacinações de reforço a cada 3-4 semanas até 16 semanas de vida.
- A American Association of Feline Practitioners (Associação Norte-americana de Clínicos de Gatos) classifica como indispensáveis as vacinas contra o FHV, o FPV e o calicivírus, recomendando a vacinação de todos os gatos,

sendo as 3 na primeira consulta já com 6 semanas de vida e a repetição a cada 3-4 semanas até 16 semanas e 1 ano depois da última vacina do filhote; os reforços contra o calicivírus devem ser dados a cada 3 anos.
• A vacinação não elimina a infecção viral em exposição subsequente, mas previne a doença clínica causada pela maioria das cepas.

COMPLICAÇÕES POSSÍVEIS
• Pneumonia intersticial — complicação mais séria; pode ser potencialmente letal.
• Infecções bacterianas secundárias dos pulmões ou das vias aéreas superiores.
• Úlceras bucais e artrite aguda costumam desaparecer sem complicações.
• A doença hemorrágica sistêmica pode ser grave e fatal.

EVOLUÇÃO ESPERADA E PROGNÓSTICO
• Doença clínica — em geral, surge 3-4 dias após a exposição.
• Assim que aparecerem os anticorpos neutralizantes (cerca de 7 dias após a exposição), a recuperação geralmente será rápida.
• O prognóstico é excelente, a menos que ocorra pneumonia grave ou doença hemorrágica sistêmica.
• Gatos recuperados — persistentemente infectados por longos períodos; eliminarão continuamente pequenas quantidades do vírus nas secreções bucais.

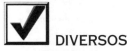

DIVERSOS

DISTÚRBIOS ASSOCIADOS
Os gatos acometidos também podem ser infectados simultaneamente pelo FHV-1, sobretudo em instituições com muitos gatos e gatis de reprodução.

FATORES RELACIONADOS COM A IDADE
Em geral, ocorre em filhotes jovens cuja imunidade materna declinou.

POTENCIAL ZOONÓTICO
Nenhum.

GESTAÇÃO/FERTILIDADE/REPRODUÇÃO
Em geral, não constitui um problema, porque a maioria das gatas já foi exposta ou vacinada antes de ficar prenhe.

SINÔNIMO(S)
Infecção pelo picornavírus felino — calicivírus felino originalmente classificado como um picornavírus; a literatura especializada mais antiga refere-se à infecção por essa denominação; não há picornavírus conhecido que infecte gatos.

VER TAMBÉM
• Bordetelose — Gatos.
• Clamidiose — Gatos.

ABREVIATURA(S)
• FHV = herpes-vírus felino.
• FPV = parvovírus felino.
• PCR = reação em cadeia da polimerase.
• RNA = ácido ribonucleico.

Sugestões de Leitura
Barr MC, Olsen CW, Scott FW. Feline viral diseases. In: Ettinger SJ, Feldman EC, eds. Veterinary Internal Medicine, 4th ed. Philadelphia: Saunders, 1995, pp. 409-439.
Gaskell RM, Dawson S, Radford AD. Feline respiratory disease. In: Greene CE, ed., Infectious Diseases of the Dog and Cat, 3rd ed. St. Louis: Saunders Elsevier, 2006, pp. 145-154.
Pedersen NC, Elliot JB, Glasgow A, et al. An isolated epizootic of hemorrhagic-like fever in cats caused by a novel and highly virulent strain of feline calicivirus. Vet Microbiology 2000, 73:281-300.
Pesavento PA, Chang K-O, Parker JSL. Molecular virology of feline calicivirus. Vet Clin North Am Small Anim Pract 2008, 38(4):775-786.
Radford AD, Addie D, Belàk, et al. Feline calicivirus infection: ABCD guidelines on prevention and management. J Feline Med Surg 2009, 11:556-564.
Richards JR, Elston TH, Ford RB, et al. The 2006 American Association of Feline Practioners Feline Vaccine Advisory Panel Report. JAVMA 2006, 229:1405-1441.
Scott FW. Virucidal disinfectants and feline viruses. Am J Vet Res 1980, 41:410-414.
Scott FW, Geissinger CM. Long-term immunity in cats vaccinated with an inactivated trivalent vaccine. Am J Vet Res 1999, 60:652-658.

Autor Fred W. Scott
Consultor Editorial Stephen C. Barr

Infecção pelo Poxvírus — Gatos

CONSIDERAÇÕES GERAIS

REVISÃO
- Membro do gênero *Orthopoxvirus*, família Poxviridae.
- Vírus DNA envelopado, resistente ao ressecamento (viável por anos), mas facilmente inativado por grande parte dos desinfetantes.
- Geograficamente limitado à Eurásia.
- Relativamente comum.
- A evidência sorológica da infecção pode chegar a 10% em gatos na Europa ocidental.

IDENTIFICAÇÃO
- Gatos — domésticos e exóticos.
- Sem predisposição etária, sexual ou racial.

SINAIS CLÍNICOS
- Lesões cutâneas — múltiplas, circulares; característica dominante; geralmente se desenvolvem na cabeça, no pescoço ou nos membros anteriores.
- Lesões primárias — pápulas crostosas, placas, nódulos, úlceras crateriformes ou áreas de celulite ou de abscessos.
- Lesões secundárias — nódulos eritematosos que sofrem ulceração e formam crosta; frequentemente disseminados; desenvolvem-se após 1-3 semanas.
- Lesões bucais — erosões, úlceras concomitantes ou isoladas (20% dos casos).
- Prurido variável.
- Sistêmicos — 20% dos casos; anorexia; letargia; pirexia; vômito; diarreia; secreção oculonasal; conjuntivite; pneumonia.

CAUSAS E FATORES DE RISCO
- Hospedeiro reservatório — roedores silvestres (ratos silvestres, camundongos, gerbos, esquilos comuns).
- Acredita-se que a infecção seja adquirida durante a caça e transmitida por roedores infectados; mais comum nos jovens adultos e caçadores ativos, quase sempre a partir do ambiente rural.
- Lesões — frequentemente se desenvolvem no local de alguma ferida por mordedura (presumivelmente infligida pela presa portadora do vírus).
- A maior parte dos casos ocorre entre os meses de agosto e outubro (hemisfério norte), época em que pequenos mamíferos silvestres atingem níveis máximos da população e são mais ativos.
- Sinais cutâneos e sistêmicos graves com prognóstico mau estão frequentemente associados à imunossupressão (iatrogênica ou coinfecção por FeLV ou FIV).
- Transmissão de gato para gato — rara; provoca apenas infecção subclínica.

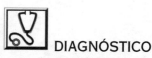

DIAGNÓSTICO

DIAGNÓSTICO DIFERENCIAL
- Infecções bacterianas e fúngicas.
- Complexo granuloma eosinofílico.
- Neoplasia — particularmente mastocitoma; linfossarcoma.
- Dermatite miliar.

HEMOGRAMA/BIOQUÍMICA/URINÁLISE
Sem contribuição.

OUTROS TESTES LABORATORIAIS
Testes sorológicos — demonstram títulos crescentes; inibição da hemaglutinação, neutralização do vírus, fixação do complemento ou ELISA; os títulos podem permanecer elevados durante meses ou anos.

DIAGNÓSTICO POR IMAGEM
N/D.

MÉTODOS DIAGNÓSTICOS
- Isolamento do vírus a partir de material da crosta — diagnóstico definitivo; 90% dos testes são positivos.
- Microscopia eletrônica de extratos da crosta, biopsia ou exsudato — fornece um rápido diagnóstico presuntivo; 70% dos testes são positivos.
- Biopsia de pele — alterações histológicas características de hiperplasia e hipertrofia epidérmicas; vesícula multilocular e ulceração; grandes corpúsculos de inclusão intracitoplasmáticos eosinofílicos.
- PCR.

TRATAMENTO

- Sem tratamento específico.
- Suporte (antibióticos, fluidos) quando houver necessidade.
- Colar elizabetano — para evitar lesão autoinfligida.

MEDICAÇÕES

MEDICAMENTO(S)
Antibióticos — evitam infecções secundárias.

CONTRAINDICAÇÕES/INTERAÇÕES POSSÍVEIS
Agentes imunossupressores (p. ex., glicocorticoides e acetato de megestrol) — totalmente contraindicados, pois podem induzir doença sistêmica fatal.

ACOMPANHAMENTO

PREVENÇÃO
- O hospedeiro reservatório natural possivelmente é representado por pequenos roedores; os gatos são infectados de forma acidental.
- Vacinas — não disponíveis; o vírus da vacínia pode ser considerado para coleções valiosas de zoológicos, mas seus efeitos em gatos não domésticos não foram pesquisados.

EVOLUÇÃO ESPERADA E PROGNÓSTICO
- A maioria dos gatos apresenta recuperação espontânea em 1-2 meses.
- A cicatrização pode ser protelada por infecção cutânea bacteriana secundária.
- O prognóstico é mau com envolvimento respiratório ou pulmonar grave.

DIVERSOS

POTENCIAL ZOONÓTICO
- Infecções humanas raras pelo poxvírus foram relacionadas ao contato com gatos infectados com lesões cutâneas; utilizar precauções básicas de higiene (luvas descartáveis) ao manipular os gatos infectados.
- A infecção costuma ser leve e transitória em seres humanos saudáveis, embora possam ocorrer infecções graves e até mesmo letais em indivíduos imunocomprometidos.
- Pode provocar lesão cutânea dolorosa e doença sistêmica grave, particularmente em pessoas muito jovens ou muito idosas com algum problema de pele preexistente e nos indivíduos imunodeficientes.
- Com a interrupção da vacinação contra varíola (com seu efeito imunológico de reatividade cruzada), pode-se esperar um aumento nas infecções humanas por poxvírus.

ABREVIATURA(S)
- ELISA = ensaio imunoabsorvente ligado à enzima.
- FeLV = vírus da leucemia felina.
- FIV = vírus da imunodeficiência felina.
- PCR = reação em cadeia da polimerase.

Sugestões de Leitura
Gaskell RM, Bennett M. Feline poxvirus infection. In: Chandler EA, Gaskell CJ, Gaskell RM, eds., Feline Medicine and Therapeutics. Oxford, UK: Blackwell Scientific, 1994, pp. 515-520.
Godfrey DR, Blundell CJ, Essbauer S, et al. Unusual presentations of cowpox infection in cats. J Small Anim Pract 2004, 45:202-205.
Schulze C, Alex M, Schirrmeier H, et al. Generalized fatal cowpox virus infection in a cat with transmission to a human contact case. Zoonoses Public Health 2007, 54:31-37.

Autor J. Paul Woods
Consultor Editorial Stephen C. Barr

Infecção pelo Vírus da Imunodeficiência Felina

CONSIDERAÇÕES GERAIS

DEFINIÇÃO
Um retrovírus complexo que causa doença por imunodeficiência em gatos domésticos; mesmo gênero (Lentivírus) que o HIV, o agente causal da AIDS em humanos.

FISIOPATOLOGIA
• A infecção compromete a função do sistema imune; a disfunção imunológica ocorre em função de alterações das citocinas, hiperativação inespecífica de linfócitos T e B, anergia imunológica e apoptose de células-T.
• A patogenicidade pode depender da cepa ou do subtipo viral; os subtipos A e B são mais comuns nos EUA.
• Infecção aguda — o vírus dissemina-se a partir do local de entrada para os tecidos linfáticos e o timo via células dendríticas, infectando primeiro os linfócitos-T e depois os macrófagos.
• O receptor primário é o CD134 felino; o vírus também utiliza receptores de quimiocinas como receptores secundários.
• Células $CD4^+$ e $CD8^+$ — ambas podem ser infectadas de forma lítica em cultura; o vírus diminui seletiva e progressivamente as células $CD4^+$ (T auxiliares); a inversão da proporção $CD4^+$:$CD8^+$ (de ~2:1 para <1:1) desenvolve-se lentamente; uma redução absoluta das células-T $CD4^+$ é observada após vários meses de infecção.
• Infecção precoce e ativação das células-T reguladoras $CD4^+CD25^+$ podem limitar a resposta imune eficaz à infecção por FIV.
• Os pacientes permanecem clinicamente assintomáticos até que a imunidade mediada por células fique comprometida — o declínio está associado a citocinas Th1 reduzidas; a função imune humoral fica comprometida nos estágios avançados da infecção.
• Macrófagos — principal reservatório do vírus nos gatos acometidos; essas células transportam o vírus para tecidos em todo o corpo; defeitos na função (p. ex., aumento da produção de TNF).
• Astrócitos e células microgliais no cérebro, bem como megacariócitos e células mononucleares da medula óssea, podem ser infectados; pode ocorrer perda neuronal.
• A coinfecção com o FeLV pode aumentar a expressão do FIV em muitos tecidos, inclusive os rins, o cérebro e o fígado.

SISTEMA(S) ACOMETIDO(S)
• Gastrintestinal — síndrome semelhante à panleucopenia.
• Hematológico/linfático/imune — perda de células-T $CD4^+$; infiltrados linfocíticos-plasmocitários nos tecidos (especialmente na gengiva e nos tecidos linfoides).
• Nervoso — alterações na função dos astrócitos e na expressão de neurotransmissores.
• Oftálmico — uveíte anterior.
• Renal/urológico — nefropatia.
• Reprodutivo — morte fetal ou infecções perinatais.
• Outros sistemas corporais — infecções secundárias.

GENÉTICA
• Nenhuma predisposição à infecção.
• Pode desempenhar um papel na evolução e na gravidade do quadro.

INCIDÊNCIA/PREVALÊNCIA
EUA e Canadá — 1,5-3% na população de gatos sadios; 9-15% na de gatos com sinais de doença clínica.

DISTRIBUIÇÃO GEOGRÁFICA
Mundial; as taxas de soroprevalência são muito variáveis.

IDENTIFICAÇÃO
Espécie
Gatos.

Idade Média e Faixa Etária
• A prevalência da infecção aumenta com a idade.
• Idade média — 5 anos no momento do diagnóstico.

Sexo Predominante
Macho — mais agressivo; comportamento errante.

SINAIS CLÍNICOS
Comentários Gerais
• Diversos em virtude da natureza imunossupressora da infecção. • É impossível a distinção clínica entre a doença associada e as imunodeficiências vinculadas ao FeLV.

Achados Anamnésicos
Doenças secundárias recidivantes, sobretudo com sinais respiratórios superiores e gastrintestinais.

Achados do Exame Físico
• Dependem da ocorrência de infecções oportunistas. • Linfadenomegalia — leve a moderada. • Gengivite, estomatite, periodontite — 25-50% dos casos. • Trato respiratório superior — rinite; conjuntivite; ceratite (30% dos casos); associados, em geral, a infecções por herpes-vírus felino e calicivírus. • Insuficiência renal crônica — glomerulonefrite imunomediada. • Diarreia persistente — 10-20% dos casos; proliferação bacteriana ou fúngica excessiva, inflamação induzida por parasitas; efeito direto da infecção pelo FIV sobre o epitélio gastrintestinal.
• Infecções crônicas, irresponsivas ou recidivantes da orelha externa e da pele — originárias de infecções bacterianas ou dermatofitose. • Febre e emaciação — especialmente no estágio final; possivelmente em decorrência de altos níveis de TNF. • Doença ocular — uveíte anterior; inflamação da parte plana; glaucoma. • Linfoma ou outra neoplasia. • Anormalidades neurológicas — alteração dos padrões normais de sono; mudanças comportamentais (andar compassado e agressividade); déficits motores e neurocognitivos; neuropatias periféricas.

CAUSAS
• Transmissão de um gato para outro; em geral, por meio de ferimentos causados por mordidas.
• Transmissão perinatal ocasional.
• Embora a transmissão sexual seja incomum, o FIV já foi detectado no sêmen.

FATORES DE RISCO
• Macho. • Comportamento errante.

DIAGNÓSTICO

DIAGNÓSTICO DIFERENCIAL
• Infecções bacterianas, parasitárias, virais ou fúngicas primárias.
• Toxoplasmose — manifestações neurológicas e oculares podem ser o resultado de infecção por *Toxoplasma*, pelo FIV ou ambos.
• Doenças neoplásicas não virais.

HEMOGRAMA/BIOQUÍMICA/URINÁLISE
• O hemograma completo pode permanecer normal.
• Anemia, linfopenia ou neutropenia — podem ser observadas; pode ocorrer neutrofilia em resposta a infecções secundárias.
• Urinálise e perfil bioquímico sérico — proteína sérica alta por causa de hipergamaglobulinemia.

OUTROS TESTES LABORATORIAIS
Sorologia
• Detecta anticorpos contra o FIV.
• ELISA — teste de triagem de rotina; *kits* para uso na clínica com placas de microtitulação para o diagnóstico laboratorial; confirma resultados positivos com exames adicionais, especialmente em gatos sadios de baixo risco ou quando o diagnóstico resultaria em eutanásia.
• *Western blot** (*immunoblot*) — exame confirmatório de amostras positivas no teste ELISA.
• Filhotes — quando esses animais têm <6 meses de vida, o resultado do teste poderá ser positivo em função da transferência passiva de anticorpos provenientes da gata positiva para o FIV; o resultado positivo do teste não indica infecção; testar novamente aos 8-12 meses de vida para determinar se há infecção.
• Os gatos vacinados exibirão resultados positivos quanto à presença de anticorpos contra o FIV.

Outros
• Isolamento ou detecção do vírus — outros métodos estão ocasionalmente disponíveis em um esquema experimental.
• RT-PCR — útil em gatos vacinados ou filhotes com anticorpos maternos; o uso é dificultado pelos resultados inconsistentes entre os laboratórios.
• Avaliação de $CD4^+$:$CD8^+$ — ajuda a determinar a extensão da imunossupressão.

ACHADOS PATOLÓGICOS
• Linfadenopatia — associada à hiperplasia folicular e infiltração paracortical maciça de plasmócitos; mais tarde, pode-se observar um misto de hiperplasia folicular e depleção ou involução folicular; nos estágios terminais, depleção linfoide é o achado predominante.
• Infiltrados linfocíticos e plasmocitários — em gengivas, linfonodos e outros tecidos linfoides, além de baço, rins, fígado e cérebro.
• Manguito perivascular, gliose, perda neuronal, com vacuolização da substância branca e células gigantes ocasionais no cérebro.
• Lesões intestinais semelhantes àquelas observadas na infecção pelo parvovírus felino (síndrome semelhante à panleucopenia felina).

TRATAMENTO

CUIDADO(S) DE SAÚDE ADEQUADO(S)
• Ambulatoriais — são suficientes para a maioria dos pacientes.
• Internação — em casos de infecções secundárias graves até que a condição se estabilize.

---

* N. T.: Também conhecido como teste da mancha ocidental.

Infecção pelo Vírus da Imunodeficiência Felina

CUIDADO(S) DE ENFERMAGEM
• Principal consideração — tratar as infecções secundárias e oportunistas.
• Terapia de suporte — fluidos parenterais e suplementos nutricionais, se necessários.

ATIVIDADE
Normal.

DIETA
• Normal.
• Diarreia, doença renal ou emaciação crônica — alimentação especial, conforme a necessidade.

ORIENTAÇÃO AO PROPRIETÁRIO
• Informar o proprietário sobre o caráter lentamente progressivo da infecção e sobre o fato de que os gatos saudáveis positivos quanto à presença de anticorpos podem continuar sadios por anos.
• Orientar o proprietário sobre a possibilidade de que os gatos com sinais clínicos tenham problemas de saúde recidivantes ou crônicos que necessitem de atendimento médico.
• Discutir a importância de manter os gatos dentro de casa para protegê-los da exposição a patógenos secundários e prevenir a disseminação do FIV.

CONSIDERAÇÕES CIRÚRGICAS
• Tratamento odontológico ou cirurgia bucal — frequentemente necessários; limpeza dos dentes, extrações dentárias, biopsia gengival.
• Biopsia ou remoção de tumores.

MEDICAÇÕES

MEDICAMENTO(S) DE ESCOLHA
• Zidovudina (Retrovir®) — 5-15 mg/kg VO a cada 12 h — agente antiviral direto; o medicamento mais eficaz contra infecção aguda; monitorizar o paciente quanto à ocorrência de efeitos tóxicos sobre a medula óssea.
• Imunomoduladores — podem aliviar alguns sinais clínicos; alfainterferona recombinante humana (Roferon®) diluída em solução fisiológica a 30 unidades/dia VO por 7 dias em semanas alternadas; pode aumentar as taxas de sobrevida e melhorar o estado clínico do paciente; omegainterferona recombinante felina em altas doses (Virbagen Omega®) a uma dose de 1 milhão de unidades/kg SC diariamente por 5 dias em 3 intervalos (dias 0-4, dias 14-18, dias 60-64); tentar também o *Propionibacterium acnes* (Immunorregulin®) na dose de 0,5 mL/gato IV, 1-2 vezes por semana, ou acemanana (Carrasyn®) a 100 mg/gato VO diariamente.
• Gengivite e estomatite — podem ser refratárias ao tratamento.
• Antibacterianos ou antimicóticos — úteis para proliferação excessiva de bactérias ou fungos; talvez haja necessidade de terapia prolongada ou altas doses; para infecções bacterianas anaeróbicas, usar o metronidazol a 7-15 mg/kg VO a cada 8-12 h ou a clindamicina a 11 mg/kg VO a cada 12 h.
• Corticosteroides ou sais de ouro — o uso criterioso, porém rigoroso, pode ajudar a controlar a inflamação imunomediada.
• Anorexia — estimulação do apetite a curto prazo: diazepam a 0,2 mg/kg IV ou oxazepam a 2,5 mg/gato VO; estimulação do apetite mais prolongada e reversão da caquexia: esteroides anabólicos ou acetato de megestrol; eficácia desconhecida em gatos positivos para o FIV.
• Corticosteroides tópicos — para uveíte anterior; a resposta a longo prazo pode ser incompleta ou fraca; inflamação da parte plana, em geral, regride espontaneamente e pode recidivar.
• Glaucoma — tratamento-padrão.
• É recomendável a vacinação anual contra vírus respiratórios e entéricos com vacinas inativadas.

CONTRAINDICAÇÕES
• Griseofulvina — evitar ou usar com extrema cautela em gatos positivos para o FIV; pode induzir à neutropenia grave; a neutropenia será reversível se o medicamento for retirado cedo o bastante; no entanto, infecções secundárias associadas à condição podem ser potencialmente letais.
• Vacinas de vírus vivo modificado — podem causar doença em gatos imunossuprimidos apesar de improvável.

PRECAUÇÕES
Corticosteroides sistêmicos — utilizar com cuidado; podem causar imunossupressão adicional.

INTERAÇÕES POSSÍVEIS
Ver a seção "Contraindicações".

ACOMPANHAMENTO

MONITORIZAÇÃO DO PACIENTE
Varia de acordo com infecções secundárias e outras manifestações da doença.

PREVENÇÃO
• Evitar o contato com gatos positivos para o FIV.
• Realizar a quarentena e testar os gatos recém-chegados antes de introduzi-los em casas onde há muitos gatos.

Vacinas
• Vacina de vírus inteiro inativado, composta de subtipo duplo (A e D) (Fel-O-Vax® contra o FIV, Fort Dodge Animal Health).
• Eficácia de 0-80% depois de 3 doses, dependendo do modelo de estudo e do sistema de desafio.
• Os ensaios com anticorpos não são capazes de distinguir entre gatos vacinados e infectados pelo FIV; a detecção do vírus pela técnica de PCR é inconsistente; um teste ELISA discriminatório recém-desenvolvido pode ser útil para determinar o estado real de infecção pelo FIV.

EVOLUÇÃO ESPERADA E PROGNÓSTICO
• Nos primeiros 2 anos após o diagnóstico ou 4,5-6 anos após o tempo estimado de infecção, cerca de 20% dos gatos morrem, porém mais de 50% permanecem assintomáticos.
• Nos estágios finais da doença (emaciação e infecções oportunistas frequentes ou graves), a expectativa de vida é ≤1 ano.

DIVERSOS

DISTÚRBIOS ASSOCIADOS
• Doença bacteriana, viral, fúngica e parasitária secundária.
• Tumores linfoides.
• Doença imunomediada.

FATORES RELACIONADOS COM A IDADE
Os filhotes podem ser positivos ao teste por causa da transferência passiva de anticorpos pela mãe.

POTENCIAL ZOONÓTICO
• Nenhum conhecido; as provas contra a transmissão do FIV para humanos são convincentes, mas não podem ser consideradas conclusivas em virtude do tempo relativamente curto em que o vírus vem sendo estudado.
• Os macacos são suscetíveis à infecção experimental; há indícios de declínio das células-T $CD4^+$.
• Transmissão potencial de patógenos secundários (p. ex., *Toxoplasma gondii*) a humanos imunocomprometidos.

GESTAÇÃO/FERTILIDADE/REPRODUÇÃO
Gatas positivas para o FIV — há relatos de abortamentos e natimortos; a transmissão para os filhotes será pouco frequente se a gata for positiva quanto à presença de anticorpos antes da concepção; a taxa de transmissão pode ser dependente do subtipo ou da cepa (> 90% para infecções experimentais com algumas cepas).

SINÔNIMO(S)
Síndrome da imunodeficiência felina.

VER TAMBÉM
Tópicos individuais sobre doenças infecciosas secundárias, doença ocular, gengivite e estomatite.

ABREVIATURA(S)
• AIDS = síndrome da imunodeficiência adquirida.
• ELISA = ensaio imunoabsorvente ligado à enzima.
• FeLV = vírus da leucemia felina.
• FIV = vírus da imunodeficiência felina.
• HIV = vírus da imunodeficiência humana.
• PCR = reação em cadeia da polimerase.
• RT-PCR = reação em cadeia da polimerase reversa via transcriptase reversa.
• TNF = fator de necrose tumoral.

Sugestões de Leitura
Harbour DA, Caney SMA, Sparkes AH. Feline immunodeficiency virus infection. In: Chandler EA, Gaskell CJ, Gaskell RM, eds., Feline Medicine and Therapeutics, 3rd ed. Oxford: Blackwell, 2004, pp. 607-620.
Levy J, Crawford C, Hartmann K, Hofmann-Lehmann R, Little S, Sundahl E, Thayer V. 2008. American Association of Feline Practitioners' feline retrovirus management guidelines. J Feline Med Surg 2008, 10:300-316.
Richards JR. Feline immunodeficiency virus vaccine: Implications for diagnostic testing and disease. Biologicals 2005, 33:215-217.
Sellon RK, Hartmann K. Feline immunodeficiency virus infection. In: Greene CE, ed., Infectious Diseases of the Dog and Cat, 3rd ed. St. Louis: Saunders Elsevier, 2006, pp. 131-143.

Autor Margaret C. Barr
Consultor Editorial Stephen C. Barr

INFECÇÃO PELO VÍRUS DA LEUCEMIA FELINA

CONSIDERAÇÕES GERAIS

DEFINIÇÃO
Um retrovírus simples (gênero Gamarretrovírus) que causa imunodeficiência e doença neoplásica em gatos domésticos.

FISIOPATOLOGIA
- Existem quatro subgrupos de FeLV — A, B, C e T; o FeLV-A é o mais transmissível, estando presente em todos os isolamentos; o FeLV-B surge da recombinação do gene *env* do FeLV-A com sequências retrovirais endógenas (50% dos isolamentos); o FeLV-C (1% dos isolamentos) origina-se de uma mutação nas sequências do gene *env*; o FeLV-T infecta apenas as células-T.
- A infecção precoce consiste em 5 estágios — (1) replicação viral nas tonsilas e nos linfonodos faríngeos; (2) infecção de alguns linfócitos-B circulantes e macrófagos que disseminam o vírus; (3) replicação nos tecidos linfoides, nas células epiteliais das criptas intestinais e nas células precursoras da medula óssea; (4) liberação de neutrófilos e plaquetas infectados da medula óssea para o sistema circulatório; e (5) infecção de tecidos epiteliais e glandulares, com subsequente eliminação do vírus pela saliva e pela urina.
- Uma resposta imune adequada interrompe a evolução no estágio 2 ou 3 (4-8 semanas após a exposição) e força o vírus a ficar latente.
- Uma viremia persistente (estágios 4 e 5) geralmente se desenvolve 4-6 semanas após a infecção, mas pode levar 12 semanas.
- Indução tumoral — ocorre quando o DNA pró-viral se integra no DNA cromossômico do gato em regiões críticas (oncogenes).
- Integração do vírus perto do gene celular *c-myc* ou de genes próximos que influenciam a expressão do *c-myc* — geralmente resulta em linfossarcoma do timo.
- Vírus do sarcoma felino — mutantes do FeLV; surgem pela recombinação entre os genes do FeLV e os do hospedeiro; as proteínas de fusão do vírus e do hospedeiro são responsáveis pela indução eficiente de fibrossarcomas.

SISTEMA(S) ACOMETIDO(S)
- Hematológico/linfático/imune — anemia; discrasias de células sanguíneas; neoplasias que se originam na medula óssea; imunossupressão, possivelmente resultante de disfunção neuroendócrina; redução absoluta nos subgrupos de células-T $CD4^+$ e $CD8^+$; queda na relação $CD4^+$:$CD8^+$.
- Nervoso — mielopatia degenerativa, neoplasias.
- Todos os outros sistemas corporais — imunossupressão com infecções secundárias ou desenvolvimento de doença neoplásica.

GENÉTICA
Nenhuma predisposição genética.

INCIDÊNCIA/PREVALÊNCIA
- Prevalência nos EUA — 2-3% na população de gatos saudáveis; taxa de infecção mundial de 1-8% em gatos sadios; 3-4 vezes maior em gatos com sinais de doença clínica.
- Declínio na prevalência norte-americana desde os anos 80 — atribuído aos programas de teste e remoção, possivelmente aos programas de vacinação.

DISTRIBUIÇÃO GEOGRÁFICA
Mundial.

IDENTIFICAÇÃO
Espécies
Gatos.

Idade Média e Faixa Etária
- Prevalência maior entre 1-6 anos de idade.
- Média — 3 anos.

Sexo Predominante
Proporção entre machos e fêmeas — 1,7:1.

SINAIS CLÍNICOS
Comentários Gerais
- Início da doença associada ao FeLV — geralmente ocorre em um período de meses a anos após a infecção.
- Doenças associadas — não neoplásicas ou neoplásicas; a maioria das doenças não neoplásicas ou degenerativas resulta de imunossupressão.
- Os sinais clínicos de imunodeficiência induzida pelo FeLV não podem ser distinguidos daqueles de imunodeficiência induzida pelo FIV.

Achados Anamnésicos
- Paciente com acesso permitido a ambientes externos.
- Membro de uma casa onde há vários gatos.

Achados do Exame Físico
- Dependem do tipo de doença (neoplásica ou não neoplásica) e da ocorrência de infecções secundárias.
- Linfadenomegalia — leve a grave.
- Trato respiratório superior — rinite, conjuntivite e ceratite (18% dos casos).
- Diarreia persistente — proliferação bacteriana ou fúngica excessiva; inflamação parasitária; efeito direto de infecção sobre as células das criptas.
- Gengivite; estomatite; periodontite.
- Infecções crônicas, irresponsivas ou recidivantes da orelha externa e da pele; abscessos.
- Febre e emaciação (42-53% dos casos).
- Linfoma — doença neoplásica associada mais comum; linfomas tímicos e multicêntricos altamente associados; linfomas diversos (de origem extranodal) envolvem com maior frequência os olhos e o sistema nervoso.
- Leucemias eritroides e mielomonocíticas — leucemias não linfoides predominantes.
- Fibrossarcomas — em pacientes coinfectados pelo vírus mutante do sarcoma; mais frequentes em gatos jovens.
- Neuropatias periféricas; ataxia progressiva.

CAUSAS
- Transmissão de um gato para outro(s) — mordidas; contato íntimo casual (auto-higienização da pelagem); bandejas sanitárias ou tigelas de água/comida compartilhadas.
- Transmissão perinatal — morte fetal e neonatal de filhotes de 80% das gatas acometidas; transmissão transplacentária e transmamária em pelo menos 20% dos filhotes sobreviventes de gatas infectadas.

FATORES DE RISCO
- Idade — os filhotes são muito mais suscetíveis à infecção do que os adultos.
- Machos — resulta do comportamento.
- Comportamento errante (vida livre).
- Muitos gatos na mesma casa.

DIAGNÓSTICO

DIAGNÓSTICO DIFERENCIAL
- FIV.
- Outras infecções — bacterianas, parasitárias, virais ou fúngicas.
- Doenças neoplásicas não virais.

HEMOGRAMA/BIOQUÍMICA/URINÁLISE
- Anemia — geralmente grave; com maior frequência, a anemia é arregenerativa; as anemias regenerativas costumam estar associadas a coinfecções por *Mycoplasma haemofelis* ou *M. haemominutum*.
- Linfopenia ou linfocitose.
- Neutropenia — ocasionalmente cíclica; pode ocorrer em resposta a infecções secundárias ou doença imunomediada.
- Trombocitopenia e anemia hemolítica imunomediada — podem ocorrer secundariamente à formação de imunocomplexos.
- Achados da urinálise e do perfil bioquímico sérico — dependem do sistema acometido e do tipo de doença.

OUTROS TESTES LABORATORIAIS
- IFA — identifica o antígeno p27 do FeLV em leucócitos e plaquetas em esfregaços fixados de sangue total ou preparados de camada leucocitária; resultados positivos indicam uma infecção produtiva em células da medula óssea; 97% dos gatos positivos no teste de IFA permanecem persistentemente infectados e virêmicos pelo resto da vida; em geral, o antígeno p27 pode ser detectado por volta de 4 semanas depois da infecção, embora possa demorar até 12 semanas para se obter um teste positivo; no caso de gatos leucopênicos, usar esfregaços da camada leucocitária, em vez de sangue total.
- ELISA — detecta o antígeno solúvel p27 do FeLV em amostras de sangue total, soro, plasma, saliva ou lágrimas; mais sensível que o IFA para detectar infecções precoces ou transitórias; um único teste positivo não pode predizer que os gatos ficarão persistentemente virêmicos; testar novamente 12 semanas depois (muitos veterinários testam com IFA nesse momento); os resultados falso-positivos são mais comuns quando se usa sangue total em vez de soro ou plasma; testes positivos com saliva ou lágrimas devem ser checados com sangue total (IFA) ou soro (ELISA).
- Alguns gatos são persistentemente positivos no teste de ELISA e negativos no teste de IFA; foi detectado material genético pró-viral do FeLV em células sanguíneas circulantes de alguns desses gatos; demonstra infecção, apesar de não haver viremia detectável associada às células.
- A vacinação contra o FeLV não interfere nos testes, pois eles detectam o antígeno e não o anticorpo.

DIAGNÓSTICO POR IMAGEM
Atrofia do timo (filhotes debilitados).

MÉTODOS DIAGNÓSTICOS
Aspiração ou biopsia de medula óssea — com eritroblastopenia (anemia arregenerativa), a medula óssea costuma exibir hipercelularidade em virtude de uma parada na diferenciação de células eritroides; pode-se observar anemia aplásica verdadeira com medula óssea hipocelular; alguns casos de anemia resultam de doença mieloproliferativa.

Infecção pelo Vírus da Leucemia Felina

ACHADOS PATOLÓGICOS
• Lesões — dependem do tipo de doença; a hipercelularidade da medula óssea frequentemente acompanha doença neoplásica.
• Infiltrados linfocíticos e plasmocitários nas gengivas, nos linfonodos, em outros tecidos linfoides, no baço, nos rins e no fígado.
• Lesões intestinais semelhantes àquelas observadas com infecção pelo parvovírus felino (síndrome semelhante à panleucopenia felina).

TRATAMENTO
CUIDADO(S) DE SAÚDE ADEQUADO(S)
• Ambulatoriais para a maioria dos gatos.
• Hospitalares — podem ser necessários com infecções secundárias graves, anemia ou caquexia, até que a condição se estabilize.
• Transfusões de sangue — suporte de emergência; talvez haja necessidade de múltiplas transfusões; a transferência passiva de anticorpos diminui o nível de antigenemia do FeLV em alguns gatos; portanto, é válida a imunização de gatos doadores de sangue com vacinas contra o FeLV.

CUIDADO(S) DE ENFERMAGEM
• Tratamento de infecções secundárias e oportunistas — providência principal.
• Terapias de suporte (p. ex., fluidos parenterais e suplementos nutricionais) podem ser úteis.

ATIVIDADE
Normal.

DIETA
• Normal.
• Diarreia, doença renal ou emaciação crônica — podem necessitar de dietas especiais.

ORIENTAÇÃO AO PROPRIETÁRIO
• Discutir a importância de se manter os gatos dentro de casa e isolados daqueles negativos para o FeLV, a fim de protegê-los da exposição a patógenos secundários e evitar a disseminação do vírus.
• Abordar a relevância de se fornecer uma nutrição satisfatória e proporcionar um manejo de rotina para o controle de infecções bacterianas, virais e parasitárias secundárias.

CONSIDERAÇÕES CIRÚRGICAS
• Biopsia ou remoção de tumores.
• Tratamento odontológico ou cirurgia bucal — limpeza dentária, extrações dentárias, biopsia gengival.

MEDICAÇÕES
MEDICAMENTO(S) DE ESCOLHA
• Zidovudina (Retrovir®, 5-15 mg/kg VO a cada 12 h) — proporciona melhora clínica, mas não elimina o vírus.
• Imunomoduladores — podem aliviar alguns sinais clínicos; a alfainterferona recombinante humana (Roferon®, diluído em solução fisiológica, 30 U/dia VO por 7 dias em semanas alternadas) pode aumentar as taxas de sobrevida e melhorar a condição clínica do paciente; *Propionibacterium acnes* (Immunoregulin®, 0,5 mL/gato IV, 1-2 vezes por semana); acemanana (Carrasyn®, 100 mg/gato/dia VO).
• Infecção por *Mycoplasma haemofelis* — suspeita em todos os gatos com anemias hemolíticas regenerativas; oxitetraciclina (Terramycin®, 15 mg/kg VO a cada 8 h, ou Liquamycin®, 7 mg/kg IM ou IV a cada 12 h) ou doxiciclina (5 mg/kg VO a cada 12 h) por 3 semanas; utilizar glicocorticoides orais a curto prazo se houver necessidade.
• Linfoma — tratado com os protocolos quimioterápicos combinados-padrão; períodos de remissão variam, em média, de 3-4 meses; alguns gatos podem permanecer em remissão por muito mais tempo.
• Doença mieloproliferativa e leucemias — mais refratárias ao tratamento; para anemia, tentar o uso de eritropoietina (Epogen®, 35-100 UI/kg SC a cada 48 h); para neutropenia, tentar o emprego de G-CSF recombinante humano (Neupogen®, 5μg/kg SC a cada 24 h).
• É recomendável a vacinação anual contra vírus respiratórios e entéricos com vacinas inativadas.

CONTRAINDICAÇÕES
Vacinas de vírus vivos modificados podem causar a doença em gatos imunossuprimidos.

PRECAUÇÕES
Corticosteroides sistêmicos — utilizar com cuidado em virtude do potencial de imunossupressão adicional.

ACOMPANHAMENTO
MONITORIZAÇÃO DO PACIENTE
Varia de acordo com as infecções secundárias e outras manifestações da doença.

PREVENÇÃO
• Evitar o contato com gatos positivos para o FeLV.
• Realizar a quarentena e testar os gatos recém-chegados antes de introduzi-los em casas onde há vários gatos.

Vacinas
• A maioria das vacinas disponíveis no mercado induz à formação de anticorpos neutralizantes do vírus, específicos para a proteína viral gp70; a eficácia relatada varia de <20% a quase 100%, dependendo do ensaio e do sistema de desafio; as vacinas de células inteiras inativadas tendem a ser as mais eficientes (a vacina recombinante que contém o vírus canarypox contra o FeLV tem eficácia semelhante sem adjuvante).
• Testar os gatos para o FeLV antes da primeira vacinação; se o teste não for feito antes da vacinação, os proprietários deverão estar cientes de que o gato já pode estar infectado.
• Vacinar os filhotes com 8-9 semanas e 12 semanas de vida; dar o reforço com 1 ano de idade; repetir a vacinação a cada 2-3 anos.

EVOLUÇÃO ESPERADA E PROGNÓSTICO
Gatos persistentemente virêmicos — mais de 50% sucumbem a doenças relacionadas 2-3 anos após a infecção.

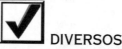

DIVERSOS
DISTÚRBIOS ASSOCIADOS
• Doença bacteriana, viral, fúngica e parasitária secundária.
• Tumores linfoides.
• Fibrossarcomas.
• Doença imunomediada.

FATORES RELACIONADOS COM A IDADE
• Filhotes recém-nascidos — a maioria (70-100%) é suscetível à infecção persistente.
• Filhotes maiores — menos de 30% são suscetíveis até as 16 semanas de vida.

POTENCIAL ZOONÓTICO
Provavelmente baixo, mas controverso — estudos relatam resultados conflitantes de anticorpos contra o FeLV em pessoas e quanto à correlação entre certas leucemias humanas e a exposição a gatos.

GESTAÇÃO/FERTILIDADE/REPRODUÇÃO
• Abortamentos, natimortos e reabsorções fetais são comuns em gatas positivas para o FeLV.
• Transmissão de gatas para os filhotes — em pelo menos 20% dos nascidos vivos.

SINÔNIMO(S)
FeLV-AIDS — um FeLV mutante que provoca o rápido desenvolvimento de doença por imunodeficiência.

VER TAMBÉM
Tópicos individuais sobre neoplasia, doenças infecciosas secundárias, doença ocular e gengivite/estomatite.

ABREVIATURA(S)
• AIDS = síndrome da imunodeficiência adquirida.
• IFA = anticorpo imunofluorescente.
• ELISA = ensaio imunoabsorvente ligado à enzima.
• FeLV = vírus da leucemia felina.
• FIV = vírus da imunodeficiência felina.
• G-CSF = fator estimulador da colônia de granulócitos.

Sugestões de Leitura
Dunham SP, Graham E. Retroviral infections in small animals. Vet Clin North Am Small Anim Pract 2008, 38:879-901.
Jarrett O, Hosie MJ. Feline leukemia virus infection. In: Feline Medicine and Therapeutics, 3rd ed. Oxford: Blackwell, 2004, pp. 597-604.
Levy JK, Crawford PC. Feline leukemia virus. In: Ettinger SJ, Feldman EC, eds., Textbook of Veterinary Internal Medicine, 6th ed. St. Louis: Elsevier, 2005, pp. 653-659.
Levy J, Crawford C, Hartmann K, Hofmann-Lehmann R, Little S, Sundahl E, Thayer V. 2008. American Association of Feline Practitioners' feline retrovirus management guidelines. J Feline Med Surg 2008, 10:300-316.
Lutz H, Addie D, Boucraut-Baralon C, Egberink H, Frumus T, Gruffydd-Jones T, Hartmann K, Hosie MJ, Lloret A, Marsillo F, Pennisi MG, Radford AD, Thiry E, Truyen U, Horzinek MC. Feline leukaemia: ABCD guidelines on prevention and management. J Feline Med Surg 2009, 11:565-574.

Autor Margaret C. Barr
Consultor Editorial Stephen C. Barr

INFECÇÃO PELO VÍRUS DA PSEUDORRAIVA

CONSIDERAÇÕES GERAIS

REVISÃO
- Doença rara, porém altamente fatal, dos cães e dos gatos; costuma ocorrer nos animais que têm contato com suínos.
- Caracterizada por morte súbita, quase sempre sem sinais característicos ou com sinais que incluem hipersalivação, prurido intenso e alterações neurológicas.
- Também conhecida como doença de Aujeszky, "prurido de louco" ou paralisia bulbar infecciosa.

IDENTIFICAÇÃO
- Cães e gatos domésticos e exóticos.
- Outros animais domésticos — suínos, bovinos, ovinos e caprinos.
- Acomete principalmente cães e gatos de criação, sem predileção racial ou etária.

SINAIS CLÍNICOS
- Morte súbita.
- Hipersalivação.
- Respiração rápida e laboriosa.
- Febre.
- Vômito.
- Neurológicos — depressão e letargia, ataxia, convulsões, relutância ao movimento, decúbito, prurido intenso e automutilação, coma e morte.

CAUSAS E FATORES DE RISCO
- Vírus da pseudorraiva (herpes-vírus suíno) — um alfa-herpes-vírus.
- Contato com suínos.
- Consumo de carne crua contaminada ou miúdos de suínos.
- Ingestão de ratos infectados.

DIAGNÓSTICO

DIAGNÓSTICO DIFERENCIAL
- Raiva — na forma furiosa, o cão ou o gato acometido atacará qualquer coisa que se movimente; sem prurido ou morte súbita; resultado positivo no teste do anticorpo imunofluorescente no cérebro.
- Cinomose — sem hipersalivação, morte súbita ou mudança na personalidade; sinais respiratórios e gastrintestinais são comuns.
- Intoxicação (por organofosforado, chumbo, estricnina, arsênico inorgânico) — sem prurido ou mudança na personalidade; histórico de exposição à toxina; sinais compatíveis com intoxicação.

HEMOGRAMA/BIOQUÍMICA/URINÁLISE
Sem alterações características.

OUTROS TESTES LABORATORIAIS
Análises sorológicas — revelam anticorpos contra o vírus da pseudorraiva caso o animal se recupere.

DIAGNÓSTICO POR IMAGEM
N/D.

MÉTODOS DIAGNÓSTICOS
- Teste do anticorpo imunofluorescente — tecido cerebral.
- Isolamento do vírus — tecidos acometidos.
- Inoculação em animal (coelho).

ACHADOS PATOLÓGICOS
- Lesões cutâneas graves — causadas por automutilação decorrente do prurido intenso.
- Exame histopatológico — células gliais e ganglionares do tecido neurológico revelam corpúsculos de inclusão intranuclear de Cowdry tipo A.
- Meningoencefalite não supurativa na medula oblonga.

TRATAMENTO

- Cães e gatos — não há nenhum tratamento eficaz conhecido.
- Ficam indicados o tratamento geral de suporte e a prevenção da autolesão.

MEDICAÇÕES

MEDICAMENTO(S)
- Nenhum específico.
- Antivirais anti-herpéticos — não avaliados para cães e gatos.
- Evolução rápida torna improvável a utilização bem-sucedida de medicamentos antivirais.

CONTRAINDICAÇÕES/INTERAÇÕES POSSÍVEIS
Nenhuma.

ACOMPANHAMENTO

PREVENÇÃO
- Evitar o contato com suínos infectados, o hospedeiro reservatório.
- Evitar o consumo de carne de porco contaminada.
- Evitar a ingestão de ratos infectados.
- Não costuma ocorrer a transmissão gato a gato e cão a cão.

EVOLUÇÃO ESPERADA E PROGNÓSTICO
- Clássica (gatos) — 60% dos casos; dura 24-36 h; quase invariavelmente fatal.
- Atípica (gatos) — 40% dos casos; dura >36 h; quase invariavelmente fatal.

DIVERSOS

POTENCIAL ZOONÓTICO
Leve potencial de infecção humana; tomar cuidado ao se tratar animais infectados e manipular tecidos e líquidos infectados.

Sugestões de Leitura
Glass CM, McLean RG, Katz JB, et al. Isolation of pseudorabies (Aujeszky's disease) virus from a Florida panther. J Wildlife Dis 1994, 30:180-184.
Gustafson DP. Pseudorabies (Aujeszky's disease, mad itch, infectious bulbar paralysis). In: Holzworth J, ed., Diseases of the Cat. Philadelphia: Saunders, 1987, pp. 242-246.
Hawkins BA, Olson GR. Clinical signs of pseudorabies in the dog and cat. A review of 40 cases. Iowa State Univ Vet 1985, 47:116-119.
Vandevelde M. Pseudorabies. In: Greene CE, ed., Infectious Diseases of the Dog and Cat, 3rd ed. St. Louis: Saunders Elsevier, 2006, pp. 183-186.

Autor Fred W. Scott
Consultor Editorial Stephen C. Barr

Infecção pelo Vírus Formador de Sincício Felino

CONSIDERAÇÕES GERAIS

REVISÃO
- Um retrovírus complexo da família Spumavirinae que infecta gatos, aparentemente com pouco ou nenhum efeito patogênico.
- Encontrado em todo o mundo; prevalência estimada, 10-70% ou mais.
- Presente em algumas populações de felinos não domésticos.
- Infecção ligada estatisticamente à poliartrite crônica progressiva; a doença não foi reproduzida por infecção experimental.
- Os gatos infectados experimentalmente apresentam glomerulonefrite ou pneumonia intersticial subclínica.
- Algumas cepas infectam as células linfoblastoides e induzem à apoptose — sugere um impacto potencial sobre a função imunológica em gatos.
- Pesquisa — baixo potencial de doença; gera nocividade ao se utilizar cultura de células originárias de tecido felino; testar os gatos e retirá-los do estudo se positivos para o FeFV.
- O potencial para uso como terapia genética ou vetor de vacina está sob investigação.

IDENTIFICAÇÃO
- Gatos — acomete mais os gatos de vida livre do que os locais com múltiplos gatos ou gatis.
- A prevalência do vírus é baixa em filhotes e aumenta com a idade.
- Não há predileção sexual clara — alguns estudos antigos revelaram que os machos eram mais provavelmente infectados do que as fêmeas; no entanto, um estudo conduzido em gatos australianos não constatou qualquer diferença entre as taxas de infecção em machos e fêmeas.
- Ocorre poliartrite crônica progressiva (possivelmente pela formação de imunocomplexos) de forma predominante em machos com 1,5-5 anos de idade.

SINAIS CLÍNICOS
- A maioria dos gatos acometidos apresenta-se saudável.
- Ligações estatísticas com doença mieloproliferativa e poliartrite crônica progressiva — na verdade, podem refletir coinfecção com FIV.
- Poliartrite crônica progressiva — articulações tumefatas; marcha anormal; linfadenopatia.

CAUSAS E FATORES DE RISCO
- Transmissão — um tanto controversa; possivelmente por meio de mordidas; gatos de vida livre correm maior risco de infecção.
- Coinfecções com FIV e FeLV — razoavelmente comuns, talvez por causa dos modos de transmissão e dos fatores de risco compartilhados; a coinfecção por FeFV não intensifica a patogênese inicial de infecções por FIV.
- Transmitido de forma eficiente de gatas infectadas para a prole, provavelmente *in utero* (ou seja, por via intrauterina).
- A alta prevalência da infecção em algumas populações de gatos sugere que o contato casual possa desempenhar um papel na transmissão; isso não foi demonstrado experimentalmente.

DIAGNÓSTICO

DIAGNÓSTICO DIFERENCIAL
Sinais de poliartrite crônica progressiva — teste para pesquisa de FIV, FeLV e doença articular séptica.

HEMOGRAMA/BIOQUÍMICA/URINÁLISE
Geralmente normais.

OUTROS TESTES LABORATORIAIS
- Sorologia — para detecção de anticorpos contra FeFV e isolamento do vírus; não está disponível com facilidade; não é particularmente útil porque a correlação entre a infecção e a doença pelo FeFV é muito tênue.
- Isolamento do vírus — a partir de linfócitos periféricos ou camada leucocitária.

MÉTODOS DIAGNÓSTICOS
- Citologia do líquido articular — em caso de poliartrite crônica progressiva; pode revelar grande quantidade de neutrófilos e grandes células mononucleares.
- Histologia — infiltrados linfoplasmocitários são comuns na presença de doença articular.

TRATAMENTO

Nenhum, exceto para a poliartrite crônica progressiva.

MEDICAÇÕES

MEDICAMENTO(S)
Poliartrite crônica progressiva — doses imunossupressoras de prednisolona (10-15 mg/gato/dia) e ciclofosfamida (7,5 mg/gato/dia por 4 dias semanalmente).

CONTRAINDICAÇÕES/INTERAÇÕES POSSÍVEIS
Medicamentos imunossupressores — ter cuidado ao utilizá-los em pacientes coinfectados com FIV ou FeLV.

ACOMPANHAMENTO

EVOLUÇÃO ESPERADA E PROGNÓSTICO
- Infecção apenas pelo FeFV — consequências adversas improváveis.
- Poliartrite crônica progressiva — em geral, é difícil de controlar; prognóstico mau em termos de recuperação a longo prazo.

DIVERSOS

DISTÚRBIOS ASSOCIADOS
- Poliartrite crônica progressiva.
- Coinfecções pelo FIV e FeLV.

SINÔNIMO(S)
- Vírus sincicial felino.
- Vírus felino espumoso.

VER TAMBÉM
- Poliartrite Erosiva Imunomediada.
- Poliartrite Não Erosiva Imunomediada.

ABREVIATURA(S)
- FeFV = vírus formador de sincício felino.
- FeLV = vírus da leucemia felina.
- FIV = vírus da imunodeficiência felina.

Sugestões de Leitura
German AC, Harbour DA, Helps CR, Gruffydd-Jones TJ. Is feline foamy vírus really apathogenic? Vet Immunol Immunopathol 2008, 123:114-118.
Greene CE. Feline foamy (syncytium-forming) virus infection. In: Greene CE, ed., Infectious Diseases of the Dog and Cat, 3rd ed. St. Louis: Saunders Elsevier, 2006, pp. 154-155.

Autor Margaret C. Barr
Consultor Editorial Stephen C. Barr

Infecção pelo Vírus Oeste do Nilo

CONSIDERAÇÕES GERAIS

REVISÃO
- Uma doença viral aguda a inaparente com manifestações neurológicas, causada pelo vírus Oeste do Nilo, um membro da família Flaviviridae, gênero *Flavivírus*. A distribuição geográfica do vírus ocorre na América do Norte, África, Ásia, sul da Europa e Austrália (vírus Kunjin).
- A via natural de infecção se dá por meio da picada de inúmeras espécies de mosquitos, dependendo da localização geográfica. A infecção produz uma viremia de baixo nível, que não é detectável por volta do sexto dia após a infecção. Já o anticorpo é detectável em torno do sétimo dia após a infecção.

IDENTIFICAÇÃO
- Infecções naturais não limitadas por espécie ou idade.
- A soroprevalência varia com a região geográfica (3-38%).

SINAIS CLÍNICOS
- Alta porcentagem de cães sem manifestação de sinais clínicos — nenhum cão experimentalmente infectado demonstrou sinais clínicos.
- Período de incubação — 2-4 dias após a infecção.
- Resposta febril — 40,3-42,2°C 3-6 dias após a infecção.
- Em cães acometidos, os sinais comuns são ataxia, depressão, anorexia, tremores, déficits proprioceptivos conscientes, crises convulsivas, fraqueza, paralisia flácida.

CAUSAS E FATORES DE RISCO
- Doença neurológica causada pelo vírus Oeste do Nilo.
- Os cães de rua têm uma probabilidade muito maior de serem soropositivos do que aqueles mantidos dentro de casa.
- Os cães errantes têm uma probabilidade muito maior de serem soropositivos do que aqueles com dono.
- A linhagem do vírus tipo 1 é mais neurovirulenta (todos os isolamentos da América do Norte) do que a linhagem tipo 2 (África).
- A oscilação anual das infecções está ligada à densidade das populações de mosquito.

DIAGNÓSTICO

DIAGNÓSTICO DIFERENCIAL
- Em um nível individual, os sinais de doença neurológica induzida pelo vírus Oeste do Nilo são indistinguíveis daqueles associados a várias infecções por "arbovírus", p. ex., encefalite equina oriental, encefalite equina venezuelana, encefalite de La Crosse.
- Outras considerações no diagnóstico diferencial — raiva, cinomose canina, neosporose, toxoplasmose, pseudorraiva, vírus da encefalomiocardite.

HEMOGRAMA/BIOQUÍMICA/URINÁLISE
- Geralmente normais.
- A amostragem seriada pode revelar uma queda nos leucócitos, mas pode permanecer dentro da normalidade.

DIAGNÓSTICO POR IMAGEM
Eletroencefalograma.

MÉTODOS DIAGNÓSTICOS
Baixos níveis de viremia tornam altamente improvável a detecção do agente na fase aguda. Se uma tentativa for feita, o teste de escolha será o PCR-RT para detecção do vírus Oeste do Nilo especificamente ou dos arbovírus em geral. Amostras séricas agudas e convalescentes devem ser coletadas para mensuração do título de IgM no teste ELISA e ensaios de neutralização viral. Para exame pós-morte — PCR-RT e/ou imuno-histoquímica.

ACHADOS PATOLÓGICOS
Lesões macroscópicas não estão presentes em um número limitado de cães submetidos à necropsia (um único caso com epicardite).
Lesões histológicas no cérebro — meningoencefalite leve, multifocal, não supurativa (infiltrados perivasculares linfocíticos a linfo-histiocíticos predominantemente na substância cinzenta).

TRATAMENTO

Terapia de suporte direcionada à redução dos sinais neurológicos.

MEDICAÇÕES

- Agentes antivirais não foram testados quanto à eficácia.
- Antipiréticos para reduzir a febre.
- Medicamentos anticonvulsivantes.

PREVENÇÃO
Embora disponíveis para equinos, as vacinas não são aprovadas para cães.

DIVERSOS

POTENCIAL ZOONÓTICO
- O vírus Oeste do Nilo é capaz de infectar inúmeras espécies, inclusive o homem; contudo, é geralmente necessário o inseto vetor para a transmissão. A viremia é muito baixa em cães infectados para servir como hospedeiro aos mosquitos hematófagos infectantes.
- É necessário tomar muito cuidado com a necropsia, já que as partículas virais infecciosas podem estar presentes em amostras teciduais.

RISCO A OUTROS ANIMAIS
O vírus não é transmitido do cão infectado para outros animais. A constatação de caso clínico de infecção pelo vírus Oeste do Nilo deve ser anotada como uma indicação de mosquitos infectados na região.

ABREVIATURAS
ELISA = ensaio imunoadsorvente ligado à enzima
PCR-RT = reação em cadeia da polimerase-transcriptase reversa ou por transcrição reversa.

RECURSOS DA INTERNET
http://npic.orst.edu/pest/mosquito/wnv.html (links para muitos outros sites).

Sugestões de Leitura
Njaa BL. Emerging viral encephalitides in dogs and cats. Vet Clin Small Anim 2008, 38:863–878.

Autor Edward J. Dubovi
Consultor Editorial Stephen C. Barr

Infecção por Astrovírus

CONSIDERAÇÕES GERAIS

REVISÃO
Uma infecção viral intestinal rara, caracterizada por enterite e diarreia.

IDENTIFICAÇÃO
- Gatos.
- Não há predisposição racial, sexual nem etária.

SINAIS CLÍNICOS
- Diarreia do intestino delgado frequentemente de coloração verde e aspecto aquoso.
- Os filhotes felinos exibem sinais mais graves.
- Pode ser grave e aguda o suficiente a ponto de provocar desidratação e anorexia.

CAUSAS E FATORES DE RISCO
- RNA vírus pequeno, não envelopado, do gênero *Astrovirus*.
- Não se conhecem detalhes a respeito da incidência/prevalência e dos fatores predisponentes.

DIAGNÓSTICO

DIAGNÓSTICO DIFERENCIAL
- Muitas causas de gastrenterite.
- Alergia alimentar.
- Ingestão de toxinas.
- Enteropatia inflamatória.
- Neoplasias.
- Parasitas intestinais.
- Infecções virais — panleucopenia, rotavírus, coronavírus entérico, calicivírus entérico.
- Infecções bacterianas — salmonelose, coliformes.
- Infecções por protozoários — *Giardia*, criptosporidiose.

HEMOGRAMA/BIOQUÍMICA/URINÁLISE
N/D.

OUTROS TESTES LABORATORIAIS
- Microscopia eletrônica das fezes — identifica as partículas do *Astrovirus*.
- O isolamento no laboratório não é uma tarefa fácil.

DIAGNÓSTICO POR IMAGEM
N/D.

MÉTODOS DIAGNÓSTICOS
Nenhum.

ACHADOS PATOLÓGICOS
Não há nenhum achado descrito; semelhantes a uma enterite branda, à rotavirose ou à coronavirose.

TRATAMENTO
- Controlar a diarreia.
- Restabelecer os equilíbrios hidreletrolíticos.

MEDICAÇÕES

MEDICAMENTO(S)
Não há medicamentos antivirais específicos para essa infecção.

CONTRAINDICAÇÕES/INTERAÇÕES POSSÍVEIS
Nenhuma.

ACOMPANHAMENTO

MONITORIZAÇÃO DO PACIENTE
Monitorizar os níveis hídricos e eletrolíticos.

PREVENÇÃO
Isolar os gatos acometidos durante a doença aguda.

COMPLICAÇÕES POSSÍVEIS
Infecções virais e bacterianas intestinais secundárias.

EVOLUÇÃO ESPERADA E PROGNÓSTICO
- A doença costuma durar <1 semana.
- Mortalidade — parece ser baixa.
- Prognóstico — bom.
- Se a diarreia persistir, pesquisar outras causas.

DIVERSOS

POTENCIAL ZOONÓTICO
A análise da sequência de *Astrovirus* de humanos e animais sugere que a transmissão homem-animal não ocorra.

Sugestões de Leitura
Barr MC, Olsen CW, Scott FW. Feline viral diseases. In: Ettinger SJ, Feldman EC, eds., Veterinary Internal Medicine. Philadelphia: Saunders, 1995, pp. 409–439.
Lukashov VV, Goudsmit J. Evolutionary relationships among Astroviridae. J Gen Virol 2002, 83:1397–1405.

Autor Fred W. Scott
Consultor Editorial Stephen C. Barr

INFECÇÃO POR CORONAVÍRUS — CÃES

CONSIDERAÇÕES GERAIS

REVISÃO
• Coronavírus entérico canino — surtos esporádicos de vômito e diarreia em cães; ampla distribuição mundial, inclusive em canídeos silvestres. • Coronavírus respiratório canino — associado ao complexo de doença respiratória infecciosa ("tosse dos canis"); também possui ampla distribuição mundial. • Infecção pelo coronavírus entérico canino — não costuma ser aparente; pode ocorrer uma enterite leve a grave, da qual a maioria dos cães se recupera; relato de óbito em filhotes jovens; restrita aos dois terços superiores do intestino delgado e aos linfonodos associados; ao contrário da infecção pelo parvovírus canino tipo 2, as células da cripta intestinal são poupadas. • Pode ocorrer uma infecção simultânea pelo parvovírus canino tipo 2; mais grave; frequentemente fatal. • Raros isolamentos podem causar doença sistêmica. • Os coronavírus sofrem rápida evolução e são altamente variáveis. As diferenças na virulência entre isolamentos individuais são prováveis.

IDENTIFICAÇÃO
• Sabe-se que apenas os cães silvestres e domésticos são suscetíveis à doença. • O coronavírus respiratório canino pode ser sazonal, sendo as infecções mais comuns no inverno. • O coronavírus canino pode causar infecções inaparentes em gatos. • Acomete todas as idades e raças.

SINAIS CLÍNICOS
• Bastante variáveis. Raramente, podem ocorrer isolamentos virulentos que causam doença sistêmica. • Adultos — a maior parte das infecções não é aparente. • Filhotes — podem desenvolver uma enterite grave e fatal. • Período de incubação —1-3 dias. • Início súbito de vômito, geralmente apenas um único episódio. • Diarreia — pode ser intensa; de coloração amarelo-esverdeada ou laranja; mole ou líquida; tipicamente fétida (sinal característico); pode persistir por alguns dias até >3 semanas; pode recidivar posteriormente. • Tosse; o coronavírus respiratório canino pode estar associado ao complexo de doença respiratória infecciosa canina. • Filhotes jovens — podem sofrer diarreia e desidratação prolongadas e graves. • Os sinais de anorexia e depressão são comuns. • A febre é rara. • Efeitos respiratórios leves. • Um isolamento de coronavírus canino identificado na Itália causou sintomas graves em um pequeno surto. Os sinais incluíram pirexia, anorexia, depressão, vômito, enterite hemorrágica, angústia respiratória e leucopenia que persistiram por >1 semana. Também ocorreram ataxia e crises convulsivas em filhotes caninos, com óbitos em 2 dias após o início dos sintomas.

CAUSAS E FATORES DE RISCO
• Coronavírus canino — estritamente relacionado com o vírus da PIF, o coronavírus entérico felino e o vírus da gastrenterite transmissível suína; não se sabe se os vírus de suínos e gatos provocam a doença natural em cães; facilmente inativado por desinfetantes comuns. • Coronavírus respiratório canino — distinto em termos genéticos e sorológicos do coronavírus canino; mais intimamente relacionado com o coronavírus bovino e o coronavírus humano OC43. • Estresse (p. ex., adestramento intensivo e lotação) — maior risco; surtos esporádicos têm ocorrido em cães que participam de exposições ou estão alojados em canis, onde as introduções de novos cães são frequentes; as lotações e as condições insalubres promovem a doença clínica. • Para o coronavírus canino, as fezes constituem a fonte primária de infecção; vírus disseminado por cerca de 2 semanas. • Para o coronavírus respiratório canino, as secreções respiratórias e os fômites são provavelmente as fontes de infecção.

DIAGNÓSTICO

DIAGNÓSTICO DIFERENCIAL
• Infecções causadas por bactérias, protozoários ou outros vírus intestinais. • Infecções causadas por outros agentes associados ao complexo de doença respiratória infecciosa. • Outras causas de doença respiratória superior leve a moderada. • Intoxicação ou intolerância alimentares.

HEMOGRAMA/BIOQUÍMICA/URINÁLISE
Normais.

OUTROS TESTES LABORATORIAIS
• Testes sorológicos — disponíveis; ainda não foram padronizados. • Títulos humorais (anticorpos) — geralmente baixos; podem não indicar infecção recente em virtude da alta taxa de infecção assintomática.

MÉTODOS DIAGNÓSTICOS
• Isolamento viral para o coronavírus entérico canino — efetuado a partir das fezes em culturas celulares felinas no início da diarreia. O isolamento viral para o coronavírus respiratório canino é difícil e, portanto, não recomendado. • PCR — com o uso de sondas específicas ao tipo e à cepa do vírus. • Imunofluorescência de cortes congelados do intestino delgado — para casos fatais; pode revelar os antígenos virais nas células de revestimento do epitélio viloso. • Microscopia eletrônica — partículas virais típicas do coronavírus canino; a interpretação requer experiência.

ACHADOS PATOLÓGICOS
• Os relatos de necropsia para o coronavírus entérico canino são limitados, exceto em casos de infecções experimentais. • Podem exibir alças dilatadas do intestino delgado, preenchidas por gás e material amarelo-esverdeado aquoso. • Macroscópicos — restritos à mucosa do intestino delgado, que pode ficar congesta ou hemorrágica; os linfonodos mesentéricos costumam estar infartados e edematosos. • Alterações microscópicas típicas — atrofia e fusão das vilosidades intestinais; aprofundamento das criptas; aumento na celularidade da lâmina própria; achatamento do epitélio, com incremento das células caliciformes. • Lesões — comumente mascaradas por autólise *post-mortem*. • A "cepa altamente patogênica" descrita na Itália causou lesões hemorrágicas nos pulmões e intestinos delgados, além de líquido abdominal serossanguinolento. Também se observaram hemorragias nos rins (infartos corticais) e linfonodos.

TRATAMENTO
• A maior parte dos cães acometidos recupera-se sem tratamento. • Para o coronavírus entérico canino, tratamento hidroeletrolítico de suporte, especialmente em casos de infecções graves com desidratação. • Para o coronavírus respiratório canino, o tratamento é o mesmo que para o complexo da doença respiratória infecciosa canina ("tosse dos canis").

MEDICAÇÕES

MEDICAMENTO(S)
Antibióticos — não costumam ser indicados, exceto em casos de enterite, sepse ou doença respiratória.

ACOMPANHAMENTO

PREVENÇÃO
• Vacinas — uso controverso; há vacinas inativadas e vivas modificadas disponíveis; aparentemente seguras; eficácia desconhecida, exceto por períodos breves (2-4 semanas) após a vacinação. Não recomendadas. Vacinas contra o coronavírus entérico canino não promovem a proteção cruzada contra o coronavírus respiratório canino. • Em canis, é essencial o rigor quanto ao isolamento e à higiene. • Coronavírus entérico canino e coronavírus respiratório canino — altamente contagiosos; disseminação rápida.

COMPLICAÇÕES POSSÍVEIS
Diarreia pelo coronavírus entérico canino — pode persistir por 10-12 dias; a recidiva é possível.

EVOLUÇÃO ESPERADA E PROGNÓSTICO
• Prognóstico — normalmente bom, exceto em casos de infecções graves de filhotes jovens. • A maioria dos casos recupera-se após alguns dias da doença. • As fezes moles ou líquidas podem persistir por várias semanas.

DIVERSOS

DISTÚRBIOS ASSOCIADOS
• Podem ocorrer infecções concomitantes pelo parvovírus canino ou por outros agentes. • Acredita-se que as infecções por outros patógenos entéricos intensifiquem a doença. • As infecções por outros patógenos respiratórios costumam estar associadas ao coronavírus respiratório canino.

ABREVIATURA(S)
• PIF = peritonite infecciosa felina. • PCR = reação em cadeia da polimerase.

Sugestões de Leitura
Decaro N, Buonavoglia C. An update on canine coronaviruses: Viral evolution and pathobiology. Vet Microbiology 2008, 132:221-234.
Erles K, Brownlie J. Canine respiratory coronavirus: An emerging pathogen in the canine infectious respiratory disease complex. Vet Clin North Am Small Anim Pract 2008, 38:815-825.

Autor John S. Parker
Consultor Editorial Stephen C. Barr

Infecção por Helicobacter

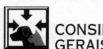

CONSIDERAÇÕES GERAIS

DEFINIÇÃO
Helicobacter spp. são bactérias microaerófilas gram-negativas e urease-positivas que variam de cocoides a curvas a espiraladas.

FISIOPATOLOGIA
Helicobacter spp. no Estômago
• A descoberta da associação do *Helicobacter pylori* com gastrite, úlceras pépticas e neoplasia gástrica fundamentalmente mudou a compreensão sobre doença gástrica em seres humanos.
• Os supostos mecanismos pelos quais o *H. pylori* altera a fisiologia gástrica em seres humanos incluem a ruptura da barreira da mucosa gástrica (em virtude da secreção de fosfolipases e citotoxinas vacuolizantes) e alterações na atividade secretora gástrica (p. ex., diminuição da secreção de somatostatina, induzindo à hipergastrinemia e hipercloridria).
• A infecção pelo *H. pylori* em seres humanos também é associada ao aumento da secreção de citocinas pró-inflamatórias, fator de necrose tumoral alfa e óxido nítrico.
• Foram isoladas várias espécies de *Helicobacter* do estômago de cães e gatos. Tipicamente, múltiplas espécies de *Helicobacter* estão presentes.
• Até o momento, o *H. pylori*, a espécie mais importante em seres humanos, só foi identificado em uma única colônia de gatos de laboratório.
• Uma possível relação entre causa e efeito de *Helicobacter* spp. com inflamação gástrica em cães e gatos não está solucionada; inflamação ou degeneração glandular acompanha a infecção em alguns cães e gatos, mas não em todos.
• Experimentos para determinar a patogenicidade do *H. pylori* em gatos SPF (livre de patógenos específicos) e de *H. pylori* e *H. felis* em cães gnotobióticos demonstraram gastrite, proliferação de folículos linfoides e respostas imunes humorais após infecção.

Helicobacter spp. no Fígado e nos Intestinos
• O papel desempenhado por *Helicobacter* spp. na doença intestinal e hepática em cães e gatos não está claro.
• Foram identificados vários microrganismos do tipo *Helicobacter* nas fezes de cães e gatos normais e diarreicos.
• *H. canis* também foi isolado do fígado de cão com hepatite multifocal ativa.

SISTEMA(S) ACOMETIDO(S)
• Gastrintestinal — estômago: infecção gástrica por *Helicobacter* spp. pode ocasionar gastrite; intestinos: pode ser observada a presença de diarreia em alguns cães com infecção pelo *H. canis*.
• Hepatobiliar — hepatite aguda foi associada à infecção por *H. canis*.

GENÉTICA
Nenhuma base genética para suscetibilidade à infecção por *Helicobacter* spp. foi estabelecida.

INCIDÊNCIA/PREVALÊNCIA
Helicobacter spp. Gástricas
• Microrganismos gástricos do tipo *Helicobacter* são altamente prevalentes em cães e gatos — 86% dos gatos de origem aleatória, 90% dos gatos de estimação clinicamente sadios, 67-86% dos cães de estimação saudáveis em termos clínicos. • Tais microrganismos do tipo *Helicobacter* foram demonstrados em amostras de biopsia gástrica em 57-76% dos gatos e 61-82% dos cães que foram levados ao veterinário por causa de vômitos recidivantes.
• Até o momento, o *H. pylori* foi identificado apenas em uma colônia de gatos de laboratório.

Helicobacter spp. Intestinais e Hepáticas
• O *H. canis* foi isolado de 4% de 1.000 cães avaliados.
• Foi relatado apenas 1 caso de hepatite associada ao *H. canis*.
• A prevalência de *H. fennelliae* e *H. cinaedi* permanece indeterminada.

DISTRIBUIÇÃO GEOGRÁFICA
• A infecção por *H. pylori* em seres humanos tem maior prevalência em países menos desenvolvidos.
• Não há informações disponíveis para cães e gatos.

IDENTIFICAÇÃO
Espécies
Cães e gatos.

Idade Média e Faixa Etária
• A infecção gástrica por *Helicobacter* spp. parece ser adquirida em uma idade jovem.
• O cão com hepatite associada ao *H. canis* tinha 2 meses de vida.

SINAIS CLÍNICOS
Achados Anamnésicos
• A infecção assintomática por *Helicobacter* é comum.
• Foram relatados, sem exceção, os sinais de vômito, anorexia, dor abdominal, perda de peso e/ou borborigmo em cães e gatos com infecções gástricas por *Helicobacter* spp.
• Diarreia em cães pode estar associada à infecção pelo *H. canis*.
• Há relatos de vômito, fraqueza e morte súbita em cão com infecção hepática por *H. canis*.

Achados do Exame Físico
• Em geral, não há nada digno de nota.
• Pode haver sinais de desidratação em decorrência da perda de líquidos e eletrólitos nos vômitos e/ou na diarreia.

CAUSAS
Helicobacter spp. Gástricas
• *H. felis*, *H. heilmannii* e *H. baculiformis* foram identificados em gatos. • *H. felis*, *H. bizzozeronii*, *H. salomonis*, *H. heilmannii*, *H. bilis*, *Flexispira rappini* e *H. cynogastricus* foram identificados em cães.

Helicobacter spp. Intestinais e Hepáticas
• *H. bilis*, *H. canis*, *H. cinaedi* e *Flexispira rappini* foram identificados nas fezes de cães normais e diarreicos. • *H. cinaedi* — foi identificado em 1 gato, mas seus significado é desconhecido. • *H. canis* — foi relatado em 1 cão com hepatite aguda.

FATORES DE RISCO
Condições sanitárias insatisfatórias e superlotação podem facilitar a disseminação da infecção.

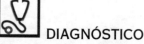

DIAGNÓSTICO

DIAGNÓSTICO DIFERENCIAL
Comentários Gerais
Altas taxas de prevalência de infecção por *Helicobacter* spp. em cães e gatos. Portanto, a exclusão de outras causas de doença gástrica e a identificação positiva de *Helicobacter* spp. são cruciais antes do diagnóstico de doença gastrintestinal atribuída à infecção por *Helicobacter* spp.

Helicobacteriose Gástrica
É imprescindível distinguir de outras causas de vômitos (doenças gastrintestinais tanto primárias como secundárias que possam causar vômitos).

Helicobacteriose Intestinal
É obrigatório diferenciar de outras causas de diarreia (doenças gastrintestinais tanto primárias como secundárias).

Helicobacteriose Hepática
É indispensável distinguir de outras causas de doença hepatobiliar.

HEMOGRAMA/BIOQUÍMICA/URINÁLISE
• Podem refletir anormalidades hidreletrolíticas secundárias a vômitos e/ou diarreia.
• Podem refletir alterações compatíveis com hepatopatia em pacientes com hepatite associada a *H. canis*.

OUTROS TESTES LABORATORIAIS
• O exame de esfregaços por impressão (decalque) da mucosa gástrica ou lavados gástricos com o uso dos corantes de May-Grünwald-Giemsa, Gram ou Diff-Quick é um teste sensível para *Helicobacter* spp. Pode ser facilmente realizado, embora não seja capaz de distinguir entre os diferentes microrganismos do tipo *Helicobacter*.
• Teste rápido da urease — requer amostra de biopsia gástrica, embora seja fácil de realizar em animais submetidos à gastroduodenoscopia.
• Foi demonstrado que o teste respiratório da ureia marcada com carbono 13 ou o exame de sangue são confiáveis para identificar os cães infectados, embora não estejam disponíveis atualmente no mercado.
• Cultura bacteriana — requer técnicas e meios especiais, apesar de ser pouco prática.
• PCR de DNA extraído de amostras de biopsia ou do suco gástrico.
• Testes sorológicos (ELISA) medem a IgG circulante no soro, mas esses testes não conseguem distinguir os diferentes microrganismos do tipo *Helicobacter*.
• A histopatologia possibilita o diagnóstico definitivo de infecção gástrica por *Helicobacter* spp., embora não seja capaz de diferenciar os diferentes microrganismos do tipo *Helicobacter*.

DIAGNÓSTICO POR IMAGEM
Radiografia e ultrassonografia abdominais costumam permanecer normais em pacientes apenas com infecção por *Helicobacter* spp.

MÉTODOS DIAGNÓSTICOS
Helicobacteriose Gástrica
• A endoscopia pode revelar nódulos superficiais que sugerem hiperplasia de folículos linfoides.
• Outros achados endoscópicos incluem espessamento difuso das pregas gástricas, achatamento da mucosa, hemorragias puntiformes e erosões.

Helicobacteriose Hepática
Biopsia/histopatologia hepática (coloração de Warthin-Starry) e cultura.

ACHADOS PATOLÓGICOS
• A identificação de microrganismos do tipo *Helicobacter* necessita da coloração especial de amostras de tecido com o corante de Warthin-

INFECÇÃO POR HELICOBACTER

Starry ou Steiner modificado. O corante H&E de rotina pode revelar microrganismos maiores do tipo *Helicobacter*, mas os menores costumam passar despercebidos.
• Doença gástrica associada a *H. spp.* — gastrite linfocítico-plasmocitária e hiperplasia de folículos linfoides; raramente há infiltrações neutrofílicas. Não há relatos de úlceras gástricas em cães e gatos.
• Hepatite associada ao *H. canis* — necrose hepatocelular; infiltração do parênquima hepático por células mononucleares, além de bactérias espiraladas a curvas predominantemente nos canalículos biliares.

TRATAMENTO

CUIDADO(S) DE SAÚDE ADEQUADO(S)
• A patogenicidade de *Helicobacter* spp. em cães e gatos ainda não está esclarecida. portanto, não há diretrizes geralmente aceitas para o tratamento.
• Atualmente, não há indicação para tratar animais assintomáticos com infecção por *Helicobacter* spp.
• A erradicação de *Helicobacter* spp. gástricas deve ser considerada apenas em cães e gatos infectados com sinais clínicos compatíveis que não podem ser atribuídos a outro processo mórbido.

CUIDADO(S) DE ENFERMAGEM
Fluidoterapia em pacientes desidratados.

DIETA
Dietas facilmente digeríveis em pacientes com sinais gastrintestinais.

ORIENTAÇÃO AO PROPRIETÁRIO
Explicar a dificuldade de se estabelecer o diagnóstico definitivo, a alta prevalência de infecções por microrganismos do tipo *Helicobacter* em cães e gatos normais, o potencial de recidiva e o potencial zoonótico, apesar de mínimo, dessas infecções.

MEDICAÇÕES

Comentários Gerais
• A terapia tripla (combinação de dois antibióticos e um antissecretor) é eficaz em seres humanos com infecção pelo *H. pylori*, com taxas de cura de aproximadamente 90%.
• A terapia combinada pode eliminar as infecções por *Helicobacter* spp. em cães e gatos de forma menos eficaz que em humanos.
• Tratar por 2-3 semanas.

MEDICAMENTO(S) DE ESCOLHA
Antibióticos (Dois com Um Antissecretor)
• Claritromicina (cães, 5 mg/kg VO a cada 12 h; gatos, 62,5 mg/gato VO a cada 12 h).
• Metronidazol (cães, 11-15 mg/kg VO a cada 12 h; gatos, 12,5 mg/kg VO a cada 12 h).
• Amoxicilina (22 mg/kg VO a cada 12 h).
• Azitromicina (5 mg/kg VO a cada 24 h).
• Tetraciclina (20 mg/kg VO a cada 8 h).

• Subsalicilato de bismuto é protetor de mucosa e antiendotoxêmico, além de ter propriedades antibacterianas fracas; não se sabe qual propriedade é responsável por seus efeitos benéficos em infecções por microrganismos do tipo *Helicobacter* (0,22 mL/kg de 130 mg/15 mL de solução de Pepto-Bismol® VO a cada 4-6 h).

Agentes Antissecretores (Um com Dois Antibióticos)
• Omeprazol (0,7-1 mg/kg VO a cada 12 h).
• Famotidina (0,5 mg/kg VO a cada 12-24 h).
• Ranitidina (1-2 mg/kg VO a cada 12 h).
• Cimetidina (5-10 mg/kg VO a cada 6-8 h).

Helicobacter spp. Intestinais e Hepáticas em Cães
A combinação de amoxicilina e metronidazol nas doses supramencionadas pode ser eficaz.

CONTRAINDICAÇÕES
Hipersensibilidade a um dos antibióticos.

MEDICAMENTO(S) ALTERNATIVO(S)
Pacientes com infecções por microrganismos do tipo *Helicobacter* e gastrite que não respondem à antibioticoterapia em geral recebem terapia imunossupressora (prednisolona, ou outros) para enteropatia inflamatória com acometimento gástrico.

ACOMPANHAMENTO

MONITORIZAÇÃO DO PACIENTE
• Testes sorológicos não são úteis para confirmar a erradicação de microrganismos gástricos do tipo *Helicobacter* — os títulos séricos de IgG podem não diminuir por até 6 meses após a eliminação da infecção.
• O teste respiratório de ureia marcada com carbono 13 e o exame de sangue foram avaliados para monitorizar a erradicação de microrganismos do tipo *Helicobacter* em cães e gatos, embora esses testes não estejam atualmente disponíveis no mercado.
• Se os vômitos persistirem ou voltarem após a interrupção da terapia combinada, talvez haja necessidade de repetir a biopsia endoscópica para determinar se a infecção foi erradicada com sucesso.

PREVENÇÃO
Evitar superlotação e más condições sanitárias.

EVOLUÇÃO ESPERADA E PROGNÓSTICO
• A eficácia dos esquemas terapêuticos empregados atualmente em cães e gatos para erradicar as infecções por *Helicobacter* spp. é questionável.
• Metronidazol (20 mg/kg VO a cada 12 h), amoxicilina (20 mg/kg VO a cada 12 h) e famotidina (0,5 mg/kg VO a cada 12 h) por 14 dias erradicaram a infecção por *Helicobacter* spp. com eficácia em 6 de 8 cães avaliados 3 dias após o tratamento, mas todos os cães foram recolonizados por volta do 28° dia após o término do tratamento.

• Claritromicina (30 mg/gato VO a cada 12 h), metronidazol (30 mg/gato VO a cada 12 h), ranitidina (20 mg/gato VO a cada 12 h) e bismuto (40 mg/gato VO a cada 12 h) por 4 dias foram eficazes para erradicar o *H. heilmannii* em 11 de 11 gatos por 10 dias, mas 2 gatos foram reinfectados 42 dias depois do tratamento.
• Amoxicilina (20 mg/kg VO a cada 8 h), metronidazol (20 mg/kg VO a cada 8 h) e omeprazol (0,7 mg/kg VO a cada 24 h) por 21 dias erradicaram transitoriamente o *H. pylori* em 6 gatos, mas todos foram reinfectados 6 semanas após o tratamento. (*Nota:* essa dose de metronidazol tem potencial de toxicidade).

DIVERSOS

DISTÚRBIOS ASSOCIADOS
Outras doenças gástricas.

FATORES RELACIONADOS COM A IDADE
Os microrganismos gástricos do tipo *Helicobacter* parecem ser adquiridos em uma idade jovem.

POTENCIAL ZOONÓTICO
• A alta prevalência de *Helicobacter* spp. em cães e gatos aumenta a possibilidade de que os animais de estimação sirvam como reservatórios para a transmissão dessas espécies de microrganismos para os seres humanos.
• *H. pylori*, *H. heilmannii* e *H. felis* foram isolados de humanos com gastrite.
• *H. fennelliae* e *H. cinaedi* foram isolados de pessoas imunocomprometidas com proctite e colite.
• *H. cinaedi* e *H. canis* também foram associados à septicemia em pessoas.
• *H. pylori* não foi identificado em cães ou gatos de estimação.

GESTAÇÃO/FERTILIDADE/REPRODUÇÃO
Evitar o uso de metronidazol e tetraciclina em animais prenhes.

SINÔNIMO(S)
• Bactéria espiral gástrica.
• Gastroespirilo.

VER TAMBÉM
• Gastrite Crônica.
• Vômito Crônico.

ABREVIATURA(S)
• ELISA = ensaio imunoabsorvente ligado à enzima.
• H&E = hematoxilina e eosina.
• PCR = reação em cadeia da polimerase.

Sugestões de Leitura
Leib MS, Duncan RB, Ward DL. Triple antimicrobial therapy and acid suppression in dogs with chronic vomiting and gastric *Helicobacter* spp. J Vet Intern Med 2007, 21:1185-1192.

Autores Jan S. Suchodolski e Jörg M. Steiner
Consultor Editorial Albert E. Jergens

Infecção por Herpes-Vírus — Cães

CONSIDERAÇÕES GERAIS

REVISÃO
- Doença sistêmica geralmente fatal em filhotes de cães, causada pelo herpes-vírus canino.
- Herpes-vírus canino — comum na população canina mundial, embora a doença seja pouco frequente; permanece latente em vários tecidos após a infecção primária; latente nos gânglios do nervo trigêmeo; pode ser excretado nas secreções nasais em intervalos imprevisíveis; a recidiva pode ser provocada por estresse ou tratamento com corticosteroide; isolado de cães com doença respiratória, mas sem ligação causal demonstrada.
- Alta mortalidade nas ninhadas; acredita-se que a regulação deficiente da temperatura corporal e os mecanismos imaturos da resposta imunológica sejam responsáveis pela suscetibilidade excepcional de filhotes de cães com menos de 2-3 semanas de vida.
- Todos os sistemas orgânicos são acometidos.
- Doença ocular em cães com mais de 3-4 semanas de vida pode ser mais comum do que se pensava.
- Fêmeas adultas não prenhes costumam ter infecções localizadas inaparentes na nasofaringe ou na genitália externa.
- Infecções transplacentárias nas últimas 3-4 semanas de gestação — mortes fetais, frequentemente com mumificação; abortamentos; nascimento de filhotes caninos mortos ou agonizantes.
- Há relatos de infecções genitais localizadas em ambos os sexos.

IDENTIFICAÇÃO
- Apenas os membros da família canina (cães, coiotes e lobos) são suscetíveis.
- A morte costuma ocorrer entre 9 e 14 dias após o nascimento; variação de 1 dia (infecção pré-natal) a cerca de 1 mês (infecção neonatal).
- Mais comumente relatada em cães de raças puras, embora não haja predominância racial.

SINAIS CLÍNICOS
- Dispneia. • Secreção nasal serosa a mucopurulenta. • Anorexia. • Fezes moles, inodoras, amarelo ou verde-acinzentadas. • Choro intenso persistente. • Sinais de encefalite.
- Respiração ofegante grave antes da morte.
- Ocasionalmente, observam-se hemorragias petequiais nas mucosas. • Período de incubação de 4-6 dias em cães neonatos. • Início súbito; a morte ocorre 12-36 h depois. • Alguns filhotes são encontrados mortos sem sinais premonitórios.
- Ocasionalmente, os filhotes com sinais leves sobrevivem, mas depois costumam desenvolver ataxia, sinais vestibulares persistentes ou cegueira.
- Fêmeas adultas podem ter lesões linfofoliculares ou hemorrágicas na vagina. • Infertilidade — há indícios de soroprevalência elevada em canis com problemas reprodutivos. • Conjuntivite — o herpes-vírus canino pode ser uma causa comum de conjuntivite idiopática adquirida. • Ceratite pelo herpes-vírus canino — apesar de relatada, a incidência é atualmente desconhecida.

CAUSAS E FATORES DE RISCO
- Herpes-vírus canino — herpes-vírus típico; há apenas um único sorotipo descrito; um vírus atípico foi isolado na Grã-Bretanha a partir de lesões semelhantes à varíola canina no trato genital e associado a lesões genitais masculinas, abortamentos e natimortos.
- Fêmeas jovens suscetíveis e seus filhotes recém-nascidos estão sob maior risco.
- Canis de reprodução fechados — herpes-vírus canino endêmico; além de a infecção ser menos comum, a maioria dos adultos é imune; cadelas reprodutoras suscetíveis recém-introduzidas também estão sob alto risco.
- Já se observou a ocorrência de surtos de abortamentos com perdas maciças de filhotes quando cadelas prenhes mantidas em lares particulares foram reunidas para dar cria.
- Em cães adultos, medicamentos imunossupressores podem provocar reativação de herpes-vírus canino latente com doença ocular transitória associada.

DIAGNÓSTICO

DIAGNÓSTICO DIFERENCIAL
- Bactérias (brucelose, coliformes ou estreptococos), toxoplasmose, substâncias tóxicas — sem lesões macroscópicas típicas do herpes-vírus canino.
- Vírus diminuto canino (parvovírus canino tipo 1) — causa doença entérica ou respiratória; sem lesões características do herpes-vírus canino.
- Vírus da cinomose e adenovírus canino tipo 1 (hepatite canina) — incomuns; sem lesões renais características do herpes-vírus canino.

HEMOGRAMA/BIOQUÍMICA/URINÁLISE
Pode ocorrer trombocitopenia.

OUTROS TESTES LABORATORIAIS
A sorologia tem pouco valor.

MÉTODOS DIAGNÓSTICOS
- Cortes de tecido congelado — colorações para imunofluorescência ou imunoperoxidase; revelam o antígeno viral na maioria dos órgãos, especialmente nas áreas de lesão.
- Culturas celulares — o isolamento viral de vários tecidos é facilmente executado, em particular dos pulmões e rins; refrigerar as amostras, não congelá-las.
- PCR em tempo real de DNA isolado das amostras de tecidos sob suspeita (p. ex., *swabs* conjuntivais).

ACHADOS PATOLÓGICOS

Macroscópicos
- Lesões características — necrose focal disseminada; hemorragia em vários órgãos.
- Rins — áreas hemorrágicas difusas, focos necróticos e infartos hemorrágicos são patognomônicos.
- Pulmões, fígado, adrenais — focos difusos de hemorragia e necrose.
- Acometimento variável do intestino delgado.
- Linfonodos e baço — aumento generalizado; achado compatível.

Histopatológicos
- Focos de necrose perivascular — com ou sem uma leve infiltração celular; rins, pulmões, fígado, baço, intestino delgado e cérebro.
- Lesões no SNC de filhotes que se recuperam — ganglioneurite não supurativa; meningoencefalite; alterações necróticas no cerebelo e na retina; inclusões intranucleares acidófilas podem ser observadas, mas não são abundantes.
- Lesões necrosantes — podem ser vistas na placenta fetal.

TRATAMENTO
- Não recomendado. • Terapia medicamentosa antiviral — em geral, não é bem-sucedida. • Soro imune obtido de cadelas recuperadas — benéfico para diminuir as mortes de filhotes quando o antissoro é administrado antes do início da doença.

MEDICAÇÕES

MEDICAMENTO(S)
N/D.

CONTRAINDICAÇÕES/INTERAÇÕES POSSÍVEIS
O uso de medicamentos imunossupressores em animais adultos pode induzir à recidiva de herpes-vírus canino latente, levando possivelmente à doença ocular (conjuntivite e/ou ceratite).

ACOMPANHAMENTO
- É possível esperar ninhadas normais de cadelas que sofreram perda de filhotes ou abortamentos.
- Existe uma vacina de subunidade inativada disponível na Europa. Seu uso é sugerido para cadelas prenhes sob risco. No entanto, faltam dados a campo a respeito de seu benefício.
- Isolar fêmeas prenhes, em especial as jovens, quando introduzidas em um canil; os adultos costumam eliminar o herpes-vírus canino latente nas secreções nasais por 1-2 semanas após o encontro com cães recém-introduzidos na criação.
- Os filhotes que sobrevivem podem sofrer surdez, cegueira, encefalopatia ou dano renal.

DIVERSOS

FATORES RELACIONADOS COM A IDADE
- Cães de todas as idades são suscetíveis.
- Ocorre doença fatal apenas em filhotes caninos infectados durante o período neonatal (1-10 dias após o nascimento).

GESTAÇÃO/FERTILIDADE/REPRODUÇÃO
Infecção das progenitoras durante as últimas 3 semanas de gestação — infecções fetais com morte e mumificação ou filhotes doentes que morrem logo após o nascimento.

ABREVIATURA(S)
- PCR = reação em cadeia da polimerase.
- SNC = sistema nervoso central.

Sugestões de Leitura
Green CE, Carmichael LE. Canine herpesvirus infection. In: Greene CE, ed., Infectious Diseases of the Dog and Cat, 3rd ed. St. Louis: Saunders Elsevier, 2006, pp. 47-53.

Autor John S. Parker
Consultor Editorial Stephen C. Barr

Infecção por Herpes-Vírus — Gatos

CONSIDERAÇÕES GERAIS

DEFINIÇÃO
Causadora de doença aguda em gatos domésticos e muitas espécies exóticas de gatos, caracterizada por espirro, febre, rinite, conjuntivite e ceratite ulcerativa.

FISIOPATOLOGIA
O FHV-1 provoca uma infecção citolítica aguda do epitélio respiratório ou ocular após exposição oral, intranasal ou conjuntival. Esse vírus intracelular passa de célula em célula e não estimula uma forte resposta imune do hospedeiro.

SISTEMA(S) ACOMETIDO(S)
- Tegumentar — pode ocorrer dermatite herpética próxima aos orifícios nasais.
- Oftálmico — frequentemente causa conjuntivite com secreção ocular serosa ou purulenta; pode ocorrer ceratite ulcerativa ou panoftalmite.
- Reprodutor — a infecção *in utero* causada por infecção de gatas prenhes pode resultar em infecções herpéticas graves em neonatos.
- Respiratório — rinite com espirro e secreção nasal serosa a purulenta; pode ocorrer traqueíte; a sinusite crônica pode ser uma sequela.

GENÉTICA
N/D.

INCIDÊNCIA/PREVALÊNCIA
- Comum, especialmente em casas com muitos gatos ou outros locais que albergam grande número de gatos, em razão da facilidade de transmissão. Os gatis e abrigos constituem a fonte de grande parte das infecções.
- Perpetuada por portadores latentes que albergam o vírus nos gânglios nervosos, sobretudo no gânglio trigêmeo.

DISTRIBUIÇÃO GEOGRÁFICA
Encontrada no mundo todo.

IDENTIFICAÇÃO
Espécies
Acomete todos os gatos domésticos e muitos gatos exóticos.

Raça(s) Predominante(s)
- Nenhuma.
- Como as raças braquicefálicas apresentam doença mais grave de córnea, é mais provável que elas sofram sequestro nessa estrutura ocular.

Idade Média e Faixa Etária
- Gatos de todas as idades.
- Os filhotes são mais suscetíveis.

Sexo Predominante
N/D.

SINAIS CLÍNICOS
Achados Anamnésicos
- Início agudo de espirro paroxístico.
- Blefarospasmo e secreção ocular.
- Anorexia — por febre alta, mal-estar generalizado ou incapacidade olfativa.
- Sinais recorrentes — portadores.
- Abortamento.

Achados do Exame Físico
- Febre — de até 41°C.
- Rinite — secreção nasal serosa, mucopurulenta ou purulenta.
- Conjuntivite — secreção ocular serosa, mucopurulenta ou purulenta.
- Rinite/sinusite crônica — secreção nasal purulenta crônica; a presença de sinusite não pode ser determinada sem a obtenção de radiografias.
- Ceratite — ulceração, descemetocele ou panoftalmite.

CAUSAS
FHV-1, do qual existe apenas 1 sorotipo.

FATORES DE RISCO
- Ausência de vacinação contra FHV-1, embora as vacinas não confiram imunidade esterilizante.
- Ambientes com inúmeros gatos, superlotação, ventilação insatisfatória, baixas condições sanitárias, nutrição deficiente ou estresse físico ou psicológico.
- Gestação e lactação.
- Doenças concomitantes, especialmente aquelas causadas por microrganismos imunossupressores ou outros microrganismos respiratórios.
- Filhotes nascidos de gatas portadoras — infectados com aproximadamente 5 semanas de vida.

DIAGNÓSTICO

DIAGNÓSTICO DIFERENCIAL
- Infecção por calicivírus felino — menos espirro, conjuntivite, ceratite ulcerativa; pode causar estomatite ulcerativa, pneumonia.
- Infecção por *Chlamydophila* felino — conjuntivite mais crônica, que pode ser unilateral; pneumonite; inclusões intracitoplasmáticas em raspados conjuntivais; responsiva a tetraciclinas ou cloranfenicol.
- Infecção bacteriana (*Bordetella*, *Haemophilus*, ou *Pasteurella*) — menor envolvimento nasocular; frequentemente responsiva a antibióticos.

HEMOGRAMA/BIOQUÍMICA/URINÁLISE
- Não são diagnósticos.
- Pode ocorrer leucopenia transitória seguida por leucocitose.

OUTROS TESTES LABORATORIAIS
- O teste de PCR feito a partir de *swabs* faríngeos e conjuntivais identificará a presença do vírus; esse teste é mais sensível do que outras modalidades diagnósticas. Pode ser transitoriamente positivo após vacinação com vírus vivo modificado de FHV-1.
- Ensaio de imunofluorescência — raspados nasais ou conjuntivais; detecção viral.
- Isolamento viral — amostra de *swab* faríngeo.
- Esfregaços conjuntivais corados — detectam os corpúsculos de inclusão intranucleares.

DIAGNÓSTICO POR IMAGEM
Radiografia — projeções ventrodorsal e rostrocaudal (tangencial ou *skyline*) de boca aberta do crânio revelam a presença de doença crônica na cavidade nasal e nos seios frontais; esse exame não é capaz de diferenciar com segurança os quadros de infecção, neoplasia e pólipos inflamatórios; ausência de achados radiográficos anormais em caso de doença aguda.

MÉTODOS DIAGNÓSTICOS
N/D.

ACHADOS PATOLÓGICOS
- Macroscópicos — secreção nasocular; edema de mucosa do epitélio das vias aéreas superiores; traqueíte; sinusite; ceratite ulcerativa; panoftalmite.
- Microscópicos — edema de submucosa; infiltração dos tecidos respiratórios superiores e conjuntivais por células inflamatórias; sinusite crônica; corpúsculos de inclusão intranucleares nas células epiteliais.

TRATAMENTO

CUIDADO(S) DE SAÚDE ADEQUADO(S)
Tratamento hospitalar — suporte nutricional e hídrico para gatos anoréxicos; evitar o contágio.

CUIDADO(S) DE ENFERMAGEM
- Tratamento ambulatorial — manter o paciente dentro de casa para evitar o estresse induzido pelo ambiente, o que pode estender a evolução da doença.
- Fluidoterapia — intravenosa ou subcutânea; para corrigir e evitar a desidratação; para afinar as secreções nasais.

ATIVIDADE
Isolar os gatos acometidos durante a fase aguda, pois tais animais são contagiosos.

DIETA
- Tratamento ambulatorial — estimular o consumo alimentar para evitar anorexia, que induz a uma cascata de consequências negativas; oferecer alimentos com paladar e odor atrativos.
- Tratamento hospitalar — alimentação enteral forçada para gatos anoréxicos; remover as secreções nasais (com isso, pode ocorrer respiração nasal) antes de iniciar a alimentação via sonda orogástrica; evitar o uso de sondas nasesofágicas por causa de rinite.

ORIENTAÇÃO AO PROPRIETÁRIO
- Informar ao proprietário sobre a natureza contagiosa da doença.
- Discutir os protocolos de vacinação adequados e a vacinação precoce de gatos em ambientes e casas com inúmeros animais dessa espécie.
- Comunicar ao proprietário o fato de que o desmame e o isolamento precoces de todos os outros gatos, exceto dos companheiros de ninhada, podem evitar as infecções.

CONSIDERAÇÕES CIRÚRGICAS
Pode haver a necessidade da implantação cirúrgica de sondas de alimentação (inseridas via esofagostomia ou gastrostomia) quando ocorre anorexia prolongada.

MEDICAÇÕES

MEDICAMENTO(S) DE ESCOLHA
- Antibióticos de amplo espectro — ampicilina (20-40 mg/kg VO a cada 8 h; 10-20 mg/kg IV, IM, SC a cada 6-8 h) ou amoxicilina (10-40 mg/kg a cada 8-12 h VO, IM, SC) para infecções bacterianas secundárias.
- Combinações de antibióticos — ampicilina ou amoxicilina e alguma fluoroquinolona (enrofloxacino [2,5 mg/kg VO, IM, IV a cada 12 h], orbifloxacino [2,5-7,5 mg/kg VO a cada 24 h], marbofloxacino [2,75-5,55 mg/kg VO a cada 24 h]) para infecções bacterianas secundárias.
- A lisina (500 mg a cada 12 h) pode ter algum efeito viricida.
- Antibióticos oftálmicos — para ceratite.

Infecção por Herpes-Vírus — Gatos

- Antivirais oftálmicos — idoxuridina, trifluridina; para úlceras herpéticas; devem ser instilados a cada 2 horas para obtenção de efeito significativo.
- Há certa evidência de que a administração de vacina intranasal 2-6 dias antes da exposição resultará na redução dos sinais clínicos. Essa medida pode ser útil em caso de surto em um ambiente repleto de gatos.

CONTRAINDICAÇÕES
- A idoxuridina oftálmica pode ser dolorosa em alguns gatos; interromper a medicação.
- Corticosteroides sistêmicos — podem induzir à recidiva em gatos cronicamente infectados.
- Corticosteroides oftálmicos — podem predispor à ceratite ulcerativa.
- Descongestionantes nasais em gotas — cloridrato de oximetazolina a 0,25%; diminuem a secreção nasal; contraindicados, pois alguns gatos rejeitam e outros sofrem rinorreia de rebote.

PRECAUÇÕES
A morte costuma advir de suporte nutricional e hídrico inadequado ou imunossupressão causada por FeLV ou FIV.

MEDICAMENTO(S) ALTERNATIVO(S)
Fanciclovir — os relatos iniciais indicam eficácia em uma dose de 15 mg/kg a cada 8-12 h VO; medicamento caro.

ACOMPANHAMENTO

MONITORIZAÇÃO DO PACIENTE
Monitorizar o apetite atentamente; hospitalizar o paciente para o fornecimento de alimentação enteral forçada em caso de anorexia.

PREVENÇÃO
Vacinas
- Vacinação de rotina com vacina de vírus vivo modificado ou vírus inativado — previne o desenvolvimento de doença grave; não impede a ocorrência de infecção e replicação viral local com doença clínica leve e disseminação viral.
- Vacinar os animais com 8-10 e 12-14 semanas de vida e fornecer reforços anuais para obtenção de máxima proteção, especialmente em populações de alto risco.
- Casas ou ambientes endêmicos com múltiplos gatos — vacinar os filhotes com uma dose de vacina intranasal com 10-14 dias de vida e, depois, por via parenteral com 6, 10 e 14 semanas de vida; isolar a ninhada de *todos* os outros gatos por volta de 3-5 semanas de vida; em seguida, utilizar o protocolo de vacinação de filhotes para evitar infecções precoces.

COMPLICAÇÕES POSSÍVEIS
- Rinite ou rinossinusite crônica com espirro e secreção nasal prolongados.
- Ceratite ulcerativa herpética.
- Sequestro de córnea que deve ser removido por via cirúrgica.
- Obstrução permanente do ducto nasolacrimal com secreção ocular crônica.

EVOLUÇÃO ESPERADA E PROGNÓSTICO
- Em geral, 7-10 dias antes da remissão espontânea, caso não ocorram infecções bacterianas secundárias.
- O prognóstico geralmente é bom se as terapias hídrica e nutricional forem adequadas.

DIVERSOS

DISTÚRBIOS ASSOCIADOS
Doenças respiratórias virais ou bacterianas simultâneas.

FATORES RELACIONADOS COM A IDADE
Mais grave em filhotes de gatos.

POTENCIAL ZOONÓTICO
Nenhum.

GESTAÇÃO/FERTILIDADE/REPRODUÇÃO
As gatas prenhes que desenvolvem a doença podem transmitir o FHV-1 aos filhotes no útero, resultando em abortamento ou doença neonatal.

SINÔNIMOS
- Coriza.
- Rinotraqueíte felina.
- Rino.

VER TAMBÉM
- Bordetelose — Gatos.
- Infecção por Calicivírus Felino.

ABREVIATURAS
- FeLV = vírus da leucemia felina.
- FHV-1 = herpes-vírus felino tipo 1.
- FIV = vírus da imunodeficiência felina.
- PCR = reação em cadeia da polimerase.

Sugestões de Leitura
Gaskell RM, Dawson S, Radford A, et al. Feline herpesvirus. Vet Res 2007, 38(2):337-354.
Maggs DJ. Update on pathogenesis, diagnosis, and treatment of feline herpesvirus type 1. Clin Tech Small Anim Pract 2005, 20(2):94-101.
Malik R, Lessels NS, Webb S, et al. Treatment of feline herpesvirus-1 associated disease. J Feline Med Surg 2009, 11(1):40-48.
Thiry E, Addie D, Belak S, et al. Feline herpesvirus infection: ABCD guidelines on prevention and management. J Feline Med Surg 2009, 11(7):547-555.

Autor Gary D. Norsworthy
Consultor Editorial Stephen C. Barr

INFECÇÃO POR OLLULANIS

CONSIDERAÇÕES GERAIS

REVISÃO
Um nematódeo tricostrongiloide — os vermes adultos são encontrados na parede gástrica de gatos, causando gastrite crônica com consequente anorexia, vômito e perda de peso.

IDENTIFICAÇÃO
• Gatos de colônia — predispostos, provavelmente por terem acesso direto ao vômito de outros gatos.
• Gatos errantes que vivem em áreas urbanas intensamente povoadas por gatos — alta incidência de infecção.
• Chitas, leões, tigres, onças cativos — suscetíveis à infecção.

SINAIS CLÍNICOS
• Vômito, anorexia, perda de peso crônicos.
• Morte causada por gastrite crônica.

CAUSAS E FATORES DE RISCO
• *Ollulanus tricuspis* — os adultos (até 1 mm de comprimento apenas) espiralam-se na mucosa gástrica, causando erosões superficiais.
• Com o passar do tempo, as erosões gástricas podem se agravar com inflamação acentuada, acúmulo de agregados linfoides e alterações fibrosas na mucosa e submucosa.
• Ovos — eclodem dentro dos vermes fêmeas com subsequente desenvolvimento das larvas em larvas L3 infectantes.
• Larvas L3 — eliminadas no conteúdo gástrico e expelidas pelo vômito; infectantes para outros gatos.
• Vermes machos e fêmeas adultos eliminados no vômito — também são capazes de infectar outros gatos.
• Infecção distribuída por toda a América do Norte, Austrália, Nova Zelândia, Europa, Argentina, Chile.
• Alemanha — até 40% dos gatos de vida livre podem estar infectados.

DIAGNÓSTICO

DIAGNÓSTICO DIFERENCIAL
• Outras causas de vômito, incluindo:
• Dieta.
• Toxinas — chumbo, etileno glicol.
• Distúrbio metabólico — diabetes melito, doença renal/hepática, acidose, intermação, hipoadrenocorticismo, hipertireoidismo.
• Anormalidades gástricas — enteropatia inflamatória, neoplasia, obstrução, gastrite atrófica, úlceras, dilatação/vólvulo, infestação parasitária como *Physaloptera*.
• Distúrbios da junção gastresofágica — hérnia hiatal.
• Distúrbios do intestino delgado — enteropatia inflamatória, neoplasia, infecção fúngica/viral, obstrução, íleo paralítico.
• Distúrbios do intestino grosso — colite, obstipação, enteropatia inflamatória.
• Distúrbios abdominais — pancreatite, gastrinoma, peritonite, esteatite, piometra, hérnia diafragmática, neoplasia.
• Distúrbios neurológicos — doença psicogênica, doença do movimento (cinetose), lesões vestibulares, traumatismo craniencefálico, neoplasia cerebral.
• Diversas — dirofilariose e cardiopatia.

HEMOGRAMA/BIOQUÍMICA/URINÁLISE
Reflete os sinais clínicos de diarreia/vômito — desidratação.

OUTROS TESTES LABORATORIAIS
• Larvas (ou ovos) — raramente encontrados nas fezes, pois são digeridos dentro do trato GI.
• Vômito — examinar em busca das larvas L3.
• O vômito pode ser induzido no gato com o medicamento xilazina (0,5 mg/kg IV, ou 1 mg/kg IM) — medida bem-sucedida em cerca de 70% dos casos.

DIAGNÓSTICO POR IMAGEM
Ultrassonografia abdominal — pode revelar espessamento gástrico; raramente se observam os parasitas.

MÉTODOS DIAGNÓSTICOS
• Visualização dos vermes por meio de endoscópio — difícil em virtude do tamanho dos vermes.
• Lavagem gástrica — fazer a coleta do lavado com salina seguida por centrifugação para precipitar as larvas L3 ou usar a técnica de Baermann.
• Histopatologia — a biopsia gástrica ocasionalmente mostra os parasitas.

TRATAMENTO

• Poucos tratamentos foram relatados.
• Fembendazol, oxfendazol e pamoato de pirantel — todos já foram utilizados, mas provavelmente são ineficazes.
• Embora os gatos possam apresentar uma melhora clínica, os parasitas não são removidos do estômago.

MEDICAÇÕES

MEDICAMENTO(S)
• Tetramisol — administrado como uma formulação a 2,5% na dose de 5 mg/kg VO em dose única; eficaz.

CONTRAINDICAÇÕES/INTERAÇÕES POSSÍVEIS
Tetramisol — a essa dose, tal medicamento não deve causar nenhum efeito colateral em gatos.

ACOMPANHAMENTO

Alertar o proprietário para ficar atento aos vômitos adicionais — tratar com outro ciclo de tetramisol se tais vômitos ocorrerem.

DIVERSOS

A infecção por *Ollulanus* foi identificada em um gato com adenocarcinoma gástrico concomitante.

ABREVIATURAS
GI = gastrintestinal.

Sugestões de Leitura
Barr SC, Bowman DD. *Ollulanus* infection. In: Canine and Feline Infectious Diseases and Parasitology. Ames, IA: Blackwell, 2006, pp. 385-387.
Bowman DD, Hendrix CM, Lindsay DS, et al. *Ollulanus tricuspis*. In: Feline Clinical Parasitology. Ames: Iowa State University Press, 2002, pp. 262-265.
Cecchi R, Wills SJ, Dean R, et al. Demonstration of *Ollulanus tricuspis* in the stomach of domestic cats by biopsy. J Comp Pathol 2006, 134:374-377.
Dennis MM, Bennett N, Ehrhart EJ. Gastric adenocarcinoma and chronic gastritis in two related Persian cats. Vet Pathol 2006, 43:358-362.

Autor Stephen C. Barr
Consultor Editorial Stephen C. Barr

Infecção por Reovírus

CONSIDERAÇÕES GERAIS

REVISÃO
- Vírus órfão entérico respiratório (reovírus) — gênero pertencente à família Reoviridae; RNA vírus não envelopado de fita dupla; isolado a partir dos tratos entérico e respiratório; não associado a qualquer doença conhecida (daí a denominação *órfão*).
- Ubíquo em termos de distribuição geográfica e faixa de hospedeiros; acomete praticamente todas as espécies de mamíferos, incluindo os seres humanos.
- Vírus — infecta células epiteliais maduras nas extremidades luminais das vilosidades intestinais; provoca destruição celular, resultando na atrofia das vilosidades (semelhante ao rotavírus e ao coronavírus).
- A perda da capacidade absortiva e a perda das enzimas da borda em escova (p. ex., dissacaridases) levam à diarreia osmótica.

IDENTIFICAÇÃO
Cães e gatos.

SINAIS CLÍNICOS
Cães
- Conjuntivite.
- Rinite.
- Traqueobronquite — papel menos importante.
- Pneumonia.
- Diarreia.
- Encefalite — rara.

Gatos
- Geralmente a doença é leve.
- Doença respiratória.
- Conjuntivite.
- Gengivite.
- Ataxia.
- Diarreia.

CAUSAS E FATORES DE RISCO
- Excretados predominantemente pelos tratos respiratório e digestório; adquiridos por inalação e ingestão oral.
- A infecção é comum; não se reproduziu doença específica.
- Outros patógenos virais — infecções observadas repetidas vezes; especula-se que o reovírus possa ter efeito imunossupressor que agrava tais infecções.

DIAGNÓSTICO

DIAGNÓSTICO DIFERENCIAL
- Enterite viral canina — parvovírus canino; coronavírus canino; astrovírus canino; calicivírus canino; herpes-vírus canino; vírus da cinomose; rotavírus canino.
- Traqueobronquite infecciosa canina — parainfluenza canina; *Bordetella bronchiseptica*; micoplasmas; adenovírus caninos tipos 1 e 2; herpes-vírus canino; vírus da cinomose; vírus da influenza canina; coronavírus respiratório canino.
- Doença respiratória superior felina — vírus da rinotraqueíte felina; calicivírus felino; *Chlamydia*; micoplasma; infecção bacteriana.

HEMOGRAMA/BIOQUÍMICA/URINÁLISE
Não contribuem para o diagnóstico.

OUTROS TESTES LABORATORIAIS
- Isolamento do vírus — efeito citopático de desenvolvimento lento.
- Histopatologia — grandes corpúsculos de inclusão intracitoplasmáticos na microscopia eletrônica.
- PCR-RT
- Microscopia eletrônica.

DIAGNÓSTICO POR IMAGEM
N/D.

MÉTODOS DIAGNÓSTICOS
N/D.

TRATAMENTO
- A importância do reovírus como patógeno é questionável.
- Nenhuma vacina foi desenvolvida.
- Outras medidas de controle são ignoradas.

MEDICAÇÕES

MEDICAMENTO(S)
N/D.

CONTRAINDICAÇÕES/INTERAÇÕES POSSÍVEIS
N/D.

ACOMPANHAMENTO
N/D.

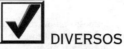

DIVERSOS

POTENCIAL ZOONÓTICO
- A infecção pode se disseminar entre indivíduos da mesma espécie ou de espécies diferentes.
- O papel (se existir algum) de que os animais funcionam como reservatório para o vírus ou como possível fonte de infecção humana é desconhecido.
- Seres humanos — desde a mais tenra idade, a grande maioria demonstra indícios sorológicos de infecção prévia pelo reovírus; não é fácil relacioná-lo com alguma doença; a maior parte das infecções deve permanecer assintomática ou mescla-se de forma imperceptível com doença respiratória e gastrintestinal sem importância da fase de bebê ou início da infância.
- Vírus candidato à terapia oncolítica do câncer (p. ex., glioma maligno).

ABREVIATURA(S)
- PCR-RT = reação em cadeia da polimerase via transcriptase reversa.

Sugestões de Leitura

Decaro N, Campolo M, Desario C, et al. Virological and molecular characterization of a mammalian orthoreovirus type 3 strain isolated from a dog in Italy. Vet Microbiology 2005, 109:19-27.

Comins C, Heinemann L, Harrington K, et al. Viral therapy for cancer "as nature intended." Clin Oncology 2008, 20:548-554.

Autor J. Paul Woods
Consultor Editorial Stephen C. Barrb

INFECÇÕES ANAERÓBIAS

CONSIDERAÇÕES GERAIS

REVISÃO
• As bactérias anaeróbias (ou seja, aquelas que necessitam de baixa tensão de oxigênio) compreendem uma grande parcela da flora normal, especialmente as existentes nas superfícies mucosas.
• Podem ser cocos ou bastonetes gram-positivos ou gram-negativos.
• Gêneros mais comuns — *Bacteroides*, *Fusobacterium*, *Actinomyces*, *Propionibacterium*, *Peptostreptococcus* (*Streptococcus* entérico), *Porphyromonas* e *Clostridium*.
• A maioria das infecções anaeróbias é polimicrobiana e contém pelo menos duas espécies de microrganismos anaeróbios distintos misturados com anaeróbios facultativos ou bactérias aeróbias (especialmente *E. coli*).
• Cada microrganismo varia quanto ao potencial de resistência à exposição ao oxigênio.
• Toxinas e enzimas nocivas podem ser elaboradas pelos microrganismos, levando à propagação da infecção para tecidos saudáveis adjacentes.
• Todos os sistemas corporais constituem um risco potencial de infecção anaeróbia.

IDENTIFICAÇÃO
Cães e gatos.

SINAIS CLÍNICOS
Comentários Gerais
• Determinados pelo sistema corporal envolvido.
• Certas áreas do corpo costumam ser mais associadas a infecções anaeróbias (proximidade das mucosas).
• O potencial de envolvimento dos anaeróbios pode ser negligenciado em um processo infeccioso, levando a confusão na interpretação dos resultados da cultura e na seleção de antibióticos.

Achados do Exame Físico
• Odor fétido associado à ferida ou secreção exsudativa. • Presença de gases nos tecidos ou nos exsudatos associados. • Alteração na cor dos tecidos, especialmente em peles de cor escura.
• Peritonite, piotórax ou piometra. • Odontopatia grave. • Feridas ou abscessos profundos que não cicatrizam conforme o previsto.

CAUSAS E FATORES DE RISCO
• Causadas geralmente pela flora corporal normal; uma solução de continuidade nas barreiras protetoras permite a invasão bacteriana.
• O surgimento de infecções na proximidade de alguma mucosa deve levantar o índice de suspeita para envolvimento anaeróbio.
• Fatores predisponentes — imunossupressão, feridas ocasionadas por mordeduras, odontopatias, fraturas abertas, cirurgias abdominais e corpos estranhos.

DIAGNÓSTICO

DIAGNÓSTICO DIFERENCIAL
• Feridas irresponsivas à terapia clínica adequada — se os resultados das culturas aeróbicas forem negativos, suspeitar de microrganismos anaeróbios.
• Gatos com feridas não cicatrizantes — efetuar teste quanto à presença de FeLV e FIV.
• Animais de meia-idade e idosos — invasão tumoral (p. ex., no trato gastrintestinal).

HEMOGRAMA/BIOQUÍMICA/URINÁLISE
• A leucocitose neutrofílica e a monocitose são comuns.
• As anormalidades bioquímicas dependem do envolvimento de órgão específico.
• Leucocitose, hipoglicemia, aumento da fosfatase alcalina e hipoalbuminemia sugerem disseminação sistêmica da infecção.

OUTROS TESTES LABORATORIAIS
• A cultura de bactérias anaeróbias é frequentemente frustrante por causa da natureza fastidiosa desses microrganismos e dos erros na manipulação e no envio de amostras.
• Meios e recipientes adequados devem estar à disposição antes da coleta da amostra; os laboratórios de diagnóstico podem fornecer a orientação.
• As amostras não devem ser refrigeradas antes do envio.
• Amostras adequadas para cultura podem incluir líquido (p. ex., pleural, peritoneal, etc.) ou tecido.

DIAGNÓSTICO POR IMAGEM
Ditado pelas condições de cada paciente (p. ex., suspeita de infecção óssea, peritonite, etc.)

MÉTODOS DIAGNÓSTICOS
• A inspeção citológica revela quantidade abundante de neutrófilos degenerados com formas morfologicamente diversas de bactérias intra e extracelulares; a presença de grandes bactérias filamentosas é sugestiva de infecções anaeróbias.
• Se não for realizada na clínica, a coloração de Gram deverá ser solicitada mediante o envio da amostra.

TRATAMENTO

• Drenagem torácica — importante em casos de piotórax (ver capítulo específico).
• Oxigênio hiperbárico — algum uso em potencial; pode ter disponibilidade limitada.

CIRURGIA
• Não deve ser adiada diante da suspeita de anaeróbios.
• Combinada com antibioticoterapia sistêmica — a melhor chance de um resultado positivo.
• Indicada geralmente em casos de complicação de piometra, osteomielite e peritonite por microrganismos anaeróbios.
• Limpar e remover as toxinas e os tecidos desvitalizados da ferida.
• Intensificar a drenagem de pus.
• Restabelecer o fluxo sanguíneo local.
• Aumentar a tensão de oxigênio.

MEDICAÇÕES

MEDICAMENTO(S)
• Antibioticoterapia isolada — pouca probabilidade de êxito; penetração insatisfatória de medicamentos em exsudatos.
• Seleção de antibióticos — basicamente empírica, pela dificuldade de isolamento dos anaeróbios e pela demora no retorno dos resultados da cultura.
• Como a maioria das infecções anaeróbias é polimicrobiana, a antibioticoterapia direcionada contra os anaeróbios e quaisquer componentes anaeróbicos têm maior probabilidade de sucesso.
• Amoxicilina com clavulanato — em muitos casos, é considerada o antibiótico de escolha; conveniente e acessível; o clavulanato aumenta a atividade contra *Bacteroides*.
• Imipeném — antibiótico betalactâmico com atividade significativa contra infecções graves e resistentes.
• Cefoxitina — uma cefalosporina com atividade confiável contra os anaeróbios.
• Clindamicina — pode ser particularmente útil contra infecções do trato respiratório; fica concentrada dentro dos leucócitos.
• Cloranfenicol — tem penetração tecidual satisfatória, embora seja bacteriostático e associado a efeitos adversos, sobretudo em gatos; a preocupação de exposição humana também limita seu uso.
• Metronidazol — útil contra todos os anaeróbios clinicamente significativos (exceto o *Actinomyces*).
• Aminoglicosídeos — uniformemente ineficazes contra os anaeróbios.
• Combinações de trimetoprima-sulfa — ineficazes; penetração insatisfatória em exsudatos.
• Quinolonas — habitualmente ineficazes, embora as quinolonas mais recentes de espectro expandido tenham atividade contra os anaeróbios (p. ex., pradofloxacino).

ACOMPANHAMENTO

MONITORIZAÇÃO DO PACIENTE
A monitorização dos parâmetros varia de acordo com a condição de cada paciente.

COMPLICAÇÕES POSSÍVEIS
A infecção localizada pode evoluir para infecção sistêmica se não for devidamente identificada e tratada.

EVOLUÇÃO ESPERADA E PROGNÓSTICO
Dependem da identificação e da resolução da causa subjacente; talvez haja necessidade de antibioticoterapia a longo prazo.

DIVERSOS

DISTÚRBIOS ASSOCIADOS
Ver a seção "Causas e Fatores de Risco".

ABREVIATURA(S)
• FeLV = vírus da leucemia felina.
• FIV = vírus da imunodeficiência felina.

Sugestões de Leitura
Hirsh DC, Jang SS. Anaerobic infections. In: Greene CE, ed., Infectious Diseases of the Dog and Cat, 3rd ed. St. Louis: Saunders Elsevier, 2006, pp. 381-388.

Autor Sharon Fooshee Grace
Consultor Editorial Stephen C. Barr

Infecções Bacterianas pelas Formas L

CONSIDERAÇÕES GERAIS

REVISÃO
Causadas por variantes bacterianas com paredes celulares ausentes ou defeituosas.

Formas bacterianas L
- Isoladas de seres humanos, animais e plantas.
- Nomeadas pelo Instituto Lister (Londres), onde foram descobertas em 1935.
- Também conhecidas como microrganismos L ou formas bacterianas com parede celular deficiente.
- Diferem do *Mycoplasma* pela falta de esterois em suas membranas (semelhantes às bactérias).
- Delicadas, frágeis, pleomórficas, esféricas e osmoticamente instáveis; equivalentes do ponto de vista estrutural a protoplastos e esferoplastos, os quais são incapazes de se dividir.
- Podem crescer e se replicar por fissão celular de forma irregular, produzindo células-filhas que diferem em termos de tamanho, conteúdo de ácido nucleico e quantidade de citoplasma.
- Formadas como uma variante espontânea das bactérias ou quando a síntese da parede celular fica inibida ou prejudicada por antibióticos (p. ex., penicilina), imunoglobulinas específicas ou enzimas lisossomais que degradam as paredes celulares.
- Podem ser induzidas praticamente a partir de todas as bactérias Gram-positivas e Gram-negativas em condições apropriadas.
- Podem se reverter à cepa de parede celular normal em hospedeiro adequado ou meio favorável.
- Compreendem tanto as formas L instáveis (que podem se reverter para bactérias dotadas de parede normal) com perda reversível de organização da parede celular em virtude das variantes fenotípicas de bactérias como as formas L estáveis (incapazes de se reverter) com perda irreversível da parede celular em função de mutações genômicas.
- Geralmente sem patogenicidade.

IDENTIFICAÇÃO
- Esporádicas em gatos e cães.
- Mais comuns em gatos de todas as idades e vida errante.

SINAIS CLÍNICOS
- Cães — artrite.
- Gatos — ferida penetrante (geralmente mordida de outro gato); ferida cirúrgica infectada; celulite; febre; artrite; sinovite.

CAUSAS E FATORES DE RISCO
- Mordeduras, arranhões ou traumatismo podem permitir que o microrganismo penetre na pele e no tecido subcutâneo.
- Reservatório ambiental desconhecido.
- Formação estimulada por tratamento do hospedeiro com antibiótico, resistência do hospedeiro, disponibilidade de local *in vivo* para estabelecimento do foco infeccioso e virulência relativamente baixa a moderada da bactéria infectante.
- Infectividade muito reduzida, mas pode reverter e exibir as propriedades patogênicas da bactéria original.

DIAGNÓSTICO

DIAGNÓSTICO DIFERENCIAL
- *Mycoplasma* — diferenciar por meio de microscopia de fase, microscopia eletrônica ou mensuração das proteínas de ligação à penicilina.
- Infecções cutâneas supurativas causadas por micobactérias, leveduras ou fungos.
- Artrite provocada por doença imunomediada, bactérias, espiroquetas, *Mycoplasma*, *Rickettsia*, *Chlamydia*, vírus ou fungo.

HEMOGRAMA/BIOQUÍMICA/URINÁLISE
- Neutrofilia com desvio à esquerda.
- Monocitose.
- Linfocitose.
- Eosinofilia.
- Leve anemia normocítica normocrômica.
- Proteína total sérica elevada.

OUTROS TESTES LABORATORIAIS
- Citologia — exsudato de lesões drenantes contém macrófagos e neutrófilos.
- Líquido articular — contagem neutrofílica elevada.
- Cultura — difícil; requer meios especiais (Hayflick); aspecto de "ovo frito" das colônias em ágar sólido (porção central embebida no ágar; crescimento vacuolizado fino na superfície do ágar).
- Microscopia óptica — difícil de demonstrar.
- Microscopia eletrônica — pode revelar microrganismos pleomórficos característicos desprovidos de parede celular em fagócitos.
- Caracterização e especificação exatas — o microrganismo precisa reverter para o estado com parede celular (pode levar anos).

DIAGNÓSTICO POR IMAGEM
Radiografias — tumefação do tecido mole periarticular; proliferação do periósteo.

MÉTODOS DIAGNÓSTICOS
N/D.

ACHADOS PATOLÓGICOS
- Biopsia — celulite piogênica; paniculite; artrite piogranulomatosa crônica; tenossinovite.
- Colorações — nem as convencionais (H&E) nem as especializadas (gram, acidorresistente, prata, PAS) revelam os microrganismos.

TRATAMENTO
- Limpeza delicada degrada os microrganismos frágeis.
- Permite que feridas abertas cicatrizem como efeito secundário.

MEDICAÇÕES

MEDICAMENTO(S)
- Sensibilidade antibiótica variável.
- Tetraciclina — 22 mg/kg VO a cada 8 h por, no mínimo, 1 semana após o desaparecimento dos sinais.
- A febre costuma cessar dentro de 24-48 h.
- Antibióticos β-lactâmicos — inibem a síntese da parede celular; portanto, não são eficazes.

CONTRAINDICAÇÕES/INTERAÇÕES POSSÍVEIS
N/D.

ACOMPANHAMENTO
As alterações artríticas persistem.

DIVERSOS
- O significado em termos de saúde pública é desconhecido.
- Ubíquo; portanto, o papel desempenhado em doença é questionável.
- Podem desempenhar um papel em infecções recidivantes ou doenças crônicas.

ABREVIATURA(S)
- H&E = hematoxilina e eosina.
- PAS = ácido periódico de Schiff.

Sugestões de Leitura
Allan EJ, Holschen C, Gumpert J. Bacterial L forms. Adv Appl Microbiol 2009, 68:1-39.
Greene CE. Mycoplasmal, ureaplasmal, and l-form infections. In: Greene CE, ed., Infectious Diseases of the Dog and Cat, 3rd ed. St. Louis: Saunders Elsevier, 2006, pp. 264-265.

Autor J. Paul Woods
Consultor Editorial Stephen C. Barr

INFECÇÕES POR ESTAFILOCOCOS

CONSIDERAÇÕES GERAIS

REVISÃO
• *Staphylococcus* — bactérias Gram-positivas, esféricas e facultativamente anaeróbicas (cocos); *staphyle* (vem do grego, que significa "cacho de uvas"), por seu arranjo microscópico característico em cachos; produzem diversas infecções caracterizadas pela formação de pus, envolvendo todos os tecidos corporais; podem produzir toxinas (superantígenos) que exercem sinais sistêmicos intensos (febre, hipotensão, choque, falência múltipla de órgãos, óbito). • Ubíquas; vivem livres no ambiente e como parasitas comensais da pele e do trato respiratório superior. • Cepas patogênicas e não patogênicas; amplo espectro de virulência, variação de hospedeiro e especificidades de locais; não são estritamente específicas em termos de hospedeiro ou local. • Cepas patogênicas — possuem toxinas e enzimas extracelulares (p. ex., coagulase, estafiloquinase, hemolisina e epidermolisinas); estafilocoagulase nas cepas mais patogênicas (p. ex., *S. aureus*, *S. intermedius*, *S. pseudintermedius*).

IDENTIFICAÇÃO
• Cães e gatos. • Muito jovens — suscetíveis por causa da imunidade incompleta em desenvolvimento. • Idosos, debilitados — suscetíveis por causa das defesas prejudicadas do hospedeiro. • Imunocomprometidos — mais suscetíveis.

SINAIS CLÍNICOS
• Febre. • Anorexia. • Dor. • Prurido. • Podem acometer todos os sistemas orgânicos. • Abscessos e infecções em pele, olhos, orelhas, sistema respiratório, trato geniturinário, esqueleto e articulações — comuns. • Cães — piodermite; otite externa; cistite; prostatite; pneumonia; abscessos; osteomielite; discospondilite; artrite; mastite; bacteremia; endocardite; infecções de feridas; síndrome do choque tóxico. • Gatos — abscessos; infecções bucais; otite externa; conjuntivite; metrite; colangio-hepatite; cistite; bacteremia.

CAUSAS E FATORES DE RISCO
• Patógenos oportunistas. • Doença — por distúrbio do equilíbrio natural hospedeiro-parasita quando os mecanismos de defesa locais e gerais ficam significantemente diminuídos (p. ex., doenças debilitantes crônicas). • Infecção secundária — alergias (atopia, alimento, pulgas); endocrinopatias (hipotireoidismo, hiperadrenocorticismo); parasitas (demodicose); seborreia. • Queimaduras ou feridas — complicações. • Transmissão — microrganismos aerógenos; portadores e contato direto (núcleos em gotículas).

DIAGNÓSTICO

DIAGNÓSTICO DIFERENCIAL
• Dermatite — alergias, seborreia, imunomediada. • Outras causas infecciosas — vírus, bactérias, fungos, *Rickettsia*, protozoários. • Neoplasia. • Doenças imunomediadas.

HEMOGRAMA/BIOQUÍMICA/URINÁLISE
• Leucogramas normais ou elevados. • Bioquímica — pode sugerir a causa subjacente (p. ex., hipotireoidismo, hiperadrenocorticismo). • Urinálise — piúria (com ou sem bacteriúria) com cistite.

OUTROS TESTES LABORATORIAIS
• Microscopia direta. • Coloração de Gram. • Citologia — neutrófilos e cocos isolados ou aos pares, cadeias curtas ou cachos irregulares. • Cultura — evitar a contaminação superficial; coletar as amostras por aspirado, lavado ou biopsia; não interpretar exageradamente um isolamento positivo; os microrganismos podem ser isolados de animais normais. • Os microrganismos sobrevivem por até 48 h nas amostras clínicas quando mantidas sob refrigeração (4°C), sobretudo nos *swabs* contendo algum meio de conservação. • Teste de suscetibilidade antibiótica (antibiograma). • Tipagem molecular com eletroforese em gel de campo pulsado.

DIAGNÓSTICO POR IMAGEM
Radiologia — lesões osteolíticas e osteoproliferativas na osteomielite; padrão pulmonar intersticial ou alveolar na pneumonia; urólitos radiodensos (estruvita).

MÉTODOS DIAGNÓSTICOS
LCS — na suspeita de meningite ou discospondilite.

ACHADOS PATOLÓGICOS
Lesão característica de abscesso — tecido necrótico, fibrina e grande número de neutrófilos.

TRATAMENTO
• Manipular e descartar de forma adequada os objetos contaminados.
• Microrganismo resistente a muitas agressões ambientais e desinfetantes comuns.
• Limpeza antibacteriana tópica de feridas e piodermites — pode ser benéfica.
• Os animais com infecção suspeita ou confirmada por *Staphylococcus aureus* resistente à meticilina devem ser isolados.

MEDICAÇÕES

MEDICAMENTO(S)
• Resistência a antibióticos — grande propensão em virtude da produção de β-lactamase, a qual inativa as penicilinas; podem transportar plasmídeos (segmentos de material genético que podem carrear genes codificadores de resistência a antibióticos) que podem ser transferidos para outras cepas de estafilococos ou espécies de bactérias.
• Histórico de tratamento antimicrobiano prévio para infecção estafilocócica — a realização de cultura e o teste de suscetibilidade antibiótica são indicados.
• Cepas não produtoras de penicilinase — penicilina G à dose de 10.000-20.000 U/kg IM, SC a cada 12-24 h ou penicilina V na dose de 8-30 mg/kg VO a cada 8 h.
• Cepas produtoras de penicilinase — usar medicamentos resistentes à penicilinase.
• Cefalosporinas de primeira geração — raramente resistentes; cefalexina na dose de 22 mg/kg VO a cada 8 h; cefadroxila à dose de 22 mg/kg VO a cada 8-12 h.
• Penicilinas sintéticas resistentes à β-lactamase — raramente resistentes; oxacilina à dose de 22-40 mg/kg VO a cada 8 h; dicloxacilina à dose de 10-25 mg/kg VO a cada 8 h e amoxicilina potencializada pelo ácido clavulânico à dose de 12,5-25 mg/kg VO a cada 8-12 h.
• Gentamicina — raramente resistente; 2-4 mg/kg IV, IM, SC a cada 8 h.
• Enrofloxacino — raramente resistente; 2,5-5 mg/kg VO, IM a cada 12 h.
• Sulfonamidas potencializadas pela trimetoprima — resistência pouco frequente; 30 mg/kg IV, VO a cada 12 h.
• Cloranfenicol — resistência pouco frequente; 40-50 mg/kg IV, IM, SC, VO a cada 8-12 h.
• Alergia à penicilina — tentar cefalosporina, clindamicina ou vancomicina.
• O *Staphylococcus* resistente à meticilina (expressa o gene mecA) ocasionalmente isolado dos cães e gatos é um problema emergente.

CONTRAINDICAÇÕES/INTERAÇÕES POSSÍVEIS
Evitar medicamentos imunossupressores.

DIVERSOS

POTENCIAL ZOONÓTICO
• Possível.
• A maior parte das pessoas e dos animais de estimação carreia sua própria flora estafilocócica patogênica; a doença não é causada por mera exposição; no entanto, a transmissão dos cães para os seres humanos é possível.
• Infecções causadas por mordidas contêm um misto de microrganismos aeróbios e anaeróbios tanto da pele do paciente como da boca do animal, incluindo *Staphylococcus*.
• O *Staphylococcus aureus* resistente à meticilina pode ser transmitido entre os animais e os seres humanos; por essa razão, os animais de estimação representam um risco de infecção aos proprietários e à equipe veterinária (do mesmo modo, portadores humanos de *Staphylococcus aureus* resistente à meticilina podem infectar os animais suscetíveis).
• A higiene das mãos é parte integrante das medidas preventivas para evitar a disseminação de *Staphylococcus aureus* resistente à meticilina entre os animais e os seres humanos, bem como entre os animais.

ABREVIATURA(S)
• LCS = líquido cerebrospinal.

Sugestões de Leitura
Cox HU. Staphylococcal infections. In: Greene CE, ed., Infectious Diseases of the Dog and Cat, 3rd ed. St. Louis: Saunders Elsevier, 2006, pp. 316-320.
Kempker R, Mangalat D, Kongphet-Tran T, Eaton M. Beware of the pet dog: A case of *Staphylococcus intermedius* infection. Am J Med Sci 2009, 338:425-427.
Leonard FC, Markey BK. Meticillin-resistant *Staphylococcus aureus* in animals: A review. Vet J 2008, 175:27-36.

Autor J. Paul Woods
Consultor Editorial Stephen C. Barr

Infecções por Estreptococos

CONSIDERAÇÕES GERAIS

REVISÃO
- *Streptococcus* — bactérias esféricas, Gram-positivas, imóveis e facultativamente anaeróbicas (cocos); crescem aos pares ou em cadeias; microrganismos comensais; flora normal do trato respiratório superior, orofaringe, trato genital inferior e pele; em condições apropriadas, são capazes de infectar todas as áreas do organismo; as infecções primárias envolvem os sistemas respiratório, circulatório, tegumentar, urogenital ou nervoso central; invasor secundário frequente dos tecidos corporais.
- Classificados pela capacidade de hemolisar as hemácias e de produzir uma zona nas placas de ágar-sangue ao redor da colônia bacteriana — α-hemolíticos (zona esverdeada de hemólise parcial); β-hemolíticos (zona clara de hemólise); γ-hemolíticos (sem alteração; não hemolíticos); os β-hemolíticos costumam ser mais patogênicos do que os α-hemolíticos que, por sua vez, são mais patogênicos do que as cepas não hemolíticas.
- As cepas hemolíticas ainda são subdivididas pelas diferenças antigênicas nos carboidratos da parede celular — sorogrupos de Lancefield A-H e K-T (p. ex., *S. canis* grupo G); é mais provável que alguns grupos estejam associados à doença, dependendo da espécie (p. ex., grupo G associado a cães e gatos; grupo A associado a seres humanos).
- Produzem exotoxinas — estreptolisinas (hemolisinas), estreptoquinases, desoxirribonucleases e hialuronidases.

IDENTIFICAÇÃO
- Cães e gatos.
- Muito jovens — mais propensos à infecção por causa da imunidade incompleta em desenvolvimento; acomete particularmente filhotes felinos nascidos de gata primípara.

SINAIS CLÍNICOS
- Variam com o local da infecção e a imunocompetência do hospedeiro.
- Fraqueza.
- Tosse.
- Dispneia.
- Febre.
- Hematêmese.
- Hematúria.
- Linfadenopatia.
- Dor.
- Cães — abscessos; septicemia; endometrite; piometra; vaginite; mastite; proctite; otite; artrite; definhamento dos filhotes; abortamento; infecção do trato urinário; pielonefrite; pneumonia; endocardite; meningoencefalite; fasciite necrosante; síndrome do choque tóxico estreptocócico; infecções de feridas; esterilidade da cadela.
- Gatos — abscessos; septicemia; peritonite; linfadenite cervical; faringite; tonsilite; artrite; pneumonia; definhamento dos filhotes; fasciite necrosante.

CAUSAS E FATORES DE RISCO
- Idade, exposição e resposta imune — importantes para determinar a doença.
- Virulência — depende dos produtos celulares, componentes da superfície e substâncias relacionadas.
- Oportunistas — feridas, traumatismo, procedimentos cirúrgicos, infecções virais ou condições imunossupressoras.
- FeLV, PIF, imunodeficiência, infecções virais respiratórias, doença do trato urinário inferior felino — condições predisponentes.
- Anticorpos maternos geralmente protegem os filhotes caninos e felinos contra doença clínica.
- Ocorre estado de portador.
- Suspeita-se de superantígenos bacterianos como a causa do envolvimento de múltiplos órgãos em síndrome do choque tóxico e fasciite necrosante.

DIAGNÓSTICO

DIAGNÓSTICO DIFERENCIAL
Outras causas infecciosas — vírus, bactérias, fungos, *Rickettsia*, protozoários.

HEMOGRAMA/BIOQUÍMICA/URINÁLISE
- Leucócitos normais ou elevados com resposta inflamatória neutrofílica com desvio à esquerda ou desvio à esquerda degenerativo.
- Cocos — podem ser encontrados nos neutrófilos circulantes em casos de sepse avassaladora.
- Bioquímica — pode sugerir as condições predisponentes.
- Urinálise — piúria (com ou sem bacteriúria) com cistite.

OUTROS TESTES LABORATORIAIS
- Microscopia direta.
- Coloração de Gram — dos exsudatos; revela cocos Gram-positivos em cadeias e isolados.
- Cultura — dos tecidos acometidos; exsudatos ou aspirados com agulha; confirma o diagnóstico.
- Teste de suscetibilidade antibiótica (antibiograma).
- PCR.

DIAGNÓSTICO POR IMAGEM
Radiografias — padrão pulmonar intersticial ou alveolar na pneumonia; urólitos radiodensos (estruvita).

ACHADOS PATOLÓGICOS
- Inflamação aguda — abscessos macro ou microscópicos.
- Septicemia — o exame pós-morte revela onfaloflebite, peritonite, hepatite, pneumonia e miocardite.

TRATAMENTO

- Fornecer cuidados satisfatórios de enfermagem.
- Reidratar.
- Drenar e irrigar o abscesso.
- Debridar o tecido necrótico.

MEDICAÇÕES

MEDICAMENTO(S)
- Penicilina — primeira escolha; penicilina G na dose de 10.000-20.000 U/kg IM, SC a cada 12-24 h ou penicilina V na dose de 8-30 mg/kg VO a cada 8 h.
- Ampicilina — 20-30 mg/kg IV, IM, SC, VO a cada 8 h; utilizada isoladamente ou em combinação com gentamicina à dose de 2-4 mg/kg IV, IM, SC a cada 8 h; para o grupo B.
- Eritromicina — 10-20 mg/kg IV, SC, VO a cada 8 h.
- Clindamicina — 11 mg/kg VO a cada 12-24 h.
- Tratamento profilático — indicado para todos os filhotes felinos nascidos de fêmeas primíparas em caso de infecção neonatal.

CONTRAINDICAÇÕES/INTERAÇÕES POSSÍVEIS
Evitar medicamentos imunossupressores.

ACOMPANHAMENTO

PREVENÇÃO
- Evitar superlotação e saneamento ambiental insatisfatório.
- Prevenção nos recém-nascidos — imersão do umbigo e do cordão umbilical em tintura de iodo a 2%.
- Prevenção nas colônias — evitar a superpopulação; manter os comedouros limpos; isolar os animais infectados.

DIVERSOS

POTENCIAL ZOONÓTICO
- Cães e gatos podem não exibir sinais clínicos com estreptococos do grupo A, mas podem servir como reservatórios para infecção humana.
- Os estreptococos isolados de pessoas costumam ser de origem humana e não de origem animal.
- Há relatos de infecções por *S. canis* em pessoas por mordidas de cães e contato de úlceras ou feridas com cães.

ABREVIATURA(S)
- FeLV = vírus da leucemia felina.
- PCR = reação em cadeia da polimerase.
- PIF = peritonite infecciosa felina.

Sugestões de Leitura
Byun J-W, Yoon S-S, Woo G-H, et al. An outbreak of fatal hemorrhagic pneumonia caused by *Streptococcus equi* subsp. *zooepidemicus* in shelter dogs. J Vet Sci 2009, 10:269-271.
Greene CE, Prescott JF. Streptococcal and other gram-positive bacterial infections. In: Greene CE, ed., Infectious Diseases of the Dog and Cat, 3rd ed. St. Louis: Saunders Elsevier, 2006, pp. 302-309.
Messer JS, Wagner SO, Baumwart RD, Colitz CM. A case of canine streptococcal meningoencephalitis diagnosed using universal bacterial polymerase chain reaction assay. JAAHA 2008, 44:205-209.
Sura R, Hinckley LS, Risatti GR, Smyth JA. Fatal necrotising fasciitis and myositis in a cat associated with *Streptococcus canis*. Vet Record 2008, 162:450-453.

Autor J. Paul Woods
Consultor Editorial Stephen C. Barr

INFECÇÕES POR MICOBACTÉRIAS

CONSIDERAÇÕES GERAIS

REVISÃO
• Micobactérias — bactérias superiores (gênero *Mycobacterium*) acidorresistentes, Gram-positivas; patógenos obrigatórios ou esporádicos em seres humanos e nos animais.
• Tuberculose — provocada por *Mycobacterium tuberculosis* (humanos), *M. bovis* (bovinos e alguns mamíferos selvagens) e *M. microti* (ratos selvagens) e semelhantes ao *M. microti*; cães e gatos expostos a hospedeiros primários esporadicamente infectados; doença disseminada ou de vários órgãos provocada por microrganismo parasitário obrigatório; rara em cães e gatos nos países desenvolvidos.
• Lepra — *M. lepraemurium* (dos roedores) e 2 microrganismos da lepra sem denominação (*M. visibilis* [nome provisório]).
• Gatos — duas síndromes — síndrome 1, que acomete gatos jovens com doença nodular localizada, envolvendo os membros com números esparsos a moderados de bacilos acidorresistentes presentes nas lesões (*M. lepraemurium*); síndrome 2, que acomete gatos idosos com lesões cutâneas generalizadas com grandes números de bacilos acidorresistentes nas lesões (espécie sem denominação com afinidade por *M. malmoense*).
• Cães — síndrome do granuloma leproide canino, provocado por *Mycobacterium* spp. sem denominação e não obtido por cultura, mas identificado por sequenciamento do DNA.
• Infecção sistêmica ou não cutânea por micobactéria não tuberculosa — grupo *M. chelonae-abscessus*, complexo *M. avium*, *M. fortuitum*, *M. genavense*, *M. kansasii*, *M. massiliense*, *M. simiae*, *M. smegmatis*, *M. thermoresistable*, *M. xenopi*; infecções esporádicas em cães e gatos; alguns pacientes com doença concomitante ou imunossupressora ou o resultado da introdução de microrganismo saprófita em tecido traumatizado; as síndromes incluem pleurite, granulomas localizados ou disseminados, doença disseminada, neurite, broncopneumonia.
• Infecções cutâneas/subcutâneas atribuídas a micobactérias de crescimento rápido — também conhecidas como paniculite micobacteriana.
• Cães e gatos — provocadas por micobactérias saprófitas do grupo *M. fortuitum*, grupo *M. chelonae-abscessus*, grupos *M. smegmatis*, *M. phlei*, complexo *M. terrae*, *M. thermoresistable*, *M. ulcerans*.

SISTEMA(S) ACOMETIDO(S)
• Respiratório. • Cutâneo/Exócrino.
• Determinado pela causa.

IDENTIFICAÇÃO
Tuberculose
• Gatos e cães de qualquer idade.
• Cães da raça Basset hound e gatos da raça Siamês são relatados como os mais suscetíveis; provas incertas (possível aberração estatística).

Lepra Felina
• Gatos adultos e filhotes de vida livre; filhotes felinos e gatos adultos jovens na síndrome 1; gatos mais idosos (média de 9 anos) na síndrome 2.

Granuloma Leproide Canino
• Há relatos de casos em cães pertencentes a raças de grande porte, mantidos no exterior da residência, com pelagem curta, especialmente das raças Boxer e Pastor alemão.

Micobacteriose Não Tuberculosa Sistêmica
• Doença esporádica que pode acometer cães e gatos de qualquer idade.

Paniculite Micobacteriana
• Gatos e cães adultos.

SINAIS CLÍNICOS
Tuberculose
• Os sinais são correlacionados com a via de exposição. • Principais locais de envolvimento — linfonodos orofaríngeos, tecidos cutâneos e subcutâneos da cabeça e das extremidades; sistema pulmonar; sistema gastrintestinal. • Cães — respiratório, especialmente tosse; é incomum a presença de dispneia. • Gatos — infecção adquirida a partir do leite contaminado: perda de peso, diarreia crônica e intestinos espessados; a partir da prática de predação: nódulos cutâneos, úlceras e trajetos drenantes. • Praticamente todos os cães e muitos gatos — linfadenopatia faríngea e cervical; ânsia de vômito (i. e., esforço improdutivo para vomitar), ptialismo ou abscesso tonsilar; linfonodos são visíveis ou firmes, fixos e sensíveis à palpação; podem ulcerar e drenar.
• Pirexia. • Depressão. • Anorexia parcial e perda de peso. • Podem ocorrer osteopatia hipertrófica ou hipercalcemia. • Doença disseminada — efusão em cavidade corporal; massas viscerais; lesões ósseas ou articulares; massas dérmicas e subcutâneas, além de úlceras; linfadenopatia e/ou abscessos; sinais do SNC; morte súbita.

Lepra Felina
• Síndrome 1 — nódulos iniciais localizados nos membros; evoluem rapidamente e podem ulcerar; evolução clínica agressiva; recidiva após excisão cirúrgica; em algumas semanas, aparecem lesões disseminadas.
• Síndrome 2 — nódulos cutâneos iniciais localizados ou generalizados que não ulceram, mas são lentamente progressivos por meses a anos.
• Micobacteriose granulomatosa multissistêmica felina — espessamento difuso da pele e envolvimento de múltiplos órgãos.

Granuloma Leproide Canino
• Um ou mais nódulos indolores bem circunscritos (2 mm-5 cm) na derme ou no subcutâneo; frequentemente na cabeça ou na orelha, embora possam ocorrer em qualquer parte do corpo; apenas as lesões muito grandes ulceram.
• Nenhum sinal sistêmico de doença.

Micobacteriose Não Tuberculosa Sistêmica
• Infecções pulmonares e sistêmicas com micobacteriose atípica raras são relatadas nos cães; nesse caso, os sinais são de tuberculose.
• Na infecção por *M. avium*, a doença é disseminada mais frequentemente.

Paniculite Micobacteriana
• Lesão cutâneo-traumática que não cicatriza com o tratamento apropriado; dissemina-se localmente pelo tecido subcutâneo (paniculite); a lesão original aumenta, formando uma úlcera profunda que drena exsudato hemorrágico oleoso; o tecido circunjacente torna-se firme; ulcerações puntiformes satélites se abrem e drenam.
• Deiscência da ferida nos locais de cirurgia.

CAUSAS E FATORES DE RISCO
Tuberculose
• Fonte de exposição — sempre um hospedeiro típico infectado.
• Cães — expostos, em geral, a uma pessoa infectada na residência (*M. tuberculosis*); a via consiste na ingestão de material infeccioso expectorado; possível exposição a aerossol; os pacientes são mais frequentemente encontrados em áreas urbanas com imigrantes vindos dos países em desenvolvimento.
• Gatos — tipicamente expostos pela ingestão de leite não pasteurizado de bovinos infectados (*M. bovis*); muito menos comum atualmente do que no passado; podem ser expostos por predação de pequenos mamíferos infectados (*M. bovis*, espécie de tuberculose indefinida).

Lepra Felina
• Na síndrome 1 — há relatos de casos em áreas costeiras temperadas e cidades portuárias; o clima frio pode facilitar o crescimento do microrganismo nas extremidades.
• Na síndrome 2 — os casos são originários de ambientes rurais e semirrurais; a idade avançada ou a imunoincompetência podem ser fator de risco. Os fatores exatos de risco permanecem indefinidos; postula-se a exposição aos roedores.

Granuloma Leproide Canino
• Possivelmente associado a picadas de mosquitos, podendo exibir oscilação sazonal; a pelagem curta pode predispor.
• É provável que a doença seja mundialmente distribuída, porém a maior parte dos casos foi relatada na Australásia e no Brasil.
• Nos Estados Unidos, há relatos de casos da Califórnia, do Havaí e da Flórida.

Micobacteriose Não Tuberculosa Sistêmica
• A maior parte dos pacientes relatados está imunossuprimida ou apresenta doenças sistêmicas concomitantes.
• Exposição — as vias de exposição na doença pulmonar e sistêmica são desconhecidas.

Paniculite Micobacteriana
• Grande parte das infecções apresenta histórico de traumatismo ou ferida cirúrgica prévia; a maior parte dos pacientes é imunocompetente.
• Traumatismo e inoculação acidental da gordura subcutânea podem resultar em infecção; histórico de possível ferimento por mordedura (doença subcutânea).
• Animais obesos podem estar sob maior risco do que os magros.

DIAGNÓSTICO

DIAGNÓSTICO DIFERENCIAL
• As infecções micobacterianas apresentam prognósticos, recomendações terapêuticas e consequências à saúde pública diferentes; no início, no entanto, podem apresentar sinais semelhantes, sobretudo lesões cutâneas. • Todas as manifestações: infecções fúngicas e outras infecções actinomicóticas devem ser consideradas.
• Paniculite: a nocardiose pode ser clinicamente idêntica.

OUTROS TESTES LABORATORIAIS
Tuberculose
Tuberculose (cães) — teste cutâneo intradérmico com derivado proteico purificado ou bacilo de Calmette-Guérin (BCG) no pavilhão auricular interno; pode produzir resultados falso-positivos em função das reações cruzadas com micobactérias não tuberculosas.

Infecções por Micobactérias

DIAGNÓSTICO POR IMAGEM
Radiografia
• Lesões torácicas, abdominais ou esqueléticas — sugerem doença infecciosa granulomatosa.
• Nenhuma lesão específica para as micobacterioses. • Lesões de tuberculose pulmonar — podem se tornar calcificadas ou cavitárias.

MÉTODOS DIAGNÓSTICOS
• Diagnóstico obtido com base na avaliação histopatológica e microbiológica do material de biopsia do tecido acometido.
• Pode ser utilizada a aspiração de material purulento de qualquer local após a desinfecção da pele sobrejacente para identificação microbiológica; talvez seja justificável o uso das técnicas de aspiração guiadas por ultrassom.
• Amostras de biopsia — não devem estar contaminadas por bactérias superficiais; precisam incorporar o centro de um foco granulomatoso.
• Esfregaços de tecidos infectados — para detecção com colorações acidorresistentes, como a carbolfucsina ou o fluorocromo (método da auramina-rodamina). Na coloração de rotina, os microrganismos coram-se negativamente, revelando "fantasmas" de bacilos dentro de macrófagos; *swabs* ou aspirados de lesões cutâneas drenantes ou linfonodos, lavado transtraqueal; escovações endoscópicas; citologia retal; decalques por impressão obtidos na biopsia cirúrgica. Esfregaços fixados pelo calor devem ser enviados juntamente com o tecido para cultura.
• Cultura — há necessidade de meios e técnicas especiais; o encaminhamento para laboratórios especializados pode ser necessário para microrganismos não tuberculosos (Mycobacterium Mycology Referral, University of Texas Health Center at Tyler, Microbiology Section).
• Metodologias por PCR — úteis para qualquer uma das infecções micobacterianas, sendo realizadas com o uso de amostras de tecidos ou líquidos; para o granuloma leproide canino e as duas síndromes de lepra felina, não há *primers* (iniciadores) disponíveis no mercado; essas metodologias, no entanto, podem ser utilizadas para identificar os microrganismos sob suspeita.

TRATAMENTO
Tuberculose
• Deve ser obtida uma permissão das autoridades locais de saúde nos casos de infecção por *Mycobacterium tuberculosis*, devendo-se sempre levar o potencial zoonótico em consideração.
• Múltiplos agentes quimioterápicos utilizados para tratar a tuberculose humana são bem-sucedidos em animais; entretanto, as infecções pelo complexo *M. avium* são de difícil tratamento.

Lepra Felina
• Antes da disseminação generalizada, as lesões individuais podem ser submetidas à excisão rigorosa com margens de segurança; tal procedimento pode ser curativo.
• O tratamento cirúrgico deve ser precedido pela terapia sistêmica.

Granuloma Leproide Canino
• A excisão é curativa; as lesões podem ser autocuráveis; a terapia antimicrobiana pode auxiliar na cicatrização.

Infecções Não Tuberculosas Subcutâneas e Sistêmicas
• O tratamento deve ser feito com base na identificação do microrganismo e no antibiograma.
• Com frequência, é justificável o uso de terapia com múltiplos medicamentos.
• O debridamento cirúrgico rigoroso pode ajudar na resolução; é recomendável a terapia antimicrobiana antes e durante a cirurgia.

MEDICAÇÕES
MEDICAMENTO(S)
Tuberculose
• Sempre fazer uso de tratamento por via oral com dois ou três medicamentos; jamais tentar tratamento com um único medicamento para nenhum microrganismo.
• Recomendação atual — fluoroquinolona (p. ex., enrofloxacino), claritromicina e rifampicina por 6-9 meses.
• Enrofloxacino, orbifloxacino, marbofloxacino, moxifloxacino e ciprofloxacino — 5-15 mg/kg VO a cada 24 h.
• Rifampicina — 10-20 mg/kg VO a cada 24 h ou dividida a cada 12 h (máximo, 600 mg/dia).
• Claritromicina — 5-10 mg/kg VO a cada 24 h.
• Isoniazida e rifampicina — combinações utilizadas; pouco se sabe sobre seu uso em gatos; 1 relato recente de tratamento (gato) com isoniazida, rifampicina e diidroestreptomicina por 3 meses relatou perda de peso, mas um desfecho bem-sucedido.
• Isoniazida — 10-20 mg/kg (até 300 mg no total) VO a cada 24 h.
• Etambutol — 15 mg/kg VO a cada 24 h.
• Pirazinamida — no lugar do etambutol; 15-40 mg/kg VO a cada 24 h.
• Diidroestreptomicina — 15 mg/kg IM a cada 24 h.

Lepra Felina
• Rifampicina — 10-20 mg/kg a cada 24 h ou dividida a cada 12 h.
• Agente possivelmente útil — claritromicina conforme descrição prévia.

Infecções Não Tuberculosas Subcutâneas e Sistêmicas
• Nesses casos, pode ser utilizado o teste de sensibilidade *in vitro* na escolha da quimioterapia.
• Entre os antibióticos relatados como eficazes contra diversos isolamentos de micobacteriose atípica estão os macrolídeos, as sulfonamidas potencializadas pela trimetoprima, as tetraciclinas, os aminoglicosídeos e as fluoroquinolonas.
• Em geral, os medicamentos contra tuberculose não são eficazes.
• A monoterapia (i. e., tratamento com um único agente) não é recomendada em virtude da resposta insatisfatória a longo prazo; portanto, é aconselhável o tratamento com dois agentes.
• Os antibióticos fluoroquinolonas, sulfonamidas potencializadas pela trimetoprima, tetraciclinas e claritromicina são úteis para alguns casos isolados.
• A resposta pode ser prevista pela espécie isolada, mas a terapia a longo prazo deve ser feita com base no antibiograma.
• O tratamento deve continuar por 2-6 meses.

• Recidivas após a interrupção do tratamento ou durante o curso terapêutico são comuns.

CONTRAINDICAÇÕES/INTERAÇÕES POSSÍVEIS
Medicamentos tradicionais contra a tuberculose — ficar alerta para quaisquer reações adversas; experiência limitada, especialmente nos gatos.

ACOMPANHAMENTO
MONITORIZAÇÃO DO PACIENTE
• Medicamentos antituberculose e contra a lepra — examinar por, no mínimo, uma vez por mês; monitorizar o paciente quanto à presença de anorexia e perda de peso.
• Obter o perfil da função hepática mensalmente.
• Instruir os proprietários a relatar imediatamente as lesões cutâneas.

PREVENÇÃO
Os clínicos conhecedores de caso de tuberculose humana em residência com cães ou gatos devem aconselhar os proprietários sobre o risco de zoonose reversa.

EVOLUÇÃO ESPERADA E PROGNÓSTICO
Tuberculose
• Reservado; atualmente, no entanto, é indefinido, já que a experiência com medicamentos modernos que se revelam mais bem tolerados por períodos prolongados é limitada.

Lepra Felina
• Reservado a mau — para a síndrome 1.
• Razoável — para a síndrome 2, especialmente se as lesões forem passíveis de excisão cirúrgica.

Granuloma Leproide Canino
• Prognóstico bom.

Infecções Não Tuberculosas Subcutâneas e Sistêmicas
• As recidivas são comuns; abordagens cirúrgicas rigorosas e múltiplos medicamentos podem melhorar o resultado.

DIVERSOS
POTENCIAL ZOONÓTICO
• Tuberculose — os animais domésticos de companhia acometidos representam riscos zoonóticos potenciais sérios aos proprietários; as autoridades de saúde pública devem ser notificadas do diagnóstico antes ou depois de morte (isso pode ser exigido por lei); não tentar o tratamento sem a concordância das autoridades de saúde pública.
• *M. tuberculosis* — maior potencial de zoonose, especialmente com lesões cutâneas drenantes.
• Transmissão da doença dos cães e gatos para os humanos — registrada muito raramente.

ABREVIATURA(S)
• DNA = ácido desoxirribonucleico.
• PCR = reação em cadeia da polimerase.

Autor Mitchell D. Song
Consultor Editorial Alexander H. Werner
Agradecimento a Carol S. Foil, autora deste capítulo na edição anterior.

Infecções por Rotavírus

CONSIDERAÇÕES GERAIS

REVISÃO
- RNA vírus não envelopado de fita dupla; *rota* vem do latim e significa "roda" por causa do formato do capsídeo; gênero inserido na família Reoviridae; relativamente resistente à destruição ambiental (solventes ácidos e lipídicos); o capsídeo duplo único protege o vírus da inativação na parte superior do trato gastrintestinal.
- Ampla gama de hospedeiros, identificados em quase todas as espécies pesquisadas.
- A causa mais significativa de gastrenterite grave em crianças com <2 anos de idade e animais jovens por todo o mundo.
- Transmissão — contaminação orofecal.
- Infecção — acomete as células epiteliais maduras nas extremidades luminais das vilosidades intestinais; causa tumefação, degeneração e descamação; as vilosidades desnudas contraem-se; resulta em atrofia vilosa com perda da capacidade absortiva e perda das enzimas da borda em escova (p. ex., dissacaridases); leva à diarreia osmótica.

IDENTIFICAÇÃO
- Cães e gatos.
- Filhotes caninos com <12 semanas de vida e, mais frequentemente, com <2 semanas de vida — diarreia.
- Filhotes felinos e gatos jovens (com <6 meses de vida) — mais suscetíveis à infecção.

SINAIS CLÍNICOS
- Cães — a maior parte das infecções é subclínica ou limitada à diarreia inespecífica aquosa a mucoide relativamente branda, anorexia e letargia; raros casos fatais relatados.
- Gatos — exibem principalmente diarreia subclínica ou leve; nas coinfecções ou em condições de estresse, pode ocorrer doença clínica mais grave.

CAUSAS E FATORES DE RISCO
- Rotavírus.
- Animais jovens com sistemas imunológicos imaturos estão sob maior risco.

DIAGNÓSTICO

DIAGNÓSTICO DIFERENCIAL
- Enterite viral canina — parvovírus canino; coronavírus canino; astrovírus canino; calicivírus canino; herpes-vírus canino; vírus da cinomose; reovírus canino.
- Enterite viral felina — parvovírus felino (vírus da panleucopenia felina); FeLV; coronavírus felino; astrovírus felino; calicivírus felino.
- Outras causas de enterite — bactérias (p. ex., *Salmonella*, *Campylobacter* e *Clostridium*); fungos; protozoários; parasitas; corpos estranhos; intussuscepção; alergias; agentes tóxicos.

HEMOGRAMA/BIOQUÍMICA/URINÁLISE
Não contribuem para a formulação do diagnóstico.

OUTROS TESTES LABORATORIAIS
- Sorologia — não recomendada; a maior parte dos animais (p. ex., 85% dos cães) carreia anticorpos gerados por exposição prévia ou derivados da transferência de imunidade passiva a partir da cadela ou da gata; é imprescindível demonstrar a diferença de 4 vezes nas amostras séricas agudas e convalescentes.
- Microscopia eletrônica direta — detecta o vírus nas fezes; método rápido; falta de sensibilidade.
- Microscopia imunoeletrônica — mais sensível e específica do que a microscopia eletrônica direta; não está comumente disponível.
- ELISA — detecta antígeno de grupo comum aos rotavírus nas fezes.
- Teste de aglutinação em látex: Rotalex® (Orion Diagnostica Oy, Espoo, Finlândia); Virogen Rotatest® (Wampole Laboratories, Cranbury, NJ).
- Isolamento do vírus.
- PCR.

DIAGNÓSTICO POR IMAGEM
N/D.

MÉTODOS DIAGNÓSTICOS
Histologia — vilosidades tumefatas do intestino delgado; infiltração leve por macrófagos e neutrófilos; vírus detectado pelo teste de anticorpo fluorescente.

TRATAMENTO
- Sintomático para diarreia — fluidos, eletrólitos e restrição alimentar.
- Antibioticoterapia — não é indicada.
- Principal proteção — provavelmente é conferida por anticorpos presentes no leite da cadela ou da gata imunes.

MEDICAÇÕES

MEDICAMENTO(S)
N/D.

CONTRAINDICAÇÕES/INTERAÇÕES POSSÍVEIS
N/D.

ACOMPANHAMENTO
N/D.

DIVERSOS

POTENCIAL ZOONÓTICO
- Os rotavírus não são específicos para o hospedeiro; portanto, os filhotes caninos ou felinos acometidos podem representar um risco potencial de saúde aos seres humanos, particularmente para bebês.
- Ter cuidado ao manipular material fecal de animais de companhia com diarreia.
- Humanos — diarreia; bebês nos países desenvolvidos: alta morbidade e baixa mortalidade (atribuída à fluidoterapia); bebês e crianças novas nos países desenvolvidos: principal causa de diarreia com risco de vida (mais de 600 mil óbitos por ano em crianças com <5 anos de idade); nos EUA, mais de 3 milhões de episódios de diarreia, ~500 mil consultas clínicas, ~600 mil internações, mas apenas 20-40 mortes por ano.

ABREVIATURA(S)
- ELISA = ensaio imunoabsorvente ligado à enzima.
- FeLV = vírus da leucemia felina.
- PCR = reação em cadeia da polimerase.

Sugestões de Leitura
Estes MK, Kapikian AZ. Rotavirus. In: Knipe DM, Howley PM, eds., Fields Virology, 5th ed. Philadelphia: Lippincott Williams & Wilkins, 2007, pp. 1917-1974.
McCaw DL, Hoskins JD. Canine viral enteritis. In: Greene CE, ed., Infectious Diseases of the Dog and Cat, 3rd ed. St. Louis: Saunders Elsevier, 2006, pp. 63-73.

Autor J. Paul Woods
Consultor Editorial Stephen C. Barr

Infertilidade das Cadelas

CONSIDERAÇÕES GERAIS

DEFINIÇÃO
Queixa à anamnese que ocorre em cadelas que apresentam ciclos anormais, falha na cópula, falha na concepção ou perda da prenhez.

FISIOPATOLOGIA
• Fertilidade normal — requer ciclo estral normal com ovulação de ovos normais no trato reprodutivo saudável e patente; fertilização por espermatozoides normais; implantação do concepto no endométrio; formação da placenta zonária normal e manutenção da prenhez na presença de elevada concentração de progesterona ao longo de todo o período de aproximadamente 2 meses de gestação.
• A interrupção de qualquer um desses processos provoca infertilidade.

SISTEMA(S) ACOMETIDO(S)
Reprodutivo.

IDENTIFICAÇÃO
• Animais de todas as idades; pode ser mais comum nos mais idosos.
• Cadelas com >6 anos de idade — mais provavelmente apresentam hiperplasia endometrial cística subjacente; podem estar predispostas à infecção uterina, além de falha na concepção ou na implantação.
• Raças caninas predispostas à insuficiência da tireoide — podem apresentar uma prevalência maior; incluem as raças Golden retriever, Doberman pinscher, Dachshund, Setter irlandês, Schnauzer miniatura, Dinamarquês, Poodle e Boxer.

SINAIS CLÍNICOS

Achados Anamnésicos
• Falha no ciclo estral.
• Ciclos muito frequentes (intervalo interestro igual ou inferior a 4 meses).
• Falha na cópula.
• Cópula normal, sem subsequente prenhez ou parto.

Achados do Exame Físico
• Exame negativo de prenhez após o acasalamento.
• Exame positivo de prenhez sem o parto subsequente.

CAUSAS
Animais adquiridos quando já adultos — possibilidade de ovário-histerectomia prévia.

Cadelas
• Inseminação na época inadequada durante o ciclo estral — mais comum.
• Infecção uterina subclínica.
• Hiperplasia endometrial cística.
• Fatores de infertilidade no macho.
• Insuficiência da tireoide.
• Hipercortisolismo.
• Anormalidade anatômica.
• Anormalidade cromossômica.
• Função ovariana anormal.
• *Brucella canis* — sempre uma possibilidade.

Gatas
• Causas semelhantes às das cadelas.
• Ausência de estímulo copulatório suficiente para induzir à ovulação.
• Infecção sistêmica viral ou protozoária.

FATORES DE RISCO
• *B. canis* (cadelas).
• Insuficiência da tireoide (cadelas).
• Hipercortisolismo (cadelas e gatas) — endógeno ou exógeno.
• Infecção viral sistêmica (cadelas e gatas) — herpes-vírus canino; FeLV; FIV.
• Infecção protozoária sistêmica (cadelas e gatas) — por exemplo, toxoplasmose.
• Qualquer condição mórbida debilitante crônica (cadelas e gatas).
• Anomalia vaginal congênita (cadelas e gatas).

DIAGNÓSTICO

DIAGNÓSTICO DIFERENCIAL

Informação da Anamnese
• Extremamente valiosa na distinção das causas.
• A paciente tem ciclos? Anestro primário = sem ciclo estral manifesto em torno dos dois anos de idade; anestro secundário = sem ciclo estral manifesto depois de um ano de ciclo normal.
• A paciente concebeu ou pariu anteriormente? Se sim, recentemente ou há quanto tempo? Qual o tamanho da ninhada? Qual a porcentagem de natimortos? Que porcentagem da ninhada foi desmamada?
• A paciente está livre de infecção sistêmica viral ou protozoária?
• A paciente é capaz de copular normalmente?
• A paciente foi acasalada com macho de fertilidade comprovada (i. e., ninhada gerada nos últimos 6 meses) no momento adequado do ciclo estral?
• A paciente ovulou durante o ciclo estral e manteve concentração de progesterona compatível com a prenhez durante toda a gestação?
• A cadela é eutireóidea?

HEMOGRAMA/BIOQUÍMICA/URINÁLISE
Geralmente normais.

OUTROS TESTES LABORATORIAIS

Teste Sorológico para B. canis (cadelas)
• Teste de aglutinação rápida em lâmina — utilizado como teste de triagem; sensível mas inespecífico (D-Tec CB, Synbiotics Corp.).
• Se os resultados forem positivos — será recomendável a reavaliação do animal por teste de imunodifusão em ágar gel (Cornell University Diagnostic Laboratory) ou cultura bacteriana de sangue total e aspirado de linfonodo.

Mensuração da Progesterona Sérica
• Deve permanecer elevada durante toda a gestação.
• Pode-se medir no momento do exame.
• Se a concentração estiver <2 ng/mL no meio da gestação e ocorrer perda da prenhez, esse quadro será indicativo de função luteal insuficiente (hipoluteodismo) [ver "Abortamento Espontâneo (Perda Gestacional Prematura) — Cadelas" e "Parto Prematuro"].
• Concentração >2 ng/mL — pode indicar cio silencioso; estro sem alterações comportamentais ou físicas evidentes; ou produção patológica de progesterona a partir de estrutura ovariana luteal, neoplasia ovariana funcional ou glândula adrenal.
• Ensaio quantitativo de progesterona (quimioluminescência, fluorescência, imunoensaio enzimático) — é importante para detectar níveis <2,0 ng/mL. Os ensaios hospitalares rápidos têm uma precisão menor, sendo capazes de detectar entre 2 e 5 ng/mL.

Cadelas
• A progesterona pode ser medida durante o proestro e estro para prever o momento da ovulação e otimizar o manejo reprodutivo.
• Concentração e ovulação — 1,0-1,9 ng/mL, provável ovulação em 3 dias (reavaliar); 2,0-2,9 ng/mL, ovulação em 2 dias; 3,0-3,9 ng/mL, ovulação em 1 dia; 4,0-10,0 ng/mL, ovulação naquele dia.
• Ótimo dia de acasalamento para o máximo tamanho da ninhada — 2 dias após a ovulação.
• Dia da ovulação desde o início do proestro ou do estro — extremamente variável; não está bem correlacionado com o comportamento em estação (ver "Acasalamento, Momento Oportuno").

Gatas
• A progesterona pode ser medida após o acasalamento para avaliar a indução da ovulação.
• Concentração >2 ng/mL — indica tecido luteal funcional.

Outros Testes
• Cultura bacteriana para pesquisa de microrganismos uterinos (cadelas e gatas) — o corrimento vaginal que se origina no útero durante o proestro ou estro é coletado diretamente por histerotomia ou cateterização transcervical ou indiretamente da vagina anterior com o uso de *swab* estéril reservado para isso.
• Teste de hormônio tireoidiano (cadelas) — pode-se medir a concentração sérica em repouso de T_3 ou T_4 e TSH canino.
• Teste sorológico — herpes-vírus canino e toxoplasmose [ver "Abortamento Espontâneo (Perda Gestacional Prematura) — Cadelas"]; FeLV, FIV e toxoplasmose [ver "Abortamento Espontâneo (Perda Gestacional Prematura) — Gatas"].
• Cariótipo (cadelas e gatas) — realizado em amostras de sangue heparinizado de pacientes com anestro primário ou persistente; atentar para anormalidades cromossômicas capazes de provocar diferenciação sexual anormal (teste realizado por Molecular Cytogenetics Laboratory, Texas A&M University; agendamento por telefone com antecedência; ver "Distúrbios do Desenvolvimento Sexual").
• Teste do cortisol sérico (cadelas e gatas) — se a concentração sérica em repouso estiver elevada, pesquisar a causa subjacente.
• Avaliação do sêmen (cães e gatos) — é recomendada a avaliação direta para descartar oligospermia ou azoospermia; alternativamente, pode-se testar o acasalamento do macho com outra fêmea para provar a fertilidade; descartar azoospermia no gato pelo encontro de espermatozoides no lavado vaginal ou em amostras de *swab* da fêmea ou na urina coletada do macho por cistocentese (ver "Infertilidade do Macho — Cães").

DIAGNÓSTICO POR IMAGEM
• Radiografia e ultrassonografia — os ovários normais e o útero não gravídico geralmente não são visíveis ao exame radiográfico; os ovários normais e o útero não gravídico serão visualizados se os equipamentos tiverem alta resolução e frequência próxima ao campo de imagem; ovários grandes podem indicar doença cística ovariana ou neoplasia; útero visível pode indicar hiperplasia endometrial cística.

INFERTILIDADE DAS CADELAS

- Métodos de contraste positivo — vaginografia em cadelas; histerografia em cadelas e gatas; realizadas antes da puberdade ou quando a paciente estiver no cio (estro); podem revelar anormalidade anatômica (p. ex., estrutura anormal e sem patência) (ver "Más-formações Vaginais e Lesões Adquiridas").
- Ultrassom — pode diagnosticar prenhez em até 20-24 dias após a ovulação; exame valioso para comprovar perda gestacional; útil para detectar hiperplasia endometrial cística e líquido intraluminal.

MÉTODOS DIAGNÓSTICOS
- Laparotomia (cadelas e gatas) — avaliar a anatomia do trato tubular e das gônadas.
- Histerotomia — para obter amostra direta de cultura uterina; biopsia do útero ou dos ovários.

TRATAMENTO
- Gatas — reprodutoras sazonais; dependem do fotoperíodo; apresentam ciclo quando expostas a longos períodos de luz solar, normalmente do final de janeiro ao meio de outubro no hemisfério norte; induzir o ciclo durante todo o ano por exposição diária à luz solar de pelo menos 12 h; para uma gata que não apresenta ciclos durante a estação fisiológica de acasalamento, questionar o proprietário sobre confinamento em casa e exposição à luz solar.
- Causa hereditária (p. ex., insuficiência da tireoide) — aconselhar o proprietário quanto à pertinência de se manter a paciente no programa de acasalamento.
- Ressecção cirúrgica de anomalias vaginais (cadelas) — pode facilitar a monta natural e a expulsão vaginal dos filhotes.
- Reparo cirúrgico de trato tubular sem patência (cadelas e gatas) — método difícil; prognóstico reservado em termos de fertilidade futura.
- Drenagem cirúrgica de cistos ovarianos (cadelas e gatas) — eficácia desconhecida.
- Ovariectomia unilateral de ovário neoplásico (cadelas e gatas) — a fertilidade futura depende do retorno à função normal do ovário remanescente e da ausência de metástase.
- Supressão do cio (estro) por um ou dois ciclos estrais — pode beneficiar as cadelas com ciclos frequentes (intervalo interestro curto).
- Prognóstico quanto à fertilidade futura — inicialmente bom, porque a causa mais comum é o manejo reprodutivo inadequado; pior com outras causas.

MEDICAÇÕES

MEDICAMENTO(S) DE ESCOLHA
- Antibióticos (cadelas e gatas) — em casos de infecção uterina; a escolha depende da cultura bacteriana e do teste de sensibilidade do útero ou do corrimento vaginal durante o proestro ou o estro.
- L-tiroxina — na insuficiência da tireoide; cadelas: 0,01-0,02 mg/kg VO a cada 12 h; prognóstico reservado em termos de fertilidade futura com retorno ao estado eutireóideo.

Tratamento com Gonadotropina
- Para indução da ovulação.
- GnRH, que provoca a liberação do LH endógeno da hipófise, ou hCG, que possui atividade semelhante ao LH.
- Gatas que não são adequadamente estimuladas a ovular no momento da cópula — GnRH (25 μg/gata IM ou hCG 250 UI/gata IM) na hora do acasalamento.
- Doença cística ovariana — gatas: GnRH (25 μg/gata IM) ou hCG (250 UI/gata IM); cadelas: GnRH (50 μg/cadela IM) ou hCG (1.000 UI/cadela, metade IV, metade IM); provoca ovulação ou luteinização do tecido ovariano cístico.
- Indução do estro (cadelas) — dietilestilbestrol (5 mg a cada 24 h VO por 9 dias ou até os sinais de proestro induzido); bromocriptina (20 μg/kg a cada 12 h VO por 21 dias); cabergolina (5 μg/kg a cada 24 h VO por até 30 dias ou até os sinais de proestro induzido); deslorrelina (implante de 2,1 mg, Ovuplant®; aplicado no vestíbulo; precisa ter um nível de progesterona <0,5 ng/mL no início; o implante é removido após a confirmação da ovulação: progesterona >10 ng/mL).
- Supressão do estro (cadelas) — acetato de megestrol (2 mg/kg VO diariamente por 8 dias se iniciado dentro dos 3 primeiros dias do proestro ou 0,5 mg/kg VO diariamente por 32 dias se instituído no anestro) ou mibolerona (a dose depende do peso corporal; 30 μg VO diariamente para cadelas que pesam de 0,5-12 kg, 60 μg diariamente para cadelas de 12-23 kg, 120 μg diariamente para cadelas de 23-45 kg, 180 μg para cadelas com mais de 45 kg e para a raça Pastor alemão e seus cruzamentos).

CONTRAINDICAÇÕES
- O tratamento com progestinas, incluindo acetato de megestrol, é contraindicado em cadelas com hiperplasia endometrial cística ou histórico de doença dependente da progesterona.
- O tratamento com mibolerona fica contraindicado em Bedlington terrier e outras raças com hepatopatia familiar.
- Todas as terapias hormonais são contraindicadas em cadelas potencialmente prenhes.

ACOMPANHAMENTO

MONITORIZAÇÃO DA PACIENTE
- L-tiroxina (cadelas) — concentrações sanguíneas de T_3 e T_4 são reavaliadas após 1 mês da suplementação para garantir a absorção adequada do medicamento e o retorno ao estado eutireóideo.
- Ultrassonografia (cadelas e gatas) — para obtenção do diagnóstico definitivo de prenhez; monitorizar a gestação.
- Teste da progesterona (cadelas e gatas).

DIVERSOS

DISTÚRBIOS ASSOCIADOS
- Infertilidade causada por endocrinopatia — sinais de anormalidade dermatológica (p. ex., alopecia com insuficiência da tireoide ou hipercortisolismo); sinais sistêmicos de doença (p. ex., polidipsia e poliúria com hipercortisolismo).
- Cadelas com anormalidade anatômica vaginal — doença do trato urinário ou vaginite persistentes ou recidivantes.

POTENCIAL ZOONÓTICO
Infecção por *B. canis* — o microrganismo será menos facilmente eliminado se os animais acometidos forem gonadectomizados; enfatizar a boa higiene.

VER TAMBÉM
Ver a seção "Causas".

ABREVIATURA(S)
- FeLV = vírus da leucemia felina.
- FIV = vírus da imunodeficiência felina.
- GnRH = hormônio liberador da gonadotropina.
- hCG = gonadotropina coriônica humana.
- LH = hormônio luteinizante.
- T_3 = tri-iodotironina.
- T_4 = tiroxina.
- TSH = hormônio tireostimulante.

Sugestões de Leitura
Johnston SD, Root Kustritz MV, Olson PN. Clinical approach to infertility in the bitch. In: Canine and Feline Theriogenology. Philadelphia: Saunders, 2001, pp. 257-273.
Johnston SD, Root Kustritz MV, Olson PN. Clinical approach to the complaint of infertility in the queen. In: Canine and Feline Theriogenology. Philadelphia: Saunders, 2001, pp. 486-495.
Meyers-Wallen VN. Abnormal and unusual estrous cycles. Theriogenology 2007, 68:1205-1210.

Autor Margaret V. Root Kustritz
Consultor Editorial Sara K. Lyle

Infertilidade dos Cães Machos

CONSIDERAÇÕES GERAIS

DEFINIÇÃO
- Fertilidade reduzida ou ausente; não implica esterilidade.
- Resulta de uma ampla variedade de problemas que impedem a liberação de número suficiente de espermatozoides para fertilizar oocistos maduros ovulados na cadela ou número excessivo de espermatozoides comprometidos em termos bioquímicos/estruturais.

FISIOPATOLOGIA
- Espermatogênese — compreende a formação e o desenvolvimento dos espermatozoides desde a espermatogônia até os espermatozoides maduros; processo cíclico, coordenado, controlado de forma hormonal; são necessários aproximadamente 70 dias para a fase completa (61,9 dias nos cães sem raça definida, bem como nas raças Poodle, Pinscher, Beagle e Labrador; no entanto, essa fase foi de 56,5 dias no Pit bull terrier). A fase testicular é de 61,9 dias, enquanto a fase epididimária, 10-14 dias; dessa forma, os problemas testiculares necessitam de, no mínimo, 70 dias para a recuperação; já os problemas epididimários exigem, pelo menos, 10-14 dias.
- Azoospermia — ejaculado completamente desprovido de espermatozoides.
- Oligozoospermia — ejaculado com baixo número de espermatozoides.
- Teratospermia — ejaculado com número normalmente elevado de espermatozoides com formato anormal.
- Causas primárias — espermatogênese comprometida ou interrompida; obstrução dos ductos de saída; inflamação geniturinária; neoplasia testicular; estresse ambiental; anormalidade congênita; disfunção endócrina.

SISTEMA(S) ACOMETIDO(S)
- Reprodutivo.
- Endócrino/metabólico.
- Musculoesquelético.
- Nervoso.

GENÉTICA
- Há uma incidência crescente de causas hereditárias substanciais de infertilidade no cão macho reprodutor.
- Criptorquidismo — trata-se de um traço autossômico recessivo poligênico hereditário limitado ao sexo em cães. Os cães criptorquídicos apresentam uma frequência elevada de hérnias inguinais/umbilicais, luxação patelar, problemas prepuciais e penianos.
- Deficiência de α-L-fucosidase — nos cães machos, foi relatado distúrbio hereditário de armazenamento lisossomal; provoca efeito deletério específico na disgenesia acrossômica e na maturação prejudicada do esperma.
- Discinesia ciliar primária — anormalidade congênita da ultraestrutura ciliar; padrões de motilidade ausente, irregular ou assincrônica de todas as células ciliadas; diagnosticada por microscopia eletrônica dos espermatozoides.
- Hipotireoidismo — nas fêmeas, alguns distúrbios da tireoide parecem ser herdados e exercem efeitos específicos sobre a ciclicidade; o efeito do hipotireoidismo sobre a fertilidade dos machos está menos claramente definido e provavelmente é mínimo.

INCIDÊNCIA/PREVALÊNCIA
Incidência verdadeira desconhecida, mas provavelmente crescente com endogamia ou consanguinidade contínua. É provável que a porcentagem seja mais alta do que a esperada, pois ainda não foi identificado o grau completo de efeitos genéticos.

IDENTIFICAÇÃO
Espécies
Cães.
Raça(s) Predominante(s)
Prevalência relativamente mais elevada de problemas específicos observados em mais raças endogâmicas com endogamia intensiva.
Idade Média e Faixa Etária
A prevalência aumenta com a idade.

SINAIS CLÍNICOS
Comentários Gerais
Queixa geral — geração de nenhum filhote; taxa de parição <75% quando acasalado no momento correto com fêmeas férteis; o proprietário suspeita da infertilidade do macho.

Achados Anamnésicos
- Idade da descida testicular.
- Idade na primeira tentativa de acasalamento.
- Temperamento do cão (muito excitado).
- Libido e comportamento no acasalamento.
- Frequência e número de acasalamentos.
- Método utilizado para sincronizar os acasalamentos.
- Tipo de sêmen utilizado (fresco, fresco estendido, resfriado estendido ou congelado).
- Capacidade de sobrevivência das células do esperma do cão ao congelamento ou resfriamento.
- Manejo do sêmen e via de inseminação.
- Tamanho da(s) ninhada(s).
- Histórico familiar de infertilidade.
- Grau de acasalamento consanguíneo.
- Estado de fertilidade das cadelas acasaladas.
- Estado da *Brucella canis* de todos os animais acasalados.
- Terapias atuais e anteriores de medicamentos e dieta, especialmente corticosteroides.
- Doença clínica ou cirúrgica prévia.

Achados do Exame Físico
- Prepúcio e pênis — palpados para identificar massas ou aderências.
- Pênis não ereto exteriorizado — para determinar se a mucosa superficial contém qualquer lesão clinicamente relevante e se o osso peniano não está lesado.
- Testículos e epidídimo — palpados e examinados, sendo observados o tamanho e a simetria do epidídimo em relação aos testículos.
- Uretra interna e próstata — palpação retal digital para determinar localização, tamanho e simetria.

CAUSAS
Sincronização incorreta do acasalamento — causa mais comum.

Congênitas
- Anormalidades cromossômicas (síndrome XXY) e reversão sexual XX (síndrome do macho XX) — machos fenotípicos com testículos hipoplásicos e sem espermatogênese; ver "Distúrbios do Desenvolvimento Sexual".
- Aplasia de células germinativas — a biopsia revela síndrome "apenas das células de Sertoli".
- Aplasia segmentar uni ou bilateral do epidídimo ou do ducto espermático — causa oligospermia ou azoospermia.

Adquiridas
- Ejaculação incompleta — redondezas não familiares; assoalho escorregadio; cadela sem estro; proprietário ou cadela dominantes presentes.
- Obstrução dos ductos eferentes, dos epidídimos ou dos ductos deferentes — leva à azoospermia se bilateral; granuloma espermático, espermatocele, inflamação aguda, estenose inflamatória crônica, aplasia segmentar, neoplasia, vasectomia anterior e tentativas de incluir os testículos em localização escrotal.
- Inflamação ou infecção dos testículos — especialmente *B. canis* e *Escherichia coli*; necessita de tratamento imediato e rigoroso para evitar a infertilidade.
- Hipotireoidismo — papel incerto; avaliar a função da tireoide em casos de qualidade insatisfatória do sêmen; pode estar associado à redução da libido.
- Hiperprolactinemia — papel incerto; avaliar os níveis de prolactina na presença de azoospermia.
- Hiperadrenocorticismo — provoca atrofia testicular e oligospermia; provavelmente reversível.
- Medicamentos — parasiticidas, corticosteroides, esteroides anabólicos, estrogênios, androgênios, progestogênios, agonistas/antagonistas do GnRH, cetoconazol, anfotericina B, alguns agentes antifúngicos podem interferir na espermatogênese ou interromper esse processo; avaliar todas as terapias tópicas e sistêmicas.
- Toxinas ambientais — contaminantes que promovem disfunção do sistema endócrino podem afetar o eixo hipotalâmico-hipofisário e a esteroidogênese gonadal; efeitos desconhecidos, mas suspeitos, nos cães.
- Traumatismo, lesão ambiental, neoplasia testicular, doença sistêmica, isquemia e estresse pelo calor — podem provocar infertilidade ou esterilidade temporária.
- Prostatopatia — parece reduzir acentuadamente a qualidade do sêmen e a libido.
- Acasalamento consanguíneo — diminui a fertilidade; sem um programa reprodutivo sério e cruzamento exogâmico com os animais fecundos normais acima, as linhagens reduzidas de fertilidade poderão não ser recuperadas.
- Orquite linfocitária — familiar em algumas raças (p. ex., Beagle e Borzoi); os animais acometidos podem ser férteis quando jovens; a fertilidade declina a uma velocidade acelerada com a idade.
- Ejaculação retrógrada — algum fluxo retrógrado para a bexiga normal.

FATORES DE RISCO
- Distúrbios congênitos que afetam a função reprodutiva — não são incomuns; tendem a ocorrer em raças selecionadas.
- Cadelas para teste de reprodutores e machos reprodutores não testados para doença infecciosa (p. ex., *B. canis* e cultura bacteriana do trato genital) antes do acasalamento.

DIAGNÓSTICO

DIAGNÓSTICO DIFERENCIAL
Antes de extensa avaliação diagnóstica no macho, determinar se as cadelas são férteis (ninhadas anteriores) e se os acasalamentos foram sincronizados de forma ideal (ver "Infertilidade na Fêmea" e "Acasalamento, Momento Oportuno").

INFERTILIDADE DOS CÃES MACHOS

HEMOGRAMA/BIOQUÍMICA/URINÁLISE
- Geralmente normais.
- Brucelose ou prostatite — alterações variáveis no leucograma (normal ou leucocitose) e na urinálise (números elevados de leucócitos); depende do curso de tempo da infecção; são possíveis resultados falso-negativos no teste para brucelose; a antibioticoterapia também pode gerar resultados falso-negativos.
- Doença sistêmica — embora possa comprometer a função reprodutiva, a infertilidade não costuma ser a primeira queixa ao exame.

OUTROS TESTES LABORATORIAIS
Perfil Endócrino
- Testosterona em repouso — machos intactos normais, 0,4-10 ng/mL; faixa mais comum, 1-4 ng/mL.
- Tecido androgênico — confirmado se a concentração sérica de testosterona aumentar 100% sobre o valor em repouso 2-3 h após a injeção de 1-2 µg/kg de GnRH ou 40 UI/kg de hCG; útil para detectar criptorquidismo bilateral.
- Baixo nível de testosterona com altos níveis de FSH e LH — indicam insuficiência testicular primária.
- Testosterona normal e FSH elevado — indicam insuficiência de compartimento germinal; nível aumentado de FSH em virtude da perda de secreção da inibina por células de Sertoli viáveis.
- Testosterona, FSH e LH baixos — indicam hipogonadismo.
- Função da tireoide — avaliada pela referência basal de T_3 e T_4, valores de TSH e teste de estimulação (ver "Hipotireoidismo").

DIAGNÓSTICO POR IMAGEM
Ultrassonografia — auxilia na identificação de lesões que alteram a arquitetura testicular e epididimária (p. ex., neoplasia, espermatocele, orquite, epididimite); avalia a próstata quanto à presença de hiperplasia, prostatite crônica, cisto, abscesso ou neoplasia (ver "Hiperplasia Prostática Benigna", "Cistos Prostáticos", "Prostatite e Abscesso Prostático" e "Prostatomegalia").

MÉTODOS DIAGNÓSTICOS
Exame da Sanidade do Acasalamento
- Fundamental para garantir a obtenção de todas as informações adequadas; sempre deve consistir em duas coletas de sêmen.
- Porções do ejaculado prostático e rico em esperma — coletadas como frações separadas com o uso de vagina artificial estéril e tubos plásticos atóxicos, graduados e estéreis na presença de cadela no cio (estro).
- Fração rica em esperma — volume; concentração, motilidade e características morfológicas das células espermáticas; exame citológico; culturas qualitativa e quantitativa.
- Fração prostática e urina (coletada por cistocentese) — exame citológico; culturas qualitativa e quantitativa.
- Resultados da cultura — devem ser correlacionados com evidência clínica e citológica de infecção ativa; evidência de inflamação se mais de 3-5 leucócitos forem observados por campo de grande aumento (especialmente na fração rica em esperma).
- Fração prostática indicativa de infecção clinicamente relevante — reavaliar por outras técnicas de amostragem que evitem contaminação a partir da mucosa peniana e do prepúcio; é possível a obtenção de resultados negativos ao exame citológico em casos de prostatite crônica.
- Ejaculado azoospérmico ou oligospérmico — coletar novamente uma hora depois e outra vez em várias ocasiões antes de se confirmar a infertilidade.

Marcadores Epididimários
Concentração da fosfatase alcalina no líquido seminal — normal: 8.000 a 40.000 U/mL; origem epididimária; poderá indicar obstrução se a concentração estiver <5.000 U/mL e se foi obtido o ejaculado completo; efeitos patológicos da obstrução serão mais facilmente observados se a fosfatase alcalina for medida em dois ejaculados coletados com intervalo de 60 min.

ACHADOS PATOLÓGICOS
- Biopsia testicular — determina o grau de espermatogênese e a integridade da barreira hematotesticular; diferencia obstrução dos ductos eferentes de hipoplasia e degeneração testiculares; permite prognóstico informado.
- Biopsia incisional — superior à aspiração ou biopsia com agulha para obter amostra diagnóstica; há necessidade de fixação em Bouin para processamento do tecido.

TRATAMENTO
ATIVIDADE
- Restrita se a atividade ou o uso supostamente estiver induzindo à hipertermia (ver "Intermação e Hipertermia").
- Nenhuma restrição para outras causas de infertilidade.

DIETA
Garantir dieta adequada e suplementação mineral; evitar a suplementação de produtos que contenham quantidades excessivas ou indefinidas de hormônios esteroides (p. ex., extratos de testículos, ovários e adrenais).

ORIENTAÇÕES AO PROPRIETÁRIO
- Informar ao proprietário que os testículos necessitarão de no mínimo 70 dias a partir da correção das causas identificadas para retornar à função.
- Enfatizar a paciência enquanto o paciente estiver sendo submetido a check-ups regulares para garantir que não haja piora da condição.

CONSIDERAÇÕES CIRÚRGICAS
Em diversos casos, a realização de nova anastomose dos ductos de saída obstruídos é bem-sucedida para produção de esperma.

MEDICAÇÕES
MEDICAMENTO(S) DE ESCOLHA
- Medicações específicas devem ser administradas por tempo suficiente e em uma dosagem que garanta a penetração tecidual. Antibióticos (selecionados com base nas características de penetração e espectro) — cloranfenicol, trimetoprima-sulfa, eritromicina e enrofloxacino; são recomendados, em geral, por no mínimo 3-4 semanas para conferir níveis adequados e contínuos dentro do trato reprodutivo.
- Ejaculação retrógrada — pseudoefedrina utilizada com sucesso limitado em humanos com esse tipo de ejaculação; 4-5 mg/kg VO a cada 8 h ou 1 e 3 h antes da coleta; fenilpropanolamina, 4-8 mg/kg VO a cada 24 h, 5 dias antes da coleta.

CONTRAINDICAÇÕES
- Trimetoprima-sulfas — contraindicadas se o animal for predisposto a ceratite seca.
- Cloranfenicol e trimetoprima-sulfas — segundo relatos, induzem a discrasias sanguíneas.
- Cloranfenicol — é associado a anorexia e vômitos, mas ainda pode ser o antibiótico de melhor penetração tecidual.

ACOMPANHAMENTO
MONITORIZAÇÃO DO PACIENTE
Reavaliar em intervalos que levem em conta a duração do ciclo espermatogênico (70 dias), mas que sejam frequentes o suficiente a ponto de permitir a detecção de condição deteriorante.

PREVENÇÃO
Evitar a exposição a extremos de temperatura ambiente (calor ou frio).

COMPLICAÇÕES POSSÍVEIS
Retorno de 10% dos casos à fertilidade após diagnóstico e tratamento apropriados.

DIVERSOS
DISTÚRBIOS ASSOCIADOS
- Infecção por brucelose — discospondilite, poliartrite, paresia posterior, febre e uveíte.
- Prostatopatia — obstipação, dificuldades de locomoção, febre, hematúria, polaciúria e disúria.
- Orquite linfocitária — tireoidite linfocítica.

FATORES RELACIONADOS COM A IDADE
- Declínio na produção diária de esperma e nas células espermáticas morfologicamente normais — com a idade.
- É difícil avaliar o efeito isolado da idade sobre a fertilidade.
- A maioria dos cães idosos e inférteis possui doenças concomitantes (p. ex., doença sistêmica ou prostática e neoplasia testicular) que têm efeitos comprovados sobre a fertilidade.

ABREVIATURA(S)
- FSH = hormônio foliculoestimulante.
- GnRH = hormônio liberador da gonadotropina.
- hCG = gonadotropina coriônica humana.
- LH = hormônio luteinizante.
- TSH = hormônio tireostimulante.

Sugestões de Leitura
Johnston SD, Root Kustritz MV, Olson PNS. Clinical approach to infertility in the male dog. In: Johnston SD, Root Kustritz MV, Olson PNS, Canine and Feline Theriogenology. Philadelphia: Saunders, 2001, pp. 370-387.

Autor Richard A. Fayrer-Hosken
Consultor Editorial Sara K. Lyle

Infestação por Trematódeos

CONSIDERAÇÕES GERAIS

REVISÃO
- A infecção por *Platynosomum concinnum* ocorre nos gatos em estados norte-americanos como Flórida, Ohio, Illinois, Havaí e em muitas outras regiões tropicais e semitropicais. Esta é a infecção mais comum por trematódeos que acometem o fígado dos animais de companhia na América do Norte.
- A infestação é adquirida a partir da ingestão de algum hospedeiro intermediário infectado (p. ex., lagarto ou rã).
- Nas áreas endêmicas, estima-se que 15-85% dos gatos com acesso a hospedeiros intermediários estejam infectados.
- *Metorchis conjunctus* também pode infectar o fígado e as estruturas biliares de gatos.
- Trematódeos relatados em cães: *Heterobilharzia americana* (América do Norte); guaxinim é o hospedeiro definitivo natural e o hospedeiro reservatório mais importante; *Metorchis conjunctus*; *Clonorchis sinensis* (China), *Schistosoma japonicum* (Filipinas), *Metorchis bilis* e *Opisthorchis felineus* (Alemanha) em cães de trenó alimentados com uma dieta que inclui peixe cru.

IDENTIFICAÇÃO
Platynosomum Concinnum
O paciente típico é um gato jovem (6-24 meses) com acesso à fauna local.

SINAIS CLÍNICOS
- Dependem da gravidade da infecção.
- A maior parte dos gatos infestados não apresenta sinais clínicos.
- Em casos de infestação grave: icterícia, emaciação, anorexia, vômito, diarreia mucoide, hepatomegalia, distensão abdominal, mal-estar, febre.

CAUSAS E FATORES DE RISCO
P. concinnum
- Os adultos residem nos ductos biliares e na vesícula biliar; o ciclo de vida necessita de dois hospedeiros intermediários e de clima tropical ou semitropical.
- Ovos embrionados — saem nas fezes dos gatos; ingeridos pelo primeiro hospedeiro intermediário: um caramujo terrestre.
- Miracídios — eclodem dos ovos no caramujo; penetram nos tecidos do hospedeiro; evoluem para esporocistos.
- Esporocistos-filhos maduros — emergem do caramujo e, em seguida, são ingeridos por um segundo hospedeiro intermediário: geralmente um camaleão (mas também gambás, lagartixas, rãs e sapos); entram nos ductos biliares e aí residem até que o hospedeiro seja ingerido como presa pelo gato.
- Cercárias — liberadas no trato digestivo superior do gato; migram para os ductos biliares, onde amadurecem e liberam os ovos em cerca de 8 semanas.
- Fatores de risco para a infecção — clima tropical ou subtropical; existência de hospedeiros intermediários adequados; acesso a algum ambiente externo ou interno/externo; habilidades bem-sucedidas de caça; consumo do hospedeiro intermediário infectado.

Metorchis conjunctus
- Gatos — pode infectar o fígado e as estruturas biliares inicialmente, provocando diarreia aquosa manchada de sangue e, mais tarde, indícios de invasão da árvore biliar; os ovos são eliminados nas fezes 17 dias a partir da infecção inicial.
- A infecção é associada a eosinofilia transitória e enzimas hepáticas elevadas.

Heterobilharzia americana
- Os ovos que contêm o miracídio completamente desenvolvido são eliminados nas fezes do hospedeiro final. Na água doce, os ovos eclodem e liberam os miracídios que penetram nos hospedeiros caramujos, onde os esporocistos se desenvolvem. As cercárias são liberadas do hospedeiro caramujo 25 dias depois da infecção; essas cercárias infectam o hospedeiro vertebrado (cão, ser humano) por penetração na pele.
- Os trematódeos adultos evoluem no fígado e migram para as veias mesentéricas; por essas veias, os ovos se disseminam para várias vísceras, incluindo fígado, pâncreas, linfonodos mesentéricos, baço e intestinos, onde desencadeiam uma inflamação granulomatosa e lesões vasculares escleróticas.
- Os ovos aparecem nas fezes 68 dias após a infecção.

Schistosoma haematobium
- Os trematódeos adultos e ovos se dispersam para órgãos esplâncnicos, incluindo fígado e pâncreas; nas veias portas ou hepáticas, os ovos e adultos são associados a focos granulomatosos fibróticos encapsulados.

DIAGNÓSTICO

DIAGNÓSTICO DIFERENCIAL
- Colangio-hepatite; lipidose hepática; carcinoma do ducto biliar; linfoma hepático e qualquer distúrbio que provoque oclusão do ducto biliar principal.
- Quadro identificado pelo encontro de ovos de trematódeos nas fezes, observando-se estruturas ovoides anecoicas com centro ecoico na árvore biliar por meio de ultrassom, exame citológico da bile ou aspirados hepáticos; o diagnóstico mais definitivo é obtido por meio do exame histopatológico de amostras de fígado, estruturas biliares ou pâncreas.

ASPECTOS CLINICOPATOLÓGICOS
Mais bem definidos para o *Platynosomum concinnum* em gatos.

HEMOGRAMA/BIOQUÍMICA/URINÁLISE
- Hemograma completo — variáveis; eosinofilia que começa 3 semanas depois da infecção; persiste por meses; nem todos os gatos infectados demonstram eosinofilia.
- Bioquímica — atividades elevadas das enzimas hepáticas, especialmente ALT e AST; a fosfatase alcalina pode permanecer normal ou apenas levemente aumentada no início.
- Bilirrubina — aumentada; acentuadamente alta em casos de doença grave avançada.
- Urinálise — bilirrubinúria.

OUTROS TESTES LABORATORIAIS
- Ácidos biliares em jejum/pós-prandiais — aumentados.
- Exame de fezes — teste diagnóstico definitivo não invasivo: os ovos de *P. concinnum* são detectados em apenas 25% dos gatos infectados.
- Recuperação de ovos nas fezes — sedimentação é a técnica mais bem-sucedida; formalina-éter ou acetato de sódio são os agentes mais confiáveis (demonstram 8 vezes mais ovos do que o exame direto de fezes).
- Pacientes com poucos parasitas (1 a 5 trematódeos) — podem liberar apenas 2-10 ovos/g de fezes; por essa razão, podem não se descobrir ovos pelo exame de fezes.
- Exames seriados de fezes — podem ser necessários.

DIAGNÓSTICO POR IMAGEM
- Radiografia abdominal — pode revelar hepatomegalia leve.
- Ultrassonografia abdominal — diferencia obstrução biliar de doença hepatocelular; demonstra uma ou mais das seguintes alterações: (1) obstrução biliar: vesícula biliar, ducto biliar comum (>2 mm) e ductos intra-hepáticos dilatados; (2) sedimento da vesícula biliar com trematódeos (estruturas hipoecoicas ovais com centro ecoico), parede da vesícula biliar levemente espessada com aparência de camada dupla (colecistite); (3) parênquima hepático hipoecoico, com áreas portais hiperecoicas proeminentes (ductos) associadas à colangio-hepatite.

MÉTODOS DIAGNÓSTICOS
- Exame de fezes — para pesquisa de ovos de trematódeos.
- Colecistocentese — revela os ovos de trematódeos.
- Biopsia hepática — exibe os sinais de infecção.

ACHADOS PATOLÓGICOS
- Macroscópicos — o fígado pode parecer grande e amarelo-esverdeado, com os ductos biliares dilatados; podem ser observados trematódeos nos ductos biliares ou na vesícula biliar; tamanho aumentado e tortuosidade dos ductos biliares ao corte transversal.
- Histopatológicos — dependem do número de trematódeos e da duração da infestação; *estágio precoce* (4-6 semanas): ductos biliares aumentados e áreas periductais infiltradas com células inflamatórias, especialmente eosinófilos; *estágio mediano* (4 meses): hiperplasia adenomatosa grave do epitélio do ducto biliar e inflamação periductal coincidente; *estágio tardio* (6 meses): tecido conjuntivo fibroso peribiliar extenso que pode causar estenose do ducto biliar.

TRATAMENTO

Internação ou tratamento ambulatorial — depende da gravidade da doença.

Paciente Internado
- Fluidos poliônicos balanceados com suplementação de cloreto de potássio — 20-40 mEq/L; administrados conforme for apropriado; escolhidos com base nos eletrólitos séricos.
- Suporte nutricional — evitar o desenvolvimento da lipidose hepática; fornecer dieta rica em proteína e densamente calórica, além de garantir a ingestão alimentar; usar sondas de alimentação, se houver necessidade, para garantir o consumo alimentar adequado em gatos inapetentes; raramente, os sinais clínicos graves podem

necessitar de nutrição parenteral; raras vezes, a encefalopatia hepática necessita de restrição proteica.
• Suplementação com vitaminas do complexo B — importante para gatos anoréxicos e doentes sob fluidoterapia; 2 mL de vitaminas solúveis do complexo B/L de fluido.

MEDICAÇÕES
MEDICAMENTO(S)
• Praziquantel — 20 mg/kg SC a cada 24 h por 3-5 dias constitui o tratamento de escolha; os ovos podem ser eliminados nas fezes por até 2 meses após o tratamento. O praziquantel à dose de 30 mg/kg VO em dose única e 50 mg/kg SC em dose única eliminou a *Heterobilharzia americana* em cão sintomático.
• Prednisolona — dose inicial para os gatos que apresentam eosinofilia: 1-2 mg/kg/dia por 2-4 semanas; em seguida, reduzir gradativamente em decréscimos de 50% a cada duas semanas.
• Ácido ursodesoxicólico — 10-15 mg/kg VO a cada 24 h; a formulação de comprimido e a dose dividida administrada juntamente com a alimentação atingem a melhor biodisponibilidade.
• Cobertura antibiótica de amplo espectro para proteger o animal contra infecção retrógrada da árvore biliar por microrganismos entéricos introduzidos pelo parasita; infecção estimulada pela morte do trematódeo nos tecidos.
• Terapia antioxidante — sugerida pela lesão tecidual necroinflamatória; vitamina E (10 UI/kg VO diariamente) e *S*-adenosilmetionina (Denosyl-SD4® tem biodisponibilidade comprovada em gatos como doador de glutationa): 20 mg/kg VO diariamente, comprimidos entéricos revestidos, até a normalização das enzimas hepáticas.
• Antieméticos — metoclopramida (0,2-0,4 mg/kg VO ou SC a cada 6-8 h ou sob infusão em velocidade constante a 1-2 mg/kg/dia); ondansetrona (0,5 mg/kg a cada 12 h IV ou VO 30 min antes da alimentação); maropitanto (1,0 mg/kg [5 mg/gato] IV, SC ou VO uma vez ao dia; por 5 dias no máximo).

CONTRAINDICAÇÕES
Prenhez — ter cuidado com a utilização de medicamento.

ACOMPANHAMENTO
MONITORIZAÇÃO DO PACIENTE
• Monitorizar os sinais clínicos, o apetite, a condição e o peso corporais, a atividade das enzimas hepáticas, o nível de bilirrubina e a sedimentação fecal.
• Ficar atento para os sinais de oclusão da árvore biliar após a administração do praziquantel.

PREVENÇÃO
• Restringir o acesso a ambientes externos em caso de parasita endêmico.
• Profilaxia com praziquantel — a cada 3 meses; pode ser necessária para os gatos de rua em climas tropicais endêmicos.

COMPLICAÇÕES POSSÍVEIS
• Morte por insuficiência hepática; doença sintomática não tratada.
• Obstrução da árvore biliar.
• Pancreatite (rara).
• Insuficiência pancreática exócrina — na infecção crônica.
• Colangite/colangio-hepatite (supurativa ou não supurativa).

EVOLUÇÃO ESPERADA E PROGNÓSTICO
Espera-se a recuperação sem complicações na maior parte dos pacientes tratados.

DIVERSOS
POTENCIAL ZOONÓTICO
Nenhum.
VER TAMBÉM
• Lipidose Hepática.
• Obstrução do Ducto Biliar.
• Síndrome Colangite/Colangio-hepatite.
ABREVIATURA(S)
• ALT = alanina aminotransferase.
• AST = aspartato aminotransferase.

Sugestões de Leitura
Tams TR. Hepatobiliary parasites. In: Sherding RG, ed., The Cat: Disease and Management. Philadelphia: Saunders, 1994, pp. 607-611.

Autor Sharon A. Center
Consultor Editorial Sharon A. Center
Agradecimento Julie Corbet-Pembleton

Inflamação Orofaríngea Felina

CONSIDERAÇÕES GERAIS

REVISÃO
- Resposta inflamatória que afeta a cavidade bucal em gatos.
- A inflamação bucal e orofaríngea é classificada pela localização como:
- Gengivite — inflamação da gengiva.
- Periodontite — inflamação de tecidos periodontais não gengivais (ou seja, o ligamento periodontal e os ossos alveolares).
- Mucosite alveolar — inflamação da mucosa alveolar (ou seja, mucosa que se encontra sobrejacente ao processo alveolar e se estende da junção mucogengival sem delimitação evidente até o sulco vestibular e o assoalho bucal).
- Mucosite sublingual — inflamação da mucosa sobre o assoalho bucal.
- Mucosite labial/bucal — inflamação da mucosa dos lábios e das bochechas.
- Mucosite caudal — inflamação da mucosa da porção caudal da cavidade bucal, delimitada medialmente por pregas palatoglossas e fauces (do latim garganta), dorsalmente pelos palatos duro e mole e, rostralmente, pela mucosa alveolar e bucal.
- Palatite — inflamação da mucosa ou do revestimento dos palatos duro e/ou mole.
- Glossite — inflamação da mucosa da superfície dorsal e/ou ventral da língua.
- Queilite — inflamação dos lábios (incluindo a área da junção mucocutânea e a pele dos lábios).
- Osteomielite — inflamação do osso mandibular e da medula óssea.
- Estomatite — inflamação do revestimento mucoso de qualquer uma das estruturas na boca; na prática clínica, o termo deve ficar reservado para descrever inflamação bucal disseminada (além de gengivite e periodontite) que também pode se estender para tecidos da submucosa.
- Tonsilite — inflamação da tonsila palatina.
- Faringite — inflamação da faringe.

IDENTIFICAÇÃO
- Gatos.
- Predisposição de raças puras — Abissínio, Persa, Himalaio, Birmanês, Siamês e Somali.

SINAIS CLÍNICOS
- Ptialismo.
- Halitose.
- Disfagia.
- Anorexia — preferência por alimento pastoso.
- Perda de peso.
- Pelo sujo e emaranhado pela falta de higiene pessoal.
- Lesões eritematosas, ulcerativas e proliferativas que afetam estruturas como gengiva, arcos glossopalatinos, língua, lábios, mucosa bucal e/ou palato duro.
- Inflamação gengival que envolve completamente o dente, comparada com gengivite, que costuma ocorrer nas superfícies bucal e labial.
- Pode se estender para os arcos glossofaríngeos e o palato.

CAUSAS E FATORES DE RISCO
- Causa desconhecida; há suspeita de etiologias bacterianas, virais e imunológicas.
- Achados significativos de calicivírus felino.
- A imunossupressão causada por FeLV ou FIV também pode levar ao surgimento de infecções pouco responsivas; a maioria dos gatos acometidos é negativa para FeLV e FIV.

DIAGNÓSTICO

DIAGNÓSTICO DIFERENCIAL
- Doença periodontal.
- Processo maligno bucal.
- Complexo granuloma eosinofílico.

HEMOGRAMA/BIOQUÍMICA/URINÁLISE
- Níveis elevados de globulina. Gamopatia policlonal secundária à produção de anticorpos após invasão bacteriana nos tecidos periodontais.
- Pode haver leucocitose e eosinofilia.

DIAGNÓSTICO POR IMAGEM
Radiografias intrabucais para avaliar a presença de doença periodontal e reabsorção dentária.

MÉTODOS DIAGNÓSTICOS
Biopsia (sobretudo de lesões unilaterais) para descartar neoplasia — principalmente carcinoma de células escamosas.

TRATAMENTO

- A terapia inicial para mucosite precoce envolve raspagem dentária supra e subgengival, bem como cuidados domésticos e tratamento (extração) para os dentes acometidos por doença periodontal de graus 1 e 2.
- Para os casos de mucosite vestibuloalveolar focal, a extração dos dentes locais geralmente culmina na resolução do quadro.
- Para estomatite caudal, a extração dos dentes distais ao canino resultou no desaparecimento da inflamação em 60% dos casos sem necessidade adicional de medicação, 20% dos casos necessitaram de controle com medicamentos e 20% não desapareceram em um único estudo publicado.
- Para auxiliar nas extrações: promova a confecção de retalhos cirúrgicos de todos os quadrantes para exposição do dente. Utilize uma broca de alta velocidade com jato de água para criar uma vala (calha) de osso onde as raízes se encontravam, removendo grande parte da gengiva queratinizada, do ligamento periodontal e do osso alveolar perirradicular. Antes de suturar, aplaine a margem alveolar para remover as bordas pontiagudas.
- Se os pacientes não responderem à extração dos dentes distais aos caninos, remova todos os dentes; ao extrair os dentes, preste atenção especial à remoção de toda substância dentária; tire radiografias intrabucais antes e depois da cirurgia; a aplicação pós-operatória de fluocinonida a 0,05% (Lidex® Gel) na margem gengival pode ajudar na cicatrização.
- Os casos refratários com extensa lesão proliferativa na porção caudal da cavidade bucal e faringe apresentam um prognóstico mais reservado.

MEDICAÇÕES

MEDICAMENTO(S)
- O uso de medicamentos e outras terapias tem sucesso limitado a longo prazo; é típica a ausência de resposta permanente à prática de higiene bucal convencional, bem como aos antibióticos, anti-inflamatórios e imunossupressores. O uso de medicamentos não deve ser considerado como o principal método de controle da inflamação orofaríngea.
- Antibióticos — clindamicina (5 mg/kg a cada 12 h), metronidazol, amoxicilina, ampicilina, enrofloxacino, tetraciclina.
- Corticosteroides — prednisona (2 mg/kg inicialmente 1 vez ao dia, seguido pela administração em dias alternados); acetato de metilprednisolona (2 mg/kg a cada 7-30 dias) também pode ajudar a controlar a inflamação.
- Sais de ouro — Solganal® (Schering) 1 mg/kg IM 1 vez por semana até a melhora (até 4 meses) e, depois, a cada 14-35 dias.
- Clorambucila 2 mg/m^2 VO em dias alternados ou 20 mg/m^2 VO em semanas alternadas.
- Lactoferrina bovina (40 mg/kg) aplicada às mucosas bucais.
- Alfainterferona ou omegainterferona 30 UI/dia de 7 em 7 dias (ou seja, 7 dias sim, 7 dias não) por tempo indefinido.
- Laser de CO_2 para diminuir o tecido inflamado.
- Ciclosporina — uma faixa terapêutica de 2-10 mg/kg/dia, dependendo da absorção do produto e da resposta do paciente; monitorizar os resultados da bioquímica e os níveis de vale.

ACOMPANHAMENTO

Monitorizar a resposta à terapia e a ocorrência de efeitos colaterais potenciais dos agentes terapêuticos.

DIVERSOS

SINÔNIMOS
- Estomatite linfocítica-plasmocitária.
- Estomatite.

ABREVIATURAS
- FeLV = vírus da leucemia felina.
- FIV = vírus da imunodeficiência felina.

RECURSOS DA INTERNET
http://www.avdc.org/Nomenclature.html

Sugestões de Leitura
Harvey CE, Emily PP. Small Animal Dentistry. St. Louis: Mosby, 1993.
Wiggs RB, Lobrise HB. Veterinary Dentistry: Principles and Practice. Philadelphia: Lippincott-Raven, 1997.

Autor Jan Bellows
Consultor Editorial Heidi B. Lobprise

INFLUENZA — CÃES

CONSIDERAÇÕES GERAIS

REVISÃO
• Uma doença viral contagiosa aguda a subaguda com uma manifestação respiratória quase exclusiva causada pelo vírus da influenza canina (CIV), um ortomixovírus com uma ligação genética direta com o vírus da influenza equina H3N8 (EUA) ou com um vírus aviário H3N2 (Coreia).
• A via natural de infecção ocorre por meio de partículas aerógenas ou contato oral com superfícies contaminadas. A replicação do vírus parece ficar restrita às células epiteliais das vias aéreas superiores e inferiores com possível envolvimento de macrófagos alveolares. A resposta humoral é detectável por volta de 8 dias após a infecção, enquanto os títulos de anticorpos permanecem detectáveis por mais de 1 ano. As respostas imunes protetoras não foram definidas.
• A atividade do CIV H3N8 foi detectada pela primeira vez em todas as regiões de corridas de galgos nos Estados Unidos em 2004. Atualmente, o vírus é enzoótico em cães que não praticam corridas em, pelo menos, três regiões dos Estados Unidos: Flórida, Colorado e a costa oriental de Connecticut à Virgínia.
• O CIV H3N2 foi detectado pela primeira vez na Coreia em 2007. A ligação genética do vírus não foi determinada, nem a extensão da doença epizoótica, definida.

IDENTIFICAÇÃO
• As infecções naturais por CIV H3N8 são atualmente limitadas aos cães.
• Todas as raças de cães são suscetíveis e não há qualquer restrição etária na suscetibilidade.
• Os galgos demonstram sinais mais graves nas infecções por CIV H3N8, mas outros fatores além da raça podem contribuir para o padrão da doença, como a cepa viral.
• As infecções por CIV H3N2 revelam sinais clínicos mais graves do que aquelas por CIV H3N8.

SINAIS CLÍNICOS
• 60-80% dos cães infectados desenvolvem sinais clínicos.
• Período de incubação de 2-4 dias após a infecção.
• Resposta febril modesta (39,4-40°C) 3-6 dias após a infecção.
• Secreção nasal clara, que pode evoluir para secreção mucoide espessa, causada mais frequentemente por colonização bacteriana secundária.
• A forma mais grave da doença exibe temperaturas mais altas com o desenvolvimento de pneumonia e aumento da frequência respiratória 6-10 dias após a infecção.
• Muitos cães desenvolvem tosse que pode persistir por várias semanas.

CAUSAS E FATORES DE RISCO
• Infecção respiratória causada pelo vírus da influenza canina.
• A maioria dos casos apresenta histórico de alojamento em grupo: canis, centros de cuidados diários e abrigos de resgate, ou contato com cães que recentemente estiveram em um alojamento.
• Como o CIV é uma infecção viral relativamente nova de cães, praticamente todos os cães são suscetíveis.

DIAGNÓSTICO

DIAGNÓSTICO DIFERENCIAL
• Em um nível individual, os sinais precoces (iniciais) de influenza canina são indistinguíveis daqueles de tosse dos canis. • A distinção de patógenos respiratórios típicos de cães é encontrada em ambientes com grupos de animais, onde 60-80% dos cães podem exibir sinais clínicos. • Mais tarde na evolução da doença, pode ocorrer o desenvolvimento de pneumonia com ou sem infecções bacterianas secundárias.

HEMOGRAMA/BIOQUÍMICA/URINÁLISE
• Geralmente normais. • O hemograma pode refletir um estresse em princípio e, depois, o desenvolvimento de pneumonia bacteriana (leucocitose, com desvio à esquerda).

OUTROS TESTES LABORATORIAIS
O teste de inibição da hemaglutinação no soro pode ser usado para avaliar a exposição ao CIV.

MÉTODOS DIAGNÓSTICOS
• Na fase aguda da doença (1-3 dias após o início dos sinais clínicos), um *swab* nasal pode ser utilizado para detectar o agente pelo teste de PCR ou isolamento viral. • Depois de mais de 7 dias do início dos sinais clínicos, o soro coletado para o teste de inibição da hemaglutinação pode determinar a exposição ao CIV. • Os testes ELISA de captura de antígeno fornecem níveis inaceitáveis de falso-negativos.

ACHADOS PATOLÓGICOS
A lesão primária causada pela infecção consiste na destruição da camada de células epiteliais ciliadas nas vias aéreas superiores com extensão para os pulmões. Áreas de consolidação pulmonar podem ser encontradas 6-10 dias após a infecção.

TRATAMENTO
• Os animais acometidos devem ser tratados para evitar a infecção de outros cães. • O período contagioso do CIV estende-se até aproximadamente 6 dias após o início dos sinais clínicos. • A tosse contínua do animal acometido que ultrapassa 6 dias não é um sinal de disseminação viral. • É fortemente recomendado o tratamento dos casos sem complicações em um esquema ambulatorial para evitar infecção nosocomial (hospitalar). • Hospitalizar apenas aqueles casos com pneumonia que necessitam de suporte de fluido IV. • Repouso forçado — por pelo menos 14-21 dias (casos sem complicações); 2 meses em casos de pneumonia. • Se os cães desenvolverem pneumonia bacteriana por *Bordetella bronchiseptica*, eles poderão permanecer contagiosos para essa bactéria mesmo depois de meses da recuperação.

MEDICAÇÕES
• Os agentes antivirais não foram testados quanto à sua eficácia. • O tratamento com antibióticos de amplo espectro pode ser necessário para evitar e controlar as infecções bacterianas secundárias — amoxicilina/ácido clavulânico, doxiciclina, ou trimetoprima-sulfadiazina. • Para os casos graves, resistentes às antibioticoterapias de primeira escolha mencionadas anteriormente, emprega-se a terapia combinada de algum aminoglicosídeo (gentamicina ou amicacina) com alguma cefalosporina (cefazolina). O enrofloxacino pode ser utilizado como medicamento alternativo ao uso da gentamicina. • Em casos graves (broncopneumonia), manter a antibioticoterapia por pelo menos 2 semanas depois da resolução radiográfica dos sinais. • Para bactérias resistentes (*B. bronchiseptica* e outras), é importante proceder à cultura e ao antibiograma para estabelecer a sensibilidade bacteriana; talvez haja necessidade da administração de antibióticos por nebulização (canamicina 250 mg; gentamicina 50 mg; polimixina B 333.000 UI) por 3-5 dias.
• Supressores da tosse (tartarato de butorfanol ou bitartarato de hidrocodona) são frequentemente eficazes na supressão de tosse seca improdutiva.
• Broncodilatadores (teofilina ou aminofilina) oferecem pouca ajuda, mas podem aliviar os sibilos.

ACOMPANHAMENTO
• Se a infecção for estabelecida em um canil, é recomendável evacuar o ambiente por 1-2 semanas e desinfetá-lo com hipoclorito de sódio (na diluição de 1:30), clorexidina ou benzalcônio.
• Os casos sem complicações devem desaparecer dentro de 10-14 dias; se o paciente continuar tossindo depois de 14 dias, deve-se questionar o diagnóstico de doença sem complicações. • Os cães que se recuperam de infecção por *B. bronchiseptica* ficam imunes por no mínimo 6 meses. • A taxa de mortalidade é altamente variável, estando muito provavelmente relacionada com o grau de infecção bacteriana secundária, a cepa do vírus e a intensidade dos cuidados veterinários. • Atualmente, há uma única vacina aprovada contra CIV H3N8 para uso em cães.

DIVERSOS

POTENCIAL ZOONÓTICO
Não há evidência para indicar que o CIV seja capaz de infectar os seres humanos.

RISCO A OUTROS ANIMAIS
Considerando-se a estreita ligação genética com o H3N8 equino, existe o potencial de que o CIV H3N8 infecte os cavalos. Os gatos podem ser infectados pelo CIV H3N8, mas nenhuma doença natural foi detectada.

ABREVIATURAS
• CIV = vírus da influenza canina. • ELISA = ensaio imunoadsorvente ligado à enzima. • PCR = reação em cadeia da polimerase.

RECURSOS DA INTERNET
www.diaglab.vet.cornell.edu/issues/civ.asp.

Sugestões de Leitura
Dubovi EJ, Njaa BL. Canine influenza. Vet Clin Small Anim 2008, 38:827-836.

Autor Edward J. Dubovi
Consultor Editorial Stephen C. Barr

Instabilidade Atlantoaxial

CONSIDERAÇÕES GERAIS

REVISÃO
- Origina-se de má-formação ou ruptura da articulação entre as duas primeiras vértebras cervicais (atlas e áxis), o que provoca compressão da medula espinal. • Pode resultar em traumatismo ou compressão da medula espinal na junção entre o atlas e o áxis, podendo causar dor cervical (cervicalgia) e/ou graus variados de ataxia proprioceptiva geral/tetraparesia atribuída ao neurônio motor superior, tetraplegia (com ou sem nocicepção) e morte por parada respiratória.

Etiologia
- Congênita: anomalia do processo odontoide do áxis (aplasia, hipoplasia ou má-formação [angulação dorsal] dessa estrutura) e de suas inserções ligamentosas. • Adquirida: pode ser uma consequência de lesão traumática.

IDENTIFICAÇÃO
- Congênita — cães da raça toy (Yorkshire terrier, Poodle toy ou miniatura, Chihuahua, Pequinês e Lulu da Pomerânia). • Idade de início — comumente antes dos 12 meses de vida. • Rara em raças caninas de grande porte, cães com >1 ano de idade e gatos. • Não há predisposição sexual.

SINAIS CLÍNICOS
- Tetraparesia ambulatória intermitente ou progressiva, geralmente associada à dor cervical — sinal mais comum.
- Os sinais variam de leves a moderados, desde tetraparesia ambulatória proprioceptiva geral/atribuída ao neurônio motor superior até tetraparesia não ambulatória proprioceptiva geral/decorrente do neurônio motor superior ou tetraplegia, dependendo do grau de compressão da medula espinal e do processo patológico secundário (i. e., edema, hemorragia ou gliose).
- Dor cervical sem déficits neurológicos concomitantes.
- Episódios de colapso secundários à fraqueza.
- Os reflexos espinais permanecem normais ou ficam exagerados com tônus muscular normal ou aumentado em todos os quatro membros.
- Pode ocorrer morte aguda quando acompanhada por traumatismo e parada respiratória (incomum).

CAUSAS E FATORES DE RISCO
- Costuma ser causada pelo desenvolvimento anormal do processo odontoide do áxis ou de suas estruturas de sustentação ligamentosa, resultando em subluxação da articulação atlantoaxial.
- Fratura do áxis.
- Os sinais clínicos frequentemente ocorrem como resultado de traumatismo leve ou insignificante (p. ex., saltos ou brincadeiras).
- Tais sinais podem ser exacerbados por atividade física, como flexão do pescoço.
- Cães da raça toy — estão sob risco de má-formação congênita do processo odontoide do áxis.

DIAGNÓSTICO

DIAGNÓSTICO DIFERENCIAL
- Os diagnósticos diferenciais são compatíveis com várias causas de mielopatias cervicais, incluindo:
- Outra má-formação congênita.
- Traumatismo.
- Meningite ou meningomielite (i. e., infecciosas ou não infecciosas [meningoencefalomielite granulomatosa]).
- Mielopatia embólica fibrocartilaginosa.
- Herniação de disco.
- Neoplasia.

HEMOGRAMA/BIOQUÍMICA/URINÁLISE
Permanecem normais.

DIAGNÓSTICO POR IMAGEM
- Radiografias simples da coluna cervical:
- Projeção lateral — deslocamento dorsocaudal do áxis em relação ao atlas, resultando em um aumento na distância entre as vértebras.
- Projeção ventrodorsal ou oblíqua — pode revelar ausência, hipoplasia ou má-formação (angulação dorsal) do processo odontoide do áxis.
- Técnicas de obtenção de imagens transversais:
- RM.
- Modalidade de imagem de escolha.
- O diagnóstico é formulado com base na observação de deslocamento dorsocaudal do áxis em relação ao atlas, conforme evidenciado pelos seguintes aspectos da articulação atlantoaxial:
- Dorsal: deslocamento do processo espinhoso do áxis.
- Ventral: aumento no tamanho da cavidade articular dos ossos occipital, atlas e áxis.
- Permite a identificação de compressão da medula espinal.
- Possibilita o reconhecimento de processo patológico secundário na medula espinal, como edema, hemorragia ou gliose, o que pode exercer um impacto sobre o prognóstico.
- TC:
- Pode permitir uma visualização detalhada de estruturas ósseas, o que possibilita a criação de imagens reconstruídas tridimensionais para ajudar o planejamento cirúrgico.
- Precauções:
- O posicionamento adequado do animal pode exigir sedação ou anestesia geral.
- A sedação ou anestesia geral carreia um risco significativo de traumatismo iatrogênico.
- É preciso ter cuidado ao posicionar os animais.
- EVITAR A FLEXÃO DO PESCOÇO.
- A flexão pode exacerbar a compressão, o que pode agravar os sinais clínicos ou provocar o óbito em função de traumatismo da medula espinal.
- Para proteger os animais contra a flexão cervical durante a recuperação, é recomendável sua monitorização rigorosa até que eles sejam capazes de sustentar a cabeça e o pescoço normalmente.

TRATAMENTO

- Antes do tratamento, deve-se buscar uma consulta com neurologista ou cirurgião especializado.
- O tratamento inadequado pode levar à deterioração irreversível da função neurológica.

CLÍNICO
- A imobilização do pescoço com colar do tipo tala é usada para estabilizar a coluna cervical em extensão.
- O material do molde em fibra de vidro é posicionado ventralmente, desde a face rostral da mandíbula até a cartilagem xifoide, e incorporado no material da bandagem, o que imobiliza a cabeça e o pescoço.
- Restrição estrita da atividade física (confinamento em gaiola) por, no mínimo, 8 semanas.
- Há necessidade de trocas frequentes da bandagem e da tala.
- Medicação adjuvante (ver adiante).

Prognóstico Geral
- Desfecho bem-sucedido observado em 62,5% dos cães.
- A melhoria do prognóstico foi associada ao quadro de início agudo e à curta duração dos sinais clínicos (<30 dias).
- A cirurgia é recomendada para tratar os animais que não melhoram ou sofrem recidiva dos sinais após tratamento clínico.

CIRURGIA
- Tratamento de escolha na maioria dos casos.
- Abordagem cirúrgica; o método ventral é o preferido.
- Abordagem ventral — há uma variedade de métodos:
- Aplicação de pino transarticular ou técnica com parafuso interfragmentário do tipo *lag screw*; as extremidades ventrais dos pinos são incorporadas em polimetilmetacrilato para evitar a migração do pino.
- Aplicação de pino transarticular e parafusos corticais ventrais ou fios de Kirschner nos corpos do atlas e do áxis ± fios de Kirschner aplicados longitudinalmente e conectados aos parafusos; as cabeças dos parafusos e os fios de Kirschner são incorporados em polimetilmetacrilato para conferir a fixação.
- Abordagem dorsal — utilizar fio ou material de sutura sintético para fixar o processo espinhoso do áxis ao arco dorsal do atlas; confere uma fixação menos rígida e pode estar associada a maior falha do implante.
- É necessária a restrição rigorosa da atividade física durante o primeiro mês do pós-operatório, seguida pelo retorno gradativo à atividade no mês seguinte.
- Medicação adjuvante (ver adiante).

Prognóstico Geral
- Varia de 63 a 91% de sucesso.
- A melhoria do prognóstico foi associada a cães jovens (<24 meses), duração dos sinais clínicos <10 meses e déficits neurológicos leves.
- Complicações:
- Falha de melhora ou agravamento dos déficits neurológicos.
- Falha/infecção do implante.
- Respiratórias — dispneia, tosse e pneumonia por aspiração.
- Morte.

MEDICAÇÕES

MEDICAMENTO(S)
- Medicação anti-inflamatória:
- Corticosteroides: prednisona a 0,5-1,0 mg/kg VO dividido 2 vezes ao dia por 2 semanas, acompanhada por um esquema de redução gradativa. O protocolo sugerido após a dose inicial: 0,5 mg/kg VO diariamente por 5 dias, seguido por 0,5 mg/kg VO em dias alternados por 5 dias.
- AINE: curso terapêutico de 1 a 4 semanas.

- Analgesia:
- Tramadol: 2-4 mg/kg VO a cada 6-8 h.
- Gabapentina: 10-20 mg/kg VO a cada 6-8 h.

CONTRAINDICAÇÕES/INTERAÇÕES POSSÍVEIS
- Corticosteroides — é preciso ter cautela ao administrá-los em associação ao tratamento clínico; podem reduzir a dor, o que resulta em aumento na atividade física e consequente traumatismo da medula espinal.
- Evitar a associação de AINEs e corticosteroides em todos os pacientes — aumenta o risco de hemorragia gastrintestinal potencialmente letal.

ACOMPANHAMENTO
- Os cães submetidos a tratamento clínico necessitam de trocas frequentes (semanais) da bandagem para traumatismo associado dos tecidos moles.
- Todos os cães devem ser reavaliados em 1 e 3 meses (no pós-operatório ou depois da remoção do colar cervical) e mensalmente até que os déficits neurológicos desapareçam ou permaneçam estáticos durante 2-3 meses.
- Talvez haja necessidade de check-ups mais frequentes para os cães que sofrem complicações ou recidiva dos sinais.
- Os animais não tratados podem sofrer deterioração da função neurológica, traumatismo agudo catastrófico da medula espinal, parada respiratória e morte.

DIVERSOS
- A reabilitação pode desempenhar um papel significativo no nível funcional neurológico final do paciente.
- Tal reabilitação só deve ser considerada em cães com >30 dias do pós-operatório ou depois da retirada do colar cervical (tala).

ABREVIATURAS
- AINE = anti-inflamatório não esteroide.
- RM = ressonância magnética.
- TC = tomografia computadorizada.

RECURSOS DA INTERNET
http://www.acvs.org/AnimalOwners/HealthConditions/SmallAnimalTopics/AtlantoaxialInstability/.

Sugestões de Leitura

Beaver DP, Ellison GW, Lewis DD. Risk factors affecting the outcome of surgery for atlantoaxial subluxation in dogs: 46 cases (1978-1998). JAVMA 2000, 216(7):1104-1109.

Fossum TW, Hedlund CS, Johnson AL, et al. Small Animal Surgery. St. Louis: Mosby-Year Book, 1997.

Havig ME, Cornell KK, Hawthorne JC, McDonnell JJ, Selcer BA. Evaluation of nonsurgical treatment of atlantoaxial subluxation in dogs: 19 cases (1992-2001). JAVMA 2005, 227(2):257-262.

McCarthy RJ, Lewis DD, Hosgood G. Atlantoaxial subluxation in dogs. Compend Contin Educ Pract Vet 1995, 17:215-226.

Platt SR, Chambers JN, Cross A. A modified ventral fixation for surgical management of atlantoaxial subluxation in 19 dogs. Vet Surg 2004, 33(4):349-354.

Sanders SG, Bagley RS, Silver GM, Moore M, Tucker RL. Outcomes and complications associated with ventral screws, pins, and polymethyl methacrylate for atlantoaxial instability in 12 dogs. JAAHA 2004, 40:204-210.

Schulz KS, Waldron DR, Fahie M. Application of ventral pins and polymethylmethacrylate for the management of atlantoaxial instability: Results in nine dogs. Vet Surg 1997, 26(4):317-325.

Shires PK. Atlantoaxial instability. In: Slatter D, ed., Textbook of Small Animal Surgery, 3rd ed. Philadelphia: Saunders, 2003.

Tomlinson J. Surgical conditions of the cervical spine. Semin Vet Med Surg Small Anim 1996, 11(4):225-234.

Autores Mathieu M. Glassman e Marc Kent
Consultor Editorial Peter K. Shires

Insuficiência Cardíaca Congestiva Direita

CONSIDERAÇÕES GERAIS

DEFINIÇÃO
Insuficiência do lado direito do coração em bombear o sangue a uma velocidade suficiente para suprir as necessidades metabólicas do paciente ou evitar o acúmulo de sangue dentro da circulação venosa sistêmica.

FISIOPATOLOGIA
• A pressão hidrostática elevada leva ao extravasamento de líquido da circulação venosa para os espaços pleural e peritoneal e, potencialmente, para o pericárdio e o interstício dos tecidos periféricos.
• Quando o extravasamento de líquido excede a capacidade dos vasos linfáticos na drenagem das áreas acometidas, desenvolvem-se efusão pleural, ascite, efusão pericárdica e edema periférico.

SISTEMA(S) ACOMETIDO(S)
Todos os sistemas orgânicos podem ser acometidos pela má distribuição sanguínea ou pelos efeitos da congestão passiva decorrente do fluxo retrógrado de sangue venoso.

GENÉTICA
• Em certas raças, alguns defeitos cardíacos congênitos apresentam base genética.
• A miocardiopatia arritmogênica do ventrículo direito parece ter uma base genética em cães da raça Boxer.

INCIDÊNCIA/PREVALÊNCIA
Comum.

DISTRIBUIÇÃO GEOGRÁFICA
Observada em qualquer lugar, mas a prevalência das causas varia com o local.

IDENTIFICAÇÃO
Espécies
Cães e gatos.

Raça(s) Predominante(s)
Varia com a causa.

Idade Média e Faixa Etária
Varia com a causa.

Sexo Predominante
Varia com a causa.

SINAIS CLÍNICOS
Comentários Gerais
• Os sinais variam com a causa subjacente e entre as espécies.
• A efusão pleural sem ascite e hepatomegalia é rara em cães com ICCD (insuficiência cardíaca congestiva direita).
• A ascite sem efusão pleural é rara em gatos com ICCD.
• Efusão pericárdica de pequeno volume sem tamponamento é relativamente comum em gatos com ICCD.
• Edema periférico intersticial é uma manifestação rara de ICCD em ambas as espécies.

Achados Anamnésicos
• Fraqueza.
• Letargia.
• Intolerância a exercícios.
• Distensão abdominal.
• Dispneia, taquipneia.

Achados do Exame Físico
• Distensão venosa jugular.
• Reflexo hepatojugular.
• Pulso jugular em alguns animais.
• Hepatomegalia.
• Ascite — comum em cães e rara em gatos com ICCD.
• Possível sopro regurgitante na região da valva atrioventricular direita (tricúspide) ou sopro de ejeção na base do coração esquerdo (estenose pulmonar).
• Em caso de efusões pleural ou pericárdica, o animal exibirá abafamento das bulhas cardíacas.
• Pulsos femorais débeis.
• Em caso de efusão pleural ou ascite grave, o animal apresentará respiração rápida e superficial.
• Edema periférico (infrequente).

CAUSAS
Insuficiência (Miocárdica) de Bombeamento do Ventrículo Direito
• Miocardiopatia dilatada (MCD) idiopática.
• Miocardiopatia arritmogênica do ventrículo direito.
• Tripanossomíase.
• Cardiotoxicidade pela doxorrubicina.
• Hipertireoidismo crônico.

Sobrecarga do Ventrículo Direito por Volume
• Insuficiência crônica das valvas atrioventriculares (mitral ± tricúspide) causada por endocardiose.
• Displasia da valva atrioventricular direita (tricúspide).

Sobrecarga do Ventrículo Direito por Pressão
• Dirofilariose.
• Doença pulmonar obstrutiva crônica com hipertensão pulmonar.
• Tromboembolia pulmonar.
• Estenose pulmonar.
• Tetralogia de Fallot.
• Tumores do ventrículo direito.
• Hipertensão pulmonar primária.

Obstáculo ao Preenchimento do Ventrículo Direito
• Efusão pericárdica (tamponamento).
• Pericardite constritiva/restritiva.
• Massas no átrio direito ou na veia cava.
• Estenose da valva atrioventricular direita (tricúspide).
• Coração direito triatriado.

Distúrbios de Ritmo
• Bradicardia, em geral bloqueio atrioventricular completo.
• Taquiarritmias, em geral taquicardia supraventricular sustentada.

FATORES DE RISCO
• Falta de profilaxia para a dirofilariose.
• Prole de um animal com defeito cardíaco congênito do lado direito.
• Condições indutoras de um aumento na demanda do débito cardíaco (p. ex., hipertireoidismo, anemia e gestação).

DIAGNÓSTICO

DIAGNÓSTICO DIFERENCIAL
• É imprescindível diferenciar de outras causas de efusão pleural e ascite; em geral, requer avaliação diagnóstica completa, incluindo-se hemograma, perfil bioquímico, pesquisa de dirofilariose, toracocentese ou abdominocentese com análise e exame citológico do líquido e, algumas vezes, ultrassonografias torácica e abdominal.
• Os animais com ascite ou efusão pleural decorrentes de insuficiência cardíaca devem apresentar distensão venosa jugular.

HEMOGRAMA/BIOQUÍMICA/URINÁLISE
• O hemograma completo costuma permanecer normal; os animais com dirofilariose podem exibir eosinofilia.
• Em virtude da congestão hepática passiva, há uma elevação leve a moderada das enzimas hepáticas (i. e., alanina aminotransferase, aspartato aminotransferase e fosfatase alcalina sérica); em geral, os níveis de bilirrubina encontram-se normais.
• Em alguns animais, observa-se azotemia pré-renal.

OUTROS TESTES LABORATORIAIS
O teste de dirofilariose pode estar positivo.

DIAGNÓSTICO POR IMAGEM
Achados Radiográficos Torácicos
• Aumento de volume do coração direito em alguns animais.
• Dilatação da veia cava caudal (diâmetro maior do que o comprimento da vértebra imediatamente acima do coração).
• Efusão pleural (particularmente em gatos).
• Hepatoesplenomegalia e possível ascite (especialmente em cães).

Ecocardiografia
• Os achados variam de acordo com a causa subjacente. Exame particularmente útil para registrar defeito congênito, massa cardíaca e efusão pericárdica.
• A ultrassonografia abdominal revela hepatomegalia com dilatação da veia hepática, inversão do fluxo (Doppler) e, possivelmente, ascite.

MÉTODOS DIAGNÓSTICOS
Achados Eletrocardiográficos
• Em caso de efusões pericárdica ou pleural, o animal apresentará complexos QRS pequenos (<1 mV) em todas as derivações do eixo frontal.
• Em caso de efusão pericárdica, há alternância elétrica ou elevação do segmento ST.
• Evidência do aumento de volume cardíaco direito (p. ex., ondas P altas [>0,4 mV] na derivação II, ondas S profundas nas derivações I, II e aVF, além de desvio do eixo para a direita).
• Arritmias atriais ou ventriculares.
• O ECG pode permanecer normal em pacientes com ICCD.

Abdominocentese
• A análise do líquido ascítico em pacientes com ICCD revela geralmente um transudato modificado com proteína total >2,5 mg/dL.

Toracocentese
• Os gatos com efusão pleural associada à ICCD podem apresentar transudato, transudato modificado ou efusão quilosa.
• Os cães com efusão pleural e ICCD podem exibir transudato ou transudato modificado.

Pressão Venosa Central
• A pressão venosa central encontra-se alta (>9 cmH$_2$O).

ACHADOS PATOLÓGICOS
• Os achados cardíacos variam com a doença.
• Hepatomegalia em animais com necrose centrolobular (condição crônica).

Insuficiência Cardíaca Congestiva Direita

TRATAMENTO

CUIDADO(S) DE SAÚDE ADEQUADO(S)
A maioria dos animais é tratada em um esquema ambulatorial, a menos que se encontrem dispneicos ou sofram colapso (p. ex., efusão pleural ou pericárdica significativa).

CUIDADO(S) DE ENFERMAGEM
A toracocentese e a abdominocentese podem ser necessárias em intervalos periódicos em pacientes que não respondem mais ao tratamento clínico ou naqueles com dispneia grave causada por efusão pleural ou ascite.

ATIVIDADE
Restringir a atividade física.

DIETA
Efetuar restrição moderada de sódio; em animais com doença avançada, indica-se a restrição rigorosa desse sal.

ORIENTAÇÃO AO PROPRIETÁRIO
• Com raras exceções (p. ex., em casos de dirofilariose, arritmias, hipertireoidismo e efusão pericárdica idiopática), a ICCD é incurável.
• A maior parte dos pacientes exibe melhora com o tratamento inicial, mas frequentemente apresenta insuficiência recidivante.

CONSIDERAÇÕES CIRÚRGICAS
• Para tratar certos defeitos congênitos (como a estenose pulmonar), fica indicada a intervenção cirúrgica ou a valvuloplastia com balão.
• A colocação do oclusor Amplatzer é recomendada para defeitos do septo atrial adequados em termos morfológicos.
• Em caso de efusão pericárdica, efetua-se a pericardiocentese ou a pericardiectomia.
• Remoção de dirofilárias do coração pela veia jugular em cães com síndrome da veia cava.

MEDICAÇÕES

MEDICAMENTO(S) DE ESCOLHA
Os medicamentos devem ser administrados somente após a formulação de um diagnóstico definitivo.

Diuréticos
• A furosemida (1-2 mg/kg a cada 8-24 h) ou outro diurético de alça constitui o diurético inicial de escolha. Os diuréticos são indicados para remover o acúmulo de líquido em excesso.
• A espironolactona (0,5-2 mg/kg VO a cada 12-24 h) aumenta a sobrevida em seres humanos com insuficiência cardíaca. Utilizar em combinação com a furosemida.

Digoxina
• Em animais com insuficiência miocárdica (p. ex., miocardiopatia dilatada), emprega-se a digoxina (cães, 0,22 mg/m^2 a cada 12 h; gatos, 0,01 mg/kg a cada 48 h).
• Também se indica a digoxina em animais com ICC e arritmias supraventriculares associadas (p. ex., taquicardia sinusal, fibrilação atrial e taquicardia atrial ou juncional).

Vasodilatadores
• Inibidores da ECA, como o enalapril (0,5 mg/kg a cada 12-24 h) ou o benazepril (0,25-0,5 mg/kg a cada 24 h), são úteis em MCD e insuficiência valvar atrioventricular crônica.
• Sildenafila (0,5-1 mg/kg VO a cada 12 h até 2-3 mg/kg a cada 8 h) pode ser benéfica no quadro de hipertensão pulmonar.

Pimobendana
• Sensibilizador dos canais de cálcio que atua como inodilatador, causando vasodilatação arterial e aumento da contratilidade do miocárdio.
• Particularmente útil em insuficiência do miocárdio.
• Dose — 0,25-0,3 mg/kg VO a cada 12 h.

CONTRAINDICAÇÕES
• Evitar o uso de diuréticos em pacientes com efusão/tamponamento pericárdico.
• Evitar o uso de vasodilatadores em pacientes com efusão pericárdica ou obstruções fixas à via de saída.

PRECAUÇÕES
• Os inibidores da ECA e os dilatadores arteriais devem ser utilizados com cautela em pacientes com possíveis obstruções à via de saída.
• Os quadros de hipertensão pulmonar, hipotireoidismo e hipoxia aumentam o risco de intoxicação pela digoxina; o hipertireoidismo diminui os efeitos da digoxina.
• É preciso ter cuidado ao se empregar os inibidores da ECA e a digoxina em pacientes nefropatas.
• Também se deve ter prudência ao usar a dobutamina em gatos.
• A espironolactona pode causar prurido facial em gatos.

INTERAÇÕES POSSÍVEIS
• A combinação de diuréticos em altas doses e inibidores da ECA pode alterar a perfusão renal e causar azotemia.
• A terapia diurética combinada aumenta o risco de desidratação e de distúrbios eletrolíticos.

MEDICAMENTO(S) ALTERNATIVO(S)
• Os pacientes irresponsivos a certos agentes terapêuticos (p. ex., furosemida, espironolactona, vasodilatadores e digoxina [se indicada]) podem se beneficiar com terapia diurética tripla pela adição de um diurético tiazídico.
• Na constatação de deficiência, efetuar a suplementação de potássio e magnésio; em animais submetidos aos inibidores da ECA ou à espironolactona, é recomendável empregar os suplementos de potássio com cautela.
• Tratar as arritmias se houver indicação clínica.
• A suplementação de taurina é indicada em casos de MCD tanto em cães como em gatos com deficiência desse aminoácido.
• A suplementação de carnitina pode ajudar alguns cães com MCD (p. ex., Cocker spaniel e Boxer).

ACOMPANHAMENTO

MONITORIZAÇÃO DO PACIENTE
• Monitorizar a função renal, os níveis dos eletrólitos, o estado de hidratação, a frequência e o esforço respiratórios, a frequência cardíaca, o peso corporal e a circunferência abdominal (cães).
• Caso se desenvolva azotemia, diminuir a dosagem do diurético. Se a azotemia persistir e o animal ainda estiver sob efeito de um inibidor da ECA, reduzir ou interromper a administração do inibidor em questão. No desenvolvimento de azotemia, baixar a dose da digoxina para evitar a intoxicação.
• Para detectar arritmias, realizar a monitorização periódica com o ECG.
• Monitorizar as concentrações da digoxina. Os valores normais ficam entre 0,5-1,5 ng/mL para uma amostra sérica obtida 8-10 h após a administração de uma dose.

COMPLICAÇÕES POSSÍVEIS
• Tromboembolia pulmonar.
• Arritmias.
• Distúrbios eletrolíticos.
• Intoxicação pela digoxina.
• Azotemia e insuficiência renal.

EVOLUÇÃO ESPERADA E PROGNÓSTICO
O prognóstico varia de acordo com a causa subjacente.

DIVERSOS

FATORES RELACIONADOS COM A IDADE
• Em animais jovens, observam-se causas congênitas.
• Em animais idosos, geralmente se constatam cardiopatias degenerativas e neoplasias.

VER TAMBÉM
• Ascite.
• Capítulos sobre Doenças Indutoras de ICCD.
• Efusão Pleural.
• Quilotórax.

ABREVIATURA(S)
• AV = atrioventricular.
• ECA = enzima conversora da angiotensina.
• ECG = eletrocardiograma.
• ICCD = insuficiência cardíaca congestiva direita.
• MCD = miocardiopatia dilatada.

Sugestões de Leitura
International Small Animal Cardiac Health Council. Recommendations for the diagnosis of heart disease and the treatment of heart failure in small animals. In: Miller MS, Tilley LP, eds., Manual of Canine and Feline Cardiology, 2nd ed. Philadelphia: Saunders, 1995.
Stickland KN. Pathophysiology and therapy of heart failure. In: Tilley LP, Smith FWK, Oyama MA, Sleeper MM, eds., Manual of Canine and Feline Cardiology, 4th ed. St. Louis: Saunders Elsevier, 2008, pp. 49-77.

Autores Francis W. K. Smith Jr. e Bruce W. Keene
Consultores Editoriais Larry P. Tilley e Francis W. K. Smith Jr.

Insuficiência Cardíaca Congestiva Esquerda

CONSIDERAÇÕES GERAIS

DEFINIÇÃO
Insuficiência do lado esquerdo do coração em bombear o sangue a uma velocidade suficiente para suprir as necessidades metabólicas do paciente ou evitar o acúmulo de sangue dentro da circulação venosa pulmonar.

FISIOPATOLOGIA
• O débito cardíaco baixo causa letargia, intolerância a exercícios, síncope e azotemia pré-renal. • A pressão hidrostática elevada induz ao extravasamento de líquido da circulação venosa pulmonar para o interstício pulmonar e os alvéolos. Quando o extravasamento de líquido excede a capacidade dos vasos linfáticos na drenagem das áreas acometidas, desenvolve-se o edema pulmonar.

SISTEMA(S) ACOMETIDO(S)
• Todos os sistemas orgânicos podem ser acometidos pela má perfusão. • Respiratório, em função do edema. • Cardiovascular.

GENÉTICA
Em certas raças, alguns defeitos cardíacos congênitos, miocardiopatias e valvulopatia cardíaca apresentam base genética.

INCIDÊNCIA/PREVALÊNCIA
Comum.

DISTRIBUIÇÃO GEOGRÁFICA
Observada em qualquer lugar, mas a prevalência das causas varia com o local.

IDENTIFICAÇÃO
Espécies
Cães e gatos.

Raça(s) Predominante(s)
Varia com a causa.

Idade Média e Faixa Etária
Varia com a causa.

Sexo Predominante
Variam com a causa.

SINAIS CLÍNICOS
Comentários Gerais
Os sinais variam com a causa subjacente e entre as espécies.

Achados Anamnésicos
• Fraqueza, letargia, intolerância a exercícios.
• Tosse (cães) e dispneia; os sinais respiratórios frequentemente pioram durante a noite e podem ser aliviados, assumindo-se a posição em estação, esternal ou com os cotovelos abduzidos (ortopneia). • Os gatos raramente tossem.

Achados do Exame Físico
• Taquipneia. • Tosse, muitas vezes suave em conjunto com taquipneia (cães). • Dispneia e taquipneia quando o animal apresenta edema pulmonar. • Crepitações e sibilos pulmonares.
• Mucosas pálidas/cinzas/cianóticas. • Tempo de preenchimento capilar prolongado. • Possíveis sopros ou ritmos de galope. • Pulsos femorais débeis.

CAUSAS
Insuficiência (Miocárdica) de Bombeamento do Ventrículo Esquerdo
• Miocardiopatia dilatada (MCD) idiopática.
• Tripanossomíase (rara). • Cardiotoxicidade por doxorrubicina (cães). • Hipotireoidismo (raro).
• Hipertireoidismo (raramente causa insuficiência da bomba cardíaca; costuma gerar insuficiência cardíaca de alto débito).

Sobrecarga do Coração Esquerdo por Pressão
• Hipertensão sistêmica. • Estenose subaórtica.
• Coarctação da aorta (rara; predisposição da raça Airedale terrier). • Tumores do ventrículo esquerdo (raros).

Sobrecarga do Coração Esquerdo por Volume
• Endocardiose da valva atrioventricular esquerda (mitral) (cães). • Displasia da valva atrioventricular esquerda (cães e gatos). • Persistência do ducto arterioso (cães). • Defeito do septo ventricular.
• Insuficiência aórtica secundária à endocardite (cães).

Obstáculo ao Preenchimento do Coração Esquerdo
• Efusão pericárdica com tamponamento.
• Pericardite restritiva. • Miocardiopatia restritiva.
• Miocardiopatia hipertrófica. • Massas atriais esquerdas (p. ex., tumores e trombos).
• Tromboembolia pulmonar. • Estenose mitral (rara).

Distúrbios de Ritmo
• Bradicardia (bloqueio AV de alto grau).
• Taquicardia (p. ex., fibrilação atrial, taquicardia supraventricular sustentada e taquicardia ventricular).

FATORES DE RISCO
Condições indutoras do débito cardíaco elevado e crônico (p. ex., hipertireoidismo, anemia e gestação).

DIAGNÓSTICO

DIAGNÓSTICO DIFERENCIAL
É imprescindível diferenciar de outras causas de tosse, dispneia e fraqueza.

HEMOGRAMA/BIOQUÍMICA/URINÁLISE
• O hemograma completo costuma permanecer normal; pode haver leucograma de estresse.
• Elevação leve a moderada das enzimas hepáticas; em geral, níveis normais da bilirrubina.
• Azotemia pré-renal em alguns animais.

OUTROS TESTES LABORATORIAIS
• Podem ser detectados distúrbios da tireoide.
• As concentrações séricas do fragmento N-terminal do pró-peptídeo natriurético cerebral são mais altas em animais com insuficiência cardíaca congestiva esquerda do que nos animais normais.

DIAGNÓSTICO POR IMAGEM
Achados Radiográficos
• Aumento de volume do coração esquerdo e das veias pulmonares. • Edema pulmonar, frequentemente na região hilar; no entanto, pode ser irregular, sobretudo em gatos; um edema pulmonar agudo pode ter início no lobo pulmonar caudal direito.

Ecocardiografia
• Os achados variam de forma acentuada com a causa, mas o aumento de volume do átrio esquerdo constitui um achado relativamente compatível em casos de edema pulmonar cardiogênico. • Teste diagnóstico de escolha para registrar defeitos congênitos, massas cardíacas e efusão pericárdica.

MÉTODOS DIAGNÓSTICOS
Achados Eletrocardiográficos
• Arritmias atriais ou ventriculares. • Evidência do aumento de volume do coração esquerdo (p. ex., ondas P largas, complexos QRS altos e amplos e desvio do eixo para a esquerda). • Podem permanecer normais.

ACHADOS PATOLÓGICOS
Os achados cardíacos variam com a doença.

TRATAMENTO

CUIDADO(S) DE SAÚDE ADEQUADO(S)
• Em geral, o tratamento é feito em um esquema ambulatorial a menos que o paciente se encontre dispneico ou gravemente hipotenso. • Sempre que possível, deve-se identificar e corrigir a causa subjacente. • Minimizar a manipulação de animais criticamente dispneicos. O estresse pode matar!

CUIDADO(S) DE ENFERMAGEM
O oxigênio é capaz de salvar a vida de pacientes criticamente dispneicos.

ATIVIDADE
Restringir a atividade física.

DIETA
Instituir uma dieta com restrição moderada de sódio. Em animais com doença avançada, indica-se a restrição rigorosa desse sal.

ORIENTAÇÃO AO PROPRIETÁRIO
Com raras exceções (p. ex., animais com distúrbios da tireoide, arritmias e cardiopatias responsivas ao tratamento nutricional), a insuficiência cardíaca congestiva esquerda (ICCE) é incurável.

CONSIDERAÇÕES CIRÚRGICAS
• Intervenções cirúrgicas como a embolização com espiral, a colocação do oclusor Amplatzer ou a valvuloplastia com balão podem beneficiar pacientes selecionados com algumas formas de valvulopatia cardíaca congênita e adquirida. No entanto, a resposta a essas intervenções varia.
• Em animais com efusão pericárdica, efetuar a pericardiocentese.

MEDICAÇÕES

MEDICAMENTO(S) DE ESCOLHA
Diuréticos
• A furosemida (1-2 mg/kg a cada 8-24 h) ou outro diurético de alça constitui o diurético inicial de escolha; os diuréticos são indicados para remover o edema pulmonar. Os animais criticamente dispneicos necessitam muitas vezes da administração IV de doses altas (4-8 mg/kg) para estabilização; se o animal ainda continuar gravemente dispneico, será possível repetir essa dose em 1 h. A administração de bólus IV na dose de 0,66 mg/kg, seguida por uma infusão em velocidade constante de 0,66 mg/kg/h por 8 h provoca uma diurese mais acentuada do que uma dose equivalente dividida em dois bólus IV administrados com intervalo de 4 h. Assim que o edema desaparecer, reduzir para uma dosagem

Insuficiência Cardíaca Congestiva Esquerda

mais baixa, porém eficaz. • A espironolactona (0,5-2 mg/kg VO a cada 12-24 h) aumenta a sobrevida em seres humanos com insuficiência cardíaca congestiva. Utilizar em combinação com a furosemida. • Os diuréticos tiazídicos podem ser adicionados à furosemida e à espironolactona em casos refratários de insuficiência cardíaca.

Digoxina
• Em animais com insuficiência miocárdica (p. ex., miocardiopatia dilatada), emprega-se a digoxina (cães, 0,22 mg/m^2 a cada 12 h; gatos, 0,01 mg/kg a cada 48 h). • Também se indica a digoxina para tratar as arritmias supraventriculares (p. ex., taquicardia sinusal, fibrilação atrial e taquicardia atrial ou juncional) em pacientes com ICC. • Em seres humanos, a digoxina não tem nenhum efeito sobre a taxa de mortalidade, mas diminui o número de internações por insuficiência cardíaca.

Venodilatadores
• Unguento de nitroglicerina (~0,6 cm/5 kg a cada 6-8 h) causa venodilatação, reduzindo as pressões de preenchimento do átrio esquerdo. • Uso para a estabilização imediata de pacientes com edema pulmonar e dispneia graves. • Podem ser úteis em animais com ICCE crônica; para evitar a tolerância, usar de forma intermitente e com intervalo de 12 h entre a última dose do primeiro dia e a primeira dose do dia seguinte.

Inibidores da ECA
• Em grande parte dos animais com ICCE, fica indicado um inibidor da ECA, como o enalapril (0,5 mg/kg a cada 12-24 h) ou o benazepril (0,25-0,5 mg/kg a cada 24 h). • Os inibidores da ECA aumentam a sobrevida e melhoram a qualidade de vida em cães com ICCE secundária à valvulopatia degenerativa e à MCD.

Inotrópicos Positivos
• Pimobendana (0,25-0,3 mg/kg VO a cada 12 h) é um sensibilizador dos canais de cálcio que dilata as artérias e aumenta a contratilidade do miocárdio. Constitui o agente terapêutico de primeira linha em casos de MCD. Útil em cães com ICC causada por valvulopatia crônica. • Dobutamina (cães, 2,5-10 µg/kg/min; gatos, 2-10 µg/kg/min) é um agente inotrópico positivo potente que pode fornecer um valioso suporte a curto prazo em pacientes acometidos por insuficiência cardíaca com contratilidade cardíaca deficiente. • Em geral, os agentes inotrópicos positivos são potencialmente arritmogênicos e, por essa razão, há necessidade de monitorização rigorosa.

Agentes Antiarrítmicos
Tratar as arritmias se houver indicação clínica.

CONTRAINDICAÇÕES
Evitar os vasodilatadores em pacientes com efusão pericárdica ou obstrução fixa à via de saída.

PRECAUÇÕES
• É preciso ter cautela ao utilizar os inibidores da ECA e os dilatadores arteriais em pacientes com possível obstrução à via de saída. • Os quadros de hipertensão pulmonar, hipotireoidismo e hipoxia aumentam o risco de intoxicação pela digoxina; o hipertireoidismo diminui os efeitos da digoxina.
• Os inibidores da ECA e a digoxina devem ser empregados com cuidado em pacientes nefropatas.
• Também se deve ter prudência ao usar a dobutamina em gatos. • A espironolactona pode causar prurido facial em gatos.

INTERAÇÕES POSSÍVEIS
• A combinação de diuréticos em altas doses e inibidores da ECA pode causar azotemia, especialmente em animais submetidos à restrição severa de sódio.
• A terapia diurética combinada aumenta o risco de desidratação e de distúrbios eletrolíticos.
• A terapia vasodilatadora combinada predispõe o animal à hipotensão.

MEDICAMENTO(S) ALTERNATIVO(S)
Dilatadores Arteriais
• A hidralazina (1-2 mg/kg VO a cada 12 h; 0,5 mg/kg VO inicialmente quando adicionado a algum inibidor da ECA) ou o anlodipino (0,05-0,2 mg/kg VO a cada 24 h) podem substituir um inibidor da ECA em pacientes intolerantes ao medicamento ou com insuficiência renal avançada. Monitorizar quanto à ocorrência de hipotensão e taquicardia; em animais com ICCE refratária, tais agentes podem ser adicionados com cautela a um inibidor da ECA.
• O nitroprusseto (1-10 µg/kg/min) é um dilatador arterial potente, que costuma ficar reservado para o suporte a curto prazo em pacientes com edema potencialmente letal.

Bloqueadores dos Canais de Cálcio
• Em pacientes com ICCE, frequentemente se emprega o diltiazem (0,5-1,5 mg/kg VO a cada 8 h) para o controle da frequência cardíaca em animais com arritmias supraventriculares não controladas pela digoxina, bem como em gatos com miocardiopatia hipertrófica.

Betabloqueadores
• Em animais com taquicardia supraventricular, miocardiopatia hipertrófica e hipertireoidismo, utilizam-se os medicamentos atenolol e metoprolol para o controle da frequência cardíaca.
• Esses agentes são utilizados isoladamente ou em combinação com um antiarrítmico de classe 1 para o controle de arritmias ventriculares; tais medicamentos deprimem a contratilidade (inotrópicos negativos) e, por essa razão, devem ser usados com cautela em pacientes com insuficiência miocárdica.
• Com base em estudos em seres humanos, os betabloqueadores podem aumentar a sobrevida em animais com MCD idiopática; o tratamento é instituído de forma mais eficiente sob a orientação de um cardiologista, iniciando-se com uma dose muito baixa e aumentando-se a dosagem gradativamente. Para tal finalidade, emprega-se com frequência o carvedilol com dose inicial de 0,1 mg/kg a cada 24 h e titulação até 0,5 mg/kg a cada 12 h.

Suplementos Nutricionais
• Na constatação de deficiência, fazer uso da suplementação de potássio e magnésio; em animais submetidos aos inibidores da ECA ou à espironolactona, é importante usar os suplementos de potássio com cautela.
• A suplementação de taurina é recomendada em casos de MCD tanto em cães (p. ex., Cocker spaniel americano) como em gatos com deficiência desse aminoácido.
• A suplementação de L-carnitina pode ajudar alguns cães com MCD.
• A coenzima Q10 tem valor potencial, com base nos resultados de ensaios de pequena escala em seres humanos com MCD.

ACOMPANHAMENTO
MONITORIZAÇÃO DO PACIENTE
• Monitorizar a função renal, os níveis dos eletrólitos, o estado de hidratação, a frequência e o esforço respiratórios, a frequência cardíaca, o peso corporal e a circunferência abdominal (cães).
• Caso se desenvolva uma azotemia, diminuir a dosagem do diurético. Se a azotemia persistir e o animal ainda estiver sob efeito de um inibidor da ECA, reduzir ou interromper a administração do inibidor em questão. No desenvolvimento de azotemia, utilizar a digoxina com cautela.
• Na suspeita de arritmias, monitorizar o ECG.
• Verificar a concentração da digoxina em intervalos periódicos. A faixa recomendada fica entre 0,5-1,5 ng/mL, 8-10 h após a dosagem.

PREVENÇÃO
• Minimizar o estresse, a atividade física e o consumo de sódio em pacientes com cardiopatia.
• A prescrição de um inibidor da ECA em uma fase precoce da cardiopatia em pacientes com MCD pode retardar a evolução da cardiopatia e adiar o início da ICC. O papel dos inibidores da ECA em animais assintomáticos com valvulopatia mitral permanece controverso.

COMPLICAÇÕES POSSÍVEIS
• Síncope. • Tromboembolia aórtica (gatos).
• Arritmias. • Distúrbios eletrolíticos.
• Intoxicação pela digoxina. • Azotemia e insuficiência renal.

EVOLUÇÃO ESPERADA E PROGNÓSTICO
O prognóstico varia com a causa subjacente.

DIVERSOS
FATORES RELACIONADOS COM A IDADE
• Em animais jovens, observam-se causas congênitas. • Em animais idosos, geralmente se constatam cardiopatias degenerativas e neoplasias.

VER TAMBÉM
• Capítulos sobre Doenças Indutoras de ICCE.
• Edema Pulmonar Não Cardiogênico.

ABREVIATURA(S)
• AV = atrioventricular.
• ECA = enzima conversora da angiotensina.
• ECG = eletrocardiograma.
• ICCE = insuficiência cardíaca congestiva esquerda.
• MCD = miocardiopatia dilatada.

Sugestões de Leitura
Atkins C, Bonagura J, Ettinger S, et al. Guidelines for the diagnosis and treatment of canine chronic valvular heart disease. J Vet Intern Med 2009, 23:1142-1150.
Stickland KN. Pathophysiology and therapy of heart failure. In: Tilley LP, Smith FWK, Oyama MA, Sleeper MM, eds., Manual of Canine and Feline Cardiology, 4th ed. St. Louis: Saunders Elsevier, 2008, pp. 49-77.

Autores Francis W. K. Smith Jr. e Bruce W. Keene
Consultores Editoriais Larry P. Tilley e Francis W. K. Smith Jr.

Insuficiência Hepática Aguda

CONSIDERAÇÕES GERAIS

DEFINIÇÃO
• Dano parenquimatoso hepático agudo tão grave a ponto de o fígado se mostrar incapaz de suprir as necessidades metabólicas. • Perda súbita de mais de 75% da massa hepática funcional, principalmente por causa de necrose hepática maciça aguda indutora de uma síndrome catastrófica em múltiplos órgãos em indivíduo previamente saudável; pode evoluir rapidamente para o óbito.

FISIOPATOLOGIA
• Necrose — secundária à má perfusão, hipoxia, medicamentos ou substâncias químicas hepatotóxicos, excesso de calor ou agentes infecciosos. • Disfunção hepática — depende do tipo de insulto e da distribuição de zona no lóbulo hepático; é acompanhada por extravasamento de enzimas e comprometimento da função hepática, levando à falência de órgãos caracterizada por coagulopatia, hemorragia entérica e início agudo de encefalopatia hepática. • Má perfusão ou hipoxia — costumam afetar a zona 3 (região pericentral ou centrolobular). • Toxinas ingeridas — afetam a zona onde ocorrem a metabolização e a geração de toxinas; variável. • Insuficiência hepática — está associada a uma miríade de desarranjos metabólicos, inclusive alterações na homeostasia da glicose, na síntese de proteínas (albumina, proteínas de transporte, pró-coagulantes e fatores anticoagulantes) e na capacidade de destoxificação; pode resultar em morte.

SISTEMA(S) ACOMETIDO(S)
• Hepatobiliar — necrose hepatocelular; insuficiência hepática e icterícia. • Nervoso — encefalopatia hepática; edema cerebral. • Gastrintestinal — vômitos; diarreia; melena; hematoquezia. • Hematológico/linfático/imune — desequilíbrios de fatores pró-coagulantes e anticoagulantes; CID. • Renal/urológico — dano aos túbulos renais por certas toxinas ou vasoconstrição fisiológica. • Estado circulatório hiperdinâmico — associado a endotoxemia, TNF e desidratação.

INCIDÊNCIA/PREVALÊNCIA
• Necrose hepática variável com distúrbios hepatobiliares primários e secundários. • É incomum uma necrose hepática grave que leve à insuficiência hepática aguda; exemplos: antibióticos à base de sulfa, ingestão de xilitol, cicádea, algas azul-esverdeadas, cogumelos *Amanita* ou intoxicação hepática por cobre em cães; diazepam em gatos.

IDENTIFICAÇÃO
Espécies
Mais comum em cães do que em gatos.
Raça(s) Predominante(s)
Raças com predisposição aparente à hepatite crônica podem exibir maior risco.

SINAIS CLÍNICOS
• Início agudo de sinais clínicos inespecíficos; letargia, inapetência, distúrbios GI (vômitos, a diarreia no intestino delgado pode ser sanguinolenta); PU/PD. • Hepatomegalia sensível. • Tendências hemorrágicas. • Icterícia. • Encefalopatia hepática. • Crises convulsivas.

CAUSAS
Medicamentos
• Ver "Hepatotoxinas". • Toxicidade relacionada com diversos medicamentos, podendo ser intrínseca (direta) ou idiossincrática (imprevisível, não relacionada com a dose) com hipersensibilidade imunomediada ou lesão metabólica.
Toxinas Biológicas
• Ver "Hepatotoxinas".
Agentes Infecciosos
• Ver "Hepatotoxinas".
Lesão Térmica
• Intermação/insolação. • Hipertermia generalizada após tratamento contra o câncer.
Hipoxia Hepática
• Doença tromboembólica, choque, CID. • Insuficiência circulatória aguda de qualquer causa.

FATORES DE RISCO
• Administração de qualquer medicamento ou substância potencialmente hepatotóxica. • Exposição a toxinas do ambiente (p. ex., cogumelo *Amanita*, aflatoxina de origem alimentar, ingestão de cicádea, algas azul-esverdeadas, adoçante artificial xilitol [goma, bala] em cães). • Indutores enzimáticos (p. ex., fenobarbital) — podem aumentar a formação de toxinas a partir de alguns xenobióticos. • Ingestão indiscriminada de substância.

DIAGNÓSTICO

DIAGNÓSTICO DIFERENCIAL
• Pancreatite ou gastrenterite agudas graves — diferenciadas pelos dados dos exames laboratoriais e pelas técnicas de diagnóstico por imagem. • Descompensação aguda de doença hepatobiliar crônica — distinguida pela revisão do prontuário clínico prévio, bem como pelos resultados dos exames de sangue, da ultrassonografia abdominal e da biopsia hepática.

HEMOGRAMA/BIOQUÍMICA/URINÁLISE
• Anemia e pan-hipoproteinemia — associadas a sangramento. • Trombocitopenia — decorrente de sangramento, CID ou hipertensão portal. • Atividade enzimática hepática — elevação aguda de ALT e AST; aumentos menores de fosfatase alcalina e GGT. • Hipoglicemia — implica prognóstico grave (especialmente em gatos). • Hipocolesterolemia — síntese prejudicada. • Concentração de ureia normal a baixa. • Hiperbilirrubinemia: inicialmente ausente. • Bilirrubinúria — sempre anormal em gatos. • Cristalúria por urato de amônio significa hiperamonemia e insuficiência hepática. • Cilindros granulares e glicosúria renal indicam lesão tubular proximal atribuída à toxicidade (p. ex., intoxicação por carprofeno, cobre ou outra substância em cães).

OUTROS TESTES LABORATORIAIS
• Ácidos biliares séricos totais — valores altos confirmam disfunção hepática ou desvio portossistêmico. • Concentração plasmática de amônia — valores altos coincidem com ácidos biliares séricos totais elevados; confirma insuficiência hepática; hiperamonemia inconsistente, mas refletida pela cristalúria por biurato de amônio. • Provas de coagulação — identificam anormalidades dos fatores de coagulação, disfunção de plaquetas, CID, níveis baixos de fibrinogênio, atividade da antitrombina ou da proteína C (e níveis baixos de colesterol), sugestivos de insuficiência hepática grave ou CID descompensada.

DIAGNÓSTICO POR IMAGEM
• Radiografia abdominal — pode identificar fígado de tamanho normal ou levemente aumentado. • Ultrassonografia abdominal — pode revelar indícios de doença não hepática (p. ex., pancreatite) e/ou alterações francas no tecido hepático compatíveis com lesão hepática crônica (p. ex., remodelagem implicada por textura hepática heterogênea ou nodularidade ou fluxo sanguíneo portal hepatofugal); descarta obstrução biliar como causa de hiperbilirrubinemia. • TC cerebral — insensível para edema cerebral precoce.

OUTROS MÉTODOS DIAGNÓSTICOS
• Biopsia hepática — necessária para confirmar a presença de necrose e caracterizar o acometimento de zona acinar. • Aspirado do fígado por agulha fina — pode identificar degeneração hepatocelular, retenção de cobre, hepatócitos displásicos observados com a ingestão de cicádea ou aflatoxina; estase biliar nos canalículos.

ACHADOS PATOLÓGICOS
• Macroscópicos — fígado levemente aumentado e mosqueado. • Microscópicos — revelam necrose; identificam acometimento zonal; podem ajudar a determinar a causa subjacente: hipoxia acarreta necrose da zona 3, enquanto certas toxinas envolvem necrose da zona 1 ou 3.

TRATAMENTO

CUIDADO(S) DE SAÚDE ADEQUADO(S)
Paciente internado — há necessidade de cuidados intensivos.

CUIDADO(S) DE ENFERMAGEM
• Adiar a inserção de cateteres centrais até que as diáteses hemorrágicas estejam controladas com vitamina K1, transfusão de plasma fresco congelado ou, então, até a disponibilidade de sangue total fresco ou plasma fresco congelado. Além de não haver vantagens, a administração profilática de plasma fresco congelado pode contribuir para o início de edema cerebral. • Fluidos — que não contenham lactato; administrados, inicialmente, a uma velocidade utilizada para reanimação; monitorizar a pressão arterial periférica e a oximetria de pulso. É comum a presença de distúrbios acidobásicos mistos. • Reposição de coloide — em casos de baixa pressão oncótica gerada por sangramento e perda de proteínas; é preferível o uso de plasma; a próxima alternativa mais eficiente é o hetamido; evitar a utilização de dextrana 70; a albumina humana pode induzir a reações alérgicas agudas fatais. • Potássio, fosfato e glicose — suplementar se pertinente; baixos níveis de fosfato, potássio e glicose agravam a encefalopatia hepática e outros sinais clínicos, dificultando os cuidados críticos de suporte. • Esquema de fluidoterapia — ajustar de acordo com as necessidades de manutenção após atingir a normovolemia; fornecer tipicamente 1/3 da taxa de manutenção normal com cristaloides poliônicos se administrados concomitantemente com coloide sintético em velocidade lenta sob infusão constante. • Suplementação de oxigênio — se a oximetria de pulso revelar uma saturação

INSUFICIÊNCIA HEPÁTICA AGUDA

≤80%. • Na suspeita de edema cerebral — elevar a cabeça em um ângulo de 30° do chão e considerar o uso de manitol. • Paciente predisposto a infecções a partir da translocação de bactérias entéricas — tratar com antimicrobianos de amplo espectro; o paciente pode não manifestar febre ou leucocitose em casos de infecção. • Sepse/síndrome da resposta inflamatória sistêmica — maiores riscos de edema cerebral. • Administração precoce de *N*-acetilcisteína — pode ser aconselhável; melhora a perfusão microvascular e a oxigenação tecidual, além de amenizar o dano oxidativo (ver adiante).

ATIVIDADE
A restrição promove a cura e a regeneração do fígado.

DIETA
• Vômitos intratáveis — suspender o alimento por VO até que estejam sob controle; usar antieméticos (ver adiante). • Quando a nutrição enteral estiver contraindicada (paciente sonolento), providenciar a nutrição parenteral parcial até que a alimentação balanceada seja instituída; aconselhável por não mais de 5 dias. • Se a nutrição enteral estiver cronicamente comprometida, estabelecer a nutrição parenteral total com cateter; usar fórmula de NPT com conteúdo normal de nitrogênio; a suplementação com aminoácidos de cadeia ramificada permanece controversa. • Alimentação enteral — refeições frequentes em pequenas quantidades para otimizar os processos de digestão e assimilação, além de minimizar a formação de toxinas entéricas que contribuem para a encefalopatia hepática. • Composição da dieta — usar conteúdo proteico normal (nitrogênio) se o paciente se mostrar tolerante; restrição moderada de proteína com encefalopatia hepática (2,5 g/kg de peso corporal); no entanto, é essencial se esforçar para manter o balanço nitrogenado positivo para a regeneração hepática. • É essencial a suplementação de vitaminas — hidrossolúveis (o dobro do normal); vitamina K1 (0,5-1,5 mg/kg SC ou IM, 3 doses em intervalos de 12 h e, em seguida, 1 vez por semana); vitamina E (10 UI/kg VO ou injetável a cada 24 h). • Probiótico/prebiótico (iogurte): podem conferir proteção contra a translocação de bactérias entéricas; fornecer uma fonte proteica láctea tolerada em cães com encefalopatia hepática.

ORIENTAÇÃO AO PROPRIETÁRIO
• Informar ao proprietário sobre o fato de que a insuficiência hepática aguda é uma condição grave e que alguns pacientes vêm a óbito mesmo com tratamento ideal. • Informar ao proprietário sobre a necessidade de se investigar uma causa subjacente para a necrose (p. ex., exposição a medicamento ou toxina), embora essa causa frequentemente não seja confirmada.

MEDICAÇÕES

MEDICAMENTO(S) DE ESCOLHA
Medicamentos para os Vômitos
• Metoclopramida — 1-2 mg/kg/dia sob infusão em velocidade constante para vômitos leves ou infrequentes; contraindicada se a espironolactona for utilizada para a mobilização de ascite. • Ondansetrona — 0,5-1,0 mg/kg IV a cada 24 h. • Clorpromazina — 0,5 mg/kg SC, IM ou por via retal, a cada 8-24 h, para vômitos intensos; assegurar primeiro a expansão volêmica.

• Maropitanto — 1,0 mg/kg SC a cada 24 h.
• Bloqueadores dos receptores histaminérgicos H_2 — famotidina (0,5 mg/kg IM ou SC a cada 12-24 h) para sangramento entérico; reservar a cimetidina (0,5 mg/kg a cada 8-12 h) para inibição intencional do citocromo P450.

Medicamentos para a Encefalopatia Hepática
• Lactulose — 0,5-2,0 mL/kg VO a cada 8 h; ou por via retal se a VO for perigosa. • Probiótico (iogurte) (ver anteriormente). • Metronidazol — 7,5 mg/kg VO a cada 12 h ou por via retal se a VO for perigosa. • Rifaximina — 5-10 mg/kg VO ou por via retal a cada 12 h (o antibiótico não absorvido altera a flora intestinal). • Neomicina — 22 mg/kg VO ou por via retal a cada 12 h.

Medicamentos para o Edema Cerebral Associado à Encefalopatia Hepática
• Manitol — 1 g/kg durante 10-20 min, administrado por meio de filtro; se não ocorrer uma rápida diurese em 1 h, medir a osmolalidade plasmática e a pressão arterial para verificar se ocorreu expansão volêmica excessiva. • Furosemida — 0,5-1,0 mg/kg IV a cada 8-24 h para aumentar a excreção de água livre e reduzir a produção de LCS; monitorizar a hidratação e o potássio sérico para evitar a desidratação e a hipocalemia (que agravam a encefalopatia hepática).

Medicamentos para a Coagulopatia
• Sangue total fresco ou plasma fresco congelado — para sangramento clinicamente significativo.

Varredores de Radicais Livres e Antioxidantes
• Para dano contínuo (lesão de membrana), lesão por reperfusão e hipoxia. • Vitamina E — 10 UI/kg VO a cada 24 h. • Vitamina C — 100-500 mg a cada 24 h; evitar em caso de concentrações hepáticas elevadas de ferro ou cobre.
• *N*-acetilcisteína — 140 mg/kg IV ou VO; para a via IV, usar solução a 10% diluída em solução fisiológica a 1:2 e administrar por meio de filtro não pirogênico de 0,25 μm; seguir com 70 mg/kg a cada 6-12 h. • *S*-adenosilmetionina (como doador de glutationa, utilizar produto biodisponível comprovado) — 20 mg/kg VO a cada 24 h com o estômago vazio; possui inúmeros benefícios, incluindo-se metabolismo intermediário relevante e síntese de glutationa, além de promover regeneração do fígado e exercer efeito antifibrótico.

Hepatoprotetores
• Silibinina (extrato de cardo leitoso) — eficácia relatada para intoxicação por *Amanita* e certas outras toxinas; utilizar o produto unido à fosfatidilcolina poli-insaturada sob a forma de complexo, 2-5 mg/kg VO a cada 24 h. • Ácido ursodesoxicólico — se houver lesão hepática crônica ou mediante a persistência de ácidos biliares elevados (10-15 mg/kg VO a cada 24 h, sendo mais bem absorvido se fornecido juntamente com o alimento).

CONTRAINDICAÇÕES
O ideal é evitar o uso de medicamentos que sejam biotransformados principalmente pelo fígado ou que alterem o fluxo sanguíneo hepático ou a atividade enzimática metabólica se possível. No entanto, isso pode ser impraticável, porque o metabolismo de muitos fármacos envolve as vias hepáticas ou a depuração biliar.

PRECAUÇÕES
A administração de sangue total armazenado ou papa de hemácias pode precipitar ou exacerbar a encefalopatia hepática por causa das altas concentrações de amônia.

INTERAÇÕES POSSÍVEIS
Metabolismo hepático comprometido.

MEDICAMENTO(S) ALTERNATIVO(S)
Tecer considerações dependendo do caso.

ACOMPANHAMENTO

MONITORIZAÇÃO DO PACIENTE
• Temperatura, pulso, respiração e estado mental — a cada 1-2 h até a estabilização. • Vigilância acentuada para detectar infecção, especialmente nosocomial associada ao uso iatrogênico de cateter.
• Peso corporal — 2 vezes ao dia para orientar a fluidoterapia; registrar o peso e a condição corporais para avaliar o balanço nitrogenado e o equilíbrio energético. • Equilíbrio acidobásico e eletrolítico (em especial de potássio e fosfato), além da glicemia — mensurar a cada 12-24 h nas primeiras 72 h.
• Atividade das enzimas hepáticas e concentração sérica de bilirrubina, colesterol e fibrinogênio — a cada 2-3 dias até que se observe uma melhora.

PREVENÇÃO
• Vacinar os cães contra o vírus da hepatite infecciosa canina. • Evitar a ingestão indiscriminada de hepatotoxinas e a exposição ambiental. • Considerar as terapias medicamentosas como toxinas potenciais.

COMPLICAÇÕES POSSÍVEIS
• Hipoglicemia. • Sangramento GI incontrolável e CID. • Encefalopatia hepática, edema cerebral, herniação cerebral. • Insuficiência hepática crônica, além de fibrose e cirrose por formação cicatricial pós-necrótica. • Insuficiência renal aguda. • Morte.

EVOLUÇÃO ESPERADA E PROGNÓSTICO
Prognóstico — depende do grau de destruição de massa hepática e da proficiência dos cuidados de suporte.

DIVERSOS

DISTÚRBIOS ASSOCIADOS
• Pancreatite. • Sepse/endotoxemia/choque.
• Diátese hemorrágica; hemorragia entérica grave; CID. • Insuficiência renal.

POTENCIAL ZOONÓTICO
Exposição a toxinas.

SINÔNIMO(S)
• Necrose hepática aguda. • Insuficiência hepática fulminante.

VER TAMBÉM
• Ascite. • Coagulopatia por Hepatopatia.
• Encefalopatia Hepática. • Capítulos sobre Hepatite. • Hepatotoxinas. • Icterícia.
• Insuficiência Renal Aguda.

ABREVIATURA(S)
• ALT = alanina aminotransferase. • AST = aspartato aminotransferase. • CID = coagulação intravascular disseminada. • GGT = γ-glutamil transferase. • LCS = líquido cerebrospinal. • NPT = nutrição parenteral total. • TNF = fator de necrose tumoral.

Autor Sharon A. Center
Consultor Editorial Sharon A. Center

Insuficiência Pancreática Exócrina

CONSIDERAÇÕES GERAIS

DEFINIÇÃO
Síndrome causada por quantidades inadequadas de enzimas digestivas pancreáticas no intestino delgado.

FISIOPATOLOGIA
• Causada muito comumente pela síntese e secreção insuficientes de enzimas pancreáticas pelo pâncreas exócrino.
• Em casos raros, pode ser causada por obstrução do ducto pancreático.
• A síntese insuficiente de enzimas digestivas pancreáticas pode ser atribuída à atrofia acinar pancreática idiopática — a causa mais comum de insuficiência pancreática exócrina em cães.
• Também pode ser decorrente de pancreatite crônica, com consequente destruição das células acinares, o que corresponde à segunda causa mais comum em cães e a causa mais comum em gatos.
• A secreção pancreática exócrina deficiente resulta em má digestão, má absorção de nutrientes e fezes moles com esteatorreia.
• A má absorção contribui para a proliferação de bactérias no intestino delgado (também conhecida como disbacteriose).

SISTEMA(S) ACOMETIDO(S)
• Gastrintestinal — comprometimento da mucosa duodenal (atrofia vilosa, infiltrados celulares inflamatórios, atividades anormais das enzimas da mucosa) e proliferação bacteriana no intestino delgado.
• Nutricional — desnutrição proteico-calórica.

GENÉTICA
Presume-se que seja hereditária em cães da raça Pastor alemão e provavelmente transmitida por um traço complexo (estudos recentes sugeriram um traço autossômico recessivo, mas isso não foi comprovado).

INCIDÊNCIA/PREVALÊNCIA
• A atrofia acinar pancreática é observada com maior frequência no Pastor alemão, porém com menor frequência em Collie de pelo áspero e Eurasiano.
• Outras causas de insuficiência pancreática exócrina podem ser constatadas em todas as raças caninas e felinas.
• Menos comum em gatos do que em cães.

DISTRIBUIÇÃO GEOGRÁFICA
• Cães — N/D.
• Gatos — N/D.

IDENTIFICAÇÃO
Espécies
Cães e gatos.

Raça(s) Predominante(s)
Pastor alemão, Collie de pelo áspero e Eurasiano.

Idade Média e Faixa Etária
• Atrofia acinar pancreática em cães jovens.
• Pancreatite crônica em cães e gatos de qualquer idade, embora seja mais comum em animais de meia-idade a idosos.

SINAIS CLÍNICOS
Comentários Gerais
• Considerar em cães jovens (faixa etária de aproximadamente 1-4 anos) da raça Pastor alemão com diarreia crônica, sugerindo má assimilação.
• Gravidade — varia; depende do tempo decorrido antes do diagnóstico e da terapia.

Achados Anamnésicos
• Perda de peso com apetite normal a aumentado.
• Diarreia ou fezes moles crônicas.
• A diarreia frequentemente se assemelha a fezes de bovino e pode ser contínua ou intermitente.
• Volumes fecais maiores do que o normal com esteatorreia.
• Flatulência e borborigmo são comuns, especialmente em cães.
• Pode exibir coprofagia e/ou pica.
• Pode ser acompanhada por poliúria/polidipsia com diabetes melito como uma sequela da pancreatite crônica.

Achados do Exame Físico
• Magreza.
• Redução da massa muscular.
• Pelagem de baixa qualidade.
• Gatos com esteatorreia podem exibir uma pelagem "suja" e engordurada em torno da região perineal, mas isso é observado na minoria dos casos.

CAUSAS
• Atrofia acinar pancreática.
• Pancreatite crônica.
• Adenocarcinoma pancreático com consequente obstrução do ducto pancreático.
• Infestação por trematódeo pancreático (*Eurytrema procyonis*) em gatos.

FATORES DE RISCO
• Raça — Pastor alemão, Collie de pelo áspero e Eurasiano.
• Qualquer condição que predisponha os cães ou gatos à pancreatite crônica.

DIAGNÓSTICO

DIAGNÓSTICO DIFERENCIAL
• Causas secundárias de diarreia crônica e perda de peso (p. ex., insuficiência hepática, insuficiência renal, hipoadrenocorticismo e hipotireoidismo em cães ou hipertireoidismo em gatos).
• Doença gastrintestinal primária (p. ex., infecciosa, inflamatória, neoplásica, mecânica ou tóxica).

HEMOGRAMA/BIOQUÍMICA/URINÁLISE
Geralmente normais.

OUTROS TESTES LABORATORIAIS
Exames Fecais Diretos/Indiretos
Negativos quanto à presença de parasitas.

Provas da Função Pancreática Exócrina — Imunorreatividade semelhante à da tripsina
• Exame diagnóstico de escolha em cães e gatos.
• Princípio do teste — a imunorreatividade sérica semelhante à da tripsina pode ser detectada por um ensaio que mede o tripsinogênio e a tripsina liberados diretamente no sangue a partir do tecido acinar pancreático; a imunorreatividade sérica semelhante à da tripsina é detectada em todos os cães e gatos normais com massa pancreática exócrina funcional.
• Concentrações séricas de imunorreatividade semelhante à da tripsina — muito reduzidas em casos de insuficiência pancreática exócrina.
• Valores da imunorreatividade semelhante à da tripsina — cães (≤2,5 µg/L) e gatos (≤8,0 µg/L).
• Os testes de imunorreatividade semelhante à da tripsina canina e felina são espécie-específicos.
• Vantagens — simples; rápidas; necessidade de amostra isolada de soro (em jejum); altamente sensíveis e específicas para insuficiência pancreática exócrina em ambas as espécies.

Provas da Função Pancreática Exócrina — Outras
• Ensaios da atividade proteolítica fecal feitos com o uso de substratos à base de caseína são utilizados para diagnosticar a insuficiência pancreática exócrina em cães e gatos.
• Contudo, a atividade proteolítica fecal é associada a resultados falso-positivos e falso-negativos e deve ser utilizada apenas em espécies exóticas para as quais um teste de imunorreatividade sérica semelhante à da tripsina não se encontra disponível.
• Outras desvantagens incluem a necessidade de coleta de múltiplas amostras fecais durante dias e a falta de disponibilidade do teste.
• Um ensaio para a mensuração da elastase fecal foi recentemente validado para o cão. No entanto, esse teste é associado a uma alta taxa de resultados falso-positivos e não pode ser recomendado nesse momento. Um resultado positivo sugestivo de insuficiência pancreática exócrina deve ser verificado pela mensuração de uma concentração da imunorreatividade sérica canina semelhante à da tripsina.

Testes de Triagem para Má Assimilação
O exame microscópico das fezes em busca de alimento não digerido, a avaliação da atividade proteolítica fecal por digestão do filme de raio X e o teste da turbidez plasmática não são confiáveis *nem* recomendados.

Níveis de Cobalamina e Folato
• Em geral, são rodados como um painel com a imunorreatividade semelhante à da tripsina.
• Utilizados para avaliar proliferação bacteriana no intestino delgado em cães e doença concomitante do intestino delgado (como enteropatia inflamatória) tanto em cães como em gatos.
• A cobalamina (vitamina B_{12}) encontra-se frequentemente diminuída em cães e gatos com insuficiência pancreática exócrina e pode levar à falha terapêutica se não for tratada.

DIAGNÓSTICO POR IMAGEM
Radiografias abdominais e ultrassonografia não são dignas de nota a menos que o paciente tenha outros distúrbios.

ACHADOS PATOLÓGICOS
• Atrofia acinar pancreática — atrofia/ausência acentuadas de tecido acinar pancreático à inspeção macroscópica em cães com atrofia acinar pancreática.
• Pancreatite crônica — ao exame microscópico, ácinos e possivelmente ilhotas eliminados e substituídos por tecido fibroso. Também pode haver uma infiltração inflamatória ativa.

TRATAMENTO

CUIDADO(S) DE SAÚDE ADEQUADO(S)
• Tratamento clínico ambulatorial.
• Pacientes com diabetes melito concomitante podem inicialmente necessitar de hospitalização para regulação da insulina por causa de hiperglicemia.

Insuficiência Pancreática Exócrina

DIETA
- A suplementação da dieta com reposição de enzimas pancreáticas constitui a base da terapia.
- O tipo da dieta não desempenha um papel no tratamento de insuficiência pancreática exócrina em cães e gatos.
- Contudo é recomendável evitar o fornecimento de dietas pobres em gorduras e ricas em fibras.
- Aproximadamente 80% de todos os cães com insuficiência pancreática exócrina e praticamente todos os gatos com esse tipo de insuficiência são deficientes em cobalamina e necessitam de suplementação dessa vitamina (cobalamina injetável pura a 250 µg/injeção em gatos e 250-1.500 µg/injeção em cães; uma vez por semana por 6 semanas, em semanas alternadas por 6 semanas e mais uma dose um mês depois, com reavaliação da concentração sérica de cobalamina um mês depois da última dose).
- Os cães gravemente desnutridos também necessitam de suplementação com tocoferol. As reservas corporais de outras vitaminas lipossolúveis provavelmente também se encontram diminuídas em cães e gatos com insuficiência pancreática exócrina, mas a suplementação não parece ser crucial.

ORIENTAÇÃO AO PROPRIETÁRIO
- Abordar a natureza hereditária na raça Pastor alemão.
- Discutir o custo da suplementação de enzimas pancreáticas e a necessidade de terapia pelo resto da vida.
- Debater a possibilidade de diabetes melito em pacientes com pancreatite crônica.

CONSIDERAÇÕES CIRÚRGICAS
Torção mesentérica relatada na raça Pastor alemão na Finlândia, mas não na América do Norte.

MEDICAÇÕES
MEDICAMENTO(S) DE ESCOLHA
- Enzimas pancreáticas em pó constituem o tratamento de escolha.
- Inicialmente — misturar a enzima em pó ao alimento a uma dose de 1 colher das de chá/10 kg de peso corporal a cada refeição; fornecer 2 refeições diárias para promover o ganho de peso.
- A pré-incubação das enzimas com o alimento *não* aumenta a eficácia da terapia enzimática oral.
- A suplementação de cobalamina será crucial se o paciente tiver deficiência dessa vitamina.
- A administração de antiácidos (famotidina, ranitidina ou omeprazol) pode melhorar a condição em pacientes irresponsivos.
- A maioria dos cães responde à terapia em 5-7 dias. Após a obtenção de uma resposta completa, a quantidade do suplemento de enzimas pancreáticas pode ser gradativamente reduzida a uma dose que impeça o retorno dos sinais clínicos.
- Antibioticoterapia oral (tilosina, 25 mg/kg VO a cada 12 h) pode ser necessária por 4-6 semanas em cães com proliferação bacteriana no intestino delgado (disbacteriose) concomitante. Contudo, na maioria dos cães, essa disbacteriose exibe resolução espontânea no início da terapia de reposição enzimática.

CONTRAINDICAÇÕES
Evitar comprimidos de enzimas pancreáticas com revestimento entérico; a dissolução de sua camada protetora é imprevisível, podendo ser constatadas respostas insatisfatórias.

MEDICAMENTO(S) ALTERNATIVO(S)
- O custo da reposição de enzimas pancreáticas é muito alto. Além disso, alguns gatos se recusam a consumir o suplemento de enzimas pancreáticas. Com frequência, esses pacientes podem ser tratados de forma bem-sucedida pela administração de pâncreas cru de bovino, suíno ou caça (animal selvagem).
- Cada colher das de chá de suplemento de enzimas pancreáticas precisa ser reposta com 28-85 g de pâncreas picado cru.
- O pâncreas cru pode ser mantido refrigerado por meses sem perder sua atividade enzimática.

ACOMPANHAMENTO
MONITORIZAÇÃO DO PACIENTE
- Semanal no primeiro mês de terapia.
- Há melhora acentuada da diarreia — a consistência fecal costuma se normalizar em 1 semana.
- Ganho de peso corporal.
- Para os cães que não respondem depois de 1 semana de terapia enzimática, é recomendável a administração de antibióticos para proliferação bacteriana no intestino delgado concomitante.
- Assim que o peso corporal e o condicionamento se normalizarem, reduzir gradualmente a dosagem diária dos suplementos enzimáticos até um nível que mantenha o peso corporal normal.

PREVENÇÃO
Não acasalar os pacientes com atrofia acinar pancreática.

COMPLICAÇÕES POSSÍVEIS
- Cerca de 20% dos cães não respondem às enzimas pancreáticas e necessitam de terapia adicional.
- A maioria dos pacientes com insuficiência pancreática exócrina tem deficiência de cobalamina e necessita de tratamento adequado.
- Alguns cães tratados com suplementos de enzimas pancreáticas desenvolvem ulcerações bucais. Em grande parte desses cães, a dose dos suplementos de enzimas pancreáticas pode ser reduzida, ao mesmo tempo em que se mantém a resposta terapêutica. Em alguns pacientes, a dose dos suplementos de enzimas pancreáticas precisa ser constantemente ajustada para evitar falha terapêutica e ulceração bucal.

EVOLUÇÃO ESPERADA E PROGNÓSTICO
- A maioria das causas é irreversível e a terapia pode ser necessária pelo resto da vida.
- Para os cães com insuficiência pancreática exócrina apenas, o prognóstico é bom com a suplementação adequada de enzimas e o tratamento de suporte.
- O prognóstico é mais reservado em pacientes com insuficiência pancreática exócrina e diabetes melito em razão da pancreatite crônica.

DIVERSOS
DISTÚRBIOS ASSOCIADOS
- Proliferação bacteriana no intestino delgado.
- Enteropatia inflamatória.
- Diabetes melito.
- Coagulopatia associada responsiva à vitamina K foi relatada em um gato.

FATORES RELACIONADOS COM A IDADE
Considerar a insuficiência pancreática exócrina em cães jovens adultos com diarreia crônica.

GESTAÇÃO/FERTILIDADE/REPRODUÇÃO
Não acasalar os animais com insuficiência pancreática exócrina supostamente atribuída à atrofia acinar pancreática.

SINÔNIMO(S)
- Atrofia pancreática juvenil.
- Atrofia acinar pancreática.

VER TAMBÉM
- Diarreia Crônica — Cães.
- Diarreia Crônica — Gatos.
- Pancreatite.

RECURSOS DA INTERNET
www.cvm.tamu.edu/gilab

Sugestões de Leitura
Batchelor DJ, Noble PJ, Taylor RH, et al. Prognostic factors in canine exocrine pancreatic insufficiency: Prolonged survival is likely if clinical remission is achieved. J Vet Intern Med 2007, 21:54-60.
Rutz GM, Steiner JM, Williams DA. Oral bleeding associated with pancreatic enzyme supplementation in three dogs with exocrine pancreatic insufficiency. JAVMA 2002, 221:1716-1718.
Steiner JM. Exocrine pancreas. In: Steiner JM, ed., Small Animal Gastroenterology. Hannover: Schlütersche-Verlagsgesellschaft mbH, 2008, pp. 283-306.
Steiner JM, Williams DA. Serum feline trypsin-like immunoreactivity in cats with exocrine pancreatic insufficiency. J Vet Intern Med 2000, 14:627-629.
Westermarck E, Wiberg M, Steiner JM, Williams DA. Exocrine pancreatic insufficiency in dogs and cats. In: Ettinger SJ, Feldman EC, eds., Textbook of Veterinary Internal Medicine, 6th ed. St. Louis: Elsevier, 2005, pp. 1492-1495.

Autor Jörg M. Steiner
Consultor Editorial Albert E. Jergens

Insuficiência Renal Aguda

CONSIDERAÇÕES GERAIS

DEFINIÇÃO
Uremia aguda é uma síndrome clínica caracterizada por início súbito de fluxo de saída renal ou insuficiência excretora; acúmulo de toxinas urêmicas; desequilíbrio hidreletrolítico e acidobásico e sinais clínicos de uremia. Dependendo da causa subjacente, a uremia aguda é potencialmente reversível se diagnosticada com rapidez e tratada de forma rigorosa. O presente capítulo refere-se à lesão renal aguda intrínseca e obstrução ureteral.

FISIOPATOLOGIA
- Lesão renal aguda pode ser desencadeada por isquemia, nefrotoxinas, infecção, obstrução prolongada do fluxo de saída da urina e doenças sistêmicas não renais graves (p. ex., pancreatite, neoplasia).
- A lesão renal aguda pode ser dividida em quatro estágios sequenciais: (1) início, (2) extensão, (3) manutenção e (4) recuperação. Do ponto de vista clínico, a transição de um estágio para o outro pode não ser claramente evidente, mas nem todos os estágios precisam estar presentes em cada paciente.
- A insuficiência excretora renal é perpetuada por múltiplos fatores, incluindo: (1) diminuição da área de superfície glomerular e da permeabilidade, (2) fluxo sanguíneo renal baixo, (3) obstrução intratubular por debris tubulares, (4) edema celular e intersticial e (5) "perda retrógrada" do filtrado renal através do epitélio tubular lesionado. A resolução ocorre por meio de regeneração e reparo renais.
- Obstrução ureteral origina-se da presença de ureterólitos, sangue inspissado (espesso) ou debris inflamatórios.

SISTEMA(S) ACOMETIDO(S)
- Endócrino/metabólico.
- Renal/urológico.
- GI.
- Nervoso.
- Respiratório.
- Musculosquelético.
- Hematológico/linfático/imune.

INCIDÊNCIA/PREVALÊNCIA
- A prevalência é mais baixa do que a de doença renal crônica.
- A prevalência pode aumentar no outono e no inverno no Hemisfério Norte com a maior exposição do animal a anticongelantes de aquecedores contendo etilenoglicol e a ambientes úmidos que favorecem a manutenção da *Leptospira*.
- A obstrução ureteral com urólitos constitui a causa mais comum de uremia aguda grave em gatos.

IDENTIFICAÇÃO
Espécies
Cães e gatos.

Raça(s) Predominante(s)
Nenhuma.

Idade Média e Faixa Etária
- O pico de prevalência ocorre entre 6-8 anos em cães e gatos.
- Os animais mais idosos estão sob maior risco.

SINAIS CLÍNICOS
Achados Anamnésicos
Início súbito de anorexia, inquietação, depressão, vômito (± sangue), diarreia (± sangue), halitose, ataxia, crises convulsivas, exposição a toxina ou medicamento conhecido, condições clínicas ou cirúrgicas recentes e oligúria/anúria ou poliúria.

Achados do Exame Físico
Condição normal do corpo e da pelagem, depressão, desidratação (super-hidratação iatrogênica), congestão da esclera, ulceração bucal, glossite, necrose da língua, hálito urêmico, hipotermia, febre, taquipneia, bradicardia, bexiga urinária não palpável e rins grandes, dolorosos, firmes e assimétricos.

CAUSAS
Hemodinâmicas/Hipoperfusão
Choque, traumatismo, tromboembolia (p. ex., CID, vasculite e reação transfusional), intermação/insolação, vasoconstrição excessiva (p. ex., administração de AINE), insuficiência adrenal, vasodilatação excessiva (p. ex., administração de inibidor da ECA ou medicamento anti-hipertensivo), anestesia prolongada, hipertensão significativa, insuficiência cardíaca.

Nefrotóxicas
Etilenoglicol, aminoglicosídeo, anfotericina B, agente quimioterápico (p. ex., cisplatina e doxorrubicina), tiacetarsamida, AINE, agentes de contraste radiográfico, metais pesados (p. ex., chumbo, mercúrio, arsênico e tálio), veneno de inseto ou de cobra, pigmento heme, cálcio, ingestão de uva ou passa (cães) e ingestão de lírio (gatos).

Doença Intrínseca e Sistêmica
Leptospirose, doença de Lyme, glomerulonefrite e arterite imunomediadas, pancreatite, septicemia, CID, insuficiência hepática, intermação/insolação, reação transfusional, endocardite bacteriana, pielonefrite, necrose cortical e linfoma. Obstrução uni ou bilateral dos ureteres (gatos).

FATORES DE RISCO
- Endógenos — doença renal crônica preexistente, desidratação, sepse, hipovolemia, hipotensão, idade avançada, doença concomitante, hiponatremia, hipocalemia, hipocalcemia e acidose.
- Exógenos — medicamentos (p. ex., furosemida, AINE, inibidor da ECA e aminoglicosídeo), anestesia prolongada, dietas acidificantes, traumatismo, falência múltipla de órgãos e temperatura ambiente elevada.

DIAGNÓSTICO

DIAGNÓSTICO DIFERENCIAL
- Azotemia pré-renal — oligúria, densidade urinária concentrada (cães, ≥1,030; gatos, ≥1,035), corrigível com repleção hídrica.
- Azotemia pós-renal — anúria, disúria, estrangúria, bexiga urinária grande, obstrução uretral e uroperitônio.
- Doença renal crônica — poliúria, polidipsia, histórico de doença crônica, perda de condição corporal e anemia.
- Pré-renal na doença renal crônica — características clínicas e laboratoriais de doença renal crônica, porém passível de correção parcial com repleção hídrica.
- Pré-renal na lesão renal aguda — uremia de início agudo, parcialmente corrigida com repleção hídrica.
- Hipoadrenocorticismo — hiponatremia, hipercalemia.
- Pancreatite — lipase sérica aumentada, dor abdominal cranial, imunorreatividade semelhante à da tripsina elevada, hiperbilirrubinemia e aumento na atividade das enzimas hepáticas.

HEMOGRAMA/BIOQUÍMICA/URINÁLISE
- Hematócrito normal ou elevado, leucocitose variável e linfopenia.
- Aumentos progressivos (moderados a graves) nos níveis de ureia, creatinina e fósforo; potássio e glicose variavelmente elevados e concentração variavelmente baixa de bicarbonato e cálcio.
- Densidade urinária (≤1,020), proteinúria leve a moderada, glicosúria; quantidade variável de cilindros celulares e/ou granulares, além de leucócitos, hemácias e células epiteliais tubulares; bacteriúria e cristalúria por oxalato de cálcio variáveis (observadas, algumas vezes, em associação com intoxicação por etilenoglicol).

OUTROS TESTES LABORATORIAIS
- É comum a constatação de acidose metabólica, embora possam ocorrer distúrbios acidobásicos mistos.
- Título *de Leptospira* — ≥1:800 a sorotipo não vacinal ou títulos crescentes.
- Concentração de etilenoglicol — positiva se o paciente estiver intoxicado; aumento da osmolalidade sérica e/ou do hiato osmolar ou aniônico.

DIAGNÓSTICO POR IMAGEM
- Radiografias simples e contrastada — os rins encontram-se normais a aumentados de volume, com contornos lisos bilaterais; rins assimétricos em gatos (síndrome do "rim grande-rim pequeno") na obstrução ureteral — procurar pequenos urólitos radiodensos no retroperitônio.
- Nefropielografia percutânea ou TC contrastada nos casos de obstrução ureteral.
- Ultrassonografia — hiperecogenicidade cortical grave sugere intoxicação pelo etilenoglicol. Hiperecogenicidade cortical moderada é sugestiva de glomerulonefrite ou nefrose. Dilatação pélvica e/ou ureteral ou densidades calcificadas apontam para obstrução ao fluxo de saída.

MÉTODOS DIAGNÓSTICOS
- Monitorização do débito urinário — ajuda não só no estabelecimento do diagnóstico, mas também na formulação do tratamento e do prognóstico: anúria; oligúria, ≤0,25 mL/kg/h (≤1 mL/kg/h durante a fluidoterapia); sem oligúria, ≥2 mL/kg/h.
- Aspirado obtido por agulha fina — pode definir o diagnóstico de linfoma como causa da renomegalia.
- Biopsia renal percutânea — ajuda a estabelecer a causa, a gravidade e a reversibilidade potencial da lesão; mais tarde, no curso da doença (4-6 semanas), esse tipo de exame pode ajudar a predizer a ocorrência de reparo renal em andamento e a permanência da lesão renal.

ACHADOS PATOLÓGICOS
Nefrose ou nefrite, glomerulonefrite, cristais de oxalato de cálcio, edema intersticial e falta de fibrose intersticial; o estágio subagudo caracteriza-se por epitélio tubular adelgaçado, fibrose e mineralização intersticiais, infiltração celular e regeneração tubular variável.

INSUFICIÊNCIA RENAL AGUDA

TRATAMENTO

CUIDADO(S) DE SAÚDE ADEQUADO(S)
Tratar como paciente internado; eliminar as causas incitantes; interromper os medicamentos nefrotóxicos; estabelecer e manter a estabilidade hemodinâmica; melhorar os desequilíbrios hídricos com risco de morte, as anormalidades bioquímicas e as toxicidades urêmicas; instituir a lavagem gástrica, induzir à êmese e administrar carvão ativado, catárticos e antídotos específicos aos pacientes com intoxicação aguda; hemodiálise/hemoperfusão precoce pode eliminar muitas toxinas.

CUIDADO(S) DE ENFERMAGEM
• Hipovolemia — corrigir os déficits hídricos estimados com solução fisiológica a 0,9% ou solução poliônica balanceada dentro de 2-4 h se o estado do paciente permitir; assim que o paciente estiver hidratado, as necessidades hídricas contínuas serão supridas com glicose a 5% para as perdas insensíveis (aproximadamente 20-25 mL/kg/dia) e solução eletrolítica balanceada equivalente à perda urinária e a outras perdas (i. e., vômito e diarreia); evitar a super-hidratação; repor as perdas sanguíneas por meio da transfusão de sangue total.
• Hipervolemia — interromper a administração de fluido e eliminar o excesso dele com administração de diuréticos ou diálise.
• Monitorizar o peso corporal por, no mínimo, 4 vezes ao dia e ajustar a dose dos fluidos para manter o peso estável assim que o paciente estiver hidratado.

DIETA
• Restringir a ingestão oral (i. e., "nada por via oral") até que o vômito desapareça. As reservas endógenas de gordura e proteína são consumidas enquanto o paciente se encontra anoréxico; as necessidades energéticas em repouso precisam ser supridas durante 3-5 dias, utilizando dietas com restrição moderada de proteína ou soluções de nutrição enteral formuladas para controlar a azotemia e atender às necessidades calóricas.
• Nutrição parenteral (animais vomitando) — supre as necessidades calóricas por meio do fornecimento de glicose e emulsão lipídica sob a forma de solução; as necessidades proteicas (cães, 2-3 g/100 kcal; gatos, 3-4 g/100 kcal) são supridas por misturas de aminoácidos.
• Nutrição enteral (animais com anorexia e sem vômito) — as necessidades calóricas e proteicas são supridas por dietas renais compostas, soluções enterais líquidas ou dietas formuladas fornecidas via sonda nasoesofágica ou tubo inserido via esofagostomia, gastrostomia ou enterostomia.

ORIENTAÇÃO AO PROPRIETÁRIO
Informar o proprietário sobre o prognóstico mau quanto à recuperação plena; ao potencial de complicações mórbidas do tratamento (p. ex., sobrecarga de fluido, sepse e falência múltipla de órgãos); às despesas com a hospitalização prolongada; às alternativas ao tratamento clínico convencional (i. e., diálise peritoneal, hemodiálise e transplante renal); ao potencial zoonótico da leptospirose.

CONSIDERAÇÕES CIRÚRGICAS
• Em casos de obstrução ureteral aguda, talvez haja necessidade de ureterotomia, ressecção e reimplante ureterais ou aplicação de *stents** ureterais
• O transplante renal pode conferir sobrevida a longo prazo para os gatos com lesão renal aguda fulminante irresponsiva.

Diálise Peritoneal ou Hemodiálise
• A diálise pode estabilizar o paciente até que se restabeleça a função renal ou se realize a cirurgia corretiva (remoção de obstrução ureteral, transplante renal); sem a diálise, a maioria dos pacientes oligúricos vem a óbito antes que ocorra o reparo renal.
• As indicações específicas incluem oligúria ou anúria graves, sobrecarga hídrica ou distúrbios eletrolíticos acidobásicos com risco de morte, ureia ≥100 mg/dL, creatinina sérica ≥10 mg/dL, evolução clínica refratária ao tratamento conservativo, estabilização perioperatória e intoxicação por toxina dializável.

MEDICAÇÕES

MEDICAMENTO(S) DE ESCOLHA
Produção Inadequada de Urina
• Garantir a repleção volêmica do paciente por meio da fluidoterapia; fornecer fluido isonático adicional para obter expansão volêmica de 3%; a falha na indução da diurese indica dano grave do parênquima ou estimativa inferior do déficit hídrico; quando repleto de líquido, administrar os diuréticos.
• Manitol hipertônico (10-20%) — 0,25-1,0 g/kg IV por 15-30 min; se eficaz, continuar a administração sob a forma de bólus IV intermitente a cada 4-6 h; quando ineficaz, interromper.
• Furosemida (alternativa ou subsequente ao manitol) — 2-6 mg/kg IV; caso seja eficaz, continuar a cada 8 h; se ineficaz, interromper.
• Dopamina — a falta de eficácia comprovada e a ocorrência de efeitos colaterais potenciais contraindicam o uso desse agente, exceto para controle da pressão arterial.
• Caso esses tratamentos falhem na indução da diurese dentro de 4-6 h, considerar a realização de diálise.

Distúrbios Metabólicos e Acidobásicos
Administrar bicarbonato se o nível sérico desse sal estiver ≤16 mEq/L; reposição do bicarbonato: mEq = déficit de bicarbonato × peso corporal (kg) × 0,3; administrar metade IV durante 30 min e o restante em 2-4 h; reavaliar o caso em seguida.

Hipercalemia
• Corrigir a desidratação com fluidos livres de potássio (NaCl a 0,9%).
• Minimizar a ingestão de potássio.
• Interromper as medicações que promovam hipercalemia (p. ex., inibidor da ECA, diuréticos poupadores de potássio).
• Diuréticos de alça: furosemida na dose de 2-4 mg/kg IV.
• Bicarbonato de sódio à dose de 1-2 mEq/kg IV, suficiente para corrigir o déficit existente desse sal, se o nível for desconhecido.
• Glicose ± insulina: 1-2 mL/kg de glicose a 50% (diluída até 25%) IV ou insulina regular a 0,1-0,2 U/kg sob a forma de bólus IV, seguida por 1-2 g de glicose/unidade de insulina.
• Gliconato de cálcio: 0,5-1,0 mL/kg de gliconato de cálcio a 10% IV durante 10-15 minutos.
• Hipercalemia refratária — diálise.

Vômito
• Reduzir a produção de ácido gástrico — famotidina (0,5 mg/kg IM, IV a cada 24 h) ou ranitidina (0,5-2 mg/kg IV a cada 8-12 h) ou omeprazol (0,5-1,0 mg/kg VO a cada 24 h [cães]).
• Protetor de mucosa — sucralfato (0,5-1 g VO a cada 6-8 h).
• Antieméticos — maropitanto (1 mg/kg SC a cada 24 h) ou ondansetrona (0,1-0,3 mg/kg IV a cada 8-12 h) ou dolasetrona (0,5 mg/kg SC, IV a cada 24 h) ou metoclopramida (0,2-0,5 mg/kg SC, IV ou IM a cada 6-8 h; 0,01-0,02 mg/kg/h sob infusão a velocidade constante).

PRECAUÇÕES
Modificar as dosagens de todos os medicamentos que exigem metabolismo ou eliminação renais.

ACOMPANHAMENTO

MONITORIZAÇÃO DO PACIENTE
Equilíbrios hidreletrolítico e acidobásico; peso corporal; pressão arterial; débito urinário; e estado clínico; diariamente.

PREVENÇÃO
• Prever o potencial de lesão renal aguda em pacientes idosos ou naqueles com doença sistêmica, sepse, traumatismo, instabilidade hemodinâmica, falência múltipla de órgãos ou sob medicamentos nefrotóxicos ou anestesia prolongada.
• Pode ser uma medida preventiva manter a hidratação, uma leve expansão volêmica com soro fisiológico e a administração de manitol.
• Monitorizar a produção urinária e a azotemia em pacientes de alto risco.

COMPLICAÇÕES POSSÍVEIS
Crises convulsivas, coma, arritmias cardíacas, hipertensão, insuficiência cardíaca congestiva, edema pulmonar, pneumonite urêmica, pneumonia por aspiração, sangramento GI, choque hipovolêmico, sepse, parada cardiopulmonar e morte.

EVOLUÇÃO ESPERADA E PROGNÓSTICO
• O prognóstico depende da causa subjacente, do grau de lesão renal e da presença de doença ou falência orgânica concomitante, bem como da idade do paciente e da resposta à terapia.
• Taxas de sobrevida de 50%, variando de 20% para intoxicação por etilenoglicol até 80% para os casos de leptospirose aguda.
• Etiologias infecciosas e obstrutivas apresentam prognóstico melhor quanto à recuperação do que causas tóxicas.
• Lesão renal aguda não oligúrica — tipicamente mais branda do que a oligúrica; a recuperação pode ocorrer em 2-6 semanas, mas o prognóstico permanece reservado a desfavorável.
• Lesão renal aguda oligúrica — implica lesão renal extensa; além de ser difícil de tratar, possui prognóstico mau quanto à recuperação sem diálise; a recuperação é sinalizada por poliúria súbita (e quase sempre excessiva) e retorno vagaroso e, possivelmente, incompleto da função renal em

---

* N. T.: Stents são dispositivos intraluminais utilizados para manter o calibre de vasos; no caso específico, para manter o lúmen do ureter.

Insuficiência Renal Aguda

4-12 semanas; a diálise prolonga a possibilidade de regeneração e reparo renais.
• Lesão renal aguda anúrica — prognóstico mau sem a diálise; recuperação frequentemente incompleta da função renal.

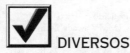

DIVERSOS

POTENCIAL ZOONÓTICO
Leptospirose — evitar o contato com a urina infectada.

GESTAÇÃO/FERTILIDADE/REPRODUÇÃO
Complicação rara da prenhez nos animais; promovida por metrite, piometra e sepse pós-parto ou hemorragia agudas.

SINÔNIMO(S)
Falência renal aguda, necrose tubular aguda, uremia aguda.

VER TAMBÉM
• Azotemia e Uremia.
• Hipercalemia.
• Hipertensão Sistêmica.
• Leptospirose.
• Ureterolitíase.

ABREVIATURA(S)
• AINE = anti-inflamatório não esteroide.
• CID = coagulação intravascular disseminada.
• ECA = enzima conversora de angiotensina.
• GI = gastrintestinal.
• TC = tomografia computadorizada.

Sugestões de Leitura
Cowgill LD, Langston C. Acute kidney injury. In: Bartges J, Polzin DJ, eds., Nephrology and Urology of Small Animals. Ames, IA: Wiley-Blackwell, 2011.

Autores Sheri J. Ross e Larry D. Cowgill
Consultor Editorial Carl A. Osborne

Insuficiência Renal Crônica

CONSIDERAÇÕES GERAIS

DEFINIÇÃO
A doença renal é considerada crônica quando presente por >3 meses. A doença renal envolve lesões funcionais ou estruturais em um ou ambos os rins, conforme detectadas por exames de sangue ou de urina, técnicas de diagnóstico por imagem ou biopsia renal. Essa definição inclui todos os casos previamente descritos pelos termos insuficiência ou falência renais, bem como as formas menos avançadas de doença renal. Os pacientes são categorizados em estágios na sequência de doença renal crônica progressiva (estágio da doença renal crônica, de acordo com a *International Renal Interest Society* [IRIS]), com base em dois ou mais valores séricos de creatinina obtidos em algumas semanas, quando o paciente estiver em jejum e bem hidratado.

FISIOPATOLOGIA
A redução de mais de ~75% na função renal resulta em diminuição na capacidade de concentração da urina (levando a poliúria e polidipsia [PU/PD]) e na retenção de produtos residuais nitrogenados do catabolismo proteico (levando à azotemia). A doença renal crônica mais avançada culmina em uremia. A produção reduzida de eritropoetina e de calcitriol pelos rins resulta em anemia hipoproliferativa e hiperparatireoidismo secundário renal, respectivamente.

SISTEMA(S) ACOMETIDO(S)
- Cardiovascular — hipertensão; pericardite urêmica.
- Endócrino/metabólico — hiperparatireoidismo secundário renal, ativação do sistema renina-angiotensina-aldosterona, deficiência da eritropoetina.
- Gastrintestinal — estomatite urêmica, halitose urêmica, cálculo dentário acentuado, náusea, vômito, anorexia, sangramento gastrintestinal, diarreia (pode ser hemorrágica).
- Hematológico/linfático/imune — anemia; diátese hemorrágica.
- Musculosquelético — osteodistrofia renal.
- Neuromuscular — crises convulsivas e outros sinais neurológicos atribuídos à hipertensão e/ou uremia; tremores musculares, emaciação muscular.
- Oftálmico — descolamento da retina, hemorragia ou edema decorrentes de hipertensão.
- Reprodutor — capacidade reprodutiva prejudicada.
- Respiratório — pneumonite urêmica.
- Cutâneo/exócrino — calcinose cutânea.

GENÉTICA
- Condição hereditária nas seguintes raças (modo de herança, conhecido ou suspeito, indicado entre parênteses):
- Gatos Abissínios (autossômico dominante, com penetrância incompleta).
- Gatos Persas (autossômico dominante).
- Bull terrier (autossômico dominante).
- Cairn terrier (autossômico recessivo).
- Pastor alemão (autossômico dominante).
- Samoieda (dominante ligado ao cromossomo X).
- Cocker spaniel inglês (autossômico recessivo).
- Displasia renal (modo de herança não esclarecido): Shih tzu, Lhasa apso, Golden retriever, Elkhound norueguês, Chow chow, Poodle standard, Wheaten terrier de pelo macio, Malamute do Alasca, Schnauzer miniatura, Kooiker holandês e, esporadicamente, em muitas outras raças.

INCIDÊNCIA/PREVALÊNCIA
- Há relatos norte-americanos de 9 casos para cada 1.000 cães examinados e 16 casos para cada 1.000 gatos examinados.
- A prevalência aumenta com a idade — em animais com >15 anos de idade, relatam-se 57 casos para cada 1.000 cães examinados e 153 casos para cada 1.000 gatos examinados.

DISTRIBUIÇÃO GEOGRÁFICA
Mundial.

IDENTIFICAÇÃO
Espécies
Cães e gatos.

Raça(s) Predominante(s)
Nenhuma.

Idade Média e Faixa Etária
A idade média ao diagnóstico é de aproximadamente 7 anos nos cães e 9 anos nos gatos. Pode acometer animais de qualquer idade, porém a prevalência aumenta com o avanço da idade.

Sexo Predominante
Nenhum.

SINAIS CLÍNICOS
Comentários Gerais
Os sinais clínicos estão relacionados com o estágio da doença renal crônica e a presença de complicações como proteinúria e hipertensão. Cães e gatos com doença renal crônica nos estágios 1 e 2 podem permanecer assintomáticos; a manifestação dos sinais clínicos tipicamente se torna aparente nos estágios 3 e 4. Um animal com doença renal crônica estável (particularmente nos estágios 3 e 4) pode descompensar, resultando em uma crise urêmica.

Achados Anamnésicos
- PU/PD (menos frequente nos gatos do que nos cães); observa-se a bandeja sanitária (caixa de areia) mais úmida; urina mais clara.
- Anorexia.
- Letargia.
- Vômito.
- Perda de peso.
- Noctúria.
- Constipação.
- Diarreia.
- Cegueira aguda — por causa da hipertensão.
- Crises convulsivas ou coma — sinais tardios.
- Os gatos também podem apresentar ptialismo e fraqueza muscular com ventroflexão cervical (por causa da miopatia hipocalêmica).

Achados do Exame Físico
- Rins pequenos e irregulares (ou rins aumentados secundariamente à doença renal policística ou linfoma).
- Desidratação.
- Caquexia.
- Letargia, fraqueza.
- Mucosas pálidas.
- Ulceração bucal.
- Halitose urêmica.
- Constipação.
- Retinopatia hipertensiva.
- Osteodistrofia renal (pode-se manifestar como dor óssea [ostealgia], particularmente no crânio).
- Temperatura corporal reduzida.

CAUSAS
- A origem é desconhecida na maior parte dos casos em virtude do diagnóstico tardio.
- Inclui doença renal familiar e congênita, nefrotoxinas, hipercalcemia, nefropatia hipocalêmica, glomerulopatias, amiloidose, pielonefrite, doença renal policística, nefrólitos, obstrução urinária crônica, medicamentos, linfoma, leptospirose (após insuficiência renal aguda) e PIF.

FATORES DE RISCO
Idade, proteinúria, hipercalcemia, hipocalemia (gatos), hipertensão, infecção do trato urinário, diabetes melito.

DIAGNÓSTICO

DIAGNÓSTICO DIFERENCIAL
- Ver o capítulo sobre poliúria/polidipsia para o diagnóstico diferencial.
- Azotemia — inclui causas de azotemia pré e pós-renal, insuficiência renal aguda e hipoadrenocorticismo.
- Azotemia pré-renal — caracterizada por azotemia com densidade urinária >1,030 nos cães e >1,035 nos gatos. O rápido declínio na azotemia após a correção dos problemas de volume/perfusão indica azotemia pré-renal. A azotemia pré-renal é um achado comum em pacientes com vômito e azotemia intrarrenal primária.
- Azotemia pós-renal — caracterizada por azotemia com obstrução ou ruptura do sistema excretor; a correção rápida da azotemia após a eliminação da obstrução apoia a azotemia pós-renal.
- Insuficiência renal aguda — diferenciada pelo tamanho normal a aumentado do rim, cilindrúria, falta de indicações de cronicidade (ausência de rins pequenos, anemia hipoproliferativa e osteodistrofia renal) e histórico de exposição recente à nefrotoxina ou a episódio hipotensivo.
- Hipoadrenocorticismo — caracterizado por hiponatremia e hipercalemia com valor de cortisol em repouso <1 μg/dL ou resposta adrenal diminuída à estimulação com ACTH.

HEMOGRAMA/BIOQUÍMICA/URINÁLISE
- Anemia hipoproliferativa.
- Ureia e creatinina elevadas.
- Hiperfosfatemia.
- Acidose metabólica (hiato aniônico normal ou elevado).
- Hipocalemia ou hipercalemia.
- Hipercalcemia ou hipocalcemia.
- Densidade urinária <1,030 nos cães e <1,035 nos gatos.
- Proteinúria.

OUTROS TESTES LABORATORIAIS
- Relação de proteína:creatinina urinárias para determinar a magnitude da proteinúria.
- Teste da microalbuminúria para fazer triagem em busca de indícios precoces de lesão glomerular.

DIAGNÓSTICO POR IMAGEM
- Radiografias abdominais podem demonstrar rins de tamanho pequeno (ou rins de tamanho grande secundários à doença renal policística ou linfoma).
- O ultrassom revela rins de tamanho pequeno e parênquima renal hiperecoico, com distinção menos aparente entre o córtex e a medula em

Insuficiência Renal Crônica

alguns animais. Animais com linfoma frequentemente apresentam renomegalia com parênquima renal hipoecoico.
• Ver também "Doenças Renais de Base Congênita e de Desenvolvimento", "Pielonefrite", "Nefrolitíase", "Hidronefrose" e "Doença Renal Policística".

MÉTODOS DIAGNÓSTICOS
• Medição da pressão arterial para detectar hipertensão.
• Mensuração da taxa de filtração glomerular pode ser útil para detectar perda da função renal antes do início de azotemia.
• Biopsia renal não é indicada em pacientes com rins de tamanho pequeno; pode ser indicada em pacientes proteinúricos com rins normais a aumentados.

ACHADOS PATOLÓGICOS
• Achados macroscópicos — rins de tamanho pequeno, com superfície nodular ou granular; a cápsula renal frequentemente se adere ao parênquima renal.
• Achados histopatológicos — variáveis. Os pacientes com doença renal crônica proteinúrica em estágio 1 podem exibir alterações compatíveis com várias formas de glomerulopatia. A avaliação completa do material de biopsia desses pacientes requer microscopia óptica, imunofluorescente e eletrônica. Em pacientes com doença renal crônica mais avançada, há alterações inespecíficas, incluindo processo de fibrose intersticial e focos de células mononucleares intersticiais; nefropatia generalizada crônica ou rins em estágio terminal.
• Os achados podem ser específicos para doenças que causam doença renal crônica em alguns pacientes com doença menos avançada.

TRATAMENTO
CUIDADO(S) DE SAÚDE ADEQUADO(S)
Pacientes com doença renal crônica compensada podem ser tratados em um esquema ambulatorial; pacientes em crise urêmica devem ser tratados com internação.

CUIDADO(S) DE ENFERMAGEM
• Pacientes em crise urêmica — corrigir os déficits hidreletrolíticos com fluidoterapia intravenosa (p. ex., solução de Ringer lactato); corrigir 50-75% das necessidades hídricas estimadas em 4-8 h para evitar lesão renal adicional decorrente de isquemia; no entanto, evitar a administração excessiva de fluido.
• Fluidoterapia subcutânea (a cada 24-48 h) pode beneficiar os pacientes (especialmente gatos) com doença renal crônica moderada a grave. Continuar a terapia apenas se houver melhora clínica.

ATIVIDADE
Sem restrição.

DIETA
• As rações destinadas a cães e gatos com doença renal crônica (p. ex., Prescription Diet k/d da Hill®) retardam o início da crise urêmica e prolongam a sobrevida em animais com doença renal crônica nos estágios 2-4. Tais rações constituem um padrão de cuidado para esses pacientes.
• As rações que contêm teor proteico reduzido e ácidos graxos ômega-3 podem ser benéficas em pacientes proteinúricos com doença renal crônica em estágio 1.
• Os componentes importantes das rações renais incluem: teor reduzido de proteína, fósforo, sódio e ácido, além de suplementação de ácidos graxos ômega-3 e antioxidantes.
• Livre acesso à água limpa e fresca a qualquer momento.

ORIENTAÇÃO AO PROPRIETÁRIO
• Cães e muitos gatos — a doença renal crônica tipicamente evolui para insuficiência renal terminal em meses a anos.
• A doença renal crônica pode não ser progressiva em alguns gatos.
• Níveis mais elevados de proteína são associados a tempos de sobrevida mais curtos. Esse efeito pode ser atenuado pela terapia para proteinúria.
• Caráter hereditário de doenças renais familiares.

CONSIDERAÇÕES CIRÚRGICAS
• Evitar a hipertensão durante a anestesia para evitar lesão renal adicional.
• Transplantes renais foram realizados com sucesso em gatos com doença renal crônica.

MEDICAÇÕES
MEDICAMENTO(S) DE ESCOLHA
Crise Urêmica
• Famotidina (0,5-1 mg/kg VO, IM, IV a cada 12-24 h) para minimizar os sintomas de náusea e vômito.
• Antieméticos (maropitanto 1 mg/kg a cada 24 h até 5 dias ou ondansetrona 0,1-0,2 mg/kg IV lento a cada 12 h) para minimizar o vômito e o apetite reduzido devido à náusea.
• Cloreto de potássio em fluidos por via IV ou gliconato de potássio VO (2-6 mEq/gato/dia), conforme a necessidade, para corrigir a hipocalemia.
• Bicarbonato de sódio para corrigir a acidose metabólica (IV para elevar o pH sanguíneo acima de 7,1).

Doença Renal Crônica Compensada
• Famotidina (cães, 0,5-1 mg/kg VO a cada 24 h; gatos, 5 mg/gato VO a cada 48 h) para minimizar a gastrite urêmica e os possíveis sintomas de náusea e inapetência.
• Antiemético (maropitanto) e gliconato de potássio conforme descrito anteriormente.
• Quelantes de fosfato intestinal (p. ex., carbonato de alumínio, 30-100 mg/kg/dia VO com as refeições), conforme a necessidade, para corrigir a hiperfosfatemia (ver "Hiperparatireoidismo Secundário Renal").
• Calcitriol (iniciar a 2 ng/kg VO a cada 24 h e monitorizar o efeito sobre o PTH e o cálcio ionizado — evitar a indução de hipercalcemia) (ver "Hiperparatireoidismo Secundário Renal").
• Darbepoetina (ver "Anemia de Doença Renal Crônica").
• Anlodipino (cães, 0,1-0,6 mg/kg VO a cada 24 h; gatos, 0,625-1,25 mg/gato VO a cada 24 h) ou inibidores da ECA (p. ex., enalapril ou benazepril, 0,5 mg/kg VO a cada 24 h), conforme a necessidade, para hipertensão. O anlodipino é mais eficaz do que os inibidores da ECA em gatos com hipertensão induzida por doença renal crônica. Se refratários à monoterapia, considerar a combinação de anlodipino e inibidor da ECA com monitorização frequente da pressão arterial.
• Inibidor da ECA (benazepril ou enalapril) para proteinúria (iniciar a 0,5 mg/kg VO a cada 24 h; pode aumentar para 1 mg/kg VO a cada 12 h, se necessário, para reduzir a proteinúria).

CONTRAINDICAÇÕES
Evitar medicamentos nefrotóxicos (aminoglicosídeos, cisplatina, anfotericina B) e corticosteroides.

PRECAUÇÕES
• Talvez haja necessidade de modificação da dose ou do intervalo entre as doses para alguns medicamentos eliminados pelos rins.
• Utilizar os inibidores da ECA com cuidado; monitorizar o paciente quanto à piora da azotemia.
• Em geral, evitar os AINEs.

INTERAÇÕES POSSÍVEIS
Cimetidina ou trimetoprima podem provocar aumentos por artefato na concentração sérica de creatinina pela redução da secreção tubular nos cães com doença renal crônica.

MEDICAMENTO(S) ALTERNATIVO(S)
• Metoclopramida (0,2-0,4 mg VO ou SC a cada 6-8 h) pode ser utilizada além dos antagonistas do receptor H_2 para tratar o vômito urêmico.
• Ranitidina (0,5-2 mg/kg VO ou IV a cada 12 h) ou cimetidina (5 mg/kg a cada 8-12 h para cães; 2,5-5 mg/kg a cada 8-12 h para gatos) podem ser usadas no lugar da famotidina.
• Hemodiálise e transplante renal estão disponíveis em hospitais de referência selecionados.

ACOMPANHAMENTO
MONITORIZAÇÃO DO PACIENTE
• Cães e gatos com doença renal crônica — monitorizar em intervalos regulares; semanalmente, no início, em pacientes submetidos ao calcitriol ou à eritropoetina; a cada 1-3 meses nos pacientes com doença renal crônica nos estágios 3 e 4 (banco de dados mínimo: perfil bioquímico e hematócrito).
• Pacientes proteinúricos — monitorizar, pelo menos, a cada 3-4 meses (banco de dados mínimo: creatinina sérica e relação de proteína:creatinina urinárias).

PREVENÇÃO
• Não acasalar os animais com doença renal familiar.
• Incluir urinálise e creatinina sérica no exame anual para cães e gatos mais idosos.

COMPLICAÇÕES POSSÍVEIS
• Hipertensão sistêmica.
• Uremia.
• Anemia.
• Infecção do trato urinário.
• Nefrolitíase e uretrolitíase.
• Cálculo dentário exuberante.

EVOLUÇÃO ESPERADA E PROGNÓSTICO
• Curto prazo — dependem da gravidade.
• Longo prazo — reservado a mau em cães (a doença renal crônica tende a ser progressiva em meses a anos); mau a bom em gatos (a doença renal crônica não evolui em alguns animais dessa espécie).

Insuficiência Renal Crônica

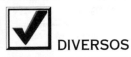
DIVERSOS

DISTÚRBIOS ASSOCIADOS
- Hipertireoidismo em gatos.
- Infecção do trato urinário.
- Hipertensão sistêmica.
- Nefrolitíase e ureterolitíase.

FATORES RELACIONADOS COM A IDADE
A função renal normal diminui com a idade.

POTENCIAL ZOONÓTICO
Nenhum.

GESTAÇÃO/FERTILIDADE/REPRODUÇÃO
Pacientes com doença renal crônica leve podem manter a prenhez; aqueles com doença moderada a grave podem ser inférteis ou apresentar abortamentos espontâneos; não é recomendado o acasalamento de pacientes do sexo feminino.

SINÔNIMO(S)
- Insuficiência renal crônica.
- Nefropatia crônica.
- Falência renal crônica.

VER TAMBÉM
- Anemia de Doença Renal Crônica.
- Azotemia e Uremia.
- Doença Renal Policística.
- Doenças Renais de Base Congênita e de Desenvolvimento.
- Hidronefrose.
- Hiperparatireoidismo Secundário Renal.
- Hipertensão Sistêmica.
- Insuficiência Renal Aguda.
- Nefrolitíase.
- Obstrução do Trato Urinário.
- Pielonefrite.
- Poliúria e Polidipsia.
- Proteinúria.

ABREVIATURA(S)
- ACTH = hormônio adrenocorticotrópico.
- AINE = anti-inflamatório não esteroide.
- ECA = enzima conversora da angiotensina.
- IRIS = International Renal Interest Society (Sociedade Internacional de Interesse Renal).
- PIF = peritonite infecciosa felina.
- PU/PD = poliúria e polidipsia.

RECURSOS DA INTERNET
www.iris-kidney.com.

Sugestões de Leitura
Polzin DJ. Chronic kidney disease. In: Ettinger SJ, Feldman EC, eds., Textbook of Veterinary Internal Medicine, 7th ed. St. Louis: Elsevier, 2010, pp. 1990-2021.
Ross SJ, Polzin DJ, Osborne CA. Clinical progression of early chronic renal failure and implications for management. In: August JR, ed., Consultations in Feline Internal Medicine. St. Louis: Elsevier, 2006, pp. 389-398.

Autor David J. Polzin
Consultor Editorial Carl A. Osborne

INSULINOMA

CONSIDERAÇÕES GERAIS

DEFINIÇÃO
Neoplasia funcional das células β das ilhotas pancreáticas que secretam quantidade excessiva de insulina, independentemente da concentração de glicose.

FISIOPATOLOGIA
A secreção excessiva de insulina leva à captação e utilização demasiadas de glicose pelos tecidos sensíveis a esse hormônio e produção hepática reduzida desse açúcar; isso causa hipoglicemia e seus sinais clínicos associados.

SISTEMA(S) ACOMETIDO(S)
• Nervoso — crises convulsivas, desorientação, comportamento anormal, colapso, polineuropatia/neuropatia periférica, paresia posterior e ataxia.
• Musculosquelético — fraqueza e fasciculações musculares.
• Gastrintestinal — polifagia e ganho de peso.

INCIDÊNCIA/PREVALÊNCIA
• Cães — incomum.
• Gatos — raro.

IDENTIFICAÇÃO
Espécies
Cães e gatos.

Raça(s) Predominante(s)
• Cães — Labrador retriever, Poodle standard, Boxer, Fox terrier, Setter irlandês, Pastor alemão, Golden retriever e Collie.
• Gatos — nenhuma; possivelmente Siamês.

Idade Média e Faixa Etária
• Cães — meia-idade a idosos; média, 10 anos; variação, 3-14 anos.
• Gatos — média, 15 anos; variação, 12-17 anos.

SINAIS CLÍNICOS
Comentários Gerais
• Frequentemente episódicos.
• Podem ou não estar relacionados com jejum, agitação, exercício e/ou ingestão de alimento.
• Os cães geralmente demonstram mais de um sinal clínico, que evoluem com o passar do tempo.

Achados Anamnésicos
• Cães — crises convulsivas focais e/ou generalizadas são mais comuns. Os achados adicionais podem incluir fraqueza, paresia posterior, colapso, fasciculações musculares, comportamento bizarro (anormal), letargia e depressão, ataxia, polifagia, ganho de peso, poliúria e polidipsia, além de intolerância ao exercício.
• Gatos — crises convulsivas, ataxia, fasciculações musculares, fraqueza, letargia e depressão, anorexia, perda de peso e polidipsia.

Achados do Exame Físico
• Geralmente dentro dos limites normais, a menos que o animal esteja em uma crise hipoglicêmica com os sinais supramencionados.
• A obesidade é um achado comum.
• Raramente, pode-se observar polineuropatia em cães (paresia à paralisia, atrofia muscular e/ou hiporreflexia).

CAUSAS
A maior parte dos cães e gatos possui carcinoma ou adenocarcinoma isolados das células β do pâncreas produtores de insulina.

Aproximadamente 50% ou mais dos cães e gatos com insulinomas desenvolverão ou apresentarão metástases.

FATORES DE RISCO
Fatores como jejum, agitação, exercício e ingestão de alimentos podem aumentar o risco de episódios hipoglicêmicos.

DIAGNÓSTICO

DIAGNÓSTICO DIFERENCIAL
• Hipoglicemia por tumor extrapancreático — hipoglicemia paraneoplásica foi registrada nos cães com inúmeros tumores, incluindo carcinoma hepatocelular, carcinoma mamário metastático, carcinoma pulmonar primário e outros; esses tumores geralmente secretam insulina ou fatores insulinossímiles.
• Realizar uma avaliação completa da hipoglicemia e descartar causas como insulina iatrogênica, hipoglicemia neonatal ou relacionada com a raça toy, ingestão de agentes hipoglicemiantes orais, insuficiência hepática, sepse, hipoadrenocorticismo, hipoglicemia do cão de caça e doenças do armazenamento de glicogênio.
• Crises convulsivas e colapso — considerar uma variedade de diferenciais, incluindo causas cardiovasculares (p. ex., síncope), metabólicas (p. ex., anemia, hepatoencefalopatia, hipocalcemia e hipoadrenocorticismo) e neurológicas (p. ex., epilepsia, neoplasia, toxina e doença inflamatória).

HEMOGRAMA/BIOQUÍMICA/URINÁLISE
• Resultados frequentemente dentro dos limites de normalidade, exceto pela hipoglicemia (<65-70 mg/dL na maioria dos pacientes).
• Normoglicemia não descarta a presença de insulinoma. Uma pequena porcentagem de pacientes pode ter normoglicemia intermitente, o que supostamente se deve à produção de hormônios contrarregulatórios (p. ex., adrenalina, glicocorticoides, glucagon).

OUTROS TESTES LABORATORIAIS
Determinação simultânea da glicose e da insulina em jejum
• Ao iniciar o jejum (os pacientes sempre devem ser internados e monitorizados de perto durante esse período em virtude do alto risco de episódios hipoglicêmicos extremos), coletar amostras sanguíneas basais e depois de hora em hora ou a cada duas horas para a determinação da glicose sérica e o armazenamento do soro. Quando a glicose sérica cair abaixo de 60 mg/dL, enviar essa amostra de soro à determinação simultânea de glicose e insulina sérica. Quando a insulina estiver elevada diante de hipoglicemia, a presença de insulinoma será altamente provável; no entanto, se a insulina estiver dentro dos limites normais diante de hipoglicemia, o insulinoma será possível. Se o valor de insulina estiver abaixo dos limites de normalidade durante a hipoglicemia, o insulinoma será improvável, embora possa haver a necessidade de múltiplas amostras.
• Fórmulas que utilizam valores hipoglicêmicos simultâneos de glicose e insulina, como a relação insulina:glicose e a relação insulina:glicose corrigida, estão caindo em desuso em função de sua baixa especificidade.

DIAGNÓSTICO POR IMAGEM
• Radiografias torácicas e abdominais — são úteis para avaliação de doença metastática e/ou causas de hipoglicemia induzidas por tumor extrapancreático, bem como de alguns outros diagnósticos diferenciais.
• Ultrassonografia — menos de 50% das massas pancreáticas são claramente identificadas por meio do exame ultrassonográfico.
• TC — técnica superior para detecção de insulinomas primários em cães; no entanto, resultados falso-positivos de metástases em linfonodos são comuns e problemáticos; essa técnica deve ser utilizada basicamente para delimitação/confirmação pré-operatória de massa pancreática primária.
• Cintilografia e TC por emissão de próton único — intermitentemente bem-sucedidas na detecção de insulinomas.
• Ultrassom intraoperatório — amplamente utilizado para detecção macroscópica de tumor oculto em insulinomas humanos; raramente relatado na medicina veterinária.

MÉTODOS DIAGNÓSTICOS
Laparotomia exploratória — indicada na suspeita de insulinoma, com base nos resultados físicos, bioquímicos e/ou imagens supramencionados.

ACHADOS PATOLÓGICOS
Ao exame histopatológico, os insulinomas pancreáticos primários em cães costumam ser carcinomas ou adenocarcinomas das células β das ilhotas pancreáticas e, ocasionalmente, adenomas; no entanto, os cães com adenomas podem subsequentemente desenvolver metástase, sugerindo a existência de limitações na delimitação do potencial de malignidade com a microscopia óptica de insulinomas. Em gatos, a maioria dos tumores é maligna, sendo comum a constatação de metástase.

TRATAMENTO

CUIDADO(S) DE SAÚDE ADEQUADO(S)
• Hospitalizar para avaliação e cirurgia desde que a hipoglicemia com risco de vida seja uma possibilidade muito real.
• Tratar como paciente de ambulatório se o proprietário recusar a cirurgia e o paciente não estiver clinicamente hipoglicêmico.

CUIDADO(S) DE ENFERMAGEM
Para episódios hipoglicêmicos de emergência, administrar a glicose a 50% (1 mL/kg IV lentamente por 1-3 min) para controlar as crises convulsivas e os sinais de hipoglicemia grave. Assim que os sinais clínicos da hipoglicemia de emergência diminuírem, prosseguir a fluidoterapia com glicose a 2,5% (aumentar para 5%, se houver necessidade, para controlar os sinais clínicos). Alternativamente, se o paciente conseguir comer, administrações frequentes de dieta apropriada (ver a seção "Dieta") podem substituir os fluidos contendo glicose em muitos pacientes.

ATIVIDADE
Restrita.

DIETA
• Fornecer 4-6 pequenas refeições diariamente.
• A dieta deve ser rica em proteína, gordura e carboidratos complexos, mas pobre em açúcares simples.

- Evitar rações semiúmidas que diluem os níveis de gordura, proteína e carboidrato mencionados anteriormente.

ORIENTAÇÃO AO PROPRIETÁRIO
O proprietário deve estar ciente dos sinais de hipoglicemia e procurar atendimento imediato, se ocorrerem.

CONSIDERAÇÕES CIRÚRGICAS
- O tratamento cirúrgico melhora o prognóstico em relação à terapia clínica isolada.
- O controle clínico é importante para evitar hipoglicemia grave antes de uma laparotomia exploratória. A maioria dos pacientes responde bem a refeições pequenas e frequentes, bem como aos corticosteroides. Em raros casos refratários, o uso de fluidos IV contendo glicose a 2,5 a 5% e/ou de glucagon pode ser necessário.
- Os objetivos da cirurgia incluem a confirmação do diagnóstico, a elucidação da presença/ausência de quaisquer metástases extrapancreáticas e/ou de outra doença e a remoção da maior quantidade possível de tecido cancerígeno.
- Na cirurgia, grande parte dos insulinomas pode ser inspecionada e/ou palpada. Caso não se consiga encontrar a massa pancreática, o uso de ultrassom intraoperatório pode ser benéfico. Em casos raros, pode-se usar o azul de metileno a 1% IV (3 mg/kg adicionados a 250 mL de NaCl a 0,9%, administrados por via IV lentamente durante 30-45 min) para delinear algum insulinoma pancreático oculto; no entanto, anemia hemolítica, pseudocianose e nefrotoxicidade hemoglobinúria são possíveis efeitos colaterais; por essa razão, o uso de rotina não é recomendado.
- Aproximadamente 15% dos cães possuem múltiplos insulinomas primários; portanto, sempre se deve examinar o pâncreas inteiro.
- Realizar biopsia dos linfonodos regionais e avaliar o fígado (e outros conteúdos abdominais) com rigor por meio da biopsia de quaisquer anormalidades. Cerca de 40-50% dos cães terão metástase. Em um único estudo, dos 14 cães com suspeita de terem metástase extrapancreática proveniente de algum insulinoma pancreático primário, apenas 8 (57%) tinham indícios histológicos de metástase. Portanto, a presença do que se parece com uma metástase deve ser avaliada por biopsia e não induzir automaticamente à eutanásia do animal durante a cirurgia.

MEDICAÇÕES
MEDICAMENTO(S) DE ESCOLHA
Tratamento de Emergência/Agudo
- Ver a seção "Cuidado(s) de Enfermagem" anteriormente.

Tratamento a Longo Prazo
- Se a terapia à base de dieta não for eficaz, pode-se lançar mão dos glicocorticoides, como a prednisona, em uma dosagem inicial de 0,25 mg/kg VO a cada 12 h; essa dose poderá ser aumentada, conforme a necessidade, para 2-3 mg/kg VO a cada 12 h.

- O diazóxido (Proglycem®) estimula os processos de gliconeogênese/glicogenólise hepáticos e inibe a secreção de insulina. Pode ser administrado à dose de 5-60 mg/kg VO a cada 12 h (iniciar com a dose baixa e aumentar conforme a necessidade) em conjunto com as modificações da dieta e/ou o uso de glicocorticoides quando esses agentes se tornarem menos eficazes. Além de ter um custo alto para alguns proprietários, pode não ser fácil encontrar o diazóxido.
- Estreptozocina é uma nitrosureia que tem como alvo semisseletivo as células β pancreáticas. Pode ser administrada à dose de 500 mg/m² lentamente por via IV em 2 h após uma diurese com NaCl a 0,9% de 3 h e seguida por uma diurese de 2 h. Esse protocolo pode ser repetido a cada 3 semanas até que a normoglicemia seja atingida. Além de ser emetogênica, a estreptozocina é hepato e/ou nefrotóxica.
- Glucagon é gliconeogênico e pode ser usado na dose de 5 ng/kg/min sob infusão a velocidade constante (até fazer efeito) para tratar hipoglicemia refratária grave aguda.
- Análogos sintéticos da somatostatina — octreotida (10-20 μg SC a cada 8-12 h) ou lantreotida (nenhuma dose determinada em espécies veterinárias) — podem ser utilizados para evitar a hipoglicemia em cães refratários aos tratamentos convencionais.

CONTRAINDICAÇÕES
Insulina.

PRECAUÇÕES
- Quando administrados isoladamente, os bólus de glicose podem precipitar crises hipoglicêmicas adicionais.
- Glicocorticoides utilizados em altas doses por períodos prolongados podem causar hiperadrenocorticismo iatrogênico.
- Diazóxido pode provocar mielossupressão, irritação gastrintestinal, anemia aplásica, cataratas, trombocitopenia e taquicardia em seres humanos.
- Estreptozocina pode causar êmese, insuficiência hepática, insuficiência renal, diabetes melito e pancreatite.

INTERAÇÕES POSSÍVEIS
A hidroclorotiazida pode potencializar o diazóxido.

ACOMPANHAMENTO
MONITORIZAÇÃO DO PACIENTE
- Orientar o proprietário a monitorar o paciente quanto ao retorno e/ou à evolução dos sinais de hipoglicemia.
- Determinações da glicose sérica no hospital são importantes para monitorar o retorno e/ou a evolução da hipoglicemia associada ao insulinoma.

COMPLICAÇÕES POSSÍVEIS
Episódios recidivantes ou progressivos de hipoglicemia.

EVOLUÇÃO ESPERADA E PROGNÓSTICO
- É mais provável que os cães submetidos à laparotomia exploratória se tornem e permaneçam normoglicêmicos por mais tempo e tenham tempos de sobrevida mais prolongados em comparação aos cães tratados por meio clínico. Mesmo na presença de doença metastática local, é provável que qualquer redução da carga tumoral melhore o controle normoglicêmico com terapias clínicas. A média de duração do controle normoglicêmico após a cirurgia é inversamente correlacionada com o estágio da doença e varia de 14 meses para aqueles cães sem indícios de metástase a apenas 2-3 meses para os outros cães com metástase nodal e/ou à distância. O tempo médio de sobrevida também é inversamente correlacionado com o estágio da doença e varia de aproximadamente 16-19 meses (variação, 2-60 meses) para cães sem indícios de metástase a 7-9 meses em cães com indícios de metástase nodal e/ou à distância. Estudos mais recentes registraram tempos médios de sobrevida até mais longos, ou seja, de 17-18 meses para todos os cães com insulinoma e 25-42 meses para aqueles submetidos a terapias clínica e cirúrgica.
- Gatos — o tempo médio de sobrevida gira em torno de 6 meses e meio; variação: 0-18 meses.

DIVERSOS
DISTÚRBIOS ASSOCIADOS
Obesidade atribuída à hiperinsulinemia.

FATORES RELACIONADOS COM A IDADE
Cães mais jovens possuem tempos de sobrevida mais curtos.

SINÔNIMO(S)
- Tumor secretor de insulina.
- Tumor de células β.
- Hiperinsulinismo.
- Tumor de células das ilhotas.
- Adenocarcinoma de células das ilhotas.
- Tumor pancreático produtor de insulina.

VER TAMBÉM
Hipoglicemia.

ABREVIATURA(S)
- TC = tomografia computadorizada.

Sugestões de Leitura
Moore AS, Nelson RW, Henry CJ, Rassnick KM, Krista O, Ogilvie GK, Kintzer P. Streptozocin for treatment of pancreatic islet cell tumors in dogs: 17 cases (1989-1999). JAVMA 2002, 221(6):811-818.
Polton GA, White RN, Brearley MJ, Eastwood JM. Improved survival in a retrospective cohort of 28 dogs with insulinoma. J Small Anim Pract 2007, 48(3):151-156.
Robben JH, Pollak YW, Kirpensteijn J, Boroffka SA, Van Den Ingh TS, Teske E, Voorhout G. Comparison of ultrasonography, computed tomography, and single-photon emission computed tomography for the detection and localization of canine insulinoma. J Vet Intern Med 2005, 19(1):15-22.

Autor Phil Bergman
Consultor Editorial Deborah S. Greco

Intermação e Hipertermia

CONSIDERAÇÕES GERAIS

DEFINIÇÃO
- Hipertermia é definida como uma elevação da temperatura corporal acima da faixa de normalidade. Embora os valores normais publicados para cães e gatos variem um pouco, aceita-se em geral que temperaturas corporais >39°C sejam anormais.
- A hipertermia pode ser categorizada em pirogênica (pirexia ou febre) e não pirogênica.
- Intermação ("choque pelo calor", choque térmico) é uma forma de hipertermia não pirogênica que ocorre quando os mecanismos de dissipação de calor do corpo não conseguem ajustar o calor excessivo. Isso pode gerar a disfunção de múltiplos órgãos. Temperaturas de 41°C sem sinais de inflamação são sugestivas de hipertermia não pirogênica.
- Hipertermia maligna é uma hipertermia familiar incomum não pirogênica que pode ocorrer secundariamente a alguns anestésicos.
- Outras causas de hipertermia não pirogênica incluem exercício excessivo, tireotoxicose e lesões hipotalâmicas.

FISIOPATOLOGIA
- O ponto de ajuste hipotalâmico sofre alteração na febre verdadeira. É mais provável que isso seja mediado pela interleucina-1 (pirogênio endógeno).
- A hipertermia não pirogênica não muda o ponto de ajuste hipotalâmico.
- A temperatura crítica que acarreta disfunção orgânica múltipla é de 42,7°C.
- Os processos fisiopatológicos primários de intermação estão relacionados com lesão térmica, o que pode levar a necrose celular, hipoxemia e desnaturação proteica.
- A intermação e suas sequelas podem causar a síndrome de resposta inflamatória sistêmica (SRIS).

SISTEMA(S) ACOMETIDO(S)
- Nervoso — dano neuronal, hemorragia parenquimatosa e edema cerebral.
- Cardiovascular — hipovolemia, arritmias cardíacas, isquemia miocárdica e necrose.
- Gastrintestinal — isquemia e ulceração da mucosa, translocação bacteriana e endotoxemia.
- Hepatobiliar — necrose hepatocelular.
- Renal/urológico — insuficiência renal aguda.
- Hematológico/linfático/imune — hemoconcentração, trombocitopenia, CID.
- Musculosquelético — rabdomiólise.

DISTRIBUIÇÃO GEOGRÁFICA
Podem ocorrer em qualquer clima, embora sejam mais comuns em ambientes quentes e/ou úmidos.

IDENTIFICAÇÃO

Espécies
- Cães ou gatos.
- Raro nos gatos.

Raça(s) Predominante(s)
- Podem ocorrer em qualquer raça.
- Animais de pelos longos.
- Raças braquicefálicas.

Idade Média e Faixa Etária
- Todas as idades podem ser acometidas, porém são mais frequentes nos extremos etários.
- Cães jovens podem ter tendência a se exercitar demais.
- Cães idosos com doença preexistente.

SINAIS CLÍNICOS

Achados Anamnésicos
- Causa subjacente identificável (dia quente, animal dentro de carro fechado ou confinado em outra área sem ventilação adequada, acidente de banho e tosa associado a gaiolas de secagem, exercício excessivo, acesso restrito à água).
- Doença subjacente predisponente: paralisia laríngea, doença obstrutiva braquicefálica, doença cardiovascular, doença neuromuscular, histórico prévio de doença relacionada com o calor.

Achados do Exame Físico
- Respiração ofegante.
- Hipersalivação.
- Hipertermia.
- Mucosas hiperêmicas.
- Mucosas pálidas.
- Cianose.
- Taquicardia.
- Disritmias cardíacas.
- Choque.
- Angústia respiratória.
- Hematêmese.
- Hematoquezia.
- Melena.
- Petéquias.
- Alterações na atividade mental.
- Crises convulsivas.
- Tremores musculares.
- Ataxia.
- Coma.
- Oligúria/anúria.
- Parada respiratória.
- Parada cardiopulmonar.

CAUSAS
- Ambiente com calor e umidade excessivos (pode ser decorrente de condições climáticas ou acidentes como ficar em ambiente fechado sem ventilação, carro ou gaiolas de secagem para banho e tosa).
- Doença das vias aéreas superiores.
- Exercício.
- Toxicose (alguns compostos que causam crises convulsivas, i. e., estricnina e metaldeído).
- Anestesia (hipertermia maligna).

FATORES DE RISCO
- Histórico prévio de doença relacionada com o calor.
- Extremos etários.
- Intolerância ao calor em virtude de má aclimatação.
- Obesidade.
- Mau condicionamento cardiopulmonar.
- Hipertireoidismo.
- Doença cardiopulmonar subjacente.
- Raças braquicefálicas.
- Pelagem espessa.
- Desidratação.

DIAGNÓSTICO

DIAGNÓSTICO DIFERENCIAL
- Se as temperaturas ultrapassarem 41°C sem indícios de inflamação, deve-se considerar o quadro de intermação.
- Respiração ofegante e hipersalivação podem não ser observadas com febre verdadeira, pois o ponto de ajuste hipotalâmico encontra-se elevado na febre.

HEMOGRAMA/BIOQUÍMICA/URINÁLISE
- Podem ajudar a identificar o processo mórbido subjacente.
- Podem ser benéficos para identificar as sequelas da hipertermia.
- As anormalidades do hemograma completo podem incluir leucograma de estresse, leucopenia, anemia, eritrócitos nucleados, trombocitopenia ou hemoconcentração.
- O perfil bioquímico pode revelar azotemia, hiperalbuminemia, elevações nas enzimas séricas (ALT, AST, CK), hipernatremia, hipercloremia, hiperglicemia, hipoglicemia, hiperfosfatemia, hipercalemia, hipocalemia, hiperbilirrubinemia.
- A urinálise pode mostrar hiperestenúria, proteinúria, cilindrúria, hemoglobinúria, mioglobinúria.

OUTROS TESTES LABORATORIAIS
- A hemogasometria pode exibir distúrbio acidobásico misto, alcalose respiratória ou acidose metabólica.
- O perfil de coagulação pode indicar prolongamento do TCA, do TP ou do TTP. Produtos de degradação da fibrina (PDF) ou dímeros D podem ser positivos. Poderá haver CID se o TP e o TTP estiverem prolongados juntamente com PDF ou dímeros D positivos e trombocitopenia. Se disponível, a mensuração da antitrombina III pode ser valiosa.
- Tromboelastografia pode registrar hiper ou hipocoagulabilidade.

DIAGNÓSTICO POR IMAGEM
- Radiografias torácicas podem ajudar a identificar doença cardiopulmonar subjacente ou fatores predisponentes.
- Radiografias e/ou ultrassonografias abdominais podem ajudar a identificar processo mórbido subjacente.
- TC ou RM podem ajudar a identificar lesão hipotalâmica.

MÉTODOS DIAGNÓSTICOS
Monitorização contínua da temperatura.

TRATAMENTO

- Proceder ao reconhecimento precoce é o segredo do sucesso terapêutico.
- Corrigir a hipertermia imediatamente; aspergir água ou imergir na água antes de levar o paciente para alguma instituição veterinária. Utilizar resfriamento por convecção com ventiladores. O resfriamento por evaporação, como a aplicação de álcool nos coxins palmoplantares, nas axilas e na região inguinal, também é uma opção.
- Interromper os procedimentos de resfriamento quando a temperatura atingir 39,4°C para evitar hipotermia.
- Providenciar suplementação de oxigênio via gaiola, máscara ou cateter nasal.
- Efetuar suporte ventilatório se necessário.
- Fornecer suporte hídrico com doses de choque de fluidos cristaloides ou coloides.
- Tratar as complicações, além dos quadros de CID, insuficiência renal e edema cerebral.
- Tratar a doença subjacente ou corrigir os fatores predisponentes.

CUIDADO(S) DE SAÚDE ADEQUADO(S)
- Os pacientes devem ser hospitalizados até que a temperatura esteja estabilizada.

- A maioria dos pacientes precisa de cuidados intensivos por vários dias.

CUIDADO(S) DE ENFERMAGEM
- Resfriamento externo; tentar evitar o gelo, pois isso pode causar vasoconstrição periférica e impedir a dissipação de calor. Uma resposta de tremor também é indesejável, pois isso gera calor.
- Fluidoterapia; podem ser administrados cristaloides isotônicos nas velocidades utilizadas para choque (90 mL/kg/h para cães; 45-60 mL/kg/h para gatos) com base na avaliação clínica. Coloides sintéticos também podem ser usados para tratar o choque (20 mL/kg em cães, 5-10 mL/kg em gatos).
- Suplementação de oxigênio: pode ser administrada via máscara, gaiola ou cânula nasal.

ATIVIDADE
Restrita.

DIETA
Nada por via oral até que o animal se encontre estabilizado.

ORIENTAÇÃO AO PROPRIETÁRIO
- Ter conhecimento dos sinais clínicos.
- Saber como resfriar os animais.
- Um episódio de intermação pode predispor a outros.

CONSIDERAÇÕES CIRÚRGICAS
Poderá ser necessário o procedimento de traqueostomia se a obstrução das vias aéreas superiores for uma causa subjacente ou fator contribuinte.

MEDICAÇÕES
MEDICAMENTO(S) DE ESCOLHA
- Não existem medicamentos específicos para hipertermia ou intermação; a terapia depende da apresentação clínica.
- Antimicrobianos profiláticos de amplo espectro podem diminuir a incidência de translocação bacteriana. Cefalosporinas de 1ª geração combinadas com fluoroquinolonas fornecem excelente cobertura dos 4 quadrantes.
- Insuficiência renal aguda — dopamina IV sob infusão a velocidade constante (2-5 μg/kg/min); furosemida IV (2-4 mg/kg conforme a necessidade).
- Edema cerebral — manitol (1 g/kg IV por 15-30 min); furosemida (1 mg/kg IV), 30 min após a infusão de manitol; corticosteroides (fosfato sódico de dexametasona [1-2 mg/kg IV]; succinato sódico de prednisona [10-20 mg/kg IV] ou metilprednisolona [15 mg/kg IV]). O uso de corticosteroides é considerado controverso em virtude dos efeitos colaterais adversos nesses pacientes.
- Arritmia ventricular — bólus de lidocaína (2 mg/kg IV) seguido por infusão intravenosa contínua (25-75 μg/kg/min) ou procainamida (6-8 mg/kg IV).
- Acidose metabólica — bicarbonato de sódio (0,3 × peso corporal [kg] × excesso de base); administrar metade sob a forma de bólus IV.
- CID — plasma fresco congelado (20 mL/kg) e heparina (50-200 U/kg SC a cada 6-8 h). A 1ª dose de heparina pode ser colocada na unidade de plasma.
- Trombocitopenia — se grave, pode ser tratada com sangue total fresco, plasma rico em plaquetas, plaquetas liofilizadas ou concentrados de plaquetas congeladas.
- Vômitos ou diarreia hemorrágicos — antibióticos de amplo espectro e antagonistas dos receptores H_2 ou inibidores da bomba de prótons combinados com sucralfato.
- Crises convulsivas — diazepam (0,5-1 mg/kg IV) ou midazolam; fenobarbital (6 mg/kg IV conforme a necessidade).

CONTRAINDICAÇÕES
- Anti-inflamatórios não esteroides não estão indicados em casos de hipertermia não pirogênica, porque o ponto de ajuste hipotalâmico não se encontra alterado.
- O uso de corticosteroides é considerado controverso na intermação em virtude dos efeitos colaterais.
- O resfriamento com gelo é contraindicado, pois pode levar à vasoconstrição periférica e dificultar a dissipação do calor.

PRECAUÇÕES
Recorrer às recomendações do fabricante.

INTERAÇÕES POSSÍVEIS
Recorrer às recomendações do fabricante.

ACOMPANHAMENTO
MONITORIZAÇÃO DO PACIENTE
- Os pacientes devem ser monitorizados de perto durante o período de resfriamento e por, no mínimo, 24 h depois do episódio. A maioria dos animais precisa ser monitorizada por vários dias, dependendo da apresentação clínica e das sequelas. Um exame físico completo deve ser feito diariamente. Além disso, os seguintes parâmetros devem ser considerados:
- Temperatura corporal.
- Peso corporal.
- Pressão arterial.
- Pressão venosa central.
- Índices de coagulação (TCA, TP, TTP, PDF).
- Eletrocardiograma.
- Auscultação torácica.
- Urinálise e débito urinário.
- Hematócrito, proteína total.
- Hemograma completo, perfil bioquímico.

PREVENÇÃO
Evitar os fatores de risco.

COMPLICAÇÕES POSSÍVEIS
- Disritmias cardíacas.
- Falência de órgãos.
- Coma.
- Crises convulsivas.
- Insuficiência renal aguda.
- CID.
- SRIS.
- Edema pulmonar — angústia respiratória aguda.
- Rabdomiólise.
- Necrose hepatocelular.
- Parada respiratória.
- Parada cardiopulmonar.

EVOLUÇÃO ESPERADA E PROGNÓSTICO
- O prognóstico depende da causa ou do processo mórbido subjacente.
- O prognóstico pode depender do tempo transcorrido entre o evento e a admissão hospitalar.
- O prognóstico é reservado, dependendo da ocorrência de complicações (insuficiência renal e CID) e da duração do episódio.
- Um episódio pode predispor o animal a outros episódios em função do dano ao centro termorregulador.

DIVERSOS
SINÔNIMO(S)
- Choque pelo calor.
- Exaustão pelo calor.
- Prostração pelo calor.
- Doença relacionada com o calor.

VER TAMBÉM
Febre.

ABREVIATURA(S)
- ALT = alanina aminotransferase.
- AST = aspartato aminotransferase.
- CID = coagulopatia intravascular disseminada.
- CK = creatina quinase.
- PDF = produtos de degradação da fibrina.
- RM = ressonância magnética.
- SRIS = síndrome de resposta inflamatória sistêmica.
- TC = tomografia computadorizada.
- TCA = tempo de coagulação ativada.
- TP = tempo de protrombina.
- TTP = tempo de tromboplastina parcial.

Sugestões de Leitura
Bruchim Y, Klement E, Saragusty J, et al. Heat stroke in dogs: A retrospective study of 54 cases (1999-2004) and analysis of risk factors for death. J Vet Intern Med 2006, 20:38-46.
Drobatz KJ, Macintire DK. Heat-induced illness in dogs: 42 cases (1976-1993). JAVMA 1996, 209:1894-1899.
Gfeller R. Heat stroke. In: Ettinger SJ, Feldman EC, eds., Textbook of Veterinary Internal Medicine, 6th ed. St. Louis: Elsevier, 2005, pp. 437-440.
Rushlander D. Heat stroke. In: Kirk RW, Bonagura JD, eds., Current Veterinary Therapy XI. Philadelphia: Saunders, 1992, pp. 143-146.
Waters JM. Hyperthermia. In: Wingfield WE, Raffe MR, eds., The Veterinary ICU Book. Jackson Hole, WY: Teton NewMedia, 2002, pp. 1130-1136.

Autor Steven L. Marks
Consultores Editoriais Larry P. Tilley e Francis W.K. Smith, Jr.

Intoxicação Alimentar pelo Salmão

CONSIDERAÇÕES GERAIS

REVISÃO
- Infecção pelo microrganismo riquetsiano *Neorickettsia helminthoeca*.
- Microrganismo — invade o epitélio do intestino delgado e o tecido linfoide associado; por fim, desenvolve-se infecção sistêmica.
- Ocorre na orla do Pacífico norte dos EUA.

IDENTIFICAÇÃO
- Cães de todas as idades.
- Sem predisposição sexual ou racial.

SINAIS CLÍNICOS
- Diarreia.
- Vômito.
- Linfadenopatia.
- Secreção oculonasal.
- Febre.

CAUSAS E FATORES DE RISCO
- Ingestão de peixe cru contendo o vetor do trematódeo ou os microrganismos *Neorickettsia helminthoeca*.
- O consumo de peixe cru em área endêmica é um fator de risco.

DIAGNÓSTICO

DIAGNÓSTICO DIFERENCIAL
- Intoxicação.
- Parvovírus canino tipo 2.
- Erliquiose.
- Cinomose.

HEMOGRAMA/BIOQUÍMICA/URINÁLISE
Sem achados específicos.

OUTROS TESTES LABORATORIAIS
N/D.

DIAGNÓSTICO POR IMAGEM
N/D.

MÉTODOS DIAGNÓSTICOS
- Coloração de Giemsa — aspirado de linfonodo enfartado; revela corpúsculos riquetsianos intracitoplasmáticos.
- Exame de fezes — revela ovos operculados do trematódeo *Nanophyetus salmincola*.

ACHADOS PATOLÓGICOS
- Alterações no tecido linfoide — tecidos aumentados e amarelados, com focos brancos proeminentes.
- Conteúdo intestinal — frequentemente contém sangue livre.

TRATAMENTO

- Internação — para pacientes agudamente enfermos.
- Tratar da mesma forma que a erliquiose canina.
- Terapia de suporte — fluidos com eletrólitos; medidas básicas para controlar a diarreia.

MEDICAÇÕES

MEDICAMENTO(S)
- Oxitetraciclina — 7,5-10 mg/kg IV a cada 12 h por 14 dias; 20 mg/kg VO a cada 12 h.
- Tetraciclina — 15-20 mg/kg VO a cada 8 h por 14 dias.
- Cloranfenicol — 40-50 mg/kg VO a cada 8 h por 14 dias.
- Praziquantel — 20-30 mg/kg SC ou VO a cada 24 h por 3 dias para matar os nematódeos.

ACOMPANHAMENTO

MONITORIZAÇÃO DO PACIENTE
Monitorizar a hidratação, os eletrólitos, o equilíbrio acidobásico e a temperatura corporal.

PREVENÇÃO
- Impedir que os animais comam peixe cru.
- Informar o proprietário sobre a necessidade de agir rapidamente e considerar outros cães que possam ter ingerido o mesmo peixe cru.

EVOLUÇÃO ESPERADA E PROGNÓSTICO
- Os animais provavelmente sucumbirão em 5-10 dias da infecção, a menos que sejam tratados.
- Com o diagnóstico e o tratamento precoces — prognóstico bom.
- Não tratados — casos quase sempre fatais.

DIVERSOS

DISTÚRBIOS ASSOCIADOS
- Agente da febre da fascíola de Elokomin — semelhante à riquétsia; provoca uma forma mais leve da doença.
- A infecção por *Nanophyetus salmincola* em si não provoca doença clínica grave.

POTENCIAL ZOONÓTICO
Nenhum risco relatado para os humanos.

RECURSOS DA INTERNET
- www.merckvetmanual.com/mvm/htm/bc/57305.htm.
- www.vetmed.wsu.edu/ClientED/salmon.asp.

Sugestões de Leitura
Gorham JR, Foreyt WJ. Salmon poisoning disease. In: Greene CE, ed., Infectious Diseases of the Dog and Cat, 3rd ed. St. Louis: Saunders Elsevier, 2006, pp. 198-203.

Autor Johnny D. Hoskins
Consultor Editorial Stephen C. Barr

INTOXICAÇÃO PELO CHUMBO

CONSIDERAÇÕES GERAIS

DEFINIÇÃO
Intoxicação (nível sanguíneo de chumbo >0,4 ppm) em virtude da exposição aguda ou crônica a alguma forma de chumbo.

FISIOPATOLOGIA
• O dano celular é atribuído à capacidade do chumbo de substituir outros cátions polivalentes (especialmente cátions divalentes, como cálcio e zinco) importantes para a homeostase celular.
• Diversos processos biológicos são acometidos, incluindo transporte de metais, metabolismo de energia, apoptose, condução de íons, adesão de células, sinalização inter e intracelular, processos enzimáticos, maturação proteica e regulação genética.

SISTEMA(S) ACOMETIDO(S)
• Gastrintestinal — mecanismo desconhecido, provável dano aos nervos periféricos.
• Hematológico/linfático/imune — interferência na síntese de hemoglobina, fragilidade aumentada e sobrevida diminuída das hemácias, liberação de reticulócitos e hemácias nucleadas da medula óssea, inibição da 5'-pirimidina nucleotidase com consequente retenção de produtos de degradação do RNA, agregação de ribossomos com subsequente formação de pontilhado basófilo.
• Nervoso — lesão capilar; alteração dos canais iônicos de membrana e das moléculas de sinalização.
• Renal/urológico — lesão às células tubulares proximais em virtude de disfunção enzimática e dano oxidativo.

GENÉTICA
N/D.

INCIDÊNCIA/PREVALÊNCIA
• A incidência real é desconhecida.
• Prevalência decrescente em cães — atribuída à eliminação das fontes.
• Prevalência estacionária a crescente em gatos — aumento da consciência e do diagnóstico.
• Maior número de casos durante os meses mais quentes.
• Prevalência mais elevada em animais jovens — maior biodisponibilidade de chumbo e barreira hematencefálica mais permeável.

DISTRIBUIÇÃO GEOGRÁFICA
• Baixa condição socioeconômica da família que possui o animal de estimação, associada à elevada concentração sanguínea de chumbo nos animais.
• Áreas de casas e edifícios mais antigos.

IDENTIFICAÇÃO
Espécies
Os cães são mais comumente acometidos que os gatos.

Raça(s) Predominante(s)
N/D.

Idade Média e Faixa Etária
Principalmente cães com <1 ano de idade.

Sexo Predominante
N/D.

SINAIS CLÍNICOS
Comentários Gerais
• Principalmente gastrintestinais e neurológicos.
• Gastrintestinais — frequentemente precedem os sinais nervosos (SNC); predominantes em casos de exposição crônica de níveis baixos.
• SNC — ocorre com maior frequência na exposição aguda, além de ser mais comum em animais mais jovens.

Achados Anamnésicos
• Histórico de reforma de casa ou edifício mais antigo ou ingestão de objetos contendo chumbo.

Achados do Exame Físico
• Vômito.
• Diarreia.
• Anorexia.
• Dor abdominal.
• Regurgitação por megaesôfago.
• Letargia.
• Histeria.
• Crises convulsivas.
• Cegueira.
• Gatos — há relatos de anormalidades vestibulares centrais como nistagmo vertical e ataxia.

CAUSAS
• Ingestão de alguma forma de chumbo — tinta e resíduos de tinta ou poeira de lixamento; baterias de automóvel; linóleo; solda; materiais e suprimentos de encanamento; compostos lubrificantes; massa de vidraceiro; papel de alcatrão; folha de chumbo; bolas de golfe; objeto com chumbo (p. ex., projéteis, anzóis de pesca e pesos de cortinas); vidro chumbado.
• Utilização de tigelas de cerâmica para alimentos ou água inadequadamente esmaltados.
• Tintas de chumbo ou poeira ou solo contaminado por esse metal são fontes comuns de exposição.

FATORES DE RISCO
• Idade inferior a 1 ano.
• Residência em áreas economicamente pobres.
• Residência em casa ou edifício antigo em reforma.

DIAGNÓSTICO

DIAGNÓSTICO DIFERENCIAL
Cães
• Cinomose.
• Encefalites infecciosas.
• Epilepsia.
• Intoxicação por brometalina, metilxantina ou micotoxina tremorgênica.
• Intoxicação por AINE.
• Intermação/insolação.
• Parasitose intestinal.
• Intussuscepção.
• Corpo estranho.
• Pancreatite.
• Hepatite infecciosa canina.

Gatos
• Doenças degenerativas do sistema nervoso ou doenças de armazenamento.
• Encefalopatia hepática.
• Encefalites infecciosas.
• Intoxicação por organofosforados, brometalina ou metilxantina.

HEMOGRAMA/BIOQUÍMICA/URINÁLISE
• Entre 5 e 40 hemácias nucleadas/100 leucócitos sem anemia.
• Ausência de hemácias nucleadas não descarta o diagnóstico.
• Anisocitose, policromasia, pecilocitose, células-alvo, hipocromasia.
• Pontilhado basófilo das hemácias; frequentemente difícil de detectar.
• Leucocitose neutrofílica.
• Gatos — há relatos de elevação da AST e fosfatase alcalina.
• Urinálise — lesão renal inespecífica branda; glicosúria; hemoglobinúria.

OUTROS TESTES LABORATORIAIS
Concentração de Chumbo
• Tóxica — sangue total antes da morte: >0,4 ppm (40 µg/dL); fígado e/ou rim após a morte: >5 ppm (peso úmido).
• Valores mais baixos — devem ser interpretados em conjunto com a anamnese e os sinais clínicos.
• Sem concentrações sanguíneas "residuais" normais de chumbo; tipicamente menores que 0,05 ppm.
• Níveis sanguíneos — não se correlacionam com a ocorrência ou a gravidade dos sinais clínicos.
• Teste de mobilização do CaNa$_2$EDTA — coletar uma única amostra de urina de 24 h; administrar o CaNa$_2$EDTA (75 mg/kg IM); coletar uma segunda amostra de urina de 24 h; na intoxicação, o chumbo na urina aumenta 10-60 vezes após a administração do EDTA (o succímer pode compreensivelmente substituir o CaNa$_2$EDTA).

DIAGNÓSTICO POR IMAGEM
Pode-se notar material radiopaco no trato gastrintestinal; não é diagnóstico.

MÉTODOS DIAGNÓSTICOS
N/D.

ACHADOS PATOLÓGICOS
• Macroscópicos — podem-se notar lascas de tinta ou objetos de chumbo no trato gastrintestinal.
• Corpúsculos de inclusão intranucleares — possivelmente observados nos hepatócitos ou nas células epiteliais tubulares renais; forma de armazenamento intracelular do chumbo; considerados patognomônicos.
• Lesões cerebrocorticais — espongiose, hipertrofia vascular, glicose, necrose neuronal, desmielinização.

TRATAMENTO

CUIDADO(S) DE SAÚDE ADEQUADO(S)
• Paciente internado — primeiro curso terapêutico de quelação, dependendo da gravidade dos sinais clínicos.
• Paciente de ambulatório — quelantes administrados por via oral.

CUIDADO(S) DE ENFERMAGEM
• Fluidos eletrolíticos balanceados — solução de Ringer simples; reposição do déficit hídrico.
• Lavagem gástrica ou irrigação intestinal total — pode estar indicada.

ATIVIDADE
N/D.

DIETA
N/D.

ORIENTAÇÃO AO PROPRIETÁRIO
• Informar o proprietário sobre o potencial de efeitos adversos do chumbo à saúde humana.

Intoxicação pelo Chumbo

- Notificar os serviços oficiais de saúde pública.
- Determinar a fonte ou origem do chumbo.

CONSIDERAÇÕES CIRÚRGICAS
Remoção de objetos de chumbo do trato gastrintestinal.

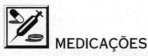

MEDICAÇÕES

MEDICAMENTO(S) DE ESCOLHA
- Esvaziamento do trato gastrintestinal — catárticos salinos; sulfato de sódio ou de magnésio (cães, 2-25 g; gatos, 2-5 g VO em solução a 20% ou menos).
- Controle das crises convulsivas — diazepam (administrado até fazer efeito; cães e gatos, 0,5 mg/kg IV) ou fenobarbital sódico (administrar em incrementos de 10-20 mg/kg IV até fazer efeito).
- Alívio do edema cerebral — manitol (0,25-2 g/kg de infusão IV lenta a 15-25% durante 30-60 min).
- Os relatos variam sobre o uso de corticosteroides para o controle do edema cerebral decorrente de intoxicação por chumbo. As tendências atuais preferem evitar os corticosteroides ou, se esses agentes forem utilizados, a dosagem deverá ser limitada para 0,5-1,0 mg/kg administrada IV lentamente.
- Há algumas provas de que os antioxidantes ou os agentes contendo tiol possam ser úteis — vitaminas C e E, ácido α-lipoico, N-acetilcisteína; não foram determinadas doses ideais.
- Vitaminas do complexo B, especialmente tiamina, também podem ser úteis; também não foram definidas doses ideais.
- Redução da carga corporal de chumbo por terapia de quelação — CaNa$_2$EDTA (cães e gatos, 25 mg/kg SC, IM, IV a cada 6 h por 2-5 dias); diluir para uma solução a 1% com glicose a 5% antes da administração; pode necessitar de múltiplos cursos terapêuticos se a concentração de chumbo no sangue estiver elevada; aguardar um período de 5 dias de repouso entre os cursos de tratamento. Succímer — alternativa ao uso de CaNa$_2$EDTA; agente quelante administrado por via oral; 10 mg/kg VO a cada 8 h durante 5 dias, seguidos por 10 mg VO a cada 12 h por 2 semanas; esperar um período de repouso de 2 semanas entre os tratamentos; pode ser administrado por via retal se os sinais clínicos como a êmese impedirem a administração oral; os gatos são tratados de forma bem-sucedida com 10 mg/kg VO a cada 8 h por 17 dias; vantagens sobre outros quelantes: pode ser administrado por VO, permitindo o tratamento como paciente de ambulatório; não aumenta a absorção do chumbo pelo trato gastrintestinal; não relatado como nefrotóxico; a quelação de elementos essenciais como o zinco e o cobre não é clinicamente significativa.

CONTRAINDICAÇÕES
- CaNa$_2$EDTA — não administrar a pacientes com comprometimento renal ou anúria; estabelecer o fluxo urinário antes da administração; não administrar por via oral.

PRECAUÇÕES
- CaNa$_2$EDTA — a segurança na gestação não foi estabelecida; teratogênico em doses terapêuticas, embora seja recomendado em detrimento ao succímer em gestantes na medicina humana.
- Succímer — a segurança na gestação não foi estabelecida; fetotóxico em doses muito maiores (100-1.000 mg/kg) que a dose terapêutica recomendada.

INTERAÇÕES POSSÍVEIS
CaNa$_2$EDTA — depleção de zinco, ferro e manganês no tratamento a longo prazo.

MEDICAMENTO(S) ALTERNATIVO(S)
N/D.

ACOMPANHAMENTO

MONITORIZAÇÃO DO PACIENTE
Chumbo do sangue — deve ser <0,1 ppm; avaliar 10-14 dias após o término da terapia de quelação.

PREVENÇÃO
- Testar tinta, poeira e solo antes do acesso do animal, se houver probabilidade de contaminação por chumbo.
- Determinar a fonte de chumbo e removê-la do ambiente do paciente.

COMPLICAÇÕES POSSÍVEIS
Ocasionalmente, sinais neurológicos permanentes (p. ex., cegueira).

EVOLUÇÃO ESPERADA E PROGNÓSTICO
- Os sinais devem melhorar drasticamente dentro de 24-48 h após o início da terapia quelante.
- Prognóstico — favorável com o tratamento.
- Crises convulsivas incontroláveis — prognóstico reservado.

DIVERSOS

DISTÚRBIOS ASSOCIADOS
N/D.

FATORES RELACIONADOS COM A IDADE
Cães com <1 ano de vida — maior biodisponibilidade de chumbo e barreira hematencefálica mais permeável.

POTENCIAL ZOONÓTICO
Nenhum; todavia, humanos no mesmo ambiente podem ficar sob risco de exposição.

GESTAÇÃO/FERTILIDADE/REPRODUÇÃO
- Passagem transplacentária — pode provocar intoxicação neonatal.
- Lactação — é improvável que o chumbo mobilizado dos ossos intoxique animais lactentes.

SINÔNIMO(S)
Plumbismo.

VER TAMBÉM
Envenenamento (Intoxicação).

ABREVIATURA(S)
- AINE = anti-inflamatório não esteroide.
- AST = aspartato aminotransferase.
- CaNa$_2$EDTA = edetato de cálcio dissódico.
- SNC = sistema nervoso central.

RECURSOS DA INTERNET
http://www.aspcapro.org/animal-poisoncontrol.php.

Sugestões de Leitura

Casteel SW. Lead. In: Peterson ME, Talcott PA, eds., Small Animal Toxicology. St. Louis: Saunders Elsevier 2006, pp. 795-805.

Knight TE, Kent M, Junk JE. Succimer for treatment of lead toxicosis in two cats. JAVMA 2001, 218:1946-1948.

Knight TE, Kumar MSA. Lead toxicosis in cats — a review. J Feline Med Surg 2003, pp. 249-255.

Morgan RV. Lead poisoning in small companion animals: An update (1987-1992). Vet Hum Toxicol 1994, 36:18-22.

Morgan RV, Moore FM, Pearce LK, et al. Clinical and laboratory findings in small companion animals with lead poisoning: 347 cases (1977-1986). JAVMA 1991, 199:93-97.

Morgan RV, Pearce LK, Moore FM, et al. Demographic data and treatment of small companion animals with lead poisoning: 347 cases (1977-1986). JAVMA 1991, 199:98-102.

Ramsey DT, Casteel SW, Fagella AM, et al. Use of orally administered succimer (meso-2,3-dimercaptosuccinic acid) for treatment of lead poisoning in dogs. JAVMA 1996, 208:371-375.

Autor Robert H. Poppenga
Consultor Editorial Gary D. Osweiler

Intoxicação pelo Lírio

CONSIDERAÇÕES GERAIS

REVISÃO
- Plantas dos gêneros *Lilium* e *Hemerocallis* — plantas ornamentais amplamente utilizadas; muito tóxicas para os gatos; incluem lírio-da-páscoa, lírio-tigre, lírio japonês, lírio rubro, inúmeros híbridos de *Lilium* e lírios diurnos.
- Ingestão de folhas ou flores — resulta em síndrome nefrotóxica grave; há relatos de que a ingestão de apenas 2-3 folhas seja letal.
- Princípio(s) tóxico(s) não elucidado(s), embora tenha(m) sido encontrado(s) na fração hidrossolúvel da planta.

IDENTIFICAÇÃO
- Gatos — intoxicação sistêmica.
- Cães — a intoxicação provoca apenas um leve desconforto gastrintestinal, mesmo após a ingestão de grandes quantidades do material vegetal.
- Não foi constatada predileção etária ou racial.

SINAIS CLÍNICOS
- Início súbito de vômito — desaparece gradualmente dentro de 2-4 h.
- Depressão e anorexia — início aproximadamente ao mesmo tempo que o vômito; persistem durante toda a síndrome.
- Poliúria e desidratação — em torno de 12-24 h; levam à insuficiência renal anúrica.
- Vômito — recidiva em torno de 36 h; acompanhado por fraqueza progressiva.
- Decúbito — por volta de 3-4 dias.
- Morte — em torno de 4-7 dias após a ingestão.

CAUSAS E FATORES DE RISCO
- Plantas — lírio-da-páscoa; lírio-tigre; lírio híbrido asiático; lírio japonês; híbridos de *Lilium*, principalmente quando utilizados em arranjos florais ou como plantas em vasos caseiros.
- Toda a ingestão de material vegetal dos gêneros *Lilium* e *Hemerocallis* pelos gatos deve ser considerada potencialmente tóxica.
- Gatos criados exclusivamente dentro de casa — são predispostos à ingestão de plantas recém-introduzidas.

DIAGNÓSTICO

DIAGNÓSTICO DIFERENCIAL
Nefrotoxinas
- Ácido acetilsalicílico e outros AINEs.
- Zinco.
- Ácido bórico.
- Etilenoglicol.
- Mercúrio.
- Antibacterianos nefrotóxicos — aminoglicosídeos.

Doenças Sistêmicas
- Manifestação aguda de insuficiência renal crônica.
- Obstrução urinária.
- Doença renal imunomediada.
- Leptospirose.
- Pielonefrite.
- Linfoma.

HEMOGRAMA/BIOQUÍMICA/URINÁLISE
- Leucograma de estresse.
- Níveis moderado a intensamente elevados de ureia, fosfato e potássio.
- Creatinina — é comum um aumento grave; geralmente, 15-29 mg/dL; pode estar na faixa de 40.
- Atividade elevada das enzimas AST, ALT e fosfatase alcalina no fim da doença.
- Proteinúria grave, glicosúria e densidade baixa; inúmeros cilindros epiteliais tubulares.
- Cristalúria — *não* provocada pela ingestão dessas plantas.
- Na ingestão de quantidades muito altas, pode ocorrer o aumento dos níveis de amilase e lipase.

OUTROS TESTES LABORATORIAIS
N/D.

DIAGNÓSTICO POR IMAGEM
N/D.

MÉTODOS DIAGNÓSTICOS
- Se possível, examinar as plantas para verificar se elas foram mastigadas.
- Submeter a planta à identificação por um profissional da área de horticultura ou especialista, se houver necessidade.

ACHADOS PATOLÓGICOS
- Macroscópicos — rins tumefatos; trato gastrintestinal vazio; edema perirrenal moderado a grave.
- Histológicos — necrose tubular renal aguda grave, com membranas basais intactas; edema intersticial leve a grave; formação intensa de cilindros nos ductos coletores; pode-se notar a evidência de figuras mitóticas no epitélio tubular remanescente.

TRATAMENTO

- Descontaminação precoce — diminui a duração e a gravidade dos sinais.
- Fluidoterapia — o início dentro de 24 h da ingestão evita a insuficiência renal anúrica; solução fisiológica intravenosa administrada 2-3 vezes como manutenção por 24 h.
- Insuficiência renal anúrica — diálise constitui o único tratamento eficaz; com 7 dias de tratamento, o paciente retorna à função renal normal.

MEDICAÇÕES

MEDICAMENTO(S)
- Descontaminação — carvão ativado (2 g/kg VO).
- Catártico — sorbitol (2,1 g/kg VO) ou sulfato de magnésio (0,5 g/kg VO).

CONTRAINDICAÇÕES/INTERAÇÕES POSSÍVEIS
- Evitar fluidos que contenham potássio.
- Evitar medicamentos eliminados por depuração renal.
- Diuréticos (manitol, fluidos hipertônicos, furosemida, tiazidas) — não são eficazes para desencadear a produção de urina após o início de anúria.

ACOMPANHAMENTO

MONITORIZAÇÃO DO PACIENTE
Acompanhamento periódico por meio da bioquímica sérica para garantir função renal normal; particularmente importante após o procedimento de diálise.

EVOLUÇÃO ESPERADA E PROGNÓSTICO
Desidratação — causada por insuficiência renal poliúrica; necessária para que a doença evolua para anúria.

DIVERSOS

VER TAMBÉM
- Envenenamento (Intoxicação).
- Insuficiência Renal Aguda.

ABREVIATURA(S)
- AINE = anti-inflamatório não esteroide.
- ALT = alanina aminotransferase.
- AST = aspartato aminotransferase.

Sugestões de Leitura
Groff RM, Miller JM, Stair EL, et al. Toxicoses and toxins. In: Norsworthy GD, ed., Feline Practice. Philadelphia: Lippincott, 1993, pp. 551-569.
Hall JO. Lily poisoning. In: Peterson ME, Talcott PA, eds., Small Animal Toxicology. Philadelphia: Saunders, 2006, pp. 806-811.

Autor Jeffery O. Hall
Consultor Editorial Gary D. Osweiler

Intoxicação por Ácido Acetilsalicílico

CONSIDERAÇÕES GERAIS

REVISÃO
• Administrada pelos proprietários aos animais para o alívio da dor e do desconforto de baixa intensidade; atualmente, é utilizada com menor frequência em função do aumento na popularidade de outros analgésicos vendidos sem receita médica.
• Ocorrem irritação e hemorragia gástricas em 10-20% dos casos.
• As doses repetidas podem produzir ulceração e perfuração gastrintestinais.
• Podem ocorrer hepatite tóxica, supressão da atividade da medula óssea e anemia, especialmente em gatos.

IDENTIFICAÇÃO
Gatos e, menos comumente, cães.

SINAIS CLÍNICOS
• Depressão.
• Vômito — pode apresentar estrias de sangue.
• Taquipneia.
• Febre.
• Fraqueza muscular e ataxia.
• Coma e óbito em 1 ou mais dias.

CAUSAS E FATORES DE RISCO
• Proprietários que empregam as diretrizes de dosagem humana para medicar os gatos — constitui a causa mais comum.
• Deficiência na capacidade de conjugação glicurônica (gatos).
• Meia-vida biológica — gatos, 44,6 h; cães, 7,5 h; responsável pelo risco mais elevado em gatos.

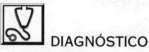

DIAGNÓSTICO

DIAGNÓSTICO DIFERENCIAL
• Sinais clínicos — não característicos.
• Histórico de ingestão de ácido acetilsalicílico ou medicamentos com esse componente em sua formulação — fator importante; a constatação de sinais dentro de 5 dias deve suscitar preocupações.
• Condição dolorosa preexistente — questionar o proprietário quanto à administração de ácido acetilsalicílico.

HEMOGRAMA/BIOQUÍMICA/URINÁLISE
• Gatos — propensos à formação dos corpúsculos de Heinz.
• Hiponatremia e hipocalemia.

OUTROS TESTES LABORATORIAIS
• Alcalose respiratória inicial, acompanhada por acidose metabólica.
• Concentrações séricas ou urinárias do ácido salicílico.
• Níveis elevados de cetonas, ácidos pirúvicos e lácticos, bem como de aminoácidos.
• Declínio na depuração renal dos ácidos sulfúrico e fosfórico.

DIAGNÓSTICO POR IMAGEM
N/D.

MÉTODOS DIAGNÓSTICOS
N/D.

TRATAMENTO

• Internação — seguir os princípios terapêuticos gerais para os casos de intoxicação.
• Correção do equilíbrio acidobásico — fluidoterapia intravenosa contínua.
• Indução do esvaziamento gástrico — realização de lavagem gástrica ou indução de êmese.
• Diálise peritoneal ou hemodiálise ou hemoperfusão — procedimentos heroicos.

MEDICAÇÕES

MEDICAMENTO(S)
• Não há nenhum antídoto específico disponível.
• Carvão ativado — 2 g/kg VO neutralizam o intestino.
• Bicarbonato de sódio — 1 mEq/kg IV alcaliniza a urina.

CONTRAINDICAÇÕES/INTERAÇÕES POSSÍVEIS
N/D.

ACOMPANHAMENTO

• É vital manter a função renal e o equilíbrio acidobásico.
• Distúrbios acidobásicos graves, desidratação intensa, hepatite tóxica, depressão da medula óssea e coma são indicativos de prognóstico mau.

DIVERSOS

Certifique-se de que o histórico de medicação com o ácido acetilsalicílico não se refere a outros analgésicos disponíveis no mercado.

Sugestões de Leitura
Oehme FW. Aspirin and acetaminophen. In: Kirk RW, ed., Current Veterinary Therapy IX: Small Animal Practice. Philadelphia: Saunders, 1986, pp. 188-189.

Autor Frederick W. Oehme
Consultor Editorial Gary D. Osweiler

INTOXICAÇÃO POR ESTRICNINA

CONSIDERAÇÕES GERAIS

REVISÃO
- Estricnina — poderoso convulsivante; toxina alcaloide; derivada das sementes de *Strychnos nux-vomica* e *S. ignatii*; utilizada para matar esquilos (lisos e listrados), camundongos, cães de pradaria, ratos, toupeiras, pequenos roedores mamíferos e predadores.
- Absorção muito rápida.
- Início dos sinais clínicos — 10 min a 2 h.
- Efeitos — bloqueia reversivelmente a ligação da glicina (neurotransmissor inibitório); resulta na estimulação de reflexos descontrolados, hiperextensão e rigidez muscular com envolvimento maior dos músculos extensores, acompanhados por crises convulsivas.
- Eliminada sob a forma de metabólitos hepáticos e como composto original na urina.
- Causa da morte — apneia e hipoxia atribuídas à rigidez dos músculos respiratórios.
- Iscas — contendo >0,5% de estricnina são limitadas para uso por aplicadores certificados; contendo <0,5% de estricnina estão disponíveis para o público em geral em alguns estados.

IDENTIFICAÇÃO
- Cães e gatos.
- Todas as idades são suscetíveis.

SINAIS CLÍNICOS
- Crises convulsivas tetânicas violentas — podem ser desencadeadas por estímulos físicos, visuais ou auditivos.
- Rigidez extensora.
- Rigidez muscular.
- Opistótono.
- Taquicardia.
- Hipertermia.
- Apneia.
- Vômito — muito raro.

CAUSAS E FATORES DE RISCO
- Intoxicação maliciosa — razoavelmente comum.
- Exposição direta às iscas — mais comum nos cães do que em outras espécies.
- Intoxicação retransmitida pela ingestão de roedores e pássaros intoxicados.
- DL_{50} — cães, 0,2 mg/kg; gatos, 0,5 mg/kg.

DIAGNÓSTICO

DIAGNÓSTICO DIFERENCIAL
- Outras substâncias tóxicas — chumbo; nicotina; anfetaminas; metaldeído; chocolate; fosfeto de zinco; micotoxinas tremorgênicas; antidepressivos; 4-aminopiridina; cocaína; piretrinas ou piretroides; 1080 (fluoracetato); cafeína; LSD; inseticidas organoclorados.
- Doenças sistêmicas — uremia; insuficiência hepática; neoplasia; hipoglicemia; encefalites; intermação/insolação; traumatismo; isquemia; tétano.

HEMOGRAMA/BIOQUÍMICA/URINÁLISE
- Creatina quinase e lactato desidrogenase elevadas.
- Mioglobinúria.
- Acidose metabólica sistêmica.

OUTROS TESTES LABORATORIAIS
- Análise do conteúdo estomacal, fígado, rim ou urina — revela a presença de estricnina; se o óbito for muito rápido, o rim e a urina serão negativos.
- Gasometria sanguínea — revela acidose.

DIAGNÓSTICO POR IMAGEM
N/D.

MÉTODOS DIAGNÓSTICOS
- CUIDADO: não induzir a uma crise convulsiva pelo estímulo; *não* é diagnóstica e pode ser letal.
- Pressão arterial — pode revelar hipertensão sistêmica.

ACHADOS PATOLÓGICOS
- Associados ao traumatismo provocado pela atividade convulsiva.
- Iscas — frequentemente encontradas no conteúdo estomacal; as iscas à base de grãos podem ser codificadas pelas cores vermelha ou verde.

TRATAMENTO

SUPORTE VITAL GERAL
- Paciente internado — pode necessitar de tratamento por até 48-72 h.
- Principais objetivos — evitar a asfixia; controlar as crises convulsivas e a rigidez muscular; pode necessitar da anestesia completa e respiração artificial.
- Manter o paciente em ambiente quieto, tranquilo e escuro.
- Banhos de água fria — no caso de hipertermia.

DESCONTAMINAÇÃO
- Diminui a duração e a gravidade dos sinais clínicos.
- Lavagem gástrica ou enterogástrica — reduz a absorção.
- Diurese fluida — aumenta a eliminação; solução fisiológica com manitol a 5% (7 mg/kg/h).
- Êmese — não induzir a menos que seja dentro de minutos da ingestão e o paciente esteja assintomático, pois isso pode desencadear crises convulsivas.

MEDICAÇÕES

MEDICAMENTO(S)
- Descontaminação — carvão ativado (2 g/kg VO); catártico (sorbitol à dose de 2,1 g/kg VO; sulfato de magnésio à dose de 0,5 g/kg VO).
- Controle das crises convulsivas — diazepam (pode não ser eficaz); pentobarbital (até fazer efeito); guaiacolato de glicerol (110 mg/kg IV, repetido conforme a necessidade); metocarbamol (150 mg/kg IV, repetido na base de 90 mg/kg conforme necessário); anestesia por inalação.
- Acidificação urinária — cloreto de amônio (150 mg/kg); aumenta a eliminação.

CONTRAINDICAÇÕES/INTERAÇÕES POSSÍVEIS
- Não induzir à êmese em pacientes sintomáticos.
- Não acidificar com o cloreto de amônio se o paciente estiver em acidose diagnosticada com base na gasometria venosa.
- Não utilizar cetamina.
- Não usar morfina.

ACOMPANHAMENTO

- Monitorizar o paciente quanto à presença de dano renal secundário por mioglobinúria e possível desenvolvimento de cilindros tubulares.
- Prognóstico — reservado até que as crises convulsivas estejam controladas; bom depois do controle dessas crises.

DIVERSOS

VER TAMBÉM
Envenenamento (Intoxicação).

ABREVIATURA(S)
- DL_{50} = dose letal de produto tóxico que provoca a morte de 50% dos animais testados.
- LSD = dietilamida do ácido lisérgico.

Sugestões de Leitura
Osweiler GD. Strychnine poisoning. In: Kirk RW, ed., Current Veterinary Therapy VIII. Philadelphia: Saunders, 1983, pp. 98–100.
Talcott PA. Strychnine. In: Peterson ME, Talcott PA, eds., Small Animal Toxicology. Philadelphia: Saunders, 2006, pp. 1076–1082.

Autor Jeffery O. Hall
Consultor Editorial Gary D. Osweiler

Intoxicação por Etanol

CONSIDERAÇÕES GERAIS

REVISÃO
- Etanol (CH_2OH) — álcool alifático de cadeia curta; altamente miscível com água; solúvel em sistemas aquosos; menos volátil que hidrocarbonetos comparáveis (p. ex., etano); solvente para medicações; principal componente de bebidas alcoólicas; metabolizado em acetaldeído.
- As formas desnaturadas podem conter outras frações tóxicas (p. ex., acetona, benzeno, cânfora, óleo de rícino, ftalatos, querosene, ácido sulfúrico, terpineol); podem complicar os efeitos.
- Concentração de álcool — expressa como prova (2 vezes a concentração em porcentagem).
- Intoxicação aguda — um volume de 5-8 mL/kg sob a forma de álcool puro é considerado a dose letal mais baixa; considerar a porcentagem de álcool no consumo de produto específico.
- Mecanismo de ação — dano às membranas celulares com comprometimento da condução nervosa de sódio e potássio.
- Pode inibir os receptores de glutamato no cérebro, com redução do GMP cíclico.

IDENTIFICAÇÃO
- Mais comum em cães.
- Sem predileção racial ou sexual.
- Os animais jovens são considerados mais suscetíveis.
- Exposição a bebidas, corantes, tintas, desinfetantes, gasolina, colutórios bucais, pinturas, perfumes e produtos farmacêuticos.

SINAIS CLÍNICOS
- SNC — predominantes; desenvolvem-se 15-30 min após a ingestão com o estômago vazio ou 1-2 h com o estômago cheio.
- Altas dosagens — ataxia; reflexos reduzidos; mudanças comportamentais; excitação ou depressão; hipotermia.
- Flatulência se a fonte for uma massa de pão.
- Poliúria e/ou incontinência.
- Sinais avançados — depressão ou narcose; frequência respiratória lenta; acidose metabólica; parada cardíaca; morte.

CAUSAS E FATORES DE RISCO
- Acidental — acesso a bebidas, produtos comerciais ou medicações derramados que contenham álcool.
- Intencional — dada pelos proprietários ou por outros; os cães podem consumir cerveja com facilidade se ela for oferecida.
- As bebidas alcoólicas provavelmente constituem a fonte mais comum — tanto acidental como intencional.
- Produtos fermentados — massa de pão, massas podres.
- Exposição dérmica — produtos que contenham álcool.

DIAGNÓSTICO

DIAGNÓSTICO DIFERENCIAL
- Outros alcoóis — metanol, isopropanol; butanol.
- Uso de drogas ou abuso de medicamentos — maconha; barbitúricos.
- Estágios iniciais de intoxicação por etilenoglicol (anticongelante).
- Solventes hidrocarbonetos halogenados ou alifáticos.
- Pesticidas — amitraz; antiparasiticidas macrolídeos.

HEMOGRAMA/BIOQUÍMICA/URINÁLISE
- Monitorizar o animal quanto à ocorrência de hipoglicemia; níveis de glicose sanguínea <60 mg/dL são considerados graves.
- Acidose metabólica provavelmente é atribuída à acidemia láctica induzida pelo etanol.

OUTROS TESTES LABORATORIAIS
- Concentrações sanguíneas de etanol — sinais clínicos de intoxicação em filhotes caninos com mais de 0,6 mg/mL e adultos com mais de 1-4 mg/mL; disponíveis em laboratórios humanos e veterinários.
- Gasometria sanguínea e hiato aniônico elevado — avaliar potencial acidose.

DIAGNÓSTICO POR IMAGEM
N/D.

MÉTODOS DIAGNÓSTICOS
N/D.

TRATAMENTO
- Carvão ativado — não é eficaz para detoxificação oral.
- Êmese ou lavagem gástrica — efetuadas com cuidado em pacientes deprimidos, com proteção das vias aéreas para evitar aspiração.
- Função respiratória deprimida — fornecer ventilação artificial.
- Fluidos IV — corrigir a desidratação.
- Acidose — administrar bicarbonato de sódio, de acordo com a gravidade da acidose.
- Parada cardíaca — terapia cardíaca (ver "Parada Cardiopulmonar").
- A depressão do SNC pode ser melhorada com o uso de ioimbina.

MEDICAÇÕES

MEDICAMENTO(S)
- Fomepizol (4-metilpirazol) — possível inibição do metabolismo de álcool (ver "Intoxicação por Etilenoglicol"), embora o uso contra etanol não tenha sido especificamente esclarecido.
- Adrenalina e bicarbonato — parada cardíaca (ver "Parada Cardiopulmonar").
- O tratamento para acidose pode incluir a administração de bicarbonato de sódio.
- Utilizar se a causa não for prontamente reversível, se o pH arterial estiver <7,2 e se os procedimentos ventilatórios não tiverem reduzido a acidemia.
- mEq de bicarbonato requerido = $0,5 \times 0,5$ de peso corporal em kg × (CO_2 total desejado em mEq/L − CO_2 mensurado em mEq/L).
- Administrar metade da dose calculada total lentamente em 3-4 h por via IV.
- Reavaliar a gasometria e o estado clínico do animal.
- Ioimbina para depressão do SNC — 0,1-0,2 mg/kg IV. Iniciar com a dose mais baixa. A meia-vida por via IV é curta (<2 h); por essa razão, pode haver a necessidade de repetição da terapia.

CONTRAINDICAÇÕES/INTERAÇÕES POSSÍVEIS
Não administrar outros depressores do SNC.

ACOMPANHAMENTO
- Monitorizar o pH sanguíneo, os gases sanguíneos, o pH urinário e o hiato aniônico — evidência de acidose.
- Recuperação dos sinais clínicos — geralmente em 8-12 h.

DIVERSOS

ABREVIATURA(S)
- SNC = sistema nervoso central.

Sugestões de Leitura
Kammerer M, Sachot E, Blanchot D. Ethanol toxicosis from ingestion of rotten apples by a dog. Vet Hum Toxicol 2001, 43(6):349-350.
Means C. Bread dough toxicosis in dogs. J Vet Emerg Crit Care 2003, 13(1):39-41.
Richardson JA. Ethanol. In: Peterson ME, Talcott PA, eds., Small Animal Toxicology, 2nd ed. St. Louis: Saunders, 2006, pp. 698-701.

Autor Gary D. Osweiler
Consultor Editorial Gary D. Osweiler

INTOXICAÇÃO POR ETILENOGLICOL

CONSIDERAÇÕES GERAIS

DEFINIÇÃO
Resulta da ingestão de substâncias que contêm etilenoglicol (p. ex., anticongelante).

FISIOPATOLOGIA
• Etilenoglicol — absorvido rapidamente a partir do trato gastrintestinal; alimento no estômago retarda a absorção.
• Toxicidade — inicialmente causa depressão do SNC, ataxia, irritação gastrintestinal e poliúria ou polidipsia; metabolizado com rapidez pela enzima hepática álcool desidrogenase em glicoaldeído, ácido glicólico; ácido glioxálico e ácido oxálico; induz a acidose metabólica grave e dano ao epitélio renal.
• Dose letal mínima — gatos, 1,4 mL/kg; cães, 6,6 mL/kg.

SISTEMA(S) ACOMETIDO(S)
• Gastrintestinal — irritação da mucosa.
• Nervoso — inebriação por etilenoglicol e glicoaldeído por causa da inibição da respiração, do metabolismo da glicose e da serotonina, bem como da alteração das concentrações de amina.
• Renal/urológico — inicialmente, diurese osmótica; depois, os metabólitos, sobretudo os cristais de oxalato de cálcio monoidratado, são diretamente citotóxicos ao epitélio tubular renal, resultando em insuficiência renal. Atualmente, acredita-se que o mecanismo de toxicidade envolva a fixação do oxalato à membrana plasmática celular e a ativação da atividade enzimática, bem como a produção de radicais livres e peroxidação lipídica, levando à necrose celular.

INCIDÊNCIA/PREVALÊNCIA
• Comum em pequenos animais.
• Taxa de fatalidade mais alta de todos os venenos; taxa de fatalidade maior em gatos do que em cães.
• Incidência semelhante em gatos e cães.

DISTRIBUIÇÃO GEOGRÁFICA
Maior incidência em áreas mais frias, onde o anticongelante costuma ser mais utilizado.

IDENTIFICAÇÃO
Espécies
Cães, gatos e muitas outras espécies, inclusive aves.
Idade Média e Faixa Etária
• Qualquer idade é suscetível (3 meses a 13 anos).
• Média — 3 anos.

SINAIS CLÍNICOS
Comentários Gerais
• Dependentes da dose.
• Quase sempre agudos.
• Causados pelo etilenoglicol não metabolizado e seus metabólitos tóxicos (frequentemente fatal).

Achados do Exame Físico
• Iniciais — observados 30 min a 12 h após a ingestão em cães; náuseas e vômitos; depressão leve a grave; ataxia e pateamento; fasciculações musculares; nistagmo; tremores da cabeça; diminuição dos reflexos de retirada e da capacidade de se erguer; poliúria e polidipsia.
• Cães — com o aumento da depressão, o paciente bebe menos, mas a poliúria continua, resultando em desidratação; os sinais do SNC diminuem transitoriamente após cerca de 12 h, mas retornam depois.
• Gatos — em geral, ficam bastante deprimidos; não apresentam polidipsia.
• Oligúria (cães, 36-72 h; gatos, 12-24 h) e anúria (72-96 h após a ingestão) — desenvolvem-se frequentemente caso não sejam tratadas.
• Pode-se observar hipotermia grave.
• Letargia grave ou coma.
• Crises convulsivas.
• Anorexia.
• Vômitos.
• Úlceras bucais.
• Salivação.
• Rins — em geral tumefatos e dolorosos, particularmente em gatos.

CAUSAS
Ingestão de etilenoglicol, o principal componente (95%) da maioria das soluções anticongelantes.

FATORES DE RISCO
Acesso ao etilenoglicol — disponibilidade disseminada; sabor um tanto desagradável; dose letal mínima pequena; falta de consciência pública da toxicidade.

DIAGNÓSTICO

DIAGNÓSTICO DIFERENCIAL
• Aguda (30 min a 12 h após a ingestão) — intoxicação por etanol, metanol e maconha; diabetes melito cetoacidótico; pancreatite; gastrenterite.
• Estágio renal — insuficiência renal aguda por nefrotoxinas (p. ex., antibióticos aminoglicosídeos, anfotericina B, quimioterápicos para câncer, ibuprofeno, plantas contendo oxalato como filodendros, plantas da família dos lírios [gatos], ciclosporina, toxicose por uvas e passas [causa hipercalcemia, ao contrário da toxicose por etilenoglicol] e metais pesados); leptospirose, nefrite tubulointersticial, doença glomerular e vascular; isquemia renal (hipoperfusão).

HEMOGRAMA/BIOQUÍMICA/URINÁLISE
• Volume globular (hematócrito) e proteína total — geralmente altos dada a desidratação.
• Leucograma de estresse — comum.
• BUN e creatinina elevados — cão, 36-48 h após a ingestão; gatos, 12 h após a ingestão.
• Pode ocorrer hiperfosfatemia transitória 3-6 h após a ingestão, em virtude dos inibidores do fosfato ferruginoso no anticongelante. Também se observa hiperfosfatemia com azotemia dada a filtração glomerular reduzida.
• Hipercalcemia se o animal tiver oligúria ou anúria.
• Hipocalcemia — ocorre em aproximadamente metade dos pacientes, dada a quelação do cálcio pelo ácido oxálico; sinais clínicos observados com pouca frequência por causa de acidose.
• Hiperglicemia — ocorre em cerca da metade dos pacientes, dados a inibição do metabolismo da glicose por aldeídos, o aumento da adrenalina e dos corticosteroides endógenos e a uremia.
• Isostenúria — por volta de 3 h após a ingestão, dada a diurese osmótica e a polidipsia induzida pela hiperosmolalidade sérica; continua nos estágios finais de toxicose por causa da disfunção renal.
• Cristalúria por oxalato de cálcio — achado compatível; apenas 3 h após a ingestão em gatos e 6 h depois em cães; a forma monoidratada é mais comum.
• pH urinário — diminui de forma consistente.
• Achados inconsistentes — hematúria; proteinúria; glicosúria.
• É possível observar cilindros granulosos e celulares, além de leucócitos, hemácias e células epiteliais renais.

OUTROS TESTES LABORATORIAIS
Hemogasometria
• Os metabólitos provocam acidose metabólica grave.
• Concentração total de CO_2, plasmática de bicarbonato e pH sanguíneo — baixos por volta de 3 h após a ingestão; acentuadamente baixos em torno de 12 h.
• PCO_2 — diminui, por causa da compensação respiratória parcial.
• Hiato aniônico — aumentado por volta de 3 h após a ingestão; picos com 6 h após a ingestão; permanece aumentado por cerca de 48 h (os metabólitos de etilenoglicol são ânions não medidos).

Outros
• Osmolalidade sérica e hiato osmolar — altos cerca de 1 h após a ingestão, paralelamente com as concentrações séricas de etilenoglicol; relacionados com a dose; em geral, permanecem altos por cerca de 18 h após a ingestão; a intoxicação por etilenoglicol é a causa mais comum de hiato osmolar elevado.
• Concentração sérica de etilenoglicol — picos 1-6 h após a ingestão; geralmente não é detectável no soro ou na urina por volta de 72 h.
• *Kits* comerciais (Pharmacol REACT EG) medem concentrações >50 mg/dL; fazer a estimativa, multiplicando-se o hiato osmolar por 6,2.
• O etilenoglicol é detectado apenas no soro ou plasma.
• Como esses *kits* não medem os metabólitos, é imprescindível utilizá-los dentro das primeiras horas após a ingestão.
• Os resultados estão disponíveis em 6 minutos, mas não devem ser lidos após 10 minutos.
• Indicados para cães e gatos. Alguns gatos podem ter toxicose em níveis abaixo de 50 mg/dL.
• Podem ser observados resultados falso-positivos com propilenoglicol (como no diazepam), glicerol, manitol e sorbitol. O etanol também pode se combinar com propilenoglicol ou glicerol até gerar um resultado falso-positivo.
• Os exames de urina, face, patas ou vômitos com a lâmpada de Wood são sugeridos por alguns para detectar a fluoresceína adicionada algumas vezes ao anticongelante. Além de inespecífico, frequentemente esse método não é considerado confiável.

DIAGNÓSTICO POR IMAGEM
Ultrassonografia — os córtices renais podem estar hiperecoicos por causa dos cristais.

MÉTODOS DIAGNÓSTICOS
• Biopsia renal — com anúria; confirma o diagnóstico.
• Exame citológico de impressões renais — em geral, diagnósticos; numerosos cristais de oxalato de cálcio.

ACHADOS PATOLÓGICOS
• Rins — geralmente se apresentam tumefatos.
• O exame dos rins à necropsia revela concentrações renais acentuadamente elevadas de cálcio.

Intoxicação por Etilenoglicol

TRATAMENTO

CUIDADO(S) DE SAÚDE ADEQUADO(S)
- Gatos — em geral, são hospitalizados.
- Cães — não costumam ser internados se apresentados em menos de 5 h após a ingestão e tratados com fomepizol; internados se intoxicados há mais de 5 h, para receberem fluidoterapia intravenosa a fim de corrigir a desidratação, aumentar a perfusão tecidual e promover a diurese.

CUIDADO(S) DE ENFERMAGEM
- Metas — impedir a absorção; aumentar a excreção; impedir o metabolismo.
- Indução de vômitos e lavagem gástrica com carvão ativado — não são recomendadas a menos que possam ser realizadas nos 30 primeiros minutos após a ingestão em virtude da rápida absorção de etilenoglicol.
- Fluidos intravenosos — corrigem a desidratação, aumentam a perfusão tecidual e promovem a diurese; acompanhados de bicarbonato por via intravenosa lenta para corrigir a acidose metabólica.
- Monitorização seriada das concentrações plasmáticas de bicarbonato — 0,3-0,5 × peso corporal (kg) × (24 – bicarbonato plasmático) = bicarbonato de sódio necessário (mEq).
- Monitorização do pH urinário em resposta à terapia.
- Azotemia e insuficiência renal oligúrica (cães) — a maior parte do etilenoglicol foi metabolizada; pouco benefício advindo da inibição da álcool desidrogenase; corrigir os distúrbios hidroeletrolíticos e acidobásicos; estabelecer a diurese; diuréticos (em particular manitol) podem ajudar; a diálise peritoneal pode ser útil; talvez seja necessário um tratamento prolongado (várias semanas) antes que a função renal seja restabelecida.

CONSIDERAÇÕES CIRÚRGICAS
Transplante renal — bem-sucedido em gatos com insuficiência renal induzida pelo etilenoglicol.

MEDICAÇÕES

MEDICAMENTO(S) DE ESCOLHA

Cães
Fomepizol (4-metilpirazol; Antizol-Vet) — inibidor eficaz da álcool desidrogenase e atóxico para o fígado; mais caro que o etanol (o custo inicial é compensado pela redução do tempo na terapia intensiva); a 5% (50 mg/mL) à dose de 20 mg/kg IV inicialmente; em seguida, 15 mg/kg IV em 12-24 h; depois, 5 mg/kg IV em 36 h.

Gatos
- Fomepizol — os gatos devem receber uma dose muito maior desse medicamento do que os cães; 125 mg/kg IV inicialmente, depois 31,25 mg/kg em 12, 24 e 36 h.
- Etanol — utilizado se o fomepizol não estiver disponível; a 20% na dose de 5 mL/kg diluídos em líquidos e administrados por gotejamento IV durante 6 h em 5 tratamentos; em seguida, mais 4 tratamentos de 8 h cada.

CONTRAINDICAÇÕES
Evitar medicamentos indutores de depressão do SNC.

PRECAUÇÕES
- Substratos competitivos (álcoois, como o etanol) — contribuem para a depressão do SNC; monitorizar a respiração.
- Gatos — em geral, apresentam hipotermia; necessitam de uma fonte externa de calor.
- Outros pirazóis — podem ser tóxicos para a medula óssea e o fígado; não substituem o fomepizol.

INTERAÇÕES POSSÍVEIS
- Fomepizol — contribui levemente para a depressão do SNC em gatos; nenhuma em cães.
- Etanol — contribui para a depressão do SNC; aumenta ainda mais a osmolalidade sérica.

MEDICAMENTO(S) ALTERNATIVO(S)
- Etanol, propilenoglicol e 1,3-butanediol — maior afinidade pela álcool desidrogenase do que o etilenoglicol; eficazes para inibir o metabolismo do etilenoglicol; podem causar depressão do SNC e aumentar a osmolalidade sérica; concentrações séricas constantes de etanol a 100 mg/dL inibem grande parte do metabolismo do etilenoglicol.
- Etanol — mesmo nos estágios iniciais, requer hospitalização por aproximadamente 3 dias; infusão intravenosa constante (de etanol e fluidos); monitorização contínua do estado respiratório e acidobásico.

ACOMPANHAMENTO

MONITORIZAÇÃO DO PACIENTE
BUN, estado acidobásico e débito urinário — monitorizados diariamente nos primeiros dias.

PREVENÇÃO
- Aumentar a consciência do proprietário quanto à toxicidade — ajuda a prevenir a exposição; proceder ao tratamento precoce dos pacientes.
- Utilizar novos produtos anticongelantes contendo propilenoglicol (relativamente atóxico).

COMPLICAÇÕES POSSÍVEIS
- Sem azotemia — em geral, não há complicações.
- Capacidade de concentração da urina — pode estar prejudicada com a azotemia; o paciente pode se recuperar.

EVOLUÇÃO ESPERADA E PROGNÓSTICO
- Sem tratamento — insuficiência renal oligúrica (cães, 36-72 h; gatos, 12-24 h); anúria por volta de 72-96 h após a ingestão.
- Cães tratados em menos de 5 h após a ingestão — prognóstico excelente com fomepizol.
- Cães tratados em até 8 h após a ingestão — a maioria se recupera.
- Cães tratados em até 36 h após a ingestão — pode ser benéfico impedir o metabolismo de qualquer resíduo de etilenoglicol.
- Gatos tratados dentro de 3 h após a ingestão — prognóstico bom.
- Se uma grande quantidade de etilenoglicol tiver sido ingerida, o prognóstico será mau, a menos que o paciente seja tratado dentro de 4 h após a ingestão.
- Pacientes com azotemia e insuficiência renal oligúrica — prognóstico mau; quase todo o etilenoglicol terá sido metabolizado.

DIVERSOS

FATORES RELACIONADOS COM A IDADE
Pacientes com menos de 6 meses de vida e insuficiência renal oligúrica às vezes não se recuperam totalmente.

SINÔNIMO(S)
Envenenamento por anticongelante.

VER TAMBÉM
- Hiperosmolaridade.
- Insuficiência Renal Aguda.

ABREVIATURA(S)
- BUN = nitrogênio ureico sanguíneo (ureia).
- SNC = sistema nervoso central.

Sugestões de Leitura
Connally HE, Hamar DW, Thrall MA. Inhibition of canine and feline alcohol dehydrogenase activity by fomepizole. Am J Vet Res 2000, 61:450-455.
Connally HE, Thrall MA, Forney SD, et al. Safety and efficacy of 4-methylpyrazole as treatment for suspected or confirmed ethylene glycol intoxication in dogs: 107 cases (1983-1995). JAVMA 1996, 209:1880-1883.
Dial SM, Thrall MA, Hamar DW. Comparison of ethanol and 4-methylpyrazole as therapies for ethylene glycol intoxication in the cat. Am J Vet Res 1994, 55:1771-1782.
Poldelski V, Johnson A, Wright S, et al. Ethylene glycol-mediated tubular injury; identification of critical metabolites and injury pathways. Am J Kidney Dis 2001, 38:239-248.
Thrall MA, Grauer GF, Connally HE, et al. Ethylene glycol. In: Talcott P, Peterson M, eds., Small Animal Toxicology, 2nd ed. Philadelphia: Elsevier Saunders, 2005, pp. 702-726.
Thrall MA, Grauer GF, Dial SM. Antifreeze poisoning. In: Bonagura JD, ed., Kirk's Current Veterinary Therapy XII. Philadelphia: Saunders, 1995, pp. 232-237.

Autor Gary D. Osweiler
Consultor Editorial Gary D. Osweiler
Agradecimento O autor deseja agradecer as colaborações feitas por Mary Anna Thrall, Gregory F. Grauer, Heather E. Connally e Sharon M. Dial às edições prévias deste capítulo.

INTOXICAÇÃO POR METALDEÍDO

CONSIDERAÇÕES GERAIS

DEFINIÇÃO
- Metaldeído é um polímero policíclico do acetaldeído, que acomete principalmente o sistema nervoso. Trata-se de um ingrediente de iscas para lesmas e caracóis, utilizado como combustível sólido em alguns fogareiros a campo e comercializado como pastilhas de chama colorida para mercadorias de festa.
- As iscas para lesmas e caracóis podem ser adquiridas sob a forma de líquidos, grânulos, pós solúveis ou péletes, o que também pode conter outros agentes tóxicos, como arsenato ou inseticidas.

FISIOPATOLOGIA
- Mecanismo exato desconhecido. Sugere-se que o metaldeído seja convertido em acetaldeído após a ingestão e que o acetaldeído seja o principal agente tóxico.
- Pode aumentar os neurotransmissores excitatórios ou diminuir os neurotransmissores inibitórios.

SISTEMA(S) ACOMETIDO(S)
- Hepatobiliar — relata-se hepatotoxicose tardia, embora não seja comum.
- Neuromuscular — provoca crises convulsivas e tremores musculares.
- Pode ocorrer falência múltipla de órgãos secundariamente a convulsões e hipertermia.

INCIDÊNCIA/PREVALÊNCIA
Dependem da localização geográfica.

DISTRIBUIÇÃO GEOGRÁFICA
Encontrada mais comumente nas regiões costeiras e baixas, as quais apresentam uma prevalência mais elevada de lesmas e caracóis do que em outras áreas.

IDENTIFICAÇÃO
Espécies
Cães (mais comum) e gatos.

SINAIS CLÍNICOS
Comentários Gerais
Pode ocorrer imediatamente após a ingestão ou demorar até 3 h.

Achados Anamnésicos
- Ansiedade e respiração ofegante são sinais clínicos precoces.
- Podem ocorrer hipersalivação e/ou vômito.
- Ataxia.
- Tremores musculares.
- Convulsões.

Achados do Exame Físico
- Crises convulsivas — podem ser intermitentes no início, mas evoluir para uma forma contínua; não evocadas necessariamente por estímulos externos.
- Entre as convulsões — podem-se notar tremores musculares e ansiedade; o animal pode se mostrar hiperestésico a ruídos, luz e/ou toque.
- Hipertermia — temperatura de até 42,2°C é comum; provavelmente provocada por atividade muscular excessiva decorrente das convulsões; pode levar à CID ou falência múltipla de órgãos se não for controlada.
- Taquicardia e hiperpneia.
- Possível nistagmo ou midríase.
- Possível hipersalivação, vômito ou diarreia.
- Ataxia antes das crises convulsivas ou entre elas.

CAUSAS
Ingestão do metaldeído.

FATORES DE RISCO
Residir em área com alta prevalência de lesmas e caracóis.

DIAGNÓSTICO

DIAGNÓSTICO DIFERENCIAL
- Intoxicação por estricnina — provoca crises convulsivas intermitentes que podem ser evocadas por estímulos externos.
- Penitrem A — micotoxina geralmente encontrada nas nogueiras inglesas mofadas ou no queijo cremoso; foi relatada em outros gêneros alimentícios; causa síndrome tremorgênica.
- Roquefortina — micotoxina encontrada no queijo azul mofado e em outros alimentos; provoca síndrome tremorgênica.
- Intoxicação pelo chumbo — pode provocar crises convulsivas, mudanças comportamentais, cegueira, vômito, diarreia.
- Rodenticida fosfeto de zinco — pode causar crises convulsivas e hiperestesia.
- Rodenticida brometalina — pode gerar crises convulsivas.
- Inseticidas organoclorados — provocam crises convulsivas na maior parte dos mamíferos.
- Inseticidas anticolinesterásicos — organofosforados e carbamatos; podem causar crises convulsivas, quase sempre acompanhadas por salivação excessiva, lacrimejamento, micção e defecação.

HEMOGRAMA/BIOQUÍMICA/URINÁLISE
- Sem características específicas ou diagnósticas.
- Aumento das atividades séricas de enzimas musculares.
- Acidose metabólica.
- É possível a constatação de alterações nos valores renais ou hepáticos, mas muito provavelmente secundária à falta de controle da hipertermia.

OUTROS TESTES LABORATORIAIS
Teste para detecção do metaldeído — vômito, conteúdo estomacal, soro, urina ou fígado. As capacidades do teste variam amplamente entre os laboratórios; por essa razão, é preciso verificar em primeiro lugar quais as amostras recomendadas.

ACHADOS PATOLÓGICOS
- As lesões não são compatíveis nem patognomônicas. • Congestão hepática, renal e pulmonar. • Hemorragias petequiais e equimóticas. • Hemorragias subendocárdicas e subepicárdicas. • Conteúdo estomacal pode apresentar odor "químico", descrito como um odor de formaldeído.

TRATAMENTO

CUIDADO(S) DE SAÚDE ADEQUADO(S)
Cuidado intensivo de emergência do paciente internado até o término das convulsões e o controle da hipertermia.

CUIDADO(S) DE ENFERMAGEM
- Controle da hipertermia com enemas retais, bolsas de água fria, fluidos, etc.
- Monitorização do paciente para evitar aspiração de vômito.
- Fluidoterapia frequentemente necessária para desidratação ou acidose.

DIETA
Não alimentar os pacientes que estão vomitando, em crise convulsiva ou intensamente sedados.

MEDICAÇÕES

MEDICAMENTO(S) DE ESCOLHA
- Não há nenhum antídoto disponível.
- Diminuir a absorção em pacientes assintomáticos ou estabilizados com eméticos, lavagem gástrica e/ou carvão ativado conforme for conveniente.
- Controlar as convulsões com diazepam, barbitúricos, anestesia geral, metocarbamol isoladamente ou em combinação, se necessário.

CONTRAINDICAÇÕES
Jamais induzir ao vômito os pacientes em crise convulsiva.

PRECAUÇÕES
Não utilizar depressores em pacientes já deprimidos.

ACOMPANHAMENTO

MONITORIZAÇÃO DO PACIENTE
Permitir a redução periódica dos anticonvulsivantes para reavaliar a condição convulsiva.

PREVENÇÃO
- Não aplicar o metaldeído em áreas acessíveis aos animais de estimação. • Alguns fabricantes coram o produto de verde ou azul para ajudar na identificação. • Alguns estados norte-americanos exigem que os fabricantes ajustem a formulação de modo a diminuir a palatabilidade aos animais de estimação.

COMPLICAÇÕES POSSÍVEIS
- É possível a ocorrência de disfunção hepática ou renal alguns dias depois da recuperação dos sinais clínicos iniciais; tais disfunções provavelmente são sequelas das convulsões e da hipertermia.
- Pneumonia por aspiração é uma preocupação em qualquer animal em crise convulsiva.
- Hipertermia pode levar à CID ou falência múltipla de órgãos. • Pode ocorrer cegueira temporária ou perda de memória.

EVOLUÇÃO ESPERADA E PROGNÓSTICO
- Prognóstico — depende principalmente da quantidade ingerida, do tempo transcorrido até o tratamento e da qualidade dos cuidados fornecidos. • O atraso no tratamento ou o uso de terapia inadequada pode resultar em morte dentro de horas da exposição.

DIVERSOS

ABREVIATURA(S)
- CID = coagulação intravascular disseminada.

Autor Konnie H. Plumlee
Consultor Editorial Gary D. Osweiler

Introdução de Novos Animais de Estimação na Família

CONSIDERAÇÕES GERAIS

DEFINIÇÃO
Introdução de novos animais de estimação em uma casa com ou sem outros animais domésticos preexistentes.

FISIOPATOLOGIA
- O estresse pode ser causado por:
  - Introdução a estranhos (animais preexistentes e familiares).
  - Divisão de recursos e espaço na casa.
  - Idade/porte/socialização/temperamento/espécie do animal preexistente e do recém-chegado.
  - Tipo de membros da família (adultos/crianças/bebês).

SISTEMA(S) ACOMETIDO(S)
- Comportamental — medo, ansiedade, agressividade.
- Gastrintestinal — inapetência, vômito, diarreia.
- Renal/Urológico — micção domiciliar.
- Cutâneo — higiene pessoal excessiva com possível alopecia e lesões de pele.

GENÉTICA
- O comportamento é uma combinação da genética e do ambiente; as influências incluem:
- Comportamento de progenitores e irmãos.
- Comportamento dos animais residentes e dos recém-chegados durante introduções prévias dentro/fora da casa.
- Ambiente onde o animal foi socializado.

INCIDÊNCIA/PREVALÊNCIA DE PROBLEMAS DURANTE AS INTRODUÇÕES
- Cão com cão — desconhecidas.
- Gato com gato — 50% das introduções iniciais podem envolver agressividade.
- Entre espécies — desconhecidas.

IDENTIFICAÇÃO
Qualquer idade, sexo, espécie ou raça.

SINAIS CLÍNICOS

Comentários Gerais
A proficiência do proprietário na leitura da linguagem corporal das espécies envolvidas é essencial para avaliar a resposta à introdução inicial e subsequentes encontros. A linguagem corporal e a conduta do proprietário também podem contribuir para os resultados.

Achados Anamnésicos
Introdução de novo animal de estimação na família.

Achados do Exame Físico
É desejável a avaliação comportamental e física completa antes das introduções. Determinar a existência de quaisquer problemas comportamentais ou médicos preexistentes.

FATORES DE RISCO
- Socialização insatisfatória e problemas comportamentais prévios no animal residente ou no recém-chegado.
- Distúrbios médicos preexistentes no animal residente ou no recém-chegado.
- Distúrbios comportamentais em membros da família.
- Falta de plano terapêutico abrangente para as introduções.
- A introdução de animais de pequeno porte ou crianças com animais de porte maior pode gerar um risco de graves lesões ou até mesmo morte em caso de agressões.

DIAGNÓSTICO

DIAGNÓSTICO DIFERENCIAL
N/D.

HEMOGRAMA/BIOQUÍMICA/URINÁLISE
N/D.

TRATAMENTO

ABORDAGEM DAS INTRODUÇÕES
A paciência é essencial; introduções mais lentas podem aumentar o sucesso. Se houver vários animais residentes, recém-chegados e membros da família, as introduções devem ser feitas em um esquema gradativo de um a um antes da introdução ao grupo. Proceder às introduções iniciais em território neutro se possível. As pessoas envolvidas devem permanecer calmas e tranquilamente encorajadoras.

Segurança e Prevenção de Problemas
- Realizar a separação do animal doméstico a menos que ele esteja participando ativamente das introduções.
- Adaptar os animais domésticos ao confinamento em uma espécie de caixote/engradado ou em um espaço com porta fechada ou cercado.
- Para todos os cães: utilizar enforcador e focinheira do tipo cesta para obtenção de controle extra.
- Para todos os gatos: utilizar coleira do tipo peitoral.
- Adestrar os animais para aceitação desses métodos com reforços positivos apenas.

Relação com o Proprietário
- Cães: resposta proficiente aos comandos de *Sit* e *Down* (sentado e deitado).
- Gatos: resposta ao comando *Touch* (tocar um alvo ou a ponta do dedo mediante pedido).
- Adestrar apenas com reforços positivos.
- Os animais de estimação devem conquistar todas as coisas (comida, atenção, brincadeiras, passeio, acesso aos móveis da casa, etc.), efetuando um simples pedido em primeiro lugar.
  - Crie uma relação previsível e de confiança entre o animal de estimação e o proprietário.
- As técnicas de punição positiva, como gritos ou punições físicas, são contraindicadas.

Mudança Comportamental

Introduções Sem Complicação
- Na ausência de problemas comportamentais ou médicos preexistentes, o simples condicionamento clássico pode ser o bastante.
- Empregar medidas de segurança e suspender todas as coisas boas (alimento, brinquedos, atenção, brincadeiras), a menos que os animais de estimação ou as pessoas que estão sendo introduzidos estejam presentes. Continuar até que a linguagem corporal adequada esteja evidente.
- Se os animais estiverem aparentemente estressados ou muito focados entre si ou na nova pessoa, os proprietários devem solicitar que o animal estressado obedeça a um pedido do tipo *Sit* ou *Touch*, para receber uma recompensa.
- Se o animal de estimação não conseguir realizar essa tarefa, a introdução está ocorrendo muito rapidamente. Mudar para os métodos de dessensibilização e contracondicionamento (adiante).

Animais com Distúrbios Comportamentais Preexistentes ou Introduções Descomplicadas, porém Malsucedidas
Em caso de problemas comportamentais durante introduções prévias, o proprietário deve proceder aos métodos de dessensibilização e contracondicionamento dos animais de estimação entre si e/ou em relação aos membros da família. Talvez haja necessidade de realizar as introduções com outros animais de estimação separadamente daquelas com novas pessoas.
- Em primeiro lugar, proceda aos métodos de dessensibilização e contracondicionamento a odores e sons enquanto os animais de estimação estão atrás de portas fechadas. Misture os odores, trocando as roupas de cama entre os animais e as pessoas.
- Coloque os comedouros em um dos lados da porta, a uma distância que permita aos animais de estimação se sintam confortáveis o suficiente para comer de forma tranquila e relaxada. Comer mais rápido do que o normal ou olhar ao redor com nervosismo enquanto se alimenta pode indicar ansiedade e, nesse caso, a distância deve ser aumentada.
- A cada refeição, diminua a distância em relação à porta em alguns centímetros até que os animais de estimação se sintam bem ao comer ao lado da porta. Os membros da família podem ficar em pé do lado de fora da porta durante as refeições. Se o animal se recusar a comer ou se alimentar com pressa, é sinal de que a distância está muito pequena. Retorne a uma distância bem-sucedida e, a cada refeição subsequente, diminua pela metade a distância da tentativa anterior.
- Em seguida, proceda aos métodos de dessensibilização e contracondicionamento a acessos visuais. *Devem ser empregadas todas as medidas de segurança.* É imprescindível que as crianças sejam supervisionadas por algum adulto todo o tempo. Se não houver um adulto para observar cada animal ou criança, é melhor prender o animal ou colocá-lo em um caixote ou engradado.
- Descubra a distância entre os animais de estimação ou entre esses animais e as pessoas em que se manifesta uma linguagem corporal relaxada e adequada. Ver adiante.
- Ofereça os petiscos favoritos ou reforços para a manifestação de uma linguagem corporal adequada em direção a outros animais de estimação ou pessoa. Se isso for bem-sucedido, diminua a distância em alguns centímetros e repita o procedimento.
- Prossiga até que os animais de estimação sejam capazes de pegar os petiscos enquanto estão próximos a outros animais e diretamente de novos membros da família.
- Mantenha todas as sessões de dessensibilização e contracondicionamento durante breves períodos (3-5 minutos) e termine com uma anotação satisfatória.
- Mantenha os animais ou estes e as pessoas separados a uma distância segura até a próxima sessão planejada.

Compreensão da Linguagem Corporal para Aumentar o Sucesso das Introduções
- Faça a leitura da linguagem corporal dos animais e de sua capacidade de apanhar petiscos/alimentos para garantir que a introdução prossiga de forma suficientemente lenta.
- Caso se observe uma linguagem corporal adequada (posição neutra da orelha/cauda, alimentação normal, postura calma/tranquila/atenciosa em relação ao proprietário), o ritmo da introdução está correto.
- Caso se observe uma linguagem corporal inadequada (agressividade — animal tenso/rígido, com olhar fixo, piloereção, vocalização/rosnada/resmungo; medo — tremor, cauda encolhida e enrolada, orelhas para trás e baixas, ausência de alimentação, fuga), o ritmo da

Introdução de Novos Animais de Estimação na Família

introdução está muito rápido. ○ Os proprietários devem redirecionar a atenção do animal doméstico com os comandos de *Sit* ou *Touch*, recompensá-lo e, depois, interromper a sessão. ○ Se esse redirecionamento não for possível, os proprietários devem remover o animal tranquilamente com o auxílio de uma coleira. Pode acontecer alguma lesão se o animal for apanhado com rapidez para a remoção. ○ A próxima sessão deve ser retomada a uma distância previamente bem-sucedida, e as futuras diminuições da distância devem ser metade da modificação anterior.

ATIVIDADE
Proporcionar a todos os animais de estimação níveis adequados de atividade em relação à sua idade, saúde e espécie. Se essa atividade for possível com os animais e/ou as pessoas recém-introduzidos de forma segura e divertida, isso servirá como um condicionamento clássico entre eles.

DIETA
• Evite mudanças na dieta durante as introduções, pois isso pode resultar em complicações (evacuação/micção domiciliar, diarreia/vômito). • É imprescindível que os animais domésticos tenham comedouros individuais. • Na ausência de agressividade relacionada com o alimento, coloque as vasilhas bem afastadas ou em locais separados, se houver aparente ansiedade dos animais na hora da alimentação; quando não há agressividade, os membros da família e as crianças supervisionadas podem colocar petiscos nas vasilhas durante a refeição. • Na presença de agressividade relacionada com o alimento, não forneça alimentação *ad libitum* (ou seja, à vontade); além disso, separe os animais domésticos e as pessoas durante as refeições com cercados ou portas trancadas.

ORIENTAÇÃO AO PROPRIETÁRIO
• É recomendável a avaliação do histórico médico e comportamental de qualquer animal recém-introduzido na casa. • É imprescindível que os proprietários permaneçam calmos durante as introduções e conheçam as formas de leitura da linguagem corporal do animal de estimação. • Os proprietários devem ser advertidos sobre o fato de que a aceitação de recém-chegados pode demorar e que comportamentos de ansiedade e/ou agressividade de baixa intensidade podem persistir por algum tempo. • A falta de progresso é motivo para o acompanhamento e, talvez, o encaminhamento do animal para um veterinário especialista em comportamento.

CONSIDERAÇÕES CIRÚRGICAS
A menos que uma introdução seja feita especificamente para fins reprodutivos, os animais domésticos devem ser castrados. O comportamento do estro (cio) pode aumentar o nível de agitação/excitação de todos os animais. É menos provável que os animais castrados tenham o comportamento de marcação territorial com a urina.

MEDICAÇÕES
MEDICAMENTO(S) DE ESCOLHA
Não haverá indicação do uso de medicamentos se os animais envolvidos apresentarem um comportamento normal antes das introduções e caso se forneçam recursos adequados e espaços suficientes na casa. Se houver comportamentos preexistentes baseados em agressividade, medo ou ansiedade ou se tais comportamentos ocorrerem durante as introduções, deve-se proceder a uma avaliação completa para formular um diagnóstico e determinar se um medicamento é indicado e, em caso afirmativo, o agente terapêutico de escolha.

PRECAUÇÕES
As medicações que alteram o comportamento podem resultar em uma reação idiossincrática ou paradoxal com níveis elevados de medo, ansiedade, excitação/agitação ou agressividade. Os proprietários devem separar os animais de forma segura e procurar orientação caso ocorram efeitos colaterais comportamentais ou médicos.

ACOMPANHAMENTO
MONITORIZAÇÃO DO PACIENTE
A monitorização será semanal se não houver distúrbios preexistentes e se o plano terapêutico for obedecido. Na presença de problemas preexistentes, talvez haja necessidade de orientação dos proprietários a cada breve sessão de introdução para determinar como eles devem proceder.

PREVENÇÃO
• Mantenha os animais separados a uma distância segura, a menos que se façam introduções supervisionadas. • Forneça recursos extras (comedouros, áreas de repouso, brinquedos, bandejas sanitárias, etc.) para acomodar os novos animais introduzidos. • Os proprietários devem permanecer calmos e, sossegadamente, elogiar ou fornecer petiscos pelo bom comportamento durante as introduções. • Proporcionar refúgio e abrigo livre de crianças e de outros animais para os recém-chegados.

COMPLICAÇÕES POSSÍVEIS
• A agressividade pode resultar em lesões graves ou morte. • Pode ocorrer anorexia em virtude do estresse ou da competição social. • A evacuação domiciliar em gatos pode ser atribuída a muitos fatores, como: falta de acesso a uma bandeja sanitária, sujeira/falta de asseio ou número insuficiente de bandejas sanitárias, modificação da dieta, ou CIF. • A evacuação domiciliar em cães pode ser causada por áreas inacessíveis para as necessidades fisiológicas, falta de adestramento doméstico, modificação da dieta ou colite induzida por estresse. • A marcação com urina pode ser atribuída a comportamento territorial e/ou ansiedade. • A ansiedade pode provocar comportamentos compulsivos, como higiene e embelezamento excessivos, automutilação ou perseguição da cauda.

EVOLUÇÃO ESPERADA E PROGNÓSTICO
• As introduções bem-sucedidas dependem da disposição do proprietário em ser paciente e de sua capacidade de fazer a leitura da linguagem corporal dos animais de estimação em busca dos primeiros sinais de angústia, desconforto ou aflição (bocejo/lambedura dos lábios/olhos arregalados/hábito de exploração/tremor/vocalização/agachamento) ou excitação/agitação (piloereção/olhar fixo/orelhas voltadas para a frente/cauda ereta). • As introduções que prosseguem lentamente e não apresentam complicações devem ser bem-sucedidas. • Se a introdução inicial for estressante ou na ocorrência de agressividade, o prognóstico quanto ao êxito diminui. • Nem todos os companheiros da casa se tornam companhias unidas e afetivas. O sucesso em algumas situações pode ser definido como animais que convivem na mesma casa sem encontros agressivos contínuos ou evidência de estresse ou ansiedade.

DIVERSOS
DISTÚRBIOS ASSOCIADOS
Problemas comportamentais prévios (agressividade ou medo em situações novas ou estressantes) podem predispor os animais a problemas futuros durante as introduções.

FATORES RELACIONADOS COM A IDADE
Ainda dentro de seus períodos de socialização, pode ser mais fácil introduzir os animais jovens com outros animais de estimação e estranhos, desde que sejam fornecidos cuidados adequados com a devida supervisão para tornar as introduções seguras sem indução ao medo.

GESTAÇÃO/FERTILIDADE/REPRODUÇÃO
Introduções estressantes durante a gestação de um animal de estimação podem afetar o comportamento tanto da mãe como da ninhada. Os animais dotados de comportamento anormal ou incapazes de se adaptar a mudanças não devem ser reproduzidos.

VER TAMBÉM
• Capítulos sobre agressividade em cães e gatos.
• Transtornos Compulsivos — Gatos.
• Transtornos Compulsivos — Cães. • Medos, Fobias e Ansiedades — Gatos. • Medos, Fobias e Ansiedades — Cães. • Evacuação Domiciliar — Gatos. • Evacuação Domiciliar — Cães. • Comportamento de Marcação Territorial e Errático — Gatos. • Comportamento de Marcação Territorial e Errático — Cães.

ABREVIATURAS
CIF = cistite (idiopática) intersticial felina.

RECURSOS DA INTERNET
• American College of Veterinary Behaviorists: http://www.dacvb.org.
• American Veterinary Society of Animal Behavior: http://avsabonline.org.
• Animal Behavior Resources Institute, Inc.: http://abrionline.org/index.php.
• Humane Society of the United States: http://www.humanesociety.org/animals/dogs/tips/introducing_new_dog.html e http://www.humanesociety.org/animals/cats/tips/introducing_new_cat.html.

Sugestões de Leitura

Beaver BV. Canine Behavior: Insights and Answers, 2nd ed. New York: Elsevier, 2008, pp. 108-192.

Beaver BV. Feline Behavior: A Guide for Veterinarians, 2nd ed. St. Louis: Saunders, 2003, pp. 100-163.

Bergman L, Gaskins L. Expanding families: Preparing for and introducing dogs and cats to infants, children, and new pets. Vet Clin North Am Small Anim Pract 2008, 38(5):1043-1063.

Levine ES, Perry P, Scarlett J, Houpt KA. Intercat aggression in households following the introduction of a new cat. Appl Anim Behav Sci 2005, 90:325-336.

Autor Lori Gaskins
Consultor Editorial Debra F. Horwitz

INTUSSUSCEPÇÃO

CONSIDERAÇÕES GERAIS

DEFINIÇÃO
• Invaginação de um segmento intestinal para dentro do lúmen do segmento adjacente.
• As intussuscepções são classificadas de acordo com sua localização dentro do trato gastrintestinal. Intussuscepções ileocólica e jejunojejunal são os tipos mais comumente encontrados nos pequenos animais. Outras que foram descritas incluem gastresofágica, duodenojejunal e cecocólica.
• O segmento invaginado dentro do lúmen da intussuscepção recebe o nome de *intussuscepto*, enquanto o segmento embainhado é chamado de *intussuscipiente*.
• É mais comum que o segmento proximal seja invaginado dentro do segmento distal.

FISIOPATOLOGIA
• O mecanismo exato da geração de intussuscepção não é conhecido.
• Muitos animais acometidos são jovens (<1 ano de idade) e apresentam histórico de enterite recente.
• A presença de irritação gastrintestinal pode fazer com que o segmento proximal passe por um estado hiperperistáltico e sofra invaginação no segmento distal mais flácido.
• A ocorrência de intussuscepção leva a uma obstrução mecânica do trato gastrintestinal. Essa obstrução pode ser parcial ou completa.
• O comprometimento vascular costuma ocorrer na intussuscepto e, ocasionalmente, pode ocorrer no intussuscipiente. O comprometimento da drenagem venosa mediante irrigação arterial intacta induz à formação de edema acentuado e à ocorrência de hemorragia intramural que, finalmente, pode evoluir para extravasamento de sangue para o lúmen intestinal.
• A persistência da intussuscepção pode levar a consequente queda na distribuição de oxigênio para a camada da mucosa. Isso pode conduzir a subsequente falha na barreira mucosa e perda de uma barreira eficaz contra as bactérias e endotoxinas que ingressam na corrente sanguínea a partir do lúmen intestinal.
• Com o tempo, o comprometimento vascular pode levar a necrose intestinal e, por fim, extravasamento de conteúdo para a cavidade peritoneal. Isso induz ao desenvolvimento de peritonite séptica.

SISTEMA(S) ACOMETIDO(S)
• Gastrintestinal — obstrução mecânica, íleo paralítico.
• Cardiovascular — a perda de líquido (vômito e diarreia) pode levar à hipovolemia.

IDENTIFICAÇÃO
Espécies
Embora sejam relatadas em cães e gatos, as intussuscepções são mais comuns em cães.

Raça(s) Predominante(s)
• Os cães da raça Pastor alemão parecem ser predispostos a intussuscepções gastresofágicas, respondendo por aproximadamente 60% dos casos relatados dessa condição. Essa raça também parece ser super-representada nos outros tipos de intussuscepções.
• Os gatos da raça Siamês podem ser predispostos.

Idade Média e Faixa Etária
• Em razão dos fatores de risco para o desenvolvimento de intussuscepção (i. e., parasitismo, enterite viral, imprudência alimentar, ingestão de corpo estranho), os animais acometidos por essa doença são frequentemente mais jovens.
• Os animais mais idosos com intussuscepção devem ser submetidos a triagem rigorosa em busca de doenças capazes de provocar uma alteração no peristaltismo, como neoplasia intestinal ou outras doenças murais.

Sexo Predominante
• Originalmente se acreditava que os machos superavam o número de fêmeas com intussuscepção gastresofágica. Relatos recentes, no entanto, contestam essa informação.
• Não há predileção sexual comprovada para outros tipos de intussuscepções em pequenos animais.

SINAIS CLÍNICOS
Comentários Gerais
• Os sinais clínicos associados à intussuscepção dependem da região anatômica desse acontecimento.
• Em geral, as intussuscepções que ocorrem em segmentos mais proximais apresentam sinais clínicos e evolução mais graves da doença.
• As intussuscepções gastresofágicas tipicamente provocam sinais clínicos mais graves do que aquelas situadas em segmentos mais distais.
• A gravidade dos sinais clínicos também depende da natureza da obstrução (parcial ou completa).

Achados Anamnésicos
• Vômitos.
• Diarreia (que pode ou não ter sangue fresco ou melena).
• Dor e/ou distensão abdominais.
• Anorexia.
• Perda de peso.
• É mais comum que esses sinais sejam de início agudo, embora possam estar ocorrendo há semanas ou meses.

Achados do Exame Físico
• Podem exibir dor/desconforto abdominais evidentes.
• Dependendo da gravidade da intussuscepção e da duração de tempo de sua existência, alguns pacientes poderão revelar sinais de comprometimento cardiovascular.
• Pode ser palpável a presença de massa em formato de salsicha no abdome. A destreza em palpar a intussuscepção é variável.
• As intussuscepções ileocólicas podem se manifestar com protrusão do intussuscepto pelo reto. Isso pode ser diferenciado de prolapso retal pela introdução de sonda ao longo da lateral do tecido sobressalente. A presença de fórnix de fundo cego indica a existência de prolapso retal e não intussuscepção.

CAUSAS
• Qualquer doença que altere a motilidade gastrintestinal pode levar à intussuscepção. As causas conhecidas incluem: enterite, cirurgia abdominal recente, doença intestinal mural e parasitismo intestinal.
• As intussuscepções ocorrem em 8-33% dos cães submetidos a transplante de aloenxerto renal e 5% daqueles submetidos a enxertos de células hematopoiéticas. A razão para isso é incerta, mas pode estar relacionada com o uso de agentes imunossupressores.

DIAGNÓSTICO

DIAGNÓSTICO DIFERENCIAL
• Qualquer doença capaz de causar vômito e diarreia.
• Algumas intussuscepções podem ser de natureza crônica; portanto, um histórico crônico de vômito e/ou diarreia não descarta uma intussuscepção. Essa lista inclui, mas não é limitada a, parasitas intestinais, enterite viral (p. ex., infecções por parvovírus), enterite bacteriana, corpos estranhos, enteropatia inflamatória, vólvulo mesentérico e neoplasia intestinal.

HEMOGRAMA/BIOQUÍMICA/URINÁLISE
• Leucograma — pode variar de normal a leucopenia (especialmente na presença de sepse ou em caso de infecção por parvovírus) até leucocitose (resposta a estresse ou em alguns pacientes sépticos).
• Hematócrito — pode estar elevado (em caso de desidratação ou gastrenterite hemorrágica subjacente) ou diminuído (em caso de hemorragia intraluminal).
• Análise bioquímica — pode revelar desarranjos eletrolíticos em razão da perda por vômito ou diarreia. Tais anormalidades podem incluir hiponatremia, hipocloridemia, hipocalemia. O animal poderá exibir azotemia (pré-renal) se estiver significativamente desidratado. Também pode estar com hipoalbuminemia em razão da perda por efusão para o lúmen intestinal. Isso pode ocorrer no caso de alterações da permeabilidade intestinal subsequentes a necrose da mucosa intestinal.
• Urinálise — pode revelar densidade elevada em resposta à desidratação.

OUTROS TESTES LABORATORIAIS
• Podem-se observar níveis elevados de lactato em razão do comprometimento vascular ao segmento intestinal.
• A gasometria pode revelar acidose metabólica secundária à desidratação e hipoperfusão. Alternadamente, se a obstrução resultar em vômito principalmente gástrico (obstrução pilórica), poderá haver uma alcalose metabólica hipoclorêmica e hipocalêmica.

DIAGNÓSTICO POR IMAGEM
• Radiografias simples podem revelar um padrão intestinal obstrutivo. O grau de distensão intestinal pode estar relacionado com o grau de obstrução.
• Radiografias simples podem ou não demonstrar indícios de massa de tecido mole compatível com a intussuscepção.
• Em casos de intussuscepção gastresofágica, pode-se observar a presença de massa de tecido mole dentro do lúmen do esôfago próximo ao hiato esofágico do diafragma. Esses achados podem ser confundidos com hérnia de hiato, embora a gravidade dos sinais clínicos tipicamente associados a uma hérnia desse tipo seja muito mais branda em comparação a uma intussuscepção gastresofágica.
• A ultrassonografia do abdome é muito útil no diagnóstico de intussuscepções abdominais. A intussuscepção aparece como uma massa

INTUSSUSCEPÇÃO

padronizada-alvo em cortes transversais e como diversas linhas paralelas em cortes longitudinais.
• Estudos contrastados do trato GI superior ou enemas de bário podem ser proveitosos para apoiar o diagnóstico de intussuscepção.

ACHADOS PATOLÓGICOS
• O exame da intussuscepção revela a invaginação de segmento do intestino no segmento adjacente.
• O exame histopatológico demonstra graus variáveis de congestão venosa, comprometimento vascular, necrose da parede intestinal e peritonite.

TRATAMENTO

CUIDADO(S) DE SAÚDE ADEQUADO(S)
Os esforços iniciais devem se concentrar na estabilização do paciente, bem como na correção da desidratação e das anormalidades eletrolíticas existentes.

CUIDADO(S) DE ENFERMAGEM
• Administração de fluido intravenoso para corrigir a desidratação, além de repor as perdas contínuas previstas por meio de vômito e diarreia.
• Tipicamente, empregam-se os cristaloides isotônicos. A escolha específica do tipo de fluido é ditada pelos desarranjos eletrolíticos.

ATIVIDADE
É recomendável a atividade controlada por 10-14 dias do pós-operatório.

DIETA
• Se o paciente exibir vômitos ativos, não fornecer nada por via oral. Se isso ocorrer no pós-operatório, o íleo paralítico poderá ser uma causa subjacente.
• A maioria dos pacientes pode ser prontamente alimentada dentro de 24 h após a correção cirúrgica.

ORIENTAÇÃO AO PROPRIETÁRIO
• Intervenção cirúrgica imediata é o tratamento recomendado para as intussuscepções.
• Enfatizar a importância da identificação e do tratamento da causa subjacente.
• As complicações podem incluir: mortalidade perioperatória, peritonite séptica, estada hospitalar prolongada até a estabilização e recidiva. Há relatos de que as taxas de recidiva sejam de 6-27%.

CONSIDERAÇÕES CIRÚRGICAS
• A correção cirúrgica deve ser realizada assim que o animal estiver estabilizado o suficiente para suportar a anestesia e o procedimento cirúrgico. A intussuscepção é uma emergência cirúrgica.
• É recomendável a realização de laparotomia exploratória de todo o abdome para ajudar na identificação de quaisquer causas subjacentes em potencial. Além disso, pode haver múltiplas intussuscepções em um único paciente.
• Algumas intussuscepções podem ser reduzidas manualmente por uma espécie de ordenha suave do intussuscepto a partir do segmento intussuscipiente. À redução, o intestino pode ou não estar viável.
• No caso em que a redução manual não seja possível ou se a viabilidade do intestino for questionável, haverá necessidade de ressecção e anastomose intestinais.
• A enteroplicatura foi proposta como um procedimento para evitar a ocorrência de recidiva. Um artigo recente identificou alguns cães que necessitaram de um segundo procedimento cirúrgico para corrigir problemas mantidos pelo procedimento de enteroplicatura. É importante ter cuidado ao se realizar esse procedimento. Em poucas palavras, as voltas criadas no intestino devem ser suaves; portanto, é preciso evitar rotações bruscas nas alças intestinais. A camada submucosa das alças intestinais adjacentes deve ser incluída nas suturas, mas o lúmen não deve ser penetrado.

MEDICAÇÕES

MEDICAMENTO(S) DE ESCOLHA
• É recomendável o uso profilático de antibióticos. A escolha de antibióticos deve ser ditada pelas bactérias encontradas.
• A redução manual de uma intussuscepção é considerada um procedimento cirúrgico limpo, enquanto as técnicas de ressecção e anastomose intestinais são consideradas um procedimento "limpo contaminado".
• Não é aconselhável a administração de antibióticos a longo prazo, exceto nos casos em que haja peritonite séptica no pré ou pós-operatório.

CONTRAINDICAÇÕES
Alguns cirurgiões acreditam que as medicações que estimulem o peristaltismo (p. ex., metoclopramida) sejam contraindicadas por facilitarem a criação de um ambiente propício para a recidiva da intussuscepção.

ACOMPANHAMENTO

MONITORIZAÇÃO DO PACIENTE
• No pós-operatório, os pacientes devem ser mantidos sob fluidos intravenosos e analgésicos.
• A maioria das recidivas ocorre nos primeiros dias da cirurgia, embora haja relatos de recidivas até 3 semanas depois da cirurgia.
• Tipicamente, ocorre deiscência intestinal 3-5 dias depois do pós-operatório. Os sinais, o diagnóstico e o tratamento de peritonite séptica são abordados em outro lugar neste livro.

PREVENÇÃO
A prevenção de muitas das causas subjacentes pode ser obtida por meio de medidas como vacinação contra parvovírus, controle de parasitas intestinais, restrição de situações em que os pacientes podem ser expostos à imprudência alimentar ou ingestão de corpo estranho.

COMPLICAÇÕES POSSÍVEIS
• Recidiva — 6-27% dos pacientes.
• Peritonite séptica — pode resultar de deiscência intestinal pós-operatória ou contaminação intraoperatória.
• Síndrome do intestino curto — é uma complicação rara que pode ocorrer com ressecções maciças (geralmente >70% em cães) do intestino delgado.

EVOLUÇÃO ESPERADA E PROGNÓSTICO
• Dependem altamente da causa subjacente, do local da intussuscepção e do estado do animal à apresentação.
• Em geral, à medida que a intussuscepção se desloca mais no sentido distal, o prognóstico melhora, já que esses pacientes não são tão clinicamente acometidos. As intussuscepções gastresofágicas têm prognóstico grave com taxas de mortalidade que chegam a 95%, enquanto as intussuscepções intestinais apresentam prognóstico bom.

DIVERSOS

DISTÚRBIOS ASSOCIADOS
• As intussuscepções podem ser associadas a parasitas intestinais, enterite viral, doenças intestinais murais.
• As intussuscepções gastresofágicas são tipicamente associadas a algum distúrbio subjacente no esôfago.

FATORES RELACIONADOS COM A IDADE
Os pacientes mais jovens são tipicamente acometidos por enterite subjacente (viral ou bacteriana) ou parasitismo intestinal, enquanto os mais idosos costumam ser mais afetados por neoplasia intestinal.

VER TAMBÉM
• Obstrução Gastrintestinal.
• Peritonite.

ABREVIATURA(S)
• GI = gastrintestinal.

Sugestões de Leitura
Applewhite AA, Cornell KK, Selcer BA. Diagnosis and treatment of intussusceptions in dogs. Compend Contin Educ Pract Vet 2002, 24:110–127.
Brown DC. Small intestines. In: Slatter D, ed., Textbook of Small Animal Surgery, 3rd ed. Philadelphia: Saunders, 2003, pp. 644–664.
Oaks MG, Lewis DD, Hosgood G, et al. Enteroplication for the prevention of intussusception recurrence in dogs: 31 cases. JAVMA 1994, 205:72–75.

Autor S. Brent Reimer
Consultor Editorial Albert E. Jergens

Laceração da Parede Atrial

CONSIDERAÇÕES GERAIS

REVISÃO
• Laceração endocárdica é um defeito linear limitado à camada endocárdica do átrio (tipicamente o átrio esquerdo) resultante da distensão da parede atrial além de seus limites elásticos. • Também poderá ocorrer uma laceração da parede atrial se a fenda ou a separação se estender através do miocárdio e do epicárdio, culminando em um defeito de espessura completa na parede atrial e hemorragia no espaço pericárdico.

FISIOPATOLOGIA
• A laceração endocárdica tipicamente resulta de aumento na pressão atrial esquerda secundária à regurgitação mitral grave; a degeneração endocárdica também pode desempenhar um papel. • Se a laceração for incompleta, a fibrina poderá selar o defeito temporariamente; isso cicatriza como uma depressão linear na superfície endocárdica ou subsequentemente se estende através do miocárdio, resultando em uma laceração completa do átrio esquerdo. • Uma laceração do átrio esquerdo resulta em sangramento superagudo no saco pericárdico, bem como no comprometimento hemodinâmico grave potencialmente letal secundário a tamponamento cardíaco agudo. • Se ocorrer uma laceração no septo interatrial, pode-se formar um defeito adquirido do septo atrial. • Raramente, também pode ocorrer laceração de qualquer um dos átrios secundária a traumatismo rombo.

SISTEMA(S) ACOMETIDO(S)
• Cardiovascular. • Respiratório.

GENÉTICA
Foi demonstrado que a predisposição à endocardiose tem um componente hereditário em algumas raças.

INCIDÊNCIA/PREVALÊNCIA
A laceração atrial é uma causa rara de efusão pericárdica hemorrágica no cão, compreendendo cerca de 2% dos casos de efusão no pericárdio.

IDENTIFICAÇÃO
Espécies
Cães; incomum em gatos.

Raça(s) Predominante(s)
• O mesmo que as raças predisponentes para endocardiose; mais comum em raças caninas de pequeno a médio porte. • As raças Poodle, Dachshund, Cocker spaniel e Pastor de Shetland podem ser super-representadas. • Se o traumatismo for a causa, qualquer raça poderá ser representada.

Idade Média e Faixa Etária
Cães de meia-idade a mais idosos estão predispostos.

Sexo Predominante
Em cães machos, observa-se uma incidência mais alta tanto de endocardiose como de laceração do átrio esquerdo.

SINAIS CLÍNICOS
Achados Anamnésicos
• Início agudo de fraqueza e colapso, que podem evoluir rapidamente para parada respiratória ou cardiopulmonar; o episódio pode suceder um período de agitação ou atividade acentuada. • O histórico de cardiopatia de longa duração com sinais de ICC é descrito em grande parte dos pacientes. • Comumente se observa piora aguda de tosse ou dispneia. • Possível histórico de traumatismo rombo.

Achados do Exame Físico
• Colapso.
• Taquicardia.
• Pulsos arteriais débeis (fracos) ou pulso paradoxal.
• Mucosas pálidas, lodosas ou cinzentas; tempo de preenchimento capilar prolongado.
• Outros sinais de cardiopatia significativa (p. ex., sopro, ritmo de galope, arritmia, tosse ou dispneia) estão tipicamente presentes.
• Sinais de insuficiência cardíaca direita (p. ex., ascite e distensão venosa jugular) também podem ser observados em determinados pacientes.
• As bulhas cardíacas podem estar abafadas; se auscultado antes da ocorrência de laceração da parede atrial, o sopro pode estar reduzido em termos de intensidade.

CAUSAS E FATORES DE RISCO
• Endocardiose da valva atrioventricular esquerda (mitral) — valvopatia crônica.
• Miocardiopatia dilatada.
• Persistência do ducto arterioso.
• Neoplasias cardíacas, mais comumente hemangiossarcoma.
• Traumatismo torácico.
• Cateterização cardíaca.

FATORES DE RISCO
• Regurgitação mitral grave, além do aumento de volume do átrio esquerdo.
• Pode ser precipitada por algum episódio de agitação, estresse ou atividade.

DIAGNÓSTICO

DIAGNÓSTICO DIFERENCIAL
• Outras causas de colapso cardiovascular agudo.
• Efusão pericárdica proveniente de outras causas (p. ex., neoplásicas e idiopáticas).
• Insuficiência cardíaca.
• Arritmias cardíacas graves.
• Infarto do miocárdio.
• Tromboembolia pulmonar.
• Outras causas de hipotensão.

HEMOGRAMA/BIOQUÍMICA/URINÁLISE
• É rara a ocorrência de anemia a menos que seja efetuado o procedimento de pericardiocentese, já que o volume de perda sanguínea é relativamente pequeno.
• Elevações nos níveis séricos de lactato, além de acidose metabólica.
• Aumento na atividade das enzimas ALT e AST em alguns pacientes.
• Azotemia pré-renal; é possível a constatação de hiponatremia ou outros desarranjos eletrolíticos.

OUTROS TESTES LABORATORIAIS
Os níveis da porção N-terminal do pró-peptídeo natriurético cerebral e da troponina-I podem estar elevados.

DIAGNÓSTICO POR IMAGEM
Achados Radiográficos
• Espera-se um aumento de volume moderado a grave no átrio esquerdo.
• A comparação com outras radiografias torácicas prévias pode revelar o arredondamento e aumento extra da silhueta cardíaca; a silhueta cardíaca globoide característica associada à efusão pericárdica pode ser mais evidente na projeção dorsoventral.
• Haverá infiltrados pulmonares intersticiais a alveolares na presença de ICC esquerda concomitante.
• Alterações como efusão pleural de pequeno volume, ascite, hepatomegalia e veia cava caudal grande podem ser observadas em virtude de ICC direita.

Achados Ecocardiográficos
• Efusão pericárdica é observada como um espaço hipoecoico entre o coração e o saco pericárdico; já o volume da efusão pericárdica identificado pode ser relativamente pequeno, pois o pericárdio permanece inelástico em função da natureza aguda do sangramento; pode ser observada a presença de coágulo sanguíneo hiperecoico linear característico dentro do saco pericárdico.
• Com frequência, a laceração real não é identificada, embora um trombo associado seja ocasionalmente visualizado dentro do átrio esquerdo.
• O tamponamento cardíaco é evidenciado por colapso diastólico do átrio e/ou do ventrículo direito.
• Sinais de endocardiose mitral avançada, incluindo espessamento e prolapso dessa valva atrioventricular esquerda, regurgitação mitral moderada a grave, aumento de volume moderado a grave do átrio esquerdo e frequentemente uma ou mais cordas tendíneas rompidas.

MÉTODOS DIAGNÓSTICOS
Achados Eletrocardiográficos
• Taquicardia sinusal.
• Arritmias atriais ou ventriculares.
• Diminuição na amplitude dos complexos QRS.
• Alternância elétrica.
• Anormalidades do segmento ST.
• Possível padrão de aumento de volume do átrio ou ventrículo esquerdos.

ACHADOS PATOLÓGICOS
• A laceração endocárdica é observada macroscopicamente como uma depressão linear pálida ou branca no endocárdio atrial.
• As lacerações da parede atrial aparecem como defeitos de espessura completa que se estendem através do endocárdio, miocárdio e epicárdio atriais; pode ou não haver trombo associado. A face caudolateral do átrio esquerdo é mais comumente acometida, com a ocorrência de muitas lacerações na junção atrioauricular.
• Em casos de lacerações agudas, observa-se efusão pericárdica hemorrágica ou trombo pericárdico.
• A endocardiose mitral caracteriza-se por folhetos espessados dessa valva atrioventricular esquerda com bordas enroladas; também pode ser observada ruptura das cordas tendíneas; são possíveis lesões de jato atriais.
• Em caso de aumento de volume grave do átrio esquerdo, espera-se uma cardiomegalia.

TRATAMENTO

• Em caso de forte suspeita de laceração do átrio esquerdo, deve-se efetuar a pericardiocentese apenas se a efusão estiver provocando um tamponamento cardíaco potencialmente letal e

LACERAÇÃO DA PAREDE ATRIAL

sintomático, pois pode ocorrer uma hemorragia extra no saco pericárdio ou exsanguinação assim que o líquido pericárdico for removido.
• Se a pericardiocentese for realizada, remover apenas uma quantidade suficiente de líquido para melhorar os sinais clínicos.
• É provável que a realização da pericardiocentese não seja uma tarefa fácil, considerando-se o pequeno volume de efusão tipicamente identificado, o aumento cardíaco grave e o pequeno porte de grande parte dos cães com ruptura do átrio esquerdo; a orientação ultrassonográfica e a monitorização eletrocardiográfica contínua são altamente recomendadas.
• Os melhores métodos para o tratamento de lacerações do átrio esquerdo não foram claramente estabelecidos; no entanto, é recomendável o tratamento médico rigoroso para reduzir a pressão atrial esquerda, utilizando redutores da pré e pós-carga, com base na experiência clínica da autora.
• Caso se forme um coágulo de fibrina sobre o defeito, o paciente poderá se estabilizar e se recuperar.

CUIDADO(S) DE ENFERMAGEM
• Administrar o oxigênio a cães com dispneia ou sinais de instabilidade hemodinâmica.
• Administrar fluidos IV ou produtos derivados do sangue apenas se houver indícios de hipovolemia; a maioria dos cães permanece em estado de sobrecarga volêmica e, com isso, a maior expansão de volume intravascular aumentará a pressão atrial esquerda e potencialmente agravará o tamponamento.

ATIVIDADE
O repouso estrito em gaiola no período agudo deve ser seguido por restrição crônica da atividade física.

ORIENTAÇÃO AO PROPRIETÁRIO
A laceração atrial esquerda tipicamente acompanha cardiopatia avançada, havendo a necessidade de terapia clínica crônica; embora o prognóstico seja reservado quanto a sobrevida após evento agudo, alguns cães com laceração atrial esquerda vivem mais de um ano depois do incidente.

CONSIDERAÇÕES CIRÚRGICAS
• O procedimento de toracotomia exploratória poderá ser considerado se a hemorragia persistir ou recidivar, embora deva ser feito com cautela, dado o estado avançado da cardiopatia tipicamente presente.
• Punção transeptal com introdução de cateter e laceração da fossa oval com balão também podem ser contempladas para descomprimir o átrio esquerdo; no entanto, isso pode resultar em insuficiência cardíaca direita ou hipoxemia por desvio da direita para a esquerda.

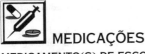

MEDICAÇÕES
MEDICAMENTO(S) DE ESCOLHA
• As lacerações atriais ocorrem secundariamente ao aumento na pressão atrial esquerda; dessa forma, a terapia clínica deve se concentrar na redução das pressões atriais esquerdas para diminuir a hemorragia contínua no espaço pericárdico e permitir a formação de coágulo de fibrina no local da laceração; isso pode ser obtido com redutores da pré-carga (p. ex., diuréticos, pasta de nitroglicerina) e/ou da pós-carga (vasodilatadores arteriais).
• A redução tanto da pré como da pós-carga precisa ser empreendida com cuidado para evitar a piora do comprometimento hemodinâmico.
• A diminuição da pós-carga pode ser alcançada por meio de doses conservadoras de nitroprussseto de sódio; uma dose inicial baixa de 0,5-1 µg/kg/min sob infusão em velocidade constante é recomendada para produzir uma queda na pressão atrial esquerda, sem precipitar uma hipotensão significativa; é aconselhável a monitorização da pressão arterial, podendo-se titular a dose para cima, conforme a necessidade, a cada 15-30 minutos até, no máximo, 10 µg/kg/min para obter a melhora nos sinais clínicos e/ou o declínio na pressão arterial de 10-15 mmHg.
• Alternativamente, o anlodipino pode ser iniciado a uma dose de 0,1-0,2 mg/kg VO a cada 24 h; a terapia crônica com esse agente pode ser implementada em animais normotensos ou hipertensos para reduzir a fração regurgitante e diminuir a pressão atrial esquerda.
• Os diuréticos devem ser usados com cuidado, se necessários, para tratar dispneia associada à ICC concomitante (p. ex., 1-2 mg/kg de furosemida por via IV, conforme a necessidade); os sinais de ICC esquerda podem se agravar à medida que o tamponamento cardíaco se resolve em virtude do aumento na pré-carga; nesse caso, poderá haver a necessidade de terapia diurética mais rigorosa.
• Pimobendana (0,2-0,3 mg/kg VO a cada 12 h) pode resultar em maior redução da pressão atrial esquerda, embora os estudos não tenham avaliado de forma específica o uso desse agente no quadro de ruptura do átrio esquerdo.
• Assim que o paciente se encontrar estabilizado, é recomendável a implementação de inibidores da ECA (p. ex., enalapril a 0,5 mg/kg a cada 12-24 h) para o controle crônico de insuficiência cardíaca concomitante.

PRECAUÇÕES
• Nesses pacientes, não se justifica uma fluidoterapia rigorosa; a expansão volêmica adicional pode aumentar a pressão atrial esquerda, agravar o tamponamento cardíaco e contribuir para o comprometimento hemodinâmico.
• Os melhores métodos para o tratamento da laceração atrial esquerda não foram claramente estabelecidos; a escolha de se realizar ou não a pericardiocentese e de se administrar ou não redutores da pré e/ou pós-carga deve ser feita com base na avaliação do estado volêmico, da pressão arterial e da estabilidade clínica do paciente.

INTERAÇÕES POSSÍVEIS
O nitroprussseto de sódio nunca deve ser administrado concomitantemente com inibidores da fosfodiesterase tipo V (p. ex., sildenafila ou tadalafila) em virtude do potencial de hipotensão sistêmica com risco de vida.

ACOMPANHAMENTO
MONITORIZAÇÃO DO PACIENTE
• É recomendável a monitorização estreita da frequência e do esforço respiratórios, da coloração das mucosas e do tempo de preenchimento capilar, bem como da qualidade do pulso e da frequência cardíaca; também é aconselhável a monitorização da pressão arterial caso se faça uso de vasodilatadores arteriais.
• O exame de acompanhamento com ecocardiografia ajuda a determinar a resolução da efusão pericárdica e a reabsorção de algum coágulo atrial ou pericárdico.
• Em seguida, recomenda-se o acompanhamento minucioso a cada 2-3 meses para verificações repetidas do líquido pericárdico e ajustes da medicação, conforme se julgar pertinente.

PREVENÇÃO
É recomendável evitar atividade física e agitação extenuantes.

COMPLICAÇÕES POSSÍVEIS
• Mesmo se a laceração se fechar, o paciente fica propenso a novas lacerações por conta da cardiopatia subjacente.
• A maioria dos cães terá ou desenvolverá ICC concomitante.

EVOLUÇÃO ESPERADA E PROGNÓSTICO
O prognóstico quanto à sobrevida é reservado a mau; no entanto, alguns animais podem viver bem por alguns meses ou mais com monitorização estrita, restrição da atividade física e tratamento clínico ideal da cardiopatia.

DIVERSOS
DISTÚRBIOS ASSOCIADOS
• ICC.
• Compressão dos brônquios do tronco principal.
• Hipertensão pulmonar.

SINÔNIMOS
• Ruptura atrial.
• Laceração atrial.

VER TAMBÉM
• Capítulos sobre ICC.
• "Efusão Pericárdica".

ABREVIATURAS
• ALT = alanina aminotransferase.
• AST = aspartato aminotransferase.
• ECA = enzima conversora de angiotensina.
• ICC = insuficiência cardíaca congestiva.

RECURSOS DA INTERNET
James Buchanan Cardiology Library: http://www.vin.com/MEMBERS/CMS/Misc/Default.aspx?id=7703.

Sugestões de Leitura
Fox PR, Sisson D, Moise S. Textbook of Canine and Feline Cardiology. Philadelphia: Saunders, 1999.
Reineke EL, Burkett DE, Drobatz KJ. Left atrial rupture in dogs: 14 cases (1990-2005). J Vet Emerg Crit Care 2008, 18:158-164.
Rush JR. Chronic valvular disease in dogs. In: Bonagura JD, Twedt DC, eds., Kirk's Current Veterinary Therapy XIV. St. Louis: Saunders Elsevier, 2009, pp. 780-786.
Sadanaga KK, MacDonald MJ, Buchanan JW. Echocardiography and surgery in a dog with left atrial rupture and hemopericardium. J Vet Intern Med 1990, 4:216-221.

Autor Suzanne M. Cunningham
Consultores Editoriais Larry P. Tilley e Francis W.K. Smith, Jr.

Lacerações da Córnea e Esclera

CONSIDERAÇÕES GERAIS

DEFINIÇÃO
• Penetrantes — ferida ou corpo estranho que penetra, mas não atravessa completamente, a córnea ou a esclera. • Perfurantes — ferida ou corpo estranho que atravessa a córnea ou a esclera por completo; maior risco de perda da visão, quando comparado às lesões penetrantes.
• Simples — envolvem apenas a córnea ou a esclera; podem ser penetrantes ou perfurantes; as outras estruturas oculares permanecem intactas.
• Complicadas — perfurante; envolvem outras estruturas, além da córnea ou da esclera; encarceramento ou prolapso uveal, vítreo ou retiniano através da ferida; catarata traumática; hifema; lacerações palpebrais.

FISIOPATOLOGIA
• Traumatismo penetrante — feridas ocasionadas por mecanismo de fora para dentro.
• Traumatismo rombo — feridas provocadas por mecanismo de dentro para fora; o olho sofre alterações súbitas em suas dimensões equatorial e axial, bem como na pressão intraocular; o ferimento real pode estar situado em outra região que não seja o ponto de impacto; frequentemente, gera muito mais danos do que o traumatismo penetrante. • Todo o corpo estranho ou parte dele que desencadeia a lesão pode ficar retido na ferida ou no olho.

SISTEMA(S) ACOMETIDO(S)
• Musculosquelético — crânio ou tecido orbital circunjacente.
• Nervoso — inconsciência ou lesão cerebral.
• Oftálmico.

INCIDÊNCIA/PREVALÊNCIA
Comum.

IDENTIFICAÇÃO
Espécies
Cães e gatos.

SINAIS CLÍNICOS
Achados Anamnésicos
• Geralmente de início agudo.
• Histórico comum de passeio por vegetação densa, tiro por armas de fogo ou outros projéteis balísticos ou arranhadura por outro gato.
• O traumatismo pode não ser observado.

Achados do Exame Físico
• Variam com os tecidos acometidos.
• Comuns — deformidades corneana, esclerótica ou palpebral; edema; hemorragia.
• Pode-se observar o corpo estranho retido.
• Muitas vezes, cicatrizam-se com rapidez; podem aparecer apenas como hematoma subconjuntival.
• Também podem ser vistos defeitos da íris, distorção da pupila, hifema, catarata, hemorragia do humor vítreo, descolamento da retina e exoftalmia.

CAUSAS
Traumatismo rombo ou penetrante.

FATORES DE RISCO
• Diminuição na acuidade visual preexistente.
• Animais jovens, ingênuos ou altamente inquietos.
• Caça ou corrida por vegetação densa.
• Brigas.

DIAGNÓSTICO

DIAGNÓSTICO DIFERENCIAL
• A anamnese ou a presença de corpo estranho retido costumam ser diagnósticos. • Em caso de não observação do evento traumático e não constatação do corpo estranho — considerar úlcera de córnea não traumática, hifema, etc.
• Ceratite ulcerativa traumática — início agudo; formatos linear, estrelado ou em V; possivelmente múltipla. • Hifema traumático — quase invariavelmente acompanhado por lesões corneanas ou escleróticas, bem como por hemorragia subconjuntival ou periocular.
• Cataratas traumáticas — é comum a ruptura da cápsula do cristalino. • Descolamento traumático da retina — quase invariavelmente acompanhado por hemorragia intraocular.

HEMOGRAMA/BIOQUÍMICA/URINÁLISE
• Em geral, não colaboram com o diagnóstico.
• Considerar como triagem pré-anestésica ou diante de possível causa não traumática.

OUTROS TESTES LABORATORIAIS
• Exame citológico, cultura aeróbia, antibiograma da ferida e do corpo estranho — recomendados mesmo que a infecção não esteja aparente; pode ser necessária a coleta da amostra sob anestesia geral no momento da cirurgia. • Levar em consideração outros testes (contagem plaquetária, perfil de coagulação, etc.) na possibilidade de causas não traumáticas.

DIAGNÓSTICO POR IMAGEM
• Ultrassonografia ocular — se os meios oculares se apresentarem opacos; pode esclarecer o grau e a natureza da doença intraocular; pode detectar a presença de corpo estranho. • Radiografias ou TC orbitais — podem ajudar a determinar o trajeto do projétil balístico; podem detectar a presença de corpo estranho.

MÉTODOS DIAGNÓSTICOS
• Determinam a natureza, a força e a direção de impacto do objeto — ajudam a identificar quais os tecidos possivelmente envolvidos. • Não aplicar pressão sobre o olho até se descartar ruptura ou laceração do bulbo ocular. • Avaliar a visão — resposta à ameaça; aversão à luz brilhante/intensa.
• Pele periocular e órbita — examinar em busca de lacerações ou deformidades; suspeitar de envolvimento do bulbo ocular se uma laceração palpebral atravessar a margem das pálpebras ou penetrar no septo da órbita; os pontos de entrada são frequentemente pequenos e cicatrizam-se com rapidez. • Motilidade ocular anormal — sugere traumatismo dos músculos extraoculares, hemorragia ou edema orbitais, corpos estranhos retidos ou dano aos nervos periféricos ou ao SNC.
• Ruptura esclerótica — considerar essa possibilidade em casos de hemorragia subconjuntival, sobretudo se a câmara anterior estiver anormalmente profunda ou superficial, se houver hemorragia do humor vítreo ou se o olho se encontrar anormalmente flácido. • Pupilas — tamanho; formato; simetria; reflexos direto e consensual à luz. • Oftalmoscopia detalhada — avalia a transparência dos meios intraoculares e a integridade do fundo ocular; descartar corpo estranho intraocular. • Teste de Seidel — se houver qualquer dúvida a respeito de extravasamento corneano ou esclerótico; utilizar uma tira de fluoresceína, seca a levemente umedecida, para tingir ou corar uma camada delgada desse corante na superfície do defeito; o humor aquoso extravasado combina-se com a cor laranja da fluoresceína, formando uma espécie de diminuto córrego verde fluorescente (mais bem observado com uma iluminação de cobalto).

ACHADOS PATOLÓGICOS
• Dependem das feridas e dos tecidos acometidos.
• Em geral, correlacionam-se estreitamente com os achados do exame físico. • Hemorragia do humor vítreo — pode se organizar em uma banda fibrosa, que exerce uma tração sobre a retina, levando ao seu descolamento. • Sarcoma pós-traumático (gatos) — pode ocorrer meses a anos após traumatismo ocular grave.

TRATAMENTO

CUIDADO(S) DE SAÚDE ADEQUADO(S)
• Depende da gravidade.
• Esquema ambulatorial — caso se garanta a integridade do bulbo ocular.

CUIDADO(S) DE ENFERMAGEM
• Sedação — considerada em pacientes inquietos ou indóceis.
• Durante os passeios — colocar um colar elizabetano e usar uma coleira peitoral ou passar o membro torácico ipsilateral através da guia, a fim de evitar a compressão cervical e o consequente aumento na pressão intraocular do olho acometido.
• Evitar o uso de retalhos (*flaps*) elaborados a partir da terceira pálpebra em pacientes com perfurações ou feridas penetrantes profundas ou extensas.

Lesões Consideradas para Tratamento Clínico
• Feridas não penetrantes, sem nenhuma sobreposição ou espaçamento da margem da lesão — usar um colar elizabetano; instilar soluções oftalmológicas tópicas de antibióticos ou de atropina.
• Feridas não perfurantes, com leve espaçamento da lesão ou margens em declive — aplicar lentes de contato terapêuticas flexíveis, além do colar elizabetano; instilar soluções oftalmológicas tópicas de antibióticos ou de atropina.
• Perfuração corneana puntiforme simples de espessura completa, com teste de Seidel negativo, que exibe a câmara anterior formada e não apresenta nenhum prolapso uveal — pacientes sedentários; utilizar lentes de contato terapêuticas flexíveis, além do colar elizabetano; instilar soluções oftalmológicas tópicas de antibióticos e de atropina; reavaliar algumas horas após a aplicação da lente e depois em 24 e 48 h.

ATIVIDADE
Geralmente, os animais ficam confinados dentro de casa (gatos) ou limitados a passeios com coleira até que a cicatrização esteja concluída. Para reduzir a pressão sobre o pescoço e o risco de aumento da pressão intraocular com extravasamento da ferida, prefere-se o uso de peitoral à coleira.

ORIENTAÇÃO AO PROPRIETÁRIO
Alertar o proprietário quanto à possibilidade da não manifestação de toda a extensão da lesão (cataratas, descolamentos da retina, infecções) até alguns dias ou semanas após o dano e à necessidade do acompanhamento prolongado.

LACERAÇÕES DA CÓRNEA E ESCLERA

CONSIDERAÇÕES CIRÚRGICAS

Lesões com Necessidade de Exploração ou Reparo Cirúrgicos
• Lacerações corneanas de espessura completa, com teste de Seidel positivo. • Feridas de espessura completa, com encarceramento ou prolapso iridianos. • Lacerações escleróticas ou corneosclerais de espessura completa. • Suspeita de retenção de corpo estranho ou ruptura da esclera posterior. • Ferida simples não perfurante com margens que se mostram moderada ou abertamente espaçadas e ainda são longas ou correspondem a mais de dois terços da espessura da córnea.

Lesões Consideradas para Exploração ou Reparo Cirúrgicos
• Lacerações corneanas pequenas de espessura completa, com teste de Seidel negativo e sem encarceramento ou prolapso do tecido uveal.
• Lacerações conjuntivais amplas. • Lacerações corneanas ou escleróticas de espessura parcial em paciente ativo.

MEDICAÇÕES

MEDICAMENTO(S) DE ESCOLHA

Antibióticos
• Feridas complicadas, aquelas com retenção de plantas e outras causadas por traumatismo rombo com desvitalização tecidual — a infecção é comum.
• Endoftalmite bacteriana — 5-7% das perfurações; muito rara em feridas penetrantes, mas não perfurantes, da córnea.
• Feridas penetrantes — antibióticos tópicos isolados (p. ex., neomicina, polimixina B e bacitracina) ou solução de gentamicina a cada 6-8 h; em geral, é suficiente.
• Feridas perfurantes com teste de Seidel negativo — ciprofloxacino sistêmico (cães, 10-20 mg/kg VO a cada 24 h), cefazolina tópica (33 mg/mL, adicionando-se cefazolina injetável às lágrimas artificiais) e gentamicina ou tobramicina fortificadas (adicionar um aminoglicosídeo injetável à solução oftalmológica comercial para atingir a concentração final de 14 mg/mL), ambas a cada 4-6 h.
• Feridas perfurantes com teste de Seidel positivo — ciprofloxacino sistêmico (cães, 10-20 mg/kg VO a cada 24 h); cefazolina tópica e gentamicina ou tobramicina fortificadas, conforme exposto acima, somente quando o defeito se tornar impermeável.

Anti-inflamatórios
• Soluções tópicas de dexametasona a 0,1% ou de acetato de prednisolona a 1% — a cada 6-12 h; assim que a ferida for suturada ou sofrer epitelização (fica negativa à coloração com fluoresceína), contanto que não haja infecção.
• Prednisona sistêmica — 0,5-1 mg/kg a cada 12-24 h; indicada em casos de feridas suturadas ou epitelizadas, quando a inflamação se mostrar grave; no envolvimento do cristalino ou de estruturas mais posteriores; em casos de infecção ou não epitelização da ferida e obrigatoriedade do controle da inflamação para preservar o olho.
• AINEs tópicos — flurbiprofeno ou um de vários outros; poderão ser utilizados se os corticosteroides tópicos forem contraindicados e o controle da inflamação for obrigatório para preservar o olho.

Midriáticos
• Solução oftalmológica de atropina a 1% — a cada 6-12 h; em casos de miose significativa ou reação da câmara anterior.

Analgésicos
• Atropina tópica ou ácido acetilsalicílico oral (cães, 10-15 mg/kg VO, a cada 12–8 h) — podem proporcionar alívio suficiente da dor.
• Carprofeno — 2,2 mg/kg VO a cada 12 h ou 4,4 mg VO a cada 24 h.
• Tramadol — iniciar com a dose de 1–2 mg/kg a cada 12 h, podendo aumentá-la até 5 mg/kg a cada 6 h ou conforme a necessidade.
• Butorfanol — cães, 0,2-0,4 mg/kg; gatos, 0,1-0,2 mg/kg IV, SC ou IM a cada 2-4 h ou conforme a necessidade; dor leve aguda; não há necessidade de sedação.
• Oximorfona — cães, 0,05-0,1 mg/kg; gatos, 0,05 mg/kg IV, SC ou IM a cada 4-6 h ou conforme a necessidade; dor grave aguda; há necessidade de sedação.
• Naloxona — 0,04 mg/kg IV, SC ou IM, para reverter o efeito de narcóticos.

CONTRAINDICAÇÕES
• Pomadas oftalmológicas tópicas — evitar em casos de perfurações com teste de Seidel positivo.
• Ciprofloxacino sistêmico — evitar em raças caninas de porte pequeno e médio entre 2-8 meses de vida, de porte grande entre 2-12 meses e de porte gigante entre 2-18 meses; potencial de dano à cartilagem articular de crescimento rápido.

PRECAUÇÕES
• Aminoglicosídeos — a aplicação tópica poderá ser irritante e impedir a reepitelização, se forem utilizados com frequência e em concentrações altas; possibilidade de intoxicação quando administrados em pacientes muito pequenos ou quando fornecidos por mais de uma via.
• As soluções tópicas poderão ser preferíveis às pomadas se a integridade da córnea for questionável.
• Atropina — pode exacerbar a ceratoconjuntivite seca e o glaucoma.
• AINEs tópicos ou sistêmicos — utilizar com cautela em casos de hifema; não se conhece a segurança dos AINE tópicos em gatos.

INTERAÇÕES POSSÍVEIS
AINEs sistêmicos — podem potencializar a nefrotoxicidade dos aminoglicosídeos; garantir a hidratação satisfatória e a função renal adequada, especialmente em cães de pequeno porte.

MEDICAMENTO(S) ALTERNATIVO(S)
Solução oftalmológica tópica de ciprofloxacino — pode ser utilizada no lugar da combinação de cefazolina tópica e algum aminoglicosídeo fortificado; alguns estreptococos são resistentes.

ACOMPANHAMENTO

MONITORIZAÇÃO DO PACIENTE
• Feridas penetrantes profundas ou extensas não submetidas ainda à sutura e feridas perfurantes — reavaliadas a cada 24-48 h durante os primeiros dias para garantir a integridade do bulbo ocular, monitorizar a presença de infecção e verificar o controle da inflamação ocular.
• Feridas penetrantes superficiais — avaliadas geralmente em intervalos de 3-5 dias até a cicatrização.
• Antibioticoterapia — alterada de acordo com os resultados da cultura e do antibiograma.

PREVENÇÃO
• É preciso ter cuidado ao se introduzir novos filhotes de cães em ambientes domésticos com gatos que possuam garras nas patas dianteiras.
• Minimizar as atividades de corrida por vegetações densas ou ter um frasco de soro fisiológico à mão para irrigar os olhos e remover os debris.
• Minimizar a exposição de cães com cegueira ou diminuição na acuidade visual à vegetação densa.

COMPLICAÇÕES POSSÍVEIS
• Perda do olho ou da visão.
• Inflamação ou dor oculares crônicas.
• Sarcoma pós-traumático — pode se desenvolver em olhos de gatos cegos que sofreram grave traumatismo; considerar o procedimento de enucleação em todos os olhos felinos traumatizados e cegos para evitar o aparecimento desse tipo de sarcoma.

EVOLUÇÃO ESPERADA E PROGNÓSTICO
• A maioria dos olhos com lacerações da córnea ou retenção de corpos estranhos também na córnea é passível de recuperação.
• Quanto mais posterior for a lesão, pior será o prognóstico quanto à manutenção da visão.
• Prognóstico mau — envolvimento esclerótico ou uveal; sem percepção luminosa; lesões perfurantes com acometimento do cristalino ou em casos de hemorragia vítrea ou descolamento da retina significativos.
• As lesões penetrantes costumam ter prognóstico melhor, quando comparadas às perfurantes.
• O traumatismo rombo carreia prognóstico pior que o penetrante.

DIVERSOS

DISTÚRBIOS ASSOCIADOS
Dependem da natureza e do grau da lesão.

GESTAÇÃO/FERTILIDADE/REPRODUÇÃO
• Corticosteroides sistêmicos — podem complicar a prenhez.
• Ciprofloxacino sistêmico — provavelmente deve ser evitado durante a prenhez.

VER TAMBÉM
• Catarata.
• Ceratite Ulcerativa.
• Descolamento da Retina.
• Hifema.
• Proptose.

ABREVIATURA(S)
• AINEs = anti-inflamatórios não esteroides.
• SNC = sistema nervoso central.
• TC = tomografia computadorizada.

RECURSOS DA INTERNET
http://dro.hs.columbia.edu/rptglobe.htm.

Sugestões de Leitura
Gilger BC, Bentley E, Ollivier FJ. Diseases and surgery of the canine cornea and sclera. In: Gerlatt KN, ed., Veterinary Ophthalmology, 4th ed. Ames, IA: Blackwell, 2007, pp. 690-752.

Autor Paul E. Miller
Consultor Editorial Paul E. Miller

Laringopatia

CONSIDERAÇÕES GERAIS

DEFINIÇÃO
• A laringe é composta de estruturas cartilaginosas que circundam a rima da glote. As funções da laringe são controlar o fluxo de ar durante a respiração, proteger as vias aéreas inferiores de aspiração durante a deglutição e controlar a fonação. • As laringopatias em cães e gatos incluem paralisia da laringe, laringite aguda, laringite obstrutiva, colapso da laringe pela síndrome braquicefálica das vias aéreas, obstrução por corpo estranho, neoplasia e traumatismo.

FISIOPATOLOGIA
• Qualquer diminuição no diâmetro da abertura da laringe aumentará a resistência ao fluxo de ar e resultará em estridor à inspiração. A redução no fluxo de ar levará à hipoxia, cianose ou angústia respiratória e declínio na troca de calor (intolerância ao calor, hipertermia). • Inflamação ou lesões das cordas vocais podem induzir à afonia ou alteração no latido ou miado.

SISTEMA(S) ACOMETIDO(S)
• Respiratório — podem ocorrer pneumonia por aspiração e hipoventilação com cianose quando a função da laringe fica comprometida.
• Cardiovascular — a hipoxia pode levar à taquicardia. • Gastrintestinal — podem ocorrer ânsia de vômito (vômito seco), regurgitação, vômito e/ou disfagia em caso de polineuropatia que provoque paralisia da laringe e disfunção do esôfago; esofagite é frequentemente associada à síndrome braquicefálica das vias aéreas. • Nervoso — podem ocorrer depressão, estupor ou coma se a obstrução grave da laringe induzir à hipertermia maligna.

GENÉTICA
• A paralisia laríngea juvenil no Bouvier des Flandres é transmitida como um traço dominante, embora a base molecular dessa doença não tenha sido elucidada. • Em paralisia da laringe associada à polineuropatia no cão Leonberger, sugere-se uma herança ligada ao cromossomo X. • Foi comprovado que nenhum outro distúrbio da laringe seja genético no cão ou gato, embora haja relatos de condições familiares e predisposições raciais.

INCIDÊNCIA/PREVALÊNCIA
• As laringopatias são muito mais comuns em cães do que em gatos. • Atualmente, a paralisia congênita da laringe é só esporádica no Bouvier des Flandres. • A paralisia idiopática da laringe é uma doença comum de cães mais idosos pertencentes a raças de grande porte; no entanto, a prevalência exata é desconhecida. • A síndrome braquicefálica das vias aéreas é uma síndrome comum nos cães da raça Buldogue francês e inglês.
• A ocorrência de traumatismo e o desenvolvimento de neoplasia na laringe são raros.

IDENTIFICAÇÃO
Espécies
Cães e gatos.

Raça(s) Predominante(s)
• O complexo paralisia laríngea/polineuropatia familiar ocorre nas raças Dálmata, Rottweiler, Leonberger e Montanhês dos Pirineus (Grande Pireneus). • A paralisia congênita da laringe é encontrada em cães das raças Bouvier des Flandres, Husky, mestiços de Husky, Pastor alemão branco e, provavelmente, Bull terrier. • A paralisia adquirida idiopática da laringe é constatada com maior frequência em raças caninas de grande porte (especialmente Labrador e Golden retrievers). • A síndrome braquicefálica das vias aéreas, como o próprio nome diz, é verificada em raças braquicefálicas de cães. • Os cães da raça Golden retriever são propensos a rabdomioma laríngeo.

Idade Média e Faixa Etária
• Paralisia congênita e familiar da laringe — o início dos sinais clínicos geralmente se dá nos primeiros meses de vida (entre 2 e 8 meses), diferentemente do Leonberger (1-9 anos) e do Pastor alemão branco (2 anos).
• Paralisia adquirida da laringe — é possível em qualquer idade, embora seja mais frequente em cães mais idosos.
• Neoplasia — cães de meia-idade a idosos, com idade média de 8 anos.

SINAIS CLÍNICOS
Achados Anamnésicos
• Respiração ofegante.
• Intolerância a exercício e calor.
• Respiração ruidosa.
• Vocalização alterada.
• Tosse ocasional.
• Casos graves — dispneia, colapso, síncope ou, até mesmo, morte súbita.
• Polineuropatia, polimiopatia ou miastenia grave — regurgitação, fraqueza, marcha anormal (o padrão de anormalidades varia).

Achados do Exame Físico
• Respiração ofegante, polipneia e estridor inspiratório em casos caninos.
• A respiração é menos ruidosa em gatos com laringopatia.
• Cianose.
• É frequente a presença de hipertermia.
• Pneumonia por aspiração — febre, crepitações à auscultação respiratória.
• Polineuropatia, polimiopatia ou miastenia grave — paraparesia ou tetraparesia com reflexos espinais diminuídos.
• Cão Leonberger com polineuropatia familiar — marcha de pisada elevada dos membros pélvicos com reflexos deprimidos dos nervos cranianos e espinais.
• Cão Rottweiler acometido pelo complexo paralisia laríngea/polineuropatia — frequentemente se observam cataratas.

CAUSAS
Paralisia da Laringe
Congênita
• Degeneração neuronal do núcleo ambíguo (Bouvier des Flandres e Husky).
• Idiopática.

Adquirida
• Idiopática.
• Polineuropatia — idiopática; familiar (complexo paralisia laríngea/polineuropatia); imunomediada.
• Miastenia grave.
• Polimiopatia — idiopática; imunomediada; infecciosa (toxoplasmose, neosporose).
• Lesão cervical ventral ou torácica cranial — neoplasia ou traumatismo com envolvimento de um ou ambos os nervos recorrentes; os exemplos incluem linfoma do nervo vago no gato e neuropatia traumática secundária à tireoidectomia.
• Laringite aguda:
  ◦ A causa frequentemente não é encontrada.
  ◦ Vírus — vírus da parainfluenza canina, herpes-vírus felino tipo 1.
  ◦ Bactérias — *Bordetella bronchiseptica*.
  ◦ Refluxo gastroesofágico.
  ◦ Laringite obstrutiva crônica idiopática (linfoplasmocitária, granulomatosa).
• Neoplasia da laringe:
  ◦ Cão — rabdomioma, rabdomiossarcoma, adenocarcinoma, carcinoma de células escamosas.
  ◦ Gato — linfoma, carcinoma de células escamosas.
• Traumatismo:
  ◦ Lesões causadas por corpos estranhos.
  ◦ Traumatismo cervical, feridas causadas por mordeduras.
  ◦ Colapso da laringe secundário à síndrome braquicefálica das vias aéreas.

FATORES DE RISCO
Com exceção da raça, não há fatores de risco para o desenvolvimento de paralisia congênita ou adquirida da laringe. Os fatores de risco para o desenvolvimento de sinais clínicos graves ou fatais em casos de paralisia da laringe incluem obesidade, temperatura quente ou úmida (especialmente em ambiente fechado como carro) e doença concomitante das vias aéreas inferiores ou dos pulmões.

DIAGNÓSTICO

DIAGNÓSTICO DIFERENCIAL
• As doenças da faringe podem ser confundidas com as da laringe, pois pode haver engasgo, estridor e tosse em ambos os grupos de doença. Não se observa disfagia em casos de laringopatia, mas esse sinal pode estar presente no caso de lesão da faringe.
• As doenças da traqueia podem ser confundidas com as da laringe em alguns casos. O sinal de tosse é mais frequente em doenças traqueais do que laríngeas, enquanto o estridor inspiratório é mais usual em laringopatias.

HEMOGRAMA/BIOQUÍMICA/URINÁLISE
• Nenhuma anormalidade é específica de qualquer problema na laringe.
• Pode haver leucocitose caso ocorra pneumonia por aspiração.
• Aumento leve a moderado nas enzimas hepáticas em caso de hipoxemia crônica.
• Hipercolesterolemia pode estar presente se houver hipotireoidismo concomitante.

OUTROS TESTES LABORATORIAIS
• Em caso de paralisia da laringe secundária à polineuropatia/polimiopatia:
• Perfil da tireoide no cão.
• Títulos de anticorpo contra *Toxoplasma gondii* (cão e gato) e *Neospora caninum* (cão).
• Títulos de anticorpo contra os receptores da colinesterase.

DIAGNÓSTICO POR IMAGEM
• Radiografias torácicas — para descartar pneumonia por aspiração como uma complicação de disfunção da laringe, outros problemas das vias aéreas inferiores que possam influenciar o prognóstico e/ou massa mediastínica como causa de paralisia da laringe.

LARINGOPATIA

- Se houver vômito/regurgitação — proceder à deglutição de bário com fluoroscopia (para identificar megaesôfago ou disfunção esofágica associados à polineuropatia ou miastenia grave, para identificar esofagite de refluxo/hérnia de hiato coexistentes em alguns casos de síndrome braquicefálica das vias aéreas).
- Ultrassonografia da faringe/laringe — para identificar possível presença de massa.

MÉTODOS DIAGNÓSTICOS

Laringoscopia
- Método de escolha para identificar paralisia, colapso, massa, traumatismo, corpo estranho ou inflamação da laringe.
- Há necessidade de anestesia geral ou sedação profunda.
- Paralisia da laringe:
  - Diagnóstico confirmado pela perda de abdução das cartilagens aritenóideas durante a inspiração profunda.
  - Geralmente bilateral, embora a paralisia unilateral seja possível no início da evolução da doença.
  - A paralisia unilateral foi descrita em gatos.
  - É possível a obtenção de resultados falso-positivos, por causa da influência exercida pela anestesia geral sobre a função da laringe. Se houver dúvida em relação ao diagnóstico, é aconselhável a administração intravenosa de cloridrato de doxapram (1-2 mg/kg) para aumentar o esforço respiratório.

Esofagoscopia
- Realizada quando se observa vômito/regurgitação para descartar esofagite de refluxo ou hérnia de hiato.

Rinoscopia Retrógrada
- Efetuada quando se suspeita de faringopatia ou no caso de síndrome braquicefálica das vias aéreas.

ACHADOS PATOLÓGICOS
Paralisia da laringe:
- Achados macroscópicos — vermelhidão, tumefação e espessamento das cartilagens aritenóideas e das pregas vocais.
- Achados histopatológicos — edema e inflamação inespecíficos da mucosa e submucosa da laringe; atrofia por desnervação dos músculos da laringe no caso de neuropatia do(s) nervo(s) laríngeo(s) recorrente(s).
- Laringite obstrutiva crônica idiopática:
  - Achados histopatológicos — inflamação linfoplasmocitária, granulomatosa ou piogranulomatosa da submucosa laríngea.

TRATAMENTO

CUIDADO(S) DE SAÚDE ADEQUADO(S)
- Paralisia:
  - Tratamento médico ambulatorial — em pacientes estáveis que aguardam pela cirurgia.
  - Emergência:
  - Sedação/anestesia.
  - Succinato de prednisolona (30 mg/kg IV e, em seguida, 15 mg/kg IV após 6 h, depois prednisolona na dose de 0,5 mg/kg VO a cada 12 h até a cirurgia).
  - Terapia de resfriamento com fluidos IV e água fria no pescoço ou álcool nos coxins palmoplantares.

CUIDADO(S) DE ENFERMAGEM
- Paralisia:
  - Evitar ambientes quentes e pouco ventilados, estresse e agitação intensa, pois tais fatores comprometem ainda mais os mecanismos normais de resfriamento e a troca apropriada de ar.
  - Evitar o uso de coleiras cervicais.
  - Evitar o ganho de peso.

ATIVIDADE
O exercício deve ser intensamente limitado em animais que sofrem de paralisia da laringe, sobretudo em temperaturas quentes.

DIETA
A perda de peso é defendida em pacientes que se encontram acima do peso ideal e apresentam paralisia da laringe.

ORIENTAÇÃO AO PROPRIETÁRIO
- Paralisia:
  - Discutir a importância da cirurgia e o risco de sua não realização (hipoxemia crônica, pneumonia por aspiração repetida, intermação/insolação, risco de sufocamento e morte).
  - Abordar as complicações potenciais da cirurgia.
  - Falar sobre o prognóstico reservado com a cirurgia em casos com polineuropatia.
  - Tratar sobre a possível herdabilidade desse problema em certas raças.
- Neoplasia:
  - Esclarecer as opções cirúrgicas/quimioterápicas.

CONSIDERAÇÕES CIRÚRGICAS
- Paralisia — cirurgia (lateralização aritenoide unilateral) é o tratamento de escolha tanto em cães como em gatos; a correção cirúrgica bilateral não é aconselhada, pois isso aumenta o risco de pneumonia por aspiração; a terapia com prednisolona por via oral (em doses anti-inflamatórias) deve ser administrada por alguns dias antes da cirurgia para diminuir o edema da laringe.
- Neoplasia — a cirurgia pode ser curativa em alguns casos, para rabdomioma, rabdomiossarcoma ou carcinoma de células escamosas; a colocação de tubo de traqueostomia pode melhorar a qualidade de vida se a excisão cirúrgica não for possível.

MEDICAÇÕES

MEDICAMENTO(S)
- Paralisia — caso o proprietário desista da cirurgia, lançar mão da terapia com prednisolona por via oral (0,5 mg/kg a cada 12 h por 1 semana e, em seguida, promover a redução gradativa da dosagem para 0,5 mg/kg a cada 48 h).
- Linfoma (principalmente em gatos) — quimioterapia (ver "Linfoma — Gatos").

PRECAUÇÕES
Tomar precauções de segurança no caso da administração de quimioterapia.

ACOMPANHAMENTO

MONITORIZAÇÃO DO PACIENTE
- Período pós-cirúrgico imediato — verificar a temperatura retal, que deve ser mantida normal.
- Monitorizar o animal quanto à ocorrência de pneumonia por aspiração (a curto e longo prazos).
- Se a cirurgia for bem-sucedida, a intolerância ao exercício e calor, bem como o sinal de estridor, deverão diminuir.

COMPLICAÇÕES POSSÍVEIS
- Paralisia — a recidiva dos sinais clínicos não será comum se a cirurgia for realizada de forma correta; é possível a ocorrência de pneumonia por aspiração, pois a laringe é colocada em uma posição aberta fixa; o risco de pneumonia por aspiração aumentará caso se efetue a lateralização aritenoide bilateral ou se coexistir a disfagia atribuída à disfunção da faringe e/ou do esôfago.
- Tumor — haverá recidiva dos sinais clínicos se a ressecção completa não for possível; também há aumento no risco de pneumonia por aspiração no período pós-operatório.

EVOLUÇÃO ESPERADA E PROGNÓSTICO
- Paralisia idiopática — prognóstico bom com a cirurgia; reservado a mau caso o proprietário desista do procedimento cirúrgico.
- Paralisia associada à disfunção esofágica — prognóstico mau.
- Tumor — prognóstico reservado a bom no caso de ressecção bem-sucedida de tumor benigno; mau no caso de carcinoma, mesmo com radioterapia; variável no caso de linfoma felino.

DIVERSOS

DISTÚRBIOS ASSOCIADOS
- Algumas vezes, a paralisia da laringe é associada à presença de massa no mediastino anterior ou na região cervical ventral.
- A coexistência de megaesôfago, fraqueza ou marcha anormal em casos de paralisia da laringe sugere polineuropatia, polimiopatia ou miastenia grave.

FATORES RELACIONADOS COM A IDADE
Paralisia congênita e familiar da laringe — início dos sinais clínicos no primeiro ano de vida.

GESTAÇÃO/FERTILIDADE/REPRODUÇÃO
Não é recomendável o acasalamento de cães acometidos por paralisia congênita da laringe ou pelo complexo paralisia laríngea/polineuropatia.

VER TAMBÉM
- Síndrome Braquicefálica das Vias Aéreas.
- Cianose.
- Miastenia Grave.

Sugestões de Leitura
Gabriel A, Poncelet L, Van Ham L, Clercx C, Braund KG, Bhatti S, Detilleux J, Peeters D. Laryngeal paralysis-polyneuropathy complex in young related Pyrenean mountain dogs. J Small Anim Pract 2006, 47:144-149.
Hammel SP, Hottinger HA, Novo RE. Postoperative results of unilateral arytenoid lateralization for treatment of idiopathic laryngeal paralysis in dogs: 39 cases (1996-2002). JAVMA 2006, 228:1215-1220.
Schachter S, Norris CR. Laryngeal paralysis in cats: 16 cases (1990-1999). JAVMA 2000, 216;1100-1103.

Autores Dominique Peeters e Cécile Clercx
Consultor Editorial Lynelle R. Johnson

Leiomioma do Estômago e dos Intestinos Delgado e Grosso

CONSIDERAÇÕES GERAIS

REVISÃO
Tumor benigno raro que surge da musculatura lisa do estômago e do trato intestinal; com a imuno-histoquímica, esses tumores podem ser reclassificados como um tumor do estroma gastrintestinal ou semelhante a ele.

IDENTIFICAÇÃO
- Os cães são mais comumente acometidos do que os gatos.
- Afeta cães e gatos de meia-idade a mais idosos (>6 anos).
- Nenhuma predisposição racial.

SINAIS CLÍNICOS
Achados Anamnésicos
- Relacionados com a localização no trato gastrintestinal.
- Estômago — vômito.
- Intestino delgado — vômito; perda de peso; borborigmos; flatulência.
- Intestino grosso e reto — tenesmo; hematoquezia; algumas vezes, prolapso retal.

Achados do Exame Físico
- Estômago — sem anormalidades específicas.
- Intestino delgado — com frequência, não há qualquer achado anormal; pode-se palpar a presença de massa mesoabdominal; ocasionalmente, verificam-se alças dolorosas e distendidas do intestino delgado.
- Intestino grosso e reto — pode-se sentir a presença de massa palpável pelo reto.

CAUSAS E FATORES DE RISCO
Desconhecidos.

DIAGNÓSTICO

DIAGNÓSTICO DIFERENCIAL
- Corpo estranho.
- Enteropatia inflamatória.
- Parasitas.
- Adenocarcinoma.
- Leiomiossarcoma.
- Tumor do estroma gastrintestinal ou semelhante a ele.
- Linfoma.
- Pancreatite.

HEMOGRAMA/BIOQUÍMICA/URINÁLISE
- Em geral, permanecem normais.
- Hipoglicemia — ocasionalmente.
- Estômago e intestino delgado — pode-se observar anemia microcítica hipocrômica (anemia ferropriva, ou seja, por deficiência de ferro).

OUTROS TESTES LABORATORIAIS
N/D.

DIAGNÓSTICO POR IMAGEM
- Ultrassonografia abdominal — pode revelar espessamento da parede do estômago ou do intestino; o leiomioma gástrico é mais comum na junção gastresofágica.
- Radiografia com contraste (estômago e intestino delgado) — pode revelar massa expansiva ocupadora de espaço.
- Radiografia com duplo contraste (intestino grosso e reto) — revela massa expansiva ocupadora de espaço.

MÉTODOS DIAGNÓSTICOS
Aspirados por Agulha Fina
Caso se observe massa ou espessamento ao exame ultrassonográfico, pode-se obter o aspirado por agulha fina para citologia a fim de descartar outros diagnósticos diferenciais; para os leiomiomas, o exame citológico é geralmente de baixo rendimento.

Trato Gastrintestinal Superior
Realizar endoscopia do trato gastrintestinal superior e biopsia da mucosa; muitas vezes, no entanto, esses métodos não são diagnósticos, porque os tumores estão situados profundamente em relação à superfície da mucosa ou distalmente ao comprimento do aparelho. Portanto, a biopsia cirúrgica quase sempre é necessária para confirmar o diagnóstico.

Intestino Grosso e Reto
Colonoscopia pode revelar a presença de massa; a biopsia da mucosa pode não ser diagnóstica por causa do revestimento do tumor por mucosa normal; a biopsia cirúrgica frequentemente é necessária. Caso se consiga palpar a massa pelo reto, poderão ser obtidas biopsias transretais.

TRATAMENTO

- Ressecção cirúrgica — tratamento de escolha; curativo se o tumor for ressecável.
- Até mesmo leiomiomas volumosos frequentemente podem ser removidos de forma bem-sucedida com margens estreitas.

MEDICAÇÕES

MEDICAMENTO(S)
Se o leiomioma for reclassificado como um tumor do estroma gastrintestinal (positivo para o gene KIT), pode-se considerar o uso de algum inibidor da tirosina quinase (fosfato de toceranibe) como terapia de acompanhamento.

CONTRAINDICAÇÕES/INTERAÇÕES POSSÍVEIS
N/D.

ACOMPANHAMENTO

- Ressecção completa — cuidado pós-operatório normal; não há necessidade de qualquer acompanhamento adicional.
- Monitorizar a glicose sanguínea no pós-operatório se o animal estiver hipoglicêmico antes da cirurgia.

DIVERSOS

DISTÚRBIOS ASSOCIADOS
Hipoglicemia — identificada como uma síndrome paraneoplásica associada.

Sugestões de Leitura
Frost D, Lasota J, Miettinen M. Gastrointestinal stromal tumors and leiomyomas in the dog: A histopathologic, immunohistochemical, and molecular genetic study of 50 cases. Vet Pathol 2003, 40:42-54.

Maas CP, ter Haar G, Van Der Gaag I, et al. Reclassification of small intestinal and cecal smooth muscle tumors in 72 dogs: Clinical, histologic, and immunohistochemical evaluation. Vet Surg 2007, 36:302-313.

McPherron MA, Withrow SJ, Seim HB, Powers BE. Colorectal leiomyoma in seven dogs. JAAHA 1992, 28:43-46.

Autor Laura D. Garrett
Consultor Editorial Timothy M. Fan

Leiomiossarcoma do Estômago e dos Intestinos Delgado e Grosso

CONSIDERAÇÕES GERAIS

REVISÃO
- Tumor maligno incomum que surge da musculatura lisa do estômago e do trato intestinal.
- Tende a ser localmente invasivo; taxa metastática acima de 50%, geralmente em locais intra-abdominais.
- Prognóstico razoável a reservado.
- No intestino grosso, o ceco costuma ser acometido.
- Análises recentes reclassificaram muitos leiomiossarcoma em tumores do estroma gastrintestinal ou semelhantes a eles; há necessidade do exame de imuno-histoquímica para diferenciar.
- Raramente, ocorrem leiomiossarcomas verdadeiros; no entanto, este capítulo referirá a esses tumores como leiomiossarcomas, pois é como eles foram caracterizados nos trabalhos de referência.

IDENTIFICAÇÃO
- Os cães são mais comumente acometidos que os gatos.
- Acomete principalmente cães e gatos de meia-idade a mais idosos (>6 anos).
- Sem predisposição racial.

SINAIS CLÍNICOS

Achados Anamnésicos
- Relacionados com o trato gastrintestinal.
- Estômago — vômito; perda de peso.
- Intestino delgado — vômito; perda de peso; diarreia; borborigmos; flatulência.
- Intestino grosso e reto — tenesmo; pode levar a prolapso retal; hematoquezia.

Achados do Exame Físico
- Estômago — inespecíficos.
- Intestino delgado — pode-se palpar a presença de massa mesoabdominal; às vezes, verificam-se alças distendidas e dolorosas do intestino delgado à palpação abdominal.
- Intestino grosso e reto — pode-se sentir a presença de massa palpável pelo reto.

CAUSAS E FATORES DE RISCO
Desconhecidos.

DIAGNÓSTICO

DIAGNÓSTICO DIFERENCIAL
- Corpo estranho.
- Enteropatia inflamatória.
- Parasitas.
- Adenocarcinoma.
- Leiomioma.
- Tumor do estroma gastrintestinal ou semelhante a ele.
- Linfoma.
- Pancreatite.

HEMOGRAMA/BIOQUÍMICA/URINÁLISE
- Geralmente normais.
- Anemia — pode ser microcítica hipocrômica (anemia ferropriva, ou seja, por deficiência de ferro).
- Leucocitose.
- Hipoglicemia — relatada como uma síndrome paraneoplásica.

DIAGNÓSTICO POR IMAGEM
- Ultrassonografia abdominal — pode revelar espessamento da parede do estômago ou do intestino.
- Radiografia com contraste positivo (estômago e intestino delgado) — revela massa expansiva ocupadora de espaço.
- Radiografia com duplo contraste (intestino grosso e reto) — revela massa expansiva ocupadora de espaço.

MÉTODOS DIAGNÓSTICOS

Aspirados por Agulha Fina
- Caso se observe massa ou espessamento ao exame ultrassonográfico, o aspirado por agulha fina com citologia pode revelar células mesenquimais com características de malignidade sugestivas de sarcoma.
- Qualquer linfonodo infartado observado à ultrassonografia pode ser submetido a aspirado por agulha fina e citologia para pesquisa de metástase.

Trato Gastrintestinal Superior
- Endoscopia e biopsia da mucosa — podem ser realizadas, mas os resultados quase sempre não são diagnósticos, pois a massa pode estar fora do alcance do aparelho em alguns tumores situados profundamente à superfície da mucosa.
- Biopsia cirúrgica — frequentemente necessária para confirmar o diagnóstico.

Intestino Grosso e Reto
- Colonoscopia — pode permitir a observação da massa; a biopsia da mucosa pode não ser diagnóstica por causa do revestimento do tumor por mucosa normal.
- Biopsia profunda — realizar, se possível.

TRATAMENTO
- Ressecção cirúrgica — tratamento de escolha.
- É menos provável que o leiomiossarcoma cecal sofra metástases.
- A cirurgia pode proporcionar uma sobrevida prolongada nos casos de massas do intestino delgado.
- Avaliar cuidadosamente o paciente em busca de metástases antes de cirurgia extensa (p. ex., linfonodos mesentéricos, fígado e pulmões).

MEDICAÇÕES

MEDICAMENTO(S)
Se o leiomiossarcoma for reclassificado como um tumor do estroma gastrintestinal (positivo para o gene KIT), pode-se considerar o uso de algum inibidor da tirosina quinase (fosfato de toceranibe) como terapia de acompanhamento.

ACOMPANHAMENTO

EVOLUÇÃO ESPERADA E PROGNÓSTICO
- Os leiomiossarcomas frequentemente sofrem metástases para o fígado; com frequência, acomete os linfonodos locais próximos.
- Uma série de casos mais antigos revelou:
  - Casos com envolvimento do intestino delgado tiveram sobrevida média de 12 meses.
  - Casos com acometimento do ceco exibiram sobrevida média de 7,5 meses, porém a maioria morreu de outras causas.
  - Casos gástricos são muito raros, mas os poucos relatados apresentavam taxa elevada de metástases e períodos curtos de sobrevida.
- Até mesmo os cães com metástase podem exibir sobrevidas prolongadas, com média relatada de 21,7 meses em um único estudo de cães com leiomiossarcoma metastático do trato GI.
- Um relato recente verificou períodos de sobrevida semelhantes entre cães com leiomioma, leiomiossarcoma, tumor do estroma gastrintestinal e tumores semelhantes a este:
  - 42 cães acometidos por tumores do intestino delgado e submetidos a tratamento cirúrgico tiveram sobrevidas de 62,6 e 52,3% em um período de 1 e 2 anos.
  - 19 cães acometidos por tumores do ceco e submetidos a tratamento cirúrgico apresentaram sobrevidas de 84,2 e 66% em um período de 1 e 2 anos.
- Ressecção completa — exame físico de rotina, radiografia torácica e ultrassonografia abdominal 1, 3, 6, 9 e 12 meses após a cirurgia.
- Ressecção incompleta — suporte sintomático para aliviar os sinais clínicos.

DIVERSOS

DISTÚRBIOS ASSOCIADOS
Hipoglicemia — relatada como uma síndrome paraneoplásica.

ABREVIATURA(S)
- GI = gastrintestinal.

Sugestões de Leitura

Cohen M, Post GS, Wright JC. Gastrointestinal leiomyosarcoma in 14 dogs. J Vet Intern Med 2003, 17:107-110.

Crawshaw J, Berg J, Sardinas JC, et al. Prognosis for dogs with nonlymphomatous, small intestinal tumors treated by surgical excisions. JAAHA 1998, 34:451-456.

Frost D, Lasota J, Miettinen M. Gastrointestinal stromal tumors and leiomyomas in the dog: A histopathologic, immunohistochemical, and molecular genetic study of 50 cases. Vet Pathol 2003, 40:42-54.

Kapatkin AS, Mullen HS, Matthiesen DT, Patnaik AK. Leiomyosarcoma in dogs: 44 cases (1983-1988). JAVMA 1992, 201:107.

Maas CP, ter Haar G, Van Der Gaag I, et al. Reclassification of small intestinal and cecal smooth muscle tumors in 72 dogs: Clinical, histologic, and immunohistochemical evaluation. Vet Surg 2007, 36:302-313.

Swann HM, Holt DE. Canine gastric adenocarcinoma and leiomyosarcoma: A retrospective study of 21 cases (1986-1999) and literature review. JAAHA 2002, 38:157-164.

Autor Laura D. Garrett
Consultor Editorial Timothy M. Fan

Leishmaniose

CONSIDERAÇÕES GERAIS

REVISÃO
- Protozoário — gênero *Leishmania*; provoca dois tipos de doença: cutânea e visceral. • Sistemas orgânicos acometidos — cutâneo: pele, hepatobiliar, baço, rins, olhos e articulações; visceral: diátese hemorrágica. • Os cães acometidos nos Estados Unidos invariavelmente adquiriram a infecção em outro país. • *L. donovani infantum* — bacia do Mediterrâneo, Portugal e Espanha; casos esporádicos na Suíça, norte da França e Holanda. • Complexo *L. donovani* ou *L. braziliensis* — áreas endêmicas das Américas do Sul e Central, bem como sul do México. • Há relatos de casos endêmicos em cães (Oklahoma e Ohio) e gatos (Texas) nos Estados Unidos. Considerada endêmica em cães de caça nos Estados Unidos. • Flebótomos como vetores — transmitem os parasitas flagelados para a pele do hospedeiro. Vetor desconhecido nos Estados Unidos. • Gatos — localiza-se com frequência na pele. • Cães — invariavelmente se dissemina por todo o organismo para a maior parte dos órgãos; insuficiência renal é a causa mais comum de morte. • Período de incubação — de 1 mês a vários anos.

IDENTIFICAÇÃO
- Cães — praticamente todos desenvolvem doença visceral ou sistêmica; 90% também apresentam envolvimento cutâneo; nenhuma predileção sexual ou racial. • Gatos — doença cutânea (rara); sem predileção sexual ou racial.

SINAIS CLÍNICOS
Viscerais
- Intolerância ao exercício. • Perda de peso grave e anorexia. • Diarreia, vômito, epistaxe e melena — menos comuns. • Cães — linfadenopatia e lesões cutâneas em 90% dos casos; emaciação; possíveis sinais de insuficiência renal (poliúria, polidipsia, vômito); neuralgia, poliartrite, polimiosite, lesões osteolíticas, e rara periostite proliferativa; aproximadamente um terço dos pacientes exibe febre e esplenomegalia.

Cutâneos
- Hiperqueratose — achado mais proeminente; descamação epidérmica excessiva, com espessamento e despigmentação, além de rachaduras e fissuras do focinho e dos coxins palmoplantares.
- Pelagem— seca; quebradiça; perda de pelos.
- Cães — podem ser observados nódulos intradérmicos e úlceras; unhas anormalmente longas ou quebradiças constituem um achado específico em alguns pacientes.
- Gatos — costumam desenvolver nódulos cutâneos (sobretudo nas orelhas).

CAUSAS E FATORES DE RISCO
- Viagem a regiões endêmicas (em geral, o Mediterrâneo), onde os cães ficam expostos a flebótomos infectados.
- Pode ocorrer a transmissão na transfusão de sangue obtido de animais infectados.
- Também pode ocorrer a transmissão *in utero* da progenitora para os filhotes.
- Pode ocorrer a transmissão entre os cães por contato direto.

DIAGNÓSTICO

DIAGNÓSTICO DIFERENCIAL
- Visceral — micoses (blastomicose, histoplasmose); lúpus eritematoso sistêmico; neoplasia metastática; cinomose; vasculite.
- Cutânea — outras causas de hiperqueratose: seborreia idiopática primária e dermatoses nutricionais (responsiva à vitamina A, responsiva ao zinco); hiperqueratose nasodigital idiopática, dermatose liquenoide-psoriasiforme, displasia epidérmica e síndrome do comedão do Schnauzer são raras e específicas de certas raças. • Biopsia cutânea — lesões hiperqueratóticas e nodulares; a existência dos microrganismos confirma o diagnóstico. • Hiperglobulinemia — diferenciar de erliquiose crônica e mieloma múltiplo.

HEMOGRAMA/BIOQUÍMICA/URINÁLISE
- Hiperproteinemia com hiperglobulinemia — quase 100% dos casos. • Hipoalbuminemia — 95% dos casos. • Proteinúria — 85% dos casos.
- Atividade enzimática hepática elevada — 55% dos casos. • Trombocitopenia — 50% dos casos.
- Azotemia — até 45% dos casos. • Leucopenia e linfopenia — 20% dos casos.

OUTROS TESTES LABORATORIAIS
- Diagnóstico sorológico disponível por IFA ou ELISA — a maioria dos testes gera reação cruzada com o *Trypanosoma cruzi* (microrganismo estreitamente relacionado); diferenciar com base nos sinais clínicos, na anamnese e na probabilidade de exposição. • PCR — exame sensível, que pode ser usado em raspados conjuntivais; entre em contato com o Laboratório Diagnóstico de Doenças Transmitidas por Vetores, Universidade do Estado da Carolina do Norte (EUA), na cidade de Raleigh.

MÉTODOS DIAGNÓSTICOS
- Culturas — realizadas em biopsias ou aspirados de pele, baço, medula óssea ou linfonodos pelos Centros Norte-americanos de Controle e Prevenção de Doenças. • Citologia e histopatologia — identificam os microrganismos intracelulares em amostras de biopsias ou aspirados (listadas anteriormente).

ACHADOS PATOLÓGICOS
- Infiltração celular (principalmente de histiócitos e macrófagos) e formas amastigotas intracelulares características — identificadas em muitos tecidos: pele, linfonodos, fígado, baço e rim. • Ulcerações da mucosa — ocasionalmente encontradas no estômago, intestino e cólon.

TRATAMENTO

- Efetuado em um esquema ambulatorial.
- Animais emaciados e cronicamente infectados — considerar a eutanásia; prognóstico muito mau.
- Dieta — proteína de alta qualidade; especial para insuficiência renal se houver necessidade. • Gatos — a remoção cirúrgica de lesões nodulares dérmicas isoladas é a melhor escola. • Orientar o proprietário sobre o potencial de transmissão zoonótica dos microrganismos presentes nas lesões para os seres humanos. • Informar o cliente sobre a impossibilidade de eliminação definitiva dos microrganismos e a ocorrência inevitável da recidiva, exigindo novo tratamento.
- Existe uma vacina disponível para cães na Europa e algumas regiões da América do Sul.

MEDICAÇÕES

MEDICAMENTO(S) DE ESCOLHA
- Estibogliconato de sódio — disponível nos Centros Norte-americanos de Controle e Prevenção de Doenças; 30-50 mg/kg IV ou SC a cada 24 h por 3-4 semanas. • Antimoniato de meglumina — 100 mg/kg IV ou SC a cada 24 h por 3-4 semanas. • Alopurinol — produz curas clínicas, embora ocorram recidivas. Mais eficiente quando utilizado em combinação com outros medicamentos (meglumina ou anfotericina B) em forma de manutenção. Dose: 7 mg/kg VO a cada 8 h por 3 meses ou 10 mg/kg/dia VO por 2-24 meses ou 20 mg/kg VO a cada 12-24 h por tempo indefinido. • Anfotericina B — 0,5-0,8 mg/kg diluída em 50 mL de glicose a 5% em água, administrada por via IV em 1 minuto a cada 48 h para uma dose total de 8-15 mg/kg.

CONTRAINDICAÇÕES/INTERAÇÕES POSSÍVEIS
- Cães gravemente doentes — iniciar os medicamentos antimoniais em doses baixas.
- Insuficiência renal — tratar antes de administrar os agentes antimoniais; o prognóstico depende da função renal no início do tratamento.
- Estibogliconato de sódio — dor no local da injeção; se esse medicamento for subdosado, poderá surgir resistência. • Anfotericina B — pode ocorrer nefrotoxicidade.

ACOMPANHAMENTO

- Eficácia do tratamento — monitorizar o paciente por meio da melhora dos sinais clínicos e da identificação dos microrganismos em biopsias repetidas. • Recidivas — alguns meses até um ano após o tratamento; reavaliar no mínimo a cada 2 meses após o término da terapia. • Recidivas — identificadas pela detecção de aumento nos níveis sanguíneos de globulina ou pelo reaparecimento dos sinais clínicos em um cão previamente em remissão. • Prognóstico quanto à cura — muito reservado.

DIVERSOS

- A leishmaniose é uma doença notificável — os casos confirmados precisam ser relatados aos Centros Norte-americanos de Controle e Prevenção de Doenças. • Orientar o proprietário sobre o potencial zoonótico dessa doença.

ABREVIATURA(S)
- ELISA = ensaio imunoabsorvente ligado à enzima. • IFA = teste de anticorpo imunofluorescente. • PCR = reação em cadeia da polimerase.

Sugestões de Leitura
Baneth G. Leishmaniasis. In: Greene CE, ed., Infectious Diseases of the Dog and Cat, 3rd ed. St. Louis: Saunders Elsevier, 2006, pp. 685-698.

Autor Stephen C. Barr
Consultor Editorial Stephen C. Barr

LEPTOSPIROSE

CONSIDERAÇÕES GERAIS

DEFINIÇÃO
- Causada por membros patogênicos do gênero *Leptospira*. • Doenças agudas e crônicas dos cães (principalmente nefrite e hepatite) e de outros animais, incluindo felinos, apesar de raramente.
- Cães — as sorovariantes que causam a doença variam de acordo com a região geográfica; as sorovariantes recentes e preocupantes dos EUA incluem *L. grippotyphosa*, *L. autumnalis* e *L. pomona*; as vacinas devem incluir as sorovariantes representativas encontradas na região.

FISIOPATOLOGIA
- *Leptospira* — penetra na pele ou nas mucosas intactas ou lesionadas com corte; invade rapidamente a corrente sanguínea (4-7 dias); dissemina-se para todas as partes do organismo (2-4 dias). • A invasão leva à febre, leucocitose, anemia transitória (hemólise), hemoglobinúria leve e albuminúria. • A febre e a bacteremia logo desaparecem. • Dano aos capilares e às células endoteliais; ocasionalmente resulta em hemorragias petequiais. • Fígado — necrose hepática e icterícia.
- Rim — leptospirúria; a *Leptospira* pode se localizar nos túbulos renais lesados; o microrganismo replica-se rapidamente nas células do epitélio tubular. • Anticorpos séricos precoces surgem quase no momento em que a bacteremia cessa. • Morte — geralmente, o resultado de nefrite intersticial, lesão vascular e insuficiência renal; pode resultar de septicemia aguda ou CID.

SISTEMA(S) ACOMETIDO(S)
- Cardiovascular — dano ao endotélio; hemorragia. • Hepatobiliar — hepatite; disfunção; necrose. • Nervoso — meningite. • Renal/urológico — nefrite intersticial focal; nefrose hemoglobinúrica; lesão/insuficiência tubular.
- Respiratório — vasculite; pneumonia intersticial.

Doença crônica
- Oftálmico — uveíte anterior. • Renal/urológico — insuficiência renal crônica. • Reprodutivo — abortamento; filhotes fracos. • Reprodutivo — *Salmonella typhimurium* e *Leptospira* são relacionadas com natimorto felino.

INCIDÊNCIA/PREVALÊNCIA
- Incidência relatada (cães) — falsamente baixa; a maior parte das infecções é inaparente e permanece sem diagnóstico. • Prevalência (cães) — cidade, 37,8%; suburbana, 18,7%.

DISTRIBUIÇÃO GEOGRÁFICA
- Mundial, especialmente em climas ou estações quentes e úmidos. • *L. canicola* e *L. icterohaemorrhagiae* — sorovariantes usuais; doença clínica nos cães; *L. canicola* é mais comum em todo o mundo; *L. icterohaemorrhagiae* é mais comum na Austrália. • *L. bratislava* — ainda precisa ser confirmada por cultura como sorovariante em cães nos EUA. • Água estagnada e solo neutro ou levemente alcalino promovem a presença no ambiente.

IDENTIFICAÇÃO
Espécies
- Cães e, raramente, gatos.

Idade Média e Faixa Etária
- Cães jovens sem anticorpos maternos passivos — maior probabilidade de apresentar a doença grave. • Cães idosos com níveis adequados de títulos de anticorpos — raramente apresentam doença clínica a menos que expostos a alguma sorovariante não contida na vacina.

Sexo Predominante
Tradicionalmente, cães machos costumam ser mais acometidos; contestado por relatos recentes.

SINAIS CLÍNICOS

Comentários Gerais
- Variam com a idade e com o estado imune, bem como com os fatores ambientais que afetam a sobrevivência da *Leptospira* e a virulência da sorovariante infectante. • Hospedeiro reservatório primário — pode disseminar sorovariante específica pela disseminação urinária; pode não apresentar sinais clínicos ou doença menos grave (nefrite intersticial difusa aguda a crônica, p. ex., *L. canicola* nos cães, com resposta humoral relativamente fraca). • Hospedeiro incidental (acidental) — doença grave aguda (p. ex., *L. icterohaemorrhagiae* nos cães com resposta humoral intensa).

Achados Anamnésicos
Doença Superaguda a Subaguda
- Febre. • Músculos doloridos. • Enrijecimento.
- Tremores. • Fraqueza. • Anorexia. • Depressão.
- Vômito. • Desidratação rápida. • Diarreia com ou sem sangue. • Icterícia. • Tosse espontânea. • Dificuldade respiratória. • PD/PU que evoluem para anúria. • Corrimento vaginal sanguinolento. • Morte — sem sinais clínicos.

Doença Crônica
- Sem doença aparente. • Febre de origem indeterminada. • PD/PU — insuficiência renal crônica.

Achados do Exame Físico
Doença Superaguda a Aguda
- Taquipneia. • Pulso irregular rápido. • Perfusão capilar deficiente. • Hematêmese. • Hematoquezia.
- Melena. • Epistaxe. • Mucosas congestas.
- Hemorragias petequiais e equimóticas disseminadas. • Relutância ao movimento, hiperestesia paraspinal, marcha rígida.
- Conjuntivite. • Rinite. • Hematúria.
- Linfadenopatia leve.

CAUSAS
- Cães — *L. canicola*, *L. icterohaemorrhagiae*, *L. pomona*, *L. grippotyphosa*, *L. copenhagenii*, *L. australis*, *L. autumnalis*, *L. ballum* e *L. bataviae*.
- Gatos — *L. canicola*, *L. grippotyphosa*, *L. pomona* e *L. bataviae*.

FATORES DE RISCO
Transmissão
- Direta — contato de hospedeiro a hospedeiro via urina infectada, corrimento pós-abortamento, feto/corrimento infectado e contato sexual (sêmen).
- Indireta — exposição (via urina) a algum ambiente contaminado (vegetação, solo, alimento, água, cama) sob condições nas quais a *Leptospira* é capaz de sobreviver.
- Agente da doença — sorovariante *Leptospira*, sendo que cada uma delas possui seus próprios fatores de virulência, dose infectante e via de exposição.
- A leptospirose nos animais de companhia é frequentemente o resultado de propagação da doença que ocorre nos animais selvagens (muitos tipos distintos de mamíferos) na área; tais animais, por sua vez, podem ser hospedeiros de manutenção de diferentes sorovariantes.

Fatores do Hospedeiro
- Vacina — a proteção é específica para a sorovariante; pode não evitar a colonização do rim e a liberação na urina; existem novas vacinas disponíveis do tipo "subunidade"; além disso, as pesquisas têm se mostrado promissoras para um antígeno pan-valente que exerceria proteção cruzada contra muitas sorovariantes.
- Animais de rua ou cães de caça — exposição das mucosas à água; exposição da pele com abrasão ou amolecida pela água aumenta o risco da infecção.

Fatores Ambientais
- Ambiente quente e úmido; estação úmida (áreas de chuvas intensas) das regiões temperadas; áreas de baixada (pantanosas, lamacentas, irrigadas); climas úmidos quentes das regiões tropicais e subtropicais.
- Variação de temperatura — de 7-10°C até 34-36°C.
- Água — o microrganismo sobrevive melhor na água estagnada do que na água corrente; pH neutro ou levemente alcalino.
- O microrganismo sobrevive 180 dias no solo úmido e por mais tempo na água estagnada.
- População animal densa — canis e ambientes urbanos; aumenta as possibilidades de exposição à urina.
- Exposição a roedores e outros animais selvagens.

DIAGNÓSTICO

DIAGNÓSTICO DIFERENCIAL
Doença Subaguda a Aguda
- Cães — dirofilariose; anemia hemolítica imunomediada; bacteremia/septicemia; vírus da hepatite infecciosa canina; herpes-vírus canino; neoplasia hepática; traumatismo; lúpus; febre maculosa das Montanhas Rochosas; erliquiose; toxoplasmose; neoplasia renal; cálculos renais.
- Gatos — micoplasmose hemotrópica; medicamentos (paracetamol); bacteremia/septicemia; doenças associadas ao FIV e FeLV; colangite; toxoplasmose; PIF; neoplasia hepática; doença autoimune; traumatismo; cálculos renais; neoplasia renal.

Doença Reprodutiva/Neonatal
- Cães — brucelose; cinomose; herpes.
- Gatos — PIF; FeLV; panleucopenia; herpes-vírus; toxoplasmose; salmonelose.

HEMOGRAMA/BIOQUÍMICA/URINÁLISE
- Hematócrito e sólidos plasmáticos totais — elevados em virtude da desidratação; raramente hematócrito baixo (hemólise).
- Leucocitose com desvio à esquerda — leucopenia inicialmente durante a fase leptospirêmica.
- Trombocitopenia.
- Elevação dos produtos de degradação da fibrina.
- Ureia e creatinina — elevadas; principalmente de origem renal.
- Alterações eletrolíticas — dependem do grau de disfunção renal e gastrintestinal.
- Hiponatremia.
- Hipocloremia.
- Hipocalemia — hipercalemia na insuficiência renal.
- Hiperfosfatemia.
- Hipoalbuminemia.

LEPTOSPIROSE

- Acidose — bicarbonato sérico baixo.
- Alanina aminotransferase, aspartato aminotransferase, lactato desidrogenase e fosfatase alcalina — elevadas.
- Proteinúria.
- Isostenúria — insuficiência renal aguda.

OUTROS TESTES LABORATORIAIS

Sorologia (Teste de Aglutinação Microscópica)
- Testar no estágio agudo e 3-4 semanas depois (soro convalescente).
- Pacientes não vacinados — os títulos podem ser baixos inicialmente (1:100-1:200); podem estar mais altos no soro convalescente (1:800-1:1600 ou mais elevados) se uma sorovariante homóloga de *Leptospira* for testada; várias sorovariantes podem sofrer reação cruzada no teste de aglutinação microscópica, especialmente se houver altos títulos contra uma única sorovariante.
- Pacientes vacinados, mais idosos com bactérias integrais — esperam-se títulos elevados (até 12-16 semanas pós-vacinação) que, em seguida, declinam para <1:400; novas vacinas de subunidades — os títulos sobem para ≥1:1600 por 12 semanas para as sorovariantes *L. canicola* e *L. icterohaemorrhagiae*; os títulos para outras sorovariantes de vacinas de subunidades são mais variáveis (*L. pomona* e *L. grippotyphosa*).
- Rodar todas as amostras séricas (agudas e convalescentes) ao mesmo tempo, se possível.

Microscopia da Urina em Campo Escuro
- Quase sempre não conclusiva.
- Difícil leitura.
- Necessita de urina recém-coletada.

Teste do Anticorpo Fluorescente na Urina
- Mais conclusivo.
- A *Leptospira* não precisa estar viável; encaminhar a urina dentro do gelo para o laboratório por encomenda urgente.
- Tratar previamente com furosemida 15 min antes da coleta de urina para aumentar a taxa de sucesso.
- Correlacionar os resultados com o histórico clínico.

Teste de PCR na Urina e no Tecido
- Promissor, mas ainda experimental.

MÉTODOS DIAGNÓSTICOS
- Cultura dos líquidos corporais antes da morte (urina, sangue, humor aquoso) e dos tecidos após a morte (rim, fígado, feto, placenta) — geralmente impraticável por causa da natureza fastidiosa (exigente) da *Leptospira*; entrar em contato com o laboratório em busca do meio de transporte adequado.
- Teste do anticorpo fluorescente — realizado em todos os tecidos encaminhados para avaliação após a morte, especialmente rim e fígado; antes da morte, é possível testar a urina.
- Corantes especiais (coloração argêntica de Warthin-Starry) — tentar a imuno-histoquímica com anticorpos monoclonais em cortes de rim, fígado e tecido fetal/placentário fixados em formalina.
- PCR — alguns laboratórios desenvolveram protocolos para amostras tanto de urina como de tecidos.

ACHADOS PATOLÓGICOS
- O grau de doença renal e hepática depende da sorovariante e da imunidade do hospedeiro.
- Gatos — apresentam, em geral, lesões menos graves.
- Cães (doença aguda) — os pulmões podem estar edematosos; rins pálidos e aumentados de volume; fígado aumentado de volume, podendo estar friável com necrose e hemorragia multifocais; o trato gastrintestinal pode estar hemorrágico.

TRATAMENTO

CUIDADO(S) DE ENFERMAGEM
- Desidratação e choque — solução intravenosa isotônica, poliônica, balanceada, parenteral (Ringer lactato).
- Hemorragia grave — talvez haja necessidade de transfusão sanguínea em associação com o tratamento para CID.
- Oligúria ou anúria — reidratar inicialmente; em seguida, administrar diurético osmótico intravenoso ou diurético tubular; o procedimento de diálise peritoneal pode ser necessário.

ORIENTAÇÃO AO PROPRIETÁRIO
Informar ao proprietário sobre o potencial zoonótico da urina contaminada dos cães acometidos e de seu ambiente.

MEDICAÇÕES

MEDICAMENTO(S) DE ESCOLHA
- Penicilina G procaína — 40.000-80.000 U/kg IM a cada 24 h ou dividida a cada 12 h até que a função do rim retorne ao normal.
- Diidroestreptomicina — 10-15 mg/kg IM a cada 12 h por 2 semanas para eliminar o microrganismo dos tecidos intersticiais renais; tentar a estreptomicina se não houver insuficiência renal. Medicamento não disponível em qualquer lugar.
- Doxiciclina — 5 mg/kg VO ou IV a cada 12 h por 2 semanas; utilizar apenas para eliminar tanto a leptospiremia como a leptospirúria.

PRECAUÇÕES
- Aminoglicosídeo — monitorizar cuidadosamente os pacientes com insuficiência renal.
- Penicilinas (cães) — ajustar as doses na insuficiência renal.

MEDICAMENTO(S) ALTERNATIVO(S)
- Ampicilina ou amoxicilina — no lugar da penicilina (ampicilina a 22 mg/kg VO a cada 6-8 h por 2 semanas; amoxicilina a 22 mg/kg VO a cada 8-12 h por 2 semanas).
- Eritromicina.

ACOMPANHAMENTO

PREVENÇÃO
- Vacinas (cães) — as vacinas de bacterina inteira contêm as sorovariantes *L. canicola* e *L. icterohaemorrhagiae* (atualmente, algumas também incluem *L. pomona* e *L. grippotyphosa*); promovem imunidade contra sorovariantes homólogas e proteção de doença clínica manifesta; podem não evitar a colonização dos rins, resultando em um estado de portador crônico; vacinas sorovariante-específicas; não promovem proteção contra outras sorovariantes presentes na natureza. As vacinas mais recentes de subunidades contêm as sorovariantes *L. pomona*, *L. icterohaemorrhagiae*, *L. grippotyphosa* e *L. canicola*; alega-se que a vacina confere proteção contra doença clínica e evita a colonização dos rins.
- Vacinas — vacinar os cães conforme as recomendações atuais do rótulo; a imunidade induzida pela bactéria dura apenas 6-8 meses, além de ser específica para a sorovariante (sem proteção cruzada fora do sorogrupo); repetir a vacinação por, no mínimo, uma vez ao ano; vacinar os cães de risco (cães de caça, de exposição ou aqueles com acesso a lagoas/poços) a cada 4-6 meses, especialmente nas áreas endêmicas.
- Canis — higienização rigorosa para evitar o contato com a urina infectada; controlar os roedores; monitorizar e remover os cães portadores até que sejam tratados; isolar os animais acometidos durante o tratamento.
- Atividade — limitar o acesso às áreas lamacentas/pantanosas, lagoas, áreas de baixada com água superficial estagnada, pastos intensamente irrigados e acesso à vida selvagem.

COMPLICAÇÕES POSSÍVEIS
- CID.
- Disfunção renal e hepática permanente.
- Uveíte.
- Abortamento.

EVOLUÇÃO ESPERADA E PROGNÓSTICO
- A maioria das infecções é subclínica ou crônica.
- Prognóstico reservado na doença grave aguda.

DIVERSOS

FATORES RELACIONADOS COM A IDADE
Doença clínica grave nos cães jovens (não vacinados ou isentos de anticorpos maternos).

POTENCIAL ZOONÓTICO
- Elevado; os microrganismos disseminam-se na urina dos animais infectados.
- Higiene rigorosa do canil e desinfecção das instalações (desinfetante à base de iodo ou soluções alvejantes estabilizadas).
- Animais agudamente infectados e animais portadores precisam ser tratados.

GESTAÇÃO/FERTILIDADE/REPRODUÇÃO
- Possível abortamento.
- Terapia antimicrobiana — considerar o efeito do medicamento sobre o feto em desenvolvimento.

ABREVIATURA(S)
- CID = coagulação intravascular disseminada.
- FeLV = vírus da leucemia felina.
- FIV = vírus da imunodeficiência felina.
- PCR = reação em cadeia da polimerase.
- PD/PU = polidipsia e poliúria.
- PIF = peritonite infecciosa felina.

Sugestões de Leitura
Greene CE, Sykes JE, Brown CA, Hartmann K. Leptospirosis. In: Greene CE, ed., Infectious Diseases of the Dog and Cat, 3rd ed. St. Louis: Saunders Elsevier, 2006, pp. 402-417.

Autor Patrick L. McDonough
Consultor Editorial Stephen C. Barr

LESÃO CEREBRAL

CONSIDERAÇÕES GERAIS

DEFINIÇÃO
- Primária — resultado de insulto inicial direto.
- Secundária — alterações da vasculatura e do tecido cerebrais que ocorrem após lesão primária.

FISIOPATOLOGIA
- Aceleração, desaceleração e forças rotacionais contribuem para a lesão primária. • Cérebro sob risco de hipoxia — altas necessidades de oxigênio e glicose; mínimo armazenamento de oxigênio; poucos capilares recrutáveis. • Forças responsáveis pelo fluxo sanguíneo cerebral — pressão de perfusão cerebral (PPC) = pressão arterial média (PAM) — pressão intracraniana (PIC).
- Sangramento, edema cerebral (vasogênico e citotóxico) e/ou vasospasmos provocam elevação da PIC, o que induz a baixo fluxo sanguíneo cerebral e isquemia, tumefação cerebral e herniação; elevações pequenas e progressivas da PIC são mais bem toleradas que aumentos pequenos e agudos. • Hipotensão, hipoxia — principais fatores que contribuem para a lesão secundária.

SISTEMA(S) ACOMETIDO(S)
- Nervoso — crises convulsivas, estupor, coma, contração espasmódica, alterações posturais.
- Cardiovascular — arritmias por disfunção dos centros cardiovasculares centrais. • Endócrino/Metabólico — alterações na liberação de ADH e na concentração de sódio; desregulação da temperatura central; insulinorresistência; depleção de cortisol por estresse prolongado. • Oftálmico — alterações na posição ocular, movimentos oculares, reflexos pupilares à luz, papiledema.
- Respiratório — padrões respiratórios anormais por disfunção dos centros reguladores; edema pulmonar neurogênico.

DISTRIBUIÇÃO GEOGRÁFICA
Mundial.

IDENTIFICAÇÃO
Espécies
Cães e gatos.

SINAIS CLÍNICOS
Achados Anamnésicos
- Determinar a causa — traumatismo; parada cardíaca; insuficiência cardíaca; hipertensão; toxinas; coagulopatias com sangramento intracraniano; comprometimento respiratório grave prolongado; hipoglicemia. • Queda na consciência — implica evolução de sangramento intracraniano, edema cerebral, isquemia.
- Atividade convulsiva — envolvimento do cérebro ou do diencéfalo.

Achados do Exame Físico
- Procurar por indícios de traumatismo.
- Insuficiência cardíaca ou respiratória — hipoxia, cianose, hipoventilação. • Má perfusão — pulso fraco, mucosas pálidas. • Sangue proveniente das orelhas ou do nariz — traumatismo com sangramento intracraniano. • Palpação do crânio — fraturas que necessitam de descompressão cirúrgica. • Hipotermia, hipertermia — efeitos sobre a perfusão e a taxa metabólica. • Bradicardia contínua com níveis normais de potássio — lesão do mesencéfalo, da ponte ou da medula. • Reflexo de Cushing — bradicardia e hipertensão ou hipotensão. • Equimose ou petéquias — problemas hemorrágicos. • Hemorragias retinianas ou vasos distendidos — hipertensão, coagulopatia. • Papiledema — edema cerebral. • Descolamento da retina — causas infecciosas, neoplásicas ou hipertensivas.

Achados do Exame Neurológico
- Podem piorar durante a ressuscitação volêmica — hipertensão, hemorragia intracraniana.
- Determinar o nível de consciência. • Situar a lesão ao córtex cerebral (melhor prognóstico), mesencéfalo/tronco encefálico, ou multifocal.
- Alterações posturais — rigidez descerebrada em caso de lesão do mesencéfalo; rigidez descerebelada em caso de lesão do cerebelo. • Déficits focais superagudos sugerem causas vasculares.

Reflexos Pupilares à Luz
- Pupilas mióticas responsivas — lesão cerebral ou diencéfalica. • Pupilas dilatadas não responsivas (uni ou bilaterais) ou pupilas fixas no ponto médio e não responsivas — lesão do mesencéfalo.
- Pupilas puntiformes — lesão da ponte ou da medula.

Nervos Cranianos
- Normais — lesão do cérebro-diencéfalo. • Perda do nistagmo fisiológico — lesão do tronco encefálico; realizar se a manipulação cervical for possível. • III par de nervos cranianos — lesão do mesencéfalo. • V e XII pares de nervos cranianos — lesão da ponte ou da medula.

Padrões Respiratórios
- Respiração de Cheyne-Stokes — lesão cerebral ou diencéfalica difusa grave. • Hiperventilação — lesão do mesencéfalo. • Respiração atáxica ou apnêustica — lesão da ponte ou da medula.

CAUSAS
- Traumatismo craniencefálico. • Hipoxia ou isquemia prolongada. • Choque prolongado, hipotensão. • Hipoglicemia grave. • Crises convulsivas prolongadas. • Hipertermia ou hipotermia grave. • Alterações na osmolalidade sérica (sódio, glicose). • Toxinas. • Neoplasia.
- Hipertensão. • Doenças inflamatórias, infecciosas, imunomediadas. • Deficiência de tiamina. • Migração parasitária.

FATORES DE RISCO
- Animais errantes de vida livre — traumatismo, toxinas. • Doença cardíaca, respiratória, hemostática coexistente. • Diabetes melito — insulinoterapia.

DIAGNÓSTICO

DIAGNÓSTICO DIFERENCIAL
Causas sistêmicas de estados alterados de consciência — doença metabólica; toxinas; medicamentos; infecção.

HEMOGRAMA/BIOQUÍMICA/URINÁLISE
- Refletem os efeitos sistêmicos de traumatismo ou hipoxemia. • Alterações no sódio sérico sugerem anormalidades do ADH central.

OUTROS TESTES LABORATORIAIS
- Gasometria arterial — hipoxemia; alterações graves do pH; hipercarbia. • Perfil de coagulação — na suspeita de trombose ou sangramento intracraniano. • Títulos de doença infecciosa.

DIAGNÓSTICO POR IMAGEM
- Radiografias do crânio — detectam fraturas.
- TC — detecta hemorragia aguda, infartos, fraturas, corpos estranhos penetrantes, herniação.
- RM — detecta edema cerebral, hemorragia, massa, doenças infiltrativas, herniação, fraturas.

MÉTODOS DIAGNÓSTICOS
- ECG — detecta arritmias. • Pressão arterial — determina a perfusão. • LCS — se a causa for desconhecida e se não houver contraindicações.

ACHADOS PATOLÓGICOS
- Edema cerebral. • Herniação. • Hemorragia.
- Infarto. • Laceração, contusão. • Hematomas.
- Fratura de crânio. • Necrose. • Apoptose.

TRATAMENTO

CUIDADO(S) DE SAÚDE ADEQUADO(S)
- Objetivos da terapia — maximizar os processos de oxigenação e ventilação; manter a pressão arterial e a PPC; diminuir a PIC; reduzir a taxa metabólica cerebral. • $PaCO_2$ — manter em 35-45 mmHg; na suspeita de PIC elevada, a hiperventilação em 32-35 mmHg pode reduzir o fluxo sanguíneo cerebral e a PIC. • PaO_2 — deve ser >50 mmHg para manter a autorregulação do fluxo sanguíneo cerebral. • Evitar o reflexo de tosse ou espirro durante a entubação ou suplementação nasal de oxigênio — pode elevar a PIC; administrar lidocaína (cães: 0,75 mg/kg IV) antes.
- Não obstruir o fluxo sanguíneo da veia jugular; o desvio de volume sanguíneo para as veias jugulares é um mecanismo compensatório durante o aumento da PIC.

CUIDADO(S) DE ENFERMAGEM
- Terapia rigorosa apenas para lesão do mesencéfalo/tronco encefálico ou sinais neurológicos deteriorantes. • A ressuscitação volêmica superzelosa pode contribuir para a formação de edema cerebral. • É recomendável o uso de técnicas de ressuscitação volêmica com pequenos volumes; utilizar a quantidade mínima para manter a pressão arterial sistólica > 90 mmHg com frequência cardíaca normal. • Utilizar apenas os cristaloides (soro fisiológico ou solução balanceada isotônica em incrementos de 20-30 mL/kg repetidos até atingir o desfecho) na suspeita de hemorragia.
- Combinação de cristaloides com coloides de alto peso molecular (hetamido a 5 mL/kg ou oxiglobina em incrementos de 3-5 mL/kg durante 5-8 minutos) na presença de hipotensão ou vasculite. • Utilizar os coloides com moderação de forma a minimizar o extravasamento para o tecido cerebral na suspeita de hemorragia. • Evitar hipertensão. • Nivelar a cabeça ou o corpo ou elevá-la em um ângulo de 20°; jamais deixá-la mais baixa que o corpo. • Proceder aos cuidados de enfermagem para evitar as complicações secundárias do decúbito. • Manter as vias aéreas desobstruídas; utilizar o procedimento de sucção e umidificar as vias aéreas se o animal estiver entubado; hiperoxigenar o paciente e considerar a administração IV ou intratraqueal de lidocaína antes de succionar para evitar dessaturação e tosse significativas. • Lubrificar os olhos. • Posicionar o animal em decúbito sobre o esterno; se o animal estiver em decúbito lateral, mudar de posição a cada 2 h para evitar congestão pulmonar hipostática. • Evitar sujeira com fezes ou urina.
- Manter a temperatura corporal central em um nível normal ou sob leve hipotermia; evitar

Lesão Cerebral

hipertermia. • Manter a hidratação do animal com solução cristaloide eletrolítica balanceada.

ATIVIDADE
Restrita.

DIETA
Iniciar a alimentação por fluxo de gotejamento/escoamento (ou seja, pouco a pouco) para suprir as demandas metabólicas elevadas.

ORIENTAÇÃO AO PROPRIETÁRIO
Os sinais neurológicos podem piorar antes de melhorar.
O grau de recuperação neurológica pode não ser evidente por vários dias, mas possivelmente >6 meses para déficits neurológicos residuais. Anormalidades sistêmicas graves contribuem para a instabilidade do SNC.

CONSIDERAÇÕES CIRÚRGICAS
Fratura de crânio com depressão cerebral, corpo estranho penetrante, ou evidência de problema cirúrgico ao exame de TC ou RM (herniação, hidrocefalia, hematoma).

MEDICAÇÕES

MEDICAMENTO(S) DE ESCOLHA

PIC elevada
• Reduzir a pressão intracraniana por meio de hiperventilação, terapia farmacológica, drenagem do LCS pelos ventrículos, ou descompressão cirúrgica.
• Furosemida na dose de 0,75 mg/kg IV: diminui a produção do LCS e reduz a PIC; utilizada em pacientes com hemorragia, insuficiência cardíaca congestiva, sobrecarga volêmica, doenças hiperosmolares, ou insuficiência renal anúrica; usar antes do manitol ou como único diurético.
• Manitol na dose de 0,1-0,5 g/kg em bólus IV repetido em intervalos de 2 h três a quatro vezes em cães e duas a três vezes em gatos; é imprescindível a administração de doses repetidas a tempo e em tempo oportuno; restabelece o fluxo sanguíneo cerebral e diminui a PIC; pode exacerbar a hemorragia.
• Salina hipertônica a 7% (2-4 mL/kg IV); pode reduzir o volume hídrico até atingir o desfecho. Considerar o uso da salina hipertônica no lugar do manitol. Pode exacerbar o edema cerebral se extravasar; combinar com coloide.
• Glicocorticosteroides em altas doses — sem benefício no tratamento agudo e nas consequências a longo prazo em seres humanos; morbidade mais elevada.
• Administração de analgésicos/sedativos (p. ex., fentanila na dose de 5 mcg/kg IV, depois 5 mcg/kg/h sob taxa de infusão contínua), conforme indicado. Evitar agentes capazes de reduzir a PPC.
• Espancamento, crises convulsivas, ou atividade motora descontrolada — podem elevar a PIC; diazepam sob taxa de infusão contínua (0,5-1 mg/kg/h), midazolam sob taxa de infusão contínua (0,2-0,4 mg/kg IV) ou propofol (3-6 mg/kg IV titulado até fazer efeito; 0,1-0,6 mg/kg/min sob taxa de infusão contínua: monitorizar a ocorrência de hipotensão).
• Dose de ataque do fenobarbital (4 mg/kg/h por três doses) se houver atividade convulsiva.
• Desmopressina (DDAVP) para hipernatremia refratária. A dosagem de emergência não foi estabelecida para os animais (seres humanos: vasopressina aquosa sob taxa de infusão contínua a 2,5 unidades/h tituladas até obter um débito urinário de 100 mL/h).
• Coma barbitúrico — em caso de aumento da PIC refratário para reduzir a taxa metabólica cerebral; administrar a dose de ataque do pentobarbital até fazer efeito (até 10 mg/kg IV durante 30 minutos; manter a 1 mg/kg/h sob taxa de infusão contínua); o paciente deve ser entubado, mantendo-se a pressão arterial, a oxigenação e a ventilação.

Outros tipos de terapia
• O resfriamento do paciente a 32-33°C pode conferir proteção cerebral quando realizado em até 6 horas da isquemia global ou lesão cerebral grave.
• Suplementação de glicose — conforme a necessidade para hipoglicemia.
• Hiperglicemia — infusão contínua de insulina regular (a dosagem para este uso não é documentada em animais; considerar a dose baixa de 0,5-1 unidade/kg/dia) para manter a glicose sérica entre 80 e 120 mg/dL após ressuscitação volêmica; monitorizar a glicemia.
• Uso de sonda para alimentação inicial por fluxo de gotejamento/escoamento; cisaprida (0,5 mg/kg a cada 8-12 h) pode promover motilidade GI.

CONTRAINDICAÇÕES
• Medicamentos que provocam hipertensão, hipotensão.
• Medicamentos que causam hiperexcitabilidade.
• Não utilizar agentes osmóticos na presença de hemorragia intracraniana.

PRECAUÇÕES
• Evitar hipotensão, hipoxemia, hipertensão, hiperglicemia, hipoglicemia, hipernatremia.
• Evitar sobrecarga volêmica intravascular.
• Não permitir que a cabeça fique em um plano abaixo do corpo.
• Não usar as veias jugulares.
• Manitol e salina hipertônica — podem agravar o estado neurológico na presença de hemorragia intracraniana.
• Hiperventilação — manter a $PaCO_2$ >25 mmHg; não realizar por períodos prolongados (>48 horas).

ACOMPANHAMENTO

MONITORIZAÇÃO DO PACIENTE
• Exames neurológicos repetidos — para detectar deterioração que justifique uma intervenção terapêutica rigorosa.
• Pressão arterial — manter a administração de fluido adequado e evitar a ocorrência de hipertensão.
• Gasometria sanguínea, oximetria de pulso, CO_2 corrente final (capnografia) — para avaliar a necessidade de suplementação de oxigênio ou ventilação.
• Glicose sanguínea — manter a 80-120 mg/dL.
• ECG — para detectar arritmias que possam afetar a perfusão, a oxigenação e o fluxo sanguíneo cerebral.
• PIC — para detectar elevações e monitorizar a resposta à terapia.

PREVENÇÃO
Manter os animais domésticos em uma área confinada ou presos com coleira.

COMPLICAÇÕES POSSÍVEIS
• Crises convulsivas.
• Herniação cerebral.
• Hemorragia intracraniana.
• Evolução de sinais cerebrocorticais para mesencefálicos.
• Desnutrição.
• Pneumonia por aspiração.
• Congestão pulmonar hipostática.
• Dissecação corneana.
• Queimadura por escaldagem de urina.
• Obstrução das vias aéreas por muco.
• Arritmias cardíacas — geralmente bradiarritmias.
• Hipotensão.
• Hipernatremia.
• Hipocalemia.
• Insuficiência respiratória.
• Déficits neurológicos residuais.
• Morte.

EVOLUÇÃO ESPERADA E PROGNÓSTICO
• Animais jovens, lesão cerebral primária mínima, e lesão secundária que consiste em edema cerebral — prognóstico melhor.
• Sem deterioração do estado neurológico por 48 horas — prognóstico melhor.
• Ressuscitação rápida da pressão arterial sistólica para >90 mmHg — melhor resultado neurológico.
• Manutenção da glicemia (80-120 mg/dL) associada a um melhor desfecho em seres humanos.
• Escore de Coma de Glasgow pode oferecer informações prognósticas.

DIVERSOS

SINÔNIMOS
• Traumatismo craniencefálico.
• Lesão cerebral traumática.

VER TAMBÉM
Estupor e Coma.

ABREVIATURAS
• ADH = hormônio antidiurético.
• ECG = eletrocardiograma.
• GI = gastrintestinal.
• LCS = líquido cerebrospinal.
• PAM = pressão arterial média.
• PIC = pressão intracraniana.
• PPC = pressão de perfusão cerebral.
• RM = ressonância magnética.
• SNC = sistema nervoso central.
• TC = tomografia computadorizada.

RECURSOS DA INTERNET
www.braininjury.com.
www.cvmbs.colostate.edu/clinsci/wing/comascor.html.
www.emedicine.com/pmr/topic212.htm.
www.traumaticbraininjury.com.

Sugestões de Leitura
Mathews K, Parent J. Head trauma. In: Mathews K, ed., Veterinary Emergency Critical Care Manual, 2nd ed. Guelph, Ontario: Lifelearn, 2006, pp. 691-701.

Autor Rebecca Kirby
Consultor Editorial Joane M. Parent

Lesão por Mordedura de Fio Elétrico

CONSIDERAÇÕES GERAIS

REVISÃO
- A lesão por mordedura de fio elétrico é um evento incomum, que ocorre quando o animal morde um fio de eletricidade.
- Embora outras causas de eletrocussão possam ocorrer, elas são raras em cães e gatos.
- As correntes elétricas domésticas são alternadas (60 Hz) ou 120 volts e perigosas.
- A lesão pode ser decorrente de termolesão ou interrupção da atividade eletrofisiológica normal do tecido excitável.
- O edema pulmonar pode ser sequela da eletrocussão; além disso, acredita-se que a fisiopatologia seja neurogênica e mediada por via central, levando à hipertensão pulmonar.
- Há relatos de formação de cataratas após a eletrocussão.

IDENTIFICAÇÃO
- Observada em cães e gatos.
- Mais comum em cães.
- Mais frequentemente constatada em animais jovens. Em relatos publicados, as idades variam de 5 meses a 1 ano e meio.
- Não há predileção racial ou sexual.
- Não há base genética.

SINAIS CLÍNICOS
- Queimaduras da gengiva, da língua e do palato.
- Pelos ou pelos tácteis (também conhecidos como vibrissas ou bigodes) chamuscados.
- Os sinais clínicos mais comuns relacionam-se à dispneia aguda.
- Tosse.
- Taquipneia.
- Ortopneia.
- Aumento no esforço respiratório.
- Cianose.
- Crepitações durante a auscultação pulmonar.
- Taquicardia.
- Tremores musculares.
- Atividade tônico-clônica.
- Colapso.

CAUSAS E FATORES DE RISCO
- Mastigação de fio elétrico.
- Idade jovem.
- Acomete principalmente cães, mas também há relatos em gatos.

DIAGNÓSTICO

DIAGNÓSTICO DIFERENCIAL
- Insuficiência cardíaca congestiva esquerda — pode ser atribuída à cardiopatia congênita ou adquirida. A presença de sopro cardíaco ou disritmia pode ajudar a diferenciar, mas as disritmias também podem ser observadas em casos de lesões por mordedura de fio elétrico.
- Histórico de intoxicação por rodenticida antagonista da vitamina K.
- Traumatismo torácico — anamnese, radiografias torácicas.
- Outras causas de edema pulmonar não cardiogênico.
- Doença do espaço pleural — ruídos pulmonares abafados à auscultação, radiografias torácicas.
- Lesões térmicas ou químicas — anamnese, exame físico, radiografias torácicas.
- Exposição ao fogo ou inalação de fumaça — anamnese, exame físico.
- Pneumonia atípica — anamnese, exame físico, radiografias torácicas.

HEMOGRAMA/BIOQUÍMICA/URINÁLISE
Podem ajudar a descartar outras causas sistêmicas de edema pulmonar não cardiogênico.

OUTROS TESTES LABORATORIAIS
A gasometria arterial pode ser útil para registrar a ocorrência de hipoxemia. Pode não ser fácil realizar esse tipo de análise em pacientes instáveis.

DIAGNÓSTICO POR IMAGEM
- As radiografias torácicas podem ajudar a distinguir entre causas cardiogênicas e não cardiogênicas do edema pulmonar.
- O padrão broncoalveolar misto generalizado costuma ser o padrão radiográfico. O edema apresenta-se frequentemente mais notável nos campos pulmonares dorsocaudais.
- A ecocardiografia pode ajudar a identificar uma cardiopatia subjacente.

MÉTODOS DIAGNÓSTICOS
- Eletrocardiograma — pode ajudar a distinguir as doenças cardiogênicas e não cardiogênicas; entretanto, também se podem observar disritmias em casos de eletrocussão e outras causas de edema pulmonar não cardiogênico.
- Ecocardiografia — deve ajudar a identificar insuficiência cardíaca como uma causa.

ACHADOS PATOLÓGICOS
- Líquido róseo e espumoso nas vias aéreas.
- Pulmões congestos e preenchidos por líquido.
- Petéquias subendocárdicas e subepicárdicas.
- Lesões bucais circunscritas de coloração cinza ou castanha pálidas.

TRATAMENTO

- Se o paciente estiver próximo a um fio/cabo sob tensão elétrica, deve-se desligar a eletricidade e removê-lo para uma área segura.
- Se o animal se apresentar inconsciente, deve-se estabelecer uma via aérea patente (desobstruída).
- Suplementação de oxigênio.
- Talvez haja necessidade de ventilação mecânica.
- Proceder à fixação de acesso venoso.

MEDICAÇÕES

MEDICAMENTO(S)
- Se o animal se encontrar em choque, tratar com cristaloides intravenosos (90 mL/kg/h em cães, 45-60 mL/kg/h em gatos) ou coloides (20 mL/kg em cães, 5-10 mL/kg em gatos)
- Na presença de edema pulmonar, administrar a furosemida (2-4 mg/kg IV). A administração desse diurético é controversa, pois se trata de uma forma de edema pulmonar não cardiogênico.
- Os corticosteroides já foram empregados, mas seu uso permanece controverso e de valor desconhecido.
- Se necessário, fornecer suporte inotrópico.
- Administrar terapia antiarrítmica, conforme a necessidade.
- Efetuar o tratamento sintomático das queimaduras bucais e cutâneas.

ACOMPANHAMENTO

MONITORIZAÇÃO DO PACIENTE
- É aconselhável monitorizar o paciente até sua estabilização.
- Exame físico.
- Também se recomenda a monitorização das lesões bucais, uma vez que elas podem impedir o animal de se alimentar.
- Eletrocardiografia.
- Pressão venosa central.
- Pressão arterial.
- Gasometria sanguínea arterial.
- Radiografias torácicas.

PREVENÇÃO
- É preciso descartar os fios elétricos danificados.
- Evitar a exposição do animal a fios elétricos.
- Adotar regras domiciliares de segurança projetadas para crianças.

COMPLICAÇÕES POSSÍVEIS
- Pode ocorrer infecção das queimaduras, mas isso não é comum.
- Fístula oronasal decorrente de queimaduras graves.

EVOLUÇÃO ESPERADA E PROGNÓSTICO
- O prognóstico baseia-se na resposta à terapia.
- O edema pulmonar pode se desenvolver de 1 a 36 h após o incidente.
- O edema pulmonar associado à eletrocussão vincula-se a uma alta taxa de mortalidade (38,5%).
- Se o paciente sobreviver nas primeiras 24 h, o prognóstico será mais favorável.
- A resolução do edema pulmonar pode levar de 3-5 dias.
- A maioria das lesões bucais desaparece.
- A inapetência relacionada às lesões bucais também desaparece.

DIVERSOS

DISTÚRBIOS ASSOCIADOS
Já se relatou a formação de cataratas em um cão, 18 meses após a eletrocussão.

Sugestões de Leitura

Brightman AH, Brogdon JD, Helper LC, Everds N. Electrical cataracts in the canine: A case report. JAAHA 1984, 20:895-898.

Drobatz KJ, Saunders HM, Pugh CR, Hendricks JC. Noncardiogenic pulmonary edema in dogs and cats: 26 cases (1987-1995). JAVMA 1995, 206:1732-1736.

Kolata RJ, Burrows CF. The clinical features of injury by chewing electrical cords in dogs and cats. JAAHA 1981, 17:219-222.

Lee-Parritz DE, Pavletic MM. Physical and chemical Injuries: Heatstroke, hypothermia, burns, and frostbite. In: Murtaugh RJ, Kaplan PM, Veterinary Emergency and Critical Care Medicine. St. Louis: Mosby Year Book, 1992, pp. 194-212.

Autor Steven L. Marks
Consultores Editoriais Larry P. Tilley and Francis W.K. Smith, Jr.

Leucemia Linfoblástica Aguda

CONSIDERAÇÕES GERAIS

REVISÃO
- Distúrbio linfoproliferativo definido pela presença de prolinfócitos e linfoblastos neoplásicos circulantes na corrente sanguínea; a maioria origina-se das células B.
- Pode ser precedida por síndrome mielodisplásica.
- Os pacientes apresentam um comprometimento da imunidade celular e humoral.
- Caracterizada por infiltração da medula óssea (e locais extramedulares) e deslocamento de células-tronco hematopoiéticas normais.
- Pode se infiltrar em outros órgãos.

IDENTIFICAÇÃO
- Cães — relação macho:fêmea, 3:2; tende a acometer animais mais jovens com idade média em torno de 5-6 anos de idade (faixa etária, 1-12 anos).
- Rara em gatos (também acomete animais mais jovens, sobretudo com infecção pelo FeLV).

SINAIS CLÍNICOS
- Frequentemente inespecíficos, podendo incluir letargia e anormalidades gastrintestinais.
- Hepatosplenomegalia.
- Linfadenomegalia.
- Hemorragias petequiais ou equimóticas.
- Outros sinais — refletem infiltração orgânica específica; qualquer órgão pode estar envolvido.

CAUSAS E FATORES DE RISCO
- Cães — radiação ionizante; vírus oncogênicos; agentes químicos incluindo quimioterapia alquilante; foram identificadas mutações de sentido trocado (*missense*) e duplicações em *tandem* em oncogenes como Flt3, c-kit e N-ras em cães com leucemia linfoblástica aguda.
- Gatos — infecção pelo FeLV.

DIAGNÓSTICO

DIAGNÓSTICO DIFERENCIAL
- Infecção aguda ou crônica — toxoplasmose; cinomose; erliquiose.
- Anemia aplásica.
- Neoplasia metastática.
- Pode ser difícil diferenciar entre o linfoma multicêntrico com envolvimento da medula óssea e presença de linfoblastos circulantes e o quadro de leucemia linfoblástica aguda. Tipicamente, o linfoma é caracterizado pela existência de doença periférica volumosa e ausência de doença sistêmica, enquanto a leucemia linfoblástica aguda exibe enfartamento nulo ou moderado dos linfonodos periféricos, esplenomegalia acentuada e sinais de doença sistêmica com início relativamente agudo.
- Outros distúrbios mieloproliferativos e leucemias.

HEMOGRAMA/BIOQUÍMICA/URINÁLISE
- Hemograma completo — anemia normocítica normocrômica arregenerativa; neutropenia; trombocitopenia; todas essas anormalidades estão presentes em mais de 75% dos casos.
- O hemograma completo também pode revelar linfocitose ou leucopenia linfoblástica.
- Perfil bioquímico sérico — atividades elevadas das enzimas hepáticas.

OUTROS TESTES LABORATORIAIS
- Exame citológico de aspirado da medula óssea — infiltração linfoblástica com números baixos de precursores mieloides e eritroides, bem como números baixos de megacariócitos; caracterizada pelo grau de envolvimento da medula óssea, tipo celular de origem e diferenciação.
- Biopsia nuclear de medula óssea com estudos imuno-histoquímicos ou bioquímicos enzimáticos — pode ser necessária para diferenciar de outros tipos de leucemia.
- Os marcadores de superfície incluem CD34 (células-tronco), CD18 (leucócitos) e CD79a (células B).
- As enzimas incluem peroxidase e éster de cloroacetato.
- Os exames de imunocitoquímica ou citometria de fluxo efetuados na amostra obtida por aspirado de medula óssea também podem caracterizar o quadro de leucemia linfoblástica aguda por meio de marcadores de superfície.
- A análise do rearranjo dos genes de receptores antigênicos por PCR pode confirmar uma população clonal expandida.
- A proteína C-reativa frequentemente se encontra elevada em pacientes com leucemia linfoblástica aguda.

DIAGNÓSTICO POR IMAGEM
Radiografia simples e ultrassonografia — quase sempre revelam hepatosplenomegalia.

MÉTODOS DIAGNÓSTICOS
Aspirado e biopsia de medula óssea.

TRATAMENTO

- Em geral, o tratamento é feito em um esquema ambulatorial a menos que haja necessidade de cuidado de suporte.
- Os pacientes encontram-se imunocomprometidos e, portanto, não devem ficar expostos à doença infecciosa.
- Transfusões — conforme indicação, para repor as hemácias, as plaquetas ou os fatores da coagulação.
- Consulte um veterinário especialista em oncologia em busca de abordagens terapêuticas atualizadas. O transplante de medula óssea pode ser uma opção imediata caso se consiga atingir uma remissão inicial com o uso de quimioterapia; esse tipo de transplante, no entanto, está disponível apenas em centros cirúrgicos seletos de oncologia veterinária.

MEDICAÇÕES

MEDICAMENTO(S)
- L-asparaginase (10.000 U/m² IM após pré-tratamento com difenidramina); utilizada geralmente como agente de indução inicial.
- Quimioterapia combinada — prednisona (20 mg/m² VO a cada 12 h), vincristina (0,5-0,7 mg/m² IV semanalmente) e ciclofosfamida (200-250 mg/m² divididos VO semanalmente); pode resultar em remissão parcial ou completa de curta duração.
- Citosina arabinosídeo (400 mg/m² semanalmente); administrar em velocidade constante de infusão por 6-8 horas; pode causar trombocitopenia ou outra mielossupressão.
- Agentes quimioterápicos mais rigorosos podem ser usados após o declínio da linfocitose e a resolução das citopenias.

CONTRAINDICAÇÕES/INTERAÇÕES POSSÍVEIS
Após a quimioterapia, pode-se observar uma síndrome de lise tumoral aguda, em que ocorre um aumento súbito nos níveis de potássio e fósforo após a liberação maciça desses elementos a partir das células cancerígenas lesionadas.

ACOMPANHAMENTO

MONITORIZAÇÃO DO PACIENTE
Monitorizar a contagem do sangue periférico e a produção da medula óssea — julgar o sucesso e a toxicidade do tratamento.

COMPLICAÇÕES POSSÍVEIS
Hemorragia por trombocitopenia — principal causa de morte nos cães.

EVOLUÇÃO ESPERADA E PROGNÓSTICO
Prognóstico grave, pois a maioria dos cães vem a óbito em algumas semanas.

DIVERSOS

GESTAÇÃO/FERTILIDADE/REPRODUÇÃO
Quimioterapia — contraindicada nas fêmeas prenhes.

ABREVIATURA(S)
- FeLV = vírus da leucemia felina.
- PCR = reação em cadeia da polimerase.

Sugestões de Leitura
Tasca S, Carli E, Caldin M, et al. Hematologic abnormalities and flow cytometric immunophenotyping results in dogs with hematopoietic neoplasia: 210 cases (2002-2006). Vet Clin Path 2009, 38(1):2-12.

Autor Kim A. Selting
Consultor Editorial Timothy M. Fan
Agradecimento Linda S. Fineman

LEUCEMIA LINFOCÍTICA CRÔNICA

CONSIDERAÇÕES GERAIS

REVISÃO
- Distúrbio linfoproliferativo incomum.
- Lentamente progressivo durante meses a anos.
- Os linfócitos neoplásicos circulantes são maduros e bem-diferenciados.
- Pode-se originar no baço ou na medula óssea.

SISTEMA(S) ACOMETIDO(S)
- Hematopoiético.
- Linfático.

IDENTIFICAÇÃO
- Mais frequente nos cães do que nos gatos.
- Cães — idade média, 10 anos (variação, 1,5-15 anos); relação macho:fêmea chega a 2:1.

SINAIS CLÍNICOS
- Inespecíficos, mas frequentemente não há nenhum sinal clínico de doença.
- Letargia, apetite diminuído, perda de peso.
- Polidipsia e poliúria.
- Linfadenomegalia, esplenomegalia.
- Febre.
- Contusões.

CAUSAS E FATORES DE RISCO
Desconhecidos.

DIAGNÓSTICO

DIAGNÓSTICO DIFERENCIAL
- Linfoma — pode apresentar uma fase leucêmica (estágio V).
- Leucemia linfoblástica aguda.
- Doenças hematológicas imunomediadas.
- Estimulação antigênica crônica (linfocitose reativa) — erliquiose, leptospirose, leishmaniose.

HEMOGRAMA/BIOQUÍMICA/URINÁLISE
- Linfocitose — faixa de 5.000-500.000 células/µL, tipicamente linfócitos pequenos e maduros.
- Em cães, mais de 60% apresentam morfologia de grande linfócito granular. Células maiores podem ser observadas, especialmente com a evolução para crise blástica (estágio avançado).
- Anemia normocítica normocrômica leve a moderada (arregenerativa).
- Contagem plaquetária normal a reduzida (menos de 20% dos casos).
- Globulinas séricas normais a levemente elevadas.

OUTROS TESTES LABORATORIAIS
- Exame citológico (aspirado da medula óssea ou biopsia de núcleo) — pode revelar números elevados de linfócitos maduros (especialmente leucemia linfocítica crônica de células B); exclusão de linhagens celulares normais nos estágios avançados.
- Imunocitoquímica, citometria de fluxo, PCR do rearranjo de receptores antigênicos para determinar a linhagem celular.
- Eletroforese de proteínas séricas para detectar os picos monoclonais.
- Proteinúria de Bence-Jones.
- Teste de Coombs direto — pode ser positivo na anemia hemolítica imunomediada secundária.
- Sorologia para pesquisa de E. canis.

DIAGNÓSTICO POR IMAGEM
Radiografia e ultrassonografia — podem revelar esplenomegalia e linfadenomegalia interna.

MÉTODOS DIAGNÓSTICOS
- Aspirado (citologia) ou biopsia (histopatologia) da medula óssea.
- Citologia ou histopatologia de linfonodo.

TRATAMENTO

- Em geral, os pacientes são tratados em um esquema ambulatorial com terapia oral.
- Esplenectomia — pode ser considerada em caso de envolvimento do baço e quando parece haver um local primário (leucemia linfocítica crônica de grande linfócito granular, medula normal) de linfócitos neoplásicos.
- O tratamento deve ser instituído quando o paciente exibir sintomas debilitantes, linfadenomegalia ou organomegalia, citopenias ou contagem de linfócitos acima de 50.000/µL (arbitrário).
- Consultar um veterinário especialista em oncologia para atualizações no tratamento.

MEDICAÇÕES

MEDICAMENTO(S)
- Clorambucila — 6 mg/m^2 VO a cada 24 h por 7-14 dias; depois, 6 mg/m^2 VO a cada 48 h e, finalmente (como manutenção) 2-3 mg/m^2 a cada 48 h, ajustado com base na resposta e no hemograma completo (cães); 2 mg a cada 3-4 dias (gatos).
- Prednisona — 20 mg/m^2 VO a cada 12 h (cães); 5-10 mg/gato a cada 24 h (gatos); em combinação com a clorambucila; pode ser gradativamente reduzida ou interrompida quando a contagem de linfócitos se normaliza.
- Agentes e protocolos quimioterápicos alternativos devem ser considerados quando se desenvolver resistência ou crise blástica com o passar do tempo — consulte um oncologista.

CONTRAINDICAÇÕES/INTERAÇÕES POSSÍVEIS
Quimioterapia — pode ter efeitos colaterais tóxicos; o clínico deve procurar orientação de um oncologista antes de iniciar o tratamento se ele não estiver familiarizado com medicamentos citotóxicos.

ACOMPANHAMENTO

Inicialmente, exame quinzenal do hemograma completo — para avaliar a resposta ao tratamento e a evolução da doença.

COMPLICAÇÕES POSSÍVEIS
Mielossupressão induzida por quimioterapia crônica; talvez haja necessidade de alterar a dosagem, dependendo das contagens de neutrófilos e plaquetas.

EVOLUÇÃO ESPERADA E PROGNÓSTICO
- Evolução variável, mas eventualmente progressiva para crise blástica ou resistência à terapia.
- O tempo médio de sobrevida com a terapia chega a 18 meses.

DIVERSOS

GESTAÇÃO/FERTILIDADE/REPRODUÇÃO
A quimioterapia é contraindicada em fêmeas prenhes.

ABREVIATURA(S)
- PCR = reação em cadeia da polimerase.

Sugestões de Leitura
Adam F, Villiers E, Watson S, et al. Clinical pathological and epidemiological assessment of morphologically and immunologically confirmed canine leukemia. Vet Comp Onc 2009, 7:181-195.
Leifer CE, Matus RE. Chronic lymphocytic leukemia in the dog: 22 cases (1974-1984). JAVMA 1986, 189:214-217.
McDonough SP, Moore PF. Clinical, hematologic, and immunophenotypic characterization of canine large granular lymphocytosis. Vet Pathol 2000, 37:637-646.
Tasca S, Carli E, Caldin M, et al. Hematologic abnormalities and flow cytometric immunophenotyping results in dogs with hematopoietic neoplasia: 210 cases (2002-2006). Vet Clin Path 2009, 38:2-12.
Vernau W, Moore PF. Na immunophenotypic study of canine leukemias and preliminary assessment of clonality by polymerase chain reaction. Vet Immunol Immunopathol 1999, 69:145-164.
Workman HC, Vernau W. Chronic lymphocytic leukemia in dogs and cats: The veterinary perspective. Vet Clin North Am Small Anim Pract 2003, 33:1379-1399.

Autor Louis-Philippe de Lorimier
Consultor Editorial Timothy M. Fan

Leucoencefalomielopatia no Rottweiler

CONSIDERAÇÕES GERAIS

REVISÃO
- Doença desmielinizante, degenerativa e progressiva, que acomete principalmente a medula espinal cervical em cães adultos da raça Rottweiler e mestiços dessa raça.
- Comprometimento da substância branca do SNC, caracterizado por síntese e/ou manutenção anormais da mielina.
- Ocorre mundialmente.
- Provavelmente exibe herança autossômica recessiva.

IDENTIFICAÇÃO
- Raça Rottweiler — ambos os sexos; início nos cães adultos de 1,5-4 anos.

SINAIS CLÍNICOS
- Início insidioso, progressivo e indolor.
- Sinais da medula espinal prevalecem apesar do processo desmielinizante disseminado: ataxia proprioceptiva e fraqueza atribuída à lesão dos neurônios motores superiores, envolvendo todos os quatro membros.
- Reflexos espinais normais a exagerados.
- Presença do reflexo extensor cruzado nos estágios finais.

CAUSAS E FATORES DE RISCO
- Desconhecidos.
- Consanguinidade.
- Doença mielinolítica.

DIAGNÓSTICO

DIAGNÓSTICO DIFERENCIAL
- Distrofia neuroaxonal e polineuropatia sensório-motora distal — distúrbios neurológicos relatados também no Rottweiler; diferenciados com base nos déficits neurológicos; distrofia neuroaxonal: os déficits relacionam-se com o cerebelo; polineuropatia sensório-motora distal: tetraparesia associada a sinais de lesão do neurônio motor inferior.
- Discospondilite, fratura ou luxação e discopatia intervertebral — dor cervical (cervicalgia); doença do disco raramente é observada em raças caninas de grande porte em idade jovem.
- Lesões compressivas cervicais como espondilomielopatia vertebral cervical (síndrome de Wobbler), cisto subaracnoide cervical e tumores da medula espinal — é difícil diferenciá-los com base apenas nos sinais clínicos; todos podem ter um início insidioso; há necessidade do exame de RM para descartar lesão expansiva ocupadora de espaço.

HEMOGRAMA/BIOQUÍMICA/URINÁLISE
Normais.

OUTROS TESTES LABORATORIAIS
N/D.

DIAGNÓSTICO POR IMAGEM
- Radiografias simples cervicais espinais permanecem normais.
- RM para descartar compressão da medula espinal das vértebras cervicais.

MÉTODOS DIAGNÓSTICOS
A análise do LCS permanece normal.

ACHADOS PATOLÓGICOS
- Desmielinização disseminada no tronco cerebral, nos pedúnculos cerebelares caudais e nas pirâmides, bem como nos nervos e tratos ópticos, estendendo-se para a medula espinal torácica; lesão mais grave na medula espinal mesocervical.
- Degeneração waleriana mínima.
- Lesões bilaterais com alguma assimetria.

TRATAMENTO

- O tratamento é ambulatorial a menos que a gravidade dos déficits neurológicos impeça o cuidado de enfermagem em casa.
- Atividade — aquilo que puder ser tolerada.
- Dieta — garantir a ingestão adequada do alimento; o paciente pode ter dificuldade para encontrar a área de alimentação.
- Estado neurológico — deteriora lenta e progressivamente; por fim, o paciente fica incapaz de caminhar ou ficar em estação.

MEDICAÇÕES

MEDICAMENTO(S)
Não há nenhum disponível.

CONTRAINDICAÇÕES/INTERAÇÕES POSSÍVEIS
N/D.

ACOMPANHAMENTO

- Exame neurológico — monitorizar mensalmente para avaliar a evolução.
- Evitar a formação de úlceras de decúbito, bem como a ocorrência de assaduras por escaldagem de urina e fezes, mantendo o paciente em uma cama limpa, seca e almofadada (p. ex., pele de carneiro sintética).
- Tetraparesia grave — dentro de 6-12 meses após o início dos sinais clínicos.
- Eutanásia — por causa da debilidade grave.

DIVERSOS

ABREVIATURA(S)
- LCS = líquido cerebrospinal.
- RM = ressonância magnética.
- SNC = sistema nervoso central.

Sugestões de Leitura
Summers BA, Cummings JF, de Lahunta A. Veterinary Neuropathology. St. Louis: Mosby, 1995, pp. 285-286.
Wouda W, van Nes JJ. Progressive ataxia due to central demyelination in rottweiler dogs. Vet Q 1986, 8:89-97.

Autor Joane M. Parent
Consultor Editorial Joane M. Parent

LINFADENITE

CONSIDERAÇÕES GERAIS

DEFINIÇÃO
- Inflamação de um ou mais linfonodos, caracterizada por migração ativa de neutrófilos, macrófagos ou eosinófilos para dentro do nodo.
- Hiperplasia linfoide não é uma forma de linfadenite.

FISIOPATOLOGIA
- Em geral, refere-se ao resultado de algum agente infeccioso que ganha acesso a algum linfonodo e estabelece a infecção; por causa da função de filtração dos linfonodos, é provável que eles sejam expostos a agentes infecciosos.
- Muitos microrganismos podem provocar inflamação; no entanto, agentes como fungos e micobactérias que residem dentro dos macrófagos e eliciam uma resposta inflamatória granulomatosa são particularmente propensos ao estabelecimento de infecção dentro dos linfonodos.
- Não infecciosa — ocorre com pouca frequência; um exemplo é a linfadenite eosinofílica que ocorre como um componente ocasional de doenças inflamatórias eosinofílicas.

SISTEMAS ACOMETIDOS
- Hemático/linfático/imune.
- Pode ser componente de doença infecciosa mais disseminada.

GENÉTICA
- Não há nenhuma base genética conhecida.
- Exceção — casos raros de imunodeficiência; por exemplo, a suscetibilidade familiar de determinados cães da raça Basset hound à micobacteriose, da qual a linfadenite consiste em uma manifestação frequente; cães da raça Rottweiler podem ser predispostos a síndromes hipereosinofílicas idiopáticas, provocando linfadenite eosinofílica.

INCIDÊNCIA/PREVALÊNCIA
- Manifestação frequente de uma série de doenças infecciosas.
- A incidência exata é desconhecida.

DISTRIBUIÇÃO GEOGRÁFICA
Mesma que aquela de infecções fúngicas sistêmicas como histoplasmose (Estados Unidos, região central) e blastomicose (Estados Unidos, região central e oriental) e, menos comumente, leishmaniose (sul e sudoeste dos Estados Unidos).

IDENTIFICAÇÃO
Espécies
Cães e gatos.

Raça(s) Predominante(s)
Nenhuma.

Idade Média e Faixa Etária
Tendo em vista sua suscetibilidade à infecção, os neonatos podem apresentar uma taxa mais elevada de ocorrência em comparação aos animais mais idosos.

Sexo Predominante
Nenhum.

SINAIS CLÍNICOS
Comentários Gerais
- Complicações da infecção em outro órgão — em geral, relacionam-se mais com esse órgão do que com o linfonodo inflamado.
- Componente de infecção sistêmica — associado à doença inflamatória sistêmica: febre, mal-estar e anorexia.

Achados Anamnésicos
- Raramente provoca aumento de linfonodo grave o suficiente a ponto de ser observado pelos proprietários.
- Sinais sistêmicos de doença inflamatória ou disfunção orgânica.

Achados do Exame Físico
- Linfonodos inflamados são tipicamente grandes e firmes, podendo ser dolorosos.
- Linfadenite bacteriana — o animal pode desenvolver abscessos dentro dos nodos que podem se abrir para o exterior e se manifestar como trajetos drenantes.
- Os animais também podem apresentar febre e outros sinais sistêmicos de infecção.

CAUSAS
Bactérias
- Ocasionalmente, relata-se grande parte das espécies patogênicas aeróbias e anaeróbias.
- Agentes mais prováveis — *Pasteurella, Bacteroides* e *Fusobacterium* spp.
- Alguns microrganismos, como *Yersinia pestis* (peste bubônica) e *Francisella tularensis* (tularemia), possuem uma afinidade particular pelos linfonodos; por essa razão, é particularmente provável que se manifestem como linfadenite, sobretudo nos gatos.
- Infecção por *Bartonella vinsonii* pode provocar linfadenite granulomatosa nos cães. As espécies de *Bartonella* podem causar hiperplasia linfoide em gatos; entretanto, os microrganismos não são detectados nas colorações de rotina.

Fungos
- As infecções por fungos costumam incluir linfadenite como única manifestação de doença sistêmica.
- Os microrganismos prováveis incluem *Blastomyces, Cryptococcus, Histoplasma, Coccidiodes* e *Sporothrix*.
- Muitos outros agentes micóticos foram ocasionalmente relatados.

Vírus
- Muitas infecções virais são implicadas por causa da hiperplasia linfoide.
- Coronavírus da PIF.
- Linfonodos mesentéricos são mais comumente acometidos.

Outros
- Protozoários — animais com toxoplasmose e leishmaniose frequentemente apresentam linfadenite, embora seja improvável que ela seja o achado clínico mais evidente.
- Algas — com frequência, a linfadenite é uma manifestação da prototecose canina.
- Não infecciosos (p. ex., associados à doença eosinofílica pulmonar ou sistêmica) — geralmente desconhecidos.

FATORES DE RISCO
- Animais com a função imune comprometida ficam suscetíveis à infecção e, portanto, à linfadenite.
- FeLV e FIV estão entre as causas mais comuns de comprometimento imunológico nos pacientes veterinários.

DIAGNÓSTICO

DIAGNÓSTICO DIFERENCIAL
- É preciso averiguar se a massa palpável ou visível realmente se trata de um linfonodo e não uma massa neoplásica ou um processo inflamatório como sialoadenite.
- Com frequência, não é possível distinguir a linfadenite de outras causas de linfadenomegalia, como hiperplasia linfoide, linfoma e neoplasia metastática, com base nos achados clínicos.
- Febre e linfonodos dolorosos provavelmente estão associados à linfadenite.
- O linfoma e a hiperplasia linfoide são causas mais comuns de aumento generalizado de linfonodos em comparação à linfadenite.

HEMOGRAMA/BIOQUÍMICA/URINÁLISE
- Embora os animais acometidos possam apresentar um leucograma inflamatório, a ausência de tais alterações não exclui o diagnóstico.
- Alguns animais com causas sistêmicas de linfadenite (p. ex., infecções fúngicas e leishmaniose) podem apresentar hiperglobulinemia acentuada.
- Eosinofilia circulante, muitas vezes grave, é um achado relativamente consistente nos animais com doenças eosinofílicas extensas e graves o suficiente a ponto de provocarem linfadenite.
- Os resultados da bioquímica podem refletir o grau de envolvimento orgânico a partir do processo mórbido subjacente.

OUTROS TESTES LABORATORIAIS
Testes sorológicos para as várias doenças fúngicas sistêmicas e possivelmente *Bartonella* spp. podem ser valiosos para a identificação, embora esses testes sejam mais bem empregados apenas quando as tentativas de demonstrar o microrganismo falharem.

DIAGNÓSTICO POR IMAGEM
Radiografia e ultrassonografia — envolvimento de nodos internos, como aqueles das cavidades torácica e abdominal, nos pacientes com doença inflamatória sistêmica; úteis para avaliar o envolvimento de outros órgãos, por exemplo, pneumonia em paciente com blastomicose ou histoplasmose.

MÉTODOS DIAGNÓSTICOS
- Citologia de aspirado obtido por agulha fina é suficiente para diagnosticar a maior parte dos casos; um simples corante hematológico tipo Romanowsky (p. ex., Diff-Quik) costuma ser adequado.
- A coloração de Gram pode ser realizada nos pacientes com suspeita de infecção bacteriana.
- Achados citológicos — proporção elevada de neutrófilos, macrófagos, eosinófilos ou alguma combinação desses tipos celulares, os quais raramente são observados nos linfonodos normais.
- Bactérias, agentes fúngicos, protozoários e algas — quase sempre estão presentes nos aspirados de linfonodos obtidos por agulha fina dos animais com essas infecções; o exame citológico frequentemente é o meio mais eficaz de detectar e identificar agentes infecciosos específicos nos animais com linfadenite de nodo isolado ou de infecção sistêmica.
- Quando o diagnóstico não for formulado pelo exame citológico, pode-se indicar a biopsia do

LINFADENITE

linfonodo; as amostras podem ser utilizadas tanto para avaliação histopatológica como para cultura.

ACHADOS PATOLÓGICOS
- Embora os linfonodos acometidos possam estar normais ao exame macroscópico, com frequência eles se encontram grandes e firmes; o grau de aumento varia amplamente e quase sempre distorce a forma do nodo.
- Linfadenite grave pode se estender através da cápsula do nodo para os tecidos adjacentes.
- À superfície de corte, os nodos acometidos frequentemente se apresentam hiperêmicos e podem apresentar nódulos mal definidos; nos exemplos extremos de linfadenite purulenta, pode ocorrer o desenvolvimento de abscessos.
- Lesões histológicas de linfadenite purulenta incluem infiltração difusa ou multifocal do nodo acometido por neutrófilos; a arquitetura corticomedular normal do nodo pode sofrer desorganização.
- Linfadenite granulomatosa — acúmulos de macrófagos ativados, envolvendo o parênquima do nodo.
- Linfadenite eosinofílica — grande número de eosinófilos tanto dentro dos seios como no parênquima cortical.
- É comum a constatação de necrose em todas as formas.

TRATAMENTO

CUIDADO(S) DE SAÚDE ADEQUADO(S)
- Como a linfadenite é mais uma lesão do que uma doença específica, nenhum grupo exclusivo de recomendações terapêuticas é adequado.
- As características da inflamação e o agente causal ditam o tratamento apropriado.

CUIDADO(S) DE ENFERMAGEM
N/D.

ATIVIDADE
N/D.

DIETA
N/D.

ORIENTAÇÃO AO PROPRIETÁRIO
N/D.

CONSIDERAÇÕES CIRÚRGICAS
N/D.

MEDICAÇÕES

MEDICAMENTO(S) DE ESCOLHA
- A terapia medicamentosa eficaz requer a identificação do agente causal.
- É provável que a linfadenite purulenta de um único linfonodo seja de causa bacteriana; nesse caso, ela poderá ser tratada com antibióticos sistêmicos de amplo espectro se nenhum microrganismo for detectado na avaliação citológica inicial.

PRECAUÇÕES
N/D.

MEDICAMENTO(S) ALTERNATIVO(S)
N/D.

ACOMPANHAMENTO

PREVENÇÃO
N/D.

EVOLUÇÃO ESPERADA E PROGNÓSTICO
N/D.

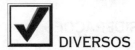

DIVERSOS

DISTÚRBIOS ASSOCIADOS
- Múltiplos linfonodos acometidos — frequentemente consistem na manifestação de infecção sistêmica que também acomete muitos outros órgãos.
- Detecção de fungos, protozoários ou algas em qualquer nodo inflamado deve alertar o médico-veterinário para a possibilidade de infecção sistêmica pelo agente encontrado.

FATORES RELACIONADOS COM A IDADE
Nenhum.

POTENCIAL ZOONÓTICO
- Peste bubônica, tularemia e microrganismos micóticos representam algum risco de infecção para seres humanos.
- As amostras obtidas dos animais acometidos devem ser manipuladas com cuidado.

GESTAÇÃO/FERTILIDADE/REPRODUÇÃO
N/D.

ABREVIATURA(S)
- FeLV = vírus da leucemia felina.
- FIV = vírus da imunodeficiência felina.
- PIF = peritonite infecciosa felina.

Sugestões de Leitura
Duncan JR. The lymph nodes. In: Cowell RL, Tyler RD, eds., Diagnostic Cytology of the Dog and Cat. Goleta, CA: American Veterinary, 1989, pp. 93–98.
Rogers KS, Barton CL, Landis M. Canine and feline lymph nodes: II: Diagnostic evaluation of lymphadenopathy. Compend Contin Educ Pract Vet 15:1493–1503.

Autores Kenneth M. Rassnick e Alan H. Rebar
Consultor Editorial A.H. Rebar

LINFADENOPATIA

CONSIDERAÇÕES GERAIS

DEFINIÇÃO
Linfonodos anormalmente grandes, generalizados ou localizados a um único nodo ou grupo de nodos regionais.

FISIOPATOLOGIA
- Pode resultar de hiperplasia e reatividade de elementos linfoides, infiltração inflamatória ou proliferação neoplásica dentro do linfonodo.
- Em virtude de sua função de filtração, os linfonodos frequentemente atuam como sentinelas da doença nos tecidos drenados por eles; a inflamação de qualquer tecido é quase sempre acompanhada por aumento dos nodos drenantes, que mais provavelmente resulta de hiperplasia linfoide reativa, mas também pode ser provocada por extensão do processo inflamatório para dentro dos nodos (linfadenite).
- Hiperplasia reativa envolve a proliferação de linfócitos e plasmócitos em resposta à estimulação antigênica; a hiperplasia isolada envolve a proliferação de linfócitos apenas, sendo um estágio precoce da hiperplasia reativa.
- Linfadenite — implica a migração ativa de neutrófilos, macrófagos ativados ou eosinófilos para dentro do linfonodo.
- Agentes infecciosos podem estar envolvidos.
- Proliferação neoplásica pode ser primária (linfoma maligno) ou metastática.

SISTEMA(S) ACOMETIDO(S)
Hemático/linfático/imune.

IDENTIFICAÇÃO
- Cães e gatos.
- Sem predileção racial, sexual ou etária.

SINAIS CLÍNICOS
- Tipicamente não provoca sinais clínicos.
- Graves — podem provocar obstrução mecânica e interferência na função de órgãos adjacentes, cujos sinais dependem do linfonodo acometido e podem incluir disfagia, regurgitação, angústia respiratória, disqueiza e tumefação (inchaço) de membro.
- Os cães e gatos podem estar sistemicamente doentes por processos mórbidos subjacentes.

CAUSAS

Hiperplasia/Reatividade Linfoide
- Infecção localizada ou sistêmica causada por agentes infecciosos de todas as categorias (i. e., bactérias, vírus, fungos, protozoários e algas) quando a infecção não envolve diretamente o nodo.
- Alguns agentes infecciosos podem produzir linfadenite de determinados linfonodos com hiperplasia concomitante de outros nodos que não estejam diretamente infectados.
- Outros agentes infecciosos (p. ex., riquétsia, *Bartonella* spp. e *Brucella canis*) — hiperplasia sem linfadenite manifesta.
- Infecção por FIV e FeLV — hiperplasia generalizada, embora possa ocorrer depleção linfoide no final do curso da doença; a linfadenite pode se desenvolver com alguma infecção secundária.
- Estímulo antigênico por outros fatores que não agentes infecciosos (p. ex., alérgenos).
- Pode se desenvolver nos animais com doença imunomediada (p. ex., LES e artrite reumatoide).

Linfadenite
- Bactérias — capazes de provocar linfadenite purulenta, a qual pode evoluir para abscedação; algumas delas (p. ex., *Mycobacterium* spp. e *Bartonella* spp.) induzem a linfadenite granulomatosa; outros agentes incluem microrganismos aeróbios e anaeróbios, *Pasteurella*, *Bacteroides*, *Fusobacterium*, *Yersinia pestis* e *Francisella tularensis*.
- Fungos — infecções sistêmicas por histoplasmose, blastomicose, criptococose e esporotricose.
- Raros — protozoários, algas e parasitas metazoários.
- Diversos linfonodos envolvidos — frequentemente representa uma manifestação de infecção sistêmica, como histoplasmose ou blastomicose.
- Apesar de ocorrer infecção primária dos linfonodos, a linfadenite costuma ser acompanhada por (e geralmente resulta de) infecção de outros tecidos que são drenados pelo nodo acometido.
- Eosinofílica — pode estar associada à inflamação alérgica do órgão drenado pelo linfonodo acometido (p. ex., pele acometida por dermatite alérgica a pulgas); pode ser encontrada em paciente com doença eosinofílica idiopática multissistêmica, como as síndromes hipereosinofílicas caninas e felinas, ou em linfonodo que drena mastocitoma.
- Com frequência, ocorrem linfadenite e hiperplasia reativa concomitantemente.

Neoplasia
- Gatos — transformação neoplásica de linfócitos pelo FeLV.
- Cães — linfoma, causa desconhecida.
- Muitos tumores que sofrem metástase para os linfonodos — causa desconhecida.

FATORES DE RISCO
- Função imune comprometida predispõe o animal à infecção e, portanto, à linfadenite.
- É provável que os animais com doenças alérgicas desenvolvam hiperplasia do linfonodo ou linfadenite eosinofílica.
- Linfoma (gatos) — infecção por FIV ou FeLV.
- Linfadenomegalia causada por neoplasias metastáticas — variam conforme o tipo de neoplasia primária.

DIAGNÓSTICO

DIAGNÓSTICO DIFERENCIAL
- Geralmente, pode-se admitir que a presença de massa em localização característica de linfonodo seja um deles; a avaliação citológica de aspirado obtido por agulha fina costuma solucionar qualquer dúvida.
- Linfonodos palpáveis em cães normais — nodos mandibular, pré-escapular, axilar, inguinal superficial e poplíteo; nodos facial, retrofaríngeo e ilíaco são palpáveis quando se encontram maiores que o normal.
- Aumento intenso de linfonodo (>5 vezes o tamanho normal) — mais provavelmente se desenvolve em pacientes com abscedação (linfadenite) e linfoma.
- Menores graus de aumento — atribuíveis à hiperplasia reativa, linfadenite ou neoplasia.
- A extensão do aumento nos pacientes com doença metastática é amplamente variável.
- Múltiplos linfonodos acometidos por todo o organismo — provavelmente são o resultado de infecção sistêmica ou linfoma que provoque linfadenite ou hiperplasia linfoide.
- Abscedação e neoplasias metastáticas acometem, em geral, um único linfonodo.

HEMOGRAMA/BIOQUÍMICA/URINÁLISE
- Citopenias — observadas em casos de linfoma, anemia de doença crônica, estresse, doença esplênica ou infiltração neoplásica da medula óssea; constatadas também em doença por riquétsia ou vírus.
- Linfocitose — sugere riquetsiose (cães) e neoplasia linfoide (cães e gatos); linfócitos atípicos no sangue ajudam a estabelecer o diagnóstico de neoplasia linfoide.
- Eosinofilia — pode ocorrer nos animais com linfadenopatia atribuída à doença cutânea alérgica ou parasitária.
- Neutrofilia com ou sem desvio à esquerda — pode se desenvolver nos pacientes com linfadenite, hiperplasia linfoide ou neoplasia.
- Hipercalcemia — relativamente comum em cães e rara em gatos com linfoma.
- Hiperglobulinemia — pode se desenvolver nos pacientes com doença inflamatória crônica ou neoplasia linfoide.

OUTROS TESTES LABORATORIAIS
- Gatos — teste para detecção do antígeno de FeLV e FIV nos animais com linfonodos grandes; os animais infectados podem ter linfoma, hiperplasia linfoide ou até linfadenite provocada por imunossupressão.
- Testes sorológicos para pesquisa de anticorpos contra agentes fúngicos sistêmicos como *Blastomyces* e *Cryptococcus* ou bactérias como *Bartonella* spp. podem ajudar a estabelecer esses diagnósticos.

DIAGNÓSTICO POR IMAGEM
- Radiografia e ultrassonografia — envolvimento dos linfonodos dentro da cavidade corporal.
- Lesões associadas ao aumento de linfonodo podem ser detectadas em outros órgãos (p. ex., pneumonia difusa nos cães com blastomicose e tumor primário nos animais com linfadenomegalia provocada por neoplasia metastática).

MÉTODOS DIAGNÓSTICOS

Exame Citológico
- Aspirados de linfonodos acometidos ajudam a determinar a categoria principal da linfadenomegalia (i. e., hiperplasia, inflamação ou neoplasia) e podem fornecer um diagnóstico específico nos pacientes com determinadas doenças infecciosas ou neoplasias; uma coloração hematológica (tipo Romanowsky) padrão (p. ex., Diff-Quik) é apropriada na maior parte dos casos.
- A coloração de Gram pode ser feita nos animais com suspeita de linfadenite bacteriana.
- Aspirados de linfonodos reativos e hiperplásicos contêm população celular mista, em que predominam pequenos linfócitos juntamente com grandes linfócitos, plasmócitos, neutrófilos ocasionais e (talvez) alguns eosinófilos e mastócitos.
- Aspirados de linfonodos acometidos por linfadenite contêm proporções elevadas de neutrófilos, macrófagos e/ou eosinófilos, dependendo da causa da inflamação; agentes

LINFADENOPATIA

infecciosos específicos, como bactérias e fungos sistêmicos, podem estar evidentes.
• Com frequência, o exame citológico representa o meio de diagnóstico nos animais com infecção fúngica sistêmica, como blastomicose e criptococose.
• Aspirados de linfonodos acometidos por linfoma tipicamente contêm proporção elevada (em geral >50%) de grandes linfócitos. Essas células costumam ser blastos com nucléolos claramente identificáveis.
• Aspirados de linfonodos contendo neoplasia metastática têm populações de células que não são observadas nos nodos normais; o aspecto de tais células varia amplamente, dependendo do tipo de neoplasia.

Outros
• Nos gatos, a hiperplasia linfoide grave já foi erroneamente diagnosticada como linfoma; portanto, é essencial a realização de biopsia para os animais com linfadenomegalia.
• Quando não for possível a formulação do diagnóstico pelo exame citológico, poderá ser necessária a realização de biopsia cirúrgica; a biopsia excisional é preferida em relação à biopsia aspirativa com agulha.
• O diagnóstico citológico de linfoma deve ser confirmado pelo exame histopatológico do linfonodo excisado para classificação precisa do tumor e para obtenção de informações prognósticas em potencial.

TRATAMENTO

• Como existem muitos processos mórbidos e agentes específicos capazes de causar linfadenomegalia, o tratamento depende do estabelecimento da causa subjacente.
• Nos animais com suspeita de linfoma, os corticosteroides não deverão ser administrados antes de se concluir os testes de estadiamento se a quimioterapia puder ser instituída.

MEDICAÇÕES

MEDICAMENTO(S) DE ESCOLHA
As medicações apropriadas variam com a causa de aumento do linfonodo.

CONTRAINDICAÇÕES
N/D.

INTERAÇÕES POSSÍVEIS
N/D.

MEDICAMENTO(S) ALTERNATIVO(S)
N/D.

ACOMPANHAMENTO

MONITORIZAÇÃO DO PACIENTE
Monitorizar o tamanho do linfonodo para avaliar a eficácia do tratamento.

DIVERSOS

DISTÚRBIOS ASSOCIADOS
• Hiperplasia do linfonodo e linfadenite quase sempre são componentes ou manifestações de doença sistêmica.
• O linfoma pode envolver outros órgãos (p. ex., fígado, baço, intestinos, rins e meninges), com diversas consequências clínicas.
• Em geral, a doença clínica nos animais com neoplasias metastáticas nos linfonodos é atribuível mais ao tumor primário do que à metástase; entretanto, são exceções: cães com carcinoma tonsilar, que podem apresentar linfonodos mandibulares maciçamente grandes, e cães com adenocarcinoma dos sacos anais, que muitas vezes apresentam linfonodos sublombares extraordinariamente grandes.

FATORES RELACIONADOS COM A IDADE
Nenhum.

POTENCIAL ZOONÓTICO
• É improvável a transmissão direta de doenças que provocam linfadenite para os seres humanos, com exceção de micose sistêmica, esporotricose, tularemia, peste e *Bartonella* spp.
• É preciso ter cuidado ao se obter aspirado por agulha fina nos animais que possam ter doença fúngica sistêmica.

GESTAÇÃO/FERTILIDADE/REPRODUÇÃO
N/D.

VER TAMBÉM
• Linfadenite.
• Linfoma — Cães.
• Linfoma — Gatos.

ABREVIATURA(S)
• FeLV = vírus da leucemia felina.
• FIV = vírus da imunodeficiência felina.
• LES = lúpus eritematoso sistêmico.

Sugestões de Leitura
Day MJ, Whitbread TJ. Pathological diagnoses in dogs with lymph node enlargement. Vet Record 1988, 136:72–73.
Duncan JR. The lymph nodes. In: Cowell RL, Tyler RD, eds., Diagnostic Cytology of the Dog and Cat. Goleta, CA: American Veterinary, 1989, pp. 93–98.
Rogers KS, Barton CL, Landis M. Canine and feline lymph nodes. II. Diagnostic evaluation of lymphadenopathy. Compend Contin Educ Pract Vet 1993, 15:1493–1503.

Autores Kenneth M. Rassnick e Alan H. Rebar
Consultor Editorial A. H. Rebar

LINFANGIECTASIA

CONSIDERAÇÕES GERAIS

DEFINIÇÃO
Distúrbio obstrutivo do sistema linfático do trato gastrintestinal, resultando em hipertensão linfática e enteropatia com perda de proteínas.

FISIOPATOLOGIA
• A obstrução linfática resulta na dilatação e ruptura de vasos lácteos intestinais, com subsequente perda do conteúdo linfático (proteínas plasmáticas, linfócitos e quilomícrons) para o lúmen intestinal.
• Embora algumas das proteínas possam ser digeridas e reabsorvidas, a perda entérica excessiva de proteínas plasmáticas acaba resultando em pan-hipoproteinemia.
• A hipoproteinemia provoca diminuição na pressão oncótica do plasma, levando à formação de edema, ascite e/ou efusão pleural em casos graves.

SISTEMA(S) ACOMETIDO(S)
• Gastrintestinal — diarreia.
• Respiratório — efusão pleural.
• Pele — edema subcutâneo.
• Sistêmico — ascite.

GENÉTICA
Há relatos de tendência familiar para enteropatia com perda de proteínas nas raças Wheaten terrier de pelo macio, Basenji, Yorkshire terrier e Lundehund norueguês, mas a causa genética real não foi identificada para qualquer uma dessas raças.

INCIDÊNCIA/PREVALÊNCIA
Incomum.

DISTRIBUIÇÃO GEOGRÁFICA
N/D.

IDENTIFICAÇÃO
Espécies
Cães.

Raça(s) Predominante(s)
Prevalência elevada nas raças Wheaten terrier de pelo macio, Basenji, Lundehund norueguês e Yorkshire terrier.

Idade Média e Faixa Etária
Pode acometer cães de qualquer idade. É mais comum em cães de meia-idade.

Sexo Predominante
Há relatos de uma prevalência aumentada nas fêmeas da raça Wheaten terrier de pelo macio; nenhuma predileção sexual foi relatada em outras raças.

SINAIS CLÍNICOS
• Sinais clínicos são variáveis.
• Diarreia — crônica, intermitente ou contínua, consistência aquosa a semissólida; entretanto, nem todos os pacientes apresentam diarreia.
• Ascite.
• Edema subcutâneo.
• Dispneia por efusão pleural.
• Perda de peso.
• Flatulência.
• Vômito.

CAUSAS
Linfangiectasia Primária ou Congênita
• Focal — acomete os linfáticos intestinais apenas.
• Anormalidades linfáticas difusas (p. ex., quilotórax, linfedema, quiloabdome e obstrução do ducto torácico).

Linfangiectasia Secundária
• Insuficiência cardíaca congestiva direita.
• Pericardite constritiva.
• Síndrome de Budd-Chiari.
• Neoplasia (linfossarcoma).

FATORES DE RISCO
N/D.

DIAGNÓSTICO

DIAGNÓSTICO DIFERENCIAL
• Linfangiectasia precisa ser diferenciada de outras causas de enteropatia com perda de proteínas.
• Também é imprescindível diferenciar a enteropatia com perda de proteínas de outras causas de hipoalbuminemia.

HEMOGRAMA/BIOQUÍMICA/URINÁLISE
• Hipoalbuminemia e hipoglobulinemia (pan-hipoproteinemia).
• Hipocolesterolemia.
• Hipocalcemia.
• Linfopenia.

OUTROS TESTES LABORATORIAIS
Testes para Diferenciar Enteropatia com Perda de Proteínas de Outras Causas de Hipoalbuminemia
• Concentração de ácidos biliares séricos (pré e pós-prandiais) — para descartar insuficiência hepática.
• Relação de proteína:creatinina urinárias — para excluir nefropatia com perda de proteínas.
• Pesquisa de sangue oculto nas fezes — para descartar perda sanguínea gastrintestinal.
• Concentração fecal do inibidor da α1-proteinase — para confirmar perda intestinal de proteína.

Testes para Diferenciar Outras Causas de Perda Proteica Excessiva no Trato GI
• Esfregaço e flutuação fecais — para descartar parasitas intestinais.
• Concentrações séricas de cobalamina e folato — para excluir proliferação bacteriana no intestino delgado e deficiência de cobalamina (apesar de não causar enteropatia com perda de proteínas, essa deficiência é um indicador de doença da porção distal do intestino delgado grave e de longa data), que podem ser associadas à perda proteica intestinal excessiva.
• Cultura fecal para o diagnóstico de patógenos entéricos específicos (i. e., *Salmonella* spp., *Campylobacter* spp. e *Yersinia* spp.) — na suspeita de etiologia infecciosa.
• Teste da enterotoxina do *Clostridium* — caso se suspeite de enterite infecciosa.
• Análise de líquido das efusões nas cavidades corporais — a efusão associada à linfangiectasia costuma ser um transudato, mas ocasionalmente há quiloabdome e quilotórax.

DIAGNÓSTICO POR IMAGEM
• Radiografias toracoabdominais simples — para descartar cardiopatia e neoplasia.
• Radiografias abdominais — para excluir enteropatia mecânica e outras causas de enteropatia com perda de proteínas.
• Ultrassom abdominal — para descartar doença intestinal mecânica e outras causas de enteropatia com perda de proteínas.
• Ecocardiografia — para excluir insuficiência cardíaca congestiva direita.

MÉTODOS DIAGNÓSTICOS
• Endoscopia permite a inspeção e a biopsia da mucosa intestinal.
• Laparotomia possibilita a visualização dos linfáticos intestinais dilatados e a biopsia dos intestinos (toda a espessura) e dos linfonodos.
• O ECG pode ajudar a avaliar o coração e descartar insuficiência cardíaca congestiva direita.

ACHADOS PATOLÓGICOS
• Achados macroscópicos à laparotomia podem incluir linfáticos dilatados que são visíveis como uma rede semelhante à malha por todo o mesentério e superfície serosa.
• Podem ser vistos pequenos nódulos amarelo-esbranquiçados e depósitos granulares espumosos adjacentes aos linfáticos.
• Achados histopatológicos incluem dilatação balonosa das vilosidades, provocada pelos vasos lácteos acentuadamente dilatados.
• As vilosidades podem estar edematosas; algumas apresentam uma aparência romba.
• Associados, geralmente, a edema da mucosa ou acúmulos difusos ou multifocais de linfócitos e plasmócitos na lâmina própria.

TRATAMENTO

CUIDADO(S) DE SAÚDE ADEQUADO(S)
• Tratados principalmente como pacientes de ambulatório.
• Podem necessitar de hospitalização caso ocorra o desenvolvimento de complicações atribuídas à hipoalbuminemia

CUIDADO(S) DE ENFERMAGEM
N/D.

ATIVIDADE
Normal.

DIETA
• Dieta pobre em gordura, porém rica em proteína de alta qualidade.
• Triglicerídeos de cadeia longa estimulam o fluxo intestinal de linfa e podem levar ao aumento na perda intestinal de proteína.
• Dietas enriquecidas com triglicerídeos de cadeia média podem ser benéficas.
• Pode-se optar pelo fornecimento de triglicerídeos de cadeia média para suplementar a gordura e aumentar a ingestão calórica.
• Fontes comerciais de triglicerídeos de cadeia média — óleo de triglicerídeos de cadeia média ou Portagen® (Mead Johnson, Evansville, IN)
• Suplementar com vitaminas lipossolúveis — A, D, E, K.
• Também podem ser utilizadas dietas elementares.

ORIENTAÇÃO AO PROPRIETÁRIO
Abordar a evolução imprevisível da doença e a resposta ao tratamento.

CONSIDERAÇÕES CIRÚRGICAS
• Quando a linfangiectasia intestinal for secundária a uma obstrução linfática identificável, considerar a cirurgia para aliviar a obstrução.
• Pericardiectomia pode ser indicada nos casos de pericardite constritiva.

LINFANGIECTASIA

- Os casos que se beneficiam da intervenção cirúrgica são raros.

MEDICAÇÕES
MEDICAMENTO(S) DE ESCOLHA
- Tentar o uso de corticosteroides se a terapia nutricional isolada não for bem-sucedida (tal terapia, no entanto, não tem a intenção de tratar a linfangiectasia, mas sim a inflamação gastrintestinal concomitante). Prednisona ou prednisolona oral na dose de 2 mg/kg a cada 12 h por 5-7 dias, seguida por 1 mg/kg a cada 12 h por no mínimo 6 semanas. Após a remissão da doença, a dosagem pode ser lentamente reduzida para a dose mais baixa, porém eficaz, no controle da doença.
- Se o animal for deficiente em cobalamina, essa vitamina deverá ser suplementada para obter a resposta terapêutica: 250-1.500 µg/cão SC uma vez por semana por 6 semanas e, em seguida, 1 dose um mês depois. Acompanhar com uma reavaliação 30 dias após a última dose.
- Na suspeita de proliferação bacteriana no intestino delgado, o paciente deverá ser tratado com tilosina na dose de 25 mg/kg a cada 12 h por 6 semanas.

CONTRAINDICAÇÕES
N/D.
PRECAUÇÕES
N/D.
INTERAÇÕES POSSÍVEIS
N/D.
MEDICAMENTO(S) ALTERNATIVO(S)
N/D.

ACOMPANHAMENTO
MONITORIZAÇÃO DO PACIENTE
- Peso corporal, indícios de sinais clínicos recidivantes (efusão pleural, ascite e/ou edema), além de concentrações séricas de proteína total, albumina e globulina.
- Os pacientes precisam ser reavaliados, dependendo da gravidade do processo patológico.

PREVENÇÃO
N/D.

COMPLICAÇÕES POSSÍVEIS
- Dificuldade respiratória pela efusão pleural.
- Depleção proteico-calórica grave.
- Diarreia intratável.

EVOLUÇÃO ESPERADA E PROGNÓSTICO
- Prognóstico reservado.
- Alguns animais não respondem ao tratamento.
- Em alguns pacientes, podem ser atingidas remissões de vários meses a mais de 2 anos.

DIVERSOS
DISTÚRBIOS ASSOCIADOS
Cães da raça Wheaten terrier de pelo macio podem apresentar nefropatia com perda de proteínas concomitante.

FATORES RELACIONADOS COM A IDADE
N/D.
POTENCIAL ZOONÓTICO
N/D.
GESTAÇÃO/FERTILIDADE/REPRODUÇÃO
N/D.
VER TAMBÉM
Enteropatia com Perda de Proteínas.
ABREVIATURA(S)
- ECG = eletrocardiograma.

Sugestões de Leitura
Kull PA, Hess RS, Craig LE, et al. Clinical, clinicopathologic, radiographic, and ultrasonographic characteristics of intestinal lymphangiectasia in dogs: 17 cases (1996-1998). JAVMA 2001, 219:197-202.
Littman MP, Dambach DM, Vaden SL, et al. Familial protein-losing enteropathy and protein-losing nephropathy in soft coated Wheaten terriers: 222 cases (1983-1997). J Vet Intern Med 2000, 14:68-80.
Melzer KJ, Sellon RK. Canine intestinal lymphangiectasia. Compend Contin Educ Pract Vet 2002, 24:953-961.

Autor Jörg M. Steiner
Consultor Editorial Albert E. Jergens

LINFEDEMA

CONSIDERAÇÕES GERAIS

REVISÃO
- Acúmulo anormal de líquido linfático rico em proteína nos espaços intersticiais, especialmente a gordura subcutânea.
- O linfedema crônico provoca fibrose tecidual.
- Pode ser congênito ou adquirido.

IDENTIFICAÇÃO
- Mais comum nos cães do que nos gatos.
- Congênito nos cães da raça Buldogue e relatado como hereditário/congênito em uma família da raça Poodle; possível predileção racial nas raças Labrador retriever e Old English sheepdog.

SINAIS CLÍNICOS

Achados Anamnésicos
- Primário/congênito — geralmente se apresenta sob a forma de tumefação periférica do membro ao nascimento ou se desenvolve nos primeiros meses.
- Começa tipicamente na extremidade distal e avança lentamente no sentido proximal.

Achados do Exame Físico
- Mais comum nos membros, especialmente nos pélvicos; pode ser uni ou bilateral.
- Menos comum na porção ventral de tórax, abdome, orelhas e cauda.
- Edema depressível não doloroso; a temperatura da área acometida permanece normal.
- A qualidade depressível se perde com a cronicidade à medida que ocorre fibrose.
- Claudicação e dor são incomuns a menos que se desenvolva celulite.

CAUSAS E FATORES DE RISCO
- Má-formação hereditária/congênita do sistema linfático — aplasia, incompetência valvular e fibrose de linfonodo.
- Produção excessiva de líquido intersticial secundária à hipertensão venosa (associada à insuficiência cardíaca congestiva e obstrução da drenagem venosa) ou aumento da permeabilidade vascular (associada a infecções, traumatismos, calor e irradiação).
- Lesão secundária a vasos linfáticos ou linfonodos — associada a traumatismos, infecções (p. ex., infecção linfática pela filária *Brugia pahangi* — sudeste da Ásia), neoplasias (p. ex., linfoma, linfangiossarcoma [raro]) e ligadura do ducto torácico (raro).

DIAGNÓSTICO

DIAGNÓSTICO DIFERENCIAL
- Edema provocado por estase venosa (p. ex., insuficiência cardíaca congestiva e cirrose); procurar por varizes, hiperpigmentação e ulceração.
- Fístulas arteriovenosas — auscultar sopro contínuo em "maquinaria"; palpar os vasos pulsáteis; confirmar com angiograma.
- Edema causado por hipoproteinemia — nefropatia ou enteropatia com perda de proteínas, insuficiência hepática, perda de soro por queimaduras ou hemorragia; verificar a concentração de proteína sérica.
- Traumatismo — rever a anamnese; procurar por contusões e lacerações.
- Neoplasia — se a tumefação for firme, obter aspirado para exame citológico.
- Celulite — pesquisar por febre, dor e tumefação quente.

HEMOGRAMA/BIOQUÍMICA/URINÁLISE
Resultados normais.

OUTROS TESTES LABORATORIAIS
N/D.

DIAGNÓSTICO POR IMAGEM
A linfografia é uma ferramenta valiosa para comprovar anormalidades dentro do sistema linfático; os melhores resultados são obtidos com injeção de meio de contraste aquoso injetado diretamente no vaso linfático. Consultar a seção de "Sugestões de Leitura" em busca da descrição detalhada dessa técnica.

MÉTODOS DIAGNÓSTICOS
N/D.

TRATAMENTO

- Não há tratamento curativo — pode-se tentar uma série de tratamentos cirúrgicos e clínicos.
- O repouso e a massagem dos membros acometidos não auxiliam.
- Tratamento conservativo — uso a prazo longo de meias compressivas, aliado ao cuidado da pele e uso de antibióticos para tratar a celulite e a linfangite; pode ser bem-sucedido em alguns pacientes.
- Métodos cirúrgicos — podem ser tentados quando os tratamentos conservativos e as medicações falham; linfangioplastia, técnicas de formação de ponte, desvios linfaticovenosos, anastomose linfática superficial e profunda, além de procedimentos excisionais; embora nenhum deles seja consistentemente benéfico, os métodos excisionais foram relatados apenas nos cães.
- Em seres humanos — a aplicação de calor de micro-ondas nas áreas acometidas parece benéfica e soma-se aos efeitos das benzopironas (ver a seção "Medicamento(s)").
- Dietas rigorosamente restritas em triglicerídeos de cadeia longa estão sendo pesquisadas nos seres humanos.

MEDICAÇÕES

MEDICAMENTO(S)
- As benzopironas diminuem o edema rico em proteína, estimulando os macrófagos a liberarem proteases; efeitos benéficos foram registrados em estudos experimentais nos cães. Rutina, 50 mg/kg VO a cada 8 h, pode ser benéfica. Um estudo conduzido em humanos demonstrou que o uso combinado de benzopironas por vias oral e tópica seja mais eficaz do que ambas isoladas.
- Diuréticos, esteroides, anticoagulantes e agentes fibrinolíticos foram utilizados, porém não confirmaram benefícios.

CONTRAINDICAÇÕES/INTERAÇÕES POSSÍVEIS
Diuréticos — inicialmente diminuem a tumefação, porém aumentam o conteúdo proteico do líquido intersticial, resultando em mais lesão e fibrose teciduais.

ACOMPANHAMENTO

- Filhotes caninos com linfedema grave podem vir a óbito.
- Resolução constatada em alguns filhotes apenas com envolvimento do membro pélvico.
- Prognóstico mau em casos de linfangiossarcoma.

DIVERSOS

Sugestões de Leitura
Fossum TW, King LA, Miller MW, et al. Lymphedema: Clinical signs, diagnosis, and treatment. J Vet Intern Med 1992, 6:312-319.
Fossum TW, Miller MW. Lymphedema: Etiopathogenesis. J Vet Intern Med 1992, 6:283-293.
Williams JH. Lymphangiosarcoma of dogs: A review. J S Afr Vet Assoc 2005, 76(3):127-131.

Autor Francis W.K. Smith, Jr.
Consultores Editoriais Larry P. Tilley e Francis W.K. Smith, Jr.

LINFOMA — CÃES

CONSIDERAÇÕES GERAIS

DEFINIÇÃO
Proliferação clonal de linfócitos neoplásicos T ou B ou não T/não B, principalmente nos linfonodos, na medula óssea e nas vísceras. A pele é ocasionalmente acometida.

FISIOPATOLOGIA
• Geralmente de origem unifocal.
• A maioria origina-se de linfócitos B, com porcentagem menor de casos com origem nos linfócitos T.
• O tipo celular T costuma ser associado à pele (linfoma cutâneo epiteliotrópico) e/ou localização mediastínica.
• Proliferação clonal rápida e elevada fração de crescimento podem ser responsáveis pelo início repentino dos sinais clínicos.

SISTEMA(S) ACOMETIDO(S)
• Hemático/linfático/imune — linfadenopatia generalizada, quase sempre periférica, com ou sem envolvimento do baço, do fígado e/ou da medula óssea e linfócitos malignos circulantes.
• Gastrintestinal — infiltração do estômago, dos intestinos e dos linfonodos associados.
• Respiratório — proliferação de linfócitos neoplásicos nos linfonodos mediastínicos, no timo ou no parênquima pulmonar.
• Cutâneo — algumas vezes, é classificado como linfoma de localização extranodal; no entanto, síndromes distintas são associadas à localização cutânea.
• Diversos (extranodais) — proliferação de linfócitos neoplásicos ou invasão por essas células na medula óssea e nos tecidos ocular, mucocutâneo, neural, renal, cardíaco e outros.

GENÉTICA
• A expressão do gene supressor tumoral ubíquo p53 nesse tipo de tumor é rara.
• É comum a hibridização citogenética em linfoma canino.
• É documentada a perda ou o ganho de cromossomos caninos.
• Imunofenótipos são significativos do ponto de vista prognóstico, sendo que os tipos celulares B são mais responsivos ao tratamento e têm prognóstico melhor.

INCIDÊNCIA/PREVALÊNCIA
Relatadas em 6-30 para cada 100.000 cães por ano.

IDENTIFICAÇÃO
Espécies
Cão.

Raça(s) Predominante(s)
• Raças Boxer, Basset hound, Golden retriever, São Bernardo, Terrier escocês, Airedale terrier e Buldogue — raças relatadas como de alto risco.
• Dachshund e Pomerânia — raças relatadas como de baixo risco.
• A raça parece determinar o risco relativo de doença das células B ou T.

Idade Média e Faixa Etária
Pacientes geralmente com 5-10 anos de idade.

SINAIS CLÍNICOS
Comentários Gerais
• Dependem da forma anatômica e do estágio da doença.

Achados Anamnésicos
• Todas as formas de linfoma podem ter achados anamnésicos inespecíficos, incluindo anorexia, letargia e perda de peso.
• Multicêntricos — linfadenopatia generalizada e indolor é mais comum; pode-se notar abdome distendido secundariamente à hepatomegalia, esplenomegalia ou ascite.
• Gastrintestinais — vômito; diarreia; anorexia; desconforto abdominal.
• Mediastínicos — tosse; dificuldade de deglutição; anorexia; salivação; respiração laboriosa; intolerância ao exercício secundária ao efeito expansivo de massa(s) e/ou efusão.
• Cutâneos — a pele pode ter lesões crônicas e irresponsivas tipo placa que se expandem e coalescem em lesões maiores.
• Extranodais — variam com a localização anatômica; oculares: fotofobia e conjuntivite; SNC: crises convulsivas; renais: dor lombar; cardíaco: intolerância ao exercício ou síncope.

Achados do Exame Físico
• Multicêntricos — linfonodo(s) grande(s), móvel(is), irregular(es), indolor(es), generalizado(s), com ou sem hepatosplenomegalia.
• Gastrintestinais — perda de peso acentuada ou massa abdominal palpável; alças intestinais espessadas; irregularidades da mucosa retal.
• Mediastínicos — dispneia; taquipneia; sons cardíacos abafados secundários à efusão pleural.
• Cutâneos — placas elevadas que podem coalescer, além de lesões irregulares e exsudativas.
• Extranodais — oculares: uveíte anterior, hemorragias retinianas e hifema; neurais: demência, crises convulsivas e paralisia; renais: renomegalia e insuficiência renal; cardíacos: arritmias.

CAUSAS
Nenhuma causa específica comprovada.

DIAGNÓSTICO

DIAGNÓSTICO DIFERENCIAL
• Doença infecciosa, neoplásica, imunomediada e inflamatória.
• Avaliação citológica e histológica, além de estadiamento completo — diferenciar de outras doenças.

HEMOGRAMA/BIOQUÍMICA/URINÁLISE
• Podem ser observadas anormalidades como anemia, linfocitose, linfopenia, neutrofilia, monocitose, blastos circulantes e trombocitopenia.
• Elevações nas atividades de ALT ou fosfatase alcalina com envolvimento hepático.
• Hipercalcemia na minoria dos pacientes (20-30%).
• Urinálise geralmente normal.

OUTROS TESTES LABORATORIAIS
Imunofenotipagem para determinar as características das células T e B.

DIAGNÓSTICO POR IMAGEM
• Radiografia torácica — pode revelar linfadenopatia esternal ou traqueobrônquica, mediastino alargado, densidades pulmonares e efusão pleural.
• Radiografia abdominal — pode revelar linfadenopatia sublombar ou mesentérica, massa intestinal, efusões abdominais e hepato(spleno)megalia.
• Ultrassonografia — linfadenopatia abdominal (obscurecida pela efusão nas radiografias), nódulos viscerais ou aspecto rendado às vísceras, como o baço.

MÉTODOS DIAGNÓSTICOS
• Citologia de aspirado por agulha fina — para confirmar o diagnóstico de linfoma maligno.
• Biopsia — para confirmar a classificação histomorfológica.
• Punção do LCS — se o paciente tiver sinais atribuídos ao SNC.
• ECG — para identificar arritmias antes da administração da doxorrubicina.

ACHADOS PATOLÓGICOS
• Secção de corte — massas esbranquiçadas homogêneas com áreas de necrose.
• População monomórfica de células neoplásicas arredondadas discretas que destroem e substituem o parênquima dos linfonodos e de órgãos viscerais ou da medula óssea.
• Há muito subtipos e classificações em uso para a forma multicêntrica.
• A imunofenotipagem é prognóstica e determinará o tipo de linfócito de origem.
• A forma cutânea pode ser categorizada como epiteliotrópica (em geral, células T) ou não epiteliotrópica (em geral, células B).
• A forma epiteliotrópica ainda pode ser categorizada como micose fungoide, síndrome de Sezary ou reticulose pagetoide.

TRATAMENTO

CUIDADO(S) DE SAÚDE ADEQUADO(S)
• Paciente internado — quimioterapia intravenosa.
• Paciente ambulatorial — após a remissão, alguns protocolos possibilitam a administração de medicamentos por via oral pelo proprietário em casa.
• Radioterapia — pode ser utilizada para tratar linfadenopatia refratária, grande envolvimento mediastínico e áreas cutâneas solitárias. A radioterapia também pode ser aplicada no SNC em casos de envolvimento neurológico refratário. Além disso, a radioterapia também está sendo usada como adjuvante à quimioterapia em alguns centros oncológicos.

CUIDADO(S) DE ENFERMAGEM
Fluidoterapia — pode beneficiar pacientes com doença avançada; pode beneficiar pacientes clinicamente enfermos, azotêmicos e/ou desidratados.

DIETA
Fornecer nutrição adequada.

ORIENTAÇÕES AO PROPRIETÁRIO
• Advertir o cliente de que a quimioterapia raramente é curativa e em geral ocorrem recidivas.
• Informar ao proprietário que os efeitos colaterais dos medicamentos quimioterápicos dependem da dose e do(s) tipo(s) utilizado(s), porém geralmente estão associados ao trato gastrintestinal e à medula óssea.
• Esclarecer ao proprietário que as taxas de resposta a grande parte dos protocolos quimioterápicos compostos por múltiplos agentes são altas (>80%).
• Notar que a qualidade de vida é boa enquanto o paciente estiver recebendo a quimioterapia e enquanto estiver em remissão.

LINFOMA — CÃES

CONSIDERAÇÕES CIRÚRGICAS
• Raramente bem-sucedidas, a menos que limitadas a um local acessível.
• A remoção de linfonodo(s) pode ser necessária para o diagnóstico em alguns casos.

MEDICAÇÕES

MEDICAMENTO(S) DE ESCOLHA
• Sempre consultar um veterinário especialista em oncologia em busca das novidades mais recentes em termos de quimioterapia eficaz, taxas de administração, precauções e efeitos colaterais.
• Quimioterapia combinada — embora existam muitos protocolos, alguns apresentam tempos superiores de remissão e de sobrevida, com possível aumento na toxicidade.
• Tratamento com agente único (doxorrubicina) — associada a tempos de remissão e de sobrevida semelhantes àqueles para algumas quimioterapias combinadas.
• Corticosteroides apenas — não recomendados como opção terapêutica isolada; entretanto, podem ser eficazes para atingir a remissão parcial em cães por curtos períodos de tempo (1-2 meses).

Protocolo com Doxorrubicina
• Administrar 30 mg/m^2 IV a cada 21 dias (1 mg/kg para animal com <10 kg) por 3-5 tratamentos além da remissão completa (4-6 tratamentos totais).

Combinação Menos Eficaz
Protocolo Quimioterápico I (COP sem Manutenção)
• Vincristina — 0,5 mg/m^2 IV no primeiro dia.
• Ciclofosfamida — 50 mg/m^2 VO do 4º ao 7º dia.
• Prednisona — 20 mg/m^2 VO a cada 12 h.
• Repetir semanalmente por 6 semanas.

Combinação Mais Eficaz
Protocolo Quimioterápico II (L-CHOP sem Manutenção)
• L-asparaginase — 10.000 UI/m^2 na semana 1.
• Prednisona — 20 mg/m^2 VO a cada 24 h por 4 semanas e, depois, reduzir gradativamente em mais 4 semanas.
• Vincristina — 0,7 mg/m^2 IV na semana 1.
• Ciclofosfamida — 250 mg/m^2 IV na semana 2.
• Vincristina — 0,7 mg/m^2 IV na semana 3.
• Doxorrubicina — 30 mg/m^2 IV na semana 4.
• Vincristina — 0,7 mg/m^2 IV na semana 6.
• Ciclofosfamida — 250 mg/m^2 IV na semana 7.
• Vincristina — 0,7 mg/m^2 IV na semana 8.
• Doxorrubicina — 30 mg/m^2 IV na semana 9.
• Vincristina — 0,7 mg/m^2 IV na semana 11.
• Ciclofosfamida — 250 mg/m^2 IV na semana 12.
• Vincristina — 0,7 mg/m^2 IV na semana 13.
• Doxorrubicina — 30 mg/m^2 IV na semana 14.
• Vincristina — 0,7 mg/m^2 IV na semana 16.
• Ciclofosfamida — 250 mg/m^2 IV na semana 17.
• Vincristina — 0,7 mg/m^2 na semana 18.
• Doxorrubicina — 30 mg/m^2 IV na semana 19.

CONTRAINDICAÇÕES
Evitar a doxorrubicina em pacientes com arritmia ou miocardiopatia preexistente.

PRECAUÇÕES
• Sempre consultar um veterinário especialista em oncologia sobre as doses, as taxas de administração e os efeitos colaterais.
• Doxorrubicina — utilizar com cuidado ou não usar de modo algum na presença de contratilidade cardíaca deficiente ou arritmias.
• L-asparaginase ou doxorrubicina — fazer tratamento prévio com difenidramina (1 mg/kg SC) 20 min antes da administração.
• Sempre utilizar um cateter e um sistema de gotejamento ao se administrar a doxorrubicina por via IV.
• Esperar maior toxicidade com doses e protocolos mais agressivos.

INTERAÇÕES POSSÍVEIS
Todos os medicamentos quimioterápicos precisam ser administrados de acordo com os protocolos publicados, porque muitos deles podem ter sobreposição dos efeitos colaterais.

MEDICAMENTO(S) ALTERNATIVO(S)
• Existem muitos protocolos de tratamento alternativo e de salvamento; consultar um veterinário especialista em oncologia.
• Lomustina (CCNU) ou dacarbazina (DTIC) — podem ser empregados nos casos refratários.
• Alguns centros combinam a quimioterapia com radioterapia.

ACOMPANHAMENTO

MONITORIZAÇÃO DO PACIENTE
• Exame físico e avaliação citológica ou histológica — todos os linfonodos não responsivos.
• Hemograma completo e contagem de plaquetas — devem ser obtidos antes de cada tratamento sucessivo. Caso se observe leucopenia ou neutropenia grave (leucócitos <2.000 células/mm^3; neutrófilos <1.000 células/mm^3), será recomendável a instituição da dosagem reduzida (20%) do agente citotóxico mais recentemente utilizado.
• Após o término das 4 primeiras semanas de terapia, consultar um veterinário especialista em oncologia se a remissão completa não tiver sido atingida.
• Ecocardiografia e ECG — periodicamente durante e após a administração da doxorrubicina para ajudar a identificar o desenvolvimento de cardiotoxicidade.

COMPLICAÇÕES POSSÍVEIS
• Leucopenia e neutropenia.
• Vômito e diarreia.
• Anorexia.
• Cardiotoxicidade — atribuída à doxorrubicina; geralmente após dose cumulativa total de 180-240 mg/m^2.
• Alopecia em certas raças caninas submetidas à doxorrubicina (Poodle, Old English sheepdog, Schnauzer, etc.).
• Sepse.
• Esfacelamento tecidual — com a dose extravasada para fora da veia.

EVOLUÇÃO ESPERADA E PROGNÓSTICO
• Duração média da primeira remissão com quimioterapia combinada ou doxorrubicina — 6-9 meses, dependendo do imunofenótipo.
• Com o uso de protocolos mais agressivos compostos por múltiplos agentes, os pacientes que atingem a remissão completa devem chegar a 90% ou mais.
• Tempo médio de sobrevida com a quimioterapia combinada é frequentemente de 9-12 meses ou mais.
• Forma mediastínica e/ou hipercalcemia — prognóstico pior.
• Linfomas de células T geralmente têm uma remissão mais curta e um prognóstico pior.
• Formas primárias do SNC, gastrintestinal difusa e cutânea em vários locais — associadas à resposta insatisfatória ao tratamento.

DIVERSOS

GESTAÇÃO/FERTILIDADE/REPRODUÇÃO
O tratamento de cadela prenhe está contraindicado.

SINÔNIMO(S)
• Linfossarcoma.
• Linfoma maligno.

VER TAMBÉM
• Hipercalcemia.
• Leucemia Linfoblástica Aguda.
• Leucemia Linfocítica Crônica.

ABREVIATURA(S)
• ALT = alanina aminotransferase.
• CCNU = 1-(2-cloroetil)-3-cicloexil-1-nitroso-ureia.
• COPLA = ciclofosfamida, vincristina (Oncovin®), prednisona e L-asparaginase.
• DTIC = (dimetiltriazeno)imidazol carboxamida.
• ECG = eletrocardiograma.
• LCS = líquido cerebrospinal.
• SNC = sistema nervoso central.

Sugestões de Leitura
Breen M, Modiano JF. Evolutionarily conserved cytogenetic changes in hematological malignancies of dogs and humans — man and his best friend share more than companionship. Chromosome Res 2008, 16:145-154.
De Lorimier LP. Updates on the management of canine epitheliotrophic cutaneous T-cell lymphoma. Vet Clin North Am Small Anim Pract 2006, 36(1):213-228.
Garrett LD, Thamm DH, Chun R, et al. Evaluation of a 6-month chemotherapy protocol with no maintenance therapy for dogs with lymphoma. J Vet Intern Med 2002, 16(6):704-709.
Morrison WB. Lymphoma in Dogs and Cats. Jackson, WY: Teton NewMedia, 2005. Rassnick KM, McEntee MC, Erb HN, et al. Comparison of 3 protocols for treatment after induction of remission in dogs with lymphoma. J Vet Intern Med 2007, 21(6):1364-1373.

Autor Wallace B. Morrison
Consultor Editorial Timothy M. Fan

LINFOMA — GATOS

CONSIDERAÇÕES GERAIS

DEFINIÇÃO
Transformação maligna de linfócitos.

FISIOPATOLOGIA
Oncogênese viral (FeLV) ou química (fumaça de cigarro) em alguns animais, embora a fisiopatologia seja desconhecida em outros.

SISTEMA(S) ACOMETIDO(S)
• Hemático/linfático/imune.
• Gastrintestinal.
• Renal/urológico (alta taxa de recidiva no SNC).
• Oftálmico.
• Nervoso.
• Cutâneo/exócrino.
• Respiratório — cavidade nasal.

GENÉTICA
N/D.

INCIDÊNCIA/PREVALÊNCIA
• Cerca de 90% dos tumores hematopoiéticos e 33% de todos os tumores nos gatos.
• Prevalência — 41,6-200 para cada 100.000 gatos.

DISTRIBUIÇÃO GEOGRÁFICA
Diferenças regionais podem estar relacionadas com diferenças nas prevalências de FeLV.

IDENTIFICAÇÃO

Espécies
Gatos.

Raça(s) Predominante(s)
Raças Siamês e Oriental são super-representadas em alguns estudos.

Idade Média e Faixa Etária
• Idade média de gatos positivos ao FeLV — 3 anos.
• Idade média de gatos negativos ao FeLV — 7 anos.
• Idade mediana de gatos com linfoma de localização extranodal — 13 anos.
• A maioria dos gatos com linfoma tipo Hodgkin tem mais de 6 anos de idade.

Sexo Predominante
Nenhum.

SINAIS CLÍNICOS

Comentários Gerais
Dependem da forma anatômica; o linfoma é o tumor mais comum da medula espinal em gatos.

Achados Anamnésicos
• Forma mediastínica — respiração com a boca aberta; tosse; regurgitação; anorexia; perda de peso.
• Forma alimentar — anorexia; perda de peso; letargia; vômito; constipação; diarreia; melena; sangue vivo nas fezes.
• Forma renal — compatível com insuficiência renal (p. ex., vômito, anorexia, polidipsia, poliúria e letargia).
• Forma nasal — secreção nasal ou epistaxe, sinais oculares, ruído respiratório, espirro, anorexia.
• Forma multicêntrica — possivelmente nenhum nos estágios iniciais; anorexia, perda de peso e depressão com a evolução da doença.
• Forma espinal — pode-se observar paresia posterior rapidamente progressiva.
• Forma cutânea — massas dérmicas pruriginosas, hemorrágicas ou alopécicas podem ser observadas.

Achados do Exame Físico
• Forma mediastínica — porção torácica cranial não compressível, dispneia, taquipneia.
• Forma alimentar — intestinos espessados ou massas abdominais.
• Forma renal — rins grandes e irregulares.
• Forma nasal — secreção nasal purulenta ou mucoide, deformidade facial, epífora, exoftalmia.
• Forma multicêntrica — linfadenomegalia generalizada.
• Todas as formas — febre; desidratação; depressão; caquexia em alguns pacientes.

CAUSAS
FeLV.

FATORES DE RISCO
• Exposição ao FeLV.
• Exposição ambiental à fumaça de cigarro (risco relativo de 2,4 vezes — risco este que aumenta linearmente de acordo com a duração e a quantidade de exposição).

DIAGNÓSTICO

DIAGNÓSTICO DIFERENCIAL
• Forma mediastínica — insuficiência cardíaca congestiva; miocardiopatia; quilotórax; piotórax; hemotórax; pneumotórax; hérnia diafragmática; doença pulmonar alérgica; timoma; carcinoma ectópico da tireoide; carcinomatose pleural; toxicidade pelo paracetamol.
• Forma alimentar — ingestão de corpo estranho; ulceração intestinal; infecção fúngica intestinal; enteropatia inflamatória; intussuscepção; linfangiectasia; outro tumor gastrintestinal.
• Forma renal — pielonefrite; amiloidose; glomerulonefrite; insuficiência renal crônica; rins policísticos.
• Forma multicêntrica — infecção micótica sistêmica; doença imunomediada; toxoplasmose; hiperplasia linfoide; reação de hipersensibilidade; peste (especificamente se houver linfadenopatia cervical proeminente como ocorre com a forma tipo Hodgkin).

HEMOGRAMA/BIOQUÍMICA/URINÁLISE
• Podem-se observar anemia (fator prognóstico negativo), leucocitose e linfoblastose.
• Pode-se constatar elevação nos níveis de ureia e creatinina, bem como na atividade das enzimas hepáticas, além de hipercalcemia (rara) e gamopatia monoclonal.
• Podem-se observar isostenúria, bilirrubinúria e proteinúria.

OUTROS TESTES LABORATORIAIS
Teste para detecção de FeLV: costuma ser negativo em gatos mais idosos e naqueles com linfoma linfocítico granular grande, renal (45%), multicêntrico (20%) ou intestinal (15%), mas geralmente positivo em gatos mais jovens e naqueles com linfoma mediastínico (85%) ou neurológico (SNC).

DIAGNÓSTICO POR IMAGEM
• Radiografia torácica — avaliar o animal quanto à presença de massa mediastínica, efusão pleural, padrões parenquimatosos pulmonares anormais (raros) e linfadenomegalia peri-hilar ou retroesternal.
• Ultrassonografia abdominal — revela alterações difusas na ecotextura de órgãos como fígado, baço e rins, além de espessamento focal dos intestinos e da parede gástrica.
• Espessamento subcapsular hipoecoico é associado a linfoma renal.
• Ao contrário dos cães, a heterogeneidade nodal não é fortemente associada a linfoma.
• Apesar do espessamento dos intestinos, a estrutura das camadas pode estar preservada.
• TC — efeito expansivo na área acometida; exame utilizado particularmente em casos de linfoma nasal.

MÉTODOS DIAGNÓSTICOS
• Exame do aspirado de medula óssea ou biopsia de núcleo.
• Aspirado ou biopsia de massa ou linfonodo.

ACHADOS PATOLÓGICOS
• Macroscópicos — provavelmente de coloração branca a acinzentada, com áreas de hemorragia e necrose.
• Citológicos — população monomórfica de células linfoides, às vezes com múltiplos nucléolos proeminentes e cromatina nuclear grosseira.
• Histopatológicos — variam; há diversos esquemas de classificação morfológica em uso.
• Linfoma nasal origina-se mais frequentemente de células-B imunoblásticas.
• Linfoma tipo Hodgkin é caracterizado por células de Reed-Sternberg e poucas células neoplásicas em um fundo composto por uma população de células-T reativas com histiócitos e granulócitos.
• Linfoma linfocítico granular grande afeta mais comumente o intestino e os linfonodos mesentéricos.
• O linfoma de células-B é mais comum no estômago (100%) e no intestino grosso (88%), enquanto o linfoma de células-T é mais usual no intestino delgado (52%).
• No linfoma GI, o acometimento de células pequenas é mais comum (2/3) do que o de células grandes (1/3).

TRATAMENTO

CUIDADO(S) DE SAÚDE ADEQUADO(S)
Como paciente de ambulatório sempre que possível. Haverá necessidade de cuidados de suporte, dependendo dos sinais clínicos.

CUIDADO(S) DE ENFERMAGEM
Fluidoterapia, estimulantes do apetite, toracocentese, etc. quando indicados pelos sinais clínicos.

ATIVIDADE
Normal.

DIETA
Sem modificação, embora seja possível a adição de ácidos graxos ômega-3 à dieta (origem do óleo de peixe).

ORIENTAÇÃO AO PROPRIETÁRIO
• Escolher um protocolo que se ajuste ao animal de estimação e ao estilo de vida do proprietário.
• Enfatizar que os efeitos colaterais são passíveis de tratamento e devem ser tratados imediatamente.
• Informar ao proprietário que o objetivo é induzir a remissão e obter boa qualidade de vida para os pacientes o maior tempo possível.

CONSIDERAÇÕES CIRÚRGICAS
- Para aliviar obstruções ou perfurações intestinais e remover massas solitárias.
- Para obter amostras para exame histopatológico.

MEDICAÇÕES
MEDICAMENTO(S) DE ESCOLHA
- Quimioterapia — usada em combinação ou como protocolo sequencial; alguns protocolos possuem períodos de indução e de manutenção.
- Existem muitas variações de protocolos combinados semelhantes, embora todos tenham a mesma eficácia.
- Linfoma de alto grau pode responder aos protocolos CHOP (ciclofosfamida, doxorrubicina, vincristina [Oncovin®], prednisona) como o protocolo da Universidade de Wisconsin-Madison (medicamentos alternados em sequências repetidas) ou COP-doxorrubicina (iniciar com o COP e, depois, finalizar o protocolo com uma sequencia de tratamentos com doxorrubicina).
- Linfoma intestinal de baixo grau pode responder à clorambucila oral (baixas doses diárias ou altas doses pulsadas) e prednisona.
- Radioterapia — pode ser empregada no linfoma localizado; não são raras recidivas fora do campo de radiação.
- Consultar um veterinário especialista em oncologia em busca das doses, dos protocolos e das melhores opções terapêuticas.

CONTRAINDICAÇÕES
Evitar a doxorrubicina em gatos com insuficiência renal preexistente, pois foi demonstrado que altas doses cumulativas sejam potencialmente nefrotóxicas.

PRECAUÇÕES
- Mielossupressão secundária à quimioterapia — mais comum em gatos positivos ao FeLV.
- Buscar orientação antes de se iniciar o tratamento caso o clínico não esteja familiarizado com o uso de medicamentos citotóxicos. Alguns agentes, como vincristina e doxorrubicina, são vesicantes e podem causar esfacelamento/necrose tecidual em caso de extravasamento da medicação para fora da veia.

INTERAÇÕES POSSÍVEIS
Nenhuma.

ACOMPANHAMENTO
MONITORIZAÇÃO DO PACIENTE
- Exame físico, hemograma completo e contagem de plaquetas — antes de cada tratamento quimioterápico e 1 semana após a administração de cada medicamento novo ou, ainda, se houver preocupação quanto a baixas contagens celulares.
- Radiografia ou técnicas avançadas de diagnóstico por imagem — conforme a necessidade, dependendo da localização do tumor primário.

PREVENÇÃO
Evitar a exposição ou o acasalamento entre felinos positivos ao FeLV.

COMPLICAÇÕES POSSÍVEIS
- Leucopenia/neutropenia.
- Sepse.
- Anorexia.
- Mais de 80% dos proprietários de animais de estimação ficam satisfeitos com a qualidade de vida do gato durante a quimioterapia.

EVOLUÇÃO ESPERADA E PROGNÓSTICO
- Dependem da resposta inicial à quimioterapia, do tipo anatômico, do *status* do FeLV e da carga tumoral.
- Sobrevida média de acordo com o tratamento (em geral, taxa de resposta de 50-70%):
- Com a prednisona isolada — 1 mês e meio a 2 meses.
- Quimioterapia com o protocolo COP/CHOP — 6-9 meses.
- Terapia de salvamento à base de doxorrubicina em casos refratários — resposta de 22% com desfecho variável.
- Sobrevida média de acordo com o *status* do FeLV:
- Negativo = 7 meses (17 meses e meio se houver baixa carga tumoral).
- Positivo = 3 meses e meio (4 meses em caso de baixa carga tumoral).
- Sobrevida média de acordo com a localização anatômica:
- Renal — negativo para o FeLV, 11 meses e meio; positivo para o FeLV, 6 meses e meio.
- Nasal — 1 ano e meio a 2 anos e meio com radiação e quimioterapia.
- A quimioterapia pode não aumentar a sobrevida em detrimento à radiação isolada.
- Doses mais altas de radiação (>32 Gy) resultam em sobrevida mais longa.
- Mediastínico — cerca de 10% dos pacientes vivem mais de 2 anos.
- Alimentar — 8 meses.
- Multicêntrico periférico — 23 meses e meio.
- Se localizado (tempo médio de remissão) — 114 semanas.
- Sobrevida média de acordo com a histologia (grau ou subtipo do tumor):
- Linfoma linfocítico de células pequenas do trato gastrintestinal com ou sem envolvimento de outras vísceras: resposta global de 95% à clorambucila e à prednisona com sobrevida média de aproximadamente 2 anos (mais longa em remissão completa *versus* parcial).
- Linfoma linfocítico granular grande: resposta de ~30% com tempo médio de sobrevida de 57 dias.
- Gatos com linfoma tipo Hodgkin podem viver bem por longos períodos de tempo, mesmo sem tratamento (meses a anos).

DIVERSOS
DISTÚRBIOS ASSOCIADOS
- Hipoglicemia (rara).
- Gamopatia monoclonal (rara).
- Hipercalcemia (10-15%).

FATORES RELACIONADOS COM A IDADE
Gatos jovens com linfoma geralmente são positivos para o FeLV.

POTENCIAL ZOONÓTICO
Nenhum.

GESTAÇÃO/FERTILIDADE/REPRODUÇÃO
Não utilizar a quimioterapia em gatas prenhes.

SINÔNIMO(S)
- Linfossarcoma.
- Linfoma maligno.

ABREVIATURA(S)
- FeLV = vírus da leucemia felina.
- GI = gastrintestinal.
- SNC = sistema nervoso central.

Sugestões de Leitura
Ettinger SN. Principles of treatment for feline lymphoma. Clin Tech Small Anim Pract 2003, 18(2):98-102.
Haney SM, Beaver L, Turrel J, et al. Survival analysis of 97 cats with nasal lymphoma: A multi-institutional retrospective study (1986-2006). J Vet Intern Med 2009, 23(2):287-294.
Kiselow MA, Rassnick KM, McDonough SP, et al. Outcome of cats with low-grade lymphocytic lymphoma: 41 cases (1995-2005). JAVMA 2008, 232(3):405-410.
Milner RJ, Peyton J, Cooke K, et al. Response rates and survival times for cats with lymphoma treated with the University of Wisconsin-Madison chemotherapy protocol: 38 cases (1996-2003). JAVMA 2005, 227(7):1118-1122.
Taylor SS, Goodfellow MR, Browne WJ, et al. Feline extranodal lymphoma: Response to chemotherapy and survival in 110 cats. J Small Anim Pract 2009, 50(11):584-592.
Wilson HM. Feline alimentary lymphoma: Demystifying the enigma. Top Companion Anim Med 2008, 23(4):177-184.

Autor Kim A. Selting
Consultor Editorial Timothy M. Fan
Agradecimento Terrance A. Hamilton

Linfoma Cutâneo Epiteliotrópico

CONSIDERAÇÕES GERAIS

REVISÃO
- Linfoma cutâneo epiteliotrópico — forma mais comum de linfoma cutâneo de células-T.
- Uma neoplasia maligna incomum de cães e gatos.
- Síndrome de Sézary — forma rara de linfoma epiteliotrópico; nessa síndrome, ocorrem lesões cutâneas, invasão de linfonodos periféricos por linfócitos neoplásicos, e leucemia simultaneamente.
- Reticulose pagetoide — forma rara de linfoma epiteliotrópico; o infiltrado linfoide fica confinado à epiderme e estruturas anexas nos estágios iniciais da doença e estende-se para a derme nos estágios tardios.

SISTEMA(S) ACOMETIDO(S)
- Hematológico/Linfático/Imunológico.
- Cutâneo/Exócrino.

IDENTIFICAÇÃO
- Cães e gatos — mais comum em cães.
- Faixa etária de 6-14 anos — média de 8,6 anos.
- Aparentemente não há predileção racial ou sexual.

SINAIS CLÍNICOS
Achados Anamnésicos
- Dermatopatia crônica — meses antes do diagnóstico.
- Raramente agudo.
- Mimetiza outras dermatoses inflamatórias.
- Prurido ausente a intenso.

Achados do Exame Físico
- Há quatro categorias clínicas de apresentação:
  - Eritrodermia esfoliativa: eritema, descamação, despigmentação, alopecia generalizadas.
  - Mucocutânea: despigmentação, eritema, erosão e ulceração que afetam as junções mucocutâneas faciais.
  - Tumoral: placas, nódulos e massas eritematosos ou escamosos solitários ou múltiplos.
  - Ulceração da cavidade bucal: ulceração grave da gengiva, do palato e/ou da língua.
- Lesões — tipicamente em toda a pele; tendência acentuada ao envolvimento das junções mucocutâneas (lábios, pálpebras, plano nasal, junção anorretal, ou vulva) ou da cavidade bucal (gengiva, palato ou língua); as lesões podem ficar limitadas às junções mucocutâneas ou à mucosa bucal.
- Eritrodermia esfoliativa; a evolução para o estágio tumoral é muito rápida em cães quando comparados aos seres humanos.
- Formas de acometimento das junções mucocutâneas e da mucosa bucal: tendem a se mesclar com a cronicidade.
- Raramente ocorre o desenvolvimento de nódulos sem um estágio de mancha ou placa preexistente (*forma d'emblee*, forma de apresentação inicial e imediata em francês).
- Ocasionalmente, o estágio nodular pode evoluir para uma forma disseminada com envolvimento de linfonodos, leucemia e, raras vezes, outros órgãos.

CAUSAS E FATORES DE RISCO
Nenhum identificado: supõe-se uma estimulação antigênica crônica.

DIAGNÓSTICO

DIAGNÓSTICO DIFERENCIAL
- Dermatofitose, demodicose, dermatite esfoliativa associada a timoma felino — alopecia, eritema, descamação.
- Dermatite alérgica e acaríase sarcóptica — prurido, eritema, descamação generalizados.
- Lúpus eritematoso cutâneo, eritema multiforme, outras doenças imunomediadas — despigmentação/ulceração mucocutâneas.
- Estomatite crônica não neoplásica — doença infiltrativa e ulcerativa da mucosa bucal.
- Histiocitoma, histiocitose cutânea, mastocitoma ou qualquer outra neoplasia cutânea — formação de nódulo ou massa.

HEMOGRAMA/BIOQUÍMICA/URINÁLISE
- Anormalidades laboratoriais — variam, dependendo do estágio e da forma do linfoma cutâneo das células T, bem como da disseminação ou não da doença.
- Células de Sézary — pequenos linfócitos neoplásicos (8-20 µm) com núcleo convoluto e aspecto cerebriforme estão presentes no sangue periférico de pacientes com a síndrome de Sézary.
- Geralmente, esses exames não são dignos de nota se apenas a pele ou a mucosa estiver acometida.

DIAGNÓSTICO POR IMAGEM
Radiografias e ultrassonografia — esses exames não costumam ser utilizados nos estágios iniciais, mas acabam sendo necessários para confirmar a presença de doença sistêmica e/ou o estadiamento do tumor.

MÉTODOS DIAGNÓSTICOS
- Raspados cutâneos e cultura fúngica — descartam os quadros de demodicose e dermatofitose, se aplicáveis.
- Biopsia cutânea — permite a formulação do diagnóstico definitivo; obter amostras de múltiplas lesões de diferentes aspectos, mas evitar lesões erodidas/ulceradas e infectadas.

ACHADOS PATOLÓGICOS
- Infiltrado de linfócitos neoplásicos — na epiderme e no epitélio de folículos pilosos e estruturas anexas; difusamente distribuído ou sob a forma de microagregados de Pautrier isolados dentro do epitélio.
- Infiltrado dérmico — polimorfo; também consiste em linfócitos malignos que obscurecem a junção dermoepidérmica; nos estágios de mancha e placa, fica limitado à superfície da derme; no estágio nodular, estende-se para a camada profunda da derme e o subcutâneo.
- Epiteliotropismo de linfócitos neoplásicos — geralmente permanece proeminente em todos os estágios.

TRATAMENTO

- O objetivo é manter uma boa qualidade de vida o máximo de tempo possível.
- A terapia costuma ser de pouco benefício.
- Raramente, os nódulos solitários podem ser submetidos à excisão cirúrgica.
- Radioterapia: radiação total da pele com feixe de elétrons ou radiação de ortovoltagem é bem tolerada e pode ser benéfica em alguns casos.

MEDICAÇÕES

MEDICAMENTO(S)
- Quimioterapia — vários protocolos utilizados com sucesso limitado a nulo.
- Lomustina (CCNU) — taxa de resposta global de 80% com remissão completa atingida em cerca de 25% dos casos (60-70 mg/m² VO a cada 3-4 semanas por 3 a 5 tratamentos em média).
- Altas doses de ácido linoleico (p. ex., óleo de girassol) — a dose de 3 mL/kg VO 2 vezes/semana demonstrou uma melhora satisfatória em 7 de 10 gatos por até 2 anos.
- Quimioterapia tópica — mecloretamina (mostarda de nitrogênio) resultou em algum êxito no tratamento de lesões precoces; no entanto, há uma falta de eficácia a longo prazo: potencial carcinogênico para o proprietário e para a equipe de veterinários.
- Corticosteroides — tópicos e/ou sistêmicos podem resultar em certo alívio sintomático.
- Retinoides — isotretinoína (3 mg/kg/dia) ou acitretina (2 mg/kg/dia) pode ser benéfica; o custo pode ser um fator limitante.
- Imiquimode — um imunomodulador tópico com efeitos antineoplásicos e antivirais pode ser útil para doença localizada. Não há relatos publicados na literatura veterinária.

CONTRAINDICAÇÕES/INTERAÇÕES POSSÍVEIS
- Dependem do protocolo quimioterápico ou terapêutico.
- Buscar orientação de um oncologista ou dermatologista veterinário antes de iniciar a terapia caso não se esteja familiarizado com os agentes citotóxicos e/ou aprender sobre os protocolos terapêuticos mais recentes.

ACOMPANHAMENTO

- Prognóstico grave.
- O tempo de sobrevida médio para os cães depende do estágio da doença no momento do diagnóstico, da escolha terapêutica e da resposta à terapia. Varia de algumas semanas a mais de 18 meses.
- Raramente, os cães e gatos podem viver por mais de 2 anos após o estabelecimento do diagnóstico.
- A morte costuma ser o resultado de eutanásia.

DIVERSOS

SINÔNIMOS
- Linfoma, epidermotrópico.
- Micose fungoide.

Sugestões de Leitura
Fontaine J, Bovens C, Bettenay S, et al. Canine cutaneous epitheliotropic T-cell lymphoma: A review. Vet Comp Onc 2009, 7:1-14.

Autor Sheila Torres
Consultor Editorial Alexander H. Werner

LIPIDOSE HEPÁTICA

CONSIDERAÇÕES GERAIS

DEFINIÇÃO
• Lipidose hepática felina — >80% dos hepatócitos acumulam triglicerídeos, resultando em colestase grave e disfunção hepática.

FISIOPATOLOGIA
• Os gatos têm uma propensão ao acúmulo de triglicerídeos nos vacúolos citosólicos dos hepatócitos. • Fatores causais — privação de energia e proteína; aumento de mobilização da gordura periférica; aumento da síntese hepática de triglicerídeos; comprometimento da β-oxidação hepática de ácidos graxos; exportação hepatocelular reduzida de triglicerídeos. • Vacúolos de triglicerídeos — distensão de hepatócitos; deslocamento de organelas para a periferia da célula; disfunção de organela; compressão dos canalículos. • Insuficiência hepática — rara encefalopatia hepática evidente.

SISTEMA(S) ACOMETIDO(S)
• Hepatobiliar — colestase intra-hepática grave; disfunção ou insuficiência hepática.
• Gastrintestinal — anorexia, vômitos.
• Hematológico/linfático/imune — hemácias de formato anormal (pecilócitos), hemólise por corpúsculos de Heinz. • Musculosquelético — emaciação de tecido periférico. • Nervoso — encefalopatia hepática, ptialismo, condição moribunda. • Renal/urológico — depleção de potássio; acúmulo de triglicerídeos nos túbulos renais.

INCIDÊNCIA/PREVALÊNCIA
É a causa mais comum de hepatopatia felina grave indutora de icterícia na América do Norte.

DISTRIBUIÇÃO GEOGRÁFICA
Mundial.

IDENTIFICAÇÃO
Espécies
Gatos e, raramente, cães.

Idade Média e Faixa Etária
• Média — 8 (1-16 anos). • Acomete principalmente adultos de meia-idade.

SINAIS CLÍNICOS
Achados Anamnésicos
• Anorexia e perda de peso. • Icterícia. • Letargia e fraqueza que evoluem para colapso. • Vômitos, diarreia ou constipação. • Ptialismo (pode refletir encefalopatia hepática ou aversão alimentar).
• Flexão ventral do pescoço (fraqueza, depleções eletrolíticas: potássio, fosfato). • Anormalidades atribuídas a doenças subjacentes.

Achados do Exame Físico
• Icterícia. • Hepatomegalia. • Desidratação.
• Fraqueza — ventroflexão do pescoço, decúbito.
• Ptialismo. • Colapso/obnubilação. • Outros, dependendo da doença subjacente ou primária; encefalopatia hepática (raramente evidente).

CAUSAS
Lipidose Hepática Idiopática
• "Idiopática" = terminologia inadequada; problemas de saúde prévios provocam anorexia ou má assimilação na maioria dos gatos.

Lipidose Hepática Secundária
• Mais de 85% dos gatos com lipidose hepática apresentam distúrbios que causam anorexia ou má assimilação; o restante tem histórico de privação alimentar. • Hepatopatia primária — anomalia vascular portossistêmica; síndrome colangite/colangio-hepatite; obstrução extra-hepática do ducto biliar; colelitíase; neoplasia. • Gastrintestinais — obstrução; neoplasia; enteropatia inflamatória; pancreatite. • Doença urogenital — nefrite intersticial crônica; sinais atribuídos ao trato urinário inferior; insuficiência renal. • Condições neurológicas. • Doenças infecciosas — toxoplasmose; PIF; doença relacionada com o FIV ou o FeLV. • Hipertireoidismo. • Deficiência de B12. • Muitas outras condições sistêmicas ou toxinas. • Protocolo para rápida perda de peso.

FATORES DE RISCO
• Obesidade. • Anorexia. • Balanço nitrogenado negativo; catabolismo. • Perda de peso rápida.
• Deficiência de B12.

DIAGNÓSTICO

DIAGNÓSTICO DIFERENCIAL
• Hepatopatia primária subjacente — síndrome colangite/colangio-hepatite, colelitíase, obstrução extra-hepática do ducto biliar ou neoplasia (especialmente linfoma diferenciado por ultrassonografia abdominal, além de aspirado e biopsia do fígado). • Anomalia vascular portossistêmica — raramente confundida; diagnóstico feito por ultrassom ou cintilografia colorretal, além de testes laboratoriais.
• Toxoplasmose hepática ou PIF — diferenciar por biopsia do fígado e sorologia. • Pancreatite — diferenciar por ultrassonografia abdominal, testes séricos (baixa imunorreatividade da lipase pancreática felina diminui a probabilidade de pancreatite; valores altos podem estar associados à inflamação local ou pancreatite; os valores de amilase e lipase são inconstantes); citologia de aspirado pancreático; inspeção e biopsia do pâncreas. • Doença gastrintestinal — enteropatia inflamatória diferenciada por biopsia intestinal endoscópica ou de espessura total; obstrução diferenciada por radiografia (simples ou contrastada) e ultrassonografia abdominais.
• Toxicidades — suspeitas com base no histórico (p. ex., diazepam, paracetamol, metimazol orais).
• Hipertireoidismo — diferenciado por meio do perfil sérico de função da tireoide.

HEMOGRAMA/BIOQUÍMICA/URINÁLISE
• Hematologia — é comum a observação de pecilócitos; anemia arregenerativa; anemia hemolítica: hipofosfatemia grave ou corpúsculos de Heinz (baixo nível de glutationa); o leucograma reflete o distúrbio subjacente. • Bioquímica — hiperbilirrubinemia; atividade elevada de fosfatase alcalina e ALT; GGT normal ou levemente elevada se não houver distúrbio necroinflamatório primário do tecido biliar ou pancreático; nível baixo de ureia; creatinina normal; glicose variável (embora a hipoglicemia seja rara); colesterol e albumina variáveis; globulinas geralmente normais (podem estar elevadas com doença inflamatória subjacente); hipocalemia (associada à falha em sobreviver e ao fenômeno da realimentação); hipofosfatemia grave (<2 mg/dL) durante as primeiras 72 h (fenômeno da realimentação). • Urinálise — é comum a constatação de lipidúria e urina não concentrada; não se observa cristalúria por biurato de amônio; depleção de potássio (alguns gatos).

OUTROS TESTES LABORATORIAIS
• Tempos de coagulação prolongados — TP, TTPA, TCA e especialmente PIAVK em >50% dos gatos testados; fibrinogênio geralmente normal; as anormalidades são corrigidas com terapia parenteral à base de vitamina K_1. • Hiperamonemia — raramente avaliada. • Ácidos biliares séricos — altos antes de hiperbilirrubinemia; determinação redundante quando o animal já está ictérico.
• Deficiência de B12 — pode aumentar a suscetibilidade à lipidose hepática.

DIAGNÓSTICO POR IMAGEM
Radiografia Abdominal Simples
• Hepatomegalia. • Podem-se observar aspectos do distúrbio subjacente.

Ultrassonografia Abdominal
• Hiperecogenicidade difusa do parênquima hepático — reflete a vacuolização lipídica hepática — hiperecogenicidade renal (vacuolização lipídica nos túbulos renais) compromete as comparações de ecogenicidade entre os órgãos. • Buscar pela causa primária indutora de lipidose hepática.

MÉTODOS DIAGNÓSTICOS
• Citologia de aspirado por agulha fina — mais de 80% dos hepatócitos revelam vacuolização citosólica; raramente, há necessidade de biopsia para confirmar a lipidose hepática. • Diagnóstico definitivo de lipidose hepática — com base no histórico, nas características clínicas, na atividade elevada da fosfatase alcalina, na ecogenicidade difusa do parênquima hepático e na vacuolização lipídica de hepatócitos ao exame citológico do aspirado; a citologia de aspirado não é capaz de excluir distúrbios hepáticos primários subjacentes (p. ex., síndrome colangite/colangio-hepatite, obstrução extra-hepática do ducto biliar e anomalia vascular portossistêmica). • Biopsia do fígado — fornece o diagnóstico definitivo de distúrbios hepáticos primários subjacentes; *realizada apenas em caso de resposta insatisfatória à terapia ou atividade elevada da GGT*; estabilizar o gato antes dos procedimentos de anestesia e biopsia para diminuir o risco de óbito. • Três doses de vitamina K1 (0,5-1,5 mg/kg SC ou IM) em intervalos de 12 h, pelo menos 12 h *antes* dos procedimentos de obtenção de amostra por aspiração, biopsia hepática, cateterização da veia jugular ou inserção de tubo alimentar para reduzir o risco de hemorragia iatrogênica.

ACHADOS PATOLÓGICOS
• Macroscópicos — hepatomegalia difusa, com superfície lisa; consistência gordurosa friável, coloração amarelo-pálido com aspecto reticulado; a amostra de biopsia flutua em formalina.
• Microscópicos — vacuolização hepatocelular difusa e grave; vacúolos grandes (macrovesiculares) ou pequenos (microvesiculares).

TRATAMENTO

CUIDADO(S) DE SAÚDE ADEQUADO(S)
• Internação — necessária para gatos em decúbito ou naqueles com ventroflexão do pescoço (por deficiência de potássio, fosfato ou tiamina). • Alta hospitalar — após a estabilização do paciente (ou seja, quando ele estiver livre de problemas) e o estabelecimento da via de nutrição enteral.
• Tratamento ambulatorial — diminui o estresse e, portanto, facilita a recuperação em alguns gatos.

Lipidose Hepática

CUIDADO(S) DE ENFERMAGEM
• Fluidos poliônicos balanceados — *evitar* a suplementação de lactato e glicose. • É importante a suplementação com cloreto de potássio — utilizar uma escala móvel (ver "Hipocalemia"). • Os suplementos de fosfato costumam ser necessários (ver "Hipofosfatemia"), especialmente após a retomada da alimentação (fenômeno da realimentação). • Raramente, há necessidade de suplementos de magnésio (utilizados se a suplementação de potássio parecer ineficaz).

Corrigir a Hipofosfatemia
• Fosfato sérico <2 mg/dL secundário à realimentação gera sinais patológicos: anorexia, vômitos, fraqueza, mionecrose, íleo paralítico, hemólise e sinais neurológicos confundidos com encefalopatia hepática. • Tratamento — dose inicial do fosfato de potássio de 0,01-0,03 mmol/kg/h IV (fosfato parenteral comercial = 3 mmol/mL de fosfato); monitorizar o fosfato sérico a cada 3-6 h; interromper quando a concentração de fosfato se estabilizar para >2 mg/dL. • **CUIDADO:** reduzir a suplementação IV com cloreto de potássio para evitar hipercalemia iatrogênica.

Corrigir a Depleção de Glutationa Hepática
• O baixo nível de glutationa hepática é confirmado em casos de lipidose hepática; no entanto, as mensurações de rotina da glutationa não estão disponíveis; há risco elevado de lesão oxidativa em decorrência da doença primária; acúmulo de lipídios; ou déficits energéticos induzidos por hipofosfatemia. • Intervenção para crise por baixos níveis de glutationa hepática ou anemia por corpúsculos de Heinz — usar *N*-acetilcisteína (140 mg/kg IV e, em seguida, 70 mg/kg IV de solução a 10% diluída a 1:2 em solução fisiológica; administrar por meio de filtro não pirogênico de 0,22-0,25 μ durante 20 min). • Quando a nutrição enteral for restabelecida, mudar para SAMe (200 mg/gato VO a cada 24 h).

ATIVIDADE
A atividade pode aumentar a motilidade gástrica quando a gastroparesia complica a alimentação (vômitos crônicos); na fase inicial de recuperação, os gatos se apresentam muito fracos.

DIETA
• Suporte nutricional — indispensável para a recuperação. • Dietas felinas ricas em proteínas e calorias — são essenciais. • Teor calórico — 50-60 kcal/kg de peso corporal ideal/dia; transição gradual para as necessidades calóricas completas em 3-5 dias; fornecer pequenas refeições várias vezes ao dia. • Alimentação forçada — costuma ser necessária. • Alimentação oral forçada — pode causar aversão alimentar. • Alimentação por tubo — feita inicialmente por meio de sonda nasogástrica, trocada para sonda esofágica após melhora do estado de hidratação e do nível de eletrólitos, além da suplementação de vitamina K1. • Evitar a realização de laparotomia para inserção de sonda gástrica; os gatos com lipidose hepática apresentam altos índices de mortalidade. • Oferecer a alimentação diária por via oral com cuidado para avaliar o interesse pela comida. • Não é recomendável o uso de dietas enterais à base de fórmulas humanas para estresse.

Suplementos
• Aumentam a sobrevida em gatos gravemente acometidos: L-carnitina de qualidade médica (ampla variabilidade em termos de biodisponibilidade; Carnitor® na dose recomendada de 250-500 mg/dia); taurina (250-500 mg/dia); tiamina (50-100 mg/dia); vitamina B12 (inicialmente, 1 mg IM ou SC em dose única): determinar as necessidades crônicas de vitamina B12 por meio de mensurações sequenciais dessa vitamina (intervalos semanais); vitaminas hidrossolúveis (o dobro da dose normal); vitamina E (10 UI/kg/dia); doadores de tiol (*N*-acetilcisteína e SAMe): conforme exposto anteriormente; gliconato de potássio (para hipocalemia): diminui os suplementos de potássio em fluidos; óleo de origem marinha no alimento (2.000 mg a cada 24 h).

ORIENTAÇÃO AO PROPRIETÁRIO
• Análises bioquímicas sequenciais são necessárias para avaliar a recuperação. • Orientação ao proprietário sobre a utilização e os cuidados relativos às sondas de alimentação. • As sondas podem permanecer no lugar por 4-6 meses. • É improvável que ocorra recidiva; a função hepática não será cronicamente comprometida.

CONSIDERAÇÕES CIRÚRGICAS
• Laparotomia exploratória e biopsia hepática (se indicadas) — inspecionar em busca de distúrbios subjacentes e fazer biopsia de órgãos como pâncreas, estômago e intestino delgado. • Evitar intervenções cirúrgicas até a correção do estado de hidratação e das depleções de eletrólitos, o alívio da anemia por corpúsculo de Heinz e o desaparecimento da coagulopatia.

MEDICAÇÕES

MEDICAMENTO(S)
• Vitamina K1 — recomendada para todos os gatos com suspeita de lipidose hepática (ver "Coagulopatia por Hepatopatia"); evitar a dosagem excessiva: hemólise oxidativa e lesão hepática. • Os medicamentos para amenizar a encefalopatia hepática não costumam ser necessários. • Controle da êmese — metoclopramida (0,2-0,5 mg/kg SC a cada 8 h, 30 min antes das refeições, ou sob infusão IV em velocidade constante na dose de 0,01-0,02 mg/kg/h ou 1-2 mg/kg/dia); dolasetrona (0,5-0,6 mg/kg a cada 24 h IV, SC, VO); ou maropitanto (1 mg/kg IV, SC, VO a cada 24 h por, no máximo, 5 dias); famotidina: para evitar o dano à porção inferior do esôfago em caso de vômito, 0,5-1,0 mg/kg a cada 12-24 h. • Antibióticos sistêmicos — conforme apropriado para infecções concomitantes.

CONTRAINDICAÇÕES/PRECAUÇÕES
• Ajustar as doses das medicações de acordo com o metabolismo hepático ou a excreção. • Evitar o uso de benzodiazepínicos e barbitúricos — podem provocar encefalopatia hepática. • Estimulantes do apetite (p. ex., diazepam, oxazepam e ciproeptadina) — não proporcionam consumo calórico confiável; podem produzir sedação; raramente causam insuficiência hepática fulminante. • Evitar o emprego de medicamentos que contenham transportador de propilenoglicol (p. ex., etomidato e diazepam) — acarretam hemólise em animais com lipidose hepática. • Ácido ursodesoxicólico — provavelmente não é benéfico em casos de lipidose hepática; pode promover deficiência de taurina (se utilizado, suplementar com esse aminoácido). • Suplementos de glicose — podem aumentar o acúmulo hepático de triglicerídeos. • Evitar a utilização de tetraciclinas e estanazolol — promovem o depósito de triglicerídeos. • Evitar anestesia com propofol (derivado fenólico) — pode provocar hemólise 12 h após a infusão em gatos com anemia por corpúsculo de Heinz; os gatos acometidos por lipidose hepática recuperam-se de forma lenta; em vez disso, utilizar anestesia inalatória.

ACOMPANHAMENTO

MONITORIZAÇÃO DO PACIENTE
• Peso e condição corporais, além do estado de hidratação e do nível de eletrólitos — é importante a realização de ajustes criteriosos nos níveis de calorias, fluidos e eletrólitos. • Bilirrubina sérica — declina em até 2 semanas após o tratamento adequado; prediz a recuperação. • Atividade das enzimas hepáticas — demora para se normalizar; não prediz a recuperação. • Alta hospitalar e retorno para casa — quando os vômitos estiverem sob controle, a gastroparesia resolvida, os valores de bilirrubina total diminuindo, o paciente deambulando e não houver problemas com a sonda de alimentação. • Alimentação com sonda — só interromper após consumo alimentar voluntário confirmado por 2 semanas.

PREVENÇÃO
• Obesidade — evitar; a redução de peso não deve exceder 2% do peso corporal por semana. • O proprietário deve verificar o consumo alimentar durante o regime de perda de peso e o estresse em casa.

COMPLICAÇÕES POSSÍVEIS
• Mau funcionamento ou obstrução da sonda de alimentação — as obstruções do tubo são aliviadas por suco de mamão, bebida não alcoólica carbonatada ou pasta líquida de enzimas pancreáticas; deixar por 15 min e então irrigar com água morna. • É rara a ocorrência de encefalopatia hepática após a introdução de suporte nutricional. • Insuficiência hepática ocasionando a morte. • Distúrbio causal subjacente intratável.

EVOLUÇÃO ESPERADA E PROGNÓSTICO
• Resposta ideal à alimentação com sonda e aos suplementos nutricionais — recuperação em 3-6 semanas. • A terapia descrita resulta em 85% de recuperação nos animais gravemente acometidos. • A doença subjacente influencia o desfecho clínico. • A lipidose hepática raramente recidiva; além disso, ela não causa disfunção hepática crônica.

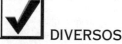

DIVERSOS

SINÔNIMO(S)
• Síndrome do fígado gorduroso. • Esteatose hepática. • Vacuolização hepática felina. • Hepatopatia vacuolar. • Degeneração vacuolar.

ABREVIATURA(S)
• FeLV = vírus da leucemia felina. • FIV = vírus da imunodeficiência felina. • PIAVK = proteínas invocadas pela ausência ou antagonismo da vitamina K. • PIF = peritonite infecciosa felina. • TCA = tempo de coagulação ativada. • TP = tempo de protrombina. • TTPA = tempo de tromboplastina parcial ativada. • SAMe = *S*-adenosilmetionina.

Autor Sharon A. Center

LIPOMA

CONSIDERAÇÕES GERAIS

REVISÃO
- Lipomas são tumores benignos dos adipócitos (células de gordura). Seu aspecto é o de adipócitos maduros sem atipia celular ou nuclear, idênticos às células que formam a gordura do adulto.
- Há relatos de que esses tumores ocorram em cerca de 16% dos cães e 12% dos gatos; entretanto, sua verdadeira incidência provavelmente é mais elevada, uma vez que muitos lipomas são diagnosticados pelo aspecto clínico sem histologia.
- Esse tumor pode ocorrer em qualquer parte do organismo, embora as regiões subcutâneas do tórax, do abdome, dos membros e das axilas possam ser mais comumente acometidas. Os lipomas também foram relatados dentro do tórax e das cavidades abdominais, bem como no útero, na vagina e na vulva.

IDENTIFICAÇÃO
- Mais comum nos cães de meia-idade a idosos; raramente observado nos gatos.
- Não existe predisposição racial, embora haja relatos de que as raças Labrador retriever, Doberman pinscher, Schnauzer miniatura, Cocker spaniel, Dachshund e Weimaraner estejam sob alto risco.
- Animais obesos podem ser mais suscetíveis.
- Cadelas são mais predispostas.
- Os lipomas nos felinos podem ocorrer com mais frequência em machos castrados.

SINAIS CLÍNICOS
- Geralmente solitários, embora possam ocorrer múltiplos lipomas no mesmo indivíduo.
- Variabilidade no tamanho, na forma (frequentemente redondos) e na velocidade de crescimento (em geral, lentos).
- Com frequência, os animais permanecem assintomáticos a menos que a massa se torne grande o suficiente a ponto de provocar dificuldades funcionais. Os lipomas aumentam por expansão e não por invasão. Também podem comprimir órgãos adjacentes quando ocorrem na cavidade torácica ou abdominal.
- À palpação, os lipomas costumam ser moles; no entanto, aqueles que se desenvolvem entre os planos musculares podem ser firmes e confundidos com lipomas infiltrativos ou sarcomas de tecido mole. A região caudal da coxa é um local comum para lipomas intermusculares (entre os músculos semimembranáceo e semitendíneo).
- Em muitos casos, o tumor está presente há muito tempo (1 ano ou mais) antes da consulta ao veterinário.

CAUSAS E FATORES DE RISCO
Desconhecidos.

DIAGNÓSTICO

DIAGNÓSTICO DIFERENCIAL
- Hemangiopericitoma.
- Lipoma infiltrativo.
- Lipossarcoma ou outros sarcomas de tecido mole (p. ex., mixossarcoma e fibrossarcoma).
- Mastocitomas.

HEMOGRAMA/BIOQUÍMICA/URINÁLISE
Normais.

OUTROS TESTES LABORATORIAIS
N/D.

DIAGNÓSTICO POR IMAGEM
Radiografia — revela a presença de tecido/massa de densidade gordurosa, circundado por estruturas com densidade de tecido mole.

MÉTODOS DIAGNÓSTICOS
Citologia de aspirado por agulha fina — revela adipócitos maduros normais; a gordura tende a coalescer em gotículas que são removidas da lâmina durante a coloração, deixando uma amostra razoavelmente acelular.

ACHADOS PATOLÓGICOS
Histologicamente compatível com o tecido adiposo normal, o que pode ser subclassificado se outros elementos teciduais estiverem presentes, por exemplo, cartilagem (condrolipoma), vasos sanguíneos (angiolipoma), elementos hematopoiéticos (mielolipoma) ou colágeno (fibrolipoma); nenhuma infiltração tumoral nas estruturas circundantes (p. ex., músculo).

TRATAMENTO

- Excisão cirúrgica é curativa, uma vez que esses tumores estão bem encapsulados.
- Lipomas intermusculares da região caudal da coxa estendem-se profundamente entre os planos musculares, mas não invadem as estruturas adjacentes; desfecho bem-sucedido com a remoção cirúrgica.
- Embora haja relatos da injeção intralesional de cloreto de cálcio a 10%, esse procedimento não é recomendado em virtude da irritação local e necrose tecidual.

MEDICAÇÕES

MEDICAMENTO(S)
Tratamento clínico é desnecessário e de eficácia improvável.

CONTRAINDICAÇÕES/INTERAÇÕES POSSÍVEIS
N/D.

ACOMPANHAMENTO

MONITORIZAÇÃO DO PACIENTE
Fazer com que o proprietário monitorize o paciente quanto à ocorrência de recidiva, que é rara e pode ser resolvida com sucesso por uma segunda cirurgia. Se o tumor recidivar, considerar a possibilidade de lipoma infiltrativo ou sarcoma de tecido mole.

PREVENÇÃO
Não há nenhuma medida preventiva específica, exceto a possibilidade de evitar a obesidade.

COMPLICAÇÕES POSSÍVEIS
N/D.

EVOLUÇÃO ESPERADA E PROGNÓSTICO
- Espera-se a cura com a excisão cirúrgica completa. Com a remoção incompleta, pode ocorrer recidiva. A cirurgia é mais bem realizada antes que o tumor interfira na função ou na mobilidade do animal. Pode ocorrer o desenvolvimento de outros lipomas primários em outros locais. Raramente, ocorre a presença de outros elementos teciduais dentro do tumor, como cartilagem, colágeno ou células hematopoiéticas; no entanto, não parece que isso exerça impacto sobre o desfecho cirúrgico ou o prognóstico.
- No caso do diagnóstico de lipossarcoma, o comportamento é semelhante ao de outros sarcomas de tecido mole; portanto, consulte a literatura especializada relevante a respeito desses tumores.

DIVERSOS

DISTÚRBIOS ASSOCIADOS
Possivelmente, obesidade.

FATORES RELACIONADOS COM A IDADE
Nenhum fator específico, exceto a predisposição geral relacionada com o avanço da idade para o desenvolvimento do tumor.

GESTAÇÃO/FERTILIDADE/REPRODUÇÃO
A cirurgia provavelmente pode ser adiada até depois do parto.

VER TAMBÉM
Lipoma Infiltrativo.

Sugestões de Leitura
Goldschmidt MH, Hendrick MJ. Tumors of the skin and soft tissues. In: Meuten DJ, ed., Tumors of Domestic Animals, 4th ed. Ames: Iowa State University Press, 2002, pp. 45-117.

Autor Anthony J. Mutsaers
Consultor Editorial Timothy M. Fan

Lipoma Infiltrativo

CONSIDERAÇÕES GERAIS

REVISÃO
- Variante invasiva e não encapsulada do lipoma que não sofre metástase.
- Neoplasia benigna que se infiltra nos tecidos moles, particularmente nos músculos, incluindo as fáscias, os tendões, os nervos, os vasos sanguíneos, as glândulas salivares, os linfonodos e as cápsulas articulares e, ocasionalmente, os ossos.
- Infiltração muscular tipicamente extensa.
- Cura cirúrgica difícil de obter.
- Ocorre com uma frequência muito menor que o lipoma.

IDENTIFICAÇÃO
- Em geral, cães de meia-idade.
- Não há predileção racial definitivamente demonstrada; Labrador retriever — possivelmente super-representado.
- Pode ser mais comum nas fêmeas do que nos machos.

SINAIS CLÍNICOS
- Massa difusa e volumosa de tecido mole.
- Clinicamente aparece como tumefação muscular localizada e/ou abdome distendido em caso de componente abdominal.
- Infiltração da musculatura pélvica, esternal e cervical lateral, bem como da coxa e do ombro — mais comum; provas recentes não sugerem previsão clara de localização.

CAUSAS E FATORES DE RISCO
Desconhecidos.

DIAGNÓSTICO

DIAGNÓSTICO DIFERENCIAL
- Sarcoma de tecido mole, particularmente lipossarcoma, hemangiopericitoma, mixossarcoma, rabdomiossarcoma e fibrossarcoma.
- Lipoma.
- Lipoma intermuscular.
- Mastocitoma.

HEMOGRAMA/BIOQUÍMICA/URINÁLISE
Normais.

OUTROS TESTES LABORATORIAIS
N/D.

DIAGNÓSTICO POR IMAGEM
- Radiografia — revela tecido adiposo denso entre as estruturas densas de tecido mole.
- Imagem por RM ou TC — permite a discriminação adequada dos tumores para o planejamento de cirurgia e/ou radioterapia; entretanto, a diferenciação entre gordura normal e lipoma infiltrativo pode ser problemática.

MÉTODOS DIAGNÓSTICOS
Exame citológico do aspirado — revela adipócitos maduros sem atipia celular ou nuclear, idênticos às células que formam a gordura do adulto.

ACHADOS PATOLÓGICOS
- Exame histológico — adipócitos bem diferenciados; pode ser indistinguível do tecido adiposo normal.
- Característica peculiar — infiltração tumoral dentro dos feixes musculares e entre eles, bem como em outros tecidos.

TRATAMENTO

CONSIDERAÇÕES CIRÚRGICAS
- A invasividade característica torna a excisão extremamente difícil; não é fácil distinguir entre o tumor e o tecido adiposo normal.
- Margens tumorais pouco definidas — podem contribuir para a constatação de alta taxa de recidiva após a excisão cirúrgica.
- 36-50% dos pacientes apresentam recidiva dentro de 3-16 meses, exceto na amputação de membro para tumor apendicular.
- Amputação de membro acometido — recomendada apenas quando o quadro afeta a qualidade de vida; o tumor traz poucos inconvenientes a menos que interfira no movimento, provoque dor relacionada à compressão ou se desenvolva em região anatômica de importância vital. Contudo, a amputação deve ser realizada antes que o crescimento da extensão proximal do tumor atravesse a margem cirúrgica acessível.

RADIOTERAPIA POR FEIXE EXTERNO
- Benéfica para controle do tumor a longo prazo — sobrevida média de 40 meses em estudo retrospectivo de 13 cães, sendo que apenas um deles (7,7%) foi submetido à eutanásia em virtude de sinais relacionados com o tumor (*versus* 26,7% tratados apenas com a cirurgia).
- O tumor pode ser estabilizado em cães com doença mensurável.
- Cirurgia citorredutiva para doença microscópica antes da radiação pode resultar no controle da doença a longo prazo.
- É improvável que a radioterapia elimine os adipócitos maduros inativos por meio mitótico, mas ela pode inibir a infiltração progressiva por lesar a microcirculação tumoral.

MEDICAÇÕES

MEDICAMENTO(S)
N/D.

CONTRAINDICAÇÕES/INTERAÇÕES POSSÍVEIS
N/D.

ACOMPANHAMENTO

MONITORIZAÇÃO DO PACIENTE
- Foco — se e quando recomendar a cirurgia e a radioterapia adjuvante para margens cirúrgicas incompletas.
- Reavaliações — esquema ditado pelo crescimento do tumor e pela escolha do tratamento.

COMPLICAÇÕES POSSÍVEIS
Efeitos colaterais agudos temporários (p. ex., dermatite úmida e alopecia) são esperados com a radioterapia. Também é recomendável a consulta com um oncologista especialista em radioterapia a respeito dos efeitos colaterais específicos relacionados com a região anatômica afetada.

EVOLUÇÃO ESPERADA E PROGNÓSTICO
O controle do crescimento tumoral a longo prazo pode ser obtido com a aplicação de radioterapia por feixe externo, isoladamente ou em combinação com a cirurgia. A ausência de potencial metastático confere um prognóstico muito bom com o controle do crescimento tumoral local. No caso do diagnóstico de lipossarcoma, o comportamento tumoral é semelhante ao de outros sarcomas de tecido mole; portanto, é aconselhável a consulta à literatura especializada relevante sobre esses tumores.

DIVERSOS

SINÔNIMO(S)
- Lipomatose.
- O lipoma infiltrativo foi referido como um lipossarcoma bem-diferenciado.

VER TAMBÉM
Lipoma.

ABREVIATURA(S)
- RM = ressonância magnética.
- TC = tomografia computadorizada.

Sugestões de Leitura
McEntee MC, Page RL, Mauldin GN, et al. Results of irradiation of infiltrative lipoma in 13 dogs. Vet Radiol Ultrasound 2000, 41:554-556.

Autor Anthony J. Mutsaers
Consultor Editorial Timothy M. Fan

Lúpus Eritematoso Cutâneo (Discoide)

CONSIDERAÇÕES GERAIS

REVISÃO
- Considerado como uma variante benigna do LES.
- Uma das doenças cutâneas imunomediadas mais comuns.
- Envolve predominantemente o plano nasal, a face e as orelhas.

IDENTIFICAÇÃO
- Cães e gatos.
- Muito incomum em gatos.
- Raças caninas predominantes — Collie, Pastor alemão, Husky siberiano, Pastor de Shetland, Malamute do Alasca, Chow chow e seus cruzamentos.
- Sem predileção etária.

SINAIS CLÍNICOS
- Sintomas inicial: despigmentação do plano nasal e/ou dos lábios.
- A despigmentação evolui para erosões e ulcerações.
- Perda da arquitetura "arredondada" normal do plano nasal.
- Podem ocorrer perda de tecido e formação de cicatriz.
- As lesões crônicas são frágeis e podem facilmente sofrer hemorragia; raras vezes, ocorre hemorragia intensa a partir de dano arteriolar.
- Também pode envolver o pavilhão auricular e a região periocular; raramente, os pés e a genitália.

CAUSAS E FATORES DE RISCO
- Mecanismo exato indeterminado; a radiação actínica pode alterar a natureza antigênica dos queratinócitos.
- Exacerbação sazonal e geográfica — associada ao aumento da radiação actínica*.

DIAGNÓSTICO

DIAGNÓSTICO DIFERENCIAL

Principais Considerações
- Outras doenças imunomediadas — pênfigo foliáceo, pênfigo eritematoso, LES.
- Reações a medicamentos.
- Dermatomiosite.
- Dermatofitose nasal.
- Piodermite mucocutânea.
- Hipersensibilidade a insetos.

Outras Considerações (Raras)
- Alergia por contato.
- Dermatose responsiva ao zinco.
- Traumatismo.
- Dermatite necrolítica superficial.
- Linfoma cutâneo epiteliotrópico de células T.
- Carcinoma de células escamosas.

HEMOGRAMA/BIOQUÍMICA/URINÁLISE
Geralmente normais a menos que sejam atribuídos a alguma causa subjacente.

OUTROS TESTES LABORATORIAIS
AAN, preparação de LE e teste de Coombs — geralmente normais ou negativos exceto em LES.

OUTROS MÉTODOS DIAGNÓSTICOS
- Biopsia e histopatologia diferenciarão o lúpus eritematoso discoide de outros distúrbios.
- Biopsias de lesões despigmentadas, erosões leves ou lesões levemente crostosas são preferíveis para o diagnóstico.

ACHADOS PATOLÓGICOS
- A histopatologia é caracterizada por dermatite de interface liquenoide com apoptose proeminente das células basais, graus variados de atrofia epidérmica, e incontinência pigmentar.
- O exame histopatológico não é capaz de diferenciar com facilidade o lúpus eritematoso discoide de piodermite mucocutânea.
- Evitar amostras de lesões ulcerativas e intensamente crostosas se possível.
- O exame imunopatológico pode ser feito, mas não costuma ser necessário.

TRATAMENTO
- Não há risco de morte, mas pode ser deformante.
- Evitar exposição solar direta e utilizar bloqueadores solares à prova d'água.

MEDICAÇÕES

MEDICAMENTO(S)
- Terapia tópica:
  - Glicocorticosteroides — inicialmente, um produto fluorado potente (p. ex., fluocinolona a 0,1%) a cada 24 h por 14 dias; em seguida, a cada 48-72 h; assim que estiver em remissão, trocar por algum produto menos potente (p. ex., hidrocortisona a 0,5% ou 2,5%) se possível.
  - Pomada de tacrolimo (a 0,1%) em princípio a cada 12-24 h e, depois, reduzir gradativamente para cada 24-72 h assim que o quadro estiver em remissão.
- Terapia sistêmica:
  - Tetraciclina e niacinamida — 250 mg de cada VO a cada 8 h para cães com <10 kg; 500 mg VO a cada 8 h para cães de porte maior.
  - Prednisona — considerar nos casos graves ou irresponsivos; 2-4 mg/kg/dia isoladamente ou em combinação com azatioprina, 2 mg/kg VO em dias alternados; reduzir a prednisona gradativamente para 0,5-1 mg/kg VO a cada 48 h para manutenção a longo prazo.
  - Ciclosporina — 5-10 mg/kg VO diariamente como terapia imunossupressora alternativa.
- Considerar antibioticoterapia sistêmica por, no mínimo, 3-4 semanas antes da terapia imunossupressora sistêmica para diferenciar de piodermite mucocutânea.
- Vitamina E — 10-20 UI/kg VO a cada 12 h; pode ajudar a reduzir a inflamação e proteger a pele.

ACOMPANHAMENTO

MONITORIZAÇÃO DO PACIENTE
- Reavaliar 14 dias após o início do tratamento quanto à resposta clínica.
- Hemograma completo e bioquímica sérica — a cada 12 meses em caso de terapia tópica e a cada 3-6 meses em caso de terapia sistêmica.
- Hemograma completo e contagem de plaquetas — a cada 2 semanas no primeiro mês; em seguida, a cada 3-6 meses enquanto estiver sendo submetido à azatioprina.

PREVENÇÃO
Os animais acometidos devem evitar a exposição à luz ultravioleta.

COMPLICAÇÕES POSSÍVEIS
- Formação de cicatriz.
- Piodermite secundária.
- Hemorragia.
- Deformação.

EVOLUÇÃO ESPERADA E PROGNÓSTICO
- Natureza progressiva, embora não costume exibir risco de morte se não for tratado.
- Com o tratamento adequado, espera-se a remissão na maior parte dos casos.
- Os casos que necessitam de terapia imunossupressora crônica apresentam um prognóstico mais reservado, embora as remissões sejam comuns com o tratamento mais rigoroso.

DIVERSOS

SINÔNIMO(S)
- Síndrome hepatocutânea.
- Eritema migratório necrolítico.
- Dermatite necrolítica superficial.

ABREVIATURA(S)
- AAN = anticorpo antinuclear.
- LE = lúpus eritematoso.
- LES = lúpus eritematoso sistêmico.

Sugestões de Leitura

Griffies JD, Mendelsohn CL, Rosenkrantz WR, et al. Topical 0.1% tacrolimus for the treatment of discoid lupus erythematosus and pemphigus erythematosus in dogs. JAAHA 2004, 40:29-41.

Rosenkrantz WS. Discoid lupus erythematosus. In: Current Veterinary Dermatology. St. Louis: Mosby, 1993.

Wiemelt SP, Goldschmidt MH, Greek JS, et al. A retrospective study comparing the histopathological features and response to treatment in two canine nasal dermatoses, DLE and MCP. Vet Dermatol 2004, 15:341-348.

Autor Dawn E. Logas
Consultor Editorial Alexander H. Werner
Agradecimento Agradecemos ao autor deste capítulo na edição anterior, Wayne Rosenkrantz.

---

* N. T.: Tipo de radiação (p. ex., a luz do Sol), cuja ação pode provocar modificações químicas em algumas substâncias ou tecidos orgânicos (como a pele).

Lúpus Eritematoso Sistêmico

CONSIDERAÇÕES GERAIS

DEFINIÇÃO
Doença autoimune polissistêmica, caracterizada pela formação de anticorpos contra uma ampla gama de autoantígenos. Anticorpos patogênicos, imunocomplexos circulantes e células T autorreativas são os principais mediadores de lesão tecidual.

FISIOPATOLOGIA
• Causa desconhecida.
• São produzidos anticorpos direcionados contra uma ampla variedade de antígenos da membrana, do citoplasma e do núcleo, resultando em hipersensibilidade do tipo III.
• Complexos antígeno-anticorpo são formados e depositados em diversos locais, incluindo vasos sanguíneos, glomérulos renais, membrana sinovial, plexo coroide e pele, resultando em hipersensibilidade do tipo III.
• Produção de células-T autorreativas provoca hipersensibilidade do tipo IV.
• Lesão tecidual é causada por ativação do complemento por imunocomplexos circulantes, infiltração de células inflamatórias e citotoxicidade direta dos autoanticorpos contra antígenos ligados à membrana.
• As manifestações clínicas dependem da localização dos imunocomplexos e da especificidade dos autoanticorpos.
• Fatores genéticos, ambientais, farmacológicos e infecciosos podem ser deflagradores da doença.

SISTEMA(S) ACOMETIDO(S)
• Musculosquelético — depósito de imunocomplexos nas membranas sinoviais.
• Cutâneo/exócrino — depósito de imunocomplexos na pele.
• Renal/urológico — depósito de imunocomplexos nos glomérulos.
• Hematológico/linfático/imune — autoanticorpos contra hemácias, leucócitos, plaquetas ou precursores da medula óssea.
• Outros sistemas orgânicos — se houver depósito de imunocomplexos ou anticorpos (músculo, nervo, olho, p. ex.).

GENÉTICA
Quadro hereditário, apesar de não ocorrer por meio de mecanismos autossômicos simples. As raças predispostas incluem Pastor alemão, Pastor de Shetland, Collie, Beagle e Poodle. Foram determinadas várias colônias de cães com elevada predisposição para LES, embora haja uma associação com o tipo de complexo de histocompatibilidade maior (alelo DLA).

INCIDÊNCIA/PREVALÊNCIA
Incomum em cães, porém raro em gatos.

DISTRIBUIÇÃO GEOGRÁFICA
N/D.

IDENTIFICAÇÃO
Espécies
Cães e gatos.

Raça(s) Predominante(s)
• Raças de médio a grande porte.
• Pastor alemão, Poodle e Beagle são super-representados.
• Cães da raça Pointer alemão de pelo curto são predispostos a lúpus eritematoso cutâneo esfoliativo.
• Collie de pelagem áspera e Pastor de Shetland são predispostos a lúpus eritematoso cutâneo vesicular.
• Gatos das raças Siamês e Persa podem estar sob alto risco de LES.

Idade Média e Faixa Etária
A idade média é de 5 anos, com variação de 6 meses a 13 anos de idade.

Sexo Predominante
Os cães machos foram super-representados em um único estudo apenas.

SINAIS CLÍNICOS
Achados Anamnésicos
• Letargia.
• Anorexia.
• Claudicação com desvio do membro.
• Lesões cutâneas.
• Febre.
• Fraqueza.
• Outros achados dependem do(s) órgão(s) acometido(s).
• O início dos sinais clínicos pode ser agudo ou insidioso.
• A doença frequentemente tem uma evolução remissiva e recidivante.
• Diferentes manifestações clínicas são, muitas vezes, sequenciais e não concomitantes.

Achados do Exame Físico
• Articulações tumefatas e/ou dolorosas — constituem o principal sinal apresentado em grande parte dos animais. As articulações frequentemente se encontram intumescidas, mas não deformadas (não erosivas).
• As lesões cutâneas podem ser simétricas ou focais — podem ser observadas alterações como eritema, descamação, ulceração, despigmentação, vesículas e/ou alopecia.
• Ulceração das junções mucocutâneas e da mucosa bucal.
• Febre persistente ou cíclica — especialmente na fase aguda.
• Linfadenopatia.
• Hepatosplenomegalia.
• Dor ou atrofia musculares.
• Sinais neurológicos.

CAUSAS
A causa definitiva não foi identificada. Células-T supressoras podem estar defeituosas em cães com LES.

FATORES DE RISCO
Exposição à luz ultravioleta pode exacerbar as lesões cutâneas.

DIAGNÓSTICO

• Diagnóstico definitivo — teste de ANA ou LE positivo (ou ambos) e dois dos principais sinais ou um dos sinais principais e dois dos menores.
• Diagnóstico provável — teste de ANA ou de células de LE positivo (ou ambos) e um dos sinais principais *ou* dois dos sinais menores.
• Sinais principais — poliartrite, glomerulonefrite, lesões cutâneas, anemia hemolítica, trombocitopenia e polimiosite.
• Sinais menores — febre de origem indeterminada, úlceras bucais, linfadenopatia periférica, pleurite, pericardite, miocardite, sinais neurológicos (crises convulsivas, neuropatia).

DIAGNÓSTICO DIFERENCIAL
• Doenças neoplásicas — podem estar associadas a imunocomplexos circulantes; o paciente pode apresentar sinais semelhantes àqueles do LES.
• É importante excluir doenças infecciosas como erliquiose, leishmaniose e bartonelose, já que o LES é tratado com medicamentos imunossupressores.

HEMOGRAMA/BIOQUÍMICA/URINÁLISE
• Hemograma completo — pode revelar anemia, leucopenia, leucocitose ou trombocitopenia; a anemia pode ser moderada e arregenerativa (p. ex., anemia de doença crônica) ou grave e regenerativa (p. ex., hemolítica).
• Bioquímica — os resultados são amplamente variáveis, dependendo do(s) órgão(s) acometido(s).
• Urinálise — relação de proteína:creatinina elevada (>1) passível de repetição com sedimento benigno e cultura negativa indica proteinúria patológica atribuída à glomerulonefrite.

OUTROS TESTES LABORATORIAIS
• Teste de ANA — detecta anticorpos direcionados contra antígenos nucleares. Podem ser observados resultados falso-positivos em cães e gatos normais, bem como naqueles com doenças infecciosas, inflamatórias ou neoplásicas ou naqueles submetidos a certos medicamentos (p. ex., penicilinas, sulfonamidas, tetraciclinas). Os anticorpos antinucleares são detectados em 10-20% dos cães com sororreatividade para *Bartonella vinsonii*, *Erhlichia canis* e *Leishmania infantum*. Também ocorrem resultados falso-negativos.
• Teste de LE — identifica material nuclear opsonizado dentro dos neutrófilos e macrófagos; o resultado positivo garante o diagnóstico do LES; teste muito demorado.
• Teste da antiglobulina direta (teste de Coombs) — identifica complemento ou anticorpo na superfície das hemácias; esse exame deve ser rodado apenas em pacientes com anemia.

DIAGNÓSTICO POR IMAGEM
• Radiografias das articulações acometidas — revelam tumefação de tecido mole, compatível com artrite não erosiva.
• Radiografias toracoabdominais — podem demonstrar hepato ou esplenomegalia.

MÉTODOS DIAGNÓSTICOS
• Artrocentese — contagem celular elevada, com neutrófilos não degenerados e monócitos, além de baixa viscosidade são achados característicos.
• Cultura bacteriana do líquido sinovial — negativa.
• Hemocultura em animais com febre — negativa.
• Biopsia de pele — em pacientes com lesões cutâneas; colocar a amostra em formalina tamponada a 10% (para exame histopatológico) ou solução de Michel (para teste de imunofluorescência).

ACHADOS PATOLÓGICOS
• Poliartrite não erosiva com infiltração das membranas sinoviais por neutrófilos e linfócitos; sem formação de pano.
• Glomerulonefrite membranosa ou membranoproliferativa.

LÚPUS ERITEMATOSO SISTÊMICO

- Dermatite de interface mononuclear com degeneração hidrópica dos queratinócitos e corpúsculos eosinofílicos arredondados representando queratinócitos basais apoptóticos.
- Vasculite e paniculite em alguns pacientes.
- Imunofluorescência — depósito de imunocomplexos ao longo da membrana basal da junção dermoepidérmica.
- A vasculite pode ser observada em qualquer órgão, especialmente o miocárdio, o pericárdio e as meninges.
- Hiperplasia linfoide reativa nos linfonodos e no baço.

TRATAMENTO

CUIDADO(S) DE SAÚDE ADEQUADO(S)
- Hospitalização — pode ser necessária para o tratamento inicial (p. ex., em paciente com crise hemolítica).
- Tratamento ambulatorial — frequentemente possível.

CUIDADO(S) DE ENFERMAGEM
O cuidado de suporte varia com os sistemas acometidos.

ATIVIDADE
- Repouso forçado — durante os episódios de poliartrite aguda.
- Evitar a exposição à luz solar na suspeita de fotossensibilização.

DIETA
É recomendável a restrição proteica, com o uso de proteína de alta qualidade e suplementação de ácidos graxos ômega-3, nos animais com glomerulonefrite.

ORIENTAÇÃO AO PROPRIETÁRIO
- Discutir a evolução progressiva e imprevisível da doença.
- Abordar a necessidade de tratamento imunossupressor a longo prazo e seus efeitos colaterais.
- Falar sobre a herdabilidade da doença.

CONSIDERAÇÕES CIRÚRGICAS
Nenhuma.

MEDICAÇÕES

MEDICAMENTO(S) DE ESCOLHA
- Corticosteroides — para controlar a resposta imune anormal e reduzir a inflamação; p. ex., prednisona (1-2 mg/kg VO a cada 12 h).
- Medicamentos imunossupressores citotóxicos — ajudam quando a prednisona falha na melhora da condição depois de 7-10 dias ou quando o paciente fica intolerante ao esteroide.
- Azatioprina (cães, 2 mg/kg VO a cada 24 h até a remissão e, depois, em dias alternados).
- Clorambucila (gatos, 0,1-0,2 mg/kg VO a cada 24 h inicialmente e, em seguida, a cada 48 h).
- Reduzir as doses de forma gradativa (não mais do que a cada 3-4 semanas) assim que a remissão for atingida.

PRECAUÇÕES
- Os gatos são suscetíveis à intoxicação pela azatioprina; por essa razão, o uso desse medicamento não é recomendado para essa espécie.
- A azatioprina e a clorambucila podem causar mielossupressão.
- O tratamento com medicamentos imunossupressores pode aumentar o risco de infecções graves.

INTERAÇÕES POSSÍVEIS
O uso concomitante de ácido acetilsalicílico e da prednisona aumenta o risco de ulceração gastrintestinal.

MEDICAMENTO(S) ALTERNATIVO(S)
- Ciclosporina — microemulsão, p. ex., Atopica® — cães, 5-10 mg/kg/dia VO divididos em 2 vezes ao dia; gatos, 0,5-3 mg/kg a cada 12 h — pode ser tentada em pacientes refratários; utilizar com cuidado e suspender mediante a ocorrência de efeitos colaterais (p. ex., gastrite, dermatite linfocitoide, papilomatose, hiperplasia gengival). É recomendada a mensuração da concentração de vale da ciclosporina.
- Ciclofosfamida (cães, 50 mg/m² VO por 4 dias consecutivos e, depois, 3 dias sem o medicamento; repetir semanalmente).
- A ciclofosfamida pode induzir à cistite hemorrágica e mielossupressão.
- Levamisol (cães, 2-5 mg/kg VO em dias alternados por 4 meses [150 mg por paciente, no máximo]) combinado com prednisona (0,5-1,0 mg/kg a cada 12 h). A prednisona é reduzida de forma gradual em 1-2 meses, enquanto o levamisol é mantido por 4 meses.

ACOMPANHAMENTO

MONITORIZAÇÃO DO PACIENTE
- Exame físico — semanal.
- Hemograma completo e análise bioquímica — para monitorar os efeitos colaterais dos medicamentos imunossupressores; no dia 7 e, em seguida, a cada 2-4 semanas.
- ANA — frequentemente permanece elevado durante a remissão, mas pode declinar à medida que o paciente apresenta melhora clínica.

PREVENÇÃO
Não acasalar os animais acometidos.

COMPLICAÇÕES POSSÍVEIS
- Insuficiência renal e síndrome nefrótica secundárias à glomerulonefrite.
- Broncopneumonia, infecção do trato urinário ou sepse secundárias à imunossupressão.

EVOLUÇÃO ESPERADA E PROGNÓSTICO
O prognóstico é reservado. A presença da anemia hemolítica e da glomerulonefrite, bem como o desenvolvimento de infecção bacteriana, justificam um prognóstico mau.

DIVERSOS

POTENCIAL ZOONÓTICO
N/D.

GESTAÇÃO/FERTILIDADE/REPRODUÇÃO
O uso de medicamentos imunossupressores citotóxicos nos animais prenhes está contraindicado.

VER TAMBÉM
- Anemia Imunomediada.
- Glomerulonefrite.
- Poliartrite Imunomediada Não Erosiva.
- Trombocitopenia Imunomediada Primária.

ABREVIATURA(S)
- ANA = anticorpo antinuclear.
- LE = lúpus eritematoso.
- LES = lúpus eritematoso sistêmico.

RECURSOS DA INTERNET
www.vin.com

Sugestões de Leitura
Bryden SL, White SD, Dunstone SM, Burrows AK, Olivry T. Clinical, histopathological, and immunological characteristics of exfoliative cutaneous lupus erythematosus in 25 German short-haired pointers. Vet Dermatol 2005, 16:239-252.
Chabanne L, Fournel C, Monier JC, Rigal D. Canine systemic lupus erythematosus: Part 1: Clinical and biologic aspects. Compend Contin Educ Pract Vet 1999, 21:135-141.
Chabanne L, Fournel C, Rigal D, Monier JC. Canine systemic lupus erythematosus: Part 2: Diagnosis and treatment. Compendium 1999, 21:402-421.
Smee NM, Harkin KR, Wilkerson MJ. Measurement of serum antinuclear antibody titer in dogs with and without systemic lupus erythematosus. JAVMA 2007, 230:1180-1183.
Smith BE, Tompkins MB, Breitschwerdt EB. Antinuclear antibodies can be detected in dog sera reactive to *Bartonella vinsonii* subsp. *Berkhoffii*, *Ehrlichia canis*, or *Leishmania infantum* antigens. J Vet Intern Med 2004, 18:47-51.
Tizard IR. Veterinary immunology: An introduction. Philadelphia: Saunders, 2000.

Autores J. Catharine Scott-Moncrieff e Mary F. Thompson
Consultor Editorial A.H. Rebar

Luxação do Cristalino

CONSIDERAÇÕES GERAIS

REVISÃO
• Deslocamento total do cristalino a partir de sua posição normal.
• Anterior — para a frente por meio da pupila em direção à câmara anterior.
• Posterior — em direção ao segmento posterior/câmara vítrea.
• Ocorre quando a cápsula do cristalino se separa a 360° das zônulas que mantêm o cristalino no lugar.
• Subluxação — separação parcial do cristalino de suas inserções zonulares; o cristalino permanece na posição normal ou quase normal na pupila.
• Luxação primária — atribuída à alteração patológica nas zônulas ciliares, incluindo o desenvolvimento anormal ou degeneração; geralmente hereditária nos cães; quase sempre bilateral.
• Luxação congênita — frequentemente associada à microfaquia (cristalino pequeno).
• Luxação secundária — causada por ruptura ou degeneração das zônulas ciliares como resultado de inflamação crônica, buftalmia (aumento de volume do globo ocular) ou neoplasia intraocular.

IDENTIFICAÇÃO
• Cães — costuma ser observada principalmente nos adultos (sobretudo daqueles de 4-9 anos de idade); raças caninas mais comumente acometidas: raças puras e mestiças de Terrier, Terrier tibetano, Border collie, Pastor alemão e alguns cães da raça Spaniel.
• Também pode ocorrer em animais idosos de raças predispostas, presumivelmente como uma condição de início tardio.
• Cães e gatos — secundária; qualquer idade/raça.

SINAIS CLÍNICOS
• Dor ocular aguda ou crônica, com congestão episcleral e edema corneano difuso, especialmente na presença de glaucoma ou em caso de luxação anterior.
• Edema corneano central — causado pelo contato do cristalino com o endotélio, resultando na ruptura mecânica das células endoteliais.
• Câmara anterior anormalmente rasa ou profunda.
• Iridodonese (tremor ou movimento anormal da íris); facodonese (tremor ou movimento anormal do cristalino).
• Crescente afáquico (área da pupila desprovida de cristalino).
• Cristalino claro malposicionado — observado, às vezes, em olho normalmente assintomático.

CAUSAS E FATORES DE RISCO
• Primário — padrão de herança incerto.
• Luxação primária e glaucoma primário — podem ocorrer simultaneamente em algumas raças (ver a seção "Identificação").
• Uveíte, sobretudo uveíte crônica induzida pelo cristalino.
• Neoplasia intraocular — pode luxar fisicamente o cristalino ou causar inflamação crônica, levando à degeneração zonular.
• Traumatismo — raras vezes, faz com que o cristalino normal sofra luxação sem sinais de uveíte grave ou hifema.

DIAGNÓSTICO

DIAGNÓSTICO DIFERENCIAL
• Uveíte, glaucoma e episclerocerattite granulomatosa nodular — também provocam dor e vermelhidão nos olhos, com edema corneano, e podem ser concomitantes.
• Buftalmia pode provocar luxação do cristalino; geralmente diferenciada da luxação primária do cristalino por meio da anamnese.
• Distrofia ou degeneração endotelial corneana — também podem causar edema de córnea, tornando difícil a observação das estruturas intraoculares; em geral, são diferenciadas da luxação primária do cristalino por meio da anamnese.
• Diagnóstico formulado com base no exame físico minucioso e na anamnese detalhada.

HEMOGRAMA/BIOQUÍMICA/URINÁLISE
Normais a menos que a luxação do cristalino seja uma sequela de alguma doença sistêmica indutora de uveíte ou disseminação de neoplasia.

DIAGNÓSTICO POR IMAGEM
• Radiografias torácicas e ultrassonografia abdominal — podem ser indicadas se a luxação for secundária à neoplasia intraocular.
• Ultrassonografia ocular — ferramenta valiosa se o edema corneano ou os meios oculares turvos impedirem o exame e a anamnese.
• Ultrassonografia de alta resolução ou biomicroscopia por ultrassom — exame *in vivo* dos 4-5 mm anteriores do globo ocular, o qual inclui resolução microscópica de todo o segmento anterior, da retina periférica e de alguns anexos.

MÉTODOS DIAGNÓSTICOS
• Exame oftalmológico completo, incluindo a tonometria.
• Para algumas raças predispostas à luxação do cristalino, existe um novo teste de DNA disponível.

TRATAMENTO

• Olhos com potencial de visão — mais bem tratados, removendo-se o cristalino com ou sem aplicação de prótese de lente intraocular no sulco ciliar. • Muitas vezes, o tratamento miótico tópico pode manter o cristalino que sofreu luxação posterior atrás da pupila, podendo adiar ou até mesmo evitar a cirurgia em alguns casos. • Olhos com cegueira irreversível podem ser tratados por meio de enucleação ou evisceração com prótese intraescleral; se secundários à neoplasia, o procedimento de enucleação será a melhor escolha para fins terapêuticos e diagnósticos.

MEDICAÇÕES

MEDICAMENTO(S)
• Iniciar os medicamentos expostos a seguir e, se o olho apresentar potencial para visão, encaminhar o paciente imediatamente a algum oftalmologista veterinário para extração intracapsular do cristalino. • Miótico tópico — análogo da prostaglandina (Xalatan®, Lumigan®, Travatan®) a cada 12 h; indicado em casos de luxação posterior ou subluxação primária; esse medicamento também reduzirá a PIO; diminui a possibilidade de glaucoma e luxação anterior. • Se a pupila for obstruída por luxação anterior do cristalino, a tropicamida pode fazer com que a pupila se dilate, liberando o cristalino e aliviando a obstrução pupilar causada pelo glaucoma; utilizar com cuidado. • Manitol — 1 g/kg IV por mais de 20 min; indicado para PIO elevada (>40 mmHg). • Inibidores da anidrase carbônica — metazolamida (2-4 mg/kg VO a cada 12 h); instituídos para reduzir a produção aquosa. • Anti-inflamatório tópico — fosfato sódico de dexametasona a 0,1% ou acetato de prednisolona a 1% (a cada 6 h).

CONTRAINDICAÇÕES/INTERAÇÕES POSSÍVEIS
• Mióticos tópicos — contraindicados se o cristalino estiver na câmara anterior. • O proprietário deve verificar a localização do cristalino antes de aplicar o miótico.

ACOMPANHAMENTO

• Luxação posterior primária submetida a tratamento clínico — a PIO deve ser verificada 24 h após o início do tratamento e com maior frequência daí em diante; assim que a PIO estiver estabilizada, examinar novamente o paciente por, no mínimo, a cada 3 meses; encaminhar para avaliação. • Monitorizar o animal quanto à ocorrência de glaucoma secundário e descolamento da retina. • Um estudo recente constatou um risco semelhante de glaucoma secundário ao se comparar a extração intracapsular do cristalino e o uso de brometo de demecário para manter o cristalino atrás da íris; nesse estudo, o tempo até a perda da visão também foi semelhante. • Se apenas um cristalino estiver envolvido no momento do exame, o outro cristalino também poderá vir a ser acometido; o oftalmologista pode optar pela extração extracapsular do cristalino por meio de facoemulsificação com colocação de lente intraocular no olho contralateral se ele ainda não estiver luxado.

DIVERSOS

ABREVIATURA(S)
• PIO = pressão intraocular.

Sugestões de Leitura
Binder DR, Herring IP, Gerhard T. Outcomes of nonsurgical management and efficacy of demecarium bromide treatment for primary lens instability in dogs: 34 cases (1990-2004). JAVMA 2007, 231(1):89-93.
Davidson MG, Nelms SR. Diseases of the canine lens and cataract formation. In: Gelatt KN, ed., Veterinary Ophthalmology, 4th ed., volume 2. Ames: Blackwell Publishing, 2007, pp. 859-887.
Nasisse MP, Glover TL. Surgery for lens instability. Vet Clin North Am Small Anim Pract 1997, 27:1175-1192.

Autor Carmen M.H. Colitz
Consultor Editorial Paul E. Miller

Luxação ou Avulsão dos Dentes

CONSIDERAÇÕES GERAIS

REVISÃO
- A luxação dentária pode ser vertical (i. e., intrusão ou extrusão) ou lateral.
- A intrusão ocorre quando o dente é tracionado no sentido apical para dentro do osso alveolar.
- A extrusão ocorre quando o dente é deslocado no sentido vertical, parcialmente para fora do alvéolo.
- Luxação lateral — o dente acometido está inclinado no sentido labial ou palatal/lingual; pode ocorrer quando um traumatismo traciona a coroa em uma direção e a raiz, na direção oposta; sempre associada à fratura da placa óssea alveolar lingual ou labial, o que confere a luxação do dente, em vez da fratura.
- Avulsão — um dente avulsionado sofreu uma luxação total a partir de seu alvéolo.

IDENTIFICAÇÃO
Cães e gatos.

SINAIS CLÍNICOS
- Intrusão — o dente parece mais curto do que o normal; não se detecta nenhuma mobilidade dentária.
- Extrusão — o dente parece mais longo do que o normal e apresenta mobilidade tanto no sentido vertical como no horizontal.
- Luxação lateral — a coroa do dente é deslocada em uma direção labial ou palatal/lingual.
- Avulsão — o dente intacto encontra-se totalmente deslocado a partir de seu alvéolo.

CAUSAS E FATORES DE RISCO
- Luxação/avulsão — costuma resultar de algum incidente traumático (p. ex., acidente automobilístico ou briga entre cães).
- O traumatismo provoca lesões periodontais, conferindo dessa forma mobilidade anormal e malposicionamento do dente.
- O dente canino superior é o mais comumente luxado/avulsionado.
- A periodontite avançada constitui fator predisponente.

DIAGNÓSTICO

DIAGNÓSTICO DIFERENCIAL
- Luxação — fratura da raiz, onde o segmento coronário é deslocado.
- Avulsão — perda de dentes, decorrente de periodontite grave.

HEMOGRAMA/BIOQUÍMICA/URINÁLISE
Sem contribuições diagnósticas.

OUTROS TESTES LABORATORIAIS
N/D.

DIAGNÓSTICO POR IMAGEM
Comentários Gerais
- As radiografias são indispensáveis.
- É imprescindível o emprego de técnicas radiográficas intrabucais e filmes radiográficos dentários.

Achados Radiográficos
- Intrusão — estreitamento do espaço do ligamento periodontal na região apical.
- Extrusão — alargamento do ligamento periodontal, especialmente na porção apical.
- Luxação lateral — alargamento e estreitamento do espaço do ligamento periodontal e fratura da placa óssea alveolar.
- Avulsão — alvéolo vazio, mas intacto.

TRATAMENTO

- Reposicionar e fixar o dente em sua posição normal; imobilizar com fios acrílicos e fios de aço — um método eficaz de se obter a estabilização e o alinhamento oclusal.
- Manipular o dente avulsionado apenas pela sua coroa e irrigá-lo delicadamente com solução salina estéril; se estiver gravemente contaminada, a raiz do dente poderá ser submetida à suave limpeza com *swabs* de gazes estéreis umedecidos com solução salina.
- É preciso manipular o dente com delicadeza e o mínimo possível; é essencial não remover o ligamento periodontal da raiz, pois há necessidade da viabilidade desse ligamento para a consolidação.
- Reposicionar o dente em seu alvéolo ósseo; em geral, não é necessário remover os coágulos sanguíneos do alvéolo; o dente é apenas posicionado firmemente em seu alvéolo ósseo e fixado nessa posição.
- As contraindicações para o reposicionamento de um dente luxado ou avulsionado são: dentes decíduos, periodontite grave, cáries ou lesões reabsortivas.
- Os dois fatores mais importantes na determinação do resultado terapêutico correspondem ao tempo de permanência do dente avulsionado fora de seu alvéolo ósseo e ao meio de armazenagem do dente durante esse período.
- Quanto mais cedo o dente avulsionado for reimplantado, melhor será o prognóstico; resultados mais favoráveis serão obtidos se o dente for reimplantado dentro de 30 min após a avulsão; não deixar o dente avulsionado secar antes do reimplante; o melhor meio para armazenar um dente avulsionado é a solução salina; caso essa solução não esteja disponível, recorrer ao leite.
- Orientar os proprietários a colocar o dente na solução salina ou no leite e levar o animal acometido o mais rápido possível ao consultório.
- O aparelho de fixação costuma ser deixado no local por 4-6 semanas; deve-se manter a higiene bucal durante esse período; emprega-se um aparelho de jato de água do tipo Water Pick® ou uma seringa de extremidade curva para remover os debris presentes entre a imobilização, os dentes e os tecidos moles; o enxágue da cavidade bucal com solução de clorexidina também é útil.
- As imobilizações são removidas com o auxílio de alicates ou brocas de alta rotação; nesse momento, o dente deverá se apresentar estável ou com pouquíssima mobilidade; obter radiografias; se o dente ainda estiver frouxo, houve falha do reimplante e o dente deverá ser extraído.

MEDICAÇÕES

MEDICAMENTO(S)
- Recomenda-se o uso de antibiótico bactericida de amplo espectro; o tempo de administração será breve se a higiene bucal for mantida.
- Caso não seja possível a aplicação de medidas de higiene bucal, os antibióticos poderão ser indicados durante todo o período de imobilização.
- O enxágue bucal diário com uma solução de gliconato de clorexidina a 0,12% diminuirá a necessidade de antibioticoterapia prolongada.

CONTRAINDICAÇÕES/INTERAÇÕES POSSÍVEIS
Nenhuma.

ACOMPANHAMENTO

- Um dente avulsionado invariavelmente desenvolve necrose pulpar; o dente deve ser submetido ao tratamento endodôntico para evitar o comprometimento periapical.
- É melhor efetuar a terapia endodôntica ao se remover a imobilização.
- É comum ocorrer reabsorção radicular externa e anquilose após o reimplante.
- Os dentes luxados frequentemente sofrem necrose pulpar; por essa razão, é preciso avaliá-los em intervalos regulares.
- Os sinais de acometimento pulpar (p. ex., manchas nos dentes ou indícios radiográficos de comprometimento periapical) são indicações para o tratamento endodôntico.

DIVERSOS

Sugestões de Leitura
Gorrel C. Emergencies. In: Veterinary Dentistry for the General Practitioner. Philadelphia: Saunders, 2004, pp. 131-155.
Gorrel C, Robinson J. Endodontic therapy. In: Crossley DA, Penman S, eds., Manual of Small Animal Dentistry. Gloucestershire, UK: BSAVA, 1995, pp. 168-181.

Autor Cecilia Gorrel
Consultor Editorial Heidi B. Lobprise

Luxação Patelar

CONSIDERAÇÕES GERAIS

DEFINIÇÃO
Deslocamento medial ou lateral da patela a partir de sua posição anatômica normal na tróclea femoral.

FISIOPATOLOGIA
• Pode ser leve a grave; diferentes graus de alterações clínicas e patológicas; classificada em graus de I-IV.
• Alterações musculoesqueléticas comuns — rotação da tíbia sobre seu eixo longitudinal; encurvamento das porções distal do fêmur e proximal da tíbia; tróclea femoral rasa ou ausente; displasia das epífises femoral e tibial; deslocamento do grupo muscular do quadríceps.

SISTEMA(S) ACOMETIDO(S)
Musculoesquelético.

GENÉTICA
• São propostas heranças recessiva, poligênica e multifocal.
• Fator hereditário em gatos da raça Devon rex.

INCIDÊNCIA/PREVALÊNCIA
• Uma das anormalidades mais comuns da articulação do joelho nos cães.
• Medial — >75% dos casos (cães de pequeno e grande porte, além de gatos).
• Envolvimento bilateral — 50% dos casos.
• Rara nos gatos, embora possa ser mais comum do que se suspeita, porque a maioria dos gatos acometidos não exibe claudicação.

IDENTIFICAÇÃO
Espécies
• Predominantemente cães.
• Raras vezes em gatos.

Raça(s) Predominante(s)
• Mais comum nas raças caninas miniatura e toy.
• Cães — raças Poodle toy e miniatura; Yorkshire terrier; Pomerânia; Pequinês; Chihuahua; Boston terrier.

Idade Média e Faixa Etária
Sinais clínicos — podem se desenvolver logo após o nascimento; em geral, depois dos 4 meses de vida.

Sexo Predominante
O risco para as fêmeas é uma vez e meia maior do que os machos.

SINAIS CLÍNICOS
Comentários Gerais
A manifestação clínica depende do grau (gravidade), da quantidade de artrite degenerativa, da cronicidade da doença e da ocorrência de outras anormalidades da articulação do joelho (p. ex., ruptura do ligamento cruzado).

Achados Anamnésicos
• Sustentação e função do membro posterior persistentes anormais nos neonatos e nos filhotes caninos.
• Pulos ocasionais ou claudicação intermitente do membro posterior — piora nos cães jovens a maduros.
• Sinais repentinos de claudicação — atribuídos a traumas menores ou ao agravamento da artropatia degenerativa nos animais maduros.

Achados do Exame Físico
• Grau I — a patela pode ser deslocada manualmente a partir da tróclea, mas retorna imediatamente à posição normal quando a pressão é liberada.
• Grau II — a patela pode ser deslocada manualmente ou sofrer luxação espontânea com a flexão da articulação do joelho; a patela permanece luxada até que seja manualmente reduzida ou até que o paciente estenda a articulação do joelho.
• Grau II — o paciente sustenta o membro acometido de forma intermitente com a articulação do joelho flexionada.
• Grau III — a patela permanece luxada a maior parte do tempo, mas pode ser reduzida manualmente com a articulação do joelho em extensão; o movimento dessa articulação resulta em nova luxação da patela.
• Grau IV — a patela fica permanentemente luxada, sendo impossível sua reposição manual; pode haver rotação de até 90° do platô tibial proximal; tróclea femoral rasa ou ausente.
• Graus III e IV — agachamento, além de postura com encurvamento de membro (joelho varo) ou fechado de frente (joelho valgo) para as luxações medial ou lateral, respectivamente; a maior parte do peso corporal é transferida para os membros anteriores.
• Dor — ocorre conforme a patela muda de posição ou se a abrasão tiver contato com osso exposto.

CAUSAS
• Congênita.
• Traumática.

FATORES DE RISCO
• Joelho varo — deslocamento lateral da porção proximal do fêmur; o músculo vasto medial traciona a patela no sentido medial.

DIAGNÓSTICO

DIAGNÓSTICO DIFERENCIAL
• Ruptura do ligamento cruzado cranial — movimento de gaveta cranial positivo; concomitante em 15-20% dos casos.
• Fratura por avulsão da tuberosidade tibial — patela alta.
• Ruptura do tendão patelar — patela alta.
• Má união e mau alinhamento de fraturas do fêmur ou da tíbia — podem resultar no deslocamento do grupo muscular do quadríceps.

DIAGNÓSTICO POR IMAGEM
• Radiografias craniocaudal e mesolateral da articulação do joelho — indicadas para todas as luxações de graus III e IV; incluem a articulação do quadril e do jarrete para detectar encurvamento e/ou torção do fêmur e da tíbia.
• Radiografias tangenciais (tipo *skyline*) da tróclea femoral — ajudam a determinar sua forma (rasa, achatada ou convexa).

MÉTODOS DIAGNÓSTICOS
• Artrocentese e análise do líquido sinovial — leve aumento nas células mononucleares (geralmente <2.000 células/mL).
• Palpação do grau de liberdade da patela — paciente acordado ou sedado se necessário.

ACHADOS PATOLÓGICOS
• Macroscópicos — lesões por desgaste da cartilagem da patela e da tróclea femoral; redundância da cápsula articular no lado oposto da luxação; fibrose e contratura no lado da luxação.
• Microscópicos — fibrilação da cartilagem e perda do conteúdo de glicosaminoglicanos; sinovite.

TRATAMENTO

CUIDADO(S) DE SAÚDE ADEQUADO(S)
• Paciente de ambulatório — todas as luxações de grau I e algumas de grau II.
• Paciente internado (cirurgia) — a maior parte das luxações de grau II e todas as luxações de graus III e IV.

CUIDADO(S) DE ENFERMAGEM
• Crioterapia (bolsas ou compressas de gelo) — iniciada imediatamente após a cirurgia; 15-20 min a cada 8 h por 3-5 dias.
• Exercícios passivos com amplitude de movimento do joelho — assim que forem tolerados pelo animal.

ATIVIDADE
Normal a restrita, dependendo da gravidade.

DIETA
Controle do peso — diminui a carga e o estresse (tensão) sobre o mecanismo de sustentação da patela.

ORIENTAÇÃO AO PROPRIETÁRIO
• Discutir sobre a herdabilidade da condição.
• Avisar o proprietário sobre o potencial de recidiva após a cirurgia.
• Informar o proprietário sobre o alto risco de doença do ligamento cruzado cranial.
• Alertar o proprietário sobre o fato de que a condição pode piorar com o tempo (p. ex., passar de grau I para grau II).

CONSIDERAÇÕES CIRÚRGICAS
• O mau alinhamento é a causa subjacente — transposição da crista tibial constitui o procedimento definitivo de realinhamento.
• A tensão do retináculo e da cápsula articular no lado da luxação impede o realinhamento — é essencial a realização de capsulotomia medial para liberação.
• A superficialidade do sulco troclear é avaliada e tratada com um dos procedimentos cirúrgicos a seguir:
• Trocleoplastia — uso de raspagem ou broca para aprofundar o sulco troclear.
• Condroplastia troclear — consiste na elevação da cartilagem hialina de superfície e na curetagem do osso esponjoso para aprofundar o sulco; em seguida, procede-se à colocação da cartilagem de volta sobre o osso exposto, apenas nos cães muito jovens.
• Sulcoplastia de recessão — consiste na remoção de uma cunha em forma de V, no aprofundamento do defeito e, depois, na recolocação da cunha; técnica preferida para a maior parte dos pacientes, pois a cartilagem de superfície basicamente permanece intacta.
• Sulcoplastia de recessão em bloco — consiste na remoção de um bloco em vez de uma cunha; essa técnica aumenta a área de superfície da cartilagem em contato com a patela.

- Transposição da tuberosidade tibial — realinha o eixo longitudinal do mecanismo do quadríceps, de forma que ele fique centralizado sobre a tróclea femoral; osteotomiza a tuberosidade tibial, deixando-a aderida distalmente; em seguida, transpõe-na em direção oposta à luxação e a estabiliza com pinos de Kirschner e, em cães de grande porte, com fio ortopédico em banda de tensão.
- Imbricação da cápsula articular e dos tecidos moles de sustentação do lado oposto da luxação — para ajudar a manter a patela no sulco.
- Osteotomias corretivas das porções distais do fêmur e proximal da tíbia — realinham o eixo longitudinal do membro posterior; indicadas, em geral, apenas nas luxações de grau IV com encurvamento e torção significativos.

MEDICAÇÕES

MEDICAMENTO(S) DE ESCOLHA
- AINE — minimizam a dor; diminuem a inflamação; meloxicam (dose de ataque de 0,2 mg/kg VO e, depois, 0,1 mg/kg diariamente VO — na fórmula líquida), carprofeno (2,2 mg/kg VO a cada 12 h), etodolaco (10-15 mg/kg VO uma vez ao dia), deracoxibe (3-4 mg/kg VO uma vez ao dia — mastigável) por 7 dias (para dor pós-operatória).

CONTRAINDICAÇÕES
Evitar os corticosteroides por causa dos efeitos colaterais potenciais e do dano à cartilagem articular associados à utilização a longo prazo.

PRECAUÇÕES
AINE — irritação gastrintestinal pode impedir seu uso.

MEDICAMENTO(S) ALTERNATIVO(S)
Medicamentos condroprotetores (p. ex., glicosaminoglicanos polissulfatados, glicosamina e sulfato de condroitina) — podem ajudar a limitar o dano e a degeneração da cartilagem.

ACOMPANHAMENTO

MONITORIZAÇÃO DO PACIENTE
- Após a trocleoplastia — estimular a utilização precoce e ativa do membro.
- Limitar o exercício a passeios de coleira por 4 semanas; evitar saltos.
- Exames anuais — para avaliar a evolução.

PREVENÇÃO
- Desestimular o acasalamento dos animais acometidos.
- Não repetir acasalamentos entre machos e fêmeas que resultem em ninhada acometida.

COMPLICAÇÕES POSSÍVEIS
Recidiva após a estabilização cirúrgica — há relatos de que ela chegue até 48%; geralmente de grau mais baixo do que a luxação original.

EVOLUÇÃO ESPERADA E PROGNÓSTICO
- Com tratamento cirúrgico — >90% dos pacientes ficam livres de claudicação e da disfunção clínica.
- Artropatia degenerativa — evidência radiográfica em quase todas as articulações acometidas do joelho após a cirurgia. O impacto clínico parece mínimo em cães de pequeno porte.

DIVERSOS

DISTÚRBIOS ASSOCIADOS
Doença do ligamento cruzado cranial.

VER TAMBÉM
Artrite (osteoartrite).

ABREVIATURA(S)
- AINE = anti-inflamatórios não esteroides.

Sugestões de leitura

Arnoczky S, Tarvin G. Surgical repair of patella luxations and fractures. In: Bojrab MJ, ed., Current Techniques in Small Animal Surgery, 4th ed. Philadelphia: Lea & Febiger, 1998, pp. 1237-1244.

Brinker WO, Piermattei DL, Flo GL. Patellar luxations. In: Brinker WO, Piermattei DL, Flo GL, eds., Handbook of Small Animal Orthopedics and Fracture Repair, 3rd ed. Philadelphia: Saunders, 1997, pp. 516-534.

Harasen G. Patellar luxation: Pathogenesis and surgical correction. Can Vet J 2006, 47(10):1037-1039.

Hayes AG, Boudrieau RJ, Hungerford LL. Frequency and distribution of medial and lateral patellar luxation in dogs: 124 cases (1982-1992). JAVMA 1994, 205(5): 716-720.

Hulse DA. Medial patellar luxation in the dog. In Bojrab MJ, ed., Disease Mechanisms in Small Animal Surgery, 2nd ed. Philadelphia: Lea & Febiger, 1993, pp. 808-817.

Johnson AL, Broaddus KD, Hauptman JG, Marsh S, Monsere J, Sepulveda G. Vertical patellar position in large-breed dogs with clinically normal stifles and large-breed dogs with medial patellar luxation. Vet Surg 2006, 35(1):78-81.

Johnson AL, Probst CW, Decamp CE, et al. Comparison of trochlear block recession and trochlear wedge recession for canine patellar luxation using a cadaver model. Vet Surg 2001, 30:140-150.

Johnson ME. Feline patellar luxation: A retrospective case study. JAAHA 1986, 22:835-838.

Kaiser S, Cornely D, Golder W, Garner MT, Wolf KJ, Waibl H, Brunnberg L. The correlation of canine patellar luxation and the anteversion angle as measured using magnetic resonance images. Vet Radiol Ultrasound 2001, 42(2):113-118.

L'Eplattenier H, Montavon P. Patellar luxation in dogs and cats: Management and prevention. Compend Contin Educ Pract Vet 2002, 24:292-298.

———Patellar luxation in dogs and cats: Pathogenesis and diagnosis. Compend Contin Educ Pract Vet 2002, 24:234-239.

Moore JA, Banks WJ. Repair of full thickness defects in the femoral trochlea of dogs after trochlear arthroplasty. Am J Vet Res 1989, 50(8):1406-1413.

Olmstead ML. Lateral luxation of the patella. In Bojrab MJ, ed., Disease Mechanisms in Small Animal Surgery, 2nd ed. Philadelphia: Lea & Febiger, 1993, pp. 818-820.

Remedios AM, Basher AW, Runyon CL, et al. Medial patellar luxation in 16 large breed dogs: A retrospective study. Vet Surg 1992, 21(1):5-9.

Roush JK. Canine patellar luxation. Vet Clin North Am 1993, 23:855-875.

Roy RG, Wallace LJ, Johnston GR, et al. A restrospective evaluation of stifle osteoarthritis in dogs with bilateral medial patellar luxation and unilateral surgical repair. Vet Surg 1992, 21(6):475-479.

Slocum B, Slocum TD. Patella luxation. In: Bojrab MJ, ed., Current Techniques in Small Animal Surgery, 4th ed. Philadelphia: Lea & Febiger, 1998, pp. 1222-1236.

Talcott KW, Goring RL, de Haan JJ. Rectangular recession trochleoplasty for treatment of patellar luxation in dogs and cats. Vet Comp Orthop Traumatol 2000, 13:39-43.

Towle HA, Griffon DJ, Thomas MW, Siegel AM, Dunning D, Johnson A. Pre- and postoperative radiographic and computed tomographic evaluation of dogs with medial patellar luxation. Vet Surg 2005, 34(3):265-272.

Wander KW, Powers BE, Schwarz PD. Cartilage changes in dogs with surgically treated medial patellar luxations. Vet Comp Orthop Traumatol 1999, 12:183-187.

Willauer C, Vasseur P. Clinical results of surgical correction of medial luxation of the patella in dogs. Vet Surg 1987, 16:31-36.

Autor Peter K. Shires
Consultor Editorial Peter K. Shires
Agradecimento O autor e os editores agradecem a contribuição de Peter D. Schwarz, que foi o autor deste capítulo em uma edição mais antiga.

Luxações Articulares

CONSIDERAÇÕES GERAIS

DEFINIÇÃO
A luxação trata-se de uma ruptura completa das superfícies articulares contíguas de uma articulação quando as estruturas de sustentação em torno da articulação estão lesionadas ou ausentes. A subluxação é uma ruptura parcial.

FISIOPATOLOGIA
• Todas as articulações sinoviais possuem uma cápsula articular que une os ossos que se articulam. A camada fibrosa dessa cápsula é um estabilizador importante da articulação. A maioria das articulações possui ligamentos adicionais que reforçam a cápsula articular para aumentar a resistência ao movimento fora da amplitude normal de movimento dessa articulação. Todas as articulações de movimento também têm um sistema de músculos e tendões que exercem forças sobre a articulação para controlar o movimento. As forças de cocontração em torno de uma articulação exercem muita influência sobre a estabilidade dessa articulação. A instabilidade ocorre quando o sistema de estabilização é lesionado ou rompido ou não se desenvolve normalmente.
• Se a frouxidão for clinicamente aparente, então o problema costuma ser descrito como luxação ou subluxação dessa articulação.
• Pode ocorrer luxação como resultado de forças traumáticas que fazem com que a articulação se mova além dos limites elásticos dos tecidos de sustentação.
• As alterações secundárias são postas em movimento pelo dano aos tecidos que gera inicialmente e, depois, mais tarde, um dano articular mais crônico.

SISTEMA(S) ACOMETIDO(S)
• Musculosquelético — principalmente o ambiente intra-articular e as estruturas de sustentação em torno da articulação, incluindo a cápsula articular, os ligamentos colaterais e as unidades musculotendíneas de sustentação.
• Neurológico — o *feedback* neurológico e a inervação para o sistema de sustentação também podem ser acometidos.

GENÉTICA
• A síndrome de hiperfrouxidão é um fator hereditário em seres humanos. Os filhotes caninos podem exibir hiperfrouxidão temporária quando confinados.
• A displasia coxofemoral é uma forma de frouxidão hereditária da articulação do coxal.
• A luxação do ombro é uma predisposição hereditária em raças de pequeno porte, como Poodles miniaturas.
• A instabilidade femoropatelar que leva à luxação medial da patela é uma doença hereditária comum em raças caninas de pequeno porte.
• A síndrome de Ehlers-Danlos é um distúrbio congênito do colágeno que induz à frouxidão articular.

INCIDÊNCIA/PREVALÊNCIA
Algumas formas de frouxidão/luxação (displasia coxofemoral e luxação patelar medial) são muito comuns.

DISTRIBUIÇÃO GEOGRÁFICA
Não observada.

IDENTIFICAÇÃO
Raça(s) Predominante(s)
• Varia com a articulação acometida.
• Articulação do coxal — as raças de grande porte exibem sinais clínicos de displasia coxofemoral com maior frequência que aquelas de porte menor, mas raças de todos os portes podem ter sinais radiográficos.
• Luxações traumáticas não são específicas à raça em qualquer articulação.
• É mais comum a ocorrência de luxação congênita do cotovelo em raças miniaturas (Poodles).
• A luxação femorotibiopatelar envolve mais comumente a ruptura de ambos os ligamentos cruzados e um dos ligamentos colaterais.
• A luxação medial da patela é mais usual em cães de pequeno porte.
• As luxações espinais ocorrem como resultado de traumatismo, com lesão associada à medula espinal.

Idade Média e Faixa Etária
• Traumáticas — qualquer idade.
• Frouxidão/luxação congênita — tipicamente observada no cão jovem, com futura manifestação de artropatia degenerativa secundária.

Sexo Predominante
Nenhum.

SINAIS CLÍNICOS
• Posição anatômica anormal de um osso em relação ao osso adjacente.
• A luxação coxofemoral é comumente craniodorsal (deslocamento da cabeça do fêmur em relação ao acetábulo).
• Usualmente, a luxação do ombro é medial.
• É comum que a luxação do cotovelo seja próximo-lateral.
• As luxações do carpo e do tarso costumam resultar em varo, valgo ou hiperextensão quando tensionadas (ou seja, submetidas a estresse).
• Em casos de luxação aguda, comumente se observam inchaço imediato, dor e não utilização do membro. Pode ocorrer a sustentação parcial do peso com luxação crônica ou subluxação.

CAUSAS
• Deslocamento traumático de tecidos normais além de seus limites elásticos.
• Estresse mínimo sobre articulações anormalmente instáveis de etiologia congênita.

FATORES DE RISCO
• Conformação anormal, que provoca aumento da tensão (estresse) sobre a articulação
• Fadiga, que causa fraqueza muscular e incoordenação
• Anormalidades neurológicas
• Acesso a veículos em movimento

DIAGNÓSTICO

DIAGNÓSTICO DIFERENCIAL
• Fraturas.
• Artropatia — imunomediada, séptica ou degenerativa.

HEMOGRAMA/BIOQUÍMICA/URINÁLISE
• Não se esperam anormalidades que estejam diretamente relacionadas com a luxação.
• Alterações induzidas por traumatismo em situações traumáticas.

OUTROS TESTES LABORATORIAIS
Artrocentese pode eliminar a artropatia não traumática.

DIAGNÓSTICO POR IMAGEM
• As radiografias confirmam o diagnóstico pelo registro do mau alinhamento anatômico.
• Em alguns casos, pode haver a necessidade de projeções obtidas sob estresse articular.

MÉTODOS DIAGNÓSTICOS
• Palpação da frouxidão/luxação (manobra de Ortolani, gaveta cranial, luxação patelar medial, frouxidão/instabilidade induzida por estresse).
• Palpação da posição do osso deslocado.

ACHADOS PATOLÓGICOS
• Hemorragia, edema e ruptura de ligamentos e da cápsula articular, induzidas por traumatismo.
• Alterações secundárias relacionadas com a artropatia degenerativa.

TRATAMENTO

CUIDADO(S) DE SAÚDE ADEQUADO(S)
Repouso, redução da mobilidade e do edema, controle da dor e estabilização da articulação ou recuperação do membro, removendo a origem da dor.

CUIDADO(S) DE ENFERMAGEM
• Imobilizar a articulação com o uso de bandagem/tala se a articulação acometida for distal às regiões inguinais ou axiais.
• Aplicar compressas frias por 5-10 minutos 4 ou 5 vezes ao dia, em princípio, para diminuir a inflamação.

ATIVIDADE
Proporcionar repouso em gaiola até a estabilização articular e, depois, retornar lentamente à função para incentivar a consolidação e o fortalecimento da sustentação de tecidos moles do membro.

DIETA
Normal.

ORIENTAÇÃO AO PROPRIETÁRIO
A prática de atividade física e o ganho de peso aumentam a probabilidade de alterações degenerativas a longo prazo.

CONSIDERAÇÕES CIRÚRGICAS
• A redução fechada sob anestesia pode ser bem-sucedida se as estruturas de sustentação estiverem intactas e se não houver nenhuma aberração anatômica.
• Na falha da redução fechada, pode-se usar uma abordagem cirúrgica aberta. Após a redução, deve ser aplicada alguma forma de estabilização cirúrgica para diminuir a possibilidade de nova luxação. Depois da sutura cirúrgica, frequentemente se utiliza uma tipoia de sustentação externa para limitar o movimento até que os tecidos em torno da articulação cicatrizem (p. ex., tipoia de Ehmer após redução de luxação craniodorsal do coxal).
• A incidência de nova luxação é alta, sobretudo no caso de luxações congênitas.
• Os procedimentos de recuperação incluem o uso de prótese articular, remoção cirúrgica dos pontos de contato entre os ossos (ostectomia da cabeça e do colo femorais), artrodese e amputação.

LUXAÇÕES ARTICULARES

MEDICAÇÕES

MEDICAMENTO(S) DE ESCOLHA
• Os AINE diminuem a síntese de prostaglandina, inibindo as enzimas cicloxigenases:
• Carprofeno (2,2 mg/kg VO ou SC a cada 12 h, ou 4,4 mg/kg VO ou SC a cada 24 h).
• Deracoxibe (1-2 mg/kg VO a cada 24 h).
• Firocoxibe (5 mg/kg VO a cada 24 h).
• Meloxicam (0,1 mg/kg VO ou SC a cada 24 h).
• Tramadol (1-4 mg/kg VO a cada 8-12 h), inibidor da recaptação de serotonina, em combinação com AINE.

CONTRAINDICAÇÕES
• Sensibilidade gastrintestinal.
• Doença renal ou hepática.

PRECAUÇÕES
Interromper os medicamentos em caso de vômito ou diarreia.

INTERAÇÕES POSSÍVEIS
• Outros AINE.
• Esteroides.

MEDICAMENTO(S) ALTERNATIVO(S)
Analgésicos.

ACOMPANHAMENTO

MONITORIZAÇÃO DO PACIENTE
• Sempre obtenha radiografias após a redução.
• Tire radiografias de acompanhamento quando a tala/tipoia for removida (tipicamente 2-4 semanas após a redução).

PREVENÇÃO
• Quintais cercados.
• Manutenção da tipoia no lugar até que ocorra a consolidação/cicatrização.

COMPLICAÇÕES POSSÍVEIS
• Nova luxação.
• Infecção pós-cirúrgica.
• Falha do implante de prótese articular.

EVOLUÇÃO ESPERADA E PROGNÓSTICO
• Espera-se o retorno da função a menos que ocorra alguma complicação.
• A alta incidência de nova luxação torna o prognóstico reservado.
• Artropatia degenerativa progressiva.

DIVERSOS

SINÔNIMOS
Deslocamento.

VER TAMBÉM
• Artrite (Osteoartrite).
• Displasia Coxofemoral.

ABREVIATURAS
AINE = anti-inflamatórios não esteroides.

Sugestões de Leitura
Alam MR, Lee JI, Kang HS, et al. Frequency and distribution of patellar luxation in dogs: 134 cases (2000 to 2005). Vet Comp Orthop Traumatol 2007, 20(1):59-64.
Duff SR, Bennett D. Hip luxation in small animals: An evaluation of some methods of treatment. Vet Record 1982, 111(7):140-143.
Evers P, Johnston GR, Wallace LJ, Lipowitz AJ, King VL. Long-term results of treatment of traumatic coxofemoral joint dislocation in dogs: 64 cases (1973-1992). JAVMA 1997, 210(1):59-64.
Harrell, A.G. 3rd. Reduction of simple lateral luxation of the elbow joint. Vet Med Small Anim Clin 1978, 73(9):1156-1157.
Laing EJ. Collateral ligament injury and stifle luxation. Vet Clin North Am Small Anim Pract 1993, 23(4):845-853.
McDonell HL. Unilateral congenital elbow luxation in a Cavalier King Charles spaniel. Can Vet J 2004, 45(11):941-943.
McLaughlin R.M. Traumatic joint luxations in small animals. Vet Clin North Am Small Anim Pract 1995, 25(5):1175-1196.

Autores Wesley J. Roach e Spencer A. Johnston
Consultor Editorial Peter K. Shires
Agradecimento Os autores e editores agradecem as contribuições de Peter K. Shires, que autorizou esse capítulo nas edições anteriores.

MÁ-ABSORÇÃO DA COBALAMINA

CONSIDERAÇÕES GERAIS

REVISÃO
- Adquirida ou hereditária.
- A absorção da cobalamina (vitamina B_{12}) requer a formação de complexos cobalamina-fator intrínseco (FI). O FI é secretado exclusivamente pelo pâncreas exócrino em gatos e pelo pâncreas exócrino e estômago em cães.
- A cobalamina é absorvida exclusivamente no íleo de cães e gatos por um mecanismo mediado por receptor.
- Na forma adquirida, a má-absorção pode ser atribuída à doença gastrintestinal envolvendo o íleo.
- A má-absorção da cobalamina também pode ocorrer secundariamente à insuficiência pancreática exócrina (IPE), devido à secreção reduzida do FI.
- A anomalia congênita envolve a má-absorção seletiva da cobalamina secundariamente à ausência do receptor para o complexo cobalamina-FI na borda em escova do íleo de Schnauzers gigantes, Border collies, Beagles e outras raças; muito rara.

IDENTIFICAÇÃO
- Adquirida:
  ∘ Se a má-absorção da cobalamina for atribuída à IPE, a identificação será a mesma que aquela para esse tipo de insuficiência (Pastor alemão, Collie de pelo áspero, Cavalier King Charles spaniel, Jack Russell terrier, Chow chow); 1-4 anos de idade — a idade depende da etiologia da IPE (atrofia acinar *versus* pancreatite crônica). A IPE é observada em gatos mais idosos secundariamente à pancreatite crônica.
  ∘ Se a má-absorção for secundária à enteropatia, cães e gatos de meia-idade a idosos estarão envolvidos.
- Hereditária:
  ∘ Os sinais aparecem com 6-12 semanas de idade em Schnauzers gigantes, mas aos 4-6 meses em Border collies. Provavelmente variável.
  ∘ Traço autossômico recessivo simples no Schnauzer gigante.

SINAIS CLÍNICOS
- Adquirida:
  ∘ Sinais clínicos atribuíveis à IPE: diarreia, aumento do apetite, subpeso, ocasionalmente vômito.
  ∘ Sinais clínicos atribuíveis à enteropatia: diarreia, perda de peso, vômito, apetite deficiente.
- Hereditária:
  ∘ Anorexia.
  ∘ Letargia.
  ∘ Falha de ganho de peso; falha de desenvolvimento.
  ∘ Raramente, estupor e encefalopatia.

CAUSAS E FATORES DE RISCO
- Adquirida:
  ∘ IPE em cães e gatos (causada por atrofia acinar ou pancreatite crônica).
  ∘ Doenças que envolvem a porção distal do íleo: enteropatia inflamatória, enteropatia responsiva aos alimentos, linfoma, outros.
  ∘ Outras doenças (gatos): doença hepatobiliar, pancreatite; muitos gatos têm doenças de vários sistemas orgânicos.
- Hereditária:
  ∘ Trato autossômico recessivo simples no Schnauzer gigante.

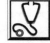

DIAGNÓSTICO

DIAGNÓSTICO DIFERENCIAL
- Outras doenças metabólicas congênitas.
- Parasitismo gastrintestinal.

HEMOGRAMA/BIOQUÍMICA/URINÁLISE
- Adquirida:
  ∘ Podem permanecer normais.
  ∘ Dependem da etiologia subjacente; hipoalbuminemia em caso de enteropatia com perda de proteínas, enzimas hepáticas elevadas em caso de colangite em gatos.
- Hereditária:
  ∘ Neutropenia leve a grave (1.760-$4.440/mm^3$) com hipersegmentação.
  ∘ Anemia arregenerativa crônica (volume globular de 21-33%) com anisocitose e poiquilocitose.
  ∘ Podem permanecer normais.

OUTROS TESTES LABORATORIAIS
- Adquirida:
  ∘ As concentrações séricas da cobalamina encontram-se baixas ou baixas a normais (abaixo de 300 ng/L).
- Todos os cães e gatos com histórico de doença gastrintestinal crônica devem ser submetidos à mensuração das concentrações séricas da cobalamina, sobretudo nos casos em que há uma resposta abaixo do ideal à terapia.
  ∘ Alterações compatíveis com a etiologia subjacente, como imunorreatividade baixa semelhante à tripsina em IPE ou imunorreatividade elevada da lipase pancreática em pancreatite.
  ∘ As concentrações séricas do ácido metilmalônico (AMM) estão acima do normal em gatos com deficiência da cobalamina.
- Hereditária:
  ∘ As concentrações séricas da cobalamina encontram-se muito baixas (geralmente indetectáveis).
  ∘ As concentrações séricas e urinárias de AMM apresentam-se acima do normal.
  ∘ Concentrações sanguíneas elevadas de amônia.
  ∘ Alterações megaloblásticas da medula óssea.

DIAGNÓSTICO POR IMAGEM
Não são úteis.

MÉTODOS DIAGNÓSTICOS
- Em casos adquiridos, os procedimentos para determinar a etiologia subjacente de hipocobalaminemia podem incluir IST, ILP, ensaio alimentar e biopsia gastrintestinal.
- Considerar a realização de biopsia gastrintestinal em animais com histórico crônico de sinais gastrintestinais e hipocobalaminemia com concentração normal de IST, especialmente se os quadros de enteropatia responsiva aos alimentos e parasitismo tiverem sido descartados.

TRATAMENTO

- É necessário o tratamento da causa subjacente (IPE, enteropatia inflamatória, etc.) na forma adquirida.
- É justificável a realização de tratamento médico ambulatorial (administração parenteral de cobalamina a longo prazo) nas formas hereditária e adquirida.

MEDICAÇÕES

MEDICAMENTO(S)
- Cianocobalamina 1.000 μg/mL, SC.
- Adquirida:
  ∘ Dosagens da cobalamina para cães e gatos.
  – Gatos, 4,5-9 kg — 250 μg.
  – Cães <4,5 kg — 250 μg.
  – Cães, 4,5-9 kg — 400 μg.
  – Cães, 9-18 kg — 600 μg.
  – Cães, 18-27 kg — 800 μg.
  – Cães, 27-36 kg — 1.000 μg.
  – Cães, 36-45 kg — 1.200 μg.
  – Cães >45 kg — 1.500 μg.
- O esquema posológico consiste em 1 dose 1 vez por semana por 6 semanas, depois 1 dose após 30 dias. Reavaliar os níveis de cobalamina 30 dias após a última dose. Talvez haja necessidade de suplementação a longo prazo.
- Hereditária:
  ∘ Cianocobalamina 0,5-1 mg SC a cada 7 dias, depois 1 vez por mês pelo resto da vida.

ACOMPANHAMENTO

Administração parenteral mensal de cobalamina

MONITORIZAÇÃO DO PACIENTE
- Medir a concentração sérica da cobalamina 1 mês depois da última administração na forma adquirida. Se a doença subjacente tiver desaparecido e as reservas de cobalamina forem repostas, os níveis dessa vitamina deverão estar acima do normal. Se a cobalamina estiver dentro da faixa de normalidade, o tratamento deverá ser mantido pelo menos mensalmente. Se os níveis estiverem abaixo do normal, haverá necessidade de avaliação adicional para determinar a doença subjacente e a suplementação de cobalamina deverá ser mantida 1 vez por semana ou em semanas alternadas.

DIVERSOS

ABREVIATURA(S)
- AMM = ácido metilmalônico. • FI = fator intrínseco. • ILP = imunorreatividade da lipase pancreática. • IPE = insuficiência pancreática exócrina. • IST = imunorreatividade semelhante à da tripsina.

RECURSOS DA INTERNET
http://vetmed.tamu.edu/gilab/research/cobalamin-information#Therapy.

Sugestões de Leitura
Batchelor DJ, Noble P-JM, Taylor RH, Cripps PJ, German AJ. Prognostic factors in canine exocrine pancreatic insufficiency: Prolonged survival is likely if clinical remission is achieved. J Vet Intern Med 2007, 21:54-60.
Ruaux CG, Steiner JM, Williams DA. Early biochemical and clinical responses to cobalamin supplementation in cats with signs of gastrointestinal disease and severe hypocobalaminemia. J Vet Intern Med 2005, 19:155-160.

Autor Krysta Deitz
Consultor Editorial Albert E. Jergens

MÁ-FORMAÇÃO ARTERIOVENOSA DO FÍGADO

CONSIDERAÇÕES GERAIS

REVISÃO
- Fístulas arteriovenosas (AV) intra-hepáticas são comunicações entre as próprias artérias hepáticas e veias portais intra-hepáticas que forçam uma circulação esplâncnica hepatofugal.
- O sangue flui da artéria hepática para o sistema porta de forma retrógrada em direção à veia cava através de múltiplos desvios portossistêmicos adquiridos.
- As fístulas AVs são raras, geralmente congênitas, mas podem ser adquiridas (lesão cirúrgica, traumatismo, neoplasia).

IDENTIFICAÇÃO
- Cães e, menos comumente, gatos.
- Manifestação relacionada com a idade (congênita): <2 anos.
- Não há raça ou sexo predominante.

SINAIS CLÍNICOS
Comentários Gerais
- Doença vaga ou aguda; são levados à consulta por sinais de hipertensão portal e desvio portossistêmico adquirido: ascite, encefalopatia hepática.

Achados Anamnésicos
- Os cães podem sofrer uma transição normal às rações de crescimento, ao contrário daqueles com anomalia vascular portossistêmica que demonstram encefalopatia hepática.
- Início agudo de ascite ou encefalopatia hepática.
- Letargia, anorexia, vômito, diarreia, perda de peso, polidipsia, demência, distensão abdominal.

Achados do Exame Físico
- Condição corporal apática e letárgica, ascite; segmento hepático aumentado de volume, com a(s) fístula(s) AV(s) raramente palpável(is).
- Ruído hepático raramente auscultável.

CAUSAS E FATORES DE RISCO
- Em geral, refletem más-formações vasculares congênitas (vasos isolados ou múltiplos) que, por sua vez, refletem na falha de diferenciação de primórdios embrionários em comum.
- Raras vezes, a má-formação arteriovenosa do fígado é secundária a traumatismo, inflamação, neoplasia, intervenções cirúrgicas ou procedimentos cirúrgicos abdominais (p. ex., biopsia do fígado).
- A hipertensão portal resulta no estabelecimento de desvio portossistêmico adquirido.

DIAGNÓSTICO

DIAGNÓSTICO DIFERENCIAL
- Sinais referentes ao SNC — distúrbios infecciosos (p. ex., cinomose); toxicidades (p. ex., chumbo); hidrocefalia; epilepsia idiopática; distúrbios metabólicos (p. ex., hipoglicemia, hipo/hipercalcemia); encefalopatia hepática (p. ex., hepatopatia grave ou anomalia vascular portossistêmica).
- Efusão abdominal — transudato puro (ascite; nefropatia ou enteropatia com perda de proteínas, hepatopatia); transudato modificado (más-formações cardíacas congênitas, insuficiência cardíaca direita, tamponamento pericárdico, obstrução supradiafragmática da veia cava, neoplasia, trombose da veia porta); hemorragia.
- Hipertensão portal — hepatopatia crônica, hepatopatia fibrosante juvenil, hipertensão portal não cirrótica ou idiopática, cirrose, trombos portais.

HEMOGRAMA/BIOQUÍMICA/URINÁLISE
- Microcitose eritrocitária (desvio portossistêmico adquirido), células-alvo.
- Hipoalbuminemia; globulina sérica normal ou baixa; atividade normal ou moderadamente elevada da fosfatase alcalina e ALT; nível baixo e variável da ureia, além de hipocolesterolemia.
- Hipostenúria ou isostenúria.
- Cristalúria por biurato de amônio.

OUTROS TESTES LABORATORIAIS
- Testes de coagulação — anormalidades variáveis, embora possam permanecer normais; proteína C baixa.
- Análise do líquido peritoneal — transudato puro (proteína total <2,5 g/dL) ou transudato modificado.
- Ácidos biliares séricos totais — em geral, valores aumentados em jejum; valores pós-prandiais sempre elevados; padrão de desvio.
- Concentração plasmática da amônia — geralmente alta.

DIAGNÓSTICO POR IMAGEM
Radiografia
- Efusão abdominal.
- Micro-hepatia ou volume normal em decorrência do amplo lobo hepático associado às fístulas AVs.
- Renomegalia.

Ultrassonografia Abdominal
- Efusão abdominal.
- Lobo hepático com extensa fístula AV em comparação à maioria dos outros lobos, que se encontram atrofiados em virtude de hipoperfusão portal.
- Estruturas tubulares anecoicas tortuosas (fístulas AVs) exibem fluxo pulsátil ou turbulento unidirecional com Doppler de fluxo colorido.
- Os ramos da artéria hepática e/ou da veia porta podem parecer tortuosos.
- Fluxo portal hepatófugo através de desvio portossistêmico adquirido.
- Renomegalia.
- Cálculos ou urólitos semelhantes à areia: bexiga urinária ou pelve renal.
- Descartar a presença de trombose portal.

Angiografia Contrastada
- Não indicada na maioria dos casos.
- Portografia venosa — confirma o desvio portossistêmico adquirido.
- Arteriografia hepática — necessária para demonstrar a comunicação AV (injeção do contraste no tronco celíaco ou na artéria mesentérica anterior).

TC Multissetorial
- Técnica contrastada não invasiva de diagnóstico por imagem da vasculatura hepática; a reconstrução tridimensional ilustra a má-formação.

Ecocardiografia
- Para descartar cardiopatia direita, doença pericárdica e oclusão da veia cava.

MÉTODOS DIAGNÓSTICOS
- Laparotomia exploratória para lobectomia/ressecção da fístula AV.
- Biopsia hepática — amostras obtidas tanto dos lobos hepáticos acometidos como daqueles inalterados; o fígado "normal" frequentemente possui uma arterialização vascular intensa (mais intensa do que aquela associada à anomalia vascular portossistêmica ou hipertensão portal não cirrótica).

TRATAMENTO

CUIDADO(S) DE SAÚDE ADEQUADO(S)
Antes da ressecção cirúrgica da fístula AV ou de embolização seletiva percutânea, efetuar a internação do paciente em casos de encefalopatia hepática e para o tratamento da ascite.

CUIDADO(S) DE ENFERMAGEM
- Dieta — restringir a ingestão de nitrogênio para amenizar a encefalopatia hepática e a hiperamonemia; limitar o consumo de sódio (ascite).
- Encefalopatia hepática — eliminar o endoparasitismo, bem como os distúrbios hídricos e eletrolíticos, tratar as infecções e instituir os tratamentos para alterar a captação e a formação entéricas de toxinas responsáveis pela encefalopatia hepática (ver "Encefalopatia Hepática").
- Ascite — mobilizar o líquido ascítico, restringindo-se a atividade física e a ingestão sódica; efetuar a abdominocentese em casos de ascite tensa que esteja prejudicando a ventilação ou a alimentação; e uso combinado de furosemida e espironolactona (ver "Hipertensão Portal" e adiante).

CONSIDERAÇÕES CIRÚRGICAS
- A ressecção do lobo hepático que contenha a fístula AV é complicada por outra má-formação vascular dentro do fígado; pode ocorrer recidiva da doença; a embolização vascular seletiva percutânea com acrilamida pode resultar em tromboembolia, melhora (pode ser temporária) ou sinais clínicos contínuos.
- Múltiplas más-formações vasculares microscópicas mantêm a hipertensão portal e o desvio portossistêmico adquirido.
- Não efetuar a ligadura do desvio portossistêmico adquirido nem realizar bandagem da veia cava.

MEDICAÇÕES

MEDICAMENTO(S)
Encefalopatia Hepática
Ver Encefalopatia Hepática.

Ascite
- Furosemida (0,5-2 mg/kg VO, IM ou IV a cada 12-24 h) — utilizada de forma mais eficiente quando associada à espironolactona.
- Espironolactona (0,5-2 mg/kg VO a cada 12 h) — iniciar com o dobro da dose como uma espécie de dose de ataque de uma única vez.
- A terapia diurética crônica deve ser individualizada até a obtenção de resposta, em intervalos de 4-7 dias.
- A ascite refratária aos diuréticos pode necessitar de abdominocentese terapêutica para iniciar a diurese ou do uso de antagonista dos receptores V_2 de vasopressina.

MÁ-FORMAÇÃO ARTERIOVENOSA DO FÍGADO

Tendências ao Sangramento
Ver Coagulopatia por Hepatopatia.

Hemorragia Gastrintestinal
• Antagonistas do receptor histaminérgico do tipo 2 (famotidina 0,5 mg/kg VO, IV ou SC a cada 12-24 h); administrar por tempo indeterminado; o sangramento e a ulceração gastrintestinais são complicações comuns a longo prazo.
• Gastroprotetor — sucralfato 0,25-0,5 g/10 kg VO a cada 8-12 h.
• Eliminar o endoparasitismo.

CONTRAINDICAÇÕES
Evitar os medicamentos que contam com a biotransformação hepática, bem como aqueles que reagem com os receptores GABA-benzodiazepínicos.

ACOMPANHAMENTO

MONITORIZAÇÃO DO PACIENTE
Bioquímica — inicialmente, em intervalos bimestrais a mensais até a estabilização do animal, depois a cada 3 meses; monitorizar o paciente quanto à presença de hipoalbuminemia, infecção e controle ideal da encefalopatia hepática.

EVOLUÇÃO ESPERADA E PROGNÓSTICO
• O prognóstico será razoável se o paciente sobreviver à ressecção cirúrgica da fístula AV.
• O paciente pode necessitar de um tratamento nutricional e clínico por tempo indefinido (encefalopatia hepática, ascite) por causa de lesões vasculares microscópicas coexistentes (todos os lobos hepáticos); o desvio portossistêmico adquirido continua necessitando de tratamento contínuo da encefalopatia hepática.

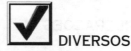

DIVERSOS

VER TAMBÉM
• Anomalia Vascular Portossistêmica Congênita.
• Ascite.
• Desvio Portossistêmico Adquirido.
• Encefalopatia Hepática.
• Hipertensão Portal.

ABREVIATURA(S)
• ALT = alanina aminotransferase.
• AV = arteriovenosa.
• GABA = ácido gama-aminobutírico.
• GI = gastrintestinal.
• SNC = sistema nervoso central.
• TC = tomografia computadorizada.

Autor Sharon A. Center
Consultor Editorial Sharon A. Center

MALOCLUSÃO ESQUELÉTICA E DENTÁRIA

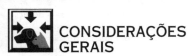

CONSIDERAÇÕES GERAIS

DEFINIÇÃO
- *Oclusão ideal*: interdigitação perfeita dos dentes superiores e inferiores.
  - Incisivos maxilares em posição rostral aos incisivos mandibulares correspondentes.
  - O canino mandibular está inclinado no sentido labial e divide o espaço entre o terceiro incisivo maxilar e o canino opostos.
  - Os pré-molares maxilares não entram em contato com os pré-molares mandibulares: as coroas dos pré-molares mandibulares ficam em posição lingual aos pré-molares maxilares; as cúspides da coroa do pré-molar mandibular dividem os espaços interdentais rostrais ao pré-molar maxilar correspondente.
  - A cúspide mesial do quarto pré-molar maxilar encontra-se em posição lateral ao espaço entre o quarto pré-molar mandibular e o primeiro molar.
- *Maloclusão*: qualquer desvio da oclusão normal descrita anteriormente, em função do posicionamento anormal de algum dente (maloclusão dentária) ou em virtude de assimetria ou desvio dos ossos que sustentam a dentição (maloclusão esquelética).

Sistema de Classificação de Ângulo Modificado de Maloclusão
- Classe 0 — oclusão normal: avaliar o alinhamento dos incisivos (mordida em tesoura), pré-molares (efeito de cisalhamento) e dentes carniceiros (alinhamento estreito dos sulcos de desenvolvimento: quarto pré-molar superior ao primeiro molar inferior).
- Classe 0, tipo 3 — o que seria considerado "normal" em raças braquicefálicas (p. ex., Boxer e Buldogue); algumas raças permitem mordida "nivelada".
- Classe 1 — neutroclusão: uma relação rostrocaudal normal dos arcos dentários maxilares e mandibulares com mau posicionamento de um ou mais dentes individuais (maloclusão dentária); mordida cruzada anterior (rostral); dente em lança (mesioversão); dentes caninos de base estreita (linguoversão); e mordida cruzada posterior (caudal).
- Classe 2 — distoclusão mandibular: uma relação rostrocaudal anormal em que o arco mandibular oclui caudalmente à sua posição normal em relação ao arco maxilar (maloclusão esquelética).
- Classe 3 — distoclusão mandibular: uma relação rostrocaudal anormal em que o arco mandibular oclui rostralmente à sua posição normal em relação ao arco maxilar (maloclusão esquelética).
- Classe 4 — maloclusão esquelética assimétrica: assimetria maxilomandibular que pode ocorrer em uma direção rostrocaudal (relação anormal unilateral), em uma direção lado a lado (perda do alinhamento na linha média) ou em um sentido dorsoventral com espaço vertical anormal entre os arcos dentários opostos (mordida aberta).
- "Mordida torcida" é um termo usado para descrever diversas anormalidades oclusais unilaterais, como nos casos em que um quadrante é alongado e o outro quadrante, encurtado.

IDENTIFICAÇÃO
Espécies
Cães e gatos.

Raça(s) Predominante(s)
Há predileção racial por determinadas maloclusões (p. ex., dentes em lança no Pastor de Shetland).

Idade Média e Faixa Etária
A maloclusão costuma ser aparente após erupção dos dentes (permanentes ou decíduos).

SINAIS CLÍNICOS
- Variam muito de acordo com o tipo, a extensão e as consequentes lesões provocadas pela maloclusão.
- Podem estar associados a mordidas abertas ou fechadas ou ao apinhamento dos dentes.
- Doença periodontal — pode resultar de apinhamento ou mau alinhamento dos dentes.
- Defeitos de tecidos moles — decorrentes de contato dentário traumático; podem ser observados no assoalho da boca e no palato; o traumatismo palatal eventualmente pode resultar na formação de fístula oronasal.
- Fraturas ou atrito (desgaste) dos dentes — podem resultar do contato dentário inadequado.

Maloclusões de Classe 1
- Mordida cruzada anterior (rostral) — incisivos maxilares deslocados no sentido palatal ou incisivos mandibulares deslocados no sentido labial.
- Caninos de base estreita — as pontas dos caninos mandibulares tocam o palato em posição lingual ao ponto de contato normal, imediatamente labial ao diastema entre o incisivo do canto e o canino maxilar (linguoversão).
- Dentes em lança — mesioversão do(s) canino(s) maxilar(es): o diastema entre o incisivo do canto e esse canino frequentemente está diminuído e pode forçar o canino mandibular para uma posição anormal. Mais comum nas raças dolicocefálicas (p. ex., Sheltie e Collie).
- Mordida cruzada posterior (caudal) — a maior parte é atribuída à inversão da relação (labial/lingual) entre os dentes carniceiros superior e inferior; mais comum nas raças dolicocéfalas (p. ex., Collie, Sheltie e algumas raças de caça visual).

CAUSAS
- Fatores congênitos ou hereditários — maloclusões esqueléticas (classes 2, 3 e 4) e predileção racial.
- Impedimento à erupção dentária — opérculo; retenção do tecido mole de revestimento.
- Erupção tardia dos dentes decíduos ou permanentes.
- Retenção (persistente) ou perda tardia dos dentes decíduos.
- Lesão traumática com envolvimento das maxilas ou dos dentes.

FATORES DE RISCO
Predisposições hereditárias.

DIAGNÓSTICO

DIAGNÓSTICO DIFERENCIAL
- Deslocamento dentário — atribuído a traumatismos, massas bucais ou outras causas.
- Obstrução mecânica — gerado por fraturas da mandíbula, dentes luxados ou subluxados ou corpos estranhos indutores de mordida aberta.
- O diagnóstico definitivo é formulado com base em achados visuais e radiográficos, bem como no Sistema de Classificação de Ângulo Modificado de Maloclusão (ver a seção "Definição").
- Examinar os padrões raciais para determinar o que pode ser aceitável para a raça.

HEMOGRAMA/BIOQUÍMICA/URINÁLISE
Geralmente normais.

DIAGNÓSTICO POR IMAGEM
- Fotografia bucal — antes, durante e depois do tratamento.
- Radiografia intrabucal — para avaliar as raízes dos dentes e a presença de anormalidades.

MÉTODOS DIAGNÓSTICOS
- Exame bucal completo — para avaliar outras anormalidade da boca.
- Impressões e moldes — para avaliação e confecção do aparelho.

TRATAMENTO

CUIDADO(S) DE SAÚDE ADEQUADO(S)
- A avaliação precisa de anormalidades de oclusão ajudará a determinar se o tratamento é justificável e que tratamento é apropriado.
- Nem toda maloclusão necessita de correção ortodôntica. Se a mordida for funcional e não traumática para o animal, o tratamento poderá ser dispensado. Além disso, a extração (ou a redução da coroa com capeamento da polpa dentária) dos dentes ofensores frequentemente pode ser uma alternativa eficaz a tratamentos ortodônticos mais clássicos. Em geral, o tratamento ortodôntico baseia-se na prevenção de trauma, desgaste ou lesão por contato inadequado com tecidos duros ou moles, devendo ser realizado apenas por indivíduo experiente.

DIETA
Dietas pastosas com aparelhos.

ORIENTAÇÃO AO PROPRIETÁRIO
Cuidados Domésticos com o Aparelho
- Examinar o aparelho duas vezes ao dia.
- Irrigar a boca com solução ou gel de higiene bucal.
- Evitar a mastigação de objetos e fornecer uma dieta pastosa até que o aparelho seja removido.

CONSIDERAÇÕES CIRÚRGICAS
Maloclusão de Classe 1 de Dente Permanente
- O tratamento envolve principalmente movimentos de inclinação dos dentes, embora a extrusão possa ser necessária para conferir retenção adequada.
- Mordida cruzada anterior (rostral) — apinhamento: odontoplastia para dentes finos (ter cuidado); barra no arco maxilar labial com braquetes ortodônticos em botão e ligaduras ou elásticos ortodônticos em cadeia para tração (para movimentar os incisivos maxilares à frente ou para extruir) é um dos melhores métodos de tratamento; barra no arco maxilar lingual com mola digital, plano de inclinação mandibular ou maxilar, aparelho com parafuso de expansão maxilar ou braquetes mandibulares e elásticos ortodônticos em cadeia são, sem exceção, possíveis modalidades de tratamento.
- Dentes caninos de base estreita — prevenção de traumatismo, dor e desconforto por contato, bem como da formação de fístula oronasal; se o caso for muito leve, a realização de gengivoplastia ou gengivectomia no diastema poderá liberar o contato; talvez haja necessidade de aparelho

Maloclusão Esquelética e Dentária

ortodôntico para ajudar a orientar um desvio mais significativo, inclinando o dente para uma localização funcional ou oclusão adequada; movimentos ortodônticos de inclinação podem ser conferidos por uma série de aparelhos diferentes, por exemplo, plano inclinado de acrílico ou de resina, parafusos de expansão, molas em W, planos de inclinação de molde metálico e planos de autoinclinação de resina (acumulados no dente).
• Dente em lança — botão ou braquetes aplicados em direção à ponta do dente canino para ser movimentado (dente-alvo) e próximos à gengiva dos dentes de âncora (quarto pré-molar superior e primeiro molar), com elástico ortodôntico em cadeia para tração aplicado entre os dois; monitorizar cuidadosamente para evitar o deslocamento do dente de âncora (a área de superfície radicular deve exceder aquela do dente-alvo).
• Mordida cruzada posterior (caudal) — na maior parte dos casos, não há necessidade de nenhum tratamento, já que a mordida é tipicamente funcional; em situações traumáticas, procede-se à extração de um dos dentes ofensores; a correção ortodôntica é demorada e cansativa, exigindo a aplicação de aparelhos ortodônticos mais avançados e o bloqueio da mordida aberta.

Maloclusão de Classes 2, 3 e 4 de Dente Permanente
• Baseia-se em medidas para proporcionar uma oclusão funcional não traumática para a saúde clínica do animal; se já estiver presente, o tratamento poderá não ser necessário.
• Pode necessitar de procedimento ortodôntico e cirúrgico avançado e, em geral, é mais bem manipulado por especialista.

Maloclusão de Classe 1 de Dente Decíduo
Extração cuidadosa e delicada do dente decíduo maloclúido para remover o impedimento físico inadequado (ortodontia interceptiva), na esperança de que o dente permanente sofra erupção na posição adequada; quando realizada no mínimo 4 semanas antes da erupção do dente permanente, taxa de sucesso >80% não é incomum.

Maloclusão de Classes 2, 3 e 4 de Dente Decíduo
Extração cuidadosa e delicada do dente decíduo maloclúido, na esperança de que as mandíbulas curtas sejam liberadas do travamento da mordida, permitindo seu crescimento (se houver potencial genético) antes da erupção dos dentes permanentes e do restabelecimento da mordida travada; quando realizada pelo menos 6 semanas antes da erupção do dente permanente, taxa de sucesso <20% é comum.

ACOMPANHAMENTO
MONITORIZAÇÃO DO PACIENTE
• Para a oclusão corrigida ficar estável, é necessário que ela seja de autorretenção ou poderá reverter para maloclusão; examinar com 2 semanas, 2 meses e 6 meses após a conclusão do tratamento para verificar se o resultado desejado se encontra estável.
• É aconselhável a obtenção de radiografias em torno de 6 meses após o tratamento e subsequente comparação com filmes radiográficos obtidos antes do tratamento, para determinar se todos os dentes ainda parecem viáveis (vivos) e para avaliar quaisquer alterações radiculares que possam ter ocorrido em virtude de pressões do dente e movimentos da raiz durante a ortodontia.

PREVENÇÃO
• Seleção cuidadosa de filhotes, com o exame clínico geral e bucal, bem como com a avaliação e o histórico dos pais, antes da aquisição.
• Cruzamento seletivo feito com base nas características preferidas da raça.
• Monitorização cuidadosa da erupção dos dentes decíduos e permanentes para detecção e tratamento precoces, se necessários.

COMPLICAÇÕES POSSÍVEIS
• Extração seletiva do dente decíduo antes da erupção do dente permanente —potencial de lesão aos botões do dente permanente subjacente por lesão direta com instrumentos de extração ou subsequente inflamação traumática, afetando o crescimento e a maturidade do dente; as lesões podem resultar em morte dos botões dentários, perda da vitalidade dos dentes à medida que sofrem erupção, displasia ou dilaceração da raiz, hipoplasia da coroa ou hipomineralização.
• Movimento ortodôntico dos dentes permanentes — diversas condições podem resultar de reabsorção da raiz, anquilose da raiz ou falta de vitalidade do dente; essas condições são raras em procedimentos ortodônticos conduzidos de forma adequada.

EVOLUÇÃO ESPERADA E PROGNÓSTICO
• O curso do tratamento pode variar com o tipo de maloclusão, bem como com a natureza e os hábitos do animal (p. ex., mastigação inadequada).
• Em geral, a maior parte dos casos demora 1-7 meses para a fase de movimento e retenção, dependendo da gravidade do quadro e da necessidade de extrusão do(s) dente(s) para a estabilização das mordidas. O prognóstico é bom a excelente em grande parte dos pacientes tratados.
• O prognóstico é razoável a bom na maioria das maloclusões sem tratamento.

• Complicações nos casos não tratados — doença periodontal; atrito ou fraturas dentárias; traumatismo aos tecidos moles; formação de fístula oronasal; ressecamento ou dessecação das superfícies dentárias expostas, resultando na coloração bege a acastanhada.
• Alguns casos NÃO necessitam de intervenção ortodôntica nem exigem esse tipo de intervenção; é aconselhável apenas uma observação de rotina para detecção e tratamento precoces de quaisquer complicações secundárias (p. ex., doença periodontal, desgaste ou dentes lascados).

DIVERSOS
DISTÚRBIOS ASSOCIADOS
• Falta de simetria da cabeça.
• Traumatismo ao tecido mole bucal.
• Dentes lascados.
• Dessecação das superfícies dentárias expostas.
• Doença periodontal.

GESTAÇÃO/FERTILIDADE/REPRODUÇÃO
Embora os animais tenham o direito clínico à oclusão correta e funcional que possa ser razoavelmente conferida pelo tratamento, regras de associações de animais, princípios de associação profissional, bem como legislação estadual e nacional, podem entrar em conflito com o direito do animal ao adequado tratamento clínico. Algumas regras de associações de criadores desqualificam os animais com modificação da aparência natural (com determinadas exceções) e os proprietários devem estar conscientes disso. Na suspeita de envolvimento hereditário, informar ao proprietário. Se o tratamento estiver sob consideração, o proprietário ou seu representante deve conhecer sua responsabilidade para informar quem quer que seja que tenha o direito de saber de tal alteração. Além disso, a possibilidade de remoção do animal do agrupamento genético por métodos adequados deve ser discutida.

RECURSOS DA INTERNET
http://www.avdc.org/Nomenclature.html.

Sugestões de Leitura
Lobprise HB. Blackwell's Five-Minute Veterinary Consult Clinical Companion—Small Animal Dentistry. Ames, IA: Blackwell, 2007 (para mais informações, incluindo técnicas e métodos diagnósticos).
Wiggs RB, Lobprise HB. Veterinary Dentistry: Principles and Practice. Philadelphia: Lippincott-Raven, 1997, pp. 457-463.

Autor Robert B. Wiggs
Consultor Editorial Heidi B. Lobprise

MÁS-FORMAÇÕES CONGÊNITAS ESPINAIS E VERTEBRAIS

CONSIDERAÇÕES GERAIS

DEFINIÇÃO
Desenvolvimento anômalo de estruturas espinais, evidentes ao nascimento ou dentro das primeiras semanas de vida.

FISIOPATOLOGIA
• Má-formação dos ossos occipitais, do atlas e do áxis; má-formação do processo odontoide; má-formação occipitoatlantoaxial; e displasia occipital — podem causar subluxação atlantoaxial com compressão e traumatismo secundários aos primeiros segmentos da medula espinal cervical.
• Outras anomalias embrionárias ou evolutivas das vértebras — hemivértebra, vértebra de transição, vértebra em bloco e vértebra em borboleta; esses defeitos geram deformidade e instabilidade do canal vertebral e, em raras ocasiões, compressão da medula espinal ou das raízes nervosas associadas.
• Disgenesia sacrococcígea — caracterizada por ausência ou desenvolvimento parcial dos segmentos sacrocaudais da medula espinal; associada frequentemente a más-formações extras (p. ex., espinha-bífida).
• Espinha-bífida — causada por falha de fusão dos arcos vertebrais; pode estar associada à protrusão da medula espinal e das meninges; com frequência, há outras más-formações ligadas a essa síndrome, como displasia espinal, disrafismo, siringomielia/hidromielia e mielodisplasia.
• Estenose espinal congênita — pode ocorrer quando más-formações vertebrais produzem um estreitamento segmentar ou difuso da medula espinal; erros inatos no crescimento esquelético, hipertrofia do ligamento amarelo e proliferação do tecido ósseo também podem contribuir para a estenose.

SISTEMA(S) ACOMETIDO(S)
Nervoso — medula espinal; raízes nervosas; e coluna vertebral (vértebras).

GENÉTICA
• Em grande parte das doenças espinais congênitas, suspeita-se de base genética com modo de herança desconhecido.
• Disgenesia sacrococcígea — traço autossômico dominante.
• Hemivértebra torácica do Pointer alemão de pelo curto — traço autossômico recessivo.

DISTRIBUIÇÃO GEOGRÁFICA
N/D.

IDENTIFICAÇÃO

Espécie(s) e Raça(s) Predominante(s)
• Má-formação dos ossos occipitais, do atlas e do áxis— mais comum em raças caninas de pequeno porte.
• Hemivértebra, vértebra de transição, vértebra em bloco e vértebra em borboleta — mais comuns em raças braquicefálicas de "cauda em parafuso" (p. ex., Buldogue francês e inglês, Pug, Boston terrier).
• Disgenesia sacrococcígea — gatos da raça Manx.
• Espinha-bífida — Buldogue e outras raças de cauda em parafuso, além de gatos Manx.
• Mielodisplasia — Weimaraner.
• Estenose espinal congênita — Doberman pinscher; raças condrodistróficas.

Idade Média e Faixa Etária
• Frequentemente silenciosa, a má-formação vertebral pode causar doença clínica durante a fase de crescimento rápido do animal (p. ex., 5-9 meses de vida).
• As anomalias da medula espinal geram doença clínica a partir do nascimento.

SINAIS CLÍNICOS
• Torção da coluna vertebral — lordose; cifose; e escoliose em casos de más-formações vertebrais.
• Ataxia e paresia associadas à compressão e ao traumatismo da medula espinal.
• Os sinais variam com o(s) segmento(s) medular(es) envolvido(s).

CAUSAS
Em grande parte das anormalidades espinais congênitas, suspeita-se de defeitos hereditários relacionados à raça, embora provavelmente haja o envolvimento de interações entre vários genes e fatores ambientais (p. ex., compostos teratogênicos e deficiências nutricionais), o que explicaria algumas dessas alterações patológicas complexas.

FATORES DE RISCO
• Compostos teratogênicos.
• Toxinas.
• Deficiências nutricionais.
• Estresse.

DIAGNÓSTICO

DIAGNÓSTICO DIFERENCIAL
• Doença metabólica (p. ex., doenças de armazenamento).
• Doença nutricional (p. ex., hipo e hipervitaminose A, deficiência de tiamina).
• Processos inflamatórios ou infecciosos de início precoce (p. ex., virais, protozoários e, raramente, bacterianos).
• Exposição a toxinas (p. ex., chumbo, organofosforados, hexaclorofeno e organoclorados).
• Traumatismo.

HEMOGRAMA/BIOQUÍMICA/URINÁLISE
Em geral, permanecem dentro dos limites de normalidade.

OUTROS TESTES LABORATORIAIS
N/D.

DIAGNÓSTICO POR IMAGEM
• Radiografias simples — na maioria dos casos, podem revelar uma ou mais más-formações das vértebras e desvio da coluna vertebral.
• Mielografia — essencial para determinar com precisão o(s) grau(s) de compressão da medula espinal quando se observam sinais neurológicos; sob fluoroscopia, podem-se obter as projeções fletidas e estendidas com extrema cautela.
• Técnicas avançadas de diagnóstico por imagem, como TC e RM — podem ser úteis para caracterizar ainda mais as estruturas circunjacentes envolvidas (p. ex., compressão de raiz nervosa espinal, hipertrofia de ligamento e hipoplasia do processo odontoide).

MÉTODOS DIAGNÓSTICOS
Análise do líquido cerebrospinal para descartar processos infecciosos/inflamatórios.

ACHADOS PATOLÓGICOS
• Más-formações congênitas múltiplas — presença frequentemente concomitante; as alterações patológicas refletem diversos processos mórbidos.
• Compressão aguda da medula espinal, secundária a uma ou mais más-formações congênitas — pode resultar em isquemia medular, hemorragia, insuflação da bainha de mielina no ponto de compressão ou traumatismo, e tumefação ou perda axonal; em casos de compressão crônica da medula espinal, certas alterações como degeneração da mielina, astrocitose e fibrose são mais proeminentes; nas regiões espinais craniais e caudais à lesão primária, pode-se observar a degeneração walleriana em vias ascendentes ou descendentes, respectivamente.
• Alterações crônicas — podem se originar de más-formações vertebrais secundárias à proliferação do tecido ósseo, ao espessamento da cápsula articular, à hipertrofia dos processos articulares e ao espessamento dos ligamentos circunjacentes à medula espinal.
• Subluxação atlantoaxial — aplasia ou hipoplasia congênitas do processo odontoide e dos ligamentos circunjacentes.
• Más-formações occipitoatlantoaxiais — fusão do atlas com o osso occipital (gatos) e angulação dorsal do processo odontoide (cães).
• Displasia occipital — anomalia do forame magno, na qual o osso occipital se apresenta parcialmente formado e a membrana de tecido fibroso recobre a porção caudal do cerebelo.
• Disgenesia sacrococcígea — aplasia ou hipoplasia das vértebras caudais.
• Espinha-bífida — fusão incompleta dos arcos vertebrais dorsais, local onde é possível a protrusão das meninges ou da medula espinal; observada mais comumente nas áreas lombar ou sacral caudais; em alguns casos, pode-se observar uma depressão secundária à falta de separação entre o neuroectoderma e outras estruturas ectodérmicas, restando uma pequena fixação entre a medula espinal ou as meninges e a pele; constatada frequentemente em casos de mielodisplasia, defeitos do canal central, siringomielia ou hidromielia e diferenciação anormal da substância cinzenta.
• Estenose espinal — as alterações patológicas observadas no interior da medula espinal costumam ser crônicas e causadas por estreitamento focal ou difuso do canal vertebral.

TRATAMENTO

CUIDADO(S) DE SAÚDE ADEQUADO(S)
• Depende da gravidade dos déficits neurológicos.
• Ambulatorial — se o animal ainda consegue andar.
• Internação — se o paciente não for capaz de caminhar ou necessitar de tratamento cirúrgico de emergência (p. ex., em casos de subluxação atlantoaxial).

CUIDADO(S) DE ENFERMAGEM
• Restrição da atividade física, combinada com fisioterapia — podem ajudar os pacientes com déficits neurológicos no período pós-operatório; em pacientes gravemente acometidos, poderá haver a necessidade de carrinhos ortopédicos.

Más-formações Congênitas Espinais e Vertebrais

- Controle da micção — pode ser essencial em casos com distúrbios da micção concomitantes à lesão espinal.

ATIVIDADE
Restrita, especialmente na presença de subluxação vertebral.

DIETA
A manutenção de um peso corporal magro limita o estresse exercido sobre a coluna vertebral.

ORIENTAÇÃO AO PROPRIETÁRIO
- Do ponto de vista clínico, muitas más-formações vertebrais congênitas são silenciosas. • Quando a má-formação congênita resulta em anormalidades neurológicas, deve-se efetuar um exame clínico completo e minucioso.
- Além disso, há suspeita de hereditariedade; dessa forma, o acasalamento deve ser realizado apenas com sérias ponderações.
- Muitos cães e gatos com comprometimento neurológico que ficam sem tratamento são submetidos à eutanásia.
- Portanto, a intervenção cirúrgica precoce é muitas vezes imprescindível para aliviar a compressão da medula espinal e evitar danos futuros.

CONSIDERAÇÕES CIRÚRGICAS
- Em geral, a descompressão cirúrgica é requerida quando a má-formação congênita leva ao estreitamento do canal vertebral e à compressão da medula espinal. Em casos de compressão medular crônica ou difusa, as respostas terapêuticas após a cirurgia são mínimas.
- Subluxação atlantoaxial — a descompressão ventral cirúrgica, combinada com a estabilização da articulação atlantoaxial com pinos ou parafusos, constitui o tratamento de escolha.
- Espinha-bífida — as meningoceles podem ser submetidas à oclusão cirúrgica para evitar o extravasamento do líquido cerebrospinal e a ocorrência de infecções; a cirurgia não costuma ser empreendida quando há o envolvimento do parênquima da medula espinal.

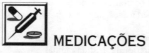

MEDICAÇÕES

MEDICAMENTO(S) DE ESCOLHA
Os corticosteroides podem ser utilizados em alguns casos, mas demonstram resultados questionáveis.

CONTRAINDICAÇÕES
Evitar o uso de esteroides em casos de infecções concomitantes.

PRECAUÇÕES
Os esteroides podem causar a ulceração gastrintestinal e inibir o crescimento ósseo.

INTERAÇÕES POSSÍVEIS
Os esteroides diminuem a resposta imunológica subsequente à vacinação.

MEDICAMENTO(S) ALTERNATIVO(S)
N/D.

ACOMPANHAMENTO

MONITORIZAÇÃO DO PACIENTE
- Exames neurológicos frequentes — indispensáveis muitas vezes para monitorizar a evolução dos sinais clínicos (p. ex., a cada 4-6 meses).
- Radiografias — repetir conforme a necessidade.

PREVENÇÃO
Evitar a reprodução dos animais acometidos.

COMPLICAÇÕES POSSÍVEIS
- Dependem do tipo e da gravidade dos sinais neurológicos. Em casos de subluxação da articulação atlantoaxial, pode ocorrer morte súbita.
- Na ocorrência de subluxação vertebral, também é possível constatar uma paralisia aguda, com traumatismo e compressão medular adicionais.
- Após descompressão/estabilização cirúrgicas, pode-se observar uma falha do implante.

EVOLUÇÃO ESPERADA E PROGNÓSTICO
- O prognóstico varia, dependendo do tipo de má-formação, do grau de compressão ou lesão medular, bem como das técnicas cirúrgicas de descompressão ou estabilização.
- Má-formação vertebral sem compressão da medula espinal — o prognóstico é bom.
- Subluxação atlantoaxial após descompressão ou estabilização cirúrgicas — o prognóstico é razoável a bom.
- Compressão da medula espinal submetida a tratamento cirúrgico — o prognóstico é razoável.
- Espinha-bífida associada à má-formação da medula espinal, neuropatia crônica apesar de tratamento cirúrgico e incontinência por lesão do neurônio motor inferior — o prognóstico é mau.

- O tratamento clínico costuma não ser suficiente para aliviar os sinais neurológicos moderados a graves, causados pela compressão medular secundária a uma ou mais más-formações vertebrais congênitas.

DIVERSOS

DISTÚRBIOS ASSOCIADOS
N/D.

FATORES RELACIONADOS COM A IDADE
N/D.

POTENCIAL ZOONÓTICO
N/D.

GESTAÇÃO/FERTILIDADE/REPRODUÇÃO
N/D.

VER TAMBÉM
- Ataxia.
- Disrafismo Espinal.
- Espondilomielopatia Cervical (Síndrome de Wobbler).
- Instabilidade Atlantoaxial.
- Paralisia.

ABREVIATURA(S)
- RM = ressonância magnética.
- TC = tomografia computadorizada.

Sugestões de Leitura
Dewey CW. Myelopathy: Disorders of the spinal cord. In: Dewey CW, ed., A Practical Guide to Canine and Feline Neurology. Ames, IA: Wiley-Blackwell, 2008, pp. 350-361, 396-398.
Jeffrey ND. Handbook of Small Animal Spinal Surgery. Philadelphia: Saunders, 1995.
Lorenz MD, Kornegay JN. Handbook of Veterinary Neurology, 4th ed. St Louis: Saunders, 2004.
Summer BA, Cummings JF, de Lahunta A. Veterinary Pathology. Philadelphia: Mosby-Year Book, 1995.

Autor Christiane Massicotte
Consultor Editorial Joane M. Parent

MÁS-FORMAÇÕES VAGINAIS E LESÕES ADQUIRIDAS

CONSIDERAÇÕES GERAIS

DEFINIÇÃO
Alteração na arquitetura anatômica, decorrente de anomalias congênitas (hímen imperfurado, septo dorsoventral, constrição himenal, fístula retovaginal, aplasia segmentar e cistos) e condições adquiridas (hiperplasia vaginal, corpos estranhos, estenoses, aderências, fístulas e neoplasias).

FISIOPATOLOGIA
Congênitas
- Desenvolvimento embriológico normal — o par de ductos paramesonéfricos (de Müller) funde-se, formando o corpo uterino, a cérvix e a vagina; o seio urogenital forma o vestíbulo, a uretra e a bexiga urinária; o hímen (constituído dos revestimentos epiteliais dos ductos paramesonéfricos e do seio urogenital, bem como de uma camada interposta de mesoderma) normalmente desaparece ao nascimento.
- Erros durante o desenvolvimento embrionário — hímens imperfurados; septos dorsoventrais; constrições himenais (incluindo estenoses vestibulovaginais); divertículo vaginal (vagina dupla, bolsa vaginal); cistos.

Adquiridas
- Formação de tecido cicatricial na vagina — resposta a traumatismo ou inflamação; em casos de cicatriz madura, podem-se observar aderências ou estenoses, que estreitam o diâmetro da vagina.
- Hiperplasia vaginal (cadelas) — resultado de uma resposta exagerada da mucosa vaginal aos estrogênios; o efeito gerado é a formação de edema, e não hiperplasia ou hipertrofia.
- Processos neoplásicos — o leiomioma extraluminal é mais comum; geralmente ocorrem em pacientes idosas; sua ocorrência não compromete o estado do ovário.

SISTEMA(S) ACOMETIDO(S)
- Reprodutivo — principal efeito: interferência com a monta natural e o parto; problema concomitante frequente: vaginite.
- Renal/urológico — as infecções ascendentes do trato urinário não são incomuns; pode-se notar incontinência urinária em conjunto com más-formações congênitas da área do hímen (a inter-relação ainda não está esclarecida, além de não ser universalmente aceita).
- Cutâneo/exócrino — em geral, observa-se dermatite perivulvar secundária à vaginite ou à incontinência urinária.

GENÉTICA
Congênita — possível suspeita de componente hereditário; não existe nenhuma evidência direta.

INCIDÊNCIA/PREVALÊNCIA
- Incidência (congênita) — desconhecida; as condições podem permanecer assintomáticas, especialmente se a fêmea nunca for usada para reprodução.
- Prevalência (septos vaginais) — em um único estudo, relata-se uma prevalência de 0,03% de todos os casos observados.

IDENTIFICAÇÃO
Espécies
Cadelas e gatas.

Raça(s) Predominante(s)
- Congênitas — nenhuma raça identificada.
- Hiperplasia vaginal — as raças de grande porte são mais predispostas.

Idade Média e Faixa Etária
- Lesão congênita (p. ex., hímen imperfurado, estenose e septos) — fêmeas jovens (<2 anos de idade) intactas ou castradas.
- Hiperplasia vaginal — fêmeas jovens (<2 anos de idade) intactas.
- Lesão adquirida (aderências e estenoses) — fêmeas de qualquer idade após a puberdade.
- Neoplasia — idade média, 10 anos; não tem nenhum efeito sobre o estado ovariano.

SINAIS CLÍNICOS
Achados Anamnésicos
- Corrimento vulvar.
- Lambedura excessiva da vulva.
- Micção frequente ou inapropriada.
- Estrangúria ou disquezia.
- Incontinência urinária.
- Atrativa aos machos.
- Recusa a monta.
- Massa nos lábios vulvares.

Achados do Exame Físico
- Geralmente normais.
- É comum verificar indícios de corrimento vaginal ou dermatite perivulvar.
- Ocasionalmente, observa-se hipoplasia vulvar.

CAUSAS
- Congênitas.
- Inflamatórias.
- Hormonais.
- Traumáticas.
- Neoplásicas.

DIAGNÓSTICO

DIAGNÓSTICO DIFERENCIAL
- Vaginite — concomitante com muitas más-formações; diferenciada por meio de vaginoscopia e vaginografia com contraste positivo.
- Infecção do trato urinário — distinguida por meio de citologia vaginal e urinálise concomitante em amostra coletada por cistocentese.
- Piometra — diferenciada por meio de hemograma completo, perfis bioquímicos e ultrassonografia abdominal.

HEMOGRAMA/BIOQUÍMICA/URINÁLISE
- Hemograma completo e bioquímica — geralmente normais.
- Urinálise — pode revelar indícios de infecção ascendente secundária do trato urinário.

DIAGNÓSTICO POR IMAGEM
Vaginografia com Contraste Positivo
- Define o fórnix vaginal até a cérvix, a uretra, a porção cranial do vestíbulo e a bexiga urinária.
- Delimita o canal cervical e o lúmen uterino em pacientes intactas durante o estro.
- Identifica estenoses, septos, hímens persistentes, massas, fístulas retovaginais, fístulas uretrovaginais, ruptura vaginal e divertículos.
- As pacientes devem permanecer em jejum por 24 horas; deve-se aplicar um enema 2 h antes do procedimento.
- Colocar a paciente sob sedação ou anestesia geral.
- Introduzir no vestíbulo um cateter de Foley com extremidade em balão; insuflar o balão; infundir meios de contraste iodados aquosos (1 mL/kg); evitar a distensão excessiva ou abaixo do ideal.
- Relação da altura máxima da vagina com a altura mínima da junção vestibulovaginal — normal >0,35; leve 0,26-0,35; moderada 0,20-0,25 e grave <0,20.
- Incontinência urinária — pode ser necessária a realização de urografia excretora para descartar a presença de ureteres ectópicos ou de colo vesical em posição intrapélvica; uretrocistoscopia.

Ultrassonografia Abdominal
- Grande parte da vagina não é acessível por conta da pelve óssea.
- Massas vaginais craniais — ocasionalmente, podem ser observadas.
- A infusão de solução salina na vagina antes do exame auxilia na inspeção; ajuda a diferenciar lesões luminais de transmurais ou extraluminais.

MÉTODOS DIAGNÓSTICOS
- A ordem de execução dos procedimentos é importante; tais procedimentos estão listados aqui conforme sua ordem de recomendação.
- Cultura vaginal — identifica infecções secundárias; recomenda-se o uso de um *swab* (Culturette®) reservado para isso para evitar a contaminação proveniente do vestíbulo e da porção caudal da vagina (ver "Corrimento Vaginal"; "Vaginite").
- Citologia vaginal — identifica a fase do ciclo estral; revela células inflamatórias ou neoplásicas (ver "Acasalamento, Momento Oportuno").
- Exame digital do vestíbulo e da porção caudal da vagina — mensura o diâmetro; identifica estenoses ou massas caudais; avalia o tamanho e a conformação da vulva; a paciente deve ser mantida em estação com apoio do abdome (sedação) ou em decúbito (anestesia).
- Vaginoscopia — identifica estenoses, aderências, septos, divertículos, massas e corpos estranhos; podem-se empregar diversos espéculos; recomenda-se o uso de um espéculo longo (16-20 cm), oco e rígido (p. ex., proctoscópio infantil) com fibra óptica ou foco halogênio de luz; deve-se equiparar o diâmetro do espéculo com o porte da paciente; é normal a existência de prega pós-cervical (obscurece a inspeção do óstio externo da cérvix); cistoscópios rígidos (utilizados para inseminação transcervical) são adequados para muitas anomalias, mas necessitam de distensão vaginal (sob anestesia geral) com salina ou ar para visualizar algumas anomalias ou lesões.
- Diagnóstico por imagem — indicado quando os resultados dos procedimentos prévios sugerem uma anormalidade anatômica; vaginografia e/ou ultrassonografia.

ACHADOS PATOLÓGICOS
Congênitas
- Hímen imperfurado — membrana fenestrada delgada, banda(s) dorsoventral(is) ou membrana espessa na junção vestibulovaginal; constitui o defeito mais comum e mais simples; o restante do trato genital permanece normal.
- Septo dorsoventral — orientado em sentido dorsoventral na vagina, cranial à junção vestibulovaginal; pode-se notar a cérvix dupla (variante mais comum); vagina dupla ou fundo uterino dividido (raro).
- Constrição himenal ou estenose vestibulovaginal — constrição moderada a grave na junção vestibulovaginal.

Más-formações Vaginais e Lesões Adquiridas

- Hipoplasia ou aplasia vaginal — estruturas como vagina, cérvix, útero e vulva podem estar ausentes ou hipoplásicas.

Adquiridas
- Estenoses e aderências — podem ser identificadas em qualquer lugar da vagina ou do vestíbulo; resultado de traumatismo e/ou inflamação prévios; é comum observar vaginite persistente; recusa a monta, distocia ou problemas com a micção como sequelas.
- Hiperplasia e prolapso vaginais.
- Neoplasia vaginal — geralmente leiomioma; costuma ser extraluminal na parede do vestíbulo; já foram relatados leiomiossarcomas, tumores venéreos transmissíveis, lipomas, mastocitomas, carcinomas epidermoides, carcinomas de células escamosas, fibromas, fibrossarcomas e carcinomas invasivos do trato urinário.
- Corpos estranhos — material de plantas, lascas de madeira e *swabs*; são ocasionalmente encontrados.

TRATAMENTO

CUIDADO(S) DE SAÚDE ADEQUADO(S)
- Em geral, o tratamento é feito em um esquema ambulatorial até que a natureza do defeito seja determinada.
- A paciente é internada para a realização de vaginografia com contraste positivo.

CUIDADO(S) DE ENFERMAGEM
Dilatação manual — com os dedos ou algum objeto rígido e liso; em pacientes com hímen imperfurado ou estenose vestibulovaginal leve, pode-se tentar tal procedimento; é possível efetuá-lo gradativamente em pacientes sedadas durante vários cursos terapêuticos; em pacientes anestesiadas, é possível executá-lo de uma única vez até a dilatação máxima; o sucesso é variável; tipicamente leva à redução, mas não à resolução completa, dos sinais clínicos; é improvável que resolva estenoses moderadas ou graves.

CONSIDERAÇÕES CIRÚRGICAS
- Ressecção, transecção, excisão — indicadas para muitas lesões congênitas (p. ex., hímen imperfurado e septos dorsoventrais pequenos) e adquiridas (pequenas estenoses ou aderências na porção caudal da vagina ou massas).
- Episiotomia — necessária geralmente para o acesso cirúrgico adequado.
- Vaginoplastia em formato de T — descrita em casos de estenose vestibulovaginal; a ressecção parece conferir as melhores chances de resolução, embora os resultados sejam variáveis.
- Ressecção completa do anel — para estenose vaginal.
- Ablação transendoscópica a laser — há um único relato desse procedimento para a correção de septo dorsoventral em uma cadela da raça Buldogue inglês que, subsequentemente, acasalou e pariu quatro filhotes por via vaginal.

- Ovário-histerectomia — indicada em pacientes sem valor reprodutivo; exibe sinais clínicos apenas durante o estro.
- Ablação da vagina (vaginectomia cranial ao orifício uretral externo) e ovário-histerectomia — também em pacientes sem valor reprodutivo; vaginite refratária, concomitante e grave em todas as fases do ciclo estral; estenose vaginal grave; tumores vaginais de base larga.

MEDICAÇÕES

MEDICAMENTO(S) DE ESCOLHA
- Vaginite concomitante — comum; em geral, desaparece com a correção do defeito anatômico; em condições graves, deve-se acelerar a resolução com o uso apropriado de terapia local e antibióticos (ver o capítulo sobre Vaginite).
- Lesões estenosadas — emprego de corticosteroides (prednisona: 1 mg/kg VO a cada 24 h), associados com a dilatação manual, na tentativa de evitar as recidivas; as taxas de recidivas são altas com ou sem o uso de esteroides.

ACOMPANHAMENTO

PREVENÇÃO
Lesões congênitas — possivelmente hereditárias, mas ainda não foram confirmadas; para uma linhagem familiar com número elevado de animais acometidos, recomenda-se a castração desses animais e de seus pais.

COMPLICAÇÕES POSSÍVEIS
- Distocia, infecções do trato urinário, incontinência e vaginite — em casos de más-formações vaginais; em pacientes irresponsivos ao tratamento.
- Estenoses e aderências — podem ser complicações pós-operatórias de procedimentos cirúrgicos planejados para a correção de anormalidades.

EVOLUÇÃO ESPERADA E PROGNÓSTICO
- Dependem da gravidade da lesão e do grau de inflamação depois do tratamento.
- Prognóstico após o tratamento de hímens imperfurados; bandas dorsoventrais curtas e estenoses ou aderências caudais — de razoável a bom quanto à melhora dos sinais clínicos; de razoável a reservado quanto à resolução completa dos sinais clínicos e ao retorno da fertilidade normal.
- Prognóstico em casos de constrições himenais, hipoplasia vaginal e estenoses ou aderências craniais graves — de reservado a mau quanto à resolução completa dos sinais clínicos e ao retorno da fertilidade normal; em casos de vaginite grave concomitante, a melhor recomendação é a ablação da vagina.

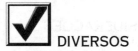

DIVERSOS

DISTÚRBIOS ASSOCIADOS
- Infecções do trato urinário.
- Vaginite.
- Incontinência urinária.

FATORES RELACIONADOS COM A IDADE
- Congênitas — mais prováveis em cadelas jovens em qualquer estado ovariano.
- Hiperplasia vaginal — mais provável em cadelas jovens intactas.
- Neoplasia da vagina ou do vestíbulo — mais provável em cadelas idosas em qualquer estado ovariano.

GESTAÇÃO/FERTILIDADE/REPRODUÇÃO
- Algumas pacientes podem ser "acasaladas" por meio de inseminação artificial; a possibilidade de parto vaginal é improvável sem a correção da anomalia.
- Alertar o proprietário quanto à provável necessidade de uma cesariana eletiva.

VER TAMBÉM
- Corrimento Vaginal.
- Hiperplasia e Prolapso Vaginais.
- Tumor Venéreo Transmissível.
- Vaginite.
- Tumores Vaginais.

Sugestões de Leitura
Crawford JT, Adams WM. Influence of vestibulovaginal stenosis, pelvic bladder, and recessed vulva on response to treatment for clinical signs of lower urinary tract disease in dogs: 38 cases (1990-1999). JAVMA 2002, 221(7):995-999.
Johnston SD, Root Kustritz MV, Olson PNS. Disorders of the canine vagina, vestibule, and vulva. In: Canine and Feline Theriogenology. Philadelphia: Saunders, 2001, pp. 225-242.
Johnston SD, Root Kustritz MV, Olson PNS. Disorders of the feline vagina, vestibule, and vulva. In: Canine and Feline Theriogenology. Philadelphia: Saunders, 2001, pp. 472-473.
Kyles AE, Vaden S, Hardie EM, Stone EA. Vestibulovaginal stenosis in dogs: 18 cases (1987-1995). JAVMA 1996, 209:1889-1893.
Lulich JP. Endoscopic vaginoscopy in the dog. Theriogenology 2006, 66(3):588-591.
Mathews KG. Surgery of the canine vagina and vulva. Vet Clin North Am Small Anim Pract 2001, 31(2):271-290.
Root MV, Johnston SD, Johnston GR. Vaginal septa in dogs: 15 cases (1983-1992). JAVMA 1995, 206:56-58.

Autor Sara K. Lyle
Consultor Editorial Sara K. Lyle

MASSAS BUCAIS

CONSIDERAÇÕES GERAIS

DEFINIÇÃO
• O crescimento da cavidade bucal pode ser benigno ou maligno.
• Quarta área mais comum de malignidade em cães e gatos.
• A maioria dos processos malignos bucais é localmente invasiva e lenta para sofrer metástase.

FISIOPATOLOGIA

Gato
• Carcinoma de células escamosas — faixa etária de 3 a 21 anos (média de 12 anos e meio); a região sublingual constitui o local mais comum; existem duas formas (tonsilar e não tonsilar); os sinais comumente apresentados incluem salivação excessiva e/ou sangramento provenientes da boca; com frequência, invade o tecido ósseo, provocando afrouxamento dos dentes; a morbidade e a mortalidade resultam de doença local e não de metástase à distância. Há uma especulação de que, possivelmente, haja uma associação viral.
• Fibrossarcomas — faixa etária de 1 a 21 anos (média de 10,3 anos); não há local de predileção específico; todos são associados à destruição tecidual local; ocasionalmente, observa-se invasão muscular e óssea.

Cão
• Epúlides são os tumores bucais benignos mais comuns; existem três tipos:
  ◦ Epúlide fibromatosa — comum em cães (e gatos); faixa etária de 1 a 17 anos (média de 7 anos e meio); existem tanto formas pedunculadas como sésseis; costumam ter superfície rosada e lisa.
  ◦ Fibroma odontogênico periférico (epúlide ossificante) — semelhante à epúlide fibromatosa, mas com matriz osteoide.
  ◦ Ameloblastoma acantomatoso (epúlide acantomatosa) — classificado como benigno, mas tende a invadir tecido ósseo adjacente, além de ser localmente agressivo.
• Melanoma maligno — o tumor maligno bucal mais comum no cão; as raças Cocker spaniel, Pastor alemão, Chow chow e cães com mucosas intensamente pigmentadas são predispostos; as massas podem ser amelanóticas; os machos são mais acometidos que as fêmeas. Ocorre em muitas regiões na cavidade bucal (o local mais comum em ordem de ocorrência é a mucosa gengival, mucosa bucal, lábios, língua e palato); além de ser localmente invasivo, sofre metástase para os pulmões e linfonodos regionais; as queixas comumente apresentadas são sangramento bucal, ptialismo ou halitose; o tamanho do tumor à apresentação é importante para a sobrevida do paciente; no cão, melanomas com <2 cm carreiam uma taxa de sobrevida melhor (média de 511 dias) do que aqueles com >2 cm (média de 164 dias); os tumores localizados rostralmente têm prognóstico melhor do que aqueles de localização distal.
• Carcinoma de células escamosas — a próxima malignidade bucal mais comum; origina-se do epitélio gengival; além de ser vermelho e ulcerado, pode ter projeções semelhantes à couve-flor; as raças caninas de grande porte são predispostas; o prognóstico depende da localização na cavidade bucal; os carcinomas localizados rostralmente carreiam um prognóstico melhor do que aqueles situados na base da língua ou nas tonsilas; as lesões nos lábios e na mucosa bucal possuem um baixo índice metastático; as lesões gengivais facilmente se infiltram no osso subjacente; as lesões na língua (em virtude do movimento) e nas tonsilas tendem a sofrer metástase e são as mais agressivas.
• Carcinoma papilar de células escamosas — um tumor de crescimento rápido em filhotes caninos (<1 ano); localizado na gengiva papilar; localmente agressivo, mas não sofre metástase; o tratamento de escolha é a excisão. Há especulação de que o carcinoma papilar de células escamosas esteja associado ao papilomavírus.
• Fibrossarcoma — a terceira malignidade bucal mais comum em cães (e a segunda mais comum em gatos); os fibrossarcomas apresentam predileção pelo maxilar de cães machos e idosos de grande porte; a gengiva é mais comumente acometida, sobretudo em torno do quarto pré-molar maxilar, seguido pelo palato duro e pela mucosa bucal; embora sejam lentamente invasivos, raramente sofrem metástase.
• Tumores do epitélio laminar dentário — originam-se de células epiteliais da lâmina dentária; formam-se a partir do epitélio dentário durante o desenvolvimento ou podem se originar de ninhos de células epiteliais que mantêm a capacidade de atuar como lâmina dentária.
• Ameloblastoma — o tumor mais comum do epitélio laminar dentário em cães; comporta-se como tumores lentamente expansíveis que ocorrem em camadas profundas dentro do osso; pode ser cístico ou sólido.
• Osteossarcoma — ocorre principalmente em cães de meia-idade de médio a grande porte. A invasão óssea local resulta em tumefação facial significativa, além de ser localmente invasivo com baixo índice metastático.
• Odontoma complexo — tumor benigno raro constituído de componentes dentários desorganizados não formadores de estruturas semelhantes a dentes. Embora não sofra metástase, esse tipo de tumor é localmente destrutivo e envolvido por cápsula cística.
• Odontoma composto — semelhante aos odontomas complexos com a exceção de que o odontoma composto é constituído de componentes dentários organizados formadores de estruturas semelhantes a dentes.
• Plasmocitoma — origem nos plasmócitos; ocorre principalmente em cães mais idosos; além de ter caráter agressivo, pode sofrer metástase.
• Outros tipos de tumor incluem carcinoma indiferenciado, linfoma, fibroma, melanocitoma, papiloma, mastocitoma, tumor de células gigantes, neurofibroma, mixofibrossarcoma e rabdomiossarcoma.

SISTEMA(S) ACOMETIDO(S)
Gastrintestinal — cavidade bucal.

GENÉTICA
N/D.

INCIDÊNCIA/PREVALÊNCIA
• As massas bucais não são raras. Variam com o tipo de massa. Ver a seção "Fisiopatologia".
• A cavidade bucal é a quarta região mais comum para a localização de tumor em cães e gatos.

DISTRIBUIÇÃO GEOGRÁFICA
Nenhuma.

IDENTIFICAÇÃO

Espécies
Cães e gatos.

Raça(s) Predominante(s)
As raças Golden retriever, Pointer alemão de pelo curto, Weimaraner, São Bernardo e Cocker spaniel são mais propensas a tumores bucais; já as raças Dachshund e Beagle são menos propensas a tumores bucais; Boxer é predisposto à hiperplasia gengival.

Idade Média e Faixa Etária
• Os animais mais idosos são acometidos com maior frequência.
• Odontoma complexo, odontoma composto, papiloma e carcinoma papilar de células escamosas costumam ocorrer em cães com menos de 2 anos de idade.

Sexo Predominante
• Os machos costumam ser mais acometidos por melanomas e fibrossarcomas bucais do que as fêmeas.
• Os osteossarcomas são mais comuns nas fêmeas que nos machos.

SINAIS CLÍNICOS

Achados Anamnésicos
• Perda de peso.
• Anorexia.
• Consegue comer apenas alimentos pastosos.
• Relutância ou dor à mastigação.
• Mastiga apenas de um lado.

Achados do Exame Físico
• Com frequência, o animal encontra-se assintomático.
• Halitose.
• Deslocamento dos dentes.
• Maloclusão.
• Hemorragia bucal.
• Disfagia.
• Salivação anormal.
• Incapacidade de abrir ou fechar a boca.
• Simetria facial anormal.
• Tumefação facial.
• Relutância ao toque da cabeça.
• Mobilidade dos dentes.
• Perda de dentes.

CAUSAS
• Desconhecidas.
• Papiloma — papilomavírus.

FATORES DE RISCO
• O carcinoma tonsilar de células escamosas ocorre dez vezes mais comumente em cães de ambientes urbanos do que nos rurais.
• Carcinoma de células escamosas — mais prevalente em cães de pelagem branca em um único estudo.
• Qualquer irritação bucal crônica (doença periodontal, tabagismo passivo) aumenta o risco de desenvolvimento de tumor bucal.
• Papilomas virais podem se tornar malignos e se transformar em carcinoma de células escamosas.
• Há relatos de que os vírus FeLV, FIV ou FSV possam desempenhar um papel no desenvolvimento de carcinoma de células escamosas.
• Alguns pesquisadores demonstraram que os gatos que utilizavam coleiras antipulgas tinham um risco 5 vezes maior de desenvolver carcinoma bucal de células escamosas do que aqueles que não faziam uso desse dispositivo preventivo.
• O tabagismo passivo pode estar associado ao desenvolvimento de carcinoma de células escamosas em gatos.
• Os cães (filhotes) imunossuprimidos são mais comumente acometidos por papilomas.

M

MASSAS BUCAIS

• Muito raramente, o ameloblastoma acantomatoso pode se transformar em carcinoma de células escamosas com radioterapia.

DIAGNÓSTICO

DIAGNÓSTICO DIFERENCIAL
• Infecção — viral/bacteriana/fúngica.
• Odontoma.
• Cisto dentígero.
• Cisto radicular.
• Granuloma apical.
• Pólipos nasofaríngeos.
• Granuloma eosinofílico.
• Calcinose circunscrita.
• Hiperplasia gengival proliferativa.
• Ulceração bucal (úlceras urêmicas, doença autoimune, síndrome do mastigador de gengiva).
• Hipercementose.
• Granuloma apical.
• Rânula.
• Tonsilite.
• Estomatite linfoplasmocitária.

HEMOGRAMA/BIOQUÍMICA/URINÁLISE
Exames utilizados para descartar outras complicações primárias ou secundárias; p. ex., anemia, uremia.

OUTROS TESTES LABORATORIAIS
O estadiamento molecular de melanomas malignos pode ser obtido, fazendo-se a triagem de aspirados de linfonodos em busca do RNAm de antígenos associados ao melanoma; tal estadiamento ajuda na detecção de doença metastática.

DIAGNÓSTICO POR IMAGEM
• Radiografias da mandíbula acometida para avaliar a presença de invasão óssea e dos pulmões para verificar a ocorrência de metástases (obter, no mínimo, três projeções: ventrodorsal, lateral direita e lateral esquerda).
• RM ou TC da área da massa para determinar a extensão e o grau da lesão.
• RM fornece informações mais precisas a respeito do tamanho das massas e da invasão de estruturas adjacentes. Como os melanomas têm um sinal hiperintenso nas imagens ponderadas em T1 e um sinal hipointenso nas imagens ponderadas em T2, o exame de RM facilita a identificação da extensão do crescimento local.
• TC fornece imagens melhores de calcificação e erosão óssea cortical. As imagens de TC podem ser acentuadas com o uso de meio de contraste (p. ex., ioexol) para delinear o tumor.

MÉTODOS DIAGNÓSTICOS
Aspirado, biopsia ou remoção cirúrgica de linfonodos regionais infartados para exame citológico e/ou histológico em busca de metástases.

ACHADOS PATOLÓGICOS
• É imprescindível a realização de biopsia; obter amostra de camadas teciduais profundas que circundam a massa; utilizar as técnicas de excisão, biopsia em cunha ou biopsia com *punch* (saca-bocado).
• A citologia também pode ser valiosa, porém não é tão definitiva quanto a histopatologia.

TRATAMENTO

CUIDADO(S) DE SAÚDE ADEQUADO(S)
• Depende do tipo de tumor.
• Tumores benignos são passíveis de tratamento a longo prazo mediante cirurgia e, algumas vezes, com radioterapia.
• Tumores malignos são tratados de forma cirúrgica, obtendo-se sucesso variável, dependendo do tipo e da localização do tumor, bem como da ocorrência de metástase à apresentação.
• Em circunstâncias avançadas, a terapia combinada (cirurgia, quimioterapia e radiação) pode proporcionar os melhores cuidados ao paciente.
• Terapias de alvo molecular fornecem aos oncologistas ferramentas para o tratamento de cânceres com maior especificidade. Essas modalidades podem ser utilizadas para classificar os tumores, auxiliar na predição do prognóstico e ajudar a determinar o plano terapêutico exato.

CUIDADO(S) DE ENFERMAGEM
• Controle da dor.
• Cuidados de suporte.

ATIVIDADE
N/D.

DIETA
O suporte nutricional é essencial em qualquer plano terapêutico. Para um suporte nutricional adequado, talvez haja necessidade da colocação de tubo via gastrostomia, esofagostomia ou tubo percutâneo via gastrostomia ou nasogástrico.

ORIENTAÇÃO AO PROPRIETÁRIO
N/D.

CONSIDERAÇÕES CIRÚRGICAS/RADIOTERÁPICAS/QUIMIOTERÁPICAS
• O diagnóstico e o tratamento precoces oferecem as melhores chances de um desfecho bem-sucedido.
• A primeira ressecção cirúrgica também confere a melhor oportunidade de ressecção completa.
• Excisão completa em bloco é o tratamento de escolha, com as margens cirúrgicas variando de 1 a 2 cm, dependendo do tipo de tumor.
• A radioterapia deve ser oferecida nos casos em que a excisão completa não é possível e/ou a massa está localizada na face caudal da cavidade bucal e impede a excisão cirúrgica completa.
• Radioterapia de megavoltagem é considerada atualmente o padrão de cuidado para o tratamento de tumores bucais; no entanto, a radioterapia de intensidade modulada é uma tecnologia relativamente nova, que está sendo adotada com rapidez.
• A quimioterapia é justificada em sarcomas bucais de células redondas ou em malignidades metastáticas de alto grau.
• Papiloma — excisão marginal é o tratamento de escolha (principalmente para avaliação histológica a fim de descartar outras formas de tumores); a maioria apresenta regressão espontânea com o tempo; no entanto, o uso de vacinas autógenas é um tratamento eficaz, especialmente quando as massas estão comprometendo a mastigação.
• Epúlide fibromatosa — a excisão marginal é o tratamento de escolha; a aplicação de crioterapia e radiação também confere sucesso a longo prazo.
• Fibroma odontogênico periférico (epúlide ossificante) — tratar da mesma forma que a epúlide fibromatosa.
• Ameloblastoma acantomatoso — a excisão com margens de, no mínimo, 1 cm costuma ser curativa; a radiação também é utilizada com êxito; a combinação de cirurgia e radiação pode ser mais eficaz (necessitando de cirurgia menos agressiva); no entanto, se a radiação não estiver prontamente disponível, a cirurgia poderá ser a única opção terapêutica; a cirurgia deve ser rigorosa, com margens de 2 cm nos casos em que as margens são pouco definidas e naqueles em que a ressecção é possível; as melhores chances de resolver o problema de forma cirúrgica estão na primeira vez; extrair qualquer dente que possa impedir a cicatrização incisional; se o tumor recidivar, sua natureza será mais agressiva; há relatos de que o ameloblastoma acantomatoso recidive como o carcinoma de células escamosas. Múltiplas injeções (10) de bleomicina (5 mg) realizadas no local do tumor foram eficazes em um pequeno número de casos relatados.
• Melanoma maligno — o prognóstico será melhor se o tumor for pequeno e se estiver localizado na parte rostral da mandíbula; se a cirurgia for a terapia escolhida, ela deverá ser rigorosa; tipicamente, são realizados os procedimentos de mandibulectomia ou maxilectomia; tempos médios de sobrevida em torno de 8 meses; a combinação de cirurgia, radiação e quimioterapia (cisplatina em doses baixas) conferiu sobrevida média de 14 meses em um único estudo; a pigmentação não afeta o prognóstico; relativamente radiorresistente; um único estudo demonstrou tempo de sobrevida média de 14 meses após a radiação isolada; o problema com o melanoma não é o tratamento da doença local, mas sim da metástase; pesquisas indicam que a vacinação é uma cura promissora. A vacina formulada com base no DNA é indicada para os melanomas malignos de estágio II-III, segundo a classificação de tumor, nodo e metástase, após a obtenção de controle cirúrgico local. Foi demonstrado que os análogos de platina utilizados isoladamente como monoterapia ou combinados com piroxicam tenham atividade antitumoral nos casos de melanoma maligno.
• Carcinoma de células escamosas — prognóstico melhor a longo prazo do que o melanoma maligno ou o fibrossarcoma no cão; poderá ser amplamente excisado por meio cirúrgico ou irradiado no cão, sobretudo se a lesão for rostral (prognóstico melhor do que aqueles localizados caudalmente); realizar maxilectomia ou mandibulectomia com margem cirúrgica livre de tumor de 2 cm como objetivo; nos cães, apenas a radiação confere taxa de sobrevida média de 15-17 meses; nos cães, o prognóstico quanto à sobrevida após o tratamento dos casos com envolvimento lingual é mau; os cães toleram o procedimento de glossotomia parcial com envolvimento de 40-60% da língua; para tumores maiores do que 2 cm ou aqueles submetidos a ressecções incompletas, os procedimentos de cirurgia, radiação e quimioterapia (mitoxantrona ou cisplatina com piroxicam) podem ser as melhores opções. Em gatos, a ressecção cirúrgica confere uma taxa de sobrevida média de 2 meses. Pode-se usar a carboplatina ou a mitoxantrona para o tratamento paliativo. A radioterapia local juntamente com aminobisfosfonato é considerada um tratamento

MASSAS BUCAIS

paliativo satisfatório para os gatos com carcinoma de células escamosas.
- Fibrossarcoma — a excisão cirúrgica com margem de, no mínimo, 2 cm resulta, em geral, em taxa de sobrevida média de 12 meses; geralmente, há necessidade de maxilectomia ou mandibulectomia; a excisão cirúrgica em combinação com radio e quimioterapia oferece o melhor prognóstico; a radiação ou a quimioterapia isoladas confere uma taxa de sobrevida média mais baixa do que somente a cirurgia; os fibrossarcomas palatinos carreiam o pior prognóstico, em função da impossibilidade de ressecção cirúrgica. A radioterapia pode ser útil após a remoção cirúrgica.
- Osteossarcoma — o ideal é a ampla remoção cirúrgica com margens de 2 cm. Nos locais de metástase, pode ocorrer recidiva. A radioterapia deve ser considerada após a cirurgia para doença microscópica. A radioterapia paliativa pode ser utilizada isoladamente.
- Plasmocitoma — raro; responde por 5% dos tumores bucais no cão; apesar de serem localmente agressivos, raramente sofrem metástase. A remoção cirúrgica é o tratamento de escolha.
- Odontoma complexo/composto — a ressecção cirúrgica em bloco será curativa se todas as estruturas forem removidas. A cirurgia pode ser muito extensa, sendo imprescindível a remoção das paredes císticas do tumor.

MEDICAÇÕES

MEDICAMENTO(S) DE ESCOLHA
Agentes quimioterápicos (ver a seção "Considerações Cirúrgicas/Radioterápicas/Quimioterápicas).

CONTRAINDICAÇÕES
N/D.

PRECAUÇÕES
N/D.

INTERAÇÕES POSSÍVEIS
N/D.

MEDICAMENTO(S) ALTERNATIVO(S)
N/D.

ACOMPANHAMENTO

MONITORIZAÇÃO DO PACIENTE
Varia com a natureza da massa.

PREVENÇÃO
Remover ou tratar qualquer irritação bucal.

COMPLICAÇÕES POSSÍVEIS
- A remoção cirúrgica de parte da língua poderá resultar em necrose avascular se a língua for transeccionada em posição imediatamente caudal à origem dos ramos dorsais das artérias linguais.
- As complicações pós-operatórias da mandibulectomia incluem deiscência da ferida, disfunção da preensão, enfraquecimento da língua, desvio medial da língua, salivação excessiva, ulceração do palato secundária à maloclusão e necrose por compressão.
- As mandibulectomias podem ser realizadas em gatos, mas resultam em maiores complicações (tumefação da língua, formação de rânula) do que nos cães. Esse tipo de cirurgia pode culminar em complicações estéticas.
- Nas primeiras semanas, a radioterapia em baixas doses pode causar diarreia, náusea, vômito e perda de pelo (a repilação costuma ser branca); altas doses geram os mesmos efeitos colaterais mencionados, bem como ulceração/necrose bucal, mucosite, cataratas (essas lesões ocorrem em quase todos os casos e são autolimitantes com os cuidados de suporte) e tumores induzidos pela radiação (principalmente em cães jovens submetidos à radioterapia para tumores responsivos a esse tipo de tratamento). Apesar de serem improváveis, podem ocorrer efeitos tardios da radiação com necrose óssea e muscular. A radioterapia de intensidade modulada confere uma distribuição mais precisa da dose e, por essa razão, está sendo rapidamente aceita como a melhor forma de radioterapia com poucos efeitos colaterais.
- As complicações da quimioterapia são variadas, dependendo do medicamento utilizado.

EVOLUÇÃO ESPERADA E PROGNÓSTICO
- É provável que os cães com margens cirúrgicas inadequadas livres do tumor tenham uma probabilidade 2,5 vezes maior de morrer do tumor do que aqueles submetidos à excisão cirúrgica completa; alguns pacientes cirúrgicos necessitam de sonda de gastrostomia para facilitar a suplementação nutricional durante o período de tratamento.
- Cães com tumores localizados em posição caudal ao primeiro pré-molar apresentavam um risco 3 vezes maior de morrer da doença do que aqueles com tumores situados em posição rostral ao primeiro pré-molar.
- A vacinação de cães com melanoma maligno parece ser curativa, além de ser oferecida em diversas regiões na América do Norte.
- O estadiamento de tumores bucais utilizando o sistema de classificação TNM (tumor primário, linfonodos distantes regionais {cervical, submandibular e parotídeo} e metástase) possibilita a formulação de um prognóstico com maior precisão; quanto mais alto o estágio (I-IV), pior será o prognóstico.
- Os fibrossarcomas possuem 4 tipos histológicos: uma malignidade de baixo grau (prognóstico melhor), uma malignidade intermediária, uma malignidade de alto grau e um fibrossarcoma de baixo grau ao exame histológico, porém alto grau em termos biológicos, que é relatado em raças caninas de grande porte (principalmente Golden retriever) e apresenta um prognóstico mau em virtude de seu rápido crescimento e metástase.

DIVERSOS

DISTÚRBIOS ASSOCIADOS
N/D.

FATORES RELACIONADOS COM A IDADE
N/D.

POTENCIAL ZOONÓTICO
Nenhum.

GESTAÇÃO/FERTILIDADE/REPRODUÇÃO
N/D.

ABREVIATURA(S)
- FeLV = vírus da leucemia felina.
- FIV = vírus da imunodeficiência felina.
- FSV = vírus do sarcoma felino.
- RM = ressonância magnética.
- TC = tomografia computadorizada.

Sugestões de leitura
Ettinger SJ, Feldman EC. Textbook of Veterinary Internal Medicine, 7th ed. St Louis: Saunders Elsevier, 2010.
Fosum T. Small Animal Surgery, 3rd ed. St Louis: Mosby Elsevier, 2007.
Harvey CE, Emily PP. Small Animal Dentistry. Philadelphia: Mosby, 1993.
Nelson RW, Couto CG. Small Animal Internal Medicine, 3rd ed. St Louis: Mosby, 2003.
Meuten DJ. Tumors in Domestic Animals. Ames: Iowa State University Press, 2002.
Wiggs RB, Lobprise HB. Veterinary Dentistry: Principles and Practice. Philadelphia: Lippincott-Raven, 1997.

Autor James M.G. Anthony
Consultor Editorial Heidi B. Lobprise

MASTITE

CONSIDERAÇÕES GERAIS

REVISÃO
- Infecção bacteriana de uma ou mais glândulas lactantes.
- Resultado de infecção ascendente, traumatismo à glândula ou disseminação hematógena.
- *Escherichia coli*, estafilococos, e estreptococos β-hemolíticos — mais comumente envolvidos.
- Infecção potencialmente letal; pode levar a choque séptico.
- Sepse — efeito direto das glândulas mamárias com envolvimento sistêmico.

IDENTIFICAÇÃO
- Cadela e gata após o parto.
- Cadela ou gata (raro) lactante pseudoprenhe.

SINAIS CLÍNICOS
Achados Anamnésicos
- Anorexia.
- Letargia.
- Negligência dos filhotes caninos e felinos.
- Falha de desenvolvimento dos filhotes de ambas as espécies.

Achados do Exame Físico
- Glândula(s) mamária(s) firme(s), tumefata(s), quente(s) e dolorosa(s), das quais pode ser espremido um líquido purulento ou hemorrágico.
- Febre, desidratação e choque séptico — com envolvimento sistêmico.
- Podem resultar em formação de abscesso ou ocorrência de gangrena da(s) glândula(s).

CAUSAS E FATORES DE RISCO
- Infecção ascendente via canais do teto.
- Traumatismo infligido pelas unhas e pelos dentes dos filhotes caninos e felinos.
- Más condições de higiene.
- Infecção sistêmica, que se origina em outra parte do corpo (p. ex., metrite).

DIAGNÓSTICO

DIAGNÓSTICO DIFERENCIAL
- Galactostase — sem doença sistêmica; exame citológico e cultura do leite auxiliam na diferenciação.
- Adenocarcinoma mamário inflamatório — a glândula acometida não produz leite; diferenciado por biopsia.

HEMOGRAMA/BIOQUÍMICA/URINÁLISE
- Leucocitose com desvio à esquerda.
- Leucopenia — com sepse.
- Hematócrito, proteína total e ureia levemente elevados — com desidratação.

DIAGNÓSTICO POR IMAGEM
- Ultrassonografia revela perda da camada de distinção do tecido normal nas glândulas.
- Doppler colorido pode ajudar no estabelecimento do prognóstico — a perda dos vasos sanguíneos em áreas inflamadas prediz uma evolução para gangrena.

OUTROS TESTES LABORATORIAIS
Cultura e sensibilidade do leite obtido das glândulas acometidas; é recomendável a realização de triagem quanto à presença de *Staphylococcus aureus* resistente à meticilina.

MÉTODOS DIAGNÓSTICOS
Leite — normalmente um pouco mais ácido do que o soro; pode ficar alcalino com a infecção; citologia: neutrófilos, macrófagos e outras células mononucleares podem ser observadas em número elevado no leite normal; observa-se a presença de grande número de bactérias livres e fagocitadas, bem como neutrófilos degenerados, na doença séptica; cultura bacteriana para identificar o microrganismo.

TRATAMENTO
- Paciente internada até a estabilização.
- Filhotes caninos e felinos — pode ser permitido que os neonatos continuem mamando a menos que as glândulas estejam necrosadas ou a fêmea esteja com doença sistêmica; afeta a escolha dos antibióticos; monitorizar o ganho de peso em neonatos: os filhotes caninos devem ganhar 10% de seu peso ao nascimento por dia, enquanto os filhotes felinos devem recuperar de 7-10 g/dia no mínimo.
- Desidratação ou sepse — fluidoterapia intravenosa.
- Correção dos distúrbios eletrolíticos e da hipoglicemia.
- Tratamento do choque, se indicado.
- Aplicação de compressas mornas e ordenha da(s) glândula(s) acometida(s) várias vezes ao dia.
- Aplicação de curativos com folhas de couve sobre as glândulas acometidas pode acelerar a resolução do quadro.
- Glândulas com abscesso ou gangrena — necessitam de debridamento cirúrgico.

MEDICAÇÕES

MEDICAMENTO(S)
- Leite ácido — bases fracas; eritromicina (10 mg/kg VO a cada 8 h, cadelas e gatas) ou lincomicina (15 mg/kg VO a cada 8 h, cadelas e gatas).
- Leite alcalino — ácidos fracos; amoxicilina ou cefalosporina (20 mg/kg a cada 8 h, cadelas e gatas).
- Leite alcalino ou ácido — cloranfenicol (40-50 mg/kg VO a cada 8 h) e enrofloxacino (2,5 mg/kg a cada 12 h).
- Pode-se fazer infusão da(s) glândula(s) acometida(s) com solução de Betadine® a 1% por meio de cânula lacrimal.
- Cabergolina (5 μg/kg VO a cada 24 h, 5-7 dias) para suprimir a lactação nas glândulas acometidas em pacientes com sepse; os neonatos devem ser criados manualmente.

CONTRAINDICAÇÕES/INTERAÇÕES POSSÍVEIS
Deixe a paciente amamentar — evitar tetraciclina, enrofloxacino e cloranfenicol; pode-se fazer uso de cefalosporinas, amoxicilina e amoxicilina com ácido clavulânico.

ACOMPANHAMENTO

MONITORIZAÇÃO DA PACIENTE
- Exame físico e hemograma completo.
- Avaliação ultrassonográfica repetida ajuda a avaliar a cura — aparecerá uma camada normal de diferenciação dos tecidos com a recuperação do quadro.

PREVENÇÃO
- Limpeza do ambiente.
- Tricotomia dos pelos ao redor das glândulas mamárias.
- Corte das unhas dos filhotes caninos e felinos.
- Medidas para garantir a amamentação dos neonatos em todas as glândulas.

COMPLICAÇÕES POSSÍVEIS
- Abscesso ou gangrena — pode causar a perda da(s) glândula(s).
- Filhotes caninos e felinos criados manualmente — requer um considerável comprometimento por parte do proprietário.

EVOLUÇÃO ESPERADA E PROGNÓSTICO
Prognóstico — bom com o tratamento.

DIVERSOS

RECURSOS DA INTERNET
England G, Yeager A, Colcannon PW. Ultrasound imaging of the reproductive tract of the bitch. In: Colcannon PW, England G, Verstegen III J, Linde-Forsberg C, eds., Recent Advances in Small Animal Reproduction. International Veterinary Information Service, Ithaca NY, www.ivis.org, última atualização: 21-Jul-2003; A1203.0703.

Sugestões de Leitura
Johnston SD, Root Kustritz MV, Olson PNS. Periparturient disorders in the bitch. In: Johnston SD, Root Kustritz MV, Olson PNS, eds., Canine and Feline Theriogenology. Philadelphia: Saunders, 2001, pp. 131-134.
Olson JD, Olson PN. Disorders of the canine mammary gland. In: Morrow DA, ed., Current Therapy in Theriogenology 2. Philadelphia: Saunders, 1986, pp. 506-509.
Trasch K, Wehrend A, Bostedt H. Ultrasonographic description of canine mastitis. Vet Radiol Ultrasound 2007, 48(6):580-584.
Wiebe VJ, Howard JP. Pharmacologic advances in canine and feline reproduction. Top Companion Anim Med 2009, 24(2):71-99.

Autor Joni L. Freshman
Consultor Editorial Sara K. Lyle

MASTOCITOMAS

CONSIDERAÇÕES GERAIS

DEFINIÇÃO
• Células redondas malignas de origem hematopoiética, contendo grânulos repletos de inúmeras substâncias vasoativas, incluindo histamina, heparina, serotonina, dopamina, triptase e quimase.
• Tumor cutâneo maligno mais comum no cão, representando aproximadamente 7-21% de todos os tumores cutâneos caninos.
• Os tumores podem afetar a derme, o subcutâneo, o baço, o fígado e os intestinos.

FISIOPATOLOGIA
• A liberação de histamina dos mastocitomas afeta uma grande variedade de tecidos.
• Como os receptores histaminérgicos H_2 estão localizados principalmente dentro do estômago, acredita-se que a histamina seja um dos estimulantes mais significativos da secreção de ácido gástrico.
• Em casos extremos, pode ocorrer a perfuração do trato gastrintestinal, levando à peritonite.
• A liberação de histamina em torno de um tumor leva à produção de pápulas, urticárias e eritemas.
• A liberação local de heparina também é comum, resultando em sangramento e subsequente equimose, o que pode ser observado ao redor do tumor.

SISTEMA(S) ACOMETIDO(S)
• Cutâneo — os mastocitomas constituem o tumor cutâneo maligno mais comum do cão.
• Gastrintestinal — em avaliação à necropsia, 35-83% dos cães com mastocitomas têm indícios de ulceração gastrintestinal.
• Hemático/linfático/imune — é comum a ocorrência de metástases para os linfonodos em tumores de alto grau. Apesar de raras, podem ocorrer metástases para a medula óssea.
• Hepatobiliar — o fígado e o baço são locais comuns de metástases à distância para mastocitomas de alto grau.

GENÉTICA
As predileções raciais específicas indicam a existência de alguma predisposição genética.

INCIDÊNCIA/PREVALÊNCIA
• Tumor cutâneo maligno mais comum no cão, representando cerca de 7-21% de todos os tumores caninos de pele.
• Os mastocitomas intestinais e viscerais primários são raros no cão.
• Segundo tumor cutâneo mais comum no gato, respondendo por 20% dos tumores cutâneos.
• Tumores esplênicos mais comuns de gatos, compreendendo metade dos mastocitomas diagnosticados nessa espécie.

IDENTIFICAÇÃO
Espécies
Cães e gatos.
Raça(s) Predominante(s)
• Cães — raças braquicefálicas, bem como Golden retriever, Labrador, Rhodesian ridgeback, Beagle, Staffordshire terrier, Weimaraner, Shar-pei e Boiadeiro australiano.
• Gatos — Siamês.

Idade Média e Faixa Etária
• Cães — animais de meia-idade, faixa de 4 meses a 18 anos de idade.
• Gatos — animais de meia-idade (8-9 anos para tipos mastocíticos cutâneos) e mais idosos (tumor intestinal e esplênico); no entanto, a forma histiocítica de mastocitomas cutâneos afeta gatos jovens com uma idade média de 2,4 anos.

Sexo Predominante
• Cães — sem predileção.
• Gatos — macho Siamês.

SINAIS CLÍNICOS
Cães
• Pode ser encontrada a presença de massa no subcutâneo ou na pele; também pode estar presente dentro de lipomas.
• Pode ser observada a formação de edema regional ou o sinal de Darier na região em torno do tumor que sofreu degranulação.
• Em cães com doença metastática, pode-se constatar linfadenopatia de linfonodos regionais.
• Histórico de evolução intermitente e regressão de tamanho.
• Sinais sistêmicos com doença local ou sistêmica avançada: vômito, anorexia, perda de peso e melena.

Gatos
• A doença visceral manifesta-se sob a forma de perda de peso crônica, anorexia, diarreia e letargia.
• Em casos de mastocitoma intestinal primário, pode-se palpar lesão expansiva focal.

CAUSAS
• Receptor tirosina quinase, mutação c-kit.
• Receptor associado ao crescimento e desenvolvimento de mastócitos.
• Foi demonstrado que até 30% dos mastocitomas contenham uma mutação no oncogene c-kit, induzindo a um receptor constitutivamente ativado e uma divisão celular descontrolada.

FATORES DE RISCO
Ver as seções "Raças Predominantes" e "Causas".

DIAGNÓSTICO

DIAGNÓSTICO DIFERENCIAL
• Formas cutâneas — tumores de anexos, basaliomas, histiocitoma, lipoma e sarcoma de tecidos moles.
• Formas viscerais — linfoma, tumores histiocíticos, histiocitomas fibrosos malignos, mieloma múltiplo, hemangiossarcoma, hemangioma e hiperplasia mieloide eritroide.
• Formas intestinais — linfoma, adenocarcinoma, leiomioma, leiomiossarcoma, tumores do estroma gastrintestinal e infecções fúngicas.

HEMOGRAMA/BIOQUÍMICA/URINÁLISE
• Anemia (regenerativa secundária à perda sanguínea gastrintestinal).
• Eosinofilia, mastocitose e trombocitopenia.
• Identificação de mastócitos circulantes é mais comum no gato com mastocitoma visceral do que no cão.
• Níveis elevados de ureia secundários a sangramento gastrintestinal e elevação dos valores hepáticos secundária à metástase.

OUTROS TESTES LABORATORIAIS
• Exame da camada leucocitária em gatos com mastocitoma visceral e intestinal.
• Aspirado e citologia de linfonodos regionais.

DIAGNÓSTICO POR IMAGEM
• Radiografias torácicas — pesquisa de metástases intratorácicas ou para linfonodos esternais.
• Ultrassonografia abdominal — avaliação visceral com ênfase em órgãos como fígado, baço e linfonodos mesentéricos.

MÉTODOS DIAGNÓSTICOS
• Exame citológico de aspirado por agulha fina para obtenção do diagnóstico definitivo.
• Biopsia (incisional ou excisional) para formulação do diagnóstico definitivo e classificação histológica do tumor.

ACHADOS PATOLÓGICOS
• Cães — escala de classificação de Patnaik:
  ○ Tumores de grau I (grau baixo) apresentam um comportamento principalmente benigno e representam ~36%.
  ○ Tumores de grau II (grau intermediário) constituem a forma mais comum e representam ~43%.
  ○ Tumores de grau III (grau elevado) correspondem à forma mais agressiva, são metastáticos e representam ~20%.
• Gatos — formas histológicas de mastocitomas cutâneos:
  ○ Forma mastocítica — tumor isolado, além de ser a forma mais comum (compacta ou difusa). Existem duas variedades histológicas de mastocitomas mastocíticos no gato:
    ○ Compactas — comportamento mais benigno.
    ○ Difusas — mais indiferenciado e agressivo.
• Forma histiocítica — múltiplas lesões sobre a cabeça e o pescoço com comportamento relativamente benigno.

TRATAMENTO

CUIDADO(S) DE SAÚDE ADEQUADO(S)
N/D.

CUIDADO(S) DE ENFERMAGEM
N/D.

ATIVIDADE
Restrita para os animais com cargas tumorais maciças (como gatos com mastocitomas viscerais ou cães com tumores volumosos) até que a massa seja submetida a tratamento apropriado.

DIETA
N/D.

ORIENTAÇÃO AO PROPRIETÁRIO
Os proprietários de cães com mastocitomas devem ser informados de que 14-17% dos cães desenvolverão outros mastocitomas. Todas as massas recentes devem ser avaliadas por um veterinário.

CONSIDERAÇÕES CIRÚRGICAS
• Recomendações convencionais (cães) — margens de 2-3 cm e um único plano fascial profundo, talvez sejam desnecessários em mastocitomas de grau II nos cães, pois a maioria das margens "sujas" não volta a crescer localmente.
• Margens estreitas (gatos) — grande parte dos tumores não voltará a crescer, seguindo margens cirúrgicas estreitas.
• Esplenectomia (gatos) — recomendada em gatos com carga tumoral visceral maciça apesar da presença de metástases.

MASTOCITOMAS

RADIOTERAPIA
• Para mastocitomas submetidos à excisão incompleta em locais não acessíveis à nova excisão cirúrgica ou nos casos em que não há possibilidade de outra cirurgia (cães).
• Pode ser utilizada em doença macroscópica, embora seja possível a ocorrência de reações sistêmicas graves (inclusive óbito).

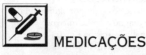

MEDICAÇÕES

MEDICAMENTO(S) DE ESCOLHA
Cães
• Vimblastina (2,3 mg/m^2 IV a cada 7 dias por 4 vezes e, em seguida, a cada 14 dias por mais 4 vezes) e prednisona (1 mg/kg VO a cada 24 h).
• Apenas vimblastina (3,5 mg/m^2 IV a cada 14 dias).
• Lomustina (50-70 mg/m^2 VO a cada 21 dias).
• Torcerinibe (2,75-3,25 mg/kg VO, dependendo da extensão da doença).
• Masitinibe (12,5 mg/kg VO a cada 24 h).

Gatos
• Lomustina (48-65 mg/m^2 VO a cada 4-6 semanas).
• Vimblastina (2 mg/m^2 IV a cada 7 dias por 4 vezes e, em seguida, a cada 14 dias por mais 4 vezes) e prednisona (1 mg/kg VO a cada 24 h).

CONTRAINDICAÇÃO E PRECAUÇÕES
• Vimblastina — utilizar com cuidado em animais com hepatopatia; esse agente também é mielossupressor e possui propriedades vesicantes.
• Lomustina — é hepatotóxica, devendo ser evitada em cães com hepatopatia subjacente; esse medicamento é extremamente mielossupressor e associado à trombocitopenia refratária. Administrar com Denamarin® (protetor hepático).
• Torcerinibe e masitinibe — podem causar úlceras gastrintestinais, mielossupressão, dor muscular e desarranjo gastrintestinal.

INTERAÇÕES POSSÍVEIS
• Torcerinibe e masitinibe devem ser utilizados com cuidado em combinação com outros medicamentos que induzam a úlceras gástricas, como prednisona ou AINE, ou nos pacientes com ulceração gástrica secundária ao mastocitoma.
• Também se deve ter cuidado com o uso da lomustina com outros agentes hepatotóxicos, como AINE.

MEDICAMENTO(S) ALTERNATIVO(S)
Tratamento sintomático — cloridrato de difenidramina (Benadryl®), prednisona, famotidina ou outros inibidores histaminérgicos H$_2$, omeprazol e sulcralfato devem ser considerados para qualquer cão ou gato com mastocitoma macroscópico.

ACOMPANHAMENTO

MONITORIZAÇÃO DO PACIENTE
Cães
• Grau I ou II — a ressecção cirúrgica completa deve ser curativa na maioria dos pacientes.
• Grau II (alto) — a ressecção cirúrgica completa deve ser avaliada a cada 3 meses por 1 ano com exame físico, ultrassonografia abdominal e avaliação de linfonodos.
• Tumores de grau elevado (grau III ou aqueles presentes em locais associados a prognóstico negativo) — exame físico, testes sanguíneos e ultrassonografia abdominal a cada 2 meses por 1 ano e, depois, a cada 6 meses por mais 2 anos.

Gatos
• Visceral ou intestinal — ultrassonografia abdominal a cada 3 meses por 1 ano.

PREVENÇÃO
N/D.

COMPLICAÇÕES POSSÍVEIS
Mielo ou hepatotoxicidade relacionadas com a quimioterapia.

EVOLUÇÃO ESPERADA E PROGNÓSTICO
• A excisão completa de mastocitomas de grau baixo na maioria dos locais é curativa.
• A excisão completa de mastocitomas de grau elevado ou aqueles localizados em áreas associadas a prognóstico mau (junções mucocutâneas, ± regiões inguinais) frequentemente necessita de terapia adjuvante com quimioterapia. Os tempos médios de sobrevida variam aproximadamente de 11-12 meses.
• A excisão incompleta de mastocitoma de grau baixo pode necessitar de terapia local adicional com alguma outra cirurgia (a cura é frequente nesse caso) ou radioterapia (85% ficam livre da doença em 3 anos).
• A excisão incompleta de mastocitoma de grau elevado necessita de terapia local adicional, além da quimioterapia sistêmica. Os tempos médios de sobrevida variam de 6 a 12 meses.
• A ocorrência de metástase regional para algum linfonodo deve ser tratada com excisão cirúrgica no momento da remoção do tumor primário. Há necessidade de quimioterapia sistêmica. Os tempos médios de sobrevida são tipicamente menores que 9 meses.
• Indícios de metástase à distância são frequentemente tratados com quimioterapia sistêmica ou terapias complementares isoladas, com sobrevida média de 4 meses ou menos.

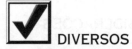

DIVERSOS

DISTÚRBIOS ASSOCIADOS
A doença progressiva e metastática tem o potencial de gerar a produção excessiva de ácido clorídrico pelas células parietais, com ulceração gástrica, melena, anemia ferropriva e perfuração gástrica associadas.

FATORES RELACIONADOS COM A IDADE
N/D.

POTENCIAL ZOONÓTICO
N/D.

GESTAÇÃO/FERTILIDADE/REPRODUÇÃO
Enquanto estiverem sob quimioterapia, os cães não deverão ser acasalados. Não há estudos a longo prazo sobre a fertilidade em cães ou gatos previamente tratados com lomustina, vimblastina ou inibidores de receptores tirosina quinase.

SINÔNIMO(S)
• Tumor de mastócitos.
• Mastocitose sistêmica.

ABREVIATURA(S)
• AINE = anti-inflamatório não esteroide.

RECURSOS DA INTERNET
• www.merckvetmanual.com/mvm/index.jsp?cfile = htm/bc/.
• www.vet.uga.edu/VPP/CLERK/Dahm/Index.php.
• www.vetmed.wsu.edu/deptsOncology/owners/mastCell.aspx.

Sugestões de Leitura
London CA, Seguin B. MCTs in the dog. Vet Clin North Am Small Anim Pract 2003, 33(3):473-489, v.
London CA, et al. Expression of stem cell factor receptor (c-kit) by the malignant mast cells from spontaneous canine mast cell tumours. J Comp Pathol 1996, 115(4):399-414.
Ogilvie GK, Moore AS, eds. Feline Oncology. Yardley, PA: Veterinary Learning Systems, 2001.
Wilcock BP, Yager JA, Zink MC. The morphology and behavior of feline cutaneous mastocytomas. Vet Pathol 1986, 23(3):320-324.
Withrow SJ, Vail DM, eds. Small Animal Clinical Oncology, 4th ed. Philadelphia: Saunders, 2007.

Autor Heather M. Wilson-Robles
Consultor Editorial Timothy M. Fan

MEDIASTINITE

CONSIDERAÇÕES GERAIS

REVISÃO
- O mediastino ocupa a porção central do tórax e, em termos anatômicos, é delimitado cranialmente pela entrada torácica, caudalmente pelo diafragma, lateralmente pela pleura mediastínica, dorsalmente pelas costelas e pela goteira paravertebral e ventralmente pelo esterno. É revestido em ambos os lados por pleura parietal, contém os principais órgãos na porção central do tórax e separa esses órgãos dos lobos pulmonares esquerdo e direito.
- Mediastinite — um processo inflamatório com envolvimento do espaço mediastínico, sendo geralmente o resultado de infecção bacteriana ou fúngica.
- Doença aguda — infecção grave pode se mostrar potencialmente letal e se disseminar para o espaço pleural; pode ocorrer o desenvolvimento de sepse.
- Crônica — além do possível desenvolvimento de granuloma ou abscesso mediastínico, pode resultar em síndrome da veia cava cranial ou abscedação interna latente crônica.
- Sistemas acometidos — sistema cardiovascular por causa da interferência no retorno venoso; sistema respiratório secundariamente ao efeito de massa intratorácica ou efusão pleural; sistema gastrintestinal por interferir na função esofágica.

IDENTIFICAÇÃO
Raro em cães e gatos.

SINAIS CLÍNICOS
- Letargia e fraqueza.
- Disfagia e regurgitação.
- Edema da cabeça, do pescoço e dos membros anteriores.
- Polipneia, dificuldade respiratória ou respiração obstruída, e tosse.
- A presença de febre deve levantar a suspeita de algum processo infeccioso.

CAUSAS E FATORES DE RISCO
- Doença aguda — geralmente resulta de perfuração esofágica, laceração traqueal, migração de corpo estranho ou ferida no pescoço; pode ocorrer o desenvolvimento de abscessos mediastínicos subsequentemente a infecções ou distúrbios neoplásicos que surgem no mediastino ou nos tecidos adjacentes.
- Doença crônica — costuma resultar de infecção bacteriana (p. ex., *Actinomyces* e *Nocardia* spp.) ou fúngica (p. ex., *Coccidioides*, *Cryptococcus*, *Blastomyces* e *Histoplasma* spp.). É possível a infecção por *Spirocerca lupi*.
- Fatores predisponentes — corpo estranho esofágico; traumatismo cervical ou torácico.

DIAGNÓSTICO

DIAGNÓSTICO DIFERENCIAL
- Pericardite, piotórax e pneumonia isolados.
- Massa mediastínica cranial — linfossarcoma; timoma, tumor da tireoide ou da paratireoide; tumor neurogênico; tumor mesenquimal; cisto mediastínico.
- Disfunção motora esofágica, hérnia hiatal deslizante.
- Distúrbios gastresofágicos, compreendendo refluxo gastresofágico, vômito crônico e outros distúrbios GI superiores.

HEMOGRAMA/BIOQUÍMICA/URINÁLISE
- Leucograma elevado com desvio à esquerda.
- Hematócrito e proteína total — podem estar elevados em virtude da depleção volêmica/desidratação.

OUTROS TESTES LABORATORIAIS
Testes laboratoriais adicionais para descartar outras causas possíveis de sinais clínicos.

DIAGNÓSTICO POR IMAGEM
- Radiografias torácicas — geralmente revelam um aumento focal ou difuso do mediastino; pode ser acompanhado por pneumotórax ou efusão pleural bilateral, dependendo do processo patológico subjacente.
- Estudo contrastado do esôfago — avaliar perfuração esofágica ou outra anormalidade; utilizar meio de contraste hidrossolúvel (i. e., ioexol ou iopamidol) diante da suspeita de perfuração.
- Ultrassonografia torácica — diferenciar entre acúmulo de líquido mediastínico (p. ex., cisto e abscesso), reação inflamatória e tumor.
- Tomografia computadorizada — exame mais definitivo do que a ultrassonografia.

MÉTODOS DIAGNÓSTICOS
- Citologia — toracocentese de qualquer efusão pleural; aspirado transtorácico por agulha fina ou biopsia com agulha de excisão de massa mediastínica de origem não cardíaca nem vascular.
- Aspirado ou biopsia guiados por ultrassom podem ser muito valiosos na amostragem precisa dos tecidos.
- Encaminhamento das amostras coletadas para cultura bacteriana aeróbia e anaeróbia, bem como para teste de sensibilidade (antibiograma).

TRATAMENTO

- Terapia antibiótica ou antifúngica, conforme indicação.
- Drenagem e debridamento de material do abscesso.
- Internação do paciente com restrição da atividade física até que a infecção esteja controlada e a condição estabilizada.
- Efusão pleural de quantidade acentuada ou piotórax de qualquer grau — tratado por meio de toracostomia com sonda.
- Soluções eletrolíticas fisiologicamente balanceadas ou nutrição parenteral —administrar por via parenteral até que a alimentação por via oral seja possível e a ingestão de água e alimento retorne ao normal ou quase normal.
- Perfuração esofágica — emergência cirúrgica; após o reparo cirúrgico, utilizar a alimentação por via parenteral ou sonda gástrica por 3-5 dias.
- Doença crônica — há necessidade de exploração cirúrgica em caso de doença associada a abscesso ou granuloma.
- Toracostomia por sonda — manter a sonda após a cirurgia por meio de sucção contínua com selo d'água ou lavagem intermitente e sucção por 5-7 dias ou até que seja removida uma quantidade desprezível de líquido.

MEDICAÇÕES

MEDICAMENTO(S)
- Antibiótico bactericida de amplo espectro — selecionado com base na cultura bacteriana e no teste de sensibilidade; deve ser administrado por via parenteral por, no mínimo, a primeira semana de tratamento e, depois, por via oral.
- Tratamento antifúngico — indicado para infecção micótica. Os agentes recomendados incluem itraconazol, fluconazol e anfotericina B; o tratamento costuma ser necessário por 3-6 meses.

CONTRAINDICAÇÕES/INTERAÇÕES POSSÍVEIS
- Antibióticos aminoglicosídeos e anfotericina B — evitar na presença de azotemia.

ACOMPANHAMENTO

MONITORIZAÇÃO DO PACIENTE
- Registro diário da temperatura.
- Hemograma — a cada 2-3 dias durante a hospitalização (em geral, 7-10 dias).
- Radiografias torácicas — em intervalos de 7-10 dias (com maior frequência se houver necessidade de drenagem).
- Antibióticos — continuar geralmente por 1 semana após o hemograma e as radiografias retornarem ao normal; com abscedação, continuar por mais 4-6 semanas.

COMPLICAÇÕES POSSÍVEIS
- Piotórax.
- Sepse.
- Fibrose mediastínica.

EVOLUÇÃO ESPERADA E PROGNÓSTICO
- Avisar os proprietários sobre o prognóstico reservado.
- Com diagnóstico precoce e tratamento rigoroso — prognóstico razoável a bom.
- Com fibrose mediastínica — prognóstico reservado a mau a longo prazo.
- Complicações identificadas — disfunção da motilidade esofágica; compressão da veia cava cranial ou caudal; paralisia do nervo laríngeo recorrente ou frênico.

DIVERSOS

ABREVIATURA(S)
- GI = gastrintestinal.

Sugestões de Leitura
Biller DS. Mediastinal disease. In: Ettinger ST, Feldman EC, eds., Textbook of Veterinary Internal Medicine, 5th ed. Philadelphia: Saunders, 2000, pp. 1094-1096.
Jergens AE. Diseases of the esophagus. In: Ettinger SJ, Feldman EC, eds., Textbook of Veterinary Internal Medicine, 6th ed. St. Louis: Elsevier, 2005, pp. 1298-1310.

Autores Lynelle R. Johnson e Neil K. Harpster
Consultor Editorial Lynelle R. Johnson

Megacólon

CONSIDERAÇÕES GERAIS

DEFINIÇÃO
Condição de aumento persistente no diâmetro do intestino grosso, associado à constipação/obstipação crônica e motilidade colônica baixa a ausente.

FISIOPATOLOGIA
- O megacólon adquirido origina-se da impactação fecal colônica crônica que leva à absorção excessiva de água das fezes e à formação de concreções fecais solidificadas.
- A distensão prolongada do cólon resulta em alterações irreversíveis na motilidade colônica, que leva à inércia colônica.
- A ausência congênita de células ganglionares colônicas (doença de Hirschsprung) não está claramente comprovada nos pequenos animais.
- A patogênese de megacólon idiopático em gatos provavelmente envolve um distúrbio da função normal da musculatura lisa do cólon.

SISTEMA(S) ACOMETIDO(S)
Gastrintestinal.

GENÉTICA
N/D.

INCIDÊNCIA/PREVALÊNCIA
Desconhecidas.

DISTRIBUIÇÃO GEOGRÁFICA
N/D.

IDENTIFICAÇÃO
Espécies
- Megacólon idiopático — gatos.
- Megacólon adquirido — cães e gatos.

Raça(s) Predominante(s)
Alguns indícios de risco aumentado nos gatos da raça Manx.

Idade Média e Faixa Etária
- Megacólon idiopático — gatos de meia-idade a idosos (idade média, 4,9 anos; faixa etária, 1-15 anos).
- Megacólon adquirido — nenhuma.

Sexo Predominante
Nenhum.

SINAIS CLÍNICOS
Achados Anamnésicos
- Megacólon idiopático — tipicamente um problema recidivante/crônico; sinais clínicos frequentemente presentes por meses a anos.
- Megacólon adquirido — os sinais podem ser agudos ou crônicos.
- Constipação/obstipação.
- Tenesmo com volume fecal pequeno ou ausente.
- Fezes endurecidas e ressecadas.
- Defecação pouco frequente.
- Pode ocorrer uma pequena quantidade de diarreia (frequentemente mucoide) após tenesmo prolongado.
- Sinais ocasionais de vômito, anorexia e/ou depressão.
- Perda de peso.

Achados do Exame Físico
- A palpação abdominal revela o cólon aumentado com massa fecal endurecida.
- O exame digital do reto pode indicar a causa subjacente (obstrutiva) e confirmar a impactação fecal.
- Desidratação.
- Pelagem emaranhada malcuidada.

CAUSAS
- Idiopático — gatos.
- Obstrução mecânica — má união de fratura pélvica, corpo estranho ou dieta inadequada (especialmente ossos), estenose (constrição), prostatopatia, hérnia perineal, neoplasia, atresia anal ou retal.
- Causas de disquezia — doença anorretal (saculite anal, abscesso do saco anal, fístula perianal, proctite), traumatismo (pelve fraturada, membro fraturado, quadril deslocado, ferida ou laceração por mordedura perianal, abscesso perineal).
- Distúrbios metabólicos — hipocalemia, desidratação grave.
- Medicamentos — vincristina, bário, antiácidos, sucralfato, anticolinérgicos.
- Doença neurológica/neuromuscular — anormalidades congênitas das vértebras caudais (especialmente dos gatos Manx), paraplegia, mielopatia, discopatia intervertebral, disautonomia, neuropatia sacral, traumatismo ao nervo sacral (p. ex., lesão por tração/fratura da cauda), traumatismo à inervação colônica.

FATORES DE RISCO
- Condições que levam à incapacidade de manter a postura (fraturas de membro e da região pélvica, doença neuromuscular, etc.) ou dor retoanal.
- Fraturas pélvicas anteriores.
- Possível associação com baixa atividade física e obesidade.
- Hérnias perineais.

DIAGNÓSTICO

DIAGNÓSTICO DIFERENCIAL
- Outras causas de massas colônicas palpáveis (p. ex., linfoma, carcinoma, intussuscepção) — distinguir com base na textura, no exame retal, no diagnóstico por imagem e na biopsia de mucosa.
- Disúria/estrangúria — excluir pela palpação da bexiga e do cólon, bem como pela urinálise.
- Tenesmo causado pela inflamação dos segmentos inferiores do intestino (colite) — descartar por meio de palpação, exame retal e diagnóstico por imagem.

HEMOGRAMA/BIOQUÍMICA/URINÁLISE
- O hemograma completo pode exibir indícios de desidratação (hematócrito e proteínas totais elevados) e leucograma de estresse.
- Podem surgir anormalidades eletrolíticas, dependendo da duração da obstipação; pode haver azotemia pré-renal com desidratação.
- Urinálise — sem alterações compatíveis; é importante não só confirmar a função renal normal nos animais desidratados, mas também descartar doença do trato urinário inferior como diagnóstico diferencial.

OUTROS TESTES LABORATORIAIS
N/D.

DIAGNÓSTICO POR IMAGEM
- Radiografias abdominais/pélvicas para identificar quaisquer causas subjacentes.
- Pode-se facilmente observar o cólon aumentado, repleto de fezes, nas radiografias abdominais simples.
- Ultrassonografia abdominal pode identificar massas murais ou obstrutivas.

MÉTODOS DIAGNÓSTICOS
Talvez haja necessidade de colonoscopia para descartar lesões obstrutivas murais ou intraluminais.

ACHADOS PATOLÓGICOS
- A dilatação mais grave ocorre tipicamente nos cólons transverso e descendente, embora toda a extensão do cólon possa estar envolvida.
- O cólon geralmente está normal do ponto de vista histológico.

TRATAMENTO

CUIDADO(S) DE SAÚDE ADEQUADO(S)
- Tratamento clínico do animal internado; a cirurgia pode ser indicada se o problema for recidivante/grave.
- Terapia clínica — restabelecer a hidratação normal, seguida pela anestesia e esvaziamento manual do cólon com o uso de enemas de água morna, gelatina hidrossolúvel e extração delicada das fezes com o dedo enluvado ou pinça de esponja; não traumatizar excessivamente a mucosa colônica.
- Continuar o tratamento a longo prazo em casa.

CUIDADO(S) DE ENFERMAGEM
- A maior parte dos pacientes requer suporte de fluidos parenterais para corrigir a desidratação.
- Administração intravenosa de soluções eletrolíticas balanceadas é a via preferida.

ATIVIDADE
- Estimular a atividade e o exercício.
- Restrição será indicada no período pós-operatório se a cirurgia for realizada.

DIETA
- Muitos pacientes necessitam de dieta produtora de poucos resíduos; dietas com fibras formadoras de volume podem piorar ou levar à recidiva da distensão fecal colônica.
- Ocasionalmente, uma dieta rica em fibras é valiosa.
- Uma dieta mais palatável do tipo de manutenção pode ser suplementada com produtos como Metamucil® ou recheio de torta de abóbora.

ORIENTAÇÃO AO PROPRIETÁRIO
- Na doença idiopática ou em casos de lesão colônica grave, o tratamento clínico frequentemente é por toda a vida e pode ser frustrante.
- A recidiva é comum.
- A cirurgia (colectomia subtotal) está indicada quando o tratamento clínico falhar.

CONSIDERAÇÕES CIRÚRGICAS
- Uma causa obstrutiva subjacente necessita de correção cirúrgica.
- Evitar a administração de enema/esvaziamento do cólon antes da colectomia subtotal.
- Colectomia subtotal com anastomose ileorretal ou colorretal — tratamento de escolha para o megacólon idiopático refratário ao tratamento clínico.
- A colectomia também pode ser necessária em casos de megacólon obstrutivo causado por alterações irreversíveis na motilidade colônica.

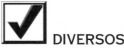

MEDICAÇÕES

MEDICAMENTO(S) DE ESCOLHA
• Pode-se melhorar a motilidade colônica nos casos menos graves com a cisaprida, medicamento GI procinético (cães, 0,1-0,5 mg/kg VO a cada 8-12 h; gatos, 2,5-10 mg/gato a cada 8-12 h).
• Amolecedores de fezes (p. ex., lactulose, 1 mL/4,5 kg VO a cada 8-12 h até fazer efeito) são recomendados em conjunto com a cisaprida e a dieta.
• Antibióticos profiláticos de amplo espectro são recomendados antes do esvaziamento do cólon e durante o período perioperatório em caso de cirurgia eletiva.

CONTRAINDICAÇÕES
• Enemas de retenção com fosfato de sódio (p. ex., Fleet; C. B. Fleet Co., Inc.) — por causa de sua associação com hipocalcemia grave.
• Óleo mineral e vaselina branca — por causa do perigo de pneumonia lipoide por aspiração fatal em virtude da falta de sabor.

PRECAUÇÕES
Laxantes comuns para tricobezoares (p. ex., Laxatone® e Cat-a-Lax®) são tipicamente ineficazes.

INTERAÇÕES POSSÍVEIS
N/D.

MEDICAMENTO(S) ALTERNATIVO(S)
Docusato de sódio pode ser utilizado como amolecedor das fezes no lugar da lactulose.

ACOMPANHAMENTO

MONITORIZAÇÃO DO PACIENTE
• Após ressecção e anastomose colônicas — verificar sinais de deiscência e peritonite por 3-5 dias.
• A deterioração clínica justifica a realização de abdominocentese e/ou lavado peritoneal para detectar extravasamento pela anastomose.
• Manter o suporte de fluidos até que o paciente seja capaz de comer e beber.

PREVENÇÃO
• Reparar as fraturas pélvicas que estreitam o canal pélvico.
• Evitar a exposição a corpos estranhos e o fornecimento de ossos.

COMPLICAÇÕES POSSÍVEIS
• Recidiva ou persistência — mais comum.
• Complicações cirúrgicas potenciais incluem peritonite, diarreia persistente, formação de estenose e recidiva da obstipação.
• Perfuração traumática do cólon é uma complicação grave de esvaziamento fecal exagerado.

EVOLUÇÃO ESPERADA E PROGNÓSTICO
• Em termos históricos, o tratamento clínico não é recompensador.
• A cisaprida parece melhorar o prognóstico em relação ao tratamento clínico em alguns pacientes, mas pode não ser suficiente nos casos graves ou de longa duração.
• Diarreia pós-operatória — esperada; tipicamente desaparece dentro de 6 semanas (80% dos gatos acometidos por megacólon idiopático e submetidos à colectomia subtotal), mas pode persistir por diversos meses; as fezes ficam mais bem formadas à medida que o íleo se adapta pelo aumento da capacidade de reservatório e de absorção da água.
• O procedimento de colectomia subtotal é bem tolerada pelos gatos; as taxas de recidiva da constipação são tipicamente baixas.

DIVERSOS

DISTÚRBIOS ASSOCIADOS
Hérnia perineal.

FATORES RELACIONADOS COM A IDADE
Condições clínicas concomitantes (p. ex., insuficiência renal crônica e hipertireoidismo) podem ocorrer no megacólon idiopático, já que muitos gatos são idosos.

POTENCIAL ZOONÓTICO
N/D.

GESTAÇÃO/FERTILIDADE/REPRODUÇÃO
• O efeito da cisaprida sobre o feto é desconhecido.
• Pacientes estariam sob alto risco de distocia se levassem a prenhez a termo.

VER TAMBÉM
• Constipação e Obstipação.
• Disquezia e Hematoquezia.
• Hérnia Perineal.

Sugestões de Leitura
Washabau RJ, Holt D. Diagnosis and management of feline idiopathic megacolon. Vet Clin North Am 1999, 29:589-603.
———. Diseases of the large intestine. In: Ettinger SJ, Feldman EC, eds., Textbook of Veterinary Internal Medicine, 6th ed. St. Louis: Elsevier, 2005, pp. 1378-1408.

Autor Albert E. Jergens
Consultor Editorial Albert E. Jergens

MEGAESÔFAGO

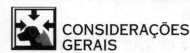

CONSIDERAÇÕES GERAIS

DEFINIÇÃO
O megaesôfago é definido como uma dilatação generalizada e difusa do esôfago com peristalse diminuída a ausente.

FISIOPATOLOGIA
• No esôfago normal, a presença de bolo alimentar na porção esofágica proximal estimula os neurônios sensoriais aferentes.
• Os sinais são transmitidos por via central, pelos nervos vago e glossofaríngeo ao trato solitário e núcleo ambíguo.
• Os impulsos motores retornam pelos neurônios eferentes do nervo vago até estimular o músculo estriado (cães) e a musculatura estriada e lisa (gatos) a fim de provocar a contração do esôfago.
• Lesões em qualquer lugar ao longo dessa via podem levar ao surgimento de megaesôfago e consequente retenção de alimento e líquidos.
• Há provas de que uma disfunção dos nervos aferentes seja a lesão mais comum em casos idiopáticos de megaesôfago.

SISTEMA(S) ACOMETIDO(S)
• Gastrintestinal — disfagia, regurgitação, perda de peso.
• Musculosquelético — fraqueza, perda de peso.
• Nervoso — polifagia, possível manifestação de distúrbio neurológico/neuromuscular sistêmico.
• Respiratório — pneumonia por aspiração.

GENÉTICA
• Forma congênita — o megaesôfago pode ser hereditário em cães da raça Fox terrier de pelo duro (autossômico recessivo) e Schnauzer miniatura (autossômico recessivo com penetrância de 60% ou autossômico dominante).
• Outras raças relatadas incluem Dachshund, Pastor alemão, Dinamarquês, Setter irlandês, Labrador retriever, Pug (uma única ninhada com quatro filhotes acometidos) e Shar-pei chinês.
• A miastenia grave pode ser congênita em Jack Russell terrier, Springer spaniel, Fox terrier de pelo macio e Samoiedo.
• Forma adquirida — muitas doenças podem ter uma associação com megaesôfago. Predisposições genéticas como tais doenças estão listadas em cada doença separadamente.

INCIDÊNCIA/PREVALÊNCIA
• Todas as formas congênitas são raras.
• A doença adquirida é incomum no cão e rara no gato.

IDENTIFICAÇÃO
Espécies
Os cães são mais comumente acometidos que os gatos.

Raça(s) Predominante(s)
• Cães — ver a seção "Genética".
• Gatos — raça Siamês e aparentados.

Idade Média e Faixa Etária
• Os casos congênitos manifestam-se logo após o nascimento ou no momento do desmame de dietas líquidas para alimentos mais sólidos.
• Os casos adquiridos podem ser observados em qualquer idade, dependendo da etiologia.

SINAIS CLÍNICOS
Achados Anamnésicos
• Os proprietários frequentemente relatam vômito; nesse caso, o veterinário precisa diferenciar vômito de regurgitação.
• Regurgitação (considerado o sinal característico); disfagia; tosse/secreção nasal com pneumonia por aspiração; apetite devorador ou inapetência; perda de peso ou crescimento deficiente; ptialismo e halitose.
• Outros sinais dependem da etiologia subjacente.

Achados do Exame Físico
• Pode-se notar tumefação no pescoço, representando uma distensão da porção esofágica cervical; ptialismo; halitose; aumento dos ruídos respiratórios; secreção nasal e febre (em caso de pneumonia concomitante); caquexia; fraqueza; perda de peso.
• Os animais devem ser cuidadosamente avaliados quanto à presença de déficits miopáticos ou neurológicos concomitantes que podem indicar doença generalizada. A atrofia muscular (se presente) pode ser focal ou generalizada.
• Deve-se dar especial atenção aos pares IX, X e XI de nervos cranianos, já que suas origens estão próximas ao núcleo ambíguo.

CAUSAS
Congênitas
Megaesôfago idiopático, miastenia grave (rara).

Adquirido/Início no Adulto
• Idiopático (mais comum).
• Doença neuromuscular — miastenia grave (25% dos casos em cães); lúpus eritematoso sistêmico; miosite/doença miopática; disautonomia (mais comum em gatos); cinomose; doença do armazenamento de glicogênio (tipo II); tétano/botulismo; dermatomiosite; dano traumático ao nervo vago (bilateral); foi identificada uma possível associação entre paralisia laríngea e megaesôfago.
• Obstrução esofágica — anomalia do anel vascular; neoplasia esofágica ou periesofágica (linfoma, leiomioma, etc.); estenose; corpo estranho; granuloma.
• Intoxicação — chumbo, tálio, anticolinesterase; acrilamida.
• Endocrinopatia — hipoadrenocorticismo, hipotireoidismo (controverso).
• Diversos — timoma, dilatação e vólvulo gástricos, hérnia de hiato, intussuscepção gastresofágica; esofagite (refluxo gastresofágico, infecção parasitária).

DIAGNÓSTICO

DIAGNÓSTICO DIFERENCIAL
• É importante distinguir regurgitação de vômito.
• Regurgitação — processo passivo; pouco a nenhum esforço abdominal; sem fase prodrômica; o material regurgitado tem quantidades elevadas de muco espesso.
• Vômito — processo ativo; fase prodrômica; o material vomitado tem uma coloração intensa de bile.
• A forma do material expelido, a presença de alimento não digerido e a duração de tempo desde a ingestão até a regurgitação ou o vômito são menos úteis para a diferenciação.

HEMOGRAMA/BIOQUÍMICA/URINÁLISE
• Podem permanecer dentro dos limites de normalidade.
• Na presença de pneumonia, pode-se observar leucograma inflamatório.
• Outras alterações podem identificar a etiologia subjacente — pontilhado basófilo nas hemácias em intoxicação por chumbo; proteinúria em caso de doença infecciosa ou inflamatória; distúrbios eletrolíticos em caso de hipoadrenocorticismo; hipercolesterolemia em caso de hipotireoidismo; CK elevada em caso de doença miopática.

OUTROS TESTES LABORATORIAIS
• Títulos de anticorpos contra os receptores da acetilcolina em todos os casos de megaesôfago (para triagem de miastenia grave generalizada ou focal).
• Teste de estimulação com ACTH ou nível de cortisol basal para pesquisa de hipoadrenocorticismo.
• Perfil de função da tireoide para hipotireoidismo (pode ser influenciado por doença concomitante).
• Níveis sanguíneos e urinários de chumbo.
• Títulos do ANA para avaliação de LES.
• Níveis sanguíneos de colinesterase em busca de intoxicação por organofosforado.

DIAGNÓSTICO POR IMAGEM
Radiografias Torácicas Simples
• Esôfago dilatado preenchido com ar, líquido ou alimento.
• Indícios de pneumonia por aspiração (broncogramas aéreos, marcas alveolares, efusão pleural).
• Deslocamento ventral da traqueia nas radiografias obtidas em projeção lateral.
• Radiografias em projeção ventrodorsal podem revelar o deslocamento lateral da traqueia.
• Indícios da etiologia subjacente: massa mediastínica, hérnia de hiato, neoplasia, etc.
• As radiografias não diferenciam os cães com megaesôfago atribuído à miastenia grave daqueles com megaesôfago causado por outras etiologias.

Esofagograma Contrastado e Fluoroscopia
• Líquido de bário ou refeição de bário pode demonstrar acúmulo anormal, motilidade deficiente ou lesões estruturais. Também se pode fazer uso do io-hexol.
• Utilizar com cuidado em animais com megaesôfago em virtude do risco de aspiração do material de contraste.
• Ter extrema cautela em pacientes com indícios radiográficos de pneumonia.
• Monitorizar os animais de perto após a obtenção das radiografias em busca de sinais de aspiração.
• Fluoroscopia — pode ser utilizada para avaliar a peristalse primária e secundária. Esse exame também pode determinar a consistência alimentar mais eficaz para tratamento a longo prazo.

Cintilografia Nuclear
• A câmera de raios gama acompanha a passagem do alimento radiomarcado pelo esôfago.
• Evita o uso de agentes de contraste e o risco de aspiração desses agentes.

MÉTODOS DIAGNÓSTICOS
• Esofagoscopia — pode ser usada não só para a recuperação de corpos estranhos, mas também para a avaliação de lesão obstrutiva, neoplasia ou esofagite sob suspeita. A neoplasia esofágica distal pode mimetizar megaesôfago idiopático e necessitar de endoscopia para o diagnóstico.

MEGAESÔFAGO

- EMG — na suspeita de doença neuromuscular, podendo ser utilizada em conjunto com biopsias dos tecidos muscular e nervoso.
- Manometria esofágica — mede as pressões intraesofágica e esfincteriana esofágica inferior (incomum).
- Testes adicionais — podem ser indicados em casos de doença do SNC: análise do LES, títulos para cinomose, TC ou RM do cérebro.
- Exame de fezes — pode indicar infecção por *Spirocerca lupi*.

ACHADOS PATOLÓGICOS
Achados macroscópicos e histopatológicos variam, dependendo da causa subjacente e da presença de fatores complicantes.

TRATAMENTO

CUIDADO(S) DE SAÚDE ADEQUADO(S)
- Deve ser instituída terapia para a etiologia subjacente (quando aplicável).
- Os aspectos mais relevantes envolvem medidas para suprir as necessidades nutricionais ou evitar a pneumonia por aspiração.

CUIDADO(S) DE ENFERMAGEM
- A pneumonia por aspiração pode exigir oxigenoterapia, nebulização/tapotagem, fluidoterapia com solução eletrolítica balanceada.
- Esses animais podem estar em decúbito e, por essa razão, necessitam de cama macia, devendo ser trocados de posição a cada 4 h. Ou, então, eles devem ser mantidos em decúbito esternal.

ATIVIDADE
Dependendo da etiologia, a restrição da atividade não será necessária.

DIETA
- As necessidades nutricionais devem ser calculadas com precisão, indicando o grau de debilidade.
- É essencial a experimentação com diferentes consistências de alimentos. Pode-se lançar mão de papas ou mingaus líquidos, pequenas bolas de carne, caldos batidos no liquidificador, etc.
- Alguns casos se beneficiam de alimentações fornecidas via gastrostomia.
- Tanto o comedouro como o bebedouro devem ser suspensos (45-90° do chão) e o animal deve ser mantido em uma posição ereta por 10-15 min após a ingestão de água ou alimento. Pode ser mais fácil conseguir uma posição ereta com o uso de uma "cadeira" específica.

ORIENTAÇÃO AO PROPRIETÁRIO
- A maioria dos casos de megaesôfago necessita de terapia pelo resto da vida, mesmo se a etiologia subjacente for encontrada. A dedicação do proprietário é muito importante para o tratamento a longo prazo.
- Grande parte dos animais vem a óbito em decorrência da pneumonia por aspiração ou por causa da evolução da doença subjacente.

CONSIDERAÇÕES CIRÚRGICAS
- A intervenção cirúrgica fica indicada para anomalias do anel vascular, fístula broncoesofágica, alguns corpos estranhos e outras lesões obstrutivas, ou timectomia.
- A dilatação com balão é indicada para os casos de estenose esofágica.
- Não é recomendável a ressecção cirúrgica do megaesôfago.

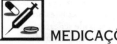

MEDICAÇÕES

MEDICAMENTO(S)
- Antibióticos para pneumonia por aspiração (selecionados idealmente com base nos resultados da cultura e do antibiograma de material obtido por lavado transtraqueal ou broncoalveolar).
- Terapia específica para a etiologia subjacente se houver indicação — agentes imunossupressores (utilizar com cuidado na presença de pneumonia) para doença imunomediada; piridostigmina para miastenia grave, suplementação de prednisona para hipoadrenocorticismo, etc.
- Bloqueadores dos receptores histaminérgicos H_2 para esofagite — ranitidina (1-2 mg/kg VO, IV a cada 12 h), cimetidina (4-10 mg/kg VO, SC, IM, IV a cada 6 h), famotidina (0,5-1 mg/kg VO, SC, IM, IV a cada 12-24 h). Em casos graves, podem ser utilizados os inibidores da bomba de prótons — omeprazol (0,5-1 mg/kg VO a cada 24 h).

Procinéticos
- Metoclopramida (0,2-0,4 mg/kg SC ou VO a cada 6-12 h) aumenta o tônus do esfíncter esofágico inferior e a motilidade gástrica e, possivelmente, esofágica.
- Cisaprida (0,5 mg/kg VO a cada 8-12 h) é mais eficaz para refluxo esofágico do que a metoclopramida; no entanto, a cisaprida pode retardar o tempo de trânsito esofágico; pode ser mais útil em gatos em virtude do aumento da musculatura lisa na porção distal do esôfago.
- Outros agentes modificadores da motilidade (p. ex., nizatidina) não foram avaliados em termos de motilidade esofágica.

PRECAUÇÕES
- A absorção de medicamentos administrados por via oral pode ficar comprometida.
- As formas injetáveis devem ser utilizadas quando aplicável.
- Se indicados, os corticosteroides precisam ser usados com cuidado em virtude do risco de pneumonia por aspiração.

ACOMPANHAMENTO

MONITORIZAÇÃO DO PACIENTE
- As radiografias torácicas devem ser repetidas mediante a suspeita de pneumonia por aspiração (febre, tosse, letargia).
- Os casos de pneumonia podem necessitar de hemograma completo, gasometria sanguínea e lavado broncoalveolar.
- Os animais devem ser avaliados e pesados regularmente para determinar a evolução da doença e garantir a ingestão nutricional adequada.

PREVENÇÃO
Caso se identifique algum corpo estranho esofágico, ele deverá ser removido o mais rápido possível.

COMPLICAÇÕES POSSÍVEIS
- Pneumonia por aspiração.
- Outras, dependendo da etiologia.

EVOLUÇÃO ESPERADA E PROGNÓSTICO
- Os casos congênitos apresentam prognóstico reservado (recuperação de 20-46%).
- Os cães da raça Schnauzer miniatura podem ter um prognóstico melhor.
- O prognóstico pode melhorar com a identificação e o tratamento da etiologia específica (p. ex., hipoadrenocorticismo, anomalia do anel vascular).
- Aproximadamente 50% dos casos de miastenia grave respondem à terapia.
- O prognóstico é mau na doença idiopática de início no adulto.
- A dedicação do proprietário é crucial.

DIVERSOS

DISTÚRBIOS ASSOCIADOS
Pneumonia por aspiração.

FATORES RELACIONADOS COM A IDADE
- Sinais de regurgitação em animais muito jovens ou ao desmame podem indicar lesão congênita.
- O prognóstico pode ser melhor em animais jovens.

POTENCIAL ZOONÓTICO
- Nenhum para megaesôfago.
- O estado de vacinação antirrábica deve ser determinado em qualquer animal com possível doença neurológica.

SINÔNIMO(S)
- Aperistalse (ausência de contrações progressivas eficazes) esofágica.
- Dilatação esofágica.

VER TAMBÉM
- Disfagia.
- Corpos Estranhos Esofágicos.
- Miastenia Grave.
- Pneumonia Bacteriana.
- Pneumonia por Aspiração.
- Regurgitação.

ABREVIATURA(S)
- ACTH = hormônio adrenocorticotrópico.
- ANA = anticorpo antinuclear.
- CK = creatina quinase.
- EMG = eletromiografia.
- LCS = líquido cerebrospinal.
- LES = lúpus eritematoso sistêmico.
- RM = ressonância magnética.
- SNC = sistema nervoso central.
- TC = tomografia computadorizada.

RECURSOS DA INTERNET
http://marvistavet.com/html/bodymegaesophagus.html.

Sugestões de Leitura
Gaynor AR, Shofer FS, Washabau RJ. Risk factors for acquired megaesophagus in dogs. JAVMA 1997, 211:1406-1412.
Jergens AJ. Diseases of the esophagus. In: Ettinger SJ, Feldman EC, eds., Textbook of Veterinary Internal Medicine, 6th ed. St. Louis: Elsevier, 2005, pp. 1298-1310.
Wray JD, Sparks AH. Use of radiographic measurements in distinguishing myasthenia gravis from other causes of canine megaoesophagus. J Small Anim Pract 2006, 47:256-263.

Autor Jo Ann Morrison
Consultor Editorial Albert E. Jergens

Melanoma Uveal em Cães

CONSIDERAÇÕES GERAIS

REVISÃO
- Melanomas das úveas anterior (p. ex., íris e corpo ciliar) e posterior (coroide).
- Representa a neoplasia intraocular primária mais comum em cães.
- Costuma ser benigno e unilateral; com frequência, apresenta comportamento ocular destrutivo.
- Acomete mais frequentemente a úvea anterior.
- Melanoma uveal anterior — índice de 4% de metástase vascular aos pulmões e às vísceras.
- Melanoma coroidal — raramente sofre metástase.

IDENTIFICAÇÃO
- Não há predisposição racial nem sexual.
- Melanoma uveal anterior — a idade média é de 8-10 anos.
- Melanoma coroidal — a idade média é de 6,5 anos.
- Faixa etária — de 2 meses a 17 anos de idade.

SINAIS CLÍNICOS
Uveal Anterior
- Massa pigmentada na esclera ou na córnea.
- Massa pigmentada visível na câmara anterior ou posterior à margem pupilar.
- Pupilar irregular.
- Uveíte.
- Glaucoma.
- Hifema.
- Sem perda da visão — a menos que ocorra a obstrução da pupila pela massa ou o desenvolvimento de glaucoma.

Coroidal
- Muitas vezes, passa despercebido em virtude da localização do tumor; geralmente constitui um achado incidental. • À fundoscopia, observa-se a presença de massa no segmento ocular posterior.
- Crescimento muito lento; raramente necessita de enucleação. • Tumor raro.

CAUSAS E FATORES DE RISCO
- Idiopáticas.
- Transformação potencial de máculas planas e pigmentadas da íris em melanomas.
- Labrador retriever jovem — presumivelmente há uma herança autossômica recessiva.

DIAGNÓSTICO

DIAGNÓSTICO DIFERENCIAL
- Proliferações não neoplásicas da úvea — as máculas da íris não se mostram em relevo.
- Hiperpigmentação difusa da íris, secundária à uveíte crônica, particularmente em Golden retriever (uveíte pigmentar/uveíte do Golden retriever) e Boxer.
- Melanose ocular em Cairn terrier.
- Cistos uveais — além de exibir transiluminação, podem se deslocar livremente dentro do olho, ao contrário dos melanomas.
- Massas granulomatosas.
- Íris bombé* (seclusão pupilar).

---

* N.T.: Trata-se da aderência total do bordo pupilar ao cristalino ou lente intraocular.

- Perfuração ocular em casos de prolapso uveal.
- Outras condições neoplásicas oculares, sobretudo melanoma conjuntival, que pode ser erroneamente interpretado como extensão extraescleral de melanoma uveal. O melanoma conjuntival costuma ser maligno e tem comportamento agressivo em cães, tornando essencial diferenciá-lo de melanoma uveal.
- Eversão da margem pupilar em função da uveíte (ectrópio uveal).

HEMOGRAMA/BIOQUÍMICA/URINÁLISE
Em geral, normais.

OUTROS TESTES LABORATORIAIS
N/D.

DIAGNÓSTICO POR IMAGEM
Ultrassonografia ocular — pode ajudar a determinar a extensão da massa.

MÉTODOS DIAGNÓSTICOS
- Biomicroscopia com lâmpada de fenda — determina o tamanho e a localização da massa.
- Transiluminação da massa.
- Tonometria.
- Oftalmoscopia indireta — com ou sem indentação escleral concomitante.
- Gonioscopia — avalia o ângulo de drenagem quanto à extensão do tumor.
- Ultrassonografia ocular — utilizada se houver opacidade da córnea e se não for possível a observação de estruturas oculares mais profundas ou, então, na suspeita de ocultamento de massa no corpo ciliar pela íris.

ACHADOS PATOLÓGICOS
- Os achados costumam ficar restritos ao bulbo ocular enucleado; a biopsia é impraticável em grande parte dos pacientes.
- Em geral, observam-se dois tipos de células — células arredondadas preenchidas com melanina; células fusiformes.
- Aspecto benigno e índice mitótico baixo (<2 figuras mitóticas por campo óptico em aumento de 10×) — são comuns.
- Índice mitótico — constitui o critério mais confiável em termos de malignidade; em geral, há 4 figuras mitóticas por campo óptico em aumento de 10× em casos de tumores malignos do ponto de vista clínico.
- Ao enviar os olhos para avaliação histológica, devem-se solicitar o clareamento dos cortes teciduais e a avaliação do índice mitótico.
- Será melhor se a avaliação histológica do bulbo ocular for feita por um patologista veterinário especializado em oftalmologia.

TRATAMENTO

- Os tumores costumam ser benignos, podendo-se optar pela monitorização a cada 3-6 meses.
- Labrador retriever jovem — o crescimento é agressivo e, portanto, exige a realização de cirurgia.
- Orientar o proprietário sobre a enucleação; muitas vezes, esse tipo de procedimento gera problemas emocionais aos donos dos animais.
- Enfatizar a natureza unilateral da condição, a possibilidade de preservação do olho contralateral e a adaptação dos animais monoculares que, embora possuam um único olho, podem viver muito bem.
- Indicações da enucleação — rápido aumento no tamanho da massa; impossibilidade de recuperação do olho; disseminação difusa da massa no espaço intraocular; dano significativo à função visual; invasão extraocular; complicações secundárias (p. ex., glaucoma, sinais de dor e hemorragia). Nota: embora o glaucoma seja um processo que causa dor (cefaleia), o proprietário frequentemente não percebe isso.
- Técnica de enucleação — utilizar uma técnica cirúrgica delicada para evitar a distribuição de células tumorais na circulação; evitar a compressão sobre o quiasma óptico, pois isso pode levar à cegueira do olho contralateral; proceder à exenteração de todo o conteúdo orbital caso se observe a extensão extraescleral do tumor.
- Outros tratamentos cirúrgicos — utilizados com pouca frequência; iridectomia setorial e iridociclectomia de pequenas massas isoladas.
- Tratamento de pequenos tumores da íris a laser.
- A vacina contra melanoma não tem eficácia conhecida; provavelmente é ineficaz em pacientes sem enucleação.

MEDICAÇÕES

MEDICAMENTO(S) OU MEDICAÇÃO ALTERNATIVA COMPLEMENTAR
Resveratrol, um antioxidante potente, inibe o crescimento do tumor uveal em dois modelos animais de melanoma uveal, além de ser uma opção benigna e desejável para manter a saúde ocular de cães acometidos.

CONTRAINDICAÇÕES/INTERAÇÕES POSSÍVEIS
N/D.

ACOMPANHAMENTO

- Radiografias ou ultrassonografias toracoabdominais pós-operatórias — aos 6 e 12 meses se o índice mitótico estiver alto ou se o paciente apresentar extensão tumoral a estruturas extraesclerais, a porções vasculares ou ao nervo óptico.
- Avaliar o local da enucleação em busca de recidiva tumoral.

DIVERSOS

Sugestões de Leitura
Cook CS, Wilkie DA. Treatment of presumed iris melanoma in dogs by diode laser photocoagulation: 23 cases. Vet Ophthalmology 1999, 2:217-225.
Wilcock BP, Peiffer RL. Morphology and behavior of primary ocular melanomas in 91 dogs. Vet Pathol 1986, 23:418-424.
Van Ginkel PR, Soesiawati R, et al. Reservatrol (a potent antioxidant) inhibits uveal melanoma tumor growth via early mitochondrial dysfunction. Invest Ophthalmol Vis Sci 2008, 49(4):1299-1306.

Autor Terri L. McCalla
Consultor Editorial Paul E. Miller

MELANOMA UVEAL EM GATOS

CONSIDERAÇÕES GERAIS

REVISÃO
- Também conhecido como melanoma difuso da íris.
- O tumor intraocular mais comum em gatos.
- Costuma se originar da superfície anterior da íris, com extensão ao corpo ciliar e à coroide.
- Tende a ser plano e difuso, mas não nodular (diferente dos melanomas intraoculares em cães).
- Inicialmente, exibe aspecto histológico e clínico benigno.
- Característica peculiar — pode desenvolver doença metastática até muitos anos depois.
- A taxa de metástase pode ser de até 63%, embora outro estudo tenha constatado lesões metastáticas em 3 de 37 casos de melanoma ocular felino (8,1%).
- A ocorrência de glaucoma secundário pode aumentar o risco de metástase.

IDENTIFICAÇÃO
- Não há predisposição sexual nem racial.
- A idade média de gatos acometidos é de 9,5 anos, embora possa acometer gatos adultos de qualquer idade.

SINAIS CLÍNICOS
Achados Anamnésicos
- Mudança de coloração da íris.
- Glaucoma secundário indutor de midríase ou buftalmia, que resultam em cegueira.

Achados do Exame Físico
- Superfície da íris — espessada, irregular e geralmente pigmentada, embora possa não estar pigmentada.
- Lesões — focais a difusas; costumam ser planas; evolução lenta; podem envolver um ou ambos os olhos.
- Doença avançada — muitas vezes, observam-se células tumorais pigmentadas no humor aquoso; espessamento homogêneo da íris.
- Pode-se notar infiltração no ângulo de drenagem, o que possivelmente resulta em glaucoma secundário.

DIAGNÓSTICO

DIAGNÓSTICO DIFERENCIAL
- Máculas na superfície da íris que não parecem se alterar com o passar do tempo — podem ser lesões pigmentadas benignas; é mais provável que sejam decorrentes de melanocitoma, uma lesão benigna.
- Heterocromia da íris — alteração congênita e não progressiva na pigmentação dessa estrutura ocular.
- Alteração difusa na cor da íris, resultante de uveíte anterior crônica. Difere de melanoma uveal pelo histórico de uveíte anterior crônica.
- Atrofia da íris — ocorre perda do estroma anterior da íris, aumentando a visualização do tecido posterior intensamente pigmentado dessa estrutura ocular. O adelgaçamento da íris é observado como orifícios de espessura completa na íris ou como defeitos de retroiluminação na íris quando a luz reflete o tapete de volta através da íris.
- Melanomas do limbo — apresentam comportamento benigno; tendem a ser massas límbicas focais, localizadas no segmento superior, planas a levemente elevadas, que não invadem o trato uveal, a menos que sejam muito extensas.

HEMOGRAMA/BIOQUÍMICA/URINÁLISE
Normais.

DIAGNÓSTICO POR IMAGEM
- Radiografias torácicas e ultrassonografia abdominal — ajudam a determinar a presença e a extensão de metástase.
- A obtenção de imagens é recomendada no período pré-cirúrgico e a cada 6 meses após o diagnóstico.

MÉTODOS DIAGNÓSTICOS
- Exame oftalmológico completo, incluindo tonometria e gonioscopia.
- Aspirado por agulha fina da superfície da íris ("a vácuo") — de valor diagnóstico questionável; não é benéfico para o estadiamento do tumor.
- Biópsia da íris — pode ser realizada, mas não é proveitosa para a classificação do estágio tumoral.
- A presença de melanócitos no ângulo iridocorneano e no plexo venoso ciliar sugere a ocorrência de disseminação de células metastáticas pelo corpo, mas essas metástases podem não ser evidenciadas até alguns anos depois.

TRATAMENTO

- Varia com a idade do gato, a extensão e a velocidade de evolução, a preferência do oftalmologista e o nível de preocupação do proprietário quanto ao potencial de malignidade.
- Gato idoso com evolução lenta — considerar apenas a realização de exames periódicos e a obtenção de fotografias seriadas para monitorizar a evolução da(s) lesão(ões).
- Gato mais jovem com doença rapidamente progressiva — contemplar o procedimento de enucleação.
- Pequenas lesões isoladas semelhantes a máculas foram aparentemente submetidas a tratamento bem-sucedido com fotoablação a laser (diodo), embora não haja estudos de acompanhamento controlados ou a longo prazo.
- Envolvimento difuso leve a moderado da íris — a maioria dos oftalmologistas prefere uma abordagem conservativa de exames periódicos e fotografias seriadas para monitorizar o crescimento da(s) lesão(ões). A enucleação será uma alternativa se a evolução puder ser documentada ou se o proprietário estiver muito preocupado com o potencial de malignidade.
- Envolvimento extenso da íris com consequente alteração no formato ou na mobilidade das pupilas, extensão para outras estruturas além da íris, invasão do ângulo de drenagem ou glaucoma secundário — sugere-se a enucleação.
- Gatos com espessamento da íris e envolvimento do ângulo iridocorneano, com ou sem glaucoma, no entanto, apresentaram tempos de sobrevida semelhantes quando comparados a gatos-controle não acometidos de idade compatível.
- Lesões avançadas que consistem em envolvimento infiltrativo da íris, incluindo o epitélio posterior e o corpo ciliar, têm diminuído os tempos de sobrevida, presumivelmente em consequência da doença metastática.
- Na enucleação, deve-se empregar uma técnica cirúrgica delicada; em seres humanos, a enucleação é associada à ocorrência de metástases.

MEDICAÇÕES

MEDICAMENTO(S)
N/D.

ACOMPANHAMENTO

MONITORIZAÇÃO DO PACIENTE
- PIO — monitorização trimestral se as opções cirúrgicas forem recusadas pelo proprietário; os leves aumentos da PIO podem ser tratados com a administração oral ou tópica de inibidores da anidrase carbônica (p. ex., dorzolamida ou brinzolamida com a instilação de 1 gota no olho acometido a cada 8 h ou metazolamida na dosagem aproximada de 6,25 mg/gato VO a cada 12-24 h); a enucleação constitui o método mais eficiente para o controle do glaucoma secundário a melanoma.
- Locais comuns de metástase — fígado, pulmões, linfonodos regionais; monitorização periódica.

EVOLUÇÃO ESPERADA E PROGNÓSTICO
- Um único estudo a longo prazo revela que os pacientes com melanoma precoce da íris não apresentam alto risco de metástase potencialmente fatal, em comparação aos animais do grupo controle; no entanto, os pacientes com lesões avançadas exibem uma redução drástica nos tempos de sobrevida.
- Lesões — focais, multifocais a difusas; geralmente planas; pigmentação em alguns meses a anos (i. e., variável); podem envolver um ou ambos os olhos.
- Doença avançada — com frequência, observam-se células tumorais pigmentadas no humor aquoso; há espessamento homogêneo da íris, o que provoca uma anormalidade no formato pupilar e alteração na mobilidade pupilar.
- Prognóstico — reservado, mesmo após a realização da enucleação; a metástase pode não se tornar evidente por alguns anos ou, então, ser diagnosticada à necropsia.

DIVERSOS

SINÔNIMO(S)
- Melanoma da íris.
- Melanoma difuso da íris.

ABREVIATURA(S)
- PIO = pressão intraocular.

Sugestões de Leitura

Dubielzig RR. Ocular neoplasia in small animals. Vet Clin North Am Small Anim Pract 1990, 20:837-848.

Kalishman JB, Chappell RJ, Flood LA, Dubielzig RR, et al. A matched observational study of survival in cats with enucleation due to diffuse iris melanoma. Vet Ophthalmology 1998, 1:25-29.

Schaffer EH, Gordon S. Feline ocular melanoma. Clinical and pathologico-anatomic findings in 37 cases. Tierarztl Prax 1993, 21(3):255-264.

Autor Carmen M.H. Colitz
Consultor Editorial Paul E. Miller

MELENA

CONSIDERAÇÕES GERAIS

DEFINIÇÃO
Presença de sangue digerido nas fezes, às quais confere aspecto enegrecido, alcatroado.

FISIOPATOLOGIA
Geralmente, resulta de sangramento GI superior, mas pode estar associada a sangue ingerido da cavidade bucal ou do trato respiratório.

SISTEMA(S) ACOMETIDO(S)
• Gastrintestinal. • Respiratório. • Coagulação.

IDENTIFICAÇÃO
• Mais comum nos cães do que nos gatos.

SINAIS CLÍNICOS
Achados Anamnésicos
• Pacientes com hemorragia do trato GI superior podem exibir vômito (de aspecto sanguinolento ou semelhante a "borra de café"), inapetência, perda de peso, fraqueza e/ou palidez de mucosa.
• Pacientes com hemorragia do trato respiratório podem apresentar epistaxe, espirros, hemoptise, palidez de mucosa, fraqueza e/ou dispneia.
• Pacientes com coagulação anormal podem revelar petéquia, equimose, palidez de mucosa, epistaxe, hematúria, hifema e/ou fraqueza.

Achados do Exame Físico
Dependem da causa subjacente.

CAUSAS
Ulceração/Erosão GI Primária
• Neoplasia — linfoma, adenocarcinoma.
• Pólipos benignos.
• Infecciosa — pitiose, doença fúngica, infestação parasitária, *Helicobacter* spp.
• Mecânica — corpo estranho.
• Inflamatória — gastrite aguda; gastropatia hemorrágica; gastrite/enterite linfoplasmocitária, eosinofílica, granulomatosa e/ou histiocítica.
• Medicamentos — AINE, corticosteroides.

Doenças Metabólicas/Outras Indutoras de Ulceração GI
• Insuficiência renal.
• Doença/insuficiência hepática.
• Pancreatite.
• Hipoadrenocorticismo.
• Neoplasia — gastrinoma, mastocitoma.
• Choque, má perfusão.

Ingestão de Sangue
• Dieta (alimentos crus).
• Lesão esofágica — neoplasia, esofagite.
• Lesão bucal ou faríngea — neoplasia, abscesso.
• Lesão nasal — neoplasia, rinite fúngica, rinite inflamatória.
• Lesão respiratória — torção de lobo pulmonar, neoplasia, pneumonia, traumatismo (indutor de hemoptise).

Coagulopatia
• Trombocitopenia.
• Disfunção plaquetária — doença de von Willebrand, trombastenia, trombopatia, AINE.
• Anormalidades de fator de coagulação — ingestão de rodenticida anticoagulante, deficiência de fator de coagulação.
• CID.

FATORES DE RISCO
Artrite ou outras condições que necessitem do uso de AINE ou corticosteroides.

DIAGNÓSTICO

DIAGNÓSTICO DIFERENCIAL
• Medicações indutoras de fezes enegrecidas — subsalicilato de bismuto, terapia oral com ferro.
• É imprescindível a distinção entre doença intestinal e extraintestinal.

HEMOGRAMA/BIOQUÍMICA/URINÁLISE
• Anemia microcítica, hipocrômica, pouco regenerativa em caso de perda crônica de sangue.
• Anemia regenerativa no início da perda sanguínea — pode ser pouco regenerativa se a perda ultrapassar 3-5 dias.
• Pan-hipoproteinemia representa perda sanguínea significante.
• Trombocitopenia, neutrofilia em alguns pacientes; pancitopenia em outros.
• Exame da bioquímica pode revelar causa extraintestinal de melena — insuficiência renal, hepatopatia, hipoadrenocorticismo.
• Urinálise pode demonstrar hematúria nos pacientes com defeitos da coagulação.

OUTROS TESTES LABORATORIAIS
• O perfil da coagulação pode revelar anormalidade nesse processo.
• O tempo de sangramento pode estar prolongado.
• O exame de fezes pode exibir alguma causa infecciosa — parasitas, *Clostridium* spp.
• O raspado retal pode demonstrar a presença de microrganismos fúngicos (*Histoplasma* spp.).
• Teste de estimulação com ACTH anormalmente baixo em casos de hipoadrenocorticismo.
• Teste da urease para *Helicobacter* spp.

DIAGNÓSTICO POR IMAGEM
• Radiografia abdominal pode revelar a presença de massa, corpo estranho ou anormalidades na forma e/ou no tamanho renal ou hepático.
• Radiografias torácicas podem identificar lesões pulmonares e/ou traqueobrônquicas.
• TC nasal pode indicar lesões intranasais.
• Ultrassonografia pode revelar a presença de massa GI, hepatopatia, pancreatite ou nefropatia.
• Série radiográfica do trato GI superior com bário pode delinear massa, ulceração ou defeito de enchimento no estômago ou intestino delgado superior.

MÉTODOS DIAGNÓSTICOS
• Endoscopia permite a visualização de massas e/ou úlceras (esofágica, gástrica e/ou duodenal), recuperação de corpos estranhos GI e coleta de amostras para biopsia.
• Rinoscopia pode permitir a visualização de lesões nasais (a retroflexão do endoscópio ou broncoscópio e a avaliação das coanas são medidas úteis).
• Broncoscopia possibilita a visualização de lesões das vias aéreas.
• Aspirado e citologia da medula óssea, conforme indicação, na presença de pancitopenia.

TRATAMENTO

• Paciente internado — a exceção pode ser um animal com parasitas intestinais.
• Tratamento da doença subjacente — insuficiência renal, hepatopatia, hipoadrenocorticismo, doença respiratória, etc.
• Reposição hídrica com soluções eletrolíticas balanceadas e suplementação de potássio.
• Transfusões com sangue total ou papa de hemácias em caso de anemia grave.
• Transfusão de sangue total ou de plasma se o paciente tiver alguma coagulopatia.
• Interrupção temporária da ingestão oral no caso de vômito. Talvez haja necessidade do uso de antieméticos.
• Pode haver a necessidade de cirurgia para ulceração gastroduodenal grave ou neoplasia.

MEDICAÇÕES

MEDICAMENTO(S) DE ESCOLHA
• Protetores de mucosa para ulceração/erosão gastroduodenal — antagonistas dos receptores H_2 (p. ex., ranitidina 2 mg/kg IV ou VO a cada 12 h ou famotidina 0,5 mg/kg IV ou VO a cada 12-24 h); sucralfato 0,5-1 g VO a cada 6-8 h; misoprostol 3-5 mcg/kg VO a cada 8 h.
• Terapia tripla na suspeita ou na confirmação de *Helicobacter* (ver "Infecção por *Helicobacter*").

CONTRAINDICAÇÕES
Evitar o uso de corticosteroides e AINE nos pacientes com ulceração/erosão gastrintestinal.

MEDICAMENTO(S) ALTERNATIVO(S)
Bloqueador da bomba Na/K-ATPase (omeprazol 0,7 mg/kg VO a cada 24 h) poderá ser utilizado se os antagonistas do receptor H_2 não tiverem sucesso ou inicialmente em caso de ulceração esofágica ou gastroduodenal grave.

ACOMPANHAMENTO

MONITORIZAÇÃO DO PACIENTE
• Mensuração diária do hematócrito até que a anemia esteja estabilizada e, depois, semanalmente.
• Avaliação do estado de hidratação diariamente se o paciente estiver vomitando.

COMPLICAÇÕES POSSÍVEIS
• Perfuração gástrica ou duodenal com consequente peritonite.
• Choque hipovolêmico e morte na perda aguda grave de sangue.

DIVERSOS

POTENCIAL ZOONÓTICO
Helicobacter spp. possuem potencial zoonótico desconhecido.

VER TAMBÉM
Doenças causais individuais — Hipoadrenocorticismo, *Helicobacter*, etc.

ABREVIATURA(S)
• ACTH = hormônio adrenocorticotrópico.
• AINE = anti-inflamatórios não esteroides.
• CID = coagulação intravascular disseminada.
• GI = gastrintestinal.
• TC = tomografia computadorizada.

Autor Lisa E. Moore
Consultor Editorial Albert E. Jergens

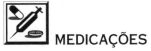

CONSIDERAÇÕES GERAIS

REVISÃO
- Tumores das meninges, mais comumente encontrados dentro do crânio sobre o cérebro.
- Em geral, são massas solitárias; ocasionalmente múltiplas (gatos).
- Podem ocorrer sob a forma de massas em forma de placas sobre o assoalho da calvária, de forma paranasal ou (raramente) em localização retrobulbar mais nos cães do que nos gatos; também se desenvolvem ao longo da medula espinal, porém com menor frequência e com predileção por local intradural extramedular.
- Comprimem o tecido adjacente, provocando edema vasogênico.
- Cães — tendem a ser mais invasivos em direção ao parênquima cerebral ou vasculatura circundante.
- Tumor mais comum do cérebro de cães e gatos.

IDENTIFICAÇÃO
- Cães e gatos.
- Cães — sem predileção racial; as raças mesocefálicas podem apresentar uma incidência mais elevada de meningiomas paranasais; a maioria tem >7 anos de idade; faixa etária de 11 semanas a 14 anos; um sarcoma meníngeo espinal foi diagnosticado em Rottweiler com 11 semanas de vida; levemente predominante nas fêmeas.
- Gatos — a maioria possui >9 anos de idade; faixa etária de 1 a 24 anos; leve predominância pelos machos.

SINAIS CLÍNICOS
- Variam com a localização do tumor.
- Tipicamente crônicos e insidiosamente progressivos em semanas a meses.
- Poderão ser agudos se a invasão vascular resultar em isquemia focal ou caso ocorra o rápido desenvolvimento de edema.
- Predominam os déficits lateralizantes.

Intracranianas
- Doença cerebral — predominante; alteração do comportamento e estado mental; déficits visuais e proprioceptivos contralaterais; crises convulsivas.
- Cães — crises convulsivas de início tardio constituem o sinal mais comumente apresentado, sem evidência de déficits ao exame neurológico (doença de área silenciosa).
- Gatos — as crises convulsivas são menos comuns que nos cães.

Intraespinais
- Ataxia e disfunção motora — variam com a localização do tumor ao longo da coluna vertebral.
- Dor cervical ou dorsal.

CAUSAS E FATORES DE RISCO
- Incertos.
- A comprovação em gatos jovens com mucopolissacaridose tipo I sugere uma relação causal.

DIAGNÓSTICO

DIAGNÓSTICO DIFERENCIAL
- Outros tumores primários (p. ex., glioma) ou secundários (p. ex., por extensão ou metástase) do SNC — maior rapidez no início e na evolução dos sinais; diferenciar por imagem do cérebro (neuroimagem).
- Granuloma *por Cryptococcus* — há relatos de que tenha o mesmo aspecto do meningioma em gatos ao exame de TC.
- Meningoencefalite granulomatosa — pode causar déficits focais progressivos nos cães.
- Meningiomas de área silenciosa — podem mimetizar encefalopatia metabólica.
- Tumores da bainha nervosa, gliomas, linfoma, meningomielite focal e discopatia intervertebral tipo II — diferenciar de síndrome da medula espinal.

HEMOGRAMA/BIOQUÍMICA/URINÁLISE
Geralmente normais.

OUTROS TESTES LABORATORIAIS
Análise do LCS — raramente realizado por causa dos resultados característicos das técnicas de diagnóstico por imagem; resultados normais ou alto teor proteico, às vezes com pleocitose neutrofílica ou mista.

DIAGNÓSTICO POR IMAGEM
- RM da cabeça — modalidade diagnóstica preferida para doença intracraniana e espinal.
- RM — frequentemente aparece como lesão expansiva (tipo massa) do cérebro ou da medula espinal difusamente acentuada por contraste, hiperintensa em imagens ponderadas em T2 e isointensa em imagens ponderadas em T1; uma "cauda" dural é um aspecto característico.
- TC — revela um realce homogêneo de lesão bem circunscrita.
- Radiografia e TC do crânio — podem revelar hiperostose da calvária adjacente ao meningioma e densidade tecidual aumentada se o tumor estiver calcificado.
- Mielografia — tipicamente revela massa intradural extramedular em casos de mielopatia; aparência de "montículo de golfe" dificulta a diferenciação de tumor da bainha nervosa sem a realização de biopsia.
- O procedimento de biopsia permanece necessário para o diagnóstico definitivo.

MÉTODOS DIAGNÓSTICOS
Eletroencefalografia — revela atividade de onda lenta e de voltagem média a elevada, indicando depressão cortical; pode apresentar formas de ondas paroxísticas características de atividade convulsiva.

TRATAMENTO

- Paciente de ambulatório, se tratado por meio clínico.
- Paciente internado — desidratação; anorexia; crises convulsivas frequentes.
- Excisão cirúrgica — necessária para o tratamento definitivo; geralmente bem-sucedida se o tumor for acessível; em cães, é mais comum a excisão parcial por causa da invasividade.
- Radioterapia — após a excisão parcial ou se a excisão não for possível; pode estar associada a tempo de sobrevida prolongado.
- Tratamento clínico — os esteroides são apenas paliativos; hidroxiureia pode estar associada a tempo de sobrevida prolongado; após excisão parcial ou pós-radiação ou como agente isolado.
- Fluidos — evitar a administração exagerada; pode exacerbar o edema cerebral e os déficits neurológicos.

MEDICAÇÕES

MEDICAMENTO(S)

Edema Cerebral
- Corticosteroides — melhoram os déficits neurológicos associados ao edema vasogênico.
- Em caso de estupor, ataxia grave ou sinais de herniação — succinato sódico de metilprednisolona (30 mg/kg IV) ou fosfato sódico de dexametasona (0,25 mg/kg IV).
- Deterioração contínua ou sem melhora — solução de manitol a 20% (0,5-2 g/kg em taxa de infusão constante por mais de 20 min).
- Uma vez estabilizado — prednisona (0,5 mg/kg a cada 12 h) ou dexametasona (0,02-0,05 mg/kg VO a cada 8 h; em seguida, reduzir gradativamente para a dose mais baixa, porém eficaz).

Crises Convulsivas
- Medicamentos antiepilépticos — obrigatórios mediante a ocorrência de 1 crise convulsiva a cada 6-8 semanas ou crises agrupadas; recomendados em qualquer atividade convulsiva.
- Fenobarbital (primeira escolha) — 2-3 mg/kg IV ou VO a cada 12 h, ou brometo de potássio a 250 mg/mL na dose de 20 mg/kg a cada 12 h em cães; zonisamida 5-10 mg/kg a cada 12 h (cães); levetiracetam 20 mg/kg a cada 8 h (cães ou gatos).
- Crises convulsivas agrupadas — diazepam (0,5 mg/kg/h em taxa de infusão constante) para tratar as crises contínuas, adicionando fenobarbital IV (2-3 mg/kg a cada 12 h) para o tratamento a longo prazo; ou levetiracetam IV (20 mg/kg a cada 8 h).

Quimioterapia
Hidroxiureia a 150 mg/kg/semana (cães) e 75 mg/kg/semana (gatos).

CONTRAINDICAÇÕES/INTERAÇÕES POSSÍVEIS
- Cloranfenicol e cimetidina — evitar com o fenobarbital, pois esses agentes retardam seu metabolismo.
- Evitar modificação da dieta enquanto o animal estiver sendo tratado com brometo de potássio — o conteúdo de cloreto do alimento afeta inversamente o nível sérico do brometo.

ACOMPANHAMENTO

- Efetuar exames neurológicos seriados — detectam melhora acentuada nos déficits dentro de 24-48 h após o início dos corticosteroides.
- Avaliar os níveis séricos de fenobarbital e brometo 3 semanas após o início da terapia; mensurar as enzimas hepáticas a cada 6 meses durante o tratamento com o fenobarbital.
- Monitorizar o hemograma completo com contagem de plaquetas a cada 1-2 semanas até a estabilização do paciente e, depois, obter o hemograma completo novamente e o perfil bioquímico a cada 3-4 meses com a administração da hidroxiureia.

Gatos
- Excisão cirúrgica — prognóstico bom; 75% dos pacientes submetidos à excisão cirúrgica são curados; a atividade convulsiva pode persistir apesar da excisão bem-sucedida.

Meningioma

- Tratamento clínico — os déficits neurológicos ficam mais graves, mas isso pode demorar muitos meses, já que os meningiomas tendem a ser de crescimento lento; a doença toracolombar evolui para paralisia e incapacidade de controlar a micção; causa retenção urinária e (possivelmente) atonia vesical e cistite.

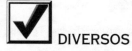

DIVERSOS

ABREVIATURA(S)
- LCS = líquido cerebrospinal.
- RM = ressonância magnética.
- SNC = sistema nervoso central.
- TC = tomografia computadorizada.

Sugestões de Leitura
Snyder JM, Shofer FS, Van Winkle TJ, Massicotte C. Canine intracranial primary neoplasia: 173 cases (1986-2003). J Vet Intern Med 2006, 20:669-75
Troxel MT, Vite CH, Van Winkle TJ, Newton AL, Tiches D, Dayrell-Hart B, Kapatkin AS, Shofer FS, Steinberg SA. Feline intracranial neoplasia: Retrospective review of 160 cases (1985-2001). J Vet Intern Med 2003, 17:850-859.

Autor Richard J. Joseph
Consultor Editorial Joane M. Parent

Meningite-arterite Responsivas a Esteroides — Cães

CONSIDERAÇÕES GERAIS

REVISÃO
• Podem ser agudas ou crônicas. • Lesões — mais notáveis no SNC, acometendo as meninges e as artérias meníngeas; além disso, há alterações vasculares em órgãos como coração, fígado, rim e sistema gastrintestinal. • Fatores genéticos — podem desempenhar algum papel; há suspeitas em colônias de cães da raça Beagle e em Nova Scotia duck tolling retriever. • Ocorrência mundial.

IDENTIFICAÇÃO
• Cães. • Raças Beagle, Montanhês de Berna, Nova Scotia duck tolling retriever e Boxer são predispostas; qualquer raça pode ser acometida.
• Acomete principalmente cães jovens adultos de ambos os sexos; faixa etária de 5-18 meses.

SINAIS CLÍNICOS
• Clássicos (agudos) — hiperestesia; rigidez cervical; marcha rígida; febre de até 42°C.
• Crônicos — déficits neurológicos que, em geral, refletem lesão na medula espinal ou multifocal.

CAUSAS E FATORES DE RISCO
• Causa desconhecida. • Achados patológicos, dados laboratoriais e resposta acentuada aos esteroides — sugerem doença imunomediada relacionada à falta de regulação na produção de IgA. • Observações epidemiológicas — a alteração na resposta imune pode ser desencadeada por algum fator ambiental, possivelmente de natureza infecciosa.

DIAGNÓSTICO

DIAGNÓSTICO DIFERENCIAL
• Forma aguda — meningite bacteriana; tumores das meninges (histiocitose, meningioma, linfossarcoma); discospondilite. • Forma crônica — meningite bacteriana; tumores das meninges (histiocitose, meningioma, linfossarcoma); encefalites virais; meningoencefalite granulomatosa; infecções por protozoários; lesões inflamatórias de origem desconhecida.

HEMOGRAMA/BIOQUÍMICA/URINÁLISE
• Forma aguda — leucocitose com neutrofilia e desvio à esquerda.
• Forma crônica — o hemograma completo não contribui para o diagnóstico.

OUTROS TESTES LABORATORIAIS
Níveis de IgA (no soro e LCS) — geralmente elevados; fortemente sugestivos do diagnóstico, sobretudo em casos de doença crônica; altos níveis séricos da proteína C-reativa.

DIAGNÓSTICO POR IMAGEM
Mielografia, RM ou TC — para excluir tumores.

MÉTODOS DIAGNÓSTICOS
Exame do LCS
• Forma aguda — elevação leve a moderada do conteúdo de proteínas; pleocitose moderada a acentuada, com células predominantemente polimorfonucleares.
• Forma crônica — nível proteico normal ou levemente elevado; pleocitose leve a moderada com população celular mista ou com predomínio de células mononucleares.

ACHADOS PATOLÓGICOS
Forma Aguda
• Meningite acentuada com infiltração de macrófagos, plasmócitos, linfócitos e números variados de células polimorfonucleares, principalmente nas meninges da região cervical.
• Lesões das artérias meníngeas — mais degenerativas com inflamação perivascular.

Forma Crônica
• Espessamento fibroso acentuado e mineralização focal das leptomeninges.
• Paredes arteriais — espessadas e estenóticas em virtude da proliferação celular da camada íntima e do processo de fibrose.

TRATAMENTO
• Paciente internado — no início, instituição de fluidoterapia e compressas de gelo são medidas úteis para a temperatura corporal elevada.
• Paciente de ambulatório — após o tratamento inicial.
• Acompanhamentos regulares — informar o proprietário sobre os efeitos colaterais do tratamento com esteroide a longo prazo.

MEDICAÇÕES

MEDICAMENTO(S)
• Sinais iniciais com pleocitose leve no LCS — AINEs; monitorizar o paciente com cuidado.
• Em caso de primeira recidiva ou agravamento dos sintomas com pleocitose maciça no LCS — começar o tratamento a longo prazo (6 meses) com prednisolona (4 mg/kg VO a cada 24 h por 1-2 dias; em seguida, reduzir de forma lenta e gradual); reavaliar o paciente (incluindo a coleta do LCS e o exame de sangue) a cada 4-6 semanas após o início do tratamento.
• Com a normalização do exame neurológico, do LCS e dos níveis séricos da proteína C-reativa — reduzir a dose do esteroide.
• Pleocitose persistente — continuar com a mesma dosagem de esteroide.
• O tratamento pode ser interrompido depois de aproximadamente 6 meses.
• Medicamentos imunossupressores se o paciente não responder bem à prednisolona isolada; usada em combinação.
• Considerar o uso de protetores gastrintestinais para evitar a formação de úlceras.

CONTRAINDICAÇÕES/INTERAÇÕES POSSÍVEIS
Corticosteroides — o tratamento em altas doses pode levar a complicações sérias; efeitos colaterais sem risco de morte (poliúria, polidipsia, polifagia e ganho de peso); não são tolerados por cerca de 5% dos cães.

ACOMPANHAMENTO

MONITORIZAÇÃO DO PACIENTE
Exames para controle clínico — a cada 4-6 semanas; incluir o exame de sangue e a coleta do LCS; mensuração dos níveis séricos da proteína C-reativa até a interrupção dos esteroides.

PREVENÇÃO
Controle rigoroso do esquema terapêutico para evitar recidivas frequentes.

COMPLICAÇÕES POSSÍVEIS
• Hemorragia subaracnoide — pode culminar em tetra ou paraplegia aguda.
• Lesões hipóxicas da medula espinal ou do cérebro — doença crônica; pode resultar em anormalidades da marcha e crises convulsivas.
• Efeitos colaterais do tratamento imunossupressor — infecções bacterianas; sangramento no trato gastrintestinal; pancreatite.

EVOLUÇÃO ESPERADA E PROGNÓSTICO
• Forma aguda — prognóstico relativamente bom nos cães jovens submetidos à terapia intensa precoce.
• Casos crônicos com recidivas frequentes — prognóstico reservado; estudos controlados mencionam que cerca de 60% dos cães são curados após o tratamento imunossupressor.

DIVERSOS

DISTÚRBIOS ASSOCIADOS
Poliartrite.

FATORES RELACIONADOS COM A IDADE
Animais idosos não toleram bem o tratamento com esteroide a longo prazo; no entanto, a condição é rara nos cães com >5 anos de idade.

SINÔNIMO(S)
• Meningite asséptica.
• Meningomielite responsiva a corticosteroide.
• Síndrome de poliarterite juvenil canina.

ABREVIATURA(S)
• AINE = anti-inflamatórios não esteroides.
• LCS = líquido cerebrospinal.
• RM = ressonância magnética.
• SNC = sistema nervoso central.
• TC = tomografia computadorizada.

Sugestões de Leitura
Anfinsen KP, Berendt M, Liste FJ, et al. A retrospective epidemiological study of clinical signs and familial predisposition associated with aseptic meningitis in the Norwegian population of Nova Scotia duck tolling retrievers born 1994-2003. Can J Vet Res 2008, 72:350-355.
Bathen-Noethen A, Carlson R, Menzel D, Mischke R, Tipold A. Concentrations of acute-phase proteins in dogs with steroid responsive meningitis-arteritis. J Vet Intern Med 2008, 22:1149-1156.
Tipold A, Schatzberg SJ. An update on steroid responsive meningitis-arteritis. J Small Anim Pract 2010, 51:150-154.

Autor Andrea Tipold
Consultor Editorial Joane M. Parent

Meningite/Meningoencefalite/Meningomielite Bacterianas

CONSIDERAÇÕES GERAIS

DEFINIÇÃO
- Meningite — inflamação das meninges.
- Meningoencefalite — inflamação das meninges e do cérebro.
- Meningomielite — inflamação das meninges e da medula espinal.

FISIOPATOLOGIA
- A infecção bacteriana do SNC costuma ocorrer por extensão direta a partir de um local extraneural infectado. Menos comumente, a infecção é introduzida por traumatismo penetrante ou corpo estranho migratório.
- A disseminação hematógena de bactérias para o SNC é rara, exceto em neonatos septicêmicos e pacientes gravemente imunossuprimidos.
- A inflamação das meninges costuma levar à inflamação secundária do cérebro ou da medula espinhal, resultando em déficits neurológicos.
- Debris inflamatórios e cicatrização podem obstruir o fluxo do LCS, levando à hidrocefalia secundária.

SISTEMA(S) ACOMETIDO(S)
- Nervoso — meninges, cérebro ou medula espinal.
- Sinais polissistêmicos — podem estar presentes quando a infecção se originar em local extraneural.

INCIDÊNCIA/PREVALÊNCIA
Raras.

IDENTIFICAÇÃO
Espécies
Cães e gatos.

Idade Média e Faixa Etária
- Qualquer idade.
- Os neonatos podem ter um risco relativamente mais alto por causa da onfaloflebite.

Sexo Predominante
Machos e fêmeas são igualmente acometidos.

SINAIS CLÍNICOS
Comentários Gerais
- Os pacientes quase sempre exibem doença sistêmica.
- Em pacientes septicêmicos, podem-se constatar os sinais de depressão, choque, hipotensão e CID.
- Os sinais do SNC podem ser profundos e rapidamente progressivos.

Achados do Exame Físico
- Pirexia.
- Rigidez e hiperestesia cervicais — especialmente nos casos de meningite.
- Déficits neurológicos — refletem a localização do parênquima envolvido (p. ex., atividade mental alterada, déficits de nervo craniano, déficits de reação postural, paresia e crises convulsivas).
- Pode-se encontrar o local extraneural da infecção bacteriana subjacente.
- Vômito.
- Bradicardia com hipertensão sistêmica sugere pressão intracraniana elevada.

CAUSAS
- Meningoencefalite — geralmente secundária à extensão local de infecção da orelha interna, dos olhos, do espaço retrobulbar, dos seios nasais ou das passagens nasais. Também pode ocorrer com fraturas traumáticas do crânio ou migração de corpos estranhos, como farpas de gramíneas e espinhos do porco-espinho.
- Meningomielite — secundária à discospondilite ou osteomielite vertebral.
- Pode ocorrer disseminação hematógena de infecção bacteriana em neonatos com onfaloflebite, pacientes imunossuprimidos ou em cães com endocardite bacteriana, prostatite, discospondilite, pneumonia ou gastrenterite.
- O local de origem nem sempre é encontrado.

FATORES DE RISCO
- Infecção bacteriana não tratada.
- Estado imunocomprometido.
- Lesão envolvendo o SNC ou estruturas adjacentes.

DIAGNÓSTICO

DIAGNÓSTICO DIFERENCIAL
Meningite Infecciosa (Não Bacteriana)
- Microrganismos fúngicos, protozoários, virais e riquetsianos podem causar meningite; os achados clínicos e laboratoriais, bem como os locais extraneurais acometidos, podem sugerir o diagnóstico específico.
- Cinomose canina, toxoplasmose, neosporose, criptococose, blastomicose, neuroborreliose, meningite riquetsiana e peritonite infecciosa felina, sem exceção, provocam doença que mimetiza meningite/meningoencefalite bacterianas.
- LCS — inflamatório com pleocitose linfocítica variável, mononuclear mista ou neutrofílica, dependendo da etiologia.
- O diagnóstico é feito pela identificação dos microrganismos no LCS ou em locais extraneurais (com o uso de exame citológico, cultura ou PCR) e por sorologia.

Meningite-Arterite Responsivas a Esteroides (Meningite Asséptica)
- Observadas, sobretudo, em cães jovens adultos (6-19 meses) de grande porte, mas cães de meia-idade e idosos são ocasionalmente acometidos.
- Beagle, Boxer, Montanhês de Berna, Pointer alemão de pelo curto, Weimaraner e Nova Scotia duck tolling retriever são predispostos; no entanto, qualquer raça pode ser acometida.
- Dor cervical sem déficits neurológicos é o sinal mais comum.
- Ocorre febre em 60-80% dos cães acometidos. Os sinais podem ter recidivas e remissões inicialmente.
- Os cães afetados permanecem normais do ponto de vista sistêmico.
- Podem ocorrer déficits neurológicos em cães cronicamente acometidos ou inadequadamente tratados.
- LCS — aumento na contagem de células nucleadas e no teor de proteínas. Nos casos agudos, observa-se pleocitose neutrofílica; já nos casos crônicos, pode haver o predomínio de células mononucleares. Resultados negativos nas culturas bacterianas.
- Aumento na concentração de IgA no soro e no LCS.
- Resposta drástica à administração de corticosteroide.

Meningoencefalomielite Granulomatosa
- Doença inflamatória idiopática do cérebro, da medula espinal e das meninges nos cães.
- Cães jovens adultos aos de meia-idade são mais frequentemente acometidos — Poodle e Terrier são predispostos; entretanto, qualquer raça pode ser acometida.
- Anormalidades neurológicas refletem o local da(s) lesão(ões).
- Dor cervical/febre em alguns cães com a forma disseminada que envolve a medula espinal cervical e as meninges.
- Sem sinais sistêmicos.
- LCS — pleocitose mononuclear mista com linfócitos, monócitos, plasmócitos e macrófagos grandes; pode incluir 20% de neutrófilos não tóxicos.
- Cultura do LCS — negativa.

Meningoencefalite Necrosante/ Leucoencefalite Necrosante
- Distúrbios inflamatórios idiopáticos do cérebro, específicos à raça e caracterizados por necrose regional com formação de áreas de cavitação.
- Os sinais refletem dano ao córtex cerebral (crises convulsivas, mudança comportamental, andar em círculo) em Pug, Maltês terrier, Chihuahua, Pequinês, Shih-tzu e Lhasa apso com meningoencefalite necrosante.
- Cães da raça Yorkshire terrier com leucoencefalite necrosante apresentam lesões no cérebro e no tronco cerebral que resultam em crises convulsivas e atividade mental anormal, bem como marcha anormal, inclinação da cabeça e anormalidades de nervo craniano.
- Sem sinais sistêmicos.
- LCS — aumento no conteúdo de proteína e na contagem de células nucleadas totais (tanto na meningoencefalite como na leucoencefalite necrosantes). Pequenos linfócitos predominam na meningoencefalite necrosante, embora seja comum a constatação de pleocitose mononuclear mista em leucoencefalite necrosante.

Neoplasia Primária do SNC
- Histórico prolongado; sinais neurológicos limitados ao SNC; resultados normais nos testes laboratoriais padrão.
- O diagnóstico é obtido por TC, RM, análise do LCS e biopsia.

HEMOGRAMA/BIOQUÍMICA/URINÁLISE
- É comum a presença de leucocitose; pode ser observado desvio à esquerda ou toxicidade.
- Indícios bioquímicos de envolvimento de outros órgãos (p. ex., fígado e rim) podem ser observados em pacientes septicêmicos. A hiperglobulinemia pode refletir infecção extraneural crônica.
- Piúria e bacteriúria em pacientes com infecção subjacente do trato urinário ou da próstata e em alguns animais bacterêmicos.

OUTROS TESTES LABORATORIAIS
- Testes sorológicos — para diferenciar doença fúngica, protozoária, riquetsiana e viral de doença bacteriana; gatos: título para toxoplasma pode ser positivo sem doença clínica.
- Exame citológico dos tecidos infectados — pele, olhos, secreção nasal, linfonodo, lavado traqueal; ajuda a identificar os microrganismos causais não bacterianos, especialmente em animais com doença fúngica.
- Hemocultura e urocultura — positivas em 30% dos cães com meningite bacteriana.

Meningite/Meningoencefalite/Meningomielite Bacterianas

DIAGNÓSTICO POR IMAGEM
- Radiografia de tórax/abdome e ultrassonografia do abdome — para identificar infecção subjacente ou outra doença significativa.
- Radiografia da coluna vertebral — discoespondilite pode ser identificada como foco de infecção.
- Radiografia/TC do crânio — podem identificar os seios nasais, a cavidade nasal ou as orelhas como o ponto inicial da infecção.
- Ecocardiografia — realizada na suspeita de endocardite valvular com base nos sinais de sopro/arritmia.
- RM — confirma a presença de inflamação do SNC e pode identificar o local extraneural de infecção (seios nasais, cavidade nasal, orelhas).

MÉTODOS DIAGNÓSTICOS
Análise do LCS
- Coleta — preocupante em animais com atividade mental reduzida, sugestiva de pressão intracraniana elevada, uma vez que o procedimento pode precipitar a ocorrência de herniação cerebral — tratar antes com manitol.
- Análise — pleocitose neutrofílica com elevada concentração proteica; os neutrófilos podem parecer tóxicos ou degenerados e, ocasionalmente, observam-se bactérias intracelulares; não é uma tarefa fácil diferenciar a meningite asséptica de bacteriana por meio citológico.
- Cultura — aeróbia ou anaeróbia; pode ser positiva (<40%) — a inoculação do LCS em caldo de enriquecimento aumenta a recuperação diagnóstica.
- Ensaio de PCR bacteriano universal no LCS pode ser utilizado para identificar o DNA de microrganismos causais em casos de cultura bacteriana negativa.

ACHADOS PATOLÓGICOS
- É possível notar empiema subdural, herniação ou material purulento na superfície do cérebro.
- Infiltração leptomeníngea supurativa difusa é comum.

TRATAMENTO
CUIDADO(S) DE SAÚDE ADEQUADO(S)
Paciente internado — tratar com rigor; com frequência, há necessidade de monitorização dos cuidados intensivos.

CUIDADO(S) DE ENFERMAGEM
Fluidoterapia e cuidados de suporte — conforme indicados para o choque.

ATIVIDADE
Restrita.

ORIENTAÇÃO AO PROPRIETÁRIO
Informar o proprietário sobre a importância do tratamento rápido e rigoroso, bem como sobre o caráter reservado do prognóstico quanto à recuperação.

MEDICAÇÕES
MEDICAMENTO(S) DE ESCOLHA
Antibióticos
- Agentes bactericidas que atingem concentrações terapêuticas dentro do LCS são os mais desejáveis — é recomendável o uso de medicamentos lipossolúveis com pequeno tamanho molecular, baixa ligação proteica e baixo grau de ionização sob pH fisiológico.
- Culturas — LCS, sangue, urina, local primário; determinar a sensibilidade aos medicamentos; caso não seja possível a obtenção das culturas, selecionar um agente de amplo espectro que penetre na barreira hematencefálica.
- Os medicamentos recomendados incluem cefalosporinas de terceira geração (moxalactam, ceftriaxona, cefotaxima), fluoroquinolonas, trimetoprima, sulfonamidas, clindamicina, doxiciclina e metronidazol.
- Agentes como penicilina, ampicilina e amoxicilina-clavulanato penetram no SNC com inflamação; uma boa opção para utilizar em combinação com algum outro antibiótico que continuará atravessando a barreira hematencefálica à medida que a inflamação desaparece.
- Administrar antibióticos por via intravenosa durante 3-5 dias para atingir altas concentrações no LCS com rapidez e, em seguida, manter sob terapia oral.
- A terapia IV imediata pode ser formulada com base na citologia; penicilina para infecções por Gram-positivos, fluoroquinolona (enrofloxacino ou ciprofloxacino) ou cefalosporina de terceira geração para infecções por Gram-negativos.

Anticonvulsivantes
- Indicados nas crises convulsivas.
- Diazepam inicialmente e, em seguida, fenobarbital.

Corticosteroides
- A maior parte do dano ao SNC se deve à inflamação — isso pode se agravar com lise bacteriana induzida pelos antibióticos.
- Pode-se administrar a dexametasona (0,2 mg/kg) antes da antibioticoterapia e, depois, a cada 12 h por 2 dias.

CONTRAINDICAÇÕES
- Aminoglicosídeos e cefalosporinas de primeira geração — não penetram na barreira hematencefálica mesmo na presença de meninges inflamadas.
- Cloranfenicol atinge altas concentrações no LCS, mas está associado a uma alta taxa de recidiva; não utilizar.

ACOMPANHAMENTO
MONITORIZAÇÃO DO PACIENTE
Monitorizar em busca de sinais do sistema nervoso, febre, leucocitose e sinais sistêmicos.

PREVENÇÃO
Tratar as infecções locais adjacentes ao SNC (p. ex., infecções dos olhos, das orelhas, dos seios nasais, do nariz e da coluna vertebral) precoce e rigorosamente para evitar extensão ao SNC.

COMPLICAÇÕES POSSÍVEIS
A lesão provocada pela inflamação do cérebro e da medula espinal ou a trombose associada podem ser irreversíveis.

EVOLUÇÃO ESPERADA E PROGNÓSTICO
- Resposta aos antibióticos — variável; prognóstico reservado.
- Muitos pacientes morrem apesar do tratamento.
- Alguns pacientes recuperam-se completamente, enquanto outros exibem déficits neurológicos residuais.
- É recomendável o tratamento por, no mínimo, 4 semanas após a resolução de todos os sinais clínicos.

DIVERSOS
VER TAMBÉM
- Encefalite.
- Meningoencefalomielite Granulomatosa.
- Meningite-Arterite Responsivas a Esteroides — Cães.

ABREVIATURA(S)
- CID = coagulação intravascular disseminada.
- LCS = líquido cerebrospinal.
- PCR = reação em cadeia da polimerase.
- PIF = peritonite infecciosa felina.
- RM = ressonância magnética.
- SNC = sistema nervoso central.
- TC = tomografia computadorizada.

Sugestões de Leitura
Kent M. Bacterial infections of the central nervous system. In: Greene CE, ed., Infectious Diseases of the Dog and Cat, 3rd ed. St. Louis: Saunders Elsevier, 2006, pp. 962-973.
Messier JS, Wagner SO, Baumwart RD, et al. A case of canine streptococcal meningoencephalitis diagnosed using universal bacterial polymerase chair reaction assay. JAAHA 2008, 44:205-209.
Radaelli ST, Platt SR. Bacterial menigoencephalomyelitis in dogs: A retrospective study in 23 cases (1990-1999). J Vet Intern Med 2002, 16:159-163.
Sturges BK, Dickinson PJ, Kortz GD, et al. Clinical signs, magnetic resonance imaging features, and outcome after surgical and medical treatment of otogenic intracranial infection in 11 cats and 4 dogs. J Vet Intern Med 2006, 20:648-656.
Tipold A. Diagnosis of inflammatory and infectious diseases of the central nervous system in dogs: A retrospective study. J Vet Intern Med 1995, 5:304-314.

Autor Susan M. Taylor
Consultor Editorial Joane M. Parent

Meningoencefalomielite Eosinofílica

CONSIDERAÇÕES GERAIS

REVISÃO
Embora a meningoencefalomielite eosinofílica possa estar associada a meningite, encefalite e mielite como resultado de infecção no SNC ou migração parasitária, na maioria dos casos, nenhuma causa subjacente pode ser encontrada. A meningoencefalomielite eosinofílica idiopática ocorre em raças caninas de grande porte, jovens às de meia-idade. A doença desaparece em grande parte dos casos após tratamento com esteroides.

IDENTIFICAÇÃO
• Cães e, raramente, gatos.
• Meningoencefalomielite eosinofílica idiopática — cães de grande porte (>25 kg) são predispostos.
• Idade média — 3 anos e meio (8 meses-13 anos).

SINAIS CLÍNICOS
• Variam com a localização do SNC e a gravidade do quadro.
• Déficits neurológicos — associados mais frequentemente ao envolvimento do crânio, porém com menor frequência ao acometimento da medula espinal e, raras vezes, dos nervos cranianos.

CAUSAS E FATORES DE RISCO
• Meningoencefalomielite eosinofílica idiopática (causa desconhecida) — maioria dos casos relatados.
• Infecciosas — *Dirofilaria immitis* e miíase por *Cuterebra* em gatos; *Neospora* sp., *Prototheca* sp., *Cryptococcus* sp., e migração de nematoides com *Baylisascaris procyonis* em cães.
• *Angiostrongylus* — cães na Austrália.
• Discopatia intervertebral provavelmente como resposta alérgica ao material do disco.

DIAGNÓSTICO

DIAGNÓSTICO DIFERENCIAL
• Não pode ser diferenciada de outras encefalites com base apenas nos sinais clínicos; é imprescindível a análise do LCS.
• Meningoencefalomielite eosinofílica idiopática — predominância de sinais cerebrais; resultados negativos de teste sorológico; pleocitose eosinofílica acentuada no LCS (20-95%); geralmente responsiva a esteroides.
• Doenças infecciosas — identificadas na presença de sinais sistêmicos e por meio de exame de sangue, avaliação de amostra fecal, análise do LCS, sorologia do soro/LCS e diagnóstico por imagem.

HEMOGRAMA/BIOQUÍMICA/URINÁLISE
• Eosinofilia periférica — incomum.
• Análise bioquímica e urinálise — geralmente normais em casos de doença idiopática; atividade enzimática hepática e creatinina quinase podem estar elevadas em casos de doenças infecciosas.

OUTROS TESTES LABORATORIAIS
• Sorologia — para descartar a suspeita de doenças infecciosas.
• Flutuação e sedimentação fecais — para descartar migração parasitária.

DIAGNÓSTICO POR IMAGEM
• Radiografia torácica e ultrassonografia abdominal — para descartar envolvimento sistêmico.
• RM — variável; observam-se lesões expansivas focais tipo massa, anormalidades difusas do parênquima, realce meníngeo difuso pós-contraste; as anormalidades dependem da causa e da localização da lesão.

MÉTODOS DIAGNÓSTICOS
Análise do LCS
• Pleocitose eosinofílica significativa quando estiver >10%.
• A presença de pleocitose eosinofílica, por si só, não é capaz de diferenciar meningoencefalomielite eosinofílica idiopática de infecção indutora de pleocitose eosinofílica no LCS.
• Meningoencefalomielite eosinofílica idiopática — contagem total de células nucleadas de 4-3.880 células/mL (média de 99 células/mL; referência <0,003) com 22-95% de eosinófilos.
• Infecções — 62-4.740 células/mL (média de 875 células/mL) com 30-95% de eosinófilos.

Teste Sorológico do LCS
• Se os eosinófilos no LCS estiverem >10%, procurar por doença parasitária e fúngica.
• Teste para dirofilariose, *N. caninum*, *T. gondii*, e *C. neoformans*.

ACHADOS PATOLÓGICOS
• A pleocitose eosinofílica no LCS não se correlaciona necessariamente com os eosinófilos observados no parênquima do SNC.
• A ampla variedade de achados patológicos pode indicar múltiplas causas ou a mesma doença submetida à biopsia em diversos momentos.

TRATAMENTO

• O paciente costuma ser internado por causa da gravidade dos sinais clínicos.
• Atividade — conforme tolerada.
• Dieta regular.

MEDICAÇÕES

MEDICAMENTO(S)
• Doença idiopática — administração de esteroide; dexametasona (0,25 mg/kg a cada 24 h por 1 dia; depois, 0,15 mg/kg a cada 24 h por 6 dias); seguir com prednisona (0,5 mg/kg a cada 24 h por 8 semanas); em seguida, "desmamar" o paciente lentamente por mais de 8 semanas a 6 meses, dependendo da resposta clínica.
• Doença protozoária — clindamicina, sulfonamidas e pirimetamina.
• Dirofilariose — a migração das microfilárias para o SNC é rara; não há nenhum tratamento disponível além do suporte.

CONTRAINDICAÇÕES/INTERAÇÕES POSSÍVEIS
• É importante diferenciar meningoencefalomielite eosinofílica idiopática de infecção, pois o tratamento difere bastante — doses imunossupressoras de esteroides *versus* tratamento contra o microrganismo causal.
• Os esteroides devem ser utilizados com cuidado se o diagnóstico ainda não foi confirmado.

ACOMPANHAMENTO

MONITORIZAÇÃO DO PACIENTE
Paciente internado — repetir o exame neurológico a cada 6 h para monitorar a evolução do quadro.

PREVENÇÃO
O tratamento com esteroides não deve ser interrompido mesmo se o animal voltar ao normal dentro de alguns dias. É obrigatório o tratamento por, no mínimo, 8 semanas, acompanhadas pela redução gradual da medicação durante o maior número de semanas possível.

COMPLICAÇÕES POSSÍVEIS
• Pode ocorrer recidiva após interrupção do medicamento.
• Garantir a dosagem adequada da medicação e retomar o tratamento por um período de tempo mais prolongado.

EVOLUÇÃO ESPERADA E PROGNÓSTICO
• Doença idiopática — prognóstico bom na maioria dos casos com tratamento precoce; a melhora costuma ser observada nas primeiras 72 h; recuperação completa em 2-6 meses. Alguns pacientes continuam se debilitando apesar do tratamento com esteroides e vêm a óbito.
• Doença protozoária — prognóstico mau a grave.
• Migração parasitária — prognóstico reservado a mau, dependendo da localização da lesão; os sinais clínicos podem desaparecer, porém as larvas frequentemente continuam migrando, podendo levar o paciente à óbito.
• Degradação de eosinófilos é tóxica para o tecido nervoso; o paciente pode apresentar déficits permanentes atribuídos não só à doença primária, mas também à morte dos eosinófilos.

DIVERSOS

FATORES RELACIONADOS COM A IDADE
A meningoencefalomielite eosinofílica idiopática é mais frequente em raças caninas de grande porte, jovens às de meia-idade (>25 kg).

VER TAMBÉM
Encefalite.

ABREVIATURA(S)
• LCS = líquido cerebrospinal.
• RM = ressonância magnética.
• SNC = sistema nervoso central.

Sugestões de Leitura
Williams JH, Köster LS, Naidoo V, et al. Review of idiopathic eosinophilic meningitis in dogs and cats, with a detailed description of two recent cases in dogs. J S Afr Vet Assoc 2008, 79(4):194-204.
Windsor RC, Sturges BK, Vernau KM, et al. Cerebrospinal fluid eosinophilia in dogs. J Vet Intern Med 2009, 23(2):275-281.

Autor Joane M. Parent
Consultor Editorial Joane M. Parent

MENINGOENCEFALOMIELITE GRANULOMATOSA

CONSIDERAÇÕES GERAIS

DEFINIÇÃO
A meningoencefalomielite granulomatosa refere-se a uma doença inflamatória que afeta o SNC de forma focal, difusa ou multifocal. É preciso ter cautela ao se diagnosticar a condição, pois a confirmação da doença só é possível por meio de análise histopatológica do tecido acometido. A meningoencefalomielite granulomatosa é o distúrbio inflamatório do SNC mais aceito e identificado no cão. Em consequência disso, diversos distúrbios virais e idiopáticos menos graves, muitas vezes, são erroneamente diagnosticados como meningoencefalomielite granulomatosa.

FISIOPATOLOGIA
• Desconhecida. Há suspeitas de uma base imunológica; também foi sugerida uma causa infecciosa.
• Foram identificadas três formas clinicopatológicas — ocular, multifocal (cérebro ou medula oblonga e espinal) e focal (foco isolado no cérebro ou na medula espinal).

SISTEMA(S) ACOMETIDO(S)
• Nervoso.
• Oftálmico.

GENÉTICA
Nenhuma base genética comprovada.

INCIDÊNCIA/PREVALÊNCIA
• Desconhecidas. Como raramente são obtidas biopsias cerebrais, é feito um diagnóstico presuntivo na maioria dos casos.
• Doença provavelmente incomum, pois foram necessários longos períodos de tempo (14-17 anos) para compilar os casos confirmados por meio histopatológico: JAVMA 1986, 188:418-422 (22 casos em 14 anos); JAVMA 1998, 212:1902-1906 (42 casos, dois deles encaminhados para instituições, em 14 anos); Vet Record 2001, 148:467-472 (20 casos em 17 anos).

DISTRIBUIÇÃO GEOGRÁFICA
Mundial.

IDENTIFICAÇÃO
Raça(s) Predominante(s)
Embora a meningoencefalomielite granulomatosa tenha sido estereotipada como uma doença de raças toy jovens aos de meia-idade (especialmente Terriers e Poodles), qualquer raça de porte médio e maior pode ser acometida.

Idade Média e Faixa Etária
• Média — 5 anos.
• Variação — 6 meses a 10 anos.

Sexo Predominante
Prevalência levemente maior em fêmeas.

SINAIS CLÍNICOS
• Os sinais dependem da forma da doença e da localização neuroanatômica.
• Forma cerebral — frequentemente resulta em atividade convulsiva.
• Forma ocular — início agudo de cegueira com pupilas dilatadas e irresponsivas.
• Forma focal — *lesão cerebral*: desorientação, mudanças comportamentais, crises convulsivas, cegueira cortical, andar em círculo compulsivo, compressão da cabeça contra objetos; *lesão do tronco cerebral*: sonolência, déficits dos nervos cranianos (mais comumente disfunção facial e vestibular), hemiparesia ipsolateral; *lesão da medula espinal*: dor cervical (cervicalgia), tetraparesia (lesões de C1-C5 ou C6-T2) ou paraparesia (lesões de T3-L3 ou L4-S2) e ataxia proprioceptiva.

CAUSAS
Desconhecidas.

FATORES DE RISCO
• Desconhecidos.
• Alguns cães desenvolvem sinais clínicos dentro de 5-10 dias da vacinação.

DIAGNÓSTICO

DIAGNÓSTICO DIFERENCIAL
• A combinação de anamnese, exame neurológico, análise do LCS e resultados do RM costuma levar a um diagnóstico correto de doença inflamatória, embora a definição da causa da inflamação possa ser problemática.
• O diagnóstico é feito somente por meio de estudos histopatológicos. Alguns cães com doença inflamatória do SNC são tratados de forma bem-sucedida, mas faltam dados a respeito desses casos. Biopsias cerebrais raramente são realizadas para confirmar o diagnóstico. É possível que alguns cães que sobrevivem à doença inflamatória do SNC tenham lesões compatíveis com meningoencefalomielite granulomatosa, mas estudos pós-morte não estão disponíveis para comprovar isso. Alternativamente, os cães que sobrevivem à doença inflamatória do SNC podem estar sofrendo de outro tipo de doença inflamatória viral ou idiopática menos grave.
• Doenças inflamatórias infecciosas — agentes virais (vírus da cinomose, outros vírus); fúngicos (*Blastomyces dermatitidis*, *Coccidioides* spp., *Cryptococcus neoformans*); riquetsiais (*Rickettsia rickettsii*); bacterianos (*Ehrlichia* spp., *E. coli*, *Streptococcus*); protozoários (*Neospora caninum*, *Toxoplasma gondii*).
• Outras doenças inflamatórias — encefalite necrosante do Yorkshire terrier, Maltês e Pug; meningite imunomediada responsiva a esteroides (Beagle, Montanhês de Berna, Nova Scotia duck tolling retriever, Weimaraner, Boxer).
• Degeneração súbita e adquirida da retina.
• Tumor cerebral — meningioma, glioma, papiloma do plexo coroide, linfoma.
• Luxação subatlantoaxial.

HEMOGRAMA/BIOQUÍMICA/URINÁLISE
• Geralmente normais.
• Hemograma completo — pode haver leucograma de estresse (leucocitose e neutrofilia segmentada com linfopenia).

OUTROS TESTES LABORATORIAIS
Teste sorológico para descartar doenças infecciosas do SNC.

DIAGNÓSTICO POR IMAGEM
RM — método de escolha; as anormalidades são variáveis e consistem em lesões expansivas solitárias, múltiplas ou circunscritas. Múltiplas áreas de realce heterogêneo de contraste são frequentes na forma multifocal da doença. Outros achados incluem efeito expansivo com desvio da linha média, hidrocefalia obstrutiva, edema da substância branca e destruição dos sulcos. Em geral, as lesões na RM são caracterizadas como hipointensas nas imagens ponderadas em T1, mas hiperintensas naquelas ponderadas em T2. Lesões necróticas são identificadas por centro de hipointensidade com realce periférico em anel.

MÉTODOS DIAGNÓSTICOS
Análise do LCS
• Faixa de referência — leucócitos (0-3 células/μL); concentração de proteína (0-30 mg/dL).
• Ajuda a confirmar a presença de doença inflamatória, mas raramente demonstra uma causa definitiva. Os itens a seguir são apenas diretrizes, pois existe uma sobreposição significativa no que diz respeito à citologia do LCS de diferentes distúrbios inflamatórios.
• Doenças inflamatórias — concentração de leucócitos e proteínas geralmente elevada.
• Meningoencefalomielite granulomatosa — em geral, pleocitose mononuclear; no entanto, pode haver pleocitose polimorfonuclear ou LCS normal.
• Bacteriana (rara em cães) — pleocitose polimorfonuclear acentuada.
• Infecções fúngicas e protozoárias — pleocitose mista (células mononucleares e polimorfonucleares); raramente se identifica algum microrganismo fúngico (*Cryptococcus neoformans* ou *Blastomyces dermatitidis*).
• Infecções virais — pleocitose mononuclear.

Biopsia Cerebral
O único método definitivo para obter o diagnóstico de meningoencefalomielite granulomatosa.

ACHADOS PATOLÓGICOS
• Característica principal — distribuição perivascular densa de infiltrados mononucleares (linfócitos, monócitos e plasmócitos).
• Ao exame macroscópico, a alteração da cor e o amolecimento do tecido acometido são algumas vezes evidentes.

TRATAMENTO

CUIDADO(S) DE SAÚDE ADEQUADO(S)
• Pacientes estáveis podem receber alta com o tratamento recomendado.
• Internação — para cães gravemente acometidos; monitorizar o paciente de perto quanto à evolução dos déficits neurológicos.
• Em casos graves, a avaliação sequencial do tamanho da pupila, da resposta pupilar à luz e da atividade mental é útil para determinar o risco de herniação.

CUIDADO(S) DE ENFERMAGEM
• Fluidos intravenosos aos pacientes anoréxicos. Tomar cuidado para não super-hidratar, pois isso exacerbaria o edema cerebral.
• Proporcionar uma gaiola almofadada para repouso dos cães com ataxia vestibular, demência grave ou atividade convulsiva.
• Os pacientes em decúbito devem ser virados com frequência (a cada 4 h).

ATIVIDADE
• Depende da gravidade da doença e da localização da lesão.
• Os pacientes atáxicos devem ficar confinados a uma gaiola almofadada para evitar lesão.

DIETA
Garantir uma ingestão calórica adequada.

Meningoencefalomielite Granulomatosa

ORIENTAÇÃO AO PROPRIETÁRIO
• Explicar para o proprietário sobre a significativa sobreposição dos sinais clínicos entre as diferentes doenças inflamatórias. Insistir com a importância de uma avaliação diagnóstica minuciosa.
• A taxa de mortalidade da meningoencefalomielite granulomatosa é claramente distorcida pelos casos graves que vão para o exame pós-morte. As biopsias cerebrais raramente são conduzidas.
• Alguns cães com doença inflamatória do SNC podem ser tratados de forma bem-sucedida. Contudo, é necessário um tratamento a longo prazo, bem como a obediência do proprietário à terapia.
• A terapia com corticosteroide pode ser necessária por tempo indefinido.

CONSIDERAÇÕES CIRÚRGICAS
N/D.

MEDICAÇÕES
MEDICAMENTO(S) DE ESCOLHA
Corticosteroides
• Dexametasona — 0,25 mg/kg IV ou VO a cada 24 h por 4 dias, seguida por prednisona a 1-2 mg/kg VO a cada 24 h por 2 semanas. Em seguida, fornecer prednisona a 1-2 mg/kg a cada 48 h por 3-4 semanas. A dose é ajustada de acordo com a resposta e os efeitos colaterais. O objetivo é encontrar a dosagem que mantém os sinais clínicos sob controle, com efeitos colaterais mínimos. Caso se observe deterioração dos sinais clínicos com a redução gradativa dos esteroides, volte imediatamente para a dose anterior que controlou os sinais.
• Para evitar ulceração gastrintestinal, combinar a esteroidoterapia com famotidina a 0,5-1 mg/kg IV ou VO a cada 12 h.
• Fenobarbital — 2 mg/kg VO a cada 12 h.

CONTRAINDICAÇÕES
• Condições provocadas por fungos, bactérias e protozoários podem ser exacerbadas pelo uso de esteroides. Portanto, é importante descartar esses distúrbios infecciosos com avaliação diagnóstica apropriada.
• Não é recomendável a utilização de esteroides em paciente tratado ou recém-tratado com AINE.

PRECAUÇÕES
A redução na terapia com corticosteroide pode resultar em recidiva dos sinais clínicos que, outra vez, podem não ser controlados como no início.

INTERAÇÕES POSSÍVEIS
N/D.

MEDICAMENTO(S) ALTERNATIVO(S)
• Azatioprina — 2 mg/kg VO a cada 24 h.
• Citosina-arabinosídeo — 50-100 mg/m² da área de superfície corporal a cada 12 h por 2-3 dias SC ou IV. Repetir o tratamento a cada 3 semanas.
• Ciclosporina — 3-7 mg/kg VO a cada 12 h.
• Leflunomida — 4 mg/kg VO a cada 24 h.
• Ciclofosfamida — 2,2 mg/kg VO a cada 48 h.
• Radioterapia — tratamento alternativo na forma focal da doença quando outras terapias falharem. Confirmar o diagnóstico com histopatologia antes de iniciar a radioterapia.

ACOMPANHAMENTO
MONITORIZAÇÃO DO PACIENTE
• Repetir o exame neurológico periodicamente (a cada 2-4 semanas).
• Avaliar o hemograma completo e o perfil bioquímico regularmente para monitorizar o paciente quanto à presença de leucopenia, trombocitopenia e função hepatorrenal caso se faça uso de terapias alternativas.
• Monitorizar a urina em pacientes submetidos a tratamento com esteroides a longo prazo — proteinúria ou infecção são consequências frequentes.

PREVENÇÃO
N/D.

COMPLICAÇÕES POSSÍVEIS
• Deterioração dos sinais clínicos apesar do tratamento rigoroso.
• Estado epiléptico, demência, herniação cerebral e morte.

EVOLUÇÃO ESPERADA E PROGNÓSTICO
• Nem todos os pacientes com doença inflamatória do SNC têm prognóstico mau.
• A meningoencefalomielite granulomatosa foi estereotipada como uma doença fatal sem provas suficientes. Não se sabe se os cães sobreviventes tinham meningoencefalomielite granulomatosa, pois raramente são feitas biopsias cerebrais.

DIVERSOS
DISTÚRBIOS ASSOCIADOS
N/D.

FATORES RELACIONADOS COM A IDADE
N/D.

POTENCIAL ZOONÓTICO
Nenhum.

GESTAÇÃO/FERTILIDADE/REPRODUÇÃO
A terapia com corticosteroide pode afetar a gestação.

SINÔNIMO(S)
• Encefalite granulomatosa.
• Meningoencefalite granulomatosa.

VER TAMBÉM
• Encefalite.
• Encefalite Secundária à Migração Parasitária.
• Meningite/Meningoencefalite/Meningomielite Bacteriana.
• Meningoencefalomielite Eosinofílica.
• Encefalite Necrosante.
• Meningite-Arterite Responsivas a Esteroides — Cães.

ABREVIATURA(S)
• AINE = anti-inflamatório não esteroide.
• LCS = líquido cerebrospinal.
• RM = ressonância magnética.
• SNC = sistema nervoso central.
• TC = tomografia computadorizada.

RECURSOS DA INTERNET
• www.ivis.org.
• www.vin.com.

Sugestões de Leitura
Adamo PF, Adams WM, Steinberg H. Granulomatous meningoencephalomyelitis in dogs. Compend Contin Educ Pract Vet 2007, 29(11):678-690.
Bagley RS. Clinical features of important and common diseases involving the intracranial nervous system of dogs and cats. In: Fundamentals of Veterinary Clinical Neurology. Ames, IA: Blackwell, 2005, pp. 134-140.
Demierre S, Tipold A, Griot-Wenk ME, et al. Correlation between the clinical course of granulomatous meningoencephalomyelitis in dogs and the extent of mast cell infiltration. Vet Record 2001, 148:467-472.
Dewey CW. Encephalopathies: Disorders of the brain. In: A Practical Guide to Canine and Feline Neurology. Ames, IA: Blackwell, 2003, pp. 142-163.
Munana KR, Luttgen PJ. Prognostic factors for dogs with granulomatous meningoencephalomyelitis: 42 cases (1982-1996). JAVMA 1998, 212:1902-1906.

Autor Carolina Duque
Consultor Editorial Joane M. Parent

MESOTELIOMA

CONSIDERAÇÕES GERAIS

REVISÃO
- Tumor raro em cães e gatos, que se origina das células mesoteliais do revestimento seroso das cavidades pleural, pericárdica ou peritoneal.
- Em cães, também há relatos de que esse tumor se origine da túnica vaginal dos testículos.

IDENTIFICAÇÃO
- Animais mais idosos — cães e gatos.
- O subtipo esclerosante é mais comum em machos.
- Os cães da raça Pastor alemão são super-representados.

SINAIS CLÍNICOS
- Efusão pleural — dispneia, taquipneia, intolerância ao exercício, tosse, ânsia de vômito, cianose.
- Efusão pericárdica — letargia, anorexia, fraqueza, colapso, angústia respiratória, intolerância ao exercício, distensão abdominal, vômito.
- Ascite — distensão e desconforto abdominais, anorexia, vômito, letargia.
- Tumefação dos testículos.
- Os sinais do subtipo esclerosante são secundários à constrição em torno dos órgãos acometidos — vômito, problemas urinários.

CAUSAS E FATORES DE RISCO
- Aumento do risco na exposição a asbesto (amianto).
- Possível aumento do risco em Golden retriever com efusão pericárdica hemorrágica idiopática.

DIAGNÓSTICO

DIAGNÓSTICO DIFERENCIAL
Outras causas de efusão — hipoproteinemia, vasculite, neoplasia (p. ex., linfoma, quimiodectoma, hemangiossarcoma, carcinomatose), causas idiopáticas, insuficiência cardíaca congestiva, hepatopatia, processos infecciosos/inflamatórios.

HEMOGRAMA/BIOQUÍMICA/URINÁLISE
N/D.

OUTROS TESTES LABORATORIAIS
N/D.

DIAGNÓSTICO POR IMAGEM
- Radiografia torácica — para identificar a efusão pleural e avaliar a silhueta cardíaca (i. e., coração globoide compatível com efusão pericárdica).
- Ecocardiografia — para identificar efusão pericárdica e descartar neoplasia cardíaca primária.
- Ultrassonografia toracoabdominal — para avaliar as efusões.
- TC — para identificar a presença de lesões expansivas tipo massa e avaliar os pulmões diante de efusão pleural.

MÉTODOS DIAGNÓSTICOS
- Citologia das efusões para descartar causas infecciosas de linfoma — não é fácil diagnosticar o mesotelioma no exame citológico, pois as células mesoteliais são tipicamente liberadas nas efusões e podem ser altamente reativas.
- Cirurgia exploratória (aberta ou via exame toracoscópico ou laparoscópico) com biopsias.
- Níveis de fibronectina nas efusões — inespecíficos para mesotelioma, mas tipicamente elevados em efusões neoplásicas.

TRATAMENTO
- Pericardiotomia ou remoção de massa se possível.
- Pericardiocentese ou toracocentese sintomática.

MEDICAÇÕES

MEDICAMENTO(S)
- Quimioterapia intracavitária:
  - Cisplatina (apenas no cão) 50-70 mg/m^2 a cada 3 semanas com diurese salina.
  - Carboplatina (gato) 180-200 mg/m^2 a cada 3-4 semanas.
  - Carboplatina (cão) 300 mg/m^2 a cada 3 semanas.
  - Mitoxantrona (cão) 5,0-5,5 mg/m^2 a cada 3 semanas.
- Quimioterapia intravenosa — doxorrubicina a 30 mg/m^2 (cão com mais de 10 kg de peso corporal) ou 1 mg/kg (cão com menos de 10 kg ou gato) ou mitoxantrona (4,5-5,5 mg/m^2 para cão e gato) uma vez a cada 3 semanas.

CONTRAINDICAÇÕES/INTERAÇÕES POSSÍVEIS
- A quimioterapia pode causar efeitos tóxicos sobre o trato gastrintestinal, a medula óssea, o coração e outros órgãos — buscar por orientação se não estiver familiarizado com agentes citotóxicos.
- A cisplatina é particularmente nefrotóxica. Não usar em gatos; provoca edema pulmonar fatal.
- A doxorrubicina pode ser nefrotóxica em gatos.

ACOMPANHAMENTO
- Exames de sangue — particularmente hemograma completo para monitorar a ocorrência de supressão da medula óssea secundária à quimioterapia e mensuração dos índices renais para monitorar a ocorrência de nefrotoxicidade se o tratamento for feito com cisplatina.
- Radiografias seriadas do tórax e/ou ultrassonografias do coração e das cavidades toracoabdominais para monitorar a recorrência das efusões e a resposta do tumor.

EVOLUÇÃO ESPERADA E PROGNÓSTICO
- Prognóstico — variável e segundo relatos de casos.
  - Cisplatina intracavitária (cães) — faixa de 8 meses a >3 anos.
  - Carboplatina intracavitária (gatos) com piroxicam — 6 meses.
  - Cirurgia aliada à cisplatina intracavitária e doxorrubicina IV — >27 meses.
  - Sobrevida relatada apenas com a cirurgia — 4-9 meses.

DIVERSOS
Não é recomendável acasalar os animais com câncer. A quimioterapia é teratogênica — não administrar em fêmeas em gestação.

ABREVIATURA(S)
- TC = tomografia computadorizada.

Sugestões de Leitura
Garrett LD. Mesothelioma. In: Withrow SJ, Vail DM, eds., Small Animal Clinical Oncology, 4th ed. Philadelphia: Saunders, 2007, pp. 804-808.

Autor Rebecca G. Newman
Consultor Editorial Timothy M. Fan

Metemoglobinemia

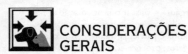

CONSIDERAÇÕES GERAIS

DEFINIÇÃO
• Teor de metemoglobina no sangue >1,5% da hemoglobina total.
• A metemoglobina difere da hemoglobina, pois a fração ferro dos grupos heme foi oxidada do estado ferroso (+2) para o estado férrico (+3).

FISIOPATOLOGIA
• Cerca de 3% da hemoglobina é oxidada a metemoglobina todos os dias nos animais normais como resultado da auto-oxidação da hemoglobina ou secundária aos oxidantes produzidos nas reações metabólicas normais.
• A metemoglobina geralmente é responsável por <1% da hemoglobina total, pois é constantemente reduzida de volta à hemoglobina por uma reação enzimática da citocromo b_5 redutase (metemoglobina redutase) dependente do NADH [dinucleotídeo nicotinamida adenina] dentro das hemácias.
• Causada pela produção aumentada da metemoglobina pelos oxidantes ou redução diminuída da metemoglobina associada à deficiência da enzima citocromo b_5 redutase da hemácia.

SISTEMA(S) ACOMETIDO(S)
• Hematológico/linfático/imune — capacidade reduzida de transporte de oxigênio pelo sangue, já que a metemoglobina não consegue se ligar ao oxigênio; se o conteúdo de metemoglobina atingir valores elevados (p. ex., >50% da hemoglobina total), diversos órgãos poderão sofrer dano hipóxico.
• Hepatobiliar — além da lesão hipóxica, o fígado pode sofrer um dano direto pelos medicamentos oxidantes metabolizados por ele.
• Renal/urológico — além da lesão hipóxica, os rins podem ser lesados caso ocorra hemólise intravascular.

IDENTIFICAÇÃO
• Cães e gatos.
• Deficiência da citocromo b_5 redutase das hemácias foi identificada nas raças caninas Chihuahua, Borzói, Setter inglês, mestiços de Terrier, Cockapoo, Coonhound, Poodle, Corgi, Pomerânia, mestiços de Pit bull e Esquimó toy, bem como nos gatos domésticos de pelo curto.

SINAIS CLÍNICOS
Causados por Via Direta
• Possivelmente não se observa qualquer sinal clínico nos animais com metemoglobinemia leve a moderada.
• Mucosas de aparência cianótica — pode ser difícil identificá-las nos animais intensamente pigmentados.
• Letargia, taquicardia, taquipneia, ataxia e estupor provocados pela hipoxia quando o conteúdo da metemoglobina exceder os 50%.
• Estado comatoso e morte quando o teor de metemoglobina ultrapassar os 80%.

Causados por Doenças Associadas
• Vômito, anorexia e diarreia são possíveis nos pacientes com intoxicação medicamentosa.
• Hemoglobinúria secundária à hemólise intravascular grave em alguns pacientes com anemia hemolítica concomitante por corpúsculos de Heinz.
• Edema subcutâneo, envolvendo especialmente a face, e salivação nos gatos com intoxicação pelo paracetamol.

CAUSAS
• Intoxicação — paracetamol, benzocaína, fenazopiridina e almíscar também podem provocar anemia hemolítica por corpúsculos de Heinz; há relatos de que o excesso de nitrito em rações para pequenos animais e a intoxicação por hidroxicarbamida provoquem metemoglobinemia sem anemia hemolítica por corpúsculo de Heinz.
• Deficiência da citocromo b_5 redutase da hemácia.

FATORES DE RISCO
• Aplicação de benzocaína à pele ou mucosa traumatizadas aumenta a probabilidade de absorção sistêmica e desenvolvimento de metemoglobinemia.
• É muito mais provável que os gatos desenvolvam metemoglobinemia significativa em termos clínicos em comparação aos cães após a administração do paracetamol.
• Metemoglobinemia secundária à deficiência da citocromo b_5 redutase é um distúrbio hereditário.

DIAGNÓSTICO

DIAGNÓSTICO DIFERENCIAL
• Tanto a baixa tensão de oxigênio no sangue como a metemoglobinemia podem gerar mucosas de aspecto cianótico e amostras sanguíneas de cor escura.
• A hipoxemia é comprovada pela mensuração de baixos níveis da PO_2 na amostra de sangue arterial.
• Suspeita-se da metemoglobinemia quando o sangue arterial com PO_2 normal ou elevada estiver escurecido.

ACHADOS LABORATORIAIS
Medicamentos Capazes de Alterar os Resultados Laboratoriais
Nenhum.

Distúrbios Capazes de Alterar os Resultados Laboratoriais
A ocorrência de hemólise na amostra poderá elevar o valor da metemoglobina, especialmente se o teste da metemoglobina não for realizado logo após a coleta da amostra.

Os Resultados Serão Válidos se os Exames Forem Realizados em Laboratório Humano?
• Sim, desde que o método para lisar as hemácias não provoque a formação da metemoglobina no animal submetido ao teste.
• Não se deve utilizar a saponina para lisar as hemácias, pois ela aumenta o valor da metemoglobina em algumas espécies.

HEMOGRAMA/BIOQUÍMICA/URINÁLISE
• Metemoglobinemia crônica secundária à deficiência da citocromo b_5 redutase pode resultar em um hematócrito levemente elevado; ao contrário, a anemia pode acompanhar a metemoglobinemia provocada por medicamentos oxidantes.
• Se for grave ou induzida por medicamentos oxidantes, podem-se observar indícios de lesão a vários órgãos (p. ex., níveis elevados de ureia e ALT).

OUTROS TESTES LABORATORIAIS
• Teste da mancha — determinar se o teor de metemoglobina do paciente é clinicamente importante: uma gota de sangue do paciente é colocada em um pedaço de papel branco absorvente e uma gota de sangue controle normal é colocada próxima à anterior. Se o conteúdo de metemoglobina for ≥10%, o sangue do paciente estará notavelmente mais acastanhado do que o vermelho brilhante do sangue controle.
• A determinação precisa do teor de metemoglobina requer que o sangue seja rapidamente enviado ao laboratório.
• O conteúdo de metemoglobina nos cães com deficiência da citocromo b_5 redutase varia de 13 a 41%; o teor de metemoglobina em seis gatos deficientes foi de 44-52%.
• O diagnóstico definitivo da deficiência da citocromo b_5 redutase é formulado, mensurando-se a atividade enzimática nas hemácias; esse ensaio é feito em alguns laboratórios de pesquisa e requer preparativos realizados antes de as amostras serem encaminhadas.

DIAGNÓSTICO POR IMAGEM
N/D.

MÉTODOS DIAGNÓSTICOS
• O sangue deve ser corado para pesquisa dos corpúsculos de Heinz caso haja indícios de intoxicação.
• A presença dos corpúsculos de Heinz indica exposição a algum medicamento oxidante que também pode provocar anemia hemolítica.

TRATAMENTO

• Leve a moderada — não há necessidade de tratamento específico para reduzir o conteúdo de metemoglobina.
• Induzida por medicamento — a utilização do medicamento deve ser interrompida; as hemácias podem converter grande parte da metemoglobina de volta à hemoglobina dentro de 24 h após a eliminação da exposição ao medicamento.
• Deficiência hereditária da citocromo b_5 redutase — os animais apresentam expectativa de vida normal e geralmente não necessitam de tratamento, embora os veterinários talvez queiram administrar uma única injeção IV de azul de metileno (ver adiante) 1 hora antes de um animal deficiente ser anestesiado para alguma cirurgia a fim de maximizar a quantidade de hemoglobina capaz de se ligar ao oxigênio.
• Devem ser administradas transfusões de sangue total aos pacientes com anemia grave e àqueles com hematócrito em rápido declínio e sinais clínicos sugestivos de um estado em deterioração.
• Hemólise intravascular grave — é recomendada a administração de fluido IV.
• Tratamento de desequilíbrios eletrolíticos e acidobásicos também pode ser indicado para pacientes com vômito ou diarreia graves, lesão renal concomitante ou choque iminente.
• A administração de oxigênio tem valor limitado, já que a metemoglobina não consegue se ligar ao oxigênio; além disso, o aumento no oxigênio dissolvido resulta apenas em um pequeno aumento no teor do oxigênio sanguíneo.

METEMOGLOBINEMIA

MEDICAÇÕES
MEDICAMENTO(S) DE ESCOLHA
• Azul de metileno — administrado lentamente durante vários minutos sob a forma de solução a 1% (1 mg/kg IV); pode ser administrado a pacientes com metemoglobinemia grave; uma resposta drástica deve ocorrer durante os 30 primeiros min do tratamento. **Cuidado:** embora essa dose possa ser repetida caso haja necessidade, o azul de metileno pode provocar anemia por corpúsculos de Heinz em gatos e cães.
• *N*-acetilcisteína será eficiente no tratamento da intoxicação pelo paracetamol nos gatos se for administrada dentro de algumas horas após a exposição; a dosagem recomendada é de 140 mg/kg VO, seguida por 70 mg/kg a cada 6 h por sete tratamentos.

CONTRAINDICAÇÕES
Nenhuma.

PRECAUÇÕES
Nos pacientes submetidos a medicamentos que provocam uma formação considerável de corpúsculos de Heinz e metemoglobinemia, o tratamento com azul de metileno pode potencializar a formação desses corpúsculos e o surgimento de anemia; consequentemente, é prudente medir o hematócrito por 3 dias após o tratamento com azul de metileno para garantir que uma anemia clinicamente relevante não se desenvolva.

INTERAÇÕES POSSÍVEIS
Nenhuma.

MEDICAMENTO(S) ALTERNATIVO(S)
Nenhum.

ACOMPANHAMENTO
MONITORIZAÇÃO DO PACIENTE
• O aspecto cianótico da pele e das mucosas deve desaparecer após a redução da metemoglobina a uma quantidade que não produza sinais clínicos.
• O sangue no teste da mancha deve aparecer vermelho brilhante após a redução da metemoglobina a valores <10% da hemoglobina total.
• Se o tratamento com azul de metileno for administrado ou os corpúsculos de Heinz estiverem presentes dentro das hemácias, o hematócrito deverá ser monitorizado rigorosamente, porque, em geral, ele não atinge seu ponto mais baixo até cerca de 3 dias após a exposição inicial ao oxidante.

COMPLICAÇÕES POSSÍVEIS
Poderão ocorrer coma e morte se o teor de metemoglobina atingir os 80% da hemoglobina total.

DIVERSOS
DISTÚRBIOS ASSOCIADOS
Anemia por corpúsculos de Heinz.

POTENCIAL ZOONÓTICO
Nenhum.

GESTAÇÃO/FERTILIDADE/REPRODUÇÃO
N/D.

VER TAMBÉM
• Anemia por Corpúsculo de Heinz.
• Toxicidade do Paracetamol.

ABREVIATURA(S)
• ALT = alanina aminotransferase.

Sugestões de Leitura
Harvey JW. The erythrocyte: Physiology, metabolism, and biochemical disorders. In: Kaneko JJ, Harvey JW, Bruss ML, Clinical Biochemistry of Domestic Animals, 6th ed. San Diego: Academic Press, 2008, pp. 173-240.

Autor John W. Harvey
Consultor Editorial A.H. Rebar

METRITE

CONSIDERAÇÕES GERAIS

REVISÃO
- Infecção uterina bacteriana que se desenvolve no período pós-parto imediato (em geral, dentro da primeira semana); ocasionalmente, desenvolve-se após abortamento ou inseminação artificial não estéril — raramente após o acasalamento natural.
- Bactérias — ascendem para o útero pela cérvix aberta; o útero pós-parto grande e flácido fornece o ambiente ideal para o crescimento; bactérias Gram-negativas (p. ex., *Escherichia coli*) são comumente isoladas.
- Infecção com potencial risco de vida; pode levar ao choque séptico.
- Acomete o útero diretamente; envolvimento sistêmico à medida que se desenvolve a sepse.
- Pode se tornar crônica e levar à infertilidade.

IDENTIFICAÇÃO
- Cadela e gata após o parto.
- Nenhuma predileção etária ou racial.

SINAIS CLÍNICOS
Achados Anamnésicos
- Corrimento vulvar de odor fétido, purulento, sanguinopurulento ou esverdeado escuro.
- Depressão.
- Anorexia.
- Negligência dos filhotes caninos e felinos.
- Produção de leite reduzida.

Achados do Exame Físico
- Febre.
- Útero grande à palpação abdominal.
- Desidratação.
- Mucosas congestas.
- Taquicardia — com sepse.

CAUSAS E FATORES DE RISCO
- Distocia.
- Manipulação obstétrica.
- Retenção de fetos ou placentas.
- Parto prolongado (ninhada grande).
- Pós-abortamento, pós-acasalamento natural ou inseminação artificial (rara).

DIAGNÓSTICO

DIAGNÓSTICO DIFERENCIAL
- Subinvolução de sítios placentários — nenhum sinal de infecção ao exame citológico da vagina.
- Eclâmpsia — diferenciada pela concentração do cálcio sérico.
- Mastite — diferenciada pelos achados do exame físico.

HEMOGRAMA/BIOQUÍMICA/URINÁLISE
- Neutrofilia com desvio à esquerda.
- Leucopenia — ocasionalmente com choque endotóxico.
- Hematócrito, proteína total, creatinina, ureia e densidade urinária elevados — secundários à desidratação.
- Enzimas hepáticas elevadas — com endotoxemia.
- Densidade urinária baixa — pode ser observada na ocorrência de endotoxemia.

OUTROS TESTES LABORATORIAIS
N/D.

DIAGNÓSTICO POR IMAGEM
- Radiografia — revela o útero grande e, possivelmente, feto(s) retido(s).
- Ultrassonografia — exibe acúmulo de líquido intrauterino, aumento dos cornos uterinos, placenta(s) retida(s) e feto(s) retido(s); mostra efusão abdominal secundária à ruptura uterina.

MÉTODOS DIAGNÓSTICOS
- Exame citológico vaginal — detecta neutrófilos degenerados com bactérias intra e extracelulares.
- Cultura vaginal anterior ou transcervical protegida — para pesquisa de microrganismos aeróbios e anaeróbios; identificar o microrganismo e seu padrão de sensibilidade antibiótica.

TRATAMENTO

- Paciente internado até que os sinais sistêmicos desapareçam.
- Desidratação — solução eletrolítica balanceada intravenosa.
- Tratamento do choque.
- Distúrbios eletrolíticos e hipoglicemia — corrigir; identificados pelo perfil da bioquímica sérica.
- Ovário-histerectomia — tratamento de escolha para feto(s) ou placenta(s) retido(s), ruptura uterina ou infecção grave e caso não haja intenção de acasalamentos futuros.
- Paciente cronicamente acometido irresponsivo ao tratamento clínico — pode-se lançar mão dos procedimentos de histerotomia e lavagem contanto que o útero não tenha áreas friáveis.
- Útero friável — isolar com compressas e manipular cuidadosamente durante a cirurgia.

MEDICAÇÕES

MEDICAMENTO(S)
- Antibióticos — iniciar com agentes de amplo espectro (por via oral se o paciente estiver estabilizado; intravenosa se o paciente estiver em choque); escolha confirmada por meio de cultura e antibiograma; continuar por, no mínimo, 14 dias.
- Amamentação planejada — amoxicilina-ácido clavulânico (cadelas, 12,5-25 mg/kg VO a cada 12 h; gatas, 62,5 mg/gata VO a cada 12 h); pode-se administrar a cada 8 h nas infecções por Gram-negativos; ou oxacilina (22-40 mg/kg VO a cada 8 h) para começar.
- Amamentação não planejada — enrofloxacino (2,5-10 mg/kg VO a cada 12 h) para começar.
- Ocitocina — 0,5-1 U/kg IM; em seguida, repetir após 1-2 h; pode-se notar uma resposta inadequada se decorreram >48 h desde o parto.
- $PGF_{2\alpha}$ — 100 µg/kg SC a cada 12 h por 5-8 dias; para esvaziar o útero; efetuar a avaliação ultrassonográfica antes da interrupção do tratamento para garantir a resolução do acúmulo de líquido no lúmen uterino.

CONTRAINDICAÇÕES/INTERAÇÕES POSSÍVEIS
- Prostaglandina — pode induzir à ruptura uterina se o tecido estiver desvitalizado.
- Ocitocina — pode não ser eficaz depois de 48 h do parto.
- Irrigação uterina — pode provocar a ruptura da parede desvitalizada.

ACOMPANHAMENTO

MONITORIZAÇÃO DO PACIENTE
- Hemograma completo, temperatura, exame citológico vaginal e sinais clínicos.
- Ultrassonografia — monitorizar o esvaziamento do líquido uterino.

COMPLICAÇÕES POSSÍVEIS
- Ovário-histerectomia — necessária quando o tratamento clínico for ineficaz.
- Ruptura uterina e peritonite — podem ocorrer com o tratamento clínico.
- Talvez os proprietários tenham de alimentar os filhotes manualmente e monitorizar o ganho de peso diário para garantir uma nutrição adequada: os filhotes caninos devem ganhar 10% do peso ao nascimento por dia, enquanto os filhotes felinos devem recuperar, no mínimo, 7-10 g/dia.

EVOLUÇÃO ESPERADA E PROGNÓSTICO
- Ovário-histerectomia — prognóstico bom quanto à recuperação; recomendada para as pacientes idosas.
- Tratamento clínico — o prognóstico quanto à recuperação depende da identificação precoce do problema pelo proprietário — bom no início; pode afetar adversamente a futura reprodução.

DIVERSOS

ABREVIATURA(S)
- $PGF_{2\alpha}$ = prostaglandina $F_{2\alpha}$.

Sugestões de Leitura
Feldman EC, Nelson RW. Periparturient diseases. In: Feldmnan EC, Nelson RW, eds., Canine and Feline Endocrinology and Reproduction. Philadelphia: Saunders, 2004, pp. 808-834.
Johnston SD, Root Kustritz MV, Olson PNS. Periparturient disorders in the bitch. In: Johnston SD, Root Kustritz MV, Olson PNS, eds., Canine and Feline Theriogenology. Philadelphia: Saunders, 2001, pp. 129-145.
Magne ML. Acute metritis in the bitch. In: Morrow DA, ed., Current Therapy in Theriogenology 2. Philadelphia: Saunders, 1986, pp. 505-506.

Autor Joni L. Freshman
Consultor Editorial Sara K. Lyle

MIASTENIA GRAVE

CONSIDERAÇÕES GERAIS

DEFINIÇÃO
Distúrbio da transmissão neuromuscular, caracterizado por fraqueza muscular e fadiga excessiva.

FISIOPATOLOGIA
Falha de transmissão na junção neuromuscular — origina-se de anormalidades estruturais ou funcionais dos receptores nicotínicos de acetilcolina (forma congênita) e da destruição mediada por autoanticorpos dos receptores da acetilcolina e das membranas pós-sinápticas (forma adquirida).

SISTEMA(S) ACOMETIDO(S)
- Neuromuscular — resultado de anormalidades ou da destruição dos receptores da acetilcolina.
- Respiratório — pode-se encontrar pneumonia por aspiração secundária a megaesôfago.

GENÉTICA
- Formas familiares congênitas — raças Jack Russell terrier, Springer spaniel, Fox terrier pelo liso; Dachshund miniatura de pelo liso, Gammel Dansk Honsehund; modo de herança autossômico recessivo.
- Adquirida — como acontece com outras doenças autoimunes, necessita de base genética apropriada para que ocorra a doença; multifatorial, envolvendo influências ambientais, infecciosas e hormonais.
- Formas familiares de miastenia grave adquirida — ocorrem nas raças Terra Nova e Dinamarquês.

INCIDÊNCIA/PREVALÊNCIA
- Congênita — rara.
- Adquirida — não é incomum em cães; rara em gatos.

DISTRIBUIÇÃO GEOGRÁFICA
Mundial.

IDENTIFICAÇÃO
Espécies
Cães e gatos.

Raça(s) Predominante(s)
- Congênita — raças Jack Russell terrier; Springer spaniel; Fox terrier de pelo liso; Dachshund miniatura de pelo liso, Gammel Dansk Honsehund.
- Adquirida — diversas raças: Golden retriever, Pastor alemão, Labrador retriever, Dachshund, Terrier escocês, Akita; além de gatos Abissínio e Somali.

Idade Média e Faixa Etária
- Congênita — 6-8 semanas de vida.
- Adquirida — idade bimodal de início; cães: 1-4 anos de idade e 9-13 anos de idade.

Sexo Predominante
- Congênita — nenhum.
- Adquirida — pode haver leve predileção pelas fêmeas no grupo etário jovem; nenhuma no grupo de idade avançada.

SINAIS CLÍNICOS
Comentários Gerais
- Adquirida — pode haver diversas apresentações clínicas, variando desde envolvimento focal dos músculos esofágicos, faríngeos e extraoculares até colapso agudo generalizado.
- Deve ser incluída no diagnóstico diferencial de qualquer cão com megaesôfago adquirido, fraqueza atribuída à lesão do neurônio motor inferior ou massa mediastínica cranial.

Achados Anamnésicos
- Regurgitação — comum; é importante diferenciar entre vômito e regurgitação.
- Mudança na vocalização.
- Fraqueza relacionada ao exercício.
- Colapso agudo.
- Fraqueza progressiva.
- Sono com os olhos abertos.

Achados do Exame Físico
- O paciente pode parecer normal em repouso.
- Salivação excessiva, regurgitação e tentativas repetidas de deglutição.
- Atrofia muscular — geralmente não encontrada.
- Dispneia — na pneumonia por aspiração.
- Fadiga ou câibra — com exercício leve.
- Exame neurológico meticuloso — achados sutis: reflexo palpebral reduzido ou ausente (pode ser fatigável); pode-se notar reflexo de ânsia de vômito fraco ou ausente; reflexos espinais em geral normais, porém fatigáveis (raramente ausentes, embora o cão se mostre incapaz de suportar seu peso).
- Ventroflexão do pescoço (gatos, incomum em cães).

CAUSAS
- Congênita.
- Imunomediada.
- Paraneoplásica.

FATORES DE RISCO
- Base genética apropriada.
- Neoplasia — particularmente o timoma.
- Tratamento com metimazol (gatos) — pode resultar em doença reversível.
- Vacinação pode exacerbar miastenia grave ativa.
- Fêmea intacta.

DIAGNÓSTICO

DIAGNÓSTICO DIFERENCIAL
- Outros distúrbios de transmissão neuromuscular — paralisia pelo carrapato; botulismo; intoxicação pela colinesterase.
- Polineuropatias agudas ou crônicas.
- Polimiopatias — incluindo a polimiosite.
- O diagnóstico depende da anamnese cuidadosa, dos exames físico e neurológico completos e dos exames laboratoriais especializados.

HEMOGRAMA/BIOQUÍMICA/URINÁLISE
- Normais.
- Creatina quinase sérica — geralmente normal; pode estar elevada em caso de miastenia grave associada a polimiosite e timoma concomitante.

OUTROS TESTES LABORATORIAIS
- Título sérico de anticorpo contra os receptores da acetilcolina — diagnóstico para a forma adquirida.
- Função da tireoide e da adrenal — podem-se observar anormalidades associadas à forma adquirida.

DIAGNÓSTICO POR IMAGEM
Radiografias torácicas — megaesôfago; massa mediastínica cranial; pneumonia por aspiração.

MÉTODOS DIAGNÓSTICOS
- Biopsia guiada pelo ultrassom da massa mediastínica cranial — pode apoiar o diagnóstico de timoma.
- Aumento espetacular na força muscular após a administração do cloreto de edrofônio (0,1 mg/kg IV) — podem-se observar respostas falso-positivas e falso-negativas.
- Reflexo palpebral reduzido ou ausente — pode retornar após a administração do cloreto de edrofônio.
- Avaliação eletrofisiológica — necessidade questionável com a disponibilidade cada vez maior do teste de anticorpo contra os receptores da acetilcolina; muitos pacientes com a forma adquirida apresentam maus riscos anestésicos.
- Eletrocardiograma — na bradicardia; bloqueio cardíaco de terceiro grau foi recentemente comprovado em alguns pacientes com a doença adquirida.

ACHADOS PATOLÓGICOS
Biopsia de massa mediastínica cranial pode revelar timoma, hiperplasia tímica ou atrofia tímica.

TRATAMENTO

CUIDADO(S) DE SAÚDE ADEQUADO(S)
- Paciente internado — até que sejam efetuadas as dosagens adequadas dos medicamentos anticolinesterásicos.
- Pneumonia por aspiração — pode necessitar de cuidado intensivo.
- Sonda inserida via gastrotomia — poderá ser necessária se o paciente for incapaz de comer ou de beber sem regurgitação significativa.

CUIDADO(S) DE ENFERMAGEM
- Oxigenoterapia, antibioticoterapia intensiva, fluidoterapia intravenosa e cuidados de suporte — geralmente necessários na pneumonia por aspiração.
- Manutenção nutricional com sonda inserida via gastrotomia — múltiplas refeições de dieta rica em calorias; cuidados satisfatórios de higiene.
- Elevação das tigelas de água e ração na presença de megaesôfago.

ATIVIDADE
Autolimitante em virtude da gravidade da fraqueza muscular e do grau de pneumonia por aspiração.

DIETA
Pode-se tentar o uso de diferentes consistências de alimento — papa; ração de consistência dura; ração de consistência mole; avaliar qual é mais bem tolerado.

ORIENTAÇÃO AO PROPRIETÁRIO
- Avisar o proprietário que, embora a doença seja tratável, a maior parte dos pacientes necessita de meses com alimentação e medicação especiais.
- Informar ao proprietário sobre o fato de que ser dedicado é importante para um desfecho favorável da miastenia grave adquirida.

CONSIDERAÇÕES CIRÚRGICAS
- Massa mediastínica cranial — timoma.
- Antes de tentar a remoção cirúrgica, estabilizar o paciente com medicamentos anticolinesterásicos e tratar a pneumonia por aspiração.
- A fraqueza pode não ser clinicamente evidente no início.

MIASTENIA GRAVE

• Suspeita de timoma — avaliar todos os pacientes para a doença adquirida antes da cirurgia.

MEDICAÇÕES
MEDICAMENTO(S) DE ESCOLHA
• Medicamentos anticolinesterásicos — prolongam a ação da acetilcolina na junção neuromuscular; brometo de piridostigmina sob a forma de comprimidos ou xarope (Mestinon® xarope, diluído meio a meio em água) na dose de 1-3 mg/kg VO a cada 8-12 h.
• Corticosteroides — 0,5 mg/kg a cada 24 h; iniciados caso haja resposta deficiente à piridostigmina ou se não houver resposta ao desafio com o cloreto de edrofônio.

CONTRAINDICAÇÕES
Evitar medicamentos que possam reduzir a margem de segurança da transmissão neuromuscular — antibióticos aminoglicosídeos; agentes antiarrítmicos; fenotiazinas; anestésicos; narcóticos; relaxantes musculares; magnésio.

PRECAUÇÕES
• Evitar grandes volumes de bário para avaliação do megaesôfago.
• Esôfago grande repleto de ar observado nas radiografias simples — o estudo com bário não é indicado.
• Evitar dosagens imunossupressoras de prednisona — pode piorar a fraqueza muscular.
• Evitar vacinações desnecessárias.

INTERAÇÕES POSSÍVEIS
N/D.

MEDICAMENTO(S) ALTERNATIVO(S)
• Azatioprina — 2 mg/kg VO pela sonda inserida via gastrostomia a cada 24 h. Reduzir para cada 48 h quando houver remissão clínica da doença.
• Micofenolato — 20 mg/kg VO a cada 12 h. Diminuir a dosagem pela metade assim que se observar uma melhora ou resolução significativa dos sinais clínicos.

ACOMPANHAMENTO
MONITORIZAÇÃO DO PACIENTE
• O retorno da força muscular deve ser evidente.
• Radiografias torácicas — avaliadas a cada 4-6 semanas para a resolução do megaesôfago.
• Títulos de anticorpo contra os receptores da acetilcolina — avaliados a cada 8-12 semanas; diminuem para a faixa normal com a remissão imune.

PREVENÇÃO
N/D.

COMPLICAÇÕES POSSÍVEIS
• Pneumonia por aspiração.
• Parada respiratória.

EVOLUÇÃO ESPERADA E PROGNÓSTICO
• Sem pneumonia grave por aspiração nem fraqueza faríngea — prognóstico bom quanto à recuperação completa; a resolução costuma ocorrer dentro de 6-8 meses.
• Presença de timoma — prognóstico reservado a menos que se realizem a remoção cirúrgica completa do tumor e o controle dos sintomas da miastenia.

DIVERSOS
DISTÚRBIOS ASSOCIADOS
• Outros distúrbios autoimunes — tireoidite; distúrbios cutâneos; hipoadrenocorticismo; trombocitopenia; anemia hemolítica; enteropatia inflamatória.
• Distúrbios do timo — timoma; hiperplasia tímica.
• Outras neoplasias.

FATORES RELACIONADOS COM A IDADE
Idade bimodal de início — 1-4 anos de idade e 9-13 anos de idade.

POTENCIAL ZOONÓTICO
N/D.

GESTAÇÃO/FERTILIDADE/REPRODUÇÃO
• Seres humanos — a fraqueza pode melhorar durante a gestação, porém piora após o parto; alguns neonatos de mães acometidas apresentam fraqueza temporária semelhante à da miastenia grave que, além de durar de alguns dias a semanas, é atribuída à transferência *in utero* de autoanticorpos da mãe.
• Comprovada em cadelas após o parto.

VER TAMBÉM
• Capítulos que tratam de doenças autoimunes.
• Megaesôfago.

RECURSOS DA INTERNET
Laboratório Neuromuscular Comparativo: http://vetneuromuscular.ucsd.edu.

Sugestões de Leitura
Shelton GD. Megaesophagus secondary to myasthenia gravis. In: Kirk WR, Bonagura JD, eds., Current Veterinary Therapy XI. Philadelphia: Saunders, 1992, pp. 580-583.
Shelton GD. Myasthenia gravis and disorders of neuromuscular transmission. Vet Clin North Am 2002, 31:189-200.
Shelton GD. Treatment of autoimmune myasthenia gravis. In: Bonagura JD, Twedt DC, eds., Current Veterinary Therapy XIV. Philadelphia: Saunders, 2009, pp. 1108-1111.
Shelton GD, Lindstrom JM. Spontaneous remission in canine myasthenia gravis: Implications for assessing human MG therapies. Neurology 2001, 57:2139-2141.

Autor G. Diane Shelton
Consultor Editorial Peter K. Shires

MICOPLASMOSE

CONSIDERAÇÕES GERAIS

DEFINIÇÃO
- Classe de Mollicutes (Latim, *mollis*, "mole"; *cutis*, "pele").
- Divididos em tipos hemotrópicos (conhecidos antigamente como *Haemobartonella* e *Eperythrozoon*), que são abordados em outro lugar, e não hemotrópicos, que estão discutidos aqui.
- Mais de 80 gêneros; três famílias: micoplasmas, ureaplasmas e acoleplasmas.
- As menores (0,2-0,3 μm) e mais simples células procariotas capazes de autorreplicação.
- Bastonetes Gram-negativos, anaeróbios facultativos e fastidiosos.
- Desprovidos de parede celular; portanto, são elásticos, altamente pleomórficos e sensíveis à lise por choque osmótico, aos detergentes, aos alcoóis e a anticorpo específico mais complemento; envolvidos por membrana celular de três camadas compostas de lipídios anfipáticos (fosfolipídios, glicolipídios, lipoglicanos, esteróis) e proteínas; a maioria deles necessita de esteróis para o crescimento.
- Diferentes das bactérias de formas L, sem parede ou com a parede defeituosa, as quais podem se reverter para a cepa de parede celular normal.
- Reproduzem-se por fissão binária; a replicação do genoma não é necessariamente sincronizada com a divisão celular, resultando em formas de brotamento e cadeias tipo rosário.
  - Genoma pequeno, tipicamente de 0,6-1,4 Mb.
  - Baixo conteúdo genômico G + C (23-40 % de mol).
  - Acredita-se que o pequeno genoma seja o resultado de evolução redutiva a partir de um ancestral Gram-positivo comum que se adapta à vida parasitária obrigatória.
- Ubíquos na natureza como parasitas, comensais ou saprófitas nos animais, vegetais e insetos; muitos são patógenos de seres humanos, animais, vegetais e insetos.

FISIOPATOLOGIA
- Com frequência, faz parte da flora residente como comensal nas mucosas dos tratos respiratório superior, digestivo e genital; a patogenicidade e o papel desempenhado na doença quase sempre são controversos.
- As espécies demonstram considerável especificidade pelo hospedeiro.
- Os mecanismos pelos quais a doença é causada são pouco compreendidos.
- Algumas espécies aderem-se às células por meio de receptores específicos; o tamanho pequeno e a natureza elástica permitem sua adaptação à forma e aos contornos das superfícies celulares do hospedeiro.
- Íntimo contato com as células do hospedeiro — necessário para assimilação de nutrientes vitais e dos fatores de crescimento (p. ex., precursores do ácido nucleico), os quais os microrganismos não são capazes de sintetizar; juntamente com a tendência de as proteínas exógenas se ligarem à membrana do micoplasma, esse contato íntimo pode fazer com que o microrganismo escape da resposta imune do hospedeiro; pode incorporar o antígeno da célula do hospedeiro na membrana do micoplasma (capeamento) em virtude da falta de parede celular; ao contrário, o antígeno proteico do micoplasma pode vir a ser incorporado na superfície da célula do hospedeiro, envolvendo com isso a célula do hospedeiro em reações imunológicas prejudiciais direcionadas contra o microrganismo.
- Produtos produzidos durante o crescimento — carboidrato, hemolisinas, enzimas proteolíticas, amônia e endonucleases capsulares; o acúmulo de metabólitos do micoplasma (i. e., H_2O_2 e NH_3) pode contribuir para os efeitos citopáticos e o dano tecidual; glicoproteínas e proteínas citotóxicas foram isoladas das membranas de várias espécies.
- Resposta imune — predominantemente humoral; como acontece com as infecções bacterianas, IgM e IgA são os primeiros anticorpos a aparecer, seguidas por IgG.
- Exsudato fibrinoso que acompanha as infecções — protege o microrganismo dos anticorpos e de medicamentos antimicrobianos; contribui para a cronicidade.
- Invasores bacterianos secundários — comuns (p. ex., ligação às células do trato respiratório resulta na destruição dos cílios, o que predispõe o paciente à infecção bacteriana secundária).

SISTEMA(S) ACOMETIDO(S)
Cães
- Respiratório — pneumonia e infecções respiratórias superiores; provocadas por *M. cynos*; associadas ao *M. canis*, *M. spumans*, *M. edwardii*, *M. feliminutum*, *M. gateae* e *M. bovigenitalium*.
- Renal/urológico — infecções dos tratos urinário e genital (p. ex., balanopostite, uretrite, prostatite, cistite, nefrite, vaginite e endometrite); causadas por *M. canis* e *M. spumans*.
- Reprodutivo — micoplasma e ureaplasma; associados a quadros de infertilidade, morte embrionária precoce, abortamentos, natimortos ou recém-nascidos fracos e mortalidade neonatal.
- Musculosquelético — artrite; por *M. spumans*.
- Gastrintestinal — associada à colite.

Gatos
- Oftálmico — conjuntivite; associada a *M. felis* (5-25%).
- Respiratório — pneumonia, associada a *M. gateae*, *M. feliminutum* e *M. felis*; infecções respiratórias superiores, associadas a *M. felis*.
- Musculosquelético — poliartrite fibrinopurulenta crônica e tenossinovite; associadas a *M. gateae* e microrganismos micoplásmicos inespecíficos.
- Renal/urológico — infecções do trato urinário.
- Reprodutivo — abortamentos e mortes fetais; associados a *M. gateae* e ureaplasmas.
- Cutâneo/exócrino — abscessos cutâneos crônicos.

INCIDÊNCIA/PREVALÊNCIA
- Habitantes frequentes das mucosas; *M. gateae* e/ou *M. felis* encontrados na cavidade bucal ou no trato urogenital de 70-80% dos gatos saudáveis.
- Taxa de isolamento nos cães doentes muito mais elevada do que nos cães normais (p. ex., pulmão, útero e prepúcio).

DISTRIBUIÇÃO GEOGRÁFICA
Ubíquo.

IDENTIFICAÇÃO
Espécies
Cães e gatos.

Idade Média e Faixa Etária
Todas as idades.

SINAIS CLÍNICOS
Comentários Gerais
- Papel patogênico controverso.

Achados Anamnésicos
- Poliartrite — claudicação intermitente crônica; relutância ao movimento; dor articular (artralgia).
- Febre.
- Mal-estar.
- Conjuntivite — uni ou bilateral.

Achados do Exame Físico
- Poliartrite — edema difuso do membro; tumefação articular; dor.
- Conjuntivite — blefarospasmo; quemose; hiperemia conjuntival; epífora; e secreção ocular serosa ou purulenta.
- Rinite leve — espirros.

CAUSAS
- Flora micoplásmica dos cães — *M. canis*, *M. spumans*, *M. maculosum*, *M. edwardii*, *M. cynos*, *M. molare*, *M. opalescens*, *M. feliminutum*, *M. gateae*, *M. arginini*, *M. bovigenitalium*, *Acholeplasma laidlawii* e ureaplasmas.
- Flora micoplásmica dos gatos — *M. felis*, *M. gateae*, *M. feliminutum*, *M. arginini*, *M. pulmonis*, *M. arthritidis*, *M. gallisepticum*, *Acholeplasma laidlawii* e ureaplasmas.

FATORES DE RISCO
- Comensais — ocasionalmente provocam infecção sistêmica associada à imunodeficiência, imunossupressão ou câncer.
- Resistência comprometida do hospedeiro — pode permitir que o microrganismo atravesse a barreira mucosa e se dissemine.
- Microrganismo pode ser oportunista — um dos fatores em um complexo causal multifatorial (p. ex., o comprometimento da depuração pulmonar pela infecção viral pode fazer com que o microrganismo estabeleça a infecção nos pulmões como patógeno oportunista secundário).
- Fatores predisponentes — estresse (p. ex., problemas reprodutivos associados a operações de superpopulação) e outros fatores (p. ex., tumores urinários e cálculos urinários).
- Taxa de isolamento do microrganismo nos cães doentes muito mais elevada do que nos cães normais.

DIAGNÓSTICO

DIAGNÓSTICO DIFERENCIAL
- Infecção respiratória superior (cães e gatos) — agentes virais (vírus da parainfluenza, cinomose, herpes-vírus, calicivírus felino, reovírus); *Chlamydia psittaci*; bactérias (*Bordetella bronchiseptica*, estafilococos, estreptococos, coliformes).
- Infecção do trato urinário (cães e gatos) — bactérias (estafilococos, estreptococos, coliformes); fungos (*Candida*); parasitas.
- Infertilidade, morte embrionária precoce, abortamentos, natimortos ou recém-nascidos fracos e mortalidade neonatal (cães) — bactérias (*Brucella*, *Salmonella*, *Campylobacter*, *E. coli*, estreptococos); vírus (herpes-vírus canino, cinomose, adenovírus canino); *Toxoplasma gondii*; endocrinopatias (deficiência de progesterona, hipotireoidismo).

Micoplasmose

- Prostatite (cães) — bactérias (*E. coli*, *Brucella canis*); fungos (*Blastomyces*, *Cryptococcus*).
- Artrite (cães e gatos) — imunomediada, bacteriana (estafilococos, estreptococos, coliformes, anaeróbios); bactérias de forma L; riquétsia (*Ehrlichia*); *Borrelia burgdorferi*; fungos (*Coccidioides*, *Cryptococcus*, *Blastomyces*); protozoários (*Leishmania*); vírus (calicivírus felino).
- Conjuntivite (gatos) — herpes-vírus felino; calicivírus felino; reovírus felino; *Chlamydia psittaci*; bactérias.

HEMOGRAMA/BIOQUÍMICA/URINÁLISE
Com Poliartrite
- Anemia leve.
- Leucocitose neutrofílica.
- Hipoalbuminemia.
- Hipoglobulinemia.
- Proteinúria resultante de glomerulonefrite por imunocomplexo.

OUTROS TESTES LABORATORIAIS
- Testes sorológicos — fixação do complemento, imunodifusão em ágar gel, ELISA; detectam o microrganismo.
- Difícil de demonstrar nos tecidos e a partir deles.
- Extremamente pleomórficos — nos esfregaços (p. ex., raspados conjuntivais) observados como cocobacilos, formas em cocos, formas em anel, espirais e filamentos.
- Colorações — pouco corados (Gram-negativos); preferidos: corantes de Giemsa ou Romanowsky.
- Teste do anticorpo fluorescente — permite o diagnóstico definitivo; isola e identifica ou detecta o microrganismo nos tecidos; é possível enviar *swabs* de algodão introduzidos em meio de caldo Hayflick ou *swabs* comercialmente disponíveis; microrganismos frágeis; refrigerar as amostras e enviar ao laboratório dentro de 48 horas; congelar para conservar por mais tempo.
- PCR de RNA ribossômico 16S.
- Eletroforese em gel com gradiente de desnaturação — utilizada para identificar os micoplasmas de difícil cultura ou de difícil diferenciação.

DIAGNÓSTICO POR IMAGEM
Poliartrite — nenhuma alteração radiográfica.

MÉTODOS DIAGNÓSTICOS
- Poliartrite — números elevados de neutrófilos não degenerados no líquido sinovial.
- Líquido prostático — células inflamatórias com cultura bacteriana negativa.

TRATAMENTO
CUIDADO(S) DE SAÚDE ADEQUADO(S)
Como paciente de ambulatório.

MEDICAÇÕES
MEDICAMENTO(S) DE ESCOLHA
- Sensíveis a antibióticos que especificamente inibem a síntese nas células procariotas.
- Tetraciclinas — 22 mg/kg VO a cada 8 h.
- Doxiciclina — 5 mg/kg VO a cada 12 h.
- Cloranfenicol — 40-50 mg/kg IV, IM, SC, VO a cada 8-12 h.
- Não há nenhum procedimento padronizado para os testes de suscetibilidade antimicrobiana *in vitro*.
- Antibiótico tópico — conjuntivite.

CONTRAINDICAÇÕES
- Pomadas esteroides tópicas — a utilização inadequada para conjuntivite pode prolongar a infecção e predispor o paciente à ulcera de córnea.
- Tetraciclinas — evitar o uso em animais com <6 meses de vida.
- Tetraciclina e cloranfenicol — evitar o emprego em fêmeas prenhes.

PRECAUÇÕES
Sulfonamidas e β-lactâmicos — inibem a síntese de peptideoglicano; microrganismo resistente por causa da ausência de paredes celulares.

MEDICAMENTO(S) ALTERNATIVO(S)
- Gentamicina.
- Canamicina.
- Espectinomicina.
- Espiramicina.
- Tilosina.
- Eritromicina.
- Nitrofuranos.
- Fluoroquinolonas.

ACOMPANHAMENTO
MONITORIZAÇÃO DO PACIENTE
Tratar por período prolongado.
PREVENÇÃO
- Não há vacinas disponíveis.
- O microrganismo é imediatamente destruído por dessecação, luz solar e desinfecção química.

EVOLUÇÃO ESPERADA E PROGNÓSTICO
Prognóstico bom nos animais dotados de sistemas imunes competentes e submetidos à antibioticoterapia apropriada.

DIVERSOS
DISTÚRBIOS ASSOCIADOS
M. pneumoniae — infecta o trato respiratório nos seres humanos no mundo todo; provoca pneumonia, bronquite ou infecção do trato respiratório superior, todas de origem micoplásmica; em geral autolimitante; raramente fatal.

FATORES RELACIONADOS COM A IDADE
Tetraciclinas — evitar em animais com <6 meses de vida.

POTENCIAL ZOONÓTICO
- Em geral, não é considerada zoonótica.
- Há relatos do desenvolvimento de tenossinovite micoplásmica supurativa em veterinário que foi arranhado por um gato que estava sendo tratado de colite.
- A especificidade dos micoplasmas pelo hospedeiro é questionável por alguns, em particular entre as espécies estritamente relacionadas de mamíferos.

GESTAÇÃO/FERTILIDADE/REPRODUÇÃO
Tetraciclina e cloranfenicol — não utilizar em fêmeas em gestação.

SINÔNIMO(S)
Microrganismos semelhantes à pleuropneumonia.

ABREVIATURA(S)
- ELISA = ensaio imunoabsorvente ligado à enzima.
- PCR = reação em cadeia da polimerase.

Sugestões de Leitura
Chalker VJ. Canine mycoplasmas. Res Vet Sci 2005, 79:1-8.
Greene CE. Mycoplasmal, ureaplasmal, and L-form infections. In: Greene CE, ed., Infectious Diseases of the Dog and Cat, 3rd ed. St. Louis: Saunders Elsevier, 2006, pp. 260-265.
Sasaki Y. Mycoplasma. In: Chan VL, Sherman PM, Bourke B, eds., Bacterial Genomes and Infectious Diseases. Totowa, NJ: Humana Press, 2006, pp. 175-190.

Autor J. Paul Woods
Consultor Editorial Stephen C. Barr

Micoplasmose Hemotrópica (Hemoplasmose)

CONSIDERAÇÕES GERAIS

REVISÃO
Destruição de hemácias e anemia causadas por fixação do parasita à superfície externa dessas células e resposta imune montada pelo hospedeiro.

IDENTIFICAÇÃO
- Cães e gatos. • A doença aguda é mais comum em gatos jovens, enquanto a forma crônica, mais comum em adultos. • Em gatos, é mais comum em machos. • As doenças aguda e crônica afetam os cães esplenectomizados e não esplenectomizados, respectivamente. • Beagles criados em canis podem estar sob alto risco de infecção. • Não há predileção sexual em cães.

SINAIS CLÍNICOS

Gatos
- Para infecção pelo *M. haemofelis*:
  ◦ Gravidade variável da doença, desde infecção inaparente (doença crônica) até depressão acentuada e morte (doença aguda).
  ◦ Febre intermitente (apenas 50% das vezes) durante a fase aguda, depressão, fraqueza, anorexia, anemia, mucosas pálidas, esplenomegalia, e (ocasionalmente) icterícia.
- Para infecção por *Candidatus M. haemominutum*:
  ◦ Geralmente resulta em infecção inaparente.
  ◦ Diminuição mínima ou nula do hematócrito.
- Para infecção por *Candidatus M. turicensis*:
  ◦ Informações limitadas a respeito da infecção natural.
  ◦ Anemia moderada após infecção experimental.

Cães
Sinais leves ou inaparentes (p. ex., mucosas pálidas e apatia) — exceto quando os cães foram esplenectomizados ou a função esplênica está alterada.

CAUSAS E FATORES DE RISCO
- Causada por bactérias previamente classificadas no gênero *Haemobartonella*; atualmente, no entanto, esses microrganismos são identificados como micoplasmas (micoplasmas hemotrópicos ou hemoplasmas) com base em determinações genéticas. • *Mycoplasma haemofelis* (previamente classificado como a forma grande da *Haemobartonella felis*), *M. haemominutum* (antigamente classificado como a forma pequena da *H. felis*) e *M. haemocanis* (anteriormente classificado como *H. canis*). • A infecção por *M. haemofelis* em gatos geralmente provoca uma doença mais grave que a infecção por *M. haemominutum*. • Gatos — anemia mais grave se infectados por FeLV. • Cães — a probabilidade de anemia grave é muito alta se submetidos à esplenectomia ou acometidos por alterações patológicas no baço.

DIAGNÓSTICO

DIAGNÓSTICO DIFERENCIAL
- Outras causas de anemia hemolítica, incluindo AHAI, babesiose (não em gatos nos Estados Unidos), citauxzoonose (gatos apenas), anemia hemolítica por corpúsculos de Heinz, anemia hemolítica microangiopática, deficiência da piruvato cinase, e deficiência da fosfofrutocinase (cães apenas). • Diferenciada de AHAI somente por meio da identificação dos parasitas no sangue (esfregaço sanguíneo corado ou ensaios espécie-específicos à base de PCR) — ambos os distúrbios (AHIM e/ou infecção por *M. haemofelis*) podem ser positivos no teste de Coombs. • As espécies de *Babesia* e *Cytauxzoon* são microrganismos protozoários que diferem em termos de morfologia desses microrganismos micoplasmais. • Novos corantes azuis de metileno usados para identificar os corpúsculos de Heinz. • Ensaios enzimáticos ou testes de DNA especializados utilizados para diagnosticar as deficiências da piruvato cinase e da fosfofrutocinase.

HEMOGRAMA/BIOQUÍMICA/URINÁLISE
- Anemia, presente com maior frequência com reticulocitose em animais com infecções clinicamente importantes — pode parecer pouco regenerativa se tiver ocorrido um declínio súbito no volume globular no início da doença ou se houver outros distúrbios concomitantes (p. ex., infecções por FeLV ou FIV em gatos).
- Autoaglutinação pode ser observada em amostras de sangue de gatos após seu resfriamento abaixo da temperatura corporal. • Leucograma total e diferencial variável de pouco auxílio diagnóstico.
- Raramente se observa leve hemoglobinemia; não há relatos de hemoglobinúria. • Às vezes, pode-se mensurar uma hiperbilirrubinemia, mas raramente ela é grave. • É observada bilirrubinúria considerável em alguns cães. • Anormalidades relacionadas com hipoxia anêmica podem ser demonstradas por meio de perfis bioquímicos, embora o perfil possa permanecer normal.
- Hipoglicemia é possível em gatos moribundos ou caso se demore para separar as células sanguíneas do plasma ou do soro.

OUTROS TESTES LABORATORIAIS
- Corantes hematológicos de rotina (p. ex., Wright-Giemsa) para identificar os microrganismos em esfregaços sanguíneos; tais esfregaços devem ser examinados em busca dos microrganismos antes do início do tratamento. • Os microrganismos podem se destacar das hemácias em sangue armazenado e coletado com EDTA. • Corantes para contagem de reticulócitos não podem ser utilizados, pois os reticulócitos puntiformes em gatos parecem semelhantes aos parasitas. • Os microrganismos devem ser diferenciados de corante precipitado, artefatos refráteis de ressecamento ou fixação, corpúsculos de Howell-Jolly pouco corados e pontilhado basofílico. • Microrganismos felinos — pequenos cocos, anéis ou bastonetes corados de azul em hemácias, frequentemente muitos parasitas para *M. haemofelis*; pequenos bastonetes ou microrganismos cocoides em baixo número para *Candidatus M. haemominutum*; parasitas não conclusivamente observados no sangue para *Candidatus M. turicensis*. • Microrganismos caninos — comumente formam cadeias de microrganismos que aparecem como estruturas filamentosas na superfície das hemácias. • A parasitemia é cíclica e, por essa razão, os microrganismos nem sempre são identificáveis no sangue (sobretudo nos gatos). • Os ensaios à base de PCR são capazes de detectar os parasitas no sangue abaixo do número necessário para formular um diagnóstico por meio de esfregaço sanguíneo corado.

MÉTODOS DIAGNÓSTICOS
- Em pacientes com anemia arregenerativa, é recomendável a realização de biopsia da medula óssea para detectar outros distúrbios (p. ex., distúrbios mieloproliferativos). • O teste de PCR de cães e gatos doadores de sangue é fortemente recomendado.

TRATAMENTO
- Sem tratamento, a mortalidade em caso de infecção por *M. haemofelis* pode chegar a 30% em gatos. • O tratamento é ambulatorial a menos que o animal esteja gravemente anêmico ou moribundo. • As transfusões sanguíneas são necessárias quando a anemia é considerada potencialmente letal. • A administração IV de fluido contendo glicose é aconselhável em animais moribundos.

MEDICAÇÕES

MEDICAMENTO(S)
- Doxiciclina (5 mg/kg VO a cada 12 h), tetraciclina (20 mg/kg VO a cada 8 h) ou oxitetraciclina (20 mg/kg VO a cada 8 h) deve ser administrada por, no mínimo, 3 semanas e até 6 semanas para eliminação da infecção. • Achados preliminares indicam que o enrofloxacino (5 mg/kg VO a cada 24 h) por 2 semanas pode ser eficaz em gatos. • Glicocorticoides, como prednisolona (1-2 mg/kg VO a cada 12 h), podem ser administrados para os animais gravemente anêmicos; diminuir a dose de forma gradual à medida que o volume globular aumenta.

CONTRAINDICAÇÕES/INTERAÇÕES POSSÍVEIS
- Há relatos de estenoses esofágicas em gatos após a administração de doxiciclina.
- As tetraciclinas podem produzir febre ou evidência de doença gastrintestinal em gatos.
- O enrofloxacino em doses acima de 5 mg/kg/dia pode causar retinotoxicidade.
- Não é recomendável o uso de cloranfenicol para tratar os gatos, pois esse antibiótico causa hipoplasia eritroide dose-dependente.

ACOMPANHAMENTO
- Examinar o animal 1 semana depois do tratamento para confirmar o aumento do volume globular.
- Alertar os proprietários sobre o fato de que os gatos podem permanecer portadores mesmo após a conclusão do tratamento, mas raramente manifestam recidiva da doença uma vez que o volume globular retorne ao normal.

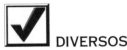

DIVERSOS

ABREVIATURAS
- AHAI = anemia hemolítica autoimune
- AHIM = anemia hemolítica imunomediada
- EDTA = ácido etilenodiaminotetracético
- PCR = reação em cadeia da polimerase

Autores Joanne B. Messick e John W. Harvey
Consultor Editorial A. H. Rebar

Micotoxicose — Aflatoxina

CONSIDERAÇÕES GERAIS

REVISÃO
Hepatotoxicidade resultante de um produto tóxico do fungo *Aspergillus flavus* e outras espécies.

IDENTIFICAÇÃO
- Embora o relato seja raro em cães, a micotoxicose por aflatoxina ocorre periodicamente em grandes surtos associados a rações.
- Há relatos apenas experimentais em gatos.
- Machos jovens e fêmeas prenhes podem ser mais suscetíveis.

SINAIS CLÍNICOS
Início Agudo
- Forma mais comum em pequenos animais.
- O rápido início dos sinais pode se desenvolver até 3 semanas após a exposição.
- Recusa precoce pelo alimento ou anorexia.
- Vômito e diarreia.
- Icterícia.
- Coagulopatia e hemorragia gastrintestinal.
- Morte inesperada sem desenvolvimento dos sinais clínicos.

Crônicos
- Anorexia ou recusa pelo alimento.
- Vômito.
- Diarreia.
- Insuficiência hepática.
- Ascite — a ocorrência é variável.

CAUSAS E FATORES DE RISCO
- Alimentos à base de grãos contaminados antes da colheita com *Aspergillus flavus*, *A. parasiticus* e outras espécies.
- Comum em vários grãos de cereais; também há relatos em amendoins, outros frutos oleaginosos, e batatas.
- Pode ocorrer após a produção em rações armazenadas em condições úmidas e quentes; alimentos expostos a elementos estragados com bolor evidente; ingestão de lixo.
- Os bolores produtores de micotoxinas crescem a temperaturas de 24-35°C e umidade de 18-20%.
- Foram observados sinais agudos em cães que ingeriram alimentos contendo 60 ppb de aflatoxina.
- Ativada em epóxido tóxico pelas enzimas hepáticas do citocromo P450.
- Alguns animais individuais são mais suscetíveis:
  - Filhotes das espécies canina e felina.
  - Machos intactos.
  - Fêmeas prenhes.

DIAGNÓSTICO

DIAGNÓSTICO DIFERENCIAL
- Leptospirose.
  - Sorologia.
- Parvovírus.
  - ELISA.
  - Sorologia.
  - Isolamento viral.
- Toxicose por rodenticida anticoagulante.
  - PIAVK para descartar toxicose por anticoagulante.
  - Triagem de rodenticida anticoagulante.
- Outras causas de hepatopatia subaguda a crônica e CID associada.

HEMOGRAMA/BIOQUÍMICA/URINÁLISE
- Níveis séricos diminuídos de proteína C, antitrombina III e colesterol.
- Hiperbilirrubinemia.
- Hipoalbuminemia.
- ALT elevada.
- Elevações variáveis nas enzimas GGT, AST e fosfatase alcalina.

OUTROS TESTES LABORATORIAIS
- TP e TTPA prolongados.
- Baixo nível de fibrinogênio em virtude de insuficiência na síntese hepática.

MÉTODOS DIAGNÓSTICOS
- Biopsia hepática.
- Histopatologia.
- Excreção rápida do metabólito da aflatoxina (Aflatoxina M1) na urina.
- Análise de amostras de alimento sob suspeita em busca de aflatoxina.
  - Com frequência, o alimento contaminado não está mais disponível.

ACHADOS PATOLÓGICOS
- Hepatomegalia com alteração gordurosa.
- Icterícia.
- Ascite.
- Hemorragia gastrintestinal.
- Petéquias multifocais e equimose.
- Alteração gordurosa microvesicular em hepatócitos.
- Necrose hepatocelular centrolobular, possível evidência de regeneração.
- Colestase canalicular.
  - Fibrose portal em ponte com proliferação dos ductos biliares.

TRATAMENTO
- Avaliação e estabilização.
- Transfusão.
- Correção de desequilíbrios hidreletrolíticos.
- Carvão ativado para exposição recente a altas doses.
- Vitaminas do complexo B e vitamina K$_1$.
- Gastroprotetores.
- Dieta limpa e não contaminada.
  - Fonte proteica de alta qualidade.

MEDICAÇÕES

MEDICAMENTO(S)
- Embora não haja nenhum antídoto específico, utilizam-se hepatoprotetores.
- N-acetilcisteína parenteral em cães gravemente acometidos.
  - Solução a 20% diluída a 1:4 com soro fisiológico e administrada por via IV lenta a uma dose de ataque de 140 mg/kg, seguida pela dose de manutenção de 70 mg/kg IV a cada 8 h.
- S-Adenosilmetionina.
  - 20 mg/kg VO diariamente sob a forma de comprimidos revestidos entéricos com o estômago vazio.

CONTRAINDICAÇÕES/INTERAÇÕES POSSÍVEIS
- Evitar medicamentos metabolizados pelo fígado para ativação.
- Evitar inseticidas organofosforados ou piretroides.

ACOMPANHAMENTO

MONITORIZAÇÃO DO PACIENTE
- No mínimo, diariamente.
- Enzimas e bioquímica sérica, incluindo colesterol.
- TP e TTPA.
- Proteína C.

PREVENÇÃO
- Evitar a utilização de gênero alimentício com mofo evidente.
- Estocar o alimento em lugar seco, limpo e fresco.
- Limpar regularmente os comedouros e os recipientes de alimentos.

COMPLICAÇÕES POSSÍVEIS
Nenhuma complicação relatada em cães e gatos.

EVOLUÇÃO ESPERADA E PROGNÓSTICO
Prognóstico — mau, mesmo com o tratamento.

DIVERSOS

FATORES RELACIONADOS COM A IDADE
Os animais jovens são mais suscetíveis à aflatoxina.

GESTAÇÃO/FERTILIDADE/REPRODUÇÃO
- Efeitos indiretos sobre o útero.
- Potencialmente teratogênica.
- Fêmeas prenhes podem ficar mais suscetíveis à intoxicação.

ABREVIATURA(S)
- ALT = alanina aminotransferase.
- AST = aspartato aminotransferase.
- CID = coagulação intravascular disseminada.
- ELISA = ensaio imunoabsorvente ligado à enzima.
- GGT = gama-glutamiltransferase.
- PIAVK = proteínas induzidas por antagonistas da vitamina K.
- TP = tempo de protrombina.
- TTPA = tempo de tromboplastina parcial ativada.

Sugestões de Leitura
Bischoff K, Garland T. Aflatoxicosis in dogs. In: Bonagura JD, Twedt DC, eds., Kirk's Current Veterinary Therapy XIV. St. Louis: Saunders, 2009, pp. 156-159.
Hooser SB, Talcott PA. Mycotoxins. In: Peterson ME, Talcott PA, eds., Small Animal Toxicology, 2nd ed. Philadelphia: Saunders, 2006, pp. 888-897.
Meerdink GL. Aflatoxin. In: Plumlee KH, ed., Clinical Veterinary Toxicology. St. Louis: Mosby, 2004, pp. 231-235.

Autor Karyn Bischoff
Consultor Editorial Gary D. Osweiler

Micotoxicose — Desoxinivalenol

CONSIDERAÇÕES GERAIS

REVISÃO
- Desoxinivalenol (vomitoxina) é uma toxina que pode ser produzida por fungos do gênero *Fusarium* em grãos como trigo, aveia, cevada e milho.
- A principal fonte de exposição para cães e gatos é pelo consumo de ração produzida com grãos contaminados por desoxinivalenol.
- Embora o mecanismo exato ainda não esteja bem definido, o desoxinivalenol pode inibir a síntese proteica celular e ativar as quinases intracelulares envolvidas na transdução de sinal. Além disso, a ingestão de desoxinivalenol pode causar recusa ao alimento, possivelmente relacionada com a suprarregulação de citocinas pró-inflamatórias, como IL-6; também pode exercer um efeito emético central com consequente indução de vômito.

IDENTIFICAÇÃO
- Cães e gatos.
- Não há predisposição racial ou sexual.
- Os sinais podem ser mais comuns em animais jovens.

SINAIS CLÍNICOS
- Cães e gatos sofrem início súbito de anorexia e vômito, o que pode resultar na perda de peso.
- O início dos sinais clínicos pode ocorrer dentro de minutos da exposição.
- Os sinais clínicos anormais também podem desaparecer rapidamente após a remoção do alimento contaminado.

CAUSAS E FATORES DE RISCO
- Os animais ficam expostos ao desoxinivalenol quando o grão contendo a micotoxina é misturado à ração completa.
- Há diferenças acentuadas entre as espécies em termos de toxicidade: suínos (mais sensíveis) > roedores > cães > gatos > aves domésticas > seres humanos > ruminantes (menos sensíveis).
- Experimentalmente, o consumo alimentar de cães das raças Beagle e Brittany fica reduzido quando as concentrações de desoxinivalenol em seu alimento estão acima de 4,5 ± 1,7 mg de desoxinivalenol/kg de alimento.
- A ingestão alimentar nos gatos sofre declínio com concentrações de desoxinivalenol superiores a 7,7 ± 1,1 mg/kg.
- Em cães e gatos, é comum a ocorrência de vômito quando a concentração de desoxinivalenol em seu alimento se encontra acima de 8 mg/kg.

DIAGNÓSTICO

DIAGNÓSTICO DIFERENCIAL
- Outras causas de inapetência e vômito.
- Infecções virais, bacterianas ou parasitárias.
- Outras intoxicações (p. ex., exposição a organofosforados/carbamatos ou etilenoglicol).
- Ingestão de plantas venenosas, provocando irritação no trato gastrintestinal.
- Ingestão de lírios pelos gatos, resultando em insuficiência renal grave.
- Outras condições clínicas, como pancreatite, neoplasia e inflamação do trato gastrintestinal.

HEMOGRAMA/BIOQUÍMICA/URINÁLISE
Esses exames podem ser utilizados para descartar outras causas de inapetência e vômito.

OUTROS TESTES LABORATORIAIS
Análise da ração quanto à presença do desoxinivalenol por cromatografia em camada fina ou cromatografia líquida de alta pressão.

DIAGNÓSTICO POR IMAGEM
Pode ser empregado para descartar outras causas de inapetência e vômito.

MÉTODOS DIAGNÓSTICOS
N/D.

ACHADOS PATOLÓGICOS
Não existem lesões macroscópicas ou microscópicas patognomônicas.

TRATAMENTO

A retirada da ração contaminada deve resultar na interrupção imediata do vômito e retorno ao consumo alimentar normal.

MEDICAÇÕES

MEDICAMENTO(S)
N/D.

CONTRAINDICAÇÕES/INTERAÇÕES POSSÍVEIS
N/D.

ACOMPANHAMENTO

MONITORIZAÇÃO DO PACIENTE
- Monitorizar o estado de hidratação e os níveis de eletrólitos em caso de vômito grave.
- Garantir o retorno do animal ao peso normal após a remoção da ração contendo desoxinivalenol.

PREVENÇÃO
Fornecer ração de alta qualidade, livre de desoxinivalenol.

EVOLUÇÃO ESPERADA E PROGNÓSTICO
O prognóstico é excelente após a remoção do alimento contendo desoxinivalenol.

DIVERSOS

FATORES RELACIONADOS COM A IDADE
Em outras espécies mais bem estudadas (p. ex., suínos), os animais jovens são mais gravemente acometidos e em concentrações mais baixas de desoxinivalenol na ração do que os adultos.

Sugestões de Leitura
Hughes DM, Gahl MJ, Graham CH, Grieb SL. Overt signs of toxicity to dogs and cats of dietary deoxynivalenol. J Anim Sci 1999, 77:693-700.
Richard JL. Some major mycotoxins and mycotoxicoses — an overview. Int J Food Microbiol 2007, 119:3-10.

Autor Stephen B. Hooser
Consultor Editorial Gary D. Osweiler

Micotoxicose — Toxinas Tremorgênicas

CONSIDERAÇÕES GERAIS

REVISÃO
- Penitrem A — produzido pelo fungo *Penicillium crustosum* (e, talvez, por outras espécies de *Penicillium*); o envenenamento por essa toxina foi relatado em cães que ingeriram pão, queijo e nozes inglesas mofados.
- Roquefortina — produzida por *Penicillium roquefortii* (e, talvez, por outras espécies de *Penicillium*); foi relatada por provocar intoxicação em cães pela ingestão de queijo mofado ou de material orgânico decomposto (compostagem).

IDENTIFICAÇÃO
- Cães e, raramente, gatos.
- Intoxicação por penitrem A e roquefortina foi relatada em cães de várias idades e raças logo após a ingestão de alimentos mofados ou de compostagem.

SINAIS CLÍNICOS
- Tremores musculares moderados a graves e crises convulsivas — começam de minutos a horas (2-4 h nos relatos de casos) após a ingestão de alimento mofado ou de compostagem.
- Os cães acometidos podem ficar hiper-responsivos aos estímulos externos.
- Sinais precoces — podem incluir respiração ofegante, hiperatividade, vômito, ataxia, incoordenação, fraqueza, taquicardia e/ou rigidez.
- Crises convulsivas ou tremores musculares prolongados — podem levar à hipertermia, hipoglicemia, desidratação e anorexia.
- Casos graves — pode resultar em morte.
- Necrose hepática — foi relatada experimentalmente.

CAUSAS E FATORES DE RISCO
- Cães (e, potencialmente, gatos) ficam expostos ao penitrem A e à roquefortina quando ingerem alimento mofado ou matéria orgânica em decomposição (compostagem).
- Experimentalmente, doses de 0,125 mg/kg de penitrem A produziram tremores dentro de 30 minutos.
- Doses de 0,5 mg/kg de penitrem A resultaram no início agudo de tremores, necrose hepática grave e morte.

DIAGNÓSTICO

DIAGNÓSTICO DIFERENCIAL
- Causas tóxicas de crises convulsivas — estricnina; inseticidas (p. ex., organofosforados, carbamatos, organoclorados, nicotina e piretroides); metaldeído; fosfeto de zinco; brometalina; metilxantinas (teobromina e cafeína), anfetaminas, cocaína.
- Causas não tóxicas de crises convulsivas — inflamação; formação congênita de mielina anormal; condições metabólicas (p. ex., encefalopatia hepática ou urêmica).

HEMOGRAMA/BIOQUÍMICA/URINÁLISE
Realizar os exames de hemograma completo, bioquímica e urinálise para avaliar o estado do paciente e para ajudar a descartar outras causas de tremores e crises convulsivas.

OUTROS TESTES LABORATORIAIS
N/D.

DIAGNÓSTICO POR IMAGEM
N/D.

MÉTODOS DIAGNÓSTICOS
- Cromatografia em camada fina ou cromatografia líquida de alta pressão — análise do vômito, conteúdo estomacal e irrigações para lavagem gástrica em busca de penitrem A ou roquefortina.
- A presença de roquefortina C no vômito ou conteúdo estomacal pode servir como um biomarcador sensível para intoxicação por penitrem A.
- Análise da bile — relatada como valiosa.

ACHADOS PATOLÓGICOS
- Não existem lesões patognomônicas associadas à intoxicação por penitrem A ou roquefortina.
- Há relatos de que doses elevadas de penitrem A provoquem dano hepático grave experimentalmente.

TRATAMENTO

- Remover o alimento ou o material orgânico contaminados.
- Induzir o vômito (se o paciente não estiver sob risco de aspiração) ou instituir a lavagem gástrica seguida pela administração de carvão ativado.
- Termorregulação, conforme indicado.

MEDICAÇÕES

MEDICAMENTO(S)
- Diazepam — para controlar as crises convulsivas.
- Barbitúricos — se os tremores e as crises convulsivas não puderem ser controlados com o diazepam.
- Bicarbonato de sódio — poderá ser necessário se houver algum desequilíbrio acidobásico.
- Outro tratamento sintomático e cuidados de suporte — conforme indicação.

CONTRAINDICAÇÕES/INTERAÇÕES POSSÍVEIS
N/D.

ACOMPANHAMENTO

MONITORIZAÇÃO DO PACIENTE
Os pacientes devem ser monitorizados quanto à ocorrência de tremores ou crises convulsivas, hipertermia, desidratação, desequilíbrios acidobásicos, lesão hepática, rabdomiólise e dificuldades respiratórias.

PREVENÇÃO
Evitar que os animais comam itens alimentares mofados, lixo ou compostagem.

COMPLICAÇÕES POSSÍVEIS
- Crises convulsivas — podem não ser controladas com o diazepam.
- Desequilíbrios acidobásicos — podem se desenvolver.
- Lesão hepática e rabdomiólise — podem ocorrer.
- Há relatos de pneumonia por aspiração como sequela do vômito e/ou da lavagem gástrica.
- A exposição poderá ser fatal se doses letais forem consumidas e absorvidas antes da instituição da descontaminação gastrintestinal e do tratamento.

EVOLUÇÃO ESPERADA E PROGNÓSTICO
- Muito bons se o tratamento rigoroso for instituído imediatamente, a toxina for removida do trato gastrintestinal e as crises convulsivas forem controladas com diazepam ou barbitúricos.
- Na maior parte dos casos clínicos, relata-se que a recuperação esteja concluída dentro de 24-48 h.
- Em alguns casos relatados, sinais de fraqueza, rigidez muscular e incoordenação persistiram, mas desapareceram lentamente em 1-2 semanas.
- Alguns casos graves foram relatados como fatais.

DIVERSOS

Sugestões de Leitura

Puschner B. Mycotoxins. Vet Clin North Am Small Anim Pract 2002, 32:409-419.

Tiwary AK, Puschner B, Poppenga RH. Using roquefortine C as a biomarker for penitrem A intoxication. J Vet Diagn Invest 2009, 21:237-239.

Young KL, Villar D, Carson TL, Imerman PM, Moore RA, Bottoff MR. Tremorgenic mycotoxin intoxication with penitrem A and roquefortine in two dogs. JAVMA 2003, 222:52-53.

Autor Stephen B. Hooser
Consultor Editorial Gary D. Osweiler

Mieloma Múltiplo

CONSIDERAÇÕES GERAIS

DEFINIÇÃO
• Neoplasia maligna rara do tecido hematopoiético derivada de uma população clonal de plasmócitos malignos na medula óssea.
• Três dentre quatro características distintivas devem estar presentes para o diagnóstico: gamopatia monoclonal; plasmócitos neoplásicos ou plasmocitose da medula óssea; lesões ósseas líticas; e proteinúria de Bence-Jones (cadeia leve). Em geral, >5% de células neoplásicas ou 10-20% de plasmócitos na medula óssea.

FISIOPATOLOGIA
• Proliferação de um único clone de plasmócitos que produz imunoglobulinas (IgA, IgG ou IgM) ou subunidades (cadeias pesada ou leve).
• Superprodução de IgM resulta em uma síndrome denominada macroglobulinemia de Waldenstrom.
• IgA ou IgG podem sofrer polimerização e aumentar a viscosidade sérica (oito a dez vezes o normal).
• Distúrbios hemorrágicos secundários aos efeitos do revestimento de plaquetas por paraproteína, trombocitopenia, viscosidade aumentada do sangue e interferência nos fatores normais de coagulação.
• Nefrotoxicidade está relacionada com o depósito proteico de amiloide ou o efeito direto da proteína sobre as células epiteliais tubulares renais.
• Hipercalcemia em alguns casos.
• Podem ocorrer citopenias.

SISTEMA(S) ACOMETIDO(S)
• Musculosquelético — múltiplas áreas de lise óssea ativa no esqueleto, incluindo a coluna vertebral (especialmente lombar), a pelve, o crânio e, ocasionalmente, os ossos apendiculares.
• Nervoso, Cardiovascular e Respiratório — possíveis anormalidades secundárias à hiperviscosidade.
• Tecidos moles — plasmócitos neoplásicos podem estar presentes em locais extraesqueléticos (p. ex., fígado, baço, linfonodos, rim, faringe, pulmão, músculo e trato gastrintestinal).

INCIDÊNCIA/PREVALÊNCIA
• Cães — prevalência relatada <1% de todos os tumores malignos; <8% dos tumores malignos hematopoiéticos; 3,6% de todos os tumores ósseos.
• Gatos — prevalência relatada <1% dos tumores hematopoiéticos.

IDENTIFICAÇÃO
Espécies
Cães e gatos.

Raça(s) Predominante(s)
Os cães da raça Pastor alemão e outras raças puras são mais frequentemente acometidas que aqueles de raças mistas.

Idade Média e Faixa Etária
Acomete principalmente cães e gatos de meia-idade ou idosos (6-13 anos).

SINAIS CLÍNICOS
Comentários Gerais
Sinais atribuídos, em geral, à infiltração e lise ósseas, aos efeitos das proteínas monoclonais produzidas pelo tumor (p. ex., hiperviscosidade e nefrotoxicidade) e à infiltração de órgão(s) pelas células neoplásicas.

Achados Anamnésicos
• Dependem da localização e da extensão da doença.
• Fraqueza.
• Claudicação.
• Dor.
• Paresia.
• Incontinência urinária.
• Epistaxe — uni ou bilateral.
• Hemorragias retinianas e cegueira.
• Sangramento proveniente de locais de punção venosa.
• Demência.
• Mal-estar.
• Respiração laboriosa.
• Poliúria.
• Polidipsia.
• Sangramento gastrintestinal.

Achados do Exame Físico
Cães
• Sangramento — especialmente do nariz ou das mucosas (36%).
• Cegueira, hemorragia da retina ou dilatação dos vasos retinianos (35%); descolamento da retina; glaucoma; uveíte anterior.
• Claudicação (47%), dor e fraqueza ósseas (60%) — em casos de lesões ósseas líticas.
• Demência, mal-estar (11%) e coma (raro).
• Polidipsia e poliúria (25%) — com hipercalcemia ou disfunção renal.
• Mucosas pálidas.
• Febre.
• Letargia.
• Hepatosplenomegalia.

Gatos
• Anorexia.
• Perda de peso.
• Mal-estar.
• Polidipsia.
• Poliúria.
• Febre.

CAUSAS
Desconhecidas.

DIAGNÓSTICO

DIAGNÓSTICO DIFERENCIAL
• Infecciosos — distúrbios bacterianos, fúngicos e parasitários.
• Pode ocorrer gamopatia monoclonal secundária a distúrbios infecciosos, como erliquiose e leishmaniose, e outras condições neoplásicas, como leucemia e plasmocitoma mucocutâneo.
• Neoplásicos — metástase para o osso a partir de carcinoma ou sarcoma ou outros tumores sólidos, como mastocitoma ou linfoma, etc.
• Imunomediados — hipergamaglobulinemia benigna; artrite reumatoide; gastrenterocolite plasmocitária.

HEMOGRAMA/BIOQUÍMICA/URINÁLISE
• Hemograma — anemia arregenerativa (70% dos cães); neutropenia (25% dos cães); trombocitopenia (30% dos cães); eosinofilia; leucemia de plasmócitos (muito rara).
• Aumento na formação de *rouleaux* nas hemácias, na viscosidade sérica ou na proteína total sérica com hipoalbuminemia (65% dos cães) e hiperglobulinemia.
• Hipercalcemia (17% dos cães; muito rara nos gatos).
• Ureia, creatinina, fosfatase alcalina ou ALT elevados.
• Proteínas de Bence-Jones — indetectáveis na urinálise de rotina (tira reagente de imersão).
• Proteinúria, isostenúria, cilindrúria, piúria, hematúria ou bacteriúria.

OUTROS TESTES LABORATORIAIS
• Eletroforese de proteínas séricas — identifica gamopatia monoclonal na região beta ou gama e, ocasionalmente, haverá uma gamopatia biclonal.
• Quantificação da imunoglobulina sérica.
• Eletroforese de proteínas urinárias — identifica as proteínas de Bence-Jones (imunoglobulina de cadeia leve); positiva em 30-40% dos cães.
• Perfil de coagulação.
• Viscosidade sérica — elevada.
• Tempo de sangramento ou testes de função plaquetária.

DIAGNÓSTICO POR IMAGEM
• Radiografia (cães) — o esqueleto axial e apendicular pode revelar lesões líticas multifocais (removidas) em 50%.
• Radiografia (gatos) — as lesões ósseas são raras embora possa haver pequenas lesões líticas puntiformes.
• Locais extraesqueléticos podem ser identificados por organomegalia.
• Ultrassonografia — detecta alterações na ecotextura de órgãos viscerais (p. ex., infiltração).

MÉTODOS DIAGNÓSTICOS
O diagnóstico depende da identificação de pelo menos três das quatro características expostas a seguir: gamopatia monoclonal; plasmócitos neoplásicos ou plasmocitose na medula óssea; lesões ósseas líticas observadas nas imagens; e proteinúria de Bence-Jones (cadeia leve). Em geral, >5% de células neoplásicas ou 10-20% de plasmócitos na medula óssea. Em gatos, foi relatada a infiltração de plasmócitos em órgãos abdominais (fígado e/ou baço) em cerca de 50% dos casos.

ACHADOS PATOLÓGICOS
• Coloração — esverdeada no tecido mole; cinza-avermelhada dentro da medula óssea.
• Camadas ou células redondas discretas isoladas com citoplasma eosinofílico, núcleos excêntricos, zona clara perinuclear e aspecto de roda de carro da cromatina nuclear.
• As células neoplásicas podem crescer entre as trabéculas ósseas ou provocar erosão e lise das trabéculas e do córtex ósseos.

TRATAMENTO

CUIDADO(S) DE SAÚDE ADEQUADO(S)
• Internação na presença de azotemia, hipercalcemia, distúrbio hemorrágico ou infecção bacteriana clinicamente importante.
• Plasmaférese, quando disponível, diminui a carga proteica; para o paciente sintomático, retirar um volume de sangue venoso, centrifugá-lo, descartar o plasma e retornar as hemácias aos fluidos intravenosos (cristaloides) para o paciente; com sinais de hiperviscosidade, realizar flebotomia e

Mieloma Múltiplo

repor por via intravenosa com volume igual de fluidos isotônicos.
• Radioterapia — pode ser utilizada em áreas isoladas com intenção curativa ou paliativa, sendo particularmente eficaz para o tratamento de dor óssea por lise.
• Consultar sempre um veterinário especialista em oncologia em busca das informações terapêuticas mais recentes.

CUIDADO(S) DE ENFERMAGEM
• Venopunção — empregar técnica asséptica e ficar preparada para o controle de hemorragia a partir do local.
• Infecção bacteriana — tratar rigorosamente com antibióticos apropriados.
• Hipercalcemia e insuficiência renal — tratar de forma adequada.

ATIVIDADE
Mieloma múltiplo — tratar como paciente imunocomprometido; tomar cuidado para evitar infecção bacteriana (p. ex., causada por feridas perfurantes em cães ou brigas de gatos).

ORIENTAÇÃO AO PROPRIETÁRIO
• Informar ao proprietário que a quimioterapia é paliativa, embora sejam possíveis remissões prolongadas.
• Avisar o proprietário sobre a possibilidade de ocorrência de recidivas.
• Discutir os efeitos colaterais, que dependem dos medicamentos utilizados.
• Informar ao proprietário que a maior parte dos pacientes desenvolve leucopenia branda com a quimioterapia.

CONSIDERAÇÕES CIRÚRGICAS
Áreas não responsivas à quimioterapia ou lesões solitárias podem ser removidas por meio cirúrgico.

RADIOTERAPIA
A radioterapia pode ser paliativa, especialmente em casos refratários. As indicações para esse tipo de terapia incluem tratamento de lesões ósseas dolorosas, compressão da medula espinal, fraturas patológicas (após estabilização de fratura) ou ampla massa de tecido mole. Consultar um oncologista especialista em radioterapia.

MEDICAÇÕES

MEDICAMENTO(S) DE ESCOLHA
• Cães — melfalana (0,1 mg/kg VO a cada 24 h por 10 dias; em seguida, 0,05 mg/kg VO a cada 24 h) e prednisona (0,5 mg/kg VO a cada 24 h por 10 dias; em seguida, 0,5 mg/kg a cada 24 h por 60 dias e, depois, interromper); a ciclofosfamida pode ser utilizada em adição à melfalana ou no lugar deste medicamento (200-300 mg/m^2 IV uma vez por semana ou 50 mg/m^2 VO a cada 24 h por 4 dias por semana).
• Gatos — melfalana (0,5 mg VO a cada 24 h por 10 dias; em seguida, 0,5 mg VO a cada 24 h) e prednisona (2,5 mg VO a cada 24 h).
• Bisfosfonatos, como pamidronato dissódico, para controlar a hipercalcemia em caso de mieloma múltiplo refratário. Não foram estabelecidas doses definitivas para cães ou gatos, mas podem ser administradas doses de 1 a 2 mg/kg diluídos em 250 mL de soro fisiológico por via IV por no mínimo 2 h com segurança. Isso pode ser repetido a cada 3 a 4 semanas.

PRECAUÇÕES
• Melfalana — medicamento muito mielossupressor, especialmente para as plaquetas.
• Ciclofosfamida — pode ser benéfica para substituir a melfalana na trombocitopenia.
• Os animais acometidos podem apresentar baixos números de neutrófilos ou linfócitos não funcionais; tomar cuidado para minimizar a exposição a agentes infecciosos (p. ex., virais, bacterianos e fúngicos).
• Empregar técnica asséptica ou muito limpa ao efetuar qualquer técnica invasiva, mesmo na coleta de sangue.
• A quimioterapia pode ser tóxica; buscar por orientação antes de iniciar qualquer tratamento caso não se esteja familiarizado com o uso de agentes citotóxicos.

MEDICAMENTO(S) ALTERNATIVO(S)
Cães — protocolo quimioterápico combinado mais rigoroso; ciclofosfamida (200 mg/m^2 IV a cada 14 dias), vincristina (0,7 mg/m^2 IV a cada 14 dias), melfalana (0,1 mg/kg VO a cada 24 h por 10 dias; em seguida, 0,05 mg/kg VO a cada 24 h) e prednisona (0,5 mg/kg VO a cada 24 h). Doxorrubicina (30 mg/m^2 IV a cada 21 dias) mais vincristina (0,7 mg/m^2 IV a cada 14 dias) e fosfato sódico de dexametasona (1 mg/kg IV uma vez por semana) também podem ser tentados como protocolo de salvamento.

ACOMPANHAMENTO

MONITORIZAÇÃO DO PACIENTE
• Hemograma completo e contagens plaquetárias — semanalmente por, no mínimo, 4 semanas; avaliar a resposta da medula óssea.
• Testes com resultados anormais — repetir mensalmente por duas vezes para avaliar a resposta ao tratamento.
• Eletroforese de proteínas — mensalmente por vários meses até que padrões proteicos normais sejam obtidos e, depois, monitorizar periodicamente quanto à ocorrência de recidiva.
• Radiografias esqueléticas anormais — repetidas mensalmente por 2 vezes e, em seguida, em meses alternados até a normalização para avaliar a resposta ao tratamento.

COMPLICAÇÕES POSSÍVEIS
• Sangramento.
• Infecções secundárias.
• Fraturas patológicas.
• Mesmo com o tratamento, pode levar alguns meses antes que os sinais clínicos desapareçam.
• Quimioterapia pode provocar leucopenia ou trombocitopenia, anorexia, alopecia, cistite hemorrágica e/ou pancreatite.

EVOLUÇÃO ESPERADA E PROGNÓSTICO
É preciso tomar um cuidado contínuo para proteger os pacientes de infecção secundária.

Cães
• Sobrevida média com agentes alquilantes e prednisona — 18 meses.
• Sobrevida média com a prednisona — 7 meses.
• Resposta completa em 43%; resposta parcial em 49%.
• Hipercalcemia, lise óssea extensa ou proteinúria de Bence-Jones — tempos de sobrevida frequentemente mais curtos.

Gatos
Sobrevida com agentes alquilantes e prednisona — 2-9 meses.

DIVERSOS

GESTAÇÃO/FERTILIDADE/REPRODUÇÃO
A quimioterapia está contraindicada nos animais em gestação.

SINÔNIMO(S)
• Mieloma de plasmócitos.
• Plasmocitoma.
• Mielocitoma.
• Mielossarcoma.
• Leucemia de plasmócitos.
• Eritrocitoma.
• Linfocitoma.
• Sarcoma de plasmócitos.

VER TAMBÉM
• Hipercalcemia.
• Insuficiência Renal Crônica.

ABREVIATURA(S)
• ALT = alanina aminotransferase.

RECURSOS DA INTERNET
http://www.vet.uga.edu/vpp/clerk/Maczuzak/index.htm

Sugestões de Leitura
Giraudel JM, Pages JP, Guelfi JF. Monoclonal gammopathies in the dog: A retrospective study of 18 cases (1986-1999) and literature review. JAAHA 2002, 38:135-147.
Matus RE, Leifer CE, MacEwan EG, Hurvitz AI. Prognostic factors for multiple myeloma in the dog. JAVMA 1986, 11:1288-1292.
Mellor PJ, Haugland S, Murphy S, et al. Myeloma-related disorders in cats commonly present as extramedullary neoplasms in contrast to myeloma in human patients: 24 cases with clinical follow-up. J Vet Intern Med 2006, 45:1376-1383.
Morrison WB. Plasma cell neoplasms. In: Morrison WB, ed., Cancer in Dogs and Cats: Medical and Surgical Management. Jackson, WY: Teton NewMedia, 2002, pp. 671-677.
Patel RT, Caceres A, French AF, et al. Multiple myeloma in 16 cats: a retrospective study. Vet Clin Path 2005, 34:341-352.

Autor Wallace B. Morrison
Consultor Editorial Timothy M. Fan

Mielomalacia (Aguda, Ascendente, Descendente)

CONSIDERAÇÕES GERAIS

REVISÃO
- Necrose isquêmica ou hemorrágica, aguda, progressiva da medula espinal após traumatismo agudo a esta medula.
- Aparece primeiro no local da lesão; em seguida, evolui tanto cranial como caudalmente.
- A morte poderá ser causada por paralisia respiratória se os nervos intercostais e frênicos forem acometidos.

IDENTIFICAÇÃO
- Qualquer idade ou raça.
- Em vista da estreita associação entre a herniação aguda de disco tipo I e a mielomalacia, as raças predispostas à primeira afecção são mais comumente acometidas.

SINAIS CLÍNICOS
- Paralisia aguda decorrente da lesão espinal — sinal clínico inicial.
- Lesão toracolombar — paralisia com reflexos espinais exagerados nos membros pélvicos.
- Percepção da dor — geralmente ausente em posição caudal à lesão.
- Malacia da medula espinal — evolui de modo a envolver os segmentos espinais lombossacros dentro de 72 h, causando arreflexia e atonia dos membros pélvicos, ânus dilatado e bexiga flácida de fácil compressão manual; segmentos torácicos e cervicais da medula espinal podem estar envolvidos 7-10 dias após o insulto inicial.
- Hemorragia subaracnóidea secundária à necrose da microvasculatura na medula espinal — pode provocar hipertermia e dor meníngea extrema.

CAUSAS E FATORES DE RISCO
- Discopatia tipo I.
- Traumatismo de vértebra(s) ou da medula espinal.

DIAGNÓSTICO

DIAGNÓSTICO DIFERENCIAL
- Não é possível diferenciá-la de traumatismo espinal.
- O diagnóstico é feito com base na paralisia dos membros pélvicos atribuída à lesão do neurônio motor superior, que evolui para paralisia devida à lesão do neurônio motor inferior e avança no sentido rostral para a linha de analgesia.

HEMOGRAMA/BIOQUÍMICA/URINÁLISE
- Geralmente normais no início.
- Acidente de trânsito — anormalidades inespecíficas relacionadas com lesão de outros órgãos.
- Após a condição ter se desenvolvido, pode ocorrer desvio à esquerda degenerativo causado por necrose maciça da medula espinal.

OUTROS TESTES LABORATORIAIS
N/D.

DIAGNÓSTICO POR IMAGEM
- Radiografia simples da coluna vertebral — indícios de hérnia de disco; fratura ou luxação vertebral.
- Mielografia — compressão medular; edema; infiltração do meio de contraste no parênquima espinal.
- RM — hiperintensidade do parênquima nas imagens ponderadas em T2, associada a outros indícios de lesão espinal.

MÉTODOS DIAGNÓSTICOS
Punção do LCS coletado da cisterna cerebelomedular — resultados inespecíficos; relacionam-se com o estágio de desenvolvimento da mielomalacia clínica ascendente/descendente; pleocitose neutrofílica quase sempre presente.

TRATAMENTO

- Não há nenhum tratamento para reverter a lesão da medula espinal.
- Agentes valiosos para o tratamento dos efeitos secundários advindos do traumatismo da medula espinal (p. ex., succinato sódico de metilprednisolona e compostos 21-aminoesteroides) — não avaliados para mielomalacia; podem ser úteis para interromper a evolução; no entanto, não há dados objetivos.
- Há hipóteses de que polímeros inorgânicos como o polietilenoglicol restabeleça a função após lesão neurológica, mas novamente não há dados objetivos disponíveis.

MEDICAÇÕES

MEDICAMENTO(S)
- A terapia é controversa.
- Alguns dados apoiam o uso de succinato sódico de metilprednisolona — 30 mg/kg IV inicialmente; em seguida, 15 mg/kg IV 2 e 6 h após a dose inicial; e, depois, 2,4 mg/kg/h por 42 h se o tratamento for instituído em até 8 h do traumatismo.
- Bloqueador histaminérgico H_2 (p. ex., cimetidina), sucralfato ou misoprostol — protegem contra úlceras gastrintestinais nos pacientes submetidos a corticosteroides.

CONTRAINDICAÇÕES/INTERAÇÕES POSSÍVEIS
- Terapia com metilprednisolona pode ser nociva se administrada 8 h ou mais depois do traumatismo.
- Aumento na incidência de infecção associado à administração da metilprednisolona em seres humanos.

ACOMPANHAMENTO

- Em alguns pacientes, a condição evolui apenas no sentido caudal; a paralisia é permanente, embora não ocorra comprometimento respiratório.
- Relatada após laminectomia descompressiva, sugerindo que a cirurgia não impede sua ocorrência.

DIVERSOS

ABREVIATURA(S)
- LCS = líquido cerebrospinal.
- RM = ressonância magnética.

Sugestões de Leitura
Kube SA, Olby NJ. Managing acute spinal cord injuries. Compend Contin Educ Pract Vet 2008, 30(9):496-504.
Olby NJ. Current concepts in the management of acute spinal cord injury. J Vet Intern Med 1999, 13:399-407.

Autor Karen Dyer Inzana
Consultor Editorial Joane M. Parent

Mielopatia — Paresia/Paralisia — Gatos

CONSIDERAÇÕES GERAIS

DEFINIÇÃO
• Mielopatia — qualquer doença que afeta a medula espinal; pode causar paralisia (perda completa dos movimentos voluntários) ou paresia (fraqueza) que pode afetar todos os quatro membros (tetraparesia/plegia), os membros pélvicos (para) apenas, os membros torácicos e pélvicos ipsilaterais (hemi), ou um único membro (mono).
• Paresia/paralisia também pode ser causada por distúrbios neuromusculares.

FISIOPATOLOGIA
• Mielopatia — pode afetar a substância cinzenta ou branca da medula espinal ou, mais frequentemente, ambas.
• Lesões dos tratos ascendentes da substância branca — afetam as modalidades sensoriais, como sensação de toque, pressão, propriocepção, dor e temperatura abaixo do nível da lesão.
• Lesões dos tratos descendentes da substância branca — afetam as vias motoras, produzindo sinais atribuídos a distúrbio do neurônio motor superior. Os corpos celulares dos neurônios motores superiores ficam localizados no cérebro; eles controlam a atividade voluntária e têm função inibitória sobre os neurônios motores inferiores. Os sinais de comprometimento do neurônio motor superior incluem paresia/paralisia, tônus muscular normal a aumentado (hipertonia) e reflexos espinais normais ou exagerados (hiper-reflexia) abaixo do nível da lesão.
• Lesões na substância cinzenta da medula espinal — afetam as funções sensório-motoras da região inervada pelos nervos, cujos corpos celulares estão situados na substância cinzenta. Os nervos motores na substância cinzenta da medula espinal também recebem o nome de neurônios motores inferiores. Os sinais de comprometimento do neurônio motor inferior incluem paresia/paralisia, tônus muscular reduzido ou ausente (hipo ou atonia), atrofia dos músculos inervados por aquele segmento, e, reflexos espinais reduzidos ou ausentes (hipo ou arreflexia).

SISTEMA(S) ACOMETIDO(S)
Nervoso.

GENÉTICA
• Doenças do armazenamento lisossomal — gangliosidose GM1/GM2, esfingomielinose (doença de Niemann-Pick), mucopolissacaridose VI (MPS VI), e glicogenose tipo IV causam paresia ou paralisia em gatos; padrão de herança autossômico recessivo.
• Distrofia neuroaxonal e atrofia muscular espinal — doenças degenerativas da medula espinal relatadas como distúrbios autossômicos recessivos.
• Siringoidromielia/mielodisplasia podem ser associadas à disgenesia sacrocaudal (sacrococcígea) — distúrbio autossômico dominante em gatos Manx.

IDENTIFICAÇÃO
Raça(s) Predominante(s)
• Gangliosidose GM1/GM2 — gatos Siamês, Korat, e doméstico de pelo curto.
• Doença do armazenamento de glicogênio tipo IV — gatos dos Bosques da Noruega.
• Siringoidromielia/mielodisplasia — gatos Manx e cruzamentos dessa raça com disgenesia sacrocaudal.
• Esfingomielinose (doença de Niemann-Pick) — gatos Siamês, Balinês, e doméstico de pelo curto.
• Mucopolissacaridose tipo VI — Siamês e doméstico de pelo curto.
• Doença idiopática do armazenamento de polissacarídeos complexos — Abissínios.
• Distrofia neuroaxonal — Siamês e doméstico de pelo curto.

SINAIS CLÍNICOS
• Os sinais clínicos variam com a localização e a gravidade da lesão.
• Lesão cervical — todos os membros ou os membros ipsilaterais são acometidos por ataxia proprioceptiva e tetraparesia/plegia, hemiparesia/plegia; reflexos e tônus normais a aumentados; ± dor no pescoço (cervicalgia); ± síndrome de Horner ipsi/bilateral; ± incontinência urinária com dificuldade de compressão vesical; aumento do tônus do esfíncter uretral e bexiga urinária tensa.
• Lesão cervicotorácica — todos os membros ou os membros ipsilaterais são acometidos por ataxia proprioceptiva e tetraparesia/plegia, hemiparesia/plegia; hipo/arreflexia, hipo/atonia e atrofia muscular nos membros torácicos com reflexos e tônus normais a aumentados nos membros pélvicos; ± dor no pescoço (cervicalgia); ± síndrome de Horner ipsi/bilateral; reflexo cutâneo do tronco ipsi/bilateral diminuído/ausente; ± incontinência urinária com dificuldade de compressão vesical; aumento do tônus do esfíncter uretral e bexiga urinária tensa.
• Lesão toracolombar — membros torácicos normais; ambos os membros pélvicos ou o membro pélvico ipsilateral são acometidos por ataxia proprioceptiva e paraparesia/plegia; reflexos e tônus normais a aumentados; ± dor toracolombar; ± reflexo cutâneo do tronco diminuído/ausente abaixo da lesão; ± sensação reduzida/ausente abaixo da lesão; ± postura de Schiff-Sherrington; ± incontinência urinária com dificuldade de compressão vesical; aumento do tônus do esfíncter uretral e bexiga urinária tensa.
• Lesão lombossacra — membros torácicos normais; os membros pélvicos ou o membro pélvico ipsilateral são acometidos por ataxia proprioceptiva e paraparesia/plegia ou monoparesia/plegia; hipo/arreflexia; hipo/atonia; atrofia muscular; ± dor regional; ± incontinência urinária e fecal, com bexiga grande e flácida de fácil compressão, tônus diminuído do esfíncter uretral; ± tônus diminuído ou ausente da cauda e do ânus; ± sensação diminuída ou ausente abaixo da lesão.

CAUSAS
• Degenerativas e/ou hereditárias — distrofia neuroaxonal ou neuronal, atrofia muscular espinal, e doenças de armazenamento (gangliosidose GM1/GM2, esfingomielinose, glicogenose tipo IV, doença idiopática do armazenamento de polissacarídeos complexos, e mucopolissacaridose tipo VI).
• Anômalas — siringoidromielia, mielodisplasia, meningocele ou meningomielocele, e síndrome da medula espinal presa frequentemente associadas à disgenesia sacrocaudal, cisto aracnoide espinal, cisto epitelial intradural espinal, cisto/seio dermoide espinal.
• Metabólicas — hipervitaminose A, hiperparatireoidismo secundário nutricional, mielopatia associada à deficiência de cobalamina.
• Neoplásicas — linfoma, neoplasia da coluna vertebral (osteossarcoma, fibrossarcoma, plasmocitoma, e condrossarcoma), meningiomas, sarcomas, tumores histiocíticos, tumores gliais, tumores neuroectodérmicos primitivos, tumores da bainha dos nervos periféricos, e tumores metastáticos.
• Inflamatórias ou infecciosas — PIF, meningomielite bacteriana, meningomielite fúngica (*Cryptococcus neoformans*, *Coccidioides immitis*, *Histoplasma capsulatum*), meningomielite por *Toxoplasma gondii*, meningomielite eosinofílica, poliomielite idiopática, e mielopatia associada ao FeLV.
• Traumáticas — fraturas/luxações vertebrais e feridas penetrantes (feridas por mordeduras, projéteis balísticos, microchips); discopatia intervertebral.
• Vasculares — isquemia ou infarto de etiologia desconhecida, embolia fibrocartilaginosa, más-formações vasculares intraósseas, e mielopatia secundária à fístula aortocaval.

FATORES DE RISCO
• Gatos de rua — sob risco de mielite traumática e infecciosa.
• Gatos FeLV-positivos — sob risco de mielopatia associada a esse vírus e linfoma.

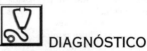

DIAGNÓSTICO

DIAGNÓSTICO DIFERENCIAL
Diferenciar de outros processos patológicos capazes de causar paresia/paralisia — neuromiopatia isquêmica causada por tromboembolia arterial, e doenças neuromusculares periféricas como neuropatia diabética, polirradiculoneurite, miopatia hipocalêmica, distrofia muscular, polimiosite, e miastenia grave.

HEMOGRAMA/BIOQUÍMICA/URINÁLISE
• Frequentemente normais.
• Várias anormalidades inespecíficas podem ser encontradas em associação com mielite infecciosa e linfoma.
• Doenças do armazenamento lisossomal — um acúmulo anormal de produtos do metabolismo celular pode ser observado dentro do citoplasma de leucócitos periféricos.

OUTROS TESTES LABORATORIAIS
• Sorologia — FeLV/FIV, *Cryptococcus neoformans*, *Coccidioides immitis*, *Histoplasma capsulatum*, e *Toxoplasma gondii*.
• Teste de aglutinação em látex — *Cryptococcus neoformans* (soro ou líquido cerebrospinal).
• Triagem metabólica com exame de urina para doenças do armazenamento lisossomal.
• Teste genético para pesquisa de doença do armazenamento de glicogênio tipo IV em gatos dos Bosques da Noruega e mucopolissacaridose tipo VI em gatos Siamês e doméstico de pelo curto.

DIAGNÓSTICO POR IMAGEM
• Radiografia espinal — pode revelar más-formações vertebrais congênitas ou adquiridas (MPS VI), discospondilite, fraturas e luxações vertebrais, tumores ósseos, e sinais radiográficos sugestivos de discopatia intervertebral.

MIELOPATIA — PARESIA/PARALISIA — GATOS

- Mielografia — pode revelar compressão extradural compatível com discopatia intervertebral ou tumor intervertebral, ou tumores intradurais extramedulares.
- TC — exame mais sensível que a radiografia para o diagnóstico de discospondilite, fraturas vertebrais, e tumores ósseos; pode revelar siringomielia e tumores intramedulares.
- RM — exame mais sensível que a TC para o diagnóstico de tumores intramedulares, doenças inflamatórias/infecciosas e vasculares, e anomalias como siringomielia, mielodisplasia, meningocele ou meningomielocele, síndrome da medula espinal presa, cisto aracnoide espinal, cisto epitelial intradural espinal, e cisto/seio dermoide espinal.

MÉTODOS DIAGNÓSTICOS

Líquido Cerebrospinal
- Para confirmar um processo inflamatório que afeta as meninges e/ou a medula espinal.
- O aumento na contagem total de células nucleadas e nas proteínas sugere um processo inflamatório que afeta as meninges e/ou a medula espinal; esse líquido deve ser avaliado quanto à presença de microrganismos fúngicos e bacterianos.
- Outros testes laboratoriais realizados no LCS — teste de aglutinação em látex para detecção de *Cryptococcus neoformans*; ELISA para *Cryptococcus neoformans* e *Histoplasma capsulatum*; PCR para coronavírus felino e *Toxoplasma gondii*; cultura bacteriana e fúngica.

Eletrodiagnóstico
Eletromiografia, velocidade de condução nervosa, estimulações repetitivas — ajudam a diferenciar paresia/paralisia causada por alguma mielopatia decorrente de distúrbios neuromusculares periféricos.

TRATAMENTO

CUIDADO(S) DE SAÚDE ADEQUADO(S)
- Avaliação emergencial e possível cirurgia — na suspeita de alguma causa traumática de paresia/paralisia.
- Tratamento médico-hospitalar — para déficits neurológicos graves, como paralisia e incontinência urinária.

CUIDADO(S) DE ENFERMAGEM
- Os gatos sem deambulação devem ficar confinados em uma espécie de caixa ou engradado acolchoado ou uma área fechada em um ambiente seco e limpo e mudados de posição a cada 6 h se eles não forem capazes de assumir uma posição esternal.
- Na presença de incontinência urinária, a bexiga urinária deverá ser comprimida a cada 6-8 horas.
- Evitar/tratar úlceras de decúbito e queimadura por escaldagem de urina.
- Tratar a constipação.
- A fisioterapia é útil não só para evitar atrofias e contraturas musculares, mas também para manter as articulações flexíveis, especialmente para reabilitação pós-operatória em casos de traumatismo vertebral ou discopatia intervertebral.

ATIVIDADE
Restrita — sobretudo na suspeita de alguma causa traumática de paresia/paralisia, mas também para prevenção de traumatismo secundário à paresia/paralisia.

ORIENTAÇÃO AO PROPRIETÁRIO
Se o gato for tratado como um paciente ambulatorial, abordar todos os aspectos dos cuidados de enfermagem e as possíveis complicações com o proprietário.

CONSIDERAÇÕES CIRÚRGICAS
Tratamento cirúrgico — para fraturas e luxações vertebrais, discopatia intervertebral, e algumas neoplasias.

MEDICAÇÕES

MEDICAMENTO(S) DE ESCOLHA
- Não recomendado(s) até que um diagnóstico seja estabelecido.
- Traumatismo espinal — succinato sódico de metilprednisolona administrado em até 8 horas da lesão na dose de 30 mg/kg sob a forma de bólus IV lento, seguido de 15 mg/kg IV, 2 e 6 horas depois, acompanhado por taxa de infusão contínua a 2,5 mg/kg/hora por 42 horas.

CONTRAINDICAÇÕES
Os corticosteroides são contraindicados na suspeita de alguma doença infecciosa; esses agentes também podem alterar os resultados dos exames de LCS, RM ou TC, dificultando a obtenção do diagnóstico.

ACOMPANHAMENTO

MONITORIZAÇÃO DO PACIENTE
Repetir o exame neurológico — em uma frequência determinada pela gravidade e evolução do estado neurológico.

COMPLICAÇÕES POSSÍVEIS
- Infecção urinária.
- Queimadura por escaldagem de urina.
- Constipação ou incontinência fecal.
- Atrofias e contraturas musculares.
- Úlceras de decúbito.

DIVERSOS

FATORES RELACIONADOS COM A IDADE
- Em gatos com <2 anos de idade, as mielopatias são frequentemente causadas por doenças anômalas ou hereditárias, inflamatórias, ou infecciosas, metabólicas, e traumáticas. PIF é a causa mais importante de mielopatia nesse grupo etário.
- Em gatos de 2-8 anos de idade, os quadros de linfoma, PIF e traumatismo são causas importantes de mielopatia.
- Em gatos com >8 anos de idade, as doenças vasculares e neoplásicas são mais comuns, especialmente linfoma e tumores vertebrais.

POTENCIAL ZOONÓTICO
As infecções por *Toxoplasma gondii* representam um potencial zoonótico.

VER TAMBÉM
- Tromboembolia Aórtica.
- Coccidioidomicose.
- Criptococose.
- Peritonite Infecciosa Felina.
- Infecção pelo Vírus da Leucemia Felina.
- Mielopatia Embólica Fibrocartilaginosa.
- Histoplasmose.
- Discopatia Intervertebral — Gatos.
- Linfoma — Gatos.
- Doenças do Armazenamento Lisossomal.
- Meningite/Meningoencefalite/Meningomielite, Bacteriana.
- Tumores da Bainha Nervosa.
- Distrofia Neuroaxonal.
- Fenômeno de Schiff-Sherrington.
- Toxoplasmose.

ABREVIATURAS
- ELISA = ensaio imunoadsorvente ligado à enzima
- FeLV = vírus da leucemia felina
- FIV = vírus da imunodeficiência felina
- LCS = líquido cerebrospinal
- MPS = mucopolissacaridose
- PCR = reação em cadeia da polimerase
- PIF = peritonite infecciosa felina
- RM = ressonância magnética
- TC = tomografia computadorizada

RECURSOS DA INTERNET
- Vite CH, Braund KG. Braund's Clinical Neurology in Small Animals: Localization, Diagnosis and Treatment. www.ivis.org.
- www.vin.com.

Sugestões de Leitura
Goncalves R, Platt S, Llabr´es-Diaz FJ, et al. Clinical and magnetic imaging findings in 92 cats with clinical signs of spinal cord disease. J Feline Med Surg 2009, 11:53-59.
Marioni-Henry K, Van Winkle TJ, Smith SH, et al. Tumors affecting the spinal cord of cats: 85 cases (1980-2005). JAVMA 2008, 232:237-243.
Marioni-Henry K, Vite CH, Newton AL, et al. Prevalence of diseases of the spinal cord of cats. J Vet Intern Med 2004, 8:851-858.

Autor Katia Marioni-Henry
Consultor Editorial Joane M. Parent

Mielopatia Degenerativa

CONSIDERAÇÕES GERAIS

DEFINIÇÃO
Mielopatia degenerativa canina é uma doença neurodegenerativa fatal e progressiva de início na fase adulta. Recentemente, foi demonstrado que essa mielopatia seja o resultado de uma mutação no gene da superóxido dismutase 1 (*SOD1*) em diversas raças. Sabe-se que as mutações desse gene causam algumas formas de esclerose lateral amiotrófica, também conhecida como doença de Lou Gehrig. Em cães mais idosos, ocorrem sinais iniciais de ataxia espástica progressiva atribuída aos neurônios motores superiores e ataxia proprioceptiva geral nos membros pélvicos. Se a eutanásia for adiada, os sinais clínicos evoluirão para tetraparesia/plegia flácida e outros sinais atribuídos aos neurônios motores inferiores.

FISIOPATOLOGIA
• Uma mutação de sentido trocado (*missense*) no éxon 2 do gene *SOD1*.
• As lesões podem representar uma axonopatia central e periférica multissistêmica.
• A predileção pela gravidade da lesão na medula espinal mesotorácica pode ser o resultado de porcentagens mais baixas de contribuições da artéria radicular e de vasos de pequeno calibre em comparação a outras regiões da medula espinal.
• A escassez de suprimento vascular na medula espinal torácica pode predispô-la a dano por distúrbios oxidativos e metabólicos.

SISTEMA(S) ACOMETIDO(S)
• Sistemas nervosos central e periférico.
• Medula espinal toracolombar no estágio inicial da doença.
• Evolui de modo a envolver a medula espinal cervical e lombar, bem como o sistema nervoso periférico mais tardiamente no curso da doença.
• Os neurônios do tronco cerebral também podem ser acometidos.
• A doença pode envolver as raízes nervosas e os gânglios radiculares dorsais.

GENÉTICA
• Muito provavelmente, possui um modo de herança autossômico recessivo.
• Em virtude da preponderância de raças caninas puras acometidas, atualmente se suspeita de uma herança familiar.
• A mutação no gene *SOD1* constitui o agente causal da mielopatia degenerativa, mas não possui penetrância completa.
• Os cães que são homozigotos para o alelo mutante estão *sob risco* de desenvolvimento de mielopatia degenerativa. Nem todos os cães que são homozigotos para a mutação desenvolverão esse tipo de mielopatia. É altamente improvável que os cães normais ou portadores em teste genético desenvolvam a mielopatia degenerativa.

INCIDÊNCIA/PREVALÊNCIA
A taxa de prevalência de mielopatia degenerativa relatada para todos os cães e coletada do Veterinary Medical Database (Banco de Dados Veterinários Norte-americanos) (1990-1999) foi de 0,19%.

DISTRIBUIÇÃO GEOGRÁFICA
Mundial.

IDENTIFICAÇÃO
Raça(s) Predominante(s)
• As raças com mielopatia degenerativa confirmada por meio de exame histopatológico e registrada na literatura especializada incluem Pastor alemão, Pembroke Welsh corgi, Chesapeake Bay retriever, Rhodesian ridgeback, Boxer, Husky siberiano, Poodle miniatura, raças mistas.
• Além disso, os autores foram capazes de confirmar a mielopatia degenerativa nas raças Montanhês de Berna, Poodle standard (padrão), Kerry blue terrier, Cardigan Wesh corgi, Golden retriever, Fox terrier de pelo duro, Esquimó americano, Wheaten terrier de pelo macio e Pug (na espera de publicação).
• Outras raças previamente relatadas com o diagnóstico presuntivo, mas sem confirmação histopatológica, incluem Terrier irlandês, Labrador retriever, Montanhês de Berna, Kuvasz, Collie, Pastor belga, Schnauzer gigante, Wheaten terrier de pelo macio e Dinamarquês.

Idade Média e Faixa Etária
• Idade média — 9 anos de idade.
• Faixa etária — mais de 5 anos de idade.

Sexo Predominante
Machos e fêmeas são igualmente acometidos.

SINAIS CLÍNICOS
Iniciais:
• Paraparesia atribuída ao neurônio motor superior.
• Ataxia proprioceptiva geral insidiosa, progressiva e assimétrica. A marcha revela uma paraparesia espástica de passadas longas.
• Déficits proprioceptivos de posicionamento da pata.
• Os reflexos espinais costumam estar presentes ou exagerados (o reflexo patelar pode estar reduzido).
• A presença de reflexo extensor cruzado é variável.
• A ausência de hiperestesia paraspinal é uma característica clínica chave.

Tardios:
• Paresia dos membros pélvicos que leva à plegia e, finalmente, evolui para tetraparesia/plegia.
• Diminuição ou ausência do reflexo patelar.
• Perda leve a moderada de massa muscular nos membros pélvicos em virtude de atrofia neurogênica.
• Reflexos espinais reduzidos nos membros pélvicos.
• ± Incontinência urinária e fecal.

Estágio Terminal:
• Tetraplegia flácida.
• Dificuldade de deglutição e com os movimentos da língua.
• Ausência dos reflexos espinais em todos os membros.
• Reflexo cutâneo do tronco reduzido a ausente.
• Emaciação muscular generalizada profunda.
• Incontinência urinária e fecal.
• A percepção sensorial permanece inalterada.

CAUSAS
• Genéticas.
• Outras causas hipotéticas incluem: distúrbios imunomediados, deficiências metabólicas, estresse tóxico e oxidativo.

FATORES DE RISCO
• O fator de risco é a homozigosidade para o alelo mutante.

• Pode haver outros fatores ambientais e genes modificadores da genética; os estudos ainda estão em andamento.

DIAGNÓSTICO

DIAGNÓSTICO DIFERENCIAL
• Discopatia intervertebral do tipo II.
• Neoplasia intramedular da medula espinal.
• Estenose lombossacra degenerativa.
• Displasia do coxal.
• Outras doenças ortopédicas coexistentes.

HEMOGRAMA/BIOQUÍMICA/URINÁLISE
• Em geral, permanecem normais.
• Realizados para descartar outra doença metabólica subjacente.
• A urinálise pode identificar indícios de infecção secundária do trato urinário.

OUTROS TESTES LABORATORIAIS
• Teste de cultura e antibiograma da urina.
• Provas de função da tireoide.
• Teste genético.

DIAGNÓSTICO POR IMAGEM
• Radiografias simples da coluna vertebral.
• Mielografia avalia a presença de doença compressiva da medula espinal.
• Mielografia combinada com TC — técnica mais sensível para avaliar lesões sob suspeita.
• RM — técnica preferida para avaliar a existência de lesões compressivas extradurais e intramedulares.

MÉTODOS DIAGNÓSTICOS
• Análise do LCS para pesquisa de doença inflamatória.
• O diagnóstico definitivo é determinado por meio de histopatologia *post-mortem* da medula espinal.

ACHADOS PATOLÓGICOS
• Os axônios e a mielina da medula espinal são acometidos em todos os funículos; lesões mais graves na porção dorsal dos funículos laterais.
• Bainhas de mielina/cilindros dos axônios vacuolizados, mais extensivamente na medula espinal mesotorácica.
• A proliferação astroglial é proeminente em áreas gravemente acometidas de distribuição da lesão.
• Em geral, a distribuição da lesão é descrita como assimétrica e descontínua. Contudo, provas mais recentes descrevem a distribuição da lesão como simétrica e contínua em cães que sobrevivem por longos períodos com mielopatia degenerativa.
• As amostras de tecido nervoso mostram perda de fibras nervosas, resultante da degeneração axonal e desmielinização secundária.
• As amostras de tecido muscular revelam grupos grandes e pequenos de fibras atróficas típicas de desnervação.

TRATAMENTO

CUIDADO(S) DE SAÚDE ADEQUADO(S)
• Cuidados de suporte
• As raças de pequeno porte podem sobreviver por mais tempo com mielopatia degenerativa, pois o proprietário é capaz de fornecer os cuidados apropriados com facilidade.

Mielopatia Degenerativa

CUIDADO(S) DE ENFERMAGEM
• Quando o cão perde a capacidade deambulatória, é preciso mantê-lo em superfícies bem acolchoadas para evitar a formação de úlceras de decúbito sobre as proeminências ósseas.
• Manter os pelos aparados, bem como a pele seca e limpa, para evitar a queimadura por escaldagem de urina secundária à incontinência.
• A urina deve ser monitorizada quanto à mudança de odor e coloração, o que pode indicar uma infecção do trato urinário.
• A fisioterapia com o uso de exercícios de amplitude de movimento e exercícios isométricos pode ajudar a manter a mobilidade dos membros e a força dos músculos.

ATIVIDADE
• Incentivar a atividade física para retardar a atrofia por desuso dos membros pélvicos.
• A prática de hidroterapia pode envolver o uso de uma esteira submersa na água.
• Um carrinho ortopédico pode ajudar na movimentação do paciente.

DIETA
• Manter uma dieta balanceada.
• Evitar o ganho de peso.

ORIENTAÇÃO AO PROPRIETÁRIO
• Informar ao proprietário sobre o prognóstico mau a longo prazo.
• O fornecimento de cuidados de enfermagem meticulosos é crucial para evitar as complicações secundárias no paciente em decúbito.

CONSIDERAÇÕES CIRÚRGICAS
Nenhuma.

MEDICAÇÕES

MEDICAMENTO(S) DE ESCOLHA
Ainda não há nenhum tratamento comprovado que seja eficaz para retardar ou deter a evolução da doença.

CONTRAINDICAÇÕES
N/D.

PRECAUÇÕES
N/D.

INTERAÇÕES POSSÍVEIS
N/D.

MEDICAMENTO(S) ALTERNATIVO(S)
• Ácido aminocaproico (500 mg/cão; 15 mg/kg VO a cada 8 h).
• Vitamina E (1.000-2.000 UI/cão a cada 24 h).
• Vitamina B_{12} (100-200 µg/cão VO a cada 24 h).

ACOMPANHAMENTO

MONITORIZAÇÃO DO PACIENTE
• Repetir os exames neurológicos.
• Avaliar a presença de retenção urinária.
• Efetuar a urinálise e a urocultura para monitorizar a existência de infecção do trato urinário.

PREVENÇÃO
• Evitar a formação de úlceras de decúbito, a retenção de urina e o ganho de peso.
• Evitar também a ocorrência de dermatite por escaldagem de urina.

COMPLICAÇÕES POSSÍVEIS
• A retenção de urina pode predispor o paciente a infecções do trato urinário.
• As úlceras de decúbito podem gerar infecções cutâneas locais.

EVOLUÇÃO ESPERADA E PROGNÓSTICO
• Ocorre paraplegia em até 6-9 meses desde o momento do diagnóstico.
• Tetraparesia pode ser evidente dentro de 1-2 anos desde o momento do diagnóstico.
• O prognóstico a longo prazo é mau.

DIVERSOS

DISTÚRBIOS ASSOCIADOS
• Outras doenças neurológicas associadas ao início em idade avançada.
• Neoplasia da medula espinal.
• Discopatia intervertebral.
• Doença ortopédica.

FATORES RELACIONADOS COM A IDADE
Os cães de idade mais avançada são comumente acometidos.

POTENCIAL ZOONÓTICO
Nenhum.

GESTAÇÃO/FERTILIDADE/REPRODUÇÃO
N/D.

SINÔNIMO(S)
• Esclerose lateral amiotrófica canina.
• Mielopatia degenerativa canina.
• Radiculomielopatia degenerativa.
• Mielopatia do Pastor alemão.

VER TAMBÉM
• Discopatia Intervertebral Cervical.
• Discopatia Intervertebral Toracolombar.
• Estenose Lombossacra e Síndrome da Cauda Equina.

ABREVIATURA(S)
• LCS = líquido cerebrospinal.
• RM = ressonância magnética.
• TC = tomografia computadorizada.

RECURSOS DA INTERNET
www.caninegeneticdiseases.net/dm

Sugestões de Leitura
Awano T, Johnson GS, Wade C, Katz ML, Johnson GC, Taylor JF, Perloski M, Long S, March PA, Olby NJ, Khan S, O'Brien DP, Lindblad-Toh K, Coates JR. Genome-wide association analysis reveals a SOD1 missense mutation canine degenerative myelopathy that resembles amyotrophic lateral sclerosis. Proc Natl Acad Sci 2009, 106:2794-2799.

Coates JR, March PA, Ogelsbee M, et al. Clinical characterization of a familial degenerative myelopathy in Pembroke Welsh Corgi dogs. J Vet Intern Med 2007, 21:1323-1331.

Dewey CW. A Practical Guide to Canine and Feline Neurology, 2nd ed. Ames, IA: Wiley-Blackwell, 2008, pp. 344-345.

March PA, Coates JR, Abyad R, et al. Degenerative myelopathy in 18 Pembroke Welsh Corgi dogs. Vet Pathol 2009, 46:241-250.

Autor Joan R. Coates
Consultor Editorial Joane M. Parent

Mielopatia Embólica Fibrocartilaginosa

CONSIDERAÇÕES GERAIS

DEFINIÇÃO
Necrose isquêmica aguda da medula espinal, causada por êmbolos fibrocartilaginosos.

FISIOPATOLOGIA
- Êmbolos — encontrados nas artérias e/ou veias espinais; a fonte possivelmente vem de material do disco intervertebral ou medula óssea do corpo vertebral.
- O mecanismo exato de entrada na vasculatura espinal é desconhecido.

SISTEMA(S) ACOMETIDO(S)
Nervoso.

GENÉTICA
N/D.

INCIDÊNCIA/PREVALÊNCIA
- Causa comum de doença da medula espinal em raças caninas não condrodisplásicas.
- Não relatada em raças condrodisplásicas.
- Rara em gatos.

DISTRIBUIÇÃO GEOGRÁFICA
N/D.

IDENTIFICAÇÃO
Espécies
Cães e gatos.

Raça(s) Predominante(s)
- Raças de porte grande e gigante — maior prevalência.
- Schnauzer miniatura e Pastor de Shetland — super-representadas; hiperlipoproteinemia e consequente hiperviscosidade são comuns nessas raças; pode contribuir para infarto da medula espinal sem êmbolos fibrocartilaginosos.

Idade Média e Faixa Etária
- A maioria dos pacientes tem 3-5 anos de idade.
- Faixa etária de 16 semanas a 10 anos.

Sexo Predominante
Leve predominância em machos.

SINAIS CLÍNICOS
Achados Anamnésicos
- No início dos sinais, é comum algum traumatismo leve ou exercício vigoroso.
- Início súbito.
- O cão acometido tipicamente chora de dor; a dor diminui em minutos a horas (na maioria dos casos).
- Sinais de paresia ou paralisia desenvolvem-se em questão de segundos, minutos ou horas.
- A condição se estabiliza em 12-24 h.

Achados do Exame Físico
N/D.

Achados do Exame Neurológico
- Déficits — geralmente lateralizados; o lado não acometido costuma estar levemente afetado ou normal; simetricamente distribuído em alguns pacientes.
- Dor — no início dos sinais e, depois, geralmente ausente; costuma ter diminuído no momento em que o animal é examinado; pode ser sentida por algumas horas em pacientes com acometimento grave.
- Qualquer nível da medula espinal pode ser acometido, dependendo da distribuição do material embólico.
- Ataxia leve a paralisia.
- Déficits do neurônio motor superior ou inferior.

- Lesão da medula espinal — unilateral ou apenas a face dorsal ou ventral da medula espinal, causando déficit do membro ipsolateral com perda sensorial, mas preservando o tônus muscular e a função motora (ou vice-versa); ou outras combinações ímpares são possíveis em pacientes com lesões focais de quadrantes.
- Se os sinais evoluírem além de 24 h, considerar a presença de outras doenças.

CAUSAS
Desconhecidas.

FATORES DE RISCO
- A prática de exercício vigoroso pode desencadear o incidente.
- Hiperlipoproteinemia.

DIAGNÓSTICO

DIAGNÓSTICO DIFERENCIAL
- Mielopatia aguda, assimétrica, indolor e não progressiva — a presença dessas características ajuda muito no diagnóstico.
- Dor no dorso e no pescoço com sinais simétricos — discopatia intervertebral; discospondilite; tumor vertebral; fratura e luxação; radiografia simples, RM, TC e/ou mielografia ajudam a confirmar o diagnóstico.
- Hemorragia parenquimatosa na medula espinal secundária à diátese hemorrágica (p. ex., causada pela ingestão de rodenticida anticoagulante, trombocitopenia ou CID) — excluir mediante exame cuidadoso em busca de evidência de hemorragia, com contagem de plaquetas e determinação dos tempos de coagulação.
- Mielite focal — diferenciada com base no histórico progressivo e na análise do LCS.

HEMOGRAMA/BIOQUÍMICA/URINÁLISE
Geralmente normais.

OUTROS TESTES LABORATORIAIS
N/D.

DIAGNÓSTICO POR IMAGEM
- Radiografia simples da coluna vertebral — geralmente normal.
- Mielografia simples e por TC — no estágio agudo, em geral, demonstra tumefação intramedular focal no local do êmbolo; depois, costuma ser normal ou mostrar uma área de atrofia medular.
- RM — técnica ideal de diagnóstico por imagem; nas imagens ponderadas em T2, pode haver uma redução na intensidade de sinal do disco e um aumento na intensidade de sinal do parênquima da medula espinal no local da lesão.

MÉTODOS DIAGNÓSTICOS
Análise do LCS
- Os resultados dependem da localização (p. ex., cisterna lombar *versus* cerebelomedular) e do momento de coleta do líquido em relação ao início dos sinais clínicos.
- Estágio agudo — pode-se observar um número elevado de hemácias e neutrófilos; alguns dias depois, só é possível ver um leve aumento de proteína.
- Às vezes normal.

ACHADOS PATOLÓGICOS
- Macroscópicos — tumefação focal na medula espinal com hemorragia.

- Microscópicos — êmbolos de fibrocartilagem em artérias e veias da medula espinal e das meninges; necrose hemorrágica e malacia nas substâncias cinzenta e branca.

TRATAMENTO

CUIDADO(S) DE SAÚDE ADEQUADO(S)
Paciente internado — para tratamento clínico imediato e procedimentos diagnósticos.

CUIDADO(S) DE ENFERMAGEM
- Manter os pacientes em decúbito em uma superfície acolchoada; virá-lo com frequência para evitar úlceras de pressão.
- Ajudar e estimular o paciente a andar o mais rápido possível.
- Auxiliar o esvaziamento vesical várias vezes ao dia, se necessário, por compressão manual ou cateterização para evitar distensão da bexiga e lesão do músculo detrusor.
- A prática de hidroterapia em piscina ou esteira subaquática pode ser útil na reabilitação.
- O uso de coleira peitoral leve com guia localizada dorsalmente destinada para cães de busca e resgate, como a Ruff Wear Web Master Dog Harness® (www.ruffwear.com), pode ser muito útil para o manejo dos cuidados de enfermagem em casa durante a recuperação.

ATIVIDADE
- Restrita até o estabelecimento do diagnóstico em caso de instabilidade da coluna vertebral gerada por outras causas, como herniação de disco intervertebral ou fratura/luxação.
- Assim que a mielopatia embólica fibrocartilaginosa for confirmada, a atividade deverá ser incentivada e não restrita.

DIETA
Normal a menos que haja hiperlipidemia; nesse caso, fornecer uma dieta pobre em gordura, como Hill's Prescription Diet r/d.

ORIENTAÇÃO AO PROPRIETÁRIO
- Informar ao proprietário sobre o fato de que a recuperação da paresia ou da paralisia é lenta e gradual, quando ocorre.
- Orientar o proprietário sobre a necessidade de cuidados de suporte consideráveis (fornecidos em casa) da maioria dos pacientes durante a recuperação.

CONSIDERAÇÕES CIRÚRGICAS
N/D.

MEDICAÇÕES

MEDICAMENTO(S) DE ESCOLHA
Succinato sódico de metilprednisolona — pode ser benéfico se administrado nas primeiras 8 h após o início dos sinais, de acordo com estudos de lesão aguda da medula espinal causada por impacto sobre a medula; 30 mg/kg IV como primeiro tratamento; em seguida, 15 mg/kg 2 e 6 h depois e, daí em diante, a cada 6 h até um curso terapêutico total de 24-48 h; administrar cada dose lentamente durante 10-15 min; a injeção muito rápida pode causar vômito. Além de ser um tratamento controverso, pode não ser eficaz.

Mielopatia Embólica Fibrocartilaginosa

CONTRAINDICAÇÕES
Analgésicos não esteroides — não administrar com succinato sódico de metilprednisolona; aumentam a probabilidade de ulceração gastrintestinal.

PRECAUÇÕES
• Succinato sódico de metilprednisolona — não é benéfico com tratamento por mais de 24-48 h e aumenta muito os efeitos adversos (p. ex., ulceração gastrintestinal).
• Dieta rica em fibras e pobre em gorduras como a Hill's Prescription Diet r/d durante e após o tratamento com esteroides diminui a ocorrência de ulceração gastrintestinal.

INTERAÇÕES POSSÍVEIS
N/D.

MEDICAMENTO(S) ALTERNATIVO(S)
N/D.

ACOMPANHAMENTO

MONITORIZAÇÃO DO PACIENTE
• Avaliações neurológicas sequenciais — durante as primeiras 12-24 h após o exame inicial.
• Estado neurológico — 2, 3 e 4 semanas após o início dos sinais clínicos.
• Incontinência urinária — urinálise e cultura bacteriana/antibiograma detectam a presença de infecção do trato urinário.

PREVENÇÃO
• A recidiva é altamente improvável, mas possível.
• Não existe nenhum método conhecido de prevenção na maioria dos casos.
• Em caso de hiperlipidemia, fornecer uma dieta com baixo teor de gordura (<10%) e óleos de peixe ômega-3 por via oral na dose de 10-30 mg/kg a cada 24 h.

COMPLICAÇÕES POSSÍVEIS
• Incontinência urinária e fecal.
• Infecção do trato urinário.
• Queimaduras causadas por escaldagem de urina e úlceras de pressão.

EVOLUÇÃO ESPERADA E PROGNÓSTICO
• Presença de percepção da dor e sinais do neurônio motor superior — o prognóstico quanto a uma melhora acentuada é bom.
• Perda de percepção da dor — prognóstico mau.
• Arreflexia de membros ou esfíncteres — quase nenhuma possibilidade de recuperação.
• Movimentos intencionais e reflexos reduzidos — é comum a recuperação funcional; é provável algum grau de déficit permanente.
• A evolução dos sinais clínicos atribuídos à lesão dos neurônios motores superior e inferior, bem como uma área aumentada de perda sensorial, indicam mielomalacia ascendente ou descendente e prognóstico sem esperança; considerar a eutanásia.
• Estado neurológico — pouca alteração nos primeiros 14 dias após o início; ocorre melhora entre 21-42 dias; remielinização completa em grande parte dos pacientes 6-12 semanas após o início; se não houver melhora após 21-30 dias, a recuperação será altamente improvável.

DIVERSOS

DISTÚRBIOS ASSOCIADOS
Distúrbios que induzem a um comprometimento da função circulatória podem predispor ou mimetizar a mielopatia embólica fibrocartilaginosa — hiperadrenocorticismo; hipotireoidismo; pressão arterial sistêmica elevada; síndrome da hiperviscosidade; hiperlipidemia; diátese hemorrágica; endocardite bacteriana.

FATORES RELACIONADOS COM A IDADE
N/D.

POTENCIAL ZOONÓTICO
N/D.

GESTAÇÃO/FERTILIDADE/REPRODUÇÃO
Administração de corticosteroides em altas doses — pode causar parto prematuro.

ABREVIATURA(S)
• CID = coagulação intravascular disseminada.
• LCS = líquido cerebrospinal.
• RM = ressonância magnética.
• TC = tomografia computadorizada.

Sugestões de Leitura
Gandini G, Cizinauska S, Lang J, et al. Fibrocartilaginous embolism in 75 dogs: Clinical findings and factors influencing the recovery rate. J Small Anim Pract 2003, 44:76-80.
Grunenfelder FI, Weishaupt D, Green R, et al. Magnetic resonance imaging findings in spinal cord infarction in three small breeds dogs. Vet Radiol Ultrasound 2005, 46:91-96.
Hawthorne JC, Wallace LJ, Fenner WR, et al. Fibrocartilaginous embolic myelopathy in miniature schnauzers. JAAHA 2001, 37:374-383.
Mikszewski JS, Van Winkle TJ, Troxel MT. Fibrocartilaginous embolic myelopathy in five cats. JAAHA 2006, 42:226-233.
Summers BA, Cummings JF, de Lahunta A. Veterinary Neuropathology. St Louis: Mosby, 1995, pp. 246-249.

Autor Allen Sisson
Consultor Editorial Joane M. Parent

Miocardiopatia — Boxer

CONSIDERAÇÕES GERAIS

REVISÃO
Miocardiopatia caracterizada mais comumente por taquiarritmias ventriculares, que podem ser acompanhadas por síncope ou morte cardíaca súbita. Uma pequena porcentagem (<5%) de pacientes desenvolve insuficiência cardíaca congestiva com disfunção sistólica, comparável à miocardiopatia dilatada observada em outras raças caninas.

IDENTIFICAÇÃO
• Cães. • Específica ao Boxer, embora raramente se observe uma apresentação clínica similar no Buldogue inglês. • Geralmente observada em cães adultos, com pelo menos 2 anos de idade. Há relatos do envolvimento de cães com até 6 meses de vida. Alguns animais acometidos podem não desenvolver os sinais clínicos até os 10 anos de idade.

SINAIS CLÍNICOS
• Os sinais clínicos são variáveis, mas costumam envolver uma das três manifestações a seguir:
• Cão assintomático com complexos ventriculares prematuros (CVP), detectados ao exame de rotina.
• Ocorrência de síncope no cão com CVP, detectados ao exame eletrocardiográfico ou à monitorização com Holter (ECG ambulante).
• Sinais de insuficiência cardíaca esquerda (p. ex., tosse e taquipneia) ou insuficiência biventricular (p. ex., ascite, taquipneia e tosse) com CVP. Essa manifestação é a menos comum.
• Antes do desenvolvimento de sinais clínicos evidentes, poderá ocorrer a morte súbita.

CAUSAS E FATORES DE RISCO
• Início no adulto, distúrbio hereditário (autossômico dominante).
• Uma mutação genética (deleção) em um gene desmossômico cardíaco é associada ao desenvolvimento da doença. Ainda não se sabe se isso é a única causa genética ou se outras mutações genéticas serão identificadas.
• Verificou-se que, pelo menos, uma família de cães da raça Boxer com CVP, dilatação ventricular e disfunção sistólica apresentou níveis reduzidos de L-carnitina no miocárdio e demonstrou certa melhora clínica quando suplementada com esse aminoácido. Ainda não foi esclarecida a relação de causa e efeito, mas a resposta a essa suplementação não ocorre em todos os cães com disfunção miocárdica.

DIAGNÓSTICO

DIAGNÓSTICO DIFERENCIAL
• Estenose aórtica — formas moderadas e graves podem estar associadas aos CVP.
• Formas raras de cardiopatia adquirida (neoplasia, endocardite).
• Doença abdominal (especialmente comprometimento esplênico) pode se associar ao desenvolvimento de CVP.
• A ecocardiografia e a ultrassonografia abdominal podem ser utilizadas para diferenciar a miocardiopatia do Boxer de outras causas de doença cardíaca e abdominal.

OUTROS TESTES LABORATORIAIS
• Atualmente, o teste genético pode ser realizado para fazer a triagem do animal quanto à presença da mutação genética (http://www.cvm.ncsu.edu/vhc/csds/vcgl/index.html) associada à miocardiopatia do Boxer. As amostras enviadas podem ser sangue em tubo de EDTA ou *swab* bucal da superfície da mucosa bucal.
• Os níveis plasmáticos da L-carnitina podem ser avaliados em cães da raça Boxer com dilatação ventricular e disfunção sistólica. Contudo, os níveis plasmáticos nem sempre refletem os níveis miocárdicos. Se os níveis no plasma não estiverem baixos, ainda será possível a presença de níveis miocárdicos reduzidos e, nesse caso, a suplementação com L-carnitina pode ser considerada.

DIAGNÓSTICO POR IMAGEM
Radiografia Torácica
• Normal na maioria dos cães acometidos.
• Os cães com dilatação ventricular e disfunção sistólica podem exibir aumento de volume cardíaco e indícios de insuficiência cardíaca (p. ex., edema pulmonar).

Ecocardiografia
• Normal em grande parte dos cães acometidos.
• Uma pequena porcentagem de cães apresenta dilatação ventricular e disfunção sistólica.

MÉTODOS DIAGNÓSTICOS
Eletrocardiograma
• Muitos cães não exibirão CVP no ECG de curta duração, já que a arritmia pode ser intermitente. Alguns cães terão um ou mais CVP positivos em um ECG breve na derivação II.
• Independentemente do caso, se houver a suspeita de doença, será recomendada a monitorização com Holter para determinar a gravidade e a complexidade da arritmia e obter um registro basal para fins comparativos logo após a instituição do tratamento. Se o Holter não estiver disponível e o cão se mostrar sintomático com CVP positivos ao ECG, a terapia deverá ser considerada.

ACHADOS PATOLÓGICOS
• Na maioria dos casos, as anormalidades macroscópicas são inespecíficas. Em uma pequena porcentagem de casos, pode-se constatar dilatação dos ventrículos esquerdo e direito.
• As anormalidades histopatológicas incluem a presença de infiltrado gorduroso e fibroso na parede livre do ventrículo direito (e, algumas vezes, do septo interventricular e do ventrículo esquerdo).

TRATAMENTO

• O objetivo terapêutico envolve a redução na quantidade de CVP, nos sinais clínicos e no risco de morte cardíaca súbita. Infelizmente, não há provas de que a terapia seja capaz de diminuir o risco de morte súbita. A decisão de iniciar a terapia no Boxer assintomático com CVP é controversa, uma vez que todos os antiarrítmicos podem agravar a arritmia. Contudo, já se constatou a morte súbita de cão com até 300 CVP/24 h. Em geral, inicia-se a terapia medicamentosa se houver mais de 1.000 CVP/24 h, sucessões significativas de taquicardia ventricular ou outros sinais de complexidade da arritmia (p. ex., bigeminia e acoplamentos) ou ainda sinais clínicos (síncope, intolerância a exercício) relacionados com os CVP.
• Os episódios de síncope e morte cardíaca súbita podem ser mais frequentemente associados ao estresse e à agitação do animal. Sempre que possível, deve-se tentar a diminuição do estresse e do esforço físico. Não há relação direta entre restrição física e sobrevivência. Alguns cães morrem enquanto adormecem. Assim, não é recomendável a restrição rigorosa da atividade física.

MEDICAÇÕES

MEDICAMENTO(S)
• As duas melhores escolhas para o tratamento da arritmia ventricular são: sotalol (1,5-3,5 mg/kg VO a cada 12 h) ou mexiletina (5-6 mg/kg VO a cada 8 h). Alguns cães continuam exibindo ectopia ventricular significativa após o tratamento com um dos medicamentos supramencionados; esses casos parecem responder bem à combinação de sotalol (1,5-3,5 mg/kg VO a cada 12 h) e mexiletina (5-6 mg/kg VO a cada 8 h). Esses medicamentos têm diferentes mecanismos de ação e parecem atuar de forma segura e complementar.
• Em cães com disfunção sistólica e insuficiência cardíaca, considerar o tratamento com furosemida (1-2 mg/kg VO a cada 12 h), enalapril (0,5 mg/kg VO a cada 12 h), pimobendana (0,25 mg/kg VO a cada 12 h), espironolactona (1-2 mg/kg VO a cada 12-24 h) e L-carnitina (50 mg/kg VO a cada 8-12 h).

CONTRAINDICAÇÕES/INTERAÇÕES POSSÍVEIS
Qualquer medicamento antiarrítmico tem o potencial de agravar uma arritmia.

ACOMPANHAMENTO

• Se possível, repetir a monitorização com Holter em 2 semanas após o início da terapia para avaliar a resposta do animal. Os cães acometidos podem ter uma variabilidade diária de 85% no número de CVP antes dos medicamentos; portanto, uma resposta satisfatória à terapia corresponderia a uma diminuição de 85% na quantidade de CVP. Contudo, nem sempre é possível atingir essa redução; nesses casos, uma melhora na complexidade da arritmia e nos sinais clínicos seria um objetivo razoável.
• Sugere-se a monitorização anual com Holter e ecocardiografia.
• É imprescindível advertir os proprietários de que os cães estão constantemente sob risco de morte súbita. No entanto, muitos cães podem ser mantidos com antiarrítmicos durante anos. Os cães com disfunção sistólica e dilatação cardíaca apresentam prognóstico mau, embora alguns desses animais demonstrem melhora e retardo na evolução do quadro quando suplementados com a L-carnitina.

Autor Kathryn M. Meurs

MIOCARDIOPATIA DILATADA — CÃES

CONSIDERAÇÕES GERAIS

DEFINIÇÃO
Caracterizada por dilatação cardíaca esquerda e direita, normalidade das valvas atrioventriculares (ou minimamente comprometidas) e das artérias coronárias, declínio significativo do estado inotrópico e ocorrência de disfunção miocárdica principalmente durante a sístole; no entanto, a disfunção diastólica progressiva com fisiologia restritiva pode representar um indicador negativo independente da sobrevida.

FISIOPATOLOGIA
• A insuficiência miocárdica leva à queda do débito cardíaco e ao desenvolvimento de ICC.
• Uma dilatação do anel AV e uma disfunção dos músculos papilares favorecem a insuficiência valvar.
• Embora sinais atribuídos ao lado esquerdo do coração costumem predominar, é comum a evidência de comprometimento grave do lado direito no final da evolução clínica.

SISTEMA(S) ACOMETIDO(S)
• Cardiovascular.
• Respiratório — edema pulmonar.
• Renal/urológico — azotemia pré-renal.
• Todos os sistemas orgânicos são acometidos pelas quedas no débito cardíaco.

GENÉTICA
Há fortes suspeitas de causa genética ou suscetibilidade hereditária em grande parte das raças e registro comprovado em outras (Cão d'água português, Boxer, e Doberman pinscher) com modos variáveis de herança. Um teste genético está disponível no mercado para pesquisa da mutação causal em cães da raça Boxer (estriatina) e Doberman pinscher (piruvato desidrogenase cinase). Essas mutações não parecem ser a causa em outras raças predispostas. A caracterização completa da correlação entre o genótipo e o fenótipo em cada raça necessitará de mais estudos.

INCIDÊNCIA/PREVALÊNCIA
Estimada em 0,5-1,1% em raças predispostas e, possivelmente, mais alta em regiões geográficas específicas.

DISTRIBUIÇÃO GEOGRÁFICA
Nenhuma, exceto em casos de miocardiopatia causada pela doença de Chagas, que está restrita ao sul dos Estados Unidos (Costa do Golfo).

IDENTIFICAÇÃO
Espécies
Cães.

Raça(s) Predominante(s)
• Doberman pinscher, Boxer.
• Raças gigantes: Scottish deerhound, Wolfhound irlandês, Dinamarquês, São Bernardo, Afghan hound, Cão Montanhês de Berna.
• Cocker spaniel, cão d'água português.

Idade Média e Faixa Etária
4-10 anos de idade.

Sexo Predominante
Acomete os machos com frequência maior que as fêmeas, em grande parte das raças, mas não em todas.

SINAIS CLÍNICOS
Achados Anamnésicos
• Respiratórios — taquipneia, dispneia, tosse.
• Perda de peso.
• Fraqueza, letargia, anorexia.
• Distensão abdominal.
• Síncope (geralmente associada a arritmias importantes).
• Alguns cães permanecem assintomáticos, apresentando a chamada miocardiopatia dilatada pré-clínica, cujo diagnóstico é controverso.
• Os parâmetros ecocardiográficos específicos à raça aliados a biomarcadores cardíacos (NT-proBNP) podem ser úteis para identificar os cães no estágio pré-clínico da doença.

Achados do Exame Físico
• Podem permanecer completamente normais na doença pré-clínica.
• Fraqueza, depressão e, possivelmente, choque cardiogênico.
• Pulso femoral hipocinético decorrente do baixo débito cardíaco.
• Déficits de pulso em casos de fibrilação atrial, contrações ventriculares ou supraventriculares prematuras, e taquicardia ventricular paroxística.
• Pulsos jugulares decorrentes de regurgitação tricúspide (valva atrioventricular direita), arritmias ou ICC direita.
• Ruídos respiratórios — abafados em casos de efusão pleural; crepitações na presença de edema pulmonar.
• Constatação de 3ª bulha cardíaca ou galope de somação.
• Os sopros de regurgitação mitral e/ou tricúspide são comuns, mas geralmente focais e tênues.
• São comuns indícios auscultatórios de arritmia cardíaca.
• Tempo de preenchimento capilar lento e possível cianose.
• Hepatomegalia com ou sem ascite.

CAUSAS
• O mecanismo primário ainda precisa ser identificado e permanece idiopático na grande maioria dos casos. A maior parte dos autores acredita que praticamente todos os casos representem anormalidades familiares de proteínas cardíacas estruturais, energéticas ou contráteis.
• Em diversas raças (inclusive Golden retriever, Boxer, Doberman pinscher e Cocker spaniel), há registros de deficiências nutricionais (taurina e/ou carnitina).
• Além disso, sugerem-se etiologias virais, protozoárias e imunomediadas.
• Hipotireoidismo e taquiarritmias persistentes (algumas vezes associadas à má-formação congênita da valva atrioventricular direita [tricúspide]) podem causar insuficiência miocárdica reversível.

DIAGNÓSTICO

DIAGNÓSTICO DIFERENCIAL
• Endocardiose.
• Cardiopatia congênita.
• Dirofilariose.
• Endocardite bacteriana.
• Tumores cardíacos e efusão pericárdica.
• Obstrução das vias aéreas: corpo estranho, neoplasia, paralisia laríngea.
• Pneumopatia primária — broncopatia, pneumonia, neoplasia, aspiração, vasculopatia (p. ex., dirofilariose).
• Efusões pleurais (p. ex., piotórax, hemotórax, quilotórax).
• Traumatismo, com consequente hérnia diafragmática, hemorragia pulmonar, pneumotórax.

HEMOGRAMA/BIOQUÍMICA/URINÁLISE
Os testes hematológicos e a urinálise de rotina costumam permanecer normais, a menos que sejam alterados por reduções graves no débito cardíaco ou elevações graves nas pressões venosas (p. ex., azotemia pré-renal, ALT elevada e hiponatremia), terapia para insuficiência cardíaca (p. ex., hipocalemia, hipocloremia e alcalose metabólica por diurese) ou doença concomitante.

OUTROS TESTES LABORATORIAIS
Biomarcadores cardíacos, inclusive NT-proBNP, encontram-se elevados em estágios pré-clínicos e clínicos da doença. Estudos clínicos que investigam o uso desses marcadores para o diagnóstico, o prognóstico e a otimização da terapia estão em andamento.

DIAGNÓSTICO POR IMAGEM
Achados Radiográficos
• Podem permanecer completamente normais na fase pré-clínica.
• É comum a constatação de cardiomegalia generalizada e sinais de ICC.
• Nos casos precoces, o aumento de volume atrial e ventricular esquerdos pode ser mais evidente.
• Em alguns casos, o grau de cardiomegalia pode ser menor do que se pode esperar com a gravidade dos sinais clínicos.
• Muitas vezes, o grau de cardiomegalia é consideravelmente menor do que seria esperado em cão com valvulopatia cardíaca primária e sinais clínicos compatíveis.
• Efusão pleural, hepatomegalia, ascite.

Achados Ecocardiográficos
• A dilatação do ventrículo esquerdo frequentemente precede os declínios evidentes nos índices da função sistólica.
• Exame diagnóstico com padrão de excelência.
• Dilatação atrial e ventricular.
• Índices ecocardiográficos da função sistólica do miocárdio (baixos índices da porcentagem do encurtamento fracional, encurtamento da área e movimento anular mitral; imagem por Doppler tecidual) podem estar reduzidos.
• Os estudos por Doppler espectral podem confirmar a velocidade e/ou a aceleração baixas do fluxo transaórtico, bem como a regurgitação mitral e/ou tricúspide.
• A evidência de enchimento restritivo do VE por meio do Doppler é um indicador independente de redução da sobrevida.

MÉTODOS DIAGNÓSTICOS
Eletrocardiografia
• Ritmo sinusal ou taquicardia sinusal, com complexos atriais ou ventriculares prematuros isolados.
• A fibrilação atrial e a taquicardia ventricular (paroxística ou sustentada) são muito comuns em cães da raça Doberman pinscher.
• Os cães da raça Boxer comumente apresentam arritmias ventriculares isoladas, sem evidência de cardiopatia funcional ou anatômica.

Miocardiopatia Dilatada — Cães

- Prolongamento do QRS (>0,06 s) e possível aumento das voltagens (R >3,0 mV na derivação II), sugerindo aumento de volume do ventrículo esquerdo.
- Pode exibir ondas R "inclinadas" em declive, com depressão do segmento ST-T, indicando doença do miocárdio ou isquemia do VE.
- Pode ainda revelar baixas voltagens (efusões pleural ou pericárdica, hipotireoidismo concomitante).

ACHADOS PATOLÓGICOS
- Dilatação de todas as câmaras cardíacas, com adelgaçamento de suas paredes.
- Leve espessamento do endocárdio, com áreas pálidas no interior do miocárdio (necrose, fibrose).
- Do ponto de vista histológico, há duas formas distintas: (1) infiltração gordurosa — tipo degenerativo observado em Boxer e Doberman pinscher e (2) outro tipo fibroso ondulante adelgaçado observado em muitas raças de porte gigante, grande e médio, incluindo alguns cães das raças Boxer e Doberman pinscher.

TRATAMENTO

CUIDADO(S) DE SAÚDE ADEQUADO(S)
Com a exceção de cães gravemente acometidos, pode-se administrar grande parte da terapia em esquema ambulatorial.

ATIVIDADE
Permitir que o cão escolha seu próprio nível de atividade.

DIETA
- Durante a terapia inicial para os sinais clínicos, é primordial simplesmente manter a ingestão calórica adequada.
- Objetivo — reduzir a ingestão de sódio na dieta para <12-15 mg/kg/dia.
- Ao se utilizar terapia cardioativa potente, tipicamente não é necessária a restrição rigorosa de sódio.
- É melhor usar as rações comerciais disponíveis no mercado.

ORIENTAÇÃO AO PROPRIETÁRIO
- Enfatizar os sinais clínicos potenciais associados à evolução da doença e aos efeitos adversos dos medicamentos.
- A monitorização da frequência respiratória em repouso frequentemente fornece informações sobre descompensação iminente.

MEDICAÇÕES

MEDICAMENTO(S) DE ESCOLHA
Primeiramente, é preciso identificar os problemas do paciente — ICC (esquerda ou direita), arritmia, hipotermia, insuficiência renal, choque.

Doença Pré-clínica
- Atualmente, não há provas de que a intervenção precoce altere a evolução da doença pré-clínica.
- O ensaio internacional PROTECT (do inglês *Prospective Trial of Cardioprotective Effect of Carperitide Treatment* [Ensaio Prospectivo do Efeito Cardioprotetor do Tratamento com Carperitida]) em andamento está avaliando a eficácia da intervenção precoce sob monoterapia com a pimobendana.
- A avaliação crítica sugere que a intervenção precoce com inibidores da ECA é de mínimo benefício em termos de sobrevida.

Estabilização Inicial
- Tratar a hipoxemia com a administração de oxigênio; evitar a perda de calor se o animal estiver hipotérmico (ambiente aquecido); fornecer fluidos IV ou SC (soro glicosado a 5% ou NaCl a 0,45% com glicose a 2,5%), somente após o controle do edema pulmonar ou a aspiração da efusão pleural.
- Na presença de edema pulmonar — furosemida (2-4 mg/kg IM ou IV, depois 1-2 mg/kg a cada 6-12 h nos primeiros 2-3 dias) ou a mesma dose diária total administrada sob a forma de infusão contínua.
- Nitroglicerina tópica a 2% durante as primeiras 24-48 h para edema pulmonar grave — aplicar ~2,5-5,0 cm a cada 8 h (ficar atento para hipotensão).
- Se houver efusão pleural significativa, efetuar a drenagem de cada hemitórax com o uso de cateter tipo borboleta de calibre 18-20.
- Na constatação de insuficiência cardíaca e choque cardiogênico graves, pode-se indicar o uso de dobutamina. Esse medicamento, por sua vez, pode predispor o animal a arritmias malignas, particularmente em cães hipóxicos. A pimobendana por via oral (ver dosagem a seguir) também pode trazer importante benefício hemodinâmico imediato (2-4 h).
- Digoxina — terapia oral (ver adiante).
- Dobutamina — infusão cautelosa de 5-10 µg/kg/min durante 24-72 h (iniciar com a dose baixa e gradativamente titular para cima com base na resposta).
- Se uma taquicardia ventricular paroxística estiver presente, administrar a lidocaína lentamente em bólus de 2 mg/kg (até 8 mg/kg no total) para a conversão de tal arritmia em ritmo sinusal. Prosseguir com a infusão de lidocaína (50-75 µg/kg/min).
- Se a lidocaína se mostrar ineficaz, administrar a procainamida lentamente em bólus IV de 2 mg/kg (até 20 mg/kg no total) para a conversão da arritmia em um ritmo sinusal. Dar continuidade com infusão de 25-50 µg/kg/min ou 8-20 mg/kg IM a cada 6 h (cuidado com pró-arritmia).

Terapia de Manutenção
- Em casos de MCD, os inibidores da ECA (enalapril, benazepril, lisinopril) são considerados a base da terapia.
- No início do esquema terapêutico, é recomendável a instituição de enalapril (0,25-0,5 mg/kg VO a cada 12 h), benazepril (0,5 mg/kg VO a cada 24 h) ou lisinopril (0,5 mg/kg VO a cada 24 h). Alguns dados sugerem que o enalapril possa prolongar o período pré-clínico.
- Para alguns cães de raças gigantes, administra-se uma dose diária de manutenção de 0,375-0,50 mg de digoxina (divididos a cada 12 h). Não exceder 0,015 mg/kg/dia nem ultrapassar 0,375 mg por dia na raça Doberman pinscher. Como a pimobendana tem substituído a digoxina como o agente inotrópico positivo de escolha, a digoxina será utilizada principalmente para o controle da resposta da frequência ventricular em caso de fibrilação atrial (ver adiante).
- Para o controle de edema pulmonar, efusão pleural ou ascite, emprega-se a furosemida (0,5-3 mg/kg VO a cada 8-24 h).
- Ao bloquear a aldosterona, a espironolactona (0,5-1 mg/kg VO a cada 24 h) diminui a mortalidade em seres humanos com insuficiência cardíaca. Em casos de insuficiência cardíaca refratária, o clínico pode lançar mão de doses mais elevadas desse diurético (1-2 mg/kg VO a cada 12 h).
- Os betabloqueadores poderão ser usados com cautela, assim que a insuficiência cardíaca estiver controlada com outros medicamentos (ver a seção "Precauções"). Se tolerável, o uso crônico desses agentes betabloqueadores pode restabelecer a função do miocárdio. O carvedilol (0,25-1,25 mg/kg VO a cada 12 h) é um α e β-bloqueador com atividade antioxidante. Iniciar com o limite inferior da faixa da dose e elevá-la gradativamente em um período de 6 semanas, se essa alteração na dosagem for tolerada. Em pacientes com MCD clínica, deve-se consultar um cardiologista antes de se empregar os betabloqueadores, pois isso pode resultar em deterioração clínica rápida e profunda.
- A pimobendana (0,25-0,3 mg/kg VO a cada 12 h) é um medicamento sensível ao cálcio e um vasodilatador inotrópico positivo que, quando adicionado à furosemida, a algum inibidor da ECA e à digoxina, melhora a categoria funcional da insuficiência cardíaca e aumenta o tempo de sobrevida no Doberman pinscher.
- O papel da carnitina e da taurina na terapia da MCD permanece controverso. Contudo, os cães da raça Cocker spaniel americano com miocardiopatia dilatada geralmente respondem de forma favorável à suplementação da taurina e L-carnitina, mas ainda necessitam de outros medicamentos cardíacos.

Arritmias
- No caso de fibrilação atrial, a lentificação na resposta da frequência ventricular é obtida por meio da administração crônica de digitálicos, combinados com atenolol (0,75-1,5 mg/kg VO a cada 12 h) ou diltiazem (Dilacor®) (2-7 mg/kg VO a cada 12 h).
- O objetivo terapêutico é obter uma frequência ventricular entre 100-140 bpm em repouso.
- A terapia exposta acima apenas controla a frequência ventricular, por meio da depressão da condução cardíaca do nodo AV; em geral, ela não converte o ritmo decorrente da fibrilação atrial em ritmo sinusal.
- Amiodarona (10-15 mg/kg VO a cada 24 h por 7-10 dias, seguida por 5-10 mg/kg VO a cada 24 h) pode controlar a resposta da frequência ventricular ou, em alguns casos, resultar em conversão da arritmia em ritmo sinusal.
- A terapia oral crônica para taquicardia ventricular inclui procainamida (8-20 mg/kg VO a cada 6-8 h), mexiletina (5-8 mg/kg VO a cada 8 h), amiodarona (5-10 mg/kg VO a cada 24 h) ou sotalol (1-2 mg/kg VO a cada 12 h).
- Se necessárias, a procainamida e a mexiletina podem ser combinadas com algum betabloqueador.

CONTRAINDICAÇÕES
Em casos de taquicardia ventricular paroxística descontrolada grave ou em animais com função renal comprometida, deve-se evitar o uso da digoxina.

PRECAUÇÕES
- Os betabloqueadores e os bloqueadores dos canais de cálcio são agentes inotrópicos negativos e podem exibir efeito adverso agudo sobre a função do miocárdio, embora inúmeros estudos em seres humanos sugiram um possível benefício na MCD pela administração crônica de betabloqueadores.

MIOCARDIOPATIA DILATADA — CÃES

- A combinação de diuréticos e inibidores da ECA pode resultar em azotemia, sobretudo em pacientes com insuficiência cardíaca grave ou disfunção renal preexistente.

INTERAÇÕES POSSÍVEIS
- Os medicamentos quinidina, amiodarona e diltiazem podem aumentar os níveis séricos da digoxina e predispõem o animal à intoxicação digitálica.
- A disfunção renal, o hipotireoidismo e a hipocalemia predispõem à intoxicação digitálica.

MEDICAMENTO(S) ALTERNATIVO(S)
- Em vez de um inibidor da ECA ou em acréscimo a esse tipo de agente (cuidado com a hipotensão), podem-se utilizar outros vasodilatadores, incluindo a hidralazina e o anlodipino.
- O papel da coenzima Q10 ainda precisa ser determinado.

ACOMPANHAMENTO

MONITORIZAÇÃO DO PACIENTE
- Os exames clínicos, as radiografias torácicas, as medições da pressão arterial, as avaliações da bioquímica sérica de rotina e os ECGs seriados são extremamente úteis.
- A repetição da ecocardiografia raramente é informativa ou indicada.
- As avaliações seriadas dos níveis séricos da digoxina (faixa terapêutica = 0,5-1 ng/mL) obtidos 6-8 h após a ingestão do comprimido e as determinações dos perfis bioquímicos séricos podem ajudar a evitar as complicações iatrogênicas.

COMPLICAÇÕES POSSÍVEIS
- Morte súbita por arritmias.
- Problemas iatrogênicos associados ao tratamento clínico (ver anteriormente).

EVOLUÇÃO ESPERADA E PROGNÓSTICO
- Sempre fatal.
- O óbito costuma ocorrer 6-24 meses após o diagnóstico.
- Tipicamente, a raça Doberman pinscher apresenta prognóstico mau, em geral com sobrevida inferior a 6 meses a partir do momento do diagnóstico (a adição da pimobendana pode aumentar substancialmente a sobrevida).
- A fibrilação atrial, a taquicardia ventricular paroxística, a evidência de enchimento restritivo do VE por meio do Doppler e a redução acentuada na porcentagem do encurtamento fracional provavelmente constituem marcadores de sobrevida curta e morte súbita.

DIVERSOS

FATORES RELACIONADOS COM A IDADE
A prevalência aumenta com a idade.

SINÔNIMO(S)
- Miocardiopatia congestiva.
- Miocardiopatia das raças gigantes.

VER TAMBÉM
- Deficiência de Carnitina.
- Deficiência de Taurina.
- Fibrilação Atrial e Flutter Atrial.
- Taquicardia Ventricular.

ABREVIATURA(S)
- AE = átrio esquerdo.
- AV = atrioventricular.
- ECA = enzima conversora de angiotensina.
- ECG = eletrocardiograma.
- ICC = insuficiência cardíaca congestiva.
- MCD = miocardiopatia dilatada.
- VE = ventrículo esquerdo.

RECURSOS DA INTERNET
Washington State University Veterinary Cardiac Genetic Laboratory: http://www.vetmed.wsu.edu/deptsVCGL/.

Sugestões de Leitura
Oyama MA. Canine cardiomyopathy. In: Tilley LP, Smith FWK, Oyama MA, Sleeper MM, eds., Manual of Canine and Feline Cardiology, 4th ed. St. Louis: Saunders Elsevier, 2008, pp. 139-150.

Autor Matthew W. Miller
Consultores Editoriais Larry P. Tilley e Francis W. K. Smith Jr.

Miocardiopatia Dilatada — Gatos

CONSIDERAÇÕES GERAIS

DEFINIÇÃO
• A miocardiopatia dilatada corresponde a uma doença do músculo cardíaco, caracterizada por insuficiência sistólica do miocárdio e dilatação do coração por sobrecarga volêmica, que leva a sinais de insuficiência cardíaca congestiva e baixo débito cardíaco. • Antes de 1987, a miocardiopatia dilatada era a segunda miocardiopatia mais comumente diagnosticada em gatos. A maioria dos gatos provavelmente sofria de miocardiopatia secundária, em função da deficiência de taurina. Hoje em dia, a miocardiopatia dilatada idiopática primária é uma causa rara de cardiopatia nessa espécie.

FISIOPATOLOGIA
Em termos histopatológicos, o miocárdio de gatos com MCD idiopática tem evidência de miocitólise, fibrose, fragmentação das miofibrilas e vacuolização. O exame macroscópico revela aumento excêntrico global de todas as quatro câmaras cardíacas. Essas alterações anatômicas são associadas a insuficiência sistólica progressiva do miocárdio, diminuição da contratilidade, redução da complacência e regurgitação secundária da valva atrioventricular esquerda (mitral) em virtude de dilatação anular dessa valva. Tipicamente, essas alterações são identificadas ao exame de ecocardiografia. A disfunção crônica do miocárdio acaba levando ao desenvolvimento de insuficiência cardíaca congestiva e sinais clínicos.

SISTEMA(S) ACOMETIDO(S)
• Cardiovascular — a MCD é uma doença primária do miocárdio, que afeta principalmente o coração e sua capacidade de manter um débito cardíaco adequado para atender às necessidades do corpo. • Musculosquelético — os gatos com MCD podem se apresentar com tromboembolia aórtica, que provoca paraparesia ou monoparesia aguda. • Renal/Urológico — os gatos com MCD e insuficiência cardíaca congestiva muitas vezes exibem má perfusão renal e comumente sofrem de azotemia pré-renal. • Respiratório — os gatos costumam se apresentar com taquipneia ou dispneia causada pela insuficiência cardíaca congestiva em casos de MCD. Esses gatos podem desenvolver edema pulmonar e efusão pleural.

GENÉTICA
Em função da experiência humana com MCD, é provável que a MCD felina apresente uma mutação genética, hereditária ou *de novo**, como a causa de sua doença. Até o momento, entretanto, nenhuma mutação definitiva foi identificada no gato. Além disso, uma avaliação genética quantitativa de um grande gatil sugeriu a existência de um fator hereditário no desenvolvimento de MCD.

INCIDÊNCIA/PREVALÊNCIA
MCD felina idiopática é um distúrbio relativamente incomum hoje em dia, já que a taurina é suplementada de forma adequada em rações para gatos. Um estudo retrospectivo europeu de 106 gatos com miocardiopatia felina de 1994 a 2001 revelou que a MCD foi diagnosticada em cerca de 10% dos casos nesse grupo. Na experiência da autora, a prevalência de MCD idiopática felina pode ser menor que 10%.

IDENTIFICAÇÃO
Espécies
Gatos.

Raça(s) Predominante(s)
Como a prevalência é baixa, as predileções raciais não são claramente definidas. Ou seja, o gato Birmanês pode ter uma incidência elevada.

Idade Média e Faixa Etária
9 anos (5-13 anos).

Sexo Predominante
Fêmeas.

SINAIS CLÍNICOS
Comentários Gerais
• Gatos com MCD idiopática geralmente apresentam sinais de insuficiência cardíaca congestiva. • Raramente, esses gatos são diagnosticados antes do início dos sinais clínicos.

Achados Anamnésicos
Sinais relacionados com o baixo débito cardíaco:
• Anorexia. • Fraqueza. • Depressão.
Sinais relacionados com a insuficiência cardíaca congestiva: ○ Dispneia. ○ Taquipneia.
Sinais relacionados com a tromboembolia:
○ Dor e paraparesia de início súbito.

Achados do Exame Físico
• A frequência cardíaca pode estar rápida, normal ou lenta. • Sopro cardíaco sistólico tênue.
• Impulso cardíaco esquerdo débil. • Ritmo de galope. • Possível arritmia. • Hipotermia. • Tempo de preenchimento capilar prolongado.
• Taquipneia. • Ruídos pulmonares abafados (efusão pleural). • Crepitações (edema pulmonar).
• Ascite. • Pulsos femorais hipocinéticos. • Possível paresia e dor nos membros pélvicos, em virtude da tromboembolia aórtica.

CAUSAS
A etiologia subjacente da miocardiopatia dilatada idiopática permanece desconhecida, embora tenha sido identificada uma predisposição genética em algumas famílias de gatos. A deficiência de taurina era uma causa comum de insuficiência miocárdica secundária antes de 1987.

DIAGNÓSTICO

DIAGNÓSTICO DIFERENCIAL
• Miocardiopatia dilatada por deficiência de taurina. Como a miocardiopatia dilatada idiopática primária e a deficiência de taurina apresentam manifestações clínicas semelhantes, deve-se admitir que os gatos com insuficiência miocárdica tenham a deficiência mencionada até que se demonstre a falta de resposta à suplementação com esse aminoácido.
• Insuficiência miocárdica secundária a doenças prolongadas congênitas ou adquiridas do ventrículo esquerdo por sobrecarga volêmica. • A miocardiopatia hipertrófica remodelada em estágio terminal pode se manifestar com um coração hipocontrátil dilatado. • Miocardiopatia arritmogênica do ventrículo direito.

HEMOGRAMA/BIOQUÍMICA/URINÁLISE
Muitos gatos apresentarão azotemia pré-renal relacionada com o baixo débito cardíaco.

OUTROS TESTES LABORATORIAIS
• Garantir que as concentrações dos hormônios tireoidianos estejam normais. • As concentrações de taurina menores que 40 nmoles/L no plasma e inferiores a 250 nmoles/L no sangue total estão abaixo do normal e são sugestivas de miocardiopatia dilatada por deficiência desse aminoácido. As análises de taurina são efetuadas em um número limitado de instituições e necessitam de manipulações especiais. • Os biomarcadores cardíacos, como peptídeo natriurético tipo B aminoterminal plasmático (NT-proBNP) e as concentrações da troponina I cardíaca (cTnI) seriam elevados em um gato com insuficiência cardíaca congestiva causada por miocardiopatia dilatada idiopática.

DIAGNÓSTICO POR IMAGEM
Achados Radiográficos
• As radiografias frequentemente revelam efusão pleural ou edema pulmonar. • Cardiomegalia generalizada.

Achados Ecocardiográficos
• Constitui a modalidade diagnóstica de escolha. • Os achados característicos incluem adelgaçamento das paredes ventriculares, aumento das dimensões terminossistólicas e terminodiastólicas do ventrículo esquerdo, aumento de volume do átrio esquerdo e encurtamento fracional baixo. • Pode ser visualizada efusão pleural e pericárdica. • Pode ser observada a presença de contraste ecocardiográfico espontâneo ou a formação de trombo.

MÉTODOS DIAGNÓSTICOS
Eletrocardiografia
• Os achados eletrocardiográficos podem permanecer normais ou revelar padrões de aumento de volume atrial ou ventricular esquerdos. • É possível a detecção de arritmias tanto ventriculares como supraventriculares.

Análise da Efusão Pleural
Tipicamente, a efusão pleural é um transudato modificado, com nível de proteína total abaixo de 4 g/dL e contagem de células nucleadas inferior a 2.500/mL. Uma efusão quilosa também pode estar presente. A análise da efusão pleural é importante para descartar outras causas desse tipo de derrame, como piotórax, peritonite infecciosa, ou linfossarcoma.

ACHADOS PATOLÓGICOS
• A proporção entre peso corporal:peso cardíaco mostra-se aumentada. • Todas as quatro câmaras cardíacas encontram-se dilatadas. As paredes ventriculares apresentam-se delgadas, enquanto o lúmen do ventrículo esquerdo se encontra dilatado. • A anatomia valvar permanece normal.
• A histopatologia revela miocitólise e fibrose do miocárdio.

TRATAMENTO

CUIDADO(S) DE SAÚDE ADEQUADO(S)
• Esses gatos costumam estar em insuficiência cardíaca congestiva e devem ser internados, tipicamente em uma unidade de terapia intensiva até a estabilização.

CUIDADO(S) DE SAÚDE ADEQUADO(S)
• A toracocentese é utilizada para ambos os fins, tanto terapêuticos como diagnósticos.

---

* N. T.: Uma nova mutação que não foi herdada de nenhum dos progenitores.

MIOCARDIOPATIA DILATADA — GATOS

- A suplementação com oxigenoterapia é benéfica em gatos com insuficiência cardíaca congestiva para diminuir o esforço respiratório.
- Se os animais estiverem hipotérmicos, recomenda-se o aquecimento externo (incubadora ou colchonete térmico).

ATIVIDADE
Manter o gato dentro de casa somente depois da alta hospitalar para reduzir o estresse. Deixar o gato ditar suas próprias atividades.

DIETA
Tipicamente, esses gatos apresentam-se anoréxicos; dessa forma, pode ser necessária a estimulação de seu apetite com muitos tipos de alimentos. Por fim, é recomendável uma dieta hipossódica.

ORIENTAÇÃO AO PROPRIETÁRIO
Alguns gatos necessitarão de toracocentese intermitente crônica para controlar a grande quantidade de efusão pleural apesar da terapia médica.

MEDICAÇÕES

MEDICAMENTO(S) DE ESCOLHA
- Para eliminar o edema pulmonar e a efusão pleural, é recomendável o uso da furosemida. A dose recomendada varia de 1-4 mg/kg a cada 8-12 h. Inicialmente, deve-se administrar esse diurético por via parenteral e depois trocar para via oral. Cronicamente, é aconselhável a dose mais baixa e eficaz da furosemida.
- No tratamento imediato da insuficiência cardíaca congestiva, pode-se aplicar a nitroglicerina (unguento a 2%) por via tópica em uma área de ~0,5-1,3 cm e utilizar os diuréticos concomitantemente para reduzir ainda mais a pré-carga. A nitroglicerina diminuirá a dose de furosemida, sendo particularmente útil em pacientes com hipotermia ou desidratação.
- Para diminuir a pré e a pós-carga, recomenda-se o enalapril ou benazepril na dose de 0,25 a 0,5 mg/kg VO a cada 24 h logo que o gato estiver apto a tomar medicamentos por essa via. Utilizar esses medicamentos com cuidado e, possivelmente, evitá-los se a creatinina estiver acima de 2,5 mg/dL.
- Pimobendana, um inodilatador, também é recomendável para fortalecer a contratilidade cardíaca e produzir alguma vasodilatação. A dose recomendada varia de 0,1-0,3 mg/kg VO a cada 12 h. A pimobendana não é aprovada atualmente para uso em gatos.
- A suplementação de taurina é aconselhável a uma dose de 250 mg VO a cada 12 h até que uma ausência de resposta a esse aminoácido pelo paciente.
- A digoxina é opcionalmente recomendada para fortalecer a contratilidade cardíaca e por seus efeitos neuro-humorais positivos na dose de 0,03 mg/gato (1/4 de um comprimido de 0,125 mg) ou 0,01 mg/kg VO a cada 48 h. A digoxina pode ser administrada concomitantemente com a pimobendana. Contudo, pode ser um problema administrar diversos comprimidos a um gato e, se surgirem essas dificuldades na administração, a pimobendana poderá ser mais eficaz que a digoxina.
- Em pacientes com sinais graves de insuficiência cardíaca congestiva e débito cardíaco baixo, pode-se fornecer a dobutamina em doses extremamente baixas. A dose varia de 0,25-5 µg/kg/min IV sob taxa de infusão contínua. É aconselhável a monitorização ECG.
- Como a doença tromboembólica é preocupante, considerar o uso de algum agente antitrombótico, como: ácido acetilsalicílico na dose de 81 mg VO a cada 72 h (com alimento); clopidogrel na dose de 17,5 mg (1/4 de comprimidos de 75 mg) VO a cada 24 h; heparina não fracionada na dose de 200 unidades/kg SC a cada 8 h; OU heparina de baixo peso molecular (p. ex., dalteperina na dose de 100 unidades/kg SC a cada 12-24 h ou enoxaparina 1 mg/kg SC a cada 12-24 h).
- Os medicamentos antiarrítmicos também podem ser necessários para controlar as arritmias supraventriculares ou ventriculares. Em caso de taquicardia supraventricular ou fibrilação atrial rápida, é recomendado o diltiazem na dose de 0,1 mg/kg IV lento; diltiazem oral de liberação não sustentada na dose de 7,5 mg/gato VO a cada 8 h; ou formulação oral de liberação sustentada (Cardizem CD®) na dose de 10 mg/kg VO a cada 24 h. Em caso de taquicardia ventricular rápida e sustentada, é recomendada a lidocaína IV lenta na dose de 0,2-0,5 mg/kg (repetir 1 ou 2 vezes no máximo) ou o sotalol VO na dose de 2 mg/kg a cada 12 h.
- Betabloqueadores, como atenolol, são úteis no tratamento de arritmias supraventriculares e ventriculares. Os betabloqueadores também são utilizados no tratamento da miocardiopatia dilatada a longo prazo em seres humanos, em função de seus efeitos miocárdicos positivos e benefícios quanto à sobrevida. A experiência clínica é limitada em casos de miocardiopatia dilatada felina; sendo assim, esses agentes terapêuticos devem ser utilizados com cuidado, uma vez que eles diminuem a contratilidade cardíaca de forma intensa. A dose recomendada varia de 3,125 a 6,25 mg VO a cada 12-24 h. Iniciar com a dose baixa e titular para cima, com base na frequência cardíaca e nos sinais clínicos.

PRECAUÇÕES
- A menos que sejam necessários para o controle imediato do ritmo cardíaco, os bloqueadores dos canais de cálcio ou os bloqueadores β-adrenérgicos podem diminuir a contratilidade e o débito cardíaco. Utilizar com cuidado.
- A terapia diurética e vasodilatadora demasiada pode causar azotemia e distúrbios eletrolíticos.
- Em caso de insuficiência renal confirmada ou sob suspeita, é recomendável reduzir a dose da digoxina.
- Os medicamentos enalapril ou benazepril devem ser utilizados com cuidado e, possivelmente, suspensos se o nível sérico de creatinina estiver acima de 3 mg/dL.
- A dobutamina pode gerar crises convulsivas e taquiarritmias cardíacas.

ACOMPANHAMENTO

MONITORIZAÇÃO DO PACIENTE
- Repetir o exame idealmente com mensuração da pressão arterial, obtenção de radiografias torácicas e análise do perfil bioquímico dentro de 1 semana para determinar a resposta à terapia.
- A monitorização da frequência respiratória em repouso em casa é útil para determinar a necessidade de ajuste da dose do diurético ou do procedimento de toracocentese.
- Efetuar a monitorização periódica dos parâmetros eletrolíticos e renais.
- É recomendável mensurar as concentrações da digoxina 2 semanas após a instituição da terapia. A faixa terapêutica gira em torno de 0,5-1,5 ng/dL, 8-12 h após a ingestão do comprimido.
- Repetir o ecocardiograma em 2-3 meses após o início da suplementação com taurina para avaliar a resposta à terapia.

PREVENÇÃO
Garantir que os gatos consumam uma dieta rica em proteínas com suplementação suficiente de taurina na dieta. Não utilizar dietas vegetarianas.

COMPLICAÇÕES POSSÍVEIS
A tromboembolia é a complicação mais temida de qualquer miocardiopatia felina.

EVOLUÇÃO ESPERADA E PROGNÓSTICO
- Apesar da terapia intensiva, esses gatos apresentam prognóstico mau.
- A insuficiência cardíaca congestiva pode ser refratária e recorrente em termos médicos apesar da terapia médica adequada.
- Não é rara a repetição da toracocentese.

DIVERSOS

DISTÚRBIOS ASSOCIADOS
Insuficiência cardíaca congestiva, tromboembolia, efusão pleural, arritmias cardíacas.

SINÔNIMOS
Cardiomiopatia.

VER TAMBÉM
- Tromboembolia Aórtica.
- Insuficiência Cardíaca Congestiva — Esquerda.
- Insuficiência Cardíaca Congestiva — Direita.

ABREVIATURAS
- MCD = miocardiopatia dilatada.

Sugestões de Leitura

Ferasin L, Sturgess CP, Cannon MJ, et al. Feline idiopathic cardiomyopathy: A retrospective study of 106 cats (1994-2001). J Feline Med Surg 2003, 5:151-159.

Fox PR, et al. Spontaneously occurring arrhythmogenic right ventricular cardiomyopathy in the domestic cat: A new animal model similar to human disease. Circulation 2000, 102:1863-1870.

Kittleson MD. Feline myocardial disease. In: Ettinger SJ, Feldman EC, eds., Textbook of Veterinary Internal Medicine, 6th ed. St. Louis: Elsevier, 2005, pp. 1082-1103.

Lawler DF, Templeton AJ, Monti KL. Evidence of genetic involvement in feline dilated cardiomyopathy. J Vet Intern Med 1993, 7:383-387.

Pion PD, Kittleson MD, Rogers QR, et al. Myocardial failure in cats associated with low plasma taurine: A reversible cardiomyopathy. Science 1987, 237:764-768.

Autor Teresa C. DeFrancesco
Consultores Editoriais Larry P. Tilley e Francis W. K. Smith Jr.

MIOCARDIOPATIA HIPERTRÓFICA — CÃES

CONSIDERAÇÕES GERAIS

REVISÃO
Miocardiopatia hipertrófica foi definida como "hipertrofia miocárdica inadequada do ventrículo esquerdo não dilatado, que ocorre na ausência de algum estímulo identificável para a hipertrofia." A miocardiopatia hipertrófica (MCH) é uma doença rara em cães, caracterizada por hipertrofia concêntrica (aumento na espessura da parede) do ventrículo esquerdo. O processo patológico primário está confinado ao coração e compromete outros sistemas orgânicos apenas na presença de insuficiência cardíaca congestiva. O aumento na espessura da parede do VE leva a um dano no enchimento ventricular (pela falta de complacência e anormalidade do relaxamento), com elevação resultante na pressão terminodiastólica do VE e na pressão do AE. A câmara atrial esquerda costuma aumentar de volume, em resposta à pressão terminodiastólica elevada do VE. Em geral, ocorre insuficiência da válvula mitral e/ou obstrução dinâmica da via de saída do VE, secundariamente às alterações estruturais e/ou funcionais do aparato mitral, causadas pelo mau alinhamento dos músculos papilares subsequente à hipertrofia.

IDENTIFICAÇÃO
- A incidência da MCH em cães é muito baixa, de tal forma que ainda faltam relatos precisos a respeito da identificação.
- Cães machos jovens (<3 anos).
- As raças Rottweiler, Dálmata, Pastor alemão e Pointer são super-representadas.
- A MCH também é encontrada com certa regularidade em cães adultos da raça Boston terrier.

SINAIS CLÍNICOS
Achados Anamnésicos
- A maioria dos animais permanece assintomática.
- Sinais de insuficiência cardíaca congestiva esquerda predominam em cães sintomáticos.
- Síncope, geralmente durante atividade física ou exercício.
- Morte súbita constitui o sinal clínico mais comumente relatado.

Achados do Exame Físico
- Sopro cardíaco sistólico.
- Ritmo de galope cardíaco.
- Sinais de insuficiência cardíaca esquerda (p. ex., tosse, dispneia, cianose, intolerância ao exercício).

CAUSAS E FATORES DE RISCO
Não se conhece a causa da miocardiopatia hipertrófica. Foram documentadas anormalidades genéticas em genes responsáveis pela codificação de proteínas contráteis do miocárdio em seres humanos e gatos, mas não em cães. Há suspeita de uma base genética, pois a maioria dos cães acometidos é jovem, mas não há confirmação.

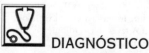

DIAGNÓSTICO

DIAGNÓSTICO DIFERENCIAL
- Hipertensão sistêmica.
- Distúrbios cardíacos infiltrativos.
- Outras causas de insuficiência cardíaca congestiva.
- Tireotoxicose.
- Displasia mitral congênita.

DIAGNÓSTICO POR IMAGEM
Radiografias
- Podem permanecer normais.
- Podem revelar aumento de volume do AE ou VE.
- Presença de edema pulmonar em cães com insuficiência cardíaca congestiva esquerda.

Ecocardiografia
- Cães com MCH grave costumam exibir espessamento acentuado da parede do ventrículo esquerdo, hipertrofia dos músculos papilares, e aumento de volume do átrio esquerdo. A hipertrofia geralmente é global, afetando todas as áreas da parede do ventrículo esquerdo, mas pode ser mais regional ou segmentar (assimétrica). As formas mais leves podem apresentar hipertrofia sutil do VE.
- Em cães com MCH, é comum o movimento anterior sistólico da valva atrioventricular esquerda (mitral), sugerindo obstrução dinâmica à via de saída do VE.

OUTROS TESTES LABORATORIAIS
Eletrocardiografia
- Pode permanecer normal.
- Há relatos de anormalidades do segmento e da onda T.
- Raramente, podem ocorrer arritmias ectópicas atriais ou ventriculares.

Pressão Arterial
- Em geral, permanece normal. Deve ser avaliada para descartar hipertensão sistêmica como a causa de hipertrofia do VE.

ACHADOS PATOLÓGICOS
- Relação anormal de peso cardíaco:peso corporal.
- Hipertrofia concêntrica do ventrículo esquerdo.
- Pode haver uma lesão de impacto sobre o septo interventricular, exibindo uma variedade de aspectos, desde uma pequena lesão opaca até uma placa espessada.
- A valva atrioventricular esquerda (mitral) por si só frequentemente se encontra espessada e alongada.
- Pode haver graus variados de aumento de volume do AE.

TRATAMENTO

O tratamento é feito em esquema ambulatorial, a menos que o animal esteja em insuficiência cardíaca congestiva. A restrição da atividade física e do sódio na dieta é benéfica.

MEDICAÇÕES

MEDICAMENTO(S)
- O tratamento será adotado apenas se houver indícios de insuficiência cardíaca congestiva ou arritmias graves ou nos pacientes com frequentes episódios de síncope.
- Em pacientes com insuficiência cardíaca congestiva esquerda, defende-se o uso de diuréticos e inibidores da ECA.
- Em cães com gradientes elevados de pressão entre VE-aorta por obstrução dinâmica à via de saída do VE, recomenda-se a administração de bloqueador β-adrenérgico ou bloqueador dos canais de cálcio; no entanto, ainda não há provas dos benefícios.
- Os bloqueadores β-adrenérgicos ou os bloqueadores dos canais de cálcio também podem melhorar a oxigenação do miocárdio, diminuir a frequência cardíaca, restabelecer a função diastólica do VE e controlar as arritmias; por essa razão, também podem ser benéficos em cães com insuficiência cardíaca congestiva esquerda.

CONTRAINDICAÇÕES/INTERAÇÕES POSSÍVEIS
- É recomendável evitar o uso dos medicamentos inotrópicos positivos, pois eles podem agravar a obstrução dinâmica à via de saída do VE.
- Também se deve evitar o uso de bloqueadores dos canais de cálcio associado a β-bloqueadores, pela possibilidade de desenvolvimento de bradiarritmias clinicamente significativas.
- Em pacientes com obstrução dinâmica à via de saída do VE, é aconselhável evitar o emprego de dilatadores arteriolares potentes. Contudo, o uso de vasodilatadores mais brandos, como os inibidores da ECA, em pacientes com insuficiência cardíaca congestiva geralmente é bem tolerado.

ACOMPANHAMENTO

- A reavaliação depende da gravidade dos sinais clínicos e, quando feita por meio de radiografias e ecocardiografia, pode ser útil para caracterizar a evolução da doença e ajustar a dose dos medicamentos.
- Em virtude da raridade desse distúrbio em cães, há poucas informações a respeito do prognóstico. Em cães com insuficiência cardíaca congestiva grave ou outras complicações, o prognóstico em geral é reservado.

DIVERSOS

ABREVIATURA(S)
- AE = átrio esquerdo.
- ECA = enzima conversora da angiotensina.
- MCH = miocardiopatia hipertrófica.
- VE = ventrículo esquerdo.

Sugestões de Leitura
Kittleson MD. Hypertrophic cardiomyopathy. In: Kittleson MD, Kienle RD, eds., Small Animal Cardiovascular Medicine. St. Louis: Mosby, 1998, pp. 347-362.
Oyama MA. Canine cardiomyopathy. In: Tilley LP, Smith FWK, Oyama MA, Sleeper MM, eds., Manual of Canine and Feline Cardiology, 4th ed. St. Louis: Saunders Elsevier, 2008, pp. 139-150.

Autor Richard D. Kienle
Consultores Editoriais Larry P. Tilley e Francis W. K. Smith Jr.

MIOCARDIOPATIA HIPERTRÓFICA — GATOS

CONSIDERAÇÕES GERAIS

DEFINIÇÃO
Hipertrofia concêntrica inadequada da parede livre ventricular e/ou do septo intraventricular do ventrículo esquerdo não dilatado. Essa miocardiopatia ocorre independentemente de outros distúrbios cardíacos ou sistêmicos.

FISIOPATOLOGIA
• A disfunção diastólica origina-se de um ventrículo esquerdo espessado e não complacente.
• Ocorre o desenvolvimento de alta pressão de enchimento do ventrículo esquerdo, levando a um aumento de volume do átrio esquerdo. • A hipertensão venosa pulmonar provoca a formação de edema pulmonar. Alguns gatos desenvolvem insuficiência biventricular (i. e., edema pulmonar, efusão pleural, efusão pericárdica de pequeno volume sem tamponamento e, raramente, ascite).
• A estase sanguínea no átrio esquerdo aumentado predispõe o paciente a tromboembolia aórtica.
• Pode ocorrer obstrução dinâmica à via de saída aórtica, além de movimento anterior sistólico (MAS) do folheto anterior da valva atrioventricular esquerda (mitral) associado à insuficiência mitral secundária.

SISTEMA(S) ACOMETIDO(S)
• Cardiovascular — insuficiência cardíaca congestiva (ICC), tromboembolia aórtica e arritmias. • Pulmonar — dispneia em caso do desenvolvimento de ICC. • Renal/Urológico — azotemia por má perfusão.

GENÉTICA
Algumas famílias de gatos foram identificadas com alta prevalência da doença, mas a doença parece ser hereditária como um traço autossômico dominante em gatos da raça Maine Coon e Ragdoll, em que foram identificadas mutações no gene responsável pela codificação da proteína C ligadora de miosina (MyBPC). A genética não foi determinada de forma definitiva em outras raças; no entanto, as mutações das raças Maine Coon e Ragdoll não foram identificadas em gatos acometidos das raças Sphynx (Esfinge), Bosques da Noruega, Bengal, Siberiano ou Britânico de pelo curto.

INCIDÊNCIA/PREVALÊNCIA
Desconhecidas, mas relativamente comuns. Estudos recentes estimam que a prevalência possa chegar até 15% da população.

IDENTIFICAÇÃO
Espécies
Gatos.

Raça(s) Predominante(s)
Há registros de uma associação familiar em gatos das raças Maine Coon, Ragdoll, Sphynx (Esfinge), Britânico e Americano de pelo curto, e Persa.

Idade Média e Faixa Etária
Varia de 5-7 anos, com relato de casos de 3 meses a 17 anos. Algumas raças de gatos, incluindo Ragdoll e Sphynx (Esfinge), podem desenvolver a doença em uma idade mais jovem (média de 2 anos de idade). A MCH é mais frequentemente uma doença de gatos jovens aos de meia-idade; sopros inexplicáveis em gatos geriátricos são mais provavelmente associados a hipertireoidismo ou hipertensão.

Sexo Predominante
Machos.

SINAIS CLÍNICOS
Achados Anamnésicos
• Dispneia. • Anorexia. • Intolerância ao exercício. • Vômitos. • Colapso. • Morte súbita. • A tosse é rara em gatos com miocardiopatia e geralmente sugestiva de pneumopatia.

Achados do Exame Físico
• Ritmo de galope (S3 ou S4). • Sopro sistólico em muitos animais. • O batimento cardíaco apical (também conhecido como choque da ponta) pode estar exagerado. • Alterações como abafamento dos sons cardíacos, falta de complacência torácica e dispneia caracterizada por respirações rápidas e superficiais podem estar associadas à efusão pleural. • Na presença de edema pulmonar, há dispneia e crepitações. • Pulso femoral débil. • Em animais com tromboembolia aórtica, observam-se paralisia aguda dos membros pélvicos com coxins palmoplantares e leitos ungueais cianóticos, extremidades frias e ausência de pulso femoral. Os êmbolos raramente acometem os membros torácicos. • Em alguns animais, verificam-se arritmias. • Os animais assintomáticos podem não exibir quaisquer sinais clínicos.

CAUSAS
• Geralmente desconhecidas — provavelmente existem múltiplas causas. • Mutações da MyBPC em alguns gatos com MCH.

Causas Possíveis
• Anormalidades da proteína contrátil (miosina) ou de outras proteínas do sarcômero (p. ex., troponina, proteínas ligantes de miosina, e tropomiosina).
• Anormalidade no acoplamento entre excitação-contração influenciado pelas catecolaminas.
• Metabolismo anormal do cálcio miocárdico.
• Anormalidade do colágeno ou de outra matriz intercelular. • Excesso do hormônio de crescimento.
• Obstrução dinâmica à via de saída do ventrículo esquerdo, o que pode contribuir para hipertrofia secundária dessa câmara cardíaca.

FATORES DE RISCO
Prole de animais com mutações familiares da MyBPC.

DIAGNÓSTICO

DIAGNÓSTICO DIFERENCIAL
• Outras formas de miocardiopatia (p. ex., miocardiopatia dilatada e restritiva).
• Hipertireoidismo. • Estenose aórtica.
• Hipertensão sistêmica. • Acromegalia. • Causas não cardíacas de efusão pleural (p. ex., piotórax, quilotórax, neoplasia).

HEMOGRAMA/BIOQUÍMICA/URINÁLISE
• Os resultados costumam permanecer normais.
• Em alguns animais, observa-se azotemia pré-renal.

OUTROS TESTES LABORATORIAIS
• Análise da MyBPC. A mutação difere para gatos das raças Maine Coon e Ragdoll. • Em gatos acima de 6 anos de idade, avaliar a concentração dos hormônios tireoidianos para descartar o hipertireoidismo. Essa endocrinopatia causa hipertrofia do miocárdio, que pode ser confundida com a MCH. • As concentrações séricas do peptídeo natriurético cerebral são mais altas em gatos com MCH do que naqueles normais, e ainda mais altas em gatos com MCH sintomática. O valor preditivo positivo desse teste para diferenciar gatos normais daqueles com MCH assintomática é desconhecido na população geral e, portanto, esse teste não deve ser usado para fazer a triagem de todos os gatos assintomáticos.

DIAGNÓSTICO POR IMAGEM
Radiografia
• As radiografias ventrodorsais frequentemente revelam um coração com aspecto de "coração de namorados", em função do aumento de volume biatrial e do ventrículo esquerdo pontiagudo. • Em determinados animais, observam-se edema pulmonar, efusão pleural ou ambos. • As radiografias podem permanecer normais em gatos assintomáticos. • As radiografias podem não ser capazes de diferenciar as várias formas de miocardiopatia.

Ecocardiografia
• Hipertrofia do septo interventricular (SIV) ou da parede posterior ventricular esquerda (espessura diastólica da parede >6 mm). • A hipertrofia pode ser simétrica (com comprometimento do SIV e da parede posterior) ou assimétrica (com envolvimento do SIV ou da parede posterior, mas não de ambos).
• Hipertrofia dos músculos papilares.
• Encurtamento fracional normal ou elevado.
• Lúmen ventricular esquerdo normal ou reduzido.
• Aumento de volume do átrio esquerdo.
• Movimento anterior sistólico da valva atrioventricular esquerda (mitral) em alguns animais. • Obstrução à via de saída do ventrículo esquerdo (alguns animais). • Trombo no átrio esquerdo (raro). • *Nota*: Há certa sobreposição entre gatos normais (especialmente aqueles submetidos à cetamina e os desidratados) e gatos com MCH branda. Correlacionar os achados ecocardiográficos com os achados físicos. A presença de aumento de volume do átrio esquerdo favorece a MCH.

MÉTODOS DIAGNÓSTICOS
Eletrocardiografia
• Em casos de insuficiência cardíaca, é comum a constatação de taquicardia sinusal (frequência cardíaca >240 bpm); no entanto, alguns gatos com insuficiência cardíaca grave e hipotermia apresentam-se bradicárdicos. • Ocasionalmente, observam-se complexos atriais e ventriculares prematuros. • A fibrilação atrial é observada em alguns casos avançados. • Com frequência, verifica-se desvio do eixo à esquerda. • O ECG não é capaz de diferenciar as várias formas de miocardiopatia. • Os gatos com MCH podem exibir um ECG normal.

Pressão Arterial Sistêmica
• O paciente encontra-se normotenso ou hipotenso.
• Avaliar a pressão arterial em todos os pacientes com hipertrofia miocárdica para descartar hipertensão sistêmica como a causa da hipertrofia.

ACHADOS PATOLÓGICOS
• Ventrículo esquerdo não dilatado, associado à hipertrofia do septo interventricular ou da parede livre ventricular esquerda. • Hipertrofia dos músculos papilares. • Aumento de volume do átrio esquerdo. • Espessamento da valva atrioventricular esquerda (mitral). • Hipertrofia miocárdica com mau alinhamento dos miócitos (desarranjo das miofibras). • Fibrose intersticial. • Formação cicatricial ou banda fibrosa miocárdica.
• Hipertrofia e estreitamento luminal das artérias coronárias intramurais.

Miocardiopatia Hipertrófica — Gatos

TRATAMENTO

CUIDADO(S) DE SAÚDE ADEQUADO(S)
Os gatos com ICC devem ser internados para o tratamento clínico inicial.

CUIDADO(S) DE ENFERMAGEM
• Minimizar o estresse. • Fornecer oxigênio em caso de dispneia. • Aquecer o ambiente se o animal estiver hipotérmico.

ATIVIDADE
Restrita.

DIETA
Restrição de sódio em animais com ICC.

ORIENTAÇÃO AO PROPRIETÁRIO
• Muitos gatos diagnosticados enquanto se encontram assintomáticos acabam desenvolvendo ICC, mas também podem desenvolver tromboembolia aórtica e sofrer morte súbita.
• Se o gato estiver sendo submetido à varfarina, minimizar o potencial de traumatismos e a subsequente hemorragia.

MEDICAÇÕES

MEDICAMENTO(S) DE ESCOLHA

Furosemida
• Dosagem — 1-2 mg/kg VO, IM, IV a cada 8-24 h.
• Os animais criticamente dispneicos muitas vezes necessitam de uma dosagem elevada (4 mg/kg IV). Se o gato ainda continuar gravemente dispneico, será possível a repetição dessa dose em 1 h. Indicada para o tratamento de edema pulmonar, efusão pleural e ascite. • Os gatos são sensíveis à furosemida e propensos à desidratação, azotemia pré-renal e hipocalemia. • Assim que o edema pulmonar desaparecer, reduzir gradativamente a dosagem para o limite mais baixo capaz de controlar o reaparecimento do edema.

Inibidores da ECA
• Dosagem — enalapril ou benazepril a 0,25-0,5 mg/kg a cada 24 h. • Ainda não estão bem definidas as indicações em gatos com MCH — atualmente, os autores utilizam esses agentes em casos de ICC.

Betabloqueadores
• Dosagem — atenolol (6,25-12,5 mg/gato VO a cada 12 h). • Os efeitos benéficos podem compreender a lentificação da frequência sinusal, a correção de arritmias atriais e ventriculares, bem como a inibição plaquetária. • Mais eficazes do que o diltiazem no controle da obstrução dinâmica à via de saída. • Seu papel em pacientes assintomáticos ainda não está esclarecido, mas os autores costumam empregar os betabloqueadores na presença de hipertrofia e obstrução dinâmica à via de saída. • Contraindicados na presença de ICC.

Diltiazem
• Dosagem — 7,5-15 mg/gato VO a cada 8 h ou 10 mg/kg VO a cada 24 h (Cardizem CD®) ou 30 mg/gato a cada 12 h (Dilacor XR®). • Os efeitos benéficos podem incluir a lentificação da frequência sinusal, a resolução das arritmias supraventriculares, a melhora do relaxamento diastólico, a vasodilatação coronariana e periférica, bem como a inibição plaquetária. • Pode diminuir a hipertrofia e as dimensões do átrio esquerdo em alguns gatos. • Seu papel em pacientes assintomáticos ainda não está determinado.

Ácido Acetilsalicílico
• Dosagem — 81 mg/gato a cada 2-3 dias em casos de aumento de volume atrial intenso.
• Deprime a agregação plaquetária, minimizando de forma esperançosa o risco de tromboembolia.
• Alertar os proprietários sobre o possível desenvolvimento de trombos apesar da administração do ácido acetilsalicílico.

Unguento de Nitroglicerina
• Dosagem — 0,6-1,3 cm/gato aplicados por via tópica a cada 6-8 h ou sob a forma de emplastro a 2,5 mg/24 h. • Frequentemente utilizado na estabilização aguda de gatos com edema pulmonar ou efusão pleural graves. • Quando administrado de modo intermitente, pode ser útil para o tratamento a longo prazo de casos refratários.

CONTRAINDICAÇÕES
Evitar os betabloqueadores em gatos com êmbolos; esses agentes causam vasoconstrição periférica. Caso o emprego dos betabloqueadores nesse quadro seja imprescindível para o controle da arritmia, selecionar um bloqueador beta-1 seletivo, como o atenolol.

PRECAUÇÕES
Utilizar os inibidores da ECA com cautela em animais azotêmicos.

MEDICAMENTO(S) ALTERNATIVO(S)

Espironolactona
• Dosagem — 1 mg/kg a cada 12-24 h.
• Utilizada em conjunto com a furosemida em gatos com ICC. • Pode causar prurido facial.

Varfarina e Heparina de Baixo Peso Molecular
• Empregadas ocasionalmente em gatos sob alto risco de tromboembolia. • Ver o capítulo sobre "Tromboembolia".

Clopidogrel (Plavix®)
Dosagem — 18,75 mg/gato/dia. Inibidor da função plaquetária, superior ao ácido acetilsalicílico em seres humanos; estudo sob andamento para avaliar a eficácia na prevenção de tromboembolia aórtica em gatos.

Betabloqueador Associado ao Diltiazem
• Os gatos que permanecem taquicárdicos sob um agente terapêutico isolado podem ser tratados de forma cautelosa com o emprego de um betabloqueador associado ao diltiazem.
• Monitorizar o paciente quanto à ocorrência de bradicardia e hipotensão.

ACOMPANHAMENTO

MONITORIZAÇÃO DO PACIENTE
• Observar atentamente o animal em busca de sinais de dispneia, letargia, fraqueza, anorexia e paralisia ou paresia dolorosa dos membros pélvicos. • Em caso de tratamento com a varfarina, monitorizar o tempo de protrombina. • Ao tratar o paciente com um inibidor da ECA ou a espironolactona, monitorizar a função renal e os eletrólitos. • Repetir o ecocardiograma em 6 meses para avaliar a eficácia do tratamento da hipertrofia. Se um betabloqueador ou o diltiazem já foi prescrito em um animal assintomático e houver indícios de hipertrofia progressiva/aumento de volume do átrio esquerdo, considerar a troca do agente para outra classe farmacológica (ou a adição de inibidor da ECA) e reavaliar o paciente 4-6 meses depois. • As avaliações ecocardiográficas que revelam diâmetros do AE >2 cm ou perda da função sistólica do VE devem incitar uma profilaxia mais rigorosa contra tromboembolia aórtica.

PREVENÇÃO
Evitar as situações indutoras de estresse que possam precipitar a ICC.

COMPLICAÇÕES POSSÍVEIS
• Insuficiência cardíaca. • Tromboembolia aórtica e paralisia. • Arritmias cardíacas/morte súbita.

EVOLUÇÃO ESPERADA E PROGNÓSTICO
• É mais provável que os animais homozigotos para mutações da MyBPC desenvolvam MCH grave e em uma idade mais precoce que os heterozigotos.
• O prognóstico varia de forma considerável, provavelmente pela existência de múltiplas causas. Em um único estudo de gatos com MCH que vivem no mínimo 24 h após a apresentação, verificaram-se:
  ○ Gatos assintomáticos: sobrevida média de 563 dias (variação: 2-3.778 dias).
  ○ Gatos com síncope: sobrevida média de 654 dias (variação: 28-1.505 dias).
  ○ Gatos com ICC: sobrevida média de 563 dias (variação: 2-4.418 dias).
  ○ Gatos com tromboembolia aórtica: sobrevida média de 184 dias (variação: 2-2.278 dias).
  ○ Uma idade mais avançada do paciente e um aumento de volume maior do átrio esquerdo predizem uma sobrevida mais curta.

DIVERSOS

DISTÚRBIOS ASSOCIADOS
Tromboembolia aórtica.

GESTAÇÃO/FERTILIDADE/REPRODUÇÃO
• Alto risco de complicações. • Evitar o uso do ácido acetilsalicílico.

VER TAMBÉM
• Acromegalia — Gatos. • Hipertensão Sistêmica.
• Hipertireoidismo. • Insuficiência Cardíaca Congestiva — Esquerda. • Sopros Cardíacos.
• Tromboembolia Aórtica.

ABREVIATURA(S)
• ECA = enzima conversora de angiotensina.
• MCH = miocardiopatia hipertrófica.
• MyBPC = proteína C ligadora de miosina.
• SIV = septo interventricular.

RECURSOS DA INTERNET
http://www.vetmed.wsu.edu/deptsVCGL/felineTests.aspx.

Sugestões de Leitura
Kienle RD. Feline cardiomyopathy. In: Tilley LP, Smith FWK, Oyama MA, Sleeper MM, eds., Manual of Canine and Feline Cardiology, 4th ed. St. Louis: Saunders Elsevier, 2008, pp. 49-77.

Autores Francis W. K. Smith Jr., Bruce W. Keene e Kathryn M. Meurs
Consultores Editoriais Larry P. Tilley e Francis W. K. Smith Jr.

Miocardiopatia Restritiva — Gatos

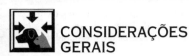

CONSIDERAÇÕES GERAIS

DEFINIÇÃO
Miocardiopatia não infiltrativa, caracterizada por disfunção diastólica (preenchimento, relaxamento), aumento de volume atrial grave, espessura normal da parede do ventrículo esquerdo e disfunção sistólica variável.

FISIOPATOLOGIA
• Pode predominar uma fibrose do endomiocárdio (forma da MCR com fibrose endomiocárdica) ou pode haver uma fibrose do miocárdio (MCR miocárdica). Além disso, as alterações miocárdicas semelhantes à MCR e as síndromes clínicas podem ser resultantes de dano ao miocárdio por outras causas (p. ex., infarto) ou um estágio terminal de outros distúrbios miocárdicos (p. ex., MCH). • A MCR miocárdica pode ser a "via final comum" ou o "resultado final" de mais de uma miocardiopatia, incluindo doenças inflamatórias ou imunomediadas. • A disfunção diastólica associada a MCR e miocardiopatias semelhantes à MCR (denominadas algumas vezes de "miocardiopatia intermediária") é frequentemente associada a insuficiência cardíaca biventricular (ICC), tromboembolia arterial e arritmias.

SISTEMA(S) ACOMETIDO(S)
• Cardiovascular. • Respiratório.

INCIDÊNCIA/PREVALÊNCIA
Pode representar 8-12% das miocardiopatias em gatos, mas a incidência é controversa em virtude dos critérios diagnósticos variáveis.

IDENTIFICAÇÃO
• Gatos. • Não há predileções raciais ou sexuais. • Gatos de meia-idade a idosos.

SINAIS CLÍNICOS
Achados Anamnésicos
• Na ausência de ICC:
  ○ Letargia. ○ Hiporexia e perda de peso.
  ○ Síncope (rara; geralmente indica arritmia grave). ○ Paresia ou paralisia (i. e., sinais de tromboembolia arterial). ○ Alguns gatos permanecem assintomáticos.
• Na presença de ICC, os sinais supramencionados se somam aos expostos a seguir:
  ○ Dispneia. ○ Taquipneia. ○ Respiração de boca aberta. ○ Cianose. ○ Distensão abdominal.

Achados do Exame Físico
• Na ausência de ICC:
  ○ Depressão. ○ Caquexia. ○ Taquicardia.
  ○ Arritmias. ○ Ritmo de galope. ○ Pode exibir sopro cardíaco sistólico.
• Na presença de ICC, os sinais supramencionados se somam aos expostos a seguir:
  ○ Taquipneia. ○ Dispneia. ○ Respiração ofegante.
  ○ Cianose. ○ Hepatomegalia ou ascite, associados à distensão venosa jugular. ○ Crepitações pulmonares. ○ Em casos de efusão pleural, observa-se o abafamento de sons cardíacos ou ruídos respiratórios. ○ Paralisia ou paresia com perda dos pulsos femorais; uma ou mais extremidades frias e dolorosas (tromboembolia arterial).

CAUSAS
• Não se conhece(m) a(s) verdadeira(s) causa(s); muitas vezes, não se consegue registrar nenhuma doença "predisponente". • As causas desencadeantes sob suspeita incluem endocardite ou miocardite, doença de pequenos vasos e outras causas de isquemia miocárdica.

DIAGNÓSTICO

DIAGNÓSTICO DIFERENCIAL
• Outras causas de sinais de ICC (p. ex., edema pulmonar, ascite e intolerância a exercícios):
  ○ Miocardiopatia hipertrófica. ○ Miocardiopatia dilatada. ○ Anormalidades cardíacas congênitas descompensadas. ○ ICC secundária à tireotoxicose ou cardiopatia hipertensiva.
• Outras causas de síncope, colapso, fraqueza e letargia:
  ○ Arritmias associadas a qualquer outra forma de cardiopatia. ○ Arritmias relacionadas com doença metabólica ou neurológica.
  ○ Anormalidade neurológica ou musculosquelética. ○ Doença metabólica ou distúrbio eletrolítico.
• Outras causas de paralisia ou paresia (tromboembolia arterial):
  ○ Qualquer forma de cardiopatia.
  ○ Anormalidade neurológica ou musculoesquelética.

HEMOGRAMA/BIOQUÍMICA/URINÁLISE
• A maioria dos testes laboratoriais não contribui para o diagnóstico de miocardiopatia restritiva.
• O perfil bioquímico (com mensuração dos eletrólitos) e a urinálise de rotina são úteis para registrar os distúrbios concomitantes ou complicantes (p. ex., azotemia pré-renal e anormalidades do potássio).

OUTROS TESTES LABORATORIAIS
Os níveis plasmáticos de taurina podem estar baixos em alguns gatos.

DIAGNÓSTICO POR IMAGEM
Achados Radiográficos Torácicos
• Cardiomegalia, com aumento desproporcional de volume atrial. • Infiltrados intersticiais ou alveolares ou efusões pleurais com distensão venosa pulmonar em casos de ICC.

Achados Ecocardiográficos
Nota: Os achados "típicos" são controversos; o diagnóstico de miocardiopatia restritiva costuma ter como base os achados ecocardiográficos a seguir (ver "Sugestões de Leitura"):
• Achados presentes em grande parte dos casos de MCR ou doenças semelhantes à MCR:
  ○ Aumento de volume biatrial grave. ○ Aumento de volume atrial, desproporcional ao grau de aumento de volume do ventrículo esquerdo.
  ○ Pode haver efusão pleural. ○ Efusão pericárdica leve a moderada pode estar presente. ○ Trombos intracardíacos ecodensos nos átrios ou aderidos às paredes atriais ou ventriculares em alguns gatos.
• Achados típicos da forma de MCR com fibrose endomiocárdica:
  ○ Parede do ventrículo esquerdo, normal ou levemente espessada. ○ Presença de ampla banda fibrosa ecogênica, unindo como ponte a parede do VE e o septo ventricular. ○ Diminuição no lúmen do ventrículo esquerdo ou estreitamento na porção média do ventrículo causada por fibrose ou bandas fibrosas. ○ Dilatação do ventrículo esquerdo, imediatamente distal à valva atrioventricular esquerda (mitral).
  ○ Evidência de obstrução sistólica mesoventricular ao nível da banda fibrosa com o uso do Doppler.
• Achados típicos de MCR miocárdica:
  ○ Anormalidades no movimento ou hipertrofia das paredes regionais, focos subendocárdicos hiperecoicos, bandas moderadoras. ○ Áreas regionais de miocárdio ecogênico, indicativas de isquemia ou banda fibrosa. ○ Evidência de disfunção diastólica com o uso do Doppler.
  ○ Espessura da parede do VE e do septo, normal a levemente aumentada. ○ Fração de encurtamento, normal a levemente reduzida.
  ○ Insuficiência valvar atrioventricular ausente ou branda, detectada por meio da ecocardiografia com Doppler.
• Achados típicos de miocardiopatias semelhantes à MCR:
  ○ Dilatação variável com paredes normais, levemente espessadas ou levemente adelgaçadas.
  ○ Insuficiência das valvas atrioventriculares esquerda (mitral) e/ou direita (tricúspide), leve a moderada. ○ Evidência de disfunção diastólica com o uso do Doppler. ○ Fração de encurtamento, baixa normal a reduzida.

MÉTODOS DIAGNÓSTICOS
Achados Eletrocardiográficos
• É comum a constatação de taquicardia sinusal, mas os gatos com ICC e desidratação graves podem ser bradicárdicos ou hipotérmicos à apresentação. • Defeitos de condução intraventricular, incluindo bloqueios de ramo do feixe de His. • Ectopias isoladas, taquicardias supraventriculares ou ventriculares paroxísticas ou sustentadas e fibrilação atrial. • Padrões de aumento de volume atrial ou ventricular.

ACHADOS PATOLÓGICOS
• MCR miocárdica: aumento do peso global do coração, aumento de volume biatrial grave, espessura da parede e tamanho do VE relativamente normais, fibrose miocárdica desigual, evidência de trombos intracavitários no átrio ou ventrículo esquerdos. • MCR endomiocárdica: fibrose e banda fibrosa endomiocárdicas graves no VE, formando frequentemente uma "ponte" entre o septo interventricular e a parede ventricular esquerda, aumento de volume biatrial grave, trombos intracavitários. Em alguns casos, pode haver evidência histopatológica de inflamação endomiocárdica.

TRATAMENTO

CUIDADO(S) DE SAÚDE ADEQUADO(S)
• Os pacientes com ICC aguda e grave devem ser internados para receber os cuidados de emergência. • Os animais levemente sintomáticos ou assintomáticos podem ser tratados em um esquema ambulatorial.

CUIDADO(S) DE ENFERMAGEM
• Os animais gravemente dispneicos devem receber oxigênio por meio de gaiola, cânula nasal ou máscara (cuidado com o estresse sobre o paciente). • As efusões pleurais potencialmente letais são reduzidas via toracocentese. • Em caso de desidratação, administrar com cautela fluidos com baixo teor de sódio (cuidado com o agravamento da ICC). • Manter o ambiente com baixo nível de

Miocardiopatia Restritiva — Gatos

estresse para diminuir a ansiedade do paciente (p. ex., proporcionar repouso em gaiola e minimizar a manipulação). • Em pacientes hipotérmicos, pode ser necessário o uso de colchonetes térmicos. • A frequência respiratória pode ser utilizada para monitorizar o sucesso da toracocentese ou da terapia diurética (a frequência respiratória deve diminuir com a terapia; os aumentos podem indicar o desenvolvimento de complicações).

ATIVIDADE
• É sugerido o repouso em gaiola para pacientes com ICC grave. • A maioria dos gatos restringirá seus próprios exercícios em caso de ICC.

DIETA
• Em caso de insuficiência cardíaca aguda, alimentar o animal manualmente, conforme a necessidade. É recomendado o fornecimento crônico de dietas hipossódicas.

ORIENTAÇÃO AO PROPRIETÁRIO
• Quando o paciente estiver pronto para receber a alta hospitalar, o proprietário deve ser orientado a respeito dos possíveis efeitos colaterais das medicações e da importância de manter uma ingestão alimentar e hídrica estável. • Os proprietários podem ser aconselhados sobre como monitorizar a frequência respiratória de seu gato em casa, com instruções para entrar em contato em caso de aumento súbito ou progressivo dessa frequência ao longo dos dias.

MEDICAÇÕES

MEDICAMENTO(S) DE ESCOLHA
Insuficiência Cardíaca Congestiva Aguda
• Administração parenteral de furosemida (0,5-2 mg/kg IV, IM, SC a cada 1-6 h). • Dobutamina (1-5 μg/kg/minuto sob a forma de infusão contínua, iniciando com a dose mais baixa e aumentando em 1-2 h) para aumentar a função diastólica e sistólica. • Aplicação tópica de unguento de nitroglicerina (a 2%, em uma área de ~0,3-0,6 cm a cada 12 h). • Oxigenoterapia por meio de gaiola, máscara, cânula nasal.
• Procedimento de toracocentese, conforme a necessidade, para aliviar a dispneia decorrente da efusão pleural. • As arritmias supraventriculares graves podem ser tratadas com o uso de diltiazem (1,5-2,5 mg/kg VO a cada 8 h) ou diltiazem de longa ação (10 mg/kg VO a cada 24 h). • A taquicardia ventricular pode desaparecer com a resolução da ICC. • A terapia imediata da taquicardia ventricular pode envolver o uso da lidocaína (0,25-0,5 mg/kg IV LENTAMENTE); monitorizar o paciente de perto em busca de sinais neurológicos de toxicidade. • Betabloqueadores (propranolol [2,5-7,5 mg VO a cada 8 h] ou atenolol [6,25-12,5 mg VO a cada 12 h]) podem ser utilizados para tratar as arritmias supraventriculares ou ventriculares, mas não até que se trate a ICC (ver o item "Contraindicações").
• Pimobendana (1,25 mg/gato VO a cada 12 h) pode ser útil para aumentar a função sistólica e diastólica em insuficiência cardíaca aguda. *Nota*: a pimobendana não é aprovada para uso clínico em gatos; além disso, os dados clínicos a respeito da segurança são limitados.

Terapia Crônica
• A furosemida é gradativamente reduzida até a dose eficaz mais baixa. • A terapia crônica com diltiazem diminui a frequência cardíaca e melhora as arritmias supraventriculares nos gatos acometidos. • É possível lançar mão dos betabloqueadores para diminuir a frequência cardíaca e tratar as arritmias supraventriculares ou ventriculares. • Os inibidores da enzima conversora de angiotensina (ECA) podem reduzir a retenção de líquido e a necessidade de diuréticos (enalapril, 0,25-0,5 mg/kg VO a cada 24-48 h; benazepril, 0,25-0,5 mg/kg VO a cada 24 h).
• Pimobendana (0,625-1,25 mg/gato VO a cada 12 h) pode ser útil para aumentar a função sistólica e diastólica e controlar a insuficiência cardíaca crônica. *Nota*: a pimobendana não é aprovada para uso clínico em gatos; além disso, os dados clínicos a respeito da segurança são limitados. • Tratar os distúrbios associados (p. ex., desidratação, hipotermia). • Ácido acetilsalicílico (80 mg VO a cada 72 h) pode ser administrado para evitar a tromboembolia, mas sua eficácia é questionável. • Clopidogrel (1/4 de um comprimido de 75 mg VO a cada 24 h) pode ser usado para diminuir a agregação plaquetária cronicamente, mas sua eficácia não é comprovada.

CONTRAINDICAÇÕES
• Betabloqueadores — bloqueio atrioventricular, ICC não tratada, bradicardia, insuficiência miocárdica e asma (especialmente os betabloqueadores não seletivos, p. ex., propranolol). • Diltiazem — bradicardia, bloqueio atrioventricular, insuficiência miocárdica e hipotensão. • Furosemida — desidratação, hipocalemia e azotemia. • Inibidores da ECA — azotemia, hipotensão e hipercalemia.

INTERAÇÕES POSSÍVEIS
• Não é recomendado o uso concomitante de betabloqueadores e diltiazem; essa associação pode levar à bradicardia, à hipotensão e ao bloqueio atrioventricular grave. • O uso de inibidores da ECA em animais desidratados ou hiponatrêmicos pode resultar em hipotensão, azotemia e hipercalemia. • A terapia crônica com ácido acetilsalicílico pode aumentar o risco de efeitos colaterais renais dos inibidores da ECA.

ACOMPANHAMENTO

MONITORIZAÇÃO DO PACIENTE
• Exames físicos seriados frequentes (intensidade mínima de estresse sobre o paciente) para avaliar não só a resposta ao tratamento, mas também a resolução do edema e das efusões pulmonares.
• Nos primeiros dias da terapia, é importante a avaliação contínua da hidratação e da função renal para evitar a ocorrência de diurese excessiva e azotemia.
• Para manter as efusões em níveis compatíveis ao conforto do animal, talvez haja necessidade de toracocenteses repetidas.
• Uma avaliação "mais pragmática" e "sem interferência" de hora em hora da frequência respiratória nas primeiras 12-24 h pode ser usada para monitorizar a eficácia da terapia de ICC.
• As radiografias podem ser repetidas em 12-24 h para monitorizar a resolução do infiltrado pulmonar.
• Durante os primeiros 3-5 dias de terapia, é aconselhável a monitorização rigorosa do nível de eletrólitos e dos valores renais (especialmente de creatinina e potássio) para detectar desidratação, insuficiência renal e hipocalemia (causada pela administração de diuréticos e anorexia) ou hipercalemia (em caso de uso dos inibidores da ECA).
• Repetir o exame físico do animal e a análise da bioquímica sanguínea depois de aproximadamente 10-14 dias de tratamento.
• A critério do clínico, repetir o ECG e as radiografias.
• Os pacientes estáveis são reavaliados a cada 2-4 meses ou em uma frequência maior diante do surgimento de complicações.

PREVENÇÃO
• Não há medidas preventivas conhecidas para MCR.
• Terapia antiplaquetária (p. ex., bissulfato de clopidogrel, ácido acetilsalicílico) ou anticoagulante (p. ex., varfarina) é recomendada para evitar as complicações tromboembólicas de MCR, mas a eficácia de tais medidas não está comprovada.

COMPLICAÇÕES POSSÍVEIS
Necrose tecidual ou perda de função nos membros acometidos por complicações tromboembólicas de MCR.

EVOLUÇÃO ESPERADA E PROGNÓSTICO
• Altamente variáveis, com base na apresentação heterogênea da doença e dos sinais clínicos.
• A maioria dos gatos com MCR e ICC vive por 3-12 meses e, alguns, até 2 anos.

DIVERSOS

DISTÚRBIOS ASSOCIADOS
Tromboembolia aórtica.

FATORES RELACIONADOS COM A IDADE
A MCR ocorre em gatos de meia-idade a idosos — um grupo etário que também está sob risco de doença cardiovascular secundária a hipertireoidismo. O hipertireoidismo deve ser descartado por meio de exames adequados em pacientes cardiovasculares felinos com ≥12 anos de idade.

SINÔNIMO(S)
• Miocardiopatia intermediária.
• Miocardiopatia de grau intermediário.

VER TAMBÉM
• Insuficiência Cardíaca Congestiva — Direita.
• Insuficiência Cardíaca Congestiva — Esquerda.
• Tromboembolia Aórtica.

ABREVIATURA(S)
• ECA = enzima conversora de angiotensina.
• ECG = eletrocardiografia.
• ICC = insuficiência cardíaca congestiva.
• MCH = miocardiopatia hipertrófica.
• MCR = miocardiopatia restritiva.

Sugestões de Leitura
Kienle RD. Feline cardiomyopathy. In: Tilley LP, Smith FWK, Oyama MA, Sleeper MM, eds., Manual of Canine and Feline Cardiology, 4th ed. St. Louis: Saunders Elsevier, 2008, pp. 151-175.

Autor Rebecca L. Stepien
Consultores Editoriais Larry P. Tilley e Francis W. K. Smith Jr.

ESPÉCIES CANINA E FELINA

MIOCARDITE

CONSIDERAÇÕES GERAIS

DEFINIÇÃO
• Inflamação do músculo cardíaco, quase sempre provocada por agentes infecciosos, que afetam os miócitos, o interstício, os elementos vasculares ou o pericárdio.
• Doenças virais, bacterianas, riquetsiais, fúngicas e protozoárias estão todas associadas à inflamação do miocárdio (i. e., miocardite).
• Agentes farmacológicos (p. ex., doxorrubicina) também podem ser uma causa.

FISIOPATOLOGIA
• Mecanismos — produção de toxina, invasão direta do tecido miocárdico e lesão miocárdica imunomediada; vasculite associada à doença sistêmica; reações alérgicas e lesão direta ao miócito provocada por agentes farmacológicos. Protozoários (p. ex., *Trypanosoma cruzi*) levam à miocardite granulomatosa; miocardite viral está associada a reações imunológicas mediadas por células.
• O envolvimento miocárdico pode ser focal ou difuso. As manifestações clínicas dependem da extensão das lesões. Envolvimento grave difuso pode levar à lesão miocárdica global e ICC; lesões discretas envolvendo o sistema de condução cardíaca podem provocar arritmias profundas.

SISTEMA(S) ACOMETIDO(S)
• O envolvimento orgânico sistêmico depende do agente causal.
• Cardiovascular — insuficiência miocárdica ou arritmias.
• Respiratório — caso se desenvolva edema pulmonar.

INCIDÊNCIA/PREVALÊNCIA
• Miocardite viral (p. ex., parvovírus, vírus da cinomose e herpes-vírus) — rara; filhotes caninos muito jovens em seus primeiros meses de vida podem ser profundamente acometidos; em uma segunda forma (por parvovírus), desenvolve-se uma miocardiopatia dilatada em cães com 5-6 meses de vida, que foram infectados durante suas primeiras semanas de vida.
• Miocardite protozoária associada ao *T. cruzi* (i. e., doença de Chagas) relatada em cães com <2 anos de idade no sudeste dos Estados Unidos. Os machos costumam ser mais acometidos do que as fêmeas. Ocasionalmente, o *Toxoplasma gondii* provoca miocardite. Animais imunossuprimidos (p. ex., gatos com vírus da leucemia felina) estão sob maior risco. *Hepatozoon canis* é relatado em cães que vivem na região do Golfo do Texas.
• Miocardite fúngica — observada principalmente em associação com infecção fúngica sistêmica; o envolvimento miocárdico varia com a prevalência regional e a prevalência da manifestação sistêmica.
• Miocardite bacteriana — pode ser provocada por sepse e bacteremia generalizadas.
• Cardiotoxicidade pela doxorrubicina — relatada em cães submetidos a doses cumulativas = 150-240 mg/m^2.
• Miocardite por espiroqueta associada à *Borrelia burgdorferi* — comprovada em 10% dos seres humanos com doença de Lyme; a incidência e a prevalência nos cães não estão bem comprovadas.

DISTRIBUIÇÃO GEOGRÁFICA
Suspeitar de miocardite associada a agentes infecciosos nos locais onde essas doenças forem endêmicas (ver adiante).

IDENTIFICAÇÃO
Espécies
Cães e gatos.
Idade Média e Faixa Etária
Miocardite viral — observada principalmente em animais com <1 ano de vida.

SINAIS CLÍNICOS
Comentários Gerais
• Relacionados com o grau e a localização do envolvimento miocárdico.
• Variam desde arritmias até ICC.
• O início de disfunção cardíaca em associação com doença sistêmica ou com a utilização de agentes farmacológicos específicos quase sempre é a principal indicação de miocardite.
Achados Anamnésicos
• Tosse, intolerância ao exercício, dispneia — associados à ICC.
• Síncope e fraqueza — associados a arritmias.
• Manifestações sistêmicas concomitantes — frequentemente observadas na miocardite infecciosa.
• Uso de agentes antineoplásicos ou outros agentes farmacológicos — associado ao início de disfunção cardíaca.
Achados do Exame Físico
• Pode-se encontrar ritmo de galope ou sopro — depende da natureza da lesão miocárdica.
• Arritmias — podem ser auscultadas.
• Febre — comum nos pacientes com infecção ativa associada à miocardite.

CAUSAS
• Vírus (p. ex., parvovírus, vírus da cinomose, herpes-vírus, vírus do Oeste do Nilo).
• Protozoários (p. ex., *Trypanosoma cruzi*, *Toxoplasma. gondii*, *Neospora caninum*, *Hepatozoon canis*, *Babesia* spp., e *Leishmania* spp.).
• Bactérias (p. ex., *Bartonella vinsonii* subespécie *Berkhoffii*).
• Fungos (p. ex., *Cryptococcus neoformans*, *Coccidioides immitis*, *Blastomyces dermatitidis*, e *Aspergillus terreus*).
• Algas (p. ex., *Prototheca* spp.)
• Doxorrubicina.

FATORES DE RISCO
• Exposição a agentes infecciosos.
• Utilização de compostos miocardiotóxicos.
• Imunossupressão.
• Doenças debilitantes.

DIAGNÓSTICO

DIAGNÓSTICO DIFERENCIAL
• Considerar sempre cardiopatia preexistente, incluindo defeitos congênitos, miocardiopatia e valvulopatia adquirida.
• Histórico de sopro cardíaco ou da presença de arritmias antes do início da doença sistêmica ajuda a diferenciar de outras doenças.
• Envolvimento orgânico extracardíaco e identificação de agentes infecciosos podem ajudar no diagnóstico.

HEMOGRAMA/BIOQUÍMICA/URINÁLISE
Anormalidades — variam, dependendo do envolvimento orgânico.

OUTROS TESTES LABORATORIAIS
• Testes sorológicos para ajudar na identificação de agente infeccioso.
• Exame citológico de efusões pericárdicas, pleurais e peritoneais para identificar o microrganismo infeccioso.
• Hemocultura para diagnosticar bacteremia.
• Troponina — os níveis podem estar elevados.

DIAGNÓSTICO POR IMAGEM
Achados Radiográficos Torácicos
• A silhueta cardíaca pode aparecer grande ou normal, dependendo da extensão de envolvimento.
• Edema pulmonar, congestão ou efusão pleural nos pacientes com ICC.
• Coração globoide em alguns animais com efusão pericárdica.
• Granuloma pulmonar pode ser encontrado nos animais com infecção miocárdica granulomatosa.
Achados Ecocardiográficos
• Refletem a extensão do dano miocárdico; poderão ser normais se as lesões forem pequenas ou afetarem principalmente o sistema de condução cardíaca.
• Efusão pericárdica em alguns pacientes; o pericárdio pode aparecer espessado e hiperecoico, dependendo da extensão de envolvimento pericárdico.
• O miocárdio pode aparecer mosqueado com áreas irregulares ou desiguais de hiperecogenicidade causadas por inflamação miocárdica, fibrose ou granulomas.
• Discinesia regional provocada pelo envolvimento focal pode ser apreciada ao exame de ecocardiografia bidimensional.
Angiografia
• Em virtude da qualidade e da natureza não invasiva da ecocardiografia, a cateterização cardíaca raramente é indicada para o diagnóstico.
• A angiografia poderá ser utilizada para detectar envolvimento de câmara cardíaca específica ou efusão pericárdica se a ecocardiografia não estiver disponível.

MÉTODOS DIAGNÓSTICOS
Achados Eletrocardiográficos
• Padrões de aumento de volume do coração em alguns pacientes — dependendo da extensão de envolvimento da câmara.
• Arritmias — incluem taquiarritmias tanto atriais como ventriculares.
• Diferenciar bloqueios e hemibloqueios dos ramos direito e esquerdo do feixe de His a partir de padrões de aumento ventricular.
• Distúrbios da condução nodal atrioventricular em alguns pacientes.
Biopsia Endomiocárdica
• Valiosa para detecção de agentes infecciosos (p. ex., protozoários e elementos fúngicos) ou infiltrados de células inflamatórias.
Pericardiocentese
• Alivia a efusão pericárdica.
• Enviar o líquido para exame citológico e possível cultura bacteriana.
Estudo com Monitor Holter
• Para detectar arritmias, frequência e gravidade.
• Para monitorizar a terapia antiarrítmica.

Miocardite

ACHADOS PATOLÓGICOS
• Câmaras cardíacas dilatadas com áreas desiguais e irregulares de hiperemia, necrose ou fibrose
• Granulomas observados ao exame macroscópico em alguns pacientes.
• Exame microscópico do miocárdio ou do pericárdio pode revelar células inflamatórias (p. ex., linfócitos, plasmócitos e macrófagos), fibrose irregular ou os próprios agentes infecciosos.
• Desprendimento de miofibras — observada em pacientes com toxicidade pela doxorrubicina.

TRATAMENTO
CUIDADO(S) DE SAÚDE ADEQUADO(S)
• Hospitalizar os pacientes com ICC para tratamento clínico inicial.
• Hospitalizar os pacientes com arritmias ventriculares graves para tratamento antiarrítmico inicial.
• Hospitalizar os pacientes com manifestações sistêmicas graves para tratamento clínico rigoroso.

ATIVIDADE
Restrita.

DIETA
Restrição de sódio se houver ICC.

ORIENTAÇÃO AO PROPRIETÁRIO
• As manifestações cardíacas podem persistir mesmo com a resolução da doença sistêmica.
• Determinadas arritmias (i. e., taquiarritmias ventriculares) podem predispor o animal à morte súbita.
• Pode não ser fácil o diagnóstico antes da morte.
• Alguns agentes infecciosos podem representar um risco à saúde pública.

CONSIDERAÇÕES CIRÚRGICAS
O bloqueio atrioventricular completo pode necessitar do implante de marca-passo.

MEDICAÇÕES
MEDICAMENTO(S) DE ESCOLHA
• Se algum agente etiológico específico for identificado, direcionar o tratamento contra ele.
• Ajustar o tratamento antiarrítmico à arritmia predominante.
• Tratar a ICC com furosemida (1-2 mg/kg VO a cada 6-12 h), enalapril (0,25-0,5 mg/kg VO a cada 12-24 h) e digoxina (0,22 mg/m^2 VO a cada 12 h) ou pimobendana (0,25 mg/kg VO a cada 12 h).

CONTRAINDICAÇÕES
Considerações relativas à saúde pública podem impedir o tratamento de algumas doenças infecciosas (i. e., *T. cruzi*).

PRECAUÇÕES
• Todos os medicamentos antiarrítmicos apresentam propriedades pró-arrítmicas e devem ser monitorizados de modo rigoroso.
• Envolvimento orgânico sistêmico (p. ex., envolvimento renal) pode necessitar de dosagens modificadas do medicamento ou da utilização de vários medicamentos cardíacos; monitorizar cuidadosamente a função sistêmica.

ACOMPANHAMENTO
MONITORIZAÇÃO DO PACIENTE
• Terapia antiarrítmica — auscultação e ECG frequentes.
• Titulação sorológica quando apropriada.
• Auscultação e radiografias de acompanhamento — tratamento da ICC.
• Hemogramas e bioquímica sérica — efeitos sistêmicos.

PREVENÇÃO
• Evitar o acasalamento de animais com histórico de vacinação deficiente.
• Evitar as áreas endêmicas se possível.
• Monitorizar o ECG e o ecocardiograma ao utilizar a doxorrubicina.

EVOLUÇÃO ESPERADA E PROGNÓSTICO
• Depende da extensão e da gravidade do envolvimento miocárdico.
• Muitas doenças fúngicas e protozoárias sistêmicas não respondem bem ao tratamento clínico.
• Pacientes com inflamação miocárdica extensa, degeneração e sinais de ICC — prognóstico muito mau.
• Pacientes com arritmias isoladas e controláveis — prognóstico bom se a causa subjacente for tratada com sucesso.

DIVERSOS
DISTÚRBIOS ASSOCIADOS
Frequentemente acompanha doença sistêmica.

FATORES RELACIONADOS COM A IDADE
Miocardite viral — mais frequentemente observada em animais com < 1 ano de vida.

POTENCIAL ZOONÓTICO
• Varia com o agente infeccioso envolvido.
• Pode ser elevado com infecções micóticas e protozoárias.

GESTAÇÃO/FERTILIDADE/REPRODUÇÃO
Algumas doenças virais (p. ex., herpes-vírus e parvovírus caninos) são transmitidas para o feto durante a prenhez.

VER TAMBÉM
• Aspergilose Disseminada.
• Babesiose.
• Bartonelose.
• Blastomicose.
• Cinomose.
• Infecção pelo Parvovírus Canino.
• Doença de Chagas (Tripanossomíase Americana).
• Coccidioidomicose.
• Criptococose.
• Hepatozoonose.
• Infecção pelo Herpes-vírus — Cães.
• Leishmaniose.
• Neosporose.
• Prototecose.
• Toxoplasmose.
• Complexos Ventriculares Prematuros.
• Taquicardia Ventricular.

ABREVIATURA(S)
• ECG = eletrocardiograma.
• ICC = insuficiência cardíaca congestiva.

Sugestões de Leitura
Breitschwerdt EB, Atkins CE, Brown TT, Kordick DL, Snyder PS. Bartonella vinsonii subsp. berkhoffii and related members of the alpha subdivision of the Proteobacteria in dogs with cardiac arrhythmias, endocarditis, or myocarditis. J Clin Microbiol 1999, 37(11):3618-3626.
Cannon AB, Luff JA, Brault AC, MacLachlan NJ, Case JB, Green EN, Sykes JE. Acute encephalitis, polyarthritis, and myocarditis associated with West Nile virus infection in a dog. J Vet Intern Med 2006, 20(5):1219-1223.
Kraus MS, Gelzer ARM, Moise S. Treatment of cardiac arrhythmias and conduction disturbances. In: Tilley LP, Smith FWK, Oyama MA, Sleeper MM, eds., Manual of Canine and Feline Cardiology, 4th ed. St. Louis: Saunders Elsevier, 2008, pp. 326-331.
Lobetti RG. Cardiac involvement in canine babesiosis. J S Afr Vet Assoc 2005, 76(1):4-8.
Schmiedt C, Kellum H, Legendre AM, Gompf RE, Bright JM, Houle CD, Schutten M, Stepien R. Cardiovascular involvement in 8 dogs with Blastomyces dermatitidis infection. J Vet Intern Med 2006, 20(6):1351-1354.

Autores Larry P. Tilley e Michael B. Lesser
Consultores Editoriais Larry P. Tilley e Francis W.K. Smith, Jr.

MIOCARDITE TRAUMÁTICA

CONSIDERAÇÕES GERAIS

REVISÃO
- Miocardite traumática é o termo aplicado à síndrome de arritmias que, algumas vezes, complica os traumatismos rombos; no entanto, constitui um termo incorreto, em virtude da maior probabilidade de as lesões miocárdicas (se presentes) assumirem a forma de necrose do que inflamação.
- Pode não ser necessária uma lesão cardíaca direta para o desenvolvimento de arritmia pós-traumática; é provável que fatores extracardíacos tenham importância etiológica.
- A prevalência de arritmias graves após traumatismo rombo é relativamente baixa, mas alguns pacientes desenvolvem distúrbios de ritmo relevantes em termos clínicos; portanto, o ritmo cardíaco de todas as vítimas de traumatismo deve ser rigorosamente avaliado.
- Em grande parte dos pacientes acometidos, ocorrem taquiarritmias ventriculares; as arritmias e bradiarritmias supraventriculares são incomuns. Muitas vezes, os ritmos ventriculares que complicam os traumatismos rombos são relativamente lentos e detectados apenas durante pausas no ritmo sinusal; tais ritmos são denominados de forma mais apropriada como ritmos idioventriculares acelerados. Os complexos QRS são amplos e bizarros; a frequência cardíaca é >100 bpm, mas geralmente <160 bpm. Em geral, esses ritmos são benignos do ponto de vista tanto elétrico como hemodinâmico.
- Taquicardias ventriculares perigosas também podem complicar os traumatismos rombos e ainda podem evoluir a partir de ritmos idioventriculares acelerados aparentemente benignos, comprometendo a perfusão e colocando o paciente sob risco de morte súbita.

IDENTIFICAÇÃO
Cães; raramente, gatos.

SINAIS CLÍNICOS

Achados Anamnésicos
- Traumatismo, decorrente muitas vezes de acidentes automobilísticos.
- As arritmias são percebidas frequentemente após 48 h do traumatismo.

Achados do Exame Físico
- As arritmias poderão ser inaparentes se a frequência de um ritmo idioventricular acelerado se equiparar à do ritmo sinusal.
- Em alguns pacientes, observam-se ritmos irregulares e rápidos.
- Em pacientes com ritmos ventriculares rápidos e pouco tolerados, verificam-se sinais de má perfusão periférica (p. ex., fraqueza, mucosas pálidas e pulsos femorais débeis).

CAUSAS E FATORES DE RISCO
- Traumatismo rombo.
- Hipóxia.
- Distúrbio autônomo.
- Desequilíbrios eletrolíticos.
- Distúrbios acidobásicos.

DIAGNÓSTICO

DIAGNÓSTICO DIFERENCIAL
- Os ritmos idioventriculares acelerados devem ser diferenciados de taquicardia ventricular.
- Ritmos idioventriculares acelerados — desencadeados geralmente por complexos ventriculares diastólicos tardios (ritmo de escape) ou por complexos de fusão; em geral, a frequência cardíaca é de 100-160 bpm.
- Taquicardia ventricular — iniciada comumente por um complexo ventricular prematuro; as frequências cardíacas excedem 160 bpm.

HEMOGRAMA/BIOQUÍMICA/URINÁLISE
- Níveis frequentemente elevados de creatina quinase, enzimas hepáticas e desidrogenase láctica, em função do traumatismo de órgãos.
- Concentrações séricas elevadas de troponina são sugestivas de necrose do miocárdio.
- Distúrbios eletrolíticos (particularmente hipocalemia e hipomagnesemia) predispõem o animal à arritmia ventricular.

OUTROS TESTES LABORATORIAIS
N/D.

DIAGNÓSTICO POR IMAGEM
Achados Radiográficos Torácicos
Em alguns pacientes, há indícios de traumatismo, incluindo pneumotórax, fraturas de costela e contusão pulmonar.

MÉTODOS DIAGNÓSTICOS
Achados Eletrocardiográficos
Arritmias ventriculares, conforme foi previamente discutido.

TRATAMENTO

- Tratar as condições extracardíacas, incluindo dor, distúrbios eletrolíticos e hipóxia, que podem predispor o animal à arritmia ventricular.
- Obter radiografias torácicas de todos os pacientes acometidos por traumatismo rombo; identificar e corrigir os distúrbios, como o pneumotórax.
- A necessidade de terapia antiarrítmica é determinada pelos sinais clínicos e pelo aspecto eletrocardiográfico da arritmia; em geral, não há necessidade de supressão farmacológica do ritmo idioventricular acelerado.
- Fornecer fluidoterapia em casos de choque.

MEDICAÇÕES

MEDICAMENTO(S)
- Tratar inicialmente os ritmos ventriculares rápidos ou aqueles associados ao comprometimento hemodinâmico com o uso de lidocaína (2 mg/kg em bólus IV); pode-se administrar o total de 8 mg/kg em 10-12 min. Iniciar a infusão de lidocaína (25-75 µg/kg/min) assim que o ritmo for estabilizado com o fornecimento desse antiarrítmico em forma de bólus.
- Se a administração de lidocaína falhar na cardioversão ao ritmo sinusal, tentar a procainamida ou, com cuidado, os β-bloqueadores (como o esmolol ou o propranolol) ou até mesmo os agentes antiarrítmicos da classe III (como a amiodarona ou o sotalol).
- Considerar a cardioversão de corrente direta enquanto o animal estiver sob anestesia ou sedação intensa, para tratar os ritmos ventriculares rápidos, instáveis em termos hemodinâmicos e irresponsivos à terapia medicamentosa.
- Os agentes antiarrítmicos não são necessariamente benignos, pois eles podem agravar as arritmias existentes e fornecer substrato para o desenvolvimento de novas arritmias (pró-arritmias); ponderar cuidadosamente o risco ou o benefício relativos em cada etapa terapêutica.

CONTRAINDICAÇÕES/INTERAÇÕES POSSÍVEIS
N/D.

ACOMPANHAMENTO

- É recomendada a monitorização eletrocardiográfica dos animais com arritmias; em geral, as arritmias que complicam traumatismos rombos são autolimitantes e desaparecem dentro de 48-72 h.
- Se a terapia antiarrítmica for considerada necessária, ela poderá ser interrompida após 2-5 dias.
- Embora as arritmias perigosas ocasionalmente compliquem os traumatismos rombos, o prognóstico costuma depender da gravidade da lesão extracardíaca.

DIVERSOS

VER TAMBÉM
- Choque Cardiogênico.
- Ritmo Idioventricular.
- Taquicardia Ventricular.

ABREVIATURA(S)
- bpm = batimentos por minuto.

Sugestões de Leitura
Abbott JA. Traumatic myocarditis. In: Bonagura JD, ed., Kirk's Current Veterinary Therapy XII. Philadelphia: Saunders, 1995, pp. 846-850.

Autor Jonathan A. Abbott
Consultores Editoriais Larry P. Tilley e Francis W.K. Smith, Jr.

MIOCLONIA

CONSIDERAÇÕES GERAIS

REVISÃO
- Contração grosseira, repetitiva, involuntária e rítmica de parte de um músculo, de um músculo inteiro ou de um grupo muscular em taxas de até 60/min.
- Pode acometer um ou diversos grupos musculares; ocorre mais comumente em músculos apendiculares ou mastigatórios.
- Pode ocorrer de modo sincrônico ou assincrônico em diversas áreas.
- Pode persistir durante o sono.
- Disfunção do SNC que envolve os neurônios motores inferiores e os interneurônios em nível segmentar da medula espinal ou do tronco cerebral.
- Um sinal clínico; apesar de relatada mais comumente na infecção pelo vírus da cinomose, a mioclonia pode ser causada por outras encefalites e processos degenerativos que acometem os neurônios motores.

IDENTIFICAÇÃO
Adquirida
- Cães e, raramente, gatos.
- Nenhuma predisposição sexual, etária ou racial.

Congênita
- Mioclonia reflexa familiar — raças Labrador retriever e Dálmata; desenvolve-se nas 3 primeiras semanas de vida.
- Degeneração esponjosa da substância branca e/ou cinzenta — cães: mioclonia dos músculos paravertebrais em cães neonatos da raça Silky terrier; Samoieda em 12 dias de vida; Saluki aos 3 meses; Labrador retriever aos 4-6 meses. Gatos — Mau egípcio aos 7 meses. Síndromes raras.

SINAIS CLÍNICOS
Achados Anamnésicos
- Na cinomose — observada após um ataque de sinais gastrintestinais, tosse e/ou secreção purulenta ocular ou nasal; persiste em repouso e até mesmo durante o sono ou leve anestesia; frequência constante em determinado paciente; o diagnóstico da cinomose pode preceder a mioclonia por meses a anos; ocorre mais frequentemente na fase crônica da cinomose.
- Na mioclonia reflexa familiar — observada quando o paciente começa a caminhar; contrações musculares intermitentes induzidas por estímulo auditivo ou tátil e pelo exercício; envolve todos os membros, o pescoço e a cabeça (p. ex., os músculos faciais e mastigatórios); paciente incapaz de se levantar sem assistência.
- Na degeneração esponjosa — é observada uma variedade de sinais clínicos, tais como tremor, espasticidade, opistótono e mioclonia.
- Mioclonia induzida pela clorambucila — relatada em gato com linfoma.

Achados do Exame Físico
- Músculos mastigatórios e apendiculares — mais frequentemente acometidos em mioclonia induzida pela cinomose; pode haver paresia do membro acometido.
- Pode-se observar a presença de outros sinais sugestivos de cinomose (p. ex., coxins palmoplantares ásperos, secreção purulenta ocular e nasal, além de coriorretinite).
- Déficits neurológicos sugestivos de lesões multifocais em alguns pacientes.
- O paciente pode estar saudável sob outros aspectos.

CAUSAS E FATORES DE RISCO
Congênitas
- Familiar na raça Labrador retriever.
- Degeneração esponjosa de causa desconhecida, mas provavelmente hereditária.
- Tratamento com clorambucila em gatos com linfoma.

Adquiridas
- Vírus da cinomose — causa mais frequente; a única doença do SNC repetidamente associada à mioclonia nos cães; cães não vacinados estão sob risco.
- Encefalite de qualquer causa — cães e gatos.
- Doença degenerativa — especialmente degeneração esponjosa.
- Descrita em cão com intoxicação pelo chumbo.

DIAGNÓSTICO

DIAGNÓSTICO DIFERENCIAL
- Mioclonia congênita — em neonatos ou durante os primeiros meses de vida em cães saudáveis sob outros aspectos. Agitação, atividade voluntária e estímulos táteis/auditivos frequentemente aumentam as contrações musculares.
- Vírus da cinomose — cão não vacinado; a mioclonia é observada antes, durante ou depois de doença aguda do SNC; com maior frequência depois, quando o animal se encontra saudável sob outros aspectos. A mioclonia envolve um membro, mais de um membro, os músculos faciais ou mastigatórios.
- "Cabeça oscilante" — raças Doberman, Labrador retriever e, frequentemente, Buldogue inglês; episódios de oscilação na cabeça como um sim ou sem direção; ocorrem de forma rara e intermitente; limitadas à cabeça; duram desde poucos segundos a minutos; o cão acometido continua sua atividade e permanece normal sob outros aspectos.
- Doença do Doberman dançarino — diferenciada com base na raça e nos movimentos observados (p. ex., o cão mantém um membro pélvico flexionado enquanto se encontra em estação; ambos os membros costumam ser acometidos, conferindo uma aparência de dançarino na postura em estação).

HEMOGRAMA/BIOQUÍMICA/URINÁLISE
- Congênita ou secundária a alguma infecção prévia pelo vírus da cinomose — normais.
- Outras formas adquiridas — poderão sugerir uma causa específica se o paciente tiver encefalomielite infecciosa; normais sob outros aspectos.

DIAGNÓSTICO POR IMAGEM
RM — pode ajudar a determinar o diagnóstico em casos de doença adquirida aguda.

MÉTODOS DIAGNÓSTICOS
Início agudo — análise do LCS, teste sorológico e diagnóstico por imagem para determinar a causa se houver outros sinais físicos ou neurológicos.

TRATAMENTO
- Encefalomielite ativa — paciente internado; estabelecer o diagnóstico e iniciar o tratamento.
- Exercício — conforme a tolerância.
- Dieta — garantir uma nutrição adequada com doença ativa do SNC; modificar, se houver necessidade, na presença de vômito ou diarreia.
- Mioclonia reflexa familiar — sinais clínicos nas raças Labrador retriever e Dálmata são graves e, em geral, incompatíveis com a qualidade de vida.

MEDICAÇÕES

MEDICAMENTO(S)
- Na cinomose crônica inativa — o tratamento quase sempre é desnecessário; pode-se obter alívio com a procainamida (125-250 mg/cão VO a cada 6-12 h).
- Há relatos de que a gabapentina seja benéfica em síndrome de tremor (10-20 mg/kg a cada 8 h).
- Clorazepato (0,6-2 mg/kg VO a cada 8 h) — mioclonia reflexa familiar; pode-se observar melhora.
- Encefalomielite ativa — tratar de acordo.

ACOMPANHAMENTO
- Monitorizar a doença do SNC.
- Em geral, a mioclonia persiste por tempo indefinido; pode ocorrer remissão espontânea.
- Infecção ativa pelo vírus da cinomose — prognóstico mau a grave.
- Cinomose crônica — a mioclonia persiste, mas o paciente permanece saudável sob outros aspectos.

DIVERSOS

SINÔNIMO(S)
Coreia canina.

ABREVIATURA(S)
- LCS = líquido cerebrospinal.
- RM = ressonância magnética.
- SNC = sistema nervoso central.

Sugestões de Leitura
Lorenz MD, Kornegay JN. Handbook of Veterinary Neurology, 4th ed. St Louis: Elsevier, 2004, pp. 276-278.

Autor Joane M. Parent
Consultor Editorial Joane M. Parent

Miopatia Inflamatória — Polimiosite e Dermatomiosite

CONSIDERAÇÕES GERAIS

DEFINIÇÃO
• Polimiosite — distúrbio no qual os músculos esqueléticos são lesionados por processo inflamatório não supurativo com infiltração linfocitária predominante. Terminologia restrita à forma imunomediada.
• Dermatomiosite — a polimiosite é associada a lesões cutâneas características.

FISIOPATOLOGIA
• Inflamação dos músculos esqueléticos — resulta em fraqueza muscular, rigidez, mialgia e atrofia.
• Inflamação muscular — pode ser o resultado de distúrbios imunomediados, infecciosos ou paraneoplásicos; pode ser uma sequela de determinadas terapias medicamentosas.

SISTEMA(S) ACOMETIDO(S)
• Cutâneo/exócrino — particularmente se relacionados com distúrbio imunomediado generalizado do tecido conjuntivo.
• Gastrintestinal — em particular os músculos faríngeos e esofágicos, porque são predominantemente compostos de musculatura esquelética nos cães.
• Neuromuscular — envolvimento muscular generalizado, incluindo músculos da mastigação e dos membros.

GENÉTICA
• Desconhecida.
• Como acontece com as doenças autoimunes em geral, deve existir uma base genética apropriada.
• Forma familiar de polimiosite autoimune em cães da raça Terra Nova.
• Dermatomiosite — relatada por ter padrão de herança autossômica dominante nos cães das raças Collie de pelo duro e Pastor de Shetland.

INCIDÊNCIA/PREVALÊNCIA
• Desconhecidas.
• Miopatias inflamatórias generalizadas — incomuns, embora a identificação possa estar crescendo.

DISTRIBUIÇÃO GEOGRÁFICA
Provavelmente mundial.

IDENTIFICAÇÃO
Espécies
Cães e, raramente, gatos.
Raça(s) Predominante(s)
• Polimiosite — diversas raças de cães e de gatos podem ser acometidas; associada às raças Terra Nova e Boxer.
• Dermatomiosite — relatada nas raças Collie de pelo duro, Pastor de Shetland e Boiadeiro australiano.
Idade Média e Faixa Etária
• Polimiosite — nenhuma predileção etária óbvia.
• Dermatomiosite — 3-5 meses de vida.
Sexo Predominante
Nenhuma predileção sexual evidente.

SINAIS CLÍNICOS
Comentários Gerais
• Polimiosite — geralmente associada à marcha rígida, mialgia variável e/ou fraqueza muscular. Podem-se observar regurgitação e megaesôfago.

• Creatina quinase sérica elevada — apoia, mas não faz o diagnóstico de miosite. Não descartar polimiosite se a creatina quinase estiver normal.
• Biopsia muscular — necessária para confirmar o diagnóstico.
Achados Anamnésicos
• Marcha enrijecida e afetada — aguda ou crônica.
• Tumefação e/ou atrofia muscular.
• Dor muscular variável.
• Fraqueza muscular generalizada e intolerância ao exercício.
• Regurgitação de alimento ou dificuldade de deglutição.
Achados do Exame Físico
• Dor variável à palpação de grupos musculares.
• Atrofia muscular generalizada, incluindo os músculos da mastigação.
• Anormalidades da marcha, incluindo marcha enrijecida e afetada.
• Exame neurológico — não se encontra anormal; pode haver um reflexo faríngeo reduzido se os músculos faríngeos estiverem acometidos.
• Dermatomiosite (cães) — lesões cutâneas típicas.

CAUSAS
• Imunomediadas.
• Infecciosas — *Toxoplasma gondii*; *Neospora canis*; doenças relacionadas com carrapatos; infecção bacteriana rara.
• Induzidas por medicamentos.
• Síndrome paraneoplásica ou pré-neoplásica.

FATORES DE RISCO
• Base genética apropriada.
• Possivelmente, infecção bacteriana ou viral prévia.
• Neoplasia, possivelmente oculta.
• Exposição a carrapatos.

DIAGNÓSTICO

DIAGNÓSTICO DIFERENCIAL
• Poliartrite — diferenciada pelo exame físico e pela avaliação do líquido articular.
• Distúrbios musculares não inflamatórios — diferenciados por biopsia muscular.
• Polineuropatia — diferenciada pelo exame neurológico, eletrofisiologia e biopsia dos músculos e nervos periféricos.
• Discopatia intervertebral crônica — diferenciada pelo exame neurológico e pela creatina quinase sérica.
• Miastenia grave — diferenciada por título positivo para o anticorpo AChR.

HEMOGRAMA/BIOQUÍMICA/URINÁLISE
Creatina quinase sérica — variavelmente elevada.

OUTROS TESTES LABORATORIAIS
• Título sérico do anticorpo antinuclear — pode ser positivo nos distúrbios do tecido conjuntivo.
• Pode-se observar hipotireoidismo concomitante.
• Troponina cardíaca I — pode ter miocardite concomitante.

DIAGNÓSTICO POR IMAGEM
• Regurgitação — avaliar radiografias torácicas quanto à presença de dilatação esofágica ou neoplasia.
• Silhueta cardíaca — avaliar o tamanho e o formato do miocárdio.
• Fraqueza faríngea — realizar estudo dinâmico para avaliar o processo de deglutição.

MÉTODOS DIAGNÓSTICOS
• Biopsia muscular — representa o único teste mais importante para diagnosticar polimiosite; é necessária a obtenção de múltiplas amostras de músculos, já que a condição pode passar despercebida se a distribuição for irregular.
• Ecocardiografia — para avaliar a função do miocárdio.
• Avaliação eletrodiagnóstica (EMG, mensuração da velocidade de condução nervosa) — realizada para determinar a distribuição do envolvimento muscular e os músculos a serem biopsiados; deve ajudar a diferenciar as causas miopáticas das neuropáticas de fraqueza muscular.

ACHADOS PATOLÓGICOS
• Tumefação ou atrofia muscular.
• Amostras de biopsia — costumam conter infiltrados de células mononucleares.
• Raros neutrófilos ou eosinófilos — podem ser notados.
• Miofibras em processo de regeneração — podem ser observadas.
• Cisto parasitário dentro das miofibras — raro.
• Condição crônica — é possível observar atrofia e fibrose extensas das miofibras.

TRATAMENTO

CUIDADO(S) DE SAÚDE ADEQUADO(S)
Tratamento ambulatorial.

CUIDADO(S) DE ENFERMAGEM
Cuidados de suporte — podem ser necessários para evitar feridas cutâneas e úlceras de decúbito nos pacientes gravemente acometidos sem deambulação.

ATIVIDADE
Deve aumentar, juntamente com a força muscular, à medida que a inflamação dos músculos diminui.

DIETA
• Megaesôfago — pode exigir a alimentação em plano elevado; tentar alimentos de consistências diferentes.
• Regurgitação grave — pode ser necessária a colocação de sonda alimentar gástrica para manter a hidratação e a nutrição.

ORIENTAÇÃO AO PROPRIETÁRIO
• Avisar o proprietário sobre a possível necessidade de terapia imunossupressora a longo prazo para um distúrbio imunomediado.
• Informar ao proprietário quanto à possível ocorrência de atrofia muscular residual e contraturas com doença crônica e fibrose extensa.
• Sugerir aconselhamento genético para distúrbios familiares.

CONSIDERAÇÕES CIRÚRGICAS
Apenas para neoplasia concomitante.

MEDICAÇÕES

MEDICAMENTO(S) DE ESCOLHA
• Corticosteroides — dosagens imunossupressoras geralmente resultam em melhora clínica da condição imunomediada; reduzir para a dosagem mais baixa em dias alternados, dose esta que mantenha a creatina quinase normal e ainda

MIOPATIA INFLAMATÓRIA — POLIMIOSITE E DERMATOMIOSITE

melhore a força e a mobilidade musculares; talvez haja necessidade de terapia a longo prazo.
• Agente infeccioso identificado — iniciar tratamento específico.
• Insuficiência miocárdica identificada — instituir terapia específica.

CONTRAINDICAÇÕES
N/D.

PRECAUÇÕES
Corticosteroides — observar o paciente quanto à ocorrência de infecção e efeitos colaterais indesejáveis; lembrar que o tratamento crônico pode levar a atrofia muscular.

INTERAÇÕES POSSÍVEIS
N/D.

MEDICAMENTO(S) ALTERNATIVO(S)
Efeitos colaterais intoleráveis dos corticosteroides — instituir a dose mais baixa desses agentes combinados com outro medicamento (p. ex., azatioprina).

ACOMPANHAMENTO

MONITORIZAÇÃO DO PACIENTE
• Creatina quinase sérica — avaliação periódica; se elevada, deve diminuir para a faixa de referência normal.
• Corticosteroides — efeitos colaterais.

PREVENÇÃO
N/D.

COMPLICAÇÕES POSSÍVEIS
• Corticosteroides — efeitos colaterais indesejáveis.
• Recidiva dos sinais clínicos — em caso de interrupção terapêutica muito precoce.
• Resposta clínica insatisfatória — dosagens inadequadas dos corticosteroides.

EVOLUÇÃO ESPERADA E PROGNÓSTICO
• Condição imunomediada — prognóstico bom a razoável.
• Distúrbio paraneoplásico associado à neoplasia oculta — prognóstico reservado.

DIVERSOS

DISTÚRBIOS ASSOCIADOS
• Outros distúrbios autoimunes concomitantes.
• Neoplasia.

FATORES RELACIONADOS COM A IDADE
N/D.

POTENCIAL ZOONÓTICO
N/D.

GESTAÇÃO/FERTILIDADE/REPRODUÇÃO
Desconhecida.

VER TAMBÉM
Miopatia Não Inflamatória — Endócrina.

ABREVIATURA(S)
• AChR = receptor de acetilcolina.
• EMG = eletromiografia.

RECURSOS DA INTERNET
Comparative Neuromuscular Laboratory: http://vetneuromuscular.ucsd.edu.

Sugestões de Leitura

Evans J, Levesque D, Shelton GD. Canine inflammatory myopathies: A clinicopathologic review of 200 cases. J Vet Intern Med 2004, 18:679-691.

Hargis AM, Haupt KH, Prieur DJ, Moore MP. A skin disorder in three Shetland sheepdogs: Comparison with familial canine dermatomyositis of collies. Compend Contin Educ Pract Vet 1985, 7:306-318.

Neravanda D, Kent M, Platt SR, Gruenenfelder FI, Shelton GD, Schatzberg SJ. Lymphoma-associated polymyositis in dogs. J Vet Intern Med 2009, 23:1293-1298.

Podell M. Inflammatory myopathies. Vet Clin North Am 2002, 31:147-167.

Shelton GD. From dog to man: The broad spectrum of inflammatory myopathies. Neuromusc Disord 2007, 17:663-670.

Warman S, Pearson G, Barrett E, Shelton GD. Dilatation of the right atrium in a dog with polymyositis and myocarditis. J Small Anim Pract 2008, 49:302-305.

Autor G. Diane Shelton
Consultor Editorial Peter K. Shires

Miopatia Inflamatória Focal — Miosite dos Músculos Mastigatórios e Extraoculares

CONSIDERAÇÕES GERAIS

DEFINIÇÃO
- Mastigatória — miopatia inflamatória focal que acomete os músculos da mastigação (músculos temporal, masseter e pterigoide) e poupa os músculos dos membros.
- Extraocular — afeta seletivamente os músculos extraoculares, poupando os músculos dos membros e da mastigação.

FISIOPATOLOGIA
- Mastigatória — suspeita de causa imunomediada atribuída a autoanticorpos contra fibras do tipo 2M e resposta clínica positiva a doses imunossupressoras de corticosteroides.
- Extraocular — suspeita de causa imunomediada devida à resposta clínica positiva aos corticosteroides.

SISTEMA(S) ACOMETIDO(S)
Neuromuscular — músculos da mastigação; músculos extraoculares.

GENÉTICA
- Desconhecida.
- Como ocorre com as doenças autoimunes em geral, deve existir base genética apropriada.
- Mastigatória — os cães da raça Cavalier King Charles spaniel apresentam uma forma familiar e podem ser acometidos com menos de 6 meses de vida.
- Extraocular — os cães da raça Golden retriever pode apresentar predisposição genética.

INCIDÊNCIA/PREVALÊNCIA
- Desconhecidas.
- Mastigatória — relativamente comum.

DISTRIBUIÇÃO GEOGRÁFICA
Provavelmente mundial.

IDENTIFICAÇÃO
Espécies
- Cães (comum).
- Gatos (rara).

Raça(s) Predominante(s)
- Diversas.
- Mastigatória — Rottweiler, Doberman, Samoieda e Cavalier King Charles spaniel desenvolvem formas graves.
- Extraocular — Golden retriever.

Idade Média e Faixa Etária
Nenhuma predisposição etária óbvia.

Sexo Predominante
Nenhuma predileção sexual evidente.

SINAIS CLÍNICOS
Comentários Gerais
Mastigatória — sinais clínicos geralmente relacionados com anormalidades do movimento da mandíbula, dor na mandíbula e atrofia dos músculos da mastigação; não é um diagnóstico "fechado"; em geral, necessita de exames laboratoriais para confirmar o diagnóstico.

Achados Anamnésicos
- Mastigatória — dor aguda ou crônica ao abrir a mandíbula; incapacidade de apanhar uma bola ou de colocar alimento na boca; músculos agudamente tumefatos (inchados); atrofia muscular progressiva.
- Extraocular — exoftalmia bilateral.

Achados do Exame Físico
- Mastigatória — dor mandibular acentuada à manipulação e/ou trismo; tumefação muscular aguda com exoftalmia; atrofia muscular com enoftalmia; incapacidade de abrir a mandíbula sob anestesia.
- Extraocular — exoftalmia bilateral; visão prejudicada.

CAUSAS
Imunomediadas.

FATORES DE RISCO
- Base genética apropriada.
- Possível infecção bacteriana ou viral prévia.
- A vacinação pode exacerbar a doença ativa.

DIAGNÓSTICO

DIAGNÓSTICO DIFERENCIAL
- Abscesso retro-orbital — passagem de sonda atrás do último molar superior.
- Doença da articulação temporomandibular — articulação anormal ao exame radiográfico.
- Polimiosite — creatina quinase sérica elevada; anormalidades generalizadas no EMG; biopsias musculares diagnósticas.
- Atrofia neurogênica dos músculos temporais — determinada por EMG e por biopsia muscular.
- Atrofia dos músculos mastigatórios causada pelos corticosteroides — histórico de utilização desses agentes terapêuticos; alterações características na biopsia muscular.
- Atrofia dos músculos mastigatórios decorrente de distúrbios endócrinos — testes de função da tireoide e da adrenal.

HEMOGRAMA/BIOQUÍMICA/URINÁLISE
Creatina quinase sérica — normal ou levemente elevada.

OUTROS TESTES LABORATORIAIS
- Biopsia muscular — teste diagnóstico de escolha para miopatia mastigatória.
- Ensaio imuno-histoquímico — demonstra a presença de autoanticorpos contra fibras do tipo 2M dos músculos mastigatórios em cortes congelados de biopsia muscular; negativo em casos de polimiosite e doença extraocular.
- ELISA — detecta a existência de autoanticorpos contra as proteínas das fibras do tipo 2M dos músculos mastigatórios.

DIAGNÓSTICO POR IMAGEM
- Radiografia das articulações temporomandibulares.
- Ultrassonografia da órbita ocular — na doença extraorbital; demonstra os músculos extraoculares tumefeitos.
- RM — para demonstração de inflamação/necrose nos músculos.

MÉTODOS DIAGNÓSTICOS
EMG — para diferenciar entre doença extraocular e polimiosite; músculos mastigatórios anormais apenas na miosite mastigatória; anormalidades generalizadas incluindo os músculos mastigatórios na polimiosite.

ACHADOS PATOLÓGICOS
Mastigatória
- Tumefação ou atrofia dos músculos mastigatórios.
- Amostra de biopsia — podem-se observar necrose das miofibras, fagocitose e infiltração de células mononucleares com distribuição multifocal e perivascular; podem-se observar atrofia das miofibras e processo de fibrose nas condições crônicas; raros eosinófilos.

Extraocular
Infiltração de células mononucleares — restrita aos músculos extraoculares.

TRATAMENTO

CUIDADO(S) DE SAÚDE ADEQUADO(S)
Tratamento ambulatorial.

CUIDADO(S) DE ENFERMAGEM
Sonda inserida via gastrostomia — pode ser necessária em restrições graves na mobilidade mandibular; necessita de boas práticas de higiene e cuidados de suporte.

ATIVIDADE
N/D.

DIETA
Mastigatória — pode necessitar de alimento líquido ou papa até que a mobilidade da mandíbula seja restabelecida; pode requerer a colocação de sonda para alimentação gástrica para facilitar a ingestão calórica e hídrica.

ORIENTAÇÃO AO PROPRIETÁRIO
- Avisar o proprietário sobre a possível necessidade de tratamento com corticosteroide a longo prazo.
- Informar ao proprietário sobre a possível ocorrência de atrofia residual dos músculos e restrição do movimento mandibular em casos de miopatia mastigatória crônica.

CONSIDERAÇÕES CIRÚRGICAS
Não há indicação de cirurgia.

MEDICAÇÕES

MEDICAMENTO(S) DE ESCOLHA
Corticosteroides — dosagens imunossupressoras, reduzidas gradativamente conforme a mobilidade da mandíbula, o sinal de tumefação e os níveis séricos da creatina quinase retornam ao normal; mantidos na dosagem mais baixa em dias alternados, capaz de evitar a restrição da mobilidade mandibular; tratada por, no mínimo, seis meses.

CONTRAINDICAÇÕES
N/D.

PRECAUÇÕES
- Corticosteroides — ficar atento quanto à ocorrência de infecção e efeitos colaterais indesejáveis.
- Os sinais clínicos podem recidivar se o tratamento for interrompido muito precocemente.

INTERAÇÕES POSSÍVEIS
N/D.

MEDICAMENTO(S) ALTERNATIVO(S)
Efeitos colaterais intoleráveis dos corticosteroides — instituir a dose mais baixa desses agentes e combinar com outro medicamento (p. ex., azatioprina).

MIOPATIA INFLAMATÓRIA FOCAL — MIOSITE DOS MÚSCULOS MASTIGATÓRIOS E EXTRAOCULARES

ACOMPANHAMENTO

MONITORIZAÇÃO DO PACIENTE
• Mastigatória — retorno da mobilidade mandibular e declínio da creatina quinase sérica.
• Extraocular — tumefação reduzida dos músculos extraoculares.

PREVENÇÃO
N/D.

COMPLICAÇÕES POSSÍVEIS
• Corticosteroides — efeitos colaterais indesejáveis.
• Recidiva dos sinais clínicos — em caso de interrupção terapêutica muito precoce.
• Resposta clínica insatisfatória — dosagens inadequadas dos corticosteroides.
• Estrabismo restritivo (miosite extraocular).
• Observar a posição da língua — podem ocorrer congestão venosa e protrusão da língua sob anestesia.

EVOLUÇÃO ESPERADA E PROGNÓSTICO
• Mastigatória — a mobilidade mandibular deve retornar ao normal a menos que a condição seja crônica e ocorra o desenvolvimento de fibrose grave; prognóstico bom se tratada precocemente com dosagens adequadas de corticosteroides.
• Extraocular — resposta satisfatória aos corticosteroides; prognóstico bom a menos em casos crônicos com estrabismo restritivo.

DIVERSOS

DISTÚRBIOS ASSOCIADOS
Outros distúrbios autoimunes concomitantes.

FATORES RELACIONADOS COM A IDADE
N/D.

POTENCIAL ZOONÓTICO
N/D.

GESTAÇÃO/FERTILIDADE/REPRODUÇÃO
Desconhecida.

SINÔNIMO(S)
• Miosite eosinofílica.
• Miosite atrófica.

VER TAMBÉM
• Miopatia Inflamatória — Polimiosite e Dermatomiosite.
• Miopatia Não Inflamatória — Endócrina.

ABREVIATURA(S)
• ELISA = ensaio imunoabsorvente ligado à enzima.
• EMG = eletromiograma.
• RM = ressonância magnética.

RECURSOS DA INTERNET
Comparative Neuromuscular Laboratory: http://vetneuromuscular.ucsd.edu.

Sugestões de Leitura
Allgoewer I, Blair M, Basher T, Davidson M. Extraocular myositis and restrictive strabismus in 10 dogs. Vet Ophthalmology 2000, 3:21-26.
Carpenter JL, Schmidt GM, Moore FM, et al. Canine bilateral extraocular polymyositis. Vet Pathol 1989, 26:510-512.
Melmed C, Shelton GD, Bergman R, Barton C. Masticatory muscle myositis: Pathogenesis, diagnosis, and treatment. Compend Contin Educ Pract Vet 2004, 26:590-605.
Nanai B, Phillips L, Christiansen J, Shelton GD. Life threatening complication associated with anesthesia in a dog with masticatory muscle myositis. Vet Surg 2009, 38:645-649.
Orvis JS, Cardinet GH III. Canine muscle fiber types and susceptibility of masticatory muscles to myositis. Muscle Nerve 1981, 4:354-359.
Podell M. Inflammatory myopathies. Vet Clin North Am 2002, 31:147-167.
Shelton GD, Cardinet GH III, Bandman E. Canine masticatory muscle disorders: A clinicopathological and immunochemical study of 29 cases. Muscle Nerve 1987, 10:753-766.

Autor G. Diane Shelton
Consultor Editorial Peter K. Shires

Miopatia Não Inflamatória – Cãibra Hereditária do Terrier Escocês

CONSIDERAÇÕES GERAIS

REVISÃO
- Distúrbio hereditário em cães da raça Terrier escocês, caracterizado por hipertonicidade ou cãibra muscular episódica.
- Não associada a qualquer alteração morfológica no músculo, no nervo periférico ou no SNC.
- É mais bem caracterizada como um distúrbio de movimento do que uma miopatia.
- Acredita-se que essa condição seja o resultado de um distúrbio do metabolismo da serotonina dentro do SNC.
- Distúrbio semelhante foi relatado em cães jovens das raças Dálmata e Labrador retriever — pode ser o resultado da baixa quantidade de receptores para o neurotransmissor glicina no SNC.
- Também ocorrem síndromes episódicas de hipertonicidade muscular em cães da raça Cavalier King Charles spaniel (síndrome de queda); tais síndromes já foram relatadas em Terrier norueguês, Bichon frisé, Border terrier, Wheaten terrier, Springer spaniel e, esporadicamente, em outras raças.

IDENTIFICAÇÃO
- Cães jovens da raça Terrier escocês, tipicamente com <1 ano de idade. Os sinais clínicos podem ser observados em filhotes com até 6-8 semanas de vida.
- Nenhuma predileção sexual conhecida.

SINAIS CLÍNICOS
- Normais em repouso e no início do exercício.
- Exercício ou agitação adicionais — abdução dos membros torácicos; arqueamento (cifose) da coluna espinal toracolombar; enrijecimento ou hiperflexão dos membros pélvicos (marcha em passo de ganso).
- O paciente pode cair, com a cauda e os membros pélvicos firmemente flexionados contra o corpo.
- Respiração — pode parar por curto período de tempo.
- Músculos faciais — podem estar contraídos.
- Sem perda de consciência.
- Variam em termos de gravidade.
- Episódios — podem durar até 30 min.

CAUSAS E FATORES DE RISCO
Condição hereditária, com provável modo de transmissão recessivo.

DIAGNÓSTICO

DIAGNÓSTICO DIFERENCIAL
- Distúrbio convulsivo — distinguido com base no histórico familiar, nos sinais clínicos típicos sem perda de consciência e na indução dos sinais com antagonistas serotoninérgicos.

HEMOGRAMA/BIOQUÍMICA/URINÁLISE
Normais.

OUTROS TESTES LABORATORIAIS
N/D.

DIAGNÓSTICO POR IMAGEM
N/D.

MÉTODOS DIAGNÓSTICOS
Os sinais clínicos podem ser induzidos, administrando-se o antagonista serotoninérgico metisergida (0,3 mg/kg VO). As cãibras são evidentes em 2 h e podem durar 8 h.

TRATAMENTO

Modificação comportamental e/ou mudanças ambientais — para eliminar situações desencadeantes (agitação, estresse); podem ser adequadas no controle dos episódios.

MEDICAÇÕES

MEDICAMENTO(S)
- Maleato de acepromazina (0,1-0,75 mg/kg IM ou VO), diazepam (0,5-1,5 mg/kg VO a cada 8 h), ou vitamina E (>125 U/kg a cada 24 h) — podem reduzir a incidência e a gravidade da cãibra do Terrier escocês.
- Fluoxetina, um inibidor seletivo da recaptação de serotonina, resultou em uma diminuição acentuada nos sinais clínicos em um único cão Terrier escocês a uma dose de 1,2 mg/kg a cada 12 h inicialmente, acompanhada por 0,8 mg/kg a cada 12 h. A melhora clínica foi mantida por >1 ano.
- Clonazepam na dose de 0,5 mg/kg a cada 8 h pode resultar em melhora de cães da raça Cavalier King Charles spaniel com síndrome de hipertonicidade (síndrome de queda).

CONTRAINDICAÇÕES/INTERAÇÕES POSSÍVEIS
- Antagonistas serotoninérgicos — aumentam a gravidade dos sinais clínicos.
- Ácido acetilsalicílico, indometacina, fenilbutazona, Banamine® (flunixina meglumina) e penicilina — podem exacerbar os sinais clínicos.

ACOMPANHAMENTO

MONITORIZAÇÃO DO PACIENTE
Não é progressiva.

PREVENÇÃO
- Não incentivar o acasalamento dos animais acometidos e aparentados.
- Não repetir os cruzamentos entre machos e fêmeas que resultem em uma prole acometida.

EVOLUÇÃO ESPERADA E PROGNÓSTICO
- Leve a moderada — prognóstico razoável a bom a longo prazo; em geral, a incapacidade é aceitável pelos proprietários; não progressiva.
- Grave — prognóstico reservado.

DIVERSOS

DISTÚRBIOS ASSOCIADOS
N/D.

FATORES RELACIONADOS COM A IDADE
N/D.

POTENCIAL ZOONÓTICO
N/D.

GESTAÇÃO/FERTILIDADE/REPRODUÇÃO
N/D.

ABREVIATURA(S)
- SNC = sistema nervoso central.

Sugestões de Leitura
Geiger KM, Klopp LS. Use of a selective serotonin reuptake inhibitor for treatment of episodes of hypertonia and kyphosis in a young adult Scottish Terrier. JAVMA 2009, 235:168-171.
Meyers KM, Clemmons RM. Scotty cramp. In: Kirk RW, ed., Current Veterinary Therapy VIII. Philadelphia: Saunders, 1983, pp. 702-704.
Shelton GD. Muscle pain, cramps and hypertonicity. Vet Clin North Am Small Anim Pract 2004, 34(6):1483-1496.

Autor Georgina Child
Consultor Editorial Peter K. Shires

Miopatia Não Inflamatória — Distrofia Muscular Hereditária Ligada ao Cromossomo X

CONSIDERAÇÕES GERAIS

REVISÃO
- Distrofia muscular é uma miopatia generalizada hereditária, progressiva e degenerativa.
- A forma mais comum em cães ocorre como resultado de uma deficiência da proteína associada à membrana muscular, a distrofina.
- O gene responsável pela codificação da distrofina está situado no cromossomo X; por essa razão, é provável que mutações recentes sejam responsáveis por casos isolados.
- A distrofia muscular atribuída à deficiência de distrofina tem um modo de herança ligado ao cromossomo X; além disso, os animais acometidos são predominantemente machos.
- Deficiência da distrofina — identificada pela primeira vez em cães da raça Golden retriever. Subsequentemente, foram relatados casos nas raças Setter irlandês, Samoieda, Rottweiler, Pastor belga, Pembroke Welsh corgi, Spaniel britânico, Pointer alemão de pelo curto, Rat terrier, Schnauzer miniatura, Labrador retriever, Malamute do Alasca, Fox terrier de pelo duro, Spitz japonês, Cavalier King Charles spaniel. São prováveis casos esporádicos em outras raças.
- Também ocorre distrofia muscular hipertrófica associada à deficiência de distrofina em gatos domésticos de pelo curto.
- A deficiência de outras proteínas associadas ao tecido muscular, p. ex., laminina alfa-2 (merosina) e sarcoglicano, foi recém-identificada em cães e gatos, mas não é necessariamente ligada ao cromossomo X (fêmeas acometidas).
- Também há relatos de distrofias musculares não classificadas em outros cães (machos e fêmeas).
- Uma miopatia hereditária e não progressiva compatível com distrofia muscular com modo de herança autossômico recessivo ocorre em gatos jovens da raça Devon Rex.
- Uma distrofia muscular congênita foi identificada em gatos jovens machos da raça Sphynx (Esfinge).

IDENTIFICAÇÃO
- Observada principalmente em cães neonatos e jovens (<1 ano).
- Descrita em gatos.
- A distrofia muscular causada por deficiência de distrofina afeta, sobretudo, machos.
- Sabe-se que diversas raças caninas são acometidas. Mais bem descrita em Golden retriever.
- Fêmeas — costumam ser portadoras de defeito do gene responsável pela codificação da distrofina, mas as fêmeas com deficiência dessa proteína podem exibir fraqueza muscular, tremores, deformidades dos membros e intolerância ao exercício.
- Pode-se observar distrofia muscular atribuída a defeitos de outras proteínas musculares ou defeitos não classificados em cães e gatos jovens machos ou fêmeas de qualquer raça.

SINAIS CLÍNICOS
Cães
- Golden retriever — intolerância ao exercício; marcha afetada; marcha saltitante dos membros pélvicos como coelho; postura plantígrada; trismo parcial; atrofia muscular (especialmente os músculos do tronco e o temporal); hipertrofia de alguns músculos (sobretudo a língua); cifose; lordose; salivação; disfagia; pneumonia por aspiração (causada pelo envolvimento faríngeo e/ou esofágico).
- Outras raças — sinais clínicos semelhantes; tais sinais também incluem vômito e megaesôfago.
- As anormalidades variam em termos de gravidade, início e evolução; podem ser observadas já com 6 semanas de vida; tendem a se estabilizar por volta dos 6 meses.
- Falta de desenvolvimento e sucção ineficaz do leite — podem ser evidentes nos filhotes caninos jovens.
- Insuficiência cardíaca — pode ocorrer em função de miocardiopatia.
- Pode ocorrer o desenvolvimento de contraturas musculares graves.
- Reflexos espinais — normais inicialmente; podem se tornar hipoativos.

Gatos
- Deficientes em distrofina — hipertrofia muscular; marcha enrijecida; rigidez cervical; intolerância ao exercício; vômito; podem-se observar nódulos calcificados na língua.
- Geralmente acomete animais jovens, mas não se mostrou aparente em um único gato até os 21 meses de vida.
- Outras miopatias hereditárias em gatos podem causar atrofia muscular; fraqueza; ventroflexão da cabeça e do pescoço; protrusão dorsal das escápulas, com os músculos tríceps braquial e cervical dorsal mais gravemente acometidos.

CAUSAS E FATORES DE RISCO
- Deficiência de distrofina — defeito hereditário do cromossomo X.
- Outras distrofias musculares podem não estar ligadas ao cromossomo X.
- Miopatia do Devon Rex — autossômica recessiva.

DIAGNÓSTICO

DIAGNÓSTICO DIFERENCIAL
Outras miopatias hereditárias, infecciosas (sobretudo por protozoários), imunomediadas ou metabólicas; distinguidas pelo exame histológico do músculo e pela demonstração da deficiência de distrofina.

HEMOGRAMA/BIOQUÍMICA/URINÁLISE
- Deficiência de distrofina — normais, exceto pela elevação acentuada na creatina quinase sérica (pode ser >10.000 U/L; aumento adicional após o exercício). Também é provável que a atividade da AST esteja elevada.
- Outras distrofias musculares — a creatina quinase pode estar normal.

OUTROS TESTES LABORATORIAIS
- Biopsia muscular — a deficiência de distrofina é demonstrada pela avaliação imuno-histoquímica de músculo recém-congelado; método diagnóstico.
- Análise imuno-histoquímica de músculo — também pode avaliar o paciente em busca de anormalidades em outras proteínas musculares, incluindo proteínas associadas à distrofina, laminina, sarcoglicano.
- Teste sorológico — pode ser justificável para descartar causas infecciosas e imunomediadas.

MÉTODOS DIAGNÓSTICOS
Eletromiografia — revela descargas repetitivas complexas.

ACHADOS PATOLÓGICOS
Exame histológico do músculo (deficiência de distrofina) — necrose e regeneração das fibras musculares; mineralização das miofibras (pode ser notável); hipertrofia das miofibras (pode haver variação no tamanho das miofibras); fibrose.

TRATAMENTO

Nenhum tratamento se mostrou eficaz.

MEDICAÇÕES

MEDICAMENTO(S)
Glicocorticoides — podem proporcionar certa melhora; razão desconhecida. Contudo, a calcificação das miofibras aumenta, o que pode ser deletério.

ACOMPANHAMENTO

MONITORIZAÇÃO DO PACIENTE
Monitorizar periodicamente quanto à ocorrência de pneumonia por aspiração ou miocardiopatia.

PREVENÇÃO
- Desestimular o acasalamento dos animais acometidos.
- Não repetir os cruzamentos entre machos e fêmeas que resultem em prole acometida.

COMPLICAÇÕES POSSÍVEIS
Complicações como pneumonia por aspiração ou miocardiopatia podem ser potencialmente letais.

EVOLUÇÃO ESPERADA E PROGNÓSTICO
- Prognóstico geral — reservado a mau, pois não existe tratamento paliativo eficaz.
- Golden retriever — os sinais tendem a se estabilizar aos 6 meses de vida.
- Outras raças caninas e gatos — evolução variável.

DIVERSOS

ABREVIATURA(S)
- AST = aspartato aminotransferase.

Sugestões de Leitura
Dickinson PJ, LeCouteur RA. Feline neuromuscular disorders. Vet Clin North Am Small Anim Pract 2004, 34(6):1307-1359.
Kornegay JN. The X-linked muscular dystrophies. In: Kirk RW, Bonagura JD, eds., Current Veterinary Therapy XI. Philadelphia: Saunders, 1992, pp. 1042-1047.
Schatzberg SJ, Shelton GD. Newly identified neuromuscular disorders. Vet Clin North Am Small Anim Pract 2004, 34(6):1497-1524.
Shelton GD, Engvall E. Muscular dystrophies and other inherited myopathies. Vet Clin North Am Small Anim Pract 2002, 32(1):103-124.

Autor Georgina Child
Consultor Editorial Peter K. Shires

Miopatia Não Inflamatória — Endócrina

CONSIDERAÇÕES GERAIS

DEFINIÇÃO
Miopatias associadas a várias endocrinopatias (incluindo hipotireoidismo, hipertireoidismo, hipoadrenocorticismo, hiperadrenocorticismo) e associadas ao uso exógeno de corticosteroides (miopatia esteroide).

FISIOPATOLOGIA

Com Disfunção Adrenal
- Excesso de glicocorticoide — metabolismo proteico muscular prejudicado; pode acelerar a degradação de proteína miofibrilar e solúvel na musculatura esquelética; diminuição do metabolismo dos carboidratos em virtude da indução de um estado resistente à insulina; pode-se notar uma elevação dos níveis de ACTH.
- Insuficiência adrenal — insuficiência circulatória; desequilíbrio hidreletrolítico; metabolismo comprometido dos carboidratos.

Com Doença Tireóidea
- Hipertireoidismo — aumento da respiração mitocondrial; degradação proteica e oxidação lipídica aceleradas; depleção do glicogênio; diminuição da captação de glicose.
- Hipotireoidismo — metabolismo energético muscular comprometido pela diminuição na degradação do glicogênio e na gliconeogênese, bem como na capacidade oxidativa e glicolítica; metabolismo prejudicado dos carboidratos estimulado pela insulina.

SISTEMA(S) ACOMETIDO(S)
- Neuromuscular — metabolismo energético prejudicado.
- Cardiovascular — metabolismo energético comprometido; distúrbios circulatórios.

GENÉTICA
N/D.

INCIDÊNCIA/PREVALÊNCIA
- Incidência exata desconhecida.
- Miopatias relacionadas com corticosteroides exógenos — comuns.
- Miopatias associadas a síndrome de Cushing e hipotireoidismo — não são incomuns.

DISTRIBUIÇÃO GEOGRÁFICA
Provavelmente mundial.

IDENTIFICAÇÃO

Espécies
- Cães — miopatia esteroide; fraqueza associada a hiperadrenocorticismo e hipoadrenocorticismo; hipotireoidismo.
- Gatos — fraqueza associada a hipertireoidismo.

Raça(s) Predominante(s)
Acomete várias raças.

Idade Média e Faixa Etária
- Miopatia esteroide — cães de qualquer idade.
- Outros distúrbios — ver doença específica.

Sexo Predominante
Nenhuma predileção sexual encontrada.

SINAIS CLÍNICOS

Comentários Gerais
Utilização de corticosteroide nos cães — músculos muito suscetíveis; atrofia muscular (particularmente os músculos da mastigação) não é rara com o uso prolongado desses agentes terapêuticos.

Achados Anamnésicos
- Fraqueza, atrofia e rigidez musculares.
- Regurgitação.
- Disfagia.
- Disfonia.

Achados do Exame Físico
- Fraqueza muscular, rigidez, cãibras e mialgia.
- Hipertrofia ou atrofia musculares.
- Pode-se não observar a presença de outros sinais clínicos de um distúrbio endócrino.

CAUSAS
- Disfunção endócrina.
- Autoimune.
- Neoplásica.

FATORES DE RISCO
N/D.

DIAGNÓSTICO

DIAGNÓSTICO DIFERENCIAL
- Miopatias inflamatórias — distinguidas por biopsia muscular.
- Miopatias não inflamatórias — diferenciadas por biopsia muscular.

HEMOGRAMA/BIOQUÍMICA/URINÁLISE
- Testes de referência basal — anormalidades compatíveis com distúrbio endócrino.
- Creatina quinase sérica — costuma permanecer normal, mas pode estar levemente aumentada em caso de necrose das fibras musculares.

OUTROS TESTES LABORATORIAIS
Testes de função da tireoide e adrenal — devem ser diagnósticos.

DIAGNÓSTICO POR IMAGEM
- Estudos dinâmicos — avaliar função faríngea e esofágica; com regurgitação e disfagia.
- Avaliação cardíaca — para gatos com hipertireoidismo.

MÉTODOS DIAGNÓSTICOS
- Biopsia muscular — é importante a caracterização do tipo de fibras em cortes recém-congelados; cortes em parafina não serão diagnósticos.
- Eletromiografia.

ACHADOS PATOLÓGICOS
- Hiperadrenocorticismo e miopatias esteroides — atrofia seletiva das fibras musculares do tipo 2; pode haver fibras lobuladas ou vermelhas rotas com miotonia associada.
- Hipoadrenocorticismo — resultados normais nas biopsias musculares.
- Hipertireoidismo (gatos) — resultados normais nas biopsias musculares.
- Hipotireoidismo — atrofia das fibras do tipo 2; pode-se notar um aumento nas fibras do tipo 1; podem-se observar depósitos positivos ao PAS e corpúsculos de bastonetes de nemalina.

TRATAMENTO

CUIDADO(S) DE SAÚDE ADEQUADO(S)
Depende(m) do distúrbio endócrino específico.

CUIDADO(S) DE ENFERMAGEM
Fisioterapia — em caso de manifestações musculosqueléticas.

ATIVIDADE
- Miopatia clínica por corticosteroide (seres humanos) — a inatividade piora a condição; atividade muscular aumentada pode evitar parcialmente a atrofia.
- Fisioterapia — pode ajudar a evitar e tratar a fraqueza e a emaciação musculares em cães submetidos a glicocorticoides.

DIETA
- Regurgitação e megaesôfago — alimentar em plano elevado.
- Disfagia e dilatação esofágica — dar o alimento com a consistência mais bem tolerada.
- Sonda alimentar gástrica — se a alimentação por via oral não for tolerada.

ORIENTAÇÃO AO PROPRIETÁRIO
Depende do distúrbio endócrino específico.

CONSIDERAÇÕES CIRÚRGICAS
Remoção da neoplasia.

MEDICAÇÕES

MEDICAMENTO(S) DE ESCOLHA
- Dependem do distúrbio endócrino específico.
- Miopatia por corticosteroide — reduzir a dosagem desse agente terapêutico ao nível mais baixo possível; usar um corticosteroide não fluorado e doses em dias alternados.
- Armazenamento de lipídios dentro das miofibras em caso de miopatia esteroide — L-carnitina (50 mg/kg VO a cada 12 h) pode melhorar a força muscular.

CONTRAINDICAÇÕES
N/D.

PRECAUÇÕES
Dependem do distúrbio endócrino específico.

INTERAÇÕES POSSÍVEIS
N/D.

MEDICAMENTO(S) ALTERNATIVO(S)
Corticosteroides fluorados, triancinolona, betametasona e dexametasona — têm maior probabilidade de produzir fraqueza muscular; utilizar dose equivalente de algum outro corticosteroide.

ACOMPANHAMENTO

MONITORIZAÇÃO DO PACIENTE
- Depende do distúrbio endócrino específico.
- Miopatia por esteroide — deve-se notar o retorno da força e da massa musculares com a redução do uso desse tipo de medicamento.

PREVENÇÃO
N/D.

COMPLICAÇÕES POSSÍVEIS
Dependem dos distúrbios endócrinos específicos.

EVOLUÇÃO ESPERADA E PROGNÓSTICO
- Miotonia associada a hiperadrenocorticismo — prognóstico mau quanto à resolução.
- Miopatia esteroide — prognóstico bom quanto ao retorno da força e da massa musculares; a recuperação pode levar semanas.
- Miopatia hipotireoidea — é comum a melhora na dor e no enrijecimento musculares.

MIOPATIA NÃO INFLAMATÓRIA — ENDÓCRINA

- Hipertireoidismo (gatos) — prognóstico bom quanto ao retorno da força muscular após a reversão do estado eutireoideo.
- Hipoadrenocorticismo — prognóstico bom quanto ao retorno da força muscular.
- Disfagia e regurgitação — podem desaparecer com o tratamento adequado.

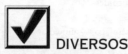
DIVERSOS
DISTÚRBIOS ASSOCIADOS
- Podem-se notar múltiplas endocrinopatias.
- Hipotireoidismo (cães) — miastenia grave concomitante.

FATORES RELACIONADOS COM A IDADE
N/D.

POTENCIAL ZOONÓTICO
N/D.

GESTAÇÃO/FERTILIDADE/REPRODUÇÃO
Desconhecida.

ABREVIATURA(S)
- ACTH = hormônio adrenocorticotrópico.
- PAS = ácido periódico de Schiff.

RECURSOS DA INTERNET
Comparative Neuromuscular Laboratory: http://vetneuromuscular.ucsd.edu.

Sugestões de Leitura
Jaggy A, Oliver JE, Ferguson DC, et al. Neurological manifestations of hypothyroidism: A retrospective study of 29 cases. J Vet Intern Med 1994; 8:328-330.
LeCouteur RA, Dow SW, Sisson AF. Metabolic and endocrine myopathies of dogs and cats. Semin Vet Med Surg Small Anim 1989, 4:146-155.
Platt SR. Neuromuscular complications in endocrine and metabolic disorders. Vet Clin North Am 2002, 31:125-146.
Rossmeisl JH, Duncan RB, Inzana KD, Panciera DL, Shelton GD. Longitudinal study of the effects of chronic hypothyroidism on skeletal muscle in dogs. Am J Vet Res 2009, 70:879-889.

Autor G. Diane Shelton
Consultor Editorial Peter K. Shires

Miopatia Não Inflamatória — Hereditária no Labrador Retriever

CONSIDERAÇÕES GERAIS

REVISÃO
- Miopatia hereditária de cães da raça Labrador retriever.
- Reconhecida mundialmente.
- Modo de herança autossômico recessivo simples.
- Mais recentemente nomeada como miopatia centronuclear ou miopatia tipo centronuclear.
- Mecanismo(s) fisiopatológico(s) ainda desconhecido(s); no entanto, foi identificada a mutação genética causal.
- Perda dos reflexos tendinosos e exame histológico do músculo — mais típicos de alguma causa neurogênica do que miopática.
- Não há nenhuma anormalidade imuno-histoquímica sugestiva de algum distúrbio de proteína muscular.
- Nenhuma alteração morfológica foi identificada no SNC ou nos nervos periféricos.

IDENTIFICAÇÃO
- Ocorre em cães da raça Labrador retriever de pelagem negra e amarela.
- Idade de início — variável (6 semanas a 7 meses); mais comumente identificada aos 3-4 meses.
- Acomete machos e fêmeas.

SINAIS CLÍNICOS
- A gravidade varia desde marcha afetada e intolerância ao exercício até fraqueza muscular intensa, marcha com o membro pélvico saltitante como coelho, ventroflexão da cabeça e do pescoço, dorso arqueado e postura articular anormal (posição em "jarrete de vaca", carpos hiperestendidos).
- Piora com o exercício, a agitação e o clima frio.
- O paciente pode entrar em colapso com o exercício forçado.
- Alguma melhora em repouso.
- Atrofia muscular generalizada — leve a grave.
- Atrofia com frequência mais proeminente do membro proximal e dos músculos mastigatórios.
- Reflexos tendinosos — normais, hipoativos ou ausentes.
- Ocasionalmente, os pacientes permanecem em decúbito ou desenvolvem megaesôfago.

CAUSAS E FATORES DE RISCO
Modo de herança autossômico recessivo.

DIAGNÓSTICO

DIAGNÓSTICO DIFERENCIAL
- Com pouca atrofia muscular — a intolerância ao exercício pode mimetizar sinais de miastenia grave, cardiopatia ou doença ortopédica.
- Com atrofia muscular acentuada — considerar outras miopatias (infecciosas, imunomediadas, metabólicas, congênitas) e distúrbios generalizados atribuídos ao neurônio motor inferior.
- Miopatia infecciosa atribuída à infecção congênita por *Neospora caninum* tem incidência mais alta em cães da raça Labrador retriever.
- Distrofia muscular congênita em cão macho causada por deficiência de distrofina também foi relatada nessa raça.
- Em um Labrador retriever macho e jovem, também foi descrita uma suposta miopatia hereditária semelhante em termos histológicos à miopatia hereditária do Dinamarquês

HEMOGRAMA/BIOQUÍMICA/URINÁLISE
Creatina quinase — normal ou leve a moderadamente elevada.

OUTROS TESTES LABORATORIAIS
Há um teste de DNA disponível no mercado para a detecção da mutação genética causal.

DIAGNÓSTICO POR IMAGEM
N/D.

MÉTODOS DIAGNÓSTICOS
- EMG — atividade espontânea, incluindo descargas repetitivas complexas, especialmente no membro proximal e nos músculos mastigatórios; pode não revelar quaisquer anormalidades em casos de doença leve.
- Exame histológico do músculo — revela variação no tamanho da fibra, atrofia angular de ambas as miofibras (tipos 1 e 2), atrofia agrupada, aumento nos núcleos centrais, degeneração e regeneração musculares, além de fibrose; pode-se notar deficiência nas miofibras do tipo 2 ou predomínio nas miofibras do tipo 1.

TRATAMENTO

- Não há nenhum tratamento específico.
- Evitar o frio, pois ele exacerba os sinais clínicos.
- Não incentivar o acasalamento dos animais acometidos, bem como de pais e ninhadas dos cães afetados.
- Não repetir cruzamentos entre machos e fêmeas que resultem em uma prole acometida.

MEDICAÇÕES

MEDICAMENTO(S)
A suplementação de L-carnitina (50 mg/kg VO 2 vezes ao dia) pode ser benéfica no restabelecimento da força muscular.

CONTRAINDICAÇÕES/INTERAÇÕES POSSÍVEIS
Nenhuma conhecida.

ACOMPANHAMENTO

- Os sinais clínicos costumam se estabilizar em aproximadamente 1 ano de idade.
- Doença leve — pode ser um animal de estimação aceitável; pode apresentar alguma melhora na tolerância ao exercício.
- Pneumonia por aspiração — risco em cães com megaesôfago.

DIVERSOS

DISTÚRBIOS ASSOCIADOS
N/D.

FATORES RELACIONADOS COM A IDADE
N/D.

POTENCIAL ZOONÓTICO
N/D.

GESTAÇÃO/FERTILIDADE/REPRODUÇÃO
N/D.

ABREVIATURA(S)
- EMG = eletromiografia.
- SNC = sistema nervoso central.

RECURSOS DA INTERNET
www.ivis.org, Labrador Retriever Hereditary Myopathy (Miopatia Hereditária do Labrador Retriever).

Sugestões de Leitura
Cosford KL, Taylor SM, Thompson L, Shelton GD. A possible new inherited myopathy in a young Labrador retriever. Can Vet J 2008, 49(4):393-397.
McKerrell RE, Braund KG. Hereditary myopathy of Labrador retrievers. In: Kirk RW, Bonagura JD, eds., Current Veterinary Therapy X. Philadelphia: Saunders, 1989, pp. 820-821.
Schatzberg SJ, Shelton GD. Newly identified neuromuscular disorders. Vet Clin North Am Small Anim Pract 2004, 34(6):1497-1524.
Shelton GD, Engvall E. Muscular dystrophies and other inherited myopathies. Vet Clin North Am Small Anim Pract 2002, 32(1):103-124.

Autor Georgina Child
Consultor Editorial Peter K. Shires

Miopatia Não Inflamatória — Metabólica

CONSIDERAÇÕES GERAIS

DEFINIÇÃO
• Miopatia associada a distúrbios do metabolismo do glicogênio, metabolismo lipídico ou fosforilação oxidativa e metabolismo da mitocôndria.
• Atualmente, pouco caracterizada na medicina veterinária.

FISIOPATOLOGIA
• Geralmente associada a defeitos enzimáticos hereditários ou adquiridos, envolvendo vias metabólicas importantes.
• Pode resultar no armazenamento de subprodutos metabólicos anormais ou anormalidades morfológicas das mitocôndrias.

SISTEMA(S) ACOMETIDO(S)
• Cardiovascular — dependência do metabolismo oxidativo para produção de energia.
• Hemático/linfático/imune — as hemácias dependem do metabolismo glicolítico.
• Nervoso — dependência do metabolismo glicolítico e oxidativo para produção de energia.
• Neuromuscular — dependência do metabolismo oxidativo para produção de energia.
• Produtos de armazenamento em outros órgãos — fígado; baço.

GENÉTICA
Indeterminada.

INCIDÊNCIA/PREVALÊNCIA
Rara, exceto as miopatias provocadas por armazenamento de lipídios.

DISTRIBUIÇÃO GEOGRÁFICA
Desconhecida; provavelmente mundial.

IDENTIFICAÇÃO
Espécies
Cães e gatos.

Raça(s) Predominante(s)
• Deficiência da fosfofrutoquinase muscular — Springer spaniel inglês, Cocker spaniel americano, Whippet.
• Deficiência de maltase ácida — Lapland.
• Deficiência de enzima desramificante — Pastor alemão, Akita, Retriever de pelo encaracolado.
• Deficiência da piruvato desidrogenase fosfatase 1 — Clumber spaniel, Sussex spaniel.
• Miopatia mitocondrial — Old English sheepdog, Yorkshire terrier e, possivelmente, Jack Russell terrier.

Idade Média e Faixa Etária
• Defeitos metabólicos hereditários — 2-3 meses.
• Defeitos metabólicos adquiridos — adultos.

Sexo Predominante
Nenhum encontrado.

SINAIS CLÍNICOS
Comentários Gerais
Pouquíssimas dessas condições foram descritas de forma adequada.

Achados Anamnésicos
• Fraqueza muscular.
• Intolerância ao exercício.
• Cãibras.
• Colapso.
• Regurgitação e/ou disfagia.
• Anormalidades esofágicas e/ou faríngeas.
• Urina escura; mioglobinúria; hemoglobinúria.
• Encefalopatia.
• Vômito.

Achados do Exame Físico
• Fraqueza relacionada com o exercício, enrijecimento e/ou cãibras.
• Exame neurológico anormal — desorientação; estupor; coma.
• Distensão abdominal — acúmulo de produto de armazenamento no fígado.
• Pode parecer normal, com sinais clínicos flutuantes.

CAUSAS
• Erro inato do metabolismo.
• Defeito metabólico adquirido.
• Infecções virais.
• Induzida por medicamento.
• Fatores ambientais.

FATORES DE RISCO
• Distúrbios hereditários.
• Base genética pertinente.
• Outros desconhecidos.

DIAGNÓSTICO

DIAGNÓSTICO DIFERENCIAL
• Miopatias inflamatórias — diferenciadas por biopsia muscular.
• Outras miopatias não inflamatórias — diferenciadas por biopsia muscular.
• Outras encefalopatias metabólicas — diferenciadas por avaliação laboratorial.

HEMOGRAMA/BIOQUÍMICA/URINÁLISE
• Níveis plasmáticos de lactato e piruvato — elevados em repouso ou após o exercício, com distúrbios de oxidação dos ácidos graxos ou do processo de fosforilação oxidativa; nenhuma elevação nos distúrbios glicolíticos.
• Níveis de creatina quinase sérica — podem estar elevados com o exercício e normais em repouso; podem ficar persistentemente elevados.
• Hipoglicemia — pode ocorrer em alguns distúrbios glicolíticos e oxidativos.
• Hiperamonemia — pode ocorrer nos defeitos do ciclo da ureia.

OUTROS TESTES LABORATORIAIS
• Quantificação dos aminoácidos plasmáticos — acúmulos anormais.
• Quantificação dos ácidos orgânicos urinários — para demonstrar a produção anormal de ácido orgânico.
• Quantificação dos níveis plasmáticos, urinários e musculares da carnitina — podem estar baixos nos distúrbios primários ou secundários desse aminoácido; baixos nas acidúrias orgânicas primárias.
• Ensaios enzimáticos específicos — dependem do defeito metabólico sob suspeita.
• Culturas de fibroblastos — estudo do defeito metabólico.
• Testes de DNA — para identificação dos cães acometidos e portadores sempre que disponíveis.

DIAGNÓSTICO POR IMAGEM
RM — avaliar o SNC; revela anormalidades nos seres humanos.

MÉTODOS DIAGNÓSTICOS
• Microscopia óptica — cortes musculares recém-congelados; demonstra os produtos de armazenamento (glicogênio, lipídio) ou a presença de mitocôndrias anormais.
• Microscopia eletrônica do músculo — revela mitocôndrias anormais, inclusões paracristalinas e acúmulo de glicogênio ou de lipídio.
• Avaliação do sistema cardiovascular — pode haver miocardiopatia concomitante.
• Outras biopsias orgânicas — em caso de organomegalia.

ACHADOS PATOLÓGICOS
• Gotículas de triglicerídeos no músculo — miopatia por armazenamento de lipídios.
• Fibras vermelhas rotas no músculo — miopatia mitocondrial.
• Depósito muscular de glicogênio — distúrbio de armazenamento do glicogênio.

TRATAMENTO

CUIDADO(S) DE SAÚDE ADEQUADO(S)
• Internação — pode necessitar de cuidados intensivos em caso de encefalopatia grave, crises convulsivas, acidemia láctica, hipoglicemia ou hiperamonemia.
• Tratamento ambulatorial — sinais clínicos relacionados apenas com o sistema neuromuscular.

CUIDADO(S) DE ENFERMAGEM
Depende do tipo e da gravidade do distúrbio.

ATIVIDADE
Restrição ao exercício — na presença de fraqueza muscular, enrijecimento ou colapso induzido pelo exercício.

DIETA
• Evitar períodos prolongados de jejum.
• Restrições — dependem do defeito subjacente.
• Terapia com vitamina e cofator — determinada pelo defeito subjacente.

ORIENTAÇÃO AO PROPRIETÁRIO
• Alertar o proprietário sobre a impossibilidade de cura de grande parte dos defeitos metabólicos, embora alguns possam ser tratados.
• Aconselhar contra acasalamento dos indivíduos acometidos.

CONSIDERAÇÕES CIRÚRGICAS
N/D.

MEDICAÇÕES

MEDICAMENTO(S) DE ESCOLHA
• Dependem da anormalidade e dos sinais clínicos.
• Miopatias por armazenamento de lipídios — L-carnitina (50 mg/kg VO a cada 12 h); riboflavina (50-100 mg VO a cada 24 h); coenzima Q10 (1 mg/kg VO a cada 24 h).
• Miopatias mitocondriais — podem se beneficiar com tratamento semelhante àquele listado para miopatias por armazenamento de lipídios.

CONTRAINDICAÇÕES
Nenhuma conhecida.

PRECAUÇÕES
Evitar jejum e exercício extenuante se precipitarem os sinais clínicos.

INTERAÇÕES POSSÍVEIS
N/D.

MIOPATIA NÃO INFLAMATÓRIA — METABÓLICA

MEDICAMENTO(S) ALTERNATIVO(S)
N/D.

ACOMPANHAMENTO

MONITORIZAÇÃO DO PACIENTE
• Miopatias por armazenamento de lipídios — retorno da força muscular; eliminação da dor muscular.
• Creatina quinase sérica elevada — deve retornar ao normal.

PREVENÇÃO
N/D.

COMPLICAÇÕES POSSÍVEIS
Comprometimento neurológico grave.

EVOLUÇÃO ESPERADA E PROGNÓSTICO
• Distúrbio intratável — prognóstico mau.
• Miopatias por armazenamento de lipídios — prognóstico bom se não houver acidemia orgânica subjacente.

DIVERSOS

DISTÚRBIOS ASSOCIADOS
• Síndrome de Cushing iatrogênica e espontânea (i. e., de ocorrência natural).
• Miopatias por armazenamento de lipídios — encontradas em alguns cães.
• Anemia hemolítica — causada por defeito metabólico subjacente.

FATORES RELACIONADOS COM A IDADE
• Erros inatos — geralmente encontrados em cães jovens.
• Defeitos adquiridos — constatados em cães adultos.

POTENCIAL ZOONÓTICO
N/D.

GESTAÇÃO/FERTILIDADE/REPRODUÇÃO
Desconhecida.

SINÔNIMO(S)
• Deficiência de maltase ácida — glicogenose tipo II.
• Doença de Cori — glicogenose tipo III.
• Distúrbios do armazenamento de glicogênio.
• Miopatias por armazenamento de lipídios.
• Miopatias mitocondriais.
• Deficiência de fosfofrutoquinase — glicogenose tipo VII.

ABREVIATURA(S)
• RM = ressonância magnética.
• SNC = sistema nervoso central.

RECURSOS DA INTERNET
• Comparative Neuromuscular Laboratory: http://vetneuromuscular.ucsd.edu.
• PennGen: http://vet.upenn.edu/researchcenters/penngen.
• VetGenLLC: http://www.vetgen.com/.

Sugestões de Leitura
Cameron JM, Maj MC, Levandovskiy V, MacKay N, Shelton GD, Robinson BH. Identification of a canine model of pyruvate dehydrogenase phosphatase 1 deficiency. Mol Genet Metab 2007, 90:15-23.
Fyfe JC. Molecular diagnosis of inherited neuromuscular disease. Vet Clin North Am 2002, 31:287-300.
Gerber K, Harvey JW, D'Agorne S, Wood J, Giger U. Hemolysis, myopathy, and cardiac disease associated with hereditary phosphofructokinase deficiency in two Whippets. Vet Clin Path 2009, 38:46-51.
Platt SR. Neuromuscular complications in endocrine and metabolic disorders. Vet Clin North Am 2002, 31:125-146.
Shelton GD. Canine lipid storage myopathies. In: Bonagura JD, Kirk RW, eds., Current Veterinary Therapy XII. Philadelphia: Saunders, 1995, pp. 1161-1163.
Shelton GD, Engvall E. Muscular dystrophies and other inherited myopathies. Vet Clin North Am 2002, 31:103-124.

Autor G. Diane Shelton
Consultor Editorial Peter K. Shires

Miopatia Não Inflamatória — Miotonia Hereditária

CONSIDERAÇÕES GERAIS

REVISÃO
• Miopatia caracterizada por contração persistente ou relaxamento tardio das fibras musculares no início do movimento ou quando estimuladas a contrair. • Pode acometer todos os músculos esqueléticos. • A miotonia pode ser congênita ou adquirida. • Miotonia congênita — atribuída a algum defeito do sarcolema e, em alguns casos, pode estar associada à condutância anormal de cloreto pela membrana muscular. • Miotonia adquirida pode estar associada à miopatia inflamatória ou não inflamatória e pode ser induzida experimentalmente pela ingestão de herbicidas 2,4D e dicamba.
• Hiperadrenocorticismo pode resultar em miopatia indutora de sinais clínicos semelhantes à miotonia.
• Neuromiotonia e mioquimia são distúrbios raros caracterizados por atividade contínua das fibras musculares que supostamente é atribuída à hiperexcitabilidade de ramificações nervosas terminais (neuromiotonia) ou hiperexcitabilidade do axônio dos neurônios motores em qualquer nível (mioquimia) e não um distúrbio muscular primário. • Neuromiotonia caracteriza-se por rigidez muscular e relaxamento tardio. • Mioquimia descreve movimentos musculares ondulantes rítmicos que produzem um movimento ondulado da pele. • A causa de neuromiotonia e mioquimia em casos relatados permanece incerta. • Foi feito um diagnóstico histológico de ataxia hereditária de cães da raça Jack Russell terrier em vários animais acometidos dessa raça com atividade contínua das fibras musculares e ataxia concomitante.

IDENTIFICAÇÃO
• Miotonia congênita — descrita nos cães jovens das raças Chow chow e Schnauzer miniatura; raramente observada em outras raças caninas. • Os sinais clínicos são observados quando os filhotes acometidos começam a andar. • Miotonia adquirida — todas as raças de qualquer idade são potencialmente suscetíveis. • Há relatos de miotonia em gatos domésticos jovens.
• Neuromiotonia e mioquimia (atividade contínua das fibras musculares) — descritas em cães jovens predominantemente da raça Jack Russell terrier no mundo todo e, raras vezes, em outras raças caninas e no gato.

SINAIS CLÍNICOS
Achados Anamnésicos
• Dificuldade de se levantar. • Rigidez após o repouso ou o início da atividade. • Pode-se notar dispneia, mudança da vocalização, disfagia e/ou regurgitação, sobretudo após a alimentação. • Pode melhorar com o exercício. • Pode ser exacerbada pelo frio. • Rigidez muscular e mioquimia observadas em cães jovens da raça Jack Russell terrier podem resultar em hipertermia potencialmente letal. Nessa raça, os sinais clínicos são episódicos, embora os cães acometidos também possam ter ataxia contínua.

Achados do Exame Físico
• Hipertrofia dos músculos da parte proximal do membro, dos músculos do pescoço, e da língua. • A língua pode se projetar da boca. • Abdução dos membros torácicos. • Marcha rígida, afetada e saltitante como coelho nos membros pélvicos. • O paciente pode cair e permanecer rígido em decúbito lateral por curtos períodos de tempo. Pode vir a ficar cianótico. • Os cães acometidos da raça Schnauzer miniatura podem ter anormalidades craniofaciais, como encurtamento mandibular.

CAUSAS E FATORES DE RISCO
• Chow chow — suspeita-se de modo de herança autossômico recessivo. • Schnauzer miniatura — modo de herança autossômico recessivo conhecido. Mutação no gene CLCN1 responsável pela codificação dos canais de cloreto C1C-1 voltagem-dependentes da musculatura esquelética. Essa mutação também foi encontrada em cão Boiadeiro australiano com miotonia hereditária.

DIAGNÓSTICO

DIAGNÓSTICO DIFERENCIAL
Outras miopatias — distinguidas não só pela identificação, mas também pelos achados clínicos, eletromiográficos e histológicos.

HEMOGRAMA/BIOQUÍMICA/URINÁLISE
• Creatina quinase — pode permanecer normal ou levemente aumentada em miotonia congênita.
• Creatinina quinase — pode estar elevada em miotonia adquirida.

OUTROS TESTES LABORATORIAIS
Há um teste de DNA disponível para detecção de alelo mutante em cães afetados e portadores da raça Schnauzer miniatura.

MÉTODOS DIAGNÓSTICOS
• Percussão dos músculos e da língua em cães conscientes e anestesiados — provoca a formação de covinhas (depressões) que se mantêm.
• Eletromiografia — miotonia caracterizada por descargas multifocais ou generalizadas de alta frequência, que aparecem e desaparecem em termos de amplitude e frequência (potenciais evocados tipo bombardeiro de mergulho), mas aumentam após a percussão muscular. Descargas mioquímicas — explosões rítmicas de alta frequência de potenciais de unidade motora isolada são achados característicos em mioquimia.

ACHADOS PATOLÓGICOS
• Histologia muscular — os achados histopatológicos em miotonia congênita podem permanecer normais ou revelar leves alterações (p. ex., hipertrofia de algumas fibras musculares, atrofia angular, núcleos centrais, variação no tamanho das fibras). • Podem ser observadas alterações degenerativas e/ou inflamatórias ao exame histológico do músculo em casos de miotonia adquirida. • Nenhuma anormalidade é encontrada na biopsia muscular em cães da raça Jack Russell terrier com neuromiotonia e mioquimia (atividade contínua das fibras musculares).

TRATAMENTO

• Não há nenhum tratamento específico.
• Desestimular atividades que resultem em hiperventilação. • Evitar exercício extenuante e agitação. • Evitar o frio. • Anestesia (indução e recuperação) — possível risco de obstrução respiratória em virtude de adução das cordas vocais ou regurgitação.

MEDICAÇÕES

MEDICAMENTO(S)
• Medicamentos estabilizantes de membrana — procainamida, quinidina, fenitoína e mexiletina; podem diminuir a gravidade dos sinais clínicos. • Há relatos de que a procainamida seja mais eficaz em cães da raça Chow chow. O tratamento pode diminuir a rigidez, o estridor e a regurgitação, embora a marcha permaneça anormal. • Também há relatos de que a procainamida de liberação estendida a 40-50 mg/kg a cada 8-12 h ou a mexiletina a 8,3 mg/kg a cada 8 h seja eficiente na raça Schnauzer miniatura. • Relata-se que o uso de procainamida a 10 mg/kg a cada 8 h ou mexiletina a 4 mg/kg a cada 12 h ou fenitoína de liberação sustentada a uma dose crescente de 50-100 mg/kg por 6 semanas, com subsequente monitorização da concentração sérica a 2-8 mg/L, diminua a frequência dos episódios de atividade contínua das fibras musculares em aproximadamente metade dos cães acometidos da raça Jack Russell terrier, mas a resposta costuma ser temporária. • Pode ser necessário o uso de anestesia e resfriamento para tratar a hipertermia em episódios de atividade contínua das fibras musculares em Jack Russell terrier.

CONTRAINDICAÇÕES/INTERAÇÕES POSSÍVEIS
A miotonia em seres humanos é agravada pelo tratamento com dantroleno, agentes bloqueadores beta-adrenérgicos, diuréticos e agentes bloqueadores neuromusculares. Agentes que contenham brometo, como brometo de potássio, podem ser contraindicados.

ACOMPANHAMENTO

PREVENÇÃO
• Chow chow e Schnauzer miniatura — condição hereditária; orientar o proprietário em relação ao acasalamento. • Teste de PCR para cães portadores da raça Schnauzer miniatura. • Desestimular o acasalamento dos animais acometidos. • Não repetir os cruzamentos entre machos e fêmeas que resultaram em prole acometida.

COMPLICAÇÕES POSSÍVEIS
• Obstrução do trato respiratório e/ou aspiração de alimento regurgitado — podem ser potencialmente letais; orientar os proprietários sobre os sintomas clínicos e o tratamento. • Hipertermia associada à atividade contínua das fibras musculares em Jack Russell terrier representa um risco de vida.

EVOLUÇÃO ESPERADA E PROGNÓSTICO
Prognóstico reservado.

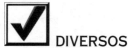

ABREVIATURA(S)
• PCR = reação em cadeia da polimerase.

Sugestões de Leitura
Vite CH. Myotonia and disorders of altered muscle cell membrane excitability. Vet Clin North Am Small Anim Pract 2002, 32(1):169-187.

Autor Georgina Child
Consultor Editorial Peter K. Shires

Mixedema e Coma Mixedematoso

CONSIDERAÇÕES GERAIS

REVISÃO
- Coma mixedematoso é uma manifestação rara potencialmente letal de hipotireoidismo grave, além de ser considerado como uma emergência endócrina.
- O desenvolvimento de coma mixedematoso requer um evento precipitante que sobrepuje os mecanismos homeostáticos normais. Nenhum evento isolado foi identificado nos animais.
- O maior desafio no coma mixedematoso é identificar a síndrome. Uma vez identificada, há necessidade de cuidados de suporte imediatos e intensivos. Há relatos de sucesso no tratamento; no entanto, as taxas de mortalidade podem ser altas.

IDENTIFICAÇÃO
- Cães, cuja maioria pertence à raça Doberman pinscher.
- Faixa etária: 5-7 anos.
- Nenhuma predileção sexual.
- Não há relatos de coma mixedematoso em gatos.

SINAIS CLÍNICOS

Achados Anamnésicos
- Os achados comuns em pacientes com coma mixedematoso são alterações no estado mental, termorregulação alterada e edema cutâneo não depressível.
- As alterações da atividade mental, causadas pela formação de edema cerebral, podem variar desde modificação no estado de alerta até coma. A depressão mental é a avaliação mais comum do estado mental. O coma não é constantemente relatado.
- Podem ser relatados outros sinais compatíveis com hipotireoidismo.
- Os pacientes podem ter sido previamente diagnosticados com hipotireoidismo.

Achados do Exame Físico
- Hipotermia sem tremor é um achado compatível com coma mixedematoso. A tiroxina amplia a função das catecolaminas, ajudando a estimular a atividade muscular associada ao tremor. O nível reduzido de T_4 diminui a capacidade de tremor.
- Extremidades frias em virtude de vasoconstrição periférica e desvio central de sangue secundário à hipotermia.
- Edema cutâneo não depressível atribuído ao depósito de glicosaminoglicanos no espaço intersticial da pele.
- Pode-se observar uma diminuição nos ruídos pulmonares e sons cardíacos, causada por efusão pleural (presente em até 50% dos casos).

CAUSAS E FATORES DE RISCO
- O coma mixedematoso origina-se de hipotireoidismo primário grave crônico não tratado.
- Segundo relatos, ambas as formas de hipotireoidismo primário (tireoidite linfocítica e atrofia tireóidea idiopática) são associadas ao desenvolvimento de coma mixedematoso.
- Um evento precipitante secundário costuma ser associado ao início de uma crise por mixedema. Eventos precipitantes podem incluir, mas não se limitam a, infecções, doença respiratória, insuficiência cardíaca e hipovolemia.
- Há relatos esporádicos sugestivos de que a exposição a temperaturas frias possa atuar como um evento precipitante, embora isso não tenha sido consistentemente relatado.

DIAGNÓSTICO

DIAGNÓSTICO DIFERENCIAL
- Fraqueza pode estar associada à doença cardiovascular, doença neurológica e outras endocrinopatias.
- Miocardiopatia dilatada se o paciente pertencer à raça Doberman pinscher.
- Hipotermia pode estar associada a choque e outras doenças cardiovasculares e endócrinas. Hipotermia associada a outros fatores que não o coma mixedematoso geralmente será acompanhada por tremor.

HEMOGRAMA/BIOQUÍMICA/URINÁLISE
- Leve anemia arregenerativa é a anormalidade mais comumente observada.
- Hipercolesterolemia. • Hipertrigliceridemia.
- Hipoglicemia. • Hiponatremia. • Hipoxemia.
- Hipercarbia. • Resultados normais na urinálise.

OUTROS TESTES LABORATORIAIS
- Testes de função da tireoide indicam hipotireoidismo grave com níveis baixos de T_4 total e T_4 livre, mas elevados de TSH.
- Tempo de sangramento da mucosa bucal apresenta-se prolongado (a hipotermia diminui a função das plaquetas).
- Análise do líquido da efusão pleural — transudato modificado.

DIAGNÓSTICO POR IMAGEM
Radiografias torácicas — constatação de efusão pleural em até 50% dos casos. Raramente se observa edema pulmonar localizado na região peri-hilar.

ACHADOS PATOLÓGICOS
As biopsias cutâneas podem demonstrar espessamento da derme, presença de mixedema e vacuolização dos músculos eretores do pelo.

TRATAMENTO
- O coma mixedematoso é uma emergência médica.
- Assim que o diagnóstico presuntivo de coma mixedematoso for feito, haverá necessidade de tratamento imediato com internação do paciente.
- Em virtude da natureza crítica e potencialmente letal do coma mixedematoso, o tratamento deverá ser instituído antes de os resultados dos testes da função tireóidea confirmarem uma suspeita clínica de mixedema.
- Estabelecimento imediato de via área patente (desobstruída) e ressuscitação de hipotensão, conforme a necessidade.
- Talvez haja necessidade de ventilação mecânica.
- Fluidoterapia IV é administrada para manter a pressão arterial e tratar os níveis reduzidos de sódio. Os pacientes com coma mixedematoso apresentam uma capacidade reduzida em eliminar a água livre.
- Administração de fluidos intravenosos: cloreto de sódio a 0,9% (20 mL/kg - bólus inicial). Reavaliar e continuar a administração desses fluidos (2,5-7 mL/kg/h). Velocidade selecionada com base nos valores de pressão arterial, ritmo cardíaco, frequência cardíaca e frequência respiratória.
- A base da terapia consiste na administração intravenosa de hormônio tireoidiano sintético.
- É imprescindível evitar o rápido reaquecimento, pois isso pode causar vasodilatação periférica, hipotensão e possível colapso cardiovascular. A correção da hipotermia deve ser passiva e feita em algumas horas.

MEDICAÇÕES

MEDICAMENTO(S)
- Tratamento imediato definitivo: levotiroxina, 5 µg/kg (0,005 mg/kg) IV a cada 12 h.
- Uma dose de reposição mais conservadora deve ser utilizada quando houver preocupação quanto à função cardíaca, especialmente com a capacidade do coração em lidar com um aumento súbito e rápido na taxa metabólica. Nesses casos, reduzir a dose da levotiroxina em 50-75%.
- Assim que a condição do paciente estiver estabilizada e o paciente for capaz de engolir, a terapia oral com levotiroxina deverá ser iniciada a uma dose de 0,02 mg/kg VO a cada 12 h.

CONTRAINDICAÇÕES/INTERAÇÕES POSSÍVEIS
- Deve ser considerada uma dose IV mais baixa da levotiroxina em pacientes com cardiopatia.
- É imprescindível evitar o rápido reaquecimento.

ACOMPANHAMENTO
- O prognóstico é grave.
- Se o paciente sobreviver ao tratamento inicial, a terapia e a monitorização recomendadas para hipotireoidismo deverão ser instituídas.
- Avaliação do paciente quanto ao potencial de algum evento precipitante subjacente.

DIVERSOS

VER TAMBÉM
Hipotireoidismo.

ABREVIATURA(S)
- T_4 = tiroxina, tetraiodotironina.
- TSH = hormônio tireostimulante.

Sugestões de Leitura
Feldman ED, Nelson RW, eds. Hypothyroidism. In: Canine and Feline Endocrinology and Reproduction, 3rd ed. St. Louis: Elsevier Saunders, 2004, pp. 86-151.
Finora K, Greco DS. Hypothyroidism and myxedema coma in veterinary medicine — physiology, diagnosis and treatment. Compend Contin Educ Pract Vet 2007, 29:19-32.
Henik RA, Dixon RM. Intravenous administration of levothyroxine for treatment of suspected myxedema coma complicated by severe hypothermia in a dog. JAVMA 2000, 216:713-717.

Autor Kevin Finora
Consultor Editorial Deborah S. Greco

Mortalidade Neonatal (Síndrome do Definhamento)

CONSIDERAÇÕES GERAIS

DEFINIÇÃO
Morte que ocorre do nascimento até 2 semanas de vida.

FISIOPATOLOGIA
• Atividade termorreguladora, respostas imunológicas e controle glicêmico inadequados conferem maior suscetibilidade a uma série de insultos, geralmente uma combinação de fatores ambientais, infecciosos, nutricionais e metabólicos.
• Hipotermia, hipoglicemia, desidratação e hipoxia — constituem prelúdios comuns.

SISTEMA(S) ACOMETIDO(S)
• Cardiovascular.
• Endócrino/metabólico.
• Hepatobiliar.
• Nervoso.
• Renal/urológico.
• Respiratório.

IDENTIFICAÇÃO
• Cães e gatos.
• Filhotes de cão e de gato com *pedigree* — mais propensos a defeitos congênitos (e hereditários).

SINAIS CLÍNICOS
Comentários Gerais
• Perdas antes do desmame — tipicamente 10-30%; cerca de 65% ocorrem durante a primeira semana; perdas maiores em gatil ou canil devem ser consideradas anormais.
• Achados do histórico e do exame físico — raramente estreitam a lista de diagnóstico diferencial, por causa do número limitado de meios com que os neonatos podem responder à doença.

Achados Anamnésicos
• Baixo peso ao nascimento, perda de peso e/ou falha no ganho de peso.
• Atividade e apetite reduzidos.
• Fraqueza.
• Os filhotes apresentam vocalização e inquietação constantes no início, embora se mostrem quietos e inativos mais tarde.
• Tendência a permanecerem isolados da mãe e do restante da ninhada.

Achados do Exame Físico
• Inespecíficos.
• Fraqueza, hipotermia (a temperatura do recém-nascido gira em torno de 35,5°C, subindo para 37-37,8°C durante a quarta semana de vida), hipoglicemia, desidratação — comuns e inter-relacionadas.
• Angústia respiratória, diarreia ou hemoglobinúria — podem ser observadas.
• Defeitos anatômicos macroscópicos — podem ser detectáveis.

CAUSAS
Não Infecciosas
• Relacionadas com a mãe — distocia ou parto prolongado; canibalismo; falha da lactação; traumatismo; falta ou excesso de atenção; nutrição inadequada, incluindo a deficiência de taurina nos filhotes felinos.
• Ambientais — qualquer fator que desestimule a amamentação e gere a hipotermia, incluindo extremos de temperatura, extremos de umidade, condições inadequadas de saneamento, superlotação e estresse.
• Nutricionais — amamentação inadequada ou ineficaz; hipoglicemia; mau funcionamento digestivo induzido pela hipotermia.
• Isoeritrólise neonatal — gata com sangue tipo B; filhote com sangue tipo A.

Defeitos Congênitos
• Defeitos anatômicos macroscópicos — mais frequentemente em filhotes de gato (cerca de 10% dos neonatos que não sobrevivem) do que em filhotes de cão.
• Anormalidades gastrintestinais — fenda palatina; agenesia ou atresia segmentar intestinal.
• Anormalidades craniofaciais — falha de fechamento da linha média, provocando herniação.
• Defeitos cardíacos — displasia valvular; defeito do septo ventricular; fístula atrioventricular.
• Defeitos respiratórios — anormalidades da parede torácica; peito (tórax) escavado; discinesia ciliar primária; deficiência do surfactante.
• Erros inatos do metabolismo — geralmente traços autossômicos recessivos.

Infecciosas
• Virais (filhotes de gato) — calicivírus felino; FeLV; FIV; herpes-vírus felino tipo 1; vírus da panleucopenia felina.
• Virais (filhotes de cão) — adenovírus canino tipo 1; vírus da cinomose; herpes-vírus canino; parvovírus canino tipo 1; vírus da influenza canina.
• Bacterianas — adquiridas principalmente via placenta, canal do parto, umbigo, feridas cutâneas ou pelos tratos gastrintestinal, respiratório ou urinário.
• Sepse neonatal — principalmente por *E. coli*, *Streptococcus* β-hemolíticos, *Staphylococcus* coagulase-positivo e microrganismos entéricos Gram-negativos.
• Respiratórias — *Bordetella bronchiseptica*; *Pasteurella multocida*.
• Entéricas — *E. coli*; *Salmonella* spp.; *Campylobacter* spp.
• *Brucella canis* — filhotes caninos.
• Parasitárias — infecção maciça pelos helmintos *Toxocara canis*, *Toxocara cati*, *Toxascaris leonina*, *Ancylostoma caninum* ou *Ancylostoma tubaeforme*; parasitas coccídios como *Toxoplasma*, *Neospora*, *Isospora*, *Cryptosporidium* ou *Giardia*.

FATORES DE RISCO
• Peso abaixo do normal ao nascimento ou falha em crescer normalmente — filhotes de gato: ganho mínimo diário de 7-10 g; filhotes de cão: devem atingir o dobro do peso em torno dos 10-12 dias; ambas as espécies: 5-10% de ganho de peso por dia geralmente é um valor aceitável.
• Distocia ou parto prolongado.
• Consanguinidade — maior incidência de genótipo homozigoto recessivo.
• Gato com sangue tipo A e gata com sangue tipo B.

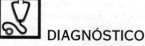

DIAGNÓSTICO

DIAGNÓSTICO DIFERENCIAL
Perdas excessivas atribuídas a uma combinação de fatores ambientais, imunológicos, nutricionais, infecciosos e metabólicos; há necessidade de detecção e correção dos problemas em cada área para evitar perdas contínuas.

HEMOGRAMA/BIOQUÍMICA/URINÁLISE
Amostras de sangue dos indivíduos acometidos não costumam ser passíveis de coleta antes da morte nem patognomônicas.

Hemograma Completo
• O estado de hidratação e a idade do paciente influenciam os resultados.
• Leve anemia normocítica normocrômica.
• As contagens leucocitárias são variáveis; podem-se notar trombocitopenia e neutrofilia (com desvio à esquerda) leve a moderada no caso de paciente séptico.

Bioquímica
• Hipoglicemia.
• Outras alterações dependem do sistema orgânico envolvido.

Urinálise
• Hemoglobinúria — com isoeritrólise neonatal.
• Bactérias — com infecção.
• Densidade urinária — >1,017 sugere hidratação inadequada.

OUTROS TESTES LABORATORIAIS
• Teste antigênico para FeLV.
• Teste humoral para FIV.
• Sorologia — *Brucella canis*; herpes-vírus canino; vírus da influenza canina; *Toxoplasma*; *Neospora*.

DIAGNÓSTICO POR IMAGEM
N/D.

MÉTODOS DIAGNÓSTICOS
• Histopatológico — exame de múltiplos tecidos coletados à necropsia.
• Triagem metabólica de amostra urinária — descartar erros inatos do metabolismo.
• Isolamento do vírus.
• Cultura bacteriana.
• Tipagem sanguínea em gatos com *pedigree*.
• Exame de fezes — parasitas.

ACHADOS PATOLÓGICOS
Pós-morte — extremamente importantes; é aconselhável a realização do exame o mais rápido possível após o óbito para minimizar a autólise; dar especial atenção aos seguintes itens:
• Estômago — desprovido de conteúdo pela falta de amamentação; considerar as causas relacionadas com a mãe (p. ex., comportamento ou lactação inadequados) ou problemas neonatais (p. ex., fraqueza, traumatismo ou anormalidade fisiológica); cheio de leite: sugere morte súbita (p. ex., traumatismo ou doença superaguda) ou disfunção gastrintestinal (temperatura corporal <35°C).
• Tamanho do timo abaixo do normal — não é patognomônico; pode ser o resultado de múltiplas causas (p. ex., infecção viral, nutrição e defeito do sistema imune).
• Petéquias — comuns; acompanhadas por hemorragia em outros sistemas orgânicos sugere coagulopatia ou septicemia.
• Urina na bexiga — implica certo grau de disfunção renal ou de cuidado inadequado por parte da mãe.
• Pulmões — devem parecer da mesma forma que dos adultos; coloração vermelho-escura homogênea típica de animal natimorto que não respirou; hemorragia, edema, congestão e coloração mosqueada anormal, porém inespecífica.
• Notar más-formações.

MORTALIDADE NEONATAL (SÍNDROME DO DEFINHAMENTO)

• Múltiplas amostras teciduais — encaminhar para o laboratório de diagnóstico; isolamento do vírus, cultura bacteriana e antibiograma, além de exame histopatológico; checar junto ao laboratório para enviar as amostras de forma adequada.

TRATAMENTO
• Corrigir qualquer deficiência subjacente na criação ou na seleção reprodutiva.
• Aquecimento — aquecer o neonato lentamente até 36-36,7°C durante várias horas, se necessário; proporcionar temperatura ambiente de 29-35°C e umidade relativa de 55-65%.
• Oxigênio — suplementar a 30-40%, em caso de necessidade.
• Fluidos intravenosos — considerar a administração de solução de glicose a 5% aquecida no caso de hipoglicemia; administrar a solução de Ringer lactato ou solução de Ringer lactato de meia potência e glicose a 2,5% (via intravenosa, intraóssea ou subcutânea) na dose de 1 mL/30 g de peso corporal.
• Não tentar alimentar o animal se a temperatura corporal estiver <35°C e se não houver reflexo de sucção; uma vez aquecido, estimular a amamentação.
• Isoeritrólise neonatal — não permitir a amamentação nas primeiras 24 h após o nascimento.

MEDICAÇÕES
MEDICAMENTO(S) DE ESCOLHA
• Antibióticos — os agentes comumente utilizados são as penicilinas (penicilina G, ampicilina, amoxicilina, amoxicilina com ácido clavulânico) e cefalosporinas de primeira geração; reduzir a dose do adulto pela metade e utilizar o mesmo intervalo posológico.

• Suplemento — fórmula de substituto (sucedâneo) do leite.
• Vitamina K$_1$ — 0,01-0,1 mg SC ou IM uma única vez.

CONTRAINDICAÇÕES
Aminoglicosídeos, tetraciclinas, fluoroquinolonas, trimetoprima-sulfonamida e cloranfenicol — evitar durante o período neonatal.

PRECAUÇÕES
A absorção, a distribuição, o metabolismo e a excreção de medicamentos em cães e gatos diferem significativamente durante as primeiras cinco semanas de vida daqueles dos adultos.

INTERAÇÕES POSSÍVEIS
N/D.

MEDICAMENTO(S) ALTERNATIVO(S)
N/D.

ACOMPANHAMENTO
MONITORIZAÇÃO DO PACIENTE
• Estado de hidratação — verificar diariamente; o ressecamento da boca e a urina de coloração amarelo-dourada indicam desidratação.
• Peso corporal — monitorizar diariamente ou em dias alternados nos neonatos em crescimento.
• Mãe — verificar se a amamentação e o cuidado estão adequados; suplementar com fórmula de substituto (sucedâneo) do leite, se necessário.

COMPLICAÇÕES POSSÍVEIS
N/D.

DIVERSOS
DISTÚRBIOS ASSOCIADOS
N/D.

FATORES RELACIONADOS COM A IDADE
N/D.

POTENCIAL ZOONÓTICO
N/D.

GESTAÇÃO/FERTILIDADE/REPRODUÇÃO
N/D.

SINÔNIMO(S)
• Síndrome da emaciação.
• Síndrome do definhamento de filhotes caninos e felinos.

ABREVIATURA(S)
• FeLV = vírus da leucemia felina.
• FIV = vírus da imunodeficiência felina.

RECURSOS DA INTERNET
• www.netcat.org/symposium/fadingkittens.html.
• www.vetmedpub.com/vetmed/article/articleDetail.jsp?id = 197291.
• www.wolfweb.com.au/acd/fadingpupsyn.html.

Sugestões de Leitura
Hoskins JD. Clinical evaluation of the kitten: From birth to eight weeks of age. Compend Contin Educ Pract Vet 1990, 12:1215-1225.
Hoskins JD. Fading puppy and kitten syndromes. Feline Pract 1993, 21:19-22.
Jones RL. Special considerations for appropriate antimicrobial therapy in neonates. Vet Clin North Am Small Anim Pract 1987, 17:577-602.
Lawler DF. Care and diseases of neonatal puppies and kittens. In: Kirk RW, Bonagura JD, eds., Current Veterinary Therapy X. Philadelphia: Saunders, 1989, pp. 1325-1333.
Lawler DF. Investigating kitten deaths in catteries. In: August JR, ed., Consultations in Feline Internal Medicine. Philadelphia: Saunders, 1991, pp. 47-54.

Autor Johnny D. Hoskins
Consultor Editorial Stephen C. Barr

Mucocele da Vesícula Biliar

CONSIDERAÇÕES GERAIS

REVISÃO
- Acúmulo de conglomerado mucoide viscoso e espesso de bile na vesícula biliar, que prejudica sua capacidade de armazenamento e sua função.
- O lodo biliar espesso expande a vesícula biliar, resultando em colecistite necrosante.

IDENTIFICAÇÃO
- Cães.
- Pastor de Shetland, Schnauzer miniatura e Cocker spaniel são super-representados.
- Adultos de meia-idade a idosos.
- Sem predominância sexual.

SINAIS CLÍNICOS

Comentários Gerais
- Sintomática ou assintomática.
- A forma assintomática é descoberta à ultrassonografia abdominal por outros problemas de saúde.

Achados Anamnésicos: Sintomáticos
- Desconforto abdominal episódico.
- Anorexia.
- Vômito.
- Poliúria e polidipsia.
- Letargia.
- Colapso: peritonite vasovagal ou biliar.

Achados do Exame Físico
- Letargia.
- Dor abdominal cranial.
- Icterícia.
- Desidratação.
- Febre.
- Pode não exibir qualquer sinal físico.

CAUSAS E FATORES DE RISCO
- Erros inatos do metabolismo lipídico, conforme observado nas raças Schnauzer miniatura e Pastor de Shetland.
- Condições clínicas associadas à hipercolesterolemia ou indutoras de dislipidemia, tais como: hipotireoidismo, hiperplasia adrenal típica ou atípica (hormônios sexuais), terapia com glicocorticoide, diabete melito, pancreatite recidivante, dieta rica em gordura para cão com algum distúrbio predisponente.
- Dismotilidade da vesícula biliar — pode desempenhar algum papel causal.
- Hipertrofia cística das glândulas da vesícula biliar produtoras de muco — comum em cães idosos; pode exercer um papel causal ou facilitador.

DIAGNÓSTICO

DIAGNÓSTICO DIFERENCIAL
Condições indutoras de estase biliar — dismotilidade da vesícula biliar; neoplasia; colélitos; pancreatite.

HEMOGRAMA/BIOQUÍMICA/URINÁLISE

Hemograma Completo
- Leucograma inflamatório — variável.
- Anemia arregenerativa — se houver inflamação crônica ou hipotireoidismo.

Bioquímica
- Atividade elevada das enzimas hepáticas — único sinal de doença em alguns cães ou pode ser observada em casos de manifestação aguda; fosfatase alcalina, GGT, ALT e AST.
- Hiperbilirrubinemia variável.
- Hipoalbuminemia em caso de ruptura da árvore biliar e ocorrência de peritonite biliar.
- Azotemia pré-renal.
- Anormalidades eletrolíticas com distúrbios hídricos e acidobásicos — atribuídos à peritonite biliar ou a vômitos excessivos.

Urinálise
- Sem características específicas.

OUTROS TESTES LABORATORIAIS
- Concentrações de triglicerídios — altas em casos de erros inatos do metabolismo lipídico, endocrinopatias, diabete melito ou pancreatite.
- Provas de coagulação — normais a menos que haja obstrução extra-hepática do ducto biliar, ruptura da árvore biliar, peritonite biliar, sepse ou CID.

DIAGNÓSTICO POR IMAGEM
- Radiografia abdominal — fígado normal ou aumentado; perda de detalhes da imagem na porção abdominal cranial em caso de peritonite focal (colecistite necrosante); presença de gás intra-hepático indica inflamação séptica com microrganismo produtor de gás (rara).
- Ultrassonografia abdominal — o fígado pode estar grande, com as bordas arredondadas; é comum um parênquima hepático hiperecoico difuso a multifocal (associado mais frequentemente à hepatopatia vacuolar); vesícula biliar distendida e, às vezes, ducto biliar comum e ducto cístico distendidos na presença de obstrução extra-hepática do ducto biliar; a interface de líquido que circunda a vesícula biliar acentua a imagem da parede e sugere colecistite ou ruptura da vesícula biliar; parede da vesícula biliar difusamente espessa com hiperecogenicidade segmentar e aspecto laminado da parede em casos de colecistite necrosante; parede de margem dupla também pode ser vista com colecistite aguda, hepatite, colangio-hepatite, dispersão de líquido para o terceiro espaço (hipoproteinemia, insuficiência cardíaca direita, insuficiência renal, pielonefrite, efusão abdominal, sobrecarga hídrica iatrogênica); a imagem ultrassonográfica típica consiste um lúmen biliar preenchido por debris ecogênicos amorfos que aparecem com um padrão estrelado ou finamente estriado, semelhante a fatias de quiuí ("sinal do quiuí"); ruptura da vesícula biliar associada à solução de continuidade na parede dessa vesícula, líquido pericolecístico ou efusão generalizada e hiperecogenicidade dos tecidos circunjacentes; pode ser difícil visualizar os ductos biliares intra-hepáticos ou, então, eles podem parecer proeminentes (colangite ascendente) ou distendidos (obstrução extra-hepática do ducto biliar); pode não ser uma tarefa fácil obter imagens de ruptura da vesícula biliar; a mucocele pode ser liberada para a cavidade abdominal, onde é possível obter a imagem de discreta "massa" livre e flutuante.
- Estudo da motilidade da vesícula biliar — indicado em casos de mucocele biliar iminente identificado de forma fortuita e volume da vesícula biliar ≥1 mL/kg de peso corporal; as mensurações sequenciais do volume dessa vesícula após a ingestão de alguma refeição (100 g) podem envolver a administração de eritomicina na dose de 1 mg/kg como agonista da motilina responsável pela contração da vesícula biliar. A vesícula biliar normal contrai-se ≥25% do volume inicial se a imagem for obtida em 15, 30, 45, 60, 90 e 120 minutos após a refeição.

MÉTODOS DIAGNÓSTICOS
- Amostra obtida por aspiração — líquido adjacente às estruturas biliares ou livre na cavidade abdominal; elucida a ruptura da árvore biliar e a presença de infecção. **Cuidado:** não realizar colecistocentese, pois isso pode causar peritonite biliar; costuma ser difícil obter amostra de conteúdo da mucocele em virtude de sua natureza espessa e viscosa.
- Laparotomia exploratória — para diagnóstico, colecistectomia e, talvez, colecistoenterostomia.
- Biopsia hepática — avalia a existência de distúrbios hepatobiliares coexistentes ou prévios. Coletar a amostra de biopsia distante da vesícula biliar para evitar a amostragem das glândulas peribiliares.
- Cultura bacteriana e antibiograma — obter amostra de efusão, da parede e do conteúdo da vesícula biliar, bem como do fígado; solicitar cultura para bactérias aeróbias e anaeróbias.
- Citologia — esfregaços por impressão da vesícula biliar, do fígado e da bile para determinação imediata de inflamação séptica supurativa e neoplasia.

ACHADOS PATOLÓGICOS
- Macroscópicos — em casos de vesícula biliar distendida, a parede pode estar eritematosa com áreas focais de necrose; peritonite focal pode ser evidente; o fígado e as estruturas extra-hepáticas biliares, em geral, parecem normais; conteúdo da vesícula biliar: verde-escuro a negro, viscoso, firme ou sólido organizado amarelo-esverdeado à superfície de corte com textura elástica. Lesões proliferativas na mucosa da vesícula biliar representam hiperplasia cística da mucosa.
- Microscópicos — infiltrado inflamatório misto e fibrose (crônica) na lâmina própria da parede da vesícula biliar, com áreas focais de necrose se houver colecistite necrosante; hiperplasia da mucosa da vesícula biliar (comum); colangite ascendente e colangio-hepatite; os hepatócitos podem demonstrar hepatopatia vacuolar (inclusões de glicogênio e/ou lipídios) (ver distúrbios associados).

TRATAMENTO
- Ambulatorial com ácido ursodesoxicólico e S-adenosilmetionina para induzir à colerese e conferir hepatoproteção — a terapia clínica não é aconselhada para solucionar uma mucocele.
- Internação — nesse caso, o tratamento depende da apresentação do paciente: com colecistite necrosante aguda grave ou síndrome determinada como achado incidental ao exame ultrassonográfico.
- Se o paciente estiver hiperlipidêmico, investigar a causa e restringir a gordura na dieta.
- Pacientes sintomáticos necessitam de cirurgia exploratória para colecistectomia e tratamento de peritonite biliar potencial.
- Colecistotomia e remoção da mucocele em caso de retenção da vesícula biliar podem levar à recidiva da mucocele biliar.
- Fluidoterapia — soluções poliônicas balanceadas para corrigir a hidratação e as anormalidades eletrolíticas.
- Ficar preparado para terapia com hemoderivado.

MUCOCELE DA VESÍCULA BILIAR

• Lavagem abdominal — durante a cirurgia caso se confirme a presença de peritonite biliar.

MEDICAÇÕES
MEDICAMENTO(S)
Antimicrobianos
• Iniciar antibióticos de amplo espectro *antes* da cirurgia: microrganismos entéricos Gram-negativos e anaeróbios são muito provavelmente oportunistas; continuar o tratamento por 8 semanas se houver complicações sépticas; ajustar os medicamentos com base nos resultados de cultura e antibiograma.

Vitamina K₁
• 0,5-1,5 mg/kg IM ou SC a cada 12 h por 3 doses — se houver icterícia; a via oral talvez seja ineficaz.

Antieméticos/Antiácidos/Gastroprotetores
• Metoclopramida, 0,2-0,5 mg/kg VO, IV ou SC a cada 6-8 h ou 1-2 mg/kg/dia em velocidade de infusão constante.
• Ondansetrona, 0,5-1,0 mg/kg VO 30 min antes da refeição, no máximo a cada 8 h, ou 0,1-0,2 mg/kg por via IV lenta a cada 6-12 h) — se o paciente estiver vomitando.
• Antagonistas dos receptores histaminérgicos H_2: famotidina, 0,5 mg/kg VO, IV, SC a cada 12-24 h.
• Sucralfato, 0,25-1,0 g VO a cada 8-12 h — para sangramento gastrintestinal.

Colerese
• Manter o estado de hidratação.
• Ácido ursodesoxicólico: efeitos coleréticos, hepatoprotetores, anti-inflamatórios e antiendotóxicos (10-15 mg/kg VO divididos a cada 12 h juntamente com o alimento; os comprimidos possuem melhor biodisponibilidade); administrar por tempo indefinido.
• *S*-adenosilmetionina pode conferir um efeito colerético; a dose pode ser mais alta do que aquela utilizada como antioxidante (ver adiante); a colerese é obtida com 40 mg/kg VO diariamente.

Antioxidantes
• Vitamina E: α-tocoferol, 10 UI/kg/dia VO juntamente com o alimento; efeitos antioxidantes, anti-inflamatórios e antifibróticos.
• *S*-adenosilmetionina: 20 mg/kg VO diariamente 2 horas antes da alimentação (Denosyl SD4® tem biodisponibilidade e eficácia comprovadas como doador de glutationa reduzida); administrada até a normalização das enzimas hepáticas ou por tempo indefinido em caso de hepatite crônica.

CONTRAINDICAÇÕES/INTERAÇÕES POSSÍVEIS
N/D.

ACOMPANHAMENTO
MONITORIZAÇÃO DO PACIENTE
Repetir os exames sequenciais de hemograma, bioquímica e técnicas de diagnóstico por imagem para monitorizar a resposta do animal ao tratamento.

COMPLICAÇÕES POSSÍVEIS
• Colangite ou colangio-hepatite.
• Peritonite biliar.
• Obstrução extra-hepática do ducto biliar.

EVOLUÇÃO ESPERADA E PROGNÓSTICO
• Prognóstico bom com cirurgia bem-sucedida, terapia colerética crônica, correção ou tratamento de condições comórbidas e modificação da dieta.
• Prever uma evolução clínica prolongada com a ruptura do trato biliar ou a presença de peritonite.
• Pode ocorrer recidiva mesmo se a vesícula biliar for removida ou em caso de retenção dessa vesícula, com ou sem a administração de terapia clínica crônica.

DIVERSOS
VER TAMBÉM
• Colecistite e Coledoquite.
• Colelitíase.
• Hepatite Crônica Ativa.
• Peritonite Biliar.
• Hepatopatia Vacuolar.

ABREVIATURA(S)
• ALT = alanina aminotransferase.
• AST = aspartato aminotransferase.
• CID = coagulação intravascular disseminada.
• GGT = γ-glutamiltransferase.

Sugestões de Leitura
Center SA. Diseases of the gallbladder and biliary tree. Vet Clin North Am Small Anim Pract 2009, 39(3):543-598.
Pike FS, Berg J, King NW, et al. Gallbladder mucocele in dogs: 30 cases (2000-2002). JAVMA 2004, 224:1615-1622.
Worley DR, Hottinger HA, Lawrence HJ. Surgical management of gallbladder mucoceles in dogs: 22 cases (1999-2003). JAVMA 2004, 225:1418-1422.

Autor Sharon A. Center
Consultor Editorial Sharon A. Center

Mucocele Salivar

CONSIDERAÇÕES GERAIS

REVISÃO
• Mucoceles salivares são cavidades não revestidas por epitélio e preenchidas com saliva que extravasou de uma glândula ou ducto salivares lesados; tais mucoceles são circundadas por tecido de granulação que se forma secundariamente à inflamação provocada pela saliva livre.
• Existem quatro pares principais de glândulas salivares: parótidas, mandibulares, sublinguais e zigomáticas. Glândulas salivares bucais menores estão localizadas no palato mole, nos lábios, na língua e nas bochechas.
• Os tipos de mucocele estão relacionados na Tabela 1. O tipo mais comum ocorre com a ruptura do ducto sublingual.

SISTEMA(S) ACOMETIDO(S)
Gastrintestinal.

IDENTIFICAÇÃO
• Três vezes mais frequente nos cães do que nos gatos.
• Todas as raças são suscetíveis. As raças comumente acometidas incluem Poodle miniatura (mucoceles faríngeas), Pastor alemão, Dachshund e Silky terrier australiano.
• Leve predisposição dos machos comparados às fêmeas.
• Sem predisposição etária.

SINAIS CLÍNICOS

Mucocele Cervical
• Massa cervical macia, flutuante, mínima ou indolor que se desenvolve de forma gradativa.
• A dor costuma se manifestar somente durante a fase de manifestação aguda da mucocele.

Rânula
• Tumefação sublingual, macia e em forma de rã (*L. rana*, uma espécie de rã).
• Com frequência, a saliva apresenta-se manchada de sangue secundariamente ao autotraumatismo ocasionado durante a alimentação.

Mucocele Zigomática
• Tumefação facial periorbital.
• Exoftalmia.
• Estrabismo divergente.
• Dor periocular.
• Neuropatia do nervo óptico relacionada com a compressão exercida pela mucocele.

Mucocele Faríngea
• Movimento anormal da língua.
• Angústia respiratória.
• Disfagia.

CAUSAS E FATORES DE RISCO
• A causa raramente é identificada. As causas sob suspeita incluem:
  ◦ Traumatismo rombo na cabeça e no pescoço (coleiras asfixiantes).
  ◦ Ferimento por mordedura.
  ◦ Corpo estranho penetrante.
  ◦ Cirurgia do canal auricular, transposição do ducto parotídeo.
  ◦ Sialólitos.
  ◦ Dirofilariose.

DIAGNÓSTICO

• O diagnóstico baseia-se na anamnese, no exame visual e na paracentese da massa.
• Determinar o local de origem com a ajuda de exame bucal, palpação, sialografia ou exploração da mucocele.

DIAGNÓSTICO DIFERENCIAL
• Sialadenite (segunda doença salivar mais comum, que geralmente envolve a glândula mandibular, quase sempre concomitante com sialoceles).
• Sialadenose.
• Neoplasia salivar (rara; as glândulas mandibulares e parótidas são mais comumente envolvidas; em geral, são carcinomas ou adenocarcinomas em cães; as neoplasias benignas são exclusivamente encontradas nos gatos).
• Sialólitos (fosfato ou carbonato de cálcio).
• Abscesso cervical.
• Infarto da glândula salivar (95% ocorrem na glândula mandibular).
• Corpo estranho.
• Hematoma.
• Linfonodos císticos ou neoplásicos.
• Mixoma ou mixossarcoma orbital.
• Cistos tonsilares.
• Cistos tireoglossos (raros, congênitos).
• Bolsa cística de Rathke e cistos branquiais (raros, congênitos).

HEMOGRAMA/BIOQUÍMICA/URINÁLISE
Raramente se observam anormalidades laboratoriais.

OUTROS TESTES LABORATORIAIS
N/D.

DIAGNÓSTICO POR IMAGEM
• Raramente necessário.
• Radiografias cervicais simples são indicadas apenas para identificar sialólitos, corpos estranhos ou neoplasia.
• Radiografias do crânio, às vezes, são valiosas para diferenciar doença neoplásica da mucocele zigomática, caso a avaliação citológica seja indeterminada.
• Sialografia (injeção de agente de contraste iodado hidrossolúvel no ducto salivar) fica reservada para os pacientes com traumatismo, cirurgias anteriores ou trajetos fistulosos drenantes.
• Ultrassonografia retrobulbar revela a presença de lesão cavitária em 75% das mucoceles zigomáticas e 50% dos abscessos retrobulbares.
• A obtenção de imagens em corte transversal pode ser valiosa para diferenciar entre doenças neoplásicas e não neoplásicas.

MÉTODOS DIAGNÓSTICOS

Paracentese Asséptica
• Diferencia as mucoceles de neoplasias, de abscessos e de sialadenite.
• O líquido aspirado é viscoso, amarelado, claro ou manchado de sangue, com baixa contagem celular. As sialoceles inflamadas caracterizam-se por inflamação plasmocítica-linfocitária crônica de baixo grau.
• A avaliação citológica (coloração de Wright) revela conglomerados difusos ou irregulares de mucina corada de rosa a violeta, grandes células fagocitárias com pequenos núcleos redondos e citoplasma espumoso, células epiteliais de glândula salivar entremeadas e neutrófilos não degenerados em pequeno número.
• Coloração com o corante específico para a mucina (p. ex., ácido periódico de Schiff) para o diagnóstico definitivo.

TRATAMENTO

• Os pacientes com angústia respiratória aguda (mucoceles faríngeas) talvez tenham de ser entubados ou submetidos à traqueostomia temporária. Antes da entubação, pode ser necessária a drenagem através da boca por meio de incisão perfurante.
• A completa excisão cirúrgica do complexo glândula-ducto envolvido e a drenagem da mucocele constituem o tratamento de escolha. A drenagem prolongada pode ser conseguida com a marsupialização das rânulas e das mucoceles faríngeas e com a colocação de drenos de Penrose nas mucoceles cervicais.

MEDICAÇÕES

MEDICAMENTO(S)
Antibióticos selecionados com base na avaliação bacteriológica se houver abscesso ou sialadenite concomitante.

CONTRAINDICAÇÕES
O tratamento não cirúrgico de mucoceles salivares com drenagem ou injeções repetidas de agentes cauterizantes ou anti-inflamatórios não promove a cura e ainda complicará a cirurgia subsequente por induzir à formação de abscesso ou fibrose.

Tabela 1.

Tipos de Mucoceles		
Tipo de Mucocele Salivar	Localização	Glândula/Ducto Envolvido
Mucocele cervical	Espaço intermandibular, ângulo da mandíbula, região cervical superior	Sublingual
Rânula	Tecidos sublinguais	Mandibular ou sublingual
Mucocele faríngea	Parede da faringe	Sublingual
Mucocele zigomática	Ventral ao bulbo ocular	Zigomática
Mucocele parótida	Ângulo da mandíbula, ventral à orelha	Parótida
Mucoceles complexas	Dependendo do envolvimento da glândula/ducto (ver anteriormente)	Dois ou mais ductos/glândulas

MUCOCELE SALIVAR

ACOMPANHAMENTO

MONITORIZAÇÃO DO PACIENTE
• Troca diária das bandagens com a colocação do dreno de Penrose.
• Os drenos de Penrose costumam ser removidos 24-72 h após a cirurgia.
• O local de drenagem deve cicatrizar por segunda intenção e contração após a marsupialização.

COMPLICAÇÕES POSSÍVEIS
• Formação de seroma (17% em caso de ressecção das mucoceles mandibulares e sublinguais).
• Infecção.
• Recidiva da mucocele (<5% em caso de ressecção completa).

EVOLUÇÃO ESPERADA E PROGNÓSTICO
• Prognóstico excelente com a excisão cirúrgica completa.
• Infecção ou injeção prévias complicam a excisão cirúrgica bem-sucedida.

DIVERSOS

DISTÚRBIOS ASSOCIADOS
Sialadenite.

SINÔNIMO(S)
• Cisto melífero.
• Cisto salivar.
• Sialocele.

Sugestões de Leitura
Dunning D. Salivary gland. In: Slatter D, ed., Textbook of Small Animal Surgery, 3rd ed. Philadelphia: Saunders, 2003, pp. 558-561.
Hedlund CS. Salivary mucoceles. In: Fossum TW, ed., Small Animal Surgery, 2nd ed. St. Louis: Mosby, 2002, pp. 302-307.
Ritter MJ, von Pfeil DJ, Stanley BJ, Hauptman JG, Walshaw R. Mandibular and sublingual sialocoeles in the dog: A retrospective evaluation of 41 cases, using the ventral approach for treatment. N Z Vet J 2006, 54(6):333-337.

Autor Susanne K. Lauer
Consultor Editorial Albert E. Jergens

Mucopolissacaridose

CONSIDERAÇÕES GERAIS

REVISÃO
- As mucopolissacaridoses são caracterizadas pelo acúmulo de GAG e resultam da função comprometida de 1 dentre 11 enzimas necessárias para a degradação normal do GAG. Quase todos esses distúrbios foram descritos em animais.
- Os GAG não degradados são armazenados nos lisossomos, resultando em disfunção tecidual e orgânica progressiva.

Tipos de MPS [mucopolissacaridoses] Relatados em Cães e Gatos
- MPS I — deficiência de α-l-iduronidase; ocorre o armazenamento de sulfato de dermatan e heparan. • MPS II — deficiência de iduronato sulfatase; observa-se o armazenamento de sulfato de dermatan e heparan; primeira MPS identificada em seres humanos. • MPS IIIA— deficiência de heparan N-sulfatase; o sulfato de heparan é armazenado. • MPS VI — deficiência de arilsulfatase B; é armazenado o sulfato de dermatan; primeira MPS identificada em um animal. • MPS VII — deficiência de β-glicuronidase; são armazenados o sulfato de dermatan, o heparan e a condroitina.

IDENTIFICAÇÃO
- Gatos — MPS I e VII, doméstico de pelo curto; MPS VI, Siamês e doméstico de pelo curto.
- Cães — MPS I, Plott hound; MPS II, Labrador retriever; MPS IIIA, Dachshund de pelo duro e cães de caça; MPS VI, Pinscher miniatura, Schnauzer miniatura e Welsh corgi; MPS VII, raças mistas e Pastor alemão. • Ambos os sexos são igualmente acometidos por MPS I, III, VI e VII; os machos são basicamente acometidos por MPS II.

SINAIS CLÍNICOS
- Nanismo (exceto gatos com MPS I).
- Osteopatia grave (disostose múltipla).
- Artropatia degenerativa, incluindo subluxação do quadril. • Dismorfia facial — mais evidente no gato Siamês, o qual normalmente possui uma face alongada em comparação a outros gatos.
- Hepatomegalia (exceto gatos com MPS VI).
- Turvamento da córnea — resultado de opacidades granulares finas no estroma corneano, de início aparente com aproximadamente 8 semanas de vida. • Aumento de volume da língua (cães). • Espessamento das válvulas cardíacas.
- Excreção urinária excessiva de GAG. • Grânulos metacromáticos (corpúsculos de Alder-Reilly) nos leucócitos sanguíneos. • A doença evolui; os sinais clínicos tornam-se aparentes com 2-4 meses de vida. • Os animais acometidos podem viver por vários anos, porém a dificuldade locomotora é progressiva. • Anormalidades esqueléticas mais graves nos gatos com MPS VI do que naqueles com MPS I; alguns gatos com MPS VI desenvolvem paresia posterior em virtude de compressão da medula espinal. • Manipulação da cabeça ou do pescoço costuma ser dolorosa.

CAUSAS E FATORES DE RISCO
- A transmissão da MPS é autossômica recessiva, exceto MPS II, a qual é recessiva ligada ao cromossomo X. • A consanguinidade aumentará o risco se o gene defeituoso estiver presente na família.

DIAGNÓSTICO

DIAGNÓSTICO DIFERENCIAL
- Grânulos metacromáticos dentro dos neutrófilos e linfócitos — são sugestivos de MPS; também são observados na gangliosidose GM_2, uma doença do armazenamento lisossomal que, ao contrário da MPS, se caracteriza por doença neurológica progressiva e morte precoce; os grânulos também podem ser encontrados nos neutrófilos de alguns gatos da raça Burmês que apresentam linfócitos normais e não têm anormalidades clínicas; muito raramente, a granulação tóxica dos neutrófilos pode ter aparência semelhante. • Turvamento da córnea — também observada em inúmeras outras doenças do armazenamento lisossomal, incluindo a deficiência de lipase ácida, as gangliosidoses GM_1 e GM_2 e manosidose; perfis das enzimas lisossomais podem ser obtidos para diagnosticar definitivamente o tipo de distúrbio de armazenamento; edema e distrofia corneanos podem apresentar aparência semelhante. • Embora o aspecto radiográfico da MPS seja característico, outros distúrbios com similaridades incluem hipotireoidismo congênito, displasia epifisária e hipervitaminose A.

HEMOGRAMA/BIOQUÍMICA/URINÁLISE
- Exame de esfregaços sanguíneos corados pelo Wright revela neutrófilos e monócitos contendo inúmeros grânulos metacromáticos distintos.
- Grânulos muito indistintos nos animais com MPS I. • Grânulos geralmente inaparentes quando corados pelo Diff-Quik. • Linfócitos ocasionais apresentam vacúolos que contêm grânulos metacromáticos, particularmente nos animais com MPS VII.

OUTROS TESTES LABORATORIAIS
- Preparações citológicas coradas pelo Wright de amostras de linfonodo, fígado, medula óssea e líquido articular revelam grânulos metacromáticos característicos dentro das células.
- A presença de GAG em excesso na urina geralmente indica MPS.
- Diagnóstico definitivo estabelecido pela mensuração da atividade das enzimas lisossomais no soro, nos grânulos de leucócitos ou no fígado congelado.

DIAGNÓSTICO POR IMAGEM
- Radiografia — baixa densidade óssea com adelgaçamento dos córtices.
- Anormalidades epifisárias — variam de leves irregularidades a grandes defeitos recortados no osso subcondral.
- Alterações articulares — achatamento do acetábulo e formação de osteófito periarticular.
- Em alguns gatos, observa-se tecido ósseo proliferativo ao redor de todas as facetas articulares das vértebras, causando a fusão das vértebras cervicais.

MÉTODOS DIAGNÓSTICOS
Laboratórios especializados podem mensurar a atividade das enzimas lisossomais em grânulos de leucócitos e detectar mutações de genes específicos em alguns distúrbios.

ACHADOS PATOLÓGICOS
Lisossomos distendidos observados nas células de muitos tecidos examinados por microscopia óptica e eletrônica.

TRATAMENTO

TRATAMENTO DEFINITIVO
- Transplante de medula óssea — após o enxertamento bem-sucedido, leucócitos normais derivados do doador fornecem a enzima ausente para vários tecidos; quando realizado em uma idade muito precoce, os animais acometidos levam vidas quase normais; não é tão valioso quando efetuado após a maturidade esquelética; além de ser um procedimento caro e com risco de vida, há necessidade de uma cria normal como doador.
- Terapia de reposição enzimática, com o uso de enzima recombinante ao nascimento, seguida pelo transplante de medula óssea, é muito eficaz nos modelos animais de MPS.
- Tanto o transplante de medula óssea como a terapia de reposição enzimática são dispendiosos e foram empregados em primeiro lugar nos modelos animais para determinar o sucesso potencial em crianças; pouquíssimos animais de proprietários foram tratados.
- A terapia genética é muito eficaz em alguns modelos animais, sendo a principal modalidade terapêutica que está sendo avaliada atualmente.

MEDICAÇÕES

MEDICAMENTO(S)
Os animais acometidos ficam suscetíveis à infecção respiratória viral e bacteriana; os antibióticos podem ser indicados.

ACOMPANHAMENTO

PREVENÇÃO
- Evitar cruzamento consanguíneo na família com histórico da doença.
- Ensaios enzimáticos devem ser realizados para diagnosticar heterozigotos.

EVOLUÇÃO ESPERADA E PROGNÓSTICO
- Prognóstico razoavelmente bom em animais tratados com transplante de medula óssea.
- Em geral, os animais não submetidos ao tratamento desenvolvem doença articular e esquelética grave e podem perder a deambulação dos 3 aos 5 anos de idade.

DIVERSOS

ABREVIATURA(S)
- GAG = glicosaminoglicano.
- MPS = mucopolissacarídeo.

Sugestões de Leitura
Haskins M, Casal M, Ellinwood NM, et al. Animal models for mucopolysaccharidoses and their clinical relevance. Acta Paediatr Suppl 2002, 91:88-97.

Autor Mary Anna Thrall
Consultor Editorial A.H. Rebar

Narcolepsia e Cataplexia

CONSIDERAÇÕES GERAIS

REVISÃO
Distúrbios do sono.

Narcolepsia
• Síndrome caracterizada por sonolência excessiva, cataplexia, paralisia do sono e alucinações hipnagógicas (sonhos antes de dormir; seres humanos). Episódios súbitos de sono paradoxal sem um período prévio de sono de ondas lentas.

Cataplexia
• Colapso súbito, episódico e espontâneo secundário à atonia completa dos músculos esqueléticos (paralisia flácida) causada por inibição dos neurônios motores inferiores da medula espinal.
• Os pacientes permanecem alertas e acompanharão com os olhos.
• Sinal clínico mais comum de narcolepsia em pequenos animais.

IDENTIFICAÇÃO
• Cães e, raramente, gatos.
• Hereditária comprovada — Labrador retriever, Dachshund e Doberman pinscher.
• Mutação gênica autossômica recessiva — o gene *canarc-1* é encontrado no cromossomo 12, responsável pela codificação do receptor de hipocretina.
• Suposta base genética para Poodle miniatura — modo de herança desconhecido.
• Para doença hereditária, os sinais clínicos aparecem entre 2 e 4 meses de vida com intensificação dos sinais em torno de 1 ano de idade. Possível desaparecimento dos sinais clínicos mais tarde.
• Pode ocorrer o desenvolvimento da forma adquirida em animais mais idosos (possível depleção da produção de hipocretina pelo hipotálamo); essa forma também pode ocorrer em qualquer raça canina ou raça mista, em qualquer idade.
• Os sinais clínicos na forma adquirida costumam persistir pelo resto da vida.

SINAIS CLÍNICOS
• Exames físico e neurológico — normais, exceto durante um episódio.
• Início — superagudo.
• Há relatos de sonolência diurna excessiva e padrões de sono fragmentados nos animais domésticos, embora a cataplexia costume ser o sinal clínico identificado pelos proprietários.
• Episódios de cataplexia — início agudo de paralisia flácida sem perda de consciência que dura alguns segundos a minutos (até 20 minutos) com retorno súbito ao normal; múltiplos episódios em 1 dia.
• Narcolepsia — movimentos oculares, contrações espasmódicas musculares e gemidos (como ocorre no sono REM) são frequentemente observados durante os episódios.
• Os pacientes costumam acordar com barulhos muito altos, carícias ou outros estímulos externos.

CAUSAS E FATORES DE RISCO
• Hereditários em algumas raças.
• Possível envolvimento do sistema imunológico na doença adquirida.
• Anormalidades de neurotransmissores — serotonina, dopamina, norepinefrina, neuropeptídeo hipocretina (orexina).
• Relatos raros com lesões pontinomedulares (tronco cerebral).
• Agitação, emoções, alimentação e anestesia geral podem induzir a episódios narcolépticos.

DIAGNÓSTICO

DIAGNÓSTICO DIFERENCIAL
• Síncope.
• Atividade convulsiva — incontinência urinária ou fecal, salivação excessiva e rigidez muscular não são características de narcolepsia em que há o predomínio de atonia. A recuperação após um evento narcoléptico é imediata.
• Crise não convulsiva (ataque com queda).
• Distúrbios neuromusculares — o início dos sinais clínicos não costuma ser tão súbito e a recuperação não tão imediata quanto em casos de narcolepsia.

HEMOGRAMA/BIOQUÍMICA/URINÁLISE
• Normais.

OUTROS TESTES LABORATORIAIS
• Teste de DNA para raças específicas (Labrador retriever, Dachshund, e Doberman pinscher).
• LCS — normal.

DIAGNÓSTICO POR IMAGEM
RM cerebral — normal.

MÉTODOS DIAGNÓSTICOS
• Observar um episódio — se uma atividade constante (alimentação, agitação, etc.) eliciar os ataques, tentar a simulação da atividade.
• Teste da cataplexia eliciada pelo alimento — colocar 10 pedaços de comida em fileira com 30-60 cm de distância; registrar o tempo necessário para o paciente comer todos os pedaços, bem como o número, o tipo e a duração de qualquer ataque ocorrente; os cães normais comem todo o alimento em <45 s e não apresentam ataques, enquanto os acometidos demoram >2 min para comer o alimento e podem ter 2-20 ataques.
• Desafio da fisostigmina (inibidor da colinesterase) para induzir cataplexia em cão acometido — administrar 0,025-0,1 mg/kg IV; repetir o teste eliciado pelo alimento 5-15 min depois da injeção; aumentar a dosagem em caso de necessidade (0,05 mg/kg; 0,075 mg/kg; 0,10 mg/kg); os efeitos de cada dose duram 15-45 min.

TRATAMENTO

• Objetivo primário — diminuir a gravidade e a frequência dos episódios catalépticos.
• Informar ao proprietário sobre o caráter não fatal da cataplexia, a não ocorrência de asfixia com o alimento nem obstrução das vias aéreas, e a ausência de sofrimento por parte do animal.
• Avisar o proprietário sobre o fato de que atividades como caça, natação e exercício sem coleira colocam o paciente em risco.
• Se os episódios forem pouco frequentes e a qualidade de vida for preservada, o tratamento deverá ser adiado e o ambiente adaptado para evitar estimulações específicas.

MEDICAÇÕES

MEDICAMENTO(S)
• Imipramina (Tofranil®) — 0,5 mg/kg VO a cada 8 h.
• Metilfenidato (Ritalin®) — 0,25 mg/kg VO a cada 12-24 h.
• Selegilina (Anipryl®) — 2 mg/kg a cada 24 h.
• Ioimbina — 50-100 µg/kg SC ou VO a cada 8-12 h.
• Também é possível a combinação — imipramida e metilfenidato.

CONTRAINDICAÇÕES/INTERAÇÕES POSSÍVEIS
• Muitos pacientes desenvolvem tolerância medicamentosa; talvez haja necessidade da troca do medicamento.
• Frequências cardíaca e respiratória elevadas, anorexia, tremores, hipertermia induzida por exercício.

ACOMPANHAMENTO

• O ato de evitar atividades incitantes pode reduzir os episódios, dispensando a necessidade de medicamentos.
• Os pacientes com a forma hereditária podem melhorar com a idade.
• O prognóstico varia com o tratamento; alguns pacientes permanecem sintomáticos.

DIVERSOS

ABREVIATURA(S)
• LCS = líquido cerebrospinal.
• RM = ressonância magnética.

RECURSOS DA INTERNET
http://med.stanford.edu/school/Psychiatry/narcolepsy/.

Sugestões de Leitura
De Lahunta A, Glass EN. Narcolepsy and cataplexy. In: Veterinary Neuroanatomy and Clinical Neurology, 3rd ed. St. Louis: Saunders Elsevier, 2009, pp. 468-472.

Autor Myléne-Kim Leclerc
Consultor Editorial Joane M. Parent
Agradecimento a T. Mark Neer por ter escrito este capítulo nas edições anteriores.

Nefrolitíase

CONSIDERAÇÕES GERAIS

DEFINIÇÃO
- Nefrólitos — urólitos localizados na pelve renal ou nos divertículos coletores do rim.
- Os nefrólitos ou seus fragmentos podem passar para os ureteres (ureterólitos).
- Os nefrólitos que não são infectados, não provocam obstrução nem sinais clínicos e não aumentam progressivamente são denominados *inativos*.

FISIOPATOLOGIA
Os nefrólitos são capazes de obstruir a pelve renal ou o ureter, predispor o animal à pielonefrite e resultar em lesão compressiva do parênquima renal, levando à insuficiência renal; ver os capítulos sobre os diferentes tipos de urólitos em busca da fisiopatologia da urolitíase; nos gatos, podem se formar nefrólitos compostos de coágulos sanguíneos mineralizados com fosfato de cálcio, secundariamente à hematúria renal crônica.

SISTEMA(S) ACOMETIDO(S)
- Renal/urológico — acomete o trato urinário, com potencial para obstrução, infecções recidivantes do trato urinário ou insuficiência renal.
- Obstrução da pelve renal ou do ureter em animal com pielonefrite — pode resultar em septicemia e, dessa forma, acometer qualquer sistema corporal.

GENÉTICA
Recorrer aos capítulos que descrevem a genética relacionada com os diferentes tipos de urólitos.

INCIDÊNCIA/PREVALÊNCIA
- Os nefrólitos recuperados de cães e gatos compõem <5% dos urólitos enviados aos centros laboratoriais de análise. A verdadeira incidência de nefrólitos provavelmente é bem mais elevada, porque muitos animais com nefrólitos permanecem assintomáticos ou não são tratados por métodos que abrangem a recuperação de urólitos, possibilitando sua análise quantitativa.
- As composições minerais de nefrólitos caninos encaminhados para análise em ordem decrescente de frequência são oxalato de cálcio (43%), estruvita (26%), purinas (p. ex., urato de amônio, urato de sódio, ácido úrico; 13%), compostos (12%), mistos (3%), cistina (1,7%), fosfato de cálcio (1,5%) e sílica (0,3%).
- As composições minerais de nefrólitos felinos encaminhados para análise em ordem decrescente de frequência são oxalato de cálcio (71%), estruvita (8%), matriz não cristalina (7%), compostos (6%), fosfato de cálcio (4%), mistos (3%), purinas (2%), cistina (0,1%) e sílica (0,04%).

IDENTIFICAÇÃO
Espécies
Cães e gatos.

Raça(s) Predominante(s)
Cães
- Nefrólitos de oxalato de cálcio — Schnauzer miniatura, Lhasa apso, Yorkshire terrier, Poodle miniatura e Shih tzu.
- Nefrólitos de estruvita — Schnauzer miniatura, Bichon frisé, Shih tzu, Yorkshire terrier, Lhasa apso, Cocker spaniel e Poodle miniatura.
- Nefrólitos de purina — Dálmata, Yorkshire terrier e Buldogue inglês.
- Nefrólitos de cistina — Terra Nova, Dachshund, Buldogue inglês, Mastiff e muitas outras.

Gatos
Doméstico de pelo curto (33%), doméstico de pelo longo (17%), Persa (8%), Siamês (6%), raça desconhecida (19%).

Idade Média e Faixa Etária
- Cães — idade média dos animais acometidos, 9 anos (faixa de 4 meses a 14 anos).
- Gatos — idade média dos animais acometidos, 8 anos (faixa de 2 meses a 18 anos).

Sexo Predominante
- Em geral, os nefrólitos nos cães são levemente mais comuns nas fêmeas (55%) do que nos machos (41%), com 4% não especificados; para os nefrólitos de estruvita, fêmeas > machos; para os nefrólitos de oxalato de cálcio, cistina e urato, machos > fêmeas.
- Nos gatos, os nefrólitos são um pouco mais comuns nas fêmeas (55%) que nos machos (45%).

SINAIS CLÍNICOS
Comentários Gerais
Muitos pacientes permanecem assintomáticos e, por essa razão, os nefrólitos são diagnosticados durante a avaliação de outros problemas.

Achados Anamnésicos
- Nenhum ou hematúria, vômito e infecção recidivante do trato urinário; disúria e polaciúria nos animais com infecção do trato urinário ou urocistólitos concomitantes.
- Sinais atribuíveis à uremia nos animais com obstrução bilateral ou insuficiência renal.
- Sinais referíveis à urolitíase do trato urinário inferior se os urólitos estiverem presentes nos tratos urinários superior e inferior.
- A chamada cólica renal com dor abdominal/lombar aguda e vômito é rara.

Achados do Exame Físico
Dor abdominal ou lombar à palpação ou sem achados significativos.

CAUSAS
- Para obtenção da extensa lista de causas, consultar os capítulos sobre cada tipo de urólito. A supersaturação da urina com minerais calculogênicos é um fator de risco para a urolitíase.
- Urolitíase por oxalato de cálcio — hipercalciúria, hipercalcemia, hipocitratúria, hiperoxalúria, hiperparatireoidismo primário, ingestão excessiva de cálcio na dieta.
- Urolitíase por fosfato de cálcio — sangramento renal crônico (gatos), hipercalcemia, hiperparatireoidismo, excesso de cálcio e fósforo na dieta, acidose tubular renal.
- Urolitíase por cistina — cistinúria.
- Urolitíase por estruvita induzida por infecção — infecção do trato urinário por microrganismos produtores de urease. Dietas ricas em proteínas que produzem grande quantidade de ureia excretada na urina também são parte integrante da etiopatogênese de urólitos de estruvita induzidos por infecção.
- Urolitíase por urato — defeito genético na conversão do ácido úrico em alantoína (Dálmatas), desvio portossistêmico.
- Urolitíase por xantina — administração de alopurinol e ingestão elevada de purina na dieta em cães predispostos à urolitíase por urato. Aparentemente constitui um erro inato do metabolismo de purina em gatos.

FATORES DE RISCO
- Urina alcalina — urólitos de estruvita e de fosfato de cálcio.
- Urina ácida — urólitos de oxalato de cálcio, de cistina, de urato e de xantina.
- Retenção de urina e formação de urina altamente concentrada.
- Infecção do trato urinário inferior — infecção ascendente e pielonefrite.
- Condições que predispõem à infecção do trato urinário (p. ex., uretrostomia perineal, ureteres ectópicos, refluxo vesicoureteral e administração exógena de esteroides ou hiperadrenocorticismo [urólitos de oxalato de cálcio]).

DIAGNÓSTICO

DIAGNÓSTICO DIFERENCIAL
- Considerar a existência de nefrólitos em qualquer paciente com insuficiência renal, infecção recidivante do trato urinário, vômito agudo (pancreatite aguda, gastroenterite aguda, obstrução intestinal ou gástrica, etc.) ou dor abdominal ou lombar (p. ex., protrusão do disco intervertebral e peritonite).
- Em geral, os nefrólitos são confirmados por meio de radiografias ou ultrassonografia; diferenciar a mineralização da pelve renal ou dos divertículos coletores da nefrolitíase verdadeira.

HEMOGRAMA/BIOQUÍMICA/URINÁLISE
- Resultados do hemograma completo — geralmente normais a menos que o paciente tenha pielonefrite; os pacientes com pielonefrite podem apresentar leucocitose e neutrofilia imatura.
- Análise da bioquímica sérica — geralmente normal a menos que a ocorrência de obstrução bilateral, pielonefrite ou lesão renal compressiva leve à insuficiência renal (azotemia com densidade urinária inadequada, hiperfosfatemia); a hipercalcemia pode contribuir para a formação de nefrólitos de oxalato de cálcio ou de fosfato de cálcio.
- Urinálise — pode revelar hematúria e cristalúria; o tipo de cristal pode indicar a composição mineral; piúria, proteinúria e bacteriúria também podem ser observadas nos animais com infecção do trato urinário.

OUTROS TESTES LABORATORIAIS
- Enviar todos os nefrólitos recuperados ou fragmentos deles para análise quantitativa. Embora a identificação definitiva do tipo de nefrólito necessite da análise quantitativa, a composição mineral frequentemente pode ser prevista com base na identificação do animal, no aspecto do exame radiográfico e nos achados da urinálise.
- Os resultados da cultura bacteriana de urina podem confirmar a infecção do trato urinário nos animais com pielonefrite concomitante.

DIAGNÓSTICO POR IMAGEM
- Podem-se detectar nefrólitos radiopacos (p. ex., fosfato de cálcio, oxalato de cálcio e estruvita) por meio de radiografias simples; os urólitos de cistina e sílica são levemente radiopacos.
- Os urólitos de purinas (urato de amônio, urato de sódio, ácido úrico, xantina, etc.) costumam ser radiotransparentes a menos que contenham uma mistura de minerais biogênicos radiodensos.

NEFROLITÍASE

- Pode-se lançar mão dos exames de ultrassonografia ou urografia excretora para confirmar a presença, o tamanho e o número de nefrólitos ou ureterólitos, independentemente da densidade radiográfica.

MÉTODOS DIAGNÓSTICOS
Após a aplicação de litotripsia extracorpórea por ondas de choque, os fragmentos do nefrólito podem ser recuperados para análise quantitativa por micção espontânea, cistoscopia, recuperação auxiliada por cateter ou uro-hidropropulsão miccional.

TRATAMENTO

CUIDADO(S) DE SAÚDE ADEQUADO(S)
Tratar os pacientes com nefrólitos inativos em um esquema ambulatorial. Os protocolos de dissolução clínica podem ser administrados em pacientes desse tipo. A remoção dos nefrólitos por meio de cirurgia ou litotripsia extracorpórea por ondas de choque necessita de hospitalização.

DIETA
A dissolução clínica dos nefrólitos necessita de dieta apropriada para o tipo específico de nefrólito. Ver a seção "Medicações".

ORIENTAÇÃO AO PROPRIETÁRIO
- Nefrólitos inativos — podem não necessitar de remoção, mas devem ser monitorizados periodicamente por meio de urinálise, urocultura e radiografia. Os nefrólitos potencialmente podem provocar obstrução em qualquer momento, o que pode resultar em hidronefrose sem sinais clínicos. Dessa forma, o tratamento conservativo e a monitorização carreiam um leve risco de lesão renal não detectada e potencialmente irreversível, o que precisa ser ponderado diante da lesão renal potencial decorrente de nefrotomia.
- Nefrólitos (especialmente urólitos metabólicos) — tendem a recidivar após a remoção; monitorizar o paciente a cada 3-6 meses.

CONSIDERAÇÕES CIRÚRGICAS
- Indicações para a remoção dos nefrólitos — obstrução, infecção recidivante, nefrólitos sintomáticos, aumento progressivo do nefrólito e rim contralateral não funcional.
- Opções de tratamento para os nefrólitos — dissolução clínica, cirurgia e litotripsia extracorpórea por ondas de choque. Nefrólitos de oxalato de cálcio, a composição mineral mais comumente detectada em nefrólitos recuperados de cães e gatos, não são responsivos à dissolução clínica. Ureterólitos ou nefrólitos que provocam obstrução completa também não são responsivos à dissolução clínica.
- Opções cirúrgicas — nefrotomia ou pielolitotomia. Como os nefrólitos são circundados pelo tecido renal, o procedimento de nefrotomia é necessário em grande parte dos cães e gatos. A remoção do nefrólito por meio da nefrolitotomia percutânea foi relatada nos cães.
- Litotripsia extracorpórea por ondas de choque — método seguro e eficaz de tratamento dos nefrólitos e ureterólitos caninos; os fragmentos do nefrólito passam pelo ureter e seguem para a bexiga, sendo eliminados pela urina.
- Litotripsia extracorpórea por ondas de choque — não é tão eficaz para o tratamento de nefrólitos e ureterólitos nos gatos em comparação com os cães.

MEDICAÇÕES

MEDICAMENTO(S) DE ESCOLHA
- Antibióticos selecionados com base na urocultura e antibiograma, conforme a necessidade; é recomendável o uso de antibióticos durante o procedimento ao se tratar os nefrólitos infectados por meio da litotripsia extracorpórea por ondas de choque ou remoção cirúrgica.
- Os protocolos de dissolução clínica ficam limitados aos urólitos de estruvita, de purina e de cistina.
- Quando praticável, o consumo de água em rações (enlatadas) com alto teor de umidade deve ser incorporado ao protocolo terapêutico. Tentar aumentar a excreção de urina com densidade <1,020 (cães) ou <1,025 (gatos).
- Os protocolos de dissolução clínica para os nefrólitos de estruvita incluem a dieta calculolítica (Prescription Diet s/d, Hill's®) e antibioticoterapia adequada (i. e., se o paciente tiver infecção do trato urinário) durante o tratamento.
- Os protocolos de dissolução clínica para os nefrólitos de purina em cães podem ser tentados por meio de dieta alcalinizante com restrição de proteína e purina (Prescription Diet Canine u/d, Hill's®), alopurinol (15 mg/kg VO a cada 12 h) e suplemento de citrato de potássio, conforme a necessidade, para manter o pH urinário em ~7,0.
- A dissolução clínica da nefrolitíase canina por cistina pode ser tentada, fazendo-se uso de dieta alcalinizante restrita em proteína (Prescription Diet Canine u/d, Hill's®), 2-MPG (Thiola®, 15 mg/kg VO a cada 12 h) e suplemento de citrato de potássio, conforme a necessidade, para manter a urina com pH de ~7,5.

CONTRAINDICAÇÕES
- Não utilizar o alopurinol sem a restrição de purina na dieta, pois essa combinação pode provocar nefrolitíase por xantina em cães predispostos à urolitíase por urato.
- Não oferecer dietas acidificantes aos pacientes azotêmicos a menos que o pH sanguíneo e o CO_2 total sejam monitorizados quanto ao desenvolvimento de acidose metabólica.

ACOMPANHAMENTO

MONITORIZAÇÃO DO PACIENTE
Radiografias abdominais (ultrassonografia para urólitos radiotransparentes), urinálise e urocultura a cada 3-6 meses para detectar recidiva do nefrólito. Cães tratados com litotripsia extracorpórea por ondas de choque — examinar a cada 2-4 semanas por meio de radiografias e ultrassonografia até que os fragmentos do nefrólito tenham passado pelo sistema excretor.

PREVENÇÃO
Eliminar os fatores predisponentes para cada tipo de urólito, aumentar o volume urinário e corrigir os fatores que contribuem para a retenção urinária.

COMPLICAÇÕES POSSÍVEIS
Hidronefrose, insuficiência renal, infecção recidivante do trato urinário e pielonefrite.

EVOLUÇÃO ESPERADA E PROGNÓSTICO
- Altamente variáveis; dependem do tipo, da localização e do tamanho do nefrólito, bem como da presença de complicações secundárias (p. ex., obstrução, infecção e insuficiência renal) e da obediência do proprietário aos protocolos de tratamento e prevenção.
- Os nefrólitos inativos podem permanecer inativos por anos, resultando em prognóstico excelente.
- Os autores obtiveram resultados excelentes com a aplicação de litotripsia extracorpórea por ondas de choque para o tratamento de cães com nefrólitos — retorno à saúde normal e prognóstico excelente.
- O prognóstico de pacientes com insuficiência renal provocada pela nefrolitíase depende da gravidade e da velocidade de evolução da insuficiência renal.
- Os nefrólitos que provocam obstrução ao fluxo de saída da urina ou estão associados a rins não funcionais não podem ser dissolvidos por meio clínico.

DIVERSOS

DISTÚRBIOS ASSOCIADOS
Hiperadrenocorticismo e administração crônica de glicocorticoides estão associados a urólitos de oxalato de cálcio e infecção do trato urinário, resultando em urolitíase por estruvita.

GESTAÇÃO/FERTILIDADE/REPRODUÇÃO
- Contraindicação para a litotripsia extracorpórea por ondas de choque.
- Ácido aceto-hidroxâmico, um inibidor da urease, é teratogênico.

SINÔNIMO(S)
Concreções renais, cálculos renais, renólitos, cálculos ou pedras no rim.

VER TAMBÉM
- Hidronefrose.
- Insuficiência Renal Crônica.
- Obstrução do Trato Urinário.
- Pielonefrite.
- Urolitíase por Cistina.
- Urolitíase por Estruvita — Cães.
- Urolitíase por Estruvita — Gatos.
- Urolitíase por Fosfato de Cálcio.
- Urolitíase por Oxalato de Cálcio.
- Urolitíase por Urato.
- Urolitíase por Xantina.

ABREVIATURA(S)
- 2-MPG = 2-mercaptopropionil-glicina.

RECURSOS DA INTERNET
www.vet.utk.edu/clinical/sacs/lithotripsy

Sugestões de Leitura
Lane IF, Labato MA, Adams LG. Lithotripsy. In: August JR, ed., Consultations in Feline Internal Medicine. St. Louis: Elsevier, 2006, pp. 407-414.

Autores Carl A. Osborne e Larry G. Adams
Consultor Editorial Carl A. Osborne

Nefrotoxicidade Induzida por Medicamentos

CONSIDERAÇÕES GERAIS

DEFINIÇÃO
Lesão renal provocada por agente farmacológico utilizado para diagnosticar ou tratar algum distúrbio clínico.

FISIOPATOLOGIA
- Os medicamentos podem provocar nefrotoxicose por interferência no fluxo sanguíneo renal, na função glomerular, na função tubular ou por inflamação intersticial.
- Muitos medicamentos são nefrotóxicos, porque são excretados principalmente pelos rins.
- A maior parte dos medicamentos nefrotóxicos provoca necrose tubular renal proximal.
- Se a lesão renal for grave, ocorrerá o desenvolvimento de insuficiência renal aguda.

SISTEMA(S) ACOMETIDO(S)
- Renal/urológico.
- Gastrintestinal — inapetência, vômito, diarreia ou melena em virtude de irritação ou ulceração gastrintestinal nos pacientes com uremia.
- Endócrino/metabólico — acidose metabólica decorrente da eliminação diminuída de ácido pelos rins e da incapacidade de reabsorção do bicarbonato filtrado nos túbulos pelos glomérulos.
- Hematológico/linfático/imune — anemia por perda sanguínea ou tempo de sobrevida reduzido das hemácias em pacientes com uremia; suscetibilidade aumentada a infecções por causa da disfunção imune em pacientes com uremia.
- Nervoso — depressão e letargia associadas ao efeito das toxinas urêmicas sobre o sistema nervoso central.
- Neuromuscular — fraqueza atribuída aos efeitos sistêmicos da uremia.
- Respiratório — taquipneia ou angústia respiratória por pneumonite urêmica ou resposta compensatória à acidose metabólica.

GENÉTICA
N/D.

INCIDÊNCIA/PREVALÊNCIA
N/D.

DISTRIBUIÇÃO GEOGRÁFICA
N/D.

IDENTIFICAÇÃO
Espécies
Cães e gatos.

Raça(s) Predominante(s)
N/D.

Idade Média e Faixa Etária
Qualquer idade; pacientes idosos são mais suscetíveis.

Sexo Predominante
N/D.

SINAIS CLÍNICOS
Achados Anamnésicos
- Poliúria e polidipsia.
- Inapetência.
- Depressão.
- Vômito.
- Diarreia.

Achados do Exame Físico
- Desidratação.
- Úlceras bucais.
- Hálito de odor fétido.

CAUSAS
Medicamentos Antimicrobianos
- Aminoglicosídeos — todos os medicamentos dessa classe são potencialmente nefrotóxicos, incluindo neomicina, gentamicina, amicacina, canamicina e estreptomicina. Devido ao uso frequente no passado, a nefrotoxicose associada ao tratamento com aminoglicosídeo era mais frequentemente relacionada com a gentamicina.
- Tetraciclinas — produtos vencidos podem provocar síndrome adquirida semelhante à de Fanconi, caracterizada por glicosúria, proteinúria e acidose tubular renal; a administração IV aos cães em dosagens elevadas (>30 mg/kg) pode causar insuficiência renal aguda.
- A administração de medicamentos com sulfa (p. ex., trimetoprima-sulfadiazina) foi associada à insuficiência renal aguda nos cães, porém nenhuma relação causal foi comprovada.

Medicamentos Antifúngicos
Anfotericina B.

Medicamentos Antineoplásicos
- Cisplatina — causa clinicamente importante de nefrotoxicose nos cães.
- Doxorrubicina — possível causa de nefrotoxicose em gatos, mas não foi bem documentada.

AINE
- Ácido acetilsalicílico, ibuprofeno, naproxeno, piroxicam, flunixino meglumina e outros podem provocar nefrotoxicose.
- Mais provavelmente causam lesão renal nos pacientes com nefropatia preexistente ou naqueles com desidratação concomitante ou outras causas de hipovolemia.

Inibidores da ECA
- Enalapril, benazepril e outros.
- Mais provavelmente causam insuficiência renal aguda em pacientes com hiponatremia, desidratação ou insuficiência cardíaca congestiva.

Agentes de Contraste Radiográfico
A administração intravenosa dos agentes de contraste radiográfico à base de iodo pode provocar insuficiência renal aguda, sobretudo em pacientes com desidratação, hipovolemia ou hipotensão associada à anestesia inalatória.

FATORES DE RISCO
- Desidratação.
- Idade avançada, provavelmente porque os pacientes mais idosos apresentam doença renal preexistente.
- Nefropatia ativa ou inativa.
- Hipoperfusão renal; as causas potenciais incluem qualquer distúrbio associado à hipovolemia (p. ex., vômito, hemorragia e hipoadrenocorticismo), baixo débito cardíaco (p. ex., insuficiência cardíaca congestiva, pericardiopatia, arritmias cardíacas e anestesia inalatória) ou vasoconstrição renal (p. ex., administração de AINE).
- Anormalidades eletrolíticas e acidobásicas, incluindo hipocalemia, hiponatremia, hipocalcemia, hipomagnesemia e acidose metabólica.
- Terapia medicamentosa concomitante — a administração da furosemida aumenta a nefrotoxicidade dos aminoglicosídeos; o tratamento com medicamentos citotóxicos (p. ex., ciclofosfamida) pode aumentar o potencial nefrotóxico dos medicamentos.
- Febre.
- Sepse.

DIAGNÓSTICO

DIAGNÓSTICO DIFERENCIAL
- Deve-se diferenciar de outras causas de insuficiência renal aguda (p. ex., intoxicação pelo etilenoglicol, ingestão de uvas/passas [cães], intoxicação pelo lírio [gatos], isquemia renal, leptospirose).
- A maior parte dos pacientes apresenta histórico de tratamento recente (i. e., nas últimas 2 semanas) com algum medicamento potencialmente nefrotóxico; pode ocorrer insuficiência renal aguda vários dias depois da interrupção de algum aminoglicosídeo.
- Determinar todos os medicamentos que foram administrados ao paciente, incluindo as preparações vendidas sem receita (p. ex., ácido acetilsalicílico, ibuprofeno e naproxeno) e medicações vendidas para utilização humana (p. ex., AINE ou inibidor da ECA).

HEMOGRAMA/BIOQUÍMICA/URINÁLISE
- Hemograma — geralmente normal a menos que existam problemas concomitantes (p. ex., hemorragia gastrintestinal associada à administração de AINE).
- Análise bioquímica — permanece normal nos estágios iniciais da nefrotoxicose induzida por medicamentos ou revela sinais compatíveis com insuficiência renal aguda, incluindo azotemia, hiperfosfatemia e acidose metabólica.
- Urinálise — pode revelar densidade urinária baixa (frequentemente <1,025), proteinúria, glicosúria ou cilindrúria.

OUTROS TESTES LABORATORIAIS
N/D.

DIAGNÓSTICO POR IMAGEM
N/D.

MÉTODOS DIAGNÓSTICOS
Pode haver indicação de biopsia renal para determinar a causa de insuficiência renal aguda e o potencial de reversibilidade, sobretudo em pacientes que não respondem favoravelmente ao tratamento conforme o esperado. A magnitude das alterações morfológicas renais pode parecer branda em comparação à magnitude da azotemia.

ACHADOS PATOLÓGICOS
A maior parte dos medicamentos nefrotóxicos causa necrose tubular renal proximal.

TRATAMENTO

CUIDADO(S) DE SAÚDE ADEQUADO(S)
- Tratar os pacientes com insuficiência renal aguda com internação.
- Tratar os pacientes sem azotemia que podem comer e beber o suficiente para manter a hidratação em um esquema ambulatorial.

CUIDADO(S) DE ENFERMAGEM
- Administrar soro fisiológico a 0,9% por via intravenosa nos pacientes com insuficiência renal; a solução de Ringer lactato pode ser utilizada, embora contenha uma pequena quantidade de potássio, o que pode não ser ideal para os pacientes com insuficiência renal aguda e hipercalemia.

NEFROTOXICIDADE INDUZIDA POR MEDICAMENTOS

• Corrigir rapidamente os déficits de hidratação (i. e., em 6-8 h) para minimizar a lesão renal adicional. Calcular o volume de fluido a ser administrado da seguinte forma: volume (mL) = peso corporal (kg) × % de desidratação × 1.000 mL.
• Além de corrigir os déficits de hidratação, administrar as necessidades de manutenção (~66 mL/kg/dia) e repor quaisquer perdas contínuas causadas por vômito e diarreia. Como um valor mínimo, admitir que os pacientes com insuficiência renal aguda estejam perdendo 3-5% de seu peso corporal por causa das perdas contínuas.

ATIVIDADE
Reduzir.

DIETA
• Os pacientes de ambulatório podem receber sua dieta habitual. Os efeitos das rações terapêuticas renais sobre cães e gatos com doença renal crônica em estágio 1 (não azotêmica) de acordo com a IRIS não foram avaliados; no entanto, elas podem ajudar a retardar a evolução para os estágios mais tardios.
• Modificar a dieta para os pacientes com insuficiência renal aguda; evitar a alimentação por via oral até que o vômito esteja controlado.
• Ao se iniciar a alimentação por via oral, fica indicada uma ração terapêutica renal (como a k/d Prescription Diet da Hill) para ajudar a controlar os sinais de uremia.
• Os pacientes que se recuperam de nefrotoxicose induzida por medicamentos podem desenvolver doença renal crônica, que deve ser tratada pelo fornecimento de ração terapêutica renal por tempo indefinido.

ORIENTAÇÃO AO PROPRIETÁRIO
• Evitar estresse desnecessário (p. ex., hospedagem em hotel ou cirurgia eletiva); proporcionar acesso ilimitado à água limpa e fresca durante todo o tempo.
• Caso se desenvolvam alguns sinais de doença, como inapetência, vômito ou diarreia, retornar o paciente de forma imediata para os cuidados veterinários, a fim de minimizar a piora da função renal.

CONSIDERAÇÕES CIRÚRGICAS
• Evitar a realização de cirurgia eletiva até que a nefropatia esteja solucionada.
• Se a cirurgia for necessária, administrar fluidos (5-20 mL/kg/h) durante a anestesia para manter a pressão sanguínea arterial média (>60 mmHg) e a perfusão renal adequadas. Monitorar o débito urinário e ajustar a velocidade de administração dos fluidos para manter a produção urinária de 1-2 mL/kg/h.

MEDICAÇÕES

MEDICAMENTO(S) DE ESCOLHA
Nenhum.

CONTRAINDICAÇÕES
Não usar a furosemida para promover a diurese nos pacientes com nefrotoxicidade por aminoglicosídeo.

PRECAUÇÕES
• Evitar os medicamentos que possam piorar a lesão renal nos pacientes com nefrotoxicose, incluindo AINE, vasodilatadores e inibidores da ECA.
• Utilizar medicamentos menos tóxicos sempre que possível (p. ex., carboplatina no lugar da cisplatina, outros antimicrobianos eficazes em vez de aminoglicosídeos).

INTERAÇÕES POSSÍVEIS
N/D.

ACOMPANHAMENTO

MONITORIZAÇÃO DO PACIENTE
• Pesar os pacientes hospitalizados várias vezes ao dia para detectar alterações no equilíbrio hídrico e ajustar a fluidoterapia de acordo.
• Realizar a análise bioquímica, incluindo a mensuração dos eletrólitos, a cada 1-2 dias para avaliar a gravidade da azotemia e detectar anormalidades eletrolíticas e acidobásicas.
• Em pacientes submetidos a aminoglicosídeos — efetuar a urinálise a cada 1-2 dias para detectar sinais precoces de nefrotoxicose, como glicosúria, proteinúria aumentada e cilindrúria; interromper o aminoglicosídeo caso se observe qualquer um desses sinais.
• Mensurar o débito urinário para determinar se o paciente está poliúrico ou oligúrico; ajustar a fluidoterapia com base nesses achados e determinar a necessidade de tratamento adicional para estimular a produção urinária. Não super-hidratar o paciente com fluidos parenterais.

PREVENÇÃO
• Evitar ou corrigir os fatores de risco que predisponham ao desenvolvimento de nefrotoxicose induzida por medicamentos.
• Administrar diurese salina a todos os cães submetidos à cisplatina.
• Evitar a utilização de medicamentos nefrotóxicos a menos que sejam necessários (p. ex., usar os aminoglicosídeos apenas se o paciente estiver com sepse avassaladora e os resultados da cultura indicarem os aminoglicosídeos como o único antimicrobiano eficaz).

• Monitorizar a concentração sérica do aminoglicosídeo e realizar urinálises frequentes enquanto se administra esse tipo de medicamento.
• Não administrar a furosemida com um aminoglicosídeo, pois é provável que essa combinação aumente a nefrotoxicidade deste último medicamento.

COMPLICAÇÕES POSSÍVEIS
• Insuficiência renal aguda.
• Doença e insuficiência renais crônicas.

EVOLUÇÃO ESPERADA E PROGNÓSTICO
• Os pacientes sem azotemia podem desenvolver insuficiência renal aguda após vários dias de exposição, especialmente aos aminoglicosídeos.
• A lesão renal provocada por medicamentos nefrotóxicos pode levar ao desenvolvimento de insuficiência renal crônica meses a anos depois da recuperação de lesão renal induzida por medicamentos.

DIVERSOS

DISTÚRBIOS ASSOCIADOS
N/D.

FATORES RELACIONADOS COM A IDADE
N/D.

POTENCIAL ZOONÓTICO
N/D.

GESTAÇÃO/FERTILIDADE/REPRODUÇÃO
N/D.

VER TAMBÉM
Insuficiência Renal Aguda.

ABREVIATURA(S)
• AINE = anti-inflamatório não esteroide.
• ECA = enzima conversora de angiotensina.
• IRIS = International Renal Interest Society.

RECURSOS DA INTERNET
www.iris-kidney.com (contém informações sobre o estadiamento de cães e gatos com doença renal crônica e as recomendações terapêuticas para cada estágio, segundo a IRIS).

Sugestões de Leitura
Behrend EN, Grauer GF, Mani I, et al. Hospital-acquired acute renal failure in dogs: 29 cases (1983-1992). JAVMA 1996, 208:537-541.
Langston C. Acute uremia. In: Ettinger SJ, Feldman EC, eds., Textbook of Veterinary Internal Medicine, 7th ed. Philadelphia: Elsevier, 2009, pp. 1969-1985.
Vaden SL, Levine J, Breitschewerdt EB. A retrospective case-control of acute renal failure in 99 dogs. J Vet Intern Med 1997, 11:58-64.

Autor S. Dru Forrester
Consultor Editorial Carl A. Osborne

Nematódeos (Ascaríase)

CONSIDERAÇÕES GERAIS

REVISÃO
- A ascaríase é causada por *Toxocara canis* (cães), *T. cati* (gatos) e *Toxascaris leonina* (cães e gatos); o *Baylisascaris* (guaxinins) pode infectar os cães.
- A transmissão transplacentária de larvas de *T. canis* dos tecidos da cadela para os filhotes resulta em infecção pré-natal e pré-patência mais curta; ocorre transmissão transmamária das larvas com ambas as espécies de *Toxocara*; nenhuma transmissão transplacentária ou transmamária ocorre com o *Toxascaris*.
- No primeiro mês de vida, os neonatos caninos infectados podem desenvolver dor abdominal e sofrer rápida deterioração antes de os ovos aparecerem nas fezes.
- Os filhotes caninos e felinos com mais idade podem adquirir a infecção pela ingestão de ovos larvados disseminados nos recintos pelas mães com infecção pós-gestacional; as progenitoras podem ser infectadas pela ingestão de estágios imaturos nas fezes ou no vômito de filhotes caninos.
- A infecção também pode ocorrer pela predação de hospedeiros vertebrados de transporte infectados por larvas infectantes latentes adquiridas pela ingestão de ovos larvados.
- Os ascarídeos adultos ocorrem no lúmen do intestino delgado; os estágios larvais de *Toxocara* spp. podem migrar pelo fígado e pulmão.
- Se forem muito numerosos, os ascarídeos robustos relativamente grandes (até 10-12 cm de comprimento) poderão distender o intestino e induzir à cólica, interferência na motilidade intestinal, incapacidade de utilizar o alimento e, raramente, ruptura intestinal.

IDENTIFICAÇÃO
- Cães e gatos.
- Particularmente importante em termos clínicos nos filhotes caninos e felinos em virtude da transmissão no útero e/ou pelo colostro/leite.

SINAIS CLÍNICOS
- Distensão abdominal ("barriga grande"); frequentemente com distensão palpável dos intestinos. • Cólica. • Fraqueza, perda da condição corporal, caquexia. • Amamentação ou apetite deficientes. • Fezes escassas. • Tosse causada pela migração das larvas pelos pulmões. • Toda a ninhada pode estar acometida.

CAUSAS E FATORES DE RISCO
- Infecção da cadela por *Toxocara* com larvas latentes nos tecidos ou infecção da gata durante o final da prenhez ou no início da lactação.
- Alimento ou ambiente contaminado por fezes.
- Acesso a hospedeiros de transporte infectados.
- Infecções entéricas concomitantes.

DIAGNÓSTICO

DIAGNÓSTICO DIFERENCIAL
- Infecção perinatal transmamária de neonatos por ancilóstomos (anemia, melena, fraqueza, letargia, mucosas pálidas, enterite) ou *Strongyloides* (diarreia); coccidiose e giardíase também provocam enterite em filhotes caninos e felinos; examinar as fezes para identificar os ovos ou as larvas.
- Pode ocorrer *Physaloptera* no vômito, mas não nas fezes de cães/gatos infectados; os ascarídeos possuem três lábios e asas cervicais; o *Physaloptera* têm colar cervical anterior.

HEMOGRAMA/BIOQUÍMICA/URINÁLISE
Geralmente normais.

OUTROS TESTES LABORATORIAIS
N/D.

DIAGNÓSTICO POR IMAGEM
N/D.

MÉTODOS DIAGNÓSTICOS
- Flutuação fecal para detectar os ovos; ovos de *Toxocara* são esféricos, com a membrana mais externa rugosa do envoltório, célula escura única (zigoto preenchendo o interior), 80-85 μm (*T. canis*), ~75 μm (*T. cati*).
- Ovos de *Baylisascaris* são semelhantes aos ovos de *T. canis*, porém menores (~76 × 60 μm), com o envoltório mais finamente rugoso.
- Ovos de *Toxascaris* são ovoides, com a membrana exterior lisa do envoltório, 1 ou 2 células de citoplasma claro sem preencher o interior; 80 × 70 μm de diâmetro.
- Achados de necropsia dos irmãos da mesma ninhada que morreram com sinais semelhantes.
- Identificação dos ascarídeos nas fezes, no vômito ou no intestino delgado pela presença de três lábios e asas cervicais, bem como pelo tamanho.

TRATAMENTO
- É realizado tratamento anti-helmíntico em um esquema ambulatorial.
- Os casos agudos graves são tratados com internação; suplementar com fluidos intravenosos.
- Milbemicina ou outro anti-helmíntico eficaz contra *T. canis* é sugerido para o tratamento (fora da indicação da bula) de *Baylisascaris* no cão.
- Alertar o proprietário sobre a possibilidade de morte súbita ou debilidade crônica.
- Tratar a cadela ou a gata com anti-helmíntico adulticida/larvicida (fembendazol) para remover os estágios intestinais e diminuir a probabilidade de transmissão para as ninhadas subsequentes.

MEDICAÇÕES

MEDICAMENTO(S)
Anti-helmínticos Adulticidas/Larvicidas
- Fembendazol 50 mg/kg VO a cada 24 h durante 3 dias.
- Milbemicina oxima 0,5 mg/kg (cães) ou 2 mg/kg (gatos) VO a cada 30 dias.
- Emodepsida (3 mg/kg)/praziquantel (12 mg/kg) por via tópica uma única vez para gatos com 8 anos de idade ou mais; repetir em 30 dias se o gato for reinfectado.

Anti-helmínticos Adulticidas
- Pirantel, 5 mg/kg (cães) ou 10-20 mg/kg (gatos, fora da indicação da bula) VO.
- Pirantel/praziquantel, dose da bula para gatos.
- Febantel/praziquantel/pirantel, dose da bula para cães.
- Ivermectina/pirantel, dose da bula para cães.
- Pamoato de pirantel 5 mg/kg (cães) ou 10-20 mg/kg (gatos, fora da indicação da bula).
- Selamectina 6 mg/kg por via tópica uma única vez (*T. catis*, gatos), fora da indicação da bula nos cães.
- Milbemicina oxima, dose da bula para cães e gatos.
- Moxidectina/imidaclopride, dose da bula por via tópica para cães e gatos.

CONTRAINDICAÇÕES/INTERAÇÕES POSSÍVEIS
N/D.

ACOMPANHAMENTO

MONITORIZAÇÃO DO PACIENTE
Repetir os exames fecais após o tratamento em filhotes caninos/felinos e/ou repetir a terapia anti-helmíntica a cada 2-3 semanas até que o animal tenha idade suficiente para receber o produto anti-helmíntico mensal, porque as larvas migratórias adquiridas da cadela ou da gata continuarão se desenvolvendo.

PREVENÇÃO
- Para minimizar a contaminação ambiental por ovos infectantes, tratar os cães/gatos infectados com o uso de anti-helmíntico, além de remover e descartar as fezes imediatamente. • Impedir que os cães/gatos cacem ou ingiram hospedeiros de transporte. • Proceder ao tratamento da cadela ou da gata com anti-helmíntico adulticida/larvicida fora da indicação da bula para remover os estágios intestinais e diminuir a transmissão vertical para a prole.

COMPLICAÇÕES POSSÍVEIS
- A transmissão transplacentária de grande número de larvas pode resultar em morte fetal ou no nascimento de filhotes caninos fracos e inviáveis.
- A infecção por grande número de ascarídeos pode causar obstrução e possível ruptura do intestino delgado.

EVOLUÇÃO ESPERADA E PROGNÓSTICO
Prognóstico bom após o tratamento anti-helmíntico; reservado em casos de infecção pré-natal grave por *T. canis*.

DIVERSOS

FATORES RELACIONADOS COM A IDADE
Maior preocupação clínica nos neonatos.

POTENCIAL ZOONÓTICO
- Quadros de larva migrans visceral, ocular ou neural, bem como problemas abdominais ou cutâneos crônicos, podem acompanhar a ingestão de ovos infectantes de *Toxocara* spp. ou *Baylisascaris* pelos seres humanos.
- O *Baylisascaris* constitui a causa mais provável de larva migrans neural.

RECURSOS DA INTERNET
- www.capcvet.org. • www.cdc.gov.

Sugestões de Leitura
Bowman DD. Georgis' Parasitology for Veterinarians, 9th ed. St. Louis: Saunders, 2009, pp. 197-198, 201-208.

Autor Julie Ann Jarvinen
Consultor Editorial Stephen C. Barr

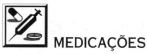

CONSIDERAÇÕES GERAIS

REVISÃO
• *Neospora caninum* — protozoário coccidiano recém-identificado e confundido anteriormente com *Toxoplasma gondii*; taquizoítas e cistos teciduais lembram o *T. gondii* à microscopia óptica.
• Cães (e coiotes) — hospedeiros definitivos: os oocistos excretados nas fezes são infectantes para outros cães e bovinos por meio da contaminação de alimentos. A neosporose é a principal causa de abortamento nos bovinos (hospedeiro intermediário).
• Doença provocada pela necrose associada a dano tecidual a partir da ruptura de cisto e invasão do taquizoíta.
• Transmissão — transplacentária, resultando em infecção congênita. Ingestão de oocistos esporulados eliminados nas fezes do cão ou cistos teciduais nos tecidos dos hospedeiros intermediários.

IDENTIFICAÇÃO
• Cães — infecções naturais (principalmente filhotes); os cães de caça são super-representados.
• Gatos — infectados por via experimental, embora tenham sido encontrados anticorpos em gatos domésticos e selvagens.

SINAIS CLÍNICOS
• Semelhantes àqueles da toxoplasmose, exceto pelo fato de que as anormalidades neurológicas e musculares predominam e quase sempre são mais graves.
• Cães jovens (<6 meses) — é mais comum uma paralisia rígida ascendente atribuída à lesão do neurônio motor inferior; distinguida de outras formas de paralisia pela atrofia muscular gradual; rigidez dos membros pélvicos (mais acometidos do que os membros torácicos); evolui para contratura rígida dos membros.
• Fraqueza cervical e disfagia, além de trismo e paralisia do nervo hipoglosso — desenvolvem-se de modo gradual; a paralisia dos músculos respiratórios acaba levando ao óbito.
• Ataxia secundária à atrofia do cerebelo.
• Cães idosos — costumam exibir envolvimento do SNC (crises convulsivas, tremores, mudanças comportamentais, cegueira), polimiosite (paralisia flácida do neurônio motor inferior), miocardite e dermatite; como acontece na toxoplasmose, praticamente qualquer órgão pode ser acometido; tremor cefálico; déficits posturais atribuídos à doença cerebelar; síndrome de Horner.
• Dermatite ulcerativa e piogranulomatosa generalizada observada nos cães sob tratamento imunossupressor para LES e linfoma.

CAUSAS E FATORES DE RISCO
N. caninum: o fornecimento de carne crua para cães pode ser um fator de risco, devendo-se evitá-lo.

DIAGNÓSTICO

DIAGNÓSTICO DIFERENCIAL
• Cães jovens — outras causas de sinais neurológicos multifocais periféricos, incluindo principalmente doenças infecciosas (toxoplasmose, cinomose); polirradiculoneurite progressiva; outras causas de doenças musculares difusas do neurônio motor inferior são raras.
• Cães idosos com doença do SNC — outras doenças infecciosas (doenças fúngicas, raiva, pseudorraiva); intoxicação (chumbo, organofosforados, carbamatos, hidrocarbonetos clorados, estricnina); encefalite não supurativa; meningoencefalite granulomatosa; doença metabólica (hipoglicemia, encefalopatia hepática).

HEMOGRAMA/BIOQUÍMICA/URINÁLISE
• Dependendo do sistema orgânico envolvido.
• Envolvimento muscular — atividades da creatina fosfoquinase e da AST podem estar elevadas.

OUTROS TESTES LABORATORIAIS
• Teste sorológico (IFA, ELISA e imunoprecipitação) — LCS ou soro.
• Anticorpos não reagem de forma cruzada com *T. gondii*.
• Detecção do microrganismo — os oocistos nas fezes devem ser diferenciados de *Hammondia* spp.
• Taquizoítas em aspirados, esfregaços ou cortes teciduais precisam ser diferenciados daqueles de *Toxoplasma* por imuno-histoquímica.
• PCR — técnica utilizada com sucesso como ferramenta diagnóstica, que distingue o *Neospora* de outros parasitas.

DIAGNÓSTICO POR IMAGEM
N/D.

MÉTODOS DIAGNÓSTICOS
LCS — leve aumento no conteúdo de proteína e no número de células nucleadas; células principalmente mononucleares; podem ser observados neutrófilos, embora alguns casos tenham grande quantidade de eosinófilos.

ACHADOS PATOLÓGICOS
• Encefalomielite não supurativa.
• Inflamação grave não supurativa das leptomeninges e do córtex do cerebelo.
• Miosite.
• Miofibrose.
• Polirradiculoneurite.
• Pneumonia, atrofia cerebelar, miocardite necrosante multifocal e dermatite nodular — foram descritas.
• Dermatite ulcerativa e piogranulomatosa.
• O *N. caninum* parece induzir a mais inflamação do que o *T. gondii*.
• Histologia — diferenciação pelo local de estabelecimento no citoplasma da célula hospedeira (não dentro de um vacúolo parasitóforo, como o *T. gondii*).
• Cistos teciduais — aqueles de *N. caninum* possuem paredes mais espessas; diferenciados de *T. gondii* por coloração imuno-histoquímica.
• Microscopia eletrônica — róptrias eletrodensas dos taquizoítas de *N. caninum*; aqueles de *T. gondii* têm forma de favo de mel.

TRATAMENTO

• Assim que ocorrer contratura muscular ou paralisia ascendente, o prognóstico quanto à melhora clínica será mau.
• A evolução da doença clínica pode ser impedida pelo tratamento.

MEDICAÇÕES

MEDICAMENTO(S)
• Ver "Toxoplasmose".
• Clindamicina — 25-50 mg/kg VO ou IM por dia, dividido em duas doses; continuar por, no mínimo, duas semanas após o desaparecimento dos sinais clínicos.

CONTRAINDICAÇÕES/INTERAÇÕES POSSÍVEIS
N/D.

ACOMPANHAMENTO

• Tratar por longo período de tempo.
• Realizar teste sorológico da mãe ou de outros cães e bovinos contactantes.

DIVERSOS

POTENCIAL ZOONÓTICO
Nenhum identificado (ao contrário do *T. gondii*).

VER TAMBÉM
Toxoplasmose.

ABREVIATURA(S)
• AST = aspartato aminotransferase.
• ELISA = ensaio imunoabsorvente ligado à enzima.
• IFA = anticorpo imunofluorescente.
• LCS = líquido cerebrospinal.
• LES = lúpus eritematoso sistêmico.
• PCR = reação em cadeia da polimerase.
• SNC = sistema nervoso central.

Sugestões de Leitura
Dubey JP, Vianna MC, Kwok OC, et al. Neosporosis in beagle dogs: Clinical signs, diagnosis, treatment, isolation and genetic characterization of Neospora caninum. Vet Parasitol 2007, 149:158-166.
Reichel MP, Ellis JT, Dubey JP. Neosporosis and hammondiosis in dogs. J Small Anim Pract 2007, 48:308-312.
Windsor RC, Sturges BK, Vernau KM, et al. Cerebrospinal fluid eosinophilia in dogs. J Vet Intern Med 2009, 23:275-281.

Autor Stephen C. Barr
Consultor Editorial Stephen C. Barr

Neurite Idiopática do Trigêmeo

CONSIDERAÇÕES GERAIS

REVISÃO
- Paralisia bilateral súbita dos ramos mandibulares do nervo trigêmeo, resultando em incapacidade de fechar a boca. As lesões são caracterizadas por extensa neurite trigeminal não supurativa, desmielinização, e rara degeneração axonal que afeta todas as porções do nervo e gânglio trigêmeo sem envolvimento do tronco encefálico.
- Também conhecida como queda da mandíbula, neuropatia trigeminal, paralisia mandibular.

IDENTIFICAÇÃO
- Principalmente cães adultos.
- Rara em gatos.

SINAIS CLÍNICOS
- Início agudo de queda da mandíbula.
- Incapacidade de fechar a boca.
- Salivação.
- Dificuldade na preensão do alimento, alimentação desorganizada (bagunçada).
- A deglutição permanece intacta quando o alimento e a água são colocados na porção caudal da boca.
- Cerca de um terço dos cães acometidos exibirão perda da sensibilidade facial.
- Poucos cães sofrem paralisia simpática da cabeça (síndrome de Horner).
- Atrofia muscular a longo prazo, dependendo do grau de envolvimento axonal.

CAUSAS E FATORES DE RISCO
Desconhecidos; suspeita-se de distúrbio autoimune.

DIAGNÓSTICO

DIAGNÓSTICO DIFERENCIAL
- Distúrbios musculosqueléticos das articulações temporomandibulares e da mandíbula — diferenciados pelo histórico de traumatismo, dor e achados do exame físico.
- Raiva — sempre se deve considerá-la em princípio até que haja prova suficiente para descartá-la.
- Encefalite com envolvimento dos núcleos motores do nervo trigêmeo bilateral.
- Neoplasia — há relatos de envolvimento de ambos os nervos mandibulares em casos de leucemia mielomonocítica, linfoma, e neurofibrossarcoma; em geral, não tem um início agudo.
- Miosite dos músculos da mastigação — a manifestação exclui esse problema caracterizado por trismo e dificuldade/incapacidade de abrir a boca.

HEMOGRAMA/BIOQUÍMICA/URINÁLISE
Geralmente normais.

OUTROS TESTES LABORATORIAIS
N/D.

DIAGNÓSTICO POR IMAGEM
RM — aumento difuso dos nervos afetados que aparecem isointensos a hiperintensos nas imagens ponderadas em T2 na presença de edema; realce do contraste nas imagens ponderadas em T1 após a administração do contraste.

MÉTODOS DIAGNÓSTICOS
- Não há exame específico.
- Radiografia do crânio, RM, análise do LCS e biopsia muscular — para descartar os diagnósticos diferenciais.

TRATAMENTO

- Recuperação em até 2-3 semanas após o início. É necessário o tratamento de suporte durante esse período.
- O tratamento é ambulatorial se o proprietário for capaz de ajudar o paciente a comer e beber.
- O paciente não consegue segurar ou deslocar o alimento e a água para a garganta, mas será capaz de engolir se o bolo alimentar for colocado na porção caudal da boca e se a mandíbula for mantida fechada manualmente. Também podem ser colocados água e alimento pastoso no canto da boca com o uso de seringa e a cabeça levemente elevada.
- Fluidos — administração subcutânea se o suporte oral for insuficiente.
- Tubos de alimentação inseridos via esofagostomia ou gastrostomia — raramente necessários para manter a ingestão alimentar adequada.

MEDICAÇÕES

MEDICAMENTO(S)
Os corticosteroides não são indicados pois não há evidência de que esses agentes melhorem a recuperação. Além disso, os efeitos colaterais (poliúria e polidipsia) podem dificultar o tratamento.

ACOMPANHAMENTO

- Distúrbio autolimitante.
- Recuperação completa em 2-3 semanas.
- Atrofia bilateral simétrica dos músculos da mastigação, mas sem trismo.

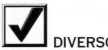

DIVERSOS

ABREVIATURAS
- LCS = líquido cerebrospinal.
- RM = ressonância magnética.

Sugestões de Leitura
Mayhew PD, Bush WW, Glass EN. Trigeminal neuropathy in dogs: A retrospective study of 29 cases (1991–2000). JAAHA 2002, 38:262–270.

Autor Mylène-Kim Leclerc
Consultor Editorial Joane M. Parent
Agradecimento T. Mark Neer por esse capítulo nas edições anteriores.

NEURITE ÓPTICA

CONSIDERAÇÕES GERAIS

REVISÃO
- Inflamação de um ou de ambos os nervos ópticos, culminando no declínio da função visual.
- Pode ser uma doença primária ou secundária à doença sistêmica do SNC, já que o nervo óptico se comunica com o espaço subaracnóideo.
- Acomete os sistemas oftálmico e nervoso.

IDENTIFICAÇÃO
- Cães e gatos.
- Primária — rara; geralmente acomete cães com >3 anos de idade.
- Secundária — varia muito de acordo com a causa.

SINAIS CLÍNICOS
Achados Anamnésicos
- Cegueira de início agudo.
- Déficits visuais parciais — frequentemente passam despercebidos.

Achados do Exame Físico
- Cegueira ou visão reduzida em um ou em ambos os olhos.
- Pupilas fixas e dilatadas — podem exibir reflexo pupilar à luz intacto, porém diminuído.
- Exame fundoscópico (fundo ocular) — tumefação do disco óptico; hemorragia focal; coriorretinite ativa ou inativa.
- Fundo frequentemente normal com doença retrobulbar ou intracraniana do nervo óptico.

CAUSAS E FATORES DE RISCO
- Idiopáticos.
- Micoses sistêmicas.
- Cinomose.
- PIF.
- Neoplasia — primária ou metastática.
- Toxoplasmose.
- *Neosporum caninum*.
- Meningoencefalomielite granulomatosa.
- Toxicidade — chumbo.

DIAGNÓSTICO

DIAGNÓSTICO DIFERENCIAL
- Cegueira cortical — reflexo pupilar à luz normal; exame normal do fundo ocular; possivelmente outros déficits neurológicos.
- SDSAR (cães) — reflexo pupilar à luz mínimo a ausente; fundo ocular normal (no início da evolução); eletrorretinograma plano.

HEMOGRAMA/BIOQUÍMICA/URINÁLISE
Sem anormalidades específicas.

OUTROS TESTES LABORATORIAIS
Testes sorológicos específicos para vírus, protozoários ou fungos.

DIAGNÓSTICO POR IMAGEM
Neuroimagem — TC e/ou RM.

MÉTODOS DIAGNÓSTICOS
- Análise do LCS.
- Eletrorretinograma — pesquisar a função da retina; normal na neurite óptica, plana na SDSAR.
- Potenciais evocados visuais — pesquisar a função do nervo óptico.

TRATAMENTO

Com base na doença subjacente.

MEDICAÇÕES

MEDICAMENTO(S)
- Depende(m) do processo mórbido primário quando identificável.
- Idiopática — prednisona a 2 mg/kg a cada 12 h por 14 dias; em seguida, 1 mg/kg a cada 12 h por 14 dias; e, então, redução gradual até a dose de manutenção.

CONTRAINDICAÇÕES/INTERAÇÕES POSSÍVEIS
N/D.

ACOMPANHAMENTO

- Monitorizar os sinais clínicos ou os potenciais evocados visuais, se disponíveis.
- Prognóstico — depende da causa subjacente.
- A cegueira pode ser permanente na neurite óptica idiopática.
- Evolução clínica — imprevisível.
- Exacerbações agudas — podem ocorrer se a medicação for inadequada.

DIVERSOS

ABREVIATURA(S)
- LCS = líquido cerebrospinal.
- PIF = peritonite infecciosa felina.
- RM = ressonância magnética.
- SDSAR = síndrome de degeneração súbita e adquirida da retina.
- SNC = sistema nervoso central.
- TC = tomografia computadorizada.

Sugestões de Leitura
Braund KG. Clinical Syndromes in Veterinary Neurology, 2nd ed. St. Louis: Mosby, 1994.

Autor David Lipsitz
Consultor Editorial Paul E. Miller

Neuropatias Periféricas (Polineuropatias)

CONSIDERAÇÕES GERAIS

DEFINIÇÃO
Doenças que acometem nervos motores, sensoriais, autônomos e/ou cranianos periféricos, em qualquer combinação.

FISIOPATOLOGIA
- Hereditária ou adquirida.
- Processo patológico primário — destruição ou degeneração das células do corno ventral (neuropatia), desmielinização primária ou degeneração do axônio (com desmielinização secundária).

SISTEMA(S) ACOMETIDO(S)
- Nervoso — principalmente o sistema nervoso periférico; possível envolvimento dos nervos cranianos.
- Outros sistemas orgânicos — muitos podem estar envolvidos no processo mórbido primário.

GENÉTICA
- A maioria é hereditária como distúrbios autossômicos recessivos.
- Atrofia muscular espinal no Spaniel britânico — distúrbio autossômico dominante.

INCIDÊNCIA/PREVALÊNCIA
- Hereditária — rara.
- Envolvimento de nervo periférico em doenças metabólicas e neoplásicas — incidência desconhecida.
- Inflamatória — incomum; paralisia do Coonhound é encontrada com maior frequência (prevalência um tanto sazonal: mais alta no outono e no início do inverno).

DISTRIBUIÇÃO GEOGRÁFICA
- Paralisia do Coonhound — América do Norte e América Central, bem como partes da América do Sul.
- Doença de desnervação distal — cães no Reino Unido; não relatada em outros lugares.

IDENTIFICAÇÃO
Espécies
Cães e gatos.

Raça(s) Predominante(s)
Hereditária
Atrofia Muscular Espinal
- Spaniel britânico, Lapland sueco, Pointer inglês, Pastor alemão, Rottweiler.
- Neuronopatia progressiva — Cairn terrier.

Axonopatias
- Neuropatia axonal gigante — Pastor alemão.
- Axonopatia progressiva — Boxer, Leonberger.
- Hiperoxalúria primária — gatos da raça Doméstico de pelo curto.
- Complexo paralisia laríngea/polineuropatia — Dálmata, Rottweiler e Pireneu.
- Polineuropatia distal — gato Sagrado da Birmânia.
- Polineuropatia sensório-motora distal — Rottweiler, Malamute do Alasca.

Desmielinização
- Neuropatia hipertrófica — Mastiff tibetano.

Doenças do Armazenamento Lisossomal
- Leucodistrofia de células globoides — West Highland branco, Cairn terrier, filhotes de gatos da raça Doméstico de pelo curto.
- Alfa-L-fucosidose — Springer spaniel.
- Gangliosidose G_{M1} tipo II — gatos da raça Siamês e mista.
- Esfingomielinose — gato Siamês, Doméstico de pelo curto.
- Lipofuscinose ceroide — Setter inglês, Chihuahua, Dachshund, gato Siamês.

Neuropatia sensorial
- Dachshund de pelo longo, Pointer inglês, Pointer alemão de pelo curto, Springer spaniel inglês, Spaniel francês e Border collie.

Adquirida
- Paralisia do Coonhound — por causa de sua utilização, o Coonhound apresenta incidência mais alta do que outras raças.
- Polineuropatia diabética clínica — mais comum em gatos do que em cães.
- Insulinomas — Pastor alemão, Boxer, Setter irlandês, Poodle standard e Collie.

Idade Média e Faixa Etária
Hereditária
- Em geral, começam com <6 meses de vida.
- Hiperquilomicronemia felina — geralmente com >8 meses.
- Hiperoxalúria felina — 5-9 meses.
- Polineuropatia distal do Rottweiler — >1 ano.
- Neuropatia axonal gigante no Pastor alemão — 14-16 meses.
- Formas intermediária e crônica de atrofia muscular espinal no Spaniel britânico heterozigoto — 6-12 meses.

Adquirida
- Secundária à neoplasia e à hipoglicemia associada ao insulinoma — animais de meia-idade a mais idosos.
- Polirradiculoneurite por *Neospora* — observada em cães com <6 meses de vida; incidência mais alta com 2-4 meses.

SINAIS CLÍNICOS
Achados Anamnésicos
Hereditária
- Maioria — lenta e progressiva; fraqueza generalizada, tremores musculares, atrofia muscular, frequentemente com postura e marcha plantígrada/palmígrada.
- Neuropatias sensoriais — automutilação ou ataxia leve a grave.
- Doenças do armazenamento lisossomal — é comum o envolvimento do SNC lentamente progressivo; ocorrem tremores da cabeça, ataxia, dismetria, crises convulsivas, cegueira, demência e depressão em conjunto com sinais generalizados atribuídos à lesão do neurônio motor inferior.
- Esfingomielinose em gatos — presente, muitas vezes, apenas com neuropatia motora e sensorial progressiva.
- Neuropatia axonal gigante do Pastor alemão — fraqueza generalizada rapidamente progressiva (<3 semanas).

Adquirida
- Evolução rápida ou lenta.
- Evolução rapidamente progressiva — marcha inicial rígida e afetada, levando à paresia ou paralisia generalizada progressiva (paralisia do Coonhound, doença de desnervação distal).
- Evolução lentamente progressiva — fraqueza generalizada e atrofia muscular; nas polineuropatias distais (neuropatia diabética, sobretudo em gatos), postura plantígrada/palmígrada.
- Disautonomia — principalmente com início agudo (<48 horas) de depressão, anorexia, regurgitação, íleo paralítico, xerostomia, ceratoconjuntivite seca, constipação, protrusão da terceira pálpebra, vômito e incontinência urinária.
- Metabólica — os proprietários relatam sinais clínicos não neurológicos associados ao defeito inicial.
- Paraneoplásica — o tumor primário pode ser clinicamente silencioso no momento da apresentação ou descoberto em radiografias torácicas ou ultrassonografia abdominal de rotina.

Achados do Exame Físico
- Motor e sensório-motor — tetraparesia a tetraplegia, hiporreflexia a arreflexia, hipotonia a atonia e atrofia muscular são achados clássicos; tremores musculares são comuns. Parestesia, especialmente em neuropatia diabética felina.
- Sensorial — déficits proprioceptivos; hipostenia a anestesia, sem atrofia muscular ou hiporreflexia (exceto no Boxer); ataxia sensorial.
- Hipotireoidismo — pode estar associado à polineuropatia generalizada, à paralisia laríngea, ao megaesôfago, à paralisia do nervo facial e à vestibulopatia periférica.
- Doenças do armazenamento lisossomal — é comum o encontro de hepatosplenomegalia.
- Paraneoplásico — pode haver indícios de neoplasia.
- Disautonomia — ressecamento nasal, xerostomia, baixa produção lacrimal, bradicardia e arreflexia anal.
- Hiperquilomicronemia felina primária — são comuns granulomas lipídicos, que podem ser palpados sob a pele e no abdome.
- Hiperoxalúria primária (gatos) — rins aumentados e doloridos à palpação abdominal.
- Anormalidades de nervo craniano (incluindo disfonia e afonia) — variável.

CAUSAS
Adquiridas
- Imunes — primárias ou secundárias; podem ser observadas em casos de LES ou outras doenças imunológicas (p. ex., polimiosite, glomerulonefrite, poliartrite e pênfigo).
- Metabólicas — diabetes melito (gatos), hipotireoidismo e insulinoma; podem estar associadas a (adeno) carcinomas, melanoma maligno, mastocitoma (tumor de mastócitos), osteossarcoma, mieloma múltiplo ou linfossarcoma.
- Infecciosas — *Neospora caninum*; FeLV; PIF.
- Agentes quimioterápicos — vincristina; vimblastina; cisplatina; colchicina.
- Tóxicas — tálio; organofosforados; tetracloreto de carbono; lindano.
- Idiopáticas.

FATORES DE RISCO
Desenvolvimento de doenças específicas associadas (metabólica, imunológica, neoplásica) ou exposição a medicações/toxinas específicas associadas ou fatores causais (saliva do guaxinim).

DIAGNÓSTICO

DIAGNÓSTICO DIFERENCIAL
- Aguda — botulismo; paralisia por carrapato; miastenia grave fulminante; mielopatias multifocais ou disseminadas agudas.

Neuropatias Periféricas (Polineuropatias)

- Crônica — polimiopatia; mielopatias multifocais ou disseminadas crônicas.

HEMOGRAMA/BIOQUÍMICA/URINÁLISE
- Testes laboratoriais padrão — não refletem a ocorrência de polineuropatia; frequentemente indicam possível doença metabólica ou neoplásica subjacente.
- Creatina quinase sérica alta — indica miopatia concomitante ou diagnóstico alternativo de polimiopatia.

OUTROS TESTES LABORATORIAIS
- Nenhum em relação à polineuropatia/polirradiculoneurite presente.
- ANA, preparação de lúpus eritematoso e teste de Coombs — ajudam no diagnóstico de doença imunológica.
- Nível baixo dos hormônios tireoidianos em teste de estimulação com TSH, T_4 baixa, T_4 livre baixa e TSH endógeno alto — hipotireoidismo.
- Relação de insulina:glicose corrigida — >30 apoia o diagnóstico de insulinoma.
- Sorologia — auxilia no diagnóstico de *N. caninum* e de infecção por FeLV/FIV.
- Enzimas lisossomais específicas baixas liberadas de leucócitos — indicam doenças específicas de armazenamento lisossomal.
- Níveis plasmáticos baixos de noradrenalina e adrenalina — disautonomia.
- Níveis séricos elevados de colesterol, triglicerídeos e lipoproteína de densidade muito baixa — hiperquilomicronemia.
- Hiperoxalúria e acidúria l-glicérica — observada na hiperoxalúria primária (gatos).
- Gamopatia monoclonal — mieloma múltiplo.

DIAGNÓSTICO POR IMAGEM
- Radiografias torácicas e abdominais — importantes no diagnóstico de megaesôfago; revela íleo paralítico, atonia vesical, constipação e esvaziamento gástrico tardio na disautonomia.
- Radiografia torácica e ultrassonografia abdominal — ajudam a pesquisar por causa neoplásica.

MÉTODOS DIAGNÓSTICOS
- Eletrofisiologia (EMG, teste de condução nervosa sensório-motora e amplitudes do potencial de ação, além de estudos da raiz nervosa ventral e dorsal) — base para o diagnóstico.
- Análise do LCS lombar — valioso no diagnóstico de envolvimento de raiz nervosa.
- Biopsia muscular — confirma a presença de desnervação.
- Biopsia de nervo periférico (distal) — caracteriza ainda mais o processo patológico.

ACHADOS PATOLÓGICOS
A distribuição da lesão ao longo dos nervos periféricos (proximal, distal ou disseminada) e o grau de degeneração axonal, desmielinização e/ou degeneração neuronal do corpo celular dependem da condição específica presente.

TRATAMENTO
CUIDADO(S) DE SAÚDE ADEQUADO(S)
- Em geral, o paciente é tratado em um esquema ambulatorial.
- Paciente internado — observar as polirradiculoneuropatias agudas de perto em busca de insuficiência respiratória na fase progressiva inicial da doença.

CUIDADO(S) DE ENFERMAGEM
- Disautonomia — pode necessitar de fluidoterapia IV intensiva e/ou alimentação parenteral.
- Fisioterapia — excelente tratamento auxiliar.

DIETA
- Em geral, não há manejo especial a menos que ocorra megaesôfago ou disfagia.
- Hiperquilomicronemia — só uma dieta pobre em gordura pode resolver a polineuropatia dentro de 2-3 meses.
- Paralisia — ter a certeza de que o paciente consegue alcançar a comida e a água.
- Regurgitação e/ou vômito (p. ex., na disautonomia) — interromper temporariamente a ingestão oral. Considerar o uso de sonda inserida via gastrostomia.
- Diabetes melito — monitorar o consumo alimentar. Nos gatos, fornecer uma dieta pobre em carboidrato, mas rica em proteína. A neuropatia diabética é frequentemente reversível com modificação da dieta e controle do diabetes.

ORIENTAÇÃO AO PROPRIETÁRIO
- Informar ao proprietário sobre o fato de que o tratamento da causa primária pode não levar à reversão dos sinais atribuídos aos nervos periféricos, e, em alguns casos, a deterioração prosseguirá. Na degeneração axonal canina, ocorre uma deterioração progressiva e implacável.

MEDICAÇÕES
MEDICAMENTOS DE ESCOLHA
- Hereditária — a maioria não é passível de tratamento.
- Adquirida — o objetivo é tratar a causa primária, com a esperança de que a polineuropatia secundária melhore ou desapareça após terapia adequada; nem sempre é bem-sucedida.
- Neuropatia desmielinizante recidivante ou progressiva crônica — mais provavelmente de origem imunológica; pode melhorar com corticoterapia imunossupressora a longo prazo (prednisona na dose de 1-2 mg/kg VO a cada 12 h), azatioprina (2,2 mg/kg VO a cada 24 h) ou ciclofosfamida (50 mg/m² a cada 48 h); a resposta é variável em cada paciente.
- Relacionada com o LES — tratar igual à polineuropatia recidivante ou progressiva crônica.
- Neoplasia — a corticoterapia imunossupressora pode melhorar a polineuropatia, sem exercer ação específica contra o tumor primário.
- Polirradiculoneurite associada ao *Neospora* — clindamicina (5,5 mg/kg VO a cada 12 h); a eficácia é questionável.
- Disautonomia — tratar de forma sintomática com fluidoterapia IV, lágrimas artificiais, metoclopramida (0,2-0,4 mg/kg VO a cada 8 h), betanecol (gatos: 0,5-2,5 mg SC a cada 12 h ou 2,5-10 mg VO a cada 6-8 h; cães: 0,5-15 mg SC a cada 12 h ou 2,5-30 mg VO a cada 6-8 h) e colírios de fisostigmina.

CONTRAINDICAÇÕES
Corticoterapia — contraindicada na polirradiculoneurite associada ao *Neospora* e na paralisia do Coonhound.

ACOMPANHAMENTO
MONITORIZAÇÃO DO PACIENTE
Repetir os exames neurológicos.

PREVENÇÃO
- Evitar o acasalamento de pacientes com doenças hereditárias ou associadas ao *Neospora* (transferência placentária do microrganismo pela cadela).
- Evitar o contato com guaxinins para cães com histórico prévio de paralisia do Coonhound. Evitar vacinações futuras na suspeita de condição associada a vacinas.

COMPLICAÇÕES POSSÍVEIS
- Hereditária — deterioração neurológica contínua, que acaba levando à incapacidade deambulatória.
- Progressiva aguda ou crônica — atrofia muscular grave; úlceras de decúbito; infecção do trato urinário; fibrose e contratura musculares; pneumonia por aspiração.

EVOLUÇÃO ESPERADA E PROGNÓSTICO
- Condições desmielinizantes — apresentam melhora mais rápida do que aquelas que envolvem degeneração axonal (a maioria), o que pode levar meses para a recuperação parcial ou completa se houver.
- Hereditária — a maioria tem prognóstico mau a reservado (exceto a hiperquilomicronemia felina).
- Polirradiculoneurite aguda (paralisia do Coonhound) — prognóstico bom a longo prazo; pode levar semanas a meses para recuperação.
- Metabólica — prognóstico razoável a bom com tratamento bem-sucedido da anormalidade metabólica primária; os insulinomas possuem alta taxa de recidiva.
- Outras adquiridas — a maioria demonstra deterioração contínua apesar do tratamento.

DIVERSOS
GESTAÇÃO/FERTILIDADE/REPRODUÇÃO
Corticosteroides em altas doses e outros agentes imunossupressores — contraindicados durante a prenhez.

ABREVIATURA(S)
- ANA = anticorpo antinuclear.
- EMG = eletromiografia.
- FeLV = vírus da leucemia felina.
- FIV = vírus da imunodeficiência felina.
- LCS = líquido cerebrospinal.
- LES = lúpus eritematoso sistêmico.
- PIF = peritonite infecciosa felina.
- SNC = sistema nervoso central.
- T_4 = tiroxina.
- TSH= hormônio tireostimulante.

RECURSOS DA INTERNET
http://www.medicine.ucsd.edu/vet neuromuscular/index.html.

Autor Paul A. Cuddon
Consultor Editorial Joane M. Parent

NEUTROPENIA

CONSIDERAÇÕES GERAIS

DEFINIÇÃO
• Contagem neutrofílica <3.000 neutrófilos/μL nos cães e <2.500 neutrófilos/μL nos gatos.
• Pode se desenvolver de forma isolada ou como componente de pancitopenia.
• Frequentemente acompanhada por desvio à esquerda e alterações tóxicas (p. ex., basofilia citoplasmática, vacuolização citoplasmática espumosa, corpúsculos de Döhle e/ou granulação tóxica).
• Certas raças, como Galgo ou Tervuren belga, normalmente podem ter uma contagem de neutrófilos abaixo do intervalo de referência em relação a outros cães.

FISIOPATOLOGIA
Resulta de um entre quatro mecanismos — (1) produção ou liberação diminuída de neutrófilos pela medula óssea, (2) desvio de neutrófilos do *pool* circulante dentro dos grandes vasos para o *pool* marginal, aderidos ao endotélio de capilares, (3) migração elevada para os tecidos a partir do sangue em função de consumo tecidual/inflamação graves e (4) destruição imunomediada.

SISTEMA(S) ACOMETIDO(S)
• Predispõe o paciente à infecção sistêmica por uma variedade de patógenos.
• Muitos sistemas corporais podem ser acometidos em qualquer combinação, dependendo do(s) local(is) de infecção.

GENÉTICA
• O modo de herança de hematopoiese cíclica canina é autossômico recessivo, envolvendo a subunidade β do complexo proteico adaptador 3 (AP3), o que redireciona o tráfego da enzima neutrófilo elastase das membranas para os grânulos.
• Um traço genético com penetrância tardia provavelmente parece explicar a neutropenia relacionada com a idade em Tervuren belga.
• A má absorção seletiva de cobalamina é um traço autossômico recessivo, resultando em neutropenia atribuída à falha de expressão do receptor para o complexo fator intrínseco-cobalamina.
• A neutropenia crônica com hiperplasia mieloide da medula óssea foi diagnosticada em filhotes aparentados da raça Border collie na Austrália e Nova Zelândia. Embora não se conheça o defeito, ele pode resultar da incapacidade dos neutrófilos em deixar a medula óssea e ingressar na circulação periférica. Há suspeitas de um modo de herança autossômico recessivo.

IDENTIFICAÇÃO
• Nada específico para infecção generalizada.
• Schnauzer, Beagle, Pastor australiano e Border collie com má absorção hereditária de cobalamina.
• Collie cinza e possivelmente Border collie com hematopoiese cíclica canina.
• Cães da raça Tervuren belga.
• Cães aparentados da raça Border collie na Austrália e Nova Zelândia com neutropenia crônica.
• Há relatos de deficiência de G-CSF em cães da raça Rottweiler com neutropenia idiopática crônica.

SINAIS CLÍNICOS
• Os animais sépticos geralmente se apresentam com sinais inespecíficos de doença, como letargia, fraqueza e inapetência. Com frequência, esses animais encontram-se febris, embora a normotermia não descarte a infecção. Outros sinais podem incluir taquicardia, mucosas congestas, tempo de preenchimento capilar prolongado e pulsos débeis (fracos), alguns dos quais estão relacionados com septicemia e choque endotóxico.
• Os Collies cinzas com hematopoiese cíclica exibem neutropenia grave a cada 12-14 dias. Ocorrem episódios de febre, diarreia, gengivite, infecção respiratória, linfadenite e artrite em associação com a neutropenia. Esses cães raramente passam de 1 ano de idade.
• Não há sinais clínicos em Tervuren belga.
• Os cães aparentados da raça Border collie na Austrália e Nova Zelândia com neutropenia crônica apresentavam infecções bacterianas recidivantes que se manifestaram como osteomielite e gastrenterite.

CAUSAS

Produção Deficiente de Neutrófilos, Morte de Células-tronco, ou Inibição
• Agentes infecciosos — cães e gatos, parvovírus, mielonecrose induzida por bactérias, e micose sistêmica; gatos, FeLV e FIV; cães, *Ehrlichia canis*, *Anaplasma phagocytophilum*.
• Medicamentos, substâncias químicas e toxinas — cães e gatos, agentes quimioterápicos e cefalosporinas; gatos, ingestão da micotoxina T-2, cloranfenicol e compostos com anel benzênico, metimazol e griseofulvina; cães, estrogênio, fenilbutazona, trimetoprima-sulfadiazina, fenobarbital.
• Falta de fatores tróficos — má absorção hereditária de cobalamina/vitamina B_{12}.
• Radiação ionizante.

Espaço Hematopoiético Reduzido Secundário à Mieloftise
• Mielonecrose.
• Mielofibrose.
• Neoplasia disseminada, leucemia e síndrome mielodisplásica.
• Doença granulomatosa disseminada (histoplasmose e criptococose).

Proliferação Cíclica de Células-tronco
• Hematopoiese cíclica hereditária.
• Tratamento com ciclofosfamida.
• Doença idiopática.
• Supressão imunomediada da granulopoiese.
• Mal comprovada em cães e gatos.

Migração Neutrofílica
• Ocorre desvio de neutrófilos do *pool* neutrofílico circulante para o *pool* neutrofílico marginal nos pacientes com endotoxemia. Acredita-se que isso seja o mecanismo por trás da neutropenia em animais septicêmicos atribuída a *Bartonella* spp. e outras bactérias. A anafilaxia é outra causa, porém incomum.

Sobrevivência Reduzida
• Infecção bacteriana grave (causa mais comum) — sepse, pneumonia, peritonite e piotórax.
• Destruição imunomediada (incomum).
• Destruição induzida por medicamentos.
• Hiperesplenismo (sequestro).

FATORES DE RISCO
• Doença hereditária — hematopoiese cíclica no Collie cinza e possivelmente no Border collie.
• Má absorção hereditária de cobalamina nas raças Schnauzer gigante, Beagle, Pastor australiano e Border collie.
• Exposição a medicamentos e substâncias químicas — superdosagem de estrogênio nos cães (pancitopenia) e cloranfenicol, além de compostos com anel benzênico nos gatos.
• Exposição a diversos agentes infecciosos — cães e gatos, infecção bacteriana avassaladora; cães, infecção aguda por *Ehrlichia canis* e infecção por parvovírus; gatos, panleucopenia, infecção por FIV/FeLV.
• Animais de meia-idade e idosos são menos eficazes em recuperar a medula óssea após agressão tóxica grave.

DIAGNÓSTICO

DIAGNÓSTICO DIFERENCIAL
• A maioria das neutropenias se deve a doenças infecciosas não bacterianas, como infecções por FeLV, FIV e parvovírus, além de micoses sistêmicas.
• Infecção bacteriana com inflamação e/ou endotoxemia acentuadas.
• Efeitos citotóxicos diretos de medicamentos e outras toxinas sobre as células-tronco mieloides e as células circulantes.
• Doença primária da medula óssea.
• Destruição imunomediada.
• A raça do cão pode levantar a suspeita de doença hereditária.

HEMOGRAMA/BIOQUÍMICA/URINÁLISE
• O diagnóstico é confirmado pela realização de hemograma completo e contagens diferenciais de leucócitos.
• Há necessidade de múltiplos hemogramas completos para confirmar a neutropenia verdadeira e/ou descartar o diagnóstico de hematopoiese cíclica.
• Urinálise com cultura bacteriana e antibiograma para avaliar a presença de infecção do trato urinário.

Fatores Capazes de Alterar Erroneamente os Resultados Laboratoriais
• Falha em misturar a amostra de sangue de forma adequada antes da amostragem para o hemograma completo (erro laboratorial).
• Obtenção de amostra de sangue a partir de cateter IV utilizado para administração de fluido (diluição da amostra).
• Coagulação parcial da amostra de sangue com encarceramento ou agregação de neutrófilos (anticoagulação deficiente).
• Pode ocorrer leuquergia/aglutinação de leucócitos no tubo após a coleta da amostra em função do revestimento dessas células por anticorpos. Isso diminuirá falsamente a contagem de leucócitos, já que os leucócitos aglomerados não são contados por analisadores automatizados de hematologia.

OUTROS TESTES LABORATORIAIS
• Teste sorológico — para descartar erliquiose, anaplasmose e parvovirose nos cães, mas panleucopenia e infecções por FIV/FeLV nos gatos.
• Demonstração de anticorpos antineutrófilos por citometria de fluxo e observação de leucoaglutinação — essencial para diagnosticar neutropenia imunomediada.
• Considerar cultura microbiológica do sangue ou de suposto(s) local(is) de infecção bacteriana ou

administração empírica de antibiótico na suspeita de infecção oculta.

DIAGNÓSTICO POR IMAGEM
Radiografia simples e ultrassonografia podem ajudar a localizar os pontos ocultos de infecção não aparentes durante o exame físico.

MÉTODOS DIAGNÓSTICOS/ACHADOS PATOLÓGICOS
• Exame de aspirado da medula óssea e biopsia de núcleo — não só para avaliar a produção de neutrófilos, mas também para excluir mieloftise, mielonecrose e mielofibrose. Os animais que se recuperam de neutropenia periférica podem ser erroneamente diagnosticados com leucemia aguda em função da alta porcentagem de mieloblastos nas medulas com desvios extremos à esquerda.
• Exame citológico de preparações — para comprovar o excesso de demanda tecidual por neutrófilos, verificar o sequestro de neutrófilos nas cavidades corporais ou entre os planos teciduais, confirmar a presença de infecção bacteriana e identificar os locais de perda imperceptível ou oculta de neutrófilos a partir de lesões na pele ou nas mucosas.
• Cultura do local da infecção ou hemocultura em animais febris.
• Exposição provocativa à administração parenteral de cobalamina/vitamina B_{12} deve reverter a anemia, a neutropenia e a hipersegmentação neutrofílica nas raças acometidas.

TRATAMENTO

CUIDADO(S) DE SAÚDE ADEQUADO(S)
• A principal preocupação é a presença ou o desenvolvimento de infecção.
• Na ausência de pirexia, antibióticos orais de amplo espectro que poupem a flora GI anaeróbica normal devem ser administrados profilaticamente em um esquema ambulatorial (sobretudo se a contagem neutrofílica estiver abaixo de 1.000 neutrófilos/μL).
• Pirexia — indica infecção atual; tratada com mais rigor; a internação é recomendada para a administração parenteral de fluidos cristaloides e antibióticos com alvo sobre bactérias anaeróbias e aeróbias até que a infecção seja contida.

MEDICAÇÕES

MEDICAMENTO(S)
• Sem febre (cães e gatos) — trimetoprima-sulfadiazina (15 mg/kg VO a cada 12 h) ou cefalexina (30 mg/kg VO a cada 12 h) ou enrofloxacino (5-20 mg/kg VO a cada 24 h; notar o potencial de toxicidade da retina nos gatos com doses >5 mg/kg).
• Com febre (cães e gatos) — ampicilina (22 mg/kg IV a cada 6-8 h) ou ampilicina + sulbactam (15 mg/kg IV a cada 8 h) ou cefazolina (20-30 mg/kg IV cada 6-8 h) ou enrofloxacino (5-10 mg/kg IV a cada 24 h; notar o potencial de toxicidade da retina nos gatos).
• Se clinicamente justificável, a cobertura anaeróbica adicional é fornecida pelo metronidazol (15 mg/kg IV a cada 12 h) e/ou alguma cefalosporina de última geração.

• rhG-CSF (cães e gatos) — 5-10 mg/kg/dia SC por 3-6 doses pode ser eficaz para estimular a produção de neutrófilos a curto prazo; no entanto, por ser uma proteína estranha, esse fator acaba eliciando a produção de anticorpos neutralizantes em 14-21 dias, o que então pode reagir de forma cruzada com G-CSF endógeno.
• A neutrofilia desaparece depois de 5 dias da interrupção do G-CSF.
• Neutropenia imunomediada — prednisolona (1-4 mg/kg VO a cada 12 h).

PRECAUÇÕES
• Manter a hidratação ao se administrar medicamentos com sulfa para evitar a cristalização renal.

ACOMPANHAMENTO

MONITORIZAÇÃO DO PACIENTE
• É mais provável que a neutropenia ocorra 7-10 dias após a administração de grande parte dos agentes quimioterápicos, embora ela possa se desenvolver mais tarde em até 2-3 semanas após a administração de lomustina e carboplatina.
• Hemogramas completos periódicos; a melhora é indicada pela elevação na contagem de leucócitos ou neutrófilos, resolução do desvio à esquerda e desaparecimento de alterações tóxicas. Essa melhora será observada após terapia antimicrobiana adequada se a sepse bacteriana foi a causa desencadeante da neutropenia.
• Durante a recuperação da neutropenia, espera-se uma leucocitose neutrofílica de rebote.
• Com a produção acelerada de neutrófilos vista na terapia com rhG-CSF, esperam-se os efeitos de toxicidade e desvio à esquerda, que não podem ser interpretados como sepse.

COMPLICAÇÕES POSSÍVEIS
Infecções secundárias.

DIVERSOS

DISTÚRBIOS ASSOCIADOS
Infecção secundária, sepse.

FATORES RELACIONADOS COM A IDADE
A recuperação da medula óssea com células hematopoiéticas é mais difícil em animais de meia-idade e idosos, por causa da redução relacionada com a idade no número de células-tronco.

GESTAÇÃO/FERTILIDADE/REPRODUÇÃO
Animais Prenhes
• Os medicamentos listados devem ser utilizados apenas se os benefícios superarem os riscos inerentes.
• Os agentes terapêuticos à base de sulfa atravessam a placenta e podem causar icterícia, anemia hemolítica e kernicterus*.

---

* N. T.: Termo usado patologicamente para descrever aumento de bilirrubina nos gânglios da base, tronco cerebral e cerebelo e, clinicamente, para descrever uma síndrome associada à hiperbilirrubinemia. Os sinais clínicos incluem atetose, espasticidade muscular ou hipotonia, olhar fixo na vertical deficiente e surdez. A bilirrubina não conjugada entra no cérebro e age como uma

• Embora a trimetoprima atravesse a placenta, não há registro de dano após a administração desse medicamento no início da gravidez; no entanto, esse agente terapêutico não deve ser usado próximo ao término da gestação por causa da inibição do ácido fólico.
• Não foram conduzidos estudos de segurança adequadamente controlados de rhG-CSF em cães e gatos (incluindo animais prenhes); a administração de altas doses (80 μg/kg/dia) de rhG-CSF em coelhos prenhes foi associada a reabsorção fetal, abortamento e hemorragia acentuada do trato geniturinário.

VER TAMBÉM
• Erliquiose.
• Infecção pelo Vírus da Imunodeficiência Felina (FIV).
• Infecção pelo Vírus da Leucemia Felina (FeLV).
• Hiperestrogenismo (Intoxicação por Estrogênio).
• Panleucopenia Felina.
• Parvovirose Canina.

ABREVIATURA(S)
• FeLV = vírus da leucemia felina.
• FIV = vírus da imunodeficiência felina.
• GI = gastrintestinal.
• rhG-CSF = fator estimulador das colônias de granulócitos humano recombinante.

Sugestões de Leitura
Brown MR, Rogers KS. Neutropenia in dogs and cats: A retrospective study of 261 cases. JAAHA 2001, 37:131-139.
Thamm DH, Vail DM. Aftershocks of cancer chemotherapy: Managing adverse effects. JAAHA 2007, 43:1-7.
Thrall MA, Baker DC, Campbell TW, DeNicola D, Fettman MJ, Lassen ED, Rebar A, Weiser G. Veterinary Hematology and Clinical Chemistry. Ames, IA: Blackwell, 2006.

Autores Jennifer L. Owen e A. Rick Alleman
Consultor Editorial A.H. Rebar
Agradecimento a Kenneth S. Latimer por suas contribuições na edição anterior desta seção.

---

neurotoxina, geralmente em associação com condições que comprometem a barreira hematencefálica (ex. sepse). Essa condição ocorre principalmente em neonatos (recém-nascidos), embora raramente possa ocorrer em adultos.

Nistagmo

CONSIDERAÇÕES GERAIS

DEFINIÇÃO
- Oscilação involuntária rítmica dos globos oculares.
- Nistagmo rítmico — mais comum; movimentos oculares lentos em uma única direção com fase de recuperação rápida na direção oposta.
- Nistagmo pendular — observado com menos frequência; caracterizado por pequenas oscilações dos olhos sem componente rápido ou lento.

FISIOPATOLOGIA
- O nistagmo é mais comumente um reflexo de disfunção vestibular.
- As projeções nervosas passam pelo tronco cerebral desde os núcleos vestibulares até os núcleos dos III, IV e VI pares de nervos cranianos, os quais inervam os músculos extraoculares. Esse sistema controla o nistagmo fisiológico, o qual confere movimentos oculares conjugados coordenados em associação com alterações na posição da cabeça. Quando esse sistema sofre algum transtorno, desenvolve-se o nistagmo rítmico independentemente do movimento da cabeça (o assim-chamado nistagmo patológico). O nistagmo pode ser de natureza horizontal, rotatório ou vertical, sendo nomeado de acordo com a direção da fase rápida do movimento.
- Nistagmo espontâneo — nistagmo patológico que ocorre quando a cabeça se encontra em uma posição normal e não está se movimentando; frequentemente desaparece depois de alguns dias.
- Nistagmo posicional — nistagmo patológico, eliciado apenas quando a cabeça é colocada em uma posição não habitual; pode ser observado com maior frequência em condições mais crônicas.
- O nistagmo rítmico deve ser diferenciado do nistagmo pendular, o qual é mais frequentemente observado como achado acidental nos gatos das raças Siamês, Birmanês e Himalaio.
- Nistagmo pendular — anormalidade congênita na qual uma porção maior do que a usual de fibras do nervo óptico se cruza no quiasma; também pode ser observado em casos de doença cerebelar e déficits visuais.

SISTEMA(S) ACOMETIDO(S)
Nervoso.

GENÉTICA
N/D.

INCIDÊNCIA/PREVALÊNCIA
Nistagmo, como sinal de vestibulopatia, é uma manifestação clínica relativamente comum em cães e gatos.

DISTRIBUIÇÃO GEOGRÁFICA
N/D.

IDENTIFICAÇÃO
Espécies
Cães e gatos.

Raça(s) Predominante(s)
Nenhuma.

Idade Média e Faixa Etária
Varia, dependendo da causa subjacente; condições neoplásicas e vestibulopatia geriátrica canina são mais comuns em animais mais idosos.

Sexo Predominante
Nenhum.

SINAIS CLÍNICOS
N/D.

CAUSAS
Vestibulopatia Periférica
- Metabólicas — hipotireoidismo.
- Neoplásicas — tumor da bainha nervosa ou tumor envolvendo os tecidos ósseos ou moles circundantes.
- Inflamatórias — otite média-interna; pólipos nasofaríngeos (gatos).
- Idiopáticas — vestibulopatia geriátrica canina; vestibulopatia idiopática felina.
- Tóxicas — por exemplo, aminoglicosídeos, iodóforos tópicos, clorexidina tópica.
- Traumatismo.

Vestibulopatia Central
- Degenerativas — distúrbios de armazenamento; degeneração neuronal; doença desmielinizante.
- Neoplásicas — tumores primários ou metastáticos.
- Nutricionais — deficiência de tiamina.
- Inflamatórias/infecciosas — virais (cinomose, peritonite infecciosa felina); bacterianas; protozoárias (toxoplasmose, neosporose); fúngicas (criptococose, blastomicose, histoplasmose, coccidioidomicose, aspergilose); riquetsiais (erliquiose, febre maculosa das Montanhas Rochosas); inflamatórias, não infecciosas (meningoencefalomielite granulomatosa, encefalite necrosante).
- Tóxicas — chumbo; hexaclorofeno; metronidazol.
- Traumatismo.
- Vasculares — hemorragia; infarto.

FATORES DE RISCO
A administração sistêmica de certos antibióticos (metronidazol, aminoglicosídeo) e a administração ótica de iodóforos e soluções de clorexidina.

DIAGNÓSTICO

DIAGNÓSTICO DIFERENCIAL
Vestibulopatia Periférica
- Nistagmo — rotatório ou horizontal, com a fase rápida direcionada longe do lado da lesão; não altera a direção.
- Outros sinais de vestibulopatia — inclinação da cabeça, ataxia, andar em círculos, queda ou rolamento e estrabismo vestibular estão frequentemente presentes e ocorrem de forma ipsolateral à lesão.
- Déficits do nervo facial ipsolateral e/ou síndrome de Horner — podem ser observados em virtude da estreita associação do VII par de nervos cranianos e da inervação simpática com o VIII par de nervos cranianos, pois eles atravessam a parte petrosa do osso temporal.

Vestibulopatia Central
- Nistagmo — pode ser horizontal, rotatório ou vertical; pode mudar de direção com diferentes posições da cabeça.
- Outros sinais de vestibulopatia — inclinação da cabeça, ataxia, andar em círculos, queda ou rolamento e estrabismo vestibular estão presentes com frequência.
- Envolvimento de outras estruturas do tronco cerebral — alterações no nível de consciência, paresia, déficits de reação postural e outros déficits dos nervos cranianos (V e VII pares são os mais comumente acometidos); os déficits são tipicamente ipsolaterais à lesão.
- Vestibulopatia paradoxal — pode ocorrer com determinadas lesões do cerebelo; nesses casos, os déficits de reação postural são ipsolaterais à lesão, enquanto a inclinação da cabeça e outros sinais vestibulares estão direcionados em posição contralateral à lesão.

HEMOGRAMA/BIOQUÍMICA/URINÁLISE
Em geral, os resultados permanecem normais.

OUTROS TESTES LABORATORIAIS
- Provas de função da tireoide — na suspeita de hipotireoidismo.
- Cultura bacteriana de amostra obtida por meio de miringotomia — se um quadro de otite média-interna for provável.
- Teste sorológico — para pesquisa de agentes infecciosos potenciais.

DIAGNÓSTICO POR IMAGEM
- Obtenção de imagens da bula timpânica para avaliar a presença de otite média-interna — as radiografias simples são de valor limitado; os exames de TC e RM são mais sensíveis.
- TC ou RM do cérebro — exames indicados nos animais com vestibulopatia central para avaliar qualquer anormalidade cerebral estrutural.

MÉTODOS DIAGNÓSTICOS
Análise do LCS — em caso de vestibulopatia central para avaliar a presença de inflamação.

ACHADOS PATOLÓGICOS
Variáveis, dependendo da causa subjacente.

TRATAMENTO

CUIDADO(S) DE SÁUDE ADEQUADO(S)
- A causa da doença e a gravidade dos sinais determinam se o animal será mais bem tratado como paciente de ambulatório ou internado.
- Como regra geral, os animais com envolvimento central necessitam de cuidados mais intensivos do que aqueles com doença periférica.

CUIDADO(S) DE ENFERMAGEM
- A fluidoterapia fica indicada nos estágios agudos da doença para os animais que apresentam anorexia e vômito.
- Os animais com disfunção vestibular grave devem ficar confinados a uma área bem acolchoada no estágio agudo da doença para minimizar o autotraumatismo secundário à desorientação.

ATIVIDADE
- Os animais devem ser alojados em superfícies antiderrapantes; é recomendável evitar a subida ou descida por escadas.
- A prática de exercícios deve ser supervisionada, com fornecimento de ajuda até que os sinais de desequilíbrio desapareçam.

DIETA
N/D.

ORIENTAÇÃO AO PROPRIETÁRIO
- Muitos animais exibem melhora logo nos primeiros dias, pois o sistema nervoso é capaz de compensar os distúrbios vestibulares que permanecem estáticos ou são lentamente progressivos, independentemente da causa.
- A compensação envolve sinais visuais e somatossensoriais (táteis), além de depender do

feedback proveniente dos trajetos vestibulares; o retorno às atividades normais deve ser incentivado para reforçar os mecanismos compensatórios.

CONSIDERAÇÕES CIRÚRGICAS
Os sinais de disfunção vestibular podem se agravar transitoriamente após um episódio anestésico; é mais provável que isso reflita uma perda de compensação.

MEDICAÇÕES
MEDICAMENTO(S) DE ESCOLHA
• Meclizina (cães: 4 mg/kg VO a cada 24 h) ou maropitanto (cães: 1 mg/kg SC ou 2 mg/kg VO a cada 24 h) — utilizados para tratar a doença do movimento (cinetose); podem aliviar os sinais de náusea e vômito associados à doença aguda.
• Diazepam (cães: 0,5 mg/kg VO a cada 8 h) — recomendado nos casos de intoxicação por metronidazol; pode ajudar a diminuir os sinais vestibulares agudos por outras causas, diminuindo a atividade em repouso dos neurônios vestibulares e aliviando o desequilíbrio nos impulsos vestibulares até o cérebro.
• O tratamento clínico específico é direcionado à causa subjacente, se alguma puder ser identificada.

CONTRAINDICAÇÕES/INTERAÇÕES POSSÍVEIS
• Evitar o uso de medicamentos ototóxicos potenciais, como os aminoglicosídeos. A toxicidade é mais provável em animais com comprometimento renal.
• Evitar a instilação tópica de medicamentos na orelha de animal com suspeita de otite média-interna, especialmente se a membrana timpânica não puder ser observada ou não estiver intacta. Tais agentes podem exacerbar os sinais vestibulares e provocar surdez.

PRECAUÇÕES
• Evitar a utilização do metronidazol em doses diárias superiores a 60 mg/kg, pois isso foi associado à disfunção vestibular nos cães.
• Pode ocorrer o desenvolvimento de disfunção vestibular após a administração de metronidazol em doses mais baixas, embora isso seja menos provável.

INTERAÇÕES POSSÍVEIS
N/D.

MEDICAMENTO(S) ALTERNATIVO(S)
N/D.

ACOMPANHAMENTO
MONITORIZAÇÃO DO PACIENTE
Repetir o exame neurológico — realizá-lo 2 semanas após o diagnóstico inicial para monitorizar a melhora ou a evolução da doença.

PREVENÇÃO
N/D.

COMPLICAÇÕES POSSÍVEIS
• Desidratação e desequilíbrio eletrolítico associados aos sinais de anorexia e vômito.
• Extensão rara da otite média-interna para o tronco cerebral adjacente.

EVOLUÇÃO ESPERADA E PROGNÓSTICO
• O prognóstico varia, dependendo da causa da vestibulopatia.
• Os animais com vestibulopatia periférica apresentam um prognóstico melhor do que aqueles com envolvimento central.
• Os déficits residuais podem persistir após a resolução do processo patológico subjacente em função do dano irreversível às estruturas neurais.

• A recidiva é possível em algumas das condições (otite média/interna, vestibulopatia geriátrica canina, vestibulopatia idiopática felina).

DIVERSOS
DISTÚRBIOS ASSOCIADOS
N/D.

FATORES RELACIONADOS COM A IDADE
N/D.

POTENCIAL ZOONÓTICO
N/D.

GESTAÇÃO/FERTILIDADE/REPRODUÇÃO
N/D.

VER TAMBÉM
• Ataxia.
• Inclinação da Cabeça.
• Otite Média e Interna.

ABREVIATURA(S)
• LCS = líquido cerebrospinal.
• RM = ressonância magnética.
• TC = tomografia computadorizada.

RECURSOS DA INTERNET
neuro.vetmed.ufl.edu/neuro/vestibular/vestib.htm.

Sugestões de Leitura
Thomas WB. Vestibular dysfunction. Vet Clin North Am Small Anim Pract 2000, 30:227-249.

Autor Karen R. Muñana
Consultor Editorial Joane M. Parent

Nocardiose

CONSIDERAÇÕES GERAIS

REVISÃO
- Infecção rara de cães e gatos.
- Microrganismo — saprófita do solo; entra no organismo pela contaminação de feridas ou por inalação respiratória.
- O sistema imune comprometido aumenta a possibilidade da infecção.

SISTEMA(S) ACOMETIDO(S)
- Linfático.
- Musculoesquelético.
- Nervoso.
- Respiratório.
- Cutâneo/exócrino.

IDENTIFICAÇÃO
Cães e gatos de qualquer raça.

SINAIS CLÍNICOS
- Dependem do local da infecção.
- Pleurais — piotórax, com consequente dispneia, emaciação e febre.
- Cutâneos — feridas crônicas que não cicatrizam; frequentemente acompanhadas por trajetos fistulosos; se extensas, podem resultar em linfadenopatia, linfonodos drenantes e osteomielite.
- Disseminados — mais comuns nos cães jovens; em geral, começam no trato respiratório; letargia, febre e perda de peso; febre cíclica pode ser uma característica; possível acometimento do SNC; pode ocorrer efusão pleural e/ou abdominal.
- Pode causar pneumonia ou piotórax em gatos.

CAUSAS E FATORES DE RISCO
- *Nocardia asteroides* (cães e gatos).
- *N. brasiliensis* (apenas gatos).
- *N. nova* (comum na Austrália; atualmente nos EUA).
- *Proactinomyces* spp. (raras).

DIAGNÓSTICO

DIAGNÓSTICO DIFERENCIAL
Cutânea
- Actinomicose.
- Micobacteriose atípica.
- Lepra.
- Abscessos de feridas causadas por mordedura.
- Trajetos drenantes resultantes de corpos estranhos.

Pleural
- Piotórax bacteriano.
- Neoplasia torácica.
- Hérnia diafragmática crônica.

Disseminada
- Peste.
- Infecções fúngicas sistêmicas.
- Peritonite infecciosa felina.

HEMOGRAMA/BIOQUÍMICA/URINÁLISE
- Leucocitose neutrofílica.
- Anemia arregenerativa — nas infecções de longa duração (anemia de doença crônica).
- Bioquímica — geralmente normal; pode-se observar hipergamaglobulinemia nas infecções de longa duração.

OUTROS TESTES LABORATORIAIS
N/D.

DIAGNÓSTICO POR IMAGEM
Radiografias — podem revelar efusão pleural ou peritoneal, pleuropneumonia ou osteomielite.

MÉTODOS DIAGNÓSTICOS
- Citologia — toracocentese ou abdominocentese para amostras; corar esses ou outros exsudatos com corantes Romanowsky, Gram ou acidorresistente modificado para o diagnóstico rápido; podem revelar cocos e bastonetes filamentosos ramificados Gram-positivos; não podem ser distinguidos de *Actinomyces* spp.
- Cultura — diagnóstica; cultura aeróbica em meio de Sabouraud.

ACHADOS PATOLÓGICOS
- *N. asteroides* — reação piogranulomatosa mais supurativa do que com *Actinomyces* spp.
- *N. brasiliensis* — reação granulomatosa com fibrose extensa.
- Apesar da presença habitual do microrganismo, não é possível distingui-lo de *Actinomyces* spp em termos histopatológicos.

TRATAMENTO

- Efusões pleurais ou peritoneais e forma disseminada — internação até a estabilização clínica do paciente e a remoção da efusão; fluidoterapia para reidratação e manutenção é frequentemente necessária.
- Antibioticoterapia a longo prazo e trajetos fistulosos drenantes — tratamento ambulatorial.
- Dieta — estimular o consumo, oferecendo alimentos com sabores e odores atrativos; é essencial o fornecimento de nutrição enteral forçada para pacientes anoréxicos internados; é preferível a alimentação com sonda orogástrica.
- Cirurgia — quando possível, a drenagem cirúrgica deve acompanhar o tratamento clínico; é importante colocar sonda de toracostomia na efusão pleural; tentar a drenagem cirúrgica, bem como o debridamento dos trajetos e linfonodos drenantes; tomar cuidado para identificar corpos estranhos.

MEDICAÇÕES

MEDICAMENTO(S)
- Identificação do microrganismo na cultura — realizar antibiograma.
- Na ausência dos exames de cultura ou na espera dos resultados — medicamentos satisfatórios de primeira escolha: sulfonamidas (p. ex., sulfadiazina na dose de 100 mg/kg IV ou VO como dose de ataque, seguida de 50 mg/kg IV ou VO a cada 12 h) e combinações de sulfonamida-trimetoprima (15-30 mg/kg VO a cada 12 h).
- Aminoglicosídeos — gentamicina (3 mg/kg IV, IM ou SC a cada 8 h); amicacina (6,5 mg/kg IV, IM, SC a cada 8 h).
- Tetraciclinas — doxiciclina (10 mg/kg VO a cada 24 h); cloridrato de tetraciclina (15-20 mg/kg VO a cada 8 h); minociclina (5-12,5 mg/kg VO a cada 12 h).
- Eritromicina — 10-20 mg/kg VO a cada 8 h; ou combinada com ampicilina (20-40 mg/kg VO a cada 8 h) ou com amoxicilina (6-20 mg/kg VO a cada 8-12 h).
- Amoxicilina ou ampicilina associada a algum aminoglicosídeo — combinação sinérgica; considerar o uso desses medicamentos em qualquer infecção grave quando a cultura não for possível ou estiver pendente.
- Período médio de tratamento é de 6 semanas; entretanto, o tratamento clínico deve se estender por várias semanas após a aparente remissão da doença.

CONTRAINDICAÇÕES/INTERAÇÕES POSSÍVEIS
- Tetraciclina (gatos) — pode provocar febre de até 41,5°C; interromper e substituir se a febre aumentar durante o tratamento.
- A combinação de sulfonamida-trimetoprima a longo prazo pode causar anorexia e mielossupressão irreversível em gatos. Evitar esses efeitos com a suplementação de folato (1 mg VO a cada 24 h).

ACOMPANHAMENTO

Monitorizar cuidadosamente quanto à ocorrência de febre, perda de peso, crises convulsivas, dispneia e claudicação no primeiro ano após o tratamento aparentemente bem-sucedido em razão do potencial de envolvimento dos ossos e do SNC.

DIVERSOS

VER TAMBÉM
Actinomicose.

ABREVIATURA(S)
- SNC = sistema nervoso central.

Sugestões de Leitura
Edwards DF. Nocardiosis. In: Greene CE, ed., Infectious Diseases of the Dog and Cat, 3rd ed. St. Louis: Saunders Elsevier, 2006, pp. 456-461.
Malik R, Krockenberger MB, O'Brien CR, et al. Nocardia infections in cats: A retrospective multi-institutional study of 17 cases. Australian Vet J 2006, 84(7):235-245.
Sivacolundhu RK, O'Hara AJ, Read RA. Thoracic actinomycosis (arcanobacteriosis) or nocardiosis causing thoracic pyogranuloma formation in three dogs. Australian Vet J 2001, 79(6):398-402.
Thomovsky E, Kerl ME. Actinomycosis and nocardiosis. Compend Contin Educ Pract Vet 2008, 10(3):4-10.

Autor Gary D. Norsworthy
Consultor Editorial Stephen C. Barr

Obesidade

CONSIDERAÇÕES GERAIS

DEFINIÇÃO
Excesso de gordura corporal, que frequentemente resulta em efeitos adversos à saúde. Até mesmo um excesso moderado na gordura corporal pode aumentar a morbidade e diminuir o tempo de vida.

FISIOPATOLOGIA
Acúmulo de tecido adiposo em função de um desequilíbrio entre a ingestão e o gasto energéticos. Os fatores que contribuem para a obesidade estão relacionados com o estilo de vida, incluindo castração, atividade restrita e acesso abundante aos alimentos. As complicações secundárias da obesidade podem ser atribuídas ao aumento dos mediadores inflamatórios e do estresse oxidativo, juntamente com resistência à insulina, induzida em indivíduos obesos.

SISTEMA(S) ACOMETIDO(S)
Adiposo/endócrino/musculoesquelético — o tecido adiposo de indivíduos obesos é infiltrado por macrófagos. Tanto os adipócitos como os macrófagos associados secretam mediadores inflamatórios e endócrinos, como fator de necrose tumoral-alfa, resistina, interleucinas, e outros. Esses compostos contribuem para a insulinorresistência ou as alterações artríticas comuns em animais obesos.

IDENTIFICAÇÃO
- Cães e gatos.
- Todas as idades, com a maior prevalência (quase 50%) em cães e gatos de meia-idade.
- Mais comum em animais de estimação castrados que vivem dentro de casa.

SINAIS CLÍNICOS
Achados Anamnésicos
- Ganho de peso.
- Pode ser relatada uma intolerância ao exercício.

Achados do Exame Físico
- Excesso na gordura corporal e no escore da condição corporal (ver a seção "Métodos Diagnósticos").

CAUSAS E FATORES DE RISCO
- A obesidade é causada por desequilíbrio entre a ingestão e o gasto energéticos, em que o consumo excede o gasto.
- Fatores como castração, oportunidades reduzidas de atividade física e idade podem diminuir o gasto.
- O fornecimento exagerado de alimentos altamente calóricos, a troca frequente de rações e o oferecimento de petiscos em excesso contribuem para a ingestão calórica excessiva.
- Hipotireoidismo, insulinoma ou hiperadrenocorticismo são causas pouco frequentes de obesidade.

DIAGNÓSTICO

DIAGNÓSTICO DIFERENCIAL
Distensão abdominal por prenhez, ascite ou neoplasia.

MÉTODOS DIAGNÓSTICOS
- O diagnóstico de obesidade é feito pela medição do peso corporal e obtenção do escore de condição corporal.
- O escore de condição corporal fornece uma avaliação semiquantitativa da composição do corpo. Isso envolve a avaliação visual e a palpação, especialmente sobre as costelas, a região lombar e a área de inserção da cauda, comparando-se com o padrão. Utilizando um sistema de 9 pontos, cada unidade acima do ideal reflete um excesso do peso corporal de aproximadamente 10-15%. Os animais com escore de condição corporal igual ou superior a 7 estão obesos.
- Mensuração do peso corporal.

TRATAMENTO

- Perda de peso, induzida pela redução no consumo calórico para um nível abaixo do gasto.
- A perda bem-sucedida de peso também requer a manutenção do peso perdido a longo prazo.
- Ambas as abordagens dependem das mudanças na forma com que o proprietário alimenta e interage com o animal de estimação.

ORIENTAÇÃO AO PROPRIETÁRIO
- O tratamento da obesidade conta não só com a obediência do proprietário, mas também com modificações na alimentação e nas interações comportamentais. As etapas direcionadas ao proprietário para um programa bem-sucedido de perda de peso incluem:
  ○ Reconhecimento do problema — muitos proprietários não admitem que seu animal de estimação esteja com sobrepeso. Utilizar um sistema de escore da condição corporal para ilustrar como o diagnóstico está sendo feito. Ensinar o proprietário como avaliar e monitorar o escore de condição corporal de seu animal.
  ○ Importância do problema — os proprietários que encaram a obesidade como um problema estritamente estético podem não ter motivação suficiente para tratá-la. Orientar os proprietários sobre o aumento no risco de doenças (p. ex., osteoartrite, diabetes melito, doenças do trato urinário inferior felino, etc.) ou a diminuição no tempo de vida para identificar a obesidade como uma condição que necessita de tratamento adequado.
  ○ Adesão do proprietário ao programa de perda de peso — determinar se os proprietários estão dispostos e aptos a fazer isso. Eles fornecerão uma dieta terapêutica? Eles dão comida da mesa? Eles conseguem fornecer medidas corretas e/ou múltiplas refeições? Eles podem aumentar o exercício do animal de estimação? Em casas com muitos animais, os proprietários alimentarão os animais separadamente?
  ○ Obediência ao programa de perda de peso — os proprietários devem receber instruções por escrito sobre as quantidades específicas a serem fornecidas, utilizando a ração acordada. O proprietário deve compreender que "xícaras" de ração se referem a um copo-medida de ~230 g. Para cães de pequeno porte e gatos, o uso de balança de cozinha ou escala em gramas para medir as recomendações dietéticas toleradas pode ajudar na precisão. Os petiscos devem ser oferecidos como parte do programa (ver adiante), já que muitos proprietários continuarão a fornecê-los.
  ○ Comunicação contínua — o acompanhamento frequente durante o programa de perda de peso ajuda o proprietário a obedecer.

DIETA
- Certos macronutrientes podem facilitar uma perda de peso mais saudável ou mais fácil:
  ○ Proteína — o aumento do teor proteico na dieta facilita a perda de gordura corporal, ao mesmo tempo em que minimiza a perda de massa corporal magra, que corresponde ao tecido metabolicamente ativo. A preservação da massa corporal magra deve ajudar no controle do peso a longo prazo, mantendo uma necessidade energética mais alta em repouso. A proteína também estimula o metabolismo, aumenta o gasto energético e contribui para a saciedade.
  ○ Fibra — a adição de fibra na dieta representa uma pequena quantidade de energia, o que ajuda a reduzir as calorias totais. Além de contribuir para a saciedade, a fibra também estimula o metabolismo do intestino e o uso de energia.
  ○ Redução do teor de gordura — a gordura é densamente calórica e, portanto, dietas pobres em gordura têm níveis mais baixos de calorias.
- Outros fatores relacionados com a dieta que podem auxiliar no controle do peso:
  ○ Carnitina — esse composto, produzido por via endógena a partir dos aminoácidos lisina e metionina, é necessário para a oxidação lipídica.
  ○ A suplementação pode ser benéfica quando a ingestão de proteína na dieta é limitada.
  ○ Isoflavonas — fitonutrientes metabolicamente ativos que estimulam o metabolismo energético. Esses compostos podem reduzir o efeito rebote sobre o peso e ajudar a manter a massa corporal magra.

Refeição Principal
- As calorias devem ser limitadas sem restrição excessiva de nutrientes essenciais. Para a perda de peso, é recomendável o uso de dieta terapêutica hipocalórica, com relação elevada de nutrientes:calorias.
- A quantidade fornecida deve visar uma perda de 1-2% no peso corporal/semana. Uma perda de peso mais rápida pode aumentar a perda de massa corporal magra e estimular o efeito rebote sobre o peso assim que a perda for atingida.
- A alimentação inicial baseia-se em 60-75% da necessidade energética de manutenção calculada, utilizando o peso corporal-alvo. O peso corporal-alvo pode ser estimado, utilizando-se o peso atual e o escore de condição corporal; ou um alvo intermediário, p. ex., pode ser selecionado o nível de 20% abaixo do peso ideal.
- Necessidade energética de manutenção média = 55 kcal/kg para gatos; 110 kcal/kg^{0,75} para cães.
- Ajustar as quantidades de alimentação mensalmente para compensar as diminuições na necessidade energética de manutenção em virtude da restrição de calorias e da perda de peso, bem como em função das diferenças individuais na necessidade energética da manutenção.
- Dietas com alto teor de umidade podem ser utilizadas para diminuir as calorias/porções. Essa abordagem parece ser mais eficaz para os gatos em comparação aos cães, pois os primeiros tendem a controlar sua ingestão com base no volume.
- Se o proprietário não estiver disposto a usar uma dieta terapêutica, deve-se evitar uma restrição calórica intensa. Um diário alimentar pode ser usado para registrar o consumo atual em um período de 3-7 dias. Na sequência, o animal de estimação deve ser alimentado com 10-20% a menos da quantidade previamente recebida.

OBESIDADE

Petiscos
- Os petiscos frequentemente fazem parte do elo proprietário-animal.
- A completa abstinência dos petiscos é um obstáculo ao cumprimento do programa de perda de peso.
- Em vez disso, oferecer uma tolerância de 10% das calorias diárias sob a forma de petiscos e fornecer uma lista de petiscos hipocalóricos adequados para cães e gatos.

ATIVIDADE
- A restrição calórica resulta em declínios compensatórios no gasto energético basal. O aumento da atividade física ajuda a compensar isso e cria oportunidades alternativas de interações proprietário-animal. Fornecer várias sugestões adequadas para cada proprietário e paciente. Por exemplo:
- Passeio de coleira para cães e gatos adestrados — por, no mínimo, 15 minutos duas vezes ao dia.
- Atividades, como *fetch* (o ato de apanhar uma bola), brinquedos interativos para gatos, ou brincar com foco luminoso de laser.
- Bolas de ração — feitas para conter petiscos ou peletes e liberá-los aleatoriamente conforme o cão ou o gato brinca com elas. O alimento contido nessas bolas deve fazer parte da tolerância calórica diária.

MEDICAÇÕES
MEDICAMENTO(S) DE ESCOLHA
Dirlotapida, aprovado apenas para uso em cães, pode causar supressão do apetite suficiente para induzir à perda de peso. A dose de partida é de 0,01 mL/kg de peso corporal uma vez ao dia, por via oral ou juntamente com a ração. Após 2 semanas, aumentar para 0,02 mL/kg por 2 semanas. Em seguida, ajustar a dose, conforme a necessidade, para atingir uma perda de peso a uma taxa de 0,7% de peso corporal/semana. Ajustar a dose mensalmente, sem exceder uma dose máxima de 0,20 mL/kg.

CONTRAINDICAÇÕES
- A dirlotapida não é indicada para uso em gatos ou outras espécies não caninas.
- Também não é indicada para uso em cães com hepatopatias ou cadelas prenhes ou lactantes.

PRECAUÇÕES/INTERAÇÕES POSSÍVEIS
- Os efeitos colaterais comuns incluem vômito, diarreia, letargia e atividade elevada das enzimas hepáticas.
- A restrição alimentar intensa induzida pelo medicamento pode induzir a deficiências nutricionais. Utilizar com uma dieta formulada para perda de peso, com alto teor de proteína.
- Não introduzir medicamento ou nova dieta ao mesmo tempo, pois a ocorrência de vômito relacionado com o medicamento e a baixa ingestão alimentar podem ser incorretamente atribuídas à dieta.
- O apetite e o peso retornarão após a interrupção do medicamento. Por isso, há necessidade de orientação ao proprietário e a instituição de plano alimentar adequado para compensar isso.

MEDICAMENTO(S) ALTERNATIVO(S)
Mitratapida (1 mL/8 kg de peso corporal) tem um mecanismo de ação semelhante, mas limita-se a um único curso terapêutico por cão.

ACOMPANHAMENTO
- Durante o programa de controle do peso, é importante a comunicação frequente com o proprietário.
- 1 semana — chamadas telefônicas da clínica para tratar qualquer problema e reforçar a importância do programa.
- Mensalmente — o paciente deve ser pesado na clínica em um esquema mensal. Se necessários, devem ser feitos ajustes nas diretrizes de tolerância alimentar nesse momento.
- Ao atingir o peso-alvo — assim que o paciente tiver alcançado o escore de condição corporal ideal, devem ser fornecidas diretrizes para manutenção do peso.
- As necessidades energéticas serão mais baixas do que eram antes da perda do peso, embora isso possa aumentar um pouco com o tempo.
- Os proprietários devem continuar medindo a quantidade de ração, monitorizando o escore de condição corporal ou o peso corporal e ajustando a tolerância alimentar, conforme a necessidade, para manter a perda.

DIVERSOS
DISTÚRBIOS ASSOCIADOS
- Osteoartrite.
- Diabetes melito ou insulinorresistência.
- Dermatoses.
- Lipidose hepática felina.
- Doenças do trato urinário inferior felino.
- Diminuição na expectativa de vida.

FATORES RELACIONADOS COM A IDADE
- A necessidade energética de manutenção diminui com a idade em cães, o que aumenta o risco de obesidade.
- Em gatos, a necessidade energética de manutenção também diminui com a idade até cerca de 10-12 anos.
- A prevalência mais elevada de obesidade ocorre entre 5 e 10 anos de idade tanto em cães como em gatos.

POTENCIAL ZOONÓTICO
N/D.

GESTAÇÃO/FERTILIDADE/REPRODUÇÃO
- A obesidade pode interferir na capacidade reprodutiva da fêmea ou na geração de prole saudável.
- Contudo, não se incentiva a restrição calórica durante a prenhez ou a lactação, pois a restrição de nutrientes pode ter efeitos adversos sobre a ninhada a longo prazo.

SINÔNIMO(S)
Excesso de peso.

Sugestões de Leitura
Cave MC, Hurt RT, Frazier TH, et al. Obesity, inflammation, and the potential application of pharmaconutrition. Nutr Clin Pract 2008, 23:16-34.
Kealy RD, Lawler DF, Ballam JM, et al. Effects of diet restriction on life span and age-related changes in dogs. JAVMA 2002, 220:1315-1320.
Laflamme DP. Development and validation of a body condition score system for cats: A clinical tool. Feline Pract 1997, 25:13-18.
———. Development and validation of a body condition score system for dogs: A clinical tool. Canine Pract 1997, 22:10-15.
———. Nutrition for aging cats and dogs and the importance of body condition. Vet Clin North Am Small Anim Pract 2005, 35(3):713-742.
Vasconcellos RS, Borges NC, Goncalves KNV, et al. Protein intake during weight loss influences the energy required for weight loss and maintenance in cats. J Nutr 2009, 139:855-860.
Wren JA, Ramudo AA, Campbell SL, et al. Efficacy and safety of dirlotapide in the management of obese dogs evaluated in two placebo-controlled, masked clinical studies in North America. J Vet Pharmacol Ther 2007, 30(Suppl 1):81-89.

Autor Dorothy P. Laflamme
Consultor Editorial Albert E. Jergens

Obstrução do Ducto Biliar

CONSIDERAÇÕES GERAIS

DEFINIÇÃO
Colestase causada por obstrução da árvore biliar na altura do ducto biliar (comum) extra-hepático (OEHDB) ou na altura dos ductos hepáticos (pode envolver um, vários ou todos os ductos, dependendo da causa subjacente).

FISIOPATOLOGIA
• Lesão hepatobiliar grave — pode ocorrer dentro de semanas do quadro de obstrução de ducto, secundária ao acúmulo de mediadores inflamatórios, ácidos biliares e constituintes biliares nocivos, efeito mecânico de distensão ductal e dano oxidativo (considerado o principal mecanismo patológico).
• Bile — pode ficar incolor (bile branca), em função da queda na secreção de bilirrubina e do aumento na produção de mucina em caso de oclusão do ducto cístico.
• Infecção bacteriana de estruturas biliares — alto risco, em virtude do comprometimento no fluxo de bile (mecanismo normal de depuração).

SISTEMA(S) ACOMETIDO(S)
Hepatobiliar.

IDENTIFICAÇÃO
Espécies
Cães e gatos.

Raça(s) Predominante(s)
Animais predispostos à pancreatite e à formação de colélitos incluindo mucocele da vesícula biliar — raças hiperlipidêmicas (p. ex., Schnauzer miniatura e Pastor de shetland); raças caninas de pequeno porte podem ser predispostas à colelitíase.

Idade Média e Faixa Etária
Animais de meia-idade a idosos.

Sexo Predominante
Nenhum.

SINAIS CLÍNICOS
Achados Anamnésicos
• Dependem do distúrbio subjacente.
• Letargia progressiva.
• Doença intermitente.
• Icterícia progressiva.
• Fezes pálidas (acólicas): OEHDB completa.
• Polifagia — a obstrução completa causa má assimilação de nutrientes.
• Tendências hemorrágicas dentro de 10 dias da OEHDB completa, mais evidente em gatos.

Achados do Exame Físico
• Dependem do distúrbio subjacente.
• Perda de peso.
• Icterícia grave.
• Hepatomegalia.
• Efeito de lesão expansiva cranial tipo massa — estruturas biliares extra-hepáticas (cães de pequeno porte e gatos).
• Fezes acólicas — a menos que ocorra sangramento entérico (a hemoglobina é uma fonte de pigmento biliar).
• Tendências hemorrágicas.
• Urina de coloração laranja.

CAUSAS E FATORES DE RISCO
• Associadas a diversos distúrbios.
• Colelitíase.
• Coledoquite.
• Neoplasia.
• Má-formação dos ductos (cistos do colédoco, doença hepatobiliar policística, formação de cistoadenoma [gatos]).
• Infestação parasitária (fascíolas/trematódeos; gatos).
• Compressão extrínseca (linfonodos, neoplasia, pancreatite, encarceramento do ducto biliar comum em hérnia diafragmática).
• Fibrose ductal (traumatismo, peritonite, pancreatite; envolvimento de ducto importante em alguns gatos com colangite/colangio-hepatite).
• Estenose ductal (traumatismo rombo, iatrogênico por manipulações ou procedimentos cirúrgicos).

DIAGNÓSTICO

DIAGNÓSTICO DIFERENCIAL
• Lesões expansivas tipo massa — tumores hepáticos primários ou metastáticos; tumores em vísceras adjacentes.
• Hepatopatia infiltrativa difusa — neoplásica, inflamatória, lipidose hepática (gatos), amiloide (raro).
• Hepatite infecciosa — bacteriana, viral, parasitária (fascíolas/trematódeos).
• Hepatite crônica "ativa" descompensada.
• Hepatopatia por armazenamento de cobre.
• Cirrose em fase terminal.
• Insuficiência hepática fulminante.
• Cistos biliares — cisto do colédoco (gatos), cistoadenoma, doença hepatobiliar policística (gatos).
• Pancreatite.
• Lipidose hepática — gatos.
• Colangite/colangio-hepatite — gatos (especialmente a forma esclerosante, que causa destruição intra-hepática de ducto biliar).

HEMOGRAMA/BIOQUÍMICA/URINÁLISE
Hemograma completo
• Anemia — arregenerativa (anemia de doença crônica) ou regenerativa (sangramento entérico) leves.
• Microcitose — incomum.
• Leucograma — variável; leucocitose neutrofílica; leucograma com desvio à esquerda em casos de sepse.
• Plasma — acentuadamente ictérico.

Bioquímica
• Enzimas hepáticas — variáveis; aumentos acentuados típicos na fosfatase alcalina e GGT; atividade elevada da ALT e AST.
• Bilirrubina total sérica — de moderada a acentuadamente alta; em geral, encontra-se em um nível menos acentuado do que quando observada em casos de hemólise ou lipidose hepática.
• Albumina — em geral, apresenta-se dentro dos limites de normalidade, exceto quando a duração da OEHDB ultrapassa 6 semanas (cirrose biliar estabelecida); nesse caso, os níveis baixos da albumina refletem a insuficiência na síntese proteica.
• Globulinas — em geral, permanecem normais.
• Glicose — costuma estar normal a menos que haja cirrose biliar (hipoglicemia) ou sepse.
• Hipercolesterolemia — comum.
• Os resultados do fracionamento da bilirrubina se sobrepõem aos achados de anemia hemolítica acentuada.

Urinálise
• Bilirrubinúria e cristais de bilirrubina.
• Ausência de urobilinogênio — a menos que ocorra sangramento entérico; teste não confiável.

OUTROS TESTES LABORATORIAIS
• Ácidos biliares séricos — sempre se encontram acentuadamente elevados; não acrescentam informações diagnósticas.
• Anormalidades de coagulação — desenvolvem-se dentro de 10 dias da OEHDB, em virtude da deficiência de vitamina K (PIAVK e TP com tempos de coagulação mais sensíveis); pode ocorrer o desenvolvimento de CID; os gatos são aparentemente predispostos.
• Exame fecal — as fezes acólicas sugerem OEHDB; mascaradas por um pequeno volume de melena; a constatação de ovos de trematódeos indica infestação por fascíolas.

DIAGNÓSTICO POR IMAGEM
• Radiografia abdominal — hepatomegalia; pode apontar a existência de lesão expansiva tipo massa na área da vesícula biliar, bem como a presença de sinais de pancreatite e, raramente, colélito(s) mineralizado(s).
• Colecistografia — raramente fornece informações práticas adicionais.
• Ultrassonografia abdominal — pode-se verificar a evidência de obstrução dentro de 72 h (ducto biliar extra-hepático distendido e tortuoso, além da distensão dos ductos biliares intra-hepáticos); é possível observar a evidência de doença subjacente ou primária (p. ex., pancreatite, lesões císticas, lesões expansivas, colélitos). Atenção: a "sedimentação" da bile na vesícula biliar e a repleção dessa vesícula são comuns em pacientes com anorexia ou em jejum — não confundir com obstrução da vesícula biliar.
• Cuidado: os ductos extra-hepáticos dos gatos são serpiginosos, quando comparados com os dos cães; sempre se recomenda a avaliação da imagem do fígado em busca de evidência da distensão dos ductos biliares intra-hepáticos (diferenciar os ductos de vasos por meio do exame com Doppler colorido).

MÉTODOS DIAGNÓSTICOS
• Citologia hepática aspirativa — indicada para incluir e considerar o quadro de lipidose hepática em gatos ou obter amostras de lesões expansivas aparentes; evitar a aspiração de trato biliar obstruído (extravasamento de bile).
• Biopsia por agulha — fortemente contraindicada; pode levar à peritonite biliar iatrogênica.
• Laparotomia — a abordagem mais eficiente; permite procedimentos como biopsia tecidual; descompressão biliar: excisão de massa, remoção de colélito(s) ou de bile inspissada (espessa); criação de anastomose biliar-entérica, conforme a necessidade.

ACHADOS PATOLÓGICOS
• Macroscópicos — ducto biliar distendido e tortuoso; vesícula biliar distendida: a causa é geralmente óbvia; obstrução com >2 semanas de duração: fígado aumentado de volume de cor verde escura ou mogno; obstrução completa e crônica de ducto cístico produz bile branca ou clara.
• Microscópicos — precoce: hiperplasia epitelial biliar e proliferação ductal biliar com inflamação intraluminal (geralmente neutrófilos); distensão crônica das estruturas biliares: desvitalização do

Obstrução do Ducto Biliar

epitélio biliar; debris necróticos e inflamação supurativa nos ductos biliares; inflamação e edema periportais mistos; necrose parenquimatosa multifocal; fibrose periductal circunferencial, e edema.

TRATAMENTO

CUIDADO(S) DE SAÚDE ADEQUADO(S)
Internação — intervenção cirúrgica em casos de OEHDB.

CUIDADO(S) DE ENFERMAGEM
• Fluidoterapia — depende das condições subjacentes (ver "Pancreatite"); reidratar e fornecer fluidos de manutenção antes da anestesia geral e da intervenção cirúrgica; suplementar os fluidos poliônicos com cloreto de potássio e fosfato; proceder a ajustes criteriosos dos eletrólitos, dependendo da condição eletrolítica.
• Vitaminas hidrossolúveis — nos fluidos intravenosos; vitaminas do complexo B (2 mL/L de fluidos poliônicos).

ATIVIDADE
Depende do estado do paciente e das tendências ao sangramento (coagulopatia).

DIETA
• Manter o balanço nitrogenado: evitar as dietas com restrição de proteínas.
• Restringir o teor de gordura — se houver má assimilação lipídica evidente causada pela falta de ácidos biliares entéricos.
• Suplementar as vitaminas lipossolúveis: vitaminas E e K são mais urgentes; as outras [vitaminas D e A] podem levar à toxicidade.

ORIENTAÇÃO AO PROPRIETÁRIO
• Informar o proprietário sobre o caráter indispensável da descompressão biliar cirúrgica, já que a OEHDB evoluirá para cirrose biliar dentro de 6 semanas; a pancreatite indutora de OEHDB é uma exceção, pois ela pode exibir resolução espontânea dentro de 2-3 semanas.
• Alertar o proprietário sobre o fato de que o êxito da cirurgia depende não só da causa subjacente, mas também dos resultados da biopsia hepática e das culturas das amostras.

CONSIDERAÇÕES CIRÚRGICAS
• Exploração cirúrgica — imperativa para o tratamento e a determinação da causa subjacente; iniciar antibioticoterapia antes da cirurgia.
• Excisão de massas; remoção de colélito(s) e bile inspissada (espessa).
• Ressecção da vesícula biliar — em casos de colecistite necrosante ou mucocele da vesícula biliar.
• Anastomose biliar-entérica — em casos de oclusão insolúvel, pancreatite fibrosante sem resolução, ou neoplasia; o estoma anastomótico deve ter pelo menos 2,5 cm de largura. A inserção de *stent** em vez de anastomose biliar-entérica pode ser complicada por infecção e obstrução desse dispositivo.
• Hipotensão e bradicardia (reflexo vasovagal) — podem ocorrer com a manipulação da árvore

---
* N. T.: Dispositivo metálico, utilizado com a finalidade de manter o lúmen de uma artéria permeável, com seu calibre próximo do normal, formando uma nova "parede" para o vaso.

biliar; ter à mão os medicamentos de emergência (anticolinérgicos) e o suporte ventilatório, para evitar o reflexo vasovagal; garantir o acesso de cateter intravenoso e a expansão do volume; utilizar fluidos coloides, se necessário; estar preparado para a ocorrência de hemorragia.
• Biopsias/amostras cirúrgicas — enviar as amostras teciduais e biliares para a realização de culturas bacterianas aeróbias e anaeróbias; enviar os tecidos para exame histopatológico; fazer preparados citológicos a partir de impressões (decalques) teciduais e esfregaços biliares; pesquisar por meio citológico a presença de infecção bacteriana, neoplasia e ovos de trematódeos.
• Microrganismos bacterianos — observados apenas em lâminas coradas com o corante do tipo Wright-Giemsa; emprega-se a coloração de Gram para caracterizar os microrganismos e orientar a escolha do antibiótico. Os microrganismos entéricos oportunistas são mais comuns.
• Colangite esclerosante (gatos) — pode se confundir clinicamente com a OEHDB (ductopenia intra-hepática); além disso, a colangite não responderá à descompressão da árvore biliar; a biopsia hepática é essencial para o diagnóstico.

MEDICAÇÕES

MEDICAMENTO(S) DE ESCOLHA
Vitamina K₁
• Fornecer 12-36 h antes da cirurgia (0,5-1,5 mg/kg IM ou SC). Administrar 3 doses em intervalos de 12 h. **Cuidado:** evitar a administração IV, pois pode causar anafilaxia. Em caso de OEHDB crônica insolúvel, administrar a vitamina K₁ por via parenteral por período de tempo prolongado, com frequência titulada utilizando a PIAVK.

Antibióticos
• Antes da cirurgia — utilizar antibióticos de amplo espectro de ação contra oportunistas gram-negativos e anaeróbios entéricos por causa de infecções biliares potenciais, pois as manipulações cirúrgicas podem precipitar a bacteremia.

Antioxidantes
• Vitamina E (acetato de α-tocoferol) — 10-100 UI/kg; uma dose oral maior que a usual (normal = 10 UI/kg/dia) é necessária em OEHDB crônica por causa da má absorção de gordura (ausência de ácidos biliares entéricos) ou utilizar o TPGS-vitamina E (preferido). Em caso de OEHDB crônica insolúvel (rara), utilizar o TPGS-vitamina E (10 UI/kg/dia VO) e a vitamina K₁ injetável (ver anteriormente).
• *S*-Adenosilmetionina (SAMe; Denosyl SD4® tem biodisponibilidade e eficácia comprovadas como doador de glutationa) — 20 mg/kg de comprimidos entéricos revestidos por via oral a cada 24 h (2 h antes da refeição); possui muitos outros benefícios.

Ácido Ursodesoxicólico
• 10-15 mg/kg VO por dia — em casos de colerese pós-cirúrgica; é essencial manter uma hidratação adequada; não é adequado antes da descompressão biliar; não foi demonstrado que esse medicamento facilite a assimilação de gordura em casos de OEHDB crônica; possui efeitos antifibróticos, antiendotóxicos, hepatoprotetores e imunomoduladores.

Preparação do Intestino antes da Cirurgia
• Essa preparação pode diminuir a endotoxemia (reduzindo a hipotensão perioperatória) e altera agudamente a flora entérica para reduzir a translocação entérica de patógenos oportunistas.
• Limpeza mecânica do cólon com água ou fluidos cristaloides.
• Medicações administradas por via oral ou por enema alto: neomicina: 22 mg/kg a cada 8 h; lactulose: 1-2 mL/kg a cada 8 h; metronidazol: 7,5 mg/kg a cada 12 h; rifaximina: 5-10 mg/kg a cada 12 h; bactérias probióticas (dose empírica do produto).
• Enrofloxacino: 2,5 mg/kg VO a cada 12 h.

Protetores Gastrintestinais
• Agentes redutores da acidez gástrica — famotidina (bloqueador dos receptores H₂) ou omeprazol (inibidor da bomba de prótons), em combinação com sucralfato para citoproteção local se os medicamentos orais forem tolerados e o sangramento entérico, identificado; alternar a administração do sucralfato com outras medicações orais para evitar as interações medicamentosas.

CONTRAINDICAÇÕES
Proporcionar a descompressão biliar antes da instituição do ácido ursodesoxicólico.

PRECAUÇÕES
Ver o item "hipotensão e bradicardia (reflexo vasovagal)" na seção "Considerações Cirúrgicas".

MEDICAMENTO(S) ALTERNATIVO(S)
N/D.

ACOMPANHAMENTO

MONITORIZAÇÃO DO PACIENTE
• Depende da condição subjacente — monitorizar especialmente em busca dos distúrbios subjacentes indutores da OEHDB; ver informações sobre as afecções próprias para esse quadro.
• Valores da bilirrubina total — refletem agudamente a descompressão biliar; os valores normalizam-se dentro de dias.
• Atividades das enzimas hepáticas — declinam lentamente.
• Hemograma completo — repetir a cada 2-3 dias inicialmente em caso de quadro séptico.
• Peritonite biliar — avaliar a circunferência abdominal, o peso corporal e o acúmulo de líquido abdominal (p. ex., por meio de palpação, ultrassonografia [método preferido] e abdominocentese).
• Determinar a necessidade de suplementação com enzimas pancreáticas, com base no local da anastomose biliar-entérica; os pacientes submetidos a colecistojejunostomias podem se beneficiar da suplementação enzimática; não se pode contar com os valores da substância imunorreativa semelhante à tripsina para estimar a suficiência exócrina pancreática nessa circunstância; avaliar a condição e o peso corporal, bem como as fezes quanto à presença de esteatorreia (sugere má assimilação lipídica); se as fezes estiverem esteatorreicas após anastomose biliar-entérica e não ictéricas, reduzir o teor de gordura da dieta e suplementá-la com enzimas pancreáticas.

PREVENÇÃO
N/D.

COMPLICAÇÕES POSSÍVEIS
• Peritonite biliar.
• Nova formação de estenose do ducto biliar — se não for desviado por via cirúrgica.
• Estenose da anastomose biliar-entérica.
• Hemorragia entérica grave em casos de OEHDB — vasculopatia entérica hipertensiva com coagulopatia por deficiência da vitamina K.
• Hemorragia durante a cirurgia.
• Hipotensão irresponsiva durante a cirurgia.
• Reflexo vasovagal — manipulações da árvore biliar.

EVOLUÇÃO ESPERADA E PROGNÓSTICO
• Dependem da doença subjacente.
• Prognóstico bom mediante a resolução da pancreatite fibrosante e da inflamação pancreática; podem ocorrer o restabelecimento da desobstrução do ducto biliar e a oclusão espontânea da anastomose biliar-entérica.
• O veterinário deve estar ciente de que a árvore biliar aparecerá distendida nas avaliações ultrassonográficas subsequentes.
• Fibrose peribiliar permanente por conta da OEHDB.
• Os gatos com colangite esclerosante podem parecer ter a OEHDB, mas eles não respondem à descompressão biliar; nesse caso, a biopsia hepática é essencial para o diagnóstico.

CONSIDERAÇÕES/PRECAUÇÕES
• Prever as tendências hemorrágicas e o reflexo vasovagal durante os procedimentos cirúrgicos.
• Sempre enviar amostras de fígado e da árvore biliar para exame histológico, bem como todos os tecidos e a bile para culturas bacterianas aeróbia e anaeróbia.

DIVERSOS
DISTÚRBIOS ASSOCIADOS
• Ver a seção "Causas e Fatores de Risco".
• A Colangite Esclerosante (gatos) confunde-se com a OEHDB.

VER TAMBÉM
• Síndrome Colangite/Colangio-hepatite.
• Mucocele da Vesícula Biliar.
• Ver a seção "Causas e Fatores de Risco".

ABREVIATURA(S)
• ALT = alanina aminotransferase.
• AST = aspartato aminotransferase.
• CID = coagulação intravascular disseminada.
• GGT = gama-glutamiltransferase.
• OEHDB = obstrução extra-hepática do ducto biliar.
• PIAVK = proteínas invocadas pela ausência ou antagonismo da vitamina K.
• TP = tempo de protrombina.
• TPGS-vitamina E = succinato de d-α-tocoferil polietilenoglicol.

Sugestões de Leitura
Center SA. Diseases of the gallbladder and biliary tree. In: Guilford WG, Center SA, Strombeck DR, et al., eds., Strombeck's Small Animal Gastroenterology, 3rd ed. Philadelphia: Saunders, 1996, pp. 860-888.
Center SA. Diseases of the gallbladder and biliary tree. Vet Clin North Am Small Anim Pract 2009, 39(3):543-598.
Center SA. Interpretation of liver enzymes. Vet Clin North Am Small Anim Pract 2007, 37(2):297-333.

Autor Sharon A. Center
Consultor Editorial Sharon A. Center

Obstrução do Trato Urinário

CONSIDERAÇÕES GERAIS

DEFINIÇÃO
Trata-se da restrição ao fluxo de urina desde os rins, passando pelo trato urinário, até o orifício uretral externo.

FISIOPATOLOGIA
• Em função de lesões com envolvimento das vias excretoras, desenvolve-se uma resistência excessiva ao fluxo de urina através do trato urinário, o que leva a aumento na pressão do espaço urinário proximal à obstrução e pode ocasionar distensão anormal desse espaço por acúmulo de urina. As consequências fisiopatológicas resultantes dependem do local, do grau e da duração da obstrução. A obstrução completa produz um estado fisiopatológico equivalente ao da insuficiência renal aguda oligúrica. • A perfuração das vias excretoras com extravasamento de urina é equivalente do ponto de vista funcional.

SISTEMA(S) ACOMETIDO(S)
• Renal/urológico.
• Sistemas gastrintestinal, cardiovascular, nervoso e respiratório à medida que a uremia se desenvolve.

IDENTIFICAÇÃO
• Cães e gatos.
• Mais comum em machos do que em fêmeas.

SINAIS CLÍNICOS

Achados Anamnésicos
• Polaciúria (comum).
• Estrangúria.
• Redução na velocidade ou no calibre do jato urinário ou ausência de fluxo urinário durante os esforços de micção.
• Hematúria macroscópica.
• Sinais de uremia que se desenvolvem quando a obstrução do trato urinário é completa (ou quase completa): letargia, apatia, diminuição do apetite e vômito.

Achados do Exame Físico
• Distensão vesical palpável excessiva (i. e., bexiga excessivamente grande ou túrgida) ou inapropriada (i. e., persistência após esforços de micção).
• Com frequência, os urólitos são palpáveis nas uretras de machos caninos obstruídos.
• Ocasionalmente, descobre-se renomegalia palpável em animais com obstrução ureteral parcial crônica, sobretudo quando a lesão é unilateral.
• Sinais de uremia grave — desidratação, fraqueza, hipotermia, bradicardia com hipercalemia moderada, taquipneia com respirações superficiais, estupor ou coma, ocorrência de crises convulsivas em fase terminal, taquicardia resultante de disritmias ventriculares induzidas por hipercalemia grave.
• Sinais de perfuração das vias excretoras — o extravasamento de urina na cavidade peritoneal causa dor e distensão abdominais; já o extravasamento de urina nos espaços periuretrais provoca dor e tumefação nos tecidos intrapélvicos ou perineais, dependendo do local da lesão uretral; febre.

CAUSAS

Causas Intraluminais
• Estruturas sólidas ou semissólidas, incluindo urólitos, tampões uretrais em gatos, coágulos sanguíneos e fragmentos teciduais esfacelados.
• Local mais comum — a uretra.
• Urolitíase — a causa mais frequente em machos caninos.
• Tampões uretrais — a causa mais usual em machos felinos.

Causas Intramurais
• Neoplasia do colo vesical ou da uretra — causa comum em cães.
• Lesões inflamatórias piogranulomatosas na uretra — observadas ocasionalmente em cães.
• A ocorrência de fibrose no local da lesão ou inflamação prévia pode causar estreitamento ou estenose, o que pode impedir o fluxo urinário ou constituir um local de alojamento de debris intraluminais.
• Distúrbios prostáticos em machos caninos.
• Nos locais de obstrução intraluminal (p. ex., uretral), podem ocorrer edema, hemorragia ou espasmo de componentes musculares, que contribuem para obstrução persistente ou recidivante ao fluxo urinário após a remoção do material intraluminal. Podem-se desenvolver alterações teciduais em virtude das lesões infligidas pelo material obstrutivo, pelas manipulações empregadas na remoção deste material ou ambos.
• Rupturas, lacerações e punções — causadas geralmente por incidentes traumáticos.

Causas Mistas
• Deslocamento da bexiga urinária para o interior de uma hérnia perineal.
• Neurogênica (ver "Retenção Urinária Funcional").

FATORES DE RISCO
• Urolitíase, particularmente em machos.
• Doença do trato urinário inferior felino, sobretudo em machos.
• Prostatopatias em cães.

DIAGNÓSTICO

DIAGNÓSTICO DIFERENCIAL
• O agachamento improdutivo repetido na bandeja sanitária por gatos com obstrução uretral pode ser erroneamente interpretado como constipação.
• Os animais cujos esforços de micção não são observados por seus proprietários podem ser examinados, em função de sinais atribuíveis à uremia sem histórico de possível obstrução.
• A avaliação de qualquer paciente com azotemia deve incluir a consideração de possíveis causas pós-renais (p. ex., obstrução urinária). Ver capítulo sobre "Azotemia e Uremia" quanto ao diagnóstico diferencial desse problema.
• Os pacientes com ruptura vesical podem exibir sinais clínicos (p. ex., anorexia, vômito, diarreia, depressão, letargia, fraqueza e colapso) e resultados dos testes laboratoriais (azotemia, hipercalemia e hiponatremia) semelhantes àqueles comumente observados em pacientes com hipoadrenocorticismo (doença de Addison).
• Assim que a existência de uma obstrução urinária for identificada, os esforços diagnósticos se concentrarão na detecção da presença e na avaliação da magnitude de anormalidades secundárias à obstrução, bem como na identificação do local, da causa e da natureza (parcial ou completa) do(s) impedimento(s) ao fluxo urinário.

HEMOGRAMA/BIOQUÍMICA/URINÁLISE
• Os resultados do hemograma costumam permanecer normais, embora se possa observar leucograma de estresse.
• A análise bioquímica revela azotemia, hiperfosfatemia, acidose metabólica, hipercalemia e redução do cálcio ionizado proporcionalmente à duração da obstrução completa.
• Os sinais de hematúria e proteinúria são comuns; a presença de cristalúria apoia o diagnóstico de urolitíase; em pacientes com neoplasia, podem-se observar células epiteliais atípicas.

OUTROS TESTES LABORATORIAIS
Os urólitos eliminados ou recuperados devem ser enviados para análise cristalográfica para a determinação de sua composição mineral.

DIAGNÓSTICO POR IMAGEM

Radiografia Abdominal
• Urólitos — são frequentemente demonstrados por meio de radiografias simples; em função do tamanho, da composição ou do local de alguns urólitos, fica difícil ou impossível observá-los.
• A uretrografia com contraste positivo constitui o método mais sensível de detecção de lesões intraluminais e intramurais na uretra; já a cistografia com duplo contraste representa o método mais sensível de detecção de lesões no lúmen e na parede vesicais.
• A obstrução do trato urinário superior (i. e., ureter ou pelve renal) pode ser detectada por meio de urografia excretora em caso de preservação satisfatória da função renal no(s) lado(s) acometido(s), de tal modo que o meio de contraste radiográfico seja excretado e fique suficientemente concentrado a ponto de ser observado em um ponto proximal à obstrução.

Ultrassonografia Abdominal
• A ultrassonografia é altamente sensível para a detecção de lesões na bexiga urinária e na uretra proximal (incluindo a próstata em cães) e obstruções no trato urinário superior (i. e., ureter ou pelve renal). O grau de sensibilidade da ultrassonografia depende da experiência do ultrassonografista.

MÉTODOS DIAGNÓSTICOS
• A eletrocardiografia pode detectar anormalidades secundárias à hipercalemia, incluindo ondas T altas, intervalo P-R prolongado, bradicardia e parada atrial.
• A cateterização transuretral tem valor diagnóstico e terapêutico. À medida que o cateter é inserido no lúmen uretral, podem-se determinar o local e a natureza do material obstrutivo. Parte desse material ou sua totalidade (p. ex., pequenos urólitos e tampões uretrais felinos) pode ser induzido a ser eliminado pela uretra no sentido distal e, sempre que possível, enviado ao laboratório para análise quantitativa. A irrigação retrógrada do lúmen uretral pode impulsionar os debris intraluminais em direção à bexiga urinária. Embora as lesões uretrais intramurais sejam algumas vezes detectadas durante a cateterização, a inserção do cateter poderá ser normal. Os animais que se mostram incapazes de urinar apesar da geração de pressão intravesical adequada (i. e., dotados de resistência excessiva ao fluxo de saída) e possuem uretras facilmente cateterizadas e irrigadas apresentam lesões intramurais ou retenção urinária funcional.
• A avaliação citológica de amostras obtidas a partir do trato urinário com o auxílio de cateteres

Obstrução do Trato Urinário

pode ser diagnóstica, particularmente em casos de carcinoma uretral ou vesical e algumas prostatopatias. Deve-se empregar massagem prostática ou manipulação física da extremidade do cateter, posicionado próximo à lesão sob suspeita, para produzir amostras ricas em células recuperadas por meio da aspiração do material ou da obtenção de lavado com solução salina em uma seringa acoplada.
• A cistoscopia pode ser útil, sobretudo em cadelas com lesões intramurais no colo vesical ou na uretra.

TRATAMENTO

CUIDADO(S) DE SAÚDE ADEQUADO(S)
• A obstrução completa constitui uma emergência médica, que pode representar um risco de vida ao animal; em geral, deve-se instituir o tratamento imediatamente.
• Obstrução parcial — não constitui necessariamente uma emergência, mas esses pacientes podem estar sob risco de desenvolver obstrução completa; se a obstrução parcial não for tratada com prontidão, poderão ocorrer danos irreversíveis ao trato urinário.
• Internar o paciente até que sua capacidade de micção seja restabelecida.
• Algumas vezes, a cirurgia é imprescindível.
• O controle e o prognóstico a longo prazo dependem da causa da obstrução.
• O tratamento envolve três componentes importantes: o combate dos desarranjos metabólicos associados à uremia pós-renal (p. ex., desidratação, hipotermia, acidose, hipercalemia e azotemia); o restabelecimento e a manutenção de alguma via patente (desobstruída) ao fluxo urinário; e a implantação de tratamentos específicos contra a causa subjacente de retenção urinária.
• O desvio urinário por meio de cistostomia com sonda é útil em casos selecionados.

CUIDADO(S) DE ENFERMAGEM
• Fornecer fluidoterapia aos pacientes com desidratação ou azotemia. Administrar fluidos por via intravenosa em casos de desarranjos sistêmicos moderados ou graves. A solução de Ringer lactato corresponde ao fluido de escolha, exceto para pacientes com hipercalemia grave (i. e., >8 mEq/L e/ou alterações eletrocardiográficas); nesses animais, a solução salina a 0,45% e a solução de glicose a 2,5% com a adição de bicarbonato de sódio (1-2 mEq/kg, administrados sob a forma de bólus lentos) constituem o fluido de escolha. A solução salina fisiológica com o acréscimo de glicose (a 2,5% por via IV) representa uma escolha alternativa de fluido para pacientes com desidratação e hipercalemia.
• É preciso combater os efeitos cardiotóxicos da hipercalemia que representarem risco imediato de vida, por meio da administração de gliconato de cálcio (2-10 mL de solução a 10% por via IV, administrado lentamente até se obter o efeito). Assim que a hipercalemia e seus efeitos forem reduzidos, deve-se empregar a solução de Ringer lactato.

MEDICAÇÕES

MEDICAMENTO(S)
Os procedimentos para o alívio da obstrução frequentemente exigem o fornecimento de sedativos ou anestésicos ou são facilitados por tal administração. Quando houver desarranjos sistêmicos substanciais, deve-se a princípio instituir a administração de fluidos e de outras medidas de suporte. Antes da anestesia e da cateterização, pode-se efetuar descompressão vesical cuidadosa por meio da cistocentese. Calcular a dosagem do sedativo ou do anestésico, utilizando o extremo inferior da faixa recomendada ou fornecer somente até a obtenção do efeito. O isoflurano é o anestésico de escolha; certamente, no entanto, outros anestésicos ou sedativos podem gerar resultados satisfatórios.

CONTRAINDICAÇÕES
Em virtude de sua excreção renal, deve-se evitar a aplicação intramuscular de cetamina em pacientes com obstrução completa. Caso não se consiga eliminar a obstrução, poderá ocorrer uma sedação prolongada.

PRECAUÇÕES
Evitar os medicamentos redutores da pressão sanguínea ou indutores de arritmias cardíacas até a resolução da desidratação e da hipercalemia.

ACOMPANHAMENTO

MONITORIZAÇÃO DO PACIENTE
• Avaliar o animal com frequência quanto à produção de urina e ao estado de hidratação, bem como ajustar a velocidade de administração dos fluidos de acordo com essa avaliação.
• Verificar a capacidade miccional adequada ou utilizar periodicamente a cateterização transuretral para combater a retenção de urina.
• A aplicação do cateter de demora com drenagem em sistema fechado será apropriada se a inserção desse dispositivo exigir a contenção química do animal ou for indevidamente traumática. Entretanto, a cateterização uretral breve e frequente representará a melhor escolha caso se consiga inserir o cateter com facilidade e repetidas vezes (i. e., em alguns cães).
• Quando o ECG indicar alterações com risco de vida, deve-se utilizar inicialmente a monitorização contínua para orientar o tratamento e avaliar a resposta terapêutica.

COMPLICAÇÕES POSSÍVEIS
• Óbito.
• Lesão das vias excretoras, enquanto se tenta aliviar a obstrução.
• Hipocalemia durante a diurese pós-obstrutiva.
• Recidiva da obstrução.

DIVERSOS

DISTÚRBIOS ASSOCIADOS
• Bradicardia secundária à hipercalemia.
• Azotemia, hiperfosfatemia e acidose metabólica.

FATORES RELACIONADOS COM A IDADE
Muitas vezes, o tratamento eficaz da causa subjacente de obstrução (p. ex., tumor e prostatopatia) não é uma tarefa fácil em cães idosos.

GESTAÇÃO/FERTILIDADE/REPRODUÇÃO
N/D.

SINÔNIMO(S)
Obstrução uretral.

VER TAMBÉM
• Azotemia e Uremia.
• Doença Idiopática do Trato Urinário Inferior dos Felinos.
• Hidronefrose.
• Hipercalemia.
• Retenção Urinária Funcional.

ABREVIATURA(S)
• ECG = eletrocardiograma.

Sugestões de Leitura
Adams LG, Syme HM. Canine ureteral and lower urinary tract diseases. In: Ettinger SJ, Feldman EC, eds., Textbook of Veterinary Internal Medicine, 7th ed. Philadelphia: Saunders, 2010, pp. 2086-2115.
Bowles MH. Unblocking the urethra of the male cat. In: Ettinger SJ, Feldman EC, eds., Textbook of Veterinary Internal Medicine, 7th ed. Philadelphia: Saunders, 2010, pp. 434-436.
Drobatz KJ. Urethral obstruction in cats. In: Bonagura JD, Twedt DC, eds., Kirk's Current Veterinary Therapy XIV, 14th ed. Philadelphia: Saunders, 2009, pp. 951-954.
Labato MA, Acierno MJ. Micturition disorders and urinary incontinence. In: Ettinger SJ, Feldman EC, eds., Textbook of Veterinary Internal Medicine, 7th ed. Philadelphia: Saunders, 2010, pp. 160-164.
Westropp JL, Buffington CAT. Lower urinary tract disorders in cats. In: Ettinger SJ, Feldman EC, eds., Textbook of Veterinary Internal Medicine, 7th ed. Philadelphia: Saunders, 2010, pp. 2069-2086.

Autor George E. Lees
Consultor Editorial Carl A. Osborne

Obstrução Gastrintestinal

CONSIDERAÇÕES GERAIS

DEFINIÇÃO
Impedância física parcial ou completa ao fluxo da ingesta e/ou secreções em direção aboral (oposta à boca) através do piloro para o duodeno (obstrução da saída gástrica) ou através do intestino delgado. As obstruções na faringe, no esôfago, no intestino grosso e no reto, bem como os distúrbios da motilidade, são abordadas em outros capítulos (consultar a seção "Ver Também").

FISIOPATOLOGIA
Obstrução ao Fluxo de Saída Gástrico
- Ocorre o acúmulo de ingesta e líquidos no estômago.
- Os vômitos resultam em perda de líquido rico em ácido clorídrico (proveniente das secreções gástricas) com subsequente alcalose metabólica hipoclorêmica.
- Também ocorrem graus variados de desidratação, comprometimento tecidual, mal-estar e perda de peso, dependendo da etiologia subjacente, da gravidade e da cronicidade.

Obstrução do Intestino Delgado
- A ingesta e os líquidos acumulam-se na área proximal à obstrução.
- Os vômitos podem resultar em desidratação significativa e desequilíbrios eletrolíticos (em particular hipocalemia), dependendo da localização (proximal *versus* distal), do tipo de obstrução (parcial ou completa), e da cronicidade.
- Dano à mucosa e isquemia intestinal podem resultar em endotoxemia e sepse.

SISTEMA(S) ACOMETIDO(S)
- Comportamental — associada a desconforto ou dor abdominal (postura de oração, mudança no temperamento).
- Cardiovascular — choque hipovolêmico; taquicardia.
- Gastrintestinal — anorexia; vômitos; diarreia; e mal-estar.
- Respiratório — pneumonia por aspiração.

GENÉTICA
Desconhecida (ver a seção "Raças Predominantes").

INCIDÊNCIA/PREVALÊNCIA
Comum.

IDENTIFICAÇÃO
Espécies
- Cães e gatos.
- Os corpos estranhos são mais comuns em cães em virtude da ingestão indiscriminada.

Raça(s) Predominante(s)
- Estenose pilórica congênita — mais comum em raças braquicefálicas (p. ex., Boxer, Boston terrier) e no gato Siamês.
- Gastropatia hipertrófica crônica adquirida — mais comum em Lhasa apso, Shih tzu, Pequinês e Poodle.
- Dilatação e vólvulo gástricos — mais comum em raças de grande porte (p. ex., Pastor alemão e Dinamarquês).

Idade Média e Faixa Etária
- Corpos estranhos — mais comuns em animais jovens, embora possam ocorrer em qualquer idade.
- Estenose pilórica — ocorre com maior frequência em animais jovens.
- Gastropatia hipertrófica crônica — mais comum em animais de meia-idade a idosos.
- Intussuscepções — mais comuns em animais jovens.

SINAIS CLÍNICOS
Achados Anamnésicos
- Vômitos — sinal característico; é importante diferenciar vômito (contrações abdominais forçadas) de regurgitação (passiva); podem ocorrer logo após a ingestão de alimento, especialmente com obstrução da saída gástrica; o vômito de alimento ingerido há mais de 8 h depois da ingestão é compatível com retenção gástrica; os sinais clínicos costumam ser mais graves em obstruções do estômago e do intestino delgado proximal; podem ser caracterizados como vômitos em jato.
- Outros sinais clínicos variáveis — anorexia; letargia; mal-estar; ptialismo; diarreia; melena; e perda de peso.
- Os animais podem continuar exibindo movimentos do intestino mesmo em caso de obstrução intestinal.
- Os proprietários devem ser questionados sobre a possível ingestão de corpo estranho por parte do animal.

Achados do Exame Físico
- O exame físico frequentemente constitui o método diagnóstico mais útil para obstrução intestinal.
- Os achados podem variar desde um animal normal até uma crise potencialmente letal — incluem desidratação, choque, corpo estranho palpável, desconforto ou dor abdominal e massa abdominal (intussuscepção ou tumor).
- Corpos estranhos lineares — é indispensável um exame sublingual minucioso para detectá-los; embora sejam mais comuns em gatos, também ocorrem em cães; sedação ou anestesia para o exame bucal e a palpação abdominal costumam ser muito úteis para o diagnóstico.

CAUSAS
Obstrução da Saída Gástrica
- Corpos estranhos.
- Estenose pilórica.
- Gastropatia hipertrófica crônica.
- Neoplasia.
- Dilatação e vólvulo gástricos.
- Gastrite ou gastrenterite granulomatosa (p. ex., pitiose).

Obstrução do Intestino Delgado
- Corpos estranhos.
- Intussuscepção.
- Hérnias (encarceradas).
- Torção ou vólvulo mesentéricos.
- Neoplasia.
- Enterite granulomatosa.
- Estenose.

FATORES DE RISCO
- Exposição a corpos estranhos e tendência a ingeri-los.
- Intussuscepção — associada a parasitismo intestinal e enterite viral.

DIAGNÓSTICO

DIAGNÓSTICO DIFERENCIAL
- Doença metabólica (p. ex., insuficiência renal, hepatopatia, diabetes melito cetoacidótica e hipoadrenocorticismo).
- Gastrenterite infecciosa (p. ex., viral, bacteriana e parasitária).
- Pancreatite.
- Peritonite.
- Toxicidade.
- Úlcera gastroduodenal.
- Gastrenterite inespecífica.
- Doença do SNC.

HEMOGRAMA/BIOQUÍMICA/URINÁLISE
- Esses testes diagnósticos são úteis para excluir outras causas dos sinais clínicos (p. ex., insuficiência renal, pancreatite, hepatopatia, hipoadrenocorticismo e cetoacidose diabética) e para avaliar o estado geral do paciente.
- Hemograma — pode revelar anemia por perda sanguínea gastrintestinal, leucocitose de estresse ou leucocitose degenerativa com desvio à esquerda ou leucopenia em virtude de lesão grave da mucosa ou perfuração intestinal com subsequente peritonite séptica.
- Perfil bioquímico e gasometria arterial — frequentemente revelam alcalose metabólica hipoclorêmica com obstrução da saída gástrica; hipocalemia e azotemia pré-renal são achados variáveis.

DIAGNÓSTICO POR IMAGEM
Radiografia Abdominal Simples
- Pode revelar a presença de corpo estranho radiopaco no estômago ou no intestino, distensão gástrica grave ou alças intestinais obstruídas com dilatação em decorrência do acúmulo de líquido e/ou gás.
- É importante diferenciar íleo adinâmico (em geral, difuso) de obstrução (em geral, segmentar).
- A interpretação das radiografias tem de ser feita dentro do contexto da anamnese, do exame físico e de outros dados laboratoriais para evitar o diagnóstico errôneo e a cirurgia desnecessária.

Radiografia Contrastada
- Estudos contrastados positivos — podem revelar esvaziamento gástrico tardio (mais de 4 h com contraste líquido e mais de 8-10 h com contraste líquido misturado ao alimento), corpos estranhos, obstrução completa e massas.
- Pneumocólon — pode ser útil na suspeita de intussuscepção ileocólica.

Ultrassonografia Abdominal
Pode ser útil para detectar corpos estranhos, obstruções (especialmente intussuscepção intestinal) e distúrbios acentuados na motilidade GI.

MÉTODOS DIAGNÓSTICOS
- Endoscopia — pode ser proveitosa não só para confirmar obstrução gástrica e intestinal proximal, mas também para obter amostras de biopsia de massas; particularmente útil com alguns tipos de corpos estranhos que podem ser retirados com esse método.
- Paracentese abdominal e análise citológica — mais sensíveis que o exame físico e as radiografias (i. e., podem detectar pequenas quantidades de efusão abdominal); podem revelar inflamação asséptica associada a comprometimento intestinal vascular (antes da perfuração) ou peritonite séptica; podem indicar a necessidade de laparotomia exploratória.

ACHADOS PATOLÓGICOS
Exame histopatológico de massas gastrintestinais indutoras de obstrução — pode revelar inflamação granulomatosa, infecção fúngica (p. ex., pitiose) e neoplasia.

Obstrução Gastrintestinal

TRATAMENTO

CUIDADO(S) DE SAÚDE ADEQUADO(S)
• Internação — para diagnóstico, cuidados clínicos iniciais de suporte e alívio da obstrução (em geral, com cirurgia).
• Cirurgia — como as obstruções intestinais agudas são consideradas como um quadro emergencial, a intervenção cirúrgica deve ser realizada o mais rápido possível após o fornecimento dos cuidados clínicos de suporte imediatos; os intestinos não toleram bem o comprometimento vascular; em geral, há necessidade de ressecção e anastomose intestinais (com aumento da morbidade associada e complicações potenciais), mas a enterotomia poderá ser bem-sucedida em caso de diagnóstico precoce.
• O atraso no diagnóstico pode resultar em necrose intestinal, perfuração e peritonite séptica.

CUIDADO(S) DE ENFERMAGEM
• Fluidos cristaloides IV — necessários para reidratação e suporte circulatório, bem como para correção de anormalidades acidobásicas e eletrolíticas; para comprometimento circulatório grave (choque), administrar fluidos cristaloides isotônicos a 90 mL/kg (cães) ou 70 mL/kg (gatos) por 1-2 h.
• Coloides (dextrana ou hetamido) — também podem ser benéficos; é necessária a avaliação frequente da hidratação e dos eletrólitos (com ajustes terapêuticos apropriados); para a obstrução da saída gástrica indutora de alcalose metabólica hipoclorêmica, o fluido de escolha é a solução fisiológica a 0,9%; caso contrário, será adequada a solução de Ringer lactato ou outra solução eletrolítica balanceada.
• Suplementação apropriada de potássio — importante.

ATIVIDADE
Restrita.

DIETA
Nada por via oral até o alívio da obstrução e a resolução dos vômitos; em seguida, fornecer dieta branda por 1-2 dias, com retorno gradual à alimentação normal.

ORIENTAÇÃO AO PROPRIETÁRIO
Alertar o proprietário sobre o fato de que os animais com tendência a ingerir corpos estranhos costumam repetir o hábito; devem-se empreender todos os esforços razoáveis para evitar o acesso deles aos corpos estranhos.

CONSIDERAÇÕES CIRÚRGICAS
Obstrução da Saída Gástrica
• Piloroplastia ou piloromiotomia — para estenose pilórica ou gastropatia hipertrófica crônica.
• Gastrotomia — para corpos estranhos que não podem ser removidos à endoscopia.
• Ressecção (p. ex., gastroduodenostomia Billroth I e gastrojejunostomia Billroth II) — para massas granulomatosas ou neoplásicas.

• Gastropexia — para dilatação e vólvulo gástricos.
Obstrução Intestinal
• Enterotomia.
• Ressecção e anastomose — na presença de isquemia e necrose intestinais.
• Lavagem peritoneal aberta — quando há perfuração e peritonite séptica.
• Enteropexia profilática — em caso de intussuscepção.

MEDICAÇÕES

MEDICAMENTO(S)
• Antibióticos parenterais de amplo espectro — com lesão significativa da mucosa ou sepse; ampicilina (20 mg/kg IV a cada 8 h) ou ticarcilina/clavulanato (50 mg/kg IV a cada 8 h) e algum aminoglicosídeo (gentamicina, 6,6 mg/kg IV a cada 24 h) ou fluoroquinolona (enrofloxacino, 5 mg/kg IV ou IM a cada 24 h).
• Glicocorticoides solúveis de ação curta — para choque; fosfato sódico de dexametasona (0,5-1 mg/kg IV) ou succinato sódico de prednisolona (5 mg/kg IV).
• Antieméticos — metoclopramida (0,2-0,5 mg/kg SC ou IV a cada 6-8 h ou 1-2 mg/kg/24 h sob infusão em velocidade constante); podem ser administrados *após* o alívio da obstrução; o maropitant pode ser usado em cães na dose de 1 mg/kg SC a cada 24 h.
• Antagonistas dos receptores H_2 (p. ex., ranitidina, 1-2 mg/kg VO, SC, IV a cada 12 h) e/ou protetores da mucosa gástrica (p. ex., sucralfato, 250 mg/gato VO a cada 8-12 h ou 250-1.000 mg/cão VO a cada 8-12 h) — podem ser utilizados em pacientes com ulceração da mucosa.

CONTRAINDICAÇÕES
Agentes procinéticos (p. ex., metoclopramida e cisaprida).

PRECAUÇÕES
Não é recomendável o uso de antibióticos aminoglicosídeos na presença de choque, desidratação ou comprometimento renal, por causa da nefrotoxicidade desses agentes em potencial.

ACOMPANHAMENTO

MONITORIZAÇÃO DO PACIENTE
• Monitorizar rigorosamente a hidratação, o hematócrito/sólidos totais e o estado eletrolítico; ajustar a fluidoterapia de acordo.
• Monitorizar o paciente em busca de sinais de peritonite no pós-operatório.

PREVENÇÃO
• Os proprietários devem ser advertidos sobre o fato de que alguns animais de estimação com tendência a ingerir corpos estranhos podem repetir o ato.

• São importantes os esforços para evitar que isso ocorra.

COMPLICAÇÕES POSSÍVEIS
• Pneumonia por aspiração.
• Peritonite séptica (necrose e perfuração intestinais, além de deiscência).
• Íleo adinâmico e/ou gastroparesia.

EVOLUÇÃO ESPERADA E PROGNÓSTICO
• Casos sem complicações — o prognóstico é bom a excelente.
• Perfuração intestinal e peritonite séptica — prognóstico inicialmente reservado.
• Gastrenterite granulomatosa obstrutiva — prognóstico reservado a mau, especialmente com pitiose.
• Torção ou vólvulo mesentéricos — prognóstico mau a grave (a maioria dos pacientes vem a óbito apesar da cirurgia).

DIVERSOS

FATORES RELACIONADOS COM A IDADE
Ver a seção "Identificação".

VER TAMBÉM
• Abdome Agudo.
• Constipação e Obstipação.
• Corpos Estranhos Esofágicos.
• Disfagia.
• Distúrbios da Motilidade Gástrica.
• Estenose Esofágica.
• Estenose Retal.
• Gastropatia Pilórica Hipertrófica Crônica.
• Hérnia de Hiato.
• Intussuscepção.
• Megacólon.
• Megaesôfago.
• Pitiose.
• Regurgitação.
• Síndrome da Dilatação e Vólvulo Gástricos.
• Vômito Agudo.
• Vômito Crônico.

ABREVIATURA(S)
• GI = gastrintestinal.
• SNC = sistema nervoso central

Sugestões de Leitura
Bjorling DE. Acute abdomen syndrome In: Morgan RV, ed., Handbook of Small Animal Practice. New York: Churchill Livingstone, 1992, pp. 483-487.
Slatter D. Textbook of Small Animal Surgery, 2nd ed. Philadelphia: Saunders, 1993.
Strombeck DR, Guilford WG. Small Animal Gastroenterology, 2nd ed. Davis, CA: Stonegate, 1990, pp. 219-223, 391-401.

Autores Steve L. Marks e Albert E. Jergens
Consultor Editorial Albert E. Jergens

Oftalmia Neonatal

CONSIDERAÇÕES GERAIS

REVISÃO
- Infecção da conjuntiva e/ou da córnea antes ou logo depois da separação das pálpebras no neonato.
- Ocorre em filhotes de cão e de gato.
- Associada a *Staphylococcus* spp. ou *Streptococcus* spp. em cães e gatos, bem como ao herpes-vírus nos gatos.
- Risco potencial à visão.
- Fonte de infecção — acredita-se que seja proveniente de uma infecção intrauterina, uma infecção vaginal da mãe por ocasião do nascimento, ou da falta de higiene no ambiente.

IDENTIFICAÇÃO
- Acomete todas as raças de cães e de gatos.
- Neonatos, antes do momento em que eles abrem as pálpebras (10-14 dias após o parto).

SINAIS CLÍNICOS
- As margens palpebrais superiores e inferiores ainda estão aderidas (ancilobléfaro fisiológico) e fazem uma saliência em virtude do acúmulo de *debris* e de secreção dentro dos fórnices conjuntivais e entre a córnea e as pálpebras.
- Pode-se notar uma secreção mucoide a mucopurulenta que sai pelo canto medial do olho.
- Estruturas como a córnea e a conjuntiva podem estar ulceradas.
- Podem-se observar aderências (simbléfaro) da conjuntiva à córnea ou a outras áreas da conjuntiva (incluindo a da membrana nictitante).
- Ocasionalmente, observa-se perfuração da córnea com prolapso da íris e colapso do globo.

CAUSAS E FATORES DE RISCO
- Infecções intrauterinas ou vaginais da mãe no momento do parto.
- Ambiente sujo para os neonatos.

DIAGNÓSTICO

DIAGNÓSTICO DIFERENCIAL
Neonatos com entrópio em que as pálpebras já se encontram separadas — pode haver secreção mucoide a purulenta; a visão da córnea pode estar embaçada; pode ter o aspecto de ancilobléfaro; diferenciado pela idade (pacientes com mais de 10-14 dias de vida) e pela possibilidade de separar as pálpebras.

HEMOGRAMA/BIOQUÍMICA/URINÁLISE
Normais a menos que haja infecção sistêmica concomitante.

OUTROS TESTES LABORATORIAIS
- Culturas da secreção ocular do neonato e/ou do corrimento vaginal da mãe — pode ajudar a diagnosticar infecção bacteriana.
- Citologia dos tecidos acometidos — pode ajudar a determinar a presença de bactérias.
- Testes do anticorpo imunofluorescente ou reação em cadeia da polimerase (gatos) — para detecção de herpes-vírus felino.

DIAGNÓSTICO POR IMAGEM
N/D.

MÉTODOS DIAGNÓSTICOS
- Exame físico completo da mãe e do neonato.
- Coloração com fluoresceína — para pesquisa de ulceração na córnea ou conjuntiva.

TRATAMENTO

- Separação das pálpebras — base do tratamento; pode ser conseguida pela tração manual, começando no canto medial, ou pela introdução no canto medial de pequena lâmina de tesoura de dissecção romba ou da extremidade romba de uma lâmina de bisturi, separando (não cortando) as pálpebras delicadamente.
- Sacos conjuntivais e córnea — lavados com solução salina tépida (morna) ou solução aquosa de iodopovidona na diluição de 1:50 para remover a secreção.
- Compressas mornas — podem ajudar na separação das pálpebras e na prevenção de nova aderência.
- Suporte sistêmico — conforme a necessidade.

MEDICAÇÕES

MEDICAMENTO(S)
- Antibióticos tópicos de amplo espectro — p. ex., neomicina, bacitracina ou polimixina B; aplicados 4 vezes ao dia por, no mínimo, 1 semana; o antibiótico deve ser escolhido com base na cultura bacteriana e no antibiograma, se disponível.
- Terapia antiviral no caso de infecção por herpes-vírus em gatos.

CONTRAINDICAÇÕES/INTERAÇÕES POSSÍVEIS
- Tetraciclina — não utilizar no neonato por causa do risco de acometimento dos ossos ou dos dentes; cloranfenicol ou ciprofloxacino tópicos são os medicamentos de escolha para *Chlamydophila*.
- Corticosteroides tópicos — contraindicados.

ACOMPANHAMENTO

MONITORIZAÇÃO DO PACIENTE
- Compressas mornas — podem ser necessárias por alguns dias para impedir novas readerências das pálpebras.
- Antibióticos tópicos — mantidos por, no mínimo, 7 dias.
- Observar as ninhadas que não foram inicialmente acometidas.
- Tratar as infecções vaginais da mãe com medicações apropriadas.

PREVENÇÃO
- Manter limpos o ambiente externo e os mamilos da mãe.
- Tratar a infecção vaginal na mãe antes do parto, se possível.

COMPLICAÇÕES POSSÍVEIS
- Ceratite grave com formação cicatricial e simbléfaro.
- Ruptura da córnea com ftise* secundária; a cegueira pode ser irreversível.

DIVERSOS

Sugestões de Leitura
Stades FC, Gelatt KN. Diseases and surgery of the canine eyelid. In: Gelatt KN, ed., Veterinary Ophthalmology, 4th ed. Ames, IA: Blackwell, 2007, pp. 563-617.
Williams MM. Neonatal ophthalmic disorders. In: Kirk RW, ed. Current Veterinary Therapy X. Philadelphia: Saunders, 1989, pp. 658-673.

Autor Simon A. Pot
Consultor Editorial Paul E. Miller
Agradecimento Stephanie L. Smedes

---

* N. T.: Diminuição; extinção; destruição.

Olho Cego "Silencioso"

CONSIDERAÇÕES GERAIS

DEFINIÇÃO
Perda da visão em um ou ambos os olhos, sem congestão vascular ocular ou outros sinais externamente aparentes de inflamação ocular.

FISIOPATOLOGIA
Resulta de anormalidades na focalização de imagens na retina, na detecção de imagens pela retina, na transmissão através do nervo óptico ou na interpretação pelo SNC.

SISTEMA(S) ACOMETIDO(S)
• Oftálmico. • Nervoso.

IDENTIFICAÇÃO
• Cães e gatos. • Qualquer idade, raça ou sexo.
• Diversas causas (p. ex., cataratas e atrofia retiniana progressiva) têm uma base genética e com frequência são altamente específicas à raça e à faixa etária. • SDSAR — tende a ocorrer em cães idosos. • Hipoplasia do nervo óptico — congênita.

SINAIS CLÍNICOS

Achados Anamnésicos
• Variam com a causa subjacente. • Colisão com objetos. • Comportamento desajeitado.
• Relutância ao movimento. • Diminuição na acuidade visual em iluminação fraca.

Achados do Exame Físico
• Variam com a causa subjacente. • Redução ou ausência de resposta à ameaça. • Diminuição nas respostas de acomodação visual.

CAUSAS
• Cataratas — em geral, todo o cristalino deve ficar opaco para produzir a cegueira completa; a opacificação incompleta pode diminuir o desempenho visual de tarefas que exigem a visão.
• Perda da capacidade de focalização do cristalino — raramente leva à cegueira completa; ocorre uma hiperopia substancial (hipermetropia) quando não se repõe a capacidade óptica da lente após a extração do cristalino ou quando o cristalino sofre luxação posterior para fora do plano pupilar e em direção ao humor vítreo. • Retina— SDSAR; APR; descolamento da retina; deficiência de taurina (gatos), toxicidade do enrofloxacino (gatos); toxicidade da ivermectina (cães, gatos).
• Nervo óptico — neurite óptica; neoplasia do nervo óptico ou dos tecidos adjacentes; traumatismo; hipoplasia do nervo óptico; toxicidade do chumbo; tração excessiva sobre o nervo óptico durante o procedimento de enucleação, resultando em traumatismo ao nervo óptico contralateral ou ao quiasma óptico (especialmente cães braquicefálicos e gatos).
• SNC (amaurose) — lesões do quiasma ou do trato óptico; radiação óptica; córtex visual. A perda da visão associada ao SNC que ocorre em um nível superior ao quiasma óptico frequentemente exibe distúrbios visuais vagos em que o paciente ainda permanece com alguma visão, mas claramente não tem uma visão normal.

FATORES DE RISCO
• Diabetes melito mal controlado — cataratas.
• Animais aparentados com cataratas ou APR de base genética. • Hipertensão sistêmica — descolamento da retina. • Hipoxia do SNC — a cegueira pode se tornar aparente após anestesia excessivamente profunda ou reanimação de uma parada cardíaca.

DIAGNÓSTICO

DIAGNÓSTICO DIFERENCIAL

Sinais
• Inflamação no segmento anterior e glaucoma — conjuntiva tipicamente congesta. • Pacientes jovens — podem não apresentar respostas à ameaça; percorrem labirintos com êxito ou acompanham visualmente movimentos com as mãos ou bolas de algodão. • Período pós-ictal — perda transitória da visão. • Atividade mental anormal — pode ser difícil determinar se um animal tem ou não acuidade visual; outras anormalidades neurológicas ajudam a situar a lesão.

Causas
• Neurite óptica, descolamento da retina, SDSAR ou hipoxia do córtex visual — perda súbita da visão (por horas a semanas). • SDSAR — muitas vezes precedida por poliúria, polidipsia, polifagia e ganho de peso. • APR — perda visual gradativa, especialmente em iluminação fraca; perda visual aparentemente aguda em mudanças repentinas no ambiente. • Catarata — histórico de opacificação e perda visuais gradativas e rapidamente progressivas em um olho "silencioso". • Hipoplasia do nervo óptico — congênita; pode ser uni ou bilateral.
• Neuropatia óptica ou doença do SNC — sinais de outras anormalidades neurológicas. • Respostas pupilares à luz — em geral, permanecem normais em casos de cataratas ou lesões do córtex visual; respostas vagarosas a ausentes em casos de doenças da retina ou do nervo óptico. • Oftalmoscopia — normal em casos de SDSAR, neurite óptica retrobulbar e lesões dos trajetos visuais superiores; anormal em casos de descolamento da retina e neuropatias da cabeça do nervo óptico.

HEMOGRAMA/BIOQUÍMICA/URINÁLISE
• Costumam permanecer normais a menos que haja uma doença sistêmica subjacente.
• Hiperglicemia ou glicosúria — possível constatação em casos de cataratas diabéticas.
• Atividade sérica elevada da fosfatase alcalina e alterações compatíveis com hiperadrenocorticismo (síndrome de Cushing) — sugerem SDSAR.
• Descolamento da retina secundário à hipertensão sistêmica (gatos) — concentrações séricas levemente altas da ureia ou da creatinina; alterações compatíveis com hipertireoidismo.

OUTROS TESTES LABORATORIAIS
• Nível sanguíneo do chumbo e sorologia para pesquisa de micoses profundas ou infecções virais — considerar na suspeita de neurite óptica (ver "Neurite Óptica"). • TSDBD — pode ajudar a descartar a síndrome de Cushing associada à SDSAR. • Anormalidades nos hormônios sexuais são comuns em pacientes com SDSAR.

DIAGNÓSTICO POR IMAGEM
• Ultrassonografia ocular — pode demonstrar o descolamento da retina (especialmente se os meios oculares estiverem opacos) ou lesão expansiva do nervo óptico.
• Radiografias cranianas simples — raras vezes informativas.
• TC ou RM — frequentemente úteis em casos de lesões da órbita ou do SNC.

MÉTODOS DIAGNÓSTICOS
• Exame oftálmico com foco de luz — em geral, permite o diagnóstico de cataratas ou de descolamentos da retina, graves o suficiente a ponto de causarem cegueira.
• Oftalmoscopia — pode revelar APR ou doença do nervo óptico; o exame normal sugere a presença de SDSAR, neurite óptica retrobulbar ou de lesão do SNC.
• Pressão sanguínea sistêmica — determinar em casos de descolamentos da retina.
• Eletrorretinografia — na dúvida quanto ao diagnóstico, esse exame diferencia as retinopatias das doenças do nervo óptico ou do SNC.
• Punção do LCS — pode ser valiosa em causas neurogênicas de perda da visão.

TRATAMENTO

• Antes de instituir o tratamento, deve-se tentar obter o diagnóstico definitivo em um esquema ambulatorial.
• Considerar o encaminhamento do animal a especialistas antes de se tentar uma terapia empírica.
• A maioria das causas não é fatal, embora seja imprescindível efetuar uma avaliação minuciosa para descartar as doenças potencialmente fatais.
• Tranquilizar o proprietário de que grande parte das causas de um olho cego "silencioso" é indolor e que os animais cegos podem levar uma vida relativamente normal e funcional.
• Alertar o proprietário sobre a necessidade de se avaliar o ambiente quanto aos possíveis riscos para um animal cego.
• Aconselhar o proprietário a não acasalar os pacientes com atrofia retiniana progressiva ou cataratas genéticas e a submeter os animais aparentados a exames.
• Descolamento da retina — recomendar restrição intensa da atividade física até que a retina esteja firmemente aderida.
• Dieta com restrição calórica — para evitar a obesidade; em virtude da redução do nível de atividade.
• Gatos com retinopatia induzida por fatores nutricionais — garantir uma dieta com níveis adequados de taurina.
• SDSAR, APR, atrofia e hipoplasia do nervo óptico — não existe nenhum tratamento eficaz.
• Cataratas, luxação do cristalino e algumas formas de descolamento da retina — o tratamento cirúrgico é o mais eficaz.

MEDICAÇÕES

MEDICAMENTO(S) DE ESCOLHA
• Dependem da causa.
• Caso o animal se recuse a uma avaliação minuciosa, se for improvável uma doença infecciosa e ainda se houver o diagnóstico provável de SDSAR ou de neurite óptica retrobulbar — considerar a prednisolona sistêmica (1-2 mg/kg/dia durante 7-14 dias, com subsequente redução gradativa da dose); pode-se efetuar a administração concomitante de cloranfenicol oral ou de outro antibiótico sistêmico de amplo espectro.

CONTRAINDICAÇÕES
Não utilizar corticosteroides sistêmicos e outros medicamentos imunossupressores em casos de

Olho Cego "Silencioso"

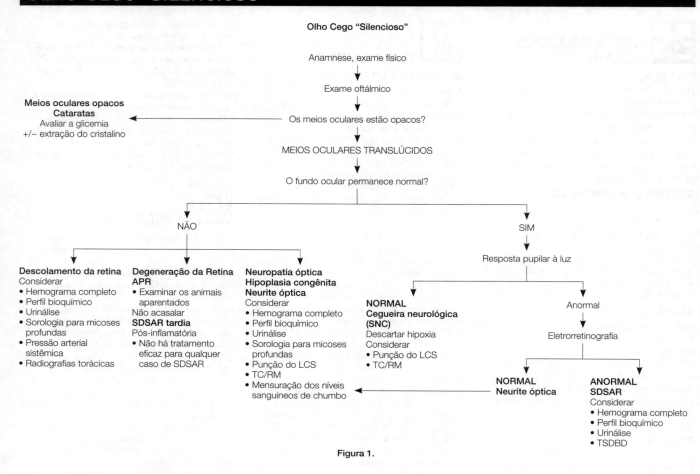

Figura 1.

neurite óptica e descolamento da retina de origem infecciosa.
PRECAUÇÕES
O pré-tratamento com corticosteroides pode mimetizar ou mascarar as alterações das enzimas hepáticas na SDSAR.
INTERAÇÕES POSSÍVEIS
N/D.
MEDICAMENTO(S) ALTERNATIVO(S)
• Flunixino meglumina (cães) — pode-se tentar uma única dose (0,5 mg/kg IV) no lugar dos corticosteroides se não forem descartadas as causas infecciosas.
• Azatioprina oral — 1-2 mg/kg/dia por 3-7 dias, com redução gradativa e subsequente da dose; pode ser utilizada para tratar os descolamentos imunomediados da retina se os corticosteroides sistêmicos não forem eficazes; realizar o hemograma completo, a contagem plaquetária e mensuração das enzimas hepáticas a cada 1-2 semanas durante as 8 primeiras semanas e depois em intervalos regulares.

 ACOMPANHAMENTO

MONITORIZAÇÃO DO PACIENTE
• Repetir os exames oftálmicos — conforme a necessidade, para garantir o controle da inflamação ocular e, se possível, a manutenção da visão.

• Recidiva da perda visual — comum em casos de neurite óptica; pode ocorrer semanas, meses ou anos após a manifestação inicial.
COMPLICAÇÕES POSSÍVEIS
• Óbito.
• Perda permanente da visão.
• Perda do olho.
• Inflamação e dor oculares crônicas.
• Obesidade decorrente da inatividade ou como sequela da SDSAR.

 DIVERSOS

DISTÚRBIOS ASSOCIADOS
• SDSAR (cães) — sinais similares aos do hiperadrenocorticismo.
• Doença neurológica — podem-se notar crises convulsivas, mudanças de comportamento ou de personalidade, andar em círculo ou outros sinais atribuídos ao SNC.
• Miocardiopatia (gatos) — deficiência de taurina.
FATORES RELACIONADOS COM A IDADE
• APR e muitas cataratas — idades de início específicas às raças.
• SDSAR — tende a ocorrer em cães mais idosos.
• Hipoplasia do nervo óptico — congênita.
POTENCIAL ZOONÓTICO
N/D.

GESTAÇÃO/FERTILIDADE/REPRODUÇÃO
Os corticosteroides e os medicamentos imunossupressores podem complicar a gestação.
ABREVIATURA(S)
• APR = atrofia progressiva da retina.
• LCS = líquido cerebrospinal.
• SDSAR = síndrome de degeneração súbita e adquirida da retina.
• TSDBD = teste de supressão com dose baixa de dexametasona.
• SNC = sistema nervoso central.
• TC = tomografia computadorizada.
• RM = ressonância magnética.
RECURSOS DA INTERNET
• Livros: http://www.petcarebooks.com/.
• Pepe the Blind Dog: http://www.pepedog.com/.
• Uma ideia original para cães cegos, mas ativos: o colete de anjo: http://angelvest.homestead.com/

Sugestões de Leitura
Maggs DJ, Miller PE, Ofri R. Fundamentals of Veterinary Ophthalmology, 4th ed. St Louis: Saunders Elsevier, 2008.
Rubin LF. Inherited Eye Disease in Purebred Dogs. Baltimore: Williams & Wilkins, 1989.

Autor Paul E. Miller
Consultor Editorial Paul E. Miller

OLHO VERMELHO

CONSIDERAÇÕES GERAIS

DEFINIÇÃO
Hiperemia das pálpebras ou da vasculatura ocular, ou hemorragia dentro do olho.

FISIOPATOLOGIA
• Dilatação ativa dos vasos oculares — em resposta à inflamação intraocular ou extraocular ou à congestão passiva.
• Hemorragia oriunda de vasos sanguíneos existentes ou recém-formados.

SISTEMA(S) ACOMETIDO(S)
Oftálmico — olho e/ou anexos oculares.

IDENTIFICAÇÃO
Cães e gatos.

SINAIS CLÍNICOS
Achados Anamnésicos
Dependem da causa.
Achados do Exame Físico
• Dependem da causa.
• Pode acometer um ou ambos os olhos.
• Resultado de doença sistêmica — são comuns anormalidades em outros sistemas orgânicos.

CAUSAS
• Praticamente todo caso se enquadra em uma ou mais das categorias a seguir:
• Blefarite.
• Conjuntivite.
• Ceratite.
• Episclerite ou esclerite.
• Uveíte anterior.
• Glaucoma.
• Hifema.
• Doença orbital — em geral, a anormalidade da órbita ocular é mais proeminente.

FATORES DE RISCO
• Doenças sistêmicas infecciosas ou inflamatórias.
• Imunocomprometimento.
• Coagulopatias.
• Hipertensão sistêmica.
• Irritação por medicamentos oftálmicos tópicos — aminoglicosídeos; pilocarpina; adrenalina.
• Neoplasia.
• Traumatismo.

DIAGNÓSTICO

DIAGNÓSTICO DIFERENCIAL
Pode ocorrer mais de uma causa simultaneamente.
Sinais Semelhantes
• Descartar as variações normais.
• Conjuntiva palpebral — normalmente mais avermelhada do que a conjuntiva bulbar.
• Um ou dois grandes vasos episclerais — podem permanecer normais se o olho estiver "silencioso" sob outros aspectos.
• Hiperemia leve transitória — com excitação (agitação), exercício e esforço.
• Síndrome de Horner — pode provocar dilatação vascular conjuntival leve; diferenciada por outros sinais e testes farmacológicos.

CAUSAS
• Vasos (conjuntivais) superficiais — originam-se próximos ao fórnix; movimentam-se juntamente com a conjuntiva; ramificam-se repetidas vezes; branqueiam com rapidez com fenilefrina tópica a 2,5% ou adrenalina a 1:100.000; sugerem distúrbios superficiais oculares (p. ex., conjuntivite, ceratite superficial e blefarite).
• Vasos (episclerais) profundos — originam-se próximos ao limbo; ramificam-se com pouca frequência; não se movimentam com a conjuntiva; branqueiam de modo lento ou incompleto com simpaticomiméticos tópicos; sugerem episclerite ou doença intraocular (p. ex., uveíte anterior ou glaucoma).
• Secreção — mucopurulenta a purulenta: típica de distúrbios da superfície ocular e blefarite; serosa ou ausente: típica de distúrbios intraoculares.
• Pálpebras tumefatas ou inflamadas — indicam blefarite.
• Opacificação da córnea, neovascularização ou retenção do corante fluoresceína — sugerem ceratite.
• Rubor aquoso ou infiltrado celular (aumento do conteúdo de proteínas ou células na câmara anterior) — confirma o diagnóstico de uveíte anterior.
• Pupila — miótica: comum em casos de uveíte anterior; dilatada: comum em casos de glaucoma; normal: em casos de blefarite e conjuntivite.
• Íris de formato ou cor anormais — sugerem uveíte anterior.
• Cristalinos com catarata ou luxação — sugerem glaucoma ou uveíte anterior.
• Pressão intraocular — elevada: diagnóstico de glaucoma; baixa: sugestiva de uveíte anterior.
• Perda de visão — sugere glaucoma, uveíte anterior ou ceratite grave.
• Glaucoma e uveíte anterior — podem complicar o quadro de hifema.

HEMOGRAMA/BIOQUÍMICA/URINÁLISE
• Tipicamente normais, exceto na uveíte anterior, no glaucoma ou no hifema secundários a doença sistêmica.
• Ver "Uveíte Anterior — Cães"; "Uveíte Anterior — Gatos"; "Hifema".

OUTROS TESTES LABORATORIAIS
Dependem da causa.

DIAGNÓSTICO POR IMAGEM
• Radiografias torácicas — considerar na uveíte anterior ou se a neoplasia intraocular for uma possibilidade.
• Radiografia ou ultrassonografia abdominais — podem ajudar a descartar causas infecciosas ou neoplásicas.
• Ultrassonografia ocular — se os meios oculares estiverem opacos; pode definir a extensão e a natureza da doença intraocular ou identificar a presença de tumor intraocular.

MÉTODOS DIAGNÓSTICOS
Tonometria — exame obrigatório em todo o paciente com olho vermelho inexplicado.
Distúrbios da Superfície Ocular
• Cultura bacteriana aeróbica e perfil de sensibilidade (antibiograma) — em casos de secreção purulenta, doença crônica ou resposta insatisfatória ao tratamento.
• Teste lacrimal de Schirmer.
• Exame citológico do tecido acometido — pálpebra; conjuntiva; córnea.
• Gatos — considerar a realização dos testes de PCR ou anticorpo imunofluorescente nos raspados de conjuntiva ou da córnea para detecção de herpes-vírus felino e *Chlamydia*; coletar amostra antes da coloração com fluoresceína para evitar resultados falso-positivos ao teste de anticorpo imunofluorescente.
• Coloração com fluoresceína.
• Biopsias da conjuntiva — em casos de conjuntivite crônica ou lesão expansiva.
• Ver doença específica — "Conjuntivite — Gatos"; "Conjuntivite — Cães"; "Blefarite"; "Ceratite".
Distúrbios Intraoculares
• Coloração pela fluoresceína.
• Ver doença específica — "Uveíte Anterior — Gatos"; "Uveíte Anterior — Cães"; "Hifema"; "Glaucoma".

TRATAMENTO

• Geralmente como paciente de ambulatório.
• Colar elizabetano — considerado para evitar autotraumatismo.
• Evitar ambientes sujos ou aqueles que possam levar a traumatismo ocular, sobretudo quando se empregam corticosteroides tópicos.
• Como existe uma estreita margem de erro, considerar o encaminhamento caso não se consiga atribuir a condição a uma das causas relacionadas ou se o clínico não conseguir descartar o glaucoma na consulta inicial ou, ainda, se o diagnóstico for tão incerto a ponto de a administração isolada de antibiótico ou corticosteroide tópicos ser questionável.
• Poucas causas são fatais; entretanto, pode ficar indicada uma avaliação diagnóstica detalhada (sobretudo em casos de uveíte anterior e hifema) para descartar doenças sistêmicas potencialmente fatais.
• Úlceras de córnea profundas e glaucoma — podem ser mais bem tratados de forma cirúrgica.

MEDICAÇÕES

MEDICAMENTO(S)
• Dependem da causa específica.
• Em geral, controlam a dor ocular, a inflamação, a infecção e a pressão intraocular.
• Ácido acetilsalicílico — 10-15 mg/kg VO a cada 8-12 h (cães); pode controlar a inflamação e a dor oculares leves, na espera dos resultados dos testes.
• Carprofeno — 2,2 mg/kg a cada 12 h ou 4,4 mg/kg a cada 24 h.
• Flunixino meglumina — 0,5 mg/kg IV uma única vez; pode ser usada em cães com inflamação ocular grave, na espera dos resultados dos testes.

CONTRAINDICAÇÕES
• Corticosteroides tópicos — contraindicados se a córnea retiver o corante fluoresceína.
• Corticosteroides sistêmicos — evitar até que causas sistêmicas infecciosas tenham sido descartadas.

PRECAUÇÕES
• Aminoglicosídeos tópicos — podem ser irritantes; podem impedir a repitelização se utilizados com frequência ou em concentrações elevadas.
• Soluções tópicas — podem ser preferidas em lugar das pomadas se a perfuração da córnea for possível.
• Atropina — pode exacerbar ceratoconjuntivite seca e glaucoma.

Olho Vermelho

• AINE — utilizar com cuidado no hifema.
INTERAÇÕES POSSÍVEIS
N/D.
MEDICAMENTO(S) ALTERNATIVO(S)
N/D.

ACOMPANHAMENTO
MONITORIZAÇÃO DO PACIENTE
• Depende da causa.
• Exames oftalmológicos repetidos — conforme a necessidade para garantir que a pressão intraocular, a dor ocular e a inflamação estejam bem controladas.
• Quanto maior o risco de perda da visão, maior a necessidade de acompanhamento rigoroso do paciente; pode requerer exame diário ou com maior frequência.

COMPLICAÇÕES POSSÍVEIS
• Morte.
• Perda do olho ou perda permanente da visão.
• Inflamação e dor oculares crônicas.

DIVERSOS
DISTÚRBIOS ASSOCIADOS
Inúmeras doenças sistêmicas.
FATORES RELACIONADOS COM A IDADE
N/D.
POTENCIAL ZOONÓTICO
Ver "Uveíte Anterior — Cães"; "Uveíte Anterior — Gatos".

GESTAÇÃO/FERTILIDADE/REPRODUÇÃO
Corticosteroides sistêmicos podem complicar a prenhez.

ABREVIATURA(S)
• AINE = anti-inflamatórios não esteroides.
• PCR = reação em cadeia da polimerase.

Sugestões de Leitura
Gelatt KN, ed. Veterinary Ophthalmology, 4th ed. Ames, IA: Blackwell, 2007.
Maggs DJ, Miller PE, Ofri R. Slatter's Fundamentals of Veterinary Ophthalmology, 4th ed. St. Louis: Saunders, 2008.

Autor Paul E. Miller
Consultor Editorial Paul E. Miller

Oligúria e Anúria

CONSIDERAÇÕES GERAIS

DEFINIÇÃO
• Oligúria — produção de quantidade anormalmente pequena de urina (a oligúria é variavelmente descrita como uma taxa de produção de urina <0,27, <0,5 ou <1,0-2,0 mL/kg/h). Em pacientes normovolêmicos ou hipervolêmicos com boa perfusão, a produção de urina <1,0 mL/kg/h indica oligúria absoluta.
• Anúria — formação de essencialmente nenhuma urina (taxa de produção de urina <0,08 mL/kg/h).

FISIOPATOLOGIA
• Ocorre oligúria fisiológica (pré-renal) quando os rins limitam a perda de água durante episódios de baixa perfusão renal para manter o equilíbrio hidreletrolítico. A osmolalidade elevada do plasma ou o baixo volume de líquido circulante efetivo estimula a síntese e a liberação do ADH. Esse hormônio atua sobre os rins para induzir à formação de pequenas quantidades de urina concentrada (a característica da oligúria fisiológica).
• A oligúria patológica (renal) resulta de comprometimento grave do parênquima renal. Os fatores incluem (1) alta resistência nos vasos glomerulares aferentes, (2) baixa permeabilidade glomerular, (3) extravasamento retrógrado do filtrado dos túbulos renais lesados, (4) obstrução intratubular renal e (5) perda extensa de néfrons, resultando em redução acentuada na quantidade do filtrado glomerular produzido.
• A anúria pode ser de origem renal ou pós-renal. Nefropatia grave ocasionalmente provoca anúria, mas a anúria verdadeira é mais indicativa de obstrução urinária. Os mecanismos são os mesmos que os da anúria patológica (p. ex., obstrução do fluxo urinário ou ruptura da via excretora).

SISTEMA(S) ACOMETIDO(S)
• Renal — incapacidade de eliminar os resíduos e a água de forma adequada; hipercalemia.
• Urológico — distensão do sistema coletor — frequentemente acompanhada por dor e/ou urgência miccional. Risco elevado de infecção do trato urinário.

IDENTIFICAÇÃO
• Cães e gatos.
• Os gatos jovens adultos têm uma incidência mais alta de anúria associada à obstrução do trato urinário.
• O risco de lesão renal aguda aumenta com a idade.

SINAIS CLÍNICOS
• Redução na quantidade de urina eliminada.
• Bexiga urinária dilatada, esforço para urinar, e frequência elevada de micção com obstrução uretral.
• Sinais sistêmicos de uremia se os sinais de oligúria/anúria persistir.

CAUSAS
• Oligúria fisiológica — hipoperfusão renal (provocada por baixo volume sanguíneo ou hipotensão) ou hipertonicidade (causada, em geral, por hipernatremia).
• Oligúria patológica — lesão renal oligúrica aguda (insuficiência renal) ou nefropatia crônica avançada.
• Anúria — obstrução completa do trato urinário, ruptura da via excretora urinária ou nefropatia primária muito grave.

FATORES DE RISCO
• Oligúria fisiológica — causas de redução no volume efetivo de líquido circulante, incluindo desidratação, baixo débito cardíaco, hipotensão.
• Oligúria e anúria patológicas causadas por nefropatia primária (fatores de risco para lesão renal aguda) — nefropatia preexistente, exposição a nefrotoxinas, desidratação, baixo débito cardíaco, hipotensão, desequilíbrio eletrolítico, acidose, idade avançada, febre, sepse, hepatopatia, falência múltipla de órgãos, traumatismo, diabetes melito, hipoalbuminemia, síndrome de hiperviscosidade.
• Anúria — urolitíase, neoplasia do trato urinário, doença idiopática do trato urinário inferior felino, distúrbio da micção, traumatismo, hematúria macroscópica.

DIAGNÓSTICO

DIAGNÓSTICO DIFERENCIAL
• Oligúria fisiológica é sugerida pelos sinais de má perfusão tecidual (p. ex., desidratação; tempo de preenchimento capilar prolongado; mucosas pálidas; pulso fraco, rápido ou irregular; extremidades frias); possível histórico de perda recente de líquido (vômito, diarreia, poliúria, hemorragia); os sinais de uremia estão tipicamente ausentes. A oligúria termina rapidamente quando a hipoperfusão renal é corrigida.
• Suspeitar de oligúria patológica e de anúria renal com a detecção de qualquer um dos fatores de risco mencionados anteriormente; o maior número de fatores de risco está associado a um maior risco de desenvolvimento de lesão renal (os fatores de risco são cumulativos). Pacientes com oligúria patológica provocada por nefropatia crônica apresentam histórico de nefropatia progressiva (incluindo poliúria de longa duração, polidipsia, apetite deficiente e perda de peso). Pacientes com nefropatia crônica estão sob risco de desenvolver lesão renal aguda. Comumente se observam sinais de uremia; além disso, a fluidoterapia e outras medidas destinadas a restaurar a perfusão renal adequada quase sempre falham em aumentar o fluxo urinário.
• Suspeitar de anúria por obstrução do trato urinário ou ruptura da via excretora em pacientes que repetidamente fazem esforço para urinar, mas não conseguem produzir urina. Esses pacientes podem ter histórico de polaciúria, disúria, estrangúria, hematúria, urolitíase, traumatismo ou manipulação do trato urinário. Nos pacientes com obstrução do trato urinário, o exame físico pode revelar aumento de volume da bexiga urinária, dor na região abdominal posterior e massas ou urólitos na uretra ou no lúmen vesical. O exame físico dos pacientes com ruptura do trato urinário pode revelar ascite, infiltração de líquido nos tecidos ao redor do trato urinário, dor na região abdominal caudal, massas ou urólitos na bexiga urinária ou na uretra ou indícios de traumatismo (p. ex., fratura pélvica). A obstrução do trato urinário provocada por obstrução urinária funcional pode ficar sob suspeita nos pacientes com aumento de volume da bexiga urinária, resistência aumentada à compressão manual vesical e sinais neurológicos com envolvimento dos membros posteriores e/ou da cauda. Podem se desenvolver sinais de uremia. O restabelecimento do fluxo urinário ou a correção de rupturas das vias excretoras restabelece com rapidez o fluxo urinário adequado.

HEMOGRAMA/BIOQUÍMICA/URINÁLISE
• As concentrações séricas da ureia e creatinina encontram-se elevadas a menos que o início da oligúria e da anúria seja muito recente.
• A hipercalemia é comum em casos de oligúria e anúria patológicas, porém menos comum e menos grave em animais com oligúria fisiológica (exceto naqueles com hipoadrenocorticismo).
• A oligúria fisiológica caracteriza-se por densidade urinária elevada (valores acima de 1,030 em cães e 1,035 em gatos). A oligúria associada a valores mais baixos da densidade urinária sugere doença do parênquima renal ou obstrução do trato urinário. Pacientes com defeitos de concentração urinária causados por outras doenças ou medicamentos são a exceção a essa regra.
• Anúria por comprometimento do parênquima renal tipicamente se caracteriza por valores da densidade urinária abaixo de 1,030 (cães) ou 1,035 (gatos). A densidade urinária nos pacientes com anúria pós-renal varia. A capacidade adequada de concentrar a urina frequentemente se perde após a obstrução do trato urinário, porém pode persistir após a ruptura da via excretora.

OUTROS TESTES LABORATORIAIS
N/D.

DIAGNÓSTICO POR IMAGEM
• Radiografias e ultrassonografias abdominais são valiosas para descartar obstrução do trato urinário e ruptura da via excretora.
• Exames de urografia excretora, uretrocistografia retrógrada, pielografia ou vaginouretrocistografia podem fornecer uma prova definitiva de obstrução do trato urinário ou ruptura da via excretora.
• A distensão da via excretora ou a detecção de urólitos dentro dos ureteres, do colo vesical ou da uretra sugere obstrução do trato urinário.
• A detecção de líquido dentro da cavidade peritoneal ou adjacente ao trato urinário garante o diagnóstico de ruptura da via excretora. O extravasamento do meio de contraste a partir do sistema coletor confirma a ruptura.

MÉTODOS DIAGNÓSTICOS
• Eletrocardiografia para determinar se o paciente apresenta hipercalemia clinicamente relevante (ver Hipercalemia).
• Uretrocistoscopia pode fornecer indícios de obstrução ou de ruptura do trato urinário.
• A colocação de sonda urinária pode fornecer informações a respeito da integridade do trato urinário inferior. Essa abordagem, no entanto, não é recomendada como método diagnóstico, pois pode gerar engano e ainda provocar traumatismo adicional e infecção iatrogênica do trato urinário.

TRATAMENTO

• Oligúria e anúria são emergências clínicas; caso não sejam tratadas, podem levar ao óbito dentro de horas a dias. A morte tipicamente resulta de uremia, hipercalemia, acidose ou sepse.
• Hipovolemia persistente pode induzir à lesão renal isquêmica.

Oligúria e Anúria

- Corrigir a hipoperfusão renal rapidamente pela administração intravenosa de soro fisiológico ou solução de Ringer lactato.
- A terapia para oligúria e anúria renais primárias costuma ficar limitada ao cuidado dos sintomas e de suporte destinado a permitir a sobrevivência do paciente por tempo suficiente para que ocorra alguma recuperação espontânea da função renal. A eliminação do fator causal pode retardar ou interromper a lesão renal adicional (p. ex., suspensão da terapia com aminoglicosídeos, correção de hipercalcemia ou restabelecimento da perfusão renal adequada); entretanto, uma vez desenvolvidas a oligúria ou a anúria patológicas, poucas nefropatias serão passíveis de tratamento específico.
- Causas pós-renais de anúria podem ser corrigidas por métodos não cirúrgicos ou cirúrgicos. Os métodos não cirúrgicos incluem a uro-hidropropulsão retrógrada de urólitos ou de tampões uretrais ou a colocação de cateteres transuretrais para restaurar o fluxo urinário de baixa pressão. Os métodos cirúrgicos podem compreender a remoção de urólitos, pólipos ou tecidos neoplásicos ou a correção cirúrgica de lacerações, estenoses ou malposicionamento dos rins, ureteres, bexiga urinária e uretra.

MEDICAÇÕES

MEDICAMENTO(S)
- Em pacientes com oligúria renal, os diuréticos são indicados após o estabelecimento da normovolemia. A diurese induzida por diurético não indica necessariamente uma melhora da função renal, mas um aumento na produção de urina facilita a terapia hidreletrolítica.
- A administração de diuréticos antes de uma perfusão renal adequada é contraproducente e pode promover lesão renal.
- Evitar desidratação induzida por diurético.
- Furosemida (2-4 mg/kg IV) quase sempre é utilizada de início em pacientes com oligúria renal. O fluxo urinário deve aumentar dentro de 1 h. Se a diurese não ocorrer depois de uma hora, a furosemida poderá ser repetida na mesma dosagem ou com o dobro da dose. Caso ocorra a diurese, esse agente terapêutico poderá ser administrado sob taxa de infusão constante a 0,25-1 mg/kg/h ou a 2-4 mg/kg IV a cada 8 h para manter a diurese.
- O manitol (0,25-1 g/kg IV) pode ser administrado sob a forma de solução a 10% ou 20% por 15-20 min. O fluxo urinário deve aumentar dentro de 1 h. Não repetir a administração do manitol se não ocorrer a diurese; ele pode provocar expansão volêmica excessiva. Caso ocorra a diurese, o manitol poderá ser mantido sob taxa de infusão constante a 1-2 mg/kg/h ou doses IV intermitentes de 0,25-0,5 g/kg a cada 4-6 h para manter a diurese. Evitar o uso desse agente terapêutico na presença de super-hidratação, edema pulmonar ou insuficiência cardíaca congestiva.
- Em cães, a dopamina (0,5-3 μg/kg/min) pode ampliar o fluxo de urina, aumentando o fluxo sanguíneo renal, a filtração glomerular e a excreção renal de sódio. Doses mais elevadas podem provocar vasoconstrição renal, taquicardia e arritmias cardíacas, sendo contraindicadas em casos de lesão renal aguda. A dopamina, em geral, é administrada concomitantemente com a furosemida. A diurese deve ocorrer dentro de 1 a 2 h. Se isso não acontecer, a dopamina deverá ser mantida até que se consiga conservar o equilíbrio hidreletrolítico sem terapia medicamentosa adicional. Se o fluxo urinário não aumentar dentro de 2 h, interromper a dopamina. A dopamina não é o tratamento apropriado para a oligúria nos gatos.
- Fenoldopam (0,1-0,6 μg/kg/min), um antagonista seletivo do receptor dopaminérgico A1, promove uma diurese tardia (4 a 6 h) em gatos normais; no entanto, sua eficácia em gatos oligúricos não foi estabelecida.

CONTRAINDICAÇÕES
Medicamentos nefrotóxicos.

PRECAUÇÕES
- Administrar os fluidos de modo criterioso aos pacientes que estejam persistentemente em oligúria ou anúria, para evitar a super-hidratação. Em pacientes com oligúria renal irresponsiva, a diálise peritoneal ou a hemodiálise podem ser necessárias para corrigir a expansão volêmica excessiva iatrogênica induzida pela fluidoterapia.
- A falha em corrigir os déficits hídricos antes de iniciar a administração de diurético pode causar hipoperfusão renal e lesão renal isquêmica adicionais.
- Usar medicamentos que necessitam de excreção renal com cuidado. Caso seja razoável esperar a resolução da oligúria ou da anúria dentro de minutos a algumas horas (p. ex., oligúria e anúria fisiológicas atribuídas à obstrução do trato urinário), podem-se utilizar as dosagens normais de medicamentos que exigem a excreção renal.
- Evitar soluções eletrolíticas que contenham mais de 4 mEq de potássio por litro em grande parte dos animais. Contudo, alguns pacientes hipocalêmicos podem necessitar da administração rigorosa de doses mais altas de potássio.
- A dopamina pode provocar arritmias cardíacas, particularmente em animais com hipercalemia. A monitorização com ECG é recomendada ao se utilizar dosagens elevadas em animais com hipercalemia.

INTERAÇÕES POSSÍVEIS
A furosemida pode promover a nefrotoxicidade associada a antibióticos aminoglicosídeos.

ACOMPANHAMENTO

MONITORIZAÇÃO DO PACIENTE
- Taxa de fluxo urinário — determinar precocemente durante o curso terapêutico do caso. Quando incerta, a cateterização transuretral intermitente deve ser considerada para determinar a produção de urina com precisão. Os cateteres devem ser colocados, utilizando-se técnica asséptica. É menos provável que a cateterização intermitente cause infecção do trato urinário do que um cateter de demora. Quanto menor o tempo de permanência do cateter, menor será o risco de infecção urinária. Utilizar um sistema de drenagem urinária fechado e estéril.
- As concentrações de creatinina, ureia e potássio devem ser reavaliadas depois de 12-24 h; os pacientes com hipercalemia grave podem necessitar de monitorização mais frequente das concentrações séricas de potássio.
- ECG deve ser realizado em intervalos adequados não só para avaliar os efeitos cardíacos do medicamentos e da hipercalemia, mas também para monitorizar a resposta ao tratamento.

PREVENÇÃO
- Evitar substâncias e medicamentos nefrotóxicos.
- Evitar desidratação e contração volêmica.

COMPLICAÇÕES POSSÍVEIS
- Hipercalemia e cardiotoxicidade associada.
- Morte induzida pela uremia.
- Desidratação.
- Super-hidratação.
- Infecção bacteriana do trato urinário e sepse.

EVOLUÇÃO ESPERADA E PROGNÓSTICO
- Oligúria e anúria constituem sinais indicativos de prognóstico mau em nefropatia aguda ou crônica; a menos que se consiga corrigir o fluxo urinário, não se espera a sobrevivência do animal.
- Anúria associada à obstrução do trato urinário é frequentemente reversível caso se consiga restabelecer a patência (desobstrução) da uretra.

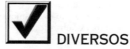

DIVERSOS

VER TAMBÉM
- Azotemia e Uremia.
- Hipercalemia.
- Insuficiência Renal Aguda.
- Insuficiência Renal Crônica.
- Nefrotoxicidade Induzida por Medicamento.
- Obstrução do Trato Urinário.

ABREVIATURA(S)
- ADH = hormônio antidiurético.
- ECG = eletrocardiograma.

Sugestões de Leitura
Cowgill LD, Langston C. Acute kidney disease. In: Bartges J, Polzin DJ, eds., Nephrology and Urology of Small Animals. Ames, IA: Wiley-Blackwell (in press).
Ross L. Acute renal failure. In: Bonagura JD, Twedt DC, eds., Kirk's Current Veterinary Therapy XIV. St. Louis: Saunders, 2009, pp. 879-882.

Autor David J. Polzin
Consultor Editorial Carl A. Osborne

ONCOCITOMA

CONSIDERAÇÕES GERAIS

REVISÃO
- Neoplasia benigna rara derivada das células oxifílicas: células neuroendócrinas atípicas que ocorrem de forma disseminada por todas as glândulas endócrinas e tecidos epiteliais.
- Localização mais comum na laringe.
- Minimamente invasivo.
- Não metastático.
- Colorações especiais demonstraram que a maioria dos oncocitomas consiste, na verdade, em rabdomiomas: tumores benignos da musculatura estriada.
- Os oncocitomas podem ocorrer nos rins.
- Existem dois relatos de caso de oncocitoma renal no cão; nenhum deles exibiu indícios de metástase. Um dos casos era bilateral e localmente invasivo na musculatura lombar; já o segundo caso era unilateral e facilmente ressecável com nefrectomia.

IDENTIFICAÇÃO
- Cães jovens a meia-idade; há apenas um único relato em gato.
- Sem predisposição racial.

SINAIS CLÍNICOS
Achados Anamnésicos
- Dependentes da localização da massa.
- Dispneia; mudança na vocalização em caso de massa laríngea.

Achados do Exame Físico
- Dispneia inspiratória.
- Massa que se projeta no lúmen da laringe ao exame sob sedação.

CAUSAS E FATORES DE RISCO
Desconhecidos.

DIAGNÓSTICO

DIAGNÓSTICO DIFERENCIAL
- Paralisia da laringe.
- Carcinoma.
- Carcinoma de células escamosas.
- Mastocitoma.
- Linfoma.

HEMOGRAMA/BIOQUÍMICA/URINÁLISE
Geralmente normais.

OUTROS TESTES LABORATORIAIS
N/D.

DIAGNÓSTICO POR IMAGEM
- Radiografia cervical lateral — avaliação do espaço laríngeo.
- Radiografia torácica — avaliação de metástase pulmonar no caso de tumor maligno.
- TC ou RM — pode permitir a delimitação completa da extensão e da origem do tumor.

MÉTODOS DIAGNÓSTICOS
- Exame da laringe sob sedação ou anestesia geral.
- Citologia da massa — possibilita a exclusão de outra neoplasia, como linfoma e mastocitoma.
- Biopsia incisional para histopatologia — necessária para o diagnóstico definitivo.

TRATAMENTO

- Ressecção cirúrgica — tratamento de escolha.
- A despeito de má localização, a maior parte dos oncocitomas (rabdomiomas) pode ser removida ("descascada") ao mesmo tempo em que se preserva a função da laringe.

MEDICAÇÕES

MEDICAMENTO(S) DE ESCOLHA
N/D.

CONTRAINDICAÇÕES/INTERAÇÕES POSSÍVEIS
N/D.

ACOMPANHAMENTO

MONITORIZAÇÃO DO PACIENTE
- Ressecção completa — cuidado pós-operatório normal; não há necessidade de qualquer acompanhamento adicional.
- Ressecção incompleta — monitorizar a recidiva dos sinais clínicos; talvez seja necessário prosseguir com uma cirurgia mais rigorosa (laringectomia completa com traqueostomia permanente).

EVOLUÇÃO ESPERADA E PROGNÓSTICO
- Prognóstico bom a excelente.
- A ressecção completa é curativa.

DIVERSOS

ABREVIATURA(S)
- RM = ressonância magnética.
- TC = tomografia computadorizada.

Sugestões de Leitura
Carlisle CH, Biery DN, Thrall DE. Tracheal and laryngeal tumors in the dog and cat: Literature review and 13 additional patients. Vet Radiol Ultrasound 1991, 32:229-235.

Autor Laura D. Garrett
Consultor Editorial Timothy M. Fan

Osteocondrodisplasia

CONSIDERAÇÕES GERAIS

REVISÃO
- Anormalidade do crescimento e do desenvolvimento da cartilagem e do osso; abrange muitos distúrbios que envolvem o crescimento ósseo.
- Resulta de ossificação endocondral anormal.
- Defeitos esqueléticos — em geral, envolvem o esqueleto apendicular; especificamente, as placas de crescimento metafisárias.
- Acondroplasia — falha de crescimento da cartilagem; caracterizada por displasia proporcional de membros curtos; evidente logo após o nascimento.
- Hipocondrodisplasia — forma menos grave de acondroplasia.
- Raças características — resulta da seleção de determinados traços desejáveis.
- Acomete os sistemas musculosquelético e, possivelmente, oftálmico.

IDENTIFICAÇÃO
- Raças acondroplásicas — Buldogue; Boston terrier; Pug; Pequinês; Spaniel japonês; Shi tzu.
- Raças hipocondroplásicas — Dachshund; Basset hound; Beagle; Welsh corgi; Dandie Dinmont terrier; Terrier escocês; Skye terrier.
- Anormalidades condrodisplásicas não selecionadas relatadas — Malamute do Alasca; Samoieda; Labrador retriever; Pointer inglês; Elkhound norueguês; Grande pirineus; Cocker spaniel; Terrier escocês; Deerhound escocês; Beagle; Poodle miniatura; Buldogue francês.
- Displasia oculosquelética — diagnosticada em Labrador retriever e Samoieda.

SINAIS CLÍNICOS
Achados Anamnésicos
- Normais do ponto de vista fenotípico ao nascimento, com retardo do crescimento identificado nos primeiros meses de vida.
- Deformidades esqueléticas óbvias.

Achados do Exame Físico
- Em geral, acomete o esqueleto apendicular; pode acometer o esqueleto axial.
- Ossos longos — parecem mais curtos do que o normal; frequentemente arqueados.
- Principais articulações (cotovelo, femorotibial, carpo, tarso) — parecem aumentadas.
- Rádio e ulna — em geral, gravemente acometidos em virtude do crescimento assincrônico.
- Arqueamento lateral dos membros anteriores.
- Articulações do carpo aumentadas.
- Deformidade valga dos pés.
- Maxila encurtada — prognatismo mandibular relativo.
- Desvios da coluna vertebral — atribuídos a hemivértebras.
- Retina — displasia; descolamento parcial a completo.

CAUSAS E FATORES DE RISCO
- Raças acondrodisplásicas e hipocondrodisplásicas — traço autossômico dominante.
- Raças condrodisplásicas não selecionadas — traço autossômico recessivo simples ou poligênico.
- Ninhadas frequentemente acometidas.

DIAGNÓSTICO

DIAGNÓSTICO DIFERENCIAL
- Fechamento prematuro das fises ulnar e radial — histórico de traumatismo; nenhum outro osso acometido; anormalidades uni ou bilaterais.
- Nanismo hipofisário.

DIAGNÓSTICO POR IMAGEM
- Radiografia dos membros acometidos — achatamento irregular da metáfise; alargamento da linha fisária; núcleos endocondrais retidos; irregularidades na ossificação do osso longo acometido; artropatia degenerativa e frouxidão articular atribuídas a tensão (estresse) anormal e sustentação do peso nos membros.
- Radiografia da coluna vertebral — hemivértebras; vértebras cuneiformes (ou seja, em forma de cunha).

MÉTODOS DIAGNÓSTICOS
Biopsia óssea da placa de crescimento — diagnóstico definitivo.

ACHADOS PATOLÓGICOS
Achados histológicos: desorganização da zona proliferativa, anormalidades dentro da zona hipertrófica, formação anormal do osso esponjoso primário e secundário.

TRATAMENTO

- Acondrodisplasia — considerada como uma anormalidade habitual em algumas raças (condrodistróficas).
- Cirurgia — geralmente de pouco benefício para condrodisplasia não selecionada.
- Osteotomia corretiva para realinhar o(s) membro(s) ou a(s) articulação(ões) — pode ter benefício limitado.

MEDICAÇÕES

MEDICAMENTO(S)
- Analgésicos e agentes anti-inflamatórios — é justificável o uso paliativo; os AINE inibem a síntese de prostaglandina via enzima ciclo-oxigenase.
- Deracoxibe (1-2 mg/kg VO a cada 24 h).
- Carprofeno (2,2 mg/kg VO a cada 12 h ou a cada 24 h).
- Etodolaco (10-15 mg/kg VO a cada 24 h).
- Meloxicam (dose de ataque de 0,2 mg/kg VO e, depois, 0,1 mg/kg VO a cada 24 h — sob a forma líquida).
- Firocoxibe (5 mg/kg VO a cada 24 h).
- Tepoxalina (dose de ataque de 20 mg/kg e, depois, 10 mg/kg VO a cada 24 h).
- Tramadol (1-4 mg/kg VO a cada 8-12 h).
- Agentes condroprotetores — glicosaminoglicanos polissulfatados, glicosamina e sulfato de condroitina; podem apresentar benefício limitado na prevenção de alterações na cartilagem articular.

ACOMPANHAMENTO

PREVENÇÃO
- Não repetir os acasalamentos entre machos e fêmeas que resultaram em filhotes acometidos.
- Desestimular o cruzamento dos animais acometidos.

COMPLICAÇÕES POSSÍVEIS
Estruturas intra-articulares e periarticulares — degeneram-se em virtude da conformação anormal do esqueleto apendicular; induz à alteração na biomecânica; resulta em má qualidade de vida.

EVOLUÇÃO ESPERADA E PROGNÓSTICO
Dependem da gravidade.

DIVERSOS

SINÔNIMO(S)
- Querubismo.
- Nanismo.

ABREVIATURA(S)
- AINE = anti-inflamatório não esteroide.

Sugestões de Leitura
Arnbjerg J, Jensen AL, Olesen AB. X-linked spondylo-epiphyseal dysplasia tarda in the Danish-Swedish farm hound. J Small Anim Pract 2007, 48(1):36-38.
Franch J, Font J, Ramis A, Lafuente P, Fontecha P, Cairo J. Multiple cartilaginous exostosis in a Golden Retriever cross-bred puppy: Clinical, radiographic and backscattered scanning microscopy findings. Vet Comp Orthop Traumatol 2005, 18(3):189-193.
Horton WA. The evolving definition of a chondrodysplasia. Pediatr Pathol Mol Med 2003, 22(1):47-52.
Jacobson LS, Kirberger RM. Canine multiple cartilaginous exostoses: Unusual manifestations and a review of the literature. JAAHA 1996, 32(1):45-51.
Martinez S, Fajardo R, Valdes J, Ulloa-Arvizu R, Alonso R. Histopathologic study of long-bone growth plates confirms the basset hound as an osteochondrodysplastic breed. Can J Vet Res 2007, 71(1):66-69.
Rorvik AM, Teige J, Ottesen N, Lingass F. Clinical, radiographic, and pathologic abnormalities in dogs with multiple epiphyseal dysplasia: 19 cases (1991-2005). JAVMA 2008, 233:600-606.
Sande RD, Bingel SA. Animal models of dwarfism. Vet Clin North Am Small Anim Pract 1982, 13:71.

Autores Wesley J. Roach e Spencer A. Johnston
Consultor Editorial Peter K. Shires
Agradecimento Os autores e editores agradecem as colaborações de Peter D. Schwarz e Peter Shires, que foram os autores deste capítulo em edições anteriores.

OSTEOCONDROSE

CONSIDERAÇÕES GERAIS

DEFINIÇÃO
Processo patológico na cartilagem em crescimento, caracterizado principalmente por distúrbio da ossificação endocondral que leva à retenção excessiva de cartilagem.

FISIOPATOLOGIA
• As células da cartilagem articular imatura e das placas de crescimento não se diferenciam normalmente.
• O processo de ossificação endocondral sofre um atraso, mas a cartilagem continua crescendo, resultando em regiões anormalmente espessas que são menos resistentes aos estresses mecânicos.
• É comum a doença bilateral.
• Articulações mais comumente acometidas — ombro (cabeça caudocentral do úmero); cotovelo (face medial do côndilo umeral); femorotibial (côndilo femoral: o lateral é mais acometido que o medial); jarrete (crista do tálus: a medial é mais acometida que a lateral).
• Outras localizações relatadas — cabeça do fêmur; margem dorsal do acetábulo; cavidade glenoide (escápula); patela; porção distal do rádio; maléolo medial; placa terminal cranial do sacro; facetas articulares vertebrais; vértebras cervicais.

Cartilagem Articular Imatura
• Nutrição mantida por difusão de nutrientes pelo líquido sinovial.
• Cartilagem espessada resulta em comprometimento do metabolismo, levando à degeneração e necrose de células pouco nutridas.
• Fissura dentro da cartilagem espessada — pode resultar de estresse mecânico; acaba levando à formação de retalho da cartilagem ou osteocondrite dissecante; pode provocar claudicação.
• Claudicação (dor) — torna-se evidente assim que o líquido sinovial estabelecer contato com o osso subcondral; influenciada por produtos de decomposição da cartilagem liberados no líquido sinovial; inflamação.

Retenção de Cartilagem nas Placas de Crescimento
• Não costuma levar à necrose, provavelmente em virtude da nutrição conferida por vasos dentro da cartilagem.
• Pode levar a deslizamento e crescimento assimétrico; mais acentuada na fise ulnar distal.

SISTEMA(S) ACOMETIDO(S)
Musculosquelético.

GENÉTICA
• Transmissão poligênica — expressão determinada pela interação de fatores genéticos e ambientais.
• Índice de herdabilidade — depende da raça; 0,25-0,45.

INCIDÊNCIA/PREVALÊNCIA
Problema frequente e grave em muitas raças caninas.

DISTRIBUIÇÃO GEOGRÁFICA
N/D.

IDENTIFICAÇÃO

Espécies
• Cães.
• Clinicamente demonstrada — equinos; suínos; frangos de corte em crescimento; perus; seres humanos.

Raça(s) Predominante(s)
Raças de porte grande e gigante — Dinamarquês, Labrador retriever, Terra Nova, Rottweiler, Montanhês de Berna, Setter inglês, Old English sheepdog.

Idade Média e Faixa Etária
• Início dos sinais clínicos — tipicamente 4-8 meses.
• Diagnóstico — geralmente 4-18 meses.
• Sintomas de artropatia degenerativa secundária — qualquer idade.

Sexo Predominante
• Ombro — machos (2:1).
• Cotovelo, femorotibial e jarrete — nenhum.

SINAIS CLÍNICOS

Comentários Gerais
Dependem da(s) articulação(ões) acometida(s) e de artropatia degenerativa concomitante.

Achados Anamnésicos
Claudicação — mais comum; início súbito ou insidioso; um ou mais membros; piora após o exercício; duração de várias semanas a meses; leve, moderada ou grave; paciente pode suportar pouco peso no membro acometido.

Achados do Exame Físico
• Dor — eliciada, em geral, à palpação por flexionar, estender ou rotacionar a articulação envolvida.
• Geralmente, há claudicação com sustentação do peso.
• Efusão articular com distensão capsular — comum na osteocondrite dissecante do cotovelo, da articulação femorotibial e do jarrete.
• Atrofia muscular — achado compatível com claudicação crônica.
• Osteocondrite dissecante do jarrete — hiperextensão da articulação tarsocrural.

CAUSAS
• Problemas de desenvolvimento.
• Relacionadas com a nutrição.

FATORES DE RISCO
• Dieta que contém três vezes a mais dos níveis recomendados de cálcio.
• Crescimento e ganho de peso rápidos.

DIAGNÓSTICO

DIAGNÓSTICO DIFERENCIAL
• Fraturas intra-articulares (osteocondrais).
• Displasia do cotovelo.
• Panosteíte.

HEMOGRAMA/BIOQUÍMICA/URINÁLISE
N/D.

OUTROS TESTES LABORATORIAIS
N/D.

DIAGNÓSTICO POR IMAGEM

Radiografia
• Projeções-padrão craniocaudais e mediolaterais — necessárias para todas as articulações envolvidas.
• Aparece sob a forma de achatamento do osso subcondral ou transparência subcondral.
• Não é capaz de diferenciar entre osteocondrose e osteocondrite dissecante.
• Esclerose do osso subjacente — comum nas lesões crônicas de osteocondrite dissecante; pode-se observar o retalho se estiver calcificado.
• Corpos calcificados dentro da articulação (articulação de camundongo) — indicam retalho cartilaginoso desalojado.
• Projeções oblíquas — podem melhorar a observação, especialmente de lesões do jarrete, do cotovelo e do ombro.
• Projeções tipo *skyline* (tangencial) das cristas talares da articulação do jarrete — ajudam a identificar lesões mediais e laterais.

TC e RM
• Técnicas valiosas para observar a extensão das lesões subcondrais.
• Não confiáveis para detectar retalho cartilaginoso solto (frouxo).

Artrografia com Contraste Positivo
• Método útil para diferenciar de osteocondrite dissecante do ombro.

MÉTODOS DIAGNÓSTICOS
• Punção da articulação e análise do líquido sinovial — confirma o envolvimento; deve-se observar um líquido de coloração amarelo-palha com viscosidade normal a reduzida; com a citologia, devem-se notar >10.000 células nucleadas/μL (um número >90% deve ser composto por células mononucleares).
• Artroscopia — minimamente invasiva; método excelente para diferenciar de osteocondrite dissecante e para o tratamento corretivo.

ACHADOS PATOLÓGICOS
• Cartilagem articular — inicialmente, pode parecer amarelada.
• Retenção da cartilagem articular, que se estende para dentro do osso subcondral, rodeada por quantidade aumentada de osso trabecular.
• Fendas entre o osso trabecular subjacente e a camada profunda degenerada e necrótica da cartilagem espessada (retida) sobrejacente.

TRATAMENTO

CUIDADO(S) DE SAÚDE ADEQUADO(S)
N/D.

CUIDADO(S) DE ENFERMAGEM
• Crioterapia (aplicação de compressa com gelo) da articulação acometida — imediatamente após a cirurgia; 5-10 min, três vezes ao dia, por 3-5 dias.
• Exercícios de amplitude de movimento — instituídos assim que o paciente puder tolerar.

ATIVIDADE
• Restrita.
• Evitar atividades concussivas rígidas (p. ex., correr no piso de concreto).

DIETA
Controle de peso — importante para reduzir a carga e, portanto, a tensão sobre a(s) articulação(ões) acometida(s).

ORIENTAÇÃO AO PROPRIETÁRIO
• Discutir a natureza hereditária da doença.
• Avisar o proprietário sobre o possível desenvolvimento de artropatia degenerativa.
• Abordar a influência da ingestão excessiva de nutrientes que promovam crescimento rápido.

Osteocondrose

CONSIDERAÇÕES CIRÚRGICAS
- Osteocondrose — condição não cirúrgica a menos que algum fragmento ósseo se desloque para um lugar clinicamente relevante; nesse caso, ficará indicada a remoção cirúrgica.
- Pode evoluir para osteocondrite dissecante à medida que o paciente cresce.
- Artrotomia ou artroscopia — indicada para a maior parte dos pacientes com osteocondrite dissecante.
- Ombro — indicada para todas as lesões de osteocondrite dissecante; método exploratório indicado para os sinais de dor e claudicação, com indícios radiográficos de osteocondrose.
- Cotovelo — indicada para todas as lesões de osteocondrite dissecante; recomendada para avaliar outras condições (ver "Displasia do Cotovelo").
- Articulação femorotibial — há controvérsias; os pacientes desenvolvem artropatia degenerativa mesmo com o procedimento; artroscopia pode melhorar a taxa de recuperação e a função a longo prazo.
- Jarrete — remover o retalho osteocondral; a realização de cirurgia é controversa; todos os pacientes desenvolvem artropatia degenerativa grave mesmo com o procedimento; tentar reimplantar o retalho ao osso subcondral subjacente, se justificável.
- Sacro — remover o fragmento em caso de impingidela das raízes nervosas da cauda equina.

MEDICAÇÕES
MEDICAMENTO(S) DE ESCOLHA
Medicamentos anti-inflamatórios (AINE) e analgésicos — podem ser utilizados para o tratamento sintomático de artropatia degenerativa associada à osteocondrite dissecante; não promove a cicatrização do retalho cartilaginoso (portanto, a cirurgia ainda é indicada).

CONTRAINDICAÇÕES
Evitar os corticosteroides em função dos efeitos colaterais potenciais e do dano à cartilagem articular associado ao uso a longo prazo.

PRECAUÇÕES
AINE — irritação gastrintestinal pode impedir seu uso.

INTERAÇÕES POSSÍVEIS
N/D.

MEDICAMENTO(S) ALTERNATIVO(S)
Medicamentos condroprotetores (p. ex., glicosaminoglicanos polissulfatados, glicosamina e sulfato de condroitina) — podem ajudar a limitar o dano e a degeneração da cartilagem; talvez ajudem a aliviar a dor e a inflamação.

ACOMPANHAMENTO
MONITORIZAÇÃO DO PACIENTE
- Monitoramento periódico até que o esqueleto do paciente esteja desenvolvido (maduro) — recomendado para avaliar a evolução do quadro para uma lesão de osteocondrite dissecante.
- Após a cirurgia de osteocondrite dissecante — restringir a atividade por 4-6 semanas; estimular o movimento ativo precoce da(s) articulação(ões) acometida(s).
- Exames anuais — recomendados para avaliar a progressão da artropatia degenerativa.

PREVENÇÃO
- Desestimular o acasalamento dos pacientes.
- Não repetir os cruzamentos entre machos e fêmeas que resultaram em filhotes acometidos.
- Ganho de peso restrito e crescimento em cães jovens — podem diminuir a incidência.

COMPLICAÇÕES POSSÍVEIS
N/D.

EVOLUÇÃO ESPERADA E PROGNÓSTICO
- Ombro — prognóstico bom a excelente quanto ao retorno à função plena; desenvolvimento de osteoartrite mínima em caso de osteocondrose e após cirurgia de osteocondrite dissecante.
- Cotovelo, articulação femorotibial e jarrete — prognóstico razoável para osteocondrose e reservado para osteocondrite dissecante; depende do tamanho da lesão (mais importante) e da presença de artropatia degenerativa, bem como da idade ao diagnóstico e tratamento; ocorre o desenvolvimento de osteoartrite progressiva mesmo depois de cirurgia.
- Sacro — prognóstico bom após remoção do fragmento.

DIVERSOS
DISTÚRBIOS ASSOCIADOS
N/D.

FATORES RELACIONADOS COM A IDADE
N/D.

POTENCIAL ZOONÓTICO
N/D.

GESTAÇÃO/FERTILIDADE/REPRODUÇÃO
N/D.

VER TAMBÉM
Displasia do Cotovelo.

ABREVIATURA(S)
- AINE = anti-inflamatório não esteroide.
- RM = ressonância magnética.
- TC = tomografia computadorizada.

Sugestões de Leitura
Fox SM, Walker AM. The etiopathogenesis of osteochondrosis. Vet Med 1993, 88:116-122.
Gielen I, van Bree H, Van Ryssen B, De Clercq T, De Rooster H. Radiographic, computed tomographic and arthroscopic findings in 23 dogs with osteochondrosis of the tarsocrural joint. Vet Record 2002, 150(14):442-447.
Gielen I, van Ryssen B, van Bree H. Computerized tomography compared with radiography in the diagnosis of lateral trochlear ridge talar osteochondritis dissecans in dogs. Vet Comp Orthop Traumatol 2005, 18(2):77-82.
Hanna FY. Lumbosacral osteochondrosis: Radiological features and surgical management in 34 dogs. J Small Anim Pract 2001, 42(6):272-278.
Kuroki K, Cook JL, Stoker AM, Turnquist SE, Kreeger JM, Tomlinson JL. Characterizing osteochondrosis in the dog: Potential roles for matrix metalloproteinases and mechanical load in pathogenesis and disease progression. Osteoarthritis Cartilage 2005, 13(3):225-234.
Kuroki K, Cook JL, Tomlinson JL, Kreeger JM. In vitro characterization of chondrocytes isolated from naturally occurring osteochondrosis lesions of the humeral head of dogs. Am J Vet Res 2002, 63(2):186-193.
Richardson DC, Zentek J. Nutrition and osteochondrosis. Vet Clin North Am Small Anim Pract 1998, 28(1):115-135.
Tomlinson JL, Cook JL, Kuroki K, Kreeger JM, Anderson MA. Biochemical characterization of cartilage affected by osteochondritis dissecans in the humeral head of dogs. Am J Vet Res 2001, 62(6):876-881.
Vandevelde B, Van Ryssen B, Saunders JH, Kramer M, Van Bree H. Comparison of the ultrasonographic appearance of osteochondrosis lesions in the canine shoulder with radiography, arthrography, and arthroscopy. Vet Radiol Ultrasound 2006, 47(2):174-184.

Autor Peter K. Shires
Consultor Editorial Peter K. Shires
Agradecimento O autor e os editores agradecem a colaboração de Peter D. Schwarz, que foi o autor deste capítulo em uma edição mais antiga.

Osteodistrofia Hipertrófica

CONSIDERAÇÕES GERAIS

DEFINIÇÃO
Doença inflamatória dos ossos que acomete filhotes de cães em fase rápida de crescimento.

FISIOPATOLOGIA
- Caracteriza-se por inflamação supurativa asséptica dentro das trabéculas metafisárias de ossos longos.
- Os ossos em fase rápida de crescimento são acometidos de forma mais grave.
- Metáfises — alargadas em virtude de tumefação perimetafisária e deposição óssea.
- Microfraturas trabeculares e separação metafisária — ocorrem em posição adjacente e paralela à fise.
- Defeito na formação óssea.
- Periostite ossificante — pode ser extensa.
- Etiologia desconhecida.

SISTEMA(S) ACOMETIDO(S)
- Gastrintestinal — diarreia.
- Musculosquelético — distribuição simétrica; a parte distal dos membros anteriores é mais gravemente acometida; pode-se notar mineralização do tecido mole em outros órgãos; junções costocondrais alargadas.
- Respiratório — pneumonia intersticial.

GENÉTICA
Suspeita de hiper-reatividade à imunoestimulação (vacinas).

INCIDÊNCIA/PREVALÊNCIA
Baixas.

DISTRIBUIÇÃO GEOGRÁFICA
N/D.

IDENTIFICAÇÃO

Espécies
Cães.

Raça(s) Predominante(s)
- Cães de grande porte em fase rápida de crescimento.
- Dinamarquês, Weimaraner — mais comum.
- Relatadas — Wolfhound irlandês, São Bernardo, Kuvasz, Setter irlandês, Doberman pinscher, Pastor alemão, Labrador retriever, Boxer e muitas outras.

Idade Média e Faixa Etária
- Acomete filhotes de 3-4 meses de vida.
- Variação do início — 2-8 meses de vida.

Sexo Predominante
Acomete mais machos do que fêmeas.

SINAIS CLÍNICOS

Comentários Gerais
Claudicação — pode ser episódica; a magnitude varia de leve até a falta de sustentação do peso; o episódio inicial pode desaparecer sem recidiva.

Achados Anamnésicos
- Dependem da gravidade do episódio.
- Os proprietários frequentemente descrevem um filhote deprimido que reluta em se mover.
- Inapetência — comum.
- Dor.

Achados do Exame Físico
- Claudicação — simétrica, mais grave nos membros anteriores.
- Metáfises — dolorosas; quentes; tumefatas distalmente às metáfises do rádio, da ulna e da tíbia.
- Pirexia — até 41,1°C.
- Inapetência.
- Depressão.
- Perda de peso.
- Desidratação.
- Diarreia.
- Caquexia.
- Debilitação.
- Manifestações de doença sistêmica — respiratória ou gastrintestinal.
- Hiperqueratose dos coxins palmoplantares.
- Anemia.

CAUSAS
Desconhecidas; foram propostas as hipóteses a seguir:

Metabólicas
- Hipovitaminose C — subestimada; pode ser observada como resultado da utilização excessiva de vitamina C disponível na formação óssea hiperativa.
- Hipocuprose — em ratos, mas não em cães.

Nutricionais
- Supernutrição e suplementação excessiva — associação inconsistente.
- Ocorrência parcial em ninhadas.
- A correção da dieta nem sempre altera a evolução da doença nem evita as recidivas.

Infecciosas
- Microrganismos bacterianos ou fúngicos — podem ser secundários quando encontrados.
- Não transmissíveis.
- Associação temporal com a vacinação contra o vírus da cinomose.
- O desenvolvimento secundário pode depender da época em que o neonato foi exposto.

FATORES DE RISCO
A vacinação contra o vírus da cinomose pode precipitar uma reação inflamatória descontrolada nos centros osteogênicos.

DIAGNÓSTICO

DIAGNÓSTICO DIFERENCIAL
- Panosteíte — sem tumefação metafisária; densidades intramedulares algodonosas em ossos longos nas radiografias.
- Metafisite/epifisite séptica — as radiografias das extremidades não são típicas de osteodistrofia hipertrófica; assimétricas; pode-se notar inflamação supurativa séptica na aspiração de lesões metafisárias/epifisárias com agulha; os achados hematológicos implicam infecção bacteriana (neutrofilia com desvio à esquerda).
- Displasia do cotovelo — sem tumefação metafisária; sem febre; dor localizada no(s) cotovelo(s); sinais radiográficos típicos.
- Osteocondrite dissecante — sem tumefação metafisária ou febre; dor localizada no ombro ou no cotovelo; defeitos subcondrais nas radiografias.
- Poliartrite séptica — inflamação supurativa séptica à artrocentese; cultura.
- Poliartrite asséptica — inflamação supurativa asséptica à artrocentese.

HEMOGRAMA/BIOQUÍMICA/URINÁLISE
- Não contribuem positivamente para o diagnóstico.
- Leucograma de estresse.
- Parâmetros séricos normais.
- Hipocalcemia incomum.

OUTROS TESTES LABORATORIAIS
N/D.

DIAGNÓSTICO POR IMAGEM
- Radiografias da parte distal dos membros — zonas radiolucentes irregulares dentro das metáfises, paralelas e adjacentes às fises; metáfises cintilantes; neoformação óssea extraperiosteal que se estende até as diáfises; mineralização de tecidos moles perimetafisários; crescimento assincrônico dos ossos pares; arco cranial; deformidade em valgo; em geral, simétricas bilaterais.
- Vértebras, ossos metacárpicos/metatársicos, costelas, escápula, úmero e mandíbula — raramente acometidos.
- Radiografias torácicas — podem revelar infiltrados intersticiais.

MÉTODOS DIAGNÓSTICOS
N/D.

ACHADOS PATOLÓGICOS
- Metáfises distais do rádio e da ulna — alterações mais graves; anormalidades semelhantes em todos os ossos longos.
- Macroscópicos — metáfises alargadas; mineralização periférica; tumefação de tecido mole.

Histológicos
- Inflamação supurativa asséptica da metáfise (osteocondrite), em especial adjacente às placas de crescimento.
- Necrose e provável falha secundária de deposição do tecido ósseo na malha trabecular de cartilagem calcificada da zona esponjosa primária.
- Microfraturas trabeculares e impactação óssea.
- Mineralização de tecidos moles perimetafisários e dos tecidos moles em outras regiões do corpo.
- Pneumonia intersticial.

TRATAMENTO

CUIDADO(S) DE SAÚDE ADEQUADO(S)
- Nenhum específico.
- De suporte — desde nenhum até cuidados intensivos para filhotes gravemente acometidos.
- Dependem da gravidade do episódio, da presença de pirexia e da capacidade do paciente em manter a hidratação normal e o apetite.

CUIDADO(S) DE ENFERMAGEM
- Alguns pacientes não ficam em estação e nem se movem e, portanto, são propensos ao desenvolvimento de úlceras de pressão; é preciso virá-los a cada 2-4 h para evitar o surgimento de feridas e a congestão hipostática do pulmão dependente.
- Fluidoterapia intravenosa para desidratação; depois, fluidoterapia de manutenção.

ATIVIDADE
- Restrita — corridas e saltos podem exacerbar a lesão metafisária e resultar em mais inflamação.
- Confinamento em uma pequena área bem acolchoada — recomendado.
- Passeios apenas com coleira.

DIETA
- Ração comercial normal para filhotes.
- Evitar suplementos.

Osteodistrofia Hipertrófica

ORIENTAÇÃO AO PROPRIETÁRIO
- Alertar o proprietário quanto à natureza recidivante da doença.
- Informar ao proprietário sobre o fato de que as deformidades ósseas sofrerão remodelagem até certo ponto com o passar do tempo, mas as deformações em arco e valgo são permanentes.
- Avisar o proprietário que quanto mais grave for a doença, mais grave será a deformidade em arco.

CONSIDERAÇÕES CIRÚRGICAS
- Nenhuma específica.
- Podem-se implementar métodos cirúrgicos de alimentação (sondas inseridas via faringostomia, esofagostomia ou gastrostomia) — para filhotes de cães debilitados que não comem nem bebem e frequentemente têm episódios recidivantes de sinais clínicos agudos.
- Osteotomia corretiva caso se desenvolva deformidade de crescimento a partir da desorganização da fise.

MEDICAÇÕES
MEDICAMENTO(S) DE ESCOLHA
- Medicamentos anti-inflamatórios — para a dor e pelos efeitos antipiréticos; pode-se tentar:
  - Ácido acetilsalicílico (10 mg/kg VO a cada 12 h).
  - Carprofeno (2,2 mg/kg IM ou VO a cada 12 h).
  - Firocoxibe (5 mg/kg VO a cada 24 h).
  - Etodalaco (10-15 mg/kg VO a cada 24 h).
  - Deracoxibe (1-2 mg/kg VO a cada 24 h) (3-4 mg/kg VO a cada 24 h, limite de 7 dias).
  - Meloxicam (cães, dose de ataque de 0,2 mg/kg VO e, em seguida, 0,1 mg/kg VO a cada 24 h; gatos, 0,1 mg/kg VO a cada 24 h — sob a forma líquida).
  - Tepoxalina (dose de ataque de 20 mg/kg e, em seguida, 10 mg/kg VO a cada 24 h).
- Analgésicos — podem ser utilizados em conjunto com medicação anti-inflamatória.
- Tramadol (1-4 mg/kg VO a cada 8-12 h).
- Prednisona (0,5-1 mg/kg VO a cada 24 h); utilizada apenas quando não houver resposta aos AINE — pode causar distúrbios do crescimento da fise.

CONTRAINDICAÇÕES
Vitamina C — pode estar contraindicada; pode acelerar a calcificação distrófica e diminuir a remodelação óssea.

PRECAUÇÕES
- Evitar o uso de agentes imunossupressores na presença de alguma infecção secundária.
- AINE — podem causar ulceração gástrica; ficar atento para os sinais de hematêmese ou melena; JAMAIS utilize em conjunto com outros AINE ou esteroides.

INTERAÇÕES POSSÍVEIS
Nenhuma.

MEDICAMENTO(S) ALTERNATIVO(S)
Nenhum.

ACOMPANHAMENTO
MONITORIZAÇÃO DO PACIENTE
Sinais de melhora — menor sensibilidade metafisária; o paciente se levanta; o apetite melhora; a pirexia desaparece.

PREVENÇÃO
N/D.

COMPLICAÇÕES POSSÍVEIS
- Caquexia.
- Deformidades em arco permanentes.
- Infecção bacteriana secundária.
- Úlceras de pressão.
- Fasciculações musculares, crises convulsivas — com hipocalcemia.
- Pode ocorrer septicemia secundária.
- Recidiva.
- Morte.

EVOLUÇÃO ESPERADA E PROGNÓSTICO
- Evolução — dias a semanas.
- Maioria dos pacientes — um ou dois episódios e recuperação.
- Alguns pacientes — parecem ter episódios recidivantes intratáveis de dor e pirexia; raramente morrem ou são submetidos à eutanásia.
- Prognóstico — em geral, bom; reservado em casos de múltiplas recidivas ou problemas secundários complicantes.
- Deformidade em arco persistente — elimina muitos filhotes de raça pura das exposições.

DIVERSOS
DISTÚRBIOS ASSOCIADOS
Nenhum comprovado.

FATORES RELACIONADOS COM A IDADE
Vacinação (vírus da cinomose).

POTENCIAL ZOONÓTICO
Nenhum.

GESTAÇÃO/FERTILIDADE/REPRODUÇÃO
Ocorre apenas em animais jovens.

SINÔNIMO(S)
- Osteopatia metafisária.
- Deficiência da vitamina C.
- Escorbuto.

VER TAMBÉM
- Displasia do Cotovelo.
- Osteocondrose.
- Panosteíte.

ABREVIATURA(S)
- AINE = anti-inflamatório não esteroide.

Sugestões de Leitura
Abeles V, Harrus S, Amgles JM. Hypertrophic osteodystrophy in six Weimaramer puppies associated with systemic signs. Vet Record 1999, 145(5):130-134.
Crumlish PT, Sweeney T, Jones B, Angles JM. Hypertrophic osteodystrophy in the Weimaraner dog: Lack of association between DQA1 alleles of the canine MHC and hypertrophic osteodystrophy. Vet J 2006, 171:308-313.
Demko J, McLaughlin R. Developmental orthopedic disease. Vet Clin North Am Small Anim Pract 2005, 35(5):1111-1135.
Foale RD, Herrtgae ME, Day MJ. Retrospective study of 25 young Weimaraners with low serum immunoglobulin concentrations and inflammatory disease. Vet Record 2003, 153:553-558.
Franklin MA, Rochat MC, Broaddus KD. Hypertrophic osteodystrophy of the proximal humerus in two dogs. JAAHA 2008, 44(6):342-346.
Harrus S, et al. Development of hypertrophic osteodystrophy and antibody response in a litter of vaccinated Weimaraner puppies. J Small Anim Pract 2002, 43:27-31.

Autores Steven M. Cogar e Spencer A. Johnston
Consultor Editorial Peter K. Shires
Agradecimento O autor e os editores agradecem as colaborações de Peter K. Shires, que foi o autor deste capítulo na edição anterior.

OSTEOMIELITE

CONSIDERAÇÕES GERAIS

DEFINIÇÃO
Inflamação aguda ou crônica do osso e de seus elementos associados de tecido mole de estruturas como medula, endósteo, periósteo e canais vasculares, causada normalmente por bactérias e raramente por fungos e outros microrganismos.

FISIOPATOLOGIA
• Extensão de infecções dos tecidos moles para os ossos — rara em pequenos animais.
• Microrganismos disseminados pela via hematógena — a partir de focos infecciosos em um local distante no corpo. As bactérias tipicamente se localizam na região metafisária de ossos longos em animais jovens e vértebras de adultos. O processo de inflamação e a formação de trombo produzem um ambiente isquêmico que promove a proliferação bacteriana.
• Inoculação direta do osso por bactérias patogênicas — via mais comum de infecção. Pode não dar início à infecção a menos que fatores teciduais locais sejam acometidos, como: vascularização deficiente em virtude de lesão concomitante dos tecidos moles ou instabilidade por fratura, necrose de tecidos ósseos ou moles, sequestro, alteração das defesas teciduais, material estranho ou implantes cirúrgicos.
• As bactérias produzem um revestimento de mucopolissacarídeo que, juntamente com as proteínas e os debris celulares do hospedeiro, forma um biofilme (película biológica), que não só protege as bactérias contra a ação de fagócitos, antibióticos e anticorpos, mas também induz algumas bactérias a se transformarem em cepas mais virulentas e mais resistentes a antimicrobianos. A adesão de bactérias a implantes e sequestros, bem como a proteção pelo biofilme, permitem novas infecções assim que a antibioticoterapia for interrompida.
• A reabsorção óssea devida à infecção e à instabilidade provoca o alargamento da lacuna da fratura e o afrouxamento do implante, contribuindo para a persistência da infecção.

SISTEMA(S) ACOMETIDO(S)
Musculosquelético.

GENÉTICA
Raças com imunodeficiência hereditária ou doenças hematógenas.

INCIDÊNCIA/PREVALÊNCIA
• Doença hematógena — 10% das infecções em cães.
• A prevalência após redução aberta e fixação interna de fraturas fechadas não é incomum. Prevalência após traumatismo e fratura aberta — desconhecida; relativamente comum.
• Discospondilite em cães e gatos adultos e doença fúngica — não é incomum.

DISTRIBUIÇÃO GEOGRÁFICA
• Actinomicose — em geral, farpas de gramíneas provocam infecções de tecido mole, não osteomielite; na osteomielite, provavelmente há algum contaminante do solo: Califórnia, Flórida, Reino Unido e Austrália.
• Blastomicose — regiões central e oriental dos Estados Unidos: região dos Grandes Lagos e vales dos rios Mississipi e Ohio.
• Coccidioidomicose — sudoeste dos Estados Unidos, México, além das Américas Central e do Sul.
• Histoplasmose — vales dos rios Ohio, Missouri e Mississipi e afluentes.

IDENTIFICAÇÃO
Espécies
Cães e gatos.
Raça(s) Predominante(s)
Raças com imunodeficiência e doenças hematógenas.
Idade Média e Faixa Etária
Infecção metafisária hematógena — cães jovens.
Sexo Predominante
Machos caninos — para infecção pós-traumática; blastomicose.

SINAIS CLÍNICOS
Comentários Gerais
• Infecções agudas de ferida pós-operatória após cirurgia ortopédica — podem ser indistinguíveis da condição aguda; podem evoluir para doença crônica.
• A maior parte dos pacientes apresenta a doença crônica no momento do exame e do diagnóstico.
Achados Anamnésicos
• Claudicação.
• Trajetos drenantes.
• Traumatismo anterior.
• Fratura ou cirurgia — doença pós-traumática.
• Fraqueza dos membros posteriores e dificuldade de se levantar — discospondilite ou osteomielite vertebral.
• Viagens para regiões endêmicas de infecções micóticas — infecções fúngicas.
Achados do Exame Físico
• Doença hematógena aguda (cães) — início repentino de doença sistêmica; tumefação dos tecidos moles sobre o local acometido; claudicação; pirexia; letargia; dor no membro.
• Condição crônica — trajetos drenantes crônicos, dor, atrofia muscular, contratura muscular.
• Fraturas não consolidadas com infecção concomitante — instabilidade, crepitação e deformidade do membro.
• Infecções fúngicas — tumefação do membro, claudicação e trajetos intermitentemente drenantes.
• Infecções ósseas da coluna vertebral — dor e déficits neurológicos (p. ex., paresia e paralisia).

CAUSAS
• Fratura aberta.
• Lesão traumática.
• Redução aberta e fixação interna de fratura fechada.
• Cirurgia ortopédica eletiva.
• Implante de prótese articular.
• Ferida por projétil balístico.
• Corpo estranho penetrante.
• Feridas por mordedura e unhada.
• Extensão de infecção do tecido mole para o osso — periodontite; rinite; otite média; paroníquia.
• Infecção hematógena.
• Estafilococos, geralmente o *S. intermedius*, causam cerca de 46-74% das infecções ósseas; com frequência, geram infecções monomicrobianas. As infecções ósseas polimicrobianas são comuns, podendo envolver aeróbios Gram-negativos, tais como: *E. coli*, *Pseudomonas*, *Proteus*, e *Klebsiella* spp.
• Isolamentos bacterianos anaeróbios podem chegar até 70% e incluem *Actinomyces*, *Clostridium*, *Peptostreptococcus*, *Bacteroides*, e *Fusobacterium*.
• Infecção fúngica geralmente resulta de disseminação hematógena — *Coccidioides immitis*; *Blastomyces dermatitidis*; *Histoplasma capsulatum*; *Cryptococcus neoformans*, *Aspergillus*.

FATORES DE RISCO
• Fratura aberta e contaminação óssea.
• Traumatismo de tecido mole.
• Feridas penetrantes.
• Migração de corpo estranho.
• Cirurgias/implantes ortopédicos.
• Aloenxerto ósseo cortical.
• Imunodeficiência.
• Infecção nosocomial.

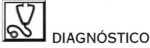

DIAGNÓSTICO

DIAGNÓSTICO DIFERENCIAL
• Panosteíte.
• Neoplasia.
• Cistos ósseos.
• União tardia de fratura em função de instabilidade.
• Osteodistrofia hipertrófica.
• Osteopatia hipertrófica.
• Infarto ósseo medular.

HEMOGRAMA/BIOQUÍMICA/URINÁLISE
• Hemograma completo — leucograma inflamatório com desvio à esquerda em caso de doença aguda.
• Pode haver hifas fúngicas na urina de pacientes sistemicamente enfermos com aspergilose.

OUTROS TESTES LABORATORIAIS
• Sorologia — confirma algumas infecções fúngicas.
• Hemoculturas em cães com suspeita de infecção hematógena.

DIAGNÓSTICO POR IMAGEM
Radiologia
• Doença aguda — arquitetura óssea normal; em caso de infecção anaeróbia, pode ser evidente a presença de gás.
• Doença crônica — sequestro (segmento avascular de osso cortical); neoformação óssea periosteal; formação de invólucro (tecido ósseo reativo circundando o sequestro); reabsorção óssea — alargamento das lacunas de fratura; adelgaçamento do córtex; osteopenia generalizada; afrouxamento do implante.
• Fistulograma — pode ajudar a identificar os sequestros ou corpos estranhos radiotransparentes.
Outras
• Ultrassonografia — localiza grandes acúmulos de líquido; orienta a amostragem do líquido por aspirado com agulha.
• Cintilografia — difosfonato de metileno marcado pelo Tc^{99m}; altamente sensível para detectar o aumento na vascularidade do osso; não é específica para osteomielite.

MÉTODOS DIAGNÓSTICOS
• Aspirados de líquido de áreas flutuantes ou biopsias de tecido com agulha Jamshidi — coletados por meio de técnicas estéreis; submetidos a culturas aeróbias e anaeróbias; possibilitam a identificação dos microrganismos; permitem a

OSTEOMIELITE

determinação da suscetibilidade *in vitro* do medicamento antimicrobiano.
• Biopsia cirúrgica aberta — indicada quando os aspirados com agulha são negativos ou quando há necessidade de debridamento para a terapia; amostras para cultura obtidas de tecido necrótico, sequestro, implantes e material estranho; exame histopatológico para confirmar a suspeita de infecção fúngica e descartar neoplasia. Solicitar o uso de corantes especiais para fungos nas amostras histopatológicas.
• Amostras de líquido e de tecido para cultura anaeróbia — colocar imediatamente em meio de transporte apropriado. Evitar a cultura de líquido purulento obtido dos trajetos drenantes — os resultados são ilusórios, pois frequentemente adquirem contaminantes da pele.
• Hemoculturas — indicadas em osteomielite hematógena aguda ou doença crônica com septicemia.

ACHADOS PATOLÓGICOS
• Sequestro ósseo — praticamente diagnóstico.
• Inflamação e necrose do osso e dos tecidos adjacentes — bactérias piogênicas.
• Exame citológico ou histopatológico de esfregaços ou cortes — induz, em geral, ao diagnóstico de infecção fúngica.

TRATAMENTO
CUIDADO(S) DE SAÚDE ADEQUADO(S)
• Paciente internado — debridamento cirúrgico, drenagem, cultura, irrigação e tratamento da ferida até que a infecção comece a se resolver; fraturas infectadas (estabilização cirúrgica).
• Paciente de ambulatório — terapia com medicamento antimicrobiano por via oral a longo prazo.

CUIDADO(S) DE ENFERMAGEM
• Depende da gravidade, da localização e do grau de lesão do tecido mole associado.
• Evitar a contaminação do patógeno para outros pacientes.
• Fisioterapia.

ATIVIDADE
Restrita — com qualquer risco de desenvolvimento de fratura patológica; com fratura não consolidada.

DIETA
Sem restrição.

ORIENTAÇÃO AO PROPRIETÁRIO
• Avisar o proprietário sobre o custo do tratamento, a probabilidade de recidiva, a possibilidade de intervenções cirúrgicas repetidas e a duração prolongada do tratamento.
• Discutir o prognóstico.

CONSIDERAÇÕES CIRÚRGICAS
• Doença crônica — debridamento cirúrgico; remoção do sequestro (sequestrectomia); estabelecimento de drenagem.
• Fratura estável infectada — deixar os implantes de fixação interna preexistentes no local durante a consolidação.
• Fratura instável infectada — remover os implantes; estabilizar com fixação esquelética externa ou interna.
• Déficits ósseos — aplicação de enxerto com osso esponjoso autólogo imediatamente ou após a infecção ter desaparecido e o tecido de granulação ter se formado na ferida.
• Grandes defeitos segmentares nos ossos longos — construção de ponte pela técnica de Ilizarov ou outro transporte de segmento ósseo.
• Infecção crônica localizada — passível de resolução por meio de amputação (cauda, dedo, membro) ou ressecção em bloco (esterno, parede torácica, mandíbula, maxila) e oclusão primária da ferida.
• Remover todos os implantes após a consolidação da fratura; bactérias albergadas por biofilme do implante podem levar à recidiva ou constituir fator patogênico para sarcoma associado à fratura.
• A cobertura do osso exposto com o uso de *flap* (retalho) muscular no início do curso terapêutico diminui acentuadamente a contaminação do osso e promove a consolidação da fratura.

MEDICAÇÕES
MEDICAMENTO(S) DE ESCOLHA
• Administrar algum antimicrobiano bactericida de amplo espectro por via IV durante 3-5 dias enquanto se aguardam os resultados da cultura e do antibiograma. O antibiótico final deve ser selecionado com base na determinação *in vitro* de suscetibilidade dos microrganismos; considerar também a possível toxicidade, a frequência, a via de administração e o custo; a maioria penetra bem no osso normal e infectado; devem ser administrados por 4-8 semanas; continuar por, no mínimo, 2 semanas após a resolução radiográfica e clínica da infecção.
• Estafilococos (cães) — geralmente *S. intermedius*, os quais são resistentes à penicilina, por causa da produção de β-lactamase; altamente suscetíveis à cloxacilina, amoxicilina-clavulanato, cefazolina e clindamicina.
• Antibióticos eficazes contra anaeróbios que também estão disponíveis para administração parenteral: ampicilina sódica, metronidazol, e clindamicina.
• Aminoglicosídeos e quinolonas (ciprofloxacino e enrofloxacino) — eficazes contra bactérias aeróbias Gram-negativas.
• Quinolonas — podem ser administradas por via oral; não são nefrotóxicas; para proteger contra a resistência, utilizar apenas em infecções provocadas por microrganismos Gram-negativos ou *Pseudomonas*, que são resistentes a outros agentes antimicrobianos orais.
• Doença crônica — liberação local contínua de medicamentos antimicrobianos por esferas de metilmetacrilato impregnadas com antibiótico ou polímeros biodegradáveis.
• Terapia antifúngica a longo prazo (meses); osteomielite fúngica — tratar por, no mínimo, 1 mês além da resolução dos sinais clínicos; p. ex., itraconazol 5-10 mg/kg VO a cada 24 h; a administração contínua pode controlar a aspergilose disseminada por até 2 anos.
• Analgésicos — narcóticos e/ou anti-inflamatórios não esteroides injetáveis são importantes para estimular a sustentação do peso e o uso do membro.

CONTRAINDICAÇÕES
Quinolonas — evitar em cães imaturos; potencial de lesão cartilaginosa.

PRECAUÇÕES
Aminoglicosídeos — podem provocar nefrotoxicidade, sobretudo em pacientes desidratados e com perdas eletrolíticas ou nefropatia preexistente.

MEDICAMENTO(S) ALTERNATIVO(S)
Identificar outros medicamentos antimicrobianos pela repetição das culturas e determinação da suscetibilidade se a infecção se tornar irresponsiva ao agente inicial.

ACOMPANHAMENTO
MONITORIZAÇÃO DO PACIENTE
• Radiografia — 2-3 semanas após a intervenção e, depois, sequencialmente, conforme a necessidade, para monitorizar a consolidação óssea, tipicamente a cada 4-6 semanas.
• Realização de nova cultura do tecido ósseo — na suspeita de infecção persistente.

COMPLICAÇÕES POSSÍVEIS
• Recidiva.
• Evolução para doença crônica.
• Neoplasia maligna — sequela rara de infecção crônica das fraturas reparadas com fixação interna.

EVOLUÇÃO ESPERADA E PROGNÓSTICO
• Resposta favorável ao tratamento em 90% dos cães acometidos, embora a recidiva seja possível, particularmente em caso de infecções crônicas.
• Infecção aguda e discospondilite bacteriana crônica — podem ser curadas com 4-8 semanas de terapia com medicamento antibacteriano se houver necrose óssea limitada e sem fratura.
• Doença crônica — a resolução apenas com medicamento antibacteriano é improvável; fornecer tratamento cirúrgico apropriado.
• A recidiva da infecção crônica em semanas, meses ou anos após o último tratamento pode necessitar de sequestrectomia repetida.
• Considerar a amputação em casos crônicos graves com perda irreversível da função do membro.

DIVERSOS
SINÔNIMO(S)
Infecção óssea.

VER TAMBÉM
Discospondilite.

Sugestões de Leitura
Bubenik LJ, Smith MM. Orthopaedic Infections. In: Slatter D, ed., Textbook of Small Animal Surgery, 3rd ed. Philadelphia: Saunders Elsevier, 2003, pp. 1862-1875.
Greene CE, Budsberg SC. Musculoskeletal infections. In: Greene CE, ed., Infectious Diseases of the Dog and Cat, 3rd ed. St. Louis: Saunders Elsevier, 2006, pp. 823-833.
Hay CW. Osteomyelitis. In: Birchard SJ, Sherding RG, eds., Saunders Manual of Small Animal Practice, 3rd ed. St. Louis: Saunders Elsevier, 2006, pp. 1210-1213.

Autor Tisha A.M. Harper
Consultor Editorial Peter K. Shires
Agradecimento a Mark M. Smith pelas colaborações como autor na edição anterior.

Osteopatia Craniomandibular

CONSIDERAÇÕES GERAIS

REVISÃO
- Doença proliferativa, não inflamatória e não neoplásica dos ossos da cabeça.
- Principais ossos acometidos — ramos mandibulares; occipital e parietal; bulas timpânicas; processos zigomáticos do temporal.
- O envolvimento simétrico bilateral é mais comum.
- Acomete o sistema musculosquelético.

IDENTIFICAÇÃO
- Raças Scottish terrier, Cairn terrier e West Highland white terrier — mais comuns.
- Labrador retriever, Dinamarquês, Boston terrier, Doberman pinscher, Setter irlandês, Buldogue inglês, Bulmastife, Pastor de Shetland e Boxer — podem ser acometidos.
- Em geral, acomete filhotes caninos em crescimento com 4-8 meses de vida.
- Não há predileção sexual.
- A castração pode aumentar a incidência.

SINAIS CLÍNICOS
Achados Anamnésicos
- Relacionam-se em geral com dor em torno da boca e dificuldade progressiva de abrir a boca.
- Dificuldades de preensão e mastigação — podem levar à inanição.

Achados do Exame Físico
- Atrofia dos músculos temporais e masseteres — comum.
- Espessamento irregular palpável dos ramos da mandíbula e/ou da região da articulação temporomandibular.
- Incapacidade de abrir completamente a mandíbula, mesmo sob anestesia geral.
- Pirexia intermitente.
- Exoftalmia bilateral.

CAUSAS E FATORES DE RISCO
- Supostamente hereditária — ocorre em determinadas raças e famílias.
- West Highland white terrier — traço autossômico recessivo.
- Scottish terrier — possível predisposição.
- Terrier jovem com doença periótica de ossos longos — monitorar em busca de doença.

DIAGNÓSTICO

DIAGNÓSTICO DIFERENCIAL
- Osteomielite — acometimento ósseo assimétrico; geralmente não é tão extensa; lise óssea; ausência de predileção racial; histórico de ferida penetrante.
- Periostite traumática — envolvimento ósseo assimétrico; não costuma ser tão extensa; histórico de traumatismo.
- Neoplasias — pacientes adultos; acometimento ósseo assimétrico; maior reação óssea lítica; doença metastática.
- Hiperostose da calvária — paciente jovem — ossos frontais, parietais e occipitais; não envolve a mandíbula; pode apresentar o envolvimento de ossos longos.

HEMOGRAMA/BIOQUÍMICA/URINÁLISE
- Fosfatase alcalina e fosfato inorgânico séricos — podem estar elevados.
- Pode-se observar hipogamaglobulinemia ou α_2-hiperglobulinemia.

OUTROS TESTES LABORATORIAIS
Sorologia — descarta agentes fúngicos; indicada em casos atípicos.

DIAGNÓSTICO POR IMAGEM
- Radiografias do crânio — revelam proliferação óssea irregular, semelhante a um rosário, da mandíbula ou das bulas timpânicas (acometimento bilateral); neoformação óssea perióstica extensa (exostoses), que afeta um ou mais ossos em torno da articulação temporomandibular; podem revelar fusão das bulas timpânicas e do processo angular da mandíbula.
- TC — pode ajudar a avaliar o envolvimento ósseo da articulação temporomandibular.

MÉTODOS DIAGNÓSTICOS
Biopsia e cultura ósseas (bacteriana e fúngica) — necessárias somente em casos atípicos; descartam neoplasia e osteomielite.

ACHADOS PATOLÓGICOS
- Biopsia óssea — revela a substituição do osso lamelar normal por um osso fibroso rústico/grosseiro e aumentado de volume, além de osteólise osteoclástica das regiões perióstica ou subperióstica.
- Medula óssea — substituída por estroma fibrovascular.
- Células inflamatórias — observadas ocasionalmente na periferia da lesão óssea.

TRATAMENTO
- Apenas paliativo.
- Excisão cirúrgica das exostoses — resulta em novo crescimento dentro de semanas.
- Dieta em forma de papa ou mingau rico em calorias e proteínas — ajuda a manter o equilíbrio nutricional.
- Colocação cirúrgica de sonda via faringostomia, esofagostomia ou gastrostomia — considerada para ajudar a manter o equilíbrio nutricional.

MEDICAÇÕES

MEDICAMENTO(S)
- Analgésicos e anti-inflamatórios — justifica-se o uso paliativo.
- AINE — inibem as enzimas ciclo-oxigenase.
- Deracoxibe (1-2 mg/kg VO a cada 24 h, mastigável).
- Carprofeno (2,2 mg/kg VO a cada 12 h ou 4,4 mg/kg a cada 24 h).
- Etodolaco (10-15 mg/kg VO a cada 24 h).
- Meloxicam (dose de ataque de 0,2 mg/kg VO, depois 0,1 mg/kg VO a cada 24 h — na forma líquida).
- Tepoxalina (dose de ataque de 20 mg/kg, depois 10 mg/kg VO a cada 24 h).
- Firocoxibe (5 mg/kg VO a cada 24 h).

ACOMPANHAMENTO

MONITORIZAÇÃO DO PACIENTE
Reavaliações frequentes — obrigatórias para assegurar a manutenção do equilíbrio nutricional e o controle da dor adequados.

PREVENÇÃO
- Não repetir o acasalamento de casais que geraram ninhadas acometidas.
- Desestimular a reprodução de animais acometidos.

EVOLUÇÃO ESPERADA E PROGNÓSTICO
- A dor e o desconforto podem diminuir na maturidade esquelética (10-12 meses de vida); as exostoses podem regredir.
- Prognóstico — depende do envolvimento dos ossos circunjacentes à articulação temporomandibular.
- Pode ser necessária a eutanásia eletiva.

DIVERSOS

SINÔNIMO(S)
Mandíbula de leão.

ABREVIATURA(S)
- AINE = anti-inflamatórios não esteroides.
- TC = tomografia computadorizada.

Sugestões de Leitura
Franch J, Cesari JR, Font J. Craniomandibular osteopathy in two Pyrenean mountain dogs. Vet Record 1998, 142(17):455-459.
Huchkowsky SL. Craniomandibular osteopathy in a bullmastiff. Can Vet J 2002, 43(11):883-885.
LaFond E, Breur GJ, Austin CC. Breed susceptibility for developmental orthopedic diseases in dogs. JAAHA 2002, 38(5):467-477.
McConnell JF, Hayes A, Platt SR, Smith KC. Calvarial hyperostosis syndrome in two bullmastiffs. Vet Radiol Ultrasound 2006, 47(1):72-77.
Padgett GA, Mostosky UV. The mode of inheritance of craniomandibular osteopathy in West Highland White terrier dogs. Am J Med Genet 1986, 25(1):9-13.
Pastor KF, Boulay JP, Schelling SH, Carpenter JL. Idiopathic hyperostosis of the calvaria in five young bullmastiffs. JAAHA 2000, 36(5):439-445.
Taylor SM, Remedios A, Myers S. Craniomandibular osteopathy in a Shetland sheepdog. Can Vet J 1995, 36(7):437-439.
Watson ADJ, Adams WM, Thomas CB. Craniomandibular osteopathy in dogs. Compend Contin Educ Pract Vet 1995, 17:911-921.

Autores Steven M. Cogar e Spencer A. Johnston
Consultor Editorial Peter K. Shires
Agradecimento Os autores e editores agradecem as contribuições feitas por Peter D. Schwarz e Peter K. Shires, que foram os autores deste capítulo nas edições anteriores.

Osteopatia Hipertrófica

CONSIDERAÇÕES GERAIS

REVISÃO
- Resulta de alterações do fluxo sanguíneo periférico e neoproliferação óssea periosteal em locais onde a concentração de oxigênio é baixa ao longo da região diafisária de ossos longos, começando muitas vezes nas falanges distais, metacarpos e metatarsos.
- Patogenia — especulativa; teorias: anoxia crônica, toxinas obscuras, hiperestrogenismo e mecanismos reflexos neurovasculares autônomos mediados pelos ramos aferentes do vago ou de nervos intercostais.
- Em geral, é considerada como uma manifestação de processo patológico intratorácico ou intra-abdominal primário.
- Acomete o sistema musculosquelético.
- Ocorre uma forma primária em seres humanos.

IDENTIFICAÇÃO
- Mais comum em cães do que em gatos.
- Idade de maior frequência — 8 anos; coincide com a incidência máxima de neoplasias.
- Idade média — 5,6 anos no caso de cães com lesões pulmonares não neoplásicas.

SINAIS CLÍNICOS
Achados Anamnésicos
- Inquietação.
- Relutância ao movimento.
- Aumento de volume da parte distal dos membros.

Achados do Exame Físico
- Claudicação, feridas/escaras e membros doloridos.
- Membros — aumentados e firmes ao toque; sem edema.
- Edema — predominantemente abaixo do nível das articulações dos cotovelos e jarretes, estendendo-se distalmente para os artelhos.

CAUSAS E FATORES DE RISCO
- Tumores pulmonares primários e metastáticos.
- Condições torácicas não neoplásicas — pneumonia; dirofilariose; cardiopatia congênita ou adquirida; corpos estranhos brônquicos; infestação esofágica por *Spirocerca lupi*; atelectasia pulmonar focal.
- Sarcoma esofágico.
- Rabdomiossarcoma embrionário da bexiga.
- Adenocarcinoma do fígado ou da próstata.
- Mesoteliomas torácicos e abdominais.

DIAGNÓSTICO

DIAGNÓSTICO DIFERENCIAL
- Osteomielite — assimétrico e, em geral, edematoso; lise; histórico de traumatismo penetrante ou infecção sistêmica.
- Neoplasia metastática — assimétrica.

HEMOGRAMA/BIOQUÍMICA/URINÁLISE
- Dependem da causa subjacente.
- Fosfatase alcalina sérica — pode estar elevada.

OUTROS TESTES LABORATORIAIS
Ultrassonografia — ajuda a identificar e diferenciar lesões primárias.

DIAGNÓSTICO POR IMAGEM
- Radiografias dos ossos longos acometidos — ampla neoformação óssea periosteal bilateral simétrica e rugosa nas regiões diafisárias; lesões em brotos projetam-se para fora do córtex e perpendicularmente ao eixo longitudinal; forma-se novo osso periosteal em torno de toda a circunferência do osso; articulações não são acometidas.
- Radiografias das cavidades torácica e abdominal — indicadas; identificam a causa subjacente.

MÉTODOS DIAGNÓSTICOS
Biopsia óssea e cultura (bacteriana e fúngica) — necessárias apenas em casos atípicos; indicadas para excluir neoplasia e osteomielite.

TRATAMENTO
- Voltado para a causa primária subjacente.
- Opções em casos selecionados — vagotomia unilateral no lado de uma lesão pulmonar; incisão através da pleura parietal; ressecção de costela subperiosteal; vagotomia cervical bilateral.

MEDICAÇÕES

MEDICAMENTO(S)
- Dependem da causa subjacente.
- Glicocorticoides (p. ex., prednisona) — podem ser usados para melhorar os sinais clínicos e diminuir a extensão do edema.
- Analgésicos — conforme a necessidade.

CONTRAINDICAÇÕES/INTERAÇÕES POSSÍVEIS
N/D.

ACOMPANHAMENTO

MONITORIZAÇÃO DO PACIENTE
- Quando a condição indica outro processo patológico — é importante reconhecer a necessidade de outros testes diagnósticos para identificar a causa primária.
- Eliminação da causa desencadeante — pode levar à regressão dos sinais clínicos.

EVOLUÇÃO ESPERADA E PROGNÓSTICO
- Alterações ósseas — podem levar vários meses para regredir.
- Prognóstico — reservado a mau devido à ocorrência comum de causas neoplásicas.

DIVERSOS

SINÔNIMO(S)
- Osteopatia pulmonar hipertrófica.
- Osteoartropatia pulmonar hipertrófica.
- Osteoartropatia hipertrófica.

Sugestões de Leitura

Anderson TP, Walker MC, Goring RL. Cardiogenic hypertrophic osteopathy in a dog with a right-to-left shunting patent ductus arteriosus. JAVMA 2004, 224(9):1464-1466, 1453.

Crumlish PT, Sweeney T, Jones B, Angles JM. Hypertrophic osteodystrophy in the Weimaraner dog: Lack of association between DQA1 alleles of the canine MHC and hypertrophic osteodystrophy. Vet J 2006, 171(2):308-313.

de Melo Ocarino N, Fukushima FB, de Matos Gomes A, Bueno DF, de Oliveira TS, Serakides R. Idiopathic hypertrophic osteopathy in a cat. J Feline Med Surg 2006, 8(5):345-348.

Demko J, McLaughlin R. Developmental orthopedic disease. Vet Clin North Am Small Anim Pract 2005, 35(5):1111-1135.

Dunn ME, Blond L, Letard D, Difruscia R. Hypertrophic osteopathy associated with infective endocarditis in an adult boxer dog. J Small Anim Pract 2007, 48(2):99-103.

Foster SF. Idiopathic hypertrophic osteopathy in a cat. J Feline Med Surg 2007, 9(2):172-173.

Foster WK, Armstrong JA. Hypertrophic osteopathy associated with pulmonary Eikenella corrodens infection in a dog. JAVMA 2006, 228(9):1366-1369.

Halliwell WH. Tumorlike lesions of bone. In: Bojrab MJ, ed., Disease Mechanisms in Small Animal Surgery. Philadelphia: Lea & Febiger, 1993, pp. 933-934.

Watrous BJ, Blumenfeld B. Congenital megaesophagus with hypertrophic osteopathy in a 6-year-old dog. Vet Radiol Ultrasound 2002, 43(6):545-549.

Autor Peter K. Shires
Consultor Editorial Peter K. Shires
Agradecimento O autor e os editores agradecem a colaboração de Peter D. Schwarz, que foi o autor deste capítulo em uma edição mais antiga.

OSTEOSSARCOMA

CONSIDERAÇÕES GERAIS

DEFINIÇÃO
Trata-se do tumor ósseo primário mais comum nos cães. Acomete tipicamente o esqueleto apendicular de raças caninas de porte grande a gigante. O comportamento biológico dessa neoplasia é maligno, com metástases pulmonares microscópicas em ≥90% dos cães no momento do diagnóstico. Essa doença é menos comum nos gatos, mas o comportamento biológico nessa espécie é menos agressivo do que nos cães.

FISIOPATOLOGIA
Implantes metálicos, genética e histórico de radioterapia prévia sobre o local são, sem exceção, associados ao desenvolvimento de osteossarcoma em cães.

SISTEMA(S) ACOMETIDO(S)
• Musculosquelético — o esqueleto apendicular (região metafisária de ossos longos) é mais comumente acometido nos cães. O osteossarcoma também pode ocorrer no esqueleto axial.
• Respiratório — essa neoplasia espalha-se por via hematógena; o local mais comum de metástase é o pulmão, mas outros locais incluem os ossos e tecidos moles, como pele, rins e fígado.

GENÉTICA
Há forte predileção racial, com certo grau de hereditariedade identificado em raças gigantes, como Deerhound escocês e Wolfhound irlandês.

INCIDÊNCIA/PREVALÊNCIA
• Cães — o osteossarcoma responde por até 85% dos tumores ósseos primários em cães, representando cerca de 5% de todos os processos malignos relatados nessa espécie.
• Gatos — o osteossarcoma constitui o tumor ósseo primário mais comum em gatos, respondendo por menos de 7% de todos os cânceres relatados nessa espécie.

IDENTIFICAÇÃO
Espécies
Cães e gatos.

Raça(s) Predominante(s)
• Cães — raças de porte grande a gigante.
• Gatos — doméstico de pelo curto.

Idade Média e Faixa Etária
• Cães — pico bimodal dos 2 aos 7 anos; ocorrência relatada em animais jovens de até 6 meses de vida.
• Gatos — idade média, 8 anos e meio; faixa, 4-18 anos.

Sexo Predominante
Cães e gatos — não há forte predileção sexual.

SINAIS CLÍNICOS
Comentários Gerais
• Como o osteossarcoma costuma ocorrer no esqueleto apendicular de cães e gatos, os achados clínicos comuns são tumefação, claudicação e dor.
• As lesões do esqueleto axial podem ser mais sutis, com tumefação localizada, massa palpável ou dor como características clínicas-chave.

Achados Anamnésicos
• Claudicação (aguda ou crônica) é o problema mais comum.
• Os sinais de osteossarcoma do esqueleto axial variam, dependendo do local da lesão.
• Outras queixas incluem inapetência e letargia.

Achados do Exame Físico
• Nos casos de osteossarcoma do esqueleto axial, é comum a presença de tumefação firme e dolorosa do local acometido.
• O grau de claudicação varia desde incapacidade parcial até total de sustentar o peso.
• Raramente, os animais se apresentarão com fratura patológica.
• Podem ser observados os sinais de tumefação nos tecidos moles sobre a área acometida e linfedema.

CAUSAS
Desconhecidas em ambas as espécies.

FATORES DE RISCO
• Cães — raças de porte grande a gigante estão sob maior risco.
• Castração em uma idade precoce.
• Implantes metálicos nos locais de reparo de fraturas.
• Histórico de exposição à radiação ionizante.
• Gatos — desconhecidos.

DIAGNÓSTICO

DIAGNÓSTICO DIFERENCIAL
• Outros tumores ósseos primários (i. e., fibrossarcoma, condrossarcoma).
• Tumores ósseos metastáticos (i. e., carcinoma prostático, mamário ou outros carcinomas).
• Processos infecciosos (i. e., osteomielite fúngica ou bacteriana).

HEMOGRAMA/BIOQUÍMICA/URINÁLISE
• Elevações da fosfatase alcalina representam um fator prognóstico mau.
• É importante realizar esses exames para avaliar o estado de saúde geral antes de iniciar a terapia.

DIAGNÓSTICO POR IMAGEM
Radiografias do Local Primário
• É recomendável a obtenção de, no mínimo, duas projeções da lesão primária (i. e., anteroposterior e lateral para os locais apendiculares de acometimento).
• Os achados típicos incluem lise óssea e neoproliferação óssea na região metafisária dos ossos longos.
• Com frequência, há tumefação significativa dos tecidos moles.
• Raramente, o osteossarcoma envolve ambos os lados de uma cavidade articular.

Radiografias Torácicas
• Sempre é aconselhável a obtenção de três projeções radiográficas do tórax (lateral direita e esquerda, além de dorsoventral), embora a doença metastática visível esteja presente em <10% dos casos no momento da consulta.
• Se metástases pulmonares forem identificadas no diagnóstico inicial, o prognóstico será mais grave.
• As lesões metastáticas tipicamente aparecem sob a forma de nódulos isolados e arredondados, com densidade de tecido mole.

Cintilografias Ósseas Nucleares
• Podem ser úteis para identificar doença metastática dos tecidos ósseo ou mole mais precocemente do que as radiografias simples.
• Esse exame não diferencia entre locais de traumatismo prévio ou inflamação e neoplasia metastática.
• Não é uma técnica comumente utilizada.

MÉTODOS DIAGNÓSTICOS
Aspirado Ósseo
• Procedimento relativamente não invasivo de alta recuperação, realizado com o uso de agulha de calibre 18 para retirar as células do local do tumor.
• A avaliação citológica pode fornecer um diagnóstico de neoplasia mesenquimal maligna.

ACHADOS PATOLÓGICOS
• Macroscópicos — destruição leve a grave do osso cortical com neoproliferação óssea.
• Histológicos — população maligna de células mesenquimais, que são arredondadas e poligonais a fusiformes. A produção de osteoide é um achado diagnóstico para osteossarcoma. Não foi demonstrado que as subclassificações em osteoblástico, condroblástico ou telangiectásico sejam consistentemente prognósticas. O osteossarcoma parosteal (justacortical) é uma variante de tecido mole raramente observada, que pode ter um comportamento biológico menos agressivo do que outras formas de osteossarcoma.

TRATAMENTO

CUIDADO(S) DE SAÚDE ADEQUADO(S)
Internação versus Tratamento Ambulatorial
• A avaliação diagnóstica é feita em um esquema ambulatorial.
• A cirurgia e o primeiro tratamento quimioterápico (se concomitante) são efetuados com o paciente internado.
• As doses subsequentes de quimioterapia são realizadas em um esquema ambulatorial.

ATIVIDADE
Restrita após a cirurgia até que tenha ocorrido cicatrização adequada.

DIETA
Não há necessidade de qualquer modificação específica da dieta, embora a perda de peso possa beneficiar os amputados em geral.

ORIENTAÇÃO AO PROPRIETÁRIO
• O prognóstico a longo prazo é mau.
• Os proprietários precisam entender que os objetivos terapêuticos são aliviar o desconforto e prolongar a vida, pois a cura é improvável.
• Além disso, os proprietários devem ficar preparados para os possíveis efeitos colaterais induzidos pela quimioterapia.

CONSIDERAÇÕES CIRÚRGICAS
Cães — Pontos Apendiculares
• O manejo cirúrgico convencional envolve a amputação do membro acometido (desarticulação do quarto anterior ou do quadril).
• Terapia de recuperação do membro está disponível em um número restrito de hospitais de referência. Essa técnica é adequada apenas para lesões radiais distais. O tumor primário é removido por meio cirúrgico, substituído por aloenxerto e estabilizado com placa óssea.
• Quimioterapia adjuvante é recomendada após qualquer procedimento cirúrgico (ver adiante).

Cães — Pontos Axiais
• Dependendo da localização, a excisão cirúrgica rigorosa e a quimioterapia adjuvante são recomendadas (ver adiante).
• O osteossarcoma mandibular pode ter um comportamento biológico menos agressivo do que em outros locais; um único estudo relatou um

Osteossarcoma

tempo médio de sobrevida de 71% em 1 ano apenas com a cirurgia. No entanto, estudos recentes sugerem que o osteossarcoma originário da mandíbula seja altamente metastático, justificando o tratamento com quimioterapia adjuvante.

Gatos — Pontos Apendiculares
• Somente a amputação é considerada apropriada.
• Tipicamente, a terapia adjuvante não é necessária.

Gatos — Pontos Axiais
• Dependendo do local da lesão, deve-se tentar a excisão cirúrgica rigorosa.
• A recidiva local parece ser a principal razão para a falha terapêutica.

Metastectomia
• O procedimento de metastectomia pulmonar foi descrito para cães com osteossarcoma.
• Os critérios de seleção para os cães serem submetidos a esse procedimento incluem longo intervalo livre de doença (>300 dias) e apenas 1-2 nódulos pulmonares ao exame de TC.

Neoplasias Inoperáveis
• Radioterapia paliativa (fracionamento grosseiro).
• O controle da dor com medicamentos anti-inflamatórios não esteroides, opioides ou bisfosfonatos pode melhorar a qualidade de vida e, assim, prolongar a sobrevida.

MEDICAÇÕES

MEDICAMENTO(S) DE ESCOLHA
Tratamento Definitivo
• Quimioterapia com medicamentos à base de platina (cisplatina ou carboplatina) ou doxorrubicina constitui o padrão atual de cuidado; é recomendável, no mínimo, 4 doses.
• Agentes como cisplatina, carboplatina ou doxorrubicina consistem no padrão de cuidado.
• Cisplatina — 70 mg/m^2 IV a cada 3 semanas. Esse medicamento deve ser administrado com diurese induzida por soro fisiológico, para evitar nefrotoxicidade: 18,3 mL/kg/h por 4 h; administrar a quimioterapia em 20 min; em seguida, continuar a diurese por mais 2 h. A cisplatina provocará vômito dentro de 2 h da administração. É imprescindível a administração de antieméticos antes da cisplatina; talvez haja necessidade da prescrição de terapia antiemética para o paciente que recebeu alta.
• Carboplatina — 300 mg/m^2 IV a cada 3 semanas.
• Doxorrubicina — na dose de 30 mg/m^2 IV a cada 3 semanas por cinco doses representa a opção terapêutica mais barata; pode ser utilizada em combinação com a cisplatina.

• A quimioterapia não é eficaz contra doença macroscópica.
• Tipicamente, a quimioterapia é instituída em até 2 semanas após a cirurgia.

CONTRAINDICAÇÕES
• Os pacientes com disfunção renal preexistente não devem ser tratados com quimioterápicos à base de platina.
• Não administrar a cisplatina aos gatos.

PRECAUÇÕES
• Evitar os cateteres e as agulhas de alumínio ou de metal, porque esse tipo de material interfere na atividade dos medicamentos contendo platina.
• Buscar por orientação antes de iniciar o tratamento se não estiver familiarizado com medicamentos citotóxicos.

MEDICAMENTO(S) ALTERNATIVO(S)
Tratamento Paliativo
• O controle da dor deve ser feito em pacientes cujos proprietários recusem o tratamento definitivo.
• A dor é controlada com o uso de agentes anti-inflamatórios não esteroides, ± tramadol (2-5 mg/kg a cada 8-12 h), ± paracetamol com codeína (0,5-2 mg/kg a cada 8-12 h), ± fentanila transdérmica (conforme as instruções da embalagem).
• Eutanásia quando a qualidade de vida declina.

ACOMPANHAMENTO

MONITORIZAÇÃO DO PACIENTE
• Monitorar o hemograma completo em busca de indícios de mielossupressão 10-14 dias após a quimioterapia.
• Doxorrubicina — efetuar exames periódicos de ecocardiografia e ECG, já que a cardiotoxicidade cumulativa pode ocorrer com ≥180 mg/m^2.
• Obter radiografias torácicas a cada 2-3 meses após a cirurgia para avaliar a presença de metástases.
• Tirar radiografias do local da cirurgia a cada 2-3 meses para monitorizar a ocorrência de recidiva local após recuperação do membro.

COMPLICAÇÕES POSSÍVEIS
• É muito provável a ocorrência de metástase; os locais de disseminação incluem pulmões, outros ossos, tecidos moles.
• Pode ocorrer osteopatia hipertrófica secundariamente a metástases pulmonares.
• Os animais submetidos à recuperação do membro podem desenvolver infecções recidivantes, recidivas locais ou falha de implantes.
• Os amputados raramente exibem complicações secundárias à artropatia degenerativa em outros membros.

EVOLUÇÃO ESPERADA E PROGNÓSTICO
Cães
• A sobrevida média gira em torno de 4 meses sem tratamento, apenas com amputação ou somente com radioterapia paliativa.
• A sobrevida média é prolongada para 10 meses com cirurgia e quimioterapia.

Gatos
• A sobrevida média é >2 anos em casos de osteossarcoma apendicular submetido à cirurgia.
• A sobrevida média é de 5 meses e meio para osteossarcoma axial que passou por intervenção cirúrgica.

DIVERSOS

GESTAÇÃO/FERTILIDADE/REPRODUÇÃO
Não acasalar os animais que estejam passando por quimioterapia.

SINÔNIMO(S)
• Sarcoma histiocítico (osso).
• Sarcoma osteogênico.

VER TAMBÉM
• Condrossarcoma do Osso.
• Fibrossarcoma do Osso.
• Hemangiossarcoma do Osso.

ABREVIATURA(S)
• ECG = eletrocardiograma.
• TC = tomografia computadorizada.

Sugestões de Leitura
Bergman PJ, MacEwen EG, Phillips B, Powers BE, Dernell WS, et al. Use of single-agent carboplatin as adjuvant or neoadjuvant therapy in conjunction with amputation for appendicular osteosarcoma in dogs. JAAHA 2009, 45:33-38.
Green EM, AdamsWM, Forrest LJ. Four fraction palliative radiotherapy for osteosarcoma in 24 dogs. JAAHA 2002, 38:445-451.
Heldmann E, Anderson MA, Wagner-Mann C. Feline osteosarcoma: 145 cases (1990-1995). JAAHA 2000, 36:518-521.
Lascelles BD, Dernell WS, Correa MT, et al. Improved survival associated with postoperative wound infection in dogs treated with limb-salvage surgery for osteosarcoma. Ann Surg Oncol 2005, 12:1073-1083.
Straw RC, Withrow SJ, Richter SL, et al. Amputation and cisplatin for treatment of canine osteosarcoma. J Vet Intern Med 1991, 5:205-210.

Autor Ruthanne Chun
Consultor Editorial Timothy M. Fan

OTITE EXTERNA E MÉDIA

CONSIDERAÇÕES GERAIS

DEFINIÇÃO
- Otite externa — inflamação do canal auditivo externo; inclui estruturas anatômicas do pavilhão auricular, canais horizontais e verticais, bem como a parede externa da membrana timpânica.
- Otite média — inflamação da orelha média; inclui estruturas anatômicas da parede medial da membrana timpânica, bula (cavidade timpânica), ossículos da orelha e tuba auditiva.
- Os termos não são diagnósticos, mas descrições de sinais clínicos.

FISIOPATOLOGIA
- Otite externa — a inflamação crônica resulta em alterações no ambiente normal do canal; o canal da orelha externa é revestido por epitélio que contém glândulas apócrinas modificadas (cerume); as glândulas aumentam de tamanho e produzem cera em excesso; a epiderme e a derme sofrem espessamento e ficam fibrosadas; as dobras espessadas do canal reduzem de modo efetivo a largura desse canal; a calcificação da cartilagem auricular é o resultado do estágio final.
- Otite média — com frequência, corresponde a uma extensão da otite externa e, muitas vezes, ocorre sem a ruptura do tímpano; pode ocorrer a partir de pólipos ou de neoplasia dentro da orelha média ou da tuba auditiva.

SISTEMA(S) ACOMETIDO(S)
- Cutâneo/exócrino.
- Nervoso.

DISTRIBUIÇÃO GEOGRÁFICA
A umidade do ambiente pode predispor à infecção.

IDENTIFICAÇÃO
Espécies
Cães e gatos.

Raça(s) Predominante(s)
- Cães com orelhas pendulares — sobretudo os das raças Spaniel e Retriever.
- Cães com canais externos hirsutos — raças Terrier e Poodle.
- Estenose do canal auditivo externo — na raça Shar-pei.

SINAIS CLÍNICOS
Comentários Gerais
- Otite média secretora primária — Cavalier King Charles spaniel.
- Otite externa — frequentemente constitui um sintoma secundário de doença subjacente.
- Infecção — com exsudato purulento e fétido.
- Inflamação — dor, prurido e eritema com ou sem exsudatos.
- Otite externa crônica (cães) — resulta em ruptura da membrana timpânica (71%) e otite média (82%).

Achados Anamnésicos
- Dor — animal arisco em relação a toque na cabeça ou recusa à abertura da boca.
- Meneios (sacudidas) de cabeça.
- Arranhões no pavilhão auricular.
- Orelhas com odor desagradável.
- Déficits do sistema vestibular periférico ou do nervo facial por extensão para a orelha interna.

Achados do Exame Físico
Otite Externa
- Vermelhidão e tumefação do canal externo, levando à estenose.
- Descamação e exsudação — podem resultar na presença de odor fétido e obstrução do canal.
- Sinais vestibulares indicam o desenvolvimento da otite média/interna.
- Surdez decorrente da obstrução.
- Exsudatos purulentos e fétidos.
- Inflamação, dor, prurido e eritema dos pavilhões auriculares e dos canais externos.
- Hematoma aural.
- Cicatriz palpável e calcificação da cartilagem auricular.
- Manutenção do pavilhão auricular em posição abaixada e/ou inclinação da cabeça para o lado acometido (se unilateral).

Otite Média
- Membrana timpânica intacta: abaulamento do tecido com evidência de líquido e/ou gás caudalmente; a membrana pode estar opaca; o líquido pode ser purulento ou hemorrágico.
- Membrana timpânica rompida: secreção em direção ao canal ou bula preenchida de debris.
- Surdez.
- Dor à palpação da bula ou à abertura da boca.
- Faringite, tonsilite ou secreção através da tuba auditiva.
- Linfadenopatia em casos graves ou crônicos.

CAUSAS
Causas Predisponentes
- As causas predisponentes alteram o ambiente do canal auditivo, facilitando o processo de inflamação e promovendo o aparecimento de infecção secundária.
  - Conformação anormal do canal externo ou relacionada com a raça (p. ex., estenose, hirsutismo e pavilhão pendular) limita o fluxo de ar adequado para o canal — ver "Raça(s) Predominante(s)".
  - Umidade excessiva (p. ex., por natação ou limpezas frequentes com soluções inadequadas); obediência exagerada do proprietário às recomendações de limpeza da orelha.
  - Reação e irritação a medicamento tópico, além de traumatismo por técnicas abrasivas de limpeza.
  - Doenças sistêmicas subjacentes produzem anormalidades no ambiente e na resposta imune do canal auditivo.

Causas Primárias
- As causas primárias desencadeiam ou causam diretamente inflamação dentro do canal auditivo:
  - Parasitas (otite externa) — *Otodectes cynotis*, *Demodex* spp., *Sarcoptes* e *Notoedres*, além de *Otobius megnini*.
  - Hipersensibilidades — atopia, alergia alimentar, alergia de contato e reação sistêmica ou local a medicamento.
  - Corpos estranhos — farpas de plantas.
  - Obstruções — neoplasia, pólipos, hiperplasia das glândulas ceruminosas e acúmulo de pelos; também podem ser um evento secundário.
  - Otite externa/média unilateral e persistente/recidivante é um quadro mais suspeito de obstrução, corpo estranho ou crescimento.
  - Distúrbios de queratinização e produção aumentada de cerume — obstrução funcional do canal auditivo.
  - Doenças autoimunes — frequentemente acometem os pavilhões auriculares; às vezes, envolvem o canal auditivo externo.
  - Otite média secretora primária.

Causas Perpetuantes
- As causas perpetuantes impedem a resolução do processo inflamatório e/ou infeccioso do canal auditivo:
  - Infecção bacteriana — *Staphylococcus pseudintermedius, Pseudomonas aeruginosa, Enterococcus* spp., *Proteus mirabilis, Streptococcus* spp., *Corynebacteria* spp., e *Escherichia coli*.
  - *Pseudomonas aeruginosa* é obtida mais comumente à cultura em casos de otite média.
  - Infecção por fungos/leveduras: *Malassezia pachydermatis, Candida albicans* e, raramente, outros fungos (*Sporothrix schenckii, Cryptococcus neoformans*).
  - Alteração crônica: estenose do canal auditivo em função de hiperplasia das glândulas ceruminosas e formação de pólipo(s), tumefação por inflamação, formação cicatricial e calcificação. A alteração crônica aumenta a retenção de debris na orelha por produção elevada de cerume e remoção diminuída por migração epidérmica e obstrução física.

DIAGNÓSTICO

HEMOGRAMA/BIOQUÍMICA/URINÁLISE
Podem indicar alguma doença subjacente primária.

OUTROS TESTES LABORATORIAIS
Teste de Alergia
- Teste com dieta hipoalergênica (ou seja, com restrição de ingrediente) para hipersensibilidade alimentar.
- Teste intradérmico para atopia.

DIAGNÓSTICO POR IMAGEM
- Radiografias das bulas timpânicas: podem estar normais; as bulas podem parecer turvas se estiverem preenchidas de exsudato; observa-se espessamento da bula e/ou da parte petrosa do osso temporal com doença crônica; presença de osteólise com osteomielite ou doença neoplásica.
- TC ou RM: evidências detalhadas da densidade de líquido ou tecido mole na bula timpânica, nos tecidos adjacentes ou na tuba auditiva; o exame de TC é mais útil para alterações ósseas, enquanto o de RM é mais proveitoso para avaliação da membrana timpânica e dos tecidos moles.

MÉTODOS DIAGNÓSTICOS
- Otoscopia direta: visualização do canal auditivo externo, da membrana timpânica e da bula (em caso de ruptura do tímpano).
- Video-otoscopia: confere a imagem ampliada do canal auditivo e a coleta mais controlada de amostra.
- Raspados cutâneos dos pavilhões auriculares: para pesquisa de parasitas.
- Biopsia cutânea: para avaliação de doença autoimune, neoplasia ou hiperplasia das glândulas ceruminosas.
- Cultura do exsudato: útil em casos de infecção persistente; mais indicada quando se observam bastonetes no exame citológico.

Otite Externa e Média

- Exame microscópico do exsudato da orelha: única ferramenta diagnóstica mais importante após o exame completo do canal auditivo.
- Aparência do exsudato: infecções por leveduras comumente produzem exsudato espesso amarelo-acastanhado; infecções por bactérias costumam gerar exsudato fino castanho-escuro; entretanto, a aparência física do exsudato não permite o diagnóstico preciso do tipo de infecção; portanto, é necessário o exame microscópico.
- As infecções dentro do canal podem sofrer alterações com o tratamento prolongado ou recorrente; dessa forma, a repetição do exame do exsudato auricular é necessária nos casos crônicos.
- Miringotomia: consiste na inserção de agulha espinal ou cateter estéril através da membrana timpânica para coleta de amostra de líquido dentro da bula com o objetivo de realizar o exame citológico e a cultura.

Exame Microscópico
- Preparações: fazer de ambos os canais (o conteúdo de cada canal pode não ser o mesmo); espalhar as amostras finamente em lâmina de microscópio; examinar as amostras sem corante e com corante de Wright modificado.
- Ácaros: diagnóstico presuntivo.
- Tipo(s) de bactérias ou leveduras: auxiliam na escolha do tratamento, além de determinar a necessidade de cultura.
- Anotar os achados (tipos de microrganismos; presença de células) no prontuário; classificar o número de microrganismos e o tipo de células presentes em uma escala padronizada (p. ex., de 0-4) para permitir a monitorização terapêutica.
- Leucócitos dentro do exsudato: indica infecção ativa; talvez haja indicação de terapia sistêmica.

TRATAMENTO

ORIENTAÇÃO AO PROPRIETÁRIO
Ensinar aos proprietários, por demonstração, o método adequado de limpar e medicar as orelhas (sobretudo o volume da medicação a ser instilada).

CONSIDERAÇÕES CIRÚRGICAS
- Indicada quando o canal se encontra com estenose ou obstrução graves ou quando se diagnostica neoplasia ou pólipo.
- Otite média grave e irresponsiva pode necessitar de osteotomia ou ablação das bulas timpânicas.

MEDICAÇÕES

MEDICAMENTO(S) DE ESCOLHA

Soluções de Limpeza
- A integridade do tímpano deve ser avaliada antes da introdução de soluções e/ou medicamentos no canal auditivo externo.
- Em caso de tímpano não intacto: irrigações com solução salina e ácido acético a 2,5% (vinagre e água na diluição de 1:1).
- Ceruminolíticos — sulfossuccinato sódico de dioctila, esqualina, propilenoglicol.
- Antissépticos — ácido acético ou gliconato de clorexidina a 0,2%. O Tris-EDTA tem propriedades antibacterianas e sinérgicas com certos antibióticos.
- Adstringentes — álcool isopropílico, ácido bórico, ácido salicílico.
- Agentes anti-infecciosos/parasiticidas são específicos para o(s) microrganismo(s) identificado(s).

Irrigação das Orelhas
- Talvez haja necessidade de sedação em casos dolorosos e para evitar traumatismo adicional ao canal auditivo.
- É recomendável o uso de soluções suaves inicialmente.
- Seringa de bulbo ou cateter de borracha vermelha de French adequadamente aparado é utilizado para irrigar a solução e remover os debris.
- Repetir a limpeza em uma frequência gradativamente decrescente durante a terapia.
- Evitar irrigações vigorosas da orelha em casos de otite média/interna.

Sistêmicos
- O exame citológico dos exsudatos ajudará a determinar o tipo de medicação sistêmica necessária.
- A inflamação perpetua a doença, exigindo terapia anti-inflamatória.
- Otite média e otite externa crônica/grave devem ser tratadas com medicação sistêmica por no mínimo 4-6 semanas.
- Antibióticos — devem ser selecionados com base nos resultados da cultura e do antibiograma em casos de otite recorrente.
  - Cocos — cefalexina (22 mg/kg a cada 12 h), amoxicilina tri-idratada/clavulanato de potássio (10-15 mg/kg a cada 12 h) e cloranfenicol (55 mg/kg a cada 8 h). Clindamicina (11 mg/kg a cada 24 a 12 h) para envolvimento ósseo.
  - Bastonetes — fluoroquinolonas: enrofloxacino (10-20 mg/kg a cada 12 h para cães; 5 mg/kg/dia para gatos), ciprofloxacino (10-25 mg/kg a cada 12 h), marbofloxacino (5,5 mg/kg/dia). Aminoglicosídeo: amicacina (20 mg/kg/dia). β-lactâmicos: ticarcilina (10-15 mg/kg a cada 12 a 8 h), imipeném, ceftazidima.
- Antifúngicos — devem ser utilizados com terapia tópica também. Cetoconazol (5 mg/kg a cada 24 a 12 h) e itraconazol (5 mg/kg/dia).
- Anti-inflamatórios — dosagens gradativamente reduzidas: prednisolona (0,5-1 mg/kg/dia), dexametasona (0,1 mg/kg/dia), triancinolona (0,1 mg/kg/dia).
- Antiparasitários — ivermectina (300 mcg/kg VO 1-2 semanas por 4 tratamentos), selamectina, moxidectina (ver "Contraindicações" adiante).

Tópicos
- Terapia tópica é fundamental para a resolução e o controle da otite externa.
- Limpar completamente o canal auditivo externo dos debris; a irrigação completa sob anestesia geral fica reservada aos pacientes que não cooperam ou para os casos graves, incluindo a otite média.
- Continuar as limpezas frequentes até que os sintomas desapareçam e, em seguida, de forma rotineira para manter o controle.
- Aplicar medicações tópicas apropriadas com frequência e em quantidade suficiente para tratar todo o canal de modo completo.
- É preciso ter cuidado ao usar medicamentos com tímpano rompido.
- As pomadas e loções podem ser oclusivas a menos que utilizadas com critério; as soluções são preferidas.
- Antibióticos — escolhidos com base na avaliação citológica, nos resultados de cultura/antibiograma e/ou utilizados de forma empírica. Gentamicina, neomicina, amicacina, enrofloxacino e sulfadiazina de prata. Além disso, pode-se optar pelo uso de cloranfenicol e tobramicina.
- Antifúngicos — imidazóis: clotrimazol, cetoconazol, miconazol, tiabendazol. Além disso, existem a nistatina e a terbinafina.
- Anti-inflamatórios — corticosteroides: dexametasona, fluocinolona, betametasona, triancinolona e mometasona.
- Antiparasitários — ivermectina, amitraz e tiabendazol.
- Resistência aos medicamentos — fazer cultura e antibiograma do exsudato auricular; recentemente, foi demonstrado que suspensões de sulfadiazina de prata sejam eficazes.

CONTRAINDICAÇÕES
- Tímpano rompido — ter cuidado com produtos tópicos de limpeza além da solução salina estéril ou ácido acético diluído e antibióticos aminoglicosídeos; o potencial de ototoxicidade é preocupante; controverso.
- Ivermectina — não aprovada pela FDA para uso por via sistêmica; as raças caninas de pastoreio apresentam sensibilidade elevada às avermectinas por conta da mutação do gene MDR1.

PRECAUÇÕES
- Ter extrema cautela ao limpar os canais auditivos externos de todos os animais com otite externa crônica e grave, porque o tímpano pode ser facilmente rompido.
- Apesar de serem geralmente temporárias, as complicações vestibulares pós-irrigação nos gatos são comuns; avisar os proprietários de possíveis complicações e efeitos residuais.

INTERAÇÕES POSSÍVEIS
- Várias medicações tópicas raramente induzem irritação por contato ou resposta alérgica; reavaliar todos os casos com piora do quadro.
- O uso de corticosteroide é controverso com otite média/interna.

ACOMPANHAMENTO

MONITORIZAÇÃO DO PACIENTE
A repetição dos exames do exsudato pode auxiliar no monitoramento da infecção.

PREVENÇÃO
- Limpeza de rotina da orelha pelo proprietário.
- Controle das doenças subjacentes.

COMPLICAÇÕES POSSÍVEIS
- Otite externa não controlada pode levar à otite média, surdez, vestibulopatia, celulite, paralisia do nervo facial, evolução para otite interna e raramente meningoencefalite.
- Complicações pós-irrigação do canal auditivo externo em gatos (sinais vestibulares) não são incomuns; os proprietários devem ser advertidos quanto aos possíveis efeitos residuais.

EVOLUÇÃO ESPERADA E PROGNÓSTICO
- Otite externa — com o tratamento adequado, a maior parte dos casos se resolve em 3-4 semanas; a falha na correção da causa primária subjacente resulta na recidiva.
- Fatores perpetuantes (p. ex., estenose do canal auditivo e calcificação da cartilagem auricular) não se resolverão e poderão resultar em recidiva.
- Otite média — pode demorar 6 semanas ou mais com antibióticos por via sistêmica até que

todos os sinais tenham desaparecido e a membrana timpânica tenha cicatrizado.
• Osteomielite da parte petrosa do osso temporal e da bula timpânica pode necessitar de 6-8 semanas de antibióticos.
• Os sinais vestibulares costumam melhorar dentro de 2-6 semanas.

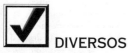 **DIVERSOS**

POTENCIAL ZOONÓTICO
• Infestações por ácaros *Sarcoptes* ou *Notoedres* podem causar prurido e dermatite passageiros em seres humanos.
• Possível transmissão de infecção por fungos (dermatofitose, esporotricose) para seres humanos.

ABREVIATURAS
• EDTA = ácido etilenodiaminotetracético.
• RM = ressonância magnética.
• TC = tomografia computadorizada.

Sugestões de Leitura
Cole LK. Systemic therapy for otitis externa and media. In: Bonagura JD, Twedt DC, eds., Kirk's Current Veterinary Therapy XIV. St. Louis: Saunders, 2009, pp. 434-436.
Logas D. Ear-flushing techniques. In: Bonagura JD, Twedt DC, eds., Kirk's Current Veterinary Therapy XIV. St. Louis: Saunders, 2009, pp. 436-438.
Mendelsohn C. Topical therapy of otitis externa. In: Bonagura JD, Twedt DC, eds., Kirk's Current Veterinary Therapy XIV. St. Louis: Saunders, 2009, pp. 428-434.

Autor Alexander H. Werner
Consultor Editorial Alexander H. Werner

Otite Média e Interna

CONSIDERAÇÕES GERAIS

DEFINIÇÃO
Inflamação das orelhas média (otite média) e interna (otite interna) mais comumente provocada por infecção bacteriana.

FISIOPATOLOGIA
• Surge com maior frequência por extensão de infecção da orelha externa através da membrana timpânica; pode se estender a partir das cavidades bucal e nasofaríngea via tuba de Eustáquio (faringotimpânica).
• Interna — também pode resultar de disseminação hematógena de alguma infecção sistêmica.

SISTEMA(S) ACOMETIDO(S)
• Gastrintestinal — afeta o paladar; decorre de lesão ao ramo parassimpático do nervo facial (cordas timpânicas), que inervam os dois terços rostrais ipsolaterais da língua.
• Nervoso — receptores vestibulococleares na orelha interna, bem como nos nervos facial, simpático (pupila) e parassimpático (glândula lacrimal) na orelha média, com possível extensão da infecção por via intracraniana.
• Oftálmico — córnea e conjuntiva, por exposição e/ou falta de produção lacrimal após lesão nervosa.

IDENTIFICAÇÃO
Espécies
Cães e gatos.

Raça(s) Predominante(s)
• Raças Cocker spaniel e outras de orelhas longas.
• Cães da raça Poodle com otite crônica ou faringite por doença dentária.

Idade Média e Faixa Etária
Qualquer idade.

SINAIS CLÍNICOS
Comentários Gerais
Dependem da gravidade e da extensão da infecção; variam de nenhum até aqueles relacionados com desconforto da bula e envolvimento do sistema nervoso.

Achados Anamnésicos
• Dor à abertura da boca; relutância para mastigar; meneios (sacudidas) de cabeça; esfregar as patas na orelha acometida.
• Inclinação da cabeça.
• O paciente pode se inclinar, mudar de direção ou rolar para o lado acometido com vestibulite periférica.
• Déficits vestibulares — persistentes, transitórios ou episódicos.
• Envolvimento bilateral — amplas excursões da cabeça, ataxia do tronco e surdez.
• Vômito e náusea — podem ocorrer durante a fase aguda.
• Lesão do nervo facial — saliva e alimento escorrendo pelos cantos da boca; incapacidade para piscar; secreção ocular.
• Anisocoria (pupila menor do lado acometido), protrusão da terceira pálpebra, enoftalmia e ptose (síndrome de Horner) — podem ser observadas.

Achados do Exame Físico
• Evidência de eritema auricular e secreção otológica, bem como de canais espessados e estenosados, indica otite externa.
• Membrana timpânica acinzentada, embaçada, opaca e saliente ao exame otoscópico indica exsudato da orelha média.
• Tártaro dentário, gengivite, tonsilite ou faringite — podem estar associados.
• Linfadenopatia mandibular ipsolateral — pode ocorrer nas infecções graves.
• Pode ser detectada dor à abertura da boca ou à palpação da bula timpânica.
• Úlcera de córnea — provocada pela incapacidade de piscar ou pelo ressecamento do olho.

Achados do Exame Neurológico
• Lesão às estruturas neurológicas associadas depende da gravidade e da localização.
• Porção vestibular do VIII par de nervos cranianos — inclinação ipsolateral da cabeça.
• Lesão bilateral do VIII par de nervos cranianos — rara; o paciente reluta a se movimentar e pode permanecer em posição agachada com amplas excursões da cabeça; nistagmo fisiológico fraco a ausente.
• Nistagmo — pode ser observado em repouso ou posicional e rotatório ou horizontal; não muda de direção.
• Estrabismo vestibular — pode-se observar desvio ventral ipsolateral do globo ocular com a extensão do pescoço.
• Podem ocorrer inclinação ipsolateral, mudança de posição, queda ou rolamento.
• Lesão do nervo facial — paresia/paralisia ipsolateral da orelha, das pálpebras, dos lábios e das narinas; a produção de lágrimas pode ficar reduzida (indicada pelo teste lacrimal de Schirmer); na paralisia crônica do nervo facial, ocorre contratura do lado acometido da face provocada por fibrose dos músculos desnervados; os déficits podem ser bilaterais.
• Cadeia simpática acometida — síndrome de Horner; sempre há miose da pupila acometida; podem-se notar protrusão da terceira pálpebra, ptose e enoftalmia.

CAUSAS
• Bactérias — agentes primários.
• Leveduras (*Malassezia* spp., *Candida* spp.) e *Aspergillus* — agentes a serem considerados.
• Ácaros — predispõem o paciente a infecções bacterianas secundárias.
• Doença unilateral — corpos estranhos, traumatismo, pólipos e tumores (p. ex., fibromas, carcinoma de células escamosas, carcinoma de glândulas ceruminosas e tumores ósseos primários).

FATORES DE RISCO
• Pólipos nasofaríngeos e neoplasia da orelha interna, média ou externa — podem predispor o paciente à infecção bacteriana.
• Irrigação vigorosa da orelha.
• Soluções de limpeza otológica (p. ex., clorexidina) — podem ser irritantes para a orelha média e interna; evitar se o tímpano estiver rompido.
• Anestesia inalatória e viagem de avião — mudança nas pressões da orelha média.

DIAGNÓSTICO

DIAGNÓSTICO DIFERENCIAL
• Sinais associados a anomalias vestibulares congênitas estão presentes desde o nascimento.
• Hipotireoidismo — pode estar associado a déficits dos VII e VIII pares de nervos cranianos; perfil anormal da tireoide (nível de T_4, T_4 livre e TSH) garante o diagnóstico.
• Vestibulopatias centrais — diferenciadas pela ocorrência de letargia, sonolência, estupor e outros sinais atribuídos ao tronco cerebral ou ao cerebelo.
• Neoplasia e pólipos nasofaríngeos — causas comuns de otite média e interna refratárias e recidivantes; diagnosticados pelo exame bucal e otológico, bem como pela obtenção de imagens da cabeça.
• Deficiência de tiamina (gatos) — sinais vestibulares centrais bilaterais; histórico de dieta exclusivamente à base de peixe ou anorexia persistente.
• Toxicidade pelo metronidazol — sinais de envolvimento cerebelar bilateral (porção vestibular) após dosagem elevada ou uso prolongado.
• Traumatismo — anamnese e evidência física de lesão.
• Vestibulopatia idiopática (cães idosos e gatos jovens a meia-idade), paralisia facial idiopática e síndrome de Horner idiopática — diagnósticos realizados por exclusão.
• *Cryptococcus* — foi relatado em associação com vestibulopatia periférica em gatos.

HEMOGRAMA/BIOQUÍMICA/URINÁLISE
• Leucocitose com desvio à esquerda — pode ser observada.
• Globulinas — podem estar elevadas se a infecção for crônica.

OUTROS TESTES LABORATORIAIS
• Hemoculturas e/ou uroculturas — podem ser positivas com fonte hematógena de infecção.
• T_4 baixa, T_4 livre com nível elevado do TSH no hipotireoidismo.

DIAGNÓSTICO POR IMAGEM
• Video-otoscopia — proporciona o exame detalhado do canal auditivo externo e da membrana timpânica; a membrana timpânica pode parecer turva na presença de exsudato na orelha média; ajuda a avaliar a integridade da membrana timpânica, permitindo a obtenção de amostras diagnósticas para os exames de citologia e cultura/antibiograma e a realização de lavagens terapêuticas do canal auditivo externo e da cavidade auricular média.
• Radiografia das bulas — não constitui um teste sensível; pode-se observar espessamento das bulas e da parte petrosa do osso temporal na doença crônica; pode-se constatar osteólise nos casos graves de osteomielite; podem estar normais.
• TC ou RM — evidência detalhada da densidade de líquido e tecido mole dentro da orelha média e extensão de envolvimento das estruturas adjacentes; o exame de TC é melhor para revelar as alterações ósseas associadas, enquanto o de RM é mais eficiente para avaliar as estruturas circunjacentes de tecido mole, incluindo o tronco cerebral e o cerebelo.

MÉTODOS DIAGNÓSTICOS
• Miringotomia — inserir uma agulha espinal (calibre 20; 6-9 cm) através do otoscópio e da membrana timpânica a fim de aspirar o líquido da orelha média para exame citológico, além de cultura e antibiograma.
• RAETC — testa a integridade funcional das vias auditivas periférica e central; detecta a perda da audição.

OTITE MÉDIA E INTERNA

- Análise do LCS — caso se observem pleocitose neutrofílica e conteúdo proteico elevado com a extensão intracraniana da infecção, fazer cultura e antibiograma.

ACHADOS PATOLÓGICOS
Exsudato purulento dentro da cavidade da orelha média, rodeado por bulas espessadas e evidência microscópica de neutrófilos degenerados com bactérias intracelulares.

TRATAMENTO

CUIDADO(S) DE SAÚDE ADEQUADO(S)
- Paciente internado — infecção debilitante grave; sinais neurológicos.
- Dar alta para os pacientes estáveis, na dependência de avaliações diagnósticas adicionais e de cirurgia, se houver indicação.

CUIDADO(S) DE ENFERMAGEM
- Fluidoterapia — se o animal não conseguir comer nem beber em função de vômitos e desorientação.
- Otite externa concomitante — fazer cultura e limpar a orelha; utilizar solução salina normal tépida (morna) se o tímpano estiver rompido; caso se faça uso de alguma solução de limpeza, acompanhar com irrigação completa com solução salina normal; secar o canal auditivo com *swab* de algodão e fazer sucção com vácuo leve; adstringentes (p. ex., Otic Domeboro® ou ácido bórico) podem ser eficazes.

ATIVIDADE
Restrita na presença de sinais vestibulares consideráveis para evitar lesão.

DIETA
- Vômito gerado por vestibulite — suspender o alimento e a água por 12-24 h.
- Desorientação grave — alimentação manual e pequenas quantidades de água com frequência; elevar a cabeça para evitar pneumonia por aspiração.

ORIENTAÇÃO AO PROPRIETÁRIO
- Informar ao proprietário sobre o fato de que a maior parte das infecções bacterianas desaparece com curso terapêutico precoce de antibióticos de amplo espectro e não sofre recidiva.
- Avisar ao proprietário sobre a possível ocorrência de sinais recidivantes, podendo haver a necessidade de drenagem cirúrgica.

CONSIDERAÇÕES CIRÚRGICAS
- Reservar a cirurgia para os pacientes que apresentam recidiva, não respondem ao tratamento ou estão piorando.
- Não confiar na gravidade dos sinais neurológicos como indicação para a intervenção cirúrgica; reservar a cirurgia para os pacientes com evidência de exsudato da orelha média, osteomielite refratária ao tratamento clínico e pólipos ou neoplasia nasofaríngeos.
- Osteotomia das bulas — permite a drenagem da cavidade da orelha média.
- Ablação da orelha pelo canal auditivo horizontal — indicada quando a otite média está associada à otite externa recidivante ou neoplasia.
- Exame citológico e cultura/antibiograma de efusão da orelha média e avaliação histopatológica de amostras de tecido anormal — realizar no momento da cirurgia.

MEDICAÇÕES

MEDICAMENTO(S) DE ESCOLHA
- Soluções antibióticas tópicas de base aquosa ou oftálmicas (em caso de ruptura da membrana timpânica) — cloranfenicol ou preparado antibiótico triplo; ou ofloxacino (Floxin®) na forma de solução otológica a cada 12 h — cães e gatos.
- Antibióticos — a longo prazo (6-8 semanas); agentes tópicos e sistêmicos são selecionados com base na cultura e no antibiograma, se disponíveis.
- Amoxicilina/ácido clavulânico (Clavamox®) — 12,5-22 mg/kg a cada 12 h VO é um bom antibiótico de primeira escolha.
- Antibióticos à base de fluoroquinolonas ou cefalosporinas de terceira geração são boas alternativas de segunda escolha ou podem ser utilizados em combinação, se os exames de cultura e antibiograma não estiverem disponíveis; enrofloxacino (Baytril® a 5-10 mg/kg a cada 24 h [cães] e 5 mg/kg a cada 24 h [gatos]) ou marbofloxacino (Zeniquin® a 5 mg/kg a cada 24 h) ou cefpodoxima (Simplicef® a 10 mg/kg a cada 12 h); clindamicina (Cleocin® a 5-30 mg/kg a cada 12 h) na suspeita de anaeróbios.
- Preparações contra náusea e enjoo — meclizina (Antivert®, Antrizine®, Bonine®, Dramamine Less Drowsy Formula®): 12,5 mg VO a cada 24 h (cães com menos de 10 kg e gatos), 25 mg VO a cada 24 h (cães com mais de 10 kg); ou citrato de maropitanto (Cerenia®) a 1 mg/kg SC ou VO (cães).

CONTRAINDICAÇÕES
- Tímpano rompido ou déficits neurológicos associados — evitar preparações de base oleosa ou irritantes da orelha externa (p. ex., clorexidina) e aminoglicosídeos, os quais são tóxicos às estruturas da orelha interna.
- Otite média ou interna — corticosteroides tópicos e sistêmicos estão contraindicados; podem exacerbar a infecção.

PRECAUÇÕES
Evitar irrigação vigorosa da orelha externa; pode causar ou exacerbar os sinais de otite média ou interna.

ACOMPANHAMENTO

MONITORIZAÇÃO DO PACIENTE
Avaliar o quadro quanto à resolução dos sinais depois de 10-14 dias ou antes disso se o paciente estiver piorando.

PREVENÇÃO
Limpeza otológica de rotina e profilaxia dos dentes — podem reduzir as possibilidades de infecção.

COMPLICAÇÕES POSSÍVEIS
- Sinais associados à lesão dos nervos vestibular (inclinação da cabeça) e facial ou síndrome de Horner (miose) — podem persistir.
- Infecções graves da orelha média/interna — podem se disseminar para o tronco cerebral.
- Osteomielite da parte petrosa do osso temporal e efusão na cavidade da orelha média — sequelas comuns de otite externa crônica grave.
- Osteotomia da bula timpânica — as complicações pós-operatórias incluem síndrome de Horner, paralisia facial e início ou exacerbação de disfunção vestibular ou surdez com infecções bilaterais.

EVOLUÇÃO ESPERADA E PROGNÓSTICO
- Otite média e interna — responsivas, em geral, ao tratamento clínico; curso terapêutico de 2 a 4 meses com antibiótico para evitar recidiva.
- Quando o tratamento clínico de otite externa for ineficaz, considerar a ressecção cirúrgica lateral da orelha.
- Sinais vestibulares — observa-se melhora em 2-6 semanas; mais rapidamente em cães de pequeno porte e gatos.

DIVERSOS

FATORES RELACIONADOS COM A IDADE
Ácaros otológicos são mais comuns em filhotes de cão e de gato.

SINÔNIMO(S)
Infecções da orelha média e interna.

VER TAMBÉM
- Inclinação da Cabeça.
- Otite Externa e Média.
- Paresia e Paralisia do Nervo Facial.
- Síndrome de Horner.

ABREVIATURA(S)
- LCS = líquido cerebrospinal.
- RAETC = resposta auditiva evocada do tronco cerebral.
- RM = ressonância magnética.
- TC = tomografia computadorizada.
- TSH = hormônio tireoestimulante.
- T_4 = tiroxina.

Sugestões de Leitura
Angus JC, Campbell KL. Uses and indications for video-otoscopy in small animal practice. Vet Clin North Am Small Anim Pract 2001, 31(4):809-828.
Garosi LS, Dennis R, Penderis J, Lamb CR, Targett MP, Cappello R, Delauche AJ. Results of magnetic resonance imaging in dogs with vestibular disorders: 85 cases (1996-1999). JAVMA 2001, 218(3):385-391.
Murphy KM. A review of techniques for the investigation of otitis externa and otitis media. Clin Tech Small Anim Pract 2001, 16:236-241.
Sturges BK, Dickinson PJ, Kortz GD, Berry WL, Vernau KM, Wisner ER, LeCouteur RA. Clinical signs, magnetic resonance imaging features, and outcome after surgical and medical treatment of otogenic intracranial infection in 11 cats and 4 dogs. J Vet Intern Med 2006, 20:648-656.

Autor Richard J. Joseph
Consultor Editorial Joane M. Parent

PANCITOPENIA

CONSIDERAÇÕES GERAIS

DEFINIÇÃO
Leucopenia, anemia arregenerativa e trombocitopenia simultâneas; não é uma doença em si, mas sim um grupo de achados laboratoriais que possivelmente resultam de múltiplas causas.

FISIOPATOLOGIA
- Os mecanismos podem incluir produção reduzida de células na medula óssea ou utilização, destruição ou sequestro periféricos aumentados; pode ocorrer um ou mais desses mecanismos conjuntamente.
- A produção diminuída ocorre quando células-tronco pluripotentes, multipotentes ou comprometidas são destruídas, sua proliferação ou diferenciação fica suprimida ou a maturação das células diferenciadas é retardada ou impedida.
- Se as células-tronco pluripotentes forem acometidas, ocorrerá o desenvolvimento de pancitopenia; se as células-tronco comprometidas estiverem envolvidas, aparecerá citopenia daquele tipo celular.
- O aumento no uso e na destruição de células tipicamente resulta na produção aumentada na medula óssea. São necessários, no mínimo, 2-3 dias antes que o aumento na produção comece a ponto de exercer efeito sobre as contagens de células do sangue periférico; além disso, o pico de produção costuma levar uma semana; portanto, a velocidade de utilização ou destruição necessária para provocar citopenia não é tão grande durante os primeiros dias da doença como é no final.
- O sequestro de células na microcirculação, especialmente aquelas do baço, do intestino e dos pulmões, pode causar citopenia do tipo celular envolvido.

SISTEMA(S) ACOMETIDO(S)
Hematológico/linfático/imune — medula óssea, baço, linfonodos e outros tecidos linfoides; dependendo da causa, esses órgãos podem ser acometidos por depleção, degeneração, necrose, hiperplasia, displasia ou discrasia celular; podem ocorrer alterações isoladas ou em combinação.

INCIDÊNCIA/PREVALÊNCIA
A pancitopenia é uma ocorrência incomum e nem sempre ocorre com as causas listadas abaixo. Um único estudo (Weiss et al., 1999) determinou uma incidência de 2,4% em cães.

DISTRIBUIÇÃO GEOGRÁFICA
A menos que a causa de pancitopenia seja atribuída a algum agente infeccioso localizado em certa região (p. ex., leishmaniose, histoplasmose), não existe nenhuma distribuição geográfica específica.

IDENTIFICAÇÃO
- Cães e gatos.
- Sem predileção etária, sexual ou racial.

SINAIS CLÍNICOS

Achados Anamnésicos
- A anamnese reflete a causa subjacente.
- Letargia ou palidez por anemia.
- Hemorragia petequial ou sangramento nas mucosas por trombocitopenia.
- Episódios febris repetidos ou infecções frequentes ou persistentes por leucopenia.

Achados do Exame Físico
- Letargia, fraqueza.
- Mucosas pálidas.
- Hemorragias petequiais.
- Hemorragia nas mucosas (p. ex., hematúria, epistaxe, hemoptise e melena).
- Febre.

CAUSAS

Doenças Infecciosas
- FeLV.
- FIV.
- Erliquiose.
- Peritonite infecciosa felina.
- Parvovírus canino e felino.
- Vírus da hepatite infecciosa canina.
- Histoplasmose.
- Leishmaniose.
- Citauxzoonose.
- Endotoxemia e septicemia (especialmente microrganismos gram-negativos ou tularemia).

Medicamentos, Substâncias Químicas e Toxinas
- Estrogênio (administração exógena, tumor de células de Sertoli (sertolinoma), tumor de células intersticiais).
- Fenilbutazona.
- Fenobarbital.
- Griseofulvina.
- Metimazol (gatos).
- Cloranfenicol.
- Sulfadiazina-trimetoprima.
- Fembendazol, albendazol.
- Captopril.
- Cefalosporinas de segunda geração.
- Medicamentos quimioterápicos (azatioprina, doxorrubicina, carboplatina, ciclofosfamida, citosina arabinosídeo, vimblastina, hidroxiureia).
- Tálio.
- Toxina T-2 do *Fusarium*.
- Radiação ionizante.

Doenças Proliferativas e Infiltrativas
- Neoplasia hematopoiética (p. ex., leucemias aguda e crônica, linfoma, tumores histiocíticos e mielodisplasia).
- Mielofibrose.
- Mieloftise.
- Osteosclerose.

Doenças Imunomediadas
- Anemia aplásica (também conhecida como pancitopenia aplásica).
- Anemia hemolítica imunomediada e trombocitopenia imunomediada (quando as células precursoras constituem o alvo do sistema imunológico).

FATORES DE RISCO
Variam com cada causa.

DIAGNÓSTICO

DIAGNÓSTICO DIFERENCIAL
- Início agudo com sinais clínicos graves — mais compatível com condições que causam necrose, destruição ou sequestro de células.
- Início lento, insidioso — mais compatível com condições que causam supressão da medula óssea.

ACHADOS LABORATORIAIS
Medicamentos capazes de alterar os resultados laboratoriais

Com frequência, os glicocorticoides provocam aumento leve a moderado na contagem de neutrófilos segmentados, o que pode mascarar a presença de neutropenia.

Distúrbios capazes de alterar os resultados laboratoriais
A técnica de flebotomia pode resultar em aglomeração das plaquetas e ocorrência de hemólise, levando à contagem plaquetária e ao hematócrito falsamente baixos, respectivamente.

HEMOGRAMA/BIOQUÍMICA/URINÁLISE
- Leucopenia — caracterizada por neutropenia com ou sem linfopenia.
- Anemia arregenerativa — a gravidade depende da duração e da causa subjacente.
- Trombocitopenia.
- Avaliação do esfregaço sanguíneo — pode revelar agentes infecciosos (p. ex., *Ehrlichia* spp. e *Histoplasma capsulatum*); pode revelar células anormais de qualquer linhagem, sugerindo doenças mieloproliferativas ou linfoproliferativas.
- Alterações tóxicas nos leucócitos — podem sugerir lesão da medula óssea (p. ex., por parvovírus ou agente químico), septicemia ou endotoxemia.
- Alterações bioquímicas — dependem do órgão e do grau de envolvimento (p. ex., pode-se observar a elevação das enzimas hepáticas em determinadas doenças infecciosas, toxinas e doenças infiltrativas).

OUTROS TESTES LABORATORIAIS
- Contagem de reticulócitos — uma resposta regenerativa à anemia sugere destruição, uso ou sequestro de hemácias; já uma resposta arregenerativa é sugestiva de supressão da medula óssea e merece exame dessa estrutura.
- Testes imunológicos para doenças infecciosas (p. ex., FeLV, FIV e *Ehrlichia* spp.)
- PCR para doenças infecciosas.

OUTROS MÉTODOS DIAGNÓSTICOS
- Exame da medula óssea — indicado quando não se consegue determinar a causa da pancitopenia por outros testes.
- Medula óssea hipercelular associada à mielodisplasia, neoplasia, mieloftise e recuperação de parvovirose.
- Medula óssea hipocelular associada à necrose, mielofibrose e supressão (p. ex., medicamentos, estrogênio e anemia aplásica)
- Se não for possível obter o aspirado da medula óssea, deve-se suspeitar de mielofibrose, necrose ou hipocelularidade acentuada; nesse caso, a biopsia de núcleo deverá ser avaliada.

ACHADOS PATOLÓGICOS
Biopsia de núcleo da medula óssea — pode-se observar a substituição do tecido hematopoiético normal por tecido necrótico, neoplásico, fibroso ou adiposo, dependendo da causa subjacente.

TRATAMENTO

- O tratamento de suporte depende da situação clínica, incluindo antibioticoterapia rigorosa e transfusões de componentes sanguíneos.
- É imperativo o tratamento da condição subjacente.

PANCITOPENIA

MEDICAÇÕES

MEDICAMENTO(S) DE ESCOLHA
O tratamento deve ser apropriado para a situação clínica (i. e., o grau em que cada população celular se encontra diminuída, a presença de febre ou infecção e diagnósticos específicos suspeitos ou estabelecidos); ver as causas específicas.

CONTRAINDICAÇÕES
• Medicamentos que podem suprimir a hematopoiese ainda mais (ver a seção "Causas").
• AINE, clopidogrel e outros medicamentos que possam interferir na função plaquetária.

PRECAUÇÕES
Em função do comprometimento do estado imunológico do paciente, os glicocorticoides e outros medicamentos imunossupressores só deverão ser utilizados quando forem absolutamente necessários e com extrema cautela.

MEDICAMENTO(S) ALTERNATIVO(S)
Fatores de crescimento hematopoiético recombinante
• CSF-G recombinante humano — 1-5 μg/kg/dia SC; estimula a produção de neutrófilos.
• Eritropoietina recombinante humana — dosagem inicial: 100 U/kg SC três vezes por semana; estimula a eritropoiese.

ACOMPANHAMENTO

MONITORIZAÇÃO DO PACIENTE
• Exame físico diário, incluindo o monitoramento frequente da temperatura corporal.
• Hemograma periódico — a frequência depende da gravidade da citopenia, da idade, da condição física geral do paciente e da causa subjacente.

PREVENÇÃO
• Castração dos machos criptorquídicos.
• Vacinação contra doenças infecciosas.
• Monitoramento frequente do hemograma em pacientes com câncer que recebem quimio ou radioterapia.

COMPLICAÇÕES POSSÍVEIS
• Hemorragia.
• Sepse.

EVOLUÇÃO ESPERADA E PROGNÓSTICO
• Depende da causa subjacente.
• Em geral, é justificável o estabelecimento de prognóstico reservado.

DIVERSOS

DISTÚRBIOS ASSOCIADOS
Infecções secundárias — em pacientes com neutropenia.

POTENCIAL ZOONÓTICO
• Tularemia.
• O proprietário pode contrair histoplasmose pela mesma fonte do paciente.

GESTAÇÃO/FERTILIDADE/REPRODUÇÃO
O estresse da doença subjacente pode provocar abortamento; ver os respectivos tópicos a respeito dos efeitos de diferentes causas sobre a prenhez.

VER TAMBÉM
• Anemia aplásica.
• Anemia arregenerativa.
• Anemia regenerativa.
• Causas específicas de pancitopenia.
• Neutropenia.
• Trombocitopenia.

ABREVIATURA(S)
• CSF-G = fator estimulante de colônia de granulócitos.
• FeLV= vírus da leucemia felina.
• FIV = vírus da imunodeficiência felina.
• PCR = reação em cadeia da polimerase.

Sugestões de leitura
Brazzell JL, Weiss DJ. A retrospective study of aplastic pancytopenia in the dog: 9 cases (1996-2003). Vet Clin Path 2006, 35:413-417.
Weiss DJ. Aplastic anemia. In: Weiss DJ, Wardrop KJ, eds., Schalm's Veterinary Hematology, 6th ed. Ames, IA: Blackwell Publishing Ltd., 2010, 256-260.
Weiss DJ. Aplastic anemia. In: Feldman BF, Zinkl JG, Jain NC, eds., Schalm's Veterinary Hematology, 5th ed. Philadelphia: Lippincott Williams & Wilkins, 2000, 212-215.
——Detecting and diagnosing the cause of canine pancytopenia. Vet Med 2002, 97:21-32.
Weiss DJ, Evanson OA. A retrospective study of feline pancytopenia. Comp Haematol Int 2000, 10:50-55.
Weiss DJ, Evanson OA, Sykes J. A retrospective study of canine pancytopenia. Vet Clin Path 1999, 28:83-88.

Autor Darren Wood
Consultor Editorial A.H. Rebar

PANCREATITE

CONSIDERAÇÕES GERAIS

DEFINIÇÃO
- Inflamação do pâncreas.
- Pancreatite aguda — inflamação do pâncreas que ocorre abruptamente com pouca ou nenhuma alteração patológica permanente.
- Pancreatite crônica — doença inflamatória contínua que é acompanhada por alteração morfológica irreversível.

FISIOPATOLOGIA
- Os mecanismos de defesa do hospedeiro normalmente evitam a autodigestão do pâncreas pelas enzimas pancreáticas; porém, em algumas circunstâncias, essas defesas naturais falham; dessa forma, ocorre autodigestão quando essas enzimas digestivas são ativadas dentro das células acinares.
- A lesão tecidual local e sistêmica é atribuída à atividade das enzimas pancreáticas liberadas e de diversos mediadores inflamatórios, como as cininas, os radicais livres e os fatores relacionados com o complemento.

SISTEMA(S) ACOMETIDO(S)
- Gastrintestinal — motilidade GI alterada (íleo paralítico) em virtude da peritonite química regional; peritonite local ou generalizada atribuída à permeabilidade vascular aumentada; enteropatia inflamatória concomitante pode ser observada nos gatos.
- Cardiovascular — arritmias cardíacas podem resultar da liberação do fator depressor do miocárdio.
- Hematológico — ocorrem ativação da cascata de coagulação e coagulopatia sistêmica por consumo (CID).
- Hepatobiliar — lesões atribuídas a quadros de choque, dano pelas enzimas pancreáticas, infiltrados celulares inflamatórios, lipidose hepática e colestase intra/extra-hepática.
- Respiratório — edema pulmonar ou efusão pleural; síndrome da angústia respiratória do adulto é uma sequela rara, mas potencialmente fatal com complicações sistêmicas.

INCIDÊNCIA/PREVALÊNCIA
- Desconhecida.
- Até 1% dos cães normais apresentam evidência histológica de pancreatite.
- Pesquisas em necropsia sugerem uma prevalência elevada nos gatos com colangite, distúrbios hepatobiliares e enteropatia inflamatória.

IDENTIFICAÇÃO
Espécies
Cães e gatos.

Raça(s) Predominante(s)
- Schnauzer miniatura. • Poodle miniatura.
- Cocker spaniel. • Gatos da raça Siamês.

Idade Média e Faixa Etária
- Pancreatite aguda é mais comum em cães de meia-idade e idosos (>7 anos); idade média à apresentação é de 6 anos e meio.
- Idade média para pancreatite aguda em gatos é de 7,3 anos.

Sexo Predominante
Cadelas.

SINAIS CLÍNICOS
Comentários Gerais
- Cães — predominantemente sinais do trato GI.
- Gatos — sinais vagos, inespecíficos e não localizados.

Achados Anamnésicos
- Letargia/depressão/anorexia — comuns em cães e gatos.
- Vômito — comum em cães, porém menos comum em gatos.
- Perda de peso — comum em gatos.
- Os cães podem apresentar dor abdominal.
- Diarreia — mais frequentemente observada em cães do que em gatos.
- Icterícia — comum em cães e gatos.

Achados do Exame Físico
- Letargia grave — ambas as espécies.
- Desidratação — comum; causada por perdas GI.
- Dor abdominal.
- Lesões expansivas podem ser palpadas tanto em cães como em gatos.
- Febre — comum nos cães; há relatos tanto de febre como de hipotermia nos gatos.
- Icterícia — mais comum nos gatos.
- Anormalidades sistêmicas menos comuns incluem angústia respiratória, distúrbios hemorrágicos e arritmias cardíacas.

CAUSAS
- Geralmente desconhecidas; as possibilidades incluem:
  ○ Fatores nutricionais (p. ex., hiperlipoproteinemia). ○ Traumatismo/isquemia pancreática. ○ Refluxo duodenal.
  ○ Medicamentos/toxinas (ver a seção "Contraindicações"). ○ Obstrução do ducto pancreático. ○ Hipercalcemia. ○ Agentes infecciosos — toxoplasmose, PIF. ○ Extensão de inflamação hepatobiliar ou intestinal felina.

FATORES DE RISCO
- Raça (ver a seção "identificação").
- Obesidade nos cães.
- Doença concomitante nos cães (p. ex., diabetes melito, hiperadrenocorticismo, insuficiência renal crônica e neoplasia).
- Administração recente de medicamento (ver a seção "Contraindicações").
- Enteropatia/hepatopatia inflamatória concomitante nos gatos.
- Ver também a seção "Causas".

DIAGNÓSTICO

DIAGNÓSTICO DIFERENCIAL
Outras causas de abdome agudo:
- Doença GI (obstrução, corpo estranho, perfuração, gastrenterite, doença ulcerosa) — excluir com base no hemograma completo/bioquímica/urinálise, diagnóstico por imagem, paracentese e endoscopia com biopsia.
- Torção esplênica — descartar por meio das técnicas de diagnóstico por imagem.
- Hipoadrenocorticismo — excluir com base no hemograma completo/bioquímica/urinálise, teste de estimulação com ACTH.
- Doença urogenital (pielonefrite, prostatite ou abscedação, piometra, ruptura ou obstrução do trato urinário, insuficiência renal aguda) — descartar com base no hemograma completo/bioquímica/urinálise, urocultura/antibiograma e diagnóstico por imagem.
- Doença hepatobiliar (colangio-hepatite) — excluir com base no hemograma completo/bioquímica/urinálise, ácidos biliares, diagnóstico por imagem e biopsia do fígado.
- Neoplasia abdominal — descartar por meio das técnicas de diagnóstico por imagem e por citologia ou biopsia.

HEMOGRAMA/BIOQUÍMICA/URINÁLISE
- Hemograma completo — nos cães, frequentemente revela hemoconcentração, leucocitose com desvio à esquerda e neutrófilos tóxicos; os gatos apresentam maior variabilidade e podem demonstrar neutrofilia (30%) e anemia arregenerativa (26%).
- Bioquímicas séricas — quase sempre apresentam azotemia pré-renal; as atividades das enzimas hepáticas (ALT, fosfatase alcalina) frequentemente se encontram elevadas por causa da isquemia hepática ou por exposição a toxinas pancreáticas; a hiperbilirrubinemia é mais comum nos gatos, sendo atribuída à lesão hepatocelular e obstrução biliar intra/extra-hepática; observa-se hiperglicemia em cães e gatos com pancreatite necrosante em virtude da hiperglucagonemia; pode-se notar hipoglicemia leve nos cães; os gatos com pancreatite supurativa podem apresentar hipoglicemia; são comuns as anormalidades de hipercolesterolemia e hipertrigliceridemia.
- Urinálise — nada digno de nota.

OUTROS TESTES LABORATORIAIS
- Atividades séricas da amilase e da lipase não são marcadores sorológicos de confiança — podem estar elevadas nos cães, porém são inespecíficas; também aumentam com doença hepática, renal ou neoplásica na ausência de pancreatite; a dexametasona pode aumentar as concentrações da lipase sérica nos cães.
- A imunorreatividade da lipase pancreática é um marcador sorológico altamente sensível e específico de inflamação pancreática no cão e no gato.
- Radiografias abdominais — podem incluir opacidade aumentada do tecido mole no compartimento abdominal cranial direito; perda do detalhe visceral ("aspecto de vidro fosco") em virtude da efusão abdominal; padrão de gás estático na parte proximal do duodeno; ângulo ampliado entre o antro pilórico e o duodeno proximal.
- Radiografias torácicas — podem revelar efusão pleural leve ou complicações pulmonares mais graves.
- Ultrassonografia abdominal — lesões expansivas sólidas ou císticas não homogêneas sugerem abscesso pancreático; pode haver massa pancreática ou ecogenicidade alterada (hipoecoica) na área do pâncreas; podem-se observar efusão peritoneal e obstrução biliar extra-hepática.
- Imunorreatividade da lipase pancreática e ultrassonografia do pâncreas em combinação apresentam a sensibilidade mais elevada para o diagnóstico de pancreatite canina e felina antes do óbito.
- Triagem em busca de hipocobalaminemia em gatos.

MÉTODOS DE DIAGNÓSTICO
- Biopsia por aspiração com agulha guiada pelo ultrassom pode confirmar a presença de inflamação, abscesso ou cisto.
- Laparoscopia com biopsia pancreática por pinça para o diagnóstico histológico.
- A avaliação histopatológica pode falhar na detecção de inflamação pancreática focal ou segmentar; por essa razão, essa ferramenta diagnóstica não pode ser usada em todos os casos.

PANCREATITE

ACHADOS PATOLÓGICOS
- Achados macroscópicos (pancreatite aguda) — tumefação leve com pancreatite edematosa; áreas amarelo-acinzentadas de necrose pancreática com quantidades variáveis de hemorragia na pancreatite necrosante.
- Achados macroscópicos (pancreatite crônica) — pâncreas diminuído de tamanho, firme, cinzento e irregular; pode conter amplas aderências nas vísceras adjacentes.
- Alterações microscópicas (pancreatite aguda) — incluem edema, necrose parenquimatosa e infiltrado celular neutrofílico nas lesões agudas.
- Alterações microscópicas (pancreatite crônica) — fibrose pancreática ao redor dos ductos, hiperplasia epitelial dos ductos e infiltrado celular mononuclear; lesões inflamatórias também podem ser observadas no parênquima hepático e na mucosa intestinal dos gatos.
- Observar a presença de doença inflamatória concomitante (inflamação linfocítico-plasmocitária) no intestino e fígado de gatos.

TRATAMENTO
CUIDADO(S) DE SAÚDE ADEQUADO(S)
- Tratamento clínico do paciente internado.
- Fluidoterapia IV rigorosa.
- Objetivos da fluidoterapia — corrigir a hipovolemia e manter a microcirculação pancreática.
- Solução eletrolítica balanceada, como a solução de Ringer lactato, é o fluido de primeira escolha para a reidratação.
- Corrigir a desidratação inicial (mL = % de desidratação × peso em kg × 1.000) e administrar por 4-6 h.
- Talvez haja necessidade de coloides (oxiglobina, hetamido).
- Após a reposição dos déficits, administrar fluidos adicionais para equilibrar as necessidades de manutenção (2,5 × o peso em kg) e as perdas contínuas (estimadas).
- Em geral, a suplementação com cloreto de potássio (KCl) é necessária por causa da perda de potássio no vômito; basear essa suplementação nos níveis séricos mensurados (utilizar 20 mEq de KCl/L do fluido IV se os níveis de potássio no soro não forem conhecidos; não administrar em uma velocidade mais rápida que 0,5 mEq/kg/h).

ATIVIDADE
Restrita.

DIETA
- Continuar a alimentar por via oral a menos que o vômito seja intratável; a alimentação mantém a integridade epitelial intestinal e minimiza a translocação bacteriana.
- Animais com vômito intermitente devem ser tratados com antieméticos — metoclopramida (infusão contínua) ou fenotiazínicos (após a correção dos déficits hídricos).
- Alimentação com cateter inserido via jejunostomia é a mais ideal, pois permite a nutrição enteral ao mesmo tempo em que se promove o repouso pancreático; a colocação do cateter via jejunostomia endoscópica percutânea foi descrita recentemente.
- Nada por via oral em animais com vômito persistente pelo menor período de tempo possível; quando o vômito não tiver ocorrido por 4-6 h, oferecer pequenas quantidades de água; se toleradas, iniciar refeições frequentes em pequenas quantidades com dieta à base de carboidrato (p. ex., arroz cozido); introduzir gradativamente uma fonte proteica de alto valor biológico como queijo *cottage* ou carne magra.
- Evitar dietas ricas em proteína e em gordura.
- Pacientes que necessitam de jejum (i. e., nada por via oral) por período prolongado podem necessitar de alimentação entérica administrada por jejunostomia ou nutrição parenteral total.

ORIENTAÇÃO AO PROPRIETÁRIO.
- Falar sobre a necessidade de hospitalização prolongada.
- Discutir as despesas do diagnóstico e do tratamento.
- Abordar as possíveis complicações a curto e a longo prazos (ver a seção "Distúrbios Associados").

CONSIDERAÇÕES CIRÚRGICAS
- Talvez haja necessidade de cirurgia para remoção de pseudocistos, abscessos ou tecido desvitalizado observado na pancreatite necrosante.
- Pode ser necessária a realização de laparotomia e de biopsia pancreática para confirmar a presença de pancreatite e/ou descartar outras doenças não pancreáticas.
- Obstrução biliar extra-hepática gerada pela pancreatite requer correção cirúrgica.

MEDICAÇÕES
MEDICAMENTO(S)
- Corticosteroides são indicados apenas no choque.
- Antieméticos de ação central indicados no vômito intratável — metoclopramida (1-2 mg/kg em 24 h), clorpromazina (0,5 mg/kg IM ou SC a cada 8 h) ou proclorperazina (0,1 mg/kg a cada 8 h). Maropitanto (Cerenia®), administrado a uma dose de 1 mg/kg SC a cada 24 h, também é útil no controle de vômito agudo em cães.
- Antibióticos se houver indícios de sepse — penicilina G (20.000 U/kg a cada 6 h), ampicilina sódica (20 mg/kg a cada 8 h) e enrofloxacino (5-20 mg/kg IV a cada 12 h nos cães).
- Analgésicos para aliviar a dor abdominal, por exemplo, buprenorfina (0,005-0,01 mg/kg IM, IV ou SC a cada 6-12 h).

CONTRAINDICAÇÕES
- Anticolinérgicos (p. ex., atropina). • Azatioprina.
- Clorotiazida. • Estrogênios. • Furosemida.
- Tetraciclinas.

PRECAUÇÕES
Usar os antieméticos fenotiazínicos apenas nos pacientes bem hidratados; esses medicamentos apresentam propriedades hipotensoras.

ACOMPANHAMENTO
MONITORIZAÇÃO DO PACIENTE
- Avaliar o estado de hidratação com rigor durante as primeiras 24 h do tratamento; realizar o exame físico e mensurar os itens como peso corporal, hematócrito, proteína plasmática total, ureia e débito urinário duas vezes ao dia.
- Avaliar a eficácia da fluidoterapia após 24 h e ajustar as velocidades de fluxo e a composição do fluido de acordo com o quadro; repetir os exames bioquímicos para avaliar o estado eletrolítico/acidobásico.
- Repetir a mensuração das concentrações plasmáticas de enzimas (imunorreatividade da lipase pancreática) depois de 7 dias para avaliar o processo inflamatório.
- Observar o paciente de perto quanto à ocorrência de complicações sistêmicas que envolvem uma variedade de sistemas orgânicos; fazer os testes diagnósticos apropriados, conforme a necessidade (ver a seção "Distúrbios Associados").
- Reduzir os fluidos de modo gradual até as necessidades de manutenção, se possível.
- Manter a alimentação oral ou a nutrição enteral conforme descrição prévia.
- Reavaliar e corrigir as concentrações séricas baixas contínuas de cobalamina.

PREVENÇÃO
- Redução do peso em caso de obesidade.
- Evitar dietas ricas em gordura.
- Evitar medicamentos que possam desencadear a doença (ver a seção "Contraindicações").

COMPLICAÇÕES POSSÍVEIS
- Falha na resposta ao tratamento de suporte.
- Condições associadas potencialmente letais.

EVOLUÇÃO ESPERADA E PROGNÓSTICO
- Bom para a maior parte dos pacientes com pancreatite edematosa; em geral, esses pacientes respondem ao tratamento sintomático apropriado.
- Mais reservado a mau para os pacientes com pancreatite necrosante e condições sistêmicas.

DIVERSOS
DISTÚRBIOS ASSOCIADOS
Com risco de morte
- Edema pulmonar (p. ex., síndrome da angústia respiratória do adulto). • Arritmias cardíacas.
- Peritonite. • CID. • Lipidose hepática felina.

Sem risco de morte
- Diabetes melito. • Insuficiência pancreática exócrina. • Colangio-hepatite felina. • Enteropatia inflamatória felina.

FATORES RELACIONADOS COM A IDADE
Mais comum em animais de meia-idade.

VER TAMBÉM
- Abdome agudo. • Insuficiência pancreática exócrina.

ABREVIATURA(S)
- ACTH = hormônio adrenocorticotrópico.
- ALT = alanina aminotransferase.
- CID = coagulação intravascular disseminada.
- GI = gastrintestinal.
- PIF = peritonite infecciosa felina.

RECURSOS DA INTERNET
www.vin.com/VIN.plx.

Sugestões de leitura
Zoran DL. Pancreatitis in cats: Diagnosis and management of a challenging disease. JAAHA 2006, 42:1-9.

Autor Albert E. Jergens
Consultor Editorial Albert E. Jergens

Paniculite

CONSIDERAÇÕES GERAIS

REVISÃO
Inflamação do tecido adiposo subcutâneo por inúmeras causas.

SISTEMA(S) ACOMETIDO(S)
Cutâneo/exócrino.

IDENTIFICAÇÃO
• Gatos — sem predileção etária, sexual ou racial. • Cães — sem predileção etária, sexual ou racial em lesões solitárias. • Paniculite nodular estéril — cadelas; as raças Dachshund e Poodle são predispostas; no entanto, pode ocorrer em qualquer raça.

SINAIS CLÍNICOS
• Incomum em cães e gatos. • Nódulos subcutâneos ou trajetos drenantes isolados ou múltiplos. • Podem ser dolorosos e flutuantes a firmes. • Dividida em tipos: lobular (envolve os lóbulos de gordura), septal (envolve os septos interlobulares de tecido conjuntivo) e difuso (envolve tanto os septos lobulares como os interlobulares). • O tipo difuso é mais usual em cães, enquanto o tipo septal é mais comum em gatos. • Lesões — costumam ocorrer sobre o tronco; podem se tornar císticas e desenvolver trajetos drenantes; podem ser dolorosas antes e logo depois da ruptura; as ulcerações quase sempre cicatrizam com a formação de crosta e cicatriz.
• Casos iniciais de doença isolada ou multifocal — os nódulos apresentam-se livremente móveis sob a pele; em geral, a pele sobrejacente ao nódulo permanece normal, mas pode ficar eritematosa ou (com menor frequência) castanha ou amarelada.
• Nódulos — variam desde alguns milímetros a vários centímetros de diâmetro; podem ser firmes e bem circunscritos ou moles e pouco definidos; à medida que aumentam de volume e se desenvolvem, os nódulos podem se fixar à camada profunda da derme (assim, a pele sobrejacente não fica livremente móvel). • A gordura envolvida pode necrosar. • Exsudato — geralmente consiste em uma pequena quantidade de secreção oleosa; amarelo-acastanhado a sanguinolento. • Lesões múltiplas (cães e gatos) — os sinais sistêmicos são comuns (p. ex., anorexia, pirexia, letargia e depressão).

CAUSAS E FATORES DE RISCO
• Infecciosas — por bactérias, fungos, micobactérias oportunistas, além de embolia infecciosa. • Imunomediadas — paniculite lúpica, eritema nodoso, ou reação medicamentosa. • Idiopáticas — paniculite nodular estéril. • Traumatismo. • Neoplásicas — mastocitoma multicêntrico, linfossarcoma cutâneo. • Corpos estranhos. • Pós-injeção — corticosteroides, vacinas, outras injeções subcutâneas. • Possível deficiência da vitamina E em gatos (esteatite).

DIAGNÓSTICO

DIAGNÓSTICO DIFERENCIAL
Processos infecciosos
• Mais comuns que a paniculite estéril/imunomediada. • A paniculite profunda é mais provável sobre os pontos de pressão. • Além disso, a piodermite profunda pode ter lesões associadas de piodermite superficial (p. ex., pápulas, pústulas e colaretes epidérmicos). • Aspirados e esfregaços por impressão (decalque) — número acentuado de neutrófilos com quantidade variável de células mononucleares e bactérias em casos de piodermite profunda. Em casos de infecções fúngicas, pode-se notar a presença dos microrganismos fúngicos, além de uma quantidade variável de células mononucleares. • Cultura/antibiograma (aeróbios e anaeróbios, bem como para infecções fúngicas profundas por micobactérias de crescimento rápido) a partir de exsudatos e amostras de biopsia.
• O procedimento de biopsia demonstra a presença de microrganismo ou infiltrado compatível com infecção. • Na suspeita de blastomicose, uma amostra de urina também poderá ser enviada para detecção do antígeno.

Cistos Cutâneos
• Geralmente indolores. • Bem demarcados. • Em geral, sem inflamação. • Aspirados — *debris* amorfos; sem células inflamatórias. • Biopsias — confirmam o diagnóstico.

Lipomas
• Moles; em geral, bem delimitados. • Sem inflamação ou trajetos drenantes. • Aspirados — lipócitos; sem células inflamatórias. • Biopsias — confirmam o diagnóstico.

Mastocitoma/Linfoma Epiteliotrópico
• Multifocais. • Podem acometer a cabeça, as pernas e as mucosas. • Quase sempre eritematosos. • Apresentações variáveis. • Aspirados — muitas vezes sugestivos. • Biopsias — confirmam o diagnóstico.

Paniculite Nodular Estéril
• Diagnóstico estabelecido pela exclusão de outras causas de paniculite. • Aspirados revelam a presença de neutrófilos e macrófagos espumosos, mas sem microrganismos. • Biopsias, culturas e outros testes diagnósticos — conforme indicados pela apresentação clínica. • Resultados negativos nas culturas de exsudato e tecido.

HEMOGRAMA/BIOQUÍMICA/URINÁLISE
• A maior parte dos casos não apresenta anormalidades. • Ocasionalmente, observa-se desvio à esquerda regenerativo ou eosinofilia.
• Leve leucocitose. • Leve anemia arregenerativa, normocítica e normocrômica.

OUTROS TESTES LABORATORIAIS
• Anticorpo antinuclear — para paniculite lúpica. • Eletroforese das proteínas séricas. • Níveis séricos de lipase/amilase.

DIAGNÓSTICO POR IMAGEM
Ultrassonografia — a pancreatite pode ser fator que contribui para o quadro (raro).

MÉTODOS DIAGNÓSTICOS
• Cultura bacteriana e antibiograma (tecido) — necessários para identificar bactérias primárias ou secundárias. • Cultura para fungos e micobactérias atípicas (tecido). • Biopsias com culturas negativas para o diagnóstico de paniculite nodular estéril.
• Colorações especiais de amostras histopatológicas — podem ajudar a identificar o agente causal.

ACHADOS PATOLÓGICOS
• Biopsias excisionais (cirúrgicas) — mais precisas do que as amostras de biopsias obtidas com saca-bocado (também conhecido como *punch*) na maior parte dos casos; as biopsias feitas com saca-bocado não fornecem amostra suficientemente profunda para fazer o diagnóstico.
• Lesões histopatológicas — necessárias para formular o diagnóstico da paniculite; para identificar necrose, fibrose ou vasculite. O uso de colorações especiais ajudará na identificação dos agentes infecciosos.

TRATAMENTO
• Lesões isoladas — excisão cirúrgica. • Lesões múltiplas — necessitam de medicações sistêmicas.

MEDICAÇÕES

MEDICAMENTO(S)
• Resultados positivos na cultura exigem tratamento antifúngico, antibacteriano ou antimicobacteriano adequado. • Paniculite nodular estéril — tratamento sistêmico com esteroides; prednisona (2,2 mg/kg diariamente) até que as lesões regridam por completo (3-6 semanas); após a remissão, reduzir a dosagem de modo gradual em 2 semanas; ocasionalmente, pode haver a necessidade de uma redução gradativa mais lenta para minimizar a possibilidade de recidiva; muitos pacientes são curados; alguns pacientes, no entanto, necessitam de tratamento em dias alternados com doses baixas para manter a remissão. • Vitamina E por via oral — pode controlar os casos leves. • Azatioprina (1 mg/kg VO diariamente) — pode ser utilizada em caso de contraindicação dos corticosteroides ou na ausência de resposta aos corticosteroides isolados.
• Tetraciclina e niacinamida podem ser eficazes em alguns cães (500 mg de cada medicamento [cães >10 kg] ou 100-250 mg de cada medicamento [cães <10 kg] VO a cada 8 h por 2-3 meses. Depois disso, pode-se tentar a redução gradual).
• Ciclosporina pode ser benéfica em alguns cães. Iniciada, em geral, a 5 mg/kg a cada 24 h por 4-8 semanas e, depois, reduzida de forma gradativa.

ACOMPANHAMENTO
• Depende do tipo e da duração do tratamento. • Monitorizar o hemograma completo, a contagem plaquetária, o perfil bioquímico e a urinálise caso se faça uso de agentes imunossupressores ou glicocorticosteroides a longo prazo.

DIVERSOS

Sugestões de Leitura
Medleau L, Hnilica KA. Small Animal Dermatology: A Color Atlas and Therapeutic Guide, 2nd ed. St. Louis: Saunders Elsevier, 2006.
Scott DW, Miller WH, Griffin CE. Muller & Kirk's Small Animal Dermatology, 6th ed. Philadelphia: Saunders, 2001.

Autor Karen A. Kuhl
Consultor Editorial Alexander H. Werner
Agradecimento a Kevin Shanley por ter escrito este capítulo na edição anterior.

PANLEUCOPENIA FELINA

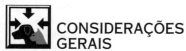

CONSIDERAÇÕES GERAIS

DEFINIÇÃO
Infecção entérica viral aguda de gatos, caracterizada por início súbito, depressão, vômitos e diarreia, além de desidratação grave e alta mortalidade.

FISIOPATOLOGIA
O vírus causador, o parvovírus felino (FPV), infecta apenas células mitóticas, causando citólise celular aguda de células em rápida divisão.

SISTEMA(S) ACOMETIDO(S)
• Gastrintestinal — destruição das células das criptas intestinais do jejuno e do íleo; enterite aguda com vômitos e diarreia; vilosidades cegas encurtadas com má absorção de nutrientes, desidratação e bacteremia secundária.
• Hematológico/linfático/imune — panleucopenia grave; atrofia do timo. • Nervoso e Oftálmico — em neonatos felinos, as células granulares em rápida divisão do cerebelo e as células da retina são destruídas; hipoplasia cerebelar com ataxia e displasia da retina. • Reprodutivo — infecção *in utero* em gatas não imunes, o que acarreta morte fetal, reabsorção fetal, abortamento, natimortos ou mumificação fetal.

GENÉTICA
N/D.

INCIDÊNCIA/PREVALÊNCIA
• Populações não vacinadas — a doença infecciosa felina mais grave e importante. • Vacinação de rotina — controle quase total da doença.
• Extremamente contagiosa. • Vírus extremamente estável, sobrevivendo por anos em locais contaminados.

DISTRIBUIÇÃO GEOGRÁFICA
Mundial em populações não vacinadas.

IDENTIFICAÇÃO
Espécies
• Família Felidae — todas, domésticas e exóticas.
• Família Canidae — suscetíveis ao parvovírus canino estreitamente relacionado; alguns canídeos exóticos podem ser suscetíveis à infecção pelo FPV.
• Mustelídeos — especialmente a marta; podem ser suscetíveis. • Procionídeos — guaxinim e quati; suscetíveis.

Raça(s) Predominante(s)
Nenhuma.

Idade Média e Faixa Etária
• Gatos de qualquer idade não vacinados e não submetidos à exposição prévia podem se infectar assim que perderem a imunidade materna por transferência passiva. • Filhotes com 2-6 meses de vida — mais suscetíveis a desenvolverem doença grave. • Adultos — geralmente apresentam infecção leve ou subclínica.

Sexo Predominante
N/D.

SINAIS CLÍNICOS
Achados Anamnésicos
• Histórico de exposição recente (p. ex., adotado de abrigo de animais). • Filhote recém-adquirido.
• Filhote com 2-4 meses de vida proveniente de lugares onde há antecedentes de panleucopenia felina. • Sem histórico de vacinação ou vacinado pela última vez quando tinha menos de 16 semanas de vida. • Início súbito, com vômitos, diarreia, depressão e anorexia completa. • O proprietário pode suspeitar de envenenamento.
• O gato pode ter desaparecido ou ter se escondido por 1 dia ou mais antes de ser encontrado. • O proprietário pode relatar que o gato deixa a cabeça cair na vasilha de água ou alimento, mas não come nem bebe.

Achados do Exame Físico
• Depressão — pode ser leve ou grave. • "Postura típica de panleucopenia" — esterno e queixo no chão, patas dobradas sob o corpo e extremidade superior das escápulas elevada acima da cabeça.
• Desidratação — surge rapidamente; pode ser grave. • Podem ocorrer vômitos e diarreia.
• Temperatura corporal — sofre, em geral, elevação leve a moderada ou depressão nos estágios iniciais da doença; torna-se gravemente subnormal à medida que o gato acometido fica moribundo.
• Dor abdominal — pode ser eliciada à palpação. • Intestino delgado — túrgido e com forma de mangueira ou flácido. • São comuns infecções subclínicas ou discretas com poucos ou nenhum sinal clínico, especialmente em adultos. • Ataxia causada por hipoplasia cerebelar — filhotes infectados *in utero* ou no período neonatal; sinais que se mostram evidentes com 10-14 dias de vida e persistem por toda a vida; hipermetria; dismetria; incoordenação com postura em base larga e cauda elevada como um "leme"; alerta, afebril e normal sob outros aspectos; às vezes, observa-se displasia da retina.

CAUSAS
Parvovírus Felino (FPV)
• DNA vírus pequeno e monofilamentar.
• Sorotipo antigênico único.
• Reatividade cruzada antigênica considerável com o parvovírus canino tipo 2 e o vírus da enterite em marta.
• Extremamente estável contra fatores ambientais, temperatura e grande parte dos desinfetantes.
• Requer uma célula em mitose para replicação.

Parvovírus Canino (CPV) Tipos 2a, 2b e 2c
• CPV-2a, CPV-2b e CPV-2c podem produzir panleucopenia felina em gatos domésticos e/ou exóticos.
• As propriedades do CPV são semelhantes àquelas do FPV.

FATORES DE RISCO
• Qualquer um que aumente a atividade mitótica das células das criptas do intestino delgado — parasitas intestinais; bactérias patogênicas.
• Secundários ou coinfecções — infecções virais respiratórias superiores.
• Idade — filhotes com 2-6 meses de vida tendem a ser acometidos mais gravemente.

DIAGNÓSTICO

DIAGNÓSTICO DIFERENCIAL
• Síndrome semelhante à panleucopenia por infecção pelo FeLV— infecção crônica; enterite crônica; panleucopenia crônica; geralmente anemia; paciente positivo para o antígeno do FeLV no sangue e/ou na saliva.
• Salmonelose — em geral, infecção subclínica; gastrenterite grave; leucograma total geralmente elevado.
• Envenenamento agudo — semelhante à doença aguda ou fulminante; depressão grave; temperatura abaixo do normal; leucograma total não deprimido intensamente.
• Muitas doenças de gatos podem causar sinais clínicos discretos, difíceis de serem diferenciados de panleucopenia felina leve; o leucograma total sempre se encontra baixo durante a infecção aguda com panleucopenia felina, mesmo nas infecções subclínicas.

HEMOGRAMA/BIOQUÍMICA/URINÁLISE
• Panleucopenia — achado mais compatível; leucogramas, em geral, entre 500-3.000 células/dL durante a doença aguda.
• Achados bioquímicos, em geral, inespecíficos.

OUTROS TESTES LABORATORIAIS
• Imunoensaio fecal para detecção de antígeno do CPV (CITE® Canine Parvovirus Test Kit, IDEXX Labs) — não aprovado para a panleucopenia felina; detecta o antígeno do PVF nas fezes.
• Tira de teste cromatográfico — fezes para FPV e CPV.
• Sorologia — amostras de soro pareadas (das fases aguda e convalescente); detecta aumento no título de anticorpo.

MÉTODOS DIAGNÓSTICOS
• Isolamento do vírus a partir de fezes ou tecidos acometidos (p. ex., timo, intestino delgado e baço).
• Microscopia eletrônica fecal — detecta partículas do parvovírus, presumivelmente o FPV.

ACHADOS PATOLÓGICOS
Macroscópicos
• Pelagem áspera.
• Desidratação grave.
• Indícios de vômitos e diarreia.
• Perda de peso.
• Intestino delgado edematoso e túrgido.
• Hemorragias petequiais ou equimóticas nas superfícies serosas e/ou mucosas do jejuno e do íleo.
• Atrofia do timo.
• Medula óssea gelatinosa ou líquida.
• Infecção *in utero* ou neonatal — hipoplasia macroscópica do cerebelo.

Microscópicos
• Criptas do intestino delgado dilatadas, com desprendimento de células epiteliais.
• Vilosidades intestinais encurtadas e cegas.
• Ausência de infiltrados linfocíticos em todos os tecidos.
• Depleção linfocítica de folículos nos linfonodos, nas placas de Peyer e no baço.
• Infecção neonatal e fetal — desorientação e depleção das células granulares e de Purkinje no cerebelo.
• Inclusões intranucleares eosinofílicas nos tecidos acometidos durante os estágios iniciais da infecção; não são observadas, em geral, no exame histopatológico de rotina dos tecidos fixados em formalina.

TRATAMENTO

CUIDADO(S) DE SAÚDE ADEQUADO(S)
• Princípios básicos do tratamento — reidratação; restabelecimento do equilíbrio eletrolítico; cuidados de suporte até o sistema imune do

PANLEUCOPENIA FELINA

paciente produzir anticorpos antivirais que neutralizem o vírus.
- Hospitalares — casos graves; hidratação e reposição de eletrólitos.
- Ambulatoriais — casos leves.

CUIDADO(S) DE ENFERMAGEM
- Fluidoterapia — essencial nos casos graves; com reposição de eletrólitos e suporte intravenoso de nutrientes, pode fazer a diferença entre a sobrevivência e a morte.
- Transfusões de sangue total — se o nível plasmático de proteínas cair para menos de 4 g/dL ou se o leucograma total estiver em menos de 2.000 células/dL.

ATIVIDADE
Manter o paciente dentro de casa durante a doença aguda — evita a contaminação do ambiente; impede que o gato se esconda.

DIETA
Suspender o alimento temporariamente até a gastrenterite aguda ser controlada.

ORIENTAÇÃO AO PROPRIETÁRIO
- Informar o proprietário sobre o fato de que todos os gatos atuais e futuros na casa precisam ser vacinados contra o FPV antes de serem expostos a ele.
- Orientar o proprietário sobre o fato de que o vírus permanecerá infectante no local por anos a menos que o ambiente possa ser adequadamente desinfetado com água sanitária.

CONSIDERAÇÕES CIRÚRGICAS
Nenhuma.

MEDICAÇÕES

MEDICAMENTO(S) DE ESCOLHA
Antibióticos de amplo espectro — para combater bacteremia secundária por bactérias intestinais.

CONTRAINDICAÇÕES
Medicações orais até que a gastrenterite tenha sido controlada.

MEDICAMENTO(S) ALTERNATIVO(S)
Nenhum.

ACOMPANHAMENTO

MONITORIZAÇÃO DO PACIENTE
- Monitorizar a hidratação e o equilíbrio eletrolítico com rigor.
- Monitorizar o hemograma completo diariamente ou pelo menos a cada 2 dias até a recuperação.
- Os gatos recuperados ficam imunes à infecção pelo FPV pelo resto da vida e não precisam mais de vacinação.

PREVENÇÃO
- Ambientes contaminados (p. ex., gaiolas, pisos e vasilhames de água e alimento) devem ser desinfetados com uma diluição de água sanitária a 1:32.
- O FPV é resistente à maioria dos desinfetantes comerciais.

Vacinas
- As vacinas contra panleucopenia felina são vacinas essenciais, devendo ser administradas a todos os gatos.
- A vacinação de rotina dos filhotes evita completamente a doença.
- Vacinas parenterais de vírus vivo modificado ou inativado.
- Vacina intranasal de vírus vivo modificado.
- Imunidade — de longa duração, talvez pelo resto da vida.
- Filhotes — vacinar já com 6 semanas de vida e, em seguida, a cada 3-4 semanas até as 16 semanas de vida; as recomendações recentes sobre as diretrizes de vacinação da American Association of Feline Practitioners (Associação Norte-americana de Clínicos Felinos) alteraram o momento de aplicação da última vacina para quando o animal tem, pelo menos, 16 semanas de vida, em vez de 12 semanas de vida, uma vez que a imunidade de origem materna em alguns filhotes pode não ter declinado até 16 semanas de vida.
- Reforços — 1 ano depois da última vacina; em seguida, repetir por não mais que a cada 3 anos.
- Não utilizar as vacinas de vírus vivo modificado em gatas prenhes.

COMPLICAÇÕES POSSÍVEIS
- Enterite crônica — fúngica ou por outra causa.
- Efeitos teratogênicos (hipoplasia cerebelar, que resulta em ataxia pelo resto da vida) — infecção do feto pelo vírus.
- Choque e outras complicações — desidratação grave e desequilíbrio eletrolítico.

EVOLUÇÃO ESPERADA E PROGNÓSTICO
- Praticamente todos os casos são agudos e duram apenas 5-7 dias.
- Se a morte não ocorrer durante a doença aguda, a recuperação em geral será rápida e sem complicações; pode levar várias semanas para que o paciente recupere o peso e a condição corporal.
- O prognóstico é reservado durante a doença aguda, especialmente se o leucograma total estiver abaixo de 2.000 células/dL.

DIVERSOS

DISTÚRBIOS ASSOCIADOS
Doenças virais do trato respiratório superior, inclusive rinotraqueíte viral felina e infecção pelo calicivírus felino.

FATORES RELACIONADOS COM A IDADE
- Clínicos — em geral, uma doença de filhotes.
- Subclínicos — geralmente em adultos.

POTENCIAL ZOONÓTICO
Nenhum.

GESTAÇÃO/FERTILIDADE/REPRODUÇÃO
- Gatas prenhes não vacinadas correm maior risco de ter a infecção.
- Os fetos quase sempre se infectam com efeitos fatais ou teratogênicos, mesmo quando a mãe tem uma infecção subclínica.
- Reabsorção fetal, abortamento, mumificação fetal, natimortos ou o nascimento de filhotes fracos e debilitados.
- Os filhotes podem exibir ataxia em função da hipoplasia cerebelar quando começam a andar.

SINÔNIMO(S)
- Cinomose felina.
- Enterite viral felina.
- Infecção pelo parvovírus felino

ABREVIATURA(S)
- CPV = parvovírus canino.
- FeLV = vírus da leucemia felina.
- FPV = parvovírus felino.

Sugestões de Leitura
Greene CE, Addie DD. Felineparvovirus infection. In: Greene CE, ed., Infectious Diseases of the Dog and Cat, 3rd ed. St. Louis: Saunders Elsevier, 2006, pp. 78-88.
Lappin MR, Veir J, Hawley J. Feline panleukopenia virus, feline herpesvirus-1, and feline calicivirus antibody responses in seronegative specific pathogen-free cats after a single administration of two different modified live FVRCP vaccines. J Feline Med Surg 2009, 11:159-162.
Richards JR, Elston TH, Ford RB, et al. The 2006 American Association of Feline Practitioners Feline Vaccine Advisory Panel Report. JAVMA 2006; 229:1405-1441.
Scott FW. Virucidal disinfectants and feline viruses. Am J Vet Res 1980, 41:410-414.
Scott FW, Geissinger CM. Long-term immunity in cats vaccinated with an inactivated trivalent vaccine. Am J Vet Res 1999, 60:652-658.
Truyen U, Addie D, Belák S, et al. Feline panleukopenia: ABCD guidelines on prevention and management. J Feline Med Surg 2009, 11:538-546.

Autor Fred W. Scott
Consultor Editorial Stephen C. Barr

PANOSTEÍTE

CONSIDERAÇÕES GERAIS

DEFINIÇÃO
Condição dolorosa autolimitante, que acomete um ou mais dos ossos longos de cães jovens pertencentes a raças de porte médio a grande. Do ponto de vista clínico, a panosteíte é caracterizada por claudicação e, ao exame radiográfico, por alta densidade da cavidade medular.

FISIOPATOLOGIA
• Causa desconhecida.
• As tentativas de isolar os microrganismos falharam.
• Aberrações metabólicas, alérgicas ou endócrinas — sem apoio.
• Dor — pode ser atribuída a distúrbio de elementos endosteais e periosteais, congestão vascular ou pressão intramedular elevada.

SISTEMA(S) ACOMETIDO(S)
Musculosquelético — claudicação de intensidade variável; pode acometer um único membro ou se tornar uma claudicação com troca do membro.

GENÉTICA
• Sem transmissão comprovada.
• Predominância da raça Pastor alemão na população acometida sugere fortemente uma base hereditária.

INCIDÊNCIA/PREVALÊNCIA
Nenhuma estimativa confiável; comum.

DISTRIBUIÇÃO GEOGRÁFICA
N/D.

IDENTIFICAÇÃO
Espécies
Cães.

Raça(s) Predominante(s)
• Pastor alemão e seus cruzamentos — afetados com maior frequência.
• Raças de médio a grande porte — mais comumente acometidas.

Idade Média e Faixa Etária
• Em geral, 5-18 meses de vida.
• Desde os 2 meses de vida até os 5 anos de idade.

Sexo Predominante
Machos.

SINAIS CLÍNICOS
Comentários Gerais
Claudicação — se nenhuma anormalidade distinta for notada ao exame físico ou nas radiografias, repetir os exames 4-6 semanas mais tarde.

Achados Anamnésicos
• Sem traumatismo associado.
• Claudicação — intensidade variável; envolve, em geral, os membros anteriores inicialmente; pode acometer os membros posteriores; pode-se observar claudicação com troca do membro; pode-se observar falta de sustentação do peso.
• Doença grave — leve depressão; inapetência; perda de peso.

Achados do Exame Físico
• Dor — à palpação profunda dos ossos longos (diáfise) em um membro acometido; característica distintiva e peculiar; palpar com firmeza ao longo de toda a haste de cada osso ao mesmo tempo em que se evita qualquer pinçamento da musculatura circundante.
• Ossos — a ulna é o osso mais comumente acometido; pode acometer o rádio, o úmero, o fêmur e a tíbia (em ordem decrescente de frequência), concomitante ou subsequentemente.
• Pode-se notar febre de baixo grau.
• Pode-se observar atrofia muscular.

CAUSAS
Desconhecidas.

FATORES DE RISCO
Cães puros da raça Pastor alemão ou seus mestiços.

DIAGNÓSTICO

DIAGNÓSTICO DIFERENCIAL
• Sempre considerar o diagnóstico de panosteíte na presença de claudicação em cão Pastor alemão ou mestiço.
• Pode ocorrer isoladamente ou em combinação com outras doenças ortopédicas juvenis.
• Osteocondrite dissecante.
• Fragmentação do processo coronoide medial.
• Não união do processo ancôneo.
• Displasia coxofemoral.
• Fraturas e lesões ligamentosas causadas por traumatismo não observado.
• Claudicação com troca do peso — artrites imunomediadas; doença de Lyme; endocardite bacteriana.
• Coccidioidomicose.
• Osteomielite bacteriana.

HEMOGRAMA/BIOQUÍMICA/URINÁLISE
• Geralmente normais.
• Pode-se notar eosinofilia no início da doença.

OUTROS TESTES LABORATORIAIS
N/D.

DIAGNÓSTICO POR IMAGEM
• Densidades radiográficas dentro da medula dos ossos longos — achados característicos; confirmam o diagnóstico.
• Lesões radiográficas iniciais, médias e tardias:
• Lesões iniciais — o padrão trabecular das extremidades das diáfises torna-se mais proeminente; pode aparecer indistinto; podem-se observar opacidades granulares.
• Lesões médias — opacidades escleróticas irregulares e dispersas inicialmente ao redor do forame nutrício, e mais tarde, por toda a diáfise; córtex alargado; periósteo espessado com opacidade aumentada.
• Lesões tardias — durante a resolução, opacidade geral diminuída do canal medular (seguindo para a normalidade); padrão trabecular grosseiro e alguma opacidade granular podem persistir; pode ser um período em que o canal medular se torna mais radiotransparente do que o normal.
• O exame de cintilografia óssea pode revelar lesões sutis que, mais tarde, se tornam mais aparentes nas radiografias de acompanhamento.

MÉTODOS DIAGNÓSTICOS
Biopsia óssea — ocasionalmente indicada para descartar neoplasia e infecções bacterianas ou fúngicas que apresentam aspecto radiográfico semelhante.

ACHADOS PATOLÓGICOS
• Biopsia ou necropsia — raramente são realizadas por conta do prognóstico excelente quanto à recuperação.
• Nenhuma lesão patológica macroscópica.
• Degeneração dos adipócitos medulares circundando o forame nutrício, seguida pela proliferação das células do estroma vascular dentro dos sinusoides medulares.
• Formação de osteoide e de novo osso endosteal — avança nos sentidos proximal e distal.
• Congestão vascular — pode acompanhar a proliferação de novo osso, estimulando secundariamente a reação endosteal e periosteal.
• Remodelagem do endósteo — ocorre durante a resolução; restabelece a arquitetura normal do endósteo e da medula.

TRATAMENTO

CUIDADO(S) DE SAÚDE ADEQUADO(S)
Paciente de ambulatório.

CUIDADO(S) DE ENFERMAGEM
Fluidoterapia de manutenção e de reposição — ocasionalmente se deve aos períodos prolongados de inapetência e pirexia.

ATIVIDADE
• Limitada — não foi demonstrado que a restrição da atividade acelere a recuperação; diminui a dor.
• Doença moderada a grave — a dor pode provocar autolimitação do movimento, levando à atrofia muscular.

ORIENTAÇÃO AO PROPRIETÁRIO
• Avisar ao proprietário que o paciente pode desenvolver outras doenças ortopédicas juvenis.
• Informar ao proprietário que os sinais de dor e claudicação podem perdurar por várias semanas.
• Alertar o proprietário que é comum a recidiva dos sinais clínicos até os 2 anos de idade.

CONSIDERAÇÕES CIRÚRGICAS
N/D.

MEDICAÇÕES

MEDICAMENTO(S) DE ESCOLHA
AINE
• Minimizam a dor; diminuem a inflamação.
• O tratamento sintomático não tem qualquer relação com a duração da doença.
• Carprofeno (2,2 mg/kg VO a cada 12 h), etodolaco (10-15 mg/kg VO a cada 24 h), meloxicam (0,2 mg/kg VO, IV ou SC no primeiro dia e, depois, 0,1 mg/kg 1 vez ao dia), deracoxibe (1-2 mg/kg VO 1 vez ao dia para osteoartrite, 3-4 mg/kg VO 1 vez ao dia para dor no pós-operatório; não exceder 7 dias), firocoxibe (5 mg/kg VO 1 vez ao dia), ácido acetilsalicílico tamponado ou dotado de revestimento entérico (10-25 mg/kg VO a cada 8 ou 12 h).
• Glicocorticoides
• Pode-se administrar a dose anti-inflamatória — prednisona (0,1-0,5 mg/kg VO).
• Efeitos colaterais potenciais bem comprovados.
• Objetivo do uso crônico — dose baixa e tratamento em dias alternados.

CONTRAINDICAÇÕES
AINE — a ocorrência de desarranjo gastrintestinal pode impedir a utilização.

PRECAUÇÕES
AINE — a maior parte provoca algum grau de ulceração gástrica.

PANOSTEÍTE

INTERAÇÕES POSSÍVEIS
AINE — não usar em combinação com os glicocorticoides; risco de ulceração do trato gastrintestinal; considerar tempos apropriados de descanso na troca de um AINE para outro.

MEDICAMENTO(S) ALTERNATIVO(S)
N/D.

ACOMPANHAMENTO

MONITORIZAÇÃO DO PACIENTE
Reavaliar a claudicação a cada 2-4 semanas para detectar problemas ortopédicos concomitantes mais graves.

PREVENÇÃO
N/D.

COMPLICAÇÕES POSSÍVEIS
N/D.

EVOLUÇÃO ESPERADA E PROGNÓSTICO
• Doença autolimitante.
• Tratamento — sintomático; parece não ter influência sobre a duração dos sinais clínicos.
• Envolvimento de múltiplos membros — comum.
• Claudicação — tipicamente dura de alguns dias a várias semanas; pode persistir por meses.
• Alguns casos apresentam dor contínua e claudicação irresponsiva à terapia. Nesses cães, recomenda-se a eutanásia.

DIVERSOS

DISTÚRBIOS ASSOCIADOS
N/D.

FATORES RELACIONADOS COM A IDADE
Acomete tipicamente cães imaturos e jovens.

POTENCIAL ZOONÓTICO
N/D.

GESTAÇÃO/FERTILIDADE/REPRODUÇÃO
Há relatos de que as fêmeas sejam mais suscetíveis à panosteíte durante o estro; nenhuma relação comprovada com os hormônios reprodutivos ou a prenhez.

SINÔNIMO(S)
• Enostose.
• Osteodistrofia fibrosa.
• Osteomielite juvenil.
• Panosteíte eosinofílica.

ABREVIATURA(S)
• AINE = anti-inflamatórios não esteroides.

Sugestões de Leitura
Halliwell WH. Tumorlike lesions of bone. In: Bojrab MJ, ed., Disease Mechanisms in Small Animal Surgery, 2nd ed. Philadelphia: Saunders, 1993, pp. 932-933.
LaFond E, Bruer GJ, Austin CC. Breed susceptibility for developmental diseases in dogs. JAAHA 2002, 38:467-477.
Muir P, Dubielzig RR, Johnson KA. Panosteitis. Compend Contin Educ Pract Vet 1996, 18:29-33.
Piermattei DL, Flo GL, DeCamp CE. Miscellaneous conditions of the musculoskeletal system. In: Handbook of Small Animal Orthopedics and Fracture Repair, 4th ed. Philadelphia: Saunders, 2006, pp. 775-778.
Schwarz T, Johnson VS, Voute L, Sullivan M. Bone scintigraphy in the investigation of occult lameness in the dog. J Small Anim Pract 2004, 45:232-237.
Trostel CT, Pool RR, McLaughlin RM. Canine lameness caused by developmental orthopedic diseases: Panosteitis, Legg-Calvé-Perthes disease, and hypertophic osteodystrophy. Compend Contin Educ Pract Vet 2003, 25(4):282-292.

Autor Larry Carpenter
Consultor Editorial Peter K. Shires

PAPILEDEMA

CONSIDERAÇÕES GERAIS

REVISÃO
- Papiledema — tumefação do disco óptico secundária a aumento da pressão intracraniana sem perda perceptível da visão.
- Também conhecido como edema do disco óptico.
- Tumefação do disco óptico também pode acompanhar outras neuropatias ópticas, como neurite óptica.
- Acomete os sistemas oftálmico e nervoso.

IDENTIFICAÇÃO
Cães e gatos.

SINAIS CLÍNICOS
Achados Anamnésicos
- Sinais cerebrais.
- O edema do disco óptico por si só não produz déficits visuais.

Achados do Exame Físico
- Sinais do SNC.
- Elevação e hiperemia da cabeça do nervo óptico.
- Turvamento da margem do disco óptico.
- Preenchimento da escavação fisiológica*.
- Reflexos pupilares à luz encontram-se normais a quase normais.

CAUSAS E FATORES DE RISCO
- Hidrocefalia.
- Encefalopatia hepática.
- Neoplasia — primária ou metastática.
- Cinomose (cães).
- PIF (gatos).
- Micoses sistêmicas.
- Toxoplasmose.
- *Neospora caninum*.
- Meningoencefalomielite granulomatosa.
- Traumatismo.

DIAGNÓSTICO

DIAGNÓSTICO DIFERENCIAL
- Neurite óptica — tipicamente exibe reflexos pupilares anormais à luz e alguma perda perceptível da visão.
- Anomalias congênitas como mielinização excessiva. Alterações não progressivas sem alterações perceptíveis no reflexo pupilar à luz ou na visão. A mielinização excessiva é comum em cães da raça Golden retriever.

HEMOGRAMA/BIOQUÍMICA/URINÁLISE
Sem anormalidades específicas.

OUTROS TESTES LABORATORIAIS
Testes sorológicos específicos para vírus, fungos ou protozoários, com base nas possíveis causas.

DIAGNÓSTICO POR IMAGEM
- Neuroimagem —TC ou RM.
- Ultrassonografia orbital.

MÉTODOS DIAGNÓSTICOS
Análise do LCS — mede a pressão intracraniana.

TRATAMENTO

- Resolver a causa da pressão intracraniana aumentada ou da doença orbital.
- Pacientes necessitam de monitorização crítica.
- Manter a $PaCO_2$ em 30-35 mmHg.

MEDICAÇÕES

MEDICAMENTO(S)
- Manitol — 1 g/kg IV por 20 min; repetido conforme a necessidade.
- Salina hipertônica 3 mL/kg IV por 10 min.
- Corticosteroides — prednisona (0,5 mg/kg VO a cada 12 h) ou fosfato sódico de dexametasona (0,25 mg/kg IV a cada 8-12 h); não são indicados para traumatismo cefálico.
- Salina hipertônica 3-4 mL/kg IV por 2-5 min.

CONTRAINDICAÇÕES/INTERAÇÕES POSSÍVEIS
- Cuidado com a herniação cerebral.
- Corticosteroides sistêmicos — não utilizar até que as causas infecciosas estejam descartadas.

ACOMPANHAMENTO

Prognóstico — depende da doença subjacente.

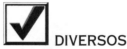

DIVERSOS

ABREVIATURA(S)
- LCS = líquido cerebrospinal.
- PIF = peritonite infecciosa felina.
- RM = ressonância magnética.
- SNC = sistema nervoso central.
- TC = tomografia computadorizada.

Sugestões de Leitura
Whiting AS, Johnson LN. Papilledema: Clinical clues and differential diagnosis. Am Fam Physician 1994, 5:1125-1134.

Autor David Lipsitz
Consultor Editorial Paul E. Miller

---

* N. T.: Pequena fossa ou depressão, localizada no cérebro (ou próximo ao mesmo), do disco óptico, por meio do qual passam os vasos retinianos centrais.

PAPILOMATOSE

CONSIDERAÇÕES GERAIS

REVISÃO
- Lesões da pele e das mucosas de cães e gatos, causadas por papilomavírus.
- As verrugas constituem a manifestação mais comum das lesões de papilomatose.
- Placas virais que, algumas vezes, evoluem para carcinoma de células escamosas ou carcinoma invasivo, são identificadas em cães e gatos.
- Carcinoma bowenoide *in situ* representa a lesão mais comum por papilomavírus em gatos.
- A maioria das verrugas em cães é exofítica*; os papilomas elevados ou invertidos não são incomuns.

SISTEMA(S) ACOMETIDO(S)
Cutâneo/exócrino.

IDENTIFICAÇÃO
Cães
- Existem dois tipos genéticos de vírus com, pelo menos, seis cepas e seis síndromes:
- Cães jovens com lesões nos coxins palmoplantares.
- Pápulas, placas, nódulos pigmentados discretos em cães jovens adultos.
- Schnauzer miniatura, Pug — placa pigmentada.
- Papilomas bucais, oculares e genitais geralmente em cães jovens.
- Papilomas cutâneos em qualquer idade.

Gatos
- A papilomatose é mais comum em gatos mais idosos; associada a imunocomprometimento (p. ex., FIV).

SINAIS CLÍNICOS
Cães
- Os papilomas cutâneos são frequentemente pedunculados, consistindo em lâminas de epitélio, dotados de até 1 cm de diâmetro e localizados em qualquer lugar.
- Os papilomas bucais em cães jovens envolvem estruturas como lábios, gengivas, línguas, palato, orofaringe e esôfago; tais papilomas interferem nos processos de preensão e deglutição; o traumatismo resulta em halitose e ptialismo intensos.
- As lesões podem ficar confinadas às regiões genitais ou palpebrais.
- Os papilomas invertidos são menos comuns e, com frequência, ficam localizados na parte ventral do abdome, têm até 2 cm e possuem um poro central.
- Placas caninas são observadas com maior frequência em cães das raças Schnauzer miniatura e Pug; raramente se transformam em carcinoma de células escamosas; as partes ventrais do abdome e as regiões internas da coxa são frequentemente envolvidas.

Gatos
- Papilomas exofíticos são extremamente raros; os papilomas mais comuns são placas pigmentadas simples, que podem evoluir para carcinoma bowenoide *in situ* ou para carcinoma invasivo.
- Com frequência, os gatos têm 10 anos de idade ou mais; podem ter outras doenças sistêmicas indutoras de imunossupressão (p. ex., FIV).

---
* N.T.: Que tende a crescer para fora, além do epitélio superficial do qual se origina.

CAUSAS E FATORES DE RISCO
- Verrugas bucais em cães que nunca tiveram esse tipo de lesão e animais recuperados imunes.
- Cães — acredita-se que os papilomas cutâneos envolvam defeitos imunológicos mediados por células.
- Gatos mais idosos e imunocomprometidos desenvolvem placas ou carcinoma bowenoide *in situ*.
- Placas caninas — base genética em algumas raças.

DIAGNÓSTICO

DIAGNÓSTICO DIFERENCIAL
Cães
- Cavidade bucal e orofaringe — epúlide fibromatoso; tumor venéreo transmissível; carcinoma de células escamosas.
- Lesões cutâneas — hiperplasia sebácea; acrocórdone**.
- Placas pigmentadas — melanocitoma.
- Papilomas invertidos — distinguir acantoma queratinizante infundibular.

Gatos
- Múltiplas lesões hiperqueratóticas e sésseis — placas ou granulomas eosinofílicos; queratoses actínicas; lesões cutâneas de FeLV; carcinoma de células escamosas multicêntrico *in situ*; carcinoma de células escamosas.

HEMOGRAMA/BIOQUÍMICA/URINÁLISE
Normais.

OUTROS TESTES LABORATORIAIS
Gatos: FeLV, FIV.

MÉTODOS DIAGNÓSTICOS
- Aspecto típico das lesões macroscópicas; a biopsia confirma o diagnóstico.
- Verrugas e placas cutâneas em cães e gatos necessitam de exame histopatológico.
- Imuno-histoquímica demonstra a presença de antígenos virais dentro das lesões; a técnica de PCR não é tão definitiva.

TRATAMENTO
- A maioria das lesões geralmente regride de forma espontânea (sobretudo as formas bucais).
- Cirurgia para remover os tumores bucais (excisão, criocirurgia ou eletrocirurgia) — em casos de oclusão (obstrução) de via aérea; incômodo para se alimentar; razões estéticas.
- Corticosteroides sistêmicos — retirar em caso de recidiva de doença bucal ou cutânea grave ou persistente.
- Doença persistente (cães) — pode-se tratar com autovacinação; usar vacina autógena ativada pelo calor; tratamento controverso.
- Gatos — diagnóstico para doenças viscerais ou causas de imunossupressão; terapia com interferona ou imiquimode (Aldara®) para placas e carcinoma bowenoide *in situ*.

** N.T.: Pequenos papilomas localizados geralmente nas faces laterais do pescoço, axilas, porção superior do tronco e pálpebras de pacientes de meia-idade ou idosos.

MEDICAÇÕES
- Interferona (omegainterferona) — 1 MU/kg por via SC 3 vezes por semana durante 4 semanas.
- Imiquimode (Aldara®) — aplicado 3 vezes por semana durante 4 semanas.

ACOMPANHAMENTO

MONITORIZAÇÃO DO PACIENTE
Monitorizar as lesões cuidadosamente para detectar os sinais (ulceração, exsudação purulenta e crescimento rápido) de transformação maligna para carcinoma de células escamosas.

PREVENÇÃO
- Separar os cães com papilomas bucais dos animais suscetíveis.
- Canis comerciais com surtos de papilomatose bucal — pode-se considerar o uso de vacinas autógenas.
- Vacina viva para papilomatose bucal em cães — há relatos de que esse tipo de vacina induza a tumores epiteliais hiperplásicos e carcinoma de células escamosas nos locais de vacinação; período de latência de 11-34 meses.

EVOLUÇÃO ESPERADA E PROGNÓSTICO
- Cães — em geral, o prognóstico é bom; período de incubação de 1-8 semanas; a regressão costuma ocorrer com 1-5 meses; as lesões podem persistir por 24 meses ou mais.
- Gatos — o prognóstico de placas e carcinoma bowenoide *in situ* a longo prazo depende basicamente das doenças concomitantes.

DIVERSOS

SINÔNIMOS
Doença de Bowen = carcinoma bowenoide *in situ*.

ABREVIATURA(S)
- FeLV = vírus da leucemia felina.
- FIV = vírus da imunodeficiência felina.
- PCR = reação em cadeia da polimerase.

Sugestões de Leitura
Gross TL, Ihrke PJ, Walder EM, Affolter VK. Skin Diseases of the Dog and Cat, 2nd ed. Oxford: Blackwell Science, 2005, pp. 157-159,567-581.
Sundberg JP. Papillomaviruses. In: Castro AE, Heuscele WP, eds., Veterinary Diagnostic Virology. St Louis: Mosby, 1992, pp. 148-150.

Autor Elizabeth R. May
Consultor Editorial Alexander H. Werner
Agradecimento aos autores da edição anterior Edward G. Clark e Suzette M. LeClerc

Parada Atrial

CONSIDERAÇÕES GERAIS

DEFINIÇÃO
Ritmo eletrocardiográfico caracterizado pela ausência de ondas P; esse distúrbio pode ser temporário (p. ex., associado à hipercalemia ou induzido por medicamentos), terminal (p. ex., associado à hipercalemia grave ou a um coração em falência) ou persistente.

Características do ECG
Parada Atrial Persistente
- Ausência de ondas P.
- Frequência cardíaca geralmente lenta (<60 bpm).
- Ritmo regular com complexos QRS do tipo supraventricular.
- A frequência cardíaca não aumenta com a administração da atropina.

Parada Atrial Hipercalêmica
- Frequência cardíaca normal ou lenta.
- Ritmo regular ou irregular.
- Os complexos QRS tendem a ser largos e se tornam cada vez mais amplos à medida que o nível de potássio se eleva; em casos de hipercalemia grave (potássio >10 mEq/L), os complexos QRS são substituídos por uma curva bifásica nivelada.
- A frequência cardíaca pode aumentar um pouco com a aplicação de atropina.

FISIOPATOLOGIA
Parada Atrial Persistente
Causada por distrofia muscular atrial; é comum o envolvimento da musculatura esquelética.

Parada Atrial Hipercalêmica
Em geral, ocorre com níveis séricos de potássio >8,5 mEq/L; o valor é influenciado pelos níveis séricos de sódio e cálcio, bem como pelo estado acidobásico. Os pacientes hipercalêmicos com parada atrial exibem a atuação do nó sinusal, mas os impulsos não ativam os miócitos atriais; assim, o ritmo associado recebe o nome de ritmo sinoventricular. Como o nó sinusal permanece funcional, o ritmo irregular pode ser decorrente da arritmia sinusal.

SISTEMA(S) ACOMETIDO(S)
Cardiovascular.

GENÉTICA
Nenhuma base genética.

INCIDÊNCIA/PREVALÊNCIA
Distúrbio rítmico raro.

DISTRIBUIÇÃO GEOGRÁFICA
Nenhuma.

IDENTIFICAÇÃO
Espécies
Cães e gatos.

Raça(s) Predominante(s)
Parada atrial persistente — mais comum em Springer spaniel inglês; acomete ocasionalmente outras raças.

Idade Média e Faixa Etária
Praticamente todos os animais com parada atrial persistente são jovens; os animais com hipoadrenocorticismo costumam estar na faixa etária jovem à meia-idade.

Sexo(s) Predominante(s)
O hipoadrenocorticismo é mais comum em fêmeas (69%).

SINAIS CLÍNICOS
Achados Anamnésicos
- Variam com a causa subjacente.
- É comum a presença de letargia; é possível a ocorrência de síncope.
- Os pacientes com parada atrial persistente podem exibir sinais de insuficiência cardíaca congestiva (ICC).

Achados do Exame Físico
- Variam com a causa subjacente.
- É comum a bradicardia.
- Os pacientes com parada atrial persistente podem apresentar emaciação muscular esquelética no antebraço e na escápula.

CAUSAS
- Hipercalemia.
- Doença atrial, muitas vezes associada à distensão dessa câmara cardíaca (p. ex., gatos com miocardiopatia).
- Miopatia atrial (parada atrial persistente).

FATORES DE RISCO
Parada Atrial Hipercalêmica
- Hipoadrenocorticismo.
- Condições indutoras de obstrução ou ruptura do trato urinário.
- Insuficiência renal oligúrica ou anúrica.

DIAGNÓSTICO

DIAGNÓSTICO DIFERENCIAL
- Fibrilação atrial lenta.
- Bradicardia sinusal com pequenas ondas P perdidas na linha basal.

HEMOGRAMA/BIOQUÍMICA/URINÁLISE
Parada Atrial Persistente
- Normais.

Parada Atrial Hipercalêmica
- Hipercalemia.
- Hiponatremia e relação de sódio:potássio <27 na ocorrência de parada atrial secundária ao hipoadrenocorticismo.
- Azotemia e hiperfosfatemia em casos de hipoadrenocorticismo, insuficiência renal e ruptura ou obstrução do trato urinário.

OUTROS TESTES LABORATORIAIS
Na suspeita de hipoadrenocorticismo, efetua-se o teste de estimulação com o ACTH.

DIAGNÓSTICO POR IMAGEM
Se houver suspeita de parada atrial persistente, lança-se mão da ecocardiografia e da eletromiografia — nesses exames, poderão ser observadas algumas anormalidades, como cardiomegalia e diminuição na contratilidade.

MÉTODOS DIAGNÓSTICOS
Biopsia de músculo esquelético em animais com parada atrial persistente.

ACHADOS PATOLÓGICOS
Parada Atrial Persistente
- Átrios bastante aumentados de volume e delgados como papel; em geral, ocorre o envolvimento biatrial, embora há relato de um caso de envolvimento apenas do átrio esquerdo.
- Emaciação muscular escapular e braquial grave em alguns cães.
- Fibrose acentuada, fibroelastose, inflamação mononuclear crônica e esteatose nos átrios e no septo interatrial.

TRATAMENTO

CUIDADO(S) DE SAÚDE ADEQUADO(S)
Parada Atrial Persistente
Não representa uma condição com risco de vida; o animal poderá ser tratado em um esquema ambulatorial.

Parada Atrial Hipercalêmica
Há risco de vida em potencial; muitas vezes, exige tratamento rigoroso.

CUIDADO(S) DE ENFERMAGEM
Em pacientes com parada atrial hipercalêmica, é necessária a fluidoterapia intensiva com solução salina a 0,9% para corrigir a hipovolemia e reduzir os níveis séricos de potássio (ver "Hipercalemia").

ATIVIDADE
Em pacientes com parada atrial persistente e sinais de ICC ou síncope, deve-se restringir a atividade física.

DIETA
N/D.

ORIENTAÇÃO AO PROPRIETÁRIO
Parada Atrial Persistente
Os sinais clínicos geralmente melhoram depois do implante de marca-passo; mesmo após a correção da frequência e do ritmo cardíacos com esse dispositivo, ainda poderão surgir sinais de ICC com possível persistência dos sintomas de fraqueza e letargia.

CONSIDERAÇÕES CIRÚRGICAS
Parada Atrial Persistente
Implante de marca-passo ventricular permanente para regular a frequência e o ritmo cardíacos.

Parada Atrial Hipercalêmica
A hipercalemia secundária à obstrução ou ruptura do trato urinário pode necessitar de intervenção cirúrgica.

MEDICAÇÕES

MEDICAMENTO(S) DE ESCOLHA
Parada Atrial Persistente
No desenvolvimento de ICC, tratar o animal com diuréticos e inibidor da ECA (p. ex., enalapril ou benazepril).

Parada Atrial Hipercalêmica
- Tratar a causa subjacente (p. ex., insuficiência renal oligúrica e hipoadrenocorticismo).
- Fluidoterapia rigorosa com solução salina a 0,9% e, possivelmente, administração de bicarbonato de sódio ou insulina com glicose, conforme se encontra discutido na seção sobre "Hipercalemia".
- Gliconato de cálcio — neutraliza os efeitos cardíacos da hipercalemia; pode ser utilizado em casos com risco de vida para restabelecer o ritmo sinusal, ao mesmo tempo em que se institui o tratamento para reduzir a concentração do potássio.

PARADA ATRIAL

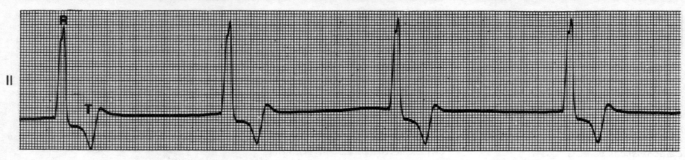

Figura 1. Parada atrial em cão com nível de potássio de 9 mEq/L. Observar a ausência de ondas P e a presença de complexos QRS amplos.

CONTRAINDICAÇÕES
Em pacientes hipercalêmicos, é fundamental evitar os fluidos com potássio em sua composição ou os medicamentos que aumentem a concentração desse íon.

PRECAUÇÕES
Os diuréticos diminuem a pré-carga e podem agravar a fraqueza em cães com parada atrial persistente e ICC a menos que tenha sido feito o implante de marca-passo.

INTERAÇÕES POSSÍVEIS
N/D.

MEDICAMENTO(S) ALTERNATIVO(S)
N/D.

 ACOMPANHAMENTO

MONITORIZAÇÃO DO PACIENTE
• Monitorizar o ECG durante o tratamento da hipercalemia e também periodicamente em animais com marca-passo ventricular permanente.
• Monitorizar os eletrólitos em pacientes com parada atrial hipercalêmica.
• Monitorizar os pacientes com parada atrial persistente em busca de sinais de ICC.

PREVENÇÃO
N/D.

COMPLICAÇÕES POSSÍVEIS
ICC em pacientes com parada atrial persistente.

EVOLUÇÃO ESPERADA E PROGNÓSTICO
Parada Atrial Persistente
Os sinais clínicos geralmente melhoram depois do implante de marca-passo. Mesmo após a correção da frequência e do ritmo cardíacos com esse dispositivo, ainda poderão surgir sinais de ICC com possível persistência dos sintomas de fraqueza e letargia. Ainda pode haver a persistência de sinais relacionados com distrofia muscular.

Parada Atrial Hipercalêmica
O prognóstico a longo prazo é excelente caso se consiga corrigir a causa subjacente e reverter a hipercalemia.

 DIVERSOS

DISTÚRBIOS ASSOCIADOS
Doenças indutoras de hipercalemia (p. ex., hipoadrenocorticismo, obstrução uretral ou laceração do trato urinário, acidose e medicamentos).

FATORES RELACIONADOS COM A IDADE
Parada atrial persistente — diagnosticada comumente em animais jovens;
Hipoadrenocorticismo — diagnosticado em geral em animais jovens aos de meia-idade.

POTENCIAL ZOONÓTICO
Nenhum.

GESTAÇÃO/FERTILIDADE/REPRODUÇÃO
N/D.

SINÔNIMO(S)
Silêncio atrial.

VER TAMBÉM
• Hipercalemia.
• Hipoadrenocorticismo (Doença de Addison).
• Obstrução do Trato Urinário.
• Toxicidade da Digoxina.

ABREVIATURA(S)
• ACTH = hormônio adrenocorticotrófico.
• ECA = enzima conversora da angiotensina.
• ECG = eletrocardiograma.
• ICC = insuficiência cardíaca congestiva.

Sugestões de Leitura
Kraus MS, Gelzer ARM, Moise S. Treatment of cardiac arrhythmias and conduction disturbances. In: Tilley LP, Smith FWK, Oyama MA, Sleeper MM, eds., Manual of Canine and Feline Cardiology, 4th ed. St. Louis: Saunders Elsevier, 2008, pp. 315-332.
Tilley LP, Smith FWK Jr. Electrocardiography. In: Tilley LP, Smith FWK, Oyama MA, Sleeper MM, eds., Manual of Canine and Feline Cardiology, 4th ed. St. Louis: Saunders Elsevier, 2008, pp. 49-77.

Autor Francis W.K. Smith, Jr.
Consultores Editoriais Larry P. Tilley e Francis W.K. Smith, Jr.

PARADA CARDIOPULMONAR

CONSIDERAÇÕES GERAIS

DEFINIÇÃO
- Interrupção da perfusão e da ventilação efetivas, em virtude da perda das funções cardíaca e respiratória coordenadas.
- Se não for identificada e corrigida, a parada cardíaca invariavelmente acompanha parada respiratória.

FISIOPATOLOGIA
- O quadro de hipoxia generalizada ou celular pode ser a causa ou a consequência de morte súbita.
- Após 1-4 minutos de obstrução das vias aéreas, os esforços respiratórios param, enquanto a circulação permanece intacta.
- Se a obstrução continuar por 6-9 minutos, os quadros de hipotensão e bradicardia graves levarão à midríase, ausência de sons cardíacos e falta de pulso palpável.
- Após 6-9 minutos, as contrações miocárdicas cessam mesmo que o ECG possa parecer normal — atividade elétrica sem pulso (denominada antigamente dissociação eletromecânica).
- A fibrilação ventricular, a assistolia ventricular e a atividade elétrica sem pulso são ritmos indicativos de interrupção da contratilidade miocárdica.

SISTEMA(S) ACOMETIDO(S)
- Todos os sistemas são acometidos, mas primeiramente aqueles que exigem o maior aporte de oxigênio e nutrientes.
- Cardiovascular.
- Renal/urológico.
- Neurológico.

IDENTIFICAÇÃO
- Cães e gatos. • Qualquer idade, raça ou sexo.

SINAIS CLÍNICOS
- Perda de consciência.
- Midríase (pupilas dilatadas).
- Cianose.
- Suspiro agônico ou ventilação ausente.
- Ausência de pulsos periféricos.
- Hipotermia.
- Ausência de sons cardíacos auscultáveis.
- Falta de resposta a estímulos.

CAUSAS
- Hipoxemia causada por desequilíbrio entre ventilação/perfusão, dano à barreira de difusão, hipoventilação ou desvio.
- Má distribuição de oxigênio, por conta de anemia ou vasoconstrição.
- Miocardiopatia — infecciosa, inflamatória, infiltrativa, traumática, neoplásica, ou embólica.
- Anormalidades acidobásicas.
- Desarranjos eletrolíticos — hipercalemia, hipocalcemia e hipomagnesemia.
- Hipovolemia.
- Choque.
- Agentes anestésicos.
- Toxemia.
- Traumatismo do SNC.
- Choque elétrico.

FATORES DE RISCO
- Doença cardiovascular.
- Doença respiratória.
- Traumatismo.
- Anestesia.
- Septicemia.
- Endotoxemia.
- Arritmias ventriculares — taquicardia ventricular, fenômeno da onda R sobre a T, complexos ventriculares multiformes.
- Aumento no tônus parassimpático — gastrenteropatias, doenças respiratórias, manipulações dos olhos, da laringe ou de vísceras abdominais.
- Crises convulsivas prolongadas.
- Manipulações cardiovasculares invasivas — pericardiocentese, cirurgia, angiografia.

DIAGNÓSTICO

O colapso cardiovascular súbito associado a débito cardíaco inadequado pode levar a graves consequências.
- A avaliação e o diagnóstico imediatos são críticos.
- Avaliação dos ABCs — vias aéreas, base respiratória e circulação.

DIAGNÓSTICO DIFERENCIAL
- Hipovolemia grave e ausência de pulsos palpáveis.
- Efusão pericárdica, débito cardíaco reduzido e sons cardíacos abafados.
- Efusão pleural com parada respiratória.
- A parada respiratória pode ser confundida com PCP.
- A obstrução das vias aéreas superiores pode evoluir rapidamente para uma PCP.

HEMOGRAMA/BIOQUÍMICA/URINÁLISE
Podem ajudar a identificar uma causa subjacente para a PCP, mas não devem fazer parte integrante da triagem inicial.

OUTROS TESTES LABORATORIAIS
- A gasometria arterial pode ser útil durante ou após os procedimentos de ressuscitação, mas não faz parte do tratamento inicial de emergência.
- A gasometria venosa pode ter mais utilidade durante a ressuscitação em comparação à arterial, pois fornece as concentrações de eletrólitos e lactato.

DIAGNÓSTICO POR IMAGEM
- As radiografias torácicas podem auxiliar na identificação do processo patológico subjacente, mas devem ser consideradas somente após a estabilização do paciente.
- A ecocardiografia pode confirmar a efusão pericárdica ou a miocardiopatia subjacente, mas não deve interferir nos procedimentos de ressuscitação.
- As radiografias ou ultrassonografias abdominais podem ser úteis assim que o paciente estiver estabilizado para identificar a doença subjacente.

MÉTODOS DIAGNÓSTICOS
Assim que uma PCP se desenvolver, a monitorização contínua do ECG, a monitorização da pressão arterial, a oximetria de pulso e a capnografia poderão ser exames proveitosos na avaliação da eficácia dos procedimentos de ressuscitação.

TRATAMENTO

- Imediatamente após o diagnóstico da PCP, deve-se instituir a ressuscitação cardiopulmonar (RCP); a RCP pode ser dividida em suportes vitais cardíacos básico e avançado.
- As recomendações atuais (2005) da American Heart Association incorporaram a desfibrilação no suporte vital básico.

SUPORTE VITAL CARDÍACO BÁSICO

A — Vias Aéreas
- Avaliação — inspecionar as vias aéreas, estendendo-se a cabeça e o pescoço do paciente e tracionando-se a língua para fora e para a frente; remover quaisquer debris (p. ex., secreções, sangue ou vômito), manualmente ou por meio de sucção.
- Estabelecer uma via aérea por meio de entubação orotraqueal ou, na presença de obstrução completa, efetuar traqueostomia de emergência.

B — Base Respiratória
- Avaliação — certificar-se de que o animal não está respirando.
- Instituir ventilação artificial — administrar dois movimentos respiratórios breves de ~2 s de duração cada e reavaliar; se não ocorrer nenhuma respiração espontânea, prosseguir com as ventilações a uma velocidade adequada para o animal em questão (frequência respiratória normal de 10 a 24 movimentos respiratórios por minuto). As pressões de pico das vias aéreas não devem ultrapassar 20 cmH$_2$O.
- As técnicas para ventilação incluem a respiração boca a boca, boca-nariz ou boca-sonda orotraqueal; essas técnicas fornecem oxigênio a ~16%; o uso do Ambu ou do ar ambiente proporciona oxigênio a 21%.
- A técnica preferida consiste na entubação orotraqueal e na ventilação com oxigênio a 100%, utilizando-se o Ambu ou um aparelho de anestesia inalatória.
- A velocidade sugerida de administração do oxigênio é de 150 mL/kg/min.

C — Circulação
- Avaliação — realizar a palpação dos pulsos periféricos e a auscultação cardíaca para confirmar a PCP.
- A massagem cardíaca externa confere, na melhor das hipóteses, ~30% do débito cardíaco normal; a massagem cardíaca interna é 2 a 3 vezes mais eficaz no restabelecimento das perfusões cerebral e coronariana.
- Os estudos hemodinâmicos em modelos animais sugerem a existência de diversos mecanismos distintos para a geração do fluxo sanguíneo (sístole artificial) durante as compressões torácicas; no transcorrer da massagem cardíaca externa, a teoria da bomba cardíaca tira vantagem da compressão direta do coração em pacientes com menos de 7 kg de peso corporal; em pacientes com mais de 7 kg, emprega-se a teoria da bomba torácica; essa técnica emprega as elevações nas pressões intratorácicas para aumentar o débito cardíaco por meio de efeitos indiretos sobre as artérias principais.

TÉCNICAS DE COMPRESSÃO/VENTILAÇÃO
- Executar as compressões torácicas com rapidez, a uma velocidade de 80-100 compressões/min; o tórax deve ser movimentado em ~30%.
- Utilizar a bomba cardíaca em pacientes com menos de 7 kg de peso corporal; com o paciente em decúbito lateral direito, efetuar as compressões diretamente sobre o coração (3°-5° espaços intercostais); isso pode ser feito, utilizando-se uma ou ambas as mãos.

Parada Cardiopulmonar

- Empregar a bomba torácica em pacientes com mais de 7 kg de peso corporal; com o paciente em decúbito lateral direito, aplicar as compressões torácicas na parte mais ampla do tórax.
- Há relatos de diferentes esquemas de compressão e ventilação.
- O objetivo é fornecer compressões (80-100/min) e ventilações (10-24/min) adequadas sem interromper as compressões para realizar as ventilações e sem tentar sincronizar as ventilações com as compressões.
- A interposição de compressões abdominais entre as compressões torácicas aumenta os fluxos sanguíneos cerebral e coronariano por meio de um incremento na pressão diastólica aórtica. Não foi demonstrado que essa técnica aumente a sobrevida.

RCP COM O TÓRAX ABERTO
- Indicada se a RCP com o tórax fechado for ineficaz ou se condições preexistentes, como tórax frouxo/oscilante, obesidade, hérnia diafragmática ou efusão pericárdica, impedirem as técnicas com o tórax fechado.
- Realizar essa RCP através de uma toracotomia esquerda na altura do quinto ou sexto espaço intercostal.
- Efetuar o procedimento de pericardiectomia.
- Para impulsionar o sangue ventricular em direção aos grandes vasos, empregam-se a superfície palmar dos dedos e o polegar; a compressão digital da aorta descendente pode ajudar a restabelecer a perfusão coronariana e cerebral.

SUPORTE VITAL CARDÍACO AVANÇADO
D — Drogas
- A seleção dos medicamentos deve ter como base o tipo de arritmia presente.
- A atropina e a adrenalina são as opções terapêuticas mais corretas e frequentes.
- Atropina — 0,05 mg/kg IV (0,54 mg/mL), ou seja, 1 mL/paciente de 10 kg.
- Adrenalina em baixas doses — 0,01 mg/kg IV (diluição de 1:10.000), ou seja, 1 mL/paciente de 10 kg.
- Outros agentes como vasopressina podem ser considerados se a terapia inicial falhar.

E — ECG
- É imperativa uma interpretação precisa do ECG.
- Avaliar as derivações do ECG.
- Minimizar a interrupção das compressões torácicas durante a leitura do ECG.

F — Controle da Fibrilação e Administração de Fluidos
- A desfibrilação é dependente do tempo; efetuá-la imediatamente.
- Administrar os fluidos com cautela a menos que hipovolemia conhecida tenha levado à PCP. Cristaloides, coloides ou produtos sanguíneos podem ser considerados, inclusive a oxiglobina.

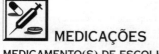

MEDICAÇÕES
MEDICAMENTO(S) DE ESCOLHA
- A seleção do medicamento deve feita com base no tipo de arritmia presente.
- Administrar os medicamentos por via venosa central, intratraqueal, intraóssea ou venosa periférica, em ordem decrescente de preferência. Os volumes devem ser dobrados em caso de administração por via orotraqueal e diluídos em soro fisiológico.
- Utilizar a via de administração intracardíaca somente como o último recurso a menos que uma RCP com o tórax aberto esteja sendo realizada. É ideal a administração do agente no ventrículo esquerdo com compressão digital concomitante da aorta descendente.

PRECAUÇÕES
Caso exista histórico conhecido de hipovolemia, utilizar apenas altas velocidades de administração de fluidos; o fornecimento excessivo de fluidos pode levar à queda na perfusão coronariana.

ACOMPANHAMENTO
MONITORIZAÇÃO DO PACIENTE
- Manter a normalidade na frequência cardíaca e na pressão arterial com o emprego de fluidos e agentes inotrópicos.
- Pressão sanguínea arterial.
- Pressão venosa central.
- Gasometria sanguínea.
- Manter a respiração por meio de ventilação artificial e suplementação de oxigênio.
- Estado neurológico — caso se desenvolvam sinais de pressão intracraniana elevada, considerar o uso de manitol, corticosteroides e furosemida.
- ECG — contínuo.
- Débito urinário.
- Temperatura corporal.
- Radiografias torácicas para avaliar os danos causados pela ressuscitação.
- Diagnosticar e corrigir os fatores indutores da PCP inicial.

PREVENÇÃO
Monitorização cautelosa de todos os pacientes criticamente enfermos.

COMPLICAÇÕES POSSÍVEIS
- Vômitos.
- Pneumonia por aspiração.
- Fraturas de costelas ou estérnebras.
- Edemas e contusões pulmonares.
- Pneumotórax.
- Insuficiência renal aguda.
- Déficits neurológicos.
- Arritmias cardíacas.

EVOLUÇÃO ESPERADA E PROGNÓSTICO
- O prognóstico depende do processo patológico subjacente.
- O rápido retorno às funções cardíaca e respiratória espontâneas melhora o prognóstico.
- O prognóstico global é mau; <10% dos pacientes recebem alta.

DIVERSOS
POTENCIAL ZOONÓTICO
N/D.

GESTAÇÃO/FERTILIDADE/REPRODUÇÃO
N/D.

SINÔNIMO(S)
- Parada cardíaca.
- Ataque cardíaco.

VER TAMBÉM
- Fibrilação Ventricular.
- Parada Ventricular (Assistolia).

ABREVIATURA(S)
- ECG = eletrocardiograma.
- PCP = parada cardiopulmonar.
- RCP = ressuscitação cardiopulmonar.
- SNC = sistema nervoso central.

Sugestões de Leitura

American Heart Association. Guidelines for cardiopulmonary resuscitation and emergency cardiovascular care. Circulation 2005, 112(24) Supplement.

Cole SG, Drobatz KJ. Cardiopulmonary resuscitation. In: Tilley LP, Smith FWK, Oyama MA, Sleeper MM, eds., Manual of Canine and Feline Cardiology, 4th ed. St. Louis: Saunders Elsevier, 2008, pp. 333-341.

Cole SG, Otto CM, Hughes D. Cardiopulmonary cerebral resuscitation in small animals—a clinical practice review (part I). J Vet Emerg Crit Care, 2002, 12(4):261-267.

Cole SG, Otto CM, Hughes D. Cardiopulmonary cerebral resuscitation in small animals—a clinical practice review (part II). J Vet Emerg Crit Care 2003, 13(1):13-23.

Haldane S, Marks SL. Cardiopulmonary cerebral resuscitation: Emergency drugs and postresuscitative care (part II). Compend Contin Educ Pract Vet 2004, 26(10):791-799.

Haldane S, Marks SL. Cardiopulmonary cerebral resuscitation: Techniques (part I). Compend Contin Educ Pract Vet 2004, 26(10):780-790.

Hofmeister EH, Brainard BM, et al. Prognostic indicators for dogs and cats with cardiopulmonary arrest treated by cardiopulmonary cerebral resuscitation at a university teaching hospital. JAVMA 2009, 235:50-57.

Plunkett SJ, McMichael M. Cardiopulmonary resuscitation in small animal medicine: An update. J Vet Intern Med 2008, 22:9-25.

Waldrop JE, Rozanski EA, et al. Causes of cardiopulmonary arrest, resuscitation management, and functional outcome in dogs and cats surviving cardiopulmonary arrest. J Vet Emerg Crit Care 2004, 14(1):22-29.

Autor Steven L. Marks
Consultores Editoriais Larry P. Tilley e Francis W.K. Smith, Jr.

Parada Sinusal e Bloqueio Sinoatrial

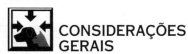

CONSIDERAÇÕES GERAIS

DEFINIÇÃO
- Parada sinusal — distúrbio da formação do impulso, causado por diminuição na velocidade ou interrupção da automaticidade espontânea do nó sinusal; falha do nó sinoatrial em iniciar um impulso no tempo esperado. O intervalo P-P não é igual a um múltiplo do intervalo P-P básico.
- Bloqueio sinoatrial — distúrbio da condução do impulso; um impulso formado dentro do nó sinusal falha na despolarização dos átrios ou o faz com demora; mais comumente, a ritmicidade básica do nó sinusal não é interrompida e a duração da pausa é um múltiplo do intervalo P-P básico. Classificado em bloqueio sinoatrial de primeiro, segundo e terceiro graus (semelhantemente aos graus do bloqueio AV). Não é fácil diagnosticar bloqueio sinoatrial de primeiro e terceiro graus a partir do ECG. O bloqueio sinoatrial de segundo grau é o mais comum: bloqueio sinoatrial Mobitz tipo I (Wenckebach) — o intervalo P-P encurta-se progressivamente antes de uma pausa; a duração da pausa é menor do que dois ciclos P-P; bloqueio sinoatrial Mobitz tipo II — a duração da pausa que ocorre após um batimento sinusal é múltiplo exato (duas, três ou quatro vezes o normal) do intervalo P-P básico.

Características do ECG
- Existe uma onda P normal para cada complexo QRS com uma pausa igual ou superior a duas vezes o intervalo P-P normal; o ritmo é regularmente irregular ou irregular com pausas (Fig. 1).
- Batimentos juncionais ou de escape ventricular — se as pausas forem significativamente prolongadas. O marca-passo subsidiário assume o ritmo com batimentos de escape normalmente a partir do tecido juncional AV ou das fibras de Purkinje.
- O ECG de superfície não é capaz de diferenciar parada sinusal de bloqueio no cão por causa da variação do intervalo R-R normal (arritmia sinusal).

FISIOPATOLOGIA
- Influências simpáticas e parassimpáticas podem alterar a despolarização espontânea do nó sinusal; o estímulo vagal da acetilcolina, que se liga aos sítios de receptores do nó sinoatrial, pode retardar a automaticidade do nó sinusal, por reduzir a inclinação da curva na fase 4 de despolarização; o estímulo simpático libera noradrenalina, que se liga aos receptores β_1 no nó sinoatrial, aumentando a velocidade de descarga nodal sinoatrial espontânea.
- Ocorre o fenômeno de inibição pós-funcionamento quando a parada sinusal acompanha uma sequência de batimentos ectópicos. O nó sinusal necessita de um período de preparo até que sua velocidade usual de automaticidade seja restabelecida.
- Doença intrínseca do nó sinusal pode afetar o equilíbrio entre o fluxo eferente parassimpático e simpático para o nó sinoatrial e sua velocidade de descarga espontânea.
- A duração da parada sinusal pode ser longa e possivelmente irreversível quando o nó sinusal fica suprimido pela taquicardia ectópica, particularmente em caso de cardiopatia subjacente grave. Parada sinusal persistente não atribuída a qualquer medicamento quase sempre indica síndrome do nó sinusal doente.

SISTEMA(S) ACOMETIDO(S)
Cardiovascular — poderão aparecer sinais clínicos de fraqueza ou síncope se a parada ou o bloqueio sinusais provocarem períodos suficientemente longos (em geral de 5 s ou mais) de assistolia ventricular sem batimentos de escape iniciados por marca-passos latentes.

GENÉTICA
- Observados em cães puros da raça Pug com estenose hereditária do feixe de His.
- Constatados em cadelas da raça Schnauzer miniatura predispostas à síndrome do nó sinusal doente.
- Cães da raça Dálmata treinados para caça, mas congenitamente surdos, apresentam, com frequência, nó sinoatrial anormal e artérias atriais múltiplas.

INCIDÊNCIA/PREVALÊNCIA
- Achado acidental normal nas raças caninas braquicefálicas, em que a inspiração provoca o aumento reflexo do tônus vagal.
- Comum nas raças caninas predispostas à síndrome do nó sinusal doente.
- Raro nos gatos.

DISTRIBUIÇÃO GEOGRÁFICA
N/D.

IDENTIFICAÇÃO
Espécies
Cães e gatos.

Raça(s) Predominante(s)
- Raças braquicefálicas.
- Raças predispostas à síndrome do nó sinusal doente (p. ex., Schnauzer miniatura, Dachshund, Cocker spaniel, Pug e West Highland white terrier).

Idade Média e Faixa Etária
Quando associados à síndrome do nó sinusal doente, acometem geralmente animais mais idosos.

Sexo Predominante
Em associação com a síndrome do nó sinusal doente, afeta fêmeas mais idosas.

SINAIS CLÍNICOS
Comentários Gerais
Em geral, não há nenhum significado clínico em si se interrompidos outra vez pela despolarização do nó sinusal ou, então, se marca-passos latentes escaparem imediatamente para evitar a assistolia ventricular.

Achados Anamnésicos
- Em geral, nenhum.
- Podem ocorrer sinais de baixo débito cardíaco (p. ex., fraqueza e síncope) na falha de disparo do nó sinoatrial em tempo oportuno se nenhum foco mais baixo de marca-passo se encarregar do ritmo.
- A morte súbita é possível com períodos prolongados de assistolia ventricular.

Achados do Exame Físico
- Podem estar normais.
- Os sons cardíacos após uma pausa podem estar mais altos do que o usual, porque os ventrículos demoram mais para se encher e ejetar uma quantidade maior de sangue.
- Frequência cardíaca extremamente baixa se a parada ou o bloqueio forem prolongados ou frequentes.
- Em caso de cardiopatia significativa — pode haver achados compatíveis com débito cardíaco baixo (p. ex., tempo de perfusão prolongado, mucosas pálidas e pulsos femorais fracos).

CAUSAS
Fisiológicas
- Estímulo vagal secundário a tosse ou irritação faríngea.
- Compressão no globo ocular ou no seio carotídeo.
- Manipulação cirúrgica.

Patológicas
- Cardiopatia degenerativa (fibrose).
- Cardiopatia dilatada.
- Miocardite aguda.
- Cardiopatia neoplásica.
- Síndrome do nó sinusal doente.
- Irritação do nervo vago secundária à neoplasia torácica ou cervical.
- Desequilíbrio eletrolítico.
- Intoxicação medicamentosa (p. ex., digoxina).

FATORES DE RISCO
- Determinados medicamentos, incluindo digitálicos, quinidina, propranolol, xilazina, acepromazina.
- Doença do trato respiratório.
- Manobras vagais.

DIAGNÓSTICO

DIAGNÓSTICO DIFERENCIAL
- Arritmia e bradicardia sinusais acentuadas.
- Nem sempre é possível diferenciar parada sinusal de bloqueio sinoatrial sem registros diretos da descarga do nó sinusal; as pausas que consistem em múltiplos exatos do intervalo de batimento dominante sugerem bloqueio sinusal.

HEMOGRAMA/BIOQUÍMICA/URINÁLISE
Anormalidades eletrolíticas séricas em alguns animais, especialmente hipercalcemia (K^+ sérico >5,7 mEq/L).

OUTROS TESTES LABORATORIAIS
N/D.

DIAGNÓSTICO POR IMAGEM
- Radiografias torácicas na suspeita de doença cardíaca ou neoplásica.
- Ecocardiografia mediante a suspeita de cardiopatia estrutural ou neoplásica.

MÉTODOS DIAGNÓSTICOS
- Teste de resposta provocativa à atropina para avaliar a função do nó sinusal. Administrar 0,04 mg/kg desse medicamento por via IM; avaliar a tira do ritmo cardíaco do ECG na derivação II 30 min mais tarde em relação à resposta ou administrar 0,04 mg/kg IV acompanhado pelo ECG em 10 min. A resolução da arritmia com a administração da atropina sugere o aumento do tônus vagal como a causa subjacente.
- Monitoramento cardíaco com o paciente em deambulação poderá revelar períodos prolongados de falha dos impulsos a partir do nó sinoatrial se os sinais de fraqueza ou síncope estiverem presentes.
- Nas pessoas, um período de parada sinusal após massagem na carótida direita que demore mais de 3 s sugere responsividade sinusal inadequada.
- Estudos eletrofisiológicos do nó sinusal.

PARADA SINUSAL E BLOQUEIO SINOATRIAL

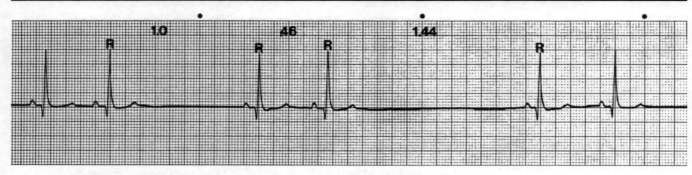

Figura 1. Parada sinusal intermitente em raça braquicefálica com distúrbio do trato respiratório superior e episódios de síncope. As pausas (1 e 1,44 s) são superiores a duas vezes o intervalo R-R normal (0,46). (De: Tilley LP: *Essentials of canine and feline electrocardiography*. 3. ed. Baltimore: Williams & Wilkins, 1992, com permissão.)

• Concentração de digoxina sérica, se aplicável; ensaio realizado 6-8 horas após a ingestão do comprimido; concentrações séricas terapêuticas são tipicamente de 0,8-1,5 ng/mL.

ACHADOS PATOLÓGICOS
Estudo histológico do nó sinoatrial pode revelar necrose, fibrose e/ou alterações degenerativas no nó sinusal.

TRATAMENTO

CUIDADO(S) DE SAÚDE ADEQUADO(S)
Parada ou bloqueio sinusais assintomáticos não necessitam de tratamento. Se houver sinais clínicos, a abordagem terapêutica dependerá da causa, do estado cardíaco subjacente e da gravidade dos sintomas. Qualquer indicação terapêutica poderá ser instituída em um esquema ambulatorial a menos que haja necessidade do implante de marca-passo, o qual necessita de internação.

CUIDADO(S) DE ENFERMAGEM
Corrigir quaisquer anormalidades eletrolíticas que possam estar contribuindo para o quadro.

ATIVIDADE
Irrestrita a menos que se desenvolvam sinais de fraqueza, síncope ou ICC.

DIETA
N/D.

ORIENTAÇÃO AO PROPRIETÁRIO
O marca-passo artificial pode ser necessário em paciente sintomático e irresponsivo ao tratamento clínico.

CONSIDERAÇÕES CIRÚRGICAS
Implante de marca-passo artificial de demanda em animais com sinais clínicos que não respondam ao tratamento.

MEDICAÇÕES

MEDICAMENTO(S) DE ESCOLHA
• Em paciente sintomático, considerar a atropina (0,04 mg/kg IV, IM), o glicopirrolato (0,005-0,01 mg/kg IV, IM) ou o isoproterenol (10 μg/kg IM, SC a cada 6 h ou diluir 1 mg em 500 mL de glicose a 5% ou solução de Ringer simples e infundir por via IV 0,5-1 mL/min [1-2 μg/min] ou até fazer efeito).
• Se o animal se mostrar responsivo aos medicamentos anticolinérgicos injetáveis (p. ex., atropina) — pode-se prescrever o brometo de propantelina por via oral (0,25-0,5 mg/kg a cada 8-12 h) ou a hiosciamina (0,003-0,006 mg/kg a cada 8 h) para tratamento em casa; também pode ser considerada a terapia broncodilatadora com aminofilina, teofilina, albuterol ou terbutalina para tratamento por via oral.

CONTRAINDICAÇÕES
Se o paciente manifestar sintomas secundários a pausas prolongadas, interromper quaisquer medicamentos que possam ser os agentes causais (p. ex., digitálicos, β-bloqueadores e bloqueadores dos canais de cálcio).

PRECAUÇÕES
Evitar medicamentos que deprimam a função do nó sinoatrial.

INTERAÇÕES POSSÍVEIS
N/D.

MEDICAMENTO(S) ALTERNATIVO(S)
Se os sinais não desaparecem com o tratamento clínico, considerar o implante de marca-passo artificial de demanda ventricular.

ACOMPANHAMENTO

MONITORIZAÇÃO DO PACIENTE
Quando indicada, procede-se à avaliação com ECG seriado periódico para determinar a eficácia terapêutica e a possível evolução para uma disritmia mais séria.

PREVENÇÃO
N/D.

COMPLICAÇÕES POSSÍVEIS
Se associados à cardiopatia primária, poderá ocorrer o desenvolvimento de ICC, havendo a necessidade de terapias adequadas.

EVOLUÇÃO ESPERADA E PROGNÓSTICO
Se a síndrome do nó sinusal doente for a causa, o paciente sintomático poderá responder bem à intervenção clínica; caso o animal se mostre pouco responsivo, o implante de marca-passo permanente poderia melhorar acentuadamente o prognóstico.

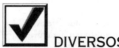
DIVERSOS

DISTÚRBIOS ASSOCIADOS
• Síndrome do nó sinusal doente.
• Arritmia sinusal.
• Bradicardia sinusal.

FATORES RELACIONADOS COM A IDADE
N/D.

POTENCIAL ZOONÓTICO
N/D.

GESTAÇÃO/FERTILIDADE/REPRODUÇÃO
N/D.

SINÔNIMO(S)
• Bloqueio sinusal.
• Pausa sinusal.

VER TAMBÉM
• Arritmia Sinusal.
• Bradicardia Sinusal.
• Síndrome do Nó Sinusal Doente.

ABREVIATURA(S)
• AV = atrioventricular.
• ECG = eletrocardiograma.
• ICC = insuficiência cardíaca congestiva.

Sugestões de Leitura
Boyett MR, Honjo H, et al. The sinoatrial node, a heterogeneous pacemaker structure. Cardiovasc Res 2000, 47(4):658-687.
Issa ZF, Miller JM, Zipes DP. Sinus node dysfuncion. In: Clinical Arrhythmology and Electrophysiology: A Companion to Braunwald's Heart Disease. Philadelphia: Saunders, 2008, pp. 118-126.
Kittleson MD, Kienle RD. Small Animal Cardiovascular Medicine. St. Louis: Mosby, 1998.
Tilley LP, Smith FWK, Oyama MA, Sleeper MM, eds., Manual of Canine and Feline Cardiology, 4th ed. St. Louis: Saunders Elsevier, 2008.
Tilley LP. Essentials of Canine and Feline Electrocardiography, 3rd ed. Baltimore: Williams & Wilkins, 1992.

Autor Deborah J. Hadlock
Consultores Editoriais Larry P. Tilley e Francis W.K. Smith, Jr.

Parada Ventricular (Assistolia)

CONSIDERAÇÕES GERAIS

DEFINIÇÃO
Ausência de complexos ventriculares no ECG ou ausência de atividade ventricular (dissociação eletromecânica).

Características do ECG
A assistolia ventricular pode se resultante de bloqueio ou parada sinoatriais graves ou de bloqueio AV de terceiro grau sem ritmo de escape juncional ou ventricular; as características eletrocardiográficas incluem:
- Presença de ondas P em pacientes com bloqueio AV completo (Fig. 1).
- Ausência de ondas P durante a assistolia em pacientes com bloqueio ou parada sinoatriais graves.
- Ausência de complexos QRS.
- Dissociação eletromecânica — registro eletrocardiográfico de ritmo cardíaco (P-QRS-T) e ausência de débito cardíaco efetivo ou pulso femoral palpável.

FISIOPATOLOGIA
A assistolia ventricular representa uma parada cardíaca; se o ritmo ventricular não for restabelecido em 3-4 min, poderá ocorrer dano cerebral irreversível.

SISTEMA(S) ACOMETIDO(S)
- Cardiovascular.
- Todos os sistemas orgânicos são acometidos pela perda da perfusão.

GENÉTICA
N/D.

INCIDÊNCIA/PREVALÊNCIA
Desconhecidas.

DISTRIBUIÇÃO GEOGRÁFICA
Nenhuma.

IDENTIFICAÇÃO
Espécies
Cães e gatos.

Raça(s) Predominante(s)
Nenhuma.

Idade Média e Faixa Etária
Desconhecidas.

SINAIS CLÍNICOS
Achados Anamnésicos
- Doença sistêmica ou cardíaca graves em muitos pacientes.
- Outras arritmias cardíacas em alguns pacientes.
- Síncope.

Achados do Exame Físico
- Não se consegue palpar nenhum pulso ventricular.
- Parada cardíaca.
- Colapso.
- Morte.

CAUSAS
- Bloqueio AV completo, com ausência de ritmo de escape ventricular ou juncional.
- Parada ou bloqueio sinusais graves.
- Hipercalcemia (Fig. 2).

FATORES DE RISCO
- Qualquer doença sistêmica (p. ex., acidose e hipercalcemia intensas) ou cardíaca graves.
- Hipoadrenocorticismo indutor de hipercalcemia.
- Ruptura ou obstrução do trato urinário, com hipercalcemia resultante.

DIAGNÓSTICO

DIAGNÓSTICO DIFERENCIAL
Descartar artefato eletrocardiográfico; reaplicar os eletrodos eletrocardiográficos e garantir o contato satisfatório com a pele e a aplicação de quantidade suficiente de álcool.

HEMOGRAMA/BIOQUÍMICA/URINÁLISE
A hipercalcemia grave constitui uma possível causa.

OUTROS TESTES LABORATORIAIS
N/D.

DIAGNÓSTICO POR IMAGEM
N/D.

MÉTODOS DIAGNÓSTICOS
Pressão arterial sistêmica — ausência de pressão passível de leitura.

ACHADOS PATOLÓGICOS
N/D.

TRATAMENTO

CUIDADO(S) DE SAÚDE ADEQUADO(S)
- A assistolia é um ritmo frequentemente fatal, que exige tratamento rigoroso imediato.
- A regulação artificial do ritmo pela implantação de marca-passo transvenoso poderá ter êxito se o miocárdio estiver mecanicamente responsivo.
- A conversão elétrica com corrente direta não será eficaz a menos que se consiga converter o ritmo em fibrilação ventricular com o uso de medicamentos.

CUIDADO(S) DE ENFERMAGEM
Tratar qualquer problema passível de tratamento, como hipotermia, hipercalcemia e distúrbios acidobásicos.

ATIVIDADE
N/D.

DIETA
N/D.

ORIENTAÇÃO AO PROPRIETÁRIO
Nenhuma.

CONSIDERAÇÕES CIRÚRGICAS
Nenhuma.

MEDICAÇÕES

MEDICAMENTO(S) DE ESCOLHA
- Instituir a reanimação cardiopulmonar.
- Adrenalina — 0,2 mg/kg IV, intratraqueal ou intralingual (dobrar a dose para a administração intratraqueal e fornecê-la com volume equivalente de soro fisiológico).
- Atropina — 0,05 mg/kg IV, intratraqueal ou intralingual (dobrar a dose para a administração intratraqueal e fornecê-la com volume equivalente de soro fisiológico).
- Bicarbonato de sódio — 1 mEq/kg IV para cada 10 min de parada cardíaca.
- A dexametasona e a dopamina podem ser úteis em pacientes com dissociação eletromecânica.

CONTRAINDICAÇÕES
Medicamentos depressores da condução dos nodos sinusal ou AV em pacientes com parada sinusal ou bloqueio cardíaco (p. ex., β-bloqueadores, bloqueadores dos canais de cálcio e digoxina).

PRECAUÇÕES
Nenhuma.

INTERAÇÕES POSSÍVEIS
Nenhuma.

MEDICAMENTO(S) ALTERNATIVO(S)
Gliconato de cálcio — pacientes com parada ventricular e hipercalcemia.

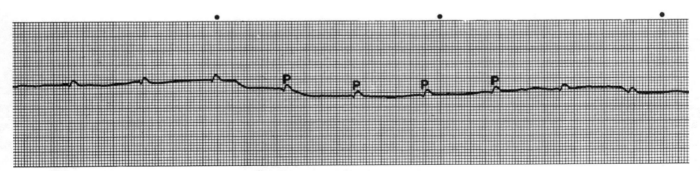

Figura 1. Assistolia ventricular em cão com bloqueio AV completo grave. Apenas as ondas P (atividade atrial) estão presentes; não há nenhuma atividade ventricular. (Derivação II, 50 mm/s, 1 cm = 1 mV.) (De: Tilley LP: *Essentials of canine and feline electrocardiography*. 3. ed., Baltimore: Williams & Wilkins, 1992, com permissão.)

PARADA VENTRICULAR (ASSISTOLIA)

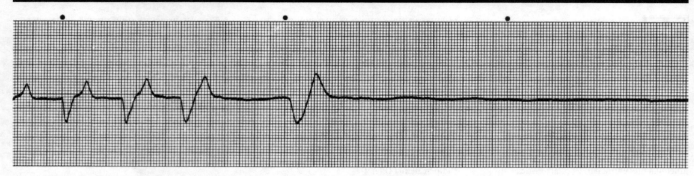

Figura 2. Assistolia ventricular em gato com hipercalemia grave (11 mEq/L) decorrente de obstrução uretral. Após quatro complexos QRS largos e bizarros (parada atrial com atraso na condução ventricular), não se observa nenhuma onda P nem complexo QRS. (Derivação II, 50 mm/s, 1 cm = 1 mV.) (De: Tilley LP: *Essentials of canine and feline electrocardiography*. 3. ed., Baltimore: Williams & Wilkins, 1992, com permissão.)

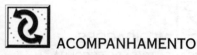

ACOMPANHAMENTO

MONITORIZAÇÃO DO PACIENTE
- Se o animal for reanimado — avaliar o hemograma completo, o perfil bioquímico e a urinálise.
- Se o animal sobreviver e se houver a suspeita de cardiopatia primária — efetuar o ecocardiograma e obter radiografias torácicas.
- ECG — monitorizar de perto e com frequência.

PREVENÇÃO
Monitorização cuidadosa de pacientes criticamente enfermos para evitar e corrigir os distúrbios acidobásicos, a hipotensão e a hipoxemia.

COMPLICAÇÕES POSSÍVEIS
- Óbito.
- CID e falência múltipla de órgãos.

EVOLUÇÃO ESPERADA E PROGNÓSTICO
Os pacientes costumam vir a óbito. Se o ritmo sinusal for restabelecido, o prognóstico geralmente ainda será reservado a mau, já que não é rara a recidiva da parada.

DIVERSOS

DISTÚRBIOS ASSOCIADOS
Nenhum.

FATORES RELACIONADOS COM A IDADE
Nenhum.

POTENCIAL ZOONÓTICO
Nenhum.

GESTAÇÃO/FERTILIDADE/REPRODUÇÃO
Nenhum.

SINÔNIMO(S)
Assistolia ventricular.

VER TAMBÉM
- Bloqueio Atrioventricular Completo (Terceiro Grau).
- Parada Cardiopulmonar.
- Parada Sinusal e Bloqueio Sinoatrial.

ABREVIATURA(S)
- AV = atrioventricular.
- CID = coagulação intravascular disseminada.
- ECG = eletrocardiograma.
- IV = intravenosa.

Sugestões de Leitura
Kraus MS, Gelzer ARM, Moise S. Treatment of cardiac arrhythmias and conduction disturbances. In: Tilley LP, Smith FWK, Oyama MA, Sleeper MM, eds., Manual of Canine and Feline Cardiology, 4th ed. St. Louis: Saunders Elsevier, 2008, pp. 315-332.
Tilley LP, Smith FWK, Jr. Electrocardiography. In: Tilley LP, Smith FWK, Oyama MA, Sleeper MM, eds., Manual of Canine and Feline Cardiology, 4th ed. St. Louis: Saunders Elsevier, 2008, pp. 49-77.

Autor Francis W.K. Smith, Jr.
Consultores Editoriais Larry P. Tilley e Francis W.K. Smith, Jr.

PARAFIMOSE, FIMOSE E PRIAPISMO

CONSIDERAÇÕES GERAIS

REVISÃO
- Fimose — incapacidade de protrusão do pênis além do orifício prepucial.
- Parafimose — o pênis projeta-se a partir do orifício prepucial, mas não consegue retornar à sua posição normal.
- Priapismo — extrusão prolongada do pênis ereto não associada a desejo sexual (excitação); pode resultar de estímulo parassimpático excessivo ou de fluxo venoso reduzido a partir do corpo cavernoso do pênis; condição relativamente incomum em cães e rara em gatos.

IDENTIFICAÇÃO
- Cães e gatos.
- Raças Pastor alemão e Golden retriever — é observada uma estenose prepucial congênita indutora de fimose; possivelmente hereditária.
- Gato Siamês — um único relato notou que 6 dentre 7 casos de priapismo eram em gatos dessa raça.

SINAIS CLÍNICOS
- Fimose — pode não ser detectada até que o paciente não tenha êxito nas tentativas de cópula; defeitos graves no neonato interferem na micção; pode provocar acúmulo de urina na cavidade prepucial, o que pode causar balanopostite, levando à septicemia.
- Parafimose — quando for de curta duração, o único sinal poderá ser a lambedura do pênis exteriorizado; após algumas horas de exposição, pode-se observar necrose isquêmica e obstrução uretral; os sinais de edema e tumefação podem tornar difícil a diferenciação do priapismo.
- Priapismo — ereção peniana persistente que dura >4 h; o bulbo da glande encontra-se firme e tumefata.

CAUSAS E FATORES DE RISCO
- Fimose — provocada por orifício prepucial anormalmente pequeno; pode ser congênita ou adquirida (p. ex., causada por lesão ou doença); pode estar associada a frênulo peniano ou prepucial persistente, uma fina faixa de tecido conjuntivo que une o pênis e o prepúcio ao longo da parte ventral da glande.
- Parafimose — associada, em geral, à ereção e/ou cópula; o pelo que circunda o orifício prepucial fica aprisionado contra a superfície do pênis, especialmente o bulbo da glande, impedindo a retração; um orifício prepucial moderadamente estenosado pode contribuir para o quadro; lesões; fraturas do osso do pênis; doença neurológica (encefalomielite, discopatia intervertebral); balanopostite; tumefação peniana (neoplasia, estrangulamento com corpo estranho); músculos prepuciais incompetentes.
- Priapismo — não isquêmico (arterial, fluxo elevado) causado por traumatismo, agentes vasoativos e distúrbios neurológicos, como cinomose canina; isquêmico (veno-oclusivo, fluxo reduzido) provocado por traumatismo durante o acasalamento, cinomose crônica, encefalomielite, tromboembolia peniana, uso de anfetamina, neoplasia peniana, abscesso perineal; causa frequentemente desconhecida; seres humanos (anemia falciforme, discrasias hematológicas, hemodiálise, fluidoterapia, terapia com heparina, medicamentos vasoativos, lesão da medula espinal, anestesia, obstrução uretral atribuída a urólitos).

DIAGNÓSTICO

DIAGNÓSTICO DIFERENCIAL
- Parafimose — exposição da glande do pênis provocada por anormalidade dos músculos retratores do pênis ou dos músculos do prepúcio, amplo orifício prepucial, prepúcio curto ou priapismo.

HEMOGRAMA/BIOQUÍMICA/URINÁLISE
- Geralmente normais.
- Fimose nos neonatos — podem-se notar a presença de balanopostite grave e indícios de septicemia (p. ex., leucocitose, neutrofilia que evolui para neutropenia, e uroculturas positivas).

OUTROS TESTES LABORATORIAIS
- Gasometria do sangue coletado diretamente do pênis (aspirado do corpo cavernoso) para diferenciar os tipos de priapismo em cães:
- Priapismo isquêmico: pH <7,25, PO_2 <30 mmHg, PCO_2 >60 mmHg.
- Priapismo não isquêmico: pH de 7,4, PO_2 >90 mmHg, PCO_2 <40 mmHg.

DIAGNÓSTICO POR IMAGEM
- Ultrassonografia — para visualização de vasos penianos ingurgitados.
- Exame neurológico acompanhado por radiografias, ressonância magnética — para avaliação da medula espinal.

TRATAMENTO

Fimose
- Aumento cirúrgico do orifício prepucial.
- Frênulo peniano persistente (cães) — remover a faixa de tecido, mantendo a glande do pênis à lâmina parietal do prepúcio.

Parafimose
- Necessita de tratamento imediato — após 24 h, a lesão do tecido e a obstrução da uretra podem necessitar de amputação do pênis; o objetivo é recolocar o pênis na posição normal.
- Cateter urinário de demora — se a patência (desobstrução) da uretra for uma preocupação.
- Remover os corpos estranhos.
- Lubrificar o pênis.
- Aplicar compressas com soluções de glicose hipertônica.
- Aumentar o orifício prepucial por via cirúrgica, se necessário.
- Segundo relatos, o procedimento de falopexia (fixação do pênis à parede abdominal) já foi bem-sucedida na correção do distúrbio.
- A castração não é eficiente, pois a parafimose não é uma doença dependente da testosterona.

Priapismo
- A aspiração do sangue peniano pode ser tanto terapêutica (alívio temporário da dor) como diagnóstica (a gasometria sanguínea pode ajudar a diferenciar os quadros isquêmicos dos não isquêmicos).
- A identificação da causa subjacente nem sempre é possível antes que ocorra isquemia do pênis; os procedimentos de amputação peniana e uretrostomia perineal costumam ser necessários em virtude da necrose isquêmica irreparável do pênis; a castração não é eficaz.
- Amputação peniana e uretrostomia perineal — indicadas para os gatos com dificuldade de micção.
- Bandagem compressiva do abdome e cateter urinário de demora — para manter o pênis dentro do prepúcio; também podem reduzir o edema localizado.

MEDICAÇÕES

MEDICAMENTO(S)
- Pomadas antibióticas — mantém o tratamento; evitam aderências entre o pênis e o prepúcio.
- Nenhum medicamento aprovado ou sem segurança comprovada.

ACOMPANHAMENTO

EVOLUÇÃO ESPERADA E PROGNÓSTICO
- Fimose — razoável a bom se identificada antes do desenvolvimento da septicemia.
- Parafimose e priapismo — reservado a mau quanto ao retorno da atividade reprodutiva; razoável a bom quanto à vida com tratamento clínico precoce bem-sucedido, falopexia, falectomia (remoção cirúrgica do pênis) parcial ou total.

DIVERSOS

Sugestões de Leitura
Feldman EC, Nelson RW. Canine and Feline Endocrinology and Reproduction, 3rd ed. Philadelphia: Saunders, 2004, pp. 954-956.
Gunn-Moore DA, Brown PJ, Holt PE, Gruffydd-Jones T. Priapism in seven cats. J Small Anim Pract 1995, 36:262-266.
Johnston SD, Root Kustritz MV, Olson PNS. Disorders of the canine penis and prepuce. In: Canine and Feline Theriogenology. Philadelphia: Saunders, 2001, pp. 356-367.
Johnston SD, Root Kustritz MV, Olson PNS. Disorders of the feline penis and prepuce. In: Canine and Feline Theriogenology. Philadelphia: Saunders, 2001, pp. 539-543.
Lavely JA. Priapism in dogs. Top Companion Anim Med 2009, 24:49-54.
Somerville ME, Anderson SM. Phallopexy for treatment of paraphimosis in the dog. JAAHA 2001, 37:397-400.

Autor Carlos R.F. Pinto
Consultor Editorial Sara K. Lyle

Paralisia

CONSIDERAÇÕES GERAIS

DEFINIÇÃO
- Paresia — enfraquecimento do movimento voluntário.
- Paralisia — ausência de movimento voluntário.
- Quadriparesia (tetraparesia) — fraqueza dos movimentos voluntários em todos os membros.
- Quadriplegia (tetraplegia) — ausência de movimentos voluntários em todos os membros.
- Paraparesia — fraqueza dos movimentos voluntários nos membros pélvicos.
- Paraplegia — ausência de movimentos voluntários em todos os membros pélvicos.
- Síndrome de Schiff-Sherrington — associada a traumatismo grave da medula espinal, abaixo da vértebra T2; quando o paciente se encontra em decúbito lateral, os membros torácicos e o pescoço ficam em extensão, com paralisia dos membros pélvicos; a função dos membros torácicos permanece normal; o prognóstico baseia-se na presença ou ausência de percepção da dor nos membros pélvicos.
- Choque espinal — associado a traumatismo grave da medula espinal, localizado geralmente próximo à coluna toracolombar; membros pélvicos paralisados, com os reflexos inicialmente arrefléxicos dos membros pélvicos, que se tornam exagerados (e mais indicativos de localização da lesão em T3-L3) depois de minutos a algumas horas do traumatismo.

FISIOPATOLOGIA
- Fraqueza — provocada por lesões no sistema dos neurônios motores superior ou inferior.
- Corpos ou núcleos celulares do sistema dos neurônios motores superiores — localizados dentro do cérebro; responsáveis por iniciar o movimento voluntário.
- Axônios provenientes desses corpos celulares — formam tratos (rubrospinal, corticospinal, vestibulospinal, reticulospinal) que descem do cérebro para fazer sinapse nos interneurônios na medula espinal.
- Axônios interneuronais — fazem sinapse nos grandes neurônios motores alfa na parte ventral da substância cinzenta da medula espinal.
- Grandes neurônios motores alfa — são corpos celulares de origem do sistema dos neurônios motores inferiores, o qual é responsável pelos reflexos espinais.
- Coleções de neurônios motores inferiores nas intumescências cervical e lombar — dão origem a axônios que formam as raízes nervosas ventrais, os nervos espinais e (por fim) os nervos periféricos que inervam os músculos dos membros.
- Avaliação dos reflexos dos membros — determina qual sistema (neurônio motor superior ou inferior) está envolvido.
- Neurônios motores superiores e seus axônios — exercem influência inibitória sobre os grandes neurônios motores alfa do sistema dos neurônios motores inferiores; mantém a normalidade no tônus muscular e nos reflexos espinais; se o sistema dos neurônios motores superiores for lesionado, os reflexos espinais não serão mais inibidos nem controlados e os reflexos se tornarão exagerados ou hiper-refléxicos.
- Grandes neurônios motores alfa ou seus processos (neurônios periféricos) — também mantêm o tônus muscular normal e os reflexos espinais normais; se o sistema dos neurônios motores inferiores for lesionado, os reflexos espinais não poderão ser eliciados (arrefléxicos) ou estarão diminuídos (hiporrefléxicos) e a emaciação muscular geralmente se apresentará grave depois de 5-7 dias da lesão.

SISTEMA(S) ACOMETIDO(S)
Nervoso.

IDENTIFICAÇÃO
Qualquer espécie.

SINAIS CLÍNICOS
Comentários Gerais
Fraqueza dos membros — início agudo ou gradual.

Achados Anamnésicos
- O proprietário pode descrever o paciente como "abatido", incapaz de se mover, caminhar ou ficar em estação.
- Muitas doenças focais compressivas da medula espinal começam com ataxia e evoluem para fraqueza e finalmente para paralisia.

Achados do Exame Físico
- Geralmente normais a menos que o processo mórbido seja sistêmico.
- Se estiver com dor, o paciente poderá refutar a manipulação durante o exame.
- Êmbolos aórticos (neuromiopatia isquêmica) — o paciente pode estar paraplégico e com arreflexia ou hiporreflexia ao exame; pulsos femorais ausentes; extremidades frequentemente frias; leitos ungueais muitas vezes cianóticos.

Achados do Exame Neurológico
- Confirmam que o problema é fraqueza ou paralisia.
- Localizam o problema nos neurônios motores superior ou inferior.
- Se os membros estiverem paralisados — provavelmente a bexiga também estará paralisada, com micção voluntária negativa.
- Tetraparesia com reflexos espinais exagerados em todos os membros — lesão localizada nos segmentos C1-C5 da medula espinal ou no cérebro.
- Tetraparesia com reflexos espinais normais ou deprimidos do membro torácico e reflexos exagerados do membro pélvico — lesão situada nos segmentos C6-T2 da medula espinal.
- Tetraparesia com reflexos espinais e tônus muscular deprimidos em todos os membros — lesão difusa, envolvendo músculos ou nervos periféricos ou, então, intumescências cervicais (segmentos C6-T2 da medula espinal) e lombares (segmentos L4-S2 da medula espinal).
- Membros torácicos normais, mas paraparesia/paraplegia com reflexos espinais exagerados do membro pélvico — lesão localizada nos segmentos T3-L3 da medula espinal.
- Membros torácicos normais, porém paraparesia/paraplegia com reflexos espinais deprimidos a ausentes do membro pélvico — lesão situada no segmento L4 da medula espinal e caudalmente.
- Normalidade do membro torácico e atividade motora do membro pélvico, porém cauda/ânus flácidos e incontinência urinária e/ou fecal — lesão localizada no segmento S2 da medula espinal e caudalmente.
- Membros torácicos normais, mas paraparesia/paraplegia e reflexos patelares deprimidos — a lesão envolve os segmentos L4-6 da medula espinal, os quais se situam nos corpos vertebrais L3-4.
- Membros torácicos normais, porém paraparesia/paraplegia, reflexos patelares exagerados e reflexos flexor e ciático fracos — se apenas a medula espinal estiver acometida (sem envolvimento da raiz), a lesão envolverá os segmentos L6-S2 da medula espinal, os quais se localizam nos corpos vertebrais L4-L6.

CAUSAS
Quadriplegia
- Neurônio motor inferior — início agudo: paralisia do Coonhound, botulismo, paralisia pelo carrapato, forma fulminante da miastenia grave, ou mioneurite por protozoário; início mais gradual: polineuropatias e polimiopatias por toxicidade, infecção, inflamação, endocrinopatia, doença metabólica, ou doença congênita/hereditária.
- Neurônio motor superior — hérnia de disco; discospondilite; embolia fibrocartilaginosa; traumatismo; neoplasia; mielite por muitas causas; más-formações da coluna ou da medula espinal.

Paraplegia
- Neurônio motor superior — hérnia de disco; discospondilite; embolia fibrocartilaginosa; neoplasia; traumatismo; más-formações congênitas da coluna ou da medula espinal; mielopatia degenerativa.
- Neurônio motor inferior — embolia fibrocartilaginosa; hérnia de disco; instabilidade lombossacra; discospondilite; traumatismo; neoplasia; espinha-bífida.

Quadriplegia com Déficits de Nervos Cranianos, Crises Convulsivas ou Estupor
- Neurônio motor superior — doenças do tronco cerebral: encefalite; neoplasia; traumatismo; acidentes vasculares; distúrbios congênitos ou hereditários.

FATORES DE RISCO
- Discopatia degenerativa — Dachshund; Poodle; Cocker spaniel e Beagle.
- Cães de caça — paralisia do Coonhound.
- Animais errantes — traumatismo da medula espinal e da coluna.
- Luxação atlantoaxial — raças toy e de pequeno porte.
- Instabilidade lombossacra — raças de grande porte; raças de trabalho; Pastor alemão.
- Espondilomielopatia cervical (síndrome de Wobbler) — raças de grande porte; Doberman pinscher; Dinamarquês.
- Siringomielia: Cavalier King Charles spaniel; Weimaraner.
- Cistos aracnoides espinais: Rottweiler; raças de pequeno porte.

DIAGNÓSTICO

DIAGNÓSTICO DIFERENCIAL
- Membros pélvicos fracos ou paralisados — ter certeza de que os pulsos femorais estão presentes e normais; êmbolos arteriais aórticos ou femorais podem levar à paraparesia ou paraplegia do neurônio motor inferior.
- Reflexos espinais — localizam a fraqueza nos segmentos cervical, toracolombar ou lombar inferior da medula espinal.
- Início agudo — ter cuidado ao movimentar o paciente em virtude da possibilidade de traumatismo.

HEMOGRAMA/BIOQUÍMICA/URINÁLISE
Geralmente normais a menos que doenças inflamatórias estejam envolvidas.

OUTROS TESTES LABORATORIAIS
• Inflamação do trato urinário — cultura bacteriana da urina pode gerar resultados positivos nos casos de discospondilite.
• Discospondilite — diagnóstico por meio de radiografia da coluna vertebral (lise do espaço do disco intervertebral); obter o título para *Brucella*; considerar a realização de hemo e urocultura.
• Fraqueza induzida pelo exercício — determinar os títulos de anticorpos contra os receptores da acetilcolina (teste para miastenia grave); verificar a concentração de creatina quinase sérica (polimiosite ou polimiopatia), a contagem de hemácias (anemia ou policitemia) e a concentração da glicose sanguínea (hipoglicemia); averiguar a presença de arritmia cardíaca e hipoxia via ECG, radiografia torácica, monitoramento com Holter e ecocardiografia; fazer biopsia muscular.
• Fraqueza do neurônio motor inferior ou dor muscular, atrofia muscular ou hipertrofia — determinar a concentração de creatina quinase para auxiliar o diagnóstico de polimiosite; fazer biopsia de tecido muscular e nervoso; avaliar os títulos séricos para *Neospora caninum* e *Toxoplasma gondii*.
• Mielite ou meningite — cão: mensurar os títulos para *N. caninum*, *T. gondii*, febre maculosa das Montanhas Rochosas, *Ehrlichia* spp. e vírus da cinomose; gato: obter os títulos séricos para *T. gondii* e *Cryptococcus neoformans* e avaliar o líquido espinal em busca de sinais do vírus da peritonite infecciosa felina e do *C. neoformans*.

DIAGNÓSTICO POR IMAGEM
• Radiografia da coluna vertebral — pode revelar hérnia de disco, discospondilite, tumor ósseo, má-formação vertebral congênita e fratura ou luxação.
• Mielografia — necessária se as radiografias simples não forem diagnósticas e quando os exames de TC ou RM não se encontram disponíveis.
• TC ou RM — têm substituído a mielografia em locais onde a tecnologia está disponível.

MÉTODOS DIAGNÓSTICOS
• Análise do LCS — realizada antes da mielografia para detectar mielite e meningite; caso se detecte um alto teor de proteína ou células, considerar a análise de título para doença infecciosa.
• Eletromiografia com agulha e velocidade de condução nervosa motora — podem auxiliar o diagnóstico e a caracterização de sinais generalizados do neurônio motor inferior.
• Biopsia de tecido muscular e nervoso — fraqueza generalizada do neurônio motor inferior.
• Obtenção de aspirado do espaço do disco intervertebral sob orientação fluoroscópica; realizar os exames de citologia e cultura para isolar algum agente infeccioso se a discospondilite for observada nas técnicas de diagnóstico por imagem.

TRATAMENTO
• Paciente internado — em caso de fraqueza ou paralisia grave até que a função vesical possa ser determinada.
• Alimentação manual — com sinais difusos do neurônio motor inferior, a deglutição pode estar acometida; a alimentação manual é feita até que o paciente consiga engolir de forma adequada.
• Alimentação em plataforma suspensa ou colocação de sonda — recomendada para animais com megaesôfago até que se resolva o problema.
• Atividade — restrita até que se consiga descartar traumatismo da coluna vertebral e hérnia de disco.
• Fisioterapia — importante para pacientes com paralisia; tonifica os músculos e mantém flexíveis as articulações.
• Cama ou leito — verificar e limpar frequentemente para evitar assadura pela urina e piodermite superficial; utilizar cama almofadada ou colchão d'água para ajudar a evitar a formação de úlceras de decúbito.
• Mudança de posição — alternar os pacientes quadriplégicos de um lado para outro quatro a oito vezes ao dia; evita a ocorrência de congestão pulmonar hipostática e a formação de úlceras de decúbito.
• Cirurgia — para hérnia de disco, fratura, algumas neoplasias e condições congênitas; quase sempre é o método mais eficaz e mais rápido para restabelecer e melhorar o estado neurológico.

MEDICAÇÕES

MEDICAMENTO(S) DE ESCOLHA
• O uso de corticosteroides até mesmo em doenças conhecidas como traumatismo da coluna vertebral ou hérnia de disco é controverso. Esses agentes podem ser úteis para aliviar a dor associada a algumas causas de paralisia da medula espinal, mas não aceleram a recuperação medular.
• Dexametasona — 0,1-0,2 mg/kg a cada 48 h para alívio da dor por duas a três doses.
• Prednisolona — 0,5-1 mg/kg a cada 12-24 h para alívio da dor por 3-5 dias.
• Brometo de piridostigmina — 0,5-3 mg/kg VO a cada 8-12 h para suspeita de miastenia grave; administrar enquanto se aguardam os resultados dos títulos.
• Sinais agudos generalizados do neurônio motor inferior — procurar por carrapatos; imersão com inseticidas adequados; se necessários.

CONTRAINDICAÇÕES
Corticosteroides — não utilizar em casos de discospondilite ou mielite/meningite por fungos ou protozoários; não usar na miastenia grave associada à pneumonia por aspiração.

PRECAUÇÕES
Corticosteroides — associados à ulceração e hemorragia gastrintestinais, cicatrização tardia de feridas e suscetibilidade aumentada a infecções.

MEDICAMENTO(S) ALTERNATIVO(S)
• AINEs — para doenças espinais associadas a desconforto ou dor óssea.
• Tramadol — 2 mg/kg a cada 12 h VO (cães ou gatos), até 4-5 mg/kg a cada 12 h (apenas para os cães) para alívio da dor. Evitar o uso com antidepressivos.
• Gabapentina — 3-10 mg/kg a cada 12 h VO para dor neuropática.
• Butorfanol — 0,2-0,6 mg/kg a cada 2-4 h para controle da dor.

ACOMPANHAMENTO

MONITORIZAÇÃO DO PACIENTE
• Exames neurológicos — diariamente para monitorizar o estado do paciente.
• Bexiga urinária — esvaziar (por compressão manual ou cateterização) três a quatro vezes ao dia para evitar superdistensão e subsequente atonia vesical; assim que a função vesical retornar, o paciente poderá ser tratado em casa.

COMPLICAÇÕES POSSÍVEIS
• Infecção do trato urinário, atonia vesical, assadura por urina e piodermite, constipação, formação de úlceras de decúbito.
• Pneumonia por aspiração — na doença generalizada do neurônio motor inferior ou em qualquer paciente quadriplégico.
• Mielomalacia — em caso de traumatismo grave da medula espinal ou hérnias de disco.
• Comprometimento ou paralisia respiratória — na mielomalacia ou doença generalizada do neurônio motor inferior.

DIVERSOS

VER TAMBÉM
• Fenômeno de Schiff-Sherrington.
• Ver a seção "Causas".

ABREVIATURA(S)
• AINE = anti-inflamatório não esteroide.
• ECG = eletrocardiograma.
• LCS = líquido cerebrospinal.
• RM = ressonância magnética.
• TC = tomografia computadorizada.

Sugestões de Leitura
Davies C, Shell L. Neurological problems. In: Common Small Animal Medical Diagnoses: An Algorithmic Approach. Philadelphia: Saunders, 2002, pp. 36-59.
de Lahunta A, Glass EN. Veterinary Neuroanatomy and Clinical Neurology, 3rd ed. Philadelphia: Saunders, 2008.
Negrin A, Schatzberg S, Platt SR. The paralyzed cat: Neuroanatomic diagnosis and specific spinal cord diseases. J Feline Med Surg 2009, 11:361-372.

Autora Linda G. Shell
Consultora Editorial Joane M. Parent

Paralisia do Carrapato

CONSIDERAÇÕES GERAIS

DEFINIÇÃO
Tetraparesia a tetraplegia flácidas atribuídas aos neurônios motores inferiores, causadas por neurotoxinas salivares (ixovotoxinas) provenientes de determinadas espécies de fêmeas de carrapatos.

FISIOPATOLOGIA
• Carrapato — injeta as neurotoxinas salivares que diminuem a velocidade de condução nervosa e a amplitude dos potenciais de ação musculares compostos, inibem a condução das terminações nervosas e interferem no mecanismo de despolarização/liberação de acetilcolina na terminação nervosa pré-sináptica, levando à redução na liberação desse neurotransmissor. Há suspeitas de que esses efeitos estejam associados à interrupção do fluxo de sódio através das membranas axonais nos nódulos de Ranvier e nas terminações nervosas.
• Infestação pelo carrapato *Ixodes holocyclus* — a neurotoxina depende fortemente da temperatura; um único carrapato adulto é suficiente para causar sinais neurológicos, mas uma grande infestação por ninfas ou larvas do carrapato *Ixodes* também pode induzir aos sinais clínicos.
• Sinais clínicos — ocorrem 6-9 dias após a fixação inicial do carrapato.
• Nem todos os animais infestados desenvolvem a paralisia causada pelo carrapato; nem todas as fêmeas de carrapatos adultas produzem a toxina.

SISTEMA(S) ACOMETIDO(S)
• Nervoso — o sistema nervoso periférico e a junção neuromuscular são os sistemas mais acometidos pelas neurotoxinas; os nervos cranianos podem vir a ser envolvidos, incluindo os nervos vagos e faciais pelos carrapatos da América do Norte e, também, os nervos trigêmeos e os do sistema nervoso simpático pelo carrapato *Ixodes* da Austrália.
• Respiratório — pode-se observar paralisia dos músculos intercostais e do diafragma; também é possível o comprometimento do centro respiratório da porção caudal do tronco encefálico (raro com os carrapatos da América do Norte; mais comum com os carrapatos *Ixodes* da Austrália).

GENÉTICA
Não apresenta nenhuma base genética.

INCIDÊNCIA/PREVALÊNCIA
• América do Norte e Austrália — um tanto sazonal (mais prevalente nos meses de verão); nas áreas mais quentes (sul dos EUA; norte da Austrália), o problema pode ocorrer durante o ano todo.
• Incidência global — baixa nos EUA; mais alta na Austrália.

DISTRIBUIÇÃO GEOGRÁFICA
• EUA— *Dermacentor variabilis*: ampla distribuição nos dois terços orientais do país e na Califórnia, bem como em Oregon; *D. andersoni*: desde a região de Cascatas até as Montanhas Rochosas; *Amblyomma americanum*: do Texas e de Missouri até a Costa do Atlântico; *A. maculatum*: temperatura e umidade elevadas das costas do Atlântico e do Golfo do México.
• Austrália — *Ixodes holocyclus*: limitado às áreas costeiras do leste australiano; associada especialmente a áreas de arbustos e cerrados (vegetações rasteiras).

IDENTIFICAÇÃO
Espécies
• Austrália — cães e gatos.
• EUA — cães; os gatos parecem ser resistentes.

Raça(s) Predominante(s)
Nenhuma.

Idade Média e Faixa Etária
Qualquer idade.

Sexo Predominante
N/D.

SINAIS CLÍNICOS
Achados Anamnésicos
• O paciente caminhou por áreas arborizadas ou abertas cerca de 1 semana antes do início dos sinais clínicos.
• Início — gradativo; começa com oscilação e fraqueza nos membros pélvicos.

Achados do Exame Neurológico
Carrapatos da América do Norte
• Assim que os sinais neurológicos aparecem, ocorre o rápido desenvolvimento de tetraparesia a tetraplegia generalizada atribuída à lesão ascendente dos neurônios motores inferiores.
• O paciente fica extremamente fraco ou até em decúbito em 1-3 dias, com hiporreflexia à arreflexia e hipotonia à atonia.
• Preservação da sensibilidade à dor.
• Disfunção dos nervos cranianos — não constitui uma característica proeminente; podem-se observar fraqueza facial e tônus mandibular reduzido; algumas vezes, ocorrem disfonia e disfagia no início da doença.
• Paralisia respiratória — incomum nos EUA; pode ocorrer em pacientes gravemente acometidos.
• Os processos de micção e defecação costumam permanecer normais.
• Não há efeitos cardiovasculares.

Carrapatos Ixodídeos
• Sinais neurológicos — muito mais graves e rapidamente progressivos; a fraqueza motora ascendente pode evoluir para tetraplegia dentro de algumas horas.
• Sialose (fluxo de saliva ou salivação), megaesôfago e vômito ou regurgitação — são achados característicos.
• Sistema nervoso simpático — pupilas midriáticas e pouco responsivas; hipertensão; taquiarritmias; pressão hidrostática capilar pulmonar elevada; edema pulmonar.
• Centro respiratório na porção caudal da medula oblonga — somado às alterações pulmonares periféricas; provoca declínio progressivo na frequência respiratória sem mudança no volume corrente, resultando em hipoxia, hipercapnia e acidose respiratória.
• Paralisia dos músculos respiratórios — muito mais prevalente; os cães e gatos evoluem para dispneia, cianose e paralisia respiratória dentro de 1-2 dias se não forem tratados.

CAUSAS
Estados Unidos
• *D. variabilis* — carrapato comum da madeira.
• *D. andersoni* — carrapato da madeira das Montanhas Rochosas.
• *A. americanum* — carrapato-estrela solitário.
• *A. maculatum* — carrapato da Costa do Golfo.

Austrália
I. holocyclus — secreta uma neurotoxina bem mais potente do que as espécies da América do Norte.

FATORES DE RISCO
Ambientes que albergam carrapatos.

DIAGNÓSTICO

DIAGNÓSTICO DIFERENCIAL
• Botulismo.
• Polineuropatia aguda.
• Polirradiculoneurite aguda (paralisia do Coonhound).
• Doença denervante distal.
• Miastenia grave fulminante.
• Mielopatia generalizada (difusa) ou multifocal.

HEMOGRAMA/BIOQUÍMICA/URINÁLISE
Normais.

OUTROS TESTES LABORATORIAIS
Gasometria sanguínea arterial — pacientes gravemente acometidos; PaO_2 baixa, $PaCO_2$ alta e pH baixo.

DIAGNÓSTICO POR IMAGEM
Radiografia torácica (carrapato *Ixodes*) — megaesôfago.

MÉTODOS DIAGNÓSTICOS
• Busca minuciosa pelo carrapato — cabeça, pescoço, corpo e membros, canais auditivos, boca, reto, vagina e prepúcio, bem como entre os dedos e os coxins podais; remover o carrapato imediatamente.
• Eletrodiagnóstico (eletromiograma) — atividade de inserção normal e ausência de atividade espontânea das miofibras (sem fibrilações e com ondas pontiagudas positivas); falta de potenciais de ação das unidades motoras; a estimulação nervosa motora é acompanhada por queda drástica na amplitude ou ausência completa dos potenciais de ação musculares compostos; haverá diminuição nas velocidades de condução nervosa motora se houver registro de potenciais de ação musculares compostos.

ACHADOS PATOLÓGICOS
N/D.

TRATAMENTO

CUIDADO(S) DE SAÚDE ADEQUADO(S)
Internação — para qualquer disfunção neurológica sugestiva de paralisia causada por carrapato; internar o animal até se encontrar e remover o carrapato ou até se efetuar o tratamento apropriado para matar os carrapatos escondidos.

CUIDADO(S) DE ENFERMAGEM
• Cuidados de suporte sob internação — essenciais até que o paciente comece a demonstrar sinais de recuperação.
• Gaiola de oxigênio — em casos de hipoventilação e hipoxia.
• Ventilação artificial — em casos de insuficiência respiratória.
• Fluidoterapia intravenosa — não costuma ser necessária a menos que a recuperação seja prolongada.

Paralisia do Carrapato

ATIVIDADE
- Manter o animal em ambiente tranquilo.
- Paralisia causada por carrapatos *Ixodes* — manter o paciente em local fresco com ar-condicionado; a toxina é sensível à temperatura; evitar a atividade física para impedir o aumento na temperatura corporal.

DIETA
Suspender a ingestão de água e alimentos se o paciente apresentar disfagia ou vômito/regurgitação.

ORIENTAÇÃO AO PROPRIETÁRIO
- Carrapatos não ixodídeos — informar o proprietário sobre o caráter essencial dos cuidados de enfermagem, embora a recuperação do paciente seja rápida após a remoção dos carrapatos (muitas vezes dentro de 24-48 h).
- Carrapatos ixodídeos — alertar o proprietário que, muitas vezes, os sinais clínicos continuam piorando, mesmo depois da remoção dos carrapatos (os sinais atribuídos aos nervos cranianos e a fraqueza frequentemente se intensificam 24-48 h após a retirada do ectoparasita); assim, é imprescindível efetuar tratamento mais rigoroso para neutralizar as toxinas.

CONSIDERAÇÕES CIRÚRGICAS
N/D.

MEDICAÇÕES

MEDICAMENTO(S) DE ESCOLHA
- EUA — caso não se consiga encontrar o carrapato, aplicar banhos de imersão com inseticidas sistêmicos como fipronil (Frontline®) ou, alternativamente, imersão do paciente em banheira com inseticida; com frequência, esses banhos constituem o único tratamento necessário.
- Austrália — é preciso neutralizar as toxinas circulantes por meio da aplicação de soro hiperimune (0,5-1 mg/kg IV), dependendo da gravidade dos sinais clínicos; em casos graves, a fenoxibenzamina, um antagonista α-adrenérgico (1 mg/kg IV diluído em solução salina e administrado lentamente durante 20 min), parece ser benéfica no alívio dos efeitos simpáticos; pode-se lançar mão da acepromazina (0,5-1 mg/kg IV) como medicamento alternativo (possui efeitos bloqueadores α-adrenérgicos).

CONTRAINDICAÇÕES
- Os medicamentos que interferem na transmissão neuromuscular são contraindicados (p. ex., tetraciclinas, aminoglicosídeos e penicilina procaína).
- Carrapatos ixodídeos — a atropina é contraindicada nos estágios avançados da doença ou em casos de bradicardia acentuada.

PRECAUÇÕES
Carrapatos ixodídeos — administrar fluidos intravenosos em uma velocidade bastante lenta, para evitar complicações futuras de congestão pulmonar.

INTERAÇÕES POSSÍVEIS
N/D.

MEDICAMENTO(S) ALTERNATIVO(S)
N/D.

ACOMPANHAMENTO

MONITORIZAÇÃO DO PACIENTE
- Carrapatos não ixodídeos — reavaliar o estado neurológico após a remoção dos carrapatos pelo menos 1 vez ao dia — deve-se observar uma rápida melhora na força muscular dos animais.
- Carrapatos ixodídeos — monitorizar o estado neurológico, bem como as funções respiratória e cardiovascular, de forma contínua e intensiva, mesmo depois da retirada dos carrapatos, em virtude dos efeitos residuais das neurotoxinas.

PREVENÇÃO
- Pesquisar de forma vigilante e atenta a presença de carrapatos após a exposição (pelo menos, a cada 2-3 dias); os sinais não ocorrem por 6-9 dias depois da fixação do ectoparasita.
- É útil a aplicação tópica de rotina de fipronil (Frontline®) ou de banhos inseticidas semanais.
- Após a exposição à neurotoxina do *Ixodes*, desenvolve-se uma imunidade adquirida de curta duração.

COMPLICAÇÕES POSSÍVEIS
Se o paciente sobreviver aos efeitos agudos da toxina, não haverá complicações a longo prazo.

EVOLUÇÃO ESPERADA E PROGNÓSTICO
- Carrapatos não ixodídeos — o prognóstico será bom a excelente se os carrapatos forem removidos; a recuperação ocorre em 1 até, no máximo, 3 dias.
- Carrapatos ixodídeos — o prognóstico frequentemente é reservado; a recuperação mostra-se prolongada; o óbito ocorre em 1-2 dias sem tratamento.

DIVERSOS

DISTÚRBIOS ASSOCIADOS
N/D.

FATORES RELACIONADOS COM A IDADE
N/D.

POTENCIAL ZOONÓTICO
Embora os seres humanos possam adquirir a doença pela picada dos mesmos carrapatos (especialmente na Austrália), a paralisia causada por esses ectoparasitas não é transmitida dos animais domésticos acometidos para o homem.

GESTAÇÃO/FERTILIDADE/REPRODUÇÃO
Desconhecido.

VER TAMBÉM
- Botulismo.
- Miastenia Grave.
- Neuropatias Periféricas (Polineuropatias).
- Paralisia do Coonhound (Polirradiculoneurite Idiopática).

Sugestões de Leitura
Atwell RB, Campbell FE, Evans EA. Prospective survey of tick paralysis in dogs. Australian Vet J 2001, 79:412-418.
Dewey CW. A Practical Guide to Canine and Feline Neurology, 2nd ed. Ames, IA: Wiley-Blackwell, 2008, pp. 549-551.
Lorenz MD, Kornegay JN. Handbook of Veterinary Neurology, 4th ed. St. Louis: Saunders Elsevier, 2004, pp. 191-192.
Malik R, Farrow BRH. Tick paralysis in North America and Australia. Vet Clin North Am Small Anim Pract 1991, 21:157-171.

Autor Paul A. Cuddon
Consultor Editorial Joane M. Parent

Paralisia do Coonhound (Polirradiculoneurite Idiopática)

CONSIDERAÇÕES GERAIS

DEFINIÇÃO
• Inflamação aguda de múltiplas raízes nervosas e nervos periféricos em cães, com ou sem histórico prévio de contato com saliva de guaxinim, vacinação, infecção gastrintestinal ou respiratória.
• Modelo animal proposto para a síndrome de Guillain-Barré em seres humanos.

FISIOPATOLOGIA
• Basicamente desconhecida — a saliva de guaxinim é associada em grande parte ao desenvolvimento dessa doença.
• Doença imunomediada que se desenvolve 7-14 dias após evento prévio oportuno (reação de hipersensibilidade tardia?).
• Acredita-se que a fisiopatologia envolva uma reação do sistema imunológico do cão a algum antígeno de reação cruzada (possível epítopo de carboidrato).

SISTEMA(S) ACOMETIDO(S)
Nervoso
• SNP — envolvimento mais grave nas raízes nervosas ventrais e nos componentes radiculares ventrais dos nervos espinais.
• Nervos cranianos — em alguns pacientes; principalmente os pares dos nervos VII e X.
• Paralisia respiratória — secundária ao envolvimento dos nervos intercostais e frênicos em determinados pacientes.

GENÉTICA
Não há nenhuma base genética comprovada.

INCIDÊNCIA/PREVALÊNCIA
• A polineuropatia mais comumente identificada em cães na América do Norte.
• Incidência baixa.

DISTRIBUIÇÃO GEOGRÁFICA
• Paralisia do Coonhound — está relacionada com a distribuição de guaxinins (p. ex., América do Norte e América Central; partes da América do Sul).
• PIAC — mundial.

IDENTIFICAÇÃO
Espécies
Cães e, muito ocasionalmente, gatos.

Raça(s) Predominante(s)
• Paralisia do Coonhound — acomete a raça Coonhound, mas qualquer raça que entre em contato com guaxinins se mostra suscetível.
• PIAC — nenhuma.

Idade Média e Faixa Etária
N/D.

Sexo Predominante
N/D.

SINAIS CLÍNICOS
Comentários Gerais
PIAC — os sinais neurológicos e a evolução patológica são os mesmos já listados, exceto quanto ao encontro inicial conhecido com o guaxinim.

Achados Anamnésicos
• Aparecem 7-14 dias após o contato com a saliva do guaxinim (por meio de mordida ou arranhadura), o receptor de uma vacinação, ou o desenvolvimento de alguma infecção respiratória ou gastrintestinal.
• Marcha espástica (rígida) em todos os membros — no início.
• Evolução rápida para tetraparesia a tetraplegia flácida, atribuída à lesão do neurônio motor inferior.
• Apetite e consumo hídrico — costumam permanecer normais
• Micção e defecção — normais. Alguns cães não urinarão no início, possivelmente em virtude de uma incapacidade de manter uma postura adequada.
• Evolução inicial — geralmente ocorre em 4-5 dias; a evolução máxima pode levar até 10 dias.

Achados do Exame Neurológico
• Simétricos em geral.
• Hiporreflexia a arreflexia generalizada, hipotonia a atonia, além de atrofia muscular neurogênica grave.
• Em alguns pacientes, os membros pélvicos são mais gravemente acometidos que os torácicos. Ocasionalmente, os pacientes podem exibir o inverso.
• Respiração — laboriosa em cães gravemente acometidos; evolução ocasional para paralisia respiratória; as alterações de afonia ou disfonia são comuns.
• Paresia facial — fechamento palpebral incompleto bilateral em muitos pacientes.
• Dor — a sensibilidade permanece intacta; a hiperestesia é comum, em virtude do envolvimento variável das raízes nervosas dorsais em caso de reação inflamatória.
• Disfunção motora — sempre predomina; em geral, até mesmo o paciente tetraplégico consegue abanar sua cauda.

CAUSAS
• Paralisia do Coonhound — contato com o guaxinim; talvez seja mais relevante o contato com a saliva do guaxinim.
• PIAC — nada comprovado; é possível que haja infecção respiratória ou gastrintestinal por vírus ou bactérias ou vacinação prévias.

FATORES DE RISCO
• Paralisia do Coonhound — essa raça tende a ser predisposta, principalmente em função da natureza de suas atividades; uma doença prévia não confere imunidade e pode aumentar o risco de recidiva; não são raros múltiplos surtos.
• PIAC — desconhecidos.

DIAGNÓSTICO

DIAGNÓSTICO DIFERENCIAL
• Outras polineuropatias agudas (a neuropatia paraneoplásica é a mais comum).
• Doença indutora de desnervação distal.
• Botulismo.
• Paralisia causada pelo carrapato.
• Envenenamento pela picada da aranha viúva-negra.
• Mielopatia generalizada (difusa) ou multifocal (envolvendo as intumescências cervical e lombossacra).

HEMOGRAMA/BIOQUÍMICA/URINÁLISE
Em geral, permanecem normais.

OUTROS TESTES LABORATORIAIS
• Imunoglobulinas séricas — em alguns pacientes, observam-se altos níveis séricos de IgG, mas não de IgM.
• Imunológicos — reação sérica à saliva do guaxinim no teste ELISA; os cães com paralisia do Coonhound apresentam reação positiva intensa, que diminui em termos de intensidade com o passar do tempo; os cães sem a doença, mas que entraram em contato com o guaxinim, também exibem reação positiva intensa; os cães com PIAC, mas sem nenhum contato com guaxinim, revelam negatividade na reação.

DIAGNÓSTICO POR IMAGEM
N/D.

MÉTODOS DIAGNÓSTICOS
Análise do LCS
• Lombar — alto conteúdo de proteínas, sem aumento no número de leucócitos, em todas as fases da doença.
• Cerebelomedular — nível levemente elevado de proteínas em pacientes examinados após as fases agudas da doença.
• O extravasamento de albumina pela barreira hematencefálica supostamente rompida constitui a principal causa do aumento proteico.
• Grande parte dos pacientes não apresenta nenhuma produção intratecal de imunoglobulinas.

Eletrodiagnóstico
• Eletromiografia (EMG) — atividade espontânea generalizada, cuja intensidade depende do momento do exame após o início da doença e da gravidade dos sinais neurológicos (EMG normal nos primeiros 4-5 dias).
• Amplitudes acentuadamente baixas do potencial de ação muscular composto após estimulação dos nervos motores.
• Ondas F — ondas tardias, indicativas da atuação dos nervos motores proximais e das raízes nervosas ventrais; anormalidades comuns: latências mínimas elevadas, proporção aumentada, amplitudes baixas.
• Velocidades de condução dos nervos motores — geralmente se encontram dentro do limite de normalidade; os pacientes com acometimento grave podem exibir valores levemente baixos.
• Função dos nervos sensoriais — comumente permanece normal.
• Essas anormalidades fornecem indícios de axonopatia periférica grave, juntamente com envolvimento e desmielinização axonais nas raízes nervosas ventrais.

ACHADOS PATOLÓGICOS
• Raízes nervosas ventrais e componentes radiculares ventrais dos nervos espinais — desenvolvem as lesões mais graves, que consistem em graus variados de degeneração axonal, desmielinizações paranodal e segmentar, bem como infiltração leucocitária (predominantemente de monócitos e macrófagos, com grupos dispersos de linfócitos e plasmócitos).
• Nervos periféricos — acometidos de modo semelhante, embora em menor escala.
• Raízes nervosas dorsais — acometidas em gravidade muito menor.

TRATAMENTO

CUIDADO(S) DE SAÚDE ADEQUADO(S)
• Internação — monitorizar os pacientes de perto na fase progressiva da doença (especialmente durante os 4 primeiros dias) quanto ao aparecimento de problemas respiratórios.

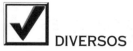
Paralisia do Coonhound (Polirradiculoneurite Idiopática)

- Comprometimento respiratório grave — cuidado intensivo; suporte ventilatório com pressão positiva, conforme a necessidade.
- Fluidoterapia intravenosa — solução de Ringer lactato; imprescindível apenas se o paciente ficar desidratado por incapacidade de alcançar e ter acesso à água.
- Esquema ambulatorial — em paciente estabilizado, após a confirmação diagnóstica inicial da doença.

CUIDADO(S) DE ENFERMAGEM
- Os pacientes costumam se mostrar capazes de se alimentar e beber se eles conseguirem alcançar o alimento e a água; muitas vezes, é preciso alimentá-los manualmente em função da paralisia.
- Fisioterapia intensiva — importante para diminuir a atrofia muscular.
- Mudança frequente de posição e cama acolchoada de boa qualidade — essenciais para evitar as úlceras de decúbito; no entanto, a atrofia muscular neurogênica grave é inevitável.

ATIVIDADE
Estimular os movimentos ao máximo possível; muitos pacientes ficam tetraplégicos.

DIETA
- Não há nenhuma restrição.
- Certificar-se de que o paciente consegue alcançar o alimento e a água.
- Fraqueza cervical — pode ser necessária a alimentação manual do paciente.

ORIENTAÇÃO AO PROPRIETÁRIO
- Informar ao proprietário sobre o caráter essencial de bons cuidados de enfermagem.
- Discutir a importância de se evitar as úlceras de decúbito e a queimadura por escaldagem de urina, além de se limitar o grau de atrofia muscular por meio de fisioterapia diligente (p. ex., movimentos passivos dos membros e natação à medida que a resistência/força do paciente começa a melhorar).
- Instruir o proprietário sobre a necessidade não só de uma cama macia e elástica (a lã e a palha são excelentes), que deve ser mantida limpa e livre de fezes e urina, mas também da mudança frequente de posição (a cada 3-4 h), da aplicação de banhos frequentes e do fornecimento de nutrição adequada para o paciente.

CONSIDERAÇÕES CIRÚRGICAS
N/D.

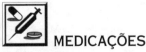
MEDICAÇÕES
MEDICAMENTO(S) DE ESCOLHA
- Não há nenhum medicamento com eficiência comprovada.
- Imunoglobulinas — 1 g/kg IV diariamente por 2 dias consecutivos ou 0,4 g/kg IV diariamente por 4-5 dias consecutivos; quando administradas na fase precoce da doença, essas proteínas podem diminuir a gravidade e/ou abreviar o tempo de recuperação.

CONTRAINDICAÇÕES
Corticosteroides — não melhoram os sinais clínicos nem abreviam a evolução da doença; podem reduzir o tempo de sobrevida em seres humanos com a síndrome de Guillain-Barré.

PRECAUÇÕES
N/D.

INTERAÇÕES POSSÍVEIS
N/D.

MEDICAMENTO(S) ALTERNATIVO(S)
N/D.

ACOMPANHAMENTO
MONITORIZAÇÃO DO PACIENTE
- Esquema ambulatorial — manter-se em contato estreito com o proprietário para verificar a ocorrência de complicações ou alterações no estado do paciente.
- Urinálise — examinar em intervalos periódicos quanto à presença de cistite em pacientes tetraplégicos ou gravemente tetraparéticos.
- O ideal é reavaliar, pelo menos, a cada 2-3 semanas.

PREVENÇÃO
- Paralisia do Coonhound — evitar o contato com guaxinins; muitas vezes, isso não é possível em função do ambiente e do uso comum dos cães Coonhound como caçadores de guaxinins.
- PIAC — se houver uma forte associação com algum evento prévio específico conhecido (p. ex., vacinação), evitar vacinações futuras.

COMPLICAÇÕES POSSÍVEIS
- Paralisia respiratória — na fase progressiva da doença.
- Úlceras de decúbito, queimadura por escaldagem de urina e cistite — comuns nos cães em decúbito crônico.

EVOLUÇÃO ESPERADA E PROGNÓSTICO
- A maioria se recupera completamente.
- Déficits neurológicos residuais leves — duração de algumas semanas em cães leve a moderadamente acometidos; duração de 3-4 meses em casos de doença grave.

DIVERSOS
DISTÚRBIOS ASSOCIADOS
N/D.

FATORES RELACIONADOS COM A IDADE
N/D.

POTENCIAL ZOONÓTICO
N/D.

GESTAÇÃO/FERTILIDADE/REPRODUÇÃO
Não se conhece o efeito sobre os fetos provenientes de cadela acometida.

SINÔNIMO(S)
Paralisia do cão Coonhound.

VER TAMBÉM
- Botulismo.
- Neuropatias Periféricas (Polineuropatias).
- Paralisia pelo Carrapato.

ABREVIATURA(S)
- ELISA = ensaio imunoabsorvente ligado à enzima.
- EMG = eletromiografia.
- LCS = líquido cerebrospinal.
- PIAC = polirradiculoneurite idiopática aguda canina.
- SNP = sistema nervoso periférico.

Sugestões de Leitura
Cuddon PA. Electrophysiologic assessment of acute polyradiculoneuropathy in dogs: Comparison with Guillain-Barr´e syndrome in people. J Vet Intern Med 1998, 12:294-303.
Cummings JF, de Lahunta A, Holmes DF, Schultz RD. Coonhound paralysis: Further clinical studies and electron microscopic observations. Acta Neuropathol 1982, 56:167-178.
Northington JW, Brown MJ. Acute canine idiopathic polyneuropathy: A Guillain-Barr´e-like syndrome in dogs. J Neurol Sci 1982, 56:259-273.

Autor Paul A. Cuddon
Consultor Editorial Joane M. Parent

Paraproteinemia

CONSIDERAÇÕES GERAIS

REVISÃO
- Presença no sangue de uma proteína anormal (paraproteína ou componente M) produzida por um único clone de células. A paraproteína pode ser composta de moléculas inteiras de imunoglobulina, subunidades, cadeias leves ou cadeias pesadas. Esse distúrbio é comumente observado nas neoplasias de plasmócitos, como o mieloma múltiplo, ou em outras doenças linfoproliferativas, como a leucemia linfocítica crônica ou o linfoma.
- Os sinais primários estão relacionados com a neoplasia subjacente e podem estar relacionados com a invasão de tecido ósseo ou a infiltração da medula óssea.
- Níveis de paraproteína sérica acentuadamente elevados podem produzir sinais de síndrome de hiperviscosidade.

SISTEMA(S) ACOMETIDO(S)
- Musculosquelético — a lise óssea causada pelas células neoplásicas podem provocar claudicação e fraturas patológicas.
- Nervoso — a lise óssea das vértebras pode provocar sinais neurológicos; desorientação, crises convulsivas, déficits de nervos cranianos ou sinais vestibulares podem estar associados à síndrome de hiperviscosidade.
- Hematológico/linfático/imune — mieloftise e destruição imunomediada secundária podem causar anemia, leucopenia ou trombocitopenia. A hemostasia pode ficar comprometida pela interferência da paraproteína na função das plaquetas e dos fatores de coagulação; produção inibida das imunoglobulinas normais leva à redução dos níveis dessas moléculas, aumentando a suscetibilidade à infecção.
- Oftálmico — a síndrome de hiperviscosidade pode provocar dilatação e tortuosidade dos vasos retinianos, descolamento da retina ou hemorragia da retina
- Cardiovascular — a síndrome de hiperviscosidade pode causar taquicardia, miocardiopatia hipertrófica, e ritmo de galope, bem como insuficiência cardíaca em gatos com maior frequência do que nos cães.
- Renal/urológico — é possível a insuficiência renal secundária à infiltração tumoral; nesse tipo de envolvimento orgânico, a síndrome de hiperviscosidade provoca hipoxia renal, proteinúria, hipercalcemia da malignidade ou infecção.

IDENTIFICAÇÃO
- Cães — meia-idade a mais idosos. • Gatos (rara) — mais idosos. • Sem predileção sexual.

SINAIS CLÍNICOS
- Letargia e fraqueza.
- Claudicação, paresia.
- Epistaxe ou sangramento gengival.
- Petéquias ou equimoses.
- Cegueira ou hemorragia retiniana.
- Poliúria e polidipsia.
- Crises convulsivas.

CAUSAS E FATORES DE RISCO
- Fatores que contribuem para o mieloma múltiplo — foram sugeridos fatores como predisposição genética, infecções virais, imunoestimulação crônica e exposição a carcinógenos.
- Vírus da leucemia felina provoca linfoma nos gatos.

DIAGNÓSTICO

DIAGNÓSTICO DIFERENCIAL
- Gamopatia monoclonal — linfoma, leucemia linfocítica crônica e aguda, erliquiose, leishmaniose, bartonelose, dirofilariose, processos inflamatórios crônicos (p. ex., piodermite), amiloidose, gastrenterite plasmocitária e PIF.
- Gamopatia policlonal — micoses sistêmicas, infecções hemoparasitárias, PIF, estomatite linfoplasmocitária (gatos), doença autoimune crônica e neoplasias (linfoma, mastocitoma).
- Sangramento — na maior parte dos casos, é atribuído à paraproteinemia e trombocitopenia; outras possibilidades: trombocitopenia/patia e vasculite imunomediadas paraneoplásicas, infecciosas ou autoimunes.
- Síndrome de hiperviscosidade — ver "Síndrome da Hiperviscosidade".

HEMOGRAMA/BIOQUÍMICA/URINÁLISE
- Anemia/leucopenia/trombocitopenia — secundária à mieloftise ou a mecanismos autoimunes; linfocitose acentuada associada à leucemia linfocítica crônica ou ao linfoma dentro da medula óssea.
- Proteína total e globulina — elevadas.
- Albumina — pode estar baixa.
- Cálcio — pode estar aumentado secundariamente à malignidade, insuficiência renal ou lise óssea.
- Ureia e creatinina — podem estar elevadas secundariamente à azotemia renal primária.
- Proteinúria — provocada por cadeias leves (i. e., proteína de Bence-Jones); não detectada nos exames de rotina; há necessidade da realização de imunoensaio ou eletroforese na amostra de urina.

OUTROS TESTES LABORATORIAIS
- Eletroforese de proteínas — para identificar pico monoclonal.
- Imunoeletroforese — ajuda a definir o tipo de gamopatia (i. e., IgG, IgA ou IgM).
- Viscosimetria — pode ajudar a definir a síndrome de hiperviscosidade.
- Teste para detecção de FIV e FeLV.
- Teste para pesquisa de doença infecciosa.

DIAGNÓSTICO POR IMAGEM
- Radiologia dos ossos acometidos — para identificar um possível local para a obtenção de aspirado ou a realização de biopsia.
- Radiografia simples do esqueleto ou cintilografia óssea — para definir a extensão das lesões líticas. As localizações mais comuns para lesões de mieloma múltiplo incluem corpos vertebrais, costelas, pelve, crânio e ossos longos proximais.
- Radiografia toracoabdominal ou ultrassonografia abdominal — em busca de indícios de linfonodos infartados ou organomegalia sugestivos de linfoma.

OUTROS MÉTODOS DIAGNÓSTICOS
- Aspirado/biopsia de medula óssea — um número de plasmócitos <5% é considerado como normal, enquanto uma quantidade >20% em cães ou >10% com atenção especial à morfologia da célula em gatos é compatível com mieloma múltiplo; mieloftise associada a outras doenças linfoproliferativas.
- Biopsia óssea de lesão lítica — raramente necessária para diagnosticar o mieloma múltiplo.
- Aspirado de linfonodo — para identificar população neoplásica de linfócitos no linfoma; para identificar amastigotas de *Leishmania* ou mórulas de *Ehrlichia*.
- Citologia ou histopatologia de órgão e imuno-histoquímica — para pesquisa de população neoplásica de células, agentes infecciosos (p. ex., imunofluorescência para coronavírus felino nos macrófagos) ou amiloide; notar: coagulopatias podem evitar métodos diagnósticos invasivos.

TRATAMENTO
- Tratamento de suporte, dependendo da manifestação da doença e do sistema orgânico acometido.
- Síndrome de hiperviscosidade — ver "Síndrome da Hiperviscosidade".
- Quimioterapia para processos neoplásicos, como mieloma múltiplo, leucemia linfocítica crônica, ou linfoma.

MEDICAÇÕES

MEDICAMENTO(S)
- Antibióticos nas infecções secundárias a imunocomprometimento.
- Ver doenças específicas em busca de medicamentos específicos.

ACOMPANHAMENTO
- Ver doenças específicas.
- Eletroforese pode ser monitorizada como indicação da resposta ao tratamento.

DIVERSOS

DISTÚRBIOS ASSOCIADOS
Incompetência imunológica.

SINÔNIMO(S)
- Gamopatia monoclonal. • Proteína M.

VER TAMBÉM
- Linfoma — Cães. • Linfoma — Gatos.
- Mieloma Múltiplo. • Síndrome da Hiperviscosidade.

ABREVIATURA(S)
- FeLV = vírus da leucemia felina.
- FIV = vírus da imunodeficiência felina.
- PIF = peritonite infecciosa felina.
- PCR = reação em cadeia da polimerase.

Sugestões de Leitura
Hohenhaus AE. Syndromes of hyperglobulinemia: Diagnosis and therapy. In: Bonagura JD, Kirk RW, eds. Kirk's Current Veterinary Therapy XII. Philadelphia: Saunders, 1995, pp. 523-530.

Autor Julie Armstrong
Consultor Editorial A.H. Rebar

PARASITAS RESPIRATÓRIOS

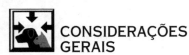
CONSIDERAÇÕES GERAIS

DEFINIÇÃO
Helmintos, artrópodes e protozoários que residem no trato respiratório ou nos vasos pulmonares de cães e gatos.

FISIOPATOLOGIA
A infestação por parasitas provoca rinite, bronquite, pneumonite ou arterite, dependendo da localização do microrganismo dentro do sistema respiratório. A invasão do parasita costuma resultar em inflamação eosinofílica.

SISTEMA(S) ACOMETIDO(S)
- Respiratório.
- Cardiovascular.
- Hepático — com a migração hepatopulmonar de alguns parasitas (*Toxocara* spp.).
- Neurológico — com a migração de parasitas para o cérebro (*Cuterebra*) ou hemorragia cerebral (*Angiostrongylus*).

INCIDÊNCIA/PREVALÊNCIA
Depende do parasita.

DISTRIBUIÇÃO GEOGRÁFICA
- *Pneumonyssoides caninum* — mundial.
- *Eucoleus boehmi* — América do Norte.
- *Linguatula serrata* — mundial.
- *Cuterebra* spp. — América do Norte.
- *Oslerus (Filaroides) osleri* — mundial.
- *Filaroides hirthi* — América do Norte.
- *Andersonstrongylus (Filaroides) milksi* — América do Norte; Europa.
- *Crenosoma vulpis* — mundial.
- *Eucoleus (Capillaria) aerophilus* — mundial.
- *Aelurostrongylus abstrusus* — mundial.
- *Paragonimus kellicotti* — América do Norte.
- *Toxoplasma gondii* — mundial.
- *Angiostrongylus vasorum* — principalmente na Europa e na América do Sul, mas com expansão mundial.
- *Toxocara* spp. — mundial.

IDENTIFICAÇÃO
Espécies
Cães e gatos.

SINAIS CLÍNICOS
Comentários Gerais
- Existem quatro categorias básicas — envolvimento das vias aéreas superiores (cavidade e seios nasais), do trato respiratório inferior (traqueia e brônquios), do parênquima pulmonar e do sistema vascular; classificadas com base na localização e no estilo de vida do parasita.
- Frequentemente insidiosos e crônicos, com poucos sinais clínicos.
- O comprometimento respiratório nem sempre é grave.

Achados Anamnésicos
- Respiratório superior — espirros; secreção nasal (serosa, sanguinolenta); espirro reverso; irritação ou fricção nasal; sinais neurológicos com *Cuterebra* spp.
- Respiratório inferior e parênquima — embora possa permanecer assintomático, pode apresentar tosse variável, taquipneia ou padrão respiratório alterado.
- Vascular — pode haver perda de peso, letargia, tosse, intolerância ao exercício.

Achados do Exame Físico
- Respiratório superior — achados semelhantes aos anamnésicos; variáveis.
- Respiratório inferior e parênquima — tosse eliciada à palpação da traqueia; ocasionalmente, auscultam-se ruídos pulmonares ásperos.
- Vascular — pode se apresentar com sinais de doença pulmonar, insuficiência cardíaca do lado direito, anemia, coagulopatia, sinais neurológicos.

CAUSAS
- Respiratório superior (cavidade e seios nasais) — *Pneumonyssoides caninum*; *Eucoleus boehmi*; *Linguatula serrata*; *Cuterebra* spp.
- Respiratório inferior (traqueia e brônquios) — cães e gatos: *Eucoleus (Capillaria) aerophilus* (raro nos gatos); cães: *Oslerus osleri*, *Filaroides hirthi*, *Andersonstrongylus milksi*, *Crenosoma vulpis*.
- Parênquima pulmonar — cães e gatos: *Paragonimus kellicotti*, *Toxoplasma gondii*; cães: *Filaroides hirthi*, *Andersonstrongylus milksi*; gatos: *Aelurostrongylus abstrusus*, *Cuterebra* spp.
- Vascular — cães e gatos: *Dirofilaria immitis*; migração de larvas de *Toxocara canis* e *cati*; cães: *Angiostrongylus vasorum*.

FATORES DE RISCO
- Dependem do parasita específico — alguns deles possuem hospedeiros intermediários ou paratênicos que precisam ser ingeridos pelo hospedeiro definitivo, colocando os animais que caçam ou vasculham lixo sob maior risco.
- *Crenosoma vulpis* — caramujos.
- *Paragonimus kellicotti* — caramujos; caranguejos; mariscos.
- *Aelurostrongylus abstrusus* — lesmas e caramujos; hospedeiros de transporte: roedores, sapos, lagartos, pássaros.
- *Linguatula serrata* — ingestão de miúdos de ovinos.
- *Toxoplasma gondii* — ingestão de pequenos mamíferos e pássaros infectados ou, menos comumente, pela ingestão de oocistos esporulados no solo ou na água.
- Residências com muitos animais em condições de vida insalubres — permitem a transmissão por contato direto ou orofecal.

DIAGNÓSTICO

DIAGNÓSTICO DIFERENCIAL
- Respiratório superior — outras causas de epistaxe, rinite ou sinusite (ver tópicos específicos).
- Respiratório inferior — bronquite aguda (não parasitária); bronquite crônica; traqueobronquite infecciosa.
- Parênquima pulmonar — doença pulmonar eosinofílica; broncopneumonia; pneumonia granulomatosa; granulomatose pulmonar.
- Vascular — outras causas de coagulopatia, insuficiência cardíaca do lado direito ou doença arterial pulmonar.

HEMOGRAMA/BIOQUÍMICA/URINÁLISE
- Hemograma completo — variável; podem-se notar eosinofilia, basofilia, neutrofilia e monocitose; pode-se observar anemia com *Angiostrongylus vasorum*.
- Bioquímica — frequentemente normal; aumento na atividade das enzimas hepáticas com alguns parasitas durante os estágios iniciais como resultado da migração pelo fígado se a carga parasitária for substancial.
- Urinálise — normal.

OUTROS TESTES LABORATORIAIS
Pode-se observar coagulopatia com *Angiostrongylus vasorum*.

DIAGNÓSTICO POR IMAGEM
Radiografias Torácicas
- Achados frequentemente inespecíficos — padrão intersticial generalizado; infiltrados peribronquiolares, com padrão nodular a alveolar.
- *Oslerus* — podem-se observar densidades nodulares de tecido mole dentro da traqueia ao nível da carina traqueal.
- *Paragonimus* — podem-se visualizar bolhas, lesões císticas ou pneumotórax causado pela ruptura das bolhas ou dos cistos.
- *Dirofilaria* — aumento de volume do lado direito do coração, artérias pulmonares tortuosas e truncadas, infiltrados pulmonares (cães). Poucas alterações cardíacas nos gatos.

MÉTODOS DIAGNÓSTICOS
Exame do esputo
Pode revelar a presença de ovos ou larvas (L-1).

Exame de Fezes
- Com frequência, há necessidade de múltiplos exames; os resultados negativos não descartam a infecção.
- Esfregaço fecal direto: *Angiostrongylus* (larvas).
- Flutuação fecal padrão: *Eucoleus aerophilus* (ovos), *Eucoleus boehmi* (ovos).
- Centrifugação com sulfato de zinco: *Aelurostrongylus* (larvas), *Oslerus osleri*, *Andersonstrongylus milksi*, *Filaroides hirthi* (larvas, ovos larvados).
- Técnica de Baermann: *Aelurostrongylus* (larvas), *Oslerus osleri*, *Andersonstrongylus milksi*, *Filaroides hirthi* (larvas, ovos), *Crenosoma* (larvas, ovos larvados), *Angiostrongylus* (larvas).
- Sedimentação: *Paragonimus* (ovos).

Rinoscopia
- Respiratório superior — exame por faringoscopia ou rinoscopia retrógrada com irrigação anterógrada de gás anestésico; quase sempre permite a visualização de ácaros nasais; obtenção de lavado nasal retrógrado e exame citológico do líquido podem ser valiosos.
- *Eucoleus boehmi* — o exame histopatológico pode revelar a presença de ovos nas camadas profundas dentro do epitélio.
- *Linguatula serrata* — diagnóstico feito por meio da observação de ovos nas secreções nasais ou em torno das narinas.

Broncoscopia
- Respiratório inferior e parênquima — raramente podem ser vistos parasitas traqueais e brônquicos, além de nódulos parasitários; ocasionalmente, os parasitas podem ser removidos para a identificação definitiva.
- Lavado traqueal ou broncoalveolar — pode permitir a identificação de larvas (*Oslerus osleri*, *Aelurostrongylus*, *Crenosoma*, *Filaroides hirthi*, *Andersonstrongylus milksi*, *Angiostrongylus*); ovos (*Eucoleus aerophilus*, *Paragonimus*); microrganismos (*Toxoplasma*).
- *Oslerus osleri* — também pode ser diagnosticado por escovação ou exame histopatológico de nódulos na carina traqueal.

Parasitas Respiratórios

ACHADOS PATOLÓGICOS
- Respiratório superior — podem ser encontrados ácaros nasais ou vermes no epitélio da cavidade e dos seios nasais.
- Respiratório inferior e parênquima — podem ser vistos nódulos pulmonares contendo parasitas por todo o parênquima ou dentro dos brônquios.
- Vascular — as alterações incluem formação de trombos e proliferação da camada íntima das paredes vasculares.
- *Cuterebra* spp. — pode ser encontrado nos cortes cerebrais quando associado a sinais neurológicos.

TRATAMENTO

CUIDADO(S) DE SAÚDE ADEQUADO(S)
Paciente de ambulatório — parasitas respiratórios superiores e inferiores; talvez haja necessidade da repetição dos exames para monitorizar a resposta.

ATIVIDADE
Repouso estrito em gaiola caso ocorra disfunção pulmonar grave com parasitas respiratórios superiores ou inferiores e com infecção parasitária vascular ou doença bolhosa associada ao *Paragonimus*.

DIETA
Sem restrições especiais.

ORIENTAÇÃO AO PROPRIETÁRIO
- Explicar que a resposta e a duração do tratamento dependem do tipo do parasita.
- Avisar o proprietário sobre o risco de recidiva em cães com estilos de vida favoráveis à transmissão de parasitas (p. ex., cães de caça, cães atletas, residências com muitos cães, gatos de rua).

CONSIDERAÇÕES CIRÚRGICAS
Cistos rompidos de *Paragonimus* geralmente necessitam de excisão cirúrgica.

MEDICAÇÕES

MEDICAMENTO(S) DE ESCOLHA
- Anti-helmínticos — poucos estudos confirmam a eficácia; a maioria dos dados não tem comprovação científica. Para o tratamento de *Dirofilaria*, ver seções específicas sobre Dirofilariose.
- *Pneumonyssoides caninum* — ivermectina na dose de 200 µg/kg SC ou VO por dois tratamentos com 3 semanas de intervalo ou uma vez por semana durante 3 semanas; **NOTA:** não indicada para utilização em cães nessa dosagem; dosagem contraindicada nas raças Collie e mestiços, bem como nos Pastores australianos, por causa da alta incidência de intoxicação; milbemicina oxima na dose de 0,5-1 mg/kg VO semanalmente durante 3 semanas; selamectina na dose de 6-24 mg/kg aplicada a cada 2 semanas por 3 tratamentos.
- *Cuterebra* — ivermectina na dose de 300 µg/kg SC ou VO em dias alternados por 3 doses combinadas com uma dose gradativamente reduzida de corticosteroides.
- *Linguatula serrata* — remoção física de microrganismos dos seios nasais.
- *Eucoleus aerophilus, Eucoleus boehmi* — ivermectina na dose de 200 µg/kg VO uma única vez; fembendazol na dose de 25-50 mg/kg a cada 12 h por 10-14 dias; muito difíceis de eliminar.
- *Oslerus osleri* — a terapia eficaz ainda não foi totalmente determinada. Considerar o uso da ivermectina na dose de 400 µg/kg SC ou VO a cada 3 semanas por 4 doses.
- *Crenosoma vulpis* — levamisol na dose de 7,5 mg/kg SC a cada 48 h (duas doses); fembendazol na dose de 50 mg/kg VO a cada 24 h por 7 dias; milbemicina oxima na dose de 0,5 mg/kg VO uma única vez.
- *Aelurostrongylus abstrusus* — fembendazol na dose de 25-50 mg/kg VO a cada 24 h por 10 dias; ivermectina na dose de 400 µg/kg SC.
- *Filaroides hirthi, Andersonstrongylus milksi* — fembendazol na dose de 50 mg/kg VO a cada 24 h por 14 dias; albendazol na dose de 50 mg/kg VO a cada 12 h por 5 dias, repetir em 3 semanas.
- *Paragonimus kellicotti* — praziquantel na dose de 25 mg/kg VO, SC a cada 8 h por 3 dias; fembendazol na dose de 25-50 mg/kg VO a cada 12 h por 14 dias.
- *Toxoplasma* — clindamicina na dose de 12,5 mg/kg VO a cada 12 h por 28 dias.
- *Angiostrongylus vasorum* — fembendazol na dose de 50 mg/kg VO a cada 24 h por 7-21 dias; milbemicina oxima na dose de 0,5 mg/kg VO semanalmente por 4 semanas; levamisol na dose de 7,5 mg/kg por 2 dias consecutivos, seguido por dois dias a 10 mg/kg e se a infecção não for eliminada, o esquema terapêutico deverá ser repetido (não indicado para uso em cães).
- Migração de larvas de *Toxocara* spp. — fembendazol na dose de 50 mg/kg VO a cada 24 h por 10 dias.
- Agentes anti-inflamatórios — as recomendações para uso concomitante de esteroides variam.

CONTRAINDICAÇÕES
Ivermectina — não aprovada para utilização em cães ou gatos a não ser para profilaxia contra dirofilariose; contraindicada em dosagens > 100 µg/kg nas raças com suscetibilidade aumentada conhecida (Collie e mestiços, além de Pastor australiano).

ACOMPANHAMENTO

MONITORIZAÇÃO DO PACIENTE
- Extrações seriadas de larvas nas fezes pela técnica de Baermann ou exame de fezes em busca de ovos — alguns anti-helmínticos podem suprimir a produção de ovos ou de larvas em algumas espécies.
- Resolução dos sinais clínicos — sugere a resposta ao tratamento; não indica a depuração completa dos parasitas.
- Eosinofilia periférica, se observada inicialmente, pode diminuir com o tratamento.
- Exame broncoscópico repetido — pode ajudar a avaliar a eficácia do tratamento nos casos de *Oslerus osleri*.

PREVENÇÃO
- Evitar atividades que predisponham a infestações (muitas vezes, isso não é praticável).
- Evitar o contato com animais silvestres reservatórios (sobretudo canídeos e felídeos selvagens).
- Considerar o tratamento profilático para dirofilariose.

COMPLICAÇÕES POSSÍVEIS
- Lesão pulmonar crônica — possível com cargas maciças e persistentes de parasitas do trato respiratório inferior.
- As infestações não costumam ser fatais; no entanto, algumas espécies podem resultar em grave dano pulmonar; *Cuterebra* spp. e *Angiostrongylus* podem causar complicações neurológicas fatais.
- *Pneumonyssoides caninum* já foi associado à dilatação e vólvulo gástricos.

EVOLUÇÃO ESPERADA E PROGNÓSTICO
- Com tratamento rigoroso — prognóstico, em geral, de razoável a excelente; variável.
- Retorno ao desempenho — depende da cronicidade da doença e do nível de lesão pulmonar crônica pelos parasitas do trato respiratório inferior.
- A recidiva é possível.

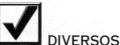

SINÔNIMO(S)
- Infestação por vermes pulmonares — *Aelurostrongylus, Eucoleus (Capillaria) aerophilus, Crenosoma, Oslerus osleri, Filaroides hirthi, Andersonstrongylus milksi*.
- Infestação por ácaros nasais — *Pneumonyssoides caninum, Pneumonyssus caninum*.
- "Dirofilariose francesa"* — *Angiostrongylus vasorum*.

VER TAMBÉM
- Dirofilariose — Cães. • Dirofilariose — Gatos.
- Pneumonia Eosinofílica.

RECURSOS DA INTERNET
- Bowman DD. Respiratory System Parasites of the Dog and Cat (Part I): Nasal Mucosa and Sinuses, and Respiratory Parenchyma: http://www.ivis.org/advances/Parasit Bowman/ddb resp/ivis.pdf. _ Bowman DD. Respiratory System Parasites of the Dog and Cat (Part II): Trachea and Bronchi, and Pulmonary Vessels: http://www.ivis.org/advances/ParasitBowman/ddb resp2/ivis.pdf.

Sugestões de Leitura
Conboy G. Natural infections of Crenosoma vulpis and Angiostrongylus vasorum in dogs in Atlantic Canada and their treatment with milbemycin oxime. Vet Record 2004, 55(1):16-18.
Denk D, Matiasek K, et al. Disseminated angiostrongylosis with fatal cerebral haemorrhages in two dogs in Germany: A clinical case study. Vet Parasitol 2009, 160(1-2):100-108.
Lacorcia L, Gaser R, Anderson BA, Beveridge I. Comparison of bronchoalveolar lavage fluid examination and other diagnostic techniques with the Baermann technique for detection of naturally occurring Aelurostrongylus abstrusus infection in cats. JAVMA 2009, 235(1):43-49.
Marks SL, Moore MP, Rishniw M. Pneumonyssus caninum: The canine nasal mite. Compend Contin Educ Pract Vet 1994, 16:577-582.

Autor Jill S. Pomrantz
Consultor Editorial Lynelle R. Johnson

---

* N. T.: Verme descrito por parasitologistas franceses.

PARESIA E PARALISIA DO NERVO FACIAL

CONSIDERAÇÕES GERAIS

DEFINIÇÃO
Disfunção do nervo facial (VII par de nervos cranianos), causando paresia (fraqueza) ou paralisia dos músculos da expressão facial, que incluem as orelhas, as pálpebras, os lábios e as narinas.

FISIOPATOLOGIA
• Centrais — comprometimento do núcleo facial dentro da medula rostral (tronco encefálico).
• Periféricas — comprometimento do nervo facial em qualquer local ao longo de sua extensão e ao nível da junção neuromuscular.

SISTEMA(S) ACOMETIDO(S)
• Nervoso — nervo facial periférico ou seu núcleo no tronco cerebral.
• Oftálmico — se os neurônios pré-ganglionares parassimpáticos que inervam as glândulas lacrimais e a glândula da terceira pálpebra e seguem com o nervo facial no sentido proximal forem acometidos, desenvolve-se ceratoconjuntivite seca por causa da falta de secreção lacrimal.

GENÉTICA
N/D.

INCIDÊNCIA/PREVALÊNCIA
Mais comum em cães do que em gatos.

DISTRIBUIÇÃO GEOGRÁFICA
N/D.

IDENTIFICAÇÃO
Espécies
Cães e gatos.

Raça(s) Predominante(s)
Paralisia idiopática — Cocker spaniel, Beagle, Pembroke Welsh corgi, Boxer, Setter inglês e gatos domésticos de pelo longo.

Idade Média e Faixa Etária
Adultos.

Sexo Predominante
N/D.

SINAIS CLÍNICOS
Comentários Gerais
• Avaliar a força do fechamento palpebral — as pálpebras devem se fechar completamente ao se passar um dedo de modo delicado sobre as pálpebras.
• Idiopáticas em muitos animais — o lado não acometido pode vir a ser afetado dentro de algumas semanas a meses; raramente, pode ocorrer de forma bilateral na primeira apresentação.
• A maioria dos pacientes com acometimento bilateral do nervo sofre de doença sistêmica associada à polineuropatia — procurar por outros déficits nervosos.
• Pode acompanhar outros sinais clínicos e/ou déficits neurológicos — sempre realizar um exame neurológico completo.
• A queda das orelhas nem sempre é evidente em cães e gatos com orelhas eretas.

Achados Anamnésicos
• O animal se suja quando come; a comida fica retida em torno da boca.
• Salivação excessiva no lado acometido.
• Assimetria facial.
• Olhos — não se fecham; o animal os esfrega com as patas; secreção ocular.

Achados do Exame Físico
• Assimetria facial — queda dos lábios e das orelhas, fissura palpebral ampla, colabamento das narinas.
• Reflexo palpebral diminuído ou ausente.
• Resposta à ameaça diminuída ou ausente.
• Impossibilidade de fechar as pálpebras.
• Salivação excessiva ou alimento que cai pela boca no lado acometido.
• Crônicos — os pacientes podem exibir contração do músculo facial e desvio da face em direção ao lado acometido em função de fibrose muscular subsequente à paralisia e desnervação.
• Teste lacrimal de Schirmer diminuído, secreção mucopurulenta do olho acometido e conjuntivite ou ceratite de exposição com ceratoconjuntivite seca concomitante.
• Alteração do estado mental (p. ex., sonolência ou estupor) e/ou anormalidades de outros nervos cranianos e distúrbios da marcha podem ser observados secundariamente à doença intracraniana (tronco encefálico).
• Espasmos hemifaciais (tétano do nervo facial) podem ser observados com pouca frequência em animais com lesões irritantes afetando o nervo facial como neurite ou otite média. Esses pacientes sofrem contração dos músculos faciais, dando um aspecto de "sorriso forçado" no lado acometido da face. No entanto, esse processo é dinâmico e, às vezes, a face parecerá normal, somente até começar o aspecto de "sorriso forçado" outra vez. Caso se observe essa apresentação clínica, é recomendável a investigação minuciosa quanto à presença de comprometimento da orelha média.
• Em pacientes com lesão talamocortical contralateral, pode-se observar paresia facial intermitente quando estiverem relaxados — pela "liberação" da influência do neurônio motor superior sobre o neurônio motor inferior (VII par de nervos cranianos).

CAUSAS
Periféricas Unilaterais
• Idiopáticas.
• Metabólicas — hipotireoidismo.
• Infecciosas — otite média-interna (cães e gatos).
• Inflamatórias — pólipos nasofaríngeos (gatos).
• Iatrogênicas — secundárias à ablação cirúrgica do canal auditivo externo ou osteotomia da bula timpânica; secundárias à limpeza otológica excessiva; reação idiossincrática a sulfonamidas potencializadas (cães).
• Neoplásicas — colesteatoma aural, carcinoma de células escamosas.
• Traumatismo — fratura da porção petrosa do osso temporal; lesão direta do nervo facial advinda de laceração ou compressão por hematoma ou outra massa.
• Tóxicas — paralisia pelo carrapato (*Dermacentor* spp., *Ixodes holocyclus*).

Periféricas Bilaterais
• Idiopáticas — raras.
• Inflamatórias — polirradiculoneurite (paralisia do Coonhound).
• Imunomediadas — polineuropatia, miastenia grave.
• Metabólicas — polineuropatia paraneoplásica (p. ex., insulinoma).
• Tóxicas — botulismo.
• Infecciosas — a borreliose de Lyme em seres humanos não foi comprovada em cães até o momento.

SNC
• Mais unilaterais.
• Infecciosas — encefalites virais, bacterianas, fúngicas, riquetsianas e protozoárias.
• Inflamatórias — meningoencefalomielite granulomatosa.
• Neoplásicas — primárias como meningioma, tumor do plexo coroide; tumor metastático como hemangiossarcoma, carcinoma, linfoma.

FATORES DE RISCO
Otites externa e média crônicas.

DIAGNÓSTICO

DIAGNÓSTICO DIFERENCIAL
• Diferenciar o envolvimento uni de bilateral.
• Procurar por outros déficits neurológicos — mudança de comportamento, distúrbio da marcha, outros déficits de nervos cranianos.
• Idiopático — diagnóstico de exclusão; provável se o paciente não tiver antecedentes ou sinais físicos de otopatia e nenhum outro déficit neurológico.
• Hipotireoidismo — com evidência clínica (p. ex., letargia, más condições da pelagem, ganho de peso, etc.).
• Otite média-interna — se houver síndrome de Horner e/ou inclinação da cabeça e/ou ceratoconjuntivite seca simultaneamente.
• Doença do SNC — em caso de sonolência, distúrbios da marcha ou outros déficits dos nervos cranianos.

HEMOGRAMA/BIOQUÍMICA/URINÁLISE
• Em geral, permanecem normais na paralisia facial idiopática.
• Hipercolesterolemia de jejum e/ou anemia arregenerativa normocítica/normocrômica — podem ser vistas na paralisia facial associada ao hipotireoidismo.
• Hipoglicemia — com insulinoma.

OUTROS TESTES LABORATORIAIS
• Indicados em pacientes com suspeita de doença subjacente.
• Relação de insulina:glicose para detectar insulinoma.
• Anticorpos contra os receptores de acetilcolina para diagnosticar miastenia grave.
• T_4 total e TSH canino para diagnosticar hipotireoidismo.

DIAGNÓSTICO POR IMAGEM
• Radiografias da bula timpânica — (quatro projeções: duas oblíquas, uma de boca aberta a 30° e outra dorsoventral) não são sensíveis para doenças da orelha média e interna.
• TC — sensível para avaliar doenças da orelha média e interna; modalidade preferida para avaliar estruturas ósseas na orelha média.
• RM — superior à TC para visualização de estruturas intracranianas; preferível para doença do SNC; intensificação de contraste do nervo facial em cães com paralisia idiopática desse nervo; quanto maior a extensão do realce, pior será o prognóstico quanto ao retorno da função.

MÉTODOS DIAGNÓSTICOS
• Teste lacrimal de Schirmer — avalia a produção de lágrimas (>15 mm em 60 segundos); sempre deve ser realizado ao se avaliar um paciente com paresia/paralisia facial.

PARESIA E PARALISIA DO NERVO FACIAL

- Teste com fluoresceína — avalia a presença de úlcera de córnea secundária à ceratoconjuntivite seca.
- Exame otoscópico — avalia a integridade da membrana timpânica e busca por indícios de otite média.
- Análise do LCS — avalia indícios de doença intracraniana; não é sensível se utilizada isoladamente; deve ser combinada com técnicas de diagnóstico por imagem (p. ex., RM).
- Eletromiografia do músculo facial — avalia a presença de desnervação e doença neuromuscular.
- Teste eletrodiagnóstico dos reflexos dos nervos facial e trigêmeo — avalia a integridade dos nervos periféricos; permite a distinção entre lesões periféricas e centrais.

ACHADOS PATOLÓGICOS
Idiopáticos — pode-se observar degeneração de fibras mielinizadas grandes e pequenas, sem evidência de inflamação.

TRATAMENTO

CUIDADO(S) DE SAÚDE ADEQUADO(S)
- Paciente ambulatorial — paralisia facial idiopática.
- Paciente internado — avaliação clínica inicial e tratamento de doença sistêmica ou neurológica (SNC) se presente.

CUIDADO(S) DE ENFERMAGEM
N/D.

ATIVIDADE
N/D.

DIETA
Não há necessidade de nenhuma alteração.

ORIENTAÇÃO AO PROPRIETÁRIO
- Avisar que os sinais clínicos podem ser permanentes; no entanto, à medida que a fibrose muscular se desenvolve, há uma "compressão" natural do lado acometido que diminui a assimetria; a salivação excessiva, em geral, cessa em 2-4 semanas.
- Informar o proprietário que o outro lado pode ser acometido.
- Discutir os cuidados com os olhos — talvez haja necessidade de lubrificar a córnea do lado acometido; poderão ser necessários cuidados adicionais se o animal for um reprodutor com exoftalmia natural; o proprietário precisa verificar regularmente se há vermelhidão, secreção ou dor.
- Informar o proprietário sobre o fato de que a maioria dos animais tolera bem esse déficit nervoso; não há impacto significativo sobre a qualidade de vida.

CONSIDERAÇÕES CIRÚRGICAS
Osteotomia da bula timpânica — pode ser indicada em pacientes com distúrbios da orelha média.

MEDICAÇÕES

MEDICAMENTO(S) DE ESCOLHA
- Tratar a doença específica, se possível (p. ex., tiroxina para hipotireoidismo).
- Doença idiopática — nenhum tratamento é requerido; a eficácia dos corticosteroides não é conhecida, embora eles sejam comumente utilizados em pessoas para tratar a paralisia de Bell.
- Reposição de lágrimas — se o resultado do teste lacrimal de Schirmer for baixo (<15 mm); indicada em pacientes com ceratoconjuntivite seca ou exoftalmia dos globos oculares.

CONTRAINDICAÇÕES
Na suspeita de doença da orelha média e na possibilidade de ruptura da membrana timpânica, não utilizar soluções otológicas tópicas de limpeza em virtude do risco de ototoxicidade.

PRECAUÇÕES
N/D.

INTERAÇÕES POSSÍVEIS
N/D

MEDICAMENTO(S) ALTERNATIVO(S)
N/D.

ACOMPANHAMENTO

MONITORIZAÇÃO DO PACIENTE
- Reavaliar precocemente em busca de indícios de úlceras de córnea.
- Avaliar mensalmente (a cada 2-3 meses) as respostas à ameaça e os reflexos palpebrais, bem como os movimentos dos lábios e das orelhas, quanto ao retorno da função, além do estado do olho acometido e do desenvolvimento de outros déficits neurológicos indicativos de doença progressiva.

PREVENÇÃO
N/D.

COMPLICAÇÕES POSSÍVEIS
- Ceratoconjuntivite seca.
- Úlceras de córnea.
- Contratura grave no lado da lesão.
- Assimetria facial permanente (apenas estética).

EVOLUÇÃO ESPERADA E PROGNÓSTICO
- Dependem da causa subjacente se uma complicação estiver presente.
- Doença idiopática — prognóstico reservado em termos de recuperação completa.
- A melhora pode levar semanas ou meses ou nunca ocorrer.
- Às vezes, desenvolve-se contratura do lábio.
- As úlceras de córnea podem perfurar e necessitar de enucleação.

DIVERSOS

DISTÚRBIOS ASSOCIADOS
N/D.

FATORES RELACIONADOS COM A IDADE
N/D.

POTENCIAL ZOONÓTICO
N/D.

GESTAÇÃO/FERTILIDADE/REPRODUÇÃO
N/D.

SINÔNIMO(S)
- Neurite facial.
- Paralisia facial.
- Neuropatia facial idiopática.

VER TAMBÉM
- Ceratite Ulcerativa.
- Ceratoconjuntivite Seca.
- Hipotireoidismo.
- Otite Média e Interna.

ABREVIATURA(S)
- LCS = líquido cerebrospinal.
- SNC = sistema nervoso central.
- RM = ressonância magnética.
- TC = tomografia computadorizada.

Sugestões de Leitura
Cook LB. Neurologic evaluation of the ear. Vet Clin North Am Small Anim Pract 2004, 34:425-435.
Schlicksup MD, Van Winkle TJ, Holt DE. Prevalence of clinical abnormalities in cats found to have nonneoplastic middle ear disease at necropsy: 59 cases (1991-2007). JAVMA 2009, 235(7):841-843.
Varejao AS, Munoz A, Lorenzo V. Magnetic resonance imaging of the intratemporal facial nerve in idiopathic facial paralysis in the dog. Vet Radiol Ultrasound 2006, 47(4):328-333.

Autor Andrea M. Finnen
Consultor Editorial Joane M. Parent
Agradecimento T. Mark Neer por ter escrito este capítulo nas edições anteriores.

PARTO PREMATURO

CONSIDERAÇÕES GERAIS

REVISÃO
Atividade inadequada do miométrio antes do período gestacional fisiológico (ou seja, pré-termo), capaz de levar ao abortamento.

IDENTIFICAÇÃO
Cadela ou gata prenhe; sem predileção etária ou racial.

SINAIS CLÍNICOS
Corrimento vulvar: hemorrágico ou loquial.

CAUSAS E FATORES DE RISCO
Desconhecidos; a genética pode desempenhar um papel; a luteólise pode resultar em parto prematuro ou contribuir para esse tipo de parto.

DIAGNÓSTICO

DIAGNÓSTICO DIFERENCIAL
- Gestação a termo, início de parto normal.
- Perda gestacional patológica (traumatismo, toxina, distúrbio de desenvolvimento, ou causas infecciosas).

HEMOGRAMA/BIOQUÍMICA/URINÁLISE
- Geralmente normais (pode estar presente uma anemia típica de gestação).
- Podem ocorrer anemia por perda sanguínea e leucograma inflamatório.

OUTROS TESTES LABORATORIAIS
Em caso de abortamento, o nível sérico de progesterona pode ficar <2 ng/mL.

DIAGNÓSTICO POR IMAGEM
- Avaliação ultrassonográfica da frequência cardíaca do feto (o estresse é evidenciado por frequências constantemente <170).
- Quando ocorre a morte fetal (Figuras 1, 2), há uma alteração no aspecto morfológico normal do útero e dos fetos.

MÉTODOS DIAGNÓSTICOS
- Tocodinamometria é um método diagnóstico; a constatação de >0-2 contrações/hora não é normal para gestação pré-termo (antes da 8ª semana).
- Ensaio quantitativo de progesterona (quimioluminescência, fluorescência, ensaio imunoenzimático) é importante para detectar níveis <2,0 ng/mL. Os ensaios hospitalares rápidos são menos precisos, entre 2 e 5 ng/mL.

TRATAMENTO

- Em seres humanos, o repouso pélvico em leito e a administração de antibióticos não contribuem para um resultado positivo, embora sejam prescritos com frequência.
- São administrados agentes tocolíticos (beta-agonistas, bloqueadores dos canais de cálcio, sulfato de magnésio, inibidores da prostaglandina sintetase).

MEDICAÇÕES

MEDICAMENTO(S)
- Tocolíticos (terbutalina 0,03 mg/kg VO a cada 6-12 h conforme a necessidade); a dose é titulada com base na monitorização uterina.
- ± Compostos progestacionais: progesterona em veículo oleoso é administrada por via IM na dose de 2 mg/kg a cada 72 h. Altrenogeste (Regu-Mate®, Hoechst-Roussel), um progestágeno sintético fabricado para uso na égua, é dosado por via oral a 0,088 mg/kg a cada 24 h. A administração exógena de progesterona deve ser utilizada apenas se o nível sérico desse hormônio estiver abaixo de 2 ng/mL.

CONTRAINDICAÇÕES/INTERAÇÕES POSSÍVEIS
- Gestação prolongada se a terbutalina ou os compostos progestacionais não forem suspensos 24-48 horas antes da devida data, calculada a partir da primeira elevação da progesterona, do pico do hormônio luteinizante, ou do 1º dia do diestro citológico (ver Acasalamento, Momento Oportuno).
- Lactação deficiente caso se faça uso de compostos progestacionais.
- Masculinização de fetos do sexo feminino se os compostos progestacionais forem utilizados. Retenção forçada de uma gestação patológica se um parto prematuro idiopático for erroneamente diagnosticado.

ACOMPANHAMENTO

- Ultrassonografia abdominal seriada.
- Tocodinamometria seriada.

DIVERSOS

Geralmente um diagnóstico por exclusão de todas as outras causas de abortamento tardio (*Brucella canis*, metrite, placentite, traumatismo, doença metabólica, coagulopatia, erro inato do metabolismo, defeitos genéticos), incitando a realização de tocodinamometria no meio do período gestacional (mesotermo) na próxima gestação.

RECURSOS DA INTERNET
www.ivis.org.

Sugestões de Leitura
Davidson AP. The diagnosis and management of premature labor in the bitch and queen. Proceedings, Society for Theriogenology Annual Meeting, August 2004.
Newman RB, Campbell BA, Stramm SL. Objective tocodynamometry identifies labor onset earlier than subjective maternal perception. Obstet Gynecol 1998, 76:1089-1093.
Root Kustritz MV. Use of supplemental progesterone in management of canine pregnancy. In: Concannon PW, England G, Verstegen III J, Linde-Forsberg C, eds., Recent Advances in Small Animal Reproduction. International Veterinary Information Service, Ithaca NY, www.ivis.org, 2001.
Scott-Moncrieff JC, Nelson RW, Bill RL, et al. Serum disposition of exogenous progesterone after intramuscular administration in bitches. Am J Vet Res 1990, 51:893-895.

Autores Autumn P. Davidson e Tomas W. Baker
Consultor Editorial Sara K. Lyle

PARVOVIROSE CANINA

CONSIDERAÇÕES GERAIS

DEFINIÇÃO
- Do ponto de vista clínico, a parvovirose canina caracteriza-se por inapetência, vômito, diarreia e perda de peso. Os casos graves da doença resultam em sepse, endotoxemia, CID e síndrome da angústia respiratória aguda.
- O parvovírus canino (CPV) original sofreu mudanças genéticas, desdobrando-se em CPV-1 e CPV-2. O CPV-2, por sua vez, desenvolveu-se ainda mais em CPV-2a (1979), CPV-2b (1984) e CPV-2c (Itália, 2001), que diferem em termos de proteínas do capsídeo e amplitude de hospedeiros.
- A doença mais grave associa-se ao CPV-2b.
- O CPV-1 pode causar uma diarreia intratável geralmente fatal em filhotes caninos neonatos.

FISIOPATOLOGIA
- O CPV apresenta uma via orofecal de infecção. Em seguida, ocorre proliferação linfoide dentro das tonsilas, dos linfonodos mesentéricos e de outros tecidos linfoides. Antes dos sinais clínicos, constata-se viremia em torno de 3-5 dias após a infecção.
- Os animais virêmicos demonstram disseminação viral nas fezes antes do aparecimento dos sinais clínicos. Tipicamente, essa eliminação fecal não dura mais do que 10 dias.
- O período de incubação é de 7-14 dias.
- Em princípio, o CPV tem como alvo as células das criptas da porção distal do duodeno e depois se estende para o jejuno.
- Os sinais clínicos começam a se manifestar por volta de 6-10 dias após a infecção.
- Os animais acometidos apresentam leucopenia e neutropenia concomitantes. Isso se deve principalmente ao aumento da demanda tecidual, ao desvio do reservatório (*pool*) circulante para o reservatório (*pool*) marginal/periférico e à depleção das reservas medulares.
- Raramente, observa-se a forma miocárdica do CPV. Essa manifestação é atribuível à infecção intrauterina ou neonatal pelo CPV-2 e tipicamente causa morte súbita.
- Os casos graves desenvolvem sepse e endotoxemia por bactérias entéricas Gram-negativas. A resposta de citocinas observada na parvovirose equivale àquela constatada em casos de sepse. A sepse provoca colapso circulatório, falência múltipla de órgãos e morte.

SISTEMA(S) ACOMETIDO(S)
- Gastrintestinal — destruição das criptas intestinais; inapetência; vômitos; diarreia osmótica, secretora, hemorrágica proveniente do intestino delgado.
- Sanguíneo/Linfático/Imune — depleção linfoide; depleção da medula óssea; destruição do timo, das placas de Peyer e do TLAI, levando à imunossupressão.
- Comportamental — letargia; depressão decorrente de desidratação, sepse, hipoglicemia.
- Cardiovascular — miocardite causadora de morte súbita; choque hipovolêmico indutor de colapso circulatório; bacteremia, septicemia, endotoxemia, hipercoagulabilidade (como alteração precoce); hipocoagulabilidade (observada em casos de CID e perdas significativas da antitrombina).
- Nervoso — depressão mental; coma por hipoglicemia, choque, hemorragia intracraniana. Não há provas de que o CPV infecte os neurônios em cães.
- Hepatobiliar — icterícia; elevação na atividade das enzimas hepáticas por colestase; endotoxemia.
- Renal/Urológico — azotemia pré-renal; azotemia renal por falência múltipla de órgãos.
- Respiratório — síndrome da angústia respiratória aguda em casos graves.

GENÉTICA
Desconhecida.

INCIDÊNCIA/PREVALÊNCIA
- A incidência diminuiu drasticamente com a vacinação.
- Ainda é observada em canis reprodutores, centros de zoonose para captura de animais errantes, abrigos de sociedades protetoras e áreas com grande quantidade de filhotes caninos imunocomprometidos ou inadequadamente vacinados.

DISTRIBUIÇÃO GEOGRÁFICA
Mundial.

IDENTIFICAÇÃO
Espécies
- Cães.
- Gatos — podem ser infectados pelo CPV-2b.

Raça(s) Predominante(s)
Rottweiler, Doberman pinscher, Pit bull, Labrador retriever, Pastor alemão, Springer spaniel inglês, cães de trenó do Alasca.

Idade Média e Faixa Etária
- A maioria dos casos é observada entre 6 semanas e 6 meses de vida.
- Os casos mais graves da doença ocorrem em filhotes mais jovens.

SINAIS CLÍNICOS
Comentários Gerais
Os filhotes com sinais de letargia, inapetência, vômitos ou diarreia devem levantar a suspeita de parvovirose canina.

Achados Anamnésicos
Os proprietários relatam em seu animal alterações como perda de vigor, inapetência, vômitos e diarreia profusa, associados à perda rápida e intensa de peso.

Achados do Exame Físico
- Taquicardia.
- As mucosas podem estar pálidas, congestas ou ictéricas.
- Desidratação.
- Dor ou desconforto à palpação abdominal.
- Os intestinos podem estar preenchidos por líquido ou, raramente, pode haver uma intussuscepção palpável.
- Os filhotes podem estar febris ou hipotérmicos.
- Podem ainda exibir vômito/diarreia na sala de exame.

CAUSAS
Infecção pelo CPV-2b.

FATORES DE RISCO
- Predisposição racial, conforme foi exposto anteriormente.
- Possíveis distúrbios imunossupressores concomitantes (p. ex., parasitismo maciço).
- Protocolo incompleto de vacinação, falha da vacinação ou interferência com os anticorpos maternos.

DIAGNÓSTICO

DIAGNÓSTICO DIFERENCIAL
- Ingestão de corpo estranho ou toxina, imprudência alimentar/alimentação inadequada.
- Parasitismo gastrintestinal (ancilóstomos, *Cryptosporidia*).
- Infecção pelo *Clostridium perfringens*.
- Infecção pelo *Campylobacter*.
- Coronavírus.
- Gastrenterite hemorrágica.
- Intussuscepção.

HEMOGRAMA/BIOQUÍMICA/URINÁLISE
- Neutropenia (tipicamente grave) e linfopenia.
- Durante a fase de recuperação, pode-se observar leucocitose.
- Além disso, é possível a constatação de enzimas hepáticas elevadas, hipoglicemia, pan-hipoproteinemia, azotemia, distúrbios eletrolíticos e indícios do envolvimento de múltiplos órgãos no exame bioquímico.

DIAGNÓSTICO POR IMAGEM
- Radiografias abdominais simples para avaliar o trato gastrintestinal em busca de possíveis corpos estranhos ou obstruções intestinais; pode-se observar íleo paralítico generalizado.
- A ultrassonografia abdominal pode revelar enfartamento dos linfonodos mesentéricos (raras vezes), bem como alças intestinais distendidas e preenchidas por líquido.

MÉTODOS DIAGNÓSTICOS
- Identificação, histórico e achados do exame físico fornecem a suspeita clínica.
- ELISA fecal — para pesquisa do antígeno viral; teste mais comumente utilizado; em função do tempo relativamente curto de eliminação viral nas fezes, pode-se notar a ocorrência de resultados falso-negativos; em casos de vacinação recente (5-15 dias após a aplicação da vacina), pode-se constatar a ocorrência de resultados falso-positivos.
- Hemograma completo concomitante — revela leucopenia e neutropenia.
- PCR em tempo real — demonstrou recentemente ser um exame altamente sensível e específico.
- Outros testes empregados com menor frequência — isolamento viral, microscopia eletrônica, cultura tecidual e sorologia por inibição da hemaglutinação.

ACHADOS PATOLÓGICOS
Macroscópicos
- A inspeção das paredes intestinais revela edema e hemorragia.
- Os intestinos podem conter um líquido aquoso e hemorrágico, além de apresentar mucosa esfacelada e necrosada.
- Tipicamente, não se observa linfadenomegalia.
- O timo pode estar atrofiado.
- Em casos de comprometimento do miocárdio, poderá haver estrias pálidas nesse músculo.

Histológicos
- As lesões intestinais microscópicas incluem necrose do epitélio das criptas; vilosidades cegas e encurtadas; e ainda colapso da lâmina própria.
- O tecido linfoide e as placas de Peyer podem estar necrosados.
- Em diversos métodos, podem-se observar os corpúsculos de inclusão viral.

PARVOVIROSE CANINA

- Como lesão cardíaca microscópica, observa-se infiltração linfocítica-plasmocitária em torno dos miócitos.
- Em casos de endotoxemia e choque concomitantes, pode haver lesões em vários órgãos.

TRATAMENTO

CUIDADO(S) DE SAÚDE ADEQUADO(S)
- A internação para os tratamentos de cuidado intensivo e de suporte aumenta significativamente a sobrevida.
- É fundamental manter o isolamento dos casos hospitalizados de outros pacientes.
- A equipe hospitalar deve ser orientada a respeito dos métodos adequados de limpeza e desinfecção para evitar a disseminação do vírus.

CUIDADO(S) DE ENFERMAGEM
- A fluidoterapia intravenosa com cristaloides representa a base do tratamento. As velocidades de administração dos fluidos devem responder às necessidades de manutenção e às perdas contínuas, que podem ser intensas.
- Em pacientes hipoalbuminêmicos, pode ser necessária a terapia com coloides.
- Também se pode lançar mão de transfusões com plasma ou soro hiperimune.

ATIVIDADE
É recomendável restringir a atividade física até que os filhotes se recuperem.

DIETA
- Em casos de vômitos prolongados, recomenda-se a suspensão do alimento e da água.
- Após 24 h sem vômitos, podem ser introduzidas pequenas quantidades de água.
- A nutrição enteral ou microenteral deve ser contemplada em casos de anorexia com 3-4 dias de duração. A nutrição enteral precoce via tubo nasoesofágico também pode melhorar o resultado clínico.
- Nos casos graves, a nutrição parenteral pode ser requerida.
- Foi demonstrado que a suplementação com glutamina restabelece a integridade do enterócito.
- Em princípio, deve-se fornecer uma dieta leve e de fácil digestibilidade (p. ex., Hill's i/d®, Purina EN®), com transição gradativa para a ração normal.

ORIENTAÇÃO AO PROPRIETÁRIO
- O vírus permanece estável no ambiente, mas pode ser destruído por uma solução alvejante (p. ex., hipoclorito de sódio ou água sanitária) na diluição de 1:30.
- A vacina não produz imunidade imediata; assim, é recomendável manter os filhotes caninos suscetíveis em isolamento.

CONSIDERAÇÕES CIRÚRGICAS
- A única indicação cirúrgica consiste no desenvolvimento raro de intussuscepção intestinal em decorrência da hipermotilidade produzida pela diarreia.
- Assim, é obrigatória a palpação abdominal diária e rigorosa.

MEDICAÇÕES

MEDICAMENTO(S) DE ESCOLHA
- Antieméticos — frequentemente necessários por conta dos vômitos prolongados; metoclopramida (0,2-0,4 mg/kg SC a cada 6-8 h ou sob taxa de infusão constante de 1-2 mg/kg/dia IV); antagonistas dos receptores serotoninérgicos (ondansetrona, 0,5-1,0 mg/kg IV a cada 12-24 h); antagonistas dos receptores da neurocinina (maropitanto 1 mg/kg SC a cada 24 h por até 5 dias consecutivos) - aprovados para uso em cães de 16 semanas ou mais.
- Bloqueadores dos receptores H_2 — podem diminuir a náusea; cimetidina (4-10 mg/kg SC, IM, IV a cada 6 h); ranitidina (1-2 mg/kg IV a cada 12 h); famotidina (0,5-1 mg/kg SC, IM, IV a cada 12-24 h).
- Antibióticos (ver a seção "Precauções") — para combater a sepse; devem ter um amplo espectro de ação, inclusive contra os microrganismos Gram-negativos; os protocolos de combinação costumam ser utilizados.
- Anti-helmínticos — podem ser usados para erradicar parasitas concomitantes.
- Analgésicos — podem ser necessários em casos graves.
- Há relatos empíricos que descrevem o uso do soro antiendotoxina de origem equina. No momento, não há estudos controlados que demonstrem benefício quanto à sobrevida do animal submetido a essa terapia.
- Estudos recentes não revelaram nenhum benefício em relação à sobrevida, utilizando o fator estimulante de colônias de granulócitos, o anti-TNF ou a proteína recombinante bactericida e indutora de aumento na permeabilidade ($rBPI_{21}$).

PRECAUÇÕES
- Em função dos riscos de defeitos sobre a cartilagem, não se recomenda o uso das fluoroquinolonas.
- Os aminoglicosídeos devem ser utilizados apenas em filhotes caninos bem hidratados.
- É preciso ter extrema cautela ao utilizar os AINE (inclusive o fluxinino meglumina [Banamine®]) em virtude da toxicidade renal.
- *Nota:* a cimetidina deve ser usada com cuidado em virtude do extenso metabolismo hepático via citocromo P450.

MEDICAMENTO(S) ALTERNATIVO(S)
Os filhotes menos gravemente acometidos podem ser tratados em um esquema ambulatorial com terapia subcutânea e/ou intraperitoneal se o proprietário tiver restrições financeiras.

ACOMPANHAMENTO

MONITORIZAÇÃO DO PACIENTE
Tipicamente, a recuperação é completa. A imunidade é prolongada e pode ser vitalícia.

PREVENÇÃO
- A vacinação mostra-se eficaz em reduzir drasticamente a incidência da doença.
- Para minimizar a interferência dos anticorpos maternos, recomendam-se as vacinas de vírus vivo modificado (de altos títulos).
- A interferência decorrente dos anticorpos maternos é a principal razão de falha vacinal. Alguns filhotes caninos podem ter anticorpos maternos até 18 semanas de vida. • Os protocolos recomendam a vacinação com 6, 9 e 12 semanas de vida.
- As raças de alto risco podem necessitar de um protocolo inicial mais prolongado, estendendo-se até 22 semanas.
- Estudos recentes indicam que a imunidade pode durar mais de 3 anos após um esquema vacinal inicial completo.

COMPLICAÇÕES POSSÍVEIS
- Sepse.
- Endotoxemia.
- Choque.
- Intussuscepção.
- CID.
- Síndrome da angústia respiratória aguda.

EVOLUÇÃO ESPERADA E PROGNÓSTICO
- A mortalidade se deve principalmente à endotoxemia.
- A terapia rigorosa aumenta a sobrevida, mas as taxas de mortalidade ainda podem chegar a 30%.

DIVERSOS

FATORES RELACIONADOS COM A IDADE
Os filhotes caninos mais jovens apresentam a forma mais grave da doença (ver anteriormente).

VER TAMBÉM
- Choque Séptico
- Diarreia Aguda
- Sepse e Bacteremia
- Vômito Agudo

ABREVIATURA(S)
- CID = coagulação intravascular disseminada
- ELISA = ensaio imunoabsorvente ligado à enzima
- TNF = fator de necrose tumoral
- PCR = reação em cadeia da polimerase
- CPV = parvovírus canino
- TLAI = tecido linfoide associado ao intestino

RECURSOS DA INTERNET
http://www.avma.org/animal_health/brochures/canine_parvo/parvo_brochure.asp

Sugestões de Leitura

McCaw D, Hoskins JD. Canine viral enteritis. In: Greene CE, ed., Infectious Diseases of the Dog and Cat, 3rd ed. St. Louis: Saunders Elsevier, 2006, pp. 63-71.

Mohr AJ, Leisewitz AL, Jacobson LS, et al. Effect of early enteral nutrition on intestinal permeability, intestinal protein loss, and outcome in dogs with severe parvoviral enteritis. J Vet Intern Med 2003:791-798.

Rewerts JM, Cohn LA. CVT update: Diagnosis and treatment of parvovirus. In: Bonagura J, ed., Kirk's Current Veterinary Therapy XIII. Philadelphia: Saunders, 2000, pp. 629-632.

Autor Jo Ann Morrison
Consultor Editorial Albert E. Jergens

Peito Escavado

CONSIDERAÇÕES GERAIS

REVISÃO
- Deformidade do esterno e das cartilagens costais que resulta no estreitamento dorsal a ventral do tórax, principalmente na face caudal.
- Podem-se notar anormalidades secundárias da função cardiovascular e respiratória por restrição ventilatória e compressão cardíaca.
- Os casos são considerados de origem congênita.
- Defeito raro.
- Defeitos cardíacos concomitantes são comuns.
- Obstrução respiratória superior em uma idade jovem pode causar gradientes respiratórios anormais e subsequente peito escavado.
- Alguns pacientes demonstram síndrome do nadador — os cães neonatos não conseguem se posicionar adequadamente e permanecem em decúbito esternal, o que pode levar à invaginação do esterno.

IDENTIFICAÇÃO
- Cães e gatos.
- Raças braquicefálicas são predispostas.
- Idade mais comum de apresentação — 4 semanas a 3 meses.
- Os casos são relatados com maior frequência em gatos machos do que nas gatas; no entanto, não se observa qualquer predisposição sexual em cães.

SINAIS CLÍNICOS
- Defeito torácico, facilmente palpado ou observado.
- Graus variados de angústia respiratória.
- Intolerância ao exercício.
- Perda de peso.
- Infecções respiratórias recidivantes.
- Tosse.
- Vômito.
- Cianose.
- Hiporexia.
- Sopros cardíacos associados à presença de defeitos cardíacos concomitantes ou à compressão do coração.
- Sons cardíacos abafados.
- Nenhuma correlação entre a gravidade dos sinais clínicos e a gravidade das anormalidades anatômicas ou fisiológicas.
- Deformidades vertebrais.
- Síndrome do nadador — os membros não fazem adução de forma adequada; deambulação prejudicada.

CAUSAS E FATORES DE RISCO
- Predisposição genética — pode haver esse tipo de predisposição.
- Etiologia desconhecida — as causas sob suspeita incluem anormalidades de pressão intrauterina, encurtamento do tendão central do diafragma, deficiência dos músculos abdominais craniais e osteogênese ou condrogênese anormal.
- Os cães predispostos a processos obstrutivos respiratórios têm maior risco que os outros.
- Os filhotes caninos criados em superfícies que provocam uma deambulação insatisfatória podem estar predispostos à síndrome do nadador.

DIAGNÓSTICO

DIAGNÓSTICO DIFERENCIAL
- Hérnia diafragmática congênita (pleuroperitoneal ou pericardioperitoneal).
- Más-formações ou colapso traqueais.
- Defeitos cardíacos congênitos.
- Edema pulmonar.
- Hemotórax.
- Piotórax.
- Pneumonia.
- Traqueobronquite/bronquite.
- Síndrome braquicefálica das vias aéreas.

DIAGNÓSTICO POR IMAGEM
Radiografias Torácicas
- Confirmam as anormalidades esqueléticas do esterno e das costelas.
- Volume torácico diminuído.
- Malposicionamento cardíaco — deslocamento cranial e à esquerda da silhueta cardíaca.
- Doença pulmonar secundária concomitante.
- Mensurar os índices frontossagitais e vertebrais para caracterizar o grau de deformidade como leve, moderado ou grave e para ajudar a predizer a resposta ao tratamento.

Ecocardiografia
- Para descartar defeitos congênitos concomitantes ou outra cardiopatia.

TRATAMENTO

- Decisão para reparar deformidades — tomada com base nos sinais clínicos. Em caso de achado incidental com sinais clínicos mínimos a ausentes, a intervenção talvez não seja indicada.
- As opções terapêuticas incluem coaptação esternal ou esternectomia parcial. A decisão é tomada com base na idade do animal e no grau de deformidade.
- A cirurgia beneficia os pacientes com angústia respiratória concomitante; benefícios desconhecidos em pacientes sem angústia respiratória, mas com deformidade moderada ou grave.
- Os pacientes assintomáticos podem desenvolver sinais mais tarde; já os pacientes com sinais clínicos da doença podem apresentar evolução.
- Filhotes caninos com a síndrome do nadador — colocar em superfícies com piso excelente; a colocação de talas nos membros anteriores e posteriores pode melhorar a adução.
- Raças braquicefálicas com obstrução aérea superior concomitante podem se beneficiar da cirurgia direcionada a esses problemas.
- Anestesia — os pacientes necessitam de monitorização constante; suporte ventilatório deve estar disponível.

MEDICAÇÕES

MEDICAMENTO(S)
Tratar as condições clínicas subjacentes ou secundárias.

CONTRAINDICAÇÕES/INTERAÇÕES POSSÍVEIS
Nenhuma.

ACOMPANHAMENTO

- Exames — ditados pelos sinais clínicos ou quando se exclui a intervenção cirúrgica.
- Não existe qualquer ação específica para evitar a doença; às vezes, pode existir o envolvimento de fatores genéticos.
- Evolução dos sinais respiratórios — pode se desenvolver nos pacientes assintomáticos ou levemente sintomáticos.
- Prognóstico — reservado a bom, dependendo da intervenção realizada em momento oportuno e por especialistas.

DIVERSOS

DISTÚRBIOS ASSOCIADOS
- Defeitos cardíacos.
- Síndrome do nadador.

Sugestões de Leitura
Boudrieau RJ, Fossum TW, Hartsfield SM, et al. Pectus excavatum in dogs and cats. Compend Contin Educ Pract Vet 1990, 12:341-355.
Sweet DC, Water DJ. Role of surgery in the management of dogs with pathologic conditions of the thorax — part II. Compend Contin Educ Pract Vet 1991, 13:1671-1677.

Autor Catriona MacPhail
Consultor Editorial Lynelle R. Johnson

PÊNFIGO

CONSIDERAÇÕES GERAIS

REVISÃO
- Grupo de dermatoses autoimunes, caracterizado por graus variáveis de ulceração e formação de crostas, além de pústulas e vesículas.
- Acomete a pele e algumas vezes as mucosas.
- Formas identificadas nos animais: pênfigo foliáceo, pênfigo eritematoso, pênfigo vulgar, pênfigo pustular pan-epidérmico (vegetante), pênfigo crônico familiar benigno canino (doença de Hailey-Hailey), pênfigo paraneoplásico.

FISIOPATOLOGIA
- Autoanticorpo ligado ao tecido direcionado contra os antígenos das células intraepidérmicas (desmogleínas) e os receptores da acetilcolina é depositado dentro dos espaços intercelulares, provocando separação celular epidérmica e arredondamento celular (acantólise).
- Gravidade da ulceração e da doença — relacionada com a profundidade de depósito do autoanticorpo no interior da pele.
- Tipos — foliáceo, vulgar, eritematoso e pustular pan-epidérmico (vegetante).
- Foliáceo — depósito de autoanticorpo nas camadas superficiais da epiderme.
- Vulgar — lesões mais graves; mediado pelo depósito do autoanticorpo imediatamente acima da zona da membrana basal; resulta na formação de úlcera mais profunda.
- Os fatores implicados na deflagração do pênfigo são fatores genéticos, hormonais, neoplásicos, farmacológicos, nutricionais, virais, emocionais (estresse) e físicos (queimaduras, radiação UV).

SISTEMA(S) ACOMETIDO(S)
Cutâneo/exócrino.

GENÉTICA
Pênfigo crônico familiar benigno (doença de Hailey-Hailey) — pode ter uma predisposição genética (genodermatose autossômica dominante em seres humanos).

INCIDÊNCIA/PREVALÊNCIA
- Grupo raro de doenças.
- Foliáceo — tipo mais comum.
- Eritematoso — relativamente comum; pode ser uma variante mais benigna do pênfigo foliáceo ou uma síndrome mista de pênfigo e lúpus eritematoso.
- Vulgar — segundo tipo mais comum; a forma mais grave.
- Pustular pan-epidérmico (vegetante) — tipo mais raro; a evolução da doença pode ser mais grave do que o foliáceo.
- Paraneoplásico — raro; os sinais clínicos variam desde lesões crostosas graves até relativamente benignas.

IDENTIFICAÇÃO
Espécies
- Foliáceo, vulgar e eritematoso — cães e gatos.
- Pustular pan-epidérmico (vegetante) — apenas cães.

Raça(s) Predominante(s)
- Foliáceo — Akita, Bearded collie, Chow chow, Dachshund, Doberman pinscher, Spitz finlandês, Terra Nova e Schipperke.
- Eritematoso — Collie, Pastor alemão e Pastor de Shetland.

Idade Média e Faixa Etária
Em geral, animais de meia-idade a idosos.

Sexo Predominante
Nenhum relatado.

SINAIS CLÍNICOS
Foliáceo
- Escamas, crostas, pústulas, colaretes epidérmicos, erosões, eritema, alopecia e hiperqueratose com formação de fissuras nos coxins palmoplantares.
- Vesículas ocasionais são transitórias.
- Envolvimento comum — cabeça, orelhas e coxins palmoplantares; quase sempre se torna generalizado.
- Não é comum a presença de lesões nas mucosas e junções mucocutâneas.
- Gatos — é comum o envolvimento dos mamilos e dos leitos ungueais.
- Às vezes, observam-se linfadenopatia, edema, depressão, febre e claudicação (se os coxins palmoplantares estiverem envolvidos); todavia, os pacientes frequentemente se encontram em bom estado de saúde.
- Dor e prurido variáveis.
- Possível infecção bacteriana secundária.

Eritematoso
- Semelhantes aos do pênfigo foliáceo.
- Lesões geralmente confinadas à cabeça, à face e aos coxins palmoplantares.
- Despigmentação mucocutânea é mais comum do que com outras formas, podendo preceder a formação de crostas.

Vulgar
- Ulceração bucal é frequente, podendo preceder as lesões cutâneas.
- Lesões ulcerativas, erosões, colaretes epidérmicos, bolhas e crostas.
- Mais grave do que os pênfigos foliáceo e eritematoso.
- Acomete as mucosas, as junções mucocutâneas e a pele; pode se tornar generalizado.
- Regiões axilares e inguinais são frequentemente envolvidas.
- Sinal de Nikolski positivo (lesão erosiva nova ou estendida criada quando se aplica uma pressão lateral à pele próxima a uma lesão existente).
- Prurido e dor variáveis.
- Anorexia, depressão e febre.
- É comum a ocorrência de infecções bacterianas secundárias.

Pustular Pan-epidérmico (Vegetante)
- Grupos de pústulas se tornam lesões papilomatosas eruptivas e massas vegetativas que exsudam.
- Não foi observado envolvimento bucal.
- Nenhuma doença sistêmica.

CAUSAS
Indeterminadas — genética e possível evento deflagrador (p. ex., infecção viral, medicamento).

FATORES DE RISCO
Indeterminados.

DIAGNÓSTICO

DIAGNÓSTICO DIFERENCIAL
Foliáceo
- Foliculite bacteriana.
- Dermatofitose.
- Demodicose.
- Candidíase.
- Distúrbios de queratinização.
- Lúpus eritematoso.
- Pênfigo eritematoso.
- Dermatose pustular subcórnea.
- Erupção medicamentosa.
- Dermatite responsiva ao zinco.
- Dermatomiosite.
- Tirosinemia.
- Micose fungoide.
- Malignidades linforreticulares.
- Necrose epidérmica metabólica.
- Pustulose eosinofílica estéril.
- Dermatose linear por IgA.

Eritematoso
- Pênfigo foliáceo.
- Lúpus eritematoso sistêmico.
- Lúpus eritematoso discoide.
- Piodermite nasal.
- Demodicose.
- Dermatofitose.
- Epidermólise bolhosa simples.
- Síndrome uveodermatológica.

Vulgar
- Penfigoide bolhoso.
- Lúpus eritematoso sistêmico.
- Necrólise epidérmica tóxica.
- Erupção medicamentosa.
- Micose fungoide.
- Neoplasia linforreticular.
- Causas de estomatite ulcerativa.
- Eritema multiforme.

Pustular Pan-epidérmico (Vegetante)
- Pênfigo vulgar.
- Foliculite bacteriana.
- Pênfigo foliáceo.
- Dermatoses liquenoides.
- Neoplasia cutânea.

HEMOGRAMA/BIOQUÍMICA/URINÁLISE
- As anormalidades são incomuns.
- Às vezes, observam-se leucocitose e hiperglobulinemia.

OUTROS TESTES LABORATORIAIS
Anticorpo antinuclear — pode ser fracamente positivo apenas no pênfigo eritematoso.

MÉTODOS DIAGNÓSTICOS
- Citologia de aspirados ou esfregaços por impressão (decalque) de pústulas ou crostas — células acantolíticas e neutrófilos; ocasionalmente com eosinófilos.
- Cultura bacteriológica — identificar infecções bacterianas secundárias.

ACHADOS PATOLÓGICOS
- Biopsias de lesão da pele ou em torno dela — acantólise e fenda intraepidérmica; formação de microabscessos ou pústulas; queratinócitos acantolíticos de superfície.
- Localização das lesões epidérmicas — varia com a doença; pênfigos foliáceo e eritematoso apresentam fenda subcórnea ou intragranular e acantólise; pênfigos vulgar e pustular pan-epidérmico (vegetante) exibem fenda suprabasilar.
- Imunopatologia da biopsia de pele via testes de anticorpo imunofluorescente ou teste imuno-histoquímico — podem demonstrar coloração positiva nos espaços intercelulares em 50-90% dos casos; os resultados podem ser influenciados pela administração concomitante ou prévia de corticosteroides (ou outro medicamento imunossupressor); imunofluorescência indireta,

PÊNFIGO

em geral, é negativa; o pênfigo eritematoso pode exibir a coloração das membranas basais e dos espaços intercelulares.

TRATAMENTO

CUIDADO(S) DE SAÚDE ADEQUADO(S)
• Terapia de suporte inicial com internação para os pacientes gravemente acometidos.
• Tratamento ambulatorial com visitas iniciais frequentes ao hospital (a cada 1-3 semanas); reduzir para a cada 1-3 meses quando se alcança a remissão e o paciente se encontra sob esquema terapêutico clínico de manutenção.

CUIDADO(S) DE ENFERMAGEM
Os pacientes gravemente acometidos podem necessitar de antibióticos e hidroterapia/embebições.

DIETA
Pobre em gordura — para evitar a pancreatite precipitada pelos corticosteroides e (possivelmente) pelo tratamento com azatioprina.

ORIENTAÇÃO AO PROPRIETÁRIO
Advertir o proprietário sobre a necessidade de o animal evitar a exposição ao sol, já que a luz ultravioleta pode exacerbar as lesões.

MEDICAÇÕES

MEDICAMENTO(S)

Pênfigo Foliáceo e Vulgar

Corticosteroides
• Prednisona ou prednisolona — 1,1-2,2 mg/kg/dia VO divididos a cada 12 h para iniciar o controle.
• Dose mínima de manutenção — 0,5 mg/kg VO a cada 48 h.
• Reduzir a dosagem gradativamente em intervalos de 2-4 semanas para 5-10 mg/semana.

Agentes Citotóxicos
• Mais da metade dos pacientes necessita da adição de outros medicamentos imunomoduladores.
• Em geral, esses agentes atuam de forma sinérgica com a prednisona, permitindo a redução da dose e dos efeitos colaterais dos corticosteroides.
• Azatioprina — 2,2 mg/kg VO a cada 24 h e, em seguida, a cada 48 h (cães); raramente utilizada em gatos em virtude do potencial de supressão acentuada da medula óssea; dose de 1 mg/kg a cada 24-48 h (gatos).
• Clorambucila — 0,2 mg/kg diariamente; melhor escolha para os gatos.
• Ciclofosfamida — 50 mg/m² VO calculada de acordo com a área de superfície corporal a cada 48 h (cães).
• Ciclosporina — 15-27 mg/kg diariamente VO; aplicação limitada.
• Dapsona — 1 mg/kg VO a cada 8 h; em seguida, conforme a necessidade (cães); aplicação limitada.

Crisoterapia
• Frequentemente utilizada em conjunto com a prednisona.
• Auranofina — 0,1-0,2 mg/kg VO a cada 12-24 h.

Pênfigo Eritematoso e Pustular Pan-epidérmico (Vegetante)
• Prednisona ou prednisolona oral — 1,1 mg/kg VO a cada 24 h; em seguida, a cada 48 h; depois, passar para a menor dose possível de manutenção; pode ser interrompida quando o quadro estiver em remissão.
• Esteroides tópicos podem ser suficientes nos casos leves.

PRECAUÇÕES
• Corticosteroides — poliúria, polidipsia, polifagia, mudanças de temperamento, diabetes melito, pancreatite e hepatotoxicidade.
• Azatioprina — pancreatite.
• Medicamentos citotóxicos — leucopenia, trombocitopenia, nefrotoxicidade e hepatotoxicidade.
• Crisoterapia — leucopenia, trombocitopenia, nefrotoxicidade, dermatite, estomatite e reações alérgicas.
• Ciclofosfamida — cistite hemorrágica.
• Imunossupressão — pode predispor o animal a infecções por *Demodex*, bem como a infecções cutâneas e sistêmicas por fungos e bactérias.

MEDICAMENTO(S) ALTERNATIVO(S)

Corticosteroides Alternativos
• Utilizar no lugar da prednisona se ocorrerem efeitos colaterais indesejáveis ou resposta insatisfatória ao tratamento.
• Metilprednisolona — 0,8-1,5 mg/kg VO a cada 12 h; para os pacientes pouco tolerantes à prednisona.
• Triancinolona — 0,2-0,3 mg/kg VO a cada 12 h; em seguida, 0,05-0,1 mg/kg a cada 48-72 h.
• Pulsoterapia com glicocorticoide — 11 mg/kg IV de succinato sódico de metilprednisolona por 3 dias consecutivos para induzir à remissão; aplicação limitada.

Esteroides Tópicos
• Creme de hidrocortisona.
• Corticosteroides tópicos mais potentes — valerato de betametasona a 0,1%, acetonida de fluocinolona, ou triancinonida a 0,1%; a cada 12 h; em seguida, a cada 24-48 h.

Diversos
Tetraciclina e niacinamida — 500 mg VO a cada 8 h (cães >10 kg); metade da dose para cães <10 kg; aplicação limitada (especialmente em caso de pênfigo eritematoso).

ACOMPANHAMENTO

MONITORIZAÇÃO DO PACIENTE
• Monitorar a resposta ao tratamento.
• Monitorar os efeitos colaterais da medicação — hematologia e bioquímica sérica de rotina, sobretudo nos pacientes sob altas doses de corticosteroides, medicamentos citotóxicos ou crisoterapia; reavaliar a cada 1-3 semanas e, em seguida, a cada 1-3 meses quando o quadro estiver em remissão.

EVOLUÇÃO ESPERADA E PROGNÓSTICO

Pênfigos Vulgar e Foliáceo
• Há necessidade de terapia com corticosteroides e medicamentos citotóxicos.
• Os pacientes podem necessitar de medicação pelo resto da vida.
• É necessária a monitorização do paciente.
• Os efeitos colaterais das medicações podem alterar a qualidade de vida.
• Podem ser fatais se não forem tratados (especialmente o pênfigo vulgar).
• Infecções secundárias provocam morbidade e possível mortalidade (sobretudo o pênfigo vulgar).

Pênfigos Eritematoso e Pustular Pan-epidérmico (Vegetante)
• Relativamente benignos e autolimitantes.
• Por fim, os corticosteroides orais podem ser reduzidos para baixas doses de manutenção; podem ser interrompidos em alguns pacientes.
• Se não forem tratados, ocorrerá o desenvolvimento de dermatose; sintomas sistêmicos são raros.
• Prognóstico razoável.

DIVERSOS

GESTAÇÃO/FERTILIDADE/REPRODUÇÃO
Evitar o uso de esteroides e medicamentos citotóxicos durante a prenhez.

Sugestões de Leitura
Ackerman LJ. Immune-mediated skin diseases. In: Morgan RV, ed., Handbook of Small Animal Practice, 3rd ed. Philadelphia: Saunders, 1997, pp. 941-943.
Angarano DW. Autoimmune dermatosis. In: Nesbitt GH, ed., Contemporary Issues in Small Animal Practice: Dermatology. New York: Churchill Livingstone, 1987, pp. 79-94.
Rosenkrantz WS. Pemphigus foliaceous. In: Griffin CE, Knochka KW, MacDonald JM, et al., eds., Current Veterinary Dermatology. St. Louis: Mosby, 1993, pp. 141-148.

Autor Karen Helton Rhodes
Consultor Editorial Alexander H. Werner

PERDA DE PESO E CAQUEXIA

CONSIDERAÇÕES GERAIS

DEFINIÇÃO
• *Perda de peso* refere-se à perda não intencional de peso corporal. Em relação ao peso corporal estável anterior, a perda aguda de 10% ou a perda crônica de 15% é considerada clinicamente importante.
• *Caquexia* equivale a um estado de perda de peso intensa e emaciação tecidual grave secundárias a alguma doença subjacente, como câncer, insuficiência cardíaca ou condições inflamatórias graves. Além da perda de gordura, os pacientes caquéticos perdem uma quantidade significativa de massa corporal magra, especialmente da musculatura esquelética.
• *Sarcopenia* corresponde a uma perda desproporcional de músculo esquelético e massa corporal magra. A sarcopenia pode ocorrer sem a perda de peso corporal.
• A perda de massa corporal magra, como ocorre em casos de caquexia e sarcopenia, contribui para a debilidade do paciente, incluindo fraqueza, fadiga e falta de ar.
• Em cães e gatos, a perda de massa corporal magra é um fator de risco significativo de mortalidade.
• A perda de peso ou a condição corporal baixa-normal é associada a uma sobrevida mais curta em pacientes com problemas cardíacos ou câncer.

FISIOPATOLOGIA
Perda de Peso
• A perda de peso pode ocorrer em função de um consumo alimentar reduzido ou um gasto energético aumentado, incluindo desgaste metabólico, resultando em balanço energético negativo.
• A ingestão alimentar diminuída ou insuficiente pode ser causada por hiporexia (apetite deficiente) secundária à doença sistêmica, doença bucal ou anosmia*; ou por acesso inadequado a nutrientes, que poderá ocorrer se o acesso ao alimento for restrito.
• A diminuição na absorção de nutrientes pode ser causada por disfagia, vômito ou regurgitação, bem como pelas síndromes de má digestão e má absorção.
• A ingestão ou absorção calórica reduzida em animais normalmente saudáveis leva a alterações compensatórias no metabolismo, como declínio no metabolismo energético e desvio para utilização de energia a partir dos lipídeos.

Caquexia
• A caquexia, com perda de gordura e massa corporal magra, ocorre secundariamente a doenças inflamatórias agudas ou crônicas, como câncer, cardiopatia, insuficiência renal, diabetes, sepse, febre crônica, etc.
• As características que diferenciam a caquexia de uma simples perda de peso incluem ativação de citocinas inflamatórias, ativação do sistema ubiquitina-proteassoma e desregulação metabólica, resultando em incremento do metabolismo energético.
• A caquexia é associada a elevações na IL-6, TNF-α e outras citocinas pró-inflamatórias; norepinefrina, epinefrina e cortisol; aumento do estresse oxidativo; e redução dos fatores anabólicos, como IGF-1 e DHEA.
• As alterações inflamatórias resultam em desregulação do apetite, resistência à insulina e degradação acentuada de proteína muscular. As citocinas inflamatórias ativam o sistema ubiquitina-proteassoma e prejudicam a síntese tecidual.
• A taxa metabólica basal elevada e as ineficiências metabólicas contribuem para a emaciação tecidual. A ocorrência de anorexia secundária ou a suspensão do alimento agrava a desnutrição proteicocalórica.
• O fornecimento de nutrição a pacientes caquéticos sem o tratamento da doença subjacente ou da desregulação metabólica raramente é bem-sucedido para corrigir a perda de tecidos corporais.

SISTEMA(S) ACOMETIDO(S)
• Todos os sistemas corporais podem ser acometidos por perda de peso, dependendo da doença subjacente e da gravidade da doença.
• A caquexia pode resultar em fraqueza muscular, fadiga e comprometimento respiratório.

IDENTIFICAÇÃO
Cães e gatos, embora seja particularmente proeminente nos animais em processo de envelhecimento.

SINAIS CLÍNICOS
Achados Anamnésicos
• Os sinais clínicos em pacientes com perda de peso incluem apetite normal, aumentado, diminuído ou ausente, febre ou outros sinais de doença sistêmica.
• A obtenção de histórico alimentar abrangente é importante para determinar a ingestão de nutrientes, o tipo de dieta e qualquer modificação da dieta, bem como a quantidade oferecida e consumida.
• As informações anamnésicas sobre a atividade diária do paciente, o ambiente, a presença de prenhez, o apetite ou os sinais de gastrenteropatia (p. ex., vômito, diarreia, consistência e coloração das fezes, disfagia e regurgitação) podem ajudar a avaliar o nível de gasto calórico ou indicar a existência de má absorção.
• Outros achados anamnésicos podem ser indicativos de doenças subjacentes, como poliúria, polidipsia, mudanças de atitude, claudicação ou intolerância ao exercício.

Achados do Exame Físico
• O exame físico deve obrigatoriamente incluir a medição do peso corporal, o escore da condição corporal e avaliação da emaciação muscular.
• Em animais obesos, pode ocorrer a perda de massa corporal magra apesar da gordura corporal em excesso; assim, esses índices devem ser avaliados separadamente.
• O peso corporal deve ser comparado diante dos dados anamnésicos para determinar a alteração do peso em porcentagem.
• O escore da condição corporal é uma avaliação semiquantitativa da composição do corpo, geralmente com base em um sistema padronizado de 5 ou 9 pontos. Esse escore da condição corporal correlaciona-se bem com a gordura do corpo.
• A emaciação muscular é avaliada por meio da palpação do corpo sobre estruturas como escápulas, crânio e asas do ílio, bem como dos músculos glúteo e vasto. Isso costuma ser avaliado de forma subjetiva em uma escala de 4 pontos.

• A avaliação adicional deve visar à detecção de qualquer anormalidade que possa estar associada a alguma doença subjacente (ver a seção "Causas").

CAUSAS
Causas Nutricionais
• Quantidade insuficiente ou qualidade insatisfatória do alimento.
• Dieta com baixo teor de calorias ou proteínas.
• Competição em lar com muitos animais de estimação.

Anorexia/Pseudoanorexia
• Incapacidade de cheirar, apreender ou mastigar os alimentos.
• Disfagia.
• Náusea.
• Regurgitação.
• Vômito.

Distúrbios de Má Absorção e Má Digestão
• Enteropatia infiltrativa e inflamatória.
• Linfangiectasia.
• Parasitismo intestinal grave.
• Declínios na função digestiva relacionados com a idade.
• Insuficiência pancreática exócrina.

Distúrbios Metabólicos
• Falência de órgãos — insuficiência cardíaca, hepática e renal.
• Hipoadrenocorticismo.
• Hipertireoidismo (especialmente gatos).
• Câncer.
• Catabolismo elevado — febre, infecção, inflamação, câncer.

Perda Excessiva de Nutrientes
• Enteropatia com perda de proteína.
• Nefropatia com perda de proteína.
• Diabetes melito.
• Lesões cutâneas extensas (p. ex., queimaduras).

Doença Neuromuscular
• Comprometimento do neurônio motor inferior.
• Doença neurológica (SNC) — associada geralmente à anorexia ou pseudoanorexia.

Uso Fisiológico Excessivo de Calorias
• Aumento da atividade física.
• Ambiente com frio extremo ou prolongado.
• Prenhez ou lactação.

FATORES DE RISCO
• Idade.
• Ver a seção "Causas".

DIAGNÓSTICO

• O diagnóstico é feito pela avaliação do escore da condição corporal e da emaciação muscular. Pode ocorrer a perda de massa corporal magra sem alteração significativa do peso (sarcopenia).
• O peso corporal deve ser comparado ao peso histórico se disponível após o ajuste de sub e super-hidratação.
• Uma vez confirmada a perda de peso ou de massa corporal magra, procurar pela causa subjacente.

DIAGNÓSTICO DIFERENCIAL
• Ver a seção "Causas".
• Determinar se a perda de peso está associada à ingestão de calorias ou absorção de nutrientes aumentada, normal ou diminuída.
• Estabelecer qual era o apetite do paciente no início da perda de peso, pois qualquer condição

---
* N. T.: Perda ou diminuição sensível do olfato.

PERDA DE PESO E CAQUEXIA

pode levar à anorexia se ela persistir por período de tempo suficientemente longo a ponto de debilitar o paciente.
• A febre sugere uma possível causa infecciosa ou inflamatória subjacente.
• A ausência de febre é mais compatível com causas metabólicas de perda de peso, como insuficiência cardíaca, renal ou hepática.

HEMOGRAMA/BIOQUÍMICA/URINÁLISE
• Os testes laboratoriais podem ser indicativos de doença subjacente.
• Nenhum teste laboratorial mede a desnutrição proteicocalórica com segurança, embora possam se observar os seguintes valores:
• Hematócrito baixo, fosfatase alcalina elevada e/ou ureia baixa com creatinina sérica normal a aumentada.

OUTROS TESTES LABORATORIAIS
• Determinados pela lista de diagnósticos diferenciais mais prováveis do clínico, com base nos achados da anamnese e do exame físico, bem como pelo banco de dados inicial.
• Efetuar os testes sorológicos em busca de FeLV e FIV em gatos com perda de peso de causa desconhecida.
• Mensurar a concentração sérica de T_4 em qualquer gato com >5 anos de idade acometido por perda de peso de causa desconhecida.
• Examinar os exames de flutuação fecal e esfregaço direto seriados para excluir parasitismo intestinal.
• Em áreas endêmicas, ou em animais com histórico de viagem, descartar parasitas urinários, bem como doenças protozoárias e fúngicas.
• Testes específicos da função de órgãos, conforme indicados pelos achados da anamnese e do exame físico, bem como pelo banco de dados inicial. Os exemplos incluem imunorreatividade sérica semelhante à da tripsina em busca de insuficiência pancreática exócrina; teste de estimulação com o ACTH para pesquisa de hipoadrenocorticismo; ácidos biliares séricos pré e pós-prandiais quanto à presença de doença hepatobiliar e relação da proteína:creatinina urinárias na suspeita de nefropatias com perda proteica.

DIAGNÓSTICO POR IMAGEM
Radiografias da região toracoabdominal ou de outras partes do corpo, bem como ultrassonografia ou ecocardiografia, podem ser indicadas, dependendo de outros achados clínicos e das causas subjacentes sob suspeita.

MÉTODOS DIAGNÓSTICOS
• Variam, dependendo dos achados diagnósticos iniciais e da causa subjacente sob suspeita da perda de peso. Ver capítulo(s) em busca das doenças específicas.
• Se houver indicações de laparotomia exploratória, considerar a colocação de sonda de alimentação nesse momento.

TRATAMENTO
• O princípio terapêutico mais importante consiste no tratamento da causa subjacente da perda de peso e no fornecimento de suporte nutricional adequado.
• É comum a ingestão proteicocalórica inadequada entre os pacientes internados.

• As necessidades calóricas devem ser calculadas como necessidades energéticas em repouso (70 kcal × $kg^{0,75}$). Quando a alimentação for iniciada, começar com o fornecimento de 50% das necessidades energéticas em repouso no dia 1 e aumentar gradativamente em 2-3 dias até suprir essas necessidades. Monitorizar o peso do corpo e a resposta do paciente, mas aumentar de forma gradual conforme a tolerância. Embora os animais não necessitem aumentar seu peso corporal, a alimentação excessiva muito rápida pode resultar em problemas metabólicos associados à síndrome de realimentação.
• A menos que contraindicado, o consumo de proteína deve ser aumentado acima dos níveis de manutenção para estimular a retenção ou o restabelecimento da massa corporal magra.

ORAL
• *Se o paciente se encontrar fisicamente capaz de ingerir, digerir e absorver os nutrientes, esta será a via preferida.*
• Para aumentar o consumo voluntário, oferecer um alimento palatável várias vezes ao dia, além de fornecer o alimento habitual do paciente, um tipo de ração úmida (a menos que o animal prefira a seca) e o alimento aquecido à temperatura corporal.
• A menos que haja contraindicações, considerar o uso de dietas formuladas com altos teores de proteínas, calorias e gorduras. Os exemplos incluem dietas terapêuticas de "cuidados críticos", bem como dietas de desempenho e crescimento.
• Os ácidos graxos ômega-3 de cadeia longa, EPA e DHA, podem reduzir os mediadores inflamatórios. Considerar as dietas enriquecidas com EPA e DHA para pacientes caquéticos ou aqueles com condições inflamatórias. Os exemplos compreendem dietas terapêuticas para artrite, problemas dermatológicos e distúrbios neoplásicos. Alternativamente, suplementar com cápsulas de óleo de peixe ricas em EPA na dose de 1 g de óleo de peixe/4,5 kg de peso corporal.
• Se os pacientes que estiverem abaixo do peso ideal se recusarem a se alimentar com as dietas terapêuticas (p. ex., dieta renal e/ou cardíaca), tentar uma marca alternativa, adicionar algum caldo ou outro flavorizante ou considerar o uso de dieta caseira. A ingestão adequada de alguma dieta de manutenção é preferível ao consumo inadequado de alguma dieta terapêutica.
• Pode-se tentar o uso de estimulantes de apetite a curto prazo (ver a seção "Medicamentos").
• A alimentação forçada raramente é eficaz, não sendo aconselhável.

ENTERAL
• *Se o paciente for incapaz ou estiver pouco disposto a ingerir o alimento, mas ainda se mostrar apto a digerir e absorver os nutrientes, esta será a via preferida.*
• É preferível a alimentação enteral o mais proximal possível no trato GI, conforme a tolerância do paciente.
• Podem ser utilizadas sondas nasesofágicas ou nasogástricas (3,5-8 French) até que os pacientes possam ser submetidos à anestesia para colocação de uma sonda mais calibrosa. Em virtude do pequeno calibre da sonda, pode-se lançar mão apenas de dietas líquidas.
• Sondas esofágicas (12-14 French para gatos, 18-22 French para cães) ou gástricas (18-22 French) podem ser inseridas com relativa rapidez, utilizando uma série de técnicas.

• É mais difícil inserir e manejar as sondas de jejunostomia ou gastrojejunostomia (5-8 French), pois elas necessitam de dietas líquidas via infusão crônica. Essas sondas podem ser adequadas para pacientes com vômito intratável.

PARENTERAL
• *Se o paciente for intolerante às alimentações enterais, esta será a via preferida.*
• A nutrição parenteral total requer um acesso venoso central reservado para isso, o que precisa ser colocado e mantido de forma asséptica para reduzir as complicações.
• As complicações do metabolismo e as síndromes de realimentação são muito comuns em pacientes catabólicos e caquéticos.
• A proteína contida em misturas parenterais deve fornecer 15-25% e 25-35% de calorias para cães e gatos, respectivamente. As calorias restantes podem ser fornecidas por meio da administração de glicose ou por uma combinação de glicose e lipídios, com até 70% das calorias não proteicas derivadas de lipídios. As vitaminas e os eletrólitos podem ser fornecidos separadamente.
• Os pacientes devem ser alimentados com cerca de 50% das necessidades energéticas em repouso no primeiro dia, aumentando-se gradativamente em 2 dias até suprir essas necessidades. É imprescindível a monitorização rigorosa dos pacientes quanto à ocorrência de complicações.

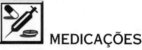

MEDICAÇÕES

MEDICAMENTO(S) DE ESCOLHA
• Dependem da causa subjacente da perda de peso; ver tópicos específicos para cada condição.
• Os estimulantes de apetite podem ser úteis, além das medicações direcionadas à condição subjacente:
• Benzodiazepínicos: diazepam (0,1-0,2 mg/kg VO a cada 12-24 h em cães; 0,05-0,10 mg/kg IV a cada 24 h para cão/gato); oxazepam (1,25-2,5 g/gato VO a cada 12-24 h; 0,3-0,4 g/kg VO a cada 12-24 h para cães); midazolam (2-5 μg/kg IV para gatos); flurazepam (0,1-0,2 mg/kg VO a cada 12-24 h para gatos).
• Propofol (1-2 mg/kg IV para cães).
• Agentes anabólicos: estanozolol (1-2 mg VO a cada 12-24 h); boldenona (5 mg SC ou IV).

CONTRAINDICAÇÕES
Ver a bula dos medicamentos em busca das peculiaridades de cada um.

PRECAUÇÕES
• Os estimulantes de apetite devem ser utilizados apenas por um período de tempo limitado (dias).
• Monitorizar o consumo alimentar para garantir uma ingestão adequada.

INTERAÇÕES POSSÍVEIS
Muitos medicamentos usados para as causas subjacentes podem causar anorexia e/ou náusea.

MEDICAMENTO(S) ALTERNATIVO(S)
• Acetato de megestrol para inibir os mediadores inflamatórios, bem como para promover o apetite e o ganho de peso.
• Clembuterol para aumentar a massa muscular.
• Ácidos graxos ômega-3 de cadeia longa para reduzir a inflamação.

Perda de Peso e Caquexia

ACOMPANHAMENTO

MONITORIZAÇÃO DO PACIENTE
• Ver as condições específicas para acompanhamento em relação à causa subjacente.
• Monitorizar o peso do corpo e o escore da condição corporal com rigor.
• O apetite e a ingestão alimentar devem ser monitorizados de perto para garantir que as necessidades nutricionais sejam supridas.

COMPLICAÇÕES POSSÍVEIS
• Ver as causas subjacentes específicas.
• Com o uso de alimentação assistida por sonda, podem ocorrer as seguintes complicações: intolerância GI com vômito e/ou diarreia; deslocamento da sonda ou regurgitação com consequente aspiração; peritonite; distúrbios metabólicos, incluindo hiperglicemia, hipofosfatemia, hipocalemia ou hipomagnesemia.
• Em caso de alimentação parenteral, pode-se observar a ocorrência de sepse; trombose; tromboflebite; distúrbios metabólicos, incluindo hiperglicemia, hiperlipidemia, azotemia, hiperamonemia, hipofosfatemia, hipocalemia ou hipomagnesemia.

DIVERSOS

DISTÚRBIOS ASSOCIADOS
Ver a seção "Causas".

FATORES RELACIONADOS COM A IDADE
A perda de massa corporal magra é mais comum em pacientes geriátricos.

POTENCIAL ZOONÓTICO
N/D.

GESTAÇÃO/FERTILIDADE/REPRODUÇÃO
A lactação pode estar associada à perda de peso em virtude do aumento no gasto calórico.

ABREVIATURA(S)
• ACTH = hormônio adrenocorticotrópico.
• DHEA = deidroepiandrosterona.
• DHA = ácido docosaexaenoico.
• EPA = ácido eicosapentaenoico.
• FeLV = vírus da leucemia felina.
• FIV = vírus da imunodeficiência felina.
• GI = gastrintestinal.
• IGF-1 = fator de crescimento insulinossímile I.
• IL-6 = interleucina-6.
• SNC = sistema nervoso central.
• TNF = fator de necrose tumoral.

RECURSOS DA INTERNET
Para encontrar um veterinário especialista em nutrição e qualificado a auxiliar na formulação de dietas de terapia ou manutenção caseiras, acesse: www.acvn.org.

Sugestões de Leitura
Chan DL, Freeman LM. Nutrition in critical illness. Vet Clin North Am Small Anim Pract 2006, 36:1225-1241.
Delaney SJ. Management of anorexia in dogs and cats. Vet Clin North Am Small Anim Pract 2006, 36:1243-1249.
Schermerhorn T. Cachexia. In: Ettinger SJ, Feldman EC, eds., Textbook of Veterinary Internal Medicine, 6th ed. St. Louis: Elsevier, 2005, pp. 78-80.
Von Wethern CJ, Wess G. A new technique for insertion of esophagostomy tubes in cats. JAAHA 2001, 37:140-144.

Autor Dorothy P. Laflamme
Consultor Editorial Albert E. Jergens
Agradecimento O autor e os editores agradecem as colaborações prévias de John Crandell, Daniel Harrington, Nathaniel C. Myers III, e Elizabeth Streeter, que foram os autores desse tópico em edições anteriores.

Perfuração da Traqueia

CONSIDERAÇÕES GERAIS

REVISÃO
A perfuração da traqueia corresponde à perda da integridade da parede traqueal, o que permite o extravasamento de ar para os tecidos circunjacentes, criando enfisema subcutâneo, pneumomediastino e, potencialmente, pneumopericárdio, pneumotórax e pneumorretroperitônio. Tal perfuração pode ser causada por traumatismos penetrante, intraluminal, ou rombo (cervical ou torácico). A gravidade pode variar desde uma perfuração pequena até a avulsão traqueal completa. Em pacientes com avulsão completa, os tecidos mediastínicos podem formar uma pseudomembrana para manter as vias aéreas desobstruídas.

SISTEMA(S) ACOMETIDO(S)
• Respiratório — decorrente do comprometimento das vias aéreas e do possível desenvolvimento de pneumotórax e pneumomediastino. • Cardiovascular — o pneumotórax e o pneumotórax de tensão podem causar o declínio no retorno venoso e no débito cardíaco. • Nervoso, musculosquelético — dependendo da gravidade da hipoxia. • Cutâneo — enfisema subcutâneo inicialmente cervical, embora possa evoluir para o corpo todo.

IDENTIFICAÇÃO
Cães e gatos — não há predileção racial, etária ou sexual.

SINAIS CLÍNICOS
• O início dos sinais clínicos pode ser imediato ou levar até 1 semana após a perfuração. • O enfisema subcutâneo e a angústia respiratória são os sinais clínicos mais comuns. • Outros sinais incluem anorexia, letargia, ânsia de vômito, ptialismo, vômito, tosse, hemoptise, estridor inspiratório e choque.

CAUSAS E FATORES DE RISCO
• Feridas cervicais penetrantes, como aquelas provocadas por mordidas ou projéteis balísticos (p. ex., armas de fogo e flechas). • Perfuração iatrogênica decorrente de lavado transtraqueal, venopunção jugular ou cirurgia cervical. • Anestesia ou entubação com falha na desinsuflação do manguito ou na estabilização da sonda endotraqueal durante o reposicionamento do paciente. A hiperinsuflação do manguito provoca ruptura da traqueia por meio de laceração linear no músculo traqueal na região da entrada torácica ou na porção intratorácica da traqueia. Isso ocorre com maior frequência durante procedimentos odontológicos e lavados endotraqueais. • O traumatismo rombo pode causar avulsão da porção intratorácica da traqueia.

DIAGNÓSTICO

DIAGNÓSTICO DIFERENCIAL
• Anestesia — barotrauma que resulta em ruptura alveolar e penumotórax. • Feridas penetrantes — a perfuração do esôfago ou as feridas cervicais por mordidas podem causar enfisema subcutâneo. • Pós-traumatismo rombo — contusões pulmonares, pneumotórax, fraturas de costela. • Outros diferenciais incluem: compressão da porção intratorácica da traqueia por massa mediastínica, hemorragia induzida por rodenticida anticoagulante, pneumotórax espontâneo, efusão pleural e fístula broncoesofágica.

HEMOGRAMA/BIOQUÍMICA/URINÁLISE
Costumam permanecer normais.

OUTROS TESTES LABORATORIAIS
A gasometria sanguínea arterial poderá revelar hipoxemia, hipercarbia e acidose respiratória se a ventilação estiver gravemente prejudicada.

DIAGNÓSTICO POR IMAGEM
• As radiografias cervicotorácicas laterais são essenciais para o diagnóstico de perfuração da traqueia. Além disso, podem-se observar alterações como enfisema subcutâneo, pneumomediastino, pneumopericárdio e pneumotórax. • Em casos de avulsão traqueal, o local de ruptura pode estar visível. • As radiografias abdominais podem demonstrar pneumorretroperitônio. • O exame de tomografia computadorizada pode ser útil na identificação do local e do grau de laceração ou ruptura da traqueia.

MÉTODOS DIAGNÓSTICOS
• A oximetria de pulso ou a gasometria sanguínea arterial podem revelar hipoxemia. • A traqueoscopia pode ser usada não só para confirmar a perfuração ou a avulsão traqueais, mas também para caracterizar a gravidade, embora possam ocorrer resultados falso-negativos.

TRATAMENTO

• É indicada a internação do paciente. • A suplementação de oxigênio a 95% durante 4 h diminuirá o enfisema subcutâneo. • Manipulação mínima para diminuir o estresse. • O tratamento clínico costuma ser apropriado em casos de perfuração iatrogênica; a maioria dos casos apresenta cicatrização espontânea. • Em caso de desenvolvimento de pneumotórax, talvez haja indicação dos procedimentos de toracocentese e até mesmo a colocação de sondas via toracostomia. • Se o paciente descompensar, ficará indicada a exploração cirúrgica. • A ruptura da traqueia secundária a traumatismo rombo ou feridas penetrantes necessita de reparo cirúrgico.
• Durante o procedimento anestésico em pacientes com avulsão traqueal, deve-se entubar apenas o segmento proximal em princípio, com a utilização de sonda endotraqueal menor que o normal. No entanto, é recomendável evitar o fornecimento de ventilação com pressão positiva para impedir a ruptura da pseudomembrana. • A abordagem em casos de perfuração da porção cervical da traqueia é feita via linha média ventral, o que pode exigir uma esternotomia mediana parcial. As áreas traqueais lesadas ocorrem frequentemente na superfície dorsolateral e devem ser submetidas ao debridamento e reparo com fio de sutura absorvível monofilamentoso 3–0 a 5–0. • Em casos de dano ou avulsão graves da traqueia, indicam-se a ressecção e a anastomose dessa estrutura. • A abordagem em casos de avulsão da porção intratorácica da traqueia costuma ser feita por meio de toracotomia lateral direita no 3º ou no 4º espaço intercostal. O segmento distal da traqueia é localizado e entubado com o uso de sonda endotraqueal estéril assim que a pseudomembrana for aberta. Após a pré-colocação das suturas, o cirurgião deverá conduzir a sonda endotraqueal do segmento cranial ao caudal.

MEDICAÇÕES

MEDICAMENTO(S)
Em casos de perfuração decorrente de feridas ocasionadas por mordeduras, fica indicada a antibioticoterapia de amplo espectro.

CONTRAINDICAÇÕES
• A sedação deve ser usada com cautela, pois pode diminuir o controle respiratório. • Os corticosteroides não são indicados a menos que haja tumefação de alta intensidade das vias aéreas anteriores.

ACOMPANHAMENTO

MONITORIZAÇÃO DO PACIENTE
• Monitorizar a frequência e o esforço respiratórios, a coloração das mucosas, o tempo de preenchimento capilar, a qualidade do pulso e a frequência cardíaca, além de realizar auscultações frequentes. • Efetuar a oximetria de pulso e/ou a gasometria sanguínea arterial. • Obter radiografias torácicas para monitorizar o grau do pneumomediastino e do pneumotórax presentes, bem como para ajudar a detectar o aparecimento de estenose traqueal.

PREVENÇÃO
• Uso de seringa de 3 mL para a insuflação do manguito em cães de pequeno porte e gatos, para evitar a hiperinsuflação desse dispositivo. • Ao reposicionar o paciente, deve-se desconectar a sonda endotraqueal do circuito anestésico. • Ao utilizar o estilete durante a entubação, deve-se evitar que ele se estenda além do término da sonda endotraqueal.

COMPLICAÇÕES POSSÍVEIS
• Estreitamento e estenose traqueais no local de perfuração ou reparo. • Paralisia da laringe por dano ao nervo laríngeo recorrente. • Deiscência do local de anastomose traqueal. • Sepse (rara). • Óbito, particularmente na indução da anestesia em casos de avulsão traqueal completa.

EVOLUÇÃO ESPERADA E PROGNÓSTICO
• A maioria dos casos responde de forma satisfatória à terapia apropriada. • Os casos de avulsão traqueal completa apresentam prognóstico reservado, em virtude de dificuldades possivelmente encontradas durante a estabilização e a anestesia; sem a cirurgia, tais casos têm prognóstico extremamente mau, decorrente da formação de estenose e do risco de morte súbita.

DIVERSOS

DISTÚRBIOS ASSOCIADOS
Quando a perfuração traqueal for causada por traumatismo rombo, poderão ocorrer contusões pulmonares, pneumotórax, fraturas de costela e hemotórax.

GESTAÇÃO/FERTILIDADE/REPRODUÇÃO
A hipoxia causada por distúrbios das vias aéreas pode resultar em angústia e óbito fetais.

Autores Lori S. Waddell e David A. Puerto
Consultor Editorial Lynelle R. Johnson

PERICARDITE

CONSIDERAÇÕES GERAIS

REVISÃO
• Distúrbio inflamatório do pericárdio parietal (saco pericárdico) e/ou visceral (epicárdio); síndromes clínicas provocadas por efusão pericárdica, pericardite constritiva, extensão inflamatória aos tecidos circunjacentes (pleural, miocárdico) ou a causa subjacente da pericardite.
• Nos cães — mais comumente observada como pericardite hemorrágica idiopática, um distúrbio inflamatório leve que pode levar à efusão e tamponamento pericárdicos com risco de morte.

IDENTIFICAÇÃO
• Cães e, raramente, gatos.
• Pericardite hemorrágica idiopática é mais comum nos cães jovens aos de meia-idade, pertencentes às raças de médio a grande porte (p. ex., Grande Pirineus, Dinamarquês, São Bernardo e Golden retriever).
• Outras dependem da causa subjacente.

SINAIS CLÍNICOS
• Gatos — raramente observada ao exame.
• Cães — os sinais costumam ser causados por débito cardíaco baixo e insuficiência cardíaca direita secundária ao tamponamento cardíaco (i. e., anorexia, fraqueza, colapso, ascite, dispneia, pulso débil (fraco), taquicardia, sons cardíacos abafados, distensão ou pulsação jugular); semelhantes àqueles observados com frequência em animais com pericardite constritiva e efusão pericárdica, as quais podem coexistir (pericardite constritiva-efusiva).
• Pulso paradoxal é o termo utilizado para pulso débil palpável com a inspiração; é fortemente sugestivo de efusão pericárdica significativa, i. e., tamponamento cardíaco.

CAUSAS E FATORES DE RISCO
• Pericardite hemorrágica idiopática — desconhecidos.
• Cães — traumatismo rombo ou penetrante e infecção bacteriana ou fúngica (p. ex., tuberculose, coccidioidomicose, actinomicose, nocardiose e infecção por *Pasteurella* spp.). A pericardite infecciosa pode resultar da migração de espinhos de porco-espinho, farpas de plantas, projéteis balísticos, etc.
• Gatos — traumatismo ou infecção (p. ex., PIF, *Staphylococcus aureus*, *Escherichia coli*, *Streptococcus*, *Actinomyces*, *Cryptococcus* e, possivelmente, *Toxoplasma*).

DIAGNÓSTICO

DIAGNÓSTICO DIFERENCIAL
• Outras causas de efusão pericárdica (p. ex., neoplasia, ruptura atrial esquerda, ICC direita, hérnia diafragmática peritoneopericárdica e cistos pericárdicos).
• Outras causas de ICC direita (p. ex., miocardiopatia, miocardite, valvulopatia tricúspide ou pulmonar, cardiopatia congênita e ICC esquerda grave).
• Outras causas de efusão abdominal (p. ex., efusão neoplásica, hemorragia e hipoproteinemia).
• Outras causas de pulsos arteriais débeis ou colapso (p. ex., miocardiopatia, choque, hipoadrenocorticismo, arritmias, trombo em sela e estenose aórtica).
• Pode estar oculto por sinais multissistêmicos relativos à doença subjacente.

HEMOGRAMA/BIOQUÍMICA/URINÁLISE
Leucocitose em alguns animais com distúrbio inflamatório sistêmico, mas não nos cães com pericardite hemorrágica idiopática.

DIAGNÓSTICO POR IMAGEM

Radiografia Torácica
• Pode sugerir efusão pericárdica (silhueta cardíaca arredondada), particularmente quando a efusão crônica permite uma expansão lenta, porém acentuada, do pericárdio; a ausência desse achado não descarta efusão pericárdica ou pericardite.
• Podem-se observar corpos estranhos radiodensos.
• Injeção intrapericárdica de gás após a pericardiocentese (pneumopericardiografia) pode revelar lesões expansivas; pode não ser uma tarefa fácil distinguir entre lesões neoplásicas e granulomas ou cistos.

Ecocardiografia
• Ecocardiografia bidimensional é o método preferido para avaliação de efusão, tamponamento cardíaco e neoplasia; o diagnóstico é feito por inspeção direta.
• Ecocardiografia Doppler pode sugerir uma fisiologia constritiva com a demonstração de uma considerável variação respiratória associada no fluxo venoso pulmonar ou no fluxo mitral de ingresso. O volume pericárdico fixo resulta em uma acentuada interdependência dos dois volumes ventriculares.

Cateterização Cardíaca
• Também não é fácil diagnosticar uma fisiologia pericárdica constritiva; esse tipo de fisiologia, no entanto, pode ser identificada pelas medidas simultâneas de pressão dos ventrículos direito e esquerdo, demonstrando a equalização da pressão dos dois lados a uma pressão diastólica final elevada. Os traçados atriais revelam uma queda rápida na pressão no início da diástole, seguida por um aumento precoce até o platô a uma pressão diastólica final elevada.

MÉTODOS DIAGNÓSTICOS

Achados Eletrocardiográficos
• Podem-se observar complexos QRS pequenos, alternância elétrica, elevação do segmento ST e arritmias. Esse exame possui baixa sensibilidade em casos de pericardite. A alteração de alternância elétrica é específica, se presente.

Análise do Líquido
• Exame citológico da efusão pericárdica — geralmente não é útil, porque não consegue diferenciar as causas mais comuns, neoplásicas e idiopáticas; pode potencialmente revelar algum agente etiológico e descartar um processo supurativo; avaliação citológica da efusão ou biopsia do pericárdio fornece o diagnóstico definitivo da pericardite.

Outros Métodos
• Na suspeita de algum agente infeccioso, fica indicada a realização de culturas aeróbias e anaeróbias da efusão.
• Exame histopatológico do pericárdio.
• Uma elevação significativa dos níveis séricos da troponina I cardíaca não é típica de efusão benigna e sugere hemangiossarcoma.

TRATAMENTO

• Pericardiocentese e pericardiectomia parcial em casos de efusão grave. Insuficiência cardíaca direita pode provocar ou resultar de efusão pericárdica; o tratamento clínico da insuficiência cardíaca é adequado no primeiro caso. A efusão atribuída à pericardite idiopática nos cães pode desaparecer após uma ou mais pericardiocenteses. Na efusão pericárdica, a exploração torácica com pericardiectomia parcial não só impede que as efusões restrinja a função cardíaca, mas também permite o debridamento cirúrgico, a obtenção de amostras para exame histopatológico, a remoção de corpos estranhos e avaliação de doença granulomatosa ou neoplásica. A pericardiectomia toracoscópica pode fornecer benefício terapêutico semelhante, mas a avaliação diagnóstica é mais limitada. A cirurgia pode ajudar a evitar subsequente doença constritiva.
• A pericardite constritiva com extenso envolvimento do epicárdio pode exigir a extirpação epicárdica para atenuar a constrição e aliviar as aderências entre o epicárdio e o pericárdio; este é procedimento difícil, com altas taxas de morbidade e mortalidade.

MEDICAÇÕES

MEDICAMENTO(S)
• Tratar a doença infecciosa com agentes quimioterápicos determinados pelo teste de cultura e antibiograma.
• É recomendável a administração de corticosteroide nos cães com pericardite hemorrágica idiopática, mas a eficácia é desconhecida; isso também é válido para a azatioprina recomendada na dose de 1 mg/kg a cada 24 h por 3 meses.

CONTRAINDICAÇÕES/INTERAÇÕES POSSÍVEIS
• A fluidoterapia exacerba a insuficiência cardíaca direita.
• Diuréticos e redutores da pré-carga — relativamente contraindicados em animais com tamponamento cardíaco.
• Os corticosteroides podem exacerbar uma infecção.

ACOMPANHAMENTO

A efusão pericárdica poderá sofrer recidiva se o pericárdio estiver intacto. Ocasionalmente, pode ocorrer efusão pleural importante do ponto de vista clínico após a pericardiectomia; nesse caso, é recomendada a realização de ecocardiografia ou radiografia torácica.

DIVERSOS

ABREVIATURA(S)
• ICC = insuficiência cardíaca congestiva.
• PIF = peritonite infecciosa felina.

PERICARDITE

Sugestões de Leitura
Chun R, Kellihan HB, Henik RA, et al. Comparison of plasma cardiac troponin I concentrations among dogs with cardiac hemangiosarcoma, noncardiac hemangiosarcoma, other neoplasms, and pericardial effusion of nonhemangiosarcoma origin. JAVMA 2010, 237(7):806-811.

Tobias AH. Pericardial disorders. In: Ettinger SJ, Feldman EC, eds., Textbook of Veterinary Internal Medicine, 6th ed. St. Louis: Elsevier, 2005, pp. 1104-1118.

Autor Donald J. Brown
Consultores Editoriais Larry P. Tilley e Francis W.K. Smith, Jr.

PERITONITE

CONSIDERAÇÕES GERAIS

DEFINIÇÃO
Processo inflamatório que envolve a serosa da cavidade abdominal.

FISIOPATOLOGIA
• Agressão à cavidade peritoneal, localizada ou generalizada, que leva ao processo inflamatório caracterizado por vasodilatação, infiltração celular, estímulo das fibras de dor e desenvolvimento de aderências.
• A extensão e a gravidade dependem do tipo da lesão.

SISTEMA(S) ACOMETIDO(S)
• Cardiovascular.
• Gastrintestinal.
• Hematológico/linfático/imune.
• Renal/urológico.

GENÉTICA
N/D.

INCIDÊNCIA/PREVALÊNCIA
N/D.

DISTRIBUIÇÃO GEOGRÁFICA
N/D.

IDENTIFICAÇÃO
Espécies
Cães e gatos.

Raça(s) Predominante(s)
Nenhuma.

Idade Média e Faixa Etária
Nenhuma.

Sexo Predominante
Nenhum.

SINAIS CLÍNICOS
Comentários Gerais
Os sinais podem ser inicialmente vagos e inespecíficos.

Achados Anamnésicos
Letargia, depressão, anorexia, vômito, diarreia.

Achados do Exame Físico
• Desconforto ou dor abdominal — localizada ou generalizada; o paciente geralmente sente dor à palpação.
• Posição de "prece" — para alívio; semelhante àquela ocasionalmente observada na pancreatite.
• É comum a presença de vômito.
• Hipotensão e choque — podem se desenvolver rapidamente.
• Taquicardia — frequentemente notada; pode ser detectada uma variedade de arritmias.
• Febre — inconstante; quando observada com outros sinais de peritonite, sugere contaminação bacteriana da cavidade abdominal.
• Perda de peso — relatada em um terço de cães e gatos com peritonite secundária.

CAUSAS
Peritonite Primária
• Incomum.
• Resulta de infecção direta por disseminação hematógena do agente causal (p. ex., PIF).

Peritonite Secundária
• Forma predominante.
• Resulta do rompimento na cavidade abdominal ou de víscera oca.
• Contaminação séptica ou química — a partir da deiscência dos locais cirúrgicos, feridas abdominais penetrantes, traumatismo abdominal rombo, pancreatite grave, piometra, abscessos hepáticos ou prostáticos; além disso, ruptura da vesícula biliar, da bexiga ou do ducto biliar.

FATORES DE RISCO
• Traumatismo.
• Cirurgia gastrintestinal.
• Abscessos não detectados do fígado, do pâncreas, da próstata e do coto uterino.

DIAGNÓSTICO

DIAGNÓSTICO DIFERENCIAL
Outras causas de dor ou distensão abdominal, sepse e choque.

HEMOGRAMA/BIOQUÍMICA/URINÁLISE
• O achado mais comum é a leucocitose neutrofílica; pode haver desvio à esquerda; desvio degenerativo à esquerda ou desenvolvimento de neutropenia podem prenunciar um prognóstico agravante.
• É comum a constatação de hemoconcentração.
• Hipoproteinemia — atribuída à exsudação da albumina.
• Hipocalemia.
• Azotemia.
• Acidose metabólica.
• Hipoglicemia — pode indicar sepse.

OUTROS TESTES LABORATORIAIS
N/D.

DIAGNÓSTICO POR IMAGEM
Ultrassonografia
Pode identificar a presença de líquido livre dentro do abdome; abscessos do pâncreas, do fígado ou da próstata e ruptura da vesícula biliar.

Radiografia
• Achados inconsistentes que dependem da causa.
• Perda do detalhe abdominal (o aspecto em "vidro fosco" sugere a presença de líquido na cavidade abdominal) — não confundir com desidratação ou ausência de gordura intra-abdominal.
• Projeção lateral em estação — pode-se observar uma linha de líquido livre.
• Projeção em decúbito lateral esquerdo com feixe horizontal — podem-se observar gases livres dentro da cavidade abdominal.
• Íleo paralítico generalizado associado aos gases abdominais livres e linha de líquido visível — podem apoiar o diagnóstico; considerar outras causas de íleo paralítico.
• Procedimentos de contraste — geralmente não são justificáveis; podem complicar o tratamento se o material de contraste entrar na cavidade abdominal; evitar o uso de bário na suspeita de perfuração gastrintestinal.

MÉTODOS DIAGNÓSTICOS
• Abdominocentese e lavagem peritoneal diagnóstica — métodos seguros e confiáveis.
• Paracentese — esvaziar a bexiga urinária; preparar de forma asséptica o local da punção (centese); utilizar agulha de calibre 22 ou cateter de Teflon para penetrar na cavidade abdominal; às vezes, algumas gotas de líquido abdominal podem ser recuperadas; se não for bem-sucedido, utilizar uma seringa de 3 mL para aplicar uma pressão negativa suave; puncionar todos os quatro quadrantes (i. e., quatro agulhas de punção separadas).
• Lavagem peritoneal diagnóstica — realizada se o líquido abdominal não for recuperado pela paracentese; esvaziar a bexiga urinária; preparar de forma asséptica o local; infundir por gravidade 20 mL/kg de solução salina estéril tépida (morna) dentro da cavidade abdominal; pode-se rolar o paciente delicadamente de um lado para o outro para aumentar a recuperação do líquido da lavagem; não é preciso recuperar toda a quantidade de fluido infundido.
• Citologia — coletar as amostras em tubos de EDTA; observar a cor e a clareza do líquido e a presença de fibrina antes de enviar ao laboratório.
• Cultura e sensibilidade — coletar amostras em tubos estéreis com anticoagulante.
• Suspeita de peritonite química — analisar o líquido abdominal quanto à presença de ureia e creatinina (para detectar extravasamento de urina), amilase (para pancreatite), fosfatase alcalina (para traumatismo intestinal) e bilirrubina (para extravasamento de bile).
• Suspeita de PIF — pode-se enviar o líquido abdominal para os exames de eletroforese de proteínas e determinação de globulina.

ACHADOS PATOLÓGICOS
N/D.

TRATAMENTO

CUIDADO(S) DE SAÚDE ADEQUADO(S)
Paciente internado — monitoramento intensivo; cuidados de suporte.

Fluidoterapia intravenosa
• Medida crítica para a correção de desequilíbrios hemodinâmicos e anormalidades eletrolíticas e acidobásicas.
• Solução eletrolítica balanceada — as soluções de Ringer lactato ou Normosol-R costumam ser aceitáveis.
• Potássio e glicose — podem necessitar de suplementação.
• Velocidade de reposição — inicialmente pode chegar a 45 mL/kg/h (gatos) e 90 mL/kg/h (cães); ajustar a velocidade com frequência à medida que o estado do paciente muda; se for suplementado com potássio, a velocidade não deverá exceder 0,5 mEq/kg/h de potássio.

CUIDADO(S) DE ENFERMAGEM
Geralmente limitados em consequência da hospitalização e do confinamento.

ATIVIDADE
N/D.

DIETA
• Ditada pela causa, quando identificada, e quaisquer condições concomitantes (p. ex., cardiopatia).
• Tubo de alimentação, se necessário, pode ser colocado para suporte nutricional (p. ex., via esofagostomia, gastrostomia e enterostomia).
• Nutrição adequada — essencial para otimizar o resultado.

ORIENTAÇÃO AO PROPRIETÁRIO
• Advertir o proprietário sobre o alto índice de morbidade e, em alguns casos, mortalidade.
• Informar o proprietário que o monitoramento extensivo e o cuidado intensivo podem ser caros.

PERITONITE

CONSIDERAÇÕES CIRÚRGICAS
- Decisão de tratar de maneira clínica ou cirúrgica — ditada pela causa (se for conhecida), pela resposta do paciente ao tratamento inicial e pela condição financeira do proprietário.
- Os casos brandos que parecem responder à terapia clínica — a cirurgia pode não ser necessária.
- Contaminação bacteriana conhecida ou peritonite química suspeita — há necessidade de intervenção cirúrgica.
- Informar aos proprietários que desistem da cirurgia sobre as possíveis consequências; mesmo com atendimento cirúrgico, muitos animais não resistem.
- Laparotomia exploratória — preparar a pele antes do amplo campo cirúrgico; caso se consiga identificar a origem da infecção, deve-se removê-la ou corrigi-la; coletar amostra de líquido para coloração de Gram; utilizar sutura monofilamentosa absorvível ou não absorvível dentro do abdome (evitar sutura multifilamentosa não absorvível e categute); antes de fechar, proceder à lavagem completa do abdome com 200-300 mL/kg de solução salina estéril, aquecida à temperatura corporal.
- Deixar o abdome aberto ou fechado — essa decisão é determinada pelo grau de contaminação, pela possibilidade de remoção de todos os debris, pela gravidade da doença e pela previsão de complicações sépticas; fechado: utilizar a sutura de rotina; aberto: fechar parcialmente e aplicar laparotomia estéril e bandagem segura; consultar algum livro de cirurgia detalhado sobre a conduta de drenagem peritoneal aberta.

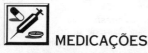

MEDICAÇÕES

MEDICAMENTO(S) DE ESCOLHA
- Antimicrobianos — de amplo espectro (contra microrganismos gram-positivos, gram-negativos, aeróbios e anaeróbios); sempre que possível, são selecionados com base na cultura e no antibiograma.
- Na espera dos resultados da cultura e do antibiograma — tentar uma combinação de aminoglicosídeo (p. ex., amicacina e gentamicina) e cefalosporina (p. ex., cefazolina) ou penicilina (p. ex., ampicilina).
- Ampicilina sódica — 22 mg/kg IV a cada 8 h.
- Gentamicina — 2-3 mg/kg IV a cada 8 h.
- Controle da dor — considerar se houver indicação.

CONTRAINDICAÇÕES
Glicocorticoides e AINES — a utilização é controversa.

PRECAUÇÕES
- Aminoglicosídeos — utilizar com cuidado se a função renal estiver comprometida.
- Hidratação adequada — essencial para aumentar a segurança desses medicamentos.

INTERAÇÕES POSSÍVEIS
N/D.

MEDICAMENTO(S) ALTERNATIVO(S)
Fluoroquinolona — enrofloxacino ou orbifloxacino; substituir no lugar de algum aminoglicosídeo, especialmente com função renal prejudicada.

ACOMPANHAMENTO

MONITORIZAÇÃO DO PACIENTE
- Equilíbrio hidreletrolítico e estado acidobásico — monitorizar com rigor.
- Frequência de monitoramento — varia de acordo com a condição do paciente e a resposta ao tratamento.
- Hemograma completo, perfil bioquímico, urinálise — a cada 1-2 dias durante os períodos de monitoramento intensivo, mesmo nos pacientes responsivos.

PREVENÇÃO
Prevenção — difícil, exceto quando fatores de risco específicos são identificados (p. ex., piometra).

COMPLICAÇÕES POSSÍVEIS
- Se a causa subjacente não for identificada e tratada, o paciente estará sob risco de complicações.
- Drenagem peritoneal aberta — herniação do conteúdo abdominal.
- Aderências.

EVOLUÇÃO ESPERADA E PROGNÓSTICO
- Prognóstico — depende da identificação rápida e do tratamento bem-sucedido da causa subjacente, bem como do acompanhamento adequado.
- Peritonite séptica — drenagem peritoneal aberta pode melhorar a sobrevida.

DIVERSOS

DISTÚRBIOS ASSOCIADOS
N/D.

FATORES RELACIONADOS COM A IDADE
N/D.

POTENCIAL ZOONÓTICO
N/D.

GESTAÇÃO/FERTILIDADE/REPRODUÇÃO
N/D.

VER TAMBÉM
Sepse e Bacteremia.

ABREVIATURA(S)
- AINE = anti-inflamatório não esteroide.
- EDTA = ácido etilenodiaminotetracético.
- PIF = peritonite infecciosa felina.

Sugestões de leitura
Costello MF, Drobatz KJDr, et al. Underlying cause, pathophysiologic abnormalities, and response to treatment in cats with septic peritonitis: 51 cases (1990-2001). JAVMA 2004, 225:897-902.
Culp WTN, Zeldis TE, Reese MS, et al. Primary bacterial peritonitis in dogs and cats: 24 cases (1990-2006). JAVMA 2009, 234:906-913.
Greenfield CL, Walshaw R. Open peritoneal drainage for treatment of contaminated peritoneal cavity and septic peritonitis in dogs and cats: 24 cases (1980-1986). JAVMA 1987, 191:100-105.

Autor Sharon Fooshee Grace
Consultor Editorial Stephen C. Barr

PERITONITE BILIAR

CONSIDERAÇÕES GERAIS

REVISÃO
Peritonite química causada pela liberação de bile na cavidade abdominal.

IDENTIFICAÇÃO
• Mais comum em cães que nos gatos. • Não há predileção etária, racial ou sexual.

SINAIS CLÍNICOS
Achados Anamnésicos
• Apresentação aguda em caso de peritonite biliar séptica. • Pode ter doença crônica em caso de peritonite biliar não séptica. • Rara ruptura biliar assintomática em virtude de encapsulação da peritonite pelo omento. • Desconforto abdominal: vago. • Letargia. • Sinais GI: anorexia, vômito, diarreia. • Perda de peso. • Distensão abdominal. • Icterícia variável. • Colapso em caso de peritonite biliar séptica.

Achados do Exame Físico
• Letargia. • Dor abdominocranial variável. • Icterícia. • Efusão abdominal. • Febre. • Choque endotóxico em caso de peritonite biliar séptica.

CAUSAS E FATORES DE RISCO
• Traumatismo a estruturas biliares. • Perfusão arterial limitada (artéria cística) à vesícula biliar. • Colecistite/coledoquite — podem se originar de mucocele da vesícula biliar; é mais comum a ocorrência de sepse em caso de colecistite necrosante. • Obstrução extra-hepática do ducto biliar — pode ser causada por neoplasia, colelitíase, pancreatite, estenose do ducto. • Peritonite biliar focal de pequeno volume — associada à colecistite; pode refletir encarceramento de bile pelo omento ou extravasamento de bile sem ruptura da árvore biliar. • Peritonite química causada pela bile — predispõe o paciente à peritonite séptica.

DIAGNÓSTICO

DIAGNÓSTICO DIFERENCIAL
• Distúrbios que promovem inflamação/desvitalização de estruturas biliares (p. ex., colecistite, coledoquite, neoplasia, traumatismo). • Distúrbios que causam obstrução extra-hepática do ducto biliar (p. ex., neoplasia, colélitos, pancreatite, estenose/fibrose do ducto). • Distúrbios que causam efusão abdominal e icterícia. • Isquemia da vesícula biliar: perda da perfusão arterial cística (traumatismo, lesão cirúrgica). • Sepse ou endotoxemia.

HEMOGRAMA/BIOQUÍMICA/URINÁLISE
• Leucograma inflamatório — em caso de colecistite necrosante ou sepse; anemia arregenerativa em caso de doença crônica. • Elevação das enzimas hepáticas, especialmente fosfatase alcalina; hiperbilirrubinemia; hipoalbuminemia; azotemia pré-renal. • Distúrbios hidroeletrolíticos e acidobásicos; é comum a presença de hiponatremia. • Bilirrubinúria.

OUTROS TESTES LABORATORIAIS
Testes de coagulação — anormais em caso de síndrome séptica, CID, ou obstrução extra-hepática crônica do ducto biliar.

DIAGNÓSTICO POR IMAGEM
• Radiografia abdominal — diminuição dos detalhes abdominais, geralmente generalizada, pode ser focal na área da vesícula biliar; efeito de massa abdominocranial; raro colélito mineralizado ou gás biliar (colecistite enfisematosa). • Radiografia torácica — rara efusão bicavitária (efusão pleural), sinais de traumatismo (p. ex., fratura de costela). • Ultrassonografia abdominal — efusão; obstrução extra-hepática do ducto biliar — vesícula biliar ou ducto biliar comum distendido; colecistite/coledoquite — vesícula biliar ou parede ductal espessa; colecistite necrosante — hiperecogenicidade da parede segmentar da vesícula biliar, além de parede laminada (representa necrose); interface líquida ao lado da vesícula biliar — realça a imagem; efeitos de massa peri-hepática/pancreática são comuns em caso de peritonite biliar; colélitos ou mucocele biliar; presença de gás nas estruturas biliares (microrganismos formadores de gás) com sombra acústica; ruptura da vesícula biliar — dificuldade na obtenção de imagem; tamanho do fígado geralmente normal; ecogenicidade variável do parênquima — reflete hepatopatia (p. ex., colangite ascendente, colangite/colangioepatite).

MÉTODOS DIAGNÓSTICOS
• Abdominocentese — proceder a avaliações físico-químicas/citológicas e culturas; otimizar a amostragem por orientação ultrassonográfica; obter amostras próximas às estruturas biliares, mas evitar a penetração das estruturas. • Citologia — esfregaços de impressão de órgãos como vesícula biliar, fígado e bile são usados para detectar infecção e neoplasia, transudato modificado ou exsudato, bile e bilirrubina fagocitadas ou livres. • Material mucinoso acelular reflete a produção biliar de mucina. • A relação de bilirrubina na efusão:soro geralmente ≥2-3:1 é uma característica útil. • Cultura e sensibilidade bacterianas aeróbias e anaeróbias — efusão, parede da vesícula biliar, fígado, conteúdo da vesícula biliar; é mais comum o encontro de microrganismos anaeróbios e oportunistas entéricos gram-negativos; infecções polimicrobianas são possíveis. • Laparotomia exploratória — adequada para obtenção do diagnóstico definitivo e formulação do tratamento; permite os procedimentos de colecistectomia, colecistenterostomia, reparo do ducto ou da vesícula biliar. • Biopsia do fígado — importante; avalia a presença de doença prévia ou coexistente.

ACHADOS PATOLÓGICOS
Dependem da causa e do local de ruptura

TRATAMENTO

• Tratamento hospitalar — a conveniência e a utilidade da cirurgia dependem do estado do paciente; atingir a normoidratação, corrigir o equilíbrio eletrolítico e acidobásico, bem como fornecer antibioticoterapia pré-operatória para obtenção da maior taxa de sobrevida. • Lavagem abdominal para reduzir o conteúdo peritoneal de bile se a cirurgia for protelada: talvez haja necessidade de ressecções e anastomoses complexas. • A necessidade de colecistectomia é decidida no momento da cirurgia.

MEDICAÇÕES

MEDICAMENTO(S)
• Antimicrobianos — em todos os pacientes, iniciar antimicrobianos de amplo espectro antes da intervenção cirúrgica; microrganismos anaeróbios e entéricos gram-negativos são mais comumente oportunistas (boas escolhas iniciais: ticarcilina, piperacilina, ou cefalosporinas de terceira geração, com enrofloxacino e metronidazol); tratamento antimicrobiano adaptado ao animal, com base nos resultados das culturas; manter por ≥ 4-8 semanas em caso de peritonite biliar séptica.
• Vitamina K_1 (0,5-1,5 mg/kg IM ou SC a cada 12 h por até 3 doses) — todos os pacientes ictéricos *antes* da cirurgia.
• Preparar o paciente para terapia com componente sanguíneo e coloide sintético.
• Antieméticos na presença de vômito — metoclopramida (0,2-0,5 mg/kg VO, SC a cada 6-8 h ou 1-2 mg/kg/24 h IV sob taxa de infusão contínua); ondansetrona (0,5-1,0 mg/kg a cada 12 h, IV ou VO, 30 minutos antes da alimentação); maropitanto (1,0 mg/kg/dia IV, SC, VO, máximo de 5 dias).
• Antagonistas dos receptores H_2 em caso de sangramento entérico — famotidina (0,5 mg/kg VO, IV, SC a cada 12-24 h); sucralfato (0,25-1,0 g VO a cada 8-12 h).
• Ácido ursodesoxicólico em caso de mucocele da vesícula biliar, colélitos, síndrome colangite/colangioepatite, ou hepatite crônica — administrar por tempo indefinido: 10-15 mg/kg/dia VO.
• Antioxidantes — vitamina E (10 UI/kg/dia); S-adenosil-l-metionina (SAMe; 20 mg/kg VO diariamente 2 horas antes da alimentação) até a normalização das enzimas, por tempo indefinido em caso de hepatite crônica ou síndrome colangite/colangioepatite, mucocele da vesícula biliar, síndrome da bile inspissada (espessa, semelhante a lodo).

ACOMPANHAMENTO

MONITORIZAÇÃO DO PACIENTE
• Testes hematológicos e bioquímicos sequenciais, bem como testes de diagnóstico por imagem.
• Repetir a abdominocentese para avaliar a presença de infecção contínua e/ou o extravasamento de bile.

COMPLICAÇÕES POSSÍVEIS
• Colangite/colangioepatite.
• Pancreatite.
• Colangite recorrente se houver necessidade de anastomose biliar-entérica.

EVOLUÇÃO ESPERADA E PROGNÓSTICO
• Prognóstico bom se a cirurgia for bem-sucedida e a infecção, eliminada.
• Mortalidade mais elevada em caso de peritonite biliar infecciosa (até 75%).
• Recuperação clínica e normalização lentas das enzimas hepáticas, mas resolução rápida da hiperbilirrubinemia.

Autor Sharon A. Center
Consultor Editorial Sharon A. Center

Peritonite Infecciosa Felina

CONSIDERAÇÕES GERAIS

DEFINIÇÃO
Doença sistêmica, imunomediada, viral de gatos domésticos e exóticos, caracterizada por início insidioso, febre irresponsiva persistente, reação tecidual piogranulomatosa, acúmulo de efusões exsudativas nas cavidades corporais e alta mortalidade.

FISIOPATOLOGIA
- O vírus da PIF replica-se localmente em células epiteliais do trato respiratório superior, da orofaringe e do trato intestinal.
- Doença imunomediada — ocorrem a produção de anticorpos antivirais e a captura do complexo vírus-anticorpo pelos macrófagos.
- O vírus é transportado dentro de monócitos/macrófagos por todo o corpo; localiza-se em várias paredes venosas e locais perivasculares.
- A replicação viral perivascular local e a subsequente reação tecidual piogranulomatosa produzem a lesão clássica.

SISTEMA(S) ACOMETIDO(S)
- Multissistêmica — lesões piogranulomatosas ou granulomatosas no omento, na superfície serosa de órgãos abdominais (p. ex., fígado, rins e intestinos), dentro de linfonodos abdominais e na submucosa do trato intestinal.
- Nervoso — podem ocorrer lesões vasculares por todo o SNC, especialmente nas meninges.
- Oftálmico — as lesões podem incluir uveíte e coriorretinite.
- Respiratório — lesões nas superfícies pulmonares; efusão pleural na forma úmida.

INCIDÊNCIA/PREVALÊNCIA
- Prevalência de anticorpos contra o FCoV — alta em grande parte das populações, sobretudo em estabelecimentos onde há muitos gatos.
- Incidência da doença clínica — baixa na maioria das populações, em especial em casas onde há apenas um gato.
- Em virtude da dificuldade no diagnóstico, no controle e na prevenção, os surtos em gatis criadores podem ser catastróficos; em gatis endêmicos, o risco de um gato positivo para o anticorpo contra o FCoV acabar desenvolvendo PIF é, em geral, <10%.

DISTRIBUIÇÃO GEOGRÁFICA
Mundial.

IDENTIFICAÇÃO
Espécie
Felina — gatos domésticos e exóticos.

Raça(s) Predominante(s)
Algumas famílias ou linhagens de gatos parecem mais suscetíveis. Chitas são particularmente suscetíveis.

Idade Média e Faixa Etária
- Maior incidência — em filhotes com 3 meses de vida a 2 anos de idade.
- A incidência diminui bruscamente depois que os gatos chegam aos 2 anos de idade.
- Gatos geriátricos podem ter uma incidência levemente elevada.

SINAIS CLÍNICOS
Comentários Gerais
- Uma ampla variedade, dependendo da virulência da cepa, da eficácia da resposta imune do hospedeiro e do sistema orgânico acometido.
- Duas formas clássicas — úmida ou efusiva, que tem como alvo as cavidades corporais; seca ou não efusiva, que acomete uma variedade de órgãos.

Achados Anamnésicos
- Início insidioso.
- Perda de peso gradual e diminuição do apetite.
- Retardo no crescimento em filhotes.
- Aumento gradativo de tamanho do abdome, conferindo aspecto em forma de barril.
- Febre persistente — flutuante; irresponsiva a antibióticos.

Achados do Exame Físico
- Depressão.
- Má condição corporal.
- Retardo do crescimento.
- Perda de peso.
- Pelagem sem brilho e áspera.
- Icterícia.
- Efusão abdominal e/ou pleural.
- Palpação do abdome — massas abdominais (granulomas ou piogranulomas) dentro do omento, na superfície de vísceras (especialmente os rins) e dentro da parede intestinal; os linfonodos mesentéricos podem estar aumentados.
- Oculares — uveíte anterior; precipitados ceráticos; alteração de cor da íris; e pupilas de formato irregular.
- Neurológicos — sinais de acometimento do tronco cerebral, da área cerebrocortical ou da medula espinal.

CAUSAS
- Coronavírus felino — existem dois tipos genômicos.
- FCoV-1 (talvez cause 85% das infecções).
- FCoV-2 (semelhante ao coronavírus canino).
- Distinção entre as formas — há grandes esforços para distinguir entre as cepas de baixa virulência ou entéricas avirulentas (FECV) e as virulentas (vírus da PIF), mas o FECV e o vírus da PIF ocorrem em ambas as formas, tipo 1 e tipo 2; dentro de cada tipo, há um espectro de vírus desde os avirulentos que produzem infecções assintomáticas até aqueles que causam PIF fatal.

FATORES DE RISCO
- Contato com gato positivo para o anticorpo contra o FCoV.
- Gatis reprodutores ou instituições com muitos gatos.
- Idade inferior a 2 anos.
- Infecção pelo FeLV.

DIAGNÓSTICO
- Forma úmida — relativamente fácil de diagnosticar ao exame clínico.
- Forma seca — difícil de obter o diagnóstico com precisão.
- Não existe um único teste laboratorial diagnóstico.

DIAGNÓSTICO DIFERENCIAL
- Febre de origem indeterminada — quando outras causas de febre tiverem sido excluídas.
- Cardiopatia indutora de efusão pleural — a efusão tem densidade e contagem celular baixas.
- Lesões de linfoma, especialmente nos rins, à palpação.
- Tumores do SNC — a maioria dos gatos é positiva ao teste para FeLV; no caso de gatos negativos para o FeLV, efetuar biopsia da lesão (se acessível) para histopatologia e imuno-histoquímica para FCoV.
- Doença respiratória — FCV, FHV, clamidiose ou várias bactérias.
- Pan-esteatite (doença da gordura amarela) — sensação e aspecto clássicos de gordura dentro da cavidade abdominal; dor à palpação abdominal; em geral, dieta exclusiva de peixe.
- Enterite causada por panleucopenia — leucopenia; ensaio fecal positivo para o antígeno do parvovírus canino.

HEMOGRAMA/BIOQUÍMICA/URINÁLISE
- Leucopenia — comum no início da infecção; mais tarde, observa-se leucocitose com neutrofilia e linfopenia.
- Pode ocorrer anemia leve a moderada.
- É comum a elevação da globulina plasmática total.
- Em geral, observam-se hiperbilirrubinemia e hiperbilirrubinúria.

OUTROS TESTES LABORATORIAIS
- Testes humorais séricos — imunoensaios, ensaios de neutralização viral; para detectar anticorpos contra FCoV; testes positivos não são diagnósticos, mas indicam apenas infecção prévia; a correlação entre a magnitude do título e a eventual confirmação da infecção não é alta.
- Ensaios de PCR — detectam o antígeno viral; a precisão dos testes positivos que se correlacionam com a doença clínica ainda está sendo avaliada.
- Ensaios de imuno-histoquímica (imunoperoxidase) — detectam o FCoV dentro de células específicas de amostras de biopsia ou cortes histopatológicos de tecidos de gatos com doenças fatais; excelentes para confirmar a causa de lesões específicas, em especial doença abdominal inflamatória que, em geral, não é diagnosticada como PIF.

DIAGNÓSTICO POR IMAGEM
- Em geral, não é necessário.
- Pode confirmar efusões abdominais e pleurais.
- Pode detectar lesões granulomatosas.

MÉTODOS DIAGNÓSTICOS
- Líquido obtido via toracocentese e abdominocentese — pálido a cor de palha; viscoso; em geral, observam-se flocos de fibrina branca; coagula se ficar estagnado; densidade geralmente elevada (1,030-1,040).
- Laparoscopia — para observar lesões específicas da cavidade peritoneal; obter amostra de biopsia para confirmação histopatológica ou imuno-histoquímica.
- Laparotomia exploratória — pode estar indicada em pacientes cujo diagnóstico será difícil se a laparoscopia não estiver disponível.

ACHADOS PATOLÓGICOS
Macroscópicos
- Variam, dependendo dos órgãos ou tecidos acometidos.
- O paciente pode estar emaciado, com pelagem áspera.

Forma Úmida
- Abdome e/ou cavidade torácica — podem conter um exsudato viscoso e espesso.

PERITONITE INFECCIOSA FELINA

- Placas piogranulomatosas brancas e grosseiras — podem estar na superfície serosa de órgãos abdominais e no omento.
- Nódulos granulomatosos — podem se projetar a partir da superfície dos rins.
- Granulomas — podem estar na parede intestinal.
- Filamentos fibrosos — podem se estender entre os órgãos.
- Fígado — pode ter lesões focais pálidas.
- Íris — pode sofrer alteração na cor.
- Córnea — pode conter precipitados ceráticos.
- SNC — pode haver lesões no cérebro e/ou na medula espinal.

Histopatológicos
- Granulomas ou piogranulomas em qualquer tecido acometido.
- Lesões — começam em torno de veias; aumentam de tamanho, envolvendo grandes porções de tecido; o aspecto microscópico é sugestivo do diagnóstico.

TRATAMENTO

CUIDADO(S) DE SAÚDE ADEQUADO(S)
Hospitalar ou ambulatorial, dependendo do estágio e da gravidade da doença, bem como da disposição e da capacidade do proprietário em fornecer bons cuidados de suporte.

CUIDADO(S) DE ENFERMAGEM
- Paracentese terapêutica — para aliviar a compressão decorrente de ascite excessiva ou de efusões pleurais.
- É importante incentivar o gato acometido a comer.

ATIVIDADE
Restringir para evitar a exposição de outros gatos, embora o maior grau de eliminação do vírus ocorra antes que o paciente exiba os sintomas.

DIETA
Qualquer alimento que estimule o paciente a comer.

ORIENTAÇÃO AO PROPRIETÁRIO
- Discutir os vários aspectos da doença, inclusive o prognóstico grave; uma vez que a PIF clínica esteja confirmada, quase 100% dos gatos acabam vindo a óbito por causa da doença.
- Informar ao proprietário sobre a alta prevalência de infecção pelo FCoV, mas a baixa incidência de doença clínica real; menos de 10% dos gatos positivos para o anticorpo contra o FCoV com menos de 2 anos de idade acabam desenvolvendo a doença clínica.

CONSIDERAÇÕES CIRÚRGICAS
- Em geral, nenhuma.
- Raramente, pode haver doença abdominal inflamatória gerada por FCoV em caso de obstrução intestinal; talvez haja necessidade de cirurgia abdominal.

MEDICAÇÕES

MEDICAMENTO(S) DE ESCOLHA
- Nenhum tratamento de rotina é eficaz.
- Pacientes com sinais generalizados e típicos quase invariavelmente morrem.
- A maioria dos gatos positivos para o FCoV tem infecção subclínica ou leve doença granulomatosa localizada que não é diagnosticada como PIF.
- Medicamentos imunossupressores (p. ex., prednisolona e ciclofosfamida) — sucesso limitado.
- Corticosteroides (injeção subconjuntival) — podem ajudar no comprometimento ocular.
- Interferonas — eficazes *in vitro*; sucesso limitado *in vivo*; há relatos de que uma interferona recombinante tenha algum sucesso no Japão.
- Antibióticos — ineficazes, porque a PIF não costuma estar associada a infecções bacterianas secundárias.

MEDICAMENTO(S) ALTERNATIVO(S)
Nenhum antiviral se mostrou eficaz.

ACOMPANHAMENTO

MONITORIZAÇÃO DO PACIENTE
Monitorizar o animal quanto ao desenvolvimento de grandes quantidades de efusão pleural.

PREVENÇÃO
- Vacina intranasal de vírus vivo modificado — disponível contra o vírus da PIF, baixa eficácia; não se pode confiar apenas na vacinação para o controle; pode tornar os gatos positivos para o anticorpo, complicando a monitorização em gatis ou colônias; em geral, a vacina contra PIF não é recomendada pelas diretrizes de vacinação da American Association of Feline Practitioners (Associação Norte-americana de Clínicos Felinos).
- Mãe/prole — o principal método de transmissão parece vir de gatas portadoras assintomáticas para suas ninhadas com 5-7 semanas de vida; depois disso, a imunidade derivada da mãe declina; interromper o ciclo de transmissão pelo desmame precoce com 4-5 semanas de vida e pelo isolamento da ninhada do contato direto com outros gatos, inclusive a mãe.
- Desinfecção de rotina — caixas de dejetos (bandejas sanitárias), jaulas/gaiolas, bem como recipientes de água e comida; inativa rapidamente o vírus; diminui a transmissão.
- Introduzir apenas gatos negativos para o anticorpo contra o FCoV em gatis ou colônias livres do vírus.
- Restringir os gatos de casa ao ambiente doméstico.

COMPLICAÇÕES POSSÍVEIS
- A efusão pleural pode exigir toracocentese.
- Obstrução intestinal em decorrência de doença abdominal inflamatória.
- Doença neurológica decorrente de lesões do SNC.

EVOLUÇÃO ESPERADA E PROGNÓSTICO
- Evolução clínica — alguns dias a vários meses.
- Prognóstico grave assim que surgem os sinais típicos; mortalidade próxima de 100%.

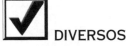

DIVERSOS

DISTÚRBIOS ASSOCIADOS
Gatos positivos para o FeLV — mais propensos ao desenvolvimento de doença clínica.

GESTAÇÃO/FERTILIDADE/REPRODUÇÃO
O vírus da PIF pode infectar fetos, resultando em morte fetal ou doença neonatal.

SINÔNIMO(S)
- Polisserosite por coronavírus felino.
- Vasculite por coronavírus felino.
- Infecção pelo coronavírus felino.

ABREVIATURA(S)
- FCoV = coronavírus felino.
- FCV = calicivírus felino.
- FECV = coronavírus entérico felino.
- FeLV = vírus da leucemia felina.
- FHV = herpes-vírus felino.
- PCR = reação em cadeia da polimerase.
- PIF = peritonite infecciosa felina.
- SNC = sistema nervoso central.

RECURSOS DA INTERNET
- Addie D. Catvirus.com. Website sobre peritonite infecciosa feline e coronavírus. http://www.dr-addie.com/.
- Cornell Feline Health Center; Apostila de Informações para o Proprietário. Peritonite Infecciosa Felina. http://www.vet.cornell.edu/fhc/brochures/fip.html.

Sugestões de Leitura

Addie D, Belák S, Boucraut-Baralon C, et al. Feline infectious peritonitis. ABCD guidelines on prevention and management. J Feline Med Surg 2009, 11:594-604.

Addie D, Jarrett O. Feline coronavirus infections. In: Greene CE, ed., Infectious Diseases of the Dog and Cat, 3rd ed. St. Louis: Saunders Elsevier, 2006, pp. 88-102.

Barr MC, Olsen CW, Scott FW. Feline viral diseases. In: Ettinger SJ, Feldman EC, eds., Veterinary Internal Medicine, 4th ed. Philadelphia: Saunders, 1995, pp. 409-439.

Brown MA, Troyer JL, Pecon-Slattery J, et al. Genetics and pathogenesis of feline infectious peritonitis virus. Emer Infect Dis 2009; 15:1445-1452.

Hartmann K, Binder C, Hirschberger J, et al. Comparison of different tests to diagnose feline infectious peritonitis. J Vet Intern Med 2003, 17:781-790.

Olsen CW. A review of feline infectious peritonitis virus: Molecular biology, immunopathogenesis, clinical aspects, and vaccination. Vet Microbiology 1993, 36:1-37

Pederson NC. A review of feline infectious peritonitis virus infection: 1963-2008. J Feline Med Surg 2009, 11:225-258.

Richards JR, Elston TH, Ford RB, et al. The 2006 American Association of Feline Practitioners Feline Vaccine Advisory Panel Report. JAVMA 2006, 229:1405-1441.

Autor Fred W. Scott
Consultor Editorial Stephen C. Barr

Persistência do Ducto Arterioso

CONSIDERAÇÕES GERAIS

DEFINIÇÃO
Patência persistente do ducto arterioso fetal, ligando a aorta descendente à artéria pulmonar.

FISIOPATOLOGIA
O ducto arterioso falha em se fechar após o nascimento, permitindo a comunicação persistente entre a aorta e a artéria pulmonar. O sangue tipicamente se desvia da esquerda para a direita. As consequências hemodinâmicas dependem da magnitude do desvio, da resistência vascular pulmonar e dos defeitos cardíacos concomitantes. Pequenos volumes de desvio são bem tolerados; volumes de desvio de moderados a grandes provocam ICC esquerda por sobrecarga de volume do ventrículo esquerdo. Com frequência muito menor, um ducto arterioso persistente calibroso (ou seja, de grande diâmetro) provoca lesão vascular pulmonar grave, resistência vascular pulmonar elevada, hipertensão pulmonar e inversão do desvio (fisiologia de Eisenmenger ou ducto arterioso persistente "reverso"), com desvio bidirecional através do ducto arterioso persistente. Os pacientes acometidos com desvio da direita para a esquerda sofrem de dessaturação arterial e policitemia deflagrada pela hipoxia.

SISTEMA(S) ACOMETIDO(S)
• Cardiovascular — sobrecarga de volume (desvio da esquerda para a direita) ou doença vascular pulmonar e policitemia (desvio da direita para a esquerda).
• Hematológico/linfático/imune — caso se desenvolva a policitemia.
• Respiratório — caso se desenvolva edema pulmonar ou hipertensão pulmonar.

GENÉTICA
Defeito geneticamente transmitido (modelo "poligênico") em muitas raças caninas, incluindo Bichon frisé, Cavalier King Charles spaniel, Chihuahua, Cocker spaniel, Collie, Springer spaniel inglês, Pastor alemão, Maltês, Poodle miniatura (e toy), Pomerânia, Pastor de Shetland e outras.

INCIDÊNCIA/PREVALÊNCIA
Segundo defeito cardíaco congênito mais comum nos cães; prevalência estimada em até 2,5 casos para cada 1.000 nascidos vivos. Má-formação muito rara nos gatos.

IDENTIFICAÇÃO

Espécies
Cães e gatos.

Raça(s) Predominante(s)
Ver a seção "Genética".

Idade Média e Faixa Etária
• A grande maioria é identificada durante a série inicial de vacinação.
• Início dos sinais relacionados com a ICC — semanas a muitos anos.

Sexo Predominante
Cães — as fêmeas predispostas em muitas raças.

SINAIS CLÍNICOS

Comentários Gerais
• Início de ducto arterioso persistente reverso — muito repentino em cães (geralmente antes dos 4 meses de vida); em geral, desenvolve-se de forma mais gradativa nos gatos.
• Não há nenhum registro significativo de que o desvio reverso se inicie após os 6 meses de vida em cães, porém os sinais relacionados com esse tipo de desvio podem passar despercebidos por algum tempo. O início dos sinais clínicos foi relatado em cães com mais de 5 anos de idade.

Achados Anamnésicos
• A maioria dos animais acometidos encontra-se assintomática na avaliação inicial.
• Angústia respiratória, tosse, intolerância ao exercício com o desenvolvimento de ICC.
• Retardo do crescimento em alguns casos.
• Ducto arterioso persistente com desvio da direita para a esquerda — fraqueza dos membros posteriores ao esforço e complicações de policitemia e hiperviscosidade (crises convulsivas ou morte súbita relacionadas com arritmias ou êmbolo da direita para a esquerda).
• Os sinais costumam ser precipitados ou agravados por exercício.

Achados do Exame Físico
• Tipicamente, ausculta-se sopro contínuo tipo maquinaria mais alto sobre a artéria pulmonar na base cardíaca craniodorsal esquerda; localizado em alguns cães; o sopro pode ser sonoro sobre o manúbrio do esterno nos cães de pequeno porte; com frequência, há um sopro sistólico concomitante de regurgitação mitral no ápice esquerdo. O sopro em filhotes de cão com <6 semanas de vida ou em gatos de qualquer idade pode ser obviamente contínuo, todavia lembra mais um sopro sistólico longo e diastólico precoce.
• Sopros altos — associados a frêmito precordial palpável.
• Pulsos arteriais — hipercinéticos (fenômeno conhecido como "golpe de aríete" ou "martelo hidráulico" [que consiste na interrupção brusca do movimento ou fluxo de água e sua consequente elevação]).
• Deslocamento caudoventral do ápice ventricular, indicando aumento de volume do ventrículo esquerdo.
• Taquipneia, angústia respiratória e crepitações inspiratórias — podem indicar ICC esquerda.
• Ritmo cardíaco rápido e irregular, com pulsos arteriais de intensidade variável caso ocorra o desenvolvimento de fibrilação atrial — isso é mais comum em cães de porte maior.
• No desvio da direita para a esquerda ("reverso"), os achados diferem — ausência de sopro contínuo, pulsos arteriais normais e impulso ventricular direito proeminente; pode haver um sopro sistólico de ejeção e uma segunda bulha cardíaca timpânica ou desdobrada; é possível a observação de pulso jugular.
• A característica típica de ducto arterioso persistente com desvio da direita para a esquerda é uma cianose distinta: mucosas craniais rosadas, porém caudais cianóticas; com policitemia secundária grave ou se houver desvio intracardíaco (defeito do septo ou persistência do forame oval), as mucosas craniais também podem estar cianóticas.

CAUSAS
Geneticamente predispostas na maior parte dos casos.

FATORES DE RISCO
Predisposição (racial) genética nos cães; os fatores de risco nos gatos são desconhecidos.

DIAGNÓSTICO

DIAGNÓSTICO DIFERENCIAL
• Os diferenciais auscultatórios principais incluem a estenose aórtica congênita com insuficiência aórtica (sopros sistólico/diastólico de vaivém) e defeito septal ventricular com prolapso da válvula aórtica em direção ao defeito (provocando sopros tanto sistólicos como diastólicos).
• Causas muito raras de sopros contínuos — fístula arteriovenosa do pulmão ou relacionada com neoplasia tireóidea, comunicação aorticopulmonar, ruptura da aorta no átrio direito ou no ventrículo direito e fístula da artéria coronária.
• Fístula(s) arterial(is) sistêmica(s) para a artéria pulmonar pode(m) resultar em achados semelhantes ao ducto arterioso persistente nas técnicas de diagnóstico por imagem; os sopros são frequentemente fracos ou ausentes.

HEMOGRAMA/BIOQUÍMICA/URINÁLISE
Geralmente normais a menos que haja desvio da direita para a esquerda; em seguida, pode haver graus variáveis de policitemia (hematócrito de 58-80%).

OUTROS TESTES SANGUÍNEOS
Ducto arterioso persistente reverso — pO_2 arterial femoral baixa em comparação à pO_2 obtida pela punção cuidadosa da artéria carótida ou braquial com o uso de agulha calibre 25. A oximetria de pulso das mucosas craniais comparada com a do reto pode comprovar a disparidade nas saturações de hemoglobina.

DIAGNÓSTICO POR IMAGEM

Achados da Radiografia Torácica
• Projeção lateral — aumento de volume do lado esquerdo do coração; tipicamente, há circulação pulmonar excessiva; com frequência, as veias pulmonares lobares são maiores do que as artérias auxiliares.
• Projeção dorsoventral (preferível para acentuar a aorta descendente) demonstra alongamento cardíaco (aumento do ventrículo esquerdo), aumento do átrio esquerdo e dilatação da aorta descendente (denominada "bossa [protuberância] ductal"); a artéria pulmonar principal encontra-se dilatada.
• ICC esquerda — distensão das veias pulmonares, aumento das densidades intersticiais/alveolares.
• Ducto arterioso persistente reverso — o coração geralmente se apresenta de tamanho normal, porém o contorno da margem cardíaca direita fica mais proeminente na projeção dorsoventral e a circulação pulmonar parece normal a reduzida; a artéria pulmonar principal e os ramos lobares proximais estão dilatados; em geral, observa-se uma bossa (protuberância) ductal na projeção dorsoventral; os campos pulmonares encontram-se claros.

Achados Ecocardiográficos
• Átrio esquerdo, ventrículo esquerdo e artéria pulmonar principal estão dilatados; o ventrículo direito está normal, exceto nos gatos; nessa espécie, é mais provável que esse ventrículo esteja hipertrofiado; a ampola ductal e o ducto distal geralmente podem ser visualizados a partir do hemitórax cranial direito e esquerdo.
• Função sistólica ventricular esquerda (fração de encurtamento) está normal a reduzida; pode estar

Persistência do Ducto Arterioso

acentuadamente diminuída em cães de grande porte com ducto arterioso persistente de longa data.
• Estudos com Doppler demonstram fluxo contínuo para a artéria pulmonar principal (a partir do ducto); frequentemente, há insuficiência pulmonar concomitante por dilatação da artéria pulmonar e regurgitação mitral provocada por dilatação cardíaca do lado esquerdo; a velocidade do fluxo transmitral e a velocidade do fluxo transaórtico estão elevadas por causa do volume aumentado e da pressão atrial esquerda; as velocidades aórticas podem estar aumentadas de forma substancial (até 2,5-3 m/s), mimetizando os achados de estenose aórtica subvalvular leve. Com frequência, é evidente uma regurgitação aórtica trivial, provavelmente por dilatação aórtica e fluxo aumentado através da válvula.
• Ducto arterioso persistente com desvio da direita para a esquerda — câmaras cardíacas esquerdas pequenas, dilatação atrial direita, hipertrofia ventricular direita e dilatação da artéria pulmonar principal e seus ramos; a ecocardiografia com contraste é valiosa para confirmar o diagnóstico; injetar solução salina na veia cefálica enquanto se obtém a imagem da aorta abdominal. O Doppler colorido e espectral cuidadosamente obtido pode identificar o desvio bidirecional de velocidade baixa através do ducto. Pode exibir regurgitação pulmonar e tricúspide de velocidade elevada, indicativa de hipertensão pulmonar.

Achados Angiográficos
• A ecocardiografia foi completamente suplantada pela angiografia para o diagnóstico.
• A demarcação angiográfica é útil para o diagnóstico diferencial de más-formações aórticas raras, arco aórtico anormal (com ducto arterioso do lado direito), fístulas arteriais sistêmicas para a artéria pulmonar, e durante os procedimentos de cateterização. A injeção do agente de contraste na aorta descendente demonstra a morfologia do ducto, informação crucial para as técnicas de oclusão ductal feitas com o uso de cateter.

MÉTODOS DIAGNÓSTICOS

Eletrocardiografia
• ECG — usado para o diagnóstico de arritmias auscultáveis.
• As anormalidades típicas incluem ondas P alargadas e ondas R altas nas derivações caudais esquerdas (II, aVF, III) e derivações precordiais esquerdas.
• Fibrilação atrial — observada raras vezes, relacionada com a dilatação acentuada do átrio esquerdo.

ACHADOS PATOLÓGICOS
• Persistência do ducto arterioso.
• Ducto arterioso persistente com desvio da esquerda para a direita — edema pulmonar, cardiomegalia (do lado esquerdo) e dilatação da aorta e da artéria pulmonar.
• Ducto arterioso persistente com desvio da direita para a esquerda — hipertrofia do ventrículo direito, dilatação da artéria pulmonar e artérias brônquicas proeminentes; o diâmetro ductal fica invariavelmente muito amplo, chegando em geral próximo ao da aorta descendente. As arteríolas pulmonares estão espessadas; pode haver arterite necrosante.

TRATAMENTO

CUIDADO(S) DE SAÚDE ADEQUADO(S)
• Tratar o edema pulmonar com furosemida e, se necessário, oxigênio, nitratos e repouso em gaiola; após a estabilização, ocluir o ducto arterioso persistente imediatamente.
• A oclusão do ducto envolve a ligadura ou oclusão cirúrgica com dispositivo oclusor de ducto canino, espiral trombogênico ou dispositivo de tampão vascular — recorrer a algum cirurgião experiente ou cardiologista para a realização desses procedimentos.
• Agendar os animais estáveis para cirurgia eletiva ou oclusão por dispositivo sem atraso; cães assintomáticos com apenas 7-8 semanas de vida não apresentam mortalidade operatória mais elevada do que os mais idosos.
• Cães com policitemia provocada por ducto arterioso persistente com desvio da direita para a esquerda — flebotomia periódica para manter o hematócrito abaixo de 65% (tipicamente 62-65%). Raras vezes, a hidroxiureia é usada para policitemia intratável.

DIETA
Normal; porém, ingestão restrita de sódio se houver ICC.

ORIENTAÇÃO AO PROPRIETÁRIO
• Cirurgia ou oclusão do ducto via transcateter — não adiar; a mortalidade será mais alta e a função do ventrículo esquerdo estará prejudicada caso ocorra o desenvolvimento de sinais clínicos.
• Após o fechamento bem-sucedido do ducto arterioso persistente e um período de convalescença de 2 semanas, o cão poderá ser tratado normalmente.

CONSIDERAÇÕES CIRÚRGICAS
• A oclusão de ducto arterioso persistente pode ser realizada através de ligadura cirúrgica pela colocação de dispositivo oclusor ou trombogênico via cateter dentro do lúmen ductal. Pacientes de porte menor (<2,5 kg) podem ser um fator limitante com os dispositivos atuais para ducto arterioso persistente, mas este nem sempre é o caso.
• De modo geral, a cirurgia pode ser efetuada dentro de 24-48 h da estabilização clínica.
• O tratamento-padrão envolve a ligadura do ducto por meio de toracotomia esquerda; a mortalidade cirúrgica e perioperatória deve estar <3% para todos os casos.
• A mortalidade com os dispositivos é até mais baixa, embora haja relatos de algumas complicações, inclusive falha na oclusão.
• Jamais corrigir o ducto arterioso persistente com desvio da direita para a esquerda de forma cirúrgica; o ventrículo direito não será capaz de ejetar contra a resistência vascular pulmonar sem a "válvula de escape" do ducto arterioso persistente.

MEDICAÇÕES

MEDICAMENTO(S) DE ESCOLHA
• Tratar o edema pulmonar com furosemida (2-4 mg/kg a cada 6-12 h VO, SC, IM ou IV, conforme a necessidade); pode ser interrompida quando o ducto arterioso persistente for ocluído.
• Quando a cirurgia não for uma opção — receitar furosemida, enalapril (0,5 mg/kg a cada 12-24 h VO) e pimobendana (0,25-0,3 mg/kg a cada 12 h VO) para controlar a ICC.
• Quando ocorrer o desenvolvimento de fibrilação atrial, adicionar digoxina e diltiazem (ver "Fibrilação Atrial" e "Flutter Atrial"). Uma alternativa é a cardioversão elétrica — uma terapia razoável, desde que o ducto possa ser fechado — nesse caso, recorra a um cardiologista.
• Para controlar a ICC grave com risco de morte — pode-se fazer uso de vasodilatadores diretos, como a hidralazina (1-2 mg/kg a cada 12 h VO) ou nitroprusseto de sódio (1-5 μg/kg/min) para diminuir o desvio da esquerda para a direita. Manter a pressão arterial sistólica em 85-90 mmHg.

CONTRAINDICAÇÕES
• No ducto arterioso persistente com desvio da esquerda para a direita — medicamentos que aumentem a resistência vascular sistêmica e a pressão arterial, exceto os necessários para anestesia e cirurgia.
• No ducto arterioso persistente com desvio da direita para a esquerda — medicamentos que induzam à vasodilatação arterial sistêmica e reduzam a pressão arterial sistêmica, incluindo medicamentos com efeitos vasodilatadores arteriais.

PRECAUÇÕES
• Medir os níveis de digoxina se prescrita.
• Monitorizar a pressão arterial, a função renal e os eletrólitos séricos para identificar problemas relacionados com terapias diurética e vasodilatadora.

MEDICAMENTO(S) ALTERNATIVO(S)
• Inibidores da prostaglandina (p. ex., indometacina) não ocluem com eficiência os ductos arteriosos persistentes nos cães.
• Considerar a hidroxiureia para tratar a policitemia grave irresponsiva à flebotomia; nem sempre é eficaz.

ACOMPANHAMENTO

MONITORIZAÇÃO DO PACIENTE
• O controle da dor é pertinente após a toracotomia e abrevia o tempo de recuperação. Considerar a aplicação de emplastro de fentanila, 8-12 h antes da indução anestésica. Instilar anestésico local (bupivacaína) na ferida cirúrgica antes do fechamento. Administrar opiáceos no pós-operatório para controlar a dor por, no mínimo, 24-48 h. A terapia analgésica após a oclusão via cateter é menos rigorosa, mas também deve ser mantida por 24-48 h.
• Pós-operatório — monitorizar os sinais vitais do paciente e a presença de dispneia, que pode estar relacionada com pneumotórax.
• Auscultação cardíaca no pós-operatório e na remoção da sutura; se os sons estiverem normais, não haverá necessidade de acompanhamento adicional nem de estudos diagnósticos. Não há base para recomendar uma reavaliação cardíaca anual de casos sem complicação que foram tratados com êxito.
• Sopro persistente contínuo indica fechamento incompleto do ducto, recanalização (descartar

Persistência do Ducto Arterioso

infecção ou migração do dispositivo) ou defeito cardíaco ou vascular concomitante.
• Sopros sistólicos são variavelmente auscultados no pós-operatório, mas devem diminuir no momento da remoção da sutura. Pesquisar novamente sopros inesperados por ecocardiografia Doppler. Quando houver apenas ligadura parcial na cirurgia, considerar o encaminhamento a algum cardiologista para oclusão com dispositivo.
• Doença súbita, febre ou sinais respiratórios agudos no pós-operatório — considerar infecção bacteriana do local da ligadura com pneumonia hematógena; há necessidade de antibioticoterapia rigorosa.
• Uma complicação não habitual é a estenose adquirida da artéria pulmonar principal e de seus ramos após cirurgia para corrigir ducto arterioso persistente.

PREVENÇÃO
Não acasalar os animais acometidos.

COMPLICAÇÕES POSSÍVEIS
• ICC esquerda.
• Arritmias cardíacas.
• Doença vascular pulmonar com hipertensão pulmonar, desvio reverso, intolerância ao exercício e policitemia.
• Morte perioperatória (por ruptura do ducto ou ocorrência de aneurisma aórtico), sangramento ou infecção.
• Recanalização do ducto.
• Embolização pulmonar ou sistêmica por deslocamento do dispositivo oclusor; hemólise por fragmentação das hemácias induzida pelo dispositivo; sepse proveniente do local cirúrgico infectado ou do dispositivo implantado.

EVOLUÇÃO ESPERADA E PROGNÓSTICO
• Raramente, os cães permanecem assintomáticos pelo resto da vida. A menos que o defeito seja ocluído, aproximadamente 50-60% dos cães morrem de ICC dentro de 1 ano do diagnóstico. O ducto arterioso persistente em cão com >3 anos deve ser avaliado caso a caso por um cardiologista.
• Cirurgia realizada antes do início de ICC moderada a grave — prognóstico excelente; cerca de 3% de mortalidade cirúrgica/perioperatória na maioria dos hospitais experientes. Índices mais baixos de mortalidade e resultados excelentes da oclusão são obtidos em hospitais *experientes* com o uso de dispositivos de oclusão ductal.
• ICC moderada a grave está relacionada com insuficiência miocárdica ventricular esquerda ou fibrilação atrial — prognóstico reservado; é recomendável o encaminhamento para um cardiologista.
• Cães com ducto arterioso persistente com desvio da direita para a esquerda podem viver por vários anos, mas frequentemente morrem de forma repentina; ocasionalmente, os cães vivem mais de 5 anos de idade (sobretudo cães da raça Cocker spaniel).
• Gatos — varia desde ICC esquerda rapidamente progressiva até o desenvolvimento gradual de doença vascular pulmonar; até pode ocorrer ICC direita com ducto arterioso persistente e doença vascular pulmonar.

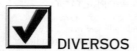

DIVERSOS

DISTÚRBIOS ASSOCIADOS
Tipicamente um defeito isolado embora possa ocorrer em conjunto com outras lesões cardíacas congênitas mais prováveis nas raças de maior porte. Ocasionalmente, uma anomalia do anel vascular é evidente, como persistência do quarto arco aórtico direito.

GESTAÇÃO/FERTILIDADE/REPRODUÇÃO
As cadelas prenhes carreiam maior risco de ICC; a prole exibe maior risco de amplo ducto arterioso persistente ou desvio reverso atribuído à doença vascular pulmonar; não acasalar os cães acometidos.

VER TAMBÉM
• Fibrilação Atrial e Flutter Atrial.
• Insuficiência Cardíaca Congestiva Esquerda.
• Sopros Cardíacos.

ABREVIATURA(S)
• ECG = eletrocardiograma.
• ICC = insuficiência cardíaca congestiva.

RECURSOS DA INTERNET
Dr. James Buchanan Cardiology Library: http://www.vin.com/library/general/JB110pda.htm,http://www.vin.com/library/general/JB103pdaRL.htm.

Sugestões de Leitura
Oyama MA, Sisson DD, Thomas WP, Bonagura JD. Congenital heart disease. In: Ettinger SJ, Feldman EC, eds., Textbook of Veterinary Internal Medicine, 6th ed. St. Louis: Elsevier, 2005, pp. 978-987.

Autor John D. Bonagura
Consultores Editoriais Larry P Tilley e Francis W.K. Smith, Jr.

PESTE

CONSIDERAÇÕES GERAIS
REVISÃO
• *Yersinia pestis* — bastonete corado bipolar Gram-negativo; pertencente à família *Enterobacteriaceae*; o reservatório inclui roedores selvagens (silvestres), esquilos terrestres, marmotas, coelhos, linces, coiotes.
• O agente causal (*Yersinia pestis*) evoluiu em sua forma atual nos últimos 20 mil anos a partir da *Yersinia pseudotuberculosis* enteropatogênica.
• Ocorre no mundo todo; o deslocamento dos animais pode resultar na ocorrência de peste em áreas não endêmicas.
• EUA — casos relatados de regiões como Novo México, Arizona, Califórnia, Colorado, Idaho, Nevada, Oregon, Texas, Utah, Washington, Wyoming e Havaí.
• Comum de maio a outubro (hemisfério norte).
• Vetores infectados (pulgas) transmitem a bactéria pela mordida. Os gatos costumam ser infectados pela ingestão de roedores infectados, e não pela mordida das pulgas de roedores.
• Bactérias — migram rapidamente dos linfáticos da pele para os linfonodos regionais; sobrevivem à fagocitose (por causa da cápsula de proteção) e multiplicam-se nos linfonodos; as células fagocitárias sofrem ruptura e o microrganismo é resistente à fagocitose adicional.
• Infecção — febre e linfadenopatia dolorida ("bubão"); a inflamação local intensa resulta em peste bubônica; bacteremia intermitente; os linfonodos podem se romper; o paciente pode se tornar septicêmico com ou sem envolvimento dos linfonodos.
• Gatos — altamente suscetíveis à infecção; doença fatal grave.
• Cães — naturalmente resistentes à infecção.
• A *Y. pestis* é um agente potencial de bioterrorismo; a ocorrência de um aglomerado de casos de pneumonia em animais de companhia pode indicar animais como sentinelas e risco de doença humana.

IDENTIFICAÇÃO
Gatos e, raramente, cães.

SINAIS CLÍNICOS
• Cães — podem demonstrar sinais febris leves e depressão.
• Gatos — são os únicos entre os carnívoros a demonstrar as formas bubônica, pneumônica e septicêmica de peste.

Bubônica (Gatos)
• Forma mais comum. • Período de incubação — 2-7 dias após a picada da pulga ou depois de ingerir roedor infectado. • A duração da doença é variável. • Bubões — cabeça e pescoço; linfadenopatia acentuada (hemorrágica, necrótica, edematosa); se o paciente sobreviver por tempo suficiente, os linfonodos formarão abscessos e sofrerão ruptura, drenando o conteúdo através de trajetos fistulosos para a pele. • Febre — 39,5-40,5°C. • Depressão. • Vômito/diarreia.
• Desidratação. • Tonsilas aumentadas de volume.
• Anorexia. • Secreção ocular. • Perda de peso.
• Ataxia. • Coma. • Úlceras bucais.

Septicêmica (Gatos)
• Rara. • Septicemia sem linfadenopatia ou formação de abscessos. • Outros sinais iguais aos da forma bubônica.

Pneumônica
• Doença grave, representando um maior risco de disseminação zoonótica para humanos contactantes.

CAUSAS E FATORES DE RISCO
• Gatos de caça ou de rua — maior risco de contato com populações de roedores selvagens e pulgas de roedores.
• Viagem a áreas endêmicas — oeste dos Estados Unidos e Havaí.
• Ambiente — domicílios ou animais com infestação maciça de pulgas; domicílios com grande população de roedores nas proximidades (p. ex., fonte de alimento no lixo ou pilhas de madeira).
• A peste está se tornando mais comum à medida que os domicílios invadem o hábitat de vidas selvagens em áreas endêmicas para essa doença.

DIAGNÓSTICO
HEMOGRAMA/BIOQUÍMICA/URINÁLISE
• Leucocitose com desvio à esquerda e alterações tóxicas acentuadas.
• Trombocitopenia — com CID.
• Alta atividade enzimática hepática e hiperbilirrubinemia.

OUTROS TESTES LABORATORIAIS
• Sorologia — Centro de Zoonoses e/ou departamento estadual de saúde; gatos e cães desenvolvem altos títulos de hemaglutinação passiva a fração 1A (cápsula antigênica) 8-12 dias após a infecção; pode-se observar um aumento de 4 vezes no título entre amostras séricas aguda e convalescente; títulos elevados persistem por >1 ano nos animais sobreviventes.
• Tempos de coagulação prolongados — com CID.

MÉTODOS DIAGNÓSTICOS
• Isolamento da cultura — por laboratório de referência; definitivo (grandes números de cocobacilos Gram-negativos com coloração bipolar); são obtidas amostras de material clínico antes da morte (abscessos, linfonodos, sangue periférico) antes do tratamento ou após a morte (linfonodos, abscessos, fígado, baço).
• Teste de anticorpo fluorescente — rápido método presuntivo para identificar animais infectados; as amostras são as mesmas que aquelas utilizadas para a cultura.

ACHADOS PATOLÓGICOS
• Gatos com doença aguda — poucas lesões; linfonodos infartados (bubões) na cabeça e no pescoço; fígado e baço aumentados de volume.
• Linfonodos — destruição da arquitetura normal; necrose hemorrágica; bactérias extracelulares.

TRATAMENTO
• Paciente internado.
• Alta mortalidade se não for tratado precocemente.
• Tratar de forma rigorosa com fluidos intravenosos para neutralizar a septicemia.
• Tratar a CID, se houver indicação.
• Tratar o paciente contra pulgas.

MEDICAÇÕES
MEDICAMENTO(S)
• Tratar todos os casos sob suspeita de forma empírica até que seja obtida a confirmação laboratorial. • Antimicrobianos sistêmicos — utilizar em todos os pacientes, exceto naqueles com envolvimento pulmonar (tais pacientes devem ser submetidos à eutanásia por causa do alto potencial zoonótico). • Tetraciclinas — oxitetraciclinas, tetraciclina, clortetraciclina; 25 mg/kg VO a cada 8 h por 10 dias; parenteral, 7,5 mg/kg a cada 12 h. • Doxiciclina — eficácia não estabelecida, mas provavelmente eficaz.
• Cloranfenicol — 30-50 mg/kg VO a cada 8 h.
• Gentamicina, trimetoprima-sulfametoxazol e canamicina — usar se outros medicamentos relacionados não puderem ser utilizados. • É necessária a coordenação com oficiais da saúde pública caso se estabeleça uma ameaça de bioterrorismo (cepas de bioengenharia de *Y. pestis* podem ser resistentes a medicamentos).

ACOMPANHAMENTO
MONITORIZAÇÃO DO PACIENTE
CID — ocorrência tardia comum na infecção se a doença não for tratada precocemente.

PREVENÇÃO
• Restringir viagens com animais de estimação para evitar áreas endêmicas. • Áreas endêmicas — manter o animal na coleira para limitar/controlar a exposição a roedores selvagens e suas pulgas; borrifar ou pulverizar o animal e a casa periodicamente para controle de pulgas. • Castrar os gatos — limita o comportamento de caça e a exposição a roedores selvagens. • Roedores — eliminar os animais e seu hábitat perto de casas e dependências (p. ex., pilhas de madeira e pilhas de lixo); armazenar os alimentos em recipiente à prova de roedores.

EVOLUÇÃO ESPERADA E PROGNÓSTICO
• Prognóstico — mau se não for tratada logo.
• A peste pneumônica tem risco maior de morte.

DIVERSOS
POTENCIAL ZOONÓTICO
• Alto; não confundir com abscessos por picada ou tularemia. • Risco de exposição via picadas de pulgas ou contato com tecido infectado no sangue.

ABREVIATURA(S)
• CID = coagulação intravascular disseminada.

Sugestões de Leitura
Gage KL, Dennis DT, Orloski KA, et al. Cases of cat-associated human plague in the western US, 1977-1998. Clin Infect Dis 2000, 30:893-900.
Gould LH, Pape J, Ettestad P, Griffith KS, Mead PS. Dog-associated risk factors for human plague. Zoonoses Public Health 2008, 55:448-454.

Autor Patrick L. McDonough
Consultor Editorial Stephen C. Barr

Petéquia, Equimose, Contusão

CONSIDERAÇÕES GERAIS

DEFINIÇÃO
Hemorragia puntiforme (petéquia) ou maior (equimose) na pele ou nas mucosas secundária à hemostasia primária anormal (mediada por plaquetas ou pela parede dos vasos); pode aparecer espontaneamente ou após traumatismo mínimo. O desenvolvimento espontâneo frequentemente ocorre nos locais de traumatismo capilar aumentado ou pressão elevada, p. ex., ventre.

FISIOPATOLOGIA
• Trombocitopenia e/ou função plaquetária defeituosa (i. e., trombocitopatia) geram um comprometimento da hemostasia primária (falha na formação de tampão plaquetário). Número de plaquetas abaixo de $50 \times 10^9/L$ é associado a um maior risco de hemorragia espontânea.
• Principais mecanismos de trombocitopenia — destruição aumentada, por exemplo, imunomediada (trombocitopenia imunomediada); produção diminuída, por exemplo, mieloftise ou mielossupressão induzida por quimioterapia; consumo aumentado, por exemplo, CID; e sequestro no baço ou no fígado, por exemplo, torção esplênica ou neoplasia.
• Principais mecanismos de trombocitopatia congênita — fator de von Willebrand deficiente ou anormal (mais comum); defeitos nas glicoproteínas da membrana plaquetária, por exemplo, trombastenia de Glanzmann em Otterhound e no Grande Pirineu (rara); defeitos nos grânulos de armazenamento das plaquetas, por exemplo, doença do *pool* de armazenamento nos gatos da raça Persa ou no Cocker spaniel americano (rara); defeitos na transdução de sinal, por exemplo, no Basset hound ou no Spitz (rara). Nota: a combinação dos dois últimos mecanismos é observada no Collie.
• Principais mecanismos de disfunção plaquetária adquirida são a inibição do metabolismo de prostaglandina induzida por medicamentos (p. ex., AINE) ou por uremia. Outras causas incluem paraproteinemia, hepatopatia, causas imunomediadas, alguns venenos de cobra e possivelmente anemia.
• Defeitos hemostáticos vasculares — causados, em geral, por permeabilidade capilar aumentada, por exemplo, febre maculosa das Montanhas Rochosas ou vasculite associada à PIF ou suporte vascular dérmico alterado, por exemplo, hiperadrenocorticismo ou síndrome de Ehlers-Danlos.

SISTEMA(S) ACOMETIDO(S)
• Gastrintestinal — melena/hematoquezia.
• Hematológico/linfático/imune — a trombocitopenia imunomediada por estar associada à anemia hemolítica imunomediada; o sangramento gastrintestinal concomitante pode causar anemia significativa.
• Neurológico — variável, dependendo da localização do sangramento.
• Oftalmológico — hemorragia da esclera/retina, glaucoma secundário e uveíte.
• Renal/urológico — hematúria.
• Respiratório — epistaxe.
• Cutâneo/exócrino — petéquia/equimose/contusão.

IDENTIFICAÇÃO
• Doberman pinscher e Terrier escocês são super-representados para a deficiência de von Willebrand. Muitas outras raças possuem a doença de von Willebrand. Note que as contusões são mais comuns que as petéquias em associação à doença de von Willebrand.
• Ver trombocitopatias específicas para distúrbios associados à raça.
• Nota: a trombocitopenia hereditária com plaquetas gigantes é observada no Cavalier King Charles spaniel; esse tipo de trombocitopenia não provoca contusão. Os cães da raça Galgo também apresentam uma contagem plaquetária menor que a normal, gerando uma leve trombocitopenia.
• Sugere-se que a trombocitopenia imunomediada tenha uma predisposição genética por causa da alta prevalência nos cães da raça Cocker spaniel, Poodle toy e Old English sheepdog. As cadelas de meia-idade também estão sob risco elevado.
• Gatos — menos comum que nos cães.

CAUSAS
Trombocitopenia
• Imunomediada — idiopática, induzida por medicamento (p. ex., antibióticos), paraneoplásica e induzida por infecção (p. ex., viral, riquetsiana, bacteriana, protozoária ou fúngica).
• Infecciosa — por exemplo, *Ehrlichia* spp. (*E. canis*, *E. ewingii*), *Anaplasma platys*, febre maculosa das Montanhas Rochosas, babesiose, leptospirose, leishmaniose, *Borrelia*, *Dirofilaria* spp., *Bartonella vinsonii*, *Mycoplasma* spp., *Histoplasma*, *Candida*, PIF, FeLV, citauxzoonose, parvovírus, herpes-vírus ou septicemia.
• Supressão da medula óssea — por exemplo, intoxicação por estrogênio ou quimioterapia.
• Relacionados com medicamentos — procainamida, sulfonamida, azatioprina, metimazol, albendazol, griseofulvina e cloranfenicol.
• Infiltração da medula óssea — doenças mieloproliferativas ou linfoproliferativas, por exemplo, mieloma múltiplo ou linfoma.
• Sequestro no fígado e/ou no baço secundário à neoplasia vascular ou torções.
• Consumo — por exemplo, CID ou extensa hemorragia recente em mucosas e serosas, como ocorre em envenenamento por rodenticida.

Trombocitopatia
• Distúrbios congênitos ou adquiridos que afetam a adesão e a agregação plaquetárias; ver a seção "Fisiopatologia".

Vasculopatia
• Vasculite secundária à infecção como febre maculosa das Montanhas Rochosas ou PIF; também em casos de vasculite imunomediada; ver doença(s) específica(s).

Deficiência de Fator de Coagulação
Os sinais clínicos não costumam estar associados à petéquia ou à equimose. É mais comum a ocorrência de hemorragia dentro de cavidades corporais, bem como hemartrose e hematomas.

FATORES DE RISCO
• A ocorrência de qualquer uma das doenças mencionadas ou predisposições raciais. A doença de von Willebrand grave é observada no Pointer alemão de pelo curto, Pastor de Shetland, Terrier escocês e Chesapeake Bay retriever.
• Histórico do uso de AINE.
• Vacinação recente é sugerida como fator de risco para trombocitopenia imunomediada.
• Doenças originárias de artrópodes.

DIAGNÓSTICO

DIAGNÓSTICO DIFERENCIAL
Não costumam ser confundidas com nada. Algumas lesões cutâneas inflamatórias podem ter aspecto semelhante à petéquia. Pode-se colocar uma lâmina de vidro sobre o local da hemorragia, aplicando-se uma pressão para branquear a pele. Se for hemorragia, ela não desaparecerá; se a lesão for secundária à inflamação, a pele branqueará.

HEMOGRAMA/BIOQUÍMICA/URINÁLISE
• As plaquetas encontram-se baixas, sendo mensuradas por contagem direta ou por estimativa em esfregaço sanguíneo bem feito. Uma única plaqueta por campo de maior aumento representa aproximadamente $15 \times 10^9/L$. Uma média de 10-30 plaquetas por campo de maior aumento corresponde à contagem normal de plaquetas. Se a contagem de plaquetas for maior do que $100 \times 10^9/L$, considerar outras causas de anormalidades da hemostasia primária.
• A fragmentação das hemácias está associada à CID ou a microangiopatias.
• *Ehrlichia morulae* ou outros hemoparasitas podem ser observados na amostra de sangue periférico.
• Os pacientes com doença mieloproliferativa ou linfoproliferativa, mielofibrose ou histórico de quimioterapia ou administração de medicamentos como estrogênios podem ter leucemia concomitante ou outras citopenias.
• Análise bioquímica — identificar doença renal ou hepática, bem como hiperglobulinemia.
• Urinálise — identificar hematúria.
• Proteinúria — pode sugerir doença imunomediada concomitante, como glomerulonefrite, e aumenta a suspeita de lúpus eritematoso sistêmico.

OUTROS TESTES LABORATORIAIS
• Estudos de coagulação (TTPA, TP, PDF, D-dímero, concentração de antitrombina III) ajudam no diagnóstico de CID. A contagem de plaquetas abaixo de $10 \times 10^9/L$ vai interferir no ensaio do TCA.
• Ensaio antigênico do fator de von Willebrand — necessário para confirmar a doença de von Willebrand.
• Testes de função plaquetária — podem ser necessários para descartar distúrbios da função plaquetária, p. ex., tempo de sangramento da mucosa bucal, tromboelastografia, agregometria plaquetária e citometria de fluxo.
• Em geral, os testes de anticorpo antiplaquetário não são recomendados, pois não são capazes de diferenciar trombocitopenia imunomediada primária da secundária.
• Eletroforese proteica sérica e urinária (procurando por proteínas de Bence-Jones) — indicada caso se observe hiperglobulinemia.
• Relação de proteína:creatinina — caso se constate a presença de proteinúria na uinálise. Uma relação elevada >1 pode ser sugestiva de glomerulonefrite concomitante.
• Teste para detecção de FeLV/FIV — causa subjacente de trombocitopenia.
• Título de anticorpo antinuclear — ajudará a diagnosticar lúpus eritematoso sistêmico se houver indícios de outra doença imunomediada.

PETÉQUIA, EQUIMOSE, CONTUSÃO

- Teste de estimulação com ACTH ou TSDBD poderão estar indicados na suspeita de hiperadrenocorticismo.
- Sorologia — ajuda a diagnosticar erliquiose, *Anaplasma platys*, *Bartonella vinsonii*, ou febre maculosa das Montanhas Rochosas.
- PCR — para infecções subjacentes como *Ehrlichia* spp., *Anaplasma platys* ou *Babesia* spp., *Mycoplasma* spp.

DIAGNÓSTICO POR IMAGEM
- Radiografia torácica em três projeções — procurar por indícios de metástase ou neoplasia primária. Identificar linfonodos aumentados ou sinais sugestivos de doença infecciosa subjacente.
- Radiografia abdominal para avaliar o tamanho do baço e do fígado. Identificar linfonodos sublombares aumentados ou massa abdominal compatível com hemangiossarcoma.
- Ultrassonografia abdominal para identificar anormalidades subjacentes da arquitetura em vários órgãos, o que sugere neoplasia, infecção ou inflamação subjacentes. Avaliar os linfonodos mesentéricos em busca de sinais de neoplasia, infecção ou inflamação.

MÉTODOS DIAGNÓSTICOS
- Tempo de sangramento da mucosa bucal será indicado se as plaquetas estiverem acima de $100 \times 10^9/L$; o tempo de sangramento da mucosa bucal prolongado sugere trombopatia. Os pacientes trombocitopênicos também apresentam esse tempo prolongado. A variação normal é menos de 4 minutos nos cães e menos de 2 minutos nos gatos.
- Os procedimentos mais invasivos são contraindicados nos pacientes com distúrbios hemorrágicos, exceto o aspirado da medula óssea e a biopsia do núcleo. Esses procedimentos estarão indicados se houver citopenias, hipergamaglobulinemia ou indícios de leucemia.
- Os procedimentos diagnósticos invasivos poderão ser realizados com menos risco se o concentrado de plaquetas puder ser administrado durante o procedimento para diminuir o risco de hemorragia.

TRATAMENTO
- Em geral, o paciente é internado até a formulação do diagnóstico definitivo.
- Minimizar a atividade para reduzir o risco de trauma menor.
- Interromper quaisquer medicamentos que possam alterar a função plaquetária; por exemplo, ácido acetilsalicílico e outros AINE.
- Interromper o medicamento que está associado à trombocitopenia imunomediada, como metimazol nos gatos ou trimetoprima-sulfa nos cães.
- Manter o volume hídrico com solução eletrolítica balanceada.
- Evitar injeções subcutâneas e intramusculares, bem como venopunção a partir da veia jugular.
- Transfusões de sangue total fresco ou de plaquetas podem ser necessárias e salvar a vida do animal antes da obtenção do diagnóstico definitivo. Garantir que as amostras de sangue sejam coletadas antes da transfusão para a realização de testes diagnósticos, como testes de coagulação, sorologia ou PCR.
- Não há nenhum tratamento específico disponível para trombopatias congênitas, a não ser o DDVAP, que pode ser utilizado na doença de von Willebrand tipo I para ajudar a controlar o sangramento. Também poderá ser administrado a doadores de sangue antes de sua coleta se o receptor precisar de cirurgia. Ver "Doença de von Willebrand" em busca de mais detalhes. As trombopatias adquiridas precisam ter a doença subjacente corrigida. O hiperadrenocorticismo pode ser tratado — ver capítulo específico. Não há tratamento para a síndrome de Ehlers-Danlos. A doença subjacente precisa ser tratada ao se tratar a vasculite. Ver capítulos específicos.

MEDICAÇÕES
MEDICAMENTO(S)
Depende do diagnóstico subjacente; p. ex.,
- Prednisona ± vincristina para trombocitopenia imunomediada.
- Doxiciclina para causas infecciosas ou até que essas causas sejam descartadas.
- Acetato de desmopressina (DDAVP) para defeitos brandos da função plaquetária, p. ex., doença de von Willebrand tipo 1.

CONTRAINDICAÇÕES
Evitar medicações injetáveis subcutâneas ou intramusculares sempre que possível.

PRECAUÇÕES
Evitar AINE e outros medicamentos que inibem a hemostasia, a não ser a heparina em casos de CID.

ACOMPANHAMENTO
Contagem plaquetária diária para pacientes com trombocitopenia até que se observe uma resposta adequada. Ver doenças específicas em busca de detalhes.

COMPLICAÇÕES POSSÍVEIS
- Morte ou morbidade causada por hemorragia no cérebro, no intestino ou em outros órgãos.
- Choque causado por hipovolemia hemorrágica.

DIVERSOS
SINÔNIMO(S)
- Diátese hemorrágica.
- Sangramento.

VER TAMBÉM
- Coagulação Intravascular Disseminada.
- Distúrbios Mieloproliferativos.
- Doença de von Willebrand.
- Hiperadrenocorticismo (Síndrome de Cushing) — Gatos.
- Hiperadrenocorticismo (Síndrome de Cushing) — Cães.
- Trombocitopatias.
- Trombocitopenia.
- Trombocitopenia Imunomediada Primária.

ABREVIATURA(S)
- ACTH = hormônio adrenocorticotrópico.
- AINE = anti-inflamatório não esteroide.
- CID = coagulação intravascular disseminada.
- DDPAV = 1-deamino-8-D-arginina vasopressina.
- FeLV = vírus da leucemia felina.
- FIV = vírus da imunodeficiência felina.
- PCR = reação em cadeia da polimerase.
- PDF = produto de degradação da fibrina.
- PIF = peritonite infecciosa felina.
- TCA = tempo de coagulação ativada.
- TP = tempo de protrombina.
- TSDBD = teste de supressão com dexametasona em baixas doses.
- TTPA = tempo de tromboplastina parcial ativada.

RECURSOS DA INTERNET
- http://www.cvm.ncsu.edu/vth/ticklab.html.
- www.diaglab.vet.cornell.edu/service/.
- www.vet.upenn.edu/penngen

Sugestões de Leitura
Brooks M, Catalfamo JL. Platelet disorders and von Willebrand's disease. In: Ettinger SJ, ed., Textbook of Veterinary Internal Medicine, 6th ed. Philadelphia: Saunders, 2005, pp. 1918-1929.
Brooks M, Catalfamo JL. Platelet dysfunction. In: Bonagura JD, Kirk RW, eds., Kirk's Current Veterinary Therapy XIII: Small Animal Practice. Philadelphia: Saunders, 2000, pp. 442-447.
Callan MB. Petechiae and ecchymoses. In: Ettinger SJ, ed., Textbook of Veterinary Internal Medicine, 6th ed. Philadelphia: Saunders, 2005, pp. 218-222.
Grindem CB. Infectious and immune-mediated thrombocytopenia. In: Bonagura JD, Kirk RW, eds., Kirk's Current Veterinary Therapy XIII: Small Animal Practice. Philadelphia: Saunders, 2000, pp. 438-442.
Russell KE, Grindem CB. Secondary thrombocytopenia. In: Feldman BF, Zinki JG, Jain NC, eds., Schalm's Veterinary Hematology. Philadelphia: Lippincott Williams & Wilkins, 2000, pp. 469-477.

Autor Julie Armstrong
Consultor Editorial A.H. Rebar

PIELONEFRITE

CONSIDERAÇÕES GERAIS

DEFINIÇÃO
Colonização microbiana do trato urinário superior, incluindo a pelve renal, os divertículos coletores, o parênquima renal e os ureteres; como a pielonefrite não costuma estar limitada à pelve e ao parênquima renais, uma expressão mais descritiva é *infecção do trato urinário superior*; este capítulo limita-se à pielonefrite bacteriana.

FISIOPATOLOGIA
• A infecção de qualquer porção do trato urinário geralmente necessita de algum comprometimento das defesas normais do hospedeiro contra infecção do trato urinário (ver os capítulos sobre infecção do trato urinário inferior); defesas normais contra infecção ascendente do trato urinário incluem barreiras de defesa da mucosa, peristaltismo ureteral, válvulas de retalho ureterovesical, fluxo unidirecional de urina e extenso aporte sanguíneo renal. A pielonefrite ocorre, em geral, pela ascensão de microrganismos, provocando infecção do trato urinário inferior. Nos cães e gatos, a disseminação hematógena dos rins não costuma causar pielonefrite. Independentemente da via de infecção, a infecção do trato urinário superior é muitas vezes acompanhada pela infecção do trato urinário inferior.
• O desenvolvimento de pielonefrite pode ser secundário à infecção de nefrólitos metabólicos. A infecção do trato urinário superior por bactérias produtoras de urease pode predispor à formação de nefrólitos por estruvita (ver Urolitíase por Estruvita — Cães).
• A obstrução de rim ou ureter infectado pode rapidamente provocar septicemia (também denominada de urossepse).

SISTEMA(S) ACOMETIDO(S)
• Renal/urológico.
• Pode provocar urossepse, afetando com isso qualquer sistema corporal.

INCIDÊNCIA/PREVALÊNCIA
• Desconhecidas.
• É provável que sua ocorrência seja muito mais comum do que sua identificação clínica, porque muitos animais com pielonefrite permanecem assintomáticos ou apresentam sinais clínicos limitados à infecção do trato urinário inferior.

IDENTIFICAÇÃO
Espécies
Detectada com maior frequência em cães do que em gatos.

Idade Média e Faixa Etária
• Cães de qualquer idade podem ser acometidos.
• Na espécie felina, a infecção do trato urinário é rara (1-3%) em animais jovens a de meia-idade. É mais comum em gatos com mais de 10 anos de idade (~10%).

Sexo Predominante
• Desconhecido; cães — infecção do trato urinário acomete mais as fêmeas do que os machos.
• Gatos — a infecção do trato urinário ocorre com uma frequência semelhante nos machos e nas fêmeas.

SINAIS CLÍNICOS
Comentários Gerais
Muitos pacientes permanecem assintomáticos ou exibem apenas sinais de infecção do trato urinário inferior.

Achados Anamnésicos
• Possivelmente nenhum.
• Poliúria/polidipsia (PU/PD).
• Dor abdominal ou lombar (incomum).
• Sinais associados à infecção do trato urinário inferior — por exemplo, disúria, polaciúria, periúria, estrangúria, hematúria e urina de odor fétido ou coloração alterada.

Achados do Exame Físico
• Nenhum.
• Dor à palpação dos rins.
• Febre.
• Um ou ambos os rins podem estar com o tamanho diminuído e/ou aumentado.

CAUSAS
Em geral, a infecção ascendente do trato urinário é causada por bactérias aeróbias; os isolamentos mais comuns são *Escherichia coli* e *Staphylococcus* spp.; outras bactérias, incluindo *Proteus*, *Streptococcus*, *Klebsiella*, *Enterobacter* e *Pseudomonas* spp., as quais frequentemente infectam o trato urinário inferior, podem ascender ao trato urinário superior. Bactérias anaeróbias, ureaplasma e fungos raramente infectam o trato urinário superior.

FATORES DE RISCO
• Ureteres ectópicos, refluxo vesicoureteral, displasia renal congênita e infecção do trato urinário inferior.
• Condições predisponentes à infecção do trato urinário — por exemplo, diabetes melito, hiperadrenocorticismo, administração exógena de esteroide, insuficiência renal, cateterização transuretral, retenção de urina, urólitos, neoplasia do trato urinário, uretrostomia perineal.
• Em gatos com doença do trato urinário inferior induzida experimentalmente, o uso de catéteres urinários permanentes combinados com a administração exógena de esteroides resultou com frequência em pielonefrite.

DIAGNÓSTICO

DIAGNÓSTICO DIFERENCIAL
• O diagnóstico clínico da pielonefrite geralmente é presuntivo, com base nos resultados dos exames de hemograma completo, bioquímica, urinálise, urocultura e técnicas de diagnóstico por imagem; o diagnóstico definitivo geralmente não é necessário para o planejamento terapêutico.
• Como muitos cães e gatos não apresentam sintomas específicos atribuíveis à pielonefrite, todo paciente com infecção do trato urinário potencialmente pode ter a pielonefrite; os melhores métodos para diferenciação entre infecção do trato urinário inferior e superior são a ultrassonografia ou a urografia excretora. Lembre-se de que a maioria dos pacientes com pielonefrite permanece assintomática.
• Considerar a possibilidade de pielonefrite como um diagnóstico de exclusão em cães e gatos com febre de origem desconhecida, PU/PD, insuficiência renal crônica e/ou dor lombar/abdominal.

HEMOGRAMA/BIOQUÍMICA/URINÁLISE
• Hemograma completo — resultados quase sempre normais em casos de pielonefrite crônica; leucocitose e neutrofilia imatura podem ser detectadas em alguns pacientes.
• Bioquímica — geralmente normal a menos que a pielonefrite crônica induza à insuficiência renal crônica (azotemia com densidade urinária inadequada).
• A urinálise revela hematúria, piúria, proteinúria, bacteriúria e cilindros leucocitários em alguns animais. Os cilindros leucocitários são diagnósticos de inflamação renal, mas infelizmente são muito raros. Observe a densidade urinária diluída nos pacientes com diabetes insípido nefrogênico, o que pode ocorrer secundariamente à pielonefrite. A ausência dessas anormalidades não descarta a pielonefrite.

OUTROS TESTES LABORATORIAIS
• Urocultura quantitativa para confirmar a infecção do trato urinário; consultar os capítulos sobre infecção do trato urinário inferior em busca da interpretação.
• Os cães com pielonefrite crônica podem apresentar resultados negativos na urocultura e necessitar de múltiplas culturas da urina para confirmar a infecção do trato urinário.

DIAGNÓSTICO POR IMAGEM
• A ultrassonografia e a urografia excretora são os melhores métodos para o diferencial presuntivo entre infecção do trato urinário superior e inferior. A ultrassonografia é mais sensível que a urografia excretora para a identificação de pielonefrite aguda leve a moderada.
• Os achados ultrassonográficos que apoiam a pielonefrite incluem dilatação da pelve renal e do ureter proximal, além de linha hiperecoica da borda da mucosa dentro da pelve renal e/ou do ureter proximal.
• A urografia intravenosa pode revelar dilatação e falta de nitidez da pelve renal com ausência de enchimento desses divertículos coletores e dilatação do ureter proximal, além de opacidade reduzida da fase de nefrograma e do meio de contraste no sistema coletor.
• Em pacientes com pielonefrite aguda, os rins podem estar aumentados de volume; já naqueles com pielonefrite crônica, os rins podem estar pequenos, com contorno superficial irregular.
• Nefrólitos concomitantes podem ser detectados em alguns pacientes por meio de radiografia simples, ultrassonografia ou urografia excretora.

MÉTODOS DIAGNÓSTICOS
• O diagnóstico definitivo requer uroculturas de material obtido da pelve ou do parênquima renais ou exame histopatológico de biopsia renal. A pielocentese pode ser realizada por via percutânea, utilizando a orientação ultrassonográfica ou durante cirurgia exploratória; pode-se obter amostra para cultura da pelve renal (ou dos nefrólitos) durante o procedimento de nefrotomia.
• Para confirmar o diagnóstico, a amostra de biopsia deve incluir o córtex e a medula renais; dessa forma, a biopsia renal deverá ser realizada por alguém familiarizado com a técnica de biopsia renal guiada por ultrassom ou por meio de cirurgia aberta e apenas se for necessária.
• As lesões renais podem ser irregulares em termos de distribuição e, portanto, a amostra de biopsia renal pode não ser representativa das lesões observadas à microscopia óptica.

PIELONEFRITE

ACHADOS PATOLÓGICOS
- Os rins acometidos por pielonefrite crônica podem exibir áreas de infarto e formação cicatricial na superfície capsular. A pelve renal e os divertículos coletores podem estar dilatados e distorcidos pelos processos de infecção e inflamação crônicas. Ocasionalmente, observa-se exsudato purulento na pelve renal.
- Os achados à microscopia óptica incluem papilite, pielite, nefrite intersticial e cilindros leucocitários no lúmen dos túbulos.

TRATAMENTO
CUIDADO(S) DE SAÚDE ADEQUADO(S)
O tratamento é feito em ambulatório, a menos que o paciente tenha septicemia ou insuficiência renal sintomática.

ATIVIDADE
Sem restrição.

DIETA
É recomendável uma dieta renal modificada (p. ex., Prescription Diet k/d da Hill®) para cães ou gatos com insuficiência renal crônica ou nefrolitíase concomitantes.

ORIENTAÇÃO AO PROPRIETÁRIO
- A pielonefrite recidivante pode ser assintomática. A pielonefrite crônica sem resolução pode levar à insuficiência renal crônica; o acompanhamento diagnóstico é importante para comprovar o desaparecimento ou a evolução da pielonefrite.
- Nos pacientes com nefrólitos, a resolução é improvável a menos que os nefrólitos sejam removidos.

CONSIDERAÇÕES CIRÚRGICAS
- A obstrução completa do trato urinário superior de paciente com pielonefrite pode evoluir rapidamente para septicemia e, portanto, deve ser considerada uma emergência médica. A causa da obstrução deve ser submetida à correção cirúrgica (ou litotripsia para os nefrólitos).
- Nefrólitos infectados — remover por meio cirúrgico, dissolver de forma clínica (estruvita) ou fragmentar com litotripsia extracorpórea por ondas de choque; utilizar antibióticos durante o procedimento para reduzir o risco de urossepse ao se manipular nefrólitos infectados.
- Em geral, a nefrectomia unilateral não é eficaz para a eliminação da suspeita de pielonefrite unilateral.

MEDICAÇÕES
MEDICAMENTO(S) DE ESCOLHA
- Escolher os antibióticos com base nos resultados da urocultura e do antibiograma.
- Os antibióticos devem ser bactericidas, atingir boas concentrações séricas e urinárias e não ser nefrotóxicos.
- Concentrações séricas e urinárias elevadas do antibiótico não garantem necessariamente altas concentrações teciduais na medula renal; portanto, pode ser difícil erradicar a pielonefrite crônica.
- Administrar os antibióticos por via oral em suas dosagens terapêuticas plenas por 4-6 semanas.
- Não utilizar medicamentos que alcancem boas concentrações na urina, porém baixas concentrações no soro (p. ex., nitrofurantoína).

CONTRAINDICAÇÕES
Não utilizar os aminoglicosídeos a menos que não existam outros medicamentos alternativos com base na urocultura e no antibiograma.

PRECAUÇÕES
A combinação de trimetoprima/sulfa pode provocar efeitos colaterais (ceratoconjuntivite seca, discrasias sanguíneas, poliartrite) quando administrada por mais de 4 semanas.

ACOMPANHAMENTO
MONITORIZAÇÃO DO PACIENTE
Submeter a urina a culturas e efetuar urinálises durante a administração de antibióticos (~5-7 dias no tratamento) e 1-4 semanas depois de terminados os antibióticos.

PREVENÇÃO
Eliminar os fatores predisponentes da infecção do trato urinário; corrigir os ureteres ectópicos.

COMPLICAÇÕES POSSÍVEIS
Insuficiência renal, pielonefrite recidivante, nefrolitíase por estruvita, septicemia, choque séptico, infecção metastática (p. ex., endocardite, poliartrite).

EVOLUÇÃO ESPERADA E PROGNÓSTICO
- Pacientes com pielonefrite aguda ou subaguda — razoável a bom, com retorno à saúde normal, a menos que o paciente também tenha nefrolitíase, insuficiência renal crônica ou alguma outra causa subjacente para infecção do trato urinário (p. ex., obstrução ou neoplasia).
- Pode não ser uma tarefa fácil resolver uma infecção crônica estabelecida da medula renal por causa da baixa penetração tecidual de antibióticos.
- Pacientes com insuficiência renal crônica provocada pela pielonefrite — prognóstico determinado pela gravidade e velocidade de evolução da insuficiência renal crônica.
- A pielonefrite recidivante será provável caso não se removam os nefrólitos infectados.

DIVERSOS
DISTÚRBIOS ASSOCIADOS
Hiperadrenocorticismo, administração exógena de glicocorticoides, insuficiência renal crônica, hipertireoidismo (gatos) e diabetes melito estão associados à infecção do trato urinário, a qual pode ascender para os ureteres e rins.

GESTAÇÃO/FERTILIDADE/REPRODUÇÃO
Utilizar antibióticos que sejam seguros para a cadela ou a gata prenhes.

SINÔNIMO(S)
Infecção do trato urinário superior, pielite.

VER TAMBÉM
- Capítulos sobre Infecção do Trato Urinário Inferior.
- Insuficiência Renal Crônica.
- Nefrolitíase.
- Obstrução do Trato Urinário.
- Urolitíase por Estruvita — Cães.
- Urolitíase por Estruvita — Gatos.

ABREVIATURA(S)
- PU/PD = poliúria/polidipsia.

Sugestões de Leitura
Bartges JW. Urinary tract infection. In: Ettinger SJ, Feldman EC, eds., Textbook of Veterinary Internal Medicine, 6th ed. St. Louis: Elsevier, 2005, pp. 1800-1808.
Neuwirth L, Mahaffey M, Crowell W, et al. Comparison of excretory urography and ultrasonography for detection of experimentally induced pyelonephritis in dogs. Am J Vet Res 1993, 54:660-669.
Senior DF. Management of difficult urinary tract infections. In: Bonagura JD, ed., Current Veterinary Therapy XIII. Philadelphia: Saunders, 2000, pp. 883-886.

Autores Carl A. Osborne e Larry G. Adams
Consultor Editorial Carl A. Osborne

PIODERMITE

CONSIDERAÇÕES GERAIS

DEFINIÇÃO
- Infecção bacteriana da pele. • Piodermite superficial — envolve a epiderme e o folículo intacto.
- Piodermite profunda — envolve a derme e, possivelmente, o subcutâneo.

FISIOPATOLOGIA
As infecções cutâneas ocorrem em casos de perda da integridade da superfície da pele, maceração da pele por exposição crônica à umidade, alteração populacional da flora bacteriana residente, comprometimento da circulação ou impacto negativo sobre a imunocompetência do paciente causado por doença sistêmica ou terapia imunossupressora.

SISTEMA(S) ACOMETIDO(S)
Pele/exócrino.

GENÉTICA
N/D.

INCIDÊNCIA/PREVALÊNCIA
- Cães — muito comum.
- Gatos — rara.

DISTRIBUIÇÃO GEOGRÁFICA
N/D.

IDENTIFICAÇÃO
Espécies
Cães e gatos.

Raça(s) Predominante(s)
- Cães — raças de pelagem curta, especialmente aquelas com dobras cutâneas excessivas.
- Pastor alemão — piodermite profunda e grave que só responde parcialmente a antibióticos e, com frequência, pode sofrer recidiva.

Idade Média e Faixa Etária
A idade de início costuma estar diretamente relacionada com a causa subjacente.

Sexo Predominante
N/D.

SINAIS CLÍNICOS
Comentários Gerais
- Superficial — geralmente envolve o tronco; a extensão das lesões pode ficar escondida pela pelagem.
- Profunda — frequentemente acomete o queixo, a ponte nasal, os pontos de pressão e os pés; pode ser generalizada e associada a sintomas de doença sistêmica, como pirexia e/ou dor.

Achados Anamnésicos
- Início agudo ou gradual.
- Prurido variável — infecção tipicamente pruriginosa; no entanto, a causa subjacente pode induzir ao prurido ou, então, a infecção estafilocócica em si pode gerar esse sinal; se associada à hipercortisolemia, a infecção poderá não ser pruriginosa.

Achados do Exame Físico
- Pápulas.
- Pústulas.
- Pápulas crostosas.
- Crostas.
- Colaretes epidérmicos.
- Manchas (máculas) eritematosas ou hiperpigmentadas circulares.
- Alopecia, pelagem com aspecto roído por traça.
- Bolhas hemorrágicas.
- Descamação.
- Liquenificação.
- Lesões em alvo.
- Abscesso.
- Furunculose, celulite.

CAUSAS
- *Staphylococcus pseudintermedius* — mais frequente.
- *Pasteurella multocida* — patógeno importante nos gatos.
- Piodermite profunda — pode ser complicada por microrganismos Gram-negativos (p. ex., *Escherichia coli*, *Proteus* spp. e *Pseudomonas* spp.).
- Raramente provocada por bactérias superiores (p. ex., *Actinomyces*, *Nocardia*, *Mycobacteria* e *Actinobacillus*).

FATORES DE RISCO
- Alergias — dermatite alérgica a pulgas; dermatite atópica; reação cutânea adversa a alimentos; dermatite alérgica por contato.
- Parasitas — especialmente *Demodex* spp.
- Infecção fúngica — dermatofitose (*Microsporum canis*, *Microsporum gypseum*, ou *Trichophyton mentagrophytes*) é mais comum.
- Endocrinopatias — hipotireoidismo; hiperadrenocorticismo; desequilíbrio dos hormônios sexuais em animais intactos.
- Imunossupressão — terapia com glicocorticoides; animais jovens.
- Seborreia — acne, síndrome do comedão do Schnauzer.
- Conformação — pelagem curta; dobras cutâneas; pele interdigital em excesso.
- Traumatismo — pontos de pressão; cuidados de embelezamento do pelo (banho e tosa); arranhões; comportamento de fuçar; fatores irritantes.
- Corpo estranho — cauda-de-raposa [planta]; farpas de gramíneas.

DIAGNÓSTICO

DIAGNÓSTICO DIFERENCIAL
- Alergia — prurido geralmente precede a erupção cutânea; no entanto, o prurido não desaparecerá com a resolução da piodermite.
- Endocrinopatia — piodermite recidivante; considerar se o prurido desaparecer com a resolução da piodermite; pode estar associada a sintomas sistêmicos.
- Dermatite alérgica a pulgas ou atopia — podem ser sazonais.
- Doenças pustulares — piodermite estafilocócica superficial; dermatofitose; demodicose; pênfigo foliáceo; e dermatose pustular subcorneal.
- Furunculose — piodermite estafilocócica profunda; infecção por bactérias superiores; demodicose; dermatofitoses; infecções fúngicas oportunistas; infecções fúngicas profundas; paniculite; e dermatose responsiva ao zinco.
- A piodermite superficial em raças de pelagem curta quase sempre é diagnosticada incorretamente como urticária, por causa do início agudo de pápulas pruriginosas e tufos foliculares que podem mimetizar as lesões de urticária.

HEMOGRAMA/BIOQUÍMICA/URINÁLISE
- Superficial — normais ou podem refletir a causa subjacente (p. ex., anemia gerada por hipotireoidismo; leucograma de estresse e elevação da fosfatase alcalina sérica atribuídos ao hiperadrenocorticismo; eosinofilia decorrente de parasitismo).
- Generalizada, profunda — pode revelar leucocitose com desvio regenerativo à esquerda e hiperglobulinemia; além disso, pode haver alterações relacionadas com a causa subjacente.

OUTROS TESTES LABORATORIAIS
N/D.

DIAGNÓSTICO POR IMAGEM
N/D.

MÉTODOS DIAGNÓSTICOS
- Raspados cutâneos, tricogramas, cultura para dermatófitos, citologia da superfície cutânea, citologia de pápula/pústula, teste alérgico intradérmico, ensaio alimentar hipoalergênico (dieta de eliminação), testes endócrinos — para identificar a causa subjacente.
- Biopsia cutânea — raramente é útil a menos que a infecção seja de natureza profunda.
- Esfregaço direto de pústula intacta — neutrófilos com bactérias intracelulares, tipicamente cocos.
- Citologia — utilizada para ajudar a diferenciar pênfigo foliáceo (queratinócitos acantolíticos) e infecções fúngicas profundas (blastomicose, criptococose) de piodermites; grãos teciduais podem identificar microrganismos filamentosos característicos de bactérias superiores.

Cultura
- Geralmente positiva para *S. pseudintermedius*.
- Outros microrganismos Gram-negativos, além de estafilococos e bactérias superiores, podem ser obtidos na cultura de lesões de piodermite profunda.
- Conteúdo de pústula intacta — resultados mais confiáveis para infecções superficiais.
- Biopsia por saca-bocado (também conhecido como *punch*) obtida com técnica estéril para cultura de tecido macerado, especialmente em caso de piodermite profunda — indicada para infecção superficial caso não se observe nenhuma pústula; é muito provável que forneça resultados falso-negativos.
- Exsudato recém-coletado de trajeto drenante ou debaixo de crosta — pode recuperar o patógeno ou, potencialmente, algum contaminante se a lesão não estiver intacta; método menos confiável.

ACHADOS PATOLÓGICOS
- Pústulas subcorneais.
- Microabscessos neutrofílicos intraepidérmicos.
- Perifoliculite.
- Foliculite.
- Furunculose.
- Dermatite nodular a difusa.
- Paniculite.
- Reação inflamatória — supurativa ou piogranulomatosa.
- Grãos teciduais dentro de piogranulomas — observados mais frequentemente com *Staphylococcus*, *Actinomyces*, *Actinobacillus* e *Nocardia*.
- Colorações especiais — usadas para identificar bactérias Gram-negativas ou microrganismos acidorresistentes.

TRATAMENTO

CUIDADO(S) DE SAÚDE ADEQUADO(S)
Geralmente em um esquema ambulatorial, exceto nos casos de piodermite profunda generalizada grave.

PIODERMITE

CUIDADO(S) DE ENFERMAGEM
- Profunda, generalizada, grave — pode necessitar de fluidos IV, antibióticos parenterais ou banhos diários com banheira de hidromassagem.
- Xampus de peróxido de benzoíla ou de clorexidina — remover os debris superficiais.
- Banhos com banheiras de hidromassagem — piodermites profundas; removem os exsudatos com crostas; estimulam a drenagem; diminuem a inflamação e aumentam a oxigenação tecidual.

ATIVIDADE
Sem restrição.

DIETA
- Dieta com nova fonte proteica ou hidrolisado proteico em caso de piodermite secundária à reação cutânea adversa a alimentos; caso contrário, forneça ração bem balanceada de alta qualidade.
- Evitar o consumo de alto teor proteico, dietas baratas de má qualidade e suplementação excessiva.

ORIENTAÇÃO AO PROPRIETÁRIO
N/D.

CONSIDERAÇÕES CIRÚRGICAS
As piodermites em dobras cutâneas podem necessitar de correção cirúrgica para evitar recidivas. Uma terapia tópica diária de manutenção pode ajudar a diminuir a gravidade e a frequência de recidivas.

MEDICAÇÕES
MEDICAMENTO(S) DE ESCOLHA
- Isolamentos de *S. pseudintermedius* — geralmente suscetíveis a cefalosporinas, cloxacilina, oxacilina, meticilina, amoxicilina-clavulanato, eritromicina, clindamicina e cloranfenicol; um pouco menos responsivos à lincomicina e trimetoprima-sulfonamida; frequentemente resistentes a amoxicilina, ampicilina, penicilina, tetraciclina e sulfonamidas.
- Amoxicilina-clavulanato — a maior parte dos isolamentos de *Staphylococcus* e *P. multocida* são suscetíveis; geralmente eficazes para infecções cutâneas nos gatos.
- Superficial — pode ser tratada inicialmente de modo empírico, fazendo uso de um dos antibióticos supramencionados.
- Recidivante, resistente ou profunda — selecionar a antibioticoterapia com base nos resultados da cultura e do antibiograma.
- Múltiplos microrganismos com sensibilidades antibióticas diferentes — escolher o antibiótico tendo como base a suscetibilidade estafilocócica.

CONTRAINDICAÇÕES
Terapia com corticosteroides — pode estimular a resistência e a recidiva mesmo quando utilizados concomitantemente com os antibióticos.

PRECAUÇÕES
- Cefalosporinas, eritromicina, lincomicina, clindamicina e oxacilina — vômito; administrar com alimento.
- Aminoglicosídeos — toxicidade renal geralmente impede o uso sistêmico prolongado.
- Trimetoprima-sulfa — ceratoconjuntivite seca, febre, hepatotoxicidade, poliartrite e anormalidades hematológicas, especialmente neutropenia.
- Cloranfenicol — utilizar com cuidado nos gatos; pode provocar leve anemia reversível nos cães; associado à anemia aplásica em seres humanos.

INTERAÇÕES POSSÍVEIS
Trimetoprima-sulfametoxazol — pode induzir a resultados falsamente diminuídos nas provas de função da tireoide.

MEDICAMENTO(S) ALTERNATIVO(S)
Bacterina (Staphage Lysate®), Staphoid AB® ou bacterinas autógenas — podem melhorar a eficácia do antibiótico e reduzir a recidiva em uma pequena porcentagem dos casos, dependendo da identificação e do tratamento bem-sucedido da causa subjacente.

ACOMPANHAMENTO
MONITORIZAÇÃO DO PACIENTE
Administrar os antibióticos por, no mínimo, 7-10 dias além da cura clínica; aproximadamente 3-4 semanas para piodermites superficiais; 6-10 semanas para piodermites profundas.

PREVENÇÃO
- Banho de rotina com xampu de peróxido de benzoíla ou de clorexidina — pode ajudar a evitar recidivas.
- Cama almofadada — pode facilitar a cura das piodermites nos pontos de pressão; considerar o uso desse tipo de cama em má cicatrização de feridas, como nos casos de hipotireoidismo.
- Aplicação tópica de gel de peróxido de benzoíla ou de pomada de mupirocina a 2% pode ser uma terapia adjuvante útil.
- A identificação e o tratamento da causa subjacente são cruciais para evitar recidiva.

COMPLICAÇÕES POSSÍVEIS
Bacteremia e septicemia.

EVOLUÇÃO ESPERADA E PROGNÓSTICO
Se a causa não for identificada e tratada de forma eficaz, será provável a ocorrência de recidiva ou a ausência de resposta.

DIVERSOS
DISTÚRBIOS ASSOCIADOS
N/D.

FATORES RELACIONADOS COM A IDADE
- Impetigo — acomete cães jovens antes da puberdade; pode estar associado a más condições de higiene; quase sempre necessita apenas de tratamento tópico.
- Dermatite pustular superficial — ocorre nos filhotes felinos; associada à "lambedura" exagerada pela gata.
- Piodermite secundária à dermatite atópica — geralmente começa entre 1 e 3 anos de idade.
- Piodermite secundária a distúrbios endócrinos — inicia, em geral, na metade da fase adulta.

POTENCIAL ZOONÓTICO
- Tuberculose cutânea — rara.
- Lepra felina — desconhecida.

GESTAÇÃO/FERTILIDADE/REPRODUÇÃO
N/D.

VER TAMBÉM
- Acne — Cães.
- Acne — Gatos.
- Fístula Perianal.
- Pododermatite.

Sugestões de Leitura
Scott DW, Miller WH, Griffin CE. Small Animal Dermatology, 6th ed. Philadelphia: Saunders, 2001.

Autor Elizabeth R. May
Consultor Editorial Alexander H. Werner

Piometra e Hiperplasia Endometrial Cística

CONSIDERAÇÕES GERAIS

DEFINIÇÃO
- Hiperplasia endometrial cística — alteração patológica progressiva no revestimento uterino mediada por via hormonal.
- Piometra — secundária à hiperplasia endometrial cística ou endometrite; desenvolve-se quando a invasão bacteriana do endométrio anormal leva ao acúmulo intraluminal de exsudato purulento.

FISIOPATOLOGIA
- Cadelas com ciclos normais — diestro de dois meses, com secreção ovariana de progesterona após cada ciclo estral.
- Exposição repetida do endométrio a altas concentrações de estrogênio, seguida por concentrações elevadas de progesterona sem prenhez — acarreta hiperplasia endometrial cística.
- Bactérias — as secreções uterinas representam um excelente meio para o crescimento desses microrganismos; ascendem a partir da vagina pela cérvix parcialmente aberta durante o proestro e o estro; flora vaginal normal; a *Escherichia coli* constitui o isolamento mais comum.

SISTEMA(S) ACOMETIDO(S)
- Reprodutivo.
- Renal/urológico.
- Hemático/linfático/imune.
- Hepatobiliar.

GENÉTICA
Nenhuma predisposição conhecida.

INCIDÊNCIA/PREVALÊNCIA
Incidência — não pode ser feita uma estimativa exata, já que a maioria das cadelas e gatas nos Estados Unidos é submetida à ovário-histerectomia eletiva.

IDENTIFICAÇÃO
Espécies
Canina e felina.

Idade Média e Faixa Etária
- Acomete geralmente animais com mais de 6 anos de idade.
- Fêmeas jovens — especialmente quando tratadas com estrogênio ou progesterona exógena.
- Cadelas — diagnosticadas, em geral, 1-12 semanas após o estro.
- Gatas — o início em relação ao estro é mais variável.
- Piometra do coto uterino nas fêmeas castradas — pode-se desenvolver a qualquer momento depois da ovário-histerectomia.

Sexo Predominante
Apenas fêmeas.

SINAIS CLÍNICOS
Achados Anamnésicos
- Cérvix fechada — sinais de doença sistêmica, que evoluem para sinais de septicemia e choque.

Achados do Exame Físico
- Útero — aumentado de volume em termos palpáveis; a palpação cuidadosa pode permitir a determinação do tamanho; a palpação muito intensa pode induzir à ruptura; com a cérvix aberta, esse órgão pode não estar grande de modo palpável.
- Corrimento vaginal — depende da desobstrução da cérvix uterina; sanguinolento a mucopurulento.
- Depressão e letargia.
- Anorexia.
- Poliúria e polidipsia.
- Vômito.
- Distensão abdominal.

CAUSAS
- Cadelas — a simples exposição repetida do endométrio ao estrogênio, seguida pela exposição à progesterona.
- Gatas — pode ser o resultado do estrogênio durante o estro, seguido pela fase progestacional, provocada pela indução da ovulação pelo coito, ovulação espontânea ou por outros estímulos (até agora indefinidos).

FATORES DE RISCO
- Fêmeas idosas nulíparas podem estar predispostas.
- Utilização farmacológica de aplicações do estrogênio (acasalamento indesejável) na metade do estro ao início do diestro.
- Nenhuma correlação com a pseudociese nas cadelas.

DIAGNÓSTICO

DIAGNÓSTICO DIFERENCIAL
- Prenhez.
- Outras causas de poliúria e polidipsia — diabetes melito; hiperadrenocorticismo; nefropatia primária.
- Vaginopatia grave.
- Hidrometra (secreção intrauterina serosa); mucometra (secreção intrauterina mucoide); hematometra (secreção intrauterina hemorrágica).

HEMOGRAMA/BIOQUÍMICA/URINÁLISE
- Neutrofilia — imatura; observada em 74% dos casos; mais grave com a cérvix fechada.
- Leve anemia normocítica e normocrômica.
- Hiperglobulinemia e hiperproteinemia.
- Azotemia.
- ALT e fosfatase alcalina — elevadas nos casos de septicemia ou desidratação grave.
- Distúrbios eletrolíticos — dependem da evolução clínica.
- Urinálise — coletar amostra por cateterização vesical (menos traumática e mais precisa em termos diagnósticos).

OUTROS TESTES LABORATORIAIS
- Exame citológico do corrimento vulvar — células polimorfonucleares degenerativas e bactérias; podem não ser distinguíveis do corrimento purulento associado à vaginopatia (p. ex., vaginite, massa vaginal, corpo estranho e anomalia anatômica vaginal).
- Exames de cultura e antibiograma do corrimento vulvar — não ajudam a confirmar o diagnóstico (as bactérias obtidas em cultura costumam fazer parte da flora vaginal normal); valiosos na determinação de antibióticos adequados.
- Teste sorológico para *Brucella canis* — teste de aglutinação rápida em lâmina utilizado para triagem; sensível, porém inespecífico. Quando positivo, reavaliar pelo teste de imunodifusão em ágar gel ou cultura bacteriana do sangue total, de aspirado de linfonodo ou do corrimento vulvar.
- Os metabólitos da prostaglandina F_2 encontram-se elevados em cadelas com piometra, em comparação àquelas com hidrometra ou mucometra.

DIAGNÓSTICO POR IMAGEM
Radiografia
- Detectar o útero grande.
- Descartar a prenhez — 45 dias após a ovulação; 43-54 dias após o acasalamento.
- Piometra — o útero pode aparecer como uma estrutura tubular distendida na porção caudal do abdome ventral.

Ultrassonografia
- Avaliar o tamanho do útero e a extensão da hiperplasia endometrial cística; a natureza do conteúdo uterino.
- Descartar a prenhez — 20-24 dias depois da ovulação.
- Parede uterina normal — não é visível como uma entidade distinta.
- Piometra ou hiperplasia endometrial cística — associada à parede uterina espessada (com ou sem áreas císticas hipoecoicas) e ao líquido luminal.
- Piometra — pode ocorrer na prenhez das cadelas (rara).

MÉTODOS DIAGNÓSTICOS
Vaginoscopia — indicada somente nas cadelas com corrimento vulvar purulento e sem aumento de volume uterino aparente; permite a determinação do local de origem do corrimento vulvar; não é possível nas gatas.

ACHADOS PATOLÓGICOS
- Endométrio (cadelas e gatas) — descrito sob a forma de paralelepípedos (ambas as condições).
- Superfície endometrial cística — recoberta por exsudato mucopurulento de odor fétido; espessada por causa do tamanho aumentado da glândula endometrial e da distensão glandular cística.

TRATAMENTO

CUIDADO(S) DE SAÚDE ADEQUADO(S)
- Paciente internada.
- Piometra — condição com risco de morte caso a cérvix esteja fechada.

CUIDADO(S) DE ENFERMAGEM
Cuidados de suporte — administração imediata de fluidos intravenosos e de antibióticos.

ORIENTAÇÃO AO PROPRIETÁRIO
- Informar ao proprietário que a ovário-histerectomia é o tratamento preferido.
- O tratamento clínico é recomendado apenas para animais valiosos em termos reprodutivos, que não se encontrem em azotemia e não tenham a cérvix fechada; avisar o proprietário que os medicamentos supressores do estro não progestacionais devem ser administrados por toda a vida, exceto quando há intenções de acasalamento.
- Esclarecer o proprietário sobre o fato de que o tratamento clínico da piometra com a cérvix fechada pode estar associado à ruptura do útero e ao desenvolvimento de peritonite (ver a seção "Contraindicações").
- Passar para o proprietário a informação de que o tratamento clínico provavelmente não cura a hiperplasia endometrial cística subjacente nas pacientes com a cérvix aberta ou fechada, mas pode permitir que algumas cadelas acometidas se reproduzam.

Piometra e Hiperplasia Endometrial Cística

CONSIDERAÇÕES CIRÚRGICAS
- Piometra (cérvix aberta ou fechada) — a ovário-histerectomia é o tratamento preferido; doença progressiva crônica.
- Piometra com a cérvix fechada — é preciso ter cuidado durante a ovário-histerectomia; o útero aumentado de volume pode estar friável.
- Ruptura do útero ou extravasamento de material purulento do coto uterino — lavagem repetida da cavidade peritoneal com solução salina estéril.

MEDICAÇÕES
MEDICAMENTO(S) DE ESCOLHA
Antibióticos
- Empíricos, dependendo dos resultados da cultura e do antibiograma.
- Todas as pacientes com piometra.
- Escolhas comuns — ampicilina (20 mg/kg VO a cada 8 h); enrofloxacino (Baytril®; 2,5 mg/kg VO a cada 12 h).

Prostaglandinas
$PGF_{2\alpha}$
- As dosagens recomendadas abaixo são apenas para o composto original; as dosagens para os compostos análogos diferem.
- Gatas — 0,1-0,5 mg/kg SC a cada 12-24 h durante 2-5 dias até que o tamanho do útero chegue próximo ao normal.
- Cadelas — 0,05-0,25 mg/kg SC a cada 12-24 h por 2-7 dias até que o útero esteja próximo do tamanho normal, conforme determinado pelos exames de palpação, radiografia ou ultrassonografia ou, então, até que nenhum líquido intrauterino seja visualizado pelo ultrassom.
- Na fase luteal (progesterona sérica > 2 ng/mL) — pode-se utilizar a dose de 0,05-0,25 mg/kg SC a cada 12 h durante 4 dias.
- Administração uma vez ao dia — causa contrações dos músculos lisos e consequente esvaziamento uterino.
- Administração duas vezes ao dia — provoca luteólise e subsequente diminuição na concentração da progesterona sérica.
- Reavaliar a paciente a cada 2-4 semanas após a interrupção; se o útero estiver aumentado de tamanho ou se a paciente ainda tiver corrimento vulvar acentuado, o protocolo poderá ser repetido.
- Ovário-histerectomia — realizada nas pacientes refratárias ao tratamento com a prostaglandina, isto é, se o útero ainda estiver aumentado de volume ou preenchido com líquido ou, então, se houver corrimento vulvar depois de duas aplicações do tratamento.

Cloprostenol
- Cadelas — 1 μg/kg SC diariamente por 7-14 dias.

Diversos
- Aglepristona (10 mg/kg SC nos dias 1, 2 e 8) — a eficácia é intensificada com o uso concomitante de prostaglandina.
- Cabergolina (5 μg/kg VO diariamente por 7-14 dias) é utilizada concomitantemente com a prostaglandina.

CONTRAINDICAÇÕES
- $PGF_{2\alpha}$ e cloprostenol com piometra de cérvix fechada — as fortes contrações do miométrio podem provocar a ruptura uterina ou forçar o exsudato purulento pelos oviductos, provocando peritonite secundária
- $PGF_{2\alpha}$ e cloprostenol em animal valioso para a reprodução — sempre descartar a prenhez antes da administração.

PRECAUÇÕES
- $PGF_{2\alpha}$ e cloprostenol — não são aprovados para uso em cadelas e gatas.
- Efeitos colaterais das prostaglandinas atribuíveis à contração da musculatura lisa incluem hipersalivação; êmese; defecação; lambedura intensa da pelagem dos flancos e da vulva (nas gatas); aparecem minutos após a injeção; desaparecem em 30-60 minutos; a gravidade diminui ao longo do esquema terapêutico; esses efeitos podem ser reduzidos diluindo-se o medicamento em volume equivalente de solução salina estéril antes da injeção subcutânea e caminhando com o animal durante 20-30 minutos depois da injeção.

MEDICAMENTO(S) ALTERNATIVO(S)
- Medicamentos que aumentem a resposta imune (p. ex., estrogênios) ou agentes não prostanoides que induzam a contratilidade do miométrio (p. ex., ocitocina e alcaloides do ergot) — não são confiáveis.
- Antibióticos — não são eficazes como tratamento único a menos que o útero se apresente com o tamanho normal e a progesterona sérica se encontre <2 ng/mL.

ACOMPANHAMENTO
MONITORIZAÇÃO DA PACIENTE
- Dar alta hospitalar quando o útero estiver próximo ao tamanho normal ou quando nenhum líquido intrauterino for visualizado pelo ultrassom e quando os sinais clínicos tiverem diminuído em termos de gravidade ou desaparecido; reavaliar depois de 2-4 semanas.
- Antibióticos — a administração é mantida por 3-4 semanas.
- Corrimento vulvar — pode persistir por até 4 semanas.
- Hemogramas completos seriados — o leucograma aumenta de forma abrupta depois da ovário-histerectomia, porque a medula óssea continua liberando neutrófilos polimorfonucleares na corrente sanguínea, os quais não conseguem mais entrar no útero.

PREVENÇÃO
- Proestro seguinte — obter amostra da parte anterior da vagina para a realização de cultura bacteriana, utilizando *swab* de cultura protegido e reservado para isso.
- Tratar a cadela com antibiótico apropriado durante 3 semanas.
- Acasalar durante o estro imediatamente após o tratamento — o útero gravídico pode ser menos suscetível à reinfecção; a cadela com hiperplasia endometrial cística subjacente possui vida reprodutiva limitada (é melhor obter o número desejado de filhotes o mais rápido possível); a cadela pode não se livrar espontaneamente da doença se deixada sem cruzamento no ciclo estral.

COMPLICAÇÕES POSSÍVEIS
A cadela pode entrar no estro logo antes do previsto após o tratamento se a terapia clínica induziu à luteólise prematura.

EVOLUÇÃO ESPERADA E PROGNÓSTICO
- Cadelas — a hiperplasia endometrial cística subjacente ainda subsiste; há predisposição à recidiva; acasalar a paciente com os machos desejados de forma sincronizada; a ovário-histerectomia é recomendada assim que a vida reprodutiva chegar ao fim; a utilização de machos subférteis não é recomendada.
- Relação de proteína: creatinina urinária superior a 10 — foi associada subsequentemente a um aumento na incidência de insuficiência renal em estágio terminal.

DIVERSOS
DISTÚRBIOS ASSOCIADOS
Piometra do coto uterino nas cadelas castradas — pode-se desenvolver a qualquer momento depois da ovário-histerectomia; pode estar associada a resquício(s) ovariano(s).

GESTAÇÃO/FERTILIDADE/REPRODUÇÃO
$PGF_{2\alpha}$ — sempre descartar a prenhez antes da administração do produto em animais valiosos para acasalamento; agente eficaz para interrupção da prenhez.

ABREVIATURA(S)
- ALT = alanina aminotransferase.
- $PGF_{2\alpha}$ = prostaglandina $F_{2\alpha}$.

Sugestões de Leitura
Fieni F. Clinical evaluation of the use of aglepristone, with or without cloprostenol, to treat cystic endometrial hyperplasia-pyovmetra complex in bitches. Theriogenology 2006, 66(6-7):1550-1556.

Hardy RM, Osborne CA. Canine pyometra: Pathophysiology, diagnosis and treatment of uterine and extrauterine lesions. JAAHA 1974, 10:245-268.

Johnston SD, Root Kustritz MV, Olson PN. Disorders of the canine uterus and uterine tubes (oviducts). In: Canine and Feline Theriogenology. Philadelphia: Saunders, 2001, pp. 206-224.

Autor Margaret V. Root Kustritz
Consultor Editorial Sara K. Lyle

PIOTÓRAX

CONSIDERAÇÕES GERAIS

DEFINIÇÃO
Acúmulo de inflamação supurativa séptica dentro da cavidade pleural.

FISIOPATOLOGIA
• Infecciosa — surge, em geral, de inoculação transpulmonar, transesofágica ou transtorácica de bactérias no espaço pleural, com subsequente pleurite supurativa.
• Cães — comumente associado a farpas de gramíneas ou outros objetos estranhos inalados e a feridas penetrantes do tórax.
• Gatos — mais comumente associado a feridas penetrantes por mordida, corpos estranhos ou, possivelmente, por extensão de pneumonia para o espaço pleural após aspiração da flora orofaríngea.
• Outras causas tanto nos cães como nos gatos — incluem extensão de discospondilite, perfuração esofágica, migração parasitária ou disseminação hematógena.

SISTEMA(S) ACOMETIDO(S)
• Respiratório.
• Hemático/linfático/imune.
• Renal/urológico — glomerulopatia com perda de proteína.

DISTRIBUIÇÃO GEOGRÁFICA
Spirocerca lupi deve ser considerado como uma causa predisponente em áreas endêmicas (África, Ásia, sudeste dos EUA).

IDENTIFICAÇÃO

Espécies
Cães e gatos.

Raça(s) Predominante(s)
• Cães — raças de caça e de esporte; especificamente, Labrador retriever, Springer spaniel e Border collie são as raças mais comumente relatadas.
• Gatos — doméstico de pelo curto.

Idade Média e Faixa Etária
Média de ~4 anos, embora haja uma ampla variação.

Sexo Predominante
Os animais machos são super-representados.

SINAIS CLÍNICOS

Comentários Gerais
• Frequentemente de início insidioso, com poucos sinais clínicos até bem tarde na evolução da doença.
• Comprometimento respiratório — em geral não é grave a menos que a doença esteja em estado avançado.
• Sinais de vômito/diarreia — podem ser a queixa principal inicial em 25% dos casos caninos.

Achados Anamnésicos
• Atividade diminuída.
• Colapso após o exercício e recuperação lenta.
• Perda de peso e anorexia parcial podem ser os únicos sinais clínicos.
• Melhora temporária com antibioticoterapia.
• Confirmar o histórico de brigas ou feridas perfurantes.

Achados do Exame Físico
• Taquipneia — em geral, aparente; pode ser leve e não associada à dificuldade respiratória.
• Caquexia — observada com frequência.
• Tosse — pode ser observada.
• Pirexia — geralmente de baixo grau, pode ser observada.
• Auscultação torácica — pode revelar sons cardíacos abafados, ruídos pulmonares diminuídos ventralmente e ruídos pulmonares amplificados dorsalmente.
• Gatos — podem apresentar poucos sinais clínicos antes do início de angústia respiratória aparentemente aguda, colapso e choque séptico; bradicardia e hipersalivação associadas a desfechos insatisfatórios.
• Lesão da parede torácica — pode não ser aparente ou estar cicatrizada no momento do exame.
• Realizar palpação e inspeção rigorosas do tórax em busca de indícios de formação cicatricial ou celulite.

CAUSAS
• Infecciosas — cães: *Actinomyces* spp., *Nocardia* spp., Anaeróbios (*Bacteroides*, *Peptostreptococcus*, *Fusobacterium*), *Corynebacterium*, *Escherichia coli*, *Pasteurella* e *Streptococcus* spp.; agentes fúngicos.
• Infecciosas — gatos: comensais bucais (p. ex., *Pasteurella multocida* e *Bacteroides* spp.) são mais comuns; anaeróbios obrigatórios (*Peptostreptococcus*, *Fusobacterium*) são comuns.
• Parasitárias — cães: ruptura esofágica de granuloma por *Spirocerca lupi*.
• Neoplásicas — raramente com tumores intratorácicos secundários a necrose tumoral.
• Torção de lobo pulmonar — ocasionalmente associada a piotórax.

FATORES DE RISCO
• Cães — de caça, testes a campo e outras atividades esportivas extenuantes ao ar livre; áreas endêmicas de *S. lupi*.
• Gatos — casas com muitos gatos, estilo de vida ao ar livre, pneumonia e infecção respiratória superior.

DIAGNÓSTICO

DIAGNÓSTICO DIFERENCIAL
• Outras efusões pleurais — quilotórax e hemotórax; exsudatos assépticos (PIF ou neoplasia); efusões transudativas; diferenciadas por exame citológico.
• Outras doenças sistêmicas devem ser consideradas na presença de achados inespecíficos.
• Em animais com sinais não localizados, devem-se considerar as doenças associadas à febre de origem desconhecida.

HEMOGRAMA/BIOQUÍMICA/URINÁLISE
• Leucocitose neutrofílica acentuada com desvio à esquerda, monocitose e anemia de doença crônica.
• Anemia regenerativa — pode ser observada em casos de hemorragia substancial na cavidade pleural.
• Hiperglobulinemia — possível em virtude de inflamação crônica.
• Hipoalbuminemia — como reagente negativo de fase aguda ou atribuída à perda renal, se a glomerulonefrite resultar de estimulação antigênica crônica.
• Fosfatase alcalina — levemente elevada por hipoxemia.
• Azotemia pré-renal — se o paciente estiver desidratado.
• Alterações orgânicas específicas — se outros órgãos estiverem secundariamente infectados (p. ex., pielonefrite e hepatite).
• Proteinúria — possível com glomerulonefropatia.

DIAGNÓSTICO POR IMAGEM
• Radiografia — efusão pleural uni ou bilateral com linhas de fissura pleural; lesões do parênquima pulmonar (consolidação, atelectasia, massas) são comuns; possíveis lesões mediastínicas.
• Ultrassonografia — efusão pleural; pode revelar quantidade acentuada de depósitos fibrinosos no espaço pleural; pode identificar massas pulmonares consolidadas, massas mediastínicas, e nódulos pulmonares abscedados ou neoplásicos.

MÉTODOS DIAGNÓSTICOS

Toracocentese
• Avaliação citológica — necessária para confirmar o diagnóstico, porque muitas efusões aparecem macroscopicamente hemorrágicas.
• Colorações de Gram — podem facilitar a identificação precoce de microrganismos patogênicos.
• Grânulos de sulfa (pequenos acúmulos de debris purulentos) no exsudato — característica de infecção por microrganismos filamentosos (p. ex., *Actinomyces* e *Nocardia*).
• Com frequência, observam-se microrganismos no exame citológico, muitas vezes dentro de neutrófilos degenerados.
• A efusão quase sempre tem odor fétido ou pútrido, especialmente nos gatos.

Microbiologia
• Submeter todas as amostras de líquido à cultura aeróbia e anaeróbia. Considerar a realização de cultura para *Mycoplasma* se as culturas-padrão forem negativas.
• Muitos dos microrganismos filamentosos, microaerófilos e anaeróbios são de crescimento lento, de forma que as culturas devem ser mantidas por mais tempo que as amostras-padrão.
• Grânulos de sulfa — a maceração pode facilitar o cultivo; contêm concentrações mais elevadas de bactérias.
• Populações bacterianas frequentemente mistas.
• Microrganismos fúngicos — a cultura depende da anamnese e da localização geográfica.
• Amostras de urina — submeter à cultura na suspeita de pielonefrite.

Esofagoscopia
• Na suspeita de *S. lupi*.

ACHADOS PATOLÓGICOS
• Pleurite fibrinosa e supurativa, com ou sem abscedação pulmonar.
• Glomerulonefrite.
• Trombose da veia cava caudal (rara).

TRATAMENTO

CUIDADO(S) DE SAÚDE ADEQUADO(S)
• Paciente internado — frequentemente durante vários dias a semanas.
• Tratar como qualquer abscesso; a drenagem é crítica, sem a qual é altamente improvável a resolução.
• Em alguns casos, há necessidade de exploração cirúrgica, debridamento e possível lobectomia.

PIOTÓRAX

CUIDADO(S) DE ENFERMAGEM
• Esvaziamento contínuo por sonda de toracostomia com sucção de baixa pressão através de sonda perfurada; utilizar sonda de grande calibre para minimizar a oclusão; continuar até que a drenagem líquida seja <2-3 mL/kg/dia e bactérias intracelulares não sejam mais observadas à coloração de Gram; a drenagem pode ser um pouco maior com sondas de borracha vermelha, porque são mais irritantes.
• Gatos — necessitam geralmente de anestesia geral para colocação da sonda.
• Cães com comprometimento respiratório grave — pode-se substituir a anestesia local e a analgesia regional pela anestesia geral.
• Radiografia torácica periódica — para garantir a colocação adequada da sonda e a ausência da formação de bolsa ou loculação de exsudatos; determinar a necessidade de colocação de sonda bilateral; registrar qualquer alteração patológica pulmonar primária que pode não estar aparente no exame inicial.
• Lavado torácico — a cada 6-8 h com solução salina estéril morna; pode ajudar a desfazer os debris consolidados. Considerar a adição de heparina (1.500 unidades/litro) ao fluido de lavagem.
• Tapotagem (percussão torácica rápida) — pode auxiliar na remoção de debris consolidados.
• Repetir a cultura bacteriana se o paciente não melhorar.

ATIVIDADE
• Paciente internado — estimular o paciente à prática de exercícios leves (10 min a cada 6-8 h); promove esforços ventilatórios e ajuda a desintegrar aderências pleurais.
• Depois da alta, aumentar gradualmente o exercício por 2-4 meses.

DIETA
• Alimento rico em calorias.
• A reposição proteica geralmente é desnecessária.

ORIENTAÇÃO AO PROPRIETÁRIO
Informar ao proprietário que o tratamento (hospitalar e ambulatorial) é demorado e dispendioso.

CONSIDERAÇÕES CIRÚRGICAS
• Cirurgia — espera-se uma taxa de cura mais elevada com a realização de procedimento cirúrgico na presença de abscesso pulmonar, fibrose pleural, torção de lobo pulmonar ou extensa loculação do pus ou em caso de envolvimento do mediastino.
• Corpo estranho identificado pela obtenção de imagens do tórax (radiografia, ultrassom, TC ou RM) — ficam indicadas a realização de toracotomia e a recuperação do corpo estranho; farpas de gramíneas são raramente encontradas, mesmo durante a cirurgia.

MEDICAÇÕES
MEDICAMENTO(S) DE ESCOLHA
Antimicrobianos
• Basicamente, a escolha é determinada pelos resultados *in vitro* do antibiograma.
• Patógeno específico sob suspeita — pode-se iniciar o tratamento antes que os resultados da cultura estejam disponíveis; escolher com base nas sensibilidades antibióticas comuns de microrganismos particulares; *Actinomyces* spp. e *Bacteroides* (não-*fragilis*) spp. quase sempre são suscetíveis à amoxicilina; *Nocardia* spp. frequentemente suscetíveis a sulfonamidas potencializadas; bactérias anaeróbias obrigatórias (incluindo *B. fragilis*) suscetíveis a amoxicilina- -ácido clavulânico, clindamicina, cloranfenicol e, em geral, metronidazol; *Pasteurella* spp. geralmente suscetíveis a penicilinas potencializadas.
• Ampicilina ou amoxicilina com inibidor da β-lactamase — boa escolha inicial para a maior parte dos pacientes; ampicilina e sulbactam (20 mg/kg IV a cada 8 h), seguidos por amoxicilina- ácido clavulânico (25 mg/kg VO a cada 8 h) quando as medicações puderem ser administradas por via oral.
• Trimetoprima-sulfa, aminoglicosídeos e quinolonas — geralmente são ineficazes.
• Ocasionalmente, há necessidade de múltiplos antibióticos.
• As dosagens são, em geral, elevadas (p. ex., amoxicilina, 40 mg/kg VO a cada 8 h) para permitir uma distribuição adequada na cavidade pleural; talvez haja necessidade de manutenção do medicamento por vários meses e, ocasionalmente, por tempo indefinido.

Analgésicos
• Necessários após toracotomia ou durante pleurocentese.
• No desconforto grave — pode-se usar emplasto de fentanila ou agentes intravenosos/ intramusculares. A eficácia da anestesia intrapleural (p. ex., bupivacaína misturada com o fluido do lavado) pode ser limitada pelas secreções purulentas.

CONTRAINDICAÇÕES
Glicocorticoides e agentes imunossupressores — evitar em caso de piotórax infeccioso.

PRECAUÇÕES
Sulfas potencializadas — podem estar associadas aos quadros de ceratoconjuntivite seca, poliartropatia, hipotireoidismo, trombocitopenia e anemia, especialmente com a utilização prolongada.

ACOMPANHAMENTO
MONITORIZAÇÃO DO PACIENTE
• Medir a produção de líquido torácico, a contagem de células no líquido pleural e a presença de bactérias para determinar o momento em que os drenos torácicos podem ser removidos. Produção decrescente de líquido, diminuição na contagem celular e ausência de bactérias geralmente observadas dentro de 4-7 dias indicam que os drenos podem ser removidos. O líquido deve ser enviado à cultura aeróbia e anaeróbia no momento da remoção do dreno.
• Avaliar as radiografias torácicas — assegurar o esvaziamento adequado do líquido.
• Antibióticos — continuar por 1 mês após o retorno do paciente ao estado clínico normal, a normalização do hemograma e a ausência de indícios radiográficos de novo acúmulo de líquido; a duração média do tratamento é de 3-4 meses, mas pode continuar por 6-12 meses ou mais.
• Avaliar o hemograma completo e as radiografias mensalmente — alterações radiográficas residuais podem ser permanentes, porém o líquido deve estar ausente.

PREVENÇÃO
Evitar atividade que predisponha o animal à doença (frequentemente essa medida não é prática).

COMPLICAÇÕES POSSÍVEIS
• Inserção incorreta da sonda de drenagem — pode impedir a drenagem adequada ou produzir pneumotórax; a colocação muito proximal (cranial) pode exercer pressão sobre as artérias e veias braquiais, resultando em edema unilateral do membro ou claudicação; laceração pulmonar durante a colocação.
• Piotórax persistente recidivante — compartimentalização do pus; interrupção prematura do tratamento; lesões pulmonares.
• Pleurite fibrosante crônica e baixo desempenho após recuperação aparente — podem ocasionalmente responder à cirurgia.
• Mediastinite persistente.

EVOLUÇÃO ESPERADA E PROGNÓSTICO
• Com tratamento rigoroso — prognóstico razoável a excelente (sobrevida de 60-90%).
• Apenas com antibioticoterapia intermitente repetida ou com drenagem inadequada — prognóstico mau.
• Retorno ao desempenho — depende da cronicidade da doença e do nível de tratamento.

DIVERSOS
DISTÚRBIOS ASSOCIADOS
• Abscedação retroperitoneal e discospondilite causada pela migração de corpo estranho pelo diafragma no espaço retroperitoneal — raramente observados.
• Glomerulonefropatia — reversível com resolução bem-sucedida do piotórax.

POTENCIAL ZOONÓTICO
Infecção fúngica durante o isolamento *in vitro*.

SINÔNIMO(S)
• Empiema.
• Pleurite supurativa.
• Pleurisia.

VER TAMBÉM
• Dispneia e Angústia Respiratória.
• Respiração Ofegante e Taquipneia.
• Efusão Pleural.
• Quilotórax.

ABREVIATURA(S)
• CID = coagulação intravascular disseminada.
• PIF = peritonite infecciosa felina.
• RM = ressonância magnética.
• TC = tomografia computadorizada.

Sugestões de Leitura
Barrs VR, Allan GS, Martin P, et al. Feline pyothorax: A retrospective study of 27 cases in Australia. J Feline Med Surg 2005, 7:211-222.
Rooney MB, Monnet E. Medical and surgical treatment of pyothorax in dogs: 26 cases (1991-2001). JAVMA 2002, 221:86-92.
Scott JA, Macintire DK. Canine pyothorax: Clinical presentation, diagnosis, and treatment. Compend Contin Educ Pract Vet 2003, 25:180-194.

Autor Catriona MacPhail
Consultor Editorial Lynelle R. Johnson

PITIOSE

CONSIDERAÇÕES GERAIS

DEFINIÇÃO
Doença infecciosa que acomete principalmente a pele ou o trato GI de cães e gatos. Causada pelo patógeno aquático *Pythium insidiosum*, microrganismo pertencente à classe dos Oomicetos.

FISIOPATOLOGIA
- Sabe-se que forma infectante do *P. insidiosum* é um zoósporo biflagelado móvel, que é liberado em ambientes de água quente e atraído quimiotaticamente para o tecido lesado e o pelo animal. Os animais provavelmente são infectados quando entram na água que contém zoósporos infectantes ou quando ingerem essa água.
- *P. insidiosum* é considerado um microrganismo mais patogênico do que oportunista, porque a imunossupressão não é pré-requisito para a infecção.
- No trato GI, a infecção pelo *P. insidiosum* provoca doença piogranulomatosa crônica, que se manifesta por espessamento transmural segmentar grave de uma ou mais áreas do estômago ou do intestino.
- Na pele, a pitiose tipicamente resulta no desenvolvimento de feridas que não cicatrizam e massas invasivas que contêm nódulos ulcerados e trajetos drenantes.

SISTEMA(S) ACOMETIDO(S)
- Formas GI e cutânea da doença são encontradas com frequência equivalente no cão. Nos gatos, os quais raramente são infectados, a forma cutânea é a mais comum. Com exceção da disseminação ocasional para os linfonodos regionais, a pitiose geralmente acomete apenas um sistema corporal em cada paciente.
- A pitiose GI acomete mais frequentemente a região do fluxo de saída gástrico, o intestino delgado proximal, a junção ileocólica ou o cólon. Muitas vezes, o mesentério circunjacente é envolvido. Raras vezes, o esôfago pode estar acometido.
- Nos cães com doença GI, eventos tromboembólicos locais induzidos por *P. insidiosum* ou por invasão vascular podem levar a isquemia da parede intestinal e perfuração do trato GI ou hemoabdome.
- Cães com pitiose cutânea são levados à consulta com maior frequência por causa de lesões cutâneas ou subcutâneas múltiplas ou solitárias envolvendo as extremidades, a inserção da cauda, a parte ventral do pescoço ou o períneo.
- Nos gatos, foram observadas lesões cutâneas ou massas subcutâneas envolvendo as regiões retrobulbar, periorbital ou nasofaríngea, a inserção da cauda ou os coxins plamoplantares. Lesões no trato GI são raras em gatos.
- O envolvimento multissistêmico é raro.

GENÉTICA
Embora os cães pertencentes a raças de grande porte sejam mais frequentemente acometidos, nenhuma predisposição genética foi comprovada.

INCIDÊNCIA/PREVALÊNCIA
- Dependem da distribuição geográfica.
- Os animais acometidos são levados à consulta com maior frequência por conta dos sinais de doença nos meses de outono ou no começo do inverno.

DISTRIBUIÇÃO GEOGRÁFICA
- A doença provocada por *P. insidiosum* ocorre principalmente nas regiões tropicais e subtropicais do mundo.
- Nos Estados Unidos, a pitiose ocorre mais frequentemente nos estados limítrofes com o Golfo do México; entretanto, foi comprovada nos estados de Oklahoma, Arkansas, Missouri, Kentucky, Tennessee, Carolinas do Norte e do Sul, Virgínia, sul de Indiana e Nova Jersey, Arizona e Califórnia.
- Fora dos Estados Unidos, a pitiose foi relatada em países como Austrália, Brasil, Birmânia, Colômbia, Costa Rica, Indonésia, Japão, Nova Guiné e Tailândia.

IDENTIFICAÇÃO

Espécies
Cães e, menos comumente, gatos.

Raça(s) Predominante(s)
- Cães pertencentes a raças de grande porte, especialmente aqueles utilizados para caça ou trabalho em testes a campo próximos a fontes de água.
- Os cães da raça Labrador retriever são superrepresentados.
- Os cães da raça Pastor alemão podem ser predispostos à pitiose cutânea.

Idade Média e Faixa Etária
É mais provável que os animais com <6 anos de idade sejam infectados.

Sexo Predominante
Os machos são acometidos com maior frequência do que as fêmeas, possivelmente por causa da exposição elevada.

SINAIS CLÍNICOS

Comentários Gerais
Os cães acometidos não costumam estar gravemente acometidos até o fim da evolução da doença.

Achados Anamnésicos
- Perda crônica de peso e ocorrência de vômito intermitente são os sinais mais comuns.
- A diarreia pode ser evidente se o cólon ou um amplo segmento do intestino delgado estiver acometido.
- Nota-se regurgitação em casos de doença esofágica rara.
- A doença cutânea caracteriza-se por nódulos que não cicatrizam, sofrem ulceração e drenam.

Achados do Exame Físico
Pitiose GI
- A emaciação é comum.
- Frequentemente, é palpável a presença de massa abdominal.
- Apesar da perda de peso grave, os cães acometidos geralmente permanecem espertos e alertas.
- Não costuma haver febre.
- Podem ocorrer sinais sistêmicos e dor abdominal com obstrução, infarto ou perfuração intestinal.

Pitiose Cutânea
- Lesões cutâneas ou subcutâneas aparecem como feridas que não cicatrizam; regiões úmidas e edematosas; ou nódulos pouco definidos que se tornam ulcerados.
- Com frequência, há múltiplos trajetos que drenam exsudato purulento ou serossanguinolento.

CAUSAS
P. insidiosum.

FATORES DE RISCO
- Exposição ambiental a áreas alagadiças, pantanosas, lagoas ou lagos contendo zoósporos infectantes.
- Atividades ao ar livre, como caça.

DIAGNÓSTICO

DIAGNÓSTICO DIFERENCIAL
Pitiose GI
- Obstrução intestinal provocada por corpo estranho ou intussuscepção crônica.
- Histoplasmose.
- Linfossarcoma gástrico ou intestinal.
- Carcinoma gástrico.
- Outra neoplasia GI.
- Enteropatia inflamatória.
- Basidiobolomicose, prototecose.
- Colite histiocítica ou idiopática.

Pitiose Cutânea
- Lagenidiose (provocada por patógenos oomicóticos do gênero *Lagenidium*).
- Zigomicose (infecções provocadas por *Basidiobolus* ou *Conidiobolus* spp.).
- Outras doenças cutâneas micóticas, como criptococose, coccidioidomicose, esporotricose, micetoma eumicótico e feoifomicose.
- Doenças cutâneas bacterianas nodulares, como actinomicose, micobacteriose, botriomicose e brucelose.
- Prototecose ou leishmaniose nodular.
- Doenças piogranulomatosas não infecciosas, como reação a corpo estranho, paniculite nodular idiopática, adenite nodular sebácea e síndrome do granuloma/piogranuloma estéril cutâneo canino.
- Neoplasia cutânea.
- Vasculite sistêmica e doença embólica cutânea.

HEMOGRAMA/BIOQUÍMICA/URINÁLISE
- Os achados laboratoriais são inespecíficos.
- Podem ocorrer eosinofilia, leucocitose e anemia de doença crônica.
- Nos cães acometidos de forma crônica, podem-se notar hiperglobulinemia e/ou hipoalbuminemia.
- Hipocalemia, hiponatremia, hipocloridemia e alcalose metabólica podem ser notadas nos cães com obstrução do fluxo gástrico de saída.
- Foi relatada hipercalcemia em um único cão acometido.
- A urinálise geralmente permanece normal.

OUTROS TESTES LABORATORIAIS
Sorologia — um teste ELISA sensível e específico encontra-se disponível no Pythium Laboratory na Universidade do Estado da Louisiana.

DIAGNÓSTICO POR IMAGEM
- Radiografia abdominal pode revelar padrão obstrutivo, espessamento da parede intestinal ou massa abdominal.
- Ultrassonografia abdominal pode revelar espessamento transmural segmentar do estômago, parte proximal do intestino delgado ou junção ileocólica. Granulomas ou linfonodos enfartados podem ficar evidentes no mesentério.

MÉTODOS DIAGNÓSTICOS
- A biopsia de lesões gastrintestinais ou cutâneas demonstra as alterações histológicas sugestivas de pitiose, porém não definitivas.

- O diagnóstico definitivo baseia-se nos exames de sorologia e cultura; as amostras de tecido devem ser encaminhadas a laboratório experiente por transporte durante a noite à temperatura ambiente.
- Uma coloração imuno-histoquímica pode ser utilizada para identificar as hifas de *P. insidiosum* nos cortes histológicos.
- O teste do PCR aninhado pode ser usado para a identificação definitiva dos isolamentos na cultura ou microrganismos nas amostras teciduais.

ACHADOS PATOLÓGICOS
- Ao exame histológico, as lesões GI e cutâneas caracterizam-se por inflamação piogranulomatosa e eosinofílica associada a amplas hifas (4-6 micrômetros), irregularmente ramificadas e raramente septadas, com paredes espessas e não paralelas.
- A predominância de eosinófilos no interior da reação inflamatória ajuda a diferenciar os quadros de pitiose e zigomicose de outras infecções micóticas.
- Os microrganismos com hifas não costumam ser visualizados nos cortes corados por hematoxilina e eosina, porém são facilmente observados na coloração argêntica.
- Os cães com lesões GI tipicamente apresentam espessamento segmentar grave de porções do estômago e/ou do intestino, frequentemente com obstrução do lúmen intestinal.
- Com frequência, nota-se linfadenopatia mesentérica, embora seja rara a presença das hifas de *P. insidiosum* no interior dos linfonodos.
- Histologicamente, a pitiose GI caracteriza-se por ulceração da mucosa, inflamação linfoplasmocitária e eosinofílica na lâmina própria, além de inflamação granulomatosa dentro da submucosa e da camada muscular.

TRATAMENTO
CUIDADO(S) DE SAÚDE ADEQUADO(S)
O tratamento de escolha é a excisão cirúrgica rigorosa de todo o tecido infectado. Infelizmente, muitos animais são levados ao veterinário muito tarde na evolução da doença, momento em que a ressecção completa não é possível.

CUIDADO(S) DE ENFERMAGEM
O cuidado de suporte deve incluir fluidos, potássio, suporte nutricional e antibióticos conforme a necessidade.

ATIVIDADE
Limitar a atividade.

DIETA
Fornecer dieta rica em calorias e altamente digestível.

ORIENTAÇÃO AO PROPRIETÁRIO
- O tratamento é dispendioso.
- O prognóstico é de reservado a mau, a menos que a ressecção completa seja possível.

CONSIDERAÇÕES CIRÚRGICAS
- Tentar uma ampla excisão cirúrgica para obter margens de 5-6 cm, mesmo se o tratamento clínico for contemplado.
- A amputação é recomendada para o tratamento de lesões nas extremidades.
- Os linfonodos mesentéricos enfartados devem ser biopsiados, embora frequentemente não contenham hifas infectantes; portanto, eles não devem ser removidos.
- Os cães quase sempre melhoram depois da ressecção das lesões obstrutivas, mesmo que uma doença significante ainda esteja macroscopicamente evidente.
- É recomendável o tratamento clínico pós-operatório com itraconazol e terbinafina (ver adiante) por 2-3 meses para reduzir a possibilidade de recidiva.
- A reavaliação da sorologia com ELISA 2-3 meses depois da cirurgia é um excelente indicador prognóstico.

MEDICAÇÕES
MEDICAMENTO(S) DE ESCOLHA
- Itraconazol (10 mg/kg VO diariamente) combinado com terbinafina (5-10 mg/kg VO diariamente) parecem ser os mais eficientes. Embora estudos controlados não tenham sido realizados, a eficácia dessa combinação provavelmente é <10% em cães com lesões não ressecáveis ou parcialmente ressecáveis.
- O tratamento clínico deve continuar por, no mínimo, 6 meses.
- Administrar o itraconazol juntamente com o alimento.

CONTRAINDICAÇÕES
Os corticosteroides frequentemente provocam uma melhora temporária nos sinais clínicos e podem ser utilizados em doses anti-inflamatórias como terapia paliativa para doença não ressecável. Contudo, o uso a longo prazo de corticosteroides nos animais submetidos a tratamento cirúrgico ou clínico com intenção de cura pode ser contraindicado.

PRECAUÇÕES
- Medicamentos azólicos não devem ser usados em animais com hepatopatia grave.
- Anorexia, enzimas hepáticas elevadas e vasculite cutânea são os efeitos adversos mais comuns do itraconazol.

INTERAÇÕES POSSÍVEIS
Antiácidos e anticonvulsivantes podem reduzir os níveis sanguíneos do itraconazol.

MEDICAMENTO(S) ALTERNATIVO(S)
- Complexo lipídico de anfotericina B demonstrou eficácia em um número limitado de cães com pitiose GI. Seu uso é recomendado quando o paciente se mostra intolerante a medicações por via oral.
- A dose do complexo lipídico de anfotericina B é de 2-3 mg/kg (cão) ou 0,5-1 mg/kg (gato) IV 3 vezes/semana por 9-12 tratamentos (dose total de 24-30 mg no cão). O medicamento deve ser diluído em glicose a 5% até uma concentração de 1 mg/mL e administrado por via IV durante 45-90 min.
- O complexo lipídico de anfotericina B não deve ser utilizado em animais azotêmicos ou hipocalêmicos.
- Efeitos colaterais, como calafrios, tremores, febre, anorexia e vômito, podem ser notados durante a infusão do complexo lipídico de anfotericina B.

ACOMPANHAMENTO
MONITORIZAÇÃO DO PACIENTE
- Sorologia com ELISA pode ser usada para monitorizar a resposta ao tratamento; a sorologia deve ser reavaliada 2-3 meses depois da cirurgia ou a cada 3 meses durante o tratamento clínico.
- A ultrassonografia abdominal é valiosa na reavaliação das lesões intestinais.
- As enzimas hepáticas devem ser avaliadas mensalmente enquanto o paciente estiver recebendo o itraconazol.
- Ureia, creatinina e potássio séricos devem ser avaliados antes da administração de cada dose do complexo lipídico de anfotericina B.

PREVENÇÃO
Monitorizar o paciente em busca dos sinais de recidiva.

COMPLICAÇÕES POSSÍVEIS
Abdome agudo e morte por trombose e perfuração GI.

EVOLUÇÃO ESPERADA E PROGNÓSTICO
- O prognóstico é de reservado a mau, a menos que a ressecção completa seja possível.
- Menos de 10% dos animais acometidos são curados apenas com o tratamento clínico.

DIVERSOS
FATORES RELACIONADOS COM A IDADE
Animais jovens são predispostos.

POTENCIAL ZOONÓTICO
As infecções em pessoas são muito raras e provêm de fonte ambiental comum. Não existem provas de transmissão direta de animais para seres humanos.

GESTAÇÃO/FERTILIDADE/REPRODUÇÃO
Antifúngicos azólicos são teratogênicos e não devem ser usados em fêmeas prenhes.

SINÔNIMO(S)
- Ficomicose. • Câncer do Pântano.

ABREVIATURA(S)
- ELISA = ensaio imunoabsorvente ligado à enzima. • GI = gastrintestinal. • PCR = reação em cadeia da polimerase.

Sugestões de Leitura

Grooters AM, Foil CS. Miscellaneous fungal infections. In: Greene CE, ed., Infectious Diseases of the Dog and Cat, 3rd ed. St. Louis: Saunders Elsevier, 2006.

Grooters AM, Gee MK. Development of a nested PCR assay for the detection and identification of Pythium insidiosum. J Vet Intern Med 2002, 16:147-152.

Grooters AM, Leise BS, Lopez MK, et al. Development and evaluation of an enzyme-linked immunosorbent assay for the serodiagnosis of pythiosis in dogs. J Vet Intern Med 2002, 16:142-146.

Autor Amy Grooters
Consultor Editorial Albert E. Jergens
Agradecimento O autor e os editores agradecem a colaboração prévia de Joseph Taboada.

PIÚRIA

CONSIDERAÇÕES GERAIS

DEFINIÇÃO
- Leucócitos (i. e., neutrófilos, eosinófilos, monócitos, linfócitos ou plasmócitos) na urina.
- Mais de cinco leucócitos por campo óptico de grande aumento geralmente é considerado anormal, porém o número de leucócitos encontrados no sedimento urinário depende do método de coleta, do volume e concentração da amostra, do grau de destruição celular após a coleta e da técnica do laboratório.

FISIOPATOLOGIA
- Grande número de leucócitos nas amostras de urina eliminada indica inflamação ativa em alguma parte ao longo do trato urogenital.
- Pode estar associada a algum processo patológico (infeccioso ou não) que provoque lesão ou morte celular; o dano tecidual evoca inflamação exsudativa caracterizada por indícios de extravasamento leucocitário (piúria) e permeabilidade vascular aumentada (hematúria e proteinúria).

SISTEMA(S) ACOMETIDO(S)
- Renal/urológico — uretra, bexiga urinária, ureteres e rins.
- Genital — prepúcio, próstata, vagina e útero.

IDENTIFICAÇÃO
Cães e gatos.

SINAIS CLÍNICOS
Comentários Gerais
- A inflamação pode provocar sinais clínicos localizados no(s) local(is) da lesão ou pode ser acompanhada por manifestações sistêmicas. Os achados do histórico e do exame físico dependem da causa subjacente, do(s) órgão(s) acometido(s), do grau de disfunção orgânica e da magnitude das respostas inflamatórias sistêmicas.
- Lesões não obstrutivas confinadas à bexiga urinária, à uretra, à vagina ou ao prepúcio raramente provocam sinais sistêmicos de inflamação. Os sinais sistêmicos podem acompanhar lesões inflamatórias generalizadas dos rins, da próstata ou do útero.

Achados do Exame Físico
Efeitos Locais da Inflamação
- Eritema das superfícies mucosas — por exemplo, vermelhidão da mucosa vaginal ou prepucial.
- Tumefação tecidual — por exemplo, renomegalia, prostatomegalia, espessamento mural da bexiga urinária ou da uretra.
- Exsudação de leucócitos e de líquido rico em proteína — por exemplo, piúria, secreção purulenta uretral ou vaginal, piometra ou abscesso prostático.
- Dor — por exemplo, resposta adversa à palpação, disúria, polaciúria e estrangúria.
- Perda da função — por exemplo, poliúria, disúria, polaciúria e incontinência urinária.

Efeitos Sistêmicos da Inflamação
- Febre.
- Depressão.
- Anorexia.
- Desidratação.

CAUSAS
Rim
- Pielonefrite — por exemplo, bacteriana, fúngica, parasitária ou micoplásmica.
- Nefrólito(s).
- Neoplasia.
- Traumatismo.
- Imunomediada.

Ureter
- Ureterite — por exemplo, bacteriana.
- Ureterólito(s).
- Neoplasia.

Bexiga Urinária
- Cistite — por exemplo, bacteriana, micoplásmica, fúngica ou parasitária.
- Urocistólito(s).
- Neoplasia.
- Traumatismo.
- Superdistensão — obstrução uretral.
- Farmacológica — ciclofosfamida.

Uretra
- Uretrite — por exemplo, bacteriana, fúngica ou micoplásmica.
- Uretrólito(s).
- Neoplasia.
- Traumatismo.
- Corpo estranho.

Próstata
- Prostatite/abscesso — por exemplo, bacteriano ou fúngico.
- Neoplasia.

Pênis/Prepúcio
- Balanopostite.
- Neoplasia.
- Corpo estranho.

Útero
- Piometra/metrite — por exemplo, bacteriana.

Vagina
- Vaginite — bacteriana, micoplásmica, viral ou fúngica.
- Neoplasia.
- Corpo estranho.
- Traumatismo.

FATORES DE RISCO
- Qualquer processo mórbido, método diagnóstico ou tratamento que altere as defesas normais do trato urinário do hospedeiro e predisponha à infecção.
- Qualquer processo mórbido, fator nutricional ou tratamento que predisponha à formação de urólitos metabólicos.

DIAGNÓSTICO

DIAGNÓSTICO DIFERENCIAL
Amostras Obtidas por Micção Espontânea
- Descartar vaginite — os sinais incluem corrimento vaginal, eritema da mucosa vaginal, lambedura da vulva e atrativa para os machos.
- Excluir piometra, metrite — os sinais compreendem corrimento vaginal, útero grande, pirexia, depressão, anorexia, poliúria, polidipsia e histórico recente de estro, parto ou administração de progestina.
- Descartar balanopostite — os sinais englobam secreção prepucial, eritema da mucosa prepucial ou peniana e lambedura do prepúcio.
- Excluir prostatite, abscesso prostático ou neoplasia prostática — os sinais abrangem secreção uretral, prostatomegalia, pirexia, depressão, disúria, tenesmo, dor abdominal caudal e marcha rígida.
- Descartar uretrite, uretrólitos, neoplasias uretrais — os sinais envolvem disúria, polaciúria, estrangúria e/ou urólitos palpáveis ou lesões expansivas na uretra.
- Excluir distúrbios inflamatórios da bexiga urinária e dos rins.

Amostras Coletadas por Cistocentese
- Descartar obstrução uretral — os sinais incluem estrangúria e anúria, além de bexiga urinária grande e superdistendida.
- Excluir distúrbios prostáticos e uretrais (ver o texto anteriormente); exsudatos purulentos prostáticos ou uretrais podem refluir para a bexiga urinária.
- Descartar cistite, urocistólitos e neoplasia vesical — os sinais podem compreender disúria, polaciúria, estrangúria e/ou urólitos palpáveis ou lesões expansivas na bexiga urinária.
- Excluir pielonefrite — os sinais podem abranger pirexia, depressão, anorexia, poliúria, polidipsia, dor renal e renomegalia.
- Descartar piúria pós-traumática — os sinais podem englobar histórico de traumatismo, incluindo causas iatrogênicas.

ACHADOS LABORATORIAIS
Medicamentos Capazes de Alterar os Resultados Laboratoriais
- Os leucócitos sofrem rápida lise na urina hipotônica ou alcalina. A administração de agentes alcalinizantes (p. ex., bicarbonato de sódio, citrato de potássio, clorotiazida ou acetazolamida) ou agentes produtores de urina hipotônica (p. ex., diuréticos e glicocorticoides) podem diminuir falsamente os números de leucócitos na urina.
- Nitrofurantoína, cefalosporinas e gentamicina podem provocar reações falso-positivas de esterase leucocitária com métodos de tiras reagentes de imersão.
- As concentrações urinárias de leucócitos podem ser baixas em pacientes com distúrbios inflamatórios que receberam medicamentos anti-inflamatórios esteroides ou não esteroides.

Distúrbios Capazes de Alterar os Resultados Laboratoriais
- Distúrbios associados à função diminuída dos leucócitos ou neutropenia absoluta podem reduzir artificialmente os valores dessas células.
- Distúrbios associados à produção de urina hipotônica ou de urina alcalina reduzem de modo artificial os valores dos leucócitos.

Fatores Diversos Capazes de Alterar os Resultados Laboratoriais
- Reação falso-negativa de esterase leucocitária nos cães quando a urina é testada pelo método da tira reagente de imersão.
- Reação falso-positiva e falso-negativa de esterase leucocitária nos gatos quando a urina é testada pelo método da tira reagente de imersão.

Os Resultados Serão Válidos se os Exames Forem Realizados em Laboratório Humano?
- Válidos se o sedimento urinário for submetido a exame microscópico; inválidos caso se faça uso apenas do método de esterase leucocitária pela tira reagente de imersão.

HEMOGRAMA/BIOQUÍMICA/URINÁLISE
- Piúria nas amostras coletadas por micção espontânea, compressão manual ou cateterização transuretral indicam lesão inflamatória envolvendo no mínimo os tratos urinário ou genital.
- Piúria em amostra coletada por cistocentese localiza o local da inflamação no trato urinário no mínimo, porém não exclui a uretra e o trato genital. Refluxos de exsudatos prostáticos para a bexiga urinária podem resultar em piúria nos pacientes com prostatopatia.
- Piúria associada a cilindros leucocitários é prova inequívoca de inflamação parenquimatosa renal.
- Lesão renal generalizada pode estar associada à leucocitose, isostenúria e azotemia concomitantes.
- Piúria associada a bactérias, fungos ou ovos de parasitas em número suficiente para serem observados pelo exame do sedimento microscópico indica que a lesão inflamatória foi provocada ou complicada por infecção do trato urinário. A detecção de bactérias no sedimento urinário pela microscopia óptica pode ser intensificada pela colocação de uma gota (20 µl) do sedimento urinário em uma lâmina de vidro, deixando secar, corando com Diff-Quik e examinando em busca de bactérias sob óleo de imersão em um aumento de 1000 vezes.
- Piúria associada a células neoplásicas indica neoplasia. O diagnóstico de neoplasia do trato urinário pelo exame citológico da urina pode ser complicado por hiperplasia e atipia de células epiteliais causada por inflamação do trato urinário ou pelas propriedades físico-químicas da urina (pH e tonicidade).

OUTROS TESTES LABORATORIAIS
- Fazer a cultura quantitativa da urina em todos os pacientes com piúria; ela representa o método mais definitivo de identificar e caracterizar infecção bacteriana do trato urinário.
- Resultados negativos da urocultura sugerem alguma causa não infecciosa de inflamação (p. ex., urólitos e neoplasia) ou inflamação associada à infecção do trato urinário provocada por microrganismos fastidiosos (p. ex., micoplasmas e vírus). Resultados falso-negativos da cultura também podem ser atribuídos à antibioticoterapia recente, manipulação incorreta da amostra ou atrasos entre a coleta e a cultura da amostra.
- Avaliação citológica do sedimento urinário, do líquido prostático, de secreção uretral ou corrimento vaginal ou biopsia de amostras obtidas por cateter ou aspirado com agulha pode ajudar a avaliar os pacientes com doença localizada dos tratos urinário ou genital. O exame citológico pode estabelecer o diagnóstico definitivo de neoplasia do trato urinário, porém os achados citológicos negativos não descartam neoplasia.

DIAGNÓSTICO POR IMAGEM
Radiografia abdominal simples, uretrocistografia e cistografia com contraste, ultrassonografia do trato urinário e urografia excretora são métodos importantes de identificar e localizar as causas subjacentes.

MÉTODOS DIAGNÓSTICOS
- Uretrocistoscopia — indicada em pacientes com lesões persistentes do trato urinário inferior para os quais o diagnóstico definitivo não foi estabelecido por outro meio menos invasivo.
- Avaliação de amostras de tecido por meio de microscopia óptica — indicada em pacientes com lesões dos tratos urinário ou genital para os quais o diagnóstico definitivo não foi estabelecido por outro meio menos invasivo; amostras de tecido podem ser obtidas por biopsia com cateter, cistoscopia e biopsia com pinça ou por laparotomia exploratória; técnicas de aspirado e biopsia com saca-bocado (também conhecido como *punch*) podem ser utilizadas para avaliar a próstata.

TRATAMENTO
- O tratamento varia, dependendo da causa subjacente e dos órgãos envolvidos.
- Piúria associada a sinais sistêmicos de doença (i. e., pirexia, depressão, anorexia, vômito, desidratação, leucocitose, poliúria e polidipsia) ou obstrução urinária justifica a avaliação diagnóstica rigorosa do paciente e o início de tratamento específico de suporte e/ou sintomático.

MEDICAÇÕES
MEDICAMENTO(S)
Dependem da causa subjacente.
CONTRAINDICAÇÕES
- Evitar os glicocorticoides ou outros agentes imunossupressores nos pacientes com suspeita de infecção dos tratos urinário ou genital.
- Evitar medicamentos potencialmente nefrotóxicos (p. ex., gentamicina) nos pacientes febris, desidratados ou azotêmicos e naqueles com suspeita de pielonefrite, septicemia ou nefropatia preexistente.

ACOMPANHAMENTO
MONITORIZAÇÃO DO PACIENTE
Avaliar a resposta ao tratamento por meio de urinálises seriadas, incluindo exame do sedimento urinário; coletar amostras da maior parte dos pacientes por cistocentese para evitar contaminação por exsudatos prepuciais ou vaginais; proceder a cateterização transuretral se os benefícios esperados superarem os riscos de infecção bacteriana iatrogênica do trato urinário.

COMPLICAÇÕES POSSÍVEIS
- Distúrbios inflamatórios infecciosos e não infecciosos do trato urinário podem provocar insuficiência renal primária, obstrução urinária, uremia, septicemia e morte.
- Piúria constitui um fator de risco potencial para a formação de matriz ou de tampões uretrais de matriz cristalina e subsequente obstrução uretral em gatos machos.

DIVERSOS
DISTÚRBIOS ASSOCIADOS
- Hematúria.
- Proteinúria.
- Bacteriúria.

SINÔNIMO(S)
Leucocitúria.

VER TAMBÉM
- Disúria e Polaciúria.
- Hematúria.
- Capítulos sobre Infecção do Trato Urinário Inferior.
- Pielonefrite.
- Proteinúria.

Sugestões de Leitura
Adams LG, Syme HM. Canine lower urinary tract disease. In: Ettinger SJ, Feldman EC, eds., Textbook of Veterinary Internal Medicine, 6th ed. St. Louis: Elsevier, 2005, pp. 1850-1874.
Bartges JW. Urinary tract infections. In: Ettinger SJ, Feldman EC, eds., Textbook of Veterinary Internal Medicine, 6th ed. St. Louis: Elsevier, 2005, pp. 1800-1808.
Kutzler MA, Yeager A. Prostatic diseases. In: Ettinger SJ, Feldman EC, eds., Textbook of Veterinary Internal Medicine, 6th ed. St. Louis: Elsevier, 2005, pp. 1809-1819.
Osborne CA, Stevens JB, Lulich JP, et al. A clinician's analysis of urinalysis. In: Osborne CA, Finco DR, eds., Canine and Feline Nephrology and Urology, 2nd ed. Baltimore: Williams & Wilkins, 1995, pp. 136-205.
Westropp JL, Buffington CAT, Chew D. Feline lower urinary tract diseases. In: Ettinger SJ, Feldman EC, eds., Textbook of Veterinary Internal Medicine, 6th ed. St. Louis: Elsevier, 2005, pp. 1828-1850.

Autores John M. Kruger, Carl A. Osborne e Cheryl L. Swenson
Consultor Editorial Carl A. Osborne

Placenta Retida

CONSIDERAÇÕES GERAIS

REVISÃO
• Cadelas — placenta retida além do período pós-parto imediato; em geral, as placentas são eliminadas depois de 15 minutos do nascimento de um filhote; pode ocorrer o desenvolvimento de metrite aguda secundária à placenta retida.
• Gatas — podem reter as placentas durante dias sem sinais de doença.
• Extremamente rara.

IDENTIFICAÇÃO
• Cadelas — rara, porém mais comum nas raças toy.
• Gatas — rara.

SINAIS CLÍNICOS
Achados Anamnésicos
• Parto recente.
• Corrimento vulvar contínuo de lóquios.
• O proprietário pode notar o número de placentas eliminado, embora essa informação nem sempre seja confiável.

Achados do Exame Físico
• Corrimento vulvar de lóquios esverdeados.
• Palpação de massa firme no útero — nem sempre possível.

CAUSAS E FATORES DE RISCO
• Raças toy.
• Tamanho grande da ninhada.
• Distocia.

DIAGNÓSTICO

DIAGNÓSTICO DIFERENCIAL
• Metrite pós-parto — o exame físico e o exame citológico vaginal não demonstram sinais de infecção em casos de placenta retida sem complicação; a metrite pode se desenvolver concomitantemente.
• Feto retido — diferenciado por meio de radiografia ou ultrassonografia.

HEMOGRAMA/BIOQUÍMICA/URINÁLISE
Geralmente normais nos casos sem complicação.

OUTROS TESTES LABORATORIAIS
Exame citológico vaginal — células epiteliais parabasais; podem-se notar eritrócitos; aglomerados de biliverdina.

DIAGNÓSTICO POR IMAGEM
Ultrassonografia — massa ecogênica, porém não fetal dentro do útero.

MÉTODOS DIAGNÓSTICOS
Laparotomia ou histerectomia — pode ser necessária para o diagnóstico.

TRATAMENTO

• Feito em um esquema ambulatorial para a cadela ou a gata com saúde.
• Instruir o proprietário a monitorar a temperatura e observar os sinais de doença sistêmica.
• Ovário-histerectomia — procedimento curativo; recomendada se não houver intenção de futuros acasalamentos.
• Remoção cirúrgica — indicada se o tratamento clínico não for bem-sucedido e se a cadela desenvolver metrite.

MEDICAÇÕES

MEDICAMENTO(S)
• Ocitocina — para condição conhecida ou suspeita em gatas e cadelas normalmente saudáveis; cadelas, 0,5 UI/kg IM até 5 UI; gatas, 0,5-1 UI IM.
• O tratamento com gliconato de cálcio (a 10%) pode preceder a ocitocina; cadelas e gatas, 0,5-1,5 mL/kg IV administrada em 15 min.
• Metrite — tratar de acordo com o quadro (ver "Metrite").

CONTRAINDICAÇÕES/INTERAÇÕES POSSÍVEIS
Não administrar medicamentos progestacionais.

ACOMPANHAMENTO

• Monitorizar a temperatura e a condição física.
• Metrite aguda (cadelas) — pode se desenvolver se a placenta não for eliminada; prognóstico de razoável a bom de recuperação com o tratamento.
• Prognóstico para futuros fins reprodutivos — bom sem metrite; razoável a mau com metrite.

DIVERSOS

VER TAMBÉM
Metrite.

Sugestões de Leitura
Feldman EC, Nelson RW. Periparturient diseases. In: Feldman EC, Nelson RW, eds., Canine and Feline Endocrinology and Reproduction, 3rd ed. Philadelphia: Saunders, 2004, pp. 808-834.

Autor Joni L. Freshman
Consultor Editorial Sara K. Lyle

PLASMOCITOMA MUCOCUTÂNEO

CONSIDERAÇÕES GERAIS

REVISÃO
• Tumor de origem plasmocitária.
• O crescimento é frequentemente rápido.
• Pode ser um subtipo de plasmocitoma extramedular que consiste em um tumor primário de origem no tecido mole, ou uma metástase de mieloma múltiplo ósseo primário.

IDENTIFICAÇÃO
• Cães e, raramente, gatos.
• Mais comum em raças mistas de cães e no Cocker spaniel.
• Idade no momento do diagnóstico (cães) — média, 9,7 anos; mediana, 10,5 anos.
• Ambos os sexos são acometidos igualmente.

SINAIS CLÍNICOS
• Em geral, trata-se de nódulo sólido elevado ou ulcerado, com 0,25-6,0 cm de diâmetro.
• Tumor dos lábios é tipicamente pequeno.
• Geralmente solitário.
• Raras vezes, polipoide.
• Boca, pés, tronco e orelhas constituem os locais comuns de acometimento.
• Ocasionalmente, ocorre com mieloma múltiplo ou linfoma, desenvolvendo-se em conjunto ou em momentos diferentes.
• Os sinais sistêmicos são raros, embora haja relato de gamopatia monoclonal.

CAUSAS E FATORES DE RISCO
Desconhecidos.

DIAGNÓSTICO

DIAGNÓSTICO DIFERENCIAL
• Outros tumores de células redondas como linfoma; mastocitoma; histiocitoma; tumor venéreo transmissível.
• Carcinoma pouco diferenciado.
• Melanoma amelanótico.
• Biopsia permitirá a distinção de outros tumores.

HEMOGRAMA/BIOQUÍMICA/URINÁLISE
Geralmente normais, a menos que o paciente tenha mieloma múltiplo ou linfoma.

OUTROS TESTES LABORATORIAIS
N/D.

DIAGNÓSTICO POR IMAGEM
• Geralmente normal.
• Tipicamente, não se identificam quaisquer indícios de metástase ou lise óssea.

MÉTODOS DIAGNÓSTICOS
• Exame macroscópico — o plasmocitoma mucocutâneo consiste geralmente em nódulos solitários, elevados, avermelhados e discretos.
• Exame citológico de aspirado por agulha fina — revela celularidade moderada a acentuada; células tumorais redondas ou poliédricas individuais com margens discretas, além de anisocitose e anisocariose proeminentes; núcleos arredondados a ovais com cromatina fina a grossa, mas sem nucléolos visíveis; citoplasma levemente basofílico.
• Exame histológico — em geral, são bem circunscritos e facilmente identificáveis. Os nódulos são densamente celulares com núcleos isolados ou múltiplos de tamanho variável e a presença de muitas mitoses; além disso, pode haver depósito de amiloide.

TRATAMENTO

• Ocasionalmente invasivo — é recomendável a excisão cirúrgica rigorosa.
• Radioterapia — deverá ser considerada se a ressecção cirúrgica resultar em desfiguração. Consultar um veterinário especialista em oncologia.

MEDICAÇÕES

MEDICAMENTO(S)
Agentes alquilantes e prednisona podem reduzir a massa tumoral; entretanto, não foi conduzida a avaliação prospectiva da eficácia contra o câncer.

CONTRAINDICAÇÕES/INTERAÇÕES POSSÍVEIS
N/D.

ACOMPANHAMENTO

MONITORIZAÇÃO DO PACIENTE
Em geral, nenhum a menos que esteja acompanhado por mieloma múltiplo ou linfoma.

EVOLUÇÃO ESPERADA E PROGNÓSTICO
Excelente em grande parte dos pacientes.

DIVERSOS

DISTÚRBIOS ASSOCIADOS
• Mieloma múltiplo.
• Linfoma — Cães.
• Gatos — pode-se notar uma amiloidose sistêmica.

VER TAMBÉM
• Amiloidose.
• Linfoma — Cães.
• Mieloma Múltiplo.

Sugestões de Leitura
Cangul IT, Wijnen M, Van Garderen E, et al. Clinico-pathological aspects of canine cutaneous and mucocutaneous plasmacytomas. J Vet Med A Physiol Pathol Clin Med 2002, 49(6):307-312.
Hargis AM. Integumentary system. In: Carlton WW, McGavin DM, eds., Thomson's Special Veterinary Pathology, 2nd ed. St. Louis: Mosby, 1995, pp. 461-511.
Morrison WB. Plasma cell neoplasms. In: Morrison WB, ed., Cancer in Dogs and Cats: Medical and Surgical Management. Jackson, WY: Teton NewMedia, 2002, pp. 671-677.
Rakich PM, Latimer KS, Weiss R, Steffens WL. Mucocutaneous plasmacytomas in dogs: 75 cases (1980-1987). JAVMA 1989, 194:803-810.

Autor Wallace B. Morrison
Consultor Editorial Timothy M. Fan

PNEUMOCISTOSE

CONSIDERAÇÕES GERAIS

REVISÃO
• *Pneumocystis carinii* — saprófita do trato respiratório mamífero, cujo ciclo de vida é concluído nos espaços alveolares; classificado como microrganismo fúngico atípico, com base na análise dos ácidos nucleicos. • Infecções — cães, clínica; gatos, subclínica; geralmente confinada ao trato respiratório; um caso relatado de doença disseminada no cão. • Transmissão da infecção — ao animal suscetível dentro da espécie; diferenças na cepa podem ser responsáveis pela falta de transmissão entre as espécies.

IDENTIFICAÇÃO
• Cães. • Nenhuma infecção clínica relatada em gatos. • Raça Dachshund com <12 meses de vida — maioria dos casos relatados; há suspeitas de ter alguma imunodeficiência congênita. • Cavalier King Charles spaniel no Reino Unido. • Doença clínica relatada em Pastor de Shetland, Cavalier King Charles spaniel, Beagle e Yorkshire terrier. • Os animais com predileção a comprometimento imunológico (p. ex., muito jovens ou muito idosos) parecem ter um risco elevado de proliferação do microrganismo.

SINAIS CLÍNICOS
• Dificuldade respiratória que evolui em 1-4 semanas. • Intolerância ao exercício — com frequência constitui a queixa principal. • Tosse. • Perda de peso gradual. • Vômito e diarreia — ocasionalmente observados. • Caquexia. • Temperatura retal normal e febre branda. • Dispneia. • Taquicardia. • Ruídos pulmonares aumentados à ausculta torácica. • Cianose — em caso de infecções graves. • Histórico prévio de infecções recidivantes, incluindo demodicose.

CAUSAS E FATORES DE RISCO
• *P. carinii*. • Humanos — risco aumentado com imunodeficiência (p. ex., HIV), estresse, terapia imunossupressora e infecção pulmonar concomitante. • Cães — fatores que afetam o risco humano podem desempenhar algum papel. • Os cães acometidos da raça Dachshund parecem ter anormalidades nas células T e B (i. e., imunodeficiência variável combinada). • Deficiência de imunoglobulina em cães da raça Cavalier King Charles spaniel (não completamente caracterizada).

DIAGNÓSTICO

DIAGNÓSTICO DIFERENCIAL
• Cardiovascular (insuficiência cardíaca congestiva, tromboêmbolos). • Alérgica (infiltrados pulmonares com eosinofilia, pneumonia ou granulomatose eosinofílica, asma bronquial). • Traumatismo (corpo estranho, gases irritantes). • Neoplasia. • Inflamação (fibrose pulmonar crônica, DPOC, faringite/tonsilite). • Parasitária (*Dirofilaria immitis*, filaroides, *Paragonimus kellicotti*, *Crenosoma vulpis*). • Agentes infecciosos (micose sistêmica, toxoplasmose, pneumonia/broncopneumonia bacteriana, pneumonia viral, tosse dos canis). • Edema pulmonar não cardiogênico. • Tromboêmbolos pulmonares.

HEMOGRAMA/BIOQUÍMICA/URINÁLISE
• Alterações geralmente inespecíficas. • Leucocitose com neutrofilia e desvio à esquerda. • Eosinofilia e monocitose. • Eritrocitose — secundária à hipoxia crônica.

OUTROS TESTES LABORATORIAIS
• Gasometria sanguínea arterial — hipoxemia; hipocapnia; aumento no pH sanguíneo e diferença na tensão do oxigênio alveoloarterial aumentada. • Testes sorológicos — não são seguros para o diagnóstico em virtude de possível imunodeficiência subjacente. • Quantificação da fração de imunoglobulina — hipogamaglobulinemia: deficiências de IgA, IgG e IgM.

DIAGNÓSTICO POR IMAGEM
Radiografia Torácica
• Alterações inespecíficas para *P. carinii*. • Leve padrão intersticial difuso com opacificação peribronquial. • Os casos mais avançados exibem opacificação maior com padrão alveolar e apagamento das margens. • Os lobos pulmonares médios são mais gravemente acometidos que os cranioventrais. • Alterações cardíacas mínimas, embora possa ocorrer o desenvolvimento de *cor pulmonale* como resultado de aumento na resistência vascular pulmonar, culminando em elevação da traqueia, aumento de volume do coração do lado direito e aumento da artéria pulmonar.

MÉTODOS DIAGNÓSTICOS
• O diagnóstico definitivo é feito pela visualização direta de *P. carinii* nos líquidos respiratórios ou amostras de biopsia. • Aspirado transtraqueal e lavado broncoalveolar — foi demonstrado que esses métodos são confiáveis para obtenção de amostras diagnósticas. • Aspirado pulmonar direto por agulha fina e biopsia do pulmão — procedimentos diagnósticos mais confiáveis; no entanto, têm maior risco de complicações. • Esfregaços por impressão (decalque) — podem ser feitos antes da fixação tecidual. • *Kits* imuno-histoquímicos disponíveis — o resultado positivo é específico e altamente diagnóstico; podem ser usados em material citológico, fixado em formalina e embebido em parafina; nota: espécies hospedeiras — foi demonstrada uma variação antigênica específica das espécies de hospedeiro, o que pode gerar resultados falso-negativos.

ACHADOS PATOLÓGICOS
• Pulmões — firmes, consolidados e castanho-pálidos ou cinzentos; líquido não espremido a partir das superfícies de corte; não sofrem colapso quando a cavidade pulmonar é aberta; podem ser observadas pequenas quantidades de líquido pleural. • Lado direito do coração — pode-se constatar certo grau de aumento. • Espaços alveolares — podem estar preenchidos com material amorfo, espumoso, eosinofílico com aparência de favo de mel; macrófagos; poucos neutrófilos; os septos podem estar espessados e fibrosos; os estágios de trofozoítas e cistos podem ser identificados. Há relatos de atrofia tecidual linfoide generalizada.

TRATAMENTO
• Internação — para administração de oxigênio a pacientes hipoxêmicos; diminuir a exposição de pacientes imunocomprometidos a outros patógenos. • Nebulização com agentes quimioterápicos pode conferir certo benefício. • Repouso em gaiola ou restrição da atividade física. • Fluido intravenoso conforme a necessidade. • Tapotagem e fisioterapia.

MEDICAÇÕES

MEDICAMENTO(S)
• Trimetoprima-sulfonamida — 15 mg/kg VO a cada 6 h por 3 semanas; medicamento de primeira escolha. • Isetionato de pentamidina — 4 mg/kg IM a cada 24 h por 3 semanas. • Carbutamida — 50 mg/kg IM a cada 12 h por 3 semanas. • Combinações de medicamentos — dapsona e pirimetamina; trimetoprima e atovaquona. • Nova opção medicamentosa potencial — caspofungina — inibidor da β-glucana sintetase que impede o desenvolvimento dos cistos — a glucana é um componente importante da parede do cisto. Não há relatos de casos em medicina veterinária. O custo elevado pode impedir o tratamento.

CONTRAINDICAÇÕES/INTERAÇÕES POSSÍVEIS
Isetionato de pentamidina — função renal prejudicada; disfunção hepática; hipoglicemia; hipotensão; hipocalcemia; urticária; distúrbios hematológicos; dor localizada no local da injeção.

ACOMPANHAMENTO

MONITORIZAÇÃO DO PACIENTE
• Gasometria sanguínea sérica, oximetria de pulso e radiografia torácica — fornecem informações prognósticas valiosas; monitorar a resposta à terapia. • Isetionato de pentamidina — verificar os níveis de ureia e glicose diariamente; interromper ou diminuir a dosagem se a azotemia ou outras complicações forem observadas. • Monitorizar o paciente quanto à resolução dos sinais de tosse e dispneia. • Evolução clínica variável.

DIVERSOS

ABREVIATURA(S)
• HIV = vírus da imunodeficiência humana.

Sugestões de Leitura
Lobetti R. Common variable immunodeficiency in miniature dachshunds affected with Pneumocystis carinii pneumonia. J Vet Diagn Invest 2000, 12:39-45.

Autor Tania N. Davey
Consultor Editorial Stephen C. Barr

Pneumonia Bacteriana

CONSIDERAÇÕES GERAIS

DEFINIÇÃO
Resposta inflamatória adquirida a bactérias virulentas no parênquima pulmonar, caracterizada pela exsudação de células e líquido para dentro das vias aéreas condutoras e dos espaços alveolares.

FISIOPATOLOGIA
- Bactérias — penetram no trato respiratório inferior, principalmente por meio de inalação ou aspiração; a penetração é menos comum por via hematógena. A infecção incita uma reação inflamatória evidente.
- Bactérias orofaríngeas — com frequência, são aspiradas; podem estar presentes por um intervalo desconhecido na árvore traqueobrônquica e no pulmão normais; têm potencial de causar ou complicar uma infecção respiratória; a presença dessas bactérias dificulta a interpretação das culturas das vias aéreas e dos pulmões.
- Árvore traqueobrônquica e carina traqueal — normalmente não são estéreis.
- Infecção respiratória — o desenvolvimento depende da complexa interação de muitos fatores: local de inoculação, número de microrganismos e sua virulência, bem como idade e resistência do hospedeiro.
- As bactérias produzem proteínas extracelulares chamadas invasinas que comprometem as defesas do hospedeiro e ajudam na disseminação dos agentes bacterianos.
- Infecções virais — alteram os padrões de colonização bacteriana; aumentam a aderência bacteriana ao epitélio respiratório; diminuem a depuração mucociliar e a fagocitose; por essa razão, permitem que as bactérias residentes invadam o trato respiratório inferior.
- Corpo estranho — inocula as bactérias em uma região pulmonar focal e leva à pneumonia obstrutiva.
- Fase exsudativa — hiperemia inflamatória; extravasamento de líquido rico em proteína para os espaços intersticial e alveolar.
- Fase da emigração leucocitária — os leucócitos se infiltram nas vias aéreas e nos alvéolos; consolidação, isquemia, necrose tecidual e atelectasia causadas por oclusão brônquica, bronquiolite obstrutiva e ventilação colateral prejudicada.

SISTEMA(S) ACOMETIDO(S)
Respiratório — infecção primária ou secundária.

GENÉTICA
Síndrome de rinite/broncopneumonia hereditária de cães da raça Wolfhound irlandês, com patogenia desconhecida.

INCIDÊNCIA/PREVALÊNCIA
Comum tanto em cães jovens como nos idosos, porém menos comum em gatos.

DISTRIBUIÇÃO GEOGRÁFICA
Disseminada.

IDENTIFICAÇÃO
Espécies
Cães e gatos.

Raça(s) Predominante(s)
Cães — raças de caça e de trabalho, bem como as esportivas e mistas com >12 kg.

Idade Média e Faixa Etária
Cães — faixa de 1 mês a 15 anos de idade; muitos casos ocorrem em cães com <1 ano de idade.

Sexo Predominante
Cães — 60% machos.

SINAIS CLÍNICOS
Achados Anamnésicos
- Tosse.
- Respiração laboriosa.
- Intolerância ao exercício.
- Anorexia e perda de peso.
- Letargia.
- Secreção nasal.

Achados do Exame Físico
- Tosse.
- Febre.
- Respiração difícil ou rápida.
- Ruídos respiratórios anormais à auscultação — intensidade ou ruídos respiratórios bronquiais aumentados, crepitações e sibilos.
- Perda de peso.
- Secreção nasal.
- Letargia.
- Desidratação.

CAUSAS
Cães
- Patógenos respiratórios primários mais comuns — *Bordetella bronchiseptica* e *Mycoplasma* spp.
- Bactérias Gram-positivas mais comuns — *Staphylococcus*, *Streptococcus* e *Enterococcus* spp.
- Bactérias Gram-negativas mais comuns — *Escherichia coli*, *Klebsiella* spp., *Pseudomonas* spp., *Pasteurella* spp.
- Bactérias anaeróbias — encontradas em abscessos pulmonares e em vários tipos de pneumonia (particularmente na pneumonia por aspiração ou corpos estranhos); relatadas com menor frequência (~20% dos casos).

Gatos
- Patógenos bacterianos — pouco documentados; *B. bronchiseptica*, *Pasteurella* spp. e *Moraxella* spp. são mais frequentemente relatadas. *Mycoplasma* spp. é considerado um patógeno primário no trato respiratório inferior.
- Estado de portador — pode existir; períodos de eliminação de *B. bronchiseptica* após estresse; as gatas infectadas podem não eliminar microrganismos antes do parto, mas começam a eliminar após o parto, servindo como fonte de infecção para os filhotes.

FATORES DE RISCO
- Infecção viral preexistente.
- Regurgitação, disfagia ou vômito.
- Defeitos funcionais ou anatômicos — paralisia laríngea, megaesôfago, fenda palatina, discinesia ciliar primária.
- Nível reduzido de consciência — estupor, coma e anestesia.
- Corpo estranho bronquial.
- Bronquiectasia.
- Terapia imunossupressora — quimioterapia, glicocorticoides, agentes imunossupressores.
- Distúrbios metabólicos graves — uremia, diabetes melito, hiperadrenocorticismo.
- Sepse.
- Idade — animais muito jovens são mais suscetíveis a infecções fatais.
- Estado de imunização.
- Ambiente — alojamento, condição higiênico-sanitária, ventilação.
- Disfunção fagocitária — FeLV e diabetes melito.
- Deficiência de complemento — rara.
- Deficiência seletiva de IgA — rara.
- Disfunção combinada de células T e células B — rara.

DIAGNÓSTICO

DIAGNÓSTICO DIFERENCIAL
- Pneumonia viral — vírus da cinomose, adenovírus, vírus da influenza, herpes-vírus.
- Pneumonia por protozoário — toxoplasmose.
- Pneumonia parasitária — capilaríase, filaroidíase.
- Pneumonia fúngica — histoplasmose, blastomicose, coccidioidomicose e criptococose.
- Pneumonia eosinofílica.
- Doença brônquica felina (asma).
- Abscesso pulmonar.
- Infecção pleural — piotórax.
- Corpo estranho bronquial.

HEMOGRAMA/BIOQUÍMICA/URINÁLISE
Leucograma inflamatório — leucocitose neutrofílica com ou sem desvio à esquerda; a ausência não descarta o diagnóstico.

OUTROS TESTES LABORATORIAIS
- Gasometria sanguínea arterial — os valores se correlacionam bem com o grau do distúrbio fisiológico; monitoramento sensível da evolução durante o tratamento; PaO_2 < 80 mmHg ao ar ambiente = hipoxemia leve a moderada; PaO_2 < 60 mmHg ao ar ambiente = hipoxemia grave.
- Considerar a realização de sorologia para pesquisa do vírus da influenza canina.
- Diagnóstico molecular está disponível para detecção de grande parte dos agentes virais.

DIAGNÓSTICO POR IMAGEM
Radiografia Torácica
- Variável — padrão broncointersticial difuso a infiltrados alveolares parciais ou completos até consolidação.
- Alterações radiográficas mais comuns — padrão alveolar caracterizado por densidades pulmonares aumentadas (margens indistintas; broncogramas aéreos ou consolidação lobar).
- Padrões pulmonares mais variáveis em gatos, como alterações intersticiais e alveolares irregulares e multifocais e/ou padrão nodular difuso.

MÉTODOS DIAGNÓSTICOS
- Exames microbiológico (culturas bacterianas aeróbias e anaeróbias, além de culturas para *Mycoplasma*) e citológico para o diagnóstico definitivo.
- Amostras — lavado transtraqueal ou endotraqueal, broncoscopia, lavado broncoalveolar (com ou sem broncoscópio) ou aspirado pulmonar com agulha fina.
- Predomínio de neutrófilos degenerados em casos de inflamação séptica (bactérias intracelulares).
- Administração recente de antibióticos — provável inflamação asséptica.
- Bactérias — nem sempre são evidentes ao exame microscópico; sempre obtenha amostras para cultura, ainda que nenhuma bactéria seja observada no exame citológico.

ACHADOS PATOLÓGICOS
- Consolidação irregular nas regiões cranioventrais.
- Pulmão consolidado — varia de vermelho-escuro a rosa acinzentado ou mais cinzento, dependendo da idade do paciente e da natureza do processo.

Pneumonia Bacteriana

- Firmeza palpável do tecido.
- Ninho de inflamação — na junção bronquiolar--alveolar.
- Precoces — bronquíolos e alvéolos adjacentes preenchidos com neutrófilos, além de uma mistura de debris celulares, fibrina e macrófagos; epitélio necrótico a hiperplásico.
- Tardios — inflamação neutrofílica, fibrinosa, hemorrágica ou necrosante, dependendo da virulência da bactéria e da resposta do hospedeiro.

TRATAMENTO

CUIDADO(S) DE SAÚDE ADEQUADO(S)
Internação do paciente — recomendável na presença de sinais multissistêmicos (p. ex., anorexia, febre alta, perda de peso e letargia).

CUIDADO(S) DE ENFERMAGEM
- Manter a hidratação sistêmica normal — importante para ajudar na depuração mucociliar e na mobilização de secreções; utilizar solução balanceada, que contém múltiplos eletrólitos.
- Nebulização com aerossol de solução salina — resultados mais rápidos se empregada com fisioterapia e antibacterianos sistêmicos.
- Fisioterapia — tapotagem da parede torácica, manipulação traqueal para estimular a tosse branda e a drenagem postural; pode intensificar a depuração das secreções; sempre fazer imediatamente após a nebulização; evitar que o paciente fique deitado em uma única posição por muito tempo.
- Oxigenoterapia — justificável para pacientes com hipoxemia ou sinais de angústia respiratória.

ATIVIDADE
Restrita durante o tratamento (paciente internado ou ambulatorial), exceto como parte da fisioterapia após o aerossol.

DIETA
- Garantir a ingestão normal com alimento rico em proteína e densamente calórico.
- Suporte nutricional enteral ou parenteral — indicado em pacientes gravemente doentes.
- Ter cuidado ao alimentar animais com megaesôfago, disfunção ou cirurgia da laringe, doença da faringe ou em decúbito.

ORIENTAÇÃO AO PROPRIETÁRIO
Avisar o proprietário de que os altos índices de morbidade e mortalidades estão associados à hipoxemia e sepse graves.

CONSIDERAÇÕES CIRÚRGICAS
Cirurgia (lobectomia pulmonar) — pode ser indicada em casos de abscesso pulmonar ou corpo estranho broncopulmonar com pneumonia secundária; poderá ser indicada se o paciente não estiver respondendo ao tratamento convencional e se a doença estiver limitada a um ou dois lobos.

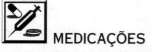

MEDICAÇÕES

MEDICAMENTO(S) DE ESCOLHA
Antimicrobianos
- Os antimicrobianos são mais bem selecionados com base nos resultados dos exames de cultura e antibiograma do lavado traqueal ou de outras amostras pulmonares.
- A antibioticoterapia empírica será justificável quando houver um risco significativo na obtenção de amostras adequadas ou se o tempo necessário para a realização da cultura gerar um atraso potencialmente letal no tratamento.
- As escolhas antimicrobianas iniciais razoáveis até a obtenção dos resultados da cultura incluem amoxicilina-clavulanato (15 mg/kg VO a cada 12 h), cefalexina (22-30 mg/kg VO a cada 12 h), enrofloxacino (cães, 5-10 mg/kg a cada 12 h ou 10-20 mg/kg a cada 24 h; gatos, 5 mg/kg a cada 24 h no máximo) ou trimetoprima-sulfonamida (15 mg/kg VO a cada 12 h).
- Cocos Gram-positivos — ampicilina (22 mg/kg VO a cada 12 h), ampicilina-sulbactam; amoxicilina; amoxicilina-clavulanato; azitromicina; cloranfenicol, eritromicina; gentamicina; trimetoprima-sulfonamida; cefalosporinas de primeira geração.
- Bastonetes Gram-negativos — enrofloxacino; cloranfenicol; gentamicina; trimetoprima-sulfonamida; amicacina; marbofloxacino; carboxipenicilinas.
- *Bordetella* — doxiciclina (5 mg/kg VO a cada 12 h); cloranfenicol; enrofloxacino; azitromicina.
- *Mycoplasma* — doxiciclina; enrofloxacino, marbofloxacino, cloranfenicol.
- Anaeróbios — amoxicilina-clavulanato; cloranfenicol; metronidazol; clindamicina; ticarcilina-clavulanato.
- Nebulização antimicrobiana para *Bordetella* — nebulização com gentamicina na dose de 5 mg/kg a cada 24 h por 5-7 dias, tipicamente como adjuvante com antimicrobianos sistêmicos.
- Continuar o tratamento por, no mínimo, 10 dias além da resolução clínica e/ou 1-2 semanas após a resolução radiográfica.

CONTRAINDICAÇÕES
- Anticolinérgicos e anti-histamínicos — podem não só engrossar as secreções, mas também inibir a mucocinese e a remoção do exsudato das vias aéreas.
- Antitussígenos — potentes agentes de ação central que inibem a mucocinese e a remoção do exsudato das vias aéreas e, consequentemente, são capazes de potencializar a infecção e a inflamação pulmonares.

INTERAÇÕES POSSÍVEIS
Evitar o uso concomitante de teofilina e fluoroquinolonas.

MEDICAMENTO(S) ALTERNATIVO(S)
- Expectorantes — recomendados por alguns clínicos; não há evidência real de que eles aumentem a mucocinese ou a mobilização das secreções.
- Broncodilatadores — recomendados por alguns clínicos para aliviar o broncospasmo.

ACOMPANHAMENTO

MONITORIZAÇÃO DO PACIENTE
- Monitorizar a frequência e o esforço respiratórios.
- O hemograma completo se normalizará.
- Gasometria sanguínea arterial — monitoramento mais sensível da evolução; a oximetria de pulso pode ser útil.
- Auscultação torácica frequente.
- Radiografias torácicas — melhoram mais lentamente do que o aspecto clínico.

PREVENÇÃO
- Vacinação — contra os agentes virais que acometem o trato respiratório superior; contra *B. bronchiseptica* se o cão estiver alojado ou for exposto a grande número de outros animais.
- Gatis — estratégias ambientais para diminuir a densidade populacional e melhorar a higiene ajudam a controlar os surtos de bordetelose.

COMPLICAÇÕES POSSÍVEIS
Pode ocorrer o desenvolvimento de sepse, mas é rara a constatação de pleuropneumonia.

EVOLUÇÃO ESPERADA E PROGNÓSTICO
- Prognóstico — bom com terapia antibacteriana rigorosa e cuidados de suporte intensivos; mais reservado em animais jovens, pacientes com imunodeficiência e naqueles debilitados ou acometidos por doença subjacente grave.
- Infecção prolongada — potencial para bronquite crônica ou bronquiectasia em qualquer paciente.
- Mortalidade — associada aos quadros de hipoxemia (baixa concentração arterial de oxigênio) e sepse graves.

DIVERSOS

DISTÚRBIOS ASSOCIADOS
- Com frequência, a pneumonia bacteriana desenvolve-se secundariamente a anormalidades funcionais ou anatômicas subjacentes — fenda palatina; hipoplasia da traqueia; discinesia ciliar primária; paralisia laríngea; megaesôfago ou outro distúrbio da motilidade esofágica.
- Bronquiectasia — trata-se tanto de um fator predisponente como uma complicação potencial.

FATORES RELACIONADOS COM A IDADE
- Filhotes de cães e de gatos — podem apresentar um prognóstico pior; filhotes de cães frequentemente desenvolvem complicações a longo prazo (p. ex., bronquite crônica).
- Problemas funcionais e anatômicos subjacentes, além de imunodeficiências — suspeitos em pacientes jovens.

GESTAÇÃO/FERTILIDADE/REPRODUÇÃO
Cadelas ou gatas infectadas por *B. bronchiseptica* — podem transmitir a infecção aos neonatos.

ABREVIATURA(S)
- FeLV = vírus da leucemia felina.

Sugestões de Leitura
Jameson PH, King LA, Lappin MR, et al. Comparison of clinical signs, diagnostic findings, organisms isolated, and clinical outcome in dogs with bacterial pneumonia: 93 cases (1986-1991). JAVMA 1995, 206:206-209.

Autores Melissa A. Herrera e Phil Roudebush
Consultora Editorial Lynelle R. Johnson

PNEUMONIA EOSINOFÍLICA

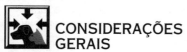

CONSIDERAÇÕES GERAIS

DEFINIÇÃO
Resposta inflamatória totalmente desenvolvida aos antígenos no parênquima pulmonar, caracterizada pela exsudação de eosinófilos e líquido dentro do interstício pulmonar, das vias aéreas condutoras e dos espaços alveolares.

FISIOPATOLOGIA
- Base imunológica — prova de apoio geralmente aceita; mecanismos envolvidos ainda não esclarecidos.
- Infiltração de eosinófilos e predomínio de células T CD4+ no líquido do lavado broncoalveolar apoiam o papel de uma resposta imunológica TH2 dominante nas vias aéreas inferiores.
- Evolução da doença — provavelmente determinada pelas características dos antígenos, pela resposta do hospedeiro e pela regulação de tal resposta.
- Três padrões mórbidos — pneumonite eosinofílica, bronquite eosinofílica e granulomatose eosinofílica pulmonar.
- Os antígenos ingressam no trato respiratório inferior por inalação ou vias hematógenas.
- Exposição crônica aos antígenos — elicia a resposta imunológica celular e humoral.
- Distúrbios pulmonares alérgicos ou por hipersensibilidade — associados à resposta humoral anormal e ao defeito imunorregulador mediado por células.
- Classes de imunoglobulinas envolvidas — IgE, IgG e outras.
- Altos números de macrófagos ativados e de linfócitos T, além de atividade deprimida das células T supressoras — alteram a imunidade mediada por célula.
- Infiltração inflamatória — do interstício pulmonar, dos espaços alveolares e da mucosa bronquial.
- Atividade de enzimas colagenolíticas — aumentada.
- Pacientes gravemente acometidos desenvolvem doença granulomatosa acentuada.
- Dirofilariose com pneumonite — as microfilárias podem ficar encarceradas na circulação pulmonar e deflagrar uma resposta imunológica.
- Mortalidade — associada à hipoxemia grave (p. ex., baixa concentração de oxigênio arterial) e (raramente) hemoptise grave.

SISTEMA(S) ACOMETIDO(S)
- Respiratório.
- Cardiovascular — pode-se observar *cor pulmonale*.

GENÉTICA
N/D.

INCIDÊNCIA/PREVALÊNCIA
N/D.

DISTRIBUIÇÃO GEOGRÁFICA
Disseminada.

IDENTIFICAÇÃO
Espécies
Cães.

Raça(s) Predominante(s)
Husky siberiano, possivelmente.

Idade Média e Faixa Etária
Pode acometer todas as idades, embora seja mais frequente em jovens adultos (4-6 anos).

Sexo Predominante
Nenhum.

SINAIS CLÍNICOS
Comentários Gerais
Extremamente variáveis, dependendo da gravidade.

Achados Anamnésicos
- Tosse — irresponsiva à terapia antibacteriana.
- Respiração laboriosa.
- Intolerância ao exercício.
- Anorexia.
- Letargia.
- Perda de peso.
- Secreção nasal.
- Febre (incomum).

Achados do Exame Físico
- Tosse áspera e úmida.
- Taquipneia ou angústia respiratória.
- Ruídos respiratórios anormais à auscultação — intensidade aumentada desses ruídos; crepitações; sibilos; podem ocorrer ruídos diminuídos.
- Perda de peso.
- Secreção nasal amarelo-esverdeada ou mucopurulenta.
- Febre (incomum).

CAUSAS
- Supostos aeroalérgenos — esporos ou hifas de fungos e actinomicetos; pólen; antígenos de insetos; deflagradores não identificados da resposta imunológica.
- Antígenos parasitários — microfilárias da dirofilária, parasitas respiratórios.

FATORES DE RISCO
- Residência em área endêmica de dirofilariose sem receber medicação preventiva.
- Ambiente empoeirado ou com mofo.
- Poluição do ar.

DIAGNÓSTICO

DIAGNÓSTICO DIFERENCIAL
- Pneumonia parasitária — capilaríase; paragonimíase; dirofilariose.
- Pneumonia fúngica — histoplasmose; blastomicose; coccidioidomicose; criptococose.
- Para pneumonite eosinofílica — pneumonia bacteriana; pneumonia viral (p. ex., vírus da cinomose e adenovírus canino); pneumonia riquetsiana (p. ex., erliquiose e febre maculosa das Montanhas Rochosas); pneumonia protozoária (p. ex., toxoplasmose); insuficiência cardíaca congestiva; bartonelose.
- Para bronquite eosinofílica — traqueobronquite infecciosa; bronquite crônica.
- Para granulomatose eosinofílica pulmonar — neoplasia (incluindo granulomatose linfomatoide); abscesso pulmonar; corpo estranho bronquial.

HEMOGRAMA/BIOQUÍMICA/URINÁLISE
- Leucograma inflamatório — leucocitose neutrofílica com ou sem desvio à esquerda, eosinofilia, basofilia ou monocitose.
- Ausência de eosinofilia — não descarta o diagnóstico.
- Hiperglobulinemia — sugere dirofilariose oculta ou estímulo antigênico crônico.

OUTROS TESTES LABORATORIAIS
Gasometria Sanguínea Arterial
- Os valores correlacionam-se bem com o grau do distúrbio fisiológico; monitorização sensível da evolução do paciente durante o tratamento.
- Hipoxemia — leve ou moderada, PaO_2 <80 mmHg no ar ambiente; grave, PaO_2 <60 mmHg no ar ambiente.

Outros
- Pesquisa de microfilárias da dirofilária e testes antigênicos — resultados positivos sugerem dirofilariose ou pneumonite eosinofílica associada à microfilária aprisionada no pulmão.
- Flutuação fecal e sedimentação fecal pela técnica de Baermann.
- Eletroforese de proteínas — pico de β-globulina (hiperbetaglobulinemia) frequentemente encontrada em caso de dirofilariose oculta.

DIAGNÓSTICO POR IMAGEM
- Os achados radiográficos dependem da extensão e da gravidade da doença.
- Radiografias torácicas — ajudam a registrar a gravidade da doença da artéria pulmonar; revelam pneumonite intersticial em cães com dirofilariose.
- Pneumonite eosinofílica — padrão intersticial linear ou miliar que se assemelha a alterações observadas no início de edema pulmonar ou pneumonia fúngica; padrão alveolar caracterizado por densidade pulmonar aumentada com margens indistintas nos pacientes gravemente acometidos; grandes artérias pulmonares tortuosas e cardiomegalia do lado direito nos pacientes com dirofilariose.
- Bronquite alérgica ou eosinofílica — padrão bronquial com brônquios espessados que se estendem para a periferia do pulmão (sinais com aparência de trilhos de trem e rosquinhas).
- Granuloma eosinofílico — lesões nodulares múltiplas de tamanhos variáveis em diferentes lobos pulmonares; densidades alveolares focais e irregulares; linfadenopatia traqueobronquial.

MÉTODOS DIAGNÓSTICOS
- Exame citológico de aspirados, lavados ou escovações — diagnóstico definitivo: inflamação eosinofílica predomina; podem-se notar outros tipos de células inflamatórias; examinar cuidadosamente as amostras em busca de fontes antigênicas (p. ex., parasitas, fungos ou neoplasia).
- Lavado transtraqueal.
- Broncoscopia; muco amarelo-esverdeado, proliferação polipoide da mucosa, colapso parcial das vias aéreas.
- Lavado broncoalveolar — com ou sem broncoscópio.
- Cultura bacteriana de líquido do lavado broncoalveolar é recomendada para descartar infecção bacteriana.
- Aspirado pulmonar por agulha fina e exame.
- Teste cutâneo intradérmico ou alérgico sorológico — raramente podem identificar os alérgenos.
- Exames fecais — flutuação de rotina, esfregaço direto, exame do sedimento e técnica de Baermann; podem ocorrer resultados negativos em virtude de eliminação intermitente.

ACHADOS PATOLÓGICOS
- Macroscópicos — lesões firmes difusas, irregulares ou nodulares; em geral, pálidas ou mosqueadas.

Pneumonia Eosinofílica

• Histopatológicos — infiltração eosinofílica, linfocítica e macrofágica das paredes alveolares e dos espaços alveolares; à medida que a doença evolui, o processo infiltrativo intersticial torna-se fibrótico com obliteração dos espaços alveolares, podendo haver granulomas dispersos dentro da fibrose intersticial. O epitélio do trato respiratório superior também pode ser envolvido por infiltração eosinofílica.

TRATAMENTO
CUIDADO(S) DE SAÚDE ADEQUADO(S)
Internação — recomendada para pacientes com sinais multissistêmicos (p. ex., anorexia, perda de peso ou letargia).
CUIDADO(S) DE ENFERMAGEM
• Desidratação — retarda a depuração mucociliar e a mobilização das secreções; manter a hidratação sistêmica normal com solução multieletrolítica balanceada.
• Suplementação de oxigênio — para angústia respiratória.
ATIVIDADE
Restrita durante o tratamento (paciente internado ou não).
DIETA
Garantir a ingestão normal.
ORIENTAÇÃO AO PROPRIETÁRIO
Advertir o proprietário sobre o fato de que as taxas de morbidade e mortalidade estão associadas à hipoxemia grave.
CONSIDERAÇÕES CIRÚRGICAS
Podem ser removidos os lobos pulmonares com granulomas grandes.

MEDICAÇÕES
MEDICAMENTOS(S) DE ESCOLHA
• Corticosteroides — prednisolona ou prednisona na dose de 2 mg/kg/dia até os sinais clínicos começarem a desaparecer (tipicamente 2-3 semanas); em seguida, diminuir de forma lenta e gradual (em meses). Com frequência, há necessidade de doses de manutenção da prednisona a longo prazo (0,125-0,5 mg/kg em dias alternados ou a cada 3 ou 4 dias).
• Após o controle adequado da doença e/ou em virtude dos efeitos colaterais de glicocorticoides sistêmicos, pode-se fazer uso dos corticosteroides inalados (p. ex., propionato de fluticasona) em conjunto com câmara de espaçamento e máscara facial.
• Terapia adulticida contra dirofilariose — em paciente positivo para dirofilariose; iniciar após a estabilização do paciente com corticosteroides e repouso.
• Itraconazol ou cetoconazol — podem ser usados com infecção broncopulmonar fúngica alérgica confirmada, que é uma condição rara; utilizar medicamentos antifúngicos apenas se a infecção por fungos for confirmada pelo exame citológico ou pela cultura.
• Hipossensibilização — injeções antialérgicas formuladas com base nos resultados de teste cutâneo intradérmico ou sorológico podem ser tentadas, mas não constituem o tratamento de escolha em grande parte dos pacientes. A maioria dos cães ainda necessita de terapia com esteroide.
CONTRAINDICAÇÕES
N/D.
PRECAUÇÕES
N/D.
INTERAÇÕES POSSÍVEIS
N/D.
MEDICAMENTO(S) ALTERNATIVO(S)
• Outros medicamentos imunossupressores (p. ex., ciclosporina) — podem ser utilizados em caso de contraindicação ou ineficácia dos corticosteroides. Não há resultados de ensaios clínicos até o momento.
• Broncodilatadores — podem ser úteis, particularmente se forem auscultados sibilos ou se for observado esforço respiratório; ver "Bronquite Crônica".

ACOMPANHAMENTO
MONITORIZAÇÃO DO PACIENTE
• Hemograma completo — mostrará a resolução da eosinofilia periférica.
• Gasometria sanguínea arterial — monitoramento mais sensível da evolução.
• Auscultação minuciosa do paciente — várias vezes ao dia.
• Radiografias torácicas — melhoram mais lentamente do que a aparência clínica.
PREVENÇÃO
• Medicamento de rotina para prevenção da dirofilariose.
• Mudança de ambiente do animal na suspeita de algum aeroalérgeno.
COMPLICAÇÕES POSSÍVEIS
Tromboembolia pulmonar — pacientes tratados com medicamentos adulticidas contra dirofilariose.
EVOLUÇÃO ESPERADA E PROGNÓSTICO
• Se o principal alérgeno for identificado e eliminado — prognóstico bom para casos leves.
• Se o alérgeno não for identificado — prognóstico bom em termos de controle; muitos pacientes necessitam de tratamento a longo prazo com esteroides.
• Infecção por dirofilariose — o prognóstico depende da gravidade dos quadros de hipertensão pulmonar, *cor pulmonale* e tromboembolia.
• Granulomatose eosinofílica — prognóstico reservado; frequentemente a doença é progressiva.

DIVERSOS
DISTÚRBIOS ASSOCIADOS
• Dirofilariose.
• Infecção fúngica broncopulmonar.
FATORES RELACIONADOS COM A IDADE
N/D.
POTENCIAL ZOONÓTICO
N/D.
GESTAÇÃO/FERTILIDADE/REPRODUÇÃO
Os corticosteroides e outros medicamentos imunossupressores estão contraindicados em animais prenhes.
SINÔNIMO(S)
• Bronquite alérgica.
• Bronquite ou broncopneumopatia eosinofílica.
• Eosinofilia pulmonar bronquítica.
• Alveolite alérgica.
• Pneumonite eosinofílica.
• Pneumonia eosinofílica.
• Pneumonite por hipersensibilidade.
• Granulomatose pulmonar eosinofílica.
• Alveolite alérgica extrínseca.
• Pneumonia por dirofilariose oculta.
• Eosinofilia pulmonar parasitária.
• Infiltrados pulmonares com eosinofilia.
VER TAMBÉM
• Dirofilariose — Cães.
• Dispneia e Angústia Respiratória.
• Granulomatose Linfomatoide.
• Parasitas Respiratórios.
• Respiração Ofegante e Taquipneia.
• Tosse.

Sugestões de Leitura
Clercx C, Peeters D. Canine eosinophilic bronchopneumopathy. Vet Clin North Am Small Anim Pract 2007, 37:917-935.
Clercx C, Peeters D, German AJ, et al. An immunologic investigation of canine eosinophilic bronchopneumopathy. J Vet Intern Med 2002, 16:229-237.
Clercx C, Peeters D, Snaps F, et al. Eosinophilic bronchopneumopathy in dogs. J Vet Intern Med 2000, 14:282-291.
Cooper ES, Schober KE, Drost WT. Severe bronchoconstriction after bronchoalveolar lavage in a dog with eosinophilic airway disease. JAVMA 2005, 227:1257-1262.

Autores Melissa A. Herrera e Phil Roudebush
Consultor Editorial Lynelle R. Johnson

PNEUMONIA FÚNGICA

CONSIDERAÇÕES GERAIS

DEFINIÇÃO
Inflamação dos tecidos pulmonar intersticial, linfático e peribrônquica causada por infecção micótica profunda.

FISIOPATOLOGIA
• Elementos fúngicos miceliais — inalados a partir de solo ou debris de plantas contaminados; os microrganismos então colonizam os pulmões.
• Fungos dimórficos como *Blastomyces dermatitidis, Histoplasma capsulatum, Coccidioides immitis* — fase de levedura à temperatura corporal. Infecções fúngicas invasivas por espécies de *Aspergillus* resultam da inalação de esporos aerógenos com o crescimento sob a forma de micélios dentro dos tecidos. • É comum a disseminação sistêmica da levedura a partir dos pulmões em cães e gatos. • Envolvimento intersticial pulmonar — pode causar hipoxia.
• Envolvimento das vias aéreas — pode causar tosse. • Imunidade mediada por células — resposta importante à infecção fúngica; leva à inflamação piogranulomatosa. • As complicações pulmonares podem incluir pneumonia intersticial, efusão pleural, formação de granuloma mediastínico, SARA e tromboembolia pulmonar.

SISTEMA(S) ACOMETIDO(S)
• Depende da doença fúngica específica (ver também capítulos que tratam de fungos específicos). • Blastomicose — cerca de 85% dos cães e gatos têm envolvimento respiratório; pneumonia intersticial, alveolar e brônquica difusa é o achado mais comum; lesões expansivas solitárias podem ser observadas, especialmente em gatos; a linfadenopatia traqueobrônquica pode contribuir para a tosse; ocasionalmente é detectada infecção nasal. • Histoplasmose — uma pneumonia intersticial difusa é comum, sobretudo em gatos; taquipneia ou dispneia são observadas em apenas 50% dos gatos e < 50% dos cães; linfadenopatia peri-hilar ou mediastínica frequentemente contribuem para a tosse.
• Coccidioidomicose — broncopneumonia ou pneumonia intersticial difusa é comum em cães, porém menos comum em gatos; linfadenopatia peri-hilar ou mediastínica também é comum.
• Criptococose — o envolvimento da cavidade nasal é mais comum; em geral, os pulmões são subclinicamente acometidos por granulomas multifocais pequenos nos cães; os sinais clínicos de doença do trato respiratório inferior não são habituais. • Aspergilose sistêmica — a pneumonia é constatada apenas em pacientes com envolvimento sistêmico e geralmente envolve o *Aspergillus terreus*; *A. fumigatus* é mais comum na rinite.

GENÉTICA
Suscetibilidades raciais podem estar relacionadas com defeitos na imunidade mediada por células.

INCIDÊNCIA/PREVALÊNCIA
Depende da distribuição geográfica.

DISTRIBUIÇÃO GEOGRÁFICA
• Blastomicose — endêmica no sudeste e no meio-oeste dos Estados Unidos ao longo dos rios Mississipi, Ohio, Missouri e Tennessee, bem como ao sul dos Grandes Lagos; também é endêmica nos estados do sul do Meio-Atlântico. • Histoplasmose — semelhante à blastomicose, porém mais amplamente distribuída; bolsões da doença no Texas, em Oklahoma e na Califórnia.
• Coccidioidomicose — sul dos Estados Unidos, do Texas à Califórnia. • Criptococose e aspergilose — esporadicamente em todos os Estados Unidos.

IDENTIFICAÇÃO
Espécies
Cães e, menos comumente, gatos.

Raça(s) Predominante(s)
• Micose sistêmica — cães pertencentes a raças de grande porte mantidos fora da residência ou utilizados para caça ou ensaios a campo; Doberman pinscher e Rottweiler podem estar predispostos à doença disseminada mais grave.
• Aspergilose sistêmica — Pastor alemão pode estar super-representado.

Idade Média e Faixa Etária
• Animais jovens (<4 anos de idade) são predispostos. • Qualquer idade pode ser acometida.

Sexo Predominante
Os machos são acometidos em uma frequência 2 a 4 vezes maior que as fêmeas.

SINAIS CLÍNICOS
Comentários Gerais
• Dependem principalmente dos sistemas envolvidos. • Doença multissistêmica aparente.

Achados Anamnésicos
• Perda de peso crônica e inapetência. • Secreção oculonasal. • Tosse — pode ser proeminente; observada de forma inconstante mesmo com doença pulmonar acentuada. • É comum a presença de dispneia ou intolerância ao exercício.
• Respiração laboriosa — mais comum em gatos; sinal de doença grave tanto em cães como em gatos. • Cegueira ou blefaroespasmo agudo — se os olhos forem acometidos. • Pápulas e nódulos cutâneos — apesar de comuns, passam frequentemente despercebidos até o aparecimento dos trajetos drenantes. • Claudicação — comum se houver envolvimento dos ossos ou desenvolvimento de osteomielite.

Achados do Exame Físico
• Depressão e emaciação — em pacientes cronicamente acometidos. • Febre — cerca de 50% dos pacientes. • Ruídos respiratórios ásperos e sonoros — comuns na auscultação. • Crepitações — podem ser proeminentes, sobretudo nos gatos.
• Tosse — pode ser induzida na palpação traqueal.
• Linfadenopatia — comum em cães com infecções fúngicas dimórficas. • Dispneia — em repouso nos casos de doença grave. • Blastomicose (cães) — múltiplos nódulos cutâneos e subcutâneos com trajetos drenantes; uveíte; é comum o descolamento granulomatoso da retina.
• Coccidioidomicose (cães) — é comum a presença de dor intensa causada por osteomielite; gatos — comumente há lesões cutâneas.
• Histoplasmose (cães) — são proeminentes os sinais de emaciação e diarreia (frequentemente sanguinolenta); gatos — observam-se lesões cutâneas. • Criptococose — é comum a existência de infecção na cavidade nasal e nos tecidos moles circunjacentes.

CAUSAS
• *Blastomyces dermatitidis* — os pulmões constituem a principal via de infecção.
• *Histoplasma capsulatum* — os pulmões e, possivelmente, o trato gastrintestinal são as principais vias de infecção. • *Coccidioides immitis* — os pulmões representam a principal via de infecção. • *Cryptococcus neoformans* e *gattii* — a cavidade nasal é a principal via de infecção com extensão direta para os olhos ou o SNC; os pulmões são uma fonte menos relevante de infecção. • *Aspergillus* spp. — a cavidade nasal e os pulmões consistem nas principais vias de infecção.

FATORES DE RISCO
• Blastomicose, histoplasmose e criptococose — exposição ambiental a solos ricos em matéria orgânica; a exposição a fezes de pássaros ou outro material fecal pode predispor o paciente à blastomicose e à criptococose; residência próxima a fontes de água é um fator de risco para blastomicose. • Coccidioidomicose — exposição ambiental a solo arenoso e alcalino após períodos de chuva; atividades externas (caça e ensaios a campo); imunossupressão (especialmente fraca imunidade mediada por células) pode contribuir para a disseminação sistêmica da infecção fúngica.
• O FeLV não parece ser um fator de risco, mas o FIV pode ser um fator de risco de pouca importância. • Prednisona — pode agravar a doença. • Quimioterapia antineoplásica.
• Neoplasia linforreticular.

DIAGNÓSTICO

DIAGNÓSTICO DIFERENCIAL
• Neoplasia metastática. • Doença pulmonar eosinofílica. • Granulomatose linfomatoide.
• Neoplasia linforreticular e histiocítica. • Doença piogranulomatosa idiopática. • PIF ou outra vasculopatia. • Pneumonia parasitária.
• Pneumonia bacteriana. • Doença brônquica crônica. • Edema pulmonar. • Tromboembolia pulmonar.

HEMOGRAMA/BIOQUÍMICA/URINÁLISE
• Leucocitose moderada com ou sem desvio à esquerda. • É comum uma linfopenia.
• Leucopenia — pode ser notada com histoplasmose. • Trombocitopenia e anemia arregenerativa são comuns. • Hiperglobulinemia e hipoalbuminemia também são anormalidades comuns. • Hipercalcemia — ocasionalmente.
• Atividade das enzimas hepáticas — a elevação é mais provável na histoplasmose. • Urinálise costuma permanecer normal. • Proteinúria — achado ocasional. • Microrganismos — podem ser observados na urina (raramente, exceto para o *Aspergillus*) se os rins ou o trato urinário inferior estiverem acometidos.

OUTROS TESTES LABORATORIAIS
• Os antígenos fúngicos podem ser detectados no soro ou na urina pelo ensaio imunoenzimático para a detecção de *Blastomyces* ou *Histoplasma* — a sensibilidade e a especificidade parecem altas. Ocorre reação cruzada entre *Blastomyces* e *Histoplasma*.
• Teste sorológico para detecção de anticorpos — produz resultados falso-positivos e falso-negativos.
• Teste de aglutinação em látex — para antígeno capsular; altamente confiável para criptococose.
• Identificação citológica ou histológica do microrganismo — diagnóstico definitivo.
• Cultura — em geral, não é necessária; pode ser difícil.

PNEUMONIA FÚNGICA

DIAGNÓSTICO POR IMAGEM
• Radiografia torácica — infiltrados peribrônquicos e intersticiais nodulares difusos; densidades nodulares podem coalescer e formar massas granulomatosas com margens indistintas; é comum a constatação de linfadenopatia traqueobrônquica; grandes granulomas focais são mais prováveis em gatos.
• Radiografia do esqueleto apendicular ou axial — osteólise com proliferação periosteal; tumefação dos tecidos moles.
• Ultrassonografia abdominal — pode revelar granulomas ou linfonodos infartados.
• Ultrassonografia ocular — pode revelar massa retrobulbar, além de uveíte posterior.

MÉTODOS DIAGNÓSTICOS
• Esfregaço por decalque (impressão) ou aspirado de nódulo cutâneo — mais provavelmente permitem a recuperação dos microrganismos.
• Aspirado pulmonar com agulha fina — possível método mais diagnóstico do que o aspirado da traqueia ou a amostra de lavado broncoalveolar.
• Aspirado ou biopsia de linfonodo.
• Punção do LCS — na criptococose.
• Exame da medula óssea ou do aspirado hepático/esplênico — na histoplasmose.
• Biopsia — pode ser necessária.

ACHADOS PATOLÓGICOS
• Inflamação piogranulomatosa.
• Microrganismos — observados, em geral, em casos de blastomicose, histoplasmose, criptococose e aspergilose; às vezes, são difíceis de encontrar na coccidioidomicose.

TRATAMENTO

CUIDADO(S) DE SAÚDE ADEQUADO(S)
• Paciente de ambulatório — se o paciente ainda estiver comendo.
• Avaliação e tratamento do paciente internado — desidratação, anorexia e hipoxia grave.

CUIDADO(S) DE ENFERMAGEM
Administração de fluidos, oxigênio e antibióticos conforme a necessidade.

ATIVIDADE
Restrita.

DIETA
• Fornecer alimento densamente calórico com proteína de alta qualidade.
• Histoplasmose acompanhada por envolvimento gastrintestinal acentuado — administrar alimento de alta digestibilidade.

ORIENTAÇÃO AO PROPRIETÁRIO
• Informar ao proprietário a probabilidade de que < 70% dos cães e uma porcentagem menor de gatos respondam ao tratamento.
• Avisar ao proprietário que, além de caro, o tratamento poderá ser necessário por mais de 2 meses.
• Aconselhar o proprietário a limpar as áreas do ambiente em que haja matéria orgânica ou fezes.

CONSIDERAÇÕES CIRÚRGICAS
Granulomas focais ou olhos granulomatosos doloridos talvez tenham de ser removidos.

MEDICAÇÕES

MEDICAMENTO(S) DE ESCOLHA
• Itraconazol — 5-10 mg/kg VO diariamente; precisa ser administrado juntamente com o alimento.
• Fluconazol — 10 mg/kg VO a cada 12 h; medicamento de escolha para criptococose e pacientes com envolvimento do trato urinário ou do SNC. Geralmente requer um tratamento mais prolongado.
• Complexo lipídico de anfotericina B — 1-2 mg/kg IV a cada 48 h por 12 tratamentos; nefrotoxicidade baixa; não há necessidade de diurese.
• Posaconazol — a dose de 5 mg/kg VO a cada 24 h juntamente com o alimento pode ser mais eficaz para aspergilose.

CONTRAINDICAÇÕES
Os corticosteroides são relativamente contraindicados, mas podem ser indicados para reduzir a inflamação durante o tratamento inicial em pacientes com dispneia grave.

PRECAUÇÕES
• Medicamentos azólicos — não usar com hepatopatia grave.
• Anfotericina B — não utilizar em pacientes azotêmicos ou desidratados; interromper a utilização com níveis de ureia > 50 mg/dL ou creatinina > 3 mg/dL.
• Itraconazol e os outros medicamentos azólicos — anorexia; aumento na atividade das enzimas hepáticas; vasculite cutânea.

INTERAÇÕES POSSÍVEIS
Antiácidos e anticonvulsivantes — podem baixar a concentração sanguínea de itraconazol.

MEDICAMENTO(S) ALTERNATIVO(S)
• Cetoconazol — 10-30 mg/kg; pode ser eficaz; incidência mais alta de efeitos colaterais; há necessidade de tratamento mais prolongado; é comum a ocorrência de recidiva.
• Anfotericina B — 0,5 mg/kg (cães) ou 0,25 mg/kg (gatos) IV 3 vezes por semana até uma dose total de 8 mg/kg se usada sozinha ou 4 mg/kg se utilizada com algum medicamento azólico (p. ex., itraconazol); administrar em 200-500 mL de glicose a 5% em água após diurese salina; melhor se utilizada com itraconazol ou cetoconazol para pacientes gravemente acometidos.
• Anfotericina B — alternativa; 0,5-0,8 mg/kg 2-3 vezes por semana; para reduzir a nefrotoxicidade, pode-se administrar por via subcutânea diluída em solução salina a 0,45%/solução de glicose a 2,5% (400 mL para gatos, 500 mL para cães < 20 kg, 1.000 mL para cães > 20 kg).
• Voriconazol — 3-4 mg/kg VO a cada 12 h para aspergilose invasiva.

ACOMPANHAMENTO

MONITORIZAÇÃO DO PACIENTE
• Enzimas hepáticas — avaliadas mensalmente enquanto o paciente estiver sendo submetido ao itraconazol, fluconazol ou cetoconazol.
• Ureia e creatinina — medir antes de cada dose de anfotericina B.
• Radiografias torácicas — reavaliar antes de interromper o tratamento.

PREVENÇÃO
Monitorizar o animal em busca de sinais de recidiva.

COMPLICAÇÕES POSSÍVEIS
• Em geral, a cegueira é permanente.
• Insuficiência renal por anfotericina B.

EVOLUÇÃO ESPERADA E PROGNÓSTICO
• Blastomicose — requer, no mínimo, 2 meses de tratamento (mais tempo com o fluconazol); 60-70% dos cães são curados pelo itraconazol; geralmente, aqueles que não são curados exibem recidiva. Os cães com dispneia ou hipoxemia apresentam um prognóstico pior.
• Outros — continuar até 1 mês após a remissão.
• Aspergilose sistêmica — o prognóstico não é tão bom quanto o de outras causas.
• Recidiva — pode ocorrer até 1 ano após o tratamento.

DIVERSOS

FATORES RELACIONADOS COM A IDADE
Animais jovens são predispostos.

POTENCIAL ZOONÓTICO
Infecções em pessoas — principalmente a partir de fonte ambiental comum; sem transmissão direta de animais para seres humanos, exceto por feridas penetrantes contaminadas pelo microrganismo.

GESTAÇÃO/FERTILIDADE/REPRODUÇÃO
• É possível a ocorrência de abortamento por infecção fúngica.
• Antifúngicos azólicos — teratogênicos; não utilizar em animais prenhes.

VER TAMBÉM
• Aspergilose. • Blastomicose.
• Coccidioidomicose. • Criptococose.
• Histoplasmose.

ABREVIATURA(S)
• FeLV = vírus da leucemia felina.
• FIV = vírus da imunodeficiência felina.
• LCS = líquido cerebrospinal.
• PIF = peritonite infecciosa felina.
• SARA = síndrome da angústia respiratória aguda.
• SNC = sistema nervoso central.

Sugestões de Leitura
Davidson A. Coccidioidomycosis and aspergillosis. In: Ettinger SJ, Feldman EC, eds., Textbook of Veterinary Internal Medicine, 6th ed. St. Louis: Elsevier, 2005, pp. 690-698.
Taboada J. Systemic mycoses. In: Morgan RV, ed., Handbook of Small Animal Practice, 5th ed. St. Louis: Saunders, 2008, pp. 1073-1086.
Taboada J, Grooters A. Systemic antifungal therapy. In: Maddison JE, Page SW, Church D, eds., Small Animal Clinical Pharmacology, 2nd ed. Edinburgh: Saunders, 2008, pp. 186-197.

Autor Joseph Taboada
Consultor Editorial Lynelle R. Johnson

PNEUMONIA INTERSTICIAL

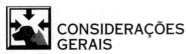

CONSIDERAÇÕES GERAIS

DEFINIÇÃO
Forma de pneumonia na qual o processo inflamatório ocorre nas paredes alveolares e no espaço intersticial.

FISIOPATOLOGIA
• Resulta de lesão aerógena ao epitélio alveolar (pneumócitos tipo I ou II) ou lesão hematógena aos capilares alveolares. A doença pode ser deflagrada por agentes infecciosos.
• Com frequência, o dano à parede alveolar ocorre secundariamente à inflamação e ao depósito de complexo antígeno-anticorpo.
• Pode ocorrer evolução de pneumonia intersticial aguda para crônica, levando à fibrose alveolar +/− acúmulo de células mononucleares no interstício e hiperplasia persistente dos pneumócitos tipo II.

SISTEMA(S) ACOMETIDO(S)
• Respiratório.
• Cardiovascular (pode desenvolver *cor pulmonale**).

INCIDÊNCIA/PREVALÊNCIA
Parcialmente compreendida.

DISTRIBUIÇÃO GEOGRÁFICA
• *Angiostrongylus vasorum* é encontrado na Europa, na Ásia e na África (raro nos Estados Unidos).
• *Leishmania chagasi* é encontrado principalmente na América do Sul e na América Central.

IDENTIFICAÇÃO
• Vírus da cinomose — cães com 3-6 meses de vida. As raças Galgo, Husky siberiano, Weimaraner, Samoieda e Malamute do Alasca são super-representadas.
• Pneumonia lipídica endógena — gatos mais idosos de ambos os sexos.
• Doença pulmonar intersticial pulmonar — animais de meia-idade a idosos das raças West Highland white terrier, ± Cairn terrier e Bull terrier.
• Doença semelhante à fibrose pulmonar idiopática felina — gatos de meia-idade a mais idosos.
• *Pneumocystis carinii* — Dachshund miniatura com < 1 ano de idade está sob risco.
• Toxoplasmose — gatos machos de meia-idade.

SINAIS CLÍNICOS
• Dependem da gravidade da doença.
• Taquipneia, tosse, dispneia, ortopneia, cianose, respiração com a boca aberta, intolerância ao exercício, ruídos respiratórios anormais na auscultação (em geral, crepitações no fim da inspiração e no começo da expiração), +/− hemoptise.
• Febre leve e secreção oculonasal estão frequentemente presentes com infecção por adenovírus canino tipo 2.
• Sinais gastrintestinais, febre, secreção oculonasal, hiperqueratose dos coxins e déficits neurológicos ou mioclonia podem ser observados na infecção pelo vírus da cinomose.
• Com frequência, animais com intoxicação pelo paraquat apresentam vômito, oligúria, diarreia e úlceras orofaríngeas (+/− hiperexcitabilidade e sinais neurológicos na fase inicial).
• Retinite, uveíte, sinais neurológicos e/ou sinais gastrintestinais podem ser observados com toxoplasmose.

CAUSAS E FATORES DE RISCO

Congênitas
• Bronquiolite obliterante com pneumonia em organização secundariamente à discinesia ciliar primária.

Metabólicas
• Pneumonite urêmica ± bronquiolite obliterante com pneumonia em organização, hepatopatia ou pancreatite em gatos.

Neoplásicas
• Bronquiectasia ou bronquiolite obliterante com pneumonia em organização, carcinoma pulmonar associado à fibrose pulmonar em gatos.

Idiopáticas
• Fibrose intersticial pulmonar e pneumonite intersticial descamativa, alguns casos de pneumonia lipídica endógena, bronquiolite obliterante com pneumonia em organização, proteinose alveolar pulmonar primária.

Inflamatórias
• A pneumonia lipídica endógena é mais comum em gatos com bronquite e bronquiectasia ou bronquiolite necrosante.

Infecciosas
• Cães — vírus da cinomose, adenovírus canino tipo 2, *Leishmania chagasi*, *Pneumocystis carinii*, *Angiostrongylus vasorum*, *Toxoplasma*.
• Gatos — toxoplasmose, FIV.

Tóxicas
• Inalação de poeiras, gases ou vapores, tiacetarsemida, aspiração de produtos à base de petróleo em gatos, proteinose alveolar pulmonar secundária, intoxicação pelo paraquat, silicose, asbestose.

Vasculares
• Tromboembolia, *larva migrans* circulante.

DIAGNÓSTICO

DIAGNÓSTICO DIFERENCIAL
• Doença das vias aéreas. • Broncopneumonia.
• Dirofilariose. • Pneumonia embólica.
• Pneumonia granulomatosa. • Neoplasia.
• Cardiopatia.

HEMOGRAMA/BIOQUÍMICA/URINÁLISE
• Podem-se observar neutrofilia, eosinofilia, linfocitose, hiperglobulinemia; pode haver policitemia em caso de hipoxemia crônica.
• Trombocitopenia imunomediada foi relatada com *Angiostrongylus vasorum*.
• Neutropenia ou enzimas hepáticas elevadas e hiperbilirrubinemia são possíveis com *Toxoplasma*.
• Enzimas hepáticas aumentadas e hiperbilirrubinemia (apenas cães) são possíveis com hepatotoxicidade atribuída à terapia com tiacetarsemida e, ocasionalmente, com intoxicação pelo paraquat.
• Azotemia grave e isostenúria com pneumonite urêmica.

OUTROS TESTES LABORATORIAIS
• Gasometria sanguínea arterial e cálculo do gradiente alveoloarterial (A-a) para avaliar o grau de comprometimento respiratório; PaO_2 < 80 mmHg indica hipoxemia de leve a moderada; PaO_2 < 60 mmHg indica hipoxemia grave; gradiente A-a > 15 indica mistura venosa.
• Testes sorológicos e outros exames para pesquisa de causas infecciosas.
• Exame de fezes para detecção de *Angiostrongylus vasorum* (técnica de Baermann).
• Análise toxicológica da urina ou do soro para diagnosticar intoxicação pelo paraquat em animais vivos.
• Teste imunodiagnóstico para exposição à *Leishmania* — a identificação citológica ou histológica de amastigotas em linfonodos ou na medula óssea é confirmatória.

DIAGNÓSTICO POR IMAGEM

Achados das Radiografias Torácicas
• Pode haver um padrão intersticial a brônquico a alveolar focal ou difuso, leve a grave, além de brônquios dilatados com bronquiectasia ou bronquiolite obliterante com pneumonia em organização.
• Aumento cardíaco do lado direito e hepatosplenomegalia na presença de hipertensão pulmonar secundária.
• Ocasionalmente se observa efusão pleural.

Tomografia Computadorizada
• Os achados da TC não estão bem descritos na literatura veterinária, mas incluem opacificação em vidro fosco, espessamento peribroncovascular e formação de bandas parenquimatosas.

OUTROS MÉTODOS DIAGNÓSTICOS
• Eletrocardiografia — podem ocorrer arritmias com hipoxia grave ou doença sistêmica.
• Biopsia aberta do pulmão é o teste diagnóstico mais definitivo.
• Lavado endotraqueal ou transtraqueal, broncoscopia com lavado broncoalveolar e/ou aspirado com agulha fina dos pulmões devem ser úteis (p. ex., podem ser observados trofozoítas ou cistos de *Pneumocystis carinii* ou *Toxoplasma* ou larvas L1 com *Angiostrongylus vasorum*); as culturas frequentemente revelam a presença de infecções bacterianas secundárias. Com proteinose alveolar pulmonar, recupera-se um material branco opaco após o lavado das vias aéreas; o exame citológico desse material demonstra uma substância granular densa com abundância de lipídios. Tal substância cora-se positivamente ao PAS.
• O ecocardiograma pode revelar indícios de hipertensão pulmonar.

ACHADOS PATOLÓGICOS
• *Angiostrongylus vasorum* — arterite trombosante e peribronquite fibrótica podem estar, além de parasitas nas arteríolas do parênquima pulmonar.
• Bronquiolite obliterante com pneumonia em organização — tampões polipoides de tecido fibroso frouxo preenchem os bronquíolos e os alvéolos; além disso, há macrófagos espumosos dentro dos alvéolos e infiltrados inflamatórios variáveis com reatividade dos pneumócitos tipo II.
• Doença pulmonar intersticial na raça West Highland white terrier — espessamento do septo alveolar em virtude do excesso de colágeno na matriz extracelular.
• Doença semelhante à fibrose pulmonar idiopática no gato — carece de inflamação e pode estar associada a carcinoma pulmonar. As alterações típicas incluem distribuição multifocal de fibrose intersticial com focos de fibroblastos/

---

* N. T.: O *cor pulmonale* é definido como uma alteração na estrutura e no funcionamento do ventrículo direito, causada por doença pulmonar (Fonte: Portal do coração).

Pneumonia Intersticial

miofibroblastos, metaplasia do epitélio alveolar e metaplasia/hiperplasia do músculo liso intersticial.
- *Leishmania chagasi* é caracterizada por pneumonite intersticial crônica e difusa, além de septos intra-alveolares espessados em alguns casos.
- Pneumonias lipídicas — lesões macroscópicas podem incluir nódulos subpleurais, parenquimatosos ou perivasculares brancos e firmes. Padrão misto de inflamação com acúmulo de macrófagos carregados de lipídios, fendas de colesterol e células gigantes multinucleadas.
- Intoxicação pelo paraquat — os pulmões encontram-se pesados, edematosos e hemorrágicos. Bolhas enfisematosas e pneumomediastino estão comumente presentes.
- Proteinose alveolar pulmonar — os espaços alveolares ficam distendidos com material proteináceo eosinofílico corado pelo PAS. Fendas de colesterol intra-alveolares e macrófagos carregados de muco com infiltrados inflamatórios mistos leves são comuns.
- Pneumonite urêmica — edema pulmonar e calcificação do músculo liso e/ou das paredes alveolares.

TRATAMENTO

- Cuidados e monitorização dos pacientes internados para aqueles com indícios de angústia respiratória. Oxigenoterapia via gaiola, intranasal, máscara ou fluxo.
- Minimizar a exposição a poeiras domésticas, vapores, fumaças químicas ou fumaça de cigarro.
- Umidificação do ar inspirado com nebulizador ou vaporizador para liquefazer as secreções.
- Proteinose alveolar pulmonar — lavado broncoalveolar terapêutico.
- Antibioticoterapia — conforme for indicado pelos resultados da cultura e do antibiograma.

ATIVIDADE
- Restrição ao exercício para os animais com esforço respiratório acentuado.
- Uso de coleira peitoral em vez de enforcador ou qualquer outra coleira de contenção.

DIETA
A perda de peso será indicada em animais obesos.

ORIENTAÇÃO AO PROPRIETÁRIO
Como ainda não foi estabelecida uma terapia específica para pneumonias intersticiais, os proprietários frequentemente são obrigados a fornecer cuidados paliativos.

CONSIDERAÇÕES CIRÚRGICAS
O diagnóstico definitivo de doença pulmonar intersticial requer a realização de exame histopatológico; tal exame será mais bem efetuado se precedido pela TC para determinar o local apropriado para a biopsia. Muitos proprietários ficam relutantes em prosseguir com métodos diagnósticos invasivos se o paciente tiver idade avançada e por causa do prognóstico mau em termos de terapia definitiva.

MEDICAÇÕES

MEDICAMENTO(S)
- Corticosteroides inalados (p. ex., fluticasona a cada 12 h) com o uso de câmara de espaçamento e máscara facial de tamanho adequado podem ser benéficos nos animais que necessitam de medicamentos anti-inflamatórios (ver adiante).
- Broncodilatadores podem ser úteis: teofilina de liberação sustentada (cão, 10 mg/kg VO a cada 12 h; gato, 15-20 mg/kg a cada 24 h), sulfato de terbutalina (cão ou gato, 0,01 mg/kg SC, IM ou IV a cada 8-12 h; cão, 0,03 mg/kg VO a cada 8-12 h; gato, 0,312-0,625 mg/gato VO a cada 8-12 h). Broncodilatadores inalatórios também podem ser utilizados da mesma forma que os corticosteroides inalados.
- *Angiostrongylus vasorum* — levamisol, 7,5 mg/kg VO a cada 24 h por 2 dias, seguido por 10 mg/kg VO a cada 24 h por 2 dias ± ácido acetilsalicílico ou corticosteroides concomitantemente. Terapias alternativas incluem fembendazol, mebendazol e ivermectina.
- Bronquiolite obliterante com pneumonia em organização — os corticosteroides foram usados com sucesso clínico em um único relato de caso (prednisona, 2,2 mg/kg VO a cada 24 h).
- Fibrose pulmonar idiopática — não há nenhuma terapia eficaz disponível. Terapia esteroide anti-inflamatória com prednisolona (0,5-1,0 mg/kg VO a cada 24-48 h é a dose frequentemente utilizada) e broncodilatadores, antitussígenos ou antibióticos se houver indicação. Não foi investigado o valor da terapia antifibrótica.
- *Leishmania chagasi* — antimoniato de meglumina na dose de 100 mg/kg IV ou SC a cada 24 h por 3-4 semanas ou estibogliconato de sódio na dose de 30-50 mg/kg IV ou SC a cada 24 h por 3-4 semanas.
- Intoxicação pelo paraquat — a indução de êmese e o uso de carvão ativado estarão indicados se a ingestão recente for conhecida. Cuidados de suporte, diurese induzida pela furosemida (mais eficaz nos primeiros 3 dias após a ingestão para aumentar a excreção), oxigenoterapia conforme a necessidade, +/- dexametasona imunossupressora, ciclofosfamida, nicotinamida, superóxido dismutase e vitamina A.

PRECAUÇÕES
A terapia imunossupressora pode exacerbar as infecções secundárias.

ACOMPANHAMENTO

MONITORIZAÇÃO DO PACIENTE
- Os proprietários devem observar a resposta clínica à terapia, bem como monitorizar a frequência e o esforço respiratórios.
- Repetir o exame físico (incluindo a auscultação do tórax), as radiografias torácicas, os testes laboratoriais e a análise de gasometria sanguínea arterial conforme indicação.

PREVENÇÃO
- Evitar a proximidade a fumaças tóxicas ou ao paraquat (não vendido legalmente nos EUA).
- Vacinar e vermifugar os animais conforme recomendação.
- Proceder ao controle apropriado de insetos.

COMPLICAÇÕES POSSÍVEIS
- Infecções pulmonares secundárias são comuns com a maioria das formas de pneumonia intersticial.
- Pode ocorrer o desenvolvimento de hipertensão pulmonar.

EVOLUÇÃO ESPERADA E PROGNÓSTICO
- Reservado em casos de *Pneumocystis carinii*, *Toxoplasma*, *Angiostrongylus vasorum*, vírus da cinomose, *Leishmania chagasi* e pneumonia lipídica endógena.
- Prognóstico mau a longo prazo em casos de fibrose pulmonar idiopática (o tempo médio de sobrevida desde o início dos sinais clínicos é de 17 meses em cães e 5 meses e meio em gatos).
- Prognóstico mau em casos de FIV e pneumonite urêmica.
- Intoxicação pelo paraquat — comumente fatal em cães.

DIVERSOS

DISTÚRBIOS ASSOCIADOS
- Adenovírus canino tipo 2 é associado algumas vezes à traqueobronquite infecciosa e pode coexistir com infecção por vírus da cinomose.
- Pneumonias infecciosas secundárias são sequelas comuns de pneumonia intersticial.
- Carcinoma pulmonar pode ser associado à fibrose pulmonar idiopática em gatos.

FATORES RELACIONADOS COM A IDADE
Animais jovens de vida livre têm maior probabilidade de sucumbir a doenças infecciosas.

POTENCIAL ZOONÓTICO
Toxoplasmose se o animal estiver liberando oocistos no ambiente.

GESTAÇÃO/FERTILIDADE/REPRODUÇÃO
É possível a ocorrência de infecção transplacentária por *Toxoplasma* e vírus da cinomose.

VER TAMBÉM
- Bronquiectasia.
- Cinomose.
- Infecção pelo Vírus da Imunodeficiência Felina (FIV).
- Leishmaniose.
- Pneumocistose.
- Toxoplasmose.

ABREVIATURA(S)
- FIV = vírus da imunodeficiência felina.
- PAS = ácido periódico de Schiff.
- TC = tomografia computadorizada.

Sugestões de Leitura
Cohn LA, Norris CR, Hawkins EC, Dye JA, Johnson CA, Williams KJ. Identification and characterization of an idiopathic pulmonary fibrosis-like condition in cats. J Vet Intern Med 2004, 18(5):632-641.
Corcoran BM, Cobb M, Martin WS, et al. Chronic pulmonary disease in West Highland white terriers. Vet Record 1999, 144:611-616.
Johnson VS, Corcoran BM, Wotton PR, Schwarz T, Sullivan M. Thoracic high-resolution computed tomographic findings in dogs with canine idiopathic pulmonary fibrosis. J Small Anim Pract 2005, 46(8):381-388.
Jones DJ, Norris CR, Samii VF, Griffey SM. Endogenous lipid pneumonia in cats: 24 cases (1985-1998). JAVMA 2000, 216:1437-1440.
Silverstein D, Greene C, Gregory C, et al. Pulmonary alveolar proteinosis in a dog. J Vet Intern Med 2000, 14(5):546-551.

Autor Deborah C. Silverstein
Consultor Editorial Lynelle R. Johnson

Pneumonia por Aspiração

CONSIDERAÇÕES GERAIS

REVISÃO
- Inflamação dos pulmões causada por inalação de ingesta oral, material regurgitado e vômito com subsequente disfunção pulmonar; desenvolve-se quando os reflexos laríngeos estão sobrecarregados ou não funcionam de forma adequada.
- Disfunção pulmonar — causada por (1) obstrução — obstrução direta das vias aéreas de pequeno calibre e obstrução indireta por broncospasmo, bem como pela produção de muco e exsudato; a obstrução das vias aéreas mais calibrosas é extremamente rara; (2) aspiração de ácido gástrico — lesiona o epitélio respiratório e o surfactante; pode causar broncospasmo e ocasionalmente SARA; (3) pneumonia bacteriana — presença de bactérias no material regurgitado, no alimento ou na flora da faringe; pode desencadear uma infecção imediata ou uma infecção secundária mais tarde na evolução da doença.

IDENTIFICAÇÃO
Cães e, menos comumente, gatos.

SINAIS CLÍNICOS
- Pode ser superaguda, aguda ou crônica.
- Tosse, taquipneia, secreção nasal ou intolerância ao exercício.
- Angústia respiratória ou cianose quando grave.
- Cianose.
- Dependendo da causa subjacente — regurgitação; vômito; disfagia; alteração da consciência (p. ex., depressão, pós-icto, demência, sedação e anestesia); estertor ou estridor.

CAUSAS E FATORES DE RISCO
- Anormalidades faríngeas — paralisia local (p. ex., idiopática, miastenia grave focal, lesão nervosa traumática); doença neuromuscular generalizada; disfunção motora cricofaríngea; más-formações anatômicas; laringoplastia pós-operatória.
- Anormalidades esofágicas — megaesôfago; esofagite de refluxo; obstrução esofágica (p. ex., massa, corpo estranho, estenose); fístula broncoesofágica.
- Alteração da consciência — sedação, anestesia; pós-icto; doença do prosencéfalo; distúrbio metabólico grave.
- Causa iatrogênica — alimentação forçada; alimentação com sonda; administração de óleo mineral.

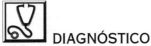

DIAGNÓSTICO

DIAGNÓSTICO DIFERENCIAL
- Pneumonia bacteriana.
- Abscesso de lobo pulmonar — consolidação pulmonar em termos de aspecto radiográfico.

HEMOGRAMA/BIOQUÍMICA/URINÁLISE
- Leucocitose neutrofílica com desvio à esquerda, embora o leucograma possa estar normal.
- Anemia arregenerativa.

OUTROS TESTES LABORATORIAIS
- Gasometria sanguínea arterial — espera-se uma hipoxemia; $PaCO_2$ geralmente baixa.
- Outros testes — considerar a pesquisa de anticorpos contra receptores da acetilcolina, testes de função da tireoide ou adrenal e mensuração da creatina quinase para avaliação de fatores predisponentes.

DIAGNÓSTICO POR IMAGEM
- Radiografia torácica — padrão broncoalveolar geralmente mais grave nos lobos pulmonares dependentes da gravidade (p. ex., craniais direito e esquerdo, além do lobo médio); poderá levar até 24 h para que o padrão se desenvolva após aspiração aguda; examinar em busca de indícios de doença esofágica ou mediastínica.
- Estudo da deglutição de contraste (ideal com a fluoroscopia) — fornece indícios de disfunção na deglutição ou no esôfago que pode predispor o paciente à aspiração. Cuidado: esse exame pode resultar em aspiração do meio de contraste.

MÉTODOS DIAGNÓSTICOS
- Lavado traqueal — coletar material para cultura bacteriana e antibiograma antes da administração de antibióticos; infecção frequentemente causada por múltiplos microrganismos com suscetibilidade imprevisível.
- Broncoscopia — indicada apenas na suspeita de obstrução de vias aéreas calibrosas com base no padrão respiratório, na auscultação ou nos achados radiográficos; remover corpo estranho e coletar amostras das vias aéreas.

TRATAMENTO

- Oxigênio — para angústia respiratória; se a angústia persistir, fornecer suporte ventilatório.
- Fluidos intravenosos — evitar a superidratação, que pode exacerbar o edema secundário.
- Ingestão oral — suspensa até que o problema primário seja identificado e tratado.
- Repouso em gaiola — para angústia respiratória.
- Não permitir que o paciente permaneça em decúbito lateral no mesmo lado por mais de 2 h.
- Assim que o paciente estiver estabilizado, a prática de exercícios leves poderá ajudar a gerar tosse produtiva e facilitar a desobstrução das vias aéreas.
- Nebulização com solução salina e tapotagem — podem facilitar a resolução da pneumonia.
- Sucção das vias aéreas — indicada somente se puder ser efetuada imediatamente após a sucção (como quando ocorre a aspiração no hospital durante a recuperação da anestesia).
- Lavagem das vias aéreas — contraindicada.

MEDICAÇÕES

MEDICAMENTO(S)
- Antibioticoterapia — é ideal suspendê-la até que uma amostra da via aérea seja coletada para citologia e cultura/antibiograma; se houver sinais de sepse ou comprometimento grave, ampicilina com sulbactam (20 mg/kg IV a cada 8 h) mais alguma fluoroquinolona IV. Ajustar a seleção dos antibióticos com base nos resultados da citologia das vias aéreas, na cultura e no antibiograma, bem como na resposta clínica; continuar por 10 dias após a resolução dos sinais clínicos e radiográficos.
- Broncodilatadores (p. ex., teofilina e terbutalina) — podem gerar uma melhora espetacular em alguns casos, embora tenham o potencial de agravar o desequilíbrio entre a perfusão e a ventilação; úteis com maior frequência em cães e gatos com aspiração aguda ou sibilos auscultáveis.
- Corticosteroides de curta ação — podem ser administrados como dose única para combater a inflamação em casos de aspiração superaguda com risco de morte.

CONTRAINDICAÇÕES/INTERAÇÕES POSSÍVEIS
- Diuréticos — geralmente contraindicados; o ressecamento das vias aéreas diminui a depuração mucociliar.
- Corticosteroides — contraindicados, em geral; predispõem o paciente à infecção.
- Antibióticos fluoroquinolona e cloranfenicol — podem prolongar a depuração dos broncodilatadores derivados de teofilina, resultando em sinais de toxicidade.

ACOMPANHAMENTO

MONITORIZAÇÃO DO PACIENTE
- Radiografias, gasometria sanguínea arterial e sinais clínicos — monitorizar a resposta ao tratamento.
- Radiografias — avaliar a cada 3-7 dias inicialmente para determinar a adequação do tratamento; depois, a cada 1-2 semanas.
- Na falta de resolução dos sinais ou em caso de piora súbita — é possível a ocorrência de recidiva da aspiração ou infecção secundária; repetir a avaliação diagnóstica, incluindo o exame de líquido do lavado traqueal ou broncoscopia.

COMPLICAÇÕES POSSÍVEIS
- É comum a ocorrência de infecção secundária.
- SARA — pode se desenvolver, particularmente após aspiração de ácido gástrico.
- É rara a formação de abscesso ou granuloma por corpo estranho.

EVOLUÇÃO ESPERADA E PROGNÓSTICO
- Prognóstico — depende da gravidade dos sinais e da capacidade de corrigir o problema subjacente.
- Aspiração aguda e grave — pode ser fatal.
- Recidiva — provável se a causa subjacente não for tratada ou caso não se consiga tratá-la.

DIVERSOS

VER TAMBÉM
- Megaesôfago.
- Pneumonia Bacteriana.
- Síndrome da Angústia Respiratória Aguda (SARA).

ABREVIATURA(S)
- SARA = síndrome da angústia respiratória aguda.

Sugestões de Leitura
Kogan DA, Johnson LR, Jandrey KE, Pollard RE. Etiology and clinical outcome in dogs with aspiration pneumonia: 88 cases (2004-2006). JAVMA 2008, 233:1748-1755.

Autor Eleanor C. Hawkins
Consultor Editorial Lynelle R. Johnson

Pneumotórax

CONSIDERAÇÕES GERAIS

DEFINIÇÃO
• Acúmulo de ar no espaço pleural; classificado como traumático ou espontâneo.
• Pneumotórax fechado — sem defeitos na parede torácica.
• Pneumotórax aberto — defeito na parede torácica, que resulta na comunicação do espaço pleural com a atmosfera.
• Pneumotórax de tensão — caso em que a pressão pleural no pneumotórax fechado excede a pressão atmosférica; gerado por transferência unidirecional de ar para dentro do espaço pleural.

FISIOPATOLOGIA
• O espaço pleural normalmente é um espaço potencial entre as pleuras visceral e parietal. Ele contém uma fina camada de líquido, que contribui para a "fixação" dos pulmões à parede torácica. O acúmulo de ar no espaço pleural rompe a vedação de tensão superficial do líquido pleural, promovendo o colapso dos pulmões e consequente afastamento desses órgãos da parede torácica.
• Pneumotórax fechado — vazamento de ar proveniente do parênquima pulmonar ou de via aérea calibrosa. A pressão pleural eleva-se proporcionalmente à quantidade de ar acumulado no espaço pleural.
• Pneumotórax de tensão — quando a pressão pleural excede a pressão atmosférica no pneumotórax fechado; tipicamente se deve a um defeito pleural ou pulmonar tipo *flap* que permite o vazamento de ar para o espaço pleural na inspiração e se fecha durante a expiração.
• Pneumotórax aberto — pode ou não estar associado à doença pulmonar; a pressão pleural iguala-se à pressão atmosférica, levando ao colapso pulmonar.
• Hipoxemia — desenvolve-se secundariamente ao colapso do parênquima pulmonar.
• Pressões intratorácicas elevadas podem reduzir o retorno venoso ao coração.
• O pneumotórax costuma ser bilateral a menos que o mediastino permaneça intacto.

SISTEMA(S) ACOMETIDO(S)
• Respiratório.
• Cardiovascular.

INCIDÊNCIA/PREVALÊNCIA
Pneumotórax traumático ocorre em >40% dos casos com traumatismo do tórax e em 11-18% dos cães e gatos levados ao veterinário por conta de trauma causado por automóvel. O pneumotórax foi relatado em ~25% dos casos com farpas de gramíneas intratorácicas e 70% dos cães com feridas torácicas por mordeduras.

IDENTIFICAÇÃO
Espécies
Cães e gatos.

Raça(s) Predominante(s)
Pneumotórax espontâneo — mais comum em cães de grande porte e tórax profundo. A raça Husky siberiano talvez seja super-representada.

SINAIS CLÍNICOS
Achados Anamnésicos
• Traumático — traumatismo recente. Anestesia e entubação recentes aumentam a possibilidade de trauma da traqueia. Toracocentese ou venopunção jugular recentes — causas iatrogênicas.
• Espontâneo — pode ou não haver histórico prévio de doença pulmonar; costuma ser agudo, embora possa ter um início lentamente progressivo.

Achados do Exame Físico
• Taquipneia.
• Angústia respiratória.
• Ortopneia.
• É comum uma respiração abdominal rápida e superficial.
• Taquicardia.
• Ruídos pulmonares reduzidos dorsalmente — pode ser difícil reconhecê-los em animais muito dispneicos.

Pneumotórax Traumático
• Sinais adicionais de traumatismo, incluindo mucosas pálidas; cianose manifesta em casos graves, choque.
• Pode ou não haver evidência de trauma torácico.
• Pneumotórax aberto — presença de traumatismo evidente na parede torácica.
• Enfisema subcutâneo em alguns casos com pneumomediastino e/ou trauma traqueal.

CAUSAS
• Traumáticas — trauma rombo, lesões torácicas ou cervicais penetrantes, pós-toracocentese ou toracotomia, perfuração esofágica, traumatismo traqueal associado ao tubo endotraqueal.
• Espontâneas — enfisema bolhoso (mais comum em cães), corpo estranho pulmonar migratório, neoplasia pulmonar, abscesso pulmonar, asma felina, pneumonia, granuloma pulmonar micótico, doença pulmonar parasitária (*Paragonimus*), cisto pulmonar congênito, bolhas pulmonares, vesículas pulmonares, enfisema bolhoso, enfisema lobar congênito.

FATORES DE RISCO
• Traumatismo.
• Toracocentese.
• Toracotomia.
• Hiperinsuflação do manguito endotraqueal.
• Doença pulmonar.
• Migração de farpas de gramíneas.

DIAGNÓSTICO

DIAGNÓSTICO DIFERENCIAL
• Efusão pleural.
• Hérnia diafragmática.
• Doença parenquimatosa pulmonar.

HEMOGRAMA/BIOQUÍMICA/URINÁLISE
Neutrofilia com desvio à esquerda se houver infecção pulmonar ou doença inflamatória.

OUTROS TESTES LABORATORIAIS
• Gases sanguíneos arteriais — podem ocorrer hipoxemia, hipocapnia ou hipercapnia.
• Sedimentação ou centrifugação-flutuação fecais com sulfato de zinco — para pesquisa de *Paragonimus*.

DIAGNÓSTICO POR IMAGEM
Radiografia Torácica
• Adiar até que o paciente esteja estabilizado; pode não ser possível a obtenção de mais de uma projeção.
• Presença de ar no espaço pleural; padrão vascular pulmonar, que não se estende à parede torácica; elevação da silhueta cardíaca e seu consequente afastamento do esterno — radiografia com feixe horizontal com o animal em decúbito lateral é a projeção mais sensível.
• Doença pulmonar pode estar mascarada pelo colapso de lobo pulmonar; talvez seja necessário repetir as radiografias após a toracocentese.
• Pneumotórax traumático — avaliar o animal em busca de outras lesões traumáticas como contusões, fratura de costelas, hérnia diafragmática, hemotórax, corpos estranhos (projéteis balísticos, pontas de flechas).
• Pneumotórax espontâneo — avaliar o paciente quanto à presença de qualquer sinal de doença parenquimatosa.

Ultrassom Torácico
• Pneumotórax evidenciado pela perda do "sinal de deslizamento".
• Em comparação às radiografias torácicas, o ultrassom tem sensibilidade de 78% e especificidade de 93% em cães após o traumatismo.

Tomografia Computadorizada Torácica
Pesquisa de pneumotórax espontâneo para ajudar a localização de doença pulmonar.

MÉTODOS DIAGNÓSTICOS
• Toracocentese — confirma o diagnóstico; remove a máxima quantidade de ar do espaço pleural.
• Broncoscopia — se houver evidência de traumatismo da traqueia ou de via aérea calibrosa.

ACHADOS PATOLÓGICOS
• Variam, dependendo da doença subjacente.
• Avaliação macroscópica — pode ser suficiente para visualizar vesículas pulmonares, lacerações dos pulmões ou das vias aéreas, doença parenquimatosa pulmonar ou massas pulmonares.
• Histopatologia — as vesículas são mais comumente encontradas no ápice e estão totalmente contidas dentro da pleura; as bolhas são revestidas por pleura, tecido pulmonar fibroso e pulmão enfisematoso.

TRATAMENTO

CUIDADO(S) DE SAÚDE ADEQUADO(S)
• Internação do paciente até a interrupção ou estabilização do acúmulo de ar.
• Os animais em angústia respiratória precisam ser submetidos à toracocentese, com a quantidade máxima de ar removido. A toracocentese pode ser realizada com cateter intravenoso conectado a equipo de extensão e válvula de escape ou via agulha tipo borboleta. A toracocentese nem sempre será necessária se o paciente estiver estabilizado.
• SEMPRE fornecer oxigenoterapia até a estabilização do paciente.
• Analgesia com medicamento tipo opioide na presença de lesões significativas após o traumatismo — utilizar o extremo inferior da faixa de dosagem de algum agonista dos receptores μ (além de conferir a melhor analgesia, esse agente pode ser revertido se houver necessidade).
• Na existência de ampla ferida aberta no tórax — cobrir com a máxima limpeza possível com bandagem hermética (uso de lubrificante/pomada estéril na periferia da ferida). Isso precisa ser acompanhado pela colocação de tubo torácico; assim que o animal estiver estabilizado, haverá necessidade de oclusão cirúrgica.

- Toracostomia com tubo — efetuada caso não se consiga estabilizar o animal com a toracocentese ou caso haja necessidade de toracocenteses repetidas nos casos de pneumotórax contínuo; colocação de tubo torácico (sob anestesia local ou geral) — o local de penetração na pele é preparado de forma asséptica no quadrante caudodorsal do tórax lateral; a incisão na pele é do mesmo tamanho que o tubo, sendo realizada sobre os espaços intercostais 11-12 ou 12-13; a pele, então, é tracionada no sentido cranial pelo assistente, para que a incisão fique sobre os espaços intercostais 7-8 ou 8-9. O tubo torácico é introduzido no espaço pleural, apontando para o sentido cranioventral; a pele, então, pode ser liberada, criando-se um túnel subcutâneo. Proceder à sutura da pele em bolsa em torno do local de inserção e fixar o tubo com o padrão de sutura chinesa tipo *finger-trap* ("armadilha de dedos"); é recomendável a obtenção de radiografias torácicas após a colocação de tubo.
- Se o pneumotórax estiver se acumulando rapidamente — realizar sucção contínua com tubo torácico via sistema de drenagem com um, dois ou três frascos e vedação submersa. Se o pneumotórax não for grave ou estiver se resolvendo — proceder à aspiração intermitente via tubo.
- Válvulas de Heimlich — válvulas unidirecionais usadas para evitar a introdução de ar dentro dos tubos torácicos. Tais válvulas são muito facilmente ocluídas com pequenas quantidades de secreções líquidas. Não recomendadas sem a observação contínua do paciente ou em animais de porte muito pequeno.
- Em situações de emergência de pneumotórax de tensão com risco de morte — considerar a realização de toracotomia de emergência para converter o problema em pneumotórax aberto; o animal pode, então, ser entubado e ventilado com pressão positiva até estabilizar.
- Pneumotórax traumático aberto — realizar a cirurgia assim que o paciente estiver estabilizado.
- Pneumotórax traumático fechado — raramente precisa de intervenção cirúrgica.
- Pneumotórax espontâneo — é recomendável a realização de intervenção cirúrgica precoce nos cães; toracotomia exploratória será frequentemente realizada via esternotomia mediana se a localização da lesão for desconhecida.

CUIDADO(S) DE ENFERMAGEM
- Fluidos intravenosos — são necessários na maioria dos casos de trauma.
- Manutenção do tubo torácico — assegurar a natureza hermética de todas as conexões (braçadeiras são excelentes para fixá-las); garantir a fixação do tubo em dois pontos para reduzir a chance de sua remoção inadvertida. Limpar o local do tubo e trocar o curativo uma vez ao dia. Não permitir que o animal mastigue o tubo torácico.

ATIVIDADE
Repouso restrito por no mínimo uma semana após a resolução do pneumotórax na tentativa de minimizar a chance de recidiva.

ORIENTAÇÃO AO PROPRIETÁRIO
- Pneumotórax traumático — discutir o possível uso de tubo torácico e a necessidade de hospitalização; alguns animais podem precisar de cirurgia.
- Pneumotórax espontâneo — é recomendável a realização de intervenção cirúrgica precoce na maioria dos casos caninos. Abordar a possibilidade de doença pulmonar subjacente, que pode tornar a resolução um desafio e a recidiva possível. Advertir o proprietário que, mesmo com a toracotomia, a origem do pneumotórax pode não ser encontrada, sendo possível a recidiva da doença.

CONSIDERAÇÕES CIRÚRGICAS
- Não utilizar ventilação com pressão positiva para pneumotórax fechado. Inserir o tubo torácico antes da ventilação ou aguardar a toracotomia antes da ventilação.
- Toracoscopia — pode permitir a visualização da lesão local; possibilita a instilação de substâncias para pleurodese.
- Toracotomia — se a lesão não for evidente, pode-se preencher o tórax com solução salina e observar bolhas como sinal de vazamento. Não é raro haver mais que uma lesão. Lobectomia pulmonar parcial ou total para lesões localizadas. Lacerações traumáticas podem ser suturadas. Em alguns casos, é possível que a localização do vazamento não seja evidente na cirurgia. O tubo de toracostomia deve ser colocado no momento da cirurgia em todos os pacientes.
- Pleurodese com abrasão mecânica da pleura ou instilação de substância inflamatória, como talco, dentro do espaço pleural (acredita-se que a taxa de sucesso seja baixa).

MEDICAÇÕES
MEDICAMENTO(S)
Uso criterioso de controle da dor.

PRECAUÇÕES
Ter cuidado com depressão respiratória excessiva com o uso de opiáceos.

ACOMPANHAMENTO
MONITORIZAÇÃO DO PACIENTE
- Frequência respiratória — o aumento sugere recidiva do pneumotórax.
- Radiografias torácicas seriadas para quantificar o acúmulo de ar.
- Oximetria de pulso se o ar exalado puder determinar o estado de oxigenação. Gases sanguíneos arteriais fornecem a melhor avaliação do estado de oxigenação na presença de doença pulmonar.
- Gases sanguíneos venosos (jugulares) centrais podem ser utilizados para avaliar o estado de ventilação via $PvCO_2$.
- Velocidade de produção de ar a partir do tubo torácico — sob drenagem contínua com sistema de sucção de 3 frascos, necessária para contar as bolhas/minuto produzidas na câmara média; em caso de aspiração intermitente, será possível a quantificação com seringa.

PREVENÇÃO
Manter o animal confinado — isso diminui a probabilidade de lesões.

COMPLICAÇÕES POSSÍVEIS
- Morte por hipoxemia e comprometimento cardiovascular.
- Colocação incorreta do tubo torácico ou traumatismo associado à toracocentese — laceração de lobo pulmonar, punção cardíaca, laceração diafragmática, trauma hepático.
- Infecção pleural por toracocentese ou drenagem torácica.

EVOLUÇÃO ESPERADA E PROGNÓSTICO
- Pneumotórax traumático — se o trauma torácico não for grave, o prognóstico será bom com toracocentese ± colocação de dreno torácico. Em casos de traumatismo grave do tórax, o paciente pode piorar apesar de todos os esforços para estabilizá-lo — geralmente por conta de contusões pulmonares graves.
- Pneumotórax espontâneo — o prognóstico depende da causa subjacente. Se houver uma única lesão focal passível de ressecção cirúrgica, o prognóstico será bom. Caso não seja possível a localização da lesão ou na presença de doença pulmonar difusa, o prognóstico será mau.

DIVERSOS
SINÔNIMO(S)
Pulmão perfurado.

VER TAMBÉM
- Dispneia e Angústia Respiratória.
- Respiração Ofegante e Taquipneia.

Sugestões de Leitura
Cooper ES, Syring RS, King LG. Pneumothorax in cats with a clinical diagnosis of feline asthma: 5 cases (1990-2000) J Vet Emerg Crit Care 2003, 13:95-101.
Lisciandro GR, Lagutchik MS, Mann KA, Voges AK, Fosgate GT, Tiller EG, Cabano NR, Bauer LD, Book BP. Evaluation of a thoracic focused assessment with sonography for trauma (TFAST) protocol to detect pneumothorax and concurrent thoracic injury in 145 traumatized dogs. J Vet Emerg Crit Care 2008, 18:258-269.
Puerto DA, Brockman DJ, et al. Surgical and nonsurgical management of and selected risk factors for spontaneous pneumothorax in dogs: 64 cases (1986-1999). JAVMA 2002, 220:1670-1674.
Scheepens ET, Peeters ME, L'eplattenier HF, Kirpensteijn J. Thoracic bite trauma in dogs: A comparison of clinical and radiological parameters with surgical results. J Small Anim Pract 2006, 47:721-726.
Schultz RM, Zwingenberger A. Radiographic, computed tomographic, and ultrasonographic findings with migrating intrathoracic grass awns in dogs and cats. Vet Radiol Ultrasound 2008, 49(3):249-255.

Autor Kate Hopper
Consultor Editorial Lynelle R. Johnson

PODODERMATITE

CONSIDERAÇÕES GERAIS

DEFINIÇÃO
Complexo inflamatório de múltiplas facetas de doenças que envolvem os pés dos cães e dos gatos.

FISIOPATOLOGIA
• Depende da causa subjacente, incluindo infecção, alergia, dermatoses autoimunes, doença endócrina ou metabólica, neoplasia e doença ambiental. • Dermatose psicogênica (causa rara).

SISTEMA(S) ACOMETIDO(S)
Cutâneo/exócrino.

INCIDÊNCIA/PREVALÊNCIA
• Cães — comum. • Gatos — rara.

IDENTIFICAÇÃO
Espécies
Cães e gatos.

Raça(s) Predominante(s)
• Raças de pelagem curta (cães) — mais comumente acometidas; raças Buldogue inglês, Dogue alemão, Basset hound, Mastife, Bull terrier, Boxer, Dachshund, Dálmata, Pointer alemão de pelo curto e Weimaraner. • Raças de pelagem longa (cães) — Pastor alemão, Labrador retriever, Golden retriever, Setter irlandês e Pequinês.
• Gatos — nenhuma.

Idade Média e Faixa Etária
• Qualquer idade. • Cães jovens: hipersensibilidade, demodicose, infecção, cistos foliculares, dermatoses autoimunes. • Cães idosos: neoplasia ou doenças sistêmicas também.

Sexo Predominante
• Caninos — machos. • Felinos — nenhum.

SINAIS CLÍNICOS
Comentários Gerais
Os achados da anamnese e do exame físico variam consideravelmente, dependendo da causa subjacente.

Achados Anamnésicos
• Anamnese — determinar o ambiente do animal e as condições gerais da criação (p. ex., dentro ou fora de casa, animal de trabalho *versus* de companhia, condições insalubres, outros animais acometidos, traumatismo, irritantes de contato, ancilóstomos), bem como a idade de início.
• Sazonalidade — sugere dermatite atópica, dermatite alérgica de contato ou dermatite irritante de contato.
• Lesões em qualquer parte do corpo.
• Lesões confinadas apenas aos pés; examinar quais os pés acometidos e as partes envolvidas (todo o pé, uma única área ou um único dedo).
• Resposta a tratamento prévio — antibióticos, antifúngicos e corticosteroides.
• Dieta, histórico de viagem e outros problemas clínicos.

Achados do Exame Físico
Infecciosos (Cães)
• Eritema e edema, além de nódulos, placas inflamatórias ("quériones" fúngicos), úlceras, fístulas, bolhas hemorrágicas ou secreção serossanguinolenta ou seropurulenta.
• Pés — podem estar macroscopicamente tumefatos; além disso, pode haver edema depressível das regiões do metacarpo e do metatarso.
• Pele — pode estar com alopecia e umidade em virtude de lambedura constante; o paciente pode apresentar certo grau de dor, prurido e paroníquia*.
• Linfonodos regionais podem estar infartados.

Infecciosos (Gatos)
• Paroníquia dolorosa, envolvendo uma ou mais unhas.
• Maior incidência de lesões nodulares, frequentemente ulceradas, em comparação aos cães.
• Coxins podais e áreas periungueais — comumente envolvidos.
• Espaços interdigitais — raramente acometidos.
• Lesões escamosas e crostosas — observadas ocasionalmente.

Alérgicos (Cães)
• Eritema e alopecia (dorsal ou ventral ou ambos), secundários ao prurido; as superfícies dorsais podem ser mais gravemente acometidas que as ventrais.
• Eritema interdigital.
• Mancha por saliva.
• Dermatite alérgica de contato — causa incomum; a dermatite das superfícies interdigitais ventrais costuma ser pior, embora toda a pata possa estar envolvida.

Alérgicos (Gatos)
• Placas pruriginosas isoladas ou múltiplas, exsudativas ou ulceradas, eosinofílicas periungueais, bem como dos dedos e espaços interdigitais.

Imunomediados (Cães)
• Crostas e ulcerações — lesões mais comuns; ocasionalmente se observam vesículas ou bolhas.
• Todos os quatro pés podem estar acometidos, especialmente os leitos ungueais e os coxins podais.
• Dermatite hiperqueratótica e erosiva dos coxins podais — achado comum no pênfigo foliáceo.

Imunomediados (Gatos)
• Lesões — geralmente envolvem o coxim podal, incluindo hiperqueratose e ulceração.
• Claudicação e paroníquia com exsudatos das pregas ungueais.

Endócrinos/Metabólicos (Cães)
• Lesões — geralmente compatíveis com infecção secundária.
• Síndrome hepatocutânea (dermatite necrolítica superficial) — condição rara; a dermatopatia precede o início dos sinais de doença interna; as lesões incluem hiperqueratose (com crostas aderentes), fissuras e ulceração dos coxins podais.

Endócrinos/Metabólicos (Gatos)
• Nódulos esbranquiçados que se assemelham à cera de vela; podem ser causados por xantomatose cutânea; observados em casos de diabetes melito.

Neoplásicos
• Cães — nódulos, variavelmente ulcerados, com descamação, eritema e despigmentação dos coxins podais; pode haver o acometimento de um único dedo (carcinoma do leito ungueal, ceratoacantoma ungueal); envolvimento de vários pés nos casos de carcinoma de células escamosas do leito ungueal; prurido variável.
• Gatos — nódulos; variavelmente ulcerados e dolorosos; destruição localizada variável, dependendo do tipo de tumor; os tumores dos coxins podais podem se desenvolver de novo ou representar um carcinoma metastático.

Ambientais (Cães e Gatos)
• Depende da causa subjacente.
• Lesões — envolvem um dos dedos ou um dos pés (corpo estranho, traumatismo) ou vários dedos (dermatite de contato irritante, intoxicação pelo tálio, alojamento em superfície áspera ou em ambiente úmido).
• Inflamação interdigital crônica, ulceração, abscesso piogranulomatoso, trajetos drenantes ou tumefação, com ou sem prurido.

Diversos
• Hiperqueratose dos coxins podais (cães) — associada a várias doenças (p. ex., dermatose responsiva ao zinco, dermatose alimentar canina genérica) e hiperqueratose digital idiopática.
• Cistos foliculares interdigitais — nódulos interdigitais, com fístulas e trajetos drenantes dorsalmente; em geral, acometem apenas os pés dianteiros; afetam o espaço interdigital lateral; histórico de recidiva e resposta insatisfatória a nula a antibióticos, com uma área de pele espessada e alopécica com comedões ventralmente.
• Nódulos sem trajetos drenantes (cães) — associados a piogranulomas estéreis em diversas raças e dermatofibrose nodular do Pastor alemão e do Golden retriever.
• Hipomelanose dos coxins podais (gatos) — associada ao vitiligo.
• Hipermelanose dos coxins podais (gatos) — associada ao lentigo simples.
• Polidactilismo e sindactilismo (gatos) — comuns em determinadas famílias.
• Mutilação e analgesia acrais — observadas nas raças Pointer (alemão de pelo curto e inglês) e Spaniel (francês e Springer inglês) — causa desconhecida; geralmente o menor da ninhada; não há tratamento conhecido; os cães costumam ser submetidos à eutanásia dentro de dias a meses do diagnóstico.

CAUSAS
Infecciosas (Cães)
• Bacterianas — *Staphylococcus pseudintermedius*, *Pseudomonas* spp., *Proteus* spp., *Mycobacterium* spp., *Nocardia* spp. ou *Actinomyces* spp.
• Fúngicas — dermatófitos, micoses intermediárias (esporotricose, micetoma) ou micoses profundas (blastomicose, criptococose).
• Parasitárias — *Demodex canis*, *Pelodera strongyloides* e ancilóstomos.
• Protozoárias — leishmaniose.

Infecciosas (Gatos)
• Bacterianas — mesmas que os cães, acrescidas de *Pasteurella* spp.
• Fúngicas — mesmas que os cães, excluindo a blastomicose.
• Parasitárias — *Neotrombicula autumnalis*, *Notoedres cati* ou *Demodex* spp.
• Protozoárias — *Anatrichosoma cutaneum*.

Alérgicas
• Cães — atopia; hipersensibilidade alimentar; dermatite de contato alérgica.
• Gatos — atopia; rara para dermatite alérgica a pulgas, hipersensibilidade alimentar ou dermatite de contato envolvendo as patas.

Imunomediadas
• Cães — pênfigo foliáceo; lúpus eritematoso sistêmico; eritema multiforme; necrólise epidérmica tóxica; vasculite; doença da aglutinina fria; pênfigo vulgar; penfigoide bolhoso;

---
* N. T.: Inflamação da pele em volta da unha.

epidermólise bolhosa adquirida; onicodistrofia lupoide simétrica.
• Gatos — pênfigo foliáceo; lúpus eritematoso sistêmico; eritema multiforme; necrólise epidérmica tóxica; vasculite; doença da aglutinina fria; pododermatite plasmocitária.

Endócrinas/Metabólicas
• Cães — hipotireoidismo; hiperadrenocorticismo; síndrome hepatocutânea (dermatite necrolítica superficial).
• Gatos — hipertireoidismo; hiperadrenocorticismo; xantomatose cutânea (secundária ao diabetes melito); pododermatite endócrina rara.

Neoplásicas
• Maior incidência nos gatos do que nos cães.
• Cães — carcinoma de células escamosas; linfoma epiteliotrópico; melanoma; mastocitoma; ceratoacantoma; papiloma invertido; adenocarcinoma écrino.
• Gatos — papiloma; epitelioma espinocelular; tricoepitelioma; fibrossarcoma; histiocitoma fibroso maligno; adenocarcinoma primário metastático do pulmão; outros carcinomas metastáticos.

Ambientais
• Cães — dermatite de contato irritante; traumatismo; pisos de concreto e de cascalho; exercício excessivo; queimadura causada pela máquina de tosa; corpos estranhos (farpas de gramíneas, pelos tipo cerdas dos cães de pelagem curta); intoxicação pelo tálio.
• Gatos — dermatite de contato irritante; corpos estranhos; intoxicação pelo tálio.

Diversas
• Cães — granuloma interdigital estéril; cisto folicular interdigital; ver a seção "Achados do Exame Físico".
• Gatos — ver a seção "Achados do Exame Físico".

FATORES DE RISCO
• Estilo de vida do animal e condições gerais da criação — influenciam o desenvolvimento.
• Excesso de exercício, alojamento em local abrasivo ou úmido, cuidado insatisfatório do pelo e/ou falta de clínica médica preventiva podem predispor um animal ou exacerbar a condição.
• Porte do corpo, conformação dos pés e raça do animal influenciam o desenvolvimento de cistos foliculares interdigitais.

DIAGNÓSTICO
DIAGNÓSTICO DIFERENCIAL
Ver as seções "Sinais Clínicos" e "Causas".

HEMOGRAMA/BIOQUÍMICA/URINÁLISE
• Dependem da causa subjacente.
• Raramente utilizados na avaliação diagnóstica inicial.

OUTROS TESTES LABORATORIAIS
• Dependem da causa subjacente.
• Testes endócrinos, sorologia ou estudos imunológicos.

DIAGNÓSTICO POR IMAGEM
• Depende da causa subjacente.

MÉTODOS DIAGNÓSTICOS
• Raspados de pele — demodicose.
• Cultura fúngica — dermatofitose.
• Esfregaço de exsudato ou pústula — infecção bacteriana ou leveduriforme.
• Biopsia — tecidos enviados para exame histopatológico, cultura bacteriana ou fúngica e potencialmente para imunopatologia.
• Cultura e antibiograma de exsudatos e/ou tecidos.
• Cães — as biopsias serão indicadas em caso de raspados de pele negativos e observação de lesões (nódulos e trajetos drenantes); as amostras obtidas da superfície ventral com trajetos drenantes podem revelar cistos foliculares e inflamação piogranulomatosa, espalhando-se para a superfície dorsal.
• Gatos — as biopsias poderão ser indicadas em todos os casos; dermatose podal é relativamente rara.
• Dieta de eliminação alimentar com restrição de algum ingrediente — hipersensibilidade alimentar.
• Teste cutâneo intradérmico — atopia.
• Testes endócrinos — hipotireoidismo, hiperadrenocorticismo, diabetes melito.

ACHADOS PATOLÓGICOS
Dependem da causa subjacente.

TRATAMENTO
CUIDADO(S) DE SAÚDE ADEQUADO(S)
Como paciente de ambulatório a menos que haja indicação de cirurgia.

CUIDADO(S) DE ENFERMAGEM
Pedilúvios, compressas quentes e/ou bandagens podem ser necessários, dependendo da causa.

ATIVIDADE
Depende da gravidade das lesões e da causa subjacente.

DIETA
Dieta hipoalergênica com restrição de ingrediente se houver indicação.

ORIENTAÇÃO AO PROPRIETÁRIO
• Depende da causa subjacente e da gravidade da condição.
• Discutir as práticas de criação e de medicina preventiva.
• Etiologias alérgicas, imunomediadas ou endócrinas podem ser controladas, mas não curadas.

CONSIDERAÇÕES CIRÚRGICAS
• Melanoma e carcinoma de células escamosas — prognóstico muito mau; o diagnóstico precoce necessita da amputação do(s) dedo(s) ou do pé.
• Infecciosas — podem se beneficiar do debridamento cirúrgico do tecido desvitalizado antes do tratamento clínico.
• Trajetos drenantes recidivantes causados por cistos foliculares interdigitais podem ser removidos com ablação a laser.

MEDICAÇÕES
MEDICAMENTO(S) DE ESCOLHA
• Depende(m) da causa subjacente e das infecções secundárias.
• Antibióticos selecionados com base na cultura e no antibiograma; por, no mínimo, 4 a 6 semanas.
• Medicações antifúngicas.
• Dosagem anti-inflamatória ou imunossupressora de corticosteroides.
• Agentes quimioterápicos.
• Terapia de reposição hormonal.
• Suplementação de zinco.
• Aminoácidos intravenosos.

PRECAUÇÕES
Dependem do protocolo terapêutico selecionado para a causa subjacente; consultar os medicamentos específicos e suas precauções.

INTERAÇÕES POSSÍVEIS
Dependem da causa subjacente e do protocolo terapêutico selecionado.

ACOMPANHAMENTO
MONITORIZAÇÃO DO PACIENTE
Depende da causa subjacente e do protocolo terapêutico selecionado.

PREVENÇÃO
• Causa ambiental — boas práticas de criação e de medicina preventiva devem evitar a recidiva.
• Causa alérgica — é importante evitar o alérgeno (ambiental ou alimentar), se possível.

COMPLICAÇÕES POSSÍVEIS
Dependem da causa subjacente e do protocolo terapêutico selecionado.

EVOLUÇÃO ESPERADA E PROGNÓSTICO
• O sucesso do tratamento depende do encontro da causa subjacente; quase sempre a causa é desconhecida; mesmo quando a causa for conhecida, o tratamento poderá ser frustrante em virtude das recidivas ou da falta de tratamentos acessíveis.
• Com frequência, a dose só pode ser controlada, mas não curada.
• Às vezes, há necessidade de intervenção cirúrgica.

DIVERSOS
FATORES RELACIONADOS COM A IDADE
Dependem da causa subjacente.

POTENCIAL ZOONÓTICO
Depende da causa subjacente; incomum.

GESTAÇÃO/FERTILIDADE/REPRODUÇÃO
Evitar a administração sistêmica de corticosteroides, antifúngicos, agentes quimioterápicos, azatioprina e certos antimicrobianos (p. ex., enrofloxacino) nas fêmeas prenhes.

Sugestões de Leitura
Gottfried SD, Popovitch CA, Goldschmidt MH, Schelling C. Metastatic digital carcinoma in the cat: A retrospective study of 36 cats (1992-1998). JAAHA 2000, 36(6):501-509.
Paradis M, de Jaham C, Page N, Sauve F, Helie P. Acral mutilation and analgesia in 13 French spaniels. Vet Dermatol 2005, 16(2):87-93.
Scott DW, Miller WH, Griffin CE. Muller & Kirk's Small Animal Dermatology, 6th ed. Philadelphia: Saunders, 2001, pp. 304-306, 431-434, 1129-1130.

Autor David Duclos
Consultor Editorial Alexander H. Werner

Poliartrite Erosiva Imunomediada

CONSIDERAÇÕES GERAIS

DEFINIÇÃO
Doença inflamatória imunomediada das articulações que resulta em erosão da cartilagem articular.

FISIOPATOLOGIA
• Patogenia — causa incitante desconhecida, pois foi extrapolada a partir das pesquisas de artrite reumatoide em seres humanos; provavelmente perpetuada pela imunidade mediada por células; predominância de linfócitos T auxiliares CD4+ e depósitos de imunocomplexos encontrados na sinóvia das articulações acometidas; leucócitos, enzimas leucocitárias, imunidade mediada por células, imunocomplexos e reações autoalérgicas são direcionadas contra os componentes da cartilagem; leva à resposta inflamatória e à ativação do complemento.
• Enzimas destrutivas — liberadas a partir de células inflamatórias, sinoviócitos e condrócitos; prejudica a cartilagem articular, induzindo a alterações erosivas.
• Poliartrite erosiva idiopática — associada à resposta antigênica anormal contra a imunoglobulina do hospedeiro, semelhantemente à artrite reumatoide humana.
• Poliartrite erosiva do Galgo e poliartrite progressiva crônica felina — antígenos "ofensores" desconhecidos.

SISTEMA(S) ACOMETIDO(S)
Musculosquelético — articulações diartrodiais.

GENÉTICA
Não conhecida por ser hereditária.

INCIDÊNCIA/PREVALÊNCIA
Rara.

IDENTIFICAÇÃO
Espécies
• Cães — poliartrite erosiva idiopática, poliartrite erosiva do Galgo.
• Gatos — poliartrite progressiva crônica felina.

Raça(s) Predominante(s)
• Raças pequenas ou *toy* (cães) — mais suscetíveis à poliartrite erosiva idiopática.
• Galgo — única raça conhecida como suscetível à poliartrite erosiva do Galgo.

Idade Média e Faixa Etária
• Poliartrite erosiva idiopática (cães) — jovens a meia-idade (8 meses de vida a 8 anos de idade).
• Poliartrite erosiva do Galgo — Galgos jovens (3-30 meses de vida) são mais suscetíveis.
• Poliartrite progressiva crônica felina (gatos) — início com 1 ano e meio a 4 anos e meio de idade.

Sexo Predominante
Poliartrite progressiva crônica felina — há relatos de que acomete apenas gatos machos.

SINAIS CLÍNICOS
Comentários Gerais
No início, as formas não erosiva e erosiva da doença inflamatória imunomediada parecem semelhantes.

Achados Anamnésicos
• Cães e gatos — rigidez simétrica inicial, especialmente após repouso, ou claudicação intermitente com troca dos membros e tumefação das articulações acometidas.
• Gatos — pode-se notar um início mais insidioso; também se pode notar claudicação com troca dos membros.
• Tumefação articular — pode ser evidente, sobretudo no carpo e no tarso.
• Geralmente, não há histórico de traumatismo.
• Também é possível observar sinais de vômito, diarreia, anorexia, pirexia, depressão e linfadenopatia.
• Frequentemente cíclica — embora pareça responder à antibioticoterapia, a poliartrite erosiva imunomediada pode sofrer remissão espontânea.

Achados do Exame Físico
• Rigidez da marcha, claudicação, amplitude de movimento diminuída, crepitação, tumefação articular e dor em uma ou mais articulações.
• Instabilidade, subluxação e luxação articulares — dependem da duração da doença.
• Claudicação — desde leve sustentação do peso até incapacidade mais grave de suportar o peso.
• Articulações diartrodiais — todas podem ser acometidas; a poliartrite erosiva idiopática e a poliartrite progressiva crônica felina acometem as articulações carpais, tarsais e falângicas; a poliartrite erosiva do Galgo costuma acometer as articulações carpais, interfalângicas proximais e tarsais, além das articulações do cotovelo, do joelho e do quadril.

CAUSAS
• Desconhecidas.
• Provável mecanismo imunológico.
• *Mycoplasma spumans* (poliartrite erosiva do Galgo) — obtido em cultura realizada em um único Galgo acometido; não isolado em outros pacientes.
• FeLV e FeFV — ligados a gatos com poliartrite progressiva crônica felina.

DIAGNÓSTICO

DIAGNÓSTICO DIFERENCIAL
• Poliartrite idiopática.
• Artrite infecciosa.
• Lúpus eritematoso sistêmico.
• Poliartrite reativa.
• Neoplasia.
• Osteoartrite — primária ou secundária.

HEMOGRAMA/BIOQUÍMICA/URINÁLISE
• Geralmente normais.
• Hemograma — podem-se notar leucocitose, neutrofilia e hiperfibrinogenemia.

OUTROS TESTES LABORATORIAIS
• Fator reumatoide — positivo somente em cerca de 25% dos pacientes com poliartrite erosiva idiopática.
• Teste de Coombs e título de anticorpo antinuclear — normais.
• Títulos séricos para *Borrelia*, *Ehrlichia* e *Rickettsia* — devem estar normais.
• Evidência sorológica de FeFV — encontrada em todos os pacientes com poliartrite progressiva crônica felina.
• Evidência sorológica de exposição ao FeLV — encontrada em 50% ou menos dos pacientes com poliartrite progressiva crônica felina.

DIAGNÓSTICO POR IMAGEM
Radiografia
• O achado mais precoce consiste em uma tumefação do tecido mole periarticular.
• Doença grave — distensão da cápsula articular; osteofitose; espessamento de tecido mole; estreitamento dos espaços articulares; esclerose subcondral; densidade óssea trabecular diminuída; anquilose óssea nas articulações gravemente acometidas.
• Radiotransparências semelhantes a cistos — observadas ocasionalmente no osso subcondral.
• Doença crônica — subluxação/luxação e deformidade articular evidente.

MÉTODOS DIAGNÓSTICOS
• Artrocentese e análise do líquido sinovial — essenciais para o diagnóstico.
• Líquido sinovial — tipicamente turvo com viscosidade normal; grande número de neutrófilos não degenerados (10.000-100.000 células/mL); enviar para os exames de cultura bacteriana e antibiograma.
• Biopsia do tecido sinovial — ajuda a formular o diagnóstico; descarta outras artrites e neoplasia.

ACHADOS PATOLÓGICOS
• Erosão da cartilagem articular — particularmente próximo à periferia nas inserções sinoviais.
• Eburnação* e esclerose do osso subcondral com perda de cartilagem em toda a espessura — doença crônica.
• Membrana sinovial — macroscopicamente espessada; podem-se observar projeções vilosas.
• Tecido de granulação (pano) — pode invadir as margens da cartilagem articular e emergir da cavidade medular até destruir a cartilagem nas regiões centrais da articulação.
• Entesiófitos — nas inserções da cápsula articular e adjacentes à articulação.
• Exame histopatológico da membrana sinovial — tipicamente revela hiperplasia sinovial vilosa, hipertrofia e infiltrado inflamatório linfoplasmocitário.
• Líquido sinovial — turvo; volume aumentado.

TRATAMENTO

CUIDADO(S) DE SAÚDE ADEQUADO(S)
Geralmente como paciente de ambulatório.

CUIDADO(S) DE ENFERMAGEM
• Fisioterapia — exercícios com amplitude de movimento, massagem e natação; pode ser indicada para doença grave.
• Bandagens e/ou talas — para evitar colapso adicional da articulação; possíveis indicações para doença grave com deambulação muito comprometida.

ATIVIDADE
Limitada para minimizar a piora dos sinais clínicos.

DIETA
Redução de peso — para diminuir a tensão exercida sobre as articulações acometidas.

ORIENTAÇÃO AO PROPRIETÁRIO
Advertir os proprietários sobre o prognóstico mau quanto à cura e resolução completa.

CONSIDERAÇÕES CIRÚRGICAS
• Tempos de cura — podem ser longos; há variação dos níveis de recuperação.

---

* N. T.: Ossificação das cartilagens articulares.

POLIARTRITE EROSIVA IMUNOMEDIADA

- Cirurgia — geralmente não recomendada como uma opção terapêutica satisfatória.
- Artroplastia — substituição total do quadril, ostectomia da cabeça femoral; pode-se considerar.
- Artrodese — em casos selecionados de dor e instabilidade articulares; carpo: geralmente produz os melhores resultados, além de ser uma boa opção de recuperação; ombro, cotovelo, joelho ou jarrete: resultados menos previsíveis.

MEDICAÇÕES

MEDICAMENTO(S) DE ESCOLHA

Poliartrite Erosiva Idiopática
- AINE (cães) — pouco recompensadores.
- Prednisona — 1,5-2,0 mg/kg VO a cada 12 h por 10-14 dias como terapia inicial; diminuir gradativamente em várias semanas para 1,0 mg/kg VO a cada 48 h se a contagem celular do líquido sinovial retornar a < 4.000 células/mL e as células mononucleares predominarem; adicionar medicamentos citotóxicos se os sinais clínicos persistirem ou se a análise do líquido sinovial estiver anormal.
- Combinação de glicocorticoides e medicamentos citotóxicos — recomendada para obtenção de efeito sinérgico; pode-se tentar o uso de ciclofosfamida, azatioprina, 6-mercaptopurina, metotrexato ou leflunomida.
- Ciclofosfamida — paciente com < 10 kg: 2,5 mg/kg; paciente de 10-50 kg: 2,0 mg/kg; paciente com > 50 kg: 1,75 mg/kg; agente administrado por via oral a cada 24 h por 4 dias consecutivos de cada semana; pode-se administrar concomitantemente com a prednisona; a dose da prednisona pode ser diminuída pela metade.
- Azatioprina ou 6-mercaptopurina — 2,0 mg/kg VO a cada 24 h por 14-21 dias e, em seguida, a cada 48 h; administrar a prednisona do mesmo modo que a ciclofosfamida, mas em dias alternados.
- Leflunomida — dose canina: 4 mg/kg VO a cada 24 h; a dosagem pode ser ajustada após vários dias para manter o nível de vale (mais baixo) de 20 μg/mL.
- Remissão — induzida, em geral, pela combinação da quimioterapia dentro de 2-16 semanas; determinada pela resolução dos sinais clínicos e pela confirmação da análise de líquido sinovial normal.
- Interromper os medicamentos citotóxicos 1-3 meses após a remissão ser obtida.
- Manutenção da remissão — a terapia com glicocorticoides em dias alternados (prednisona 1,0 mg/kg VO) é geralmente bem-sucedida; em caso de recidiva dos sinais clínicos ou da efusão sinovial, talvez haja necessidade de terapia com medicamento citotóxico a longo prazo; se os sinais clínicos não recidivarem em 2-3 meses, pode-se interromper o glicocorticoide; se os sinais clínicos recidivarem após a interrupção do glicocorticoide, instituir novamente o tratamento.
- Aurotiomalato (crisoterapia) — 1 mg/kg IM semanalmente; alivia os sintomas de forma bem-sucedida.

Poliartrite Erosiva do Galgo
- O tratamento é pouco recompensador.
- Antibióticos, AINE, glicocorticoides, medicamentos citotóxicos e glicosaminoglicanos polissulfatados (Adequan®) — falham em induzir a remissão.

Poliartrite Progressiva Crônica Felina
- O tratamento pode ajudar a retardar a evolução.
- Prednisona (2 mg/kg a cada 12 h) e ciclofosfamida (2,5 mg/kg a cada 24 h) — tipicamente utilizadas como foi descrito para poliartrite erosiva idiopática.

CONTRAINDICAÇÕES
- Medicamentos citotóxicos — não utilizar na presença de infecções crônicas ou mielossupressão (gatos com poliartrite progressiva crônica felina).
- Crisoterapia — não usar com doença renal em virtude da nefrotoxicidade.

PRECAUÇÕES
- Glicocorticoides — a utilização a longo prazo pode levar à síndrome de Cushing.
- Medicamentos citotóxicos — frequentemente induzem à mielossupressão; monitorizar o hemograma completo: se a contagem de leucócitos estiver < 6.000 células/mL e a de plaquetas, < 125.000 células/mL, interromper por 1 semana e, então, instituir novamente três quartos da dose quando as contagens retornarem ao normal.
- Em geral, as tiopurinas causam mielossupressão em 2-6 semanas; ciclofosfamida, em vários meses.
- Ciclofosfamida — limitar o uso para < 4 meses; pode desenvolver cistite hemorrágica estéril; interromper imediatamente na ocorrência de sintomas.
- A leflunomida requer um nível plasmático de vale para a monitorização; provoca necrose intestinal para cães em dosagens mais altas.

INTERAÇÕES POSSÍVEIS
Nenhuma conhecida.

MEDICAMENTO(S) ALTERNATIVO(S)
Ver a seção "Medicamento(s) de Escolha".

ACOMPANHAMENTO

MONITORIZAÇÃO DO PACIENTE
- O tratamento geralmente é frustrante e requer reavaliação frequente.
- Deterioração clínica — requer alteração na escolha ou na dosagem do medicamento ou intervenção cirúrgica.
- É importante tentar induzir à remissão; permitir que a doença fique latente sem controle aumentará o risco de artropatia degenerativa secundária.

EVOLUÇÃO ESPERADA E PROGNÓSTICO
- Provável evolução.
- Prognóstico mau a longo prazo.
- Não se espera a cura; a remissão é o objetivo.

DIVERSOS

VER TAMBÉM
Poliartrite Não Erosiva Imunomediada.

ABREVIATURA(S)
- AINE = anti-inflamatório não esteroide.
- FeFV = vírus formador de sincício felino,
- FeLV = vírus da leucemia felina.

Sugestões de Leitura

Beale BS. Arthropathies. In: Bloomberg MS, Taylor RT, Dee J, eds., Canine Sports Medicine and Surgery. Philadelphia: Saunders, 1998, pp. 517-532.

Goring RL, Beale BS. Immune mediated arthritides. In: Bojrab MJ, ed., Disease Mechanisms in Small Animal Surgery. Philadelphia: Lea & Febiger, 1993, pp. 742-750.

Hanna FY. Disease modifying treatment for feline rheumatoid arthritis. Vet Comp Orthop Traumatol 2005, 18(2):94-99.

Jacques D, Cauzinille L, Bouvy B, Dupre G. A retrospective study of 40 dogs with polyarthritis. Vet Surg 2002, 31(5):428-434.

Kaplan M, Kamanli A, Kalkan A, Kuk S, Gulkesen A, Ardicoglu O, Demirdag K. Toxocariasis seroprevalence in patients with rheumatoid arthritis. Turkiye Parazitol Derg 2005, 29(4):251-254.

Pedersen NC, Morgan JP, Vasseur PB. Joint diseases of dogs and cats. In: Ettinger SJ, Feldman EC, eds., Textbook of Veterinary Internal Medicine — Diseases of the Dog and Cat, 5th ed. Philadelphia: Saunders, 2000, pp. 1862-1886.

Ralphs SC, Beale BS. Canine idiopathic erosive polyarthritis. Compend Contin Educ Pract Vet 2000, 22:671-677, 703.

Ralphs SC, Beale BS, Whitney WO, Liska W. Idiopathic erosive polyarthritis in six dogs. Vet Comp Orthop Traumatol 2000, 13:191-196.

Autor Peter K. Shires
Consultor Editorial Peter K. Shires
Agradecimento O autor e os editores agradecem as colaborações de Brian Beale e Deanna Worley, que foram os autores deste capítulo em uma edição mais antiga.

Poliartrite Não Erosiva Imunomediada

CONSIDERAÇÕES GERAIS

DEFINIÇÃO
Doença inflamatória imunomediada das articulações que não causa alteração erosiva; inclui poliartrite idiopática, LES, poliartrite associada à doença crônica (doença infecciosa crônica, neoplásica ou enteropática), síndrome poliartrite-polimiosite, síndrome de polimiosite, síndrome poliartrite-meningite, poliartrite nodosa, amiloidose renal familiar em cães da raça Shar-pei chinês, sinovite linfocítica-plasmocitária, poliartrite de início juvenil em Akitas e a forma proliferativa de poliartrite progressiva crônica felina.

FISIOPATOLOGIA
- Patogenia — envolve reação de hipersensibilidade tipo III; depósito de imunocomplexos dentro da membrana sinovial; resposta inflamatória e subsequente ativação do complemento, levando a sinais clínicos de artrite.
- LES — o material nuclear de várias células torna-se antigênico, induzindo à formação de autoanticorpos (anticorpo antinuclear).

SISTEMA(S) ACOMETIDO(S)
Musculoesquelético — articulações diartrodiais.

GENÉTICA
Não conhecida por ser hereditária.

INCIDÊNCIA/PREVALÊNCIA
- Idiopática — mais comum em cães.
- A forma relacionada com infecção crônica pode ser erroneamente diagnosticada como idiopática.
- Outras formas raras.

DISTRIBUIÇÃO GEOGRÁFICA
N/D.

IDENTIFICAÇÃO
Espécies
Cães e gatos.

Raça(s) Predominante(s)
- Idiopática — raças caninas de porte grande (mais comum) e pequeno; rara em gatos; Pastor alemão, Doberman pinscher, Retriever, Spaniel, Pointer, Poodle toy, Lhasa apso, Yorkshire terrier e Chihuahua são super-representadas.
- LES — tendência a acometer cães pertencentes às raças de grande porte; Collie, Pastor alemão, Poodle, Terrier, Beagle e Pastor de Shetland.
- Secundária à administração de medicamentos à base de sulfa — sensibilidade aumentada no Doberman pinscher.
- Síndrome poliartrite-meningite — relatada no Weimaraner, Pointer alemão de pelo curto, Boxer, Montanhês de Berna, Beagle, Rottweiler e Akita japonês.
- Amiloidose e sinovite — características proeminentes da síndrome que acomete cães jovens da raça Shar-Pei.
- Poliartrite de início juvenil relatada em Akitas.
- Sinovite linfocítica-plasmocitária no Pastor alemão e em outras raças caninas de grande porte.

Idade Média e Faixa Etária
Cães — jovens a meia-idade.

Sexo Predominante
Poliartrite progressiva crônica felina — gatos machos apenas.

SINAIS CLÍNICOS
Comentários Gerais
No início, as formas não erosiva e erosiva da doença inflamatória imunomediada parecem semelhantes.

Achados Anamnésicos
- Cães e gatos — início agudo; claudicação de um único membro ou de múltiplos membros.
- Claudicação — pode trocar de um membro para outro.
- Geralmente sem histórico de traumatismo.
- Também se podem notar vômito, diarreia, anorexia, pirexia, poliúria ou polidipsia.
- Também é possível notar sinais associados a doença sistêmica ou infecções (piometra, prostatite ou discospondilite) ou doença neoplásica.
- Frequentemente cíclica — embora pareça responder à antibioticoterapia, a poliartrite não erosiva imunomediada pode sofrer remissão espontânea.
- A doença pode se desenvolver quando o paciente está sendo tratado com antibióticos (contendo enxofre).

Achados do Exame Físico
- Rigidez da marcha, claudicação, amplitude de movimento diminuída, crepitação, tumefação articular e dor em uma ou mais articulações.
- Claudicação — desde leve sustentação do peso até incapacidade mais grave de suportar o peso.
- Articulações diartrodiais — todas podem ser acometidas; geralmente joelho, cotovelo, carpo e tarso.
- Foco de infecção localizada crônica (piometra, prostatite).

CAUSAS
- Desconhecidas na maioria dos casos.
- Provável mecanismo imunológico.
- Crônica — associada ao estímulo antigênico juntamente com meningite concomitante, doença gastrintestinal, neoplasia, infecção do trato urinário, periodontite, endocardite bacteriana, dirofilariose, piometra, otite média ou externa crônica, infecções fúngicas e infecções crônicas por *Actinomyces* ou *Salmonella*.
- Pode ocorrer secundariamente à reação de hipersensibilidade, envolvendo o depósito de complexos medicamento-anticorpo nos vasos sanguíneos da sinóvia; antibióticos suspeitos incluem sulfas, cefalosporinas, lincomicina, eritromicina e penicilinas.
- FeLV e FeFV — ligados à poliartrite progressiva crônica felina.

FATORES DE RISCO
N/D.

DIAGNÓSTICO

DIAGNÓSTICO DIFERENCIAL
- Poliartrite erosiva precoce.
- Artrite infecciosa.
- Traumatismo de articulação.
- Polimiosite.

HEMOGRAMA/BIOQUÍMICA/URINÁLISE
- Geralmente normais.
- Hemograma — pode revelar leucocitose, neutrofilia e hiperfibrinogenemia.
- Anormalidades hematológicas (p. ex., trombocitopenia e anemia hemolítica) — observadas em apenas 10-20% dos pacientes com LES.

OUTROS TESTES LABORATORIAIS
- Preparação positiva de lúpus eritematoso ou teste positivo de anticorpo antinuclear — cães com LES.
- Títulos séricos (*Borrelia*, *Ehrlichia* e *Rickettsia*) — devem estar normais.
- Evidência sorológica de FeFV — encontrada em todos os pacientes com poliartrite progressiva crônica felina.
- Evidência sorológica de exposição ao FeLV — encontrada em 50% ou menos dos gatos com poliartrite progressiva crônica felina.

DIAGNÓSTICO POR IMAGEM
- Principal alteração radiográfica — distensão capsular da articulação.
- Pode-se observar entesiofitose em caso de doença prolongada ou recidivante.

MÉTODOS DIAGNÓSTICOS
- Artrocentese e análise do líquido sinovial — essenciais para o diagnóstico.
- Líquido sinovial — tipicamente aparece turvo com viscosidade normal; grande aumento do número de neutrófilos não degenerados (20.000-200.000 células/mL); enviar para os exames de cultura bacteriana e antibiograma.
- Biopsia sinovial — pode ajudar no diagnóstico.
- Procurar por fonte de infecção crônica.

ACHADOS PATOLÓGICOS
- Cápsula articular — pode estar espessada; efusão sinovial.
- Hipertrofia e hiperplasia sinoviais — associadas ao infiltrado de células mononucleares.
- Neutrófilos — observados nos tecidos sinoviais em virtude da quimiotaxia.

TRATAMENTO

CUIDADO(S) DE SAÚDE ADEQUADO(S)
Geralmente como paciente de ambulatório.

CUIDADO(S) DE ENFERMAGEM
- Fisioterapia — exercícios com amplitude de movimento e natação; pode ser indicada para doença grave.
- Bandagens e/ou talas — para evitar colapso adicional da articulação; possíveis indicações para doença grave com deambulação comprometida.

ATIVIDADE
Limitada para minimizar a piora dos sinais clínicos.

DIETA
Redução de peso — para diminuir a tensão exercida sobre as articulações acometidas.

ORIENTAÇÃO AO PROPRIETÁRIO
Advertir o proprietário sobre o prognóstico mau quanto à cura e resolução completa se a causa primária não for encontrada.

CONSIDERAÇÕES CIRÚRGICAS
Remover a fonte de infecção quando aplicável (piometra, etc.); nesses casos, não há necessidade de outra terapia.

MEDICAÇÕES

MEDICAMENTO(S) DE ESCOLHA
- Eliminar as causas subjacentes se possível — doença crônica; antibiótico indutor da lesão.
- Terapia típica — ensaio terapêutico inicial com glicocorticoides; se a resposta for insatisfatória,

POLIARTRITE NÃO EROSIVA IMUNOMEDIADA

utilizar quimioterapia combinada (glicocorticoides e medicamentos citotóxicos).
• Remissão completa — alcançada geralmente em 2-16 semanas; determinada pela resolução dos sinais clínicos e pela confirmação da análise de líquido sinovial normal.
• Taxa de recidiva — 30-50% assim que a terapia for interrompida.
• Prednisona — 1,5-2,0 mg/kg VO a cada 12 h por 10-14 dias como tratamento inicial; contagem celular do líquido sinovial < 4.000 células/mL e predomínio de células mononucleares: diminuir gradativamente em várias semanas para 1,0 mg/kg VO a cada 48 h; persistência dos sinais clínicos ou análise de líquido sinovial anormal: adicionar agentes citotóxicos; sem sinais clínicos após 2-3 meses de terapia em dias alternados: interromper.
• Combinação de glicocorticoides e medicamento citotóxico — recomendada para obtenção de efeito sinérgico; pode-se tentar a ciclofosfamida ou a tiopurina (azatioprina ou 6-mercaptopurina).
• Ciclofosfamida — paciente com < 10 kg: 2,5 mg/kg; paciente de 10-50 kg: 2,0 mg/kg; paciente com > 50 kg: 1,75 mg/kg; agente administrado VO a cada 24 h por 4 dias consecutivos de cada semana; administrado concomitantemente com a prednisona (conforme descrição anterior; alguns clínicos reduzem a dose total de esteroide pela metade).
• Azatioprina ou 6-mercaptopurina — 2 mg/kg VO a cada 24 h por 14-21 dias e, em seguida, a cada 48 h; administrado concomitantemente com a prednisona da mesma forma que a ciclofosfamida, mas em dias alternados.
• Leflunomida — pode ser utilizada sinergicamente com azatioprina, prednisona e ciclofosfamida (4,0 mg/kg a cada 24 h para cães). Após vários dias, ajustar a dose para níveis plasmáticos de vale (mais baixos) de 20 μg/mL.
• Interromper os medicamentos citotóxicos 1-3 meses após a remissão ser obtida.
• Manutenção da remissão — a terapia com glicocorticoide em dias alternados (prednisona, 1,0 mg/kg VO), em geral, é bem-sucedida; em caso de recidiva dos sinais clínicos ou da neutrofilia sinovial: talvez haja necessidade de terapia com medicamento citotóxico a longo prazo; se os sinais clínicos não recidivarem após 2-3 meses: pode-se interromper o glicocorticoide;

se os sinais clínicos recidivarem após a interrupção do glicocorticoide: continuar o tratamento.

Poliartrite Progressiva Crônica Felina
• O tratamento pode retardar a evolução.
• Prednisona (2 mg/kg a cada 12 h) e ciclofosfamida (2,5 mg/kg) — utilizadas tipicamente conforme descrição prévia.

CONTRAINDICAÇÕES
• Não usar medicamentos citotóxicos na presença de infecções crônicas ou mielossupressão (gatos com poliartrite progressiva crônica felina).
• Evitar o uso de glicocorticoides com AINE como ácido acetilsalicílico, carprofeno, etodolaco e deracoxibe, já que isso pode resultar em ulceração gástrica.

PRECAUÇÕES
• Glicocorticoides — a utilização a longo prazo pode levar à síndrome de Cushing iatrogênica.
• Medicamentos citotóxicos — frequentemente induzem à mielossupressão; monitorizar o hemograma semanalmente (ver "Poliartrite Erosiva Imunomediada").
• A leflunomida pode causar necrose intestinal com superdosagem.

INTERAÇÕES POSSÍVEIS
Nenhuma conhecida.

MEDICAMENTO(S) ALTERNATIVO(S)
Ver a seção "Medicamento(s) de Escolha".

ACOMPANHAMENTO

MONITORIZAÇÃO DO PACIENTE
Deterioração clínica — indica a necessidade de mudança na escolha ou na dosagem do medicamento.

PREVENÇÃO
N/D.

COMPLICAÇÕES POSSÍVEIS
N/D.

EVOLUÇÃO ESPERADA E PROGNÓSTICO
• Recidiva — observada de forma intermitente.
• LES e poliartrite progressiva crônica felina — é comum a evolução; prognóstico reservado.
• Outras formas — prognóstico bom.

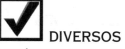

DIVERSOS

DISTÚRBIOS ASSOCIADOS
N/D.

FATORES RELACIONADOS COM A IDADE
N/D.

POTENCIAL ZOONÓTICO
N/D.

GESTAÇÃO/FERTILIDADE/REPRODUÇÃO
N/D.

ABREVIATURA(S)
• AINE = anti-inflamatórios não esteroides.
• FeFV = vírus formador de sincício felino.
• FeLV = vírus da leucemia felina.
• LES = lúpus eritematoso sistêmico.

Sugestões de Leitura
Beale BS. Arthropathies. In: Bloomberg MS, Taylor RT, Dee J, eds., Canine Sports Medicine and Surgery. Philadelphia: Saunders, 1998, pp. 517-532.
Choi E, Shin I, Youn H, Lee C. Development of canine systemic lupus erythematosus model. J Vet Med A Physiol Pathol Clin Med 2004, 51(7-8):375-383.
Goring RL, Beale BS. Immune mediated arthritides. In: Bojrab MJ, ed., Disease Mechanisms in Small Animal Surgery. Philadelphia: Lea & Febiger, 1993, pp. 742-750.
Hastings D. Suggested treatment for polyarthritis in dogs. JAVMA 2004, 225(1):29.
Pedersen NC, Morgan JP, Vasseur PB. Joint diseases of dogs and cats. In: Ettinger SJ, Feldman EC, eds., Textbook of Veterinary Internal Medicine — Diseases of the Dog and Cat, 5th ed. Philadelphia: Saunders, 2000, pp. 1862-1886.
Santos M, Marcos R, Assuncao M, Matos AJ. Polyarthritis associated with visceral leishmaniasis in a juvenile dog. Vet Parasitol 2006, 141(3-4):340-344.

Autor Peter K. Shires
Consultor Editorial Peter K. Shires
Agradecimento O autor e os editores agradecem as colaborações de Brian S. Beale e Scott P. Hammel, que foram os autores deste capítulo em uma edição mais antiga.

POLICITEMIA

CONSIDERAÇÕES GERAIS

DEFINIÇÃO
Aumento nos valores de hematócrito, concentração de hemoglobina e contagem de hemácias acima dos intervalos de referência por conta de uma elevação relativa, transitória ou absoluta no número de hemácias circulantes.

FISIOPATOLOGIA
- O número de hemácias circulantes é influenciado por alterações no volume plasmático, taxa de destruição ou de perda de hemácias, contração esplênica, secreção de eritropoetina e taxa de produção pela medula óssea.
- A eritropoiese também é influenciada pelos hormônios do córtex adrenal, da tireoide, dos ovários, dos testículos e da hipófise anterior; o hematócrito normal é mantido por uma alça endócrina.
- Classificada como relativa, transitória ou absoluta.
- Relativa — desenvolve-se quando uma redução no volume plasmático, provocada geralmente por desidratação, produz um aumento relativo nas hemácias circulantes.
- Transitória — causada pela contração esplênica, a qual injeta hemácias concentradas na circulação; como a contração esplênica é uma resposta momentânea à adrenalina, esse tipo de policitemia não costuma ser uma consideração diagnóstica relevante.
- Absoluta — caracteriza-se por um aumento absoluto na massa de hemácias circulantes como resultado do incremento na produção da medula óssea; primária ou secundária a um aumento na produção de eritropoetina.
- Absoluta primária (policitemia rubra vera) — distúrbio mieloproliferativo caracterizado pela produção descontrolada, mas ordenada, de números excessivos de hemácias maduras.
- Absoluta secundária — provocada pela liberação fisiologicamente pertinente de eritropoetina resultante de hipoxemia crônica ou pela produção inadequada e excessiva de eritropoetina ou substâncias semelhantes a esta em animal com SaO_2 normal.

SISTEMA(S) ACOMETIDO(S)
- Cardiovascular, respiratório, nervoso, renal/urológico — hiperviscosidade e má perfusão/oxigenação dos tecidos, os quais estão diretamente relacionados com o hematócrito elevado, sobretudo valores >60-70%.
- Animais com policitemia absoluta apresentam volume sanguíneo expandido, enquanto aqueles com policitemia relativa (desidratação) exibem volume reduzido; ambos os tipos podem comprometer a perfusão e a oxigenação teciduais.

DISTRIBUIÇÃO GEOGRÁFICA
- Os intervalos de referência para o hematócrito, a concentração de hemoglobina e a contagem de hemácias variam com a região geográfica e a raça do animal.
- Os animais que vivem em altitudes >6.000 pés possuem valores mais altos desses índices do que aqueles que residem ao nível do mar.

IDENTIFICAÇÃO
Espécies
Cães e gatos.

Raça(s) Predominante(s)
- Raças braquicefálicas apresentam valores do hematócrito mais elevados em comparação às normocefálicas.
- Raças grandes e excitáveis são propensas à contração esplênica.
- Os animais da raça Galgo tipicamente apresentam valores elevados do hematócrito; a faixa normal é de 50-65%.

Idade Média e Faixa Etária
Policitemia primária e absoluta — gatos, 6-7 anos; cães, 7 anos ou mais.

Sexo Predominante
Gatos machos e cadelas.

SINAIS CLÍNICOS
Comentários Gerais
Variam com o grau da policitemia.

Achados Anamnésicos
- Transitórios — excitação (agitação) ou exercício vigoroso.
- Absolutos — letargia, anorexia, epistaxe, crises convulsivas, hiperemia das mucosas.

Achados do Exame Físico
- Relativos — desidratação provocada por vômito, diarreia ou falta de ingestão hídrica e oligúria.
- Absolutos — letargia, baixa tolerância aos exercícios, mudança comportamental, mucosas de cor vermelho tijolo ou cianóticas, espirros, epistaxe bilateral, dilatação e tortuosidade dos vasos retinianos e sublinguais, além de comprometimento cardiopulmonar.
- Absolutos primários — graus variáveis de esplenomegalia, hepatomegalia, trombose e hemorragia; ocasionalmente, ocorrem crises convulsivas.
- Absolutos secundários causados por hipoxia tecidual — sinais clínicos de hipoxemia provocados por pneumopatia crônica, cardiopatia ou anomalia com desvio da direita para a esquerda ou hemoglobinopatia.
- Absolutos secundários causados por secreção inadequada de eritropoetina — sinais associados a neoplasia, lesão renal expansiva ou distúrbio endócrino.

CAUSAS
- Relativas (comuns) — vômito, diarreia, ingestão hídrica diminuída, diurese, nefropatia, hiperventilação e desvio da água do plasma para o interstício ou o lúmen gastrintestinal.
- Transitórias — excitação (agitação), ansiedade, crises convulsivas e contenção.
- Absoluta primária — distúrbio mieloproliferativo raro.
- Absoluta secundária provocada por hipoxia tecidual — pneumopatia crônica, cardiopatia ou anomalia com desvio da direita para a esquerda, altitude elevada, conformação braquicefálica da raça, metemoglobinemia e comprometimento do aporte sanguíneo renal.
- Absoluta secundária causada pela secreção inadequada de eritropoetina (rara) — cisto ou tumor renal, hidronefrose, hiperadrenocorticismo, hipertireoidismo, feocromocitoma, fibrossarcoma nasal, neoplasia hepática, schwanoma extradural, leiomiossarcoma cecal, hiperandrogenismo, administração terapêutica de eritropoetina recombinante.

FATORES DE RISCO
Nenhum.

DIAGNÓSTICO

DIAGNÓSTICO DIFERENCIAL
- Hematócrito e proteína plasmática total moderadamente elevados com desidratação concomitante — sugerem policitemia relativa.
- Absoluta secundária — causada por doenças indutoras de hipoxemia crônica ou por lesões renais expansivas, distúrbios endócrinos e neoplasias produtoras de eritropoetina ou substância semelhante a esta, independentemente de hipoxia, além de histórico da administração de eritropoetina.
- Policitemia vera — diagnosticada pela eliminação de outras causas.

HEMOGRAMA/BIOQUÍMICA/URINÁLISE
A avaliação começa com a obtenção do hemograma completo e a mensuração da proteína plasmática total. Quadros concomitantes de anemia, hipoproteinemia, desidratação, bem como os efeitos de diluição da fluidoterapia, podem influenciar a interpretação dos valores de hematócrito e da proteína plasmática total; outros testes são selecionados, conforme indicação.

OUTROS TESTES LABORATORIAIS
- Determinações da SaO_2 e da eritropoetina — diagnosticam policitemia absoluta.
- Ensaios hormonais — permitem a avaliação de disfunção endócrina; as amostras de eritropoetina podem ser enviadas para algum laboratório clínico humano; a amostra de controle obtida de animal normal (não doador de sangue) também deve ser encaminhada.
- Há uma extensa sobreposição nos valores da eritropoetina entre os animais normais e os

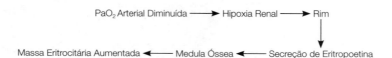

Figura 1.

POLICITEMIA

acometidos; em alguns animais com policitemia absoluta secundária, foram relatados valores da eritropoetina baixos ou normais. Laboratórios da Universidade da Pensilvânia e do Tennessee estabeleceram intervalos de referência para a eritropoetina em cães e gatos.

DIAGNÓSTICO POR IMAGEM
Radiografia e ultrassonografia são utilizadas para detectar doença cardiopulmonar e lesões expansivas dos rins e outras neoplasias.

MÉTODOS DIAGNÓSTICOS
Oximetria de pulso é realizada para determinar a saturação de oxigênio do sangue.

ACHADOS PATOLÓGICOS
• Policitemia vera — congestão vascular generalizada, trombose arterial, esplenomegalia variável e medula óssea difusamente vermelha com gordura reduzida como achados macroscópicos.
• Os achados microscópicos incluem medula hiperplásica com relação mieloide/eritroide normal ou reduzida e conteúdo diminuído de ferro.

TRATAMENTO
CUIDADO(S) DE SAÚDE ADEQUADO(S)
• Relativa — reidratação com fluidos IV apropriados para a causa primária; avaliação da função renal, do sistema gastrintestinal, do estado acidobásico e do equilíbrio eletrolítico é importante para a seleção do fluido.
• Absoluta — é recomendada a flebotomia (20 mL/kg de 1 a vários dias) para reduzir a massa eritrocitária até um hematócrito de 55%; o volume sanguíneo deve ser reposto concomitantemente com fluidos isotônicos para evitar a hipotensão, o colapso cardiovascular e a trombose.
• Secundária provocada pela produção inadequada de eritropoetina — flebotomia combinada com a identificação e a remoção da fonte de eritropoetina.
• Secundária causada por hipoxemia — flebotomia e hidroxiureia. O hematócrito elevado é uma resposta compensatória apropriada; sendo assim, a flebotomia pode ser um procedimento perigoso; se indicada, remover o sangue em uma velocidade mais lenta (5 mL/kg); talvez haja necessidade de um hematócrito mais alto (60-65%) para manter a vida do animal até que a causa da hipoxemia possa ser corrigida.

• Policitemia vera — flebotomia (20 mL/kg) e hidroxiureia; a frequência do sangramento e a dosagem da hidroxiureia devem ser ajustadas para manter o hematócrito de 55% nos cães e de 45% nos gatos.

CUIDADO(S) DE ENFERMAGEM
Oxigenoterapia pode estar indicada em pacientes com cianose, baixa saturação arterial de oxigênio, doença cardiopulmonar grave ou fraqueza após flebotomia.

ATIVIDADE
É recomendável evitar o exercício excessivo durante a flebotomia.

DIETA
Dieta normal com livre acesso à água.

ORIENTAÇÃO AO PROPRIETÁRIO
• Os pacientes precisam ser observados quanto à ocorrência de mudanças na atividade, como fraqueza, dificuldade respiratória, episódios hemorrágicos ou indícios de infecção sistêmica.
• Em caso de prescrição de agentes quimioterápicos, deverá ser discutida a segurança pessoal com a manipulação e a administração desses medicamentos. Tais agentes podem causar alterações na pigmentação da pele e esfacelamento das unhas.

CONSIDERAÇÕES CIRÚRGICAS
Se houver a necessidade de cirurgia, será imprescindível a monitorização da saturação de oxigênio com a oximetria de pulso para evitar hipoxemia.

MEDICAÇÕES
MEDICAMENTO(S) DE ESCOLHA
• Policitemia vera — hidroxiureia (40-50 mg/kg VO divididos 2 vezes ao dia, cães; 30 mg/kg a cada 24 h, gatos).
• Policitemia secundária à hipoxemia — hidroxiureia (40-50 mg/kg VO a cada 48 h).

CONTRAINDICAÇÕES
A flebotomia pode estar contraindicada nos pacientes com hipoxemia.

PRECAUÇÕES
• A remoção do sangue em uma velocidade rápida pode provocar hipotensão e colapso cardiovascular.
• Os efeitos adversos da hidroxiureia incluem hipoplasia da medula óssea com trombocitopenia, anemia e neutropenia, além de alopecia, alterações na pigmentação cutânea e esfacelamento das unhas.
• Há relatos de metemoglobinemia e anemia hemolítica em gatos tratados com hidroxiureia.

INTERAÇÕES POSSÍVEIS
Nenhuma.

MEDICAMENTO(S) ALTERNATIVO(S)
Policitemia vera — clorambucila (0,2 mg/kg VO a cada 24 h, cães e gatos) ou bussulfano (2-4 mg/m² VO a cada 24 h, cães).

ACOMPANHAMENTO
MONITORIZAÇÃO DO PACIENTE
• Hematócrito, proteína plasmática total, débito urinário e peso corporal 2-3 vezes ao dia nos animais gravemente desidratados até que a hidratação normal seja mantida.
• Pacientes que estão sendo tratados de policitemia vera por quimioterapia — monitorizar semanalmente quanto à presença de alterações no hematócrito, nos leucócitos e nas plaquetas durante o tratamento inicial; em seguida, mensalmente para o ajuste da quimioterapia e a realização de flebotomia periódica.
• Fica indicada a avaliação periódica das reservas de ferro na medula óssea ou os níveis desse elemento químico no soro para detectar deficiências.

COMPLICAÇÕES POSSÍVEIS
• Hiperviscosidade nos pacientes com policitemia absoluta, especialmente policitemia vera, pode levar a trombose, infarto ou hemorragia.
• A quimioterapia pode provocar supressão da medula óssea.
• Os pacientes com policitemias absolutas podem desenvolver deficiência de ferro como resultado da flebotomia e da eritropoiese ativa.

EVOLUÇÃO ESPERADA E PROGNÓSTICO
• Policitemia relativa: a identificação e a correção da causa primária com fluidoterapia apropriada resultam na recuperação do paciente com prognóstico razoável a bom, dependendo da causa primária.
• Policitemia absoluta secundária atribuída à hipoxemia: a evolução clínica e o prognóstico são determinados pela gravidade da lesão indutora de hipoxemia. O restabelecimento da função cardíaca ou a melhora de pneumopatia inflamatória e a redução no hematócrito com melhora na saturação

Tabela 1

	Policitemia Relativa	Policitemia Absoluta		
Mecanismo	Desidratação	Mieloproliferativa Primária	Secundária à Hipoxemia	Secundária ao Excesso de Eritropoetina
Hematócrito	Aumento	Acentuado Aumento >60%	Acentuado Aumento >60%	Acentuado Aumento >60%
Proteína plasmática total	Aumento	Normal	Normal	Normal
SaO₂		Normal >90%	Diminuição <<90%	Normal >90%
Eritropoetina		Normal/diminuída	Aumento	Aumento
Medula óssea		Hiperplasia eritroide		
Outros	Azotemia pré-renal	Leucócitos aumentados Plaquetas aumentadas		

POLICITEMIA

de oxigênio aumentam a qualidade de vida. O prognóstico permanece reservado.
• Policitemia absoluta secundária atribuída à secreção inadequada da eritropoetina: se a fonte tecidual da secreção excessiva de eritropoetina puder ser identificada (tumor, cisto renal, endocrinopatia) e removida ou corrigida, a policitemia desaparecerá com prognóstico bom a razoável, dependendo da causa.
• Policitemia absoluta primária: apesar de responsivo ao tratamento, esse distúrbio mieloproliferativo requer monitorização quanto à ocorrência de alterações nos valores do hemograma completo e nos indícios clínicos de hemorragia, trombose e atividade diminuída. O prognóstico é reservado.

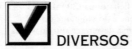

DIVERSOS

GESTAÇÃO/FERTILIDADE/REPRODUÇÃO
A hidroxiureia pode interromper ou inibir a espermatogênese.

SINÔNIMO(S)
Eritrocitose.

VER TAMBÉM
• Policitemia Vera.
• Síndrome de Hiperviscosidade.

ABREVIATURA(S)
• SaO_2 = saturação arterial de oxigênio.

Sugestões de Leitura
Cook SM, Lothrop CD. Serum erythropoietin concentrations measured by radioimmunoassay in normal, polycythemic, and anemic dogs and cats. J Vet Intern Med 1994, 8:18-25.
Hasler AH, Giger U. Serum erythropoietin values in polycythemic cats. JAAHA 1996, 12:294-301.
Mackin A. Serum erythropoietin assays. J Vet Intern Med 1994, 8:314-315.
Moore KW, Stepien RL. Hydroxyurea for treatment of polycythemia secondary to right-to-left shunting patent arteriosus in 4 dogs. J Vet InternMed 2001, 15:418-421.
Sato K, Hikasa Y, Morita T, Shimada A, Ozaki K, Kagota K. Secondary erythrocytosis associated with high plasma erythropoietin concentrations in a dog with cecal leiomyosarcoma. JAVMA 2002, 220:486-490.

Autor Peter MacWilliams
Consultor Editorial A.H. Rebar

POLICITEMIA VERA

CONSIDERAÇÕES GERAIS

REVISÃO
Distúrbio mieloproliferativo que resulta em viscosidade sanguínea elevada secundária a aumento na massa eritrocitária.

IDENTIFICAÇÃO
• Cães e gatos.
• Principalmente animais idosos.

SINAIS CLÍNICOS
• Início gradual; evolução crônica.
• Depressão.
• Anorexia.
• Fraqueza.
• Polidipsia e poliúria.
• Eritema da pele e das mucosas.
• Vasos sanguíneos retinianos dilatados e tortuosos.
• Uveíte.
• Hepatosplenomegalia (rara).

CAUSAS E FATORES DE RISCO
Desconhecidos.

DIAGNÓSTICO

DIAGNÓSTICO DIFERENCIAL
• Desidratação grave.
• Neoplasia renal.
• Pielonefrite crônica.
• Hiperadrenocorticismo.
• Estimulação androgênica.
• Hipoventilação induzida por doença pulmonar.
• Cardiopatia com desvios da direita para a esquerda.

HEMOGRAMA/BIOQUÍMICA/URINÁLISE
• Hematócrito elevado.
• Aumento absoluto na massa eritrocitária.
• Possível azotemia pré-renal.
• Leucocitose em 50% dos cães.

OUTROS TESTES LABORATORIAIS
• PaO_2 — normal.
• Concentração de eritropoetina sérica — costuma ser baixa a nula (zero) e, frequentemente, se sobrepõe com aquela relatada em outras causas de policitemia.
• Exame citológico da medula óssea e biopsia central.

DIAGNÓSTICO POR IMAGEM
• Radiografia — avalia os rins e o sistema cardiopulmonar.
• Ultrassonografia abdominal — avalia os rins e as adrenais.
• Ecocardiografia — avalia a existência de desvios cardíacos da direita para a esquerda.

MÉTODOS DIAGNÓSTICOS
• Biopsia da medula óssea.
• Eletrocardiografia — avalia a presença de cardiopatia.

TRATAMENTO

• Flebotomia e reposição concomitante com fluidos isotônicos intravenosos — alívio rápido dos sinais durante a crise clínica.
• Hidroxiureia — inibe a síntese intracelular de DNA e retarda a proliferação da medula óssea.
• Consultar um veterinário especialista em oncologia em busca das recomendações mais atuais.

MEDICAÇÕES

MEDICAMENTOS
Hidroxiureia — 40-50 mg/kg VO divididos duas vezes ao dia; titular de acordo com a resposta e a toxicidade (cães e gatos).

CONTRAINDICAÇÕES/INTERAÇÕES POSSÍVEIS
Hidroxiureia — potencialmente mielossupressora; é recomendável a monitorização sanguínea frequente.

ACOMPANHAMENTO

Efetuar reavaliações periódicas com hemograma completo, contagem plaquetária e perfil bioquímico seriados não só para monitorizar os efeitos tóxicos da hidroxiureia sobre a medula óssea e outros órgãos, mas também para avaliar a evolução da doença e/ou a remissão do estado clínico.

DIVERSOS

VER TAMBÉM
Policitemia.

RECURSOS DA INTERNET
http://www.vet.uga.edu/vpp/clerk/strait/index.htm.

Sugestões de Leitura
Hamilton TA. The leukemias. In: Morrison WB, ed., Cancer in Dogs and Cats: Medical and Surgical Management. Jackson, WY: Teton NewMedia, 2002, pp. 693-700.
Morrison WB. Polycythemia. In: Ettinger SJ, Feldman EC, eds., Textbook of Veterinary Internal Medicine, 4th ed. Philadelphia: Saunders, 1995, pp. 197-199.
Weiss DJ, Aird B. Cytologic evaluation of primary and secondary myelodysplastic syndromes in the dog. Vet Clin Pathol 2001, 30:67-75.

Autor Wallace B. Morrison
Consultor Editorial Timothy M. Fan

Polifagia

CONSIDERAÇÕES GERAIS

REVISÃO
Aumento da ingestão alimentar.

FISIOPATOLOGIA
- Falha na assimilação ou perda de nutrientes (p. ex., síndromes de má digestão/má absorção como a insuficiência pancreática exócrina).
- Incapacidade de utilização de nutrientes (p. ex., diabetes melito, dietas de má qualidade e parasitas gastrintestinais).
- Hipoglicemia (p. ex., insulinoma e dosagem excessiva de insulina).
- Aumento na taxa ou demanda metabólica (p. ex., hipertireoidismo, ambientes frios, prenhez e lactação).
- Comportamentos psicológicos ou aprendidos (p. ex., dietas palatáveis, competição e medicamentos como anticonvulsivantes ou glicocorticoides).

SISTEMA(S) ACOMETIDO(S)
- Cardiovascular — a obesidade pode piorar um quadro de cardiopatia clínica.
- Sistema nervoso central — tumores do cérebro, especialmente do hipotálamo, podem causar polifagia.
- Cutâneo — animais obesos, sobretudo gatos, são suscetíveis à dermatite.
- Musculosquelético — pacientes que se encontram acima do peso ideal ficam suscetíveis à artrite e a outros problemas ortopédicos.
- Respiratório — a obesidade exacerba a dispneia nos pacientes com doença respiratória.

IDENTIFICAÇÃO
Cães e gatos.

SINAIS CLÍNICOS
Achados Anamnésicos
- Comer com maior frequência e/ou em maior quantidade que a normal.
- São possíveis os comportamentos de busca excessiva por alimento ou furto de comida.
- Pode ocorrer perda de peso com determinados estados mórbidos (p. ex., insuficiência pancreática exócrina, diabetes melito e hipertireoidismo).
- PU/PD ocorre em alguns pacientes (diabetes melito, hipertireoidismo, hiperadrenocorticismo).

Achados do Exame Físico
Os pacientes podem exibir gordura corporal excessiva, mas aqueles com algum problema clínico subjacente (p. ex., insuficiência pancreática exócrina, diabetes melito e hipertireoidismo) podem ser magros.

CAUSAS E FATORES DE RISCO
Fisiológicas
- Prenhez.
- Lactação.
- Crescimento.
- Resposta ao ambiente frio.
- Aumento da atividade física.

Patológicas
- Diabetes melito.
- Hipertireoidismo — gatos.
- Hiperadrenocorticismo — cães.
- Insuficiência pancreática exócrina.
- Parasitas gastrintestinais.
- Insulinoma.
- Dosagem excessiva de insulina.
- Linfangiectasia.
- Tumor hipofisário secretor do hormônio do crescimento.
- Megaesôfago.
- Enterite linfocítica-plasmocitária — gatos; rara.
- Neoplasias do cérebro — raras.
- Neoplasias gastrintestinais — raras.

Iatrogênicas
- Corticosteroides.
- Progestinas.
- Benzodiazepínicos.
- Anticonvulsivantes.
- Alimento palatável/alimentação exagerada.
- Dietas de má qualidade.
- Competição pelo alimento.

DIAGNÓSTICO

DIAGNÓSTICO DIFERENCIAL
PU/PD (jornadas excessivas para a área onde se encontram o alimento e a água) — diferenciar por meio da observação.

HEMOGRAMA/BIOQUÍMICA/URINÁLISE
- Neutrofilia, monocitose, linfopenia e eosinopenia em casos de hiperadrenocorticismo e nos pacientes submetidos a corticosteroides.
- Hiperglicemia em casos de diabetes melito, tumores hipofisários secretores do hormônio do crescimento (gatos, diabetes melito insulinorresistente) e hiperadrenocorticismo (leve).
- Hipercolesterolemia em casos de ingestão recente de alimento, hiperadrenocorticismo e diabetes melito, bem como nos pacientes submetidos a corticosteroides.
- Atividade elevada da fosfatase alcalina e da ALT em casos de hiperadrenocorticismo (cães), hipertireoidismo (gatos) e diabetes melito, bem como nos pacientes submetidos a corticosteroides.
- Hipoproteinemia em casos de enteropatias com perda de proteínas (p. ex., linfangiectasia e doença intestinal inflamatória).
- Hipoglicemia nos pacientes com insulinoma ou dosagem excessiva de insulina.
- Baixa densidade urinária em casos de diabetes melito, hipertireoidismo e hiperadrenocorticismo, bem como nos pacientes submetidos a corticosteroides.
- Glicosúria, possivelmente cetonúria, em casos de diabetes melito.

OUTROS TESTES LABORATORIAIS
- Exame de fezes para descartar a presença de parasitas gastrintestinais.
- Imunorreatividade sérica semelhante à da tripsina para diagnosticar insuficiência pancreática exócrina.
- T_4 sérica total para descartar hipertireoidismo (gatos); teste de supressão da tireoide com T_3 na suspeita de hipertireoidismo embora a T_4 sérica total permaneça normal.
- Teste de supressão com dexametasona em baixas doses ou teste de estimulação com ACTH para diagnosticar hiperadrenocorticismo; mensurar o nível plasmático de ACTH ou efetuar o teste de supressão com dexametasona em altas doses para diferenciar hiperadrenocorticismo dependente da hipófise de tumor adrenal caso o hiperadrenocorticismo seja confirmado pelo teste de supressão com dexametasona em baixas doses ou pelo teste de estimulação com ACTH.
- Níveis séricos de insulina nos pacientes hipoglicêmicos para descartar insulinoma.

DIAGNÓSTICO POR IMAGEM
- Radiologia abdominal pode demonstrar hepatomegalia associada a hiperadrenocorticismo, diabetes melito e administração de corticosteroide.
- A ultrassonografia abdominal pode revelar massa adrenal ou adrenomegalia bilateral (hiperadrenocorticismo), hepatomegalia (hiperadrenocorticismo, diabetes melito ou administração de corticosteroide), espessamento da parede intestinal ou ruptura de camada desta parede (enteropatia inflamatória, linfoma, linfangiectasia) e massas pancreáticas (insulinoma).
- A RM pode ser usada para visualizar a presença de neoplasia do hipotálamo.

MÉTODOS DIAGNÓSTICOS
Endoscopia com biopsia do trato gastrintestinal superior para descartar doenças gastrintestinais.

TRATAMENTO

- Em geral, o paciente é submetido a tratamento clínico em um esquema ambulatorial.
- É mais provável que a polifagia sem ganho de peso ou com perda de peso seja atribuída a algum problema clínico; avaliar o animal antes de restrições ou manipulações da dieta.
- Uma vez excluídas as causas patológicas de polifagia, limitar a quantidade de alimento disponível, fornecer dieta com restrição calórica e/ou aumentar a atividade física na presença de obesidade ou ganho de peso:
  ○ Os proprietários precisam medir o alimento fornecido para avaliar o consumo com precisão.
  ○ Alguns cães podem se beneficiar com a adição de dietas volumosas de baixa caloria, como ervilhas enlatadas.
  ○ O fornecimento de pequenas refeições 2 a 3 vezes ao dia pode ser benéfico para alguns pacientes, desde que o alimento total fornecido permaneça o mesmo que aquele requerido para o estágio de vida e o nível de atividade a fim de promover a perda de peso ou evitar o ganho de peso.
- O ato de afastar o animal de estimação durante o preparo e o consumo das refeições de humanos permite diminuir o comportamento de pedinte, evitando que o animal consiga obter mais comida.
- Dispositivos para reduzir a velocidade de ingestão alimentar podem ser benéficos em alguns cães, como brinquedos dispensadores de ração que necessitam de manipulação para obter a porção diária.
- Se houver problemas sociais dentro da casa que influenciem o consumo alimentar, todos eles deverão ser tratados:
  ○ Alimentar todos os cães em locais separados, de preferência sem contato visual.
  ○ Ter múltiplos comedouros à disposição em uma casa com inúmeros gatos.
- A necessidade calórica diária do animal de porte médio pode ser estimada pela fórmula 30 × peso (kg) + 70.
- Brinquedos mastigáveis podem ser usados como um substituto da alimentação.

MEDICAÇÕES

MEDICAMENTO(S)
- Consultar as doenças específicas em busca de detalhes sobre o tratamento.

- Polifagia induzida por medicamento — tentar reduzir ou interromper o agente terapêutico em questão.
- Na suspeita de algum transtorno alimentar compulsivo, pode-se lançar mão de medicamentos como a clomipramina ou a amitriptilina (1-3 mg/kg VO a cada 12 h).
- O agente dirlotapida (Slentrol®) é um inibidor seletivo de proteína de transferência de triglicerídeo microssomal que bloqueia o agrupamento e a liberação de quilomícrons (classe de lipoproteínas) para a corrente sanguínea, deflagrando com isso a liberação do peptídeo YY* e a diminuição do apetite. Esse medicamento pode ser usado em cães obesos a uma dose de 0,2 mL/kg.

ACOMPANHAMENTO
MONITORIZAÇÃO DO PACIENTE
- Monitorizar o peso corporal nos pacientes com causas não patológicas de polifagia.
- Avaliar a obediência ao esquema de alimentação e à mensuração do alimento para diminuir o consumo e promover a perda de peso.

COMPLICAÇÕES POSSÍVEIS
- Obesidade na polifagia não patológica.
- Se o proprietário responder ao comportamento de pedinte do animal, a ingestão calórica não será diminuída.
- Perda de peso/emaciação nas causas patológicas de polifagia.
- Piora do processo mórbido respiratório ou cardiovascular no paciente obeso.

DIVERSOS
DISTÚRBIOS ASSOCIADOS
Obesidade.
GESTAÇÃO/FERTILIDADE/REPRODUÇÃO
Resposta fisiológica normal à prenhez.

SINÔNIMO(S)
- Hiperfagia.
- Distúrbio alimentar.
- Transtorno alimentar.

VER TAMBÉM
Obesidade.

ABREVIATURA(S)
- ACTH = hormônio adrenocorticotrópico.
- ALT = alanina aminotransferase.
- PU/PD = poliúria/polidipsia.
- T_3 = tri-iodotironina.
- T_4 = tiroxina.

Sugestões de Leitura
Monroe WE. Anorexia and polyphagia. In: Ettinger SJ, Feldman EC, eds., Textbook of Veterinary Internal Medicine. Philadelphia: Saunders, 1995, pp. 18-21.

Autor Katherine A. Houpt
Consultor Editorial Debra F. Horwitz

---

* N. T.: Inibidor do apetite.

Polioencefalomielite — Gatos

CONSIDERAÇÕES GERAIS

DEFINIÇÃO
- Meningoencefalomielite não supurativa de causa desconhecida.
- Há suspeita, mas sem comprovação, de associação com o vírus da doença de Borna.
- Os neurônios na medula espinal torácica parecem preferencialmente acometidos.
- Também se observam lesões na medula espinal cervical e lombar, bem como no tronco cerebral e no cérebro.
- A degeneração axonal e a desmielinização nos funículos ventral e lateral da medula espinal são secundárias à necrose neuronal.

IDENTIFICAÇÃO
- Gatos domésticos de pelo curto e algumas raças puras.
- Faixa etária — 2 meses de vida a 6 anos e meio de idade.
- Fêmeas são mais comumente acometidas do que machos.

SINAIS CLÍNICOS
- Variam com a localização da lesão no SNC.
- Incoordenação crônica e progressiva dos membros posteriores ou dos quatro membros.
- Crises convulsivas em alguns pacientes.

CAUSAS E FATORES DE RISCO
Há suspeita, mas sem comprovação, de causa viral.

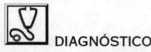

DIAGNÓSTICO

DIAGNÓSTICO DIFERENCIAL
- PIF.
- Toxoplasmose.
- Infecção fúngica.
- Infecção bacteriana.

HEMOGRAMA/BIOQUÍMICA/URINÁLISE
- As alterações laboratoriais não são bem caracterizadas.
- Alterações inespecíficas (p. ex., leucopenia e anemia arregenerativa) são raras.

OUTROS TESTES LABORATORIAIS
N/D.

DIAGNÓSTICO POR IMAGEM
N/D.

MÉTODOS DIAGNÓSTICOS
- Pleocitose mononuclear com teor proteico leve a moderadamente elevado no LCS (poucos dados).
- Títulos de anticorpos no soro ou no LCS — não avaliados totalmente.
- Foi desenvolvido um ensaio de PCR-RT duplex em tempo real; seu uso, no entanto, no diagnóstico da doença clínica ainda não foi descrito.

TRATAMENTO

Não foi tentado em nenhum dos casos relatados.

MEDICAÇÕES

MEDICAMENTO(S)
- Nenhuma terapia medicamentosa foi utilizada nos casos relatados.
- Como as lesões não são supurativas, a terapia com esteroides pode aliviar os sinais clínicos, pelo menos temporariamente.

CONTRAINDICAÇÕES/INTERAÇÕES POSSÍVEIS
N/D.

ACOMPANHAMENTO

N/D.

DIVERSOS

ABREVIATURA(S)
- LCS = líquido cerebrospinal.
- PCR-RT = reação em cadeia da polimerase via transcriptase reversa.
- PIF = peritonite infecciosa felina.
- SNC = sistema nervoso central.

Sugestões de Leitura
Berg A-L. Borna disease in cats. In: Bonagura JD, ed., Kirk's Current Veterinary Therapy XIII. Philadelphia: Saunders, 2000, pp. 976-978.
Kamhieh S, Flower RLP. Borna disease vírus (BDV) infection in cats: A concise review based on current knowledge. Vet Q 2006, 28:65-73.
Lundgren AL. Feline non-suppurative meningoencephalomyelitis: A clinical and pathological study. J Comp Pathol 1992, 107:411-425.

Autor Karen Dyer Inzana
Consultor Editorial Joane M. Parent

PÓLIPOS NASAIS E NASOFARÍNGEOS

CONSIDERAÇÕES GERAIS

REVISÃO
- Crescimentos inflamatórios não neoplásicos, que surgem do epitélio e geralmente de um pedículo.
- Nasais — incomuns; originam-se dos ossos etmoturbinados; são de natureza inflamatória em cães e gatos.
- Nasofaríngeos — relativamente comuns; originam-se da base do revestimento epitelial da bula timpânica ou da tuba auditiva (também conhecida como trompa de Eustáquio); quando os pólipos se estendem para a nasofaringe, eles são conhecidos como pólipos nasofaríngeos; também conhecidos como pólipos da orelha média, pólipos aurais ou auriculares, ou pólipos inflamatórios benignos.

IDENTIFICAÇÃO
- Pólipos nasais — cães e gatos de idade média a mais idosos.
- Pólipos nasofaríngeos — tipicamente filhotes felinos e gatos adultos jovens, mas também podem ser observados em gatos mais idosos (meses-15 anos) e, raras vezes, em cães.

SINAIS CLÍNICOS

Pólipos Nasais
- Secreção nasal mucopurulenta crônica.
- Respiração ruidosa — estertor.
- Congestão e/ou secreção nasal.
- Espirros ou epistaxe.
- Fluxo aéreo nasal reduzido, geralmente unilateral.
- Geralmente irresponsivos a antibióticos.

Pólipos Nasofaríngeos
- Estridor inspiratório.
- Ânsia de vômito.
- Cianose.
- Mudança da vocalização.
- Disfagia.
- Otite crônica irresponsiva.
- Inclinação da cabeça.
- Nistagmo.
- Ataxia.
- Síndrome de Horner.

CAUSAS E FATORES DE RISCO
Desconhecidos — suspeita de processos congênitos ou resposta a processos inflamatórios crônicos.

DIAGNÓSTICO

DIAGNÓSTICO DIFERENCIAL
- Complexo de doença respiratória superior felina.
- Estenose nasofaríngea.
- Otite externa ou média crônica.
- Corpo estranho nasal ou nasofaríngeo.
- Paralisia laríngea.
- Neoplasia nasal — linfoma, adenocarcinoma nasal.
- Neoplasia laríngea — carcinoma de células escamosas, linfoma, adenocarcinoma.
- Neoplasia aural — adenocarcinoma ceruminoso.

HEMOGRAMA/BIOQUÍMICA/URINÁLISE
N/D.

OUTROS TESTES LABORATORIAIS
N/D.

DIAGNÓSTICO POR IMAGEM
- Radiografias do crânio — densidade de tecido mole dentro de estruturas como cavidade nasal, nasofaringe, bula timpânica, canal auditivo externo; 25% de resultados falso-negativos.
- TC e RM — melhor sensibilidade para cavidade nasal ou massas nasofaríngeas.

MÉTODOS DIAGNÓSTICOS
- Exame visual da nasofaringe e da laringe, além de palpação digital do palato mole — todos sob anestesia geral, com o uso de gancho de castração, espelho odontológico e laringoscópio.
- Rinoscopia caudal com fibra óptica flexível — para examinar a nasofaringe dorsal, as coanas e a cavidade nasal caudal.
- Rinoscopia rostral com fibra óptica rígida — para examinar a cavidade nasal.
- Exame otoscópico profundo.
- Aspirado por agulha fina e/ou biopsia.
- Citologia e histopatologia.

TRATAMENTO

- Biopsia excisional para pólipos nasais.
- Remoção de pólipos nasofaríngeos por tração via cavidade bucal.
- Osteotomia ventral da bula timpânica em casos de pólipos nasofaríngeos para liberação do pedículo e remoção do revestimento epitelial.
- Cirurgia — tratamento de escolha: excisão pela cavidade bucal para os pólipos nasofaríngeos ou rinotomia para os pólipos nasais; é imperativa a excisão completa da raiz e da base do pólipo para evitar recidivas.
- Osteotomia concomitante da bula timpânica — pode evitar a recidiva dos pólipos nasofaríngeos. Recomendável em caso de envolvimento evidente da bula timpânica.

MEDICAÇÕES

MEDICAMENTO(S)
- Utilizar medicamentos antimicrobianos adequados na presença de infecção nasal ou otológica secundária.
- Considerar o curso anti-inflamatório de corticosteroides após remoção de pólipos nasofaríngeos por tração; há relatos de diminuição da taxa de recidiva.

CONTRAINDICAÇÕES/INTERAÇÕES POSSÍVEIS
N/D.

ACOMPANHAMENTO

- A remoção incompleta do pólipo e do pedículo pode resultar em recidiva.
- Pode ocorrer síndrome de Horner após a remoção do pólipo por tração ou osteotomia ventral da bula timpânica.
- Apesar de geralmente transitória, pode-se desenvolver paresia/paralisia facial ou síndrome vestibular após osteotomia da bula timpânica.
- Prognóstico excelente com a remoção completa.

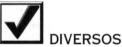

DIVERSOS

ABREVIATURA(S)
- RM = ressonância magnética.
- TC = tomografia computadorizada.

Sugestões de Leitura

Anderson DM, Robinson RK, White RA. Management of inflammatory polyps in 37 cats. Vet Record 2000, 147:684-687.

Kudnig ST. Nasopharyngeal polyps in cats. Clin Tech Small Anim Pract 2002, 17:174-177.

Veir JK, Lappin MR, Foley JE, Getzy DM. Feline inflammatory polyps: Historical, clinical, and PCR findings for feline calicivirus and feline herpes virus-1 in 28 cases. J Feline Med Surg 2002, 4(4):195-199.

Autor Catriona MacPhail
Consultor Editorial Lynelle R. Johnson

PÓLIPOS RETOANAIS

CONSIDERAÇÕES GERAIS

REVISÃO
A maior parte dos pólipos retoanais consiste em crescimentos benignos localizados na parte distal do reto. A avaliação histopatológica tipicamente revela adenomas, embora as lesões possam sofrer transformação maligna.

IDENTIFICAÇÃO
- Cães e, raramente, gatos.
- Meia-idade a idosos.
- Sem predileção racial ou sexual.

SINAIS CLÍNICOS
- Hematoquezia.
- Fezes cobertas com muco.
- Tenesmo.
- Disquezia.
- Massa(s) amolecida(s), bem vascularizada(s), friável(is) e frequentemente ulcerada(s) podem ser observadas ou palpadas por via retal.
- Geralmente isolados, embora possam ocorrer múltiplos pólipos.
- Podem ser massas pedunculadas ou sésseis de base larga.

CAUSAS E FATORES DE RISCO
Desconhecidos.

DIAGNÓSTICO

DIAGNÓSTICO DIFERENCIAL
- Carcinoma *in situ* e adenocarcinoma.
- Outras neoplasias — leiomioma, linfoma, papiloma.
- Proctite.
- Pitiose.
- Prolapso retal incompleto.

HEMOGRAMA/BIOQUÍMICA/URINÁLISE
Geralmente normais.

OUTROS TESTES LABORATORIAIS
N/D.

DIAGNÓSTICO POR IMAGEM
N/D.

MÉTODOS DIAGNÓSTICOS
- Palpação retal.
- Inspeção direta pelo ânus.
- Colonoscopia — recomendada para avaliar todo o reto e o cólon em busca de pólipos adicionais.
- Exame citológico de aspirado ou de raspado do pólipo pode auxiliar o diagnóstico inicial.
- Exame histopatológico do tecido excisado é necessário para formular o diagnóstico definitivo e avaliar se a excisão foi completa.

ACHADOS PATOLÓGICOS
- Pólipo adenomatoso.
- Hiperplasia adenomatosa.
- Carcinoma *in situ*.

TRATAMENTO

- A excisão cirúrgica é o tratamento de escolha.
- A maior parte dos pólipos pode ser exteriorizada diretamente pelo ânus e removida pela ressecção submucosa.
- Ocluir o defeito da mucosa com suturas absorvíveis, evitando o comprometimento do diâmetro do lúmen.
- Lesões que não são passíveis de exteriorização podem ser removidas por via transanal com eletrocirurgia mediante orientação endoscópica ou podem ser expostas diretamente por abordagem retal dorsal.
- Um único estudo em cães revelou uma melhora significativa dos sinais clínicos após a administração de piroxicam, embora o acompanhamento a longo prazo não esteja disponível. Inúmeros AINE foram avaliados em seres humanos com resultados mistos (ver a seção "Recursos da Internet").

MEDICAÇÕES

MEDICAMENTO(S)
- É recomendável o uso de antibióticos perioperatórios apropriados (p. ex., cefoxitina sódica [30 mg/kg IV]).
- Amolecedores fecais podem ajudar a diminuir o tenesmo — docusato de sódio (cães, 50-200 mg VO a cada 8-12 h; gatos, 50 mg VO a cada 12-24 h) ou docusato de cálcio (cães, 50-100 mg VO a cada 12-24 h; gatos, 50 mg VO a cada 12-24 h).
- Amolecedor alternativo de fezes — lactulose (1 mL/4,5 kg VO a cada 8 h até fazer efeito).

CONTRAINDICAÇÕES/INTERAÇÕES POSSÍVEIS
N/D.

ACOMPANHAMENTO

MONITORIZAÇÃO DO PACIENTE
- Examinar o local de incisão 14 dias após a cirurgia e, novamente, em 3 e 6 meses para garantir a ausência de recidiva ou estenose.
- A partir daí, realizar exame duas vezes ao ano para avaliar a recidiva.

COMPLICAÇÕES POSSÍVEIS
- Recidiva.
- Estenose retal (rara).

EVOLUÇÃO ESPERADA E PROGNÓSTICO
- Cães com adenomas simples focais apresentam prognóstico bom com baixa taxa de recidiva.
- Cães com lesões múltiplas e/ou difusas (envolvimento de >50% da circunferência da parede retal) exibem taxas muito maiores de recidiva.

DIVERSOS

VER TAMBÉM
- Adenocarcinoma dos Sacos Anais.
- Disquezia e Hematoquezia.
- Prolapso Retal e Anal.

ABREVIATURA(S)
- AINE = anti-inflamatório não esteroide.

RECURSOS DA INTERNET
http://www.jr2.ox.ac.uk/Bandolier/band129/b129-6.html. Este site revisa os resultados mistos de ensaios clínicos utilizando diversos AINE em seres humanos.

Sugestões de Leitura
Hedlund CS, Fossum TW. Surgery of the perineum, rectum, and anus. In: Fossum TW, ed., Small Animal Surgery, 3rd ed. St. Louis: Mosby, 2007, pp. 498-527.
Zoran DL. Rectoanal disease. In: Ettinger SJ, Feldman EC, eds., Textbook of Veterinary Internal Medicine, 6th ed. St. Louis: Elsevier, 2005, pp. 1408-1420.

Autor Eric R. Pope
Consultor Editorial Albert E. Jergens

POLIÚRIA E POLIDIPSIA

CONSIDERAÇÕES GERAIS

DEFINIÇÃO
• Poliúria — produção urinária maior que a normal (cães, >45 mL/kg/dia; gatos, >40 mL/kg/dia). • Polidipsia — consumo hídrico maior que o normal (cães, >90 mL/kg/dia; gatos >45 mL/kg/dia).

FISIOPATOLOGIA
• Os volumes de urina produzida e o consumo de água são controlados por interações entre os rins, a hipófise e o hipotálamo. A osmolalidade plasmática (principalmente a concentração de sódio) é o principal parâmetro monitorizado por esse sistema de controle. Receptores de volume existentes dentro dos átrios cardíacos e do arco aórtico também influenciam a sede e a produção de urina. A poliúria pode ocorrer quando a quantidade de hormônio antidiurético (ADH) funcional sintetizada no hipotálamo ou liberada pela hipófise posterior é limitada ou quando os rins deixam de responder normalmente ao ADH. Ocorre polidipsia quando o centro da sede no hipotálamo anterior é estimulado.
• Na maior parte dos pacientes, a polidipsia mantém a hidratação como uma resposta compensatória à poliúria. O plasma do paciente torna-se relativamente hipertônico e ativa os mecanismos da sede. Ocasionalmente, a polidipsia é o processo primário, enquanto a poliúria, a resposta compensatória. Em seguida, o plasma do paciente torna-se relativamente hipotônico por causa da ingestão excessiva de água, mas a secreção do ADH é reduzida, resultando na poliúria.

SISTEMA(S) ACOMETIDO(S)
• Urológico — repleção/tamanho da bexiga urinária. • Cardiovascular — volume circulante. • Endócrino/metabólico — a hipófise e o hipotálamo desempenham um papel na compensação à poliúria ou polidipsia.

IDENTIFICAÇÃO
• Cães e gatos. • Doenças congênitas em muitas raças (p. ex., diabetes insípido central, diabetes insípido nefrogênico, anomalias portovasculares e determinadas nefropatias).
• Hipoadrenocorticismo e algumas causas de polidipsia primária acometem predominantemente cães jovens. • Insuficiência renal, hiperadrenocorticismo, hipertireoidismo e distúrbios neoplásicos com envolvimento da hipófise e do hipotálamo afetam, sobretudo, cães e gatos de meia-idade e mais idosos.

CAUSAS
• Poliúria primária atribuída à resposta renal comprometida ao ADH — insuficiência renal, hiperadrenocorticismo (cães), hipertireoidismo (gatos), pielonefrite, leptospirose, hipoadrenocorticismo, piometra, insuficiência hepática, hipercalcemia, hipocalemia, exaustão de solutos da medula renal, restrição de proteína na dieta, medicamentos, diabetes insípido nefrogênico congênito. • Poliúria primária causada por diurese osmótica — diabetes melito, glicosúria renal primária, diurese pós-obstrutiva, alguns diuréticos (p. ex., manitol e furosemida), ingestão ou administração de grandes quantidades de soluto (p. ex., cloreto de sódio ou glicose) e hipersomatotropismo. • Poliúria primária atribuída à deficiência de ADH — idiopática, traumática, neoplásica ou diabetes insípido central de origem congênita; alguns medicamentos (p. ex., álcool e fenitoína). • Polidipsia primária — problema comportamental, pirexia, dor ou doença orgânica do centro da sede no hipotálamo anterior de origem neoplásica, traumática ou inflamatória.

FATORES DE RISCO
• Nefropatia ou hepatopatia. • Administração de diuréticos, corticosteroides e anticonvulsivantes. • Dietas pobres em proteína destinadas à dissolução de urólitos de estruvita nos cães.

DIAGNÓSTICO

DIAGNÓSTICO DIFERENCIAL
Diferenciar os Sinais Semelhantes
• Diferenciar a poliúria do aumento anormal na frequência de micção (polaciúria). A polaciúria frequentemente está associada à disúria, estrangúria ou hematúria. Pacientes com poliúria eliminam grandes quantidades de urina; já os pacientes com polaciúria, com frequência, eliminam pequenas quantidades de urina. Confirmar a poliúria/polidipsia pela mensuração da ingestão hídrica ou do débito urinário em um período de 24 h (é utilizado o período de coleta de 3–5 dias para diminuir os erros na medição do volume urinário).
• Alternativamente, o ato de medir a densidade urinária pode fornecer indícios da capacidade adequada de concentração da urina (cães, ≥1,030; gatos, ≥1,035), o que descarta poliúria/polidipsia persistente.

Diferenciar as Causas
• Insuficiência renal, hiperadrenocorticismo e diabetes melito são causas comuns de poliúria/polidipsia nos cães. Insuficiência renal, hipertireoidismo e diabetes melito são causas comuns de poliúria/polidipsia nos gatos.
• Caso estejam associadas à perda de peso progressiva — considerar insuficiência renal, diabetes melito, hipertireoidismo, insuficiência hepática, piometra, pielonefrite, hipoadrenocorticismo e hipercalcemia induzida por malignidade.
• Se estiverem associadas à diminuição do apetite — considerar nefropatia, pielonefrite, hipercalcemia induzida por malignidade, hepatopatia, hipoadrenocorticismo.
• Caso estejam associadas à polifagia — considerar diabetes melito, hipertireoidismo, hiperadrenocorticismo e acromegalia.
• Se estiverem associadas à alopecia bilateral e a outros problemas cutâneos — considerar hiperadrenocorticismo e outros distúrbios endocrinológicos.
• Caso estejam associadas ao hálito urêmico e à estomatite urêmica — considerar doença renal avançada.
• Se estiverem associadas ao vômito — considerar nefropatia, hipoadrenocorticismo, pielonefrite, insuficiência hepática, hipercalcemia, hipocalemia, hipertireoidismo e diabetes melito; ocasionalmente, ocorre vômito ou regurgitação após o consumo rápido de grande quantidade de água.
• Caso estejam associadas a mal-estar e/ou fraqueza — nefropatia, hipoadrenocorticismo, piometra, hipercalcemia, diabetes melito, hepatopatia, hipocalemia, hiperadrenocorticismo.
• Se estiverem associadas a nódulos palpáveis da tireoide — considerar hipertireoidismo.
• Caso estejam associadas à retinopatia hipertensiva — considerar insuficiência renal, hipertireoidismo, diabetes melito e hiperadrenocorticismo.
• Se estiverem associadas a estro recente (nos últimos dois meses) em fêmea intacta de meia-idade — considerar piometra.
• Caso estejam associadas à distensão abdominal — considerar insuficiência hepática, hiperadrenocorticismo, piometra e síndrome nefrótica.
• Se estiverem associadas à linfadenopatia, massa nos sacos anais ou outro processo neoplásico — considerar hipercalcemia da malignidade.
• Caso estejam associadas a distúrbio comportamental ou neurológico — considerar insuficiência hepática, polidipsia primária ou diabetes insípido central.
• Se estiverem associadas à polidipsia acentuada, em que os pacientes procuram e consomem água de qualquer fonte quase de forma contínua — considerar polidipsia primária, diabetes insípido central e diabetes insípido nefrogênico.
• Caso o paciente esteja sendo submetido à medicação, considerar poliúria/polidipsia induzida por medicamentos (esteroides, diuréticos, anticonvulsivantes).
• Se o paciente estiver consumindo alguma dieta destinada à prevenção ou dissolução de urólitos ou dieta rica em sal, considerar poliúria/polidipsia induzida pela dieta.
• A poliúria/polidipsia pode ser o primeiro sinal de doença em muitas condições mórbidas.

HEMOGRAMA/BIOQUÍMICA/URINÁLISE
• A urinálise é útil para confirmar poliúria, diferenciar diurese hídrica de diurese por soluto e identificar infecção do trato urinário.
• A concentração sérica de sódio ou a osmolalidade pode ajudar a diferenciar poliúria primária da polidipsia primária. É preferível a mensuração da osmolalidade sérica; a osmolalidade sérica calculada não é um substituto aceitável.
• Hipernatremia relativa ou osmolaridade sérica elevada sugere poliúria primária (os valores tipicamente tendem a ou excedem o limite superior da variação normal).
• Hiponatremia ou baixa osmolaridade sérica sugere polidipsia primária (os valores tipicamente tendem a ou declinam abaixo da variação normal), exceto nos animais com hipoadrenocorticismo, os quais apresentam hiponatremia e poliúria primária.
• Azotemia é um achado típico de causas renais para poliúria/polidipsia, mas também pode indicar desidratação resultante de polidipsia compensatória inadequada.
• Concentrações de ureia inesperadamente baixas sugerem insuficiência hepática.
• O aumento na atividade das enzimas hepáticas é compatível com hiperadrenocorticismo (especialmente quando o valor da fosfatase alcalina excede o da ALT), hipertireoidismo, insuficiência hepática, piometra e diabetes melito. A administração de alguns medicamentos que promovem poliúria/polidipsia (p. ex., anticonvulsivantes e corticosteroides) também pode elevar a atividade das enzimas hepáticas.
• Hiperglicemia persistente é compatível com diabetes melito.

POLIÚRIA E POLIDIPSIA

- Hipercalemia, particularmente se associada à hiponatremia, sugere hipoadrenocorticismo ou tratamento com diuréticos poupadores de potássio.
- Hipercalcemia induz à poliúria somente quando resultar de aumento na concentração do cálcio ionizado (não do cálcio ligado à proteína).
- Hipercalcemia e hipocalemia podem provocar ou ocorrer em associação com outras doenças indutoras de poliúria/polidipsia (p. ex., insuficiência renal crônica pode estar associada a ambas; hipoadrenocorticismo pode estar associado à hipercalcemia).
- Hipoalbuminemia apoia causas renais ou hepáticas de poliúria/polidipsia.
- Neutrofilia é compatível com pielonefrite, piometra, hiperadrenocorticismo e administração de corticosteroide.
- Valores da densidade urinária entre 1,001 e 1,003 sugerem polidipsia primária, diabetes insípido central ou diabetes insípido nefrogênico congênito.
- Glicosúria dá respaldo ao diagnóstico de diabetes melito ou glicosúria renal.
- Piúria, cilindros leucocitários e/ou bacteriúria devem incitar a consideração de pielonefrite.

OUTROS TESTES LABORATORIAIS

- Teste de estimulação com ACTH ou teste de supressão com dexametasona para descartar hiperadrenocorticismo nos cães de meia-idade a mais idosos, nos quais os achados iniciais não expliquem a poliúria/polidipsia.
- Concentração da tiroxina para excluir hipertireoidismo nos gatos de meia-idade e idosos.
- Ácidos biliares (em jejum e pós-prandiais) para descartar desvio portossistêmico ou insuficiência hepática.
- Urocultura — a pielonefrite crônica não pode ser descartada de forma conclusiva pela ausência de piúria ou de bacteriúria.
- Exame citológico do aspirado de linfonodo pode fornecer indícios de linfoma, o qual induz à poliúria pela nefrotoxicidade hipercalcêmica ou pela infiltração direta dos tecidos renais.
- Título ou PCR para *Leptospira* para excluir leptospirose.
- Teste de resposta ao ADH para descartar diabetes insípido central.
- Teste de privação de água (para avaliar a capacidade de produzir o ADH e responder a esse hormônio) é controverso em virtude de considerações humanas; usar de forma seletiva.

DIAGNÓSTICO POR IMAGEM

Radiografia abdominal simples e ultrassonografia podem fornecer indícios de distúrbios renais (p. ex., nefropatias primárias e obstrução urinária), hepáticos (p. ex., micro-hepatia, anomalias vasculares portais e infiltrado hepático), adrenais (p. ex., massa adrenal ou hipertrofia adrenal bilateral sugestiva de hiperadrenocorticismo) ou uterinos (p. ex., piometra) que podem contribuir para poliúria/polidipsia.

MÉTODOS DIAGNÓSTICOS

Teste de Privação de Água com Resposta ao ADH (ver o Apêndice II)

- Diferencia diabetes insípido central da polidipsia primária e diabetes insípido nefrogênico. Descartar outras causas de poliúria/polidipsia antes de realizar esse teste. Alguns consideram o teste de privação de água um exame perigoso e desumano e, por isso, sugerem a não realização desse teste e o encaminhamento do animal direto para a administração de ADH a fim de descartar o diabetes insípido central. A administração do ADH aos pacientes com polidipsia primária pode ser arriscada.
- Mais valioso para os pacientes com poliúria/polidipsia e hipostenúria acentuadas.
- O teste de privação de água está contraindicado nos pacientes desidratados e azotêmicos, mas o teste de resposta ao ADH pode ser realizado com segurança nesses pacientes.
- Os pacientes que concentram a urina de forma adequada em resposta à privação de água apresentam produção suficiente de ADH e resposta renal satisfatória a esse hormônio. Se outras causas forem descartadas, presume-se que a polidipsia primária esteja presente.
- Os pacientes que deixam de concentrar a urina de maneira adequada em resposta aos testes de privação de água devidamente elaborados, porém concentram mais a urina em resposta à administração exógena do ADH têm diabetes insípido central.
- Os pacientes que deixam de concentrar a urina adequadamente em resposta à privação de água e também deixam de concentrar mais a urina em resposta à administração exógena do ADH sofrem de diabetes insípido nefrogênico.

TRATAMENTO

- As consequências clínicas graves serão raras se o paciente tiver livre acesso à água e estiver disposto a bebê-la e apto para isso. Até que o mecanismo da poliúria esteja compreendido, não incentivar os proprietários a limitar o acesso à água. Direcionar o tratamento à causa subjacente.
- Os pacientes com poliúria devem ter livre acesso à água a menos que estejam vomitando. Se os pacientes com poliúria estiverem vomitando, administrar fluidos de manutenção para reposição por via parenteral após a coleta de amostras apropriadas para avaliação inicial desses animais. Fornecer também fluidos por via parenteral quando outras condições limitarem a ingestão oral ou se a desidratação persistir apesar da polidipsia.
- Basear a seleção do fluido no conhecimento da causa subjacente para a perda hídrica. Na maior parte dos pacientes, a solução de Ringer lactato é fluido de reposição aceitável.
- Quando a desidratação resultou da suspensão da água ou quando a urina estiver hipostenúrica, o fornecimento de água por via oral ou a administração parenteral de glicose a 5% em água pode ser preferível à solução de Ringer lactato.
- Polidipsia primária — tratar por meio da restrição gradual do consumo de água até um volume diário normal. Pode ser necessária a redução da ingestão hídrica ao longo de dias a semanas para evitar comportamentos indesejáveis como aumento dos latidos, consumo da própria urina ou outros padrões de comportamento bizarro. Monitorizar rigorosamente o paciente para evitar desidratação iatrogênica. O sal (1 g/30 kg a cada 12 h) ou o bicarbonato de sódio (0,6 g/30 kg a cada 12 h) podem ser administrados por via oral para ajudar a restabelecer o gradiente de soluto da medula renal. Considerar a modificação comportamental se apenas a restrição de água não for bem-sucedida.

ORIENTAÇÃO AO PROPRIETÁRIO

Não suspender a água de pacientes com poliúria, pois isso pode resultar em uma desidratação potencialmente perigosa.

MEDICAÇÕES

MEDICAMENTO(S) DE ESCOLHA
Variam com a causa subjacente.

CONTRAINDICAÇÕES
Não administrar o ADH (nem qualquer um de seus análogos sintéticos, como o DDAVP) aos pacientes com polidipsia primária por causa do risco de induzir à intoxicação hídrica.

PRECAUÇÕES
Até que os quadros de insuficiência renal e hepática sejam descartados como causas potenciais de poliúria/polidipsia, é preciso ter cuidado ao administrar qualquer medicamento eliminado por essas vias.

ACOMPANHAMENTO

MONITORIZAÇÃO DO PACIENTE
- Estado de hidratação pela avaliação clínica da hidratação e avaliação seriada do peso corporal.
- Ingestão hídrica e débito urinário — fornecem uma base de referência valiosa para avaliar a adequação da hidratação.

COMPLICAÇÕES POSSÍVEIS
Desidratação e, em casos graves, choque hipovolêmico e/ou hipernatremia.

DIVERSOS

DISTÚRBIOS ASSOCIADOS
- Infecção bacteriana do trato urinário — como consequência de cateterização transuretral.
- Pode se desenvolver incontinência urinária nos cães com disfunção concomitante do esfíncter uretral, presumivelmente por causa da elevação do enchimento vesical associada à poliúria.

VER TAMBÉM
- Doenças Renais de Natureza Congênita e de Desenvolvimento. • Diabetes Insípido. • Diabetes Melito. • Síndrome de Fanconi. • Insuficiência Hepática Aguda. • Hiperadrenocorticismo (Síndrome de Cushing) — Gatos.
- Hiperadrenocorticismo (Síndrome de Cushing) — Cães. • Hipercalcemia. • Hipertireoidismo.
- Hipoadrenocorticismo (Doença de Addison).
- Hipocalemia. • Leptospirose. • Pielonefrite.
- Piometra e Hiperplasia Endometrial Cística.
- Insuficiência Renal Aguda. • Insuficiência Renal Crônica. • Obstrução do Trato Urinário.

ABREVIATURA(S)
- ACTH = hormônio adrenocorticotrópico.
- ADH = hormônio antidiurético. • ALT = alanina aminotransferase. • DDAVP = 1-desamino-8-d-arginina (vasopressina). • PCR = reação em cadeia da polimerase.

Autor David J. Polzin
Consultor Editorial Carl A. Osborne

Problemas Comportamentais Maternos

CONSIDERAÇÕES GERAIS

DEFINIÇÃO
Comportamento materno anormal excessivo na ausência de neonatos ou comportamento materno deficiente na presença de neonatos da própria fêmea. O último caso é mais comum nos cães, enquanto o primeiro, nos gatos.

FISIOPATOLOGIA
A fisiopatologia de um tipo de comportamento materno excessivo, a pseudociese, parece ser os níveis elevados de progesterona após o estro nas cadelas não submetidas a cruzamento, seguida por queda abrupta nesses níveis. A fisiopatologia da recusa em aceitar os filhotes pelas fêmeas após a cesariana consiste no declínio de fatores incluindo a ocitocina necessária durante o período sensível para aceitação do neonato. A fisiopatologia de outros tipos de comportamento materno deficiente é desconhecida.

SISTEMA(S) ACOMETIDO(S)
Comportamental.

GENÉTICA
Embora não exista predisposição genética identificada, a predisposição na raça Jack Russel terrier indica a possível existência de algum componente genético. Há modelos genéticos de comportamento materno deficiente nas fêmeas de camundongos. Os genes responsáveis pelo comportamento materno deficiente nos camundongos são transmitidos por via paterna. Se isso for verdade em cães e gatos, seria de se esperar que as mães que rejeitam seus filhotes tenham desempenhado seus papéis normais de mãe, mas suas avós podem ter sido deficientes. A base genética deve ser pesquisada em cães e gatos.

INCIDÊNCIA/PREVALÊNCIA
A incidência do comportamento materno deficiente não foi determinada, mas parece ser baixa (i. e., menos de 1% dos casos na prática comportamental). O comportamento materno nas cadelas e nas gatas que não têm filhotes é mais comum.

DISTRIBUIÇÃO GEOGRÁFICA
N/D.

IDENTIFICAÇÃO
Espécies
Cães e gatos.

Raça(s) Predominante(s)
Comportamento materno deficiente pode ser mais comum na raça Jack Russel terrier e Cocker spaniel, embora não haja estudo quantitativo sobre isso.

Idade Média e Faixa Etária
Não há idade específica sob risco, mas as fêmeas primíparas e as cadelas mais idosas parecem estar sob risco de comportamento materno deficiente.

Sexo Predominante
Fêmeas em geral, mas alguns machos podem permitir um comportamento de sucção.

SINAIS CLÍNICOS
Comportamento Materno Deficiente
Comportamento materno ausente; a mãe simplesmente abandona sua cria. É mais provável que isso ocorra após a cesariana.

Comportamento Materno Fraco
- A mãe permanece com a cria, porém não permite que os filhotes mamem.
- Em outros casos, a mãe pode demonstrar um resgate inadequado dos filhotes, uma limpeza insuficiente dos mesmos ou falha em estimular a evacuação.
- Em outra forma de comportamento materno deficiente, a cadela leva os filhotes de um lugar para outro sem soltá-los, ou na forma mais extrema, mata alguns deles ou todos eles.

Comportamento Materno Anormal
- A cadela ou a gata pode deixar os filhotes mamar, porém os mata ao nascimento ou alguns dias depois. Ocasionalmente, a cadela, ou mais raramente a gata, abandona ou ataca seus filhotes se eles mudaram de odor ou de aparência. Uma fêmea pode ser importunada por outro animal ou outras pessoas e redirecionar sua agressividade para os filhotes.
- Uma cadela pode acidentalmente eviscerar ou até mesmo ingerir os filhotes por completo enquanto ingere as membranas fetais e o cordão umbilical. Isso deve ser distinto da lambedura normal, que pode ser muito vigorosa e até desalojar o filhote de uma teta.

Agressividade Materna
As gatas com filhotes podem ficar agressivas com outros animais, especialmente cães residentes na mesma casa. As cadelas podem se mostrar agressivas com seres humanos pouco familiares ou até mesmo familiares (conhecidos), sobretudo se estiverem com hipocalcemia.

Comportamento Materno Excessivo
- A cadela com pseudociese ou castrada durante a fase lútea tardia do ciclo estral adota, tenta amamentar e protege objetos inanimados (animais de pelúcia ou até coleiras). A cadela com pseudoprenhez pode apresentar desenvolvimento mamário e entrar em processo de lactação.
- A gata recém-castrada pode roubar os filhotes de uma gata lactante. Depois da castração, as gatas também podem entrar em lactação se forem sugadas.

CAUSAS E FATORES DE RISCO
- A presença de filhotes de gato em ambiente de gata recém-castrada é fator de risco para o comportamento materno excessivo e roubo de filhotes.
- O risco de transporte excessivo de filhotes caninos, agressividade redirecionada ou até mesmo canibalismo aumentará se houver outros cães ou muitas pessoas presentes na área do ninho.
- Fêmeas primíparas ou aquelas submetidas à cesariana estão sob maior risco em relação às multíparas ou aquelas que exibem parto normal.
- Outro fator de risco corresponde a uma ninhada grande de filhotes de gatos ou prole enferma.

DIAGNÓSTICO

DIAGNÓSTICO DIFERENCIAL
- O diferencial mais importante fica entre o comportamento materno anormal primário e o comportamento materno deficiente secundário à mastite ou metrite.
- A tetania da lactação pode resultar em comportamento agressivo embora esse comportamento raramente seja direcionado aos filhotes e ocorra mais tarde, durante a lactação, e não durante o parto.

HEMOGRAMA/BIOQUÍMICA/URINÁLISE
Geralmente normais a menos que outras condições clínicas estejam presentes. Os níveis sanguíneos de cálcio estarão baixos se a cadela estiver sofrendo de tetania da lactação.

OUTROS TESTES LABORATORIAIS
Apenas conforme indicado pelas condições metabólicas da cadela ou da gata.

DIAGNÓSTICO POR IMAGEM
Apenas conforme indicado por outros problemas.

MÉTODOS DIAGNÓSTICOS
N/D.

ACHADOS PATOLÓGICOS
A presença de leite nas glândulas mamárias das fêmeas com comportamento materno excessivo.

TRATAMENTO

CUIDADO(S) DE SAÚDE ADEQUADO(S)
Cuidado de saúde normal.

CUIDADO(S) DE ENFERMAGEM
N/D.

ATIVIDADE
N/D.

DIETA
- Dieta adequada para cadelas e gatas lactantes a fim de suprir as demandas energéticas.
- Dietas restritas para pseudociese para desestimular a lactação e diminuir a produção de leite.
- No caso de comportamento materno deficiente, a cadela ou a gata deve ser alimentada *ad libitum* (i. e., à vontade) para estimular a lactação.

ORIENTAÇÃO AO PROPRIETÁRIO
Comportamento Materno Anormal ou Deficiente
- A cadela que está carregando seus filhotes ou apresentando agressividade redirecionada a eles deve ficar isolada em área silenciosa e escura. A cadela que morde seus filhotes deve ser amordaçada. O proprietário deve estimular a evacuação dos filhotes, já que a fêmea amordaçada não consegue fazer isso. O colar elizabetano inibe o canibalismo nas gatas.
- A cadela deve ser assistida no parto e os filhotes, removidos temporariamente se ela os estiver mordendo além de cortar o cordão umbilical.
- As cadelas e gatas com comportamento materno deficiente podem apresentar o mesmo comportamento com ninhadas subsequentes.

Comportamento Materno Excessivo
- As gatas que tenham filhotes roubados devem ser separadas da mãe natural e dos filhotes.
- Os objetos adotados devem ser removidos da cadela pseudoprenhe.
- A ingestão alimentar deve ser restrita para inibir a lactação.

Agressividade Materna contra Animais ou Seres Humanos
O melhor tratamento para agressividade materna excessiva é separar os gatinhos; o desmame isolado não é suficiente, porque só a presença dos filhotes pode manter ou até reinstalar a agressividade

Problemas Comportamentais Maternos

materna em gata separada de seus filhotes por várias semanas.

CONSIDERAÇÕES CIRÚRGICAS
• Adiar a castração por 4 meses após o estro para evitar o comportamento materno pós-castração e sua agressividade acompanhante.
• A castração evita comportamento materno excessivo futuro na ausência de filhotes.

MEDICAÇÕES

MEDICAMENTO(S) DE ESCOLHA
Comportamento Materno Excessivo
• Mibolerona (Cheque drops®) era o medicamento de escolha para cadelas com pseudociese ou para aquelas que apresentam comportamento materno e lactação após a castração. A dose é de 16 µg/kg VO uma vez ao dia por 5 dias. A mibolerona inibe a prolactina e dessa forma inibe a lactação. No entanto, esse medicamento não está mais disponível exceto em algumas farmácias de manipulação.
• Bromocriptina (Parlodel®) pode ser utilizada para inibir a prolactina. A dose é de 10 µg/kg por 10 dias. Esse medicamento não deve ser administrado a animais prenhes.
• Cabergolina é um antagonista da prolactina que tem se mostrado eficaz para o tratamento de pseudociese em cães. A dose é de 5 µg/kg 1 vez ao dia VO por 4–6 dias. Alguns animais podem necessitar de mais de um curso terapêutico. Esse medicamento não está disponível no mercado na América do Norte.

CONTRAINDICAÇÕES
Não utilizar mibolerona nas gatas, pois esse agente possui estreita margem de segurança nessa espécie. Além disso, ela não deve ser administrada a cães da raça Bedlington terrier.

PRECAUÇÕES
A mibolerona pode provocar masculinização nas fêmeas, podendo incluir comportamento sexual masculino, hipertrofia do clitóris, vulvovaginite e incontinência urinária. A bromocriptina pode causar vômitos gastrintestinais, sedação e hipotensão, bem como abortamento.

INTERAÇÕES POSSÍVEIS
• Caso se faça uso de tranquilizantes, é preciso ter cuidado para que os filhotes de cães ou gatos não fiquem sedados.
• Não utilizar estrogênios ou progestagênios ao mesmo tempo que a mibolerona.

MEDICAMENTO(S) ALTERNATIVO(S)
Geralmente, não há necessidade de outros medicamentos.

Comportamento Materno Deficiente
• Ocitocina pode ser administrada por via parenteral na dose de 1–5 unidades ou por spray nasal (Syntocinon®).
• Como a prolactina parece ser necessária para o comportamento materno em outras espécies, pode-se utilizar algum bloqueador dopaminérgico, como a acepromazina (0,55–2,2 mg/kg VO). A dopamina inibe a liberação de prolactina; portanto, um bloqueador dopaminérgico aumentaria os níveis de prolactina.

CONTRAINDICAÇÕES
Não administrar a ocitocina a animais prenhes ou em combinação com agentes simpaticomiméticos.

ACOMPANHAMENTO

MONITORIZAÇÃO DO PACIENTE
Os filhotes de cães ou de gatos das fêmeas que demonstrem comportamento materno deficiente devem ser monitorizados diariamente para verificar se eles estão ganhando peso.

PREVENÇÃO
• Colocar a fêmea lactante em locais silenciosos e confortáveis, longe de ruídos e de distúrbios de outros animais ou pessoas.
• Não cruzar novamente fêmeas que demonstrem comportamento materno deficiente. Determinar se qualquer outra fêmea filha de fêmea com comportamento materno anormal também apresentou esse tipo de comportamento. Em outras espécies, o comportamento materno deficiente é um gene transmitido por via paterna; o pai deve contribuir para o gene do comportamento materno deficiente. As filhas de mães que rejeitam não rejeitarão, porém as filhas de seus irmãos podem fazê-lo.
• O comportamento materno deficiente pode ocorrer em cada ninhada; não cruzar novamente.

COMPLICAÇÕES POSSÍVEIS
• Perda da cria.
• Com frequência, os filhotes de cães e de gatos criados manualmente apresentam comportamento social anormal ou deficiente. Isso se deve em parte ao período insuficiente de amamentação e às consequências da falta de lambedura materna, o que afeta adversamente a resposta ao estresse e o comportamento reprodutivo.

EVOLUÇÃO ESPERADA E PROGNÓSTICO
• O comportamento materno excessivo, em geral, desaparece no momento do desmame normal (6–8 semanas).
• Pode ocorrer o comportamento materno deficiente em cada ninhada.

DIVERSOS

DISTÚRBIOS ASSOCIADOS
N/D.

FATORES RELACIONADOS COM A IDADE
N/D.

POTENCIAL ZOONÓTICO
N/D.

GESTAÇÃO/FERTILIDADE/REPRODUÇÃO
• Considerar particularmente a utilização de medicamentos e o efeito da doença sobre o feto.
• Não acasalar cães com histórico de comportamento materno deficiente.

SINÔNIMO(S)
Falta de instinto materno.

RECURSOS DA INTERNET
http://www.ivis.org/advances/BehaviorHoupt/houpt-aberent/chapter.

Sugestões de Leitura
Connolly PB. Reproductive behavior problems. In: Horwitz D, Mills D, Heath S, eds., BSAVA Manual of Canine and Feline Behavioural Medicine. Gloucestershire, UK: BSAVA, 2002, pp. 128–143.
Hart BL, Hart LA, Bain MJ. Canine and Feline Behavior Therapy, 2nd ed. Ames, IA: Blackwell, 2006.
Houpt KA. 2000. Maternal behavior and its aberrations. In: Houpt KA, ed., Recent Advances in Companion Animal Behavior Problems. International Veterinary Information Service (www.ivis.org).
Houpt KA, Concannon PW. Sexual and maternal behavior in cats. In: Ackerman L, ed., Cat Behavior and Training. Neptune City, NJ: TFH Publications, 1996.
Misner TL, Houpt KA. 1998. Animal behavior case of the month. JAVMA 1998, 213:1260–1262.

Autor Katherine A. Houpt
Consultor Editorial Debra F. Horwitz

Problemas Comportamentais Pediátricos — Cães

CONSIDERAÇÕES GERAIS

DEFINIÇÃO
Na maioria das vezes, esses problemas incluem comportamentos que são normais e comuns à maior parte dos filhotes, mas inaceitáveis para a família. Eles necessitam de certo grau de mudanças por meio de adestramentos e ajustes para se tornarem aceitáveis. Os problemas de adestramento incluem mastigação destrutiva, brincadeiras de morder, saltar/pular nas pessoas e subir em balcões ou móveis.

SISTEMA(S) ACOMETIDO(S)
Comportamental.

GENÉTICA
É provável que os níveis de atividade e os comportamentos de filhotes caninos jovens sejam semelhantes aos de seus progenitores. Alguns problemas podem ser mais comuns em determinadas raças, como indisciplina, problemas relacionados com atividade em raças caninas de trabalho, hábito de escavação pelos terriers, etc.

INCIDÊNCIA/PREVALÊNCIA
Comum à maior parte dos filhotes caninos.

DISTRIBUIÇÃO GEOGRÁFICA
Pode ser mais frequente nas áreas urbanas ou em ambientes onde as oportunidades de exercício estão menos disponíveis.

IDENTIFICAÇÃO
Espécies
Cães.

Raça(s) Predominante(s)
Raças de trabalho selecionadas pelos altos níveis de energia.

Idade Média e Faixa Etária
Dos 4 aos 9 meses de vida embora possam persistir até o final do segundo ano.

Sexo Predominante
Frequência e intensidade um pouco elevadas em cães machos.

SINAIS CLÍNICOS
Mastigação Destrutiva
O animal mastiga e destrói os móveis e os pertences dos membros da família. Em princípio, tal comportamento ocorre na presença dessas pessoas, mas pode ficar mais limitado a períodos de ausência do dono, uma vez que o animal tenha sido apanhado e punido diversas vezes.

Brincadeiras de Morder
O animal morde as mãos, as pernas e/ou as roupas. Em geral, as mordidas são inibidas, mas podem provocar lesões em virtude dos dentes de leite (decíduos) afiados. Pode haver rosnados e latidos, mas geralmente com um tom mais alto do que aquele associado a tipos mais graves de agressão, como o medo ou a agressividade possessiva. Os ataques de brincadeiras costumam ser deflagrados por algum movimento de um dos membros da família, mas podem ser bastante espontâneos, sem provocação ou estímulo aparente.

Saltar/Pular nas Pessoas
O animal pula e coloca as patas nas pessoas da família e/ou em visitas. Isso ocorre tipicamente durante saudações ou cumprimentos e quando o animal se encontra agitado, mas pode ocorrer quando o animal deseja atenção ou alguma coisa que a pessoa esteja segurando.

Subir em Balcões ou Móveis
O animal sobe em móveis e balcões para explorar e ter acesso a objetos a fim de mastigar ou comer. Ele também pode pular na mobília durante as brincadeiras para receber atenção ou descansar.

CAUSAS
Gerais
Níveis inadequados de controle, manejo, supervisão, adestramento, exercício e/ou estímulo mental por parte do proprietário podem ser as causas subjacentes desses problemas.

Mastigação Destrutiva
• Erupção dentária. • Brincadeira.
• Comportamento exploratório. • Comportamento de escape. • Brinquedos insuficientes ou desinteressantes. • Intolerância ao confinamento.
• Fome, alimento derramado no carpete ou na mobília. • Predação (camundongos ou outros pequenos mamíferos nas paredes ou no chão).

Brincar de Morder
Brincadeiras grosseiras, provocando e incitando o animal a morder as mãos e os pés.

Pular/Saltar nas Pessoas
• Longos períodos de confinamento, especialmente em ambiente muito pequeno. • Saudações ou cumprimentos exagerados pelos membros da família e pelas visitas. • Brincadeiras grosseiras.
• Oportunidades insuficientes para interação social. • Adestramento insuficiente.

Subir em Balcões ou Móveis
• Brinquedos insuficientes ou desinteressantes.
• Objetos ou alimentos tentadores deixados sobre os balcões ou móveis. • Desejo de interação social.
• Ausência de superfície confortável no chão onde repousa.

FATORES DE RISCO
Ver a seção "Causas".

DIAGNÓSTICO

DIAGNÓSTICO DIFERENCIAL
Mastigação Destrutiva
A ansiedade da separação pode ocorrer nos cães jovens, embora seja mais comum nos adultos. O animal tipicamente apresenta sinais significativos antes da partida e com saudações muito efusivas. O comportamento destrutivo ocorre praticamente toda vez que o animal perde o acesso a um ou mais membros da família e, em geral, é direcionado aos caminhos de saída ou aos pertences pessoais dos familiares.

Brincadeiras de Morder
• Agressividade por medo — o comportamento agressivo é acompanhado por sinais de medo e/ou submissão (postura corporal rebaixada, orelhas e cauda caídas, retração vertical das comissuras bucais). O comportamento ocorre quando o animal fica em uma situação entendida como ameaçadora. O rosnado pode ter uma intensidade mais elevada e ser acompanhado por uivos e ganidos. • Agressividade possessiva — o comportamento ocorre em situações específicas em que haja competição por algum prêmio. O animal tipicamente se enrijece e se debruça sobre o objeto protegido. Também pode ser observado um aumento na velocidade de ingestão alimentar ou rápida preensão de algum objeto firmemente à boca. O rosnado apresenta um tom mais acentuado. Pode ocorrer piloereção, assim como investida, dentada e mordida. • Encefalite viral, toxicose — a mordida costuma ser acompanhada por outros sinais mórbidos.

HEMOGRAMA/BIOQUÍMICA/URINÁLISE
N/D a menos que haja sinais concomitantes de doença.

MÉTODOS DIAGNÓSTICOS
N/D a menos que haja sinais concomitantes de doença.

TRATAMENTO

CUIDADO(S) DE SAÚDE ADEQUADO(S)
O paciente é tratado em um esquema ambulatorial.

CUIDADO(S) DE ENFERMAGEM
O encaminhamento a um adestrador para adestramento de obediência pode ser benéfico.

ATIVIDADE
• Praticar exercícios os mais vigorosos possíveis que estejam dentro dos parâmetros de saúde aceitáveis para o indivíduo.
• *Correr atrás de objeto jogado* é um excelente exercício para o animal e para lembrá-lo de que o proprietário tem controle sobre os recursos. Também ajuda os membros da família a recuperar objetos do animal dos quais ele não deveria ter a posse. Utilizando dois objetos, o ato de atirar um e segurar o outro para depois atirar assim que o animal retornar com o primeiro objeto pode ajudar a manter a continuidade da brincadeira em cães que talvez não soltem o brinquedo.

DIETA
• Fornecer quantidade suficiente de alimento nos melhores horários para manter o animal saciado, a fim de diminuir sua motivação para subir em móveis, mexer no lixo, guardar comida ou mastigar objetos inanimados. O uso de um brinquedo tipo *dispenser* para ração pode ocupar o filhote e ser um adjuvante útil para a mastigação de brinquedos.
• Orientar a família que a decisão sobre a quantidade de alimento a ser fornecido não pode ser determinada exclusivamente pelas recomendações de idade/peso listadas pelo fabricante da ração; além disso, as necessidades nutricionais podem variar consideravelmente entre os filhotes.

ORIENTAÇÃO AO PROPRIETÁRIO
Geral
• Discutir os princípios relevantes da utilização de recompensas e punição, incluindo o momento oportuno, a consistência, o valor e a intensidade. Enfatizar ao proprietário que gritos ou punições físicas devem ser evitados. Os membros da família devem ser aconselhados a jamais bater no animal, golpear seu nariz, sacudi-lo pela nuca, rolá-lo sobre seu dorso ou espremer seus lábios contra os dentes a fim de que ele pare de colocar a boca ou de morder. Essas abordagens podem aumentar a gravidade do problema, arruinar a ligação com o animal e levar a problemas mais sérios, como o medo e a agressividade. Por outro lado, os membros da família devem constantemente prestar atenção e recompensar comportamentos aceitáveis.

Problemas Comportamentais Pediátricos — Cães

- Orientar a família a ensinar o animal a se sentar sob voz de comando, fazendo uso de adestramento com atrativos alimentares tipo iscas.
- Ensinar a família como supervisionar de forma adequada.
- Abordar o confinamento e como adestrar o animal para aceitá-lo.

Mastigação Destrutiva
- Fornecer brinquedos interessantes.
- Experimentar diferentes tipos de brinquedos para descobrir as preferências do animal.
- Oferecer brinquedos onde pequenas quantidades de alimento possam ser socadas ou escondidas para torná-los mais atrativos.
- Recompensar a mastigação aceitável com elogios e fornecer petiscos para o animal quando ele morder seus próprios brinquedos.
- Manter os objetos proibidos fora do alcance.
- Fechar as portas e utilizar portinholas de bebês para restringir o acesso aos objetos.
- Borrifar os objetos que precisam ser protegidos com substâncias seguras de sabor desagradável e aversivo.
- Utilizar um alarme disparado pelo movimento para manter o animal longe dos objetos que necessitam de proteção.
- Interromper qualquer mastigação inaceitável com um "não" ríspido, com o ruído de uma lata sacudida, com o "sibilo" de uma lata de ar comprimido ou uma corneta. Qualquer um desses métodos de interrupção deve ser empregado com certa atenção ao temperamento do animal. Tais métodos devem ser de intensidade mínima, para que o comportamento seja interrompido imediatamente, mas não seja eliciada uma reação de medo por parte do animal.
- Supervisão rigorosa ou confinamento seguro podem ser necessários até por volta dos 2 anos de idade.

Brincar de Morder
- Providenciar muitos exercícios para reduzir a reatividade e a impulsividade.
- Sempre ter brinquedos à disposição para jogar para cima e distrair o animal. Utilizar brinquedos atados com alimentos para distrair a atenção do animal e mantê-lo ocupado.
- Deixar o animal amarrado quando ele estiver fora de controle e a família não puder dedicar o tempo necessário para moldar o comportamento ou esgotá-lo com exercício.
- Evitar os brinquedos que estimulem as brincadeiras de morder as mãos e os pés.
- Ter o controle do animal, controlando os recursos e fazendo-o sentar antes de receber brinquedos, alimentos, brincadeiras e atenção.
- Ignorar qualquer comportamento social intrometido por parte do filhote, como ganir, latir ou bater com os pés para chamar a atenção.
- Dizer "Ai" bem alto e se afastar do animal para interromper imediatamente qualquer mordida rude durante a brincadeira.
- Correções físicas devem ser evitadas, pois podem provocar medo, ansiedade e agressão.
- Usar coleira e enforcador, conforme a necessidade, para obtenção de maior controle.
- O filhote deve estar matriculado em aulas próprias para sua faixa etária (8 a 10 semanas de vida).

Pular/Saltar nas Pessoas
- Evitar brincadeiras e jogos que incentivem o animal a pular nas pessoas.
- Ensinar o animal a se sentar sob comando de voz.
- Toda vez que o animal se aproximar para chamar a atenção ou se dirigir a alguém, coloque rapidamente um pequeno petisco ou brinquedo diante de sua boca e mande-o sentar.
- Se possível, ignore completamente o animal quando ele estiver pulando.
- Se o animal saltar, o comportamento poderá ser interrompido com um ruído agudo (ver a seção "Mastigação Destrutiva" anteriormente) ou, então, um enforcador poderá ser usado para aumentar o controle e evitar os saltos.
- É extremamente importante que todos os membros da família sejam unânimes em reagir a esse problema e moldar o comportamento do animal e que, na verdade, ninguém esteja incentivando esse tipo de comportamento.

Subir em Balcões ou Móveis
- Manter o alimento e objetos de interesse longe de balcões e da mobília durante o período inicial de adestramento.
- Supervisionar constantemente ou colocar o animal em área segura de confinamento.
- Fornecer brinquedos interessantes para promover o estímulo mental e manter o animal focado nos objetos do chão.
- Manter o animal bem alimentado, para que ele não passe fome e provavelmente desvie sua atenção de mesas e balcões.
- Utilizar alarmes acionados pelo movimento ou pequenas caixas com ar para ensinar o animal a se manter longe dos móveis e balcões quando não supervisionado.
- Fornecer cama apropriada no chão.

MEDICAÇÕES

MEDICAMENTO(S) DE ESCOLHA
- Em geral, não há indicação de medicamentos.
- Em raras ocasiões, uma pequena quantidade de fenotiazina (p. ex., acepromazina) ou um anti-histamínico (p. ex., difenidramina) podem ser considerados para a leve sedação durante visitas de amigos ou quando o animal ainda não está sob controle.

MEDICAMENTO(S) ALTERNATIVO(S)
Foi demonstrado que coleiras com ferormônios acalmam os filhotes e aumentam o aprendizado.

ACOMPANHAMENTO

MONITORIZAÇÃO DO PACIENTE
- Consultas de acompanhamento precisam ser marcadas, considerando-se cada caso.
- Acompanhamentos por telefone em aproximadamente 10 dias, 20 dias e 6 semanas após a consulta inicial costumam ser valiosos.
- Algum membro treinado da equipe de apoio pode desempenhar um papel importante em auxiliar o acompanhamento junto ao proprietário.

PREVENÇÃO
- Providenciar quantidade adequada de supervisão e de confinamento.
- Iniciar o adestramento de obediência com recompensa de alimento em casa com 7-8 semanas de vida. Matricular em aulas para filhotes com 8-10 semanas de vida.
- Praticar grande quantidade de exercício físico e estímulo mental.
- Fornecer informações sobre os comportamentos e as necessidades do animal jovem normal (especialmente estímulo mental e físico) durante as várias fases de crescimento, de forma que a família saiba o que esperar e o que fazer.
- Sugerir o uso de brinquedos seguros e interessantes.
- Abordar as estratégias de supervisão e de confinamento.

COMPLICAÇÕES POSSÍVEIS
- Roupas e objetos da casa estragados.
- O alimento da família é ingerido pelo animal.
- Corpos estranhos/obstruções intestinais.
- Pequenas lesões cutâneas por mordidas em brincadeiras.
- Um hóspede é derrubado e se machuca.
- Elo fragilizado com o animal e possível abandono em um abrigo.

EVOLUÇÃO ESPERADA E PROGNÓSTICO
O prognóstico, em geral, é bom. A frequência e a intensidade dos comportamentos diminuirão com a idade. Saltar nas pessoas e morder de brincadeira, em geral, poderão ser rapidamente controlados se a família for unânime no adestramento. A tendência a mastigar ocasionalmente os pertences da família ou explorar os balcões em busca de alimento e outros objetos pode durar até 12-24 meses de vida, quando o animal se torna adulto do ponto de vista comportamental e menos ativo.

DIVERSOS

Sugestões de Leitura

American Animal Hospital Association. Behavior pamphlets (Playbiting, Destructive Puppy Behavior, Leadership and Control, and more). Lakewood, CO: American Animal Hospital Association, 2009.

Denenberg S, Landsberg G. Effects of dog-appeasing pheromones on anxiety and fear in puppies during training and on long-term socialization. JAVMA 2008, 233(12):1874-1882.

Dunbar I. Sirius Puppy Training, DVD. Berkeley, CA: James & Kenneth Publishers, 2006.

Hunthausen W. Preventive behavioural medicine for dogs. In: Horwitz DF, Mills D, eds., BSAVA Manual of Canine and Feline Behavioural Medicine, 2nd ed. Gloucestershire, UK: BSAVA, 2009.

Hunthausen W, Seksel K. Preventative behavioural medicine. In: Horwitz D, Mills D, Heath S, eds., BSAVA Manual of Canine and Feline Behavioural Medicine. Gloucestershire, UK: BSAVA, 2002, pp. 49-60.

Landsberg GL, Hunthausen WL, Ackerman L. Handbook of Behavior Problems of the Dog and Cat, 2nd ed. Philadelphia: Elsevier Saunders, 2003.

McConnell P. Dog Play—Understanding Play between Dogs and between Dogs and People, DVD. Black Earth, WI: McConnell Publishing, 2009.

Scidmore K, McConnell PB. Puppy Primer. Black Earth, WI: Dog's Best Friend, Ltd., 1996.

Autor Wayne Hunthausen
Consultor Editorial Debra F. Horwitz

Problemas Comportamentais Pediátricos — Gatos

CONSIDERAÇÕES GERAIS

DEFINIÇÃO
- Comportamentos indesejáveis exibidos por filhotes de gato entre o nascimento e a puberdade.
- Esses comportamentos podem incluir mordida, arranhão, brincadeira excessiva e/ou destrutiva e medo, além de comportamentos defensivos.

FISIOPATOLOGIA
- A maior parte dos problemas comportamentais pediátricos refere-se a comportamentos normais típicos da espécie.
- Falta ou privação de interações sociais apropriadas, estimulação ambiental e até mesmo nutrição podem contribuir e/ou levar a comportamentos anormais ou indesejáveis.

SISTEMA(S) ACOMETIDO(S)
Comportamental.

GENÉTICA
São apoiadas influências paternas sobre a cordialidade dos gatos em relação às pessoas.

IDENTIFICAÇÃO
Espécie
Gatos.

Idade Média e Faixa Etária
Em geral, 8–52 semanas de vida.

SINAIS CLÍNICOS
Comentários Gerais

Agressividade por Brincadeira
- Contém elementos predatórios e dentro da espécie, incluindo perseguição, caça, ataque, bote, golpe e mordida. A brincadeira pode ser solitária, com objetos, ou social, incluindo algum outro filhote ou, se este não estiver disponível, outro animal ou pessoa.
- Durante brincadeiras normais, as mordidas são inibidas e as garras não se encontram completamente estendidas.

Brincadeira Excessiva e/ou Destrutiva
- Alto nível de brincadeiras solitárias que frequentemente resultam em dano a itens da casa e interrupção do sono do proprietário.

Arranhões
- Uso das garras para arranhar superfícies que podem incluir itens de casa e pessoas.
- Os arranhões constituem um comportamento normal para a manutenção da garra e como forma de marcação territorial.
- Esse comportamento normal torna-se problemático para o dono do animal de estimação quando os objetos arranhados incluem paredes, móveis, carpetes, cortinas e outros itens domésticos.

Comportamentos de Medo
- Incluem o ato de se esconder, chiar e arranhar, além de comportamentos antissociais.

Achados Anamnésicos

Brincadeira Agressiva Direcionada às Pessoas ou a Outros Animais de Estimação da Casa
- Ataques espontâneos pelo filhote direcionados contra pessoas ou outros animais de estimação da casa.
- Emboscadas são comuns e ocorrem sem vocalizações. As mordidas costumam ser inibidas, mas podem atravessar a pele; além disso, podem ocorrer leves arranhões com as garras.

Brincadeira Agressiva Desinibida Direcionada às Pessoas
- Sinais semelhantes aos de cima, porém mais intensos. • As mordidas não são tão inibidas e, em geral, causam solução de continuidade na pele.

Brincadeira Normal Direcionada a Objetos na Residência
- Ataques de brincadeira solitária que incluem corrida intensa pela mobília da casa. • Destruindo objetos ou esfregando-se com as costas debaixo dos móveis. • Pancadas em objetos, removendo-os de superfícies horizontais.

Arranhões
- Evidência de itens arranhados na casa ou lesões por arranhadura nos membros da família.

Medo e Comportamentos Defensivos Atribuídos à Falta de Experiência Anterior
- Nenhuma exposição a seres humanos entre 3-7 semanas de vida. • Os comportamentos associados ao medo incluem, por exemplo, pupilas dilatadas, piloereção, posturas defensivas, chiados, busca por esconderijos, fuga, agressividade na presença de pessoas.

Medo e Comportamentos Defensivos Relacionados com Traumatismo Anterior
- Normal até que enfrente algum evento traumático, por exemplo, abuso, ataque de outro animal.

Medo e Comportamentos Defensivos Relacionados com Técnicas de Correção
- Normal até que seja "corrigido" por uma pessoa, por exemplo, espancamento, choque elétrico, pancada no nariz, gritos ou perseguição.
- Os filhotes, então, manifestam sinais comportamentais típicos de posturas defensivas, chiados, fuga, busca por esconderijos, pupilas dilatadas, piloereção na presença do proprietário ou em resposta a correções aparentemente leves.

CAUSAS

Brincadeira Agressiva Direcionada a Pessoas ou Outros Gatos na Residência
- Comportamento normal típico da espécie, mas sem interação social apropriada com companheiros da mesma espécie o comportamento pode se tornar desinibido e nocivo. • Os proprietários podem incentivar a brincadeira interativa indevida, promovendo a atividade lúdica com partes do corpo humano, como dedos, mãos e pés.
- Falta de outras saídas para brincadeiras mais adequadas.

Brincadeira Normal Direcionada a Objetos na Residência
- Comportamento normal típico da espécie.

Medo e Comportamentos Defensivos Atribuídos à Falta de Experiência Anterior
- Exposição mínima ou ausente a pessoas quando o filhote se encontra entre 3 e 7 semanas de vida.

Medo e Comportamentos Defensivos Relacionados com Traumatismo Anterior
- Evento traumático precoce.

Medo e Comportamentos Defensivos Relacionados com Técnicas de Correção
- Normal até que seja "corrigido" por uma pessoa, por exemplo, espancamento, choque elétrico, pancada no nariz, gritos ou perseguição.

FATORES DE RISCO

Brincadeira Agressiva Direcionada às Pessoas
- O único gato jovem na residência, filhote órfão criado manualmente.
- Nenhuma saída pertinente é fornecida para brincadeira e exploração normais.
- Incentivo de brincadeiras inadequadas por parte do proprietário.

Brincadeira Normal Direcionada a Objetos na Residência
- Falta de estímulos ambientais, incluindo a ausência de brinquedos, além de pouca brincadeira interativa com pessoas ou outros animais.
- Único filhote ou animal de estimação da casa.

Arranhões
- Ausência de materiais apropriados para arranhar.

Medo e Comportamentos Defensivos
- Falta de socialização adequada com pessoas, técnicas de correção e outra(s) experiência(s) traumática(s).

DIAGNÓSTICO

DIAGNÓSTICO DIFERENCIAL

Agressividade por Brincadeira a Pessoas
- Diferenciar brincadeira normal de agressividades mais sérias por brincadeiras desinibidas. O prognóstico depende dos fatores mencionados anteriormente.

Brincadeiras Excessivas/Comportamentos Destrutivos
- Sem diferenciais.

Arranhões
- Manutenção da unha, marcação ou relacionados com brincadeiras.

Medo e Comportamentos Defensivos
- Doenças do sistema nervoso central, p. ex., doenças anômalas, infecciosas, tóxicas.

HEMOGRAMA/BIOQUÍMICA/URINÁLISE
- Filhotes extremamente amedrontados podem apresentar níveis elevados de cortisol, ACTH e glicose.

TRATAMENTO

ATIVIDADE
Muitos problemas comportamentais pediátricos podem ser aliviados ou reduzidos pelo enriquecimento do ambiente do filhote, fornecendo brinquedos móveis e uma variedade de brinquedos, alternando-os regularmente; engajando o animal em brincadeiras interativas; permitindo o acesso do filhote a janelas teladas, caixas, sacos de papel; oferecendo uma variedade de superfícies atrativas para arranhar; e, possivelmente, trazendo um novo filhote para casa.

DIETA
Sem dúvida, a nutrição influencia o desenvolvimento do sistema nervoso e o comportamento, mas sua especificidade é incerta. É recomendável o fornecimento de dietas *Premium* no período pré-natal e para os filhotes.

ORIENTAÇÃO AO PROPRIETÁRIO
Na maioria dos casos, esses problemas são comportamentos normais do filhote julgados pelos proprietários como anormais ou excessivos e inadequados para seu estilo de vida.

Problemas Comportamentais Pediátricos — Gatos

Brincadeira Agressiva Direcionada às Pessoas
• O tratamento mais eficiente é adquirir outro filhote do mesmo porte e temperamento.
• Proporcionar e incentivar muitos exercícios regulares e brincadeiras interativas. • Identificar as circunstâncias ou situações em que podem ocorrer os ataques e ficar preparado para redirecionar a brincadeira para algum outro objeto (p. ex., lançar um pedaço de papel amassado ou outro brinquedo próprio para a espécie felina para o filhote perseguir, caçar, dar o bote e agarrar). • Não incentivar correções ou punições físicas. Orientar o proprietário a não espancar, chutar ou bater nele ou no nariz com os dedos. • Pode-se utilizar algum estímulo que chame a atenção como um instrumento para punir, como o ruído sibilante de uma lata de ar comprimido ou um esguicho de uma pistola ou garrafa d´água. • Pare de brincar com o filhote na presença de comportamentos inadequados. Pode-se usar um ruído ou chiado que chame a atenção para distrair o filhote e, então, o proprietário deverá interromper todas as brincadeiras, afastando-se do filhote e ignorando-o.
• O ato de aparar as extremidades das unhas com frequência ajuda a diminuir as lesões.

Brincadeira Agressiva Direcionada a Outros Gatos na Residência
• Adquirir outro filhote do mesmo porte e temperamento do filhote problemático. • Se a aquisição de outro filhote estiver fora de cogitação, o filhote problemático e o gato mais idoso deverão ter acesso restrito um ao outro. • Técnicas de punição que chamam a atenção provavelmente afetariam o gato mais idoso de forma aversiva.
• Proceder a brincadeiras interativas com o filhote em um esquema diário e regular, utilizando brinquedos ou objetos próprios para ele.

Brincadeira Agressiva Desinibida Direcionada às Pessoas
• Os tratamentos são semelhantes àqueles utilizados para brincadeiras agressivas normais.
• É útil colocar o filhote em um programa do tipo "trabalhar para ganhar", em que ele precisa responder ao proprietário em um formato de comando, resposta e recompensa.

Brincadeira Normal Excessiva e/ou Destrutiva e Arranhões
• Afastar os objetos valiosos, frágeis ou perigosos.
• Fornecer brinquedos apropriados para o filhote.
• Realizar brincadeiras interativas com o filhote, utilizando brinquedos ou objetos em um esquema regular e diário. • Armadilhas ou objetos autoativados de punição podem ser utilizados para manter o filhote afastado de alguns objetos ou áreas selecionadas. O uso excessivo de tais itens pode resultar em uma ansiedade generalizada.
• Fornecer postes de superfícies variáveis e garantir que eles sejam longos o suficiente para o gato se esticar e arranhar. • Aparar as extremidades das unhas com frequência ou aplicar protetores de unhas.

Medo e Comportamentos Defensivos Atribuídos à Falta de Experiência Anterior ou por Traumatismo Prévio
• Exposição gradual a pessoas sem forçar qualquer interação. • Em geral, o filhote deve ser mantido em locais onde ele se sinta confortável e onde consiga sair da vista das pessoas, tendo consciência da presença delas de forma contínua e muito frequente. • O contracondicionamento geralmente é necessário. No início, o alimento pode ser colocado na área de esconderijo ou próximo a ela. De forma gradativa, o alimento é colocado mais longe do esconderijo e mais próximo do lugar onde a pessoa está parada (imóvel). Não deve ser feita qualquer tentativa de apanhar o filhote. Algumas vezes, diversas variáveis podem ser manipuladas, dependendo da intensidade do medo desse filhote. O alimento pode ser deixado progressivamente mais longe do esconderijo, onde as pessoas realizam suas atividades normais. O alimento pode eventualmente ser colocado no colo da pessoa. Alimentos/petiscos bem mais preciosos podem ser oferecidos ao redor das pessoas. Brinquedos presos em fios ou cordas podem ser usados para atrair os filhotes a brincar. Por fim, o filhote pode aceitar carícias e depois se deixar apanhar. • Deixar o filhote fazer avanços — e não a pessoa — e evitar amedrontá-lo é um princípio importante a ser lembrado.

Medo e Comportamentos Defensivos Relacionados com Técnicas de Correção
• Identificar e interromper comportamentos inadequados de punição por parte das pessoas.
• Identificar os estímulos que eliciam os comportamentos de medo e/ou defensivos.
• Empregar as técnicas de mudança comportamental semelhantes às citadas anteriormente.

MEDICAÇÕES
MEDICAMENTO(S)
Nenhum medicamento é necessário a menos que o medo e a ansiedade sejam extremos. Ver também "Medos, Fobias e Ansiedades — Gatos".

ACOMPANHAMENTO
MONITORIZAÇÃO DO PACIENTE
• Depois de 2, 4 e 8 semanas da consulta inicial, é recomendável acompanhar por telefone ou durante as consultas subsequentes.
• Ter a certeza de que os proprietários não estão aplicando técnicas aversivas. Tais procedimentos podem induzir o filhote ao medo e à agressividade.

PREVENÇÃO
• Os problemas de comportamento de filhote são frequentemente o resultado das expectativas não realistas e das más interpretações dos comportamentos felinos normais por parte dos proprietários.
• A maioria dos problemas comportamentais dos filhotes pode ser evitada ou redirecionada.
• Entre 3 e 7 semanas de vida, os filhotes devem experimentar interações positivas com pessoas para diminuir os comportamentos de medo, bem como para desenvolver elos sociais adequados com os humanos.
• Entre 4 e 18 meses, é útil expor o filhote a companheiros tolerantes (e brincalhões) da mesma espécie, para que ele aprenda uma inibição eficaz de mordidas e brincadeiras.
• Orientar os membros da família a evitar qualquer atrito e brincadeiras de partes do corpo com os filhotes.
• As correções punitivas devem ser abordadas e desestimuladas.
• Fornecer orientação na forma de aconselhamento verbal, panfletos, vídeos, livros ou listas sobre esses assuntos nas consultas de rotina ou naquelas agendadas para os filhotes.

EVOLUÇÃO ESPERADA E PROGNÓSTICO
Comportamentos Lúdicos (Brincadeiras) Normais Direcionados às Pessoas, a Outros Gatos e a Objetos da Casa
• Protocolos terapêuticos adequadamente adotados devem resultar na redução ou na resolução do problema. À medida que o filhote cresce, muitos desses comportamentos começam a diminuir.

Brincadeira Agressiva Desinibida Direcionada às Pessoas
• Prognóstico reservado, pois muitos desses filhotes amadurecem e sua agressividade torna-se mais grave e nociva. Um prognóstico melhor é dado àqueles casos que são descobertos precocemente e recebem orientação apropriada.

Arranhões
• Em geral, se esse comportamento for desviado com sucesso e recompensado pelo uso de superfícies adequadas para arranhar, o prognóstico será bom; no entanto, à medida que o filhote amadurece, os comportamentos diminuem. Há alguns casos individuais que, ocasionalmente, apresentam alto impulso para arranhar; nesses casos, há necessidade de controle a longo prazo.

Medo e Comportamentos Defensivos Atribuídos à Falta de Experiência Anterior ou Relacionados com Traumatismo Prévio
• Pode demorar meses, e até mesmo anos, para acostumar o filhote com as pessoas; os filhotes terão variações no grau de adaptação; alguns deles talvez nunca fiquem confortáveis junto às pessoas.
• Quanto mais prolongado for o intervalo entre as 3 semanas de vida e a falta de exposição às pessoas, pior será o prognóstico.
• Quanto mais intenso o traumatismo anterior, pior será o prognóstico.

Medo e Comportamentos Defensivos Relacionados com Técnicas de Correção
• Poderão se resolver rapidamente se as correções não forem utilizadas com frequência, se elas não forem graves e se os proprietários seguirem a orientação de substituir essas técnicas de punição por procedimentos redirecionados apropriados à base de recompensas.

DIVERSOS
FATORES RELACIONADOS COM A IDADE
Medo e Comportamentos Defensivos Atribuídos à Falta de Experiência Anterior
Depois do nascimento, parece haver um período sensível, de 3-7 semanas, durante o qual o filhote precisa ser exposto para evitar reações de medo e respostas defensivas contra as pessoas.

ABREVIATURA(S)
• ACTH = hormônio adrenocorticotrópico.

Autor Kelly Moffat
Consultor Editorial Debra F. Horwitz
Agradecimento Victoria L. Voith

Problemas do Ombro, Ligamento e Tendão

CONSIDERAÇÕES GERAIS

DEFINIÇÃO
Compõem a maioria das causas de claudicação na articulação do ombro dos cães, excluindo as lesões da osteocondrite dissecante.

FISIOPATOLOGIA
Tenossinovite Bicipital
- Lesão por esforço do tendão do bíceps braquial.
- Mecanismo da lesão — traumatismo direto; traumatismo indireto (mais comum).
- Alterações patológicas — desde o rompimento parcial do tendão até alterações inflamatórias crônicas, incluindo a calcificação distrófica.
- Proliferação do tecido conjuntivo fibroso e aderências entre o tendão e a bainha — limitam o movimento; causam dor.

Contratura Fibrótica do Músculo Infraespinal
- Distúrbio musculotendíneo primário — não se trata de uma neuropatia.
- Tecido fibroso — substitui a musculatura normal.
- Perda de elasticidade e função.
- Degeneração e atrofia do músculo acometido.
- Rompimento muscular parcial — provavelmente provocado por lesões repetitivas por esforço.

Outras
- Ruptura do tendão de origem do bíceps braquial — lesão por esforço ou rompimento das fibras tendinosas na junção com o tubérculo supraglenoide da escápula ou próximo a ele.
- Mineralização do tendão do músculo supraespinal — depósitos granulares entre as fibras do tendão; causa desconhecida; provavelmente o resultado de lesão repetitiva por esforço.
- Avulsão ou fratura do tendão do músculo supraespinal — o osso sofre avulsão a partir do tubérculo maior da porção proximal do úmero.

SISTEMA(S) ACOMETIDO(S)
Musculosquelético.

INCIDÊNCIA/PREVALÊNCIA
Causa comum de claudicação do membro anterior.

IDENTIFICAÇÃO
Espécies
Cães.

Raça(s) Predominante(s)
Cães pertencentes a raças de porte médio a grande.

Idade Média e Faixa Etária
- Cães maduros do ponto de vista esquelético com ≥ 1 ano de idade.
- Geralmente 3-7 anos de idade.

SINAIS CLÍNICOS
Achados Anamnésicos
- Tenossinovite bicipital — início, em geral, insidioso; frequentemente vários meses de duração; pode ser um incidente traumático como a causa incitante; claudicação sutil intermitente que piora com o exercício.
- Ruptura do tendão de origem do bíceps braquial — semelhante à tenossinovite bicipital; pode apresentar início agudo em virtude de um evento traumático conhecido; geralmente claudicação sutil crônica, que se agrava com a atividade física.
- Mineralização do tendão do músculo supraespinal — em geral, início insidioso; claudicação crônica que piora com a atividade.
- Avulsão/fratura do tendão do músculo supraespinal — semelhante à mineralização do tendão do músculo supraespinal.
- Contratura fibrótica do músculo infraespinal — costuma ter início repentino durante o período de exercício fora de casa (p. ex., caça); a claudicação e a sensibilidade do ombro desaparecem de forma gradativa dentro de 2 semanas; o problema resulta em claudicação persistente e crônica 3-4 semanas mais tarde, a qual não é particularmente dolorosa.

Achados do Exame Físico
- Tenossinovite bicipital — fase de oscilação curta e limitada da marcha, atribuída à dor à extensão e flexão do ombro; dor inconsistentemente demonstrada à manipulação do ombro; a dor fica mais evidente, aplicando-se compressão digital profunda sobre o tendão na região do sulco intertubercular enquanto se flexiona o ombro e se estende o cotovelo simultaneamente.
- Ruptura do tendão do músculo bíceps braquial — semelhante.
- Mineralização do tendão do músculo supraespinal — semelhante; as manipulações frequentemente não produzem dor; pode-se palpar tumefação firme sobre o tubérculo maior.
- Avulsão ou fratura do tendão do músculo supraespinal — semelhante à mineralização do tendão do músculo supraespinal.
- Contratura fibrótica do músculo infraespinal — em geral não é dolorosa à manipulação; nem sempre é possível a rotação interna (pronação) da articulação do ombro; quando forçada, a face caudal da escápula eleva o tronco; quando o paciente se encontra em estação — cotovelo aduzido; pata aduzida e rotacionada para fora; quando o paciente está deambulando — o membro inferior oscila em um arco lateral (circundução) conforme a pata é impulsionada; atrofia acentuada do músculo infraespinal à palpação.

CAUSAS
- Traumatismo direto ou indireto — provavelmente.
- Lesão repetitiva por esforço (traumatismo indireto) — mais comum.

FATORES DE RISCO
- Exaustão e/ou fadiga.
- Mau condicionamento antes de realizar atividades atléticas.
- Obesidade.

DIAGNÓSTICO

DIAGNÓSTICO DIFERENCIAL
- Luxação ou subluxação da articulação do ombro — histórico de traumatismo com início agudo de claudicação; quase sempre claudicação grave com dor acentuada à manipulação da articulação do ombro.
- Osteossarcoma da parte proximal do úmero — claudicação progressiva com graus variáveis de dor à manipulação do ombro; podem-se notar tumefação e sensibilidade da parte proximal do úmero.
- Tumor da bainha nervosa do plexo braquial — claudicação lenta, insidiosa, progressiva durante meses; atrofia acentuada dos músculos com doença crônica; pode-se sentir massa firme profunda na região axilar, que fica dolorosa à palpação digital.

DIAGNÓSTICO POR IMAGEM
Radiologia
- Necessária para diferenciação.
- Projeções craniocaudais e mediolaterais necessárias para todos os pacientes.

Tenossinovite Bicipital
- Em geral, as radiografias permanecem normais em lesões recentes.
- Projeção mediolateral (doença crônica) — podem-se observar reação óssea no tubérculo supraglenoide, calcificação distrófica do tendão bicipital, esclerose do assoalho do sulco intertubercular e osteófitos no sulco intertubercular.

Ruptura do Tendão de Origem do Músculo Bíceps Braquial
- Doença crônica — pode-se observar reação óssea irregular no tubérculo supraglenoide.

Mineralização do Tendão do Músculo Supraespinal
- Projeção mediolateral — focos calcificados no tendão, craniais e imediatamente mediais ao tubérculo maior da parte proximal do úmero.
- Projeção tangencial ou *skyline* da região intertubercular da parte proximal do úmero — elimina a sobreposição; permite a distinção de calcificação do tendão do bíceps braquial.
- Quase sempre bilateral ao exame radiográfico, mas raramente produz claudicação bilateral.

Avulsão/Fratura do Tendão do Músculo Supraespinal
- Semelhante à mineralização do tendão do músculo supraespinal.
- Fragmento ósseo por avulsão — pode-se observar como um defeito no tubérculo maior do úmero; em geral, não é tão denso do ponto de vista radiográfico quanto aquele identificado na mineralização do tendão do músculo supraespinal.

Contratura Fibrótica do Músculo Infraespinal
- Normal ao exame radiográfico.

Ultrassonografia e RM
- Podem ajudar a identificar lesões musculares, tenossinovite bicipital e ruptura do tendão de origem do bíceps braquial.
- Úteis para determinar a localização de densidades calcificadas próximas ao sulco intertubercular.

MÉTODOS DIAGNÓSTICOS
- Punção articular e exame do líquido sinovial — identificam doença intra-articular; o líquido deve ter coloração amarelo-palha, com viscosidade normal a reduzida; avaliação citológica: <10.000 células nucleadas/µL (>90% são células mononucleares).
- Exploração artroscópica da articulação do ombro — diagnostica tenossinovite bicipital e ruptura do tendão de origem do bíceps braquial; confirma a falta de doença intra-articular.

ACHADOS PATOLÓGICOS
- Tenossinovite bicipital — mineralização do tendão do bíceps; osteofitose no sulco intertubercular; sinovite proliferativa; e aderências fibrosas entre o tendão do bíceps e sua bainha sinovial; ao exame histológico, observam-se proliferação sinovial, edema, fibrose, mineralização distrófica e infiltração linfocítico-plasmocitária do tendão e da sinóvia.

Problemas do Ombro, Ligamento e Tendão

- Ruptura do tendão da origem do bíceps braquial — ruptura parcial a completa do tendão do bíceps em sua inserção no tubérculo supraglenoide, sinovite proliferativa e aderências fibrosas entre o tendão do bíceps e sua bainha sinovial; ao exame histológico, observam-se proliferação sinovial, edema, fibrose e mineralização distrófica ocasional.
- Mineralização do tendão do músculo supraespinal — o tendão frequentemente parece normal, mas a incisão longitudinal revela inúmeros bolsões de debris mineralizados dentro das fibras; ao exame histológico, degeneração estromal condromucinosa do tendão com múltiplos focos de mineralização distrófica.
- Avulsão da inserção tendínea do músculo supraespinal — o tendão quase sempre parece normal, mas a incisão longitudinal revela fragmento(s) ósseo(s) circundado(s) por cápsula de tecido fibroso; em geral, observa-se defeito ósseo correspondente no tubérculo maior.

TRATAMENTO

CUIDADO(S) DE SAÚDE ADEQUADO(S)
- Paciente de ambulatório — diagnóstico precoce.
- Paciente internado — doença grave e crônica necessita de intervenção cirúrgica.
- Tenossinovite bicipital — 50-75% de sucesso com o tratamento clínico; requer cirurgia com indícios de alterações crônicas e falha do tratamento clínico.
- Ruptura do tendão de origem do bíceps braquial geralmente requer cirurgia.
- Mineralização do tendão do músculo supraespinal — pode ser um achado acidental; necessita de cirurgia após exclusão de outras causas de claudicação e tratamento clínico.
- Avulsão ou fratura do tendão do músculo supraespinal — quase sempre necessita de cirurgia por causa da irritação persistente do tendão pelo fragmento ósseo.
- Contratura fibrótica do músculo infraespinal — necessita de cirurgia.

CUIDADO(S) DE ENFERMAGEM
- Crioterapia (aplicação de bolsas de gelo) — imediatamente após a cirurgia; ajuda a reduzir a inflamação e a tumefação no local da cirurgia; realizada por 5-10 min a cada 8 h por 3-5 dias.
- Massagem regional e exercícios com amplitude de movimento — melhoram a flexibilidade; diminuem a atrofia muscular.

ATIVIDADE
- Tratamento clínico — necessita do confinamento estrito por 4-6 semanas; atividade; o retorno prematuro ao normal provavelmente exacerba os sinais e induz ao estado crônico.
- Pós-cirurgia — depende do método realizado.

DIETA
Controle do peso — diminui a carga aplicada à articulação dolorosa.

CONSIDERAÇÕES CIRÚRGICAS
- Tenossinovite bicipital — recomendada em caso de resposta insatisfatória ao tratamento clínico e doença crônica; objetivo: eliminar o movimento do tendão do bíceps dentro da bainha sinovial inflamada, realizando uma tenodese do tendão bicipital; tenodese artroscópica; ou tenodese aberta e refixação à face lateral proximal do úmero.
- Ruptura do tendão de origem do bíceps braquial — fixa novamente o tendão à face lateral proximal do úmero utilizando um parafuso e arruela com travamento ou passando o tendão por um túnel ósseo e suturando-o ao tendão do músculo supraespinal.
- Mineralização do tendão do músculo supraespinal — incisar longitudinalmente o tendão; remover os depósitos de cálcio.
- Avulsão ou fratura do tendão do músculo supraespinal — remover o(s) fragmento(s) ósseo(s).
- Contratura fibrótica do músculo infraespinal — tenotomia e excisão de parte do tendão de inserção; com frequência, percebe-se um estalido distinto após a excisão da última aderência, o que permite a completa amplitude de movimento da articulação do ombro.

MEDICAÇÕES

MEDICAMENTO(S) DE ESCOLHA

Tenossinovite Bicipital
- Injeção intra-articular de corticosteroide — tratamento inicial de escolha.
- Tratamento sistêmico (AINE ou esteroides) — não tão eficiente.
- Não injetar em uma articulação séptica; realizar análise completa do líquido sinovial se houver alguma dúvida.
- Acetato de prednisolona — 20-40 mg, dependendo do porte.
- Claudicação acentuadamente melhorada, porém não eliminada — aplicar uma segunda injeção em 3-6 semanas.
- Resolução incompleta — cirurgia recomendada.

AINE e Analgésicos
- Podem ser utilizados para o tratamento sintomático; minimizam a dor e diminuem a inflamação.
- Deracoxibe (3-4 mg/kg VO a cada 24 h, mastigável).
- Carprofeno (2,2 mg/kg VO a cada 12 ou 24 h).
- Etodolaco (10-15 mg/kg VO a cada 24 h).
- Meloxicam (dose de ataque de 0,2 mg/kg VO e, em seguida, 0,1 mg/kg VO a cada 24 h — na forma líquida).
- Tepoxalina (dose de ataque de 20 mg/kg e, depois, 10 mg/kg VO a cada 24 h).

CONTRAINDICAÇÕES
- Evitar os corticosteroides por causa dos efeitos colaterais potenciais e lesão da cartilagem articular associada à utilização a longo prazo.
- Injeção direta de corticosteroide no tendão do bíceps — pode promover rompimento adicional do tendão e consequente ruptura.

PRECAUÇÕES
AINE — a irritação gastrintestinal pode impedir a utilização.

MEDICAMENTO(S) ALTERNATIVO(S)
Medicamentos condroprotetores (p. ex., glicosaminoglicanos polissulfatados, glicosamina e sulfato de condroitina) — podem ajudar a limitar a lesão e a degeneração associadas da cartilagem.

ACOMPANHAMENTO

MONITORIZAÇÃO DO PACIENTE
A maior parte dos pacientes necessita de, no mínimo, 1-2 meses de reabilitação após o tratamento.

EVOLUÇÃO ESPERADA E PROGNÓSTICO
- Tenossinovite bicipital submetida a tratamento clínico — com frequência bem-sucedida depois de um ou dois tratamentos (50-75% dos casos) sem alterações crônicas.
- Tenossinovite bicipital tratada por via cirúrgica — resultados bons a excelentes (90% dos casos); a recuperação à função plena pode demorar 2-8 meses.
- Tenodese do tendão do bíceps braquial cirurgicamente realizada — prognóstico bom a excelente; >85% dos pacientes apresentam melhora no retorno à função.
- Mineralização do tendão do músculo supraespinal submetida à intervenção cirúrgica — prognóstico bom a excelente; recidiva possível, porém rara.
- Avulsão ou fratura do tendão do músculo supraespinal cirurgicamente tratada — prognóstico bom a excelente; recidiva possível, porém rara.
- Contratura fibrótica do músculo infraespinal submetida a tratamento cirúrgico — prognóstico bom a excelente; pacientes retornam de modo uniforme à função normal do membro.

DIVERSOS

ABREVIATURA(S)
- AINE = anti-inflamatórios não esteroides.
- RM = ressonância magnética.

Sugestões de Leitura
Laitinen OM, Flo GL. Mineralization of the supraspinatus tendon in dogs: A long-term follow-up. JAAHA 2000, 36(3):262-267.
Rivers B, Wallace L, Johnston GR. Biceps tenosynovitis in the dog: Radiographic and sonographic findings. Vet Comp Orthop Traumatol 1992, 5:51-57.
Schaefer SL, Forrest LJ. Magnetic resonance imaging of the canine shoulder: An anatomic study. Vet Surg 2006, 35(8):721-728.

Autor Peter K. Shires
Consultor Editorial Peter K. Shires
Agradecimento O autor e os editores agradecem a contribuição de Peter D. Schwarz, que foi o autor deste capítulo em uma edição mais antiga.

Prolapso da Glândula da Terceira Pálpebra (Olho de Cereja)

CONSIDERAÇÕES GERAIS

REVISÃO
- Glândula da terceira pálpebra — aderida normalmente por ligação fibrosa à periórbita abaixo da terceira pálpebra.
- Fixação fraca — várias raças de cães e gatos; predispõe os animais a prolapso uni ou bilateral.

IDENTIFICAÇÃO
- Cães e gatos.
- Cães — geralmente nos jovens (6 meses a 2 anos de idade); raças comuns: Cocker spaniel, Buldogue, Beagle, Bloodhound, Lhasa apso, Mastiff, Shih tzu, outras raças braquicefálicas.
- Gatos — raro; ocorre nas raças Birmanês e Persa.

SINAIS CLÍNICOS
- Massa oval hiperêmica que se projeta da parte de trás da borda principal da terceira pálpebra.
- Pode ser uni ou bilateral.
- Podem-se observar sinais concomitantes de epífora, conjuntiva hiperêmica ou blefarospasmo.
- Tumefação e hiperemia adicionais provocadas por irritação ambiental e ressecamento da glândula exposta.

CAUSAS E FATORES DE RISCO
- Fraqueza congênita da ligação da glândula da terceira pálpebra.
- Hereditariedade desconhecida.

DIAGNÓSTICO

DIAGNÓSTICO DIFERENCIAL
- Cartilagem da terceira pálpebra enrolada ou invertida — observada nas raças Weimaraner, Dogue alemão, Pointer alemão de pelo curto e outras raças nas quais a cartilagem em forma de T da terceira pálpebra fica enrolada para fora da superfície do olho, em vez de se amoldar à superfície da córnea.
- Neoplasia da terceira pálpebra — observada geralmente nos animais mais idosos; pode-se constatar carcinoma de células escamosas, linfoma ou fibrossarcoma; pode ter um adenoma ou adenocarcinoma como origem; fica indicada uma pequena biopsia incisional nos pacientes mais idosos (>7-9 anos) para diferenciar.
- Prolapso da gordura orbital — pode-se dissecar anteriormente entre a conjuntiva e o bulbo ocular; ocasionalmente ocorre no canto medial e mimetiza a glândula prolapsada da terceira pálpebra.

HEMOGRAMA/BIOQUÍMICA/URINÁLISE
N/D.

OUTROS TESTES LABORATORIAIS
N/D.

DIAGNÓSTICO POR IMAGEM
N/D.

MÉTODOS DIAGNÓSTICOS
N/D.

TRATAMENTO

- Reposição cirúrgica da glândula (técnica de imbricação) — ver a seção "Sugestões de Leitura".
- Excisão da glândula — evitar; a glândula produz até 50% do filme lacrimal aquoso; coloca o paciente sob risco substancial de desenvolvimento de ceratoconjuntivite seca conforme envelhece.
- Colar elizabetano — recomendado para evitar autotraumatismo.

MEDICAÇÕES

MEDICAMENTO(S)
Medicações anti-inflamatórias tópicas, como corticosteroides (na ausência de úlcera de córnea) ou agentes anti-inflamatórios não esteroides — podem ser utilizados antes e depois da cirurgia para diminuir a tumefação (inchaço).

CONTRAINDICAÇÕES/INTERAÇÕES POSSÍVEIS
N/D.

ACOMPANHAMENTO

- Recidiva — 5-20%, dependendo do procedimento cirúrgico; incentiva-se a reposição da glândula ao local de origem.
- Quando unilateral, avisar o proprietário sobre a possibilidade de prolapso da outra glândula e a inexistência de método ou medicamento preventivo.

DIVERSOS

SINÔNIMO(S)
Olho de cereja.

Sugestões de Leitura
Hendrix DVH. Canine conjunctivitis and nictitating membrane. In: Gelatt KN, ed., Veterinary Ophthalmology, 4th ed. Ames, IA: Blackwell, 2007, pp. 662-689.
Maggs DJ. Third eyelid. In: Maggs DJ, Miller PE, Ofri R, Slatter's Fundamentals of Veterinary Ophthalmology, 4th ed. St. Louis: Saunders, 2008, pp. 151-156.

Autor Brian C. Gilger
Consultor Editorial Paul E. Miller

Prolapso Retal e Anal

CONSIDERAÇÕES GERAIS

REVISÃO
• Eversão de uma ou mais camadas do reto pelo ânus.
• O prolapso anal (prolapso incompleto) é uma protrusão da mucosa anorretal pelo orifício anal externo.
• O prolapso retal (prolapso completo) é uma invaginação de camada dupla de toda a espessura do tubo retal pelo orifício anal.

IDENTIFICAÇÃO
• Cães e gatos (especialmente da raça Manx).
• Qualquer idade, sexo ou raça.
• Prevalência elevada em cães jovens parasitados e em gatos com diarreia.

SINAIS CLÍNICOS
• Tenesmo persistente.
• Prolapso incompleto — protrusão de uma parte da circunferência da mucosa retal que tipicamente parece pior logo após a defecação e depois desaparece.
• O prolapso completo aparece sob a forma de massa hiperêmica tubular que se projeta a partir do ânus.
• Prolapsos crônicos podem ser de coloração azul-escura ou enegrecida ou a mucosa pode estar ulcerada.

CAUSAS E FATORES DE RISCO
• Distúrbios gastrintestinais que provocam diarreia e tenesmo, como parasitose, colite/ enterite, constipação/obstipação, corpo estranho retal, desvio e divertículo retais, proctite e tumores retais ou anais.
• Distúrbios urogenitais, como cistite, urolitíase, prostatite, hipertrofia prostática e distocia.
• Tenesmo após cirurgia perineal, retal ou urogenital (p. ex., herniorrafia perineal).

DIAGNÓSTICO

DIAGNÓSTICO DIFERENCIAL
• Intussuscepção prolapsada — descartar pela introdução do dedo ou de sonda romba entre a massa e o ânus (a sonda não deve penetrar mais de 1-2 cm antes de entrar em contato com o fórnix; se a sonda passar 5-6 cm com facilidade, a suspeita será de intussuscepção prolapsada) ou por ultrassonografia abdominal (prestar atenção para o aumento das camadas intestinais).
• Neoplasia — descartar por palpação, aspirado com agulha fina e citologia e/ou biopsia e histopatologia.

HEMOGRAMA/BIOQUÍMICA/URINÁLISE
• Geralmente normais.
• Pode haver leucograma inflamatório ou de estresse.

OUTROS TESTES LABORATORIAIS
Exame de fezes pode confirmar a parasitose.

DIAGNÓSTICO POR IMAGEM
• Radiografia e ultrassonografia abdominais — em geral normais.
• Radiografia abdominal — pode demonstrar corpo estranho, prostatomegalia, cálculos císticos ou distensão fecal colônica.
• Ultrassonografia abdominal — pode revelar prostatomegalia, cálculos císticos, espessamento da parede vesical ou intussuscepção.

MÉTODOS DIAGNÓSTICOS
• Exame do reto para palpar hérnia perineal.
• A colonoscopia pode ajudar na avaliação de prolapso recidivante em busca de alguma causa subjacente.

ACHADOS PATOLÓGICOS
Avaliar a viabilidade do tecido prolapsado pela aparência da superfície e pela temperatura do tecido — o tecido vital aparece tumefato e hiperêmico, além de exibir exsudação de sangue vivo a partir da superfície de corte; já o tecido desvitalizado aparece roxo-escuro ou enegrecido, mas exibe a exsudação de sangue cianótico escuro a partir da superfície de corte; ulcerações podem estar presentes.

TRATAMENTO

• É imprescindível a identificação e o tratamento da causa subjacente.
• Tratamento clínico conservativo — reposicionar delicadamente o tecido prolapsado pelo ânus, fazendo uso de lubrificantes e massagem suave; agentes osmóticos podem auxiliar se houver tumefação grave.
• A utilização de anestesia epidural pode facilitar o tratamento e aliviar o desconforto.
• Aplicar sutura em bolsa de tabaco para ajudar a retenção e evitar a recidiva aguda; colocar a sutura de forma frouxa o suficiente para dar espaço à defecação.
• Reduzir o esforço para defecação com amolecedores de fezes.
• É recomendável o procedimento de colopexia para os prolapsos viáveis recidivantes ou se o tenesmo (esforço) persistir após ressecção e anastomose retais.
• Quando o prolapso não for redutível e/ou estiver desvitalizado, haverá necessidade de ressecção e anastomose retais.

MEDICAÇÕES

MEDICAMENTO(S) DE ESCOLHA
• Anestésicos/analgésicos apropriados, conforme a necessidade.
• Considerar a anestesia epidural para facilitar a cirurgia e reduzir o esforço para defecação no pós-operatório.
• É recomendado o uso de antibióticos perioperatórios adequados (p. ex., cefoxitina sódica [30 mg/kg IV]) para anastomose com ressecção.
• Agentes tópicos para auxiliar na redução — solução de glicose a 50% e KY Jelly® (lubrificante).
• Amolecedores de fezes — docusato de sódio (cães, 50-200 mg VO a cada 8-12 h; gatos, 50 mg VO a cada 12-24 h) ou lactulose (solução ou xarope a 10 g/15 mL, na dose de 1 mL/4,5 kg a cada 8-12 h até fazer efeito); continuar por 2-3 semanas após a remoção da sutura em bolsa de tabaco.
• Fornecer dieta pobre em resíduos até que a sutura em bolsa de tabaco seja removida.

CONTRAINDICAÇÕES/INTERAÇÕES POSSÍVEIS
N/D.

ACOMPANHAMENTO

MONITORIZAÇÃO DO PACIENTE
• Remover a sutura em bolsa de tabaco em 3-7 dias.
• Examinar o paciente quanto à formação de estenose retal se os esforços para defecação persistirem depois da anastomose.

COMPLICAÇÕES POSSÍVEIS
• Recidiva — especialmente se a causa subjacente não for eliminada.
• Pós-operatório — pode incluir infecção, deiscência da anastomose dentro de 5-7 dias do pós-operatório ou estenose retal.
• Incontinência fecal após a ressecção (incontinência sensorial resultante da remoção dos receptores na parede retal).

DIVERSOS

DISTÚRBIOS ASSOCIADOS
Parasitose intestinal.

VER TAMBÉM
• Colite e Proctite.
• Disquezia e Hematoquezia.
• Intussuscepção.

Sugestões de Leitura
Aronson L. Rectum and anus. In: Slatter D, ed., Textbook of Small Animal Surgery, 3rd ed. Philadelphia: Saunders, 2003, pp. 682-708.
Hedlund CS, Fossum TW. Rectal prolapse. In: Fossum TW, ed., Small Animal Surgery, 3rd ed. St. Louis: Mosby, 2007, pp. 524-527.

Autor Eric R. Pope
Consultor Editorial Albert E. Jergens

PROLAPSO URETRAL

CONSIDERAÇÕES GERAIS

REVISÃO
- Ocorre quando o revestimento de mucosa da porção distal da uretra sofre prolapso através do orifício uretral externo.
- Os sistemas acometidos incluem o urinário, o reprodutor (algumas vezes, pode ocorrer sangramento apenas durante a ereção peniana) e o sanguíneo/linfático/imunológico (a perda sanguínea pode ser grave o suficiente a ponto de causar anemia, especialmente em raças caninas de pequeno porte).
- As uretras prolapsadas frequentemente aparecem como massa congesta em formato de ervilha, que se projeta a partir da extremidade distal do pênis. Muitas vezes, tal prolapso associa-se a graus variados de hemorragia. A lambedura excessiva pode resultar em danos traumáticos adicionais à mucosa uretral exposta.

IDENTIFICAÇÃO
- Cães e, raramente, gatos.
- Mais comum em Buldogue inglês, Boston terrier e Yorkshire terrier.
- Idade média, 18 meses; faixa etária, de 4 meses a 5 anos.
- Relatada em cães machos, mas extremamente rara em gatos machos.

SINAIS CLÍNICOS
Achados Anamnésicos
- Sangramento intermitente ou persistente vindo da uretra, independentemente da micção.
- Lambedura intermitente ou persistente do pênis.
- Também pode haver disúria e polaciúria causadas por distúrbios concomitantes.

Achados do Exame Físico
- Massa de coloração vermelha a púrpura, do tamanho de uma ervilha e em formato de rosquinha, que se projeta a partir da extremidade distal do pênis.
- Em casos de sangramento intenso, observam-se mucosas pálidas.
- Pode ocorrer necrose da uretra prolapsada secundariamente a ressecamento ou traumatismo autoinduzido pela lambedura.
- Na bexiga urinária ou na uretra, podem-se detectar urólitos palpáveis.

CAUSAS E FATORES DE RISCO
- Pode resultar de excitação sexual e/ou distúrbios não relacionados (p. ex., infecções, urólitos, neoplasia) do trato urinário inferior.
- O aumento na pressão intra-abdominal secundário à disúria associada a urocistólitos pode ser um fator predisponente.
- Outras causas propostas incluem o desenvolvimento anormal da uretra com aumento sobreposto na pressão intra-abdominal, em consequência da síndrome braquicefálica das vias aéreas, de disúria ou da atividade sexual. Essa elevação na pressão intra-abdominal pode prejudicar o retorno venoso sanguíneo pelas veias pudendas, predispondo os cães suscetíveis ao ingurgitamento do corpo esponjoso circunjacente à uretra distal.
- Predisposição racial (Buldogue e Boston terrier).
- A anatomia uretral anormal associada ao aumento na pressão intra-abdominal secundário à síndrome obstrutiva das vias aéreas anteriores, qualquer causa de disúria persistente e/ou a excitação sexual podem ser fatores de risco.

DIAGNÓSTICO

DIAGNÓSTICO DIFERENCIAL
- Prostatopatia.
- Persistência do frênulo peniano.
- Fraturas do osso peniano.
- Balanopostite.
- Uretrite.
- Doença testicular.
- Uretrólitos.
- Coagulopatia.
- Neoplasia uretral.

HEMOGRAMA/BIOQUÍMICA/URINÁLISE
- Hemograma completo — pode revelar anemia regenerativa.
- Bioquímicas séricas — geralmente normais.
- Pode não se detectar hematúria significativa na urina coletada por cistocentese, mas uma amostra urinária obtida por micção espontânea pode revelar hematúria.
- Urocultura e antibiograma.

OUTROS TESTES LABORATORIAIS
O perfil de coagulação pode descartar coagulopatia.

DIAGNÓSTICO POR IMAGEM
- Radiografias abdominais simples — úteis para descartar urólitos radiodensos e avaliar a próstata.
- Cistografia com duplo contraste e uretrografia com contraste positivo — proveitosos para excluir urólitos radiotransparentes, outros distúrbios uretrais e prostatopatia.
- Ultrassonografia abdominal — benéfica para avaliar a próstata e a bexiga urinária.

MÉTODOS DIAGNÓSTICOS
- Ejaculação — útil para avaliar a uretra no momento da ereção peniana; alguns prolapsos uretrais estão presentes apenas durante essa ereção.
- A avaliação dos ejaculados também pode facilitar o exame do líquido prostático em busca de indícios de prostatopatia.

TRATAMENTO
- Pode não ser necessário se o prolapso uretral permanecer assintomático ou estiver associado apenas a sangramento episódico.
- Se o prolapso uretral estiver presente apenas durante a ereção peniana, deve-se considerar o procedimento de castração antes da tentativa de remoção cirúrgica do tecido prolapsado; a administração de dietilestilbestrol por 3-6 semanas após a cirurgia pode diminuir a frequência das ereções.
- Considerar a realização de cirurgia em pacientes com sangramento excessivo, dor ou ulceração e/ou necrose extensas do tecido prolapsado. Também se deve contemplar a cirurgia em casos de recidivas associadas ao tratamento clínico.
- Foram obtidos resultados satisfatórios por meio da redução manual do prolapso, acompanhada por uretropexia, utilizando um instrumento cirúrgico sulcado (conhecido como tenta-cânula) que reduz a uretra prolapsada ao mesmo tempo em que orienta a colocação de suturas. Os instrumentos sulcados (ou seja, as tenta-cânulas) são frequentemente incluídos nos pacotes-padrão de instrumentos para castração ou podem ser adquiridos a baixo custo em grande parte das empresas de material médico.
- Se a cirurgia for imprescindível, poderá ser necessário o uso de colar elizabetano ou de dispositivos similares de contenção para evitar o traumatismo induzido pela lambedura no local cirúrgico.
- A técnica cirúrgica com laser de CO_2 pode melhorar a hemostasia, bem como a visualização e a acurácia do cirurgião. Além disso, essa técnica pode diminuir a tumefação (inchaço) do pós-operatório. Antes de realizar o procedimento, inserir um cateter apropriado no lúmen uretral para evitar a transecção acidental da uretra com o laser. Ao realizar o procedimento, não utilizar superpulsos, pois eles podem reduzir a hemostasia. A escolha de um tamanho maior (0,8 mm) para a ponta do laser pode melhorar a hemostasia.
- Nos gatos machos, se o tratamento clínico da causa subjacente ou a redução cirúrgica do prolapso uretral não forem bem-sucedidos, talvez seja necessário considerar a realização de uretrostomia perineal como técnica de recuperação.
- Independentemente do tratamento escolhido, avisar o proprietário sobre a possibilidade de recidiva, sobretudo caso não se consiga encontrar e/ou corrigir o prolapso uretral.
- Como as raças braquicefálicas estão sob risco de apresentar tal problema, é preciso ter cautela na seleção do protocolo anestésico; durante a anestesia, é recomendável a monitorização cuidadosa dos cães pertencentes a essas raças para garantir a manutenção da oxigenação adequada.

MEDICAÇÕES

MEDICAMENTO(S)
- A uretrite bacteriana justifica o uso de antibióticos apropriados.
- Pode ser necessário o uso de dietilestilbestrol por 3-6 semanas após a cirurgia para reduzir a frequência das ereções.

CONTRAINDICAÇÕES/INTERAÇÕES POSSÍVEIS
Em virtude da possibilidade de supressão da medula óssea, é preciso considerar as relações de risco:benefício antes de se administrar os estrogênios, especialmente se os pacientes já estiverem anêmicos.

ACOMPANHAMENTO

MONITORIZAÇÃO DO PACIENTE
Monitorizar o animal por, no mínimo, 7-10 dias após a cirurgia, em busca de indícios de hemorragia grave ou recidiva do prolapso uretral.

PREVENÇÃO
Se o prolapso uretral estiver associado à ereção peniana, avisar os proprietários a evitar o contato de seus animais com cadelas ou outras situações que possam induzir a essa ereção.

COMPLICAÇÕES POSSÍVEIS
Alertar os proprietários sobre a possibilidade de ocorrência de recidiva pós-cirúrgica do prolapso,

PROLAPSO URETRAL

especialmente na falta de detecção, eliminação ou controle da causa subjacente.

EVOLUÇÃO ESPERADA E PROGNÓSTICO
• O prolapso uretral pode persistir sem sequelas significativas. Portanto, alguns cães podem não necessitar de terapia.
• Outros cães podem não apresentar qualquer problema depois da castração e/ou da correção cirúrgica do prolapso uretral.

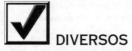

DIVERSOS
DISTÚRBIOS ASSOCIADOS
• É comum a ocorrência de uretrite concomitante.
• A urolitíase concomitante pode ser uma causa predisponente.

Sugestões de Leitura
Fossum TW. Urethral prolapse. In: Small Animal Surgery, 3rd ed. St. Louis: Mosby Elsevier, 2007, pp. 687-689.

Kirsch JA, Hauptman JG, Walshaw RA. Urethropexy technique for surgical treatment of urethral prolapse in the male dog. JAAHA 2002, 38:381-384.

Osborne CA, Sanderson SL. Medical management of urethral prolapse in male dogs. In: Bonagura JD, Kirk RW, eds., Current Veterinary Therapy XII. Philadelphia: Saunders, 1995, pp. 1027-1029.

Autores Sherry L. Sanderson e Carl A. Osborne
Consultor Editorial Carl A. Osborne

PROPTOSE

CONSIDERAÇÕES GERAIS

REVISÃO
- Deslocamento anterógrado do bulbo ocular, com as pálpebras aprisionadas posteriormente ao globo ocular.
- Frequentemente associada a traumatismo cefálico e, em geral, ocorre de forma superaguda.
- Potencial risco de perda da visão.
- Pode provocar bradicardia secundária à tração dos músculos retrobulbares e ao reflexo oculocardíaco associado (regulado pelos nervos vago e trigêmeo).

IDENTIFICAÇÃO
- Mais comum nas raças braquicefálicas em virtude de características como proeminência dos olhos, órbitas relativamente rasas e fissuras palpebrais amplas.
- Pode ocorrer em qualquer espécie ou raça se a força traumática for suficientemente grave.

SINAIS CLÍNICOS
Comentários Gerais
Bulbo ocular em posição anterior às pálpebras.

Possíveis Sinais Clínicos Concomitantes
- Hemorragia subconjuntival ou intraocular.
- Anormalidades no tamanho das pupilas — midríase (dilatação) ou miose (constrição).
- Inflamação intraocular (uveíte).
- Desvio/estrabismo do bulbo ocular.
- Ulceração e/ou ressecamento da córnea.
- Fraturas da órbita óssea ou de outras partes do crânio.
- Ruptura do bulbo ocular.
- Traumatismo encefálico.
- Traumatismo do olho contralateral.
- Choque.
- Outros sinais associados ao traumatismo.

CAUSAS E FATORES DE RISCO
- Traumatismo — causa primária; força relativamente menor (restrição) nas raças braquicefálicas; geralmente força intensa nas raças dolicocefálicas e mesocefálicas.
- Lesão retrobulbar invasiva — rara.

DIAGNÓSTICO

DIAGNÓSTICO DIFERENCIAL
- Buftalmia — aumento do bulbo ocular; raramente aguda; as pálpebras ainda permanecem posicionadas corretamente, mas podem ser incapazes de fechar completamente sobre o bulbo.
- Exoftalmia — deslocamento anterógrado do bulbo ocular; as pálpebras permanecem posicionadas corretamente, mas podem ser incapazes de fechar completamente sobre o bulbo; pode ser aguda; raramente superaguda; o olho pode não sofrer retropulsão em virtude do efeito de massa (p. ex., neoplasia, miosite, abscesso ou celulite) nos tecidos retrobulbares.

HEMOGRAMA/BIOQUÍMICA/URINÁLISE
Normais a menos que haja anormalidades relacionadas com o traumatismo.

DIAGNÓSTICO POR IMAGEM
Radiografias ou TC do crânio — podem revelar fraturas ocasionadas por traumatismo.

TRATAMENTO
- Manter a córnea lubrificada.
- Avaliar o estado geral do paciente e estabilizá-lo antes de realizar a cirurgia do bulbo ocular.

Reposicionamento do Bulbo Ocular
- Fazer com a maior segurança possível.
- Efetuar sob sedação e anestesia local ou, caso o paciente se encontre estável, sob anestesia geral.
- Cantotomia lateral — pode aliviar a tensão sobre as pálpebras e permitir o reposicionamento mais fácil do bulbo ocular; nem sempre necessária.
- Apreender as margens palpebrais com pinças oftalmológicas (p. ex., pinças de Von Graefe ou de Allis) ou ganchos de estrabismo/músculo e, depois, tracionar as pálpebras para frente e para longe do bulbo ocular, ao mesmo tempo em que se protege e se traciona delicadamente o bulbo ocular de volta à órbita (um cabo de lâmina de bisturi lubrificado pode realizar essa função).
- Colocar duas ou três suturas de colchoeiro de tarsorrafia temporária com *stents**; suturar a ferida cirúrgica da cantotomia lateral.
- Fluoresceína — não se esquecer de corar a córnea antes de fechar as suturas da tarsorrafia.
- Se o nervo óptico estiver totalmente seccionado ou se o bulbo ocular estiver rompido, infectado ou ressecado, a enucleação poderá ser melhor opção do que o reposicionamento.

MEDICAÇÕES

MEDICAMENTO(S)
- Antibióticos de amplo espectro sistêmicos e tópicos — até que as suturas sejam removidas.
- Corticosteroides sistêmicos — costumam ser utilizados pelo menos no início; podem ser mantidos em uma base crônica se houver tumefação periorbital e retrobulbar acentuada.
- Corticosteroides tópicos — podem ser usados em caso de inflamação intraocular (uveíte) ou hifema associados, contanto que não existam úlceras de córnea ou da conjuntiva.
- Atropina tópica — para inflamação ou hemorragia intraoculares; alivia o espasmo ciliar e diminui o risco de sinéquias.

CONTRAINDICAÇÕES/INTERAÇÕES POSSÍVEIS
- Corticosteroides tópicos — não utilizar com ulcerações.
- Corticosteroides sistêmicos — não usar com infecção retrobulbar.

ACOMPANHAMENTO

MONITORIZAÇÃO DO PACIENTE
Remoção da sutura — costuma ser realizada de forma sequencial e não de uma única vez, começando 10-14 dias após o reposicionamento.

---

* N. T.: Dispositivo metálico utilizado com a finalidade de manter o lúmen de uma artéria permeável, com seu calibre próximo do normal, formando uma nova "parede" para o vaso.

A integridade do bulbo, da córnea e da visão é avaliada 10-14 dias após a cirurgia.

COMPLICAÇÕES POSSÍVEIS
- Cegueira.
- A maior parte dos pacientes mantém um estrabismo dorsolateral e leve deslocamento anterógrado da face medial do bulbo ocular em função da ruptura dos músculos oblíquo inferior e reto medial. Isso pode melhorar com o tempo por conta dos processos de fibrose e contração teciduais.
- Produção diminuída de lágrimas — efetuar os testes lacrimais de Schirmer após a remoção da sutura.
- Desnervação da córnea causadora de ceratite neutrófica com ulceração crônica e sensibilidade corneana reduzida.
- Ceratite por exposição em virtude do deslocamento anterógrado do bulbo ocular, da produção reduzida de lágrimas e/ou da desnervação da córnea (diminuição do reflexo de piscar).
- Glaucoma.
- Tísica do bulbo.

EVOLUÇÃO ESPERADA E PROGNÓSTICO
- A maior parte dos olhos acometidos pode ser recuperada; a maioria provocada por traumatismo significativo ficará cega (mais comum nas raças dolicocefálicas do que nas braquicefálicas).
- Em caso de dano tecidual extenso, avulsão de mais de dois músculos extraoculares, fraturas da face e/ou órbita e ruptura da córnea ou esclera — prognóstico grave quanto à visão e recuperação do bulbo ocular em termos de estética.
- Vasos retinianos e nervo óptico normais, PIO normal e curto período de tempo desde a ocorrência até o reparo — prognóstico relativamente favorável para manter a visão.
- Resposta positiva à ameaça ou reflexo pupilar à luz direto ou consensual originário do olho lesado — prognóstico bom quanto à manutenção da visão.
- Tamanho da pupila no momento da lesão — não é necessariamente um indicador prognóstico exato; a midríase pode ser o resultado do traumatismo ao nervo óptico (caso seja permanente, isso resultará em cegueira) ou lesão ao nervo oculomotor (não afeta a visão).
- Miose — não indica necessariamente um prognóstico bom para a visão; a uveíte constitui a causa mais provável (se a uveíte for suficientemente grave, ocorrerá constrição pupilar, mesmo com lesão da retina ou do nervo óptico).

DIVERSOS

VER TAMBÉM
Doenças Orbitais (Exoftalmia, Enoftalmia e Estrabismo).

ABREVIATURA(S)
- PIO = pressão intraocular.
- TC = tomografia computadorizada.

Sugestões de Leitura
Maggs DJ, Miller PE, Ofri R. Slatter's Fundamentals of Veterinary Ophthalmology, 4th ed. St. Louis: Saunders, 2008.

Autor Simon A. Pot
Consultor Editorial Paul E. Miller
Agradecimento Stephanie L. Smedes

Prostatite e Abscesso Prostático

CONSIDERAÇÕES GERAIS

DEFINIÇÃO
Prostatite Aguda
Infecção da próstata canina por bactérias, micoplasmas e/ou fungos com sinais sistêmicos de febre, anorexia, letargia, dor e exsudato inflamatório no líquido prostático. A presença de abscedação é variável e ocorreu em 15 dentre 25 cães com prostatite em um único estudo. Os abscessos ocasionalmente se rompem dentro da cavidade peritoneal, provocando sepse, choque e morte.

Prostatite Crônica
Infecção subclínica (recente ou a longo prazo) da próstata canina na ausência de abscesso prostático e sinais polissistêmicos. Os animais acometidos permanecem assintomáticos, exceto pela presença de exsudato inflamatório no líquido prostático, o que provoca infertilidade. A prostatite crônica pode ocorrer depois da prostatite aguda ou independentemente dela.

FISIOPATOLOGIA
• A condição patológica predisponente consiste na hipertrofia prostática benigna (HPB) macro e/ou microscópica, que ocorre sob a influência da di-hidrotestosterona (DHT) em mais de 80% dos machos caninos intactos com mais de 5 anos de idade.
• A HPB caracteriza-se por alvéolos prostáticos grandes e bem vascularizados com formato irregular, além de invaginações ramificantes do epitélio com microcistos contendo líquido prostático sanguinolento; quando infectadas, essas invaginações podem se transformar em abscessos.
• A infecção da próstata canina hipertrofiada desenvolve-se mais comumente a partir da ascensão da flora uretral normal — raramente de bactérias originárias do sangue e/ou de feridas penetrantes responsáveis pela introdução de bactérias ou fungos no escroto. A próstata do macho canino intacto secreta constantemente o líquido prostático, o qual fica depositado na uretra prostática e, em seguida, flui tanto para a bexiga urinária como para fora da extremidade da uretra peniana. Na prostatite, o líquido prostático que contém sangue, exsudato inflamatório e bactérias ou fungos é depositado na bexiga urinária e liberado de forma intermitente pela extremidade do pênis.

SISTEMA(S) ACOMETIDO(S)
• Gastrintestinal — tenesmo em caso de compressão do reto pelo aumento de volume da próstata.
• Hemático/linfático/imune — neutrofilia madura ou imatura na prostatite aguda.
• Polissistêmico — choque séptico no caso de rompimento de abscesso prostático, taquicardia, má perfusão tecidual, temperatura elevada e peritonite focal ou generalizada.
• Renal/urológico — disúria em caso de compressão da uretra pelo aumento de volume da próstata; depósito de líquido prostático com exsudato inflamatório na bexiga urinária.
• Reprodutivo — dor no momento da cópula e diminuição na libido; infertilidade causada pelo líquido prostático infectado no ejaculado.

GENÉTICA
Nenhuma base genética conhecida.

INCIDÊNCIA/PREVALÊNCIA
Elevada nos machos caninos intactos acima de 5 anos de idade. A infecção é relatada em 40% dos cães com prostatopatia.

IDENTIFICAÇÃO
Espécies
Cães.
Raça(s) Predominante(s)
Todas as raças e mestiços.
Idade Média e Faixa Etária
Meia-idade; faixa etária média, 7 a 11 anos.
Sexo Predominante
Machos caninos intactos; pode ocorrer secundariamente à neoplasia prostática em cães castrados.

SINAIS CLÍNICOS
Prostatite Aguda
• Letargia/depressão.
• Anorexia.
• Tenesmo.
• Disúria.
• Pirexia.
• Dor à palpação prostática ou abdominal caudal.
• Secreção uretral sanguinolenta.
• Marcha rígida dos membros posteriores.
• Choque séptico (raro).

Prostatite Crônica
• Assintomática.
• Tenesmo.
• Disúria.
• Secreção uretral sanguinolenta.

CAUSAS
• Infecção da próstata hipertrofiada pela flora uretral ascendente, incluindo *Escherichia coli*, *Staphylococcus* spp., *Streptococcus* spp., *Proteus mirabilis*, *Klebsiella* spp., *Enterobacter* spp., *Hemophilus* spp., *Pseudomonas* spp., *Pasteurella* spp., bactérias anaeróbias e *Mycoplasma* (mais comum).
• Infecção da próstata hipertrofiada em caso de infecção bacteriana sistêmica, incluindo *Brucella canis*.
• Infecção local ou sistêmica de ferida penetrante por *Blastomyces dermatitidis*.

FATORES DE RISCO
• Idade avançada.
• Presença de testículos funcionais nos cães acometidos.
• HPB e, menos comumente, neoplasia prostática.
• Histórico de administração de androgênio ou de estrogênio.
• Comprometimento dos mecanismos de defesa do hospedeiro.

DIAGNÓSTICO

DIAGNÓSTICO DIFERENCIAL
• HPB sem infecção, distinguida pela cultura do sêmen.
• Cistos prostáticos, diferenciados pelo ultrassom e pela cultura do sêmen.
• Neoplasia prostática, distinguida pelo ultrassom e biopsia tecidual.
• Massa ou abscesso abdominal, diferenciados pela obtenção de imagens do abdome.

HEMOGRAMA/BIOQUÍMICA/URINÁLISE
• As anormalidades no hemograma completo em casos de prostatite aguda e abscedação incluem neutrofilia imatura e neutrófilos tóxicos; pode ocorrer neutropenia imatura com sepse. A maior parte dos cães com prostatite crônica apresenta hemograma normal.
• As anormalidades na bioquímica sérica são variáveis em casos de prostatite aguda. A maior parte dos cães com prostatite crônica apresenta bioquímicas séricas normais.
• As anormalidades na urinálise incluem hematúria, exsudato purulento e microrganismos causais; tais anormalidades não surgem de infecção primária do trato urinário, mas sim do depósito de líquido prostático infectado na bexiga urinária.

OUTROS TESTES LABORATORIAIS
• Exame macroscópico, citologia e cultura do sêmen total ou da (terceira) fração do líquido prostático do sêmen ou do líquido coletado na massagem da próstata revelam exsudato inflamatório com a presença de bactérias aeróbias e anaeróbias, além de *Mycoplasma* ou fungos. O líquido prostático normal deve conter menos de 100.000 unidades bacterianas formadoras de colônia por mL e menos de 5 leucócitos por campo óptico de grande aumento após a centrifugação do líquido.
• Embora a infecção por *Brucella canis* seja rara, tendo em vista o potencial zoonótico dessa infecção, é recomendável a sorologia para pesquisa desse microrganismo em todos os cães com suspeita de prostatite, com acompanhamento da cultura do sêmen caso a sorologia seja positiva.

DIAGNÓSTICO POR IMAGEM
Radiografia simples do abdome caudal, uretrocistografia retrógrada e ultrassonografia prostática estão indicadas para avaliar o tamanho e a ecotextura da próstata, bem como a presença de lesões prostáticas cavitárias. A próstata estará aumentada de volume caso seu diâmetro craniocaudal máximo, mensurado em uma linha paralela à linha que une o promontório sacral com a face anterior do púbis na radiografia lateral exceda 70% do comprimento da distância entre o promontório sacral e a face anterior do púbis.

MÉTODOS DIAGNÓSTICOS
• Coleta e avaliação do líquido prostático no plasma seminal e coleta do líquido prostático por massagem da próstata nos cães relutantes a ejacular.
• Aspirado percutâneo da próstata por agulha fina guiada pelo ultrassom.

ACHADOS PATOLÓGICOS
• A patologia macroscópica da próstata infectada inclui aumento de volume, perda variável de simetria da rafe mediana dorsal e presença variável de abscessos repletos de líquido dentro da glândula ou em sua superfície. O aumento pode ser focal, multifocal ou difuso.
• Infecção bacteriana ou fúngica provoca inflamação supurativa (bacteriana) ou granulomatosa (fúngica) da glândula. As lesões inflamatórias podem ser focais, multifocais ou difusas. Os abscessos contêm acúmulos de exsudato líquido purulento.
• Não se recomenda a biopsia da próstata infectada, porque a obtenção de imagem e o exame do líquido prostático são diagnósticos; além disso, a biopsia pode resultar na disseminação da infecção para os tecidos adjacentes.

PROSTATITE E ABSCESSO PROSTÁTICO

TRATAMENTO

CUIDADO(S) DE SAÚDE ADEQUADO(S)
• Prostatite aguda, abscesso prostático e ruptura de abscessos prostáticos dentro da cavidade peritoneal são emergências potencialmente letais que podem levar o animal a choque séptico e morte. Os pacientes acometidos devem ser internados e submetidos à coleta imediata de amostras diagnósticas (sangue, urina, sêmen e imagem).
• Os cães com prostatite crônica podem ser considerados pacientes de ambulatório para os métodos de diagnóstico, e submetidos a tratamento específico quando os resultados dos exames laboratoriais estiverem disponíveis.

CUIDADO(S) DE ENFERMAGEM
• Cães com prostatite aguda ou abscesso prostático devem receber antibioticoterapia intravenosa.
• Na suspeita de ruptura de abscesso e peritonite, administrar fluidoterapia intravenosa para choque séptico.

ATIVIDADE
É recomendável evitar o acasalamento até que as bactérias tenham sido eliminadas do líquido prostático.

ORIENTAÇÃO AO PROPRIETÁRIO
• É recomendada a castração dos cães com prostatite aguda e/ou abscesso prostático, uma vez que esse procedimento cirúrgico induz à involução permanente da próstata.
• Se houver a necessidade de manutenção do potencial reprodutivo, será recomendável o tratamento a longo prazo ou intermitente com a finasterida para induzir à involução prostática; é aconselhável a reavaliação de rotina em intervalos de 2-3 meses para a realização de cultura e citologia do sêmen, bem como para a obtenção de imagens da próstata. A HPB não só sofre recidiva com o passar do tempo nos machos caninos intactos após a interrupção do tratamento com a finasterida, mas também aumenta o risco de recidiva da prostatite.

CONSIDERAÇÕES CIRÚRGICAS
• O tratamento cirúrgico de abscessos prostáticos deve ser adiado até depois do início da terapia antimicrobiana e da involução prostática; a involução está associada à resolução dos abscessos, tornando muitas vezes a cirurgia desnecessária.
• A castração fica recomendada para induzir à involução prostática nos cães com prostatite que estão fora da reprodução; a castração deve ser adiada até depois da identificação e do tratamento (por, no mínimo, 1 semana) do agente bacteriano/fúngico causal; alternativamente, a involução clínica da próstata pode ser induzida com a finasterida.
• Procedimentos como colocação de drenos de Penrose, marsupialização, prostatectomia parcial e utilização de aspirador cirúrgico ultrassônico são defendidos para o tratamento de abscessos prostáticos nos cães; todavia, esses procedimentos são associados à elevada porcentagem de sequelas adversas a curto e a longo prazos, incluindo recidiva do abscesso. A drenagem cirúrgica com subsequente envolvimento da cavidade pelo omento é associada a menos sequelas adversas entre os tratamentos cirúrgicos.

MEDICAÇÕES

MEDICAMENTO(S)
Erradicando a Infecção
• A escolha do agente antimicrobiano é feita com base nos achados da cultura e antibiograma do líquido prostático, na solubilidade lipídica do antibiótico (o que aumenta sua capacidade de se difundir pelo líquido prostático em concentrações terapêuticas) e na avaliação do estado agudo ou crônico da infecção.
• Os antibióticos de escolha em casos de prostatite crônica são aqueles que sabidamente se difundem pelo tecido prostático normal em concentrações terapêuticas, incluindo o cloranfenicol, a eritromicina, as fluoroquinolonas e a trimetoprima. Na prostatite aguda, admite-se que a barreira hematoprostática tenha se rompido e que quase todo o antibiótico penetrará no parênquima prostático em concentrações terapêuticas.
• O tratamento antibiótico emergencial nos cães com prostatite aguda e/ou abscesso, administrado depois da coleta do líquido prostático para realização de cultura, é a combinação de amoxicilina/clavulanato (25 mg/kg VO a cada 8 h) com enrofloxacino (5 mg/kg VO a cada 12 h).

Induzindo à Involução Prostática
• O tratamento de escolha para induzir à involução permanente da próstata é a castração.
• Alternativamente, a finasterida (um inibidor da 5 α-redutase na dose de 0,1-1 mg/kg VO a cada 24 h) por 2-4 meses induz à involução do parênquima prostático, bem como de abscessos e cistos epiteliais difusos.
• A finasterida impede a conversão da testosterona em DHT, provocando por meio disso a involução prostática sem afetar adversamente a libido ou a espermatogênese.
• A HPB recidiva após a interrupção do tratamento com a finasterida.

CONTRAINDICAÇÕES
Estrogênios e androgênios provocam metaplasia escamosa prostática e HPB, respectivamente.

PRECAUÇÕES
O tratamento a longo prazo com trimetoprima pode levar à ceratoconjuntivite seca e/ou hipotireoidismo.

ACOMPANHAMENTO

MONITORIZAÇÃO DO PACIENTE
• Repetir a avaliação da cultura e citologia do sêmen, bem como da imagem da próstata.
• Os intervalos entre as reavaliações variam com a gravidade dos sinais clínicos, a presença de abscesso, a escolha entre castração ou tratamento com a finasterida para involução prostática e a utilização do cão em programa reprodutivo. Isso varia em intervalos de 1-8 semanas, com reavaliação recomendada antes do acasalamento.
• Continuar a monitorização do paciente até que o cão tenha sido castrado.

PREVENÇÃO
A castração é recomendada para induzir à involução prostática, promover a resolução da HPB e evitar a recidiva.

COMPLICAÇÕES POSSÍVEIS
• Ocorrência de recidiva da infecção caso a involução prostática não seja induzida.
• A drenagem cirúrgica do abscesso é associada a muitas complicações, incluindo incontinência urinária, abscedação recidivante, hipoproteinemia, edema escrotal, anemia, sepse e choque.

EVOLUÇÃO ESPERADA E PROGNÓSTICO
• O prognóstico é bom a excelente, exceto no caso de ruptura de abscessos prostáticos na cavidade peritoneal, com consequente peritonite.
• A castração evita a recidiva e melhora o prognóstico.
• O tratamento cirúrgico de abscessos prostáticos está associado a complicações e a um prognóstico pior em comparação à indução clínica/cirúrgica da involução prostática.

DIVERSOS

DISTÚRBIOS ASSOCIADOS
Em caso de infecção do líquido prostático, materiais como sangue, exsudato inflamatório e microrganismos podem refluir para a bexiga urinária, os quais, se detectados em amostra de urina coletada por cistocentese, podem ser erroneamente interpretados como infecção primária do trato urinário.

POTENCIAL ZOONÓTICO
Raro. Microrganismos como *Brucella canis* e *Blastomyces dermatitidis* foram isolados da urina de cães com infecção prostática; no entanto, não há relatos de infecção em seres humanos nessas fontes.

VER TAMBÉM
• Choque Séptico.
• Cistos Prostáticos.
• Disúria e Polaciúria.
• Hematúria.
• Hiperplasia Prostática Benigna.
• Peritonite.

ABREVIATURA(S)
• DHT = di-hidrotestosterona.
• HPB = hipertrofia prostática benigna.

Sugestões de Leitura
Root Kustritz MV. Collection of tissue and culture samples from the canine reproductive tract. Theriogenology 2006, 66:567-574.
Smith J. Canine prostatic disease: A review of anatomy, pathology, diagnosis, and treatment. Theriogenology 2008, 70:375-383.

Autor Margaret V. Root Kustritz
Consultor Editorial Carl A. Osborne

PROSTATOMEGALIA

CONSIDERAÇÕES GERAIS

DEFINIÇÃO
Aumento de volume anormal da próstata, determinado por palpação retal ou abdominal ou por radiografia abdominal ou ultrassonografia prostática. O aumento pode ser simétrico ou assimétrico, doloroso ou não. O tamanho normal da próstata varia com a idade, o porte, o estado de castração e a raça; por essa razão, a determinação do aumento é subjetiva.

FISIOPATOLOGIA
O aumento pode se originar de hiperplasia ou hipertrofia das células epiteliais (p. ex., hiperplasia prostática benigna), neoplasia do epitélio ou estroma prostático, alteração cística dentro do parênquima prostático ou infiltração de células inflamatórias (p. ex., prostatite bacteriana aguda e crônica e abscesso prostático).

SISTEMA(S) ACOMETIDO(S)
• Renal/urológico. • Reprodutivo.

IDENTIFICAÇÃO
• Cães. • Tipicamente observada nos machos de meia-idade a mais idosos.

SINAIS CLÍNICOS
• Pode não haver nenhum. • Esforço para defecação. • Fezes em forma de fita. • Disúria. • Obstrução do fluxo uretral.

CAUSAS
• Hiperplasia prostática benigna.
• Metaplasia escamosa.
• Adenocarcinoma.
• Carcinoma de células de transição.
• Sarcoma.
• Neoplasia metastática.
• Prostatite bacteriana aguda.
• Abscesso prostático.
• Prostatite bacteriana crônica.
• Cisto prostático.

FATORES DE RISCO
• A castração diminui o risco de hiperplasia prostática benigna e prostatite bacteriana.
• O risco de adenocarcinoma pode ser triplicado em cães castrados.

DIAGNÓSTICO

DIAGNÓSTICO DIFERENCIAL
• Hiperplasia prostática benigna — tipicamente provoca aumento simétrico indolor da próstata; não é encontrada em cães castrados.
• Neoplasia primária ou metastática — tipicamente provoca aumento assimétrico doloroso da próstata; perda de peso, diminuição do apetite, fraqueza dos membros posteriores são observadas em alguns pacientes; suspeitar de neoplasia nos cães castrados.
• Prostatite bacteriana aguda — resulta tipicamente no aumento simétrico ou assimétrico leve a moderado da próstata com dor prostática; febre, diminuição do apetite, fraqueza dos membros posteriores e dor abdominal são observadas em alguns pacientes.
• Prostatite bacteriana crônica — sinais semelhantes àqueles observados nos animais com prostatite aguda ou àqueles relacionados com infecção recidivante do trato urinário inferior (p. ex., disúria e hematúria); sinais sistêmicos são menos comuns do que na prostatite bacteriana aguda; prostatite bacteriana é rara em cães castrados.
• Abscesso prostático — pode resultar em sinais semelhantes àqueles nos pacientes com prostatite aguda ou crônica; a ruptura do abscesso provoca febre e dor abdominal caudal.
• Cistos prostáticos — podem ser associados a massa abdominal caudal palpável, esforço para urinar ou esforço para defecação; o paciente também pode permanecer assintomático.

HEMOGRAMA/BIOQUÍMICA/URINÁLISE
• Hemograma completo normal em pacientes com hiperplasia prostática benigna.
• Leucocitose em pacientes com prostatite bacteriana aguda e crônica (ocasionalmente), abscesso prostático e neoplasia prostática (ocasionalmente).
• Bilirrubina e fosfatase alcalina elevadas em alguns pacientes com abscesso prostático.
• Urinálise — pode estar normal.
• Hematúria em pacientes com hiperplasia prostática benigna.
• Piúria, hematúria, proteinúria e bacteriúria em pacientes com prostatite bacteriana.
• Piúria, hematúria, proteinúria e, ocasionalmente, células neoplásicas nos cães com neoplasia prostática.

OUTROS TESTES LABORATORIAIS
A concentração sérica de esterase prostática pode estar elevada em cães com hiperplasia prostática benigna.

DIAGNÓSTICO POR IMAGEM
Achados Radiográficos
• Prostatomegalia.

Achados Ultrassonográficos
• Abscesso ou cisto — lesões hipoecoicas ou anecoicas com realce distal.
• Prostatite bacteriana aguda — ecogenicidade prostática uniforme.
• Hiperplasia prostática benigna — ecogenicidade prostática uniforme; pequenos cistos repletos de líquido em alguns pacientes.
• Prostatite bacteriana crônica — hiperecogenicidade focal ou difusa.
• Neoplasia prostática — áreas focais a multifocais de ecogenicidade coalescente e sombreamento acústico (caso ocorra mineralização distrófica).

MÉTODOS DIAGNÓSTICOS
• Exame do líquido prostático obtido pela ejaculação ou por massagem prostática pode revelar alterações similares àquelas observadas na urinálise.
• Cultura bacteriana do líquido prostático tipicamente revela > 100.000 unidades formadoras de colônias de bactérias/mL em cães com prostatite bacteriana.
• Biopsia da próstata por agulha com orientação ultrassonográfica permite a visualização da área a ser amostrada e aumenta a probabilidade de obtenção de amostra diagnóstica; tomar cuidado para evitar a ruptura iatrogênica do abscesso prostático.

TRATAMENTO

• Varia com a causa da prostatomegalia.
• Castração cirúrgica — indicada em cães sintomáticos com hiperplasia prostática benigna e após o desaparecimento da infecção aguda em cães com prostatite bacteriana.
• Drenagem cirúrgica — indicada em cães com abscesso prostático ou grandes cistos prostáticos.

MEDICAÇÕES

MEDICAMENTO(S) DE ESCOLHA

Hiperplasia Prostática Benigna
Se a castração não for aceitável, os medicamentos expostos a seguir poderão produzir uma resposta temporária:
• Finasterida (0,1-0,5 mg/kg/dia VO por até 4 meses).
• Acetato de megestrol (0,11 mg/kg VO diariamente durante 3 semanas).
• Medroxiprogesterona (3 mg/kg SC).

Prostatite Bacteriana
• Escolher os antibióticos com base no teste de sensibilidade antibacteriana (antibiograma) do patógeno isolado e na capacidade de difusão do antibiótico pelo líquido prostático em concentrações terapêuticas. Boas escolhas recentes incluem trimetoprima-sulfa, cloranfenicol e enrofloxacino.

Carcinoma Prostático
• A quimioterapia não se mostrou benéfica.

PRECAUÇÕES
A administração de acetato de megestrol ou de medroxiprogesterona a longo prazo pode provocar diabetes melito.

ACOMPANHAMENTO

MONITORIZAÇÃO DO PACIENTE
• Radiografias abdominais ou ultrassonografia prostática para avaliar a eficácia do tratamento em casos de hiperplasia prostática benigna, carcinoma prostático ou prostatite bacteriana.
• Urocultura e cultura do líquido prostático para avaliar a eficácia do tratamento em pacientes com prostatite bacteriana.

COMPLICAÇÕES POSSÍVEIS
• Obstrução uretral.
• Obstrução retal.

DIVERSOS

VER TAMBÉM
• Adenocarcinoma Prostático.
• Cistos Prostáticos.
• Hiperplasia Prostática Benigna.
• Prostatite e Abscesso Prostático.

Sugestões de Leitura
Smith J. Canine prostatic disease: A review of anatomy, pathology, diagnosis, and treatment. Theriogenology 2008, 70:375-383.

Autores Margaret V. Root Kustritz e Jeffrey S. Klausner
Consultor Editorial Carl A. Osborne

Prostatopatia no Cão Macho Reprodutor

CONSIDERAÇÕES GERAIS

REVISÃO
- A próstata é a única glândula sexual acessória no cão; facilmente palpada pelo reto como uma glândula oval bilobada com septo mediano.
- A enzima 5-α redutase em células epiteliais prostáticas metaboliza a testosterona sérica em DHT; a DHT, por sua vez, estimula o crescimento da glândula prostática.

Hiperplasia Prostática Benigna
- Hiperplasia e hipertrofia estromais e glandulares difusas, dependentes de hormônio. • Pode ocorrer hiperplasia cística no final do processo patológico.
- Patogênese desconhecida; os fatores que contribuem para o quadro incluem a alteração associada à idade na relação intraprostática de estrogênio:androgênio, o que potencializa a resposta hiperplásica, e o crescimento DHT-permissivo da próstata. • Efeitos clínicos mínimos ou ausentes em grande parte dos cães. • Torna a próstata mais suscetível à infecção ascendente e subsequente desenvolvimento de prostatite bacteriana.

Prostatite/Abscesso Prostático
- Inflamação/infecção da próstata; abscesso da próstata. • Associados à infecção bacteriana; podem ser agudos ou crônicos. • A formação de abscesso é geralmente secundária à prostatite bacteriana crônica. • Podem ser associados à HPB ou cistos de retenção. • A glândula prostática e o trato urinário são normalmente estéreis. • A colonização bacteriana tipicamente ocorre via patógenos do trato urinário; é possível a disseminação hematógena. • Os microrganismos comumente isolados incluem *E. coli*, *Proteus vulgaris*, *Streptococci* sp., *Staphylococci* sp.; infecção bacteriana concomitante do trato urinário nem sempre é observada em caso de prostatite bacteriana crônica. • *Brucella canis* pode ser associada à prostatite aguda ou crônica (ver Brucelose). • Há relatos de prostatite fúngica (*Blastomyces* e *Cryptococcus*).

Cistos Prostáticos
- Formados dentro do parênquima prostático em consequência de hiperplasia glandular/cística coalescente e oclusão ductular (cistos de retenção) ou fora da próstata (cistos paraprostáticos). • A exposição a estrogênio induz à alteração escamosa estratificada do epitélio prostático; a subsequente oclusão ductular contribui para a formação de cisto (ver Sertolinoma). • Os cistos paraprostáticos ficam aderidos à próstata, sendo revestidos por epitélio secretor e variáveis em termos de tamanho; os cistos maiores podem ser detectados por palpação transabdominal; quase sempre estéreis.

Neoplasia Prostática
- O adenocarcinoma prostático é mais comum; outros tipos de tumores incluem fibrossarcoma, leiomiossarcoma e carcinoma de células escamosas.
- O carcinoma de células de transição da próstata surge da uretra prostática e invade a glândula prostática. • A HPB não é um fator de risco de neoplasia prostática. • O desenvolvimento de tumor não é dependente de androgênio; portanto, a castração não é uma medida protetora. • Os tumores são tipicamente detectados após disseminação metastática, já que os sinais clínicos ocorrem no final do processo patológico e a triagem precoce não está disponível. • É comum a ocorrência de metástase óssea em caso de adenocarcinoma, tipicamente para coluna lombossacra ou pelve; é típica uma reação fibrosante intraprostática com algumas áreas de ossificação e hiperplasia.

IDENTIFICAÇÃO

Incidência/Prevalência
- HPB: incidência elevada; 50% dos cães intactos exibem evidência histológica por volta dos 5 anos de idade, > 95% em torno dos 9 anos de idade.
- Prostatite/abscesso prostático: considerados comuns; cerca de 40% dos cães com cistos prostáticos têm evidência de infecção bacteriana.
- Cistos prostáticos: prevalência em torno de 14%; 42% desses tinham evidência de infecção bacteriana. • Neoplasia: baixa; faixa de prevalência de 0,2-0,6% na população geral, e 5-7% dos cães com prostatopatia.

Idade Média e Faixa Etária
- HPB: início microscópico por volta dos 5 anos de idade. • Prostatite/abscesso prostático: qualquer idade; mais comuns no adulto (> 6 anos). • Cistos prostáticos: mais comuns depois dos 8 anos de idade. • Neoplasia: a idade média é de 10 anos.

SINAIS CLÍNICOS

Comentários gerais
- Cães com prostatopatia exibem sinais clínicos sobrepostos:
  - Assintomático ◦ Disquesia, tenesmo, constipação, fezes em forma de fita ◦ Secreção uretral/prepucial sanguinolenta ◦ Disúria, hematúria, estrangúria ◦ Hemospermia.

Hiperplasia Prostática Benigna
- Se leve, geralmente silenciosa em termos clínicos
- Hematúria e hemospermia são os sinais mais comuns

Prostatite – Aguda
- Doença sistêmica (vômito, febre, inapetência)
- Piúria • Marcha de pernas rígidas

Prostatite – Crônica
- Infecção recorrente/crônica do trato urinário
- Marcha rígida • Infertilidade

Cisto Prostático
- Ver HPB, anteriormente • Se infectado, observam-se os sinais associados à prostatite

Neoplasia Prostática
- Emaciação • Disquesia • Distúrbio locomotor dos membros posteriores • Dor lombossacra

Achados do Exame Físico

Hiperplasia Prostática Benigna
- Próstata grande e não dolorosa, com aumento de volume simétrico.

Prostatite – Aguda
- Febre. • Desidratação. • Sinais de sepse. • Dor abdominal caudal. • Próstata normal a aumentada, assimétrica, dolorosa.

Prostatite – Crônica
- Próstata simétrica, não dolorosa, firme e de tamanho normal. • Pode ter áreas flutuantes (cistos focais) à palpação.

Cisto Prostático
- Próstata com aumento de volume simétrico e áreas flutuantes; cistos grandes podem dificultar a palpação retal; o aumento prostático pode ser detectado via palpação transabdominal. • Sinais externos de feminização se a formação de cisto (cistos de retenção) for atribuída à exposição a estrogênio (p. ex., Sertolinoma).

Neoplasia Prostática
- Próstata grande, assimétrica, dolorosa e irregular.
- Dor retal, abdominal, lombossacra. • Massa abdominal palpável. • Linfadenopatia (sublombar).

CAUSAS E FATORES DE RISCO

HPB
- Idade e *status* sexual constituem os principais fatores de risco.

Prostatite
- HPB e/ou cistos prostáticos • Cães reprodutores podem ter maior risco de exposição a *Brucella canis*.

Metaplasia Escamosa
- Exposição a estrogênio. • Sertolinoma.

Cisto Paraprostático
- Idade. • Exposição a estrogênio.

Neoplasia Prostática
- Idade. • Risco levemente mais baixo em cães machos intactos.

DIAGNÓSTICO

DIAGNÓSTICO DIFERENCIAL

Hematúria
- Infecção do trato urinário. • Trombocitopenia.
- Traumatismo peniano. • Neoplasia do trato urinário (carcinoma de células de transição).

Tenesmo
- Doença do cólon. • Doença do reto.

Distúrbio Locomotor/Marcha dos Membros Posteriores
- Artrite. • Discopatia degenerativa. • Doença neuromuscular. • Síndrome da cauda equina.

HEMOGRAMA/BIOQUÍMICA/URINÁLISE

Hiperplasia Prostática Benigna
- Tipicamente normais com exceção de hematúria.

Prostatite – Aguda
- Leucocitose e neutrofilia (com ou sem imaturidade e sinais de toxicidade).
- Hipoalbuminemia. • Piúria. • Bacteriúria.
- Hematúria.

Prostatite – Crônica
- Hemograma completo tipicamente normal; ocasionalmente leucocitose. • Piúria. • Bacteriúria.
- Hematúria.

Cisto Prostático
- Anemia (em caso de formação de cisto atribuída a hiperestrogenismo). • Perfil bioquímico e urinálise tipicamente normais.

Neoplasia Prostática
- Leucocitose e neutrofilia. • Fosfatase alcalina elevada. • Piúria. • Hematúria. • Ao exame do sedimento urinário, podem ser observadas células atípicas.

OUTROS TESTES LABORATORIAIS
- Cultura do líquido prostático: proceder à cultura da terceira fração do ejaculado; a dor causada por prostatopatia ativa pode interferir na ejaculação; abordagem alternativa: massagem/lavado prostático via cateterização uretral e massagem prostática com o dedo pelo reto.
- Cultura da urina: via cistocentese antepúbica; coletar antes de proceder à massagem/lavado da próstata ou coleta do sêmen.

Prostatopatia no Cão Macho Reprodutor

- Comparação dos resultados das culturas urinárias e prostáticas para identificar aqueles casos com populações bacterianas mistas na próstata *versus* bexiga/uretra.
- A prostatite é confirmada se o crescimento bacteriano do líquido prostático for ≥ 2 $\log_{10}$ a mais do que o crescimento correspondente da uretra/urina.
- Avaliação do sêmen: pode permanecer normal ou ficar hemospérmico em caso de HPB; neutrófilos, bactérias fagocitadas, grau variável de motilidade reduzida dos espermatozoides e teratospermia em caso de prostatite bacteriana.
- Teste sérico para detecção de marcadores prostáticos específicos não tem valor diagnóstico ou prognóstico no cão.

DIAGNÓSTICO POR IMAGEM
- Ultrassonografia abdominal: método preferido para diagnóstico por imagem; detecta o tamanho da glândula e a homogeneidade do tecido; identifica a presença de anormalidades focais do parênquima, como cistos ou abscessos; perda de homogeneidade do tecido (prostatite ou neoplasia); avalia os linfonodos regionais e as estruturas paraprostáticas (cistos paraprostáticos).
- Radiografia abdominal: identifica os processos de mineralização, linfadenopatia sublombar, ou metástases ósseas compatíveis com neoplasia; o grau de prostatomegalia não é correlacionado com qualquer prostatopatia específica.
- A mineralização em cães castrados tem um valor preditivo positivo de 100% para neoplasia; já a falta de mineralização prostática em cães intactos com prostatomegalia tem um valor preditivo negativo de 96% para neoplasia.
- Cistouretrograma retrógrado: avalia compressão da uretra ou identifica extravasamento do contraste.

MÉTODOS DIAGNÓSTICOS
- Lavado prostático: cultura e avaliação citológica do líquido prostático.
- Aspirado com agulha fina guiado por ultrassom: a avaliação citológica pode distinguir entre HPB, prostatite e neoplasia; a aspiração de infecções ativas pode se disseminar para os tecidos periprostáticos e subcutâneos; a aspiração de cistos raramente confere resolução clínica.
- Biopsia transabdominal guiada por ultrassom: fornece o diagnóstico definitivo de HPB, prostatite, neoplasia prostática.

TRATAMENTO
- A colocação temporária de sonda uretral de demora pode beneficiar aqueles animais com dor intensa ou obstrução uretral.
- Analgesia.
- Amolecedores fecais e dietas com pouco teor de resíduos para facilitar a defecação.

HIPERPLASIA PROSTÁTICA BENIGNA
- O tratamento fica indicado para cães sintomáticos.
- A castração é um procedimento curativo.
- O agente finasterida é o tratamento médico de escolha em animais de reprodução; diminui o peso e o diâmetro da próstata; a próstata retorna ao tamanho que se encontrava antes do tratamento 8 semanas após a interrupção da terapia; tipicamente usada para reduzir os sinais clínicos, permitindo a geração de reservas de sêmen congelado; castrar quando doses desejadas de sêmen forem armazenadas.

PROSTATITE – AGUDA
- Antibióticos selecionados com base nos resultados da cultura e do antibiograma; a barreira hematoprostática não permanece intacta em caso de prostatite aguda; administrar por, no mínimo, 3 semanas; registrar os resultados negativos na cultura do líquido prostático antes e, 1-2 semanas depois, da interrupção da antibioticoterapia.

PROSTATITE – CRÔNICA
- Antibióticos selecionados com base nos resultados da cultura e do antibiograma, bem como em sua capacidade de penetração através da barreira hematoprostática (enrofloxacino, trimetoprima, cloranfenicol, eritromicina, doxiciclina).
- Administrar por, no mínimo, 6 semanas; repetir a cultura da urina e do líquido prostático em 1 semana e antes de interromper a medicação para registrar a ausência de crescimento bacteriano.
- Caso se obtenha um resultado positivo na cultura, manter a administração de antibiótico adequado 4 semanas depois da primeira cultura negativa; repetir a cultura em 1 semana e 1 mês depois da terapia para avaliar o retorno da infecção.
- A castração é recomendada para casos refratários.

CISTO PROSTÁTICO
- A castração constitui o tratamento de escolha.
- A finasterida pode ser útil se o cisto estiver associado à HPB.
- Remover a fonte de estrogênio na presença de metaplasia escamosa.
- Grandes cistos solitários: são aconselháveis os procedimentos cirúrgicos de marsupialização e castração.
- Cistos paraprostáticos: podem ser submetidos à excisão cirúrgica.
- Aspiração e drenagem de cistos: não associadas à resolução; o líquido deve ser submetido à cultura.

NEOPLASIA PROSTÁTICA
- Metástase – típica no momento do diagnóstico.
- A diferenciação entre adenocarcinoma e carcinoma de células de transição determinará os agentes quimioterápicos adequados (ver Adenocarcinoma, Próstata, e Carcinoma de Células de Transição).
- A urina deve ser submetida à cultura para avaliação de infecção do trato urinário.
- Um ensaio com piroxicam sempre deve ser tentado com ou sem quimioterapia.

ORIENTAÇÃO AO PROPRIETÁRIO
- Teste regular para detecção de *Brucella canis* em animais de reprodução.
- Congelamento pró-ativo de sêmen em uma idade jovem antes do início de prostatopatia/HPB.

MEDICAÇÕES
MEDICAMENTO(S)
- Finasterida (0,1 mg/kg VO a cada 24 h até, no máximo, 5 mg VO a cada 24 h): inibidor da 5-α redutase; inibe a conversão intraprostática de testosterona em DHT, reduzindo com isso a DHT prostática sem alterar as concentrações séricas de testosterona; provoca a diminuição do volume do sêmen, mas não altera sua qualidade; agente terapêutico adequado para uso em cães machos reprodutores.
- Antimicrobianos: o medicamento utilizado e a duração variam com os resultados da cultura e o processo patológico; p. ex., enrofloxacino (2,5-5 mg/kg VO a cada 12 h) por 3-6 semanas.
- Piroxicam (0,3 mg/kg VO a cada 24 h): AINE com eficácia contra carcinoma de células de transição; também pode ser benéfico para adenocarcinoma.

PRECAUÇÕES
- Estrogênios e progestágenos reduzem a massa prostática via feedback negativo sobre as concentrações séricas de testosterona; no entanto, os efeitos colaterais tóxicos são comuns e, portanto, o uso desses hormônios não é seguro nem recomendado.
- Os AINE podem ser associados à disfunção hepática e/ou renal, ulcerações GI; os pacientes devem ser monitorizados quanto à ocorrência de reações adversas.
- O uso de trimetoprima-sulfa pode ser associado à ceratoconjuntivite seca e necrose hepática; também é recomendável a monitorização dos pacientes quanto à ocorrência de reações adversas.

ACOMPANHAMENTO
MONITORIZAÇÃO DO PACIENTE
- Repetir as culturas do líquido prostático para registrar a eficácia antimicrobiana conforme descrito anteriormente.
- A avaliação do sêmen deve ser realizada 70 dias depois da resolução da doença em qualquer cão que está sendo utilizado para fins reprodutivos.
- Repetir a ultrassonografia abdominal para avaliar a resposta prostática ao tratamento.
- Os cães positivos para brucelose não devem ser usados para reprodução.

EVOLUÇÃO ESPERADA E PROGNÓSTICO
- HPB é geralmente responsiva à finasterida.
- Prostatite crônica é mais refratária a tratamento médico; nesse caso, a castração pode ser indicada.
- O prognóstico é mau em caso de neoplasia prostática.

DIVERSOS
DISTÚRBIOS ASSOCIADOS
- Sertolinoma. • Infertilidade. • Infecção recorrente do trato urinário.

POTENCIAL ZOONÓTICO
- *Brucella canis*

ABREVIATURAS
- AINE = anti-inflamatório não esteroide.
- DHT = diidrotestosterona.
- GI = gastrintestinal.
- HPB = hiperplasia prostática benigna.

Autor Sophie A. Grundy
Consultor Editorial Sara K. Lyle

PROTEINÚRIA

CONSIDERAÇÕES GERAIS

DEFINIÇÃO
- Proteína urinária detectada por análise com fita reagente de imersão, relação de proteína:creatinina urinárias (≥0,4 em gatos ou ≥0,5 em cães), relação de albumina:creatinina urinárias (provavelmente >30 mg/kg) ou conteúdo de proteína na urina de 24 h (>20 mg/kg). A relação de proteína:creatinina urinárias de 0,2-0,4 em gatos e 0,2-0,5 em gatos é limítrofe.
- Microalbuminúria é a presença anormal de concentrações baixas de albumina na urina (1-30 mg/dL) que estejam abaixo do limite de detecção das fitas reagentes urinárias padrão.

FISIOPATOLOGIA
- Pré-renal: maior do que a distribuição normal de proteínas plasmáticas de baixo peso molecular para os glomérulos.
- Renal, glomerular: perda excessiva de proteínas de peso molecular maior (p. ex., albumina) através da membrana basal glomerular secundariamente à permeabilidade seletiva do glomérulo.
- Renal, tubular: reabsorção tubular reduzida de proteínas.
- Pós-renal: exsudação de sangue ou plasma para o trato urinário inferior.

SISTEMA(S) ACOMETIDO(S)
- Renal/urológico — proteinúria glomerular crônica provoca lesão tubular progressiva que resulta em insuficiência renal.
- Cardiovascular — hipertensão sistêmica é comum em casos de glomerulopatia.
- Hematológico/linfático/imune — proteinúria glomerular grave pode levar à formação de edema e/ou ao desenvolvimento de um estado hipercoagulável; a hipercoagulação é gerada por diversos mecanismos, incluindo hiperfibrinogenemia, anormalidades plaquetárias e perda de antitrombina III; a patogenia do edema envolve a retenção renal primária de sódio e a queda da pressão oncótica plasmática.

GENÉTICA
Foram descritas nefropatias familiares associadas à proteinúria glomerular em diversas raças de cães; o modo de herança foi estabelecido em apenas alguns cães: Samoieda (ligado ao cromossomo X), Cocker spaniel inglês (autossômico recessivo), Bull terrier (autossômico dominante), Dálmata (autossômico dominante), cão Montanhês de Berna (suspeita de traço autossômico recessivo), Spaniel britânico (autossômico recessivo). Doberman pinscher, Bullmastiff, Terra Nova, Rottweiler, Pembroke Welsh corgi, Beagle, Shar-pei, Foxhound inglês, Wheaten terrier de pelo macio e outros.

INCIDÊNCIA/PREVALÊNCIA
- Em um estudo com dados de urinálise obtidos de 500 cães, a prevalência da proteinúria foi de aproximadamente 19%.
- A prevalência de microalbuminúria foi de 25% em 3.041 cães e 25% em 1.243 gatos. A prevalência aumentava com o avanço da idade.

IDENTIFICAÇÃO
Espécies
- Cães e, menos comumente, gatos.

Raça(s) Predominante(s)
Proteinúria glomerular pode ser a manifestação inicial de várias nefropatias familiares (ver a seção "Genética").

Idade Média e Faixa Etária
Doenças familiares tendem a ocorrer em animais mais jovens; a proteinúria glomerular adquirida é mais provável em pacientes mais idosos.

Sexo Predominante
Provavelmente varia com as diferentes doenças.

SINAIS CLÍNICOS
- Variam com a causa subjacente e com a gravidade da proteinúria.
- Pacientes com proteinúria glomerular permanecem frequentemente assintomáticos ou exibem sinais atribuíveis às doenças subjacentes; muitos sofrem perda de peso e apresentam letargia; podem ter edema ou distensão abdominal. Os animais com tromboembolia pulmonar podem exibir dispneia aguda.
- Pacientes com distúrbios do trato urinário inferior podem ter disúria, polaciúria, micção imprópria e/ou hematúria.
- Pode haver ulceração bucal (se o paciente estiver urêmico), edema ou efusão cavitária ou, então, alterações na qualidade do pulso (em casos tromboembólicos).

CAUSAS
Proteinúria Pré-renal
- Proteinúria por sobrecarga — capacidade reabsortiva tubular excedida por grandes quantidades de proteínas plasmáticas de baixo peso molecular no filtrado glomerular (p. ex., hemólise ou rabdomiólise excessivas, produção neoplásica de paraproteínas ou proteínas de Bence-Jones).

Proteinúria Renal
- Proteinúria funcional — exercício extenuante, febre, hipotermia, crises convulsivas ou congestão venosa; causas pouco documentadas de proteinúria nos cães e nos gatos.
- Glomerulonefrite (p. ex., membranoproliferativa e proliferativa), glomerulonefropatia (p. ex., nefropatia membranosa), doença de alterações mínimas, nefrite hereditária, amiloidose, glomerulosclerose segmentar focal, glomerulosclerose.
- Em geral, a amiloidose resulta em proteinúria grave, embora os cães com outras glomerulopatias (p. ex., nefropatia membranosa, nefrite hereditária) também possam apresentar proteinúria intensa.
- Disfunção tubular que resulta em falha de reabsorção proteica tubular é associada à proteinúria leve a moderada.

Proteinúria Pós-renal
- Hemorragia ou inflamação do trato urogenital.

FATORES DE RISCO
- Doenças inflamatórias crônicas (p. ex., infecciosas e imunomediadas) e neoplásicas podem levar ao desenvolvimento de glomerulonefrite ou amiloidose. Os exemplos incluem dirofilariose, erliquiose, borreliose, babesiose, infecções bacterianas crônicas (p. ex., endocardite e piodermite), piometra, bartonelose, FIV, mastocitoma, linfossarcoma, hiperadrenocorticismo e lúpus eritematoso sistêmico.
- Hipertensão sistêmica.
- Hiperlipidemia crônica (p. ex., Schnauzer miniatura).
- Mielomas múltiplos podem produzir paraproteínas que resultam em proteinúria de Bence-Jones.

DIAGNÓSTICO

DIAGNÓSTICO DIFERENCIAL
Diferenciar proteinúria pré-renal, pós-renal e tubular renal de causas glomerulares.

HEMOGRAMA/BIOQUÍMICA/URINÁLISE
- Os testes com a fita reagente urinária e com o ácido sulfossalicílico permitem a avaliação qualitativa e semiquantitativa do teor de proteína na urina. Os resultados de ambos os testes são influenciados pela concentração urinária e precisam ser interpretados no contexto da gravidade urinária. Proteína urinária baixa (traços ou +1) pode ser normal em amostra urinária concentrada.
- A fita reagente carece de especificidade (cão, 69%; gato, 31%) e de sensibilidade (cão, 54%; gato, 60%).
- A contaminação com compostos de amônio quaternário gera resultados falso-positivos no teste colorimétrico (azul de tetrabromofenol) com a tira reagente urinária. Resultados falso-positivos do teste também ocorrem quando a urina se encontra altamente alcalina (pH >8-9) ou quando a fita reagente fica imersa na urina por período de tempo prolongado.
- Concentrações baixas das proteínas de Bence-Jones ou gamaglobulinas podem não ser detectadas pelas fitas reagentes urinárias.
- Os resultados do teste turbidimétrico com ácido sulfossalicílico ficam falsamente aumentados por meios de contraste radiográfico, penicilinas, sulfissoxazol ou pelo timol (como preservativo urinário).
- Os resultados do teste com ácido sulfossalicílico ficam falsamente diminuídos pela urina muito alcalina e aumentados na urina não centrifugada.
- Se a proteinúria for detectada por esses métodos, o sedimento urinário deverá ser avaliado quanto à presença de hematúria, piúria e/ou bacteriúria. A hematúria sozinha tipicamente não aumenta o conteúdo de albumina na urina acima de uma variação desprezível (i. e., >1 mg/dL) ou da relação de proteína:creatinina urinárias acima de 0,4 até que haja alteração visível de cor na urina. Em um estudo sobre os efeitos da inflamação na determinação da proteína urinária, 67% dos cães com graus variáveis de piúria apresentavam concentrações desprezíveis da albumina urinária (< 1 mg/dL) e 81% apresentavam relações de proteína:creatinina urinárias normais (< 0,4).
- Para determinar se a proteinúria é persistente, repetir o teste de triagem da proteína urinária em pacientes proteinúricos que, no início, apresentam sedimento urinário normal ou foram tratados para inflamação ou hemorragia do trato urinário.
- Se a proteinúria for transitória e o sedimento urinário permanecer normal, considerar a presença de proteinúria funcional ou resultados falso-positivos do teste.
- Embora nem todos os animais com glomerulopatia sejam hipoalbuminêmicos, deve-se suspeitar de proteinúria glomerular quando a proteinúria e a hipoalbuminemia forem

PROTEINÚRIA

concomitantes. À medida que a doença evolui, podem se desenvolver alterações clinicopatológicas compatíveis com glomerulopatia.

OUTROS TESTES LABORATORIAIS
• A proteína urinária deve ser quantificada pela relação de proteína:creatinina urinárias, pela relação de albumina:creatinina urinárias ou pela determinação da proteína urinária de 24 h nos cães e nos gatos que apresentam hipoalbuminemia e/ou repetidamente são positivos nos testes da fita reagente urinária ou do ácido sulfossalicílico na ausência de hemorragia ou inflamação do trato urinário inferior. A relação de proteína:creatinina urinárias é preferida para a quantificação, porque muito se sabe sobre o uso desse teste. Do ponto de vista técnico, ele é mais fácil de realizar do que as coletas de urina de 24 h.
• Poucos indícios apoiam a existência de doença tubular primária quando uma grande quantidade de albuminúria é detectada por eletroforese. Nessa situação, é preciso tentar identificar alguma doença subjacente.
• Microalbuminúria pode ser detectada nos cães com o uso de imunoensaio no ponto de cuidado ou quantificada com algum imunoensaio. A microalbuminúria é um indicador precoce de proteinúria. Se a microalbuminúria for detectada por meio de um desses testes, o teste deverá ser repetido em 2-4 semanas. Caso seja repetidamente positivo e se a concentração estiver aumentando, o paciente poderá estar sob risco de glomerulopatia e deverá ser minuciosamente avaliado em busca de alguma causa subjacente.

DIAGNÓSTICO POR IMAGEM
Ultrassonografia e radiografias podem revelar a presença de processo mórbido infeccioso, inflamatório ou neoplásico subjacente ou, então, indícios de doença do trato urinário inferior. O ultrassom pode fornecer informações sobre alterações estruturais sugestivas de nefropatia primária (p. ex., perda da distinção corticomedular, hiperecogenicidade e margem superficial irregular) ou indícios de doença do trato urinário inferior.

MÉTODOS DIAGNÓSTICOS
É necessária a realização de biopsia renal para diagnosticar a glomerulopatia de forma específica quando não se consegue identificar alguma doença subjacente ou quando a proteinúria persiste por vários meses após o tratamento da doença subjacente.

TRATAMENTO

CUIDADO(S) DE SAÚDE ADEQUADO(S)
A maior parte dos pacientes com proteinúria pode ser tratada em um esquema ambulatorial. A internação pode ser necessária durante a escolha da avaliação diagnóstica (p. ex., biopsia renal) ou quando houver complicações associadas à uremia em pacientes com proteinúria glomerular.

CUIDADO(S) DE ENFERMAGEM
A aplicação de fisioterapia e a prática de exercício podem limitar a formação de edema nos pacientes com proteinúria glomerular e hipoalbuminemia. Para esses pacientes, é recomendável evitar o confinamento em gaiola.

DIETA
Na suspeita de glomerulopatia, fornecer uma dieta com teor moderadamente reduzido de proteína e sódio, mas rica em ácidos graxos ômega-3 (dietas formuladas para nefropatias).

MEDICAÇÕES

MEDICAMENTO(S) DE ESCOLHA
Um inibidor da enzima conversora de angiotensina (ECA) deve ser administrado aos cães e, possivelmente, aos gatos com proteinúria glomerular. Se uma redução significativa na proteinúria (ver "Monitorização do Paciente") não for atingida com algum inibidor da ECA, adicionar um bloqueador dos receptores de angiotensina ao protocolo terapêutico. O uso de antagonistas da aldosterona no tratamento de proteinúria precisa de mais investigações, mas pode ser indicado aos pacientes com concentrações elevadas de aldosterona após tratamento com algum inibidor da ECA ou bloqueador dos receptores de angiotensina. Os animais com hipertensão concomitante frequentemente necessitam da adição de algum bloqueador dos canais de cálcio (p. ex., anlodipino) ou algum outro agente anti-hipertensivo para controlar tanto a hipertensão como a proteinúria.

PRECAUÇÕES
Os medicamentos que ficam altamente ligados à albumina podem apresentar um efeito alterado na presença de hipoalbuminemia. O uso de varfarina como anticoagulante deve ser evitado. Em casos de hipoalbuminemia ou de insuficiência renal crônica, podem ser necessárias doses mais elevadas de furosemida para mobilizar o edema com eficácia; entretanto, essas dosagens devem ser utilizadas com extrema cautela.

ACOMPANHAMENTO

MONITORIZAÇÃO DO PACIENTE
• Utilizar a relação de proteína:creatinina urinárias para avaliar a evolução da glomerulopatia. A resposta ao tratamento deve ser avaliada alguns meses depois da resolução de qualquer doença subjacente.
• Monitorizar concomitantemente a creatinina sérica. Proteinúria reduzida ou albuminúria diminuída podem refletir uma função renal em processo de deterioração.
• Como a relação de proteína:creatinina urinárias pode variar, talvez haja necessidade de duas a cinco avaliações seriadas para avaliar a resposta ao tratamento ou a evolução em pacientes com proteinúria glomerular e relação de proteína:creatinina urinárias > 4; uma única mensuração pode ser adequada em cães com relação de proteína:creatinina urinárias <4.
• Alterações significativas nas relações de proteína:creatinina urinárias são maiores que 35% em cães com relações de proteína:creatinina urinárias muito altas (próximas a 12), variando até >80% em cães com relações de proteína:creatinina urinárias mais baixas (próximas a 0,5) e >90% em gatos.

PREVENÇÃO
Cães e gatos adultos devem ser submetidos a urinálises anuais, incluindo a determinação da proteína urinária. Repetir os testes em 2-4 semanas se a proteinúria for detectada. Os pacientes com proteinúria ou microalbuminúria persistente de origem glomerular devem ser avaliados de forma mais detalhada em busca de causas subjacentes de lesão glomerular. Causas subjacentes potenciais devem ser eliminadas ou tratadas. Se a proteinúria persistir, se as causas subjacentes potenciais forem tratadas de modo apropriado ou se as causas subjacentes não forem identificadas e se o paciente estiver em estágio 1, 2 ou 3 de doença renal crônica, o cão ou o gato deverá ser avaliado via biopsia renal e tratado de forma adequada.

COMPLICAÇÕES POSSÍVEIS
• Edema. • Tromboembolia. • Hipertensão sistêmica. • Doença renal progressiva. • Má cicatrização de feridas.

EVOLUÇÃO ESPERADA E PROGNÓSTICO
• Variam com a causa da proteinúria.
• Proteinúria pós-renal e pré-renal deve desaparecer após a resolução das causas desencadeantes.
• A maior parte das doenças associadas à proteinúria tubular renal é progressiva.
• Embora as glomerulopatias sejam frequentemente progressivas, a taxa de evolução é variável, havendo relatos de remissões espontâneas. Os animais com proteinúria glomerular persistente podem desenvolver dano tubular renal que resulta em insuficiência renal com consequente uremia e morte. Alguns cães vêm a óbito após a detecção inicial da proteinúria, enquanto outros permanecem vivos por anos.

DIVERSOS

DISTÚRBIOS ASSOCIADOS
Proteinúria maciça pode estar associada à hipoalbuminemia, hipoglobulinemia (rara), hipercolesterolemia, antitrombina III reduzida, trombocitose e hiperfibrinogenemia.

FATORES RELACIONADOS COM A IDADE
Glomerulopatias familiares devem ser consideradas em animais jovens com proteinúria de origem glomerular.

GESTAÇÃO/FERTILIDADE/REPRODUÇÃO
Alguns agentes utilizados no tratamento de doenças associadas à proteinúria podem ser contraindicados na prenhez.

VER TAMBÉM
• Amiloidose. • Azotemia e Uremia.
• Glomerulonefrite. • Hematúria.
• Hipoalbuminemia. • Síndrome Nefrótica.
• Piúria.

ABREVIATURA(S)
• ECA = enzima conversora de angiotensina.
• FIV = vírus da imunodeficiência felina.

Sugestões de Leitura
Lees GE, Brown SA, Elliot J, et al. Assessment and management of proteinuria in dogs and cats: 2004 ACVIM forum consensus statement (small animal). J Vet Intern Med 2005, 19:377.

Autor Shelly L. Vaden
Consultor Editorial Carl A. Osborne

PROTOTECOSE

CONSIDERAÇÕES GERAIS

REVISÃO
- *Prototheca wickerhamii* e *P. zopfii* — algas (Clorophyta) azul-esverdeadas aclorofiladas unicelulares que provocam doença nos animais de sangue quente.
- Seres humanos e gatos — costumam sofrer infecção localizada da pele ou do trato gastrintestinal.
- Cães — a ocorrência de colite constitui geralmente o primeiro sinal.

SISTEMA(S) ACOMETIDO(S)
- Cutâneo/exócrino.
- Gastrintestinal.
- Nervoso.
- Oftálmico.

IDENTIFICAÇÃO
- Cães — jovens adultos pertencentes às raças de médio a grande porte, bem como as raças Boxer e Collie, são super-representados.
- As fêmeas são acometidas com maior frequência.
- Gatos — incomum, forma geralmente cutânea.

SINAIS CLÍNICOS
Achados Anamnésicos
Cães
- Diarreia intermitente e crônica do intestino grosso com sangue fresco.
- Perda de peso crônica.
- Cegueira de início agudo.
- Doença neurológica, surdez, crises convulsivas, ataxia.
- Lesões cutâneas.

Gatos
- Ulceração crônica da pele ou das mucosas com poucos sinais sistêmicos.

Achados do Exame Físico
Cães
- É mais comum o envolvimento gastrintestinal, ocular ou neurológico.
- Perda de peso e debilidade graves.
- Colite hemorrágica.
- Cegueira atribuída a coriorretinite e/ou descolamento da retina.
- SNC — depressão, ataxia, sinais vestibulares e/ou paresia.
- Pele — úlceras e crostas nas extremidades e nas superfícies mucosas.

Gatos
- Grandes nódulos cutâneos nos membros ou na face.

CAUSAS E FATORES DE RISCO
- Cães — geralmente *P. zopfii*; também pode ocorrer infecção por *P. wickerhamii*.
- Gatos — usualmente *P. wickerhamii*.
- Base desconhecida para a patogenicidade de *Prototheca*, provavelmente inoculação traumática a partir de fontes contaminadas.
- Microrganismos — o nicho ecológico corresponde a esgoto tratado ou não; sobrevivem como contaminantes de água, solo e alimento; ocasionalmente isolados de amostras fecais recém-coletadas de indivíduos saudáveis.
- Cães e seres humanos — a depressão na imunidade mediada por células pode predispor a infecções gastrintestinais e disseminadas por *P. zopfii*. A administração de corticosteroide pode ser um fator de risco em seres humanos.
- Gatos — não há nenhum fator predisponente conhecido.

DIAGNÓSTICO

DIAGNÓSTICO DIFERENCIAL
- Sistêmico — micoses sistêmicas, pitiose.
- Cutâneo — micoses sistêmicas e subcutâneas; micobacterioses.

HEMOGRAMA/BIOQUÍMICA/URINÁLISE
- Cães — frequentemente normais; dependem do sistema orgânico acometido; o microrganismo é ocasionalmente observado no sedimento urinário.
- Gatos — quase sempre normais.

OUTROS TESTES LABORATORIAIS
Punção do LCS — pleocitose com células mononucleares; teor proteico aumentado; presença de microrganismos.

MÉTODOS DIAGNÓSTICOS
Citologia
- Teste diagnóstico definitivo mais comum; utilizar a solução de iodo de Gram.
- Aspirados de mucosa retal ou colônica, humor vítreo, pele ou LCS.
- Microrganismos — unicelulares e não pigmentados, com paredes ovais ou arredondadas; as paredes celulares quase sempre aparecem dobradas; a característica diagnóstica é a formação de endósporo com septação interna em dois planos.

Histopatologia
- Amostras de biopsia — a identificação dos microrganismos pode ser diagnóstica; colorações especiais (metenamina argêntica de Gomori, PAS, Giemsa) ou imuno-histoquímica.
- Microrganismos — 3-30 µm de diâmetro. *P. wickerhamii* é redondo com esporângios (7-13 µm) com até 50 esporangiósporos esféricos. *P. zopfii* costumam ser ovais ou cilíndricos e produzem esporângios (14-25 µm) com até 20 esporangiósporos.

Cultura
- Crescem em ágar sangue ou ágar dextrose Sabouraud (sem cicloeximida) a 25-37°C, formando colônias lisas de cor branca ou creme dentro de 48 h.
- Identificação específica por meio de ágars seletivos ou testes bioquímicos em cultura (sensibilidade a clotrimazol, testes de assimilação de açúcar e álcool) ou com imuno-histoquímica.

ACHADOS PATOLÓGICOS
Cães
- Pequenos focos granulomatosos ou úlceras hemorrágicas — podem ser encontrados em muitos órgãos, especialmente os rins.
- Espessamento nodular da mucosa gastrintestinal com ulceração.
- Focos inflamatórios inespecíficos que circundam os microrganismos ou piogranulomas — mal organizados; misturados com outras células inflamatórias.

Gatos
- Massas cutâneas — localizadas; estendem-se profundamente para os tecidos subcutâneos; consistem em inflamação granulomatosa e inflamação celular mista; compostas principalmente por microrganismos.

TRATAMENTO
- Cães — excisão cirúrgica e terapia medicamentosa combinada.
- Gatos — a excisão de massas cutâneas localizadas é a principal modalidade terapêutica.

MEDICAÇÕES

MEDICAMENTO(S)
- Anfotericina B — utilização para doença localizada após a excisão cirúrgica; 0,25-0,5 mg/kg IV 3 vezes por semana ou até a dose total de 8 mg/kg; ou formulação lipídica a 1 mg/kg em dias alternados até a dose cumulativa de 12 mg/kg; a administração concomitante de tetraciclina ou amicacina pode conferir efeito sinérgico; formulações lipídicas podem ser mais eficazes e menos tóxicas para a doença cutânea; eficácia relatada para doença ocular.
- Cetoconazol, fluconazol e itraconazol — podem ser utilizados em conjunto com a anfotericina B, como tratamento de consolidação ou como agentes únicos para doença com menor risco de morte.
- Tratamentos alternativos — clotrimazol (localmente para *P. wickerhamii*); iodeto de potássio.
- Anfotericina B sob a forma de creme ou clotrimazol sob a forma de enemas para colite.

ACOMPANHAMENTO

EVOLUÇÃO ESPERADA E PROGNÓSTICO
- Difícil erradicá-la com tratamento medicamentoso.
- O protocolo terapêutico não está bem definido.
- Cães — prognóstico reservado a grave (sobrevida média de 4 meses).
- Gatos — prognóstico razoável a bom para a doença cutânea se a excisão completa das lesões for possível.

DIVERSOS

POTENCIAL ZOONÓTICO
Nenhum registrado.

ABREVIATURA(S)
- LCS = líquido cerebrospinal.
- PAS = ácido periódico de Schiff.
- SNC = sistema nervoso central.

RECURSOS DA INTERNET
http://aem.asm.org/cgi/reprint/25/6/981.

Sugestões de Leitura
Greene CE. Protothecosis. In: Greene CE, ed., Infectious Diseases of the Dog and Cat, 3rd ed. St. Louis: Saunders Elsevier, 2006, pp. 659-665.

Autor Mitchell D. Song
Consultor Editorial Alexander H. Werner
Agradecimento a Carol S. Foil por ter escrito este capítulo em edição anterior.

Protrusão da Terceira Pálpebra

CONSIDERAÇÕES GERAIS

DEFINIÇÃO
Protrusão (elevação) anormal da terceira pálpebra.

FISIOPATOLOGIA
- Cães — o movimento da terceira pálpebra é passivo.
- Gatos — há um controle nervoso simpático parcial da terceira pálpebra.
- Resulta da presença de massa orbital expansiva, que impulsiona a terceira pálpebra no sentido anterógrado, além de enoftalmia, desnervação simpática ocular ou dor ocular (oftalmalgia).

SISTEMA(S) ACOMETIDO(S)
- Oftálmico — terceira(s) pálpebra(s); órbita(s); bulbo(s) ocular(es).
- Nervoso — sistema nervoso autônomo.

IDENTIFICAÇÃO
Ver a seção "Causas".

SINAIS CLÍNICOS
- Pode não haver nenhum sinal.
- Podem ser associados à condição primária — exoftalmia; enoftalmia; blefarospasmo; síndrome de Horner.
- Uni ou bilateral — dependendo da causa.

CAUSAS

Unilateral

Blefarospasmo
- Condição ocular dolorosa — úlcera de córnea; glaucoma; uveíte; ou corpo estranho ocular.
- Pode causar a retração do bulbo ocular e a elevação secundária da terceira pálpebra.

Massa Orbital Expansiva
- Trata-se, com frequência, de abscesso ou neoplasia.
- Pode deslocar a terceira pálpebra no sentido anterior.
- Em geral, causa exoftalmia.
- Abscesso — observado geralmente em pacientes jovens; costuma ter início agudo; dor à palpação.
- Neoplasia — constatada, em geral, em pacientes idosos; início gradual; muitas vezes, é indolor (ver "Doenças Orbitais" [Exoftalmia, Enoftalmia, Estrabismo]).

Enoftalmia
- Bulbo ocular — recua na órbita, fazendo com que a terceira pálpebra pareça elevada.
- Unilateral — pode ser causada por traumatismo, atrofia da gordura orbital e inflamação; em gatos, pode ser secundária à neoplasia orbital (ver "Doenças Orbitais").

Microftalmia ou Atrofia do Bulbo
- Bulbos oculares pequenos — fazem com que a terceira pálpebra pareça elevada.
- Microftalmia — congênita; pode ser idiopática; hereditária em raças específicas (anomalia do olho do Collie); pode resultar da ingestão de toxinas (griseofulvina em gatas prenhes).
- Atrofia do bulbo — ocorre em casos de dano grave ao bulbo ocular (uveíte, glaucoma ou traumatismo graves); o corpo ciliar falha em produzir o humor aquoso; produção diminuída; bulbo ocular pequeno e fibrosado, decorrente de inflamação crônica.

Outras
- Síndrome de Horner — os sinais clínicos desenvolvem-se após desnervação simpática; elevação da terceira pálpebra; enoftalmia; ptose (queda da pálpebra superior); miose (ver "Síndrome de Horner").
- Neoplasia da terceira pálpebra — o adenocarcinoma da glândula da terceira pálpebra e o carcinoma de células escamosas das pálpebras são as mais comuns.
- Olho de cereja — ver "Prolapso da Glândula da Terceira Pálpebra (Olho de Cereja)".
- Eversão ou enrolamento da cartilagem da terceira pálpebra — observados nas raças Weimaraner, Dinamarquês, Pointer alemão de pelo curto e outras; a cartilagem em formato de T da terceira pálpebra enrola-se para fora da superfície ocular, em vez de se amoldar à superfície corneana.
- Simbléfaro — aderências pós-inflamatórias entre a terceira pálpebra e a córnea ou a conjuntiva. Comum em gatos que sofreram inflamação da superfície ocular antes da abertura das pálpebras.

Bilateral

Exoftalmia
- Lesões expansivas de ambas as órbitas.
- Costuma ser causada por lesões inflamatórias (p. ex., miosite eosinofílica e polimiosite extraocular).

Conformacional
- Específica a determinadas raças — Doberman pinscher e Pointer.
- Órbitas profundas e terceira(s) pálpebra(s) proeminente(s).
- Não é patológica.
- Não há necessidade de tratamento.

Plasmoma
- Espessamento e hiperemia imunomediados da margem livre da terceira pálpebra.
- Observado quase exclusivamente no Pastor alemão.
- Pode estar associado a ceratite superficial crônica (pano).

Outras
- Blefarospasmo.
- Enoftalmia — causada por desidratação, atrofia bilateral da gordura orbital secundária à caquexia grave e miosite crônica dos músculos da mastigação.
- Síndrome de Haw (gatos) — elevação bilateral idiopática da terceira pálpebra; todos os outros aspectos do exame oftalmológico permanecem normais; costuma desaparecer em 3-4 semanas, sem tratamento.
- Disautonomia (síndrome de Key-Gaskell) — elevação bilateral da terceira pálpebra; pupilas dilatadas irresponsivas; ceratoconjuntivite seca; mucosas secas; anorexia; letargia; regurgitação; megaesôfago; bradicardia; megacólon; distensão vesical (ver "Disautonomia").
- Tranquilizantes — muitos deles (p. ex., acepromazina) causam elevação bilateral da terceira pálpebra.
- Fadiga — pode induzir à elevação transitória da terceira pálpebra, especialmente em cães propensos ao ectrópio.

FATORES DE RISCO
Dependem da causa.

DIAGNÓSTICO

DIAGNÓSTICO DIFERENCIAL
- Causas mais comuns de início agudo da condição unilateral — dor ocular (p. ex., úlcera de córnea e uveíte); inflamação orbital (p. ex., abscesso orbital e celulite).
- Paciente de meia-idade ou idoso com condição indolor e unilateral — provável neoplasia da terceira pálpebra ou da órbita.
- Todos os pacientes — é imprescindível descartar olho pequeno (microftalmia ou atrofia do bulbo) e síndrome de Horner.
- Causas prováveis da condição bilateral — doença sistêmica (p. ex., desidratação, caquexia e disautonomia); associadas a anormalidades conformacionais.
- Prolapso da glândula da terceira pálpebra — intumescimento da face medial (bulbar) da pálpebra mencionada; entretanto, a terceira pálpebra propriamente dita costuma permanecer normal.

HEMOGRAMA/BIOQUÍMICA/URINÁLISE
- Leucocitose e desvio à esquerda — em casos de processos inflamatórios orbitais.
- Exame de sangue — geralmente frustrante na diferenciação das causas.

OUTROS TESTES LABORATORIAIS
Disautonomia — confirmada não só por mensuração das concentrações urinárias e plasmáticas de catecolaminas, mas também por testes farmacológicos do sistema nervoso autônomo.

DIAGNÓSTICO POR IMAGEM
- Radiografia torácica — indicada em todos os pacientes com síndrome de Horner, para descartar causas intratorácicas de desnervação simpática; e também naqueles com suspeita de neoplasia, para pesquisar doenças metastáticas.
- Ultrassonografia orbital — recomendada para ajudar a localizar massa orbital sob suspeita e definir sua natureza (p. ex., maciça ou cística).
- TC ou RM — definem ainda mais as massas orbitais suspeitas ou conhecidas.
- Radiografias do crânio — raramente revelam sinais de doença orbital, a menos que a lesão seja muito grande e destrutiva.

MÉTODOS DIAGNÓSTICOS
- Exame oftalmológico completo.
- Biomicroscópio com lâmpada de fenda ou alguma outra fonte de aumento — recomendados para ajudar a localizar qualquer anormalidade ocular em potencial.
- Todos os pacientes com a condição unilateral — examinar com cuidado ambas as superfícies da terceira pálpebra e do fundo-de-saco conjuntival em busca de corpo estranho ou simbléfaro.
- Testes farmacológicos — localizam a(s) lesão(ões) associada(as) à síndrome de Horner (ver "Síndrome de Horner").
- Cirurgia exploratória e biopsia — podem constituir os únicos meios de se obter o diagnóstico definitivo, diante da suspeita de massas na terceira pálpebra ou na órbita.

Citologia
- Na suspeita de lesões expansivas — massa na terceira pálpebra ou na órbita; aspirado por agulha fina; pode ajudar a formular o diagnóstico.
- Aspirado por agulha fina, não orientado por ultrassom — tentar apenas se a massa estiver situada em posição anterior ao equador do olho.
- Aspirado por agulha fina, guiado por ultrassom — em casos de massas posteriores ao olho; ajuda a evitar estruturas retrobulbares delicadas.

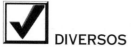

- Raspados da terceira pálpebra (Pastor alemão com suspeita de plasmoma) — revelam plasmócitos e linfócitos.

TRATAMENTO
- Depende da causa.
- Afecção dolorosa — remover a causa da irritação (p. ex., corpo estranho); tratar a condição ocular primária.
- Celulite e abscesso orbitais — em geral, respondem de forma satisfatória à drenagem e administração sistêmica de antibióticos.
- Neoplasias orbitais — costumam exigir a ampla excisão cirúrgica por meio de exenteração (extirpação) orbital; se a excisão for incompleta, poderá haver a necessidade de modalidades terapêuticas adjuvantes (p. ex., radio ou quimioterapia).
- Olhos microftálmicos — geralmente não há necessidade de nenhum tratamento; remover os bulbos oculares em casos de dor ou propensão à conjuntivite recidivante.
- Olhos traumatizados cegos — proceder à enucleação para evitar a formação de sarcomas intraoculares (gatos).
- Síndrome de Horner — tratar a causa, se esta for conhecida (~50% dos cães e gatos acometidos); caso contrário, a síndrome apresentará resolução espontânea em 4-12 semanas sem tratamento.
- Remoção cirúrgica de toda a terceira pálpebra — indicada em casos de neoplasias da terceira pálpebra; se as margens cirúrgicas não estiverem livres de neoplasia, também poderá ser necessário o emprego de modalidades terapêuticas complementares (p. ex., radio ou quimioterapia).
- Radioterapia periocular — pode resultar em ceratite grave, ressecamento ocular e cataratas; antes de instituir o tratamento, deve-se discutir com o proprietário a possibilidade de enucleação se o olho estiver no campo do feixe de radiação.
- Exenteração orbital — poderá ser justificável se a massa se estender em direção à órbita.
- Plasmomas — controlados geralmente pela aplicação tópica de medicamentos; não há cura; informar o proprietário sobre a provável necessidade de alguma forma de terapia pelo resto da vida do paciente; corticosteroides tópicos (dexametasona a 0,1% ou acetato de prednisolona a 1%; a cada 6 h inicialmente; reduzidos para cada 24 h quando a lesão estiver aparentemente resolvida); ciclosporina tópica a 1% em veículo oleoso (a cada 12 h) também é eficaz.
- Síndrome de Haw — costuma desaparecer em 3-4 semanas sem tratamento.
- Disautonomia —ver "Disautonomia".

MEDICAÇÕES
MEDICAMENTO(S) DE ESCOLHA
Ver a seção "Tratamento".
CONTRAINDICAÇÕES
Corticosteroides tópicos — uso proibido na presença de úlcera de córnea.
PRECAUÇÕES
N/D.
INTERAÇÕES POSSÍVEIS
N/D.
MEDICAMENTO(S) ALTERNATIVO(S)
N/D.

ACOMPANHAMENTO
MONITORIZAÇÃO DO PACIENTE
Neoplasias malignas — obter radiografias torácicas a cada 3-6 meses para monitorizar o animal em busca de metástases.
COMPLICAÇÕES POSSÍVEIS
- Neoplasias — possível invasão ou infecção de estruturas orbitais adjacentes (p. ex., olhos, órbitas, seios orbitais e cavidade craniana); possíveis metástases (aproximadamente 90% são malignas) para locais distantes (em geral, tórax ou fígado).
- Perda da visão — decorrente da própria lesão, da elevação da pálpebra e/ou do tratamento (p. ex., radioterapia ou exenteração).

DIVERSOS
DISTÚRBIOS ASSOCIADOS
N/D.
FATORES RELACIONADOS COM A IDADE
- Pacientes de meia-idade a idosos — sob risco de doenças neoplásicas da terceira pálpebra e da órbita.
- Pacientes jovens — sob risco de anormalidades congênitas; acometidos com maior frequência por condições inflamatórias da terceira pálpebra, em comparação a animais idosos.
POTENCIAL ZOONÓTICO
N/D.
GESTAÇÃO/FERTILIDADE/REPRODUÇÃO
N/D.
SINÔNIMO(S)
- Elevação da terceira pálpebra.
- Síndrome de Haw (gatos).
VER TAMBÉM
- Doenças Orbitais (Exoftalmia, Enoftalmia e Estrabismo).
- Ectrópio.
- Entrópio.
- Prolapso da Glândula da Terceira Pálpebra (Olho de Cereja).
- Síndrome de Horner.
ABREVIATURA(S)
- RM = ressonância magnética.
- TC = tomografia computadorizada.

Sugestões de Leitura
Hendrix DVH. Canine conjunctivitis and nictitating membrane. In: Gelatt KN, ed., Veterinary Ophthalmology, 4th ed. Ames, IA: Blackwell, 2007, pp. 662-689.
Sharp NH, Nash AS, Griffiths IR. Feline dysautonomia (the Key-Gaskell syndrome): A clinical and pathological study of forty cases. J Small Anim Pract 1985, 25:599-615.

Autor Brian C. Gilger
Consultor Editorial Paul E. Miller

PRURIDO

CONSIDERAÇÕES GERAIS

DEFINIÇÃO
A sensação que provoca o desejo de coçar, arranhar, esfregar, morder ou lamber. O prurido é indicação de pele inflamada.

FISIOPATOLOGIA
• A sensação de coceira é conduzida pelas fibras A-delta e fibras C do sistema nervoso periférico até a raiz dorsal da medula espinal. Os axônios, alguns dos quais se entrecruzam, ascendem via trato espinotalâmico lateral e fazem sinapse no tálamo caudal e, depois, seguem para o córtex sensorial. Nesse nível, outros fatores podem modificar a percepção de prurido.

SISTEMA(S) ACOMETIDO(S)
• Cutâneo/exócrino.
• Comportamental.

IDENTIFICAÇÃO
Variável, dependendo da etiologia subjacente.

SINAIS CLÍNICOS
• O ato de se arranhar, lamber, morder, esfregar ou mastigar.
• Indícios de autotraumatismo e inflamação cutânea.
• Em gatos, a alopecia sem inflamação pode ser o único sinal.

CAUSAS
• Parasitárias — pulgas, *Sarcoptes*, *Demodex*, *Otodectes*, *Notoedres*, *Cheyletiella*, *Trombicula*, piolhos, *Pelodera*, migração endoparasitária.
• Alérgicas — parasitas, atopia, alimentos, contato, medicamentos, hipersensibilidade bacteriana, hipersensibilidade à *Malassezia*.
• Bacterianas/fúngicas — *Staphylococcus* e *Malassezia pachydermatis*; raramente dermatófitos (*Trichophyton* é mais pruriginoso do que outros dermatófitos).
• Diversos — seborreia primária e secundária, calcinose cutânea, neoplasia cutânea, dermatose imunomediada e endocrinopatia variavelmente pruriginosa; doenças psicogênicas também podem estar associadas a prurido.

DIAGNÓSTICO

DIAGNÓSTICO DIFERENCIAL
• O prurido frequentemente causa alopecia.
• Alopecia sem prurido pode acompanhar endocrinopatias. Alguns animais se lambem excessivamente sem o conhecimento do proprietário.
• Demodicose, dermatofitose, piodermite bacteriana, dermatite por *Malassezia*, dermatoses imunomediadas, seborreia, algumas neoplasias cutâneas e doenças raras (p. ex., leishmaniose) podem provocar alopecia com graus variáveis de inflamação e de prurido.
• Anamnese é primordial para determinar os testes diagnósticos.
• Prurido grave que mantém o paciente e o proprietário acordados sugere escabiose, alergia/infestação por pulgas, alergia alimentar ou dermatite por *Malassezia*. Todas, com exceção da última, apresentam início agudo.
• Atopia não complicada é uma doença responsiva a esteroide que se manifesta de forma sazonal, mas pode evoluir para prurido não sazonal de regiões como face, pés, orelhas, membros anteriores, axilas e porção caudal do corpo.
• Os animais alérgicos a pulgas e alimentos são predispostos à atopia e podem revelar sinais semelhantes.

HEMOGRAMA/BIOQUÍMICA/URINÁLISE
N/D.

OUTROS TESTES LABORATORIAIS
N/D.

DIAGNÓSTICO POR IMAGEM
N/D.

MÉTODOS DIAGNÓSTICOS

Procedimentos Diversos
• Raspados cutâneos, citologia epidérmica e culturas para dermatófitos (com identificação microscópica) são muito úteis para identificar doenças primárias ou coexistentes provocadas por parasitas ou outros microrganismos.
• Lâmpada de Wood não deve ser utilizada como único meio de diagnosticar ou excluir dermatofitose em virtude do grande número de falso-negativos e interpretações incorretas da fluorescência.
• A realização de biopsia da pele terá utilidade em caso de lesões incomuns associadas ao prurido e na suspeita de dermatose imunomediada ou quando os achados do histórico e do exame físico não se correlacionarem.

Teste Alérgico
• Existem dois métodos distintos para o teste alérgico: intradérmico e sorológico. A repetibilidade do teste sorológico tem melhorado ao longo dos anos em muitos laboratórios, mas o teste intradérmico é considerado o exame com padrão de excelência e o método preferido para o teste de alergia. O uso combinado de ambos os testes pode ser proveitoso. A presença de resultados positivos não diagnostica que a alergia seja a única causa ou até mesmo uma causa que contribui para o prurido. Os resultados devem ser cuidadosamente correlacionados com o histórico e o exame físico do paciente.
• O teste cutâneo permite a identificação de imunoglobulina (sistêmica e localizada) associada a alérgenos individuais. Os testes sorológicos comerciais para alergia mensuram a IgE sérica, mas não a IgE localizada encontrada na pele. Alguns exames de sangue estão em desvantagem, porque avaliam grupos ou combinações de alérgenos ou podem não demonstrar resultados passíveis de repetição.
• Depois da correlação das reações positivas identificadas no teste alérgico com o histórico, pode-se formular a solução de imunoterapia alérgeno-específica (extrato alergênico). Essa solução contém uma mistura de alérgenos específicos. A combinação exata de alérgenos é diferente para cada paciente, baseando-se no histórico do paciente, nos resultados positivos do teste alérgico e na experiência clínica do veterinário (ou do laboratório) no tratamento de alergias. A concentração da solução de imunoterapia (extrato alergênico) também pode variar com o tipo de teste realizado e influenciar a taxa de sucesso.

Ensaios de Cursos Terapêuticos
• A terapia para escabiose ou o uso de dieta hipoalergênica pode ser adequada em alguns animais. Pode não ser uma tarefa fácil diagnosticar a escabiose canina; além disso, os raspados cutâneos são frequentemente negativos. Com frequência, é necessário um curso terapêutico com selamectina, solução de enxofre, ivermectina e outros medicamentos para descartar essa doença. O uso da ivermectina é contraindicado em Collie, Pastor de Shetland, Old English sheepdog, outras raças de pastoreio e mestiços dessas raças.
• Há vários testes disponíveis para o diagnóstico de alergia alimentar, mas os testes sorológicos não são recomendados para essa finalidade; portanto, deve-se conduzir um ensaio alimentar de forma adequada e correta. Durante o período de teste, é recomendável o fornecimento de dietas com novas fontes proteicas, escolhidas com base no histórico do paciente, ou dietas à base de hidrolisado. O ensaio alimentar deve ser mantido até a melhora do cão ou por um período de 8-10 semanas. Se o animal melhorar com o ensaio alimentar, a dieta original deverá ser reintroduzida e o paciente, monitorizado quanto ao retorno do prurido em 7-14 dias. O prurido pode retornar em questão de horas. O desafio com a dieta original é uma parte crítica do teste, mas demonstra que a melhora não foi uma coincidência. Em determinadas regiões geográficas, é preferível realizar o ensaio alimentar durante a estação mais fria, período em que os alérgenos aerógenos são menos prevalentes, uma vez que os pacientes com alergia alimentar podem ter atopia concomitante.

TRATAMENTO
• Pode haver mais de uma doença contribuindo para o prurido.
• É comum a ocorrência de infecções secundárias.
• O uso de contenção mecânica, como colar elizabetano, pode ser útil, mas raramente é praticável em tratamento a longo prazo.

MEDICAÇÕES

MEDICAMENTO(S) DE ESCOLHA

Terapia Tópica
• Esse tipo de terapia é valiosa em pacientes com prurido leve. Para áreas localizadas, o uso de sprays, loções e cremes é mais adequado. Se o prurido envolver muitas áreas, os xampus constituem o método preferido de aplicação.
• Farinha de aveia coloidal é comum em todas as formas de terapia tópica. A duração do efeito costuma ser inferior a 2 dias.
• Anti-histamínicos tópicos podem ser encontrados isoladamente ou em combinação com outros ingredientes. Não foi demonstrado que eles tenham efeito benéfico.
• Anestésicos tópicos podem oferecer apenas um duração muito curta de efeito.
• Xampus antimicrobianos ajudam a controlar as infecções bacterianas que causam prurido. No entanto, alguns xampus antibacterianos como aqueles que contêm peróxido de benzoíla ou iodo podem causar aumento do prurido pelo ressecamento excessivo.
• Solução de enxofre é levemente antipruriginosa, além de ser antiparasitária, antibacteriana e antifúngica.

- Os corticosteroides tópicos provavelmente constituem a medicação tópica mais útil. Se utilizados em excesso, esses agentes podem causar efeitos colaterais localizados e sistêmicos. A hidrocortisona é o corticosteroide tópico mais fraco e mais comum. Corticosteroides mais potentes, como betametasona, costumam ser mais eficazes e mais caros, além de ter mais efeitos colaterais. Um *spray* de triancinolona (Genesis®) é quase tão eficaz quanto os corticosteroides sistêmicos. Alguns medicamentos de corticosteroides tópicos contêm outros ingredientes (p. ex., álcool) e podem agravar a pele irritada.
- Em alguns animais, a aplicação de qualquer substância, inclusive água, pode resultar em um aumento na intensidade do prurido; no entanto, a água fria é frequentemente calmante para a pele.

Terapia Sistêmica
- A terapia é complexa e depende da etiologia. Os glicocorticosteroides bloqueiam múltiplas vias, mas, em função de seus efeitos colaterais, deve-se considerar os medicamentos que ajudam a bloquear as vias individuais do prurido. O rápido início de ação e o fácil ajuste da dose permitem que os glicocorticosteroides sejam utilizados de forma intermitente/pulsada e também como terapia crônica. Para os pacientes acometidos por atopia por mais de alguns meses durante o ano, a imunoterapia alérgeno-específica é adequada e oferece a oportunidade de obter uma cura permanente. A intervenção precoce é associada a uma taxa de sucesso mais alta.
- Ciclosporina (5 mg/kg/dia inicialmente) pode ser muito útil no tratamento de atopia, embora os efeitos colaterais gastrintestinais sejam comuns; além disso, esse medicamento é contraindicado se o paciente tiver histórico de neoplasia maligna. Outros efeitos colaterais potenciais incluem papiloma oral, hiperplasia gengival e hirsutismo. Ao contrário dos corticosteroides, a ciclosporina não pode ser utilizada para alívio rápido e requer administração a longo prazo.
- Anti-histamínicos, que incluem medicamentos como hidroxizina e difenidramina (cada um na dose de 1 mg/kg a cada 12 h) e clorfeniramina (0,5 mg/kg a cada 12 h) bloqueiam apenas uma única via que leva à inflamação e ao prurido.
- Ácidos graxos estão disponíveis sob a forma de pós, líquidos e cápsulas. Esses agentes bloqueiam a formação de mediadores inflamatórios, mas podem necessitar de 6-8 semanas de uso para obtenção do máximo efeito. Os ácidos graxos funcionam melhor como preventivos para o prurido. Também ajudam a diminuir o ressecamento ou a descamação da pele.
- Medicamentos modificadores de comportamento também pode ser úteis no controle do prurido. A amitriptilina (1-2 mg/kg a cada 12 h) tem efeitos anti-histaminérgicos potentes em cães e pode ser tão benéfica quanto os anti-histamínicos no tratamento de prurido induzido por alergia. Os efeitos colaterais são semelhantes aos dos anti-histamínicos. A fluoxetina (1 mg/kg a cada 24 h) já foi usada com êxito para tratar apenas alguns cães com dermatite acral por lambedura. O diazepam também pode ser benéfico em alguns casos, embora possa causar hepatotoxicidade aguda em gatos.

CONTRAINDICAÇÕES
- Em alguns casos, a aplicação de qualquer produto tópico, incluindo água e produtos contendo álcool, iodo e peróxido de benzoíla, exacerbará o prurido.
- A água fria pode ser calmante para a pele.
- Nos casos de prurido causado por alguma etiologia infecciosa, deve-se evitar o uso de corticosteroides.

PRECAUÇÕES
- Os corticosteroides constituem a classe de medicamentos mais comumente utilizada para o controle do prurido, embora possuam efeitos colaterais significativos e potenciais a longo prazo. Para ajudar a diminuir os efeitos colaterais com o uso prolongado, deve-se evitar a administração diária de corticosteroides orais (incluindo prednisona ou metilprednisona). O uso a curto prazo raramente causa problemas graves. É recomendável evitar o emprego de corticosteroides nos casos com histórico de pancreatite, diabetes melito, calcinose cutânea, demodicose, dermatofitose e outras doenças infecciosas.
- A ciclosporina evita esses efeitos colaterais, mas tem suas próprias contraindicações e efeitos colaterais.

INTERAÇÕES POSSÍVEIS
N/D.

MEDICAMENTO(S) ALTERNATIVO(S)
- Em casos raros, podem ser prescritos medicamentos imunossupressores alternativos, como azatioprina.
- Em função dos efeitos colaterais profundos potenciais, esses medicamentos devem ficar reservados nos casos em que todos os outros tratamentos falharam.

ACOMPANHAMENTO
MONITORIZAÇÃO DO PACIENTE
- É imperativa a monitorização do paciente, bem como a comunicação com o cliente.
- Muitas doenças não relacionadas diferentes podem contribuir para o prurido; assim, o controle de uma única doença não significa que outras causas não possam permanecer.
- Múltiplas etiologias, como dermatite por *Malassezia*, alergia à picada de pulga, atopia e piodermite, estão comumente presentes em um único paciente. A eliminação dessas causas pode não ser suficiente para reduzir o prurido de forma significativa. Os animais com alergia a alimentos e inalantes passam bem durante a época do inverno só com o uso de dieta hipoalergênica até exibirem prurido durante os meses mais quentes em associação com atopia.
- Os pacientes submetidos à medicação crônica devem ser avaliados a cada 3-12 meses quanto aos possíveis efeitos colaterais, bem como à ocorrência de novos fatores que contribuam para o quadro.

COMPLICAÇÕES POSSÍVEIS
- A frustração do proprietário é comum em função da natureza crônica do prurido.
- Raspados de pele e outros testes que podem ser negativos ou normais durante a avaliação original devem ser repetidos se os sintomas retornarem.
- As complicações também são comuns com o uso crônico de corticosteroide.

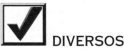

DIVERSOS
Sugestões de Leitura

Griffin CE, Hillier A. The ACVD task force on canine atopic dermatitis XXIV: Allergen-specific immunotherapy. In: Olivry T, ed., The American College of Veterinary Dermatology Task Force on Canine Atopic Dermatitis. Veterinary Immunology and Immunopathology Special Issue. Volume 81. London: Elsevier, 2001.

Scott DW, Miller WH, Griffin CE. Muller and Kirk's Small Animal Dermatology, 6th ed. Philadelphia: Saunders, 2001.

Sousa CA. Glucocorticoids in veterinary dermatology. In: Bonagura JD, Twedt DC, eds., Kirk's Current Veterinary Therapy XIV. St. Louis: Elsevier, 2008.

Autor W. Dunbar Gram
Consultor Editorial Alexander H. Werner

PSEUDOCIESE

CONSIDERAÇÕES GERAIS

DEFINIÇÃO
- Alterações físicas e comportamentais, resultantes de mudanças comportamentais normais durante o diestro e início do anestro na cadela não prenhe.
- Alterações físicas, hormonais e comportamentais após acasalamento não fértil ou ovulação espontânea na gata.

FISIOPATOLOGIA
- O perfil hormonal de cadela prenhe e não prenhe é muito semelhante após a ovulação.
- Todas as cadelas em ciclo reprodutivo passam por um diestro prolongado (>2 meses) com predomínio da progesterona após a ovulação.
- Ocorre o desenvolvimento das glândulas mamárias sob a influência de progesterona.
- Galactorreia (produção excessiva e excreção inapropriada do leite) é observada após uma elevação no nível sérico da prolactina no final do diestro; com hipotireoidismo grave, é atribuída à hiperprolactinemia resultante.
- Acredita-se que as pseudocieses na cadela ocorram como um resquício de um período em evolução quando as fêmeas de uma matilha ciclariam ao mesmo tempo, mas apenas alguns indivíduos dominantes ficariam prenhes. Os membros não prenhes da matilha ficavam disponíveis para cuidar dos filhotes das fêmeas mais dominantes.
- Qualquer evento que resulta em uma queda abrupta no nível sérico de progesterona pode levar a uma pseudociese clinicamente evidente, incluindo ovariectomia ou ovário-histerectomia durante o diestro e término do tratamento exógeno com progestina.
- As gatas que ovulam espontaneamente ou após o acasalamento, mas não ficam prenhes, sofrem um período de 6 a 7 semanas de diestro em virtude das concentrações elevadas de progesterona; algumas gatas desenvolvem uma pseudociese clinicamente evidente durante esse período.

SISTEMA(S) ACOMETIDO(S)
- Reprodutivo.
- Comportamental.
- Endócrino.

GENÉTICA
N/D.

INCIDÊNCIA/PREVALÊNCIA
- Muito comum em cadelas (>60% das cadelas em ciclo reprodutivo).
- Com frequência, ocorre ovulação espontânea na gata (35-85%), dependendo da presença de outras gatas e do macho.

IDENTIFICAÇÃO
Espécies
Cadelas e gatas.

Raça(s) Predominante(s)
Nenhuma.

Idade Média e Faixa Etária
Qualquer idade.

Sexo Predominante
Somente as fêmeas.

SINAIS CLÍNICOS
Comentários Gerais
- Embora todas as cadelas em ciclo reprodutivo tenham um perfil hormonal semelhante de progesterona e prolactina durante o diestro e início do anestro, a magnitude dos sinais clínicos associados à pseudociese é variável.
- Algumas cadelas sofrem pseudocieses evidentes e repetidas, enquanto outras têm pseudocieses ocasionais ou não evidentes.
- A magnitude dos sintomas pode variar durante cada pseudociese na mesma cadela.

Achados Anamnésicos
- Estro há 2-3 meses (cadela).
- Estro há ~ 40 dias (gata).
- Ovário-histerectomia ou ovariectomia há 3-4 dias.
- Desenvolvimento das glândulas mamárias.
- Galactorreia.
- Ganho de peso.
- Alteração comportamental, incluindo formação de ninho, comportamento materno direcionado a neonatos não aparentados, filhotes felinos, brinquedos ou outros objetos, além de agressividade e letargia.
- Inapetência.
- Distensão abdominal (rara).

Achados do Exame Físico
- Hipertrofia das glândulas mamárias.
- Galactorreia — o líquido pode ser desde claro a leitoso até castanho.

CAUSAS
- Declínio na concentração sérica de progesterona e elevação na concentração sérica de prolactina.
- Queda nas concentrações séricas de progesterona, causada por ovariectomia ou ovário-histerectomia durante o diestro.
- Interrupção do tratamento com progestina exógena.
- Hiperprolactinemia — pode ser atribuída a hipotireoidismo grave.

FATORES DE RISCO
- Ovário-histerectomia ou ovariectomia durante o diestro.
- Tratamento com progestina exógena.
- Não exerce impacto sobre a fertilidade futura.

DIAGNÓSTICO

DIAGNÓSTICO DIFERENCIAL
- Prenhez.
- Neoplasia mamária.
- Hiperplasia mamária (gatas).
- Piometra.
- Outras causas de distensão abdominal (organomegalia, ascite).
- Hipotireoidismo.
- Tumor hipofisário indutor de hiperprolactinemia (rara).

HEMOGRAMA/BIOQUÍMICA/URINÁLISE
- Anemia normocítica normocrômica — diminuição de 17-21% no volume globular (hematócrito) durante o final do diestro.
- Hipercolesterolemia — aumento de 75-94% durante o diestro.

OUTROS TESTES LABORATORIAIS
Elevação das concentrações séricas de progesterona se o exame for feito durante o diestro.

DIAGNÓSTICO POR IMAGEM
- Achados ultrassonográficos — aumento de volume uterino; exame realizado 25 dias depois do acasalamento; pode ser utilizado para avaliar a fase da prenhez e o acúmulo de líquido uterino.
- Achados radiográficos — normais; exame efetuado 54 dias após o acasalamento; pode ser usado para avaliar a presença de esqueletos fetais e o acúmulo de líquido uterino.

MÉTODOS DIAGNÓSTICOS
N/D.

ACHADOS PATOLÓGICOS
N/D.

TRATAMENTO

CUIDADO(S) DE SAÚDE ADEQUADO(S)
- Em geral, não há necessidade de tratamento.
- Tratamento ambulatorial para a provisão de cuidados médicos.

CUIDADO(S) DE ENFERMAGEM
- Evitar a autoestimulação das glândulas mamárias com o uso de colar elizabetano.
- Os proprietários podem aplicar compressas frias sobre as glândulas mamárias para diminuir a atividade dessas glândulas.
- SNA = sistema nervoso autônomo.

ATIVIDADE
Aumentar a atividade em cadelas e gatas sedentárias para intensificar o gasto calórico e diminuir as calorias disponíveis para lactação.

DIETA
Diminuir o consumo calórico por vários dias para reduzir a energia disponível para lactação.

ORIENTAÇÃO AO PROPRIETÁRIO
- Informar o proprietário sobre o fato de que as pseudocieses são normais em cadelas e não exercem impacto sobre a fertilidade futura.
- Orientar os proprietários de gatas sobre o possível desenvolvimento de piometra após ovulações espontâneas.

CONSIDERAÇÕES CIRÚRGICAS
- Ovariectomia ou ovário-histerectomia — se não houver interesse reprodutivo da cadela ou da gata.
- Realizar os procedimentos de ovariectomia ou ovário-histerectomia durante o anestro sempre que possível.

MEDICAÇÕES

MEDICAMENTO(S) DE ESCOLHA
Cabergolina 1,5-5 µg/kg uma vez ao dia por 5-7 dias — agonista dopaminérgico que reduzirá a produção e a liberação de leite por inibir a secreção de prolactina.

CONTRAINDICAÇÕES
Os agonistas dopaminérgicos (cabergolina, bromocriptina) provocarão abortamento se forem administrados à cadela ou gata prenhe, já que a prolactina é luteotrófica. Os medicamentos que suprimem a prolactina finalizarão a prenhez por reduzir a progesterona e ainda podem causar parto prematuro (abortamento).

PRECAUÇÕES
- A incidência de vômito com a administração da cabergolina será reduzida se ela for fornecida com alimento.

- As alterações na cor da pelagem em cadelas serão possíveis se o tratamento for feito por mais de 14 dias.

INTERAÇÕES POSSÍVEIS
Evitar o uso de acepromazina e metoclopramida; ambos os medicamentos podem promover a lactação e reduzir a eficácia da cabergolina.

MEDICAMENTO(S) ALTERNATIVO(S)
- Bromocriptina 10 μg/kg VO a cada 8-12 h por 5-7 dias. Reduzir a dose e administrar com alimento mediante a ocorrência de vômito.
- A terapia com diazepam a curto prazo pode ser útil para cadelas com sinais comportamentais extremos.
- Mibolerona 16 μg/kg VO a cada 24 h por 5-7 dias para reduzir os sintomas de pseudociese. Também pode ser usada a 2,6 μg/kg/dia, começando pelo menos 1 mês antes do próximo cio para suprimir o estro em cadelas, o que evitará a recidiva. Os efeitos colaterais e os riscos terapêuticos deverão ser expostos e explicados; além disso, é recomendável que os proprietários assinem um termo de consentimento informado antes do tratamento. Não fornecer a gatas.

 ACOMPANHAMENTO

MONITORIZAÇÃO DO PACIENTE
Fazer com que os proprietários monitorizem as glândulas mamárias em busca de inflamação e alteração da cor da secreção láctea, o que pode indicar mastite.

PREVENÇÃO
- Ovariectomia ou ovário-histerectomia durante o anestro sempre que possível.
- Supressão do estro.

COMPLICAÇÕES POSSÍVEIS
Mastite com significativa hipertrofia das glândulas mamárias, além de galactostase e infecção ascendente.

EVOLUÇÃO ESPERADA E PROGNÓSTICO
- Em geral, desaparece em 2-4 semanas sem tratamento.
- Resolução em 5-7 dias com agonista dopaminérgico ou mibolerona.
- Pode recidivar após qualquer ovulação.

 DIVERSOS

DISTÚRBIOS ASSOCIADOS
N/D.

FATORES RELACIONADOS COM A IDADE
N/D.

POTENCIAL ZOONÓTICO
N/D.

GESTAÇÃO/FERTILIDADE/REPRODUÇÃO
- A tendência ao desenvolvimento de pseudocieses não exerce impacto sobre a fertilidade.
- As cadelas e gatas devem ser avaliadas quanto à possibilidade de gestação antes do tratamento de pseudociese.

SINÔNIMO(S)
- Pseudoprenhez.
- Prenhez falsa.
- Pseudogestação.

RECURSOS DA INTERNET
- Gobello C, Concannon PW, Verstegen J. Canine pseudopregnancy: A review. In: Concannon PW, England G, Verstegen III J, Linde-Forsberg C, eds., Recent Advances in Small Animal Reproduction. International Veterinary Information Service, Ithaca NY, www.ivis.org; A1215.0801.
- Marti JA. Clinical aspects of mammary disease in the bitch and queen. Proceedings of the Southern European Veterinary Conference & Congreso Nacional AVEPA, 2009. International Veterinary Information Service, Ithaca, NY, www.ivis.org/proceedings/sevc/2009/eng/arus1.pdf.

Sugestões de Leitura
Gudermuth DF, Newton L, Daels P, Concannon PW. Incidence of spontaneous ovulation in young, group-housed cats based on serum and faecal concentrations of progesterone. J Repro Fert Suppl. 1997, 51:177-184.
Johnston SD, Root Kustritz MV, Olson PNS. Disorders of the mammary glands of the bitch. In: Canine and Feline Theriogenology. Philadelphia: Saunders, 2001, pp. 243-256.
Lawler DF, Johnston SD, Hegstad RL, Keltner DG, Owens SF. Ovulation without cervical stimulation in domestic cats. J Repro Fert Suppl. 1993, 47:57-61. Verstegen-Onclin K, Verstegen J. Endocrinology of pregnancy in the dog: A review. Theriogenology 2008, 70:291-299.

Autor Milan Hess
Consultor Editorial Sara K. Lyle

PSEUDOCISTOS PERIRRENAIS

CONSIDERAÇÕES GERAIS

REVISÃO
- Cisto renal capsulogênico, cisto capsular, pseudocisto pararrenal, hidronefrose capsular, cisto perirrenal e pseudocisto perirrenal são termos utilizados para descrever a renomegalia causada pelo acúmulo de líquido entre o rim e sua cápsula circundante. Um ou ambos os rins estão acometidos.
- O tecido adjacente ao acúmulo de líquido não é revestido por epitélio secretor; daí o nome de "pseudocisto".

IDENTIFICAÇÃO
- Acomete principalmente gatos machos idosos (> 8 anos).
- Quando detectada em gatos jovens, a doença costuma ser unilateral.
- Raros nos cães; a diferença na prevalência entre as espécies pode estar relacionada com a rede proeminente de veias subcapsulares que caracterizam os rins dos felinos.

SINAIS CLÍNICOS
- Os animais podem permanecer assintomáticos.
- É comum a observação de um abdome indolor e aumentado de volume.
- Sinais de insuficiência renal concomitante em alguns pacientes.

CAUSAS E FATORES DE RISCO
- A causa de acúmulo perirrenal de líquido é parcialmente compreendida.
- O acúmulo de líquido do pseudocisto é um processo dinâmico e não estático.
- A avaliação citológica e bioquímica do líquido do pseudocisto pode ajudar a entender os mecanismos fisiopatológicos.
- Pode ocorrer o acúmulo de líquido com características de transudato por causa da alta pressão hidrostática capilar ou por obstrução linfática. Alguns gatos apresentam indícios de fibrose renal à microscopia óptica. No entanto, não se sabe se a contração parenquimatosa renal progressiva oclui os vasos linfáticos e sanguíneos, promovendo a transudação do líquido.
- O acúmulo perirrenal de transudato também pode resultar da ruptura de cistos renais.
- O acúmulo de urina perirrenal pode indicar rompimento da pelve renal ou do ureter proximal.
- O acúmulo de sangue nos pseudocistos pode ser resultante de traumatismo externo, cirurgia, erosão neoplásica de vasos sanguíneos, ruptura de aneurismas, coagulopatias ou paracentese.

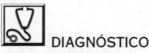

DIAGNÓSTICO

DIAGNÓSTICO DIFERENCIAL
- As causas da renomegalia incluem neoplasia renal, hidronefrose, doença renal policística (comum), peritonite infecciosa felina e nefrite micótica ou bacteriana (menos comum).
- A formação de ascite e o aumento de volume de outros órgãos abdominais podem causar distensão indolor do abdome.

HEMOGRAMA/BIOQUÍMICA/URINÁLISE
- Resultados não dignos de nota a menos que o paciente desenvolva insuficiência renal.
- Azotemia e densidade urinária inadequadamente baixa (<1,035) indicam insuficiência renal concomitante.

OUTROS TESTES LABORATORIAIS
N/D.

DIAGNÓSTICO POR IMAGEM
- A renomegalia é comumente detectada por meio de radiografias simples.
- Os exames de urografia excretora e ultrassonografia podem ser utilizados para determinar se o parênquima renal subjacente está normal ou não. Rins pequenos sob um espaço intracapsular anormalmente amplo preenchido por líquido constituem um achado comum.

MÉTODOS DIAGNÓSTICOS
O exame citológico do líquido do pseudocisto pode fornecer indícios do processo patológico subjacente que resulta no acúmulo de líquido (p. ex., transudação, hemorragia, obstrução linfática, inflamação, etc.) ou em complicações secundárias (p. ex., infecção). Concentrações de creatinina mais altas no líquido do pseudocisto em comparação ao soro são compatíveis com ruptura do trato urinário.

TRATAMENTO
- Os pseudocistos perirrenais não têm risco de morte imediato.
- Alguns animais não precisam de tratamento.
- Muitos pacientes necessitam de avaliação diagnóstica adicional e tratamento para insuficiência renal concomitante.
- Os procedimentos de capsulectomia ou fenestração pseudocística (remoção de pelo menos um corte de 1 cm × 1 cm da cápsula para minimizar o fechamento espontâneo da fenestração) costumam estar associados à melhora da distensão abdominal e ao deslocamento do órgão abdominal. Entretanto, a evolução da doença renal geralmente prossegue sem trégua.
- A omentalização cirúrgica do pseudocisto também é utilizada no tratamento da distensão abdominal.
- A resposta a longo prazo é desconhecida.
- Evitar o procedimento de nefrectomia para preservar a função renal ao máximo.
- A descompressão por paracentese, com o uso de agulha e seringa, confere alívio temporário.
- Se os pseudocistos voltarem a ser preenchidos (frequentemente em 1-2 semanas), a paracentese poderá ser repetida.

MEDICAÇÕES

MEDICAMENTO(S)
Considerar o uso de antimicrobianos adequados (i. e., antibiótico lipossolúvel escolhido com base na suscetibilidade antimicrobiana) se o pseudocisto vier a ser infectado.

CONTRAINDICAÇÕES/INTERAÇÕES POSSÍVEIS
N/D.

ACOMPANHAMENTO
- Monitorizar os pacientes periodicamente (a cada 2-6 meses) quanto ao desenvolvimento e à evolução de insuficiência renal.
- O prognóstico a curto prazo parece favorável com ou sem a descompressão do pseudocisto nos pacientes sem indícios de disfunção renal.
- O prognóstico a longo prazo não é conhecido, pois não se sabe se os pseudocistos perirrenais estão associados a lesões subjacentes no parênquima renal que podem ser progressivas.
- A sobrevida do paciente está relacionada com o grau e a evolução da disfunção renal.

DIVERSOS

Sugestões de Leitura
Beck JA, Bellenger CR, Lamb WA, et al. Perirenal pseudocysts in 26 cats. Australian Vet J 2000, 78:166-171.
Lulich JP, Osborne CA, Polzin DJ. Cystic diseases of the kidney. In: Osborne CA, Finco DR, eds., Canine and Feline Nephrology and Urology. Philadelphia: Williams & Wilkins, 1995, pp. 460-483.
Ochoa VB, DiBartola SP, Chew DJ, et. al. Perinephric pseudocysts in the cat: A retrospective study and review of the literature. J Vet Intern Med 1999, 13:47-55.

Autores Jody P. Lulich e Carl A. Osborne
Consultor Editorial Carl A. Osborne

PTIALISMO

CONSIDERAÇÕES GERAIS

DEFINIÇÃO
- Produção e secreção excessivas de saliva.
- Pseudoptialismo é a liberação em excesso de saliva que se acumulou na cavidade bucal em virtude de incapacidade de deglutição.

FISIOPATOLOGIA
- A saliva é constantemente produzida e secretada na cavidade bucal pelas glândulas salivares (parótidas, sublinguais, mandibulares, zigomáticas).
- A produção de saliva aumenta quando os núcleos salivares do tronco cerebral são estimulados.
- Centros superiores no SNC também podem excitar ou inibir os núcleos salivares.
- Estímulos gustativos e táteis na cavidade bucal aumentam a produção de saliva.
- Pode ocorrer hipersalivação fisiológica normal com a expectativa da alimentação, a hipertermia e o ato de ronronar (gatos).
- A produção de saliva pode ser acentuada em distúrbios gastrintestinais ou neurológicos (SNC).

SISTEMA(S) ACOMETIDO(S)
- Gastrintestinal.
- Hepático.
- Nervoso/neuromuscular.
- Renal/urológico.

IDENTIFICAÇÃO

Espécies
Cães e gatos.

Raça(s) Predominante(s)
- As raças Yorkshire terrier, Maltês terrier, Boiadeiro australiano, Schnauzer miniatura e Wolfhound irlandês apresentam incidência relativamente mais elevada de desvio portossistêmico congênito.
- O megaesôfago é hereditário nas raças Fox terrier de pelo duro e Schnauzer miniatura; predisposições familiares foram relatadas nas raças Pastor alemão, Terra Nova, Dinamarquês, Setter irlandês, Shar-pei, Galgo e raças do tipo Retriever, bem como em gatos da raça Siamês.
- Hérnia congênita de hiato foi identificada na raça Shar-pei.
- Raças gigantes, como São Bernardo, Dinamarquês e Mastiff, tipicamente exibem salivação excessiva em virtude da conformação do lábio inferior.

Idade Média e Faixa Etária
- É mais provável que anormalidades congênitas (p. ex., desvio portossistêmico) sejam diagnosticadas em animais mais jovens.
- Também pode ser mais provável que os animais jovens tenham ingerido substâncias tóxicas ou cáusticas ou algum corpo estranho.

SINAIS CLÍNICOS

Achados Anamnésicos
- Anorexia — observada mais frequentemente nos pacientes com lesões bucais, doença gastrintestinal e doença sistêmica.
- Alterações no comportamento alimentar — pacientes com doença bucal ou disfunção de nervos cranianos podem se recusar a ingerir alimentos duros, mastigar apenas do lado não acometido (em caso de lesões unilaterais), manter a cabeça e o pescoço em posição usual enquanto comem ou deixar cair o alimento apreendido.
- Outras mudanças comportamentais — irritabilidade, agressividade e reclusão são comuns, sobretudo nos pacientes com condição dolorosa.
- Disfagia — poderá ser observada se houver incapacidade de deglutição.
- Náusea — pode estar presente pelo aumento na deglutição.
- Regurgitação — nos pacientes com doença esofágica.
- Vômito — secundário à doença gastrintestinal ou sistêmica.
- Perda de peso — como resultado de muitos dos achados expostos anteriormente.
- Esfregar o pé na face ou no focinho — pacientes com desconforto ou dor bucais.
- Sinais neurológicos — pacientes expostos a toxinas ou medicamentos cáusticos, aqueles com encefalopatia hepática, outros com distúrbios convulsivos ou outra doença intracraniana.

Achados do Exame Físico
- Doença periodontal.
- Gengivite/estomatite causadas por toxinas, infecção, doença imunomediada ou deficiência nutricional.
- Massa na cavidade bucal — neoplasia ou granuloma.
- Glossite causada por ulceração, massa ou corpo estranho.
- Lesões da orofaringe podem ser atribuídas a inflamação, ulceração, massa ou corpo estranho.
- Sangue na saliva sugere sangramento da cavidade bucal, da faringe ou do esôfago.
- Halitose costuma ser provocada por doença da cavidade bucal, mas também pode ser o resultado de doença esofágica e/ou gástrica.
- Dor facial pode ser observada em casos de doença da cavidade bucal ou da faringe.
- Disfagia pode ser provocada por doença bucal, faríngea ou neurológica ou, então, por linfonodos retrofaríngeos anormalmente grandes.
- Déficits de nervos cranianos — lesões do nervo trigêmeo (V par de nervo craniano) podem causar salivação em virtude da incapacidade de fechar a boca; paralisia do nervo facial (VII par de nervo craniano) pode provocar salivação do lado acometido; lesões dos nervos glossofaríngeo (IX par de nervo craniano), vago (X par de nervo craniano) e hipoglosso (XII par de nervo craniano) podem causar a perda do reflexo orofaríngeo ou incapacidade de deglutição.
- Queilite ou acne — salivação persistente pode levar a lesões dermatológicas.

CAUSAS

Distúrbio de Conformação dos Lábios
- Mais comum em raças caninas gigantes.

Doenças Bucais e Faríngeas
- Traumatismo bucal.
- Corpo estranho (p. ex., corpo estranho linear, como vareta ou agulha de costura).
- Neoplasia.
- Abscesso.
- Gengivite ou estomatite — secundárias à doença periodontal, infecção bacteriana, viral (p. ex., FeLV ou FIV) ou fúngica, doença imunomediada (p. ex., estomatite linfoplasmocitária, pênfigo vulgar), uremia, ingestão de agente cáustico, plantas tóxicas, efeitos de radioterapia sobre a cavidade bucal ou queimaduras (p. ex., aquelas causadas por mordedura de fio elétrico).
- Distúrbios neurológicos ou funcionais que afetam o centro de deglutição ou doença estrutural orofaríngea.

Doenças da Glândula Salivar
- Sialadenite.
- Sialolitíase.
- Sialedenose (aumento idiopático).
- Mucocele salivar.
- Fístula da glândula salivar.
- Corpo estranho.
- Neoplasia.
- Infarto.
- Doença imunomediada (rara).

Distúrbios Esofágicos ou Gastrintestinais
- Corpo estranho esofágico.
- Neoplasia esofágica.
- Esofagite.
- Refluxo gastresofágico.
- Hérnia de hiato.
- Megaesôfago.
- Dilatação/vólvulo gástrico.
- Úlcera gástrica.
- Gastrenterite.

Distúrbios Metabólicos
- Hepatoencefalopatia (especialmente nos gatos) — causada por desvio portossistêmico congênito ou adquirido ou por insuficiência hepática.
- Hipertermia.
- Uremia.

Distúrbios Neurológicos
- Raiva — a diminuição da deglutição provoca aumento da salivação.
- Pseudorraiva nos cães.
- Botulismo.
- Tétano.
- Disautonomia.
- Distúrbios indutores de disfagia.
- Distúrbios causadores de paralisia do nervo facial ou mandíbula caída.
- Distúrbios geradores de crises convulsivas — durante uma crise, pode ocorrer ptialismo por causa da descarga autônoma ou da deglutição reduzida da saliva; além disso, o ptialismo pode ser exacerbado por mastigação vigorosa e ruidosa da mandíbula.
- Náusea associada à vestibulopatia.
- Ansiedade.

Medicamentos e Toxinas
- Aqueles que sejam cáusticos (p. ex., produtos de limpeza doméstica e algumas plantas domiciliares comuns).
- Anestesia pode induzir à esofagite de refluxo.
- Medicamentos orais, otológicos ou oftalmológicos com sabor desagradável (especialmente em gatos).
- Aqueles que induzem à hipersalivação, incluindo compostos organofosforados, medicamentos colinérgicos, inseticidas contendo ácido bórico, piretrinas e inseticidas piretroides, ivermectina (cães), fluidos contendo derivados do ácido benzoico (gatos), clozapina (dibenzodiazepínico tricíclico), cafeína e medicamentos ilícitos, como anfetaminas, cocaína e opiáceos.
- Veneno de animais (p. ex., viúvas-negras, monstros-de-gila [réptil venenoso com patas, *Heloderma suspectum*] e escorpiões norte-americanos).
- Secreções de sapo e salamandra.
- Consumo ou preensão de plantas (p. ex., poinsétia, pinheiros de Natal, cogumelos *Amanita*) podem provocar aumento da salivação.

Ptialismo

DIAGNÓSTICO

DIAGNÓSTICO DIFERENCIAL
- A diferenciação das causas de ptialismo e de pseudoptialismo requer a obtenção de histórico completo, incluindo o estado vacinal, medicações atuais, possível exposição a toxinas e duração do ptialismo.
- É possível distinguir a salivação associada à náusea (sinais de depressão, estalo com os lábios e ânsia de vômito) da disfagia pela observação do paciente.
- Exame clínico completo (com especial atenção para a cavidade bucal e o pescoço) e o exame neurológico são críticos; usar luvas para o exame quando a exposição à raiva for possível.

HEMOGRAMA/BIOQUÍMICA/URINÁLISE
- Hemograma completo — frequentemente normal; leucocitose nos pacientes com doença imunomediada, inflamatória ou infecciosa.
- Leucograma de estresse — comum nos animais que ingeriram agente cáustico ou organofosforado.
- Gatos infectados pelo FeLV podem apresentar leucopenia e anemia arregenerativa.
- Possível microcitose com desvios portossistêmicos.
- Análise bioquímica — geralmente normal, exceto nos pacientes com nefropatia (azotemia, hiperfosfatemia) e hepatoencefalopatia (atividades das enzimas hepáticas possivelmente elevadas, ureia reduzida, albumina diminuída, colesterol diminuído, bilirrubina aumentada e glicose reduzida).
- O ptialismo acentuado pode resultar em hipocalemia e acidose pela perda de saliva rica em potássio e bicarbonato.
- Em pacientes com desvio portossistêmico, pode-se observar urolitíase por urato.

OUTROS TESTES LABORATORIAIS
- Na suspeita de hepatoencefalopatia, mensuração dos ácidos biliares em jejum e pós-prandiais e/ou da amônia em jejum.
- Teste sorológico para FeLV e FIV nos gatos com lesões bucais.
- Título dos anticorpos contra o receptor da acetilcolina na suspeita de miastenia grave focal como causa de megaesôfago.
- Concentração sérica de colinesterase na suspeita de intoxicação por organofosforado.
- Teste do anticorpo fluorescente no tecido cerebral após a morte diante da suspeita de raiva.

DIAGNÓSTICO POR IMAGEM
- Radiografia simples de estruturas como cavidade bucal, pescoço e tórax ao se suspeitar de corpo estranho, anormalidade estrutural ou neoplasia.
- Radiografias abdominais ± ultrassonografia abdominal podem ajudar a diagnosticar as causas de vômito; também pode ser útil para o diagnóstico de nefro ou hepatopatia.
- Avaliação ultrassonográfica, venografia portal ou cintilografia portal podem ajudar a diagnosticar algum desvio portossistêmico.
- Avaliação fluoroscópica da deglutição pode ser valiosa nos pacientes com disfagia; considerar a deglutição de bário; no entanto, tomar extremo cuidado com animais que estejam regurgitando.
- RM ou TC para suspeita de lesões intracranianas.
- O exame de TC da cabeça pode ser mais sensível que as radiografias, sobretudo na suspeita de corpo estranho ou neoplasia.

MÉTODOS DIAGNÓSTICOS
- Biopsia e histopatologia das lesões mucocutâneas — incluindo possivelmente o teste de imunofluorescência quando se suspeitar de doença imunomediada (p. ex., pênfigo vulgar).
- Aspirado por agulha fina de lesões bucais e linfonodos regionais.
- Biopsia e histopatologia de lesão bucal, glândula salivar ou massa.
- Considerar a realização de esofagoscopia ou gastroscopia ao se suspeitar de lesões distais à cavidade bucal.

ACHADOS PATOLÓGICOS
Variam de acordo com a condição subjacente.

TRATAMENTO

CUIDADO(S) DE SAÚDE ADEQUADO(S)
- Tratar a causa subjacente (consultar as seções referentes a condições específicas).
- Tratamento sintomático para reduzir o fluxo de saliva — geralmente desnecessário; além disso, pode ser de pouco valor para o paciente e ainda mascarar outros sinais da causa subjacente e, com isso, retardar o diagnóstico; recomendado apenas quando a hipersalivação for prolongada e grave e, se possível, após o diagnóstico da causa subjacente.

CUIDADO(S) DE ENFERMAGEM
- Para ajudar a evitar o surgimento de dermatite úmida, pode-se aplicar vaselina sobre as áreas da face constantemente úmidas por saliva.
- Soluções adstringentes aplicadas por 10 min a cada 8-12 h podem ser utilizadas para tratar as áreas de dermatite úmida.

DIETA
- Suplementação nutricional (sondas de esofagostomia, de gastrostomia, etc.) pode ser necessária nos pacientes com ptialismo e anorexia secundários a causas bucais, gastrintestinais ou metabólicas.
- Aos pacientes com encefalopatia ou nefropatia, podem ser recomendadas dietas com restrição proteica.

ORIENTAÇÃO AO PROPRIETÁRIO
Depende do processo patológico subjacente.

CONSIDERAÇÕES CIRÚRGICAS
Os procedimentos cirúrgicos variam, dependendo da causa subjacente; foi descrita a ligadura do ducto da glândula parótida.

MEDICAÇÕES

MEDICAMENTO(S) DE ESCOLHA
- Os medicamentos anticolinérgicos podem ser administrados de forma sintomática para reduzir o fluxo de saliva; atropina (0,05 mg/kg SC conforme a necessidade) ou glicopirrolato (0,01 mg/kg SC conforme a necessidade).
- Fluidos cristaloides podem ser administrados por via IV ou SC para o tratamento da desidratação provocada pelo ptialismo prolongado ou grave.
- Fenobarbital (2 mg/kg VO a cada 12 h) é eficaz no tratamento de hipersialose idiopática.
- Terapia anticonvulsivante fica indicada para atividade convulsiva.

ACOMPANHAMENTO

MONITORIZAÇÃO DO PACIENTE
- Depende da causa subjacente (ver a seção "Causas").
- Monitorizar continuamente a hidratação, o peso corporal, os eletrólitos séricos e o estado nutricional, sobretudo nos animais com disfagia ou anorexia.

COMPLICAÇÕES POSSÍVEIS
- Acidose metabólica.
- Dermatite úmida.
- Desidratação.
- Hipocalemia.
- Pneumonia por aspiração.

DIVERSOS

POTENCIAL ZOONÓTICO
Raiva.

SINÔNIMO(S)
- Baba.
- Hipersalivação.
- Sialorreia.

VER TAMBÉM
- Disfagia.
- Doença periodontal.
- Encefalopatia Hepática.
- Estomatite.
- Esofagite.
- Megaesôfago.

ABREVIATURA(S)
- FeLV = vírus da leucemia felina.
- FIV = vírus da imunodeficiência felina.
- RM = ressonância magnética.
- SNC = sistema nervoso central.
- TC = tomografia computadorizada.

Sugestões de Leitura
Cornelius LM. Ptyalism. In: Lorenz MD, Cornelius LM, Small Animal Medical Diagnosis, 2nd ed. Philadelphia: Lippincott, 1993, pp. 247-252.
Gibbon KJ, Trepanier LA, Delaney FA. Phenobarbital-responsive ptyalism, dysphagia, and apparent esophageal spasm in a German shepherd puppy. JAAHA 2004, 40:230-237.
Lurye J. Diseases of salivary glands. In: Morgan RV, Handbook of Small Animal Practice, 5th ed. St. Louis: Elsevier Saunders, 2008, pp. 319-327.
Marretta SM. Ptyalism. In: Ettinger SJ, Feldman EC, eds., Textbook of Veterinary Internal Medicine, 6th ed. St. Louis: Elsevier, 2005, pp. 123-126.

Autor Valerie J. Parker
Consultor Editorial Albert E. Jergens

QUEILETIELOSE

CONSIDERAÇÕES GERAIS

REVISÃO
- Dermatopatia parasitária contagiosa de cães, gatos e coelhos, causada por ácaros superficiais de *Cheyletiella* spp (*C. yasguri, C. blakei, C. parasitovorax*).
- Os sinais de descamação e prurido leves podem mimetizar outras dermatoses mais comuns.
- Podem ocorrer lesões (zoonóticas) em seres humanos.

SISTEMA(S) ACOMETIDO(S)
- Cutâneo/Exócrino.

IDENTIFICAÇÃO
- Cães e gatos.
- Mais grave em animais jovens.
- Os cães das raças Cocker spaniel e Poodle, bem como os gatos de pelo longo, podem ser portadores inaparentes.

SINAIS CLÍNICOS

Achados Anamnésicos
- Os gatos podem exibir comportamento bizarro, meneios de cabeça ou auto-higienização/lambedura excessiva.
- Prurido — geralmente de ausente a leve, mas pode ser intenso, dependendo do estado imunológico do animal e de sua resposta à infestação.
- Somente depois do desenvolvimento de lesões em seres humanos (pseudoescabiose), pode-se suspeitar da infestação.

Achados do Exame Físico
- Descamação — sinal clínico mais importante; difusa ou semelhante a placas; mais grave em animais cronicamente infestados e debilitados.
- Frequentemente denominada de "caspas andantes" em função do tamanho grande do ácaro e da descamação excessiva da pele.
- A prevalência varia de acordo com a região geográfica em virtude da suscetibilidade do ácaro a inseticidas comuns utilizados no controle de pulgas e das diferenças no clima.
- Alguns países podem ter baixa ou nenhuma incidência do ácaro.
- Lesões — comumente se observa orientação dorsal; a cabeça pode ser acometida em gatos.
- A irritação cutânea subjacente pode ser mínima.
- Os gatos podem exibir alopecia simétrica bilateral.

CAUSAS E FATORES DE RISCO
- Os ácaros *Cheyletiella* são considerados parcialmente específicos ao hospedeiro nas seguintes espécies:
  - Cães — *C. yasguri*.
  - Gatos — *C. blakei*.
  - Coelhos — *C. parasitovorax*.
- A queiletielose deve ser considerada em todos os animais que exibem descamação, com ou sem prurido, especialmente em animais jovens ou naqueles que vivem em comunidades.
- O contágio ocorre por contato direto ou por meio de fômites.
- Fontes comuns de infestação — abrigos de animais, canis ou gatis de reprodução e estabelecimentos de banho e tosa.
- Os ácaros adultos fêmeas podem sobreviver transitoriamente no ambiente por até 10 dias.
- Os ovos podem ser encontrados nos pelos eliminados.
- Em determinados animais, pode ocorrer o desenvolvimento de hipersensibilidade aos alérgenos do ácaro, produzindo sinais clínicos de prurido (semelhantes a infestações por ácaros *Sarcoptes* e *Notoedres*).

DIAGNÓSTICO

DIAGNÓSTICO DIFERENCIAL
- Distúrbios de queratinização.
- Dermatite alérgica a pulgas.
- Infestação por ácaros *Sarcoptes* spp.
- Atopia.
- Hipersensibilidade alimentar.
- Endocrinopatia.
- Dermatofitose.

HEMOGRAMA/BIOQUÍMICA/URINÁLISE
Geralmente normais.

OUTROS TESTES LABORATORIAIS
- Exame de debris epidérmicos com uma lente ou microscópio — muito eficaz no diagnóstico de infestação.
- A quantidade de ácaros pode ser baixa; a concentração de debris para exame aumenta a probabilidade de diagnóstico.
- Coleta de debris — feita com o uso de pente antipulga (muito eficaz), raspado cutâneo, pelos arrancados, preparação em fita adesiva de acetato, coleta de escamas, e flotação fecal.
- Os ácaros *Cheyletiella* são grandes e podem ser visualizados com uma simples lupa; as escamas e os pelos podem ser examinados sob baixo aumento; não há necessidade de coloração. O encontro de ovos do ácaro também é diagnóstico.
- Para o diagnóstico definitivo de casos sob suspeita (nos quais não se conseguiu identificar os ácaros), pode ser indispensável a constatação de resposta ao uso de inseticidas.

TRATAMENTO
- É imprescindível tratar todos os animais do ambiente doméstico ao mesmo tempo.
- Para facilitar o tratamento, recomenda-se a tosa dos pelos longos (caso se opte pelo tratamento tópico).
- Base do tratamento — banhos semanais durante 6-8 semanas para remover as escamas, seguidos pela aplicação de inseticida.
- Aplicação de soluções sulfuradas — gatos e cães adultos, filhotes caninos e felinos, bem como coelhos.
- Sprays e talcos antipulgas — nem sempre são eficazes.
- Tratamento do ambiente com limpezas frequentes e sprays inseticidas — importante para eliminar as fontes de reinfestação.
- Tratamento — manter por no mínimo 6-8 semanas para evitar reinfestação a partir dos ovos eliminados.
- Pentes, escovas e utensílios de banho e tosa — descartá-los ou desinfetá-los completamente antes da reutilização.

MEDICAÇÕES

MEDICAMENTO(S)
- Aplicação de amitraz — uso em cães apenas; intervalos quinzenais por 4 vezes.
- Spray de fipronil — intervalos de 2 semanas por 4 vezes; não deve ser utilizado em coelhos (uso não aprovado pela FDA).
- Ivermectina — altamente eficaz (300 μg/kg SC 3 vezes em intervalos quinzenais); cães, gatos e coelhos com mais de 3 meses de vida; as formulações *pour-on* têm demonstrado eficácia em gatos (500 μg/kg 2 vezes em intervalos quinzenais) (uso não aprovado pela FDA).
- Selamectina (Revolution®) — 3 aplicações a cada 2-4 semanas (uso não aprovado pela FDA).
- Fórmula tópica de imidacloprida/moxidectina (Advantage-Multi®) (uso não aprovado pela FDA).
- Milbemicina oxima (Interceptor®) — 1 vez por semana por 4 semanas.
- Moxidectina (Cydectin®) — injeção subcutânea a cada 2 semanas por 3 vezes (uso não aprovado pela FDA — cães).
- Doramectina (Dectomax®) — injeção subcutânea semanal por 3 vezes (uso não aprovado pela FDA — cães).

CONTRAINDICAÇÕES/INTERAÇÕES POSSÍVEIS
- Ivermectina, moxidectina, doramectina — não são aprovadas pela FDA para uso em cães, gatos ou coelhos; assim, a participação e o consentimento do proprietário são fundamentais antes da aplicação; diversas raças caninas (p. ex., Collie, Sheltie e Pastor australiano) revelam sensibilidade elevada e, por essa razão, não devem ser tratadas com a ivermectina.
- A selamectina pode ser utilizada com segurança nas raças caninas supramencionadas.
- Evitar a ingestão de ivermectinas em cães sensíveis (mutação do gene MDR1).
- O fipronil é contraindicado em coelhos.

ACOMPANHAMENTO
- As falhas terapêuticas necessitam de reavaliação minuciosa em busca de outras causas de prurido e descamação.
- A reinfestação pode indicar o contato com um portador assintomático ou a presença de uma fonte não identificada de ácaros (p. ex., cama ou canil/gatil tipo pensão não submetidos a tratamento, animais selvagens).

DIVERSOS

POTENCIAL ZOONÓTICO
Em áreas de contato com o animal de estimação, pode-se desenvolver uma erupção cutânea papular pruriginosa nos seres humanos.

Sugestões de Leitura
Patel A, Forsythe P. In: Small Animal Dermatology. Philadelphia: Saunders, 2008.

Autores Guillermina Manigot e Alexander H. Werner
Consultor Editorial Alexander H. Werner

QUILOTÓRAX

CONSIDERAÇÕES GERAIS

DEFINIÇÃO
- Acúmulo de quilo no espaço pleural.
- Quilo — líquido que é rico em triglicerídeos, se origina dos vasos linfáticos do intestino e desemboca no sistema venoso no tórax.
- Efusão pseudoquilosa — efusão que contém menos triglicerídeos e mais colesterol em comparação ao soro.
- Linfangiectasia torácica — vasos linfáticos dilatados e tortuosos encontrados em muitos animais com quilotórax.
- Pleurite fibrosante — condição na qual o espessamento pleural leva à constrição dos lobos pulmonares; quando grave, essa condição resulta em restrição acentuada na ventilação; pode ser causada por qualquer exsudato pleural crônico, porém a maioria costuma estar associada a quilotórax e piotórax.

FISIOPATOLOGIA
- Alteração do fluxo por meio do ducto torácico com consequente extravasamento de quilo — pode ser atribuída ao aumento de pressão ou permeabilidade dentro do ducto torácico ou obstrução venosa a jusante.
- Com frequência, há linfangiectasia torácica (vasos linfáticos dilatados).
- Pode ser causado por qualquer doença ou processo que eleve as pressões venosas sistêmicas.
- Causas cardíacas — pericardiopatia, miocardiopatia, dirofilariose, outras causas de insuficiência cardíaca direita.
- Causas não cardíacas — neoplasia (especialmente linfoma mediastínico em gatos), torção dos lobos pulmonares, hérnia diafragmática, granuloma venoso, trombo venoso.
- Com menor frequência, ocorre ruptura/traumatismo do ducto torácico — por cirurgia (toracotomia) ou não (p. ex., atropelamento por carro).
- Idiopática.

SISTEMA(S) ACOMETIDO(S)
- Respiratório — os quadros de efusão quilosa ou pleurite fibrosante interferem na capacidade de expansão dos pulmões.
- Pode haver sinais sistêmicos secundários à angústia respiratória (p. ex., diminuição do apetite, perda de peso).

GENÉTICA
Desconhecida.

INCIDÊNCIA/PREVALÊNCIA
Desconhecidas.

DISTRIBUIÇÃO GEOGRÁFICA
Mundial.

IDENTIFICAÇÃO
Espécies
Cães e gatos.

Raça(s) Predominante(s)
- Cães — Afghan hound e Shiba inu.
- Gatos — Raças asiáticas (p. ex., Siamês e Himalaio).

Idade Média e Faixa Etária
- Pode acometer qualquer idade.
- Gatos — é mais comum em gatos mais idosos do que nos jovens; isso pode sugerir uma associação com neoplasia.
- Cães da raça Afghan hound — desenvolvem o quadro quando chegam à meia-idade.
- Cães da raça Shiba inu — desenvolvem ainda quando jovens (<1-2 anos de idade).

Sexo Predominante
Nenhum identificado.

SINAIS CLÍNICOS
Comentários Gerais
- Os sinais clínicos variam, dependendo da velocidade de acúmulo do líquido e do volume da efusão pleural.
- Em geral, não se manifestam até que ocorra dano acentuado à ventilação.
- Muitos pacientes parecem apresentar a condição por períodos prolongados antes do diagnóstico; provavelmente, esses animais reabsorvem o quilo em uma velocidade que impede dano respiratório evidente.

Achados Anamnésicos
- Os pacientes costumam ser examinados para avaliação de taquipneia, dificuldade respiratória (dispneia) ou tosse.
- Tosse — pode ter ocorrido há meses antes do exame.
- Taquipneia.
- Letargia.
- Anorexia e perda de peso.
- Intolerância ao exercício.

Achados do Exame Físico
- Variam com a causa da efusão.
- Sons cardíacos e ruídos pulmonares abafados na face ventral.
- Aumento nos ruídos broncovesiculares, particularmente nos campos pulmonares dorsais.
- Mucosas pálidas ou cianose.
- Arritmia.
- Sopro cardíaco.
- Sinais de insuficiência cardíaca direita (p. ex., pulsos jugulares, ascite, hepatomegalia).
- Diminuição na compressibilidade da porção torácica anterior (cranial) — comum em gatos com massa mediastínica cranial.

CAUSAS
- Massas mediastínicas anteriores (craniais) — linfoma; timoma.
- Cardiopatias — dirofilariose; miocardiopatia; efusão pericárdica.
- Torção dos lobos pulmonares.
- Obstrução venosa — granuloma, trombos.
- Anormalidade congênita do ducto torácico.
- Cirurgia cardíaca ou torácica.
- Idiopáticas — causa mais comum.

FATORES DE RISCO
Desconhecidos.

DIAGNÓSTICO

DIAGNÓSTICO DIFERENCIAL
- Outras causas de efusão pleural — neoplasia, piotórax, insuficiência cardíaca, PIF.

HEMOGRAMA/BIOQUÍMICA/URINÁLISE
- Frequentemente normais.
- Linfopenia e hipoalbuminemia — podem ser anormalidades encontradas.

OUTROS TESTES LABORATORIAIS
Teste de dirofilariose.

Análise do Líquido
- Essa análise classifica o líquido como exsudato.
- A cor dependerá do conteúdo de gordura da dieta e da presença de hemorragia concomitante — costuma ter aspecto de branco leitoso a opaco, podendo variar de amarelo a rosa.
- O conteúdo de proteínas varia, mas o alto conteúdo de lipídios tornará o índice de refração impreciso.
- Contagem total de células nucleadas — em geral, <10.000 células/μL.
- Triglicerídeos no líquido — níveis mais altos em comparação ao soro.
- Colesterol no líquido — níveis mais baixos em comparação ao soro.

Citologia
- Colocar a amostra em um tubo de EDTA para permitir que a contagem das células seja realizada.
- Em princípio, o líquido é constituído principalmente por linfócitos pequenos, neutrófilos e macrófagos contendo lipídio.
- Efusões crônicas contêm menos linfócitos em função da perda contínua e mais neutrófilos não degenerados em virtude da inflamação causada por múltiplas toracocenteses ou irritação do revestimento pleural por quilo.
- Linfócitos anormais — sugestivos de neoplasia subjacente.

DIAGNÓSTICO POR IMAGEM
Radiografias Torácicas
- Em paciente estável, obter duas a quatro projeções — efusão pleural.
- A projeção dorsoventral é associada a menos estresse que a ventrodorsal em animal com dificuldade respiratória.
- Repetir as radiografias após o procedimento de toracocentese para avaliar as causas subjacentes da efusão ou evidências de pleurite fibrosante; se colabados, os lobos pulmonares não parecem se reexpandir após a remoção do líquido pleural, ou se a angústia respiratória persistir com apenas uma quantidade mínima de líquido, suspeitar de doença subjacente do parênquima pulmonar ou da pleura (p. ex., pleurite fibrosante).

Ultrassonografia/Ecocardiografia
- Esses exames devem ser realizados antes da toracocentese se o paciente estiver estável — o líquido atua como uma janela acústica, acentuando a visualização das estruturas torácicas.
- Avaliar as causas subjacentes — detectar anormalidades na estrutura e na função cardíaca, além de pericardiopatias e massas mediastínicas.

Linfangiografia por TC
- Pode quantificar os ramos do ducto torácico com maior precisão que a linfangiografia por radiografias simples, embora isso não seja comprovado.
- Em cães, injetar por via percutânea 1-2 mL de material de contraste não iônico nos linfonodos mesentéricos com o uso de orientação ultrassonográfica.
- Obter imagens por TC torácica helicoidal antes e depois da injeção dos meios de contraste.
- Pode registrar a localização e o aspecto do ducto torácico e de seus linfáticos tributários; pode vir a ser útil para o planejamento cirúrgico (não confirmado).

ACHADOS PATOLÓGICOS
- Vasos linfáticos (incluindo o ducto torácico) — dificuldade de identificação à necropsia.

QUILOTÓRAX

- Pleurite fibrosante — os pulmões podem aparecer contraídos; as pleuras (visceral e parietal) encontram-se difusamente espessas.
- Pleurite fibrosante — do ponto de vista histológico, caracteriza-se por um espessamento pleural difuso moderado a acentuado por tecido conjuntivo fibroso com infiltrados moderados constituídos por linfócitos, macrófagos e plasmócitos.

TRATAMENTO

CUIDADO(S) DE SAÚDE ADEQUADO(S)
- Animais dispneicos — toracocentese imediata; a remoção até de pequenas quantidades de efusão pleural pode melhorar a ventilação de forma acentuada.
- Identificar e tratar a causa subjacente, se possível.
- Tratamento clínico — geralmente em esquema ambulatorial com toracocentese intermitente, conforme a necessidade, com base nos sinais clínicos (ver a seção "Medicações").
- Sondas torácicas — colocar *apenas* em pacientes com suspeita de quilotórax secundário a traumatismo (muito raro), nos casos com acúmulo rápido de líquido ou após a cirurgia.
- Optar pela cirurgia — se o tratamento clínico não solucionar o problema em 2-3 meses (ver a seção "Considerações Cirúrgicas").

CUIDADO(S) DE ENFERMAGEM
- Os pacientes submetidos a múltiplas toracocenteses raramente podem desenvolver distúrbios eletrolíticos (hiponatremia, hipercalemia) que talvez necessitem de correção por meio de fluidoterapia.
- Toracocenteses — realizar sob condições assépticas para diminuir o risco de infecção iatrogênica; a profilaxia antibiótica não costuma ser necessária caso se empregue a técnica apropriada.

ATIVIDADE
Em geral, os pacientes restringem sua própria atividade física à medida que o volume do líquido pleural aumenta ou caso desenvolvam uma pleurite fibrosante.

DIETA
- Baixo teor de gorduras — pode diminuir a quantidade de lipídios na efusão, o que possivelmente aumenta a capacidade de reabsorção do líquido pelo paciente a partir da cavidade torácica; não é uma medida curativa; pode ajudar no tratamento por facilitar a reabsorção.
- Triglicerídeos de cadeia média — são transportados pelo ducto torácico em cães e, portanto, não são mais recomendados.

ORIENTAÇÃO AO PROPRIETÁRIO
- Informar ao proprietário que nenhum tratamento específico interromperá a efusão em todos os pacientes com a forma idiopática da doença.
- Avisar o proprietário quanto à possibilidade de resolução espontânea da condição em certos pacientes após algumas semanas ou meses.

CONSIDERAÇÕES CIRÚRGICAS
Ligadura do Ducto Torácico e Pericardiectomia
- Recomendada em pacientes irresponsivos ao tratamento clínico.
- O ducto costuma ter múltiplos ramos na porção torácica caudal — local onde se efetua a ligadura; a falha na oclusão de todos os ramos resulta em efusão pleural contínua.
- Executar o procedimento sempre em conjunto com a cateterização de algum vaso linfático mesentérico para a realização da linfangiografia ou a aplicação de corante; a injeção do azul de metileno no cateter mesentérico facilita enormemente a visualização e a oclusão completa de todos os ramos.
- O espessamento do pericárdio pode evitar a formação de comunicações linfático-venosas — realizar a pericardiectomia simultaneamente com a ligadura do ducto torácico; há relatos de até 100% de sucesso quando ambas as técnicas são realizadas; pode haver a necessidade de uma segunda cirurgia se todos os ramos não forem ocluídos.

Outras
- Em caso de ligadura do ducto torácico malsucedida — pode-se considerar a cirurgia de desvio pleuroperitoneal ou pleurovenoso, embora o material fibrinoso possa ocluir o desvio facilmente.
- Pleurite fibrosante extensa — torna a cirurgia mais difícil, mas parece não ter relevância em termos de prognóstico caso se consiga interromper o acúmulo do líquido.

MEDICAÇÕES

MEDICAMENTO(S) DE ESCOLHA
- Rutina — 50-100 mg/kg VO a cada 8 h; acredita-se que esse medicamento aumente a remoção de proteínas pelos macrófagos, o que promove a absorção do líquido; parece ocorrer o desaparecimento completo da efusão em alguns pacientes; no entanto, há necessidade de mais estudos para determinar se a resolução ocorre de forma espontânea ou em reposta a essa terapia.
- Somatostatina (octreotida) — uma substância de ocorrência natural que inibe as secreções gástricas, pancreáticas e biliares e prolonga o tempo de trânsito gastrintestinal, diminui a secreção jejunal e estimula a absorção gastrintestinal de água; em casos de quilotórax traumático, a redução das secreções gastrintestinais pode ajudar na cicatrização do ducto torácico por diminuir o fluxo linfático por esse ducto; já se constatou o desaparecimento do líquido pleural em cães e gatos com quilotórax idiopático submetidos à octreotida, mas o mecanismo de ação é desconhecido; octreotida (Sandostatin®; 10 mcg/kg SC a cada 8 h por 2-3 semanas) é um análogo sintético da somatostatina que tem uma meia-vida prolongada e efeitos colaterais mínimos.
- Terapia imunossupressora (p. ex., ciclosporina) — pode ser benéfica em casos selecionados.

CONTRAINDICAÇÕES
Cardiopatia ou neoplasia — tratar a causa subjacente e não a efusão em si (além da dirofilariose em gatos, cuja ligadura do ducto torácico pode ser benéfica durante a eliminação da infecção por dirofilárias).

ACOMPANHAMENTO

MONITORIZAÇÃO DO PACIENTE
- Monitorar o animal quanto à presença de sinais de recorrência de efusão pleural (taquipneia, respiração laboriosa, angústia respiratória) — realizar a toracocentese, conforme a necessidade.
- Resolução (espontânea ou pós-cirúrgica) — reavaliar periodicamente por vários anos para detectar recidiva.

COMPLICAÇÕES POSSÍVEIS
- Pleurite fibrosante — complicação grave mais comum de doença crônica.
- Infecção iatrogênica com múltiplas toracocenteses — é importante utilizar uma técnica asséptica.
- Imunossupressão — causada por depleção de linfócitos; pode ocorrer em pacientes submetidos a toracocenteses repetidas e frequentes.

EVOLUÇÃO ESPERADA E PROGNÓSTICO
- Pode exibir resolução espontânea ou pós-cirúrgica.
- Casos sem tratamento ou de doença crônica — podem resultar em pleurite fibrosante grave e dispneia persistente.
- Eutanásia — praticada com frequência em pacientes irresponsivos à cirurgia ou ao tratamento clínico.

DIVERSOS

DISTÚRBIOS ASSOCIADOS
Anormalidades linfáticas difusas (p. ex., linfangiectasias intestinal, hepática e pulmonar e ascite quilosa) — podem ser observadas; possivelmente agravam o prognóstico.

FATORES RELACIONADOS COM A IDADE
Os pacientes jovens podem exibir um prognóstico mais satisfatório quando comparados com os animais idosos, em virtude da associação de neoplasias com a idade avançada.

ABREVIATURA(S)
- EDTA = ácido etilenodiamino tetracético.
- PIF = peritonite infecciosa felina.
- TC = tomografia computadorizada.

Sugestões de Leitura
Carrobi B, White RAS, Romanelli G. Treatment of idiopathic chylothorax in 14 dogs by ligation of the thoracic duct and partial pericardiectomy. Vet Record 2008, 163(25):743-745.
Esterline ML, Radlinsky MG, Biller DS, et al. Comparison of radiographic and computed tomography lymphangiography for identification of the canine thoracic duct. Vet Radiol Ultrasound 2005, 46:391-395.
Fossum TW, Mertens MM, Miller MW, et al. Thoracic duct ligation and pericardectomy for treatment of idiopathic chylothorax. J Vet Intern Med 2004, 18:307-310.
Johnson EG, Wisner ER, Kyles A, Koehler C, Marks SL. Computed tomographic lymphography of the thoracic duct by mesenteric lymph node injection. Vet Surg 2009, 38(3):361-367.
Radlinsky MG, Mason DE, Biller DS, Olsen D. Thoracoscopic visualization and ligation of the thoracic duct in dogs. Vet Surg 2002, 31:138-146.

Autores Jill S. Pomrantz e Theresa Fossum
Consultor Editorial Lynelle R. Johnson

Quimiodectoma

CONSIDERAÇÕES GERAIS

REVISÃO
• Quimiodectomas são tumores que se originam das células quimiorreceptoras (como aquelas existentes nos corpos aórtico e carotídeo).
• Outros nomes — tumores do corpo aórtico, paraganglioma cardíaco, APUDoma, e tumor do corpo glômico.
• Em cães, os tumores do corpo aórtico são mais comuns (80-90%) que os do corpo carotídeo (10-20%).

IDENTIFICAÇÃO
• Raro em gatos.
• Cães — de 6 a 15 anos de idade.
• Pode acometer quaisquer raças, mas as braquicefálicas são predispostas, especialmente Boxer, Boston terrier e Buldogue inglês.
• Os machos são predispostos a tumores do corpo aórtico, mas não há predileção sexual em casos de tumores do corpo carotídeo.

SINAIS CLÍNICOS
• Letargia, anorexia, fraqueza, colapso, tosse, angústia respiratória, intolerância a exercícios, distensão abdominal, vômitos, morte súbita.
• Tumor do corpo carotídeo — podem ser observados sinais como massa cervical, regurgitação, dispneia, síndrome de Horner, paralisia laríngea.
• Podem ser associados a alterações como efusão pericárdica e tamponamento cardíaco — sons cardíacos abafados, má qualidade do pulso, taquicardia, taquipneia, pulsos débeis, tempo de preenchimento capilar lento, ascite.
• Podem estar relacionados com efusão pleural — diminuição dos ruídos respiratórios ventralmente, além de cianose.
• Arritmias cardíacas com déficits de pulso.

CAUSAS E FATORES DE RISCO
Hipoxemia crônica pode desempenhar um papel no desenvolvimento dessa doença em raças braquicefálicas.

DIAGNÓSTICO

DIAGNÓSTICO DIFERENCIAL
• Outras massas localizadas na base do coração (ou seja, hemangiossarcoma, timoma, carcinoma ectópico da tireoide, abscesso, granuloma).
• Efusão pericárdica idiopática.
• Pericardite.
• Miocardiopatia.
• Insuficiência valvular.

HEMOGRAMA/BIOQUÍMICA/URINÁLISE
• Tipicamente normais, embora 36% dos pacientes possam exibir eritrócitos nucleados sem anemia.

OUTROS TESTES LABORATORIAIS
N/D.

DIAGNÓSTICO POR IMAGEM
• Radiografias torácicas — avaliam a presença de massa na região da base do coração, efusão pericárdica, lesões metastáticas nos pulmões.
• Ultrassonografia abdominal — possibilita a avaliação do abdome em busca de metástase.
• Ecocardiografia — permite a obtenção de imagens de massas, além da aorta e das artérias/veias pulmonares.

MÉTODOS DIAGNÓSTICOS
• Biopsia de massa.
• ECG — se houver evidência de arritmia, poderão ser observadas alterações como complexos QRS de baixa amplitude na presença de efusão pericárdica ou pleural, ou alternância elétrica em caso de efusão pericárdica.

TRATAMENTO

TUMORES DO CORPO AÓRTICO
• Remoção cirúrgica de massa — se possível.
• Foi demonstrado que o procedimento de pericardiectomia subfrênica prolonga a sobrevida.
• Pericardiocentese ou toracocentese sintomática.

TUMORES DO CORPO CAROTÍDEO
• Remoção cirúrgica se possível — discutir com o proprietário sobre o possível desenvolvimento de síndrome de Horner e paralisia da laringe no pós-operatório.

AMBOS
• Possível papel desempenhado pela quimioterapia (doxorrubicina) e radioterapia.

MEDICAÇÕES

MEDICAMENTO(S)
O papel da quimioterapia nessa doença ainda não foi publicado.

CONTRAINDICAÇÕES/INTERAÇÕES POSSÍVEIS
• A quimioterapia pode causar toxicidades sobre o trato GI, a medula óssea e o coração, além de outras toxicidades — buscar orientação se não houver familiaridade com os agentes citotóxicos.
• Não utilizar a doxorrubicina em cães com insuficiência cardíaca congestiva.

ACOMPANHAMENTO

MONITORIZAÇÃO DO PACIENTE
Radiografias torácicas seriadas para monitorização da evolução do tumor e da ocorrência de metástase.

EVOLUÇÃO ESPERADA E PROGNÓSTICO
• Tumores do corpo carotídeo tratados com cirurgia — tempo de sobrevida média de 25 meses e meio.
• Tumores do corpo aórtico — animais tratados com pericardiectomia apresentam tempo de sobrevida média de 730 dias *vs.* animais não submetidos a esse procedimento (tempo de sobrevida média = 42 dias).

DIVERSOS

GESTAÇÃO/FERTILIDADE/REPRODUÇÃO
Não é recomendável cruzar os animais com câncer. A quimioterapia é teratogênica e, portanto, não deve ser administrada a animais prenhes.

VER TAMBÉM
Efusão Pericárdica.

ABREVIATURAS
ECG = eletrocardiograma.
GI = gastrintestinal.

Sugestões de Leitura
Morrison WB. Nonpulmonary intrathoracic cancer. In: Morrison WB, ed., Cancer in Dogs and Cats: Medical and Surgical Management. Jackson, WY: Teton NewMedia, 2002, pp. 513-525.

Autor Rebecca G. Newman
Consultor Editorial Timothy M. Fan

RABDOMIOMA

CONSIDERAÇÕES GERAIS

REVISÃO
- Tumor benigno, extremamente raro, da musculatura estriada, que ocorre apenas com a metade da frequência de seu correlativo maligno.
- Cardíaco — local usual; provavelmente congênito; não apresenta potencial de transformação maligna.
- Extracardíaco — muito raro; relatado na língua e na laringe nos cães e no pavilhão auricular nos gatos adultos de orelha branca.

IDENTIFICAÇÃO
- Cães e gatos.
- Extracardíaco — acomete, sobretudo, animais de meia-idade.
- Sem predileções sexuais ou raciais identificadas.

SINAIS CLÍNICOS
- Cardíaco — em geral, nenhum; raramente, há sinais de insuficiência cardíaca congestiva direita.
- Extracardíaco — tumefação localizada.

CAUSAS E FATORES DE RISCO
Desconhecidos.

DIAGNÓSTICO

DIAGNÓSTICO DIFERENCIAL
Localização no Coração
- Rabdomiossarcoma.
- Linfoma.
- Hemangioma ou hemangiossarcoma.
- Fibroma ou fibrossarcoma.
- Condroma.
- Mixoma.
- Mixofibroma.
- Mesotelioma.
- Neurofibroma.
- Teratoma.
- Lipofibroma.
- Linfangioendotelioma.
- Sarcoma misto de células fusiformes.

Localização na Musculatura Esquelética
- Rabdomiossarcoma.
- Lipoma ou lipossarcoma.
- Mastocitoma.
- Fibrossarcoma.
- Hemangioma ou hemangiossarcoma.
- Doença inflamatória não neoplásica.

Localização na Língua
- Papiloma escamoso ou carcinoma de células escamosas.
- Mioblastoma de células granulares.
- Rabdomiossarcoma.
- Melanoma maligno.
- Mastocitoma.
- Fibrossarcoma.
- Plasmocitoma ou linfoma.
- Hemangioma ou hemangiossarcoma.

Localização na Laringe
- Oncocitoma.
- Rabdomiossarcoma.
- Plasmocitoma extramedular.
- Osteossarcoma.
- Condrossarcoma.
- Fibrossarcoma.
- Mastocitoma.
- Carcinoma de células escamosas.
- Linfoma.

HEMOGRAMA/BIOQUÍMICA/URINÁLISE
Normais.

OUTROS TESTES LABORATORIAIS
N/D.

DIAGNÓSTICO POR IMAGEM
- Radiografia — revela, em geral, densidade de tecido mole; não é um exame proveitoso para as formas extracardíacas.
- Ecocardiografia (cardíaca) — pode revelar a presença de massa pedunculada ou infiltrativa, acometendo mais frequentemente os ventrículos cardíacos; o septo interventricular parece ser o local mais comum.

MÉTODOS DIAGNÓSTICOS
- ECG — pode-se notar a existência de arritmias.
- Biopsia — necessária para a confirmação histológica do diagnóstico.
- Exame citológico do aspirado — ocasionalmente sugere neoplasia mesenquimal, mas não costuma fornecer um diagnóstico definitivo.

ACHADOS PATOLÓGICOS
- Marcadores imuno-histoquímicos úteis — vimentina, actina, desmina e mioglobina; diferenciam entre neoplasias do músculo estriado e neoplasias de outras células fusiformes.
- Doença embrionária — a actina é considerada o marcador mais confiável, porque os rabdomioblastos embrionários se coram positivos para a actina antes de se corarem positivos para a desmina.
- Pode não ser fácil diferenciar de outras neoplasias de células granulares eosinofílicas (p. ex., oncocitoma da laringe).
- Microscopia eletrônica de transmissão também pode ser valiosa para diferenciar rabdomioma e oncocitoma.

TRATAMENTO
- Cardíaco — nenhum.
- Extracardíaco — excisão cirúrgica.
- Glossectomia parcial envolvendo 40-60% da língua é bem tolerada pelos cães.
- Ao contrário de outros tumores laríngeos, os rabdomiomas são minimamente invasivos e podem ser removidos com sucesso com a preservação da função.

MEDICAÇÕES

MEDICAMENTO(S)
N/D.

CONTRAINDICAÇÕES/INTERAÇÕES POSSÍVEIS
N/D.

ACOMPANHAMENTO
- Avaliar mensalmente nos 3 primeiros meses; em seguida, em intervalos de 3-6 meses durante mais um ano.
- Cardíaco — pode ocorrer o desenvolvimento de descompensação cardíaca que evolui para insuficiência cardíaca congestiva.

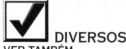

DIVERSOS

VER TAMBÉM
- Rabdomiossarcoma.
- Rabdomiossarcoma da Bexiga Urinária.

ABREVIATURA(S)
- ECG = eletrocardiograma.

Sugestões de Leitura
Mansfield CS, Callanan JJ, McAllister H. Intra-atrial rhabdomyoma causing chylopericardium and right-sided congestive heart failure in a dog. Vet Record 2000, 147:264-267.
O'Hara AJ, McConnell M, Wyatt K, et al. Laryngeal rhabdomyoma in a dog. Australian Vet J 2001, 79:817-821.

Autor Anthony J. Mutsaers
Consultor Editorial Timothy M. Fan

RABDOMIOSSARCOMA

CONSIDERAÇÕES GERAIS

REVISÃO
- Tumor maligno derivado da musculatura estriada (variedade adulta) ou das células mesenquimais pluripotentes embrionárias (variedade juvenil).
- Tumor de músculo estriado mais comum nos animais, embora represente <1% das neoplasias espontâneas.
- Apresenta tipicamente características de crescimento difuso e infiltrativo.
- Relatado nas localizações laríngea, lingual e cardíaca.
- Podem ocorrer metástases agressivas e disseminadas para órgãos como pulmões, fígado, baço, rins e adrenais.
- Nos gatos, foi relatado como sarcoma relacionado ao local de injeção.

IDENTIFICAÇÃO
- Cães e gatos.
- Variedade adulta — animais de meia-idade a idosos.
- Variedade juvenil — cães jovens.
- Sem predileção sexual ou racial.

SINAIS CLÍNICOS
- Massa grande e difusa de tecido mole, geralmente de músculo esquelético.
- Pode sofrer metástase dentro do músculo primário (múltiplos nódulos).
- Na forma cardíaca, podem ocorrer sinais de insuficiência cardíaca congestiva direita.

CAUSAS E FATORES DE RISCO
Desconhecidos.

DIAGNÓSTICO

DIAGNÓSTICO DIFERENCIAL

Localização na Musculatura Esquelética
- Fibrossarcoma.
- Mastocitoma.
- Rabdomioma.
- Lipoma, lipoma infiltrativo ou lipossarcoma.
- Hemangiossarcoma.

Localização na Laringe
- Carcinoma de células escamosas.
- Adenocarcinoma.
- Carcinoma indiferenciado.
- Osteossarcoma.
- Condrossarcoma.
- Fibrossarcoma.
- Mixocondroma.
- Leiomioma.
- Oncocitoma.
- Melanoma.

Localização na Língua
- Carcinoma de células escamosas.
- Mioblastoma de células granulares.
- Rabdomioma.
- Fibrossarcoma.
- Mastocitoma.
- Plasmocitoma ou linfoma.
- Melanoma maligno.
- Hemangioma/hemangiossarcoma.

Localização no Coração
- Hemangiossarcoma.
- Quimiodectoma.
- Rabdomioma.
- Tumor ectópico da tireoide.
- Tumor ectópico da paratireoide.
- Linfoma.
- Neoplasia metastática.

HEMOGRAMA/BIOQUÍMICA/URINÁLISE
- Geralmente normais.
- Pode causar hipoglicemia.

OUTROS TESTES LABORATORIAIS
N/D.

DIAGNÓSTICO POR IMAGEM
- Radiografia, TC ou RM revela a presença de massa densa de tecido mole.
- Ecocardiografia (cardíaca) — pode indicar a existência de massa pedunculada ou infiltrativa.

MÉTODOS DIAGNÓSTICOS
- Exame citológico — revela a neoplasia mesenquimal maligna; geralmente não fornece o diagnóstico definitivo (necessita do exame histopatológico).
- ECG — pode-se notar a ocorrência de arritmias.

ACHADOS PATOLÓGICOS
- Existem duas variedades com base nas características histomorfológicas.
- Adulto — células tumorais grandes, pleomórficas e alongadas, que possuem estriação cruzada e citoplasma eosinofílico.
- Juvenil — características embrionárias e alveolares.
- Microscopia eletrônica de transmissão — pode ser necessária para o diagnóstico definitivo.
- Exame imuno-histológico — talvez seja requerido para o diagnóstico definitivo; marcadores úteis: actina, desmina e mioglobina.

TRATAMENTO

- Excisão cirúrgica — difícil por causa da natureza invasiva.
- Glossectomia parcial envolvendo 40-60% da língua é bem tolerada pelos cães.
- Para tumores da laringe, talvez haja necessidade de laringectomia total com traqueostomia permanente.
- Amputação de algum membro acometido — pode ser um método adequado para o tratamento de doença local.
- Radioterapia — pode ser valiosa para tumores localizados, de baixo grau/bem diferenciados, particularmente como tratamento adjuvante, se ainda houver doença microscópica no pós-operatório.
- Consultar um veterinário especialista em oncologia para falar sobre as opções terapêuticas.

MEDICAÇÕES

MEDICAMENTO(S)
- Quimioterapia — pode representar um tratamento paliativo; nenhum esquema específico foi avaliado.
- Procurar por orientação antes de iniciar o tratamento caso não se esteja familiarizado com o uso de agentes citotóxicos.

CONTRAINDICAÇÕES/INTERAÇÕES POSSÍVEIS
Quimioterapia — pode ser mielossupressora e provocar intoxicação gastrintestinal; é muito importante monitorizar o paciente com rigor.

ACOMPANHAMENTO

Exame físico, radiografia torácica e ultrassonografia abdominal — mensalmente por 3 meses; depois, a cada 3-6 meses.

DIVERSOS

VER TAMBÉM
- Rabdomioma.
- Rabdomiossarcoma da Bexiga Urinária.

ABREVIATURA(S)
- ECG = eletrocardiograma.
- RM = ressonância magnética.
- TC = tomografia computadorizada.

Sugestões de Leitura
Lascelles BDX, McInnes E, Dobson JM, et al. Rhabdomyosarcoma of the tongue in a dog. J Small Anim Pract 1998, 39:587-591.
Perez J, Perez-Rivero A, Montoya A, et al. Right-sided heart failure in a dog with primary cardiac rhabdomyosarcoma. JAAHA 1998, 34:208-211.

Autor Anthony J. Mutsaers
Consultor Editorial Timothy M. Fan

RABDOMIOSSARCOMA DA BEXIGA URINÁRIA

CONSIDERAÇÕES GERAIS

REVISÃO
• Tumor maligno derivado das células mioblásticas pluripotentes ou estriadas de origem mesenquimal que circundam os ductos de Müller ou de Wolff em desenvolvimento.
• Também podem ser denominados de rabdomiossarcomas "botrioides" em virtude do aspecto em forma de cacho de uva.
• Metástase — ocorre disseminação para os linfonodos e órgãos viscerais; prevalência não claramente definida.
• Constitui <1% de todos os tumores da bexiga urinária.

IDENTIFICAÇÃO
• Cães e, muito raramente, gatos.
• A maior parte deles ocorre nas cadelas pertencentes a raças de grande porte com <18 meses de vida.
• Raça São Bernardo — pode estar super-representada.

SINAIS CLÍNICOS
• Predominantemente compatíveis com doença do trato urinário inferior.
• Hematúria.
• Estrangúria.
• Polaciúria.
• Possível retenção urinária.

CAUSAS E FATORES DE RISCO
Desconhecidos.

DIAGNÓSTICO

DIAGNÓSTICO DIFERENCIAL
• Cistite bacteriana.
• Urocistolitíase.
• Carcinoma de células de transição.
• Carcinoma de células escamosas.
• Fibroma ou fibrossarcoma.
• Linfoma.
• Pólipos vesicais.
• Uretrite granulomatosa.

HEMOGRAMA/BIOQUÍMICA/URINÁLISE
• Exames de sangue — costumam permanecer normais.
• Urinálise — geralmente revela hematúria.
• Exame citológico do sedimento urinário — pode-se encontrar pleomorfismo celular e estriações cruzadas compatíveis com o rabdomiossarcoma.

OUTROS TESTES LABORATORIAIS
Os testes disponíveis no mercado para detecção do antígeno tumoral da bexiga não serão úteis, pois foram concebidos para o carcinoma de células de transição. Também se observam resultados falso-positivos na presença de hematúria.

DIAGNÓSTICO POR IMAGEM
• Ultrassonografia da bexiga ou cistouretrografia de contraste duplo.
• Pielografia intravenosa — avaliar a existência de qualquer massa no trígono vesical; avaliar os ureteres e a pelve renal.

MÉTODOS DIAGNÓSTICOS
O diagnóstico é confirmado a partir de amostras histopatológicas obtidas na cirurgia exploratória ou na cistoscopia.

ACHADOS PATOLÓGICOS
• Marcadores imuno-histoquímicos úteis — vimentina, actina, desmina e mioglobina; diferenciam entre neoplasias de músculo estriado e outras neoplasias de células fusiformes.
• As informações ultraestruturais obtidas a partir da microscopia eletrônica de transmissão também podem ser valiosas.

TRATAMENTO
• A excisão cirúrgica é recomendada, embora seja difícil por causa do caráter invasivo.
• Ressecção cirúrgica — pode ser facilitada pela injeção de solução salina na submucosa da bexiga urinária para ajudar a estabelecer um plano de dissecção.
• A colocação de *stent* na uretra ou o procedimento de cateterização transabdominal podem ser utilizados para tratar uma possível obstrução.

MEDICAÇÕES

MEDICAMENTO(S)
• Quimioterapia adjuvante — recomendável; não só auxilia no controle ou na eliminação da doença neoplásica residual após a ressecção cirúrgica, mas também combate o desenvolvimento de doença metastática.
• Não foram relatados os resultados com a quimioterapia em ensaios controlados.
• Ciclo de 21 dias — utilizado com sucesso em um único cão; doxorrubicina (30 mg/m² IV no dia zero) e ciclofosfamida (75 mg/m² VO nos dias 3, 4, 5 e 6); administrar o total de quatro ciclos; o crescimento de célula tumoral indica uma clara evidência de resistência à quimioterapia. Consultar um veterinário especialista em oncologia em busca de mais recomendações terapêuticas.

CONTRAINDICAÇÕES/INTERAÇÕES POSSÍVEIS
A quimioterapia pode ser tóxica; buscar por orientação antes de iniciar o tratamento caso não se esteja familiarizado com o uso de agentes citotóxicos.

ACOMPANHAMENTO
• Avaliar a cada 21 dias durante a quimioterapia e, depois, a cada 3 meses; envolve a realização de exame físico, hemograma completo, perfil bioquímico sérico e urinálise.
• Radiografia torácica e ultrassonografia abdominal — a cada 3 meses durante o primeiro ano após a cirurgia.

DIVERSOS

DISTÚRBIOS ASSOCIADOS
• Osteopatia hipertrófica — ocasionalmente.
• É comum a ocorrência de cistite bacteriana concomitante; escolher os antibióticos com base na cultura bacteriana e no antibiograma.

SINÔNIMO(S)
• Rabdomiossarcoma botrioide (i. e., aspecto semelhante a cacho de uvas).
• Rabdomiossarcoma embrionário.

VER TAMBÉM
• Rabdomioma.
• Rabdomiossarcoma.

Sugestões de Leitura
Kuwamura M, Yoshida M, Yamate J, et al. Urinary bladder rhabdomyosarcoma (sarcoma botryoides) in a Young Newfoundland dog. J Vet Med Sci 1998, 60:619-621.

Autor Anthony J. Mutsaers
Consultor Editorial Timothy M. Fan

Raiva

CONSIDERAÇÕES GERAIS

DEFINIÇÃO
Poliencefalite viral grave, invariavelmente fatal, dos animais de sangue quente, incluindo os seres humanos.

FISIOPATOLOGIA
Vírus — penetra no organismo através de ferida (geralmente a partir da mordida de um animal raivoso) ou via mucosas; replica-se nos miócitos; dissemina-se para a junção neuromuscular e feixes neurotendíneos; percorre o SNC via líquido intra-axonal dentro dos nervos periféricos; difunde-se por todo o SNC; por fim, espalha-se de modo centrífugo dentro dos neurônios periféricos, sensoriais e motores.

SISTEMA(S) ACOMETIDO(S)
• Nervoso — encefalite clínica, paralítica ou furiosa.
• Glândulas salivares — contêm grandes quantidades de partículas virais infectantes, que são liberadas na saliva.

GENÉTICA
Nenhuma.

INCIDÊNCIA/PREVALÊNCIA
• Incidência da doença nos animais infectados — elevada (aproxima-se de 100%).
• Prevalência — baixa de modo geral; pode ser significante nas áreas enzoóticas; especialmente elevada em países subdesenvolvidos, onde a vacinação de cães e gatos não é uma rotina.

DISTRIBUIÇÃO GEOGRÁFICA
• Mundial.
• Exceções — Nova Zelândia, Havaí, Japão, Islândia e partes da Escandinávia.
• Cepas adaptadas a certas espécies — distribuições geográficas específicas dentro dos países endêmicos.

IDENTIFICAÇÃO
Espécies
• Todos os mamíferos de sangue quente, incluindo cães, gatos e seres humanos.
• EUA — cinco cepas endêmicas nas populações de raposas, guaxinins, gambás, coiotes e morcegos insetívoros; todas as cinco cepas podem ser transmitidas a cães e gatos.

Raça(s) Predominante(s)
Nenhuma.

Idade Média e Faixa Etária
Nenhuma, embora os animais adultos que entram em contato com animais selvagens estejam sob maior risco.

Sexo Predominante
Nenhum.

SINAIS CLÍNICOS
Comentários Gerais
• Muito variáveis; uma apresentação atípica constitui a regra e não a exceção.
• Três estágios progressivos da doença — prodrômico; furioso; e paralítico; 90% dos gatos raivosos apresentam a forma furiosa.

Achados Anamnésicos
• Mudança de atitude — solidão; apreensão, nervosismo, ansiedade; timidez ou agressividade não usual.
• Comportamento errático — mordidas ou estalos; lambedura ou mastigação no local da ferida; mordeduras na gaiola/jaula; andar a esmo e sem destino; excitabilidade; irritabilidade; indocilidade.
• Desorientação.
• Musculares — incoordenação; crises convulsivas; paralisia.
• Alteração no tom do latido.
• Excesso de salivação ou de espuma na boca.

Achados do Exame Físico
• Todos ou alguns dos achados da anamnese.
• Paralisia mandibular e laríngea, com a mandíbula caída.
• Incapacidade de engolir.
• Hipersalivação.
• Febre.
• Pupilas dilatadas — irresponsivas à luz; anisocoria.

CAUSAS
Vírus da raiva — vírus RNA de fita simples, envelopado e em formato de projétil balístico; gênero *Lyssavirus*; família *Rhabdoviridae*.

FATORES DE RISCO
• Exposição a animais selvagens, especialmente gambás, guaxinins, morcegos e raposas.
• Falta de vacinação adequada contra a raiva.
• Feridas por mordedura ou arranhões de cães, gatos ou animais selvagens não vacinados.
• Exposição a aerossóis em cavernas de morcegos.
• Animal imunocomprometido — utilização de vacina antirrábica de vírus vivo modificado.

DIAGNÓSTICO

DIAGNÓSTICO DIFERENCIAL
• A raiva deve ser seriamente considerada em qualquer cão ou gato que apresente alterações não habituais de humor ou comportamento ou que mostre sinais neurológicos inexplicáveis;
CUIDADO: manipular com cuidado considerável para evitar a possível transmissão do vírus para indivíduos que cuidem ou tratem do animal.
• Qualquer doença neurológica — tumor cerebral; encefalite viral.
• Ferida na cabeça — identificar as lesões por ferimentos.
• Paralisia da laringe.
• Asfixia.
• Infecção pelo vírus da pseudorraiva.

HEMOGRAMA/BIOQUÍMICA/URINÁLISE
Sem alterações hematológicas ou bioquímicas características.

OUTROS TESTES LABORATORIAIS
N/D.

DIAGNÓSTICO POR IMAGEM
N/D.

MÉTODOS DIAGNÓSTICOS
• LCS — podem ser observados aumentos mínimos no conteúdo de proteínas e na contagem de leucócitos.
• Teste de imunofluorescência direta do tecido nervoso — teste rápido e sensível; coletar o cérebro, a cabeça ou todo o corpo de pequeno animal que tenha morrido ou sido sacrificado; refrigerar a amostra imediatamente; enviar a laboratório oficial (ou seja, aprovado pelo estado) para o diagnóstico da raiva; **CUIDADO:** tomar extremo cuidado ao coletar, manipular e enviar essas amostras.
• Teste de imunofluorescência direta do tecido dérmico — biopsia de pele da área das vibrissas sensoriais do maxilar, incluindo folículos pilosos subcutâneos profundos; teste aprovado para o diagnóstico em seres humanos; resultado preciso se positivo, embora o resultado negativo não descarte a raiva.
• Título de anticorpos contra a raiva — um título sorológico de 0,5 UI/mL é considerado adequado para proteção em pessoas e animais vacinados.

ACHADOS PATOLÓGICOS
• Alterações macroscópicas — geralmente ausentes, apesar da doença neurológica notável.
• Alterações histopatológicas — poliencefalite aguda a crônica; aumento gradual na gravidade do processo inflamatório não supurativo no SNC à medida que a doença evolui; grandes neurônios dentro do cérebro podem conter as clássicas inclusões intracitoplasmáticas (corpúsculos de Negri).

TRATAMENTO

CUIDADO(S) DE SAÚDE ADEQUADO(S)
Rigorosamente como paciente internado.

CUIDADO(S) DE ENFERMAGEM
Administrar com extremo cuidado.

ATIVIDADE
• Confinar em área segura de quarentena com sinalização clara indicando suspeita de raiva.
• Corredores ou jaulas/gaiolas devem ficar trancados; apenas pessoas designadas devem ter acesso.
• Fornecer água e alimento sem abrir as portas da gaiola/jaula ou do corredor.

DIETA
Ração úmida pastosa; a maior parte dos pacientes não se alimenta.

ORIENTAÇÃO AO PROPRIETÁRIO
• Informar o proprietário de forma minuciosa sobre a seriedade da raiva para o animal e sobre o potencial zoonótico.
• Questionar o proprietário sobre qualquer exposição humana (p. ex., contato, mordedura) e alertar as pessoas sobre a importância em procurar um médico imediatamente.
• A autoridade local de saúde pública deve ser notificada.

CONSIDERAÇÕES CIRÚRGICAS
• Em geral, nenhuma.
• Biopsia cutânea — pode ajudar a estabelecer o diagnóstico antes da morte; deve ser confirmado pela identificação a partir do tecido neurológico (SNC).

MEDICAÇÕES

MEDICAMENTO(S) DE ESCOLHA
• Não há tratamento.
• Se houver certeza quanto ao diagnóstico, fica indicada a eutanásia do animal.

CONTRAINDICAÇÕES
Nenhuma.

RAIVA

PRECAUÇÕES
N/D.

INTERAÇÕES POSSÍVEIS
N/D.

MEDICAMENTO(S) ALTERNATIVO(S)
N/D.

ACOMPANHAMENTO

MONITORIZAÇÃO DO PACIENTE
• Todos os pacientes com suspeita de raiva devem ser isolados de forma segura e monitorizados quanto ao desenvolvimento de qualquer alteração de humor, mudança de atitude ou presença de sinais clínicos que possam sugerir o diagnóstico.
• Um cão ou gato aparentemente saudável que morda ou arranhe uma pessoa deve ser monitorizado por um período de 10 dias; se não houver nenhum sinal de doença no animal dentro desse período, a pessoa não sofreu exposição ao vírus; cães e gatos não eliminam o vírus por mais de 3 dias antes do desenvolvimento da doença clínica.
• Um cão ou gato não vacinado que seja mordido ou exposto a animal raivoso conhecido deve ficar de quarentena por até 6 meses ou de acordo com os regulamentos locais ou estaduais.

PREVENÇÃO
• Vacinas (cães e gatos) — vacinar de acordo com as recomendações padronizadas e as exigências locais e estaduais; todos os cães e gatos com qualquer exposição potencial a animais selvagens ou a outros cães; vacinar após 12 semanas de vida; em seguida, 12 meses mais tarde; e, então, a cada 3 anos, usando a vacina aprovada para esse período*; utilizar apenas vacinas inativadas ou de vetores recombinantes para os gatos.
• Países livres da raiva — cães e gatos que entram nesses países devem ficar em quarentena por longos períodos, geralmente de 6 meses.
• Desinfecção — qualquer área, gaiola/jaula, comedouro ou instrumento contaminados devem ser rigorosamente desinfetados; utilizar a diluição de 1:32 (120 mL por ~4 litros) de alvejante doméstico [Cândida®, por exemplo] para inativar o vírus com rapidez.

COMPLICAÇÕES POSSÍVEIS
Decorrentes de paralisia ou mudanças de atitude.

EVOLUÇÃO ESPERADA E PROGNÓSTICO
• Prognóstico — grave; quase invariavelmente fatal.
• Todos os cães e gatos com infecção clínica sucumbirão dentro de 1-10 dias do início dos sinais clínicos; frequentemente dentro de 3-4 dias.

DIVERSOS

DISTÚRBIOS ASSOCIADOS
Nenhum.

FATORES RELACIONADOS COM A IDADE
Nenhum.

POTENCIAL ZOONÓTICO
• Extremo.
• Os seres humanos devem evitar a mordida de animal raivoso ou de animal assintomático que esteja incubando a doença.
• Os casos de raiva devem ficar estritamente em quarentena e confinados para prevenir a exposição aos seres humanos e a outros animais.
• Regulamentos estaduais e locais devem ser seguidos cuidadosa e completamente.

GESTAÇÃO/FERTILIDADE/REPRODUÇÃO
Infecção durante a prenhez será fatal à mãe.

ABREVIATURA(S)
• LCS = líquido cerebrospinal.
• SNC = sistema nervoso central.

RECURSOS DA INTERNET
www.cdc.gov/rabies/.

Sugestões de Leitura
Barr MC, Olsen CW, Scott FW. Feline viral diseases. In: Ettinger SJ, Feldman EC, eds., Veterinary Internal Medicine. Philadelphia: Saunders, 1995, pp. 409-439.
Frymus T, Addie D, Belák S, et al. Feline rabies: ABCD guidelines on prevention and management. J Feline Med Surg 2009, 11:585-593.
Greene CE, Rupprecht CE. Rabies and other Lyssavirus infections. In: Greene CE, ed., Infectious Diseases of the Dog and Cat, 3rd ed. St. Louis: Saunders Elsevier, 2006, pp. 167-183.
Leslie M, Auslander M, Conti L, et al. Compendium of animal rabies prevention and control, 2006. JAVMA 2006, 228:858-864.
Richards JR, Elston TH, Ford RB, et al. The 2006 American Association of Feline Practioners Feline Vaccine Advisory Panel Report. JAVMA 2006, 229:1405-1441.

Autor Fred W. Scott
Consultor Editorial Stephen C. Barr

---

* N. T.: Informação referente aos países do hemisfério Norte. No Brasil, a vacinação contra a raiva começa a partir de 4 meses de vida; o reforço deve ser anual.

Reabsorção dos Dentes em Felinos (Reabsorção Odontoclástica)

CONSIDERAÇÕES GERAIS

DEFINIÇÃO
Reabsorções dentárias de etiologia desconhecida.

FISIOPATOLOGIA
• Até o momento, a causa de reabsorção dos dentes em felinos é desconhecida; as células chamadas odontoclastos, encontradas nos defeitos, fazem com que a estrutura dentária se dissolva.
• Os odontoclastos aderem-se à superfície lacunar do tecido dentário intacto; conforme a reabsorção evolui, um tecido de reparação semelhante a osso ou cimento cobre a dentina escavada; o tecido de granulação inflamado frequentemente ocupa os defeitos na coroa do dente. • Grande parte da reabsorção ocorre na raiz; pode ocorrer reabsorção tanto interna como externa; com o tempo, a remodelagem substitui o tecido da dentina por tecidos semelhantes a osso ou cimento que, ao exame radiográfico, aparecem como ancilose.

SISTEMA(S) ACOMETIDO(S)
Gastrintestinal — cavidade bucal.

INCIDÊNCIA/PREVALÊNCIA
• Quase 50% dos gatos com mais de 5 anos de idade terão, pelo menos, um único dente acometido por reabsorção. • A prevalência aumenta com o avanço da idade.

IDENTIFICAÇÃO
Espécies
Gatos.

Raça(s) Predominante(s)
Possivelmente gatos Asiático de pelo curto, Siamês, Persa e Abissínio.

SINAIS CLÍNICOS
Achados Anamnésicos
• A maioria dos gatos acometidos não revela sinais clínicos; alguns exibem hipersalivação ou dificuldade de mastigação; outro gatos apanham e largam o alimento (especialmente ração dura) durante a refeição; outros manifestam um chiado ou assobio enquanto mastigam. • Alguns gatos apresentam mudanças de comportamento — reclusivo ou agressivo.

Achados do Exame Físico
• Um aplicador com extremidade de algodão aplicado sobre a reabsorção dentária sob suspeita (estágios 2-4) geralmente causa dor evidenciada por espasmos mandibulares. • A reabsorção dos dentes pode ocorrer acima ou abaixo da margem gengival; a maioria delas é observada primeiramente na superfície labial ou bucal próxima à junção cimento-esmalte, onde a gengiva livre encontra a superfície do dente, embora as lesões radiculares geralmente precedam as reabsorções; a formação de cálculo e a presença de gengiva hiperplásica podem mascarar a lesão. • A reabsorção dentária pode ser encontrada em qualquer dente; os dentes mais comumente acometidos são os terceiros pré-molares e molares mandibulares, seguidos pelos terceiros e quartos pré-molares maxilares. • Sob anestesia geral, as lesões são examinadas com um explorador dental delicado que ajuda a identificar as lesões subgengivais coronais ao osso alveolar; a área de furcação é um local frequente e o examinador deve distinguir uma lesão reabsortiva de doença limitada à perda óssea alveolar.

Classificação de Reabsorção Dentária
• Estágio 1 (Reabsorção dentária 1): perda leve de tecido duro do dente (cimento ou cimento e esmalte).
• Estágio 2 (Reabsorção dentária 2): perda moderada de tecido duro do dente (cimento ou cimento e esmalte com perda da dentina que não se estende até a cavidade pulpar).
• Estágio 3 (Reabsorção dentária 3): perda profunda de tecido duro do dente (cimento ou cimento e esmalte com perda da dentina que se estende para a cavidade pulpar); a maior parte do dente conserva sua integridade.
• Estágio 4 (Reabsorção dentária 4): perda extensa de tecido duro do dente (cimento ou cimento e esmalte com perda da dentina que se estende para a cavidade pulpar); grande parte do dente perdeu sua integridade.
  ○ Reabsorção dentária 4a: a coroa e a raiz são igualmente acometidas.
  ○ Reabsorção dentária 4b: a coroa é mais gravemente acometida que a raiz.
  ○ Reabsorção dentária 4c: a raiz é mais gravemente acometida que a coroa.
• Estágio 5 (Reabsorção dentária 5): os resquícios de tecido duro do dente são visíveis apenas como radiopacidades irregulares, mas o revestimento gengival está completo. Essa classificação baseia-se na hipótese de que a reabsorção dentária seja um problema progressivo.
• Ver *Diagnóstico por Imagem* em busca de outro esquema de classificação (Tipo 1-3).

CAUSAS
• A etiologia é desconhecida; provavelmente multifatorial.
• O foco atual de pesquisas está voltado para as causas nutricional (p. ex., ingestão elevada de vitamina D), inflamatória e hereditária.
• Hiper-reatividade a células inflamatórias, placa dentária e/ou cálculo; endotoxinas; prostaglandinas, citocinas e proteinases estão sob investigação.

DIAGNÓSTICO

DIAGNÓSTICO DIFERENCIAL
• Síndrome de estomatite linfocítica-plasmocitária.
• Outro tipo de lesão reabsortiva (Tipo I) pode ser observado nos casos em que a doença periodontal resultou em retração da gengiva e exposição da raiz. Essas superfícies radiculares expostas podem revelar ampla reabsorção externa, mas não haverá envolvimento radicular extra (reabsorção odontoclástica).

DIAGNÓSTICO POR IMAGEM
• A radiologia intrabucal é essencial na formulação do diagnóstico definitivo e na elaboração do tratamento. • O aspecto radiográfico varia desde defeitos radiolúcidos (radiotransparentes) minúsculos do dente principalmente na junção cimento-esmalte até ancilose com reabsorção óssea alvéolo-radicular por substituição. • A reabsorção dentária também é classificada como Tipo 1-3, com base no aspecto radiográfico do dente e do espaço do ligamento periodontal. • Tipo 1 — uma radiotransparência focal ou multifocal está presente no dente com radiopacidade normal sob outros aspectos e espaço normal do ligamento periodontal. • Tipo 2 — estreitamento ou desaparecimento do espaço do ligamento periodontal em pelo menos algumas áreas e radiopacidade reduzida de parte do dente. • Tipo 3 — características de ambos os tipos (1 e 2) estão presentes no mesmo dente. Um dente com esse aspecto exibe não só áreas de normalidade e estreitamento ou perda do espaço do ligamento periodontal, mas também há radiotransparência focal ou multifocal no dente e radiopacidade reduzida em outras áreas do dente.

TRATAMENTO

DIETA
Adicione água à dieta para amolecê-la.

ORIENTAÇÃO AO PROPRIETÁRIO
A escovação diária dos dentes pode ajudar a controlar a formação de placa.

CONSIDERAÇÕES CIRÚRGICAS
• Lesões de estágio 1 — observa-se um defeito superficial; a lesão é minimamente sensível, pois não penetrou na dentina; a terapia envolve a limpeza e o polimento minuciosos dos dentes; os procedimentos de gengivectomia e odontoplastia são terapias adjuvantes.
• Lesões de estágio 2 — penetram na dentina; frequentemente necessitam de extração via exposição de retalho ou redução da coroa e fechamento da gengiva (adiante).
• Lesões de estágio 3 — invadem o sistema endodôntico; exigem a extração via exposição de retalho ou redução da coroa (adiante).
• Lesões de estágio 4 — a coroa está erodida ou fraturada, permanecendo parte dela; a gengiva cresce sobre os fragmentos radiculares, produzindo uma lesão sanguinolenta sensível à inserção de sonda periodontal; talvez haja necessidade de extração adicional (adiante).
• Lesões de estágio 5 — a coroa desapareceu, mas restaram fragmentos radiculares escassos; promova o debridamento de qualquer área inflamada. Se o ligamento periodontal estiver evidente (Tipos 1 e 3), o dente deverá ser submetido à extração cirúrgica via exposição de retalho.
• Se o ligamento periodontal não estiver evidente por causa de substituição da raiz (Tipo 2), a coroa poderá ser reduzida abaixo da gengiva com o uso de broca de alta velocidade arrefecida por água, seguida pelo fechamento da gengiva sobre a raiz.

MEDICAÇÕES
Nenhuma.

DIVERSOS

SINÔNIMOS
• Erosão da linha cervical. • Erosão dentária subgengival crônica. • Lesões reabsortivas odontoclásticas externas. • Lesões reabsortivas odontoclásticas felinas. • Erosão bucocervical idiopática. • Lesões cervicais (ou seja, na região do colo do dente). • Lesões reabsortivas subgengivais.

Autores Jan Bellows e Alexander M. Reiter
Consultor Editorial Heidi B. Lobprise

REAÇÕES ALIMENTARES (GASTRINTESTINAIS) ADVERSAS

CONSIDERAÇÕES GERAIS

DEFINIÇÃO
- Reações alimentares adversas abrangem distúrbios com alguma base imunológica (alergia alimentar), reação não imunológica (intolerância alimentar) e reações tóxicas (intoxicação alimentar).
- As reações alimentares adversas podem estar associadas a vômito e/ou diarreia em cães e gatos. Em um sentido prático, os quadros de alergia e intolerância alimentares podem ter sinais, diagnósticos e tratamentos semelhantes e, portanto, talvez não sejam facilmente distinguíveis.
- A alergia alimentar é uma causa comum de sinais cutâneos, como prurido, e ocasionalmente pode estar associada a sinais gastrintestinais.

FISIOPATOLOGIA
- A patogênese da alergia alimentar envolve eventos imunológicos complexos: ruptura na barreira da mucosa intestinal, desregulação das respostas imunes, e perda de tolerância oral. A maioria das alergias alimentares deve-se a reações de hipersensibilidade tipo 1. Os principais alérgenos alimentares incluem as proteínas de leite, ovos, carne bovina, frango e vegetais (milho, trigo e soja).
- A intolerância alimentar pode ser atribuída a reações idiossincráticas a ingredientes ou aditivos alimentares, reações farmacológicas a compostos na dieta, defeitos ou deficiências nas vias metabólicas necessárias para utilização do alimento, ou reações tóxicas a ingredientes alimentares ou alimentos estragados.
- As reações tóxicas a alimentos podem ocorrer quando um gênero alimentício é ingerido em grandes quantidades (p. ex., intoxicação por cebola).
- O alimento que está estragado ou que contém microrganismos ou suas toxinas podem produzir uma ampla variedade de sinais clínicos e gravidade.

SISTEMA(S) ACOMETIDO(S)
- Dermatológico.
- Endócrino/Metabólico.
- Gastrintestinal.

GENÉTICA
- Alergia alimentar hereditária é observada em Wheaten terriers de pelo macio.
- Enteropatia sensível ao glúten é vista principalmente em Setters irlandeses.
- Siameses e gatos mestiços dessa raça podem estar sob alto risco de reações alimentares (gastrintestinais).
- As especificidades de uma base genética não são bem definidas.

INCIDÊNCIA/PREVALÊNCIA
Mais comuns em gatos que nos cães.

DISTRIBUIÇÃO GEOGRÁFICA
N/D.

IDENTIFICAÇÃO
- Cães e gatos de qualquer idade ou raça e ambos os sexos podem ser acometidos.
- Os cães da raça Setter irlandês são predispostos à enteropatia sensível ao glúten; esses animais tendem a exibir os sinais clínicos por volta de 4-7 meses de vida.
- Os cães acometidos por enteropatias crônicas e responsivos à dieta tendem a ser jovens adultos.

SINAIS CLÍNICOS

Comentários Gerais
- Intolerância alimentar costuma causar diarreia (proveniente do intestino delgado ou grosso), vômito, flatulência, anorexia e desconforto abdominal.
- Alergia alimentar é uma causa comum de sinais cutâneos, como prurido, que pode estar associado a sinais gastrintestinais.

Achados Anamnésicos
- Intolerância alimentar aguda pode acompanhar o fornecimento de um novo gênero alimentício, uma nova fonte alimentar ou uma mudança da dieta.
- O proprietário pode relatar a interrupção dos sinais clínicos no estado de jejum ou em alguns dias após ensaio alimentar com dieta de eliminação.

Achados do Exame Físico
Em geral, o exame físico é inespecífico, mas pode revelar desconforto e distensão abdominais, flatulência ou má condição corporal.

CAUSAS
- Reações idiossincráticas a aditivos alimentares — corantes, conservantes (BHA [butilidroxianisol], glutamato monossódico, nitrato de sódio, dióxido de enxofre, etc.), temperos/condimentos, propileno glicol, etc.
- Reações farmacológicas — substâncias vasoativas (ou seja, histamina), agentes psicoativos, estimulantes (ou seja, teobromina, cafeína), etc.
- Deficiências ou defeitos metabólicos — defeitos enzimáticos da borda em escova (ou seja, deficiência da lactase), erros inatos do metabolismo, aminopeptidase N (em enteropatia sensível ao glúten).
- Reações tóxicas a alimentos ou comida estragada — temperos/condimentos, toxicidade do oxalato, toxicidade da lectina, aflatoxicose, N-propil dissulfeto*, ergotismo, botulismo, alimentação inadequada ou imprudência alimentar, etc.

FATORES DE RISCO
- Cães jovens da raça Setter irlandês suscetíveis à enteropatia sensível ao glúten podem estar sob maior risco de desenvolvimento da doença se expostos a esse ingrediente em uma idade precoce.
- Há suspeita de suscetibilidade genética do hospedeiro em Wheaten terriers.

DIAGNÓSTICO

DIAGNÓSTICO DIFERENCIAL
- Enteropatia inflamatória, parasitismo, insuficiência pancreática exócrina, e diarreia responsiva a antibióticos são capazes de produzir sinais semelhantes àqueles de reações alimentares adversas.
- Um diagnóstico presuntivo de reação alimentar adversa é feito mediante a resolução dos sinais clínicos enquanto se fornece uma dieta de eliminação com uma nova fonte proteica em sua composição.
- Algumas vezes, tenta-se o uso de dietas caseiras; no entanto, essas tentativas não são planejadas para administração a longo prazo.

* N. T.: Toxina presente no alho e na cebola.

- Os sinais gastrintestinais frequentemente melhoram em alguns dias, sobretudo em gatos.

HEMOGRAMA/BIOQUÍMICA/URINÁLISE
Em geral, normais; ocasionalmente, os animais com alergia alimentar podem ter eosinofilia.

OUTROS TESTES LABORATORIAIS
- Poucos testes diagnósticos são específicos.
- Os testes diagnósticos são realizados para descartar outros diagnósticos diferenciais e tratar os fatores indutores de complicação.
- Os níveis séricos de folato e cobalamina em jejum são úteis para avaliar a presença de hipocobalaminemia e a distribuição do comprometimento da mucosa do intestino delgado.
- Descartar o quadro de insuficiência pancreática exócrina pelo ensaio de imunorreatividade semelhante à da tripsina sérica.
- A detecção de imunoglobulinas séricas antígeno-específicas não é geralmente recomendada, pois essas imunoglobulinas não são consideradas confiáveis em animais.

DIAGNÓSTICO POR IMAGEM
- Os exames de radiografias ou ultrassonografia do abdome podem ser úteis para excluir os diagnósticos diferenciais.
- A avaliação com Doppler (ultrassom) pode detectar alterações no fluxo sanguíneo através das artérias celíaca e mesentérica cranial de cães.

MÉTODOS DIAGNÓSTICOS
- Oferecer uma dieta de eliminação durante, pelo menos, 2 semanas em gatos e 3-4 semanas em cães com sinais gastrintestinais.
- Após a melhora do animal sob uma dieta de exclusão, utilizar a exposição provocativa a ingredientes isolados sequenciais para identificar uma intolerância alimentar com precisão. Apesar de ser considerada como uma medida excelente em termos técnicos, ela geralmente é impraticável no ambiente clínico.
- Em geral, a alimentação exclusiva com uma nova fonte proteica por tempo indefinido é necessária para evitar recidiva clínica.
- Efetuar o exame de urinálise e mensurar a relação de proteína:creatinina urinária (se indicada) em Wheaten terriers alérgicos para fazer a triagem de perda proteica glomerular concomitante.

ACHADOS PATOLÓGICOS
- Em casos de alergia alimentar, podem ser observadas as alterações de atrofia vilosa e enterite linfocítica-plasmocitária leve.
- Biopsia endoscópica da mucosa pode confirmar a presença de inflamação intestinal em animais com alergia alimentar.

TRATAMENTO

CUIDADO(S) DE SAÚDE ADEQUADO(S)
Tratar geralmente em um esquema ambulatorial.

CUIDADO(S) DE ENFERMAGEM
N/D.

ATIVIDADE
Sem restrições.

DIETA
- Fornecer uma dieta com nova fonte proteica, conforme descrição prévia.

Reações Alimentares (Gastrintestinais) Adversas

- Os gatos costumam ser sensíveis a mais de um ingrediente alimentar.
- Existem inúmeras rações comerciais de alta qualidade disponíveis no mercado para uso em cães e gatos.
- Se essa abordagem for utilizada, é recomendável a avaliação dos ingredientes das várias dietas disponíveis para determinar se existe qualquer padrão capaz de ajudar a identificar o(s) ingrediente(s) ofensor(es).

ORIENTAÇÃO AO PROPRIETÁRIO
Alertar contra o fornecimento de restos de comida ou a variação de uma dieta fixa.

CONSIDERAÇÕES CIRÚRGICAS
N/D.

MEDICAÇÕES

MEDICAMENTO(S) DE ESCOLHA
- Geralmente nenhuma medicação é utilizada.
- Os problemas associados (p. ex., diarreia responsiva a antibióticos ou enteropatia inflamatória) talvez necessitem de terapia médica conforme sugerido nas seções específicas para esses problemas.

CONTRAINDICAÇÕES
N/D.

PRECAUÇÕES
N/D.

INTERAÇÕES POSSÍVEIS
N/D.

MEDICAMENTO(S) ALTERNATIVO(S)
N/D.

ACOMPANHAMENTO

MONITORIZAÇÃO DO PACIENTE
- Avaliar a eficácia da dieta de eliminação, observando-se a melhora dos sinais clínicos.
- Considerar a repetição do exame em busca de doença primária da mucosa (enteropatia inflamatória) se os animais forem irresponsivos à terapia nutricional.

PREVENÇÃO
- É recomendado evitar o(s) ingrediente(s) alimentar(es) ofensor(es).
- Se nenhum ingrediente específico for identificado, é aconselhável a adesão a uma dieta de exclusão fixa.

COMPLICAÇÕES POSSÍVEIS
Diarreia responsiva a antibióticos e enteropatia inflamatória.

EVOLUÇÃO ESPERADA E PROGNÓSTICO
- O prognóstico quanto à recuperação completa é excelente na maioria dos casos se as recomendações alimentares forem rigorosamente respeitadas.
- Wheaten terriers com alergia alimentar apresentam um prognóstico reservado quanto à recuperação completa.

DIVERSOS

DISTÚRBIOS ASSOCIADOS
Diarreia responsiva a antibióticos e enteropatia inflamatória podem estar associadas a reações alimentares adversas.

FATORES RELACIONADOS COM A IDADE
A gravidade de enteropatia sensível ao glúten em filhotes suscetíveis de Setter irlandês pode ser reduzida, evitando-se os cereais que contenham esse ingrediente.

POTENCIAL ZOONÓTICO
N/D.

GESTAÇÃO/FERTILIDADE/REPRODUÇÃO
N/D.

SINÔNIMOS
Intolerância alimentar, alergia alimentar, sensibilidade alimentar.

VER TAMBÉM
- Diarreia Aguda.
- Diarreia Responsiva a Antibióticos.
- Diarreia Crônica — Gatos.
- Diarreia Crônica — Cães.
- Insuficiência Pancreática Exócrina.
- Gastrenterite Eosinofílica.
- Gastrenterite Linfoplasmocitária.
- Enteropatia Sensível ao Glúten em Setters irlandeses.
- Enteropatia inflamatória.

RECURSOS DA INTERNET
Veterinary Information Network (Rede de Informações Veterinárias): www.vin.com/VIN.plx.

Sugestões de Leitura
Guilford WG. Food sensitivity in cats with chronic idiopathic gastrointestinal problems. J Vet Intern Med 2001, 15:7-13.
Roudebush P. Adverse reactions to foods: Allergies versus intolerance. In: Ettinger SJ, Feldman EC, eds., Textbook of Veterinary Internal Medicine, 6th ed. St. Louis: Elsevier, 2005, pp. 566-570.

Autor Albert E. Jergens
Consultor Editorial Albert E. Jergens

REAÇÕES ALIMENTARES DERMATOLÓGICAS

CONSIDERAÇÕES GERAIS

DEFINIÇÃO
- Reações adversas a alimentos, com envolvimento da pele.
- Associadas à ingestão de uma ou mais substâncias.

FISIOPATOLOGIA
- A patogenia não é completamente compreendida.
- Reações imediatas e tardias a ingredientes específicos registrados; presume-se que as reações imediatas sejam de hipersensibilidade do tipo I e as tardias, do tipo III ou IV.
- Intolerância alimentar — reação idiossincrásica não imunológica; envolve efeitos metabólicos, tóxicos ou farmacológicos de ingredientes agressores.
- Reação alimentar adversa é a expressão mais comumente utilizada, mas não distingue entre reações imunológicas e idiossincrásicas.
- Alguns relatos associam as reações alimentares adversas a uma predisposição elevada de atopia.

SISTEMA(S) ACOMETIDO(S)
- Cutâneo/exócrino.
- Gastrintestinal.
- Nervoso.

GENÉTICA
N/D.

INCIDÊNCIA/PREVALÊNCIA
- Aproximadamente 5% de todas as dermatites e 10-15% das dermatites alérgicas em cães e gatos resultam de reações alimentares adversas.
- 20-30% dos cães alérgicos aos alimentos apresentam atopia ou hipersensibilidade à picada de pulga concomitante.
- Terceira doença cutânea pruriginosa mais comum em cães; segunda mais comum em gatos.
- As porcentagens variam muito de acordo com os clínicos e a localização geográfica.

DISTRIBUIÇÃO GEOGRÁFICA
N/D.

IDENTIFICAÇÃO
Espécies
Cães e gatos.

Raça(s) Predominante(s)
Nenhuma relatada.

Idade Média e Faixa Etária
Qualquer idade.

Sexo Predominante
Nenhum.

SINAIS CLÍNICOS
Comentários Gerais
- Sintomas semelhantes a outras reações de hipersensibilidade.
- O prurido constitui o principal sinal clínico.

Achados Anamnésicos
- Prurido em qualquer local do corpo.
- Geralmente não sazonais.
- Resposta precária a doses anti-inflamatórias de glicocorticoides.
- Vômitos e/ou diarreia concomitantes.
- Borborigmo excessivo, flatulência e movimentos intestinais frequentes.
- Associação muito rara de sinais neurológicos (crises convulsivas) com hipersensibilidade alimentar.

Achados do Exame Físico
- Dermatite por *Malassezia*.
- Foliculite bacteriana secundária.
- Otite externa.
- Placas.
- Pústulas.
- Eritema.
- Crostas.
- Descamação.
- Alopecia autoinduzida.
- Escoriação.
- Liquenificação.
- Hiperpigmentação.
- Urticária.
- Angioedema.
- Dermatite piotraumática.

CAUSAS
- Reações imunomediadas (hipersensibilidade alimentar) — resultam da ingestão e da subsequente apresentação de uma ou mais glicoproteínas (alérgenos) ao sistema imunológico antes ou depois da digestão; pode ocorrer sensibilização na mucosa gastrintestinal após a absorção da substância ou ambas.
- Reações não imunomediadas (intolerância alimentar) — resultam da ingestão de alimentos com altos níveis de histamina ou substâncias que induzam a histamina diretamente ou por meio de fatores liberadores dela.

FATORES DE RISCO
- Desconhecidos.
- Parasitas intestinais ou infecções intestinais possam causar dano à mucosa intestinal, resultando na absorção anormal de alérgenos e subsequente sensibilização.

DIAGNÓSTICO

DIAGNÓSTICO DIFERENCIAL
- Hipersensibilidade à picada de pulgas — limitada, em geral, à metade caudal do corpo; frequentemente sazonal.
- Atopia — associada a prurido de regiões como face, pés, axila, virilha e períneo; geralmente sazonal; se o prurido ocorrer pela primeira vez antes dos 6 meses de vida ou depois dos 6 anos de idade, então será mais provável que o quadro se trate de hipersensibilidade alimentar do que de atopia; 20-30% dos cães com reações adversas aos alimentos também apresentam dermatite atópica.
- Reações medicamentosas — histórico de administração de medicamentos antes do desenvolvimento dos sinais e melhora após a retirada do medicamento sob suspeita.
- Escabiose — prurido geralmente específico a regiões como orelhas, cotovelos e jarretes; ácaros nos raspados de pele e resposta à terapia específica.

HEMOGRAMA/BIOQUÍMICA/URINÁLISE
N/D.

OUTROS TESTES LABORATORIAIS
Testes alérgicos (séricos) *in vitro*; não completamente sensível nem específico; discrepância significativa entre os laboratórios; atualmente, não há padrão que permita as comparações entre as técnicas; não recomendados como o único teste diagnóstico para alergia alimentar ou atopia.

DIAGNÓSTICO POR IMAGEM
N/D.

MÉTODOS DIAGNÓSTICOS
- Não existe um único teste laboratorial disponível para ajudar o clínico a confirmar ou refutar a presença de sensibilidade alimentar.
- O diagnóstico baseia-se na exclusão dietética sob a forma de ensaios alimentares com restrição do ingrediente.

Dieta de Eliminação
- Teste definitivo para reações alimentares adversas.
- Adaptada a cada paciente.
- A dieta tem de ser restrita a uma nova fonte de proteína e carboidrato.
- A maioria dos pacientes melhora dentro de 6-8 semanas.
- Os ensaios alimentares devem ser mantidos por até 10 semanas a menos que ocorra uma melhora antes disso.

Desafio e Teste Provocativo
- Usados se o paciente melhorar com a dieta de eliminação.
- Desafio — oferecer ao paciente a dieta original; um retorno dos sinais confirma que essa dieta contém algum ingrediente incitante; o período de desafio deve durar até o retorno dos sinais clínicos, mas sem ultrapassar 10 dias.
- Provocação (teste provocativo) — se o desafio tiver confirmado a presença de alguma reação alimentar adversa, acrescentar ingredientes isolados à dieta de eliminação; os ingredientes a serem testados incluem uma ampla variedade de carnes (bovina, frango, peixe, suína, cordeiro), grãos (milho, trigo, soja, arroz), ovos e laticínios; o período de provocação para cada ingrediente deverá durar até 10 dias ou menos se os sinais surgirem antes disso (os cães costumam desenvolver sinais em 1-2 dias); os resultados orientam a escolha das rações comerciais que não contenham a(s) substância(s) agressora(s).

ACHADOS PATOLÓGICOS
- Biopsias cutâneas — não são diagnósticas; ajudam a confirmar ou eliminar outros diagnósticos diferenciais.
- Achados histopatológicos — variáveis; achados comuns sugerem hipersensibilidade; pode haver foliculite bacteriana secundária ou dermatite por *Malassezia*.

TRATAMENTO

Evitar a(s) substância(s) agressora(s).

CUIDADO(S) DE SAÚDE ADEQUADO(S)
Ambulatorial.

CUIDADO(S) DE ENFERMAGEM
N/D.

ATIVIDADE
Nenhuma alteração.

DIETA
Evitar quaisquer substâncias alimentícias que provocaram o retorno dos sinais clínicos durante a fase de provocação do diagnóstico.

Reações Alimentares Dermatológicas

ORIENTAÇÃO AO PROPRIETÁRIO
• Explicar os princípios envolvidos em cada fase dos testes dietéticos diagnósticos.
• Orientar os proprietários a eliminar petiscos, brinquedos mastigáveis, vitaminas e outras medicações aromatizadas (p. ex., preventivo de dirofilariose), que possam conter ingredientes da dieta prévia do paciente.
• Animais que vivem soltos fora de casa devem ser confinados para evitar os hábitos de fuçar e caçar.
• Aconselhar todos os membros da família a aderir ao protocolo dietético com restrição do ingrediente específico.

CONSIDERAÇÕES CIRÚRGICAS
N/D.

MEDICAÇÕES

MEDICAMENTO(S) DE ESCOLHA
• Antipruriginosos sistêmicos — podem ser úteis durante as 2-3 primeiras semanas do ensaio alimentar para controlar a automutilação.
• Antibióticos ou antifúngicos — proveitosos para foliculite bacteriana secundária ou dermatite por *Malassezia*.

CONTRAINDICAÇÕES
• Antibióticos conhecidos por seus efeitos anti-inflamatórios (p. ex., tetraciclina, doxiciclina, eritromicina e sulfas potencializadas por trimetoprima) podem confundir a resposta aos ensaios alimentares.
• A administração de glicocorticoides e anti-histamínicos precisa ser interrompida por, no mínimo, 10-14 dias durante o ensaio alimentar para permitir a avaliação correta da resposta do animal.

PRECAUÇÕES
N/D.

INTERAÇÕES POSSÍVEIS
• Vitaminas e preventivos mastigáveis para dirofilariose podem conter substâncias alimentares agressivas.
• Todos os petiscos e brinquedos mastigáveis precisam ser removidos durante o ensaio alimentar.

MEDICAMENTO(S) ALTERNATIVO(S)
Nenhum.

ACOMPANHAMENTO

MONITORIZAÇÃO DO PACIENTE
Examinar o paciente, além de avaliar e registrar o prurido e os sinais clínicos a cada 3-4 semanas.

PREVENÇÃO
• Evitar a ingestão de quaisquer proteínas incluídas na dieta prévia.
• Petiscos e brinquedos mastigáveis devem ser limitados a substâncias seguras conhecidas (p. ex., maçãs e legumes).

COMPLICAÇÕES POSSÍVEIS
Outras causas de prurido precisam ser eliminadas ou controladas para permitir a avaliação precisa dos efeitos exercidos pelos antígenos alimentares sobre os sinais clínicos.

EVOLUÇÃO ESPERADA E PROGNÓSTICO
• O prognóstico será bom se os ingredientes alimentares forem a única causa do prurido e os ingredientes agressores forem evitados.
• Raramente um cão ou gato pode desenvolver hipersensibilidade a novas substâncias, o que talvez exija um novo ensaio com dieta de eliminação.
• Quaisquer outras hipersensibilidades (à picada de pulgas ou atopia) também precisam ser tratadas.
• Uma resposta parcial à dieta de eliminação sugere uma reação alimentar combinada com atopia ou com alguma outra causa de prurido.

DIVERSOS

DISTÚRBIOS ASSOCIADOS
• Foliculite bacteriana superficial.
• Dermatite por *Malassezia*.
• Otite externa.
• Dermatite atópica.

FATORES RELACIONADOS COM A IDADE
Nenhum, exceto as faixas etárias durante as quais os sintomas de alergia alimentar se desenvolvem com maior frequência.

POTENCIAL ZOONÓTICO
Nenhum.

GESTAÇÃO/FERTILIDADE/REPRODUÇÃO
N/D.

SINÔNIMO(S)
• Reações adversas aos alimentos.
• Alergia alimentar.
• Hipersensibilidade alimentar.
• Intolerância alimentar.

VER TAMBÉM
• Dermatite Atópica.
• Dermatite de Contato.
• Dermatite por *Malassezia*.
• Hipersensibilidade a Picada de Pulga e Controle de Pulgas.
• Otite Externa e Média.
• Piodermite.

Sugestões de Leitura
Ermel RW, Kock M, Griffey SM, Reinhart GA, Frick OL. The atopic dog: A model for food allergy. Lab Anim Sci 1997, 47(1):40-49.
Foster AP, Knowles TG, Moore AH, Cousins PD, Day MJ, Hall EJ. Serum IgE and IgG responses to food antigens in normal and atopic dogs, and dogs with gastrointestinal disease. Vet Immunol Immunopathol 2003, 92(3-4):113-124.
Hillier A, Griffin CE. The ACVD task force on canine atopic dermatitis (X): Is there a relationship between canine atopic dermatitis and cutaneous adverse food reactions? Vet Immunol Immunopathol 2001, 81(3-4):227-231.
Jeffers JG, Meyer EK, Sosis EJ. Responses of dogs with food allergies to single-ingredient dietary provocation. JAVMA 1996, 209(3):608-611.
Verlinden A, Hesta M, Millet S, Janssens GP. Food allergy in dogs and cats: A review. Crit Rev Food Sci Nutr 2006, 46(3):259-273.

Autor David Duclos
Consultor Editorial Alexander H. Werner

REAÇÕES À TRANSFUSÃO SANGUÍNEA

CONSIDERAÇÕES GERAIS

REVISÃO
• Classificadas como agudas ou tardias, imunomediadas ou não. • As reações graves costumam ocorrer durante ou logo após a transfusão. • Pode ocorrer com qualquer produto sanguíneo, incluindo soluções à base de hemoglobina carreadoras de oxigênio.

IDENTIFICAÇÃO
• Cães e gatos. • Não há sexo predominante.
• Todas as idades podem ser acometidas.

SINAIS CLÍNICOS
Reação Hemolítica Aguda
• Inquietação. • Febre. • Taquicardia. • Vômitos.
• Tremores. • Fraqueza. • Incontinência.
• Colapso. • Choque. • Oligúria. • Perda na eficácia da transfusão.

Reação Hemolítica Tardia
Perda na eficácia da transfusão — em geral, não há nenhum sinal clínico.

Reação Não Hemolítica Aguda
• Reação anafilática — febre, urticária, eritema, edema facial e prurido. • Transfusão de sangue contaminado — septicemia aguda, febre e choque.
• Sobrecarga circulatória/transfusão rápida — vômitos, distensão das veias jugulares, dispneia, tosse, cianose e insuficiência cardíaca congestiva.
• Toxicidade do citrato — hipocalcemia, depressão do miocárdio e fraqueza. • Hiperamonemia — encefalopatia. • Hipotermia — tremores e comprometimento da função plaquetária.

CAUSAS E FATORES DE RISCO
Os gatos de raças puras e os cães recém-transfundidos têm um risco maior de sofrerem reações transfusionais graves do que outros animais.

Hemólise Aguda
• Incompatibilidade do grupo sanguíneo.
• Formação de autoanticorpos (particularmente em gatos). • Transfusão de hemácias danificadas e hemolisadas (após aquecimento, congelamento ou dano mecânico excessivos).

Hemólise Tardia
• Reação imune aos antígenos eritrocitários secundários; ocorre após 3-14 dias.

Reação Não Hemolítica Aguda
• Anafilaxia e reação imune a componentes dos doadores, como os leucócitos ou as plaquetas, os antígenos do complexo de histocompatibilidade maior ou do plasma, resultando na liberação de mediadores inflamatórios e pirogênios.
• Transfusão de sangue contaminado — ausência de condições assépticas de coleta e armazenamento.
• Sobrecarga circulatória — transfusão rápida; volume excessivo de sangue em animais de pequeno porte ou em pacientes com insuficiência cardíaca ou insuficiência renal oligúrica.
• Toxicidade do citrato — após sobrecarga circulatória, particularmente em animais de pequeno porte ou em hepatopatas.
• Hiperamonemia — concentração elevada de amônia em sangue armazenado; importante apenas em hepatopatas.
• Hipotermia — transfusão rápida de sangue refrigerado a animais de pequeno porte ou já hipotérmicos.

Reação Não Hemolítica Tardia
• Transmissão de doença de origem hematógena — uso de doador infectado (DNA de *Mycoplasma hemofelis* encontrado em 10% dos doadores ativos em um único estudo).
• Doença enxerto contra hospedeiro associada à transfusão — complicação rara, mas >90% fatal advinda da transfusão de componentes sanguíneos que contenham linfócitos-T de doadores imunocompetentes. Ainda não foi claramente relatada em pacientes caninos ou felinos.

DIAGNÓSTICO

DIAGNÓSTICO DIFERENCIAL
• Hemólise — descartar a presença de doença hemolítica fulminante avançada (ensaio de hemaglutinação indireta, *Babesia*, *Mycoplasma hf.*) e o emprego de sangue hemolisado.
• Febre, hipotensão — excluir doenças infecciosas e inflamatórias subjacentes.

HEMOGRAMA/BIOQUÍMICA/URINÁLISE
Hemoglobinemia, leucocitose, bilirrubinemia, hemoglobinúria e bilirrubinúria.

OUTROS TESTES LABORATORIAIS
• Repetir o teste de reação cruzada para confirmar a incompatibilidade.
• Cultura bacteriana ou coloração de Gram de sangue contaminado podem constatar a presença de microrganismos.
• PCR para detecção de *Mycoplasma hemofelis* em gatos.

TRATAMENTO

• Interromper a transfusão imediatamente.
• Administrar fluidos para manter a pressão arterial e o fluxo sanguíneo renal; para hipotensão, utilizar cristaloides isotônicos como solução de Ringer lactato (50-90 mL/kg/h, com administração de 30% da dose e subsequente reavaliação).
• Terapia de suporte adicional em casos de CID, choque ou tromboembolia (ver capítulos a respeito desses quadros).

MEDICAÇÕES

MEDICAMENTO(S)
• Contra hemólise — corticosteroides de ação rápida, como o succinato sódico de prednisolona (11 mg/kg em uma única dose) ou o fosfato sódico de dexametasona (2,2 mg/kg em uma única dose); heparina (300 U/kg SC a cada 6 h; não utilizar em animais com sangramento).
• Contra urticária e febre — difenidramina (1-2 mg/kg); prednisolona (2-4 mg/kg); prosseguir com a transfusão mais tarde, se clinicamente indicada.
• Contra septicemia — antibióticos IV de amplo espectro, enquanto se aguardam os resultados da cultura bacteriana (p. ex., cefalotina/enrofloxacino); heparina.
• Contra sobrecarga volêmica — furosemida (2-4 mg/kg IV), suplementação de oxigênio.

ACOMPANHAMENTO

MONITORIZAÇÃO DO PACIENTE
• Avaliar a atitude, a temperatura, os sinais vitais, os ruídos pulmonares, o VG, os sólidos totais e a coloração do plasma antes, durante e depois da transfusão. • Em caso de reações hemolíticas agudas ou septicemia, monitorizar a PVC e o débito urinário. • Na suspeita de tromboembolia pulmonar, examinar frequentemente as radiografias torácicas e gasometrias sanguíneas arteriais.

PREVENÇÃO
• Registrar com rigor a ocorrência de qualquer reação transfusional no prontuário médico do paciente.
• Testes antes da transfusão:
  ○ Fazer a triagem de doadores quanto à presença de doença infecciosa.
  ○ Obter a tipagem sanguínea de doadores e receptores.
  ○ Utilizar cartões/membranas de tipagem (Rapid Vet-H, DMS Laboratories Inc., Flemington, NJ; Quick Test, Alvedia, Lyon, França).
  ○ Realizar o teste de compatibilidade: testes de aglutinação em gel (Rapid Vet-H companion animal crossmatch test, DMS Laboratories, Inc., Flemington, NJ).
• Seguir os protocolos-padrão de transfusão (p. ex., uso de doadores saudáveis; bem como técnicas adequadas de coleta, armazenamento e administração).
• Inicialmente, transfundir a 1 mL/min.

COMPLICAÇÕES POSSÍVEIS
• A hemólise fulminante pode causar insuficiência renal aguda, tromboembolia pulmonar, tromboembolia em múltiplos órgãos, CID e arritmias cardíacas. • A sobrecarga volêmica pode levar à insuficiência cardíaca. • Parada cardíaca.

EVOLUÇÃO ESPERADA E PROGNÓSTICO
• Evolução aguda em grande parte dos animais.
• Prognóstico bom em animais estáveis, mas reservado em animais gravemente comprometidos ou quando não se identifica o problema logo no início. • Os gatos com tipo sanguíneo B submetidos à transfusão de sangue incompatível exibem prognóstico mais grave.

DIVERSOS

ABREVIATURA(S)
• CID = coagulação intravascular disseminada.
• PVC = pressão venosa central.
• PCR = reação em cadeia da polimerase.
• VG = volume globular (hematócrito).

Sugestões de Leitura
Hohenhaus AE, Rentko V. Blood transfusions and blood substitutes, In: Di Bartola SP, ed., Fluid Therapy in Small Animal Practice, 3rd ed. St. Louis: Saunders, 2006, pp. 574-581.
Tocci LJ, Ewing PJ. Increasing patient safety in veterinary transfusion medicine: An overview of pretransfusion testing. J Vet Emerg Crit Care 2009, 19:66-73.

Autor Jörg Bucheler
Consultor Editorial A.H. Rebar

Realojamento Bem-Sucedido de Cães e Gatos de Abrigo

CONSIDERAÇÕES GERAIS

DEFINIÇÃO
Os abrigos de animais realojam milhões de cães e gatos por ano. O realojamento bem-sucedido começa com alguém que deseja adotar um cão ou gato de abrigo; tal realojamento é concluído quando essa pessoa faz um compromisso vitalício de cuidar do bem-estar, bem como das saúdes física e comportamental, do animal. Os donos de abrigos de animais, os veterinários e as comunidades devem trabalhar juntos para fornecer orientação e recurso aos proprietários de pequenos animais na tentativa de realojar os cães e gatos de abrigo com sucesso.

FISIOPATOLOGIA
• Embora milhões de animais sejam adotados por ano, nem todas as adoções são bem-sucedidas. Alguns animais adotados são devolvidos ao abrigo, dados a familiares ou amigos, ou abandonados.
• Muitos fatores influenciam o sucesso, ou a falta dele, do processo de adoção, incluindo:
  ○ O conhecimento, a experiência e o treinamento do indivíduo responsável pela adoção.
  ○ Os recursos disponíveis para auxiliar esse indivíduo.
  ○ A saúde física e comportamental do animal adotado.
• As pessoas que adotam os animais geralmente formam um vínculo com seu novo animal de estimação nos primeiros dias a meses da adoção.
• Preparar o indivíduo responsável pela adoção a respeito do que esperar e o que fazer quando o inesperado acontece pode aumentar a probabilidade de que o animal seja mantido na nova casa.

SISTEMA(S) ACOMETIDO(S)
Comportamental – os animais são frequentemente entregues a abrigos por causa de problemas comportamentais subjacentes, como comportamento indisciplinado, evacuação/micção domiciliar, arranhadura da mobília, agressividade, e ansiedade da separação. Muitos desses problemas também podem ocorrer na nova casa e devem ser tratados para garantir um realojamento bem-sucedido.

INCIDÊNCIA/PREVALÊNCIA
Aproximadamente 10-20% dos 60 milhões de cães e 75 milhões de gatos nos Estados Unidos são adquiridos de abrigos ou organizações de resgate.

IDENTIFICAÇÃO
Espécies
Cães e gatos.

Raça(s) Predominante(s)
Nenhuma raça específica é super-representada entre os animais de abrigo. Embora a maioria dos cães entregues a abrigos seja de raças mistas, cerca de 30% dos cães são de raças puras.

Idade Média e Faixa Etária
Animais de todas as idades, desde recém-nascidos a geriátricos, são entregues a abrigos. A maioria dos cães tem menos de 2 anos de idade, enquanto grande parte dos gatos entregues tem menos de 3 anos de idade.

Sexo Predominante
Nenhum sexo é super-representado.

SINAIS CLÍNICOS
Achados Anamnésicos
• Os animais recém-adotados podem exibir padrões comportamentais compatíveis com estresse:
  ○ Diminuição do apetite, diarreia.
  ○ Atividade reduzida ou aumentada e comportamento de refúgio ou reclusivo.
  ○ Os animais também podem exibir problemas comportamentais comuns como evacuação/micção domiciliar, ansiedade da separação, vocalização excessiva, arranhadura da mobília, medo ou agressividade contra pessoas ou outros animais, ou comportamento indisciplinado.
• Avaliações do comportamento:
  ○ Muitos abrigos realizam testes de avaliação do comportamento em cães e/ou gatos na tentativa de determinar a adequabilidade do animal para adoção e/ou se há necessidade de qualquer reabilitação comportamental. Essas informações podem estar disponíveis e ser incluídas na papelada de adoção.
  ○ Esses testes tentam avaliar as tendências comportamentais de um animal em uma gama de circunstâncias, incluindo:
    – Sociabilidade (interesse em interagir com as pessoas)
    – Manipulação (contato com pés e boca, carícias, abraços, beliscões)
    – Comportamento em relação a brinquedos, alimentos, e outros objetos valiosos (ou seja, artigos mastigáveis de couro cru).
    – Exposição a objetos novos e exposição a cães e gatos.
  ○ Embora esses testes forneçam informações potencialmente valiosas sobre o comportamento do animal recém-adotado, é importante notar que não existe nenhum teste utilizado atualmente em abrigos que tenha se mostrado, em periódicos especializados, altamente preditivo do comportamento do animal em uma casa. Dessa forma, embora as informações possam ser precisas, esses testes não garantem a presença ou ausência de problemas comportamentais. Quando os problemas são identificados em um teste de avaliação, o animal pode ou não ser tratado com um programa de mudança comportamental ou adotado com (ou sem) divulgação completa do problema, mas sem tratamento.
  ○ Os indivíduos responsáveis pela adoção recebem níveis variados de orientação em relação ao tratamento e manejo do problema, desde nenhuma orientação até aconselhamentos extensos e consultas de acompanhamento.
  ○ Como alguns dos problemas potencialmente identificados em um teste de comportamento podem ser muito graves, é importante que o clínico revise esses achados e reitere-os ao proprietário.

Achados do Exame Físico
Como o histórico do animal recém-adotado não é conhecido, é imprescindível a realização de exames físico completo e comportamental. É preciso ter cuidado no exame de animais recém-adotados na tentativa de reduzir o risco de agressividade aos veterinários, secundariamente a um problema médico doloroso ou experiências adversas prévias em hospitais veterinários. Na maioria dos animais recém-adotados, o exame físico não é digno de nota.

CAUSAS
• Problemas comportamentais: os problemas de comportamento foram citados como a principal causa de abandono de cães em abrigos e a segunda causa de abandono de gatos.
• Problemas domésticos: ser incapaz de encontrar uma casa onde os animais são permitidos, mudar para um novo local onde os animais não são permitidos, alergias a animais de estimação, e mudanças na dinâmica familiar são, sem exceção, razões comuns de abandono.
• Problemas financeiros: perda de um emprego ou perda de uma casa por execução de hipoteca, por exemplo, pode exigir o abandono do animal por questões econômicas.
• Problemas médicos: os animais podem ser abandonados em abrigos por causa do custo exageradamente alto do tratamento de problemas médicos agudos ou crônicos.
• Superpopulação: o acasalamento não planejado e/ou irresponsável resulta no nascimento de muitos cães e gatos. Quando os proprietários não conseguem encontrar uma casa para os animais, eles os abandonam em abrigos ou os deixam soltos nas ruas.

FATORES DE RISCO
São fatores de risco para a ocorrência de abandono em abrigos:
• Posse de mais de um animal de estimação.
• Presença de crianças na casa.
• Pouco conhecimento sobre a biologia e o comportamento do animal.
• Cada animal adotado deve ser avaliado em um esquema individual (ou seja, caso a caso).
• Os animais não são mantidos em novas casas quando as condições ambientais associadas à posse do animal se tornam opressoras ou incontroláveis.

DIAGNÓSTICO

DIAGNÓSTICO DIFERENCIAL
Os fatores que resultam em um realojamento bem-sucedido ou malsucedido são complexos, mas frequentemente estão relacionados com o vínculo da pessoa responsável pela adoção com o animal de estimação. Como não é fácil avaliar a força desse vínculo, o clínico deve contar com a identificação e o tratamento dos problemas que tornam a posse do animal mais desafiadora.

HEMOGRAMA/BIOQUÍMICA/URINÁLISE
N/D a menos que os problemas médicos sejam evidentes no momento da adoção.

OUTROS TESTES LABORATORIAIS
A obtenção de breve histórico comportamental orientará o clínico a determinar se o animal precisa de intervenção comportamental. As intervenções médicas dependem dos resultados dos achados do exame físico.

TRATAMENTO

CUIDADO(S) DE SAÚDE ADEQUADO(S)
• O estresse associado à mudança de ambiente resulta em modificação do comportamento. Os proprietários devem ser avisados de que o comportamento do animal recém-adotado provavelmente mudará nas primeiras semanas.

Realojamento Bem-Sucedido de Cães e Gatos de Abrigo

Muitos animais são calmos ou mais dominados do que é normal para sua personalidade.
• Gatos: os gatos medrosos devem ser confinados em um ambiente com comida, água, bandeja sanitária, local de refúgio e outro lugar confortável para dormir. As tigelas de água e comida devem ficar próximas ao lugar de refúgio para aumentar a probabilidade de que eles comam. A exposição a áreas da casa deve ser gradativamente permitida à medida que o gato se sente mais à vontade.
• Cães: os indivíduos responsáveis pela adoção devem fornecer ao animal um programa estruturado, além de atividade física regular e adestramento básico.
• Assim que os animais se adaptam a seu novo ambiente, eles frequentemente começam a exibir comportamentos mais "normais", como destruição, latido, arranhadura dos móveis e comportamento indisciplinado. Avisar os proprietários sobre essas mudanças potenciais ajuda-os a se preparar e a lidar com elas.

ATIVIDADE
• A prática regular de exercício é importante para manter a saúde comportamental do animal. É recomendável o fornecimento de diretrizes aos proprietários para a realização dos exercícios ideais, considerando-se o estado de saúde, a personalidade e a fase de vida do animal.
• Os proprietários podem necessitar de orientação sobre as modalidades lúdicas adequadas para a espécie e a idade do animal adotado.

DIETA
• Os proprietários devem alimentar seu animal recém-adotado com a dieta que era fornecida no abrigo e, depois, proceder lentamente à transição para uma dieta recomendada pelo veterinário em um período de 5-7 dias.
• Os animais inapetentes devem receber rações altamente palatáveis, como ração enlatada aquecida, comida/papinha de bebê, ou frango/arroz misturados com a dieta normal. Quando já existem outros animais na casa, o recém-chegado deve ter um local seguro e separado para comer, distante dos outros animais.
• Ao adotar um cão, os proprietários devem ser orientados sobre as interações adequadas enquanto o animal se alimenta e saber que, no início, ele talvez fique muito ansioso e protetor durante os horários das refeições.

ORIENTAÇÃO AO PROPRIETÁRIO
• É recomendável que os proprietários recebam orientação a respeito dos problemas potenciais dos animais recém-adotados.
• Com frequência, os animais recém-adotados apresentam-se inapetentes. Apesar de ser uma resposta potencialmente normal ao estresse, a inapetência por mais de 2 dias deve resultar em um telefonema à clínica veterinária para garantir a inexistência de qualquer problema médico subjacente.
• Os novos proprietários devem ser avisados de que muitos problemas são o resultado de medos e ansiedades associados à adaptação à nova casa.
• Os problemas comportamentais potenciais pós-adoção incluem comportamento destrutivo, evacuação/micção domiciliar, medo/refúgio, ansiedade da separação, e agressividade.
• Fornecer às pessoas que desejam adotar um animal uma lista de recursos para tratar e prevenir problemas, tais como:
• Horários e políticas de emergência de clínicas veterinárias.
• Websites com informações sobre cuidados de saúde e comportamento.
• Contatos de adestrador de cães, pensão e/ou estabelecimento de cuidados diários, clínica local de emergência, além de veterinário especialista em comportamento ou com certificado.

MEDICAÇÕES
MEDICAMENTO(S) DE ESCOLHA
N/D.

MEDICAMENTO(S) ALTERNATIVO(S)
Feromônios (Feliway® para gatos e Dog Appeasing Pheromone® para cães) podem ser úteis para reduzir o estresse e a ansiedade associados à mudança de ambiente e ao realojamento. Os difusores devem ser plugados no(s) ambiente(s) onde o animal gasta a maior parte de seu tempo.

ACOMPANHAMENTO
MONITORIZAÇÃO DO PACIENTE
As consultas de acompanhamento ou os contatos telefônicos em 1 mês, 3 meses, 6 meses e 12 meses proporcionam a intervenção precoce na tentativa de tratar os problemas antes que eles se tornem graves. O coordenador do acompanhamento deve fazer perguntas pontuais e específicas sobre o comportamento e a saúde do animal.

PREVENÇÃO
• O realojamento bem-sucedido começa com a tomada de decisão informada do proprietário ao escolher um animal do abrigo. Os abrigos frequentemente têm informações disponíveis sobre o histórico do animal, bem como dados sobre a avaliação e o exame realizados no abrigo, o que pode ajudar os indivíduos responsáveis pela adoção a selecionar um animal adequado para sua casa e seu estilo de vida.
• Os veterinários devem recomendar a adoção de animais de abrigos e grupos de resgate que forneçam uma avaliação abrangente do animal no momento do abandono, além de adestramento, reabilitação comportamental e programas de acompanhamento para garantir o sucesso da adoção.
• É recomendável que os proprietários não só adquiram conhecimento sobre os cuidados básicos e adestramento dos animais, mas também procurem ajuda de um profissional no *início* de algum problema. Muitas vezes, o atraso na avaliação e no tratamento torna o tratamento ainda mais difícil.

COMPLICAÇÕES POSSÍVEIS
Problemas médicos ou comportamentais preexistentes potenciais e/ou expectativas não realistas a respeito do tempo e do esforço necessários para o cuidado adequado de um animal podem impedir que os proprietários se apeguem ao animal de abrigo e se comprometam a mantê-lo.

EVOLUÇÃO ESPERADA E PROGNÓSTICO
O prognóstico para um animal cuidadosamente selecionado de abrigo ou grupo de resgate respeitável e conceituado é muito bom; no entanto, os animais podem desenvolver problemas médicos ou comportamentais, independentemente do local de sua aquisição.

DIVERSOS
DISTÚRBIOS ASSOCIADOS
Os distúrbios associados incluem evacuação/micção domiciliar, comportamento destrutivo, comportamento indisciplinado, arranhadura da mobília, agressividade, medo, e ansiedade da separação.

FATORES RELACIONADOS COM A IDADE
É mais provável que os animais mais jovens tenham problemas como comportamento destrutivo e indisciplinado que os mais idosos.

GESTAÇÃO/FERTILIDADE/REPRODUÇÃO
N/D.

VER TAMBÉM
• Capítulos sobre Agressividade.
• Comportamentos Destrutivos.
• Vocalização Excessiva.
• Introdução de Novos Animais de Estimação na Família.
• Síndrome de Ansiedade da Separação.
• Comportamentos Indisciplinados: Saltar, Cavar, Perseguir, Furtar.

RECURSOS DA INTERNET
www.apdt.com/petowners.
www.avma.org/bluedog.
www.bestfriends.org/theanimals.
www.hsus.org/pets/pet_care/our_pets_for_life_program.
www.vet.ohio-state.edu/indoorcat.

Sugestões de Leitura
Landsberg G, Hunthausen W, Ackerman L. Handbook of Behavior Problems of the Dog and Cat, 2nd ed. Philadelphia: Elsevier Saunders, 2003.
Miller L, Zawistowski S, eds. Shelter Medicine for Veterinarians and Staff. Ames, IA: Blackwell, 2004.
Sternberg S. Successful Dog Adoption. Indianapolis: Wiley, 2003.

Autor Sheila D'Arpino
Consultor Editorial Debra F. Horwitz

Refluxo Gastresofágico

CONSIDERAÇÕES GERAIS

REVISÃO
- Refluxo de líquido gástrico ou intestinal para o lúmen do esôfago.
- Incidência desconhecida; é provável que seja mais comum do que sua identificação clínica.
- O relaxamento transitório do esfíncter gastresofágico ou a ocorrência de vômitos crônicos pode permitir o refluxo de sucos gastrintestinais para o lúmen esofágico. Uma pequena quantidade de refluxo gastresofágico é um fenômeno normal em cães e gatos.
- Ácido gástrico, pepsina, tripsina, bicarbonato e sais biliares são, sem exceção, nocivos para a mucosa esofágica com o contato prolongado.
- A esofagite resultante de refluxo pode variar desde uma leve inflamação da mucosa superficial até uma ulceração grave envolvendo a submucosa e a muscular da mucosa.

IDENTIFICAÇÃO
- Cães e gatos; machos ou fêmeas.
- Não há relato de predominância racial.
- Pode estar associado à hérnia congênita de hiato, vista na raça Shar-pei chinesa.
- Ocorre em qualquer idade; animais mais jovens podem estar sob maior risco de refluxo por causa da imaturidade de desenvolvimento do esfíncter gastresofágico.
- Animais jovens com hérnia congênita de hiato podem estar sob risco elevado.

SINAIS CLÍNICOS
Achados Anamnésicos
- Regurgitação.
- Hipersalivação.
- Dor à deglutição — odinofagia.
- Anorexia.

Achados do Exame Físico
- Em geral, não há nada digno de nota.
- Febre e hipersalivação — com esofagite ulcerativa grave.

CAUSAS E FATORES DE RISCO
- Anestesia com relaxamento do tônus do esfíncter esofágico inferior.
- Retenção de conteúdo gástrico.
- Ingestão de corpo estranho com esofagite.
- Hérnia de hiato.
- Vômitos crônicos com esofagite.

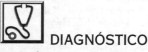

DIAGNÓSTICO

DIAGNÓSTICO DIFERENCIAL
- Doença bucal ou faríngea.
- Ingestão de agente cáustico.
- Corpo estranho esofágico.
- Tumor esofágico.
- Megaesôfago — idiopático; miastenia grave; anomalia do anel vascular.
- Hérnia de hiato.
- Intussuscepção gastresofágica.

HEMOGRAMA/BIOQUÍMICA/URINÁLISE
Geralmente normais.

OUTROS TESTES LABORATORIAIS
N/D.

DIAGNÓSTICO POR IMAGEM
- Radiografia simples do tórax — em geral, não há nada digno de nota; pode haver ar na parte distal do esôfago (achado inespecífico).
- Radiografia contrastada com bário — revela refluxo gastresofágico em alguns animais, mas não em todos; pneumonia por aspiração pode ser evidente nas partes pendentes dos pulmões.

MÉTODOS DIAGNÓSTICOS
- Esofagoscopia — o melhor meio de confirmar alterações de mucosa, compatíveis com esofagite por refluxo — superfície irregular da mucosa com hiperemia ou sangramento ativo na porção distal do esôfago. Nessa porção distal próxima ao esfíncter esofágico inferior, pode-se observar o acúmulo de secreções gastroduodenais refluídas.
- Radiografia — exame de pouco valor na confirmação de refluxo gastresofágico.

TRATAMENTO

- Geralmente ambulatorial.
- Não é necessário restringir a atividade.
- Casos moderados a graves — pode-se retirar o alimento por 1-2 dias; depois disso, refeições frequentes com baixos teores de gordura e pobres em proteína; a gordura da dieta diminui a pressão sobre o esfíncter gastresofágico e retarda o esvaziamento gástrico; a proteína estimula a secreção de ácido gástrico e pode precipitar o refluxo gastresofágico.

MEDICAÇÕES

MEDICAMENTO(S)
- Suspensão oral de sucralfato (0,5-1 g VO a cada 8 h).
- Agentes antissecretores de ácido gástrico — cimetidina (5-10 mg/kg VO a cada 8 h); ranitidina (1-2 mg/kg VO a cada 12 h); famotidina (0,5 mg/kg VO, SC, IV a cada 12-24 h); omeprazol (0,7 mg/kg VO a cada 24 h).
- Agentes procinéticos — cisaprida (0,1-0,5 mg/kg VO a cada 12 h); ranitidina (1-2 mg/kg VO, IV, SC a cada 8-12 h); metoclopramida (0,5 mg/kg VO a cada 6-8 h).

CONTRAINDICAÇÕES/INTERAÇÕES POSSÍVEIS
A suspensão de sucralfato pode interferir na absorção de outros medicamentos (p. ex., cimetidina, ranitidina, omeprazol e cisaprida).

ACOMPANHAMENTO

- Os pacientes raramente necessitam de endoscopia de acompanhamento.
- Pode ser conveniente em muitos animais simplesmente para monitorizar os sinais clínicos.
- Considerar a realização de endoscopia em pacientes irresponsivos aos tratamentos clínicos empíricos.
- Os proprietários devem evitar o fornecimento de alimentos ricos em gordura, que podem promover a retenção gástrica e exacerbar o refluxo.
- As complicações mais importantes são esofagite e formação de estenose.

DIVERSOS

DISTÚRBIOS ASSOCIADOS
Hérnia de hiato.

FATORES RELACIONADOS COM A IDADE
Pode ser mais grave em animais mais jovens por causa da imaturidade de desenvolvimento do mecanismo do esfíncter gastresofágico.

POTENCIAL ZOONÓTICO
N/D.

GESTAÇÃO/FERTILIDADE/REPRODUÇÃO
N/D.

Sugestões de Leitura
Han E. Diagnosis and management of reflux esophagitis. Clin Tech Small Anim Pract 2003, 18:231-238.
Jergens AE. Diseases of the esophagus. In: Ettinger SJ, Feldman EC eds., Textbook of Veterinary Medicine, 7th ed. Philadelphia: Saunders, 2009.
Sellon RK, Willard MD. Esophagitis and esophageal strictures. Vet Clin North Am Small Anim Pract 2003, 33:945-967.

Autor Albert E. Jergens
Consultor Editorial Albert E. Jergens

REGURGITAÇÃO

CONSIDERAÇÕES GERAIS

DEFINIÇÃO
Movimento retrógrado passivo do conteúdo esofágico em direção à faringe ou à cavidade bucal.

FISIOPATOLOGIA
A regurgitação resulta da perda de contrações esofágicas normais. No esôfago normal, a presença de um bolo alimentar no esôfago proximal estimula neurônios sensoriais aferentes. Os sinais são transmitidos centralmente, via nervos vago e glossofaríngeo, até o trato solitário e o núcleo ambíguo. Impulsos motores retornam via nervo vago até estimular a musculatura estriada (cães) e a musculatura lisa e estriada (gatos) para provocar a contração esofágica. Lesões em qualquer parte ao longo dessa via podem levar à regurgitação.

SISTEMA(S) ACOMETIDO(S)
- Gastrintestinal — disfagia, perda de peso.
- Respiratório — pneumonia por aspiração.
- Musculosquelético — fraqueza, perda de peso.
- Nervoso — polifagia.

GENÉTICA
A regurgitação atribuída a megaesôfago pode ser hereditária em cães das raças Fox terrier de pelo duro (autossômico recessivo) e Schnauzer miniatura (autossômico recessivo com penetrância de 60% ou autossômico dominante).

INCIDÊNCIA/PREVALÊNCIA
N/D.

DISTRIBUIÇÃO GEOGRÁFICA
N/D.

IDENTIFICAÇÃO

Espécies
Cães (mais comumente) e gatos.

Raça(s) Predominante(s)
- Fox terrier de pelo duro, Schnauzer miniatura. Outras raças predispostas incluem Dinamarquês, Pastor alemão, Setter irlandês, Labrador retriever, Terra Nova, Shar-pei.
- Gato Siamês e aparentados.

Idade Média e Faixa Etária
- Casos congênitos manifestam-se logo após o nascimento ou ao desmame de alimentos líquidos para sólidos.
- Casos adquiridos podem ser observados em qualquer idade, dependendo da etiologia.

Sexo Predominante
Não foi identificada qualquer predileção sexual.

SINAIS CLÍNICOS

Comentários Gerais
- Os proprietários frequentemente relatam vômito; o veterinário deve diferenciar o vômito da regurgitação. A filmagem dos eventos pelo proprietário pode ser útil.
- Regurgitação — processo passivo; pouco a nenhum esforço abdominal; sem fase prodrômica; o material regurgitado possui quantidades aumentadas de muco espesso.
- Vômito — processo ativo; é identificada a fase prodrômica; o material vomitado possui coloração biliar aumentada.
- A forma do material expelido (i. e., semelhante a tubo), a presença de alimento não digerido e a duração do tempo desde a ingestão até a regurgitação ou o vômito são aspectos de menor utilidade para a diferenciação.

Achados Anamnésicos
- Vômito (conforme entendido pelo proprietário).
- Disfagia.
- Tosse.
- Apetite voraz.
- Perda de peso.
- Outros sinais, dependendo da etiologia subjacente.

Achados do Exame Físico
- Pode-se notar tumefação cervical.
- Ptialismo.
- Halitose.
- Ruídos respiratórios aumentados.
- Secreção nasal e febre (se houver pneumonia concomitante).
- Caquexia.
- Fraqueza.

CAUSAS

Faríngeas Congênitas
- Fenda palatina ou palato curto.
- Acalasia cricofaríngea.
- Miastenia grave.

Esofágicas Congênitas
- Arco aórtico direito persistente.
- Megaesôfago.
- Doença do armazenamento de glicogênio.
- Divertículo esofágico.
- Fístula broncoesofágica.

Faríngeas Adquiridas
- Corpos estranhos.
- Neoplasia.
- Raiva.
- Intoxicação (botulismo).
- Miopatia/neuropatia.

Esofágicas Adquiridas
- Megaesôfago.
- Miastenia grave.
- Estenose.
- Neoplasia.
- Hipoadrenocorticismo.
- Hipotireoidismo.
- Hérnia de hiato.
- Intussuscepção gastresofágica.
- Refluxo gastresofágico.
- Massas periesofágicas.
- Disautonomia.
- Miopatia/neuropatia.
- Corpos estranhos.
- Doença granulomatosa.
- Intoxicação (chumbo).
- Idiopática.
- Dilatação e vólvulo gástricos.
- Infecção parasitária (*Spirocerca lupi*).
- Fístula broncoesofágica.

FATORES DE RISCO
Possível risco de refluxo gastresofágico com anestesia geral; a esofagite resultante pode levar à regurgitação.

DIAGNÓSTICO

DIAGNÓSTICO DIFERENCIAL
- A regurgitação é um sinal clínico, não um diagnóstico, sendo uma indicação de doença esofágica.
- É importante diferenciar vômito de regurgitação.

HEMOGRAMA/BIOQUÍMICA/URINÁLISE
- Sem alterações patognomônicas para regurgitação.
- Pode-se observar leucograma inflamatório na presença de pneumonia por aspiração.
- Mais valiosos para avaliação das possíveis etiologias subjacentes: por exemplo, alterações eritrocitárias na intoxicação pelo chumbo, CK elevada na miopatia, hipercalemia e hiponatremia no hipoadrenocorticismo, hipercolesterolemia no hipotireoidismo.

OUTROS TESTES LABORATORIAIS
Tais exames elucidam etiologias de distúrbios adquiridos indutores de regurgitação e incluem teste da estimulação com o ACTH ou mensuração do nível basal de cortisol (hipoadrenocorticismo); sorologia da tireoide (hipotireoidismo); nível de anticorpos contra o receptor da acetilcolina (miastenia grave); níveis sanguíneos de chumbo (intoxicação).

DIAGNÓSTICO POR IMAGEM
- Radiografia torácica e cervical — evidência do esôfago preenchido com gás, líquido ou ingesta em caso de megaesôfago; também pode revelar pneumonia por aspiração, neoplasia, corpos estranhos, hérnia de hiato, etc.
- Estudos contrastados — tanto o bário líquido como o alimento revestido por bário para avaliação de distúrbios obstrutivos. Também se pode fazer uso do io-hexol. CUIDADO: os estudos contrastados podem aumentar o risco de pneumonia por aspiração com regurgitação.
- Fluoroscopia — para pesquisa de disfunção da faringe e distúrbios da motilidade esofágica.
- Outros estudos de imagem incluem cintilografia e manometria para avaliação da motilidade e ultrassom para detecção de massas faríngeas ou cervicais.
- TC cervical e torácica também pode ser utilizada.

MÉTODOS DIAGNÓSTICOS
- A esofagoscopia pode ser valiosa em casos de esofagites, estenoses, anomalias do anel vascular, neoplasias e corpos estranhos.
- Eletromiografia (EMG) e biopsias de nervo/músculo podem ser usadas para o diagnóstico de neuropatia ou miopatia.
- Lavado transtraqueal ou broncoalveolar na presença ou suspeita de pneumonia por aspiração.

ACHADOS PATOLÓGICOS
Achados macro e microscópicos dependem da etiologia subjacente e da presença de fatores complicantes.

TRATAMENTO

CUIDADO(S) DE SAÚDE ADEQUADO(S)
- Deve-se instituir o tratamento para a etiologia subjacente.
- Os aspectos mais importantes são atender às necessidades nutricionais e tratar ou prevenir a pneumonia por aspiração.

CUIDADO(S) DE ENFERMAGEM
- A pneumonia por aspiração pode necessitar de oxigenoterapia, nebulização/tapotagem, fluidoterapia com solução eletrolítica balanceada.
- Esses animais podem se encontrar em decúbito e necessitam de cama macia. Além disso, eles devem

REGURGITAÇÃO

ser mantidos em decúbito esternal ou trocados de lado de 4 em 4 horas.

ATIVIDADE
Dependendo da etiologia, não é necessária a restrição da atividade.

DIETA
• É essencial a experimentação com consistências alimentares diferentes. Podem ser utilizadas papas líquidas, pequenas bolas de carne ou pastas batidas no liquidificador.
• Alguns casos beneficiam-se com a alimentação por gastrostomia, embora a regurgitação ainda possa ocorrer.
• Tanto o alimento como a água devem ficar em posição elevada, mas o animal também deve ser mantido em estação por 10-15 minutos após comer ou beber.
• A quantidade de quilocalorias recomendadas deve ser calculada e a dieta monitorizada, para que as necessidades energéticas básicas sejam atendidas.

ORIENTAÇÃO AO PROPRIETÁRIO
• A maior parte dos casos de regurgitação atribuída a megaesôfago necessita de tratamento pelo resto da vida, mesmo que uma etiologia subjacente seja encontrada. A dedicação do proprietário é importante para o manejo a longo prazo.
• Grande parte dos animais sucumbe à pneumonia por aspiração ou regurgitação intratável.

CONSIDERAÇÕES CIRÚRGICAS
• A intervenção cirúrgica fica indicada para anomalias do anel vascular, acalasia cricofaríngea, fístula broncoesofágica e outros distúrbios.
• A disfunção esofágica é permanente na maioria dos casos.
• A dilatação com balão é indicada nos casos de estenose esofágica.

MEDICAÇÕES

MEDICAMENTO(S) DE ESCOLHA
• Antibióticos para pneumonia por aspiração (de amplo espectro ou escolhidos com base nos resultados da cultura e do antibiograma do lavado transtraqueal ou broncoalveolar).
• Terapia específica para a etiologia subjacente, se indicada.

• Procinéticos — metoclopramida (0,2-0,4 mg/kg SC ou VO a cada 6-12 h) aumenta o tônus do esfíncter esofágico inferior e a motilidade gástrica. Cisaprida (0,5 mg/kg VO a cada 8-12 h) é mais eficaz para o refluxo esofágico do que a metoclopramida; entretanto, a cisaprida diminui o tempo de trânsito esofágico; pode ser mais útil em gatos em virtude do aumento na contração da musculatura lisa no esôfago distal.
• Outros agentes modificadores da motilidade (p. ex., nizatidina) não foram avaliados para a motilidade esofágica.
• Bloqueadores H_2 para esofagite — ranitidina (1-2 mg/kg VO, IV a cada 12 h), cimetidina (4-10 mg/kg VO, SC, IM, IV a cada 6 h), famotidina (0,5-1 mg/kg VO, SC, IM, IV a cada 12-24 h). Inibidores da bomba de prótons podem ser utilizados em casos graves — omeprazol (0,5-1 mg/kg VO a cada 24 h).

CONTRAINDICAÇÕES
N/D.

PRECAUÇÕES
• A absorção de medicamentos administrados por via oral pode ficar comprometida.
• As formas injetáveis devem ser utilizadas quando aplicável.

INTERAÇÕES POSSÍVEIS
N/D.

MEDICAMENTO(S) ALTERNATIVO(S)
N/D.

ACOMPANHAMENTO

MONITORIZAÇÃO DO PACIENTE
• Os animais com pneumonia por aspiração devem ser submetidos a radiografias torácicas e hemogramas completos até a resolução do quadro ou se houver suspeita de recidiva.
• Os animais devem ser monitorizados e pesados para avaliar o escore da condição corporal e garantir a ingestão calórica adequada.

PREVENÇÃO
N/D.

COMPLICAÇÕES POSSÍVEIS
• Pneumonia por aspiração.

• Outras, dependendo da presença de diferentes doenças (p. ex., hipotireoidismo).

EVOLUÇÃO ESPERADA E PROGNÓSTICO
• Os animais mais idosos com megaesôfago idiopático apresentam um prognóstico mau.
• Pneumonia por aspiração é a causa típica de morte ou de eutanásia.

DIVERSOS

DISTÚRBIOS ASSOCIADOS
• Pneumonia por aspiração.
• Megaesôfago.

FATORES RELACIONADOS COM A IDADE
Os animais jovens podem recuperar alguma função esofágica com terapia adequada, dependendo da etiologia.

POTENCIAL ZOONÓTICO
Nenhum.

GESTAÇÃO/FERTILIDADE/REPRODUÇÃO
N/D.

VER TAMBÉM
• Disautonomia (Síndrome de Key-Gaskell).
• Disfagia.
• Esofagite.
• Megaesôfago.
• Miastenia Grave.
• Pneumonia Bacteriana.

ABREVIATURA(S)
• ACTH = hormônio adrenocorticotrópico.
• CK = creatina quinase.
• TC = tomografia computadorizada.

Sugestões de Leitura
Guilford G. Approach to clinical problems in gastroenterology. In: Strombeck's Small Animal Gastroenterology, 3rd ed. Philadelphia: Saunders, 1996, pp. 50-58.
Guilford G, Strombeck D. Diseases of swallowing. In: Strombeck's Small Animal Gastroenterology, 3rd ed. Philadelphia: Saunders, 1996, pp. 211-235.

Autor Jo Ann Morrison
Consultor Editorial Albert E. Jergens

RENOMEGALIA

CONSIDERAÇÕES GERAIS

DEFINIÇÃO
Um ou ambos os rins anormalmente grandes, detectados por palpação abdominal ou diagnóstico por imagem.

FISIOPATOLOGIA
Os rins podem ficar anormalmente grandes por causa de infiltração celular anormal (p. ex., inflamação, infecção e neoplasia), obstrução do trato urinário, necrose tubular aguda ou desenvolvimento de pseudocistos ou cistos renais.

SISTEMA(S) ACOMETIDO(S)
- Endócrino/metabólico — acidose metabólica atribuída à eliminação reduzida de ácido pelos rins e incapacidade de recuperar o bicarbonato.
- Gastrintestinal — inapetência, vômito, diarreia ou melena gerados por irritação ou ulceração gastrintestinais em pacientes com uremia.
- Hemático/linfático/imune — anemia por perda sanguínea ou tempo de sobrevida diminuído das hemácias em pacientes com uremia; suscetibilidade aumentada a infecções por disfunção imune nos pacientes com uremia, além de produção prejudicada de eritropoetina.
- Hepatobiliar — pode ocorrer renomegalia bilateral em pacientes com desvios portossistêmicos.
- Nervoso — depressão e letargia associadas ao efeito das toxinas urêmicas sobre o sistema nervoso central.
- Renal/urológico — um ou ambos os rins anormalmente grandes. Se um único rim estiver aumentado de volume, o rim contralateral poderá ficar anormalmente pequeno em função de doença relacionada ou não. Alternativamente, o rim contralateral pode sofrer aumento compensatório. O paciente virá a óbito antes de ambos os rins se tornarem extremamente aumentados.
- Respiratório — taquipneia ou angústia respiratória causadas por pneumonite urêmica ou resposta compensatória à acidose metabólica.

IDENTIFICAÇÃO
- Cães e gatos.
- Doença renal policística, uma causa de renomegalia, ocorre em várias raças de cães (Bull terrier, Cairn terrier, e West Highland white terrier) e gatos (Persa, outros).
- O modo de herança é autossômico dominante em cães Bull terrier e gatos Persa, mas autossômico recessivo nas raças Cairn terrier e West Highland white terrier.

SINAIS CLÍNICOS

Achados Anamnésicos
- O animal pode permanecer assintomático, sobretudo se apenas um rim estiver acometido.
- Letargia. • Perda de apetite. • Perda de peso.
- Vômito. • Diarreia. • Poliúria e polidipsia.
- Alteração na cor da urina. • Aumento de volume abdominal. • Claudicação (raramente) por causa da osteopatia hipertrófica associada à neoplasia renal.

Achados do Exame Físico
- Aumento de volume abdominal. • Massa abdominal. • Dor abdominal. • Um ou ambos os rins grandes à palpação. • Um rim aumentado de volume; outro rim anormalmente pequeno.
- Desidratação. • Mucosas pálidas. • Úlceras bucais. • Hálito de odor fétido.

CAUSAS E FATORES DE RISCO

Distúrbios do Desenvolvimento/Adquiridos
- Hidronefrose — pode provocar renomegalia uni ou bilateral em cães e gatos; desenvolve-se secundariamente à obstrução ureteral (p. ex., urolitíase, estenoses ureterais e neoplasia no trígono vesical) e a ureteres ectópicos.
- Doença renal policística — causa renomegalia bilateral em gatos e quase sempre leva à insuficiência renal crônica; pode ser mais comum nos gatos da raça Persa e doméstico de pelos longos.
- Hematoma — ocorre secundariamente a traumatismo; causa rara de renomegalia em cães e gatos.
- Hipertrofia compensatória — gera renomegalia unilateral e ocorre secundariamente à anormalidade do outro rim (p. ex., hipoplasia renal, displasia renal ou nefrectomia).

Neoplásicos
- Linfoma — ocorre com maior frequência nos gatos e provoca renomegalia bilateral; alguns pacientes apresentam renomegalia unilateral.
- Carcinoma renal — tumor renal mais comum dos cães; frequentemente provoca renomegalia unilateral; muito maligno e rapidamente metastático para locais distantes, como os pulmões.
- Nefroblastoma — também denominado tumor de Wilms; tumor renal congênito que acomete cães jovens, embora possa não ser diagnosticado até que o paciente esteja com uma idade muito mais avançada; o comportamento biológico varia; geralmente é unilateral.
- Sarcomas — provocam, em geral, renomegalia unilateral e têm comportamento maligno.
- Cistadenocarcinoma — tumor renal bilateral que ocorre em cães da raça Pastor alemão; quase sempre associado a lesões cutâneas (i. e., dermatofibrose nodular).

Infecciosos/Inflamatórios
- Amiloidose.
- Leptospirose (cães).
- Peritonite infecciosa felina.
- Infecção pelo vírus da leucemia felina predispõe os gatos ao desenvolvimento de linfoma renal.
- Abscesso renal — abscesso localizado dentro do parênquima renal costuma causar renomegalia unilateral em cães e gatos.

Tóxicos
- Intoxicação pelo etilenoglicol — pode ocasionar renomegalia bilateral secundária à tumefação tubular renal e infiltração renal por cristais de oxalato de cálcio.
- Outras toxinas que podem causar lesão renal aguda (p. ex., uvas/passas, lírios).

DIAGNÓSTICO

DIAGNÓSTICO DIFERENCIAL
- É imprescindível distinguir a renomegalia de outras massas abdominais.
- A confirmação pode necessitar de métodos de diagnóstico por imagem ou do procedimento de laparotomia exploratória.

HEMOGRAMA/BIOQUÍMICA/URINÁLISE
- Azotemia, hiperfosfatemia e capacidade de concentração urinária inadequadamente baixa.
- Leucocitose — causas infecciosas, inflamatórias e neoplásicas de renomegalia.
- Anemia arregenerativa — doença renal crônica ou distúrbios inflamatórios.
- Hiperglobulinemia — distúrbios infecciosos ou inflamatórios (p. ex., peritonite infecciosa felina).
- Hematúria e proteinúria — neoplasia renal.
- Policitemia e leucocitose extrema raramente acompanham algumas neoplasias renais.
- Raramente se observam células neoplásicas na urina dos pacientes com neoplasia renal.

OUTROS TESTES LABORATORIAIS
- Fazer o teste do vírus da leucemia felina nos gatos na suspeita de linfoma renal.
- Realizar a eletroforese das proteínas séricas para distinguir entre hiperglobulinemia policlonal e monoclonal.
- Avaliar os títulos pareados para *Leptospira* spp. com 3-4 semanas de intervalo em cães com suspeita de leptospirose.

DIAGNÓSTICO POR IMAGEM

Achados Radiográficos
- Radiografias abdominais simples são indicadas para confirmar a renomegalia e identificar as possíveis causas de obstrução ureteral (p. ex., ureterólitos radiopacos).
- Os rins aumentados de volume observados em projeção ventrodorsal encontram-se com >3 a 3,5 vezes o comprimento da segunda vértebra lombar nos gatos ou nos cães, respectivamente.
- Urografia excretora para confirmar a presença de renomegalia, hidronefrose e massas expansivas dos rins.
- Pielografia anterógrada pode ser necessária para excluir obstrução ureteral em alguns gatos.
- Radiografia torácica é indicada para detectar metástases em pacientes com neoplasia renal.

Achados Ultrassonográficos
- Úteis para diferenciar as causas de renomegalia, incluindo doença renal policística, pseudocistos perirrenais, hidronefrose, neoplasia, abscesso e hematoma subcapsular.
- Inflamação aguda (p. ex., leptospirose, intoxicação pelo etilenoglicol) pode estar associada a aumento da ecogenicidade cortical, efusão perinéfrica ou banda medular de ecogenicidade aumentada.

MÉTODOS DIAGNÓSTICOS
- O exame citológico do aspirado por agulha fina pode confirmar a presença de cisto, abscesso e/ou neoplasia renais (linfoma). Em virtude do potencial de "disseminação" das células neoplásicas na parede abdominal, deve-se evitar o aspirado por agulha fina na suspeita de outros tumores renais (p. ex., carcinoma renal).
- Se nenhum diagnóstico definitivo for obtido pela avaliação citológica dos aspirados renais, poderá haver indicação de biopsia renal.

TRATAMENTO
- Diagnosticar e tratar a causa subjacente da renomegalia.
- O tratamento costuma ser feito em um esquema ambulatorial a menos que o paciente esteja

RENOMEGALIA

desidratado ou apresente insuficiência renal descompensada.
• Uma dieta renal terapêutica é indicada para prolongar o tempo de sobrevida de cães e gatos com doença renal crônica quando o nível sérico de creatinina exceder 2 mg/dL. A maioria dos pacientes aceitará a ração renal se a transição for gradativa em um período de 4 semanas; isso é particularmente crítico para os gatos.
• Se o paciente estiver saudável sob outros aspectos, fornecer a dieta normal e permitir a prática habitual de exercícios.
• Se o animal não conseguir manter a hidratação, administrar solução eletrolítica balanceada por via IV ou SC.
• Se o paciente apresentar desidratação ou perdas contínuas de líquido, como vômito ou diarreia, administrar fluidos por via IV para corrigir os déficits de hidratação, manter as necessidades diárias de líquido e repor as perdas contínuas.

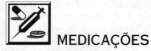 MEDICAÇÕES

MEDICAMENTO(S)
Variam com a causa.

CONTRAINDICAÇÕES/INTERAÇÕES POSSÍVEIS
Evitar os agentes nefrotóxicos.

 ACOMPANHAMENTO

MONITORIZAÇÃO DO PACIENTE
• Fazer o exame físico e pesar o paciente para avaliar o estado de hidratação.
• Outros exames (hemograma completo, perfil bioquímico sérico, urinálise, mensuração da pressão arterial) são indicados, dependendo da causa subjacente e da presença de outras condições (p. ex., anemia, azotemia, hipertensão, proteinúria).

COMPLICAÇÕES POSSÍVEIS
• Doença renal crônica, dependendo da causa subjacente da renomegalia.
• Síndromes paraneoplásicas associadas a tumores renais produtores de substâncias semelhantes a hormônios.

 DIVERSOS

DISTÚRBIOS ASSOCIADOS
N/D.

FATORES RELACIONADOS COM A IDADE
N/D.

POTENCIAL ZOONÓTICO
A leptospirose pode ser disseminada pelo contato com a urina infectada.

GESTAÇÃO/FERTILIDADE/REPRODUÇÃO
N/D.

VER TAMBÉM
• Doença Renal Policística.
• Hidronefrose.
• Intoxicação por Etilenoglicol.
• Leptospirose.
• Linfoma — Gatos.
• Obstrução do Trato Urinário.
• Peritonite Infecciosa Felina (PIF).

Sugestões de Leitura
Cuypers MD, Grooters AM, Williams J, et al. Renomegaly in dogs and cats. Part I: Differential diagnosis. Compend Contin Educ Pract Vet 1997, 19:1019-1033.

Autor S. Dru Forrester
Consultor Editorial Carl A. Osborne

Respiração Ofegante e Taquipneia

CONSIDERAÇÕES GERAIS

DEFINIÇÃO
- Taquipneia corresponde ao aumento da frequência respiratória.
- Respiração ofegante é uma respiração rápida e superficial de boca aberta, que não costuma estar associada a problemas de troca gasosa.

FISIOPATOLOGIA
- A frequência, o ritmo e o esforço respiratórios são controlados pelo centro respiratório no tronco encefálico em resposta a inúmeras vias aferentes, de origem tanto central como periférica. Tais vias incluem o córtex cerebral, os quimiorreceptores centrais e periféricos, a estimulação de mecanorreceptores nas vias aéreas que detectam os processos de insuflação e desinsuflação pulmonar, a estimulação de receptores irritantes das vias áreas, a estimulação de fibras-C nos alvéolos e vasos sanguíneos pulmonares que detectam congestão intersticial, e barorreceptores que detectam alterações na pressão arterial.
- Podem ocorrer taquipneia e respiração ofegante em resposta à estimulação de qualquer uma das vias de receptores mencionadas anteriormente.

SISTEMA(S) ACOMETIDO(S)
Respiratório.

IDENTIFICAÇÃO
- Cães e gatos; sem predileção etária ou sexual.
- Os cães mais idosos de grande porte são predispostos à respiração ofegante associada à paralisia da laringe.
- Os cães braquicefálicos são propensos à respiração ofegante em virtude de obstrução das vias aéreas superiores.

SINAIS CLÍNICOS
Achados Anamnésicos
- Os pacientes com doença respiratória ou cardíaca primária geralmente apresentam tosse ou intolerância a exercício associada.
- Causas não respiratórias — queixas clínicas associadas à doença primária, p. ex., PU/PD e polifagia em caso de hiperadrenocorticismo, sinais intermitentes de hipertensão sistêmica ou arritmia cardíaca em caso de feocromocitoma.

Achados do Exame Físico
- Pode ser observada síndrome braquicefálica (narinas estenóticas, estertores respiratórios associados a alongamento do palato mole ou eversão sacular).
- O estridor pode ser evidente à inspiração em caso de laringopatia, mas nem sempre é óbvio.
- Doença do parênquima pulmonar — pode exibir crepitações à auscultação; ruídos respiratórios ásperos são comuns, mas podem ser normais.
- Edema pulmonar cardiogênico — arritmia ou sopro cardíaco, taquicardia, ritmo de galope, hipotermia, mucosas pálidas, baixo tempo de preenchimento capilar.
- Doença do espaço pleural — ruídos respiratórios diminuídos: ventralmente — líquido; dorsalmente — ar.
- Doença da parede torácica — traumatismo visível e/ou palpável.
- Doenças não respiratórias — os achados dependerão de outras doenças, p. ex., mucosas pálidas em caso de anemia, hepatomegalia em caso de hiperadrenocorticismo.
- Outros sinais podem indicar traumatismo.

CAUSAS E FATORES DE RISCO
Respiração ofegante
- Dor, ansiedade, hipertermia.
- Síndrome braquicefálica das vias aéreas.
- Doença do sistema nervoso central com controle ventilatório anormal.
- Comprometimento cardiovascular (choque), hipertensão, arritmia.
- Terapia medicamentosa (opioides), acidose metabólica.
- Laringopatia.
- Excesso de cortisol ou norepinefrina.
- Pode ser um padrão comportamental normal em alguns cães.

Taquipneia
- Hipoxemia, hipercapnia, hipotensão, hipertermia, anemia, acidose, inflamação.
- Doença das vias aéreas — irritante inalado, doença alérgica, broncoconstrição, compressão das vias aéreas, infecção das vias aéreas.
- Doença intersticial — edema, hemorragia, inflamação, neoplasia.
- Laringe — paralisia, edema, colapso, corpo estranho, neoplasia, inflamação, traumatismo, formação de malha/rede de tecido.
- Porção cervical da traqueia — colapso, estenose, traumatismo, corpo estranho, neoplasia, parasitas.
- Doença do parênquima pulmonar — edema (cardiogênico ou não cardiogênico), pneumonia ou pneumonite, neoplasia (primária ou metastática), hemorragia.
- Tromboembolia pulmonar — AHIM, enteropatia/nefropatia com perda de proteínas, cardiopatia, neoplasia, dirofilariose.
- Efusão pericárdica.
- Efusão pleural ou pneumotórax, hérnia diafragmática.
- Distensão abdominal — organomegalia; neoplasia, gestação; obesidade; ascite; dilatação/torção gástrica.
- Doença do SNC — compressão ou infarto próximo ao centro respiratório.
- Acidose metabólica — cetose diabética, diarreia, uremia, acidose tubular renal.

DIAGNÓSTICO

DIAGNÓSTICO DIFERENCIAL
- Taquipneia sem dispneia — pode ser sugestiva de algum problema não respiratório.
- Estertor e estridor são ruídos característicos de comprometimento das vias aéreas superiores — a auscultação sobre a traqueia pode ajudar a diferenciar os ruídos provenientes das vias aéreas superiores e inferiores.
- Auscultação e percussão torácicas — muito úteis para diferenciar doença pleural (ruídos pulmonares abafados/atenuados, percussão maciça) e doença parenquimatosa (ruídos respiratórios normais ou ásperos).
- Insuficiência cardíaca congestiva — sopro, taquicardia, má qualidade do pulso, pulsos jugulares, hipotermia, crepitações à auscultação, coriza nasal.

HEMOGRAMA/BIOQUÍMICA/URINÁLISE
- Anemia — pode causar taquipneia não respiratória.
- Policitemia — hipoxia crônica.
- Leucograma inflamatório — pneumonia, piotórax.
- Eosinofilia — doença alérgica ou parasitária.
- Trombocitose — hiperadrenocorticismo predispõe à tromboembolia pulmonar; alternativamente, pode indicar anemia por deficiência de ferro (ferropriva).
- Relação sódio:potássio <27 — pode ser observada em caso de efusões quilosas pleurais ou abdominais.
- Atividade elevada da fosfatase alcalina — hiperadrenocorticismo predispõe à respiração ofegante e tromboembolia pulmonar.
- Hipoproteinemia — pode sugerir doença com perda de proteínas que pode predispor à tromboembolia pulmonar.
- Proteinúria — pode predispor à tromboembolia pulmonar.
- Hiperglicemia, glicosúria, e cetonúria — podem indicar cetoacidose como causa de taquipneia.

OUTROS TESTES LABORATORIAIS
- Teste de dirofilariose.
- Exames fecais se indicados.
- Teste de supressão com dexametasona em baixas doses para avaliar a função do córtex da adrenal, se indicado.
- Análise do líquido pleural.
- Oximetria de pulso ou exame de gasometria arterial — pode ajudar a diferenciar causas pulmonares e não respiratórias.
- Saturação da hemoglobina com oxigênio <95% apoia a presença de hipoxemia.
- PaO_2 — pressão parcial de oxigênio dissolvido no sangue arterial; normoxemia: PaO_2 80-120 mmHg (ar ambiente, nível do mar), hipoxemia: PaO_2 <80 mmHg; hiperoxemia: PaO_2 >120 mmHg; FiO_2 — fração de oxigênio inspirado varia de 0,21 (ar ambiente) a 1,0; relação PaO_2/F_IO_2 — mensuração da eficiência pulmonar; PaO_2/FiO_2 ≤500 — eficiência pulmonar normal; 300-500 — ineficiência leve; 200-300 — ineficiência moderada; <200 — ineficiência grave. A redução na eficiência pulmonar é mais comumente atribuída à doença do parênquima pulmonar.
- $PaCO_2$ — pressão parcial de CO_2 dissolvido no sangue arterial; mensuração da ventilação; $PaCO_2$ normal = 40 mmHg (cão); 31 mmHg (gato). Hipercapnia = hipoventilação = ventilação minuto alveolar reduzida. Hipocapnia = hiperventilação = ventilação minuto alveolar aumentada. A hipoventilação pode ser atribuída à obstrução das vias aéreas superiores, doença do espaço pleural, doença da parede torácica e distensão abdominal; a fadiga dos músculos respiratórios causada por um período prolongado de taquipneia pode levar à hipoventilação.
- A gasometria arterial pode revelar acidose metabólica como uma causa.
- Teste de coagulação — na suspeita de hemotórax e/ou hemorragia pulmonar.

DIAGNÓSTICO POR IMAGEM
- Radiografia cervicotorácica: *laringopatia* — o aumento da densidade pode sugerir a presença de edema. Também pode haver lesão expansiva tipo massa dos tecidos moles, estreitamento das grandes vias aéreas, linfadenopatia, anormalidades intraluminais. *Pneumonia* — infiltrados alveolares; pneumonia por aspiração geralmente com distribuição cranioventral ou lobos médios acometidos. *Edema pulmonar cardiogênico* — sombra cardíaca aumentada, distensão venosa

Respiração Ofegante e Taquipneia

pulmonar, átrio esquerdo aumentado de tamanho com infiltrados pulmonares peri-hilares em cães; os infiltrados podem ser de qualquer distribuição em gatos. *Edema pulmonar não cardiogênico* — distribuição caudodorsal. SARA — infiltrados alveolares simétricos difusos. *Anormalidades vasculares pulmonares* — tromboembolia pulmonar, dirofilariose. *Doença do espaço pleural* — pneumotórax, efusão pleural, lesões expansivas tipo massa, hérnias diafragmáticas. *Doença da parede torácica* — fraturas de costela, neoplasia.
• Ultrassonografia torácica: avaliação da distribuição de efusão pleural (excelente como guia para toracocentese). Identificação de massa pulmonar — serve como guia para aspiração com agulha fina; avaliação do mediastino. A ausência do "sinal de deslizamento" pode ser usada para identificar pneumotórax.
• Ecocardiografia: avalia a função cardíaca na suspeita de edema pulmonar cardiogênico ou efusão pleural; o aumento da pressão arterial pulmonar e a sobrecarga do ventrículo direito podem apoiar o diagnóstico de tromboembolia pulmonar; permite a visualização de massas na base do coração e descarta o quadro de efusão pericárdica.
• Ultrassonografia abdominal: avaliação de distensão abdominal e do tamanho da glândula adrenal.
• Angiografia vascular pulmonar: exame com padrão de excelência para o diagnóstico de tromboembolia pulmonar.
• Cintilografia da perfusão: embora o desequilíbrio entre ventilação e perfusão seja sugestivo de tromboembolia pulmonar, raramente esse exame é realizado; o resultado anormal na cintilografia da perfusão apoia a presença de tromboembolia pulmonar.
• Talvez haja necessidade de neuroimagem (SNC).

MÉTODOS DIAGNÓSTICOS
• Laringoscopia/nasofaringoscopia — para avaliar a função da laringe e visualizar a presença de corpos estranhos e massas; permite a visualização da região caudal da nasofaringe com o uso de gancho utilizado para exteriorização de útero/ovário e espelho odontológico.
• Broncoscopia — avalia as vias aéreas de pequeno e grande calibre; permite a obtenção de biopsias; possibilita a realização de lavagem broncoalveolar para exames de citologia e cultura.
• Toracocentese — análise e cultura do líquido.

TRATAMENTO
CUIDADO(S) DE SAÚDE ADEQUADO(S)
• Fornecer cuidados hospitalares em casos potencialmente letais; a terapia depende da causa subjacente.

• Administrar oxigênio e verificar se a taquipneia desaparece — isso apoiaria o diagnóstico de problema respiratório primário.
• Paralisia da laringe — utilizar sedação para reduzir o esforço respiratório. Verificar a temperatura corporal com frequência e resfriar os pacientes ativamente conforme a necessidade, já que a hipertermia aumentará o esforço respiratório. Doença grave das vias aéreas superiores exige entubação para estabilização do paciente; caso não se consiga a cura imediata do problema, fica indicada a colocação de tubo de traqueostomia temporária. Remover corpos estranhos; realizar excisão/biopsia cirúrgicas de massas; fazer correção cirúrgica de paralisia laríngea e síndrome braquicefálica; administrar medicamentos anti-inflamatórios para edema de laringe.
• Doença das vias aéreas inferiores — broncodilatadores (terbutalina); oxigenoterapia até a estabilização do paciente; pode haver a necessidade de corticosteroides sistêmicos para estabilizar os gatos com broncoconstrição aguda.
• Doença do parênquima pulmonar — oxigenoterapia, antibióticos em caso de pneumonia; tratar distúrbios de coagulação; edema cardiogênico requer o uso de furosemida ± vasodilatadores. Edema não cardiogênico necessita da administração de oxigênio, podendo exigir ventilação com pressão positiva se a oxigenoterapia sozinha não for adequada para estabilizar o paciente.
• Doença do espaço pleural — toracocentese para punção de ar e líquido; remover o máximo possível. Colocar um tubo torácico se houver necessidade de punções torácicas repetidas para manter o paciente estável.
• Distensão abdominal — drenar ascite apenas conforme a necessidade para manter o paciente confortável; aliviar a distensão gástrica.
• Doenças não respiratórias — tratar o problema primário.

CUIDADO(S) DE ENFERMAGEM
• Fornecer a oxigenoterapia via gaiola, cânula nasal, colar elizabetano coberto por envoltório plástico*, máscara, ou mecanismo de fluxo tipo *flow-by*. Umidificar a fonte de oxigênio em caso de oxigenoterapia nasal por mais de algumas horas.
• Manter o animal em decúbito esternal e mudá-lo de posição a cada 3-4 horas em caso de intolerância à posição de decúbito lateral. Monitorizar a temperatura regularmente, pois a hipertermia agravará a dificuldade respiratória.

ATIVIDADE
Conforme tolerância pela doença primária.

DIETA
Se a obesidade for uma causa que contribui para o problema, utilizar dieta de redução de peso.

ORIENTAÇÃO AO PROPRIETÁRIO
• A anestesia deve ser cuidadosamente adaptada ao paciente. É essencial garantir uma via aérea patente (desobstruída), além de ser importante uma rápida indução intravenosa.
• Na suspeita de paralisia da laringe, preparar o paciente para correção cirúrgica no momento do diagnóstico. Alertar os proprietários quanto à probabilidade elevada de pneumonia por aspiração como complicação em cães com laringopatia.

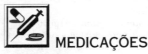

MEDICAMENTO(S)
Varia com a causa subjacente (ver "Cuidados de Saúde Adequados").

ACOMPANHAMENTO
Verificar a frequência respiratória em repouso em casa.

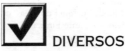

VER TAMBÉM
• Acidose, Metabólica.
• Síndrome da Angústia Respiratória Aguda.
• Asma, Bronquite — Gatos.
• Síndrome Braquicefálica das Vias Aéreas.
• Insuficiência Cardíaca Congestiva, Esquerda.
• Capítulos sobre Diabetes Melito.
• Laringopatias.
• Capítulos sobre Pneumonia.
• Pneumotórax.
• Edema Pulmonar, Não Cardiogênico.

ABREVIATURAS
• AHIM = anemia hemolítica imunomediada.
• PU/PD = poliúria/polidipsia.
• SARA = síndrome da angústia respiratória aguda.
• SNC = sistema nervoso central.

Sugestões de Leitura
Forney S. Dyspnea and tachypnea. In: Ettinger SJ, Feldman EC, eds., Textbook of Small Animal Internal Medicine, 7th ed. Philadelphia: Saunders Elsevier, 2010, pp. 253-255.
Mandell DC. Respiratory distress in cats. In: King LG, Textbook of Respiratory Disease in Dogs and Cats. Philadelphia: Saunders, 2004, pp. 12-17.

Autores Kate Hopper e Lynelle R. Johnson
Consultor Editorial Lynelle R. Johnson

---

* N. T.: Para criar um ambiente rico em oxigênio.

RETENÇÃO URINÁRIA FUNCIONAL

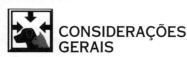

CONSIDERAÇÕES GERAIS

DEFINIÇÃO
Micção incompleta, não associada à obstrução urinária.

FISIOPATOLOGIA
Distúrbio da fase de eliminação da urina; a micção incompleta origina-se de falha neurogênica e/ou miogênica. Isso leva à hipocontratilidade da bexiga urinária (atonia do músculo detrusor) e/ou resistência indevidamente excessiva ao fluxo de saída (obstrução urinária funcional).

SISTEMA(S) ACOMETIDO(S)
• Renal/urológico. • Endócrino/metabólico.
• Nervoso.

DISTRIBUIÇÃO GEOGRÁFICA
• Mundial. • Disautonomia: Europa (Grã-Bretanha, Escandinávia) e Estados Unidos (Meio-Oeste), além de casos esporádicos em Dubai, Nova Zelândia e Venezuela.

IDENTIFICAÇÃO
Espécies
Cães e gatos.

Raça(s) Predominante(s)
• Raças condrodistróficas com discopatia intervertebral. • Gatos Manx com lesões espinais sacrais congênitas. • Cães de grande porte (Pastor alemão) com síndrome adquirida da cauda equina. • Labrador retriever, Pointer alemão de pelo curto, Pastor alemão com disautonomia.

Idade Média e Faixa Etária
Cães jovens adultos com obstrução urinária funcional.

Sexo Predominante
Mais comum em machos que em fêmeas.

SINAIS CLÍNICOS
Comentários Gerais
Os sinais incluem anormalidades primárias e secundárias de disfunção miccional.

Achados Anamnésicos
• Histórico de tentativas frequentes de micção, esforço para urinar ou simplesmente ausência de micção. • Jato urinário atenuado, interrompido ou prolongado. • O extravasamento de urina ocorre quando a pressão na bexiga urinária excede a pressão de fechamento da saída uretral (incontinência por transbordamento ou paradoxal). • Vômito, letargia, dor abdominal em casos de ruptura ou inflamação do trato urinário.

Achados do Exame Físico
• Uretra normal à palpação retal.
• A bexiga urinária permanece distendida à palpação e/ou identifica-se a presença de urina residual inapropriada (normal: 0,2-0,4 mL/kg) após tentativas de micção.
• Exame neurológico anormal (ver a seção "Diagnóstico Diferencial").
• Distensão e dor abdominais ou sinais de azotemia pós-renal em casos associados à ruptura do trato urinário.
• Incontinência urinária por transbordamento.

CAUSAS
Hipocontratilidade Vesical do Músculo Detrusor (Atonia do Detrusor)
• Desenvolve-se mais comumente como sequela de distensão vesical excessiva.
• Pode ter obstrução urinária prévia ou disfunção neurológica.
• As causas neurogênicas incluem lesões dos nervos pélvicos, bem como da medula espinal sacral e suprassacral.
• As lesões da medula espinal sacral (p. ex., más-formações congênitas, compressão da cauda equina, discopatia lombossacra e fraturas/deslocamentos vertebrais) podem resultar em bexiga superdistendida e flácida com baixa resistência ao fluxo de saída (bexiga atribuída à lesão do neurônio motor inferior).
• As lesões da medula espinal suprassacral (p. ex., protrusão de disco intervertebral, fraturas da coluna vertebral e neoplasias compressivas) podem culminar em bexiga firme e distendida de difícil compressão manual (bexiga atribuída à lesão do neurônio motor superior).
• A disautonomia pode levar à atonia do detrusor com retenção urinária.
• Os distúrbios eletrolíticos e outros distúrbios metabólicos associados à fraqueza muscular generalizada podem comprometer a contratilidade do músculo detrusor.
• Hiperadrenocorticismo canino pode causar poliúria, distensão vesical e leve retenção urinária.
• Os medicamentos indutores de graus variados de falha miogênica incluem antidepressivos tricíclicos, bloqueadores dos canais de cálcio, agentes anticolinérgicos e opioides.

Obstrução Urinária Funcional
• Ocorre quando a resistência excessiva ou inapropriada ao fluxo de saída impede a eliminação completa da urina durante a contração vesical.
• Em pacientes com lesões espinais suprassacrais (tipicamente T3-L3) ou distúrbios mesencefálicos, a resistência uretral ao fluxo de saída perde o estímulo inibitório e permanece inapropriadamente excessiva ou falha na coordenação com as contrações vesicais (dissinergia do músculo detrusor-esfíncter uretral). A condição é associada a lesões sacrais e neuropatias locais.
• Algumas vezes, idiopática.
• Pode-se observar resistência uretral demasiada, atribuída normalmente aos componentes musculares lisos ou estriados da uretra (uretrospasmo), subsequente à obstrução uretral ou em decorrência de cirurgia uretral ou pélvica, inflamação uretral ou prostatopatia.

FATORES DE RISCO
• Doença do trato urinário inferior dos felinos.
• Obstrução uretral. • Cirurgia pélvica ou uretral.
• Medicamentos anticolinérgicos. • Analgesia epidural.

DIAGNÓSTICO

DIAGNÓSTICO DIFERENCIAL
• Quando não se observa nenhuma eliminação de urina, será imprescindível diferenciar as causas de disfunção uretral ao fluxo de saída de oligúria, anúria e ruptura do trato urinário.
• A disfunção ao fluxo de saída também precisa ser diferenciada de obstrução anatômica (física e mecânica). Os sinais clínicos associados à obstrução urinária incluem polaciúria, estrangúria e hematúria; os pacientes com obstrução mecânica podem eliminar algumas gotas de urina após longos períodos de esforço.
• Os achados neurológicos em cães com lesões supraespinais que comprometem a micção englobam paralisia ou paresia dos membros pélvicos e, algumas vezes, torácicos, hiper-reflexia dos membros acometidos, bem como dor cervical, toracolombar e lombar. Além de distendida e firme, a bexiga urinária costuma ser de difícil compressão. Em pacientes com lesões crônicas ou parciais, pode ocorrer micção reflexa, caracterizada por contrações involuntárias e incompletas do músculo detrusor com espasticidade ao fluxo de saída.
• Os achados neurológicos em cães com lesões sacrais que afetam a micção incluem paresia dos membros pélvicos com hiporreflexia, diminuição do tônus anocaudal, perda sensorial perineal e depressão dos reflexos bulboespinosos. A dor lombossacra pode ser o único sinal. Tipicamente, a bexiga encontra-se distendida e flácida, sendo de fácil compressão.
• A presença de jato de urina que pode ser iniciado, mas abruptamente interrompido, é típica de dissinergia idiopática do músculo detrusor-esfíncter uretral. A palpação manual pode confirmar as contrações do músculo detrusor, que persistem após o término do fluxo e possivelmente sugerem volume residual elevado de urina.
• Em pacientes em fase de convalescença subsequente à obstrução urinária, a incapacidade de eliminar a urina pode se originar de nova obstrução, resistência uretral (funcional) excessiva ou atonia do músculo detrusor causada por hiperdistensão vesical. Caso se consiga comprimir a bexiga urinária com palpação abdominal suave, haverá grandes possibilidades de atonia do músculo detrusor. Caso se encontre alguma resistência à compressão manual e se consiga descartar a presença de obstrução uretral por meio de exame ou cateterização transuretral, será provável a obstrução funcional.
• Os sinais clínicos que acompanham a retenção urinária em pacientes com disautonomia podem incluir midríase, prolapso da terceira pálpebra, xerostomia (ressecamento da boca), regurgitação ou vômito, megaesôfago, tônus anal reduzido ou ausente, diarreia ou constipação e bradicardia.

HEMOGRAMA/BIOQUÍMICA/URINÁLISE
• Os resultados dos testes descartam causas metabólicas de doença neuromuscular; tais resultados também podem ser utilizados para detectar a gravidade da azotemia pós-renal.
• A urinálise pode revelar infecção do trato urinário, traumatismo ou inflamação.

DIAGNÓSTICO POR IMAGEM
• Radiografias simples e ultrassonografia para descartar urólitos obstrutivos, traumatismo pélvico, doença lombossacra, massas abdominais caudais.
• Cistouretrografia ou vaginouretrografia contrastadas ou, ocasionalmente, cistouretroscopia para excluir lesões obstrutivas.
• Mielografia, epidurografia, TC ou RM para localizar lesões neurológicas.

MÉTODOS DIAGNÓSTICOS
• Exame neurológico — os exames do tônus anal e caudal, bem como da sensibilidade perineal e dos reflexos bulboesponjosos fornecem uma avaliação das funções da medula espinal caudal e dos nervos periféricos.

Retenção Urinária Funcional

- Cateterização transuretral — pode ser necessária para descartar obstrução uretral; os cateteres devem passar com facilidade em animais sem obstrução mecânica e naqueles com compressão uretral extramural (p. ex., causada por massa lisa no colo vesical, prostatomegalia ou massa abdominal caudal).
- O diagnóstico de disautonomia é formulado com base em testes farmacológicos sistemáticos de respostas autônomas.
- Procedimentos urodinâmicos — podem ser utilizados para confirmar a atonia do músculo detrusor ou a obstrução funcional da uretra ou para comprovar a dissinergia do músculo detrusor-esfíncter uretral; a arreflexia do detrusor pode ser confirmada por meio de estudos cistometrográficos; a resistência uretral inapropriada ou o espasmo uretral são ocasionalmente registrados por meio da perfilometria* uretral em repouso; a combinação de cistometria com mensurações da pressão uretral ou estudos do fluxo urinário é necessária para registrar uma dissinergia.

ACHADOS PATOLÓGICOS
Atonia do Músculo Detrusor
- A hiperdistensão prévia da bexiga urinária não costuma ser discernível ao exame macroscópico.
- Hipoplasia ou aplasia das vértebras caudais e várias lesões da medula espinal sacral (cobertura anormal, meningomieloceles, lipomas intradurais) em alguns gatos Manx.
- Microscopia óptica de tecidos apropriados em casos crônicos: degeneração disseminada das células musculares lisas, dos axônios colinérgicos e dos nervos intrínsecos.

Obstrução Uretral Funcional
- Várias doenças neurológicas suprassacrais (p. ex., discopatia intervertebral, embolia fibrocartilaginosa).
- Uretrite.
- Prostatite.

TRATAMENTO
CUIDADO(S) DE SAÚDE ADEQUADO(S)
Em geral, o paciente é internado até que a função miccional adequada retorne ao normal.

CUIDADO(S) DE ENFERMAGEM
- Tratar o quadro de azotemia, bem como os desequilíbrios eletrolíticos e acidobásicos associados à retenção aguda de urina (rara).
- Identificar a presença de infecção do trato urinário e tratá-la de modo apropriado.
- Manter baixa repleção vesical por meio da cateterização intermitente ou fixação de cateter de demora ou ainda por compressão manual frequente.

ORIENTAÇÃO AO PROPRIETÁRIO
Orientar os proprietários sobre o fato de que a função vesical completa pode não retornar ao normal. Monitorar o paciente em busca de sinais de obstrução completa, uremia e infecção do trato urinário.

CONSIDERAÇÕES CIRÚRGICAS
Considerar as opções cirúrgicas para recuperação da patência (desobstrução) uretral em alguns pacientes; talvez haja necessidade de uretrostomia perineal em gatos machos com resistência uretral distal intratável.

MEDICAÇÕES
MEDICAMENTO(S) DE ESCOLHA
Atonia do Músculo Detrusor
- Betanecol (5-25 mg/cão VO a cada 8-12 h; 1,25-5 mg/gato a cada 8-12 h) — agente colinérgico; pode aumentar o impulso contrátil do músculo detrusor em bexigas parcialmente desnervadas ou agudamente superdistendidas. • Metoclopramida (cão e gato, 0,2-0,5 mg/kg VO a cada 8 h) — antagonista dopaminérgico; pode estimular a contração do músculo detrusor. • Cisaprida (cão, 0,5 mg/kg VO a cada 8 h; 1,25-5 mg/gato a cada 8-12 h) — agente procinético da musculatura lisa; pode promover o esvaziamento da bexiga.

Obstrução Uretral Funcional
- Prazosina (cão, 1 mg/15 kg VO a cada 12-24 h; gato, 0,25-0,5 mg/gato VO a cada 12-24 h ou 0,03 mg/kg IV) ou fenoxibenzamina (cão, 0,25-0,5 mg/kg VO a cada 12-24 h; gato, 1,25-7,5 mg/gato VO a cada 12-24 h) — antagonistas α-adrenérgicos diminuem a contração da musculatura lisa na uretra; costumam ser mais eficazes em cães do que em gatos.
- Diazepam (cão, 2-10 mg/cão VO a cada 8 h; gato, 1-2,5 mg/gato VO a cada 8 h ou 0,5 mg/kg IV) — relaxa a musculatura estriada do esfíncter uretral externo. • Acepromazina (cão, 0,5-2 mg/kg VO a cada 6-8 h; gato, 1-2 mg/kg VO a cada 6-8 h) — tranquilizante fenotiazínico e relaxante muscular geral com efeitos bloqueadores α-adrenérgicos sobre o tônus uretral; pode ser eficaz em gatos com resistência uretral excessiva.
- Dantroleno (cão, 1-5 mg/kg VO a cada 8-12 h; gato, 0,5-2 mg/kg VO a cada 8 h ou 1 mg/kg IV) — outro relaxante da musculatura estriada; parece ser eficaz na redução da resistência uretral distal em gatos. • Baclofeno (cão, 5-10 mg/cão VO a cada 8 h) — inibidor dos reflexos espinais; atua como relaxante da musculatura esquelética; avaliação clínica limitada em cães e gatos.

CONTRAINDICAÇÕES
- O baclofeno é contraindicado em gatos.
- A acepromazina, a fenoxibenzamina e a prazosina têm efeitos vasodilatadores — utilizar com cuidado em pacientes com depleção volêmica ou azotemia, bem como naqueles com cardiopatia.
- Acepromazina e diazepam — podem causar sedação; usar com cautela em pacientes letárgicos.

PRECAUÇÕES
- Confirmar um fluxo de saída adequado para a urina antes de se administrar o betanecol, já que esse agente pode aumentar a contração muscular do colo vesical e da uretra proximal. Efetuar pré-tratamento com α-agonistas (p. ex., fenoxibenzamina e prazosina).
- A prazosina pode causar uma potente hipotensão de "primeira dose"; para minimizar o risco, a dosagem inicial deve ser a metade da dose total.
- Hepatopatia aguda — descrita como uma complicação rara da administração oral do diazepam em gatos.

INTERAÇÕES POSSÍVEIS
A administração concomitante de cisaprida pode acentuar o efeito sedativo do diazepam.

ACOMPANHAMENTO
MONITORIZAÇÃO DO PACIENTE
- Reavaliar o volume urinário residual por meio da palpação vesical ou da cateterização transuretral periódica.
- Suspender as medicações lentamente após a correção das causas primárias e a ocorrência de função miccional adequada por vários dias.
- Realizar urinálise e urocultura seriadas para detectar infecção do trato urinário em pacientes com retenção crônica de urina.

COMPLICAÇÕES POSSÍVEIS
- Infecção do trato urinário.
- Lesão e atonia permanentes do músculo detrusor; rupturas vesical ou uretral.

EVOLUÇÃO ESPERADA E PROGNÓSTICO
- Prognóstico bom para atonia aguda do músculo detrusor causada por hiperdistensão, lesões neurológicas reversíveis agudas, obstrução funcional aguda associada a distúrbios uretrais irritantes ou obstrução em processo de resolução — a recuperação frequentemente ocorre dentro de 1 semana.
- Prognóstico razoável a mau para atonia crônica do músculo detrusor ou obstrução funcional crônica — a função urinária costuma se recuperar à medida que a função motora dos membros se recupera. Se a obstrução funcional for responsiva aos α-agonistas, poderá haver a necessidade de administração prolongada.

DIVERSOS
DISTÚRBIOS ASSOCIADOS
- Infecção do trato urinário. • Azotemia.

GESTAÇÃO/FERTILIDADE/REPRODUÇÃO
O betanecol é contraindicado.

SINÔNIMO(S)
- Disfunção miccional. • Neuropatia vesical.
- Bexiga neuropática. • Dissinergia reflexa, dissinergia do músculo detrusor-esfíncter uretral.
- Uretrospasmo.

VER TAMBÉM
- Azotemia e Uremia. • Disúria e Polaciúria.
- Discopatia Intervertebral Toracolombar.
- Doença Idiopática do Trato Urinário Inferior dos Felinos. • Estenose Lombossacra e Síndrome da Cauda Equina. • Obstrução do Trato Urinário.
- Prostatite e Abscesso Prostático.

ABREVIATURA(S)
- RM = ressonância magnética.
- TC = tomografia computadorizada.

Sugestões de Leitura
Labato MA. Micturition disorders. In: Ettinger SJ, Feldman EC, eds., Textbook of Veterinary Internal Medicine, 6th ed. St. Louis: Elsevier, 2005, pp. 105-109.

Autor Steffen O. Sum
Consultor Editorial Carl Osborne
Agradecimento O autor e o editor agradecem a colaboração de Índia F. Lane pela elaboração prévia deste capítulo e de Jeanne A. Barsanti pela revisão.

---
* N. T.: Perfil pressórico.

RINITE E SINUSITE

CONSIDERAÇÕES GERAIS

DEFINIÇÃO
• Rinite — inflamação do epitélio nasal.
• Sinusite — inflamação dos seios paranasais. Envolve o seio frontal e o recesso maxilar nos cães, mas os seios frontal e esfenopalatino nos gatos.
• A cavidade nasal se comunica diretamente com os seios paranasais; portanto, a rinite e a sinusite frequentemente ocorrem em conjunto (rinossinusite).

FISIOPATOLOGIA
A inflamação e a irritação estimulam a secreção glandular serosa na mucosa nasal. Com a cronicidade, infecções bacterianas oportunistas desenvolvem-se na mucosa nasal comprometida, fazendo com que a secreção se torne mucoide ou mucopurulenta. O processo inflamatório pode levar à destruição dos ossos turbinados e erosão da vasculatura (resultando em epistaxe).

SISTEMA(S) ACOMETIDO(S)
• Respiratório — geralmente indica doença do trato respiratório superior. Ocasionalmente, pode-se observar secreção nasal em caso de doença das vias aéreas inferiores.
• Nervoso — doença fúngica e neoplásica podem invadir o cérebro via destruição da placa cribriforme.
• Ocular — epífora com inflamação dos ductos nasolacrimais. Conjuntivite, ceratite e/ou ulcerações da córnea na rinite viral. Coriorretinite na cinomose ou em infecção por *Cryptococcus*.
• Cavidade bucal — calicivírus, FeLV, FIV estão associados à estomatite, glossite, faucite. Possíveis abscessos da raiz dentária ou fístula oronasal.

INCIDÊNCIA/PREVALÊNCIA
• Rinossinusite bacteriana primária é rara.
• Gatos — os quadros de rinossinusite crônica são comuns.
• Cão — neoplasia, rinite inflamatória, doença fúngica são comuns.

IDENTIFICAÇÃO
Espécies
Cães e gatos.

Raça(s) Predominante(s)
• Gatos braquicefálicos são mais propensos à rinite crônica e, possivelmente, rinite fúngica.
• Cães dolicocéfalos são mais propensos à infecção por *Aspergillus* e a tumores nasais.

Idade Média e Faixa Etária
• Gatos — rinossinusite viral aguda e pólipos nasofaríngeos são mais comuns em filhotes felinos jovens (6-12 semanas).
• Doenças congênitas (fenda palatina) são mais usuais em animais jovens.
• Neoplasia e doença dentária são mais comuns em animais mais idosos.
• Corpos estranhos são mais habituais em cães jovens.

Sexo Predominante
Não há predileção sexual.

SINAIS CLÍNICOS
Achados Anamnésicos
• Espirros, secreção nasal, epistaxe.
• A secreção costuma ser serosa inicialmente e depois se torna mucoide, mucopurulenta, serossanguinolenta ou hemorrágica.
• Secreção unilateral sugere corpo estranho, abscesso da raiz dentária, neoplasia ou infecção fúngica. Também pode haver rinite inflamatória idiopática com sinais unilaterais.
• Secreção bilateral é mais comum em casos de rinossinusite viral ou bacteriana, rinite inflamatória, doença faríngea ou anormalidades congênitas.
• Deformidade facial — geralmente em doença neoplásica ou fúngica.
• Espirro reverso é mais comum nos cães, enquanto a inapetência é mais comum nos gatos.

Achados do Exame Físico
• Verificar fluxo aéreo nasal diminuído, uni ou bilateral.
• Avaliar a cavidade bucal em busca de abscessos da raiz dentária, fístula oronasal ou úlceras.
• Possível aumento na sensibilidade traqueal ou tosse.
• Procurar por epífora, conjuntivite, síndrome de Horner (comprometimento da orelha média).
• Exame do fundo ocular — possível coriorretinite.

CAUSAS
Cães

Causas Incitantes Primárias
• Doença fúngica — *Aspergillus fumigatus* é o agente mais comum. *Penicillium* spp., *Rhinosporidium seeberi*, *Blastomyces dermatitidis*, *Cryptococcus neoformans* são causas raras.
• Abscessos da raiz dentária.
• Corpo estranho.
• Anormalidades congênitas, como fenda palatina ou discinesia ciliar primária.
• Causas parasitárias — ácaros nasais (*Pneumonyssoides caninum*), *Capillaria aerophagia*.
• Neoplasia intranasal — adenocarcinoma é a mais comum (31,5%). Outros tumores incluem linfoma, condrossarcomas ou osteossarcomas.
• Rinite imunomediada — a rinite alérgica é rara, porém a rinite linfoplasmocitária idiopática é mais comum.
• Outras doenças infecciosas incluem cinomose ou *Bordetella bronchiseptica*; o microrganismo *Bartonella* não foi associado à rinite.
• Traumatismo local pode provocar deformidade dos ossos ou turbinados e predispõe à rinite crônica.

Causas Secundárias
• Doença das vias aéreas inferiores (broncopneumonia) ou vômito pode provocar sinais de rinite.
• Epistaxe pode estar relacionada com hipertensão, trombocitopenia, trombocitopatia ou, raramente, outras coagulopatias, além de possível traumatismo.

Gatos

Causas Incitantes Primárias
• Infecções virais — herpes-vírus 1 e calicivírus respondem por 90% das infecções agudas.
• Infecções bacterianas — *Bordetella bronchiseptica* pode ser um patógeno primário nos gatos, porém seu significado nesses animais é incerto. *Bartonella* não está associada.
• Neoplasia — adenocarcinoma e linfoma são as mais comuns.
• Doença fúngica — *Cryptococcus neoformans* é o agente mais comum, mas considerar também *Aspergillus* e *Penicillium* (raro nos gatos).
• Pólipos nasofaríngeos nos gatos jovens.
• Redes/estenoses nasofaríngeas — congênitas ou secundárias à infecção crônica ou traumatismos.
• Abscesso da raiz dentária.
• Corpos estranhos.
• Anormalidades congênitas incluem fenda palatina.

Causas Secundárias
• Epistaxe atribuída à coagulopatia ou hipertensão.
• Aspiração de vômito para dentro da nasofaringe.

FATORES DE RISCO
• Raças dolicocéfalas — doença fúngica.
• Gatos braquicefálicos — rinossinusite.

DIAGNÓSTICO

DIAGNÓSTICO DIFERENCIAL
Descartar as causas secundárias de rinite, incluindo coagulopatia, hipertensão, doença das vias aéreas inferiores, vômito crônico.

HEMOGRAMA/BIOQUÍMICA/URINÁLISE
• O hemograma é inespecífico — pode apresentar leucocitose, neutrofilia, eosinofilia com agentes infecciosos. Anemia regenerativa na perda sanguínea grave por coagulopatia. Anemia arregenerativa em caso de doença crônica ou neoplasia. Trombocitopenia observada nas coagulopatias ou perda sanguínea grave.
• Bioquímica sérica e urinálise permanecem tipicamente normais.

OUTROS TESTES LABORATORIAIS
• Testes sorológicos para FeLV e FIV.
• Teste de aglutinação em látex para o antígeno capsular criptocócico.
• Títulos para *Aspergillus* — são possíveis resultados falso-negativos.
• Perfil da coagulação na presença de epistaxe.

DIAGNÓSTICO POR IMAGEM
• Radiografia — radiografias torácicas se houver suspeita de doença das vias aéreas inferiores, neoplasia ou doença fúngica.
• Radiografias dentárias são altamente sensíveis para detectar doença periodontal.
• Radiografias do crânio são valiosas, porém não diferenciam entre rinite inflamatória, infecção fúngica e doença neoplásica. A perda de estruturas turbinadas pode ser observada em todas as causas. As projeções ventrodorsais de boca aberta ou intrabucais proporcionam uma avaliação superior da cavidade nasal e evitam a sobreposição da mandíbula.
• Ocasionalmente se observam pólipos nasofaríngeos dentro da nasofaringe.
• TC/RM — técnicas superiores à radiografia simples na avaliação da extensão da doença e na determinação da integridade da placa cribriforme. Também são valiosas na avaliação da presença de doença em estruturas como palato, meato nasofaríngeo, seio maxilar, tecidos periorbitais e canal auditivo médio.

MÉTODOS DIAGNÓSTICOS
Pressão Arterial
• Avaliar a presença de hipertensão em caso de epistaxe.

Aspirado de Linfonodo
• Conforme indicação.

Citologia
• *Swab* nasal pode revelar o agente *Cryptococcus*.

Rinite e Sinusite

Cultura
- A utilidade da cultura é controversa — a maioria dos animais apresenta infecção bacteriana secundária. Os patógenos bacterianos potenciais são mais comumente isolados em gatos com rinossinusite do que nos saudáveis.
- A cultura fúngica de lesão tipo placa visualizada à endoscopia ajuda no diagnóstico. É menos provável que amostras coletadas às cegas sejam proveitosas.

Endoscopia
- O otoscópio avalia apenas a cavidade nasal rostral. O endoscópio rígido pode ser direcionado para os turbinados etmoides, enquanto o endoscópio flexível proporciona boa visualização no sentido rostral e pode ser retrofletido na nasofaringe para visualizar as coanas nasais caudais.
- A biopsia dirigida é possível com o uso de endoscópio rígido e flexível. Outras técnicas incluem biopsias centrais ou com pinça às cegas. A hemorragia excessiva pode ser controlada com adrenalina tópica na diluição de 1:100.000.

Cirurgia
- A rinotomia exploratória constitui a ferramenta diagnóstica mais invasiva, mas pode ser mais valiosa para biopsias difíceis, remoção de corpo estranho ou retirada de massa.

ACHADOS PATOLÓGICOS
A inflamação crônica provoca reabsorção dos turbinados, além de ulceração e necrose da mucosa. Infiltrado linfoplasmocitário indica cronicidade, enquanto infiltrado neutrofílico costuma ser indício de componente agudo. Neoplasia e fungo também provocam destruição ou lise óssea.

TRATAMENTO

CUIDADO(S) DE ENFERMAGEM
A umidificação do ambiente pode ajudar a umidificar e mobilizar as secreções nasais. Aplicar infusão intranasal de solução salina, caso tolerada. Limpeza das narinas.

DIETA
Alimentos amolecidos ou mornos em caso de diminuição do apetite.

ORIENTAÇÃO AO PROPRIETÁRIO
Sinais de rinite crônica em cães e gatos podem ser variavelmente controlados, porém raramente são eliminados.

CONSIDERAÇÕES CIRÚRGICAS
- A rinotomia fica reservada para obtenção de biopsia ou remoção de corpo estranho/massa. Raramente, esse procedimento apresenta vantagem sobre a endoscopia.
- A cirurgia é útil para remoção de pólipo(s) e doença nasal relacionada com os dentes.

MEDICAÇÕES

MEDICAMENTO(S)

Antibióticos
- Esses agentes ajudam a controlar a rinite bacteriana secundária; entretanto, não resolverão a doença. A seleção dos antibióticos é basicamente empírica (os isolamentos comuns incluem *Staphylococcus*, *Streptococcus*, *Bacillus*, *E. coli* e *Pasteurella multocida*). Com frequência, há necessidade do uso a longo prazo.
- *Chlamydophila rhinitis*. Pode ser necessária a terapia com doxiciclina a longo prazo (5 mg/kg VO a cada 12 h por 6-8 semanas). O cloranfenicol também é eficaz contra *Chlamydophila* (cães: 50 mg/kg VO a cada 12 h, gatos: 12,5-20 mg/kg VO a cada 12 h).

Antifúngicos
- Ver os capítulos sobre "Criptococose" e "Aspergilose" em busca de uma discussão detalhada a respeito do tratamento.

Alfainterferona Humana
- Inédito até esse momento — 30 UI VO a cada 24 h.

L-lisina
- Inibe a replicação do FHV tipo 1; pode ser valiosa — 250-500 mg VO a cada 12 h.

Agentes Anti-inflamatórios
- Agentes anti-inflamatórios não esteroides (piroxicam, carprofeno, deracoxibe) estão sendo utilizados como tratamento paliativo para tumores nasais (via inibição da COX-2), como agente isolado ou em conjunto com a quimioterapia.

Esteroides
- Utilizar em caso de rinite alérgica — prednisolona na dose de 1 mg/kg dividida por via VO a cada 12 h.
- Considerar o uso em caso de rinossinusite crônica em gatos ou rinite linfoplasmocitária em cães em doses anti-inflamatórias.

Anti-histamínicos
- A eficácia é discutível — clemastina, 1,34 mg VO a cada 12 h para gatos e cães de pequeno porte, 2,68 mg VO a cada 12 h para raças caninas de médio a grande porte ou hidroxizina, 2,2 mg/kg VO a cada 8-12 h.

Antiparasitários
- Ivermectina 300 µg/kg VO ou SC uma vez por semana por 3-4 vezes ou milbemicina oxima 1 mg/kg VO uma vez por semana por 3 semanas para o tratamento dos ácaros nasais.

CONTRAINDICAÇÕES
Evitar a utilização crônica de esteroides em virtude do risco de imunossupressão.

PRECAUÇÕES
- Os AINE podem provocar ulceração GI.
- As tetraciclinas podem manchar os dentes dos animais jovens.

INTERAÇÕES POSSÍVEIS
É contraindicado uso concomitante de AINE e corticosteroides.

ACOMPANHAMENTO

MONITORIZAÇÃO DO PACIENTE
Avaliação clínica e monitorização quanto à ocorrência de recidivas.

PREVENÇÃO
As vacinações nos filhotes de gato podem diminuir a gravidade e a duração da infecção viral.

COMPLICAÇÕES POSSÍVEIS
- Extensão da invasão fúngica ou neoplásica para o cérebro.
- Será possível a ocorrência de crises convulsivas e outros sinais neurológicos se a terapia antifúngica tópica for utilizada quando a placa cribriforme não estiver intacta.

EVOLUÇÃO ESPERADA E PROGNÓSTICO
- Dependem da etiologia e da extensão da doença.
- Rinite viral/bacteriana aguda — apresenta prognóstico bom; já a rinite crônica tem prognóstico reservado quanto ao controle dos sinais.
- Fúngica — prognóstico razoável a reservado, dependendo da invasividade e da resposta à terapia.
- Neoplásica — 3-5 meses sem tratamento. A expectativa de vida pode se estender até 9-23 meses com a radioterapia.

DIVERSOS

POTENCIAL ZOONÓTICO
Os microrganismos *Cryptococcus*, *Aspergillus* e *Penicillium* são transmissíveis aos seres humanos via ambiente compartilhado. Não há transmissão direta.

GESTAÇÃO/FERTILIDADE/REPRODUÇÃO
Cetoconazol, itraconazol e flucitosina são teratogênicos.

VER TAMBÉM
- Capítulo sobre Aspergilose.
- Secreção Nasal.
- Criptococose.
- Epistaxe.
- Estertor e Estridor.
- Parasitas Respiratórios.
- Pólipos Nasais e Nasofaríngeos.

ABREVIATURA(S)
- FeLV = vírus da leucemia felina.
- FHV = herpes-vírus felino.
- FIV = vírus da imunodeficiência felina.
- GI = gastrintestinal.
- RM = ressonância magnética.
- TC = tomografia computadorizada.
- AINE = anti-inflamatório não esteroide.

Sugestões de Leitura
Johnson LR, Foley JE, De Cock HE, et al. Assessment of infectious organisms associated with chronic rhinosinusitis in cats. JAVMA 2005, 227(4):579-585.
Russo M, Lamb CR, Jakovljevic S. Distinguishing rhinitis and nasal neoplasia by radiography. Vet Radiol Ultrasound 2000, 41(2):118-124.
Tasker S, Knottenbelt CM, Munro EA. Aetiology and diagnosis of persistent nasal disease in the dog: A retrospective study of 42 cases. J Small Anim Pract 1999, 40(10):473-478.

Autor Carrie J. Miller
Consultor Editorial Lynelle R. Johnson

RINOSPORIDIOSE

CONSIDERAÇÕES GERAIS

REVISÃO
- Infecção crônica rara das mucosas dos cães, resultando em uma reação fibromixoide que se desenvolve em crescimentos polipoides; tais crescimentos podem ser isolados ou múltiplos e frequentemente se projetam através da narina. Relatada em dois gatos; há raros relatos em cavalos, vacas e seres humanos.
- O sistema respiratório é acometido.
- Distribuição mundial.
- Áreas endêmicas — Argentina, Venezuela, Uganda, Cuba, Brasil, Irã, Sri Lanka e Índia.
- EUA — a maior parte das infecções foi relatada nos estados do sul.

IDENTIFICAÇÃO
- Relatada em 13 cães, 7 dos quais eram machos.
- Nenhuma predileção racial aparente.
- Relatada em dois gatos.

SINAIS CLÍNICOS
- Cavidade nasal anterior — localização mais comum.
- Espirros, epistaxe e respiração estertorosa — mais proeminentes.
- Massa — frequentemente observada fazendo protrusão a partir da narina; em geral, única e polipoide; pode ser lobulada ou séssil; a superfície pode apresentar massas carnosas superficiais brancas ou amareladas.
- Seres humanos — locais relatados: vagina, pênis, saco conjuntival e orelhas.

CAUSAS E FATORES DE RISCO
- *Rhinosporidium seeberi*, atualmente, é classificado como um dos cinco protistas na classe composta por *Dermatocystidium*, agente roseta (*Sphaerothecum destruens*), *Ichthyophonus*, *Psorospermium*, *Rhinosporidium seeberi*.
- Há suspeitas de que a água doce estagnada, a água estagnada e o ambiente árido (poeira) aumentem a probabilidade de ocorrência.

DIAGNÓSTICO

DIAGNÓSTICO DIFERENCIAL
- Neoplasia nasal.
- Pólipo inflamatório nasal.

HEMOGRAMA/BIOQUÍMICA/URINÁLISE
Geralmente normais.

OUTROS TESTES LABORATORIAIS
Nenhum.

DIAGNÓSTICO POR IMAGEM
Radiografias da cavidade nasal — geralmente normais; massa que se localiza na cavidade nasal anterior e não invade os ossos turbinados.

MÉTODOS DIAGNÓSTICOS
- Esfregaços por decalque (impressão) — revelam microrganismos a partir da massa nasal; utilizar os corantes novo azul de metileno, H&E ou PAS. Os microrganismos têm 6–8 µm de tamanho e são redondos a ovais. Em muitos microrganismos, observa-se um grande núcleo.
- Histopatologia — esporos e esporângios (o saco em que os esporos são produzidos) geralmente podem ser observados com H&E, PAS, azul de toluidina de Gridley e corante de Grocott. Nas áreas onde os esporângios se rompem, é comum a ocorrência de inflamação neutrofílica purulenta.

ACHADOS PATOLÓGICOS
Histopatologia
- Exame da massa — hiperplasia papilomatosa; ulceração do epitélio; estroma fibrovascular.
- A identificação do microrganismo é diagnóstica.
- Será observada uma intensa reação inflamatória se os microrganismos forem liberados nos tecidos circundantes.

TRATAMENTO

- É importante o fornecimento de bons cuidados de enfermagem; tipicamente não se relatam anorexia e desidratação.
- O confinamento em gaiola ou outro meio de restrição ao exercício é uma medida valiosa se ocorrer epistaxe.
- A excisão cirúrgica da massa constitui o tratamento de escolha; abordagem pelas narinas externas ou por rinotomia; a falha na remoção de toda a massa provavelmente resultará em novo crescimento.

MEDICAÇÕES

MEDICAMENTO(S)
- Os agentes cetoconazol e itraconazol já foram utilizados, mas são constantemente ineficazes, pois a rinosporidiose não se trata de uma doença fúngica.
- Dapsona — utilizada para tratar seres humanos; relato de uso em um único cão (1,1 mg/kg VO a cada 8-12 h) com resposta favorável, embora não haja cura; entretanto, possui efeitos colaterais graves.

CONTRAINDICAÇÕES/INTERAÇÕES POSSÍVEIS
Dapsona (cães) — hepatotoxicidade; anemia; neutropenia; trombocitopenia; sinais gastrintestinais; reações cutâneas.

ACOMPANHAMENTO

Se a abordagem cirúrgica for pelo orifício nasal externo, monitorizar rigorosamente o paciente quanto à ocorrência de novos crescimentos; não é fácil remover toda a massa.

DIVERSOS

POTENCIAL ZOONÓTICO
O microrganismo é infeccioso para os seres humanos, mas não há risco conhecido de transmissão direta para os humanos pela manipulação de cães infectados. O microrganismo pode ser adquirido em seres humanos pela mesma fonte que os cães.

ABREVIATURA(S)
- H&E = hematoxilina e eosina.
- PAS = ácido periódico de Schiff.

Sugestões de Leitura
Abbitt B. Rhinosporidiosis. Texas Vet 2008, 70(3):44.
Breitschwerdt EB, Castellano MC. Rhinosporidiosis. In: Greene CE, ed., Infectious Diseases of the Dog and Cat. Philadelphia: Saunders, 1998, pp. 402-404.
Caniatti M, Roccabianca P, Scanziani E, et al. Nasal rhinosporidiosis in dogs: Four cases from Europe and a review of the literature. Vet Record 1998, 142:334-338.
Wallin LL, Coleman GD, Froeling J, Parker GA. Rhinosporidiosis in a domestic cat. Med Mycol 2001, 39:139-141.
Wilson RB, Pope RW, Sumrall R. Canine rhinosporidiosis. Compend Contin Educ Pract Vet 1989, 11:730-732.

Autor Gary D. Norsworthy
Consultor Editorial Stephen C. Barr

Ritmo Idioventricular

CONSIDERAÇÕES GERAIS

DEFINIÇÃO
Se a condução dos impulsos do marca-passo do nó sinusal para os ventrículos estiver bloqueada ou a frequência dos impulsos diminuída, as regiões inferiores do coração assumirão automaticamente o papel de marca-passo para os ventrículos, o que resultará em complexos ventriculares de escape (Fig. 1) ou em um ritmo idioventricular (Fig. 2).

Características do ECG
- Uma série de batimentos de escape ventriculares com frequência cardíaca <65 bpm em cães e <100 bpm em gatos; frequências cardíacas de 65-100 bpm em cães e 100-160 bpm em gatos costumam ser designadas como *ritmo idioventricular acelerado*.
- As ondas P podem estar ausentes ou anteceder os complexos QRS ectópicos, ficar ocultas dentro desses complexos ou acompanhá-los.
- As ondas P não têm relação com os complexos QRS.
- Configuração do QRS — largo e bizarro; semelhante à do complexo ventricular prematuro.

FISIOPATOLOGIA
- Pode ser relevante do ponto de vista hemodinâmico com velocidades ventriculares lentas.
- Não ocorre em animais sadios.
- Marca-passos subsidiários parecem descarregar mais rapidamente em gatos que em cães.

SISTEMA(S) ACOMETIDO(S)
Cardiovascular.

GENÉTICA
N/D.

INCIDÊNCIA/PREVALÊNCIA
Desconhecidas.

DISTRIBUIÇÃO GEOGRÁFICA
N/D.

IDENTIFICAÇÃO
Espécies
Cães e gatos.

Raças Predominantes
- Parada atrial em cães da raça Springer Spaniel inglês e gatos da raça Siamês.
- Cães das raças Pug, Schnauzer miniatura e Dálmata são propensos a anormalidades de condução cardíaca.

Idade Média e Faixa Etária
N/D.

Sexo Predominante
N/D.

SINAIS CLÍNICOS
Achados Anamnésicos
- Alguns animais permanecem assintomáticos.
- Fraqueza.
- Letargia.
- Intolerância ao exercício.
- Síncope.
- Insuficiência cardíaca.

Achados do Exame Físico
- Ritmo irregular associado a déficits de pulso.
- Variação nas bulhas cardíacas.
- Possíveis ondas "em canhão" intermitentes nos pulsos venosos jugulares (com bloqueio AV).

CAUSAS
- Não constitui uma doença primária — trata-se do resultado secundário de uma doença primária.
- O ritmo de escape é um mecanismo de segurança para manter o débito cardíaco.

Causas de Bradicardia Sinusal e Parada Sinusal
- Aumento do tônus vagal (pressão intracraniana elevada, pressão ocular alta).
- Medicamentos — digoxina, tranquilizantes, propranolol, quinidina e anestésicos.
- Doença de Addison.
- Hipoglicemia.
- Insuficiência renal.
- Hipotermia.
- Hipercalemia.
- Hipotireoidismo.

Causas de Bloqueio AV
- Congênito.
- Neoplasia.
- Fibrose.
- Doença de Lyme.

FATORES DE RISCO
N/D.

DIAGNÓSTICO

DIAGNÓSTICO DIFERENCIAL
- Taquicardia ventricular — cães exibem frequência cardíaca > 100 bpm e gatos > 150 bpm.
- Frequência cardíaca lenta em animais com bloqueio do ramo direito do feixe de His, bloqueio do ramo esquerdo do feixe de His ou bloqueio fascicular anterior esquerdo; os animais com esses distúrbios apresentam ondas P associadas a complexos QRS.

HEMOGRAMA/BIOQUÍMICA/URINÁLISE
- Sem achados específicos.
- O exame de sangue completo pode sugerir alguma anormalidade metabólica.

OUTROS TESTES LABORATORIAIS
- Intoxicação medicamentosa.
- Título de Lyme em animais com bloqueio AV completo.

DIAGNÓSTICO POR IMAGEM
O ecocardiograma pode revelar cardiopatia estrutural.

MÉTODOS DIAGNÓSTICOS
Eletrocardiografia.

ACHADOS PATOLÓGICOS
Dependem da causa subjacente.

TRATAMENTO

CUIDADO(S) DE SAÚDE ADEQUADO(S)
- O ritmo idioventricular é um escape ou mecanismo de segurança para manter o débito cardíaco; *não* instituir um tratamento para suprimir esse ritmo de escape, mas sim direcioná-lo ao processo mórbido primário, permitindo que o ritmo de escape assuma o controle como marca-passo do coração.
- O tratamento sintomático visa aumentar a frequência cardíaca.

CUIDADO(S) DE ENFERMAGEM
Pode(m) ser necessário(s) para a doença subjacente.

ATIVIDADE
Os animais sintomáticos podem necessitar de repouso em gaiola.

DIETA
Sem modificações ou restrições a menos que sejam necessárias para tratar a condição subjacente.

ORIENTAÇÃO AO PROPRIETÁRIO
Informar o proprietário sobre a necessidade de procurar e tratar a causa subjacente de forma específica.

CONSIDERAÇÕES CIRÚRGICAS
Talvez haja necessidade da implantação de marca-passo.

MEDICAÇÕES

MEDICAMENTO(S) DE ESCOLHA
- Atropina ou glicopirrolato costumam ser indicados para bloquear o tônus vagal ou aumentar a frequência cardíaca.
- Se esses medicamentos não forem eficazes, poderá ser necessário o uso de isoproterenol, dopamina, dobutamina ou marca-passo artificial.

CONTRAINDICAÇÕES
Lidocaína, procainamida, quinidina, propranolol, diltiazem ou qualquer outro fármaco que diminua a frequência cardíaca ou reduza a contratilidade.

PRECAUÇÕES
A atropina é brevemente vagotônica logo após a injeção e pode provocar uma exacerbação temporária do distúrbio.

INTERAÇÕES POSSÍVEIS
N/D.

MEDICAMENTO(S) ALTERNATIVO(S)
N/D.

ACOMPANHAMENTO

MONITORIZAÇÃO DO PACIENTE
- ECG seriados podem mostrar o desaparecimento da lesão ou a evolução para bloqueio cardíaco completo.
- Pode ser necessária a obtenção de perfis sanguíneos seriados para monitorar o progresso do processo mórbido primário.
- Ecocardiogramas seriados podem revelar a melhora do quadro ou o aparecimento de alterações progressivas na estrutura cardíaca.

PREVENÇÃO
N/D.

COMPLICAÇÕES POSSÍVEIS
Bradicardia prolongada pode causar insuficiência cardíaca congestiva secundária ou perfusão renal inadequada.

EVOLUÇÃO ESPERADA E PROGNÓSTICO
- A arritmia pode diminuir quando o processo primário for corrigido.
- O prognóstico será reservado se a condição estiver associada a distúrbio cardíaco ou metabólico; mau se a frequência não for

RITMO IDIOVENTRICULAR

aumentada por meios farmacológicos ou caso não se consiga identificar e tratar a causa subjacente.

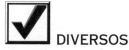 **DIVERSOS**

DISTÚRBIOS ASSOCIADOS
N/D.

FATORES RELACIONADOS COM A IDADE
N/D.

POTENCIAL ZOONÓTICO
N/D.

GESTAÇÃO/FERTILIDADE/REPRODUÇÃO
N/D.

VER TAMBÉM
- Parada Atrial.
- Bloqueio AV Completo.

ABREVIATURA(S)
- AV = atrioventricular.
- bpm = batimentos por minuto.
- ECG = eletrocardiograma.

RECURSOS DA INTERNET
www.vetgo.com/cardio

Sugestões de Leitura
Kittleson MD. Electrocardiography. In: Kittleson MD, Kienle RD, eds., Small Animal Cardiovascular Medicine. St. Louis: Mosby, 1998, pp. 72-94.

Tilley LP. Essentials of Canine and Feline Electrocardiography, 3rd ed. Baltimore: Williams & Wilkins, 1992, pp. 152, 222.

Tilley LP, Smith FWK, Jr. Electrocardiography. In: Tilley LP, Smith FWK, Oyama MA, Sleeper MM, eds., Manual of Canine and Feline Cardiology, 4th ed. St. Louis: Saunders Elsevier, 2008, pp. 49-77.

Autores Larry P. Tilley e Naomi L. Burtnick
Consultores Editoriais Larry P. Tilley e Francis W.K. Smith, Jr.

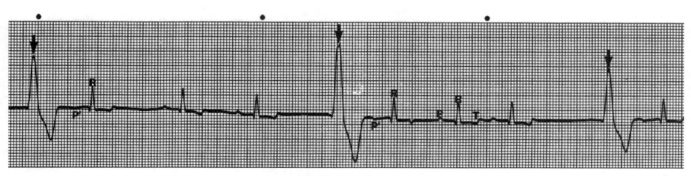

Figura 1. Complexos de escape ventricular (setas) durante várias fases no ritmo sinusal dominante em um cão durante anestesia. A frequência sinusal aumentada (não ilustrada) após a anestesia parou; 0,5 cm = 1 mV. (De: Tilley LP. *Essentials of canine and feline electrocardiography*. 3.ed. Baltimore: Williams & Wilkins, 1992, com permissão.)

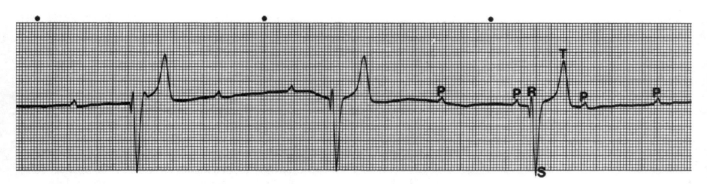

Figura 2. Bloqueio cardíaco completo. As ondas P ocorrem em uma frequência de 120, independentemente da frequência ventricular de 50. A configuração do QRS é um padrão de bloqueio do ramo direito do feixe de His. A frequência regular e o QRS estável indicam que o foco de resgate provavelmente está próximo da junção AV. (De: Tilley LP. *Essentials of canine and feline electrocardiography*. 3.ed. Baltimore: Lippincott Williams & Wilkins, 1992, com permissão.)

Ruptura Muscular (Laceração Muscular)

CONSIDERAÇÕES GERAIS

REVISÃO
Um músculo normal pode ser estirado, pinçado ou lesionado diretamente, resultando na ruptura da fibra, no enfraquecimento e na separação imediata ou tardia das porções não lesadas. Alternativamente, a estrutura muscular pode ficar comprometida por condições sistêmicas ou iatrogênicas, mas a atividade normal pode provocar ruptura muscular. A ruptura pode ser completa ou incompleta, podendo ocorrer no meio da substância ou na junção musculotendínea. O estágio agudo caracteriza-se por reação inflamatória típica que se torna crônica com maturação do colágeno, ligação cruzada, fibrose e desenvolvimento de aderência com o passar do tempo. Com frequência, a fase aguda passa despercebida, já que os sinais podem ser temporários e responder bem ao repouso. Os efeitos crônicos são quase sempre progressivos e irresponsivos à terapia de suporte.

IDENTIFICAÇÃO
• Os músculos dos membros e da mastigação são as principais estruturas acometidas.
• A lesão traumática é indiscriminada, embora determinadas atividades possam predispor a esse tipo de lesão por causa da exposição.
• As rupturas que aparentemente não estão relacionadas com o traumatismo parecem acometer os cães de trabalho de meia-idade a idosos, sem predileção sexual relatada.
• Os gatos são acometidos com menos frequência do que os cães.

SINAIS CLÍNICOS
Lesão Aguda
• Claudicação imediata, caracterizada pelo músculo específico acometido.
• Tumefação, calor e dor localizados.
• Em geral, manifestam-se por alguns dias a uma semana.

Fase Crônica (caso se desenvolva)
• Progressiva.
• Indolor.
• Geralmente associada a tecido cicatricial que impede a função normal de uma extremidade.

CAUSAS E FATORES DE RISCO
• Traumatismo.
• Superextensão.
• Miosite.
• Degenerativa (etiologia desconhecida).
• Miopatia secundária a condições clínicas como a doença de Cushing.
• Fator de risco aparente para os cães consiste em envolvimento na caça, em trilhas ou atividades semelhantes em ambientes externos.

Análise da Marcha e Achados do Exame Físico
• Vários distúrbios resultarão em anormalidades características da marcha e dor eliciada à manipulação de membro específico — alguns dos quais estão listados abaixo.
• Lesão do músculo psoas:
  ○ Dor à rotação interna com extensão ou abdução do membro pélvico.
  ○ Dor à palpação do trocanter menor do fêmur acometido.
  ○ Marcha curta e agitada.
• Contraturas dos músculos grácil, semimembranáceo e semitendíneo:
  ○ Esses animais tipicamente não têm dor à palpação dos músculos grácil, semitendíneo ou semimembranáceo.
  ○ Palpação de faixa fibrosa na área do músculo acometido também é aparente.
  ○ Passo encurtado com rotação medial da pata, rotação interna da articulação do jarrete (társica) e rotação externa do calcâneo, com rotação interna da articulação do joelho (femorotibiopatelar) na fase tardia do passo anterógrado.
• Contratura do músculo infraespinal:
  ○ Claudicação significativa do membro torácico com circundução do membro acometido.
  ○ Adução acentuada do cotovelo/abdução notável dos pés; à flexão do cotovelo, a porção distal do antebraço sofrerá desvio lateral.
  ○ Faixa fibrosa será aparente à palpação do músculo infraespinal.
• Contratura do quadríceps:
  ○ Tipicamente ocorre com falta de uso/imobilização de membro após fixação de fratura do fêmur em cães jovens sem fisioterapia apropriada.
  ○ O paciente será incapaz de flexionar a articulação do joelho (femorotibiopatelar).
• Lesões do mecanismo de Aquiles:
  ○ Claudicação sem sustentação do peso com tumefação de tecido mole proximal ao calcâneo.
  ○ Hiperflexão do tarso.
  ○ Hiperflexão dos dedos se o flexor superficial dos dedos não estiver acometido.
• Lesão/fibrose do músculo sartório:
  ○ Relatos escassos na literatura veterinária.
  ○ Membro pélvico indolor e sem sustentação do peso
  ○ Faixa fibrosa palpável na área do músculo sartório.
  ○ Marcha agitada curta, caracterizada por incapacidade de estender o quadril.

DIAGNÓSTICO

DIAGNÓSTICO DIFERENCIAL
• Disfunção neurológica — identificada por anormalidades neurológicas.
• Ruptura de tendão — rompimento visível ou palpável nessa estrutura.
• Fratura por avulsão na origem ou na inserção — evidência radiográfica de defeito e translocação de fragmento ósseo.
• Luxação/subluxação — evidência palpável ou radiográfica de instabilidade ou de mau alinhamento articular.

HEMOGRAMA/BIOQUÍMICA/URINÁLISE
Sem achados específicos à lesão.

OUTROS TESTES LABORATORIAIS
• CPK pode estar elevada nos casos agudos.
• Não existem testes específicos conhecidos disponíveis.

DIAGNÓSTICO POR IMAGEM
Achados Radiográficos
• Tumefação do tecido mole pode estar evidente nos estágios precoces.
• Pode ocorrer calcificação do músculo na área traumatizada em situações crônicas.
• Fraturas por avulsão e calcificação do tendão de inserção ou origem podem ser observadas às radiografias.

Achados Ultrassonográficos
• Tumefação local e perda da orientação normal das fibras musculares podem ser observadas no ponto da lesão nos casos agudos.
• Tecido cicatricial e áreas contraídas de tecido fibroso podem ser observados no músculo nos casos crônicos — notados como focos hiperecoicos no ventre muscular de interesse.
• Diferenças mensuráveis entre os lados normal e anormal podem ser úteis para comprovar o local do músculo acometido.

Estudos por Imagem de Corte Transversal
• Achados de TC — gera melhor contraste tecidual do que os exames supramencionados, embora ainda seja limitado a um plano axial de imagem.
• Achados de RM — edema e hemorragia provocam modificação no sinal, que pode ser diferenciada de alterações atribuídas à substituição do músculo por tecido fibroso. Isso permite a localização do problema e ajuda a identificar o tipo de problema.

MÉTODOS DIAGNÓSTICOS
Biopsia Muscular
A presença de tecido fibroso e a perda de células musculares podem ser comprovadas. Pode ser impossível diferenciar atrofia por desuso de atrofia neurológica e de fibrose induzida por lesão sem evidências corroboradoras.

TRATAMENTO

• Não existe evidência comprovada que apoie um único meio "melhor" para o tratamento das lesões musculares agudas, visando a prevenção de contratura fibrosa e aderências. Em geral, acredita-se que o cuidado imediato após a lesão deve envolver repouso e aplicação local de frio, seguida depois de horas (24-48 h) pelo calor e fisioterapia passiva (movimento). Imobilização rigorosa e estrita (com gesso ou gaiola) é potencialmente contraindicada, pois isso pode estimular a contratura e a fibrose musculares, levando à debilidade irreversível a longo prazo. Atividade leve ou sem a sustentação do peso é apropriada por um período prolongado de tempo (4-6 semanas). Medicamentos analgésicos e anti-inflamatórios devem ser recomendados por vários dias a semanas. A cirurgia pode ser realizada dentro de alguns dias depois da lesão para reparar ruptura muscular aguda óbvia que resulte em separação dos segmentos musculares lesados. Uma parte essencial do reparo muscular consiste no alívio eficaz da tensão sobre o músculo lesado, de forma que a cicatrização possa ocorrer sem ruptura à medida que a função retorna ao normal. Dispositivos ortopédicos internos ou externos podem ser necessários para conferir o alívio eficaz da tensão. Os proprietários devem estar conscientes da possibilidade de problemas relacionados com a cicatrização que afetem a marcha do paciente a longo prazo.
• Assim que a lesão muscular se tornar crônica e ser associada à contratura ou a aderências, o tratamento será direcionado à recuperação da função. A liberação cirúrgica das aderências ou faixas de tecido fibroso frequentemente é

Ruptura Muscular (Laceração Muscular)

acompanhada por alívio sintomático instantâneo. A prevenção de nova aderência e contratura progressiva é muito menos recompensadora.
• Lesões musculares específicas apresentam prognósticos amplamente díspares. As contraturas dos músculos infraespinal e psoas respondem bem à excisão cirúrgica do tendão de inserção. As contraturas dos músculos grácil, semimembranáceo e semitendíneo apresentam taxa de recidiva de 100% após a ressecção cirúrgica. A contratura do quadríceps possui taxa igualmente desanimadora de falha após a cirurgia.
• Lesões musculares que cicatrizaram em um estado alongado apresentam prognóstico melhor em termos de restabelecimento cirúrgico da função do que músculos contraídos. A lesão mais comum por alongamento envolve os músculos do tendão calcâneo. A hiperflexão do jarrete pode ser submetida à reconstrução cirúrgica, para fazer com que esses animais retornem à função relativamente normal. Isso costuma ser obtido pelo encurtamento do tendão de Aquiles e não pela junção muscular ou musculotendínea lesada.

MEDICAÇÕES

MEDICAMENTO(S)
Nenhum específico. Medicamentos anti-inflamatórios podem ser indicados nas situações agudas.

CONTRAINDICAÇÕES/INTERAÇÕES POSSÍVEIS
A imobilização do músculo lesado em uma posição que permita o desenvolvimento de aderências nas proximidades do osso frequentemente resultará em contraturas por fraturas.

ACOMPANHAMENTO

MONITORIZAÇÃO DO PACIENTE
Monitorização da amplitude de movimento repetitiva e exame de reavaliação.

PREVENÇÃO
Controle inflamatório precoce e fisioterapia passiva sem sustentação do peso, acompanhados por repouso estrito em gaiola, podem ser benéficos.

COMPLICAÇÕES POSSÍVEIS
Contratura do músculo e substituição do tecido muscular por tecido fibroso.

EVOLUÇÃO ESPERADA E PROGNÓSTICO
Específicos para o músculo e para o tipo da lesão.

DIVERSOS

DISTÚRBIOS ASSOCIADOS
Hipermobilidade articular, deformidades angulares do membro, anormalidades articulares de flexão/extensão.

FATORES RELACIONADOS COM A IDADE
Fraturas da placa de crescimento em cães jovens, particularmente fraturas de Salter-Harris da porção distal do fêmur, estão associadas à contratura do quadríceps.

ABREVIATURA(S)
• CPK = creatino quinase.
• RM = ressonância magnética.
• TC = tomografia computadorizada.

Sugestões de Leitura
Vaughan LC. Muscle and tendon injuries in dogs. J Small Anim Pract 1979, 20:711-736.

Autores Mathieu M. Glassman e Michael Weh
Consultor Editorial Peter K. Shires

SALMONELOSE

CONSIDERAÇÕES GERAIS

DEFINIÇÃO
Doença bacteriana, causada por muitos sorotipos diferentes de *Salmonella*, que provoca enterite, septicemia e abortamentos.

FISIOPATOLOGIA
• *Salmonella* — bactéria Gram-negativa que coloniza o intestino delgado (íleo). A partir daí, adere-se aos enterócitos e os invade. Acaba penetrando e se multiplicando na lâmina própria e nos linfonodos mesentéricos locais, com a consequente produção de citotoxina (morte celular) e enterotoxina (aumenta o AMPc). Ocorrem o processo de inflamação e a síntese de prostaglandina, resultando em diarreia secretora e esfacelamento da mucosa.
• Gastrenterite não complicada — os microrganismos são interrompidos no estágio de invasão do linfonodo mesentérico; o paciente apresenta apenas diarreia, vômito e desidratação.
• Bacteremia e septicemia após a gastrenterite — doença mais grave; podem resultar em infecções extraintestinais focais (abortamento, artropatia) ou endotoxemia; podem levar a infarto orgânico, trombose generalizada, CID e morte.
• Alguns pacientes se recuperam da forma septicêmica, mas sofrem recuperação prolongada como resultado de seu estado debilitado.

SISTEMA(S) ACOMETIDO(S)
• Gastrintestinal — enterocolite; inflamação, esfacelamento da mucosa, diarreia secretora.
• Doença sistêmica (p. ex., bacteremia, infecções focais e septicemia) — infarto de múltiplos órgãos, trombose, abscessos, meningite, osteomielite, abortamento.

GENÉTICA
A suscetibilidade genética não é bem conhecida.

INCIDÊNCIA/PREVALÊNCIA
• Não se conhece a incidência real.
• A maior parte das infecções é subclínica.
• Cães — a doença clínica é observada com maior frequência em animais jovens e em fêmeas prenhes; pesquisa com *swab* fecal/retal de animais domésticos de companhia clinicamente normais, canis de hospedagem e hospitais veterinários revela incidências de 30%, 16,7% e 21,5%, respectivamente. Comum nos cães da raça Galgo de corrida e cães de corrida com trenó em função da dieta à base de carne crua; a presença de *Salmonella* não implica necessariamente a ocorrência de infecção, mas pode refletir uma transferência ou transmissão passageira.
• Gatos — apresentam uma resistência natural elevada; animais hospitalizados estressados estão sob alto risco, particularmente quando tratados com algum agente antimicrobiano por via oral antes dos procedimentos de castração ou tratamento odontológico ou retirada das garras; pesquisa fecal de gatos normais e gatos de colônias de pesquisa apresenta incidências de 18% e 10,6%, respectivamente. É mais provável que gatos de abrigos apresentem *Salmonella* nas fezes; pandemia de salmonelose em aves canoras migrantes (em geral *typhimurium*) na primavera cria epidemia nos gatos caçadores de aves.
• Novos perigos são observados com a tendência de fornecer dietas comerciais à base de carne crua (particularmente frango) a cães e gatos; microrganismos como *Campylobacter* spp., além de *Salmonella* spp. e *Clostridium perfringens*, são frequentemente encontrados em dietas cruas.

DISTRIBUIÇÃO GEOGRÁFICA
Mundial.

IDENTIFICAÇÃO
Espécies
Cães e gatos.

Idade Média e Faixa Etária
• Cães — a doença clínica se manifesta nos filhotes de cão neonatos/imaturos e nas cadelas prenhes; praticamente todos os cães adultos portadores permanecem normais do ponto de vista clínico.
• Gatos — os adultos são altamente resistentes.

SINAIS CLÍNICOS
Comentários Gerais
Gravidade da doença — desde doença subclínica (estado de portador: *Salmonella* liberada nas fezes) até casos clínicos leves, moderados e graves em cães e gatos neonatos e em adultos estressados; as infecções subclínicas são mais comuns do que a doença clínica (rara).

Achados Anamnésicos
• Diarreia.
• Vômito.
• Febre.
• Mal-estar.
• Anorexia.
• Corrimento vaginal/abortamento — cadelas.
• Doença febril crônica — febre persistente, anorexia, mal-estar sem diarreia.

Achados do Exame Físico
• Estados de portador assintomático — sem sinais clínicos.
• Gastrenterite — anorexia; mal-estar/letargia; depressão; febre (39-40°C); diarreia com muco e/ou sangue; desidratação progressiva; dor abdominal; tenesmo; mucosas pálidas; linfadenopatia mesentérica; perda de peso.
• Gastrenterite com bacteremia e septicemia, choque séptico ou endotoxemia —mucosas pálidas; fraqueza; colapso cardiovascular; taquicardia; taquipneia.
• Infecções extraintestinais focais — conjuntivite; útero/abortamento; celulite; piotórax.
• Gatos — podem apresentar síndrome de doença febril crônica (sem sinais gastrintestinais); febre persistente; doença prolongada com sinais clínicos vagos e inespecíficos; e leucograma com desvio à esquerda.
• Pacientes em processo de recuperação — podem apresentar diarreia intermitente crônica por 3-4 semanas; podem eliminar a *Salmonella* nas fezes por 6 semanas ou mais.

CAUSAS
• Qualquer um dos mais de 2.000 sorotipos de salmonelas.
• Não é incomum haver dois ou mais sorotipos simultâneos em um hospedeiro animal.

FATORES DE RISCO
Agente da Doença
• Sorotipo de *Salmonella* — fatores de virulência, dose infectante e via de exposição.
• Fatores relacionados com o hospedeiro que aumentam a suscetibilidade.
• Idade — cães e gatos neonatos/jovens; sistema imunológico imaturo.
• Estado geral de saúde — animais jovens ou adultos debilitados: outra doença concomitante, parasitismo; animais jovens: trato gastrintestinal imaturo, flora microbiana normal pouco desenvolvida.
• Desarranjo da flora bacteriana normal gastrintestinal (gatos adultos) — tratamento antimicrobiano; exposição subsequente a salmonelas durante a hospitalização.

Fatores Ambientes
• A coprofagia dissemina a infecção.
• Ração desidratada (seca) para os animais de estimação — conhecida por albergar salmonelas; rações semiúmidas (p. ex., trituradas e biscoitos para cães) geralmente não se encontram sob risco.
• Petiscos caninos originários de orelha de suíno contaminados com *Salmonella*.
• Carne de cavalo fornecida a felídeos exóticos.
• Novos perigos são observados com a tendência de fornecer dietas comerciais à base de carne crua (particularmente frango) a cães e gatos; microrganismos como *Campylobacter* spp., além de *Salmonella* spp., são frequentemente encontrados em dietas cruas.
• Hábitos de auto-higienização — podem resultar na pelagem contaminada com *Salmonella*, o que contamina as jaulas/gaiolas ou os corredores por onde passam os animais, bem como os bebedouros e comedouros.
• População densa — colônias de pesquisa, animais de hospedagem/pensão; animais de abrigos/agrupados em currais; superpopulação doméstica; condições insalubres; exposição a outros animais infectados (ou portadores) — desenvolvimento de *Salmonella* no ambiente; ciclo orofecal mais eficiente; grandes chances de exposição fecal; fatores estressantes.

Animais de Caça e Errantes
• Hábito de fuçar por alimento — exposição a lixo, alimento/água contaminados, animais mortos.
• Exposição a outros animais infectados (ou portadores).
• Exposição a carne crua contaminada.

Animais Hospitalizados
• Exposição nosocomial (mais estresse) ou ativação (por estresse) de infecção preexistente assintomática (estado de portador) por *Salmonella*, especialmente nos animais tratados com medicamentos antimicrobianos.

Gatos Vacinados
• Morte dos filhotes (provavelmente infectados de forma subclínica pela *Salmonella*) depois da vacinação, com títulos elevados após vacina viva modificada contra panleucopenia.

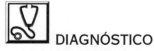
DIAGNÓSTICO

DIAGNÓSTICO DIFERENCIAL
• Gastrenterite aguda — vômito, diarreia, enterite infecciosa; diferenciar por meio de sorologia e/ou cultura.
• Gastrenterite viral — panleucopenia felina, FeLV, FIV, coronavírus entérico felino, coronavírus entérico canino, parvovírus canino, rotavírus, cinomose.
• Gastrenterite bacteriana — *E. coli*, *Campylobacter jejuni*, *Yersinia enterocolitica*.
• Síndrome de proliferação bacteriana — *Clostridium difficile*, *Clostridium perfringens*.
• Parasitas — helmintos (ancilóstomos, ascarídeos, tricúris, estrongiloides); protozoários (*Giardia*,

SALMONELOSE

Coccidia, *Cryptosporidia*); riquétsias; intoxicação alimentar pelo salmão.
• Gastrite aguda — erosões ou úlceras.
• Desconforto induzido pela dieta — exagero alimentar, alterações abruptas, inanição, sede, alergia ou intolerância alimentar, imprudências (corpo estranho, lixo).
• Sofrimento induzido por medicamento ou toxina.
• Distúrbios extraintestinais/doença metabólica.

HEMOGRAMA/BIOQUÍMICA/URINÁLISE
• Hemograma completo — variável; depende dos estágios da doença. • Neutropenia inicialmente.
• Desvio à esquerda com neutrófilos tóxicos.
• Anemia arregenerativa. • Linfopenia.
• Trombocitopenia. • Hipoalbuminemia.
• Distúrbios eletrolíticos.

MÉTODOS DIAGNÓSTICOS
• Cultura bacteriana fecal/retal — positiva; é necessário o uso de meios de cultura especiais.
• Leucócitos fecais — positivos. • Hemoculturas — positivas nos pacientes com bacteremia.
• Líquido articular — pode ser positivo à cultura.
• Estados subclínicos de portador — crônicos; cultura fecal intermitente positiva (>6 semanas).
• **NOTA:** a utilização de antimicrobianos em pacientes antes da coleta de amostras pode gerar resultados falso-negativos na cultura.

ACHADOS PATOLÓGICOS
• Lesões macroscópicas — apenas nos pacientes gravemente acometidos. • Culturas do íleo, linfonodo mesentérico, fígado/baço e medula óssea — positivas.

TRATAMENTO

CUIDADO(S) DE SAÚDE ADEQUADO(S)
• Tratamento ambulatorial — para gastrenterite não complicada (sem bacteremia) e estados de portador. • Internação — em casos de bacteremia/septicemia e gastrenterite nos animais neonatos/imaturos que ficam rapidamente debilitados pela diarreia.

CUIDADO(S) DE ENFERMAGEM
Varia de acordo com a gravidade da doença — avaliar as porcentagens de desidratação, peso corporal, perdas líquidas contínuas, choque, hematócrito/proteína total, eletrólitos, estado acidobásico.

Gastrenterite Não Complicada
• Cuidados de suporte — reposição hidreletrolítica. • Solução isotônica poliônica balanceada (solução de Ringer lactato) por via parenteral. • Fluidos por via oral — soluções de glicose hipertônica; na diarreia secretora.
• Transfusões de plasma — se a albumina sérica estiver <2 g/dL.

Animais Neonatos, Idosos e Debilitados
• Transfusões de plasma. • Cuidados de suporte — conforme descrito anteriormente.

ATIVIDADE
• Isolar os pacientes internados — todos os pacientes nos estágios agudos podem eliminar grande quantidade de salmonelas nas fezes.
• Restringir a atividade, com repouso em gaiola/jaula, monitorar e proporcionar um ambiente aquecido — animais doentes de forma aguda,

bacterêmicos/septicêmicos e cronicamente doentes.

DIETA
Restringir o alimento por 24-48 h; introduzir de modo gradual dieta altamente digestível e pobre em gordura.

ORIENTAÇÃO AO PROPRIETÁRIO
Instruir o proprietário a lavar as mãos com frequência e restringir o acesso ao paciente nos estágios agudos da doença; grande número de salmonelas pode ser eliminado nas fezes.

MEDICAÇÕES

MEDICAMENTO(S) DE ESCOLHA

Estado de Portador Assintomático
• Antimicrobianos — contraindicados.
• Medicamentos quinolônicos — foi demonstrado que esses agentes eliminam os estados de portador nos seres humanos; são necessários ensaios mais controlados nos animais.

Gastrenterite Não Complicada
• Antimicrobianos — não são indicados.
• Adsorventes e protetores intestinais de ação local.

Animais Neonatos, Idosos e Debilitados
• Glicocorticoides — foi comprovado que eles reduzem a mortalidade no choque endotóxico.
• Terapia antimicrobiana — indicada; há necessidade de cultura e antibiograma/CIM para avaliar os problemas de resistência ao medicamento. • Trimetoprima-sulfa — 15 mg/kg VO ou SC a cada 12 h. • Enrofloxacino — 5 mg/kg VO ou IM a cada 12 h; norfloxacino — 22 mg/kg VO a cada 12 h. • Cloranfenicol — cães: 50 mg/kg VO, IV, IM ou SC a cada 8 h; gatos: 50 mg/kg no total VO, IV, IM ou SC a cada 12 h.

PRECAUÇÕES
• Cloranfenicol e trimetoprima-sulfa — utilizar com cuidado nos pacientes neonatos e prenhes.
• Fluoroquinolonas — evitar a utilização em animais prenhes, neonatos ou em crescimento (cães de porte médio com <8 meses de vida; raças de porte grande ou gigante <12-18 meses de vida) por causa dos efeitos adversos de artropatia em cães de 4-28 meses de vida; não administrar doses superiores a 5 mg/kg nem por via IV em gatos.

ACOMPANHAMENTO

MONITORIZAÇÃO DO PACIENTE
• Cultura fecal — repetir mensalmente por alguns meses para avaliar o desenvolvimento do estado de portador. • Outros animais — monitorar quanto à ocorrência de disseminação secundária da infecção. • Orientar o proprietário a entrar em contato com o veterinário se o paciente apresentar sinais de doença recidivante.

PREVENÇÃO
• Manter os animais saudáveis — nutrição adequada; não fornecer carne crua; vacinar contra outras doenças infecciosas; limpar e desinfetar frequentemente as gaiolas/jaulas, corredores, bebedouros e comedouros; estocar de modo adequado os alimentos e os utensílios utilizados para alimentação. • Reduzir a superlotação — em currais, abrigos, canis, gatis e colônias de pesquisa.

• Recém-chegados — isolar e fazer a triagem; monitorizar as doenças antes de misturar com outros animais. • Vacina viva atenuada experimental mostra-se promissora, especialmente para os cães de corrida. • É importante proteger os animais em tratamento com medicamentos antimicrobianos da exposição ao ambiente contaminado com salmonela (p. ex., hospital veterinário).

COMPLICAÇÕES POSSÍVEIS
• Não é raro que ocorra a disseminação da infecção dentro da residência para outros animais ou para os seres humanos. • Desenvolvimento de infecção crônica com diarreia. • Recidiva da doença com o estresse.

EVOLUÇÃO ESPERADA E PROGNÓSTICO
• Gastrenterite não complicada — prognóstico excelente; frequentemente autolimitante; os pacientes se recuperam com bons cuidados de enfermagem. • Animais recuperados podem eliminar a *Salmonella* intermitentemente durante meses ou por mais tempo como portador recuperado. • Animais neonatos, idosos, estressados — podem desenvolver septicemia e doença sistêmica; pode ser grave e debilitante; poderá levar à morte se não forem tratados.

DIVERSOS

FATORES RELACIONADOS COM A IDADE
A doença clínica frequentemente é observada em animais neonatos e idosos.

POTENCIAL ZOONÓTICO
• Potencial elevado, sobretudo em crianças, idosos, imunossuprimidos e usuários de medicamentos antimicrobianos. • A *Salmonella* isolada de filhotes felinos com enterite é resistente a vários medicamentos. • Animais doentes de forma aguda eliminam grande quantidade de salmonelas nas fezes. • Os hábitos de auto-higienização permitem a rápida contaminação da pelagem dos animais e do ambiente. • Há necessidade de isolamento do animal.

GESTAÇÃO/FERTILIDADE/REPRODUÇÃO
• Pode complicar a doença. • Abortamento — pode ser sequela da infecção. • Terapia antimicrobiana — levar em conta o efeito sobre o feto.

ABREVIATURA(S)
• CID = coagulação intravascular disseminada.
• CIM = concentração inibitória mínima.
• FeLV = vírus da leucemia felina.
• FIV = vírus da imunodeficiência felina.

Sugestões de Leitura
Dow SW, Jones RL, Henik RA, Husted PW. Clinical features of salmonellosis in cats: six cases (1981-1986). J Am Vet Med Assoc 1989;194:1464-1466.
Greene CE. Salmonellosis. In: Greene CE, ed. Infectious diseases of the dog and cat. Philadelphia: Saunders, 1998:235-240.
Morse EV, Duncan MA. Canine salmonellosis: prevalence, epizootiology, signs, and public health significance. J Am Vet Med Assoc 1975;167:817-820.

Autor Patrick L. McDonough
Consultor Editorial Stephen C. Barr

Sarcoma Associado à Vacina

CONSIDERAÇÕES GERAIS

DEFINIÇÃO
O sarcoma associado à vacina é um tipo de tumor que se desenvolve no local de aplicação de vacina ou injeção. Os gatos são as espécies que quase sempre estão associadas a essa condição após vacinação contra o vírus da raiva e o FeLV. Também há relatos de que os cães e furões estejam sob risco desse tipo de tumor após vacinação antirrábica. Outros tipos de vacinas injetáveis e produtos não vacinais foram ocasionalmente associados ao desenvolvimento de sarcoma em gatos.

FISIOPATOLOGIA
• Embora a fisiopatologia não seja conhecida, acredita-se que a inflamação local seja um evento antecedente.
• A falta de regulação do ciclo celular que regula o gene p53 está envolvida no desenvolvimento de grande parte dos tumores.
• Esses tumores também expressam o receptor do PDGF de forma excessiva, o que pode causar a transformação de fibroblastos normais em sarcoma.
• O FeLV e o FIV não estão envolvidos na patogenia desses tumores.
• Os relatos iniciais concentravam-se nos adjuvantes vacinais que continham alumínio como agente etiológico potencial.
• No entanto, o papel do alumínio não está claro, porque nem todos os adjuvantes usados nas vacinas associadas à formação de sarcoma contêm alumínio.

SISTEMA(S) ACOMETIDO(S)
• Acomete principalmente os tecidos subcutâneos, a pele e a musculatura associada.
• Ocorre metástase em ~25% dos pacientes.

GENÉTICA
N/D.

INCIDÊNCIA/PREVALÊNCIA
Após a vacinação contra a raiva e o vírus da leucemia felina, estima-se a prevalência entre 1 e 10 casos para cada 10.000 gatos.

IDENTIFICAÇÃO
• Os gatos constituem as principais espécies acometidas e todos eles são suscetíveis.
• O sarcoma também foi relatado em cães (muito raro) e furões (prevalência desconhecida).

SINAIS CLÍNICOS
• As lesões ocorrem no local da vacinação. Muitas vezes, tais lesões assemelham-se a granulomas pós-vacinais inicialmente; no entanto, essas lesões podem persistir e/ou aumentar de tamanho.
• Além do rápido crescimento, esses tumores são altamente invasivos.
• Relata-se que as taxas de metástase sejam de 22,5-24%.
• Há relatos de metástase aos pulmões, aos linfonodos regionais e à pele.
• As lesões avançadas são volumosas, fixas e, ocasionalmente, ulceradas.

CAUSAS
• A vacinação contra o FeLV ou a raiva representa a causa predominante em gatos; muito raramente, no entanto, a vacinação antirrábica é relatada como a causa em cães e furões.
• Raras vezes, a injeção de agentes não vacinais foi associada ao desenvolvimento de sarcoma.

FATORES DE RISCO
• O risco aumenta de acordo com a frequência e a quantidade de vacinações aplicadas.
• O risco de formação do sarcoma após uma única vacinação injetável na região cervical/interescapular é 50% mais alto do que em gatos não submetidos à vacinação.
• O risco de gatos submetidos a duas vacinações nesse local é 127% maior e o risco envolvido com três ou quatro aplicações de vacinas é 175% maior do que naqueles gatos que não recebem vacinações na região cervical/interescapular.

DIAGNÓSTICO

DIAGNÓSTICO DIFERENCIAL
• Granuloma ou outras neoplasias.
• É vital a distinção entre um sarcoma vacinal e um granuloma.
• Deve-se admitir a natureza maligna das lesões até que se prove o contrário.

HEMOGRAMA/BIOQUÍMICA/URINÁLISE
Geralmente permanecem inalterados.

OUTROS TESTES LABORATORIAIS
• É recomendável a realização dos testes para detecção de FeLV e FIV.
• Aspirado e citologia de linfonodos regionais drenantes.

DIAGNÓSTICO POR IMAGEM
• Para a pesquisa de metástase à distância, devem-se obter três projeções radiográficas do tórax.
• As imagens de TC (com contraste) geralmente demonstram mais invasividade aos tecidos normais que circundam o tumor macroscopicamente visível; tal tumor pode ser determinado pelo exame físico e facilitar o planejamento terapêutico.
• As imagens de RM são superiores às de TC para determinar a distribuição e a invasividade da lesão, bem como o plano terapêutico.

MÉTODOS DIAGNÓSTICOS
• Registrar a localização, o formato e o tamanho de todas as massas que ocorrem nos locais da injeção.
• As massas que aparecem nos locais da vacinação, persistem por mais de 3 meses, são maiores que 2 cm de diâmetro ou aumentam de tamanho 1 mês depois da injeção devem ser submetidas à biopsia. Também é recomendável a realização de biopsia de lesões avançadas antes do tratamento definitivo.
• Sempre se deve planejar a biopsia, de modo que as cirurgias subsequentes consigam remover a lesão e o local biopsiado por completo.
• É aconselhável a biopsia incisional ou aspirativa (com agulha), para que qualquer tentativa de cura por cirurgias subsequentes inclua o trajeto da biopsia.
• A citologia de aspirado por agulha fina pode fornecer um diagnóstico presuntivo preliminar.

ACHADOS PATOLÓGICOS
O fibrossarcoma constitui o tipo mais comum de sarcoma associado a vacinas, embora ocorram outros tipos de sarcoma.

TRATAMENTO

• O tratamento eficiente pode não ser uma tarefa fácil em casos de doença avançada ou metastática ou caso se faça um simples debridamento em vez de uma cirurgia rigorosa.
• A obtenção da TC contrastada antes da realização de cirurgia rigorosa por algum cirurgião especialista resulta em um período de tempo substancialmente maior até a primeira recidiva, em comparação à cirurgia feita por um clínico geral.
• A aplicação de radioterapia antes ou depois da cirurgia definitiva também aumentará a sobrevida do paciente de forma considerável.
• A quimioterapia pode não aumentar a sobrevida da maioria dos pacientes.
• Sempre se deve consultar um médico-veterinário e oncologista especialista em radioterapia a respeito das recomendações terapêuticas mais recentes. Sempre que possível, é melhor optar pelo tratamento com um cirurgião-veterinário especialista em cirurgias contra o câncer.

ORIENTAÇÃO AO PROPRIETÁRIO
• Não se deve vacinar o animal excessivamente.
• Obter um termo de consentimento informado por escrito e ainda discutir os riscos da vacinação com os proprietários.

CONSIDERAÇÕES CIRÚRGICAS
• A realização de intervenção cirúrgica rigorosa por cirurgião com formação profissional especializada em cirurgia oncológica é vital para aumentar a sobrevida global do paciente e o período de tempo até a recidiva.
• A obtenção da TC e/ou RM antes da cirurgia ajudará a planejar o procedimento cirúrgico e a radioterapia.
• Em virtude da possível disseminação de células cancerígenas para outros locais, deve-se evitar o uso de drenos cirúrgicos dependentes da gravidade.

MEDICAÇÕES

Quimioterápicos, incluindo a administração intravenosa de carboplatina (200-240 mg/m^2), doxorrubicina (25 mg/m^2) ou ifosfamida (900 mg/m^2), podem diminuir a velocidade de crescimento do tumor primário e a taxa de metástases regionais e/ou à distância associadas.

CONTRAINDICAÇÕES
N/D.

PRECAUÇÕES
N/D.

INTERAÇÕES POSSÍVES
N/D.

MEDICAMENTO(S) ALTERNATIVO(S)
N/D.

ACOMPANHAMENTO

Reavaliar o animal em intervalos apropriados.

Sarcoma Associado à Vacina

PREVENÇÃO
- Avaliar os riscos de exposição a doenças e compará-los aos riscos de formação de sarcoma associado a vacinas.
- Não vacinar o paciente de forma exagerada.
- Vacinar o animal contra a raiva, a panleucopenia, o herpes-vírus tipo 1 e as caliciviroses por não mais que a cada 3 anos.
- A vacinação contra o FeLV é aconselhável apenas para os gatos com mais de 16 semanas de vida que não ficam presos em ambientes internos fechados isentos desse vírus (i. e., aos gatos com livre acesso à rua).
- Evitar a aplicação de outras vacinas a menos que haja um risco de exposição comprovado.

COMPLICAÇÕES POSSÍVEIS
É provável a ocorrência de recidivas e/ou o aparecimento de novas lesões.

EVOLUÇÃO ESPERADA E PROGNÓSTICO
- O encaminhamento a um cirurgião especialista é altamente recomendado.
- Também é altamente aconselhada a aplicação de radioterapia adjuvante.
- Relata-se que o tempo médio até a primeira recidiva seja de 66 dias após cirurgia efetuada por médico-veterinário de referência *versus* 274 dias depois de intervenção realizada por cirurgião especialista.
- Também se relata que o tempo médio até a primeira recidiva depois de excisão radical seja de 325 dias *versus* 79 dias depois de excisão local.
- Diversos estudos relatam que a radioterapia antes ou depois da realização de cirurgia rigorosa aumentará a sobrevida e estenderá o tempo até a primeira recidiva.

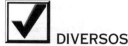

DIVERSOS

DISTÚRBIOS ASSOCIADOS
Nenhum.

FATORES RELACIONADOS COM A IDADE
Nenhum.

POTENCIAL ZOONÓTICO
Nenhum.

SINÔNIMO(S)
Sarcoma no local da injeção.

VER TAMBÉM
Capítulos sobre Fibrossarcoma.

ABREVIATURA(S)
- FeLV = vírus da leucemia felina.
- FIV = vírus da imunodeficiência felina.
- PDGF = fator de crescimento derivado de plaquetas.
- RM = ressonância magnética.
- TC = tomografia computadorizada.

RECURSOS DA INTERNET
http://www.avma.org/vafstf/.

Sugestões de Leitura
Cohen M, Wright JC, Brawner WR, et al. Use of surgery and electron beam irradiation, with or without chemotherapy, for treatment of vaccine-associated sarcomas in cats: 78 cases (1996-2000). JAVMA 2001, 219(11):1582-1589.

Eckstein C, Guscetti F, Roos M, et al. A retrospective analysis of radiation therapy for the treatment of feline vaccine-associated sarcoma. Vet Comp Onc 2009, 7(1):54-68.

Kobayashi T, HauckML, Dodge R, et al. Preoperative radiotherapy for vaccine associated sarcoma in 92 cats. Vet Radiol Ultrasound 2002, 43(5):473-479.

Munday JS, Stedman NL, Richey LJ. Histology and immunohistochemistry of seven ferret vaccination-site fibrosarcomas. Vet Pathol 2003, 40:288-293.

Poirier VJ, Thamm DH, Kurzman ID, et al. Liposome-encapsulated doxorubicin (Doxil) and doxorubicin in the treatment of vaccine-associated sarcoma in cats. J Vet Intern Med 2002, 16(6):726-731.

Rassnick KM, Rodriguez CO, Khanna C, et al. Results of a phase II clinical trial on the use of ifosfamide for treatment of cats with vaccine-associated sarcomas. Am J Vet Res 2006, 67(3):517-523.

Richards J, Elston T, Ford RB, et al. The 2006 Report of the American Association of Feline Practitioners Feline Vaccine Advisory Panel. JAVMA 2006, 229:1405-1441.

Richards JR, Starr RM, Childers HE, et al. Vaccine-associated feline sarcoma task force: Round table discussion—the current understanding and management of vaccine-associated sarcomas in cats. JAVMA 2005, 226:1821-1842.

Vascellari M, Melchiotti E, Bozza MA, et al. Fibrosarcomas at presumed sites of injection in dogs: Characteristics and comparison with non-vaccination site fibrosarcomas and feline postvaccinal fibrosarcomas. J Vet Med 2003, 50:286-291.

Autor Wallace B. Morrison
Consultor Editorial Timothy M. Fan

Sarcoma De Células Sinoviais

CONSIDERAÇÕES GERAIS

REVISÃO
- Trata-se de uma neoplasia maligna que supostamente surge de células precursoras mesenquimais primitivas fora da membrana sinovial das articulações e da bolsa. Essas células precursoras possuem a capacidade de se diferenciar em células epiteliais ou fibroblásticas; portanto, o tumor pode apresentar componentes neoplásicos tanto epiteliais como mesenquimais.
- A doença é mais comumente observada no esqueleto apendicular, afetando sobretudo o cotovelo, o joelho e as regiões escapuloumerais. O sarcoma de células sinoviais deve ser diferenciado por meio do exame imuno-histoquímico de sarcoma histiocítico, que apresenta comportamento biológico mais agressivo e prognóstico pior.

IDENTIFICAÇÃO
- Cães — qualquer raça de ambos os sexos; idade média de 9 anos.
- Gatos — raramente relatado.

SINAIS CLÍNICOS
- Claudicação lentamente progressiva.
- Massa palpável.
- Perda de peso.
- Anorexia.
- A evolução clínica pode ser prolongada por meses a anos.

CAUSAS E FATORES DE RISCO
Desconhecidos.

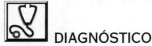

DIAGNÓSTICO

DIAGNÓSTICO DIFERENCIAL
- Outra neoplasia primária (p. ex., sarcoma histiocítico, condrossarcoma, osteossarcoma).
- Neoplasia metastática (p. ex., carcinoma prostático).
- Outras osteopatias primárias (p. ex., osteoartrite, osteomielite).

HEMOGRAMA/BIOQUÍMICA/URINÁLISE
Sem anormalidades compatíveis.

OUTROS TESTES LABORATORIAIS
N/D.

DIAGNÓSTICO POR IMAGEM
- Radiografias da lesão primária revelam envolvimento tanto ósseo como articular; é comum um aumento na opacidade do tecido mole dentro e em torno das articulações envolvidas; pode-se notar reação periosteal.
- Radiografias torácicas devem ser obtidas para pesquisa de metástase.
- É recomendável a realização de ultrassonografia abdominal para avaliar os linfonodos intra-abdominais em animais com tumores nos membros pélvicos.

MÉTODOS DIAGNÓSTICOS
- Biopsia e imuno-histoquímica para diferenciar de sarcoma histiocítico (esse tipo de sarcoma é CD18+).
- Linfonodos regionais devem ser palpados, com subsequente obtenção de aspirados por agulha fina se possível.

TRATAMENTO
- Ampla excisão cirúrgica (i. e., amputação).
- Sobrevida média em torno de 32 meses (faixa de 0-74 meses).

MEDICAÇÕES

MEDICAMENTO(S)
- Ainda não foi descrito um protocolo quimioterápico definitivo para sarcoma de células sinoviais.
- Controle da dor com AINE, conforme a necessidade.

CONTRAINDICAÇÕES/INTERAÇÕES POSSÍVEIS
N/D.

ACOMPANHAMENTO

MONITORIZAÇÃO DO PACIENTE
Monitorizar o paciente quanto à ocorrência de recidiva local e metástase pulmonar a cada 2-3 meses no primeiro ano e, depois, a cada 6 meses.

EVOLUÇÃO ESPERADA E PROGNÓSTICO
- Doença localizada — prognóstico excelente.
- Doença metastática — vários critérios histológicos (p. ex., índice mitótico elevado, alta porcentagem de necrose tumoral e alto pleomorfismo nuclear) pode conferir um prognóstico pior.

DIVERSOS

GESTAÇÃO/FERTILIDADE/REPRODUÇÃO
Não acasalar os animais que estejam recebendo quimioterapia.

ABREVIATURA(S)
- AINE = anti-inflamatórios não esteroides.

Sugestões de Leitura
Craig LE, et al. Diagnosis and prognosis of synovial tumors in dogs: 35 cases. Vet Pathol 2002, 39:66-73.

Autor Ruthanne Chun
Consultor Editorial Timothy M. Fan

SARNA NOTOÉDRICA

CONSIDERAÇÕES GERAIS

REVISÃO
• Uma dermatopatia parasitária altamente contagiosa não sazonal com prurido intenso em gatos, causada pelo ácaro *Notoedres cati*.
• O ácaro está intimamente relacionado com *Sarcoptes scabiei var. canis*.
• Os ácaros cavam túneis através da pele, provocando prurido intenso.

IDENTIFICAÇÃO
• Gatos domésticos de todas as idades e ambos os sexos.
• Embora seja razoavelmente específico ao hospedeiro, o *Notoedres cati* também pode produzir sintomas em cães, chitas, guaxinins, coelhos, quatis, civetas, linces, ocelotes, raposas e seres humanos.
• Todos os gatos contactantes geralmente desenvolvem sinais clínicos.
• Enzoótica em áreas localizadas — sobretudo grandes populações de gatos selvagens.
• Transmissão por contato direto: o ácaro tem um período de vida muito curto no ambiente.

SINAIS CLÍNICOS
• Prurido intenso não sazonal.
• Após a exposição, o prurido inicial pode ser leve, mas evolui para grave.
• O período de incubação pós-exposição de aproximadamente 5-6 semanas antes do ataque explosivo de prurido intenso pode indicar soroconversão e resposta de hipersensibilidade aprendida (IgG, além de respostas humorais e mediadas por células).
• Raros indivíduos não apresentam soroconversão e, portanto, podem não desenvolver prurido intenso.
• Ocorre o desenvolvimento de pápulas e crostas nos pavilhões auriculares, disseminando-se para pálpebras, face e pescoço (por essa razão, também é conhecida como "sarna da cabeça").
• Evolui para os pés e o períneo e, em seguida, para o corpo inteiro.
• O autotraumatismo intenso leva ao aparecimento de lesões secundárias.
• A pele fica espessa, liquenificada e coberta por crostas de cor cinza-amarelada.
• Se não for tratada, também ocorre o desenvolvimento de grandes placas de lesões e alopecia sobre todo o corpo.
• Ao contrário da escabiose canina, grande número de ácaros está presente na pele.
• Frequentemente se desenvolve linfadenopatia periférica.

CAUSAS E FATORES DE RISCO
Contato estreito com outros gatos.

DIAGNÓSTICO

DIAGNÓSTICO DIFERENCIAL
• Atopia.
• Alergia alimentar.
• Foliculite bacteriana.
• Dermatofitose.
• Demodicose.
• Dermatite por *Malassezia*.
• *Cheyletiellosis*.
• Trombiculose (bichos-de-pé).
• Dermatite otodécica.
• Pênfigo foliáceo.
• Pênfigo eritematoso.
• Lúpus eritematoso sistêmico.

HEMOGRAMA/BIOQUÍMICA/URINÁLISE
N/D.

OUTROS TESTES LABORATORIAIS
N/D.

DIAGNÓSTICO POR IMAGEM
N/D.

MÉTODOS DIAGNÓSTICOS
Raspado cutâneo superficial — é relativamente fácil encontrar os ácaros.
Ácaro menor que o *S. scabiei*, com ânus dorsal, estrias de "identificação" concêntricas dorsais típicas e apenas dois pares de pernas dianteiras que se projetam a partir da linha corporal.
Não há um teste sérico (ELISA) disponível para detecção de anticorpo antiácaro.

TRATAMENTO

• Ao utilizar imersões acaricidas (escabicidas), todo o gato deverá ser tratado.
• As falhas terapêuticas ocorrerão se o produto não for aplicado na face e nas orelhas.
• É recomendável o tratamento de todos os gatos contactantes.
• A resposta costuma ser rápida se todos os animais contactantes forem tratados.
• Pode ser recomendada a limpeza minuciosa do ambiente em que vive o gato.
• Antibióticos sistêmicos — talvez sejam necessários para resolver o problema de foliculite bacteriana secundária.

MEDICAÇÕES

MEDICAMENTO(S) DE ESCOLHA
• Imersão de todo o corpo com soluções sulfuradas 1 vez por semana durante 6-8 semanas. Talvez haja necessidade de tricotomia.
• Ivermectina — eficaz: 0,2-0,3 mg/kg SC a cada 2 semanas por 2 a 3 tratamentos.
• Enxágue com amitraz (125-250 ppm) semanalmente por, no mínimo, 3 tratamentos.
• Doramectina 0,2-0,3 mg/kg SC em dose única.
• Selamectina — uso não constante na bula (ou seja, fora da indicação terapêutica); aplicada a cada 2 semanas por 3 aplicações.

CONTRAINDICAÇÕES/INTERAÇÕES POSSÍVEIS
• O enxágue com amitraz pode causar sedação.
• A solução sulfurada tem odor desagradável, além de manchar pelos, roupas e joias.

ACOMPANHAMENTO

PREVENÇÃO
Pode ocorrer reinfestação se o contato com animais infestados continuar; é imprescindível determinar a fonte da infestação (se possível) e tratar todos os gatos contactantes.

COMPLICAÇÕES POSSÍVEIS
• Os tratamentos escabicidas tópicos são mais propensos à falha por causa de aplicação incompleta da solução terapêutica.
• Ocorrerá infestação persistente se nem todos os animais contactantes forem tratados.

EVOLUÇÃO ESPERADA E PROGNÓSTICO
A resposta à terapia é rápida, desde que todos os animais contactantes sejam tratados; com frequência, os sintomas são significativamente reduzidos em até 2 semanas de tratamento.
Não há desenvolvimento de imunidade por infestações repetidas; é provável que os sinais clínicos após uma reinfestação sejam mais rápidos em virtude da exposição prévia e do desenvolvimento de hipersensibilidade.

DIVERSOS

POTENCIAL ZOONÓTICO
• O ácaro *Notoedres cati* é zoonótico.
• As pessoas em contato direto com algum gato acometido podem desenvolver uma erupção cutânea papular e pruriginosa nos braços, no tórax ou no abdome.
• As lesões em seres humanos costumam ser transitórias e exibem resolução espontânea 10 dias depois do tratamento do(s) animal(is) acometido(s).

ABREVIATURAS
ELISA = ensaio imunoadsorvente ligado à enzima.

Sugestões de Leitura
Scott DW, Miller WH, Griffin CE. Muller & Kirk's Small Animal Dermatology, 6th ed. Philadelphia: Saunders, 2001, pp. 483-484.

Autor Liora Waldman
Consultor Editorial Alexander H. Werner

SARNA SARCÓPTICA

CONSIDERAÇÕES GERAIS

REVISÃO
Doença cutânea parasitária dos cães, não sazonal, intensamente pruriginosa, altamente contagiosa, provocada por ácaros *Sarcoptes scabiei* var. canis.

FISIOPATOLOGIA
• Os ácaros cavam túneis através do estrato córneo e provocam prurido intenso por irritação mecânica, bem como pela produção de substâncias irritantes e alergênicas, que causam reação de hipersensibilidade nos cães sensibilizados. • Reação de hipersensibilidade complexa, que envolve resposta imune humoral e mediada por célula, além de imunocomplexos circulantes.

SISTEMA(S) ACOMETIDO(S)
Cutâneo/exócrino.

IDENTIFICAÇÃO
• Acomete cães de todas as idades e raças. • Todos os cães contactantes costumam ser acometidos. • Prurido passageiro em outras espécies de hospedeiros contactantes (gatos, seres humanos).

SINAIS CLÍNICOS
• Prurido intenso não sazonal. • Em geral, ocorre a formação de crostas na lateral dos cotovelos e nas margens dos pavilhões auriculares; os condutos auditivos não são acometidos. • Ocorre o desenvolvimento de erupção cutânea papular eritematosa nos pavilhões auriculares, cotovelos, jarretes, parte ventral do abdome e tórax; os cães gravemente acometidos apresentam alopecia e crostas generalizadas, além de prurido intenso. • Raros indivíduos não sofrem soroconversão e, portanto, podem não desenvolver prurido intenso. • Doses-padrão de anti-histamínicos e antiinflamatórios de esteroides podem não reduzir o prurido. • Após a exposição, o prurido inicial pode ser leve, mas evolui para intenso. • O período de incubação após exposição de aproximadamente 5-6 semanas antes do início de prurido intenso pode indicar soroconversão e resposta de hipersensibilidade aprendida. • O autotraumatismo intenso leva a lesões secundárias. • A pele fica espessada, liquenificada e coberta por crosta amarelo-acinzentada. • Sobre todo o corpo, desenvolvem-se amplas placas de lesões e alopecia se não forem tratadas. • O número de ácaros é muito baixo em grande parte dos casos acometidos. • Indivíduos imunocomprometidos podem albergar um número maior de ácaros. • Frequentemente se desenvolve linfadenopatia periférica.

CAUSAS E FATORES DE RISCO
• Exposição a cães infectados 2-6 semanas antes do desenvolvimento dos sintomas. • Contato estreito com outros cães, sobretudo nos abrigos para animais, canis de hospedagem, tosadores, parques de cães e consultórios veterinários. • Residência em áreas infestadas por raposas ou coiotes.

DIAGNÓSTICO

DIAGNÓSTICO DIFERENCIAL
• Atopia e alergia alimentar. • Foliculite bacteriana. • Demodicose. • Dermatofitose. • Dermatite por *Malassezia*. • *Cheyletiella*. • Trombiculose (trombiculídeos). • Dermatite de contato. • Dermatite por *Pelodera*. • Dermatite otodécica. • Dirofilariose.

OUTROS TESTES LABORATORIAIS
ELISA — técnica disponível para identificar os cães infestados por *Sarcoptes*.

MÉTODOS DIAGNÓSTICOS
• Resposta ao tratamento escabicida — método mais comum para diagnosticar a escabiose. • Reflexo otopodal positivo — o ato de friccionar a margem da orelha entre o polegar e o indicador deve induzir o cão a se arranhar e se coçar com a perna traseira. • Raspados cutâneos superficiais — positivos em apenas 20% dos casos de escabiose; é extremamente difícil encontrar os ácaros, os ovos ou as pelotas de fezes; resultados falso-negativos são comuns. • Flutuação fecal — pode revelar os ácaros ou os ovos. • A resposta ao tratamento pode ser um critério necessário para estabelecimento do diagnóstico presuntivo.

TRATAMENTO

• Todo cão com prurido não sazonal deve ser tratado com algum escabicida (mesmo se os resultados do raspado cutâneo forem negativos) para descartar definitivamente a sarna sarcóptica. • Quando se utilizam banhos de imersão escabicidas, todo o cão deve ser tratado; as falhas terapêuticas ocorrerão se o produto não for aplicado na face e nas orelhas. • Todos os cães contactantes devem ser tratados, porque podem ser portadores assintomáticos. • Por causa da reação de hipersensibilidade aos ácaros da sarna, pode demorar algumas semanas para que o prurido desapareça. • Os ácaros *Sarcoptes* costumam morrer rapidamente no ambiente; entretanto, há relatos de que os ácaros sobrevivam por até 3 semanas. Portanto, pode-se recomendar a limpeza completa e minuciosa do ambiente onde vive o cão.

MEDICAÇÕES

MEDICAMENTO(S) DE ESCOLHA
• Selamectina — indicada para o tratamento da sarna quando aplicada a cada 30 dias; a aplicação a cada 2 semanas por, no mínimo, três tratamentos pode ser mais eficaz. • Ivermectina — eficaz; 0,2-0,4 mg/kg SC ou VO a cada 1-2 semanas por 3 a 4 tratamentos (por, no mínimo, 1 mês); ver a seção "Contraindicações/Interações Possíveis". • Milbemicina — pode ser eficaz quando utilizada na dose de 0,75 mg/kg VO a cada 24 h ou 2 mg/kg VO a cada semana durante 3 semanas. • Doramectina — 0,2-0,6 mg/kg SC ou IM a cada semana por 3-6 tratamentos. • Combinação de imidacloprida/moxidectina — pode ser eficaz quando aplicada duas vezes em intervalo de 4 semanas. • Banho de imersão com amitraz (250 ppm) — eficaz quando utilizado semanalmente por, no mínimo, três tratamentos. • Banhos de imersão alternativos — solução de enxofre a 2-3% ou mercaptometil ftalimida (fosmet); aplicar semanalmente e continuar por, no mínimo, 6 semanas. • Terapia antisseborreica tópica em conjunto com o tratamento escabicida — ajuda a acelerar a resolução clínica das lesões descamativas e crostosas. • Antibióticos sistêmicos — podem ser necessários para resolver a piodermite secundária. • Prednisona ou prednisolona — 1 mg/kg por 3 dias ou mais se necessário para aliviar o prurido e a automutilação.

CONTRAINDICAÇÕES/INTERAÇÕES POSSÍVEIS
• Não usar ivermectina nos cães positivos para dirofilariose ou pertencentes às raças Collie, Pastor de Shetland, Old English sheepdog, Pastor australiano e seus cruzamentos — risco elevado de intoxicação pela ivermectina nas raças de pastoreio. • Evitar a ingestão de avermectinas tópicas em cães de pastoreio e seus cruzamentos em virtude da possível mutação no gene MDR1.

ACOMPANHAMENTO

• A resposta ao tratamento pode demorar 4-6 semanas. • Os tratamentos escabicidas tópicos são mais propensos a falhar por causa da aplicação incompleta da solução terapêutica. • Poderá ocorrer reinfecção se o contato com animais infectados continuar.

COMPLICAÇÕES POSSÍVEIS
Cerca de 30% dos cães com infecções por *Sarcoptes* também reagirão aos antígenos dos ácaros da poeira doméstica nos testes cutâneos intradérmicos, sugerindo que a alergia a esse tipo de ácaro possa ser uma possível sequela da infecção por escabiose.

DIVERSOS

POTENCIAL ZOONÓTICO
• A sarna sarcóptica é zoonótica. As pessoas que entram em contato estreito com um cão acometido podem desenvolver erupção cutânea papular pruriginosa nos braços, no tórax ou no abdome (áreas que frequentemente entram em contato com os cães). • As lesões desaparecem espontaneamente 10 dias após o tratamento do(s) cão(ães) acometido(s).

ABREVIATURA(S)
• ELISA = ensaio imunoabsorvente ligado à enzima.

Sugestões de Leitura
Fourie LJ, Heine J, Horak IG. The efficacy of an imidacloprid/moxidectin combination against naturally acquired Sarcoptes scabiei on dogs. Australian Vet J 2006, 84:17-21.
Lower KS, Medleau L, Hnilica KA. Evaluation of an enzyme-linked immunosorbent assay (ELISA) for the serological diagnosis of sarcoptic mange in dogs. Vet Dermatol 2001, 12:315-320.
Scott DW, Miller WH, Griffin CE. Muller & Kirk's Small Animal Dermatology, 6th ed. Philadelphia: Saunders, 2001, pp. 476-483.

Autores Liora Waldman e Alexander H. Werner
Consultor Editorial Alexander H. Werner

SCHWANOMA

CONSIDERAÇÕES GERAIS

REVISÃO
Schwanomas são tumores de origem na bainha nervosa, que surgem das células de Schwann. A expressão tumor da bainha de nervos periféricos foi proposta para incluir schwanomas, neurofibromas e neurofibrossarcomas, porque esses tumores surgem da mesma célula. É importante notar que os schwanomas são agrupados com vários outros sarcomas de tecidos moles (p. ex., hemangiopericitoma e fibrossarcoma) para fins prognósticos e terapêuticos, pois o comportamento biológico desse grupo de tumores é semelhante.

IDENTIFICAÇÃO
- Cães — idade média de 10 anos, sem predileção sexual, nenhuma predisposição racial conhecida.
- Gatos — raramente acometidos.

SINAIS CLÍNICOS
Variam, dependendo da localização do tumor, que pode ser periférica (p. ex., pele ou língua) ou mais central (p. ex., região axilar).

CAUSAS E FATORES DE RISCO
Nenhum identificado.

DIAGNÓSTICO

DIAGNÓSTICO DIFERENCIAL
- Outra neoplasia (p. ex., mastocitoma ou linfoma).
- Doença ortopédica.
- Outra doença neurológica (p. ex., discopatia intervertebral).

HEMOGRAMA/BIOQUÍMICA/URINÁLISE
Os resultados costumam permanecer normais.

OUTROS TESTES LABORATORIAIS
Análise do LCS geralmente é pouco recompensadora em animais com sinais neurológicos centrais.

DIAGNÓSTICO POR IMAGEM
- Radiografia simples raramente é útil.
- Mielografia pode ser valiosa nos casos de envolvimento da raiz nervosa ventral ou dorsal.
- TC ou RM fornece as melhores informações sobre a extensão e a localização da doença.

MÉTODOS DIAGNÓSTICOS
Eletromiografia revela consistentemente a atividade elétrica espontânea anormal nos músculos do membro acometido.

TRATAMENTO

- A excisão cirúrgica constitui o tratamento de escolha.
- É provável que a aplicação de radioterapia após ressecção cirúrgica incompleta resulte em um excelente resultado em longo prazo.
- A excisão de massa distal ainda pode resultar em um membro funcional; na maioria dos casos, há necessidade de amputação.
- O procedimento de laminectomia é necessário em casos de envolvimento da raiz nervosa; é comum a ocorrência de recidiva local.

MEDICAÇÕES

MEDICAMENTO(S)
- Quimioterapia — não há nenhum tratamento quimioterápico bem-sucedido descrito.
- Corticosteroides — podem ajudar a reduzir o edema peritumoral e aliviar temporariamente os sinais clínicos.

CONTRAINDICAÇÕES/INTERAÇÕES POSSÍVEIS
N/D.

ACOMPANHAMENTO

EVOLUÇÃO ESPERADA E PROGNÓSTICO
- É comum a ocorrência de recidiva após excisão cirúrgica incompleta (até 72% dos casos).
- Quanto mais distal for o tumor, melhor será a possibilidade de cura cirúrgica.
- Para os tumores que envolvem o plexo braquial ou lombossacral, o intervalo médio livre da doença é de 7 meses e meio.
- Para os tumores que acometem as raízes nervosas dorsais ou ventrais, o intervalo médio livre da doença é de 1 mês.
- Os tumores de alto grau histológico (p. ex., grau 3) podem sofrer metástases para linfonodos regionais ou pulmões.

DIVERSOS

ABREVIATURA(S)
- LCS = líquido cerebrospinal.
- RM = ressonância magnética.
- TM = tomografia computadorizada.

Sugestões de Leitura
Chase D, et al. Outcome Following Removal of Canine Spindle Cell Tumours in First Opinion Practice: 104 Cases. J Small Anim Pract 2009, 50:568-574.

Autor Ruthanne Chun
Consultor Editorial Timothy M. Fan

Secreção Nasal

CONSIDERAÇÕES GERAIS

DEFINIÇÃO
Pode ser serosa, mucoide, mucopurulenta, purulenta, manchada de sangue ou com sangue vivo (epistaxe); pode conter restos alimentares.

FISIOPATOLOGIA
• Secreções — produzidas pelas células mucosas do epitélio e das glândulas submucosas; produção aumentada em virtude de hipertrofia e hiperplasia glandulares por irritação da mucosa nasal causada por estímulos infecciosos, mecânicos, químicos ou inflamatórios.
• Xeromicteria — "ressecamento nasal"; dano ao nervo facial secundário à doença na orelha média pode diminuir as secreções serosas provenientes das glândulas nasais laterais, levando à secreção mucoide compensatória; geralmente unilateral com hiperqueratose unilateral do plano nasal, ± ceratoconjuntivite seca.

SISTEMA(S) ACOMETIDO(S)
• Respiratório — mucosa do trato respiratório superior, incluindo as cavidades nasais, os seios nasais e a nasofaringe; doença do trato respiratório inferior também pode resultar em secreções provenientes das vias aéreas superiores.
• Gastrintestinal — podem ser observados sinais em casos de distúrbios de deglutição ou doenças esofágicas ou gastrintestinais quando as secreções forem forçadas para a nasofaringe.
• Hemático/linfático/imune — secreção manchada de sangue ou epistaxe atribuídas a defeitos das plaquetas ou hemostáticos.
• Oftálmico — pode haver ceratoconjuntivite seca ipsolateral se houver dano nervoso decorrente de doença na orelha média.

IDENTIFICAÇÃO
• Cães e gatos.
• Animais jovens — fenda palatina; pólipos nasais; discinesia ciliar; deficiência de imunoglobulinas.
• Animais mais idosos — tumores nasais; odontopatia primária (abscesso de raiz dentária).
• Cães de caça — corpo estranho.
• Cães dolicocefálicos — aspergilose, neoplasia nasal.

SINAIS CLÍNICOS

Achados Anamnésicos
• Espirros — relatados frequentemente como problema concomitante.
• Espirro reverso — pode ser encontrado concomitantemente em caso de envolvimento nasofaríngeo.
• É importante conhecer tanto a característica inicial como a atual da secreção, bem como se ela teve início de forma uni ou bilateral.
• Estertor — com frequência, os proprietários relatam uma respiração ruidosa, especialmente quando o animal está dormindo.
• Resposta à antibioticoterapia anterior é comum em virtude de infecção bacteriana secundária.

Achados do Exame Físico
• Secreções ou corrimentos ressecados no pelo do focinho ou dos membros anteriores.
• Pode-se notar uma redução do fluxo aéreo nasal, particularmente em casos de neoplasia nasal ou infecção fúngica no gato.
• Comprometimento patológico concomitante dos dentes, da nasofaringe ou das vias aéreas inferiores.
• Envolvimento ósseo — com tumor ou abscesso do quarto pré-molar; pode ser detectado sob a forma de tumefação da face ou do palato duro ou ainda como dor secundária à osteomielite fúngica ou bacteriana ou neoplasia.
• Despigmentação da mucosa da cartilagem alar nasal — observada em casos de aspergilose nasal canina.
• Linfadenomegalia mandibular — neoplasia, infecção fúngica, odontopatia.
• Pólipo — pode ser visível ao exame otoscópico ou pela tração do palato mole para baixo ao exame bucal.
• Coriorretinite — pode ser observada na cinomose ou na criptococose.

CAUSAS
• Unilateral — quase sempre associada a processos não sistêmicos; corpo estranho; doença relacionada com os dentes; infecções fúngicas; tumor nasal; dano ao nervo facial, levando à xeromicteria.
• Bilateral — agentes infecciosos (p. ex., rinotraqueíte viral felina ou calicivírus felino, herpes-vírus canino, cinomose e infecção bacteriana secundária); deficiência de IgA; irritante aerógeno; alergia; discinesia ciliar; rinite linfoplasmocitária ou hiperplásica.
• Unilateral que evolui para bilateral — *Aspergillus*; tumor nasal.
• Uni ou bilateral — epistaxe; corpo estranho; doença extranasal; parasitas nasais; rinite inflamatória.
• Doenças extranasais — pneumonia crônica, vômitos crônicos.

FATORES DE RISCO
• Odontopatia.
• Corpos estranhos.
• Infecciosos — animal vacinado inadequadamente; situações de canil, exposição a outros animais.
• Aspergilose nasal.
• Distúrbio de trombócitos — trombocitopenia ou trombocitopatia: imune primária ou secundária à doença infecciosa (i. e., riquetsiose) ou neoplasia.
• Defeito de coagulação atribuído à intoxicação por rodenticidas.
• Ácaros nasais — cães criados em canil.
• Imunossupressão, utilização crônica de corticosteroide e infecção por FIV ou FeLV.
• Pneumonia crônica de baixo grau.
• Vômitos crônicos.
• Otite crônica (dano a nervo facial).

DIAGNÓSTICO

DIAGNÓSTICO DIFERENCIAL
É importante diferenciar corrimento nasal, secreções ou crostas de doenças que ocorrem nas junções mucocutâneas, como pênfigo, vasculite ou leishmaniose.

Causas de Diagnóstico Diferencial
• Serosa — leve irritação; distúrbios virais e parasitários (p. ex., ácaros nasais).
• Mucoide — alergia; irritantes aerógenos inespecíficos; condição neoplásica inicial.
• Purulento (ou mucopurulento) — infecção secundária bacteriana ou fúngica, neoplasia.
• Serossanguinolento a epistaxe — tumor nasal e aspergilose; após episódios violentos ou paroxísticos de espirros; coagulopatia, distúrbio plaquetário e hipertensão sistêmica.

HEMOGRAMA/BIOQUÍMICA/URINÁLISE
Resultados inespecíficos para qualquer causa em particular, embora possam detectar problemas concomitantes; parte de uma avaliação completa antes da realização de anestesia geral para procedimentos diagnósticos.

OUTROS TESTES LABORATORIAIS
• Testes sorológicos — ajudam a diagnosticar doenças fúngicas ou riquetsiais.
• Estudos de coagulação — determinam os números e a função das plaquetas, bem como o perfil de coagulação.
• Quantificação de imunoglobulinas — diagnostica deficiência de IgA.

DIAGNÓSTICO POR IMAGEM

Radiografia do Crânio
• Anestesiar e posicionar o paciente com cuidado.
• Realizar antes os procedimentos de rinoscopia e sondagem periodontal, que podem provocar sangramento nasal e alterar a densidade radiográfica.
• Projeção lateral — detecta qualquer reação periosteal sobre o osso nasal; notar alterações macroscópicas nos dentes maxilares, na cavidade nasal e nos seios frontais; avaliar a coluna de ar que delineia a nasofaringe para defeitos de preenchimento.
• Projeções ventrodorsal e intrabucal com a boca aberta (utilizando filme radiográfico) — excelentes para avaliar as cavidades nasais e os ossos turbinados.
• Projeção rostrocaudal — avalia cada seio frontal (reação do periósteo e defeito de preenchimento).
• TC e RM — a TC é superior à radiografia para a formulação do diagnóstico; ambas as técnicas ajudam a detectar a extensão das alterações ósseas ou o envolvimento neurológico (SNC) associados a tumores nasais, rinite fúngica ou otite crônica.

Radiografia Dentária
• Projeções oblíquas laterais (utilizar tela com filme de alta velocidade ou radiografia digital) — melhor para detectar anormalidades nos dentes maxilares.
• Filme dental intrabucal, sem tela, ultraveloz — fornece excelentes detalhes de distúrbios nasais e odontológicos.

Radiografia Torácica
• Pode revelar áreas de infiltrados alveolares em paciente com pneumonia crônica ou *situs inversus*[*] em alguns cães com discinesia ciliar primária.

MÉTODOS DIAGNÓSTICOS
• Rinoscopia — indicada em casos de secreção nasal crônica ou recidivante; epistaxe aguda; avaliar as porções tanto anterior como posterior; pode estar contraindicada nos distúrbios de sangramento.
• Exame citológico nasal — é mais comum o encontro de inflamação inespecífica.
• Cultura fúngica — difícil de interpretar; são comuns resultados falso-positivos e falso-negativos.
• Cultura bacteriana pode ser útil na suspeita de microrganismos resistentes, mas exige amostragem nasal profunda sob anestesia.
• Biopsia da cavidade nasal — indicada em casos de secreção nasal crônica ou anormalidades

---

[*] N. T.: *Situs Inversus* (também conhecido por *situs transversus* ou *situs oppositus*) é uma condição congênita em que os órgãos do tórax e do abdome estão localizados em posição oposta de onde eles seriam normalmente encontrados.

SECREÇÃO NASAL

visualizadas; há necessidade de múltiplas amostras para garantir a representação adequada; pode-se realização microscopia eletrônica na suspeita de discinesia ciliar.
- Broncoscopia — indicada se houver histórico de tosse com secreção nasal.
- Sondagem periodontal de todos os dentes superiores — efetuar após o procedimento de rinoscopia; o sulco gengival normal: cães, ≤4 mm; gatos, ≤1 mm.
- Pressão arterial, plaquetas e perfil de coagulação na epistaxe.
- Teste lacrimal de Schirmer, exame otoscópico ou TC — avaliar a presença de possível dano ao nervo facial por otite crônica.
- Cintilografia e microscopia eletrônica de transmissão da traqueia — para confirmar discinesia ciliar primária.

TRATAMENTO
- Paciente de ambulatório — hidratação, nutrição, aquecimento e higiene adequados (manter as narinas limpas) — importantes em casos de espirro e secreção nasal crônicos. Priorizar a terapia local (rinossoros, nebulização nasal).
- Paciente internado — para qualquer tratamento cirúrgico, além de terapia tópica para aspergilose.

MEDICAÇÕES
MEDICAMENTO(S)
- Infecção bacteriana secundária — antibióticos; escolher um bom espectro de ação contra Gram-positivos (p. ex., amoxicilina, Clavamox®, clindamicina, azitromicina, cefalosporinas).
- Tentar secar as secreções nasais serosas — descongestionantes (efedrina na dose de 10-50 mg totais VO a cada 8-12 h até, no máximo, 4 mg/kg, para cães; 2-4 mg/kg a cada 8-12 h, para gatos); vasoconstritores tópicos (neosinefrina a 0,25-0,5% a cada 8-24 h ou oximetazolina a 0,25% a cada 24 h), mas por um período de tempo limitado — menos de 1 semana — já que esses agentes não tratam qualquer causa e podem induzir a dano à mucosa nasal.
- Rinite associada a problemas de dentes — antibióticos; procedimentos odontológicos conforme indicação.
- Corpo estranho — remoção, antibióticos.
- Parasitas nasais — ivermectina (300 µg/kg VO ou SC semanalmente por 3 semanas) ou milbemicina (nos cães da raça Collie e aparentados na dose de 1 mg/kg VO semanalmente por 3 semanas) para o tratamento de *Pneumonyssoides*; fembendazol (50 mg/kg VO a cada 24 h por 10 dias) para tratar *Eucoleus* (nematódeo nasal).
- Inflamação inespecífica — prednisolona (1-2 mg/kg VO a cada 12-24 h) ou piroxicam (0,3 mg/kg VO a cada 24-48 h).
- Aspergilose nasal canina — tratamento tópico com enilconazol ou clotrimazol.
- Criptococose ou esporotricose felina — itraconazol (5-10 mg/kg VO a cada 24 h) ou fluconazol (50 mg/gato a cada 12 h).
- Aspergilose felina — terapia tópica com itraconazol, voriconazol ou posaconazol.
- Neoplasia — radio e quimioterapia.
- Xeromicteria — administração oral de pilocarpina oftálmica na tentativa de estimular as secreções nasais.

CONTRAINDICAÇÕES
- Efedrina — nos pacientes cardíacos.
- Ivermectina — nos cães das raças Collie e aparentados.

PRECAUÇÕES
- Itraconazol — anorexia, náusea, vômito e enzimas hepáticas elevadas.
- Fenômeno de rebote — relatado com o uso exagerado de vasoconstritores nasais tópicos.

ACOMPANHAMENTO
MONITORIZAÇÃO DO PACIENTE
- Secreção nasal e espirros — observar alterações na frequência, no volume e nas características.
- Repetir a rinoscopia — indicada para assegurar a resposta adequada ao tratamento da rinite fúngica.
- Reavaliar os exames de radiografias torácicas ou broncoscopia — monitorizar a resposta ao tratamento da pneumonia crônica.

COMPLICAÇÕES POSSÍVEIS
- Perda do apetite — especialmente nos gatos.
- Extensão da doença primária (p. ex., infecção fúngica e tumor) para regiões como boca, olho ou cérebro.
- Angústia respiratória — em casos de obstrução nasal.
- Envolvimento da placa cribriforme em cães com aspergilose — o dano ao SNC durante terapia com medicamento tópico é um risco.

DIVERSOS
DISTÚRBIOS ASSOCIADOS
- Sinusite.
- Odontopatia.
- Causas secundárias — coagulopatia, pneumonia, doença cricofaríngea, megaesôfago.

FATORES RELACIONADOS COM A IDADE
Pacientes de meia-idade a idosos — as secreções nasais são frequentemente associadas a problemas dentários ou condições neoplásicas.

POTENCIAL ZOONÓTICO
N/D.

GESTAÇÃO/FERTILIDADE/REPRODUÇÃO
A segurança dos medicamentos mais recomendados não foi estabelecida nas fêmeas prenhes.

VER TAMBÉM
- Aspergilose Nasal.
- Criptococose.
- Discinesia Ciliar Primária.
- Epistaxe.
- Estenose Nasofaríngea.
- Pólipos Nasais e Nasofaríngeos.
- Rinite e Sinusite.
- Tumores Nasais.

ABREVIATURA(S)
- FeLV = vírus da leucemia felina.
- FIV = vírus da imunodeficiência felina.
- RM = ressonância magnética.
- SNC = sistema nervoso central.
- TC = tomografia computadorizada.

Sugestões de Leitura
Doust R, Sullivan M. Nasal discharge, sneezing and reverse sneezing. In: King LG, ed., Textbook of Respiratory Disease in Dogs and Cats. Philadelphia: Saunders, 2004, pp. 17-29.
McKiernan BC. Sneezing and nasal discharge. In: Ettinger SJ, Feldman EC, eds., Textbook of Veterinary Internal Medicine, 4th ed. Philadelphia: Saunders, 1994, pp. 79-85.

Autores Cécile Clercx e Brendan C. McKiernan
Consultor Editorial Lynelle R. Johnson

SEMINOMA

CONSIDERAÇÕES GERAIS
REVISÃO
- Tumor solitário, unilateral, geralmente benigno dos testículos, embora haja raros relatos de variantes malignas.
- Em geral, tem <2 cm de diâmetro; frequentemente difícil de palpar no início da evolução da doença.
- Representa o segundo tipo de tumor testicular mais comum em cães.
- Pode ser diagnosticado em 1 de cada 9 cães com >4 anos de idade; 71% não são detectados pelo exame físico.
- Surgem dos túbulos seminíferos e costumam ser clinicamente silenciosos.
- Um terço é encontrado em testículo criptorquídico; tumores extraescrotais mais comuns no testículo direito.

IDENTIFICAÇÃO
- Geralmente, acomete cães machos idosos.
- Idade média, 10 anos.
- Sem predisposição racial.
- Gatos — extremamente raro.

SINAIS CLÍNICOS
- Geralmente ausentes, embora possa haver o sinal de dor causada pela compressão de um tumor em expansão.
- Massa testicular palpável em 29% dos casos.
- Raramente associado à feminização pelo excesso de estrogênio (ver "Sertolinoma" e "Tumores das Células Intersticiais do Testículo").
- As variantes malignas sofrerão metástase.

CAUSAS E FATORES DE RISCO
Criptorquidismo.

DIAGNÓSTICO
DIAGNÓSTICO DIFERENCIAL
- Sertolinoma.
- Tumor das células de Leydig (intersticiais) do testículo.

HEMOGRAMA/BIOQUÍMICA/URINÁLISE
Geralmente normais a menos que haja indícios de síndrome de feminização no macho.

OUTROS TESTES LABORATORIAIS
N/D.

DIAGNÓSTICO POR IMAGEM
- Em geral, não são necessários.
- Ultrassonografia — tumores com < 3 cm de diâmetro costumam ser hipoecoicos; > 5 cm de diâmetro exibem geralmente padrão ecogênico misto.

MÉTODOS DIAGNÓSTICOS
- Castração.
- Exame histopatológico.

TRATAMENTO
- Castração.
- Radioterapia — relatada como eficaz nos pacientes com metástase regional.

MEDICAÇÕES
MEDICAMENTO(S)
A quimioterapia com carboplatina ou cisplatina é aconselhável em seres humanos com seminoma maligno, embora esse tratamento não seja descrito em cães.

CONTRAINDICAÇÕES/INTERAÇÕES POSSÍVEIS
N/D.

ACOMPANHAMENTO
PREVENÇÃO
N/D.

COMPLICAÇÕES POSSÍVEIS
Nenhuma provável.

EVOLUÇÃO ESPERADA E PROGNÓSTICO
- Após a castração — recuperação geralmente completa; prognóstico excelente.
- Em geral, benigno; ocasionalmente ocorre metástase para linfonodos regionais, órgãos viscerais, pulmões e outros locais; por essa razão, é necessário o estadiamento completo em casos de seminoma.

DIVERSOS
DISTÚRBIOS ASSOCIADOS
- Prostatopatia.
- Adenoma perianal.
- Hérnia perineal.

VER TAMBÉM
- Sertolinoma.
- Tumor das Células Intersticiais do Testículo.

Sugestões de Leitura
Grieco V, Riccardi E, Greppi GF, et al. Canine testicular tumours: a study on 232 dogs. J Comp Pathol 2008, 138(2-3):86-89.
McDonald RK, Walker M, Legendre AM, et al. Radiotherapy of metastatic seminoma in the dog. J Vet Intern Med 1988, 2:103-107.
Morrison WB. Cancers of the reproductive tract. In: Morrison WB, ed., Cancer in Dogs and Cats: Medical and Surgical Management. Jackson, WY: Teton NewMedia, 2002, pp. 555-564.
Spugnini EP, Bartolazzi A, Ruslander D. Seminoma with cutaneous metastases in a dog. JAAHA 2000, 36:253-256.

Autor Wallace B. Morrison
Consultor Editorial Timothy M. Fan

SEPSE E BACTEREMIA

CONSIDERAÇÕES GERAIS

DEFINIÇÃO
• Bacteremia — consiste na presença de microrganismos bacterianos viáveis na corrente sanguínea.
• Sepse — resposta inflamatória sistêmica à infecção bacteriana (p. ex., febre e hipotensão).
• Os termos não são sinônimos apesar de serem frequentemente utilizados de forma intercambiável.

FISIOPATOLOGIA
• Liberação de microrganismos bacterianos na corrente sanguínea — pode ocorrer de forma transitória, intermitente ou contínua.
• A resposta mais crítica do hospedeiro para a eliminação da bacteremia — fornecida pelo sistema fagocítico mononuclear do baço e do fígado; a ativação leva à liberação de inúmeros mediadores celulares (citocinas), dos quais alguns são benéficos e outros são nocivos; podem levar à morte do hospedeiro.
• Neutrófilos — relativamente mais importantes para a defesa contra infecção extravascular.
• Bacteremia — pode ocorrer como um evento transitório e subclínico ou se intensificar para uma sepse manifesta quando o sistema imune estiver sobrepujado; geralmente de significado mais patológico quando a corrente sanguínea é invadida a partir de pontos de drenagem venosa ou linfática.

SISTEMA(S) ACOMETIDO(S)
Cardiovascular
• Com o desenvolvimento superagudo da septicemia — débito cardíaco aumentado ou reduzido, resistência vascular sistêmica diminuída e permeabilidade vascular aumentada; por fim, desenvolve-se hipotensão refratária, levando à falência múltipla de órgãos e morte.
• Endocardite — pode se desenvolver; a presença apenas da bacteremia não é suficiente para a indução; múltiplos fatores, envolvendo tanto o hospedeiro como o microrganismo bacteriano, devem ser favoráveis para a adesão bacteriana às válvulas cardíacas.

Hemático/Linfático/Imune
• Distúrbios de coagulação e tromboembolia.
• Rim e miocárdio especialmente propensos à embolização séptica.
• Na bacteremia crônica — a estimulação antigênica do sistema imune pode levar à deposição de imunocomplexos.

Endócrino
• Foi relatada uma síndrome de insuficiência adrenal relativa em cães com sepse.

Outros
• Respiratório.
• Gastrintestinal.
• Hepatobiliar.

IDENTIFICAÇÃO
Espécies
• Cães e gatos.
• Não há relatos de predisposição etária, sexual ou racial.
• Cães machos pertencentes a raças de grande porte — predispostos à endocardite bacteriana e discospondilite.

SINAIS CLÍNICOS
Comentários Gerais
• O desenvolvimento pode ser agudo ou ocorrer de maneira vaga ou episódica.
• Variável, podendo envolver múltiplos sistemas orgânicos.
• Podem ser confundidos com os da doença imunomediada.
• Clínicos — mais graves quando houver o envolvimento de microrganismos Gram-negativos.
• Cães — os sinais mais precoces costumam ser atribuídos ao trato gastrintestinal.
• Gatos — o sistema respiratório é mais comumente envolvido.

Achados Anamnésicos
• É essencial a obtenção de histórico completo e detalhado; os achados anamnésicos são altamente variáveis, dependendo da causa subjacente.

Achados do Exame Físico
• Febre intermitente ou persistente; em um único estudo, a hipotermia era mais comum que a febre em gatos.
• Claudicação.
• Depressão.
• Taquicardia; em um único estudo, a bradicardia era mais comum que a taquicardia.
• Sopro cardíaco.
• Fraqueza.

CAUSAS
• Cães — microrganismos Gram-negativos (sobretudo *E. coli*) são mais comuns; cocos Gram-positivos e anaeróbios obrigatórios também importantes; há relatos de infecção polimicrobiana em cerca de 20% dos cães com hemoculturas positivas.
• Gatos — patógenos da corrente sanguínea geralmente bactérias Gram-negativas da família Enterobacteriaceae ou anaeróbios obrigatórios; *E. coli* e *Salmonella* são os microrganismos Gram-negativos mais comuns obtidos à cultura.
• *Pseudomonas aeruginosa* — isolamento raro das hemoculturas de animais.

FATORES DE RISCO
• Superagudos — piometra e ruptura do trato gastrintestinal são mais frequentemente associados.
• Início mais demorado — infecções da pele, do trato urinário superior, da cavidade bucal e da próstata.
• Hiperadrenocorticismo, diabetes melito, insuficiência hepática ou renal, esplenectomia, malignidade e queimaduras — fatores predisponentes.
• Estado imunodeficiente — quimioterapia, FIV, esplenectomia; risco particular.
• Glicocorticoides — considerados como importantes fatores de risco para a bacteremia; permitem maior multiplicação das bactérias nos tecidos extravasculares.
• Cateter intravenoso — proporciona acesso venoso rápido para as bactérias.
• Cateteres urinários de demora (i. e., permanentes) — podem representar um fator predisponente.
• Exame do reto.

DIAGNÓSTICO

DIAGNÓSTICO DIFERENCIAL
• Considerar outras causas de febre, sopro cardíaco, artralgia ou dorsalgia ou hipotensão.

• Os sinais clínicos de bacteremia mais crônica podem ser confundidos com doença imunomediada.

HEMOGRAMA/BIOQUÍMICA/URINÁLISE
• Leucocitose neutrofílica com desvio à esquerda e monocitose associada — anormalidades hematológicas mais comuns.
• Neutropenia — pode se desenvolver.
• Hipoalbuminemia e fosfatase alcalina elevada (até 2 vezes o limite superior de normalidade) — até 50% dos cães acometidos.
• Hipoglicemia — cerca de 25% dos cães acometidos; em um único estudo, o achado de hiperglicemia foi mais comum que o da hipoglicemia em gatos; no entanto, outro relato constatou mais gatos com hipoglicemia.

OUTROS TESTES LABORATORIAIS
• Na suspeita da sepse induzida pelo cateter — enviar a ponta do cateter para cultura.
• Urocultura — pode ser valiosa; a cultura positiva não determina se o trato urinário é a fonte primária ou secundária da infecção.
• Parâmetros de coagulação — devem ser monitorizados em grande parte dos casos.

DIAGNÓSTICO POR IMAGEM
Pode identificar a fonte da bacteremia (p. ex., piometra, próstata) ou órgãos secundariamente infectados (p. ex., discospondilite).

MÉTODOS DIAGNÓSTICOS
Hemocultura
Indicações
• Qualquer paciente que desenvolva febre (ou hipotermia), leucocitose (especialmente com desvio à esquerda), neutropenia, claudicação com desvio do membro, início recente ou alteração de sopro cardíaco ou qualquer sinal de sepse que não possa ser explicado.
• Essencial para confirmar a suspeita de bacteremia e para otimizar o tratamento do paciente; um único estudo de animais criticamente doentes relatou que cerca de 75% dos gatos e 50% dos cães tiveram hemoculturas positivas.
• Achados clínicos — não confiáveis para discriminar entre tipos específicos de bactérias.

Diretrizes
• Terapia antimicrobiana atual — não impede a coleta de hemoculturas; informar ao laboratório que o paciente está recebendo antibióticos; algumas medidas podem ser tomadas para inativar determinados medicamentos.
• Culturas anaeróbias — talvez haja necessidade de frascos especiais.
• Conjuntos (pares) de amostras — informar ao laboratório que, de cada par de frascos enviados, um é para cultura aeróbia e outro para cultura anaeróbia.
• Coletar no mínimo dois (e, de preferência, três) conjuntos de amostras — aumenta as chances de obtenção de cultura positiva e facilita a interpretação dos resultados.
• Volume — quanto maior o volume de sangue coletado, maiores serão as chances de se obter culturas positivas; com frequência, apenas alguns microrganismos estão presentes por mililitro de sangue; 10 mL de sangue por cultura é a quantidade recomendada; pode não ser possível para cães de pequeno porte e gatos; ter uma variedade de frascos de cultura à disposição (incluindo 25, 50 e 100 mL); pequenos frascos são valiosos para pacientes de pequeno porte, a fim de

SEPSE E BACTEREMIA

manter uma relação apropriada do sangue para o caldo de cultura.
• Momento oportuno de coleta — para a maior parte dos pacientes, é suficiente coletar três culturas em um período de 24 h; para pacientes criticamente doentes, coletar três culturas em um período de 2 h.

Coleta
• Frascos — aquecer à temperatura ambiente; aplicar álcool ou iodo à tampa de borracha.
• Paciente — fazer tricotomia; desinfetar minuciosamente a pele antes da venopunção para evitar a contaminação; esfregar álcool a 70% e, em seguida, aplicar antisséptico à base de iodo; deixar por, no mínimo, 1 min em contato com a pele.
• Coleta do sangue — utilizar luva estéril, palpar a veia; coletar o sangue em seringa estéril; esvaziar todo o ar da seringa; adaptar nova agulha antes de inocular o sangue nos frascos.
• Amostras — manter os frascos de cultura à temperatura ambiente para o transporte ao laboratório.

Meios de Cultura
• Meio comercial com caldo nutriente de múltiplos usos — recomendado.
• Meio que garanta o crescimento tanto de aeróbios como de anaeróbios — ideal.
• Frequentemente o laboratório que processa a cultura fornece os frascos para essa finalidade.

Interpretação dos Resultados
• Cultura positiva isolada — não é possível diferenciar bacteremia real de contaminação da amostra.
• São desejáveis duas ou mais culturas positivas identificadas como o mesmo microrganismo.
• Estafilococos coagulase-negativos, estreptococos α-hemolíticos e *Acinetobacter* — provavelmente se referem à contaminação.
• *Enterobacteriaceae*, *Bacteroidaceae*, *Pseudomonas aeruginosa*, *Staphylococcus aureus*, *Staphylococcus intermedius*, estreptococos β-hemolíticos e leveduras — quase sempre indicam bacteremia significativa do ponto de vista clínico.
• Resultados negativos de duas ou três culturas sucessivas — em geral eliminam a bacteremia atribuída a patógenos comuns; algumas bactérias menos comuns podem demorar várias semanas para crescer.

ACHADOS PATOLÓGICOS
Variam com a causa subjacente.

TRATAMENTO
CUIDADO(S) DE SAÚDE ADEQUADO(S)
• Sucesso — necessita de identificação precoce do problema e intervenção rigorosa; é essencial a monitorização cuidadosa, porque o estado do paciente pode se alterar rapidamente.
• Hipotensão — fluidos intravenosos; fluidos isotônicos (p. ex., solução de Ringer lactato) a uma taxa de até 90 mL/kg/h nos cães e 55 mL/kg/h nos gatos; ter cuidado quando a hipoalbuminemia ou a permeabilidade vascular aumentada forem uma preocupação.
• Expansores de volume (p. ex., hidroxietilamido) — podem ajudar a manter a pressão oncótica.
• Na hipoglicemia — pode-se adicionar glicose aos fluidos intravenosos.
• Eletrólitos e equilíbrio acidobásico — corrigir as anormalidades.
• Fontes externas de infecção — dar atenção especial aos cuidados de feridas e às trocas de bandagens.
• Fontes internas de infecção (p. ex., piometra ou ruptura do intestino) — é essencial proceder à intervenção cirúrgica.

CUIDADO(S) DE ENFERMAGEM
Conforme for pertinente para a situação de cada paciente.

DIETA
Suporte nutricional — fornecer por meio de alimentação assistida ou colocação de tubo.

ORIENTAÇÃO AO PROPRIETÁRIO
O prognóstico deve ser abordado junto ao proprietário.

CONSIDERAÇÕES CIRÚRGICAS
Qualquer foco de infecção identificável, como abscesso, deve ser localizado e removido sempre que possível.

MEDICAÇÕES
MEDICAMENTO(S) DE ESCOLHA
• Antibióticos — selecionados, em geral, antes de os resultados da cultura e do antibiograma estarem disponíveis; tratamento empírico aceitável enquanto se aguardam os resultados; não adiar o tratamento.
• Antimicrobianos — administrar por via intravenosa; direcionar o tratamento de forma a incluir todos os possíveis microrganismos bacterianos (Gram-positivos e negativos; aeróbios e anaeróbios).
• Se o paciente não estiver em choque — uma boa escolha é a cefalosporina de primeira geração; cães e gatos: administrar cefazolina na base de 40 mg/kg IV como dose de ataque; em seguida, 20-30 mg/kg IV a cada 6-8 h (cães e gatos).
• Aminoglicosídeos — acrescentar ao protocolo se uma terapia mais rigorosa for justificável; administrar gentamicina na base de 2-4 mg/kg IV a cada 8 h (cães e gatos).

CONTRAINDICAÇÕES
Glicocorticoides e AINE — valiosos no tratamento de choque séptico; não aumentam a sobrevida a menos que administrados nas primeiras horas do início; podem complicar o quadro clínico nos órgãos potencialmente isquêmicos (p. ex., trato gastrintestinal e rins).

PRECAUÇÕES
Aminoglicosídeos — utilizar com cuidado na presença de comprometimento renal.

ACOMPANHAMENTO
MONITORIZAÇÃO DO PACIENTE
• Terapia com aminoglicosídeo — monitorizar a função renal.
• Pressão arterial e ECG — monitorizar, se houver indicação.

COMPLICAÇÕES POSSÍVEIS
Falência múltipla de órgãos.

EVOLUÇÃO ESPERADA E PROGNÓSTICO
A bacteremia é associada a uma alta taxa de mortalidade; o óbito é causado por hipotensão, distúrbios eletrolíticos e acidobásicos e choque endotoxêmico.

DIVERSOS
DISTÚRBIOS ASSOCIADOS
• Suspeita de discospondilite (cães) — talvez haja necessidade de triagem para *Brucella canis*.
• Ver a seção "Fatores de Risco" em busca de possíveis doenças subjacentes.

SINÔNIMO(S)
• Choque séptico.
• Septicemia.

VER TAMBÉM
• Abscedação.
• Choque Séptico.
• Endocardite Infecciosa.
• Infecções Anaeróbias.

ABREVIATURA(S)
• AINE = anti-inflamatório não esteroide.
• ECG = eletrocardiograma.
• FIV = vírus da imunodeficiência felina.

Sugestões de Leitura
Bellhorn TL, Macintire DK. Bacterial translocation: Clinical implications and prevention. Compend Contin Educ Pract Vet 2002, 32:1165-1178.
Burkitt JM, Haskins SC, Nelson RW, et al. Relative adrenal insufficiency in dogs with sepsis. J Vet Intern Med 2007, 21:226-231.
Morresey PR. Synthesis of proinflammatory mediators in endotoxemia. Compend Contin Educ Pract Vet 2001, 23:829-836.
Purvis D, Kirby R. Systemic inflammatory response syndrome: Septic shock. Vet Clin North Am Small Anim Pract 1994, 24:1225-1247.

Autor Sharon Fooshee Grace
Consultor Editorial Stephen C. Barr

Sequestro de Córnea — Gatos

CONSIDERAÇÕES GERAIS

REVISÃO
- Sequestro de córnea é uma necrose focal de coagulação da área do estroma semelhante à placa, castanho-clara a preta, localizada geralmente nas regiões axial e paraxial. • Causado em geral por ulceração crônica, traumatismo ou exposição da córnea. • Sinônimos: ceratite negra.

IDENTIFICAÇÃO
- Gatos — qualquer raça, idade; acomete mais comumente os de meia-idade. • As raças braquicefálicas (Persa, Himalaio) e a siamesa são predispostas. • Os gatos *colorpoints* podem ter predisposição genética.

SINAIS CLÍNICOS
- Áreas uni a bilaterais, arredondadas a ovais focais e de tamanho variável de manchas na córnea, variando de uma cor castanho-dourada translúcida (inicialmente) até preta opaca (crônica). • Com frequência, o animal exibe uma úlcera de córnea crônica não cicatrizante. • Vascularização e edema de córnea. • Muitas vezes, o animal teve episódios prévios de ceratoconjuntivite por herpes-vírus felino tipo 1 (FHV-1). • Blefarospasmo e/ou secreção ocular (clara a mucoide ou mucopurulenta preto-acastanhada). • Hiperemia e quemose conjuntivais. • Pupila miótica. • Pode permanecer estático por longos períodos ou evoluir com rapidez. • Com a cronicidade do processo, a vascularização da córnea pode resultar em extrusão da placa.

CAUSAS E FATORES DE RISCO
- Embora a causa exata seja desconhecida, acredita-se que o sequestro de córnea envolva irritação mecânica crônica ou ulceração corneana com subsequente necrose e ressecamento dessa estrutura ocular. • Os fatores de risco propostos incluem ulceração crônica da córnea, irritação mecânica crônica da córnea, triquíase ou entrópio, conformação braquicefálica, lagoftalmia (piscar incompleto), ceratoconjuntivite seca, distúrbios qualitativos do filme lacrimal (deficiência de lipídios ou mucina), infecção por FHV-1, uso tópico de medicamentos (corticosteroides) e traumatismo iatrogênico (ceratotomia em grade).

DIAGNÓSTICO

DIAGNÓSTICO DIFERENCIAL
- Perfuração da córnea/prolapso da íris — a íris protruída é carnosa e de coloração amarela a castanho-clara. • Corpo estranho na córnea — em geral evidente. • Pigmentação da córnea — rara em gatos. • Neoplasia da córnea — ocorre melanocitoma no limbo, tipicamente indolor.

HEMOGRAMA/BIOQUÍMICA/URINÁLISE
Sem anormalidades específicas.

OUTROS TESTES LABORATORIAIS
- Teste lacrimal de Schirmer — valores muitos baixos sugerem ceratoconjuntivite seca, mas alguns gatos normais podem ter valores baixos.
- Cultura e citologia da córnea para descartar infecção corneana secundária na presença de ulceração ou infiltrado celular inflamatório nessa estrutura ocular.
- Corante de fluoresceína para determinar se a córnea está ulcerada.
- Tempo de ruptura do filme lacrimal — o tempo normal de ruptura do filme lacrimal corado pela fluoresceína é de 21 segundos. O tempo de ruptura do filme lacrimal pode estar reduzido em gatos com sequestros de córnea ou infecção por FHV-1 devido à deficiência de mucina no filme lacrimal ou secundário à doença corneana.
- Histopatologia da córnea para confirmar o diagnóstico e avaliar a totalidade da excisão.
- A córnea necrótica acelular é invadida por células inflamatórias.
- PCR "aninhado" para detecção do DNA do FHV-1 — de valor limitado, pois os gatos saudáveis normais podem carrear esse vírus e ter resultados positivos no teste de PCR.
- Biopsia conjuntival para avaliação da densidade das células caliciformes — o número das células caliciformes pode estar diminuído, secundariamente à inflamação conjuntival e/ou FHV-1.

TRATAMENTO
- Fatores como profundidade da lesão, grau de dor ocular e condição financeira do proprietário são importantes no desenvolvimento de um plano terapêutico.
- Tratamento médico — fornecimento de cuidados de suporte enquanto se aguarda que o sequestro se esfacele espontaneamente.
- Embora o tratamento médico evite a cirurgia, a dor ocular pode persistir por meses e levar à perfuração da córnea.

CONSIDERAÇÕES CIRÚRGICAS
- Ceratectomia lamelar é o procedimento de escolha. Se realizada no início do curso da doença, essa cirurgia pode aliviar a dor ocular com rapidez e promover uma cicatrização mais rápida da córnea; além disso, pode impedir que a lesão envolva o estroma corneano mais profundo.
- É recomendável a realização de procedimentos adjuvantes de aplicação de enxerto na córnea se ≥50% do estroma corneano tiver sido excisado. As opções incluem enxerto conjuntival pediculado; aplicação de enxerto com materiais biológicos sintéticos, autógenos ou heterólogos; e transposição corneoscleral.
- Tratamento pós-operatório da úlcera de córnea com antibiótico tópico de amplo espectro, pomada de atropina e suplemento de lágrima.

MEDICAÇÕES

MEDICAMENTO(S)
- Administração tópica de cloridrato de oxitetraciclina com polimixina B (Terramicina®) ou bacitracina-neomicina-polimixina B a cada 6-8 h como profilaxia.
- Pomada tópica de sulfato de atropina a 1% a cada 12-24 h para melhorar o conforto ocular do paciente e evitar a formação de sinequias posteriores. Evitar o uso de solução tópica de atropina, pois seu gosto amargo pode causar salivação profusa em gatos.
- Lubrificantes tópicos a cada 6-8 h para reduzir a irritação mecânica e evitar o ressecamento corneano; também podem impedir a evolução de sequestros precoces não ulcerados. Gel de hialuronato de sódio (Hylashield®), gel de carbômer (Lubrithal®), gel de carboximetilcelulose (Celluvisc®), hipromelose (GenTeal®).
- Terapia antiviral tópica e/ou sistêmica adjuvante nos casos em que o histórico ou os sinais clínicos são compatíveis com infecção por FHV-1.
- Alfainterferona 2b tópica (1.000-3.000 unidades/mL) a cada 6-8 h. Há relatos breves e casuais de melhora clínica em casos de sequestros de córnea, particularmente naqueles relacionados com infecção por FHV-1.

CONTRAINDICAÇÕES/INTERAÇÕES POSSÍVEIS
Antibióticos tópicos (neomicina) podem ser irritantes e causar conjuntivite química.

ACOMPANHAMENTO

MONITORIZAÇÃO DO PACIENTE
- Se o paciente for submetido a tratamento médico, examinar semanalmente para monitorizar a organização do sequestro corneano e a ocorrência de complicações associadas ao esfacelamento do sequestro.
- Se tratado por meio de ceratectomia, o olho deverá ser reavaliado a cada 7-10 dias até que o defeito da córnea tenha sofrido reepitelização (que, em geral, ocorre em até 7-14 dias).
- Os sequestros de córnea podem recorrer ou ocorrer no olho contralateral. A recorrência é mais provável em gatos com valores baixos nos testes lacrimais de Schirmer, naqueles acometidos por lesões de espessura completa ou nos casos em que a ceratectomia não resultou em excisão completa do tecido corneano pigmentado ou a causa predisponente não foi tratada.

COMPLICAÇÕES POSSÍVEIS
- Pode ocorrer perfuração da córnea se o sequestro se esfacelar, deixando um defeito de espessura completa, e/ou se o esfacelamento resultar na formação de uma úlcera profunda do estroma corneano que se torna malácica ou infectada.

DIVERSOS

DISTÚRBIOS ASSOCIADOS
- Ulceração de córnea — gatos.
- Anormalidades de conformação das pálpebras (triquíase, entrópio, etc.).

ABREVIATURAS
- FHV-1 = herpes-vírus felino tipo 1.
- PCR = reação em cadeia da polimerase.

Sugestões de Leitura
Featherstone HJ, Sansom J. Feline corneal sequestra: A review of 64 cases (80 eyes) from 1993 to 2000. Vet Ophthalmology 2004, 7(4):213-227.
Stiles J, Townsend WM, Gelatt KN. Feline ophthalmology. In: Gelatt KN, ed., Veterinary Ophthalmology, 4th ed. Ames, IA: Blackwell, 2007, pp. 1095-1164.

Autor Anne Gemensky Metzler
Consultor Editorial Paul E. Miller

Sertolinoma

CONSIDERAÇÕES GERAIS

REVISÃO
- Terceiro tumor testicular mais comum nos cães, ligado ao criptorquidismo.
- Relata-se que entre 10 e 14% dos casos são malignos e sofrem metástases para os linfonodos regionais e outros órgãos toracoabdominais.
- Foi registrada em grande parte das espécies, embora seja rara em outras espécies que não o cão.
- Em cães, 50% dos sertolinomas estão localizados nos testículos retidos na cavidade abdominal.

IDENTIFICAÇÃO
- Cães machos idosos.
- Gatos — extremamente raro.

SINAIS CLÍNICOS
- Aumento de volume unilateral do testículo afetado com atrofia do testículo não acometido.
- Síndrome de feminização — ginecomastia; galactorreia; atrofia do pênis; prepúcio penduloso; atrativo para outros cães machos; permanência na posição de fêmea para urinar.
- Metaplasia escamosa da próstata e prostatomegalia — ocasionalmente.
- Alterações dermatológicas — alopecia não pruriginosa; afinamento da pelagem; hiperpigmentação.
- Massa abdominal — se o paciente for criptorquídico.
- Possível localização inguinal.

CAUSAS E FATORES DE RISCO
Testículos criptorquídicos têm uma probabilidade 13-13,6 vezes maior de desenvolver neoplasia do que aqueles localizados no escroto.

DIAGNÓSTICO

DIAGNÓSTICO DIFERENCIAL
- Tumor de células intersticiais.
- Seminoma.
- Hiperadrenocorticismo.
- Hipotireoidismo.
- Mais provavelmente possui localização abdominal do que outros tumores testiculares; a temperatura testicular elevada na localização abdominal pode destruir as células espermatogênicas e deixar as células de Sertoli desreguladas.

HEMOGRAMA/BIOQUÍMICA/URINÁLISE
Anemia arregenerativa, leucopenia e trombocitopenia associadas ao hiperestrogenismo.

OUTROS TESTES LABORATORIAIS
- Concentração sérica elevada de estradiol em grande parte dos pacientes.
- Concentração sérica alta de progesterona na maior parte dos animais.

DIAGNÓSTICO POR IMAGEM
Ecotextura variável ao exame ultrassonográfico.

MÉTODOS DIAGNÓSTICOS
Castração e exame histopatológico de tecido apropriado.

TRATAMENTO

Castração.

MEDICAÇÕES

MEDICAMENTO(S)
N/D.

CONTRAINDICAÇÕES/INTERAÇÕES POSSÍVEIS
N/D.

ACOMPANHAMENTO

MONITORIZAÇÃO DO PACIENTE
N/D.

PREVENÇÃO
N/D.

COMPLICAÇÕES POSSÍVEIS
Nenhuma a menos que associadas à cirurgia ou ao excesso de estrogênio.

EVOLUÇÃO ESPERADA E PROGNÓSTICO
- Bom na maior parte dos pacientes.
- Reservado caso ocorra o desenvolvimento de citopenias por causa do hiperestrogenismo.

DIVERSOS

DISTÚRBIOS ASSOCIADOS
- 25-29% dos cães com sertolinoma desenvolvem síndrome de feminização do macho.
- Cerca de 70% dos tumores testiculares intra-abdominais nos cães estão associados à síndrome de feminização do macho.
- Hiperestrogenismo pode provocar falha hematopoiética.

SINÔNIMO
Tumor de células de Sertoli.

VER TAMBÉM
Hiperestrogenismo (Toxicidade do Estrogênio)

Sugestões de Leitura
Acland HM. Reproductive system: Male. In: Carlton WW, McGavin MD, eds., Thomson's Special Veterinary Pathology. St. Louis: Mosby, 1995, pp. 544-560.
Grieco V, Riccardi E, Greppi GF, et al. Canine testicular tumours: A study on 232 dogs. J Comp Pathol 2008, 138(2-3):86-89.
Metzger FL, Hattel AL, White DG. Hematuria, hyperestrogenemia, and hyperprogesteronemia due to a sertoli-cell tumor in a bilaterally cryptorchid dog. Canine Pract 1993, 18:32-35.
Morrison WB. Cancers of the reproductive tract. In: Morrison WB, ed., Cancer in Dogs and Cats: Medical and Surgical Management. Jackson, WY: Teton NewMedia, 2002, pp. 555-564.
Sherding RG, Wilson GP 3rd, Kociba GJ. Bone marrow hypoplasia in eight dogs with Sertoli cell tumor. JAVMA 1981, 178(5):497-501.

Autor Wallace B. Morrison
Consultor Editorial Timothy M. Fan

SÍNCOPE

CONSIDERAÇÕES GERAIS

DEFINIÇÃO
Perda temporária da consciência e do tônus vascular, associada à perda do tônus postural, com recuperação espontânea.

FISIOPATOLOGIA
A perfusão cerebral inadequada, bem como a distribuição insuficiente de oxigênio e de substratos metabólicos, levam à perda da consciência e do tônus motor; a perfusão cerebral prejudicada pode resultar de alterações no tônus vasomotor, de doença cerebral e do baixo débito cardíaco provocados por cardiopatia estrutural ou arritmias.

SISTEMA(S) ACOMETIDO(S)
• Cardiovascular.
• Nervoso.

IDENTIFICAÇÃO
Espécies
Cães e gatos.

Raça(s) Predominante(s)
• Síndrome do nó sinusal doente — raças Cocker spaniel, Schnauzer miniatura, Pug, Dachshund.
• Arritmias ventriculares — raças Boxer e Pastor alemão.

Idade Média e Faixa Etária
Mais comum nos animais idosos.

CAUSAS
Causas Cardíacas
• Bradiarritmias — bradicardia sinusal, parada sinusal, bloqueio AV de segundo grau, bloqueio AV completo, parada atrial.
• Taquiarritmias — taquicardia ventricular, taquicardia supraventricular, fibrilação atrial.
• Débito cardíaco baixo (não arrítmico) — miocardiopatia, endocardiose das valvas atrioventriculares, estenose subaórtica, estenose pulmonar, dirofilariose, embolia pulmonar, tumor cardíaco, tamponamento cardíaco.

Instabilidade Neurológica e Vasomotora
• Síncope vasovagal — o estresse e a agitação emocionais podem provocar estimulação simpática elevada, levando a taquicardia e hipertensão transitórias, o que é acompanhado pelo aumento compensatório no tônus vagal; esse aumento, por sua vez, leva à vasodilatação excessiva sem elevação compensatória na frequência cardíaca e no débito cardíaco; quase sempre ocorre bradicardia.
• Síncope situacional — é aquela associada à tosse, defecação, micção e deglutição.
• Hiperatividade do seio carotídeo pode provocar hipotensão e bradicardia — frequentemente a causa de síncope quando se puxa a coleira de um cão.

Causas Diversas
• Medicamentos que afetam o nível da pressão arterial e a regulação do tônus autônomo.
• Hipoglicemia, hipocalcemia e hiponatremia (rara).
• Síndromes de hiperviscosidade (p. ex., policitemia e paraproteinemia) provocam sedimentação do sangue e comprometimento da perfusão cerebral (rara).

FATORES DE RISCO
• Cardiopatia.
• Síndrome do nó sinusal doente.

• Terapia medicamentosa — vasodilatadores (p. ex., bloqueadores dos canais de cálcio, inibidores da ECA, hidralazina e nitratos), fenotiazinas (p. ex., acepromazina), antiarrítmicos e diuréticos.

DIAGNÓSTICO

DIAGNÓSTICO DIFERENCIAL
Sinais Diferenciais
• Deve-se diferenciar de outros estados de alteração da consciência, incluindo crises convulsivas e narcolepsia (distúrbio do sono).
• As crises convulsivas frequentemente estão associadas a um período prodrômico e pós-ictal; a síncope ocorre sem aviso, mas o animal costuma exibir recuperação rápida e espontânea. Ao contrário da síncope, a atividade convulsiva geralmente está associada mais à atividade muscular tônico-clônica do que à flacidez.
• Como a síncope, a narcolepsia ocorre de forma súbita, resulta em flacidez muscular e se resolve espontaneamente. Ao contrário da síncope, a narcolepsia pode durar minutos e ser interrompida por meio de ruídos altos ou estímulos externos estridentes.
• Também é preciso diferenciar de outras causas de colapso, como doença musculosquelética e doença neuromuscular (p. ex., miastenia grave) que não estejam associadas à perda da consciência.

Causas Diferenciais
• Síncope com agitação ou estresse sugere síncope vasovagal.
• Síncope com tosse, micção ou defecação aponta para síncope situacional.
• Síncope com exercício indica estados de baixo débito associados a arritmias ou cardiopatia estrutural.
• A presença de sopro apoia a existência de cardiopatia, mas não confirma uma causa cardíaca para a síncope.

HEMOGRAMA/BIOQUÍMICA/URINÁLISE
• Geralmente normais.
• Hipoglicemia ou distúrbio eletrolítico em alguns animais.

OUTROS TESTES LABORATORIAIS
• Se o animal estiver hipoglicêmico, medir a concentração da insulina na mesma amostra sanguínea. Calcular a relação de glicose:insulina corrigida para descartar insulinoma.
• Se o animal estiver com hiponatremia ou hipercalemia, considerar o teste de estimulação com ACTH.
• Na suspeita de baixo débito cardíaco, descartar dirofilariose oculta.

DIAGNÓSTICO POR IMAGEM
Ecocardiografia
Pode detectar cardiopatia estrutural capaz de reduzir o débito cardíaco.

MÉTODOS DIAGNÓSTICOS
• O proprietário precisa monitorizar a frequência cardíaca durante todo o episódio de síncope.
• Eletroencefalograma, tomografia computadorizada da cabeça, punção do líquido cerebrospinal (LCS) se houver suspeita de origem neurológica (SNC).

Achados Eletrocardiográficos
• ECG após o exercício pode revelar arritmia intermitente.

• Monitoramento com Holter (registro eletrocardiográfico de 24 horas) ou utilização de registrador de evento (de alça) — valioso para avaliar causas arrítmicas.
• Massagem no seio carotídeo com ECG e monitoramento da pressão arterial são úteis na avaliação da sensibilidade carotídea.

TRATAMENTO

CUIDADO(S) DE SAÚDE ADEQUADO(S)
• Evitar ou interromper as medicações que provavelmente precipitam a síncope.
• Tratar em um esquema ambulatorial a menos que haja evidência de cardiopatia relevante.

ATIVIDADE
Ver a seção "Orientação ao Proprietário".

ORIENTAÇÃO AO PROPRIETÁRIO
• Minimizar os estímulos que precipitam os episódios.
• Baixo débito cardíaco — minimizar a atividade.
• Vasovagal — minimizar a agitação e o estresse.
• Tosse — remover a coleira.

CONSIDERAÇÕES CIRÚRGICAS
Implante de marca-passo para síndrome do nó sinusal doente e bloqueio AV avançado e parada atrial persistente.

MEDICAÇÕES

MEDICAMENTO(S) DE ESCOLHA
Bradiarritmias
• Corrigir as causas metabólicas.
• Anticolinérgicos (p. ex., atropina, brometo de propantelina, sulfato de hiosciamina).
• Simpaticomiméticos (p. ex., isoproterenol e broncodilatadores).
• Implante de marca-passo em alguns pacientes.

Taquiarritmias
• Arritmias atriais — administrar digoxina, β-bloqueador ou diltiazem.
• Arritmias ventriculares — administrar lidocaína, mexiletina, sotalol ou β-bloqueador.

Baixo Débito Cardíaco
• Instituir o tratamento para melhorar o débito cardíaco, o que varia com a cardiopatia específica.

Vasovagal
• Teofilina ou aminofilina — ocasionalmente úteis; o mecanismo de ação nesse quadro é incerto.
• β-bloqueadores (p. ex., atenolol, propranolol e metoprolol) podem evitar indiretamente a estimulação vagal pelo bloqueio da resposta simpática inicial.
• Anticolinérgicos podem enfraquecer a resposta vagal.

PRECAUÇÕES
Medicamentos que reduzam a pressão arterial.

ACOMPANHAMENTO

MONITORIZAÇÃO DO PACIENTE
Monitoramento com ECG ou Holter para avaliar a eficácia da terapia antiarrítmica.

SÍNCOPE

PREVENÇÃO
Ver a seção "Orientação ao Proprietário".

COMPLICAÇÕES POSSÍVEIS
• Morte.
• Traumatismo quando ocorrer o colapso.

EVOLUÇÃO ESPERADA E PROGNÓSTICO
A maioria das causas não cardíacas não apresenta risco de morte; as causas cardíacas podem ser tratadas, embora a síncope nos pacientes com cardiopatia possa sugerir maior risco de mortalidade.

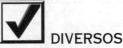

DIVERSOS

SINÔNIMO(S)
Desmaio.

VER TAMBÉM
• Crises Convulsivas (Convulsões, Estado Epiléptico) — Cães.
• Crises Convulsivas (Convulsões, Estado Epiléptico) — Gatos.
• Miastenia Grave.
• Narcolepsia e Cataplexia.

ABREVIATURA(S)
• ACTH = hormônio adrenocorticotrópico.
• AV = atrioventricular.
• ECA = enzima conversora de angiotensina.
• ECG = eletrocardiograma.
• SNC = sistema nervoso central.

RECURSOS DA INTERNET
http://www.vetmed.wsu.edu/deptsVCGL/holter.

Sugestões de Leitura
Calkins H, Zipes DP. Hypotension and syncope. In: Zipes DP, Libby P, Bonow RO, Braunwald E, eds., Braunwald's Heart Disease: A Textbook of Cardiovascular Medicine, 7th ed. Philadelphia: Elsevier Saunders, 2005, pp. 909–920.
Rush JE. Syncope and episodic weakness. In: Fox PR, Sisson D, Moise NS, eds., Textbook of Canine and Feline Cardiology, 2nd ed. Philadelphia: Saunders, 1999, pp. 446–455.

Autor Francis W.K. Smith, Jr.
Consultores Editoriais Larry P. Tilley e Francis W.K. Smith, Jr.

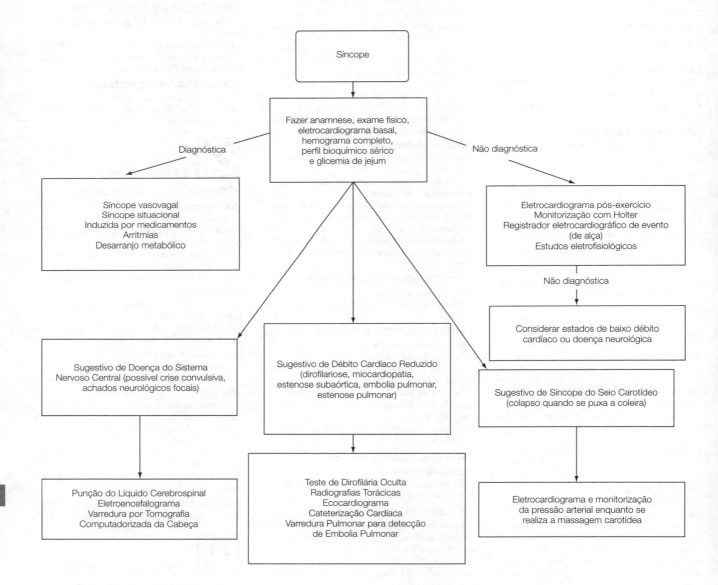

Figura 1. Algoritmo para síncope.

SÍNDROME BRAQUICEFÁLICA DAS VIAS AÉREAS

CONSIDERAÇÕES GERAIS

DEFINIÇÃO
Obstrução parcial das vias aéreas superiores, causada por qualquer combinação dos fatores expostos a seguir: estenose das narinas, palato mole excessivamente longo, sáculos laríngeos evertidos e colapso laríngeo em raças braquicefálicas de cães e gatos. Com frequência, também se diagnostica o quadro concomitante de traqueia hipoplásica, o que pode agravar a angústia respiratória.

FISIOPATOLOGIA
• Em cães normais, as vias aéreas superiores respondem por 50-70% da resistência aérea total.
• As raças braquicefálicas apresentam uma resistência elevada das vias aéreas superiores em função de estenose das narinas, formação aberrante das conchas nasais e presença de turbinados nasofaríngeos; além disso, os ossos do crânio são encurtados em termos de comprimento, mas normais em termos de largura. Os tecidos moles não são proporcionalmente reduzidos, resultando no estreitamento das passagens aéreas e no excesso de tecido. • O aumento na resistência das vias aéreas gera pressões aéreas mais negativas, que podem culminar em eversão secundária dos sáculos laríngeos, maior alongamento do palato e colapso da laringe. • O recrutamento de músculos dilatadores da faringe (esterno-hióideo) torna-se necessário para manter a desobstrução (patência) das vias aéreas. Secundariamente ao relaxamento desses músculos incumbidos pela dilatação da faringe, pode ocorrer apneia do sono (respiração desordenada durante o sono).

SISTEMA(S) ACOMETIDO(S)
• Respiratório — angústia respiratória, hipoxemia, hipercarbia, hipertermia, pneumonia por aspiração, edema pulmonar não cardiogênico causado por obstrução das vias aéreas.
• Cardiovascular — colapso cardiovascular em caso de obstrução aérea completa ou hipertermia grave. • Gastrintestinal — pode resultar em relutância para comer ou beber; além disso, o aumento na resistência das vias aéreas pode exacerbar os quadros de hérnia hiatal, refluxo gastroesofágico e esofagite.

GENÉTICA
• Ainda não se identificaram quaisquer genes específicos. • Defeito hereditário de desenvolvimento dos ossos do crânio no formato da cabeça braquicefálica, perpetuado pela reprodução seletiva.

INCIDÊNCIA/PREVALÊNCIA
• Comum em raças caninas braquicefálicas.
• Gatos — é menos comum que o quadro seja grave o bastante a ponto de necessitar tratamento.

DISTRIBUIÇÃO GEOGRÁFICA
Mundial.

IDENTIFICAÇÃO
Espécies
Cães e gatos.

Raça(s) Predominante(s)
• Cães — raças braquicefálicas (é mais comum no Buldogue inglês — até 55% da raça; Buldogue francês, Pug, Boston terrier também são comumente acometidos). • Gatos — Persa e Himalaio.

Idade Média e Faixa Etária
• Jovens adultos, diagnosticados principalmente por volta dos 2-3 anos de idade. • Se diagnosticados depois dos 4 anos de idade, procurar por doença concomitante ou circunstâncias exacerbadoras. • Há relatos de colapso da laringe em filhotes de raças braquicefálicas com até 6-7 meses de vida.

Sexo(s) Predominante(s)
Não há predisposição sexual.

SINAIS CLÍNICOS
Achados Anamnésicos
• Roncos, estridores, estertores. • Taquipneia e, frequentemente, uma respiração ofegante. • Tosse e engasgos. • Dificuldade de se alimentar e engolir (disfagia). • Ptialismo, regurgitação e vômito.
• Ocasionalmente, observam-se síncope e episódios de colapso.

Achados do Exame Físico
• Estridores e estertores. • Estenose das narinas — colapso medial da cartilagem nasal lateral.
• Aumento no esforço respiratório — retração das comissuras labiais, respiração com a boca aberta ou respiração ofegante constante, elevação na frequência respiratória, abdução dos membros torácicos, incremento no componente respiratório abdominal, recrutamento dos músculos respiratórios acessórios. • Em caso de angústia respiratória grave, pode-se observar movimento abdominal paradoxal, colapso intrínseco dos espaços intercostais, ortopneia e cianose. • Pode haver hipertermia.

CAUSAS
• Defeitos hereditários ou congênitos na conformação. • Alongamento do palato mole — relatado em mais de 90% dos casos cirúrgicos em cães. • Estenose das narinas — descrita em cerca de 50% dos casos em cães. Representa o defeito mais comum em gatos. • Formação aberrante das conchas nasais rostrais e caudais.
• Presença de turbinados nasofaríngeos recém-relatados (20% dos cães braquicefálicos e gatos).
• Laringopatia — eversão dos sáculos laríngeos (mais de 50% dos cães) e/ou colapso da laringe (cerca de 10% dos cães). • Hipoplasia da traqueia, principalmente no Buldogue.

FATORES DE RISCO
• Raça.
• Obesidade — agrava a obstrução das vias aéreas, está relacionada com resultados pós-operatórios insatisfatórios e pode contribuir para a ocorrência de refluxo gastresofágico e o desenvolvimento de pneumonia por aspiração.
• Agitação e/ou climas quentes e úmidos — o aumento da respiração ofegante pode levar à formação de edema nas vias aéreas, ao maior comprometimento do lúmen e à hipertermia.
• Atividade física — os cães frequentemente se mostram intolerantes ao exercício, em função do comprometimento das vias aéreas e da hipoxia.
• Sedação — o relaxamento dos músculos faríngeos, do palato e dos dilatadores da faringe pode gerar obstrução completa das vias aéreas.
• Infecção respiratória ou pneumopatia concomitante — levará a um maior comprometimento respiratório.
• Endocrinopatia (hipotireoidismo e hiperadrenocorticismo) — pode agravar o ganho de peso e gerar uma respiração excessivamente ofegante.

DIAGNÓSTICO

DIAGNÓSTICO DIFERENCIAL
• Corpos estranhos na nasofaringe, laringe ou traqueia. • Infecções — infecção do trato respiratório superior, abscessos nasofaríngeos.
• Obstruções neoplásicas da nasofaringe, glote, laringe ou traqueia. • Paralisia da laringe.
• Mucocele da faringe. • Pólipo ou cisto nasofaríngeo.

HEMOGRAMA/BIOQUÍMICA/URINÁLISE
• Hemograma completo — comumente normal, mas podem ocorrer policitemia em casos de hipoxia crônica e leucocitose em casos de infecção concomitante ou estresse acentuado.

OUTROS TESTES LABORATORIAIS
• Gasometria sanguínea arterial — para determinar o grau de hipercarbia, a presença de acidose respiratória e a intensidade da hipoxia, bem como a resposta à suplementação com oxigênio. • Oximetria de pulso — método rápido e não invasivo, que mensura a porcentagem de saturação de oxigênio da hemoglobina.

DIAGNÓSTICO POR IMAGEM
Achados Radiográficos
• Se o animal estiver estabilizado, recomenda-se a obtenção de radiografias cervicais e torácicas. • As radiografias cervicais podem revelar um palato mole espessado e alongado, bem como uma possível hipoplasia da traqueia. • As radiografias torácicas podem exibir pneumonia por aspiração, edema pulmonar, insuficiência cardíaca e presença de ar no esôfago, além de uma traqueia hipoplásica (DT/ET = diâmetro traqueal na altura da entrada torácica/distância da entrada torácica, o que corresponde à distância do esterno até a superfície ventral da T1). Uma relação <0,13 no Buldogue e <0,16 em outras raças braquicefálicas é sugestiva de hipoplasia da traqueia.

Fluoroscopia
Pode fornecer informações a respeito do grau de obstrução dinâmica da faringe pelo palato e por doença concomitante, como colapso da traqueia (incomum em cães braquicefálicos).

MÉTODOS DIAGNÓSTICOS
Laringoscopia/Faringoscopia
• Realizada sob anestesia geral; em função do risco de obstrução das vias aéreas, o proprietário deverá estar preparado para prosseguir com a intervenção cirúrgica se o veterinário julgar necessário. • O palato mole excessivamente alongado estende-se mais do que apenas alguns milímetros além da extremidade da epiglote e pende sobre a glote. • O palato mole frequentemente se encontra espessado e inflamado; além disso, pode haver inflamação e edema das cartilagens aritenoides. • O uso de endoscópio flexível com projeção retrofletida da nasofaringe pode revelar os turbinados nasofaríngeos. • Os sáculos laríngeos evertidos são diagnosticados por meio da observação de duas massas lisas, arredondadas e brilhantes na metade ventral da abertura da laringe — esses sáculos muitas vezes dificultam a visualização das pregas vocais.

Traqueoscopia
• Pode revelar traqueia hipoplásica, com sobreposição dos anéis dorsais e da membrana

Síndrome Braquicefálica das Vias Aéreas

dorsal dessa estrutura. • Também é possível diagnosticar o colapso da traqueia.

TRATAMENTO

CUIDADO(S) DE SAÚDE ADEQUADO(S)
• Em relação aos pacientes com sinais clínicos significativos, recomenda-se a intervenção cirúrgica. • O quadro emergencial de angústia respiratória grave exige intervenção imediata, incluindo a suplementação com oxigênio e o uso cauteloso de medicamentos ansiolíticos. • Se o animal estiver hipertérmico, é imprescindível resfriá-lo com água fria e posicioná-lo em frente a um ventilador (aumenta a perda de calor por convecção). Na presença de hipertermia extrema (>41,1°C), deve-se administrar a fluidoterapia IV na velocidade de choque. • Em caso de obstrução completa das vias aéreas, efetuar imediatamente a entubação orotraqueal e/ou a traqueostomia temporária. • Para reduzir a inflamação, pode-se administrar a dexametasona por via IV na dose de 0,1 mg/kg.

CUIDADO(S) DE ENFERMAGEM
• Os pacientes necessitam monitorização por um período de 24 h, em virtude do risco de obstrução aérea aguda e óbito. • É fundamental monitorizar a frequência e o esforço respiratórios, a frequência cardíaca, a qualidade do pulso, a coloração das mucosas, o tempo de preenchimento capilar, a temperatura e outros parâmetros físicos, antes e depois da cirurgia. • É possível realizar a monitorização da oximetria de pulso e da gasometria sanguínea arterial, dependendo da gravidade da condição. • Além de minimizar a manipulação e o estresse sobre o animal, administra-se a fluidoterapia intravenosa na velocidade de manutenção. • Efetuam-se ainda a oxigenoterapia e o resfriamento, conforme a necessidade.

ATIVIDADE
• Em geral, autolimitante.

DIETA
• A todos os cães que se encontram acima do peso ideal, recomenda-se um programa de emagrecimento. • Para os pacientes obesos e estáveis, essa perda de peso é recomendável antes da cirurgia.

ORIENTAÇÃO AO PROPRIETÁRIO
• A orientação de como se evitar os fatores de risco é decisiva. • Os proprietários devem ser informados de que os cães com síndrome braquicefálica das vias aéreas estão sob alto risco anestésico e, em casos de obesidade, risco elevado de cardiopatia ou pneumonia por aspiração. • Os proprietários também devem estar cientes de que a cirurgia corretiva muitas vezes restabelece as vias aéreas, mas não resulta em uma passagem aérea completamente normal.

CONSIDERAÇÕES CIRÚRGICAS
• Com o paciente estabilizado, efetua-se geralmente a avaliação do palato mole alongado sob anestesia geral. • Uma traqueostomia temporária pode ser colocada em prática para facilitar a exposição ou tratar a obstrução das vias aéreas. • A correção de estenose das narinas pode ser feita por meio de ressecção cuneiforme da cartilagem e do plano nasais dorsolaterais. A hemorragia é temporariamente controlada por meio de compressão, seguida por oclusão da ferida cirúrgica com 3 ou 4 suturas de material absorvível 3-0 ou 4-0. • Com o uso de tesouras, laser de dióxido de carbono ou dispositivo bipolar de selagem, promove-se a ressecção do palato mole alongado, em uma extensão que permita o contato com a extremidade da epiglote e o centro do palato mole. • O procedimento de saculectomia é realizado com o uso das pinças de Allis para preensão tecidual e tesouras curvas para aparação (corte) de todo tecido das mucosas. • Em caso de grave colapso da laringe, pode ser necessária a traqueostomia permanente.

MEDICAÇÕES

MEDICAMENTO(S)
• Administração de dexametasona a 0,1 mg/kg IV a cada 12 h por 12-24 h no pré ou pós-operatório para diminuir o edema e a inflamação. • Enquanto se aguardam os resultados da cultura e do antibiograma, fica indicado o uso de antibióticos de amplo espectro na presença de pneumonia por aspiração. • Omeprazol a 0,7 mg/kg a cada 24 h, cisaprida a 0,2 mg/kg a cada 8 h e hidróxido de magnésio a 1 mL/kg após as refeições ou sucralfato a cada 12 h resultaram em melhora clínica em 91% dos cães com esofagite, gastrite e/ou duodenite concomitantes, confirmadas por meio de avaliação endoscópica.

CONTRAINDICAÇÕES
O uso excessivo de esteroides pode levar a respiração ofegante, ganho de peso e ulceração gastrintestinal — alterações capazes de exacerbar os sinais da síndrome braquicefálica das vias aéreas.

PRECAUÇÕES
Para o alívio da ansiedade, da agitação ou do medo, deve-se empregar a sedação com extrema cautela, em virtude do risco de obstrução das vias aéreas superiores com o relaxamento muscular.

ACOMPANHAMENTO

MONITORIZAÇÃO DO PACIENTE
• No pós-operatório, o paciente requer monitorização por um período de 24 h para verificar a presença de tumefação e obstrução das vias aéreas, o que exigiria uma traqueostomia temporária.

PREVENÇÃO
• Seleção de cães sem alterações conformacionais graves pelos criadores — pode não ser uma tarefa fácil, pois os padrões raciais favorecem essas anormalidades estruturais. • Evitar os fatores de risco, principalmente o ganho de peso.

COMPLICAÇÕES POSSÍVEIS
• Hipertermia e intermação/insolação. • Pneumonia por aspiração. • Óbito em cerca de 10% dos pacientes, em consequência do comprometimento das vias aéreas. • As complicações pós-operatórias mais comuns correspondem à formação de edema (tumefação) e à obstrução das vias aéreas nas primeiras 24 h, que podem exigir a traqueostomia temporária. • Dificuldade respiratória contínua após a cirurgia corretiva. • Ressecção excessiva do palato, resultando em aspiração nasal de conteúdo alimentar por incapacidade de fechamento da nasofaringe durante a deglutição.

EVOLUÇÃO ESPERADA E PROGNÓSTICO
• O prognóstico é bom quanto ao restabelecimento da respiração (80% dos casos apresentam resultados bons a excelentes), mas as vias aéreas ainda estão longe do normal. • O prognóstico é melhor para as demais raças caninas, exceto o Buldogue inglês, e para os cães submetidos à correção concomitante de estenose das narinas e alongamento do palato mole. • Sem a cirurgia, o prognóstico é mau em virtude da evolução contínua dos componentes adquiridos da síndrome braquicefálica das vias aéreas. • É recomendável evitar os fatores de risco por toda a vida.

DIVERSOS

DISTÚRBIOS ASSOCIADOS
• Pneumonia por aspiração.
• Intermação/insolação.
• Hérnia hiatal.
• Traqueia hipoplásica.

FATORES RELACIONADOS COM A IDADE
• Os cães mais idosos podem exibir um desfecho pós-operatório mais grave, mas a maioria dos cães manifesta certa melhora.

GESTAÇÃO/FERTILIDADE/REPRODUÇÃO
O aumento de volume abdominal pode comprometer ainda mais a função respiratória da cadela prenhe, por reduzir o volume corrente devido à pressão exercida sobre o diafragma.

VER TAMBÉM
Estertor e Estridor.

RECURSOS DA INTERNET
http://www.acvs.org/AnimalOwners/HealthConditions/SmallAnimalTopics/BrachycephalicSyndrome/.

Sugestões de Leitura
Ginn JA, Kumar MSA, McKiernan BC, Powers BE. Nasopharyngeal turbinates in brachycephalic dogs and cats. JAAHA 2008, 44(5):243-249.
Monnet E. Brachycephalic airway syndrome. In: Slatter D, ed., Textbook of Small Animal Surgery, 3rd ed. Philadelphia: Saunders, 2003, pp. 808-813.
Poncet CM, Dupre GP, Freiche VG, Bouvy BM. Long-term results of upper respiratory syndrome surgery and gastrointestinal tract medical treatment in 51 brachycephalic dogs. J Small Anim Pract 2006, 47(3):137-142.
Poncet CM, Dupre GP, Freiche VG, Estrada M, Poubanne Y, Bouvy BM. Prevalence of gastrointestinal tract lesions in brachycephalic dogs with upper respiratory syndrome: Clinical study in 73 cases (2000-2003). J Small Anim Pract 2005, 46:273-279.
Riecks TW, Birchard SJ, Stephens JA. Surgical correction of brachycephalic syndrome in dogs: 62 cases (1991-2004). JAVMA 2007, 230(9):1324-1328.

Autores David A. Puerto e Lori S. Waddell
Consultor Editorial Lynelle R. Johnson

SÍNDROME COLANGITE E COLANGIO-HEPATITE

CONSIDERAÇÕES GERAIS

DEFINIÇÃO
• Colangite — inflamação da árvore biliar.
• Colangio-hepatite — inflamação das estruturas biliares e do parênquima hepático circunjacente.
• Síndrome colangite/colangio-hepatite (SCCH) — do ponto de vista histológico, é classificada como supurativa ou não supurativa (linfoplasmocitária, linfocítica), granulomatosa ou linfoproliferativa (transição para linfoma).

FISIOPATOLOGIA
• Distúrbios prévios ou coexistentes — inflamação ou obstrução da árvore biliar extra-hepática, pancreatite, enteropatia inflamatória, nefrite intersticial crônica (gatos). • Colangite bacteriana — a colestase é permissiva à infecção. • Inflamação aguda ou crônica — desencadeia hiperplasia epitelial biliar. • Inflamação crônica — pode resultar em estruturas biliares (distróficas) mineralizadas. • Forma supurativa — costuma produzir culturas bacterianas positivas ou exibir bactérias ao exame citológico em decalques teciduais ou na bile. • Forma não supurativa — imunomediada. • Colangite esclerosante — inflamação indutora de involução/destruição dos ductos biliares, presumivelmente imunomediada — induz à ductopenia de canais biliares de tamanho pequeno e médio. • Forma piogranulomatosa — secundária a mecanismos infecciosos ou imunes (cães). • Forma linfoproliferativa — especula-se que seja um estágio de transição de inflamação para neoplasia.

SISTEMA(S) ACOMETIDO(S)
• Hepatobiliar — fígado e sistema biliar.
• Gastrintestinal — pâncreas e intestino.

INCIDÊNCIA/PREVALÊNCIA
Forma não supurativa — hepatopatia crônica mais comum do gato.

IDENTIFICAÇÃO
Espécies
Gatos (comum) e cães (raro).

Raça(s) Predominante(s)
Possivelmente, gatos pertencentes às raças Himalaio, Persa e Siamês.

Idade Média e Faixa Etária
• Forma supurativa — faixa etária, 0,4-16 anos; principalmente em gatos jovens aos de meia-idade.
• Forma não supurativa — faixa etária, 2-17 anos; especialmente gatos de meia-idade.

Sexo Predominante
• Forma supurativa — os machos felinos são predispostos. • Forma não supurativa — nenhum.

SINAIS CLÍNICOS
Comentários Gerais
• Forma supurativa — doença grave de início agudo frequentemente em menos de 5 dias; associada a OEHDB. • Forma não supurativa — duração maior que 3 semanas (meses a anos).

Achados Anamnésicos
• Forma supurativa — doença aguda; febre; anorexia; vômito; colapso. • Forma não supurativa — doença cíclica; sinais crônicos vagos, incluindo letargia, vômito, anorexia e perda de peso; ductopenia (gatos) — polifágicos em virtude do fluxo biliar reduzido que compromete a assimilação de nutrientes, gerando fezes acólicas e esteatorreia por privação da captação de substâncias lipossolúveis (p. ex., vitamina K_1, ácidos graxos essenciais, vitamina E).

Achados do Exame Físico
• Forma supurativa — febre, dor abdominal; presença de icterícia ou não; desidratação; choque.
• Forma não supurativa — hepatomegalia; espessamento das alças intestinais em casos de enteropatia inflamatória; icterícia variável; efusão abdominal rara. • Ductopenia (gatos) — pelagem de aparência descuidada; alopecia toracoabdominal lateral variável; fezes acólicas variáveis.

CAUSAS
Forma Supurativa
• Infecção bacteriana — mais comum em gatos: *E. coli*, *Enterobacter*, *Enterococcus*, *Streptococcus* β-hemolíticos, *Klebsiella*, *Actinomyces*, *Clostridia* e *Bacteroides*; raramente, também pode estar associada à toxoplasmose; em cães: microrganismos oportunistas entéricos; casos raros com *Campylobacter*, *Salmonella* e *Leptospirose*, entre outros.
• Pode representar uma sequela de OEHDB ou outras causas de colestase mecânica.

Forma Não Supurativa
• Distúrbios concomitantes — colecistite; colelitíase; pancreatite; OEHDB; enteropatia inflamatória; nefrite intersticial crônica em gatos também.

FATORES DE RISCO
• Forma supurativa — OEHDB; colestase; infecções em outros locais.
• Não supurativa — em gatos: enteropatia inflamatória; pancreatite; OEHDB, nefrite intersticial crônica.

DIAGNÓSTICO

DIAGNÓSTICO DIFERENCIAL
• Lipidose hepática felina — pode ser um quadro coexistente; anormalidades enzimáticas semelhantes e icterícia, mas atividade mínima da GGT a menos que haja inflamação biliar ou pancreatite concomitante.
• OEHDB — icterícia acentuada, bem como atividades enzimáticas elevadas da fosfatase alcalina, GGT e transaminases; níveis altos do colesterol; evidência ultrassonográfica dessa obstrução.
• Pancreatite — pode desencadear a SCCH em gatos; lipemia; níveis elevados de colesterol e bilirrubina; IST, lipase e amilase inconsistentemente altas; características ultrassonográficas compatíveis; atividade da lipase pancreática espécie-específica implica inflamação pancreática (mas pode refletir enteropatia inflamatória).
• Forma linfoproliferativa e linfoma — pode envolver os intestinos com espessamento das alças intestinais ou o estômago; infiltrados periportais e características clínicas semelhantes à SCCH; podem exibir blastos circulantes em alguns casos; do ponto de vista histológico, as lesões hepáticas podem ser caracterizadas por meio de coloração imuno-histoquímica.
• Icterícia associada à septicemia — hiperbilirrubinemia frequentemente desproporcional ao grau de elevação das enzimas hepáticas.
• Doença policística (gatos das raças Himalaio e Persa) — níveis normais ou aumentos modestos das enzimas hepáticas; fibrose peribiliar grave e progressiva; pode ocorrer inflamação multifocal, mas secundariamente não supurativa.

HEMOGRAMA/BIOQUÍMICA/URINÁLISE
Hemograma Completo
• A constatação de pecilócitos é comum em gatos com hepatopatia grave; anemia arregenerativa em casos de doença crônica; hemólise por corpúsculo de Heinz em gatos gravemente enfermos.
• Forma supurativa — leucocitose neutrofílica com desvio à esquerda, neutrófilos tóxicos.
• Forma não supurativa — os achados do hemograma podem permanecer normais; distúrbios linfoproliferativos ou linfoma podem apresentar contagem elevada de linfócitos circulantes com ou sem morfologia celular anormal.

Bioquímica Sérica
• Achados compatíveis — níveis altos das enzimas fosfatase alcalina, GGT, AST, ALT; níveis ainda mais altos na SCCH não supurativa.
• Achados variáveis — teores elevados de ácidos biliares, bilirrubina e colesterol, dependendo da gravidade do quadro, do grau de colestase, das doenças coexistentes e da disfunção hepática.

OUTROS TESTES LABORATORIAIS
• IST e ILPf — podem estar altas em casos de pancreatite e enterite.
• Vitamina B12 — em gatos: os valores baixos indicam má absorção grave no intestino delgado (distúrbios infiltrativos: enteropatia inflamatória, linfoma; disfunção pancreática), antibióticos orais crônicos.
• Testes de coagulação — TP, TTPA, TCA, PIAVK (índice mais sensível em casos de coagulopatia induzida pela vitamina K_1) normais ou elevados.
• Culturas bacterianas aeróbias e anaeróbias — amostras hepáticas e biliares.

DIAGNÓSTICO POR IMAGEM
• Radiografias torácicas — linfadenopatia esternal sugere inflamação abdominal, enquanto linfadenopatia generalizada, linfoma.
• Radiografias abdominais — hepatomegalia em caso de SCCH não supurativa; pode não ser constatada nenhuma anormalidade; raramente, observam-se colélitos mineralizados ou estruturas biliares.
• Ultrassonografia abdominal — hepatomegalia; alterações ecogênicas nas estruturas biliares; colelitíase; sedimentação/depósito biliar; espessamento na parede da vesícula biliar (colecistite, edema, infiltração); lesões parenquimatosas focais (abscesso, inflamação, neoplasia); linfadenopatia (peripancreática, hepática peri-hilar, ou mesentérica) indicativa de inflamação pancreática, hepática ou intestinal ou neoplasia; hiperecogenicidade do parênquima hepático (lipidose hepática felina, inflamação, fibrose concomitantes); cistos (doença policística, cistadenoma). *Nota*: ausência de lesões ultrassonográficas em alguns gatos com SCCH ou doença policística (micropolicística) grave.

OUTROS MÉTODOS DIAGNÓSTICOS
Citologia de Aspirado por Agulha Fina
• Aspirado hepático — amostra para cultura na suspeita de SCCH supurativa ou para implicar o quadro de lipidose hepática felina; a citologia revela bactérias não observadas geralmente ao

Síndrome Colangite e Colangio-Hepatite

exame histopatológico. *Nota*: o exame citológico inclui a lipidose hepática felina, mas não é confiável para o diagnóstico da forma não supurativa; é comum a vacuolização hepatocelular em gatos doentes antes do desenvolvimento pleno da lipidose hepática.
• Colecistocentese — pode revelar supuração, bactérias, ovos de trematódeos ou neoplasias. A bile normal é desprovida de células e tem um aspecto amorfo azul com o corante de Wright-Giemsa.

Biopsia Percutânea
• Biopsia aspirativa guiada por ultrassom — pode erroneamente diagnosticar a SCCH em função da pequena quantidade de amostra; exige no mínimo 15 tríades portais para a obtenção do diagnóstico preciso; utilizar uma agulha de calibre 18 e coletar pelo menos 4 amostras.
• A imprecisão com os métodos de biopsia aspirativa e biopsia de apenas um único lobo hepático reflete o envolvimento diferencial de lobo hepático e o tamanho da amostra.
• Em gatos, podem ocorrer complicações subsequentes à biopsia (colapso vasovagal em virtude de traumatismo biliar) e amostragens não intencionais de tecidos não hepáticos, mesmo em exames guiados por ultrassom.

Laparoscopia
• Permite a inspeção direta da vesícula biliar, da porta hepática, do pâncreas, bem como dos linfonodos peri-hepáticos e peripancreáticos; além disso, possibilita a biopsia de múltiplos lobos hepáticos, pâncreas e colecistocentese.
• Na OEHDB — evitar a laparoscopia.

Laparotomia
• Suspeita de OEHDB — método recomendado.
• Permite a inspeção de estruturas biliares; a descompressão biliar; a anastomose entérica biliar; bem como a biopsia do fígado, das estruturas biliares, linfonodos, pâncreas, dos intestinos e dos linfonodos, além da colecistocentese.

AMOSTRAGEM DE TECIDO
• Na suspeita de SCCH não supurativa, realizar também biopsia do intestino e pâncreas.

GENÉTICA MOLECULAR
• O teste genético para doença policística felina pode ser adequado.

ACHADOS PATOLÓGICOS
• Forma supurativa — tumefação hepática, com bordas rombas e manchas focais; pode-se observar uma vesícula biliar eritematosa, necrosada ou de parede espessada (colecistite); esteatonecrose peripancreática e saponificação gordurosa (pancreatite); linfadenopatia peri-hepática e peripancreática; confirmação da OEHDB.
• Forma não supurativa — fígado normal a aumentado de volume e firme (pequeno em casos de doença crônica avançada); bordas rombas; irregularidade variável da superfície.
• Coloração amarela ou pálida e textura friável em casos de lipidose hepática felina concomitante.

TRATAMENTO

CUIDADO(S) DE SAÚDE ADEQUADO(S)
Internação
• Forma supurativa com doença febril aguda, dor abdominal, leucograma com desvio à esquerda — requer o suporte de hidratação, o uso de antibióticos bactericidas (inicialmente com base na citologia aspirativa e na coloração de Gram); avaliar a presença de OEHDB ou colecistite, *antes* de cirurgia: manter a antibioticoterapia por >4-8 semanas; fornecer terapia com coleréticos (ácido ursodesoxicólico, SAMe) até a normalização das enzimas hepáticas.
• Gatos sintomáticos com a forma não supurativa — fluidoterapia conforme a necessidade; avaliações diagnósticas; biopsia hepática (24 h *antes* da biopsia, administrar a vitamina K1 a 0,5-1,5 mg/kg IM a cada 12 h por 3 doses).
• Ambas as formas da SCCH (gatos) — podem necessitar de transfusões sanguíneas, associadas à cirurgia ou à biopsia.
• Fluidos poli-iônicos — suplementar com vitaminas solúveis do complexo B (2 mL/L), cloreto de potássio e fosfato de potássio, conforme a necessidade; evitar a suplementação de glicose (ver "Lipidose Hepática").

Tratamento Ambulatorial
• Forma supurativa — após o tratamento de uma crise aguda.
• Forma não supurativa — após a resolução de uma crise aguda, fornecer terapias imunomoduladoras, antioxidantes e hepatoprotetoras pelo resto da vida.

ATIVIDADE
Restrita, enquanto o animal permanecer sintomático.

DIETA
Suporte nutricional — para evitar a lipidose hepática felina, fornecer uma ração balanceada para gatos rica em proteínas e calorias, suplementada com vitaminas hidrossolúveis; dieta hipoalergênica (restrita em antígenos) em casos de enteropatia inflamatória concomitante; dietas com restrição de gorduras em casos de ductopenia grave, má absorção lipídica ou pancreatite crônica indutoras de má digestão; pode haver a necessidade da colocação de sondas de alimentação (inseridas preferencialmente via esofagostomia, mas por via jejunal em casos de pancreatite sintomática); raramente requer nutrição parenteral.

ORIENTAÇÃO AO PROPRIETÁRIO
Enfatizar a natureza crônica da forma não supurativa e a necessidade de terapia vitalícia.

CONSIDERAÇÕES CIRÚRGICAS
• Colecistectomia — em casos de colecistite.
• Colecistenterostomia — pode ser necessária em pacientes com OEHDB.
• Remoção de colélito(s).

MEDICAÇÕES

MEDICAMENTO(S)
Antibióticos contra a Forma Supurativa
• Bactericidas — direcionados contra os microrganismos oportunistas entéricos; Clavamox® (62,5 mg/gato VO a cada 12 h) ou enrofloxacino (2,5 mg/kg/a cada 12 h), associados ao metronidazol (7,5 mg/kg VO a cada 12 h) inicialmente.
• Enterococos resistentes — vancomicina (10 mg/kg a cada 12 h sob infusão IV lenta durante 7-10 dias).
• Modificar a seleção inicial ou empírica de antibióticos, com base nos resultados da cultura e do antibiograma.

Imunomodulação para a Forma Não Supurativa
• Glicocorticoides — prednisolona (cães: 2 mg/kg/dia; gatos: 4 mg/kg/dia) durante 14-21 dias; reduzir a dose de forma lenta e gradual até uma dosagem eficaz mais baixa e fornecer em dias alternados; a terapia crônica costuma ser necessária.
• Metronidazol — combinado à prednisolona, visa à imunomodulação mediada por células (ver dosagem exposta acima), especialmente em casos de enteropatia inflamatória.
• Gatos com ductopenia confirmada — necessitam de terapia mais rigorosa; resposta insatisfatória à azatioprina e toxicidade por esse agente terapêutico; a experiência clínica sugere a combinação de prednisolona, metronidazol com metotrexato em pulsos (0,4 mg como *dose total*, dividida em três no primeiro dia [ou seja, 0,13 mg totais, administrados à 0 h, às 12 h e 24 h] e repetida em intervalos semanais); pode-se fornecer tal combinação pelas vias oral, IV, IM (as vias parenterais exigem redução da dose pela metade); o folato (ácido folínico) a 0,25 mg/kg/dia deve ser administrado concomitantemente. No lugar do metotrexato pode-se usar a clorambucila na dose de ataque de 1-2 mg/gato, a cada 24 h por 3 dias e, depois, a cada 3 dias.
• Em caso de infiltrados linfoproliferativos ou neoplásicos, utilizar protocolos quimioterápicos desenvolvidos para linfoma entérico.

Antioxidantes
• Vitamina E (acetato de α-tocoferol, 10-30 UI/kg VO) — em função da má absorção lipídica, administrar altas doses em casos de OEHDB ou ductopenia crônica (ver Obstrução do Ducto Biliar para a forma hidrossolúvel da vitamina E).
• SAMe (Denosyl SD4® tem biodisponibilidade comprovada); 20 mg/kg de comprimido revestido entérico VO a cada 24 h, duas horas antes da refeição; muitos efeitos benéficos, inclusive anti-inflamatórios, atingiram remissão em gatos com a forma não supurativa da SCCH sem destruição do ducto.

Outros
• Ácido ursodesoxicólico — efeitos imunomoduladores, hepatoprotetores, coleréticos, antifibróticos e antioxidantes; 10-15 mg/kg/dia VO divididos com o alimento para obtenção da melhor biodisponibilidade; preferem-se os comprimidos às cápsulas (biodisponibilidade); pode-se formular uma suspensão aquosa (refrigerar).
• Suplementação vitamínica com tiamina (B1) [50-100 mg VO a cada 24 h por no mínimo 3 dias, seguida pela suplementação de vitaminas hidrossolúveis] e cianocobalamina (B12) [0,25-1,0 mg SC]; na suspeita de má absorção intestinal, utilizar as concentrações plasmáticas iniciais e sequenciais da vitamina B12 para justificar o tratamento e titular a frequência da dose (p. ex., alguns gatos necessitam de injeções semanais e, depois, mensais).

CONTRAINDICAÇÕES
Ajustar as doses dos medicamentos, com base na função hepática e na colestase.

SÍNDROME COLANGITE E COLANGIO-HEPATITE

ACOMPANHAMENTO

MONITORIZAÇÃO DO PACIENTE
Forma não supurativa — inicialmente, monitorizar os níveis das enzimas hepáticas e da bilirrubina em intervalos de 7-14 dias; em casos de remissão, realizar avaliações trimestrais; as mensurações séricas de ácidos biliares são complicadas pelo ácido ursodesoxicólico (detectado por meio de análises).

PREVENÇÃO
Controlar a enteropatia inflamatória.

COMPLICAÇÕES POSSÍVEIS
- A forma supurativa pode evoluir para a forma não supurativa e SCCH esclerosante.
- Diabetes melito em 30% dos gatos com SCCH esclerosante, quando tratados com prednisolona.
- Lipidose hepática felina em casos de ingestão nutricional inadequada e, em alguns gatos, induzida pela glicocorticoterapia.

EVOLUÇÃO ESPERADA E PROGNÓSTICO
- Forma supurativa — pode ser curada.
- Forma não supurativa — é possível a remissão crônica em longo prazo (registros >8 anos).

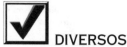

DIVERSOS

DISTÚRBIOS ASSOCIADOS
- Pancreatite.
- Lipidose hepática.
- Hepatopatia policística.
- Linfoma.
- Doença linfoproliferativa.
- Colangiocarcinoma — pode se desenvolver em alguns gatos com a forma não supurativa crônica.

VER TAMBÉM
- Colecistite e Coledoquite.
- Colelitíase.
- Enteropatia Inflamatória.
- Lipidose Hepática.
- Obstrução do Ducto Biliar.
- Pancreatite.

ABREVIATURA(S)
- ALT = alanina aminotransferase.
- AST = aspartato aminotransferase.
- GGT = γ-glutamiltransferase
- ILPf = imunorreatividade da lipase pancreática felina.
- IST = imunorreatividade semelhante à da tripsina.
- OEHDB = obstrução extra-hepática do ducto biliar.
- PIAVK = proteínas invocadas pela ausência ou antagonismo da vitamina K.
- SAMe = S-adenosil-l-metionina.
- SCCH = síndrome colangite/colangio-hepatite.
- TCA = tempo de coagulação ativada.
- TP = tempo de protrombina.
- TTPA = tempo de tromboplastina parcial ativada.

Sugestões de Leitura
Center SA. Diseases of the gallbladder and biliary tree. Vet Clin North Am Small Anim Pract 2009, 39(3):543-598.

Autor Sharon A. Center
Consultor Editorial Sharon A. Center

Síndrome da Angústia Respiratória Aguda (SARA)

CONSIDERAÇÕES GERAIS

DEFINIÇÃO
Síndrome de início agudo de insuficiência respiratória (SARA), caracterizada por infiltrados pulmonares bilaterais difusos em radiografia torácica dorsoventral, sem indício de aumento na pressão hidrostática, edema pulmonar cardiogênico ou sobrecarga por líquido. A SARA se deve a uma reação inflamatória avassaladora difusa da membrana alveolocapilar em resposta a algum insulto inflamatório pulmonar ou sistêmico. Essa síndrome pode ser dividida em duas categorias com base na gravidade. A forma menos grave recebe o nome de lesão pulmonar aguda; esse tipo de lesão é definido como uma relação entre PaO_2/FIO_2 <300; já a SARA é definida como uma relação entre PaO_2/FIO_2 <200.

FISIOPATOLOGIA
- A SARA se deve a algum insulto inflamatório difuso que provoca dano disseminado às células epiteliais alveolares e endoteliais, resultando em comprometimento na troca gasosa. Esse insulto inflamatório pode ser deflagrado por doença pulmonar primária ou ser de origem extrapulmonar. Os mecanismos de lesão incluem dano celular deflagrado por ativação neutrofílica, disfunção endotelial e mediadores pró-inflamatórios. Acredita-se que o dano seja exacerbado por lesão pulmonar induzida por ventilador, associada à hiperdistensão e abertura cíclica dos alvéolos e ao colapso de alvéolos atelectásicos.
- Fase exsudativa precoce — as primeiras 12-24 h são tipificadas por aumento na permeabilidade da membrana alveolocapilar; ocorrem a formação de líquido edematoso rico em proteínas e a infiltração de leucócitos no interstício e nos alvéolos. Os neutrófilos exacerbam o dano pela liberação adicional de citocinas e mediadores inflamatórios.
- As células epiteliais alveolares do tipo I morrem. A inundação dos alvéolos e a disfunção do surfactante levam ao colapso e à consolidação alveolares com o desenvolvimento de hipoxemia grave.
- Microtrombos na vasculatura pulmonar, vasoconstrição pulmonar hipóxica e liberação de vasoconstritores endógenos induzem à hipertensão arterial pulmonar, o que pode levar à insuficiência cardíaca direita.
- Fase membranosa hialina — a formação de membrana hialina nos espaços alveolares ocorre 3-7 dias após o insulto inicial.
- Fase fibroproliferativa — se o paciente sobreviver aos 3-7 dias iniciais, ocorrerão a proliferação de células epiteliais alveolares do tipo 2 e o processo de fibrose pulmonar.
- Em seres humanos e cães, foi relatada uma forma idiopática de SARA associada à pneumonia intersticial aguda ou fibrose pulmonar idiopática.

SISTEMA(S) ACOMETIDO(S)
- Respiratório.
- Cardiovascular — insuficiência cardíaca direita secundária à hipertensão pulmonar; o comprometimento hemodinâmico pode estar associado à ventilação mecânica rigorosa.

GENÉTICA
Foi descoberto que alguns seres humanos são mais propensos ao desenvolvimento de SARA em comparação a outros em virtude de polimorfismos genéticos específicos. Isso, no entanto, não foi investigado na população veterinária.

INCIDÊNCIA/PREVALÊNCIA
Desconhecidas.

IDENTIFICAÇÃO
Espécies
Cães e gatos.

Raça(s) Predominante(s)
Em um grupo de cães aparentados da raça Dálmata, foi relatada uma forma familiar de SARA; essa forma é clinicamente indistinguível da SARA.

Idade Média e Faixa Etária
Desconhecidas.

Sexo Predominante
Desconhecido.

SINAIS CLÍNICOS
Achados Anamnésicos
- Início agudo de angústia respiratória em pacientes com doença subjacente significativa.
- Ao desenvolver a SARA, o animal é frequentemente hospitalizado por conta da doença primária.

Achados do Exame Físico
- Angústia respiratória grave.
- Crepitações (se presentes) audíveis bilateralmente à auscultação.
- Febre — depende da doença subjacente.
- Cianose em casos mais graves.
- Sinais pertinentes ao processo patológico primário.

CAUSAS
Causas Pulmonares Primárias
- Pneumonia por aspiração.
- Pneumonia.
- Contusão pulmonar.
- Afogamento por um triz.
- Inalação de fumaça.

Causas Extrapulmonares
- Resposta inflamatória sistêmica grave.
- Sepse.
- Neoplasia.
- Pancreatite.
- Traumatismo e choque graves.
- Envenenamento grave por picada de abelha.

FATORES DE RISCO
- Síndrome da resposta inflamatória sistêmica.
- Sepse.
- Gravidade da doença.
- Transfusões múltiplas.
- Distúrbios patológicos coexistentes.

DIAGNÓSTICO

DIAGNÓSTICO DIFERENCIAL
- Insuficiência cardíaca congestiva esquerda.
- Sobrecarga por líquido.
- Pneumonia difusa.
- Hemorragia pulmonar.

HEMOGRAMA/BIOQUÍMICA/URINÁLISE
- Leucocitose ou leucopenia.
- Outras alterações dependem do processo patológico subjacente.

OUTROS TESTES LABORATORIAIS
- Gasometria arterial — relação baixa entre PaO_2/FIO_2 (na qual a PaO_2 é mensurada em mmHg, enquanto a FIO_2 corresponde a 0,21-1,0). Relação normal entre PaO_2/FIO_2 = 500; a comparação com essa relação permite a avaliação da gravidade da doença pulmonar e possibilita a comparação direta de gases sanguíneos obtidos em uma FIO_2 diferente. A $PaCO_2$ é frequentemente baixa; a hipercapnia tende a ser um desenvolvimento tardio (pré-terminal).
- Comparação entre o nível das proteínas totais do líquido edematoso das vias aéreas e o das proteínas totais do soro — uma relação <0,5 é indicativa de baixo teor proteico e edema pulmonar causado por pressão hidrostática elevada (p. ex., insuficiência cardíaca), enquanto uma relação >0,7 é sugestiva de alto teor proteico e edema pulmonar gerado por aumento na permeabilidade (p. ex., SARA e pneumonia).

DIAGNÓSTICO POR IMAGEM
Radiografia Torácica
- Infiltrados pulmonares bilaterais.
- A doença clínica pode anteceder a gravidade dos sinais radiográficos em até 12-24 h.
- Pode não ser uma tarefa fácil a distinção com o edema cardiogênico. A silhueta cardíaca costuma permanecer normal na SARA.

Ecocardiografia
- Tentativa de descartar uma causa cardiogênica para o edema pulmonar.
- Pode ser capaz de estimar o grau de hipertensão pulmonar.

MÉTODOS DIAGNÓSTICOS
Cateterização arterial pulmonar para mensurar a pressão de oclusão da artéria pulmonar (POAP) com o objetivo de excluir uma causa cardiogênica para o edema; por definição, a lesão pulmonar aguda e a SARA são associadas à POAP ≤18 mmHg.

ACHADOS PATOLÓGICOS
Macroscopia
Os pulmões estão escurecidos e pesados, mas exsudam líquido quando seccionados.

Histopatologia
- Fase aguda — congestão vascular pulmonar com líquido edematoso e acúmulo de células inflamatórias no interstício e nos alvéolos; dano ao epitélio, formação de membrana hialina, microtrombos, microatelectasia.
- Fase proliferativa — hiperplasia dos pneumócitos do tipo 2, infiltração mononuclear intersticial, organização de membranas hialinas e fibroproliferação.

TRATAMENTO

CUIDADO(S) DE SAÚDE ADEQUADO(S)
- Não há terapia específica. Os objetivos gerais consistem em manter a oxigenação tecidual e minimizar a lesão pulmonar iatrogênica, ao mesmo tempo em que se trata a doença subjacente.
- Oxigenoterapia — fornecer não mais do que o necessário para manter a PaO_2 >60-80 mmHg,

Síndrome da Angústia Respiratória Aguda (SARA)

visando a minimização da toxicidade pelo oxigênio.
• A ventilação com pressão positiva é essencial no tratamento de pacientes com SARA. Esse tipo de ventilação é indicado em pacientes que se apresentam hipoxêmicos apesar da oxigenoterapia, naqueles que necessitam de níveis elevados de oxigênio inspirado por períodos prolongados ou em outros com esforço respiratório sob risco de exaustão. É recomendável o uso de estratégias de proteção pulmonar que envolvem ventilação com pressão positiva e PEFP moderada a elevada, volumes correntes baixos e hipercapnia permissiva na tentativa de minimizar a lesão pulmonar induzida pelo ventilador. Foi descoberto que volumes correntes de 6 mL/kg aumentam significativamente a sobrevida em pacientes humanos acometidos pela SARA, quando comparados aos volumes correntes de 12 mL/kg.
• As manobras ventilatórias para o recrutamento de alvéolos colapsados e os altos níveis da PEFP podem gerar um comprometimento hemodinâmico significativo e, nesse caso, os pacientes devem ser submetidos à monitorização direta constante da pressão sanguínea arterial.
• O cuidado intensivo de suporte do sistema cardiovascular e de outros sistemas orgânicos é vital, já que esses pacientes estão sob alto risco de sofrerem da síndrome de falência múltipla de órgãos.

CUIDADO(S) DE ENFERMAGEM
• Monitorização rigorosa da temperatura, especialmente no uso da gaiola de oxigênio, uma vez que os animais dispneicos podem ficar hipertérmicos com facilidade.
• Os pacientes submetidos à ventilação exigem mudanças frequentes de posição e fisioterapia; o cuidado bucodentário regular com solução diluída de clorexidina é muito importante para reduzir a colonização bucal como fonte de sepse, ao passo que a sucção frequente da sonda endotraqueal é necessária para evitar a oclusão. Para evitar o dano à traqueia, a insuflação cautelosa do manguito e a mudança de posição do manguito endotraqueal com regularidade são medidas recomendáveis.
• Monitorização da pressão sanguínea, em decorrência da propensão dos pacientes sépticos à hipotensão.
• A fluidoterapia é relevante para manter o sistema cardiovascular e a normovolemia, ao mesmo tempo em que se evita a sobrecarga por líquido.

ATIVIDADE
Se o animal não for anestesiado para ventilação, deve-se buscar o confinamento estrito em gaiola.

DIETA
O suporte nutricional é importante, mas desafiador. A alimentação entérica é desejável, em comparação à nutrição parenteral; no entanto, é preciso considerar o alto risco de regurgitação e aspiração no paciente em decúbito.

ORIENTAÇÃO AO PROPRIETÁRIO
Os proprietários precisam ser informados a respeito do prognóstico reservado e dos altos custos da terapia.

CONSIDERAÇÕES CIRÚRGICAS
A doença subjacente pode necessitar de cirurgia.

MEDICAÇÕES
MEDICAMENTO(S) DE ESCOLHA
• Não há terapia medicamentosa específica.
• Antibióticos para a doença subjacente, se necessários.
• Agentes vasoativos para manter a pressão sanguínea.
• Medicamentos anestésicos para produzir a ventilação com pressão positiva.
• Analgesia, quando conveniente.
• Corticosteroides em baixas doses — o uso permanece controverso com relatos conflitantes de eficácia para doses baixas de esteroides no início ou final da SARA.

MEDICAMENTO(S) ALTERNATIVO(S)
A furosemida pode produzir dilatação venosa pulmonar e restabelecer a função pulmonar, sendo administrada sob a forma de bólus intermitente de 1 mg/kg IV a cada 6-12 h ou sob infusão em velocidade constante a 0,2 mg/kg/h IV.

ACOMPANHAMENTO
MONITORIZAÇÃO DO PACIENTE
Gasometria arterial, oximetria de pulso, dióxido de carbono corrente final, radiografias torácicas, pressão sanguínea arterial, ECG, temperatura, débito urinário, hemograma completo, perfis de coagulação, bioquímica sérica, hemoculturas, monitorização em busca de outra disfunção orgânica.

PREVENÇÃO
• Terapia rigorosa dos processos mórbidos primários para diminuir o insulto inflamatório ao pulmão.
• Monitorização cardiovascular intensiva e suporte de animais criticamente doentes para assegurar a perfusão tecidual adequada.
• Manejo cuidadoso dos animais em decúbito para reduzir a possibilidade de aspiração, sobretudo se o paciente apresentar doença neurológica ou distúrbio das vias aéreas superiores, que diminuem a capacidade de proteção da via aérea.

COMPLICAÇÕES POSSÍVEIS
• Síndrome da falência múltipla de órgãos — insuficiência renal aguda, CID e doença gastrintestinal são as disfunções orgânicas mais comumente observadas.
• Barotrauma — pode resultar em pneumotórax. Acredita-se que a incidência seja menor com estratégias ventilatórias baseadas em um volume corrente mais baixo.
• Pneumonia associada ao ventilador — os pacientes sob ventilação com pressão positiva apresentam um risco elevado de pneumonia; nesse caso, pode ser difícil diferenciar de agravamento da lesão pulmonar inicial. Em pacientes debilitados, deve-se considerar a realização de culturas das vias aéreas.
• A intoxicação pelo oxigênio pode ser inevitável em virtude da gravidade da hipoxemia apesar da ventilação com pressão positiva. A toxicidade por esse gás é indistinguível da SARA ao exame histopatológico, tornando impossível a determinação da incidência desse problema.

EVOLUÇÃO ESPERADA E PROGNÓSTICO
• A mortalidade em pacientes humanos permanece em 40-70%.
• A mortalidade em pacientes veterinários provavelmente chega a 100%.

DIVERSOS
DISTÚRBIOS ASSOCIADOS
Síndrome da resposta inflamatória sistêmica, síndrome da falência múltipla de órgãos, sepse.

SINÔNIMO(S)
• Choque pulmonar.
• Edema pulmonar por alto nível proteico.
• Insuficiência respiratória hipoxêmica aguda.
• Pneumonia intersticial aguda.
• Síndrome da angústia respiratória do adulto.

VER TAMBÉM
• Dispneia e Angústia Respiratória.
• Edema Pulmonar Não Cardiogênico.
• Respiração Ofegante e Taquipneia.
• Sepse e Bacteremia.

ABREVIATURA(S)
• CID = coagulação intravascular disseminada.
• PEFP = pressão expiratória final positiva.
• POAP = pressão de oclusão da artéria pulmonar (conhecida antigamente como capilar pulmonar em cunha [PCPC]).
• SARA = síndrome da angústia respiratória aguda.

RECURSOS DA INTERNET
http://www.ardsnet.org.

Sugestões de Leitura
Marino PL. Acute respiratory distress syndrome. In: The ICU Book, 2nd ed. Baltimore: Williams & Wilkins, 1998, pp. 371-387.
Parent C, King LG, Van Winkle TJ, Walker LM. Respiratory function and treatment in dogs with acute respiratory distress syndrome: 19 cases (1985-1993). JAVMA 1996, 208:1428-1433.
Syrja P, Saari S, Rajamaki M, Saario E, Jarvinen A-K. Pulmonary histopathology in Dalmatians with familial acute respiratory distress syndrome (ARDS). J Comp Pathol 2009, 141(4):254-259.
Ware LB, Bernard GR. Acute lung injury and acute respiratory distress syndrome. In: Textbook of Critical Care, 5th ed. Philadelphia: Elsevier Saunders, 2005, pp. 571-579.
Ware LB, Matthay MA. The acute respiratory distress syndrome. N Engl J Med 2000, 342:1334-1349.

Autor Kate Hopper
Consultor Editorial Lynelle R. Johnson

Síndrome da Fragilidade Cutânea Felina

CONSIDERAÇÕES GERAIS

REVISÃO
- Distúrbio de causas multifatoriais caracterizado por pele extremamente frágil.
- Tende a ocorrer em gatos idosos que possam ter hiperadrenocorticismo concomitante, diabetes melito ou uso excessivo de acetato de megestrol ou outros compostos progestacionais ou ocorre sob a forma de síndrome paraneoplásica.
- Um número pequeno de gatos não apresenta alterações bioquímicas.

SISTEMA(S) ACOMETIDO(S)
- Cutâneo/exócrino.
- Endócrino/metabólico.

IDENTIFICAÇÃO
- Doença de ocorrência natural que tende a ser identificada em gatos idosos.
- Casos iatrogênicos não apresentam predileção etária.
- Não há predileção racial ou sexual.

SINAIS CLÍNICOS
Achados Anamnésicos
- Início gradual de sinais clínicos.
- Alopecia progressiva (nem sempre presente).
- Frequentemente associada a sinais clínicos de perda de peso, pelagem opaca, hiporexia e falta de vigor (apatia).

Achados do Exame Físico
- A pele fica acentuadamente fina e lacera com a manipulação normal.
- A pele raramente sangra após lacerar.
- Podem ser observadas múltiplas lacerações (antigas e recentes) ao exame de perto.
- Também se pode notar alopecia parcial a completa da região do tronco.
- Associados, algumas vezes, à cauda de rato, às pregas da orelha, ao aspecto de barril.

CAUSAS E FATORES DE RISCO
- Hiperadrenocorticismo — dependente da hipófise ou da adrenal.
- Iatrogênica — secundária a uso excessivo de corticosteroide ou agente progestacional.
- Diabetes melito — raro a menos que associado a hiperadrenocorticismo.
- Possivelmente idiopática ou síndrome paraneoplásica.

DIAGNÓSTICO

DIAGNÓSTICO DIFERENCIAL
- Astenia cutânea.
- Síndrome paraneoplásica felina — neoplasia pancreática, lipidose hepática, colangiocarcinoma.

HEMOGRAMA/BIOQUÍMICA/URINÁLISE
- De pouco significado diagnóstico na maioria dos casos.
- Aproximadamente 80% dos gatos com hiperadrenocorticismo sofrem de diabetes melito concomitante (hiperglicemia, glicosúria).

OUTROS TESTES LABORATORIAIS
- Teste de estimulação com ACTH — 70% dos gatos com hiperadrenocorticismo apresentam resposta exagerada.
- TSDBD — em 15-20% dos gatos normais, os níveis de cortisol podem não baixar; tipicamente não suprimidos em casos de hiperadrenocorticismo e doença não adrenal.
- TSDAD — gatos normais revelam quedas nas concentrações de cortisol; tipicamente diminuído com doenças não adrenais; considerado por muitos clínicos como o melhor teste de triagem para hiperadrenocorticismo; não é confiável para diferenciar entre tumores adrenais e causas de hiperadrenocorticismo dependentes da hipófise, porque ambas as condições não mostram supressão.
- Níveis endógenos de ACTH — a variação normal na maioria dos laboratórios é de 20-100 pg/mL.

DIAGNÓSTICO POR IMAGEM
- Ultrassonografia abdominal — massas adrenais, em geral, são pequenas até o estágio terminal da doença.
- TC e RM — pode ser difícil visualizar pequenos tumores hipofisários; a RM pode ser mais bem-sucedida.

MÉTODOS DIAGNÓSTICOS
N/D.

ACHADOS PATOLÓGICOS
Exame histopatológico — sugestivo, mas não diagnóstico; a epiderme e a derme encontram-se delgadas; fibras de colágeno adelgaçadas são evidentes.

TRATAMENTO

- Deve-se excluir doença metabólica subjacente.
- Muitos pacientes estão debilitados e necessitam de cuidados de suporte.
- Correção cirúrgica das lacerações — é inútil, porque o tecido não é capaz de suportar a tensão das suturas.
- Proteger a pele com roupas próprias para gatos; diminuir as atividades que possam traumatizar a pele; remover bordas afiadas do ambiente; evitar danos pela interação com outros animais.
- Hiperadrenocorticismo — a adrenalectomia é o tratamento preferido.
- Radioterapia com cobalto-60 — sucesso variável no tratamento de tumores da hipófise.

MEDICAÇÕES

MEDICAMENTO(S)
- Tratamento clínico — pode ser útil no preparo do paciente para realizar a cirurgia e minimizar as complicações pós-operatórias (p. ex., infecções e má cicatrização de feridas).
- Não há tratamento clínico eficaz conhecido para o hiperadrenocorticismo felino.
- o,p'-DDD (mitotano) — 12,5-50 mg/kg VO a cada 12 h; resposta duvidosa; os efeitos colaterais incluem anorexia, vômitos e diarreia.
- Cetoconazol (Nizoral®) — 10-15 mg/kg VO a cada 12 h; resposta variável.
- Metirapona — 65 mg/kg VO a cada 12 h; observa-se uma melhora clínica mais frequentemente com esse medicamento do que com outros.

CONTRAINDICAÇÕES/INTERAÇÕES POSSÍVEIS
Hiperadrenocorticismo — monitorizar o gato diabético com rigor; ajustar a insulina para evitar hipoglicemia quando os níveis de cortisol caírem.

ACOMPANHAMENTO

Os pacientes encontram-se, em geral, bastante debilitados, tornando qualquer forma de tratamento arriscada; em todos os casos, é necessária monitorização estrita.

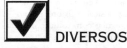

DIVERSOS

ABREVIATURA(S)
- ACTH = hormônio adrenocorticotrópico.
- o,p'-DDD = 1,1-(o,p'-diclorodifenil)-2,2-dicloroetano.
- TSDAD = teste de supressão com dexametasona em altas doses.
- TSDBD = teste de supressão com dexametasona em baixas doses.
- RM = ressonância magnética.
- TC = tomografia computadorizada.

Sugestões de Leitura
Gross TL, Ihrke PJ, Walder EJ. Veterinary Dermatopathology. Philadelphia: Mosby, 1992.
Helton Rhodes K. Cutaneous manifestations of hyperadrenocorticism. In: August JR, ed., Consultations in Feline Internal Medicine. Philadelphia: Saunders, 1997, pp. 191-198.

Autor Karen Helton Rhodes
Consultor Editorial Alexander H. Werner

SÍNDROME DE ANSIEDADE DA SEPARAÇÃO

CONSIDERAÇÕES GERAIS

DEFINIÇÃO
Os cães (e, ocasionalmente, os gatos) podem manifestar uma reação de angústia quando separados da pessoa ou das pessoas a quem estão mais ligados, geralmente seu(s) proprietário(s). A separação pode ser real (o dono, de fato, saiu) ou percebida (o animal de estimação está apenas longe do dono). A angústia resultante pode ser evidenciada por episódios de destruição, vocalização e evacuação/micção. A ansiedade da separação é um subconjunto de problemas relacionados com a separação que podem ter diferentes motivações subjacentes, incluindo medo, ansiedade, ligação exagerada com o(s) proprietário(s) e falta de interações ou estímulos adequados.

FISIOPATOLOGIA
Desconhecida.

SISTEMA(S) ACOMETIDO(S)
• Comportamental — tentativas de fuga, uivos, choro, depressão. • Cardiovascular — taquicardia. • Endócrino/metabólico — níveis aumentados de cortisol, hiperglicemia induzida pelo estresse. • Gastrintestinal — inapetência, desarranjo gastrintestinal. • Musculosquelético — traumatismo autoinduzido, resultante das tentativas de fuga. • Nervoso — estimulação adrenérgica/noradrenérgica excessiva. • Respiratório — taquipneia. • Cutâneo/exócrino — dermatite acral por lambedura.

GENÉTICA
Nada conhecido.

INCIDÊNCIA/PREVALÊNCIA
Especula-se que 7-28% dos cães de companhia sentem algum grau da síndrome de ansiedade da separação.

IDENTIFICAÇÃO
Espécies
Principalmente em cães; possível nos gatos.

Idade Média e Faixa Etária
Qualquer idade, mais comumente nos cães com >6 meses de vida; pode aumentar em termos de prevalência naqueles com >8 anos de idade.

SINAIS CLÍNICOS
Comentários Gerais
Fatores isolados como destruição, vocalização e evacuação/micção na ausência do proprietário não são diagnósticos para a ansiedade da separação.

Achados Anamnésicos
• Destruição, vocalização (choros, uivos, latidos) e evacuação/micção dentro de casa são mais comumente relatados. A destruição tem como alvo as janelas e as portas e/ou posses do proprietário. • Outros sinais incluem depressão comportamental, anorexia, salivação, busca por esconderijos, sacudidas, respiração ofegante, caminhadas, tentativas de evitar a saída do proprietário e autotraumatismo decorrente de lesões por lambedura. Ocasionalmente se notam diarreia e vômito. • Pode haver sinais de forte elo animal-proprietário: comportamentos excessivos por busca de atenção e comportamentos de seguir o dono. • Com frequência, os proprietários relatam comportamento excessivo, agitado e prolongado do animal durante a saudação ao retorno. • O(s) comportamento(s) de angústia da separação ocorre(m) independentemente do tempo de ausência do proprietário e tendem a aparecer dentro dos 30 min da partida do proprietário. • Deflagradores específicos podem desencadear a reação de ansiedade, como agitar chaves, vestir roupas para sair, fazer malas ou carregar o carro. • Podem ocorrer em cada saída e na ausência ou apenas com saídas atípicas ou passeios após o trabalho, à tarde ou nos finais de semana; o padrão inverso também pode ser observado. • Em gatos, os problemas de evacuação/micção na ausência do dono podem estar ligados à ansiedade relacionada com a separação.

Achados do Exame Físico
• Geralmente normais. • Lesões provocadas nas tentativas de fuga ou em atividades destrutivas. • Lesões cutâneas por lambedura excessiva. • Casos raros de desidratação por salivação ou diarreia atribuídas ao estresse.

CAUSAS
Causas específicas são desconhecidas. Especula-se que os fatores causais incluam:
• Socialização indevida à partida e ausência do proprietário. • Falta de interações adequadas entre o animal e seu dono. • Contato prolongado com seres humanos sem aprender a ficar sozinho. • Separação precoce inadequada ou incompleta da cadela (Escola Francesa de Comportamento). • Episódios traumáticos durante a ausência do proprietário. • Declínio cognitivo.

FATORES DE RISCO
• Os fatores de risco sob suspeita, mas não comprovados, incluem a adoção a partir de abrigos humanitários, períodos prolongados de tempo com a pessoa preferida, como durante férias ou doença, hospedagem em hotel, apego quando filhote. • Animais geriátricos parecem estar super-representados. • Possível correlação entre a ansiedade da separação e as fobias por ruídos, como aquelas por trovões e relâmpagos.

DIAGNÓSTICO

DIAGNÓSTICO DIFERENCIAL
• Vocalização — reação a influências externas, exibições territoriais ou medos. • Comportamentos destrutivos — ocorrem tanto na presença como na ausência do proprietário (p. ex., exibições territoriais destrutivas em janelas e portas; destruição atribuída a estímulos produtores de medo, como ruídos e tempestades). • Evacuação domiciliar: adestramento inadequado, doença, disfunção endócrina, declínio cognitivo. • Lambedura causada por problemas dermatológicos primários. • Problemas gerados por medo, que mimetizam comportamentos de ansiedade da separação. • Frustração por barreira — cães incapazes de ficar confinados em gaiolas de transporte ou atrás de obstáculos, mas que ficam bem se não estiverem presos. • Síndrome de disfunção cognitiva.

HEMOGRAMA/BIOQUÍMICA/URINÁLISE
As anormalidades, se presentes, sugerem diagnóstico alternativo ou doença clínica concomitante.

MÉTODOS DIAGNÓSTICOS
• Filmagem do animal de estimação quando ele estiver sozinho em casa para confirmar o diagnóstico. • Questionários voltados para o declínio cognitivo são aconselháveis para cães geriátricos. • Biopsias cutâneas diante da suspeita de problema dermatológico primário. • Punção do LCS para identificar processos infecciosos ou inflamatórios. • Endoscopia com biopsias se os sinais gastrintestinais forem persistentes.

TRATAMENTO

ATIVIDADE
A prática regular e diária de exercícios e brincadeiras programados é benéfica.

DIETA
Não há necessidade de qualquer mudança na dieta a menos que haja diarreia.

ORIENTAÇÃO AO PROPRIETÁRIO
Comentários Gerais
Estabelecer expectativas realistas sobre a duração do tratamento e a necessidade de modificação comportamental para obter uma resolução bem-sucedida do problema. Um comportamento problemático pode demorar semanas a meses para desaparecer, dependendo da gravidade e da duração do problema. Os componentes do tratamento incluem os seguintes pontos:

Adestramento de Independência
• Ensinar o cão a ser mais independente do(s) proprietário(s). • Toda a atenção está na recepção do proprietário — o proprietário começa e termina as sessões de atenção. • Nenhuma atenção para os pedidos do animal. • O animal de estimação precisa aprender a realizar uma tarefa, como "senta!". • Diminui o comportamento de seguir o proprietário enquanto este se encontra em casa. • Ensinar o cão a permanecer tranquilo em outro local fora de onde está o proprietário.

Alteração do Valor Preditivo das Pistas antes da Partida
• Apresentação dos indícios antes da partida (pegando as chaves, caminhando para a porta) sem deixar o local. Repetir as pistas 2-4 vezes por dia, até que o cão não responda aos indícios com comportamentos ansiosos (respiração ofegante, caminhadas a esmo, acompanhamento ou vigilância aumentada). • O objetivo é dissociar os indícios das partidas e diminuir a resposta ansiosa.

Contracondicionamento
• Ensinar o cão a sentar/ficar perto da porta típica de saída. • Aumentar gradualmente a distância entre o cão e o proprietário em direção à porta. • O proprietário caminha lentamente em direção à porta, aumentando o tempo fora em cada período de teste. • Eventualmente, os elementos da partida, como a abertura e o fechamento da porta, são adicionados. • Por fim, o proprietário fica do lado de fora da porta e retorna.

Contracondicionamento Clássico
• Deixar o cão com petisco alimentar palatável ou brinquedo recheado de alimento no momento da saída. • Associar a partida com algo agradável e prazeroso.

Alteração da Rotina de Partida e Retorno
• Ignorar o animal por 15-30 min antes da partida e após o retorno. • Depois de retornar, atender o

Síndrome de Ansiedade da Separação

animal apenas quando ele estiver calmo e silencioso; entretanto, pode permitir que o cão saia para evacuar ou urinar.

Partidas e Ausências Planejadas Gradativas
• Começar depois que o cão estiver habituado e respondendo a indícios anteriores à partida.
• Utilizar ausências curtas para ensinar o cão a ficar sozinho em casa. • As partidas devem ser suficientemente breves para não eliciar uma resposta de angústia da separação. • Objetivo — o animal aprende sobre a constância de retorno do proprietário e enfrenta a partida e a ausência sem ansiedade. • As saídas devem ser iguais às partidas verdadeiras (o proprietário deve efetuar todos os componentes da partida, incluindo sair com o carro, caso isso faça parte de sua rotina de partida). O proprietário deixará um indício seguro (rádio ou televisor ligados, toque de campainha) apenas nas partidas planejadas (isso não deve ser usado nas saídas em que o tempo de ausência não esteja controlado, como as saídas para o trabalho). • As saídas iniciais devem ser muito curtas, de 1-5 min.
• A duração da ausência é aumentada lentamente em intervalos de 3-5 min se nenhum dos sinais de angústia ficar evidente no intervalo mais curto.
• O aumento no intervalo deve ser variável, intercaladando saídas curtas (1-3 min) com outras mais prolongadas (5-20 min). • Caso ocorram destruição, evacuação/micção ou vocalização, a saída foi muito prolongada. Utilizar um vídeo para ajudar na ansiedade do animal de estimação. • Se as saídas e as ausências forem mantidas mesmo na presença de comportamentos angustiantes, o cão irá piorar. • Fitas de áudio para a vocalização podem ajudar a monitorizar a evolução do comportamento. • Assim que o animal puder ser deixado por 2-3 h em saída planejada, ele quase sempre poderá ser deixado durante todo o dia. • O indício é lentamente suprimido com o passar do tempo ou pode ser utilizado de modo indefinido.

Arranjos e Preparativos para o Animal durante Novo Adestramento e Ausência do Proprietário
• Não permitir mais atividade destrutiva, se possível. • O ato de mesclar ou eliminar os indícios desencadeadores de partida pode ajudar a diminuir as respostas ansiosas. • Preparativos para cuidados diários do cão ou tratadores de animais.
• Condicionamento gradual para uma gaiola de transporte. • As gaiolas de transporte não são recomendadas, a menos que o cão já esteja adestrado para isso e seja deixado confortavelmente em uma delas.

CONSIDERAÇÕES CIRÚRGICAS
Se o animal estiver sendo submetido a medicamentos, deve-se ter cuidado antes de administrar a anestesia.

MEDICAÇÕES

MEDICAMENTO(S) DE ESCOLHA
Cloridrato de Clomipramina (Clomicalm®)
• Antidepressivo tricíclico — aprovado para uso no tratamento de ansiedade da separação nos cães.
• Aprovada para os cães com >6 meses de vida.
• Dosagem: 2-4 mg/kg como dose diária total (cão). Administrada como dose única ou dividida e fornecida 2 vezes ao dia. Deve ser dada diariamente, não em um esquema "conforme a necessidade".
• Pode levar 2-4 semanas antes que o efeito comportamental seja evidente.
• Efeitos colaterais — vômito, diarreia e letargia.

Cloridrato de Fluoxetina (Reconcile®)
• Inibidor seletivo de recaptação da serotonina — aprovado para uso no tratamento de ansiedade da separação em cães.
• Dosagem: 1-2 mg/kg (cães) administrados 1 vez ao dia.
• Administrar em conjunto com um plano de mudança comportamental.
• Efeitos colaterais: letargia, diminuição do apetite, perda de peso, e vômito.

CONTRAINDICAÇÕES
• A clomipramina e a fluoxetina não devem ser utilizadas em conjunto com inibidores da monoamina oxidase (MAO), como o amitraz e a selegilina, nem dentro de 14 dias antes ou depois de algum inibidor da MAO.
• Utilizar a clomipramina com cuidado em pacientes que apresentam distúrbios de condução cardíaca.
• É aconselhável ter cautela ao usar em conjunto com medicamentos ativos no SNC, incluindo a anestesia geral e os medicamentos neurolépticos, anticolinérgicos e simpatomiméticos para cães sob clomipramina ou fluoxetina.
• Deve ser observado um intervalo de descanso de 6 semanas após a interrupção da terapia com fluoxetina antes da administração de qualquer medicamento que possa interagir com esse inibidor seletivo de recaptação da serotonina.
• A fluoxetina não deve ser usada em cães com epilepsia ou histórico de crises convulsivas ou sob medicamentos que diminuem o limiar convulsivo (fenotiazinas).
• É recomendável que os clínicos leiam as bulas em busca das contraindicações.

PRECAUÇÕES
• Não foram conduzidos estudos para determinar os efeitos da medicação em pacientes com menos de 6 meses de vida.
• Não foram realizados estudos para avaliar a interação da fluoxetina com antidepressivos tricíclicos.
• A modificação comportamental indevidamente aplicada pode, na verdade, aumentar a ansiedade.
• O confinamento em gaiola poderá resultar em lesões físicas graves para o animal se ele tentar escapar e só deve ser recomendado com cautela para aqueles animais já adestrados para isso.
• Animais irresponsivos podem ter outras ansiedades concomitantes, como fobias a ruídos e tempestades.

INTERAÇÕES POSSÍVEIS
Síndrome serotoninérgica com inibidores da MAO e inibidores seletivos de recaptação da serotonina em combinação com a clomipramina.

MEDICAMENTO(S) ALTERNATIVO(S)
• Antidepressivos tricíclicos (ATC) como a amitriptilina (cão: 1-2 mg/kg a cada 12 h).
• Benzodiazepínicos como o alprazolam para pânico no momento da saída do proprietário (cão: 0,01-0,1 mg/kg a cada 8-12 h).
• Feromônio apaziguador de cães. Análogo sintético de feromônios apaziguadores naturais da cadela lactante, a qual acalma os filhotes; usada para acalmar os cães em situações de medo, estresse e ansiedade, como a ansiedade da separação e as fobias a ruídos; disponível como difusor elétrico e coleira.

ACOMPANHAMENTO

MONITORIZAÇÃO DO PACIENTE
É necessário um acompanhamento satisfatório do proprietário para monitorizar tanto o plano terapêutico comportamental como a medicação, se for prescrita. O acompanhamento semanal é mais eficiente nos estágios iniciais para avaliar a eficácia do plano de tratamento e a obediência às instruções por parte do proprietário. Assim que o cão se tornar mais independente, se habituar a indícios anteriores à partida e ficar mais calmo nas saídas e nos retornos, poderão ser implementadas partidas gradativas planejadas.

PREVENÇÃO
Ensinar os animais a permanecer sozinhos em casa, tornando-os independentes.

COMPLICAÇÕES POSSÍVEIS
• Lesões durante as tentativas de escape.
• Comportamentos contínuos de destruição e evacuação/micção abalam o elo homem-animal e, muitas vezes, resultam em abandono.
• Outras ansiedades indutoras de sinais que mimetizam a angústia da separação; se não for identificado e tratado, o problema poderá piorar.

EVOLUÇÃO ESPERADA E PROGNÓSTICO
A ansiedade da separação frequentemente responde bem à modificação comportamental com ou sem medicação. Alguns casos graves podem ser muito resistentes ao tratamento. Outros distúrbios comportamentais concomitantes podem tornar a resolução mais difícil. O tratamento medicamentoso isolado raramente é curativo na maior parte dos distúrbios comportamentais. De forma realista, pode-se esperar que o tratamento medicamentoso diminua a ansiedade à saída do proprietário, mas ainda é preciso ensinar o cão a ficar sozinho durante as ausências de seu dono.

DIVERSOS

DISTÚRBIOS ASSOCIADOS
Outras condições de ansiedade, incluindo fobias a ruídos, ansiedade generalizada, medos e transtornos compulsivos.

FATORES RELACIONADOS COM A IDADE
Problema comportamental comum em cães mais idosos.

SINÔNIMO(S)
• Ansiedade da separação. • Ligação exagerada.

VER TAMBÉM
• Síndrome de Disfunção Cognitiva.
• Vocalização Excessiva.

ABREVIATURA(S)
• ATC = antidepressivo tricíclico.
• ISRS = inibidor seletivo de recaptação da serotonina.
• LCS = líquido cerebrospinal.
• MAO = monoamina oxidase.
• SNC = sistema nervoso central.

Autor Debra F. Horwitz
Consultor Editorial Debra F. Horwitz

SÍNDROME DE CHEDIAK-HIGASHI

CONSIDERAÇÕES GERAIS

REVISÃO
- Distúrbio hereditário autossômico recessivo de gatos da raça Persa, caracterizado por anormalidades na morfologia de células e na formação de pigmento.
- Amplos grânulos intracitoplasmáticos em leucócitos e melanócitos circulantes, formados pela fusão de grânulos preexistentes.
- A deficiência nas reservas de armazenamento de ADP, ATP, magnésio e serotonina resulta da falta de grânulos densos das plaquetas.
- Em função do dano à agregação plaquetária e à reação de liberação, ocorre um aumento na duração do sangramento a partir de traumatismos, venopunções ou cirurgias de pequeno porte.
- Normalidade nos tempos de coagulação.
- Depressão da quimiotaxia.
- Ausência de alterações nas taxas de infecção.
- Leve diminuição na contagem neutrofílica, mas dentro dos limites de referência.

IDENTIFICAÇÃO
- Gatos da raça Persa com pelagem de coloração azul-fumaça diluída e íris amarelo-esverdeadas (e tigres brancos).
- Não ocorre em cães.
- Determinadas raposas árticas com pelagem de coloração azul ou pérola.

SINAIS CLÍNICOS
Achados Anamnésicos
Sangramento prolongado a partir de traumatismos, venopunções ou cirurgias de pequeno porte.

Achados do Exame Físico
- Reflexo vermelho do fundo ocular (ausência de pigmento coroidal).
- Pelagem de coloração azul-fumaça diluído e íris amarelo-esverdeadas.
- Fotofobia (blefarospasmo e epífora) em luz intensa.

CAUSAS E FATORES DE RISCO
Doença genética.

DIAGNÓSTICO

DIAGNÓSTICO DIFERENCIAL
Diluição na cor da pelagem.

HEMOGRAMA/BIOQUÍMICA/URINÁLISE
Esfregaço sanguíneo corado por Romanowsky — leucócitos, especialmente neutrófilos, que contêm corpúsculos de inclusão citoplasmáticos de coloração rosa a magenta com 2 µm de diâmetro.

OUTROS TESTES LABORATORIAIS
Nenhum.

DIAGNÓSTICO POR IMAGEM
N/D.

MÉTODOS DIAGNÓSTICOS
Nenhum.

TRATAMENTO
- Fornecer ácido ascórbico (vitamina C) não só para aumentar a concentração do GMPc, mas também para melhorar as funções celular e plaquetária (em gatos, não há nenhum estudo controlado).
- A transfusão de plasma rico em plaquetas e coletado de gatos saudáveis normalizará temporariamente o tempo de sangramento nos animais acometidos.

MEDICAÇÕES

MEDICAMENTO(S)
Ácido ascórbico (100 mg VO a cada 8 h).

CONTRAINDICAÇÕES/INTERAÇÕES POSSÍVEIS
Nenhuma.

ACOMPANHAMENTO

MONITORIZAÇÃO DO PACIENTE
Nenhuma.

PREVENÇÃO
- Advertir o proprietário sobre o potencial de sangramento prolongado após traumatismos, venopunções ou cirurgias de pequeno porte.
- Oferecer aconselhamento genético para eliminar a síndrome de Chediak-Higashi de animais utilizados com fins reprodutivos.
- Castrar os animais acometidos e portadores ou aconselhar o proprietário a não cruzá-los.

COMPLICAÇÕES POSSÍVEIS
Tempo de sangramento prolongado.

EVOLUÇÃO ESPERADA E PROGNÓSTICO
Expectativa de vida normal.

DIVERSOS

ABREVIATURA(S)
- ADP = difosfato de adenosina.
- ATP = trifosfato de adenosina.
- GMPc = monofosfato cíclico de guanosina.

Sugestões de Leitura
August JR. Consultations in Feline Internal Medicine, 2nd ed. Philadelphia: Saunders, 1994.
Cowles BE, Meyers KM, Wardrop KJ, Menard M, Sylvester D. Prolonged bleeding time of Chediak-Higashi cats corrected by platelet transfusion. Throm Haemost 1992, 67:708-712.

Autor Kenneth S. Latimer
Consultor Editorial A. H. Rebar

Síndrome de Dilatação e Vólvulo Gástricos

CONSIDERAÇÕES GERAIS

DEFINIÇÃO
- Síndrome de cães em que o estômago se dilata e subsequentemente rotaciona em torno de seu eixo curto.
- Também conhecida pelo acrônimo DVG.

FISIOPATOLOGIA
- O mecanismo exato envolvido no desenvolvimento de DVG é pouco compreendido.
- O vólvulo pode ocorrer em qualquer direção, mas a grande maioria ocorre no sentido horário quando o animal se encontra em decúbito dorsal e o cirurgião está visualizando o paciente pela face caudal.
- Os fatores que supostamente contribuem para o quadro incluem ingestão de grande quantidade de alimento ou água, esvaziamento gástrico tardio e atividade pós-prandial excessiva. Contudo, esses fatores não ocorrem em todos os casos de DVG.
- Subsequentemente à rotação gástrica, continua ocorrendo o acúmulo de gás e líquido, que ficam encarcerados dentro do lúmen gástrico. Ocorre, então, a distensão progressiva do estômago.
- Conforme o estômago se torna progressivamente distendido, a pressão intra-abdominal aumenta. Isso leva à compressão dos vasos sanguíneos complacentes do abdome, incluindo a veia cava caudal e a veia porta. A queda no fluxo sanguíneo através desses vasos importantes induz ao declínio do retorno venoso e ao desenvolvimento de choque hipovolêmico.
- A má perfusão pode levar a efeitos sistêmicos, como falência dos órgãos, cascatas inflamatórias locais e sistêmicas, além de coagulação intravascular disseminada.

SISTEMA(S) ACOMETIDO(S)
- Gastrintestinal — a perfusão diminuída pode levar à necrose isquêmica do estômago. Em virtude da demanda metabólica mais elevada, a mucosa fica predisposta aos efeitos da isquemia.
- Cardiovascular — o declínio significativo no retorno venoso ao coração resulta em um estado hipovolêmico. Isso conduz à redução no débito cardíaco, o que pode gerar hipoxia orgânica e dano/morte tecidual. A perfusão reduzida do miocárdio, bem como a geração de mediadores inflamatórios, podem induzir a arritmias cardíacas, particularmente contrações ventriculares prematuras.
- Hematológico/linfático/imune — é comum a ocorrência de lesão esplênica, via avulsão dos vasos gástricos curtos, torção ou infarto do baço.

GENÉTICA
Nenhuma predisposição genética direta foi confirmada; no entanto, os cães que possuem parentes de primeiro grau com histórico de DVG estão sob alto risco de desenvolvimento dessa síndrome.

INCIDÊNCIA/PREVALÊNCIA
Há relatos de que a taxa de incidência para raças caninas de porte grande e gigante gire em torno de 6%.

IDENTIFICAÇÃO
Espécie
Cães.

Raça(s) Predominante(s)
- Qualquer raça de grande porte e tórax profundo.
- Dinamarquês.
- Pastor alemão.
- Raramente relatada em raças de porte menor e tórax profundo, como Dachshund e Pequinês.

Idade Média e Faixa Etária
Qualquer idade; o risco aumenta com o avanço da idade.

SINAIS CLÍNICOS
Achados Anamnésicos
- Vômito, que frequentemente evolui para ânsia de vômito improdutiva ou "vômito seco".
- Comportamento ansioso.
- Distensão e dor abdominais.
- Colapso.
- Ptialismo.
- Depressão.

Achados do Exame Físico
- Possível distensão abdominal; entretanto, o estômago distendido pode estar contido pelas costelas e, nesse caso, essa distensão não é observada.
- Taquicardia.
- Taquipneia ou dispneia.
- Pulsos débeis (fracos) e mucosas pálidas com tempo de preenchimento capilar prolongado são sugestivos de hipovolemia.

CAUSAS
- Desconhecidas.
- Provavelmente tem origem multifatorial, incluindo fatores anatômicos, genéticos e ambientais.

FATORES DE RISCO
- Tipicamente ligados à atividade física pós-prandial.
- Predisposição anatômica em cães de tórax profundo, particularmente raças de porte grande e gigante.
- Também se acreditava que o comedouro em local rebaixado incentivasse a aerofagia, o que poderia levar à DVG. Recentemente, foi identificado que a ingestão alimentar em comedouro SUSPENSO seja um fator de risco para o desenvolvimento de DVG.
- O fato de ter algum parente de primeiro grau com histórico de DVG e a velocidade mais rápida de ingestão alimentar também foram identificados como fatores de risco associados ao desenvolvimento dessa síndrome.
- É possível que o animal tenha neoplasia gastrintestinal, pois isso pode causar distúrbios de motilidade, bem como retenção gástrica de alimento e/ou ar.

DIAGNÓSTICO

DIAGNÓSTICO DIFERENCIAL
- Outras doenças que provocam distensão abdominal aguda e, potencialmente, diminuição do fluxo circulatório incluem peritonite séptica, hemoabdome, vólvulo intestinal ou gastrenterite aguda.
- "Timpanismo alimentar" é o nome comumente empregado para dilatação gástrica sem vólvulo concomitante. Isso costuma ocorrer em cães que sofrem congestão alimentar.

HEMOGRAMA/BIOQUÍMICA/URINÁLISE
- Hemograma completo — possivelmente se observam leucograma de estresse, hemoconcentração, trombocitopenia.
- Bioquímica — é comum o encontro de anormalidades eletrolíticas. Pode-se observar azotemia (pré-renal) causada por hipovolemia.
- Urinálise — pode-se verificar o aumento na densidade urinária em caso de hipovolemia.

OUTROS TESTES LABORATORIAIS
Foi constatado que a concentração plasmática de lactato seja um marcador útil para a predição de necrose gástrica subjacente, bem como para o estabelecimento do prognóstico. Os níveis plasmáticos médios de lactato em cães com necrose gástrica eram significativamente maiores (6,6 mmol/L) do que naqueles sem esse tipo de necrose (3,3 mmol/L). A sobrevida de cães com níveis plasmáticos de lactato <6,0 mmol/L era de 99%, em comparação à sobrevida de 58% experimentada por cães com níveis de lactato >6,0 mmol/L.

DIAGNÓSTICO POR IMAGEM
- Com frequência, há necessidade de estabilização adequada antes da obtenção de radiografias.
- Radiografia abdominal — a incidência abdominal lateral direita é a modalidade de escolha. Tipicamente, essa imagem revela compartimentalização do estômago, sinal considerado como patognomônico.
- Projeção dorsoventral — pode ser útil para confirmar a doença.

MÉTODOS DIAGNÓSTICOS
- É muito raro que ainda haja incertezas depois da obtenção de radiografias simples, embora elas possam persistir.
- Pode-se tentar com CUIDADO uma série radiográfica do trato GI superior com contraste positivo, pois esses pacientes estão sob alto risco de aspiração.

ACHADOS PATOLÓGICOS
- A torção esplênica pode ser um achado concomitante.
- O estômago em si fica edematoso e sofre congestão vascular e infarto, o que pode levar à necrose.

TRATAMENTO

CUIDADO(S) DE SAÚDE ADEQUADO(S)
- Essa síndrome é uma emergência!
- Os pacientes devem ser hospitalizados para avaliação clínica completa e tratamento rigoroso de insuficiência cardiovascular.
- Diversas abordagens de fluidoterapia são empregadas, com base na condição clínica do paciente e na preferência pessoal do veterinário. Pode-se lançar mão de fluidos cristaloides e/ou coloides. Se a terapia cristaloide for escolhida, será administrada uma dose de 90 mL/kg de solução isotônica em 30-60 min. A administração é feita através de locais de acesso venoso cefálico ou jugular.
- Subsequentemente à estabilização cardiovascular, é recomendável a realização de descompressão gástrica.
- A entubação orogástrica é o método preferido para efetuar a descompressão do estômago. Na tentativa de facilitar a entubação orogástrica,

Síndrome de Dilatação e Vólvulo Gástricos

pode-se fazer uso de medicamentos que poupam o sistema cardiovascular. É comum que o veterinário encontre grande resistência à passagem pelo hiato esofágico. A sonda lubrificada pode ser torcida ou reposicionada para facilitar a passagem. Também pode-se tentar diferentes posições do paciente (sentado, em estação, etc.) para facilitar a introdução da sonda.

- Nos casos em que a entubação orogástrica não é bem-sucedida, pode-se tentar o procedimento de gastrocentese percutânea. É localizado um ponto de timpanismo máximo que tipicamente corresponde a uma área do estômago preenchida por gás. Nessa área, o veterinário introduz uma agulha ou cateter calibroso no estômago. O gás tipicamente eliciará um ruído audível durante o escape. É preciso esperar um período de tempo considerável para obter a descompressão gástrica com o uso dessa técnica.
- Após a estabilização do paciente e a descompressão do estômago, fica indicada a intervenção cirúrgica. Nos casos raros em que o paciente se mostra irresponsivo às tentativas de estabilização, pode-se efetuar o procedimento cirúrgico imediatamente.

ATIVIDADE
É recomendável a restrição da atividade física por aproximadamente 2 semanas do pós-operatório.

DIETA
- É aconselhável a retomada do consumo oral de alimento assim que se obter a recuperação plena do paciente.
- Até o momento, o papel desempenhado pela altura do comedouro na ocorrência e na recidiva dessa síndrome é incerto.

ORIENTAÇÃO AO PROPRIETÁRIO
É recomendável orientar os proprietários de cão de porte grande e gigante que não tenham consciência dos sinais clínicos de dilatação e vólvulo gástricos.

CONSIDERAÇÕES CIRÚRGICAS
- A intervenção cirúrgica deve ser realizada o mais rápido possível no paciente estável ou naquele cujos esforços diligentes de estabilização se mostraram ineficazes.
- O procedimento cirúrgico tem três objetivos principais: (1) reposição anatômica do estômago (e do baço, se aplicável); (2) avaliação da viabilidade do órgão; (3) prevenção de recidiva.
- Uma vez reposicionados, o estômago e o baço deverão ser avaliados. Se houver áreas desvitalizadas, deverá ser feita a remoção via gastrectomia parcial e/ou esplenectomia.
- A prevenção de recidiva é obtida por meio de gastropexia permanente. Como existem inúmeras técnicas descritas para a realização de gastropexia, a escolha da técnica é feita principalmente com base na preferência do cirurgião.

MEDICAÇÕES

MEDICAMENTO(S) DE ESCOLHA
- É indicado o uso de antibióticos no período perioperatório. Dependendo da gravidade e da evolução da doença, a cirurgia em si pode ser uma intervenção limpa, limpa/contaminada, contaminada ou suja. Muitas vezes, é quase impossível apurar essa informação antes de a cirurgia ser realizada.
- A escolha do antibiótico deve ser feita com base nos patógenos potenciais as quais o paciente pode ser exposto. Doença moderada a grave pode expor o hospedeiro a patógenos entéricos em virtude de perfuração de víscera(s) ou perda das barreiras da mucosa normal à translocação hematógena de bactérias a partir do trato gastrintestinal. Para esses pacientes, a cefoxitina sódica (30 mg/kg IV a cada 6-8 h) pode ser uma opção adequada. Para os pacientes em que não ocorreu penetração no trato gastrintestinal, a cefazolina sódica (22 mg/kg IV a cada 2 h no período intraoperatório) é suficiente.
- Protetores gástricos podem ser implementados para minimizar ou evitar as ulcerações gastrintestinais.

CONTRAINDICAÇÕES
- O uso de alguns coloides sintéticos (p. ex., hetamido de hidroxietila) foi relacionado com a interrupção na formação do coágulo primário e, por essa razão, pode não ser apropriado em certos pacientes com DVG, como aqueles com coagulopatia subjacente como CID concomitante.
- Se possível, é aconselhável evitar o uso de medicamentos que deprimem significativamente a função cardiovascular (p. ex., acetilpromazina).

PRECAUÇÕES
Os pacientes podem descompensar agudamente a qualquer momento, em particular sob intervenção anestésica.

MEDICAMENTO(S) ALTERNATIVO(S)
Atualmente não se conhece a eficácia da administração de corticosteroides em pacientes acometidos por DVG.

ACOMPANHAMENTO

MONITORIZAÇÃO DO PACIENTE
- Cuidados de enfermagem — alguns pacientes podem necessitar da provisão de cuidados em decúbito por vários dias antes da recuperação plena.
- Controle adequado da dor.
- No pós-operatório, é comum a ocorrência de contrações ventriculares prematuras. Tais contrações resultam de hipoperfusão do miocárdio e consequente dano por isquemia ou de insulto ou retirada do baço. É recomendável a monitorização do ritmo cardíaco.
- Monitorizar o débito urinário e a função renal no pós-operatório.

PREVENÇÃO
- É preconizada a elevação do comedouro.
- Evitar a atividade física após a ingestão de água ou alimento.
- Se possível, diminuir a velocidade de consumo das refeições.
- Fornecem múltiplas refeições em pequenas quantidades várias vezes ao dia.

COMPLICAÇÕES POSSÍVEIS
- A dilatação gástrica pode recidivar, mesmo após a realização da gastropexia. A recidiva do vólvulo com o procedimento adequado de gastropexia é extremamente rara.
- A falha em remover o tecido gástrico necrosado pode resultar em subsequente perfuração do estômago e surgimento de peritonite séptica.
- Também podem ocorrer arritmias cardíacas (particularmente complexos ventriculares prematuros), CID e ulceração gástrica.

EVOLUÇÃO ESPERADA E PROGNÓSTICO
- A crescente conscientização dos proprietários de cães, aliada ao aumento na compreensão dos eventos fisiopatológicos complexos associados à DVG, reduziram significativamente a taxa de mortalidade vinculada a essa doença nos últimos 30 anos.
- O prognóstico em cães submetidos a tratamento adequado e não acometidos por necrose gástrica é excelente, com taxa de sobrevida relatada de 98%. Já os cães com necrose gástrica exibem prognóstico mais reservado, com taxa de sobrevida relatada de 66%.
- Um único artigo científico relatou uma taxa de sobrevida global em curto prazo de 83,8%. Os indicadores prognósticos negativos incluíram os quadros de hipotensão, CID e peritonite, bem como a necessidade da realização de esplenectomia e gastrectomia parcial.

DIVERSOS

FATORES RELACIONADOS COM A IDADE
Tipicamente se observa uma taxa mais alta de DVG em cães de meia-idade a idosos.

SINÔNIMOS
- Timpanismo.
- Torção gástrica.

VER TAMBÉM
- Capítulos sobre Choque.
- Sepse e Bacteremia.

ABREVIATURA(S)
- CID = coagulação intravascular disseminada.
- DVG = síndrome de dilatação e vólvulo gástricos.
- GI = gastrintestinal.

Sugestões de Leitura

Beck JJ, Staatz AJ, Pelsue DH, et al. Risk factors associated with short-term outcome and development of perioperative complications in dogs undergoing surgery because of gastric dilatation-volvulus: 166 cases (1992-2003). JAVMA 2006, 229:1934-1939.

de Papp E, Drobatz KJ, Hughes D. Plasma lactate concentration as a predictor of gastric necrosis and survival among dogs with gastric dilatation-volvulus: 102 cases (1995-1998). JAVMA 1999, 215:49-52.

Fossum TW. Surgery of the stomach. In: Fossum TW, ed., Small Animal Surgery, 2nd ed. St. Louis: Mosby, 2002, pp. 337-369.

Glickman LT, Glickman NW, Schellenberg DB, et al. Non-dietary risk factors for gastric dilatation-volvulus in large and giant breed dogs. JAVMA 2000, 217:1492-1499.

Autor S. Brent Reimer
Consultor Editorial Albert E. Jergens

Síndrome de Disfunção Cognitiva

CONSIDERAÇÕES GERAIS

DEFINIÇÃO
Síndrome associada ao processo de envelhecimento cerebral, que leva a alterações na consciência, à diminuição na responsividade a estímulos, bem como a déficits de aprendizado e memória. Também pode haver sinais progressivos de ansiedade com o envelhecimento. Nos estágios precoces, observam-se sinais sutis, conhecidos como declínio cognitivo.

FISIOPATOLOGIA
• É incerto o fato de que as alterações estejam associadas aos sinais clínicos de declínio cognitivo.
• Redução nos neurônios, diminuição de volume dos lobos frontais, aumento de volume dos ventrículos cerebrais e depósitos neurotóxicos, incluindo lipofuscina, ubiquitina e β-amiloide.
• Os radicais livres tóxicos (espécies reativas de oxigênio) aumentam com a idade, em consequência da doença crônica e dos fatores indutores de estresse, do declínio na eficiência mitocondrial relacionado com a idade e do decréscimo nos mecanismos de depuração.
• Correlações possíveis entre a quantidade de β-amiloide no córtex cerebral e o declínio na capacidade cognitiva. O aumento nos radicais livres tóxicos também parece estar correlacionado ao declínio cognitivo. • O comprometimento do fluxo sanguíneo vascular cerebral e a ocorrência de infartos podem contribuir para o quadro. • Há um comprometimento da neurotransmissão. Pode haver um declínio dos neurotransmissores (colina e catecolaminas) e da transmissão colinérgica.

SISTEMA(S) ACOMETIDO(S)
• Comportamental. • Nervoso.

GENÉTICA
Pode haver uma correlação genética em relação à distribuição do β-amiloide e à idade de início do acúmulo.

INCIDÊNCIA/PREVALÊNCIA
• Os sinais clínicos de disfunção cognitiva foram identificados em mais de 50% dos cães e gatos com >11 anos de idade. • Um total de 28% dos cães entre 11-12 anos e 68% dos cães entre 15-16 anos pode revelar ao menos um sinal clínico.
• Quadro progressivo — mais de 50% dos cães com, no mínimo, um sinal clínico manifestam sinais adicionais após 12 meses.

IDENTIFICAÇÃO
Espécies
Cães e gatos.

Idade Média e Faixa Etária
• A prevalência aumenta com o avanço da idade.
• O teste neuropsicológico em cães é capaz de identificar o declínio na memória e no aprendizado já com 6 anos de idade. • Os sinais clínicos em gatos podem se desenvolver em uma idade um pouco mais avançada; ainda não se realizou o teste neuropsicológico nos animais dessa espécie. • Os déficits podem passar despercebidos pelos proprietários dos animais de estimação até alguns anos mais tarde, exceto em cães adestrados a executar tarefas mais especializadas (p. ex., audição, visão, detecção de drogas e provas de agility).

SINAIS CLÍNICOS
Achados Anamnésicos
A maioria dos sinais clínicos pode ser classificada em 5 categorias:
• Desorientação, incluindo o fato de se sentir perdido no próprio ambiente familiar, confusão mental e incapacidade de percorrer trajetos habituais e conhecidos (p. ex., correr para o lado errado da porta). • Pode haver mudanças nas interações com seres humanos ou outros animais (possível declínio nas brincadeiras, aumento/diminuição no interesse por carinho ou elevação na irritabilidade). • Alterações no ciclo de sono-vigília (desorientação temporal), incluindo vigília ou vocalização noturnas e possivelmente sonolência durante o dia. • O adestramento doméstico e outros comportamentos previamente aprendidos podem se deteriorar. Podem ocorrer evacuação/micção domiciliar, falta de resposta a comandos já aprendidos ou menor competência à execução de tarefas aprendidas (p. ex., provas de agility, capacidade produtiva). • O nível de atividade também pode ser alterado — inatividade, além de menor interesse com as atividades exploratórias, a auto-higienização ou até mesmo a alimentação. À medida que o distúrbio evolui, os níveis de atividade podem aumentar com sinais de inquietação, marcha compassada, perambulação sem destino ou distúrbios compulsivos, como lambedura excessiva. • A ansiedade e a agitação também podem aumentar em animais domésticos com disfunção cognitiva.

Achados do Exame Físico
Pode-se notar a ausência de anormalidades específicas, especialmente associadas à disfunção cognitiva. No entanto, pode-se observar outros distúrbios médicos relacionados com a idade.

CAUSAS
• Além de não se conhecer a causa exata, nem todos os animais são acometidos. • Há alterações degenerativas relacionadas com a idade, mas fatores genéticos podem predispor os animais de estimação ao desenvolvimento de disfunção clínica significativa. • A dieta e o enriquecimento nutricional podem ser medidas parcialmente preventivas. • Ver a seção "Fisiopatologia".

FATORES DE RISCO
• Doenças ou estresses crônicos ou recidivantes podem levar ao incremento no acúmulo das espécies reativas de oxigênio. • Distúrbios que comprometem o aporte sanguíneo vascular cerebral (p. ex., hipertensão sistêmica e anemia).

DIAGNÓSTICO

DIAGNÓSTICO DIFERENCIAL
• É preciso descartar qualquer distúrbio clínico ou processo mórbido que afete o comportamento ou a atitude mental do animal de estimação.
• Afecções dolorosas (p. ex., artrite e odontopatia) podem induzir ao aumento na irritabilidade ou ao medo de ser manipulado. • Caso a mobilidade seja acometida, o animal de estimação pode ficar ainda mais agressivo em vez de se afastar ou pode se mostrar menos apto a acessar sua área de evacuação. • A diminuição nas acuidades visual ou auditiva pode levar ao declínio na responsividade ou ao aumento na reatividade a estímulos. • As doenças do trato urinário podem causar micção inapropriada ou contribuir para essa prática.
• Falência de órgãos, tumores e doenças imunes também podem influenciar o comportamento.
• As endocrinopatias, como o hipotireoidismo, podem levar a mudanças comportamentais, que variam desde letargia até agressividade. Os animais com hiperadrenocorticismo podem exibir alteração nos ciclos de sono-vigília, letargia, evacuação/micção domiciliar, respiração ofegante e polifagia. O hipertireoidismo em gatos pode provocar aumento na irritabilidade e na atividade física.
• As doenças que comprometem o sistema nervoso central ou sua circulação por via direta (tumores) ou indireta (p. ex., anemia) também exercem influência sobre o comportamento.

HEMOGRAMA/BIOQUÍMICA/URINÁLISE
• Normais em casos de síndrome de disfunção cognitiva, embora os processos patológicos concomitantes sejam comuns em animais idosos.
• Exames utilizados para fazer a triagem de outras doenças em animais idosos com sinais comportamentais.

OUTROS TESTES LABORATORIAIS
Normais em casos de síndrome de disfunção cognitiva.

DIAGNÓSTICO POR IMAGEM
• Usados para descartar causas orgânicas/estruturais primárias. • Demonstram maior relevância quando há anormalidades no exame neurológico ou em casos de início súbito, mas provavelmente apresentam menor valor diagnóstico na presença de sinais clínicos lentamente progressivos. • Os animais de estimação com disfunção cognitiva podem exibir aumento no volume dos ventrículos cerebrais e declínio global na massa cerebral, mas esses achados isolados não são diagnósticos.

MÉTODOS DIAGNÓSTICOS
• Pode haver a necessidade da realização de endoscopias, radiografias, ultrassonografias e de outros procedimentos diagnósticos especializados para descartar outras causas dos sinais clínicos.
• Na suspeita de disfunção sensorial como a causa dos sinais clínicos, ficam indicados testes adicionais, como o teste de resposta evocada auditiva do tronco encefálico (RAETE) ou o encaminhamento a um oftalmologista.
• Uma tentativa terapêutica pode ser o uso de outro auxílio diagnóstico, por exemplo, para determinar os efeitos do controle da dor sobre a resolução dos sinais clínicos.

ACHADOS PATOLÓGICOS
A avaliação dos depósitos de β-amiloide pode ser indicativa do grau de disfunção cognitiva. Esse tipo de avaliação é praticável apenas em amostras de necropsia em laboratórios especializados.

TRATAMENTO

CUIDADO(S) DE SAÚDE ADEQUADO(S)
Feito em um esquema ambulatorial.

CUIDADO(S) DE ENFERMAGEM
Depende do tipo e da gravidade dos sinais clínicos da disfunção cognitiva.

ATIVIDADE E ADESTRAMENTO
• Manter a prática de exercícios físicos, atividades lúdicas, adestramentos, esforços e outras atividades

SÍNDROME DE DISFUNÇÃO COGNITIVA

de rotina, tanto quanto for possível para a idade e a saúde do animal de estimação.
• Foi comprovado que a manutenção dos estímulos físicos e mentais diminui ou retarda a evolução do declínio cognitivo.

DIETA E SUPLEMENTOS NUTRICIONAIS
• Selecionada com base na avaliação da saúde do animal de estimação.
• Caso o estado de saúde do animal não exija uma dieta terapêutica especial, ficará recomendado o uso de dieta sênior com eficácia comprovada no restabelecimento da função cognitiva.
• Foi demonstrado que a linha de rações Prescription Diet b/d da Hills® melhora a memória, a capacidade de aprendizado e os sinais clínicos da síndrome de disfunção cognitiva. A dieta é suplementada com antioxidantes (p. ex., vitaminas E e C, selênio, betacaroteno, flavonoides e carotenoides) na forma de frutas e vegetais, ácidos graxos ômega-3 (ácido eicosapentaenoico [EPA] e ácido docosaexaenoico [DHA]), além de carnitina e ácido lipoico, que podem melhorar a integridade das mitocôndrias.
• Foi demonstrado que uma nova ração para cães (Purina ONE Vibrant Maturity 7+), formulada com base no conhecimento de fornecer aos neurônios em processo de envelhecimento uma fonte de energia alternativa a partir de triglicerídeos de cadeia média, melhora significativamente a função cognitiva em animais de estimação idosos.
• Alguns suplementos naturais podem ajudar a melhorar os sinais clínicos ou retardar o declínio da disfunção cognitiva. Um suplemento contendo fosfatidilserina, resveratrol, vitaminas B6 e E, e gingko biloba (Senilife®, CEVA Animal Health), apoequorina (Neutricks®, Quincy Animal Health) e SAMe (Novifit®, Virbac Animal Health) demonstraram alguma evidência de eficácia.

ORIENTAÇÃO AO PROPRIETÁRIO
• Além de ser necessária a terapia vitalícia, pode ser imprescindível o emprego de medicamentos concomitantes se o animal de estimação apresentar múltiplos problemas.
• Qualquer mudança na saúde ou no comportamento do animal deve ser relatada imediatamente, já que isso pode ser atribuído à disfunção cognitiva ou ao surgimento de novos problemas de saúde.
• Levando-se em consideração a saúde e o estado cognitivo do animal de estimação, o proprietário deve ser orientado sobre quaisquer limitações que podem ser superadas.

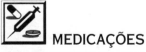

MEDICAÇÕES
MEDICAMENTO(S) DE ESCOLHA
Selegilina
• Aprovada para o uso em cães na América do Norte.
• Nos cães, a inibição da monoamina oxidase (MAO) tipo B pode contribuir para o aumento na transmissão dopaminérgica, levar à diminuição nos radicais livres e exercer efeito neuroprotetor.
• Cães: dose de 0,5-1 mg/kg VO diariamente pela manhã, com manutenção se demonstrar eficácia.
• Reavaliar os sinais clínicos quanto à melhora após 1-2 meses.
• Os efeitos colaterais podem incluir: desarranjo gastrintestinal e inquietação ocasionais, bem como comportamento repetitivo com doses mais elevadas.

Propentofilina
• Sem autorização para o uso na América do Norte, mas aprovada em outros países.
• Derivado metilxatínico.
• Visa inibir a agregação de plaquetas e a formação de trombos, tornar as hemácias mais complacentes e aumentar o fluxo sanguíneo.
• Uso indicado para o tratamento de entorpecimento e letargia em cães idosos.
• Pode reforçar o aporte de oxigênio ao SNC sem ampliar a demanda de glicose.
• Cães: dose de 3 mg/kg VO a cada 12 h.

Comentários Gerais a Respeito dos Gatos
• Não há nenhum agente terapêutico aprovado para o tratamento da síndrome de disfunção cognitiva.
• A selegilina é utilizada fora da indicação da bula (na dose de 0,5-1 mg/kg/dia) e pode ser eficaz em gatos com ansiedade, responsividade diminuída a estímulos, atividade e vocalização noturnas, bem como auto-higienização e apetite reduzidos.

CONTRAINDICAÇÕES
• Não se deve empregar a selegilina juntamente com inibidores da MAO, como o amitraz e os narcóticos, ou com agentes α-adrenérgicos, como a fenilpropanolamina, a adrenalina, os inibidores seletivos de recaptação da serotonina (p. ex., fluoxetina) ou os antidepressivos tricíclicos (p. ex., clomipramina).
• Antes de se iniciar a selegilina, há necessidade de um fracasso completo de 2 semanas após o uso de grande parte dos antidepressivos tricíclicos e 6 semanas após o emprego da fluoxetina.

PRECAUÇÕES
• Selecionar os medicamentos com efeitos sedativos e anticolinérgicos mínimos.
• É imprescindível levar em consideração as interações medicamentosas em potencial, já que os animais com idade mais avançada podem necessitar de diversos medicamentos.

INTERAÇÕES POSSÍVEIS
Ver a seção "Contraindicações".

MEDICAMENTO(S) ALTERNATIVO(S)
• Intensificação do sistema noradrenérgico com medicamentos, como a adrafanila e a modafinila, para melhorar o estado de alerta e a atividade exploratória.
• Com base em pesquisas preliminares em outras espécies, pode-se considerar o emprego de medicamentos anti-inflamatórios, terapias de reposição hormonal e extrato de gingko biloba.
• Os medicamentos utilizados em seres humanos com a doença de Alzheimer para estimular a transmissão colinérgica podem ser úteis, mas a dose e a farmacocinética em cães não foram determinadas. Os efeitos colaterais potenciais incluem: náusea, vômito, diarreia e distúrbios do estado de sono-vigília.
• Os agentes ansiolíticos (p. ex., buspirona), os medicamentos indutores do sono (p. ex., benzodiazepínicos) ou os antidepressivos (p. ex., fluoxetina) também podem ser levados em consideração para o tratamento de ansiedade e apatia (mas não em conjunto com a selegilina).
• Os suplementos naturais também podem ajudar a normalizar os ciclos de sono-vigília ou diminuir a ansiedade (melatonina, valeriana, l-treanina, α-casozepina, e Harmonease* [fabricante: VPL]).

ACOMPANHAMENTO
MONITORIZAÇÃO DO PACIENTE
• Caso se dispense o uso de medicamento ou dieta, será preciso avaliar a resposta à terapia após 30-60 dias, ajustar a dose do medicamento ou modificar o tratamento se a melhora for insuficiente.
• Caso o animal de estimação permaneça estável, recomenda-se a realização de avaliações clínicas duas vezes por ano aos pacientes mais idosos a menos que surjam outros problemas antes de a reavaliação ser oportuna.

PREVENÇÃO
• A manutenção de um ambiente estimulante e da prática de atividades físicas próprias à idade e à saúde do animal de estimação pode ajudar a evitar ou retardar o início do declínio cognitivo.
• A intervenção precoce é o melhor método de lentificar a evolução do quadro ou evitar as complicações da doença.

EVOLUÇÃO ESPERADA E PROGNÓSTICO
• Na maioria dos casos, a dieta e os medicamentos devem controlar os sinais clínicos e retardar a evolução.
• Em função do avanço na idade do animal, o declínio cognitivo pode progredir, sendo provável o surgimento de outros problemas concomitantes de saúde apesar da intervenção médica.

DIVERSOS
SINÔNIMO(S)
• Demência. • Distúrbios cognitivos e afetivos relacionados com a idade, incluindo a síndrome de confusão mental, a depressão involutiva e a distimia. • Senilidade.

ABREVIATURA(S)
• MAO = monoamina oxidase. • REATE = resposta evocada auditiva do tronco encefálico. • SAMe = dissulfato tosilato de S-adenosil-L-metionina. • SNC = sistema nervoso central.

Sugestões de Leitura
Landsberg, GM, Araujo J. Behavior problems in geriatric pets. Vet Clin North Am Small Anim Pract 2005, 35:675-698.
Landsberg GM, DePorter T, Araujo JA. Clinical signs and management of anxiety, sleeplessness and cognitive dysfunction in the senior pet. Vet Clin N Am Sm Anim Pract, in press, 41 (3) May 2011.
Landsberg GM, Hunthausen W, Ackerman L. Handbook of Behaviour Problems of the Dog and Cat, 2nd ed. Philadelphia: Elsevier Saunders, 2003.
Nielson JC, Hart BL, Cliff KD, Ruehl WW. Prevalence of behavioral changes associated with age-related cognitive impairment in dogs. JAVMA 2001, 218(11):1787-1791.

Autores Gary Landsberg e Sagi Denenberg
Consultor Editorial Debra F. Horwitz

---
* N. T.: Medicamento não disponível no Brasil – no lugar dele, podemos optar por florais de Bach.

SÍNDROME DE FANCONI

CONSIDERAÇÕES GERAIS

REVISÃO
Conjunto de anormalidades que surgem do defeito no transporte tubular renal de água, sódio, potássio, glicose, fosfato, bicarbonato e aminoácidos; a reabsorção tubular renal comprometida provoca excreção urinária excessiva desses solutos. Essa síndrome reflete uma lesão nos túbulos renais proximais.

IDENTIFICAÇÃO
Espécies
Cães.

Raça(s) Predominante(s)
Embora seja esporadicamente relatada em várias raças, a síndrome de Fanconi idiopática afeta, sobretudo, a raça Basenji (cerca de 75% dos casos). Na América do Norte, 10-30% dos cães da raça Basenji são acometidos. Presume-se que essa síndrome seja hereditária nessa raça, mas o modo de herança não é conhecido.

Idade Média e Faixa Etária
Idade ao diagnóstico: 10 semanas-11 anos. Os cães acometidos da raça Basenji costumam ter >2 anos de idade; a maioria desenvolve sinais clínicos a partir de 4 a 7 anos de idade.

Sexo Predominante
Não há predileção sexual.

SINAIS CLÍNICOS
• Variam, dependendo da gravidade das perdas de solutos específicos e do desenvolvimento de insuficiência renal.
• Perda de aminoácidos e glicose — em geral, não está associada a outros sinais clínicos além de poliúria e polidipsia (sinais clínicos mais comuns).
• Perda de peso, frequentemente apesar de um apetite normal.
• Letargia variável.
• Pode exibir apetite reduzido.
• Má condição corporal.
• Em animais jovens, pode ocorrer um crescimento anormal (raquitismo).

CAUSAS E FATORES DE RISCO
• Hereditária em cães da raça Basenji.
• Síndrome de Fanconi adquirida já foi relatada em cães tratados com gentamicina, estreptozotocina, ácido maleico (experimental), amoxicilina e petiscos de carne de frango desidratada; também relatada como secundária a hipoparatireoidismo primário.

DIAGNÓSTICO

DIAGNÓSTICO DIFERENCIAL
Glicosúria renal primária — também causa glicosúria na ausência de hiperglicemia; a documentação de aminoacidúria, proteinúria discreta ou acidose metabólica hiperclorêmica com hiato aniônico normal sugere síndrome de Fanconi.

HEMOGRAMA/BIOQUÍMICA/URINÁLISE
• Hemograma geralmente normal.
• Hipocalemia em cerca de 1/3 dos casos.
• Acidose metabólica hiperclorêmica.
• Azotemia caso ocorra o desenvolvimento de insuficiência renal.
• Podem ocorrer hipofosfatemia e hipocalcemia em animais jovens acometidos em crescimento.
• Densidade urinária, em geral, baixa (1,005-1,018); é comum a constatação de proteinúria discreta; pode haver cetonúria.
• Com frequência, a glicosúria na ausência de hiperglicemia constitui o primeiro indício da síndrome de Fanconi e antecede os sinais clínicos.

OUTROS TESTES LABORATORIAIS
Acidose metabólica hiperclorêmica (ou seja, hiato aniônico normal) atribuída à perda de bicarbonato na urina com pH urinário <5,5. O pH urinário encontra-se >6,0 em anormalidades dos túbulos renais distais e esta é uma diferença diagnóstica chave entre anormalidades dos túbulos renais proximais (síndrome de Fanconi) e distais. Não ocorre a perda de bicarbonato pela urina a menos que se administre uma dose de ataque desse sal.

DIAGNÓSTICO POR IMAGEM
Radiografia — cães jovens em crescimento podem ter características de raquitismo e deformidades angulares dos membros; os pacientes adultos podem exibir densidade óssea diminuída.

MÉTODOS DIAGNÓSTICOS
Estudos da depuração urinária para documentar a excreção excessiva de solutos como aminoácidos e eletrólitos são necessários para a confirmação. Não é recomendável avaliar os animais com menos de 8 semanas de vida, pois pode ocorrer um resultado falso-positivo. Uma amostra de urina de 24 h pode ser enviada para o Centro de Teste de Doença Genética Metabólica da Universidade da Pensilvânia para fazer a triagem de aminoacidúria e acidúria láctica. A reabsorção fracional de aminoácidos em cães acometidos varia de 50 a 96% (faixa normal, 97-100%).

ACHADOS PATOLÓGICOS
Pode ocorrer necrose papilar renal como um achado tardio. Também há relatos de cariomegalia das células tubulares.

TRATAMENTO

• Suspender a administração de qualquer medicamento que possa causar a síndrome de Fanconi ou tratar uma intoxicação específica.
• Nenhum tratamento reverterá os defeitos do transporte em cães com a doença hereditária ou idiopática.
• Como o número e a gravidade dos defeitos de transporte variam muito entre os animais acometidos, os tratamentos para hipocalemia, acidose metabólica, insuficiência renal ou raquitismo precisam ser individualizados. Os tratamentos para hipocalemia, insuficiência renal e raquitismo serão discutidos em outras partes deste livro.
• Instituir o tratamento para acidose metabólica se a concentração sanguínea de bicarbonato estiver <12 mEq/L; grandes doses de agentes alcalinizantes podem ser necessárias, porque a diminuição na capacidade de reabsorção tubular proximal resulta em perda urinária acentuada de bicarbonato; a meta da terapia alcalina é manter a concentração sanguínea de bicarbonato entre 12-18 mEq/L.
• Cães jovens em crescimento podem necessitar de vitamina D e/ou suplementação com cálcio e fósforo.

MEDICAÇÕES

MEDICAMENTO(S)
Utilizar, de preferência, citrato de potássio (1 mEq = 108 mg) a 50-500 mg/kg a cada 12 h (1 a >10 mEq/kg/dia; iniciar com uma dose baixa) ou bicarbonato de sódio (1 mEq = 84 mg) a 80-300 mg/kg a cada 8-12 h (1 a >10 mEq/kg/dia; iniciar com uma dose baixa), conforme a necessidade (com base nas mensurações dos gases sanguíneos e eletrólitos) em pacientes com acidose metabólica. Essas doses são muito mais altas que aquelas necessárias em anormalidades dos túbulos renais distais.

CONTRAINDICAÇÕES
• Evitar medicamentos que sejam nefrotóxicos ou tenham o potencial de causar síndrome de Fanconi (ver a seção "Causas e Fatores de Risco").
• Evitar o uso de cloreto de potássio, já que os pacientes acometidos são hiperclorêmicos.

ACOMPANHAMENTO

• Monitorizar a bioquímica sérica em intervalos de 10-14 dias para avaliar o efeito do tratamento e a ocorrência de qualquer alteração nos parâmetros (especialmente BUN, creatinina e concentração de potássio); como a terapia com bicarbonato pode agravar a perda renal de potássio, monitorizar regularmente a concentração sérica deste último elemento; assim que o animal estiver estabilizado, monitorizar a bioquímica sérica em intervalos de 2-4 meses. • A evolução clínica varia; alguns cães permanecem estáveis por anos; outros desenvolvem rapidamente insuficiência renal progressiva em poucos meses; a causa de morte, em geral, é uma insuficiência renal aguda, quase sempre associada à acidose metabólica grave.
• Alguns cães (18% em um único estudo) desenvolveram crises convulsivas ou outros sinais neurológicos vários anos depois do diagnóstico.

DIVERSOS

VER TAMBÉM
• Hipocalemia. • Insuficiência Renal Aguda.
• Insuficiência Renal Crônica.

RECURSOS DA INTERNET
• Centro de Teste de Doença Genética Metabólica da Universidade da Pensilvânia: http://www.vet.upenn.edu/Portals/0/media/MetabolicPamphlet08.pdf.
• Protocolo terapêutico sugerido para cães com síndrome de Fanconi idiopática: www.basenjiclub.com/old/fanconiprotocol2003.

Sugestões de Leitura
Kerl ME. Renal tubular diseases. In: Ettinger SJ, Feldman EC, eds., Textbook of Veterinary Internal Medicine, 6th ed. St.Louis: Elsevier, 2005, pp. 1824-1828.

Autor João Felipe de Brito Galvão e Stephen P. DiBartola
Consultor Editorial Carl A. Osborne

SÍNDROME DE HIPERESTESIA FELINA

CONSIDERAÇÕES GERAIS

DEFINIÇÃO
- Distúrbio idiopático de gatos, caracterizado por agitação paroxística, espasmos focais dos músculos epaxiais, vocalização e mordedura ou lambedura intensa do dorso, da cauda e dos membros pélvicos.
- Também foi chamada neurodermatite, síndrome da pele torcida, neurite, epilepsia psicomotora e dermatose pruriginosa do gato Siamês.

FISIOPATOLOGIA
Desconhecida.

SISTEMA(S) ACOMETIDO(S)
- Comportamental.
- Nervoso.
- Neuromuscular.
- Cutâneo/Exócrino.

IDENTIFICAÇÃO

Espécie
Felina.

Raça(s) Predominante(s)
Gatos Siamês, Abissínio, Birmanês e Himalaio podem ser predispostos, embora possa se desenvolver em qualquer raça.

Idade Média e Faixa Etária
- Os sinais podem ocorrer em qualquer idade.
- Mais comum — 1-5 anos de idade.

SINAIS CLÍNICOS
- Episódios de contração espasmódica da pele no dorso, com oscilação violenta da cauda, vocalização e mordedura ou lambedura intensa dos flancos e da região pélvica.
- É frequentemente evidenciado o sinal de midríase (pupilas dilatadas); além disso, o gato pode parecer agitado, correndo freneticamente pelo ambiente.
- Os episódios duram de alguns segundos a minutos. Entre eles, os gatos tipicamente se mostram normais, mas podem não gostar de ser acariciados no dorso.
- Com frequência, o exame físico geral não revela quaisquer anormalidades, além da possível alopecia e dos pelos rompidos sobre a região lombar devido à automutilação. Como muitos gatos sentem desconforto à palpação da musculatura toracolombar, a manipulação da área pode eliciar um episódio. Nenhum déficit neurológico foi observado.

CAUSAS E FATORES DE RISCO
- Não se sabe se essa síndrome é a manifestação de um problema comportamental subjacente, um distúrbio convulsivo atípico ou uma neuropatia sensorial localizada ou miopatia indutora de hiperestesia. Especula-se que a causa seja multifatorial ou que a síndrome não seja uma entidade patológica distinta com uma única causa, mas pode se desenvolver graças a uma variedade de fatores distintos.
- Os gatos que tendem a ser nervosos ou hiperexcitáveis foram descritos como os de maior risco; estresses ambientais podem servir como fator de deflagração.

DIAGNÓSTICO

DIAGNÓSTICO DIFERENCIAL
- Problemas dermatológicos que causam prurido — parasitários (p. ex., pulgas, *Notoedres* e *Cheyletiella*), fúngicos (p. ex., dermatofitose) ou alérgicos (p. ex., parasitas, inalantes e alimentos); avaliar o paciente em busca de indícios de dermatite subjacente; os raspados cutâneos e as culturas fúngicas podem ajudar a confirmar o diagnóstico.
- Doenças da coluna vertebral que levam à dor espinal — degenerativas (doença de disco intervertebral), inflamatórias (discospondilite, meningite local), neoplásicas ou traumáticas; a radiografia da coluna vertebral é útil para avaliar anormalidades que possam causar dor localizada; outros métodos diagnósticos (p. ex., mielografia, sorologia para pesquisa de agentes infecciosos, análise do LCS) podem ser necessários.
- Doenças do prosencéfalo que induzem a alterações comportamentais e/ou crises convulsivas — metabólicas (encefalopatia hepática), infecciosas/ inflamatórias (vírus da leucemia felina, vírus da imunodeficiência felina, peritonite infecciosa felina, criptococose, toxoplasmose), neoplásicas, vasculares; a avaliação diagnóstica completa, inclusive a tolerância aos ácidos biliares, sorologia para causas infecciosas de encefalite, análise do LCS e imagens do cérebro, pode ser indicada para detectar a doença cerebral subjacente.
- Problemas comportamentais — transtorno compulsivo; diagnóstico por exclusão.

HEMOGRAMA/BIOQUÍMICA/URINÁLISE
- Frequentemente normais.
- O aumento no nível de globulina foi relatado em alguns gatos.

OUTROS TESTES LABORATORIAIS
Nenhum é necessário.

DIAGNÓSTICO POR IMAGEM
Não é necessário além daquele para excluir os diagnósticos diferenciais.

MÉTODOS DIAGNÓSTICOS
- O diagnóstico é formulado com base nos achados anamnésicos e clínicos característicos, bem como por exclusão de outras doenças que possam causar sinais clínicos semelhantes.
- Atualmente, não há exame nem conjunto de exames que confirmem um diagnóstico definitivo.
- EMG — revelou indícios de atividade espontânea anormal nos músculos epaxiais toracolombares em um único estudo feito com gatos acometidos.
- Biopsia muscular — em gatos com alterações EMG; pode revelar inúmeros vacúolos dentro dos músculos epaxiais, com anticorpos marcados característicos semelhantes aos descritos na miosite/miopatia com corpúsculos de inclusão em seres humanos.

TRATAMENTO

- Ambulatorial.
- Eliminar alterações do ambiente que possam precipitar os episódios.
- A modificação comportamental foi bem-sucedida em reduzir as manifestações clínicas em alguns gatos.
- Nos casos graves de automutilação, talvez seja necessário o uso de colar elizabetano ou a aplicação de bandagem na cauda.

MEDICAÇÕES

MEDICAMENTO(S)
- Vários agentes farmacológicos são recomendados, dependendo da causa subjacente sob suspeita.
- A prednisolona é indicada na suspeita de dermatite pruriginosa.
- Os medicamentos anticonvulsivantes são frequentemente utilizados. O fenobarbital (1-2 mg/kg VO a cada 12 h) é o mais eficaz, mas não controla de forma bem-sucedida os episódios em todos os gatos. A gabapentina (5-10 mg/kg VO a cada 12 h) também pode ser utilizada por suas propriedades anticonvulsivantes, bem como para tratamento de dor neuropática.
- Inibidores seletivos de recaptação da serotonina (fluoxetina 0,5-2,0 mg/kg VO a cada 24 h), antidepressivos tricíclicos (clomipramina 0,5-1,0 mg/kg VO a cada 24 h) ou benzodiazepínicos (lorazepam 0,125-0,50 mg VO a cada 8-24 h) são recomendados na suspeita de algum transtorno comportamental primário.
- Carnitina e coenzima Q10 — em caso de miopatia subjacente.
- A resposta terapêutica é variável. Em gatos responsivos, a terapia frequentemente prossegue pelo resto da vida, pois é comum o retorno dos ataques após a suspensão dos medicamentos.

ACOMPANHAMENTO

MONITORIZAÇÃO DO PACIENTE
Para os gatos submetidos ao fenobarbital — verificar as concentrações séricas do medicamento em 2-3 semanas; repetir o hemograma completo e o perfil bioquímico em intervalos de 6-12 meses para monitorizar os efeitos adversos.

PREVENÇÃO
Evitar quaisquer estresses ambientais conhecidos.

EVOLUÇÃO ESPERADA E PROGNÓSTICO
O prognóstico depende da identificação da causa subjacente e da resposta à medicação, bem como da frequência e gravidade dos episódios.

DIVERSOS

ABREVIATURA(S)
- EMG = eletromiografia.
- LCS = líquido cerebrospinal.

Sugestões de Leitura
Ciribassi J. Feline hyperesthesia syndrome. Compend Contin Educ Pract Vet 2009, 31:116-132.

Autor Karen R. Muñana
Consultor Editorial Joane M. Parent

Síndrome de Hiperviscosidade

CONSIDERAÇÕES GERAIS

REVISÃO
- Trata-se de uma variedade de sinais clínicos causados por alta viscosidade sanguínea.
- Resulta tipicamente de uma concentração acentuadamente elevada de proteínas plasmáticas, embora possa resultar (raras vezes) da contagem de eritrócitos ou leucócitos extremamente alta.
- Observada com maior frequência como uma síndrome paraneoplásica, associada em geral ao mieloma múltiplo e a outros tumores linfoides ou leucemia.
- A proteína plasmática total pode ultrapassar 10 g/dL, com gamopatia monoclonal revelada pelo exame de eletroforese das proteínas séricas.
- Sinais clínicos causados pela redução do fluxo sanguíneo através dos vasos de calibre menor, alto volume plasmático e coagulopatia associada.
- Os sistemas acometidos incluem hematológico/linfático/imune, oftálmico e nervoso.

IDENTIFICAÇÃO
- Os cães são acometidos com maior frequência que os gatos.
- Não há predominância sexual nem racial.
- Mais comum em animais mais idosos em virtude do aumento na incidência de processos neoplásicos.

SINAIS CLÍNICOS
Achados Anamnésicos
- Sem sinais compatíveis.
- Anorexia.
- Letargia.
- Depressão.
- Poliúria e polidipsia.
- Cegueira, ataxia e crises convulsivas.
- Tendências hemorrágicas.

Achados do Exame Físico
- Déficits neurológicos, inclusive crises convulsivas e desorientação.
- Taquicardia e taquipneia se houver insuficiência cardíaca congestiva por sobrecarga volêmica.
- Epistaxe ou outro sangramento de mucosa.
- Hepatomegalia/esplenomegalia/linfadenopatia.
- Déficits visuais associados a congestão dos vasos da retina, hemorragia ou descolamento da retina e papiledema.

CAUSAS E FATORES DE RISCO
- Mieloma múltiplo e plasmocitomas (IgM > IgA > IgG).
- Leucemia linfocítica ou linfoma.
- Policitemia acentuada (hematócrito >65%).
- Inflamação atípica crônica com gamopatia monoclonal (p. ex., erliquiose em cães).
- Doença autoimune crônica (p. ex., lúpus eritematoso sistêmico e artrite reumatoide) — muito rara.

DIAGNÓSTICO

DIAGNÓSTICO DIFERENCIAL
- Outra doença neurológica inexplicável ou distúrbios hemorrágicos.
- Policitemia apropriada (p. ex., desvio cardíaco da direita para a esquerda).
- Hiperviscosidade é uma síndrome, e não o diagnóstico definitivo.

HEMOGRAMA/BIOQUÍMICA/URINÁLISE
- Anemia arregenerativa (em pacientes sem policitemia como uma causa de hiperviscosidade), trombocitopenia ou leucopenia.
- Hiperproteinemia (proteína plasmática total >9 g/dL) e hiperglobulinemia (>5 g/dL).
- Azotemia e hipercalcemia se a hiperviscosidade for causada por uma síndrome paraneoplásica.
- Isostenúria e proteinúria acentuada.

OUTROS TESTES LABORATORIAIS
- Alta concentração de IgG, IgA e IgM, conforme detectado pela radioimunodifusão.
- Viscosidade plasmática ou sérica alta (>3 em relação à água).
- Prolongamento nos tempos de protrombina ou de tromboplastina parcial ativada.

DIAGNÓSTICO POR IMAGEM
É possível a constatação de hepatosplenomegalia, cardiomegalia e lesões osteolíticas (associadas ao mieloma múltiplo).

MÉTODOS DIAGNÓSTICOS
- Infiltrado plasmocitário ou linfoide, revelado pela biopsia de medula óssea.
- Proteinúria de Bence-Jones em pacientes com mieloma múltiplo.

TRATAMENTO

CUIDADO(S) DE SAÚDE ADEQUADO(S)
- Geralmente, tratar de forma ambulatorial.
- Tratar a doença subjacente.
- Flebotomia (15-20 mL/kg) com reposição volêmica com fluido cristaloide.
- Plasmaférese (10-15 mL/kg), se disponível.

CUIDADO(S) DE ENFERMAGEM
De acordo com a doença subjacente.

MEDICAÇÕES

MEDICAMENTO(S)
- Providenciar tratamento para a condição neoplásica ou inflamatória subjacente.
- Ver em outros capítulos a terapia medicamentosa para a causa subjacente (p. ex., plasmocitomas, leucemia linfocítica, linfoma, erliquiose e policitemia).

CONTRAINDICAÇÕES/INTERAÇÕES POSSÍVEIS
- Evitar o uso de medicações que possam aumentar o volume vascular, inclusive os coloides sintéticos (p. ex., hetamido); não tentar corrigir o baixo nível compensatório de albumina.
- Evitar medicações que alteram a função plaquetária (p. ex., AINE).

ACOMPANHAMENTO

MONITORIZAÇÃO DO PACIENTE
- Monitorizar as proteínas plasmáticas ou séricas com frequência como uma espécie de marcador da eficácia terapêutica.
- Obter hemograma completo, perfil bioquímico e urinálise para monitorizar outras anormalidades laboratoriais.

DIVERSOS

VER TAMBÉM
- Erliquiose.
- Leucemia Linfocítica Crônica.
- Linfoma — Cães.
- Linfoma — Gatos.
- Mieloma Múltiplo.
- Plasmocitoma Mucocutâneo.
- Policitemia.

ABREVIATURA(S)
- AINE = anti-inflamatório não esteroide.

Sugestões de Leitura
Hohenhaus AE. Syndromes of hyperglobulinemia: Diagnosis and therapy. In: Kirk RW, ed., Current Veterinary Therapy XII. Philadelphia: Saunders, 1995, pp. 523-530.

Autor Elizabeth A. Rozanski
Consultor Editorial A.H. Rebar

SÍNDROME DE HORNER

CONSIDERAÇÕES GERAIS
REVISÃO
- Desnervação simpática do olho.
- Via anatômica muito importante.
- Acomete os sistemas nervoso e oftálmico.

Hipotálamo
↓
Tronco cerebral/medula cervical
Segmentos espinais de T1-T3
e raízes nervosas
↓
Tronco vagossimpático
↓
Gânglio cervical cranial
↓
Orelha média
↓
Ramo oftálmico (V par de nervos cranianos)
↓
Nervo ciliar longo
↓
Músculo dilatador da íris
↓
Outras fibras: músculo liso na periórbita, pálpebra superior e terceira pálpebra

Figura 1

IDENTIFICAÇÃO
- Idiopática — um único estudo sugere que machos da raça Golden retriever com 4-13 anos de idade estão sob maior risco.
- Idiopática — cães, 50-93%; gatos, 45%.
- Outras causas — N/D.

SINAIS CLÍNICOS
- Miose.
- Protrusão da terceira pálpebra.
- Ptose (queda) da pálpebra superior.
- Enoftalmia.
- Otite — possível.
- Outras anormalidades neurológicas — possíveis.

CAUSAS E FATORES DE RISCO
Ver Tabela 1.

DIAGNÓSTICO
DIAGNÓSTICO DIFERENCIAL
Uveíte anterior — pressão intraocular geralmente baixa; rubor aquoso.

DIAGNÓSTICO POR IMAGEM
- Ver Tabela 1.
- Radiografias da coluna vertebral e mielograma — podem revelar a lesão da medula espinal.
- Radiografias torácicas — podem apontar a causa da lesão ao tronco simpático (p. ex., traumatismo e tumor mediastínico).
- Radiografias do crânio — podem demonstrar problema na orelha média.
- TC e RM — podem ajudar a identificar lesão no tronco cerebral, massa retrobulbar ou problema na orelha média.
- Ultrassonografia — da região orbital; pode exibir massa retrobulbar.

MÉTODOS DIAGNÓSTICOS
- Ver Tabela 1.
- Punção do LCS — investigar doença no cérebro e na medula espinal.
- Eletromiografia — pesquisar por avulsão do plexo braquial.
- Testes farmacológicos — ver "Anisocoria".

TRATAMENTO
Tratar a doença subjacente.

MEDICAÇÕES
MEDICAMENTO(S)
- Dependem da causa subjacente.
- Idiopática — nenhum.

ACOMPANHAMENTO
- Depende da gravidade da doença subjacente.
- Idiopática — a recuperação parcial ou completa pode levar até 4 meses.

DIVERSOS
ABREVIATURA(S)
- LCS = líquido cerebrospinal.
- NMI = neurônio motor inferior.
- NMS = neurônio motor superior.
- RM = ressonância magnética.
- TC = tomografia computadorizada.

Sugestões de Leitura
ShamirMH, Ofri R. Comparative neuro-ophthalmology. In: Gelatt KN, ed., Veterinary Ophthalmology, 4th ed. Ames, IA: Blackwell, 2007, pp. 1406-1469.

Autor David Lipsitz
Consultor Editorial Paul E. Miller

Tabela 1.

Resumo de lesões que resultam em síndrome de Horner			
Localização	*Causas*	*Sinais Neurológicos Associados*	*Plano Diagnóstico*
Tronco cerebral	Traumatismo; neoplasia; doenças infecciosas; processos inflamatórios; distúrbios vasculares	Alterações do estado mental; defeitos motores ipsolaterais; déficits de nervos cranianos ipsolaterais	TC ou RM; análise do LCS
Medula espinal cervical	Traumatismo; disco; neoplasia; embolia fibrocartilaginosa	Hemiparesia/paralisia ipsolaterais; tetraparesia/paralisia; NMS; membros torácicos/pélvicos	Radiografias da coluna vertebral; análise do LCS; mielograma, RM
Medula espinal de T1-T3	Traumatismo; disco; neoplasia; embolia fibrocartilaginosa	NMI: membro(s) torácico(s); NMS: membro(s) pélvico(s)	Radiografias da coluna vertebral; análise do LCS; mielograma, RM
Raízes ventrais de T1-T3	Avulsão do plexo braquial; tumor da bainha nervosa	Lesão do plexo braquial ipsolateral; perda ipsolateral do reflexo do panículo	Exame neurológico; eletromiografia; RM
Tronco simpático, gânglio cervical cranial	Traumatismo; neoplasia mediastínica; traumatismo iatrogênico-cirúrgico	Unilaterais: nenhum; Bilaterais: disfunção laríngea/faríngea	Radiografias torácicas; ultrassonografia do pescoço, RM
Orelha média	Traumatismo; neoplasia; otite média/interna; pólipo nasofaríngeo (gato)	Vestibulopatia periférica ipsolateral; paralisia do nervo facial ipsolateral	Exame otológico; radiografias ou TC da bula timpânica; RM; miringotomia
Retrobulbar	Traumatismo; neoplasia; abscesso	Variáveis: nenhum ou acometimento dos nervos cranianos II, III, IV, V, VI	TC ou RM; ultrassonografia da órbita

Síndrome de Tremor Generalizado (Síndrome do Cão Tremedor)

CONSIDERAÇÕES GERAIS

REVISÃO
Tremor de todo o corpo.

IDENTIFICAÇÃO
- Cães.
- Raças de pequeno a médio porte (<15 kg), cães jovens adultos (<5 kg), independentemente da coloração da pelagem.
- Cães com pelagens brancas (p. ex., Maltês e West Highland white terrier) — super-representados do ponto de vista histórico.
- Ambos os sexos são acometidos.

SINAIS CLÍNICOS
- Tremor corporal difuso.
- Inicialmente, pode ser confundida com sinais de apreensão ou hipotermia.

CAUSAS E FATORES DE RISCO
Mais frequentemente associada à doença inflamatória leve do SNC.

DIAGNÓSTICO

DIAGNÓSTICO DIFERENCIAL
Ingestão de micotoxina, crises convulsivas.

HEMOGRAMA/BIOQUÍMICA/URINÁLISE
Geralmente normais.

OUTROS TESTES LABORATORIAIS
N/D.

DIAGNÓSTICO POR IMAGEM
N/D.

OUTROS MÉTODOS DIAGNÓSTICOS
Análise do LCS coletado pela cisterna cerebelomedular — leve pleocitose monocítica ou linfocitária com teor normal de proteínas; o LCS pode permanecer normal.

TRATAMENTO

Paciente ambulatorial ou internado, dependendo da gravidade dos sinais clínicos.

MEDICAÇÕES

MEDICAMENTO(S)
- Doença responsiva a esteroides; prednisolona ou prednisona (1-2 mg/kg divididos a cada 12 h) nas primeiras 1-2 semanas.
- Dependendo da resposta clínica, reduzir a dosagem de forma gradativa (geralmente, em 4-6 meses); avaliar periodicamente quanto à ocorrência de deterioração clínica; se a dosagem for reduzida com muita rapidez, os sinais clínicos poderão recidivar, necessitando de reindução da dose inicial.
- Muitos pacientes não necessitam de tratamento adicional.

CONTRAINDICAÇÕES/INTERAÇÕES POSSÍVEIS
Corticosteroides — podem estar contraindicados em caso de encefalite infecciosa.

ACOMPANHAMENTO

MONITORIZAÇÃO DO PACIENTE
Avaliações semanais por cerca de 1 mês; em seguida, mensalmente, até que os corticosteroides sejam interrompidos.

PREVENÇÃO
N/D.

COMPLICAÇÕES POSSÍVEIS
N/D.

EVOLUÇÃO ESPERADA E PROGNÓSTICO
- Os sinais clínicos costumam desaparecer em 3-7 dias após o início do tratamento com esteroides.
- Em alguns pacientes, a recidiva necessita da retomada dos corticosteroides.
- Para manter a remissão, uma pequena porcentagem dos pacientes necessita dos corticosteroides em doses baixas, em dias alternados, por tempo indefinido.

DIVERSOS

SINÔNIMO(S)
- Cerebelite idiopática.
- Síndrome do tremor.

VER TAMBÉM
Tremores.

ABREVIATURA(S)
- LCS = líquido cerebrospinal.
- SNC = sistema nervoso central.

Sugestões de Leitura
Bagley RS, Kornegay JN, Wheeler SJ, et al. Generalized tremors in Maltese: Clinical findings in seven cases. JAAHA 1993, 29:141-145.
Wagner SO, Podell M, Fenner WR. Generalized tremors in dogs: 24 cases (1984-1995). JAVMA 1997, 211:731-735.

Autor Rodney S. Bagley
Consultor Editorial Joane M. Parent

SÍNDROME DE WOLFF-PARKINSON-WHITE

CONSIDERAÇÕES GERAIS

DEFINIÇÃO
• Ocorre pré-excitação ventricular quando os impulsos originários no nó sinoatrial ou no átrio ativam uma porção dos ventrículos de forma prematura por uma via acessória, sem passar pelo nó AV; o restante dos ventrículos é ativado normalmente pelo sistema de condução usual.
• A síndrome de WPW consiste na pré-excitação ventricular com episódios de taquicardia supraventricular paroxística (Figs. 1 e 2).

Características Eletrocardiográficas de Pré-excitação Ventricular
• Frequência e ritmo cardíacos normais.
• Ondas P normais.
• Intervalo P-R curto (cães, <0,06 s; gatos, <0,05 s).
• Aumento na amplitude do QRS (cães de pequeno porte, >0,05 s; cães de grande porte, >0,06 s; gatos, >0,04 s), frequentemente com *slurring* [ausência de segmento ST, ou seja, a onda R segue o registro eletrocardiográfico direto na onda T] ou *notching* [fenestração ou chanfradura da onda R] do ramo ascendente da onda R (onda delta).

Características Eletrocardiográficas de Pré-excitação Ventricular com a Síndrome de WPW
• Frequência cardíaca extremamente rápida (cães, muitas vezes com >300 bpm; gatos, próxima aos 400-500 bpm).
• A identificação das ondas P pode não ser uma tarefa fácil.
• Os complexos QRS podem permanecer normais, exibir aumento na amplitude com ondas delta ou, então, ficar bastante largos e bizarros, dependendo do circuito.
• A condução costuma ser de 1:1 (i. e., 1 onda P para cada complexo QRS).

FISIOPATOLOGIA
• Pode estar associada a defeitos cardíacos congênitos ou adquiridos em cães ou gatos.
• Também pode estar relacionada com miocardiopatia hipertrófica em gatos.
• Ocorre comprometimento hemodinâmico durante os episódios de taquicardia supraventricular com a síndrome de WPW.

SISTEMA(S) ACOMETIDO(S)
Cardiovascular.

INCIDÊNCIA/PREVALÊNCIA
Desconhecidas.

IDENTIFICAÇÃO
Espécies
Cães e gatos.

SINAIS CLÍNICOS
Achados Anamnésicos
• Ausentes em animais com pré-excitação ventricular.
• Síncope em pacientes com a síndrome de WPW.

Achados do Exame Físico
• Ausentes em animais com pré-excitação ventricular.
• Taquicardia em animais com a síndrome de WPW.

CAUSAS
Cardiopatia Congênita
• Defeito congênito limitado ao sistema de condução.
• Defeito do septo atrial em cães ou gatos.
• Displasia da valva atrioventricular direita (tricúspide) em cães.

Cardiopatia Adquirida
• Miocardiopatia hipertrófica em gatos.

DIAGNÓSTICO

DIAGNÓSTICO DIFERENCIAL
• Pré-excitação ventricular — diferenciar de outras causas de encurtamento dos intervalos P-R (p. ex., febre, hipertireoidismo e anemia); essas condições não produzem ondas delta.
• Síndrome de WPW com complexos estreitos — diferenciar de outras arritmias supraventriculares (p. ex., taquicardia atrial, flutter atrial e fibrilação atrial); a síndrome de WPW é identificada com mais facilidade após a conversão para frequência e ritmo cardíacos normais.
• Síndrome de WPW alternante — não deve ser confundida com bigeminismo ventricular.
• Síndrome de WPW com complexos largos — é imprescindível diferenciá-la de taquicardia ventricular.
• Intervalo P-R curto — poderá estar correlacionado com um complexo QRS normal se a via anômala se desviar do nó AV e se unir ao feixe de His (i. e., síndrome de Lown-Ganong-Levine).

HEMOGRAMA/BIOQUÍMICA/URINÁLISE
Normais.

OUTROS TESTES LABORATORIAIS
Normais.

DIAGNÓSTICO POR IMAGEM
A ecocardiografia pode revelar cardiopatias estruturais.

MÉTODOS DIAGNÓSTICOS
Eletrocardiografia.

ACHADOS PATOLÓGICOS
• Os achados patológicos variam de acordo com a causa subjacente.
• Existe a possibilidade de não haver nenhuma lesão cardíaca.

TRATAMENTO

CUIDADO(S) DE SAÚDE ADEQUADO(S)
• Pré-excitação ventricular sem taquicardia — não há necessidade de tratamento.
• A síndrome de WPW requer a conversão do ritmo por meio de pressão dos olhos ou do seio carotídeo, choque por corrente direta (o tratamento mais eficaz) ou medicamentos.

ATIVIDADE
Em casos da síndrome de WPW, pode ser preciso limitar a atividade física até que as taquicardias supraventriculares sejam controladas.

ORIENTAÇÃO AO PROPRIETÁRIO
WPW — explicar a necessidade de identificar e tratar a causa subjacente, além da terapia direcionada para a taquicardia supraventricular.

CONSIDERAÇÕES CIRÚRGICAS
Ablação por cateter com o uso de corrente de radiofrequência — consiste em uma técnica relativamente recente, que confere a destruição ou a remoção das vias acessórias por meio de cateter transvenoso posicionado no local da via; pode constituir uma alternativa de escolha à terapia medicamentosa vitalícia.

MEDICAÇÕES

MEDICAMENTO(S) DE ESCOLHA
• Em seres humanos, empregam-se diversos medicamentos; as opiniões diferem em relação aos agentes terapêuticos de escolha.
• Lidocaína em bólus IV (2 mg/kg), acompanhada por gotejamento IV (25-75 µg/kg/min em velocidade de infusão constante — apenas nos cães).
• Esmolol (cães e gatos, 50-100 mg/kg em bólus; 50-200 µg/kg/min em velocidade de infusão constante).
• Propranolol (gatos, 2,5-5 mg VO a cada 8-12 h; cães, 0,2-1 mg/kg VO a cada 8 h) ou atenolol (gatos, 6,2-12,5 mg VO a cada 24 h; cães, 0,25-1 mg/kg VO a cada 12 h).
• O diltiazem pode ser eficaz (gatos, 1-2,5 mg/kg VO a cada 8 h; cães, 0,5-1,5 mg/kg VO a cada 8 h).

CONTRAINDICAÇÕES
• Digitálicos, verapamil e propranolol — podem ser contraindicados; como esses medicamentos retardam a condução através do nó AV, podem favorecer a condução através das vias anômalas.
• Gatos — o propranolol e o atenolol constituem os agentes de escolha.

ACOMPANHAMENTO

MONITORIZAÇÃO DO PACIENTE
ECG seriado.

COMPLICAÇÕES POSSÍVEIS
Nenhuma esperada.

EVOLUÇÃO ESPERADA E PROGNÓSTICO
Dependem da gravidade da causa subjacente; a maioria dos pacientes com a síndrome de WPW responde à terapia para taquicardia supraventricular — prognóstico favorável.

DIVERSOS

ABREVIATURA(S)
• AV = atrioventricular.
• bpm = batimentos por minuto.
• ECG = eletrocardiograma.
• WPW = Wolff-Parkinson-White.

RECURSOS DA INTERNET
www.vetgo.com/cardio

Sugestões de Leitura
Al-Khatib SM, Pritchett ELC. Clinical features of Wolff-Parkinson-White syndrome. Am Heart J 1999, 138:403-413.

SÍNDROME DE WOLFF-PARKINSON-WHITE

Hill BL, Tilley LP. Ventricular preexcitation in seven dogs and nine cats. JAVMA 1985, 187:1026-1031.

Kittleson MD. Electrocardiography. In Kittleson MD, Kienle RD, eds., Small Animal Cardiovascular Medicine. St. Louis: Mosby, 1998, pp. 72-94.

Kraus MS, Gelzer ARM, Moise S. Treatment of cardiac arrhythmias and conduction disturbances. In: Tilley LP, Smith FWK, Oyama MA, Sleeper MM, eds., Manual of Canine and Feline Cardiology, 4th ed. St. Louis: Saunders Elsevier, 2008, pp. 315-332.

Tilley LP. Essentials of Canine and Feline Electrocardiography, 3rd ed. Baltimore: Williams & Wilkins, 1992. Wright KN. Assessment and treatment of supraventricular tachyarrhythmias. In: Bonagura JD, ed., Kirk's Current Veterinary Therapy XIII. Philadelphia: Saunders, 2000, pp. 726-729.

Autores Larry P. Tilley e Naomi L. Burtnick
Consultores Editoriais Larry P. Tilley e Francis W.K. Smith, Jr.

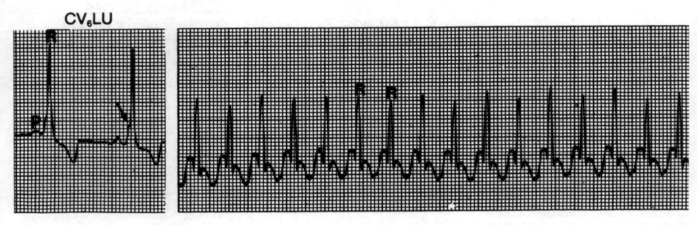

Figura 1. Síndrome de Wolff-Parkinson-White (canina). A pré-excitação ventricular está representada pelo intervalo P-R curto, pelo complexo QRS largo e pela onda delta (seta) na derivação CV$_6$LU. A atividade paroxística da taquicardia supraventricular está exibida na derivação II (registro longo). (De: Tilley LP: *Essentials of canine and feline electrocardiography*. 3. ed., Baltimore: Lippincott Williams & Wilkins, 1992, com permissão.)

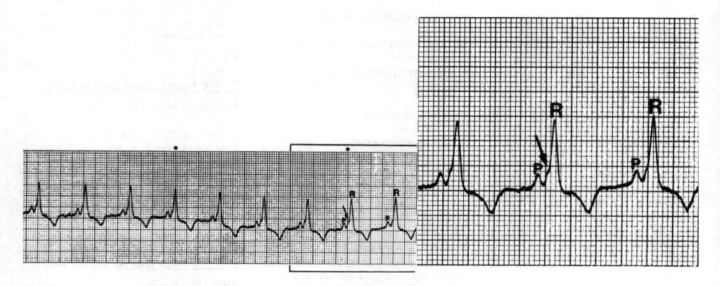

Figura 2. Pré-excitação ventricular em gato com episódios de desmaio. As ondas P apresentam-se normais, mas o intervalo P-R encontra-se curto e o complexo QRS, largo; também há ondas delta (setas). (De: Tilley LP: *Essentials of canine and feline electrocardiography*. 3. ed., Baltimore: Lippincott Williams & Wilkins, 1992, com permissão.)

SÍNDROME DO INTESTINO IRRITÁVEL

CONSIDERAÇÕES GERAIS

DEFINIÇÃO
Distúrbio caracterizado por sinais intermitentes crônicos de disfunção colônica e/ou dismotilidade na ausência de patologia gastrintestinal estrutural ou diagnóstico alternativo.

FISIOPATOLOGIA
• Há hipóteses da existência de uma relação psicossomática entre o comportamento do paciente e as respostas dos sistemas nervosos autônomo e entérico. • As causas interativas potenciais podem incluir motilidade colônica anormal, deficiência de fibra na dieta, intolerâncias alimentares, estresse/ansiedade, doença gastrintestinal concomitante.

SISTEMA(S) ACOMETIDO(S)
Gastrintestinal.

INCIDÊNCIA/PREVALÊNCIA
• Embora a incidência de síndrome do intestino irritável seja desconhecida, o autor acredita que ela seja menor que 5%.

IDENTIFICAÇÃO
Espécies
Cães (incomum); gatos (raro).
Raça(s) Predominante(s)
Qualquer raça pode ser acometida; considera-se que cães de trabalho ou raças caninas individuais sejam mais suscetíveis ao estresse.

SINAIS CLÍNICOS
Achados Anamnésicos
• São muito comuns sinais intermitentes crônicos de doença do intestino grosso, incluindo a eliminação frequente de pequenas quantidades de fezes e de muco, além de disquezia e constipação; os sintomas podem se alternar. • Também podem ocorrer dor abdominal, íleo paralítico segmentar (timpanismo), vômito e náusea.
Achados do Exame Físico
• Frequentemente não são dignos de nota. • A dor abdominal pode ser evidente.

CAUSAS
Desconhecidas.

FATORES DE RISCO
• Estresse (p. ex., mudanças na casa, modificação da dieta, ansiedade da separação) pode estar associado a episódios sintomáticos. • Em muitos cães, o estresse parece não desempenhar qualquer papel.

DIAGNÓSTICO

• Formulado com base na exclusão de todas as outras causas potenciais de sinais atribuídos ao intestino grosso. • Reservado para os pacientes submetidos a uma avaliação diagnóstica completa, incluindo biopsias gastrintestinais, vermifugação terapêutica (particularmente contra tricúris), dietas com alto teor de fibras (solúveis e/ou insolúveis) e brandas sem resolução dos sinais.

DIAGNÓSTICO DIFERENCIAL
Causas de Doença do Intestino Grosso
• Tricúris. • Colite inflamatória. • Pólipos retais. • *Clostridium perfringens*. • Colite associada à *Escherichia coli* aderente invasiva. • Diarreia do intestino grosso responsiva a fibras. • Imprudência alimentar (coloproctite induzida por corpo estranho) ou intolerância alimentar. • *Giardia*. • Histoplasmose. • Pitiose. • Neoplasia colorretal. • Inversão cecal. • Enteropatia causada pelo glúten. • Saculite anal. • Megacólon (pseudo-obstrução colorretal).
Doenças com Sinais Semelhantes
• Disúria/estrangúria — excluir por meio de observação, urinálise e técnicas de diagnóstico por imagem. • Prostatopatia — descartar com exame retal e técnicas de diagnóstico por imagem.

HEMOGRAMA/BIOQUÍMICA/URINÁLISE
Normais.

OUTROS TESTES LABORATORIAIS
Exame coprológico direto, flutuação fecal e citologia do raspado fecal/retal — normais.

DIAGNÓSTICO POR IMAGEM
• Estudos radiográficos simples e contrastados do abdome — normais ou podem revelar distensão gasosa luminal segmentar. • Ultrassonografia abdominal — normal.

MÉTODOS DIAGNÓSTICOS
• A colonoscopia geralmente é normal. • Amostras de biopsia da mucosa coletadas a partir de múltiplas áreas no cólon e no reto permanecem normais.

ACHADOS PATOLÓGICOS
• Normais. • Enteropatia crônica concomitante (p. ex., enteropatia inflamatória) pode estar presente e necessita de um controle bem-sucedido antes de se prosseguir com o diagnóstico e o tratamento da síndrome do intestino irritável.

TRATAMENTO

CUIDADO(S) DE SAÚDE ADEQUADO(S)
Tratamento clínico ambulatorial.

ATIVIDADE
O aumento na atividade física de rotina pode estimular mais a função colônica normal e reduzir o nível de estresse do animal de estimação.

DIETA
O consumo de dieta altamente digestível com fibra solúvel adicionada frequentemente é útil; se aumentada, a fibra solúvel não é útil; depois, tentar um aumento de fibra insolúvel; pode resultar em uma melhora variável.

ORIENTAÇÃO AO PROPRIETÁRIO
• A resposta ao tratamento é variável.
• Minimizar o estresse.

MEDICAÇÕES

MEDICAMENTO(S) DE ESCOLHA
• A terapia medicamentosa pode variar desde vários dias até o resto da vida.
• O autor acredita que a maioria dos casos de síndrome do intestino irritável em cães envolva hipermotilidade (espasmódica) gastrintestinal e o medicamento de escolha mais comum é o Librax® (um antiespasmódico com ansiolítico).
• Iniciar com o extremo mais baixo da faixa posológica.
Modificadores da Motilidade
• Antidiarreicos opiáceos melhoram os sinais clínicos pelo aumento da segmentação rítmica.
• Loperamida 0,1-0,2 mg/kg VO a cada 8-12 h.
• Difenoxilato 0,05-0,2 mg/kg VO a cada 8-12 h.
Combinações de Antiespasmódico-Tranquilizante-Ansiolítico
• Utilizadas para aliviar os sinais de ansiedade, cólicas abdominais, timpanismo e angústia.
• Librax® — clordiazepóxido (ansiolítico) e brometo de clidínio (anticolinérgico), 0,1-0,25 mg de clidínio/kg VO a cada 8-24 h.
• Darbazine® — isopropamida (anticolinérgico) e proclorperazina (tranquilizante), 0,14-0,22 mg/kg SC a cada 12 h VO.
• Aminopentamida, 0,01-0,02 mg/kg VO, IM, SC.
Antieméticos Parenterais
• Se a náusea e o vômito impedirem a utilização de medicamento por via oral, administrar antieméticos por via parenteral por 1-2 dias.
• Maropitanto, 1 mg/kg SC a cada 24 h em cães.
• Proclorperazina, 0,1-0,5 mg/kg a cada 6-24 h SC ou IM.
Antagonistas Serotoninérgicos
• Ramosetrona é um potente antagonista seletivo dos receptores da serotonina (5-HT3) que se mostrou útil em pessoas com síndrome do intestino irritável; no entanto, nenhum relato foi encontrado além do teste experimental em cães normais.

CONTRAINDICAÇÕES
• Opiáceos — disfunção respiratória, encefalopatia hepática, constipação e/ou debilidade grave.
• Anticolinérgicos — cardiopatia, nefropatia, hipertensão, constipação e/ou hipertireoidismo.

ACOMPANHAMENTO

MONITORIZAÇÃO DO PACIENTE
O proprietário deve monitorar a consistência das fezes e observar sinais de constipação, disquezia e desconforto abdominal.

PREVENÇÃO
Minimizar qualquer fator indutor de estresse capaz de desencadear um episódio.

COMPLICAÇÕES POSSÍVEIS
Passar despercebido por um diagnóstico correto/alternativo constitui o principal risco ao se considerar a síndrome do intestino irritável.

EVOLUÇÃO ESPERADA E PROGNÓSTICO
• Deve-se observar a melhora nas fezes, a redução no muco e o alívio da disquezia e da angústia abdominal dentro de 1-2 dias do início da medicação.
• Em alguns cães, os sinais clínicos desaparecem completamente após o tratamento; outros apresentam sinais clínicos episódicos em longo prazo.

Autor Mark E. Hitt
Consultor Editorial Albert E. Jergens

SÍNDROME DO NÓ SINUSAL DOENTE

CONSIDERAÇÕES GERAIS

DEFINIÇÃO
Distúrbio de formação do impulso dentro do nó sinusal e condução para fora desse nó; a disfunção de marca-passos subsidiários e de outros segmentos do sistema de condução cardíaca frequentemente coexiste com a disfunção do nó sinusal.

Características do ECG
- As arritmias observadas na síndrome do nó sinusal doente incluem qualquer uma das anormalidades a seguir ou todas elas: bradicardia sinusal inapropriada, pausa sinusal (representando parada sinusal ou bloqueio da saída sinoatrial), ritmo atrial ectópico lento ou períodos alternantes de bradiarritmias sinusais e taquicardia supraventricular (Fig. 1).
- Sequências paroxísticas de taquicardia supraventricular podem se alternar com períodos prolongados de inércia do nó sinusal e com frequência inércia do nó AV também, produzindo a síndrome de taquicardia-bradicardia, uma variante da síndrome do nó sinusal doente.
- As ondas P e os complexos QRS geralmente permanecem normais.
- As ondas P podem estar anormais ou ausentes com ritmo ectópico atrial lento ou ritmo de escape juncional.

FISIOPATOLOGIA
- As manifestações do ECG podem preceder o desenvolvimento dos sinais clínicos.
- Em geral, os sinais clínicos resultam da falha dos marca-passos subsidiários em gerar ritmos de escape quando ocorre disfunção do nó sinusal.
- As manifestações clínicas comuns refletem os declínios transitórios na perfusão de órgãos, particularmente a perfusão diminuída do cérebro e da musculatura esquelética.
- Raramente ocorre o desenvolvimento de insuficiência cardíaca congestiva.

SISTEMA(S) ACOMETIDO(S)
- Cardiovascular.
- Sistemas nervoso, musculoesquelético e renal podem ser secundariamente acometidos por causa da hipoperfusão.

GENÉTICA
Pode ser hereditária nos cães das raças Schnauzer miniatura e West Highland white terrier.

IDENTIFICAÇÃO

Espécies
Cães.

Raça(s) Predominante(s)
- Schnauzer miniatura (pode ser hereditária).
- Comumente observada no Cocker spaniel, no Dachshund e no West Highland white terrier.

Idade Média e Faixa Etária
A maioria dos cães tem >6 anos de idade.

Sexo Predominante
Fêmeas.

SINAIS CLÍNICOS

Achados Anamnésicos
- Os sinais clínicos variam desde um quadro assintomático até fraqueza, síncope, colapso e/ou crises convulsivas.
- A morte súbita é pouco frequente.

Achados do Exame Físico
- A frequência cardíaca pode estar anormalmente rápida ou anormalmente lenta.
- Podem ser notadas pausas.
- Alguns pacientes parecem normais.

CAUSAS
- Idiopática.
- Familiar na raça Schnauzer miniatura.
- Doença metastática.
- Doença isquêmica.

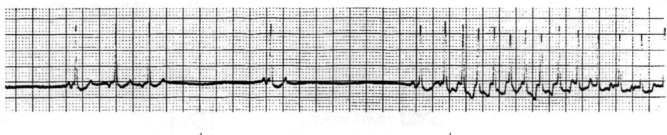

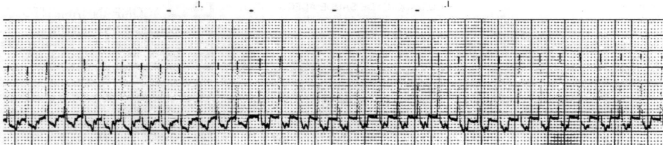

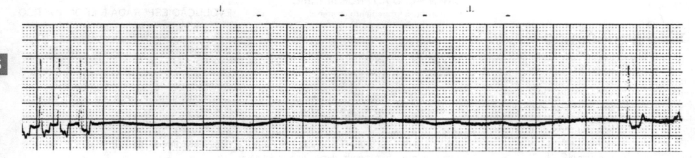

Figura 1. Tira de ritmo contínuo do ECG na derivação II (25 mm/s), registrado a partir de um cão com síndrome do nó sinusal doente, revelando um ritmo atrial ectópico interrompido por várias pausas breves. A terceira pausa inicia uma sequência paroxística de taquicardia supraventricular (250 batimentos/min), seguida por assistolia (6,6 s) finalizada por um complexo de escape juncional.

SÍNDROME DO NÓ SINUSAL DOENTE

DIAGNÓSTICO

DIAGNÓSTICO DIFERENCIAL
- Cães saudáveis podem apresentar bradicardia sinusal (frequência tão baixa quanto 30 batimentos/min) e pausas sinusais (chegando até 3,5 s) normalmente durante o sono.
- Bradicardia e parada sinusal atribuídas ao tônus vagal normal ou aumentado.
- Induzida por medicamentos (digitálicos, antagonistas α-adrenérgicos, agonistas α_2-adrenérgicos, antagonistas dos canais de cálcio, cimetidina, opioides).
- Crises convulsivas ou síncope em virtude de doença não cardíaca.
- Parada atrial secundária à hipercalemia ou doença atrial.
- Fraqueza gerada por doenças neurológicas, musculosqueléticas ou metabólicas.

HEMOGRAMA/BIOQUÍMICA/URINÁLISE
Normais.

DIAGNÓSTICO POR IMAGEM
As raças propensas à síndrome do nó sinusal doente também são predispostas à valvulopatia degenerativa; a ecocardiografia é utilizada para confirmar a presença de doença significativa das válvulas na presença de sopro cardíaco.

MÉTODOS DIAGNÓSTICOS
- Teste de resposta à atropina — indicado nos cães com bradicardia sinusal, parada sinusal e bloqueio da saída sinoatrial. Administrar atropina (0,04 mg/kg IM) e avaliar o ECG 20-30 min depois. A resposta normal (positiva) é um aumento >50% na frequência cardíaca com o desaparecimento das pausas; os cães com síndrome do nó sinusal doente geralmente exibem ausência de resposta ou resposta incompleta à atropina.
- Teste eletrofisiológico do tempo de recuperação do nó sinusal e do tempo de condução sinoatrial.
- Registro ambulatório do ECG de 24 h (monitor Holter) ou monitorização do evento para correlacionar os sinais clínicos com a arritmia.

ACHADOS PATOLÓGICOS
Variam com a causa.

TRATAMENTO

CUIDADO(S) DE SAÚDE ADEQUADO(S)
- Raramente a hospitalização é necessária, exceto para a realização do teste eletrofisiológico ou para o implante de marca-passo.
- Não tratar os animais assintomáticos.

ATIVIDADE
Evitar exercícios vigorosos e situações estressantes.

DIETA
Não há necessidade de modificação.

ORIENTAÇÃO AO PROPRIETÁRIO
O proprietário deve estar consciente de que o tratamento clínico frequentemente é ineficaz.

CONSIDERAÇÕES CIRÚRGICAS
- É necessária a colocação de marca-passo permanente para os cães que deixam de responder ao tratamento clínico e para aqueles que apresentem efeitos colaterais inaceitáveis da medicação.
- Em geral, o marca-passo permanente é necessário para os cães com síndrome de taquicardia-bradicardia.

MEDICAÇÕES

MEDICAMENTO(S)
- Não tratar os animais assintomáticos.
- Os cães sintomáticos são agrupados naqueles que apresentam principalmente bradicardia, parada sinusal e/ou bloqueio da saída sinoatrial e aqueles com taquicardia supraventricular seguida por parada sinusal.
- Cães sintomáticos responsivos à atropina com bradicardia ou parada sinusal — agentes anticolinérgicos (propantelina: cães de pequeno porte 3,75-7,5 mg VO a cada 8-12 h, cães de porte médio 15 mg VO a cada 8 h, cães de grande porte 30 mg VO a cada 8 h; hiosciamina: 0,003-0,006 mg/kg a cada 8 h).
- Cães com bradicardia e parada sinusal — pode-se tentar a teofilina (Theo-Dur®, 20 mg/kg VO a cada 12 h), a terbutalina (0,2 mg/kg VO a cada 8-12 h) ou a hidralazina (1-2 mg/kg VO a cada 8-12 h) se os medicamentos anticolinérgicos forem ineficazes (evitar a hidralazina em paciente hipotenso).
- Cães com bradicardia-taquicardia cujos sinais clínicos se devam à taquicardia ou à parada sinusal induzida pela taquicardia — pode-se administrar a digoxina (0,005 mg/kg VO a cada 12 h) ou o atenolol (0,5-1 mg/kg VO a cada 12-24 h) na tentativa de suprimir a taquicardia supraventricular (monitorizar com rigor quanto à exacerbação da bradicardia).

CONTRAINDICAÇÕES
Evitar os medicamentos que possam agravar a disfunção do nó sinusal (p. ex., antagonistas β-adrenérgicos, agentes bloqueadores dos canais de cálcio, fenotiazínicos, agentes antiarrítmicos de classes I e III, opioides, cimetidina e agonistas α_2-adrenérgicos).

PRECAUÇÕES
- As tentativas de tratar clinicamente a síndrome de bradicardia-taquicardia sem implante prévio de marca-passo carreiam um risco significativo, porque os medicamentos utilizados para controlar a taquicardia supraventricular podem piorar as bradiarritmias e vice-versa.
- É comum a ocorrência de efeitos adversos da medicação anticolinérgica (constipação, dificuldade de micção, ceratoconjuntivite seca, êmese).

ACOMPANHAMENTO

MONITORIZAÇÃO DO PACIENTE
- ECG nos pacientes assintomáticos — para detectar a evolução da doença.
- ECG nos pacientes submetidos a tratamento clínico ou com implante do marca-passo.

COMPLICAÇÕES POSSÍVEIS
- Raramente a queda na perfusão cerebral ou renal resulta em disfunção renal crônica ou dano ao SNC.
- A presença de valvulopatia significativa tem implicações quanto ao tipo de marca-passo permanente selecionado.

EVOLUÇÃO ESPERADA E PROGNÓSTICO
- Bom, após o implante de marca-passo nos animais sem insuficiência cardíaca congestiva.
- Tratamento clínico — frequentemente ineficaz; os efeitos benéficos iniciais quase sempre não se mantêm.

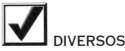

DIVERSOS

SINÔNIMO(S)
- Síndrome de bradicardia-taquicardia.
- Disfunção do nó sinusal.
- Síndrome de taquicardia-bradicardia.

VER TAMBÉM
- Bradicardia Sinusal.
- Parada Sinusal e Bloqueio Sinoatrial.
- Taquicardia Supraventricular.

ABREVIATURA(S)
- AV = atrioventricular.
- ECG = eletrocardiograma.
- SNC = sistema nervoso central.

Sugestões de Leitura

Belic N, Talano JV. Current concepts in sick sinus syndrome: I. Anatomy, physiology, and pharmacologic causes. Arch Intern Med 1985, 145:521-523.

Belic N, Talano JV. Current concepts in sick sinus syndrome: II. ECG manifestation and diagnostic and therapeutic approaches. Arch Intern Med 1985, 145:722-726.

Reiffel JA. Normal sinus rhythm and its variants. In: Podrid PJ, Kowey PR, eds., Cardiac Arrhythmia — Mechanisms, Diagnosis, and Management. Baltimore: Williams & Wilkins, 1995, pp. 752-767.

Tilley LP. Essentials of Canine and Feline Electrocardiography, 3rd ed. Baltimore: Williams & Wilkins, 1992.

Weiss AT, Rod JL, Gotsman MS, et al. Hydralazine in the management of symptomatic sinus bradycardia. Eur J Cardiol 1982, 65:841-845.

Autor Janice McIntosh Bright
Consultores Editoriais Larry P. Tilley e Francis W.K. Smith, Jr.

Síndrome do Vômito Bilioso

CONSIDERAÇÕES GERAIS

REVISÃO
• Entidade clínica associada a vômito intermitente crônico de bile que, supostamente, resulta do refluxo de conteúdo intestinal (bile) para o estômago. A motilidade gastrintestinal aboral normal, juntamente com um piloro funcional, evita o refluxo da bile e de outros conteúdos intestinais de volta para o estômago. Se houver refluxo de bile para o estômago, ela é rapidamente removida por contrações peristálticas subsequentes. A bile que permanece no lúmen gástrico, juntamente com o ácido gástrico e a pepsina, pode subsequentemente causar dano à mucosa gástrica. Há suspeitas de que o refluxo de bile seja secundário a alterações na motilidade gastrintestinal normal.
• Os sinais clínicos frequentemente ocorrem de madrugada, sugerindo que o jejum prolongado ou a inatividade gástrica possam modificar os padrões normais de motilidade, com consequente refluxo de bile.

IDENTIFICAÇÃO
• Costuma ser observada em cães, mas raramente em gatos.
• A maioria dos pacientes é de meia-idade ou mais idosa.
• Não há predisposição racial, etária ou sexual.

SINAIS CLÍNICOS
• Vômitos intermitentes e crônicos apenas de bile, associados ao estômago vazio. Em geral, ocorrem no final da noite ou no início da manhã. Podem ser diários, mas costumam ser mais intermitentes. Entre os episódios, o paciente parece normal em todos os outros aspectos.
• Em geral, os resultados do exame físico não são dignos de nota.

CAUSAS E FATORES DE RISCO
• Causa desconhecida (idiopática).
• Há suspeitas de hipomotilidade gástrica primária ou motilidade peristáltica intestinal anormal (em direção à boca) como as prováveis causas subjacentes.
• As condições indutoras de gastrite ou duodenite podem ser responsáveis pela alteração na motilidade gastrintestinal proximal e levar ao refluxo de bile. Pesquisar a presença de *Giardia*, enteropatia inflamatória, neoplasia intestina, ou obstruções como possíveis etiologias.
• Cirurgia prévia de ressecção ou abertura pilórica também aumentará o risco de refluxo enterogástrico.

DIAGNÓSTICO

DIAGNÓSTICO DIFERENCIAL
• Muitos distúrbios gastrintestinais ou não podem causar vômitos crônicos. É recomendável excluir a giardíase, já que os sinais dessa doença podem mimetizar aqueles de vômito bilioso idiopático.
• A enteropatia inflamatória pode resultar no refluxo de bile.
• Descartar também obstrução intestinal ou obstruções parciais.

HEMOGRAMA/BIOQUÍMICA/URINÁLISE
Os resultados costumam permanecer normais.

OUTROS TESTES LABORATORIAIS
Exame fecal para detectar *Giardia* ou outros parasitas.

DIAGNÓSTICO POR IMAGEM
• O estudo contrastado com bário pode revelar o esvaziamento gástrico tardio.
• O fornecimento de bário juntamente com as refeições, os marcadores radiopacos ou o uso de cápsulas especiais de radiotelemetria para avaliação da motilidade (Smartpill®) podem demonstrar o atraso na motilidade gástrica.

MÉTODOS DIAGNÓSTICOS
• Com frequência, os achados endoscópicos permanecem normais.
• Pode haver indícios de bile no estômago ou gastrite na região antral.
• A endoscopia é útil para descartar gastropatias ou duodenopatias estruturais ou inflamatórias.

TRATAMENTO
• Em geral, a síndrome do vômito bilioso não é um distúrbio debilitante grave caso se descarte a presença de problemas importantes, como gastrite, enteropatia inflamatória ou neoplasia gastrintestinal.
• Os casos idiopáticos de vômito bilioso geralmente são submetidos a tratamento sintomático em um esquema ambulatorial.
• Alimentar o animal com múltiplas refeições, incluindo uma no final da tarde, muitas vezes promove o desaparecimento dos sinais clínicos. O alimento possivelmente atua como um tampão à bile refluída ou, de alguma forma, pode intensificar a motilidade gastrintestinal.
• Se a mudança da dieta falhar, deve-se considerar o tratamento clínico.

MEDICAÇÕES

MEDICAMENTO(S)
• As escolhas incluem agentes protetores da mucosa gástrica contra a bile refluída ou agentes pró-cinéticos gástricos para melhorar a motilidade.
• Muitas vezes, uma única dose à tarde pode ser o bastante para evitar os sinais clínicos, caso eles ocorram nesse período.
• Os protetores da mucosa gástrica compreendem diversos antiácidos ou o sucralfato (1 g/25 kg).
• Os bloqueadores da produção de ácido gástrico, como a cimetidina (5 mg/kg a cada 8 h), a ranitidina (2 mg/kg a cada 8 h), a nizatidina (5 mg/kg a cada 24 h), podem ser benéficos. Tanto a ranitidina como a nizatidina também apresentam efeitos pró-cinéticos gástricos e podem ser benéficos.
• Os agentes pró-cinéticos gástricos específicos abrangem a metoclopramida (0,2-0,4 mg/kg VO a cada 6-8 h) e a cisaprida (0,1 mg/kg VO a cada 8-12 h). No momento, a cisaprida está disponível apenas em farmácias de manipulação.
• A eritromicina (0,5-1 mg/kg a cada 8 h) administrada em doses fisiológicas estimula a motilidade gástrica por meio da ativação de receptores da motilina e também pode solucionar os sinais clínicos.

CONTRAINDICAÇÕES/INTERAÇÕES POSSÍVEIS
• Os agentes pró-cinéticos gástricos não devem ser administrados em pacientes com obstrução gastrintestinal.
• A metoclopramida é contraindicada durante a administração concomitante de fenotiazínicos e narcóticos, bem como em animais epilépticos; além disso, esse antiemético pode causar nervosismo, ansiedade/inquietação ou depressão.
• A cisaprida pode ocasionar vômitos, diarreias ou cólicas abdominais.
• A eritromicina pode provocar vômitos.

ACOMPANHAMENTO
• A maioria dos pacientes responde a um dos tratamentos anteriores, e uma resposta clínica apoia o diagnóstico.
• A falha na resposta sugere outro fator subjacente ou causal.

DIVERSOS

DISTÚRBIOS ASSOCIADOS
Refluxo gastresofágico.

VER TAMBÉM
• Distúrbios da Motilidade Gástrica ou Gastrintestinal.
• Refluxo Gastresofágico.

Sugestões de Leitura
Hall JA, Twedt DC, Burrows CF. Gastric motility in dogs. Part 2: Disorders of gastric motility. Compend Contin Educ Pract Vet 1990, 12:1373–1390.
Hall JA, Washabau RJ. Diagnosis and treatment of gastric motility disorders. Vet Clin North Am Small Anim Pract 1999, 29:377–395.
Webb C, Twedt DC. Canine gastritis. Vet Clin North Am Small Anim Pract 2003, 33(5):969–985.

Autor David C. Twedt
Consultor Editorial Albert E. Jergens

SÍNDROME DOS OVÁRIOS REMANESCENTES

CONSIDERAÇÕES GERAIS

REVISÃO
- Síndrome dos ovários remanescentes é a presença de sinais comportamentais e/ou físicos de ciclo estral em cadela ou gata submetida a ovário-histerectomia prévia.
- Provocada pela presença de tecido ovariano residual funcional.
- Há relatos de que a síndrome dos ovários remanescentes seja responsável por 17% de todas as complicações pós-ovário-histerectomia.

IDENTIFICAÇÃO
- Cadelas e gatas; mais comum nas gatas.
- Sem predisposição racial ou distribuição geográfica.
- Geralmente, ocorrem sinais de estro meses a anos após a ovário-histerectomia, embora possam começar dentro de dias depois da cirurgia.

SINAIS CLÍNICOS
Cadelas
Influência do Estrogênio
- Atração por parte dos machos.
- Tumefação (inchaço) da vulva.
- Corrimento vaginal mucoide a sanguinolento.
- Interação passiva com os machos.
- Cauda em bandeira.
- Podem permitir a cópula.
- Os sinais do proestro duram em média 9 dias; os sinais do estro também duram em média 9 dias; o intervalo médio entre os sinais dos ciclos estrais é de 7 meses.
- Os sinais costumam ser cíclicos ou periódicos (i. e., a cada 6 meses).

Influência da Progesterona
- Vulva proeminente em comparação às pacientes submetidas à ovário-histerectomia completa.
- Aumento de volume do coto uterino.
- Pode ocorrer o desenvolvimento de piometra do coto uterino.

Gatas
Influência do Estrogênio
- Vocalização.
- Lordose.
- Inquietação.
- Fricção da face.
- Rolam pelo chão.
- Desvio da cauda e mudança de apoio das pernas traseiras.
- Podem permitir a cópula.
- Demonstram sinais comportamentais típicos do estro de forma cíclica (poliéstrica estacional).
- O estro dura 2-19 dias, seguido pelo interestro, que dura de 8-10 dias a menos que ocorreram os processos de ovulação e luteinização; nesse caso, o interestro é de, no mínimo, 45 dias.

Influência da Progesterona
- Aumento do volume do coto uterino.
- Pode ocorrer o desenvolvimento de piometra do coto uterino.

CAUSAS E FATORES DE RISCO
- Falha da remoção completa de ambos os ovários.
- Sem correlação com a idade na ovário-histerectomia, dificuldade da cirurgia, obesidade do paciente ou experiência do cirurgião.
- A presença de tecido ovariano anatomicamente anormal (fragmentação no ligamento largo) é possível, porém mais comum nas gatas.
- Ovário supranumerário (raro).
- Em termos experimentais, a funcionalidade retorna ao tecido ovariano removido de seu suprimento vascular e recolocado dentro ou sobre a parede abdominal lateral, o mesentério ou a superfície serosa.

DIAGNÓSTICO

DIAGNÓSTICO DIFERENCIAL
- Inflamação ou infecção do trato geniturinário.
- Hemorragia vaginal por corpo estranho (farpa de gramínea).
- Traumatismo.
- Granuloma do coto uterino secundário à doença local (reação a corpo estranho [material de sutura ou farpa de gramínea]).
- Neoplasia de porção remanescente do trato tubular (leiomioma ou leiomiossarcoma do coto uterino).
- Neoplasia de resquício ovariano (tumor de células da granulosa, carcinoma, luteoma, teratoma funcional).
- Neoplasia do trato urinário (carcinoma de células de transição).
- Anomalias vasculares do trato geniturinário.
- Coagulopatia.
- Administração exógena de estrogênio (como aquela para incompetência do esfíncter associada à incontinência urinária).
- Exposição à terapia de reposição hormonal transdérmica humana (mais comumente em cães pequenos de colo).
- Fonte extraovariana endógena de estrogênio: doença adrenal (rara).

HEMOGRAMA/BIOQUÍMICA/URINÁLISE
- Geralmente normais.
- Anemia por perda sanguínea crônica se a hemorragia vaginal for profunda; rara a menos que haja neoplasia ovariana concomitante, cistos foliculares, coagulopatia ou outra doença sistêmica.
- É possível a constatação de pancitopenia no caso de intoxicação por estrogênio.
- Pode ocorrer leucograma de estresse e isostenúria subsequentemente à piometra de coto uterino.

OUTROS TESTES LABORATORIAIS
- Observação dos sinais comportamentais e físicos do estro juntamente com a citologia vaginal e/ou a mensuração das concentrações séricas de progesterona ou estradiol, confirmando a presença de tecido ovariano funcional.
- Citologia vaginal: cornificação da mucosa vaginal é um ensaio biológico para as concentrações elevadas do estradiol plasmático (ver "Acasalamento, Momento Oportuno").
- Citologia vaginal (cadela): cornificação das células epiteliais é, em geral, >90% durante o estro (células superficiais e picnóticas ou anucleares).
- Citologia vaginal (gata): cornificação das células epiteliais varia de 10-40%; o clareamento (ausência de debris e aglomerados celulares) ocorre em 90% dos esfregaços durante o estro.
- Progesterona sérica (cadela): concentrações séricas de progesterona >2 ng/mL (mensuradas 1-3 semanas após o estro comportamental) são compatíveis com tecido lúteo funcional. GnRH (50 μg IM), hCG (400 UI IV) ou hCG (1.000 UI [1/2 IV, 1/2 IM]) podem ser utilizados para tentar induzir a ovulação ou a luteinização para fins diagnósticos; a concentração sérica da progesterona é medida 2-3 semanas mais tarde. Nota: o tecido ovariano patológico pode não ser responsivo a nenhum desses hormônios.
- Progesterona sérica (gata): a ovulação e/ou a luteinização são estimuladas mais comumente por estímulo do coito durante o estro comportamental, mas a concentração sérica da progesterona é medida 2-3 semanas depois; concentrações séricas da progesterona após a estimulação >2 ng/mL são compatíveis com estimulação adequada do coito e presença de tecido lúteo funcional. GnRH (25 μg IM) pode ser usado para tentar induzir a ovulação ou a luteinização para fins diagnósticos; a concentração sérica da progesterona é medida 2-3 semanas depois. O tecido ovariano patológico pode não ser responsivo.
- Estradiol sérico: os níveis de pico que deflagram o estro comportamental variam de 20 a >70 pg/mL; as concentrações séricas do estradiol são confirmatórias para o diagnóstico da síndrome dos ovários remanescentes com base na citologia vaginal.
- Ensaio do hormônio luteinizante (Witness LH, Synbiotics Inc.): embora não haja estudos controlados, o ensaio de LH deve ser positivo (>1 ng/mL) em cadela gonadectomizada. Ao se obter um resultado positivo, repetir em 2 horas. Se ambos os resultados forem positivos, a cadela foi submetida à gonadectomia. O resultado negativo no teste (<1 ng/mL) é encontrado nas cadelas intactas. O ensaio é aprovado para uso na cadela, embora provavelmente seja aplicável nas gatas, desde que os animais desta espécie sejam expostos a 14 horas de luz/dia.
- A citologia do corrimento vulvar pode ser supurativa caso exista granuloma ou piometra de coto uterino.
- Teste provocativo da adrenal (pré e pós-estimulação com ACTH).

DIAGNÓSTICO POR IMAGEM
Ultrassonografia
- Pode ser utilizada para apoiar o diagnóstico de síndrome dos ovários remanescentes, formulado com base no exame citológico e nos perfis hormonais.
- O tecido ovariano remanescente só pode ser visualizado durante a fase folicular (estruturas císticas anecoicas) ou na fase lútea (estruturas císticas hipo ou isoecoicas).
- A obtenção de imagem ultrassonográfica de tecido ovariano ectópico requer habilidade técnica, sendo mais eficientemente realizada com transdutor linear de alta frequência (8-10 mHz). Os resquícios ovarianos que contêm estruturas foliculares ou luteais frequentemente produzem um realce distal em virtude de seu conteúdo líquido, isso pode ser usado para situá-los em posição caudolateral ao rim ipsolateral.
- Avaliar a região dorsal à bexiga urinária em busca de resquício uterino, o que pode aumentar de volume sob influência hormonal ou em caso de doença.
- Avaliar as adrenais quanto ao tamanho e formato normais. As glândulas adrenais caninas normais medem ≤0,51-0,74 cm em corte sagital.

MÉTODOS DIAGNÓSTICOS
- Laparotomia exploratória — a remoção do tecido ovariano residual confirma e resolve o problema.

SÍNDROME DOS OVÁRIOS REMANESCENTES

- A identificação do tecido ovariano residual é facilitada pela presença de corpos lúteos ou de folículos; agendar o procedimento durante as épocas de progesterona elevada ou durante o estro comportamental. Ao contrário da ovário-histerectomia de rotina, essa laparotomia é facilitada por influência hormonal.
- Histopatologia — sempre encaminhar o tecido ovariano visível; se nenhum tecido ovariano visível for identificado, encaminhar todo o tecido residual nos pedículos ovarianos. Isso ajuda a confirmar o diagnóstico e a fazer a triagem quanto à presença de processo maligno. Enviar o tecido examinado de coto uterino para culturas aeróbias e anaeróbias, bem como para exame histopatológico (influência hormonal, resposta inflamatória, malignidade).

TRATAMENTO

- Deve ser considerado o encaminhamento a um cirurgião certificado.
- Remoção cirúrgica do tecido ovariano residual.
- Remoção cirúrgica de coto uterino significativamente acometido.
- Apesar de não ser um método curativo, o ato de restringir a exposição à luz para <8 horas por dia pode suprimir os sinais de estro em algumas, mas não todas, gatas com tecido ovariano.

MEDICAÇÕES

MEDICAMENTO(S)

- Compostos progestacionais ou androgênicos para suprimir a atividade ovariana folicular — não são recomendados por causa dos efeitos colaterais indesejáveis (neoplasia mamária, diabetes, comportamento indesejável, hepatopatia, dermatopatia).
- A imunocontracepção ou a administração de agonista do GnRH representará uma alternativa viável ou terapia adjuvante à laparotomia quando aperfeiçoada e comercialmente disponível nos Estados Unidos.

ACOMPANHAMENTO

COMPLICAÇÕES POSSÍVEIS

- A remoção do tecido lúteo funcional pode induzir a sinais de pseudociese em cadelas e gatas no pós-operatório (ver "Pseudociese").
- O uso de agentes antiprolactina (cabergolina) por via oral pode ser considerado.

EVOLUÇÃO ESPERADA E PROGNÓSTICO

- A remoção bem-sucedida do tecido ovariano remanescente deve resultar na interrupção dos sinais clínicos de estro/diestro.
- Terapia adjuvante para piometra (antibióticos sistêmicos, cuidados de suporte), conforme indicação.
- Terapia adjuvante para neoplasia ovariana funcional, conforme indicação.

DIVERSOS

VER TAMBÉM

- Acasalamento, Momento Oportuno.
- Pseudociese.

ABREVIATURA(S)

- FSH = hormônio foliculoestimulante.
- GnRH = hormônio liberador da gonadotropina.
- hCG = gonadotropina coriônica humana.
- LH = hormônio luteinizante.

Sugestões de Leitura

Baker TW. The bitch and queen: Intact female scanning. In: What's That: A Beginner's Guide to Veterinary Abdominal Ultrasound. Lakewood, CO: AAHA Press, 2009, pp. 31-34.

Davidson AP, Baker TW. Reproductive ultrasound of the bitch and queen. Top Companion Anim Med 2009, 24(2):55-63.

Davidson AP, Feldman EC. Ovarian and estrous cycle abnormalities. In: Ettinger SJ, Feldman EC, eds., Textbook of Veterinary Internal Medicine, 6th ed. St. Louis: Elsevier, 2005, pp. 1649-1655.

Johnston SD, Root Kustritz MV, Olson PN. Disorders of the canine ovary. In: Canine and Feline Theriogenology. Philadelphia: Saunders, 2001, pp. 193-205.

Johnston SD, Root Kustritz MV, Olson PN. Disorders of the feline ovary. In: Canine and Feline Theriogenology. Philadelphia: Saunders, 2001, pp. 453-462.

Kustritz MV. Theriogenology question of the month: Cause of post-estral vaginal discharge. JAVMA 2008, 232(6):841-843.

Miller DM. Ovarian remnant syndrome in dogs and cats: 46 cases (1988-1992). J Vet Diagn Invest 1995, 7:572-574.

Autores Autumn P. Davidson e Tomas W. Baker
Consultor Editorial Sara K. Lyle

SÍNDROME HIPEREOSINOFÍLICA

CONSIDERAÇÕES GERAIS

REVISÃO
- Eosinofilia idiopática persistente com infiltração de múltiplos órgãos, causando disfunção e frequentemente óbito.
- Supostamente causada por reação grave a algum antígeno não identificado ou falta de regulação do controle imunológico na produção de eosinófilos.
- Dano a órgãos causado por efeitos exercidos não só por produtos granulares de eosinófilos, mas também por citocinas derivadas dessas células e liberadas nos tecidos a partir de células ativadas e/ou necróticas.
- Locais comuns de infiltração — trato gastrintestinal (especialmente intestino e fígado), baço, medula óssea, pulmões (principalmente cães) e linfonodos (sobretudo os mesentéricos).
- Outros locais de infiltração são relatados com menor frequência.
- Mais comum em gatos do que em cães; na espécie canina, a raça Rottweiler é possivelmente super-representada.
- Não se sabe se essa doença é uma entidade patológica distinta de leucemia eosinofílica ou se isso tem importância.

IDENTIFICAÇÃO
- Gatos — pode ocorrer com maior frequência em fêmeas domésticas de pelo curto e meia-idade do que em outros.
- Cães — rara, embora a raça Rottweiler possa ser predisposta.

SINAIS CLÍNICOS
- Letargia.
- Anorexia.
- Vômitos e diarreia intermitentes.
- Hepatosplenomegalia.
- Perda de peso que leva à emaciação.
- Espessamento intestinal (difuso ou segmentar) geralmente indolor.
- Linfadenopatia mesentérica e possivelmente periférica.
- Lesões expansivas tipo massa causadas por inflamação granulomatosa e infiltração eosinofílicas envolvendo linfonodos e/ou órgãos.
- Menos frequentemente — febre, prurido e crises convulsivas.

CAUSAS E FATORES DE RISCO
- Desconhecidas; no entanto, acredita-se que seja uma reação intensa a algum estímulo antigênico subjacente, mas não identificável.
- Gatos — a enterite eosinofílica pode ser uma forma precoce.
- Não se sabe se a síndrome hipereosinofílica idiopática é uma doença distinta de leucemia eosinofílica ou se a diferenciação é clinicamente relevante.

DIAGNÓSTICO

DIAGNÓSTICO DIFERENCIAL
- Causas de eosinofilia reativa — parasitismo, reações alérgicas ou de hipersensibilidade, doença infecciosa, doença imunomediada, infecções fúngicas e neoplasia; nessas condições, no entanto, a eosinofilia costuma ser limitada em termos de magnitude e permanecer confinada a algum órgão específico.
- Leucemia eosinofílica — diferenciar por critérios: a leucemia eosinofílica tende a ter (1) eosinófilos imaturos observados em grande número na circulação e maior porcentagem no leucograma diferencial; (2) a anemia é mais comum e frequentemente mais grave; (3) a relação mieloide:eritroide na medula óssea é maior (>10:1) com mais formas blásticas/imaturas e maturação desordenada; (4) os infiltrados teciduais consistem em eosinófilos imaturos e podem revelar um padrão sinusoidal no fígado, sem fibrose; (5) em gatos, foram relatadas massas semelhantes a cloromas nos rins.

HEMOGRAMA/BIOQUÍMICA/URINÁLISE
- Leucocitose com eosinofilia acentuada, possivelmente com desvio à esquerda na série eosinofílica (não relatada de forma habitual); a contagem de eosinófilos maduros varia de 3.200 a >130.000 células/μL.
- Basofilia.
- Leve anemia.
- Em casos de dano ou disfunção de órgãos, podem ser observadas anormalidades compatíveis no hemograma completo, no perfil bioquímico e na urinálise.

OUTROS TESTES LABORATORIAIS
Descartar causas identificáveis de eosinofilia — flutuação fecal, teste para dirofilária, visualização/cultura fúngica e biopsia.

DIAGNÓSTICO POR IMAGEM
- Irregularidades na mucosa intestinal e espessamento dos intestinos observados em radiografias contrastadas e ultrassonografia.
- A infiltração de órgãos pode ser visualizada em radiografias simples e/ou ultrassonografia.

MÉTODOS DIAGNÓSTICOS
- Aspiração e/ou biopsia da medula óssea.
- Biopsia de órgão acometido ou massa.

ACHADOS PATOLÓGICOS
- Baço — infiltrados eosinofílicos na polpa vermelha, às vezes na polpa branca.
- Trato gastrintestinal — infiltrados eosinofílicos na mucosa e na submucosa do intestino delgado, às vezes no cólon e no estômago.
- Medula óssea — hipercelularidade, hiperplasia eosinofílica (até 40% de todas as células nucleadas consistem em eosinófilos), ausência de anormalidades morfológicas, maturação ordenada e alta relação mieloide:eritroide (média de 7,27:1).
- Linfonodos — hiperplasia reativa, além de infiltração de cordões e seios medulares por eosinófilos.
- Coração — infiltrados eosinofílicos no miocárdio e no endocárdio; processo de fibrose e formação de trombos.
- Outros achados (menos frequentes) — infiltrados eosinofílicos na pele, no fígado, nos pulmões, etc.

TRATAMENTO
- Utilizar terapia de manutenção em longo prazo para controlar ou reduzir a eosinofilia e o dano aos órgãos.
- Tratar a disfunção/insuficiência orgânica específica, conforme a indicação.
- A concentração sérica elevada de IgE prevê uma resposta satisfatória ao tratamento com prednisona, além de um prognóstico melhor.

MEDICAÇÕES

MEDICAMENTO(S)
- Corticosteroides — prednisona, 1-3 mg/kg/dia inicialmente; em seguida, administrar em dias alternados se a eosinofilia for suprimida; caso a eosinofilia retorne, voltar a administrar a dose diária mais elevada.
- Quimioterápicos — tentar o emprego desses agentes se a eosinofilia for resistente a esteroides, mas o pequeno número de casos relatados com a descrição dessas terapias impede a recomendação de seu uso.
- Hidroxiureia — administrar para reduzir a contagem de eosinófilos se não estiver normal ou quase normal depois de 7-14 dias de tratamento com esteroides; é mais provável seu uso em longo prazo caso se mostre eficaz em conjunto com esteroides.
- Ciclosporina A — suprime a produção de fatores hematopoiéticos para eosinófilos pelas células T.
- Vincristina e agentes alquilantes, como a clorambucila, são eficazes em seres humanos.
- Mesilato de imatinibe também é eficiente em pessoas.
- Diminuir a dosagem ou interromper o tratamento em caso de mielossupressão ou trombocitopenia.

CONTRAINDICAÇÕES/INTERAÇÕES POSSÍVEIS
Ocorrem toxicidades medicamentosas específicas para cada agente, em especial a mielossupressão.

ACOMPANHAMENTO
- Realizar a monitorização seriada da contagem de eosinófilos (nem sempre é indicativa de infiltrados teciduais) e da mielossupressão caso se faça uso de agentes quimioterápicos.
- Monitorizar os sinais clínicos (p. ex., anorexia, letargia, vômitos e diarreia) e quaisquer anormalidades físicas.
- Outros testes para função de órgãos específicos (p. ex., ácidos biliares).

DIVERSOS

Sugestões de Leitura
James FE, Mansfield CS. Clinical remission of idiopathic hypereosinophilic syndrome in a rottweiler. Australian Vet J 2009, 87:330-333.

Autor Craig A. Thompson
Consultor Editorial A.H. Rebar

SÍNDROME NEFRÓTICA

CONSIDERAÇÕES GERAIS

DEFINIÇÃO
A presença concomitante de proteinúria, hipoalbuminemia, hipercolesterolemia e ascite, além de edema subcutâneo ou outros locais extravasculares de acúmulo de líquido.

FISIOPATOLOGIA
• A glomerulopatia pode levar à perda grave de proteínas pela urina. Uma perda superior a 3,5 g de albumina/dia em seres humanos frequentemente resulta em síndrome nefrótica, embora não se conheça a gravidade da hipoalbuminemia ou da proteinúria necessárias para que essa complicação se desenvolva em cães e gatos. • A perda persistente de proteínas resulta em baixa pressão oncótica plasmática e hiperaldosteronismo, levando à retenção de sódio, retenção secundária de água e, finalmente, ascite e edema. • Em alguns casos, mecanismos intrarrenais, independentes de aldosterona, podem contribuir para a retenção de sódio, ou algum "fator de permeabilidade vascular" não identificado pode provocar o aumento da perda de proteína pelo glomérulo e da perda de líquido pela vasculatura sistêmica. • A hipercolesterolemia origina-se do acúmulo de lipoproteínas de alto peso molecular ricas em colesterol em função do catabolismo diminuído e da síntese hepática aumentada. • Outras complicações concomitantes de glomerulopatia que estão frequentemente presentes incluem hipertensão, hipercoagulabilidade, emaciação muscular e perda de peso. • Ocorrem hipercoagulabilidade e tromboembolia secundariamente a alterações como trombocitose leve, hipersensibilidade plaquetária relacionada com hipoalbuminemia, perda urinária de antitrombina, fibrinólise alterada e concentração elevada de fatores de coagulação de alto peso molecular. A antitrombina normalmente inibe os fatores de coagulação II, VII, IX, X, XI e XII.

SISTEMA(S) ACOMETIDO(S)
• Renal/urológico — proteinúria persistente, em princípio, sem sedimento urinário ativo. Com a natureza progressiva da doença e a perda dos néfrons, ocorrem azotemia e insuficiência renal crônica. • Cardiovascular — edema dependente, ascite, hipercolesterolemia/hiperlipidemia, hipertensão, hipercoagulabilidade e doença tromboembólica.

GENÉTICA
Há relatos de glomerulopatias familiares em várias raças (ver os capítulos sobre "Glomerulonefrite e Amiloidose"); no entanto, é menos provável que essas doenças resultem em síndrome nefrótica em comparação às nefropatias não familiares com perda proteica.

INCIDÊNCIA/PREVALÊNCIA
• A síndrome nefrótica é uma complicação incomum de glomerulopatia. • Pode ser mais comum que a síndrome nefrótica seja secundária a glomerulopatias que induzam à perda maciça de proteína (i. e., glomerulopatia membranosa, amiloidose).

IDENTIFICAÇÃO
Espécies
Cães e gatos.

Raça(s) Predominante(s)
Nenhuma raça parece estar sob risco elevado de sofrer síndrome nefrótica como complicação de glomerulopatia.

Idade Média e Faixa Etária
• Provavelmente exibe a mesma distribuição etária geral que cães e gatos com glomerulopatia. • Idade média de cães com glomerulonefrite = 6,5-7 anos; faixa, 0,8-17 anos. • Gatos com glomerulonefrite — idade média à apresentação = 4 anos. • A maioria dos cães e gatos com amiloidose renal tem mais de 5 anos de idade.

Sexo Predominante
Nenhum identificado.

SINAIS CLÍNICOS
Achados Anamnésicos
• Edema subcutâneo depressível e/ou ascite são as queixas mais comuns à apresentação.
• Ocasionalmente, os sinais associados a alguma doença infecciosa, inflamatória ou neoplásica subjacente podem ser a principal razão pela qual os proprietários buscam pelo atendimento veterinário. O edema ou a ascite que passaram despercebidos pelo proprietário podem ser detectados pelo exame físico ou pelas técnicas de diagnóstico por imagem. • Raras vezes, os cães podem desenvolver dispneia aguda, respiração ofegante grave, fraqueza ou colapso em virtude de efusão pleural ou pericárdica, edema pulmonar ou tromboembolia pulmonar.

Achados do Exame Físico
• Edema subcutâneo dependente depressível ou ascite.
• Complicações de hipertensão: hemorragia ou descolamento da retina, papiledema, arritmias e/ou sopros secundários à hipertrofia do ventrículo esquerdo.
• Dispneia e/ou cianose em cães com efusão pleural ou tromboembolia pulmonar.

CAUSAS
• As glomerulopatias podem ocorrer secundariamente a condições inflamatórias crônicas (p. ex., infecção, neoplasia ou doenças imunomediadas).
• Não se sabe se a síndrome nefrótica é uma consequência direta de proteinúria grave, independentemente do tipo de glomerulopatia, ou se há necessidade de fatores adicionais para resultar em extravasamento de líquido e hipercolesterolemia.

FATORES DE RISCO
Ver a seção "Causas".

DIAGNÓSTICO

DIAGNÓSTICO DIFERENCIAL
Proteinúria
• A causa mais comum é uma doença inflamatória do trato urinário pós-glomerular (p. ex., cistite/pielonefrite bacterianas, urolitíase, insuficiência renal tubular ou neoplasia do trato urinário inferior); a inflamação do trato urinário costuma estar associada (mas nem sempre) a sedimento urinário ativo — números elevados de hemácias, leucócitos, células epiteliais, cilindros e bactérias estão presentes com frequência.
• Hiperglobulinemia secundária a gamopatias monoclonais ou policlonais pode causar proteinúria, particularmente quando analisada por meio do teste turbidimétrico com o ácido sulfossalicílico (teste de Bumin).
• Nefropatias com perda de proteína tipicamente resultam em proteinúria com sedimento urinário inativo (embora possa haver cilindros hialinos); a realização de biopsia renal é o único meio preciso de distinguir os vários tipos de glomerulopatia.

Hipoalbuminemia
Pode estar associada à produção diminuída de albumina (hepatopatia grave) ou à perda aumentada de albumina (nefro e enteropatias, ambas com perda de proteína).

HEMOGRAMA/BIOQUÍMICA/URINÁLISE
• Proteinúria persistente e significativa com sedimento urinário inativo é uma indicação de nefropatias com perda de proteína.
• Hipoalbuminemia e hipercolesterolemia são comuns em animais com glomerulopatia e, por definição, são componentes essenciais da síndrome nefrótica.
• Com a doença avançada, podem ocorrer anormalidades compatíveis com insuficiência renal. A azotemia pode preceder a perda da capacidade de concentração urinária.

OUTROS TESTES LABORATORIAIS
Relação de Proteína:Creatinina Urinárias
• Utilizada para confirmar e quantificar a gravidade da proteinúria.
• A magnitude da proteinúria pode ser usada para avaliar a resposta à terapia ou a evolução da doença.

Eletroforese de Proteínas
• A eletroforese de proteínas séricas e urinárias pode ajudar a identificar a fonte da proteinúria.
• Pode haver imunoglobulinas de cadeia leve (proteínas de Bence-Jones) na urina em casos de malignidade linfoide.

DIAGNÓSTICO POR IMAGEM
• Radiografia — o achado mais comum é a perda dos detalhes abdominais em função da ascite. Podem ser detectadas alterações como efusão pleural (rara), edema pulmonar (muito raro) ou efusão pericárdica (muito rara).
• Ultrassonografia abdominal — geralmente revela grandes quantidades de líquido peritoneal e retroperitoneal. Nas glomerulopatias, pode-se observar uma leve renomegalia.

MÉTODOS DIAGNÓSTICOS
Fica indicada a realização de biopsia renal na presença de proteinúria persistente e significativa com sedimento urinário inativo. A avaliação histopatológica do tecido renal estabelecerá o diagnóstico (p. ex., o subtipo de glomerulopatia presente) e ajudará na formulação do prognóstico. Considerar a biopsia renal somente depois da conclusão de testes menos invasivos (hemograma completo, perfil bioquímico sérico, urinálise, quantificação da proteinúria) e da avaliação da capacidade de coagulação sanguínea.

TRATAMENTO

CUIDADO(S) DE SAÚDE ADEQUADO(S)
• A maior parte dos pacientes com síndrome nefrótica pode ser tratada em um esquema ambulatorial.

SÍNDROME NEFRÓTICA

- Os pacientes gravemente azotêmicos ou hipertensos ou aqueles com doença tromboembólica podem necessitar de hospitalização.

CUIDADO(S) DE ENFERMAGEM
- Abdominocentese — reversar para os pacientes com angústia respiratória ou desconforto abdominal causados por efusão pleural ou ascite. Na maioria dos pacientes, a remoção de líquido aumenta a velocidade de acúmulo de líquido e contribui para as anormalidades eletrolíticas pela retirada de grandes quantidades de sódio.
- Transfusão de plasma — não é indicada para o tratamento de rotina de hipoalbuminemia. Há necessidade de grandes quantidades de plasma para aumentar significativamente as concentrações séricas de albumina; no entanto, a proteína transfundida tem uma meia-vida relativamente curta.
- Aplicação intravenosa de albumina humana — deve ser considerada apenas nos casos muito raros em que os pacientes desenvolvem complicações potencialmente letais em função do acúmulo de líquido (p. ex., edema pulmonar; efusão pleural).
- Se a fluidoterapia intravenosa for necessária em pacientes com síndrome nefrótica para o tratamento de desidratação ou para o estabelecimento de diurese assim que ocorrer o desenvolvimento de azotemia, deverão ser utilizados fluidos alcalinizantes hipossódicos (i. e., cloreto de sódio a 0,45%). Talvez haja necessidade de velocidades mais lentas de administração para evitar o agravamento do acúmulo de líquido extravascular.

ATIVIDADE
Não se sabe se o nível de atividade deve ser modificado em pacientes com síndrome nefrótica. A restrição da atividade pode ser benéfica por causa da possibilidade de doença tromboembólica, enquanto o aumento da atividade pode ser útil para mobilizar o líquido extravascular e promover a reabsorção.

DIETA
- Dietas com teor reduzido de sódio, mas com proteínas de alta qualidade e em baixa quantidade, são recomendadas atualmente. As "rações renais" disponíveis no mercado atendem a esses critérios.
- Níveis normais ou elevados de proteína na dieta podem contribuir para a evolução da doença renal por causar hiperfiltração glomerular, aumento da proteinúria e, subsequentemente, glomerulosclerose. Assim, a terapia nutricional deve incluir uma quantidade reduzida (não restrita) de proteínas de alta qualidade.

ORIENTAÇÃO AO PROPRIETÁRIO
- Se não for possível identificar e corrigir a causa subjacente, as glomerulopatias geralmente evoluirão para insuficiência renal crônica.

- A realização de biopsia é necessária para diferenciar entre os vários subtipos de glomerulopatia e para otimizar os protocolos terapêuticos.
- Assim que ocorrer o desenvolvimento de azotemia e insuficiência renal, o prognóstico frequentemente será mau em função da rápida evolução da(s) doença(s) subjacente(s).

MEDICAÇÕES

MEDICAMENTO(S)
Ver o capítulo sobre "Glomerulonefrite" em busca das recomendações terapêuticas gerais.

Edema e Ascite
- Promover a redução de sódio na dieta.
- Reservar a abdominocentese e os diuréticos para os pacientes com angústia respiratória ou desconforto abdominal. O uso exagerado dos diuréticos pode provocar desidratação e descompensação renal aguda.
- Os pacientes que necessitam de terapia de manutenção com diuréticos para acúmulo persistente e grave de líquido extravascular devem ser tratados com algum antagonista da aldosterona (espironolactona na dose de 1-2 mg/kg VO a cada 12 h), com baixas doses de diuréticos de alça (i. e., furosemida na dose de 0,5-2 mg/kg VO a cada 8-12 h) conforme a necessidade.
- As transfusões de plasma ou albumina conferem apenas benefício temporário. Tais transfusões não são recomendadas quando o risco da terapia supera o benefício.

Proteinúria
- Inibidores da enzima conversora de angiotensina (p. ex., enalapril na dose de 0,5 mg/kg VO a cada 12 h) devem ser utilizados para diminuir a gravidade da proteinúria (ver o capítulos sobre "Glomerulonefrite"). Como a proteinúria pode ser tóxica para os túbulos renais, a terapia com inibidor da ECA deve ser instituída no momento do diagnóstico a menos que haja azotemia grave.
- Terapia anticoagulante (ácido acetilsalicílico na dose de 0,5 mg/kg VO a cada 12 h), para reduzir o risco de tromboembolia, deve ser benéfica uma vez que a albumina sérica declina abaixo de 2,0-2,5 g/dL.

PRECAUÇÕES
- As doses de medicamentos altamente ligados a proteínas (p. ex., ácido acetilsalicílico) podem necessitar de ajuste em pacientes hipoalbuminêmicos; lembre-se que as concentrações da albumina sérica podem se alterar com o tratamento ou com a evolução da doença.
- Usar inibidores da ECA com cuidado em pacientes moderada a acentuadamente azotêmicos (i. e., creatinina sérica >5,0 mg/dL).

- Os diuréticos devem ser usados com extrema cautela em pacientes com síndrome nefrótica por causa do risco de causar ou agravar a azotemia.

INTERAÇÕES POSSÍVEIS
Ver a seção "Precauções".

ACOMPANHAMENTO

MONITORIZAÇÃO DO PACIENTE
Relação de proteína:creatinina urinárias; níveis de ureia, creatinina e albumina, além de concentrações eletrolíticas; pressão arterial; e peso corporal. Idealmente, os exames de reavaliação devem ser programados em 1, 3, 6, 9 e 12 meses após o início do tratamento.

COMPLICAÇÕES POSSÍVEIS
- Insuficiência ou falência renal crônica.
- Tromboembolia pulmonar.

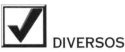

DIVERSOS

DISTÚRBIOS ASSOCIADOS
- Amiloidose.
- Glomerulonefrite.
- Glomerulopatia.
- Hipertensão.
- Hipercoagulabilidade.

GESTAÇÃO/FERTILIDADE/REPRODUÇÃO
Risco provavelmente elevado nas pacientes com hipoalbuminemia e/ou hipertensão graves.

VER TAMBÉM
- Amiloidose.
- Glomerulonefrite.
- Proteinúria.

ABREVIATURA(S)
- ECA = enzima conversora de angiotensina.

Sugestões de Leitura
Cook AK, Cowgill LD. Clinical and pathologic features of protein-losing glomerular disease in the dog: A review of 137 cases (1985-1992). JAAHA 1996, 32:313-322.
Grauer GF. Glomerulonephritis. Semin Vet Med Surg Small Anim 1992, 7:187-197.
Grauer GF, Greco DS, Getzy DM, et al. Effects of enalapril versus placebo as a treatment for canine idiopathic glomerulonephritis. J Vet Intern Med 2000, 14:562-533.
Jacob F, Polzin DJ, Osborne CA, et al. Evaluation of the association between initial proteinuria and morbidity rate or death in dogs with naturally occurring chronic renal failure. JAVMA 2005, 226:393-400.

Autores Barrak M. Pressler e Gregory F. Grauer
Consultor Editorial Carl A. Osborne

Síndrome Tipo-Sjögren

CONSIDERAÇÕES GERAIS

REVISÃO
• Doença autoimune sistêmica, caracterizada por ceratoconjuntivite seca, xerostomia e adenite linfoplasmocitária.
• Mecanismo básico desconhecido; entretanto, foram identificados autoanticorpos direcionados contra tecidos glandulares.
• Associada a outras doenças autoimunes ou imunomediadas, como a artrite reumatoide e o pênfigo.

IDENTIFICAÇÃO
• Incidência mais elevada em diversas raças caninas — Buldogue inglês, West Highland white terrier e Schnauzer miniatura.
• Doença crônica de cães adultos.
• Gatos não são acometidos.

SINAIS CLÍNICOS
Achados Anamnésicos
• Início no adulto.
• Conjuntivite e ceratite.
• Ceratite seca é a característica clínica mais proeminente.

Achados do Exame Físico
• Blefarospasmo.
• Hiperemia conjuntival.
• Lesões corneanas (desde opacidade até ulceração).
• Gengivite.
• Estomatite.

CAUSAS E FATORES DE RISCO
• Possível predisposição genética nas raças com incidência elevada.
• Desenvolve-se concomitantemente com outras doenças imunomediadas e autoimunes.

DIAGNÓSTICO

DIAGNÓSTICO DIFERENCIAL
• Outras causas de ceratoconjuntivite seca — cinomose, traumatismo e intoxicação medicamentosa.
• Ceratoconjuntivite seca associada a outras doenças imunomediadas — atopia, tireoidite linfocítica, polimiosite, lúpus eritematoso sistêmico, artrite reumatoide e doenças penfigoides.

HEMOGRAMA/BIOQUÍMICA/URINÁLISE
Normais.

OUTROS TESTES LABORATORIAIS
• Hipergamaglobulinemia revelada pela eletroforese de proteínas séricas.
• Teste do anticorpo antinuclear positivo.
• Teste positivo para célula de lúpus eritematoso.
• Teste do fator reumatoide positivo.
• Teste positivo para autoanticorpos por fluorescência indireta.

DIAGNÓSTICO POR IMAGEM
N/D.

MÉTODOS DIAGNÓSTICOS
Teste lacrimal de Schirmer (0-5 mm/min).

ACHADOS PATOLÓGICOS
• Alterações histopatológicas nas glândulas salivares — adenite linfoplasmocitária.
• Biopsia conjuntival — revela a presença de conjuntivite.

TRATAMENTO

• Voltado para o controle da ceratoconjuntivite seca.
• Qualquer doença concomitante deve ser submetida a tratamento clínico.
• Pode incluir a administração de medicamentos anti-inflamatórios ou imunossupressores.
• O tratamento cirúrgico da ceratoconjuntivite seca é indicado nos animais irresponsivos à terapia clínica.

MEDICAÇÕES

MEDICAMENTO(S)
• Preparações lacrimais tópicas.
• Antibióticos tópicos apropriados para infecção bacteriana secundária.
• Medicamentos imunossupressores ou anti-inflamatórios.
• Para o tratamento clínico mais rigoroso e intervenção cirúrgica, ver "Ceratoconjuntivite Seca".

CONTRAINDICAÇÕES/INTERAÇÕES POSSÍVEIS
O uso de esteroides tópicos em pacientes com ceratoconjuntivite seca aguda pode provocar ulceração da córnea e, portanto, não é recomendado.

MEDICAÇÕES

• Reavaliar os pacientes semanalmente até que a ceratoconjuntivite seca esteja controlada.
• Pode haver indicação de monitorização extra para tratar doença subjacente ou concomitante.
• Medicamentos imunossupressores — monitorizar os pacientes em semanas alternadas em busca de possíveis efeitos colaterais.
• Prognóstico é variável e depende da existência de doença concomitante.

DIVERSOS

VER TAMBÉM
Ceratoconjuntivite Seca.

Sugestões de Leitura
Quimby FW, Schwartz RS, Poskitt T, et al. A disorder of dogs resembling Sjögren's syndrome. Clin Immunol Immunopathol 1979, 12:471-476.

Autor Paul W. Snyder
Consultor Editorial A. H. Rebar

Síndrome Uveodermatológica

CONSIDERAÇÕES GERAIS

REVISÃO
- Síndrome rara, semelhante à síndrome de Vogt-Koyanagi-Harada em seres humanos.
- Os sinais clínicos refletem a melanina como o alvo da inflamação.

FISIOPATOLOGIA
Reações de hipersensibilidade mediada por células e presença de anticorpos antimelanina foram demonstradas em seres humanos; postula-se o envolvimento de mecanismos semelhantes em cães.

SISTEMA(S) ACOMETIDO(S)
- Cutâneo/exócrino.
- Nervoso.
- Oftálmico.

IDENTIFICAÇÃO
- Cães.
- As raças Akita, Samoieda, Husky siberiano, Malamute do Alasca e Chow chow são predispostas.
- Não há predileção sexual.
- A idade média de início é de 6 meses-6 anos.

SINAIS CLÍNICOS
- Uveíte de início súbito (fotofobia, inflamação conjuntival, dor).
- Cegueira com a evolução.
- Leucodermia concomitante ou subsequente do nariz, dos lábios e das pálpebras.
- Leucotriquia concomitante ou subsequente do focinho e das regiões periorbitais.
- Áreas como coxins palmoplantares, escroto, vulva, ânus e cavidade bucal também podem sofrer despigmentação.
- Sintomas neurológicos (meningoencefalite, perda auditiva) são possíveis, porém raríssimos.

CAUSAS E FATORES DE RISCO
- O mecanismo exato é desconhecido.
- Muito provavelmente se trata de um distúrbio autoimune.
- Possível componente viral.
- A exposição à luz solar pode exacerbar os sintomas.

DIAGNÓSTICO

DIAGNÓSTICO DIFERENCIAL
- Pênfigo foliáceo.
- Pênfigo eritematoso.
- Lúpus eritematoso discoide.
- Lúpus eritematoso sistêmico.
- Vitiligo.
- Neoplasia — linfoma epiteliotrópico.
- Inúmeras dermatoses inflamatórias e infecciosas podem causar despigmentação.

HEMOGRAMA/BIOQUÍMICA/URINÁLISE
Normais.

OUTROS TESTES LABORATORIAIS
ANA — lúpus eritematoso sistêmico.

DIAGNÓSTICO POR IMAGEM
N/D.

MÉTODOS DIAGNÓSTICOS
- A biopsia cutânea é necessária para o diagnóstico, especialmente quando correlacionada com doença ocular.
- É fortemente recomendada a interpretação da amostra tecidual por algum dermatopatologista.
- Também há fortes recomendações para consulta oftalmológica.

ACHADOS PATOLÓGICOS
As lesões iniciais revelam um padrão de interface liquenoide com histiócitos grandes e incontinência pigmentar pronunciada; é rara a presença de uma degeneração hidrópica das células da camada basal da epiderme.

TRATAMENTO

- Para evitar a formação de sinéquias posteriores e glaucoma secundário, cataratas ou cegueira, recomenda-se a instituição rápida e rigorosa da terapia imunossupressora.
- Exames da retina constituem o método mais relevante de monitorização da evolução do quadro; a melhora das lesões dermatológicas pode não refletir o processo patológico contínuo da retina.

MEDICAÇÕES

MEDICAMENTO(S)
- Recomendam-se altas doses iniciais de prednisona (1,1-2,2 mg/kg VO a cada 12-24 h) e azatioprina (1,5-2,5 mg/kg VO a cada 24 h); em casos de uso crônico, devem-se reduzir gradativamente a dosagem e a frequência de administração para um esquema em dias alternados.
- A azatioprina pode ser interrompida depois de alguns meses de terapia, embora a prednisona possa ser necessária por tempo indefinido.
- Alguns casos podem melhorar com o uso inicial de prednisona isolada, mas a ocorrência de sequelas potenciais decorrentes do atraso na instituição de uma terapia rigorosa justifica o uso adicional de azatioprina.
- Os casos refratários podem necessitar do uso de ciclosporina sistêmica; com a combinação de ciclosporina e outros agentes imunossupressores, podem ocorrer infecções oportunistas graves por microrganismos não considerados tipicamente patogênicos.
- Na presença de uveíte anterior, pode ser indicado o emprego de esteroides e cicloplégicos tópicos ou subconjuntivais.

CONTRAINDICAÇÕES/INTERAÇÕES POSSÍVEIS
N/D.

ACOMPANHAMENTO

MONITORIZAÇÃO DO PACIENTE
- Efeitos colaterais potenciais da prednisona e azatioprina — anemia, leucopenia, trombocitopenia, níveis séricos elevados da fosfatase alcalina, vômito e pancreatite.
- Bioquímicas séricas e hemogramas completos quinzenais, incluindo contagens de plaquetas inicialmente; os exames serão menos frequentes à medida que a dose e a frequência das medicações forem gradativamente reduzidas.
- Exames semanais ou quinzenais, incluindo as avaliações da retina em princípio. Os exames da retina constituem um meio importante para a monitorização da doença, já que a melhora nas lesões dermatológicas pode não indicar uma melhora nas lesões retinianas.

EVOLUÇÃO ESPERADA E PROGNÓSTICO
- Geralmente bom para os sintomas dermatológicos.
- Reservado quanto à visão a menos que o tratamento seja instituído rapidamente e se mostre eficaz.

DIVERSOS

VER TAMBÉM
- Dermatoses — Distúrbios Despigmentantes.
- Lúpus Eritematoso Cutâneo.
- Lúpus Eritematoso Sistêmico.
- Linfoma Cutâneo Epiteliotrópico.
- Pênfigo.

ABREVIATURA(S)
- ANA = anticorpo antinuclear.

Sugestões de Leitura
Laus J, Sousa M, Cabral V, Mamede F, Tinucci-Costa M. Uveodermatologic syndrome in a Brazilian fila dog. Vet Ophthalmology 2004, 7:193-196.
Scott DW, Miller WH, Griffin CE. Small Animal Dermatology, 6th ed. Philadelphia: Saunders, 2001.
Sigle K, McLellan G, Haynes J, Myers R, et al. Unilateral uveitis in a dog with uveodermatological syndrome. Sci Reports 2006, 228:543-548.

Autores W. Dunbar Gram e Marlene Pariser
Consultor Editorial Alexander H. Werner

Síndromes Mielodisplásicas

CONSIDERAÇÕES GERAIS

REVISÃO
- Categoria de doenças caracterizadas por anemias arregenerativas ou citopenias e aspectos displásicos no sangue ou na medula óssea.
- Síndromes mielodisplásicas primárias originam-se de uma expansão clonal de alguma célula-tronco pluripotente geneticamente alterada.
- Em cães, as síndromes mielodisplásicas secundárias estão associadas a neoplasia (linfoma, mieloma múltiplo), exposição a medicamentos ou toxinas, doença imunomediada, infecções ou exposição à radiação ionizante.
- Em gatos, as síndromes mielodisplásicas secundárias são tipicamente associadas à infecção pelo FeLV.

IDENTIFICAÇÃO
- Cães e, menos comumente, gatos.
- Síndromes mielodisplásicas primárias tipicamente acometem cães mais idosos.

SINAIS CLÍNICOS
- Letargia.
- Intolerância ao exercício.
- Depressão.
- Anorexia.
- Febre.
- Mucosas pálidas.
- Sopro cardíaco causado pela anemia.

CAUSAS E FATORES DE RISCO
- Virais — FeLV, FIV, parvovírus.
- Neoplasia — linfoma, mieloma múltiplo.
- Autoimunes — anemia hemolítica imunomediada, trombocitopenia imunomediada.
- Medicamentos — quimioterápicos, estrogênio, cloranfenicol, cefalosporinas, fenilbutazona, trimetoprima-sulfadiazina, quinidina, tiacetarsamida, griseofulvina, albendazol.
- Deficiência de ferro, deficiência de ácido fólico.
- Intoxicação pelo chumbo.
- Infecciosos — erliquiose, septicemia bacteriana e endotoxemia.

DIAGNÓSTICO

DIAGNÓSTICO DIFERENCIAL
- É preciso diferenciar entre síndromes mielodisplásicas primárias e secundárias.
- Outras causas de anemias arregenerativas — anemia de doença crônica, insuficiência renal crônica, doenças mieloproliferativas, doenças linfoproliferativas, mielofibrose.

HEMOGRAMA/BIOQUÍMICA/URINÁLISE
Anemia arregenerativa, citopenias.

OUTROS TESTES LABORATORIAIS
Para diagnosticar causas subjacentes de síndromes mielodisplásicas secundárias — títulos humorais/antigênicos virais, níveis de ferro, títulos contra carrapatos, teste de Coombs.

DIAGNÓSTICO POR IMAGEM
- Conforme a necessidade, para descartar causas secundárias de síndromes mielodisplásicas.
- Radiografia abdominal — avalia o paciente em busca de corpos estranhos de chumbo.
- Ultrassonografia abdominal — avalia o animal quanto à presença de massas abdominais compatíveis com testículos retidos ou sertolinomas.

MÉTODOS DIAGNÓSTICOS
Biopsia ou aspirado da medula óssea.

TRATAMENTO
- Internação ou tratamento ambulatorial.
- Em caso de síndromes mielodisplásicas secundárias — tratar a causa subjacente (p. ex., interromper medicamento, tratar infecção subjacente).
- Para animal neutropênico — limitar a exposição a outros animais doentes.
- Em pacientes anêmicos — efetuar transfusões sanguíneas.

MEDICAÇÕES

MEDICAMENTO(S)
- Para neutropenia — antibióticos de amplo espectro e filgrastim (3-5 μg/kg SC a cada 24 h em cães e gatos).
- Para anemia — eritropoietina 35-50 U/kg SC 3 vezes por semana.
- Há relatos do uso de agentes quimioterápicos para síndromes mielodisplásicas primárias — hidroxiureia, citosina arabinosídeo, prednisona, ciclosporina A, vincristina.
- Alfainterferona (gatos com FeLV).

ACOMPANHAMENTO
- Monitorização seriada com hemograma completo para avaliar a resolução das citopenias.
- O prognóstico depende do tipo de síndrome mielodisplásica (primária ou secundária).

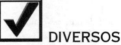

DIVERSOS

GESTAÇÃO/FERTILIDADE/REPRODUÇÃO
- Não usar quimioterapia em animais prenhes ou lactentes.
- Não é recomendável o acasalamento de animais com câncer.

VER TAMBÉM
- Infecção pelo Vírus da Imunodeficiência Felina.
- Infecção pelo Vírus da Leucemia Felina.
- Distúrbios Mieloproliferativos.

ABREVIATURA(S)
- FeLV = vírus da leucemia felina.
- FIV = vírus da imunodeficiência felina.

Sugestões de Leitura
Weiss DJ. New insights into the physiology and treatment of acquired myelodyplastic syndromes and aplastic pancytopenia. Vet Clin Small Anim 2003, 33:1317-1334.

Autor Rebecca G. Newman
Consultor Editorial Timothy M. Fan

SÍNDROMES PARANEOPLÁSICAS

CONSIDERAÇÕES GERAIS

DEFINIÇÃO
- Anomalia clínica resultante de ações não invasivas de algum tumor. Geralmente resulta da secreção anormal de produto hormonal ou semelhante a hormônio (tipo ou quantidade hormonal) que provoca uma resposta clínica inadequada.
- A fisiopatologia depende inteiramente de como o alvo do produto hormonal responde ao estímulo inadequado (ver Tab. 1).
- Os sistemas acometidos variam, dependendo da resposta do alvo hormonal.
- A maioria é considerada rara.
- Relata-se hipercalcemia em até 20% dos cães com linfoma.
- Cerca de 75% dos seres humanos com câncer tem algum distúrbio paraneoplásico durante a evolução de sua doença.

IDENTIFICAÇÃO
Qualquer cão ou gato com câncer maligno (mais comum) ou benigno (raro) ao exame histológico.

SINAIS CLÍNICOS
- Variam com o tipo de tumor e os sistemas orgânicos acometidos, mas incluem:
- Alopecia (síndrome paraneoplásica felina).
- Anemia.
- Caquexia.
- Rubor cutâneo.
- Síndrome diencefálica.
- Coagulação intravascular disseminada.
- Eosinofilia.
- Ulceração gastroduodenal.
- Hipercalcemia.
- Osteopatia hipertrófica.
- Hipoglicemia.
- Mielofibrose.
- Leucocitose neutrofílica.
- Dermatofibrose nodular.
- Policitemia.
- Dermatite necrolítica superficial.
- Trombocitopatia.
- Trombocitopenia.
- Trombocitose.

CAUSAS E FATORES DE RISCO
Secreção inadequada de hormônio ou peptídeo semelhante a hormônio por algum tumor e os efeitos exercidos sobre o tecido-alvo.

DIAGNÓSTICO

DIAGNÓSTICO DIFERENCIAL
Varia com a síndrome.

HEMOGRAMA/BIOQUÍMICA/URINÁLISE
Valiosos na identificação e no monitoramento de várias das síndromes relatadas.

OUTROS TESTES LABORATORIAIS
Níveis de cálcio ionizado e paratormônio (PTH) — avaliar os pacientes com hipercalcemia; a hipercalcemia da malignidade costuma ser caracterizada por altos níveis de cálcio ionizado e baixos níveis de PTH.

DIAGNÓSTICO POR IMAGEM
- Radiografas — detectam osteopatia hipertrófica.
- Técnicas avançadas de diagnóstico por imagem (TC ou RM) — detectam tumor oculto.

MÉTODOS DIAGNÓSTICOS
Biopsia — para diagnosticar lesões cutâneas paraneoplásicas.

TRATAMENTO
- Depende do tumor subjacente e das manifestações clínicas da síndrome paraneoplásica.
- O princípio usual é tratar a neoplasia subjacente do que tentar controlar os sinais clínicos da síndrome paraneoplásica. Algumas vezes, será pertinente tentar o controle dos sinais clínicos como tratamento paliativo se o controle do tumor primário for impossível.

MEDICAÇÕES

MEDICAMENTO(S)
Depende do tipo de tumor subjacente.

ACOMPANHAMENTO

MONITORIZAÇÃO DO PACIENTE
Tal como é feita para o tipo de tumor subjacente.

DIVERSOS

ABREVIATURA(S)
- PTH = paratormônio.
- RM = ressonância magnética.
- TC = tomografia computadorizada.

Sugestões de Leitura

Morrison WB. Paraneoplastic syndromes and the tumors that cause them. In: Morrison WB, ed., Cancer in Dogs and Cats: Medical and Surgical Management. Jackson, WY: Teton NewMedia, 2002, pp. 731-744.

Turek MM. Cutaneous paraneoplastic syndromes in dogs and cats: A review of the literature. Vet Dermatol 2003, 14:279-296.

Weller RE. Paraneoplastic disorders in dogs with hematopoietic tumors. Vet Clin North Am Small Anim Pract 1985, 15(4):805-816.

Autor Wallace B. Morrison
Consultor Editorial Timothy M. Fan

Tabela 1

Síndromes Paraneoplásicas e Tumores que as Causam

Síndrome	Tumor Primário Associado (Cão)	Tumor Primário Associado (Gato)	Mecanismo Principal
Alopecia	Carcinoma adrenal		Cães: devido ao excesso de produção do cortisol; mais frequentemente associada ao hiperadrenocorticismo. Gatos: mecanismo desconhecido
Alopecia (alopecia paraneoplásica felina)		Carcinoma do pâncreas e carcinoma da árvore biliar. Pode ser complicada por infecções por *Malassezia* spp. e infestações por pulgas	Ver "Adenocarcinoma do Pâncreas"; "Hiperadrenocorticismo (Síndrome de Cushing)"; e "Alopecia Paraneoplásica Felina"
Caquexia	Muitos	Muitos	Diversos desarranjos metabólicos provavelmente provocados por citocinas e hormônios (p. ex., fator de necrose tumoral, interferonas, interleucinas, insulina, hormônio do crescimento); podem resultar de alterações no metabolismo de lipídios, proteínas e carboidratos, que geram perda líquida de energia apesar da ingestão calórica adequada; vias metabólicas anaeróbias das células cancerígenas podem desempenhar um papel em alguns casos; outras causas de caquexia em pacientes com câncer incluem obstrução intestinal, inapetência, má absorção, má digestão e perda externa de nutrientes em efusão, na urina ou em exsudatos. Ver "Perda de Peso e Caquexia"
Síndrome do rubor cutâneo	Feocromocitoma; mastocitoma	Não há relatos	Liberação inadequada de substâncias vasoativas, como a histamina, provoca rubor paroxístico da pele

SÍNDROMES PARANEOPLÁSICAS

(Continuação)

Síndrome	Tumor Primário Associado (Cão)	Tumor Primário Associado (Gato)	Mecanismo Principal
Síndrome diencefálica	Astrocitoma	Não há relatos	O tumor está presente na região cerebral do diencéfalo; o excesso de hormônio do crescimento resulta em uma drástica perda de peso (sem acromegalia) a despeito da ingestão calórica adequada; podem ser observados outros sinais hipotalâmicos (p. ex., adipsia, incapacidade de manter a temperatura corporal)
Coagulação intravascular disseminada	Hemangiossarcoma; carcinoma; outros	Doença mieloproliferativa inflamatória	Ver "Coagulação Intravascular Disseminada"
Eosinofilia	Fibrossarcoma; carcinoma mamário	Carcinoma de células de transição da bexiga; mastocitomas; linfossarcoma	Pode ser devido à estimulação de precursores eosinofílicos por produtos como as interleucinas 2, 3 e 5, além do fator estimulante da colônia granulocítica-macrofágica
Dermatite esfoliativa (dermatite esfoliativa associada a timoma felino)	Não há relatos	Timoma	Provavelmente devido à indução de linfócitos-T autorreagentes
Síndrome de feminização	Tumores testiculares — especialmente sertolinomas		Acredita-se que a síndrome paraneoplásica se deva ao hiperestrogenismo ou a algum desequilíbrio relativo entre testosterona e estrogênio, não complicado por mielossupressão
Febre	Muitos	Muitos	Envolve o reajuste do "ponto de ajuste" hipotalâmico pelas citocinas (p. ex., interleucina 1, fator de necrose tumoral, outras indutoras da síntese local de prostaglandina [PGE$_2$] dentro do hipotálamo) que coordenam os componentes autônomos, endócrinos e comportamentais da resposta febril Ver "Febre"
Ulceração gastroduodenal	Neoplasia pancreática de outras células que não das ilhotas; mastocitoma	Mastocitoma	Secreção inadequada de gastrina (tumor de células não pertencentes às ilhotas pancreáticas) ou secreção excessiva de histamina (mastócito)
Hipercalcemia	Linfoma; carcinoma das glândulas apócrinas dos sacos anais; mieloma múltiplo; outros	Linfoma; mieloma múltiplo; outros	Cães com linfossarcoma e carcinoma das glândulas apócrinas: envolve o excesso da proteína relacionada com o paratormônio (PTH) Gatos: mecanismo não explorado Ver "Hipercalcemia"
Osteopatia hipertrófica	Tumores metastáticos e primários do pulmão	Tumores metastáticos e primários do pulmão	Caracterizado por rápido crescimento de novo osso periosteal em padrão linear nodular ou liso nas radiografias; o mecanismo exato é desconhecido, porém envolve parcialmente o estímulo aferente neural e o aumento do fluxo sanguíneo para as extremidades; impulsos aferentes que percorrem os nervos vago e intercostal a partir da lesão para o SNC podem desencadear essa síndrome. Nota: a osteopatia hipertrófica também é associada a muitos distúrbios não cancerígenos do tórax, como pneumopatia inflamatória, persistência do ducto arterioso da direita para a esquerda, abscesso pulmonar, dirofilariose, hipertensão sistêmica, endocardite valvular e espirocercose.
Síndrome de hiperviscosidade	Tumor secretor de imunoglobulina (p. ex., mieloma múltiplo e linfoma)	Tumor secretor de imunoglobulina	Acompanha o acúmulo de grandes imunoglobulinas ou pequenas imunoglobulinas polimerizadas no sangue, que resultam em diminuição do fluxo sanguíneo por conta do aumento na viscosidade. Ver "Mieloma Múltiplo" e "Paraproteinemia"
Hipoglicemia	Insulinoma; tumores benignos e malignos da musculatura lisa; grandes tumores mesenquimais	Insulinoma	Geralmente envolve a utilização excessiva de glicose ou a produção demasiada de insulina ou fatores insulinossímiles Ver "Insulinoma"
Distúrbios gerados por imunocomplexos	Leucemia linfocítica; eritrocitose primária	Linfoma	Secundário à ativação do imunocomplexo antígeno-anticorpo; a glomerulonefrite é o problema mais identificado
Miastenia grave	Timoma; outros	Massa mediastínica	O mecanismo exato é desconhecido Ver "Miastenia Grave".
Mielofibrose	Tumores pancreáticos de outras células que não das ilhotas; linfossarcoma; síndromes mielodisplásicas	Síndromes mielodisplásicas; infecção pelo vírus da leucemia felina	Ver "Síndromes Mielodisplásicas"
Leucocitose neutrofílica	Fibrossarcoma; outros	Carcinoma	Produção de peptídeo estimulante de granulócitos e monócitos é a provável causa
Dermatofibrose nodular	Cistadenoma ou cistadenocarcinoma renal principalmente em Pastor alemão e mestiços. Também foi relatada em um único cão da raça Golden retriever	Não há relatos	O mecanismo é desconhecido, mas envolve a proliferação de fibroblastos. A propensão ao desenvolvimento é hereditária em um padrão autossômico dominante. Também parece ser ligada ao cromossomo 5 em cães. Os tumores renais costumam ser lentamente progressivos e quase sempre bilaterais
Pênfigo	Linfoma mediastínico	Não há relatos	Autoimunidade contra antígenos-alvo (periplaquina e envoplaquina) na pele

SÍNDROMES PARANEOPLÁSICAS

	(Continuação)		
Síndrome	*Tumor Primário Associado (Cão)*	*Tumor Primário Associado (Gato)*	*Mecanismo Principal*
Síndrome dos nervos periféricos	Vários	Não há relatos	Mecanismo desconhecido, mas geralmente subclínico e secundário a alterações na mielinização
Policitemia	Sarcoma e carcinoma renais; outros	Não há relatos	Secreção inadequada de eritropoetina ou peptídeos semelhantes à eritropoetina Ver "Policitemia e Policitemia Vera"
Dermatite necrolítica superficial (necrose epidérmica metabólica, síndrome hepatocutânea, eritema migratório necrolítico)	Neoplasia hepática; neoplasia pancreática (glucagonoma)	Neoplasia pancreática (glucagonoma)	Muitos nomes são utilizados para descrever entidades clínicas semelhantes; observada geralmente em pacientes com hepatopatia e, menos comumente, em tumores pancreáticos secretores de glucagon; conhecida algumas vezes como síndrome do glucagonoma; o mecanismo exato é incerto; pode-se observar intolerância à glicose ou diabetes melito associado
Trombocitopatia	Tumores secretores de imunoglobulina	Tumores secretores de imunoglobulina	Moléculas de imunoglobulina inibem a agregação normal de plaquetas Ver "Trombocitopatias"
Trombocitopenia	Hemangiossarcoma	Linfoma	Trombocitopenia, imunomediada primária ou secundária à mieloftise Ver "Trombocitopenia"
Trombocitose	Distúrbios mieloproliferativos	Distúrbios mieloproliferativos	Superprodução de citocinas que estimulam a produção de trombopoetina (p. ex., interleucinas 1, 3, 6 e 11)

Siringomielia e Má-Formação Tipo Chiari

CONSIDERAÇÕES GERAIS

REVISÃO
- Má-formação tipo Chiari — distúrbio caracterizado por desequilíbrio de tamanho entre o cérebro (muito grande) e o crânio (muito pequeno) que leva à compressão do cerebelo e do tronco encefálico e ao deslocamento das estruturas neurais em direção ao forame magno, obstruindo o fluxo do LCS. Uma consequência disso é a siringomielia — quadro em que se desenvolvem cavidades preenchidas por líquido dentro da medula espinal. • O principal sinal clínico é a dor, atribuída à obstrução da pressão de pulso do LCS e/ou ao dano ao corno dorsal da medula espinal e/ou aos tratos espinotalâmicos.

IDENTIFICAÇÃO
- Cães das raças *toys*, especialmente Cavalier King Charles spaniel, Brussel Griffon, Maltês, Yorkshire terrier, Chihuahua; mais prováveis nos exemplos miniaturas do tipo da raça. • Staffordshire bull terrier. • Cães dos 5 meses de vida aos de meia-idade são predispostos. • Não há predisposição de sexo ou cor.

SINAIS CLÍNICOS
Achados Anamnésicos
- Comportamento recluso. • Choro — quando salta, fica agitado ou se levanta ou, até mesmo, durante a defecação. • Dor — intermitente e, com frequência, pior à noite. • Sensibilidade e/ou arranhadura do ombro, orelha, pescoço ou esterno. • Comportamento de arranhadura enquanto caminha, frequentemente sem contato com a pele. Pode ser deflagrado por coleira, toque, movimento ou agitação. • Fricção da orelha e face.

Achados do Exame Físico
- Podem permanecer normais. • Dor espinal variável. • Sensibilidade ao toque, sobretudo de orelhas, membros, esterno e pescoço. • Escoliose cervicotorácica, ataxia, fraqueza (casos graves).

CAUSAS E FATORES DE RISCO
- Má-formação tipo Chiari/Siringomielia — hereditariedade moderadamente alta (H^2 da siringomielia = 0,37). • Siringomielia — possível herança epistática (genes em dois ou mais lócus interagem para produzir a doença). • A siringomielia pode se desenvolver secundariamente a qualquer obstrução do fluxo do LCS (p. ex., cisto aracnoide, tumor do tronco encefálico, processo inflamatório).

DIAGNÓSTICO

DIAGNÓSTICO DIFERENCIAL
Dor Espinal/Fraqueza/Ataxia
- Discopatia intervertebral — início agudo, dor localizada persistente. • Encefalites — dor com sinais neurológicos rapidamente progressivos. • Subluxação atlantoaxial — movimento restrito do pescoço; tetraparesia e dor atribuídas à lesão do neurônio motor superior. Pode ocorrer em conjunto com má-formação tipo Chiari e siringomielia. • Discospondilite — febre e neutrofilia no início; dor constante.

Arranhadura
- Doença de pele — em siringomielia, não há lesões cutâneas.

Posição Anormal da Cabeça
- Descartar disfunção vestibular causada por doença da orelha interna, do VIII par de nervos cranianos ou de estrutura intracraniana.

DIAGNÓSTICO POR IMAGEM
Radiografias do Crânio e Pescoço
- Valor limitado; podem sugerir alterações características de má-formação tipo Chiari (base do crânio curta, alongamento compensatório do osso parietal, encurtamento do osso supraoccipital, que conferem à parte posterior do crânio uma aparência em formato de cone). Em caso de siringomielia ampla, o canal vertebral pode ser expandido, particularmente na região C2. Imagens cervicais para descartar outras anomalias vertebrais, como subluxação atlantoaxial.

Ressonância Magnética
- Para estabelecer a causa de siringomielia, ou seja, má-formação tipo Chiari ou outras causas de obstrução do LCS. • Má-formação tipo Chiari — deslocamento do cerebelo e da medula oblonga em direção ao forame magno com oclusão e pouco a nenhum LCS em torno das estruturas neurais; ventriculomegalia. • Siringomielia — formação de cavidades, contendo líquido, na medula espinal, particularmente na região C1-C4. Os cães com siringomielia cervical frequentemente apresentam siringomielia mais caudal. • Restringir o exame de RM à região cervical pode subestimar a gravidade. • Largura transversal máxima da siringomielia — indicador de dor; 95% dos cães da raça Cavalier King Charles spaniel com largura máxima da siringomielia ≥0,66 cm apresentam sinais clínicos. • Siringomielia de largura estreita pode permanecer assintomática e ser um achado incidental.

MÉTODOS DIAGNÓSTICOS
LCS — para descartar doenças inflamatórias; o conteúdo de proteína pode estar elevado.

TRATAMENTO

- Principal objetivo — alívio da dor. • A cirurgia pode proporcionar o maior sucesso a longo prazo, mas tem alta taxa de falha (~50% dos casos deterioram-se por volta de 2 anos e meio do pós-operatório). • O tratamento cirúrgico visa restabelecer o fluxo do LCS, descomprimindo o forame magno pela remoção parcial do osso supraoccipital e do arco neural de C1. • Tratamento médico inicial — tratar a dor, reduzindo a pressão do LCS; em caso de resposta satisfatória, reconsiderar a cirurgia. Se o alívio da dor estiver inadequado, adicionar ou trocar para um AINE. Se ainda inadequado, adicionar um analgésico neurogênico. Por fim, os corticosteroides podem ser eficazes para casos irresponsivos. • Acupuntura pode ser uma terapia adjuvante útil.

MEDICAÇÕES

MEDICAMENTO(S)
- Medicamentos que reduzem a pressão do LCS — diuréticos, p. ex., furosemida na dose de 1-2 mg/kg a cada 12 h (acetazolamida não é recomendada por conta dos efeitos adversos); inibidores da bomba de prótons (omeprazol na dose de 0,5-1,5 mg/kg a cada 24 h); ou antagonistas dos receptores H2 (cimetidina na dose de 5-10 mg/kg a cada 8 h). • AINE — seguir a dosagem da bula. • Analgésicos neurogênicos — gabapentina na dose de 10-20 mg/kg a cada 12 ou 8 h ou pregabalina na dose de 5 mg/kg a cada 12 h em caso de comprometimento do corno dorsal da medula espinal. • Corticosteroides — utilizar a menor dose possível capaz de controlar os sinais clínicos, começando com 0,5 mg/kg de prednisolona ou metilprednisolona diariamente; suspender os AINE.

CONTRAINDICAÇÕES/INTERAÇÕES POSSÍVEIS
- Em caso de má-formação tipo Chiari/Siringomielia, podem ocorrer crises convulsivas; a associação direta não foi comprovada; pode ser uma epilepsia idiopática concomitante. • A ocorrência de surdez é comum em cães da raça Cavalier King Charles spaniel com má-formação tipo Chiari/Siringomielia; a associação direta não foi comprovada. Esses cães com má-formação tipo Chiari podem ser mais predispostos à efusão da orelha média. • A má-formação tipo Chiari/Siringomielia não aumenta o risco anestésico.

ACOMPANHAMENTO

- Reavaliar o êxito do controle da dor e o estado neurológico do paciente a cada 1-3 meses. • Não há necessidade de restrição da atividade física, embora se possam evitar algumas atividades; a prática de higiene e embelezamento pessoais pode não ser tolerada. • Pode ser útil não só suspender a tigela de ração, mas também remover as coleiras do pescoço. • A evolução da doença é variável. Alguns cães permanecem estáveis ou sofrem deterioração mínima ao longo dos anos. Outros adquirem deficiência grave por dor e déficits neurológicos dentro de meses de observação dos primeiros sinais clínicos. • É recomendável a obtenção periódica de hemograma completo/bioquímica sérica se o animal estiver recebendo medicação.

DIVERSOS

ABREVIATURAS
- LCS = líquido cerebrospinal.
- RM = ressonância magnética.
- AINE = anti-inflamatório não esteroide.

RECURSOS DA INTERNET
- http://igitur-archive.library.uu.nl/dissertations/2007-0320-201201/UUindex.html.
- http://www.veterinary-neurologist.co.uk.

Sugestões de Leitura
Rusbridge C. Chiari-like malformation with syringomyelia in the Cavalier King Charles spaniel: Long term outcome after surgical management. Vet Surg 2007, 36:396-405.
Rusbridge C. Syringomyelia: Current concepts in pathogenesis, diagnosis and treatment. J Vet Intern Med 2006, 20:469-479.

Autor Clare Rusbridge
Consultor Editorial Joane M. Parent

Sopros Cardíacos

CONSIDERAÇÕES GERAIS

DEFINIÇÃO
Vibrações provocadas por distúrbio do fluxo sanguíneo.

Sincronização dos Sopros
- Sopros sistólicos ocorrem entre S1 e S2 (sístole).
- Sopros diastólicos ocorrem entre S2 e S1 (diástole).
- Sopros contínuos e tipo vaivém ocorrem por todo o ciclo cardíaco ou em grande parte dele.
- Os sopros contínuos geralmente são acentuados próximos a S2, enquanto os sopros de vaivém costumam estar ausentes próximos a S2.

Escala de Graduação para os Sopros
- Grau I — escassamente audível.
- Grau II — suave, porém facilmente auscultado. Não se propaga para longe do ponto de intensidade máxima.
- Grau III — sonoridade intermediária; auscultado com maior facilidade a certa distância a partir do ponto de intensidade máxima do tórax; a maior parte dos sopros relevantes do ponto de vista hemodinâmico é no mínimo de grau III.
- Grau IV — sopro sonoro que se irradia amplamente, incluindo muitas vezes o lado oposto do tórax.
- Grau V — muito sonoro, audível ao simples contato do estetoscópio com o tórax; frêmito palpável.
- Grau VI — muito alto, audível sem o contato do estetoscópio com o tórax; frêmito palpável.

Configuração
- Sopros em platô apresentam sonoridade uniforme e são típicos de sopros regurgitantes como os de insuficiência das valvas atrioventriculares esquerda e direita (mitral e tricúspide, respectivamente) e do defeito do septo ventricular.
- Sopros crescendo-decrescendo ficam mais altos e, em seguida, mais baixos e são típicos de sopros de ejeção como os de estenose das válvulas atrioventriculares (aórtica e pulmonar) e do defeito do septo atrial.
- Sopros decrescendo começam altos e, depois, ficam mais suaves e são típicos de sopros diastólicos como os de insuficiência aórtica ou pulmonar e estenose mitral ou tricúspide.

Localização
Cães
- Área mitral — quinto espaço intercostal esquerdo na junção costocondral.
- Área aórtica — quarto espaço intercostal esquerdo acima da junção costocondral.
- Área pulmonar — segundo ao quarto espaços intercostais esquerdos na borda esternal.
- Área tricúspide — terceiro ao quinto espaços intercostais direitos próximos à junção costocondral.

Gatos
- Área mitral — quinto ao sexto espaços intercostais esquerdos a um quarto de distância ventrodorsal do esterno.
- Área aórtica — segundo ao terceiro espaços intercostais esquerdos, imediatamente acima da área pulmonar.
- Área pulmonar — segundo ao terceiro espaços intercostais esquerdos, entre um terço à metade de distância ventrodorsal do esterno.
- Área tricúspide — quarto ao quinto espaços intercostais direitos, a um quarto de distância ventrodorsal do esterno.

FISIOPATOLOGIA
- Distúrbio do fluxo sanguíneo, associado ao aumento do fluxo pelas valvas/válvulas normais ou anormais ou à vibração de estruturas por esse fluxo.
- Distúrbios de fluxo associados à obstrução ao fluxo de saída ou fluxo anterógrado por valvas/válvulas estenosadas ou por um grande vaso dilatado.
- Distúrbios de fluxo associados a fluxo regurgitante por uma valva/válvula incompetente, defeito septal ou ducto arterioso persistente.

SISTEMA(S) ACOMETIDO(S)
Cardiovascular.

IDENTIFICAÇÃO
Cães e gatos.

SINAIS CLÍNICOS
Relacionam-se com a causa do sopro.

CAUSAS
Sopros Sistólicos
- Endocardiose mitral e tricúspide.
- Miocardiopatia e insuficiência da valva AV.
- Sopros de fluxo fisiológico.
- Anemia.
- Displasia mitral e tricúspide.
- Movimento anterior sistólico da mitral.
- Obstrução dinâmica ao fluxo de saída do ventrículo direito.
- Estenose subaórtica dinâmica.
- Defeito do septo atrial.
- Defeito do septo ventricular.
- Estenose pulmonar.
- Estenose aórtica.
- Tetralogia de Fallot.
- Endocardite mitral e tricúspide.
- Hipertireoidismo.
- Dirofilariose.

Sopros Contínuos ou Tipo Vaivém
- Persistência do ducto arterioso.
- Defeito do septo ventricular com regurgitação aórtica.
- Estenose aórtica com regurgitação aórtica.

Sopros Diastólicos
- Estenose mitral e tricúspide.
- Endocardite aórtica e pulmonar.

FATORES DE RISCO
Cardiopatia.

DIAGNÓSTICO

DIAGNÓSTICO DIFERENCIAL
Sinais Diferenciais
- É preciso diferenciá-los de outros sons cardíacos anormais — sons de desdobramento, sons de ejeção, ritmos de galope e estalidos.
- Também é imprescindível diferenciá-los de sons pulmonares anormais e fricções pleurais; auscultar para verificar se a sincronização do som anormal se correlaciona com a respiração ou com o batimento cardíaco.

Causas Diferenciais
- Mucosas pálidas apoiam o diagnóstico de sopro anêmico.
- Localização e irradiação do sopro e sincronização durante o ciclo cardíaco podem ajudar a determinar a causa; ver o algoritmo.

HEMOGRAMA/BIOQUÍMICA/URINÁLISE
- Anemia nos animais com sopros anêmicos.
- Policitemia nos animais com defeitos congênitos de desvio da direita para a esquerda.
- Leucocitose com desvio à esquerda nos animais com endocardite.

OUTROS TESTES LABORATORIAIS
N/D.

DIAGNÓSTICO POR IMAGEM
- Radiografia torácica — útil para avaliar o tamanho cardíaco e a vasculatura pulmonar na esperança de determinar a causa e o significado do sopro.
- Ecocardiografia — recomendada quando se suspeita de alguma causa cardíaca e quando não se conhece a natureza do defeito.
- Às vezes, há necessidade de estudos com Doppler para confirmar a causa do sopro.

MÉTODOS DIAGNÓSTICOS
- A eletrocardiografia pode ser valiosa na avaliação dos padrões de aumento cardíaco em animais com sopros.
- Hemoculturas e sorologia para *Bartonella* na suspeita de endocardite.

TRATAMENTO
- Como paciente de ambulatório a menos que a insuficiência cardíaca seja evidente.
- Tomar as decisões com base na causa do sopro e nos sinais clínicos associados.
- Não há nenhuma indicação para sopro isolado.

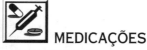

MEDICAÇÕES

MEDICAMENTO(S)
N/D.

CONTRAINDICAÇÕES
N/D.

PRECAUÇÕES
N/D.

INTERAÇÕES POSSÍVEIS
N/D.

ACOMPANHAMENTO

MONITORIZAÇÃO DO PACIENTE
Sopros sistólicos de ejeção de baixo grau em filhotes de cão podem ser fisiológicos; a maior parte deles desaparece em torno dos 6 meses de idade. Se o sopro ainda estiver presente depois dos 6 meses, proceder às técnicas de diagnóstico por imagem.

COMPLICAÇÕES POSSÍVEIS
Se o sopro estiver associado à cardiopatia estrutural, poderão ser observados sinais de insuficiência cardíaca congestiva (p. ex., tosse, dispneia e ascite) ou intolerância ao exercício.

SOPROS CARDÍACOS

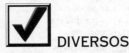

DIVERSOS

DISTÚRBIOS ASSOCIADOS
N/D.

FATORES RELACIONADOS COM A IDADE
• Sopros presentes desde o nascimento são associados, em geral, a defeito congênito ou sopro de fluxo fisiológico.
• Sopros adquiridos em cães geriátricos pertencentes a raças de pequeno porte costumam estar associados à valvulopatia degenerativa.
• Sopros adquiridos em raças caninas de grande porte são associados geralmente à miocardiopatia dilatada.
• Sopros adquiridos em gatos geriátricos são associados, em geral, a miocardiopatia ou hipertireoidismo.

POTENCIAL ZOONÓTICO
Nenhum.

GESTAÇÃO/FERTILIDADE/REPRODUÇÃO
Os sopros em filhotes caninos e felinos podem refletir algum defeito congênito e, com isso, influenciam a tomada de decisões sobre o acasalamento desse animal ou a repetição do cruzamento.

VER TAMBÉM
Ver a seção "Causas".

ABREVIATURA(S)
• AV = atrioventricular.
• S1 = primeira bulha cardíaca.
• S2 = segunda bulha cardíaca.

Sugestões de Leitura
Smith FWK, Jr., Keene BW, Tilley LP. Rapid Interpretation of Heart and Lung Sounds. St Louis: Saunders Elsevier, 2006.

Autores Francis W. K. Smith, Jr., e Robert L. Hamlin
Consultores Editoriais Larry P. Tilley e Francis W. K. Smith, Jr.

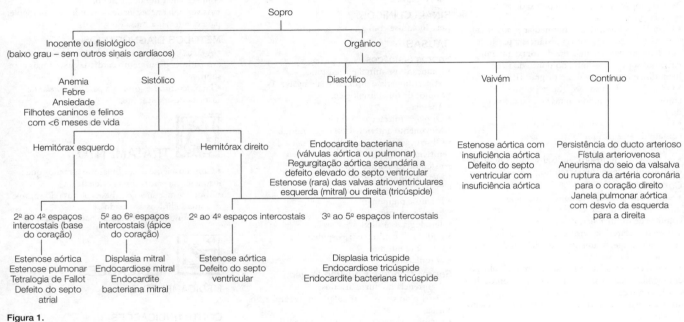

Figura 1.

Subinvolução dos Sítios Placentários

CONSIDERAÇÕES GERAIS

REVISÃO
- Falha ou retardo da involução uterina normal depois do parto (isso normalmente requer 12-15 semanas para estar concluída).
- Falha de massas eosinofílicas de colágeno nos sítios placentários em se esfacelar 3-4 semanas depois do parto.
- Falha de células trofoblásticas fetais em involuir (isso normalmente ocorre em até 2 semanas); em vez disso, elas invadem os tecidos endometriais e miometriais glandulares profundos maternos.
- Causa — desconhecida; não se suspeita de base hormonal ou uterina em função da coexistência de sítios placentários não acometidos e subinvoluídos no mesmo útero.

IDENTIFICAÇÃO
- Apenas cadelas.
- É mais comum em cadelas com <3 anos de idade.
- Incidência maior na primeira ninhada.
- Sem predileções raciais.

SINAIS CLÍNICOS

Achados Anamnésicos
- As pacientes são levadas à consulta 6-12 semanas depois do parto.
- Corrimento vulvar serossanguinolento >6 semanas do pós-parto.
- Sem sinais sistêmicos.

Achados do Exame Físico
- Corrimento vulvar serossanguinolento.
- Estruturas esféricas firmes dentro do útero à palpação abdominal.

CAUSAS E FATORES DE RISCO
- Desconhecidas.
- Hormonais — improváveis, porque apenas alguns dos sítios placentários podem estar envolvidos.
- Doença uterina — improvável, por causa da elevada prevalência na primeira ninhada.

DIAGNÓSTICO

DIAGNÓSTICO DIFERENCIAL
- Metrite — diferenciada pela citologia vaginal e pelo exame físico.
- Vaginite — distinguida pela citologia vaginal.
- Neoplasia vaginal — diferenciada pelos exames de citologia e endoscopia vaginais.
- Neoplasia uterina — distinguida pela ultrassonografia ou por laparotomia exploratória.
- Cistite — diferenciada pela citologia vaginal e por urinálise obtida via cistocentese.
- Coagulopatia — distinguida pelos tempos de coagulação.
- Traumatismo.
- Estímulo estrogênico endógeno — cadela com intervalo entre os estros extremamente encurtado.
- Estímulo estrogênico exógeno — medicamentos administrados por via oral ou contato com cremes de reposição hormonal na pele do proprietário.

HEMOGRAMA/BIOQUÍMICA/URINÁLISE
Geralmente normais.

OUTROS TESTES LABORATORIAIS
Sorologia negativa para *Brucella canis*.

DIAGNÓSTICO POR IMAGEM
Ultrassonografia uterina — espessamento focal da parede uterina; líquido ecogênico no lúmen.

MÉTODOS DIAGNÓSTICOS
- Exame citológico vaginal — essencial para o diagnóstico; revela eritrócitos e células epiteliais parabasais; podem-se notar células trofoblásticas patognomônicas (polinucleadas e intensamente vacuolizadas).
- Cultura vaginal anterior protegida — se o exame citológico vaginal ou o hemograma apoiarem o diagnóstico de metrite secundária.

ACHADOS PATOLÓGICOS
- Macroscópicos — sítios caracterizados por área hemorrágica espessada que pode ser nodular.
- Histopatológicos — para obtenção do diagnóstico definitivo; massas eosinofílicas de colágeno com trofoblastos que se estendem para o miométrio.

TRATAMENTO
- Geralmente em um esquema ambulatorial.
- Remissão espontânea — ocorre em grande parte dos pacientes antes ou no próximo ciclo; em geral, não é justificável a terapia clínica.
- Clínico — para o desenvolvimento raro da anemia, metrite ou peritonite.
- Pacientes gravemente acometidos — podem necessitar de transfusão de sangue (raros).
- Alertar o proprietário quanto à rara possibilidade de hemorragia excessiva; instruir o proprietário a monitorizar a coloração das mucosas.
- Ovário-histerectomia — curativa; tratamento de escolha se o acasalamento futuro não for desejado.
- Curetagem cirúrgica de sítios subinvoluídos — também pode ser realizada; eficácia desconhecida.

MEDICAÇÕES

MEDICAMENTO(S)
Geralmente não são bem-sucedidos.

CONTRAINDICAÇÕES/INTERAÇÕES POSSÍVEIS
- Ocitócicos — podem provocar ruptura uterina.
- Medicamentos progestacionais — aumentam o risco de metrite, a qual pode mimetizar a piometra.

ACOMPANHAMENTO

MONITORIZAÇÃO DO PACIENTE
- Coloração da mucosa e quantidade do corrimento.
- Hematócrito — caso a anemia seja uma preocupação.
- Alterações na cor ou no odor do corrimento e exame citológico e cultura vaginais — para diagnosticar infecção secundária.

COMPLICAÇÕES POSSÍVEIS
Infecção, anemia por perda sanguínea ou ruptura uterina — raras.

EVOLUÇÃO ESPERADA E PROGNÓSTICO
- Resolução espontânea — o resultado usual na maioria dos casos.
- Recidiva — não é esperada.
- Prognóstico quanto à reprodução futura — excelente com a resolução espontânea.

DIVERSOS

Sugestões de Leitura

Johnston SD. Subinvolution of placental sites. In: Kirk RW, ed. Current veterinary therapy IX. Philadelphia: Saunders, 1986:1231-1233.

Johnston SD, Root Kustritz MY, Olson PNS. Periparturient disorders in the bitch. In: Johnston SD, Root Kustritz MY, Olson PNS, eds. Canine and feline theriogenology. Philadelphia: Saunders, 2001:129-145.

Wheeler SL. Subinvolution of placental sites in the bitch. In: Morrow DA, ed. Current therapy in theriogenology 2. Philadelphia: Saunders, 1986:513-515.

Autor Joni L. Freshman
Consultor Editorial Sara K. Lyle

SURDEZ

CONSIDERAÇÕES GERAIS

DEFINIÇÃO
• Perda da capacidade auditiva em uma ou ambas as orelhas. • Existem duas formas: ○ Surdez sensório-neural — causada por dano a receptores presentes em estruturas como cóclea, nervo coclear ou vias auditivas no sistema nervoso central. ○ Surdez condutiva — causada por incapacidade de conduzir a vibração sonora desde as estruturas auriculares externas até as internas.

FISIOPATOLOGIA
Surdez Sensório-neural
• Degeneração coclear relacionada com a raça de cães e gatos neonatos — está intimamente associada a genes de pigmentação merle e malhada. Os alelos recessivos desses genes alteram a capacidade de os melanócitos da crista neural popular regiões do corpo, incluindo pele, pelo, íris, tapete ocular e porções da cóclea. A ausência de melanócitos na estria vascular da cóclea é associada à degeneração pós-natal precoce. • Degeneração coclear adquirida — causada por infecção crônica, ototoxicidade, neoplasia, exposição crônica a ruídos sonoros ou perda de células ciliadas e nervos ganglionares relacionada com a idade (presbiacusia*).
• Degeneração do sistema nervoso central — deve ser obrigatoriamente bilateral e extensa para interromper os trajetos auditivos no tronco encefálico, causando déficits neurológicos adicionais.
Surdez Condutiva
• Defeitos congênitos no canal auditivo externo, na membrana timpânica ou nos ossículos da orelha que transmitem a vibração na orelha média são raros. • Defeitos adquiridos que resultam em estenose do canal auditivo externo, ruptura da membrana timpânica, fusão dos ossículos originam-se mais comumente de otite crônica.

SISTEMA(S) ACOMETIDO(S)
Nervoso — orelha interna.

GENÉTICA
Não se conhece a genética de surdez congênita.

INCIDÊNCIA/PREVALÊNCIA
• Cães com um único alelo merle — 3,5%. • Cães com dois alelos merles ("merle duplo") — 25%; não há teste genético para o gene malhado.
• Prevalência de surdez congênita em uma ou ambas as orelhas está disponível para as seguintes raças: Leopardo da Catahoula — 63%; Dachshund colorido — 55%, Dálmata — 30%, Jack Russell terrier — 16%, Boiadeiro australiano — 15%, Bull terrier — 11%, Setter inglês — 8%, Cocker spaniel inglês — 7%, Border collie — 2,8%, Whippet — 1,3%.

DISTRIBUIÇÃO GEOGRÁFICA
Prevalência mais baixa de surdez neonatal em cães da raça Dálmata na Europa.

IDENTIFICAÇÃO
• Degeneração coclear congênita relacionada com a raça foi descrita em mais de 80 raças caninas. Com a exceção de Doberman pinscher e Shropshire terrier, todas as raças possuem uma grande quantidade de pigmentação branca associada aos genes merle ou malhado. • Surdez sensório-neural congênita presente por volta de 6 semanas de vida.
• Nenhuma associação com sexo ou genes de pigmentação da pelagem não relacionados ao merle ou malhado. • Cães com íris de cor azul apresentam uma incidência mais alta de surdez congênita.
• Gatos de raças mistas com pelagem branca e íris azul — alta incidência de surdez. Os gatos brancos de raça pura que carreiam o gene siamês para olhos azuis têm uma incidência mais baixa de surdez congênita. • Pode ocorrer surdez adquirida em qualquer raça ou idade de cão. A presbiacusia é comum em cães geriátricos.

SINAIS CLÍNICOS
• Para os proprietários, é difícil determinar a surdez unilateral. Raramente, os cães têm dificuldade de localizar o som. • Em casos de doença bilateral, os animais não respondem a sinais auditivos, como à chamada pelo nome ou ao barulho do prato de comida. Com frequência, eles são facilmente surpreendidos. Podem exibir uma resposta acentuada à vibração e a sinais visuais.

CAUSAS
Surdez Sensório-neural
• Provável etiologia genética em neonatos. • Dano adquirido à cóclea e ao nervo coclear — processo infeccioso, neoplasia do labirinto ósseo ou de nervo, traumatismo, distúrbio sistêmico, ou aplicação tópica de medicamentos ou toxinas (antibióticos — aminoglicosídeos, polimixina, eritromicina, vancomicina, cloranfenicol; antissépticos — etanol, clorexidina, cetrimida; antineoplásicos — cisplatina; diuréticos — furosemida; metais pesados — arsênico, chumbo, mercúrio; diversos — agentes ceruminolíticos, propilenoglicol, salicilatos); pólipos na orelha média.
Surdez Condutiva
• Otite externa e outras doenças do canal auditivo externo (p. ex., estenose do canal, neoplasia, ou ruptura do tímpano). • Otite média.

FATORES DE RISCO
• Coloração de pelagem merle, malhada ou branca. • Otite externa, média ou interna crônica.
• Uso de medicamentos ototóxicos.

DIAGNÓSTICO

DIAGNÓSTICO DIFERENCIAL
• Idade precoce de início — sugere causas congênitas em raças predispostas. • Uso de medicamentos ototóxicos ou otopatia crônica — indicam causas adquiridas. • Avaliar o animal quanto à presença de doença cerebral.

HEMOGRAMA/BIOQUÍMICA/URINÁLISE
Em geral, permanecem normais.

OUTROS TESTES LABORATORIAIS
• Cultura bacteriana e antibiograma do canal auditivo em casos de otites externa.
• Miringotomia** com cultura de aspirados em casos de otites média ou interna.

DIAGNÓSTICO POR IMAGEM
• Radiografias da bula timpânica e do crânio — não são exames sensíveis para otite média nem para otite interna. • TC/RM — técnicas sensíveis para otopatia média e interna.

MÉTODOS DIAGNÓSTICOS
RAETC — teste eletrofisiológico para medir a resposta elétrica da cóclea e das vias auditivas no cérebro a algum estímulo auditivo; exame confiável para identificar os cães com doença unilateral ou perda auditiva parcial; útil para diferenciar surdez sensório-neural e condutiva.

ACHADOS PATOLÓGICOS
• Surdez congênita — degeneração da estria vascular com subsequente colapso das estruturas membranosas do labirinto auditivo. O labirinto ósseo permanece intacto. • Surdez adquirida — relacionada com a doença primária, como otite ou neoplasia. • Ototoxicidade e presbiacusia — degeneração das células ciliadas auditivas, além de perda das células ganglionares e da estria vascular.

TRATAMENTO

ORIENTAÇÃO AO PROPRIETÁRIO
Os animais surdos podem ser funcionais, mas necessitam de paciência, adestramento especializado e proteção extra contra o tráfego de veículos.

CONSIDERAÇÕES CIRÚRGICAS
• Direcionadas às causas adquiridas; a surdez congênita é irreversível. • Otites externas, médias ou internas — as abordagens clínicas ou cirúrgicas dependem dos resultados da cultura e do antibiograma, bem como da resposta aos antibióticos e dos achados das técnicas de diagnóstico por imagem. • Condução auditiva — pode melhorar à medida que as otites externas ou médias desaparecerem.

MEDICAÇÕES

MEDICAMENTO(S) DE ESCOLHA
• Não há nenhum medicamento específico para surdez congênita. • Tratar as otites com base nos resultados da cultura e do antibiograma.

PRECAUÇÕES
• Aminoglicosídeos ou outros medicamentos ototóxicos — utilizar com cuidado. • Tratamento tópico do canal auditivo externo — evitar se a membrana timpânica estiver rompida.

ACOMPANHAMENTO

MONITORIZAÇÃO DO PACIENTE
Monitorizar o animal, conforme a necessidade, para o tratamento de otite.

COMPLICAÇÕES POSSÍVEIS
Os cães surdos necessitam de ambientes protegidos e adestramentos específicos para serem animais funcionais.

DIVERSOS

GESTAÇÃO/FERTILIDADE/REPRODUÇÃO
Os cães homozigotos para o gene merle recessivo são frequentemente cegos e estéreis.

ABREVIATURA(S)
• RAETC = resposta auditiva evocada do tronco cerebral. • RM = ressonância magnética. • TC = tomografia computadorizada.

Autor Karen Dyer Inzana
Consultor Editorial Joane M. Parent
Agradecimento T. Mark Neer

---

* N. T.: Diminuição auditiva relacionada ao processo de envelhecimento.

** N. T.: Incisão na membrana do tímpano para drenagem de pus ou líquido.

TAQUICARDIA SINUSAL

CONSIDERAÇÕES GERAIS

DEFINIÇÃO
Distúrbio de formação do impulso sinusal; aceleração do nó sinoatrial além de sua frequência normal de descarga (Fig. 1).

Características do ECG
- Cães — frequência cardíaca >160 bpm (raças toy >180 bpm; raças de porte gigante >140 bpm; filhotes >220 bpm).
- Gatos — frequência cardíaca >240 bpm.
- O ECG revela ritmo regular com uma possível variação pequena no intervalo R-R.
- Onda P de origem sinusal (pode apresentar pico) para cada complexo QRS com intervalo P-R constante.
- Ondas P podem ser parcial ou completamente fundidas com as ondas T precedentes.
- Geralmente apresentam início e término graduais.

FISIOPATOLOGIA
- A despolarização diastólica acelerada de fase 4 das células do nó sinusal geralmente é responsável pela taquicardia sinusal.
- Efeito adrenérgico aumentado ou inibição colinérgica acentuada resulta na alta taxa de formação do impulso sinusal; alterações na frequência cardíaca geralmente envolvem ação recíproca das divisões simpática e parassimpática do sistema nervoso autônomo.

SISTEMA(S) ACOMETIDO(S)
Cardiovascular — débito cardíaco = frequência cardíaca × volume sistólico. As alterações na frequência cardíaca afetam a pré-carga, a pós-carga e a contratilidade, que determinam o volume sistólico; a taquicardia grave pode comprometer o débito cardíaco. Frequências rápidas abreviam o tempo de enchimento diastólico e, particularmente nas cardiopatias, a frequência cardíaca aumentada pode deixar de compensar o volume sistólico diminuído, resultando em queda no débito cardíaco e no fluxo sanguíneo coronário. Taquicardias crônicas podem provocar dilatação cardíaca.

GENÉTICA
N/D.

INCIDÊNCIA/PREVALÊNCIA
- Arritmia benigna mais comum no cão e no gato.
- Distúrbio do ritmo mais comum no paciente durante o pós-operatório.

DISTRIBUIÇÃO GEOGRÁFICA
Nenhuma.

IDENTIFICAÇÃO
Espécies
Cães e gatos.
Raça(s) Predominante(s)
Nenhuma.
Idade Média e Faixa Etária
Nenhuma.
Sexo Predominante
Nenhum.

SINAIS CLÍNICOS
Comentários Gerais
Frequentemente não exibe nenhum sinal clínico, porque a condição é uma resposta compensatória a uma variedade de estresses fisiológicos ou fisiopatológicos.
Achados Anamnésicos
O significado clínico depende da causa subjacente. Em geral, a taquicardia sinusal não produz quaisquer sintomas. Se associada à cardiopatia primária, podem ser relatados os sinais de fraqueza, intolerância a exercício ou síncope.
Achados do Exame Físico
- Frequência cardíaca elevada.
- Pode permanecer normal sob outros aspectos se não estiver associada a condição patológica.
- Mucosas pálidas quando associada à anemia ou ICC.
- Pode haver febre.
- Sinais de ICC (p. ex., dispneia, tosse, cianose e ascite) quando a taquicardia sinusal estiver associada à cardiopatia primária.

CAUSAS
Fisiológicas
- Exercício.
- Dor.
- Contenção.
- Agitação.

Patológicas
- Febre.
- ICC.
- Doença pulmonar crônica.
- Choque.
- Efusão pericárdica.
- Anemia.
- Infecção.
- Hipoxia.
- Tromboembolia pulmonar.
- Hipotensão.
- Hipovolemia.
- Feocromocitoma funcional.
- Hipertireoidismo.

Farmacológicas
- Atropina.
- Adrenalina.
- Cetamina.
- Telazol.
- Quinidina.
- Broncodilatadores xantínicos.
- β-agonistas.
- Anestesia leve.

FATORES DE RISCO
- Medicações para a tireoide.
- Cardiopatias primárias.
- Inflamação.
- Prenhez.
- Anestesia.

DIAGNÓSTICO

DIAGNÓSTICO DIFERENCIAL
Deve-se diferenciar da taquicardia atrial, do flutter atrial com bloqueio AV 2:1 e da taquicardia juncional AV; à medida que a frequência sinusal aumenta, a onda P aparece mais próxima da onda T do batimento anterior. Com frequências muito rápidas, fica difícil distinguir esta condição de outra taquicardia supraventricular patológica.

HEMOGRAMA/BIOQUÍMICA/URINÁLISE
- Hematócrito baixo se o paciente estiver anêmico.
- Leucocitose com desvio à esquerda se os processos de inflamação ou infecção forem as causas.

OUTROS TESTES LABORATORIAIS
- Concentração sérica elevada de T_4 ou de T_4 livre (gatos) quando secundária ao hipertireoidismo.
- Teste de supressão com T_3 ou teste de resposta ao TRH se os valores de T_4 estiverem normais e se houver suspeita de hipertireoidismo.
- Coleta de amostra de urina de 24 h para análise de catecolaminas e seus metabólitos no diagnóstico do feocromocitoma embora os valores normais ainda não tenham sido estabelecidos; o teste de provocação para induzir à hipertensão com histamina e glucagon ou hipotensão com fentolamina pode ser valioso, mas não é prático.
- Monitorização de 24 h com Holter.
- Estudos eletrofisiológicos cardíacos.

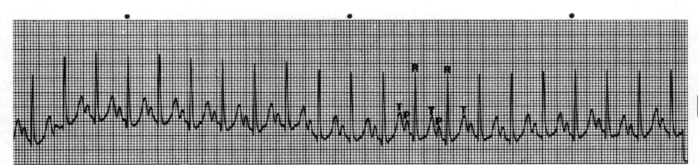

Figura 1 Taquicardia sinusal na frequência de 272 bpm em cão em choque. O ritmo é sinusal por causa da normalidade das ondas P e da relação P-R, bem como da regularidade do ritmo. (De: Tilley LP: Essentials of canine and feline electrocardiography. 3. ed. Baltimore: Williams & Wilkins, 1992, com permissão.)

TAQUICARDIA SINUSAL

DIAGNÓSTICO POR IMAGEM
• Radiografias torácicas para avaliar indícios de cardiopatia primária.
• Ecocardiograma para avaliar qualquer cardiopatia estrutural.
• Varredura da tireoide para avaliar hipertireoidismo.
• Ultrassom e angiografia abdominais para avaliar massa adrenal.
• TC e RM muito sensíveis para detectar massas adrenais.

MÉTODOS DIAGNÓSTICOS
• Considerar a manobra vagal não farmacológica para diferenciar de outras taquiarritmias supraventriculares; a compressão no globo ocular ou no seio carotídeo pode interromper a taquicardia supraventricular ectópica. Na taquicardia sinusal, as manobras vagais produzem uma diminuição gradual e transitória na velocidade da frequência cardíaca, se ocorrer. Menos comumente, graus variáveis de bloqueio AV (em geral, de primeiro grau ou de Wenckebach) podem ocorrer de modo transitório. Recomenda-se a monitorização com ECG durante essas manobras vagais.
• Um golpe precordial pode ser utilizado para diferenciar a taquicardia sinusal de outra taquicardia supraventricular. A taquicardia sinusal não será acometida, ao passo que a taquicardia supraventricular pode parar por no mínimo um ou dois batimentos.
• Mensuração seriada da pressão sanguínea arterial pode comprovar a hipertensão em pacientes com hipertireoidismo, feocromocitoma ou nefropatia.

ACHADOS PATOLÓGICOS
• Nenhum quando associada à causa fisiológica ou farmacológica. • Os achados patológicos dependem do processo mórbido primário.

TRATAMENTO

CUIDADO(S) DE SAÚDE ADEQUADO(S)
• Identificar e corrigir a causa subjacente, sempre que possível. • Independentemente de internação ou de tratamento ambulatorial, os cuidados dependem do estado clínico do paciente e da doença primária, se houver alguma (p. ex., se houver ICC, tratar como paciente de ambulatório a menos que o animal esteja dispneico ou gravemente hipotenso).

CUIDADO(S) DE ENFERMAGEM
Depende(m) da associação ou não com doença específica.

ATIVIDADE
É recomendável a restrição ao exercício se houver cardiopatia sintomática.

DIETA
Em geral, recomenda-se a restrição do sódio quando houver hipertensão e ICC.

ORIENTAÇÃO AO PROPRIETÁRIO
Discutir a importância de tratar qualquer doença primária de forma adequada, com intervenção clínica ou cirúrgica.

CONSIDERAÇÕES CIRÚRGICAS
• Tireoidectomia — opção terapêutica no hipertireoidismo (gatos).
• A remoção do tumor é o tratamento definitivo para os pacientes com feocromocitoma.

MEDICAÇÕES

MEDICAMENTO(S) DE ESCOLHA
• Estabelecer a causa subjacente e tratá-la adequadamente; em geral, a terapia antiarrítmica específica fica restrita a pacientes com ICC ou aqueles com cardiopatia secundária a hipertireoidismo ou hipertensão. • Cães — caso a ICC seja a causa, administrar digoxina e/ou pimobendana juntamente com diurético e inibidor da enzima conversora de angiotensina (ECA). Se a taquicardia sinusal persistir apesar da digoxina, considerar a adição de algum bloqueador dos canais de cálcio (p. ex., diltiazem na dose de 0,5-1,5 mg/kg VO a cada 8 h) ou β-bloqueador (p. ex., atenolol na dose de 0,25-1 mg/kg, sotalol na dose de 1-2 mg/kg) depois que a congestão estiver controlada.
• Gatos — caso a taquicardia sinusal esteja associada a hipertireoidismo sem ICC, um β-bloqueador (p. ex., atenolol na dose de 6,25-12,5 mg/gato VO a cada 12 h) pode reduzir a frequência cardíaca. Considerar a digoxina (0,008-0,01 mg/kg VO a cada 48 h, gato de porte médio, é preferível o uso de comprimidos) caso haja hipertireoidismo crônico acompanhado de ICC ou para o tratamento da miocardiopatia dilatada primária. Se a taquicardia sinusal estiver acompanhada de miocardiopatia hipertrófica, administrar atenolol (6,25-12,5 mg/gato VO a cada 12 h) ou diltiazem (1,75-2,4 mg/kg VO a cada 8 h) ou utilizar a forma de liberação sustentada do diltiazem (XR ou CD, 10 mg/kg VO a cada 24 h).

CONTRAINDICAÇÕES
Evitar medicamentos como a atropina ou as catecolaminas (adrenalina) que podem aumentar ainda mais a frequência cardíaca.

PRECAUÇÕES
β-bloqueadores podem potencialmente agravar os sinais de congestão e reduzir o débito cardíaco nos pacientes com disfunção sistólica.

INTERAÇÕES POSSÍVEIS
Consultar a bula do fabricante para medicamentos específicos.

MEDICAMENTO(S) ALTERNATIVO(S)
• Quando associada à efusão pericárdica, evitar a terapia medicamentosa e realizar a pericardiocentese.
• Se associada a determinado medicamento (p. ex., hidralazina e broncodilatadores), interromper a medicação ou ajustar a dose. • Quando associada à hipovolemia, repor o volume hídrico.

ACOMPANHAMENTO

MONITORIZAÇÃO DO PACIENTE
Depende da doença específica — na ICC, ECG seriado, radiografias torácicas, ureia, creatinina e eletrólitos séricos; no hipertireoidismo, T_4 sérica seriada, hemograma completo e bioquímica sanguínea.

PREVENÇÃO
Minimizar o nível de estresse, a atividade física e o sódio da dieta se houver cardiopatias.

COMPLICAÇÕES POSSÍVEIS
• Fraqueza ou síncope quando associada a baixo débito cardíaco. • Desenvolvimento de ICC se houver taquicardia sinusal persistente associada à cardiopatia.

EVOLUÇÃO ESPERADA E PROGNÓSTICO
• A taquicardia sinusal costuma desaparecer com a correção da causa subjacente. • Prognóstico mau apesar do tratamento se a taquicardia sinusal estiver associada a ICC. • Prognóstico favorável quanto à remissão da taquicardia sinusal quando o hipertireoidismo estiver controlado por meio clínico, cirúrgico ou com iodo radioativo.

DIVERSOS

DISTÚRBIOS ASSOCIADOS
Ver a lista de causas patológicas e fisiológicas.

POTENCIAL ZOONÓTICO
Nenhum.

GESTAÇÃO/FERTILIDADE/REPRODUÇÃO
• Aumento do débito cardíaco no final da prenhez (terço final), basicamente em virtude da frequência cardíaca acelerada. • Prenhez de múltiplos fetos em mulheres, associada à frequência cardíaca ainda mais elevada; aumento na suscetibilidade a arritmias, incluindo taquicardia sinusal.

SINÔNIMO(S)
Taquicardia sinusal inapropriada.

VER TAMBÉM
• Feocromocitoma. • Fibrilação Atrial e Flutter Atrial. • Hipertireoidismo. • Insuficiência Cardíaca Congestiva Direita. • Insuficiência Cardíaca Congestiva Esquerda. • Taquicardia Supraventricular.

ABREVIATURA(S)
• AV = atrioventricular. • bpm = batimentos por minuto. • ECG = eletrocardiograma. • ICC = insuficiência cardíaca congestiva. • RM = ressonância magnética. • TC = tomografia computadorizada. • T_3 = tri-iodotironina. • T_4 = tiroxina. • TRH = hormônio liberador da tirotropina.

RECURSOS DA INTERNET
Sístole prematura sinusal: http://www.chestjournal.org/content/64/1/111.full.pdf?ck = nck.

Sugestões de Leitura
Foe P. Unexplained preoperative tachycardia; is it an important issue? Can J Anesth 2005, 52(8):789-794.
Kittleson MD, Kienle RD. Small Animal Cardiovascular Medicine. St. Louis: Mosby, 1998.
Libby P, Bonow R, Mann D, Zipes D. Braunwald's Heart Disease: A Textbook of Cardiovascular Medicine, 8th ed. Philadelphia: Saunders, 2008.
Miller MS, Tilley LP, Smith FWK, Fox PR. Electrocardiography. In: Fox PR, Sisson D, Moise NS, eds., Textbook of Canine and Feline Cardiology, 2nd ed. Philadelphia: Saunders, 1999, pp. 67-106.
Morillo CA, Klein GJ, Thakur RK, et al. Mechanism of inappropriate sinus tachycardia: Role of sympathovagal balance. Circulation 1994, 90:873-877.

Autor Deborah J. Hadlock
Consultores Editoriais Larry P. Tilley e Francis W.K. Smith, Jr.

TAQUICARDIA SUPRAVENTRICULAR

CONSIDERAÇÕES GERAIS

DEFINIÇÃO
Despolarizações prematuras supraventriculares repetitivas que se originam de outro local além do nó sinusal, como o miocárdio atrial ou o tecido nodal atrioventricular.

Características do ECG
• Frequência cardíaca — rápida, 150-350 bpm nos cães. A frequência mais baixa da taquicardia supraventricular depende do porte do paciente. Os cães de porte menor tipicamente apresentam frequências mais altas do nó sinusal do que os de porte maior.
• O ritmo é geralmente bastante regular (intervalo R-R é constante) e pode ser contínuo, embora possa haver sequências breves frequentes ou infrequentes de taquicardia supraventricular, a assim-chamada taquicardia supraventricular paroxística. Raramente, o ritmo durante a taquicardia será irregular, sugerindo automaticidade anormal como etiologia.
• Em geral, os complexos QRS são típicos de complexos sinusais normais, estreitos e com eixo elétrico médio normal. Em alguns casos, a presença de bloqueio de ramo do feixe de His ou de condução ventricular aberrante concomitante torna difícil, se não impossível, a diferenciação entre taquicardia supraventricular e taquicardia ventricular pelo exame do ECG.
• As ondas P podem permanecer normais ou ficar anormais, mas tipicamente diferem em termos de configuração das ondas P sinusais. As ondas P podem ficar embutidas na onda T anterior e, dessa forma, não ser visualizadas.
• A condução atrioventricular costuma permanecer normal (1:1), embora possam ocorrer vários níveis de bloqueio AV funcional de segundo grau em frequências atriais mais elevadas (2:1, 3:1, 4:1, etc.).

FISIOPATOLOGIA
• A taquicardia supraventricular pode ser primária (idiopática) ou secundária a outras cardiopatias, em geral aquelas que provocam um aumento de volume dos átrios.
• Pode resultar de mecanismo reentrante ou de automaticidade anormal em um foco ectópico. Tipicamente, a taquicardia supraventricular reentrante produz um ritmo bastante regular; a taquicardia supraventricular atribuída a algum foco automático no miocárdio atrial pode produzir um ritmo irregular.
• A maior parte dos casos nos cães responde a medicamentos que alteram especificamente a condução e a refratariedade no tecido nodal AV, sugerindo a reentrada no nó AV como o mecanismo fisiopatológico.
• Estudos eletrofisiológicos recentes revelaram que determinada taquicardia supraventricular nos cães está relacionada com uma via acessória congênita entre os átrios e os ventrículos — via esta que faz com que os impulsos elétricos sigam livremente entre os átrios e os ventrículos sem atravessar o nó AV e sem atrasar a condução; nesses pacientes, a taquicardia supraventricular é provocada pela reentrada através da via acessória e do nó AV.

SISTEMA(S) ACOMETIDO(S)
• Cardiovascular — pode ocorrer o desenvolvimento de ICC secundária à insuficiência progressiva do miocárdio, associada à frequência cardíaca cronicamente elevada (a assim-chamada insuficiência miocárdica induzida por taquicardia).
• Neuromuscular — síncope ou fraqueza episódica generalizada, atribuídas ao declínio do débito cardíaco e à distribuição reduzida de oxigênio.

GENÉTICA
Com base nos dados clínicos, suspeita-se que a raça Labrador retriever tenha uma predisposição genética à via acessória congênita.

IDENTIFICAÇÃO
Espécies
Cães e, raramente, gatos.
Raça(s) Predominante(s)
A raça Labrador retriever está super-representada na literatura especializada.

SINAIS CLÍNICOS
Comentários Gerais
• Os sinais clínicos podem estar relacionados com a causa subjacente.
• Os cães com taquicardia supraventricular lenta ou taquicardia supraventricular paroxística infrequente não apresentam sinais clínicos.
• Os cães com taquicardia supraventricular rápida (frequência cardíaca, em geral, >300 bpm) normalmente exibem fraqueza ou síncope episódicas.

Achados Anamnésicos
• Em geral, os proprietários não têm consciência da arritmia. • Tosse ou anormalidades na respiração em cães com ICC. • Fraqueza ou síncope episódicas.

Achados do Exame Físico
• Ritmo cardíaco rápido, frequentemente regular. Nos cães com taquicardia supraventricular paroxística, no entanto, o ritmo pode estar normal e regular durante o exame físico.
• Pode haver indícios de má perfusão periférica — mucosas pálidas, tempo de preenchimento capilar prolongado e pulsos fracos.
• Pode não haver outros sinais além da frequência cardíaca rápida.
• Os achados podem refletir alguma condição cardíaca subjacente (p. ex., sopro cardíaco).

CAUSAS
• Valvulopatia crônica. • Miocardiopatia. • Cardiopatia congênita. • Neoplasia cardíaca. • Distúrbios sistêmicos. • Pré-excitação ventricular. • Distúrbios eletrolíticos. • Intoxicação pela digoxina. • Idiopática.

FATORES DE RISCO
• Cardiopatia. • Genéticos na raça Labrador retriever.

DIAGNÓSTICO

DIAGNÓSTICO DIFERENCIAL
• Taquicardia sinusal. • Flutter atrial. • Fibrilação atrial. • Taquicardia ventricular (a taquicardia supraventricular com bloqueio do ramo direito do feixe de His ou condução aberrante pode se parecer como taquicardia ventricular; a resolução da arritmia após a administração de lidocaína geralmente confirma a taquicardia ventricular).

DIAGNÓSTICO POR IMAGEM
• Ecocardiografia (incluindo estudos com Doppler) pode ajudar a caracterizar o tipo e a gravidade dos distúrbios cardíacos subjacentes. A ecocardiografia também é importante para avaliar a função do miocárdio em pacientes com taquicardia supraventricular idiopática.
• Quando observado ao ecocardiograma durante explosões de taquicardia supraventricular, o ventrículo esquerdo geralmente apresenta diâmetro sistólico final normal e diâmetro diastólico final pequeno, resultando em fração de encurtamento reduzida por causa do enchimento inadequado.
• Em geral, há um aumento atrial esquerdo ou direito nos cães com taquicardia supraventricular secundária a outros distúrbios cardíacos.

MÉTODOS DIAGNÓSTICOS
• O registro do ECG a longo prazo com o paciente em deambulação (Holter) pode detectar taquicardia supraventricular paroxística nos casos de síncope inexplicável. Esse exame geralmente é útil apenas se a síncope estiver ocorrendo de forma regular em um período de 24 a 48 h. Os monitores Holter também podem ajudar a caracterizar a velocidade e a frequência da taquicardia supraventricular sustentada, sendo valiosos para avaliar a eficácia da terapia.
• Registradores de evento (de alça) podem detectar taquicardia supraventricular paroxística em pacientes com episódios infrequentes de síncope (< a cada 24-48 h).
• Taquicardia supraventricular sustentada deve ser diferenciada de taquicardia sinusal, porque as duas arritmias apresentam implicações e tratamentos diferentes. Um golpe precordial pode ajudar a diferenciar a taquicardia sinusal da taquicardia supraventricular quando a frequência cardíaca estiver na faixa de 150-250 bpm; esse golpe geralmente interromperá uma taquicardia supraventricular por no mínimo 1 ou 2 batimentos, enquanto a frequência da taquicardia sinusal não diminuirá. A manobra vagal (p. ex., compressão no globo ocular ou massagem no seio carotídeo) pode interromper abruptamente a taquicardia supraventricular, mas só retarda a taquicardia sinusal de modo gradual.

TRATAMENTO

CUIDADO(S) DE SAÚDE ADEQUADO(S)
• Os pacientes assintomáticos podem ser tratados em um esquema ambulatorial; já os pacientes com taquicardia supraventricular sustentada ou sinais de insuficiência cardíaca congestiva devem permanecer hospitalizados até sua estabilização.
• A taquicardia supraventricular é uma emergência médica nos cães que apresentam fraqueza e colapso; as intervenções não farmacológicas que podem interromper a taquicardia supraventricular incluem manobras vagais, golpe precordial e cardioversão elétrica.
• As manobras vagais são quase sempre malsucedidas, embora possam ser usadas inicialmente por causa de sua facilidade de aplicação e da natureza não invasiva.
• A aplicação de um golpe precordial é capaz de interromper com êxito (>90% das vezes) a taquicardia supraventricular nos cães, mas essa manobra pode interromper o ritmo apenas por um breve período. Outras vezes, o ritmo permanece invertido. Para efetuar um golpe precordial, o cão é colocado em decúbito lateral direito e o batimento apical esquerdo, localizado. Essa região,

TAQUICARDIA SUPRAVENTRICULAR

então, é submetida a um "golpe" com a mão fechada enquanto se registra o ECG.
• Nos pacientes em que o golpe precordial não é bem-sucedido (ver adiante), é necessária a instituição de terapia médica de emergência.

CUIDADO(S) DE ENFERMAGEM
Tratar a ICC e corrigir quaisquer distúrbios eletrolíticos ou acidobásicos subjacentes.

ATIVIDADE
Restrita até que a arritmia seja controlada.

DIETA
Restrição leve a moderada de sódio na dieta no caso de ICC.

ORIENTAÇÃO AO PROPRIETÁRIO
Os proprietários devem observar os pacientes de perto em busca de sinais de baixo débito cardíaco, como fraqueza e colapso.

CONSIDERAÇÕES CIRÚRGICAS
Considerar a ablação por meio de cateter transvenoso para os pacientes com vias acessórias.

MEDICAÇÕES
MEDICAMENTO(S) DE ESCOLHA
Tratamento de Emergência
Administrar um dos seguintes medicamentos:
• Bloqueadores dos canais de cálcio — verapamil (0,05 mg/kg em bólus IV por 3-5 min até 3 vezes) ou diltiazem (0,05-0,25 mg/kg IV por 5-15 min).
• Bloqueadores β-adrenérgicos — esmolol (0,25-0,5 mg/kg administrado lentamente em bólus IV, seguido por infusão em velocidade constante de 50-200 μg/kg/min); insuficiência miocárdica moderada a grave é uma contraindicação relativa à administração desses medicamentos nessas doses.
• Métodos de cardioversão elétrica ou estimulação eletrofisiológica intracardíaca podem ser considerados em casos extremos.

Tratamento a Longo Prazo
• Digoxina — administrar em dose de manutenção por via oral ou dobrar a dose de manutenção no primeiro dia para gerar uma concentração sérica terapêutica mais rapidamente; contraindicada nos pacientes com vias acessórias.
• Bloqueador β-adrenérgico — atenolol (0,2-1 mg/kg VO a cada 12-24 h) pode ser administrado

contanto que o paciente não tenha insuficiência miocárdica moderada a grave subjacente.
• Diltiazem é o bloqueador dos canais de cálcio de escolha para o controle de taquicardia supraventricular a longo prazo. A dosagem necessária para controlar a taquicardia supraventricular não foi relatada no cão. O diltiazem é usado com maior frequência para controlar a frequência ventricular em pacientes com fibrilação atrial na dosagem de 0,5-1,5 mg/kg VO a cada 8 h. Em nossa clínica, geralmente começamos com essa faixa de dosagem, embora quase sempre seja necessário aumentar a dose para 2-3 mg/kg VO a cada 8 h para controlar o efeito da taquicardia supraventricular.
• Agentes antiarrítmicos de classe I como a quinidina e a procainamida podem ser tentados quando os medicamentos mencionados anteriormente forem ineficazes ou quando a taquicardia supraventricular for supostamente atribuída mais a um ritmo automático do que reentrante. A taquicardia supraventricular provocada por algum foco atrial automático pode produzir um ritmo irregular e ser refratária ao tratamento medicamentoso convencional. Quando a taquicardia supraventricular for atribuída a alguma via acessória, esses medicamentos serão mais eficazes.

CONTRAINDICAÇÕES
Evitar o uso de bloqueadores dos canais de cálcio em combinação com β-bloqueadores; pode ocorrer o desenvolvimento de bradiarritmias clinicamente significativas.

PRECAUÇÕES
Os bloqueadores dos canais de cálcio e os bloqueadores β-adrenérgicos possuem propriedades inotrópicas negativas e devem ser utilizados com cuidado em cães com insuficiência miocárdica comprovada.

MEDICAMENTO(S) ALTERNATIVO(S)
Tratamento de emergência — adenosina intravenosa (1-12 mg rapidamente por via IV). A adenosina é muito cara, além de ter vida curta; propranolol (0,02 mg/kg em bólus IV lento até uma dose total de 0,1 mg/kg). O propranolol tem uma meia-vida longa após administração IV e também possui efeitos significativos de bloqueio β2; em geral, esse medicamento não é recomendado a menos que não haja nenhuma alternativa disponível.

ACOMPANHAMENTO
MONITORAÇÃO DO PACIENTE
Monitoramento por ECG seriado ou Holter.

COMPLICAÇÕES POSSÍVEIS
Síncope e ICC.

EVOLUÇÃO ESPERADA E PROGNÓSTICO
A maioria é controlada de forma eficaz com medicação.

DIVERSOS
DISTÚRBIOS ASSOCIADOS
Vias acessórias em alguns pacientes.

FATORES RELACIONADOS COM A IDADE
Nos cães jovens sem indícios de cardiopatia estrutural, suspeitar de taquicardia reentrante com envolvimento de alguma via acessória.

SINÔNIMO(S)
• Taquicardia atrial. • Taquicardia juncional.

VER TAMBÉM
Fibrilação Atrial e Flutter Atrial.

ABREVIATURA(S)
• AV = atrioventricular. • bpm = batimentos por minuto. • ICC = insuficiência cardíaca congestiva.
• ECG = eletrocardiograma.

Sugestões de Leitura
Kittleson MD. Diagnosis and treatment of arrhythmias (dysrhythmias). In: Kittleson MD, Kienle RD, eds., Small Animal Cardiovascular Medicine. St. Louis: Mosby, 1998, pp. 449-494.
Kraus MS, Gelzer ARM, Moise S. Treatment of cardiac arrhythmias and conduction duisturbances. In: Tilley LP, Smith FWK, Oyama MA, Sleeper MM, eds., Manual of Canine and Feline Cardiology, 4th ed. St. Louis: Saunders Elsevier, 2008, pp. 315-332.
Wright KN. Assessment and treatment of supraventricular tachyarrhythmias. In: Bonagura JD, ed., Kirk's Current Veterinary Therapy XIII. Philadelphia: Saunders, 1999, pp. 726-730.

Autor Richard D. Kienle
Consultores Editoriais Larry P. Tilley e Francis W.K. Smith, Jr.

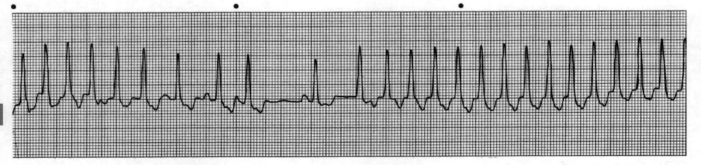
Figura 1 Nó sinusal com complexo atrial prematuro e taquicardia supraventricular paroxística. O início e o término abruptos da taquicardia ajudam a distingui-la da taquicardia sinusal (derivação II, 50 mm/s, 1 cm = 1 mV). (De: Tilley LP: *Essentials of canine and feline electrocardiography*. 3. ed. Baltimore: Williams & Wilkins, 1992, com permissão.)

TAQUICARDIA VENTRICULAR

CONSIDERAÇÕES GERAIS

DEFINIÇÃO
A taquicardia ventricular pode ocorrer em corações normais do ponto de vista estrutural (arritmias hereditárias) ou ser uma consequência de anormalidades do miocárdio associadas a quadros de miocardiopatia, valvulopatia significativa ou miocardite. Até o momento, não existe terapia clínica disponível que, sabidamente, evita a morte súbita em animais acometidos por taquiarritmias ventriculares.

Características do ECG
- Três ou mais contrações ventriculares prematuras sucessivas.
- Pode ser intermitente (paroxística) ou contínua; frequência cardíaca >150 bpm com ritmo regular.
- Complexos QRS — tipicamente largos e bizarros.
- Se houver ondas P visíveis — elas estarão desassociadas dos complexos QRS.
- Alterações eletrocardiográficas específicas à raça — a taquicardia ventricular em cães da raça Boxer é tipicamente positiva nas derivações ventrocaudais (derivações II, III e aVF) ou exibem um padrão de bloqueio de ramo esquerdo do feixe de His. A taquicardia ventricular em Doberman pinscher e Pastor alemão tem características tanto polimórficas como monomórficas.

FISIOPATOLOGIA
Arritmia potencialmente letal, pois pode se degenerar em fibrilação ventricular, resultando em morte súbita. Esse tipo de arritmia, em geral, indica miocardiopatia ou distúrbio metabólico/eletrolítico subjacente; os mecanismos incluem aumento na automaticidade, reentrada e pós-despolarizações tardias.

SISTEMA(S) ACOMETIDO(S)
Sistema cardiovascular, com efeitos secundários sobre outros sistemas, em virtude da má perfusão.

GENÉTICA
- Miocardiopatia arritmogênica do ventrículo direito na raça Boxer e miocardiopatia dilatada com taquicardia ventricular na raça Doberman pinscher são hereditárias como traços autossômicos dominantes.
- As arritmias ventriculares e a morte cardíaca súbita são hereditárias em Pastor alemão; o modo de herança é poligênico em função de alguma anormalidade em um gene importante com modificadores.

INCIDÊNCIA/PREVALÊNCIA
Arritmia comum em cães, mas incomum em gatos.

DISTRIBUIÇÃO GEOGRÁFICA
Nenhuma.

IDENTIFICAÇÃO

Espécies
Cães e gatos.

Raça(s) Predominante(s)
Observada comumente em cães de grande porte com miocardiopatia, sobretudo Boxer e Doberman pinscher. Cães da raça Pastor alemão com morte cardíaca súbita.

Idade Média e Faixa Etária
- Acomete todos os grupos etários caso não se trate de uma taquicardia ventricular específica à raça.
- Os cães da raça Boxer com miocardiopatia arritmogênica costumam se apresentar com 4-6 anos de idade, embora a frequência e a gravidade da arritmia, em geral, aumentem com o passar do tempo.
- Os cães da raça Doberman pinscher com miocardiopatia oculta tipicamente desenvolvem arritmias ventriculares, que começam com 3-6 anos de idade, embora também possa ocorrer muito mais tarde; a frequência e a gravidade da arritmia geralmente aumentam com o passar do tempo.
- Os cães da raça Pastor alemão desenvolvem arritmias ventriculares com 12-16 semanas de vida, mas a frequência e a gravidade das arritmias aumentam até 24-30 semanas de vida. Após 8 meses de vida, a gravidade da arritmia estabiliza-se ou começa a diminuir.

SINAIS CLÍNICOS

Achados Anamnésicos
- Síncope.
- Fraqueza.
- Intolerância a exercícios.
- Morte súbita.
- Podem permanecer assintomáticos.

Achados do Exame Físico
- Podem se mostrar normais se a arritmia for paroxística ou estiver ausente durante o exame.
- Pode-se auscultar uma taquicardia paroxística ou contínua.
- Os pulsos femorais podem variar ou ser fracos durante uma sucessão de taquicardia ventricular.
- Pode haver sinais de insuficiência cardíaca congestiva (ICC) ou sopro, dependendo da causa da arritmia.

CAUSAS
- Miocardiopatia.
- Defeitos congênitos (especialmente estenose subaórtica).
- Valvulopatia crônica.
- Dilatação e vólvulo gástricos.
- Miocardite traumática ou infecciosa.
- Intoxicação por digitálicos.
- Hipertireoidismo (gatos).
- Neoplasia cardíaca.
- Pancreatite.

FATORES DE RISCO
- Hipocalemia, hipercalemia.
- Hipomagnesemia.
- Distúrbios acidobásicos.
- Hipoxemia.
- Neoplasia (p. ex., hemangiossarcoma cardíaco ou esplênico).

DIAGNÓSTICO

DIAGNÓSTICO DIFERENCIAL
Taquicardia supraventricular com bloqueio de ramo do feixe de His. Caso se consigam identificar as ondas P, deve-se buscar a associação entre essas ondas e os complexos QRS. Se houver um intervalo P-R constante, o ritmo será supraventricular com bloqueio de ramo do feixe de His. Se não houver nenhuma associação entre as ondas P e os complexos QRS, o ritmo provavelmente será uma taquicardia ventricular. Caso não seja possível a identificação das ondas P em função de uma frequência rápida (P "embutida" na onda T anterior), a administração de lidocaína pode resultar na lentificação da frequência da taquicardia ventricular e na identificação das ondas P, se presentes. O término da taquiarritmia após a administração de lidocaína apoia o diagnóstico de taquicardia ventricular. Caso não se observe qualquer efeito com a lidocaína, a administração de esmolol pode resultar na lentificação da taquicardia supraventricular com bloqueio de ramo do feixe de His, de modo que as ondas P associadas aos complexos QRS possam ser identificadas.

HEMOGRAMA/BIOQUÍMICA/URINÁLISE
- A hipocalemia e a hipomagnesemia predispõem o animal à taquicardia ventricular e atenuam a resposta aos agentes antiarrítmicos de classe I (p. ex., lidocaína, procainamida, mexiletina e quinidina).
- Se a arritmia for secundária à pancreatite, haverá altos níveis de amilase e lipase.

OUTROS TESTES LABORATORIAIS
- Se a arritmia for secundária ao hipertireoidismo, haverá altos níveis de T_4 (gatos).
- Aumento da troponina I cardíaca em casos de miocardite. A troponina cardíaca é um biomarcador altamente sensível e específico de lesão do miocárdio.

DIAGNÓSTICO POR IMAGEM
A ecocardiografia pode revelar a presença de cardiopatia estrutural.

MÉTODOS DIAGNÓSTICOS
- ECG.
- Registro eletrocardiográfico deambulatório (Holter) a longo prazo ou registro eletrocardiográfico de evento — para a detecção de arritmias ventriculares intermitentes em pacientes com síncope ou fraqueza inexplicáveis.

ACHADOS PATOLÓGICOS
Variam de acordo com a causa subjacente.

TRATAMENTO

CUIDADO(S) DE SAÚDE ADEQUADO(S)
- A maioria dos pacientes com taquicardia ventricular intermitente pode ser avaliada com segurança em busca de doenças subjacentes (ecocardiograma, testes laboratoriais); no entanto, é preciso estabelecer uma base de referência real da quantidade e da qualidade da arritmia por meio do exame de Holter de 24 h antes de se iniciar a terapia.
- Em um animal instável (i. e., em decúbito lateral, fraco ou com episódios frequentes de síncope), talvez haja necessidade de tratamento intravenoso imediato em ambiente hospitalar com monitorização ECG contínua. Assim que a arritmia estiver controlada e o paciente se encontrar estável do ponto de vista hemodinâmico, deverá ser instituída a medicação por via oral. É necessário um acompanhamento com Holter de 24 h para avaliar a eficácia e os possíveis efeitos pró-arrítmicos da terapia antiarrítmica.

CUIDADO(S) DE ENFERMAGEM
Variam de acordo com a causa subjacente.

ATIVIDADE
- Em termos gerais, não há benefício conhecido para a restrição ao exercício.

TAQUICARDIA VENTRICULAR

- Os cães da raça Boxer tendem a ter uma incidência elevada de taquicardia ventricular durante momentos de agitação; dessa forma, os proprietários devem conhecer quais as situações específicas a serem evitadas em alguns casos.

DIETA
N/D.

ORIENTAÇÃO AO PROPRIETÁRIO
Alertar o proprietário quanto ao potencial de morte súbita.

CONSIDERAÇÕES CIRÚRGICAS
- Sempre que possível, determinar a causa da arritmia e tratá-la antes de induzir o paciente à anestesia geral.
- Avaliar se a taquicardia ventricular é passível de correção com uma dose-teste de lidocaína; em caso afirmativo, tratar com a lidocaína, seja em forma de bólus ou em velocidade de infusão constante, conforme a necessidade.
- A pré-medicação com acepromazina (0,02-0,05 mg/kg) eleva o limiar de fibrilação ventricular.
- Evitar o uso de medicamentos pró-arrítmicos, como agonistas alfa-2 (xilazina e medetomidina) e tiopental.
- Em pacientes inadequadamente sedados com arritmias ventriculares, não se recomendam as induções com máscara, pois o aumento do tônus simpático durante esse tipo de indução pode agravar a arritmia.
- É necessária a monitorização ECG contínua enquanto o animal se encontra anestesiado.

MEDICAÇÕES

MEDICAMENTO(S) DE ESCOLHA
Corrigir qualquer hipocalemia ou hipomagnesemia, se possível, antes de instituir a terapia clínica.

Cães
- Taquicardia ventricular aguda potencialmente letal — administrar a lidocaína lentamente em bólus IV de 2 mg/kg (até 8 mg/kg no total) para converter a taquicardia ventricular em ritmo sinusal; prosseguir com infusão de lidocaína em velocidade constante, a 30-80 µg/kg/min.
- Se a lidocaína falhar — administrar a procainamida lentamente em bólus IV de 2 mg/kg (até 20 mg/kg no total) para converter a taquicardia ventricular em ritmo sinusal; prosseguir com infusão de procainamida a 20-50 µg/kg/min ou 8-20 mg/kg IM a cada 6 h.
- Em casos de taquicardia ventricular refratária, pode-se combinar a lidocaína com a procainamida em infusões de velocidade constante.
- Se o paciente não responder à lidocaína ou à procainamida, recomenda-se a administração de bólus IV lentos de esmolol (um β-bloqueador de ação curta) a 0,05-0,1 mg/kg a cada 5 min até uma dose cumulativa de 0,5 mg/kg, ou 50-200 µg/kg/min em infusão de velocidade constante.
- A combinação de esmolol com procainamida pode causar uma queda significativa no débito cardíaco e na hipotensão.
- Taquicardia ventricular crônica em paciente estável — administrar o sotalol (1-2 mg/kg VO a cada 12 h), pois geralmente a monoterapia com mexiletina não é muito eficaz; no entanto, uma combinação de mexiletina (5-8 mg/kg VO a cada 8 h) com algum β-bloqueador como o atenolol (0,25-0,5 mg/kg VO a cada 12 h) ou sotalol (1-2 mg/kg VO a cada 12 h) pode ser mais eficaz para taquicardia ventricular refratária, especialmente em cães da raça Boxer.
- Em cães da raça Pastor alemão, a combinação de mexiletina e sotalol é a mais eficaz. A monoterapia com sotalol deve ser evitada em função de seus efeitos pró-arrítmicos nessa raça.

Gatos
- Utilizar a lidocaína com cuidado e apenas em casos de taquicardia ventricular contínua; nos gatos, é comum a ocorrência de neurotoxicidade (crises convulsivas). Usar um décimo da dosagem utilizada nos cães. • Nos gatos, prefere-se o atenolol (6,25-12,5 mg VO a cada 12 h).

CONTRAINDICAÇÕES
Evitar o uso de atropina e catecolaminas (p. ex., adrenalina e dopamina) até que a arritmia esteja controlada.

PRECAUÇÕES
- Em animais com ICC, devem-se empregar os β-bloqueadores com cautela. É recomendável a monitorização por meio de ecocardiograma para verificar o agravamento da função do miocárdio em virtude do β-bloqueio.
- O sotalol, quando utilizado como agente único, e outros medicamentos que prolongam a duração do potencial de ação podem agravar a taquicardia ventricular em cães da raça Pastor alemão com arritmias ventriculares hereditárias.

INTERAÇÕES POSSÍVEIS
A quinidina e a amiodarona elevam os níveis da digoxina.

MEDICAMENTO(S) ALTERNATIVO(S)
- Considerar a amiodarona, 10 mg/kg a cada 12 h por 1 semana (dose de ataque) e, depois, 5 mg/kg a cada 24 h (dose de manutenção) em casos de arritmias refratárias em cães. Embora a amiodarona seja um antiarrítmico potente, seus benefícios precisam ser ponderados diante de seu início de ação lento e de seus efeitos adversos, que incluem hepatotoxicidade, distúrbios gastrintestinais e discrasias sanguíneas em cães. É preciso ter cautela ao se considerar a terapia com amiodarona por causa de seus efeitos adversos. Os sinais de intoxicação incluem anorexia, vômito, letargia e elevação das enzimas hepáticas. A hepatopatia por amiodarona é reversível após a redução da dosagem ou a interrupção do medicamento. Os sinais clínicos evidentes de toxicidade desaparecem dentro de alguns dias do término da amiodarona. A atividade das enzimas hepáticas gradativamente retorna ao normal dentro de 3 meses após a interrupção da amiodarona ou a diminuição da dose.
- É recomendada a monitorização da bioquímica sérica seriada, já que os aumentos na atividade das enzimas hepáticas geralmente precedem o início dos sinais clínicos de intoxicação pela amiodarona. As enzimas hepáticas devem ser mensuradas 7 dias depois da dose de ataque e uma vez por mês durante a terapia de manutenção.
- Contemplar o sotalol (10-20 mg/gato a cada 12 h) em casos de arritmias refratárias em gatos.

ACOMPANHAMENTO

MONITORIZAÇÃO DO PACIENTE
- O aparelho Holter constitui o método de escolha para monitorizar a gravidade da arritmia e a eficácia da terapia antiarrítmica; o objetivo da terapia antiarrítmica é reduzir a frequência da ectopia ventricular em >85%.
- Pode-se lançar mão dos ECGs seriados e da telemetria — no entanto, tais exames não são tão úteis quanto a monitorização com Holter, pois é possível a ocorrência esporádica de complexos ventriculares prematuros e taquicardia ventricular paroxística ao longo do dia.
- Os níveis séricos da digoxina devem ser mensurados após 1 semana 8-10 h depois da ingestão do comprimido em pacientes submetidos a essa medicação.

PREVENÇÃO
- Corrigir os fatores predisponentes, como a hipocalemia, a hipomagnesemia, a hipoxia do miocárdio e a intoxicação por digoxina.
- Em cães da raça Boxer, devem-se restringir os níveis significativos de estresse ou agitação, pois o aumento no tônus simpático pode exacerbar a arritmia.

COMPLICAÇÕES POSSÍVEIS
- Síncope.
- Morte súbita.

EVOLUÇÃO ESPERADA E PROGNÓSTICO
- Se a causa for metabólica — a condição poderá se resolver, apresentando prognóstico bom.
- Se a condição estiver associada à cardiopatia — o prognóstico será reservado, porque a cardiopatia subjacente é provavelmente crônica e progressiva e, portanto, as arritmias também podem se agravar com o passar do tempo; a presença de taquicardia ventricular significativa aumenta o risco de morte súbita.
- Se a taquicardia ventricular estiver associada a hemangiossarcoma (cardíaco ou esplênico) — o desfecho a longo prazo será grave.
- Aproximadamente 50% dos cães da raça Pastor alemão com mais de 10 séries de taquicardia ventricular em 24 h morrem de forma súbita.
- Se os cães chegaram a 18 meses de vida, a probabilidade de morte súbita diminui.
- Ao contrário dos cães da raça Boxer com miocardiopatia arritmogênica do ventrículo direito, os da raça Doberman pinscher com taquicardia ventricular e miocardiopatia dilatada podem morrer de forma súbita durante o primeiro episódio de síncope.

DIVERSOS

DISTÚRBIOS ASSOCIADOS
N/D.

FATORES RELACIONADOS COM A IDADE
N/D.

POTENCIAL ZOONÓTICO
Nenhum.

GESTAÇÃO/FERTILIDADE/REPRODUÇÃO
N/D.

VER TAMBÉM
- Arritmias Ventriculares e Morte Súbita em Pastor Alemão.
- Complexos Ventriculares Prematuros.
- Doença de Chagas (Tripanossomíase Americana).
- Miocardite.
- Toxicidade da Digoxina.

TAQUICARDIA VENTRICULAR

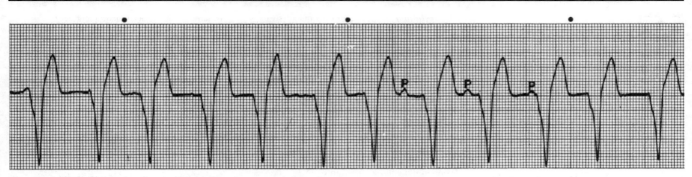

Figura 1 Taquicardia ventricular. Os complexos QRS largos e bizarros ocorrem em uma frequência de 160 batimentos/min, sem nenhuma relação com as ondas P. Há mais complexos QRS do que ondas P. A taquicardia ventricular deve ser tratada o mais rápido possível. Sempre se devem corrigir as anormalidades acidobásicas e eletrolíticas. (De: Tilley LP: *Essentials of canine and feline electrocardiography*. 3. ed., Baltimore: Williams & Wilkins, 1992, com permissão.)

ABREVIATURA(S)
- bpm = batimentos por minuto.
- ECG = eletrocardiograma.
- ICC = insuficiência cardíaca congestiva.
- T_4 = tiroxina.

Sugestões de Leitura

Gelzer AR, Kraus MS, Rishniw M, Hemsley SA, Möise NS. Combination therapy with mexiletine and sotalol supresses inherited ventricular arrhythmias in German shepherd dogs better than mexiletine or sotalol monotherapy: a randomized cross-over study. J Vet Cardiol 2010, 12(2):93-106.

Kraus MS, Ridge LG, Gelzer ARM, Pariaut R, Moise NS, Calvert C. Toxicity in Doberman pinscher dogs with ventricular arrhythmias treated with amiodarone. J Vet Intern Med 2005, 19(3):407.

Meurs KM, Spier AW, Miller MW, et al. Familial ventricular arrhythmias in boxers. J Vet Intern Med 1999, 13:437-439.

Meurs KM, Spier AW, Wright NA, et al. Comparison of the effects of four antiarrhythmic treatments for familial ventricular arrhythmias in boxers. JAVMA 2002, 221(4):522-527.

Moise NS, Gilmour RF, Jr., Riccio ML, Flahive WF, Jr. Diagnosis of inherited ventricular tachycardia in German shepherd dogs. JAVMA 1997, 210(3):403-410.

Tilley LP. Essentials of Canine and Feline Electrocardiography, 3rd ed. Baltimore: Williams & Wilkins, 1992.

Autores Marc S. Kraus e Anna R.M. Gelzer
Consultores Editoriais Larry P. Tilley e Francis W.K. Smith, Jr.

Tênias (Cestodíase)

CONSIDERAÇÕES GERAIS

REVISÃO
- Infecções por tênias adultas do intestino delgado, incluindo espécies de *Taenia*, (especialmente *T. pisiformis* dos cães e *T. taeniaeformis* dos gatos), *Dipylidium caninum*, *Echinococcus* spp. e *Mesocestoides* dos cães e gatos.
- Infecção adquirida pela ingestão de hospedeiro intermediário contendo larvas de tênias. *Taenia*, *Echinococcus* e *Mesocestoides* são adquiridos por predação de coelhos, roedores, pássaros, etc. O *Dipylidium caninum* é adquirido pela ingestão de pulgas adultas (ou piolhos).
- As tênias adultas não geram nenhum dano aparente ao hospedeiro a não ser prurido anal.
- Cestodíase larval peritoneal, causada por infecção do peritônio por larvas de *Mesocestoides*, é potencialmente fatal.
- Larvas e adultos de *Mesocestoides* podem se multiplicar de forma assexuada dentro do hospedeiro.

IDENTIFICAÇÃO
Cães e gatos.

SINAIS CLÍNICOS
- Segmentos isolados ou cadeias de segmentos, móveis ou secos, cor branca a creme, de *Taenia* e *Dipylidium* visíveis no períneo ou nas fezes; os segmentos de *Mesocestoides* são menores, mais numerosos e semelhantes a sementes de gergelim; os segmentos de *Echinococcus* são muito pequenos para serem visualizados.
- Arrastamento ou fricção do ânus no solo por causa do prurido perianal.
- Cestodíase larval peritoneal — distensão abdominal (ascite), anorexia, letargia.

CAUSAS E FATORES DE RISCO
- *Taenia*, *Echinococcus*, *Mesocestoides* — pela ingestão de vísceras de hospedeiros intermediários, como pássaros, répteis, coelhos, roedores, ovinos; tipicamente envolve o acesso a ambientes externos.
- Infecções por *Dipylidium* — pulgas (ou piolhos) no hospedeiro e/ou no ambiente.

DIAGNÓSTICO

DIAGNÓSTICO DIFERENCIAL
- Tênias adultas — impactação dos sacos anais.
- Cestodíase larval peritoneal — outras causas de ascite.

HEMOGRAMA/BIOQUÍMICA/URINÁLISE
Cestodíase larval peritoneal — há relatos de leucocitose e hipoalbuminemia.

OUTROS TESTES LABORATORIAIS
N/D.

DIAGNÓSTICO POR IMAGEM
Cestodíase larval peritoneal — ultrassonografia e radiografia abdominais.

MÉTODOS DIAGNÓSTICOS
- Exame de flutuação fecal para detectar os ovos; podem ocorrer resultados falso-negativos.
- Espremer os segmentos entre duas lâminas de vidro para liberar os ovos, adicionar uma gota de água e examinar sob microscopia em busca dos ovos.
- *Dipylidium* — pressionar uma fita adesiva contra a pele da região perianal para coletar os aglomerados de ovos e, em seguida, aplicar a fita a uma lâmina de microscópio; cada ovo do aglomerado tem ~50 μm de diâmetro e cor amarelo-pálida, além de conter um embrião hexacanto com três pares de ganchos.
- *Taenia*, *Echinococcus* — cada ovo (e não os aglomerados) tem formato esférico, cor castanha, ~30-35 μm de diâmetro e contém um embrião hexacanto.
- *Mesocestoides* — cada ovo (e não os aglomerados) tem formato oval, parede delgada e contém um embrião hexacanto.
- Cestodíase larval peritoneal — efetuar abdominocentese ou laparotomia para obter o líquido peritoneal; detectar as larvas nesse líquido por meio de microscopia ou PCR-RFLP.

TRATAMENTO
- Realizar tratamento anti-helmíntico ambulatorial para infecção intestinal por tênias adultas.
- Discutir a necessidade de controle de pulgas (ou piolhos) para evitar a recidiva de *Dipylidium*.
- Cestodíase larval peritoneal — além do tratamento anti-helmíntico, talvez haja necessidade de lavagem peritoneal ou cirurgia para remover o líquido ascítico e as larvas.

MEDICAÇÕES

MEDICAMENTO(S)
- Fembendazol na dose de 50 mg/kg VO a cada 24 h por 3 dias para *Taenia* adulta nos cães.
- Praziquantel na dose de 2,5-7,5 mg/kg VO, SC ou IM.
- Praziquantel/pamoato de pirantel — dose da bula para os gatos.
- Praziquantel/pamoato de pirantel/febantel — dose da bula para os cães, para *Taenia*, *Echinococcus*, *Mesocestoides* (fora da indicação da bula) e *Dipylidium*.
- Epsiprantel na dose de 5,5 mg/kg VO para os cães e 2,8 mg/kg VO para os gatos, para *Taenia*, *Dipylidium*.
- Emodepsida (3 mg/kg)/praziquantel (12 mg/kg), por via tópica uma única vez em gatos para infecção por *Taenia*, *Dipylidium*.
- Cestodíase larval peritoneal — praziquantel, 5 mg/kg SC repetida em 2 semanas, pode trazer a cura; fembendazol, 50-100 mg/kg VO a cada 24 h por 4-8 semanas (fora da indicação da bula); proporciona remissão clínica, mas frequentemente não leva à cura.

CONTRAINDICAÇÕES/INTERAÇÕES POSSÍVEIS
Não utilizar praziquantel ou epsiprantel para filhotes caninos ou felinos com <4 semanas de vida.

ACOMPANHAMENTO

MONITORIZAÇÃO DO PACIENTE
- Para infecção por tênias adultas, efetuar exame em busca de segmentos e/ou ovos de tênias após o tratamento; a remoção incompleta de *Mesocestoides* adultos pode resultar na repopulação do intestino por multiplicação assexuada.
- Para cestodíase larval peritoneal — realizar ultrassonografia e/ou abdominocentese para detectar recidiva; além de a eliminação ser difícil, as larvas podem repopular a cavidade peritoneal por multiplicação assexuada.

PREVENÇÃO
- Implementar o controle de pulgas (ou piolhos) para evitar a recidiva de infecção por *Dipylidium*.
- Evitar a prática de caçar presas e o ato de vasculhar lixo para impedir a ingestão de hospedeiros intermediários vertebrados e, consequentemente, a recidiva de infecção por *Taenia*, *Echinococcus* ou *Mesocestoides*.

EVOLUÇÃO ESPERADA E PROGNÓSTICO
- O tratamento anti-helmíntico eliminará as formas adultas de *Taenia*, *Echinococcus* e *Dipylidium*, mas frequentemente ocorre nova infecção.
- A remoção incompleta de *Mesocestoides* adultos por meio de tratamento anti-helmíntico pode resultar em recidiva da infecção na ausência de reinfecção como resultado de multiplicação assexuada por adultos.
- O tratamento de cestodíase larval peritoneal proporciona remissão clínica, mas com frequência não leva à cura; além de serem difíceis de eliminar, as larvas de *Mesocestoides* podem repopular a cavidade peritoneal por multiplicação assexuada.

DIVERSOS

POTENCIAL ZOONÓTICO
- Crianças podem estar sob risco de infecções por *Dipylidium* pela ingestão de pulgas adultas; nas crianças, os segmentos de tênias podem ser confundidos com nematódeos (*Enterobius*).
- A ingestão de ovos de *Echinococcus* pode provocar doença hidática em seres humanos.
- Pode ocorrer infecção de humanos por *Mesocestoides* adultos; a infecção não é adquirida a partir de cães ou gatos, mas sim por ingestão de hospedeiros intermediários vertebrados.

ABREVIATURA(S)
- PCR-RFLP = método de polimorfismo no comprimento de fragmentos de restrição, com base na reação em cadeia da polimerase.

RECURSOS DA INTERNET
- www.capcvet.org.
- www.cdc.gov.

Sugestões de Leitura
Bowman DD. Georgis' Parasitology for Veterinarians, 9th ed. St. Louis: Saunders, 2009, pp. 131-147, 149-151.
Caruso KJ, James MP, Fisher D, et al. Cytologic diagnosis of peritoneal cestodiasis in dogs caused by Mesocestoides sp. Vet Clin Path 2003, 32:50-60.
Crosbie PR, Boyce WM, Platzer EG, et al. Diagnostic procedures and treatment of eleven dogs with peritoneal infections caused by Mesocestoides spp. JAVMA 1998, 213:1578-1583.

Autor Julie Ann Jarvinen
Consultor Editorial Stephen C. Barr

TÉTANO

CONSIDERAÇÕES GERAIS

REVISÃO
• *Clostridium tetani* — bastonete obrigatório, anaeróbio, formador de esporos e Gram-positivo, encontrado no solo e como parte da flora bacteriana normal do trato intestinal de mamíferos, com predileção por feridas contaminadas, necróticas, anaeróbias (punção, cirurgia, lacerações, queimaduras, crioulceração, fraturas abertas, abrasões). • Esporos germinativos — produzem exotoxinas potentes, a tetanospasmina (toxina tetânica), nas feridas; resistentes aos desinfetantes e aos efeitos da exposição ambiental.

IDENTIFICAÇÃO
• Cães — ocasionalmente. • Gatos — raras vezes (sobretudo em casos de tétano localizado).

SINAIS CLÍNICOS
Achados Anamnésicos
• Aparecem alguns dias a alguns meses após a penetração dos esporos na ferida (fratura, cirurgia e punção). • Ferida — muitas vezes necrótica, mas pode sofrer cicatrização com o passar do tempo.

Achados do Exame Físico
Os sinais clínicos iniciais mais comuns em cães acometidos são anormalidades oculares e faciais.

Localizado
• Leve rigidez dos músculos ou do membro próximo ao local de inoculação (i. e., da ferida) dos esporos. • Rigidez dos membros (pélvicos); marcha rígida; fraqueza e incoordenação brandas. • Pode exibir resolução espontânea — reflete uma imunidade parcial contra a tetanospasmina. • Pode apresentar sinais prodrômicos a generalizados — quando uma quantidade suficiente de toxina ganha acesso ao SNC.

Progressivo/Generalizado
• Cauda — esticada; tetania progressiva dos músculos a ponto de manifestar a aparência de cavalete. • Convulsões (clônicas) — membros; o corpo todo (opistótono); dor durante as contrações. • Dificuldade respiratória — dispneia. • Dificuldade de abertura das mandíbulas — trismo (mandíbula travada). • Dificuldade de alimentação — disfagia. • Olhos — retração das pálpebras (visão sardônica); prolapso da terceira pálpebra à palpação da cabeça; recuo dos bulbos oculares na órbita (enoftalmia). • Testa franzida/preguiçada. • Orelhas eretas. • Aparência de sorriso largo e forçado — retração da comissura labial. • Salivação. • Febre, micção dolorosa (disúria) e constipação — podem ser observados. • Espasmos musculares tetânicos — decorrentes de estímulos (movimentos súbitos, sons, toques). • Óbito — durante espasmo dos músculos laríngeos e respiratórios (asfixia aguda fatal).

CAUSAS E FATORES DE RISCO
• Feridas sem curativos (p. ex., punções, cirurgia, fraturas ósseas compostas) — porta de entrada para os esporos. • Animais de rua — maiores oportunidades de sofrer ferimentos.

DIAGNÓSTICO

DIAGNÓSTICO DIFERENCIAL
• Intoxicações que mimetizam o tétano — envenenamento por chumbo e estricnina. • Reação distônica a agentes neurolépticos (atropina, acepromazina). • Raiva. • Meningoencefalite. • Polimiosite imunomediada. • Traumatismo da coluna vertebral. • Hipocalcemia. • Procurar por: lesão/traumatismo nos pés (coxins palmoplantares, unhas, espaços interdigitais), além de corpos estranhos em conjunto com feridas penetrantes.

HEMOGRAMA/BIOQUÍMICA/URINÁLISE
• Leucopenia inicial; alteração para leucocitose moderada; em seguida, retorno gradual aos valores normais. • AST e CPK — podem exibir algum aumento; resultado de danos musculares durante os estágios mais tardios da doença. • Urinálise — permanece basicamente normal; elevação nos níveis da mioglobina proveniente dos músculos lesados por excitação constante.

OUTROS TESTES LABORATORIAIS
• Sorologia — muitas vezes, os anticorpos antitetânicos não são detectáveis no soro. • Cultura — das feridas; em geral, a cultura em busca do *C. tetani* é frustrante; é imprescindível o uso de meio de transporte anaeróbio (não refrigerar). • Soro — para detecção da toxina (por meio da neutralização em camundongo). • Culturas do LCS e do sangue em busca de patógenos bacterianos de meningite.

TRATAMENTO

• Internação — é importante o fornecimento de cuidados satisfatórios e constantes de suporte e de enfermagem; período prolongado (3-4 semanas). • Alimentação — os pacientes frequentemente apresentam dificuldade de preensão do alimento, exceto quando recebem auxílio; prestar particular atenção à consistência dos alimentos que o animal ingere com facilidade; pode ser necessária a colocação de sonda via gastrotomia; a alimentação forçada ou o fornecimento de alimento por meio de sonda gástrica podem exacerbar o estado tetânico e, por essa razão, não são recomendados. • Hidratação — manter o consumo oral de água; se estiver inadequado, administrar fluidos intravenosos balanceados. • Manter o paciente em local escuro e tranquilo; não perturbá-lo. • Manter o paciente em cama macia; evitar a formação de úlceras de decúbito. • Vias aéreas e ventilação — avaliar; talvez haja necessidade da realização de entubação endotraqueal; mais tarde, pode ser imprescindível a prática de traqueostomia.

MEDICAÇÕES

MEDICAMENTO(S)
Sedação
• Para o controle dos espasmos reflexos e das convulsões. • Fenotiazínicos — são os medicamentos de escolha; clorpromazina; com ou sem barbitúricos (p. ex., fenobarbital). • Frequência cardíaca — pode declinar ao se empregar os fenotiazínicos em combinação; se a frequência estiver <60 batimentos/min, deve-se reverter a bradicardia com glicopirrolato. • Diazepam — medicamento alternativo utilizado no lugar do fenobarbital.

Antitoxina tetânica
• Inicialmente, testar quanto a reações de hipersensibilidade. • Imunoglobulina tetânica humana — administrar 500-3.000 U por via IM em múltiplos locais, especialmente próximo à ferida; ou usar a antitoxina tetânica equina (10.000 U por via IV). • Administrar toxoide tetânico adsorvido por via intramuscular.

Antibióticos
• Não surtem efeito contra a toxina já ligada aos nervos. • Metronidazol: cão, 15 mg/kg a cada 12 h ou 12 mg/kg a cada 8 h VO; gato, 10-25 mg/kg a cada 24 h VO. • Penicilina — administrar por vias sistêmica e local na ferida; 20.000 UI/kg a cada 12 h por 5 dias; usar penicilina cristalina no primeiro dia e penicilina procaína depois.

CONTRAINDICAÇÕES/INTERAÇÕES POSSÍVEIS
• Evitar o uso de glicocorticoides e atropina. • Evitar o emprego de narcóticos — causam depressão do centro respiratório.

ACOMPANHAMENTO

MONITORIZAÇÃO DO PACIENTE
• Evitar as úlceras de decúbito e as paralisias dos nervos periféricos — movimentar com cuidado os pacientes estabilizados. • Monitorizar a pressão arterial e o ECG. • Possível broncopneumonia. • Possível constipação.

PREVENÇÃO
• Vacinação — toxoide tetânico. • Evitar traumatismo das feridas cutâneas — limpar as passagens regulares dos animais e remover os arames em jardins, vidros, etc. • Tratamento da ferida — irrigação precoce e minuciosa de toda a ferida com peróxido de hidrogênio (i. e., água oxigenada); debridamento e drenagem, particularmente em feridas propensas ao tétano. • Penicilina — administrar por, no mínimo, 3 dias em casos de feridas profundas contaminadas.

EVOLUÇÃO ESPERADA E PROGNÓSTICO
• Talvez seja mais provável que os cães mais jovens com tétano desenvolvam sinais clínicos graves. • O prognóstico quanto à sobrevida em cães com tétano será bom caso não se desenvolvam anormalidades nos valores de frequência cardíaca ou pressão arterial. • Prognóstico — depende de uma série de fatores; quanto maior a quantidade de toxina ligada aos nervos, pior será o prognóstico; observa-se melhora com a remoção de fontes adicionais de toxina (debridamento e limpeza da ferida). • Curso da recuperação — lento; exige a reabilitação para recuperar o uso pleno dos membros; a maioria recupera-se em 1 semana; alguns apresentam curso de 3-4 semanas; a doença não tratada costuma ser fatal.

DIVERSOS

POTENCIAL ZOONÓTICO
Nenhum, embora os esporos tetânicos sejam ubíquos no meio ambiente.

ABREVIATURA(S)
• AST = aspartato aminotransferase. • CPK = creatino fosfoquinase. • ECG = eletrocardiograma. • LCS = líquido cerebrospinal. • SNC = sistema nervoso central.

Sugestões de Leitura
Greene CE. Tetanus. In: Greene CE, ed., Infectious Diseases of the Dog and Cat, 3rd ed. St. Louis: Saunders Elsevier, 2006, pp. 395-402.

Autor Patrick L. McDonough
Consultor Editorial Stephen C. Barr

Tetralogia de Fallot

CONSIDERAÇÕES GERAIS

REVISÃO
- Má-formação cardíaca congênita que consiste em DSV, estenose pulmonar, acavalamento/sobreposição da aorta e hipertrofia do ventrículo direito (Fig. 1). O DSV costuma ser amplo, com uma área equivalente ou superior à abertura da válvula aórtica. A anormalidade básica de desenvolvimento consiste provavelmente no desvio cranial de algum componente do septo infundibular; os outros defeitos são secundários.
- As alterações hemodinâmicas são determinadas principalmente pelo tamanho do DSV e pela gravidade da obstrução à via de saída do ventrículo direito. Um DSV amplo possibilita o equilíbrio das pressões ventriculares esquerda e direita, sendo a direção do desvio sanguíneo determinada pela relação entre a resistência vascular periférica e a resistência à ejeção ventricular direita. Uma obstrução grave à via de saída do ventrículo direito resulta em desvio da direita para a esquerda com cianose e eritrocitose compensatória como características clínicas proeminentes.
- Trata-se de um defeito congênito incomum, embora seja a má-formação cardíaca congênita mais usual indutora de cianose em cães e gatos.

IDENTIFICAÇÃO
- Cães e gatos — incomum em ambos.
- Predisposição das raças Buldogue inglês e Keeshond.

SINAIS CLÍNICOS
Achados Anamnésicos
- Fraqueza. • Síncope. • Respiração encurtada.

Achados do Exame Físico
- Em grande parte dos pacientes, verifica-se um sopro sistólico de ejeção na base cardíaca esquerda, causado por obstrução à via de saída do ventrículo direito; alguns animais com hiperviscosidade e estenose pulmonar grave não apresentam sopros cardíacos. • Cianose — observada na maioria dos pacientes; o grau da cianose depende da direção e do volume do desvio. Se a obstrução à via de saída do ventrículo direito for leve, a direção do desvio sanguíneo poderá ser da esquerda para a direita; nesse caso, a cianose não estará presente e a fisiopatologia será a de um DSV isolado. • Os pulsos arteriais costumam permanecer normais.
- Raras vezes ocorre insuficiência cardíaca congestiva, possivelmente em virtude da desembocadura do ventrículo direito no esquerdo, impedindo o desenvolvimento de pressões ventriculares direitas suprassistêmicas.

CAUSAS E FATORES DE RISCO
Congênitas; uma série contínua de defeitos conotruncais que incluem a tetralogia de Fallot é hereditária em cães da raça Keeshond; é provável que o modo de herança seja oligogênico. Os fatores genéticos são provavelmente importantes em termos etiológicos para o desenvolvimento do distúrbio de ocorrência natural/espontânea.

DIAGNÓSTICO

DIAGNÓSTICO DIFERENCIAL
- Todas as formas de estenose pulmonar, estenose aórtica, defeito do septo ventricular e defeito do septo atrial podem causar sopros de ejeção na base cardíaca esquerda.
- Os pacientes com estenose pulmonar grave e desvio da direita para a esquerda na altura do átrio podem exibir achados semelhantes ao exame físico.
- Outros desvios anatômicos da direita para a esquerda (PDA ou DSV com resistência vascular pulmonar elevada) tipicamente não geram sopros cardíacos; em casos de PDA com desvio sanguíneo da direita para a esquerda, observa-se cianose diferencial (as mucosas da cabeça encontram-se róseas, enquanto aquelas das porções caudais do corpo se apresentam cianóticas).

HEMOGRAMA/BIOQUÍMICA/URINÁLISE
- Em caso de desvio da direita para a esquerda, há eritrocitose compensatória.

DIAGNÓSTICO POR IMAGEM
Achados Radiográficos do Tórax
- Graus variados de aumento de volume do ventrículo direito.
- A porção ascendente da aorta pode estar proeminente.
- Os vasos pulmonares encontram-se pequenos.

Achados Ecocardiográficos
- Hipertrofia do ventrículo direito.
- Observação direta do DSV amplo.
- Sobreposição do DSV pela aorta.
- Infundíbulo estreito e/ou válvula pulmonar anormal.
- Evidência da estenose pulmonar ao exame com Doppler.
- A ecocardiografia contrastada tipicamente delineia um desvio sanguíneo da direita para a esquerda.

Angiocardiografia
- Revela o DSV, a hipertrofia do ventrículo direito, a estenose pulmonar e a direção do desvio sanguíneo.
- A angiografia não seletiva pode confirmar o diagnóstico em pacientes com menos de ~10 kg.

MÉTODOS DIAGNÓSTICOS
Achados Eletrocardiográficos
- Em grande parte dos cães e gatos há um padrão típico de hipertrofia do ventrículo direito.

Oximetria
- Utilizada para confirmar a dessaturação periférica da hemoglobina.

TRATAMENTO
- A maioria dos pacientes pode ser tratada em um esquema ambulatorial.
- É recomendável a restrição da atividade física.
- Tratar a eritrocitose por meio de flebotomia periódica para manter o hematócrito entre 62-68%.
- Já foram realizados procedimentos cirúrgicos paliativos que intensificam o fluxo sanguíneo pulmonar.
- A correção cirúrgica definitiva exige o desvio cardiopulmonar.

MEDICAÇÕES

MEDICAMENTO(S)
Os antagonistas não seletivos dos receptores β-adrenérgicos, como o propranolol, podem ser utilizados como paliativos; tais agentes atuam como inotrópicos negativos, limitando com isso a obstrução dinâmica à via de saída do ventrículo direito, e também evitam a queda fisiológica na resistência vascular periférica que ocorre durante os exercícios. Esses efeitos hemodinâmicos servem para limitar o desvio da direita para a esquerda. O propranolol também pode exibir efeito favorável sobre a curva de dissociação da oxiemoglobina.

CONTRAINDICAÇÕES/INTERAÇÕES POSSÍVEIS
Os vasodilatadores são contraindicados.

ACOMPANHAMENTO
- Monitorizar o hematócrito a cada 1-3 meses.
- Não é aconselhável a reprodução dos animais acometidos. • As sequelas potenciais são: endocardite bacteriana, complicações neurológicas associadas à eritrocitose, arritmias e morte súbita.
- O prognóstico é mau; a maioria dos pacientes com sinais clínicos vive menos de 1 ano; no entanto, há relatos de pacientes que sobreviveram por mais de 3 anos.

DIVERSOS

ABREVIATURA(S)
- DSV = defeito do septo ventricular.
- PDA = persistência do ducto arterioso.

Sugestões de Leitura
Kittleson MD. Tetralogy of Fallot. In: Kittleson MD, Kienle RD, eds., Small Animal Cardiovascular Medicine. St. Louis: Mosby, 1998, pp. 240-247.

Autor Jonathan A. Abbott
Consultores Editoriais Larry P. Tilley e Francis W.K. Smith, Jr.

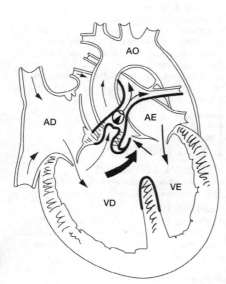

Figura 1 Tetralogia de Fallot clássica. AD = átrio direito, AE = átrio esquerdo, VD = ventrículo direito, VE = ventrículo esquerdo, AO = aorta. (De Roberts W. *Adult congenital heart disease*. Philadelphia: F.A. Davis Co., 1987, com permissão.)

TIMOMA

CONSIDERAÇÕES GERAIS

REVISÃO
- Origina-se do epitélio tímico, mas raramente sofre metástase.
- Infiltrado por linfócitos maduros.
- Pode ser associado à miastenia grave.
- Classificado como invasivo ou não.

IDENTIFICAÇÃO
- Raro em cães e gatos.
- Mais comum em raças caninas de médio e grande porte.
- Cães — idade média, 9 anos.
- Gatos — idade média, 10 anos.

SINAIS CLÍNICOS
- Provenientes da presença física do tumor — tosse, taquipneia, dispneia.
- Secundários à obstrução da veia cava cranial — tumefação da cabeça, do pescoço ou dos membros torácicos.
- Síndromes paraneoplásicas — fraqueza muscular e megaesôfago (causados por miastenia grave), poliúria e polidipsia (secundárias à hipercalcemia), polimiosite, doença cutânea.

CAUSAS E FATORES DE RISCO
N/D.

DIAGNÓSTICO

DIAGNÓSTICO DIFERENCIAL
- Linfoma (principal exclusão).
- Cisto branquial.
- Carcinoma ectópico da tireoide.
- Quimiodectoma.
- Vários subtipos de sarcoma.
- Mesotelioma.
- Granuloma não neoplásico, abscesso ou cisto.

HEMOGRAMA/BIOQUÍMICA/URINÁLISE
- Linfocitose — ocasionalmente.
- Síndrome paraneoplásica — hipercalcemia, anemia aplásica, hipogamaglobulinemia.

OUTROS TESTES LABORATORIAIS
Mensuração dos títulos de anticorpos contra os receptores da acetilcolina para confirmar a miastenia grave.

DIAGNÓSTICO POR IMAGEM
- Radiografias torácicas tipicamente revelam a presença de massa mediastínica cranial com desvio dorsal da traqueia, mas podem exibir efusão pleural ou megaesôfago.
- TC ou RM podem ser utilizadas antes de toracotomia para o planejamento cirúrgico, embora essas técnicas não sejam capazes de predizer a facilidade de ressecção.
- Ultrassonografia da massa — os timomas podem ser cavitários ou císticos, enquanto os linfomas são homogêneos.

MÉTODOS DIAGNÓSTICOS
- Aspirado por agulha fina guiado por ultrassom e citologia da massa: caracterizada por linfócitos pequenos, mastócitos ocasionais e possível população epitelial (*vs.* uma população pura de linfoblastos com linfoma).
- Teste do Tensilon® — avaliar a presença de miastenia grave em pacientes com sinais de fraqueza muscular, disfagia ou regurgitação.
- Talvez haja necessidade de biopsia para confirmar o diagnóstico.

TRATAMENTO

- Excisão cirúrgica — constitui o tratamento de escolha, embora a excisão seja possível em 70% dos casos; tende a ser altamente invasivo e de difícil ressecção em cães, porém menos invasivo e de mais fácil remoção em gatos; utilizar abordagem intercostal em casos de massas pequenas e esternotomia em casos de massas volumosas.
- Cães com miastenia grave e pneumonia por aspiração apresentam um prognóstico mais grave com a cirurgia.
- Radioterapia — potencialmente benéfica por reduzir o componente linfoide da massa (benefício de >75% dos casos); tempo de sobrevida médio: 248 dias em cães e 720 dias em gatos.

MEDICAÇÕES

MEDICAMENTO(S)
- Quimioterapia — há pouca informação disponível.
- Prednisona (20 mg/m² VO a cada 48 h) e ciclofosfamida (50-100 mg/m² VO a cada 48 h) — usadas em número bastante limitado de pacientes.
- Miastenia grave — tratar com prednisona e medicamentos anticolinesterásicos até que se consiga remover o tumor.

CONTRAINDICAÇÕES/INTERAÇÕES POSSÍVEIS
Medicamentos imunossupressores — não usar para o tratamento de miastenia grave associada à pneumonia por aspiração.

ACOMPANHAMENTO

- Radiografias torácicas — a cada 3 meses; monitorizar quanto à recidiva.

EVOLUÇÃO ESPERADA E PROGNÓSTICO
- Cura — possível se o tumor for passível de ressecção cirúrgica; mais de 80% dos pacientes vivos em 1 ano se o tumor for ressecável e se não houver megaesôfago associado; sobrevida média >1.800 dias para gatos e quase 800 dias para cães. 10-20% apresentam recidiva e podem responder favoravelmente a uma segunda cirurgia.
- Prognóstico — mau, quando não se consegue efetuar a ressecção do tumor, embora alguns cães e gatos tenham uma sobrevida prolongada apesar da ausência de terapia, provavelmente um resultado da natureza indolente do tumor.
- Pacientes com alta proporção de linfócitos no tumor têm um prognóstico mais favorável.

DIVERSOS

DISTÚRBIOS ASSOCIADOS
Tumores não tímicos concomitantes, polimiosite e outras doenças autoimunes — 20-40% dos pacientes.

VER TAMBÉM
Miastenia Grave.

Sugestões de Leitura
Gores BR, Berg, J, Carpenter JL, et al. Surgical treatment of thymoma in cats: 12 cases (1987-1992). JAVMA 1994, 204(11):1782-1785.
Smith AN, Wright JC, Brawner WR, Jr, et al. Radiation therapy in the treatment of canine and feline thymomas: A retrospective study (1985-1999). JAAHA 2001, 37(5):489-496.
Zitz JC, Birchard SJ, Couto GC, et al. Results of excision of thymoma in cats and dogs: 20 cases (1984-2005). JAVMA 2008, 232(8):1186-1192.

Autor Kim A. Selting
Consultor Editorial Timothy M. Fan
Agradecimentos Terrance A. Hamilton

TORÇÃO DE LOBO PULMONAR

CONSIDERAÇÕES GERAIS

REVISÃO
- Torção de lobo(s) pulmonar(es) no hilo, com oclusão ou estreitamento do brônquio, dos vasos linfáticos, da veia e (finalmente) das artérias.
- Lobos acometidos — o lobo médio direito é o mais comumente acometido (sobretudo em cães de grande porte); outros lobos podem sofrer torção isoladamente ou em pares. Ocasionalmente, ocorre torção na área mesolobar. Cães da raça Pug — é mais comum o envolvimento do lobo cranial esquerdo.
- No início, o lobo fica ingurgitado com sangue, o que provoca seu aumento de volume; na sequência, podem ocorrer infarto e necrose; tipicamente ocorre o desenvolvimento de efusão pleural hemorrágica; também é possível o surgimento de quilotórax.
- Sobreviventes crônicos — pode-se notar encolhimento e fibrose do lobo.

IDENTIFICAÇÃO
- Cães e, menos comumente, gatos.
- Mais comum em raças de grande porte com tórax profundo, embora as raças de pequeno porte também possam ser acometidas.
- Raça Afghan (quilotórax).
- Qualquer idade.
- Síndrome espontânea no Pug com idade igual ou inferior a 4 anos.
- Mais comum em machos.

SINAIS CLÍNICOS
- Taquipneia, além de angústia respiratória aguda ou crônica.
- Letargia.
- Anorexia.
- Febre.
- Dor.
- Ortopneia.
- Tosse, hemoptise.
- Ânsia de vômito.
- Macicez torácica ventral.
- Taquicardia.
- Mucosas pálidas.
- Cianose.
- Choque.

CAUSAS E FATORES DE RISCO
- Incoerentemente associada a distúrbios preexistentes (p. ex., traumatismo, neoplasia e quilotórax; asma/bronquite no gato).
- Cirurgia torácica ou diafragmática.
- Espontânea ou idiopática.

DIAGNÓSTICO

DIAGNÓSTICO DIFERENCIAL
- Contusão pulmonar ou atelectasia.
- Hérnia diafragmática.
- Abscesso ou infarto pulmonar.
- Neoplasia, granulomatose linfomatoide.
- Coagulopatia.
- Pneumonia, formação de êmbolo ou trombose.
- Insuficiência cardíaca congestiva.
- Efusão pleural não complicada e atelectasia compressiva.
- Granuloma fúngico ou por corpo estranho.
- Consolidação lobar ou obstrução bronquial por corpo estranho.
- Esteatite felina.

HEMOGRAMA/BIOQUÍMICA/URINÁLISE
São comuns as alterações de neutrofilia e anemia. A ocorrência de neutropenia pode carrear um prognóstico pior.

OUTROS TESTES LABORATORIAIS
Análise do líquido pleural — efusão pleural tipicamente hemorrágica com hematócrito e leucograma semelhantes ao do sangue periférico, mas com deficiência de plaquetas; com a cronicidade ou as efusões preexistentes, a efusão pode ser um transudato modificado ou exibir natureza quilosa.

DIAGNÓSTICO POR IMAGEM
Radiografia
- Opacificação de lobo acometido com perda de vasos lobares visíveis ou truncamento do brônquio.
- Inicialmente, pode revelar broncogramas aéreos com estreitamento proximal ou desorientação do brônquio torcido. Pequenas bolhas de gás com "aspecto de esponja" podem estar dispersas em todo o lobo acometido (padrão gasoso vesicular); observadas em 85% dos casos de uma sequência radiográfica.
- Efusão pleural progressiva — sugerida pela partição ventral e fissuras interlobares.
- Consolidação e tumefação ocasional do lobo torcido com possível deslocamento ou rotação do coração, da traqueia ou da carina traqueal. O desvio do mediastino pode ser contralateral ou ipsolateral. Outros lobos podem estar deslocados.
- A toracocentese gera benefícios terapêuticos e pode melhorar a visualização das estruturas intratorácicas.

Ultrassonografia
- A ultrassonografia torácica antes da remoção do líquido frequentemente confere uma melhor resolução das estruturas internas.
- Periferia hipoecoica com focos reverberantes dispersos na região central.
- Margens arredondadas dos lobos.

Tomografia Computadorizada
A realização de tomografia computadorizada pré-operatória pode ser útil. Esse exame necessita de apneia induzida por hiperventilação ou respiração presa.

MÉTODOS DIAGNÓSTICOS
- Toracocentese — obter líquido pleural para análise (transudato modificado, exsudato, hemorragia, ou possível efusão quilosa).
- Broncoscopia — pode revelar oclusão ou torção do brônquio associado.
- Exploração cirúrgica — para diagnóstico definitivo e tratamento.

TRATAMENTO

- Realização de toracocentese ou colocação de dreno torácico, conforme a necessidade.
- Administração de fluido intravenoso como terapia de suporte.
- Oxigenoterapia e tratamento do choque — quando indicados.
- Anestesia — requer suporte ventilatório adequado; monitorizar o paciente cuidadosamente.
- Remoção cirúrgica do(s) lobo(s) envolvido(s) — único tratamento eficaz; não destorcer o lobo e tentar recuperá-lo (pode levar à recidiva ou necrose); são defendidos os procedimentos de ligadura *in situ* dos vasos ou grampeamento com pinças atraumáticas; inspecionar atentamente as estruturas torácicas remanescentes em busca de quaisquer anormalidades; fazer cultura e exame patológico da amostra excisada.
- Pós-cirurgia — monitorização; cuidado de suporte; tubo de drenagem. Pode ocorrer a torção de um segundo lobo pulmonar.

MEDICAÇÕES

MEDICAMENTO(S)
- Antibióticos — no pós-operatório.
- Tratamento do choque — quando indicado.
- Controle da dor.

CONTRAINDICAÇÕES/INTERAÇÕES POSSÍVEIS
N/D.

ACOMPANHAMENTO

- Observar o paciente quanto à recidiva de efusão pleural.
- Edema pulmonar por reexpansão — pode ser um problema grave (sobretudo em gatos) se grandes volumes de líquido pleural forem retirados com rapidez ou se os pulmões cronicamente comprimidos forem submetidos à insuflação aguda na cirurgia.
- Radiografias torácicas — antes de dar alta; conforme a necessidade daí em diante.
- Prognóstico — razoável a bom se não permanecer nenhuma anormalidade subjacente.

DIVERSOS

Sugestões de Leitura
D'Anjou M, Tidwell AS, Hecht S. Radiographic diagnosis of lung lobe torsion. Vet Radiol Ultrasound 2005, 46:478-484.
Dye TL, Teague HD, Poundstone ML. Lung lobe torsion in a cat with chronic feline asthma. JAAHA 1998, 34:493-495.
Murphy KA, Brisson BA. Evaluation of lung lobe torsion in pugs: 7 cases (1991-2004). JAVMA 2006, 228:86-90.
Neath PJ, Brockman DJ, King LG. Lung lobe torsion in dogs: 22 cases (1981-1999). JAVMA 2000, 217(7):1041-1044.

Autor Bradley L. Moses
Consultor Editorial Lynelle R. Johnson

TORÇÃO ESPLÊNICA

CONSIDERAÇÕES GERAIS

REVISÃO
- Pode ocorrer como uma entidade isolada ou em associação com a síndrome de dilatação e vólvulo gástricos.
- Aguda ou crônica.
- Fisiopatologia — desconhecida.
- Sistemas acometidos — hemático/linfático/imune e cardiovascular.
- A torção esplênica isolada é rara.

IDENTIFICAÇÃO
- Mais comum nos cães pertencentes às raças de grande porte, com tórax profundo, como Pastor alemão, Poodle standard e Dinamarquês.
- Sem predileção sexual.

SINAIS CLÍNICOS
Achados Anamnésicos
- Agudos — colapso cardiovascular e dor abdominal.
- Crônicos — anorexia intermitente, vômito, perda de peso e, possivelmente, hemoglobinúria.

Achados do Exame Físico
- Mucosas pálidas, taquicardia e outros sinais de hipoperfusão.
- Massa abdominal palpável (baço).

CAUSAS E FATORES DE RISCO
- Raças caninas de grande porte e tórax profundo.
- Estiramento anterior dos ligamentos gastresplênico, frenicosplênico e esplenocólico (p. ex., dilatação e vólvulo gástricos prévios).
- Histórico de dilatação gástrica.
- Exercício excessivo, rolamento e ânsia de vômito podem contribuir para a ocorrência de torção esplênica.
- Nervosismo e ansiedade foram associados a um aumento no risco de dilatação e vólvulo gástricos.

DIAGNÓSTICO

DIAGNÓSTICO DIFERENCIAL
- Outras doenças esplênicas (p. ex., neoplasia e doença imunomediada).
- Doença gastrintestinal aguda com dor abdominal.

HEMOGRAMA/BIOQUÍMICA/URINÁLISE
- Anemia.
- Trombocitopenia.
- Leucocitose.
- Valores elevados das enzimas hepáticas.
- Hemoglobinúria.

OUTROS TESTES LABORATORIAIS
Teste de coagulação — CID (prolongamento nos tempos de protrombina e de tromboplastina parcial, além de aumento dos produtos de degradação da fibrina) por causa do consumo acelerado.

DIAGNÓSTICO POR IMAGEM
Radiografia Abdominal
- Pode ser observada massa cranial ou mesoabdominal.
- O baço pode exibir uma localização anormal.

Ultrassonografia Abdominal
- Congestão esplênica/ausência de fluxo sanguíneo para o baço.
- Veias esplênicas dilatadas.
- Infarto esplênico.

MÉTODOS DIAGNÓSTICOS
ECG — pode revelar arritmias ventriculares.

ACHADOS PATOLÓGICOS
Congestão e infarto esplênicos.

TRATAMENTO

- Trata-se de emergência cirúrgica.
- Após a estabilização cardiovascular adequada, deve-se realizar o procedimento de esplenectomia sem distorcer o pedículo esplênico.
- Também é recomendável a realização de gastropexia permanente por causa da associação com a síndrome de dilatação e vólvulo gástricos.
- Amostra esplênica deve ser encaminhada para exame histopatológico.
- Após a esplenectomia, ficam indicados o suporte hídrico e a monitorização cardiovascular.

MEDICAÇÕES

MEDICAMENTO(S)
- Não há necessidade de medicamentos específicos.
- É aconselhável o alívio da dor pós-operatória.
- Heparina (não fracionada ou de baixo peso molecular) ou transfusão de plasma (raramente em virtude do porte do paciente) podem ser consideradas caso se comprovem os quadros de CID e coagulopatia.

CONTRAINDICAÇÕES/INTERAÇÕES POSSÍVEIS
Nenhuma.

ACOMPANHAMENTO
A correção cirúrgica é considerada um procedimento curativo.

DIVERSOS

ABREVIATURA(S)
- CID = coagulação intravascular disseminada.
- ECG = eletrocardiograma.

Sugestões de Leitura
Neath PJ, Brookman DJ, Saunders HM. Retrospective analysis of 19 cases of isolated torsion of the splenic pedicle in dogs. J Small Anim Pract 1997, 38:337–392.
Stoneham A, Henderson A, O'Toole T. Resolution of severe thrombocytopenia in two standard poodles with surgical correction of splenic torsion. JVECCS 2006, 16:131–135.

Autor Elizabeth A. Rozanski
Consultor Editorial A.H. Rebar

TOSSE

CONSIDERAÇÕES GERAIS

DEFINIÇÃO
• Um reflexo de defesa súbito e frequentemente repetitivo que ajuda a limpar as vias aéreas calibrosas do excesso de secreções, irritantes, partículas estranhas e microrganismos ou remover material estranho das vias aéreas superiores.
• O reflexo da tosse consiste em três fases: inalação, exalação forçada contra uma glote fechada, e expulsão violenta de ar a partir dos pulmões após a abertura da glote, acompanhada em geral por um ruído súbito. A tosse pode acontecer de forma voluntária ou involuntária, embora se suponha que ela seja basicamente involuntária em cães e gatos.

FISIOPATOLOGIA
• Um reflexo fisiológico em animais saudáveis que protege as vias aéreas inferiores contra inalação de partículas estranhas e ajuda a remover as partículas que ficaram presas no muco; atua em conjunto com o mecanismo de depuração mucociliar.
• A via da tosse inclui os receptores da tosse, compostos por nervos sensoriais nas vias aéreas, nervo vago, centro da tosse e músculos efetores.
• A via da tosse pode ser estimulada por fatores mecânicos ou químicos. Os deflagradores endógenos incluem secreções e inflamação das vias aéreas, enquanto os exógenos abrangem fumaça e material estranho aspirado.
• Os receptores da tosse compreendem receptores de estiramento pulmonar de adaptação rápida (sensíveis a estímulos mecânicos), situados na mucosa da árvore traqueobrônquica (especialmente laringe e traqueia), e fibras-C pulmonares/bronquiais, mais sensíveis à estimulação química. Os mecanismos e as vias da tosse são muito complexos e não completamente compreendidos, até mesmo em seres humanos.

SISTEMA(S) ACOMETIDO(S)
• Respiratório — tosse de qualquer origem pode ser um fator incitante para o agravamento ou a precipitação de sinais associados a colapso traqueal em raças suscetíveis.
• Cardiovascular — aumento de volume do ventrículo direito ou comprometimento da função desse ventrículo pode se originar de algum distúrbio respiratório, causando dano tecidual, lesão hipóxica e/ou vasoconstrição pulmonar hipóxica crônica (*cor pulmonale*).

IDENTIFICAÇÃO
• Cães e gatos de todas as idades e raças.
• Sinal clínico muito mais comum em cães do que em gatos.
• A tosse de origem traqueal é menos comum em gatos do que em cães.
• As predisposições etária, racial e sexual variam com a causa incitante.

SINAIS CLÍNICOS
• A tosse deve ser diferenciada de sinais semelhantes, como espirro reverso, vômito seco, ânsia de vômito.
• A descrição da tosse pode ser útil na identificação das estruturas anatômicas envolvidas nos cães (ou seja, tosse grasnante é típica de colapso traqueal, enquanto tosse sonora e áspera, acompanhada por ânsia de vômito no final, caracteriza tosse de origem traqueal ou bronquial; a tosse úmida fraca é ouvida em casos de pneumonia moderada a grave).
• A tosse pode ser descrita como seca ou úmida, produtiva, grasnante, curta ou áspera, fraca ou sonora, acompanhada por vômito seco ou ânsia de vômito.
• A tosse pode ser eliciada por tração na coleira (origem laríngea ou traqueal), agravada por exercício ou excitação (colapso traqueal) ou ocorrer após um período de repouso (tosse causada por insuficiência cardíaca).
• Pode ser acompanhada por estertor ou estridor (origem laríngea ou traqueal) ou dispneia (muitas áreas).

CAUSAS

Doenças do Trato Respiratório Superior
• Diversas condições sinonasais provocam extensão da inflamação e/ou secreções na faringe e/ou laringe e podem levar à "síndrome de tosse das vias aéreas superiores", conhecida previamente como "síndrome de gotejamento pós-nasal".
• Laringopatia (inflamação, paralisia, tumor, granuloma, colapso).
• Traqueopatia (inflamação, infecção, corpo estranho, colapso, estenose, tumor).

Doenças do Trato Respiratório Inferior (Doença Traqueobrônquica ou Broncopulmonar)
• Inflamatórias (gatos: síndrome de bronquite felina; cães: bronquite crônica, broncopneumopatia eosinofílica).
• Infecciosas — bacterianas, virais (cinomose, tosse dos canis [cães]; FeLV, FIV, PIF, calicivírus, herpes-vírus [gatos]), parasitárias (*Filaroides* spp. [cães], *Aerulostrongylus abstrusus* [gatos], *Paragonimus kellicotti* [cães, gatos], *Dirofilaria immitis* [cães, gatos], *Capillaria aerophilia* [cães], *Crenosoma vulpis* [cães], protozoárias (toxoplasmose [gatos]; pneumocistose [cães]), fúngicas (blastomicose, histoplasmose, coccidioidomicose, criptococose, aspergilose).
• Neoplásicas (primárias, metastáticas, compressão causada por enfartamento dos linfonodos).
• Químicas ou traumáticas (aspiração, afogamento por um triz, vapores tóxicos, corpo estranho, traumatismo, hemorragia).
• Distúrbios crônicos de origem desconhecida (fibrose pulmonar intersticial).

Outras Doenças
• Doenças cardiovasculares (edema pulmonar, aumento de volume do átrio esquerdo, tumor na base do coração, embolia).
• Refluxo gastresofágico.
• Compressão das estruturas respiratórias por órgãos adjacentes (cardiomegalia, megaesôfago, enfartamento de linfonodos hilares).
• Edema pulmonar não cardiogênico (múltiplas causas).
• Inalação passiva de fumaça.
• Reação medicamentosa adversa — brometo de potássio em gatos.

FATORES DE RISCO

Fatores raciais
• Raças toys e miniaturas estão sob risco de colapso traqueal.
• Raças de terrier apresentam risco de fibrose pulmonar.
• As raças Husky, Rottweiler, Labrador e Jack Russell terrier exibem risco de broncopneumopatia eosinofílica.
• As raças gigantes têm risco de miocardiopatia dilatada.
• A raça Labrador retriever, bem como as de grande porte, demonstra risco de paralisia laríngea.
• Os gatos Siameses evidenciam risco de síndrome de bronquite felina.

Fatores ambientais
• Os gatos de pelo longo que raramente são penteados apresentam episódios periódicos de ânsia de vômito, tosse e vômito de bolas de pelo (tricobezoar).

Medicamentos
• Brometo de potássio em gatos.

Área geográfica (ou histórico de viagem)
• Certas doenças são comuns em regiões específicas (p. ex., dirofilariose, angiostrongilose).

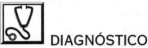

DIAGNÓSTICO

DIAGNÓSTICO DIFERENCIAL
• Sinais semelhantes.
• A tosse pode ser confundida com outros sinais, como espirro, espirro reverso, vômito seco, respiração ofegante, ânsia de vômito e vômito. A presença de ânsia de vômito terminal é frequentemente mal-interpretada como vômito.

HEMOGRAMA/BIOQUÍMICA/URINÁLISE
A obtenção de banco de dados mínimo pode sugerir infecção bacteriana aguda (leucocitose com desvio à esquerda) ou doença eosinofílica das vias aéreas (eosinofilia periférica).

OUTROS TESTES LABORATORIAIS
• Teste de filtro para microfilárias e/ou teste sorológico para filárias — pesquisam dirofilariose.
• Título humoral sérico — toxoplasmose, FIV, PIF, cinomose.
• Perfil de coagulação — para qualquer paciente que se apresente com tosse associada à epistaxe ou hemoptise.
• Testes para avaliação de possível hiperadrenocorticismo (causa potencial de tromboembolia pulmonar).

DIAGNÓSTICO POR IMAGEM
• Radiografias torácicas — constituem a primeira etapa antes de qualquer teste diagnóstico adicional; fornecem informações básicas sobre estruturas como vias aéreas intratorácicas, parênquima pulmonar, espaço pleural, mediastino e sistema cardiovascular.
• Fluoroscopia — útil para investigar doenças com suspeita de obstrução dinâmica (colapso traqueal, colapso bronquial, broncomalacia).
• Ecocardiografia — método proveitoso na suspeita de insuficiência ou disfunção cardíaca.
• Ultrassonografia torácica — em caso de efusão pleural ou na suspeita de massa pulmonar ou mediastínica.

MÉTODOS DIAGNÓSTICOS
• A endoscopia permite a visualização de anormalidades estáticas (tumor, granuloma, mucosa anormal, secreções excessivas) e dinâmicas (paralisia laríngea, colapso aéreo dinâmico) nas vias aéreas.
• Na presença de infiltrados bronquiais e/ou alveolares — as amostras de vias aéreas inferiores podem ser obtidas para fins diagnósticos (citologia, culturas bacterianas/micológicas) por meio de lavado broncoalveolar ou traqueal.

- Biopsia transtorácica (aspirado por agulha fina) ou toracoscopia — permitem a obtenção de amostra quando a infiltração intersticial é proeminente.
- Toracocentese — possibilita a amostragem de líquido pleural, podendo ser realizada sob orientação ultrassonográfica.
- Oximetria de pulso e determinação dos gases sanguíneos (gasometria).
- Testes de função pulmonar — necessitam de materiais sofisticados e/ou técnicos experientes, que não se encontram prontamente disponíveis em clínicas particulares.

TRATAMENTO

- Em geral, o paciente é tratado em um esquema ambulatorial.
- O método terapêutico mais bem-sucedido da tosse envolve o tratamento e a resolução da causa subjacente em vez do uso de medicamentos que suprimam os sinais.
- Se a tosse crônica estiver relacionada com inflamação aguda ou crônica, prefere-se a terapia anti-inflamatória àquela supressora da tosse.
- O uso de supressores da tosse deve ser limitado aos casos em que a causa da tosse não pode ser tratada nem resolvida por meios médicos e também àqueles em que a tosse excessiva leva à exaustão do paciente ou à insônia dos proprietários, bem como ao agravamento da doença.

MEDICAÇÕES
MEDICAMENTO(S) DE ESCOLHA
Terapia Antimicrobiana
- Indicada para traqueobronquite infecciosa ou broncopneumonia.

Terapia Anti-inflamatória
- Indicada em síndrome de bronquite felina, bronquite crônica canina ou broncopneumopatia eosinofílica canina.
- Prednisolona por via oral na dose de 0,5 mg/kg a cada 12 h em cães e gatos, com subsequente redução gradativa e progressiva para a cada 48 h.
- Nebulização de fluticasona ou budesonida na dose de 100-200 μg a cada 12 h com o uso de inalador dosimetrado, incluindo um espaçador com máscara facial e válvula inspiratória.

Anti-histamínicos
- Antagonistas dos receptores H_1.
- Podem ser úteis na suspeita de traqueíte ou bronquite alérgica e/ou quando a leve sedação for um efeito colateral positivo.

Antitussígenos
- Hidrocodona (apenas em cães): 0,22 mg/kg VO a cada 12 h.
- Butorfanol (apenas em cães): 0,5 mg/kg VO a cada 12 h.
- Não há antitussígenos disponíveis para gatos.

Broncodilatadores
Teofilina (para Cães e Gatos)
- A farmacocinética depende da formulação e da espécie. Existem formulações de liberação lenta.
- Os efeitos benéficos da teofilina incluem relaxamento da musculatura lisa dos brônquios, melhora na contração do diafragma e, provavelmente, alguns efeitos anti-inflamatórios.
- Os efeitos colaterais estão relacionados com os efeitos inotrópicos e cronotrópicos, bem como com o aumento da pressão arterial; também pode causar náusea, diarreia, arritmias e agitação/excitação do SNC.

β2-Agonistas (basicamente para Gatos)
- Podem ser administrados por meio de injeção, comprimido, xarope, nebulização ou inalador; em casos de emergência, são administrados por via IV. Existem medicamentos de ação curta (salbutamol, terbutalina, fenoterol) ou ação prolongada (salmeterol, formoterol).
- Podem ser administrados temporariamente para promover um alívio imediato e passageiro, mas não a longo prazo; possuem efeito limitado.
- Os efeitos colaterais incluem ressecamento da boca, taquicardia, náusea. A inalação regular de albuterol racêmico e S-albuterol (mas não do R-albuterol) induz à inflamação das vias aéreas tanto em gatos saudáveis como nos asmáticos.

Expectorantes
- Guaifenesina — é incluída em algumas preparações farmacológicas, embora o benefício não tenha sido amplamente estudado ou comprovado.

CONTRAINDICAÇÕES
Os agentes antitussígenos são estritamente contraindicados quando a tosse é necessária para remover as secreções das vias aéreas, ou seja, em doenças infecciosas ou inflamatórias dessas vias.

PRECAUÇÕES
Ver os efeitos colaterais dos respectivos medicamentos.

INTERAÇÕES POSSÍVEIS
Teofilina — a eliminação desse medicamento pode ser inibida por outros agentes terapêuticos, como fluoroquinolonas, aumentando o risco de intoxicação por esse broncodilatador.

ACOMPANHAMENTO
MONITORIZAÇÃO DO PACIENTE
- A tosse aguda deve receber tratamento adequado a fim de evitar a evolução para um quadro crônico, o que levaria a lesões possivelmente irreversíveis.
- Os distúrbios indutores de tosse crônica podem, algumas vezes, ser apenas aliviados, mas não curados; comunicar-se com o proprietário para garantir um tratamento bem-sucedido da tosse.

COMPLICAÇÕES POSSÍVEIS
- Agravamento do colapso traqueal.
- Evolução para bronquite crônica, doença pulmonar obstrutiva crônica, enfisema pulmonar, remodelagem bronquial e parenquimatosa irreversível, bronquiectasia.
- A tosse aguda e grave pode levar a quadros de síncope, fratura de costela ou pneumotórax.
- Disfunção cardíaca do lado direito.

DIVERSOS
FATORES RELACIONADOS COM A IDADE
- Em cães com distúrbios anatômicos de origem hereditária (p. ex., discinesia ciliar primária) ou congênita, os sinais podem começar no início da vida.
- É mais provável que os filhotes caninos e felinos sofram de doença infecciosa.
- Distúrbios inflamatórios afetam adultos de meia-idade.
- Insuficiência cardíaca e tumores são mais frequentes em animais mais idosos.

GESTAÇÃO/FERTILIDADE/REPRODUÇÃO
- Cães acometidos por discinesia ciliar primária.
- Possível diminuição da fertilidade (em ambos os sexos de cães), já que os cílios do trato urogenital e as células flageladas podem ser acometidos.
- Suspeita de hereditariedade em algumas raças (p. ex., Bichon frisé, Old English sheepdog).

VER TAMBÉM
- Asma e Bronquite — Gatos.
- Bronquite Crônica.
- Colapso Traqueal.
- Espirro, Espirro Reverso, Ânsia de Vômito.
- Hipoxemia.
- Insuficiência Cardíaca Congestiva Esquerda.
- Parasitas Respiratórios.
- Pneumonia Bacteriana.
- Pneumonia Eosinofílica.
- Secreção Nasal.

ABREVIATURA(S)
- FeLV = vírus da leucemia felina.
- FIV = vírus da imunodeficiência felina.
- PIF = peritonite infecciosa felina.
- SNC = sistema nervoso central.

Sugestões de Leitura
Anderson-Wessberg K. Coughing. In: King L, Textbook of Respiratory Medicine. Philadelphia: Saunders, 2003, pp. 189–192.
Bolser DC, Poliacek I, Jakus J, Fuller DD, Davenport PW. Neurogenesis of cough, other airway defensive behaviors and breathing: A holarchical system? Respiratory Physiology & Neurobiology 2006, 152:255–265.
Rozanski AE, Rush JE. Acute and chronic cough. In: Ettinger SJ, Feldman EC, eds., Textbook of Veterinary Internal Medicine, 6th ed. St. Louis: Elsevier, 2005, pp. 189–195.

Autores Cécile Clercx e Dominique Peeters
Consultor Editorial Lynelle R. Johnson

Toxicidade da Digoxina

CONSIDERAÇÕES GERAIS

REVISÃO
Comum na clínica veterinária, em função do índice terapêutico estreito da digoxina e da prevalência de dano renal em pacientes idosos com cardiopatia.

IDENTIFICAÇÃO
- Cães e gatos.
- Mais comum em pacientes geriátricos.

SINAIS CLÍNICOS
Achados Anamnésicos
- Anorexia.
- Vômito.
- Diarreia.
- Letargia.
- Depressão.

Achados do Exame Físico
A frequência cardíaca pode variar de bradicardia grave a taquicardia grave.

CAUSAS E FATORES DE RISCO
- Nefropatias — prejudicam a eliminação da digoxina.
- Pneumopatias crônicas — resultam em hipoxia e distúrbios acidobásicos.
- Obesidade — caso não se calcule a dosagem considerando o peso corporal magro.
- Hipocalemia, hipercalcemia, hipomagnesemia e hipoxia predispõem o animal a arritmias.
- Medicamentos e distúrbios que alteram o metabolismo ou a eliminação da digoxina (p. ex., quinidina e hipotireoidismo).
- Digitalização IV rápida.
- Superdosagem ou ingestão acidental do medicamento fornecido pelo proprietário.
- Administração de diurético indutor de hipocalemia.

DIAGNÓSTICO

DIAGNÓSTICO DIFERENCIAL
- Arritmias e distúrbios de condução — podem refletir cardiopatia estrutural e não a toxicidade da digoxina.
- Anorexia — comum em animais com insuficiência cardíaca.

HEMOGRAMA/BIOQUÍMICA/URINÁLISE
Os animais com hipocalemia, hipercalcemia, hipomagnesemia e insuficiência renal são predispostos à intoxicação pela digoxina.

OUTROS TESTES LABORATORIAIS
- Considerar a avaliação do estado tireóideo.
- Obter a concentração sérica da digoxina 8-10 h após uma dosagem oral — a faixa terapêutica é de 0,5-1,5 ng/mL. Um estudo recente em seres humanos verificou que níveis de digoxina superiores a 1 mg/mL estão associados à mortalidade elevada; nem todos os pacientes com concentrações >1,5 ng/mL apresentam sinais de toxicidade; alguns pacientes com valores dentro do limite de normalidade exibem sinais de toxicidade, especialmente se estiverem hipocalêmicos. O autor visa atingir um nível de digoxina entre 0,5 e 1 ng/mL.

DIAGNÓSTICO POR IMAGEM
N/D.

MÉTODOS DIAGNÓSTICOS
Achados Eletrocardiográficos
- Distúrbios de condução — bloqueio atrioventricular (AV), arritmias e depressão do segmento ST em alguns pacientes.
- Digoxina — pode causar qualquer arritmia.

TRATAMENTO

- Interromper a administração da digoxina até que os sinais de toxicidade desapareçam (24-72 h); reavaliar a necessidade da medicação; se necessário, retomar o tratamento em uma dosagem selecionada com base na concentração sérica da digoxina.
- Manter a hidratação e corrigir qualquer distúrbio eletrolítico (particularmente hipocalemia) com a administração parenteral de fluidos.
- Suspender os medicamentos que retardam o metabolismo ou a eliminação da digoxina (p. ex., quinidina, verapamil e amiodarona).
- Arritmias graves (taquicardia ventricular) e distúrbios de condução — podem ser potencialmente letais; exigem internação para o tratamento e a monitorização.

MEDICAÇÕES

MEDICAMENTO(S)
- Tratar as bradiarritmias clinicamente importantes, com a administração de atropina ou a implantação de marca-passo transvenoso temporário.
- Tratar as arritmias ventriculares relevantes do ponto de vista clínico, com lidocaína ou fenitoína; este último medicamento também reverte o bloqueio AV de alto grau.
- Os anticorpos ligantes de digoxina (p. ex., Digibind®) promovem a queda rápida da concentração desse glicosídeo em animais criticamente doentes; o uso desses produtos é limitado na clínica veterinária por seu custo exorbitante.
- Suplementação da tiroxina diante da confirmação de hipotireoidismo.

CONTRAINDICAÇÕES/INTERAÇÕES POSSÍVEIS
- Evitar ou interromper os medicamentos que retardam a eliminação ou o metabolismo da digoxina (p. ex., quinidina, verapamil e diltiazem).
- Evitar os medicamentos capazes de piorar os distúrbios de condução (p. ex., β-bloqueadores e bloqueadores dos canais de cálcio).
- Os medicamentos antiarrítmicos da classe 1A (p. ex., quinidina e procainamida) podem agravar o bloqueio AV.

ACOMPANHAMENTO

- Monitorizar com frequência a função renal e os eletrólitos em pacientes submetidos à digoxina; reduzir a dose desse glicosídeo caso se desenvolva nefropatia.
- Monitorizar periodicamente a concentração sérica da digoxina.
- Efetuar também a monitorização periódica do ECG para avaliar a presença de arritmias ou distúrbios de condução que possam sugerir toxicidade da digoxina.
- Realizar a monitorização frequente do peso corporal; alterar a dosagem da digoxina de acordo com esse peso; os pacientes com ICC muitas vezes perdem peso.

DIVERSOS

VER TAMBÉM
- Bloqueio Atrioventricular Completo (Terceiro Grau).
- Bloqueio Atrioventricular de Primeiro Grau.
- Bloqueio Atrioventricular de Segundo Grau — Mobitz Tipo I.
- Bloqueio Atrioventricular de Segundo Grau — Mobitz Tipo II.
- Taquicardia Ventricular.

ABREVIATURA(S)
- AV = atrioventricular.
- ECG = eletrocardiograma.
- ICC = insuficiência cardíaca congestiva.

Sugestões de Leitura
Opie LH, Gersh BJ. Acute and chronic heart failure: Positive inotropes, vasodilators and digoxin. In: Opie LH, Gersh BJ, eds., Drugs for the Heart: Expert Consult. Philadelphia: Elsevier Saunders, 2009, pp. 160-197.

Autor Francis W. K. Smith Jr.
Consultores Editoriais Larry P. Tilley e Francis W. K. Smith Jr.

TOXICIDADE DA VITAMINA D

CONSIDERAÇÕES GERAIS

DEFINIÇÃO
Trata-se de um distúrbio hipercalcêmico, resultante da ingestão de formulações de rodenticidas contendo vitamina D em sua composição, suplementação excessiva dessa vitamina na dieta, ingestão de metabólitos análogos da vitamina D utilizados para o tratamento de psoríase e outros distúrbios humanos imunomediados ou dietas ricas em vitamina D.

FISIOPATOLOGIA
- O colecalciferol é metabolizado em 25-hidroxicolecalciferol no fígado. O 25-hidroxicolecalciferol, por sua vez, é metabolizado em diversos metabólitos no rim, incluindo o calcitriol, o metabólito mais potente em termos de aumento na absorção intestinal e reabsorção óssea de cálcio sob condições fisiológicas.
- O 1,25-di-hidroxicolecalciferol é o metabólito ativo do colecalciferol sob condições fisiológicas.
- Sob condições tóxicas, o 25-hidroxicolecalciferol constitui o metabólito circulante ativo predominante.
- O calcipotriol (Dovonex®), um análogo do calcitriol, não necessita de ativação; por ter uma meia-vida curta de 100 minutos, esse composto análogo possui ação imediata, porém limitada.
- O calcitriol (25-hidroxicolecalciferol) e o calcipotriol aumentam a absorção intestinal de cálcio, estimulam a reabsorção óssea e intensificam a absorção de cálcio nos túbulos renais distais, resultando em hipercalcemia (cálcio sérico >12,5 mg/dL).
- O fósforo sérico também sofre aumento (>8 mg/dL).
- O resultado final é a mineralização metastática e distrófica de tecidos moles, o que resulta na fisiopatologia dos tecidos acometidos.

SISTEMA(S) ACOMETIDO(S)
- Musculosquelético — desmineralização; tremores musculares.
- Renal/urológico — calcificação, necrose tubular proximal e insuficiência renal.
- Gastrintestinal — anorexia; mineralização; êmese; hematêmese; constipação; aumento da secreção ácida gástrica.
- Cardiovascular — mineralização, arritmias.
- Nervoso — crises convulsivas ou depressão.
- Respiratório — mineralização; dispneia.

INCIDÊNCIA/PREVALÊNCIA
- Toxicose por rodenticidas à base de colecalciferol — causa mais comum de intoxicação pela vitamina D em cães e gatos.
- Intoxicação por vitamina D_3 em virtude do excesso dessa vitamina em rações comerciais foi responsável pela doença em muitos cães em janeiro de 2000 e novamente em abril de 2006 nos EUA. Isso levou à retirada das rações do mercado.
- Calcipotriol (Dovonex®, medicamento utilizado contra psoríase) — principal causa de toxicidade por análogos da vitamina D em cães. As pomadas contêm 50 µg/g de calcipotriol.
- Filhotes caninos e felinos lactentes podem ser intoxicados por meio do leite.
- Não se conhece a incidência global da toxicidade da vitamina D.

IDENTIFICAÇÃO
Espécies
- Cães e gatos.
- Outras espécies, particularmente exóticas.

Idade Média e Faixa Etária
- Acomete todas as idades; os cães mais jovens (<6 meses de vida) e os gatos são os mais sensíveis.

SINAIS CLÍNICOS
Comentários Gerais
- Calcipotriol — os sinais desenvolvem-se em 6-12 h após a ingestão.
- Rodenticidas à base de colecalciferol — os sinais desenvolvem-se em 12-36 h após a ingestão.

Achados Anamnésicos
- Vômito.
- Depressão do SNC.
- Fraqueza.
- Anorexia.
- Polidipsia.
- Poliúria.
- Diarreia.
- Melena.
- Hematêmese.
- Perda de peso corporal.
- Constipação.
- Crises convulsivas.
- Tremores musculares.

Achados do Exame Físico
- Depressão.
- Vômito.
- Diarreia.
- Hematêmese.
- Hematoquezia.
- Poliúria.
- Polidipsia.
- Dor renal à palpação.
- Hemorragia gastrintestinal.
- Dor abdominal.
- Sialorreia.
- Lesões erosivas orofaríngeas.
- Bradicardia; contrações ventriculares prematuras.
- Dispneia.

CAUSAS
- Ingestão de rodenticidas à base de colecalciferol ou análogos do calcitriol (p. ex., calcipotriol), suplementação excessiva de vitamina D na dieta ou dietas malformuladas com excesso dessa vitamina.
- Rodenticidas à base de colecalciferol (0,075%) — incluem Quintox®, Rampage®, Ortho Rat-B-Gone® e Ortho Mouse B-Gone®; uma dose tóxica única é de 2-3 mg/kg de peso corporal em cães; uma dose letal única é de 13 mg (520.000 UI)/kg de peso corporal.
- A ingestão de 1,8-3,6 µg de calcipotriol/kg de peso corporal é tóxica para os cães.
- Em cães, a ingestão diária de vitamina D_3 além da recomendação dietética máxima de 1,43 kUI/1.000 kcal de energia metabolizável pode causar toxicose crônica.
- Em gatos, a ingestão crônica de dietas que contenham concentrações de vitamina D_3 acima do nível máximo recomendado de 2,5 kUI/1.000 kcal de energia metabolizável é tóxica para os animais dessa espécie.
- Em um surto alimentar no ano de 2006, foram encontradas concentrações de vitamina D_3 entre 1,51 e 2,67 kUI/1.000 kcal de energia metabolizável.

FATORES DE RISCO
- Nefropatias, cardiopatias ou neuropatias (SNC) preexistentes.
- Neoplasia.
- Hiperparatireoidismo primário.
- Hipoadrenocorticismo.
- Doenças granulomatosas (p. ex., blastomicose).
- Hipercalcemia juvenil.
- Idade — animais jovens são mais suscetíveis.
- Hipercalcemia idiopática felina.

DIAGNÓSTICO

DIAGNÓSTICO DIFERENCIAL
- Outros distúrbios hipercalcêmicos, incluindo linfossarcoma e outras malignidades, hipoadrenocorticismo, insuficiência renal crônica, hiperparatireoidismo primário e lesões granulomatosas em tecidos moles. Como a toxicose pela vitamina D e por seus análogos suprime o PTHi, é possível diferenciá-la das doenças mencionadas. Em outras condições, o PTHi encontra-se normal ou aumentado.
- Hipercalcemia juvenil.
- Toxicidade por rodenticidas anticoagulantes e AINE — atribuível à hematêmese e melena.

HEMOGRAMA/BIOQUÍMICA/URINÁLISE
- Cálcio — hipercalcemia (cálcio sérico total >12,5 mg/dL, cálcio ionizado >6,0 mg/dL). A hipercalcemia é imediata (2-3 h) e transitória (declinará ao normal em 24 h após a ingestão) em caso de ingestão de calcipotriol. Em casos de toxicidade por rodenticidas à base de colecalciferol, a hipercalcemia ficará evidente 12 h após a ingestão e persistirá por semanas se não for tratada.
- Hiperfosfatemia (>8 mg/dL).
- Hipocalemia.
- Azotemia.
- Hipostenúria, proteinúria e glicosúria.
- Acidose metabólica.
- Calcipotriol — as outras anormalidades observadas incluem hipoalbuminemia, atividade elevada das enzimas fosfatase alcalina, ALT e AST, além de trombocitopenia, TTPA prolongado e concentração aumentada de fibrinogênio.

OUTROS TESTES LABORATORIAIS
- Atualmente, não existem testes confirmatórios em casos de intoxicação por calcipotriol. A 25-hidroxivitamina D e o calcitriol séricos permanecem normais.
- A relação de cálcio:fósforo no córtex renal de cães que vieram a óbito encontra-se no limite de 0,4-0,9 para todas as intoxicações relacionadas com a vitamina D.
- A concentração cortical renal da 25-hidroxivitamina D >80 nmol/L apoia o diagnóstico de toxicose por colecalciferol.
- A concentração biliar da 25-hidroxivitamina D >100 nmol/L apoia o diagnóstico de toxicose por colecalciferol.
- Em ingestões agudas de uma única vez, a concentração sérica da 25-hidroxivitamina D está aumentada em pelo menos 10 vezes o normal (limites de normalidade: cães, 60-215 nmol/L; gatos, 65-170 nmol/L) em casos de toxicose por colecalciferol.
- Em intoxicações crônicas, a concentração sérica de 25-hidroxivitamina D pode aumentar de 1,5 a 5 vezes acima dos valores normais.

Toxicidade da Vitamina D

- A 1,25-di-hidroxivitamina D sérica sofre apenas um aumento transitório, sendo de valor diagnóstico limitado.
- Cálcio ionizado aumentado (>6,0 mg/dL).
- PTHi diminuído (os valores normais são de 3-17 e 0-4 pmol/L em cães e gatos, respectivamente).
- Relação de Na/K normal.

DIAGNÓSTICO POR IMAGEM
Ultrassonografia — hiperecogenicidade dos rins, da parede gástrica e dos pulmões.

MÉTODOS DIAGNÓSTICOS
- ECG — pode revelar bradicardia, taquicardia sinusal e complexos ventriculares prematuros.
- Endoscopia — pode revelar a mucosa gástrica erosiva/hemorrágica.

ACHADOS PATOLÓGICOS
- Mineralização difusa da parede gástrica e dos intestinos; hemorragia na mucosa gástrica; mineralização do palato mole, das glândulas salivares e de outros tecidos moles.
- Necrose e mineralização do miocárdio (especialmente dos átrios) e dos vasos sanguíneos calibrosos, além de degeneração miocárdica.
- Mineralização do mesângio e da cápsula glomerulares, bem como das membranas basais dos túbulos renais.
- Necrose tubular.
- Mineralização dos pulmões.

TRATAMENTO

CUIDADO(S) DE SAÚDE ADEQUADO(S)
- Calcipotriol — recomenda-se o tratamento de emergência; a doença caracteriza-se por hipercalcemia transitória aguda com mineralização maciça dos tecidos moles; o prognóstico é reservado, havendo necessidade de internação.
- Colecalciferol — assim que ocorrer a manifestação dos sinais clínicos (geralmente 24-36 h após a ingestão), a descontaminação gástrica não constituirá um procedimento digno de nota, já que a absorção já estará concluída.
- Todos os casos de toxicose por vitamina D exigem a internação por, no mínimo, 48 h após a ingestão para monitorização rigorosa do paciente.

Eméticos
- Em casos de ingestão de calcipotriol, a administração de eméticos é obrigatória. Esse composto é altamente tóxico. Os eméticos também são recomendados se o animal de estimação for pego ingerindo um produto rodenticida à base de colecalciferol antes da manifestação dos sinais clínicos.
- Administração por via oral de xarope de ipeca (cães, 1-2 mL/kg; gatos, 3,3 mL/kg) ou peróxido de hidrogênio (5-25 mL/5 kg). Se o vômito não tiver ocorrido dentro de 15-20 min, deve-se repetir a dose uma única vez.
- Apomorfina (0,25 mg por via subconjuntival).

CUIDADO(S) DE ENFERMAGEM
- Corrigir a desidratação e os desequilíbrios eletrolíticos (hipocalemia).
- Estimular a calciurese com a fluidoterapia — fortemente recomendada para todos os pacientes.
- Diálise peritoneal com dialisado isento de cálcio — em casos de azotemia e hipercalcemia graves.
- Transfusão sanguínea — em casos de anemia grave ou hipovolemia.
- Antibioticoterapia — para evitar infecção bacteriana secundária, em função da ruptura na barreira de defesa do intestino.
- Alimentação parenteral — recomendada para dar repouso ao intestino e superar a anorexia.

DIETA
Oferecer dietas com baixos teores de cálcio e fósforo.

ORIENTAÇÃO AO PROPRIETÁRIO
- Alertar o proprietário a manter todos os produtos rodenticidas em locais inacessíveis aos animais de estimação.
- Avisar o proprietário a deixar todos os medicamentos fora do alcance dos animais.
- Advertir o proprietário sobre a gravidade e o tratamento dispendioso da toxicidade pela vitamina D, em função da necessidade habitual de terapia prolongada e internação.

MEDICAÇÕES

MEDICAMENTO(S) DE ESCOLHA
- Bifosfonatos (p. ex., pamidronato dissódico) — para tratar a hipercalcemia.
- Calcitonina do salmão — para tratar a hipercalcemia.

Descontaminação do Trato Gastrintestinal
- Em 6 h após a ingestão da vitamina D.
- Eméticos e carvão ativado associados a catárticos osmóticos.
- Cães — apomorfina a 0,02-0,04 mg/kg por vias IV, IM, SC ou subconjuntival.
- Gatos — xilazina a 0,4-0,5 mg/kg por via IV.
- Carvão ativado em pó (1-4 g/kg) combinado com algum catártico salino (sulfato de magnésio ou de sódio, 250 mg/kg) — por via oral ou sonda gástrica.

Redução da Hipercalcemia
- Pamidronato dissódico (Aredia®; Ciba-Geigy, Tarrytown, NY) — 1,3-2,0 mg/kg em cloreto de sódio a 0,9%, administrado por meio de infusão IV lenta em 2-4 h; repetir uma única vez 3-4 dias depois; a associação com a calcitonina do salmão não é recomendada, pois isso não tem efeitos benéficos adicionais.
- Calcitonina do salmão — 4-6 UI por via IM ou SC a cada 6 h até a estabilização do nível de cálcio; em virtude da eficácia limitada e da possível refratariedade dos pacientes, recomenda-se a combinação de calcitonina com corticosteroides ou o aumento da dose em até 10-20 UI/kg.
- Prednisolona — cães e gatos: 2-6 mg/kg IM a cada 12 h.
- Furosemida — cães: 2-6 mg/kg; gatos: 1-4 mg/kg SC, IV ou IM a cada 8-12 h.

Controle das Crises Convulsivas
- Diazepam — 0,5 mg/kg IV, repetir conforme a necessidade.

Controle das Arritmias Ventriculares Clinicamente Significativas
- Lidocaína — 50 µg/kg/min.

Proteção Gastrintestinal
- Sucralfato — 1 g de suspensão VO a cada 6 h.
- Famotidina — 15 mg IV a cada 12 h.

Antieméticos
- Metoclopramida — 6 mg SC a cada 8 h.

PRECAUÇÕES
- Doses supraterapêuticas de pamidronato dissódico — podem agravar a insuficiência renal.
- Calcitonina do salmão — associada a efeitos colaterais: anorexia, anafilaxia e êmese.
- Xilazina — pode agravar a depressão respiratória e resultar em bradicardia mediada pelo nervo vago; a ioimbina (0,1 mg/kg IV) é o antídoto da xilazina.
- Terapia prolongada com a prednisolona — pode resultar em supressão adrenocortical; reduzir as doses gradativamente em um período de 2-4 semanas.

ACOMPANHAMENTO

MONITORIZAÇÃO DO PACIENTE
- Acompanhamento da terapia com o pamidronato — níveis séricos de cálcio e ureia; mensurados em 24, 48 e 72 h após a exposição; na presença de hipercalcemia, recomenda-se a diurese com fluidos; se a hipercalcemia ainda persistir, deve-se repetir a infusão de pamidronato 72 ou 96 h após a primeira infusão, monitorando-se os níveis séricos de cálcio e ureia a cada 48 h.
- Acompanhamento da terapia com a calcitonina — níveis séricos de cálcio e ureia; monitorizar a cada 24 h e continuar o ajuste da dose até que o cálcio retorne ao normal (24-48 h para o calcipotriol ou 2-4 semanas para o colecalciferol).
- O calcipotriol causa hipercalcemia a curto prazo (24-48 h) com mineralização maciça dos tecidos moles; exige fluidoterapia e terapia de suporte rigorosas a longo prazo; a hipercalcemia induzida pelo colecalciferol é persistente, necessitando de tratamento prolongado e cuidados de suporte.

PREVENÇÃO
- Manter os rodenticidas e os medicamentos fora do alcance dos animais domésticos.
- Evitar o fornecimento de dietas ricas em vitamina D.

COMPLICAÇÕES POSSÍVEIS
- Insuficiência renal crônica — incapacidade de concentração da urina.
- Infecção bacteriana secundária — decorrente de dano intestinal.
- Lesões renais, cardiovasculares e gastrintestinais subclínicas — em virtude da mineralização.

EVOLUÇÃO ESPERADA E PROGNÓSTICO
- Calcipotriol — a menos que se institua uma terapia rigorosa imediatamente, o prognóstico será reservado, em função da natureza superaguda da condição e da mineralização maciça associada dos tecidos moles.
- Colecalciferol — depende da gravidade e da duração da hipercalcemia; na presença de hipercalcemia irresponsiva acentuada e na ocorrência de mineralização grave antes do início da terapia, o prognóstico será mau.
- Evolução usual — 2-4 semanas.

DIVERSOS

FATORES RELACIONADOS COM A IDADE
Distinguir da hipercalcemia juvenil normal.

TOXICIDADE DA VITAMINA D

GESTAÇÃO/FERTILIDADE/REPRODUÇÃO
Efeitos teratogênicos — o calcipotriol e a vitamina D têm efeitos antiproliferativos e potencial de teratogênese.

SINÔNIMO(S)
- Toxicose por colecalciferol.
- Toxicose por calcipotriol.
- Toxicose por análogos da vitamina D.
- Toxicose por Dovonex®.

ABREVIATURA(S)
- AINE = anti-inflamatório não esteroide.
- ALT = alanina aminotransferase.
- AST = aspartato aminotransferase.
- ECG = eletrocardiografia.
- PTHi = paratormônio intacto.
- SNC = sistema nervoso central.
- TTPA = tempo de tromboplastina parcial ativada.

Sugestões de Leitura

Morrow CK, Volmer PA. Cholecalciferol. In: Plumlee KH, Clinical Veterinary Toxicology. St. Louis: Mosby, 2004, pp. 448-451.

Murphy MJ. Rodenticides. Vet Clin North Am Small Anim Pract 2002, 32(2):469-484.

Rumbeiha WK. Cholecalciferol. In: Peterson ME, Talcott PA, eds., Small Animal Toxicology, 2nd ed. St. Louis: Saunders, 2006, pp. 629-642.

Rumbeiha WK, Braselton WE, Nachreiner R, et al. The post-mortem diagnosis of cholecalciferol toxicosis: A novel approach and differentiation from ethylene glycol toxicosis. J Vet Diagn Invest 2000, 12:426-432.

Rumbeiha WK, Fitzgerald SD, Kruger JM, et al. Use of pamidronate disodium to reduce cholecalciferol-induced toxicosis in dogs. Am J Vet Res 2000, 61:9-13.

Saedi N, Horn R, Muffoletto B, Wood A. Death of a dog caused by calcipotriene toxicity. J Am Acad Dermatol 2007, April, pp. 712-713.

Autor Wilson K. Rumbeiha
Consultor Editorial Gary D. Osweiler

Toxicidade das Piretrinas e dos Piretroides

CONSIDERAÇÕES GERAIS

REVISÃO
- Inseticidas.
- Piretrinas — naturais; derivadas do *Chrysanthemum cinerariaefolium* e espécies de vegetais relacionados.
- Piretroides — sintéticos; incluem acrinatrina, aletrina, bartrina, bifentrina, bioresmetrina, cismetrina, cipermetrina, dimetrina, deltametrina, ciflutrina, cifalotrina, cifenotrina, esfenvalerato, fenpropatrina, fenvalerato, flumetrina, fluvalinato, permetrina, fenotrina, teflutrina, tetrametrina, tralometrina e etofenprox (éter).
- Acometem o sistema nervoso — prolongam reversivelmente a condutância do sódio nos axônios dos nervos, resultando em descargas nervosas repetitivas.

IDENTIFICAÇÃO
As reações adversas ocorrem com maior frequência nos gatos; nos cães de pequeno porte; e nos animais jovens, idosos, doentes, anêmicos ou debilitados. Raramente, podem ocorrer reações por exposição secundária quando os gatos interagem estreitamente, por meio de contato direto ou práticas de higienização, com cães submetidos a tratamento com permetrina sob a forma de *spot-on*.

SINAIS CLÍNICOS
- Resultam de reações de hipersensibilidade alérgica imunomediada e anafiláticas, reações idiossincrásicas com base genética e reações neurotóxicas; pode ser um desafio diferenciá-las.
- Leves — hipersalivação; sacudidas dos pés; fasciculação das orelhas; leve depressão; vômito; diarreia.
- Moderados a graves — vômito e diarreia prolongados; depressão acentuada; ataxia; tremores musculares (devem ser diferenciados das sacudidas dos pés e da fasciculação das orelhas).
- Superdosagem dérmica ou oral extrema — pode produzir crises convulsivas ou morte.
- Gatos — são particularmente sensíveis aos piretroides. Com base nos dados publicados do Animal Poison Control Center (APCC, Centro norte-americano de controle de envenenamento em animais) da American Society for the Prevention of Cruelty to Animals (ASPCA, Sociedade norte-americana para prevenção de crueldade aos animais), os gatos, ao serem tratados com produtos que contenham permetrina concentrada comercializados para utilização em cães, tipicamente desenvolvem tremores musculares, ataxia, crises convulsivas, hipertermia e morte dentro de horas se a toxicidade não for tratada.
- Reações alérgicas — urticária; hiperemia; prurido; anafilaxia; choque; angústia respiratória; morte (raramente).

CAUSAS E FATORES DE RISCO
- Gatos — mais sensíveis; vias metabólicas menos eficientes, hábitos prolongados de higienização e pelagens longas capazes de reter grandes quantidades do produto aplicado de forma tópica.
- Pacientes com temperaturas corporais abaixo do normal após o banho, anestesia ou sedação — predispostos aos sinais clínicos.

DIAGNÓSTICO

DIAGNÓSTICO DIFERENCIAL
- Histórico de exposição (quantidade e frequência de utilização do produto), tipo e gravidade dos sinais clínicos, bem como início e duração desses sinais — devem ser compatíveis antes de se fazer um diagnóstico presuntivo.
- Má aplicação de produtos contra pulgas contendo permetrina destinados somente para os cães nos gatos.
- Intoxicação por compostos organofosforados, carbamato ou D-limoneno.
- Estricnina, metaldeído, micotoxinas tremorgênicas, metilxantinas, anfetaminas, hiperdosagem de agentes serotoninérgicos, intoxicação por álcool a partir de *spray* à base de álcool isopropílico.

OUTROS TESTES LABORATORIAIS
- Piretrinas — os testes analíticos para detecção em líquidos ou tecidos geralmente não se encontram disponíveis.
- Piretroides — alguns compostos podem ser detectados nos tecidos, especialmente no pelo, para confirmar a exposição. A análise do pelo quanto à presença de permetrina pode ser valiosa quando a gravidade do evento adverso em gatos for muito maior do que o previsto com base na aplicação do produto relatado. Os gatos com crises convulsivas ou tremores generalizados após a aplicação relatada de produto contra pulgas aprovado para os animais dessa espécie são suspeitos de exposição ou má aplicação de algum produto contendo permetrina destinado apenas para cães.

TRATAMENTO

- Reações adversas (salivação, sacudidas dos pés e fasciculação das orelhas) — frequentemente leves e autolimitantes; tais reações desaparecem com a observação e o cuidado veterinário limitado ou nulo.
- Paciente saturado com produtos em forma de *spray* — secar com toalha morna; escovar.
- Sinais leves contínuos — banhar em casa com detergente comum suave (evitar a hipotermia rigorosamente).
- Evolução para tremores e ataxia — hospitalização.
- Paciente gravemente acometido — recomenda-se o suporte de fluido intravenoso com solução eletrolítica balanceada.
- Manutenção da temperatura corporal normal — medida crítica. É crítico banhar o animal depois da estabilização (tremores sob controle) com detergente líquido e água morna.

MEDICAÇÕES

MEDICAMENTO(S)
- Tremores ou crises convulsivas — especialmente para os gatos expostos à permetrina; metocarbamol (Robaxin-V® injetável na dose de 55-220 mg/kg IV, sem exceder 330 mg/kg/dia; administrar metade da dose IV lentamente, aguardar até que o paciente relaxe e continuar a administração até fazer efeito; não ultrapassar a velocidade de injeção de 2 mL/min e começar com a dose mais baixa inicialmente).
- Diazepam em dosagens baixas é usado para controlar hiperestesia mínima. O controle das crises convulsivas é obtido com pentobarbital, propofol (3-6 mg/kg IV ou 0,1 mg/kg/min sob taxa de infusão constante) e anestésicos inalatórios. O metocarbomol continua sendo o agente de escolha e também pode ser usado por via oral para o tratamento de tremores leves (50-100 mg/kg a cada 8 h; tempo de início de 30 min).
- Carvão ativado (2 g/kg VO) raramente é benéfico ou recomendado. A maioria das formulações é composta de líquidos rapidamente absorvidos, contendo água, vários álcoois ou solventes de hidrocarbonetos.
- Eméticos — raramente justificados; a maior parte das formulações é constituída por líquidos rapidamente absorvidos, contendo água, vários álcoois ou solventes de hidrocarbonetos; não utilizar em caso de exposição a solvente de hidrocarboneto (potencial de aspiração); se os antieméticos forem indicados, o vômito deverá ser induzido com peróxido de hidrogênio a 3% (2,2 mL/kg, máximo de 45 mL) após a alimentação quando o paciente se encontrar assintomático e se estiver dentro de 1-2 h da ingestão.

CONTRAINDICAÇÕES/INTERAÇÕES POSSÍVEIS
- Sulfato de atropina — não é antídoto; evitar; pode provocar taquicardia, estimulação do SNC, desorientação, sonolência, depressão respiratória e até crises convulsivas.

ACOMPANHAMENTO

PREVENÇÃO
- Aplicação adequada (ou seja, de acordo com o rótulo) de produtos para controle de pulgas — diminui enormemente a incidência de reações adversas; corrigir a dose de grande parte dos produtos sob a forma de *spray*: 1 a 2 borrifadas de *spray* típico com gatilho por quilo de peso.
- Redução da salivação pelos gatos sensíveis (*sprays*) — espargir na escova de embelezamento; escovar a pelagem regularmente.
- Líquidos — o termo *banho de imersão* é comum; nunca submergir o animal; aplicar sobre o corpo; passar a esponja até recobrir as áreas secas.
- Produtos para instalações — não aplicar por via tópica a menos que recomendado para tal utilização; após a aplicação na casa ou em áreas externas, não deixar o animal naquele local até que o produto tenha secado e o ambiente tenha sido ventilado.
- Não aplicar produtos destinados apenas para cães nos gatos.
- Não usar produtos de permetrina sob a forma de *spot-on* nos cães em residências onde os gatos se higienizam ou dormem em contato físico com os cães.

EVOLUÇÃO ESPERADA E PROGNÓSTICO
- Hipersalivação — pode recidivar depois de vários dias da utilização de produto para controle de pulgas quando o paciente (especialmente gatos) cuida da própria pelagem.
- A maior parte dos sinais clínicos (leves a graves) desaparece dentro de 24-72 h.

DIVERSOS

Sugestões de Leitura
Hansen SR, Villar D, Buck WB, et al. Pyrethrins and pyrethroids in dogs and cats. Compend Contin Educ Pract Vet 1994, 16:707-713.

Autores Steven R. Hansen e Elizabeth A. Curry-Galvin
Consultor Editorial Gary D. Osweiler

TOXICIDADE DO PARACETAMOL

CONSIDERAÇÕES GERAIS

DEFINIÇÃO
Resulta da superdosagem do paciente pelo proprietário, em consequência do fornecimento de analgésicos e antipiréticos contendo paracetamol e vendidos sem prescrição médica.

FISIOPATOLOGIA
Quando os mecanismos normais de biotransformação para a detoxificação (glicuronidação e sulfatação) se encontram diminuídos, a oxidação mediada pelo citocromo P450 produz um metabólito tóxico eletrofílico (*N*-acetil benzoquinona imina), que se conjuga com a glutationa e se liga de forma tóxica a proteínas hepáticas.

Cães
• Prescrição de ≥150-200 mg/kg — quantidade suficiente de metabólito eletrofílico gerada por meio da via do citocromo P450 para que a ligação eritrocitária de glutationa produza metemoglobinemia e se ligue às proteínas hepáticas.
• Causa hepatotoxicidade dose-dependente.

Gatos
• Menor capacidade de glicuronidação; capacidade mais limitada de eliminação do paracetamol que os cães.
• As vias de biotransformação de glicuronidação e sulfatação ficam saturadas.
• Produzem o metabólito tóxico do citocromo P450 em doses muito mais baixas que os cães.
• São intoxicados com doses baixas de até 50-60 mg/kg (o que corresponde, muitas vezes, a uma dose tão baixa quanto à metade de um comprimido); isso leva a uma ligeira depleção da glutationa eritrocitária, produzindo metemoglobinemia de rápido desenvolvimento, em consequência da peculiaridade da molécula de hemoglobina felina dotada de oito grupos sulfidrílicos sensíveis à oxidação.
• A hepatotoxicose de desenvolvimento mais lento pode não se manifestar completamente antes do desenvolvimento de metemoglobinemia fatal.

SISTEMA(S) ACOMETIDO(S)
• Hematológico/linfático/imunológico — as hemácias são lesadas pela depleção da glutationa, o que confere a oxidação da hemoglobina em metemoglobina.
• Hepatobiliar — necrose hepática.
• Cardiovascular (gatos) — edema na face, nos pés e (em menor grau) nos membros torácicos, por um mecanismo indefinido.

GENÉTICA
Gatos — deficiência genética na via de conjugação por glicuronidação os torna vulneráveis.

INCIDÊNCIA/PREVALÊNCIA
• Toxicidade medicamentosa mais comum em gatos; consideravelmente menos frequente em cães.
• Medicamentos vendidos sem prescrição médica — representam a quarta causa mais comum de exposições tóxicas em pequenos animais.

DISTRIBUIÇÃO GEOGRÁFICA
N/D

IDENTIFICAÇÃO

Espécies
Maior frequência em gatos do que em cães.

Raça(s) Predominante(s)
N/D

Idade Média e Faixa Etária
N/D

Sexo(s) Predominante(s)
N/D

SINAIS CLÍNICOS

Comentários Gerais
Relativamente comum — por conta do uso crescente em seres humanos.

Achados Anamnésicos
• Depressão.
• Taquipneia.
• Mucosas escurecidas.
• O proprietário pode se lembrar das precauções quanto à administração de paracetamol em gatos após fornecer uma dose ao seu animal de estimação.

Achados do Exame Físico
• Podem aparecer 1-4 h após a administração.
• Depressão progressiva.
• Salivação.
• Vômito.
• Dor abdominal.
• Taquipneia e cianose — refletem a metemoglobinemia.
• Edema — face, pés e, possivelmente, membros torácicos; após algumas horas.
• Urina "cor de chocolate" — hematúria e metemoglobinúria; especialmente em gatos.
• Óbito.

CAUSAS
Superdosagem pelo paracetamol.

FATORES DE RISCO
• Deficiências nutricionais de glicose e/ou sulfato.
• Administração simultânea de outros medicamentos depressores da glutationa.

DIAGNÓSTICO

DIAGNÓSTICO DIFERENCIAL
• Nitritos.
• Fenacetina.
• Nitrobenzeno.
• Compostos fenólicos e cresólicos.
• Sulfetos.
• Histórico de exposição — importante para diferenciar o quadro decorrente dos medicamentos formadores de metemoglobina.

HEMOGRAMA/BIOQUÍMICA/URINÁLISE
• Metemoglobinemia e atividades séricas progressivas crescentes das enzimas hepáticas — características.
• Corpúsculos de Heinz (gatos) — proeminentes nas hemácias.
• Hematúria e/ou hemoglobinúria.

OUTROS TESTES LABORATORIAIS
• Concentração sérica do paracetamol — elevada ao máximo em 1-3 h após a ingestão; a queda é dependente da dose em gatos (aproximadamente 1/10 da velocidade de eliminação plasmática de cães).
• Nível sanguíneo da glutationa — baixo.

DIAGNÓSTICO POR IMAGEM
N/D

MÉTODOS DIAGNÓSTICOS
N/D

ACHADOS PATOLÓGICOS
• Metemoglobinemia.
• Edema pulmonar.
• Congestão hepática e renal.
• Cães — necrose hepática centrolobular; icterícia em casos crônicos.

TRATAMENTO

CUIDADO(S) DE SAÚDE ADEQUADO(S)
• Em caso de metemoglobinemia — é preciso avaliar o animal imediatamente.
• Na presença de urina de coloração escura ou sangrenta ou icterícia — internação.

CUIDADO(S) DE ENFERMAGEM
• Manipulação delicada — imperativo para os pacientes clinicamente acometidos.
• Indução de êmese e lavagem gástrica — úteis dentro de 4-6 h após a ingestão.
• Anemia, hematúria ou hemoglobinúria — podem exigir transfusão de sangue total.
• Fluidoterapia — manter a hidratação e o equilíbrio eletrolítico.
• Água — à vontade.
• Alimento — oferecido 24 h após o início do tratamento.

ATIVIDADE
Restrita.

DIETA
N/D

ORIENTAÇÃO AO PROPRIETÁRIO
• Avisar o proprietário que o tratamento em pacientes clinicamente acometidos pode ser prolongado e caro.
• Informar ao proprietário que os pacientes com lesão hepática podem necessitar de tratamento prolongado e caro.

CONSIDERAÇÕES CIRÚRGICAS
N/D

MEDICAÇÕES

MEDICAMENTO(S) DE ESCOLHA
• Carvão ativado — 2 g/kg VO; imediatamente após a conclusão da êmese e da lavagem gástrica.
• *N*-acetilcisteína (Mucomyst®) — 140 mg/kg como dose de ataque VO, IV; em seguida, 70 mg/kg VO, IV, a cada 4 h por cinco a sete tratamentos.

CONTRAINDICAÇÕES
Medicamentos que contribuem para a metemoglobinemia ou a hepatotoxicidade.

PRECAUÇÕES
Medicamentos que necessitam passar por processos extensos de biotransformação ou metabolismo hepático — utilizá-los com cautela; espera-se que suas meias-vidas sejam prolongadas.

INTERAÇÕES POSSÍVEIS
Os medicamentos que exigem a ativação ou metabolismo pelo fígado apresentam eficácia reduzida.

MEDICAMENTO(S) ALTERNATIVO(S)
• Outros medicamentos doadores de enxofre — em caso de indisponibilidade da *N*-acetilcisteína; sulfato de sódio (50 mg de solução a 1,6%/kg IV a

Toxicidade do Paracetamol

cada 4 h durante seis vezes); o uso eficaz requer um tratamento conscencioso.
- S-adenosil-l-metionina (SAMe) como doador de glutationa — uma dose de ataque (40 mg/kg VO) de sal estável de SAMe, acompanhada por uma dose de manutenção (20 mg/kg VO) a cada 24 h por 7 dias; reservada para cães capazes de manter medicamentos orais e com função hepática adequada para metabolizar a SAMe.
- Solução de azul de metileno a 1% — 8,8 mg/kg IV a cada 2-3 h por duas a três vezes; combate a metemoglobinemia sem induzir a uma crise hemolítica.
- Ácido ascórbico — 125 mg/kg VO a cada 6 h por seis vezes; apenas reduz a metemoglobinemia lentamente.

ACOMPANHAMENTO

MONITORIZAÇÃO DO PACIENTE
- Monitorização clínica contínua da metemoglobinemia — vital para um tratamento eficaz; determinação laboratorial da porcentagem da metemoglobinemia a cada 2-3 h.
- Determinação da atividade sérica das enzimas hepáticas (ALT, fosfatase alcalina) a cada 12 h; monitorização do dano hepático.
- Nível sanguíneo da glutationa — fornece indícios da eficácia da terapia de reposição sulfidrílica.

PREVENÇÃO
- Jamais administrar paracetamol aos gatos.
- Dispensar especial atenção à dose de paracetamol em cães.

COMPLICAÇÕES POSSÍVEIS
Necrose hepática e fibrose resultante — podem comprometer a função hepática a longo prazo em pacientes recuperados.

EVOLUÇÃO ESPERADA E PROGNÓSTICO
- Metemoglobinemia rapidamente progressiva — sinal grave.
- Concentrações de metemoglobina ≥50% — prognóstico grave.
- Aumento progressivamente crescente das enzimas hepáticas séricas em 12-24 h após a ingestão — preocupação séria.
- Espera-se a persistência dos sinais clínicos em 12-48 h; o óbito pode ocorrer a qualquer momento por uma possível metemoglobinemia.
- Os cães e os gatos submetidos a um tratamento imediato que reverta a metemoglobinemia e evite a necrose hepática excessiva — podem se recuperar totalmente.
- Cães — pode ocorrer o óbito por necrose hepática em alguns dias.
- Gatos — ocorre o óbito como resultado da metemoglobinemia em 18-36 h após a ingestão.

DIVERSOS

CONDIÇÕES ASSOCIADAS
N/D

FATORES RELACIONADOS COM A IDADE
Cães jovens de pequeno porte e gatos — maior risco do fornecimento (em dose única) de medicamentos contendo paracetamol pelo proprietário.

POTENCIAL ZOONÓTICO
Nenhum.

GESTAÇÃO/FERTILIDADE/REPRODUÇÃO
Impõe mais estresse e maior risco aos animais expostos.

SINÔNIMO(S)
- Paracetamol
- Tylenol®

VER TAMBÉM
Envenenamento (Intoxicação)

ABREVIATURA(S)
ALT = alanina aminotransferase

RECURSOS DA INTERNET
http://www.aspca.org/pet-care/poison-control/.

Sugestões de Leitura
Hjelle JJ, Grauer GF. Acetaminophen induced toxicosis in dogs and cats. J Am Vet Med Assoc 1986;188:742-746.
Oehme FW. Aspirin and acetaminophen. In: Kirk RW, ed., Current veterinary therapy IX. Small animal practice. Philadelphia: Saunders, 1986:188-189.
Rumbeiha WK, Oehme FW. Methylene blue can be used to treat methemoglobinemia in cats without inducing Heinz body hemolytic anemia. Vet Hum Toxicol 1992;34:120-122.
Savides MC, Oehme FW, Leipold HW. Effects of various antidotal treatments on acetaminophen toxicosis and biotransformation in cats. Am J Vet Res 1985;46:1485-1489.
Savides MC, Oehme FW, Nash SL, Leipold HW. The toxicity and biotransformation of single doses of acetaminophen in dogs and cats. Toxicol Appl Pharmacol 1984;74:26-34.
Wallace KP, Center AS, Hickford FH, Warner KL, Smith S. S-adenosyl-L-methionine (SAMe) for treatment of acetaminophen toxicity in a dog. JAAHA 2002,38(3):246-54.

Autor Frederick W. Oehme
Consultor Editorial Gary D. Osweiler

TOXICIDADE DO RODENTICIDA BROMETALINA

CONSIDERAÇÕES GERAIS

REVISÃO
- A brometalina é um rodenticida neurotóxico que produz efeitos acentuados sobre o sistema nervoso.
- O modo de ação da brometalina consiste no desacoplamento da fosforilação oxidativa. Isso resulta na formação de edema cerebral e no aumento de pressão do líquido cerebrospinal.
- As doses tóxicas são de aproximadamente 2,5 e 0,3 mg/kg em cães e gatos, respectivamente.
- Foi constatado que a dose letal média (DL_{50}) oral de isca de brometalina em pó seja de 3,7 e 0,54 mg/kg em cães e gatos, respectivamente.
- Os nomes comerciais incluem Vengeance®, Assault®, Trounce®, No Pest Rat & Mice Killer®, CyKill®, Fastrac®, e outros.
- Nome químico: N-metil-2,4-dinitro-N-[2,4,6-tribromofenil]-6-[trifluorometil]benzenamina.

IDENTIFICAÇÃO
- Cães e gatos. Outras espécies podem ser acometidas.
- Não foram observadas predileções raciais.
- Qualquer idade pode ser afetada. As iscas de rodenticida são consumidas com maior frequência por animais mais jovens (<1 ano de idade).

SINAIS CLÍNICOS
- A ingestão de doses supraletais de brometalina ($\geq DL_{50}$) pode resultar em um início agudo de excitação do sistema nervoso central, tremores musculares, e crises convulsivas.
- A ingestão de doses mais baixas de brometalina (<DL_{50}) culmina em uma síndrome tardia que se desenvolve dentro de 2-7 dias da ingestão; no entanto, podem ocorrer atrasos de até 2 semanas.
- Os sinais clínicos comuns observados incluem anorexia, ataxia progressiva, paresia, paralisia dos membros posteriores, depressão moderada a grave do sistema nervoso central, tremores musculares finos e crises convulsivas motoras focais ou generalizadas.
- Com frequência, observam-se rigidez extensora dos membros anteriores (postura de Schiff-Sherrington) e posturas descerebradas semelhantes.
- Em caso de envenenamento leve, os sinais clínicos podem desaparecer em até 1-2 semanas do início desses sinais, embora possam persistir por até 4-6 semanas em alguns animais. O prognóstico é bastante reservado em animais gravemente acometidos.

CAUSAS E FATORES DE RISCO
- Ingestão de rodenticidas contendo brometalina.
- Pode ocorrer envenenamento secundário de gatos pela ingestão de roedores envenenados pela brometalina.

DIAGNÓSTICO

DIAGNÓSTICO DIFERENCIAL
Síndromes neurológicas produzidas por traumatismo, neoplasia, distúrbios vasculares cerebrais, bem como por agentes infecciosos e outros agentes tóxicos.

HEMOGRAMA/BIOQUÍMICA/URINÁLISE
Não são previstas alterações nos eletrólitos séricos e na bioquímica sérica de rotina.

OUTROS TESTES LABORATORIAIS
- O diagnóstico depende (1) da presença de um histórico de exposição a uma dose potencialmente tóxica de um rodenticida à base de brometalina, (2) do desenvolvimento de sinais clínicos compatíveis, (3) da presença de vacuolização difusa da substância branca e (4) da confirmação analítica de resíduos de brometalina nos tecidos.
- As anormalidades eletroencefalográficas (EEG) podem incluir atividade de picos e picos-e-ondas, depressão acentuada da voltagem, e atividades anormais de ondas lentas de voltagem elevada.
- O líquido cerebrospinal obtido de cães envenenados por brometalina geralmente revela normalidade em termos de citologia, concentração de proteína, densidade e contagem celular.

DIAGNÓSTICO POR IMAGEM
Neuroimagem (RM ou TC) pode revelar edema cerebral generalizado.

ACHADOS PATOLÓGICOS
- Em geral, as lesões ficam confinadas ao sistema nervoso central.
- Pode ocorrer evidência macroscópica de edema cerebral; no entanto, isso é relativamente leve.
- As alterações histopatológicas envolvem degeneração esponjosa (vacuolização da substância branca) na substância branca do cérebro, cerebelo, tronco encefálico, medula espinal e nervo óptico em virtude da formação de edema da mielina.
- Confirmação química analítica de resíduos de brometalina em tecido fresco congelado de gordura, fígado, rim e cérebro.
- A brometalina já foi detectada em amostras de fígado e cérebro humanos fixadas em formalina por cromatografia gasosa acoplada à espectrometria de massa.

TRATAMENTO

- É justificável o tratamento precoce rigoroso com carvão ativado e um catártico por via oral para reduzir a absorção gastrintestinal do rodenticida.
- Muitos animais que se recuperam da toxicose por brometalina exibem anorexia prolongada e podem necessitar de suplementação alimentar para manter a ingestão calórica.
- Uso de colchões ou almofadas na gaiola para reduzir o risco de formação de úlceras de decúbito em animais nessa condição.

MEDICAÇÕES

MEDICAMENTO(S)
- Descontaminação do trato gastrintestinal, incluindo indução precoce de êmese seguida da administração repetida de carvão ativado (0,5-1 mg/kg VO) e um catártico osmótico (sulfato de sódio, 125 mg/kg VO), deve ser administrada a cada 4-8 horas por, no mínimo, 2-3 dias.
- Controle do edema cerebral com manitol (250 mg/kg a cada 6 h IV), dexametasona (2 mg/kg, a cada 6 h IV) e furosemida (1-2 mg/kg, a cada 6 h IV).
- Diazepam (1-2 mg/kg, conforme a necessidade, IV) e/ou fenobarbital (5-15 mg/kg, conforme a necessidade, IV) podem ser administrados para abolir os tremores musculares e as crises convulsivas graves.

CONTRAINDICAÇÕES/INTERAÇÕES POSSÍVEIS
- São contraindicações para o uso de manitol: doença renal, edema pulmonar, desidratação e hemorragia intracraniana.
- Animais submetidos à terapia com manitol podem ficar desidratados durante o tratamento.
- A reidratação de alguns animais está associada a um agravamento dos sinais clínicos, possivelmente em virtude do edema cerebral e pulmonar de rebote. Além de ser importante, a manutenção da hidratação pode ser realizada com segurança por meio da administração de fluidos orais.

ACOMPANHAMENTO

- A recuperação de um envenenamento leve pode demorar várias semanas.
- O prognóstico é mau para os animais gravemente acometidos.
- Evitar a ingestão contínua do rodenticida.

DIVERSOS
Há relatos de retransmissão da toxicidade vinda do consumo de animais envenenados pela brometalina.

ABREVIATURAS
- EEG = eletroencefalograma.
- RM = ressonância magnética.
- TC = tomografia computadorizada.

RECURSOS DA INTERNET
http://www.fluoridealert.org/pesticides/epage.bromethalin.effects.htm.

Sugestões de Leitura
Dorman DC, Parker AJ, Dye JA, Buck WB. Bromethalin neurotoxicosis in the cat. Prog Vet Neurol 1990, 1:189-196.
Dorman DC, Parker AJ, Dye JA, Buck WB. Bromethalin toxicosis in the dog. Part I: Clinical effects. JAAHA 1990, 26:589-594.
Dorman DC, Parker AJ, Dye JA, Buck WB. Bromethalin toxicosis in the dog. Part II: Selected treatments for the toxic syndrome. JAAHA 1990, 26:595-598.
Pasquale-Styles MA, Sochaski MA, Dorman DC, Krell WS, Shah AK, Schmidt CJ. Fatal bromethalin poisoning. J Forensic Sci 2006, 51:1154-1157.

Autor David C. Dorman
Consultor Editorial Gary D. Osweiler

TOXICIDADE DO VENENO DE LACERTÍLIOS

CONSIDERAÇÕES GERAIS

REVISÃO
- Lacertílios* venenosos — encontrados apenas no sudoeste dos Estados Unidos e no México; *Heloderma suspectum* (monstro do rio Gila) e *H. horridum* (lagarto frisado mexicano); mordedura firme; libera o veneno das glândulas no maxilar inferior por ação de mordedura agressiva com dentes sulcados; não agressivo; raros envenenamentos de animais.
- Componentes do veneno — pouco caracterizados em comparação a outros venenos; sem evidência de coagulação alterada na vítima.

IDENTIFICAÇÃO
Cães e gatos.

SINAIS CLÍNICOS
Achados Anamnésicos
- Início súbito de dor.
- Mordedura — geralmente na face, especialmente no lábio inferior; o lacertílio ainda pode ficar aderido ao paciente (sinal patognomônico).

Achados do Exame Físico
- Sangramento do local da mordedura.
- Pode-se notar hipotensão.
- Local da mordida extremamente doloroso.
- Tumefação localizada.
- Ptialismo — salivação excessiva.
- Lacrimejamento excessivo.
- Micção e defecação frequentes.
- Pode-se observar afonia nos gatos.

CAUSAS E FATORES DE RISCO
Atividades em ambientes externos.

DIAGNÓSTICO

DIAGNÓSTICO DIFERENCIAL
- Traumatismo.
- Mordedura de cobra venenosa — em geral, há menos picadas; depressão e anormalidades da coagulação são mais proeminentes.

HEMOGRAMA/BIOQUÍMICA/URINÁLISE
N/D.

OUTROS TESTES LABORATORIAIS
N/D.

DIAGNÓSTICO POR IMAGEM
N/D.

MÉTODOS DIAGNÓSTICOS
Eletrocardiografia — pode ser detectada a presença de arritmias.

TRATAMENTO

- Remover o lacertílio — colocar um instrumento com alavanca entre os maxilares; empurrar para parte traseira da boca do lacertílio; uma chama mantida abaixo da mandíbula do lacertílio quase sempre libera a preensão.
- Paciente internado — monitorar e tratar a hipotensão, conforme a necessidade, com fluidoterapia cristaloide.
- Local da mordedura — irrigar com lidocaína; sondar para identificar e remover fragmentos dos dentes do lacertílio (se não forem removidos, eles formarão sequestros e abscessos); embeber com solução de Burrow ou solução semelhante a cada 8 h.

MEDICAÇÕES

MEDICAMENTO(S)
- Controle da dor — pode-se fazer uso de narcóticos (se grave).
- São indicados antibióticos de amplo espectro.

CONTRAINDICAÇÕES/INTERAÇÕES POSSÍVEIS
- Corticosteroides — não costumam ser utilizados pelo autor; outros autores divergem sobre o valor desses agentes terapêuticos.
- Anti-histamínicos — não são úteis nesse caso.

ACOMPANHAMENTO

- ECG — monitorar o paciente quanto à presença de arritmias.
- Local da mordedura — monitorar em busca de infecção.

DIVERSOS

Sugestões de Leitura
Peterson ME. Poisonous lizards. In: Peterson ME, Talcott PA, eds., Small Animal Toxicology, 2nd ed. St. Louis: Saunders, 2006, pp. 812-816.

Autor Michael E. Peterson
Consultor Editorial Gary D. Osweiler

---

* N. T.: Compreendem os lagartos, os camaleões e as lagartixas, répteis de corpo alongado, com a cabeça curta e unida ao corpo por um pequeno pescoço.

TOXICIDADE DO XILITOL

CONSIDERAÇÕES GERAIS

REVISÃO
- Xilitol — um álcool de açúcar de 5 carbonos, utilizado como adoçante; presente em algumas gomas de mascar sem açúcar, balas, pastas de dentes, colutórios bucais e produtos de panificação. Também está disponível sob a forma de pó granulado para os processos de cozimento e fornada.
- A ingestão por cães pode causar vômito, fraqueza, ataxia, crises convulsivas, hipocalemia, hipofosfatemia, e hipoglicemia em virtude do excesso da liberação de insulina.
- Podem ser observadas elevações leves a moderadas de ALT em até 4 horas da ingestão.
- Pode ocorrer insuficiência hepática com elevação das enzimas hepáticas, hiperbilirrubinemia e coagulopatia em doses >5 g/kg.
- Doses >0,075-0,1 g/kg de xilitol podem causar hipoglicemia.

IDENTIFICAÇÃO
- Cães — sem predileção de raça, idade, ou sexo.
- Gatos — toxicidade não estabelecida.

SINAIS CLÍNICOS
- Podem se desenvolver em até 15-30 minutos da exposição; com gomas de mascar sem açúcar, a hipoglicemia pode ser adiada por até 12 horas.
- É comum a ocorrência de vômito.
- Letargia progressiva, fraqueza, ataxia, colapso, e crises convulsivas.
- A insuficiência hepática pode ser acompanhada por vômito e hemorragia disseminada, incluindo petéquias, equimose e sangramento gastrintestinal/abdominal.
- Os sinais clínicos de hipoglicemia podem não ser evidentes antes do início da insuficiência hepática.

CAUSAS E FATORES DE RISCO
Ingestão de xilitol ou produtos contendo esse adoçante.

DIAGNÓSTICO

DIAGNÓSTICO DIFERENCIAL
Hipoglicemia
- Dosagem excessiva de insulina.
- Agentes hipoglicemiantes à base de sulfonilureia.
- Insulinoma (tumor de células-β pancreáticas).

Insuficiência Hepática Aguda
- Paracetamol.
- Aflatoxina.
- Algas azuis e verdes.
- Amanita e cogumelos hepatotóxicos semelhantes.
- Ferro.
- Palmeira de salgueiro (*Cycad* spp.).
- Leptospirose.

HEMOGRAMA/BIOQUÍMICA/URINÁLISE
- Hipoglicemia.
- Hipocalemia.
- Hipofosfatemia.
- Atividade elevada das enzimas ALT, AST e fosfatase alcalina — o aumento pode ser adiado por até 24-48 horas.
- Bilirrubinemia.
- Trombocitopenia.

OUTROS TESTES LABORATORIAIS
- TP/TTP prolongado.
- Aumento de produtos de degradação da fibrina, D-dímeros e/ou redução do fibrinogênio.

DIAGNÓSTICO POR IMAGEM
N/D.

MÉTODOS DIAGNÓSTICOS
N/D.

ACHADOS PATOLÓGICOS
- Necrose hepática grave.
- Hemorragia disseminada.

TRATAMENTO
- Descontaminação — êmese se o paciente permanecer assintomático; é improvável que o carvão ativado seja benéfico.
- Monitorizar o paciente em intervalos de 1-2 horas quanto à ocorrência de hipoglicemia e hipocalemia e, então, corrigir conforme a necessidade.
- Monitorizar as alterações hepáticas.

MEDICAÇÕES

MEDICAMENTO(S)
- Dextrose — 0,5-1 g/kg IV seguida por taxa de infusão contínua a 2,5-5% — considerar o início com doses >0,1 g/kg.
- Cloreto de potássio — suplementar em fluidos se o nível de potássio estiver abaixo de 2,5 nmol/L.

CONTRAINDICAÇÕES/INTERAÇÕES POSSÍVEIS
Nenhuma.

ACOMPANHAMENTO
- Monitorizar os níveis de glicose por, no mínimo, 24 horas.
- Monitorizar os níveis de enzimas hepáticas, bilirrubina, TP/TTP e plaquetas por, pelo menos, 72 horas.
- Prognóstico bom em caso de hipoglicemia não complicada, com elevações leves a moderadas de ALT; reservado a mau caso ocorra necrose hepática grave.

DIVERSOS

VER TAMBÉM
- Insuficiência Hepática, Aguda.
- Hipoglicemia.
- Envenenamento (Intoxicação).

ABREVIATURAS
- ALT = alanina aminotransferase.
- AST = aspartato aminotransferase.
- TP = tempo de protrombina.
- TTP = tempo de tromboplastina parcial.

Sugestões de Leitura
Dunayer EK. Hypoglycemia associated with xylitol gum ingestion in a dog. Vet Hum Toxicol 2004, 46(2):87-88.
Dunayer EK. New findings on the effects of xylitol ingestion in dogs. Vet Med 2006, 101(12):791-796.
Dunayer EK, Gwaltney-Brant SM. Acute hepatic failure and coagulopathy associated with xylitol ingestion in eight dogs. JAVMA 2006, 229(7):1113-1117.

Autor Eric K. Dunayer
Consultor Editorial Gary D. Osweiler

TOXICIDADE DO ZINCO

CONSIDERAÇÕES GERAIS

REVISÃO
- Intoxicação ocasionada pela ingestão de objetos contendo zinco.
- Causa irritação gastrintestinal e anemia hemolítica; pode provocar falência múltipla de órgãos (p. ex., renal, hepática, pancreática e cardíaca), CID e parada cardiopulmonar.

IDENTIFICAÇÃO
Relatada com maior frequência em cães jovens de pequeno porte (ou seja, com <12 kg); também pode ocorrer em todas as espécies de todos os portes.

SINAIS CLÍNICOS
- Anorexia. • Vômito. • Diarreia. • Letargia.
- Depressão. • Mucosas pálidas.
- Hemoglobinemia. • Hemoglobinúria. • Icterícia.
- Fezes de coloração laranja. • Taquicardia.

CAUSAS E FATORES DE RISCO
- Há uma variedade de compostos de zinco com biodisponibilidades diferentes: carbonato de zinco e gliconato de zinco (suplementos alimentares), cloreto de zinco (desodorantes), piritiona de zinco (xampu), acetato de zinco (pastilhas para garganta), óxido de zinco (bloqueador solar, Desitin®, loção de calamina), sulfeto de zinco (tintas), zinco metálico (moedas).
- Metais: liga de cobre e zinco.
- Intoxicações resultantes da ingestão de material contendo zinco: moedas norte-americanas cunhadas após 1982 (fonte mais comum); porcas de parafusos; pinos; grampos; metal galvanizado (p. ex., pregos); peças provenientes de tabuleiro de jogos; zíperes; brinquedos diversos; joias.
- Preparações dermatológicas contendo zinco geralmente causam apenas irritação gastrintestinal.
- O ambiente ácido dentro do estômago promove lixiviação do zinco a partir da substância ingerida, permitindo a absorção desse elemento químico.

DIAGNÓSTICO

DIAGNÓSTICO DIFERENCIAL
- Inúmeras causas de hemólise, anemia hemolítica imunomediada, *Babesia*, intoxicação por cebola e alho.
- Toxicose por bolinhas de naftalina (naftaleno).
- Síndrome da veia cava.
- Paracetamol.
- Veneno de coral.
- Algumas espécies de cogumelos.
- Veneno de víbora.
- Superidratação.
- Emissão do odor de gambá.
- Picadas da aranha reclusa-marrom.
- Muitas causas infecciosas e inflamatórias de distúrbio gastrintestinal.

HEMOGRAMA/BIOQUÍMICA/URINÁLISE
- Anemia hemolítica, com possível formação de corpúsculos de Heinz.
- Ocorrerá regeneração se houver tempo suficiente para isso: contagem elevada de hemácias nucleadas, pontilhado basofílico, policromasia, aumento dos reticulócitos.
- Células-alvo.
- Esferocitose — anormalidade branda; incompatível.
- Leucocitose com neutrofilia.
- Hemoglobinemia.
- Bilirrubinemia.
- Altos níveis das enzimas hepáticas AST e fosfatase alcalina; são menos comuns as elevações da GGT e ALT.
- Enzimas pancreáticas elevadas — amilase e lipase — podem indicar falência múltipla de órgãos.
- Proteinúria.
- Pigmentúria (hemoglobina, bilirrubina).
- Azotemia (altos níveis de ureia e creatinina) — rara.

OUTROS TESTES LABORATORIAIS
- Os níveis séricos de zinco frequentemente ultrapassam 5 ppm (faixa normal aproximada em cães e gatos: 0,7-2 ppm).
- O sangue deve ser coletado em tubos não contaminados por zinco.
- Perfil de coagulação — pode indicar CID (TP e TTP prolongados, hipofibrinogenemia, trombocitopenia e níveis elevados dos PDF).
- É indicada a monitorização frequente do hematócrito, pois o declínio nesse índice pode ser rápido.

DIAGNÓSTICO POR IMAGEM
- Obtenção de imagens abdominais — *pode* revelar a presença de objeto(s) metálico(s) no trato gastrintestinal.
- Muitas vezes, o objeto de zinco já foi eliminado (pelo vômito ou pelas fezes) no momento em que o paciente é atendido.

MÉTODOS DIAGNÓSTICOS
ECG — pode revelar arritmias e anormalidades do segmento ST.

TRATAMENTO

- Rápida remoção do objeto de zinco por meio de endoscopia ou laparotomia/gastrotomia — procedimento imperativo.
- Fluidoterapia intravenosa — para manter a hidratação e a diurese, pois a ocorrência de insuficiência renal aguda é uma sequela grave.
- Hemólise intravascular grave — talvez haja necessidade de transfusão de sangue/papa de hemácias, além de substâncias carreadoras de oxigênio (Oxyglobin® [oxiglobina]).
- Informar o proprietário sobre os riscos da ingestão de objetos contendo zinco (especialmente moedas norte-americanas cunhadas depois de 1982).

MEDICAÇÕES

MEDICAMENTO(S)
- O uso de terapia quelante pode *não* ser justificável assim que a fonte de zinco em excesso for removida — os níveis de zinco declinam com relativa rapidez (em alguns a vários dias) pela excreção na bile, nas secreções pancreáticas e na urina.
- EDTA cálcico — 100 mg/kg SC, diluídos em solução de glicose a 5% e divididos em quatro doses diárias (tratamento semelhante ao da intoxicação por chumbo) se a melhora clínica do paciente ou a redução do zinco sanguíneo não acompanhar a remoção dos objetos de zinco.
- Penicilamina — 110 mg/kg/dia VO, divididos a cada 6-8 h por 5-14 dias (tratamento semelhante ao da intoxicação por chumbo) — esse medicamento, em geral, é utilizado com menos frequência que o EDTA cálcico.
- Heparina — 150 U/kg SC a cada 6 h; para CID.
- Antagonistas dos receptores H_2 (p. ex., cimetidina, ranitidina, famotidina), inibidores da bomba de prótons (p. ex., omeprazol) e antiácidos utilizados isoladamente ou em combinação — podem ajudar a reduzir a atividade gástrica e a taxa de liberação do zinco.
- Antieméticos.

CONTRAINDICAÇÕES/INTERAÇÕES POSSÍVEIS
Evitar os antibióticos aminoglicosídeos e outras nefrotoxinas em potencial — risco de insuficiência renal aguda.

ACOMPANHAMENTO

MONITORIZAÇÃO DO PACIENTE
- ECG — monitorizar o paciente em busca de indícios de arritmias e alterações do segmento ST.
- Perfil de coagulação, hematócrito, eritrograma, amilase, lipase, ureia, creatinina, fosfatase alcalina, AST e ALT — monitorizar durante as primeiras 72 h após a remoção do zinco.
- Monitorizar os níveis séricos de zinco.

EVOLUÇÃO ESPERADA E PROGNÓSTICO
- Falência múltipla de órgãos (p. ex., renal, hepática), CID, doença pancreática, parada cardiopulmonar — consequências potenciais.
- Rápida remoção da fonte de zinco — pode proporcionar uma melhora progressiva em 48-72 h; a recuperação plena é possível.

DIVERSOS

VER TAMBÉM
Envenenamento (Intoxicação).

ABREVIATURA(S)
- ALT = alanina aminotransferase.
- AST = aspartato aminotransferase.
- CID = coagulação intravascular disseminada.
- ECG = eletrocardiograma.
- EDTA = ácido etilenodiaminotetracético.
- GGT = gama-glutamiltransferase.
- PDF = produtos da degradação da fibrina.
- TP = tempo de protrombina.
- TTP = tempo de tromboplastina parcial.

Sugestões de Leitura
Dziwenka MM, Coppock R. Zinc. In: Plumlee KH, ed., Clinical Veterinary Toxicology. St. Louis: Elsevier Mosby, 2004, pp. 221-230.
Gurnee CM, Drobatz KJ. Zinc intoxication in dogs: 19 cases (1991-2003). JAVMA 2007, 230(8):1174-1179.
Talcott PA. Zinc poisoning. In: Peterson ME, Talcott PA, eds., Small Animal Toxicology. St. Louis: Elsevier Saunders, 2006, pp. 1094-1100.

Autor Patricia A. Talcott
Consultor Editorial Gary D. Osweiler

TOXICIDADE DOS AGENTES ANTI-INFLAMATÓRIOS NÃO ESTEROIDES

CONSIDERAÇÕES GERAIS

DEFINIÇÃO
- Toxicidade secundária à ingestão aguda ou crônica de algum AINE.
- AINE — classificados como ácidos carboxílicos (ácido acetilsalicílico, indometacina, sulindaco, ibuprofeno, naproxeno, carprofeno, ácido meclofenâmico e flunixino meglumina) ou ácidos enólicos (fenilbutazona, dipirona, piroxicam); inibidores da COX-2 (deracoxibe e firocoxibe).

FISIOPATOLOGIA
- Ação — analgésica, antipirética e anti-inflamatória pela inibição da ciclo-oxigenase; diminuem a produção de prostaglandinas que atuam como mediadores da inflamação.
- Bem absorvidos por via oral.
- Depuração — varia muito entre as espécies; eliminados lentamente nos cães e nos gatos.
- Metabolizados no fígado em metabólitos ativos ou inativos.
- Excretados nos rins via filtração glomerular e secreção tubular.

SISTEMA(S) ACOMETIDO(S)
- Gastrintestinal — erosões e úlceras.
- Hemático/linfático/imune — podem-se notar distúrbios de sangramento secundários à agregação plaquetária diminuída.
- Hepatobiliar — lesão hepatocelular idiossincrática.
- Renal/urológico — insuficiência renal aguda; nefrite intersticial aguda.

GENÉTICA
- As diferenças das espécies em termos de absorção, excreção e metabolismo de diferentes agentes são notáveis; evitar a extrapolação de dados de outras espécies ou dosagens.
- O uso de AINE fora da indicação da bula pode resultar em efeitos adversos significativos, sobretudo em gatos.
- Os AINE de venda livre (especialmente o ibuprofeno e o naproxeno) são causas comuns de toxicose por esses agentes terapêuticos em cães e gatos. O naproxeno apresenta meia-vida extremamente longa nos animais domésticos e, portanto, a exposição a esse medicamento implica alto risco de efeitos adversos significativos.

INCIDÊNCIA/PREVALÊNCIA
Está entre as dez toxicoses mais comuns relatadas para o Centro Norte-americano de Controle de Intoxicações de Animais.

DISTRIBUIÇÃO GEOGRÁFICA
N/D.

IDENTIFICAÇÃO
- Cães e gatos.
- Sem predileções por raça, idade ou sexo.

SINAIS CLÍNICOS
Comentários Gerais
- Irritação gastrintestinal — geralmente se desenvolve dentro de algumas horas.
- Envolvimento renal ou ulceração gastrintestinal — pode demorar vários dias.

Achados Anamnésicos
- Evidência do consumo acidental de medicação do proprietário.
- Letargia.
- Anorexia.
- Vômito — com ou sem sangue.
- Diarreia.
- Icterícia.
- Melena.
- Colapso e morte súbita — podem ocorrer secundariamente à perfuração de úlcera gástrica.
- Poliúria, polidipsia e oligúria.
- Ataxia, crises convulsivas, coma — podem ocorrer com grandes ingestões.

Achados do Exame Físico
- Depressão.
- Mucosas pálidas.
- Abdome doloroso.
- Desidratação.
- Febre.
- Taquicardia.
- Icterícia.

CAUSAS
Exposição acidental ou administração inadequada.

FATORES DE RISCO
- Animais predispostos à nefropatia — idade avançada; doença renal, hepática ou cardiovascular preexistente; hipotensão; outras doenças e/ou medicações concomitantes.
- Histórico prévio de úlcera ou sangramento gastrintestinal.

DIAGNÓSTICO

DIAGNÓSTICO DIFERENCIAL
Outras condições (clínicas ou toxicológicas) que causam efeitos gastrintestinais e renais; o diagnóstico baseia-se no histórico de exposição e nos sinais clínicos compatíveis.

HEMOGRAMA/BIOQUÍMICA/URINÁLISE
- Anemia — regenerativa ou arregenerativa, dependendo da duração do sangramento.
- Leucocitose — associada à úlcera gástrica perfurada e consequente peritonite.
- Ureia e creatinina — podem estar elevadas secundariamente à azotemia pré-renal ou lesão renal primária.
- Enzimas hepáticas elevadas — ocasionalmente.
- Monitorizar o débito urinário em busca de indícios de oligúria; monitorizar o paciente quanto à presença de glicosúria, proteinúria e cilindros.

OUTROS TESTES LABORATORIAIS
N/D.

DIAGNÓSTICO POR IMAGEM
N/D.

MÉTODOS DIAGNÓSTICOS
Endoscopia — verificar a existência de ulceração gastrintestinal.

ACHADOS PATOLÓGICOS
- Irritação, ulceração ou hemorragia gastrintestinais com possível perfuração gástrica e peritonite.
- Necrose tubular ou papilar renal ou nefrite intersticial.

TRATAMENTO

CUIDADO(S) DE SAÚDE ADEQUADO(S)
- Paciente de ambulatório — com sinais clínicos leves (no caso de baixa dose ingerida); tratado em casa com medicação apropriada, dieta e medidas sintomáticas.
- Paciente internado — no caso de alta dose ingerida; potencial de toxicose renal; sinais clínicos relativamente graves (vômito frequente, vômito sanguinolento, melena, anemia ou indícios de envolvimento renal); tratamento rigoroso para evitar complicações potencialmente letais.

CUIDADO(S) DE ENFERMAGEM
- Fluidoterapia — restabelecer a hidratação quando houver vômito de intensidade moderada a intensa; administração de, no mínimo, duas vezes a taxa de manutenção com envolvimento renal potencial ou conhecido (ver "Insuficiência Renal Aguda").
- Se o paciente estiver gravemente anêmico, talvez haja indicação de transfusão de sangue.

ATIVIDADE
N/D.

DIETA
- Vômito — nada por via oral.
- Vômito resolvido — começar com dieta branda, pobre em proteína.

ORIENTAÇÃO AO PROPRIETÁRIO
- Enfatizar a importância de entrar em contato com o médico veterinário ou com o Centro de Controle de Intoxicações de Animais da Sociedade Norte-americana para a Prevenção de Crueldade aos Animais sempre que um animal for exposto a algum AINE não prescrito.
- Informar ao proprietário que os cães e, particularmente, os gatos apresentam baixa tolerância aos AINE.
- Com a prescrição de algum AINE, instruir o proprietário não só a observar o animal quanto à ocorrência de efeitos adversos ou idiossincrásicos, mas também a interromper o medicamento e entrar em contato com a clínica se ocorrerem tais efeitos.

CONSIDERAÇÕES CIRÚRGICAS
A intervenção cirúrgica pode ser necessária para úlcera gástrica perfurada.

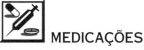
MEDICAÇÕES

MEDICAMENTO(S) DE ESCOLHA
Ingestão Recente
- Ingestão dentro de algumas horas e sem vômito — induzir à êmese (apomorfina ou peróxido de hidrogênio) a menos que o paciente apresente crises convulsivas ou depressão neurológica (SNC) acentuada.
- Após a êmese — administrar carvão ativado (1-2 g/kg VO) e algum catártico (sulfato de magnésio ou de sódio na dose de 1/4 de colher das de chá [aproximadamente 1 mL]/5 kg ou sorbitol a 70% na dose de 3 mL/kg) se não houver diarreia.
- Repetir o carvão ativado — usar metade da dose original para os AINE que sofrem recirculação entero-hepática.

Antagonistas do Receptor H_2
- Para desarranjo ou ulceração gastrintestinais.
- Eficazes principalmente para o tratamento de úlceras por dosagem excessiva aguda ou administração crônica após a suspensão do medicamento.
- A ranitidina ou a famotidina podem ser as melhores escolhas, pois a cimetidina pode inibir

Toxicidade dos Agentes Anti-Inflamatórios Não Esteroides

enzimas microssomais responsáveis pela metabolização de alguns AINE.
• Ranitidina — cães, 2 mg/kg VO, IV a cada 8 h; gatos, 2,5 mg/kg IV a cada 12 h ou 3,5 mg/kg VO a cada 12 h.
• Famotidina — cães, 0,5-1,0 mg/kg VO, SC, IV ou IM a cada 12-24 h; gatos, 0,5 mg/kg VO, SC, IV ou IM a cada 12-24 h.
• Cimetidina — 5-10 mg/kg VO, IV, IM a cada 6-8 h.

Outros
• Sucralfato — cães, 0,5-1 g VO a cada 8-12 h; gatos, 0,25 g VO a cada 8 h; liga-se às proteínas na base da úlcera; estimula a secreção de muco e de bicarbonato.
• Misoprostol — 1-3 µg/kg VO a cada 8 h; análogo da PGE_2; evita o sangramento e a ulceração gastrintestinais; promove a cicatrização durante o uso crônico nos seres humanos e nos cães tratados com ácido acetilsalicílico.
• Omeprazol — pacientes com >20 kg, 1 cápsula (20 mg) diariamente; pacientes com <20 kg, metade da cápsula; pacientes com <5 kg, um quarto da cápsula; potente inibidor da secreção ácida gástrica; bloqueia a etapa final de produção do ácido clorídrico.
• Dopamina — pode ser indicada na insuficiência renal aguda.
• Terapia anticonvulsivante padrão — diazepam, pentobarbital, fenobarbital, se necessários.
• Duração do tratamento — depende da meia-vida do agente particular ingerido.

CONTRAINDICAÇÕES
Evitar a utilização concomitante de corticosteroides ou múltiplos AINE em conjunto; contraindicados na prenhez (efeito abortifaciente).

PRECAUÇÕES
Pacientes que fazem uso de outros medicamentos nefroativos ou nefrotóxicos (p. ex., aminoglicosídeos e inibidores da ECA) — encontram-se sob maior risco de desenvolvimento de nefropatia por AINE.

INTERAÇÕES POSSÍVEIS
AINE — altamente ligados à proteína; podem ser influenciados pelo uso concomitante de outros medicamentos altamente ligados à proteína.

MEDICAMENTO(S) ALTERNATIVO(S)
N/D.

ACOMPANHAMENTO

MONITORIZAÇÃO DO PACIENTE
• Débito urinário — monitorizar o paciente de forma meticulosa quanto à ocorrência de oligúria; examinar a presença de cilindros, proteína e glicose.
• Fezes e vômito — avaliar em busca de sangramento gastrintestinal (pode não se desenvolver durante vários dias).
• Ureia e creatinina — mensurar duas vezes ao dia durante vários dias (a extensão completa do dano renal pode não ser evidente de imediato).

PREVENÇÃO
• Conservar os medicamentos fora do alcance dos animais de estimação.
• Desestimular os proprietários a medicar o animal de estimação sem a supervisão de um veterinário.
• Antes de iniciar o tratamento, examinar os pacientes de alto risco com testes laboratoriais apropriados.

COMPLICAÇÕES POSSÍVEIS
• Perfuração de úlcera gástrica e desenvolvimento de peritonite.
• Insuficiência renal aguda e crônica irreversível.

EVOLUÇÃO ESPERADA E PROGNÓSTICO
• Desarranjo ou ulceração gástricos — costumam exibir plena recuperação com o tratamento apropriado.
• Efeitos renais — geralmente reversíveis com o tratamento precoce e rigoroso.
• Hepatopatias agudas — em geral se resolvem com terapia sintomática após a interrupção do medicamento.

DIVERSOS

DISTÚRBIOS ASSOCIADOS
N/D.

POTENCIAL ZOONÓTICO
N/D.

GESTAÇÃO/FERTILIDADE/REPRODUÇÃO
• Exposição durante a prenhez — risco de efeitos cardiopulmonares e renais sobre o feto.
• Pode prolongar a prenhez, sobretudo se administrado durante o último terço e antes do início do parto.

VER TAMBÉM
• Envenenamento (Intoxicação).
• Insuficiência Renal Aguda.
• Toxicidade do Ácido Acetilsalicílico.

ABREVIATURA(S)
• AINE = anti-inflamatórios não esteroides.
• COX-2 = cicloxigenase 2
• ECA = enzima conversora de angiotensina.
• PGE_2 = prostaglandina E2.
• SNC = sistema nervoso central.

RECURSOS DA INTERNET
http://www.aspcapro.org/animal-poisoncontrol.php.

Sugestões de Leitura
Dunayer E. Ibuprofen toxicosis in dogs, cats, and ferrets. Vet Med July 2004, pp. 580-586.
Johnston SA, Budsburg SC. Nonsteroidal anti-inflammatory drugs and corticosteroids in the management of canine osteoarthritis. Vet Clin North Am Small Anim Pract 1997, 27:841-862.
Kore AC. Toxicology of nonsteroidal anti-inflammatory drugs. Vet Clin North Am Small Anim Pract 1990, 20:419-431.

Autor Judy Holding
Consultor Editorial Gary D. Osweiler

TOXICIDADE PELA IVERMECTINA

CONSIDERAÇÕES GERAIS

REVISÃO
- Intoxicação — cães submetidos à dosagem fora da especificação da bula (≥10-15 vezes a dosagem recomendada).
- Ivermectina — liga-se aos canais de íon cloreto dependentes de glutamato nas células nervosas e musculares dos invertebrados, causando subsequente paralisia e morte do parasita. Também interage com outros canais de cloreto dependentes de ligando, incluindo aqueles dependentes do GABA.
- Sensibilidade — Collies e algumas outras raças são mais sensíveis a altas doses de ivermectina. Essa sensibilidade foi associada a uma deleção hereditária do gene ABCB1 responsável pela codificação de uma bomba proteica transmembrana chamada glicoproteína-P. Acredita-se que a glicoproteína-P transporte a ivermectina para fora do tecido cerebral e para dentro da circulação.

IDENTIFICAÇÃO
- Cães.
- Cães da raça Collie — mais comumente acometidos.
- Cães homozigotos para a deleção do gene ABCB1 também são acometidos; cães heterozigotos podem reagir com doses mais altas. A mutação do gene ABCB1 foi encontrada em Pastor de Shetland, Pastor australiano, Old English sheepdog, Pastor alemão, Whippet de pelo longo, Silken windhound e uma variedade de cães de raças mistas.
- Não há predileção etária ou sexual.

SINAIS CLÍNICOS
- Midríase.
- Depressão.
- Salivação.
- Vômito.
- Ataxia.
- Tremores.
- Desorientação.
- Fraqueza, decúbito.
- Falta de responsividade.
- Cegueira.
- Bradicardia.
- Hipoventilação.
- Coma.
- Morte.

CAUSAS E FATORES DE RISCO
- Uso fora das recomendações em dosagem elevada.
- Sensibilidade racial — ver anteriormente.

DIAGNÓSTICO
- Com base na anamnese e nos sinais clínicos.
- Nenhum teste específico é útil para confirmar o diagnóstico.

DIAGNÓSTICO DIFERENCIAL
- Superdosagens de outros compostos de ivermectina — milbemicina, moxidectina, e selamectina.
- Outras substâncias tóxicas ou doenças com envolvimento do SNC.

HEMOGRAMA/BIOQUÍMICA/URINÁLISE
N/D.

OUTROS TESTES LABORATORIAIS
Gasometria sanguínea arterial — pode revelar $PaCO_2$ elevada e PaO_2 baixa provocadas pela depressão respiratória e hipoventilação.

DIAGNÓSTICO POR IMAGEM
N/D.

MÉTODOS DIAGNÓSTICOS
Fisostigmina — 1 mg IV; o retorno temporário (30-40 min) à consciência ou a recuperação do estado de alerta e da atividade muscular após a administração garante, mas não confirma, o diagnóstico; não acelera a recuperação; não indicada para tratamento; a administração do glicopirrolato em primeiro lugar pode evitar a bradicardia grave.

TRATAMENTO
- Principal — cuidados de suporte e tratamento sintomático.
- Fluidoterapia adequada, manutenção do equilíbrio eletrolítico, suporte nutricional e prevenção de complicações secundárias — objetivos importantes.
- Suporte nutricional — instituir precocemente, de preferência dentro de 2-3 dias da exposição; depressão grave do SNC ou coma podem durar semanas.
- Para o paciente em decúbito, são importantes medidas como alternância frequente da posição do paciente, uso de cama adequada, aplicação de fisioterapia, cuidados atenciosos de enfermagem e outras medidas terapêuticas padrão.
- Aplicação de lubrificantes oculares.
- Ventilação mecânica — pode ser necessária em caso de depressão respiratória.

MEDICAÇÕES

MEDICAMENTO(S)
- Não existe nenhum agente de reversão conhecido.
- Atropina ou glicopirrolato — podem ser administrados, conforme a necessidade, para tratar a bradicardia.

CONTRAINDICAÇÕES/INTERAÇÕES POSSÍVEIS
- Outros medicamentos que sabidamente provocam intoxicação em cães com a mutação do gene ABCB1: loperamida, doxorrubicina, vincristina e vimblastina.
- Não utilizar a ivermectina juntamente com cetoconazol.

ACOMPANHAMENTO
- Prognóstico e desfecho final — dependem da sensibilidade do animal individualmente e da raça, da quantidade do medicamento ingerido ou injetado, da rapidez de desenvolvimento dos sinais clínicos, da resposta ao tratamento de suporte e do estado de saúde geral do paciente.
- A convalescença pode ser prolongada (várias semanas); em muitos casos aparentemente sem esperança, cuidados de suporte satisfatórios resultaram na recuperação completa.

DIVERSOS

VER TAMBÉM
- Dirofilariose — Cães.
- Envenenamento (Intoxicação).

ABREVIATURA(S)
- GABA = ácido gama-aminobutírico.
- SNC = sistema nervoso central.

Sugestões de Leitura
Mealy KL. Canine ABCB1 and macrocyclic lactones: Heartworm prevention and pharmacogenetics. Vet Parasit 2008, 158:215-222.
Paul AJ, Tranquilli WJ. Ivermectin. In: Kirk RW, ed., Current Veterinary Therapy X. Philadelphia: Saunders, 1989, pp. 140-142.

Autor Allan J. Paul
Consultor Editorial Gary D. Osweiler

TOXICIDADE PELO FERRO

CONSIDERAÇÕES GERAIS

REVISÃO
- Ferro — elemento essencial aos organismos vivos; pode ser letal quando ingerido em grandes quantidades.
- Fontes de grandes concentrações de ferro prontamente ionizável — polivitamínicos; suplementos minerais dietéticos; suplementos para gravidez humana; alguns tipos de aquecedores de mão.
- Superdosagem — perda das limitações mucosas normais da absorção do ferro; corrosivo à mucosa gastrintestinal.
- Ferro circulante superior à capacidade total de ligação do ferro — muito reativo; provoca dano oxidativo a qualquer tipo celular.
- Dano às mitocôndrias — perda do metabolismo oxidativo.
- Sistemas primários acometidos — gastrintestinal; hepático; cardiovascular; nervoso.

IDENTIFICAÇÃO
- Cães; possivelmente em outras espécies.
- Todas as idades são suscetíveis.

SINAIS CLÍNICOS
Comentários Gerais
- Histórico — geralmente indica a ingestão de comprimidos.
- É improvável o desenvolvimento de sinais clínicos em pacientes que permanecem assintomáticos por 6-8 h.
- Ocorre em quatro estágios.

Estágio I (0-6 h)
- Vômito.
- Diarreia.
- Depressão.
- Hemorragia gastrintestinal.
- Dor abdominal.

Estágio II (6-24 h)
- Recuperação aparente.

Estágio III (12-96 h)
- Vômito.
- Diarreia.
- Depressão.
- Hemorragia gastrintestinal.
- Choque.
- Tremores.
- Dor abdominal.
- Acidose metabólica.

Estágio IV (2-6 semanas)
- Obstrução gastrintestinal por formação de estenose.

CAUSAS E FATORES DE RISCO
- Geralmente associados à ingestão de comprimidos contendo ferro.
- Cães — provavelmente ingerem grande quantidade de comprimidos, em virtude do comportamento alimentar relativamente indiscriminado.
- Dose tóxica (cães) — >20 mg/kg de ferro elementar.
- Ferro metálico e óxido de ferro (ferrugem) — não prontamente ionizável; não associado a intoxicações.
- Ter cuidado ao se calcular a ingestão do ferro; os sais de ferro em suplementos e medicações variam quanto ao teor de ferro elementar (entre 12 e 63%).

DIAGNÓSTICO

DIAGNÓSTICO DIFERENCIAL
Outras causas de gastrenterite.

HEMOGRAMA/BIOQUÍMICA/URINÁLISE
- Leucocitose.
- Hiperglicemia.
- AST, ALT, fosfatase alcalina e bilirrubina sérica normais a elevadas.

OUTROS TESTES LABORATORIAIS
Acidose metabólica.

Análise Sérica para Ferro Total e Capacidade Total de Ligação do Ferro
- Capacidade de ligação normal — 3-4 vezes o ferro sérico.
- Ferro sérico superior à capacidade total de ligação do ferro — indica intoxicação; há necessidade de tratamento; monitorizar em 2-3 h e em 5-6 h após a ingestão e nos pacientes assintomáticos (as taxas de absorção variam com a dissolução do comprimido, e as concentrações do ferro sérico mudam rapidamente).

DIAGNÓSTICO POR IMAGEM
Radiografia — comprimidos contendo ferro intacto podem ser radiopacos; é possível a visualização de bezoares de comprimidos aderidos à mucosa esofágica/gástrica.

MÉTODOS DIAGNÓSTICOS
- Análise do ferro nos tecidos após a morte — frequentemente ineficaz por causa da natureza reativa do ferro livre e da distribuição sistêmica da ligação reativa.
- Análise do conteúdo gastrintestinal ou estomacal — pode ajudar a comprovar elevadas exposições ao ferro.

ACHADOS PATOLÓGICOS
Lesões primárias macroscópicas — hemorragia no trato gastrintestinal e fígado; hepatomegalia.

TRATAMENTO
- Corrigir o choque hipovolêmico — fluidos intravenosos.
- Corrigir a acidose — adição de bicarbonato aos fluidos intravenosos.

DESCONTAMINAÇÃO E PROTEÇÃO
- Evitar lesão gastrintestinal e sistêmica adicional — remoção do ferro não absorvido do estômago; diminui a duração e a gravidade dos sinais.
- Tratar a lesão gastrintestinal — demulcentes gástricos ou sucralfato para a lesão gastrintestinal grave.
- Êmese — induzida para o paciente assintomático.
- Lavagem gástrica ou enterogástrica — reduz a absorção; realizada quando a êmese for contraindicada ou quando os bezoares de comprimidos forem identificados.
- Gastrotomia de emergência — indicada se a lavagem falhar em remover os comprimidos ou bezoares aderidos.

QUELAÇÃO
- Quelar o excesso de ferro sistêmico.
- Mesilato de deferoxamina — quelante do ferro.
- Duração do tratamento — até que a capacidade total de ligação do ferro seja maior do que a do ferro sérico.

MEDICAÇÕES

MEDICAMENTO(S)
- Mesilato de deferoxamina — 15 mg/kg/h em infusão IV ou 40 mg/kg IM a cada 4-6 h ou 40 mg/kg IV lenta a cada 4-6 h; para quelação; indicado quando o ferro sérico exceder a capacidade total de ligação do ferro.
- Sucralfato — 0,5-1 g VO a cada 8-12 h; para proteção gastrintestinal.

CONTRAINDICAÇÕES/INTERAÇÕES POSSÍVEIS
- Carvão ativado — não se liga ao ferro.
- Lavagem gástrica — contraindicada com hematêmese em virtude do alto risco de perfuração.
- Deferoxamina intravenosa — deve ser administrada lentamente ou pode precipitar arritmias cardíacas.
- Deferoxamina — teratogênica; utilizar em pacientes prenhes apenas se os benefícios superarem os riscos.

ACOMPANHAMENTO
- Enzimas hepáticas — monitorizadas até por 24 horas após o controle do ferro circulante em excesso.
- Instruir o proprietário a observar o animal quanto aos indícios de obstrução gastrintestinal por 4-6 semanas após a intoxicação.

DIVERSOS

VER TAMBÉM
- Acidose Metabólica.
- Envenenamento (Intoxicação).

ABREVIATURA(S)
- ALT = alanina aminotransferase.
- AST = aspartato aminotransferase.

Sugestões de Leitura
Greentree WF, Hall JO. Iron toxicosis. In: Bonagura JD, ed., Kirk's Current Veterinary Therapy XII. Philadelphia: Saunders, 1983, pp. 240-242.
Hall JO. Iron. In: Peterson ME, Talcott PA, eds., Small Animal Toxicology. Philadelphia: Saunders, 2006, pp. 777-784.

Autor Jeffery O. Hall
Consultor Editorial Gary D. Osweiler

TOXICOSE POR AMITRAZ

CONSIDERAÇÕES GERAIS

REVISÃO
- Amitraz — acaricida formamidínico; aplicado por via tópica para o controle de carrapatos, ácaros e piolhos.
- Produtos com amitraz em sua composição (para cães) — são formulados como um concentrado emulsificável a 19,9% em frascos de 10,6 mL para diluição e aplicação como solução embebida em esponja; como coleira de 27,5 g e 62,5 cm ou 18,5 g e 45,7 cm impregnada com uma solução a 9,0%; como um componente a 14,34% para aplicação *spot-on* de frascos com ~0,65 mL, 1,27 mL, 3,21 mL, 5,11 mL ou 6,39 mL, dependendo do porte do animal*.
- Sistema(s) acometido(s) — nervoso; endócrino/metabólico (células β do pâncreas); gastrintestinal.
- Sinais clínicos — mais associados com efeitos agonistas α_2-adrenorreceptores.
- Após a administração oral de dose elevada (cães) — a concentração plasmática atinge seu máximo em aproximadamente 6 h; a meia-vida de eliminação é longa, em torno de 24 h; os metabólitos são excretados na urina.
- Ingestão de coleiras impregnadas com amitraz de liberação prolongada — ocorrem tanto a liberação constante como a exposição sistêmica contínua até que os fragmentos da coleira sejam eliminados nas fezes.
- Toxicose — ocorre geralmente após a ingestão de coleiras impregnadas, a aplicação tópica de soluções inadequadamente diluídas ou a administração oral ou aplicação tópica de soluções em animal de porte errado.
- Podem ocorrer reações idiossincráticas.

IDENTIFICAÇÃO
- Anamnese completa — costuma identificar o uso por via tópica ou na forma de coleiras.
- Cães — comum, em função do uso mais frequente.
- Gatos — mais sensíveis que os cães embora a espécie felina seja menos provavelmente envolvida.
- Predominância em animais idosos e pertencentes às raças toy.

SINAIS CLÍNICOS
Achados Anamnésicos
Desenvolvimento agudo após a exposição (tópica ou oral).

Achados do Exame Físico
- Depressão de leve a grave.
- Ataxia.
- Bradicardia.
- Vômito.
- Hiper/hipotermia.
- Hiperglicemia.
- Hipotensão.
- Poliúria.
- Estase gastrintestinal.
- Midríase.
- Óbito (o prognóstico é tipicamente bom com o tratamento).

CAUSAS E FATORES DE RISCO
- Ingestão de coleiras ou pedaços de coleiras impregnadas.

---
* N. T.: Os produtos comercializados no Brasil podem ter outra apresentação.

- Aplicação dérmica direta inadequada.
- Ingestão de produto não diluído.
- Subsequentemente à aplicação de soluções diluídas e aplicadas de forma adequada — menos comum.
- Animais idosos, doentes, pertencentes às raças toy ou debilitados — podem ser predispostos.

DIAGNÓSTICO

DIAGNÓSTICO DIFERENCIAL
- Medicamentos de abuso (agentes psicoativos) e de prescrição — maconha; opioides; barbitúricos; benzodiazepínicos; fenotiazínicos; medicamentos anti-hipertensivos; relaxantes da musculatura esquelética; antidepressivos (tricíclicos e ISRS) e outros medicamentos ou substâncias químicas depressivas.
- Ivermectinas, avermectinas, milbemicinas — geralmente uma dose muito alta ou excepcionalmente uma raça sensível.
- Alcoóis — etanol; etilenoglicol (anticongelante); metanol (líquido para limpeza de para-brisas); álcool isopropílico (álcool de fricção para assepsia).
- Paralisia causada pelo carrapato, botulismo, traumatismo craniano, diabetes, hiperadrenocorticismo, hipotireoidismo, anemia grave, insuficiência cardíaca e choque anafilático — depressão ou fraqueza acentuadas.

HEMOGRAMA/BIOQUÍMICA/URINÁLISE
- Hiperglicemia — comum, relacionada com a inibição de insulina.
- Aumento das enzimas hepáticas — incomum.

DIAGNÓSTICO POR IMAGEM
Radiografia abdominal — pode revelar uma fivela de coleira no trato gastrintestinal.

MÉTODOS DIAGNÓSTICOS
Identificam o amitraz no pelo ou no conteúdo gastrintestinal — há métodos analíticos descritos; são úteis apenas para comprovar a exposição; não há dados disponíveis que correlacionem a concentração aos sinais clínicos.

ACHADOS PATOLÓGICOS
Exposição prolongada a altas doses — aumento de peso do fígado; leve expansão dos hepatócitos; adelgaçamento das zonas fasciculada e reticular; hiperplasia discreta da zona glomerulosa das adrenais.

TRATAMENTO
- Internação — pacientes gravemente acometidos.
- Leve sedação após a aplicação correta de soluções embebidas em esponjas — frequentemente transitória; pode não precisar de tratamento.
- Sinais brandos após a aplicação tópica — esfregar o local manualmente com um detergente de lavar louça, utilizando luvas; enxaguar com quantidades abundantes de água tépida (morna); instituir os cuidados de suporte inespecíficos (p. ex., fluidos intravenosos, manutenção de temperatura corporal normal e suporte nutricional); monitorizar o paciente em 1-2 dias até a constatação de melhora.
- Possível ingestão de coleira — recuperação desse corpo estranho por via endoscópica — a remoção de grandes fragmentos do estômago pode ser benéfica; inúmeros pedaços diminutos costumam estar situados em todo o trato gastrintestinal, tornando a remoção impraticável.

MEDICAÇÕES

MEDICAMENTO(S)
Ingestão de Coleiras, Paciente Assintomático
- Eméticos — peróxido de hidrogênio USP** a 3% (2,2 mL/kg VO; máximo de 45 mL, após o fornecimento de refeição úmida); não se recomendam a apomorfina e, particularmente, a xilazina.
- Não se comprovou que o carvão ativado seja eficaz.
- Dieta formadora de volume à base de pão integral, lactulose e abóbora.
- Enema de água tépida da torneira (5-10 mL/kg); esse tipo de enema estimulará a motilidade GI e ajudará na passagem de fragmentos da coleira por meio do trato GI.

Depressão Acentuada
- Talvez haja necessidade de reversão farmacológica dos efeitos α_2-adrenérgicos.
- Ioimbina (Yobine®) — 0,11 mg/kg IV, administrada lentamente; reverte a depressão e a bradicardia em minutos; melhora a motilidade GI; o objetivo é manter o paciente em um estado de depressão em baixo nível, com frequência cardíaca, pressão arterial, temperatura corporal e glicemia normais.
- Ingestões de coleiras — monitorizar o paciente quanto à recidiva dos sintomas; doses adicionais da ioimbina podem ser necessárias, até que os fragmentos da coleira apareçam nas fezes.
- Atipamezol (Antisedan®) — 0,05 mg/kg IM; há relatos de reversão dos sinais clínicos dentro de 10 min; a dose pode ser repetida conforme a necessidade; representa um medicamento alternativo mediante a indisponibilidade da ioimbina.
- Ioimbina e atipamezol — podem necessitar da administração repetida (conforme a necessidade) possivelmente a cada 4-8 h, porque a meia-vida nos cães é curta e a meia-vida de eliminação do amitraz é mais prolongada.
- Não usar a atropina para reverter a bradicardia; o uso é contraindicado por causa da potencialização da estase GI.

CONTRAINDICAÇÕES/INTERAÇÕES POSSÍVEIS
Ioimbina e atipamezol — a administração excessiva pode resultar em apreensão, estimulação do SNC e, raramente, crises convulsivas.

ACOMPANHAMENTO
- Temperatura corporal, pressão arterial, glicose sérica e frequência cardíaca — são parâmetros importantes.
- Observação estrita quanto à recidiva dos sinais clínicos — necessária por 24-72 h.
- Ioimbina e atipamezol — exigem a repetição da dose em casos graves, pois os efeitos de reversão diminuem antes da passagem dos fragmentos da

---
** N. T.: Segundo a farmacopeia dos Estados Unidos.

TOXICOSE POR AMITRAZ

coleira pelas fezes ou antes da eliminação do amitraz do corpo.

• Não se esperam efeitos adversos em longo prazo.

DIVERSOS

Os animais idosos, doentes ou debilitados podem levar mais tempo para se recuperar por completo.

ABREVIATURA(S)

• GI = gastrintestinal.

• ISRS = inibidor seletivo de recaptação da serotonina.

• SNC = sistema nervoso central.

RECURSOS DA INTERNET

http://www.aspcapro.org/animal-poison-control-center-articles.php.

Sugestões de Leitura

Grossman MR. Amitraz toxicosis associated with ingestion of an acaricide collar in a dog. JAVMA 1993, 203:55-57.

Hugnet C, Buronfosse F, Pineau X, et al. Toxicity and kinetics of amitraz in dogs. Am J Vet Res 1996, 57:1506-1510.

Autor Steven R. Hansen
Consultor Editorial Gary D. Osweiler

TOXICOSE POR ANFETAMINA

CONSIDERAÇÕES GERAIS

DEFINIÇÃO
Toxicose gastrintestinal, neurológica, neuromuscular e cardíaca agudas como resultado do consumo excessivo de anfetamina ou algum derivado.

FISIOPATOLOGIA
• A anfetamina e seus derivados pertencem à classe de estimulantes do SNC feniletilaminas. Várias substituições da estrutura básica da feniletilamina são responsáveis por muitos compostos farmacêuticos e ilícitos encontrados hoje em dia.
• A anfetamina é um agente simpaticomimético relacionado com a norepinefrina em termos estruturais.
• Ação central — estimula os centros corticais, incluindo o córtex cerebral, o centro respiratório medular e os sistemas ativadores reticulares.
• Ação periférica — estimula diretamente os α e β-receptores e também estimula a liberação de norepinefrina das reservas em terminações nervosas adrenérgicas.
• A anfetamina pode diminuir a velocidade de metabolismo das catecolaminas por inibição da monoamina oxidase.
• As anfetaminas são bem-absorvidas por via oral e atingem níveis plasmáticos de pico em 1-3 horas.
• Tanto a meia-vida, que varia de 7-34 horas, como a velocidade de excreção de anfetamina inalterada na urina, são dependentes do pH urinário, sendo que meias-vidas mais curtas estão associadas à urina mais ácida.
• A dose letal média (DL_{50}) oral do sulfato de anfetamina em cães é de 20-27 mg/kg e para o sulfato de metanfetamina, 9-11 mg/kg.
• Os sinais clínicos podem ser observados em doses abaixo de 1 mg/kg.
• A anfetamina e seus derivados são utilizados em seres humanos para tratar TDA/TDAH, narcolepsia e obesidade.
• O uso ilícito de anfetaminas em seres humanos também é preponderante.

SISTEMA(S) ACOMETIDO(S)
• Cardiovascular — a estimulação é mais comum: taquicardia e hipertensão.
• Gastrintestinal — anorexia, vômito, diarreia.
• Nervoso — a estimulação é mais comum; é rara a ocorrência de depressão.
• Neuromuscular — estimulação: tremores musculares e crises convulsivas.
• Oftálmico — midríase.
• Respiratório — estimulação: taquipneia.

GENÉTICA
N/D.

INCIDÊNCIA/PREVALÊNCIA
N/D.

DISTRIBUIÇÃO GEOGRÁFICA
N/D.

IDENTIFICAÇÃO
Espécies
Cães e gatos, embora seja mais prevalente em cães; outras espécies.
Raça(s) Predominante(s)
N/D.
Idade Média e Faixa Etária
N/D.
Sexo Predominante
N/D.

SINAIS CLÍNICOS
Achados Anamnésicos
• Comportamento anormal — geralmente hiperatividade, ansiedade ou estimulação, anorexia, batimento cardíaco rápido, respiração ofegante; indícios ou comprovação de exposição pelo proprietário ou cuidador.
• O início dos sinais clínicos tipicamente começa dentro de 30 minutos a 6 horas após a ingestão.

Achados do Exame Físico
• Nervoso — hiperatividade, agitação, inquietação, balanço cefálico, estimulação, andar em círculo, vocalização, desorientação, hiperestesia, ataxia, letargia ou depressão (menos comum).
• Cardiovascular — taquicardia ou bradicardia (menos comum, podendo ser reflexa), hipertensão.
• Neuromuscular — fasciculação ou tremores musculares, crises convulsivas.
• Gastrintestinal — vômito, diarreia, anorexia, sialorreia.
• Respiratório — taquipneia.
• Oftálmico — midríase com resposta pupilar à luz possivelmente baixa ou ausente.
• Outros — hipertermia.

CAUSAS
Ingestão ou administração acidental, intoxicação maliciosa.

FATORES DE RISCO
Lares com crianças ou adultos que atualmente tomam anfetamina ou algum derivado receitado ou ilícito.

DIAGNÓSTICO

DIAGNÓSTICO DIFERENCIAL
• Estricnina.
• Inseticidas organoclorados.
• Metilxantina.
• 4-aminopiridina.
• Metaldeído.
• Fenilpropanolamina.
• Albuterol.
• Nicotina.
• Micotoxinas tremorgênicas.
• Hipernatremia.
• Pseudoefedrina, fenilefrina.
• 5-fluoruracila.
• Ma huang, guaraná ou efedra.

HEMOGRAMA/BIOQUÍMICA/URINÁLISE
• Hemograma — coagulopatia intravascular disseminada secundária à hipertermia grave (rara).
• Bioquímica —
• Azotemia: pré-renal — secundária à desidratação; renal — secundária à rabdomiólise e mioglobinúria (rara).
• Elevação das enzimas hepáticas — secundária a crises convulsivas e/ou hipertermia (rara).
• Hipoglicemia.
• Urinálise — evidência de mioglobinúria, densidade urinária (alta — azotemia pré-renal; isostenúria — insuficiência renal).

OUTROS TESTES LABORATORIAIS
• Eletrólitos — desequilíbrios secundários a sinais gastrintestinais.
• Estado acidobásico — pode ocorrer acidose.
• Triagem de medicamentos de venda livre na urina — ficar atento para falso-positivos ou negativos. Verificar o manual do usuário em busca de mais informações.
• As anfetaminas estão presentes no sangue, na urina e na saliva; verificar junto ao laboratório diagnóstico veterinário local ou hospital humano quanto à disponibilidade e envio de amostra adequada.

DIAGNÓSTICO POR IMAGEM
N/D.

MÉTODOS DIAGNÓSTICOS
• Eletrocardiograma em busca da presença de qualquer taquiarritmia ou, menos comumente, bradiarritmia.
• Pressão arterial — identificação de hipertensão.

ACHADOS PATOLÓGICOS
À necropsia, a presença de anfetaminas pode ser encontrada no conteúdo gástrico, urina, plasma, fígado, rim ou músculo.

TRATAMENTO

CUIDADO(S) DE SAÚDE ADEQUADO(S)
A maioria dos casos necessita de tratamento emergencial do paciente em unidade de terapia intensiva.

CUIDADO(S) DE ENFERMAGEM
• Fluidoterapia intravenosa para corrigir desidratação e desequilíbrios eletrolíticos, bem como para ajudar a manter a função renal e promover a excreção de anfetaminas. Utilizar a pressão arterial para ajudar a orientar a velocidade de administração do fluido.
• Fluidos intravenosos frios, ventiladores, banhos de água fria para hipertermia.

ATIVIDADE
Minimizar a atividade e os estímulos.

DIETA
Suspender a alimentação em caso de acometimento moderado a grave. Fornecer dietas brandas por alguns dias após a exposição caso se observem sinais gastrintestinais significativos.

ORIENTAÇÃO AO PROPRIETÁRIO
Em caso de exposição, o proprietário deve imediatamente entrar em contato com o veterinário local ou centro de intoxicação veterinária.

CONSIDERAÇÕES CIRÚRGICAS
N/D.

MEDICAÇÕES

MEDICAMENTO(S) DE ESCOLHA
Descontaminação
• Induzir êmese — em caso de exposição recente e se o animal doméstico ainda não estiver sintomático.
• Apomorfina — 0,04 mg/kg IV, subconjuntival.
• Peróxido de hidrogênio a 3% - 2,2 mL/kg, dose máxima 45 mL.
• Lavagem gástrica em caso de ingestão extremamente volumosa ou se o paciente já estiver sintomático.
• Carvão ativado com algum catártico.

Toxicose por Anfetamina

Sinais neurológicos (SNC) de Estimulação
- Acepromazina — 0,05-1,0 mg/kg IV ou IM.
- Clorpromazina — 10-18 mg/kg IV.
- Ciproeptadina (antagonista serotoninérgico): cães, 1,1 mg/kg por via oral ou retal; gatos, 2-4 mg/gato.

Sinais Cardiovasculares
- Taquiarritmia — β-bloqueadores, como propranolol 0,02-0,04 mg/kg IV ou metoprolol.
- Contrações ventriculares prematuras — lidocaína: cães a 2-4 mg/kg IV (até, no máximo, 8 mg/kg por um período de 10 minutos). Gatos — iniciar com 0,1-0,4 mg/kg e aumentar com cuidado para 0,25-0,75 mg/kg IV lentamente se não houver resposta. De acordo com relatos, os gatos são muito sensíveis à lidocaína; portanto, é necessária a monitorização rigorosa se esse medicamento for utilizado.

Promover a Eliminação
Ácido ascórbico ou cloreto de amônio — para acidificação urinária a fim de promover a eliminação da anfetamina; entretanto, utilizar apenas se a mensuração do estado acidobásico for possível.

CONTRAINDICAÇÕES
- Embora o diazepam tenha sido utilizado com êxito para tratar as exposições à anfetamina, há evidências de que os benzodiazepínicos possam intensificar os sinais neurológicos.
- Acidificação urinária se a monitorização do estado acidobásico não for possível ou na presença de mioglobinúria.
- Indução de êmese em um paciente sintomático.

PRECAUÇÕES
N/D.

INTERAÇÕES POSSÍVEIS
- As anfetaminas inibem o metabolismo de bloqueadores adrenérgicos (doxazosina, fenoxibenzamina, prazosina, terazosina), fenobarbital e fenitoína.
- As anfetaminas potencializam o metabolismo de anticoagulantes cumarínicos, inibidores da monoamina oxidase, analgésicos opioides e antidepressivos tricíclicos.

MEDICAMENTO(S) ALTERNATIVO(S)
Fenobarbital, pentobarbital e propofol para sinais de estimulação do SNC.

ACOMPANHAMENTO

MONITORIZAÇÃO DO PACIENTE
Monitorizar no hospital até a resolução dos sinais clínicos.
Se gravemente acometido, monitorizar os valores hepáticos e renais a cada 24 horas por 72 horas ou até a resolução.

PREVENÇÃO
Todos os medicamentos e drogas ilícitas sempre devem ser mantidos fora do alcance dos animais domésticos.

COMPLICAÇÕES POSSÍVEIS
Insuficiência renal aguda secundária à mioglobinúria ou CID (rara).

EVOLUÇÃO ESPERADA E PROGNÓSTICO
- A evolução esperada dos sinais clínicos é de 12-72 horas, dependendo da dose, da eficácia de descontaminação e tratamento, bem como da taxa de eliminação.
- Prognóstico — a maioria dos pacientes tem prognóstico bom com cuidados veterinários imediatos e adequados. Crises convulsivas ou hipertermia grave podem ser um indicador prognóstico mau.

DIVERSOS

DISTÚRBIOS ASSOCIADOS
N/D.

FATORES RELACIONADOS COM A IDADE
N/D.

POTENCIAL ZOONÓTICO
Animais de estimação expostos a produtos residuais de seres humanos que tomam anfetaminas ou derivados podem ficar sintomáticos.

GESTAÇÃO/FERTILIDADE/REPRODUÇÃO
Sabe-se que as anfetaminas são teratogênicas em seres humanos. Foi descoberto que esses medicamentos atravessam a placenta em animais e também podem ser encontrados no leite.

SINÔNIMOS
- Nomes comerciais comuns de medicamentos de anfetamina e seus ingredientes ativos: Adderall® (anfetamina e dextroanfetamina); Ritalin®, Metadate®, Concerta® (metilfenidato); Daytrana® (emplastro transdérmico de metilfenidato); Focalin® (dexmetilfenidato); Vyvanse® (lisdexanfetamina), Cylert® (pemolina), Adipex-P® (fentermina), Dexedrine® (dextroanfetamina).
- Nomes de rua para drogas ilícitas à base de anfetamina: *ice* (gelo), *glass* (cristal), *crank* (manivela), *speed* (velocidade), *upper* (estimulante), êxtase, *meth* (metanfetamina) e muitos outros.

VER TAMBÉM
- Antidepressivos — Toxicose por Inibidores Seletivos de Recaptação da Serotonina (ISRS).
- Antidepressivos — Toxicose por Antidepressivos Tricíclicos (ATC).
- Toxicose por Pseudoefedrina.
- Envenenamento pela Estricnina.

ABREVIATURAS
- CID = coagulação intravascular disseminada.
- SNC = sistema nervoso central.
- TDA = transtorno do déficit de atenção.
- TDAH = transtorno do déficit de atenção com hiperatividade.

RECURSOS DA INTERNET
http://www.aspcapro.org/animal-poison-control-center-articles.php

Sugestões de Leitura
Cudia SP, Poppenga RH, Birdsall WJ. Pemoline toxicosis in a dog. JAVMA 1998, 212(1):74-76.
Mckinney PE, Palmer RB. Amphetamines and derivatives. In: Brent J, et al., eds., Critical Care Toxicology. Philadelphia: Elsevier, 2005, pp. 761-775.
Teitler JB. Evaluation of a human on-site urine multi drug test for emergency use with dogs. JAAHA 2009, 45(2):59-66.
Volmer PA. "Recreational" drugs. In: Peterson ME, Talcott PA, eds., Small Animal Toxicology. St. Louis: Elsevier, 2006, pp. 276-280.
Volmer PA. Human drugs of abuse. In: Bonagua JD, Twedt DC, eds., Current Veterinary Therapy XIV. St. Louis: Elsevier, 2009, pp. 144-145.

Autor Kirsten E. Waratuke
Consultor Editorial Gary D. Osweiler

Toxicose por Benzodiazepínicos e Soníferos

CONSIDERAÇÕES GERAIS

DEFINIÇÃO
• Toxicose causada pela ingestão de soníferos ou ansiolíticos comumente utilizados em medicina humana e veterinária.
• Medicamentos da classe dos benzodiazepínicos — incluem alprazolam (Xanax®), clonazepam (Klonopin®), diazepam (Valium®), lorazepam (Ativan®), e midazolam (Versed®).
• Classe das imidazopiridinas — incluem zaleplona (Sonata®) e zolpidem (Ambien®).

FISIOPATOLOGIA
• Os benzodiazepínicos e as imidazopiridinas ligam-se a receptores próximos ao receptor GABA/canal de cloreto nos neurônios; tais medicamentos potencializam o efeito do GABA, o que aumenta a abertura do canal de cloreto, levando à hiperpolarização dos nervos e à diminuição da excitação.
• As imidazopiridinas ligam-se próximos ao subgrupo de receptores responsável pela sedação, enquanto os benzodiazepínicos se ligam a todos os subgrupos de receptores e, dessa forma, não só mediam a sedação, mas também têm propriedades anticonvulsivantes e ansiolíticas.
• Podem ocorrer reações paradoxais; em relação ao diazepam, tais reações são tipicamente descritas como excitação, irritabilidade e comportamento aberrante em gatos e excitação em cães, cujo efeito esperado é o controle das crises convulsivas ou a sedação.
• Ambas as classes de medicamentos são bem-absorvidas por via oral e possuem rápido início de ação, frequentemente menos de 30 minutos.
• A duração de ação depende do medicamento e pode durar de horas a dias.
• Ambas as classes apresentam amplas margens de segurança; as exposições letais são raras se um único agente estiver envolvido.
• Benzodiazepínicos — os sinais podem ser observados com doses terapêuticas; no entanto, os medicamentos têm uma ampla margem de segurança, com a dose letal mínima sendo aproximadamente 1.000 vezes a dose terapêutica. Os gatos podem desenvolver insuficiência hepática idiopática com dosagem oral crônica de diazepam e clonazepam.
• Zaleplona — com base em uma revisão da base de dados da Antox da ASPCA/APCC: em cães, doses >0,11 mg/kg foram associadas a inquietação e hiperatividade; em gatos, doses >1,25 mg/kg provocaram reações paradoxais.
• Zolpidem — com base em uma revisão da base de dados da Antox da ASPCA/APCC: em cães, dosagens >0,2 mg/kg podem causar sedação leve e ataxia; doses >0,6 mg/kg podem causar reações paradoxais. Em gatos, foram observados sinais de reações paradoxais com dose de 0,34 mg/kg ou maior.

SISTEMA(S) ACOMETIDO(S)
• Gastrintestinal — vômito.
• Hepático — necrose e insuficiência agudas em gatos sob diazepam ou clonazepam.
• Nervoso — depressão do SNC e/ou reações paradoxais, ataxia, coma.
• Respiratório — depressão.

GENÉTICA
N/D.

INCIDÊNCIA/PREVALÊNCIA
A exposição é comum por serem medicamentos comumente prescritos.

DISTRIBUIÇÃO GEOGRÁFICA
Nenhuma.

IDENTIFICAÇÃO
Espécies
Cães e gatos — toxicidade aguda; gatos — possível insuficiência hepática idiopática com dosagem oral crônica de diazepam ou clonazepam.

Raça(s) Predominante(s)
Nenhuma.

Idade Média e Faixa Etária
Nenhuma.

Sexo Predominante
Nenhum.

SINAIS CLÍNICOS
Comentários Gerais
• Os benzodiazepínicos podem causar sedação com praticamente qualquer exposição (mesmo com doses terapêuticas).
• As imidazopiridinas provocam sedação com baixas doses, mas a probabilidade de reação paradoxal aumenta com doses crescentes, especialmente em cães.

Achados Anamnésicos
• Evidência de ingestão acidental do medicamento.
• Uso terapêutico do medicamento.
• Letargia.
• Ataxia.
• Sedação.
• Agitação.
• Achados do Exame Físico
• Depressão.
• Ataxia.
• Sedação.
• Hipotermia.
• Agitação.
• Hipertermia (secundária à agitação).
• Taquicardia.
• Icterícia (em gatos com insuficiência hepática idiopática).

CAUSAS
Exposição acidental, administração inadequada, ou uso terapêutico.

FATORES DE RISCO
• Animais mais jovens e mais idosos.
• Animais com distúrbios preexistentes.

DIAGNÓSTICO

DIAGNÓSTICO DIFERENCIAL
• Depressão do SNC — barbitúricos, ivermectina, etileno glicol, alcoóis (p. ex., etanol, metanol), maconha, opioides e antidepressivos (baixas doses).
• Reações paradoxais — anfetaminas, pseudoefedrina, metilxantinas, cocaína, fenilpropanolamina e síndrome serotoninérgica.

HEMOGRAMA/BIOQUÍMICA/URINÁLISE
• Não se esperam quaisquer anormalidades em dosagens excessivas agudas.
• Em gatos com insuficiência hepática idiopática, observam-se níveis elevados das enzimas hepáticas e da bilirrubina.

OUTROS TESTES LABORATORIAIS
• Os benzodiazepínicos podem ser detectados no sangue, na urina e no fígado; podem ser usados kits de triagem de medicamentos de venda livre para confirmar a exposição.
• As imidazopiridinas podem ser detectadas em líquidos e tecidos, mas tais ensaios não são facilmente disponíveis.

DIAGNÓSTICO POR IMAGEM
N/D.

MÉTODOS DIAGNÓSTICOS
N/D.

ACHADOS PATOLÓGICOS
Não se esperam alterações macroscópicas ou histológicas.

TRATAMENTO

CUIDADO(S) DE SAÚDE ADEQUADO(S)
• Tratamento ambulatorial — a maioria dos animais levemente acometidos pode ser tratada em casa com confinamento (para evitar lesões por quedas) e medidas para minimizar a estimulação.
• Tratamento hospitalar — para os animais que estão em coma ou exibem reações paradoxais.

CUIDADO(S) DE ENFERMAGEM
• Fluidos intravenosos.
• Monitorizar e controlar a temperatura corporal.
• Fornecer uma boa cama para os pacientes em decúbito, mudando-os de posição com frequência.
• Minimizar a estimulação sensorial, sobretudo em caso de reações paradoxais.

ATIVIDADE
Restringir a atividade física até a recuperação do animal para evitar a ocorrência de lesões.

DIETA
Os gatos com insuficiência hepática podem necessitar de alimentação forçada ou com tubo para provisão dos cuidados de suporte.

ORIENTAÇÃO AO PROPRIETÁRIO
• Conscientizar todos os proprietários sobre o armazenamento adequado de todos os medicamentos.
• Na prescrição de diazepam ou clonazepam aos gatos, fazer com que o proprietário monitorize seu animal de perto durante a primeira semana.

CONSIDERAÇÕES CIRÚRGICAS
N/D.

MEDICAÇÕES

MEDICAMENTO(S) DE ESCOLHA
• Acepromazina 0,025-0,05 mg/kg IV/IM, conforme a necessidade, para controlar as reações paradoxais.
• Ciproeptadina 1,1 mg/kg VO ou por via retal para cães; 2-4 mg/gato para controle das reações paradoxais.
• Flumazenil — um agente de reversão de benzodiazepínicos — 0,01 mg/kg IV a cada 1-2 h conforme a necessidade.

Toxicose por Benzodiazepínicos e Soníferos

• Pode ser usado para reverter tanto a sedação excessiva como a reação paradoxal.
• Contudo, o flumazenil pode causar crises convulsivas; por essa razão, o uso desse medicamento costuma ficar restrito a casos potencialmente letais.

CONTRAINDICAÇÕES
Não administrar outros benzodiazepínicos para controlar as reações paradoxais.

PRECAUÇÕES
N/D.

INTERAÇÕES POSSÍVEIS
Cuidado ao utilizar outros medicamentos depressivos (p. ex., barbitúricos, fenotiazinas), pois os benzodiazepínicos e soníferos podem potencializar os efeitos depressores desses agentes.

MEDICAMENTO(S) ALTERNATIVO(S)
N/D.

ACOMPANHAMENTO

MONITORIZAÇÃO DO PACIENTE
Temperatura, pulso e respiração, pressão arterial, esforço respiratório.

PREVENÇÃO
Manter os medicamentos fora do alcance de cães e gatos.

COMPLICAÇÕES POSSÍVEIS
Não se esperam complicações a longo prazo.

EVOLUÇÃO ESPERADA E PROGNÓSTICO
• O prognóstico para dosagens excessivas agudas é excelente com cuidados sintomáticos.
• O prognóstico para insuficiência hepática aguda em gatos sob diazepam é mau.

DIVERSOS

DISTÚRBIOS ASSOCIADOS
N/D.

FATORES RELACIONADOS COM A IDADE
• Animais jovens e aqueles com hepatopatia preexistente podem ter sinais prolongados em virtude da capacidade reduzida de eliminação dos medicamentos.
• Animais mais jovens podem ser mais propensos a reações paradoxais.

POTENCIAL ZOONÓTICO
Nenhum.

GESTAÇÃO/FERTILIDADE/REPRODUÇÃO
Os benzodiazepínicos são considerados teratogênicos.

VER TAMBÉM
• Toxicose por Anfetamina.
• Antidepressivos — Toxicose por Inibidores Seletivos de Recaptação da Serotonina.
• Antidepressivos — Toxicose por Antidepressivos Tricíclicos.
• Toxicose por Etanol.
• Intoxicação pelo Etileno Glicol.
• Toxicidade da Ivermectina.

ABREVIATURAS
• ASPCA/APCC = American Society for the Prevention of Cruelty to Animals/Animal Poison Control Center.
• GABA = ácido gama-aminobutírico.
• SNC = sistema nervoso central.

RECURSOS DA INTERNET
http://www.aspcapro.org/animal-poison-control.php.

Sugestões de Leitura
Center SA, Elston TH, Rowland PH, et al. Fulminant hepatic failure associated with oral administration of diazepam in 11 cats. JAVMA 1996, 209(3):618-625.
Plumb DC. Veterinary Drug Handbook, 6th ed. Ames, IA: Blackwell, 2008.

Autor Eric K. Dunayer
Consultor Editorial Gary D. Osweiler

Toxicose por Beta-2 Agonistas Inalatórios

CONSIDERAÇÕES GERAIS

REVISÃO
- A toxicose por beta-2 agonistas inalatórios ocorre quando os cães mastigam e perfuram inaladores pressurizados contendo albuterol (salbutamol) ou outros beta-agonistas utilizados para fins terapêuticos em caso de broncodilatação.
- A perda de seletividade beta-2 com a dosagem excessiva resulta em estimulação beta-1 (taquicardia).
- O aumento das catecolaminas soma-se à estimulação neurológica e cardiovascular, podendo causar translocação intracelular significativa de potássio e fósforo.
- Os propulsores de clorofluorocarbono podem sensibilizar o miocárdio a contribuir para o potencial de arritmias.

SISTEMA(S) ACOMETIDO(S)
- Comportamental — hiperatividade, apreensão, nervosismo, inquietação.
- Cardiovascular — taquicardia sinusal, outras arritmias.
- Endócrino/metabólico — hipocalemia, hipofosfatemia.
- Gastrintestinal — vômito brando.
- Musculosquelético — tremores.
- Nervoso — ansiedade, apreensão em princípio, depressão com depleção de catecolaminas.
- Neuromuscular — tremores.
- Respiratório — taquipneia.

IDENTIFICAÇÃO
- A toxicose é tipicamente observada em cães em virtude de sua predileção por alimentação inadequada ou imprudência alimentar.
- Mais comum em filhotes de cães.

SINAIS CLÍNICOS
- Taquicardia e outras arritmias.
- Letargia e depressão.
- Hiperatividade, apreensão, nervosismo, inquietação.
- Taquipneia.
- Vômito.
- Tremores.

CAUSAS E FATORES DE RISCO
- Perfuração de inaladores contendo beta-2 agonistas.
- Os animais de estimação propensos à alimentação inadequada com acesso a inaladores são suscetíveis.

DIAGNÓSTICO

DIAGNÓSTICO DIFERENCIAL
- Medicamentos à base de anfetaminas, como aqueles utilizados para TDAH (p. ex., Adderall®, Concerta®, Focalin®, Metadate®, Ritalin®, Strattera®, Vyvanse®).
- Simpaticomiméticos (p. ex., fenilpropanolamina, pseudoefedrina, fenilefrina, efedrina).
- Metilxantinas (p. ex., cafeína, teobromina).
- Metaldeído.

HEMOGRAMA/BIOQUÍMICA/URINÁLISE
- Hipocalemia.
- Hipofosfatemia.

OUTROS TESTES LABORATORIAIS
N/D.

DIAGNÓSTICO POR IMAGEM
N/D.

MÉTODOS DIAGNÓSTICOS
ECG para confirmar e monitorizar a presença de taquiarritmias.

ACHADOS PATOLÓGICOS
N/D.

TRATAMENTO

- Tratamento hospitalar — iniciar a administração de medicamentos e os cuidados de emergência o mais rápido possível após a exposição.
- Há necessidade de cuidados de enfermagem — suporte de fluido.
- Para alteração da atividade — repouso em gaiola e ambiente tranquilo.
- Nada por via oral na presença de vômito.
- Discutir com o proprietário o momento da apresentação do animal em relação à exposição; nos pacientes com manifestação tardia e prolongada, a estimulação neurológica (SNC) e cardiovascular não tratada pode representar um maior risco de arritmias mais graves e recuperação mais lenta em virtude da depleção de catecolaminas.
- Não há considerações anestésico-cirúrgicas.

MEDICAÇÕES

MEDICAMENTO(S)
- Diazepam para ansiedade, nervosismo, tremores: 0,5 mg/kg IV ou 1 mg/kg por via retal, repetir conforme a necessidade.
- Propranolol para taquicardia, hipocalemia: Cães, 0,02-0,06 mg/kg IV até fazer efeito.
- Suplementação de cloreto de potássio: Até 0,5 mEq de potássio/kg/h IV no máximo, com base no grau de déficit de potássio e conforme a necessidade.
- Fosfato de potássio (raramente necessário para tratar a hipofosfatemia): 0,01-0,03 mM/kg/h IV até fazer efeito se o fósforo sérico estiver abaixo de 1 mg/dL.
- Lidocaína para arritmias ventriculares: Cães, 2-4 mg/kg IV (até uma dose máxima de 8 mg/kg por um período de 10 minutos). Gatos, 0,25-0,75 mg/kg IV lentamente.

CONTRAINDICAÇÕES/INTERAÇÕES POSSÍVEIS
N/D.

ACOMPANHAMENTO

MONITORIZAÇÃO DO PACIENTE
- Eletrólitos (potássio, fósforo) a cada 12 h até a recuperação completa.
- NOTA: há um potencial de hipercalemia de rebote durante a recuperação com suplementação rigorosa.
- Eletrocardiografia.
- Avaliação do estado mental.

PREVENÇÃO
Ter cuidado em relação ao acesso a inaladores para cães.

COMPLICAÇÕES POSSÍVEIS
- Raramente fatal. A taquicardia sinusal é de longe o achado mais comum, mas uma taquicardia grave persistente pode resultar em hipoxia do miocárdio e arritmias mais graves.
- A depleção de catecolaminas pode resultar em um período de fraqueza e depressão assim que os efeitos de estimulação declinarem.
- A cardiopatia preexistente pode aumentar o potencial de arritmias potencialmente letais ou outras sequelas cardíacas.

EVOLUÇÃO ESPERADA E PROGNÓSTICO
Prognóstico excelente com tratamento imediato e adequado em paciente saudável sob outros aspectos.

DIVERSOS

DISTÚRBIOS ASSOCIADOS
Nenhum.

FATORES RELACIONADOS COM A IDADE
Nenhum.

POTENCIAL ZOONÓTICO
Nenhum.

GESTAÇÃO/FERTILIDADE/REPRODUÇÃO
- Como o albuterol atravessa a placenta, espera-se que os efeitos da dosagem excessiva sejam semelhantes para o feto. Hipoxia com comprometimento cardíaco na cadela pode representar um maior risco para os fetos.
- Como a toxicose supostamente se resolve em até 24 horas com nenhum efeito a longo prazo, não há efeitos adversos esperados em relação à fertilidade.

ABREVIATURAS
- ECG = eletrocardiograma.
- SNC = sistema nervoso central.
- TDAH = transtorno de déficit de atenção com hiperatividade.

RECURSOS DA INTERNET
Mensching D, Volmer PA. Breathe with Ease when Managing Beta-2 Agonist Inhaler Toxicoses in Dogs. Veterinary Medicine, junho de 2007, 369-373. PDF disponível online: http://www.aspcapro.org/animal-poison-control/veterinary-resources/animal-poison-control-center.html.

Sugestões de Leitura
Rosendale M. Bronchodilators. In: Plumlee KH, ed., Clinical Veterinary Toxicology. St. Louis: Mosby/Elsevier, 2004, pp. 305-307.

Autor Donna Mensching
Consultor Editorial Gary D. Osweiler

Toxicose por Chocolate

CONSIDERAÇÕES GERAIS

DEFINIÇÃO
Toxicose gastrentérica, neurológica e cardíaca aguda, causada pela ingestão excessiva de alcaloides metilxantínicos, presentes no chocolate. A teobromina constitui a maior fração de metilxantinas em produtos de chocolate e adubo de grãos de cacau. Uma concentração mais baixa de cafeína também está presente.

FISIOPATOLOGIA
- As metilxantinas são variavelmente absorvidas (<1 h para cafeína a 10 h para teobromina) e, após o metabolismo pelo fígado, podem ser excretadas na bile e reabsorvidas (ciclo entero-hepático).
- A meia-vida de excreção da teobromina é estimada em 17 h.
- Atravessa a placenta e a barreira hematoencefálica; pode ser reabsorvido por meio da parede da bexiga urinária.
- Inibição da fosfodiesterase — aumenta o AMPc, o que potencializa os efeitos das catecolaminas (aumenta sua liberação) e eleva o cálcio intracelular.
- As metilxantinas provocam vasoconstrição, aumento na força de contração do miocárdio e dos músculos esqueléticos, estimulação do SNC e crises convulsivas, broncodilatação e taquicardia.
- Dosagens tóxicas para alcaloides metilxantínicos:
- Teobromina
  - DL_{50} (cão) 250-500 mg/kg.
  - DL_{50} (gato) 200 mg/kg.
- Cafeína
  - DL_{50} (cão) 140 mg/kg.
  - DL_{50} (gato) 80-150 mg/kg.
- Advertência: 1/10 da DL_{50} ainda pode ser uma dose letal para alguns animais.

SISTEMA(S) ACOMETIDO(S)
- Cardiovascular — aumento na contratilidade miocárdica e taquiarritmias; taquicardia, hipertensão, contrações ventriculares prematuras.
- Gastrintestinal — início precoce de vômito e diarreia; podem ser mediados pelo SNC; podem resultar até mesmo da administração parenteral de alcaloides metilxantínicos.
- Metabólico — hipocalemia, hipertermia.
- Nervoso — estimulação; intensificação no estado de alerta e na hiperatividade reflexa; tremores; crises convulsivas tônico-clônicas.
- Renal/Urológico — poliúria, polidipsia.
- Respiratório — taquipneia, hipoxia, cianose, insuficiência respiratória.

INCIDÊNCIA/PREVALÊNCIA
- Cães — está entre as 20 intoxicações mais comuns descritas na literatura especializada recente, pelas clínicas de pequenos animais, bem como pelos Animal Poison Centers e Human Poison Control Centers (Centros Norte-americanos de Controle de Intoxicação em Animais e Seres Humanos).
- Mais comum em época de férias e feriados — fácil acesso a produtos com chocolate e doces.
- Comprimidos estimulantes contendo cafeína, até 200 mg/comprimido — fonte ocasional.

DISTRIBUIÇÃO GEOGRÁFICA
Cães urbanos e domésticos — podem exibir maior risco, em função da proximidade aos produtos à base de chocolate.

IDENTIFICAÇÃO
Espécies
- Os cães são mais frequentemente intoxicados com base em sua proximidade a produtos contendo metilxantina, capacidade em consumir grandes doses, hábitos alimentares indiscriminados, e meia-vida mais longa da teobromina em cães (meia-vida da teobromina de 17,5 h *versus* 4,5 h para cafeína).
- Os gatos raramente são acometidos.
- Outras espécies são provavelmente acometidas, mas têm acesso mais limitado ao chocolate; as cascas dos grãos de cacau podem ser uma fonte de intoxicação para cavalos e aves domésticas.

Raça(s) Predominante(s)
Cães de pequeno porte — podem estar sob maior risco, em virtude da quantidade de chocolate disponível em relação ao peso corporal.

Idade Média e Faixa Etária
- Filhotes caninos e cães jovens — maior probabilidade de ingestão de grandes quantidades de alimentos fora do habitual.
- Animais jovens são tipicamente mais comprometidos em virtude do metabolismo e da excreção.

SINAIS CLÍNICOS
Achados Anamnésicos
- Consumo recente confirmado de chocolate ou casca de cacau.
- Evidência de recipientes mastigados ou resquícios de embalagens de produtos de chocolate.
- Vômito e diarreia — com frequência, são os primeiros sinais descritos; surgem 2-4 h após a ingestão.
- Inquietação inicial e atividade acentuada ou nervosismo.
- Poliúria — pode decorrer da ação diurética.
- Hematúria ocasionalmente.
- Sinais avançados — rigidez; agitação; crises convulsivas; hiper-reflexia.

Achados do Exame Físico
- Sinais prodrômicos de vômito e diarreia, acompanhados por uma combinação de estimulação do SNC e taquicardia (frequentemente extrema).
- Hipertermia.
- Hiper-reflexia.
- Rigidez muscular.
- Crises convulsivas tônico-clônicas.
- Midríase.
- Taquipneia.
- Taquicardia.
- Hipotensão.
- Sinais avançados — indutores de insuficiência cardíaca, fraqueza, coma e óbito.
- Óbito — ocorre 12-48 h após a ingestão.

CAUSAS
- Geralmente algum tipo de chocolate processado (usado em doces e confeitaria) — contém concentrações elevadas de teobromina e cafeína.
- Dose letal mínima de cafeína e teobromina (cães) — 100-200 mg/kg.
- Potencialmente letal (cães).
- 5 g de chocolate de confeitaria fornece 20 mg de cafeína e 80 mg de teobromina (100 mg no total).
- Um cão de 20 kg pode ser intoxicado por 5 g/kg × 20 kg = 100 g de chocolate.
- O chocolate ao leite fornece apenas 2 mg de alcaloides por grama (50 g de chocolate/kg de peso corporal) ou quase 58 mg/kg, o que seria aproximadamente 1200 mg para um cão de 20 kg (quantidade improvável).
- Há relatos de intoxicação de cães pelo consumo de cascas de grãos de cacau utilizadas como adubo.

FATORES DE RISCO
- Chocolate — altamente palatável e atrativo; muitas vezes é de fácil acesso e encontra-se desprotegido nas casas e cozinhas.
- Alcaloides metilxantínicos — fácil e rapidamente absorvidos; apenas uma pequena quantidade fica ligada (20%) a proteínas plasmáticas.

DIAGNÓSTICO

DIAGNÓSTICO DIFERENCIAL
- Alcaloides convulsivantes ou excitatórios — estricnina; anfetamina; nicotina; 4-aminopiridina; cocaína; antidepressivos tricíclicos; síndrome serotoninérgica.
- Iscas de metaldeído para lesmas e caracóis.
- Intoxicação aguda por brometalina.
- Intoxicação por fosfeto de zinco.
- Pesticidas convulsivantes — organoclorados (p. ex., clordano, lindano) e piretrinas.
- Micotoxinas tremorgênicas — penitrem A; aflatrem; roquefortina.
- Medicamentos psicogênicos agudos — LSD; glória da manhã.
- Toxicose pelo fluoracetato (rara).
- Glicosídeos cardioativos — *Digitalis* spp.; *Nerium oleander*.
- Hipomagnesemia e hipocalcemia.

HEMOGRAMA/BIOQUÍMICA/URINÁLISE
- Hiper e hipoglicemia — ambas as anormalidades foram observadas e, portanto, não constituem um indicador confiável.
- Hipocalemia.
- Densidade urinária baixa e proteinúria — achados ocasionais.

OUTROS TESTES LABORATORIAIS
Ensaio de metilxantina
- Conteúdo gástrico, plasma e urina.
- Meia-vida de eliminação (cães) — 17,5 h (teobromina); a concentração plasmática ou sérica detectável deve persistir por 3-4 dias.
- Estável em amostras coletadas por 2 semanas.
- As concentrações de teobromina no soro de cães intoxicados podem variar de 100 a 300 mg/L.

MÉTODOS DIAGNÓSTICOS
ECG — revela taquicardia sinusal, contrações ventriculares prematuras e taquiarritmia ventricular.

ACHADOS PATOLÓGICOS
- Conteúdo gástrico ou intestinal — pode-se observar uma quantidade pequena ou grande de chocolate.
- Gastrenterite — achados inespecíficos.
- Tipicamente não há lesões microscópicas detectáveis ou distintas.
- Lesões renais microscópicas — descritas, mas inconsistentes; caracterizadas por degeneração hialina, picnose e cariorrexe, potencialmente por má perfusão renal.

TOXICOSE POR CHOCOLATE

Tabela 1.

Concentrações comparativas de cafeína e teobromina		
Fontes de cafeína	Quantidade (mg/g)	Quantidade (mg/ounces)*
Grãos de café	10-20	284-570
Café pingado	90-100 mg/xícara de 180 mL	15 mL
Refrigerantes à base de cola	60-90 mg/lata de 360 mL	5-8
Chocolate de confeitaria	Até 4	Até 112
Chocolate amargo	1,3	36
Chocolate ao leite	0,2	6
Cacau	Até 1,5	46
Cascas de grãos de cacau	5-8,5	142-240
Guaraná	30-50	850-1.400
Comprimidos estimulantes	200 mg/comprimido	—
Analgésicos de venda livre	60 mg/comprimido	—
Fontes de teobromina	Quantidade (mg/g)	Quantidade (mg/ounces)
Grãos de cacau	10-50	280-1.400
Chocolate de confeitaria	14-16	398-454
Chocolate ao leite	1,5-2	46-57
Cascas de grãos de cacau	5-9	142-256
Adubo de grãos de cacau	2-30	57-852
Cacau em pó	14-29	398-832

Para converter mg/g em mg/ounces, multiplique por 28,4 g/ounces.

TRATAMENTO

CUIDADO(S) DE SAÚDE ADEQUADO(S)
• Relatado(s) por telefone— tentar determinar o tipo e a quantidade de exposição; se isso não for possível, recomenda-se o encaminhamento ao hospital como um quadro de emergência toxicológica em potencial.
• Controlar as crises convulsivas.
• Desintoxicação (se as crises convulsivas estiverem controladas) com o uso de êmese inicialmente, lavagem gástrica e carvão ativado.
• Administrar carvão ativado diariamente por até 3 dias para diminuir o ciclo entero-hepático dos alcaloides. Em geral, apenas a primeira dose do carvão deve conter um catártico.
• Controlar a hipertermia.
• Tratar a taquicardia (ver a seção de "Medicamentos").
• Sondagem urinária ou eliminação frequente de urina para reduzir a reabsorção de metilxatinas pela bexiga urinária.
• Fornecer fluidoterapia IV para evitar desidratação, promover diurese, e evitar hipernatremia.

CUIDADO(S) DE ENFERMAGEM
Fluidoterapia — corrigir os distúrbios eletrolíticos causados por vômito, conforme a necessidade.

ATIVIDADE
Evitar o estresse e a agitação — podem precipitar a hiper-reflexia ou as crises convulsivas.

DIETA
• Paciente agudamente acometido — não fornecer alimentos. • Período de convalescença — dieta branda por vários dias para permitir a recuperação do quadro de gastrenterite.

ORIENTAÇÃO AO PROPRIETÁRIO
Alertar o proprietário quanto aos riscos da ingestão de chocolate.

CONSIDERAÇÕES CIRÚRGICAS
Raramente, forma-se uma massa ou concreção de chocolate que deve ser removida por meio cirúrgico.

MEDICAÇÕES

MEDICAMENTO(S) DE ESCOLHA
• Induzir a êmese — *apenas se o paciente não estiver convulsionando*; apomorfina (0,03 mg/kg IV); xarope de ipeca (1-2 mL/kg VO); peróxido de hidrogênio a 3% (1-3 mL/kg VO).
• Lavagem gástrica — realizada somente antes do início do vômito e de outros sinais clínicos em caso de ineficácia dos eméticos, controle das crises convulsivas e colocação de sonda endotraqueal.
• Assim que o vômito estiver controlado — carvão ativado (0,5-1,0 g/kg VO); adsorve os alcaloides remanescentes no trato gastrintestinal, repetido em intervalos de 3 a 6 h por 1-2 dias para evitar novo ciclo entero-hepático.
• Catártico osmótico — sulfato de sódio (0,25 g/kg VO) ou sorbitol a 70% a 1-3 mL/kg VO; promove a eliminação gastrintestinal do chocolate.
• Hiperatividade e crises convulsivas — controladas com diazepam (0,5 mg/kg IV a cada 10-20 min em até quatro vezes ou infusão IV a 0,5-1 mg/kg/h).
• Taquicardia ventricular (cães) — lidocaína (sem adrenalina), 1-2 mg/kg IV seguidos por 0,03-0,05 mg/kg/min por meio de gotejamento IV. A lidocaína NÃO É RECOMENDADA em gatos.
• Arritmias refratárias graves — metoprolol ou propranolol (0,02-0,06 mg/kg IV; não exceder a velocidade de 1 mg/min); prefere-se o metoprolol, embora ele possa ser de difícil obtenção; pode-se empregar a terapia por via oral assim que o paciente se encontrar estabilizado (metoprolol a 0,2-0,4 mg/kg VO a cada 12 h; propranolol a 0,2-1 mg/kg VO a cada 8 h); monitorizar o ECG e ficar atento quanto à ocorrência de hipotensão (uma sequela a esse tratamento).
• Em raros casos de bradicardia, utilizar atropina a 0,02-0,04 mg/kg IV, IM, ou SC.

CONTRAINDICAÇÕES
• Não utilizar a adrenalina simultaneamente com a lidocaína.
• Evitar a eritromicina e os corticosteroides, pois tais agentes diminuem a excreção das metilxantinas.
• Não usar a lidocaína em gatos acometidos.

PRECAUÇÕES
• Os efeitos podem persistir por mais tempo do que a vida efetiva dos agentes terapêuticos.
• Manter o paciente sob observação até que a administração do medicamento não seja mais necessária.
• Metilxantinas — atravessam a placenta; excretadas no leite.

MEDICAMENTO(S) ALTERNATIVO(S)
• Controle alternativo de hiper-reflexia e rigidez muscular pode ser obtido com metocarbamol (50-220 mg/kg IV lentamente).
• Em caso de resposta inadequada ao diazepam — considerar o emprego do fenobarbital (30 mg/kg IV, administrados em 5-10 min).
• Crises convulsivas refratárias — pentobarbital (3-15 mg/kg IV lentamente, conforme a necessidade).

ACOMPANHAMENTO

MONITORIZAÇÃO DO PACIENTE
• ECG — arritmias.
• Ficar atento à nefrose branda a moderada em pacientes convalescentes.

PREVENÇÃO
Avisar os proprietários sobre os riscos toxicológicos do chocolate.

COMPLICAÇÕES POSSÍVEIS
Animais prenhes ou lactentes — risco de teratogênese de recém-nascidos ou estimulação de neonatos lactentes.

EVOLUÇÃO ESPERADA E PROGNÓSTICO
• Evolução esperada — 12-36 h, dependendo da dosagem e da eficácia da desintoxicação e do tratamento.
• Pacientes tratados com êxito — costumam apresentar completa recuperação.

Toxicose por Chocolate

• Prognóstico — bom se a desintoxicação oral ocorrer dentro de 2-4 h após a ingestão; reservado em casos de sinais avançados de crises convulsivas e arritmias.

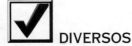

DIVERSOS

FATORES RELACIONADOS COM A IDADE
Os animais jovens são tipicamente mais comprometidos em virtude do metabolismo e da excreção.

POTENCIAL ZOONÓTICO
Embora não seja transmissível, os seres humanos e os cães podem ter acesso a fontes semelhantes.

GESTAÇÃO/FERTILIDADE/REPRODUÇÃO
Metilxantinas são teratogênicas em animais de laboratório.

VER TAMBÉM
• Antidepressivos — Toxicose por Inibidores Seletivos de Recaptação da Serotonina (ISRS).
• Antidepressivos — Toxicose por Antidepressivos Tricíclicos.
• Envenenamento (Intoxicação).
• Envenenamento pela Estricnina.
• Intoxicação pelo Metaldeído.

ABREVIATURAS
• ECG = eletrocardiograma.
• SNC = sistema nervoso central.

RECURSOS DA INTERNET
http://www.aspcapro.org/animal-poison-control.php.

Sugestões de Leitura
Albretsen JC. Methylxanthines. In: Plumlee K, ed., Veterinary Clinical Toxicology. St. Louis: Mosby, 2004, pp. 322-326.
Carson T. Methylxanthines. In: Peterson M, Talcott P, eds., Small Animal Toxicology. St. Louis: Saunders, 2006, pp. 845-852.
Drolet P, Arendt TD, Stowe CM. Cacao bean shell poisoning in 2 dogs. JAVMA 1984, 185:902-904.
Glauberg A, Blumenthal HP. Chocolate toxicosis in a dog. JAAHA 1983, 19:246-248.
Luiz JA, Heseltine J. Five common toxins ingested by dogs and cats. Compend Contin Educ Pract Vet 2008, 30:578-587.

Autor Gary D. Osweiler
Consultor Editorial Gary D. Osweiler

TOXICOSE POR METFORMINA

CONSIDERAÇÕES GERAIS

REVISÃO
- A metformina é um medicamento hipoglicemiante (biguanida) indicado para o tratamento de diabetes melito insulinoindependente (tipo 2) em seres humanos.
- O agente pode ser potencialmente útil no tratamento adjuvante de diabetes melito insulinoindependente em gatos; no entanto, o uso é controverso.
- A toxicidade causa sinais gastrintestinais e letargia.

IDENTIFICAÇÃO
- Cães e gatos.
- Não há predileções raciais, etárias ou sexuais.

SINAIS CLÍNICOS
Cães
- Sinal comum: vômito.
- Possíveis sinais: letargia, depressão, anorexia e hipotermia.

Gatos
- Sinal frequente: vômito.
- Possíveis sinais: letargia, diarreia e vocalização.

CAUSAS E FATORES DE RISCO
Ingestão de metformina em preparações compostas de um único ingrediente, bem como em combinação com outros agentes antidiabéticos.

DIAGNÓSTICO

DIAGNÓSTICO DIFERENCIAL
Outros irritantes do trato gastrintestinal.

HEMOGRAMA/BIOQUÍMICA/URINÁLISE
- Azotemia relatada em seres humanos em virtude de insuficiência renal aguda em casos de acidose láctica por biguanida; não relatada em toxicidades de animais.
- Não há relatos de hipoglicemia.

OUTROS TESTES LABORATORIAIS
- Gasometria arterial – a acidose láctica é rara, mas possível com grandes ingestões (um cão da raça Shih tzu que ingeriu 167,2 mg/kg de metformina desenvolveu acidose láctica, vômito e hipotermia. Além de não ter desenvolvido hipoglicemia, o cão se recuperou completamente com o tratamento).
- A cromatografia líquida de alto desempenho pode identificar a presença de metformina no plasma; os níveis do medicamento não são clinicamente úteis.

DIAGNÓSTICO POR IMAGEM
N/D.

MÉTODOS DIAGNÓSTICOS
N/D.

ACHADOS PATOLÓGICOS
N/D.

TRATAMENTO
- Induzir a êmese nas primeiras 2-3 horas de exposição.
- O carvão ativado deve ser considerado apenas em casos de exposição muito grande.
- Efetuar tratamento de suporte para os sinais gastrintestinais.
- Tratar a acidose láctica se presente.

MEDICAÇÕES

MEDICAMENTO(S)
- Metoclopramida 0,1-0,4 mg/kg VO, SC, ou IM a cada 6 h.
- Sucralfato 0,5-1 g VO a cada 8-12 h para cães e 0,25-0,5 g VO a cada 8-12 h para gatos.
- Famotidina 0,5 mg/kg VO, SC, ou IM a cada 12-24 h para cães e gatos.
- Ranitidina 0,5-2 mg/kg VO, SC, ou IM a cada 8-12 h para cães e 2,5 mg/kg IV a cada 12 h ou 3,5 mg/kg VO a cada 12 h para gatos.
- Omeprazol 0,5-1 mg/kg VO a cada 24 h para cães e 0,7 mg/kg VO a cada 24 h para gatos.
- Bicarbonato: se o bicarbonato sérico ou o CO_2 total não estiver disponível: 2-3 mEq/kg IV durante 30 minutos se o paciente tiver perfusão tecidual reduzida ou insuficiência renal e não tiver cetoacidose diabética. Deve ser utilizado de forma criteriosa.

CONTRAINDICAÇÕES/INTERAÇÕES POSSÍVEIS
- A administração concomitante de cimetidina pode reduzir a excreção urinária de metformina por competição pelos sistemas de transporte catiônico orgânico tubular renal.
- O fabricante afirma que outros agentes catiônicos que sofrem secreção tubular considerável (p. ex., amilorida, digoxina, morfina, procainamida, quinidina, quinina, ranitidina, triantereno, trimetoprima, e vancomicina) podem reduzir a excreção urinária de metformina.

ACOMPANHAMENTO

MONITORIZAÇÃO DO PACIENTE
N/D.

PREVENÇÃO
N/D.

COMPLICAÇÕES POSSÍVEIS
N/D.

EVOLUÇÃO ESPERADA E PROGNÓSTICO
Prognóstico bom se não ocorrer acidose láctica.

DIVERSOS

DISTÚRBIOS ASSOCIADOS
N/D.

FATORES RELACIONADOS COM A IDADE
N/D.

POTENCIAL ZOONÓTICO
N/D.

GESTAÇÃO/FERTILIDADE/REPRODUÇÃO
- Não há evidência de dano ao feto ou comprometimento da fertilidade durante estudos reprodutivos em ratos e coelhos submetidos a dosagens de 600 mg/kg de cloridrato de metformina 1 vez ao dia.
- Até o momento, não há estudos adequados e controlados feitos com o uso de cloridrato de metformina em gestantes.

VER TAMBÉM
Envenenamento (Intoxicação).

RECURSOS DA INTERNET
http://chem.sis.nlm.nih.gov/chemidplus/.
http://www.aspcapro.org/animal-poison-control.php.

Sugestões de Leitura

AHFS Drug Information. American Society of Health-System Pharmacists, 2008, pp. 3181-3194.

Animal Poison Control Center database (October 2001–October 2009). Jacqueline BH. Metformin overdose in dogs and cats. Toxicology Brief, April 2007, pp. 231-234.

Plumb DC. Veterinary Drug Handbook, 5th ed. Ames: Iowa State University Press, 2005, pp. 716-717.

Autor Hany Youssef
Consultor Editorial Gary D. Osweiler

Toxicose por Monóxido de Carbono

CONSIDERAÇÕES GERAIS

REVISÃO
• Monóxido de carbono — gás inodoro, incolor, não irritante, produzido pela combustão ineficaz de combustíveis carbonáceos. • As fontes comuns desse gás são incêndios, escapamentos de automóveis e vazamento de carvão, óleo ou gás natural/fornos de propano. • Absorvido no sangue, formando a carboxiemoglobina e reduzindo o oxigênio, o que causa hipoxia cerebral e cardíaca. • A concentração letal gira em torno de 1.000 ppm (0,1%). • A afinidade de CO pela hemoglobina é de aproximadamente 240 vezes a do oxigênio. • A carboxiemoglobina não é capaz de se ligar ao oxigênio e também diminui a capacidade de liberação de oxigênio pela hemoglobina remanescente por desviar a curva de oxiemoglobina para a esquerda. • O principal efeito consiste em hipoxia celular aguda, levando à morte. • Os sobreviventes podem sofrer necrose cardíaca e dano cerebral, resultantes da hipoxia intensa e prolongada.

IDENTIFICAÇÃO
• Cães e gatos são quase igualmente suscetíveis. • As exposições ao mau funcionamento de aquecedores no inverno podem afetar seres humanos e animais de estimação que convivem no mesmo espaço. • Outras áreas de alto risco são canis aquecidos que utilizam aquecedores não ventilados de gás ou querosene em instalações pouco ventiladas.

SINAIS CLÍNICOS
Achados Anamnésicos
• Exposição a escapamento de automóveis ou a vapores provenientes de aquecedores à base de monóxido de carbono. • O funcionamento de um motor em uma garagem fechada por 5 a 10 minutos pode produzir concentrações letais. • Incêndios em edifícios geram altas concentrações de CO que podem levar ao óbito.

Achados do Exame Físico
Exposição Aguda
• Sinais agudos evoluem dentro de minutos a horas. • Sonolência, letargia e fraqueza são sinais agudos precoces. • Taquicardia e taquipneia são achados físicos comuns. • Dispneia e crises convulsivas clônicas podem preceder depressão respiratória. • Surdez, incoordenação e coma sinalizam um desfecho fatal. • Diminuição na excitabilidade cardíaca, hipotensão, arritmia e acidose. • Pele e mucosas de coloração vermelho-cereja são sinais clássicos antes do óbito, mas nem sempre são aparentes.

Exposição crônica
• Exposição crônica pode causar náusea, vômito, acidose e tosse; pode mimetizar "gripe" ou doença infecciosa. • Baixa tolerância a exercícios. • Distúrbios da marcha, bem como dos reflexos posturais e proprioceptivos. • Pode ocorrer surdez de persistência variável em sobreviventes.

CAUSAS & FATORES DE RISCO
• Combustão incompleta dos combustíveis carbonáceos. • Má ventilação ou saídas de ventilação ou chaminés entupidas. • Gases provenientes da combustão automotiva em garagem fechada ou sistema defeituoso de combustão. • Sistemas defeituosos de calefação ou sem abertura para o escape de gás, aquecedores de água a gás ou aquecedores de ambiente a gás ou a querosene. • Incêndios — a concentração do monóxido de carbono pode chegar até 10% na atmosfera de um edifício em chamas. • Animais com dano às funções cardíaca ou pulmonar. • Animais prenhes no final da gestação podem abortar, mas demonstram apenas efeitos mínimos na mãe.

DIAGNÓSTICO

DIAGNÓSTICO DIFERENCIAL
• Intoxicação por barbitúrico, etanol, etilenoglicol, hidrocarbonetos de petróleo, chumbo; toxicose por gás cianeto ou sulfeto de hidrogênio.
• Inalação de fumaça.

HEMOGRAMA/BIOQUÍMICA/URINÁLISE
• É recomendável a obtenção de banco de dados mínimo, incluindo hemograma completo, perfil bioquímico sérico, urinálise, gasometria e hiato aniônico.
• Creatina cinase — elevada em função de isquemia muscular.
• Os exames de ECG e oximetria de pulso são recomendados se disponíveis. Notar que a oximetria de pulso pode superestimar a quantidade de hemoglobina saturada.

OUTROS TESTES LABORATORIAIS
• Carboxiemoglobina no sangue total — expressa em porcentagem de hemoglobina na forma de carboxiemoglobina; pode retornar aos níveis normais dentro de algumas horas após a interrupção na exposição ao monóxido de carbono.
• Análise de carboxiemoglobina está disponível em muitos laboratórios hospitalares humanos e alguns laboratórios diagnósticos veterinários.
• pH sanguíneo — mais baixo que o normal, secundariamente à acidose metabólica.
• PaO_2 — normal, mas não indicativa de saturação de oxiemoglobina.

MÉTODOS DIAGNÓSTICOS
ECG — alterações das ondas ST-T, compatíveis com hipoxia/anoxia do miocárdio, podem estar presentes.

TRATAMENTO

• Restaurar a oxigenação adequada ao cérebro e ao coração.
• Fornecer suplementação de oxigênio a 100% por meio de tubo endotraqueal — promove uma recuperação 4 vezes mais rápida mediante a alta afinidade de CO em se ligar à hemoglobina; oxigênio hiperbárico (geralmente indisponível em medicina veterinária) promove uma conversão até mesmo mais rápida de carboxiemoglobina em oxiemoglobina.
• O uso de oxigênio a 100% deve ser limitado para ≤18 h para evitar toxicose por esse gás.
• É importante a rápida instituição da terapia para evitar dano permanente ao SNC (malacia, desmielinização) e necrose do miocárdio.
• Providenciar ar fresco, manter as vias aéreas patentes (desobstruídas) e fornecer respiração artificial, se necessário.
• Fluidos de suporte não só para corrigir acidose, mas também para manter o fluxo sanguíneo e a boa perfusão do cérebro.

MEDICAÇÕES

MEDICAMENTO(S)
A oxigenoterapia imediata a 100%, conforme descrito, constitui o principal agente terapêutico.

CONTRAINDICAÇÕES/INTERAÇÕES POSSÍVEIS
• Evitar o uso de depressores respiratórios.
• O uso de oxigênio a 100% deve ser limitado para ≤18 h para evitar toxicose por esse gás.
• Os animais sobreviventes podem sofrer neurotoxicidade tardia, de gravidade variável.

ACOMPANHAMENTO

• Resposta significativa à terapia — deve ser observada em 1-4 h, dependendo dos danos celulares atribuídos à hipoxia.
• Sinais moderados a graves que persistem por 24 h ou mais sugerem um prognóstico mau.
• Monitorizar as funções cardíaca, pulmonar e neurológica, bem como restringir a atividade física por 2 semanas.
• Sinais neurológicos — podem aparecer dentro de alguns dias até 6 semanas após aparente recuperação.
• Eliminar a fonte de monóxido de carbono; é recomendável a utilização de detectores domésticos desse gás para evitar novas exposições.

DIVERSOS

POTENCIAL ZOONÓTICO
Estão sob risco os seres humanos presentes no mesmo ambiente saturado com monóxido de carbono.

GESTAÇÃO/FERTILIDADE/REPRODUÇÃO
Monóxido de carbono — diminui a capacidade carreadora de oxigênio do sangue materno; atravessa a placenta, ocasionando hipoxia fetal, abortamento ou dano neurológico ao feto.

Sugestões de Leitura
Berent AC, Todd J, Sergeeff J, Powell, LL. Carbon monoxide toxicity: A case series. J Vet Emerg Crit Care 2005, 15(2):128-135.
Fitzgerald KT. Carbon monoxide. In: Peterson ME, Talcot PA, eds., Small Animal Toxicology. St. Louis: Saunders, 2006, pp. 619-628.
Gorman D, Drewry A, Huang Y, et al. The clinical toxicology of carbon monoxide. Toxicology 2003, 187:25-38.

Autor Gary D. Osweiler
Consultor Editorial Gary D. Osweiler

Toxicose por Organofosforado e Carbamato

CONSIDERAÇÕES GERAIS

DEFINIÇÃO
• Resulta da exposição a compostos organofosforados ou carbamatos. De 2003 a 2005, o Centro Norte-americano de Controle de Intoxicações da Sociedade Norte-americana para a Prevenção da Crueldade contra os Animais experimentou um declínio de 46% nas chamadas telefônicas a respeito de organofosforados. Essa redução provavelmente está relacionada aos cancelamentos de vários registros e à aprovação de novas fórmulas, efetuados pela Agência Norte-americana de Proteção Ambiental. Os produtos cancelados frequentemente permanecem por anos nas casas e nos comércios. As perguntas sobre carbamato aumentaram 15% durante o mesmo período.
• Produtos animais — organofosforado: clorpirifós, cumafós, citioato, diazinon, fanfur, fention, fosmet e tetraclorvinfós; carbamato: carbaril e propoxur (muitos produtos animais contendo fosmet, tetraclorvinfós, carbaril, clorpirifós, diazinon [todos] foram suspensos).
• Produtos agrícolas, de gramados e para jardins — organofosforado: acefato, clorpirifós, diazinon, dissulfoton, fonofós, malation, paration, terbufós e outros; carbamato: carbofurano e metomil (mesmo comentário acima sobre os produtos ambientais).

FISIOPATOLOGIA
• Provoca efeitos no sistema nervoso pela inibição da colinesterase, a qual inclui a acetilcolinesterase, a pseudocolinesterase e outras esterases.
• Acetilcolinesterase — normalmente hidrolisa o neurotransmissor acetilcolina no tecido nervoso, nas hemácias e no músculo, resultando no término da transmissão nervosa.
• Pseudocolinesterase — encontrada no plasma, no fígado, no pâncreas e no tecido nervoso, principalmente nos gatos.
• Inibição da colinesterase — permite o acúmulo da acetilcolina no receptor pós-sináptico; provoca estímulo dos órgãos efetores; a reativação espontânea após a ligação de composto organofosforado é muito lenta e, com o avançar da idade, fica praticamente inexistente; reversível após a ligação com o carbamato.

SISTEMA(S) ACOMETIDO(S)
Nervoso — resulta da estimulação predominante de vias parassimpáticas; também pode resultar de estimulação simpática; a acetilcolina estimula os receptores nicotínicos do sistema nervoso somático (músculo esquelético), os receptores parassimpáticos nicotínicos pré-ganglionares e muscarínicos pós-ganglionares (músculo cardíaco, pupila, vasos sanguíneos, músculos lisos no pulmão e trato gastrintestinal, glândulas exócrinas) e os receptores simpáticos nicotínicos pré-ganglionares (adrenal e, indiretamente, músculo cardíaco, pupila, vasos sanguíneos, músculos lisos no pulmão e trato gastrintestinal, glândulas exócrinas).

GENÉTICA
• Animais com atividade colinesterásica inerentemente baixa — mais suscetíveis à depressão pela colinesterase.
• Atividade da colinesterase — mais facilmente inibida nos gatos do que nos cães.

INCIDÊNCIA/PREVALÊNCIA
Comum nos pequenos animais.

DISTRIBUIÇÃO GEOGRÁFICA
Mais comum em áreas de elevada prevalência de pulgas e atividade agrícola intensa.

IDENTIFICAÇÃO
Espécies
• Cães e gatos.
• Os gatos são mais suscetíveis.

Raça(s) Predominante(s)
Cães magros (p. ex., cães de caça visual e raças de corrida) e gatos magros de pelos longos — mais suscetíveis à inibição da colinesterase por causa da falta de gordura; muitos compostos organofosforados e metabólitos ficam armazenados na gordura e são liberados lentamente na circulação.

Idade Média e Faixa Etária
Animais jovens — intoxicados mais provavelmente pela baixa capacidade de destoxificação.

Sexo Predominante
Machos intactos são mais suscetíveis a alguns organofosforados.

SINAIS CLÍNICOS
Comentários Gerais
• Estimulação parassimpática — geralmente predomina.
• Estimulação simpática — pode resultar na falta de sinais específicos esperados; podem-se notar sinais opostos àqueles esperados.

Achados Anamnésicos
• Histórico clínico — frequentemente revela aplicações maciças ou repetidas de inseticidas contra pulgas e carrapatos; indícios de exposição a produto agrícola ou de casa e jardim.
• Inseticidas carbamatos (metomil e carbofurano) — podem provocar o rápido início de crises convulsivas, insuficiência respiratória e morte; tratar rigorosamente sem demora.
• Inseticidas organofosforados (gatos, especialmente clorpirifós) — anorexia crônica, fraqueza muscular e espasmos musculares, com ou sem episódios de intoxicação aguda, os quais podem durar de dias a semanas.

Achados do Exame Físico
• Hipersalivação.
• Vômito.
• Diarreia.
• Miose.
• Bradicardia.
• Depressão.
• Ataxia.
• Tremores musculares.
• Crises convulsivas.
• Hipertermia.
• Dispneia.
• Insuficiência respiratória.
• Morte.
• O paciente pode não apresentar todos os sinais.
• Estimulação simpática — sinais invertidos.

CAUSAS
• Utilização exagerada, uso indevido ou utilização de múltiplos inseticidas inibidores da colinesterase.
• Uso impróprio ou incorreto dos inseticidas organofosforados nos gatos (p. ex., imersões contendo organofosforados indicadas apenas para os cães ou aplicação inadequada nos gatos).
• Aplicação dérmica intencional de inseticidas para a casa ou para o jardim.

FATORES DE RISCO
• Exposição concomitante a múltiplos produtos contendo organofosforados e/ou carbamatos.
• Exposição a pisos umedecidos com produtos de estabelecimentos à base de organofosforados.
• Diluição incorreta dos inseticidas.

DIAGNÓSTICO

DIAGNÓSTICO DIFERENCIAL
• Histórico de exposição, quantidade da exposição e presença de sinais clínicos — devem ser compatíveis com a intoxicação.
• Exposição a outros produtos inseticidas — piretrina/piretroides (pulgas e carrapatos); D-limoneno (cítrus para pulgas e carrapatos); fipronil (pulgas e carrapatos); imidacloprida (pulgas).
• Outros pesticidas — estricnina; fluoracetato (1080); 4-aminopiridina (avicida); metaldeído (isca para caramujos); fosfeto de zinco/alumínio (rodenticida); brometalina (rodenticida).
• Outros intoxicantes — chocolate; cafeína; cocaína; anfetamina; micotoxinas tremorgênicas.

HEMOGRAMA/BIOQUÍMICA/URINÁLISE
N/D.

OUTROS TESTES LABORATORIAIS
Atividade da Colinesterase
• Reduzida para <25% do normal no sangue total, na retina ou no cérebro — sugere exposição a algum composto inibidor da colinesterase; é imprescindível comparar aos valores normais de referência para determinada espécie gerados pelo mesmo laboratório.
• Resultados do teste — devem ser interpretados no contexto da quantidade de exposição, dos sinais clínicos e do momento de seu início.
• Uso de laboratórios experientes na manipulação de amostras animais.
• Clorpirifós — os animais expostos experimentalmente podem permanecer normais do ponto de vista clínico, sem atividade colinesterásica detectável.
• Inibição do carbamato — a reativação pode ocorrer durante o transporte, o armazenamento e o teste da amostra, produzindo resultados falso-negativos.

DIAGNÓSTICO POR IMAGEM
N/D.

MÉTODOS DIAGNÓSTICOS
• Teste de resposta à atropina — administrar esse agente anticolinérgico em dose pré-anestésica a 0,02 mg/kg IV. A resposta antimuscarínica (taquicardia, midríase) sugere a falta de exposição à anticolinesterase.
• Detecção dos inseticidas — tecido (p. ex., cérebro, fígado, rim e gordura); conteúdo do estômago; trato gastrintestinal; pele ou pelagem; resultados negativos não descartam a intoxicação.
• Pode-se encontrar pedaços dos recipientes mastigados no trato gastrintestinal.

ACHADOS PATOLÓGICOS
• Lesões histopatológicas — raras; provavelmente não há lesões características em intoxicação aguda.
• Neuropatia tardia — não costuma estar associada a compostos organofosforados disponíveis no mercado.

Toxicose por Organofosforado e Carbamato

TRATAMENTO

CUIDADO(S) DE SAÚDE ADEQUADO(S)
• Paciente de ambulatório — sinais leves decorrentes da exposição a coleiras e talcos contra pulgas e carrapatos; tratados pela simples remoção da coleira ou escovação da pelagem para retirar o excesso de talco.
• Paciente internado — salivação contínua, tremores ou dispneia.

CUIDADO(S) DE ENFERMAGEM
• Cuidados básicos — estabilização; descontaminação; tratamento com atropina como antídoto (e cloreto de pralidoxima para a intoxicação por organofosforado); cuidados de suporte.
• Controle da atividade convulsiva e/ou dos tremores.
• Oxigênio — caso seja necessário, até que a respiração retorne ao normal.
• Fluidoterapia — pode ser necessária nos gatos com anorexia.
• Banho (exposição dérmica) — utilizar detergente comum; enxaguar com quantidades abundantes de água.

ATIVIDADE
N/D.

DIETA
Gatos com anorexia crônica — manter as necessidades nutricionais e hídricas.

ORIENTAÇÃO AO PROPRIETÁRIO
• Enfatizar a importância de seguir as instruções contidas no rótulo do inseticida.
• Avisar o proprietário sobre o fato de que os gatos com anorexia e fraqueza crônicas podem necessitar de dias a semanas de cuidados de suporte para a completa recuperação.

CONSIDERAÇÕES CIRÚRGICAS
N/D.

MEDICAÇÕES

MEDICAMENTO(S) DE ESCOLHA
• Diazepam (0,05-1 mg/kg IV até fazer efeito) é utilizado inicialmente para as crises convulsivas. Pentobarbital (5-15 mg/kg IV até fazer efeito) é adicionado para atividade convulsiva persistente. Fenobarbital (3-30 mg/kg IV até fazer efeito, dosagem baixa nos gatos) ou propofol (3-6 mg/kg IV ou 0,1 mg/kg/min sob taxa de infusão contínua). Todos podem ser utilizados para crises convulsivas refratárias.
• Sulfato de atropina — 0,2 mg/kg, um quarto IV e o restante SC, conforme a necessidade; administrado imediatamente; repetido apenas conforme a necessidade para controlar os sinais clínicos potencialmente letais advindos da estimulação muscarínica.
• Cloreto de pralidoxima (Protopam®) — 10-15 mg/kg IM, SC a cada 8-12 h até a recuperação; interromper após três doses na ausência de resposta; diminui as fasciculações musculares; mais benéfico contra os inseticidas organofosforados quando iniciado após 24 horas da exposição; até mesmo depois de vários dias da exposição dérmica, esse agente pode estimular a retomada da alimentação por gatos com anorexia (com ou sem tremores); se refrigerados e envolvidos por papel de alumínio, os frascos reconstituídos podem ser usados com sucesso por até duas semanas.
• Ingestão de solução inseticida líquida — evite a indução de êmese; há risco de aspiração, porque muitas soluções contêm solventes hidrocarbonetos.
• Na ausência de sinal clínico, solvente líquido *não* digerido e ingestão muito recente — induzir à êmese com peróxido de hidrogênio a 3% (2,2 mL/kg VO até, no máximo, 45 mL) após o fornecimento de refeição úmida.
• Esvaziamento do estômago para o paciente com sinais clínicos — efetuar lavagem gástrica, mantendo o paciente entubado, sob anestesia, com sonda gástrica calibrosa; em seguida, administrar carvão ativado (2 g/kg VO) contendo sorbitol como catártico em papa aquosa.
• Diarreia — não administrar produtos contendo o sorbitol.

CONTRAINDICAÇÕES
Tranquilizantes fenotiazínicos podem potencializar a intoxicação pelo organofosforado.

PRECAUÇÕES
Atropina — evitar o uso exagerado; pode provocar taquicardia, estimulação do SNC, crises convulsivas, desorientação, sonolência e depressão respiratória.

INTERAÇÕES POSSÍVEIS
N/D.

MEDICAMENTO(S) ALTERNATIVO(S)
N/D.

ACOMPANHAMENTO

MONITORIZAÇÃO DO PACIENTE
Monitorizar a frequência cardíaca e a respiração, bem como a ingestão hídrica e calórica.

PREVENÇÃO
• Seguir rigorosamente as instruções contidas no rótulo do inseticida.
• Evitar o uso em animais doentes ou debilitados.
• Evitar o uso simultâneo de produtos à base de organofosforados e carbamatos.

COMPLICAÇÕES POSSÍVEIS
N/D.

EVOLUÇÃO ESPERADA E PROGNÓSTICO
• Fraqueza e anorexia induzidas pela exposição crônica a inseticida organofosforado (em gatos sob exposição ao clorpirifós) — pode durar de 2-4 semanas; a maior parte dos pacientes recupera-se completamente com cuidados rigorosos de enfermagem.
• Intoxicação aguda submetida a tratamento imediato — prognóstico bom.

DIVERSOS

DISTÚRBIOS ASSOCIADOS
N/D.

FATORES RELACIONADOS COM A IDADE
Os animais jovens apresentam baixa capacidade de destoxificação.

POTENCIAL ZOONÓTICO
Nenhum.

GESTAÇÃO/FERTILIDADE/REPRODUÇÃO
N/D.

VER TAMBÉM
Envenenamento (Intoxicação).

ABREVIATURA(S)
• SNC = sistema nervoso central.

Sugestões de Leitura
Fikes JD. Feline chlorpyrifos toxicosis. In: Kirk RW, Bonagura JD, eds., Current Veterinary Therapy XI. Philadelphia: Saunders, 1992, pp. 188-191.
Fikes JD. Organophosphate and carbamate insecticides. Vet Clin North Am Small Anim Pract 1990, 20:353-367.

Autores Steven R. Hansen e Elizabeth A. Curry-Galvin
Consultor Editorial Gary D. Osweiler

TOXICOSE POR PSEUDOEFEDRINA

CONSIDERAÇÕES GERAIS

REVISÃO
Síndrome resultante da exposição a níveis excessivos de pseudoefedrina.

IDENTIFICAÇÃO
Qualquer espécie pode ser acometida, mas os cães são mais comumente envolvidos em dosagens excessivas acidentais.

SINAIS CLÍNICOS
• Midríase, respiração ofegante, hipertermia, agitação/hiperatividade, taquicardia, hipertensão são comuns. Outros sinais incluem vômito, vocalização, tremores, desorientação ou letargia.
• São possíveis os sinais de balanço cefálico, arritmias sinusais, hemorragia escleral ou atividade semelhante à crise convulsiva. Esses sinais podem ser acompanhados por colapso agudo.
• Os sinais de intoxicação aguda podem persistir por 1-3 dias, dependendo da dose de pseudoefedrina ingerida.
• Os casos graves podem evoluir para CID, mioglobinuremia/úria com lesão renal secundária, ou disfunção permanente do SNC.

CAUSAS E FATORES DE RISCO
• A pseudoefedrina é um sal sintético de efedrina e uma amina simpaticomimética indireta.
• A pseudoefedrina estimula indiretamente os receptores α-adrenérgicos e, em menor grau, os receptores β-adrenérgicos.
• Doses >1 mg/kg podem resultar em agitação, hiperatividade e respiração ofegante.
• Balanço cefálico, CID ou mioglobinúria indicam uma intoxicação grave e apresentam um prognóstico mais reservado.

DIAGNÓSTICO

DIAGNÓSTICO DIFERENCIAL
Outros estimulantes do SNC e simpaticomiméticos: anfetaminas, cocaína, antidepressivos serotoninérgicos, fenilpropanolamina, metilxantinas, efedra.

HEMOGRAMA/BIOQUÍMICA/URINÁLISE
• Na maioria dos casos não se espera quaisquer alterações clinicopatológicas específicas.
• Em casos graves, podem ocorrer CID, mioglobinemia, mioglobinúria ou azotemia.

OUTROS TESTES LABORATORIAIS
A urina ou o soro de pacientes com toxicose por pseudoefedrina pode dar um resultado positivo em teste para detecção de anfetamina em kits de teste para medicamentos de venda livre ou em triagens farmacológicas de hospitais humanos.

TRATAMENTO

• Tratar os sinais graves ou potencialmente letais em primeiro lugar.
• Controlar a estimulação do SNC primeiro e, depois, tratar a estimulação cardiovascular, pois a pressão arterial e a frequência cardíaca podem diminuir significativamente assim que os sinais neurológicos (SNC) estiverem controlados.
• Para crises convulsivas, utilizar os medicamentos propofol, pentobarbital, ou fenobarbital; considerar o uso de gás anestésico para casos refratários.
• Para agitação, hiperatividade ou outra estimulação do SNC, utilizar acepromazina ou clorpromazina.
• A ciproeptadina foi usada com algum sucesso para tratar disforia, vocalização, e hipertermia.
• Propranolol (ou outro β-bloqueador) pode ser considerado em pacientes com taquicardia sustentada.
• Talvez haja necessidade de medidas externas de resfriamento para pacientes hipertérmicos.
• A administração intravenosa de fluidos ajuda na estabilização dos efeitos cardiovasculares, no suporte da função renal, e na excreção de pseudoefedrina e seus metabólitos.
• Monitorizar a frequência e o ritmo cardíacos, a temperatura corporal e a pressão arterial. Em pacientes gravemente acometidos, monitorizar a função renal, os parâmetros de coagulação, a hidratação e os eletrólitos.
• Descontaminação gastrintestinal (indução de êmese, administração de carvão ativado) pode ser considerada em pacientes que ingeriram >1 mg/kg de pseudoefedrina e não estão exibindo sinais clínicos significativos.

MEDICAÇÕES

MEDICAMENTO(S)
• Propofol 0,1-0,6 mg/kg/min IV.
• Pentobarbital 30 mg/kg IV até fazer efeito.
• Fenobarbital 3-4 mg/kg IV.
• Acepromazina 0,05-1,0 mg/kg IM ou IV; iniciar com a dose baixa e titular para cima conforme a necessidade.
• Clorpromazina 0,5-1,0 mg/kg IV ou IM; iniciar com a dose baixa e titular para cima conforme a necessidade.
• Ciproeptadina 1,1 mg/kg VO ou via retal a cada 6 h (cães); 2-4 mg VO ou via retal (gatos).
• Propranolol 0,02-0,06 mg/kg IV a cada 6-8 horas conforme a necessidade.
• Eméticos – peróxido de hidrogênio a 3% na dose de 2,2 mL/kg VO (45 mL no máximo), podendo ser repetida uma vez se a primeira dose não for bem-sucedida; apomorfina triturada e diluída com soro fisiológico e instilada no saco conjuntival, enxaguar o olho após a êmese, ou 0,03 mg/kg IV.
• Carvão ativado na dose de 1-3 g/kg suspenso em 50-200 mL de água.

CONTRAINDICAÇÕES/INTERAÇÕES POSSÍVEIS
É recomendável evitar o uso de diazepam para controlar a estimulação do SNC, pois esse medicamento pode induzir a um efeito disfórico nesses pacientes e agravar a excitação neurológica.

ACOMPANHAMENTO
Insuficiência renal resultante de mioglobinúria pode necessitar de acompanhamento e cuidados prolongados.

DIVERSOS

As exposições a Ma-huang (efedrina) e anfetamina em animais são tratadas do mesmo modo que a toxicose por pseudoefedrina.

ABREVIATURAS
CID = coagulação intravascular disseminada.
SNC = sistema nervoso central.

Sugestões de Leitura
Means C. Ma huang: All natural but not always innocuous. Vet Med 1999, 94:511-512.

Autor Sharon Gwaltney-Brant
Consultor Editorial Gary D. Osweiler

Toxicose por Uvas e Passas

CONSIDERAÇÕES GERAIS

REVISÃO
Síndrome resultante da ingestão de uvas ou passas (*Vitis* spp.).

IDENTIFICAÇÃO
- Os cães constituem a única espécie em que a toxicose foi bem descrita.
- Não se observa predisposição racial, sexual ou etária.
- Embora haja relatos breves e incidentais de toxicose em gatos e ferrets (furões), não há dados para confirmar tal toxicose.

SINAIS CLÍNICOS
- Vômito em até 24 horas da ingestão; o vômito frequentemente contém uvas ou passas ingeridas.
- Podem ocorrer diarreia, anorexia, letargia e dor abdominal.
- Dentro de 24 horas a alguns dias, ocorre desidratação com oligúria ou anúria.
- A morte é causada por insuficiência renal anúrica ou eutanásia.

CAUSAS E FATORES DE RISCO
- O mecanismo de toxicidade e o princípio tóxico desses alimentos são desconhecidos.
- Há relatos de que as quantidades de uvas e passas capazes de causar toxicose variam de 2,8-9,6 g/kg e 11-31 g/kg, respectivamente.
- Nem todas as exposições de cães a uvas ou passas resultarão em insuficiência renal.

DIAGNÓSTICO

DIAGNÓSTICO DIFERENCIAL
Outras causas de insuficiência renal aguda — etilenoglicol, toxicose por metais pesados, antibióticos nefrotóxicos (p. ex., aminoglicosídeos), toxicose por medicamentos anti-inflamatórios não esteroides, hemoglobinúria, mioglobinúria, leptospirose, borreliose e toxicose por vitamina D.

HEMOGRAMA/BIOQUÍMICA/URINÁLISE
- Pode ocorrer o desenvolvimento de hipercalcemia, hiperfosfatemia, níveis elevados de creatinina e nitrogênio ureico sanguíneo em até 24-48 horas da ingestão.
- Também há relatos de hipercalemia, hiperamilasemia, hiperlipasemia e ALT elevada.
- Isostenúria, hipostenúria, proteinúria, hematúria e glicosúria são relatadas.
- Pode ocorrer a formação de cilindros granulosos na urina.

OUTROS TESTES LABORATORIAIS
A histopatologia dos rins revela degeneração e necrose tubulares renais difusas agudas.

TRATAMENTO

- Descontaminação gastrintestinal (indução de êmese, administração de carvão ativado) deve acompanhar a ingestão de uvas ou passas pelos cães.
- É recomendável a diurese hídrica (2 vezes a manutenção) por, no mínimo, 48 horas ou por mais tempo caso ocorra o desenvolvimento de insuficiência renal. A escolha do fluido pode variar com a circunstância, mas o cloreto de sódio a 0,9% é o mais comumente recomendado.
- Monitorizar os valores da bioquímica sérica, particularmente os valores renais, por, no mínimo, 72 horas ou por mais tempo caso ocorra o desenvolvimento de insuficiência renal.
- Corrigir os desequilíbrios hídricos (p. ex., desidratação).
- Monitorizar as entradas e saídas de líquido.
- Diuréticos (p. ex., furosemida, manitol, dopamina) caso ocorra o desenvolvimento de oligúria ou anúria.
- Pode haver a necessidade de hemodiálise ou diálise peritoneal em pacientes anúricos.

MEDICAÇÕES

MEDICAMENTO(S)
Eméticos — peróxido de hidrogênio a 3% na dose de 2,2 mL/kg VO (45 mL no máximo), podendo ser repetido uma vez se a primeira dose não for bem-sucedida; apomorfina triturada e diluída com soro fisiológico estéril e instilada no saco conjuntival, enxaguar o olho após êmese, ou 0,03 mg/kg IV.

Tratamento de Insuficiência Renal Oligúria ou Anúrica
- Manitol na dose de 0,25-0,5 g/kg de solução a 20-25% IV por 15-20 minutos, repetir a cada 4-6 h ou administrar sob a forma de infusão contínua de solução a 8-10% por 12-24 horas.
- Furosemida na dose de 2 mg/kg IV, repetir a 4 mg/kg se não ocorrer diurese em até 1 hora; utilizar com dopamina para obtenção dos melhores resultados.
- Dopamina na dose de 0,5-3 mcg/kg/minuto.

CONTRAINDICAÇÕES/INTERAÇÕES POSSÍVEIS
N/D.

ACOMPANHAMENTO

- Em cães que desenvolvem insuficiência renal, monitorizar os valores renais até que eles retornem ao normal.
- Alguns cães podem desenvolver lesão renal irreversível que necessita de tratamento pelo resto da vida.

DIVERSOS

ABREVIATURAS
ALT = alanina aminotransferase

RECURSOS DA INTERNET
Orientação ao cliente: há um artigo sobre toxicose por uvas e passas em cães (The Wrath of Grapes) disponível em http://aspcapro.org/animal-poison-control/documents/grapes.pdf.

Sugestões de Leitura
Eubig PA, et al. Acute renal failure in dogs after ingestion of grapes or raisins: A retrospective evaluation of 43 dogs (1992-2002). J Vet Intern Med 2005, 19:663-674.
Mazzaferro EM, et al. Acute renal failure associated with raisin or grape ingestion in 4 dogs. J Vet Emerg Crit Care 2004, 14:203-212.
Mostrom MS. Grapes and raisins. In: Peterson M, Talcott PA, eds., Small Animal Toxicology, 2nd ed. St. Louis: Saunders, 2006, pp. 727-731.

Autor Sharon Gwaltney-Brant
Consultor Editorial Gary D. Osweiler

Toxicose por Veneno de Aranha — Família da Reclusa-Castanha

CONSIDERAÇÕES GERAIS

REVISÃO
- Família da reclusa-castanha — *Loxosceles* spp.; tamanho corporal de 8-15 mm; pernas com 2-3 cm de comprimento; padrão do cefalotórax em forma de violino, com o pescoço do violino se estendendo caudalmente; ativa à noite.
- Distribuição — encontrada por toda a região meio-oeste da Costa do Golfo dos EUA até o vale do rio Mississípi, incluindo também a parte sul de Wisconsin. Algumas espécies são encontradas nas regiões oriental e sul da Califórnia, ocidental do Arizona e sul do Novo México.
- Mordidas — costumam ocorrer quando a aranha é capturada no leito; induz a aracnidismo necrótico, uma lesão dermatonecrótica indolente mediada pela enzima esfingomielinase D, além de provocar hemólise direta dos eritrócitos, agregação plaquetária, insuficiência renal, coagulopatia e morte.

IDENTIFICAÇÃO
Cães e gatos.

SINAIS CLÍNICOS
- Os sinais clínicos não são completamente definidos em envenenamentos caninos e felinos.
- Em seres humanos:
  ○ Dor local e sensação de ardência (pode durar de 6-8 h); acompanhadas por prurido e ferida.
- Lesão-alvo clássica — área isquêmica com escara central enegrecida em um fundo eritematoso irregular; depois de 2-5 semanas, a escara central pode se desprender, deixando uma úlcera profunda que não cicatriza e, em geral, poupa o tecido muscular.
- Menos comum — anemia hemolítica e hemoglobinúria nas primeiras 24 h.
- Outras possíveis manifestações sistêmicas nos primeiros 2-3 dias depois do envenenamento — febre; calafrios; erupção cutânea; fraqueza; leucocitose; náusea; artralgia.
- Os envenenamentos em áreas de tecido adiposo desenvolvem lesões mais significativas.

CAUSAS E FATORES DE RISCO
Mordida da aranha pertencente à família da reclusa-castanha.

DIAGNÓSTICO

Com frequência, a mordida da aranha pertencente à família da reclusa-castanha é erroneamente diagnosticada em regiões norte-americanas que não possuem populações endêmicas dessa aranha.

DIAGNÓSTICO DIFERENCIAL
- Infecção bacteriana ou micobacteriana.
- Úlcera de decúbito.
- Queimadura de terceiro grau.
- Anemia hemolítica.
- Icterícia.
- Trombocitopenia.
- Erliquiose.
- Hemoparasitismo.

HEMOGRAMA/BIOQUÍMICA/URINÁLISE
- Anemia.
- Leucocitose.
- Trombocitopenia.
- Hemoglobinúria.

OUTROS TESTES LABORATORIAIS
Perfil da coagulação — pode revelar tempos de coagulação prolongados.

DIAGNÓSTICO POR IMAGEM
N/D.

MÉTODOS DIAGNÓSTICOS
N/D.

TRATAMENTO

- Cuidados de rotina da ferida — pode necessitar de cuidados de suporte rigorosos.
- Cuidados de suporte — fluidoterapia; tratamento presuntivo de superinfecção bacteriana; (raramente) transfusão de sangue.
- Envenenamento local brando — geralmente responde a compressas frias, já que a atividade da esfingomielinase D depende da temperatura.
- Lesões necróticas — podem necessitar de debridamento após o eritema ter desaparecido.
- Envenenamento grave — pode exigir a aplicação de enxerto cutâneo depois de a lesão atingir a maturidade completa.

MEDICAÇÕES

MEDICAMENTO(S)
- Antibióticos — evitam a ocorrência de infecção secundária.
- Oxigênio hiperbárico — alguns indícios sugerem que o tratamento com esse tipo de oxigênio possa ser benéfico em modelos de animais por reduzir o tamanho da lesão cutânea.
- Dapsona — obtiveram-se resultados variados em diversos estudos. Dose utilizada de 1 mg/kg a cada 8 h por 10 dias; medicamento indicado para as lesões dermatonecróticas; inibidor de leucócitos; supostamente minimiza o componente inflamatório do envenenamento; repetir se necessário. A eficácia contra o envenenamento pela reclusa-castanha não foi estudada em cães e gatos.

CONTRAINDICAÇÕES/INTERAÇÕES POSSÍVEIS
- Não utilizar o calor — exacerba o problema.
- Dapsona — pode causar hipersensibilidade e metemoglobinemia em pacientes com deficiência da glicose-6-fosfatase (G6PD).
- Excisão cirúrgica precoce pode gerar um defeito maior do que apenas o cuidado de suporte.
- Anti-histamínicos, colchicina, anticoagulantes, nitroglicerina tópica, altas doses de vitamina C, choque elétrico e esteroides foram propostos para o tratamento, embora tenham se mostrado ineficazes.

ACOMPANHAMENTO

Monitorizar semanalmente o local da ferida até a cicatrização.

Sugestões de Leitura
Peterson ME. Spider envenomation: Brown recluse. In: Peterson ME, Talcott PA, eds., Small Animal Toxicology, 2nd ed. St. Louis: Saunders, 2006, pp. 1071-1075.

Autor Michael E. Peterson
Consultor Editorial Gary D. Osweiler

Toxicose por Veneno de Aranha — Viúva-Negra

CONSIDERAÇÕES GERAIS

REVISÃO
- Aranha viúva-negra — *Latrodectus* spp.; as fêmeas são tóxicas; 2-2,5 cm de comprimento; cor negra brilhante; marca de ampulheta vermelha ou alaranjada na parte ventral do abdome; a fêmea imatura é castanha, com tiras vermelhas a alaranjadas que se modificam para a forma de ampulheta à medida que a aranha escurece até ficar negra e envelhece.
- Mordidas — podem ser secas (sem veneno injetado).
- Variação — gênero encontrado em todos os Estados norte-americanos, exceto no Alasca; frequentemente encontradas ao redor de prédios e habitação humana.
- Veneno — contém α-latrotoxina, uma potente neurotoxina; abre os canais seletivos de cátions no terminal nervoso pré-sináptico; provoca liberação maciça de acetilcolina e noradrenalina, as quais geram espasmos musculares contínuos.

IDENTIFICAÇÃO
Cães e gatos.

SINAIS CLÍNICOS
Achados Anamnésicos
- Geralmente de início súbito.
- Pode demorar vários dias em caso de envenenamento leve.

Achados do Exame Físico
Cães
- Fasciculações musculares progressivas.
- Dor intensa.
- Cãibra de grandes massas musculares.
- Rigidez abdominal sem hipersensibilidade.
- Inquietação acentuada, com contorção de dor e espasmos.
- São previstos os sinais de hipertensão e taquicardia.
- Pode-se notar broncorreia, hipersalivação, hiperestesia, hipersensibilidade dos linfonodos, entorpecimento, tumefação facial (expressão de *Latrodectus*).
- Possível rabdomiólise.

Gatos
- Paralisia precoce e acentuada.
- Dor intensa, que se manifesta por gritos e vocalizações sonoras.
- Salivação e inquietação excessivas.

- Vômito — não é raro que o animal vomite a aranha.
- Diarreia.
- Tremores e cãibras musculares.
- Ataxia e incapacidade de permanecer em estação — torna-se adinâmico e atônico.
- Colapso respiratório.
- Morte sem o antídoto.

CAUSAS E FATORES DE RISCO
- Muito jovens ou idosos — risco aumentado.
- Hipertensão sistêmica — risco elevado.

DIAGNÓSTICO

DIAGNÓSTICO DIFERENCIAL
- Dorsalgia por discopatia.
- Abdome agudo.

HEMOGRAMA/BIOQUÍMICA/URINÁLISE
- Leucocitose.
- Creatina quinase elevada — nos espasmos musculares graves.
- Albuminúria.

OUTROS TESTES LABORATORIAIS
Resultados normais na pesquisa de sangue oculto nas fezes.

DIAGNÓSTICO POR IMAGEM
Radiografias abdominais normais.

MÉTODOS DIAGNÓSTICOS
N/D.

TRATAMENTO
- Paciente internado — para fornecimento dos cuidados de suporte.
- Monitorizar o estado respiratório.

MEDICAÇÕES

MEDICAMENTO(S)
- Antídoto — (Lyovac® [*Latrodectus*], origem equina) — 1 frasco misturado com 100 mL de solução cristaloide por via IV, administrado lentamente com monitoramento da face interna do pavilhão auricular em busca de indícios de hiperemia (indicador de resposta alérgica); a dose costuma ser suficiente para constatação de uma resposta dentro de 30 min; com a utilização adequada, as reações são raras. Em caso de reação alérgica, interromper o antídoto; administrar difenidramina; depois de 5-10 min, reiniciar o antídoto em uma velocidade mais baixa.
- Estudos sugerem que os benzodiazepínicos sejam mais eficazes do que os relaxantes musculares para o tratamento de dor muscular (mialgia) relacionada com o envenenamento pela aranha viúva-negra.
- Espasmos musculares e dor intensa são controlados pela administração intravenosa atenta de narcóticos ou de benzodiazepínicos na dose mais baixa e eficaz para evitar a ocorrência de depressão respiratória; metocarbamol (Robaxin®) alivia os espasmos musculares, mas não tem efeito sobre a hipertensão ou a depressão respiratória.
- Hipertensão intratável — nitroprusseto de sódio.
- Um antídoto novo (Aracmyn® – Instituto Bioclon, México) concluiu três ensaios clínicos de fase humana, mas ainda não foi aprovado para uso em seres humanos. Além de ter origem equina (antídoto Fab₂*), é muito menos provável que esse produto deflagre uma reação alérgica.

CONTRAINDICAÇÕES/INTERAÇÕES POSSÍVEIS
Fluidos intravenosos na hipertensão.

ACOMPANHAMENTO
- Monitorização semanal do local da ferida até a cicatrização.
- Prognóstico — incerto durante alguns dias; os casos em gatos costumam ser fatais sem o antídoto.
- Fraqueza, fadiga e insônia — podem persistir por meses.

DIVERSOS

Sugestões de Leitura
Peterson ME. Spider envenomation: Black widow. In: Peterson ME, Talcott PA, eds., Small Animal Toxicology, 2nd ed. St. Louis: Saunders, 2006, pp. 1063-1069.

Autor Michael E. Peterson
Consultor Editorial Gary D. Osweiler

---

* N. T.: Produzido a partir da fração Fab₂ de imunoglobulinas.

TOXICOSE POR VENENO DE COBRA — CORAIS

CONSIDERAÇÕES GERAIS

REVISÃO

Cobras Corais
- Há duas subespécies clinicamente importantes na América do Norte — *Micrurus fulvius fulvius*, a cobra-coral do leste (Carolina do Norte ao norte; sul da Flórida ao sul; a oeste do Rio Mississípi) e *M. fulvius tenere*, cobra-coral do Texas (oeste do Mississípi; em Arkansas, Louisiana e Texas).
- Família Elapidae — presas frontais fixas.
- Padrão de cor — faixas completas circundando o corpo; vermelhas, amarelas e negras; diferenciadas da cobra-real tricolor não venenosa pelo arranjo das faixas: se as faixas de cores amarela (cuidado) e vermelha (perigo) se tocarem, elas ficam evidentes; cabeça relativamente pequena; parte frontal da cabeça é negra; pupilas arredondadas.

Mordidas
- Relativamente raras em virtude do comportamento recluso e dos hábitos noturnos da cobra.
- Frequentemente ocorrem no lábio.
- Início dos sinais clínicos pode demorar várias horas (até 18 h) após o envenenamento.
- As vítimas desenvolvem paralisia bulbar.
- Principal causa da morte — colapso respiratório.
- Os envenenamentos por *M. fulvius tenere* parecem menos graves do que por *M. fulvius fulvius*.

IDENTIFICAÇÃO
Cães e gatos.

SINAIS CLÍNICOS
- Paralisia bulbar — acomete os nervos motores cranianos, o trato respiratório e os músculos esqueléticos; quadriplegia flácida aguda.
- Salivação — provocada pela disfagia.
- Dispneia.
- Disfonia.
- Reflexos espinais hiporreflexivos.

CAUSAS E FATORES DE RISCO
Tamanho da cobra.

DIAGNÓSTICO

DIAGNÓSTICO DIFERENCIAL
- Miastenia grave.
- Botulismo.
- Polirradiculoneurite.
- Paralisia por picada do carrapato.

HEMOGRAMA/BIOQUÍMICA/URINÁLISE
- Hemólise — apenas nos cães.
- Protuberâncias nas hemácias.
- Pode-se notar a elevação da creatina quinase.
- Hemoglobinúria — apenas nos cães.

OUTROS TESTES LABORATORIAIS
N/D.

DIAGNÓSTICO POR IMAGEM
N/D.

MÉTODOS DIAGNÓSTICOS
N/D.

TRATAMENTO

- Paciente internado — hospitalizado por, no mínimo, 48 h.
- Não há antiveneno específico disponível (*M. fulvius*). No entanto, ocorre reação cruzada protetora com os seguintes antídotos: Coralmyn® [antídoto Fab₂ de origem equina] (Instituto Bioclon, México), antídoto de cobra-coral da Costa Rica (Instituto Clodomiro Picado, Costa Rica) e antídoto de cobra-tigre *Notechis scutatus* da Austrália (CSL Limited, Parkville, Victoria, Austrália).
- Primeiros-socorros — geralmente evitar; a medida mais eficaz é o transporte rápido a uma instituição veterinária para administração do antídoto; a técnica australiana para mordidas de cobras da família Elapidae consiste na aplicação de curativo compressivo no membro mordido com bandagem tipo gelo para diminuir o fluxo de sangue e a absorção do veneno.
- **CUIDADO:** não esperar o início dos sinais clínicos para iniciar o tratamento.
- Na falta de disponibilidade do antídoto — fornecer suporte ventilatório por vários dias em estabelecimentos de cuidados críticos.

MEDICAÇÕES

MEDICAMENTO(S)
- Antídoto reativo de *M. fulvius* (ver a seção "Tratamento") — indicado se a anamnese citar a interação recente com cobra-coral; evidência de feridas puntiformes; sinais clínicos compatíveis com o envenenamento pela cobra-coral; administrar 1-2 frascos; pode haver a necessidade de frascos adicionais (técnica idêntica à do antídoto contra picada de víbora).
- Antibiótico de amplo espectro por 7-10 dias.

CONTRAINDICAÇÕES/INTERAÇÕES POSSÍVEIS
- Corticosteroides — não são indicados.
- Observar as mesmas precauções esboçadas para a administração do antídoto contra víbora (ver "Toxicose por Veneno de Cobra — Víboras").

ACOMPANHAMENTO

- Sinais clínicos acentuados podem durar de uma semana a uma semana e meia.
- A recuperação completa pode demorar meses à medida que os receptores se regeneram.

DIVERSOS

VER TAMBÉM
Toxicose por Veneno de Cobra — Víboras.

Sugestões de Leitura
Peterson ME. Snake bite: Coral snakes. In: Peterson ME, Talcott PA, eds., Small Animal Toxicology, 2nd ed. St. Louis: Saunders, 2006, pp. 1039-1048.

Autor Michael E. Peterson
Consultor Editorial Gary D. Osweiler

Toxicose por Veneno de Cobra — Víboras

CONSIDERAÇÕES GERAIS

REVISÃO
- Víboras com fosseta loreal — *Crotalus* spp. (cascavéis), *Sistrurus* spp. (cascavéis anãs e massassauga) e *Agkistrodon* spp. (trigonocéfala [cabeça-de-cobre] e mocassins d'água boca-de-algodão); presas retráteis; fosseta que atua como sensor de calor entre a narina e o olho; cabeça triangular.
- Extensão — espalhada por todo o continente dos EUA.
- Toxicidade — considerada hemotóxica; várias espécies possuem subpopulações com componentes neurotóxicos letais (p. ex., cascavel Mojave); classificação geral de gravidade: (1) cascavéis, (2) mocassins, (3) trigonocéfalas.
- Veneno — enzimas: hialuronidase e fosfolipase A (provocam lesão tecidual local) e outras que interferem na cascata da coagulação (geram defeitos importantes na coagulação); polipeptídeos não enzimáticos: acometem os sistemas cardiovascular e respiratório.
- Mordida — 85% das vítimas apresentam valores laboratoriais alterados e tumefação clinicamente importante; hipotensão grave gerada pelo acúmulo de sangue dentro dos vasos esplâncnicos (cães) ou pulmonares (gatos); perda de líquido do compartimento vascular secundário ao edema periférico grave.

IDENTIFICAÇÃO
Cães e gatos.

SINAIS CLÍNICOS
Comentários Gerais
Podem ser protelados por 8 h após o envenenamento.

Achados Anamnésicos
- Ambientes externos, meio rural.
- O proprietário vê a mordida ou ouve o ruído da cobra.

Achados do Exame Físico
- Feridas puntiformes na cabeça e nos membros torácicos em grande parte dos animais.
- Tumefação tecidual local e dor ao redor da mordida.
- Hematoma, com possível necrose e esfacelamento do tecido no local da mordida.
- Equimose e petéquias dos tecidos e das mucosas.
- Hipotensão e choque.
- Taquicardia.
- Respiração superficial.
- Depressão e letargia.
- Náusea e salivação excessiva.

CAUSAS E FATORES DE RISCO
Associados à Cobra
- Relação de fração peptídica tóxica:fração enzimática — mais elevada na primavera; mais baixa no outono; elevada nas cobras muito jovens.
- Quantidade de veneno produzido desde a última mordida.
- Agressividade e motivação da cobra.

Associados à Vítima
- Local da mordida — mordidas na língua e no torso* são mais preocupantes.
- Tamanho da vítima.

---
* N. T.: Parte do corpo formada pelo tórax, abdome e bacia.

- Tempo decorrido entre a mordida e o início do tratamento.
- Nível de atividade da vítima após a mordida — a atividade aumenta a absorção do veneno.

DIAGNÓSTICO

DIAGNÓSTICO DIFERENCIAL
- Angioedema secundário a envenenamento por inseto.
- Traumatismo rombo.
- Ferida penetrante.
- Mordida de animal.
- Penetração de corpo estranho.
- Abscesso drenante.

HEMOGRAMA/BIOQUÍMICA/URINÁLISE
- Hemoconcentração.
- Protuberâncias nas hemácias nas primeiras 24 h.
- Trombocitopenia.
- Hipocalcemia.
- Elevação da creatina quinase.
- Hematúria ou mioglobinúria.

OUTROS TESTES LABORATORIAIS
Testes de coagulação — podem-se notar TCA, TP e TTP prolongados, além de PDF elevados.

DIAGNÓSTICO POR IMAGEM
N/D.

MÉTODOS DIAGNÓSTICOS
ECG — pode-se detectar arritmia ventricular, sobretudo nos animais gravemente deprimidos.

TRATAMENTO

- Reação tecidual em torno do local da mordida — não é um indicador confiável de intoxicação sistêmica.
- Localização da mordida — pode afetar a absorção do veneno; mordidas na língua e no torso são mais preocupantes.
- Medidas de primeiros-socorros — acalmar o paciente; transportá-lo rapidamente para algum estabelecimento veterinário.
- A aplicação de antídoto é o único tratamento específico comprovado (ver a seção "Medicamentos").
- Fluidos intravenosos — corrigir a hipotensão.

MEDICAÇÕES

MEDICAMENTO(S)
- Antídoto (Crotálico polivalente, origem equina, IgG total) — 1 frasco misturado com 200 mL de fluidos cristaloides administrados lentamente por via IV com monitorização rigorosa da parte interna do pavilhão auricular quanto ao início de hiperemia (indicador de possível reação alérgica); as reações são muito mais comuns em virtude das proteínas extrínsecas contidas no frasco terapêutico.
- Antídoto (Crofab®, antídoto Fab$_1$ polivalente de origem ovina) concluiu os ensaios clínicos em cães e foi bem-sucedido em gatos. Há uma possibilidade muito menor de reações por conta das partículas de anticorpos purificadas. Foi enviada para aprovação do Departamento de Agricultura Norte-americano. O antídoto contra víbora foi o único aprovado nos EUA para seres humanos.
- Antídoto (Antivipmyn®, antídoto Fab$_2$ polivalente de origem equina — Instituto Bioclon, México) encontra-se em fase de ensaio clínico para cães. Há uma possibilidade muito menor de reações por conta das partículas de anticorpos purificadas.
- Sempre lavar e enxaguar o frasco de antídoto após a remoção inicial do mesmo; o segundo enxágue pode aumentar a coleta do antídoto em 30%.
- Reação alérgica — interromper o antídoto; administrar difenidramina; depois de 5 min, restabelecer a infusão do antídoto em uma velocidade mais lenta.
- Podem ocorrer recidivas dos sinais clínicos ou anormalidades de coagulação com qualquer antídoto; se o problema de coagulopatia inicial tiver desaparecido com o uso do antídoto, poderá ocorrer recidiva nos próximos dias, embora raramente ela seja tão grave quanto no início. Não há casos registrados de sangramento clínico com subsequente coagulopatia; no entanto, o clínico deve ficar atento para a possibilidade.

CONTRAINDICAÇÕES/INTERAÇÕES POSSÍVEIS
- **CUIDADO:** em animais submetidos a β-bloqueadores, o início da anafilaxia pode ser mascarado; portanto, a condição pode estar mais avançada no momento da identificação, sendo mais difícil de tratá-la com eficácia.
- Corticosteroides — sem valor.
- DMSO — aumenta a absorção e a disseminação do veneno.
- Heparina — não utilizar.
- Atualmente existe no mercado uma vacina contra cascavel para cães. No entanto, sua eficácia é desconhecida; até o momento existem apenas indícios sem comprovação científica ou verificação experimental. Portanto, essa vacina não é recomendada até que haja dados disponíveis sobre sua eficácia, revisados por especialistas.

ACOMPANHAMENTO

- Exames laboratoriais repetidos — 6 h após admissão no hospital.
- Sinais clínicos — podem durar uma semana a uma semana e meia.

DIVERSOS

ABREVIATURA(S)
- DMSO = dimetilsulfóxido.
- ECG = eletrocardiograma.
- PDF = produtos da degradação da fibrina.
- TCA = tempo de coagulação ativado.
- TP = tempo de protrombina.
- TTP = tempo de tromboplastina parcial.

Sugestões de Leitura
Peterson ME. Snake bite: North American pit vipers. In: Peterson ME, Talcott PA, eds., Small Animal Toxicology, 2nd ed. St. Louis: Saunders, 2006, pp. 1017–1038.

Autor Michael E. Peterson
Consultor Editorial Gary D. Osweiler

TOXICOSE POR VENENO DE SAPO

CONSIDERAÇÕES GERAIS

REVISÃO
- Há duas espécies de particular interesse — o sapo do rio Colorado (*Bufo alvarius*) e o sapo marinho (*B. marinus*); o último é mais tóxico; ambos podem ser fatais.
- Sapos — são mais ativos durante os períodos de alta umidade (a estação chuvosa [monção] no final do verão no sudoeste árido em relação aos sapos do rio Colorado); a maior parte dos contatos ocorre no final da tarde, à noite ou de madrugada.
- Toxina — produzida pelas glândulas parótidas; ato defensivo; absorvida rapidamente pelas mucosas da vítima; contém diversos componentes importantes: indolalquilaminas (semelhantes à droga ilícita denominada LSD), glicosídeos cardíacos e esteróis não cardíacos.

IDENTIFICAÇÃO
Acomete principalmente cães; raras vezes, ocorre em furões e gatos.

SINAIS CLÍNICOS
Comentários Gerais
Início rápido.

Achados Anamnésicos
- Choro e fricção das patas na boca.
- Ataxia ou marcha rígida.
- Crises convulsivas.

Achados do Exame Físico
- Sialorreia profusa.
- Hiperexcitabilidade com vocalização.
- Mucosas bucais de coloração vermelho-tijolo.
- Hipertermia.
- Colapso.
- Arritmia cardíaca ventricular acentuada — menos comum em casos de intoxicação pelo sapo do rio Colorado.
- Cianose.
- Dispneia.

CAUSAS E FATORES DE RISCO
- Residência em áreas próximas ao hábitat dos sapos.
- Ambiente externo úmido e quente.
- Animais errantes.

DIAGNÓSTICO

DIAGNÓSTICO DIFERENCIAL
Substâncias cáusticas ou outros agentes irritantes bucais.

HEMOGRAMA/BIOQUÍMICA/URINÁLISE
Pode-se notar hipercalemia.

OUTROS TESTES LABORATORIAIS
N/D.

DIAGNÓSTICO POR IMAGEM
N/D.

MÉTODOS DIAGNÓSTICOS
Eletrocardiograma — pode revelar arritmias ventriculares.

TRATAMENTO

- Intoxicação por sapos marinhos — quadro de emergência clínica; é comum a ocorrência de óbito.
- Descontaminação — lavar a boca do animal com quantidades abundantes de água por 5-10 min.
- Hipertermia (>40,6°C) — dar um banho frio; remover o paciente do banho assim que a temperatura chegar a 39,4°C.
- É imprescindível a realização de uma rápida avaliação da atividade cardíaca.

MEDICAÇÕES

MEDICAMENTO(S)
- Atropina — 0,04 mg/kg IM, SC; diminui a quantidade de salivação; ajuda a evitar a aspiração; utilizar em casos de bradicardia, bloqueio cardíaco ou outras alterações do nó sinoatrial, em consequência dos efeitos (semelhantes aos digitálicos) da toxina; não recomendada na presença de taquicardia grave.
- Esmolol ou propranolol — o esmolol tem ação muito curta e pode ser usado como uma dose de teste. Se a arritmia responder ao tratamento, será utilizado o propranolol por causa de sua duração de ação muito mais longa (horas; ver a seção "Contraindicações/Interações Possíveis"); talvez haja necessidade de uma administração rápida para combater as taquiarritmias; a administração pode ser repetida em 20 min; pode ser necessária uma infusão intravenosa contínua para arritmias persistentes.
- Esmolol 0,05-0,1 mg/kg IV a cada 5 min por uma dose máxima de 0,5 mg/kg.
- Propranolol 0,02 mg/kg IV lentamente, conforme a necessidade, até a dose máxima de 1 mg/kg.
- Anestesia com pentobarbital (cães) — aumenta a tolerância à intoxicação.
- Em casos com arritmias graves, pode-se indicar o tratamento com fragmentos Fab* de anticorpos específicos contra a digoxina (muito caro).

CONTRAINDICAÇÕES
- Cardiopatia ou asma brônquica — o paciente pode não tolerar o uso de β-bloqueadores, como esmolol e propranolol. Utilizar uma dose de teste do esmolol (duração de ação muito curta) e monitorizar rigorosamente antes de usar o propranolol (duração de ação muito mais longa).
- Anestésicos (p. ex., pentobarbital) — podem provocar a depressão da função do miocárdio já comprometido; dessa forma, é preciso ter cautela.

ACOMPANHAMENTO

- Monitorização eletrocardiográfica contínua — recomendada até a recuperação plena do paciente.
- Intoxicação por sapos do rio Colorado — os pacientes costumam se recuperar 30 min após o tratamento; se o animal for tratado, o óbito será relativamente incomum; não subestimar o risco de internação secundária.
- Intoxicação por sapos marinhos — quadro de emergência clínica; o óbito é comum.

DIVERSOS

Sugestões de Leitura
Peterson ME, Roberts BK. Toads. In: Peterson ME, Talcott PA, eds., Small Animal Toxicology, 2nd ed. St. Louis: Saunders, 2006, pp. 1083-1093.

Autor Michael E. Peterson
Consultor Editorial Gary D. Osweiler

---

* N. T.: Do inglês *Fragment antigen binding* (fragmento de ligação ao antígeno).

Toxicoses por Hidrocarboneto de Petróleo

CONSIDERAÇÕES GERAIS

DEFINIÇÃO
- Os hidrocarbonetos de petróleo constituem um grupo bastante diversificado de produtos derivados ou sintetizados a partir do óleo cru (petróleo bruto).
- Certos hidrocarbonetos que não têm origem no petróleo, como a terebintina e o óleo de linhaça, são, em termos toxicológicos, semelhantes o suficiente para serem considerados produtos à base de petróleo de peso molecular similar.
- Embora a intoxicação por óleo cru seja um problema relevante na vida selvagem e nos grandes animais, o envenenamento de pequenos animais resulta mais comumente da exposição a produtos comerciais refinados. Estes incluem misturas diversas como combustíveis, solventes, lubrificantes e ceras. Para complicar ainda mais a tarefa do clínico, existe o fato de que solventes à base de petróleo são utilizados frequentemente como carreadores "inertes" para outros tóxicos potenciais (p. ex., pesticidas, tintas e medicações).
- Do ponto de vista teórico, cada um das centenas de compostos que constituem até mesmo um produto relativamente simples como a gasolina tem suas próprias características físicas, químicas e toxicológicas, mas cada uma delas deve ser considerada no tratamento clínico do envenenamento. Na prática, entretanto, a maioria dos produtos derivados de petróleo pode ser "agrupada" em algumas categorias relativamente amplas, com base na volatilidade, na viscosidade e nos aditivos químicos. As misturas com altos pontos de ebulição (baixa volatilidade), como o asfalto, o óleo mineral e as ceras, são relativamente atóxicas. Os produtos com pontos relativamente baixos de ebulição, como o benzeno ou a terebintina, são aspirados com mais facilidade e, portanto, mais prováveis de causar pneumonite química. Em geral, os produtos mais voláteis também tendem a ser mais lipofílicos e, por isso, mais prontamente absorvidos por via sistêmica. Os produtos com alto conteúdo de hidrocarboneto aromático também estão mais predispostos à toxicidade sistêmica.
- A estocagem em recipientes inadequados e a falha na remoção de derramamentos são causas comuns de exposição nos animais de estimação. Os gatos podem ingerir quantidades significativas de gasolina ou outros hidrocarbonetos durante sua auto-higienização após contaminação tópica. Os animais de estimação frequentemente são envenenados por remédios populares que contêm gasolina, querosene e outros solventes como tônicos ou vermífugos. O uso de gasolina ou outros solventes na tentativa de remover material pegajoso da pelagem do animal também pode resultar em envenenamento.

FISIOPATOLOGIA
- Em geral, os efeitos com maior risco de morte aguda gerados pela ingestão de hidrocarbonetos resultam da pneumonite induzida por aspiração.
- A viscosidade e a tensão superficial são fortes determinantes do potencial pneumotóxico. A baixa viscosidade permite que os hidrocarbonetos penetrem ainda mais nas vias aéreas menos calibrosas. A baixa tensão superficial aumenta sua tendência a "umedecer" as superfícies pulmonares. Por exemplo, a aspiração de apenas 0,1 mL de hidrocarboneto de baixa viscosidade (p. ex., hexano) pode produzir pneumonite grave, ao passo que o produto de alta viscosidade (p. ex., óleo de motor) pode não penetrar nas vias aéreas principais.
- A inalação de vapores de hidrocarboneto (em contraste ao líquido aspirado) pode comprometer a função imune pulmonar.
- A exposição tópica a solventes à base de hidrocarboneto (p. ex., destilados de petróleo e terebintina) pode resultar na irritação e até mesmo na necrose da pele e da córnea.
- A toxicidade sistêmica é possível após exposição oral ou tópica. Embora não haja dados quantitativos prontamente aplicáveis aos pequenos animais, a toxicidade sistêmica foi relatada em seres humanos após exposição tópica ou inalação e deve ser considerada ao se avaliar os animais de estimação submetidos a uma exposição tópica maciça. Isso é particularmente importante nos pequenos animais (p. ex., filhotes de cães e de gatos, bem como roedores), que possuem uma proporção relativamente alta da área de superfície corporal em relação à massa corporal. A absorção sistêmica e, portanto, a toxicidade também são intensificadas por fatores como pelo longo, que aprisiona o produto contra a pele.

SISTEMA(S) ACOMETIDO(S)
- Cardíaco.
- Cutâneo.
- Gastrintestinal.
- Nervoso.
- Respiratório.

INCIDÊNCIA/PREVALÊNCIA
Na experiência do autor, a incidência de envenenamentos de pequenos animais tem diminuído nos últimos anos; contudo, os hidrocarbonetos de petróleo continuam sendo a principal causa de mortes por intoxicação não farmacológica em crianças.

IDENTIFICAÇÃO
Espécies
Cães e gatos.

SINAIS CLÍNICOS
Comentários Gerais
- A pneumonite é a complicação mais séria associada à ingestão de hidrocarbonetos de petróleo mais voláteis (p. ex., gasolina). Os sinais atribuíveis ao sistema respiratório costumam ocorrer dentro de alguns minutos a 1-2 h após a ingestão. Os sistemas nervoso central e gastrintestinal também podem ser acometidos, mas a morte geralmente resulta de insuficiência respiratória.
- Se ocorrer aspiração simultaneamente com a ingestão, haverá asfixia, tosse, ânsia de vômito e vários graus de dispneia. A lesão direta de componentes das vias aéreas e a ocorrência de broncospasmos podem resultar em hipoxia. A cianose também pode se desenvolver imediatamente à medida que o oxigênio alveolar é deslocado pelo vapor do hidrocarboneto.
- Há provas restritas de que *alguns* hidrocarbonetos sensibilizam o miocárdio às catecolaminas e podem precipitar arritmias.

Achados Anamnésicos
- Os sinais de envenenamento por hidrocarboneto raramente são característicos o bastante a ponto de permitir o diagnóstico sem pelo menos um forte índice de suspeita a partir do histórico. O histórico de (possível) exposição é essencial para o diagnóstico de intoxicação por hidrocarboneto.
- O envolvimento respiratório, quando presente, geralmente é progressivo nas primeiras 24-48 horas e depois desaparece de forma gradativa 3-10 dias após a exposição. É improvável o desenvolvimento de doença respiratória em animais que permanecem completamente assintomáticos por 6-12 horas após a ingestão.
- Os pacientes humanos relatam uma sensação de queimação na boca e na faringe imediatamente após a ingestão de gasolina. Os animais parecem sofrer os mesmos sintomas após ingerir hidrocarbonetos, além de babar, movimentar os maxilares, sacudir a cabeça e passar as patas no focinho.

Achados do Exame Físico
- Observadores atentos podem notar o odor característico de hidrocarboneto no hálito ou na pelagem do animal.
- A febre geralmente ocorre em 3-4 h após a aspiração, embora possa ocorrer em menos de uma hora ou em mais de 24 h.
- As propriedades irritantes dos produtos à base de petróleo podem resultar em vômito, cólica e diarreia após a exposição oral. A gravidade e, na verdade, a presença de tais sinais dependem da dose e de cada hidrocarboneto individualmente. Os hidrocarbonetos alifáticos pesados (p. ex., óleo mineral) podem produzir uma leve diarreia, mas nada mais do que isso. Os hidrocarbonetos mais leves (p. ex., gasolina) têm mais probabilidade de gerar cólica e vômito.
- Os animais intoxicados manifestam vertigem, ataxia e confusão mental. Os hidrocarbonetos produzem depressão e narcose na maioria dos casos, mas tremores e convulsões também foram relatados em alguns. Se a dose for muito alta, o animal poderá entrar em coma e morrer antes de exibir sinais de pneumonite, embora isso seja muito raro.
- Podem ocorrer arritmias e síncope como resultado da sensibilização do miocárdio às catecolaminas endógenas. A sensibilização miocárdica pode persistir por mais de 24-48h após a aparente recuperação dos efeitos neurológicos de intoxicação.

DIAGNÓSTICO

DIAGNÓSTICO DIFERENCIAL
- Várias doenças infecciosas, toxinas e/ou lesões podem resultar em sinais respiratórios semelhantes à aspiração de hidrocarboneto. Entretanto, apenas processos muito agudos (p. ex., traumatismo e quilotórax) demonstram rapidez semelhante de início.
- O vasto espectro de efeitos neurológicos ocasionalmente observado na intoxicação por hidrocarboneto pode ser confundido com aquele de intoxicação aguda por etilenoglicol ou por medicamento.

HEMOGRAMA/BIOQUÍMICA/URINÁLISE
- A urina e o soro serão negativos quanto à presença de etilenoglicol; a osmolalidade sérica permanecerá normal.
- Embora o hemograma completo possa indicar estresse, isso geralmente não ocorre no início da evolução do problema.

TOXICOSES POR HIDROCARBONETO DE PETRÓLEO

OUTROS TESTES LABORATORIAIS
• O teste de mancha simples envolve a mistura do vômito ou do conteúdo gástrico vigorosamente com água tépida (morna). Se houver gasolina ou outros destilados de petróleo, eles flutuarão na superfície. É preciso ter cuidado para distinguir entre produtos de petróleo e lipídios da dieta. O primeiro geralmente tem odor característico.
• A maioria dos produtos de petróleo mais leves que o querosene, se isolados e absorvidos em papel toalha, evapora com relativa rapidez e possui odor característico.
• A análise química da ingesta ou dos tecidos após a morte é útil na medicina legal (forense), mas não é prática para a avaliação clínica do caso agudo. Se a análise química for conduzida, coletar amostras o mais rápido possível e congelar em recipientes herméticos para evitar perdas causadas pela volatilização.

DIAGNÓSTICO POR IMAGEM
Os achados radiográficos são típicos de pneumonia por aspiração e consistem em densidades peri-hilares delicadas e infiltrados extensos nas porções ventrais dos pulmões. Tais achados pioram em 3-4 dias e depois melhoram de forma gradativa. Nem todos os animais com sinais radiográficos de aspiração de hidrocarboneto desenvolvem sinais respiratórios, mas as alterações radiográficas costumam persistir após a resolução dos sinais clínicos.

ACHADOS PATOLÓGICOS
• Se ocorreu aspiração, as principais lesões serão no trato respiratório. As lesões pulmonares são bilaterais e tipicamente envolvem as porções caudoventrais do pulmão. As lesões mais precoces incluem hiperemia, edema e hemorragia dentro das vias aéreas. O material estranho pode ser macroscopicamente visível nas vias aéreas menos calibrosas. Mais tarde, há broncospasmo, enfisema e atelectasia. Pneumatoceles, pneumotórax e enfisema subcutâneo resultam do colapso das vias aéreas. Pode haver ulcerações na mucosa da traqueia e nas vias aéreas mais calibrosas.
• Ocasionalmente, desenvolve-se pneumonia bacteriana, podendo resultar em abscesso.
• A toxicidade sistêmica muito ocasionalmente resulta em necrose hepática, miocárdica e/ou tubular renal se o animal sobreviver por >24 h.

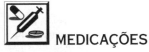

TRATAMENTO
CUIDADO(S) DE SAÚDE ADEQUADO(S)
• Em todos os casos de ingestão não complicada (i.e, não contaminada com alguma outra substância mais tóxica) de hidrocarboneto de petróleo, o principal objetivo é minimizar o risco de aspiração.
• Se a quantidade ingerida foi pequena e, particularmente, se o hidrocarboneto ingerido é conhecido por ser um dos produtos mais viscosos e menos voláteis (p. ex., óleo de motor e graxa), o repouso em gaiola e a observação podem ser tudo que é necessário.
• Se o volume ingerido foi substancial e o produto envolvido é conhecido por causar toxicidade sistêmica (p. ex., benzeno), o uso de carvão ativado fica indicado nas primeiras 4-6 h após a exposição. Estudos retrospectivos em crianças indicam que a lavagem não é benéfica.
• Se o produto contém outras substâncias altamente tóxicas (p. ex., pesticida), a descontaminação gástrica pode estar indicada, apesar do risco de aspiração. Se a lavagem for tentada, será essencial tomar precauções para evitar possível aspiração do conteúdo gástrico. Os eméticos estão contraindicados, exceto como último recurso para remover algum outro constituinte altamente tóxico (p. ex., pesticida) do trato gastrintestinal.
• Os efeitos respiratórios devem ser tratados de forma sintomática. Suplementação de oxigênio, pressão positiva contínua das vias aéreas e ventilação mecânica devem ser utilizadas sempre que houver necessidade. Entretanto, como o pneumomediastino, a pneumatocele e o pneumotórax são complicações comuns da pneumonite por hidrocarboneto, os sistemas de pressão positiva devem ser empregados com cautela. Além disso, visto que os pulmões são a principal via de eliminação sistêmica de hidrocarbonetos voláteis, os sistemas fechado ou semifechado devem ser esvaziados com frequência.
• A exposição tópica pode ser tratada, banhando o animal delicadamente com água morna e xampu suave. Se o pelo estiver particularmente pesado ou emaranhado, poderá ser necessário tosar as áreas contaminadas para evitar absorção sistêmica e minimizar a lesão cutânea.
• O tratamento sintomático das queimaduras por petróleo pode envolver a aplicação de antibacterianos tópicos ou outros agentes conforme a necessidade.
• Os hidrocarbonetos muito viscosos (p. ex., piche e ceras) também podem ser removidos com detergentes suaves. Como eles não são prontamente absorvidos, geram apenas irritação estética e cutânea, além de não serem difíceis de remover. Os materiais lipofílicos (p. ex., manteiga, banha de porco e removedor para as mãos de mecânicos) também podem ser úteis, mas a utilização de solventes não é recomendada.

CUIDADO(S) DE ENFERMAGEM
O repouso em gaiola fica indicado, tanto por seus efeitos benéficos sobre o processo de cicatrização como para minimizar os efeitos das catecolaminas induzidas pela agitação sobre o miocárdio potencialmente sensibilizado.

ORIENTAÇÃO AO PROPRIETÁRIO
Apesar de o serviço público advertir há décadas sobre os perigos dos produtos químicos domésticos, muitos proprietários de animais insistem em armazenar e utilizar produtos à base de petróleo de forma indevida. A consulta de animal exposto, intoxicado ou não, dá ao clínico uma ótima oportunidade de reforçar a necessidade de manter tais produtos fora do alcance de animais e crianças.

MEDICAÇÕES
MEDICAMENTO(S)
• No passado, o óleo mineral ou vegetal oral era recomendado para aumentar a viscosidade dos hidrocarbonetos de petróleo e, consequentemente, diminuir o risco de aspiração. Contudo, estudos retrospectivos em crianças sugerem que tal tratamento, na verdade, aumenta a probabilidade de pneumonia por aspiração e, por isso, a utilização desses óleos não é mais recomendada.
• A utilização de rotina de antibióticos é de valor questionável. A pneumonite por hidrocarboneto é basicamente de origem não bacteriana. Em um único estudo experimental em que foi administrada uma dose intratraqueal de querosene em cães, a administração parenteral de ampicilina e dexametasona não diminuiu a frequência respiratória nem as lesões pulmonares radiográficas, macroscópicas ou microscópicas. Entretanto, dadas as consequências potencialmente graves de complicações bacterianas e a inclinação relativamente pequena para o uso de antibióticos, pode ser prudente empregar alguma forma de profilaxia antimicrobiana caso tenha ocorrido vômito.
• Os corticosteroides são associados a números elevados de culturas pulmonares positivas em estudos retrospectivos e, por essa razão, são contraindicados.
• O broncospasmo pode ser tratado com β_2-agonistas.

PRECAUÇÕES
Induzir a êmese apenas como último recurso e exclusivamente nos casos em que exista um elevado grau de certeza de que deixar o material estranho no intestino represente um risco maior do que a aspiração.

ACOMPANHAMENTO
MONITORIZAÇÃO DO PACIENTE
Monitorizar o paciente por 3-4 dias para garantir que o hidrocarboneto ingerido foi removido do trato gastrintestinal e não ocorreram sequelas pulmonares.

EVOLUÇÃO ESPERADA E PROGNÓSTICO
Embora a diversidade dessa classe de produtos impeça qualquer prognóstico absoluto, a maioria das exposições a hidrocarbonetos responde de forma satisfatória à terapia conservativa de suporte.

DIVERSOS
Sugestões de Leitura
Raisbeck MF. Petroleum hydrocarbons. In: Peterson ME, Talcott PA, eds., Small Animal Toxicology. Philadelphia: Saunders, 2006, pp. 986-989.
Reese E, Kimbrough RD. Acute toxicity of gasoline and some additives. Environ Health Perspect 1993, 101:115-131.
Seymour FK, Henry JA. Assessment and management of acute poisoning by petroleum products. Hum Exp Toxicol 2001, 20:551-562.

Autor Merl F. Raisbeck
Consultor Editorial Gary D. Osweiler

Toxoplasmose

CONSIDERAÇÕES GERAIS

DEFINIÇÃO
Toxoplasma gondii — parasita protozoário coccídeo intracelular obrigatório que infecta quase todos os mamíferos; os felídeos são os hospedeiros definitivos; todos os outros animais de sangue quente (homeotérmicos) são hospedeiros intermediários.

FISIOPATOLOGIA
• Gravidade e manifestação — dependem da localização e do grau de lesão tecidual causada pelos cistos teciduais.
• Infecção — adquirida por meio da ingestão de cistos teciduais ou oocistos; os microrganismos disseminam-se para órgãos extraintestinais por via hematógena ou linfática; resulta em necrose focal de muitos órgãos (coração, olhos, SNC).
• A infecção disseminada aguda raramente é fatal.
• Doença crônica — formação de cistos teciduais; doença de baixo grau; não costuma ser aparente do ponto de vista clínico a menos que quadros de imunossupressão ou doença concomitante permitam a proliferação do microrganismo, induzindo a uma resposta inflamatória aguda.
• Doença clínica — frequentemente associada a outras infecções indutoras de imunossupressão grave (p. ex., cinomose, PIF e FeLV).

SISTEMA(S) ACOMETIDO(S)
• Multissistêmicos — em geral, os mesmos em cães e gatos.
• Oftálmico — cerca de 80% dos gatos acometidos apresentam indícios de inflamação intraocular, mais comumente uveíte.

INCIDÊNCIA/PREVALÊNCIA
• Em torno de 30% dos gatos e até 50% das pessoas são sorologicamente positivos ao *T. gondii*.
• A maioria dos animais permanece assintomática.

DISTRIBUIÇÃO GEOGRÁFICA
Mundial.

IDENTIFICAÇÃO
Espécies
Os gatos são mais comumente sintomáticos do que os cães.

Idade Média e Faixa Etária
Em um único estudo, a idade média foi de 4 anos e a variação, de 2 semanas a 16 anos.

Sexo Predominante
Machos felinos — mais comum.

SINAIS CLÍNICOS
Comentários Gerais
• Determinados principalmente pelo local e pela extensão dos danos ao órgão envolvido.
• Aguda — no momento da infecção inicial.
• Crônica — reativação da infecção encistada; causada por imunossupressão.

Achados Anamnésicos
• Sinais inespecíficos de letargia, depressão e anorexia.
• Perda de peso.
• Febre.
• Secreção ocular, fotofobia, pupilas mióticas (gatos).
• Angústia respiratória.
• Neurológicos — ataxia; crises convulsivas; tremores; paresia/paralisia; déficits dos nervos cranianos.
• Trato digestório — vômito; diarreia; dor abdominal; icterícia.
• Filhotes felinos natimortos.

Achados do Exame Físico
Gatos
• Mais grave em filhotes infectados por via transplacentária, que podem nascer mortos ou morrer antes do desmame.
• Filhotes sobreviventes — anorexia; letargia; febre alta irresponsiva a antibióticos; refletem necrose/inflamação dos pulmões (dispneia, ruídos respiratórios aumentados), do fígado (icterícia, aumento de volume abdominal decorrente de ascite) e do SNC (encefalopatia).
• Respiratórios e gastrintestinais (pós-natais) — mais comuns; anorexia; letargia; febre alta irresponsiva a antibióticos; dispneia; perda de peso; icterícia; vômito; diarreia; efusão abdominal.
• Neurológicos (pós-natais) — observados em <10% dos pacientes; cegueira; estupor; incoordenação; andar em círculos, torcicolo; anisocoria; crises convulsivantes.
• Sinais oculares (pós-natais) — comuns; uveíte (rubor aquoso, hifema, midríase); irite; descolamento da retina; iridociclite; precipitados ceráticos.
• Evolução rápida — pacientes agudamente acometidos com envolvimento do SNC e/ou do sistema respiratório.
• Evolução lenta — pacientes com reativação da infecção crônica.

Cães
• Jovens — geralmente a infecção é generalizada; febre; perda de peso; anorexia; tonsilite; dispneia; diarreia; vômito.
• Idosos — tendem a apresentar infecções localizadas; associadas principalmente aos sistemas neural e muscular.
• Neurológicos — muito variáveis; em geral, refletem inflamação neurológica difusa; crises convulsivas; tremores; ataxia; paresia; paralisia; fraqueza muscular; e tetraparesia.
• Oculares — raros; semelhantes aos sinais encontrados em gatos.
• Envolvimento cardíaco — embora possa ocorrer, não costuma ser aparente em termos clínicos.

CAUSAS
T. gondii.

FATORES DE RISCO
Imunossupressão — pode predispor o animal à infecção ou à reativação: FeLV, FIV, PIF, micoplasma hemotrópico, cinomose e glicocorticoides, quimioterapia ou pós-transplante renal.

DIAGNÓSTICO

DIAGNÓSTICO DIFERENCIAL
Gatos
• Doença intraocular (uveíte anterior) — PIF; FeLV; FIV; imunomediada; traumatismo; induzida pelo cristalino; úlcera de córnea com uveíte reflexa.
• Dispneia (sinais respiratórios) — asma; cardiogênica; pneumonia (bacteriana, fúngica, parasitária); neoplasia; dirofilariose; pleuropatia (efusões); hérnia diafragmática; lesão da parede torácica.
• Neurológico (causas de meningoencefalite) — virais (PIF, raiva, pseudorraiva); fúngicas (criptococose, blastomicose, histoplasmose); parasitárias (cuterebríase, coenurose, migração aberrante de dirofilárias); bacterianas; doença idiopática (poliencefalomielite felina).

Cães
• Associada muitas vezes a outras doenças imunossupressoras — por exemplo, podem ser observados sinais de cinomose.
• Neurológico — geralmente em cães muito jovens; diferenciar de *Neospora caninum* (ambos produzem doença neurológica [SNC] e neuromuscular).
• Considerar outras condições indutoras de sinais multifocais — toxicidade infecciosa ou inflamatória; doença metabólica.

HEMOGRAMA/BIOQUÍMICA/URINÁLISE
Hemograma Completo (Gatos)
• A maioria revela leve anemia normocítica normocrômica.
• Leucopenia — cerca de 50% dos pacientes com doença grave; principalmente em função da linfopenia.
• Neutropenia — isolada ou associada à linfopenia e desvio à esquerda degenerativo.
• Leucocitose — pode ocorrer durante a recuperação.

Bioquímica
• ALT e AST — aumento acentuado em grande parte dos pacientes.
• Hipoalbuminemia.
• Gatos — icterícia observada em cerca de 25% dos pacientes; em casos de pancreatite, observa-se com frequência o declínio brando nas concentrações séricas do cálcio; os níveis da amilase não são confiáveis.

Urinálise (Gatos)
• Proteinúria branda — pequena proporção dos pacientes.
• Bilirrubinúria — especialmente em casos de icterícia.

OUTROS TESTES LABORATORIAIS
Sorologia
• Títulos séricos de IgM, IgG e antígeno — consistem na informação mais definitiva obtida a partir de uma única amostra; determinam o tipo de infecção (ativa, recente, crônica) com amostra de acompanhamento coletada 3 semanas mais tarde.
• IgM — único teste sorológico de escolha para o diagnóstico de infecção ativa; níveis elevados 2 semanas após a infecção (em geral, coincidem com o início dos sinais clínicos); persistem por, no máximo, 3 meses e, em seguida, declinam; título prolongado: reativação ou atraso na mudança de classe dos anticorpos para IgG (resultado de imunossupressão por infecção pelos FeLV ou FIV ou terapia com esteroides).
• IgG — os títulos sobem 2-4 semanas após a infecção; persistem por >1 ano; um único título elevado não é diagnóstico de infecção ativa; o aumento de quatro vezes na titulação em um período de 3 semanas sugere infecção ativa.
• Antígeno — positivo 1-4 semanas após a infecção; como o antígeno permanece positivo durante as infecções ativas ou crônicas persistentes, ele não acrescenta muitos dados aos resultados dos títulos de anticorpos.
• Pode ser formulado um diagnóstico presuntivo de doença clínica antes do óbito com base nos parâmetros clínicos e sorológicos: (a) indícios sorológicos de infecção recente ou ativa — títulos

TOXOPLASMOSE

elevados de IgM, alteração de quatro vezes nos títulos de IgG, (b) exclusão de outras causas da síndrome clínica, e (c) resposta benéfica aos medicamentos contra *Toxoplasma*.
• PCR — técnica utilizada para verificar a presença de *T. gondii* em amostras biológicas; disponível em vários laboratórios.

DIAGNÓSTICO POR IMAGEM
Radiografias — podem-se observar: padrão misto de infiltrados pulmonares intersticiais e alveolares irregulares, efusões pleurais e abdominais, além de hepatomegalia.

MÉTODOS DIAGNÓSTICOS
• LCS — contagem elevada de leucócitos (tanto células mononucleares como neutrófilos) e de proteínas em pacientes encefalopáticos.
• Citologia — o microrganismo raramente é detectado em líquidos corporais durante a infecção aguda (LCS, efusões pleurais e peritoneais); o lavado broncoalveolar é eficaz na identificação dos microrganismos em gatos acometidos com sinais de envolvimento pulmonar.
• Exame fecal — a avaliação com solução de açúcar de Sheather pode ser diagnóstica; a liberação fecal de oocistos raramente ocorre durante a doença clínica; os oocistos podem ser detectados nos exames de rotina em gatos assintomáticos, mas são morfologicamente indistinguíveis de *Hammondia* spp. e *Besnoitia*; diferenciar os microrganismos por meio da inoculação em camundongos.

ACHADOS PATOLÓGICOS
• Focos necróticos — até 1 cm; mais comuns no fígado, no pâncreas, nos linfonodos mesentéricos e nos pulmões; necrose cerebral (áreas de descoloração de 1 cm).
• Úlceras e granulomas — podem ser observados no estômago e no intestino delgado.

TRATAMENTO

CUIDADO(S) DE SAÚDE ADEQUADO(S)
• Em geral, os animais são tratados em um esquema ambulatorial.
• Internação — em casos de pacientes acometidos por doença grave, que não conseguem manter níveis adequados de nutrição e hidratação.
• Confinamento — para pacientes com sinais neurológicos.

CUIDADO(S) DE ENFERMAGEM
Desidratação — fluidos intravenosos.

ORIENTAÇÃO AO PROPRIETÁRIO
• Gatos — prognóstico reservado em pacientes que necessitam de terapia; a resposta terapêutica é inconsistente.
• Neonatos e animais gravemente imunocomprometidos — prognóstico mais grave.

MEDICAÇÕES

MEDICAMENTO(S) DE ESCOLHA
• Clindamicina — 25-50 mg/kg VO ou IM diariamente, divididos em duas doses, por no mínimo 2 semanas após a remissão dos sinais clínicos.
• Colírio de prednisona a 1% — a cada 8 h por 2 semanas em casos de uveíte; uso concomitante.

PRECAUÇÕES
Clindamicina — anorexia, vômito e diarreia (dependentes da dose).

MEDICAMENTO(S) ALTERNATIVO(S)
• Sulfadiazina (30 mg/kg VO a cada 12 h) em combinação com pirimetamina (0,5 mg/kg VO a cada 12 h) por 2 semanas; podem causar depressão, anemia, leucopenia e trombocitopenia, especialmente em gatos.
• Ácido folínico (5 mg/dia) ou levedura de cerveja (100 mg/kg/dia) — para corrigir a supressão da medula óssea causada pela terapia com sulfadiazina/pirimetamina.

ACOMPANHAMENTO

MONITORIZAÇÃO DO PACIENTE
Clindamicina
• Examinar o paciente 2 dias após o início do tratamento — os sinais clínicos (febre, hiperestesia, anorexia, uveíte) devem começar a desaparecer; a uveíte deve exibir resolução completa dentro de 1 semana.
• Examinar o paciente 2 semanas após o início do tratamento — avaliar os déficits neuromusculares; devem apresentar resolução parcial (alguns déficits são permanentes em decorrência de danos neurológicos [SNC] ou neuromusculares periféricos).
• Examinar o paciente 2 semanas após a resolução dos sinais clínicos relatada pelo proprietário — avaliar a suspensão do tratamento; alguns déficits neuromusculares são permanentes.

PREVENÇÃO
Gatos
• Dieta — evitar a ingestão de carne crua, ossos, vísceras ou leite não pasteurizado (especialmente leite de cabra); ou os vetores mecânicos (moscas, baratas); fornecer apenas carne bem passada.
• Comportamento — evitar os hábitos de vida livre para a caça de presas (pássaros, roedores) ou a entrada em galpões onde os animais de produção são alojados.

EVOLUÇÃO ESPERADA E PROGNÓSTICO
• Prognóstico — reservado; resposta variada aos medicamentos utilizados no tratamento.
• Aguda — a terapia imediata e rigorosa é muitas vezes bem-sucedida.
• Déficits residuais (especialmente neurológicos) — não podem ser previstos antes do final da terapia.
• Doença ocular — em geral, é responsiva à terapia apropriada.
• Doença muscular ou neurológica grave — geralmente causa debilidade crônica.

DIVERSOS

DISTÚRBIOS ASSOCIADOS
• Cães jovens — cinomose.
• Gatos — FeLV, PIF e FIV; a infecção pelo FIV não influencia o desfecho clínico ou a capacidade do animal em montar uma resposta imune protetora à subsequente reinfecção; transplante renal.

FATORES RELACIONADOS COM A IDADE
A doença é pior em neonatos.

POTENCIAL ZOONÓTICO
• Considerável.
• Gatos — animais saudáveis com título positivo de anticorpos representam um pequeno risco aos seres humanos; já os animais sem título de anticorpos apresentam um risco maior de virem a ser infectados, liberando oocistos nas fezes e constituindo perigo aos seres humanos.
• Evitar o contato com oocistos ou cistos teciduais — não fornecer carne crua; lavar as mãos e as superfícies (tábuas de corte) após o preparo de carnes cruas; ferver a água de bebida se a fonte não for confiável; manter as caixas de areia cobertas para evitar a defecação dos gatos; usar luvas ao trabalhar em jardins; lavar as mãos e os vegetais antes das refeições para evitar o contato com os oocistos nos solos contaminados; esvaziar as bandejas sanitárias dos gatos diariamente (os oocistos necessitam de pelo menos 24 h para se tornarem infectantes); desinfetar as bandejas sanitárias com água fervente; controlar a população de gatos vadios/errantes, evitando a contaminação do ambiente por oocistos.
• Mulheres gestantes — evitar todo e qualquer contato com gatos que estejam excretando oocistos nas fezes; evitar o contato com solos e bandejas sanitárias de gatos; não manipular nem comer carnes cruas (para matar o microrganismo, deve-se proceder ao cozimento a 66°C).

GESTAÇÃO/FERTILIDADE/REPRODUÇÃO
• Parasitemia durante a prenhez — disseminação do microrganismo ao feto; isso provavelmente não acontece a menos que a primeira infecção da fêmea ocorra durante a prenhez (assim como ocorre em seres humanos).
• A transmissão placentária é rara.

ABREVIATURA(S)
• ALT = alanina aminotransferase.
• AST = aspartato aminotransferase.
• FeLV = vírus da leucemia felina.
• FIV = vírus da imunodeficiência felina.
• LCS = líquido cerebrospinal.
• PCR = reação em cadeia da polimerase.
• PIF = peritonite infecciosa felina.
• SNC = sistema nervoso central.

Sugestões de Leitura
Dubey JP, Lappin MR. Toxoplasmosis and neosporosis. In: Greene CE, ed., Infectious Diseases of the Dog and Cat, 3rd ed. St. Louis: Saunders Elsevier, 2006, pp. 754-775.
Schatzberg SJ, Haley NJ, Barr SC, et al. Use of a multiplex polymerase chain reaction assay in the antemortem diagnosis of toxoplasmosis and neosporosis in the central nervous system of cats and dogs. Am J Vet Res 2003, 64:1507-1513.

Autor Stephen C. Barr
Consultor Editorial Stephen C. Barr

Transtornos Compulsivos — Cães

CONSIDERAÇÕES GERAIS

DEFINIÇÃO
• Sequência repetitiva, exagerada e/ou sustentada (contínua), relativamente invariável, de movimentos, que pode ou não ser derivada de comportamentos normais de preservação (p. ex., auto-higienização, alimentação e caminhada); no entanto, tal comportamento aparentemente se manifesta sem estímulo, finalidade ou função, muitas vezes com contextos/alvos não habituais.
• Grupo heterogêneo de comportamentos — categorizados como distúrbios locomotores (movimentos giratórios, perseguição da cauda, andar em círculo, corridas contra cercas/grades, andar compassado, perseguição de luz/sombra); bucais (lambedura, sucção/mordedura de objeto/parte do corpo [p. ex., flanco, cauda, membro], pica [apetite depravado]); ou alucinatórios ("caçar moscas imaginárias", checar a extremidade traseira (posterior), ficar estático/paralisado, manter um olhar fixo) com ou sem respostas vocais e afetivas.

FISIOPATOLOGIA
• Indeterminada; provavelmente associados a alterações na função neurotransmissora do SNC: principalmente da serotonina; a dopamina e as endorfinas também são implicadas. • Diferentes transtornos compulsivos podem, de preferência, envolver diferentes regiões do cérebro.
• Conflito ou frustração motivacional parece deflagrar os comportamentos em contextos específicos associados à hiperexcitação (altos níveis de excitação/agitação); com o passar do tempo, com o conflito repetido/mantido, o comportamento torna-se independente dos estímulos originais de deflagração, sendo exibido em diversos contextos, na ausência aparente de estímulo.

SISTEMA(S) ACOMETIDO(S)
• Comportamental — medo, ansiedade, agressividade. • Cardiovascular — taquicardia. • Endócrino/metabólico — sinais causados por suprarregulação do eixo hipotalâmico-hipofisário-adrenal. • Gastrintestinal — inapetência, gastrenterite, obstrução por corpo estranho. • Sanguíneo/linfático/imune — leucograma de estresse. • Musculosquelético — perda de peso, lesão autoinfligida. • Respiratório — taquipneia. • Cutâneo/Exócrino — abrasões/lacerações; feridas/infecções cutâneas secundárias a autotraumatismo.

GENÉTICA
• Provável predisposição/suscetibilidade genética: maior do que a ocorrência esperada entre os parentes de primeira geração (embora as manifestações possam diferir). • Certas raças são super-representadas para transtornos compulsivos específicos.

IDENTIFICAÇÃO
Espécies
Cães.
Raça(s) Predominante(s)
• Cães: Bull terrier — movimentos giratórios, paralisação; Pastor alemão — movimentos giratórios, perseguição da cauda; Dinamarquês, Pointer alemão de pelo curto — comportamentos autodirecionados com a boca, corridas contra cercas/grades, alucinações; Doberman — sucção do flanco/cobertor; Schnauzer miniatura — verificação da parte traseira (posterior); Border collie — perseguição de luz/sombra.

Idade Média e Faixa Etária
Podem se apresentar em qualquer idade; geralmente se desenvolvem desde o início da maturidade social (6 meses) até a maturidade social (12-24 meses).

Sexo Predominante
Alguns transtornos compulsivos podem ser mais comuns em machos.

SINAIS CLÍNICOS
Comentários Gerais
• Há uma ampla variedade de manifestações possíveis: os comportamentos podem ser repetitivos ou estáticos (p. ex., paralisação).
• Os sinais podem ou não ser observados durante o exame. As descrições feitas pelo proprietários podem não ser claras; utilizar filmagens para auxiliar no diagnóstico e no planejamento terapêutico.

Achados Anamnésicos
• Pode haver outros sinais de ansiedade/diagnósticos comportamentais concomitantes (p. ex., ansiedade da separação, medos, agressividade) e/ou histórico de estresse (p. ex., estimulação inadequada, punição, mudança de horários, rotina ou casa). • O comportamento se manifesta primeiramente como parte de alguma brincadeira ou em situações de alto nível de excitação/agitação ou estresse; por fim, acaba ocorrendo em inúmeros contextos sem deflagradores identificáveis.
• Certos comportamentos de transtorno compulsivo manifestam-se em situações com pouca ou nenhuma estimulação externa ou evidência de estímulo (p. ex., sucção de cobertor).
• Ocorre com ou sem a presença do proprietário. Se o animal receber punição frequente pelo comportamento, isso pode dificultar a detecção quando o proprietário estiver em casa. • Indicações de transtorno compulsivo — o comportamento é ritualizado, muitas vezes de forma exagerada e, com o tempo, aumenta em termos de frequência, intensidade e duração. • Pode ser difícil ou impossível interromper o comportamento (mesmo com contenção física). • O comportamento pode interferir nas funções normais do cão, como alimentação, sono, interações sociais.

Achados do Exame Físico
• Podem não ser dignos de nota.
• Pode haver lesões autoinfligidas, claudicação, más condições corporais; manchas de saliva, alopecia, inflamação, feridas/infecções de gravidade variada (especialmente em regiões como cauda, membros anteriores, extremidades distais); desgaste/dano excessivos do dente.
• O comportamento do transtorno compulsivo pode ser observado durante o exame físico.

CAUSAS
Não há causas diretas.

FATORES DE RISCO
• Estresse secundário a ambiente (p. ex., confinamento em canil — movimentos giratórios), tratamento, doença, outros.
• Reforço do comportamento pelo proprietário ou ambiente.
• Doença ou dor — podem aumentar a ansiedade ou ser a causa primária do comportamento.
• Anormalidades sensoriais (p. ex., déficits visuais) podem contribuir para o quadro.

DIAGNÓSTICO

DIAGNÓSTICO DIFERENCIAL
• Dermatopatia (p. ex., atopia). • Gastrenteropatia (p. ex., enteropatia inflamatória). • Doença metabólica/endócrina (p. ex., síndrome de Cushing). • Neuropatia (p. ex., neoplasia do prosencéfalo). • Doença ortopédica (p. ex., artropatia degenerativa). • Qualquer distúrbio indutor de anormalidades sensoriais (disestesia, parestesia; p. ex., neuropatia sensorial). • Outros comportamentos problemáticos: comportamentos de desalojamento ou conflito, busca por brincadeira e atenção, e comportamentos secundários à falta de estimulação. • Com frequência, há necessidade de métodos diagnósticos intensivos para descartar causas físicas do comportamento, especialmente em casos de automutilação.

HEMOGRAMA/BIOQUÍMICA/URINÁLISE
• Os resultados costumam ficar dentro da faixa normal de referência dos laboratórios — úteis para triagem quanto ao estado de saúde geral; adequados antes do uso de medicamentos fora da indicação da bula. • Há relatos de aumento do hematócrito, colesterol, triglicerídeo.

OUTROS TESTES LABORATORIAIS
Diversos; específicos para os diagnósticos diferenciais.

DIAGNÓSTICO POR IMAGEM
• TC e RM — excluem encefalopatias estruturais.
• Radiografia, ultrassonografia — descartam várias anormalidades subjacentes. • Ecocardiografia — exclui ansiedade induzida por cardiopatia.

MÉTODOS DIAGNÓSTICOS
• Não há nenhum método diagnóstico específico para transtorno compulsivo. • Indicações com base em outros diagnósticos diferenciais (p. ex., biopsia).

TRATAMENTO

Nem todo comportamento repetitivo é anormal, podendo representar um mecanismo benéfico para lidar com alguma situação. Se o comportamento não for nocivo nem interferir nas funções normais do paciente, nem na saúde e nem no elo homem-animal, a intervenção pode ser desnecessária ou contraindicada.

CUIDADO(S) DE SAÚDE ADEQUADO(S)
• Em geral, o tratamento é feito em um esquema ambulatorial a menos que os pacientes com automutilação e lesão autoinfligida graves necessitem de proteção do ambiente até que os medicamentos sejam eficazes (dias a semanas); a internação pode exacerbar o transtorno compulsivo. • Sedação — medida provisória, mas necessária para interromper a automutilação grave; aumenta a suspeita de anormalidade física subjacente. • Tratar os distúrbios físicos associados (primários ou secundários) de forma intensiva.
• Fazer uso da combinação de modificação ambiental, mudança comportamental e tratamento farmacológico. • Intervenção farmacológica — implementar precocemente; a redução da ansiedade facilita a terapia comportamental. • Modificação ambiental —

ESPÉCIES CANINA E FELINA

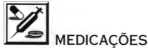

TRANSTORNOS COMPULSIVOS — CÃES

reduzir o estresse e a ansiedade; identificar e remover as fontes (p. ex., deflagradores do comportamento de transtorno compulsivo) e/ou iniciar os exercícios de dessensibilização e contracondicionamento. • Punição — contraindicada em todos os contextos; aumenta a ansiedade, podendo agravar o comportamento e estimular sua manifestação em secreto.
• Proporcionar interações estruturadas e constantes, além de rotina, em todos os casos, com quantidade suficiente de exercícios; enriquecimento/estimulação mental adequados para a espécie e o animal individualmente (com base no bom senso clínico); em geral, inclui adestramento lúdico interativo e à base de recompensa. • Mudança comportamental — ensinar o paciente a relaxar em diversos cenários ambientais; ensinar também um comportamento calmo e desejável, incompatível com aquele estereotipado vinculado a um comando verbal (p. ex., para o comportamento de andar em círculo, ensinar o animal a deitar com a cabeça e o pescoço esticados em resposta ao comando "Head down" [Cabeça para baixo]). Em alguns casos, uma coleira cervical (p. ex., Gentle Leader, Halti) deixada no cão (quando o proprietário está em casa) nas situações problemáticas pode permitir que o proprietário faça uso de uma orientação física delicada e suave em conjunto com incentivo/comando verbais para interromper o comportamento e redirecioná-lo de forma mais eficaz. • Incentivar o proprietário a identificar as situações em que ocorre o transtorno compulsivo e a prevê-lo antecipadamente, engajando o animal de estimação em uma atividade incompatível com o comportamento em questão; se o comportamento ocorrer, deve-se interrompê-lo imediatamente, redirecionando o animal para um comportamento alternativo com posterior recompensa (alimento, brincadeira ou outro reforço). • Fazer com que os proprietários monitorizem os comportamentos por meio de vídeos e diários para uma avaliação objetiva da resposta à terapia. As respostas podem ocorrer na frequência de manifestação (número de ataques) ou na intensidade dos ataques ou, possivelmente, ambas. Uma conversa sobre a escala de classificação e a forma de julgamento das alterações ajuda na avaliação da resposta terapêutica. • Evitar bandagens, coleiras, ataduras e engradados, pois tais medidas aumentam a angústia, não tratam o problema comportamental e ainda podem agravá-lo. Utilizá-los o mais brevemente possível e necessários para garantir a cicatrização de feridas.

ATIVIDADE
Depende das particularidades do caso.

DIETA
Depende das particularidades do caso.

ORIENTAÇÃO AO PROPRIETÁRIO
• É improvável que o problema seja curado; em geral, necessita de tratamento vitalício (i. e., pelo resto da vida).
• Orientar o proprietário a identificar todos os comportamentos e linguagens corporais associados à ansiedade.

CONSIDERAÇÕES CIRÚRGICAS
Amputação — evitar; é provável que o problema continue mesmo na ausência da parte do corpo acometida.

MEDICAÇÕES

MEDICAMENTO(S) DE ESCOLHA
• ATC e ISRS — atuam por meio de efeitos serotoninérgicos sobre o SNC. • Tratar, em geral, com o extremo inferior da faixa de dosagem por 4-6 semanas; aumentar gradativamente a dose em caso de ineficácia e na ausência de eventos adversos. • ISRS: fluoxetina 1-2 mg/kg a cada 24 h; sertralina 1-3 mg/kg a cada 24 h; paroxetina 1-2 mg/kg a cada 24 h. • ATC: a clomipramina é o agente mais serotoninérgico (mais eficaz, com menos efeitos colaterais) — 2-3 mg/kg a cada 12 h. • Se os sintomas desaparecerem, continuar a medicação por ≥1 mês e, depois, reduzir a dose para em uma frequência não superior a 25% por semana. É comum a recidiva.

CONTRAINDICAÇÕES
• Comprometimento hepático ou renal — para medicamentos metabolizados por esses órgãos.
• Anomalias de condução cardíaca — ATC. • Ter extremo cuidado ao se combinar agentes serotoninérgicos (p. ex., tramadol); risco de síndrome serotoninérgica (pode ser fatal). • Não utilizar ISRS ou ATC em até 2 semanas após o uso de inibidores da MAO (p. ex., selegilina, amitraz).

PRECAUÇÕES
• Todos os medicamentos listados são utilizados fora da indicação da bula nos Estados Unidos.
• Superdosagem dos ATC — distúrbios profundos de condução cardíaca. • Superdosagem de ATC/ISRS — síndrome serotoninérgica. • Efeitos colaterais mais comuns de ISRS e ATC: letargia, alteração do apetite; menos comuns: ansiedade/reatividade acentuada; os efeitos colaterais graves podem exigir a interrupção do medicamento.

INTERAÇÕES POSSÍVEIS
Os ISRS inibem de forma competitiva as enzimas do sistema citocromo P450: podem aumentar os níveis de varfarina, muitos ATC, alguns benzodiazepínicos e anticonvulsivantes, além de outros medicamentos; averiguar a compatibilidade e ajustar a dose se necessário.

MEDICAMENTO(S) ALTERNATIVO(S)
• Feromônios sintéticos podem diminuir a ansiedade: feromônio apaziguador de cães.
• L-Teanina pode reduzir a ansiedade (ver a bula em busca da dosagem). • ATC de segunda linha terapêutica, p. ex., amitriptilina 1-6 mg/kg a cada 12 h. • Selegilina (inibidor da MAO) 0,5-1 mg/kg a cada 24 h: pode ser eficaz em alguns casos.
• Antagonistas narcóticos (p. ex., naltrexona, naloxona), antipsicóticos (p. ex., tioridazina, haloperidol): risco de eventos adversos graves, eficácia controversa, falta de ansiólise; uso não recomendado em vista das alternativas disponíveis.

ACOMPANHAMENTO

MONITORIZAÇÃO DO PACIENTE
• Hemograma completo, bioquímica, T_4 (os ATC podem reduzir artificialmente os níveis séricos desse hormônio) e urinálise — semestral a anual se o paciente estiver sob tratamento crônico; ajustar as dosagens de acordo com os exames. • Os medicamentos podem levar 8-12 semanas ou mais para fazer efeito sobre os transtornos compulsivos; o primeiro sinal de eficácia pode ser uma mudança na duração/frequência do ataque. • As recidivas são comuns durante situações de estresse; tratar com aumento na intensidade de modificação do comportamento, além da adição de ansiolíticos de ação mais breve a curto prazo (p. ex., benzodiazepínicos).

PREVENÇÃO
Monitorização dos animais com os parentes acometidos; identificação e intervenção precoces.

COMPLICAÇÕES POSSÍVEIS
Lesão dermatológica/musculosquelética; distúrbios gastrintestinais.

EVOLUÇÃO ESPERADA E PROGNÓSTICO
• Os transtornos compulsivos sem tratamento sempre evoluem. • Redução de >50% no transtorno compulsivo em aproximadamente dois terços dos casos com medicamentos adequados e modificações comportamental/ambiental.

DIVERSOS

DISTÚRBIOS ASSOCIADOS
• Enteropatia inflamatória. • Dermatite acral por lambedura.

GESTAÇÃO/FERTILIDADE/REPRODUÇÃO
• Os medicamentos listados não foram avaliados ou são contraindicados em animais prenhes; portanto, deve-se evitar o uso. • Os animais acometidos não devem ser acasalados.

SINÔNIMO(S)
Transtorno obsessivo-compulsivo (TOC).

VER TAMBÉM
Dermatite acral por lambedura.

ABREVIATURA(S)
• ATC = antidepressivo tricíclico. • ISRS = inibidor seletivo de recaptação da serotonina.
• MAO = monoamina oxidase. • RM = ressonância magnética. • SNC = sistema nervoso central. • TC = tomografia computadorizada. T_4 = tireoxina.

Sugestões de Leitura
Crowell-Davis SL, Murray T. Veterinary Psychopharmacology. Ames, IA: Blackwell, 2006.
Denerolle P, White SD, Taylor TS, Vandenabeele SIJ. Organic diseases mimicking acral lick dermatitis in six dogs. JAAHA 2007, 43:215-220.
Irimajiri M, Luescher AU, Douglass G, Robertson-Plouch C, Zimmermann A, Hozak R. Randomized, controlled clinical trial of efficacy of fluoxetine for treatment of compulsive disorders in dogs. JAVMA 2009, 235(6):705-709.
Luescher AU. Diagnosis and management of compulsive disorders in dogs and cats. Vet Clin North Am Small Anim Pract 2003, 33:253-267.
Overall KL, Dunham AE. Clinical features and outcome in dogs and cats with obsessive-compulsive disorder: 126 cases (1989-2000). JAVMA 2002, 221:1445-1452.

Autor Mary P. Klinck
Consultor Editorial Debra F. Horwitz
Agradecimento Karen L. Overall

Transtornos Compulsivos — Gatos

CONSIDERAÇÕES GERAIS

DEFINIÇÃO
• Padrões comportamentais repetitivos e exagerados, relativamente invariáveis, derivados com frequência de comportamentos normais, mas fora de contexto e sem função aparente. Executados para a exclusão de outros comportamentos normais ou para o detrimento do animal. • Controversos quanto à sua classificação e interpretação; quando não se consegue identificar uma causa (i. e., em casos idiopáticos), esse título pode incluir outros comportamentos, como dermatite/alopecia psicogênica, vocalização repetitiva, andar compulsivo e sucção ou mastigação de tecidos.

FISIOPATOLOGIA
• Diagnóstico por exclusão; é imprescindível descartar as causas fisiopatológicas antes que a formulação do diagnóstico seja possível. A fisiopatologia subjacente pode envolver a atuação de neurotransmissores centrais, como serotonina, dopamina e β-endorfinas. • Pode representar uma resposta comportamental ao confinamento, a evento específico indutor de ansiedade ou a condições ambientais indefinidas (p. ex., conflito, estresse, ansiedade e frustração); com o passar do tempo, pode se tornar um comportamento fixo e independente do ambiente. • Os comportamentos podem ser de autorreforço — podem fazer com que alguns animais lidem com afecções que não atendam às suas necessidades específicas da espécie. • O proprietário pode reforçar o comportamento, fornecendo alimentos ou dando maior atenção ao gato em resposta ao transtorno compulsivo.

SISTEMA(S) ACOMETIDO(S)
• Comportamental. • Cutâneo/exócrino — dermatite/alopecia psicogênica.
• Musculoesquelético — vocalização repetitiva, andar compulsivo. • Gastrintestinal — mastigação de tecidos, sucção de lã.

GENÉTICA
Não foi identificada nenhuma relação genética específica, embora os correlatos raciais sugiram um componente hereditário.

INCIDÊNCIA/PREVALÊNCIA
Desconhecida, incomum.

DISTRIBUIÇÃO GEOGRÁFICA
Nenhuma.

IDENTIFICAÇÃO
Espécies
Gatos.

Raça(s) Predominante(s)
Gato Siamês, Birmanês e outras raças asiáticas, bem como os mestiços — super-representados para os transtornos de vocalização repetitiva e mastigação de tecidos.

Idade Média e Faixa Etária
Idade de início de aproximadamente 24 meses (faixa etária de 12-49 meses).

Sexo Predominante
Nenhum; ambos os sexos são igualmente acometidos.

SINAIS CLÍNICOS
Comentários Gerais
• Tais comportamentos, uma vez desencadeados, poderão aumentar rapidamente em termos de frequência se forem reforçados de algum modo pelo proprietário, seja por meio da alimentação ou da atenção dispensada. • A resposta ou reação do proprietário ao comportamento constitui parte integrante significativa da anamnese.

Achados Anamnésicos
• Dermatite/alopecia psicogênica — desde a auto-higienização com lambedura excessiva até a exclusão de outras atividades; o animal de estimação pode se esconder a fim de evitar repreensão ou punição (resposta negativa) do proprietário; a duração do problema é variável; o início pode coincidir com alguma modificação do ambiente (p. ex., mudança de casa ou inclusão de um novo membro na família). • Andar compulsivo — o comportamento pode começar de forma intermitente e aumentar em frequência; o início pode ocorrer em um período de confinamento (p. ex., acesso limitado à rua). • Vocalização repetitiva. • Sucção e mastigação de tecidos — alguns pacientes demonstram preferências ao tipo ou à textura de tecidos específicos, como a lã; podem ainda mastigar ou ingerir o tecido, além de triturá-lo com seus dentes molares; os animais podem se tornar peritos em encontrar o tipo de tecido preferido.

Achados do Exame Físico
• Alopecia psicogênica — focal, parcial e bilateral; ocorre mais comumente nas regiões da virilha, do ventre e das faces mediais ou caudais da coxa; aparência cutânea variável (normal ou anormal; eritematosa a esfoliada). • Andar compulsivo — tipicamente dentro dos limites de normalidade; descartar anormalidades neurológicas.
• Vocalização repetitiva — caracteristicamente dentro dos limites de normalidade, descartar hipertensão. • Sucção/mastigação de tecidos — geralmente dentro dos limites de normalidade; pode ocorrer inflamação ou obstrução gastrintestinais secundárias.

CAUSAS
• Não identificadas. • Descartar as causas orgânicas antes de se presumir uma base psicogênica.

FATORES DE RISCO
• Predisposição dos gatos por alterações nos arredores. • Descritos mais comumente em gatos domésticos.

DIAGNÓSTICO

DIAGNÓSTICO DIFERENCIAL
Descartar os diferenciais clínicos, incluindo crises convulsivas psicomotoras, antes de formular um diagnóstico comportamental. É necessária a realização de anamnese detalhada.

Alopecia Psicogênica
• Distúrbios cutâneos — especialmente aqueles associados a prurido. • Ectoparasitas, como pulgas.
• Dermatite fúngica. • Dermatite bacteriana.
• Dermatite alérgica — incluindo alergia alimentar. • Neoplasia cutânea. • Complexo granuloma eosinofílico. • Distúrbios do sistema nervoso. • Ruptura de disco intervertebral e neurite associada. • Síndrome de hiperestesia felina. • Dor.

Andar Compulsivo
• Comportamento sexual normal. • Frustração de barreira, secundária a confinamento. • Distúrbios do sistema nervoso. • Dor crônica. • Lesões cerebrais focais — tumor; acidente vascular.
• Distúrbio convulsivo. • Distúrbios metabólicos e endócrinos. • Deficiência de biotina.
• Encefalopatia hepática. • Hipertireoidismo.
• Intoxicação pelo chumbo. • Insuficiência renal.
• Deficiência de tiamina. • Síndrome de hiperestesia.

Vocalização Repetitiva
• Comportamento sexual normal. • Surdez.
• Hipertireoidismo. • Intoxicação pelo chumbo.
• Hipertensão.

Sucção/Mastigação de Tecido
• Intoxicação pelo chumbo. • Hipertireoidismo.
• Deficiência de tiamina.

HEMOGRAMA/BIOQUÍMICA/URINÁLISE
Obtenção de banco de dados mínimo para descartar anormalidades metabólicas. Nenhuma anormalidade médica compatível está associada a transtornos compulsivos.

OUTROS TESTES LABORATORIAIS
Alopecia Psicogênica
• Raspados cutâneos, culturas fúngicas e bacterianas, além de biopsias cutâneas.

Andar Compulsivo
• Análise do LCS — se indicada por exame neurológico anormal. • T_4 sérico.

Vocalização Repetitiva
• Análise do LCS — se indicada por exame neurológico anormal.
• Mensuração da pressão arterial.
• T_4 sérico.

Sucção/Mastigação de Tecido
• Nível sérico de chumbo — se indicado em casos de pica (apetite depravado).
• T_4 sérico.

DIAGNÓSTICO POR IMAGEM
• TC ou RM — se indicadas por anormalidades constatadas ao exame neurológico.
• Obtenção de imagens da tireoide — se indicada por níveis séricos questionáveis dos hormônios tireoidianos.

MÉTODOS DIAGNÓSTICOS
Alopecia psicogênica
• Exame microscópico dos pelos.
• Raspados cutâneos, culturas fúngicas e bacterianas, biopsias cutâneas, exames em busca de ectoparasitas, e testes alérgicos intradérmicos — descartam distúrbio dermatológico.
• Pode-se experimentar uma dieta de eliminação (hipoalergênica).

ACHADOS PATOLÓGICOS
Alopecia Psicogênica
• Exame microscópico dos pelos — tipicamente, as diáfises encontram-se rompidas por completo e em comprimentos variáveis, em consequência do traumatismo provocado pela lambedura.

TRATAMENTO

CUIDADO(S) DE SAÚDE ADEQUADO(S)
Cuidados de suporte.

CUIDADO(S) DE ENFERMAGEM
Sucção/Mastigação de Tecido
Criar um "lugar seguro" para os momentos em que o gato for deixado sozinho ou sem o tecido do tipo preferido.

TRANSTORNOS COMPULSIVOS — GATOS

Tabela 1.

Medicamentos e dosagens utilizados no tratamento de transtorno compulsivo felino.				
Medicamento	Classe Medicamentosa	Dosagem Oral em Gatos	Frequência	Efeitos Colaterais
Fluoxetina	ISRS	0,5-1,0 mg/kg	a cada 24 h	Diminuição do apetite, sonolência
Paroxetina	ISRS	0,25-0,50 mg/kg	a cada 24 h	Constipação
Clomipramina	ATC	0,25-0,50 mg/kg	a cada 24 h	Sonolência
Amitriptilina	ATC	0,25-1,0 mg/kg	a cada 24 h	Sonolência
Buspirona	Azapirona	0,5-1,0 mg/kg	a cada 12 h	Efeitos colaterais GI (raros)

ATIVIDADE
Aumentar as oportunidades de brincadeiras e interações sociais com o uso dos métodos preferidos pelo gato acometido.

DIETA
Sucção/mastigação de tecido: o aumento no conteúdo de fibra na dieta pode ser útil.

ORIENTAÇÃO AO PROPRIETÁRIO
• Identificar e remover os fatores responsáveis pela deflagração do comportamento, se aplicável.
• Não recompensar o comportamento.
• Orientar o proprietário a ignorar o comportamento ao máximo possível; distrair o gato e iniciar um comportamento aceitável.
• Aconselhar o proprietário a observar os detalhes referentes ao horário, lugar e meio social, para que se possa planejar um comportamento alternativo (brincadeiras ou alimentação ou brinquedo que dispense o alimento) antes do desencadeamento do comportamento compulsivo.
• Informar ao proprietário de que a punição associada ao tom de voz, movimento e toque aumenta a imprevisibilidade do ambiente do animal, pode aumentar o medo ou o comportamento agressivo do paciente e ainda romper o elo homem-animal. A punição é contraindicada em gatos que sofrem de comportamento compulsivo.
• Redução do estresse ambiental — aumentar a previsibilidade dos eventos domésticos (alimentação, brincadeiras, exercícios e momentos sociáveis com o proprietário); eliminar ao máximo possível os eventos imprevisíveis; o confinamento é contraindicado.

CONSIDERAÇÕES CIRÚRGICAS
Os gatos com hipertireoidismo podem ser tratados com tireoidectomia.

MEDICAÇÕES

MEDICAMENTO(S) DE ESCOLHA
• Os medicamentos anticompulsivos podem ser úteis. Duas classes de medicamentos são representadas por ISRS e ATC por seus efeitos sobre o sistema de neurotransmissão serotoninérgica (Tab. 1).
• Objetivo — utilizar os medicamentos até se obter o controle do comportamento por 2 meses; tentar a suspensão gradual. O tratamento deve ser retomado ao primeiro sinal de recidiva; pode ser vitalício.
• Os medicamentos estão listados com a dosagem utilizada para tratar o comportamento e os efeitos colaterais comuns.
• Os antagonistas de β-endorfinas podem ser eficazes, mas sua meia-vida de eliminação curta torna o uso desses agentes impraticável.

CONTRAINDICAÇÕES
• ISRS — hiporexia (diminuição do apetite), constipação, sedação.
• ATC — efeitos colaterais anti-histamínicos e anticolinérgicos (semelhantes aos da atropina); contraindicados em casos de anormalidades cardiovasculares (distúrbios de condução cardíaca), glaucoma, bem como retenções urinária e fecal.
• A via transdérmica não parece produzir níveis medicamentosos satisfatórios.

PRECAUÇÕES
• Uso abusivo de medicamentos — os agentes psicotrópicos apresentam potencial de abuso humano; tomar medidas sensatas de precaução para assegurar que as prescrições para os pequenos animais não sejam utilizadas de forma abusiva pelos seres humanos.
• ATC — a superdosagem (p. ex., ingestão de um frasco de pílulas) por animais de estimação ou seres humanos pode causar distúrbios cardíacos fatais; não há antídoto; geralmente são bem tolerados, embora haja inúmeros efeitos colaterais potenciais, incluindo efeitos anticolinérgicos (semelhantes aos da atropina) e anti-histamínicos; utilizar com cautela em pacientes com retenções urinária ou fecal.
• Uso de medicamentos fora da indicação da bula — não há nenhum agente aprovado pela FDA para o tratamento desses transtornos em gatos; informar ao proprietário sobre a natureza experimental desses tratamentos e os riscos envolvidos; registrar essa argumentação no prontuário médico ou com um termo de consentimento assinado ou formulário específico de liberação.
• Efeitos colaterais — fornecer instruções por escrito, juntamente com os efeitos colaterais comuns (p. ex., os ATC podem causar sedação até que se desenvolva uma tolerância ao medicamento); instituir os agentes psicotrópicos e monitorizar o paciente na presença do proprietário.

INTERAÇÕES POSSÍVEIS
Não utilizar os ATC nem os ISRS listados com inibidores da monoamina oxidase, como o amitraz e o L-deprenil®.

MEDICAMENTO(S) ALTERNATIVO(S)
• Fenobarbital na suspeita de distúrbio convulsivo.
• Deprenil® (selegilina) em caso de disfunção cognitiva.
• L-triptofano como precursor da serotonina.

ACOMPANHAMENTO

MONITORIZAÇÃO DO PACIENTE
• Antes de iniciar o tratamento, registrar a frequência de ataques estereotipados que ocorrem a cada semana, para que a evolução possa ser monitorizada.
• O tratamento bem-sucedido requer uma lista de exames de acompanhamento; um esquema recomendado consiste em telefonemas 1 semana após a consulta inicial e agendamento de consultas de retorno 4-6 semanas depois. Se a melhora for evidente, o esquema terapêutico deverá ser mantido; a melhora progressiva e contínua pode ocorrer durante as próximas 4-6 semanas. Se não houver qualquer melhora, deve-se considerar a lista de diagnósticos diferenciais ou o uso de medicamento alternativo.
• Os programas de modificação ambiental e/ou os medicamentos psicoativos devem ser ajustados de acordo com a resposta do paciente.
• Se o medicamento não for eficaz após o ajuste da dosagem, selecionar um agente pertencente à outra classe medicamentosa.

PREVENÇÃO
Criar um ambiente enriquecido (i. e., repleto de distrações) para os gatos.

COMPLICAÇÕES POSSÍVEIS
• Falha terapêutica.
• É fundamental que se tenham expectativas realistas do quadro; é improvável o controle imediato de um problema de longa duração.

EVOLUÇÃO ESPERADA E PROGNÓSTICO
Com o tratamento, o prognóstico quanto à melhora do paciente é bom; estima-se que dois terços dos pacientes respondem à satisfação do proprietário. O tratamento imediato melhora o prognóstico, pois o desfecho é adversamente influenciado pela duração do problema.

DIVERSOS

DISTÚRBIOS ASSOCIADOS
Comportamento de fuga ou agressividade direcionada contra o proprietário — se o proprietário punir o paciente quando este manifestar um comportamento estereotipado.

GESTAÇÃO/FERTILIDADE/REPRODUÇÃO
• Não acasalar os animais que exibem comportamento compulsivo.
• ATC — contraindicados em animais prenhes.

ABREVIATURA(S)
• ISRS = inibidor seletivo de recaptação da serotonina.
• ATC = antidepressivo tricíclico.

Autor Barbara L. Sherman
Consultor Editorial Debra F. Horwitz

Traqueobronquite Infecciosa Canina (Tosse dos Canis)

CONSIDERAÇÕES GERAIS

DEFINIÇÃO
Qualquer doença respiratória contagiosa dos cães que se manifeste por tosse.

FISIOPATOLOGIA
A patogenia geralmente envolve lesão ao epitélio respiratório por infecção viral, acompanhada pela invasão do tecido lesionado por bactérias, fungos, micoplasmas, parasitas ou outros microrganismos virulentos, resultando em mais lesões e sinais clínicos.

SISTEMA(S) ACOMETIDO(S)
Respiratório — primariamente acometido a menos que a doença evolua para sepse.

GENÉTICA
N/D.

INCIDÊNCIA/PREVALÊNCIA
Ocorre mais comumente em locais onde existam grupos de cães de idades e suscetibilidades variadas, quase sempre sob condições higiênicas aquém das ideais.

DISTRIBUIÇÃO GEOGRÁFICA
Mundial.

IDENTIFICAÇÃO
Espécies
Cães.

Raça(s) Predominante(s)
Nenhuma.

Idade Média e Faixa Etária
• Mais grave em filhotes de 6 semanas a 6 meses de vida.
• Pode se desenvolver em cães de todas as idades e, frequentemente, com doença subclínica preexistente das vias aéreas (p. ex., anomalia congênita, bronquite crônica e bronquiectasia).

Sexo Predominante
Nenhum.

SINAIS CLÍNICOS
Comentários Gerais
• Relacionados com o grau de lesão do trato respiratório e a idade do cão acometido.
• Podem ser inexistentes, leves ou graves com pneumonia.
• Muitos agentes virais, bacterianos e micoplasmas se disseminam com rapidez dos cães aparentemente saudáveis para outros no mesmo ambiente; os sinais geralmente se iniciam cerca de 4 dias após a exposição ao(s) agente(s) infectante(s).

Achados Anamnésicos
• Não complicados — a tosse em animais saudáveis sob outros aspectos é um sinal característico; pode ser seca e entrecortada, suave e seca, úmida e entrecortada ou paroxística, seguida por ânsia de vômito ou expectoração de muco; fatores como agitação, exercício, mudanças de temperatura ou umidade do ar inspirado e compressão cervical delicada (p. ex., da coleira) sobre a traqueia induzem a um ataque de tosse.
• Graves — inapetência a anorexia; a tosse (quando notada) é úmida e produtiva; pode-se observar letargia, anorexia, dispneia e intolerância ao exercício.

Achados do Exame Físico
• Não complicados — tosse facilmente induzida por compressão da traqueia; ruídos pulmonares frequentemente normais; animais saudáveis sob outros aspectos.
• Graves — pode-se detectar febre constante, de baixo grau ou flutuante (39,4-40°C); também se pode detectar o aumento na intensidade de ruídos pulmonares normais, crepitações ou (menos frequentemente) sibilos.

CAUSAS
• Virais — vírus da cinomose; CAV-2; parainfluenza canina; CAV-1; coronavírus respiratório canino, reovírus canino tipos 1, 2 ou 3; herpes-vírus canino tipo 1; vírus da influenza canina.
• CAV-2 e parainfluenza canina — podem lesionar o epitélio respiratório a tal ponto que a invasão por diversas bactérias e diversos micoplasmas provoca doença grave das vias aéreas.
• Bacterianas — *Bordetella bronchiseptica*, sem outros patógenos respiratórios, produz sinais clínicos indistinguíveis daqueles de outras causas bacterianas; *Pseudomonas, Escherichia coli, Klebsiella, Pasteurella, Streptococcus, Mycoplasma* e outras espécies igualmente prováveis.

FATORES DE RISCO
• Condições higiênicas abaixo das ideais e superlotação — observadas em alguns *pet shops*, abrigos de sociedades humanitárias e estabelecimentos de pesquisas, além de canis de hospedagem (tipo hotel para cães) e adestramento.
• Doença subclínica coexistente das vias aéreas — anomalias congênitas; bronquite crônica; bronquiectasia.

DIAGNÓSTICO

DIAGNÓSTICO DIFERENCIAL
• Nos cães em bom estado do ponto de vista sistêmico — bronquite parasitária, traqueobronquite irritante, corpo estranho na traqueia, colapso traqueal.
• Nos cães com sinais sistêmicos de pneumonia — inúmeros microrganismos que infetam os pulmões.
• O diagnóstico de traqueobronquite infecciosa geralmente é estabelecido de forma provisória em cão com estado de vacinação inadequado e histórico de exposição a algum cão potencialmente infectado.
• Ver "Tosse".

HEMOGRAMA/BIOQUÍMICA/URINÁLISE
• Leucopenia leve inicialmente — (5.000 a 6.000 células/dL) — pode ser detectada; sugere causa viral.
• Leucocitose neutrofílica com desvio à esquerda — frequentemente encontrada em casos de pneumonia grave.
• Perfil bioquímico sérico e urinálise — geralmente normais.

OUTROS TESTES LABORATORIAIS
Gasometria sanguínea arterial — pode ser valiosa na pneumonia.

DIAGNÓSTICO POR IMAGEM
• Radiografias — nada digno de nota na doença não complicada; valiosa, a princípio, para descartar causas não infecciosas de tosse.
• Radiografias torácicas — casos graves: podem demonstrar padrão pulmonar intersticial e alveolar com distribuição cranioventral típica de pneumonia bacteriana; pode-se observar padrão intersticial difuso típico de pneumonia viral; pode-se notar padrão pulmonar misto (p. ex., combinação de padrões alveolar, intersticial e peribronquial).

MÉTODOS DIAGNÓSTICOS
• Na suspeita de doença grave — realizar lavado transtraqueal ou lavado traqueobrônquico via broncoscopia.
• Padrão de sensibilidade antimicrobiana das bactérias obtidas em cultura — a identificação ajuda acentuadamente no fornecimento de um plano terapêutico eficiente.

ACHADOS PATOLÓGICOS
• Parainfluenza canina — provoca pouco a nenhum sinal clínico; 6-10 dias após a exposição, os pulmões de cães infectados podem conter hemorragias petequiais uniformemente distribuídas sobre as superfícies; detectado por imunofluorescência nas células epiteliais colunares dos brônquios e bronquíolos 6-10 dias após a exposição ao aerossol.
• CAV-2 — lesões confinadas ao sistema respiratório; grandes corpúsculos de inclusão intranucleares encontrados nas células do epitélio bronquial e células do septo alveolar; os sinais clínicos tendem a ser leves e de curta duração; as lesões persistem por, no mínimo, um mês após a infecção.
• Vírus da influenza canina — caracterizado por infecção secundária por *Mycoplasma* e hemorragia pulmonar.
• Bordetelose e infecção bacteriana grave — evidência de bronquite, traqueíte e rinite purulentas com hiperemia e aumento dos linfonodos bronquiais, mediastínicos e retrofaríngeos; pode-se observar grande número de microrganismos Gram-positivos ou negativos no muco do epitélio traqueal e brônquico.

TRATAMENTO

CUIDADO(S) DE SAÚDE ADEQUADO(S)
• Paciente ambulatorial — fortemente recomendado na doença não complicada.
• Paciente internado — forte recomendação para doença complicada e/ou pneumonia.

CUIDADO(S) DE ENFERMAGEM
Administração de fluido — indicada para doença complicada e/ou pneumonia.

ATIVIDADE
Repouso forçado — por, no mínimo, 14-21 dias na doença não complicada e, pelo menos, durante a evidência radiográfica de pneumonia em cães gravemente acometidos.

DIETA
Ração comercial seca ou enlatada de boa qualidade.

ORIENTAÇÃO AO PROPRIETÁRIO
• Incitar o proprietário a isolar o paciente de outros animais; os cães infectados podem transmitir o(s) agente(s) antes do início dos sinais clínicos e depois disso até que ocorra o desenvolvimento de imunidade.

TRAQUEOBRONQUITE INFECCIOSA CANINA (TOSSE DOS CANIS)

- Informar ao proprietário sobre o fato de que os pacientes com a doença não complicada devem responder ao tratamento em 10-14 dias.
- Esclarecer ao proprietário que, uma vez disseminada a infecção em um canil, ela poderá ser controlada pelo esvaziamento da instalação por 1-2 semanas e sua desinfecção com substâncias químicas comumente utilizadas, como hipoclorito de sódio (na diluição de 1:30), clorexidina e benzalcônio.

CONSIDERAÇÕES CIRÚRGICAS
N/D.

MEDICAÇÕES
MEDICAMENTO(S) DE ESCOLHA
- Amoxicilina/ácido clavulânico (12,5-25 mg/kg VO a cada 12 h) ou doxiciclina (5 mg/kg VO a cada 12 h) — tratamento inicial da doença não complicada.
- Cefalosporina de primeira geração (cefazolina, 20-35 mg/kg IV, IM a cada 8 h) com gentamicina (2-4 mg/kg IV, IM, SC a cada 6-8 h) ou amicacina (6,5 mg/kg IV, IM, SC a cada 8 h) ou enrofloxacino (2,5-5 mg/kg VO, IM, IV a cada 12 h) — geralmente são eficazes na doença grave.
- Terapia antimicrobiana — continuar por, no mínimo, 10 dias além da resolução radiográfica.
- *B. bronchiseptica* e outras espécies resistentes — alguns antimicrobianos podem não atingir concentrações terapêuticas adequadas no lúmen do trato respiratório inferior e, por esse motivo, a administração oral ou parenteral pode apresentar eficácia limitada; a nebulização com canamicina (250 mg), gentamicina (50 mg) ou polimixina B (333.000 UI) pode eliminar as espécies quando administrada diariamente por 3-5 dias. Utilizar em conjunto com antibióticos sistêmicos em cães com doença parenquimatosa.
- Butorfanol (0,55 mg/kg VO a cada 8-12 h) ou bitartarato de hidrocodona (0,22 mg/kg VO a cada 6-8 h) — supressão eficaz de tosse seca improdutiva não associada à infecção bacteriana.
- Broncodilatadores (p. ex., teofilina de liberação estendida, 10 mg/kg VO a cada 12 h) — podem ser utilizados para controlar o broncospasmo (evidenciado clinicamente por sibilos).

CONTRAINDICAÇÕES
- Não utilizar supressores da tosse em pacientes com pneumonia.
- Não usar teofilina na dose padrão em combinação com enrofloxacino.

PRECAUÇÕES
Nenhuma.

INTERAÇÕES POSSÍVEIS
Fluoroquinolonas e derivados da teofilina — o uso concomitante provoca concentração plasmática alta e possivelmente tóxica da teofilina.

MEDICAMENTO(S) ALTERNATIVO(S)
Nenhum.

ACOMPANHAMENTO
MONITORIZAÇÃO DO PACIENTE
- Doença não complicada — deve responder ao tratamento em 10-14 dias; se o paciente continuar tossindo 14 dias ou mais depois do estabelecimento de plano terapêutico adequado, questionar o diagnóstico de doença não complicada.
- Doença grave — repetir a radiografia torácica até no mínimo 14 dias além da resolução de todos os sinais clínicos.

PREVENÇÃO
A liberação do(s) agente(s) causal(is) da traqueobronquite infecciosa nas secreções respiratórias dos cães é, sem dúvida, responsável pela persistência desse problema em canis, abrigos para animais, instalações de hospedagem e hospitais veterinários.

Vacinas Virais e Bacterianas
- Disponíveis para controlar os principais agentes envolvidos.
- Vacina contra *B. bronchiseptica* e parainfluenza canina — os filhotes podem ser vacinados por via intranasal já com 2-4 semanas de vida sem interferência dos anticorpos maternos e, depois, submetidos a reforço anual; é permitida a vacinação de cães adultos com vacina intranasal em dose única (ao mesmo tempo que seus filhotes ou quando receberem suas vacinações anuais).
- Vacina parenteral inativada contra *B. bronchiseptica* — administrada em duas doses com 2-4 semanas de intervalo; é recomendada a vacinação inicial dos filhotes com 6-8 semanas de vida ou em torno disso; revacinar aos 4 meses de vida.
- Existe vacina inativada disponível contra influenza canina.

COMPLICAÇÕES POSSÍVEIS
N/D.

EVOLUÇÃO ESPERADA E PROGNÓSTICO
- Evolução natural da doença não complicada se não for tratada — 10-14 dias; a simples restrição ao exercício e a prevenção de agitação abreviam a evolução.
- Evolução típica da doença grave — 2-6 semanas; os pacientes que vieram a óbito quase sempre desenvolveram pneumonia grave com envolvimento de múltiplos lobos pulmonares.

DIVERSOS
DISTÚRBIOS ASSOCIADOS
Pode acompanhar outras anomalias do trato respiratório.

FATORES RELACIONADOS COM A IDADE
Mais grave em filhotes de 6 semanas a 6 meses de vida e naqueles de *pet shops* comerciais e abrigos de sociedades humanitárias.

POTENCIAL ZOONÓTICO
Nenhum.

GESTAÇÃO/FERTILIDADE/REPRODUÇÃO
Risco elevado em cadelas submetidas a tratamento clínico extenso; particularmente arriscado para os filhotes em desenvolvimento.

SINÔNIMO(S)
Tosse dos canis — doença não complicada.

ABREVIATURA(S)
- CAV = adenovírus canino.

RECURSOS DA INTERNET
www.cdc.gov/flu/canine/.

Sugestões de Leitura
Bemis DA. Bordetella and Mycoplasma respiratory infection in dogs. Vet Clin North Am Small Anim Pract 1992, 22:1173-1186.
Erles K, Dubovi E, Brooks HW, Brownlie J. Longitudinal study of viruses associated with canine infectious respiratory disease. J Clin Micro 2004, 42:4524-4529.
Ford RB. Canine infectious tracheobronchitis. In: Greene CE, ed., Infectious Diseases of the Dog and Cat, 3rd ed. St. Louis: Saunders Elsevier, 2006, pp. 54-61.
Hoskins JD, Taboada J. Specific treatment of infectious causes of respiratory disease in dogs and cats. Vet Med 1994, 89:443-452.
Radhakrishnan A, Drobatz KJ, Culp WT, et al. Community-acquired infectious pneumonia in puppies: 65 cases (1993-2002). JAVMA 2007, 230:1493-1497.

Autor Johnny D. Hoskins
Consultor Editorial Lynelle R. Johnson

Traumatismo da Coluna Vertebral

CONSIDERAÇÕES GERAIS

DEFINIÇÃO
• O traumatismo da coluna vertebral é causado pela aplicação de forças exógenas sobre as vértebras, os discos intervertebrais, as estruturas de sustentação tendíneas e ligamentares associadas, bem como a medula espinal. • Os sinais clínicos podem incluir hiperestesia regional, paresia dos membros e/ou ataxia proprioceptiva geral, para ou tetraplegia, perda de nocicepção, retenção urinária, e incontinência fecal.

FISIOPATOLOGIA
• Na coluna vertebral normal, os sistemas passivos (ossos, ligamentos), ativos (tendões, músculos) e neurais são responsáveis pela estabilidade.
• Compressão, curvatura lateral, torção e forças de cisalhamento podem resultar em falha desses sistemas, levando à fratura ou subluxação da coluna vertebral.
• Em alguns casos, uma lesão significativa da medula espinal pode estar presente sem instabilidade ou fratura. Herniação de disco traumática, lesões penetrantes associadas ao canal vertebral, e mielopatia vascular pós-traumática são quadros pelos quais isso pode ocorrer.
• Muito comumente, os animais são avaliados após traumatismo da coluna vertebral em virtude da presença de sinais atribuídos à medula espinal.
• A lesão da medula espinal ocorre por causa de mecanismos primários e secundários.
• A lesão primária origina-se de eventos mecânicos, como compressão, concussão, contusão e laceração da medula espinal.
• A lesão secundária corresponde à cascata bioquímica que ocorre após os eventos primários. Tal cascata consiste em estresse oxidativo, inflamação, excitotoxicidade, lesão vascular e outros processos.

SISTEMA(S) ACOMETIDO(S)
• Nervoso.
• Musculoesquelético.
• Outros sistemas, possivelmente em função do traumatismo exógeno.

INCIDÊNCIA/PREVALÊNCIA
• Fraturas e luxações vertebrais representaram 6% de todas as mielopatias felinas e 7% de todos os casos neurológicos caninos em dois estudos monocêntricos.
• A incidência de lesão traumática da medula espinal sem fratura/luxação é desconhecida.

DISTRIBUIÇÃO GEOGRÁFICA
Dados não disponíveis.

IDENTIFICAÇÃO
Espécies
Cães e gatos.

Raça(s) Predominante(s)
Os dados limitados sobre fratura/luxação vertebral sugerem que os cães de médio e grande porte são comumente acometidos.

Idade Média e Faixa Etária
Um único relato retrospectivo sobre fratura/luxação vertebral indicou que os cães e gatos acometidos eram jovens (idade média de 2 anos; faixa etária de 0,25-15 anos).

Sexo Predominante
Os machos parecem super-representados.

SINAIS CLÍNICOS
Comentários Gerais
• A maioria avassaladora de cães com traumatismo da coluna vertebral tem lesão da medula espinal.
• Podem ocorrer lesões concomitantes do sistema nervoso periférico (p. ex., traumatismo do plexo braquial) ou central (p. ex., traumatismo craniencefálico). • Do mesmo modo, frequentemente se identificam anormalidades associadas a outros sistemas corporais.

Achados Anamnésicos
• Paresia e ataxia ou para/tetraplegia de início agudo. • Sinais clínicos sugestivos de hiperestesia (vocalização, relutância a se mover, coluna arqueada). • Letargia e hiporexia (apetite deficiente).

Anormalidades do Exame Neurológico
• A lesão da medula espinal costuma ser classificada como C1-C5, C6-T2, T3-L3, L4-Cd5, multifocal, ou difusa, com base no exame neurológico. • Lesão focal da medula espinal é mais comum. • Anormalidades da marcha — em >90% dos animais; podem incluir ataxia proprioceptiva geral, paresia e perda de movimento voluntário. • Do mesmo modo, anormalidades nos reflexos espinais e nas reações posturais são comuns e refletem o(s) segmento(s) da medula espinal lesado(s). • Hiperestesia regional. • Animais com lesão grave da medula espinal podem ter ausência de nocicepção. • A ausência de nocicepção profunda é um indicador prognóstico negativo, com taxas de recuperação após fratura/luxação vertebral toracolombar tradicionalmente em <5%.

Anormalidades do Exame Físico
• Contusões pulmonares e fraturas de costelas.
• Fraturas ósseas pélvicas e apendiculares. • Feridas cutâneas. • Lesão cerebral traumática. • Lesão de órgãos abdominais.

CAUSAS
• Acidente de automóvel é a causa mais comum de traumatismo da coluna vertebral. • Outras etiologias incluem queda (frequente em gatos), feridas por projéteis balísticos e mordidas de animais.

FATORES DE RISCO
Os animais que vivem na rua, aqueles que passeiam sem coleira e outros que não ficam presos nos cabos de *pick-ups*, por exemplo, são provavelmente super-representados.

DIAGNÓSTICO

DIAGNÓSTICO DIFERENCIAL
• Outras doenças neurológicas, como herniação de disco, mielopatia embólica fibrocartilaginosa, meningomielite, discospondilite, e neoplasia da coluna vertebral, devem ser consideradas. • Lesões ortopédicas, como fratura apendicular ou lesões ligamentares, podem ocasionalmente ser confundidas com traumatismo da coluna vertebral. É recomendável a realização de ambos os exames, neurológico e ortopédico.

HEMOGRAMA/BIOQUÍMICA/URINÁLISE
• Pode haver alterações em caso de lesão significativa a outros sistemas corporais. • Anemia, achados compatíveis com desidratação (p. ex., hipernatremia), creatinina cinase elevada e hematúria são, sem exceção, comumente observados.

DIAGNÓSTICO POR IMAGEM
Radiografia
• Sensibilidade de 70% e alta especificidade para detecção de fratura/luxação vertebral. • Outros diagnósticos diferenciais, como discospondilite, podem ser descartados em caso de estudo radiográfico normal. • Radiografias vertebrais não permitem a visualização da medula espinal e exibem poucos detalhes de tecidos moles.

Mielografia
• Exame capaz de delimitar compressão extradural da medula espinal, utilizado na tomada de decisões para abordagens cirúrgicas após lesão dessa medula. • Além de invasiva, a mielografia não permite a visualização direta do parênquima da medula espinal e ainda carece dos detalhes teciduais obtidos por estudos avançados de diagnóstico por imagem. • Pode não detectar compressão lateralizada da medula espinal de forma tão eficaz quanto as modalidades avançadas de diagnóstico por imagem.

Técnicas Avançadas de Diagnóstico por Imagem
• As clínicas mais modernas utilizam os exames de TC e/ou RM para avaliar lesão da medula espinal.
• TC — técnica que exibe padrão de excelência para avaliar os ossos da coluna vertebral e também pode ser utilizada para visualizar material de disco mineralizado e hemorragia extradural. • RM — pode ser usada para visualizar a coluna vertebral óssea, mas fornece mais detalhes dos tecidos moles que a TC; constitui o único meio para descartar certos diagnósticos diferenciais, como mielopatia embólica fibrocartilaginosa, e fornece informações prognósticas a respeito da recuperação.

MÉTODOS DIAGNÓSTICOS
• LCS — a análise desse líquido frequentemente não é digna de nota; em alguns casos graves, o conteúdo da proteína total, a contagem de células nucleadas e a contagem de hemácias podem estar aumentadas. • Anormalidades do LCS em caso de lesão da medula espinal não são específicas à etiologia. • O LCS é coletado como um exame adjuvante e não como um substituto das técnicas avançadas de diagnóstico por imagem.

ACHADOS PATOLÓGICOS
• Os achados macroscópicos podem incluir evidência de luxação/fratura vertebral, hemorragia extradural, extrusão de disco, tumefação (inchaço) da medula espinal, eritema/hemorragia dural/subaracnoide e mielomalacia. • As anormalidades histopatológicas dentro da medula espinal podem englobar necrose, desmielinização, zonas de infarto da medula espinal, hemorragia do parênquima e esferoides axonais.

TRATAMENTO

CUIDADO(S) DE SAÚDE ADEQUADO(S)
• É recomendado o tratamento emergencial na unidade de terapia intensiva para todos os animais imediatamente após lesão. • Talvez haja necessidade de tratamento cirúrgico se as técnicas de diagnóstico por imagem sugerirem compressão significativa da medula espinal ou instabilidade expressiva da coluna vertebral. • O tratamento médico pode ser selecionado para os animais que

TRAUMATISMO DA COLUNA VERTEBRAL

ainda conservam a deambulação ou carecem de evidência de instabilidade/compressão.

CUIDADO(S) DE ENFERMAGEM
- Antes da realização do exame de diagnóstico por imagem, os animais devem ser imobilizados em uma maca para evitar exacerbação da lesão.
- Os animais com achados sugestivos de instabilidade da coluna vertebral nas técnicas de diagnóstico por imagem devem ser imobilizados até a estabilização cirúrgica.
- Os cães sem deambulação necessitam de cama acolchoada, mudança frequente de posição e esvaziamento da bexiga urinária.
- A fluidoterapia é necessária em caso de desidratação.
- A reabilitação física que consiste em exercícios com amplitude de movimento, estimulação elétrica dos músculos, sustentação ativa do peso e uso de esteira subaquática (subimersa) pode ser benéfica. A reabilitação física que envolve mobilização significativa deve ser realizada somente depois do tratamento da instabilidade da coluna vertebral.

• ATIVIDADE
- Restrição rigorosa do exercício por 4 semanas para todos os animais submetidos à cirurgia da coluna vertebral. Os animais com fraturas e instabilidade podem necessitar de repouso rigoroso por 6-8 semanas.
- Os animais submetidos a tratamento médico e sem instabilidade/fratura da coluna vertebral podem necessitar de períodos mais curtos de repouso, dependendo do processo patológico subjacente sob suspeita.

ORIENTAÇÃO AO PROPRIETÁRIO
Em geral, acredita-se que o resultado seja bom para os animais que sofreram lesão traumática da medula espinal com nocicepção intacta, desde que se selecione a terapia adequada.

CONSIDERAÇÕES CIRÚRGICAS
- A cirurgia é recomendada para os animais com resultados nas técnicas avançadas de diagnóstico por imagem que apoiam a presença de compressão significativa da medula espinal ou instabilidade expressiva da coluna vertebral (p. ex., subluxação, violação de múltiplos compartimentos das unidades vertebrais).
- Para estabilizar a coluna vertebral, podem ser utilizados grampos, pinos e metilmetacrilato, além de várias placas.
- Pode haver a necessidade de descompressão sem estabilização nos casos em que há hemorragia extradural significativa ou material de disco.

MEDICAÇÕES

MEDICAMENTO(S) DE ESCOLHA
- *Analgésicos opioides* são comumente utilizados para aliviar hiperestesia associada ao traumatismo (tramadol na dose de 3-5 mg/kg VO a cada 8-6 h).
- *Agentes anti-inflamatórios não esteroides* produzem analgesia e efeitos anti-inflamatórios, que podem ser benéficos. O carprofeno costuma ser utilizado na dose de 2,2 mg/kg VO a cada 12 h.
- *Antagonistas de receptores alfa* podem relaxar o esfíncter uretral interno e facilitar a micção em casos de disfunção vesical por lesão do neurônio motor inferior e superior. A prazosina pode ser administrada na dose de 1 mg/15 kg VO a cada 8-12 h.
- *Agonistas muscarínicos* estimulam a contratilidade do detrusor e podem permitir a eliminação da urina em cães com problemas vesicais atribuídos à lesão do neurônio motor inferior. O cloreto de betanecol é administrado na dose de 5-15 mg/cão VO a cada 8-12 h.

CONTRAINDICAÇÕES
- Os *glicocorticoides* continuam sendo comumente utilizados na medicina veterinária para traumatismo da coluna vertebral. Foi demonstrado que só a administração de succinato sódico de metilprednisolona em altas doses em até 8 horas da lesão seja benéfica em seres humanos.
- No entanto, não foi demonstrado que o succinato sódico de metilprednisolona e outros glicocorticoides sejam benéficos em cães com lesão da medula espinal, embora as pesquisas sejam basicamente retrospectivas. Comumente se identificam efeitos adversos no quadro de lesão da medula espinal associada a disco.

PRECAUÇÕES
- Os AINE podem resultar em úlceras gástricas nos animais com lesão da medula espinal.
- Os glicocorticoides podem causar ulceração gástrica, vômito, ulceração colônica, e infecções do trato urinário (especialmente a dexametasona).
- Os α-antagonistas podem culminar em hipotensão e sinais gastrintestinais em altas doses.
- O agonismo muscarínico não é sugerido em animais que apresentam disfunção vesical por lesão do neurônio motor superior e não estejam recebendo bloqueio-α. Os agonistas muscarínicos podem resultar em sialorreia, defecação/micção involuntárias, e bradicardia.

INTERAÇÕES POSSÍVEIS
Não é recomendável a combinação de glicocorticoides e AINE, pois isso aumenta drasticamente o risco de efeitos adversos gastrintestinais.

MEDICAMENTO(S) ALTERNATIVO(S)
Muitos medicamentos, como polietilenoglicol e ilomostate, estão sendo atualmente investigados como tratamentos médicos para lesão da medula espinal.

ACOMPANHAMENTO

MONITORIZAÇÃO DO PACIENTE
- Para monitorizar a evolução, é fortemente sugerida a obtenção do escore de lesão da medula espinal com escala validada, com base no exame físico diário.
- A escala de Frankel modificada, a escala de lesão da medula espinal do Texas e o escore motor dos membros pélvicos de 14 pontos são três sistemas validados e utilizados em cães.

PREVENÇÃO
Os animais que vivem dentro de casa e são atentamente monitorizados têm um risco mais baixo de lesão exógena da medula espinal.

COMPLICAÇÕES POSSÍVEIS
- São possíveis complicações a ataxia e a paresia crônicas, bem como a falha para recuperar a deambulação voluntária.
- Alguns animais podem ter incontinência urinária e/ou fecal, sobretudo na ausência de deambulação.
- Os animais sem deambulação estão sob risco de úlceras de pele e infecções do trato urinário.

EVOLUÇÃO ESPERADA E PROGNÓSTICO
- Os animais com nocicepção intacta têm um prognóstico bom quanto à recuperação deambulatória caso se efetue o tratamento adequado.
- Os animais que exibem ausência de nocicepção e apresentam fratura ou luxação vertebral têm um prognóstico muito mau quanto à recuperação deambulatória voluntária (< 5%), mas a literatura especializada sobre esse assunto é limitada.
- Os cães sem fratura/luxação que carecem de nocicepção podem ter consequências funcionais piores que aqueles com herniação de disco não traumática, mas os dados sobre esse subgrupo de cães com lesão traumática da medula espinal são limitados.

DIVERSOS

DISTÚRBIOS ASSOCIADOS
Os animais que apresentam lesão traumática da medula espinal frequentemente têm lesão em outros sistemas corporais.

FATORES RELACIONADOS COM A IDADE
Os animais mais jovens parecem mais comumente acometidos.

GESTAÇÃO/FERTILIDADE/REPRODUÇÃO
- Levar uma gestação a termo pode ser um grande desafio para os animais com lesão grave da medula espinal.
- A lesão da medula espinal pode afetar a capacidade de engravidar.

SINÔNIMOS
Mielopatia traumática.

VER TAMBÉM
- Mielopatia — Paresia/Paralisia — Gatos.
- Dor no Pescoço e Dorso. • Paralisia.

ABREVIATURAS
- AINE = anti-inflamatório não esteroide.
- LCS = líquido cerebrospinal.
- RM = ressonância magnética.
- TC = tomografia computadorizada.

Sugestões de Leitura
Bali MS, Lang J, Jaggy A, et al. Comparative study of vertebral fractures and luxations in dogs and cats. Vet Comp Orthop Traumatol 2009, 22:47-53.
Bruce CW, Brisson BA, Gyselinck K. Spinal fracture and luxation in dogs and cats. Vet Comp Orthop Traumatol 2008, 21:280-284.
Levine GJ, Levine JM, Budke CM, et al. Description and repeatability of a newly validated spinal cord injury scale for dogs. Prev Vet Med 2009, 89:121-127.
Olby N, Levine J, Harris T, et al. Long-term functional outcome of dogs with severe injuries of the thoracolumbar spinal cord: 87 cases (1996-2001). JAVMA 2003, 222:762-769.
Selcer RR, Bubb WJ, Walker TL. Management of vertebral column fractures in dogs and cats: 211 cases (1977-1985). JAVMA 1991, 198:1965-1968.

Autor Jonathan M. Levine
Consultor Editorial Joane M. Parent

TREMORES

CONSIDERAÇÕES GERAIS

DEFINIÇÃO
Movimentos rítmicos, oscilatórios e involuntários de todo o corpo ou de parte dele.

FISIOPATOLOGIA
• Movimento anormal causado pela contração alternada ou sincrônica de músculos antagônicos reciprocamente inervados.
• Contração sincrônica — a força ou a duração da contração são levemente distintas nos músculos opostos, resultando em movimentos bifásicos de um lado para outro.

SISTEMA(S) ACOMETIDO(S)
• Nervoso.
• Musculosquelético — fraqueza ou dor muscular.

IDENTIFICAÇÃO
• Cães e gatos.
• A idade depende da causa.

Cães
• Síndrome de tremor generalizado — cães jovens (<5 anos), pertencentes a raças de porte médio a pequeno (<15 kg), independentemente da cor da pelagem.
• Hipomielinização — 6-8 semanas de vida; Chow chow, Springer spaniel, Samoieda, Weimaraner e Dálmata.
• Tremor transitório idiopático da cabeça — Doberman pinscher, Buldogue inglês e Labrador retriever.

SINAIS CLÍNICOS
• Localizados ou generalizados.
• Localizados — envolvem com maior frequência a cabeça e os membros pélvicos.

CAUSAS

Tremor da Cabeça
• Anormalidades cerebelares — causas degenerativas; congênitas; inflamatórias; imunomediadas; tóxicas.
• Idiopáticas — as raças Doberman pinscher e Buldogue inglês são super-representadas.
• Genéticas.
• Inflamatórias — encefalites.
• Traumatismo.
• Administração de medicamentos — doxorrubicina; difenidramina; metoclopramida.

Tremor dos Membros Pélvicos
• Pode ser um sinal de fraqueza ou dor na área lombossacra.
• Metabólicas — insuficiência renal; hipoparatireoidismo; hipoglicemia.
• Lesões compressivas na medula espinal ou nas raízes nervosas — estenose lombossacra; síndrome da cauda equina; tumor da medula espinal; discospondilite.
• Neuropatia periférica; anormalidades da junção neuromuscular; miopatia.
• Má perfusão aos músculos pélvicos — ducto arterioso persistente com desvio da direita para a esquerda; outras doenças cardiopulmonares.
• Desconhecidas — membros pélvicos em cães mais idosos (tremor senil).

Tremor Generalizado
• Hipomielinização.
• Intoxicações — organofosforados; hexaclorofeno; brometalina; endectocida tópico contendo moxidectina e imidacloprida.
• Neuropatia degenerativa — doença de armazenamento; doença de Lafora; encefalopatia espongiforme.
• Síndrome de tremor generalizado idiopático — "síndrome do cão branco sacudidor".

FATORES DE RISCO
• Qualquer encefalite ou neuropatia degenerativa — doença de armazenamento e encefalopatia espongiforme.
• Tratamento com doxorrubicina, difenidramina ou metoclopramida.

DIAGNÓSTICO

DIAGNÓSTICO DIFERENCIAL
• Diferenciar tremor de arrepio, miotonia, mioclonia, fraqueza, tetania, mioclonia reflexa e crises convulsivas.
• O tremor costuma exibir movimentos mais consistentes, rítmicos, de um lado para outro e de amplitude semelhante, que persistem durante todo o estado de vigília e param durante o sono, quando comparado com agitação, arrepio, miotonia e mioclonia.
• Fraqueza — o tremor associado à fraqueza ocorre geralmente quando os músculos são forçados a se exercitar (p. ex., durante posturas em estação, caminhadas e corridas).
• Tetania — em geral, corresponde a uma extensão mais contínua dos membros e dos músculos faciais, sem um ciclo de extensão-flexão dos movimentos.
• Crises convulsivas — de curta duração; podem estar associadas a distúrbios autônomos (p. ex., micção, defecação e salivação) e alterações de consciência.
• Mioclonia reflexa — Labrador retriever e Dálmata; caracterizada por episódios prolongados de rigidez extensora com estímulos táteis ou auditivos e exercícios voluntários.

Localizados na Cabeça
• Avaliar os déficits neurológicos adicionais, sugestivos de doença cerebelar; com frequência, o tremor na cabeça como no tremor intencional representa um sinal clínico de doença cerebelar; esse tremor se agrava quando o paciente tenta movimentar a cabeça com o objetivo de alcançar algo; também pode envolver o corpo todo; os sinais de ataxia e dismetria ajudam a determinar o diagnóstico neuroanatômico.
• Condição idiopática — específica às raças (p. ex., Doberman pinscher e Buldogue inglês); o paciente costuma ser jovem no início; esporádica; ocorre em uma frequência de 2-4 Hz; direção dos movimentos de cima para baixo (movimento de "sim") ou de um lado para outro (movimento de "não"); origem anatômica desconhecida; pequena porcentagem de cães apresenta encefalite.

Localizados nos Membros Pélvicos
• Doenças da medula espinal lombossacra, cauda equina e nervos periféricos associados; doenças musculosqueléticas.

Generalizados
• Filhote canino (6-8 semanas) — anormalidade congênita de mielinização; verificar as incidências raciais.
• Cão jovem adulto — avaliar o histórico de exposição a toxinas; considerar a síndrome de tremor generalizado, sobretudo em animais com pelagem branca.

HEMOGRAMA/BIOQUÍMICA/URINÁLISE
• Geralmente permanecem normais, com doença cerebral primária associada.
• Localizados na cabeça ou nos membros pélvicos — avaliar o animal quanto à presença de doença metabólica oculta; pode-se encontrar hipoglicemia, hipocalcemia e função renal anormal.
• Algumas miopatias são caracterizadas por altos níveis de creatina quinase.

OUTROS TESTES LABORATORIAIS
N/D.

DIAGNÓSTICO POR IMAGEM
• Localizados nos membros pélvicos — radiografia simples, TC e RM; revelam anormalidades lombossacras, espinais ou vertebrais.
• Generalizados — em casos de hipomielinização, a RM pode revelar a ausência de mielina; na síndrome de tremor generalizado, a RM costuma permanecer normal; os cães da raça Maltês podem exibir hidrocefalia; no entanto, a importância desse achado é incerta.

MÉTODOS DIAGNÓSTICOS
• Análise do LCS — sensível, mas inespecífica; na síndrome de tremor generalizado, observa-se leve pleocitose mononuclear, com concentração proteica normal; o LCS também pode estar normal; em outras encefalites que envolvem o cerebelo, os resultados variam com a causa e a duração da doença.
• Eletromiografia dos membros pélvicos — pode ajudar a diagnosticar doença neuromuscular em caso de tremor localizado nesses membros.
• RAETC — para avaliar as vias auditivas centrais; útil para examinar a função do tronco cerebral na presença de doença neurológica (SNC).

TRATAMENTO
• Tratar a doença primária subjacente.
• Fornecido em um esquema ambulatorial a menos que o tratamento cirúrgico seja indicado (doença lombossacra que exija descompressão e estabilização).
• Evitar agitação e exercício — podem agravar muitos tremores.
• Tremor generalizado de origem cerebral primária — o paciente pode perder peso; monitorizar o peso e modificar a ingestão oral de acordo com ele.
• A maioria das causas em cães adultos é passível de tratamento.
• Doenças neurológicas degenerativas (p. ex., doença de armazenamento e encefalopatia espongiforme) — não há nenhum tratamento disponível.
• Hipomielinização — em geral, não é tratável; algumas raças melhoram com a maturidade (p. ex., Chow chow).
• Tremor idiopático da cabeça — não há nenhum tratamento eficaz disponível; tremor benigno de ocorrência esporádica; possui poucas consequências à saúde.
• Induzidos por medicamentos — considerar o uso de agente terapêutico alternativo.
• Suspeita de intoxicação — afastar o paciente de exposições futuras; consultar um centro de controle de envenenamentos em busca do possível antídoto.

TREMORES

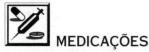

MEDICAÇÕES

MEDICAMENTO(S) DE ESCOLHA
- Geralmente, são irresponsivos aos relaxantes musculares ou anticonvulsivantes (p. ex., fenobarbital ou diazepam).
- Corticosteroides — dose imunossupressora para tratar os casos de síndrome de tremor generalizado.
- Antibióticos — em casos de discospondilite; selecionar com base nos resultados da cultura e do antibiograma da lesão, do sangue ou da urina.
- Doenças cerebelares — dependem do diagnóstico.
- Gabapentina — 5-20 mg/kg até a cada 8 h pode ser útil no tratamento de alguns tremores.

CONTRAINDICAÇÕES
Medicamentos simpaticomiméticos — podem agravar a condição.

PRECAUÇÕES
N/D.

INTERAÇÕES POSSÍVEIS
N/D.

MEDICAMENTO(S) ALTERNATIVO(S)
N/D.

ACOMPANHAMENTO

MONITORIZAÇÃO DO PACIENTE
- Monitorizar a doença primária.
- Corticosteroides para a síndrome de tremor generalizado — monitorizar inicialmente em intervalos semanais para avaliar a resposta terapêutica.

COMPLICAÇÕES POSSÍVEIS
N/D.

DIVERSOS

DISTÚRBIOS ASSOCIADOS
N/D.

FATORES RELACIONADOS COM A IDADE
N/D.

POTENCIAL ZOONÓTICO
N/D.

GESTAÇÃO/FERTILIDADE/REPRODUÇÃO
N/D.

SINÔNIMO(S)
- Agitação.
- Arrepio.

VER TAMBÉM
- Degeneração Cerebelar.
- Hipomielinização.
- Ver também a seção "Causas".

ABREVIATURA(S)
- LCS = líquido cerebrospinal.
- RAETC = resposta auditiva evocada do tronco cerebral.
- RM = ressonância magnética.
- TC = tomografia computadorizada.

Sugestões de Leitura
De Lahunta A, Glass E. Veterinary Neuroanatomy and Clinical Neurology, 3rd ed. St. Louis: Saunders Elsevier, 2009, pp. 206-220.
Lorenz MD, Kornegay JN. Handbook of Veterinary Neurology, 4th ed. St. Louis: Saunders Elsevier, 2004, pp. 265-281.
Wagner SO, Podell M, Fenner WR. Generalized tremors in dogs: 24 cases (1984-1995). JAVMA 1997, 211:731-735.

Autor Rodney S. Bagley
Consultor Editorial Joane M. Parent

TRICOMONÍASE

CONSIDERAÇÕES GERAIS

REVISÃO
- Protozoário flagelado móvel entérico em formato de pera, semelhante à *Giardia* — habita o intestino grosso de cães, gatos e seres humanos.
- Uma espécie, o *Tritrichomonas foetus*, provoca diarreia em gatos.
- Coinfecção com *Giardia* — comum.

IDENTIFICAÇÃO
Gatos jovens — geralmente com menos de 1 ano (faixa etária: 3 meses-13 anos).

SINAIS CLÍNICOS
Gatos
- Diarreia intermitente do intestino grosso.
- A diarreia ocasionalmente contém sangue e muco.
- Ânus — pode ficar edematoso, eritematoso e doloroso em filhotes de gatos.
- Prolapso retal — torna-se grave na presença de irritação anal.
- Diarreia — apresenta melhora com antibioticoterapia, mas exibe recorrência quando o tratamento é interrompido.
- A duração média da diarreia é de aproximadamente 9 meses, com desaparecimento na maioria dos gatos por volta de 2 anos.
- É comum a persistência da infecção após o desaparecimento da diarreia.

CAUSAS E FATORES DE RISCO
- *Pentatrichomonas hominis* (família: Trichomonadidae) — habita o intestino grosso de cães, gatos e seres humanos.
- Não patogênico em cães e gatos — exceto muito raramente nos casos em que pode se tornar um patógeno oportunista.
- *Tritrichomonas foetus* — provoca diarreia em gatos. Infecções experimentais de gatos com isolamentos bovinos de *T. foetus* (que causam infertilidade e abortamento no gado) sugerem que o parasita isolado causador de diarreia do intestino grosso em gatos seja diferente do *T. foetus* isolado que afeta os bovinos.
- Prevalência de *T. foetus* em gatos — ~30% em gatos de exposição, mas muito baixa em gatos selvagens ou domésticos.
- Fatores patogênicos indutores do desenvolvimento de diarreia em gatos infectados — flora bacteriana endógena, adesão do parasita ao epitélio do hospedeiro, e elaboração de citotoxina e enzima.
- Colonização do íleo terminal, ceco e cólon pelos parasitas — induz à diarreia do intestino grosso.
- Alta densidade populacional (gatis, abrigos) — pode ser um fator de risco de infecção.

DIAGNÓSTICO

DIAGNÓSTICO DIFERENCIAL
Gatos
Imprudência alimentar/alimentação inadequada; enteropatia inflamatória; neoplasia (especialmente linfoma GI); medicamentos (antibióticos); toxinas (chumbo); parasitas (criptosporidiose, *Giardia*, ancilóstomos, nematódeos); agentes infecciosos (PIF, salmonelose, proliferação bacteriana GI, clostrídios); disfunção de órgãos sistêmicos (renal, hepático, pancreático, cardíaco); distúrbio metabólico (hipertireoidismo).

HEMOGRAMA/BIOQUÍMICA/URINÁLISE
Geralmente normais — podem refletir a diarreia.

OUTROS TESTES LABORATORIAIS
- Esfregaço fecal direto — baixa sensibilidade.
- Método — diluir as fezes frescas em salina (50:50), colocar em lâmina, cobrir com lamínula, examinar sob microscópio com aumento de 40× da objetiva e condensador abaixado para aumentar o contraste.
- Diferenciação de *Giardia* (disco ventral côncavo, movimento anterógrado espiral) — *T. foetus* possui movimento anterógrado rítmico (espasmódico), além de ser em formato de fuso (fusiforme) e ter membranas ondulantes.
- Trofozoítas de *T. foetus* — não são observados no exame de flotação fecal.
- Trofozoítas de *T. foetus* — não sobrevivem sob refrigeração.
- Coprocultura para pesquisa do protozoário — utilizar sistema de cultura interno (In Pouch TF®, Biomed Diagnostics, San Jose, CA).
- Método — inocular com 0,05 g de fezes frescas, incubar à temperatura ambiente e examinar diariamente em busca de trofozoítas móveis durante 12 dias.
- *Giardia* e *P. hominis* — não crescem após 24 horas no sistema de cultura In Pouch®.
- PCR — técnica disponível no mercado e mais sensível que a coprocultura em gatos.

DIAGNÓSTICO POR IMAGEM
N/D.

MÉTODOS DIAGNÓSTICOS
N/D.

TRATAMENTO

- Essencial para descartar doença coexistente (criptosporidiose, giardíase), especialmente se a diarreia persistir após tratamento específico.
- O tratamento pode diminuir a gravidade da diarreia, mas também pode prolongar o tempo de resolução desse sinal clínico.

MEDICAÇÕES

MEDICAMENTO(S)
- *P. hominis* — metronidazol (20 mg/kg, VO a cada 12 h por 7 dias).
- *T. foetus* — todas as tentativas de tratamento farmacológico falharam até o momento.

CONTRAINDICAÇÕES/INTERAÇÕES POSSÍVEIS
- Os glicocorticoides podem exacerbar a doença clínica.
- Altas doses de metronidazol (geralmente >30 mg/kg) por períodos extensos podem causar sinais neurológicos.

ACOMPANHAMENTO

- A maioria dos gatos exibe resolução espontânea da diarreia, mas isso pode levar anos (faixa: 4 meses-2 anos).
- As recidivas da diarreia são comuns e frequentemente precipitadas por mudanças da dieta, estresse de viagem e tratamentos de outros distúrbios.

DIVERSOS

POTENCIAL ZOONÓTICO
A possível transmissão zoonótica deve ser abordada com o proprietário.

ABREVIATURAS
- GI = gastrintestinal.
- PCR = reação em cadeia da polimerase.
- PIF = peritonite infecciosa felina.

Sugestões de Leitura
Foster DM, Gookin JL, Poore MF, et al. Outcome of cats with diarrhea and *Tritrichomonas foetus* infection. JAVMA 2004, 15:888-892.
Gookin JL, Stebbins ME, Hunt E, et al. Prevalence of and risk factors from feline *Tritrichomonas foetus* and *Giardia* infection. J Clin Microbiol 2004;42:2707-2710.
Stockdale HD, Dillon AR, Newton JC, et al. Experimental infection of cats (Felis catus) with *Tritrichomonas foetus* isolated from cattle. Vet Parasitol 2008, 154:156-161.

Autor Stephen C. Barr
Consultor Editorial Stephen C. Barr

TRICURÍASE

CONSIDERAÇÕES GERAIS

REVISÃO
- O verme *Trichuris* ocorre no ceco de cães (*T. vulpis*) e gatos (*T. felis*). No entanto, a tricuríase felina é rara nos EUA.
- O ciclo de vida é direto; a infecção é adquirida pela ingestão de ovos larvados presentes em ambientes contaminados por fezes; os ovos infectantes podem persistir no ambiente por meses a anos.
- A infecção pode permanecer assintomática ou causar diarreia sanguinolenta e inflamação do intestino grosso.
- Os sinais clínicos podem ocorrer antes do período de patência, ou seja, antes que os ovos sejam eliminados nas fezes; o período pré-patente gira em torno de 70-90 dias.
- Não ocorre migração extraintestinal.

IDENTIFICAÇÃO
- Cães e gatos de qualquer idade, raça e sexo.
- Raramente observada em gatos nos EUA.

SINAIS CLÍNICOS
- Variam desde um quadro assintomático a grave.
- Diarreia intermitente do intestino grosso que, frequentemente, contém muco e sangue fresco (hematoquezia) nas fezes.
- Diarreia sanguinolenta com desidratação, anemia e perda de peso em casos graves.
- Podem ocorrer sinais clínicos antes da detecção de ovos nas fezes.
- Debilidade aguda a crônica.

CAUSAS E FATORES DE RISCO
- Ingestão de ovos infectantes (larvados) de tricúris provenientes do ambiente contaminado por fezes de cão infectado.
- No ambiente, ocorre o acúmulo de ovos, que persistem infectantes por meses a anos, sobretudo no solo e corredores sujos em áreas úmidas e com sombra.
- O retorno do cão a um ambiente contaminado por ovos infectantes após tratamento anti-helmíntico resultará em recidiva da infecção.

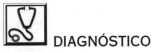

DIAGNÓSTICO

DIAGNÓSTICO DIFERENCIAL
- Infecções bacterianas (por espiroquetas) do ceco.
- Infecções por ancilóstomos — identificar ovos nas fezes; os sinais incluem anemia, mucosas pálidas e melena, e não sangue fresco nas fezes.
- Infecções por capilárias (*Pearsonema*, *Eucoleus*) — os ovos têm aspecto semelhante, porém são menores com superfície rugosa; infectam os tratos urinários ou respiratórios, respectivamente, e não o trato GI; geralmente assintomáticas.
- Pseudo-hipoadrenocorticismo secundário em tricuríase grave com acidose metabólica, hiponatremia, hipercalemia e desidratação; resposta normal à estimulação com ACTH em casos de tricuríase.

HEMOGRAMA/BIOQUÍMICA/URINÁLISE
Geralmente normais; em casos muito graves, podem ocorrer hiponatremia, hipercalemia e acidose metabólica.

OUTROS TESTES LABORATORIAIS
Teste de estimulação com ACTH em casos graves com distúrbios eletrolíticos para diferenciar tricuríase de hipoadrenocorticismo.

DIAGNÓSTICO POR IMAGEM
N/D.

MÉTODOS DIAGNÓSTICOS
- Flutuação fecal centrífuga em solução de açúcar (densidade específica >1,2) constitui o método preferido.
- Diferenciar os ovos de *Trichuris* (coloração castanha, formato ovoide ou semelhante a limão, com opérculos bipolares proeminentes, envoltório liso e uma única célula dentro do ovo, ~90 × 45 µm) dos ovos semelhantes de capilárias (menores com superfície rugosa do envoltório).

TRATAMENTO
- Tratamento ambulatorial com anti-helmíntico na maioria dos casos.
- Os casos graves com desidratação e distúrbios eletrolíticos necessitam de internação com fluidoterapia e anti-helmíntico.

MEDICAÇÕES

MEDICAMENTO(S)
- Fembendazol na dose de 50 mg/kg VO a cada 24 h por 3 dias; repetir mensalmente por três vezes; uso fora da indicação da bula em gatos.
- Febantel/praziquantel/pamoato de pirantel — usar a dose da bula VO em cães.
- Milbemicina oxima — 0,5 mg/kg VO a cada 30 dias em cães.
- Moxidectina/imidacloprida — utilizar a dose da bula em cães.

CONTRAINDICAÇÕES/INTERAÇÕES POSSÍVEIS
A correção muita rápida da hiponatremia em casos graves pode resultar em mielinólise iatrogênica.

ACOMPANHAMENTO

MONITORIZAÇÃO DO PACIENTE
Repetição do exame coprológico em busca dos ovos de tricúris e/ou repetição do tratamento anti-helmíntico em 3 semanas e 3 meses após a terapia inicial ou uma vez por mês durante 3 meses até detectar e eliminar os adultos recém-amadurecidos.

PREVENÇÃO
- Remoção e descarte imediatos das fezes para evitar contaminação ambiental por ovos infectantes.
- Tratamento anti-helmíntico de cães infectados para evitar a eliminação de ovos e a contaminação do ambiente.

EVOLUÇÃO ESPERADA E PROGNÓSTICO
Prognóstico bom após instituição do tratamento e implementação de medidas preventivas.

DIVERSOS

POTENCIAL ZOONÓTICO
Foram diagnosticados casos relativamente raros de infecção em seres humanos por *T. vulpis*, com base nas diferenças morfológicas entre os ovos de tricúris humano, *T. trichiura*, e aqueles de *T. vulpis*.

ABREVIATURA(S)
- ACTH = hormônio adrenocorticotrópico.
- GI = gastrintestinal.

RECURSOS DA INTERNET
www.capcvet.org.

Sugestões de Leitura
Bowman DD. Georgis' Parasitology for Veterinarians, 9th ed. St. Louis: Saunders, 2009, pp. 224-225.

Autor Julie Ann Jarvinen
Consultor Editorial Stephen C. Barr

Triquinose

CONSIDERAÇÕES GERAIS

REVISÃO
- Infecção por nematódeo — adultos infectam o intestino delgado de uma ampla variedade de carnívoros (incluindo cães e pessoas) e onívoros (porcos), causando doença GI leve.
- Larvas — ficam sequestradas na musculatura esquelética em todo o corpo.
- De grande importância zoonótica — os seres humanos adquirem a infecção pela ingestão de carne malcozida contendo larvas sequestradas provenientes de uma ampla variedade de animais (porcos, ursos, focas, cavalos).
- Causa miosite grave e, algumas vezes, morte em seres humanos.
- Na China — o consumo de carne de cães é uma fonte importante de triquinose em seres humanos.
- Distribuição mundial.

IDENTIFICAÇÃO
- Cães de caça (incluindo aqueles que caçam raposas) — alta taxa de infecção.
- Filhotes caninos — mais suscetíveis à infecção que os cães mais idosos.

SINAIS CLÍNICOS
- Leve desarranjo GI — vômito, diarreia.
- Mialgia, rigidez muscular — leves e raramente observadas.
- Infecção cardíaca — pode resultar em síncope causada por distúrbios de condução.
- Lesão cutânea ulcerativa não cicatrizante no gato.

CAUSAS E FATORES DE RISCO
- *Trichinella spiralis* — os cães e gatos tornam-se infectados pela ingestão de larvas L1 sequestradas no músculo de outros animais. *Trichinella nativa* — relatada como a causa de lesão cutânea ulcerativa não cicatrizante no gato.
- Fontes de infecção — principalmente gatos: roedores selvagens capturados ou carcaças de carnívoros; cães: raposas, gambás, guaxinins e porcos selvagens.
- Larvas L1 — sofrem muda em adultos no intestino delgado.
- Vermes adultos — produzem grande número de "pré-larvas", que são injetadas na mucosa intestinal.
- Pré-larvas — migram pelos vasos linfáticos inicialmente e, depois, pela corrente sanguínea até os músculos esqueléticos, onde se espiralam e se desenvolvem em L1 em estruturas semelhantes a cistos.
- Larvas L1 — permanecem infectantes no músculo por meses a anos.
- Cães — são necessárias pouquíssimas larvas apenas para infecção.
- Ingestão de grande número de larvas — resulta no mesmo grau de sequestração muscular como infecções muito pequenas, porque a maioria das larvas infectantes passa direto para o trato GI sem se desenvolver em adultos em grandes infecções.
- Taxa de infecção em cães — mais alta que nos porcos em alguns estudos.

DIAGNÓSTICO

DIAGNÓSTICO DIFERENCIAL
Outras causas de gastrenterite transitória leve — imprudência alimentar/alimentação inadequada; enteropatia inflamatória precoce; medicamentos (antibióticos); parasitas (giardíase, tricomoníase, tricúris); agentes infecciosos; corpo estranho parcial (tricobezoares em gatos).

HEMOGRAMA/BIOQUÍMICA/URINÁLISE
Hemograma completo — eosinofilia durante o estágio agudo da infecção; pode persistir por várias semanas em infecções graves.

OUTROS TESTES LABORATORIAIS
- Identificação dos pequenos adultos nas fezes (fêmea 3 mm, macho 1,5 mm) — talvez haja necessidade de exame coprológico coletado com o passar do tempo.
- Adultos e larvas nas fezes — diferenciados das larvas de *Crenosoma*, *Angiostrongylus*, e *Filaroides* pela estrutura no esôfago denominada esticossoma (tanto adultos como larvas), pelos lobos copulatórios (machos) e pela presença de pré-larvas dentro do útero (fêmeas).
- As pré-larvas podem ser identificadas no sangue (100 μm, opostas às larvas de *Dirofilaria immitis* e *Dipetalonema reconditum* de ~300 μm) — pela técnica de Knott modificada.

DIAGNÓSTICO POR IMAGEM
N/D.

MÉTODOS DIAGNÓSTICOS
Biopsia muscular — método diagnóstico de escolha; larvas L1 com estrutura característica no esôfago denominada esticossoma em "cistos".

TRATAMENTO
- Não há tratamento específico requerido para os sinais do trato GI ou mialgia.
- Albendazol — foi demonstrado que esse medicamento reduz significativamente as formas larvais nos músculos.
- Em função da eficácia do albendazol, é provável que o fembendazol seja eficaz sem efeitos colaterais.

MEDICAÇÕES

MEDICAMENTO(S)
- Fembendazol na dose de 50 mg/kg VO a cada 24 h por 10 dias.
- Albendazol na dose de 50 mg/kg VO a cada 12 h por 7 dias.

CONTRAINDICAÇÕES/INTERAÇÕES POSSÍVEIS
Albendazol — foi demonstrado que esse medicamento provoca mielossupressão em cães e gatos nessas doses.

ACOMPANHAMENTO
Ao utilizar o albendazol, deve-se monitorizar o hemograma completo quanto à presença de sinais de pancitopenia.

DIVERSOS

ABREVIATURAS
GI = gastrintestinal.

Sugestões de Leitura
Darrigrand RA, Bowman DD, Frongillo M, et al. Treatment of experimentally induced trichinosis in dogs and cats. Am J Vet Res 1993, 54:1303-1305.
Saari S, Airas N, Nareaho A, et al. A nonhealing ulcerative skin lesion associated with *Trichinella nativa* infection in a cat. J Vet Diagn Invest 2008, 20:839-843.
Sleeper MM, Bissett S, Craig L. Canine trichinosis presenting with syncope and AV conduction disturbance. J Vet Intern Med 2006, 20:1228-1231.

Autor Stephen C. Barr
Consultor Editorial Stephen C. Barr

TROMBOCITOPATIAS

CONSIDERAÇÕES GERAIS

REVISÃO
- Defeitos hereditários ou adquiridos, que podem comprometer qualquer uma das principais funções das plaquetas, incluindo a atividade pró-coagulante. • Os animais acometidos tipicamente apresentam contagens plaquetárias normais, mas exibem sangramento espontâneo ou excessivo; o sangramento de mucosas constitui o sinal clínico mais comum. • Os animais trombocitopênicos com trombocitopatia concomitante manifestarão sangramento mais excessivo do que o esperado para a contagem plaquetária.

IDENTIFICAÇÃO
- Os defeitos adquiridos são as trombocitopatias mais comuns observadas em animais de companhia. Tais defeitos ocorrem em todas as raças e todas as idades. • Os defeitos hereditários da função plaquetária podem ser diagnosticados em todas as idades, embora possam aparecer pela primeira vez em animais jovens no momento em que ocorre sangramento excessivo com a perda dos dentes decíduos. • Os defeitos hereditários são distúrbios raros que foram descritos nas seguintes raças/espécies:
    ○ Trombastenia de Glanzmann tipo I — cães das raças Otterhound e Grande Pireneu.
    ○ Doenças da reserva de armazenamento — síndrome de Chediak-Higashi em gatos da raça Persa; grânulos delta em Cocker spaniel americano; Collie cinza com hematopoiese cíclica.
    ○ Trombocitopatia (deficiência de CalDAG-GEFI) em cães das raças Basset hound, Spitz e Landseer.
    ○ Síndrome de Scott em Pastor alemão.

SINAIS CLÍNICOS
- Frequentemente, observa-se leve sangramento mucocutâneo espontâneo, como epistaxe, petéquias e sangramento gengival. • Em certos animais, pode ocorrer sangramento prolongado durante ou após procedimentos diagnósticos ou cirúrgicos.

CAUSAS E FATORES DE RISCO

Adquiridas por Medicamentos
- Os AINEs (p. ex., ácido acetilsalicílico) inibem a função plaquetária por impedir a formação do tromboxano A_2, um agonista plaquetário potente. Esse efeito é menos pronunciado ou até mesmo ausente com os antagonistas mais seletivos da ciclo-oxigenase-2 (p. ex., meloxicam e deracoxibe). • Sulfonamidas potencializadas e soluções de hidroxietila de amido suprimem a função das plaquetas em cães. • Penicilinas, tetraciclinas, agentes anestésicos/sedativos e anti-histamínicos provocam trombocitopenia e/ou defeitos da função plaquetária em seres humanos — no entanto, esses efeitos não foram registrados em cães e gatos.

Secundárias à Doença Sistêmica
- Coagulopatia intravascular disseminada, uremia, anemia, hepatopatia (colestase e desvios adquiridos ou hereditários), erliquiose, leishmaniose, trombocitopenia imunomediada, cardiopatia e distúrbios neoplásicos (neoplasias hematopoiéticas e não hematopoiéticas).

Hereditárias
- Doença de von Willebrand — trata-se de uma deficiência (Tipo I e III) ou defeito qualitativo (Tipo II) do fator de von Willebrand. • Trombocitopatia hereditária dos cães das raças Basset hound, Spitz e Landseer — defeitos de transdução de sinal atribuídos a mutações de CalDAG-GEFI. • Cães das raças Otterhound e Grande Pireneu com trombastenia de Glanzmann tipo I — defeito plaquetário causado por mutação no receptor da glicoproteína IIb-IIIa (integrina $\alpha_{IIb}\beta_3$) na superfície das plaquetas. • Doença da reserva de armazenamento: síndrome de Chediak-Higashi e deficiência da reserva de armazenamento do ADP em grânulos delta — defeito de agregação provocado pela falta de nucleotídeos de adenina. • Síndrome de Scott em cães da raça Pastor alemão — deficiência plaquetária de pró-coagulante (falha em externalizar a fosfatidilserina na superfície das plaquetas e incapacidade dessas células em manter um agrupamento eficaz dos complexos de coagulação).

DIAGNÓSTICO

HEMOGRAMA/BIOQUÍMICA/URINÁLISE
- Anemia em casos de sangramento grave; regenerativa ou arregenerativa. • Em cães com trombocitopatias hereditárias, as contagens plaquetárias tipicamente permanecem normais; em alguns cães da raça Otterhound, observam-se contagens plaquetárias baixas com plaquetas bizarras e gigantes. • Perfil bioquímico — sem alterações específicas.

OUTROS TESTES LABORATORIAIS
- Uso de analisador da função plaquetária (PFA-100®) e mensuração do fator de von Willebrand por imunoensaio — em animais com suspeita dessa doença. • Testes da função plaquetária — em laboratórios especializados. Os testes mais comuns são a agregação das plaquetas e a citometria de fluxo. • Testes de coagulação (tromboelastografia, TP e TTPA) — para descartar a coagulopatia como uma causa de hemorragia; o TTPA pode estar prolongado em alguns animais com doença de von Willebrand. • Teste genético de animais portadores.

MÉTODOS DIAGNÓSTICOS
Tempo de sangramento de mucosas — para confirmar os defeitos da função plaquetária; o tempo normal de sangramento da mucosa bucal, mensurado por meio de uma incisão de 5 mm de comprimento por 1 mm de profundidade com uma lanceta de mola (Tripplet®, Helena Laboratories, Beaumont, TX), é <4-5 min em cães e <2-3 min em gatos.

TRATAMENTO
- Transfusão de plaquetas — 20 mL/kg (mínimo de 10 mL/kg) de plasma rico em plaquetas ou plasma fresco congelado (contém partículas de plaquetas) ou 1 unidade de concentrado plaquetário ou crioprecipitado/10 kg (mínimo de 1 unidade/30 kg), dependendo da condição. • Transfusão de sangue total ou de papa de hemácias para a correção da anemia. • Em animais com distúrbios adquiridos da função plaquetária, tratar o processo patológico subjacente ou retirar o agente agressor. • Procedimentos cirúrgicos eletivos devem ser evitados ou acompanhados por produtos adequados de transfusão. • Evitar fluidoterapia excessiva. • Restringir a atividade física durante algum episódio hemorrágico.

MEDICAÇÕES

MEDICAMENTO(S)
- Acetato de desmopressina [DDAVP] (1 µg/kg SC ou IV diluído em 20 mL de solução salina e administrado por 10 min) em cães com a doença de von Willebrand durante os episódios hemorrágicos (se for eficaz, o efeito durará de 2-3 h). • A desmopressina (3 µg/kg SC) melhora o tempo de sangramento em cães com trombocitopatia atribuída ao ácido acetilsalicílico e à hepatopatia. Além disso, esse agente é benéfico em muitas trombocitopatias em seres humanos; dessa forma, pode-se contemplar seu uso em cães com outras trombocitopatias. • Administrar a desmopressina ao doador 30 min antes da coleta do sangue destinado à transfusão de cães com a doença de von Willebrand ou trombocitopatia.

ACOMPANHAMENTO
- É preciso tomar precauções especiais ao se efetuar procedimentos cirúrgicos nesses animais. • Conscientizar o proprietário sobre a possibilidade de episódios hemorrágicos recidivantes em animais com defeitos hereditários da função plaquetária, embora episódios fatais não sejam comuns. • Caso se identifique algum defeito hereditário, o animal não deverá ser utilizado para fins reprodutivos.

DIVERSOS

VER TAMBÉM
- Doença de von Willebrand. • Trombocitopenia.

ABREVIATURA(S)
- ADP = difosfato de adenosina. • AINE = anti-inflamatório não esteroide. • DDAVP = 1-desamino-8-D-arginina vasopressina. • TP = tempo de protrombina. • TTPA = tempo de tromboplastina parcial ativada.

Sugestões de Leitura
Brooks MB, Catalfamo JL. Platelet dysfunction. In: Bonagura JD, Twedt DC, Kirk's Current Veterinary Therapy XIV. St. Louis: Elsevier, 2009, pp. 292-296.
Fry, MM. Acquired platelet dysfunction. In: Weiss DJ, Wardrop KJ, Schalm's Veterinary Hematology, 6th ed. Ames, IA: Wiley-Blackwell, 2010, pp. 626-632.

Autores Inge Tarnow e Annemarie T. Kristensen
Consultor Editorial A.H. Rebar
Agradecimento O autor e os editores agradecem a colaboração prévia do Dr. Anthony C.G. Abrams-Ogg

TROMBOCITOPENIA

CONSIDERAÇÕES GERAIS

DEFINIÇÃO
Contagem de plaquetas abaixo do limite inferior da faixa de referência, que varia de acordo com o método de contagem dessas células. Grau de trombocitopenia — Grau 1: 100.000/μL até o limite inferior da faixa de referência; Grau 2: 50.000-99.000/μL; Grau 3: 25.000-49.000/μL; Grau 4: <25.000/μL.

FISIOPATOLOGIA
• As plaquetas são produzidas por megacariócitos na medula óssea e liberadas na corrente sanguínea, onde circulam por até 7 dias. • A trombocitopenia é causada por um ou mais dos seguintes fatores: declínio na produção, aumento no sequestro, utilização, destruição (perda) de plaquetas. • A trombocitopenia também pode resultar em hemorragia espontânea ou excessiva.

SISTEMA(S) ACOMETIDO(S)
• A hemorragia pode ocorrer em qualquer sistema orgânico. • Hemorragia clínica — identificada mais comumente nos sistemas cutâneo/exócrino e gastrintestinal, seguidos pelos sistemas renal/urológico e respiratório; identificada com menor frequência nos sistemas oftálmico, nervoso e reprodutor.

INCIDÊNCIA/PREVALÊNCIA
• A trombocitopenia é uma anormalidade hematológica comum. • Hemorragia grave atribuída à trombocitopenia é incomum (cães) ou rara (gatos) na clínica geral.

IDENTIFICAÇÃO
Espécies
Cães e gatos.
Raça(s) Predominante(s)
• Trombocitopenia assintomática hereditária com macroplaquetas — descrita em Cavalier King Charles spaniel. • Trombocitopenia branda assintomática hereditária — descrita em cães Galgos.

SINAIS CLÍNICOS
Comentários Gerais
• Trombocitopenia de Grau 1 não aumenta o risco de hemorragia. • Pode ocorrer hemorragia cirúrgica acentuada em casos de trombocitopenia de Grau 2. • Com trombocitopenia de grau 3, pode ocorrer hemorragia espontânea microscópica. • Risco leve, moderado e grave de hemorragia clínica espontânea com contagens plaquetárias de <25.000/μL, <10.000/μL e <5.000/μL, respectivamente (trombocitopenia de Grau 4). • Esses valores são diretrizes somente por causa da variação nos métodos de contagem das plaquetas e da imprecisão de baixas contagens dessas células. • Defeito da função plaquetária, doença de von Willebrand, coagulopatia, vasculite ou sepse concomitantes aumentam o risco de hemorragia. • Os cães com trombocitopenia imunomediada apresentam risco inferior de hemorragia para uma dada contagem plaquetária. • Os gatos exibem um risco mais baixo de hemorragia, quando comparados com os cães.
Achados Anamnésicos
• Sangramentos espontâneos ou excessivos nas mucosas, na pele, na cavidade nasal, bem como nos tratos gastrintestinal e urinário. • Letargia e colapso (anemia hemorrágica). • Dispneia e tosse (hemorragia do trato respiratório). • Sinais clínicos da doença primária.
Achados do Exame Físico
• Petéquias e equimoses na pele e nas mucosas. • Sangramento persistente oriundo de feridas e locais de venopunção. • Melena, hematoquezia, hematêmese. • Hematúria. • Hemorragias oculares. • Hepatosplenomegalia. • Mucosas pálidas. • Fraqueza. • Dispneia, hemoptise. • Sopro cardíaco. • Sinais neurológicos. • Sangramento excessivo no estro (cio). • Sinais clínicos da doença primária.

CAUSAS
• Declínio na produção — hereditário; neoplasia na medula óssea; sertolinoma; agentes infecciosos; imunomediada; medicamentos; radiação. A trombocitopenia varia de leve a grave e pode ser uma anormalidade hematológica isolada ou uma característica de pancitopenia.
• Aumento no sequestro — esplenomegalia; uma trombocitopenia grave não é comum.
• Aumento no uso — CID; trombose local; vasculite; trombocitopenia grave é incomum.
• Aumento na destruição — trombocitopenia imunomediada primária ou secundária à neoplasia; agentes infecciosos; inflamação asséptica; medicamentos. Corresponde à causa mais comum de trombocitopenia grave em cães.
• Aumento na perda — as hemorragias decorrentes de intoxicação por antagonismo da vitamina K podem resultar em trombocitopenia leve a moderada; já as hemorragias atribuídas a trauma maior podem culminar em trombocitopenia branda a grave após restauração volêmica.

FATORES DE RISCO
• Potencialmente qualquer infecção — agentes infecciosos comumente associados à trombocitopenia: FeLV; FIV; cinomose, parvovirose; *Ehrlichia canis*; *E. chaffeensis*, *E. ewingii*; *Anaplasma platys*; *A. phagocytophilum*; febre maculosa das Montanhas Rochosas; leptospirose; sepse bacteriana; histoplasmose; *Cytauxzoon felis*; *Babesia canis*, *B. gibsoni*; *Hepatozoon canis*; *Leishmania* spp.; *Theileria* spp.; dirofilariose; *Angiostrongylus vasorum* e larva migrans aberrante.
• Potencialmente qualquer inflamação não infecciosa, p. ex., vasculite.
• Potencialmente qualquer neoplasia — as neoplasias identificadas com maior frequência incluem o hemangiossarcoma, o carcinoma da tireoide, o linfoma e as leucemias agudas.
• Terapia citotóxica — mielossupressão previsível; a lomustina causa trombocitopenia cumulativa.
• Potencialmente qualquer medicamento — os medicamentos com risco conhecido de indução de mielossupressão ou trombocitopenia imunomediada imprevisíveis compreendem os estrogênios, os compostos de ouro, a fenilbutazona, o fenobarbital (cães), o cloranfenicol, a griseofulvina, a propiltiouracila e o metimazol (gatos); já os medicamentos com relatos de reações idiossincrásicas que induzem à mielossupressão englobam as cefalosporinas e o albendazol (cães, gatos), o fembendazol, as sulfonamidas, os inibidores da ECA (cães) e a ribavirina.
• Vacinação dentro de 1 mês — em casos de trombocitopenia imunomediada.
• Toxinas e venenos — zinco, *Autumn crocus* (mielossupressão); micotoxinas; xilitol (lesão hepática aguda — CID); picada de cobra.
• Hipertermia — CID.

DIAGNÓSTICO

DIAGNÓSTICO DIFERENCIAL
• Erro de mensuração decorrente da formação de agregados plaquetários — ocorre muito provavelmente em casos de venopunção traumática e em gatos. Apesar de rara, pode ocorrer a formação de aglomerados plaquetários induzidos pelo EDTA.
• Erro de contagem.
• Hemorragia local — descartar traumatismo, ulceração gastrintestinal, distúrbios primários intranasais e oftálmicos, bem como distúrbios dos tratos urinário e reprodutivo.
• Doença de von Willebrand — petéquias, equimoses e hemorragias oculares não são usuais.
• Coagulopatia — petéquias, hemorragia gastrintestinal e epistaxe são incomuns; tumefações subcutâneas e articulares, hemotórax e hemoabdome podem estar presentes.

HEMOGRAMA/BIOQUÍMICA/URINÁLISE
• Confirmar a trombocitopenia descrita por um analisador hematológico por exame microscópico de esfregaço sanguíneo; examinar a chanfradura dos agregados plaquetários; estimar a contagem de plaquetas a partir da monocamada eritrocitária, em que cerca de 50% das células estão em contato; cada campo microscópico em óleo de imersão corresponde a 15.000-25.000 plaquetas/μL.
• O volume plaquetário médio e a amplitude de distribuição de plaquetas são inversamente relacionados com a contagem dessas células e não costumam auxiliar na diferenciação das causas de trombocitopenia. Do mesmo modo, as alterações de morfologia das plaquetas são inespecíficas.
• Plaquetócrito (análogo ao hematócrito) reflete a massa de plaquetas. Um analisador quantitativo da camada leucocitária calcula o número de plaquetas a partir da massa dessas células e pode ser o melhor método para o diagnóstico de trombocitopenia patológica em cão da raça Cavalier King Charles spaniel.
• Anemia regenerativa — descartar hemorragia ou anemia hemolítica imunomediada concomitante com trombocitopenia imunomediada.
• Neutrofilia e desvio à esquerda — excluir sepse, inflamação asséptica e estimulação inespecífica de granulopoiese.
• Eosinofilia — descartar dirofilariose e outras infecções por helmintos.
• Anemia arregenerativa e neutropenia concomitantes — a trombocitopenia provavelmente se deve ao declínio na produção.
• Esquistócitos — excluir CID.
• *B. canis*, *B. gibsoni* e *C. felis* nas hemácias, *A. platys* nas plaquetas, *E. canis* e *E. chaffensis* nos monócitos, *E. ewingii* e *A. phagocytophilum* nos neutrófilos.
• Anormalidades no perfil bioquímico e na urinálise refletem a doença primária.

OUTROS TESTES LABORATORIAIS
• Antígeno do fator de von Willebrand — descartar a doença de von Willebrand.

- TP, TTPA, TCA — resultados prolongados aumentam a probabilidade de CID; o TP normal descarta antagonismo da vitamina K.
- Produtos de degradação da fibrina e D-dímero — o resultado positivo aumenta a probabilidade de CID ou trombose local.
- Culturas de órgãos anormais, sangue e urina — descartam sepse bacteriana ou fúngica.
- Sorologia e PCR — para pesquisa de microrganismos infecciosos; ver capítulos específicos.
- Flutuação fecal e técnica de Baermann — em busca de larvas parasitárias.
- Testes dos anticorpos antiplaquetários e antimegacariocíticos — os resultados negativos ajudam a descartar a trombocitopenia imunomediada.
- Teste de Coombs — o resultado positivo aumenta a probabilidade de anemia hemolítica imunomediada concomitante.
- Teste do anticorpo antinuclear — o resultado positivo aumenta a probabilidade de LES.
- Testes de função das plaquetas — difíceis de realizar na presença de trombocitopenia; ver "Trombocitopatias".
- Citometria de fluxo — para plaquetas reticuladas imaturas (análogo à contagem de reticulócitos).

DIAGNÓSTICO POR IMAGEM
As técnicas de diagnóstico por imagem são usadas para identificar esplenomegalia, hepatomegalia, neoplasias, focos infecciosos e hemorragia interna.

MÉTODOS DIAGNÓSTICOS
Biopsia da medula óssea — para descartar a diminuição na produção plaquetária: neoplasia na medula óssea, histoplasmose, interrupção da maturação, aplasia medular, mielofibrose e necrose medular; não há nenhum achado específico que inclua ou exclua a hipoplasia megacariocítica imunomediada; baixa recuperação diagnóstica se as únicas anormalidades hematológicas forem a trombocitopenia indutora de sangramento e a anemia regenerativa (provável trombocitopenia imunomediada).

TRATAMENTO
CUIDADO(S) DE SAÚDE ADEQUADO(S)
- Tratamento do distúrbio primário.
- Transfusão das plaquetas — 20 mL/kg (mínimo de 10 mL/kg) de sangue total fresco, plasma rico em plaquetas ou plasma fresco congelado (contém partículas de plaquetas) ou 1 unidade de concentrado plaquetário ou crioprecipitado/10 kg (mínimo de 1 unidade/30 kg, sendo que 1 unidade canina se refere ao produto derivado de uma unidade de 450 mL de sangue total); transfundir em casos de hemorragias críticas ou com objetivos profiláticos em casos de contagem plaquetária <5.000-10.000/μL; talvez haja necessidade de transfusões a cada 1-3 dias se a trombocitopenia grave persistir; procedimento bastante útil quando a trombocitopenia se deve ao declínio na produção ou à perda de plaquetas e nos casos em que se prevê uma rápida resolução; menos útil em casos de esplenomegalia e CID; e menos útil ainda em casos de trombocitopenia imunomediada. São preparados concentrados de plaquetas caninos frescos, armazenados à temperatura ambiente, criopreservados e liofilizados.
- Transfusão de sangue total ou de papa de hemácias para a correção da anemia — o sangramento decorrente da trombocitopenia é pior na presença de anemia.
- Não proceder à drenagem de hematomas a menos que eles sejam a causa do problema (p. ex., compressão da traqueia).

CUIDADO(S) DE ENFERMAGEM
- Minimizar as injeções IM e SC. Aplicar compressão prolongada após injeções IV, cateterizações IV e procedimentos invasivos. Impedir a venopunção jugular. A biopsia da medula óssea é um procedimento seguro.
- Evitar fluidoterapia excessiva.

DIETA
Evitar rações duras em casos de trombocitopenia grave por conta do risco de sangramento gengival.

ORIENTAÇÃO AO PROPRIETÁRIO
Caso não se consiga identificar e tratar a causa subjacente da trombocitopenia grave, ocorrerá uma falha terapêutica em função da possibilidade limitada em se fornecer transfusões plaquetárias prolongadas.

MEDICAÇÕES
MEDICAMENTO(S) DE ESCOLHA
- Ver capítulos específicos em busca das doenças indutoras de trombocitopenia.
- Antibióticos (para doenças infecciosas) têm efeitos desprezíveis sobre a função das plaquetas em cães e gatos.
- Hemorragia do SNC — dexametasona (0,25 mg/kg IV ou VO a cada 8-24 h).
- Acepromazina — tem efeitos insignificantes sobre a função das plaquetas em cães e gatos, mas pode ser usada para sedar os animais a fim de diminuir o risco de hemorragia associada à atividade excessiva.

CONTRAINDICAÇÕES
Evitar o uso de AINE que interferem na função plaquetária — para obtenção de analgesia, preferem-se os opioides. Se houver a necessidade do emprego de AINE, utilizar os inibidores da ciclo-oxigenase-2 mais seletivos (p. ex., deracoxibe).

PRECAUÇÕES
- A heparina (utilizada em casos de CID) pode agravar as hemorragias decorrentes de trombocitopenia.
- A corticoterapia pode exacerbar infecções e promover ulcerações gastrintestinais.

MEDICAMENTO(S) ALTERNATIVO(S)
- Oprelvecina (interleucina-11 recombinante humana; Neumega®; Wyeth, Philadelphia, PA) — 50 μg/kg SC a cada 24 h por, no máximo, 2 semanas; muito útil para estimular a produção de plaquetas quando a trombocitopenia é causada por terapia citotóxica; após 2 semanas, há um provável risco de formação de anticorpos neutralizantes; tem alto custo.
- Carbonato de lítio — não recomendado.
- Ácido aminocaproico — inibidor da plasmina; experiência clínica restrita; contraindicado em casos de CID; dose descrita para mielopatia degenerativa em cães: cerca de 12,5-15 mg/kg VO a cada 8 h; a dosagem humana é aproximadamente 10 vezes maior que a dos cães.

ACOMPANHAMENTO
MONITORIZAÇÃO DO PACIENTE
- Magnitude do sangramento — o controle da hemorragia clínica constitui o parâmetro mais importante para monitorizar e avaliar a eficácia do tratamento. • Contagens das plaquetas — diariamente até a estabilização do paciente e, depois, em intervalos semanais até o retorno dessas células aos valores normais. • Perfis seriados de coagulação — em caso de suspeita de CID.

DIVERSOS
DISTÚRBIOS ASSOCIADOS
- Se a trombocitopenia for decorrente da produção plaquetária reduzida, poderá haver anemia e neutropenia concomitantes. • A trombocitopenia imunomediada pode ser uma anormalidade isolada ou estar associada a outros distúrbios imunomediados.

FATORES RELACIONADOS COM A IDADE
Variam com a causa — por exemplo, FeLV em gatos mais jovens; trombocitopenia imunomediada em cães de meia-idade; neoplasia em cães mais idosos.

POTENCIAL ZOONÓTICO
A trombocitopenia pode ser atribuída a uma infecção zoonótica (p. ex., leptospirose).

VER TAMBÉM
- Anemia Imunomediada. • Coagulação Intravascular Disseminada. • Esplenomegalia. • Hifema. • Pancitopenia. • Petéquia, Equimose, Contusão. • Torção Esplênica. • Trombocitopatias. • Trombocitopenia Imunomediada Primária. • Vasculite Sistêmica. • Capítulos específicos para várias doenças infecciosas.

ABREVIATURA(S)
- AINE = anti-inflamatório não esteroide.
- CID = coagulação intravascular disseminada.
- EDTA = ácido etilenodiaminotetracético.
- FeLV = vírus da leucemia felina.
- FIV = vírus da imunodeficiência felina.
- LES = lúpus eritematoso sistêmico.
- PCR = reação em cadeia da polimerase.
- SNC = sistema nervoso central.
- TCA = tempo de coagulação ativada.
- TP = tempo de protrombina.
- TTPA = tempo de tromboplastina parcial ativada.

RECURSOS DA INTERNET
- www.ivis.org. • www.veterinarypartner.com.

Sugestões de Leitura
Botsch V, Küchenhoff H, Hartmann K, Hirschberger J. Retrospective study of 871 dogs with thrombocytopenia. Vet Record 2009, 164:647-651.
Jordan HL, Grindem CB, Breitschwerdt EB. Thrombocytopenia in cats: A retrospective study of 41 cases. J Vet Intern Med 1993, 7:261-265.

Autor Anthony C. G. Abrams-Ogg
Consultor Editorial A. H. Rebar
Agradecimento O autor e os editores agradecem as colaborações prévias do Dr. William J. Reagan

TROMBOCITOPENIA IMUNOMEDIADA PRIMÁRIA

CONSIDERAÇÕES GERAIS

DEFINIÇÃO
- Destruição imunomediada de plaquetas, sem causa identificável.
- Em casos de trombocitopenia imunomediada secundária, doenças infecciosas, neoplasias, vacinações ou medicamentos deflagram a produção de anticorpos.

FISIOPATOLOGIA
- Autoanticorpos contra plaquetas resultam na destruição prematura dessas células por macrófagos, principalmente no baço por um mecanismo Tipo II (citotoxicidade dependente de anticorpos).
- Na trombocitopenia imunomediada secundária, anticorpos ligados às plaquetas podem ser aqueles ligados aos antígenos plaquetários alterados durante a evolução da doença ou outros ligados a antígenos estranhos ou imunocomplexos.
- Os autoanticorpos podem ser direcionados contra megacariócitos, impedindo com isso a responsividade da medula.
- É possível a inibição da função plaquetária mediada por anticorpos.
- A causa da falta de regulação imunológica e da produção de autoanticorpos é desconhecida.

SISTEMA(S) ACOMETIDO(S)
- Cutâneo.
- Trato gastrintestinal.
- Respiratório.
- Oftálmico.
- Urinário.
- SNC.

GENÉTICA
A autoimunidade é frequentemente identificada em raças caninas específicas e, muitas vezes, tem base familiar, sugerindo uma forte influência genética.

PREVALÊNCIA
- Cerca de 5% dos casos de trombocitopenia canina.
- Rara (ou raramente diagnosticada) em gatos.

IDENTIFICAÇÃO
Espécies
- Comum em cães.
- Rara em gatos.

Predileções Raciais e Familiares
Cocker spaniel, Poodle, Old English sheepdog, Setter irlandês; qualquer raça pode ser acometida.

Idade Média e Faixa Etária
- Principalmente em cães de meia-idade.
- Faixa etária descrita em cães: 0,3-15 anos (média de 5 anos); em gatos: 0,7-12 anos (média de 6 anos).

Sexo Predominante
Cadelas, castradas ou intactas, são predispostas.

SINAIS CLÍNICOS
Achados Anamnésicos
- Com frequência, os cães são levados à consulta em função de hemorragia (superficial) de início agudo.
- A perda crônica de sangue atribuída à trombocitopenia imunomediada é muito rara.
- Ocasionalmente, há histórico de letargia, fraqueza e inapetência.
- Os gatos são levados ao veterinário por conta de letargia, inapetência e hemorragia (superficial).
- Os casos assintomáticos podem ser detectados durante check-ups de rotina ou triagens pré-cirúrgicas.
- Perguntas específicas: histórico de medicações/viagens ou uso de vacinação (a aplicação de vacinas nas últimas 4 semanas pode indicar reações vacinais).

Achados do Exame Físico
- Principalmente sangramento superficial.
- Petéquias/equimoses das mucosas e da pele.
- Sangramento gengival.
- Melena, hematêmese, hematoquezia.
- Epistaxe.
- Hemorragia ocular.
- Hematúria.
- Algumas vezes, hematomas.
- Hemorragia prolongada após traumatismo ou venopunção.
- Mucosas pálidas atribuídas à anemia por perda sanguínea ou a choque hemorrágico.
- Sinais neurológicos (raros) gerados por sangramento do SNC.
- Febre e leve linfadenomegalia não são usuais.
- Ocasionalmente, há esplenomegalia à palpação.

DIAGNÓSTICO

Baseia-se nos seguintes aspectos:
- Em geral, trombocitopenia grave.
- Resultado positivo no teste de anticorpos ligados às plaquetas (se disponível).
- Resposta à terapia imunossupressora.
- Exclusão meticulosa de doenças subjacentes ou deflagradores potenciais.

DIAGNÓSTICO DIFERENCIAL
- Erro de mensuração gerado por formação de aglomerados plaquetários; particularmente em gatos, as baixas contagens de plaquetas são muitas vezes incorretas (em virtude da tendência à formação de agregados e plaquetas de tamanho grande).
- Declínio na produção:
- Doenças infecciosas; vacinação nas últimas semanas; medicamentos/toxinas; radiação; distúrbios primários da medula óssea; resposta imunomediada contra megacariócitos; macrotrombocitopenia hereditária de Cavalier King Charles spaniel.
- Trombocitopenia ou pancitopenia isoladas. A trombocitopenia pode ser grave, dependendo da doença subjacente.
- Aumento no sequestro em baço aumentado de volume:
- P. ex., distúrbios inflamatórios, neoplasias; torção esplênica.
- Trombocitopenia leve a moderada a menos que outros mecanismos contribuam para o quadro (p. ex., utilização de plaquetas em casos de hemangiossarcoma).
- Aumento na utilização ou no consumo:
- CID; trombose local; vasculite/dano vascular com ou sem CID.
- Hemorragia grave: pode resultar em trombocitopenia leve a moderada após ressuscitação volêmica.
- Aumento na destruição (causa mais comum de trombocitopenia grave):
  ○ Trombocitopenia imunomediada primária.
  ○ Trombocitopenia imunomediada secundária a doenças infecciosas (anaplasmose, erliquiose, febre maculosa das Montanhas Rochosas, bartonelose, babesiose, leishmaniose, dirofilariose, infecção por *Angiostrongylus*, infecções bacterianas; FeLV, FIV, PIF, cinomose, hepatite infecciosa); inflamação estéril (em gatos, necrose do tecido adiposo, etc.); doenças neoplásicas (linfoma, leucemia, hemangiossarcoma, etc.); medicamentos/toxinas (vacinas, sulfonamidas, cefalosporinas, fenobarbital, AINE); transfusões de sangue; LES.

HEMOGRAMA/BIOQUÍMICA/URINÁLISE
- Trombocitopenia frequentemente grave (<30-40.000/μL), alto risco de sangramento espontâneo; cães e gatos podem permanecer assintomáticos.
- Exame de esfregaço sanguíneo: é possível anemia causada por perda sanguínea/anemia hemolítica imunomediada concomitante.
- O leucograma pode estar normal; leucocitose leve a moderada em um terço dos cães (em virtude de estresse/inflamação), raramente leucopenia. Algumas vezes, há monocitose, neutrofilia com/sem desvio à esquerda, linfopenia, eosinofilia, eosinopenia.
- Neutropenia concomitante pode indicar mielopatia primária ou doença infecciosa.
- Teste de coagulação geralmente normal; se anormal, considerar CID e testes adicionais.
- Resultados bioquímicos inespecíficos para trombocitopenia imunomediada. Ocasionalmente, observa-se leve aumento das enzimas hepáticas; raras vezes, há hiperbilirrubinemia causada por reabsorção de hematoma; hipoproteinemia/hipoalbuminemia atribuídas à perda sanguínea. Hiperglobulinemia pode indicar doença subjacente (p. ex., erliquiose, leishmaniose, PIF).
- Hematúria micro ou macroscópica.

OUTROS TESTES LABORATORIAIS
- Não existe teste imunodiagnóstico com padrão de excelência para trombocitopenia imunomediada amplamente disponível. Nenhum teste é capaz de diferenciar trombocitopenia imunomediada primária e secundária; a trombocitopenia imunomediada primária é um diagnóstico de exclusão.
- Foram avaliados testes diretos para detectar anticorpos ligados às plaquetas. Os ensaios de citometria de fluxo realizados em laboratórios especializados parecem ter sensibilidade e especificidade satisfatórias.
- A imunofluorescência de megacariócitos não é muito sensível.
- Teste imunodiagnóstico complementar, como teste de Coombs ou título de anticorpo antinuclear, na suspeita de anemia hemolítica imunomediada ou LES.
- Selecionar outros testes para excluir a lista de diagnóstico diferencial mencionada anteriormente para trombocitopenia (sorologia e/ou PCR para pesquisa de doenças infecciosas; microbiologia de urina e sangue, etc.).

MÉTODOS DIAGNÓSTICOS
- A avaliação da medula óssea não será indicada se o diagnóstico for aparentemente fácil e se houver resposta à terapia em alguns dias; indicada em caso de neutropenia ou anemia arregenerativa concomitantes, células nucleadas atípicas ou falha terapêutica.

TROMBOCITOPENIA IMUNOMEDIADA PRIMÁRIA

- O número de megacariócitos costuma permanecer normal ou estar aumentado; é rara a ocorrência de hipoplasia megacariocítica.
- É possível a obtenção de aspirado de linfonodos infartados por agulha fina; nenhum órgão deve ser aspirado em virtude do alto risco de sangramento intenso (caso contrário, os produtos de plaquetas devem estar disponíveis).

TRATAMENTO

CUIDADO(S) DE SAÚDE ADEQUADO(S)
- Os casos não complicados com baixo risco de sangramento e obediência satisfatória ao tratamento por parte do proprietário podem ser tratados em um esquema ambulatorial.
- Os pacientes com trombocitopenia grave apresentam risco muito elevado de sangramento e justificam confinamento estrito (p. ex., repouso em gaiola).
- Transfusão de produtos de plaquetas: 10-20 mL/kg de sangue fresco total, 1 unidade de plasma rico em plaquetas derivado de sangue total ou concentrado de plaquetas (cerca de 8×10^{10} plaquetas) por 10 (-30) kg em casos com hemorragia crítica. As plaquetas podem ser destruídas rapidamente, mas protegem contra hemorragias catastróficas até que uma terapia específica seja benéfica.
- Células de papa de hemácias ou (de preferência) sangue total fresco para corrigir anemia por perda sanguínea.
- Tratamento de hipovolemia com soluções cristaloides (os coloides podem prejudicar a função das plaquetas).

CUIDADO(S) DE ENFERMAGEM
- Não aplicar nenhuma injeção IM ou SC. Aplicar pressão prolongada após injeções IV e procedimentos invasivos (p. ex., aspiração de linfonodo). Evitar cistocentese e venopunção jugular. O aspirado da medula óssea é seguro.
- Cuidados intensivos de enfermagem em pacientes com hemorragia moderada a grave, hipovolemia, sinais atribuídos ao SNC, etc.

CONSIDERAÇÕES CIRÚRGICAS
- Alto risco de sangramento em cães com trombocitopenia grave.
- Talvez haja necessidade de transfusões peri e intraoperatórias (plaquetas).
- A esplenectomia é uma opção controversa para casos refratários irresponsivos à terapia clínica.

MEDICAÇÕES

MEDICAMENTO(S)
- Corticosteroides — metilprednisolona a 10-20 mg/kg IV uma única vez; prednisolona (cães: 1-1,5 mg/kg a cada 12 h; gatos: 1,5-2 mg/kg a cada 12 h inicialmente); raramente, a dexametasona é utilizada (0,1-0,5 mg/kg a cada 24 h).
- Considerar o uso de antibióticos (potencial de infecção oculta subjacente; predisposição à infecção por falta de regulação imunológica); doxiciclina se alguma doença oriunda de carrapatos não for excluída.
- Protetores GI (sucralfato e/ou antagonistas dos receptores histaminérgicos H_2 e/ou inibidores da bomba de prótons) para evitar ou tratar ulceração GI.
- Outros agentes imunossupressores são utilizados quando a prednisolona falha, só controla a doença em doses persistentemente elevadas, provoca efeitos colaterais inaceitáveis e para o controle de casos refratários/recidivantes a longo prazo. A maioria desses agentes não é eficaz no tratamento agudo; há poucos estudos controlados disponíveis.
- Tratamento agudo em cães: vincristina (0,02 mg/kg IV, uma única vez) ou imunoglobulinas humanas (0,5-1 g/kg IV por 6 horas, uma única vez) em combinação com prednisolona conduziram a um aumento mais rápido nas contagens de plaquetas em comparação à prednisolona isolada.
- Outros medicamentos imunossupressores para controle a longo prazo: ciclosporina (5 mg/kg a cada 24 a 12 h), azatioprina (inicialmente 2 mg/kg a cada 24 h), leflunomida (3-4 mg/kg a cada 24 h), danazol (5-10 mg/kg a cada 12 h) em combinação com prednisolona. Gatos: clorambucila (0,1-0,2 mg/kg a cada 24 h).
- Assim que a contagem das plaquetas estiver na faixa de normalidade, a dose inicial da prednisolona será reduzida de forma gradativa para aproximadamente um quarto a um quinto a cada 2 semanas, trocando por fim para uma terapia em dias alternados. Reduzir a dose lentamente durante cerca de 6 meses caso não ocorra qualquer recidiva.

PRECAUÇÕES
- Interromper quaisquer medicações desnecessárias (podem induzir à trombocitopenia imunomediada secundária).
- Corticosteroides: ulceração GI; hiperadrenocorticismo iatrogênico.
- Imunossupressão: predispõe a infecções oportunistas.
- Medicamentos citotóxicos: supressão da medula óssea.
- A redução muito rápida da dose após a remissão pode predispor o animal à recorrência. É mais difícil controlar as recidivas.

ACOMPANHAMENTO

MONITORIZAÇÃO DO PACIENTE
- Mensurações do hematócrito 2-3 vezes ao dia em casos com hemorragia grave (risco de perda sanguínea [GI] potencialmente letal).
- Mensuração diária da contagem de plaquetas até que estejam acima de 50.000/µL; em seguida, no intervalo de poucos dias até que as contagens dessas células se normalizem. Depois, a cada 1-3 semanas durante o período de redução gradativa da dose dos medicamentos.
- Hemograma completo e perfil bioquímico a cada 2-4 semanas.
- Urinálise microbiológica a cada 4-6 semanas em virtude do risco de infecções secundárias.

PREVENÇÃO
- Utilizar as vacinas de forma criteriosa. O papel desempenhado na recorrência é incerto.
- Minimizar o estresse que pode desencadear a recorrência.

COMPLICAÇÕES POSSÍVEIS
- A ocorrência de sangramento excessivo pode ser fatal; morte espontânea, p. ex., em virtude de sangramento no pericárdio ou no SNC.
- Efeitos colaterais dos medicamentos (ulceração GI, hábito de Cushing, infecções oportunistas, supressão da medula óssea).

EVOLUÇÃO ESPERADA E PROGNÓSTICO
- A contagem das plaquetas geralmente aumentará para >50.000/µL 5-7 dias após o início do tratamento (após 1-15, média de 5 dias, em 24 de 25 cães).
- Vincristina ou imunoglobulinas humanas em adição à prednisolona conduziram a um aumento mais rápido no nível das plaquetas.
- Poucos cães jamais atingem níveis plaquetários normais.
- O diagnóstico deve ser reconsiderado mediante a falha de resposta à terapia.
- 5 de 19 cães (26%) recidivaram após 19-286 dias (média de 66 dias); as causas de recidiva foram a redução da dose da prednisolona e a falta de obediência ao tratamento por parte do proprietário.
- Caso ocorram recidivas, deve-se adicionar um segundo agente imunossupressor; além disso, é aconselhável uma redução mais gradativa da dose, conduzindo o animal a um esquema posológico em dias alternados, possivelmente pelo resto de sua vida.
- 29 de 30 cães (97%) sobreviveram durante os primeiros 14 dias; o prognóstico parece favorável com terapia intensiva, incluindo produtos sanguíneos/plaquetários, conforme a necessidade.
- A taxa de mortalidade em gatos é de 15% (2/13).

DIVERSOS

DISTÚRBIOS ASSOCIADOS
Cerca de um terço dos cães com trombocitopenia imunomediada primária também apresenta anemia hemolítica imunomediada (síndrome de Evans).

SINÔNIMO(S)
- Trombocitopenia autoimune.
- Púrpura trombocitopênica idiopática/autoimune.

VER TAMBÉM
- Anemia Imunomediada.
- Coagulação Intravascular Disseminada.
- Trombocitopenia.

ABREVIATURA(S)
- AINE = anti-inflamatório não esteroide.
- CID = coagulação intravascular disseminada.
- FeLV = vírus da leucemia felina.
- FIV = vírus da imunodeficiência felina.
- GI = gastrintestinal.
- LES = lúpus eritematoso sistêmico.
- PCR = reação em cadeia da polimerase.
- PIF = peritonite infecciosa felina.
- SNC = sistema nervoso central.

Sugestões de Leitura
Putsche J, Kohn B. Primary immune-mediated thrombocytopenia in 30 dogs (1997-2003). JAAHA 2008, 44:250-257.
Wondraschek C, Weingart C, Kohn B. Primary immune-mediated thrombocytopenia in cats. JAAHA 2010, 46:12-19.

Autor Barbara Kohn
Consultor Editorial A. H. Rebar

Tromboembolia Aórtica

CONSIDERAÇÕES GERAIS

DEFINIÇÃO
A tromboembolia aórtica origina-se de trombo ou coágulo sanguíneo que é desalojado no interior da aorta, causando uma grave isquemia aos tecidos supridos por esse segmento da aorta.

FISIOPATOLOGIA
- A tromboembolia aórtica é mais comumente associada a doenças do miocárdio em gatos, miocardiopatia hipertrófica com maior frequência. Especula-se que o fluxo sanguíneo anormal (estase) e um estado hipercoagulável contribuam para a formação do trombo dentro do átrio esquerdo. O coágulo sanguíneo, então, forma um êmbolo distalmente à aorta. O local mais comum de embolização corresponde à trifurcação da aorta caudal (membros pélvicos). Outros locais menos comuns compreendem os membros torácicos, os rins, o trato gastrintestinal ou o cérebro.
- Nos cães, a tromboembolia aórtica está tipicamente relacionada com neoplasia, sepse, endocardite infecciosa, síndrome de Cushing, nefropatia com perda de proteínas ou outros estados hipercoaguláveis.

SISTEMA(S) ACOMETIDO(S)
- Cardiovascular — a maioria dos gatos acometidos apresenta cardiopatia e insuficiência cardíaca esquerda avançadas.
- Nervoso/musculosquelético — uma isquemia grave em direção aos músculos e nervos supridos pelo segmento ocluído da aorta provoca dor e paresia variáveis. No(s) membro(s) envolvido(s), ocorrem anormalidades da marcha ou paralisia.

GENÉTICA
Miocardiopatia hipertrófica, uma doença associada comum, é provavelmente hereditária. Além disso, há relatos de uma família de gatos domésticos de pelo curto com miocardiopatia hipertrófica remodelada em que todos morreram de tromboembolia aórtica.

INCIDÊNCIA/PREVALÊNCIA
- Na população felina geral, ainda não se conhece a prevalência da tromboembolia aórtica. Em dois estudos amplos de gatos com miocardiopatia hipertrófica, 12-16% deles apresentaram-se com sinais de tromboembolia aórtica. Em dois estudos retrospectivos de gatos com tromboembolia aórtica, apenas 11-25% deles tinham indícios prévios de cardiopatia.
- Rara nos cães.

DISTRIBUIÇÃO GEOGRÁFICA
N/D.

IDENTIFICAÇÃO
Espécies
Gatos, mas raramente nos cães.

Raça(s) Predominante(s)
Os gatos de raças mistas são mais comumente acometidos. Em um único estudo, as raças puras Abissínio, Birmanês e Ragdoll foram super-representadas.

Idade Média e Faixa Etária
A distribuição etária é de 1-20 anos. A idade média é de aproximadamente 8 anos.

Sexo(s) Predominante(s)
Os machos são mais comumente acometidos do que as fêmeas (2:1).

SINAIS CLÍNICOS
Achados Anamnésicos
- As queixas mais comuns são paralisia e dor de início agudo.
- Claudicação ou anormalidade da marcha.
- É habitual a constatação de taquipneia ou angústia respiratória.
- Normalmente se observam vocalização e ansiedade.
- Cerca de 15% dos gatos podem exibir vômitos antes da tromboembolia aórtica.

Achados do Exame Físico
- Em geral, verifica-se paraparesia ou paralisia dos membros pélvicos, associada a sinais atribuíveis à lesão do neurônio motor inferior. Com menor frequência, ocorre monoparesia de um dos membros torácicos.
- Dor, sobretudo, à palpação dos membros.
- Algumas horas após a embolização, o músculo gastrocnêmio torna-se frequentemente firme.
- Ausência ou diminuição dos pulsos femorais.
- Leitos ungueais e coxins podais cianóticos ou pálidos.
- Taquipneia ou dispneia.
- É comum a presença de hipotermia.
- Sopro cardíaco, arritmias ou ritmo de galope (nem sempre presente).

CAUSAS
- Miocardiopatia (todos os tipos).
- Hipertireoidismo.
- Neoplasia.
- Sepse (cães).
- Hiperadrenocorticismo (cães).
- Nefropatia com perda de proteínas (cães).

FATORES DE RISCO
Especula-se que o aumento de volume acentuado do átrio esquerdo, o contraste ecocardiográfico espontâneo ("fumaça") ou a presença de trombo intracardíaco, observados no exame ecocardiográfico, possam ser fatores de risco.

DIAGNÓSTICO

DIAGNÓSTICO DIFERENCIAL
Paresia dos membros pélvicos, secundariamente a outras causas, como neoplasia espinal, traumatismo, mielite, infarto fibrocartilaginoso ou protrusão de disco intervertebral. Essas condições com lesão medular resultante apresentam-se com sinais de comprometimento do neurônio motor superior, enquanto os pacientes com tromboembolia aórtica exibem sinais referentes ao envolvimento do neurônio motor inferior.

HEMOGRAMA/BIOQUÍMICA/URINÁLISE
- Altos níveis da creatina quinase, em consequência da lesão muscular.
- Atividades elevadas da aspartato aminotransferase e da alanina aminotransferase, como resultado de danos muscular e hepático.
- Hiperglicemia secundária ao estresse.
- Leves aumentos nas concentrações de ureia e de creatinina, resultantes do baixo débito cardíaco e dos possíveis êmbolos renais.
- Desarranjos eletrolíticos, atribuídos ao baixo débito cardíaco e dano muscular, como hipocalcemia, hiponatremia, hiperfosfatemia e hipercalemia, não são incomuns.
- As alterações do hemograma completo e da urinálise são inespecíficas.

OUTROS TESTES LABORATORIAIS
O perfil de coagulação disponível na rotina clínica tipicamente não revela anormalidades significativas, pois a hipercoagulabilidade se origina de plaquetas hiperagregáveis.

DIAGNÓSTICO POR IMAGEM
Achados Radiográficos
- Cardiomegalia é comum em gatos.
- Edema pulmonar e/ou efusão pleural em aproximadamente 50% dos gatos.
- Raras vezes observa-se a presença de massa nos pulmões, sugestiva de neoplasia.

Achados Ecocardiográficos
- Alterações compatíveis com miocardiopatia. A miocardiopatia hipertrófica é a mais comum, seguida por miocardiopatia restritiva ou não classificada e, depois, pela miocardiopatia dilatada.
- A maior parte dos casos (>50%) exibe um grave aumento de volume do átrio esquerdo, i. e., uma relação atrial esquerda:aórtica de 2,0 ou mais.
- Pode-se observar a presença de trombo no átrio esquerdo ou a formação de contraste ecocardiográfico espontâneo ("fumaça").

Achados Ultrassonográficos Abdominais
- Pode ser capaz de identificar o trombo na aorta caudal.
- Tipicamente, essa modalidade de diagnóstico por imagem não costuma ser necessária para se obter o diagnóstico.

Achados Angiográficos
- A técnica de angiografia não seletiva deve identificar um defeito de preenchimento negativo na aorta caudal, representativo do trombo.
- Esse teste não costuma ser necessário para se alcançar o diagnóstico.

MÉTODOS DIAGNÓSTICOS
Eletrocardiografia
- Os ritmos mais comumente diagnosticados na tromboembolia aórtica incluem o ritmo sinusal e a taquicardia sinusal, enquanto os distúrbios rítmicos menos comuns compreendem a fibrilação atrial, as arritmias ventriculares, as arritmias supraventriculares e a bradicardia sinusal.
- Em geral, observam-se um padrão de aumento de volume do ventrículo esquerdo e a presença de distúrbios de condução nessa câmara cardíaca (bloqueio fascicular anterior esquerdo).

ACHADOS PATOLÓGICOS
- O trombo é tipicamente identificado na trifurcação aórtica caudal.
- Ocasionalmente, observa-se a existência de trombo no átrio esquerdo.
- Também se pode constatar a presença de êmbolos nos rins, no trato gastrintestinal, no cérebro e em outros órgãos.

TRATAMENTO

CUIDADO(S) DE SAÚDE ADEQUADO(S)
Em princípio, os gatos com tromboembolia aórtica devem ser internados, pois a maioria apresenta insuficiência cardíaca congestiva concomitante e necessita de medicamentos injetáveis, além de terem dor e angústia consideráveis.

CUIDADO(S) DE ENFERMAGEM
- A fluidoterapia é utilizada com cautela, pois a maioria dos gatos apresenta miocardiopatia

TROMBOEMBOLIA AÓRTICA

avançada. Se estiver em insuficiência cardíaca congestiva, a fluidoterapia IV pode não ser necessária.
• Caso o animal se apresente com insuficiência cardíaca congestiva, a suplementação de oxigênio ou o procedimento de toracocentese poderão ser benéficos.
• Inicialmente, é recomendável manipular os membros acometidos o mínimo possível. Entretanto, à medida que ocorre a reperfusão, a fisioterapia (extensão e flexão passivas dos membros) poderá acelerar a recuperação plena.
• Nos membros acometidos, não se deve efetuar nenhuma venopunção.
• Esses gatos acometidos podem ter dificuldade de colocação postural durante a micção; consequentemente, poderá ser necessária a compressão vesical manual para evitar a distensão excessiva da bexiga ou a queimadura da pele por urina.

ATIVIDADE
É aconselhável a restrição da atividade física e do estresse.

DIETA
Inicialmente, grande parte dos gatos apresenta-se anoréxica. É fundamental estimulá-los com qualquer tipo de dieta e mantê-los sob a ingestão constante de alimentos para evitar a ocorrência de lipidose hepática.

ORIENTAÇÃO AO PROPRIETÁRIO
• Os proprietários devem ser conscientizados a respeito do prognóstico mau, tanto a curto como a longo prazo.
• A maioria dos gatos apresenta recidivas na formação de êmbolos. Grande parte dos que sobrevivem a um episódio inicial deve ser submetida a algum tipo de terapia anticoagulante, o que exigirá reavaliações frequentes e um estilo de vida domiciliar.
• Quase todos os gatos que sobrevivem a um episódio inicial recuperam completamente a função dos membros; entretanto, se a isquemia for grave e prolongada, poderão ocorrer esfacelamento/necrose de segmentos das extremidades distais ou déficits neurológicos persistentes. Em um único estudo, cerca de 15% dos gatos exibiram anormalidades neuromusculares permanentes depois de sobreviverem ao evento embólico inicial.

CONSIDERAÇÕES CIRÚRGICAS
• Tipicamente, não se recomenda a embolectomia cirúrgica, uma vez que esses pacientes são candidatos cirúrgicos de alto risco em função da cardiopatia grave.
• A trombectomia reolítica foi usada com sucesso limitado em um pequeno número de gatos com tromboembolia aórtica.

MEDICAÇÕES
MEDICAMENTO(S) DE ESCOLHA
• A terapia trombolítica, como a estreptoquinase, a uroquinase e o ativador de plasminogênio tecidual, é amplamente utilizada em seres humanos e raramente em gatos. Esses medicamentos são de alto custo e carreiam um risco significativo de complicações hemorrágicas; tais agentes não demonstraram uma melhora na eficácia terapêutica e, por essa razão, seu emprego é raro na clínica geral.
• A heparina não fracionada representa o medicamento preferido na clínica geral. Apesar de não exercer qualquer efeito sobre o coágulo estabelecido, ela evita a ativação extra da cascata de coagulação. Inicialmente, administra-se uma dose de 100-200 unidades/kg IV, seguida por 200-300 unidades/kg SC a cada 8 h. Alternativamente, é possível administrá-la a uma dose de 25-35 unidades/kg/hora sob infusão em velocidade constante, caso exista qualquer preocupação quanto a uma biodisponibilidade satisfatória pela via SC. Em seguida, titula-se a dose para prolongar o TTPA em aproximadamente o dobro.
• Teoricamente, o ácido acetilsalicílico é benéfico durante e após um episódio de tromboembolia, em virtude de seus efeitos antiplaquetários. A dose nos gatos é um comprimido de 81 mg VO a cada 48 ou 72 h. Os efeitos de vômito e diarreia não são incomuns. Alguns especialistas defendem uma minidose de 5 mg/gato a cada 72 h. As recomendações posológicas antitrombóticas para os cães variam de 0,5-2 mg/kg a cada 24 h. Sempre se deve administrar o ácido acetilsalicílico juntamente com o alimento.
• O clopidogrel é um medicamento antiagregação plaquetária. A dose nos gatos é de 18,75 mg/gato (1/4 do comprimido de 75 mg) VO a cada 24 h, enquanto a dose nos cães gira em torno de 1 mg/kg a cada 24 h. Esse agente terapêutico pode ser usado em combinação ou no lugar do ácido acetilsalicílico.
• A buprenorfina é utilizada para analgesia e sedação a uma dose de 0,005-0,02 mg/kg IV, SC ou VO a cada 6-8 h. Para uma analgesia mais forte, utilize a fentanila ou a hidromorfona.
• A acepromazina pode ser utilizada com cuidado por suas propriedades sedativas e vasodilatadoras a uma dose de 0,01-0,02 mg SC a cada 8-12 h.
• A varfarina, um antagonista da vitamina K, é o anticoagulante mais amplamente utilizado em seres humanos e foi proposta para a prevenção de recidivas de embolização em gatos que sobrevivem ao primeiro episódio. A dose inicial é de 0,25-0,5 mg/gato VO a cada 24 h. É recomendável administrá-la simultaneamente com a heparina por 3 dias. Em seguida, é preciso ajustar a dose para prolongar o TP em cerca do dobro de seu valor basal ou até atingir uma relação normalizada internacional (RNI) de 2,0-4,0. O tratamento a longo prazo com a varfarina pode representar um grande desafio, em virtude da frequência de ajustes na dose e de monitorização, além dos efeitos adversos como o sangramento.
• Recentemente, a heparina de baixo peso molecular foi proposta para a prevenção da tromboembolia aórtica felina a longo prazo. Essa heparina de baixo peso molecular apresenta uma relação mais previsível entre a dosagem e a resposta do que a varfarina e não necessita de ajustes na dose nem de monitorização. A heparina também exibe um risco mais baixo de complicações hemorrágicas. A principal desvantagem da heparina de baixo peso molecular é representada pelo alto custo do medicamento e pela via injetável de administração. As duas heparinas de baixo peso molecular utilizadas na tromboembolia aórtica felina são: a dalteparina 100 unidades/kg SC a cada 12-24 h e a enoxaparina 1 mg/kg SC a cada 12-24 h. Não se conhece a melhor dose. A heparina de baixo peso molecular costuma ser iniciada a cada 24 h em virtude do custo. Alguns estudos sugerem a necessidade de uma posologia a cada 6 h para níveis sanguíneos estáveis, embora isso possa aumentar o risco de sangramento.

CONTRAINDICAÇÕES
N/D.

PRECAUÇÕES
• A terapia anticoagulante com heparina, varfarina ou medicamentos trombolíticos pode gerar complicações hemorrágicas.
• Evitar o uso de β-bloqueador não seletivo (como o propranolol), já que ele pode acentuar a vasoconstrição periférica.

INTERAÇÕES POSSÍVEIS
A varfarina pode interagir com outros medicamentos, o que pode potencializar seus efeitos anticoagulantes.

MEDICAMENTO(S) ALTERNATIVO(S)
N/D.

ACOMPANHAMENTO
MONITORIZAÇÃO DO PACIENTE
• A monitorização eletrocardiográfica enquanto o gato estiver hospitalizado é útil para detectar lesões por reperfusão e alterações ECG relacionadas com a hipercalemia.
• A monitorização periódica dos eletrólitos e dos parâmetros renais pode ser benéfica para otimizar o controle da cardiopatia.
• O exame diário dos membros é necessário para avaliar a resposta clínica do paciente. Inicialmente, é aconselhável a mensuração do TTPA uma vez ao dia para titular a dose da heparina.
• Caso se faça uso da varfarina, o TP ou a RNI deverá ser mensurado aproximadamente 3 dias após o início da terapia e depois em intervalos semanais, até se obter o efeito anticoagulante desejado. Em seguida, é possível mensurá-los 3-4 vezes ao ano ou durante uma alteração no esquema terapêutico.

PREVENÇÃO
Em virtude da alta taxa de reembolização, torna-se altamente recomendável a realização de medidas preventivas com a administração de ácido acetilsalicílico, clopidogrel, varfarina ou heparina de baixo peso molecular.

COMPLICAÇÕES POSSÍVEIS
• A terapia anticoagulante pode levar ao sangramento.
• Em casos de isquemia prolongada, podem surgir déficits neurológicos permanentes ou anormalidades musculares nos membros pélvicos.
• Insuficiência cardíaca congestiva recidivante ou morte súbita.
• Lesões por reperfusão e morte geralmente associadas a arritmias hipercalêmicas.

EVOLUÇÃO ESPERADA E PROGNÓSTICO
• A evolução esperada é de dias a semanas para uma recuperação completa da função dos membros.
• O prognóstico geralmente é mau. Em dois estudos amplos, cerca de 60% dos gatos foram submetidos à eutanásia ou vieram a óbito durante o episódio tromboembólico inicial. O prognóstico a longo prazo varia entre 2 meses a alguns anos; no entanto, a média é de alguns meses com o tratamento. Os indicadores de um prognóstico mais desfavorável incluem hipotermia (<37°C) e

Tromboembolia Aórtica

insuficiência cardíaca congestiva. Um único estudo demonstrou um tempo médio de sobrevida de 77 dias em gatos com insuficiência cardíaca congestiva e 223 dias naqueles sem esse tipo de insuficiência.
• Os indicadores de um prognóstico melhor incluem normotermia, acometimento de um único membro e presença de função motora ao exame inicial.
• A recidiva da tromboembolia aórtica é comum.

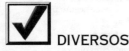 **DIVERSOS**

DISTÚRBIOS ASSOCIADOS
Ver a seção "Causas e Fatores de Risco".

FATORES RELACIONADOS COM A IDADE
N/D.

POTENCIAL ZOONÓTICO
Nenhum.

GESTAÇÃO/FERTILIDADE/REPRODUÇÃO
N/D.

SINÔNIMO(S)
• Tromboembolia em sela.
• Tromboembolia sistêmica.

VER TAMBÉM
• Miocardiopatia Dilatada — Gatos.
• Miocardiopatia Hipertrófica — Gatos.
• Miocardiopatia Restritiva — Gatos.

ABREVIATURA(S)
• ECG = eletrocardiografia.
• RNI = relação normalizada internacional.
• TTPA = tempo de tromboplastina parcial ativada.
• TP = tempo de protrombina.

Sugestões de Leitura
Cole SG, Drobatz KJ. Emergency management and critical care. In: Tilley LP, Smith FWK, Oyama MA, Sleeper MM, eds., Manual of Canine and Feline Cardiology, 4th ed. St. Louis: Saunders Elsevier, 2008, pp. 342-355.
Laste NJ, Harpster NK. A retrospective study of 100 cats with feline distal aortic thromboembolism: 1977-1993. JAAHA 1995, 31:492-500.
Smith CE, et al. Use of low molecular weight heparin in cats: 57 cases (1999-2003). JAVMA 2004, 225:1237-1241.
Smith SA. Feline arterial thromboembolism: An update. Vet Clin North Am Small Anim Pract 2004, 34:1245-1271.
Smith SA. Arterial thromboembolism in cats: Acute crisis in 127 cases (1992-2001) and long-term management with low dose aspirin in 24 cases. J Vet Intern Med 2003, 17:73-83.

Autor Teresa C. DeFrancesco
Consultores Editoriais Larry P. Tilley e Francis W.K. Smith, Jr.

TROMBOEMBOLIA PULMONAR

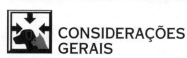

CONSIDERAÇÕES GERAIS

DEFINIÇÃO
Desenvolve-se quando algum trombo se aloja na árvore arterial pulmonar e obstrui o fluxo sanguíneo para a parte do pulmão irrigada por aquela artéria.

FISIOPATOLOGIA
• Tromboêmbolos pulmonares associados à dirofilariose ocorrem *in situ* nos vasos pulmonares; na maior parte dos outros casos, a origem do trombo é incerta.
• Pontos potenciais de origem incluem o átrio direito, a veia cava, as veias jugulares e as veias femorais ou mesentéricas; esses trombos venosos são conduzidos pela corrente sanguínea para os pulmões, onde se alojam na circulação pulmonar.
• Acredita-se que o fluxo sanguíneo anormal (estase), a lesão endotelial vascular e a coagulabilidade alterada (estado hipercoagulável) predisponham à formação de trombo.
• Na maioria dos pacientes a tromboembolia pulmonar é uma complicação de outro processo mórbido primário.

SISTEMA(S) ACOMETIDO(S)
• Cardiovascular — pode resultar em hipertensão pulmonar, levando ao aumento e à insuficiência do ventrículo direito, bem como à redução do débito cardíaco.
• Respiratório — o fluxo sanguíneo pulmonar reduzido leva à hipoxemia arterial e dispneia.

INCIDÊNCIA/PREVALÊNCIA
• Desconhecida — a probabilidade de tromboembolia pulmonar aumenta nos animais com coagulação anormal ou doença sistêmica grave.
• Diagnóstico raro nos cães e nos gatos; provavelmente subdiagnosticada em função dos sinais clínicos inespecíficos, da falta de suspeita clínica e da escassez de testes diagnósticos definitivos não invasivos.

IDENTIFICAÇÃO
Espécies
Cães e gatos.

Raça(s) Predominante(s)
Sem predisposição; a doença pode ser mais comum nos cães de médio e grande portes.

Idade Média e Faixa Etária
• Mais frequentemente observada em cães de meia-idade a mais idosos.
• Há relatos de distribuição etária bimodal na espécie felina, com pico de ocorrência em gatos com menos de 4 anos e mais de 10 anos de idade.

SINAIS CLÍNICOS
Achados Anamnésicos
• Com frequência, refletem a doença primária.
• Ocasionalmente, constituem a razão para o exame inicial; em tais pacientes, dispneia superaguda, anorexia, síncope ou colapso, tosse ou hemoptise, fraqueza, intolerância ao exercício e incapacidade para dormir ou se sentir confortável podem ser queixas anamnésicas.

Achados do Exame Físico
• Taquipneia e dispneia na maior parte dos animais; ruídos pulmonares adventícios (casuais) em alguns animais.
• Taquicardia, pulsos arteriais fracos, distensão venosa jugular, mucosas pálidas ou cianóticas, atraso no tempo de preenchimento capilar, sopro cardíaco do lado direito e desdobramento ou aumento na intensidade da segunda bulha cardíaca em animais gravemente acometidos.

CAUSAS
• Dirofilariose.
• Neoplasia.
• Hiperadrenocorticismo (síndrome de Cushing) ou administração de corticosteroide.
• Nefropatia com perda de proteínas (perda renal de antitrombina) ou enteropatia com perda de proteínas.
• Cardiopatia.
• Anemia hemolítica imunomediada.
• Pancreatite.
• Traumatismo ou cirurgia ortopédica.
• Sepse.
• Coagulopatia intravascular disseminada.
• Hepatopatia.

FATORES DE RISCO
• Coagulopatia, especialmente qualquer estado hipercoagulável.
• As doenças relacionadas na seção "Causas" estão associadas.
• Administração de estrogênio e viagem de avião podem ser fatores etiológicos em seres humanos.

DIAGNÓSTICO

DIAGNÓSTICO DIFERENCIAL
• Outras doenças indutoras de dispneia e hipoxemia significativas do ponto de vista clínico sem achados radiográficos profundos incluem obstrução das vias aéreas superiores, paralisia da laringe e processo mórbido difuso das vias aéreas (p. ex., inalação de toxina e pneumonia intersticial).
• Obstrução das vias aéreas superiores frequentemente se manifesta sob a forma de dispneia inspiratória; os ruídos respiratórios quase sempre ficam mais altos sobre a traqueia ou a laringe.
• Deve-se levar o diagnóstico em consideração no paciente com início agudo de dispneia e doença sabidamente associada à tromboembolia pulmonar.

HEMOGRAMA/BIOQUÍMICA/URINÁLISE
• Hemograma completo — pode permanecer normal; pode-se observar trombocitopenia em até 50% dos cães com tromboembolia pulmonar; também pode ocorrer o aparecimento de leucocitose.
• Perfil bioquímico — os resultados muitas vezes refletem a doença subjacente.
• Urinálise — os resultados frequentemente refletem a doença subjacente; avaliar o paciente quanto à presença de proteinúria.

OUTROS TESTES LABORATORIAIS
• Gasometria sanguínea arterial frequentemente revela hipoxemia arterial (PaO_2 quase sempre <65 mmHg) e $PaCO_2$ baixa com alcalose respiratória.
• Acidose metabólica e respiratória pode se desenvolver nos pacientes gravemente acometidos.
• Dímeros-D originam-se da degradação de fibrina de ligação cruzada e são indicadores de trombose fisiológica ou patológica. O teste de Dímeros-D desempenha um papel fundamental nos algoritmos diagnósticos para tromboembolia pulmonar em seres humanos; no entanto, a utilidade desses dímeros-D para o diagnóstico de tromboembolia pulmonar em pacientes veterinários é incerta. Os níveis plasmáticos de dímeros-D podem estar inconsistentemente elevados em cães com tromboembolia pulmonar; no entanto, um nível baixo de dímeros-D não exclui a possibilidade de tromboembolia pulmonar.
• Tromboelastografia é uma técnica que fornece uma avaliação global da coagulação e de trombólise; pode ser útil para o diagnóstico de hipercoagulabilidade sistêmica, mas não se encontra amplamente disponível.
• O perfil de coagulação pode revelar produtos de degradação da fibrina elevados, fibrinogênio anormal ou alterações no TP de um estágio e TTP ativada.
• Sorologia para dirofilariose deve ser realizada em qualquer animal com suspeita de tromboembolia pulmonar.
• Biomarcadores cardíacos — níveis cardíacos de troponina I e NT-pro-BNP podem estar elevados.

DIAGNÓSTICO POR IMAGEM
Achados Radiográficos Torácicos
Podem estar normais ou revelar artéria pulmonar aumentada ou interrompida, cardiomegalia, padrões pulmonares intersticiais e alveolares, efusão pleural de pequeno volume ou áreas de hipertransparência regional (sinal de Westermark).

Achados Ecocardiográficos
Aumento do ventrículo direito, segmento dilatado da artéria pulmonar, achatamento do septo interventricular, tamanho diminuído da cavidade ventricular esquerda, velocidade elevada dos jatos de regurgitação tricúspide ou pulmonar fornecem indícios de hipertensão arterial pulmonar em alguns pacientes; raramente um trombo aparece na imagem do coração direito ou em segmentos da artéria pulmonar principal.

Tomografia Computadorizada, Achados Angiográficos e Estudos com Radionuclídeos
• Um ou mais desses exames costumam ser necessários para o diagnóstico definitivo.
• Angiografia por TC é o método com padrão de excelência para o diagnóstico de tromboembolia pulmonar.
• Angiografia não seletiva por TC espiral pode revelar defeitos de enchimento intraluminal criados por êmbolos, infiltrados pulmonares cuneiformes periféricos ou efusão pleural.
• Cateterização cardíaca do lado direito com angiografia pulmonar pode permitir a identificação de defeitos de enchimento intraluminal ou regiões de fluxo sanguíneo pulmonar reduzido.
• Angiografia não seletiva com o uso de técnicas radiográficas convencionais possui baixo nível de sucesso diagnóstico.
• Varreduras combinadas de ventilação e perfusão com radioisótopos permitem a identificação de regiões pulmonares bem ventiladas que não recebem fluxo sanguíneo.

MÉTODOS DIAGNÓSTICOS
Eletrocardiografia
• *Cor pulmonale* agudo — desvio do eixo para a direita, P pulmonar, desvio do segmento ST, ondas T grandes.
• Arritmias.

Tromboembolia Pulmonar

ACHADOS PATOLÓGICOS
- Trombos nos ramos principais das artérias pulmonares.
- Alguns pacientes apresentam múltiplos trombos menores nos pequenos vasos das artérias pulmonares, que acabaram levando à disfunção respiratória acentuada e morte.
- É comum a existência de doença pulmonar concomitante como pneumonia, edema pulmonar, neoplasia pulmonar ou fibrose intersticial.

TRATAMENTO
CUIDADO(S) DE SAÚDE ADEQUADO(S)
Tratar os pacientes com tromboembolia pulmonar comprovada como pacientes internados até que a hipoxemia esteja solucionada.

CUIDADO(S) DE ENFERMAGEM
- Administrar fluidos intravenosos com cuidado a menos que haja depleção volêmica preexistente; tais fluidos podem contribuir para o desenvolvimento de insuficiência cardíaca congestiva direita.
- Administrar oxigênio caso exista dispneia e/ou PaO_2 <65 mmHg; a resposta à oxigenoterapia é variável.

ATIVIDADE
Restrita para evitar piora da hipoxemia ou síncope.

ORIENTAÇÃO AO PROPRIETÁRIO
- Alertar o proprietário sobre o fato de que a doença quase sempre é fatal; é provável a ocorrência de outros episódios a menos que se identifique e se corrija alguma causa subjacente; a morte súbita não é incomum.
- O tratamento com medicações anticoagulantes tradicionais pode levar a complicações hemorrágicas, exigindo reavaliações frequentes dos tempos de coagulação (p. ex., TP e TTP) para o sucesso terapêutico; as heparinas de baixo peso molecular são mais seguras e exigem menos monitorização, mas são associadas a um custo maior; a administração de anticoagulante pode ser necessária por vários meses mesmo após a resolução da doença causal.

CONSIDERAÇÕES CIRÚRGICAS
Requer desvio cardiopulmonar ou cateteres especializados e não está disponível na maior parte das instituições; mesmo quando disponível, a extrapolação da literatura humana sugere uma mortalidade cirúrgica provavelmente alta.

MEDICAÇÕES
MEDICAMENTO(S) DE ESCOLHA
- Sempre identificar e tratar a doença subjacente; caso seja improvável que isso seja bem-sucedido, esforços intensos para o tratamento da tromboembolia pulmonar provavelmente serão inúteis.
- A heparina não fracionada pode ajudar a evitar o desenvolvimento de outros trombos; baixas dosagens provavelmente são inadequadas para o tratamento inicial; indica-se a dosagem de 200-300 unidades/kg SC a cada 8 h ou, alternativamente, um bólus de 200 unidades/kg IV seguido por infusão em velocidade constante a 15-30 unidades/kg/h ajustados para manter o TTP em 1,5-2 vezes o valor basal.
- A administração de medicamento trombolítico (p. ex., uroquinase, estreptoquinase ou ativador do plasminogênio tecidual) também pode ser valiosa nos casos instáveis do ponto de vista hemodinâmico; esses medicamentos são dispendiosos e carreiam um risco elevado de complicações hemorrágicas.
- Varfarina — pode ser considerada para o tratamento a longo prazo (0,1 mg/kg a cada 24 h), com ajustes da dosagem para manter o TP em 1,5-2 vezes o valor basal; os animais precisam ser heparinizados antes da terapia com a varfarina para evitar a fase hipercoagulável inicial.
- As heparinas de baixo peso molecular são provavelmente associadas a menos complicações hemorrágicas do que a heparina não fracionada ou a varfarina, necessitam de menos monitorização intensiva e são mais adequadas para o tratamento em longo prazo.
- Foram demonstrados efeitos tromboprofiláticos para a dalteparina (150 unidades/kg SC a cada 12 h) na ausência de tempos de sangramento prolongados ou efeitos adversos; a enoxaparina foi usada na dose de 1 mg/kg SC a cada 12 h. O custo desses medicamentos pode ser um fator limitante para seu uso.

PRECAUÇÕES
Varfarina — interage com muitos outros medicamentos; o grau de anticoagulação pode se alterar depois da administração desses agentes; ou com modificações da dieta. A titulação da dose pode ser difícil nos pacientes com doenças que resultem em coagulopatia. Rever o mecanismo de ação e a farmacologia dos medicamentos antitrombóticos antes de utilizá-los.

ACOMPANHAMENTO
MONITORIZAÇÃO DO PACIENTE
- Gasometria sanguínea arterial seriada e/ou oximetria de pulso — pode ajudar a determinar uma melhora na função respiratória. • Verificar o TP a cada 3 dias inicialmente para ajustar a dosagem da varfarina a fim de atingir níveis de TP acima de 1,5-2 vezes o valor basal. É recomendável o uso de relações normalizadas internacionais para minimizar os efeitos da variabilidade nas preparações de tromboplastina sobre os resultados do TP. Conferir semanalmente depois se obter uma dosagem eficaz (tipicamente não antes de 2 semanas).

PREVENÇÃO
- A prática de atividade física passiva ou a aplicação de fisioterapia podem melhorar o fluxo de sangue venoso e evitar o desenvolvimento de trombos venosos nos pacientes imóveis com doença sistêmica grave. • O ácido acetilsalicílico (0,5-5 mg/kg VO a cada 12-24 h) pode desempenhar algum papel preventivo, embora seja inadequado como tratamento. • Clopidogrel (1-2 mg/kg VO a cada 24 h) é um agente antiplaquetário alternativo que pode exercer certo papel na prevenção. Uma única dose de ataque, de até 10 mg/kg, pode ser administrada para a rápida inativação de plaquetas em casos com trombose ativa. • A heparina pode ser administrada para os animais predispostos ao desenvolvimento da tromboembolia pulmonar (200 unidades/kg IV inicialmente e 75-200 unidades/kg SC a cada 4-8 h). • Alternativamente, a dalteparina (150 unidades/kg SC a cada 12 h) pode ser utilizada para tromboprofilaxia.

COMPLICAÇÕES POSSÍVEIS
Podem surgir complicações hemorrágicas significativas do ponto de vista clínico nos pacientes tratados com medicamentos anticoagulantes. Pode ocorrer sangramento a partir de qualquer sistema orgânico. Prever o sangramento ativo ou a anemia que necessite de transfusões de sangue ou de plasma e ter os produtos derivados do sangue prontamente disponíveis.

EVOLUÇÃO ESPERADA E PROGNÓSTICO
Geralmente reservado a mau; depende da resolução da causa desencadeante. Para doenças irreversíveis (p. ex., algumas neoplasias e nefropatia avançada com perda de proteínas), o prognóstico em longo prazo é mau; é um pouco melhor para os pacientes com tromboembolia decorrente de traumatismo ou sepse.

DIVERSOS
DISTÚRBIOS ASSOCIADOS
Ver a seção "Causas e Fatores de Risco".

SINÔNIMOS
Embolia pulmonar.

VER TAMBÉM
- Anemia Imunomediada. • Coagulação Intravascular Disseminada. • Dirofilariose — Cães. • Dirofilariose — Gatos. • Hiperadrenocorticismo (Síndrome de Cushing) — Cães. • Hiperadrenocorticismo (Síndrome de Cushing) — Gatos. • Sepse e Bacteremia. • Síndrome Nefrótica.

ABREVIATURA(S)
- NT-pro-BNP = porção N-terminal do pró-peptídeo natriurético cerebral. • TC = tomografia computadorizada. • TP = tempo de protrombina. • TTP = tempo de tromboplastina parcial.

Sugestões de Leitura
Goggs R, Benigni L, Fuentes VL, et al. Pulmonary thromboembolism. J Vet Emerg Crit Care 2009, 19:30-52.
Hackner SG. Pulmonary thromboembolism. In: Bonagura JD, Twedt DC, eds., Kirk's Current Veterinary Therapy XIV. St. Louis: Saunders Elsevier, 2009, pp. 689-697.
Johnson LR, Lappin MR, Baker DC. Pulmonary thromboembolism in 29 dogs: 1985-1995. J Vet Intern Med 1999, 13:338-345.
MacDonald KA, Johnson LR. Pulmonary hypertension and pulmonary thromboembolism. In: Ettinger SJ, Feldman EC, eds., Textbook of Veterinary Internal Medicine, 6th ed. St. Louis: Elsevier, 2005, pp. 1284-1288.
Schermerhorn T, Pembleton-Corbett JR, Kornreich B. Pulmonary thromboembolism in cats. J Vet InternMed 2004, 18:533-535.

Autores Suzanne M. Cunningham e John E. Rush
Consultores Editoriais Larry P. Tilley e Francis W.K. Smith, Jr.

TULAREMIA

CONSIDERAÇÕES GERAIS

REVISÃO
• *Francisella tularensis* — pequeno cocobacilo Gram-negativo; o tipo A, mais virulento, é encontrado em coelhos e carrapatos; o tipo B, disseminado pela água, é constatado em roedores e carrapatos; na América do Norte, é verificado principalmente em lagomorfos selvagens (coelhos de cauda de algodão, coelhos americanos, coelhos da neve) e roedores (toupeiras, esquilos, ratos almiscarados, castores); parasita intracelular facultativo; sobrevive e cresce em granulomas e/ou abscessos hepáticos. • Pico de ocorrência — final da primavera; meses de junho a agosto (EUA); dezembro (EUA). • Hemisfério Norte — ausente no Reino Unido, bem como na África, América do Sul e Austrália; nos EUA, a maioria dos casos é encontrada nos seguintes Estados: Missouri, Alasca, Oklahoma, Dakota do Sul, Tennessee, Kansas, Colorado, Illinois, Utah e Maine. • Um número crescente de surtos de tularemia em regiões da Europa fora das áreas endêmicas clássicas nos últimos anos despertou novo interesse por essa rara doença infecciosa. • Infecção — ingestão de tecido ou líquidos corporais de mamífero infectado ou água contaminada; animal picado por artrópode hematófago (carrapato), moscas, ácaros, mosquitos-pólvora, pulgas ou outros mosquitos; poucas bactérias são necessárias para infectar os gatos por meio da pele, das vias aéreas ou da conjuntiva; um número maior de bactérias é necessário para infectar o animal por meio do trato gastrintestinal.
• Contato com a pele — o microrganismo multiplica-se localmente (pápula) 3-5 dias após o contato; causa ulceração 2-4 dias depois; dissemina-se por via linfática até os linfonodos regionais e a corrente sanguínea; resulta em septicemia (pulmão, fígado, baço, linfonodos, medula óssea). • Ingestão — pode envolver linfadenopatia dos linfonodos cervicais e mesentéricos, acompanhada por disseminação septicêmica; distribuição das lesões para a face, a cavidade bucal, as tonsilas, os intestinos e os linfonodos. • Doença aguda — desenvolve-se 2-7 dias após o contato com o microrganismo. • A tularemia tem alta taxa de infecção relacionada com aerossol, baixa dose infecciosa e capacidade de induzir à doença fatal.
• *F. tularensis* é considerada com um possível agente de bioterrorismo; a ocorrência de um grupo de casos de pneumonia em animais de companhia pode indicar a presença de animais como sentinelas e o risco potencial de doença em seres humanos.

IDENTIFICAÇÃO
• Gatos — ocasionalmente. • Cães — raramente.

SINAIS CLÍNICOS
• Início súbito de anorexia, letargia, febre (40-41°C). • Enfartamento dos linfonodos submandibulares e cervicais palpáveis.
• Sensibilidade abdominal, linfonodos mesentéricos palpáveis, hepatomegalia — dependendo do estágio da doença. • Placas ou úlceras brancas multifocais ao longo dos arcos glossopalatinos e da língua. • Icterícia.

CAUSAS E FATORES DE RISCO
• Microrganismos — todos os biogrupos da *Francisella* são capazes de infectar os gatos, mas podem diferir em termos de virulência; alguns gatos podem ter uma leve infecção. • Gatos caçadores ou errantes em áreas endêmicas.
• Animais selvagens infectados na área das atividades de caça. • Exposição a parasitas hematófagos infectados.

DIAGNÓSTICO

DIAGNÓSTICO DIFERENCIAL
• Qualquer estado patológico agudo que se manifesta por linfadenopatia aguda, mal-estar, ulceração bucal com consequências fatais — considerar a tularemia. • Pseudotuberculose (*Yersinia pseudotuberculosis*) — em geral, causa vômito e diarreia.

HEMOGRAMA/BIOQUÍMICA/URINÁLISE
• Inicialmente, apresenta panleucopenia grave; em seguida, exibe leucocitose com desvio à esquerda, neutrófilos tóxicos, trombocitopenia.
• Hiperbilirrubinemia. • Hiponatremia.
• Hipoglicemia. • Alanina aminotransferase — elevada. • Bilirrubinúria. • Hematúria.

OUTROS TESTES LABORATORIAIS
Soroaglutinação em tubo ou ELISA — possível; há dificuldades de realização, exceto em laboratórios de referência; nem todos os animais respondem necessariamente à infecção em termos sorológicos.

MÉTODOS DIAGNÓSTICOS
• Esfregaço direto — lesão ou biopsia; a observação do microrganismo na coloração de Gram não é uma tarefa fácil. • Isolamento em cultura — deve ser feito por laboratórios de referência; amostras de sangue, líquido pleural ou aspirado de linfonodos, aplicados em meios de cultura contendo cisteína ou cistina; não é recuperável em meios de cultura de rotina; as bactérias não necessitam de CO_2 para o crescimento. **CUIDADO:** é preciso ter um cuidado extremo ao se trabalhar com amostras infectadas ou isolamentos. • Teste de imunofluorescência direta — materiais clínicos ou tecidos; permite a avaliação rápida do estado de infecção.

ACHADOS PATOLÓGICOS
• Placas ou úlceras brancas multifocais ao longo dos arcos glossopalatinos e da língua. • Ulceração bucal e tonsilar. • Linfadenopatia dos linfonodos cervicais, retrofaríngeos ou submandibulares com abscedação. • Lesões intestinais difusas.
• Linfadenopatia mesentérica, hepatosplenomegalia e icterícia.

TRATAMENTO

• Internação com o fornecimento de bons cuidados de enfermagem. • O tratamento precoce é importante para evitar a alta mortalidade.
• Tratar o paciente contra os ectoparasitas.

MEDICAÇÕES

MEDICAMENTO(S)
Tratar todos os casos de forma empírica até se obter a confirmação laboratorial.

Gatos
• Há poucas informações disponíveis sobre a eficácia dos antimicrobianos, em função da alta mortalidade de pacientes não submetidos ao tratamento precoce. • O tratamento precoce com a amoxicilina (20 mg/kg VO a cada 8 h por 5-7 dias ou 20 mg/kg IM ou SC a cada 12 h por 5 dias) em combinação com a gentamicina (4,4 mg/kg IM ou SC a cada 12 h e, depois, a cada 24 h, até a obtenção de uma resposta clínica ou até 7 dias) mostra-se bem-sucedido. • As fluoroquinolonas (p. ex., ciprofloxacino) têm se revelado promissoras como um novo agente terapêutico em potencial.

ACOMPANHAMENTO

MONITORIZAÇÃO DO PACIENTE
Monitorizar o paciente quanto à presença de CID — pode ocorrer no final da infecção.

PREVENÇÃO
• Viagem com os animais de estimação — evitar as áreas endêmicas. • Áreas endêmicas — confinamento dos animais para controlar a exposição e a ingestão de animais selvagens e seus ectoparasitas (carrapatos); controle dos ectoparasitas por meio da nebulização ou pulverização periódicas de inseticidas nos animais e nas pastagens. • Castração de gatos — para limitar o comportamento de caça e a exposição a animais selvagens. • Tomar medidas de precaução para restringir a contaminação dos alimentos e da água com carcaças de animais selvagens infectados.

EVOLUÇÃO ESPERADA E PROGNÓSTICO
O prognóstico é mau se o animal não for tratado precocemente; o prognóstico também é mau se os linfonodos mesentéricos estiverem palpáveis.

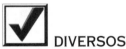

DIVERSOS

POTENCIAL ZOONÓTICO
• Alto. • Todas as pessoas que entram em contato com o paciente ou com os líquidos corporais devem usar máscara facial, luvas e aventais para evitar a infecção. • Isolar os pacientes. • Em áreas de doença emergente, a posse de gatos representa risco aos seres humanos. • As mordidas e os arranhões também representam risco aos seres humanos.
• Não confundir a tularemia com os abscessos provocados por mordidas em gatos ou com a peste.

SINÔNIMO(S)
• Febre do coelho. • Febre gerada por moscas do veado. • Doença do mercador.

ABREVIATURA(S)
• CID = coagulação intravascular disseminada.
• ELISA = ensaio imunoabsorvente ligado à enzima.

Sugestões de Leitura
Foley JE, Nieto NC. Tularemia. Vet Microbiology 2010, 140:332-338.
Valentine BA, DeBey BM, Sonn RJ, Stauffer LR, Pielstick LG. Localized cutaneous infection with Francisella tularensis resembling ulceroglandular tularemia in a cat. J Vet Diagn Invest 2004, 16:83-85.
Woods JP, Panciera RJ, Morton RJ, Lehenbauer TW. Feline tularemia. Compend Contin Educ Pract Vet 1998, 20:442-457.

Autor Patrick L. McDonough
Consultor Editorial Stephen C. Barr

Tumor das Células Basais (Basalioma)

CONSIDERAÇÕES GERAIS

REVISÃO
- Tumor originário do epitélio basal da pele.
- Abrange tumores benignos (p. ex., epitelioma basal e tumor basaloide) e malignos (p. ex., carcinoma basocelular).
- A ocorrência de metástase é rara com as formas benignas e incomum com as malignas.

IDENTIFICAÇÃO
- Tumor cutâneo mais comum em gatos (15-26%) e o segundo a terceiro tumor cutâneo mais comum em cães (4-12%).
- Idade média — cães: 6-9 anos; gatos: 10-11 anos.
- As predileções raciais incluem Cocker spaniel, Poodle e o gato Siamês.

SINAIS CLÍNICOS
- Massa intradérmica saliente firme, bem circunscrita, solitária e, muitas vezes, alopécica, tipicamente localizada na região cefálica, cervical ou escapular.
- Pode variar muito em termos de tamanho, desde poucos milímetros até muitos centímetros de diâmetro.
- Basaliomas em gatos — com frequência são intensamente pigmentados e, ocasionalmente, císticos ou ulcerados.

CAUSAS E FATORES DE RISCO
- Raça (ver "Identificação").
- Ao contrário dos basaliomas em seres humanos, a exposição à luz ultravioleta não parece desempenhar um papel em animais domésticos.

DIAGNÓSTICO

DIAGNÓSTICO DIFERENCIAL
- Outros tumores cutâneos — mastocitoma; melanoma; hemangioma; hemangiossarcoma; histiocitoma.
- Cistos intradérmicos.

HEMOGRAMA/BIOQUÍMICA/URINÁLISE
Permanecem normais.

OUTROS TESTES LABORATORIAIS
N/D.

DIAGNÓSTICO POR IMAGEM
N/D.

MÉTODOS DIAGNÓSTICOS
- A avaliação citológica de amostra obtida por aspirado com agulha fina revela células redondas com citoplasma basofílico; ocasionalmente, observa-se uma alta taxa mitótica apesar da natureza benigna.
- É necessário o exame histopatológico para obtenção do diagnóstico definitivo. Quando altamente pigmentado, a imuno-histoquímica pode ser um exame necessário para diferenciar de melanoma.

ACHADOS PATOLÓGICOS
- Padrões celulares histológicos — variam desde um aspecto sólido a cístico até um formato de tira.
- Células tumorais — podem conter pigmentação melânica; podem ainda exibir um discreto estroma eosinofílico.

TRATAMENTO

- A excisão cirúrgica constitui o tratamento de escolha e, em geral, é uma medida curativa para os tumores completamente ressecáveis.
- Os procedimentos de criocirurgia ou plesioterapia com estrôncio-90 podem ser utilizados para lesões menores (<1 cm).

MEDICAÇÕES

MEDICAMENTO(S)
N/D.

CONTRAINDICAÇÕES/INTERAÇÕES POSSÍVEIS
N/D.

ACOMPANHAMENTO

- A excisão cirúrgica completa é geralmente curativa e associada a um prognóstico excelente.
- A maioria dos tumores fica localmente confinada e não sofre metástase; nesse caso, não há necessidade de acompanhamento a longo prazo.

DIVERSOS

Sugestões de Leitura

Carpenter JL, Andrews LK, Holzworth J. Tumors and tumor-like lesions. In: Holzworth J, ed., Diseases of the Cat: Medicine and Surgery. Philadelphia: Saunders, 1987, pp. 406-596.

Cowell RL, Tyler RD, Meinkoth JH. Diagnostic Cytology and Hematology of the Dog and Cat. St Louis: Mosby, 1999, pp. 40-42.

Pakhrin B, Kang MS, Bae IH, et al. Retrospective study of canine cutaneous tumors in Korea. J Vet Sci 2007, 8:229-236.

Ramos-Vara JA, Miller MA, Johnson GC, et al. Melan A and S100 protein immunohistochemistry in feline melanomas: 48 cases. Vet Pathol 2002, 39:127-132.

Thomas RC, Fox LE. Tumors of the skin and subcutis. In: Morrison WB, ed., Cancer in Dogs and Cats: Medical and Surgical Management. Jackson, WY: Teton NewMedia, 2002, pp. 469-488.

Autor Louis-Philippe de Lorimier
Consultor Editorial Timothy M. Fan
Agradecimento O autor e o editor agradecem a contribuição prévia de Phyllis Glawe

TUMOR DE CÉLULAS INTERSTICIAIS DO TESTÍCULO

CONSIDERAÇÕES GERAIS

REVISÃO
Tumor benigno do testículo que surge das células de Leydig (intersticiais).

IDENTIFICAÇÃO
• Corresponde ao tumor testicular mais comum em cães, mas raro em gatos.
• Geralmente acomete cães idosos.

SINAIS CLÍNICOS
• Em geral, não há nenhum sinal a menos que associado à secreção de estrogênio, causando feminização e hipoplasia da medula óssea (ver "Sertolinoma").
• Massas tumorais esféricas discretas isoladas ou múltiplas (geralmente de 1 a 2 cm) dentro de um único testículo.
• Com frequência, os tumores são de coloração castanha a laranja.

CAUSAS E FATORES DE RISCO
• Geralmente desconhecidos.
• Criptorquidismo — pode predispor ao desenvolvimento desse tipo de tumor.

DIAGNÓSTICO

DIAGNÓSTICO DIFERENCIAL
• Sertolinoma.
• Seminoma.
• Hiperadrenocorticismo — com feminização.
• Hipotireodismo — com feminização.

HEMOGRAMA/BIOQUÍMICA/URINÁLISE
• Geralmente normais a menos que o excesso de estrogênio provoque hipoplasia da medula óssea (raro).
• Várias citopenias — com excesso de estrogênio (raro).

OUTROS TESTES LABORATORIAIS
• Concentração elevada de estradiol sérico.
• Concentração baixa de testosterona sérica.

DIAGNÓSTICO POR IMAGEM
Ultrassonografia — tumores com <3 cm de diâmetro tendem a ser hipoecoicos; tumores com >5 cm tendem a apresentar padrões ecogênicos mistos.

MÉTODOS DIAGNÓSTICOS
N/D.

TRATAMENTO

Castração e exame histopatológico de tecido apropriado.

MEDICAÇÕES

MEDICAMENTO(S)
• Nenhum a menos que haja hipoplasia da medula óssea, que induz à citopenia perigosa.
• Fatores estimulantes de colônia hematopoiéticos recombinantes — podem ser úteis no tratamento de hipoplasia da medula óssea.

CONTRAINDICAÇÕES/INTERAÇÕES POSSÍVEIS
N/D.

ACOMPANHAMENTO

MONITORIZAÇÃO DO PACIENTE
Nenhuma monitorização é necessária, salvo diante de hipoplasia da medula óssea.

COMPLICAÇÕES POSSÍVEIS
Citopenias causadas por excesso de estrogênio.

EVOLUÇÃO ESPERADA E PROGNÓSTICO
Em geral, são excelentes.

DIVERSOS

DISTÚRBIOS ASSOCIADOS
Prostatopatia — com tumor testicular.

VER TAMBÉM
Sertolinoma.

Sugestões de Leitura
Morrison WB. Cancers of the reproductive tract. In: Morrison WB, ed., Cancer in Dogs and Cats: Medical and Surgical Management. Jackson, WY: Teton NewMedia, 2002, pp. 555-564.
Suess RP, Barr SC, Sacre BJ, et al. Bone marrow hypoplasia in a feminized dog with an interstitial cell tumor. JAVMA 1992, 200:1346-1348.

Autor Wallace B. Morrison
Consultor Editorial Timothy M. Fan

Tumor Venéreo Transmissível

CONSIDERAÇÕES GERAIS

REVISÃO
- Tumor de ocorrência natural, transmitido sexualmente.
- Parece ser mais comum em regiões de clima temperado e grandes cidades.

IDENTIFICAÇÃO
Acomete cães intactos, de ambos os sexos.

SINAIS CLÍNICOS
- Massa tumoral avermelhada, friável, lobulada na mucosa da vagina ou do pênis.
- A mucosa bucal também pode ser acometida.
- Os proprietários podem relatar gotejamento de sangue vindo do prepúcio ou da vagina ou lambedura excessiva da área genital.
- Pode-se notar a protrusão do tumor.

CAUSAS E FATORES DE RISCO
- Transplante direto de células tumorais em mucosas escoriadas/esfoladas, transmitidas pelo coito ou por via oral.
- Cães intactos de vida livre — estão sob maior risco do que a média.

DIAGNÓSTICO

DIAGNÓSTICO DIFERENCIAL
- Outras neoplasias (p. ex., carcinoma de células escamosas; linfoma cutâneo).
- Hiperplasia vaginal.

HEMOGRAMA/BIOQUÍMICA/URINÁLISE
- Em geral, não são dignos de nota.
- Análise de urina coletada por micção espontânea revela hematúria e células anormais em alguns pacientes.

OUTROS TESTES LABORATORIAIS
N/D.

DIAGNÓSTICO POR IMAGEM
- Radiografias torácicas, embora esse tipo de tumor raramente sofra metástase.
- Aspirados de linfonodos regionais.
- Ultrassonografia abdominal para avaliar os linfonodos mesentéricos.

MÉTODOS DIAGNÓSTICOS
- Palpação cuidadosa dos linfonodos regionais.
- Exame de lâminas com esfregaços obtidos por impressão (decalque) ou aspirados tumorais revela camadas homogêneas de células arredondadas a ovais com nucléolos proeminentes, citoplasma escasso e múltiplos vacúolos citoplasmáticos claros.
- Biopsia fornece o diagnóstico definitivo.

TRATAMENTO
- Embora possa regredir espontaneamente, o tratamento ainda é recomendado, pois a remissão espontânea não é confiável.
- Excisão cirúrgica de tumores é, muitas vezes, seguida por recidiva.
- Radioterapia isolada pode ser curativa.
- Tratamento clínico é frequentemente curativo.

MEDICAÇÕES

MEDICAMENTO(S)
- Sulfato de vincristina (0,5-0,7 mg/m^2 IV uma vez por semana por 2 semanas além da resolução completa da doença macroscópica).
- Em caso de remissão parcial ou nula, pode-se tentar a administração de doxorrubicina (30 mg/m^2 IV a cada 3 semanas).

CONTRAINDICAÇÕES/INTERAÇÕES POSSÍVEIS
- Mielossupressão secundária à administração de vincristina ou doxorrubicina.
- Doxorrubicina pode ser cardiotóxica; usar com cautela, assim que a dose cumulativa de 150 mg/m^2 for atingida.
- Ocorrência de esfacelamento/necrose tecidual se houver extravasamento perivascular durante a administração de vincristina ou doxorrubicina.
- Buscar a orientação de especialistas antes de se iniciar o tratamento caso não se esteja familiarizado com o uso dos medicamentos citotóxicos.

ACOMPANHAMENTO

MONITORAÇÃO DO PACIENTE
Obter hemograma completo e contagem plaquetária antes de cada tratamento quimioterápico.

PREVENÇÃO
- Castração.
- Evitar que os animais tenham o hábito de vida livre.

COMPLICAÇÕES POSSÍVEIS
- É possível a ocorrência de recidiva tumoral após excisão cirúrgica incompleta ou reexposição.
- A doença metastática é incomum, embora haja relatos de que ela ocorra nos linfonodos regionais, nos olhos e na medula espinal.

EVOLUÇÃO ESPERADA E PROGNÓSTICO
A maioria dos casos de TVT apresenta resposta terapêutica (principalmente à quimio ou radioterapia) e prognóstico excelentes.

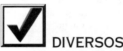

POTENCIAL ZOONÓTICO
Nenhum.

GESTAÇÃO/FERTILIDADE/REPRODUÇÃO
- Não é recomendável o tratamento de fêmeas prenhes com quimioterapia.
- Os animais podem ser infectados pelo TVT durante o coito.

ABREVIATURA(S)
- TVT = tumor venéreo transmissível.

Sugestões de Leitura
Scarpelli KC, et al. Predictive factors for the regression of canine transmissible venereal tumors during vincristine therapy. Vet J 2008, 22 de dezembro; apenas fonte *online* disponível.

Autor Ruthanne Chun
Consultor Editorial Timothy M. Fan

TUMORES CEREBRAIS

CONSIDERAÇÕES GERAIS

DEFINIÇÃO
• Os tumores cerebrais de cães ou gatos podem ser classificados como primários ou secundários, dependendo do tipo de célula de origem.
• Os tumores cerebrais primários originam-se de células normalmente encontradas dentro do cérebro e das meninges, incluindo o neuroepitélio, os tecidos linfoides, as células germinativas, as células endoteliais e os tecidos malformados.
• Os tumores secundários são neoplasias que chegam ao cérebro por metástase hematógena a partir de um tumor primário localizado fora do sistema nervoso ou neoplasias que afetam o cérebro por invasão local, ou extensão, a partir de tecidos adjacentes não neurais, como osso.
• As neoplasias da hipófise (adenomas ou carcinomas) e os tumores originários dos nervos cranianos (p. ex., tumor da bainha dos nervos trigêmeo, oculomotor ou vestibulococlear) são considerados tumores cerebrais secundários.

FISIOPATOLOGIA
• Os tumores cerebrais resultam em disfunção cerebral por causar tanto efeitos primários, como infiltração de tecido nervoso ou compressão de estruturas anatômicas adjacentes, como efeitos secundários, como hidrocefalia.
• Efeitos primários adicionais incluem interrupção da circulação cerebral, ou necrose local, o que pode culminar em maior dano ao tecido neural.
• Os efeitos secundários mais importantes de um tumor cerebral primário envolvem distúrbio da dinâmica de fluxo do líquido cerebrospinal (LCS), aumento da pressão intracraniana (PIC), formação de edema cerebral, ou herniação do cérebro.
• Os efeitos secundários costumam ser mais difusos ou generalizados em suas manifestações clínicas e podem "mascarar" a localização precisa de uma lesão intracraniana focal.

SISTEMA(S) ACOMETIDO(S)
Nervoso (cérebro).

GENÉTICA
Uma incidência excepcionalmente alta de meningiomas foi relatada em gatos com mucopolissacaridoses tipo I.

INCIDÊNCIA/PREVALÊNCIA
• Os tumores cerebrais parecem ser mais comuns em cães do que em outras espécies domésticas.
• Em cães, foi relatada uma taxa de incidência de tumores cerebrais de 14,5/100.000 da população de risco.
• Os locais mais comuns de ocorrência da neoplasia em cães imaturos (com menos de 6 meses de vida), em ordem decrescente, são o sistema hematopoiético, o cérebro e a pele.
• Em gatos, foi relatada uma incidência de aproximadamente 3,5/100.000 da população.

IDENTIFICAÇÃO
Raça(s) Predominante(s)
• Os meningiomas ocorrem com maior frequência em raças caninas dolicocefálicas.
• Os tumores de células gliais e os tumores da hipófise costumam ocorrer em raças caninas braquicefálicas.
• As raças caninas que são super-representadas incluem Boxer, Golden retriever, Doberman pinscher, Terrier escocês, e Old English sheepdog.
• Parece não haver uma predisposição racial para o desenvolvimento de tumores cerebrais em gatos.

Idade Média e Faixa Etária
• Os tumores cerebrais ocorrem em cães e gatos de qualquer idade.
• Mais frequentes em cães mais idosos, com maior incidência naqueles com mais de 5 anos de idade.

Sexo Predominante
Os gatos machos mais idosos parecem ser mais suscetíveis a meningiomas.

SINAIS CLÍNICOS
• Variam com a localização do tumor.
• O sinal clínico mais frequentemente identificado associado a algum tumor cerebral de cão ou gato é a ocorrência de crises convulsivas, particularmente se a primeira crise ocorrer depois dos 5 anos de idade.
• Outros sinais clínicos associados com frequência a algum tumor cerebral são alterações de comportamento e do estado mental, déficits visuais, andar em círculo, ataxia, inclinação da cabeça, e hiperestesia espinal cervical.
• Os sinais resultantes de uma doença em uma determinada localização no sistema nervoso são semelhantes, independentemente da causa exata.
• Com base na identificação, no histórico e nos resultados dos exames físico completo e neurológico, é possível localizar um problema no cérebro e, em alguns casos, determinar a localização aproximada.

CAUSAS
• Indeterminadas.
• Fatores nutricionais, ambientais, genéticos, químicos, virais, traumáticos e imunológicos podem ser considerados.

FATORES DE RISCO
Incertos.

DIAGNÓSTICO

DIAGNÓSTICO DIFERENCIAL
As categorias de doenças que podem resultar em sinais clínicos semelhantes àqueles de um tumor cerebral incluem distúrbios congênitos, infecções, distúrbios imunológicos e metabólicos, toxicidades, distúrbios nutricionais, traumatismos, distúrbios vasculares, degenerações, e distúrbios idiopáticos.

HEMOGRAMA/BIOQUÍMICA/URINÁLISE
O principal objetivo na realização desses exames é eliminar as causas extracranianas para os sinais de disfunção cerebral.

OUTROS TESTES LABORATORIAIS
N/D.

DIAGNÓSTICO POR IMAGEM
• Radiografias simples do tórax e ultrassonografia do abdome — para descartar um processo maligno primário em qualquer outro lugar do corpo.
• Radiografias do crânio — de valor limitado; pode detectar a presença de neoplasias do crânio ou da cavidade nasal que envolvam o cérebro por extensão local.
• Ocasionalmente, o processo de lise ou hiperostose do crânio pode acompanhar um tumor cerebral primário (p. ex., meningioma de gatos) ou pode haver mineralização dentro de uma neoplasia, visível ao exame radiográfico.
• O exame de TC proporciona uma determinação precisa da presença, da localização, do tamanho e das relações anatômicas de muitas neoplasias intracranianas.
• As imagens obtidas por RM são superiores àquelas da TC em certas regiões cerebrais (p. ex., o tronco encefálico).

MÉTODOS DIAGNÓSTICOS
Análise do LCS
• A análise do LCS pode ajudar a descartar causas inflamatórias de disfunção cerebral: em alguns casos, pode apoiar um diagnóstico de tumor cerebral.
• A coleta do LCS deve ser feita com cuidado, pois o aumento da PIC pode estar presente em associação a um tumor cerebral e alterações da pressão associadas à coleta do LCS podem induzir à herniação cerebral.
• Em geral, a coleta do LCS é protelada até que o diagnóstico avançado por imagem tenha sido concluído para avaliar fatores como a presença de edema ou hemorragia cerebral.
• O aumento no conteúdo de proteína e uma contagem normal a elevada de leucócitos no LCS geralmente são considerados como alterações "típicas" de uma neoplasia cerebral.

Biopsia
• A avaliação citológica das preparações de esfregaço feito a partir de tecido coletado por biopsia, fixado rapidamente em álcool a 95% e corado com hematoxilina-eosina, pode ser feita dentro de minutos da coleta da biopsia.
• A biopsia tecidual continua sendo o único método disponível para o diagnóstico definitivo do tipo de tumor cerebral em cães ou gatos, sendo uma consideração essencial antes de qualquer tipo de terapia.
• A biopsia nem sempre é empreendida por conta de considerações práticas, como custo e morbidade.
• Os sistemas de biopsia estereotáxica guiada por TC representam um meio relativamente rápido e extremamente preciso de biopsia tumoral, com baixa taxa de complicações.

ACHADOS PATOLÓGICOS
• A classificação de tumores do SNC em cães e gatos baseia-se principalmente nas características do tipo celular constituinte, do comportamento patológico, do padrão topográfico e das alterações secundárias presentes dentro e em volta do tumor.
• O meningioma é a neoplasia intracraniana mais comum de cães e gatos.
• A classificação do subgrupo glial de tumores neuroepiteliais baseia-se no tipo celular predominante (p. ex., astrócito ou oligodendrócito).

Cães
• Tumores embrionários foram consolidados sob um único termo "tumores neuroectodérmicos primitivos" (ou TNEP) para se ajustar à sua natureza anaplásica.
• Os tumores cerebrais que surgem das células linforreticulares foram tradicionalmente agrupados sob o título de reticulose ou linfoma histiocítico.
• Os tumores do crânio que afetam o cérebro por extensão local incluem osteossarcoma, condrossarcoma, e osteocondrossarcoma multilobular.
• Os tumores secundários mais frequentemente observados de cães englobam extensão local de adenocarcinoma nasal; metástases de

adenocarcinoma mamário, prostático, ou pulmonar; metástases de hemangiossarcoma; e extensão de adenoma ou carcinoma hipofisário.
• Podem ocorrer tumores das bainhas nervosas originários dos nervos cranianos (particularmente dos nervos oculomotor e trigêmeo) em cães.

Gatos
• Os meningiomas que envolvem múltiplas regiões intracranianas (inclusive o terceiro ventrículo) são relativamente comuns em gatos.
• Tumores cerebrais primários, exceto os meningiomas, ocorrem com pouca frequência em gatos.
• Os tumores relatados incluem astrocitoma, ependimoma, oligodendroglioma, papiloma do plexo coroide, meduloblastoma, linfoma, neuroblastoma olfatório, e gangliocitoma.
• O linfoma do cérebro pode ser primário ou secundário ou, então, um aspecto de linfoma multicêntrico de gatos.
• Os tumores secundários, cuja ocorrência foi relatada nos cérebros de gatos, envolvem macroadenomas e macrocarcinomas hipofisários, além de carcinoma metastático.
• A extensão local pode ocorrer a partir de tumores da cavidade da orelha média (p. ex., carcinoma de células escamosas), da cavidade nasal (p. ex., adenocarcinoma nasal) ou do crânio (p. ex., osteossarcoma).

TRATAMENTO
CUIDADO(S) DE SAÚDE ADEQUADO(S)
• Além dos esforços gerais para manter a homeostasia, os principais objetivos da terapia para um tumor cerebral são controlar os efeitos secundários, como PIC elevada ou edema cerebral, e erradicar o tumor ou reduzir seu tamanho.
• Atualmente, há três métodos terapêuticos disponíveis para aplicação em tumores cerebrais em cães e gatos: cirurgia, radioterapia e quimioterapia.

Cirurgia
• A intervenção neurocirúrgica é uma consideração essencial no tratamento de tumores cerebrais em cães ou gatos, seja para excisão completa, remoção parcial ou biopsia.
• Meningiomas, em particular aqueles localizados sobre as convexidades cerebrais ou nos lobos frontais do cérebro, podem ser completamente (ou quase completamente) removidos por meio de cirurgia, sobretudo em gatos.
• Os tumores primários da calota craniana (conhecida como calvária) também podem ser removidos por meio cirúrgico antes de outros tipos de terapia.

Radioterapia
• A radiação pode ser usada isoladamente ou em combinação com outros tratamentos para tumores cerebrais primários ou secundários.
• Para o sucesso da radioterapia, é essencial o planejamento terapêutico cuidadoso por um radioterapeuta qualificado e experiente.

Quimioterapia
O uso de carmustina (BCNU) ou lomustina (CCNU) pode resultar em redução do tamanho do tumor e na melhora dos sinais clínicos em cães com tumores de células gliais.
A citosina-arabinosídeo (ARA-C) já foi usada por via intratecal em cães para tratar linfoma do SNC.

MEDICAÇÕES
MEDICAMENTO(S) DE ESCOLHA
• Os glicocorticoides podem ser usados para redução do edema e, em alguns casos (p. ex., linfoma), para retardo do crescimento tumoral. Alguns animais com tumor cerebral demonstram uma melhora drástica nos sinais clínicos por semanas ou meses com manutenção da glicocorticoterapia.
• Os medicamentos fenobarbital ou brometo constituem as melhores opções terapêuticas para controle das crises convulsivas generalizadas.
• O manitol é o medicamento mais adequado para redução eficaz da PIC elevada.

ACOMPANHAMENTO
MONITORIZAÇÃO DO PACIENTE
• Exames neurológicos seriados.
• Exames seriados de TC ou RM.
COMPLICAÇÕES POSSÍVEIS
• Pneumonia por aspiração causada por depressão dos reflexos de deglutição associada ao aumento da PIC.
• Crises convulsivas.

EVOLUÇÃO ESPERADA E PROGNÓSTICO
• Existem poucos dados a respeito dos tempos de sobrevida de cães ou gatos acometidos por tumor cerebral e submetidos apenas à terapia paliativa (ou seja, terapia para controlar os efeitos secundários de algum tumor sem uma tentativa de erradicar o tumor). Os resultados de um único estudo indicam uma sobrevida média e mediana de 81 e 56 dias, respectivamente, após o diagnóstico de tumor cerebral primário por TC em 1 de cada 8 cães.
• Os resultados de vários estudos confirmam que o prognóstico de cães ou gatos com tumor cerebral primário pode melhorar significativamente por meio de remoção cirúrgica, radiação e quimioterapia, isoladamente ou em combinação.

DIVERSOS
DISTÚRBIOS ASSOCIADOS
Os cães submetidos ao tratamento de algum tumor cerebral podem desenvolver um segundo tipo de tumor em qualquer outro local do corpo.
ABREVIATURAS
• LCS = líquido cerebrospinal.
• PIC = pressão intracraniana.
• RM = ressonância magnética.
• SNC = sistema nervoso central.
• TC = tomografia computadorizada.

Sugestões de Leitura
LeCouteur RA, Withrow SJ. Tumors of the nervous system. In: Withrow SJ, Vail DM, eds., Small Animal Clinical Oncology, 4th ed. Philadelphia: Saunders, 2007, pp. 659-685.
Tomek A, Cizinauskas S, Doherr M, Gandini G, Jaggy A. Intracranial neoplasia in 61 cats: Localisation, tumour types and seizure patterns. J Feline Med Surg 2006, 8(4):243-253.
Troxel MT, Vite CH, Van Winkle TJ, Newton AL, Tiches D, Dayrell-Hart B, Kapatkin AS, Shofer FS, Steinberg SA. Feline intracranial neoplasia: Retrospective review of 160 cases (1985-2001). J Vet Intern Med 2003, 17(6):850-859.
Vernau KM, Higgins RJ, Bollen AW, Jimenez DF, Anderson JV, Koblik PD, eCouteur RA. Primary canine and feline nervous system tumors: Intraoperative diagnosis using the smear technique. Vet Pathol 2001, 38:47-57.

Autor Richard A. LeCouteur
Consultor Editorial Joane M. Parent

TUMORES DA BAINHA NERVOSA

CONSIDERAÇÕES GERAIS

REVISÃO
- Tumores dos nervos periféricos, dos nervos espinais, ou das raízes nervosas.
- O tumor maligno da bainha dos nervos periféricos é a denominação recomendada para esses tumores, no lugar de schwanoma, neurilemoma ou neurofibroma, pois a determinação da célula de origem é frequentemente impossível.
- A maioria dos tumores (80%) ocorre no membro torácico de cães.
- Aproximadamente 50% dos tumores são localizados na região do plexo ou dos nervos periféricos, enquanto os outros 50% na região das raízes nervosas.

IDENTIFICAÇÃO
- Cães — não há predisposição racial ou sexual.
- Idade média em cães — 7,9 anos; incomuns em cães com menos de 3 anos de idade.
- Raros em gatos.

SINAIS CLÍNICOS
- Claudicação progressiva crônica dos membros torácicos.
- Atrofia muscular (atrofia neurogênica) frequentemente presente, mais grave do que aquela observada em distúrbios ortopédicos.
- Pode ser observada uma redução do tônus muscular e do reflexo flexor.
- A palpação axilar detecta a presença de massa em menos de 30% dos casos.
- Ocasionalmente, há dor axilar à palpação.
- É possível a observação de síndrome de Horner em tumores que envolvem as raízes nervosas de T1-T3.
- Se o tumor comprimir a medula espinal, podem ser observadas alterações como ataxia, paresia e déficits proprioceptivos assimétricos.
- O reflexo cutâneo do tronco pode estar baixo a ausente no lado acometido.
- Em tumores lombossacrais, a palpação retal pode ser útil para detecção de massa.
- Ocasionalmente, observa-se automutilação.

CAUSAS E FATORES DE RISCO
Em alguns casos, foi identificada mutação no oncogene *neu*.

DIAGNÓSTICO

DIAGNÓSTICO DIFERENCIAL
- Distúrbios ortopédicos que causam claudicação dos membros torácicos ou pélvicos. Diferenciar por meio de exame ortopédico, radiografias ou cintilografia e resposta a repouso e medicamentos anti-inflamatórios. A gravidade da atrofia muscular também é útil na diferenciação.
- Compressão lateralizada das raízes nervosas por discopatia intervertebral, doença lombossacra, ou neoplasia espinal. Discopatia intervertebral e doença lombossacra costumam ser associadas à dor espinal. Há necessidade das técnicas avançadas de diagnóstico por imagem (TC ou RM) para distinguir essas doenças.
- Neuropatia traumática ou avulsão parcial do plexo braquial — diferenciadas pelo histórico (início agudo) e pelos achados das técnicas de diagnóstico por imagem.
- Neoplasia secundária dos nervos — linfoma, sarcoma histiocítico, condrossarcoma. Há necessidade de biopsia aspirativa com agulha fina ou biopsia central para diferenciar esses distúrbios.

OUTROS TESTES LABORATORIAIS
- Análise do LCS — achados inespecíficos.
- Citologia — a biopsia com agulha fina guiada por ultrassom pode fornecer amostra diagnóstica. Os aspectos citológicos do tumor maligno da bainha dos nervos periféricos são característicos de um sarcoma de tecidos moles.

DIAGNÓSTICO POR IMAGEM
- Radiografias simples — radiografias simples bem-posicionadas podem permitir a visualização de forame intervertebral aumentado de volume; com maior frequência, são pouco recompensadoras.
- Ultrassom — muitas vezes é capaz de identificar a presença de massa nos casos em que a palpação axilar não é recompensadora. O paciente deve ser submetido à sedação para permitir o melhor posicionamento e a biopsia aspirativa com agulha fina guiada por ultrassom. A ecogenicidade do tumor é variável.
- Mielografia — se a neoplasia tiver invadido o canal vertebral, pode-se observar um padrão intradural extramedular. Em virtude da localização das neoplasias, a mielografia é diagnóstica em aproximadamente 50% dos cães.
- TC e RM — possibilitam a visualização de tumores proximais ou distais nos membros. A hiperintensidade de sinal nas imagens ponderadas em T2 representa o padrão mais comum do exame de ressonância magnética. Os tumores malignos da bainha dos nervos periféricos costumam exibir realce do contraste em ambos os exames. Em função da alta caracterização de tecidos moles, a RM constitui a modalidade diagnóstica de escolha.

MÉTODOS DIAGNÓSTICOS
- Eletromiografia — comumente utilizada para diferenciar entre atrofia neurogênica e atrofia muscular por desuso. Os potenciais de fibrilação e as ondas agudas positivas são sugestivos de atrofia muscular neurogênica.
- Velocidade de condução nervosa — as velocidades de condução podem estar prolongadas com amplitude reduzida.
- Onda F, onda H e potenciais do corno dorsal da medula espinal — avaliam a porção radicular do nervo e podem ser úteis para diferenciar uma lesão que afeta predominantemente a raiz sensorial ou motora.

TRATAMENTO
- A ressecção cirúrgica seguindo os princípios da cirurgia oncológica é o tratamento recomendado.
- A amputação é geralmente requerida para minimizar as chances de recorrência local.
- Os procedimentos de hemilaminectomia ou laminectomia dorsal podem ser necessários para permitir a ressecção da região da raiz nervosa.
- Corticosteroides orais, como dexametasona ou prednisona, podem conferir a melhora clínica pela redução do edema peritumoral.
- Radioterapia — pode ser usada para tumores não passíveis de ressecção ou nos casos em que a cirurgia é contraindicada. Também pode ser utilizada no pós-operatório para diminuir as chances de recorrência local.

MEDICAÇÕES

MEDICAMENTO(S)
- Quimioterapia — a terapia metronômica (ciclofosfamida 10 mg/m^2 e piroxicam 0,3 mg/kg) pode ser usada para tumores da bainha nervosa submetidos à ressecção parcial em cães.
- Dexametasona 0,1-0,25 mg/kg a cada 24 h ou prednisona 0,5-1 mg/kg a cada 12-24 h pode ser usada para proporcionar melhora a curto prazo.
- Gabapentina 5-20 mg/kg a cada 8-12 h pode ser utilizada para analgesia em casos de dor neuropática.

CONTRAINDICAÇÕES/INTERAÇÕES POSSÍVEIS
Não é recomendável o uso de corticosteroides em conjunto com medicamentos anti-inflamatórios não esteroides.

ACOMPANHAMENTO
- Os tumores da bainha nervosa são localmente invasivos, mas raras vezes sofrem metástases.
- A recorrência local pós-operatória é comum (até 72% dos casos).

DIVERSOS

ABREVIATURAS
- LCS = líquido cerebrospinal
- RM = ressonância magnética
- TC = tomografia computadorizada

Sugestões de Leitura
Brehm DM, Vite CH, Steinberg HS, et al. A retrospective evaluation of 51 cases of peripheral nerve sheath tumor in the dog. JAAHA 1995, 31:349-359.
da Costa RC, Parent JM, Dobson H, et al. Ultrasound-guided fine needle aspiration in the diagnosis of peripheral nerve sheath tumors in 4 dogs. Can Vet J 2008, 49:77-81.
Kraft S, Ehrhart EJ, Gall D, et al. Magnetic resonance imaging characteristics of peripheral nerve sheath tumors of the canine brachial plexus in 18 dogs. Vet Radiol Ultrasound 2007, 48:1-7.

Autor Ronaldo Casimiro da Costa
Consultor Editorial Joane M. Parent

Tumores das Glândulas Mamárias — Cadelas

CONSIDERAÇÕES GERAIS

DEFINIÇÃO
Tumores benignos ou malignos das glândulas mamárias em cadelas.

FISIOPATOLOGIA
- Aproximadamente 50% dos tumores são malignos.
- Cerca de 50% das pacientes apresentam múltiplos tumores na cadeia mamária.
- Alguns animais terão tumores malignos associados a alguns tipos benignos.
- Carcinoma inflamatório — subtipo muito agressivo; caracterizado por crescimento rápido, textura firme, envolvimento difuso, eritema, edema de extremidades, alteração da cor e dor; a paciente pode estar anêmica, ter leucocitose e desenvolver CID; o tumor pode ser confundido com mastite, abscesso ou celulite; prognóstico mau.
- Conexões linfáticas — existentes entre as sequências direita e esquerda das glândulas; em geral, as glândulas craniais drenam para os linfonodos axilares, as glândulas caudais drenam para os linfonodos inguinais e as glândulas entre elas drenam variavelmente para um ou ambos os tipos de linfonodos; conexões plexiformes ajudam a explicar a ocorrência de metástase linfática contra o fluxo de linfa previsto.
- Alguns tumores drenarão direta ou indiretamente para os linfonodos esternais.
- Influência hormonal — sugerida pela menor incidência nas cadelas castradas em uma idade precoce (ver a seção "Prevenção").

SISTEMA(S) ACOMETIDO(S)
- Reprodutivo.
- Metástases — respiratório, nervoso e outros sistemas.

GENÉTICA
- Frequente mutação e superexpressão do gene p53.
- Superexpressão frequente do gene C-erb B2 em tipos malignos.
- Relatos de mutações do gene BRCA 1 em alguns tumores mamários em cadelas.

INCIDÊNCIA/PREVALÊNCIA
Fêmeas — 198,8 para cada 100.000.

DISTRIBUIÇÃO GEOGRÁFICA
Semelhante em todo o mundo.

IDENTIFICAÇÃO

Espécies
Cães.

Raça(s) Predominante(s)
As raças Poodles toy e miniatura, Springer spaniel inglês, Spaniel britânico, Cocker spaniel, Setter inglês, Boxer, Pointer inglês, Pastor alemão, Maltês, Doberman e Yorkshire terrier foram variavelmente relatadas por terem um alto risco.

Idade Média e Faixa Etária
- Idade média — cerca de 10,5 anos (faixa etária de 1-15 anos).
- Rara nas cadelas com <5 anos.

Sexo Predominante
Fêmeas; extremamente raro nos machos.

SINAIS CLÍNICOS

Achados Anamnésicos
Em geral, trata-se de massas isoladas ou múltiplas de crescimento lento, associadas ao mamilo.

Achados do Exame Físico
- Massas isoladas ou múltiplas — cerca de 50% das pacientes apresenta múltiplos tumores.
- As massas mamárias podem estar ulceradas.
- Podem ser livremente móveis — implica comportamento benigno.
- Podem estar fixados à pele ou à parede corporal — implica comportamento maligno.

CAUSAS
Desconhecidas; provavelmente hormonais.

FATORES DE RISCO
- Evidência circunstancial — incrimina o tratamento com progestinas e estrogênios combinados, prolactina e hormônio do crescimento.
- Obesidade de início precoce nas cadelas — pode aumentar o risco do desenvolvimento de tumores mamários.

DIAGNÓSTICO

DIAGNÓSTICO DIFERENCIAL
- Lipoma.
- Mastocitoma.
- Hiperplasia mamária.
- Mastite.

HEMOGRAMA/BIOQUÍMICA/URINÁLISE
Geralmente normais.

OUTROS TESTES LABORATORIAIS
N/D.

DIAGNÓSTICO POR IMAGEM
- Radiografia torácica — pode detectar metástase, sendo aconselhável a obtenção de três projeções.
- Radiografia abdominal — pode detectar metástase para os linfonodos ilíacos (sublombares).
- TC — é mais sensível para a detecção de metástase pulmonar do que as radiografias simples.

MÉTODOS DIAGNÓSTICOS
- Exame de preparações citológicas — frequentemente confuso; a inflamação pode mimetizar os critérios de malignidade. Tomar as decisões sempre com base no exame histopatológico e não citológico.
- Biopsia excisional — diagnóstico definitivo.

ACHADOS PATOLÓGICOS
- Macroscópicos — associados à inflamação considerável; pode-se encontrar ulceração.
- Histopatológicos — 50% benignos; 42% adenocarcinoma; 4% carcinoma inflamatório; 4% sarcoma.
- Mutações do gene p53 e superexpressão da proteína codificada por esse gene podem ser indicadores úteis de comportamento maligno acentuado e prognóstico mau.
- Foi demonstrado que os índices de proliferação celular avaliados pelo marcador Ki-67 tenham valor prognóstico, além de se correlacionarem com malignidade e baixa sobrevida.
- A expressão de receptores estrogênicos varia com o tamanho e a malignidade do tumor e, no futuro, pode se tornar um dado prognóstico.

TRATAMENTO

CUIDADO(S) DE SAÚDE ADEQUADO(S)
- Cirurgia — principal modalidade terapêutica.
- Quimioterapia — pode ser eficaz; indicada na presença de indícios histológicos de invasão linfática ou vascular.

CUIDADO(S) DE ENFERMAGEM
N/D.

ATIVIDADE
N/D.

DIETA
N/D.

ORIENTAÇÃO AO PROPRIETÁRIO
- Orientar o proprietário sobre o fato de que um caroço na mama nunca deve ser deixado no local em observação.
- Informar ao proprietário que a intervenção cirúrgica precoce é a melhor opção.
- Aconselhar a castrar antes do primeiro cio.

CONSIDERAÇÕES CIRÚRGICAS
- Excisão local (p. ex., mastectomia simples, regional ou unilateral) com margens amplas e profundas (no mínimo 2 cm em todas as direções) — pode ser tão eficaz quanto a mastectomia bilateral radical em termos de intervalo livre da doença.
- A realização de ovário-histerectomia em cadelas intactas no momento da mastectomia pode aumentar a sobrevida.

MEDICAÇÕES

MEDICAMENTO(S) DE ESCOLHA
- Consultar sempre um veterinário especialista em oncologia em busca de informações atualizadas a respeito de quimioterapia adjuvante.
- Doxorrubicina — 30 mg/m^2 IV cada 21 dias.

CONTRAINDICAÇÕES
Doxorrubicina — insuficiência miocárdica.

PRECAUÇÕES
A quimioterapia pode ser tóxica; buscar por orientação antes do tratamento caso não se esteja familiarizado com agentes citotóxicos.

INTERAÇÕES POSSÍVEIS
Doxorrubicina — os efeitos colaterais incluem mielotoxicidade, vômito e diarreia, pancreatite e lesão cardíaca.

MEDICAMENTO(S) ALTERNATIVO(S)
- Tamoxifeno — valioso em alguns seres humanos com câncer de mama; além de ser ineficaz nos cães, apresenta graves efeitos colaterais (p. ex., piometra); não usar nas cadelas.
- Estão sendo conduzidos protocolos experimentais como quimioterapia inalatória para carcinoma metastático; portanto, deve-se consultar um médico oncologista para explorar as opções quimioterápicas alternativas disponíveis atualmente.

ACOMPANHAMENTO

MONITORIZAÇÃO DA PACIENTE
Exame físico e radiografias torácicas — 1, 3, 6, 9 e 12 meses após o tratamento.

PREVENÇÃO
- Castrada antes do primeiro ciclo estral — risco de 0,5% em comparação com a cadela intacta.

- Castrada antes do segundo ciclo estral — risco de 8% em comparação com a cadela intacta.
- Castrada após o segundo estro — risco de 26% em comparação com a cadela intacta.
- Castrada após os 2 anos e meio de idade — sem efeito poupador sobre o risco.

COMPLICAÇÕES POSSÍVEIS
- Ocorrência de infecção ou deiscência da sutura com a cirurgia.
- Mielossupressão com a quimioterapia.
- CID com alguns tipos de tumores (especialmente carcinomas inflamatórios).
- Metástase à distância e morte na ausência de tratamento.

EVOLUÇÃO ESPERADA E PROGNÓSTICO
- Sobrevida média após a mastectomia em casos de adenocarcinoma tubular — 24,6 meses.
- Sobrevida média após a mastectomia em casos de carcinoma sólido — 6 meses e meio.
- Tumor benigno — prognóstico excelente após a mastectomia.
- Carcinoma com < 5 cm de diâmetro — em geral, exibe prognóstico bom se a excisão for completa.
- O envolvimento dos linfonodos regionais confirmado por exame histopatológico exerce um efeito prognóstico negativo (somente a palpação é muito imprecisa).
- Classificação histológica, crescimento intravascular e presença de necrose afetam o prognóstico.
- A presença de receptores estrogênicos e/ou receptores progestágenos afeta adversamente o prognóstico.

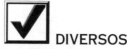

DIVERSOS

DISTÚRBIOS ASSOCIADOS
- Osteopatia hipertrófica.
- Metástase para os pulmões e para o SNC.

FATORES RELACIONADOS COM A IDADE
N/D.

POTENCIAL ZOONÓTICO
Nenhum.

GESTAÇÃO/FERTILIDADE/REPRODUÇÃO
N/D.

ABREVIATURA(S)
- CID = coagulação intravascular disseminada.
- SNC = sistema nervoso central.
- TC = tomografia computadorizada.

RECURSOS DA INTERNET
http://www.vet.uga.edu/vpp/clerk/mccarthy/index.htm

Sugestões de Leitura
Allen SW, Mahaffey EA. Canine mammary neoplasia: Prognostic indicators and response to surgical therapy. JAAHA 1989, 25:540.546.

de las Mulas JM, Mill Lan Y, Dios R. A prospective analysis of immnohistochemically determined estrogen α and progesterone receptor expression and host and tumor factors as predictors of disease-free period in mammary tumors of the dog. Vet Pathol 2005, 42:200.212.

Morrison WB. Canine and feline mammary tumors. In: Morrison WB, ed., Cancer in Dogs and Cats: Medical and Surgical Management. Jackson, WY: Teton NewMedia, 2002, pp. 565.572.

Nieto A, Pena L, Perez-Alenza MD, et al. Immunohistologic detection of estrogen receptor alpha in canine mammary tumors: Clinical and pathologic associations and prognostic significance. Vet Pathol 2000, 37:239.247.

Philibert JC, Snyder PW, Glickman N, et al. Influence of host factors on survival in dogs with malignant mammary gland tumors. J Vet Intern Med 2003, 17:102.106.

Soremno K. Canine mammary gland tumors. Vet Clin Small Anim 2003, 33:573.596.

Zuccari DAPC, Santana AE, Cury P, et al. Immunocytochemical study of Ki-67 as a prognostic marker in canine mammary neoplasia. Vet Clin Path 2008, 33:23.28.

Autor Wallace B. Morrison
Consultor Editorial Timothy M. Fan

Tumores das Glândulas Mamárias — Gatas

CONSIDERAÇÕES GERAIS

DEFINIÇÃO
Tumores benignos e malignos da glândula mamária nas gatas.

FISIOPATOLOGIA
- 5-15% dos tumores são benignos do ponto de vista histológico, sendo a maioria constituída por adenomas ou fibroadenomas simples, embora também haja relatos de papilomas intraductais e tumores complexos.
- 85-95% dos tumores são malignos, mas grande parte deles consiste em carcinomas; os sarcomas são raros (ver a seção "Achados Patológicos").
- Os carcinomas inflamatórios raramente são diagnosticados. Tais tumores são carcinomas anaplásicos com consideráveis infiltrados de células inflamatórias, estando associados a ulceração, edema e dor locais extensos, bem como rápida ocorrência de metástase.
- A metástase para os pulmões é identificada em até 70% dos gatos, enquanto a metástase para os linfonodos regionais, em até 50%. Outros locais de metástase incluem órgãos como fígado, baço, rins, glândulas adrenais, pleura, peritônio, coração, tireoide e osso. À necropsia, a metástase é identificada em >90% dos gatos.

SISTEMA(S) ACOMETIDO(S)
- Reprodutivo — glândulas mamárias.
- As metástases podem afetar qualquer sistema orgânico, sobretudo os sistemas respiratório e linfático.

GENÉTICA
A alta incidência dos tumores mamários em gatos da raça Siamês sugere algum componente genético para essa doença, mas não foram identificados genes específicos até o momento.

INCIDÊNCIA/PREVALÊNCIA
- Terceira neoplasia mais comum nos gatos (depois de tumores hematopoiéticos e cutâneos).
- A incidência estimada é de 12,8-25,4 para cada 100.000 gatos.

IDENTIFICAÇÃO
Espécies
Gatos.

Raça(s) Predominante(s)
- Gatos domésticos de pelo curto e longo costumam ser mais acometidos, mas isso provavelmente reflete a popularidade dessas raças e não uma predileção verdadeira.
- Os gatos da raça Siamês apresentam o dobro do risco de outras raças para o desenvolvimento de tumores mamários.

Idade Média e Faixa Etária
- Média — 10-12 anos.
- Variação — 9 meses a 23 anos; a maioria tem > 5 anos de idade.
- Os gatos da raça Siamês tendem a desenvolver tumores mamários em uma idade mais jovem, mas a incidência começa a atingir o platô em torno dos 9 anos de idade.

Sexo Predominante
- Predomínio nas fêmeas.
- Embora o estado reprodutivo intacto aumente o risco de tumores mamários (ver a seção "Fatores de Risco"), a maioria dos gatos diagnosticados com tumores mamários é castrada.
- 1-5% dos carcinomas mamários ocorrem em gatos machos.

SINAIS CLÍNICOS
Achados Anamnésicos
- Grande parte dos gatos é levada à consulta veterinária para avaliação de massa abdominal ventral palpável.
- Os gatos com doença metastática avançada podem ser levados ao veterinário por causa de sinais gerais de doença (p. ex., letargia ou anorexia) ou por sinais atribuíveis a um local específico de metástase (p. ex., dispneia por metástase pulmonar ou efusão pleural).
- A duração dos sinais clínicos pode variar de dias a vários meses.

Achados do Exame Físico
- As massas mamárias podem ser discretas ou infiltrativas, moles ou firmes. Massas menores muitas vezes são livremente móveis, enquanto massas maiores podem se aderir à musculatura abdominal subjacente.
- A pele sobrejacente pode permanecer intacta, mas frequentemente se encontra ulcerada.
- O mamilo associado pode estar inflamado e exsudar líquido seroso.
- Qualquer glândula pode ser acometida, embora as duas glândulas caudais sejam mais comumente acometidas. Os lados esquerdo e direito são afetados em uma frequência equivalente.
- Até metade dos gatos apresentarão múltiplos tumores acometendo as glândulas no mesmo lado e/ou no lado oposto.
- Pode haver linfadenopatia axilar ou inguinal (reativa ou metastática).
- Como as células tumorais se disseminam via vasos linfáticos, podem se formar cadeias lineares (tipo rosário) de nódulos tumorais nos vasos linfáticos dentro do tecido mamário.
- Os gatos com carcinomas inflamatórios apresentam-se com ulceração, eritema, dor e edema graves na porção abdominal ventral e nos membros pélvicos.

CAUSAS
Desconhecidas.

FATORES DE RISCO
- Em comparação a gatos intactos, os castrados com <6 meses de vida têm uma probabilidade 11 vezes menor de desenvolver carcinomas mamários, enquanto os castrados com 6-12 meses de vida têm uma probabilidade 7 vezes menor.
- Não há nenhum efeito protetor evidente quando os gatos são castrados com >12 meses de vida.
- Progestinas exógenas (p. ex., acetato de medroxiprogesterona) aumentam o risco de desenvolvimento de tumores mamários benignos e malignos em gatos machos e fêmeas. Em um único estudo, 8 de 22 gatos machos com carcinomas mamários tinham histórico de terapia com progestina exógena.
- Não foi demonstrado que a paridade afete o desenvolvimento de tumores mamários.

DIAGNÓSTICO

DIAGNÓSTICO DIFERENCIAL
- Hiperplasia fibroepitelial — especialmente em gatas intactas jovens (<2 anos), além de gatos mais idosos ou castrados submetidos a progestinas exógenas.
- Mastite.
- Outros tumores cutâneos ou subcutâneos.
- Linfadenopatia inguinal ou axilar (reativa ou neoplásica).
- Hérnia inguinal.
- Coxim gorduroso inguinal grande/proeminente.

HEMOGRAMA/BIOQUÍMICA/URINÁLISE
- Geralmente não revelam alterações dignas de nota.
- Anemia de doença crônica e/ou secundária à sangramento crônico em caso de massa ulcerada.
- Pode haver leucograma inflamatório, sobretudo se a massa estiver ulcerada.

OUTROS TESTES LABORATORIAIS
O perfil de coagulação é recomendado para gatos com suspeita de carcinomas inflamatórios em função da alta incidência de coagulopatia intravascular disseminada secundária.

DIAGNÓSTICO POR IMAGEM
- É recomendável a obtenção de radiografias torácicas em três projeções para fazer a triagem de metástase pulmonar e/ou efusão pleural. As metástases pulmonares são mais comumente associadas a nódulos intersticiais mal definidos ou padrão pulmonar difuso, embora ocasionalmente se observem nódulos intersticiais bem definidos.
- A realização de ultrassonografia abdominal é recomendada para fazer a triagem dos linfonodos ilíacos mediais e outros órgãos viscerais abdominais em busca de metástases.
- O ultrassom também pode ser utilizado para tentar visualizar os linfonodos axilares ou inguinais não palpáveis, bem como para pesquisar por pequenas massas adicionais dentro das glândulas mamárias.

MÉTODOS DIAGNÓSTICOS
- O exame citológico pode ser útil para descartar outras malignidades não mamárias. Contudo, esse exame não tem utilidade para distinguir entre massas mamárias benignas e malignas.
- É necessária a avaliação histopatológica para obter o diagnóstico definitivo. Como a maioria dos tumores mamários são malignos, o exame histopatológico costuma ser realizado em tecido removido durante mastectomia radical (ver a seção "Tratamento"). Biopsias incisionais são recomendadas com rotina apenas para gatos que apresentam doença em estágio avançado, mas não são candidatos à cirurgia local rigorosa.
- Todo o tecido removido precisa ser enviado para avaliação histopatológica. Isso permite não só a obtenção de um diagnóstico mais preciso, mas também a avaliação das margens cirúrgicas quanto à eficácia da excisão.
- Os linfonodos drenantes ipsolaterais (axilares e inguinais) devem ser removidos durante a mastectomia radical e enviados separadamente para exame histopatológico, mesmo se estiverem normais do ponto de vista macroscópico.
- O exame citológico do líquido pleural pode ser útil para confirmar metástases intratorácicas.

ACHADOS PATOLÓGICOS
- Os subtipos histológicos mais comuns são carcinomas tubulopapilares, cribriformes e sólidos.
- Não foi consistentemente demonstrado que o subtipo histológico afete o prognóstico, embora existam algumas provas de que os carcinomas tubulopapilares tenham um prognóstico melhor.
- O grau do tumor, com base no grau de formação de túbulos, pleomorfismo nuclear e celular, índice mitótico, é preditivo da sobrevida após a cirurgia.

TUMORES DAS GLÂNDULAS MAMÁRIAS — GATAS

- A invasão vascular e linfática é associada a estágio clínico mais avançado e intervalo livre de doença mais curto após o tratamento.
- Os sarcomas mamários são raros, mas potencialmente lentos para metastatizar.

TRATAMENTO

CUIDADO(S) DE SAÚDE ADEQUADO(S)
- É recomendável a realização de cirurgia para gatos com doença macroscópica confinada às glândulas mamárias com ou sem envolvimento dos linfonodos regionais.
- A quimioterapia adjuvante (pós-operatória) é recomendada após o gato ter se recuperado da cirurgia.
- A quimioterapia pode ser utilizada como uma modalidade terapêutica isolada para gatos com doença local não cirúrgica e/ou metástase à distância.
- A radioterapia pode ser considerada para melhorar o controle local após a cirurgia ou para tratar a doença local não passível de ressecção de forma paliativa.
- Para gatos com doença local não ressecável ou metástase macroscópica ou quando o proprietário recusa a terapia definitiva, é aconselhável a implantação de terapia paliativa.

ORIENTAÇÃO AO PROPRIETÁRIO
- Enfatizar os benefícios da ovário-histerectomia precoce (<6 meses de vida) em gatos não destinados a fins reprodutivos.
- Salientar a importância da detecção precoce e do tratamento rigoroso.

CONSIDERAÇÕES CIRÚRGICAS
- É recomendado o procedimento de mastectomia radical da(s) cadeia(s) mamária(s) acometida(s). Isso diminui significativamente o risco de recidiva tumoral local, bem como a recidiva nos vasos linfáticos que passam pelo tecido mamário.
- Mastectomias radicais bilaterais costumam ser submetidas a estadiamento com 2-4 semanas de intervalo; no entanto, alguns estudos sugerem que a mastectomia radical unilateral é suficientemente eficaz para controlar a doença local em um subgrupo de pacientes.
- Os linfonodos inguinais e axilares devem ser removidos ao mesmo tempo, independentemente se estiverem com o tamanho normal.
- Em gatos com doença metastática avançada, pode-se considerar a mastectomia local paliativa para remover algum tumor ulcerado ou infeccionado.

MEDICAÇÕES

MEDICAMENTO(S) DE ESCOLHA
- Doxorrubicina (25 mg/m² IV a cada 3 semanas) isoladamente ou em combinação com ciclofosfamida (100 mg/m² IV ou VO divididos durante 4 semanas).
- Mitoxantrona, carboplatina e docetaxel podem exibir atividade contra esses tumores.
- Consultar um oncologista em busca das recomendações quimioterápicas atuais.
- Analgésicos e antibióticos paliativos devem ser considerados para gatos com tumores dolorosos e/ou ulcerados.

CONTRAINDICAÇÕES
Utilizar a doxorrubicina com cuidado em gatos com insuficiência renal ou hepática.

PRECAUÇÕES
Se o clínico não estiver familiarizado com a quimioterapia, consultar um oncologista antes da administração.

INTERAÇÕES POSSÍVEIS
Radioterapia de megavoltagem e doxorrubicina — consultar um oncologista.

MEDICAMENTO(S) ALTERNATIVO(S)
- Imunomoduladores inespecíficos, como levamisol, vacinas bacterianas e tripeptídeo muramil encapsulado por lipossoma, não demonstraram qualquer benefício.
- Tamoxifeno e outros moduladores seletivos de receptores estrogênicos não foram avaliados em termos de segurança ou eficácia.

ACOMPANHAMENTO

MONITORIZAÇÃO DA PACIENTE
- É recomendável a realização de exame físico completo mensalmente nos 3 primeiros meses e, em seguida, a cada 2-3 meses. A palpação da linha de incisão prévia, das glândulas mamárias remanescentes e dos linfonodos regionais deve ser enfatizada durante o exame.
- É necessária a obtenção de radiografias torácicas em três projeções a cada 2 meses para a detecção de metástases.

PREVENÇÃO
Ovário-histerectomia antes dos 6 meses de vida pode reduzir o risco de desenvolvimento de carcinoma mamário em 11 vezes.

COMPLICAÇÕES POSSÍVEIS
Pode ocorrer o rápido desenvolvimento de efusão pleural maligna e consequente dispneia potencialmente letal.

EVOLUÇÃO ESPERADA E PROGNÓSTICO
- A maioria dos gatos vem a óbito por recidiva local e/ou metástase.
- O tamanho do tumor é fortemente preditivo do prognóstico. Para tumores com ≤2 cm de diâmetro, a sobrevida média é de >4 anos e meio (14 meses em machos). Para tumores de 2-3 cm e >3 cm de diâmetro, essa sobrevida é de 1-2 anos (5-6 meses em machos) e 4-6 meses (1-2 meses em machos), respectivamente.
- O procedimento de mastectomia radical diminui significativamente o risco de recidiva tumoral local. O impacto na sobrevida não é tão consistente, por causa da alta taxa de metástase associada a esse tipo de tumor.
- Em estudos retrospectivos, a quimioterapia adjuvante não promoveu uma melhora constante no intervalo ou na sobrevida livre de doença. Contudo, a quimioterapia tem se mostrado eficaz contra tumores mamários felinos (ver adiante), mas considerando-se a alta taxa metastática desses tumores, o tratamento quimioterápico adjuvante ainda é fortemente recomendado.
- Para gatos com doença em estágio avançado tratados com quimioterapia isolada, as taxas de resposta giram em torno de 50%. Os tempos de sobrevida são de 6-12 meses para gatos que exibem uma resposta positiva ao tratamento, mas inferior a 6 meses nos casos irresponsivos.

DIVERSOS

FATORES RELACIONADOS COM A IDADE
Ver a seção "Identificação".

GESTAÇÃO/FERTILIDADE/REPRODUÇÃO
- Dada a possível contribuição genética para essa doença, particularmente na raça Siamês, não é recomendável o acasalamento dos gatos acometidos.
- A quimioterapia não é recomendada em gatas prenhes, sobretudo durante os estágios iniciais da gestação.

Sugestões de Leitura
MacEwen EG, Hayes AA, Harvey HJ, Patnaik AK, Mooney S, Passe S. Prognostic factors for feline mammary tumors. JAAHA 1984, 185:201-204.
McNeill CJ, Sorenmo KU, Shofer FS, Gibeon L, Durham AC, Barber LG, Baez JL, Overley B. Evaluation of adjuvant doxorubicin-based chemotherapy for the treatment of feline mammary carcinoma. J Vet Intern Med 2009, 23:123-129.
Novosad CA, O'Brien MG, McKnight JA, Charney SC, Selting KA, Graham JC, Correa SS, Rosenberg MP, Gieger TL. Retrospective evaluation of adjuvant doxorubicin for the treatment of feline mammary gland adenocarcinoma: 67 cases. JAAHA 2006, 42:110-120.
Overley B, Shofer FS, Goldschmidt MH, Sherer D, Sorenmo KU. Association between ovariohysterectomy and feline mammary carcinoma. J Vet Intern Med 2005, 19:560-563.
Skorupski KA, Overley B, Shofer FS, Goldschmidt MH, Miller CA, Sorenmo KU. Clinical characteristics of mammary carcinoma in male cats. J Vet Intern Med 2005, 19:52-55.

Autor Dennis B. Bailey
Consultor Editorial Timothy M. Fan

Tumores dos Folículos Pilosos

CONSIDERAÇÕES GERAIS

REVISÃO
- Dois tipos principais — tricoepitelioma, que surge de queratinócitos na bainha radicular externa do folículo piloso ou tanto da bainha como da matriz do pelo; pilomatrixoma, que surge da matriz do pelo.
- Ambos os tipos — em geral são benignos; existem alguns relatos publicados de pilomatrixomas malignos.
- Cerca de 5% de todos os tumores cutâneos em cães, mas raros em gatos.

IDENTIFICAÇÃO
- Cães e gatos.
- Idade — em geral >5 anos.
- Sem predisposição sexual.
- Tricoepitelioma — comum em cães; raro em gatos; Golden retriever, Basset hound, Pastor alemão, Cocker spaniel, Setter irlandês, Springer Spaniel inglês, Schnauzer miniatura e Poodle standard podem ser predispostos; gatos da raça Persa.
- Pilomatrixoma — incomum em cães e gatos; Kerry blue terrier e Poodle podem ser predispostos; nenhuma predominância racial conhecida em gatos.

SINAIS CLÍNICOS
- Geralmente se trata de uma massa solitária.
- Tricoepitelioma — comum nas regiões torácica lateral e lombodorsal (cães) e na cabeça (gatos).
- Pilomatrixoma — comum em locais como dorso, ombros, flancos, cauda e membros.
- Massas dermoepiteliais firmes, arredondadas, elevadas, bem-circunscritas, frequentemente sem pelos ou ulceradas; podem ter a superfície cinzenta (tricoepiteliomas) ou lobuladas com áreas calcárias brancas (pilomatrixomas).

CAUSAS E FATORES DE RISCO
Desconhecidos.

DIAGNÓSTICO

DIAGNÓSTICO DIFERENCIAL
Distinguir de outros tumores, incluindo aqueles de células basais e escamosas, queratoacantoma, e de cistos de inclusão epidérmica.

HEMOGRAMA/BIOQUÍMICA/URINÁLISE
Em geral, normais.

OUTROS TESTES LABORATORIAIS
N/D.

DIAGNÓSTICO POR IMAGEM
N/D.

MÉTODOS DIAGNÓSTICOS
- Aspirado por agulha fina e citopatologia.
- Biopsia tecidual e histopatologia.

ACHADOS PATOLÓGICOS
- Citologia em aspirado por agulha fina — células basaloides e fantasmas sugestivas de pilomatrixoma em cães.
- Tricoepitelioma — varia quanto ao grau de diferenciação e local de origem (bainha radicular ou matriz do pelo); cistos córneos, ausência de desmossomos e diferenciação de estruturas semelhantes a folículos pilosos e formação de pelo são comuns.
- Pilomatrixoma — caracteriza-se por proliferação variável de células basofílicas que se assemelham a células da matriz do pelo e células completamente queratinizadas, fracamente eosinofílicas com núcleo central que não se cora (células sombreadas); é comum a presença de calcificação.

TRATAMENTO

Excisão completa — curativa.

MEDICAÇÕES

MEDICAMENTO(S)
Isotretinoína (1 mg/kg a cada 24 h VO) foi utilizada com sucesso para controlar múltiplos pilomatrixomas em um único cão.

CONTRAINDICAÇÕES/INTERAÇÕES POSSÍVEIS
N/D.

ACOMPANHAMENTO

- Monitorizar o paciente quanto à ocorrência de recidiva local.
- O prognóstico, em geral, é excelente; há relatos isolados de doença metastática com pilomatrixoma maligno canino.

DIVERSOS

Sugestões de Leitura

Abramo F, Pratesi F, Cantile C, et al. Survey of canine and feline follicular tumours and tumour-like lesions in central Italy. J Small Anim Pract 1999, 40:479-481.

Masserdotti C, Ubbiali FA. Fine needle aspiration cytology of pilomatricoma in three dogs. Vet Clin Path 2002, 31(1):22-25.

Rodríguez F, Herráez P, Rodríguez E, et al. Metastatic pilomatrixoma associated with neurological signs in a dog. Vet Record 1995, 137:247-248.

Scott DW, Miller WM, Griffin CE. Neoplastic and nonneoplastic tumors. In: Muller & Kirk's Small Animal Dermatology, 5th ed. Philadelphia: Saunders, 1995, pp. 1008-1016.

Toma S, Noli C. Isotretinoin in the treatment of multiple benign pilomatrixomas in a mixed-breed dog. Vet Dermatol 2005, 16(5):346-350.

Autor Louis-Philippe de Lorimier
Consultor Editorial Timothy M. Fan
Agradecimento O autor e os editores agradecem a colaboração prévia de Joanne C. Graham

Tumores Malignos Indiferenciados da Cavidade Bucal

CONSIDERAÇÕES GERAIS

REVISÃO
- Tumor raro, altamente agressivo e de crescimento rápido na região do palato duro, dos dentes molares superiores ou da maxila e da órbita em cães jovens.
- A maioria é altamente invasiva para o osso e não encapsulada, com superfície lisa a levemente nodular (confundidas como benignas); pode vir a sofrer ulceração.
- Biopsia — revela um processo maligno indiferenciado de histogênese indeterminada.
- Altamente metastático.
- É comum a constatação de linfadenopatia cervical.

IDENTIFICAÇÃO
- Cães.
- É principalmente uma doença de raças de grande porte.
- Todos os cães têm <2 anos de idade; faixa etária, 6-22 meses.
- Sem predileção sexual.

SINAIS CLÍNICOS
Achados Anamnésicos
- Salivação excessiva.
- Halitose.
- Disfagia, hiporexia.
- Secreção bucal sanguinolenta.
- Perda de peso.

Achados do Exame Físico
- Massa bucal.
- Perda dentária.
- Deformidade facial, exoftalmia.
- Linfadenopatia cervical — ocasionalmente.
- Dor à palpação ou abertura da boca.

CAUSAS E FATORES DE RISCO
Nenhum identificado.

DIAGNÓSTICO

DIAGNÓSTICO DIFERENCIAL
- Outro processo maligno bucal agressivo.
- Ameloblastoma acantomatoso.
- Abscesso.

HEMOGRAMA/BIOQUÍMICA/URINÁLISE
Podem estar normais.

OUTROS TESTES LABORATORIAIS
- Avaliação citológica do tumor primário e dos linfonodos drenantes — pode fornecer o diagnóstico presuntivo.
- Exame histopatológico compatível com tumor indiferenciado sem aspectos morfológicos característicos de origem mesenquimal ou epitelial.

DIAGNÓSTICO POR IMAGEM
- Radiografia do crânio — detecta invasão óssea profunda à massa.
- Radiografia do tórax — detecta metástase pulmonar.
- Técnicas avançadas de diagnóstico por imagem (TC ou RM) — definem a extensão local e regional da doença.

MÉTODOS DIAGNÓSTICOS
- Palpar cuidadosamente os linfonodos regionais (mandibulares e retrofaríngeos).
- Biopsia tecidual ampla e profunda (abaixo do osso) — necessária para diferenciar de outras malignidades bucais.

TRATAMENTO

DIETA
Alimentos moles e pastosos — podem ser recomendados para evitar ulceração tumoral ou após excisão bucal radical.

CONSIDERAÇÕES CIRÚRGICAS
Excisão cirúrgica radical — costuma ser ineficaz em função da presença de doença local extensa ou de metástase ao diagnóstico; se tentada, devem-se deixar margens de, no mínimo, 2 cm de tecidos ósseo e mole normais; além disso, a excisão deve ser idealmente planejada com a ajuda de alguma técnica avançada de diagnóstico por imagem com realce de contraste.

RADIAÇÃO
- Não há relatos em termos de eficácia.
- A maior parte dos tumores indiferenciados é pouco responsiva à radioterapia de megavoltagem.
- Pode ser considerada como tratamento paliativo (protocolo hipofracionado).

MEDICAÇÕES

MEDICAMENTO(S)
- Quimioterapia — eficácia não relatada; a maior parte dos tumores indiferenciados é pouco responsiva à quimioterapia sistêmica.
- Controle local temporário (paliativo) com aplicação intralesional de cisplatina (cães).
- É obrigatório o controle da dor com múltiplas modalidades terapêuticas analgésicas (AINE, opioide, analgésico adjuvante, bisfosfonato se houver osteólise).

CONTRAINDICAÇÕES/INTERAÇÕES POSSÍVEIS
A quimioterapia pode ser tóxica; buscar a orientação de um veterinário especialista em oncologia antes de iniciar o tratamento caso não haja familiaridade com medicamentos citotóxicos.

ACOMPANHAMENTO

A maioria dos cães apresenta disseminação metastática detectável no momento do diagnóstico; em geral, eles são submetidos à eutanásia dentro de 30 dias do diagnóstico, pois o crescimento do tumor é progressivo e descontrolado, resultando em baixa qualidade e condição de vida.

DIVERSOS

ABREVIATURA(S)
- AINE = anti-inflamatório não esteroide.
- RM = ressonância magnética.
- TC = tomografia computadorizada.

Sugestões de Leitura

Frazier DL, Hahn KA. Cancer chemotherapeutics. In: Hahn KA, Richardson RC, eds., Cancer Chemotherapy, a Veterinary Handbook. Baltimore: Williams & Wilkins, 1995, pp. 77-150.

Morrison WB. Cancers of the head and neck. In: Morrison WB, ed., Cancer in Dogs and Cats: Medical and Surgical Management. Jackson, WY: Teton NewMedia, 2002, pp. 489-496.

Patnaik AL, Lieberman PH, Erlandson RA, et al. A clinicopathologic and ultrastructural study of undifferentiated malignant tumors of the oral cavity in dogs. Vet Pathol 1986, 23:170-175.

Autor Louis-Philippe de Lorimier
Consultor Editorial Timothy M. Fan
Agradecimento O autor e os editores agradecem a colaboração prévia de Kevin A. Hahn

Tumores Melanocíticos Bucais

CONSIDERAÇÕES GERAIS

REVISÃO
• Invasão local progressiva de melanócitos neoplásicos dentro da cavidade bucal de cães e, menos comumente, de gatos. • Emergem da mucosa bucal (gengiva, palato, língua) e podem crescer com rapidez. • Em geral, exibem uma superfície não encapsulada, elevada, pigmentada ou não, friável, irregular, ulcerada e/ou necrosada; frequentemente invadem o osso. • Neoplasia bucal mais comum em cães; terceira neoplasia mais comum em gatos. • É comum a ocorrência de metástase (taxa metastática de 80% em cães); tipicamente acometem linfonodos regionais e pulmões, embora muitos outros locais possam ser envolvidos. • O óbito é provocado por recidiva local ou doença metastática.

IDENTIFICAÇÃO
• Os cães são mais acometidos que os gatos. • A idade média é de 10-12 anos. • Não há predileção sexual clara. • As raças super-representadas incluem Cocker spaniel, Poodle miniatura, Retriever e Chow chow (língua).

SINAIS CLÍNICOS
Achados Anamnésicos
• Salivação excessiva. • Halitose. • Disfagia. • Secreção bucal sanguinolenta. • Perda de peso.
Achados do Exame Físico
• Massa bucal (até um terço é pouco pigmentado). • Perda de dentes. • Deformidade facial. • Ocasionalmente, linfadenomegalia regional. • Dor ou desconforto.

CAUSAS E FATORES DE RISCO
Raças super-representadas.

DIAGNÓSTICO

DIAGNÓSTICO DIFERENCIAL
• Outros tumores bucais. • Epúlide. • Hiperplasia gengival. • Abscesso de raiz dentária.

HEMOGRAMA/BIOQUÍMICA/URINÁLISE
Geralmente normais.

DIAGNÓSTICO POR IMAGEM
• Radiografia do crânio de alta definição ou radiografias dos dentes — avaliam a presença de alterações osteolíticas. • Técnicas avançadas de diagnóstico por imagem como TC ou RM — fornecem imagens mais detalhadas (especialmente do maxilar) e permitem o planejamento terapêutico (cirurgia ou radioterapia). • Radiografias torácicas — avaliam os pulmões em busca de metástases. • Ultrassonografia abdominal — para concluir o estadiamento clínico do tumor e pesquisar metástases ocasionais à distância no abdome.

MÉTODOS DIAGNÓSTICOS
• Biopsia tecidual ampla e profunda — necessária para obter o diagnóstico definitivo por meio do exame de histopatologia. As biopsias sempre devem ser obtidas de dentro da boca, e não através da pele (isso comprometeria o controle local com cirurgia). • Aspirado por agulha fina e citologia de linfonodos regionais (mandibulares e retrofaríngeos) são recomendados para avaliar as metástases regionais mesmo se esses linfonodos estiverem normais em termos de tamanho e consistência à palpação.

ACHADOS PATOLÓGICOS
• Imunocitoquímica (p. ex., Melan-A, S-100, HMB-45, vimentina) — pode ajudar a confirmar o diagnóstico, especialmente em caso de tumores amelanocíticos (cerca de um terço dos casos).
• Exame histopatológico — sua descrição deve incluir o índice mitótico (mitoses por 10 campos ópticos de grande aumento), o grau de atipia/diferenciação, a invasividade e as margens cirúrgicas em caso de biopsia excisional.

TRATAMENTO

CIRURGIA
• Excisão cirúrgica radical em bloco — necessária (p. ex., mandibulectomia ou maxilectomia); bem tolerada por grande parte dos pacientes; margens cirúrgicas de, no mínimo, 2 cm; a sobrevida é melhor quando as margens estão livres de células neoplásicas. • Remoção cirúrgica dos linfonodos responsáveis pela drenagem do local — recomendável na confirmação ou na suspeita de metástase e sem evidência de doença metastática à distância (p. ex., pulmão).

RADIAÇÃO
Três a seis frações mais amplas de radioterapia de megavoltagem, uma a duas vezes por semana — conferem boa taxa de resposta (>75%) e podem oferecer um controle a longo prazo em tumores inoperáveis.

MEDICAÇÕES

MEDICAMENTO(S)
• A carboplatina foi descrita para melanoma bucal em cães, com taxa de resposta de aproximadamente 30%. Segundo relatos casuais, outros medicamentos utilizados incluem dacarbazina e lomustina.
• Nenhuma quimioterapia eficaz foi descrita nos gatos.
• Há relatos de que a cisplatina intralesional (em matriz de colágeno) promova o controle local em 50% dos cães tratados em um estudo-piloto.
• Piroxicam pode desempenhar um pequeno papel no alívio da dor e na redução do progresso tumoral.
• São recomendadas múltiplas modalidades terapêuticas analgésicas para controle da dor e do desconforto.

IMUNOTERAPIA
• Foram tentadas muitas imunoterapias com sucesso variado.
• Existe uma vacina terapêutica disponível que envolve a injeção de DNAc humano (xenogênico) responsável pela codificação de uma proteína melanocítica-específica, a tirosinase, e resulta em uma intensa resposta imunológica.
• A vacina de tirosinase é aprovada para o tratamento pós-operatório de melanomas malignos bucais em estágios II e III, resultando em um aumento no tempo de sobrevida, com efeitos colaterais mínimos.

CONTRAINDICAÇÕES/INTERAÇÕES POSSÍVEIS
Buscar por orientação de algum oncologista antes de iniciar o tratamento se não estiver familiarizado com agentes citotóxicos.

ACOMPANHAMENTO

MONITORIZAÇÃO DO PACIENTE
São recomendáveis a realização de exame físico e a obtenção de radiografias torácicas a cada 2 meses para monitorizar a recidiva tumoral local e as metástases à distância.

COMPLICAÇÕES POSSÍVEIS
Efeitos colaterais iniciais da radiação, como mucosite ou dermatite, podem se originar de protocolos hipofracionados.

EVOLUÇÃO ESPERADA E PROGNÓSTICO
• Dependem do estágio da doença; prognóstico mais favorável na doença em estágio I.
• Excisão cirúrgica completa (linfonodos locais e regionais quando positivos) é essencial para melhorar o prognóstico. O tempo médio de sobrevida com a cirurgia isolada varia de acordo com o estágio:
  ○ Estágio I — mais de 18 meses.
  ○ Estágios II e III — 5-9 meses; o prognóstico de melanoma bucal canino em estágios II e III sobe para mais de 18 meses com o uso adjuvante da vacina de tirosinase xenogênica recombinante.
  ○ Estágio IV — menos de 3 meses.
• Sobrevida com a radioterapia isolada (cães) — 5-8 meses.
• Prognóstico geral nos gatos — mau; na maioria dos casos, os tumores exibem invasividade local e são tardiamente diagnosticados durante a evolução da doença; muitas vezes, a causa do óbito é atribuída à evolução local da doença.

DIVERSOS

ABREVIATURA(S)
• RM = ressonância magnética.
• TC = tomografia computadorizada.

Sugestões de Leitura
Farrelly J, Denman DL, Hohenhaus AE, et al. Hypofractionated radiation therapy of oral melanoma in five cats. Vet Radiol Ultrasound 2004, 45:91-93.
Proulx DR, Ruslander DM, Dodge RK, et al. A retrospective analysis of 140 dogs with oral melanoma treated with external beam radiation. Vet Radiol Ultrasound 2003, 44:352-359.
Rassnick KM, Ruslander DM, Cotter SM, et al. Use of carboplatin for treatment of dogs with malignant melanoma: 27 cases (1989-2000). JAVMA 2001, 218:1444-1448.
Williams LE, Packer RA. Association between lymph node size and metastasis in dogs with oral malignant melanoma: 100 cases (1987-2001). JAVMA 2003, 222:1234-1236.

Autor Louis-Philippe de Lorimier
Consultor Editorial Timothy M. Fan

TUMORES MELANOCÍTICOS DA PELE E DOS DEDOS

CONSIDERAÇÕES GERAIS

DEFINIÇÃO
Neoplasia benigna ou maligna que surge dos melanócitos e melanoblastos (células produtoras de melanina) na epiderme.

FISIOPATOLOGIA
- Localmente invasivo.
- Quando maligno — ocasionalmente invade o tecido ósseo (p. ex., terceira falange) e sofre metástase para linfonodos, pulmões ou outros locais.

SISTEMA(S) ACOMETIDO(S)
- Cutâneo.
- Locais metastáticos — linfonodos, pulmões, ossos e vísceras.

GENÉTICA
Desconhecida.

INCIDÊNCIA/PREVALÊNCIA
- Cães — em torno de 10% de todos os tumores de pele.
- Gatos — menos de 5% de todos os tumores de pele.

DISTRIBUIÇÃO GEOGRÁFICA
Nenhuma.

IDENTIFICAÇÃO
Espécies
Os cães são mais acometidos que os gatos.

Raças Predominante(s)
- Cães — raças terriers (Terrier escocês, Boston terrier, Airedale terrier, Terrier irlandês, Schnauzer), Cocker e Springer spaniels, Setter irlandês, Chow chow, Chihuahua, raças retrievers e Doberman pinscher.
- Gatos — nenhuma.

Idade Média e Faixa Etária
- Cães — 9 anos.
- Gatos — 10-12 anos.

Sexo Predominante
- Cães — os machos podem ser levemente predispostos.
- Gatos — nenhum.

SINAIS CLÍNICOS
Achados Anamnésicos
- Massa cutânea de crescimento lento ou rápido.
- Claudicação se o dedo estiver envolvido.

Achados do Exame Físico
- Massa pigmentada ou não (amelanótica), geralmente solitária.
- Desenvolve-se em qualquer local, embora possa ser mais comum na face, no tronco, nos pés e no escroto em cães; já nos gatos, ocorre mais comumente na cabeça, no dedo, no pavilhão auricular e no nariz.
- Linfonodos regionais — podem estar infartados.
- Doença avançada — pode apresentar dispneia ou ruídos pulmonares ásperos por causa da metástase pulmonar.

CAUSAS
Desconhecidas.

FATORES DE RISCO
- Desconhecidos.
- Ao contrário de hemangiossarcoma cutâneo ou conjuntival e carcinoma de células escamosas, a exposição crônica à luz ultravioleta não é um fator de risco para tumores melanocíticos cutâneos em animais de estimação.

DIAGNÓSTICO

DIAGNÓSTICO DIFERENCIAL
Exame histopatológico ± imuno-histoquímica — podem distinguir o melanoma amelanótico de tumores de células distintas pouco diferenciados (mastocitomas, linfoma), vários sarcomas (p. ex., sarcoma histiocítico) e carcinomas.

HEMOGRAMA/BIOQUÍMICA/URINÁLISE
Geralmente normais.

OUTROS TESTES LABORATORIAIS
Marcadores imuno-histoquímicos — podem ajudar a diferenciar o melanoma (especialmente amelanótico) de outros tumores; o melanoma pode corar positivamente com vimentina, S-100, enolase neurônio-específica, HMB-45 e Melan-A (marcador mais específico, porém um pouco menos sensível).

DIAGNÓSTICO POR IMAGEM
- Radiografia torácica é recomendável para a detecção de metástases à distância.
- Técnicas avançadas de diagnóstico por imagem (TC) são mais sensíveis para detectar metástases menores.
- A radiografia da lesão é recomendada para determinar se houve envolvimento do osso subjacente, sobretudo em casos de melanoma do dedo (terceira falange). A ocorrência de osteólise é muito menos comum no melanoma do leito ungueal (em torno de 10%) do que no carcinoma de células escamosas (ao redor de 75%).

MÉTODOS DIAGNÓSTICOS
- Exame citológico do aspirado obtido por agulha fina (de massa primária, linfonodo drenante, outros).
- Presença de grânulos intracelulares (melanina) de coloração castanha em forma de bastão em células de vários tamanhos e formas.
- O pigmento pode estar ausente no caso do melanoma amelanótico.
- Podem ser observados macrófagos (melanófagos) com grandes vacúolos intracitoplasmáticos contendo melanina fagocitada.
- Observa-se maior atipia (p. ex., nucléolo grande e único, além de figuras mitóticas) em tumores malignos.
- Os linfonodos drenantes devem ser avaliados por meio do exame citológico, independentemente de seu tamanho ou aspecto clínico.

ACHADOS PATOLÓGICOS
Macroscópicos
- Massas — variam em termos de cor e aparência; podem estar ulceradas e friáveis quando malignas.
- Lesões benignas — são, em geral, de crescimento lento; têm coloração castanha a negra; variam desde máculas e placas até nódulos firmes em forma de cúpula, com 0,5-2 cm de diâmetro, bem delimitadas.
- Lesões malignas — são, em geral, de crescimento rápido; amelanótico a castanho-escuro, cinza ou negro, frequentemente maiores do que 2 cm de diâmetro e mais invasivas nos tecidos circunjacentes.
- Melanomas do dedo e das junções mucocutâneas — tendem a ser malignos.

Achados Histopatológicos
- Com frequência, não é fácil distinguir lesões benignas das malignas, porque ambas podem ter células que variam em termos de tamanho (p. ex., epitelioides, fusiformes, dendríticas e mistas), grau de pigmentação e morfologia do citoplasma.
- Lesões malignas — geralmente exibem alto índice mitótico; pleomorfismo nuclear e nucleolar (mais atipia, menos diferenciação); são invasivas aos tecidos circunjacentes; o tipo amelanótico pode representar um desafio diagnóstico; colorações imuno-histoquímicas e especiais podem ser particularmente úteis. Os marcadores de proliferação podem ajudar a predizer o comportamento do tumor.

TRATAMENTO

CUIDADO(S) DE SAÚDE ADEQUADO(S)
O paciente deve ser internado se for submetido à cirurgia a menos que as lesões sejam pequenas e superficiais.

CUIDADO(S) DE ENFERMAGEM
- Administração de fluido — indicada durante a anestesia.
- Melanoma do dedo — pode necessitar da aplicação de bandagem na parte distal do membro após a cirurgia.
- Controle da dor — analgesia multimodal (de preferência, durante e depois da cirurgia) é obrigatória com cirurgias agressivas.

ATIVIDADE
- Depende da localização do tumor.
- Em geral, restrita até que as suturas sejam removidas e todas as feridas cirúrgicas estejam cicatrizadas.

DIETA
Normal.

ORIENTAÇÃO AO PROPRIETÁRIO
- Discutir a necessidade da remoção cirúrgica precoce.
- Não se aconselha a abordagem de esperar para ver.
- Alertar o proprietário sobre o fato de que o melanoma maligno pode sofrer metástase no início da evolução da doença; portanto, o prognóstico é reservado.
- Em casos de melanoma maligno, é recomendável o uso de terapia adjuvante e a repetição do estadiamento clínico.

CONSIDERAÇÕES CIRÚRGICAS
- Ampla excisão cirúrgica — tratamento de escolha.
- Amputação do dedo — em caso de acometimento do leito ungueal.
- Linfadenectomia do linfonodo drenante — indicada mediante a confirmação ou suspeita de metástase e na ausência de indícios de disseminação detectável à distância.

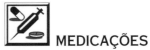

MEDICAÇÕES

MEDICAMENTO(S) DE ESCOLHA
- Quimioterapia adjuvante — recomendada em casos de melanoma maligno, excisão cirúrgica

TUMORES MELANOCÍTICOS DA PELE E DOS DEDOS

incompleta, massa não passível de ressecção ou na presença de metástase.
• Os medicamentos com certa eficácia relatada incluem carboplatina (cães e gatos), dacarbazina (DTIC) (cães), doxorrubicina e lomustina. Em geral, a taxa de resposta é inferior a 30%.

CONTRAINDICAÇÕES
Doxorrubicina — cardiotóxica; contraindicada em cardiopatia indutora de redução na contratilidade.

PRECAUÇÕES
Os veterinários que administram os quimioterápicos devem seguir as diretrizes publicadas sobre o uso desses medicamentos com segurança e devem estar familiarizados com os efeitos colaterais potenciais.

INTERAÇÕES POSSÍVEIS
Nenhuma relatada.

MEDICAMENTO(S) ALTERNATIVO(S)
• Piroxicam pode desempenhar um pequeno papel no controle da dor e do tumor.
• Analgesia multimodal é recomendável para controlar a dor e o desconforto.

ACOMPANHAMENTO

MONITORAÇÃO DO PACIENTE
• Avaliar o animal em busca de indícios de recidiva local e metástase regional — a cada 3 meses após a cirurgia ou mais cedo se o proprietário achar que a massa tumoral está retornando; ou se o paciente não estiver normal sob outros aspectos.
• Radiografia torácica — no momento da reavaliação e depois periodicamente.

PREVENÇÃO
Nenhuma.

COMPLICAÇÕES POSSÍVEIS
Nenhuma.

EVOLUÇÃO ESPERADA E PROGNÓSTICO
Cães
• Aproximadamente 25% dos tumores melanocíticos cutâneos são relatados como malignos. Melanomas no dedo, nos coxins palmoplantares, no escroto e nas junções mucocutâneas têm uma probabilidade maior de serem malignos.
• Sobrevida média em casos de melanomas cutâneos benignos, >24 meses.
• Sobrevida em casos de melanomas cutâneos malignos ou melanomas dos dedos, 10-12 meses.
• Há diferenças raciais no prognóstico em alguns estudos — a maioria dos melanomas cutâneos em Doberman pinscher e Schnauzer miniatura se comporta de forma benigna, enquanto uma grande parte dos melanomas cutâneos em Poodle miniatura se comporta de forma maligna.

Gatos
• Há relatos de que 35-50% dos melanomas sejam malignos.
• A sobrevida média em casos de melanoma da pele ou do dedo não é relatada com frequência; 4,5 meses após a cirurgia em um único estudo de 57 gatos.

DIVERSOS

DISTÚRBIOS ASSOCIADOS
Nenhum.

FATORES RELACIONADOS COM A IDADE
Nenhum.

POTENCIAL ZOONÓTICO
Nenhum.

GESTAÇÃO/FERTILIDADE/REPRODUÇÃO
N/D.

SINÔNIMO(S)
• Benigno — nevo melanocítico; melanocitoma.
• Maligno — melanossarcoma (raramente utilizado).

ABREVIATURA(S)
• DTIC = (dimetiltriazeno)-imidazol-carboxamida.

Sugestões de Leitura
Bergman PJ, Wolchok JD. Of mice and men (and dogs): Development of a xenogeneic DNA vaccine for canine oral malignant melanoma. Cancer Ther 2008, 6:817-826.
Henry CJ, Brewer WG Jr., Whitley EM, et al. Canine digital tumors: A veterinary cooperative oncology group retrospective study of 64 dogs. J Vet Intern Med 2005, 19(5):720-724.
Luna LD, Higginbotham ML, Henry CJ. Feline non-ocular melanoma: A retrospective study of 23 cases (1991-1999). J Feline Med Surg 2000, 2:173-181.
Marino DJ, Matthiesen DT, Stefanacci JD, Moroff SD. Evaluation of dogs with digit masses: 117 cases (1981-1991). JAVMA 1995, 207:726-728.
Smith SH, Goldschmidt MH, McManus PM. A comparative review of melanocytic neoplasms. Vet Pathol 2002, 39:651-678.
Spangler WL, Kass PH. The histologic and epidemiologic bases for prognostic considerations in canine melanocytic neoplasia. Vet Pathol 2006, 43(2):136-149.
Wobeser BK, Kidney BA, Power BE, et al. Diagnoses and clinical outcomes associated with surgically amputated canine digits submitted to multiple veterinary diagnostic laboratories. Vet Pathol 2007, 44:355-361.

Autor Louis-Philippe de Lorimier
Consultor Editorial Timothy M. Fan

Tumores Miocárdicos

CONSIDERAÇÕES GERAIS

REVISÃO
- Tumores miocárdicos primários e metastáticos são tumores raros em cães e gatos.
- Incidência de 0,19% em cães e 0,03% em gatos.
- Os tumores primários relatados incluem hemangiossarcoma, carcinoma ectópico da tireoide, linfoma, rabdomioma, rabdomiossarcoma, timoma, mesotelioma, condrossarcoma, osteossarcoma, fibrossarcoma, mixoma, mixossarcoma, lipoma, tumor da bainha de nervos periféricos, tumor de células granulares.

IDENTIFICAÇÃO
- Cães e gatos, porém menos comuns em gatos.
- Em cães, acometem qualquer idade, embora sejam mais comuns entre 7 e 15 anos.
- Possível incidência elevada em animais castrados.
- Alta incidência nas raças Saluki, Buldogue francês, Water spaniel irlandês, Retriever de pelo plano, Golden retriever, Boxer, Afghan hound, Setter inglês, Terrier escocês, Boston terrier, Buldogue, Pastor alemão.

SINAIS CLÍNICOS
- Colapso súbito.
- Distensão abdominal.
- Intolerância ao exercício.
- Dispneia.
- Anorexia.
- Vômito.
- Diarreia.
- Morte aguda.

CAUSAS E FATORES DE RISCO
Desconhecidos.

DIAGNÓSTICO

DIAGNÓSTICO DIFERENCIAL
- Efusão pericárdica idiopática.
- Pericardite.
- Miocardiopatia.
- Insuficiência cardíaca.
- Valvulopatia.
- Tumores da base do coração.

HEMOGRAMA/BIOQUÍMICA/URINÁLISE
Anemia em alguns pacientes.

OUTROS TESTES LABORATORIAIS
N/D.

DIAGNÓSTICO POR IMAGEM
- Radiografia torácica — pode revelar um coração globoide sugestivo de efusão pericárdica, massas na área dos átrios ou lesões metastáticas nos pulmões.
- Ecocardiografia — utilizada para o encontro de massas primárias — valor preditivo positivo e negativo de 92 e 64%, respectivamente.

MÉTODOS DIAGNÓSTICOS
- Pericardiocentese e avaliação do líquido — método proveitoso para o diagnóstico de linfoma.
- Citologia e pH da efusão pericárdica têm utilidade limitada para diferenciar condições neoplásicas e não neoplásicas.
- ECG — pode estar normal ou exibir uma variedade de arritmias; podem-se observar alternância elétrica e complexos pequenos em casos de efusão pericárdica.
- Biopsia cirúrgica de massa, se possível.

TRATAMENTO

- Remoção cirúrgica de massa, se possível.
- Pericardiectomia — pode conferir alívio da efusão pericárdica.
- Abordar a preocupação de morte súbita com o proprietário.

MEDICAÇÕES

MEDICAMENTO(S)
- Tratamento das arritmias — lidocaína (cães) a 2-4 mg/kg IV (até, no máximo, 8 mg/kg em um período de 10 min), sob infusão IV em velocidade constante a 27-75 mcg/kg/min; mexiletina (cães) a 5-8 mg/kg VO a cada 8-12 h; sotalol a 1-2 mg/kg VO a cada 12 h.
- A quimioterapia depende do tipo de tumor (ver capítulos sobre Linfoma e Hemangiossarcoma).

CONTRAINDICAÇÕES/INTERAÇÕES POSSÍVEIS
A quimioterapia pode apresentar toxicidades do trato gastrintestinal, da medula óssea, do coração e outras — procurar orientação antes do tratamento se não estiver familiarizado com agentes citotóxicos.

ACOMPANHAMENTO

- Ecocardiogramas seriados — para monitorar a resposta do tumor à quimioterapia.
- Radiografia torácica e ultrassonografia abdominal — para monitorar a evolução de doença metastática.
- ECG — para monitorar a resposta a agentes antiarritmogênicos.
- Exames de sangue — particularmente hemograma completo para monitorar a ocorrência de mielossupressão secundária à quimioterapia.
- Prognóstico — reservado a ruim.

DIVERSOS

GESTAÇÃO/FERTILIDADE/REPRODUÇÃO
- Não é recomendável acasalar os animais com câncer.
- Quimioterapia teratogênica — não administrar a animais prenhes.

VER TAMBÉM
- Hemangiossarcoma do Coração.
- Linfoma — Gatos.
- Linfoma — Cães.

ABREVIATURA(S)
ECG = eletrocardiograma.

Sugestões de Leitura
Kisseberth WC. Neoplasia of the heart. In: Withrow SJ, Vail DE, eds., Small Animal Clinical Oncology, 4th ed. Philadelphia Saunders, 2007, pp. 809-814.

Autor Rebecca G. Newman
Consultor Editorial Timothy M. Fan

TUMORES OVARIANOS

CONSIDERAÇÕES GERAIS

REVISÃO
- Tumores de células epiteliais (carcinoma), de células germinativas (disgerminoma e teratoma) e do estroma do cordão sexual (tumor de células da granulosa, tumor de células de Sertoli-Leydig, tecoma e luteoma).
- Cadelas — raros (0,5-1,2% dos tumores); 40% carcinomas, 10% tumor de células germinativas e 50% do cordão sexual.
- Gatas — raros (0,7-3,6% dos tumores); 15% de células germinativas e 85% do cordão sexual.
- É comum a ocorrência de metástase.
- Alguns tumores produzem hormônios.

IDENTIFICAÇÃO
- Cadelas e gatas.
- Animais de meia-idade a idosos.
- O teratoma desenvolve-se em pacientes jovens.

SINAIS CLÍNICOS
- Alopecia simétrica bilateral; pancitopenia; masculinização.
- Ascite ou efusão pleural — ocasionalmente.
- Outros sinais associados aos efeitos expansivos do tumor.

CAUSAS E FATORES DE RISCO
- Estado sexual intacto.
- Raças caninas: Pointer, Buldogue inglês, Boxer, Pastor alemão e Yorkshire terrier estão sob risco.

DIAGNÓSTICO

DIAGNÓSTICO DIFERENCIAL
- Outras causas de efusão abdominal.
- Outras massas mesoabdominais.

HEMOGRAMA/BIOQUÍMICA/URINÁLISE
- Sem anormalidades compatíveis.
- Pancitopenia em cães com tumores funcionais.

OUTROS TESTES LABORATORIAIS
Progesterona sérica — níveis >2 mg/mL com tumores funcionais.

DIAGNÓSTICO POR IMAGEM
- Radiografia abdominal — pode revelar a existência de massa mesoabdominal uni ou bilateral no polo caudal do rim ou a presença de efusão; também pode ser observada a mineralização do tumor.
- Ultrassonografia abdominal — confirma os achados radiográficos abdominais.
- Radiografia torácica — pode revelar a ocorrência de metástase.

MÉTODOS DIAGNÓSTICOS
- Avaliação citológica do líquido pleural ou abdominal — pode ser diagnóstica de efusão maligna.
- Avaliação citológica do tumor — as células tumorais podem facilmente se implantar na parede corporal via aspirado por agulha fina. Portanto, quase sempre é recomendada a biopsia excisional durante o aspirado da massa por agulha fina.
- Citologia vaginal — revela cornificação epitelial induzida por estrogênio em casos de tumores funcionais.
- Exame histopatológico — necessário para o diagnóstico definitivo.

TRATAMENTO

- Ovário-histerectomia — tratamento de escolha para massa solitária.
- É possível o transplante peritoneal durante a remoção cirúrgica; por essa razão, é necessária a troca das luvas e dos instrumentos cirúrgicos durante o procedimento.

MEDICAÇÕES

MEDICAMENTO(S)
- Quimioterapia — há poucas informações a respeito para cadelas e gatas; não há nenhuma terapia-padrão.
- Ciclofosfamida, clorambucila, lomustina e bleomicina — tratamento bem-sucedido em uma única paciente (cadela).
- Cisplatina — relato de tratamento bem-sucedido em três cadelas.

CONTRAINDICAÇÕES/INTERAÇÕES POSSÍVEIS
Cisplatina — não usar nas gatas; não utilizar nas cadelas com nefropatia.

ACOMPANHAMENTO

- Radiografia torácica e abdominal — a cada 3 meses; monitorizar quanto à ocorrência de recidiva e metástase.
- Ovário-histerectomia — prevenção.
- Prognóstico — reservado.
- Quimioterapia — tem o potencial de prolongar a sobrevida.

DIVERSOS

DISTÚRBIOS ASSOCIADOS
- Piometra.
- Cistos ovarianos.
- Hiperplasia endometrial cística.

Sugestões de Leitura

Morrison WB. Cancer of the reproductive tract. In: Morrison WB, ed., Cancer in Dogs and Cats: Medical and Surgical Management. Jackson, WY: Teton NewMedia, 2002, pp. 555-564.

Patnaik AK, Greenlee PG. Canine ovarian neoplasms: A clinicopathologic study of 71 cases including histology of 12 granulosa cell tumors. Vet Pathol 1987, 24:509-514.

Autor Heather M. Wilson-Robles
Consultor Editorial Timothy M. Fan
Agradecimento O autor e os editores agradecem a colaboração prévia de Terrance A. Hamilton

TUMORES UTERINOS

CONSIDERAÇÕES GERAIS

REVISÃO
- Tumores raros provenientes da musculatura lisa uterina e dos tecidos epiteliais.
- Constituem 0,3-0,4% dos tumores em cadelas e 0,2-1,5% em gatas.
- Cadelas — os tumores uterinos costumam ser benignos; 85-90% são leiomiomas; 10% são leiomiossarcomas; outros tipos (p. ex., carcinoma, fibroma, fibrossarcoma, lipoma, plasmocitoma, hemangiossarcoma) são raros.
- Gatas — os tumores uterinos, em geral, são malignos (adenocarcinoma); incluem leiomioma, leiomiossarcoma, fibrossarcoma, fibroma, lipoma e tumor dos ductos müllerianos (adenossarcoma).
- Metástase — pode ocorrer nas formas malignas.

IDENTIFICAÇÃO
- Cadelas e gatas.
- Não há relato de predisposição racial.
- Os animais de meia-idade a mais idosos são geralmente acometidos.
- Síndrome de Birt-Hogg-Dube em cães da raça Pastor alemão foi associada a leiomiomas uterinos, cistadenocarcinomas renais e dermatofibrose nodular.

SINAIS CLÍNICOS
- Cadelas — com frequência, os tumores uterinos são silenciosos do ponto de vista clínico e descobertos ao acaso; observam-se corrimento vaginal; piometra; infertilidade; compressão de órgãos abdominais ou sinais de metástase secundária.
- Gatas — corrimento vaginal (pode ser hemorrágico); ciclos estrais anormais; poliúria; polidipsia, vômito; distensão abdominal; infertilidade; prolapso uterino; sinais relacionados com a doença metastática.

CAUSAS E FATORES DE RISCO
- Estado sexual intacto.
- Mutação do gene BHD na raça Pastor alemão.

DIAGNÓSTICO

DIAGNÓSTICO DIFERENCIAL
- Piometra.
- Outras massas abdominais mesocaudais (meso-hipogástricas).

HEMOGRAMA/BIOQUÍMICA/URINÁLISE
Não há anormalidades específicas.

OUTROS TESTES LABORATORIAIS
N/D.

DIAGNÓSTICO POR IMAGEM
- Radiografias abdominais — podem detectar a presença de massa abdominal mesocaudal (meso-hipogástrica).
- Radiografias torácicas — são recomendadas para pesquisa de metástase.
- Ultrassonografia — pode revelar a existência de massa uterina.
- TC/RM — permitem a delimitação de massa e avaliação de doença metastática.

MÉTODOS DIAGNÓSTICOS
- Avaliação citológica — em casos de efusão abdominal.
- Exame histopatológico — necessário para o diagnóstico definitivo.

TRATAMENTO

Ovário-histerectomia — constitui o tratamento de escolha.

MEDICAÇÕES

MEDICAMENTO(S)
Doxorrubicina, cisplatina, carboplatina, epirrubicina — escolhas racionais para o tratamento paliativo de malignidades ou metástases.

CONTRAINDICAÇÕES/INTERAÇÕES POSSÍVEIS
- Doxorrubicina — monitorizar com cautela as pacientes com cardiopatia subjacente; considerar a provisão de tratamento prévio, bem como a realização de ecocardiogramas e eletrocardiogramas seriados.
- Cisplatina — não deve ser usada em cadelas com nefropatia preexistente; não utilizar sem diurese apropriada e concomitante; uso proibido em gatas (fatal).
- A quimioterapia pode ser tóxica; caso não se esteja familiarizado com o emprego desses agentes, deve-se buscar orientação especializada.

ACOMPANHAMENTO

MONITORIZAÇÃO DA PACIENTE
- Malignos — considerar a obtenção de radiografias toracoabdominais a cada 3 meses.
- Hemograma, perfil bioquímico e urinálise (em casos de uso da cisplatina) — efetuá-los antes de cada tratamento quimioterápico.

EVOLUÇÃO ESPERADA E PROGNÓSTICO
Prognóstico — excelente (cura) nas formas benignas; reservado nas formas malignas; mau na presença de metástases; desconhecido após a quimioterapia.

DIVERSOS

DISTÚRBIOS ASSOCIADOS
Síndrome de Birt-Hogg-Dube em cães da raça Pastor alemão foi associada a leiomiomas uterinos.

ABREVIATURA(S)
- BHD = Birt-Hogg-Dube.
- RM = ressonância magnética.
- TC = tomografia computadorizada.

Sugestões de Leitura
Klein MK. Tumors of the female reproductive system. In: Withrow SJ, MacEwen EG, eds., Small Animal Clinical Oncology, 2nd ed. Philadelphia: Saunders, 1996, pp. 347-355.
Morrison W n: Morrison WB, ed., Cancer in Dogs and Cats: Medical and Surgical Management. Jackson, WY: Teton NewMedia, 2002, pp. 555-564.

Autor Heather M. Wilson
Consultor Editorial Timothy M. Fan
Agradecimento O autor e os editores agradecem a colaboração prévia de Renee Al-Sarraf

Tumores Vaginais

CONSIDERAÇÕES GERAIS

REVISÃO
- Correspondem ao segundo grupo mais comum de tumores reprodutivos, representando 2,4-3% de todos os tumores em cadelas.
- Cadelas — 86% são tumores benignos da musculatura lisa, frequentemente pedunculados (p. ex., leiomioma, fibroleiomioma e fibroma); também há relatos de lipoma, tumor venéreo transmissível, mastocitoma, carcinoma de células escamosas, leiomiossarcoma, hemangiossarcoma, osteossarcoma ou disseminação de carcinomas primários do trato urinário.
- Cadelas — podem ser um achado incidental à necropsia.
- Gatas — são extremamente raros; os tumores costumam ter origem na musculatura lisa.
- Influência hormonal — pode desempenhar um papel no desenvolvimento de leiomiomas, fibromas ou tumores polipoides.

IDENTIFICAÇÃO
- Cadelas — idade média, 10,2-11,2 anos; raça Boxer; cadelas nulíparas.
- Gatas — não há dados disponíveis.

SINAIS CLÍNICOS
Cadelas
- Extraluminais — massa perineal de crescimento lento; corrimento vulvar; disúria; polaciúria; lambedura vulvar; distocia.
- Intraluminais — protrusão de massa a partir da vulva (frequentemente durante o estro); corrimento vulvar; estrangúria; disúria; tenesmo.

Gatas
- Massa firme.
- Constipação.

CAUSAS E FATORES DE RISCO
- Fêmeas intactas.
- As cadelas nulíparas costumam ser mais acometidas.

DIAGNÓSTICO

DIAGNÓSTICO DIFERENCIAL
- Prolapso vaginal.
- Neoplasia uretral.
- Prolapso uterino.
- Hipertrofia do clitóris.
- Pólipo vaginal.
- Abscesso vaginal.
- Hematoma vaginal.

HEMOGRAMA/BIOQUÍMICA/URINÁLISE
Não há anormalidades compatíveis.

OUTROS TESTES LABORATORIAIS
N/D.

DIAGNÓSTICO POR IMAGEM
- Radiografia torácica — recomendada; para avaliar a presença de metástases.
- Radiografia abdominal — pode detectar a disseminação cranial da massa.
- Ultrassonografia, vaginografia e uretrocistografia — podem auxiliar na delimitação da massa.
- TC/RM — permitem a delimitação definitiva do tumor, avaliam a viabilidade da cirurgia e averiguam a existência de metástase.

MÉTODOS DIAGNÓSTICOS
- Vaginoscopia com exame citológico de material aspirado — pode ajudar a determinar o tipo celular.
- Biopsia com exame histopatológico — frequentemente necessária para a obtenção do diagnóstico definitivo.

ACHADOS PATOLÓGICOS
- Intraluminais — parede vestibular; protrusão em direção à vulva; podem ocorrer como massas isoladas ou múltiplas.
- Extraluminais — teto vestibular; provocam abaulamento do períneo.

TRATAMENTO

- Excisão cirúrgica e ovário-histerectomia concomitante — constituem o tratamento de escolha.
- Radioterapia pós-operatória — pode ser benéfica em casos de sarcoma, tumores benignos submetidos à ressecção parcial, ou mastocitomas.
- Cirurgia a laser com radioterapia — há relatos breves ou pouco divulgados.

MEDICAÇÕES

MEDICAMENTO(S)
- Terapia pós-operatória — ainda não se estabeleceu nenhum protocolo-padrão.
- Doxorrubicina, cisplatina ou carboplatina — escolhas racionais para o tratamento paliativo de neoplasias malignas ou metástases.
- Piroxicam — pode ser particularmente útil para aqueles cães com tumores urinários primários que se estendem para a vagina e com carcinomas.

CONTRAINDICAÇÕES/INTERAÇÕES POSSÍVEIS
- Doxorrubicina — monitorar a paciente com rigor em casos de cardiopatia subjacente; considerar a realização de tratamento prévio e ecocardiograma/ECG seriados.
- Cisplatina — não deve ser usada em gatas (fatal); também não é recomendável o uso em cadelas nefropatas; sempre se deve empregá-la com diurese apropriada e concomitante.
- A quimioterapia pode ser tóxica; caso não se esteja familiarizado com o uso dos agentes quimioterápicos, deve-se buscar orientação de algum especialista no assunto.
- Piroxicam não deve ser utilizado com outros AINE ou prednisona, devendo-se evitá-lo em animais com nefro ou hepatopatia subjacente. Também não é aconselhável o emprego do piroxicam em combinação com a cisplatina.

ACOMPANHAMENTO

MONITORIZAÇÃO DA PACIENTE
- Radiografias toracoabdominais — considerar a obtenção a cada 3 meses se o tumor for maligno.
- Hemograma completo (doxorrubicina, cisplatina, carboplatina), perfil bioquímico (cisplatina, piroxicam), urinálise (cisplatina, piroxicam) — realizar esses exames antes de cada tratamento quimioterápico.

EVOLUÇÃO ESPERADA E PROGNÓSTICO
- Prognóstico — bom em casos de excisão completa; reservado em casos de excisão incompleta; mau na presença de metástases e em casos de tumor de células escamosas ou carcinoma.
- Recidiva — 15% (leiomioma), sem a realização de ovário-histerectomia concomitante.

DIVERSOS

Gatas — há relatos concomitantes de ovários císticos e adenocarcinoma das glândulas mamárias.

ABREVIATURA(S)
- AINE = anti-inflamatório não esteroide.
- ECG = eletrocardiograma.
- RM = ressonância magnética.
- TC = tomografia computadorizada.

Sugestões de Leitura
Manithaiudom K, Johnston SD. Clinical approach to vaginal/vestibular masses in the bitch. Vet Clin North Am Small Anim Pract 1991, 21:509-521.
Morrison WB. Cancers of the reproductive tract. In: Morrison WB, ed., Cancer in Dogs and Cats: Medical and Surgical Management. Jackson, WY: Teton NewMedia, 2002, pp. 555-564.

Autor Heather M. Wilson
Consultor Editorial Timothy M. Fan
Agradecimento O autor e os editores agradecem a colaboração prévia de Renee Al-Sarraf

ÚLCERA GASTRODUODENAL

CONSIDERAÇÕES GERAIS

DEFINIÇÃO
Úlceras gastroduodenais são lesões que se estendem através da mucosa e para a camada muscular da mucosa.

FISIOPATOLOGIA
• As úlceras gastroduodenais resultam de um ou vários fatores que alteram, danificam ou superam os mecanismos normais de defesa e reparo da barreira da mucosa gástrica.
• Os fatores que envolvem a barreira da mucosa gástrica e protegem o estômago contra a formação de úlcera incluem a camada de bicarbonato e muco sobre as células epiteliais, as células epiteliais gástricas, o fluxo sanguíneo na mucosa gástrica, a restituição e o reparo de células epiteliais e as prostaglandinas produzidas pelo trato gastrintestinal.
• Os fatores que causam dano à barreira da mucosa e predispõem à formação de úlcera gastroduodenal incluem a inibição da capacidade de autorreparo das células epiteliais, a redução do suprimento sanguíneo na mucosa e/ou o aumento da secreção de ácido gástrico.

SISTEMA(S) ACOMETIDO(S)
• Gastrintestinal — o fundo e o antro gástricos são os locais mais comuns de ulceração; esses locais parecem ser mais suscetíveis aos AINE e aos glicocorticoides; os gastrinomas (raros), em geral, provocam a formação de úlcera no duodeno proximal.
• Cardiovascular/hematológico — hemorragia aguda pode resultar em anemia e subsequente taquicardia, sopro sistólico e/ou hipotensão.

INCIDÊNCIA/PREVALÊNCIA
A incidência real é desconhecida.

IDENTIFICAÇÃO
Espécies
Cães e, menos comumente, gatos.

Raça(s) Predominante(s)
• Cães atletas de elite apresentam maior incidência de ulceração, erosão e/ou hemorragia gástricas durante exercício físico extenuante e contínuo.

Idade Média e Faixa Etária
Todas as idades.

Sexo Predominante
Os cães machos exibem alta incidência de carcinoma gástrico.

SINAIS CLÍNICOS
Comentários Gerais
Alguns animais podem permanecer assintomáticos apesar de úlcera gastroduodenal significativa.

Achados Anamnésicos
• Vômitos: sinal clínico mais comum.
• Pode haver hematêmese.
• Pode haver melena.
• Dor na porção cranial do abdome — o paciente pode arquear o dorso ou ficar na "postura de prece".
• Anorexia.
• Letargia.
• Perda de peso.
• Fraqueza, palidez e/ou colapso se ocorrer anemia grave ou perfuração/peritonite.

Achados do Exame Físico
• O exame físico pode permanecer normal.
• Melena ao exame do reto com o dedo.
• Mucosas pálidas e fraqueza se houver anemia significativa.
• Pode haver perda de peso e caquexia.
• Taquicardia, hipotensão e tempo de preenchimento capilar prolongado se houver choque hipovolêmico ou perfuração e peritonite séptica; pode haver hipertermia e distensão abdominal com perfuração e peritonite séptica.

CAUSAS
Medicamentos
AINE, glicocorticoides.

Doenças Gastrintestinais
• Enteropatia inflamatória.
• Neoplasia bucal, esofágica, gástrica ou duodenal.
• Corpo estranho bucal, esofágico, gástrico ou duodenal.
• Hiperacidez gástrica.
• Dilatação e vólvulo gástricos.
• Intussuscepção.
• Obstrução ao fluxo de saída pilórico.

Doenças Infecciosas
• Parasitismo gastrintestinal. • Riquetsioses.
• Pitiose. • Infecção por *Helicobacter*.
• Gastrenterite viral, fúngica ou bacteriana.

Doenças Metabólicas
• Insuficiência renal. • Hepatopatia.
• Hipoadrenocorticismo. • Pancreatite.

Toxicidade
• Intoxicação por metais pesados (arsênico, zinco, tálio, ferro ou chumbo).
• Intoxicação por plantas (diefenbáquia, sagueiro, cogumelo, mamona).
• Intoxicação por substâncias químicas (fenol, etilenoglicol, agentes corrosivos, cremes para psoríase — análogos da vitamina D).
• Intoxicação por pesticidas/rodenticidas (colecalciferol).

Neoplasia
• Mastocitose. • Gastrinoma. • APUDoma.

Doenças Neurológicas
• Traumatismo craniano.
• Mielopatia.

Estresse/Doenças Clínicas Importantes
• Sepse.
• Choque.
• Doença grave.
• Queimaduras.
• Intermação/insolação.
• Cirurgia de grande porte.
• Traumatismo.
• Hipo ou hipertensão.
• Doença tromboembólica.
• Exercício extenuante e contínuo.

FATORES DE RISCO
• Administração de medicamentos ulcerogênicos — AINE ou glicocorticoides.
• Pacientes criticamente enfermos.
• Choque hipovolêmico ou séptico.

DIAGNÓSTICO

DIAGNÓSTICO DIFERENCIAL
• Doença esofágica (neoplasia, esofagite, corpo estranho) — diferenciar por meio de radiografia simples, contrastada e/ou endoscopia.
• Trombocitopenia (imunomediada, paraneoplásica, infecciosa) — identificada no hemograma completo.
• Coagulopatias (CID, envenenamento por rodenticida anticoagulante) — detectadas no perfil de coagulação.
• Hemoptise — as radiografias torácicas podem revelar a presença de doença das vias aéreas ou dos pulmões.
• Regurgitação ou vômitos de sangue deglutido em decorrência de doenças extragastrintestinais (p. ex., orofaríngeas, nasofaríngeas ou cutâneas, bem como do trato urogenital e dos sacos anais).
• A administração de Pepto-Bismol® pode gerar fezes de coloração negra semelhantes a alcatrão.

HEMOGRAMA/BIOQUÍMICA/URINÁLISE
• Se a perda sanguínea for aguda (3-5 dias) — haverá anemia arregenerativa (normocítica, normocrômica, com reticulocitose mínima).
• Em caso de perda sanguínea com mais de 7 dias de duração — observa-se anemia regenerativa (macrocítica, com reticulocitose mínima).
• Se a perda sanguínea for crônica — o animal exibirá anemia por deficiência de ferro (microcítica, hipocrômica, além de reticulocitose variável, com ou sem trombocitose).
• Pode haver trombocitopenia.
• Pode haver pan-hipoproteinemia com hemorragia digestiva.
• Pode haver neutrofilia madura ou neutrofilia com desvio à esquerda em casos de sepse e/ou perfuração de úlcera gastroduodenal.
• A relação entre a ureia e a creatinina pode estar elevada nos casos de hemorragia gastrintestinal.

OUTROS TESTES LABORATORIAIS
• A pesquisa de sangue oculto nas fezes pode ser positiva — o cão deve ser submetido à dieta sem carne por 3 dias antes do teste.
• Flutuação fecal — para verificar se há parasitismo gastrintestinal.
• Ácidos biliares — se houver suspeita de hepatopatia.
• Teste de estimulação com ACTH — na suspeita de hipoadrenocorticismo.
• Níveis de gastrina — se as causas mais comuns tiverem sido excluídas.

DIAGNÓSTICO POR IMAGEM
• Radiografia abdominal pode identificar a presença de corpo estranho ou massa gástrico(a) ou duodenal, pancreatite, pneumoperitônio, efusão ou alterações compatíveis com doença renal ou hepática.
• Radiografia contrastada (de preferência, gastrograma com duplo contraste) pode identificar a existência de úlcera gastroduodenal ou doença neoplásica.
• Ultrassonografia abdominal pode identificar alterações como massa gástrica ou duodenal, espessamento ou alteração das camadas da parede gástrica ou duodenal, úlcera gástrica e/ou linfadenopatia abdominal.

MÉTODOS DIAGNÓSTICOS
• Endoscopia — método diagnóstico mais definitivo; permite a coleta de amostras de biopsia a partir das ulcerações gástricas e/ou duodenais.
• Abdominocentese pode revelar peritonite séptica.
• Obter aspirados com agulha ou amostras de biopsia de massas cutâneas ou intra-abdominais e dos linfonodos para identificar doenças.
• Cintilografia nuclear pode situar o sangramento gastrintestinal.

ÚLCERA GASTRODUODENAL

ACHADOS PATOLÓGICOS
- Inflamação e hemorragia gastroduodenais.
- Úlceras podem ter mais necrose, microtrombos e hemorragia, além de penetração mais profunda que as erosões.

TRATAMENTO

CUIDADO(S) DE SAÚDE ADEQUADO(S)
- Tratar quaisquer causas subjacentes.
- Tratar o paciente em um esquema ambulatorial se a causa for identificada e eliminada, se os vômitos não forem excessivos e se o sangramento gastroduodenal for mínimo.
- Pacientes internados — aqueles com sangramento gastroduodenal grave e/ou úlcera perfurada, vômitos excessivos e/ou choque.

CUIDADO(S) DE ENFERMAGEM
- Fluidos intravenosos para manter a hidratação, a perfusão da mucosa gástrica e/ou o tratamento do choque.
- Talvez haja necessidade de transfusões (de sangue total ou papa de hemácias) em pacientes com hemorragia gastroduodenal grave.
- Nos casos graves de hematêmese — interromper o sangramento gastrintestinal; pode-se tentar a lavagem com água gelada (deixar 10-20 mL/kg no estômago por 15-30 min) ou com noradrenalina (8 mg/500 mL) diluída em água gelada.

ATIVIDADE
Restrita.

DIETA
- Suspender a ingestão oral se houver vômitos.
- Quando a alimentação for retomada, fornecer pequenas quantidades várias vezes ao dia.
- É recomendável o fornecimento de dieta altamente digerível com teor baixo a moderado de gordura (o alto conteúdo de gordura na dieta atrasa o esvaziamento gástrico) e nível baixo de fibra.

ORIENTAÇÃO AO PROPRIETÁRIO
- Os AINE só devem ser administrados a animais de estimação sob a orientação de um veterinário.
- A administração de AINE pode resultar em ulcerações e perfurações gastroduodenais.
- Os efeitos adversos dos AINE podem ser reduzidos pelo fornecimento do remédio juntamente com o alimento e pela administração concomitante de análogo sintético da prostaglandina (p. ex., misoprostol).

CONSIDERAÇÕES CIRÚRGICAS
O tratamento cirúrgico fica indicado em casos de falha do tratamento clínico depois de 7-10 dias, falta de controle da hemorragia, ocorrência de perfuração da úlcera gastroduodenal e/ou identificação de tumor potencialmente ressecável.

MEDICAÇÕES

MEDICAMENTO(S) DE ESCOLHA
- Os antagonistas dos receptores histaminérgicos (H_2) inibem de forma competitiva a secreção de ácido gástrico (cimetidina, 5-10 mg/kg VO, SC, IV a cada 8 h [cão e gato]; ranitidina, 0,5-2 mg/kg SC, VO, IV a cada 8-12 h [cão e gato]; famotidina, 0,5 mg/kg VO, IV a cada 12-24 h [cão e gato]; nizatidina, 5 mg/kg VO a cada 24 h [cão]). Os antagonistas dos receptores H_2 diferem em termos de potência e duração de ação. A famotidina é o agente mais potente, seguido de ranitidina e, depois, cimetidina. Tratar por, no mínimo, 6-8 semanas. Pode ocorrer hipersecreção ácida gástrica de rebote quando os bloqueadores dos receptores H_2 forem interrompidos; esse efeito rebote, no entanto, pode ser minimizado pela redução gradativa da dose, assim como sua interrupção.
- Os antiácidos neutralizam a acidez gástrica e alguns induzem à síntese local de protetores de mucosa, mas precisam ser dados por pelo menos 4 a 6 vezes/dia para serem eficazes.
- A suspensão de sucralfato (0,5-1 g VO a cada 6-8 h) protege o tecido ulcerado (citoproteção) não só por se ligar aos locais ulcerados, à pepsina e aos sais biliares, mas também por estimular a síntese de prostaglandinas. A ligação é maior nas úlceras duodenais do que nas gástricas.
- Antibiótico(s) com atividade contra bactérias Gram-negativas e anaeróbios entéricos deve(m) ser administrado(s) por via parenteral na suspeita de ruptura na barreira da mucosa gastrintestinal ou na presença de pneumonia por aspiração.
- Antieméticos (clorpromazina, 0,5 mg/kg a cada 6-8 h SC, IM, IV [cão e gato]; proclorperazina, 0,1-0,5 mg/kg a cada 6-8 h SC, IM [cão e gato]; ondansetrona, 0,5 mg/kg IV a cada 12 h [cão]; 0,2 mg/kg IV a cada 12 h [gato]; metoclopramida, 1 mg/kg/24 h sob infusão em velocidade constante [cão e gato]; maropitanto, 1 mg/kg SC a cada 24 h por 5 dias [cão]; 2 mg/kg VO a cada 24 h por 5 dias [cão]) são administrados se os vômitos ocorrerem com frequência ou resultarem em perda significativa de líquido.
- Omeprazol (0,7 mg/kg VO a cada 24 h [cão]) — inibidor mais potente da secreção de ácido gástrico; tratamento de escolha para gastrinomas com indícios de metástase ou doença não ressecável e doença gastroduodenal irresponsiva à terapia com bloqueador dos receptores H_2.

INTERAÇÕES POSSÍVEIS
- Os bloqueadores dos receptores H_2 impedem a captação do omeprazol pelas células oxínticas.
- O sucralfato pode alterar a absorção de outros medicamentos. Por essa razão, esse medicamento deve ser administrado com o estômago vazio 2 h antes ou depois de outros agentes terapêuticos orais.
- Os antiácidos podem alterar a absorção oral e a eliminação renal de outros medicamentos.

MEDICAMENTO(S) ALTERNATIVO(S)
- O misoprostol, análogo sintético da prostaglandina (3 µg/kg VO a cada 8-12 h) com ações antissecretoras e citoprotetoras, ajuda a impedir e tratar as úlceras induzidas por AINE.
- Pode haver alguma eficácia no tratamento de ulcerações gastroduodenais decorrentes de outras causas.

ACOMPANHAMENTO

MONITORIZAÇÃO DO PACIENTE
- A melhora em alguns casos pode ser avaliada pela resolução dos sinais clínicos; os valores de hematócrito, proteína total, sangue oculto fecal e ureia podem ajudar a detectar perda sanguínea contínua.
- É recomendável repetir a avaliação endoscópica nos casos avançados para ajudar a determinar a duração adequada da terapia.

PREVENÇÃO
- Evitar o uso de irritantes gástricos (p. ex., AINE e corticosteroides).
- Uso concomitante de misoprostol ou inibidor da bomba de prótons com AINE; os inibidores da bomba de prótons podem ser preferíveis, porque também são terapêuticos.
- Administrar os AINE juntamente com o alimento.
- Inibidores seletivos da COX 2 ou duplos da LOX/COX podem ter menos efeitos gastrintestinais adversos do que os AINE não seletivos.

COMPLICAÇÕES POSSÍVEIS
Hemorragia, perfuração da úlcera e/ou peritonite séptica.

EVOLUÇÃO ESPERADA E PROGNÓSTICO
- Varia com as causas subjacentes.
- Úlceras gastroduodenais secundárias à administração de AINE, enteropatia inflamatória ou hipoadrenocorticismo — o prognóstico pode ser bom a excelente, dependendo da gravidade da doença.

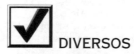

DIVERSOS

DISTÚRBIOS ASSOCIADOS
Anemia.

FATORES RELACIONADOS COM A IDADE
Neoplasias são mais comuns em animais idosos.

POTENCIAL ZOONÓTICO
O potencial zoonótico da infecção por *Helicobacter* spp. é controverso.

VER TAMBÉM
- Hematêmese.
- Melena.

ABREVIATURA(S)
- ACTH = hormônio adrenocorticotrópico.
- AINE = anti-inflamatórios não esteroides.
- CID = coagulação intravascular disseminada.
- COX = ciclo-oxigenase.
- LOX = lipo-oxigenase.

Sugestões de Leitura
Liptak JM, Hunt GB, Barrs VRD, et al. Gastroduodenal ulceration in cats: Eight cases and a review of the literature. J Feline Med Surg 2002, 4:27-42.
Neiger R. Gastric ulceration. In: Bonagura JD, Twedt DC, eds., Kirk's Current Veterinary Therapy XIV. St. Louis: Elsevier Saunders, 2009, pp. 497-501.
Simpson KW. Diseases of stomach. In: Ettinger SJ, Feldman EC, eds., Textbook of Veterinary Internal Medicine, 6th ed. St. Louis: Elsevier, 2005, pp. 1310-1331.

Autor Jocelyn Mott
Consultor Editorial Albert E. Jergens

ULCERAÇÃO BUCAL

CONSIDERAÇÕES GERAIS

DEFINIÇÃO
Perda focal ou multifocal da integridade da mucosa das camadas epiteliais superficiais em áreas específicas da cavidade bucal — ulceração da mucosa bucal.

FISIOPATOLOGIA
A ulceração da mucosa bucal geralmente coincide com inflamação orofaríngea. A inflamação oral e orofaríngea é classificada de acordo com a localização em:
• Gengivite — inflamação da gengiva.
• Periodontite — inflamação dos tecidos periodontais não gengivais (i. e., o ligamento periodontal e o osso alveolar).
• Mucosite alveolar — inflamação da mucosa alveolar (i. e., mucosa que reveste o processo alveolar e se estende a partir da junção mucogengival, sem delimitação evidente em relação ao sulco vestibular e ao assoalho bucal).
• Mucosite sublingual — inflamação da mucosa sobre o assoalho da boca.
• Mucosite labial/bucal — inflamação da mucosa de lábios e bochechas.
• Mucosite caudal — inflamação da mucosa da cavidade bucal caudal, delimitada medialmente pelas pregas e fauces palatoglossas, dorsalmente pelos palatos duro e mole e rostralmente pela mucosa alveolar e bucal.
• Palatite — inflamação da mucosa que reveste os palatos duro e/ou mole.
• Glossite — inflamação da mucosa da superfície dorsal e/ou ventral da língua.
• Queilite — inflamação dos lábios (incluindo a área da junção mucocutânea e a pele dos lábios).
• Osteomielite — inflamação do osso e da medula óssea.
• Estomatite — inflamação do revestimento mucoso de qualquer uma das estruturas da boca; em termos clínicos, o uso desse termo deve ficar reservado para a descrição de inflamação bucal disseminada (além de gengivite e periodontite), que também pode se estender para os tecidos da submucosa (p. ex., a mucosite caudal acentuada que se estende para os tecidos submucosos pode ser denominada de "estomatite caudal").
• Tonsilite — inflamação da tonsila palatina.
• Faringite — inflamação da faringe.

SISTEMA(S) ACOMETIDO(S)
Gastrintestinal — cavidade bucal.

GENÉTICA
N/D.

DISTRIBUIÇÃO GEOGRÁFICA
Nenhuma.

IDENTIFICAÇÃO

Espécies
Cães e gatos.

Raça(s) Predominante(s)
• Estomatite ulcerativa (também conhecida como estomatite periodontal ulcerativa crônica) — Maltês, Cavalier King Charles spaniel, Cocker spaniel, Bouvier des Flandres.
• Estomatite linfocítica-plasmocitária felina — pode ter predileção por gatos das raças Somali e Abissínio (ver "Inflamação Orofaríngea Felina").
• Osteomielite idiopática — pode ter predileção pela raça Cocker spaniel; complicação associada à estomatite periodontal ulcerativa crônica.

Idade Média e Faixa Etária
Nenhuma.

Sexo Predominante
Nenhum.

SINAIS CLÍNICOS
• Halitose.
• Gengivite.
• Faringite.
• Bucite/ulceração da mucosa bucal.
• Ptialismo (saliva espessa e viscosa/pegajosa).
• Dor.
• Anorexia.
• Ulceração da mucosa — "úlceras do beijo" comuns na estomatite ulcerativa.
• Placa — com ou sem cálculo dentário.
• Osso exposto, necrótico — em casos de osteíte alveolar e osteomielite idiopática.
• Alterações do comportamento secundárias à sensibilidade bucal.
• Formação de cicatriz nas margens laterais da língua — na estomatite periodontal ulcerativa crônica.
• Nota: às vezes, esses sinais começarão após a limpeza de rotina dos dentes em paciente anteriormente "normal"; eles provavelmente acabariam acontecendo, mas só foram exacerbados pela manipulação e estimulação antigênica da cavidade bucal.

CAUSAS

Metabólicas
• Diabetes melito.
• Hipoparatireoidismo.
• Hipotireoidismo.
• Nefropatia — uremia.

Nutricionais
• Desnutrição proteico-calórica.
• Deficiência de riboflavina.

Neoplásicas
• Cão — melanoma maligno; carcinoma de células escamosas; fibrossarcoma; ameloblastoma acantomatoso; epúlide benigna ulcerada.
• Gato — carcinoma de células escamosas; fibrossarcoma; melanoma maligno.

Imunomediadas
• Pênfigo vulgar — 90% possuem envolvimento bucal.
• Penfigoide bolhoso — 80% apresentam acometimento da boca.
• Lúpus eritematoso sistêmico — 50% exibem comprometimento bucal.
• Lúpus eritematoso discoide.
• Induzida por medicamento — necrólise epidérmica tóxica, eritema multiforme.
• Vasculite imunomediada.

Infecciosas
• Retrovírus — FeLV/FIV.
• Calicivírus — gato.
• Herpes-vírus — gato.
• Leptospirose — cão.
• Doença periodontal — cão e gato.

Traumáticas
• Corpo estranho — osso ou fragmentos de madeira.
• Choque por fio elétrico.
• Maloclusão.
• Doença do mastigador gengival — mastigação crônica da bochecha.

Tóxicas/Químicas
• Ingestão de substâncias químicas cáusticas.
• Tálio.

Idiopáticas
• Granuloma eosinofílico — gatos, Husky siberiano, Samoieda.
• Complexo de estomatite felina — gatos.
• Estomatite ulcerativa — cães; alérgica, reação de hipersensibilidade à placa.
• Osteomielite idiopática — cães.

FATORES DE RISCO
N/D.

DIAGNÓSTICO

DIAGNÓSTICO DIFERENCIAL
• Anamnese e exame bucal — corpos estranhos; maloclusões; queimaduras químicas, tóxicas e elétricas.
• Condições idiopáticas — sinais clínicos; anamnese; predisposições raciais; resposta ao tratamento.

HEMOGRAMA/BIOQUÍMICA/URINÁLISE
• Hiperglicemia na presença de diabetes melito; hipocalcemia em caso de hipoparatireoidismo; azotemia e isostenúria em nefropatia; leucocitose com infecções.
• Condições crônicas podem ter níveis elevados de proteína sérica total e globulina em virtude do estímulo antigênico crônico; T_4 pode estar diminuído secundariamente.

OUTROS TESTES LABORATORIAIS
• T_4 — pode estar baixo em paciente hipotireóideo ou secundariamente à inflamação crônica.
• T_4 livre — pode ser a melhor avaliação de uma função real da tireoide.
• Sorologia — teste para pesquisa de FeLV/FIV; títulos para infecções específicas.
• Culturas — em geral, são inespecíficas; contaminantes da flora bucal.

DIAGNÓSTICO POR IMAGEM
Radiografia — ajuda a determinar o envolvimento do tecido ósseo e o grau da osteomielite idiopática.

MÉTODOS DIAGNÓSTICOS
Biopsia/citologia — neoplasia, doença imunomediada e inflamação crônica resultam no predomínio de linfócitos e plasmócitos (complexo de estomatite felina e estomatite ulcerativa em cães).

ACHADOS PATOLÓGICOS
O exame histopatológico tipicamente revela inflamação inespecífica: neutrófilos, macrófagos e linfócitos, com níveis variados de perda da integridade do epitélio da mucosa.

TRATAMENTO

CUIDADO(S) DE SAÚDE ADEQUADO(S)
• Terapia de suporte — dieta pastosa; fluidos; hospitalização nos casos graves.
• Controle da dor — analgésicos tópicos/curativos protetores de úlceras, narcóticos orais, inibidores de recaptação da serotonina, antagonistas da NMDA*, gabapentina.

---

* N. T.: Anestésicos que atuam como antagonistas do receptor N-metil d-aspartato.

ULCERAÇÃO BUCAL

- Suporte nutricional — através de sonda alimentar inserida via faringostomia ou esofagostomia.
- Estomatite ulcerativa canina — cuidado meticuloso e contínuo em casa, para evitar o acúmulo de placa; limpeza dos dentes inicialmente e com frequência; terapia periodontal; extração dos dentes acometidos.
- Doença subjacente metabólica ou de outra natureza — tratar a doença sistêmica de forma apropriada.

ORIENTAÇÃO AO PROPRIETÁRIO
- Alertar o proprietário sobre o caráter reservado do prognóstico e da possível necessidade de tratamento prolongado e/ou extrações futuras. Avisar também sobre o fato de que a resposta à terapia depende da causa subjacente.
- Na estomatite ulcerativa canina ou no complexo de estomatite felina, incentiva-se o fornecimento de qualquer nível de cuidados em casa (prática de escovação ou aplicação de antimicrobianos tópicos). Cuidado: esses pacientes podem ter bocas muito sensíveis e dolorosas.

CONSIDERAÇÕES CIRÚRGICAS
- Selecionar as extrações (parcial, caudal ou toda a boca) — podem ser indicadas nas condições idiopáticas crônicas (p. ex., estomatite ulcerativa canina e complexo de estomatite felina) para remover a fonte da reação (placa/dentes).
- Remoção de toda a estrutura dentária — importante no tratamento com extração para o complexo de estomatite felina.
- Retirada do osso necrótico/avascular, fechamento com retalho gengival e antibióticos de amplo espectro — indicados na osteomielite idiopática; monitorizar o paciente quanto à ocorrência de recidiva.

MEDICAÇÕES

MEDICAMENTO(S) DE ESCOLHA
- Antimicrobianos — tratar infecções bacterianas primárias e secundárias; podem ser utilizados de forma intermitente entre as limpezas para assistência terapêutica; no entanto, o proprietário deve ser alertado quanto à possibilidade do surgimento de resistência com o uso crônico; clindamicina (11 mg/kg VO a cada 12 h); amoxicilina-clavulanato (12,5-25 mg/kg VO a cada 12 h); tetraciclina (10-22 mg/kg VO a cada 8 h).
- Medicamentos anti-inflamatórios/imunossupressores — o conforto do paciente deve ser ponderado mediante os efeitos colaterais potenciais advindos do uso de corticosteroides a longo prazo; prednisona (0,5-1 mg/kg VO a cada 12-24 h, reduzir a dosagem gradativamente).
- Protetores de mucosa — nas agressões químicas; sucralfato (1 g/25 kg VO a cada 8 h); cimetidina (5-10 mg/kg VO a cada 8-12 h).
- Analgésicos — depois da extração; carprofeno (0,5 mg/kg VO a cada 12-24 h); hidrocodona (0,22 mg/kg VO a cada 8-12 h); tramadol (2,2 mg/kg VO a cada 8-12 h).
- Terapia tópica — solução ou gel de clorexidina (antibacteriano): CHX (VRx Products, Harbor City, CA) ou CET Oral Hygiene Rinse (Virbac, Fort Worth, TX); gliconato de zinco/ácido ascórbico: MaxiGuard gel® (Addison Biologicals, Fayette, MO); dióxido de cloro estabilizado para halitose: Oxyfresh Pet Oral Hygiene Solution (Oxyfresh Worldwide, Spokane, WA).

CONTRAINDICAÇÕES
- Não utilizar esses medicamentos em pacientes com hipersensibilidades conhecidas.
- Os corticosteroides estão contraindicados em animais com infecções fúngicas sistêmicas.

PRECAUÇÕES
- Alguns antimicrobianos podem causar desarranjo gastrintestinal.
- Evitar os corticosteroides nos pacientes que já podem estar imunocomprometidos (i. e., aqueles com FeLV ou FIV).

INTERAÇÕES POSSÍVEIS
Nenhuma.

MEDICAMENTO(S) ALTERNATIVO(S)
Nenhum.

ACOMPANHAMENTO

MONITORIZAÇÃO DO PACIENTE
Exame frequente da cavidade bucal para avaliar a resolução ou recidiva.

PREVENÇÃO
Fornecimento de cuidados meticulosos em casa para evitar o acúmulo de placa.

COMPLICAÇÕES POSSÍVEIS
N/D.

EVOLUÇÃO ESPERADA E PROGNÓSTICO
- A resposta à terapia depende da causa subjacente, podendo haver a necessidade de tratamento prolongado e/ou extrações futuras.
- A inflamação pode levar de 4-6 semanas para desaparecer depois das extrações em virtude da retenção de placa nas suturas e na língua.
- Em gatos acometidos pelo complexo de estomatite felina após extrações parcial (pré-molares e molares) e total dos dentes: 60% apresentam melhora significativa, 25% exibem alguma melhora, e 15% são refratários.

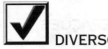

DIVERSOS

DISTÚRBIOS ASSOCIADOS
Nenhum.

FATORES RELACIONADOS COM A IDADE
Nenhum conhecido.

POTENCIAL ZOONÓTICO
Nenhum.

GESTAÇÃO/FERTILIDADE/REPRODUÇÃO
Evitar medicamentos com interações adversas conhecidas em fêmeas prenhes ou fetos em desenvolvimento.

SINÔNIMO(S)
- Estomatite ulcerativa.
- Estomatite de Vincent.
- Estomatite necrosante.

ABREVIATURA(S)
- FeLV = vírus da leucemia felina.
- FIV = vírus da imunodeficiência felina.
- NMDA = receptor N-metil d-aspartato.
- T_4 = tiroxina.

RECURSOS DA INTERNET
http://www.avdc.org/Nomenclature.html.

Sugestões de Leitura
Harvey CE. Veterinary Dentistry. Philadelphia: Saunders, 1985.
Lobprise HB. Blackwell's Five-Minute Veterinary Consult Clinical Companion — Small Animal Dentistry. Ames, IA: Blackwell, 2007 (em busca de mais assuntos, incluindo técnicas e métodos diagnósticos).
Manfra Maretta S, Brine E, Smith CW, et al. Idiopathic mandibular and maxillary osteomyelitis and bone sequestra in Cocker spaniels. In: Proceedings of the Veterinary Dental Forum, Denver, CO, 1997; sponsored by the American Veterinary Dental College, Academy of Veterinary Dentistry, and the American Veterinary Dental Society.
Smith MM. Oral and salivary gland disorders. In: Ettinger SJ, ed., Textbook of Veterinary Internal Medicine, 5th ed. Philadelphia: Saunders, 2000, pp. 1114-1121.
Wiggs RB, Lobprise HB. Veterinary Dentistry: Principles and Practice. Philadelphia: Lippincott-Raven, 1997.

Autor R. Michael Peak
Consultor Editorial Heidi B. Lobprise
Agradecimento O autor e os editores agradecem as colaborações prévias do Dr. Jan Bellows, que foi o autor deste capítulo em edições anteriores.

URETER ECTÓPICO

CONSIDERAÇÕES GERAIS

REVISÃO
• Anomalia congênita do sistema urinário. O(s) orifício(s) ureteral(is) encontra(m)-se em posição inadequada caudal ao trígono vesical (i. e., colo vesical distal, uretra, vagina, vestíbulo, útero ou próstata), resultando em incontinência urinária.
• Uma causa comum de incontinência urinária em cadelas jovens. Menos comum em cães adultos.
• Trata-se de uma diferenciação anômala dos ductos mesonéfricos e metanéfricos, resultando em interrupção inadequada no desenvolvimento do ureter.
• Cães — >95% formam um túnel intramural a partir do trígono vesical no sentido caudal, atravessando a uretra na submucosa.
• Gatos — descrito como um ureter extramural, em que a bexiga urinária é completamente desviada e o ureter se comunica distalmente no trato geniturinário.
• Comumente associado a múltiplas anomalias do trato urinário: >75% apresentam incompetência no mecanismo do esfíncter uretral concomitante, >90% exibem resquício paramesonéfrico persistente, infecções crônicas do trato urinário (6%), hidroureter (34-50%), hidronefrose (15-27%), bexigas uretrais/intrapélvicas curtas (21%).

IDENTIFICAÇÃO
• Cães e gatos.
• Cadelas jovens com incontinência urinária (frequentemente). Há relatos pouco frequentes em cães machos e gatos; em cães, a relação é de 20:1 para fêmeas:machos.
• Algumas raças caninas podem ser predispostas: Golden retriever, Labrador retriever, Husky Siberiano, Terra Nova, Poodles miniatura e toy, Terriers.

SINAIS CLÍNICOS
• Incontinência contínua ou intermitente desde o nascimento.
• Micção normal em alguns animais.
• Infecções crônicas do trato urinário.
• O quadro pode permanecer assintomático em cães machos; tipicamente, observam-se hidroureter/hidronefrose.

CAUSAS E FATORES DE RISCO
Predisposição racial (ver a seção "Identificação").

DIAGNÓSTICO

DIAGNÓSTICO DIFERENCIAL
• Incompetência no mecanismo do esfíncter uretral — perfilometria da pressão uretral com cistoscopia para descartar a presença de ureter ectópico concomitante.
• Micção inapropriada — incontinência por urgência, "bexiga hiperativa", adestramento inadequado, mudanças comportamentais (micção consciente *versus* incontinência).
• Infecção do trato urinário — pode causar polaciúria e incontinência por urgência.
• Formação de uma espécie de exsudato vaginal — extravasamento após micção quando a paciente se levanta de uma posição em decúbito.
• Hidroureter/hidronefrose congênita — cães machos com ureter ectópico frequentemente exibem continência urinária.
• Uretra curta/síndrome da bexiga intrapélvica — cistoscopia e cistouretrograma.

HEMOGRAMA/BIOQUÍMICA/URINÁLISE
A densidade urinária, bem como as concentrações séricas de ureia ou creatinina, devem permanecer normais; no entanto, podem estar anormais com anomalias concomitantes (p. ex., displasia renal).

OUTROS TESTES LABORATORIAIS
Urocultura bacteriana e antibiograma — coletar a urina por meio de cistocentese.

DIAGNÓSTICO POR IMAGEM
• Cistoscopia (sensibilidade de 96%): método diagnóstico de escolha.
• Tomografia computadorizada helicoidal (sensibilidade de 91%): exame mais preciso que a radiografia padrão.
• Ultrassonografia do trato urinário (sensibilidade de 60-91%) pode fornecer o diagnóstico exato e informações anatômicas do trato urinário superior.
• Urografia excretora (sensibilidade de 50-75%) aliada a cistograma com contraste positivo ou pneumocistograma, acompanhado por vaginouretrograma (fêmea) ou uretrograma (macho); tais exames podem diagnosticar hidroureter/hidronefrose associado, ureterocele, e/ou rins ausentes ou anormais.
• Uretrografia retrógrada (sensibilidade de 47%).

MÉTODOS DIAGNÓSTICOS
• Cistouretrovaginoscopia — permite o diagnóstico definitivo de ureter ectópico, síndrome do ureter curto, localização do orifício ectópico no trato geniturinário; identifica múltiplas fenestrações e/ou calhas.
• Perfilometria da pressão uretral — pode detectar incompetência concomitante no mecanismo do esfíncter uretral, embora o ureter ectópico intramural possa confundir os resultados e, portanto, não deve orientar o tratamento de ureter ectópico concomitante.

TRATAMENTO
• Cirúrgico: neoureterostomia (com ou sem dissecção/reconstrução do trato distal), reimplantação ureteral ou ureteronefrectomia; as taxas de complicação variam entre 14 e 25%, incluindo estenoses ureterais, extravasamento, infecção.
• Ablação à laser guiada por cistoscopia: realizada apenas em caso de ureter ectópico intramural; método diagnóstico e terapêutico ao mesmo tempo; acessa todo o trato ureteral de forma minimamente invasiva; trata os defeitos vaginais concomitantemente.
• Jamais considere o procedimento de ureteronefrectomia se uma função renal ipsolateral significativa ainda permanecer.
• Alertar os proprietários de que a incontinência poderá continuar em ~45-70% dos pacientes após a cirurgia. Muitos pacientes ficam continentes com a adição de medicamentos, o aumento dos agentes formadores de volume ou a colocação de esfíncter uretral artificial.
• Alguns filhotes caninos com incompetência do mecanismo do esfíncter uretral tornam-se continentes após seu primeiro ciclo estral.

MEDICAÇÕES

MEDICAMENTO(S)
• Fazer uso de medicamentos se a incontinência persistir após a cirurgia.
• Fenilpropranolamina: um α-bloqueador (1-1,5 mg/kg VO a cada 8 h) restabelecerá a continência após cirurgia/terapia à laser em 10-20% dos cães, melhorando os níveis de continência até 50-60%.
• Dietilestilbestrol: inicialmente 0,1-0,3 mg/kg a cada 24 h por 7 dias, depois 1 vez por semana; 0,1-1 mg VO por 3-5 dias, depois 1 mg por semana. Titular gradativamente para a dose mais baixa e eficaz. O dietilestilbestrol é potencialmente tóxico para a medula óssea e pode causar discrasias sanguíneas. Em alguns casos, o paciente pode vir a óbito por anemia aplásica. Em determinados cães, uma combinação de estrogênio e fenilpropranolamina pode ser mais eficiente.
• Em cães machos incontinentes, administra-se propionato de testosterona (2,2 mg/kg IM a cada 2-3 dias) ou metiltestosterona (0,5 mg/kg/dia) inicialmente para verificar se a terapia de reposição hormonal será eficaz. Para uma ação mais prolongada, pode-se usar o cipionato de testosterona (2,2 mg/kg IM a cada 30 dias).
• A terapia com hormônios reprodutivos não é aconselhável em animais imaturos.

OUTROS
• Injeções transuretrais de agente formador de volume na submucosa: após cirurgia/ablação à laser, pode melhorar a continência em ~60-65% dos casos.
• Após cirurgia/ablação à laser, a colocação de esfíncter uretral artificial (conhecido como oclusor hidráulico) pode restabelecer a continência em ~80%.

ACOMPANHAMENTO

EVOLUÇÃO ESPERADA E PROGNÓSTICO
• Cães — apenas com cirurgia ou ablação à laser, as taxas de continência variam de 25 a 55%, o que sobe para 60% com os medicamentos, 65% com a injeção de agente formador de volume e ~80% com a colocação de oclusor hidráulico (estudos preliminares).
• É preciso ter cuidado na avaliação de hidroureter/hidronefrose após a cirurgia, pois há relatos de estenoses ureterais; tais estenoses, por sua vez, podem resultar em perda permanente do rim ipsolateral.

DIVERSOS

DISTÚRBIOS ASSOCIADOS
Hidronefrose, hidroureter, ureterocele, bexiga pélvica, resquício paramesonéfrico persistente, septo vaginal, displasia renal, agenesia renal, incompetência no mecanismo do esfíncter uretral, uretra curta/bexiga intrapélvica.

VER TAMBÉM
• Incontinência Urinária. • Bexiga Pélvica.

Autor Allyson C. Berent
Consultor Editorial Carl A. Osborne

Ureterolitíase

CONSIDERAÇÕES GERAIS

REVISÃO
Trata-se da ocorrência de urólito (cálculo) dentro do ureter; a maioria dos ureterólitos origina-se na pelve renal e, portanto, costuma ocorrer em associação com nefrólitos. Muitos urólitos que adentram o ureter prosseguem até a bexiga urinária sem impedimento, mas os urólitos podem causar obstrução parcial ou completa do ureter, resultando em dilatação do ureter proximal e da pelve renal com subsequente destruição do parênquima renal.

IDENTIFICAÇÃO
• Cães e gatos.
• As predisposições raciais, etárias e sexuais variam de acordo com o tipo de nefrólito.

SINAIS CLÍNICOS
• Inicialmente, podem ser assintomáticos.
• Dor (cólica ureteral) durante a passagem de ureterólitos ou após obstrução ureteral aguda.
• Renomegalia se a obstrução ureteral induzir à hidronefrose.
• A síndrome do "rim grande" e "rim pequeno" está sendo identificada em uma frequência crescente em gatos, em que ocorreu previamente a obstrução de um único ureter, resultando em diminuição do rim no estágio final; ocorrem sinais de insuficiência renal e hidronefrose em virtude da obstrução do rim funcional remanescente.
• A obstrução ureteral unilateral resultará em azotemia e sinais clínicos urêmicos apenas quando a função do rim contralateral estiver comprometida.
• Pode haver sinais atribuídos à infecção do trato urinário inferior ou septicemia concomitantemente com a ureterolitíase.
• Pode ocorrer a ruptura ureteral, resultando em extravasamento e acúmulo de urina no espaço retroperitoneal.
• Os gatos com obstrução ureteral distal podem ter sinais de disúria e polaciúria.

CAUSAS E FATORES DE RISCO
• Ver os capítulos sobre cada tipo de urólito, em relação à lista de causas.
• Grande parte dos ureterólitos em cães e gatos são compostos por oxalato de cálcio. Os cães podem formar nefrólitos de estruvita e subsequente ureterólitos por conta da infecção por bactérias produtoras de urease. Os gatos podem ter ureterólitos obstrutivos compostos por coágulos sanguíneos inspissados (espessos).
• O tratamento prévio de nefrólitos por meio de litotripsia extracorpórea por ondas de choque (LEOC), a dissolução clínica ou a cirurgia para a remoção dos nefrólitos podem ser fatores de risco adicionais.

DIAGNÓSTICO

DIAGNÓSTICO DIFERENCIAL
• Considerar em todos os casos de insuficiência renal, renomegalia uni ou bilateral, dor abdominal ou acúmulo de líquido no espaço retroperitoneal. A obstrução ao fluxo de urina para ambos os rins não produzirá a mesma magnitude de renomegalia que a obstrução unilateral, porque o paciente perecerá como resultado da doença bilateral antes que ocorram as alterações nos rins.
• As radiopacidades que são detectadas por radiografias abdominais simples e podem ser confundidas com ureterólitos incluem material fecal particulado no cólon, mamilos das glândulas mamárias, peritoneólitos, linfonodos calcificados, colecistólitos e mineralização da pelve renal.
• Pode não ser uma tarefa fácil diferenciar os ureterólitos radiotransparentes de coágulos sanguíneos ureterais. Outras causas de obstrução ureteral incluem tumores intraluminais, ureteroceles, estenoses ureterais (após cirurgia ou traumatismo) e compressão extraluminal. Podem ocorrer hidrouréter e hidronefrose por ectopia ureteral, pielonefrite e obstrução do orifício ureteral na altura do trígono vesical, mais comumente em virtude de carcinoma das células de transição da bexiga.

HEMOGRAMA/BIOQUÍMICA/URINÁLISE
Esses testes avaliam a função renal e fazem a triagem em busca de doenças concomitantes antes do tratamento da ureterolitíase. A urinálise, a concentração sérica de cálcio e a excreção fracional de eletrólitos podem permitir a estimativa da composição do urólito, enquanto se aguardam os resultados da análise definitiva.

OUTROS TESTES LABORATORIAIS
• Submeter todos os ureterólitos recuperados à análise quantitativa para determinar as estratégias preventivas apropriadas.
• Os pacientes (exceto as raças Dálmata e Buldogue) com cálculos de urato devem ser avaliados quanto à presença de desvios portossistêmicos.

DIAGNÓSTICO POR IMAGEM
• Radiografia simples — os ureterólitos radiopacos podem ser observados com esse tipo de radiografia. Se ocorrerem obstrução e hidronefrose, a renomegalia poderá ser evidenciada. Em caso de ruptura ureteral, poderá haver extravasamento do meio de contraste para o espaço retroperitoneal. Os urólitos pequenos podem não ser observados nas radiografias, mesmo que sejam radiopacos.
• Radiografia contrastada — na suspeita de ureterólitos sem a possibilidade de comprovação, a realização da urografia excretora poderá ajudar a identificar o local da obstrução e também distinguirá a ruptura ureteral de hemorragia retroperitoneal. Em muitos casos, os túbulos renais lesados não concentram o contraste de forma adequada, resultando na delimitação insatisfatória do ureter; nesses casos, a injeção de contraste por nefropielocentese pode ser útil.
• Ultrassonografia — ferramenta valiosa para a detecção de hidronefrose ou hidrouréter. Também se podem observar alterações sugestivas de pielonefrite por meio do ultrassom. A dilatação da porção proximal do ureter pode ser traçada até o ureterólito, permitindo com isso sua inspeção direta. Os ureterólitos presentes nas porções média ou distal do ureter são observados com menor frequência à ultrassonografia.
• Tomografia computadorizada antes e depois da injeção IV de contraste — pode ser utilizada para confirmar ureterólitos obstrutivos se houver suspeita, mas sem confirmação, por outras modalidades de diagnóstico por imagem.

MÉTODOS DIAGNÓSTICOS
• A cintilografia nuclear isolada não deve ser usada para determinar a preservação ou a remoção cirúrgica do rim.
• A uro-hidropropulsão miccional pode ser realizada para recuperar os ureterólitos que tenham passado espontaneamente para a bexiga.

ACHADOS PATOLÓGICOS
Alterações renais macroscópicas — dilatação progressiva das pelves e dos cálices renais; em casos avançados, o rim pode ser transformado em uma estrutura cística de parede delgada com uma camada fina de parênquima cortical atrófico; é típico encontrar uma dilatação ureteral proximal ao local da obstrução.

TRATAMENTO

• Remover os ureterólitos que estejam causando obstrução (i. e., ocasionando hidronefrose ou hidrouréter) ou que não sofreram deslocamento nas radiografias sequenciais.
• Em cães, os ureterólitos são tratados com êxito por meio da LEOC. Os urólitos de oxalato de cálcio de gatos são intrinsecamente resistentes à cominuição via litotripsia por ondas de choque; portanto, essa modalidade terapêutica não é tão bem-sucedida nessa espécie.
• As técnicas cirúrgicas recomendadas para a remoção dos ureterólitos variam de acordo com o local de obstrução, a presença ou a ausência de infecção e o grau de função do rim associado. Na existência de ureterólitos nas porções média e distal do ureter, pode-se efetuar a ureteroneocistotomia: o ureter proximal à obstrução é submetido à excisão e reimplante na bexiga. Os ureterólitos presentes no ureter proximal são removidos por meio de ureterotomia. É recomendável a colocação concomitante de cateter por meio de nefrostomia. O desempenho dos procedimentos de ureterotomia ou ureteroneocistotomia exige experiência em técnicas microcirúrgicas, particularmente em gatos. A ureteronefrectomia pode ser conveniente quando a função do rim contralateral permanece normal ou na presença de hidronefrose ou pielonefrite graves no rim acometido.
• A colocação de *stent** ureteral para desviar os ureterólitos obstrutivos alivia a obstrução e provoca dilatação ureteral passiva. Os *stents* ureterais podem ser colocados por meio cirúrgico em cães e gatos ou através de cistoscopia em cadelas.

MEDICAÇÕES

MEDICAMENTO(S)
• A dissolução clínica é basicamente ineficaz para os ureterólitos.
• Alguns centros médicos para o tratamento de pedras nos rins têm sucesso na dissolução de nefrólitos de estruvita induzidos por infecção.

---

* N. T.: Dispositivo metálico, utilizado com a finalidade de manter o lúmen de alguma artéria permeável, com seu calibre próximo do normal, formando uma nova "parede" para o vaso. No caso, o *stent* foi colocado no ureter.

URETEROLITÍASE

- A terapia direcionada à prevenção da doença recidivante é imperativa após o alívio da obstrução.
- Para os ureterólitos que não estejam causando obstrução grave ou problemas funcionais renais sérios, esperar que o ureterólito passe do ureter para a bexiga urinária e seja espontaneamente eliminado na urina pode dispensar a necessidade de cirurgia ureteral.

CONTRAINDICAÇÕES/INTERAÇÕES POSSÍVEIS
- A terapia clínica destinada a promover a dissolução ou evitar a recidiva de urólitos não é totalmente benigna. Alguns pacientes não toleram a concentração elevada de sal (modificação da ração canina), a restrição de proteína, a acidificação ou os procedimentos terapêuticos relacionados que possam ser solicitados. É preciso tomar um cuidado especial em pacientes com altas demandas metabólicas, como naqueles em fases de crescimento ou lactação, e em outros com insuficiência cardíaca congestiva ou insuficiência renal.
- As tentativas de prevenção de um tipo de urólito podem promover a formação de um segundo tipo.

ACOMPANHAMENTO

MONITORIZAÇÃO DO PACIENTE
Após a remoção bem-sucedida dos ureterólitos, reavaliar o animal a cada 3-6 meses quanto à recidiva de urólitos e para garantir a colaboração do proprietário com as medidas preventivas; a realização de urinálise, radiografias (ou ultrassonografia) e urocultura costuma ser apropriada para a monitorização do paciente.

PREVENÇÃO
- Eliminação dos fatores predisponentes ao desenvolvimento de urolitíase.
- A terapia específica depende da composição mineral do urólito.

COMPLICAÇÕES POSSÍVEIS
Hidronefrose, insuficiência renal, infecção recidivante do trato urinário, pielonefrite, sepse, ruptura ureteral.

EVOLUÇÃO ESPERADA E PROGNÓSTICO
Altamente variáveis; na presença de doença unilateral, na preservação de função adequada do rim contralateral e na prevenção de recidivas, o prognóstico será bom.

DIVERSOS

ABREVIATURA(S)
- LEOC = litotripsia extracorpórea por ondas de choque.

Sugestões de Leitura
Kyles AE, Hardie EM, Wooden BG, et al. Management and outcome of cats with ureteral obstruction: 153 cases (1984-2002). JAVMA 2005, 226:937-944.

Autor Larry G. Adams
Consultor Editorial Carl A. Osborne
Agradecimento O autor e os editores agradecem a colaboração prévia de Harriet M. Syme.

Urolitíase por Cistina

CONSIDERAÇÕES GERAIS

REVISÃO
- Formação de urólitos, compostos de cistina no trato urinário.
- Ocorre em casos de cistinúria, um erro inato do metabolismo caracterizado pelo transporte anormal de cistina e de outros aminoácidos (incluindo ornitina, lisina e arginina) pelos túbulos renais.
- Cistina é filtrada livremente nos glomérulos e a maior parte sofre reabsorção ativa nos túbulos proximais.
- O comprometimento na absorção intestinal desses aminoácidos não foi associado a quaisquer estados de deficiência nutricional em cães, presumivelmente por não serem aminoácidos essenciais.
- A menos que o consumo proteico seja intensamente restrito, os cães cistinúricos não apresentam anormalidades detectáveis associadas à perda de aminoácidos. A perda excessiva de arginina na urina predispõe os gatos à encefalopatia hiperamonêmica. Alguns cães cistinúricos podem ter carnitinúria.
- O mecanismo exato de formação dos urólitos de cistina não é conhecido. Como nem todos os cães e gatos cistinúricos formam urólitos, a cistinúria constitui mais um fator predisponente do que uma causa primária de urolitíase por cistina. A cistina é relativamente insolúvel em urina ácida, porém fica mais solúvel em urina alcalina.
- Também não se conhece o modo preciso de herança da cistinúria canina. Antigamente, considerava-se que esse distúrbio genético era ligado ao sexo em todas as raças acometidas. Contudo, foi relatado há pouco tempo que a cistinúria em cães da raça Terra Nova tem padrão de herança autossômico recessivo simples. Nessa raça, os pais de cães cistinúricos são cistinúricos ou portadores, embora as ninhadas possam ser cistinúricas, portadores cistinúricos ou normais. Os resultados de um conjunto de dados indicam que a cistinúria canina seja geneticamente heterogênea.

IDENTIFICAÇÃO
- Cães — afeta principalmente os machos adultos (idade média, 5 anos; faixa etária, de 3 meses a 14 anos de idade), mas também pode acometer as fêmeas. Ocorre em mais de 70 raças, incluindo Dachshund, Buldogue inglês, Terra Nova, Labrador retriever, Staffordshire bull terrier e Welsh corgi. Os urólitos de cistina podem ser detectados em machos e fêmeas da raça Terra Nova com menos de 1 ano de idade.
- Gatos — compromete particularmente os machos e as fêmeas adultos (idade média ao diagnóstico, 3,5 anos; faixa etária, de 4 meses a 12 anos de idade); costuma ser mais identificada nas raças domésticas de pelo curto e nos siameses.

SINAIS CLÍNICOS
- Dependem da localização, do tamanho e da quantidade de urólitos; os animais acometidos podem permanecer assintomáticos.
- Os sinais típicos da presença de urocistólitos incluem polaciúria, disúria e hematúria.
- Os sinais característicos da existência de uretrólitos englobam polaciúria, disúria e, algumas vezes, eliminação de pequenos urólitos lisos à micção. A obstrução completa ao fluxo urinário pode resultar em uremia pós-renal que pode evoluir para uremia.
- Os nefrólitos são tipicamente assintomáticos, mas podem estar associados a manifestações de hidronefrose e insuficiência renal.

CAUSAS E FATORES DE RISCO
- A cistinúria representa um fator de risco.
- Predisposição racial.
- Em cães jovens e adultos (de meia-idade) com histórico prévio de urolitíase por cistina — ocorrerá recidiva dentro de 6-12 meses após a cirurgia a menos que se forneça uma terapia profilática.
- Formação de urólitos — intensificada por urina ácida, urina concentrada, bem como por micção parcial e pouco frequente.

DIAGNÓSTICO

DIAGNÓSTICO DIFERENCIAL
- Os urólitos mimetizam outras causas de polaciúria, disúria, hematúria e/ou obstrução do fluxo urinário.
- Diferenciar de outros tipos de urólitos por meio de urinálise, radiografia e análise quantitativa de urólitos eliminados pela micção ou coletados.

HEMOGRAMA/BIOQUÍMICA/URINÁLISE
- Os cristais de cistina são hexaédricos e insolúveis em ácido acético. • O teste do cianeto-nitroprussiato da urina é positivo.

OUTROS TESTES LABORATORIAIS
- Perfis de aminoácidos na urina — revelam quantidades anormais de cistina e, em alguns cães e gatos, lisina, arginina, ornitina e outros aminoácidos.
- Análise mineral quantitativa dos urólitos.
- Teste de DNA.

DIAGNÓSTICO POR IMAGEM
- Radiografia — a radiodensidade dos urólitos de cistina é semelhante à dos urólitos de estruvita e sílica, inferior à dos urólitos de oxalato e fosfato de cálcio e superior à dos urólitos de urato de amônio; quando os urólitos de cistina forem suficientemente grandes, eles poderão ser detectados por meio de radiografias simples.
- Ultrassonografia — pode detectar os urólitos de cistina, mas não fornece informações confiáveis sobre sua radiodensidade ou seu formato.

MÉTODOS DIAGNÓSTICOS
Uretrocistoscopia — usada para detectar uretrólitos e urocistólitos de cistina.

TRATAMENTO
- Dissolução clínica de urólitos por uma combinação de N-(2-mercaptopropionil)-glicina (2-MPG) e dieta terapêutica; a Prescription Diet Canine u/d da Hill diminui a excreção urinária de cistina, promove a formação de urina alcalina e reduz a concentração urinária; essa dieta é utilizada em conjunto com a 2-MPG para a dissolução dos urólitos e, muitas vezes, se mostra eficaz quando utilizada isoladamente na prevenção da recidiva dos urólitos de cistina.
- Remoção dos urocistólitos pequenos por meio de uro-hidropropulsão miccional ou cirurgia.

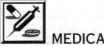

MEDICAÇÕES

MEDICAMENTO(S)
Alcalinizantes Urinários
- Considerar o uso em pacientes que apresentam urina ácida, apesar da dieta terapêutica e do controle das infecções do trato urinário por bactérias urease-positivas. • Os dados obtidos de estudos em seres humanos cistinúricos sugerem que a presença de sódio na dieta possa acentuar a cistinúria; assim, o citrato de potássio possivelmente é preferível ao bicarbonato de sódio como alcalinizante urinário. Fornecer uma quantidade suficiente de citrato de potássio (40-75 mg/kg VO a cada 12 h) para manter um pH urinário de 7,5. • Acetazolamida — usada em seres humanos; não foi avaliada em cães ou gatos.

Medicamentos com Tiol em sua Composição
- A 2-MPG diminui a concentração urinária de cistina pela combinação com a cisteína e subsequente formação do complexo cisteína-2-MPG, que se mostra mais solúvel do que a cistina.
- Para a dissolução dos urólitos de cistina em cães, pode-se administrar a 2-MPG (Thiola-Mission Pharmacal) na dosagem de 15-20 mg/kg VO a cada 12 h, associada à dieta terapêutica. Em nosso hospital, o tempo médio de dissolução foi de 78 dias (variação, de 11-211 dias). • Se a dieta terapêutica não for ideal, pode-se fornecer a 2-MPG em dosagem inferior (5-10 mg/kg VO a cada 12 h) para evitar a recidiva dos urólitos de cistina em cães.
- Os efeitos adversos induzidos pela 2-MPG são raros em cães e incluem: anemia esferocítica reversível positiva ao teste de Coombs, trombocitopenia, proteinúria glomerular, miopatia, agressividade e aumento na atividade das enzimas hepáticas. • A eficácia e a segurança da 2-MPG ainda não foram avaliadas em gatos cistinúricos.

ACOMPANHAMENTO
- Prevenção da recidiva com o controle da dieta ou a administração da 2-MPG. • Monitorização da dissolução dos urólitos em intervalos de 30 dias por meio da urinálise, bem como por radiografia (simples ou contrastada) ou ultrassonografia.
- Embora os urólitos de cistina tendam à recidiva, isso não ocorre em todos os cães e gatos cistinúricos. • Em alguns cães mais idosos, a frequência de recidiva declina em consequência de queda na magnitude da cistinúria.

DIVERSOS

ABREVIATURA(S)
- 2-MPG = N-(2-mercaptopropionil)-glicina.

Sugestões de Leitura
Bannasch D, Henthorn PS. Changing paradigms in the diagnosis of inherited defects associated with urolithiasis. Vet Clin North Am 2009, 39:111-125.

Autores Carl A. Osborne, Jody P. Lulich, e Lisa K. Ulrich
Consultor Editorial Carl A. Osborne

UROLITÍASE POR ESTRUVITA — CÃES

CONSIDERAÇÕES GERAIS

DEFINIÇÃO
Formação de concreções policristalinas (i. e., urólitos, cálculos ou pedras), compostas de fosfato amônio-magnésio (também conhecido como estruvita) no trato urinário.

FISIOPATOLOGIA
Estruvita Induzida por Infecção
• A urina precisa estar supersaturada com fosfato amônio-magnésio para que ocorra a formação dos urólitos de estruvita. A supersaturação da urina por fosfato amônio-magnésio pode estar associada a diversos fatores, incluindo infecções do trato urinário por microrganismos produtores de urease, urina alcalina, predisposição genética e dieta.
• Se os animais forem acometidos por infecções do trato urinário causadas por microrganismos produtores de urease (sobretudo as espécies de *Staphylococcus*, *Proteus* e *Ureaplasma*) e se sua urina contiver quantidade suficiente de ureia, o resultado será uma combinação única de elevações concomitantes nas concentrações de amônio (NH_4^+), fosfato (PO_4^{3-}) e carbonato (CO_3^{2-}) em ambiente alcalino. Tais condições favorecem a formação de urólitos que contenham estruvita ($MgNH_4PO_4 \cdot 6H_2O$), apatita de cálcio [$Ca_{10}(PO_4)6(OH)_2$] e apatita de carbonato [$Ca_{10}(PO_4)6CO_3$].
• O consumo de proteína na dieta em níveis acima das necessidades diárias para o anabolismo resulta na formação de ureia a partir do catabolismo de aminoácidos.
• A magnitude da hiperamonúria, da hipercarbonatúria e da alcalúria mediadas pela urease microbiana depende da quantidade de ureia (o substrato da urease) na urina.
• A excreção urinária anormal de minerais, em consequência do aumento na taxa de filtração glomerular, do declínio na reabsorção tubular ou do incremento na secreção tubular, não é necessária para o início e o crescimento dos urólitos de estruvita induzidos por infecção; no entanto, as anormalidades metabólicas e anatômicas podem induzir indiretamente à formação dos urólitos de estruvita pela predisposição às infecções do trato urinário.

Estruvita Estéril
• Nessa espécie, pode haver o envolvimento de fatores nutricionais ou metabólicos na gênese dos urólitos estéreis de estruvita.
• A urease microbiana não está envolvida na formação dos urólitos estéreis de estruvita.

SISTEMA(S) ACOMETIDO(S)
Renal/urológico.

GENÉTICA
• A alta incidência dos urólitos de estruvita em algumas raças de cães, como o Schnauzer miniatura, sugere tendência familiar. Há hipóteses de que o Schnauzer miniatura suscetível apresente aumento na suscetibilidade à infecção do trato urinário em virtude de alguma anormalidade hereditária nas defesas locais do trato urinário do hospedeiro.
• Em uma família de Cocker spaniel inglês, foram encontrados urólitos estéreis de estruvita.

INCIDÊNCIA/PREVALÊNCIA
Os urólitos de estruvita respondem por aproximadamente 40% das pedras que envolvem o trato urinário inferior canino e 33% daquelas que acometem o trato urinário superior.

DISTRIBUIÇÃO GEOGRÁFICA
Ubíqua.

IDENTIFICAÇÃO
Espécies
Cães (ver o capítulo sobre "Urolitíase por Estruvita — Gatos").

Raça(s) Predominante(s)
• Schnauzer miniatura, Shih tzu, Bichon frisé, Poodle miniatura, Cocker spaniel e Lhasa apso.
• Qualquer raça pode ser acometida.

Idade Média e Faixa Etária
• Idade média, 6 anos (variação, de <1 a >19 anos de idade).
• Em cães imaturos (<12 meses de vida), a maioria dos urólitos compõe-se de estruvita induzida por infecção.

Sexo Predominante
É mais comum em fêmeas (~85%) do que em machos (~15%), o que possivelmente se relaciona com a maior tendência ao desenvolvimento de infecção bacteriana do trato urinário pelas fêmeas.

SINAIS CLÍNICOS
Comentários Gerais
• Alguns cães permanecem assintomáticos.
• Os sinais clínicos dependem da localização, do tamanho e da quantidade de urólitos.

Achados Anamnésicos
• Os sinais típicos de urocistólitos incluem polaciúria, disúria e hematúria; algumas vezes, pequenos urólitos lisos são eliminados na urina.
• Os sinais característicos de uretrólitos compreendem polaciúria e disúria; ocasionalmente, pequenos urólitos lisos também são eliminados na micção.
• Os nefrólitos podem estar associados a manifestações de insuficiência renal. A obstrução do fluxo urinário com infecção bacteriana do trato urinário pode resultar em pielonefrite e septicemia.

Achados do Exame Físico
• Os urólitos podem ser palpados na bexiga urinária e na uretra (por exame retal).
• A obstrução da uretra pode levar a aumento de volume da bexiga urinária.
• A obstrução de um ureter pode provocar o aumento de volume do rim associado.
• A obstrução completa do fluxo urinário associada à infecção bacteriana pode causar infecção ascendente do trato urinário, sinais de insuficiência renal e sinais de septicemia.

CAUSAS
• Distúrbios do trato urinário predisponentes a infecções por bactérias produtoras de urease, patógenos fúngicos ou ureaplasma em pacientes cuja urina contém grande quantidade de ureia.
• As causas específicas de urólitos estéreis de estruvita não são conhecidas.

FATORES DE RISCO
• A exposição exógena ou endógena a altas concentrações de glicocorticoides predispõe os animais à infecção bacteriana do trato urinário.
• Retenção anormal de urina.
• A urina alcalina diminui a solubilidade da estruvita.

DIAGNÓSTICO

DIAGNÓSTICO DIFERENCIAL
• Os urólitos mimetizam outras causas de polaciúria, disúria, hematúria e/ou obstrução do fluxo urinário.
• Diferenciar de outros tipos de urólitos por meio de identificação do animal, exame retal, urinálise, urocultura, radiografia e análise quantitativa de urólitos eliminados ou coletados.

HEMOGRAMA/BIOQUÍMICA/URINÁLISE
• A obstrução completa do fluxo urinário pode causar azotemia pós-renal (p. ex., elevação nos níveis de ureia, creatinina e fósforo).
• Os cristais de fosfato amônio-magnésio tipicamente se assemelham a prismas incolores e ortorrômbicos (ou seja, possuem três eixos desiguais, que sofrem intersecção nos ângulos retos). Tais cristais podem exibir seis ou mais faces e frequentemente apresentam extremidades oblíquas.

OUTROS TESTES LABORATORIAIS
• Cultura bacteriana quantitativa da urina, coletada de preferência por cistocentese.
• Cultura bacteriana das porções internas dos urólitos de estruvita induzidos por infecção.
• Análise mineral quantitativa de urólitos coletados durante a micção, por meio da uro-hidropropulsão miccional, por aspiração com cateter urinário ou por cistoscopia.

DIAGNÓSTICO POR IMAGEM
• Os urólitos de estruvita são radiopacos e podem ser detectados por meio de radiografias simples.
• A ultrassonografia é capaz de detectar urólitos, mas não fornece nenhuma informação sobre a densidade ou o formato desses urólitos.
• Determinar de forma precisa a localização, o tamanho e a quantidade de urólitos; o tamanho e a quantidade não representam um índice confiável da provável eficácia da terapia de dissolução.

TRATAMENTO

CUIDADO(S) DE SAÚDE ADEQUADO(S)
• A uro-hidropropulsão retrógrada é indicada para deslocar os cálculos uretrais e restabelecer a patência (desobstrução) uretral, enquanto a uro-hidropropulsão miccional, para eliminar os cálculos vesicais.
• A litotripsia por ondas de choque e/ou a cirurgia exigem curtos períodos de hospitalização.
• A dissolução clínica dos urólitos de estruvita é uma estratégia conduzida em esquema ambulatorial.

DIETA
• Os urocistólitos e os nefrólitos de estruvita (estéreis e induzidos por infecção) podem ser dissolvidos pelo fornecimento de dieta calculolítica (Hill's Prescription Diet Canine s/d).
• Manter a dieta calculolítica por mais 1 mês após a evidência radiográfica da dissolução dos urólitos.
• Evitar o uso de dietas com restrição de proteínas em pacientes com desnutrição proteica e calórica. A dieta calculolítica é elaborada para a terapia de dissolução a curto prazo (semanas a meses), e não para a terapia profilática a longo prazo (meses a

Urolitíase por Estruvita — Cães

anos). Se as dietas com restrição proteica forem utilizadas, será preciso monitorizar o paciente em busca de indícios de desnutrição proteica. Evitar o fornecimento prolongado da dieta calculolítica a cães imaturos.

ORIENTAÇÃO AO PROPRIETÁRIO
- Caso se faça uso da dieta terapêutica, deve-se limitar o acesso do animal a outros tipos de alimentos e petiscos.
- O tratamento a curto prazo com dieta calculolítica e a administração de antibióticos têm se mostrado eficientes na dissolução dos urólitos de estruvita.
- A posologia da antibioticoterapia e o esquema da terapia nutricional devem ser obedecidos.

CONSIDERAÇÕES CIRÚRGICAS
- Os ureterólitos não se mostram passíveis de dissolução. Por essa razão, deve-se considerar a realização da cirurgia ou da litotripsia extracorpórea por ondas de choque em casos de ureterólitos persistentes associados à morbidade.
- A dissolução clínica dos uretrólitos também não é possível. Se houver a possibilidade de passagem dos uretrólitos em toda a extensão da uretra, será considerada a realização de uro-hidropropulsão miccional. Alternativamente, deve-se considerar a litotripsia ou promover o deslocamento dos uretrólitos em direção à bexiga urinária por meio da uro-hidropropulsão retrógrada.
- Os uretrólitos imóveis podem necessitar de uretrotomia ou uretrostomia.
- Os nefrólitos indutores de obstrução do fluxo urinário ou associados à disfunção renal não são dissolvidos por meio clínico.
- Em casos de obstrução do fluxo urinário pela presença de urólitos e/ou na identificação radiográfica (ou por outros meios) de anormalidades passíveis de correção e predisponentes à recidiva da infecção do trato urinário, deve-se ponderar a realização de correção cirúrgica.

MEDICAÇÕES

MEDICAMENTO(S)
- A dissolução de urocistólitos ou nefrólitos induzidos por infecção por meio da dieta exige a administração oral de antibióticos apropriados, selecionados com base nos resultados da cultura bacteriana quantitativa e do antibiograma. Administrar os antibióticos em dosagens terapêuticas até a ausência de evidências radiográficas de urólitos e a confirmação laboratorial de erradicação da infecção do trato urinário.
- Os pacientes com urocistólitos de estruvita induzidos por infecção associados à infecção bacteriana persistente por bactérias produtoras de urease e refratários à dissolução por meio de dietas e antibióticos podem ser submetidos ao ácido acetoidroxâmico (Lithostat®, Mission Pharmacal, 12,5 mg/kg VO a cada 12 h), um inibidor da urease que bloqueia a hidrólise da ureia em amônia.

CONTRAINDICAÇÕES
O ácido acetoidroxâmico é teratogênico e, portanto, não deve ser administrado em cadelas prenhes.

PRECAUÇÕES
- A poliúria induzida pela dieta reduzirá a concentração dos medicamentos antimicrobianos na urina; tal fato deve ser levado em consideração ao se calcular as dosagens antimicrobianas.
- Em alguns cães, a administração prolongada do ácido acetoidroxâmico em doses mais elevadas induz a anormalidades no metabolismo da bilirrubina.
- Doses mais altas do ácido acetoidroxâmico podem levar a uma anemia hemolítica reversível.

ACOMPANHAMENTO

MONITORIZAÇÃO DO PACIENTE
Deve-se monitorizar a taxa de dissolução dos urólitos em intervalos mensais por meio de urinálise, urocultura, ultrassonografia e/ou radiografia simples ou contrastada.

PREVENÇÃO
- A urolitíase por estruvita induzida por infecção pode ser evitada com a erradicação e o controle das infecções do trato urinário por bactérias produtoras de urease.
- É possível evitar a recidiva de urólitos estéreis de estruvita com o uso de dietas acidificantes e restritas em magnésio (Hill's Prescription Diet Canine c/d) ou de acidificantes urinários.
- Monitorizar os pacientes submetidos à acidificação urinária em busca de cristalúria por oxalato de cálcio. Em caso de desenvolvimento de cristalúria persistente por oxalato de cálcio, deve-se modificar o protocolo terapêutico.
- Em pacientes sob risco de cristalúria tanto por estruvita como por oxalato de cálcio, deve-se concentrar o tratamento na prevenção dos urólitos de oxalato de cálcio — se houver recidiva, os urólitos de estruvita poderão ser dissolvidos por meio clínico; já os urólitos recidivantes de oxalato de cálcio não se mostram passíveis de dissolução.

COMPLICAÇÕES POSSÍVEIS
- Há riscos e benefícios associados ao fornecimento de dietas estruvitolíticas. Nem todos os pacientes estão qualificados para a utilização da dieta terapêutica, incluindo aqueles com (1) acúmulo anormal de líquidos, (2) insuficiência renal primária azotêmica e (3) predisposições à pancreatite (especialmente Schnauzer miniatura com hiperlipidemia).
- Os urocistólitos podem passar pela uretra de machos caninos e obstruí-la, sobretudo se o paciente apresentar disúria persistente. A obstrução uretral pode ser tratada por meio da uro-hidropropulsão retrógrada ou litotripsia.
- A disúria pode ser minimizada pelo tratamento antimicrobiano das infecções bacterianas do trato urinário e pela administração oral de agentes anticolinérgicos.
- Os cães que não consomem as necessidades diárias da dieta calculolítica podem desenvolver graus variados de desnutrição calórica e proteica. É possível evitar tal ocorrência por meio do cálculo apropriado das necessidades nutricionais diárias e do ajuste na quantidade de ração fornecida, com base em exames físicos seriados.
- A poliúria associada à dieta resultará na eliminação de um volume maior de urina. Isso talvez se associe a graus variados de incontinência urinária em cadelas castradas com predisposição à incontinência responsiva a estrogênios.

EVOLUÇÃO ESPERADA E PROGNÓSTICO
- Em nosso hospital, o tempo médio para a dissolução de urocistólitos induzidos por infecção foi de aproximadamente 3 meses (variação de 2 semanas a 7 meses). O tempo médio para a dissolução dos nefrólitos de estruvita induzidos por infecção foi de 6 meses (variação, 2-10 meses). O tempo médio para a dissolução dos urocistólitos estéreis de estruvita foi de 6 semanas (variação, 4-12 semanas).
- O declínio na concentração sérica da ureia (em torno de 10 mg/dL) e a densidade urinária baixa (1,004-1,014) indicam a obediência às recomendações nutricionais.
- Se os urólitos aumentarem de tamanho durante o fornecimento da dieta terapêutica ou não começarem a diminuir de tamanho depois de aproximadamente 4-8 semanas de tratamento clínico apropriado, métodos alternativos deverão ser levados em consideração. A dificuldade em induzir a dissolução completa dos urólitos pela criação de uma urina subsaturada com estruvita deve suscitar os seguintes fatores: (1) erro na identificação do componente mineral, (2) diferença na composição mineral do núcleo dos urólitos, em comparação às outras porções do urólito, e (3) desobediência do proprietário às recomendações terapêuticas.

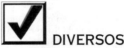

DIVERSOS

DISTÚRBIOS ASSOCIADOS
Qualquer doença que predisponha o animal à infecção bacteriana do trato urinário.

FATORES RELACIONADOS COM A IDADE
Os urólitos de estruvita induzidos por infecção representam a forma mais comum de urólito em cães imaturos. Os urólitos desenvolvem-se como resultado de infecção microbiana do trato urinário.

GESTAÇÃO/FERTILIDADE/REPRODUÇÃO
- O ácido acetoidroxâmico é teratogênico.
- A dieta calculolítica não é destinada para a manutenção da prenhez.

SINÔNIMO(S)
- Cálculos de fosfato.
- Cálculos por infecção.
- Cálculos de urease.
- Cálculos de fosfato triplo.

Sugestões de Leitura
Osborne CA, Lulich JP, Bartges JW, et al. Canine and feline urolithiasis: Relationship of etiopathogenesis to treatment and prevention. In: Osborne CA, Finco DR, eds., Canine and Feline Nephrology and Urology. Baltimore: Williams & Wilkins, 1995, pp. 798-888.

Autores Carl A. Osborne, Jody P. Lulich, e David J. Polzin
Consultor Editorial Carl A. Osborne

UROLITÍASE POR ESTRUVITA — GATOS

CONSIDERAÇÕES GERAIS

DEFINIÇÃO
Os urólitos de estruvita e os tampões uretrais de estruvita apresentam diferenças físicas e etiopatogênicas; dessa forma, esses termos não devem ser empregados como sinônimos. Os urólitos de estruvita são concreções policristalinas compostas principalmente de fosfato amônio-magnésio e pequenas quantidades de matriz. Já os tampões uretrais de estruvita em gatos costumam ser constituídos de quantidades abundantes de matriz misturada com cristais (especialmente fosfato amônio-magnésio). Alguns tampões uretrais são compostos basicamente de matriz orgânica, tecido esfacelado, sangue e/ou reagentes inflamatórios.

FISIOPATOLOGIA
• Ver o capítulo sobre "Urolitíase por Estruvita — Cães". • A forma mais comumente encontrada de tampões uretrais de ocorrência natural em gatos contém quantidades relativamente grandes de matriz, além de minerais, sobretudo de estruvita. Os fatores de risco associados à formação de cristais de fosfato amônio-magnésio contidos nos tampões uretrais são semelhantes àqueles relacionados com a formação dos urólitos de estruvita. A prevenção ou o controle desses fatores de risco devem minimizar a recidiva do componente de estruvita dos tampões uretrais. As causas específicas e a composição da matriz do tampão uretral ainda não foram classificadas. Uma hipótese é que a formação da matriz do tampão segue o início de infecções do trato urinário, sobretudo daquelas causadas por vírus.

SISTEMA(S) ACOMETIDO(S)
Renal/urológico — trato urinário superior e inferior.

INCIDÊNCIA/PREVALÊNCIA
• A prevalência dos urólitos felinos de estruvita, enviados para o Centro de Urólitos em Minnesota (EUA), declinou de 78% em 1981 para 33% em 2002, mas em seguida aumentou para 48% em 2005. Em comparação, os urólitos compostos principalmente de oxalato de cálcio aumentaram de cerca de 2% em 1981 para 55% em 2002, mas depois diminuíram para 40% em 2005. Essas mudanças drásticas na frequência de ocorrência da composição mineral de urólitos felinos correm paralelamente às alterações na composição de dietas industrializadas. • Atualmente, a estruvita representa quase 50% de todos os tipos de urólitos no trato urinário inferior dos felinos. Desses, 95% são estéreis. • Em cerca de 8% dos nefrólitos em gatos, detectou-se a presença de estruvita. • Desde 1981, a estruvita continua sendo o mineral mais comum (85%) em tampões uretrais de matriz cristalina.

IDENTIFICAÇÃO
Espécies
Gatos (ver o capítulo sobre "Urolitíase por Estruvita — Cães").

Idade Média e Faixa Etária
• A idade média no momento do diagnóstico gira em torno de 7 anos (variação, <1 a 22 anos de idade). • Os urólitos estéreis de estruvita não acometem os gatos imaturos; nesses gatos, pode ocorrer a formação de urólitos de estruvita induzidos por infecção.

Sexo Predominante
• Os urólitos de estruvita são mais comuns em fêmeas (55%) do que em machos (45%).
• Os tampões uretrais de estruvita afetam principalmente os machos.

SINAIS CLÍNICOS
Comentários Gerais
• Os gatos acometidos podem permanecer assintomáticos.
• Dependem da localização, do tamanho, da quantidade e da causa de urólitos.

Achados Anamnésicos
• Os sinais típicos de urocistólitos incluem polaciúria, disúria e hematúria.
• Os sinais característicos de uretrólitos compreendem polaciúria, disúria e, algumas vezes, eliminação de pequenos urólitos lisos.
• Em alguns gatos com obstrução do fluxo urinário, constatam-se sinais de azotemia pós-renal (p. ex., anorexia e vômito).
• Em certo número de gatos com nefrólitos, verificam-se manifestações de insuficiência renal (poliúria e polidipsia).
• Em gatos com tampões uretrais de estruvita, observam-se sinais típicos de obstrução do fluxo urinário (p. ex., disúria, bexiga urinária grande e dolorida, além de sinais de azotemia pós-renal).

Achados do Exame Físico
• Em determinados gatos com urocistólitos, nota-se parede vesical espessada, firme e contraída.
• A detecção de urocistólitos por meio da palpação não é confiável, porque é um método insensível.
• Os tampões uretrais ou os uretrólitos podem ser detectados por exame da uretra peniana e da porção distal do pênis.
• A obstrução do fluxo urinário resulta no aumento de volume da bexiga e em sinais de azotemia pós-renal.

CAUSAS
Ver a seção "Fisiopatologia".

FATORES DE RISCO
• Os fatores de risco envolvidos na formação de urólitos estéreis de estruvita incluem a composição mineral, bem como o teor de energia e umidade das dietas; os alimentos formadores de metabólitos alcalinizantes da urina; a quantidade da dieta consumida; os esquemas de alimentação *ad libitum* (ou seja, à vontade) *versus* horários de refeições programadas; a formação de urina concentrada; e a retenção de urina.
• Os prováveis fatores de risco para a formação de urólitos de estruvita induzidos por infecção compreendem as infecções do trato urinário por patógenos microbianos produtores de urease, as anormalidades nas defesas locais do hospedeiro que permitem as infecções bacterianas do trato urinário (incluindo as uretrostomias perineais) e a quantidade de ureia (o substrato da urease) excretada na urina.
• O pequeno diâmetro normal da porção distal da uretra de machos felinos os predispõe à obstrução por tampões e uretrólitos.

DIAGNÓSTICO

DIAGNÓSTICO DIFERENCIAL
• Os urólitos mimetizam outras causas de polaciúria, disúria, hematúria e/ou obstrução do fluxo urinário.
• É preciso diferenciar os urólitos de estruvita e os tampões uretrais de outros tipos de urólitos por meio de identificação do animal, urinálise, urocultura, radiografia, ultrassonografia, cistoscopia e análise quantitativa de urólitos ou tampões eliminados ou coletados.

HEMOGRAMA/BIOQUÍMICA/URINÁLISE
• A obstrução completa do fluxo urinário pode causar azotemia pós-renal (p. ex., elevação nos níveis de ureia, creatinina e fósforo).
• Os cristais de fosfato amônio-magnésio tipicamente se assemelham a prismas incolores e ortorrômbicos (ou seja, possuem três eixos desiguais, que sofrem intersecção nos ângulos retos). Com frequência, tais cristais apresentam três a oito faces.

OUTROS TESTES LABORATORIAIS
• A realização pré-terapêutica de uroculturas bacterianas quantitativas (de preferência com amostras obtidas por meio de cistocentese) revela infecções bacterianas do trato urinário em apenas ~1-3% dos pacientes acometidos de 2 a 7 anos de idade.
• Na prática clínica, a análise mineral quantitativa constitui o padrão de exame aceito para urólitos e tampões uretrais coletados durante a micção, por meio da uro-hidropropulsão miccional, por aspiração com cateter urinário ou por cistoscopia.
• Pode ser valiosa a cultura bacteriana das porções internas dos urólitos coletados na urina de pacientes com infecção por microrganismos produtores de urease.

DIAGNÓSTICO POR IMAGEM
Radiografia
• Urólitos de estruvita — são radiopacos; possivelmente detectados por meio de radiografias simples; alguns tampões uretrais de estruvita podem ser detectados por radiografias simples.
• O tamanho e a quantidade de urólitos não representam um índice confiável da provável eficácia da terapia de dissolução.
• A uretrocistografia contrastada ajuda a identificar o(s) local(is) de obstrução e estenose uretrais.

Ultrassonografia
• Detecta a localização, o tamanho e a quantidade de urólitos, mas não indica o grau de radiodensidade nem o formato dos urólitos.

MÉTODOS DIAGNÓSTICOS
A cistoscopia revela a localização, a quantidade, o tamanho e o formato de uretrólitos e urocistólitos.

ACHADOS PATOLÓGICOS
Os tampões uretrais podem conter hemácias, leucócitos, células epiteliais de transição, bactérias e/ou vírus, além de matriz e minerais.

TRATAMENTO

CUIDADO(S) DE SAÚDE ADEQUADO(S)
• A uro-hidropropulsão retrógrada é indicada para eliminar os cálculos uretrais, enquanto a lavagem, para remover os tampões uretrais.
• A uro-hidropropulsão miccional para eliminar os cálculos vesicais e uretrais e/ou a cirurgia exigem curtos períodos de hospitalização.
• A dissolução clínica dos urólitos de estruvita é uma estratégia conduzida em esquema ambulatorial.

Urolitíase por Estruvita — Gatos

ATIVIDADE
Caso se faça uso da dieta terapêutica, não se deve incentivar a prática de atividades em ambientes externos.

DIETA
- O tratamento de urólitos estéreis de estruvita com dieta adequada (a ração modelo é representada pela Hill's Prescription Diet Feline s/d) tipicamente resulta na dissolução dentro de 2-4 semanas de terapia. Por essa razão, essa dieta terapêutica tornou-se o tratamento padrão na prática clínica.
- Os urocistólitos de estruvita induzidos por infecção podem ser dissolvidos pelo fornecimento de dieta calculolítica (Hill's Prescription Diet Feline s/d) e antimicrobianos apropriados.
- Manter a dieta terapêutica por mais 1 mês após a evidência radiográfica da dissolução dos urólitos.
- A cristalúria por estruvita pode ser minimizada pelo oferecimento de dietas com acidificantes urinários e restritas em magnésio.
- As rações enlatadas (úmidas) ajudam a reduzir a concentração urinária de metabólitos calculogênicos e promovem o aumento na frequência da micção normal.

ORIENTAÇÃO AO PROPRIETÁRIO
- Caso se utilize a dieta terapêutica, deve-se limitar o acesso do animal a outros tipos de alimentos e petiscos.
- O tratamento a curto prazo (semanas a meses) com dieta calculolítica (Hill's Feline s/d) e antibióticos, conforme a necessidade, é eficaz na dissolução dos urólitos de estruvita induzidos por infecção.
- É imprescindível que os proprietários de gatos com urocistólitos de estruvita induzidos por infecção obedeçam à posologia da antibioticoterapia.
- Evitar o fornecimento de dietas calculolíticas a gatos imaturos.

CONSIDERAÇÕES CIRÚRGICAS
- Os ureterólitos não se mostram passíveis de dissolução. Por essa razão, deve-se considerar a realização de cirurgia em casos de ureterólitos persistentes associados à morbidade.
- A dissolução clínica dos uretrólitos também não é possível. Nesse caso, deve-se contemplar a execução de uro-hidropropulsão miccional para remover os uretrólitos ou os tampões uretrais. Alternativamente, deve-se promover o deslocamento dos uretrólitos em direção à bexiga urinária por meio da uro-hidropropulsão retrógrada.
- Os uretrólitos imóveis, os tampões uretrais recidivantes ou as estenoses da uretra distal podem exigir o procedimento de uretrostomia perineal.
- Considerar a litotripsia a laser para urocistólitos e/ou uretrólitos.
- Em casos de obstrução do fluxo urinário pela presença de urólitos e/ou na identificação radiográfica (ou por outros meios) de anormalidades passíveis de correção e predisponentes à recidiva da infecção do trato urinário, deve-se ponderar a realização de correção cirúrgica.
- Antes de se considerar a correção cirúrgica, os urólitos e os tampões uretrais deverão ser localizados.
- Para comprovar a remoção de todos os urólitos, fica indicada a obtenção de radiografias imediatamente após a cirurgia.

MEDICAÇÕES

MEDICAMENTO(S)
- A dissolução de urocistólitos induzidos por infecção por meio da dieta exige a administração oral de antibióticos apropriados, selecionados com base nos resultados da cultura bacteriana e do antibiograma. Administrar os antibióticos em dosagens terapêuticas até a erradicação da infecção do trato urinário e a ausência de indícios radiográficos de urólitos.
- A tolteridina pode ser considerada como um agente anticolinérgico e antiespasmódico para minimizar a hiperatividade do músculo detrusor da bexiga urinária e a incontinência de urgência; a dose empírica sugerida é de 0,05 mg/kg VO a cada 12 h.

CONTRAINDICAÇÕES
Não fornecer acidificantes urinários a pacientes azotêmicos ou gatos imaturos.

PRECAUÇÕES
Os pacientes com azotemia estão sob maior risco de manifestar reações adversas aos medicamentos.

ACOMPANHAMENTO

MONITORIZAÇÃO DO PACIENTE
Avaliar a taxa de dissolução do urólito em intervalos mensais por meio da urinálise, urocultura, radiografia simples ou contrastada ou ultrassonografia.

PREVENÇÃO
- A recidiva de urólitos estéreis de estruvita pode ser evitada com o uso de dietas acidificantes e restritas em magnésio ou acidificantes urinários. Não se devem administrar acidificantes urinários associados às dietas acidificantes.
- Considerar o uso de dieta acidificante modificada com alto teor de umidade e restrição de magnésio não suplementada com sódio (Prescription Diet c/d Multicare Feline) para minimizar a recidiva de cristalúria por estruvita e/ou oxalato de cálcio e de urólitos desses minerais.
- Monitorizar com cuidado os pacientes submetidos à acidificação urinária em busca de cristalúria por oxalato de cálcio. Em caso de desenvolvimento de cristalúria persistente por oxalato de cálcio, deve-se modificar o protocolo terapêutico.
- Em pacientes sob risco de cristalúria tanto por estruvita como por oxalato de cálcio, deve-se concentrar o tratamento na prevenção dos urólitos de oxalato de cálcio. Os urólitos de estruvita são suscetíveis à dissolução clínica; já os urólitos recidivantes de oxalato de cálcio não se mostram passíveis de dissolução.
- A urolitíase de estruvita induzida por infecção pode ser evitada por meio da erradicação e do controle das infecções do trato urinário. O emprego de dietas acidificantes com restrição de magnésio não será necessário caso se consiga erradicar os microrganismos produtores de urease.

COMPLICAÇÕES POSSÍVEIS
- Os urocistólitos podem passar pela uretra de machos felinos e obstruí-la, sobretudo se o paciente estiver com disúria persistente. A obstrução uretral pode ser tratada por meio da uro-hidropropulsão retrógrada.
- A colocação de cateter transuretral de demora aumenta o risco da indução iatrogênica de infecção bacteriana do trato urinário e/ou estenose da uretra.

EVOLUÇÃO ESPERADA E PROGNÓSTICO
Em nosso hospital, o tempo médio para a dissolução dos urocistólitos estéreis em gatos foi de 1 mês (variação, de 2 semanas a 5 meses). O tempo médio para a dissolução dos urocistólitos de estruvita induzidos por infecção foi de 10 semanas (variação, 9-12 semanas).

DIVERSOS

DISTÚRBIOS ASSOCIADOS
Qualquer doença que predisponha o animal à infecção bacteriana do trato urinário.

FATORES RELACIONADOS COM A IDADE
Em gatos imaturos, os urólitos de estruvita induzidos por infecção são os mais comuns, enquanto os urólitos estéreis dessa composição mineral são raros.

SINÔNIMO(S)
- Doença urológica felina.
- Doença do trato urinário inferior dos felinos.
- Síndrome urológica felina.

VER TAMBÉM
- Infecção do Trato Urinário Inferior.
- Nefrolitíase.
- Urolitíase por Estruvita — Cães.

Sugestões de Leitura

Osborne CA, Kruger JM, Lulich JP, et al. Feline lower urinary tract diseases. In: Ettinger SJ, Feldman EC, eds., Textbook of Veterinary Internal Medicine, 5th ed. Philadelphia: Saunders, 1999, pp. 1710-1747.

Osborne CA, Lulich JP, Kruger JM, et al. Feline urethral plugs: Etiology and pathophysiology. Vet Clin North Am 1996, 26:233-254.

Osborne CA, Lulich JP, Thumchai R, et al. Diagnosis, medical treatment, and prognosis of feline urolithiasis. Vet Clin North Am 1996, 26:589-628.

Osborne CA, Lulich JP, Thumchai R, et al. Feline urolithiasis: Etiology and pathophysiology. Vet Clin North Am 1996, 26:217-232.

Autores Carl A. Osborne, John M. Kruger, e Jody P. Lulich
Consultor Editorial Carl A. Osborne

Urolitíase por Fosfato de Cálcio

CONSIDERAÇÕES GERAIS

REVISÃO
- Formação de urólitos de fosfato de cálcio no trato urinário e condições clínicas associadas.
- Os urólitos de fosfato de cálcio representam <0,5% dos urólitos de cães e gatos enviados à análise laboratorial no Centro de Análise de Urólitos de Minnesota.
- Os urólitos de fosfato de cálcio costumam ser chamados urólitos de apatita.
- Hidroxiapatita é a forma mais comum, seguida por bruxita (fosfato de cálcio di-idratado). Carbonato de apatita, whitlockite (fosfato tricálcico) e fosfato de ortocálcio são incomuns.
- Nos rins, é encontrada uma porcentagem maior de urólitos de fosfato de cálcio em comparação à bexiga.
- Os urólitos de fosfato de cálcio, excluindo a bruxita, não possuem um formato característico. Já os urólitos de bruxita são tipicamente arredondados e lisos.
- A coloração dos urólitos de fosfato de cálcio costuma ser creme ou castanha. Os coágulos sanguíneos mineralizados com fosfato de cálcio são tipicamente pretos.

IDENTIFICAÇÃO
- Cães e gatos. • Raramente detectada em animais com menos de 1 ano de idade. • Não há outras tendências distinguíveis em relação a fatores como raça, idade e sexo em cães ou gatos.

SINAIS CLÍNICOS
- Dependem da localização, do tamanho e da quantidade de urólitos.
- Alguns pacientes apresentam-se assintomáticos.
- Tipicamente, ocorrem polaciúria, disúria, hematúria e obstrução uretral.
- Os animais com nefroureterólitos costumam permanecer assintomáticos, mas podem exibir hematúria persistente ou sinais atribuíveis à insuficiência renal concomitante (principalmente os gatos).

CAUSAS E FATORES DE RISCO
- Fosfato de cálcio — costuma ser um componente secundário dos urólitos de estruvita e oxalato de cálcio.
- Urólitos puros de fosfato de cálcio — estão associados geralmente a distúrbios metabólicos, como hiperparatireoidismo primário, acidose tubular renal, bem como excesso de cálcio e fósforo na dieta.
- Os nefrólitos, os urocistólitos e os uretrólitos constituídos de coágulos sanguíneos mineralizados com fosfato de cálcio sugerem mineralização tecidual distrófica, em contraste com mineralização metastática, que reflete o metabolismo anormal de cálcio e fósforo.
- Outros fatores de risco incluem concentração urinária, suplementos à base de vitamina D, hipercalciúria, suplementação mineral e urina alcalina (hidroxiapatita e carbonato de apatita).

DIAGNÓSTICO

DIAGNÓSTICO DIFERENCIAL
- Outras causas comuns de hematúria, disúria e polaciúria, com ou sem obstrução uretral, englobam infecção e neoplasia, ambas do trato urinário.
- O fosfato amônio de magnésio, o oxalato de cálcio, a cistina e a sílica constituem outros urólitos radiopacos.
- A mineralização metastática ou distrófica do parênquima do trato urinário pode se assemelhar aos urólitos.

HEMOGRAMA/BIOQUÍMICA/URINÁLISE
- Em geral, os resultados não são dignos de nota.
- Raramente se detectam anormalidades como hipercalcemia ou azotemia; em alguns animais com obstrução completa do fluxo urinário, observa-se azotemia pós-renal.
- A análise do sedimento urinário revela a presença de cristais amorfos em alguns pacientes; as bruxitas (fosfato de cálcio di-idratado) correspondem a cristais alongados, retangulares e em formato de ripa de madeira.

OUTROS TESTES LABORATORIAIS
- É necessária a análise quantitativa dos urólitos recuperados para confirmar a composição mineral.
- As concentrações séricas do paratormônio, do peptídeo relacionado ao paratormônio e do hidroxicolecalciferol podem ajudar no estabelecimento das causas subjacentes.

DIAGNÓSTICO POR IMAGEM
- Os urólitos de fosfato de cálcio são radiopacos e, frequentemente, detectados por meio de radiografias simples.
- A ultrassonografia pode detectar os urólitos de fosfato de cálcio.

OUTROS MÉTODOS DIAGNÓSTICOS
A detecção dos urólitos de fosfato de cálcio na uretra e na bexiga pode ser feita por cistoscopia.

TRATAMENTO
- A dissolução clínica dos urólitos de fosfato de cálcio permanece uma meta para o futuro.
- Considerar a remoção cirúrgica de urólitos do trato urinário inferior que não podem ser removidos por procedimentos minimamente invasivos (p. ex., uro-hidropropulsão miccional, recuperação com instrumento endoscópico em forma de cesta, litotripsia intracorpórea, cistotomia laparoscópica).
- Evitar a realização de uretrostomias desfigurantes, fazendo uso de uro-hidropropulsão retrógrada para conduzir os uretrólitos em direção à bexiga ou de litotripsia para fragmentar os uretrólitos.
- O procedimento de litotripsia por ondas de choque é uma alternativa à realização de cirurgia para remoção de nefrólitos, ureterólitos e urocistólitos em cães.
- A correção do hiperparatireoidismo ou de outras causas de hipercalcemia deve minimizar a nova formação de urólitos.

MEDICAÇÕES

MEDICAMENTO(S)
Não há medicamentos eficazes disponíveis para a dissolução dos urólitos de fosfato de cálcio.

CONTRAINDICAÇÕES/INTERAÇÕES POSSÍVEIS
N/D.

ACOMPANHAMENTO

MONITORIZAÇÃO DO PACIENTE
- É uma prática-padrão obter radiografias após a cirurgia para verificar a remoção completa do urólito.
- Realizar radiografias ou ultrassonografias abdominais a cada 3-5 meses para aumentar a detecção precoce da recidiva de urólitos e evitar a necessidade de repetição da cirurgia.
- Os urólitos pequenos são removidos com facilidade por meio da uro-hidropropulsão miccional ou da cateterização.

PREVENÇÃO
- Uma ração enlatada (ou seja, com alto teor de umidade) formulada para evitar a formação dos urólitos de fosfato de cálcio pode ajudar na prevenção da recidiva.
- A Prescription Diet Canine U/D (Produto da Hills para pequenos animais) é formulada para reduzir a excreção de cálcio, possui níveis restritos de fósforo e diminui a formação de urina concentrada.
- Em virtude do alto teor de umidade dos alimentos enlatados e de sua tendência em promover a diluição da urina, as rações enlatadas são mais eficazes do que as secas na prevenção da recidiva.
- Evitar a acidificação ou alcalinização excessiva da urina.

DIVERSOS

SINÔNIMO(S)
Urólitos de apatita.

Sugestões de Leitura
Kruger JM, Osborne CA, Lulich JP. Canine calcium oxalate uroliths: Etiopathogenesis, diagnosis, management. Vet Clin North Am Small Anim Pract 1999, 29:141-159.
Lulich JP, Osborne CA, Bartges JW, et al. Canine lower urinary tract disorders. In: Ettinger S, Feldman EC, eds., Textbook of Veterinary Internal Medicine, 5th ed. Philadelphia: Saunders, 2000, pp. 1747-1781.
Osborne CA, Lulich JP, Kruger JM, et al. Canine calcium phosphate uroliths: Causes, detection, and prevention. In: Hand MS, Thatcher CD, Remillard RL, Roudebush P, Novotny BJ, eds., Small Animal Clinical Nutrition, 5th ed. Topeka, KS: Mark Morris Institute, 2010, pp. 871-880.

Autores Hasan Albasan, Jody P. Lulich, e Carl A. Osborne
Consultor Editorial Carl A. Osborne

Urolitíase por Oxalato de Cálcio

CONSIDERAÇÕES GERAIS

DEFINIÇÃO
Corresponde à formação de urólitos de oxalato de cálcio no trato urinário e distúrbios clínicos associados.

FISIOPATOLOGIA
Presença de hipercalciúria, hiperoxalúria, hipocitratúria e deficiência de inibidores do crescimento de cristais.

Hipercalciúria
Em cães, acredita-se que a hipercalciúria normocalcêmica resulte da hiperabsorção intestinal de cálcio (assim denominada hipercalciúria absortiva: tipo 1 — independente da dieta; tipo 2 — dependente da dieta; e tipo 3 — hipervitaminose D induzida por fosfatúria) ou da reabsorção tubular renal reduzida de cálcio (assim denominada hipercalciúria por escoamento renal). A hipercalciúria hipercalcêmica origina-se da filtração glomerular excessiva de cálcio mobilizado, o qual supera os mecanismos reabsortivos tubulares renais normais (assim denominada hipercalciúria reabsortiva, por haver reabsorção óssea demasiada associada a concentrações séricas elevadas de cálcio).

Hiperoxalúria
Em seres humanos, a hiperoxalúria é vinculada a anormalidades hereditárias de síntese excessiva de oxalato (i. e., hiperoxalúria primária), consumo exagerado de alimentos contendo altas quantidades de oxalato ou de precursores desse sal, deficiência de piridoxina e distúrbios associados à má absorção de lipídios. A falta de bactérias responsáveis pela degradação de oxalato no intestino pode aumentar a quantidade absorvida desse sal a partir da dieta e a quantidade excretada na urina.

Hipocitratúria
O citrato urinário inibe a formação dos urólitos de oxalato de cálcio. Em virtude da formação de complexos com íons de cálcio para compor o sal de citrato de cálcio relativamente solúvel, o citrato diminui a quantidade de cálcio disponível para se ligar ao oxalato. Em cães normais, a acidose é associada a uma baixa excreção urinária de citrato, enquanto a alcalose promove a excreção desse sal na urina.

Deficiência de Inibidores do Crescimento de Cristais
Além da concentração urinária de minerais calculogênicos, as proteínas de alto peso molecular na urina, como a nefrocalcina e a osteopontina, possuem enorme capacidade de acentuar a solubilidade do oxalato de cálcio. Estudos preliminares da urina coletada de cães com urólitos de oxalato de cálcio revelaram que a nefrocalcina possuía menos resíduos de ácido carboxiglutâmico, em comparação à nefrocalcina isolada da urina de cães normais.

Fornecimento de Dietas Promotoras da Acidificação Urinária
Estudos epidemiológicos relatam que as dietas elaboradas para promover acidúria constituem um fator de risco comum em gatos. Em diversas espécies, a urina ácida é associada à hipercalciúria (mobilização óssea, aumento na filtração de cálcio, diminuição na reabsorção tubular renal) e hipocitratúria (aumento na reabsorção tubular renal).

SISTEMA(S) ACOMETIDO(S)
Renal/urológico.

INCIDÊNCIA/PREVALÊNCIA
Em cães, o oxalato de cálcio responde por aproximadamente 41% dos urólitos removidos do trato urinário inferior e por 45% daqueles removidos do trato urinário superior. Em gatos, o oxalato de cálcio representa cerca de 40% dos urólitos removidos do trato urinário inferior e 70% daqueles coletados do trato urinário superior.

DISTRIBUIÇÃO GEOGRÁFICA
Ubíqua.

IDENTIFICAÇÃO
Espécies
Cães e gatos.

Raça(s) Predominante(s)
- Cães — descrita em muitas raças. Seis raças representam 60% dos casos: Schnauzer miniatura, Lhasa apso, Yorkshire terrier, Bichon frisé, Shih tzu e Poodle miniatura.
- Gatos — Himalaio, Fold escocês, Persa, Ragdoll e Birmanês estão sob maior risco.

Idade Média e Faixa Etária
- Cães — 8,5 ± 3 anos; 60%, 6-11 anos.
- Gatos — 97%, >2 anos; 53%, 7-15 anos.

Sexo Predominante
Acomete principalmente machos caninos (73%) e machos felinos (55%).

SINAIS CLÍNICOS
Comentários Gerais
- Alguns animais apresentam-se assintomáticos.
- Dependem da localização, do tamanho e da quantidade de urólitos.
- Os animais com nefrólitos permanecem tipicamente assintomáticos, mas podem exibir hematúria persistente.
- Em gatos com insuficiência renal crônica, ocorre frequentemente obstrução ureteral associada à alteração microrrenal contralateral, hidronefrose ipsolateral e início agudo de uremia.

Achados Anamnésicos
- Os sinais típicos de urocistólitos ou uretrólitos incluem polaciúria, disúria e hematúria.
- Os nefroureterólitos são comuns em gatos com insuficiência renal crônica.

Achados do Exame Físico
- Detecção dos urocistólitos por meio de palpação abdominal ou uretral; a ausência de urólitos à palpação não exclui a presença deles.
- Aumento de volume da bexiga urinária em casos de obstrução uretral completa (mais comum em gatos).
- Os urocistólitos com contornos irregulares não costumam causar obstrução uretral completa.

CAUSAS
Ver a seção "Fisiopatologia".

FATORES DE RISCO
- Fornecimento de suplementos de cálcio por via oral, independentemente das refeições.
- O excesso de proteína e vitamina D na dieta promove hipercalciúria.
- A adição de oxalato (p. ex., chocolate e amendoim) e ácido ascórbico na dieta favorece a hiperoxalúria.
- A exposição exógena ou endógena a uma concentração elevada de glicocorticoides, o oferecimento de dietas promotoras da formação de urina ácida e a administração de furosemida provocam hipercalciúria.
- As dietas com deficiência de piridoxina ([vitamina B_6], como comida caseira) geram hiperoxalúria.
- O consumo de rações secas está associado a um risco mais alto de formação de urólito de oxalato de cálcio, em comparação às dietas enlatadas de alto teor de umidade.

DIAGNÓSTICO

DIAGNÓSTICO DIFERENCIAL
- Outras causas comuns de hematúria, disúria e polaciúria, com ou sem obstrução uretral, incluem infecção e neoplasia, ambas do trato urinário, além de doença idiopática do trato urinário inferior dos felinos.
- Outros urólitos radiopacos usuais englobam aqueles compostos de fosfato amônio-magnésio, fosfato de cálcio, cistina e sílica (cães).

HEMOGRAMA/BIOQUÍMICA/URINÁLISE
- Os resultados não costumam ser dignos de nota.
- A avaliação do sedimento urinário pode revelar cristais de oxalato de cálcio, mas a ausência de cristalúria não exclui a possibilidade da existência de urólitos.
- Hipercalcemia ou azotemia (raros em cães, porém mais comuns em gatos).

OUTROS TESTES LABORATORIAIS
Análise mineral quantitativa de urólitos.

DIAGNÓSTICO POR IMAGEM
- Os urólitos de oxalato de cálcio com >3 mm de diâmetro são radiopacos e facilmente detectados por meio de radiografia simples.
- Para verificar a presença de obstrução ureteral, há necessidade dos exames de urografia intravenosa, pielografia contrastada ou ultrassonografia.

TRATAMENTO

CUIDADO(S) DE SAÚDE ADEQUADO(S)
- Em um esquema ambulatorial, pode-se efetuar a uro-hidropropulsão retrógrada para impulsionar os cálculos uretrais de volta à bexiga urinária ou a uro-hidropropulsão miccional e recuperação em cesto com cateterização para remover os cálculos vesicais pequenos. A uro-hidropropulsão miccional é contraindicada em pacientes com obstrução uretral.
- A litotripsia a laser, a litotripsia por ondas de choque e a intervenção cirúrgica exigem breves períodos de internação.

ATIVIDADE
Reduzida durante o período de reparo tecidual após a cirurgia.

DIETA
- Não há relatos de dissolução dos urólitos de oxalato de cálcio com o emprego de dietas especiais. Estudos epidemiológicos apoiam o fornecimento de rações úmidas que promovam a formação de urina menos ácida (pH >6,3) para minimizar a formação de oxalato de cálcio.
- Algumas vezes, a hipercalcemia em gatos sem indícios de hiperparatireoidismo ou malignidade é

UROLITÍASE POR OXALATO DE CÁLCIO

minimizada pelo uso da Hill's Prescription Diet Feline w/d.

ORIENTAÇÃO AO PROPRIETÁRIO
- A remoção dos urólitos não altera os fatores responsáveis por sua formação; é necessário eliminar ou minimizar os fatores de risco para diminuir a recidiva.
- Cerca de 50% dos cães com concentração sérica normal de cálcio formam os urólitos novamente dentro de 2 anos.
- Os pacientes com hipercalcemia tipicamente apresentam recidiva dos urólitos em velocidade muito mais rápida que os outros.

CONSIDERAÇÕES CIRÚRGICAS
- Considerar a remoção cirúrgica dos urólitos de pacientes no trato urinário inferior caso não se consiga removê-los por meio de procedimentos minimamente invasivos (p. ex., uro-hidropropulsão miccional, recuperação em cesto com cateterização, litotripsia intracórporea, cistotomia laparoscópica, minicistotomia assistida por cistoscopia).
- Evitar a realização de uretrostomias desfigurantes, utilizando a uro-hidropropulsão retrógrada para impulsionar os uretrólitos em direção à bexiga urinária ou fazendo uso da litotripsia para fragmentar os uretrólitos.
- A litotripsia por ondas de choque constitui tratamento alternativo à cirurgia para a remoção de nefrólitos, ureterólitos e cálculos vesicais em cães.
- Contemplar a realização de paratireoidectomia em pacientes com hiperparatireoidismo primário e hipercalcemia.
- Para minimizar a nova formação de urólitos sobre o ninho da sutura, utilizar padrões de sutura que minimizem sua exposição no lúmen da bexiga urinária.

MEDICAÇÕES
MEDICAMENTO(S) DE ESCOLHA
Não existem medicamentos disponíveis que promovam a dissolução dos urólitos de oxalato de cálcio com eficácia.

PRECAUÇÕES
Os esteroides e a furosemida promovem calciúria.

ACOMPANHAMENTO
MONITORIZAÇÃO DO PACIENTE
- As radiografias pós-cirúrgicas são essenciais para verificar a remoção completa do urólito.
- Para evitar a necessidade de repetição da cirurgia, devem-se avaliar as radiografias abdominais a cada 3-5 meses a fim de se detectar precocemente a recidiva do urólito. Os urólitos pequenos são removidos com facilidade por meio da uro-hidropropulsão miccional ou por recuperação em cesto com cateterização.

PREVENÇÃO
- Se o paciente estiver hipercalcêmico, deve-se corrigir a causa subjacente. Considerar o fornecimento da ração Prescription Diet w/d para os gatos com hipercalciúria idiopática; administrar citrato de potássio para minimizar a acidúria.
- Se o paciente estiver normocalcêmico, deve-se considerar o emprego de uma dieta com teores reduzidos de oxalato e de proteína que não promova a formação de urina ácida (Hill's Prescription Diet Canine u/d; há diversas dietas disponíveis no mercado para gatos; no entanto, não foram realizados estudos que comprovem sua eficácia). Idealmente, a dieta deve conter uma quantidade adicional de água (rações enlatadas) e citrato, além de ter níveis adequados de fósforo e magnésio. Evitar a suplementação com as vitaminas C e D.
- Reavaliar o paciente 2-4 semanas após o início da dieta terapêutica para verificar a diluição apropriada da urina (densidade <1,020 para cães e <1,030 para gatos), o pH adequado da urina (≥6,5) e a melhora da cristalúria. Não se devem utilizar amostras urinárias coletadas ou armazenadas de forma inapropriada (p. ex., urina coletada pelos proprietários, refrigerada ou contaminada com debris) para monitorizar a eficácia terapêutica. Para promover a formação de urina menos concentrada, deve-se considerar o uso de rações enlatadas ou a adição de água em todos os tipos de alimento. Se a urina estiver ácida, deve-se pensar na adição de citrato de potássio (75 mg/kg VO a cada 12 h); ajustar a dosagem para se atingir o pH entre 6,5 e 7,5. A vitamina B_6 (2-4 mg/kg VO a cada 24-48 h) pode ajudar a minimizar a excreção de oxalato, especialmente em animais alimentados com dietas caseiras ou deficientes em piridoxina.
- *Oxalobacter formigenes* é uma bactéria intestinal que ingere o oxalato como seu único nutriente. Por metabolizar o oxalato da dieta no intestino, uma menor quantidade de ácido oxálico fica disponível para absorção, diminuindo o volume desse sal excretado na urina. Para preservar as populações saudáveis de *Oxalobacter* intestinal, deve-se evitar o uso prolongado ou indiscriminado de antimicrobianos.

COMPLICAÇÕES POSSÍVEIS
- Os urocistólitos podem passar pela uretra e obstruí-la em cães e gatos machos, particularmente se o paciente estiver sofrendo com disúria.
- Os cães que não consomem suas necessidades diárias da dieta de prevenção dos urólitos podem desenvolver graus variados de desnutrição calórica e proteica.
- Em alguns pacientes, desenvolve-se hiperlipidemia associada à dieta. Os cães da raça Schnauzer miniatura com hiperlipidemia hereditária são predispostos à pancreatite ao consumir a dieta de prevenção; nesse caso, pode-se utilizar a Hill's Prescription Diet Canine w/d como alternativa. Essa dieta deve ser suplementada com citrato de potássio, conforme a necessidade, para manter o pH urinário entre 6,5 e 7,5.

EVOLUÇÃO ESPERADA E PROGNÓSTICO
- Cerca de 50% dos cães com concentração sérica normal de cálcio apresentam recidiva na formação dos urólitos em 2 anos. O tratamento para minimizar as recidivas é útil. Os pacientes com hipercalcemia persistente tipicamente exibem nova formação de urólitos em uma velocidade mais rápida.
- Pelo menos 10% dos gatos apresentam recidiva dos cálculos em 2 anos.

DIVERSOS
DISTÚRBIOS ASSOCIADOS
Qualquer condição que predisponha o animal à hipercalciúria (p. ex., hiperadrenocorticismo, acidemia, hipervitaminose D e hiperparatireoidismo) ou hiperoxalúria (p. ex., deficiência de vitamina B_6, hiperoxalúria hereditária, bem como ingestão de chocolate e amendoim).

FATORES RELACIONADOS COM A IDADE
Rara em animais jovens (com <1 ano de idade).

GESTAÇÃO/FERTILIDADE/REPRODUÇÃO
O uso de dietas para evitar a formação de urólitos de oxalato de cálcio não é apropriado em animais prenhes.

SINÔNIMO(S)
Urolitíase por oxalato.

VER TAMBÉM
Cristalúria.

Sugestões de Leitura

Appel S, Lefebvre SL, Houston DM, et. al. Evaluation of risk factors associated with suture-nidus cystoliths in dogs and cats. JAVMA 2008, 233;1889-1895.

Kyles AE, Hardie EM, Wooden BG, et al. Management and outcome of cats with ureteral obstruction: 153 cases (1984-2002). JAVMA 2005, 226:937-944.

Lulich JP, Adams LG, Grant D, et. al. Changing paradigms in the treatment of uroliths by lithotripsy. Vet Clin North Am Small Anim Pract 2009, 39:143-160.

Lulich JP, Osborne CA. Upper tract urolith: Questions, answers, questions. In: August JR, ed., Consultations in Feline Internal Medicine, Volume 5. St. Louis: Elsevier Saunders, 2006, pp. 399-406.

Lulich JP, Osborne CA, Thumchai R, et al. Management of canine calcium oxalate urolith recurrence. Compend Contin Educ Pract Vet 1998, 20:178-189.

Lulich JP, Osborne CA, Sanderson SL, et al. Voiding urohydropropulsion: Lessons from 5 years of experience. Vet Clin North Am 1999, 29:283-292.

Autores Jody P. Lulich e Carl A. Osborne
Consultor Editorial Carl A. Osborne

Urolitíase por Urato

CONSIDERAÇÕES GERAIS

DEFINIÇÃO
Urólitos compostos de ácido úrico, urato de sódio ou urato de amônio.

FISIOPATOLOGIA
• A diminuição na conversão do ácido úrico em alantoína gera alta concentração sérica e urinária do ácido úrico.
• Os pacientes com desvio portossistêmico podem desenvolver urólitos de urato de amônio em virtude do dano ao metabolismo do ácido úrico e da amônia.

GENÉTICA
Os cães da raça Dálmata apresentam predisposição racial à formação da urolitíase por urato.

INCIDÊNCIA/PREVALÊNCIA
Corresponde a aproximadamente 5-8% dos urólitos recuperados de cães e gatos.

IDENTIFICAÇÃO
Espécies
Cães e gatos.

Raça(s) Predominante(s)
Dálmata, Buldogue inglês e raças sob risco de ter desvio portossistêmico (p. ex., Yorkshire terrier).

Idade Média e Faixa Etária
• A idade média em pacientes sem desvios portossistêmicos é de 3 anos e meio (faixa, 0,5 a >10 anos).
• A idade média em pacientes com desvios portossistêmicos é <1 ano (faixa, 0,1 a >10 anos).

Sexo Predominante
• Mais comum em cães machos sem desvios portossistêmicos.
• Em cães com desvios portossistêmicos ou gatos, não há predileção sexual.

SINAIS CLÍNICOS
Achados Anamnésicos
Hematúria, disúria, polaciúria. Possível encefalopatia hepática em pacientes com desvios portossistêmicos.

Achados do Exame Físico
• Obstrução uretral.
• Alguns pacientes apresentam-se assintomáticos.

CAUSAS
Descartar desvio portossistêmico.

FATORES DE RISCO
• Consumo elevado de purina (carne glandular).
• Acidúria persistente em animais predispostos.

DIAGNÓSTICO

DIAGNÓSTICO DIFERENCIAL
Outras causas de doença do trato urinário inferior ou superior.

HEMOGRAMA/BIOQUÍMICA/URINÁLISE
• Acidúria, cristalúria por urato, azotemia em pacientes com obstrução do fluxo urinário.
• Baixos níveis de ureia em pacientes com desvio portossistêmico.

OUTROS TESTES LABORATORIAIS
Provas de função hepática, como mensuração dos ácidos biliares, revelam resultados anormais em pacientes com desvios portossistêmicos.

DIAGNÓSTICO POR IMAGEM
• Os urólitos de urato podem ser radiotransparentes; talvez haja necessidade da realização de pielograma intravenoso para detectar os nefrólitos ou de cistografia com duplo contraste para detectar os urocistólitos. Micro-hepatia em pacientes com desvios portossistêmicos.
• A ultrassonografia pode revelar urólitos pequenos e desvios portossistêmicos.

MÉTODOS DIAGNÓSTICOS
Biopsia hepática; mensuração dos ácidos biliares e da amônia sanguínea.

ACHADOS PATOLÓGICOS
Em pacientes com desvios portossistêmicos, a biopsia hepática pode revelar atrofia e/ou displasia.

TRATAMENTO

CUIDADO(S) DE SAÚDE ADEQUADO(S)
Em casos de obstrução uretral ou ureteral, pode ser imprescindível a internação do paciente. Os urólitos de urato podem ser dissolvidos em um esquema ambulatorial.

CUIDADO(S) DE ENFERMAGEM
Fluidoterapia para corrigir a desidratação.

ATIVIDADE
Geralmente sem restrições, exceto em período pós-cirúrgico.

DIETA
Para a dissolução e a prevenção, fica indicado o fornecimento de dieta alcalinizante urinária com baixos teores de purina e altos teores de umidade.

ORIENTAÇÃO AO PROPRIETÁRIO
A recidiva dos urólitos é possível. Portanto, há necessidade da elaboração de algum plano para minimizar a recidiva.

CONSIDERAÇÕES CIRÚRGICAS
• Cistotomia, uretrotomia ou nefrotomia para a remoção dos urólitos.
• Ligadura do desvio portossistêmico.

MEDICAÇÕES

MEDICAMENTO(S)
Para a dissolução dos urólitos, emprega-se o alopurinol (15 mg/kg VO a cada 12 h), um inibidor da xantina oxidase (ver Fig. 2).

CONTRAINDICAÇÕES
Os glicocorticoides e outros agentes imunossupressores podem promover hiperuricosúria.

PRECAUÇÕES
Além de ser contraindicado em pacientes com insuficiência renal, o alopurinol não é eficaz em animais com desvios portossistêmicos.

INTERAÇÕES POSSÍVEIS
Ocorrência de erupções cutâneas com o uso de alopurinol e ampicilina.

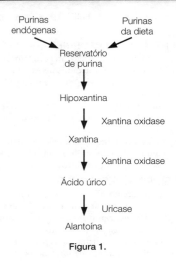

Figura 1.

ACOMPANHAMENTO

MONITORIZAÇÃO DO PACIENTE
Ver Figura 3.

PREVENÇÃO
Dieta alcalinizante urinária com baixos teores de purina e altos teores de umidade.

COMPLICAÇÕES POSSÍVEIS
• Obstrução uretral.
• Na falta de medidas preventivas, torna-se provável a recidiva dos urólitos.

EVOLUÇÃO ESPERADA E PROGNÓSTICO
• A dissolução clínica leva, em média, 4 semanas em caso de obediência satisfatória ao tratamento.
• No entanto, a dissolução clínica não costuma ser bem-sucedida em casos de desvio portossistêmico.

DIVERSOS

DISTÚRBIOS ASSOCIADOS
Desvio portossistêmico.

GESTAÇÃO/FERTILIDADE/REPRODUÇÃO
Em animais prenhes ou lactantes, não se recomenda o fornecimento de dietas hipoproteicas (i. e., com baixos níveis de proteína/purina).

Sugestões de Leitura
Bartges JW, Osborne CA, Felice LJ. Canine xanthine uroliths: Risk factor management. In: Kirk RW, Bonagura JD, eds., Current Veterinary Therapy XI. Philadelphia: Saunders, 1992, pp. 900-905.
Osborne CA, Lulich JP, Thumchai R, et al. Diagnosis, medical treatment, and prognosis of feline urolithiasis. Vet Clin North Am Small Anim Pract 1996, 26: 589-628.

Autor Joseph W. Bartges
Consultor Editorial Carl A. Osborne

Urolitíase por Urato

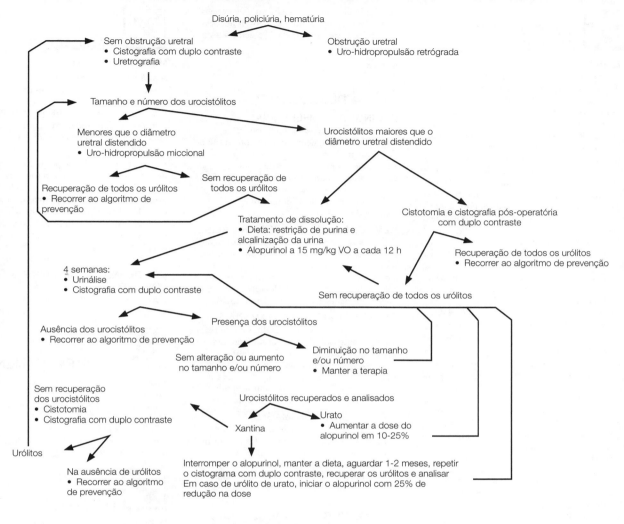

Figura 2. Algoritmo para o tratamento de urocistolitíase por urato.

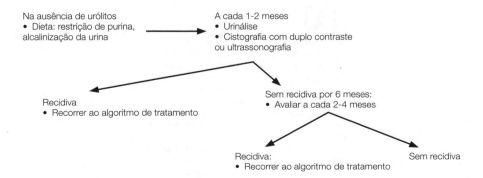

Figura 3. Algoritmo para a prevenção de urocistolitíase por urato.

Urolitíase por Xantina

CONSIDERAÇÕES GERAIS

REVISÃO
- A xantina, um produto de degradação do metabolismo da purina, é convertida em ácido úrico pela enzima xantina oxidase. O dano espontâneo (deficiência enzimática) ou induzido por medicamentos (alopurinol) à xantina oxidase acaba resultando em hiperxantinemia e xantinúria.
- Em casos de xantinúria de ocorrência espontânea, é provável a existência de defeito familiar ou congênito na atividade da xantina oxidase. Em gatos (quantidade = 75), ainda não se identificou uma predisposição racial. Em cães da raça Cavalier King Charles spaniel, postula-se a ocorrência de um modo de herança autossômico recessivo.
- Em cães, a xantinúria adquirida representa uma complicação comum do tratamento da urolitíase por urato ou da leishmaniose com alopurinol. O consumo de dietas com altos teores de purina aumenta o risco de xantinúria em pacientes tratados com alopurinol.
- Como a xantina é a forma menos solúvel das purinas excretadas na urina, a xantinúria pode estar associada à formação de urólitos de xantina.

IDENTIFICAÇÃO
- Cães e gatos. A xantinúria de ocorrência espontânea costuma ser mais observada em gatos do que em cães.
- Em cães, a xantinúria induzida pelo alopurinol pode comprometer qualquer raça, idade ou sexo. Em cães jovens da raça Cavalier King Charles spaniel, observam-se xantinúria de ocorrência espontânea e urólitos de xantina.
- Em gatos, os urólitos de xantina acometem principalmente machos e fêmeas adultos (idade média no momento do diagnóstico = 2,9 anos; faixa = de 4 meses a 12 anos). Tais urólitos são identificados com maior frequência nas raças domésticas felinas de pelo curto e nas de pelo longo.

SINAIS CLÍNICOS
- Os sinais clínicos dependem da localização, do tamanho e da quantidade de urólitos. Os animais acometidos podem permanecer assintomáticos.
- Os sinais típicos de urocistólitos incluem polaciúria, disúria e hematúria.
- Os sinais característicos de uretrólitos englobam polaciúria, disúria e, ocasionalmente, eliminação de pequenos urólitos lisos de coloração amarela. A obstrução completa do fluxo urinário pode resultar em uremia pós-renal.
- Os nefrólitos são tipicamente assintomáticos, mas podem estar associados a manifestações de hidronefrose e insuficiência renal.

CAUSAS E FATORES DE RISCO
- A xantinúria constitui um fator de risco para a formação de urolitíase por xantina.
- A predisposição racial canina pode incluir o Cavalier King Charles spaniel.
- Em gatos jovens e adultos (meia-idade) com histórico prévio de urolitíase por xantina, os urólitos frequentemente apresentam recidivas dentro de 3 a 12 meses após sua remoção a menos que se institua uma terapia profilática.
- A formação de urólitos é acentuada por alguns fatores, como: pH urinário ácido, urina altamente concentrada, micção parcial e pouco frequente.
- Em animais submetidos a quantidades excessivas de alopurinol, a xantinúria é intensificada pela falha na restrição apropriada de precursores de purina na dieta.

DIAGNÓSTICO

DIAGNÓSTICO DIFERENCIAL
- Os urólitos mimetizam outras causas de polaciúria, disúria, hematúria e/ou obstrução do fluxo urinário.
- Diferenciar de outros tipos de urólitos, especialmente urato de amônio, por meio dos exames de urinálise, radiografia e análise quantitativa de urólitos eliminados ou recuperados.

HEMOGRAMA/BIOQUÍMICA/URINÁLISE
A microscopia óptica não é capaz de distinguir entre os cristais de xantina no sedimento urinário muitas formas de urato de amônio ou urato amorfo. Todos esses cristais costumam ser de coloração castanha ou amarelo-acastanhada e podem formar esférulas de tamanho variado.

OUTROS TESTES LABORATORIAIS
- Para a diferenciação entre urólitos de xantina e urólitos compostos de urato de amônio, urato de sódio e ácido úrico, é necessária a realização de espectroscopia por infravermelho.
- Para a detecção de xantina, hipoxantina e de outros metabólitos da purina, a urina é submetida à cromatografia líquida de alta pressão.

DIAGNÓSTICO POR IMAGEM
- Radiografia — a radiodensidade dos urólitos puros de xantina é semelhante à dos tecidos moles; por esse motivo, a detecção por meio de radiografias simples não é confiável.
- Os exames de ultrassonografia, cistografia com duplo contraste e urografia intravenosa auxiliam na detecção dos urólitos e em sua localização.

OUTROS MÉTODOS DIAGNÓSTICOS
- A uretrocistoscopia pode detectar os uretrólitos e os urocistólitos de xantina.
- Pequenos urólitos podem ser recuperados para análise por aspiração via sonda transuretral ou uro-hidropropulsão miccional.

TRATAMENTO
- Ainda não foram desenvolvidos protocolos clínicos que promovam a dissolução consistente dos urólitos de xantina.
- Remoção de urocistólitos pequenos por meio da uro-hidropropulsão miccional.
- A cirurgia continua sendo o método mais confiável na remoção de urólitos ativos maiores, presentes no trato urinário inferior.
- A redução nos fatores de risco da dieta minimiza o crescimento adicional dos urólitos existentes.
- Enquanto se aguarda o resultado de estudos mais avançados, os gatos com urólitos de xantina de ocorrência espontânea devem receber rações enlatadas próprias para insuficiência renal, na tentativa de aumentar o volume urinário, minimizar os precursores de purina e diminuir a formação de urina ácida.
- As uretrostomias perineais podem minimizar a recidiva da obstrução uretral em machos felinos.

MEDICAÇÕES

MEDICAMENTO(S)

Alcalinizantes Urinários
- Considerar em pacientes com urina ácida, apesar da dieta terapêutica.
- Para manter o pH urinário em 7,0-7,5, deve-se fornecer uma quantidade suficiente de citrato de potássio ou bicarbonato de sódio.

Alopurinol
- Ao se tratar a urolitíase por urato em cães, deve-se ajustar a dose do alopurinol de acordo com a magnitude da concentração de ácido úrico na urina e da quantidade de purinas na dieta (ver o capítulo sobre "Urolitíase por Urato").
- Em cães, os urólitos induzidos pelo alopurinol podem sofrer dissolução ao se interromper a terapia com esse agente, ao mesmo tempo em que se mantém a dieta com baixos níveis de purina.

CONTRAINDICAÇÕES/INTERAÇÕES POSSÍVEIS
Não fornecer o alopurinol em cães ou gatos com urólitos de xantina de ocorrência espontânea.

ACOMPANHAMENTO
- Monitorizar a dissolução dos urólitos em intervalos mensais por meio dos exames de urinálise, radiografia contrastada ou ultrassonografia.
- Embora os urólitos de xantina de ocorrência espontânea tenham tendência à recidiva, isso não ocorre em todos os cães e gatos xantinúricos.

DIVERSOS

DISTÚRBIOS ASSOCIADOS
- Urolitíase por urato.
- Nefrolitíase.

VER TAMBÉM
- Cristalúria.
- Urolitíase por Urato.

Sugestões de Leitura
Bartges JW, Osborne CA, Felice LJ. Canine xanthine uroliths: Risk factor management. In: Kirk RW, Bonagura JD, eds., Current Veterinary Therapy XI. Philadelphia: Saunders, 1992, pp. 900-905.
Osborne CA, Lulich JP, Lekcharoensuk C, et al. Feline xanthine urolithiasis: A newly recognized cause of feline lower urinary tract disease. In: Proceedings 21st Annual ACVIM Forum, Charlotte, North Carolina, 2003, pp. 781-782.
Tsuchida S, Kagi A, Koyama H. Xanthine urolithiasis in a cat: A case report and evaluation of a candidate gene for xanthine dehydrogenase. J Feline Med Surg 2007, 9:505-508.

Autores Carl A. Osborne e Joseph W. Bartges
Consultor Editorial Carl A. Osborne

Uveíte Anterior – Cães

CONSIDERAÇÕES GERAIS

DEFINIÇÃO
• Inflamação dos tecidos da úvea anterior, incluindo a íris (irite), o corpo ciliar (ciclite) ou ambos (iridociclite). • Pode estar associada à inflamação concomitante da úvea posterior e da retina (coroidite; coriorretinite). • Pode ser uni ou bilateral.

FISIOPATOLOGIA
• O aumento na permeabilidade da barreira hematoaquosa, relacionado com etiologias infecciosas, imunomediadas, traumáticas ou outras causas, permite a entrada de proteínas plasmáticas e componentes celulares sanguíneos no humor aquoso. • A ruptura da barreira hematoaquosa é desencadeada e mantida por inúmeros mediadores químicos, como histamina, prostaglandinas, leucotrienos, serotonina, cininas e complemento.

SISTEMA(S) ACOMETIDO(S)
• Oftalmológico. • Outros sistemas também podem ser acometidos pelo processo patológico subjacente.

INCIDÊNCIA/PREVALÊNCIA
• Condição relativamente comum. • A incidência e a prevalência reais não são conhecidas.

DISTRIBUIÇÃO GEOGRÁFICA
A localização geográfica pode influenciar a incidência de certas causas infecciosas de uveíte.

IDENTIFICAÇÃO
Espécies
Cães.

Raça(s) Predominante(s)
• Na maioria das causas, não há predisposição racial. • Uveíte associada a cistos iridociliares em cães da raça Golden retriever (também conhecida como uveíte do Golden retriever). • Alta incidência de síndrome uveodermatológica em cães das raças Husky siberiano, Akita, Samoieda e Pastor de Shetland.

Idade Média e Faixa Etária
• Qualquer idade pode ser acometida. • Idade média em casos de síndrome uveodermatológica — 2,8 anos. • Idade média em uveíte do Golden retriever — 8,6 anos.

SINAIS CLÍNICOS
Achados Anamnésicos
• Olho vermelho — em decorrência de hiperemia conjuntival e rubor ciliar. • Turbidez ocular — em virtude de edema corneano, rubor aquoso, hipópio, etc. • Dor/sensibilidade ocular — manifesta-se por blefarospasmo, fotofobia ou fricção ocular. • Perda da visão — variável.

Achados do Exame Físico
A importância do exame físico completo em cães com uveíte não pode ser superestimada.

Achados Oftalmológicos
• Desconforto ocular — manifesta-se por blefarospasmo, fotofobia e fricção ocular.
• Secreção ocular — em geral, serosa; algumas vezes, mucoide a mucopurulenta. • Hiperemia conjuntival — costuma acometer tanto a conjuntiva bulbar como a palpebral. • Edema de córnea — difuso; leve a grave. • Precipitados ceráticos — agregados multifocais de células inflamatórias aderidas ao endotélio corneano; mais notável na porção ventral. • Rubor aquoso e celularidade — turbidez do humor aquoso, em função do aumento no conteúdo proteico e nos debris celulares suspensos; mais bem observada com o auxílio de um feixe luminoso estreito e brilhante, emitido por meio da câmara anterior.
• Rubor ciliar — congestão de vasos ciliares anteriores perilimbais profundos. • Vascularização profunda da córnea — distribuição pericorneana (borda em escova). • Miose e/ou resistência à dilatação farmacológica. • Tumefação da íris.
• PIO reduzida — é compatível com uveíte, mas não constitui um achado constante. • Sinequia posterior — aderências entre a face posterior da íris e a superfície anterior do cristalino. • Presença de fibrina na câmara anterior. • Hipópio ou hifema — acúmulos de leucócitos ou hemácias, respectivamente, na câmara anterior; em geral, esses acúmulos repousam em sentido horizontal na face ventral da câmara, mas podem ser difusos.
• As alterações crônicas podem incluir: rubeose irídica, hiperpigmentação da íris, catarata secundária, luxação do cristalino, afastamento da pupila, íris arqueada, glaucoma secundário e atrofia do globo ocular.

CAUSAS
• Infecciosas — micóticas (*Blastomyces dermatitidis, Cryptococcus neoformans, Coccidiodes immitis, Histoplasma capsulatum*); protozoárias (*Toxoplasma gondii, Neospora caninum, Leishmania donovani*); riquetsianas (*Ehrlichia canis, Rickettsia rickettsii*); bacterianas (*Leptospira* spp., *Bartonella* spp., *Brucella canis, Borrelia burgdorferi*, qualquer septicemia bacteriana); algas (*Prototheca* spp.); virais (adenovírus, cinomose, raiva, herpes); parasitárias (filariase ocular, larva migrans ocular).
• Imunomediadas — reação às proteínas do cristalino (em decorrência de catarata ou traumatismo dessa estrutura ocular); síndrome uveodermatológica; reação pós-vacinal à vacina contra o adenovírus canino; vasculite.
• Neoplásicas — tumores oculares primários (especialmente melanoma uveal, adenoma/adenocarcinoma iridociliar); metástase em direção ao trato uveal (a ocorrência de metástase é mais comum no linfoma).
• Metabólicas — hiperlipidemia; hiperviscosidade; hipertensão sistêmica.
• Diversos — idiopática; traumatismo; uveíte do Golden retriever; ceratite ulcerativa; abscesso do estroma corneano; esclerite; instabilidade/luxação do cristalino; doença dentária/periodontal; toxemia de qualquer causa.

FATORES DE RISCO
Não há fatores específicos; a imunossupressão e a localização geográfica podem aumentar a incidência de certas causas infecciosas de uveíte; predisposições raciais, conforme listadas anteriormente, devem ser consideradas.

DIAGNÓSTICO

DIAGNÓSTICO DIFERENCIAL
• Conjuntivite — a vermelhidão limita-se à hiperemia conjuntival (i. e., sem rubor ciliar); a secreção ocular costuma ser mais espessa e mais abundante do que na uveíte; o desconforto pode ser aliviado pela instilação de anestésicos tópicos.
• Glaucoma — o aumento na PIO é a característica mais compatível dessa doença; outros sinais podem incluir dilatação das pupilas (midríase), estrias de Haab e buftalmia.
• Luxação do cristalino — o edema de córnea pode estar situado no local de contato entre o cristalino e o endotélio ou pode ser difuso em consequência de uveíte e/ou glaucoma associados; a luxação do cristalino é altamente associado à raça.
• Ceratite ulcerativa — a coloração da córnea pela fluoresceína detecta a presença das úlceras; o edema corneano associado às úlceras apresenta-se confinado à região ulcerada ou mostra-se mais grave no local dessa ulceração; a secreção ocular é frequentemente mais espessa e mais abundante do que na uveíte; o desconforto pode ser parcialmente aliviado por meio de anestésicos tópicos.
• Distrofia ou degeneração do endotélio corneano — há edema difuso da córnea, mas a PIO permanece normal; em geral, não há sinais de hiperemia conjuntival e de desconforto ocular.
• Síndrome de Horner — os sinais de miose, enoftalmia e protrusão da membrana nictitante são similares em ambas as condições, mas a síndrome de Horner não exibe dor nem secreção ocular; o quadro de ptose associado à síndrome de Horner distingue-se do blefarospasmo, já que o último processo é mais ativo; uma hiperemia conjuntival secundária pode ser observada na síndrome de Horner, mas tanto a córnea como a câmara anterior apresentam-se translúcidas; os sinais clínicos da síndrome de Horner desaparecem após a aplicação tópica de fenilefrina a 1-10%.

HEMOGRAMA/BIOQUÍMICA/URINÁLISE
Com frequência, permanecem normais; pode haver alterações relacionadas com a doença subjacente.

OUTROS TESTES LABORATORIAIS
• A sorologia em busca das doenças infecciosas listadas na seção "Causas" pode ser pertinente, dependendo do índice de suspeita de etiologia infecciosa.
• Os sinais clínicos que levantam a suspeita de doença sistêmica, como letargia, pirexia, perda de peso, tosse, linfadenopatia, etc., justificam a realização de testes sorológicos para a pesquisa de doenças infecciosas.

DIAGNÓSTICO POR IMAGEM
• Radiografia torácica — pode revelar indícios do processo patológico causal (p. ex., micoses sistêmicas; neoplasia metastática).
• Ultrassonografia abdominal — pode ser justificável em caso de alta suspeita de doença neoplásica metastática.
• Ultrassonografia ocular — indicada se a opacidade dos meios oculares impedir o exame direto; além disso, esse exame pode demonstrar a presença de neoplasia intraocular ou descolamento da retina.

MÉTODOS DIAGNÓSTICOS
• Tonometria — PIO baixa é compatível com uveíte; a elevação na PIO indica a existência de glaucoma (doença primária ou secundária à uveíte).
• Aspirados de linfonodos — na existência de nodos enfartados palpáveis, indica-se a obtenção de aspirado para avaliação citológica.
• Centese (punção) ocular — na ocorrência de descolamento da retina, a citologia de aspirado sub-retiniano poderá revelar os agentes causais; em geral, a centese da câmara anterior é frustrante.

Uveíte Anterior – Cães

ACHADOS PATOLÓGICOS
- Macroscópicos — ver achados do exame físico.
- Histopatológicos — edema de córnea; vascularização periférica do estroma corneano profundo; precipitados ceráticos; membrana fibrovascular pré-iridiana; sinequia anterior periférica; sinequia posterior; entrópio ou ectrópio uveais; acúmulo de leucócitos no corpo ciliar, bem como na íris, esclera e coroide (infiltrados linfocíticos, plasmocitários, supurativos ou granulomatosos, dependendo da etiologia); catarata secundária; com envolvimento do segmento posterior no processo inflamatório; membrana ciclítica; bandas de tração vítrea e descolamento da retina podem estar presentes.

TRATAMENTO

CUIDADO(S) DE SAÚDE ADEQUADO(S)
Em geral, o tratamento do paciente em um esquema ambulatorial é suficiente.

CUIDADO(S) DE ENFERMAGEM
Nenhum.

ATIVIDADE
- Na maioria dos casos, não se indicam quaisquer modificações.
- A diminuição na exposição à luz pode aliviar o desconforto.

DIETA
Não há indicação de mudanças.

ORIENTAÇÃO AO PROPRIETÁRIO
- Instruir acerca das doenças sistêmicas em potencial, indutoras dos sinais oftalmológicos, e enfatizar a importância da realização de testes diagnósticos apropriados.
- Além do tratamento sintomático da uveíte, a terapia da doença subjacente (quando possível) é soberana para a obtenção de um resultado positivo.
- Informar o proprietário sobre as possíveis complicações e salientar a diminuição na probabilidade de complicações pela obediência às recomendações terapêuticas e ao acompanhamento.

CONSIDERAÇÕES CIRÚRGICAS
Ausentes na maioria dos casos. Os casos específicos que necessitam de intervenção cirúrgica compreendem a remoção de cristalinos rompidos, a retirada de cataratas indutoras de uveíte (se o prognóstico for favorável quanto ao êxito da cirurgia) e o tratamento cirúrgico de glaucoma secundário.

MEDICAÇÕES

MEDICAMENTO(S) DE ESCOLHA

Corticosteroides

Tópicos
- Acetato de prednisolona a 1% — aplicar 2-8 vezes ao dia, dependendo da gravidade da doença; reduzir gradativamente o medicamento à medida que a afecção desaparece.
- Dexametasona a 0,1% — aplicar 2-8 vezes ao dia, dependendo da gravidade da doença; diminuir a medicação de forma gradual conforme o problema se resolve.
- Outros corticosteroides tópicos (p. ex., betametasona e hidrocortisona) são consideravelmente menos eficazes no tratamento da inflamação intraocular.
- Diminuir gradualmente a frequência do tratamento em algumas semanas, conforme se observa a melhora da condição; a interrupção abrupta dos corticosteroides tópicos pode resultar no efeito rebote da inflamação ocular.

Subconjuntivais
- Acetonida de triancinolona — 4-6 mg por meio de injeção subconjuntival.
- Metilprednisolona — 3-10 mg por meio de injeção subconjuntival.
- Muitas vezes, não são necessários.
- Indicados somente nos casos graves em uma única aplicação, seguida por anti-inflamatórios tópicos e/ou sistêmicos.

Sistêmicos
- Prednisona — 0,5-2,2 mg/kg/dia inicialmente; reduzir de modo gradativo a dose após 7-10 dias.
- Utilizar apenas se as causas infecciosas sistêmicas de uveíte tiverem sido descartadas.

Medicamentos Anti-inflamatórios Não Esteroides (AINE)

Tópicos
- Menos eficazes do que os corticosteroides tópicos.
- Flurbiprofeno — aplicar 2-4 vezes ao dia, dependendo da gravidade da doença.
- Diclofenaco — aplicar 2-4 vezes ao dia, dependendo da gravidade da doença.

Sistêmicos
- Não utilizar concomitantemente com corticosteroides sistêmicos; evitar na presença de hifema.
- Ácido acetilsalicílico — 10-25 mg/kg VO a cada 12 h.
- Carprofeno — 2,2 mg/kg VO a cada 12 h ou 4,4 mg/kg VO a cada 24 h.
- Tepoxalina — 10 mg/kg VO a cada 24 h.
- Meloxicam — 0,2 mg/kg VO a cada 24 h.

Midriáticos/Cicloplégicos Tópicos
- Sulfato de atropina a 1% — aplicar 1-4 vezes ao dia, dependendo da gravidade da doença. Usar a frequência mais baixa, suficiente para manter a pupila dilatada e o alívio ocular; diminuir gradualmente o medicamento à medida que a afecção desaparece.

CONTRAINDICAÇÕES
- Evitar o uso de medicamentos mióticos (p. ex., pilocarpina e brometo de demecário), inclusive das prostaglandinas tópicas (p. ex., latanoprosta), na presença de uveíte.
- Os corticosteroides tópicos e subconjuntivais são absolutamente contraindicados na existência de ceratite ulcerativa.
- Em cães com hipertensão sistêmica ou infecções sistêmicas, é recomendável evitar o uso dos corticosteroides sistêmicos.

PRECAUÇÕES
Considerando-se a possibilidade de glaucoma secundário, recomendam-se a aplicação tópica criteriosa da atropina e a monitorização periódica da PIO.

INTERAÇÕES POSSÍVEIS
Não é recomendável o uso concomitante dos corticosteroides sistêmicos e dos AINE.

MEDICAMENTO(S) ALTERNATIVO(S)
N/D.

ACOMPANHAMENTO

MONITORIZAÇÃO DO PACIENTE
Reavaliar o paciente em 3-7 dias, dependendo da gravidade da doença. Nessa reavaliação, a PIO deverá ser monitorizada para detectar a presença de glaucoma secundário. A frequência das reavaliações subsequentes é ditada pela gravidade da doença e pela resposta ao tratamento.

PREVENÇÃO
N/D.

COMPLICAÇÕES POSSÍVEIS
- Em decorrência da etiologia sistêmica da uveíte, poderão ocorrer muitas complicações sistêmicas, inclusive o óbito.
- Entre as complicações oftalmológicas, destacam-se: catarata secundária; glaucoma secundário; luxação do cristalino; descolamento da retina; atrofia do bulbo ocular.

EVOLUÇÃO ESPERADA E PROGNÓSTICO
Extremamente variáveis; dependem da doença subjacente e da resposta terapêutica.

DIVERSOS

POTENCIAL ZOONÓTICO
Na maioria dos casos, não há risco zoonótico. Algumas formas de infecção sistêmica indutora de uveíte podem representar um pequeno risco a proprietários imunocomprometidos.

GESTAÇÃO/FERTILIDADE/REPRODUÇÃO
Evitar os corticosteroides sistêmicos. Em virtude da possibilidade de absorção sistêmica, os corticosteroides tópicos também podem representar um risco, particularmente no caso de aplicação frequente em cães de pequeno porte.

SINÔNIMO(S)
Iridociclite.

VER TAMBÉM
Olho Vermelho.

ABREVIATURA(S)
- AINE = anti-inflamatório não esteroide.
- PIO = pressão intraocular.

Sugestões de Leitura
Cullen C, Webb A. Ocular manifestations of systemic diseases. Part 1: The dog. In: Gelatt KN, ed., Veterinary Ophthalmology, 4th ed. Ames, IA: Blackwell, 2007, pp. 1470-1537.
Hendrix D. Diseases and surgery of the canine anterior uvea. In: Gelatt KN, ed., Veterinary Ophthalmology, 4th ed. Ames, IA: Blackwell, 2007, pp. 812-858.
Miller P. Uvea. In: Maggs DJ, Miller PE, Ofri R, Slatter's Fundamentals of Veterinary Ophthalmology, 4th ed. St. Louis: Saunders, 2008, pp. 203-229.

Autor Ian P. Herring
Consultor Editorial Paul E. Miller

UVEÍTE ANTERIOR – GATOS

CONSIDERAÇÕES GERAIS

DEFINIÇÃO
• Inflamação dos tecidos da úvea anterior, incluindo a íris (irite), o corpo ciliar (ciclite) ou ambos (iridociclite). • Pode estar associada à inflamação concomitante da úvea posterior e da retina (coroidite; coriorretinite). • Pode ser unil ou bilateral.

FISIOPATOLOGIA
• O aumento na permeabilidade da barreira hematoaquosa, relacionado com etiologias infecciosas, imunomediadas, neoplásicas, traumáticas ou outras causas, permite a entrada de proteínas plasmáticas e de componentes celulares sanguíneos no humor aquoso. • A ruptura da barreira hematoaquosa é desencadeada e mantida por inúmeros mediadores químicos, como histamina, prostaglandinas, leucotrienos, serotonina, cininas e complemento.

SISTEMA(S) ACOMETIDO(S)
• Oftalmológico. • Outros sistemas também podem ser acometidos pelo processo patológico subjacente.

INCIDÊNCIA/PREVALÊNCIA
• Condição relativamente comum. • A incidência e a prevalência reais não são conhecidas.

DISTRIBUIÇÃO GEOGRÁFICA
A localização geográfica pode influenciar a incidência de certas causas infecciosas de uveíte.

IDENTIFICAÇÃO
Espécies
Gatos.
Idade Média e Faixa Etária
• Idade média — 7-9 anos. • Qualquer idade pode ser acometida.
Sexo(s) Predominante(s)
Os machos intactos/castrados são mais comumente acometidos do que as fêmeas.

SINAIS CLÍNICOS
Achados Anamnésicos
• Turvamento ocular — em virtude de edema corneano, rubor aquoso, hipópio, etc. • Dor/sensibilidade ocular — manifesta-se sob a forma de blefaroespasmo, fotofobia ou fricção ocular; essa dor costuma ser menos pronunciada nos gatos do que nos cães. • Olho vermelho — em decorrência de hiperemia conjuntival e eritema ciliar; na maioria dos casos, é menos intenso do que nos cães. • Perda da visão — variável.
Achados do Exame Físico
A importância do exame físico completo em gatos com uveíte não pode ser superestimada.
Achados Oftalmológicos
• Desconforto ocular — manifesta-se sob a forma de blefaroespasmo e fotofobia. • Secreção ocular — em geral, serosa; algumas vezes, mucoide a mucopurulenta. • Hiperemia conjuntival — costuma acometer tanto a conjuntiva bulbar como a palpebral. • Edema de córnea — difuso; pode ser leve a grave. • Precipitados ceráticos — agregados multifocais de células inflamatórias aderidas ao endotélio corneano; mais notável na porção ventral. • Rubor aquoso e celularidade — turbidez do humor aquoso, em função do aumento no conteúdo proteico e nos debris celulares suspensos; mais bem observada com o auxílio de um feixe luminoso estreito e brilhante, emitido por meio da câmara anterior. • Eritema ciliar — congestão de vasos ciliares anteriores perilimbais profundos. • Vascularização profunda da córnea — distribuição pericorneana (borda em escova). • Miose e/ou resistência à dilatação farmacológica. • Tumefação da íris — pode ser generalizada ou nodular. • PIO reduzida é compatível com uveíte anterior, mas não é um achado uniforme. • Sinequia posterior — aderências entre a face posterior da íris e a superfície anterior do cristalino. • Presença de fibrina na câmara anterior. • Hipópio ou hifema — acúmulos de leucócitos ou hemácias, respectivamente, na câmara anterior; em geral, esses acúmulos se assentam no sentido horizontal na face ventral da câmara, mas podem ser difusos. • As alterações crônicas podem incluir: rubeose irídica, hiperpigmentação da íris, catarata secundária, luxação do cristalino, afastamento da pupila, íris arqueada, glaucoma secundário e bulbo ocular atrofiado.

CAUSAS
• Infecciosas — micóticas (*Blastomyces* spp., *Cryptococcus neoformans*; *Coccidiodes immitis*; *Histoplasma capsulatum*); protozoárias (*Toxoplasma gondii*); bacterianas (*Bartonella* spp., *Mycobacterium* spp. ou qualquer septicemia bacteriana); virais (FIV, FeLV, coronavírus felino; herpes-vírus tipo 1); parasitárias (oftalmomiíase; larva migrans ocular).
• Idiopáticas — uveíte linfocítica-plasmocitária.
• Imunomediadas — reação às proteínas do cristalino (em decorrência de catarata ou traumatismo do cristalino).
• Neoplásicas — tumores oculares primários (especialmente melanoma difuso da íris, sarcoma ocular); metástase em direção ao trato uveal (particularmente linfoma).
• Metabólicas — hiperlipidemia; hiperviscosidade; hipertensão sistêmica.
• Diversos — traumatismo; ceratite ulcerativa; abscesso do estroma corneano; toxemia de qualquer causa.

FATORES DE RISCO
Não há fatores específicos; a imunossupressão e a localização geográfica podem aumentar a incidência de certas causas infecciosas de uveíte.

DIAGNÓSTICO

DIAGNÓSTICO DIFERENCIAL
• Conjuntivite — a vermelhidão limita-se à hiperemia conjuntival (i. e., sem eritema ciliar); a secreção ocular costuma ser mais espessa e mais abundante do que na uveíte; o desconforto pode ser aliviado pela instilação de anestésicos tópicos.
• Glaucoma — o aumento na PIO é a característica mais compatível dessa doença; outros sinais podem incluir dilatação das pupilas (midríase), estrias de Haab e buftalmia.
• Ceratite ulcerativa — a coloração da córnea pela fluoresceína detecta a presença das úlceras; o edema corneano associado às úlceras apresenta-se confinado à região ulcerada ou mostra-se mais grave no local dessa ulceração; a secreção ocular é frequentemente mais espessa e mais abundante do que na uveíte; o desconforto pode ser aliviado por meio da instilação de anestésicos tópicos.
• Síndrome de Horner — os sinais de miose, enoftalmia e protrusão da membrana nictitante são similares em ambas as condições, mas a síndrome de Horner não exibe dor nem secreção ocular; o quadro de ptose associado à síndrome de Horner distingue-se do blefaroespasmo, já que o último processo é mais ativo; uma hiperemia conjuntival secundária pode ser observada na síndrome de Horner, mas tanto a córnea como a câmara anterior apresentam-se translúcidas; os sinais clínicos da síndrome de Horner desaparecem após a aplicação tópica de fenilefrina oftálmica a 1-10%.

HEMOGRAMA/BIOQUÍMICA/URINÁLISE
• Hemograma completo — frequentemente normal; pode haver alterações relacionadas com a doença subjacente.
• Bioquímica — muitas vezes normal; a anormalidade mais comum em gatos com uveíte é a elevação das proteínas séricas (geralmente, em função da gamopatia policlonal).
• Urinálise — comumente normal; pode haver alterações relacionadas com a doença subjacente.

OUTROS TESTES LABORATORIAIS
• Títulos séricos para o FeLV/FIV.
• Títulos para o coronavírus — apesar de inespecíficos em relação à PIF, tais títulos podem influenciar o índice de suspeita dessa doença.
• Títulos de IgM e IgG para o *Toxoplasma gondii* no soro e/ou no humor aquoso.
• Sorologia para *Bartonella* spp., PCR (soro ou humor aquoso) e/ou hemocultura.

DIAGNÓSTICO POR IMAGEM
• Radiografia torácica — pode revelar indícios do processo patológico causal (p. ex., infiltrados relacionados com a doença infecciosa; evidência de doença neoplásica metastática).
• Ultrassonografia ocular — indicada se a opacidade dos meios oculares impedir o exame direto; pode demonstrar a presença de neoplasia intraocular ou o deslocamento da retina.

MÉTODOS DIAGNÓSTICOS
• Tonometria — a PIO baixa é compatível com uveíte; a elevação na PIO indica a existência de glaucoma (doença primária ou secundária à uveíte).
• Centese (punção) ocular — na ocorrência de descolamento da retina, a citologia de aspirado sub-retiniano poderá revelar os agentes causais; pode-se efetuar a centese da câmara anterior para a pesquisa dos títulos de IgM e IgG para o *Toxoplasma gondii* ou a *Bartonella* no humor aquoso.

ACHADOS PATOLÓGICOS
• Macroscópicos — ver achados do exame físico.
• Histopatológicos — edema de córnea; vascularização periférica do estroma corneano profundo; precipitados ceráticos; membrana fibrovascular pré-iridiana; sinequia anterior periférica; sinequia posterior; entrópio ou ectrópio uveais; acúmulo de leucócitos no corpo ciliar, bem como na íris, esclera e coroide (infiltrados linfocítico-plasmocitários, supurativos ou granulomatosos, dependendo da etiologia); catarata secundária; com envolvimento do segmento posterior no processo inflamatório; membrana ciclítica; bandas de tração vítrea e descolamento da retina podem estar presentes.
• O achado histopatológico mais comum é representado por um infiltrado linfoplasmocitário na íris e no corpo ciliar (difuso ou nodular).

Uveíte Anterior – Gatos

TRATAMENTO

CUIDADO(S) DE SAÚDE ADEQUADO(S)
Em geral, o tratamento do paciente em esquema ambulatorial é suficiente.

ATIVIDADE
Na maioria dos casos, não se indicam quaisquer modificações.

DIETA
Não há indicação de mudanças.

ORIENTAÇÃO AO PROPRIETÁRIO
- Instruir acerca das doenças sistêmicas em potencial indutoras de sinais oftalmológicos e enfatizar a importância da realização de testes diagnósticos apropriados.
- Além do tratamento sintomático da uveíte, a terapia da doença subjacente (sempre que possível) é soberana para a obtenção de um resultado positivo.
- Informar o proprietário sobre as possíveis complicações e salientar a diminuição na probabilidade de complicações pela obediência às recomendações terapêuticas e ao acompanhamento.

CONSIDERAÇÕES CIRÚRGICAS
- Nenhuma na maioria dos casos.
- Os casos específicos que necessitam de intervenção cirúrgica compreendem a remoção de cristalinos rompidos e o tratamento cirúrgico de glaucoma secundário.
- A uveíte crônica indutora do glaucoma secundário comumente exige a enucleação dos globos oculares acometidos.
- Em casos de uveíte relacionada com o melanoma difuso da íris ou outros tumores intraoculares primários, recomenda-se a prática de enucleação nos gatos.

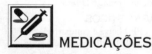

MEDICAÇÕES

MEDICAMENTO(S)

Corticosteroides

Tópicos
- Acetato de prednisolona a 1% — aplicar 2-8 vezes ao dia, dependendo da gravidade da doença; reduzir gradativamente o medicamento à medida que a afecção desaparece.
- Dexametasona a 0,1% — aplicar 2-8 vezes ao dia, dependendo da gravidade da doença; reduzir gradativamente o medicamento à medida que a afecção desaparece.
- Outros corticosteroides tópicos (p. ex., betametasona e hidrocortisona) são consideravelmente menos eficazes no tratamento da inflamação intraocular.
- Diminuir gradualmente a frequência do tratamento, conforme se observa a melhora da condição; a interrupção abrupta dos corticosteroides tópicos pode resultar no efeito rebote da inflamação intraocular.

Subconjuntivais
- Acetonida de triancinolona — 4 mg por meio de injeção subconjuntival.
- Metilprednisolona — 4 mg por meio de injeção subconjuntival.
- Muitas vezes, não são necessários.
- Indicados somente nos casos graves em uma única aplicação, seguida por anti-inflamatórios tópicos e/ou sistêmicos.

Sistêmicos
- Prednisona — 1-3 mg/kg/dia inicialmente; reduzir de forma gradativa a dose após 7-10 dias.
- Utilizar apenas se as causas infecciosas sistêmicas de uveíte tiverem sido descartadas.

Medicamentos Anti-inflamatórios Não Esteroides

Tópicos
- Flurbiprofeno — aplicar 2-4 vezes ao dia, dependendo da gravidade da doença.
- Diclofenaco — aplicar 2-4 vezes ao dia, dependendo da gravidade da doença.

Sistêmicos
- Meloxicam — 0,2 mg/kg IV, SC, VO 1 única vez e, em seguida, 0,05 mg/kg IV, SC, VO a cada 24 h por 2 dias e, depois, 0,025 mg/kg a cada 24-48 h. Em virtude dos possíveis efeitos renais, limitar a duração de uso para 4-6 dias.

Midriáticos/Cicloplégicos Tópicos
- Sulfato de atropina a 1% — aplicar 1-4 vezes ao dia, dependendo da gravidade da doença. Usar a frequência mais baixa, suficiente para manter a pupila dilatada e o alívio ocular; diminuir gradualmente o medicamento à medida que a afecção desaparece. Por causar menos salivação, é preferível o uso de pomada ao da solução em gatos.

CONTRAINDICAÇÕES
- Evitar o uso de medicamentos mióticos (p. ex., pilocarpina), inclusive das prostaglandinas tópicas (p. ex., latanoprosta) na presença de uveíte.
- Os corticosteroides tópicos e subconjuntivais são absolutamente contraindicados na existência de ceratite ulcerativa.
- Em gatos com hipertensão sistêmica, é recomendável evitar o uso dos corticosteroides (particularmente, os sistêmicos). Evitar os AINE sistêmicos em gatos com doença renal.

PRECAUÇÕES
Dada a possibilidade de glaucoma secundário, recomendam-se a aplicação tópica criteriosa da atropina e a monitorização periódica da PIO.

INTERAÇÕES POSSÍVEIS
Não é recomendável o uso concomitante de corticosteroides sistêmicos e medicamentos anti-inflamatórios não esteroides.

ACOMPANHAMENTO

MONITORIZAÇÃO DO PACIENTE
Reavaliar o paciente em 3-7 dias, dependendo da gravidade da doença. Nessa reavaliação, a PIO deverá ser monitorizada para detectar a presença de glaucoma secundário. A frequência das reavaliações subsequentes é ditada pela gravidade da doença e pela resposta ao tratamento.

COMPLICAÇÕES POSSÍVEIS

Complicações Sistêmicas
Ocorrem em consequência da etiologia sistêmica da uveíte.

Complicações Oftalmológicas
- Glaucoma secundário — complicação comum da uveíte crônica em gatos.
- Catarata secundária.
- Luxação do cristalino.
- Descolamento da retina.
- Atrofia do bulbo ocular.

EVOLUÇÃO ESPERADA E PROGNÓSTICO
- Para os olhos acometidos, o prognóstico é reservado, dependendo da doença subjacente e da resposta terapêutica.
- É mais provável que os gatos com doença subjacente tratável (p. ex., toxoplasmose) tenham um resultado favorável em termos oftalmológicos, em comparação àqueles com uveíte linfocítica-plasmocitária idiopática ou outra afecção subjacente intratável (p. ex., PIF e FIV).

DIVERSOS

FATORES RELACIONADOS COM A IDADE
- É mais provável que os gatos mais jovens sejam diagnosticados com etiologia infecciosa.
- Os gatos com idade mais avançada têm maior risco de uveíte linfocítica-plasmocitária idiopática e causas neoplásicas intraoculares.

POTENCIAL ZOONÓTICO
- Na maioria dos casos, não há risco zoonótico.
- Algumas formas de infecção sistêmica indutora de uveíte podem representar um pequeno risco a proprietários imunocomprometidos.

GESTAÇÃO/FERTILIDADE/REPRODUÇÃO
Evitar os corticosteroides sistêmicos. Em virtude da absorção sistêmica, os corticosteroides tópicos também podem representar um risco, particularmente em caso de aplicação frequente.

SINÔNIMO(S)
Iridociclite.

VER TAMBÉM
- Síndrome de Horner.
- Olho Vermelho.

ABREVIATURA(S)
- AINE = anti-inflamatório não esteroide.
- FeLV = vírus da leucemia felina.
- FIV = vírus da imunodeficiência felina.
- PIF = peritonite infecciosa felina.
- PIO = pressão intraocular.

Sugestões de Leitura
Colitz CM. Feline uveitis: Diagnosis and treatment. Clin Tech Small Anim Pract 2005, 20:117-120.
Cullen C, Webb A. Ocular manifestations of systemic diseases. Part 2: The cat. In: Gelatt KN, ed., Veterinary Ophthalmology, 4th ed. Ames, IA: Blackwell, 2007, pp. 1538-1587.
Miller P. Uvea. In: Maggs DJ, Miller PE, Ofri R, Slatter's Fundamentals of Veterinary Ophthalmology, 4th ed. St. Louis: Saunders, 2008, pp. 203-229.
Stiles J, Townsend WM. Feline ophthalmology. In: Gelatt KN, ed., Veterinary Ophthalmology, 4th ed. Ames, IA: Blackwell, 2007, pp. 1095-1164.

Autor Ian P. Herring
Consultor Editorial Paul E. Miller

VAGINITE

CONSIDERAÇÕES GERAIS

DEFINIÇÃO
Inflamação da vagina.

FISIOPATOLOGIA
• Vaginite juvenil: desconhecida, mas possivelmente atribuída a desequilíbrios do epitélio glandular da mucosa vaginal jovem.
• Vaginite primária de início no adulto: *Brucella canis* ou herpes-vírus canino. • Vaginite secundária de início no adulto: sequela de anomalia congênita, atrofia vaginal pós-ovário-histerectomia, terapia medicamentosa, corpo estranho, neoplasia, infecção do trato urinário, incontinência urinária, doença sistêmica, como diabetes melito.

SISTEMA(S) ACOMETIDO(S)
Reprodutor.

INCIDÊNCIA/PREVALÊNCIA
• Incidência de 0,7% em um único estudo.
• Vaginite primária — muito rara.

IDENTIFICAÇÃO
Espécies
Principalmente cadelas.

Idade Média e Faixa Etária
• Vaginite juvenil: acomete animais pré-púberes com menos de 1 ano de idade, variando de 8 semanas de vida a 1 ano. • Vaginite de início no adulto: afeta animais com mais de 1 ano de idade, variando de 1 a 16 anos.

SINAIS CLÍNICOS
Achados Anamnésicos
Vaginite Juvenil
• Pode não haver histórico significativo.
• Corrimento vulvar — observado com maior frequência após a micção. • Irritação vaginal.
• Formação de crostas na pelagem em torno da região vulvar. • Cadela que se arrasta na posição sentada para aliviar o prurido anal. • Lambedura vulvar excessiva. • Prurido perivulvar.
• Incapacidade de ser adestrada.

Vaginite de Início no Adulto
• Corrimento vulvar. • Lambedura vulvar excessiva. • Polaciúria. • Dor durante a micção.
• Poliúria/polidipsia. • Prurido. • Incontinência urinária. • Infertilidade.

Achados do Exame Físico
• Corrimento vulvar: mucoide a purulento, escasso a copioso (abundante). • Hiperemia vulvar.
• Hiperemia vestibular. • Dermatite perivulvar.
• Exame de palpação com os dedos — para identificação de estenoses e hímens na junção vaginovestibular, irregularidade granular da mucosa, especialmente da parede oposta à papila uretral. • Vaginoscopia — hiperemia difusa da mucosa vaginal e vestibular, folículos linfoides proeminentes, exsudatos luminais, eritema da papila uretral ou fossa clitoriana; presença de corpos estranhos, neoplasias ou anormalidades congênitas.

CAUSAS
• Vagina pré-púbere.
• Vulva infantil.
• Infecções do trato urinário.
• Incontinência urinária ou fecal.
• Corpo estranho.
• Neoplásicas — tumor venéreo transmissível; leiomioma.
• Bacterianas — *Brucella canis*, *E. coli*, *Streptococcus*, *Staphylococcus intermedius*, *Pasteurella*, *Chlamydia*, *Pseudomonas*, *Mycoplasma*.
• Virais — herpes-vírus canino.
• Anomalias congênitas, incluindo estenoses vaginovestibulares, vulva invertida.
• Traumatismo vaginal.
• Hematoma vaginal.
• Abscesso vaginal.
• Doença sistêmica — diabetes melito.
• Intoxicação por zinco.
• Androgênios exógenos ou endógenos.

FATORES DE RISCO
• Alteração da flora vaginal normal, causada pela administração de antibióticos exógenos.
• Hipertrofia do clitóris secundária a androgênios exógenos ou endógenos (hermafroditas).
• Vulva invertida ou rebaixada.
• Obesidade.
• Conformação anormal.
• Traumatismo vaginal.

DIAGNÓSTICO

DIAGNÓSTICO DIFERENCIAL
• Corrimento hemorrágico ou serossanguinolento é normal durante o proestro, podendo continuar no estro.
• Leve exsudato purulento pode ser normal no início do diestro; ao exame citológico, observam-se neutrófilos e células epiteliais não cornificadas.
• Corrimento mucoso é normal durante a prenhez.
• Corrimento pós-parto é normal por até 6-8 semanas; corrimento inodoro de coloração castanho-escura ou hemorrágico; a presença de quantidades substanciais é normal por até 4 semanas.
• Subinvolução dos sítios placentários — corrimento hemorrágico que dura por mais de 6-8 semanas no pós-parto.
• Cistouretrite.
• Corpo estranho.
• Piometra.
• Metrite.
• Placenta(s) retida(s).
• Hipertrofia do clitóris.
• Morte embrionária ou fetal.
• Contaminação por fezes ou urina, em decorrência de anomalia congênita ou condição adquirida.
• Dermatite perivulvar.
• Contaminação por urina em casos de ureter ectópico.
• Incontinência secundária a "hipoestrogenismo".
• Distúrbio de diferenciação sexual.
• Neoplasia vaginal.
• Traumatismo vaginal.
• Hematoma vaginal.
• Abscesso vaginal.
• Neoplasia ovariana.
• Intoxicação por zinco.

HEMOGRAMA/BIOQUÍMICA/URINÁLISE
• Os resultados costumam permanecer dentro dos limites de normalidade.
• Vaginite de início no adulto: os exames podem indicar infecção do trato urinário, hematúria ou doença sistêmica (como diabetes melito), até apontar a causa subjacente.
• A urinálise pode indicar urina diluída em filhotes caninos jovens (achado normal).

OUTROS TESTES LABORATORIAIS
• Sorologia para *Brucella canis*: teste de aglutinação rápida em lâmina (D-Tec CB, Synbiotics Corp., 800-228-4305); teste de imunodifusão em ágar gel (Cornell University Diagnostic Laboratory); cultura bacteriana do sangue total ou aspirado de linfonodo.
• Concentração sérica de progesterona — determina se a paciente se encontra no estro ou na fase lútea (≥2 ng/mL).

DIAGNÓSTICO POR IMAGEM
Ultrassonografia
• Descarta o útero como a fonte de qualquer corrimento vaginal.
• Permite a detecção de massas: neoplasia, granuloma ou corpo estranho; a distensão da vagina com soro fisiológico pode ajudar na visualização.

Radiografia Contrastada — Vaginograma/Uretrograma/Cistograma/Pielograma Intravenoso
• Identificam conformação ou estrutura anormais (p. ex., neoplasia ou corpo estranho) dentro da vagina.
• Descartam estenoses vestibulovaginais, bem como fístulas retovaginais e uretrovaginais.
• Excluem os diferenciais e ajudam a localizar o problema.

MÉTODOS DIAGNÓSTICOS
Cultura Vaginal e Antibiograma
• Efetuar antes de qualquer outro procedimento diagnóstico.
• Utilizar *swab* reservado para isso a fim de obter amostra da porção cranial da vagina.
• 74% dos casos de vaginite de início no adulto são positivos para crescimento bacteriano, dos quais 64% revelam culturas puras.
• Os microrganismos mais comuns são *E. coli*, *Streptococcus* spp., e *Staphylococcus intermedius*.
• Outros microrganismos incluem *Mycoplasma*, *Pasteurella*, *Pseudomonas*, *Chlamydia*.
• Lembrete: como a vagina não é um ambiente estéril, a cultura de cadelas normais resulta no crescimento da flora normal; portanto, é essencial o uso de exame citológico vaginal e outras ferramentas diagnósticas para interpretação dos resultados da cultura.

Exame Citológico Vaginal
• Sempre realizado em conjunto com a cultura vaginal.
• Vaginite juvenil: geralmente se observam leucócitos polimorfonucleares ± bactérias.
• Vaginite de início no adulto: indicativa, em geral, de inflamação séptica.
• Avalia as células epiteliais quanto ao grau de cornificação — presença de cornificação sob a influência de estrogênio.
• Determina a natureza do corrimento — inflamatório, sanguinolento, presença de material fecal.

Vaginoscopia
• Faz uso de cistouretroscópio rígido, gastroscópio pediátrico ou proctoscópio para visualização da vagina.
• Permite a observação de anomalias: hímen persistente, neoplasia, corpo estranho, traumatismo, abscesso e avaliação da mucosa vaginal.

VAGINITE

- Identifica a origem do corrimento vaginal — uterina, vaginal, vestibular ou uretral.
- Possibilita a remoção de corpo estranho ou a biopsia de massa vaginal.

Outros
- Exame vaginal com o dedo do examinador — pode ser a melhor ferramenta diagnóstica para identificação de estenoses no trajeto posterior.
- Biopsia e exame histopatológico de massa vaginal.
- Urocultura e sensibilidade — identificam infecções ascendentes/concomitantes.

TRATAMENTO

CUIDADO(S) DE SAÚDE ADEQUADO(S)
- Correção/remoção da causa subjacente.
- Em geral, o tratamento é feito em um esquema ambulatorial.
- Talvez haja necessidade de tratamento cirúrgico para remoção de corpos estranhos ou massas ou para correção de anomalias estruturais.
- Prevenção de automutilação — uso de colar elizabetano.

ATIVIDADE
Sem modificações.

DIETA
Sem alterações.

ORIENTAÇÃO AO PROPRIETÁRIO
Gerais
- *Brucella canis* — as pacientes positivas devem ser isoladas. É recomendável a eutanásia em função do potencial zoonótico e da falta de tratamento eficaz.
- É imprescindível a remoção de estrogênios e androgênios exógenos do ambiente.

Vaginite Juvenil
- Geralmente desaparece sem tratamento. Recomendar paciência.
- Deve se resolver após o primeiro ciclo estral, se não antes. Talvez seja necessário que a paciente passe por um único ciclo estral antes da ovário-histerectomia eletiva.

Vaginite de Início no Adulto
- Em geral, ocorre secundariamente à causa subjacente.
- Costuma desaparecer após a correção da causa incitante.
- Caso não se consiga identificar a causa primária, será alta a probabilidade de recuperação espontânea sem tratamento.

CONSIDERAÇÕES CIRÚRGICAS
- Correção de anomalia estrutural.
- Remoção de corpo estranho.
- Retirada de massa vaginal.
- Episioplastia.
- Em casos refratários, pode ser realizado o procedimento de vaginectomia.

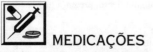

MEDICAÇÕES

MEDICAMENTO(S) DE ESCOLHA
Vaginite Juvenil
- Sem tratamento para cadelas nos casos não complicados.
- A antibioticoterapia é justificável em pacientes com desconforto excessivo (dor ou lambedura vulvar demasiada) e/ou infecções do trato urinário.
- A seleção de antibiótico é feita com base na cultura e no antibiograma.

Vaginite de Início no Adulto
- A seleção de antibiótico sistêmico é feita com base na cultura vaginal cranial positiva e no antibiograma; tratar por 4 semanas.
- Os AINE podem ser utilizados para ajudar a diminuir a inflamação.
- Doses anti-inflamatórias de corticosteroides podem ser úteis para reduzir a inflamação e o desconforto, mas os efeitos colaterais são menos desejáveis e podem resultar em subsequente infecção.
- Dietilestilbestrol — para vaginite idiopática ou recorrente em cadelas castradas; ajuda a restabelecer a integridade da mucosa normal, aumenta a cornificação do epitélio vaginal e promove a normalização da abóbada vaginal; utilizar a dose mais baixa, porém eficaz; 0,5 mg para cadelas com menos de 9 kg ou 1 mg para cadelas com mais de 9 kg, por via oral uma vez ao dia por 7 dias e, em seguida, reduzir a dose gradativamente em 2-4 semanas e manter sob a dose mais baixa, mas ainda eficaz, potencialmente pelo resto da vida.

CONTRAINDICAÇÕES
- A antibioticoterapia nas pacientes pode resultar em alteração da flora normal e desenvolvimento de infecção secundária ao tratamento.
- Duchas vaginais com agentes antibióticos/antissépticos podem ser irritantes à mucosa da vagina e agravar a condição.
- A administração de corticosteroides pode agravar a infecção concomitante do trato urinário.

PRECAUÇÕES
O fornecimento de estrogênios pode aumentar o risco de piometra em animais intactos.

INTERAÇÕES POSSÍVEIS
Os efeitos da hidrocortisona podem ser potencializados com a terapia estrogênica concomitante.

MEDICAMENTO(S) ALTERNATIVO(S)
- Vaginite juvenil pode ser tratada com dietilestilbestrol para induzir ao estro em casos refratários, embora não haja registro dos efeitos a longo prazo.
- Lenços umedecidos/infantis podem ser utilizados para limpar a região perivulvar.

ACOMPANHAMENTO

MONITORIZAÇÃO DO PACIENTE
Vaginite Juvenil
- Reavaliar se os sintomas se tornaram mais graves ou intoleráveis.
- Reavaliar após o primeiro ciclo estral.

Vaginite de Início no Adulto
- Reavaliar se os sintomas não desaparecerem após a remoção da causa subjacente.
- Efetuar nova cultura 5-7 dias após a interrupção da antibioticoterapia ou se os sintomas persistirem apesar da terapia.

PREVENÇÃO
- Adiar a ovário-histerectomia eletiva até depois do primeiro ciclo estral nos casos de vaginite juvenil.
- Evitar o uso de antibióticos em casos não justificáveis.
- Manter níveis satisfatórios de peso e condição corporais.
- Evitar a aplicação de duchas vaginais.
- Evitar a utilização de terapia androgênica exógena.

EVOLUÇÃO ESPERADA E PROGNÓSTICO
- Vaginite juvenil — início com 6 semanas a 6-12 meses de vida; dura de dias a meses, mas tipicamente é intermitente; costuma desaparecer com o tempo ou depois do primeiro ciclo estral.
- Vaginite de início no adulto — normalmente se resolve após remoção/tratamento da causa incitante; a antibioticoterapia pode acelerar a resolução em casos justificáveis, enquanto os AINE podem ajudar a resolver a inflamação.

DIVERSOS

DISTÚRBIOS ASSOCIADOS
Dermatite perivulvar.

FATORES RELACIONADOS COM A IDADE
Vaginite juvenil pode estar presente em cadelas pré-púberes, geralmente com menos de 1 ano de idade.

POTENCIAL ZOONÓTICO
Brucella canis — deve ser descartada, apesar de ser uma causa rara de vaginite.

GESTAÇÃO/FERTILIDADE/REPRODUÇÃO
- A vaginite durante a prenhez é rara, mas pode resultar em infecção ascendente e subsequente abortamento. A resolução da vaginite pode resultar em prognóstico bom em termos de fertilidade se a causa subjacente não afetar o prognóstico quanto à fertilidade.
- Anomalias estruturais, como hímen persistente, podem impedir a ocorrência de acasalamentos naturais ou predispor a distocia se a cadela for submetida à inseminação artificial.
- A formação cicatricial secundária a traumatismo pode culminar em excesso de tecido fibroso e diminuição da distensibilidade vaginal.

VER TAMBÉM
- Brucelose. • Metrite. • Piometra e Hiperplasia Endometrial Cística. • Placenta Retida.
- Subinvolução dos Sítios Placentários. • Más-formações Vaginais e Lesões Adquiridas.

ABREVIATURA(S)
- AINE = anti-inflamatório não esteroide.

Sugestões de Leitura
Bjurstrsm L, Linde-Forsberg C. Long-term study of aerobic bacteria of the genital tract in breeding bitches. Am J Vet Res 1992, 53:665-669.
Johnson CA. Diagnosis and treatment of chronic vaginitis in the bitch. Vet Clin North Am 1991, 21:523-531.
Johnston SD, Root Kustritz MV, Olson PNS. Disorders of the canine vagina, vestibule, and vulva. In: Canine and Feline Theriogenology. Philadelphia: Saunders, 2001, pp. 225-242.
Parker NA. Clinical approach to canine vaginitis: A review. Theriogenology 1998, 112-115.

Autores Leeah R. Chew e Beverly J. Purswell
Consultor Editorial Sara K. Lyle

VASCULITE CUTÂNEA — CÃES

CONSIDERAÇÕES GERAIS

REVISÃO
Inflamação da parede dos vasos sanguíneos, com infiltração neutrofílica (leucocitoclástica/não leucocitoclástica), linfocítica, raramente eosinofílica, granulomatosa ou mista.

FISIOPATOLOGIA
Reações dos tipos III (por depósito de imunocomplexos) e I (imediata).

SISTEMA(S) ACOMETIDO(S)
Cutâneo/exócrino.

IDENTIFICAÇÃO
• Cães e gatos. • Pode acometer qualquer idade, raça ou sexo. • Muito menos comum em gatos do que em cães. • As raças Dachshund, Collie, Pastor de Shetland, Pastor alemão e Rottweiler podem ser predispostas. • Varia dependendo da causa.

SINAIS CLÍNICOS
• Púrpura palpável. • Bolhas hemorrágicas ou urticária. • Alopecia focal com formação cicatricial e descamação. • Necrose e úlceras puntiformes. • Acrocianose. • Compromete as extremidades (patas, pavilhões auriculares, lábios, cauda e mucosa bucal) e pode ser dolorosa. • Anorexia, depressão, pirexia, edema depressível nas extremidades, poliartropatia e miopatia — dependem da causa subjacente.

CAUSAS E FATORES DE RISCO
• Idiopáticas. • Induzidas por medicamentos. • Induzidas por vacinas (sobretudo a antirrábica). • Reação alimentar adversa. • Doenças originárias de carrapatos — febre maculosa das Montanhas Rochosas, erliquiose, doença de Lyme. • Infecção bacteriana, fúngica e viral subjacente. • Processo metabólico subjacente (p. ex., diabetes). • Doença autoimune. • Neoplasias.

DIAGNÓSTICO

DIAGNÓSTICO DIFERENCIAL
• Ver a seção "Causas e Fatores de Risco". • Seborreia da margem auricular. • Queimaduras químicas e térmicas. • Necrólise epidérmica tóxica. • Eritema multiforme. • Dermatite eosinofílica. • Lúpus eritematoso sistêmico. • Penfigoide bolhoso. • Pênfigo vulgar. • Sepse.

HEMOGRAMA/BIOQUÍMICA/URINÁLISE
Normais a menos que haja lúpus eritematoso sistêmico ou processo metabólico subjacente.

OUTROS TESTES LABORATORIAIS
• Sepse, coagulação intravascular disseminada, lúpus eritematoso sistêmico, febre maculosa das Montanhas Rochosas e artrite reumatoide — as anormalidades podem ser constatadas em exames apropriados. • Considerar a realização de testes sorológicos para pesquisa de doenças parasitárias e infecciosas em áreas de alto risco. • Considerar a execução de testes imunodiagnósticos — título do ANA, teste de Coombs e testes da aglutinina fria.

MÉTODOS DIAGNÓSTICOS
• Raspados cutâneos — em busca de demodicose (em casos de sepse secundária).
• Biopsia de lesão precoce — enviar o material para algum dermatopatologista; os achados dependem da causa subjacente, mas costumam incluir infiltrados neutrofílicos (leucocitoclásticos/não leucocitoclásticos), linfocíticos, eosinofílicos, granulomatosos ou mistos nos vasos e em torno deles; processo de necrose vascular e trombos de fibrina podem ser proeminentes; podem ocorrer hemorragia e edema perivasculares.
• Vasculite — devem-se efetuar culturas representativas (p. ex., sangue, urina, pele, etc.) se os exames de hemograma completo, perfil bioquímico ou urinálise se mostrarem compatíveis com doença sistêmica.
• Títulos séricos em busca de infecções riquetsiais para descartar doenças originárias de carrapatos.

TRATAMENTO

• Doença subjacente — constitui a prioridade no tratamento clínico.
• Sem anormalidades sistêmicas — tratar o paciente em um esquema ambulatorial, sem modificações no consumo de água ou alimento.
• Doença sistêmica — é recomendável a internação do paciente.
• Fornecer ao proprietário um prognóstico reservado até que se descubra a causa; o prognóstico baseia-se na causa.
• Lesões individuais (focais) podem ser submetidas à excisão cirúrgica.

MEDICAÇÕES

MEDICAMENTO(S)
• Os medicamentos listados são para vasculite canina.
• Primeira linha terapêutica enquanto se aguardam os resultados histopatológicos e quando não se suspeita de nenhuma reação medicamentosa — antibióticos.
• Qualquer processo patológico subjacente deve ser identificado e devidamente tratado.
• Doença imunomediada com vasculite concomitante — prednisolona (2-4 mg/kg a cada 24 h e reduzir gradativamente de acordo com a resposta).
• Na falta de causa subjacente conhecida ou na ineficácia da prednisolona isolada — dapsona (1 mg/kg VO a cada 24 h) ou sulfassalazina (15-22 mg/kg VO a cada 8-12 h).
• Pentoxifilina 10 mg/kg VO a cada 8 h (Trental®) pode ter menos efeitos colaterais do que os medicamentos genéricos.
• Agentes imunossupressores alternativos (p. ex., clorambucila e a azatioprina) podem diminuir a necessidade e/ou a dosagem de corticosteroides.
• Ciclosporina também pode ser considerada.
• Tetraciclina e niacinamida 500 mg de cada a cada 8 h para cães com >10 kg ou 250 mg VO a cada 8 h para aqueles com <10 kg.

CONTRAINDICAÇÕES/INTERAÇÕES POSSÍVEIS
• Dapsona e sulfassalazina — não são recomendadas em casos de nefropatia, hepatopatia, discrasia sanguínea ou ceratoconjuntivite seca preexistentes; utilizar com cuidado em gatos; podem deslocar os medicamentos altamente ligados a proteínas (p. ex., metotrexato, varfarina, fenilbutazona, diuréticos tiazídicos, salicilatos, probenecida e fenitoína); biodisponibilidade diminuída por antiácidos; podem reduzir a biodisponibilidade do ácido fólico ou da digoxina; os níveis sanguíneos podem ser reduzidos na administração concomitante de sulfato ferroso ou de outros sais de ferro.
• Pentoxifilina — pode aumentar os tempos de protrombina; pode diminuir a pressão arterial; também pode causar agitação.

ACOMPANHAMENTO

• Pacientes submetidos à prednisolona, sulfassalazina ou dapsona — monitorizar inicialmente a cada 2 semanas por meio de hemograma completo, perfil bioquímico e urinálise; caso se descubra alguma doença subjacente específica, monitorizar o animal de forma apropriada.
• Com o uso da sulfassalazina ou dapsona, é recomendável a monitorização do paciente com o teste lacrimal de Schirmer a cada 2 semanas inicialmente.
• Com os agentes imunossupressores alternativos, deve-se monitorizar o paciente quanto à ocorrência de mielossupressão e hepatotoxicidade.
• Caso não se encontre nenhuma doença subjacente, o tratamento da vasculite não será tarefa fácil e o prognóstico será reservado.
• As terapias imunossupressoras sempre devem ser reduzidas para a dose terapêutica mais baixa possível.

DIVERSOS

GESTAÇÃO/FERTILIDADE/REPRODUÇÃO
• Corticosteroides e dapsona — não utilizar em fêmeas prenhes.
• Sulfassalazina — usar durante a prenhez apenas em casos de absoluta necessidade.
• Todos os medicamentos devem ser usados com cuidado em fêmeas prenhes e animais reprodutores.

ABREVIATURA(S)
• ANA = anticorpo antinuclear.

Sugestões de Leitura
Campbell KL, ed., Small Animal Dermatology Secrets. Philadelphia: Hanley & Belfus, 2004.
Greek JS. New therapeutics in dermatology. Vet Med 1996, 91(11):1021-1024.
Marsella R, Nicklin CF, Munson JW, Roberts SM. Pharmacokinetics of pentoxyfilline in dogs after oral and intravenous administration. Am J Vet Res 2000, 61(6):631-637.
Scott DW, MillerWH, Griffen CE. Muller & Kirk's Small Animal Dermatology, 6th ed. Philadelphia: Saunders, 2001.
Nichols PR, Morris DO, Beale KM. A retrospective study of canine and feline cutaneous vasculitis. Vet Dermatol 2001, 12(5):255-264.

Autor Karen A. Kuhl
Consultor Editorial Alexander H. Werner

Vasculite Sistêmica

CONSIDERAÇÕES GERAIS

REVISÃO
• Inflamação dos vasos sanguíneos, causada por lesão endotelial ou extensão de inflamação ou infecção adjacentes. • O dano endotelial por agente infeccioso, infestação parasitária, endotoxina ou deposição de imunocomplexos desencadeia um processo de inflamação local, o acúmulo de neutrófilos e a ativação do complemento. Os neutrófilos liberam enzimas lisossomais, levando à necrose da parede dos vasos, trombose e hemorragia. Em seres humanos e cães com poliarterite nodosa, a proliferação da camada íntima dos vasos, bem como a degeneração e a necrose da parede dos vasos, predominam e levam à hemorragia, trombose e necrose dos vasos envolvidos e dos tecidos adjacentes em grande parte dos pacientes. • Vasculite não dérmica (p. ex., nos rins, no fígado e em superfícies serosas das cavidades corporais) pode ser o mecanismo indutor do desenvolvimento de sinais clinicamente aparentes de doença sistêmica (p. ex., poliartrite e proteinúria), sem causar lesões externas evidentes.

IDENTIFICAÇÃO
Cães e gatos.

SINAIS CLÍNICOS
Achados Anamnésicos
• Administração de medicamentos provocadores (p. ex., penicilina, sulfonamidas, estreptomicina e hidralazina) em animais sensibilizados. • Histórico de vacinação recente. • Exposição a carrapatos. • Profilaxia insatisfatória contra a dirofilariose em áreas endêmicas.

Achados do Exame Físico
• Tumefação. • Ulceração. • Necrose da pele acometida, especialmente de mucosas, junções mucocutâneas, margens dos pavilhões auriculares e coxins palmoplantares. • Os sinais sistêmicos refletem o envolvimento de órgãos (p. ex., fígado, rins e SNC). • Sinais sistêmicos de doença (p. ex., letargia, linfadenopatia, pirexia, sinais vagos de dor e perda de peso). • Poliarterite juvenil em cães da raça Beagle, caracterizada por episódios recidivantes de febre (>40°C) e dor cervical que persistem por 3-7 dias. • Lesões cutâneas de poliarterite nodosa (nódulos subcutâneos — menos comuns em cães do que em pessoas). • Sinais associados à doença infecciosa ou imunomediada subjacente (p. ex., trombocitopenia e poliartropatia). • Exame oftalmológico — uveíte anterior, congestão da esclera, hifema.

CAUSAS E FATORES DE RISCO
Infecciosas
• Parasitárias (i. e., coração e artérias pulmonares) — *Dirofilaria immitis*, *Angiostrongylus vasorum*, *Leishmania* spp. • Virais — por exemplo, peritonite infecciosa felina e coronavirose canina. • Riquetsiais — por exemplo, febre maculosa das Montanhas Rochosas e erliquiose. • Bacterianas — sepse.

Imunomediadas
• Lúpus eritematoso sistêmico. • Artropatia semelhante à artrite reumatoide. • Reação medicamentosa semelhante ao lúpus. • Hipersensibilidades do tipo III (p. ex., a alimentos, sulfonamidas e penicilina).

• Poliarterite juvenil em Beagle. • Granulomatose de Wegener (rara). • Poliarterite nodosa. • Neoplasia. • Uremia.

DIAGNÓSTICO

DIAGNÓSTICO DIFERENCIAL
• O desenvolvimento de sinais cutâneos após a administração de medicamentos sugere uma reação medicamentosa (que, geralmente, não é imediata, mas pode se desenvolver depois de dias ou semanas). • Vasculite associada à poliartropatia e pirexia implica uma causa imune ou infecciosa. • A distribuição de lesões cianóticas ou necrosadas (nariz, orelhas, dedos, extremidade da cauda, prepúcio) e o histórico de exposição ao frio apontam para a doença da hemaglutinina fria.

HEMOGRAMA/BIOQUÍMICA/URINÁLISE
Os resultados dependem da doença subjacente.

OUTROS TESTES LABORATORIAIS
• Os testes sorológicos podem auxiliar no diagnóstico de doenças infecciosas (i. e., riquetsioses, leishmaniose). • Títulos do ANA — revelam resultados positivos em pacientes com LES, mas também podem exibir positividade naqueles com outras doenças sistêmicas. • Teste positivo quanto à presença de dirofilárias ocultas em animais com dirofilariose. • Infestação por *Angiostrongylus* diagnosticada por meio de exame de fezes e exame citológico de lavado traqueal.

DIAGNÓSTICO POR IMAGEM
As radiografias ajudam no diagnóstico de dirofilariose e da infestação por *Angiostrongylus*.

MÉTODOS DIAGNÓSTICOS
• A biopsia cutânea de amostra obtida da borda da lesão em desenvolvimento pode ser diagnóstica em casos de vasculite, mas pode não revelar a causa. • O teste de imunofluorescência da amostra de biopsia cutânea pode descartar pênfigo e doenças penfigoides. • Na suspeita de reação alérgica, a resolução dos sinais clínicos com a interrupção de medicamentos ou alimentos sob suspeita apoiará o diagnóstico.

TRATAMENTO

• Em geral, a terapia envolve a resolução do problema subjacente e os cuidados de suporte. • Em casos de condições subjacentes intratáveis ou desconhecidas — glicocorticoides, imunossupressores (p. ex., ciclofosfamida e azatioprina) e outros medicamentos (p. ex., dapsona e sulfassalazina) são ocasionalmente eficazes, mas ainda não há relatos de ensaios clínicos quanto à eficácia desses agentes nos animais.

MEDICAÇÕES

MEDICAMENTO(S)
• Vasculite infecciosa ou imunomediada — tratar a causa subjacente (ver condições específicas); cuidados de suporte.

• Reações medicamentosas semelhantes ao lúpus — interromper o medicamento; cuidados de suporte.
• Hipersensibilidade do tipo III — também se deve suspender o medicamento; cuidados de suporte.
• Poliarterite nodosa — glicocorticoides e ciclofosfamida (valor desconhecido).
• Vasculite "idiopática" — se outras causas tiverem sido descartadas, administrar a dapsona (1 mg/kg VO a cada 8 h por 14 dias, depois 1 mg/kg VO a cada 12 h por 14 dias e, em seguida, 1 mg/kg VO a cada 24 h; por fim, pode ser reduzida para a cada 48 h a fim de manter a remissão); medicamento alternativo — sulfassalazina (45 mg/kg VO a cada 8 h). Ainda não se comprovou de maneira satisfatória a eficácia de nenhum desses medicamentos. Em um número limitado de casos, empregou-se a pentoxifilina em doses de 400 mg a cada 24-48 h. As doses imunossupressoras de corticosteroides podem ser úteis em casos idiopáticos.

CONTRAINDICAÇÕES/INTERAÇÕES POSSÍVEIS
• Não administrar a sulfassalazina em pacientes sensíveis às sulfonamidas.
• A pentoxifilina é um derivado metilxantínico e pode diminuir a pressão arterial.

ACOMPANHAMENTO

• Pacientes submetidos ao tratamento com a dapsona — monitorar o hemograma completo e as enzimas hepáticas em virtude dos efeitos colaterais (p. ex., anemia hemolítica, metemoglobinemia e hepatopatia).
• Pacientes submetidos ao tratamento com a sulfassalazina — monitorar o paciente quanto à ocorrência de ceratoconjuntivite seca, discrasia sanguínea e hepatopatia.

DIVERSOS

VER TAMBÉM
• Lúpus Eritematoso Sistêmico. • Pênfigo.
• Vasculite Cutânea — Cães.

ABREVIATURA(S)
• ANA = anticorpo antinuclear.
• LES = lúpus eritematoso sistêmico.
• SNC = sistema nervoso central.

Sugestões de Leitura
Morris DO, Beale KM. Cutaneous vasculitis and vasculopathy. Vet Clin North Am Small Anim Pract 1999, 29(6):1325-1335.
Nichols PR, Morris DO, Beale KMA. Retrospective study of canine and feline cutaneous vasculitis. Vet Dermatol 2001, 12(5):255-264.

Autor Francis W.K. Smith, Jr.
Consultores Editoriais Larry P. Tilley e Francis W.K. Smith, Jr.
Agradecimento O autor e os editores gostariam de agradecer as colaborações de Jean S. Greek, que foi o autor deste capítulo na edição anterior.

VESTIBULOPATIA GERIÁTRICA — CÃES

CONSIDERAÇÕES GERAIS

DEFINIÇÃO
Distúrbio não progressivo de início agudo do sistema vestibular periférico em cães mais idosos.

FISIOPATOLOGIA
• Desconhecida.
• Suspeita-se de fluxo anormal da endolinfa nos canais semicirculares da orelha interna, secundariamente a distúrbios na produção, na circulação ou na absorção desse líquido.
• Possível intoxicação dos receptores vestibulares ou inflamação da porção vestibular do nervo vestibulococlear (VIII par de nervos cranianos).
• Frequentemente denominada de forma incorreta como acidente vascular cerebral, a vestibulopatia geriátrica não tem localização central nem origem vascular ou isquêmica.

SISTEMA(S) ACOMETIDO(S)
Nervoso — sistema vestibular periférico.

GENÉTICA
N/D.

INCIDÊNCIA/PREVALÊNCIA
Doença comum, esporádica e adquirida de cães mais idosos.

DISTRIBUIÇÃO GEOGRÁFICA
N/D.

IDENTIFICAÇÃO
Espécies
Cães.

Raça(s) Predominante(s)
• Não há relato de nenhuma raça predisponente.
• Parece ocorrer com maior frequência em raças de médio a grande porte.

Idade Média e Faixa Etária
Geriátricos; os pacientes costumam ter >8 anos de idade.

Sexo Predominante
N/D.

SINAIS CLÍNICOS
Comentários Gerais
• Sinais de disfunção vestibular periférica de início agudo, em geral unilateral, mas ocasionalmente bilateral.
• Se os sinais vestibulares forem graves, os sinais clínicos (sobretudo a marcha) não deverão ser incorretamente atribuídos à localização central (SNC).

Achados Anamnésicos
• Início súbito de desequilíbrio, desorientação, relutância em se manter em estação e (geralmente) inclinação da cabeça e movimentos irregulares dos olhos.
• Podem ser precedidos ou acompanhados por náusea e vômito.

Achados do Exame Físico
• Inclinação da cabeça — inclinação leve a acentuada; inclinada para o lado da lesão; ocasionalmente, a doença é bilateral com movimentos laterais erráticos da cabeça, sem inclinação da cabeça ou com leve inclinação na direção do lado mais gravemente acometido.
• Nistagmo anormal (em repouso) — é comum nos estágios precoces da doença; é horizontal ou rotatório, com a fase rápida sempre na direção oposta à inclinação da cabeça; em casos de doença bilateral, há um nistagmo anormal geralmente leve ou ausente e nistagmo fisiológico ou movimentos oculares conjugados diminuídos a ausentes.
• Desorientação e ataxia vestibular leves a acentuadas, com tendência ao encurvamento ou à queda na direção da inclinação da cabeça.
• A força muscular e a propriocepção permanecem normais; em casos de doença grave, o paciente pode demonstrar relutância para se manter em estação e ainda ter outros problemas (p. ex., displasia coxofemoral), o que dificulta a avaliação da marcha; em casos de doença bilateral, o animal pode apresentar postura em base larga.

CAUSAS
Desconhecidas.

FATORES DE RISCO
N/D.

DIAGNÓSTICO

DIAGNÓSTICO DIFERENCIAL
• Diferenciada de outras causas de déficits vestibulares, principalmente pelo início agudo e, em geral, pela rápida melhora sem tratamento específico.
• Otite média e interna — pode exibir paresia ou paralisia do nervo facial (VII par de nervos cranianos) ipsolateral, surdez e/ou síndrome de Horner concomitantes; a presença de otite externa em casos de ruptura da membrana timpânica apoia o diagnóstico de otite média e interna.
• Medicamentos ototóxicos — descartados por meio da anamnese.
• Traumatismo — pode causar alterações agudas similares; diferenciado por meio da anamnese e dos resultados do exame físico.
• Neuropatia hipotireóidea — em geral, não é tão aguda no início nem tão grave; pode estar associada a sinais clínicos de hipotireoidismo e possível déficit do VII par de nervos cranianos.

HEMOGRAMA/BIOQUÍMICA/URINÁLISE
• Geralmente normais.
• Pode haver hemoconcentração secundária à desidratação.
• Os distúrbios concomitantes não relacionados (p. ex., nefropatia e hepatopatia) associados ao estado geriátrico podem causar outras anormalidades laboratoriais.

OUTROS TESTES LABORATORIAIS
N/D.

DIAGNÓSTICO POR IMAGEM
• Em geral, não há necessidade de qualquer exame.
• Radiografias das bulas timpânicas: as radiografias normais não descartam comprometimento dessas estruturas.
• TC ou RM (são preferidas às radiografias) — podem ser necessárias para descartar outras causas, como otite média e interna.

MÉTODOS DIAGNÓSTICOS
• RAETC — para avaliar a porção coclear do VIII par de nervos cranianos; pode ajudar a pesquisar otite média e interna, já que apenas a porção vestibular do VIII par de nervos cranianos é acometida na vestibulopatia geriátrica.
• A surdez, no entanto, pode estar presente como uma alteração senil não relacionada.

ACHADOS PATOLÓGICOS
Nenhum relatado.

TRATAMENTO

CUIDADO(S) DE SAÚDE ADEQUADO(S)
• Doença leve — pode ser tratada geralmente em um esquema ambulatorial.
• Doença grave — os pacientes que não conseguem se mover ou necessitam de terapia de suporte com fluidos intravenosos devem ser internados durante os estágios iniciais da doença.

CUIDADO(S) DE ENFERMAGEM
• Fornecer tratamento de suporte, incluindo a administração de fluidos intravenosos (se necessários) para reidratação.
• Manter os pacientes em decúbito em ambiente quente e seco, utilizando acolchoados macios e absorventes e, se necessário, sonda urinária.
• Doença grave — inicialmente, pode haver a necessidade de fisioterapia, incluindo manipulação passiva dos membros e movimentação do corpo para lados alternados.

ATIVIDADE
Restringir a atividade física, conforme a necessidade, de acordo com o grau de desorientação e ataxia vestibular.

DIETA
• Em geral, não há necessidade de nenhuma modificação.
• Náusea, vômito e desorientação grave — a princípio, deve-se suspender o consumo de alimentos e, depois, fornecer alimentação supervisionada.

ORIENTAÇÃO AO PROPRIETÁRIO
Tranquilizar o proprietário sobre o fato de que, embora os sinais clínicos iniciais possam ser alarmantes e incapacitantes, o prognóstico é excelente quanto à rapidez na melhora e na recuperação.

CONSIDERAÇÕES CIRÚRGICAS
N/D.

MEDICAÇÕES

MEDICAMENTO(S) DE ESCOLHA
• Sedativos — em casos graves de desorientação e ataxia; diazepam (2-10 mg/cão VO ou IV a cada 8 h), acepromazina (0,02-0,05 mg/kg IM, SC, IV até, no máximo, 2 mg).
• Medicamentos antieméticos ou agentes utilizados contra a cinetose — benefício questionável; dimenidrinato (4-8 mg/kg VO, IM, IV a cada 8 h), cloridrato de meclizina (25 mg VO a cada 24 h).
• Glicocorticoides — não são recomendados, pois não alteram a evolução da doença; além disso, podem exacerbar problemas concomitantes (p. ex., desidratação).
• Antibióticos — são aconselhados caso não se consiga descartar a possibilidade de otite média e interna; trimetoprima-sulfa (15 mg/kg VO a cada 12 h ou 30 mg/kg VO a cada 12-24 h); cefalosporina de primeira geração (p. ex., cefalexina na dosagem de 10-30 mg/kg VO a cada 6-12 h); amoxicilina/ácido clavulânico (12,5 mg/kg VO a cada 12 h).

CONTRAINDICAÇÕES
N/D.

Vestibulopatia Geriátrica — Cães

PRECAUÇÕES
N/D.

INTERAÇÕES POSSÍVEIS
N/D.

MEDICAMENTO(S) ALTERNATIVO(S)
N/D.

ACOMPANHAMENTO

MONITORIZAÇÃO DO PACIENTE
• Exame neurológico do paciente ambulatorial — repetir 2-3 dias depois para confirmar a estabilização e a melhora inicial.
• A alta do paciente internado é recomendada quando ele se mostrar capaz de caminhar, além de voltar a comer e beber.

PREVENÇÃO
N/D.

COMPLICAÇÕES POSSÍVEIS
• Desequilíbrios hidreletrolíticos e descompensação de insuficiência renal (se presente) — podem resultar em vômitos e/ou consumo insuficiente de água e alimentos.
• Úlceras de decúbito/feridas por abrasão.

EVOLUÇÃO ESPERADA E PROGNÓSTICO
• A melhora dos sinais clínicos inicia-se dentro de 72 h, não só com a resolução do vômito, mas também com a recuperação do nistagmo e da ataxia vestibular.
• Inclinação da cabeça e ataxia — a melhora significativa costuma ocorrer em 7-10 dias; se não houver nenhuma melhora, devem-se pesquisar outras causas de vestibulopatia periférica; uma leve inclinação da cabeça pode persistir.
• A maioria dos pacientes examinados deve retornar ao normal dentro de 2-3 semanas.
• Recidiva — apesar de incomuns, podem ocorrer episódios repetidos de vestibulopatia geriátrica no mesmo lado ou no lado oposto da lesão; pode ocorrer um breve retorno dos sinais clínicos com estresse (p. ex., anestesia).

DIVERSOS

DISTÚRBIOS ASSOCIADOS
N/D.

FATORES RELACIONADOS COM A IDADE
Apenas os cães geriátricos são acometidos (idade média sugerida de 12 anos e meio).

POTENCIAL ZOONÓTICO
N/D.

GESTAÇÃO/FERTILIDADE/REPRODUÇÃO
N/D.

SINÔNIMO(S)
• Doença vestibular periférica canina idiopática benigna.
• Doença/síndrome vestibular idiopática canina.
• Doença vestibular periférica canina idiopática.
• Síndrome vestibular do cão idoso.

VER TAMBÉM
• Inclinação da Cabeça.
• Otite Média e Interna.

ABREVIATURA(S)
• RAETC = resposta auditiva evocada do tronco cerebral.
• RM = ressonância magnética.
• SNC = sistema nervoso central.
• TC = tomografia computadorizada.

Sugestões de Leitura
de Lahunta A, Glass E. Veterinary Neuroanatomy and Clinical Neurology, 3rd ed. St. Louis: Saunders Elsevier, 2009, pp. 328-329.
Dewey CW. A Practical Guide to Canine and Feline Neurology, 2nd ed. Ames, IA: Wiley-Blackwell, 2008, pp. 272-273.
Lorenz MD, Kornegay JN. Handbook of Veterinary Neurology, 4th ed. St. Louis: Saunders Elsevier, 2004, p. 226.
Munana KR. Head tilt and nystagmus. In: Platt SR, Olby NJ, eds., BSAVA Manual of Canine and Feline Neurology, 3rd ed. Gloucestershire, UK: BSAVA, 2004, p. 161.
Thomas WB. Vestibular dysfunction. Vet Clin North Am Small Anim Pract 2000, 30:227-249.

Autor Susan M. Cochrane
Consultor Editorial Joane M. Parent

Vestibulopatia Idiopática — Gatos

CONSIDERAÇÕES GERAIS

DEFINIÇÃO
Distúrbio não progressivo de início agudo do sistema vestibular periférico em gatos.

FISIOPATOLOGIA
• Desconhecida. • Suspeita-se de um fluxo anormal da endolinfa nos canais semicirculares da orelha interna, secundariamente a algum distúrbio na produção, na circulação ou na absorção desse líquido. • Possível intoxicação dos receptores vestibulares ou inflamação da porção vestibular do nervo vestibulococlear (VIII par de nervo craniano).

SISTEMA(S) ACOMETIDO(S)
Nervoso — sistema vestibular periférico.

INCIDÊNCIA/PREVALÊNCIA
• Doença adquirida esporádica. • Não há nenhum dado descrito.

IDENTIFICAÇÃO
Espécies
Gatos.

Idade Média e Faixa Etária
Qualquer idade; raramente observada em gatos com <1 ano de idade.

SINAIS CLÍNICOS
Comentários Gerais
Limitados aos sinais clínicos associados a distúrbios vestibulares periféricos.

Achados Anamnésicos
Início súbito e grave de desorientação, queda e rolamento, inclinação, vocalização e postura agachada, com tendência ao pânico quando é erguido do chão.

Achados do Exame Físico
• Inclinação da cabeça — sempre em direção ao lado da lesão; ocasionalmente, a doença é bilateral, apresentando excursões amplas da cabeça de um lado para outro, sem inclinação da cabeça ou com leve inclinação em direção ao lado mais gravemente acometido. • Nistagmo em repouso — costuma ser horizontal, mas pode ser rotatório com a fase rápida sempre na direção oposta à inclinação da cabeça; em casos de doença bilateral, o nistagmo anormal é geralmente leve ou ausente, enquanto o nistagmo fisiológico ou os movimentos oculares conjugados se encontram diminuídos a ausentes. • Ataxia vestibular, com tendência ao rolamento e à queda em direção à inclinação da cabeça. • Preservação da força muscular e da propriocepção normal; em casos de doença bilateral, o paciente pode apresentar relutância à deambulação, preferindo permanecer em postura agachada e possível postura em base larga.

CAUSAS
• Desconhecidas. • Infecção prévia do trato respiratório superior (anterior) — suspeita em alguns pacientes; a relação ainda não foi confirmada; em dados limitados obtidos à necropsia, não há indícios de inflamação.

FATORES DE RISCO
Há relatos de aumento no número de casos no verão e no início do outono (hemisfério norte), possivelmente após surtos de doença respiratória superior; no entanto, a doença pode ocorrer ao longo do ano.

DIAGNÓSTICO

DIAGNÓSTICO DIFERENCIAL
• O diagnóstico é formulado com base no início agudo de sinais vestibulares periféricos que melhoram rapidamente sem tratamento específico.
• Otite média e interna (p. ex., bacteriana e parasitária) — pode exibir paresia ou paralisia concomitante do nervo facial (VII par de nervo craniano) ipsolateral, síndrome de Horner, surdez, ruptura da membrana timpânica, otite externa e/ou alterações radiográficas na bula timpânica; os sinais não costumam ser autolimitantes.
• Pólipo(s) nasofaríngeo(s) — podem causar sinais vestibulares periféricos unilaterais ou, muito menos comumente, bilaterais; pode(m) ter o envolvimento concomitante da bula timpânica; os sinais não costumam ser tão agudos e graves no início, nem autolimitantes. • Ingestão do lagarto da cauda azul — sudeste dos Estados Unidos; acredita-se que isso produza uma síndrome vestibular periférica, aguda e unilateral semelhante; também se observam vômito, salivação, irritabilidade e tremor; a maioria dos pacientes recupera-se sem tratamento específico.
• Intoxicação por aminoglicosídeos, especialmente a estreptomicina — pode causar síndrome vestibular periférica aguda uni ou bilateral e/ou perda auditiva; diferenciada por meio da anamnese quanto ao uso desses medicamentos.

HEMOGRAMA/BIOQUÍMICA/URINÁLISE
Normais.

DIAGNÓSTICO POR IMAGEM
• Em geral, não há necessidade. • Radiografias das bulas timpânicas — radiografias normais não descartam comprometimento da bula. • TC ou RM — ocasionalmente necessárias para excluir outras causas, como otite média e interna, além de pólipo(s) nasofaríngeo(s).

MÉTODOS DIAGNÓSTICOS
RAETC — pode ajudar a descartar outras causas (p. ex., otite média e interna; pólipo(s) nasofaríngeo(s)); em casos de vestibulopatia idiopática, a audição não deve ser acometida, já que a doença fica limitada à porção vestibular do VIII par de nervo craniano.

ACHADOS PATOLÓGICOS
Não há nenhum achado descrito.

TRATAMENTO

CUIDADO(S) DE SAÚDE ADEQUADO(S)
• Em geral, o tratamento é feito em um esquema ambulatorial. • Internação — os pacientes gravemente acometidos podem exigir a hospitalização para o fornecimento dos cuidados de suporte.

CUIDADO(S) DE ENFERMAGEM
• Doença leve — fornecer apenas tratamento de suporte. • Doença grave — pode necessitar de fluidos intravenosos ou subcutâneos; manter o paciente em gaiola bem-acolchoada e ambiente tranquilo.

ATIVIDADE
Restrita de acordo com o grau de desorientação e ataxia.

DIETA
• No início, o paciente pode apresentar relutância em comer e beber, possivelmente em virtude da desorientação e/ou da náusea.

ORIENTAÇÃO AO PROPRIETÁRIO
Tranquilizar o proprietário sobre o fato de que, apesar de os sinais clínicos iniciais serem alarmantes e frequentemente incapacitantes, o prognóstico é excelente quanto à recuperação rápida e completa.

MEDICAÇÕES

MEDICAMENTO(S) DE ESCOLHA
• Sedativos — em casos graves de desorientação e rolamento; diazepam (1-5 mg/gato VO a cada 8-12 h) e acepromazina (0,02-0,05 mg/kg IM, SC, IV).
• Agentes antieméticos e medicamentos contra a cinetose (doença do movimento) — benefício questionável; p. ex., cloridrato de meclizina a 12,5 mg VO a cada 24 h. • Glicocorticoides — não alteram a evolução da doença; portanto, não são recomendados. • Antibióticos — o uso desses agentes é recomendável caso não se consiga descartar a possibilidade de otite média e interna no diagnóstico diferencial; trimetoprima-sulfa (15 mg/kg VO a cada 12 h); alguma cefalosporina de primeira geração (p. ex., cefalexina na dosagem de 10-30 mg/kg VO a cada 6-12 h); amoxicilina/ácido clavulânico (Clavamox® 62,5 mg/gato VO a cada 12 h, Claviseptin® 12,5 mg/kg VO a cada 12 h).

ACOMPANHAMENTO

MONITORIZAÇÃO DO PACIENTE
• Exame neurológico do paciente ambulatorial — repetir em aproximadamente 72 h para confirmar a estabilização e a melhora inicial.
• Paciente internado — pode receber alta quando se mostrar capaz de caminhar e voltar a comer e beber.

EVOLUÇÃO ESPERADA E PROGNÓSTICO
• Melhora acentuada dos sinais clínicos, sobretudo do nistagmo em repouso dentro de 72 h, com restabelecimento progressivo da marcha e da inclinação da cabeça. • Os pacientes costumam retornar ao normal dentro de 2-3 semanas.
• Inclinação da cabeça — último sinal a desaparecer; uma leve inclinação residual pode permanecer. • Se os sinais não melhorarem rapidamente, o clínico deverá pesquisar outras causas de vestibulopatia. • Raramente ocorre recidiva.

DIVERSOS

ABREVIATURA(S)
• RAETC = resposta auditiva evocada do tronco cerebral.
• RM = ressonância magnética.
• TC = tomografia computadorizada.

Autor Susan M. Cochrane
Consultor Editorial Joane M. Parent

Vocalização Excessiva

CONSIDERAÇÕES GERAIS

REVISÃO
• Vocalização incontrolável, excessiva ou observada em momentos impróprios do dia ou da noite ou, então, incômoda para proprietários, vizinhos ou outros animais de estimação. • Muitas vezes, o latido é um comportamento canino normal que pode ser inaceitável para os proprietários. O latido parece ter evoluído em cães domésticos como um meio de comunicação social, pois muitas formas caninas de latido não são observadas em lobos. Os seres humanos são capazes de identificar a motivação que está por trás de grande parte das formas de latido. • Dor, doença ou ansiedade pode levar a desconforto ou induzir à vocalização como forma de chamar a atenção. A síndrome da disfunção cognitiva pode ocasionar vocalização excessiva e despertar noturno tanto em cães como em gatos. • O declínio da audição pode estar associado à vocalização excessiva.

IDENTIFICAÇÃO
• Cães e gatos. • Raças orientais de gatos podem ser mais propensas. • Raças caninas de trabalho e de caça podem ter propensão a latir demais. • Animais de estimação propensos à perda auditiva e síndrome de disfunção cognitiva. • Gatos intactos durante o estro e a cópula.

SINAIS CLÍNICOS
Subjetivos — relacionados com a intensidade, a duração, a hora do dia ou o ambiente.

CAUSAS E FATORES DE RISCO
• Clínica — doença, dor, síndrome de disfunção cognitiva. • Ansiedade ou conflito. • Latido de alarme — resposta a novos estímulos. • Territorial — resposta de aviso (alerta) ou guarda. • Comportamento reforçado. • Vocalização por desconforto (p. ex., uivos ou ganidos) — separação da mãe ou do grupo social. • Rosnado — pode estar associado a exibições agonistas. • Comportamentos estereotipados ou transtornos compulsivos — cães. • Cruzamento — sexual (gatos). • Raça — genética.

DIAGNÓSTICO

DIAGNÓSTICO DIFERENCIAL
• Latidos durante condições de ansiedade: ocorrem durante a ausência do proprietário ou em resposta a estímulos específicos. • Latidos devidos a comportamento territorial: ocorrem quando o proprietário está presente ou ausente. • Problemas de saúde.

HEMOGRAMA/BIOQUÍMICA/URINÁLISE
Para descartar distúrbios subjacentes.

OUTROS TESTES LABORATORIAIS
T_4 — gatos.

DIAGNÓSTICO POR IMAGEM
Se houver suspeita de distúrbio clínico ou neurológico.

MÉTODOS DIAGNÓSTICOS
• Teste da RAETC na suspeita de deficiência auditiva. • Diagnóstico comportamental para determinar estímulos incitantes com base na anamnese detalhada e precisa; observação do animal, do proprietário e das interações entre ambos; filmar o comportamento, se disponível.

TRATAMENTO

Comentários Gerais
• O tratamento deve ser individualizado para o animal, o ambiente onde ele vive e o tipo de problema. • Estabelecer um programa para tratar a causa subjacente e os fatores agravantes. • Produtos como enforcadores, alarmes ativados pelos latidos, coleiras de citronela ativadas pelos latidos e dispositivos dissociadores como alarmes ou esguichos de água podem ser usados para que o animal se aquiete, o que, então, pode ser reforçado; é melhor utilizá-los na presença do proprietário. • Pode-se optar pela desvocalização como último recurso; esse procedimento, no entanto, não trata a causa subjacente e o problema ainda pode recidivar no pós-operatório.

Modificação do Comportamento
• Evitar o reforço. A retirada do estímulo pode ser um reforço. Se o proprietário der algum tipo de atenção, inclusive punição insuficientemente aversiva, a vocalização poderá ser reforçada. • Adestramento baseado em recompensa — ensina os animais a responder a comandos básicos ("Sit" [sente-se], "Down" [deite-se], "Mat" [role]). • Adestrar os cães para que fiquem quietos à voz de comando (considerar o controle com enforcador). • Os proprietários precisam ficar calmos. A ansiedade por parte do proprietário, as repreensões verbais e as punições podem aumentar a ansiedade do animal e potencializar o latido. • Substituição da resposta — ensinar uma resposta apropriada ao estímulo (p. ex., sentar quieto). • Dessensibilização e contracondicionamento — para ansiedade subjacente, deve-se expor o animal ao estímulo incitante em um nível baixo (abaixo do limiar de resposta) e associar um reforço agradável, como um alimento ou petisco, ao estímulo para mudar a resposta emocional para um comportamento calmo ou positivo. Em seguida, avançar para um estímulo gradualmente mais intenso. • Evitar a punição. Os dispositivos que interrompem ou inibem a vocalização podem ajudar a manter o animal quieto, o que, então, pode ser reforçado. Não recomendados para latido relacionado com ansiedade, pois podem aumentar essa inquietação.

Modificação do Ambiente
Fazer adaptações para minimizar a exposição aos estímulos que incitam a vocalização.

MEDICAÇÕES

MEDICAMENTO(S)
• Uso de analgésicos na suspeita de alguma condição dolorosa. • Benzodiazepínicos a curto prazo ou conforme a necessidade quando se espera uma situação de ansiedade ou para induzir o sono (cão: diazepam, 0,5-2,2 mg/kg VO, conforme a necessidade, até a cada 8 h; gato: oxazepam, 0,2-0,5 mg/kg VO, conforme a necessidade, até a cada 12 h). • Sedativos como a acepromazina (0,5-2,2 mg/kg VO conforme a necessidade) podem ser eficazes para tranquilizar o animal antes da exposição a estímulos (p. ex., passeios de carro e fogos de artifício), mas não diminuem a ansiedade e podem aumentar a sensibilidade a ruídos e a vocalização em alguns cães. • Antidepressivos tricíclicos ou inibidores seletivos de recaptação da serotonina para terapia a longo prazo em casos de ansiedade excessiva e crônica ou transtornos compulsivos; combinar com a modificação do comportamento. Clomipramina — cão: 1-3 mg/kg VO a cada 12 h; gato: 0,5 mg/kg VO a cada 24 h; fluoxetina: cão: 1-2 mg/kg VO a cada 24 h; gato: 0,5 mg/kg VO a cada 24 h. • Na presença de síndrome de disfunção cognitiva, tratar com selegilina, dieta e suplementos (ver "Síndrome de Disfunção Cognitiva"). • Utilizar produtos naturais que podem reduzir o medo ou a ansiedade (p. ex., feromônio, Feliway®, Anxitane® [l-teanina], alfa-casozepina e Harmonease®).

CONTRAINDICAÇÕES/INTERAÇÕES POSSÍVEIS
• Rever as contraindicações para qualquer medicamento utilizado. • Não utilizar os antidepressivos tricíclicos nem os inibidores seletivos de recaptação da serotonina em combinação ou com inibidores da monoamina oxidase, inclusive produtos à base de amitraz e selegilina.

ACOMPANHAMENTO

MONITORIZAÇÃO DO PACIENTE
• Modificar o programa com base na resposta. • Medicamentos, coleiras ativadas pelo latido, dispositivos dissociadores e enforcadores poderão ser acrescentados.

PREVENÇÃO
• Adestramento de obediência, com enforcador, para ficar quieto ao comando (cães). • Evitar reforço de comportamento impróprio. • Acostumar o animal a uma variedade de estímulos e ambientes durante o desenvolvimento. • Socializar o animal com diversas pessoas e outros animais ao longo do desenvolvimento.

COMPLICAÇÕES POSSÍVEIS
• A ansiedade do proprietário e as repreensões verbais podem agravar o problema. • Reforço intermitente agrava o problema.

EVOLUÇÃO ESPERADA E PROGNÓSTICO
• Variável — com base no diagnóstico, no ambiente, no animal e nas expectativas do proprietário. • A maioria pode melhorar com o tempo, mas não é eliminada. • É inviável esperar eliminar toda a vocalização.

DIVERSOS

VER TAMBÉM
• Transtornos Compulsivos — Cães.
• Transtornos Compulsivos — Gatos.
• Síndrome de Ansiedade da Separação.
• Síndrome de Disfunção Cognitiva.

ABREVIATURA(S)
• RAETC = resposta auditiva evocada do tronco cerebral.
• T_4 = tiroxina.

Autores Gary Landsberg e Sagi Denenberg
Consultor Editorial Debra F. Horwitz

VÔMITO AGUDO

CONSIDERAÇÕES GERAIS

DEFINIÇÃO
- Expulsão reflexa e forçada de conteúdo gástrico pela cavidade bucal.
- Os vômitos agudos são definidos como aqueles de duração curta (<5-7 dias) e frequência variável.

FISIOPATOLOGIA
- Trata-se de um conjunto complexo de atividades reflexas sob controle hormonal e neurológico central, que envolve a coordenação das musculaturas gastrintestinal, abdominal e respiratória.
- Os vômitos agudos frequentemente são precedidos por sinais prodrômicos de náusea, o primeiro estágio do vômito que pode incluir depressão, tremor, busca por esconderijos ou locais confortáveis, sialorreia, lambedura dos lábios, deglutição frequente, bocejo e ânsia (vômito seco).
- No primeiro estágio, há um aumento da saliva com bicarbonato para lubrificar o esôfago e neutralizar a acidez gástrica.
- Isso é acompanhado por diminuição da motilidade gastresofágica e aumento da motilidade retrógrada do intestino delgado proximal.
- O estágio 2 consiste na presença de ânsia (vômito seco), que corresponde a contrações forçadas dos músculos abdominais e do diafragma com consequente pressão intratorácica negativa e pressão intra-abdominal positiva para facilitar o deslocamento do conteúdo gástrico pela boca.
- No estágio 3, o conteúdo gástrico é expelido. Há uma alteração na pressão intratorácica de negativa para positiva pela força gerada pelos músculos abdominais e pelo diafragma. Concomitantemente, a respiração é inibida, com consequente fechamento da nasofaringe e da glote para evitar aspiração.
- O vômito ocorre quando o centro emético na medula oblonga é estimulado por mecanismos humorais ou neurais.
- A estimulação de receptores de estiramento, quimiorreceptores e osmorreceptores localizados em todo o trato GI, sistema hepatobiliar, sistema geniturinário, peritônio e pâncreas são exemplos de ativação neural (o duodeno possui a maior parte dos receptores).
- Os estímulos humorais são mediados pela zona deflagradora dos quimiorreceptores; com uma barreira hematencefálica mais permeável, uma variedade de medicamentos e toxinas também pode estimular o centro emético.
- Os gatos possuem receptores dopaminérgicos pouco desenvolvidos na zona deflagradora dos quimiorreceptores e, portanto, são pouco responsivos à apomorfina.
- Como os centros nervosos superiores podem induzir a vômitos psicogênicos, os impulsos vindos do aparelho vestibular (doença do movimento [cinetose] e vestibulopatia) podem estimular o centro emético.

SISTEMA(S) ACOMETIDO(S)
- Cardiovascular — taquicardia induzida por hipovolemia, mucosas pálidas e pulsos fracos; a hipocalemia pode causar arritmias.
- Gastrintestinal — esofagite por refluxo.
- Metabólico — distúrbios eletrolíticos e acidobásicos (p. ex., hipocalemia, hiponatremia, hipocloremia e alcalose metabólica), azotemia pré-renal e desidratação.
- Respiratório — pneumonia por aspiração, rinite por refluxo de ingesta em direção à nasofaringe.
- Nervoso — depressão.

IDENTIFICAÇÃO
Não há predileção etária, racial ou sexual.

SINAIS CLÍNICOS
Achados Anamnésicos
- Vômitos variáveis de alimento e/ou líquido (límpido ou manchado de bile ou sangue).
- Ingestão de corpo estranho.
- Letargia e perda do apetite variáveis; podem ocorrer diarreia e/ou melena.

Achados do Exame Físico
- Podem incluir desidratação (p. ex., mucosas secas, turgor cutâneo reduzido, olhos afundados, mucosas pálidas, taquicardia, pulsos fracos), alças intestinais preenchidas por líquido, ruídos intestinais excessivos, dor abdominal (localizada [p. ex., corpo estranho, pancreatite, pielonefrite e hepatopatia] *versus* difusa [p. ex., peritonite, enterite grave]) ou massa abdominal (p. ex., corpo estranho, intussuscepção e torção visceral).
- Ao exame retal, pode-se notar diarreia ou melena.
- Em vômitos decorrentes de causas infecciosas e inflamatórias, pode-se observar febre.

CAUSAS
- Reações alimentares adversas — imprudências (consumo rápido de alimento e ingestão de corpo estranho); intolerâncias (p. ex., mudança súbita da dieta e alergias).
- Medicamentos — antibióticos, anti-inflamatórios (corticosteroides e AINE), quimioterápicos, digitálicos, narcóticos, xilazina, tiacetarsamida.
- Inflamação gastrintestinal — enterite infecciosa: agentes virais (parvovírus, vírus da cinomose, coronavírus), bactérias (*Salmonella*, *Campylobacter*, *Helicobacter* spp.); gastrenterite hemorrágica.
- Úlceras gastroduodenais.
- Obstrução gastrintestinal — corpos estranhos, intussuscepção, neoplasia, vólvulo, íleo paralítico, constipação, hipertrofia da mucosa.
- Doença sistêmica — uremia, insuficiência hepática, sepse, acidose, desequilíbrio eletrolítico (hipocalemia, hipocalcemia, hipercalcemia).
- Distúrbios abdominais — pancreatite, peritonite, piometra.
- Endocrinopatia — hipoadrenocorticismo, cetoacidose diabética.
- Neuropatia — distúrbios vestibulares, meningite, encefalite, traumatismo craniano (SNC).
- Parasitismo — ascarídeos, *Giardia*, *Physaloptera*, *Ollulanus tricuspis* (gatos), intoxicação alimentar por salmão (cães).
- Toxinas — chumbo, etilenoglicol, zinco, micotoxinas, plantas domésticas.
- Diversos — anafilaxia, intermação (insolação), doença do movimento (cinetose), dor, febre.

DIAGNÓSTICO

DIAGNÓSTICO DIFERENCIAL
Diferenciação de Sinais Clínicos Semelhantes
- O vômito geralmente envolve sialorreia e ânsia, bem como contrações vigorosas dos músculos abdominais e do diafragma.
- Sempre é preciso diferenciá-lo de regurgitação (que corresponde à expulsão passiva, ou seja, sem esforço de líquido ou alimento a partir do esôfago ou da cavidade faríngea) e de disfagia (dificuldade de deglutição, observada durante a alimentação ou a ingestão de líquidos).
- Os animais que estão vomitando ainda podem apresentar distúrbios indutores de regurgitação; além disso, os vômitos frequentes podem levar à esofagite por refluxo e à regurgitação.

Diferenciação das Causas
- Classificar os pacientes como casos críticos ou não.
- Se não houver nenhum sinal de vômitos graves (p. ex., desidratação, letargia, febre, anorexia ou dor abdominal), pode-se avaliar o animal apenas com a anamnese e o exame físico completos.
- Na presença de indicadores de vômitos intensos, na intensificação da frequência dos vômitos ou na falta de resolução dos sinais clínicos em 2-3 dias, deve-se obter um banco de dados mínimo (incluindo hemograma completo, análise bioquímica, urinálise e radiografias abdominais simples) na tentativa de se descobrir a causa primária.

HEMOGRAMA/BIOQUÍMICA/URINÁLISE
- Em casos de vômitos não críticos, os resultados do hemograma, do perfil bioquímico e da urinálise permanecem tipicamente normais.
- Anemia com pan-hipoproteinemia é observada em casos de ulceração gástrica e sangramento graves.
- Desidratação — pode-se observar uma hemoconcentração (hematócrito e proteína total elevados).
- Pode-se notar leucograma de estresse.
- Causas infecciosas ou inflamatórias — pode-se verificar leucograma inflamatório.
- A densidade urinária permite a diferenciação entre a azotemia pré-renal e as causas renais de vômitos.
- Hepatopatias agudas — pode-se constatar aumento das enzimas hepáticas e da bilirrubina sérica.
- Pancreatite — possivelmente ocorre elevação da lipase, da amilase e das enzimas hepáticas.
- Hiponatremia, hipercalemia, hipoglicemia e azotemia — sugerem hipoadrenocorticismo.
- Hiperglicemia com glicosúria e cetonúria — indica diabetes melito cetoacidótica.

OUTROS TESTES LABORATORIAIS
Quando indicados, efetuar exames de sangue adicionais para a pesquisa de doenças específicas (p. ex., nível sanguíneo de chumbo, análise do etilenoglicol, teste de estimulação com o ACTH para hipoadrenocorticismo, bem como testes de imunorreatividade da lipase pancreática canina ou de imunorreatividade da lipase pancreática felina em casos de pancreatite).

DIAGNÓSTICO POR IMAGEM
- As radiografias abdominais simples permanecem frequentemente normais, embora se possa observar a presença de corpos estranhos radiodensos, íleo paralítico segmentar ou distensão gástrica indicativa de vólvulo ou obstrução do fluxo de saída; em casos de pancreatite ou peritonite, pode-se perder o contorno (a silhueta) da serosa (aspecto em "vidro fosco"); a ocorrência de efeito expansivo ou nebulosidade no quadrante cranial direito ou a presença persistente de gases na porção descendente do duodeno podem indicar pancreatite.

Vômito Agudo

- Para avaliação de corpos estranhos radiotransparentes, obstrução, intussuscepção ou vólvulo, pode-se lançar mão de radiografias contrastadas.
- O emprego de ultrassonografia abdominal também é possível para observar obstrução, intussuscepção ou pancreatite.

MÉTODOS DIAGNÓSTICOS
A endoscopia pode ser útil para avaliar o animal quanto à presença de ulceração gastroduodenal, além de corpos estranhos duodenais proximais e gástricos.

TRATAMENTO

CUIDADO(S) DE SAÚDE ADEQUADO(S)
- A causa mais frequente de vômitos agudos é a imprudência alimentar.
- A recuperação de vômitos não críticos costuma ser rápida e espontânea.

CUIDADO(S) DE ENFERMAGEM
- Os pacientes com vômitos não críticos são tratados em um esquema ambulatorial, deixando-se o trato gastrintestinal repousar e mantendo-se o animal em jejum absoluto (i. e., nada por via oral) durante 12-24 h.
- Os pacientes com vômitos críticos devem ser internados e tratados em princípio com jejum absoluto por via oral, juntamente com a administração de fluidos cristaloides intravenosos, ao mesmo tempo em que se efetuam os testes diagnósticos adicionais.

ATIVIDADE
É recomendável a restrição da atividade física até que o vômito seja interrompido.

DIETA
- Se os vômitos desaparecerem, oferecer inicialmente pequenas quantidades de água ou cubos de gelo; se os vômitos não apresentarem recidiva, prosseguir com uma fonte de carboidratos e proteínas simples, pobre em gordura e facilmente digestível, como queijo tipo *cottage* desnatado ou carne branca (frango sem a pele) e arroz na proporção de 1:3. • Caso não ocorra a recidiva dos vômitos, deve-se habituar o paciente de volta à dieta normal em 4-5 dias.

ORIENTAÇÃO AO PROPRIETÁRIO
Os proprietários devem ser orientados sobre os riscos do fornecimento de restos de comida ou outros petiscos a seus animais de estimação, mantendo-os particularmente distantes de petiscos ricos em gordura. Eles também devem limitar o acesso do animal ao lixo e supervisioná-lo enquanto ele está brincando para evitar a ingestão de corpos estranhos.

CONSIDERAÇÕES CIRÚRGICAS
A intervenção cirúrgica deve ser considerada na presença de corpos estranhos ou obstruções de qualquer tipo, bem como em casos de peritonite ou vólvulo.

MEDICAÇÕES

MEDICAMENTO(S) DE ESCOLHA
- Pode-se fazer uso dos antieméticos em pacientes com vômitos graves indutores de distúrbios eletrolíticos e/ou acidobásicos ou esofagite por refluxo.
- Há diversos antieméticos disponíveis tanto para cães como para gatos — os derivados fenotiazínicos que atuam na zona deflagradora dos quimiorreceptores e no centro do vômito incluem a clorpromazina (0,5 mg/kg SC a cada 8 h) e a metoclopramida, um antagonista dopaminérgico e modificador da motilidade que atua na zona deflagradora dos quimiorreceptores e nos receptores locais do intestino (0,2-0,5 mg/kg VO ou SC a cada 6-8 h, ou 1-2 mg/kg/dia sob infusão em velocidade constante); em casos de doença do movimento, podem-se usar os antagonistas dos receptores H_1 que atuam sobre a zona deflagradora dos quimiorreceptores (p. ex., difenidramina a 2-4 mg/kg VO, IM, a cada 6-8 h) apenas para os cães; maropitanto, um antagonista da neurocinina 1 (1 mg/kg SC a cada 24 h ou 2 mg/kg VO a cada 24 h) apenas para os cães.
- Pacientes com ulceração — podem-se usar antagonistas dos receptores H_2, como a ranitidina (1-2 mg/kg VO, SC, IV, a cada 12 h), que também aumenta o esvaziamento gástrico, e/ou o sucralfato [protetor da mucosa gástrica] (250 mg/gato VO a cada 6-12 h, 250-1.000 mg/cão VO a cada 6-12 h) como uma pasta líquida.
- Febre ou lesão da mucosa (hematêmese, melena) — pode-se indicar a administração de antibióticos (p. ex., ampicilina e metronidazol).

CONTRAINDICAÇÕES
- É preciso utilizar os fenotiazínicos com cuidado em pacientes desidratados, em virtude da possível hipotensão decorrente de seu efeito antagonista sobre os receptores alfa; esses agentes também podem diminuir o limiar convulsivo e, por essa razão, é recomendável evitá-los em epilépticos.
- Os anticolinérgicos não devem ser utilizados, pois podem causar atonia gástrica e íleo paralítico intestinal, o que pode exacerbar os vômitos.
- Em função de seus efeitos procinéticos, a metoclopramida não deve ser usada em pacientes com obstrução gastrintestinal; deve-se utilizá-la com cuidado em casos de pancreatite, porque os efeitos sobre a perfusão esplâncnica permanecem questionáveis.
- Maropitanto deve ser usado com cautela em pacientes hepatopatias e apenas por 5 dias no máximo.

PRECAUÇÕES
É preciso ter cuidado ao se utilizar os antieméticos, pois tais agentes podem suprimir os vômitos e mascarar doenças progressivas ou dificultar os meios relevantes de monitorização da resposta à terapia primária.

INTERAÇÕES POSSÍVEIS
Agentes como anticolinérgicos e opioides podem anular o efeito da metoclopramida.

MEDICAMENTO(S) ALTERNATIVO(S)
- Cisaprida.
- Famotidina.
- Dolasetrona.

ACOMPANHAMENTO

MONITORIZAÇÃO DO PACIENTE
- Em casos de aumento na frequência dos vômitos ou na ocorrência de complicações sérias, os animais deverão ser internados para o tratamento e a obtenção de dados apropriados.
- Se o vômito persistir por mais de 7 dias apesar da terapia conservadora, deve-se prosseguir com a realização de testes apropriados para vômitos crônicos.

PREVENÇÃO
- Os animais devem ser alimentados com uma dieta regular de alta qualidade.
- Os proprietários devem tentar controlar a alimentação indiscriminada e monitorizar a ingestão de corpo estranho.

COMPLICAÇÕES POSSÍVEIS
- Pneumonia por aspiração.
- Esofagite.
- Ver a seção "Sistemas Acometidos".

EVOLUÇÃO ESPERADA E PROGNÓSTICO
- O jejum absoluto (i. e., nada por via oral), seguido por dieta branda, geralmente controlará os vômitos não críticos.
- Os corpos estranhos GI apresentam prognóstico bom após recuperação endoscópica ou remoção cirúrgica.

DIVERSOS

DISTÚRBIOS ASSOCIADOS
Ver a seção "Sistema(s) Acometido(s)".

FATORES RELACIONADOS COM A IDADE
É mais provável que os animais jovens ingiram corpos estranhos e adquiram doenças virais, bacterianas e parasitárias.

POTENCIAL ZOONÓTICO
Algumas espécies de *Giardia*, *Salmonella* e *Campylobacter* podem ser infecciosas para os seres humanos.

GESTAÇÃO/FERTILIDADE/REPRODUÇÃO
O misoprostol — uma prostaglandina sintética utilizada com maior frequência no tratamento ou na prevenção de ulcerações gástricas — é contraindicado em fêmeas prenhes.

VER TAMBÉM
- Diarreia Aguda.
- Úlcera Gastroduodenal.

ABREVIATURA(S)
- ACTH = hormônio adrenocorticotrópico.
- AINE = anti-inflamatório não esteroide.
- GI = gastrintestinal.
- SNC = sistema nervoso central.

Sugestões de Leitura
Hall JA, Washabau RJ. Gastric prokinetic agents. In: Kirk's Current Veterinary Therapy XIII. Philadelphia: Saunders, 2000, pp. 614-617.
Simpson KW. Diseases of the stomach. In: Ettinger SJ, Feldman EC, eds., Textbook of Veterinary Internal Medicine, 6th ed. St. Louis: Elsevier, 2005, pp. 1310-1331.
Twedt DC. Vomiting. In: Ettinger SJ, Feldman EC, eds., Textbook of Veterinary Internal Medicine, 6th ed. St. Louis: Elsevier, 2005, 132-136.

Autor Erin Portillo
Consultor Editorial Albert E. Jergens

VÔMITO CRÔNICO

CONSIDERAÇÕES GERAIS

DEFINIÇÃO
Vômitos persistentes que duram mais de 5-7 dias ou vômitos que ocorrem de forma intermitente por vários dias/semanas. Essa condição não é responsiva a tratamento sintomático.

FISIOPATOLOGIA
Os vômitos ocorrem quando o centro do vômito, localizado na medula oblonga, é ativado por meio de estimulação humoral ou neural de vários receptores periféricos sensíveis a substâncias químicas, inflamações e alterações na osmolalidade. Uma segunda causa importante de vômitos consiste na estimulação da zona deflagradora de quimiorreceptores, responsiva a metabólitos tóxicos, certos medicamentos e toxinas hematógenas.

SISTEMA(S) ACOMETIDO(S)
- Endócrino/metabólico — desidratação, distúrbios eletrolíticos e acidobásicos.
- Cardiovascular — a hipovolemia ou os distúrbios eletrolíticos e acidobásicos podem causar arritmias.
- Gastrintestinal — refluxo gastresofágico, esofagite e subsequente estenose esofágica.
- Respiratório — pneumonia por aspiração.
- Neurológico — alteração da atividade mental.

IDENTIFICAÇÃO
- Cães e gatos.
- É mais provável que os animais jovens ingiram corpos estranhos; os corpos estranhos lineares são mais comuns em gatos.
- Predisposições raciais confirmadas ou suspeitas — as raças braquicefálicas são propensas à obstrução do fluxo de saída pilórico, secundária à hipertrofia da mucosa; os cães Basenji, Pastor alemão e Shar-pei são suscetíveis a enteropatias inflamatórias; os cães da raça Rottweiler têm tendência ao granuloma eosinofílico gástrico; a raça Airedale terrier tende a ter carcinoma pancreático; os cães das raças Beagle, Bedlington terrier, Cocker spaniel, Doberman pinscher, Labrador retriever, Skye terrier e Poodle standard têm propensão à hepatite crônica.

SINAIS CLÍNICOS

Achados Anamnésicos
- Vômito de alimento, líquido límpido ou manchado com bile, hematêmese, hiporexia ou anorexia, pica, melena, polidipsia e distensão abdominal — são típicos de gastropatia.
- Diarreia e perda de peso acentuada — são sinais mais característicos de enteropatia.
- Fraqueza, poliúria ou icterícia — sinais relacionados com outras doenças metabólicas subjacentes.

Achados do Exame Físico
- Perda de peso e más condições da pelagem podem indicar desnutrição crônica.
- A palpação abdominal pode revelar distensão, dor, alças intestinais espessadas ou massas.
- Mucosas pegajosas e pele em tenda mantida por tempo prolongado na presença de desidratação; mucosas pálidas se o paciente estiver anêmico.
- O exame retal pode detectar diarreia, hematoquezia ou melena.

CAUSAS

Doença Esofágica
- Hérnia de hiato.
- Refluxo gastresofágico.
- Esofagite distal.

Doença Infecciosa
- Gastrite relacionada com o *Helicobacter*.
- Histoplasmose.
- Pitiose.
- Proliferação bacteriana no intestino delgado.
- Parasitas gástricos — *Physaloptera* spp.
- Parasitismo intestinal.

Doenças Metabólicas
- Nefropatia.
- Doença hepatobiliar.
- Hipoadrenocorticismo.
- Pancreatite crônica.
- Cetoacidose diabética.
- Acidose metabólica.
- Distúrbios eletrolíticos — hipo/hipercalemia, hiponatremia, hipercalcemia.

Enteropatia Inflamatória
- Linfocítica, plasmocitária, eosinofílica ou granulomatosa.
- Gastrite, enterite ou colite.

Gastrenteropatia Obstrutiva
- Corpo estranho.
- Estenose pilórica congênita.
- Gastropatia hipertrófica pilórica crônica.
- Intussuscepção.

Doença Neoplásica
- Linfossarcoma, adenocarcinoma, fibrossarcoma gastrintestinais, além de tumor das células do estroma gastrintestinal.
- Adenocarcinoma pancreático.
- Tumor pancreático secretor de gastrina (gastrinoma).
- Mastocitose sistêmica.

Neuropatia
- Edema cerebral.
- Tumores do SNC.
- Encefalite/meningoencefalite.
- Vestibulopatia.

Distúrbios de Motilidade
- Dilatação pós-gástrica.
- Distúrbios pós-cirúrgicos — gástricos, duodenais.
- Desequilíbrios eletrolíticos.

Diversos
- Induzidos por medicamentos (p. ex., AINE, glicocorticoides, antibióticos e antifúngicos).
- Intolerância/alergia alimentar.
- Toxicidade.

Causas Adicionais em Gatos
- Parasitárias — dirofilariose, *Ollulanus tricuspis*, giardíase.
- Inflamatórias — colecistite, colangio-hepatite.
- Metabólicas — hipertireoidismo.
- Funcionais — constipação/obstipação.

FATORES DE RISCO
Doença associada à raça (ver a seção "Identificação").

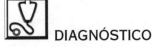

DIAGNÓSTICO

DIAGNÓSTICO DIFERENCIAL
- Inicialmente, os vômitos precisam ser diferenciados de regurgitação.
- Regurgitação constitui um movimento retrógrado passivo, em direção à cavidade oronasal, de líquido e alimento não digerido que ainda não chegou ao estômago. Além disso, a regurgitação ocorre sem um componente abdominal, situando com isso a doença no esôfago.
- Vômito é frequentemente precedido por inquietação, náusea, salivação e deglutição repetida.
- Os pacientes com vômitos também podem regurgitar em função da esofagite secundária.
- Vômito de alimento ou alimento parcialmente digerido é mais comum em casos de gastropatia primária, enquanto o vômito de bile é mais provavelmente de origem intestinal.

HEMOGRAMA/BIOQUÍMICA/URINÁLISE
- Os hemogramas completos costumam permanecer normais em casos de gastropatia primária.
- A ocorrência de sangramento gastrintestinal crônico pode causar anemia arregenerativa, muitas vezes com características de deficiência de ferro (microcitose, hipocromasia, trombocitose).
- O sangramento gastrintestinal agudo possivelmente gera anemia regenerativa ou arregenerativa, dependendo da gravidade e da duração.
- Também pode ocorrer anemia arregenerativa secundariamente a doenças metabólicas ou inflamatórias crônicas.
- Enteropatia inflamatória, pancreatite crônica, colangio-hepatite e colecistite podem provocar leucocitose neutrofílica e monocitose.
- A eosinofilia pode decorrer de gastrenterite eosinofílica, insuficiência adrenocortical e parasitismo gastrintestinal.
- A trombocitopenia foi relatada em casos de enteropatia inflamatória.
- A desidratação aumenta o hematócrito e a proteína total.
- Bioquímica fornece informações diagnósticas e terapêuticas; os resultados normais descartam doença metabólica como a etiologia subjacente.
- Os desequilíbrios eletrolíticos e acidobásicos refletem a gravidade das perdas e podem ajudar a localizar a doença.
- A alcalose metabólica hipoclorêmica, frequentemente com hipocalemia, indica perda substancial de conteúdo gástrico, mais compatível com obstrução ao fluxo de saída gástrico.
- A hipercalemia no paciente com vômito sugere hipoadrenocorticismo ou insuficiência renal oligúrica ou anúrica; ocasionalmente, a enterite causada por tricuríase ou infecção bacteriana (salmonelose) mimetiza o hipoadrenocorticismo.
- A acidose metabólica é comum em pacientes desidratados e naqueles com insuficiência renal, cetoacidose diabética e gastrenterite grave com diarreia.
- O aumento na atividade das enzimas hepáticas, a hipoalbuminemia, a hiperbilirrubinemia, a hipoglicemia ou a concentração baixa de ureia sugerem hepatopatia.
- A hiperglicemia e a glicosúria são características diagnósticas de diabetes melito.
- A hiperglobulinemia pode revelar inflamação ou infecção crônicas.
- Ocorrem hipoalbuminemia, linfopenia e hipomagnesemia, secundariamente à enteropatia com perda de proteína causada por enteropatias infiltrativas, como gastrenterite linfocítica

VÔMITO CRÔNICO

plasmocitária, neoplasia, histoplasmose ou linfangiectasia intestinal primária.
• Em casos de linfangiectasia, também se pode observar hipocolesterolemia.
• A urinálise é empregada para descartar causas não gastrintestinais de vômitos crônicos, como insuficiência renal e cetoacidose diabética.
• Urina ácida em pacientes com hipocalemia, hipocloremia e alcalose indica perda considerável de conteúdo gástrico, assim como ocorreria em casos de obstrução ao fluxo de saída gástrico.

OUTROS TESTES LABORATORIAIS
• O teste de estimulação com o ACTH ou o nível de cortisol abaixo do normal em repouso é usado para confirmar o hipoadrenocorticismo.
• A imunorreatividade da lipase pancreática pode ajudar a confirmar a pancreatite.
• A mensuração da concentração dos ácidos biliares auxilia na confirmação de doenças hepatobiliares.

DIAGNÓSTICO POR IMAGEM
• Radiografias abdominais simples ajudam a identificar corpos estranhos, distensão gastrintestinal com líquido ou gás, bem como deslocamento, mau posicionamento e/ou alterações de formato ou tamanho de órgãos abdominais.
• Radiografias torácicas simples são utilizadas para avaliar doenças infecciosas ou metastáticas pulmonares.
• Radiografias contrastadas abdominais auxiliam na identificação de corpos estranhos, massas ou doenças infiltrativas na parede gastrintestinal, ulceração da mucosa, retardo no esvaziamento gástrico e distúrbios de motilidade.
• Ultrassonografia abdominal ajuda a identificar anormalidades parenquimatosas de órgãos como fígado, vesícula biliar, rins, pâncreas e trato GI.
• TC e RM avaliam de forma mais aprofundada as anormalidades parenquimatosas de órgãos abdominais.

MÉTODOS DIAGNÓSTICOS
• Gastroduodenoscopia — permite a inspeção direta do lúmen gástrico e intestinal para identificar lesões macroscópicas da mucosa e presença de corpos estranhos; além disso, representa um método minimamente invasivo de biopsia para avaliar doenças microscópicas.
• Laparoscopia ou laparotomia exploratória é utilizada para procedimentos diagnósticos e terapêuticos mais amplos.

TRATAMENTO
• O tratamento específico deve ser direcionado à eliminação da causa subjacente em conjunto com terapia de suporte.
• Se os vômitos persistirem, deve-se interromper o consumo oral de água e alimentos por algumas horas.
• Utilizar a fluidoterapia não só para repor os déficits, mas também para suprir as perdas de manutenção e contínuas.
• Caso não se conheça o estado acidobásico ou na presença de alcalose metabólica hipoclorêmica, deve-se usar a solução fisiológica a 0,9%.
• Em casos de acidose metabólica, recomenda-se o uso da solução de Ringer lactato.

• Em casos de hipocalemia, emprega-se a suplementação com potássio; para a reposição e a manutenção, pode-se adicionar com segurança uma quantidade de 20 mEq de cloreto de potássio/L de fluido; utilizar concentrações mais altas na presença de hipocalemia grave.
• Os pacientes debilitados e aqueles em más condições nutricionais podem necessitar de nutrição parenteral ou enteral.
• Em pacientes com suspeita de alergia alimentar ou com enteropatia inflamatória, deve-se adotar uma dieta que contenha uma única fonte proteica nova.
• Aos pacientes gravemente anêmicos com indícios de sangramento gastrintestinal ativo, proceder à transfusão sanguínea.
• Caso se observe hemorragia incontrolável, obstrução ou perfuração, indica-se o tratamento cirúrgico.

MEDICAÇÕES
MEDICAMENTO(S)
• Os medicamentos antissecretores, como os bloqueadores dos receptores H_2 (p. ex., cimetidina, ranitidina, famotidina) ou os inibidores das bombas de prótons, como o omeprazol (mais potente) — ranitidina (2 mg/kg VO, IV a cada 12 h); omeprazol (0,7 mg/kg VO a cada 24 h).
• Protetores como o sucralfato (0,5-1 g/cão VO a cada 8-12 h; 0,25 g/gato VO a cada 8-12 h) para acelerar a cicatrização da mucosa gástrica; podem ser utilizados juntamente com os agentes antissecretores nos pacientes com indícios de sangramento do trato GI superior (p. ex., hematêmese ou melena).
• Antibióticos — indicados para tratar gastrite associada ao *Helicobacter* e proliferação bacteriana no intestino delgado e também como adjuvantes dos corticosteroides no tratamento da enteropatia inflamatória.
• Tratamento sugerido da gastrite associada ao *Helicobacter* — amoxicilina (20 mg/kg VO a cada 8 h) em combinação com omeprazol (0,7 mg/kg VO a cada 24 h) e metronidazol (10 mg/kg VO a cada 12 h por 21 dias); pode-se utilizar a claritromicina (7,5 mg/kg VO a cada 12 h) com amoxicilina e metronidazol (conforme exposto anteriormente) como uma terapia alternativa para os gatos.
• Metronidazol — pode ser usado a 10 mg/kg VO a cada 12 h em combinação com corticosteroides para tratar a enteropatia inflamatória.
• Enteropatia responsiva a antibióticos — tetraciclina, metronidazol, amoxicilina e tilosina, além de corrigir a causa subjacente.
• Utilizar os corticosteroides em conjunto com mudanças na dieta e o metronidazol para tratar a enteropatia inflamatória confirmada por meio de biopsia; também se pode lançar mão de azatioprina, clorambucila ou ciclosporina em pacientes com resposta insatisfatória aos corticosteroides isolados ou para diminuir a dosagem de esteroides necessária para controlar os sintomas.
• Para o tratamento de retardo no esvaziamento gástrico não associado à doença obstrutiva, pode-se fazer uso de agentes procinéticos, como a metoclopramida ou a eritromicina.

• O pamoato de pirantel é eficaz em casos de *Physaloptera*; já o fembendazol é eficiente contra *Ollulanus*.
• Os animais com sangramento gastrintestinal crônico que desenvolvem anemia hipocrômica microcítica podem necessitar de suplementação com ferro.
• O tratamento cirúrgico e/ou quimioterápico contra neoplasias depende do tipo e da localização do tumor.
• Uma hipersecreção paraneoplásica de ácido gástrico, como ocorre em casos de mastocitose e tumores pancreáticos secretores de gastrina, é tratada de forma mais satisfatória com medicamentos antissecretores, como o omeprazol, para diminuir a gastrite, as úlceras gástricas e os vômitos crônicos.
• Reservar os antieméticos para os pacientes com vômitos persistentes irresponsivos ao tratamento da doença subjacente; os fenotiazínicos (p. ex., clorpromazina) bloqueiam tanto a zona deflagradora dos quimiorreceptores como o centro do vômito; clorpromazina (0,5 mg/kg SC, IM a cada 6-8 h).
• Agentes procinéticos (p. ex., metoclopramida) — a metoclopramida (0,2-0,5 mg/kg IV, IM, VO a cada 6-8 h) também bloqueia a zona deflagradora dos quimiorreceptores; esse medicamento também pode ser utilizado sob a forma de infusão em velocidade contínua na dose de 1-2 mg/kg/dia em pacientes internados.
• Os vômitos causados por quimioterapia são tratados de forma mais eficiente com a ondansetrona (0,5-1 mg/kg IV, VO), administrada 30 min antes do tratamento quimioterápico.

PRECAUÇÕES
• Não administrar bloqueadores alfa-adrenérgicos, como clorpromazina, a pacientes desidratados, pois tais agentes podem provocar hipotensão.
• É preciso utilizar os antieméticos com cautela, pois esses agentes podem mascarar o problema subjacente.
• A metoclopramida pode causar depressão, inquietação, agitação e outras mudanças comportamentais, particularmente em gatos.
• Os corticosteroides são imunossupressores e representam um fator de risco para o desenvolvimento de ulceração gastrintestinal; deve-se ter cuidado ao se tratar a enteropatia inflamatória com corticosteroides em dosagens altas ou por períodos prolongados.
• A azatioprina e a clorambucila são mielotóxicas; portanto, recomenda-se a obtenção de hemograma completo para a pesquisa de neutropenia e trombocitopenia a cada 2 semanas durante os dois primeiros meses de tratamento e, depois, mensalmente.
• A ciclosporina pode exacerbar o vômito e a diarreia quando utilizada em altas doses; usar com cuidado em pacientes com doença renal.
• Não usar os anticolinérgicos como antieméticos, pois eles podem causar atonia e retenção gástricas, o que possivelmente exacerba os vômitos.
• A metoclopramida e a cisaprida são contraindicadas em pacientes com obstrução gastrintestinal.

INTERAÇÕES POSSÍVEIS
A cimetidina e a ranitidina interferem no metabolismo hepático de teofilina, fenitoína e varfarina e, portanto, não devem ser utilizadas em conjunto com esses medicamentos.

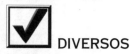

DIVERSOS

POTENCIAL ZOONÓTICO

O *Helicobacter heilmanii* e o *H. felis* podem ter potencial zoonótico; tais microrganismos foram isolados de seres humanos com gastrite crônica, mas a maioria deles teve contato próximo com cães ou gatos.

ABREVIATURA(S)
- ACTH = hormônio adrenocorticotrópico.
- AINE = anti-inflamatório não esteroide.
- GI = gastrintestinal.
- RM = ressonância magnética.
- SNC = sistema nervoso central.
- TC = tomografia computadorizada.

Sugestões de Leitura

Guilford WG, Center SA, Williams DA, Meyer DJ. Chronic gastric diseases. In: Strombeck's Small Animal Gastroenterology, 3rd ed. Philadelphia: Saunders, 1996, pp. 275-302.

Simpson K. Diseases of the stomach. In: Ettinger SJ, Feldman EC, eds., Textbook of Veterinary Internal Medicine, 6th ed. St. Louis: Elsevier, 2005, pp. 1310-1331.

Autor John M. Crandell
Consultor Editorial Albert E. Jergens

CONTEÚDO DOS APÊNDICES

Apêndice I	Valores de Referência para Testes Laboratoriais
Tabela I-A	Valores Hematológicos Normais
Tabela I-B	Valores Bioquímicos Normais
Tabela I-C	Tabela de Conversão para Unidades Hematológicas
Tabela I-D	Tabela de Conversão para Unidades Bioquímicas Clínicas

Apêndice II — Testes Endócrinos
Tabela II-A — Protocolos Para Testes da Função Endócrina
Tabela II-B — Testes do Sistema Endócrino
Tabela II-C — Tabela de Conversão para Unidades de Análise Hormonal

Apêndice III — Valores Normais Aproximados para Mensurações Comuns em Cães e Gatos

Apêndice IV — Valores Normais para o Eletrocardiograma Canino e Felino

Apêndice V — Toxicoses Clínicas — Sistemas Acometidos e Efeitos Clínicos

Apêndice VI — Agentes Tóxicos e seus Antídotos Sistêmicos — Dosagens e Métodos Terapêuticos

Apêndice VII — Riscos de Intoxicação Provenientes de Casa ou do Jardim, para Animais de Companhia
Tabela VII-A — Plantas Tóxicas — Sinais Clínicos, Antídotos e Tratamentos
Tabela VII-B — Toxicidade Relacionada a Ervas Medicinais
Tabela VII-C — Produtos de Limpeza e seus Sinais Clínicos — Antídotos e Tratamentos

Apêndice VIII — Manejo da Dor
Tabela VIII-A — Dosagens Recomendadas e Indicações de Opioides Parenterais
Tabela VIII-B — Dosagens Recomendadas e Indicações de Opioides Receitáveis
Tabela VIII-C — Dosagens Recomendadas e Indicações de AINE Parenterais
Tabela VIII-D — Dosagens Recomendadas e Indicações de AINE Receitáveis
Tabela VIII-E — Dosagens e Indicações de Medicamentos Selecionados Utilizados para o Tratamento da Dor Neuropática

Apêndice IX — Formulário de Medicamentos para Consulta em 5 Minutos

Apêndice X — Tabelas de Conversão
Tabela X-A — Tabela de conversão do Peso para Área de Superfície Corporal (em Metros Quadrados) para Cães
Tabela X-B — Valores Equivalentes Aproximados para Graus Fahrenheit e Celsius
Tabela X-C — Fatores de Conversão das Unidades de Peso

APÊNDICE I

VALORES DE REFERÊNCIA PARA TESTES LABORATORIAIS

Tabela I-A

Valores Hematológicos Normais			
Testes	Unidades	Cães	Gatos
Leucócitos	10 × 3/mm³	6-17	5,5-19,5
Eritrócitos	10 × 6/mm³	5,5-8,5	6-10
Hemoglobina	g/dL	12-18	9,5-15
Hematócrito	%	37-55	29-45
Volume corpuscular médio	fL	60-77	41-54
Hemoglobina corpuscular média	pg	19,5-26	13,3-17,5
Concentração de hemoglobina corpuscular média	%	32-36	31-36
Contagem de plaquetas (automatizada)	10 × 3/mm³	200-500	150-600
Contagem de plaquetas (manual)	10 × 3/mm³	164-510	230-680
Neutrófilos	% absoluta	60-77 3.000-11.500	35-75 2.500-12.500
Bastonetes	% absoluta	0-3 0-510	0-3 0-585
Linfócitos	% absoluta	12-30 1.000-4.800	20-55 1.500-7.000
Monócitos	% absoluta	3-10 180-1.350	1-4 0-850
Eosinófilos	% absoluta	2-10 1.000-1.250	2-12 0-1.500
Basófilos	% absoluta	0-1 0-100	0-1 0-100
Contagem de reticulócitos Corrigida Absoluta	% % /mm³	0,5-1,5 0-1 0-80.000	0-1 0-1 0-50.000

De Abbott Cell Dyne 3500; IDEXX Veterinary Services.
É importante ressaltar que os valores normais variam entre laboratórios.

Tabela I-B

Valores Bioquímicos Normais			
Testes	Unidades	Cães	Gatos
Nitrogênio ureico sanguíneo (BUN)	mg/dL	7-27	15-34
Creatinina	mg/dL	0,4-1,8	0,8-2,3
Colesterol	mg/dL	112-328	82-218
Glicose	mg/dL	60-125	70-150
Fosfatase alcalina	UI/L	10-150	0-62
Alanina aminotransferase (ALT)	UI/L	5-60	28-76
Aspartato aminotransferase (AST)	UI/L	5-55	5-55
Proteína total	g/dL	5,1-7,8	5,9-8,5
Albumina	g/dL	2,6-4,3	2,4-4,1
Globulina	g/dL	2,3-4,5	3,4-5,2
Relação albumina-globulina		0,75-1,9	0,6-1,5
Sódio	mEq/L	141-156	147-156
Potássio	mEq/L	4-5,6	3,9-5,3
Relação sódio-potássio		27-40	>27
Cloreto	mEq/L	105-115	111-125
CO_2 total	mEq/L	17-24	13-25
Hiato aniônico	mEq/L	12-24	13-27

(continua)

Valores de Referência para Testes Laboratoriais (continuação)

Tabela I-B

Valores Bioquímicos Normais (*continuação*)			
Testes	*Unidades*	*Cães*	*Gatos*
Cálcio	mg/dL	7,5-11,3	7,5-10,8
Fósforo	mg/dL	2,1-6,3	3-7
Bilirrubina total	mg/dL	0-0,4	0-0,4
Bilirrubina direta	mg/dL	0-0,1	0-0,1
Bilirrubina indireta	mg/dL	0-0,3	0-0,3
Lactato desidrogenase (LDH)	UI/L	50-380	46-350
Creatinoquinase (CK ou CPK)	UI/L	10-200	64-440
γ-Glutamiltransferase (GGT)	UI/L	0-10	1-7
Ácido úrico	mg/dL	0-2	0-1
Amilase	UI/L	500-1.500	500-1.500
Lipase	U/L	100-500	10-195
Magnésio	mEq/L	1,8-2,4	1,8-2,4
Triglicérides	mg/dL	20-150	20-90
Ácidos biliares:			
Jejum	μmol/L	0-5	0-5
Pós-prandiais	μmol/L	<25	<15
Aleatórios	μmol/L	<25	<15
Ferro total	μg/dL	33-147	33-134
Capacidade de ligação do ferro insaturado	μg/dL	127-340	105-205
Capacidade de ligação do ferro total	μg/dL	282-386	169-325

De Hitachi Chemistry Analyzer model 747 IDEXX Veterinary Services.
É importante ressaltar que os valores normais variam entre laboratórios.

Tabela I-C

Tabela de Conversão para Unidades Hematológicas				
	Valores de Exemplo		*Fatores de Conversão*	
Analisado	*Tradicional*	*SI**	*De Tradicional para SI*	*De SI para Tradicional*
Hemoglobina	15 g/dL	150 g/L	10	0,1
Hematócrito	45%	0,45 L/L	0,01	100
Eritrócitos	$6 \times 10^6/mm^3$	$6 \times 10^{12}/L$	10^6	10^{-6}
VCM	75 μ^3	75 fL	Sem alteração	Sem alteração
HCM	25 μg	25 pg	Sem alteração	Sem alteração
CHCM	33 g/dL	330 g/L	10	0,1
Leucócitos	$15 \times 10^3/mm^3$	$15 \times 10^9/L$	10^6	10^{-6}
Plaquetas	$250 \times 10^3/mm^3$	$250 \times 10^9/L$	10^6	10^{-6}

*Sistema Internacional de Unidades.
Adaptado de *Appendices*. In: Bonagura JD, ed., Kirk's Current Veterinary Therapy XIII. Philadelphia: Saunders, 2000, p. 1209 (com permissão).

VALORES DE REFERÊNCIA PARA TESTES LABORATORIAIS (CONTINUAÇÃO)

Tabela I-D

Tabela de Conversão para Unidades Bioquímicas Clínicas			
Analisado	Unidade Tradicional (com exemplos)	Fator de Conversão	Unidade do SI (com exemplos)
Ácidos biliares (totais)	0,3-2,3 µg/mL	2,45	0,74-5,64 µmol/L
Ácido fólico	3,5-11 µg/L	2,265	7,93-24,92 nmol/L
Ácido úrico	3,6-7,7 mg/dL	59,44	214-458 µmol/L
Alanina aminotransferase	0-40 U/L	1	0-40 U/L
Albumina	2,8-4 g/dL	10	28-40 g/L
Amilase	200-800 U/L	1	200-800 U/L
Amônia	10-80 µg/dL	0,5871	5,9-47 µmol/L
Aspartato aminotransferase	0-40 U/L	1	0-40 U/L
Bilirrubina	0,1-0,2 mg/dL	17,1	2-4 µmol/L
Cálcio	8,8-10,3 mg/dL	0,2495	2,20-2,58 mmol/L
Chumbo	150 µg/dL	0,04826	7,2 µmol/L
Cloreto	95-100 mEq/L	1	95-100 mmol/L
Cobre	70-140 µg/dL	0,1574	11-22 µmol/L
Colesterol	100-265 mg/dL	0,0258	2,58-5,85 mmol/L
Cortisol	2-10 µg/dL	27,59	55-280 nmol/L
Creatinina	0,6-1,2 mg/dL	88,40	50-110 µmol/L
Creatinoquinase	0-130 U/L	1	0-130 U/L
D-xilose	30-40 mg/dL	0,06666	2-2,71 mmol/L
Dióxido de carbono	22-28 mEq/L	1	22-28mmol/L
Ferro	80-180µg/dL	0,1791	14-32µmol/L
Fibrinogênio	200-400 mg/dL	0,01	2-4 g/L
Fosfatase alcalina	30-150 U/L	1	30-150 U/L
Fósforo	2,5-5 mg/dL	0,3229	0,80-1,6 mmol/L
Glicose	70-110 mg/dL	0,05551	3,9-6,1 mmol/L
Lactato	5-20 mg/dL	0,1110	0,5-2 mmol/L
Lipase, Cherry-Crandall (30°C)	0-160 U/L	1	0-160 U/L
Lipase, Sigma-Tietz (37°C)	≤1 ST U/dL	280	≤280 U/L
Lipídios (totais)	400-850 mg/dL	0,01	4-8,5 g/L
Magnésio	1,8-3 mg/dL	0,4114	0,8-1,2 mmol/L
Mercúrio	≥1 µg/dL	49,85	≤50 nmol/L
Osmolalidade	280-300 mOsm/kg	1	280-300 mmol/kg
Potássio	3,5-5 mEq/L	1	3,5-5 mmol/L
Proteína (total)	5-8 g/dL	10	50-80 g/L
Sódio	135-147 mEq/L	1	135-147 mmol/L
Testosterona	4-8 mg/mL	3,467	14-28 nmol/L
Tireoxina	1-4 µg/dL	12,87	13-51 nmol/L
Triglicérides	10-500 mg/dL	0,0113	0,11-5,65 mmol/L
Ureia	10-20 mg/dL	0,3570	3,6-7,1 nmol/L
Urobilinogênio	0-4 mg/dL	16,9	0-6,8 µmol/L
Vitamina A	90µg/dL	0,03491	3,1 µmol/L
Vitamina B_{12}	300-700 ng/L	0,738	221-516 pmol/L
Vitamina E	5-20 mg/L	2,32	11,6-46,4 µmol/L
Zinco	75-120 µg/dL	0,1530	11,5-18,5 µmol/L

De *Appendices*. In: Bonagura JD, ed., Kirk's Current Veterinary Therapy XIII. Philadelphia: Saunders, 2000, p.1214 (com permissão).

ESPÉCIES CANINA E FELINA

1341

APÊNDICE II

TESTES ENDÓCRINOS

Tabela II-A

Protocolos para Testes da Função Endócrina

DISTÚRBIOS DA GLÂNDULA ADRENAL

TESTE DE ESTIMULAÇÃO COM ACTH

Cães
Administrar 20 UI de ACTH gel por via IM ou 0,25 mg de ACTH sintético pelas vias IV ou IM (Cortrosyn®, Organon Pharmaceuticals, West Orange, NJ).

ACTH GEL
Amostras de soro devem ser obtidas antes e 2 horas depois da injeção do ACTH para análise do cortisol.

ACTH sintético
Amostras de soro devem ser obtidas antes e 1 hora depois da injeção do ACTH para análise do cortisol.

Gatos
Administrar 0,125 mg de ACTH sintético por via IV.
Amostras de soro devem ser obtidas antes e 1 hora depois da injeção do ACTH para análise do cortisol.

Interpretação

Triagem para Síndrome de Cushing
Uma resposta exagerada ao estímulo com ACTH é compatível com a síndrome de *Cushing*. Valores de corte normais elevados diferem levemente entre laboratórios.

Triagem para Hipoadrenocorticismo
Resultados pré e pós-cortisol <1 μg/dL (30 nmol/L) são compatíveis com o hipoadrenocorticismo.
Monitorização do Mitotano ou Cetoconazol.

Tratamento para a Síndrome de Cushing
Resultados pré e pós-cortisol devem estar dentro dos limites normais basais de cortisol.

TESTE DE SUPRESSÃO COM DOSE BAIXA DE DEXAMETASONA (TSDBD)

Cães
Administrar 0,015 mg/kg de dexametasona (Azium®, Schering-Plough, Union, NJ) pelas vias IV ou IM. Obtenha amostras de soro antes e 4 e 8 horas depois da injeção de dexametasona para análise do cortisol.

Gatos
Administrar 0,1 mg/kg de dexametasona pelas vias IV ou IM. Obtenha amostras de soro antes e 4 e 8 horas depois da injeção de dexametasona para análise do cortisol.

Interpretação
Três padrões básicos.

Ausência de Supressão
Todos os valores de cortisol permanecem acima de 1 μg/dL (30 nmol/L). Esse padrão é compatível com a síndrome de *Cushing*.

Supressão
Valores de cortisol ficam abaixo de 1 μg/dL (30 nmol/L) nas amostras coletadas 4 e 8 horas após a administração. Esse padrão sugere que o animal não tem síndrome de *Cushing*.

Escape da Supressão
Valores de cortisol ficam abaixo de 1 μg/dL (30 nmol/L) na amostra coletada 4 horas após a administração e ficam acima de 1 μg/dL na amostra coletada 8 horas após a administração. Esse padrão é compatível com a síndrome de *Cushing* dependente da hipófise.

Teste de supressão com dose alta de dexametasona (TSDAD)
Administrar 1 mg/kg de dexametasona (Azium®) pelas vias IV ou IM. Obter amostras de soro antes e 4 e 8 horas depois da injeção de dexametasona para análise do cortisol.

Interpretação
Qualquer resultado de cortisol abaixo de 1,5 μg/dL (45 nmol/L), em qualquer momento das 8 horas de duração do teste é considerado supressão. A supressão após uma dose alta de dexametasona é compatível com a síndrome de *Cushing* dependente da hipófise. A ausência de supressão (todos os valores permanecem acima de 1,5 μg/dL) é diagnóstica de tumor hipofisário ou adrenal.

DISTÚRBIOS DE TIREOIDE

TESTE DE ESTIMULAÇÃO COM TSH
Administrar 0,5 U/kg de TSH (dose máxima de 5 U) por via IV. Obter amostras de soro antes e 6 horas depois da injeção de TSH para determinação do T_4.

Interpretação
Níveis de T_4 pós-TSH <3 μg/dL (35 nmol/L) são compatíveis com hipotireoidismo.

TESTE DE ESTIMULAÇÃO COM TRH
Administrar 0,1 mg/kg de TRH por via IV. Obter amostras de soro antes e 4 horas depois da injeção do TRH para a determinação do T_4.

Interpretação
O aumento da concentração de T_4 <50% após a administração do TRH é compatível com hipotireoidismo.

TESTE DE SUPRESSÃO DA TIREOIDE COM T_3
Obter uma amostra sanguínea para a determinação do T_4 e do T_3. O soro deve ser removido e mantido sob refrigeração ou congelamento. Administrar T_3 (Cytomel®, SmithKline Beecham, Philadelphia, PA) por via oral na dosagem de 25 μg/gato a cada 8 horas por 2 dias. Na manhã do terceiro dia, administre 25 μg de T_3 e depois de 2-4 horas obter uma segunda amostra sanguínea para a determinação de T_3 e T_4. As amostras de soro basal (1º dia) e pós-oral de T_3 devem ser enviadas ao laboratório simultaneamente para evitar variação entre análises.

Interpretação
Uma concentração sérica de T_4 após administração de T_3 >1,5 μg/dL (20 nmol/L) é compatível com hipertireoidismo.

GASTRINOMA

TESTE DE ESTIMULAÇÃO DA SECRETINA
Administrar 2 U/kg de secretina por via IV. Obter amostras sanguíneas antes da administração da secretina e depois de 2, 5, 10, 15 e 30 minutos. Avaliar as amostras quanto à gastrina.

Interpretação
Os cães com gastrinomas apresentam elevação nos níveis de gastrina após a injeção da secretina. Em três casos relatados, dois cães apresentaram aumento nos níveis de gastrina duas vezes maior que os valores basais 5 minutos após a injeção da secretina, e um cão teve elevação nos níveis de gastrina 1, 4 vez maior que os valores basais 5 minutos após a injeção da secretina. Os cães normais apresentam queda nos níveis da gastrina depois da administração da secretina.

TESTE DE DESAFIO COM O CÁLCIO
Administrar 2 mg/kg de gliconato de cálcio por via IV no período de 1 minuto ou na dosagem de 5 mg/kg na forma de infusão IV ao longo de várias horas.
Obter uma amostra sanguínea antes da administração do cálcio e depois de 15, 30, 60, 90 e 120 minutos. Avaliar as amostras quanto à gastrina.

Interpretação
Dois pacientes relatados com gastrinoma apresentaram a duplicação no nível de gastrina 60 minutos após a infusão do cálcio.

DISTÚRBIOS DOS HORMÔNIOS SEXUAIS

TESTE DE ESTIMULAÇÃO COM GnRH
Administrar 0,5-1,0 μg/kg de GnRH por via IM. Obter amostras sanguíneas antes da administração do GnRH e 1 hora depois. Avaliar as amostras quanto à testosterona.

Interpretação
Os cães normais apresentam níveis basais de testosterona entre 0,5 e 5 ng/mL. Após a administração do GnRH, os níveis de testosterona elevam-se acima de 5 ng/mL. Os animais com hipoandrogenismo apresentam valores mais baixos.

TESTE DE ESTIMULAÇÃO COM HCG
Administrar 44 UI/kg de hCG por via IM. Obter amostras sanguíneas antes da administração do hCG e 4 horas depois. Avaliar as amostras quanto à testosterona.

Interpretação
Os cães normais apresentam níveis basais de testosterona entre 0,5 e 5 ng/mL. Após a administração do hCG, os níveis de testosterona sobem acima de 5 ng/mL. Os animais com hipoandrogenismo apresentam valores mais baixos.

DIABETES INSÍPIDO

TESTE MODIFICADO DE PRIVAÇÃO DE ÁGUA
Para descartar outras causas de poliúria e polidipsia (especialmente hiperadrenocorticismo). Iniciar a restrição hídrica 3 dias antes da privação abrupta de água.

TESTES ENDÓCRINOS (CONTINUAÇÃO)

Tabela II-A

Protocolos para Testes da Função Endócrina (continuação)

Dia 1 130-165 mL/kg/dia
Dia 2 100-125 mL/kg/dia
Dia 3 65-70 mL/kg/dia (necessidades normais para manutenção)
Na manhã do quarto dia, suspender o fornecimento de água e alimentos e, então, dê início ao teste. Pesar o paciente e esvaziar sua bexiga. O peso deve ser monitorizado em intervalos de 1 a 2 horas. Monitorizar o animal quanto à ocorrência de desidratação e depressão. Quando houver a perda de 5% do peso corporal ou o desenvolvimento de azotemia, esvazie a bexiga e avalie a densidade urinária. Nesse momento, deve-se considerar a determinação plasmática da vasopressina.

Interpretação
Se a densidade urinária estiver >1,025 (cães) ou >1,030 (gatos), interromper o teste. O paciente não apresenta diabetes insípido. Se a densidade urinária não estiver >1,025 (cães) ou >1,030 (gatos), administrar 0,55 U/kg de vasopressina aquosa por via IM (dose máxima de 5 U). Esvaziar a bexiga e avaliar a densidade urinária aos 30, 60 e 120 minutos após a administração da vasopressina. Se a densidade urinária aumentar <10%, indica-se a presença de diabetes insípido nefrogênico; se a densidade urinária aumentar de 10-50%, indica-se a presença de diabetes insípido central parcial; se a densidade urinária aumentar de 50-800%, indica-se a presença de diabetes insípido central completo.

Tabela II-B

Testes do Sistema Endócrino[*]			
Hormônio	*Unidade*	*Cães*	*Gatos*
Aldosterona[†] (plasma)			
Basal	pmol/L	14-957	194-388
Pós-ACTH	pmol/L	197-2.103	277-721
Cortisol (soro ou plasma, urina)			
Basal	nmol/L	25-125	15-150
Pós-ACTH	nmol/L	200-550	130-450
Após dose baixa de dexametasona (0,01 ou 0,015 mg/kg)	nmol/L	≤40	≤40
Após dose alta de dexametasona (0,1 ou 1 mg/kg)[‡]	nmol/L	≤40	≤40
Hormônio adrenocorticotrópico, basal (ACTH, plasma)	pmol/L	2-15	1-20
Insulina, basal (soro)	pmol/L	35-200	35-200
Paratormônio intacto[†] (soro)	pmol/L	2-13	0-4
Progesterona (soro ou plasma, fêmea)	mmol/L	≤3 em anestro, proestro 50-220 em diestro, gestação	≤3 em anestro, proestro 50-220 em diestro, gestação
Relação de cortisol-creatinina na urina	× 10⁻⁶	8-24,[†] 10[§]	–
Supressão com tri-iodotironina (T3)[*]	nmol/L	–	≤20
Testosterona (soro ou plasma, macho)	nmol/L	1-20	1-20
Tiroxina (T_4, soro)			
Basal	nmol/L	12-50	10-50
Após a administração do hormônio estimulante da tiroxina (TSH)	nmol/L	>45	>45
Tri-iodotironina, basal (T_3, soro)	nmol/L	0,7-2,3	0,5-2

[*] Preparado com assistência de ME Peterson, The Animal Medical Center, New York, NY. A menos que indicados de outra forma, os valores desta tabela são adaptados de Kemppainen RJ, Zerbe CA. Common endocrine diagnostic tests: normal values and interpretations. In: Kirk RW, ed., Current Veterinary Therapy X. Philadelphia: Saunders, 1989, pp.961-968. Determinações hormonais variam entre os laboratórios. O laboratório responsável pela análise deve fornecer os valores de referência. Antes de enviar as amostras para as determinações hormonais, consulte o laboratório para informações quanto às especificações da amostra, ao uso de anticoagulantes e à conservação da amostra. As condições gerais de amostragem foram discutidas em Reimers TJ. Guidelines for collection, storage, and transport of samples for hormone assay. In: Kirk RW, ed., Current Veterinary Therapy X. Philadelphia: Saunders, 1989, pp.968-973. Os fatores que influenciam as concentrações séricas dos hormônios tireóideos e adrenocorticais em cães foram discutidos em Reimers TJ, Lawler DF, Sutaria PM, et al. Effects of age, sex, and body size on serum concentrations of thyroid and adrenocortical hormones in dogs. Am J Vet Res 1990, 51:454.
[†] Fornecido por RF Nachreiner, Animal Health Diagnostic Laboratory, Endocrine Diagnostic Section, Michigan State University.
[‡] Esse teste é utilizado após a confirmação da hiperfunção adrenocortical. É utilizado para diferenciar tumor da adrenal (no qual não se observa supressão) de casos dependentes da hipófise (nos quais ocorre supressão, porém de forma variável).
[§] De Stolp R, Rijnberk A, Meiher JC, Croughs RJM. Urinary corticoids in the diagnosis of canine hyperadrenocorticism. Res Vet Sci 1983, 34:141. Rijnberk A, van Wees A, Mol JA. Assessment of two tests for the diagnosis of canine hyperadrenocorticism. Vet Record 1988, 122:178-180.
[*] De Peterson ME, Ferguson DC. Thyroid diseases. In: Ettinger SJ, ed., Textbook of Veterinary Internal Medicine: Diseases of the Dog and Cat, 3. ed. Philadelphia: Saunders, 1989, pp. 1632-1675.
De Appendices. Em: Bonagura JD, ed., Kirk's Current Veterinary Therapy XIII. Philadelphia: Saunders, 2000, p.1223 (com autorização).

TESTES ENDÓCRINOS (CONTINUAÇÃO)

Tabela II-C

Tabela de Conversão para Unidades de Análise Hormonal				
Unidade		*Fatores de Conversão*		
Hormônio	*Tradicional*	*SI*	*De Tradicional para SI*	*De SI para Tradicional*
Aldosterona	ng/dL	pmol/L	27,7	0,036
β-endorfina	pg/mL	pmol/L	0,289	3,43
Corticotropina (ACTH)	pg/mL	pmol/L	0,22	4,51
Cortisol	μg/dL	mmol/L	27,59	0,36
Epinefrina	pg/mL	pmol/L	5,46	0,183
Estrogênio (estradiol)	pg/mL	pmol/L	3,67	0,273
Gastrina	pg/mL	ng/L	1	1
Glucagon	pg/mL	ng/L	1	1
Hormônio do crescimento (GH)	ng/mL	μg/L	1	1
Hormônio estimulante de α-melanócitos (α-MSH)	pg/mL	pmol/L	0,601	1,66
Insulina	μU/mL	pmol/L	7,18	0,139
Norepinefrina	pg/mL	nmol/L	0,006	169
Polipeptídeo intestinal vasoativo (PIV)	pg/mL	pmol/L	0,301	3,33
Polipeptídeo pancreático (PP)	mg/dL	mmol/L	0,239	4,18
Progesterona	ng/mL	mmol/L	3,18	0,315
Prolactina	ng/mL	μg/L	1	1
Renina	ng/mL/hr	ng/L/sec	0,278	3,6
Somatostatina	pg/mL	pmol/L	0,611	1,64
Testosterona	ng/mL	nmol/L	3,47	0,288
Tiroxina (T_4)	μg/dL	nmol/L	12,87	0,078
Tri-iodotironina (T_3)	ng/dL	nmol/L	0,0154	64,9

Colaboração de ME Peterson, The Animal Medical Center, New York, NY.
De *Appendices*. In: Bonagura JD. ed., Kirk's Current Veterinary Therapy XIII. Philadelphia: Saunders, 2000, p. 1223 (com permissão).

APÊNDICE III

VALORES NORMAIS APROXIMADOS PARA MENSURAÇÕES COMUNS EM CÃES E GATOS

	Cães	Gatos
Frequência cardíaca (bpm)	60-180	140-220
Tempo de preenchimento capilar	<2 s	<2 s
Temperatura corporal	37,5-39,2°C	38,1-39,2°C
Pressão arterial média (mmHg)	90-120	100-150
Volume sanguíneo (mL/kg)	75-90	47-66
Débito cardíaco		
(mL/kg/min)	100-200	167 ± 39
(L/M^2/min)	4,72 ± 1,09	
Resistência sistêmica		
(mmHg/mL/kg/min)	0,64 ± 0,16	
(dinas/s/cm)	2.162 ± 458	
Pressão arterial pulmonar média (mmHg)	14 ± 3	
Pressão venosa central (cm H_2O)	3 ± 4	
Pressão de oclusão da artéria pulmonar (mmHg)	5 ± 2	
Débito urinário	1-2 mL/kg/h	1-2 mL/kg/h
Frequência respiratória (movimentos respiratórios/min)	10-30	24-42
Ventilação minuto (mL/kg/min)	170-350	200-350
Distribuição de oxigênio		
(mL/kg/min)	29 ± 8	
(mL/M^2/min)	815 ± 234	
Consumo de oxigênio		
(mL/kg/min)	4-11	
(mL/M^2/min)	198 ± 53	3-8
PO_2 arterial (mmHg)	85-105	100-115
SO_2 arterial	>95	>95
PCO_2 arterial (mmHg)	30-44	28-35
pH arterial	7,36-7,46	7,34-7,43
Bicarbonato (mEq/L)	20-25	17-21
Déficit de base (mEq/L)	0 a -4	-1 a -8
Proteínas plasmáticas totais (g/dL)	6-8	6,8-8,3
Albumina (g/dL)	2,5-3,5	1,9-3,9
Volume globular (hematócrito) (%)	37-55	29-48
Hemoglobina (g/dL)	12-18	9-15,1
Sódio (mEq/L)	145-154	151-158
Potássio (mEq/L)	4,1-5,3	3,6-4,9
Cloreto (mEq/L)	105-116	113-121
CO_2 Total (mEq/L)	16-26	15-21

Adaptado de Aldrich J, Haskins SC. Monitoring the critically ill patient. In: Current Veterinary Therapy XII. Philadelphia: Saunders, 1995, pp. 98-105 (com permissão).

APÊNDICE IV

VALORES NORMAIS PARA O ELETROCARDIOGRAMA CANINO E FELINO

Frequência

Cães	60-140 bpm para raças gigantes	
	70-160 bpm para cães adultos	
	Até 180 bpm para raças *toy*	
	Até 220 bpm para filhotes	
Gatos	Variação: 120-240 bpm	
	Média: 197 bpm	

Ritmo

Cães	Ritmo sinusal normal	
	Arritmia sinusal	
	Marca-passo sinoatrial migratório	
Gatos	Ritmo sinusal normal	
	Taquicardia sinusal (reação fisiológica à agitação)	

Mensurações (Derivação II, 50 mm/s, 1 cm = 1 mV)

Cães	Onda P	Largura: máximo de 0,04 s; 0,05 s em raças gigantes
		Altura: máximo de 0,4 mV
	Intervalo PR	Largura: 0,06-0,13 s
	Complexo QRS	Largura: máximo de 0,05 s em raças pequenas
		máximo de 0,06 s em raças grandes
		Altura da onda R*: máximo de 3,0 mV em raças grandes
		máximo de 2,5 mV em raças pequenas
	Segmento ST	Sem depressão: não mais que 0,2 mV
		Sem elevação: não mais que 0,15 mV
	Onda T	Pode ser positiva, negativa ou bifásica
		Não superior a 1/4 da amplitude da onda R
		Variação da amplitude ± 0,05-1 mV em qualquer derivação
	Intervalo Q-T	Largura: 0,15-0,25 s na frequência cardíaca normal; varia de acordo com a frequência cardíaca (frequências mais rápidas apresentam intervalos Q-T mais curtos e vice-versa)
Gatos	Onda P	Largura: máximo de 0,04 s
		Altura: máximo de 0,2 mV
	Intervalo PR	Largura: 0,05-0,09 s
	Complexo QRS	Largura: máximo de 0,04 s
		Altura da onda R: máximo de 0,9 mV
	Segmento ST	Sem depressão ou elevação
	Onda T	Pode ser positiva, negativa ou bifásica - mais frequentemente positiva
		Amplitude máxima de 0,3 mV
	Intervalo Q-T	Largura: 0,12-0,18 s na frequência cardíaca normal (variação de 0,07-0,20 s); varia de acordo com a frequência cardíaca (frequências mais rápidas apresentam intervalos Q-T mais curtos e vice-versa)

Eixo Elétrico Médio (plano frontal)

Cães	+40 a +100 graus
Gatos	0 a +160 graus (não é válido em muitos gatos)

Derivações torácicas precordiais (valores de especial importância)

Cães	CV_5RL (rV_2): onda T positiva, onda R não superior a 3 mV
	CV_6LL (V_2): onda S não superior a 0,8 mV, onda R não superior a 3 mV*
	CV_6LU (V_4): onda S não superior a 0,7 mV, onda R não superior a 3 mV*
	V_{10}: complexo QRS negativo, onda T negativa, exceto em Chihuahuas
Gatos	CV_6LL (V_2): onda R não superior a 1 mV
	CV_6LU (V_4): onda R não superior a 1 mV
	V_{10}: onda T negativa, R/Q não superior a 1 mV

*Valores não válidos para cães magros, de tórax profundo com menos de 2 anos de idade.
Fonte: Tilley LP. *Essentials of Canine and Feline Electrocardiography*, 3.ed. Baltimore: Williams & Wilkins, 1992, com permissão.

APÊNDICE V

TOXICOSES CLÍNICAS — SISTEMAS ACOMETIDOS E EFEITOS CLÍNICOS

Neurotoxinas

Excitação ou estimulação do sistema nervoso
  Aminopiridina
  Anfetamina
  Cafeína
  Chumbo
  Cianeto
  Cicuta aquática (*Cicuta spp.*)
  Esporão do centeio (*Claviceps spp.*)
  Estricnina
  Fenóis e clorofenóis
  Fluoroacetato
  Inseticidas organoclorados
  Inseticidas organofosforados
  Menispermo (*Menispermum canadense*)
  Metaldeído
  Micotoxinas
  Nicotina
  Teobromina
  Teofilina
Depressão, coma
  Álcoóis
  Anti-histamínicos
  Barbitúricos
  Chumbo
  Derivados da morfina
  Hidrocarbonetos alifáticos
  Hidrocarbonetos aromáticos
  Hidrocarbonetos halogenados
  Mercúrio
  Monóxido de carbono
  Salicilatos
  Venenos de cobra
Perda do controle motor
  Curare
  Castanheira-da-índia (*Aesculus spp.*)
  Chumbo
  Dissulfeto de carbono
  Esporão do centeio
  Etilenoglicol
  Hexaclorofeno
  Nicotina
  Organofosforados
  Toxina botulínica
  Triaril fosfatos
Estimulação autônoma
  Atropina
  Cogumelo agário das moscas (*Amanita muscaria*)
  Inseticidas carbamatos
  Inseticidas organofosforados
Mudanças comportamentais
  Alcaloides de beladona
  Chumbo
  Derivados do ópio
  Dietilamida do ácido lisérgico (LSD)
  Esporão do centeio
  Fósforo
  Inseticidas organoclorados
  Ipomeia
  Maconha
  Medicamento estimulante extraído do mescal
  Noz-moscada
  Pervinca
  Sulfonamidas

Agentes Tóxicos Cardiovasculares

Taquicardia e arritmias
  Adrenalina
  Anfetamina
  Antibióticos aminoglicosídeos
  Atropina
  Cafeína
  Cianeto
  Dinitrofenol
  Fluorocarbonetos
  Nicotina
  Tálio
Bradicardia
  Bário
  Cila vermelha
  Digitálicos
  Glicosídeos cardíacos
  Morfina
  Oleandro
  Opiáceos
Dano ao miocárdio
  Amanita phalloides
  Bário
  Fósforo
  Monóxido de carbono
  Oleandro
  Tálio

Agentes Tóxicos Gastrintestinais

Estomatite, faringite
  Ácidos e álcalis
  Aldeídos
  Destilados do petróleo
  Detergentes
  Fenol
  Sais de cromo
  Sais de mercúrio
Salivação
  Amanita muscaria
  Amônia
  Cresol
  Metaldeído
  Nicotina
  Organofosforados
  Tálio
Boca seca
  Anfetamina
  Anti-histamínicos
  Atropina
  Beladona
  Opiáceos
Gastrenterites
  Amanita spp.
  Antimônio
  Arsênico
  Bário

Bismuto
Cantaridina
Chumbo
Cogumelos
Detergentes, sabões, desinfetantes
Ferro
Fosfeto de zinco
Fósforo
Herbicidas fenóxicos
Mercúrio
Óleo de cróton
Plantas (ver Apêndice VII)
Sais de cobre
Tálio
Toxinas digitálicas
Toxinas do *estafilococo*

Hepatotoxinas

Acetaminofeno
Aflatoxina
Algas azul-esverdeadas
Amanita phalloides
Cobre
Derivados do alcatrão de hulha
Destilados do petróleo
Ferro
Fósforo
Hidrocarbonetos halogenados

Nefrotoxinas

Nefrotoxinas inadvertidas
  Aldeídos
  Cogumelos *Amanita*
Necrose vascular
  Chumbo
  Esporão do centeio
  Mercúrio
  Selênio

Agentes Tóxicos Respiratórios

Alérgenos
Amônia
Cloro
Gasolina, querosene
Herbicida *Paraquat*
Inseticidas organofosforados
Ozônio
Poluentes do ar (dióxido de nitrogênio, dióxido de enxofre)
Rodenticida de alfa-naftiltioureia
Tálio

Agentes Tóxicos Oculares

Midríase
  Atropina
  Beladona
  Cogumelos *Amanita*
  Metanol
Miose
  Heroína
  Morfina
  Nicotina
  Organofosforados

TOXICOSES CLÍNICAS — SISTEMAS ACOMETIDOS E EFEITOS CLÍNICOS (CONTINUAÇÃO)

Neuropatia óptica
  Arsenicais
  Arsênico
  Bismuto
  Cádmio
  Chumbo
  Cresóis
  Destilados do petróleo
  Dicromato
  Etilenoglicol
  Fenóis
  Hidrocarbonetos halogenados
  Mercúrio
  Ocratoxinas
  Óleos voláteis (p. ex., óleo de poejo ou óleo de zimbro)
  Oxalatos
  Tálio
  Terebintina
Medicamentos nefrotóxicos
  Acetaminofeno
  Anfotericina B
  Bacitracina
  Canamicina
  Gentamicina
  Neomicina
  Polimixina B
  Sulfonamidas
  Vancomicina

Agentes Tóxicos Sanguíneos

Metemoglobina
  Acetaminofeno

  Azul de metileno
  Clorato
  Cobre
  Derivados de anilina
  Nitrito
  Nitrobenzeno
Hemólise
  Acetaminofeno*
  Anilina
  Arsina
  Azul de metileno*
  Cebolas
  Cloratos
  Cobre
  Folhas vermelhas de bordo
  Nitrobenzeno
  Terebintina
  Venenos de cobra
Anemia aplásica, leucopenia, trombocitopenia
  Agentes citostáticos
  Arsenicais
  Ácido acetilsalicílico
  Benzeno
  Cloranfenicol
  Estrogênios
  Fenilbutazona
  Tolueno
  Tricloroetileno
Coagulopatia
  Aflatoxina
  Ácido acetilsalicílico
  Mercúrio

  Metanol
  Rodenticidas cumarínicos
  Tálio
  Vitamina A

Sinais Clínicos Gerais

Febre
  Atropina
  Chumbo
  Dinitrofenol
  Inseticidas organoclorados
  Metaldeído
  Monóxido de carbono
Hipotermia
  Álcool
  Arsênico
  Barbitúricos
  Fenóis
  Heroína
  Morfina
  Oxalatos
Cianose
  Dióxido de carbono
  Nitrito
  Paraquat
  Sulfeto de hidrogênio
Coloração rósea da pele
  Arsênico
  Cianeto
  Mercúrio
  Monóxido de carbono
  Tálio

*Especialmente em gatos
De Osweiler G. A brief guide to clinical toxicosis in small animals. In: Kirk RW, ed., Current Veterinary Therapy IX. Philadelphia: Saunders, 1986, pp. 132-135 (com permissão).

APÊNDICE VI

AGENTES TÓXICOS E SEUS ANTÍDOTOS SISTÊMICOS — DOSAGENS E MÉTODOS TERAPÊUTICOS

Agente Tóxico	Antídoto Sistêmico	Dosagem e Método Terapêutico
Agentes colinérgicos	Sulfato de atropina	0,02-0,04 mg/kg, conforme a necessidade
Agentes colinérgicos e inibidores da colinesterase (organofosforados, alguns carbamatos; mas não carbaril, morfina, succinilcolina ou carbam piloxima)	Cloreto de pralidoxima (2-PAM)	Solução a 5%; administrar 20-50 mg/kg IM ou por meio de injeção IV lenta (0,2-1 mg/kg; dose máxima de 500 mg/min), repetir conforme a necessidade; o 2-PAM alivia o efeito nicotínico e regenera a colinesterase; os tranquilizantes fenotiazínicos são contraindicados
Agentes produtores de metemoglobinemia (nitritos, cloratos)	Azul de metileno (não recomendado para gatos)	Solução a 1% (concentração máxima); administrar 8,8 mg/kg (0,9 mL/kg) por meio de injeção IV lenta e repetir, se houver necessidade; para evitar a queda na pressão sanguínea em casos de envenenamento por nitrito, pode-se utilizar um medicamento simpatomimético (efedrina ou adrenalina)
Alucinógenos (LSD, cloridrato de fenciclidina [PCP])	Diazepam (Valium®, Roche)	Conforme a necessidade — evita a depressão respiratória (2-5 mg/kg)
Anfetaminas	Clorpromazina	1 mg/kg IM ou IV; administrar apenas a metade da dose caso barbitúricos tenham sido administrados; bloqueia a excitação
Anticoagulantes derivados da cumarina	Vitamina K1 (AquaMEPHYTON® cápsulas de 5 mg ou emulsão a 1%, Merck)	Administrar 3-5 mg/kg SC ou VO ao dia junto com ração úmida enlatada; tratar por 7 dias em casos de anticoagulantes do tipo varfarina; tratar por 21-30 dias em casos de rodenticidas anticoagulantes de segunda geração; a terapia oral é mais eficaz do que a parenteral
	Sangue total fresco, plasma fresco ou plasma fresco congelado	Transfusão sanguínea, 10-25 mL/kg, conforme a necessidade
Arsênico, mercúrio e outros metais pesados, exceto cádmio, chumbo, prata, selênio e tálio	Dimercaprol (BAL®, Hynson, Wescott & Dunning)	Solução a 10% em óleo; administrar para pequenos animais a dosagem de 2,5-5 mg/kg IM a cada 6 h por 2 dias, depois a cada 12 h durante os próximos 10 dias ou até a recuperação (Nota: em casos de envenenamento agudo grave, deve-se fornecer a dose de 5 mg/kg somente no primeiro dia.)
	D-Penicilamina (Cuprimine®, Merck)	Desenvolvida para os casos de envenenamento crônico por mercúrio; atualmente, parece ser o medicamento mais promissor; não há relatos sobre a dosagem em animais; administrar 3-4 mg/kg a cada 6 h
Atropina, alcaloides de beladona	Salicilato de fisostigmina	0,1-0,6 mg/kg (não utilizar neostigmina)
Barbitúricos	Doxapram	Solução a 2%; administrar para pequenos animais apenas a dosagem de 3-5 mg/kg IV (0,14-0,25 mL/kg); repetir conforme a necessidade. (Nota: a citação acima é segura apenas em casos de depressão leve; em animais com níveis mais profundos de depressão, é preferível o fornecimento de suporte ventilatório [e oxigênio].)
Brometos	Cloretos (sais de sódio ou amônio)	0,5-1 g VO ao dia por vários dias; aceleram a excreção dos agentes tóxicos
Chumbo	Edetato dissódico de cálcio (EDTACa)	A dose máxima segura é de 75 mg/kg por 24 h (apenas em casos graves); o EDTA está disponível em solução a 20%; para gotejamento IV, deve-se diluir o medicamento em glicose a 5% até a concentração de 0,5%; para administração IM, deve-se adicionar procaína a uma solução a 20% para obter a concentração de 0,5% de procaína.
	EDTA e BAL	O BAL é disponível como solução a 10% em óleo (a) Em casos graves (envolvimento do SNC com >100 µg de chumbo para 100 g de sangue total), administrar BAL na dosagem de 4 mg/kg apenas como dose inicial; prosseguir após 4 h e administrar BAL e EDTA (12,5 mg/kg) a cada 4 h por 3-4 dias por via IM em locais diferentes; interromper por 2 ou 3 dias e depois repetir o tratamento por mais 3-4 dias; (b) Em casos subagudos com >100 µg de chumbo para 100 g de sangue total, administrar o EDTA na dosagem de 50 mg/kg por 24 h durante 3-5 dias.
	Penicilamina (Cuprimine®)	Pode ser utilizada após qualquer tratamento (a ou b) na dosagem de 100 mg/kg por dia por via oral durante 1-4 semanas
	Cloridrato de tiamina	Experimental para tratar os sinais do SNC; 5 mg/kg IV a cada 12 h por 1-2 semanas; administrar lentamente e observar as reações desagradáveis
Cianeto	Metemoglobina (o nitrito de sódio é utilizado para formar metemoglobina)	Solução a 1% de nitrito de sódio; a dosagem é de 16 mg/kg IV (1,6 mL/kg)

ESPÉCIES CANINA E FELINA

AGENTES TÓXICOS E SEUS ANTÍDOTOS SISTÊMICOS — DOSAGENS E MÉTODOS TERAPÊUTICOS (CONTINUAÇÃO)

Agente Tóxico	Antídoto Sistêmico	Dosagem e Método Terapêutico
Cianeto	Tiossulfato de sódio	Acompanhar com solução a 20% de tiossulfato de sódio na dosagem de 30-40 mg/kg (0,15-0,2 mL/kg) IV; se o tratamento for repetido, deve-se utilizar apenas o tiossulfato de sódio. (Nota: ambas as soluções podem ser administradas simultaneamente conforme o esquema a seguir: 0,5 mL/kg de uma combinação que consiste em 10 g de nitrito de sódio, 15 g de tiossulfato de sódio em água destilada a quantidade suficiente para 250 mL; a dosagem pode ser repetida uma única vez; se houver necessidade de tratamento adicional, deve-se administrar apenas a solução de tiossulfato de sódio a 20% na dose de 0,2 mL/kg.)
Cila vermelha	Sulfato de atropina, propranolol, cloreto de potássio	Semelhante ao método terapêutico para os digitálicos e oleandro
Cobre	D-Penicilamina (Cuprimine®)	Ver "Arsênico"
Colecalciferol	Calcitonina (Calcimar®, Rhone-Poulenc Rorer)	4 UI/kg SC ou IM a cada 8-12 h
Curare	Metilsulfato de neostigmina	Solução: 1:5.000 ou 1:2.000 (1 mL= 0,2 ou 0,5 mg/mL): a dosagem é de 0,005 mg/5 kg SC; acompanhar com a injeção IV de atropina (0,04 mg/kg)
	Cloreto de edrofônio (Tensilon®, Roche)	Solução a 1%: administrar 0,05-1 mg/kg IV
	Suporte ventilatório	
Estricnina e brucina	Pentobarbital	Administrar por via IV até fazer efeito; em geral, há necessidade de doses mais altas do que as necessárias para anestesia; deve-se colocar o animal em ambiente aquecido e tranquilo
	Amobarbital	Administrar por via IV lentamente até fazer efeito; a duração da sedação costuma ser de 4-6 h
	Metocarbamol (Robaxin®, AH Robins)	Solução a 10%; em média, a primeira dose é de 149 mg/kg IV (variação, 40-300 mg); repetir metade da dose, conforme a necessidade
	Guaiacolato de glicerila	110 mg/kg IV de solução a 5%; repetir conforme a necessidade
	Diazepam (Valium®)	2-5 mg/kg; para o controle das convulsões
Estrôncio	Sais de cálcio	Dose usual do borogluconato de cálcio
	Cloreto de amônio	0,2-0,5 g VO 3-4 vezes ao dia
Fenotiazínicos	Cloridrato de metanfetamina (Desoxyn®, Abbott)	0,1-0,2 mg/kg; pode ser necessário tratamento contra o choque hipovolêmico
	Cloridrato de difenidramina	Em casos de depressão do SNC, administra-se a dose de 2-5 mg/kg IV para tratar os sinais extrapiramidais
Fitotoxinas e toxina botulínica	As antitoxinas não estão disponíveis comercialmente (pode-se tentar obtê-las por meio dos Centros de Controle de Doenças)	Conforme indicação das antitoxinas específicas; exemplos de fitotoxinas: ricina, abrina, robina, crotina
Fluoreto	Borogliconato de cálcio	3-10 mL de solução a 5-10%
Fluoroacetato (composto 1080)	Monoacetato de glicerila (monoacetina, Sigma)	0,1-0,5 mg/kg IM por hora durante várias horas (total de 2-4 mg/kg) ou diluído (solução a 0,5-1% IV; risco de hemólise); a monoacetina está disponível apenas em lojas de produtos químicos
	Acetamida	Os animais poderão ser protegidos se a acetamida for administrada antes ou simultaneamente com o composto 1080 (experimental)
	Pentobarbital	Pode proteger contra a dose letal (experimental). (Nota: em geral, todos os tratamentos são frustrantes.)
Glicosídeos digitálicos, oleandro e sapos do gênero Bufo	Cloreto de potássio	Cães: administrar 0,5-2 g VO em doses divididas ou, em casos graves, aplicar uma solução diluída por via IV por meio de gotejamento lento (nesse caso, a monitorização com ECG é essencial)
	Difenilidantoína	25 mg/min IV até o controle das arritmias ventriculares
	Propranolol (β-bloqueador)	0,5-1 mg/kg IV ou IM, conforme a necessidade, para controlar as arritmias cardíacas (nesse caso, a monitorização com ECG é fundamental)
	Sulfato de atropina	0,02-0,04 mg/kg, conforme a necessidade, para o controle dos efeitos colinérgicos e das arritmias
Heparina	Sulfato de protamina	Solução a 1%; administrar 1-1,5 mg por meio de injeção IV lenta para antagonizar cada 1 mg de heparina; diminuir a dose à medida que aumenta o intervalo entre a injeção da heparina e o início do tratamento (após 30 minutos, administrar apenas 0,5 mg)

AGENTES TÓXICOS E SEUS ANTÍDOTOS SISTÊMICOS — DOSAGENS E MÉTODOS TERAPÊUTICOS (CONTINUAÇÃO)

Agente Tóxico	Antídoto Sistêmico	Dosagem e Método Terapêutico
Inibidores da colinesterase	Sulfato de atropina	0,2 mg/kg, repetir conforme a necessidade para atropinização; tratar primeiramente a cianose (se presente); bloqueia apenas os efeitos muscarínicos: para a obtenção de efeito prolongado, pode-se injetar a atropina em veículo oleoso. Evite a intoxicação por atropina!
Metaldeído	Diazepam (Valium®)	2-5 mg/kg IV para controlar os tremores
	Triflupromazina	0,2-2 mg/kg IV
	Pentobarbital	Administrar até fazer efeito
Metanol	Etanol	Administrar 1,1 g/kg (4,4 mL/kg) de solução a 25% IV; depois, fornecer 0,5 g/kg (2 mL/kg) a cada 4 h por 4 dias; para evitar ou corrigir a acidose, pode-se utilizar o bicarbonato de sódio na dosagem de 0,4 g/kg IV; também se pode lançar mão do carvão ativado na dosagem de 5 g/kg VO em até 4 horas da ingestão
Monóxido de carbono	Oxigênio	Oxigênio puro sob pressão normal ou alta; respiração artificial; transfusão sanguínea
Morfina e medicamentos relacionados	Cloridrato de naloxona (Narcan®, Endo)	0,1 mg/kg IV; não repetir se a respiração não permanecer satisfatória
	Tartarato de levarlofano (Lorfan®, Roche)	Administrar 0,1-0,5 mL por via IV de solução contendo 1 mg/mL (Nota: utilizar qualquer um dos antídotos apenas em casos de envenenamento agudo. Pode-se indicar o suporte ventilatório. Também se recomenda o carvão ativado.)
Oxalatos	Cálcio	Solução a 10% de gliconato de cálcio IV; administrar 3-20 mL (para controlar a hipocalcemia)
Paracetamol	N-acetilcisteína (Mucomyst®, Apothecon)	150 mg/kg como dose de ataque VO ou IV, depois 50 mg/kg a cada 4 h por 17-20 doses adicionais
Picada de aranha		
Viúva-negra	Antivenin® (Merck)	Precaução: origem equina; administrar por via IV sem diluir
	Dantroleno sódico (Dantrium®, Norwich-Eaton)	Em casos de sinais neurológicos, administrar 1 mg/kg IV, seguido de 1 mg/kg VO a cada 4 h
Marrom-reclusa	Dapsona	1 mg/kg a cada 12 h por 10 dias
Picada de cobra		
Cascavel, *copperhead*, cobra *mocassim* aquática	Antiveneno (*Crotalidae*) Polivalente (Wyeth), *Crotalidae* Trivalente (Fort Dodge)	Precaução: origem equina; administrar 1-2 frascos IV, lentamente, diluídos em 250-500 mL de solução salina ou solução de Ringer lactato; administrar também os anti-histamínicos; os corticosteroides são contraindicados
Cobra coral	Cobra coral (Wyeth)	Precaução: origem equina; pode ser utilizado igual ao antiveneno de *Crotalidae*
Plantas		Tratar os sinais conforme a necessidade (ver Apêndice VII)
Sais de ferro	Mesilato de desferroxamina (Desferal®, Ciba)	Ainda não se estabeleceu a dosagem para os animais; a dosagem para os seres humanos é de 5 g de solução a 5% por VO, depois 20 mg/kg IM a cada 4-6 h; em casos de choque, a dosagem é de 40 mg/kg por gotejamento IV durante período de 4 h; pode ser repetida em 6 h, depois 15 mg/kg por gotejamento a cada 8 h
Tálio	Difeniltiocarbazona	Cães: 70 mg/kg VO a cada 8 h por 6 dias; acelera a eliminação, mas é parcialmente tóxica
	Azul da Prússia	0,2 mg/kg VO, dividido em 3 doses diárias
	Cloreto de potássio	Administrar simultaneamente com a tiocarbazona ou com o azul da Prússia, na dosagem de 2-6 g VO, divididos em doses diárias

IM = intramuscular; IV = intravenosa; VO = via oral; SC = subcutânea; ECG = eletrocardiograma; SNC = sistema nervoso central.
De Bailey EM, Jr, Garland T. Toxicologic emergencies. In: Murtaugh RJ, Kaplan PM, eds., Veterinary Emergency and Critical Care Medicine. St. Louis: Mosby, 1992, pp. 443-446.

ESPÉCIES CANINA E FELINA

APÊNDICE VII

GARY D. OSWEILER

RISCOS DE INTOXICAÇÃO PROVENIENTES DE CASA OU DO JARDIM, PARA ANIMAIS DE COMPANHIA

Tabela VII-A

Plantas Tóxicas — Sinais Clínicos, Antídotos e Tratamentos		
Planta e Características	*Sinais Clínicos*	*Antídotos e Tratamentos*
Açafrão-de-outono (*Colchicum autumnale*) Planta doméstica A planta inteira é tóxica, sobretudo os bulbos e é estável ao calor	Sensação de queimação na garganta e na boca, sede, náusea, vômito, diarreia hemorrágica, convulsões, arritmias cardíacas, hipotensão, choque. A toxina é excretada lentamente. Com o tempo, pode ocorrer supressão da medula óssea.	Provocar vômitos se a ingestão for recente e assintomática; doses repetidas de carvão ativado. Fluidos; analgésicos e protetores gastrintestinais (p. ex., sucralfato) para aliviar a cólica e a diarreia. Eritropoietina tem sido recomendado (100 UI/kg SC) para mielossupressão.
Acônito (*Aconitum spp.*) Planta ornamental perene de jardim A planta inteira é tóxica	Salivação, náusea, êmese, diarreia, irregularidades cardíacas, depressão respiratória.	Descontaminação gastrintestinal, reposição hídrica e eletrolítica. Tratamento semelhante aos casos de superdosagem por glicosídeos digitálicos, com cuidado na administração de potássio.
Amarílis (*Hippeastrum spp.*) Planta de jardim ou vaso Os bulbos são a parte mais tóxica, as folhas nem tanto	Náusea, anorexia, vômito, diarreia, hipotensão, depressão, falência hepática, tremores; possíveis convulsões ou menos comumente depressão. Avaliar exames hematológicos e demais exames séricos para monitorizar o prognóstico.	Êmese ou lavagem gástrica se logo após ingestão; carvão ativado, fluidos e tratamento de suporte para casos avançados. Antieméticos e protetores gastrintestinais no caso de gastrenterite persistente.
Azaleia (*Rhododendron spp.*) Planta de jardim, decorativa As folhas e as flores são tóxicas (grayanotoxinas) O mel produzido a partir do néctar das flores é tóxico	Sensação de queimação na boca, salivação, êmese, diarreia, fraqueza muscular, visão debilitada, bradicardia ou taquicardia, arritmia, hipotensão. Dedaleira, oleandro, ou teixo são diagnósticos diferenciais. EMERGÊNCIA.	Não utilizar eméticos se os sinais estão em progressão. Usar carvão ativado. Há necessidade de reposição hídrica e suporte respiratório. Atropina ou glicopirrolato podem aliviar a bradicardia. Lidocaína ou procainamida para taquicardia persistente. Use antieméticos (maropitant ou ondansetrona) e bloqueadores de receptores H2, omeprazol, ou sucralfato para os sinais gastrintestinais. Caso necessite fluidos IV, fazê-lo com cautela.
Azevinho inglês (*Illex spp.*) Planta decorativa O fruto é tóxico	Náusea, vômito, diarreia; os sinais são mais prováveis de aparecer no período das festas de fim de ano; são geralmente leves a moderados e podem ser autolimitados.	Fluido e reposição eletrolítica se ocorrerem vômitos ou diarreia. Tratamento caseiro (p. ex., preencha o estômago alimentando com pão); não alimente por 1 a 2 horas.
Batata-irlandesa (*Solanum tuberosum*) Vegetal de jardim Pele verde e brotos são tóxicos	Vômito, diarreia, salivação, ataxia, tremores musculares, fraqueza, bradicardia, hipotensão. Os sinais podem variar desde aqueles semelhantes aos causados pela atropina até aqueles relacionados à inibição da colinesterase.	Descontaminação gastrintestinal. Se os sinais semelhantes aos causados pela atropina predominarem, deve-se utilizar a fisostigmina. Na presença de salivação e diarreia, deve-se usar a atropina com cautela. Use os antídotos conforme os efeitos, com cuidado, baseado nas condições do animal.
Cadeia de ouro (*Laburnum anagyroides*) Árvore decorativa com longas cadeias de flores amarelas A planta inteira é tóxica	Os alcaloides quinolizidínicos se ligam aos receptores nicotínicos e muscarínicos. Êmese, depressão, fraqueza, incoordenação, midríase e taquicardia são os sinais principais.	Descontaminação gastrintestinal com lavagem ou êmese, acompanhada pela administração de carvão ativado.
Cálmia (*Kalmia spp.*) Planta nativa dos bosques e das montanhas do leste e do sudeste dos EUA As folhas e as flores são tóxicas O mel do néctar também é tóxico	Irritação bucal, salivação, vômito em jato, diarreia, fraqueza, distúrbios visuais, bradicardia, hipotensão, bloqueio AV.	Os eméticos são contraindicados. Usar carvão ativado, reposição de fluido e suporte respiratório conforme necessário.
Castanheiro-da-índia (*Aesculus spp.*) Árvore decorativa ou florestal; folhas em forma de palmas As castanhas e as ramas são as partes mais tóxicas	Gastrenterite, diarreia, desidratação, desbalanço eletrolítico. Pode haver ataxia ou párese ocasionalmente. Normalmente não é fatal e os animais se recuperam após desintoxicação ou remoção da fonte desencadeante.	Reposição hídrica e eletrolítica, demulcentes e terapia para gastrenterite.
Cinamomo (*Melia azedarach*) Árvore ornamental de clima de áreas temperadas a subtropicais O fruto é a parte mais tóxica	Salivação, anorexia, vômitos, diarreia seguido por fraqueza, ataxia e convulsões.	Descontaminação agressiva antes do aparecimento dos sinais clínicos. Lavagem com carvão ativado. Reposição de fluido e eletrólitos, anticonvulsivantes a cuidados de suporte. Ioimbina se ocorrer disfunção autonômica.
Dafne (*Daphne mezereum*) Arbusto decorativo A planta inteira é tóxica	Formação de vesículas e edema nos lábios e cavidade bucal, salivação, sede, dor abdominal, êmese, diarreia hemorrágica.	Reposição hídrica e eletrolítica, analgésicos.
Dedaleira (*Digitalis purpurea*) Planta de jardim A planta inteira é tóxica, especialmente as folhas	Náusea, êmese, dor abdominal, diarreia, bradicardia, arritmia com intervalo P-R prolongado e hipocalemia	Descontaminação gastrintestinal com carvão ativado ou catárticos salinos. Tratar a hipocalemia e administrar lidocaína em casos de arritmias ventriculares. *Ver também* Oleandro.
Delfínio ou espora (*Delphinium spp.*) Planta de jardim, montanhas; alta com flores azuis As sementes são mais tóxicas do que as folhas	Tremor, ataxia, fraqueza, salivação.	Desintoxicação gastrintestinal; administração de fisostigmina para o tratamento dos sinais muscarínicos.

Riscos de Intoxicação Provenientes de Casa ou do Jardim, para Animais de Companhia (continuação)

Tabela VII-A

Plantas Tóxicas — Sinais Clínicos, Antidotos e Tratamentos (*continuação*)		
Planta e Características	*Sinais Clínicos*	*Antídotos e Tratamentos*
Ervilha do rosário ou feijão rogatório (*Abrus precatorius*) Nativa das ilhas caribenhas As sementes (quando rompidas ou mastigadas) são altamente tóxicas Sua importação para os EUA é ilegal	Náusea, vômito, diarreia, fraqueza, taquicardia, possível insuficiência renal, coma, óbito.	Êmese ou lavagem, acompanhadas pela administração de carvão ativado, demulcentes, fluidos e eletrólitos. Vitamina C pode aumentar a sobrevida
Estramônio ou figueira-brava (*Datura stramonium*) Erva daninha anual, mas algumas espécies são ornamentais (*Datura metel*) A planta inteira é tóxica, mas as sementes constituem a parte mais tóxica e acessível	Sede, distúrbios da visão, delírio, midríase, atonia gastrintestinal. Sinais semelhantes aos casos de superdosagem por atropina Baixo risco para animais pequenos exceto pelo acesso às sementes ou aos extratos, usados como droga recreacional.	Medicamentos parassimpaticomiméticos (p. ex., fisostigmina); sintomáticos e cuidados de suporte.
Filodendro (*Monstera* e *Philodendron spp.*) Planta doméstica As folhas são de leve a moderadamente tóxicas	Irritação imediata e dolorosa, edema de lábios, boca, língua e garganta devido ao oxalato insolúvel contido; segundo relatos, é nefrotóxica aos gatos, porém a confirmação deste efeito é mínima.	A aplicação de líquidos refrescantes ou demulcentes na boca pode ajudar a aliviar os sinais clínicos.
Fumo (*Nicotiana tabacum*) Planta de jardim, erva daninha, cigarros A planta inteira é tóxica	Início rápido de salivação, náusea, êmese, tremores, incoordenação e ataxia, seguidos por colapso e insuficiência respiratória, bradicardia e fibrilação atrial	Fornecer ventilação assistida e suporte vascular. Após o suporte respiratório, proceder à descontaminação do trato gastrintestinal com lavagem e carvão ativado. Terapia cardíaca conforme necessário (atropina para bradicardia; β-bloqueadores para hipertensão/taquicardia), anticonvulsivantes ou sedativos conforme necessário; evitar antiácidos uma vez que condições alcalinas promovem maior absorção.
Glicínia (*Wisteria spp.*) Trepadeira lenhosa ou arbusto com flores azuis a brancas A planta inteira é tóxica	Náusea, dor abdominal, vômitos prolongados.	Tratar com antieméticos e terapia de reposição de fluidos.
Hera inglesa (*Hedera helix*) Planta doméstica Os frutos e as folhas são tóxicos	Salivação, sede, êmese, gastrenterite, diarreia, dermatite	Tratamento dos sinais sintomatologicamente e prover cuidados de suporte para os sinais gastrintestinais.
Ipomeia (*Ipomoea purpurea* e *Ipomoea tricolor*) Planta anual cultivada em vaso e no jardim As sementes constituem a parte mais tóxica Ocasionalmente, utilizada como alucinógeno	Náusea, midríase, comportamento anormal, excitabilidade, tremores, reflexos diminuídos, diarreia, hipotensão. Raramente relatado. O autor tem documentado um caso clínico em cão.	Carvão ativado; manter o animal num ambiente escuro e calmo; tranquilização com diazepam conforme necessário. A fração tóxica (ácido lisérgico ou alcaloides ergotamínicos) são excretados rapidamente e os sinais clínicos são um tanto quanto passageiros.
Íris ou lírio-roxo (*Iris spp.*) Flor perene de jardim O rizoma é a parte mais tóxica	Cólica, náusea, hipersalivação, vômito, diarreia.	Reposição de fluidos e eletrólitos.
Jasmim-amarelo (*Gelsemium sempervirens*) Climas brandos a subtropicais As flores amarelas em formato de trombeta crescem em plantas trepadeiras sempre verdes	Fraqueza, convulsões, paresia ou paralisia, falência respiratória.	Terapia sintomática e de suporte respiratório. Descontaminação gastrintestinal e terapia de reposição de fluidos.
Lantana (*Lantana camara*) Planta tanto selvagem quanto de jardim cultivada em áreas de climas temperados a tropicais brandos; flores de coloração laranja brilhante, amarelas, vermelhas e rosa As folhagens e as bagas imaturas são tóxicas	Fraqueza, letargia, vômito, diarreia, midríase, dispneia. Os sinais avançados são coléstase, bilirrubinemia e fotossensibilização.	Descontaminação gastrintestinal, fluidos e suporte respiratório. Proteger contra a luz solar e tratamento para a insuficiência hepática.
Lírio, incluindo o lírio-da-páscoa, o lírio asiático (*Lilium spp.*), o hemerocale (*Hemerocallis spp.*) (*Ver* cap. sobre Envenenamento por lírio)	Depressão, oligúria, insuficiência renal em gatos, como consequência de necrose tubular tóxica.	Descontaminação gastrintestinal imediata e terapia de suporte para insuficiência renal. A toxina responsável pelo quadro é desconhecida até o presente.
Lírio-do-vale (*Convallaria majalis*) Planta ornamental de jardim As sementes e as flores são mais tóxicas que as folhas	Cólica, vômito, diarreia, bradicardia, arritmia.	Descontaminação gastrintestinal com lavagem e carvão ativado. Evitar o uso de eméticos. Utilizar a lidocaína para o tratamento das arritmias ventriculares; tratar como se fosse um quadro de superdosagem por outros glicosídeos digitálicos, incluindo a correção da hipercalemia.

RISCOS DE INTOXICAÇÃO PROVENIENTES DE CASA OU DO JARDIM, PARA ANIMAIS DE COMPANHIA (CONTINUAÇÃO)

Tabela VII-A

Plantas Tóxicas — Sinais Clínicos, Antídotos e Tratamentos (continuação)		
Planta e Características	Sinais Clínicos	Antídotos e Tratamentos
Mamona (*Ricinus communis*) Planta anual de jardim, arbusto ou planta ornamental que cresce até 2 m As sementes medem 1 cm, são mosqueadas com cores claras e escuras e altamente tóxicas	O período latente pode durar várias horas; cólica, êmese, diarreia intensa e hemorrágica, sede, tremores musculares, colapso súbito. Danos potenciais ao fígado e rins. Os sinais aparecem com maior probabilidade se a semente é mastigada. Prejudica a síntese proteica levando à morte celular disseminada.	Êmese se logo após a infestação; carvão ativado e catárticos a menos que a diarreia já esteja presente; fluidos e eletrólitos para desidratação uso de protetores gastrintestinais é indicado; monitorização de hemograma e exames séricos a fim de ajustar a terapêutica de suporte de acordo com os resultados. Algumas publicações recomendam o uso de glicocorticoide baseado em resultados de experimentos laboratoriais em animais. O prognóstico para casos em progressão clínica é reservado.
Nabo-selvagem (*Arisaema triphyllum*) Florestas e jardins de zonas temperadas A planta inteira é tóxica	Glossite, faringite, inflamação bucal, edema, salivação. Muitos dos sinais podem ser locais devido ao oxalato insolúvel nele contido.	Irrigação bucal com água. A aplicação de líquidos refrescantes ou demulcentes na boca pode aliviar os sinais clínicos.
Narciso, abrótea, junquilho (*Narcissus spp.*) Bulbo ornamental de jardim O bulbo é a parte mais tóxica	Náusea, vômito, hipotensão, diarreia; ocasionalmente óbito se uma grande quantidade de bulbos for ingerida.	Lavagem gástrica, carvão ativado, reposição de fluidos, tratamento de suporte para gastrenterite.
Oleandro (*Nerium oleander*) Planta arbustiva ornamental com 1-3 m de altura A planta inteira é tóxica Outras plantas com glicosídeos cardíacos semelhantes incluem *Kalanchoe spp.*; estrela de Belém; oleandro amarelo (*Thevetia peruviana*)	As toxinas são glicosídeos cardiotóxicos similares aos digitálicos. Náusea, sinais precoces de vômito, cólica, diarreia, bradicardia ou taquicardia e arritmia com hipercalcemia desenvolvida logo após a ingestão (1-3 horas); EMERGÊNCIA O prognóstico depende da dosagem e terapêutica efetiva precoce.	Lavagem gástrica ou indução de êmese; carvão ativado ou catárticos salinos. Tratar como se fosse um caso de superdosagem por glicosídeos digitálicos, incluindo a correção da hipercalemia. Monitorizar o potássio sérico e os índices renais. Utilizar a lidocaína, procainamida ou outros medicamentos apropriados para a arritmia e superdosagem por digitálicos. Protetores gastrintestinais devem ser usados se necessário. Digoxina imune FAB (Digibind 60 mg/kg IV) tem se mostrado eficaz em cães.
Palmeira Cica ou Sagu (incluem *Cycas spp.*, *Zamia spp.* e *Macrozamia spp.*) Principalmente no sul dos Estados Unidos e Havaí Suas toxinas são os glicosídeos cicasina e metilazometanol Todas as partes são tóxicas, porém a maior concentração está nas sementes (castanha)	Os efeitos são hepatobiliares, gastrintestinais e neurológicos. Os cães possuem maior probabilidade de envenenamento. O início dos sintomas podem se dar em menos de 1 hora até 3 dias após a ingestão. Sinais incluem vômito, diarreia, letargia, icterícia, anorexia, dor abdominal, ascite e sinais neurológicos que variam de ataxia e fraqueza até coma e convulsões.	Êmese logo após a ingestão, carvão ativado a cada 6 horas por 3 dias. Monitorização de exames séricos para falência hepática. Não há antídoto disponível. Realizar cuidados de suporte agressivamente com fluidoterapia, vitaminas do complexo B, controle de convulsões, protetores gastrintestinais, vitamina K1 e transfusão sanguínea caso necessário. Hepatoprotetores como SAMe (S-adenosil-L-metionina) também são recomendados.
Poinsétia ou bico-de-papagaio (*Euphorbia pulcherrima*) Planta de jardim ou de vaso, cultivada especialmente no Natal	Irritação bucal; pode causar vômito, diarreia e dermatite. A seiva do tronco e as folhas são de leve a moderadamente irritantes ou tóxicas.	Utilizar demulcentes e fluidos para evitar a desidratação. Lavar a boca com água; oferecer pequenas quantidades de leite, iogurte ou outros produtos que contenham cálcio para se ligar aos cristais de oxalato.
Rosa-do-Natal (*Helleborus niger*) Planta doméstica e de jardim A planta inteira é tóxica	Dor bucal e abdominal, náusea, vômito, cólica, diarreia, arritmia cardíaca, hipotensão, bloqueio cardíaco.	Lavagem gástrica ou êmese; carvão ativado ou catárticos salinos para descontaminação do trato gastrintestinal.
Ruibarbo (*Rheum rhaponticum*) e trevo (*Oxalis spp.*) Planta de jardim; planta ornamental Cru ou enlatado As folhas são ricas em oxalatos solúveis	Hipersalivação, vômito, diarreia logo após a ingestão, possível tetania hipocalcêmica. Sinais gastrintestinais podem retroceder, mas a insuficiência renal se desenvolve a partir da nefrose causada pelo oxalato insolúvel. Resultados laboratoriais mostram hipocalcemia, uremia e cristais de oxalato na urina.	A descontaminação gastrintestinal precoce (êmese, carvão ativado) é importante. Usar demulcentes e efetuar a reposição de fluidos para a gastrenterite. Cálcio IV somente se a hipocalcemia for confirmada. Tratar a possível nefrose por oxalato com fluidoterapia apropriada e monitorização da função renal.
Teixo (*Taxus cuspidata* e *Taxus baccata*) Plantas decorativas sempre verdes com duas agulhas planas ordenadas A planta inteira (exceto os frutos maduros) é tóxica	A taxina é um alcaloide cardiotóxico; causa retardo da condução atrioventricular, alargando o complexo QRS e deprimindo as ondas p; bloqueio dos canais de sódio e cálcio. Colapso agudo ou morte súbita podem ocorrer. Tremor, fraqueza, dispneia, bradicardia, fibrilação ventricular, arritmia e bloqueio cardíaco podem aparecer.	Descontaminação gastrintestinal deve ser realizada prontamente após a ingestão. Sintomáticos e terapia de suporte da função respiratória e cardiovascular de acordo com os efeitos (atropina ou glicopirrolato para bradicardia; lidocaína ou procainamida para taquicardia ou disritmias ou perfusão diminuída).
Tremoço (*Lupinus spp.*) Planta ornamental de jardim As sementes são mais tóxicas que as folhas	Salivação, ataxia, convulsões, dispneia.	Descontaminação gastrintestinal, anticonvulsivantes para controle das convulsões.
Trombeta-de-anjo (*Brugmansia spp.* ou *Datura spp.*) Planta de jardim anual com flores brancas em formato de trombeta A planta inteira é tóxica, principalmente as sementes	Sede, atonia gastrintestinal, distúrbios da visão e pupilas dilatadas, delírio, comportamento alterado. Nota: tanto *Datura spp.* quanto *Brugmansia spp.* são alcaloides parassimpatolíticos semelhantes a atropina. *Datura spp.* é comum nos Estados Unidos, mas *Brugmansia spp.* é importada.	Medicamentos parassimpaticomiméticos (fisostigmina) usado com cautela para evitar depressão respiratória. Controlar o comportamento alterado caso necessário com diazepam ou fenobarbital.

Riscos de Intoxicação Provenientes de Casa ou do Jardim, para Animais de Companhia (continuação)

Tabela VII-A

Plantas Tóxicas — Sinais Clínicos, Antídotos e Tratamentos (continuação)		
Planta e Características	Sinais Clínicos	Antídotos e Tratamentos
Urtiga (*Urtica dioica*) Erva daninha de jardins Os pelos sobre as folhas contêm toxinas que penetram na pele ao contato	Irritação e dor bucais, tumefação e edema do nariz e das regiões perioculares ou de outras áreas de contato na pele.	Os anti-histamínicos e analgésicos podem controlar os sinais relevantes. Terapia de suporte com anti-inflamatórios locais ou sistêmicos pode ser usada para o tratamento das áreas de contato acometidas.
Visco (*Phoradendron spp.*) Brotos parasitários em outras árvores As folhas, os caules e as bagas são moderadamente tóxicos	Êmese, cólica, diarreia, hipovolemia e colapso ocasional são esporadicamente reportados. Tentativas experimentais de envenenamento são amplamente negativas. O acesso pelos animais domésticos é esperado nos lares no período de férias, com seus efeitos mais provavelmente sendo no trato gastrintestinal.	Reposição de fluido e eletrolítica; podem-se utilizar demulcentes ou protetores gastrintestinais para gastrenterite.

APÊNDICE VII

CHARLOTTE MEANS

RISCOS DE INTOXICAÇÃO PROVENIENTES DE CASA OU DO JARDIM, PARA ANIMAIS DE COMPANHIA (CONTINUAÇÃO)

Tabela VII-B

Toxidade Relacionada a Ervas Medicinais						
Classe	Princípio Tóxico	Gênero e Espécie	Nomes Comuns	Sinais Clínicos	Resumo do Tratamento	Utilização Popular
Simpatomiméticos	Efedrina, pseudoefedrina, sinefrina	*Ephedra sinica, Sida cordifolia, Citrus aurantium*	Ma Huang, malva comum indiana, laranja amarga	Hipertermia, hipertensão, taquicardia, tremores, convulsões, alucinações, agitação, síndrome da serotonina	Descontaminação, monitorizar sistemas cardiovascular e nervoso central. Acepromazina para agitação, ciproeptadina para síndrome da serotonina, propranolol como β-bloqueador	Emagrecedor, levantamento de peso, "*Ecstasy*" floral, descongestionante
Metilxantinas	Cafeína, teobromina	*Camellia sinensis, Paullinia cupana, Cola acuminata, Theobroma cacao*	EGCG (chá verde), guaraná, cacau, cola, noz de cola, chocolate	Agitação, hiperatividade, poliúria, polidipsia, arritmias cardíacas, tremores, convulsões	Descontaminação, diurese por fluidoterapia, monitorizar sistemas cardiovascular e nervoso central, controlar arritmias, tremores e convulsões, cuidados de suporte/ sintomáticos	Emagrecedor, "NoDoz" floral
Hipoglicêmicos	Ácido alfalipoico, canela	Ácido alfalipoico (ALA), *Cinnamomum cassia*	Ácido tióctico, canela	Ptialismo, vômito, hipoglicemia, enzimas hepáticas ou renais aumen- -tadas, óbito (ALA)	Monitorizar glicemia, controlar hipoglicemia, controlar enzimas hepáticas	Tratamento do diabetes, envenenamento pelo fungo (cogumelo) manita (ALA)
Síndrome da Serotonina	5-hidroxitriptofano (5-HTP)	*Griffonia simplicifolia*	5-http	Vômito, diarreia, tremores, convulsões, ataxia, hiperestesia, depressão	Descontaminação, diazepam para tremores ou convulsões, ciproeptadina é um antagonista específico	Depressão, cefaleias, insônia, obesidade
Alergênicos	Arabinogalactano	*Echinacea purpúrea*	Pinha púrpura	Vômito, diarreia	Cuidados de suporte/ sintomáticos	Auxílio no tratamento de resfriados e gripes, imunoestimulante
Anticoagulantes	Hidroxicumarina, bisabolol	*Matricaria recutita, Chamaemelum nobile*	Camomila	Vômito, diarreia, letargia, epistaxe ocasional, hematoma (felinos)	Controlar coagulação, cuidados de suporte e sintomáticos, muito raramente transfusão sanguínea	Sedativo, úlceras gastrintestinais
Inibidores da MAO	Hipericina	*Hypericum perforatum*	Mosto de São João	Depressão, vômito, diarreia, tremores ocasionais, convulsões	Descontaminação, cuidados de suporte e sintomáticos, ciproeptadina para a síndrome da serotonina	Antidepressivo, insônia
Sedativos	Valepotriatos	*Valeriana officinalis*	Valeriana	Letargia, sedação	Geralmente cuidados caseiros, prevenir traumatismos	Sedativo, auxílio para dormir
Óleos essenciais	Óleo de melaleuca, pulegona, mentofurano	*Melaleuca alternifolia, Mentha pulegium*	Óleo da árvore-de-chá, óleo de poejo	Oral: vômito, diarreia, depressão do SNC, hepatotoxicidade, pneumonia por aspiração Cutâneo (como *spot-on*): paresia transitória	Cutâneo: banho Oral: fluidoterapia, N-acetilcisteína, controlar enzimas hepáticas nas ingestões de poejo. Controlar dor, promover termorregulação se necessário	Germicida, infecções fúngicas, antisséptico, controle de pulgas

RISCOS DE INTOXICAÇÃO PROVENIENTES DE CASA OU DO JARDIM, PARA ANIMAIS DE COMPANHIA (CONTINUAÇÃO)

Tabela VII-B

Toxidade Relacionada a Ervas Medicinais (*continuação*)						
Classe	*Princípio Tóxico*	*Gênero e Espécie*	*Nomes Comuns*	*Sinais Clínicos*	*Resumo do Tratamento*	*Utilização Popular*
Glicosaminoglicanos polissulfatados	PSGAG	Glicosamina, sulfato de condroitina	Adequan e muitas outras marcas	Oral: vômito, diarreia, polidipsia. IM: prolongamento transitório de TP e TTPa, agregação plaquetária reduzida, diátese	Controlar vômito e diarreia, estabilizar enzimas hepáticas em casos de ingestão abundante. Coagulopatias apenas são esperadas com doses injetáveis maiores, controlar parâmetros de coagulação	Artrite, condroprotetor
Detergentes catiônicos	Compostos de amônia quaternária	Taranja (*Citrus decumana*)	Extrato de semente de taranja	Sialorreia, vômito ± sangue, fraqueza, anorexia, hipertermia, irritação ou ulceração oral/ esofagiana, eritema cutâneo, dor, ulceração	Diluição, pasta de sucralfato, bloqueadores H2, fluidoterapia, suporte nutricional, antibiótico de largo espectro, controlar dor.	Desinfetante, antifúngico
Agentes bloqueadores alfa-2-adrenérgicos	Agentes bloqueadores alfa-2-adrenérgicos	*Pausinystalia yohimbine*	Ioimbina	Hiperatividade, agitação, tremores, convulsões, vômito, diarreia, dor abdominal, hipotensão	Monitorizar glicose, pressão sanguínea, controlar agitação, tremores, convulsões. Fluidoterapia e glicose quando necessário	Hipertensão, angina, "Viagra floral"
Salicilatos	Salicilato de metila	*Gaultheria procumbens*	Extrato de gaultéria	Distúrbios gastrintestinais, úlceras gastrintestinais, hipertermia, hepatotoxicidade, coagulopatias, coma	Protetores gastrintestinais, fluidoterapia, controlar acidose, protetores hepáticos, controlar parâmetros de coagulação	

Leitura sugerida:
DerMarderosian A, Beutler JA. The Review of Natural Products, 3. ed. St. Louis: Facts and Comparisons Group, 2002.
Means C. Selected herbal hazards. Vet clin North Am Small Anim Pract 2002, 32(2):367-382.
Wynn SG, Fougere BJ. Veterinary Herbal medicine. St. Louis: Mosby, 2007, pp. 513-514.

ESPÉCIES CANINA E FELINA

APÊNDICE VII

ANITA M. KORE

RISCOS DE INTOXICAÇÃO PROVENIENTES DE CASA OU DO JARDIM, PARA ANIMAIS DE COMPANHIA (CONTINUAÇÃO)

Tabela VII-C

Produtos de Limpeza e seus Sinais Clínicos — Antídotos e Tratamento

Os produtos domésticos geralmente são misturas químicas complexas de compostos orgânicos e inorgânicos voltados para usos específicos. Quando um animal é exposto a esse produto, é importante obter, se possível, as seguintes informações: nome comercial completo, ingredientes do produto e suas concentrações, diluição do produto ao qual o animal teve contato, sinais clínicos e sua progressão em relação ao tempo de exposição e qualquer tratamento feito pelo proprietário do animal. É útil instruir o proprietário a trazer o recipiente original do produto em questão, se possível.

A informação dos ingredientes e a toxicologia clínica de um produto específico podem se obtidas de centros de controle de intoxicação animal e humano, centros de emergência médica e serviços telefônicos de informação sobre a segurança do fabricante do produto. Muitos produtos comerciais possuem, como parte de suas bulas, informações específicas e números de telefone do fabricante.

Nome do Agente (Tipo Químico)	Sinais Clínicos	Antídotos/Tratamento/Cuidados Posteriores
Sabões (sais e ácidos graxos): Sabões em barra, sabões líquidos para lavagem de mãos	Os sabões geralmente possuem baixa toxicidade oral. Alguns podem exibir conteúdo considerável de álcalis livres, apresentando, desta forma, possível risco corrosivo. Os óleos essenciais usados como fragrâncias em sabões em barra podem causar irritação gastrintestinal. Irritação gastrintestinal - náusea, vômito, diarreia.	O tratamento envolve o uso de demulcentes e diluentes como leite ou água. A indução do vômito pode ser considerada se o volume ingerido exceder 20 g de sabão/kg de peso corporal e o sabão não for alcalino (não corrosivo) ou se o vômito espontâneo não ocorreu em 30 minutos após a ingestão. Se ocorrer vômito excessivo ou diarreia, devem ser iniciados tratamento sintomático e esforços para controlar o equilíbrio hidroeletrolítico.
Detergentes não iônicos (alquil etoxilato, etanóis polietoxi-fenoxi-alquil e estearato de polietilenoglicol): Detergentes para lavagem manual de louça, xampus e alguns detergentes para lavagem de roupas	A maior parte dos detergentes não iônicos possuem baixo poder irritante e, assim, baixa toxicidade. A ingestão de detergentes não iônicos normalmente resulta apenas em vômito e diarreia. As exposições oculares geralmente não produzem liquefação extensa do epitélio corneal.	Dependendo da via de exposição, os tratamentos para exposições a detergentes não iônicos devem incluir ingestão de diluentes como leite ou água, lavagem de olhos expostos com volume abundante de água ou lavagem radical do detergente da pele e pelame. Se ocorrer vômito prolongado, deve-se iniciar o tratamento sintomático e os cuidados para controlar o equilíbrio hidroeletrolítico.
Surfactantes aniônicos (hidrocarbonatos sulfonados ou fosforilados de cadeia curta, p. ex., alquil-sulfato de sódio, alquil-sulfonatos de sódio, dioctilsulfossuccinato de sódio, lauril sulfato de sódio, tetrapropileno sulfonado de benzeno e alquil sulfonato de benzeno). Muitos destes materiais contêm estruturantes alcalinos, como fosfato de sódio, carbonato de sódio, metassilicato de sódio ou silicato de sódio: Detergentes para lavagens de roupas, detergentes para lava-louças, alguns xampus.	A maior parte dos detergentes aniônicos possui reduzida ou moderada capacidade tóxica. Os produtos para lava-louças são considerados os mais tóxicos devido à sua maior alcalinidade, colocando-os sob risco de corrosivos. Os detergentes aniônicos ingeridos são bem absorvidos pelo trato gastrintestinal e podem ser absorvidos completamente pela pele irritada ou danificada. Pode ocorrer hemólise intravascular na presença dos detergentes aniônicos. A exposição cutânea prolongada ou repetida aos detergentes aniônicos pode resultar em irritação. Foi relatada que a exposição ocular aos detergentes para lava-louças provoca erosão e opacidade corneal. A ingestão de detergentes aniônicos frequentemente resulta em vômito, diarreia e desconforto gastrintestinal. A maioria das exposições causa indisposição, mas não é fatal.	É aconselhável a administração oral de leite ou água para diluir o detergente. Deve ser administrado carvão ativado se grandes quantidades forem ingeridas e ocorrer corrosão do trato gastrintestinal. Na exposição ocular, os olhos devem ser lavados com volume abundante de água. Para a exposição cutânea, é recomendada lavagem e enxague radicais. Se ocorrer vômito prolongado, devem ser instituídas medidas para o tratamento sintomático e controle do equilíbrio hidroeletrolítico. O paciente deve ser controlado para se evitar o desenvolvimento de hemólise. Se a hemólise ocorrer, é recomendada fluidoterapia e alcalinização urinária, no sentido de se prevenir as lesões nos túbulos renais oriundas da precipitação de hemoglobina. Adicionalmente, a função renal deve ser monitorizada. Em pacientes que ingeriram detergentes para lava-louças, deve-se examinar a cavidade bucal, orofaringe e esôfago em busca de lesões corrosivas. O tratamento para essas corrosões deve ser iniciado como descrito anteriormente na seção sobre corrosões.
Detergentes catiônicos (compostos de amônia quaternária com grupos substitutos aril ou alquil, p.ex.): Amaciantes de roupa, germicidas e sanitizantes	Salivação profusa, vômito com possível hematêmese, fraqueza muscular, fasciculações, depressão respiratória e do sistema nervoso central, febre, convulsões, colapso e coma. As ingestões de detergentes catiônicos normalmente resultam em lesões corrosivas das mucosas da cavidade bucal, língua, faringe e esôfago. O choque pode se desenvolver mais cedo ou à medida que a intoxicação progride. A perda de pelos e as ulcerações cutâneas são frequentemente vistas nos felinos; em caninos, são relatadas lesões inflamatórias dos coxins após exposição aos compostos de amônia quaternária. A exposição ocular pode resultar em efeitos clínicos de leve desconforto a lesões corneais graves, dependendo da concentração do detergente.	O tratamento da ingestão requer a administração de leite, água ou clara de ovo. O vômito não deve ser induzido quando a concentração do detergente catiônico do produto consumido for maior que 7,5%. A diluição oral pode ser acompanhada pela administração de carvão ativado e catártico salino. A esofagoscopia para a avaliação do grau de lesão corrosiva é adequada se não estiver presente estridor, disfagia ou ptialismo. Os cuidados gerais de suporte incluem controle da respiração, ingestão calórica adequada (p.ex., utilização de sonda gastresofágica percutânea [GEP]) e tratamento de qualquer convulsão que possa acontecer. Os pacientes deverão ser estritamente controlados quanto ao surgimento de choque. A pele exposta deverá ser gentilmente lavada, porém de forma completa, com sabão e água. Os olhos deverão ser totalmente avaliados e lavados com solução salina isotérmica durante 20-30 minutos. As úlceras corneais, se presentes, deverão ser pronta e persistentemente tratadas.

Riscos de Intoxicação Provenientes de Casa ou do Jardim, para Animais de Companhia (continuação)

Tabela VII-C

Produtos de Limpeza e seus Sinais Clínicos — Antídotos e Tratamento (*continuação*)		
Nome do Agente (Tipo Químico)	*Sinais Clínicos*	*Antídotos/Tratamento/Cuidados Posteriores*
Ácidos corrosivos (ácido hidroclórico [muriático], sulfúrico, nítrico ou fosfórico, bissulfito de sódio, soluções aquosas de halogenados livres [p.ex., cloretos, brometos ou iodados]): Compostos antirraquitismo, limpadores de louças sanitárias, fluidos de limpeza de cilindros de armas, fluidos de baterias de automóveis e agentes de limpeza para piscinas.	Os ácidos produzem, tipicamente, uma lesão necrótica coagulante localizada. As queimaduras por ácido raramente penetram na espessura completa da mucosa. O contato com ácidos fortes imediatamente induz dor intensa, de forma que muitos animais não ingerem volumes significativos. As queimaduras corrosivas das mucosas aparecem primeiramente com aspecto branco leitoso ou acinzentado, tornando-se negras e podendo se enrugar devido à formação de cicatriz. As estenoses podem se formar várias semanas após a lesão inicial. O animal pode vocalizar ou se tornar depressivo; alguns animais manifestam dor, expressa pela ofegação. Pode ser observada incapacidade de deglutir. Outros efeitos são hematêmese, dor abdominal, polidipsia, edema de epiglote com dispneia secundária e possível choque. A pneumonite secundária ocorre por exposição ou aspiração de vapores ácidos. Se ocorrer exposição ocular ou cutânea, podem surgir queimaduras graves. As exposições oculares são extremamente dolorosas e podem conduzir à necrose conjuntival e/ou corneal. A extensão da lesão corneal pode não ser prontamente evidente. Os ácidos tendem a penetrar no olho mais vagarosamente que as substâncias alcalinas.	O tratamento consiste na imediata dissolução da exposição utilizando água ou leite. As tentativas de neutralizar a queimadura por meios químicos são contraindicadas. A lavagem gástrica é contraindicada em ingestão cáustica e o carvão é ineficaz para adsorver cáusticos. Após a administração de um diluente, o animal deve receber cuidados de suporte. A fluidoterapia normalmente está indicada. Se estiver presente edema grave de faringe, uma sonda endotraqueal ou de traqueostomia deverá ser utilizada para garantir uma respiração desobstruída. O acometimento do esôfago é menos comum nas exposições com ácidos que nas ingestões de álcalis (ver bases corrosivas abaixo). A terapia para o choque pode ser necessária; o colapso circulatório não corrigido pode ocasionar insuficiência renal, lesões isquêmicas em órgãos vitais e morte rápida. A pele afetada deve ser agressivamente lavada com volumes abundantes de água e os olhos expostos devem ser lavados com salina estéril por pelo menos 30 minutos. Os anestésicos tópicos são úteis para conforto do paciente nas manipulações.
Bases corrosivas (hidróxido de sódio e potássio, lixívia ou potassa, carbonato de sódio e potássio, amônia e hidróxido de amônia, permanganato de potássio): Limpadores de tubulações, produtos de lavagem, limpadores líquidos e produtos para limpeza de sanitários	Produtos alcalinos causam necrose de liquefação imediata após contato. As lesões tendem a ser mais profundas e mais penetrantes que as causadas por materiais acidificantes. Podem ocorrer queimaduras de todas as camadas esofagianas. Outros sinais clínicos são similares àqueles descritos para ácidos corrosivos.	Diluição da exposição com leite ou água, da mesma forma usada para ácidos corrosivos. Cuidados de suporte, semelhante aos usados para ácidos corrosivos. Endoscopia cuidadosa com uma sonda flexível é útil nas primeiras 12-24 horas após ingestão. Interromper o procedimento ao primeiro sinal de lesão à mucosa esofagiana. A avaliação radiográfica é alternativa. Às vezes a ressecção cirúrgica dos tecidos lesados é indicada. Os esteroides são recomendados para reduzir a estenose das queimaduras circunferenciais dos álcalis. O tratamento com esteroides deve ser iniciado nas primeiras 48 horas e ser acompanhado por antibioticoterapia profilática. Os antibióticos são especificamente indicados em animais com perfurações. Os pacientes gravemente afetados podem requerer a colocação de uma sonda (GEP) para suporte nutricional. É útil controlar o equilíbrio acidobásico, a gasometria e os eletrólitos séricos. Pode ser necessária terapia para choque; o colapso circulatório não corrigido pode ocasionar insuficiência renal, lesões isquêmicas em órgãos vitais e morte rápida. A exposição da pele e olhos é tratada da mesma forma que a citada para ácidos corrosivos.

Riscos de Intoxicação Provenientes de Casa ou do Jardim, para Animais de Companhia (continuação)

Tabela VII-C

Produtos de Limpeza e seus Sinais Clínicos — Antídotos e Tratamento (continuação)		
Nome do Agente (Tipo Químico)	*Sinais Clínicos*	*Antídotos/Tratamento/Cuidados Posteriores*
Desinfetantes — fenólicos (clorofenóis, fenilfenol)	A DL_{50} oral de fenol em caninos é de aproximadamente 0,5 g/kg de peso vivo. Os felinos são mais sensíveis que caninos ao fenol e produtos fenólicos. O fenol na concentração maior que 5% resultou em queimaduras orais; concentrações acima de 1% produziram queimaduras cutâneas. A exposição ocular e cutânea aos fenóis geralmente é acompanhada por um curto intervalo de dor intensa seguida por anestesia local. As lesões cutâneas necróticas coagulantes parecem se tornar brancas e, depois, desenvolvem escaras secas nos próximos dias. A exposição ocular aos compostos fenólicos produz queimaduras graves e lesões penetrantes na córnea. A exposição oral aos compostos fenólicos produz queimaduras corrosivas da boca, orofaringe e esôfago. Os sinais clínicos iniciais são vômito, ptialismo, apreensão, hiperatividade, ataxia e respiração ofegante. À medida que a síndrome clínica avança, podem se desenvolver fasciculações, choque, arritmias cardíacas, metemoglobinemia e coma. Os danos renais e hepáticos ocorrem nas próximas 12-24 horas. A alcalose respiratória ocorre secundariamente devido à estimulação respiratória mediada centralmente.	As intoxicações decorrentes da exposição aos desinfetantes fenólicos são emergências médicas. A diluição da exposição aos fenóis com água é controversa porque tal diluição pode aumentar a absorção sistêmica. Podem ser administrados demulcentes gastrintestinais (leite ou ovos). A gravidade dos danos à mucosa da orofaringe deve ser atestada antes que a lavagem gástrica seja realizada. Se danos graves da mucosa estiverem presentes, a lavagem gástrica e a indução de vômito são contraindicadas. O carvão ativado e uma solução salina catártica podem ser administrados se os danos à mucosa forem leves ou não estiverem presentes. Para a exposição cutânea, utilizar polietilenoglicol ou glicerol nas áreas afetadas, seguido por um detergente líquido para louças e lavagem completa com água. Usar luvas de borracha grossas e roupas de proteção. Após a lavagem final, podem ser aplicadas compressas mergulhadas em uma solução de bicarbonato de sódio 0,5% nas áreas lesadas. Para exposições oculares, os olhos devem ser lavados com solução salina isotérmica por 20-30 minutos. Avaliar as erosões corneais. É necessário tratamento de suporte agressivo - equilíbrio acidobásico, função cardiovascular, função renal e função hepática devem ser cuidadosamente monitorizados. O choque e a depressão respiratória são fatores complicadores e requerem cuidados de fluidoterapia e suporte respiratório. A N-acetilcisteína pode limitar a toxicidade hepática e renal. Se estiver presente metemoglobinemia, pode ser utilizado azul de metileno ou ácido ascórbico.
Desinfetantes — alvejantes (hipoclorito de sódio, hipoclorito de cálcio, ácido diclorodimetil-hidantoína, peróxido de sódio, perborato de sódio): desodorizantes, purificadores de água, alvejantes para lavanderias, químicos para piscinas	A intoxicação por hipoclorito é resultante dos seus efeitos corrosivos na pele e nas mucosas. Os alvejantes caseiros clorados são irritantes brandos ou moderados, geralmente não estando associados à destruição tecidual significativa. Foram relatadas queimaduras orofaríngeanas, esofagianas e gástricas. As soluções mais concentradas de hipoclorito e pós alvejantes podem produzir queimaduras corrosivas. Os efeitos tóxicos comuns dos alvejantes clorados caseiros são irritação da orofaringe, ptialismo, vômito e dor abdominal. O animal exposto pode exalar odor de cloro e o clareamento dos pelos pode ser visto. As reações sistêmicas são raras e secundárias às lesões de tecidos e mucosas. A inalação dos vapores ou pós de produtos alvejantes clorados iniciam irritação pulmonar, tosse, ânsias de vômito e dispneia. Os produtos alvejantes não clorados possuem baixa toxicidade. O peróxido de sódio pode provocar gastrite moderada e vômito. Os alvejantes que contêm perborato de sódio são decompostos a peróxido e borato; esses alvejantes são mais alcalinos e, desta forma, irritantes. Eles também produzem efeitos sistêmicos oriundos do ácido bórico.	O tratamento consiste na diluição imediata da exposição com leite ou água. As áreas de contato cutâneo devem ser lavadas com sabão e enxaguadas com volume abundante de água. Devido ao fato da baixa incidência das lesões esofagianas pela ingestão de alvejantes clorados caseiros, a decisão de realizar endoscopia deve estar baseada nos sinais clínicos do paciente e na necessidade de prognóstico. Os animais com disfagia, dispneia ou queimaduras esofagianas significativas devem ser submetidos à endoscopia avaliativa cuidadosa e tratados adequadamente para a presença de lesões corrosivas.

RISCOS DE INTOXICAÇÃO PROVENIENTES DE CASA OU DO JARDIM, PARA ANIMAIS DE COMPANHIA (CONTINUAÇÃO)

Tabela VII-C

Produtos de Limpeza e seus Sinais Clínicos — Antídotos e Tratamento (*continuação*)

Nome do Agente (Tipo Químico)	Sinais Clínicos	Antídotos/Tratamento/Cuidados Posteriores
Desinfetantes — óleos de pinho e aguarrás	A DL_{50} dos óleos de pinho variam de 1 a 2,5 mL/kg de peso vivo. Os felinos são mais sensíveis que outras espécies à intoxicação por óleos de pinho. Os óleos de pinho irritam diretamente as mucosas, produzindo eritema de orofaringe, boca e pele. A exposição ocular provoca blefaroespasmo acentuado, epífora, fotossensibilidade e eritema de conjuntiva e esclera. A ingestão resulta em náusea, ptialismo, vômito sanguinolento e dor abdominal. Os efeitos sistêmicos incluem fraqueza, depressão do sistema nervoso central, ataxia, hipotensão e depressão respiratória. A toxicidade pulmonar ocorre por aspiração durante ingestão ou vômito, ou mesmo devido à pneumonite química oriunda da absorção do óleo de pinho pelo trato gastrintestinal, com subsequente deposição no pulmão. Pode ocorrer mioglobinúria, necrose hepática e insuficiência renal aguda após ingestões acentuadas.	Deverá ocorrer imediata diluição com leite, clara de ovo ou água após a ingestão de desinfetantes à base de óleo de pinho. Devido ao início rápido da depressão e o perigo de pneumonia por aspiração, a indução de vômito geralmente está contraindicada; mesmo a lavagem gástrica com a instalação de sonda endotraqueal com manguito oferece riscos. A diluição deve ser seguida pela administração de carvão ativado e um catártico salino ou osmótico. Tornam-se cruciais os cuidados de suporte e sintomáticos, consistindo em manutenção da perfusão renal e do equilíbrio eletrolítico e acidobásico. Os animais com exposição cutânea devem ser lavados com sabão e depois enxaguados com volume abundante de água, tão cedo quanto possível após a exposição.
Acetona: Removedores de esmalte para unhas, vernizes, colas, cimento para borrachas	As ingestões maiores que 2-3 mL/kg podem ser tóxicas. Os sintomas de exposição incluem depressão do SNC, odor característico de acetona na respiração e concentração elevada de cetonas urinárias. Após exposição branda, pode ocorrer depressão do SNC, ataxia e vômito. Estupor e coma estão presentes nas exposições graves. Podem estar presentes hiperglicemia e cetonemia com acidose.	O tratamento eficaz consiste, basicamente, em cuidados sintomáticos e de suporte. As ingestões recentes, ou seja, até duas horas, em um paciente com o reflexo faríngeo intacto, podem ser favorecidas pelo vômito após a administração oral de carvão ativado e um catártico. A fluidoterapia intravenosa contendo bicarbonato de sódio ajudará a controlar a acidose associada.
Isopropanol: Álcool para polimento	A dose tóxica relatada para o isopropanol (álcool para polimento) é de 1 mL/kg, mas volumes menores como 0,5 mL/kg podem causar efeitos adversos. Os sinais de intoxicação se desenvolvem em 30-60 minutos, como ataxia, vômito, hematêmese e estupor, que progride para depressão respiratória e do SNC, hipotensão grave, acidose moderada, coma e perda dos reflexos dos tendões profundos nos casos graves.	O tratamento envolve a indução de vômito se a ingestão ocorreu em até duas horas e o animal está relativamente assintomático no momento da consulta. A administração de carvão ativado é de pouco valor. Deve ser administrada fluidoterapia intravenosa com bicarbonato de sódio e o estado acidobásico e eletrolítico controlado. A hemodiálise é eficaz para a reversão da hipotensão grave e coma que ocorrem com o isopropanol.
Metanol: Limpadores de para-brisas automotivos, produtos anticongelantes lacrados	A dose letal de metanol oral em caninos é de 4-8 mL/kg. Os sinais clínicos da intoxicação por metanol em caninos são depressão do SNC, ataxia, hipotermia, depressão respiratória e coma. Os caninos e felinos não desenvolvem cegueira em virtude da intoxicação por metanol.	O tratamento é similar àquele sugerido para a intoxicação por isopropanol.

ESPÉCIES CANINA E FELINA

APÊNDICE VIII

LEIGH A. LAMONT, KURT A. GRIMM E WILLIAM J. TRANQUILLI

MANEJO DA DOR

Tabela VIII-A

Dosagens Recomendadas e Indicações de Opioides Parenterais			
Opioide	*Dose/Via/Duração*	*Indicações*	*Comentários*
Butorfanol (injetável)	Cão: 0,2-0,4 mg/kg IM, IV ou SC Gato: 0,2-0,4 mg/kg; IM, IV ou SC Duração: 1-3 h	Dor branda a moderada	Sedação branda ou nula; depressão ventilatória leve.
Buprenorfina (injetável)	Cão: 0,005-0,03 mg/kg IM, IV ou SC Gato: 0,005-0,03 mg/kg IM, IV ou SC Duração: 3-8 h	Dor branda a moderada	Pode ser difícil antagonizá-la, início do efeito 15-30 minutos.
Morfina (injetável)	Cão: 0,2-1 mg/kg IM ou SC; 0,05-0,5 mg/kg IV Gato: 0,05-0,2 mg/kg IM ou SC Duração: 3-6 h	Dor moderada a grave	Sedação; depressão respiratória; bradicardia; náusea; hipotermia; disforia em gatos sem dor ou com alta dosagem; a administração IV rápida pode causar liberação de histamina.
Hidromorfona (injetável)	Cão: 0,05-0,2 mg/kg IM, IV ou SC Gato: 0,05-0,2 mg/kg IM, IV ou SC Duração: 3-6 h	Dor moderada a grave	Efeitos colaterais semelhantes aos observados com a morfina, porém com menos vômito e sem liberação de histamina. Pode estar associada a hipertermia em gatos.
Fentanil (injetável)	Cão: 0,002-0,01 mg/kg IV ou IM Gato: 0,001-0,005 mg/kg IV ou IM Duração: 1/2-2 h	Dor moderada a grave; para analgesia prolongada, é necessária a administração em VCI	Sedação; depressão respiratória; bradicardia; náusea; duração inadequada da analgesia após única aplicação IV em bolus ou após injeção IM.

VCI = velocidade constante de infusão.

Tabela VIII-B

Dosagens Recomendadas e Indicações de Opioides Receitáveis			
Opioide	*Dose/Via/Duração*	*Indicações*	*Comentários*
Codeína (comprimidos)	Cão: 1,0-2,0 mg/kg VO Gato: 0,1-1,0 mg/kg VO (ver Comentários) Duração: 4-8 h	Dor branda a moderada	Efeitos colaterais mínimos; quando associada com paracetamol, evitar em cães com doença hepática ou anemia com corpúsculos de Heinz; *não usar em combinação com paracetamol em gatos.*
Butorfanol (comprimidos)	Cão: 0,5-1,0 mg/kg VO Gato: 0,5-1,0 mg/kg VO Duração: 2-4 h	Dor branda a moderada	Sedação branda ou ausente; depressão ventilatória leve.
Tramadol (comprimidos de liberação imediata)	Cão: 2,0-5,0 mg/kg VO a cada 8-12 h	Dor branda a moderada	Sedação, ansiedade, retenção urinária.

Tabela VIII-C

Dosagens Recomendadas e Indicações de AINE Parenterais			
AINE	*Dose/Via/Duração*	*Indicações*	*Comentários*
Carprofeno (injetável)	Cão: 2,0-4,0 mg/kg IV, SC a cada 24 h Gato: 1,0 mg/kg SC (dose única)	Dor branda a moderada	Primariamente usado no pré-operatório antes de ser transformado em formulação oral; irritação GI e função renal alterada.
Meloxicam (injetável)	Cão: 0,2 mg/kg inicialmente IM, IV ou SC; 0,1 mg/kg SC posteriormente Gato: 0,1-0,2 mg/kg inicialmente IM, SC (dose única apenas por bula) Duração: 24 h	Dor branda a moderada	Pode ser misturado à dieta; irritação GI e função renal alterada.
Cetoprofeno (injetável)	Cão: 1,0-2,0 mg/kg inicialmente IM, IV ou SC; 0,5-1,0 mg SC posteriormente Gato: 1,0-2,0 mg/kg inicialmente IM, IV ou SC; 0,5-1,0 mg/kg SC posteriormente Duração: 24 h	Dor branda a moderada; aprovado no Canadá para cães e gatos e nos Estados Unidos para equinos	Irritação GI e função renal alterada. A dosagem não deve exceder cinco dias para cães e três dias para gatos.

GI = gastrintestinal; AINE = anti-inflamatórios não esteroides.

MANEJO DA DOR (CONTINUAÇÃO)

Tabela VIII-D

Dosagens Recomendadas e Indicações de AINE Receitáveis			
AINE	*Dose/Via/Duração*	*Indicações*	*Comentários*
Carprofeno (comprimidos e mastigáveis)	Cão: 4,4 mg/kg VO ou dividido a cada 12 h Gato: 1,0 mg/kg VO (dose única) Duração: 12-24 h	Dor branda a moderada; aprovado para uso em cães com osteoartrite ou dor pós-operatória	Toxicidade associada ao uso crônico em gatos por causa da meia-vida variável; pode causar irritação GI e função renal alterada em alguns pacientes.
Deracoxibe (comprimidos mastigáveis)	Cão (dor pós-operatória): 3,0-4,0 mg/kg VO a cada 24 h conforme necessário por sete dias Cão (osteoartrite): 1,0-2,0 mg/kg VO a cada 24 h para tratamentos acima de sete dias ou em longo prazo Duração: 24 h	Dor e inflamação associadas à osteoartrite. Dor pós-operatória e inflamações associadas à cirurgia ortopédica em cães com osteoartrite. Aprovado nos Estados Unidos para dor pós-operatória em cães com peso igual ou maior que 1,8 kg	Irritação GI e função renal alterada.
Firocoxibe (comprimidos mastigáveis)	Cão: 5,0 mg/kg VO a cada 24 h	Dor e inflamação associadas à osteoartrite e à dor pós-operatória	Irritação GI e função renal alterada.
Tepoxalina (comprimidos liofilizados rapidamente desintegrados por via oral)	Cão: 10-20 mg/kg inicialmente VO; 10 mg/kg posteriormente Gato: não usado Duração: 24 h	Dor e inflamação brandas a moderadas; aprovado para cães nos Estados Unidos; administração pré-operatória não recomendada	Irritação GI e função renal alterada. Inibidor simultâneo das enzimas 5-LO e COX; recomendam-se sete dias de abstinência do medicamento quando for trocar para outro AINE.
Etodolaco (comprimidos)	Cão: 10-15 mg/kg VO Gato: não usado Duração: 24 h	Dor branda a moderada; aprovado para cães nos Estados Unidos	Hipoproteinemia; irritação GI e função renal alterada. Associado à CCS em um pequeno número de cães.
Ácido acetilsalicílico (comprimidos)	Cão: 10-25 mg/kg VO Gato: 10-15 mg/kg VO Duração: 8-12 h para cães, 24-72 h para gatos	Dor e inflamação brandas a moderadas	Irritação GI e função renal alterada; mais provável em altas doses.
Meloxicam (solução oral líquida, comprimidos)	Cão: 0,2 mg/kg inicialmente VO; 0,1 mg/kg VO posteriormente Gato: 0,1-0,2 mg/kg inicialmente VO; 0,05-0,1 mg/kg VO posteriormente (reduzir à dose mínima efetiva) Duração: 24 h	Dor branda a moderada; aprovado para cães no Canadá	Irritação GI e função renal alterada; pode ser associado com alimentos. Meloxicam não deve ser administrado aos gatos por mais que cinco dias.
Cetoprofeno (comprimidos)	Cão: 1,0-2,0 mg/kg inicialmente VO; 0,5-1,0 mg/kg VO posteriormente Gato: 1,0-2,0 mg/kg inicialmente VO; 0,5-1,0 mg/kg VO posteriormente Duração 24 h	Dor branda a moderada; aprovado no Canadá para cães e gatos e nos Estados Unidos para equinos	Irritação GI e função renal alterada. Limitar a administração a cinco dias para cães e gatos.
Paracetamol (comprimidos e suspensão líquida oral)	Cão: 10-15 mg/kg VO Gato: contraindicado Duração (em cães): 8-12 h	Dor branda a moderada; baixa ação anti-inflamatória	Tóxico para gatos; geralmente administrado em associação com codeína para cães (ver Preparações analgésicas orais).

GI = gastrintestinal; AINE = anti-inflamatório não esteroide; CCS = ceratoconjuntivite seca.

Tabela VIII-E

Dosagens e Indicações de Medicamentos Selecionados Utilizados para o Tratamento da Dor Neuropática			
Medicamento	*Dose/Via*	*Duração (VO)*	*Comentários*
Cetamina (antagonista NMDA)	Cão: 0,1-1,0 mg/kg IM, SC ou VO Gato: 0,1-1,0 mg/kg IM ou SC	4-6 h 4-6 h	Baixas doses potencializam analgésicos pós-operatórios. Não utilizar na hipertensão intracraniana.
Amantadina (antagonista NMDA)	Cão: 3,0-5,0 mg/kg VO Gato: 3,0-5,0 mg/kg VO	24 h 24 h	Usado para potencializar ou prolongar analgesia. Eficaz quando combinada com um AINE para o controle da dor associada à osteoartrite em cães.
Amitriptilina (antidepressivo tricíclico)	Cão: 1,0 mg/kg VO Gato: 2,5-10 mg/gato VO	12-24 h 24 h	Usado para potencializar ou prolongar analgesia.
Gabapentina (anticonvulsivante)	Cão: 1,0-15 mg/kg VO Gato: 1,0-15 mg/kg VO	24 h 24 h	Usualmente associado a poucos efeitos colaterais. Tem revelado bons resultados em estudos com seres humanos e animais

Para selecionar e administrar adequadamente um analgésico adjuvante, o veterinário deve estar seguro da farmacologia clínica da droga. As seguintes informações sobre a droga são necessárias: (1) indicação aprovada, (2) contraindicação (p.ex., como analgésico) amplamente aceita na prática médica veterinária, (3) efeitos colaterais comuns e efeitos adversos potencialmente graves, (4) características farmacocinéticas e (5) manual de dosagem específica para dor.
NMDA = N-metil-D-aspartato.

ESPÉCIES CANINA E FELINA

APÊNDICE IX

MARK PAPICH

Formulário de Medicamentos para Consulta em 5 Minutos

Nome do Princípio Ativo (Comercial e Outros Nomes)	Farmacologia e Indicações	Efeitos Colaterais e Precauções	Informações de Dosagem e Comentários	Formulações	Dosagem (Exceto em Casos Indicados, a Dosagem é a Mesma para Cães e Gatos)
2-PAM	Ver Cloreto de pralidoxima.				
5-Fluoruracila (Fluorouracil)	Agente antineoplásico. Antimetabólico. A ação se dá pela inibição da síntese de ácidos nucleicos.	Provoca leucopenia leve e trombocitopenia. Toxicidade do SNC. Não utilizar em gatos.	Usada em protocolos antineoplásicos. Consultar protocolos de tratamento antineoplásico para dosagens e esquemas precisos.	Frasco com 50 mg/mL.	Cães: 150 mg/m^2 IV, uma vez por semana. Gatos: não utilizar.
6-Aminosalicílico, ácido	Ver Mesalamina, Olsalazina	-	-	-	-
6-Mercaptopurina (Purinethol)	Agente antineoplásico. Antimetabólito inibidor da síntese das purinas em células cancerosas.	Muitos dos efeitos colaterais comuns à terapia antineoplásica são possíveis - e muitos deles inevitáveis - inclusive supressão da medula óssea e anemia. Não usar em gatos.	Agente usado para tratamento de várias formas de câncer, inclusive leucemia e linfoma. Consultar o protocolo antineoplásico para o regime específico.	Comprimidos de 50 mg.	Cães: 50 mg/m^2 a cada 24h VO. Gatos: não usar.
Acepromazina (PromAce e diversas formulações genéricas)	Tranquilizante fenotiazínico. Inibe a ação da dopamina como um neurotransmissor. Usada para sedação e como pré-anestésico.	As fenotiazinas podem causar sedação como efeito colateral comum. Podem causar bloqueio α-adrenérgico. Em alguns indivíduos, produz efeitos colaterais extrapiramidais.	Geralmente é usada como pré-anestésico em associação com outras drogas. Nesses casos, a dose é, em geral, de 0,02-0,2 mg/kg, IM, SC ou IV.	Comprimidos com 5, 10 e 25 mg; injetável com 10 mg/mL.	Cães: 0,5-2,2 mg/kg VO a cada 6-8h, ou 0,02-0,1 mg/kg IV, IM, SC. Não exceder a dose total de 3 mg em cães. Gatos: 1,13-2,25 mg/kg VO a cada 6-8h, ou 0,02-0,1 mg/kg IM, SC, IV.
Acetato de medroxiprogesterona (Depo-Provera [injeção]; Provera [comprimidos])	Hormônio progestágeno. Derivado da acetoxiprogesterona. Em animais, uso como tratamento hormonal progestágeno para controle do ciclo estral. Também usado no tratamento de alguns problemas de comportamento e afecções dermatológicas (p.ex., urina em borrifo em gatos e alopecia).	Os efeitos adversos são: polifagia, polidipsia, supressão adrenal (gatos), maior risco de diabetes, piometra, diarreia e maior risco de neoplasia.	Os estudos clínicos em animais enfatizaram principalmente o uso na reprodução e os efeitos com o uso para problemas de comportamento. Em comparação com acetato de megestrol, o acetato de medroxiprogesterona pode causar menos efeitos colaterais.	Injeção de suspensão contendo 150, 400 mg/mL; comprimidos de 2,5, 5, 10 mg.	1,1-2,2 mg/kg q7d IM. Uso para problemas de comportamento: injeção SC de 10-20 mg/kg. Para doença prostática em cães, usar 3-5 mg/kg IM, SC.
Acetato de megestrol (Ovaban)	Hormônio progestágeno	O uso prolongado pode causar efeitos adversos, inclusive maior risco de neoplasia e diabetes.	Evitar o uso crônico. Não deve ser usado para controle de problemas de comportamento ou em tratamentos dermatológicos.	Comprimidos de 5 mg.	Cadelas - proestro: 2 mg/kg a cada 24h VO durante 8 dias; anestro: 0,5 mg/kg a cada 24h VO durante 30 dias; comportamento: 2-4 mg/kg a cada 24h durante 8 dias (reduzir a dose para manutenção). Gatas - terapia dermatológica ou urina em borrifo: 2,5-5 mg/gato a cada 24h VO durante uma semana; em seguida, reduzir para 5 mg 1 ou 2×/semana; supressão do estro: 5 mg/gata/dia durante 3 dias; em seguida, 2,5-5 mg 1×/semana durante 10 semanas.

CONSULTA VETERINÁRIA EM 5 MINUTOS

Formulário de Medicamentos para Consulta em 5 Minutos

Nome do Princípio Ativo (Comercial e Outros Nomes)	Farmacologia e Indicações	Efeitos Colaterais e Precauções	Informações de Dosagem e Comentários	Formulações	Dosagem (Exceto em Casos Indicados, a Dosagem é a Mesma para Cães e Gatos)
Acetato de metilprednisolona (Depo-Medrol)	Forma de depósito de metilprednisolona. Absorção lenta a partir do local da injeção IM, promovendo efeitos glicocorticoides durante 3-4 semanas em alguns animais. Agente usado para terapia intralesional, terapia intra-articular e problemas inflamatórios.	Com o uso de corticosteroides, muitos efeitos adversos são possíveis. Em gatos, problemas cardiovasculares (insuficiência cardíaca congestiva) foram associados ao uso desses agentes. A longo prazo, o uso crônico de acetato de metilprednisolona pode causar efeitos adversos.	Deve-se avaliar cuidadosamente o uso do acetato de metilprednisolona, porque uma injeção causará efeitos glicocorticoides que persistirão por vários dias e até semanas.	Suspensão contendo 20 ou 40 mg/mL para injeção.	Cães: 1 mg/kg (ou 20-40 mg/cão) IM a cada 1-3 semanas. Gatos: 10-20 mg/gato IM a cada 1-3 semanas.
Acetilcisteína (Mucomyst)	Diminui a viscosidade das secreções. Usada como agente mucolítico nos olhos e em soluções para nebulização bronquial. Como é doadora de grupo sulfidrila, é empregada como antídoto para intoxicações (p. ex.: intoxicação por paracetamol em gatos).	Pode causar sensibilização em casos de administração prolongada. Pode reagir com certos materiais dos equipamentos nebulizantes.	Disponível como agente para reduzir a viscosidade das secreções respiratórias, mas é mais comumente usada como tratamento para intoxicações.	Solução a 20%.	Antídoto: 140 mg/kg (dose de ataque) e depois 70 mg/kg IV a cada 4h ou 5 doses VO. Olho: solução tópica 2% a cada 2h.
Ácido acetilsalicílico (diversas formulações genéricas e comerciais [Bufferin, Ascriptin])	Droga anti-inflamatória não esteroidal (AINE). Considera-se a ação anti-inflamatória causada pela inibição das prostaglandinas. Usada como droga analgésica, anti-inflamatória e antiplaquetária.	Margem terapêutica estreita. Altas doses frequentemente causam vômito. Outros efeitos colaterais do sistema GI podem incluir ulceração e sangramento. Os gatos são sensíveis à intoxicação aos salicilatos em virtude da baixa capacidade de depuração. Usar cautelosamente em pacientes com coagulopatias por causa da inibição plaquetária.	As doses analgésica e anti-inflamatória são, principalmente, empíricas. As doses antiplaquetárias são menores por causa dos efeitos prolongados do ácido acetilsalicílico nas plaquetas. Na administração de ácido acetilsalicílico, o fornecimento de formulações tamponadas ou a mistura aos alimentos diminui a irritação estomacal. As formulações entéricas protegidas não são recomendadas para cães e gatos.	Comprimidos com 81 e 325 mg.	Analgesia moderada: (cães) 10 mg/kg a cada 12h. Anti-inflamatório: Cães: 20-25 mg/kg a cada 12h. Gatos: 10-20 mg/kg a cada 48h. Antiplaquetário: Cães: 5-10 mg/kg a cada 8-24h. Gatos: 81 mg a cada 48-72h.
Ácido valproico (Depakene [ácido valproico]; Depakote [divalproex] [Epival é marca canadense])	Anticonvulsivante. Uso (geralmente em combinação com fenobarbital) no tratamento das convulsões refratárias em animais. A ação é desconhecida, mas pode aumentar as concentrações de GABA no SNC.	Não foram relatados efeitos adversos em animais; no entanto, foi relatada a ocorrência de insuficiência hepática em humanos. Pode-se observar sedação em alguns animais. Não usar em fêmeas prenhes. Interações farmacológicas: pode causar sangramento, se usado com medicamentos inibidores das plaquetas.	Ácido valproico está listado nesta tabela com divalproex. Divalproex se compõe de ácido valproico e valproato sódico. Doses orais equivalentes de divalproex sódico e de ácido valproico fornecem quantidades equivalentes do íon valproato.	Comprimidos de 125, 250, 500 mg (Depakote); cápsulas de 250 mg; xarope contendo 50 mg/mL (Depakene).	Cães: 50-250 mg/cão (dependendo do porte) a cada 8h VO. Para formulações de liberação retardada, começar com 250 mg/cão a cada 12h VO e aumentar para 500 mg/cão a cada 12h, se houver necessidade. Gatos: não há dose estabelecida.
ACTH	Ver Corticotropina.	-	-	-	-
Adequan	Ver Glicosaminoglicano polissulfatado (PSGAG).	-	-	-	-

ESPÉCIES CANINA E FELINA

Formulário de Medicamentos para Consulta em 5 Minutos					
Nome do Princípio Ativo (Comercial e Outros Nomes)	Farmacologia e Indicações	Efeitos Colaterais e Precauções	Informações de Dosagem e Comentários	Formulações	Dosagem (Exceto em Casos Indicados, a Dosagem é a Mesma para Cães e Gatos)
Albendazol (Valbazen)	Droga antiparasitária benzimidazólica. Inibe a absorção de glicose pelos parasitos.	Nas doses aprovadas existe grande margem de segurança. Os efeitos colaterais podem incluir anorexia, letargia e toxicidade para a medula óssea. Em altas doses tem sido associado com toxicidade para a medula óssea. Os efeitos colaterais podem ocorrer quando é administrado por mais de cinco dias.	Utilizado principalmente como anti-helmíntico, mas também tem demonstrado eficiência contra giardíase.	Suspensão com 113,6 mg/mL; creme com 300 mg/mL.	25-50 mg/kg VO a cada 12h por 3 dias. Para giardíase, usar 25 mg/kg a cada 12h por 2 dias.
Albuterol (Proventil, Ventolin)	Agonista de receptores β_2-adrenérgicos. Broncodilatador. Estimula os receptores β_2 a relaxarem a musculatura lisa bronquial. Também pode inibir a liberação de mediadores inflamatórios, especialmente os mastócitos.	Em altas doses pode causar estimulação excessiva dos receptores β-adrenérgicos (taquicardia, tremores). Podem ocorrer arritmias em doses tóxicas. Evitar o uso em animais prenhes.	As doses são principalmente extrapoladas da dose usada para seres humanos. Estudos bem controlados sobre sua eficácia em medicina veterinária não estão disponíveis. O início da ação é de 15-30 minutos; sua duração é de até 8 horas.	Comprimidos com 2, 4 e 5 mg; xarope com 2 mg/5 mL.	20-50 mcg/kg a cada 6-8h ao dia ou até o máximo de 100 mcg/kg a cada 6h.
Alopurinol (Lopurin, Zyloprim)	Diminui a produção de ácido úrico por meio da inibição das enzimas responsáveis pela sua síntese. Também usado na leishmaniose.	Pode causar reações cutâneas (hipersensibilidade).	Utilizado em seres humanos principalmente para o tratamento de gota. Usado em animais para diminuir a formação de urólitos de ácido úrico.	Comprimidos com 100 e 300 mg.	10 mg/kg a cada 8h, depois reduzir para 10 mg/kg VO a cada 24h. Para leishmaniose, usar 10 mg/kg VO a cada 12h por pelo menos quatro meses.
Alprazolam (Xanax)	Tranquilizante benzodiazepínico.	Sedação excessiva; excitação paradoxal.	Geralmente combinado com anestésicos e outros sedativos.	Comprimidos com 0,25; 0,5; 1 e 2 mg.	Cães: 0,025-0,1 mg/kg VO a cada 8h. Gatos: 0,125 mg por animal VO, a cada 8h.
Alumínio, gel de carbonato (Basaljel)	Antiácido (neutraliza acidez estomacal) e aglutinante de fosfato no intestino.	Geralmente seguro. Pode interagir com outras drogas administradas por via oral.	Doses antiácidas são indicadas para neutralizar a acidez estomacal, porém, a duração da supressão ácida é curta.	Cápsulas (equivalente a 500 mg de hidróxido de alumínio).	10-30 mg/kg VO a cada 8h (com alimentos).
Alumínio, gel de hidróxido (Amphojel)	Antiácido (neutraliza acidez estomacal) e aglutinante de fosfato no intestino.	Geralmente seguro. Pode interagir com outras drogas administradas por via oral.	Doses antiácidas são indicadas para neutralizar a acidez estomacal, porém, a duração da supressão ácida é curta.	Suspensão oral com 64 mg/mL; comprimidos com 600 mg.	10-30 mg/kg VO a cada 8h (com alimentos).
Amicacina (Amiglyde-V [veterinário] e Amikin [humano])	Droga antibacteriana da classe dos aminoglicosídeos (inibe a síntese de proteínas). O mecanismo é similar ao dos outros aminoglicosídeos (ver Gentamicina, sulfato), mas pode ser mais ativa que gentamicina.	Pode causar nefrotoxicidade em altas doses ou em terapias prolongadas. Também pode provocar ototoxicidade e vestibulotoxicidade.	Doses diárias são indicadas para maximizar a relação pico: CIM. Considerar a necessidade de monitoração em terapia prolongada.	Injetável com 50 e 250 mg/mL.	Cães: 15-30 mg/kg IV, IM, SC a cada 24h. Gatos: 10-14 mg/kg IV, IM, SC a cada 24h.
Aminopentamida (Centrine)	Droga antidiarreica. Anticolinérgica (bloqueia a acetilcolina nas sinapses parassimpáticas).	Usar com cuidado em animais com estase GI ou quando as drogas anticolinérgicas são contraindicadas (p. ex., glaucoma).	As dosagens indicadas são baseadas nas recomendações do fabricante.	Comprimidos com 0,2 mg; injetável com 0,5 mg/mL.	Cães: 0,01-0,03 mg/kg IM, SC, VO a cada 8-12h. Gatos: 0,1 mg/animal IM, SC, VO a cada 8-12h.

1365

Nome do Princípio Ativo (Comercial e Outros Nomes)	Farmacologia e Indicações	Efeitos Colaterais e Precauções	Informações de Dosagem e Comentários	Formulações	Dosagem (Exceto em Casos Indicados, a Dosagem é a Mesma para Cães e Gatos)
Amiodarona (Cordarone)	Agente antiarrítmico classe III com propriedades bloqueadoras de canais de potássio; indicada para arritmias atriais e ventriculares refratárias graves.	O efeito mais comum em cães é a redução do apetite. Também de importância é o intervalo QT aumentado. Outros efeitos adversos incluem: bradicardia, insuficiência cardíaca crônica (ICCr), hipotensão, bloqueio atrioventricular (BAV), disfunção tireoidiana, fibrose pulmonar e hepatotoxicidade. Toxicidade cardíaca aguda foi observada em cães.	Usada para taquicardia ventricular instável hemodinamicamente e recidivante; demora semanas para atingir níveis terapêuticos. Tipicamente, doses de ataque são administradas, seguidas pela dose de manutenção. Doses seguras para aplicações injetáveis não foram estabelecidas.	Comprimidos com 200 mg; injetável com 50 mg/mL.	Cães: início com 10-15 mg/kg VO a cada 12h por uma semana, depois 5-7 mg/kg a cada 12h por duas semanas. Doses de manutenção são de 7,5 mg/kg VO a cada 24h. Gatos: não foi estabelecida dose segura.
Amitraz (Mitaban)	Droga antiparasitária para ectoparasitos. Usada no tratamento de ácaros, incluindo *Demodex*. Inibe a monoaminoxidase nos ácaros.	Causa sedação em cães (α_2-agonista), podendo ser revertida pela ioimbina ou atipamezol. Quando são utilizadas altas doses, outros efeitos colaterais relatados incluem prurido, poliúria e polidipsia (PU/PD), bradicardia, hipotermia, hiperglicemia e convulsões (raramente).	Inicialmente, deveria ser utilizada a dosagem indicada pelo fabricante. Entretanto, nos casos refratários, essa dose tem sido excedida para produzir eficácia aumentada.	Banhos concentrados com 10,6 mL (19,9%).	Usar 10,6 mL para 7,5 litros de água (solução a 0,025%). Utilizar 3-6 tratamentos tópicos, com intervalos de 14 dias. Para casos refratários, essa dose tem sido excedida para produzir eficácia aumentada. As dosagens usadas incluem concentrações a 0,025, 0,05 e 0,1%, aplicadas duas vezes por semana e uma solução a 0,125% aplicada em metade do corpo, diariamente, por quatro semanas a cinco meses.
Amitriptilina, cloridrato (Elavil)	Droga antidepressiva tricíclica. Inibe a apreensão de serotonina e outros transmissores nas terminações dos nervos pré-sinápticos. Usada em animais para tratar diversos distúrbios comportamentais, como ansiedade. Utilizada em gatos para o tratamento de cistite idiopática crônica.	Múltiplos efeitos colaterais estão associados com antidepressivos tricíclicos, como os efeitos antimuscarínicos (boca seca, frequência cardíaca aumentada) e anti-histamínicos (sedação). Doses altas podem produzir cardiotoxicidade e risco de morte. Em felinos podem ocorrer sedação, redução dos hábitos higiênicos e ganho de peso.	As dosagens são empíricas. Não existem provas de eficácia disponíveis para animais. Há evidências do sucesso no tratamento de cistite idiopática em gatos. A clomipramina é preferida no tratamento de distúrbios comportamentais.	Comprimidos com 10, 25, 50, 75, 100 e 150 mg; injetável com 10 mg/mL.	Cães: 1-2 mg/kg VO a cada 12-24h. Gatos: 5-10 mg/gato/dia VO; na cistite: 2 mg/kg/dia (2,5-7,5 mg/gato/dia).
Amlodipina, besilato (Norvasc)	Droga bloqueadora dos canais de cálcio, pertencente à classe da diidropiridina. Diminui o afluxo de cálcio na musculatura lisa cardíaca e vascular. Possui maior efeito como vasodilatadora. Em cães e gatos, é útil no tratamento da hipertensão.	Pode causar hipotensão e bradicardia. Usar com cautela quando associada com outros vasodilatadores.	Em felinos, a eficácia foi obtida com a dose de 0,625 mg/gato uma vez ao dia. Se o gato for de maior tamanho (> 4,5 kg) ou refratário, aumentar a dose (J Vet Int Med 12:157-162, 1998).	Comprimidos com 2,5, 5 e 10 mg.	Cães: 2,5 mg/cão ou 0,1 mg/kg uma vez ao dia, VO. Gatos: 0,625 mg/gato VO, inicialmente, uma vez ao dia, aumentando, se necessário, para 1,25 mg/gato (média de 0,18 mg/kg).
Amônia, cloreto (formulação genérica)	Acidificante urinário.	Não usar em pacientes com acidose sistêmica. Pode não ser palatável quando adicionado a algum alimento para animais.	As dosagens são estipuladas para maximizar o efeito acidificante na urina.	Disponível como cristais.	Cães: 100 mg/kg VO a cada 12h. Gatos: 800 mg/gato (aproximadamente 1/3 a 1/4 de uma colher das de sopa) misturado ao alimento diário.

ESPÉCIES CANINA E FELINA

Formulário de Medicamentos para Consulta em 5 Minutos					
Nome do Princípio Ativo (Comercial e Outros Nomes)	*Farmacologia e Indicações*	*Efeitos Colaterais e Precauções*	*Informações de Dosagem e Comentários*	*Formulações*	*Dosagem (Exceto em Casos Indicados, a Dosagem é a Mesma para Cães e Gatos)*
Amoxicilina (Amoxi-Tabs, Biomox e outras marcas [Omnipen, Principen e Totacilin são especialidades humanas])	Antibiótico β-lactâmico. Inibe a síntese das células da parede da bactéria. Geralmente apresenta amplo espectro de ação. Usada em diversas infecções em todas as espécies.	Em geral é bem tolerada. É possível a ocorrência de reações alérgicas. Pode ocorrer diarreia com o uso oral.	As dosagens indicadas variam de acordo com a suscetibilidade bacteriana e a localização da infecção. Geralmente são necessárias doses mais altas e frequentes para os casos de infecções por Gram-negativos.	Comprimidos com 50, 100, 150, 200 e 400 mg; cápsulas com 250 e 500 mg; suspensão oral com 50 mg/mL (formulações humanas).	6,6-20 mg/kg VO a cada 8-12 horas.
Amoxicilina + clavulanato de potássio (Clavamox)	Antibiótico β-lactâmico + inibidor de β-lactamase (clavulanato/ácido clavulânico).	Similar à amoxicilina.	Similar à amoxicilina.	Comprimidos com 62,5, 125, 250 e 375 mg; suspensão com 62,5 mg/mL.	Cães: 12,5-25 mg/kg VO a cada 12h. Gatos: 62,5 mg/gato VO a cada 12h. Considerar a administração dessas doses a cada oito horas em caso de infecções por Gram-negativos.
Ampicilina (Omnipen, Principen, outros [formulações humanas])	Antibiótico β-lactâmico. Inibe a síntese da parede das células da bactéria.	Usar com cautela em animais alérgicos às drogas similares à penicilina.	As dosagens indicadas variam de acordo com a suscetibilidade bacteriana. Em comparação com a amoxicilina, possui 50% a menos de absorção quando administrada por via oral. Geralmente são necessárias doses mais altas e frequentes para os casos de infecções por Gram-negativos.	Comprimidos com 250 e 500 mg; frascos com 125, 250 e 500 mg de ampicilina sódica triidratada; injetável, frascos com 10 e 25 g.	Ampicilina sódica: 10-20 mg/kg IV, IM, SC a cada 6-8h ou 20-40 mg/kg VO a cada 8h. Ampicilina tri-hidratada: Cães: 10-50 mg/kg IM, SC a cada 12-24h. Gatos: 10-20 mg/kg IM, SC a cada 12-24h.
Ampicilina + Sulbactam (Unasyn)	Ampicilina mais um inibidor de β-lactamase (sulbactam). O sulbactam possui atividade similar à do clavulanato.	Similar à ampicilina.	Similar à amoxicilina + clavulanato.	Combinação injetável de 2:1. Frascos com 1, 5 e 3 g.	10-20 mg/kg IV, IM a cada 8h.
Ampicilina tri-hidratada (Polyflex)	Antibiótico β-lactâmico. Inibe a síntese da parede das células da bactéria.	Usar com cautela em animais alérgicos às drogas similares à penicilina.	A absorção é lenta e pode não ser suficiente para infecções agudas graves.	Injetável, frascos com 10 e 25 mg.	Cães: 10-50 mg/kg IM, SC a cada 12-24h. Gatos: 10-20 mg/kg IM, SC a cada 12-24h.
Anfotericina B (Fungizone)	Droga antifúngica. Fungicida para fungos sistêmicos, que causa danos à membrana do microrganismo.	Causa nefrotoxicidade relacionada com a dose utilizada. Também provoca febre, flebite e tremores.	Administrar por via IV, na forma de infusão lenta, diluída em fluidos e com rigoroso monitoramento da função renal. No momento do preparo da solução IV, não misturar com soluções eletrolíticas (usar glicose 5%, por exemplo); administrar fluidos de NaCl antes da terapia.	Injetável, frascos com 50 mg.	0,5 mg/kg IV a cada 48h (infusão lenta); para uma dose cumulativa, podem-se usar doses de 4-8 mg/kg.
Anfotericina B, formulação lipossomal (ABLC, Abelcet)	As mesmas indicações para a anfotericina B convencional. As formulações lipossomais podem ser usadas em altas doses, já que a margem de segurança é maior. O custo é muito maior que das formulações convencionais.	A toxicidade renal é um efeito relacionado à dosagem.	Altas doses podem ser utilizadas quando comparada à anfotericna B convencional. Diluir em solução aquosa de glicose 5% até a concentração de 1 mg/mL e administrar, por via IV, em 1-2 horas.	100 mg/20 mL em formulação lipídica.	Cães: 2-3 mg/kg IV três vezes por semana, por 9-12 tratamentos, até a dose acumulada de 24-27 mg/kg. Gatos: 1 mg/kg IV três vezes por semana, por 12 tratamentos.
Antiácidos	Ver Alumínio, gel de hidróxido; Magnésio, hidróxido; Cálcio, carbonato.	-	-	-	-

Consulta Veterinária em 5 Minutos

			Formulário de Medicamentos para Consulta em 5 Minutos		
Nome do Princípio Ativo (Comercial e Outros Nomes)	Farmacologia e Indicações	Efeitos Colaterais e Precauções	Informações de Dosagem e Comentários	Formulações	Dosagem (Exceto em Casos Indicados, a Dosagem é a Mesma para Cães e Gatos)
Apomorfina, cloridrato (formulação genérica)	Droga emética. Provoca vômito por liberação de dopamina ou efeitos diretos na zona do gatilho dos quimiorreceptores.	Produz vômito antes que ocorram efeitos colaterais graves. Usar com cautela em gatos com suspeita de sensibilidade aos opiáceos.	Consultar o Centro de Informações sobre Intoxicações ou o farmacêutico local. Não é tão eficaz em gatos como nos cães.	Comprimidos com 6 mg.	0,03-0,05 mg/kg IV, IM; 0,1 mg/kg SC; ou solução 0,25 mg para instilação oftálmica (dissolver o comprimido de 6 mg em 1-2 mL de salina).
Ascórbico, ácido (Vitamina C)	Vitamina. Utilizada como acidificante.	Toxicidade apenas em doses muito altas.	Principalmente usada como suplemento nutricional, mas doses altas têm sido utilizadas para o tratamento de determinadas doenças.	Formulações variadas, incluindo o ascorbato de sódio 250 mg/mL.	100-500 mg/animal/dia (dieta suplementar) ou 100 mg/animal a cada 8h (acidificação urinária).
Atenolol (Tenormin)	Bloqueador β-adrenérgico. Relativamente seletivo para receptores β_1. Usado principalmente como antiarrítmico ou para outras condições cardiovasculares para reduzir a taxa sinusal.	Bradicardia e bloqueio cardíaco são possíveis. Pode produzir broncoespasmo em pacientes sensíveis.	As precauções de dosagem são similares às outras drogas β-bloqueadoras. O atenolol é descrito como menos afetado pelas alterações do metabolismo hepático que outros β-bloqueadores.	Comprimidos com 25, 50 e 100 mg; suspensão oral com 25 mg/mL.	Cães: 6,25-12,5 mg/cão a cada 12h (ou 0,25-1 mg/kg a cada 12-24h), VO. Gatos: 6,25-12,5 mg/gato VO a cada 12h.
Atipamezol (Antisedan)	Antagonista α_2. Usado para reverter agonistas α_2, como a dexmedetomidina e xilazina.	Seguro. Pode causar excitação inicial em alguns animais imediatamente após a reversão.	Quando utilizado para reverter a dexmedetomidina, usar o mesmo volume da própria dexmedetomidina.	Injetável com 5 mg/kg.	Injetar o mesmo volume aplicado de dexmedetomidina. Variação das doses = 0,32 mg/kg para pequenos animais a 0,14 mg/kg para cães de grande porte.
Ativado, carvão	Ver Carvão ativado.	-	-	-	
Atracúrio (Tracrium)	Agente bloqueador neuromuscular (não despolarizante). Compete com a acetilcolina na terminação final da placa nervosa. Usada principalmente durante a anestesia ou outras condições em que é necessário inibir as contrações musculares.	Produz depressão e paralisia respiratória. As drogas bloqueadoras neuromusculares não possuem efeitos na analgesia.	Administrar apenas em situações em que o controle cuidadoso da respiração é possível. As dosagens podem necessitar de individualização para obter melhor efeito. Não misturar com soluções alcalinizantes ou solução de Ringer lactato.	Injetável com 10 mg/mL.	0,2 mg/kg IV inicialmente; depois 0,15 mg/kg a cada 30 minutos (ou infusão IV a 4-9 mcg/kg/min).
Atropina (diversas formulações genéricas)	Agente anticolinérgico (bloqueia o efeito da acetilcolina no receptor muscarínico), parassimpatolítico. Usada principalmente como adjuvante da anestesia ou de outros procedimentos para aumentar a frequência cardíaca e reduzir as secreções respiratória e gastrintestinal. Também usada como antídoto para a intoxicação por organofosforados.	Agente anticolinérgico potente. Não usar em pacientes com glaucoma, íleo paralítico, gastroparesia ou taquicardia. Os efeitos colaterais da terapia incluem xerostomia, íleo, constipação, taquicardia, retenção de urina.	Usada comumente como adjuvante da anestesia ou de outros procedimentos. Não misturar com soluções alcalinas.	Injetável com 400, 500 e 540 mcg/mL; injetável com 15 mg/mL.	0,02-0,04 mg/kg IV, IM, SC a cada 6-8h; 0,2-0,5 mg/kg (se necessário) para intoxicações por organofosforados e carbamatos.

ESPÉCIES CANINA E FELINA

1369

		Formulário de Medicamentos para Consulta em 5 Minutos			
Nome do Princípio Ativo (Comercial e Outros Nomes)	Farmacologia e Indicações	Efeitos Colaterais e Precauções	Informações de Dosagem e Comentários	Formulações	Dosagem (Exceto em Casos Indicados, a Dosagem é a Mesma para Cães e Gatos)
Azatioprina (Imuran)	Droga imunossupressiva do grupo das tiopurinas. Atua por inibição da função do linfócito T. Essa droga é metabolizada em 6-mercaptopurina, que responde pelos efeitos imunossupressores. Utilizada para tratar diversas enfermidades autoimunes.	A principal preocupação é a supressão da medula óssea. Particularmente, os gatos são sensíveis. Há alguma correlação entre o desenvolvimento de pancreatite e a administração conjunta com corticosteroides.	Normalmente usada em combinação com outras drogas imunossupressivas (como os corticosteroides) para tratar doenças imunomediadas. As doses de 2,2 mg/kg, em gatos, produzem intoxicação.	Comprimidos com 50 mg; injetável com 10 mg/mL.	Cães: 2 mg/kg VO a cada 24h inicialmente, depois 0,5-1,0 mg/kg a cada 48h. Gatos (usar com cautela): 0,3 mg/kg VO a cada 24h inicialmente, depois a cada 48h, com cuidadoso monitoramento.
Azitromicina (Zithromax)	Antibiótico do grupo das azalidas. Mecanismo de ação similar aos macrolídeos (eritromicina), inibindo a síntese proteica bacteriana por meio da inibição ribossomal. O espectro é voltado para Gram-positivos.	O vômito é mais provável de ocorrer em altas doses. Pode ocorrer diarreia em alguns pacientes.	A azitromicina pode ser mais bem tolerada que a eritromicina. A diferença principal de outros antibióticos é a alta concentração intracelular alcançada.	Cápsulas com 250 mg; comprimidos com 250 e 600 mg; suspensão oral com 100 ou 200 mg/5 mL; frascos de solução injetável com 500 mg.	Cães: 5-10 mg/kg VO diariamente por 5-7 dias, depois intervalando para cada 48h. Gatos: 5-10 mg/kg VO diariamente por 7 dias, depois intervalando para cada 48h.
AZT (Azidotimidina)	Ver Zidovudina.	-	-	-	-
Azul de metileno a 0,1% (genérico, também chamado novo azul de metileno)	Antídoto para intoxicação. Uso no tratamento da metemoglobinemia. Azul de metileno funciona como agente redutor, reduzindo metemoglobina em hemoglobina.	Azul de metileno pode causar anemia com corpos de Heinz em gatos, mas seu uso é seguro nas doses terapêuticas listadas nesta tabela.	A comparação dos efeitos quanto à intoxicação apenas foi realizada em estudos experimentais.	Solução a 1% (10 mg/mL).	1,5 mg/kg IV 1 vez; administrar lentamente.
Bactrim (sulfametoxazol + trimetoprima)	Ver Trimetoprima-combinações de sulfonamidas.	-	-	-	-
BAL (antilevisita britânica)	Ver Dimercaprol.	-	-	-	-
Benazepril (Lotensin)	Inibidor da enzima conversora da angiotensina (ECA). Usada para hipertensão e insuficiência cardíaca. A ação é similar ao enalapril e captopril.	Similar aos do enalapril e captopril.	A dosagem é baseada no uso autorizado em cães na Europa e no Canadá. Monitorar a função renal e os eletrólitos 3-7 dias após o início da terapia e periodicamente durante sua manutenção.	Comprimidos de 5, 10, 20 e 40 mg.	Cães: 0,25-0,5 mg/kg VO a cada 24h. Gatos (hipertensão sistêmica e doença renal): 0,5-1 mg/kg VO a cada 24h, ou 2,5 mg/gato VO diariamente, até o máximo de 5 mg/gato VO diariamente.
Betametasona (Celestone)	Corticosteroide potente e de longa ação. Os efeitos anti-inflamatórios e imunossupressores são, aproximadamente, 30x mais evidentes que os do cortisol. Os efeitos anti-inflamatórios ocorrem por inibição das células inflamatórias e supressão da expressão dos mediadores inflamatórios. É usada para o tratamento das doenças inflamatórias e imunomediadas.	Os efeitos colaterais dos corticosteroides são muitos e incluem polifagia, poliúria/polidipsia e supressão do eixo hipotálamo-hipófise-adrenal (HHA). Os efeitos adversos incluem ulceração gastrintestinal, hepatopatia, diabetes, hiperlipidemia, redução do hormônio tireoidiano, diminuição da síntese proteica, cicatrização de feridas e imunossupressão.	Os efeitos anti-inflamatórios são observados na dosagem e 0,1-0,2 mg/kg e os efeitos imunossupressores, na dosagem de 0,2-0,5 mg/kg.	Comprimidos com 600 mcg (0,6 mg); injetável, na forma de fosfato sódico, com 3 mg/mL.	Efeitos anti-inflamatórios: 0,1-0,2 mg/kg VO a cada 12-24h. Efeitos imunossupressores: 0,2-0,5 mg/kg VO a cada 12-24h.

Formulário de Medicamentos para Consulta em 5 Minutos

Nome do Princípio Ativo (Comercial e Outros Nomes)	Farmacologia e Indicações	Efeitos Colaterais e Precauções	Informações de Dosagem e Comentários	Formulações	Dosagem (Exceto em Casos Indicados, a Dosagem é a Mesma para Cães e Gatos)
Betanecol, cloreto	Agonista colinérgico, muscarínico. Parassimpatomimético. Estimula a motilidade gástrica e intestinal, mas usada principalmente para aumentar a contração da bexiga.	Doses altas de agonistas colinérgicos aumentarão a motilidade do trato GI, causando desconforto abdominal e diarreia. Pode provocar depressão circulatória em animais sensíveis.	Administrar injeções SC apenas, *nunca* IV. As doses são oriundas da extrapolação de doses humanas ou por métodos empíricos. Não há estudos de eficácia bem controlados disponíveis em pacientes veterinários.	Não se apresenta mais disponível comercialmente. Entretanto, pode ser obtido em farmácias de manipulação.	Cães: 5-15 mg/cão VO a cada 8h. Gatos: 1,25-5 mg/gato VO a cada 8h.
Bicarbonato de sódio (NaHCO₃) (genérico, Soda Mint)	Agente alcalinizante. Antiácido. Uso no tratamento da acidose sistêmica, ou para alcalinização da urina. Aumenta as concentrações plasmáticas e urinárias de bicarbonato.	Os efeitos adversos são atribuídos à atividade alcalinizante. Interações farmacológicas: quando administrado VO, pode ocorrer interação para diminuição da absorção de outros medicamentos (uma lista parcial incluiria agentes anticolinérgicos, cetoconazol, fluoroquinolonas, tetraciclinas).	Quando esse agente for usado para acidose sistêmica, as doses devem ser ajustadas com base nas determinações dos gases sanguíneos, ou na avaliação da acidose. As doses variam, dependendo do problema subjacente (ver seção sobre doses). Notar que: solução a 8,5% = 1 mEq/mL de NaHCO₃.	Comprimidos de 325, 520, 650 mg; injeção de várias concentrações (4,2-8,4%); a solução a 8,4% é equivalente a 1 mEq/mL.	Acidose: 0,5-1 mEq/kg IV. Insuficiência renal: 10 mg/kg a cada 8-12h VO. Alcalinização da urina: 50 mg/kg a cada 8-12h VO (1 col. chá pesa aproximadamente 2 g). Antiácido: 2-5 g; misturar com o alimento ou na água.
Bisacodil (Dulcolax)	Laxante/catártico. Atua por estimulação local da motilidade GI, mais provavelmente por irritação do intestino delgado. Utilizado principalmente como laxante ou para procedimentos em que há necessidade de evacuação intestinal.	Evitar o uso em pacientes com doença renal. Evitar a superdosagem.	Disponível como comprimidos isentos de prescrição. As doses são oriundas da extrapolação de doses humanas ou por métodos empíricos. Não há estudos de eficácia bem controlados disponíveis em pacientes veterinários. O início da ação ocorre após 1 hora.	Comprimidos com 5 mg.	5 mg/animal VO a cada 24h.
Bismuto, subsalicilato (Pepto-Bismol)	Agente antidiarreico e protetor GI. A ação antiprostaglandina do salicilato pode ser benéfica para a enterite. O bismuto é eficaz no tratamento de infecções causadas por bactérias do grupo das espiroquetas (gastrite por *Helicobacter*).	Os efeitos adversos não são comuns; entretanto, o salicilato é absorvido sistematicamente e a superdosagem deve ser evitada em animais que não toleram salicilatos (como cães e gatos sensíveis ao ácido acetilsalicílico). Os proprietários devem ser alertados que o bismuto descolore as fezes.	Disponível como comprimidos isentos de prescrição. As doses são oriundas da extrapolação de doses humanas ou por métodos empíricos. Não há estudos de eficácia bem controlados disponíveis em pacientes veterinários.	Suspensão oral: 262 mg/15 mL ou 525 mg/mL em formulação concentrada; comprimidos com 262 mg.	1-3 mL/kg/dia (em doses divididas) VO.
Bleomicina (Blenoxane)	Agente antibiótico antineoplásico. Usado no tratamento de diversos sarcomas e carcinomas. O mecanismo exato de ação é desconhecido, mas pode se ligar ao DNA e evitar a síntese.	Causa reação no local de aplicação. Provoca toxicidade pulmonar em seres humanos, bem como febre e calafrios, mas os efeitos colaterais não foram bem documentados em espécies animais.	Solução injetável normalmente usada em combinação com outros agentes antineoplásicos. Consultar protocolos antineoplásicos para detalhes com relação ao uso.	Injetável, frascos com 15 U.	Cães; 10 U/m² IV ou SC por 3 dias, depois 10 U/m² semanalmente (dose cumulativa máxima de 200 U/m²).
Brometo de neostigmina e Metilsulfato de neostigmina (Prostigmin; Stiglyn)	Anticolinesterásico. Inibidor da colinesterase. Inibe a degradação da acetilcolina na sinapse. Agente antimiastênico. Uso principalmente no tratamento da miastenia grave, ou como antídoto para o bloqueio neuromuscular causado por medicamentos bloqueadores neuromusculares.	Os efeitos adversos estão ligados aos efeitos farmacológicos do agente, isto é, estimulação colinérgica excessiva (efeitos muscarínicos). Os efeitos adversos são: diarreia, salivação, problemas respiratórios, vômito, efeitos do SNC, contrações musculares; ou no tratamento de *overdose*.	Comparativamente a outros agentes dessa classe (p.ex., piridostigmina), esses produtos geram efeitos muscarínicos mais severos. Quando um desses agentes é injetado para diagnóstico ou tratamento da miastenia, é recomendável usar atropina para contrabalançar os efeitos colaterais.	Comprimidos de 15 mg (brometo de neostigmina); injeção: 0,25, 0,5 mg/mL (metilsulfato de neostigmina).	2 mg/kg/dia VO (em doses divididas, até o efeito desejado). Injeção - antimiastênico: 10 mcg/kg IM, SC, conforme a necessidade; antídoto para bloqueio neuromuscular: 40 mcg/kg IM ou SC; meio diagnóstico auxiliar para miastenia grave: 40 mcg/kg IM ou 20 mcg/kg IV.

Formulário de Medicamentos para Consulta em 5 Minutos

Nome do Princípio Ativo (Comercial e Outros Nomes)	Farmacologia e Indicações	Efeitos Colaterais e Precauções	Informações de Dosagem e Comentários	Formulações	Dosagem (Exceto em Casos Indicados, a Dosagem é a Mesma para Cães e Gatos)
Brometo de pancurônio (Pavulon)	Bloqueador neuromuscular não despolarizante (ver Atracúrio).	Precauções similares às para o atracúrio.	Similar ao atracúrio.	Injeção: 1, 2 mg/mL.	0,1 mg/kg IV, ou começar com 0,01 mg/kg e adicionar doses de 0,01 mg/kg a cada 30 min.
Brometo de piridostigmina (Mestinon, Regonol)	Anticolinesterase. O mesmo que para neostigmina, exceto que piridostigmina tem ação mais prolongada. Usar no tratamento da toxidez anticolinérgica e no tratamento da miastenia grave.	Os efeitos adversos são causados pela excessiva atividade anticolinesterásica. Os sinais são atribuídos à acetilcolina. Interações farmacológicas: tendo em vista que esse produto contém brometo, usar com cautela em pacientes já sendo medicados com essa substância (p.ex., brometo de potássio para convulsões).	O mesmo que para a neostigmina, exceto que os efeitos adversos podem persistir por mais tempo.	Xarope contendo 12 mg/mL; comprimidos de 60 mg; injeção: 5 mg/mL.	Antimiastênico: 0,02-0,04 mg/kg q2h IV, ou 0,5-3 mg/kg a cada 8-12h VO Antídoto para bloqueio muscular: 0,15-0,3 mg/kg IM, IV.
Brometo de potássio (KBr)	Anticonvulsivante. Ação anticonvulsivante: pela estabilização das membranas dos neurônios. De ordinário, brometo é usado em pacientes refratários ao fenobarbital, ou adicionado ao tratamento com esse último agente.	Os efeitos adversos estão ligados a níveis elevados de brometo. Os sinais de toxicose são: depressão do SNC, fraqueza, ataxia. Considerar o uso de brometo de sódio em pacientes com hipoadrenocorticismo. Em comparação com cães, os efeitos adversos são mais comuns em gatos. Efeitos colaterais respiratórios similares à asma foram relatados em alguns gatos.	Geralmente o brometo é administrado em combinação com fenobarbital. Monitorar as concentrações séricas de brometo, para ajuste da dose. Concentrações plasmáticas efetivas devem se situar entre 1-2 mg/mL, mas, se o agente for usado isoladamente (sem fenobarbital), talvez haja necessidade de concentrações mais elevadas, de 2-4 mg/mL. Dietas ricas em cloreto provocarão meia-vida mais curta e a necessidade de doses mais elevadas. Brometo de sódio pode substituir brometo de potássio. Notar que 30 mg/kg de brometo de potássio equivalem a 20 mg/kg de brometo elementar.	Geralmente preparado como solução oral. (Não há formulação comercializada, mas pode ser preparada em uma farmácia de manipulação.)	Dose inicial de rotina: 30-40 mg/kg a cada 24h VO. Se administrada sem fenobarbital, usar doses mais elevadas de até 40-50 mg/kg, com monitoração das concentrações plasmáticas. Dose de ataque IV rápida: 800 mg/kg (brometo de sódio) administrada ao longo de 8 h (IV lenta). Dose de ataque oral rápida: 400-600 mg/kg VO dividida ao longo de 3-4 dias. Dose de ataque oral lenta (60 dias): 60 mg/kg/dia (30 mg/kg a cada 12h) VO durante 60 dias; em seguida, monitorar o nível sanguíneo.
Brometo de propantelina (Pro-Banthine)	Medicamento anticolinérgico (antimuscarínico). Bloqueia os receptores da acetilcolina, gerando efeitos parassimpaticolíticos (efeitos similares aos da atropina). Uso na redução da contração da musculatura lisa e da secreção do trato GI. Uso também no tratamento de efeitos cardiovasculares vagomediados.	Os efeitos adversos são atribuídos ao excesso de efeitos anticolinérgicos (antimuscarínicos). Tratar *overdoses* com fisostigmina. Usar com cautela no tratamento de doenças gastrintestinais.	Propantelina não foi avaliada em estudos clínicos em animais, mas frequentemente este é o medicamento de escolha para a terapia oral, em casos em que seja desejável um efeito anticolinérgico.	Comprimidos de 7,5, 15 mg.	0,25-0,5 mg/kg a cada 8-12h VO.

Nome do Princípio Ativo (Comercial e Outros Nomes)	Farmacologia e Indicações	Efeitos Colaterais e Precauções	Informações de Dosagem e Comentários	Formulações	Dosagem (Exceto em Casos Indicados, a Dosagem é a Mesma para Cães e Gatos)
Budesonida (Enterocort)	Corticosteroide. A budesonida é um corticosteroide de longa ação. Ela é programada para ser liberada localmente - nos intestinos - após administração oral. Apenas uma pequena fração é absorvida sistemicamente. A budesonida é utilizada para tratar a doença inflamatória intestinal.	Não foram relatados efeitos colaterais significativos. Entretanto, uma pequena absorção sistêmica pode causar efeitos glicocorticoides nos animais (como supressão das adrenais).	As cápsulas são indicadas para uso humano. Quando administrada para animais, não romper a proteção externa da droga para não comprometer a absorção intestinal.	Cápsulas com 3 mg.	0,125 mg/kg VO a cada 6-8h. O intervalo de doses pode ser aumentado a cada 12 horas quando o quadro nosológico melhorar.
Bunamidina, cloridrato (Scolaban)	Usada como agente anticestódeo. Principalmente utilizada contra infestação por cestodas em cães e gatos. O mecanismo de ação consiste na alteração da integridade do tegumento protetor do parasito.	Podem ocorrer vômito e diarreia após o uso. Evitar o uso em animais jovens.	Não fracionar comprimidos. Administrar comprimidos com o estômago vazio. Não fornecer alimentos por até 3 horas após a administração da droga.	Comprimidos com 400 mg.	20-50 mg/kg VO, em dose única.
Bupivacaína, cloridrato (Marcaína e formulações genéricas)	Anestésico local. Inibe a condução nervosa por meio do bloqueio dos canais de sódio. A ação é mais longa e potente que a da lidocaína ou outros anestésicos locais.	Os efeitos adversos em casos de infiltração local são raros. Doses altas são absorvidas sistemicamente e podem causar sinais neurológicos (tremores e convulsões). Depois da administração epidural de doses muito altas, é possível que ocorra paralisia respiratória.	Usada para infiltração local ou infusão no espaço epidural. Alguns adicionam 0,1 mEq de bicarbonato de sódio a cada 10 mL da droga para aumentar o pH, diminuir a dor da injeção e acelerar o início da ação. Usar imediatamente após a mistura com o bicarbonato.	Soluções injetáveis com 2, 5 e 5 mg/mL.	1mL de uma solução a 0,5% para 10 cm de epidural.
Buprenorfina, cloridrato (Buprenex [Vetergesic no Reino Unido])	Analgésico opioide. Agonista parcial de receptores μ e antagonista de receptores κ. É 25-50 vezes mais potente que a morfina. A buprenorfina provoca menos depressão respiratória que os outros opioides.	Os efeitos colaterais são similares aos dos outros agonistas opioides, exceto que pode causar menor depressão respiratória. A dependência, em uso crônico, pode ser menos intensa que a dos agonistas puros.	Usada para analgesia, muitas vezes em combinação com outros analgésicos ou em conjunto com anestesia geral. A sua ação é mais longa que a da morfina. É parcialmente reversível pela naloxona.	Solução com 0,3 mg/mL.	Cães: 0,006-0,02 mg/kg IV, IM, SC a cada 4-8h. Gatos: 0,005-0,01 mg/kg IV, IM a cada 4-8h. Administração bucal em gatos: 0,01-0,02 mg/kg a cada 12h.
Buspirona (BuSpar)	Agente ansiolítico. Atua pela ligação aos receptores de serotonina. Em medicina veterinária tem sido usada principalmente para o tratamento contra demarcação de território por jatos de urina em gatos.	Alguns gatos demonstram agressividade aumentada; outros revelam maior afeição pelos proprietários.	Algumas provas de eficácia sugerem a sua efetividade no tratamento de demarcação territorial por jatos de urina em gatos. Apresenta menor frequência de falhas na ação quando comparada a outras drogas.	Comprimidos com 5 e 10 mg.	Cães: 2,5-10 mg/cão VO a cada 12-24h ou 1 mg/kg VO a cada 12h. Gatos: 2,5-5 mg/gato VO a cada 24h (em alguns gatos, pode ser aumentada para 5-7,5 mg/gato, 2 vezes ao dia).
Bussulfano (Myleran)	Agente antineoplásico. É um agente alquilante bifuncional que atua quebrando o DNA das células tumorais. Usado principalmente para neoplasia linforreticular.	A leucopenia é o efeito colateral mais grave.	Normalmente utilizada em combinação com outros agentes antineoplásicos. Consultar protocolos específicos para mais detalhes.	Comprimidos com 2 mg.	3-4 mg/m^2 VO a cada 24h.

ESPÉCIES CANINA E FELINA

Formulário de Medicamentos para Consulta em 5 Minutos

Nome do Princípio Ativo (Comercial e Outros Nomes)	Farmacologia e Indicações	Efeitos Colaterais e Precauções	Informações de Dosagem e Comentários	Formulações	Dosagem (Exceto em Casos Indicados, a Dosagem é a Mesma para Cães e Gatos)
Butorfanol, tartarato (Torbutrol, Torbugesic)	Analgésico opioide. Agonista para receptores κ e antagonista fraco para receptores μ. O butorfanol é utilizado em analgesia pós-operatória, dor crônica e como agente antitussígeno.	Os efeitos colaterais são similares aos de outras drogas analgésicas opioides. A sedação é comum em doses analgésicas. A depressão respiratória pode ocorrer em altas doses. Foram observados efeitos disfóricos com o uso de algumas drogas agonistas/antagonistas.	Geralmente utilizada em combinação com agentes anestésicos ou em conjunto com outras drogas analgésicas.	Comprimidos com 1, 5 e 10 mg; injetável com 10 mg/mL.	Cães: (antitussígeno) 0,055 mg/kg SC a cada 6-12h ou 0,55 mg/kg VO; (pré--anestésico) 0,2-0,4 mg/kg IV, IM, SC (com acepromazina); (analgésico) 0,2-0,4 mg/kg a cada 2-4h. Gatos: (analgésico) 0,2-0,4 mg/kg IV, SC a cada 2-6h ou 1,5 mg/kg VO a cada 4-8h.
Cálcio, carbonato (muitas marcas disponíveis; Titralac, Tums, formulações genéricas)	Usado como suplemento oral de cálcio para a hipocalcemia. Utilizado como antiácido para tratar a hiperacidez gástrica e as úlceras GI. Neutraliza os ácidos estomacais. Também utilizado como ligante de fosfato intestinal na hiperfosfatemia.	Poucos efeitos colaterais. São possíveis concentrações aumentadas de cálcio. *Interações com outras drogas:* evitar o uso com fluoroquinolonas orais (p. ex.: ciprofloxacina, enrofloxacina), pois pode reduzir sua absorção.	As doses são principalmente derivadas da extrapolação de doses humanas. Quando usadas como suplementos de cálcio, as doses devem ser ajustadas de acordo com as concentrações séricas de cálcio.	Muitos comprimidos ou suspensão oral, por exemplo, comprimidos de 650 mg (contendo 260 mg de íon cálcio).	Quelante de fosfato: 60-100 mg/kg/dia em doses divididas VO. Suplementação de cálcio: 70-180 mg/kg/dia juntamente com o alimento.
Cálcio, citrato (Citracal [isentos de prescrição])	Suplemento de cálcio. Usado no tratamento da hipocalcemia, como ocorre no hipoparatireoidismo.	A hipercalcemia é possível com o excesso de suplementação.	As doses devem ser ajustadas de acordo com a concentração sérica de cálcio.	Comprimidos com 950 mg (contendo 200 mg de íon cálcio).	Cães: 20 mg/kg/dia VO (com as refeições). Gatos: 10-30 mg/kg VO a cada 8h (com as refeições).
Cálcio, cloreto (formulação genérica)	Suplemento de cálcio. Usado em situações críticas de suplementação como repositor eletrolítico ou cardiotônico.	É possível ocorrer superdosagem com cálcio. Não administrar soluções IV por via SC ou IM em virtude do risco de provocar necrose tissular.	A solução injetável possui 27,2 mg de íon cálcio (1,36 mEq) por mL. Normalmente usada em situações de emergência. As aplicações intracardíacas podem ser realizadas, mas evitar aplicações no miocárdio.	Solução a 10% (100 mg/mL).	0,1-0,3 mL/kg IV (lentamente).
Cálcio, dissódico EDTA	Ver Edetato dissódico de cálcio.				
Cálcio, gluconato (Kalcinate e formulações genéricas)	Suplemento de cálcio. Usado no tratamento da hipocalcemia, como ocorre no hipoparatireoidismo. Usado na deficiência eletrolítica.	A hipercalcemia é possível com o excesso de suplementação.	A solução injetável possui 97 mg (9,5 mg de íon cálcio (0,47 mEq) por mL. Os comprimidos de 500 mg contêm 45 mg de íon cálcio. Não administrar soluções IV por via SC ou IM em virtude do risco de provocar necrose tissular.	Injetável a 10% (100 mg/mL).	0,5-1,5 mL/kg IV (lentamente).
Cálcio, lactato (formulação genérica)	Suplemento de cálcio.	A hipercalcemia é possível com o excesso de suplementação.	O lactato de cálcio contém 130 mg de íon cálcio por grama.	Comprimidos isentos de prescrição médica.	Cães: 0,5-2 g/cão/dia VO (em doses divididas). Gatos: 0,2-0,5 g /gato/dia VO (em doses divididas).
Calcitriol (Rocaltrol, Calcijex)	Usado para tratar a deficiência de cálcio e doenças como a hipocalcemia associada ao hipoparatireoidismo. Também utilizada para reduzir os níveis de hormônios parati--reoidianos em pacientes com hiperparatireoidismo secundário renal. Não é indicada como suplemento de vitamina D. Atua aumentando a absorção de cálcio no intestino.	A superdosagem pode provocar hipercalcemia.	As doses devem ser ajustadas para cada paciente, de acordo com a resposta e a monitoração da concentração plasmática (hipoparatireoidismo) ou níveis da paratireoide (hiperparatireoidismo secundário renal).	Disponível na forma injetável (Calcijex) e de cápsulas (Rocaltrol); cápsulas com 0,25-0,5 mcg; injetável com 1 ou 2 mcg/mL.	Cães: 2,5-3,5 ng/kg VO a cada 24h. Gatos: 0,25 mcg/gato a cada 48h. Hiperparatireoidismo secundário renal: 2,5-3,5 ng/kg VO a cada 24h.

Formulário de Medicamentos para Consulta em 5 Minutos

Nome do Princípio Ativo (Comercial e Outros Nomes)	Farmacologia e Indicações	Efeitos Colaterais e Precauções	Informações de Dosagem e Comentários	Formulações	Dosagem (Exceto em Casos Indicados, a Dosagem é a Mesma para Cães e Gatos)
Canamicina (Kantrim)	Antibiótico aminoglicosídeo com amplo espectro de atividade.	Compartilha das mesmas propriedades que os demais aminoglicosídeos (ver Amicacina, Gentamicina).	Ver Gentamicina.	Injetável com 200 e 500 mg/mL.	10 mg/kg a cada 12h ou 20 mg/kg a cada 24h IV, IM, SC.
Captopril (Capoten)	Inibidor da enzima conversora de angiotensina (ECA). Inibe a conversão de angiotensina I em angiotensina II. Geralmente usada para tratar hipertensão e insuficiência cardíaca congestiva.	Em casos de doses excessivas, é possível que ocorra hipotensão. Pode causar azotemia em alguns pacientes, especialmente quando é administrada com diuréticos potentes (furosemida). *Interações com outras drogas:* usar cuidadosamente com diuréticos e suplementos de potássio. Os AINE podem reduzir os efeitos anti-hipertensivos.	Avaliar os pacientes com cautela para evitar a hipotensão. Como ocorre com todos os inibidores de ECA, deve-se avaliar os eletrólitos e a função renal a cada 3-7 dias depois de iniciada a terapia e durante o transcorrer desta. Em muitos animais, o uso do captopril tem sido substituído pelo enalapril e benazepril.	Comprimidos com 25 mg.	Cães: 0,5-2 mg/kg VO a cada 8-12h. Gatos: 3,12-6,25 mg/gato VO a cada 8h.
Carbimazol (Neomercazole)	Droga antitireoidiana convertida a metimazol.	Similar ao metimazol, talvez com menos efeitos GI.	Usada na Europa. A experiência clínica nos EUA é limitada.	Disponível na Europa, mas não nos EUA.	Gato: 5 mg/gato VO a cada 8h (indução), seguido por 5 mg/gato VO a cada 12h.
Carboplatina (Paraplatin)	Agente antineoplásico. Utilizada para o tratamento de diversos carcinomas. Interrompe a replicação do DNA em células tumorais por meio da ligação cruzada. Usada para o tratamento de carcinoma de células escamosas e outros carcinomas, melanomas, osteossarcomas e outros sarcomas. A sua ação é similar à da cisplatina.	A toxicose dose-limitada é a mielossupressão. Pode causar anemia, leucopenia ou trombocitopenia. A carboplatina pode induzir à toxicidade renal. Quando comparada à cisplatina, é menos emetogênica e nefrotóxica. Em gatos, causa neutropenia e trombocitopenia dose-limitante (menos intensas aos 17 dias).	Disponível para reconstituição injetável. Não usar com *kits* de administração que contenham alumínio, por causa da incompatibilidade. Geralmente é administrada em protocolos antineoplásicos específicos.	Injetável, frasco com 50 e 150 mg.	Cães: 300 mg/m² IV a cada 3-4 semanas. Gatos: 200-227 mg/m² IV a cada 4 semanas, por 4 tratamentos.
Carprofeno (Rymadil; Zenecarp no Reino Unido); Novox (formulação genérica)	AINE. Usado para o tratamento da dor e da inflamação, particularmente quando associadas à osteoartrite. Demonstrou ser seguro e eficaz no uso pré-operatório do controle da dor cirúrgica, seja por via IV ou VO. A ação do carprofeno pode se dar por meio da inibição da ciclo--oxigenase, apesar de ser uma droga relativamente poupadora de COX-1. Outros mecanismos também podem explicar sua eficácia.	Os efeitos colaterais mais comuns em pacientes clínicos foram GI (vômito, náusea e diarreia). Outros efeitos adversos são mais raros e incluem hepatotoxicose idiossincrática. Se ocorrerem, os sinais de toxicidade hepática aparecem em 2-3 semanas após o início da terapia. O uso pré-operatório não afetou negativamente a função renal ou os tempos de sangramento. Evitar o uso conjunto de carprofeno com outros AINE ou corticosteroides.	As dosagens são baseadas na investigação de campo do laboratório responsável pela droga e seus dados de registros nos EUA. Os ensaios clínicos foram conduzidos com pacientes caninos com osteoartrite e pacientes cirúrgicos. O carprofeno injetável pode ser administrado duas horas antes do procedimento cirúrgico.	Comprimidos com 25, 75 e 100 mg (convencionais e mastigáveis); solução injetável com 50 mg/mL.	Cães: 4,4 mg/kg/dia VO, administrados uma vez ao dia ou divididos 2 vezes ao dia, na dosagem de 2,2 mg/kg a cada 12h; 4,4 mg/kg/dia SC, administrados uma vez ao dia ou 2,2 mg/kg a cada 12h. Gatos: 4 mg/kg em injeção única.
Carvão ativado (Acta-Char, Charcodote, Toxiban, formulações genéricas)	Adsorvente. Usado principalmente para adsorver drogas e toxinas no intestino e para prevenir a sua absorção.	Não é absorvido sistemicamente. A sua administração é segura.	Disponível em variadas formas; normalmente utilizada como tratamento de envenenamento. Muitas preparações comerciais contêm sorbitol, o qual age como agente palatabilizante e promove a catarse intestinal.	Suspensão oral.	1-4 g/kg VO (grânulos); 6-12 mL/kg (suspensão).

ESPÉCIES CANINA E FELINA

Formulário de Medicamentos para Consulta em 5 Minutos

Nome do Princípio Ativo (Comercial e Outros Nomes)	Farmacologia e Indicações	Efeitos Colaterais e Precauções	Informações de Dosagem e Comentários	Formulações	Dosagem (Exceto em Casos Indicados, a Dosagem é a Mesma para Cães e Gatos)
Carvedilol (Coreg)	β-bloqueador não seletivo com propriedades antioxidantes e α-bloqueadora; indicado para hipertensão sistêmica e suprarregulação de receptores β em animais com insuficiência miocárdica.	Bradicardia, ICC em virtude da depressão miocárdica inicial. É possível a ocorrência de efeitos adversos dos β-bloqueadores não seletivos, incluindo fraqueza e broncoespasmo.	A dosagem inicial típica é de 0,2 mg/kg a cada 12h, depois gradualmente aumentada até 0,4 mg/kg. Se os sinais de insuficiência cardíaca piorarem em dosagens mais altas, reduzir até a dose mais bem tolerada previamente. A absorção oral é altamente variável em cães.	Comprimidos com 3,125; 6,125; 12,5 e 25 mg.	Cães: 0,2-0,4 mg/kg VO a cada 12h. Se não houver insuficiência cardíaca, a dose poderá ser aumentada, lentamente, para 1,5 mg/kg PO a cada 12h, com base nos estudos farmacocinéticos. Gatos: dosagem não estabelecida.
Cáscara sagrada (muitas marcas [p. ex.: Nature's Remedy])	Estimulante catártico. Acredita-se que sua ação ocorra por estimulação local da motilidade intestinal. Usada como laxante para tratar a constipação ou evacuar o intestino para procedimentos.	A superdosagem pode causar perdas eletrolíticas.	Disponível em diversas formulações sem prescrição médica.	Comprimidos de 100 e 325 mg.	Cães: 1-5 mg/kg/dia VO. Gatos: 1-2 mg/gato/dia VO
Cefadroxila (Cefa-Tabs, Cefa-Drops)	A cefadroxila é um antibiótico cefalosporínico de 1ª geração.	A cefadroxila é conhecida por causar vômito após administração oral em cães.	O espectro da cefadroxila é similar ao das outras cefalosporinas de 1ª geração. Para os testes de sensibilidade, usar a cefalotina como droga-padrão.	Suspensão oral com 50 mg/mL; comprimidos com 50, 100, 200 e 1.000 mg. A disponibilidade em algumas formulações orais é inconsistente.	Cães: 22 mg/kg a cada 12h, até 30 mg/kg VO a cada 12h. Gatos: 22 mg/kg VO a cada 24h.
Cefalexina (Keflex e formulações genéricas)	A cefalexina é uma cefalosporina de 1ª geração.	Similares àqueles das demais cefalosporinas.	Embora não seja aprovada para uso veterinário, alguns testes em cães com piodermite se revelaram eficazes.	Cápsulas com 250 e 500 mg; comprimidos com 250 e 500 mg; suspensão oral com 100 mg/mL ou com 125 e 250 mg/5 mL.	10-30 mg/kg VO a cada 6-12h; para piodermite, 22-35 mg/kg VO a cada 12h.
Cefazolina sódica (Ancef, Kefzol e formulações genéricas)	A cefazolina é um antibiótico cefalosporínico de 1ª geração.	Os efeitos colaterais são raros.	Cefalosporina de 1ª geração comumente usada como droga injetável para profilaxia em cirurgias, bem como na terapia aguda em infecções graves.	Injetável, 50 e 100 mg/50 mL.	20-30 mg/kg IV, IM a cada 8h. Para uso cirúrgico: 22 mg/kg a cada 2h durante a cirurgia.
Cefepima (Maxipime)	Cefalosporina de 4ª geração com espectro mais amplo que as outras classes.	Efeitos colaterais similares àqueles das demais cefalosporinas.	Esquemas de dosagens são baseados em estudos farmacocinéticos em cães.	Injetável, frasco com 500 mg e 2 g.	Cães: 40 mg/kg IM, IV a cada 6h.
Cefixima (Suprax)	A cefixima é uma cefalosporina de 3ª geração.	Similares àqueles das demais cefalosporinas.	Apesar de não aprovada para uso veterinário, os estudos farmacocinéticos em cães forneceram as dosagens recomendadas.	Suspensão oral com 20 mg/mL e comprimidos com 200 e 400 mg.	10 mg/kg VO a cada 12h; para cistite: 5 mg/kg VO a cada 12-24h.
Cefotaxima sódica (Claforan)	A cefotaxima é uma cefalosporina de 3ª geração. É usada quando é encontrada resistência aos outros antibióticos ou quando a infecção se localiza no sistema nervoso central.	Similares àqueles das demais cefalosporinas.	As cefalosporinas de 3ª geração são usadas quando se encontram resistências às cefalosporinas de 1ª e 2ª gerações.	Injetável, frascos com 500 mg, 1, 2 e 10 g.	Cães: 50 mg/kg IV, IM, SC a cada 12h. Gatos: 20-80 mg/kg IV, IM a cada 6h.
Cefotetana dissódica (Cefotan)	A cefotetana é uma cefalosporina de 2ª geração.	Similares àqueles das demais cefalosporinas.	Cefalosporina de 2ª geração similar à cefoxitina, mas podendo apresentar meia-vida longa em cães.	Injetável, frascos com 1, 2 e 10 g.	30 mg/kg IV, SC a cada 8h.

Formulário de Medicamentos para Consulta em 5 Minutos					
Nome do Princípio Ativo (Comercial e Outros Nomes)	Farmacologia e Indicações	Efeitos Colaterais e Precauções	Informações de Dosagem e Comentários	Formulações	Dosagem (Exceto em Casos Indicados, a Dosagem é a Mesma para Cães e Gatos)
Cefovecina (Convenia)	Cefalosporina de 3ª geração usada para injeções em cães e gatos. Possui meia-vida muito longa quando comparada às demais cefalosporinas.	Os efeitos colaterais podem incluir problemas GI transitórios.	Os intervalos entre doses normalmente são a cada 14 dias em cães e gatos, ou uma aplicação única.	Injetável, frasco com 80 mg/mL.	Cães e gatos: 8 mg/kg SC em aplicação injetável única ou repetida a cada 14 dias.
Cefoxitina sódica (Mefoxin)	A cefoxitina é uma cefalosporina de 2ª geração. Pode assumir atividade aumentada contra bactérias anaeróbias.	Similares àqueles das demais cefalosporinas.	Cefalosporina de 2ª geração, normalmente utilizada quando se deseja combater bactérias anaeróbias.	Injetável, frascos com 1, 2 e 10 g.	30 mg/kg IV a cada 6-8h.
Cefpodoxima proxetil (Simplicef)	Cefalosporina oral de 3ª geração. Sua atividade inclui bastonetes Gram-negativos e estafilococos.	Os efeitos colaterais mais comuns são vômito e diarreia.	Aprovada para infecções de pele e tecidos moles em cães.	Comprimidos com 100 e 200 mg.	Cães: 5-10 mg/kg VO a cada 24h. Gatos: dosagem não estabelecida.
Ceftazidima (Fortaz, Ceptaz, Tazicef)	Cefalosporina de 3ª geração. A ceftazidima possui maior ação contra *Pseudomonas aeruginosa* que outras cefalosporinas.	Similares àqueles das demais cefalosporinas.	Cefalosporina de 3ª geração. Pode ser reconstituída com lidocaína a 1% para administração IM.	Frascos com 0,5; 1; 2 e 6 g, reconstituída para 280 mg/mL.	Cães e gatos: 30 mg/kg IV, IM a cada 6h. Cães: 30 mg/kg SC a cada 4-6h.
Ceftiofur (Naxcel [ceftiofur sódico]; Excenel [cloridrato de ceftiofur])	O espectro do ceftiofur se assemelha ao de muitas cefalosporinas de 3ª geração.	Similares àqueles das demais cefalosporinas. Não substitui a forma ácida cristalina livre (Exceede) para o Naxcel.	Disponível em forma de pó para a reconstituição antes da administração. Após a reconstituição, permanece estável por 7 dias se for refrigerado, 12 horas se ficar em temperatura ambiente ou 8 semanas se congelado.	Injetável, 50 mg/mL.	2,2-4,4 mg/kg SC a cada 24h (para infecções do sistema urinário).
Cetamina (Ketalar, Ketavet, Vetalar)	Agente anestésico. Antagonista de receptores NMDA. O mecanismo exato de ação não é conhecido, mas parece agir como um agente dissociativo. Na maioria dos animais é rapidamente metabolizada e eliminada.	Provoca dor à aplicação IM. Foram relatados tremores, espasmos e estados convulsivos. Aumenta o débito cardíaco quando comparada com outros agentes anestésicos. Não usar em animais com lesão craniana em virtude da possível elevação da pressão do LCE.	Muitas vezes é usada em combinação com outros anestésicos ou adjuntos anestésicos como xilazina, acepromazina ou diazepam. As doses IV geralmente são menores que as doses IM.	Solução injetável com 100 mg/mL.	Cães: 5,5-22 mg/kg IV, IM (recomenda-se o uso associado de um sedativo ou tranquilizante). Gatos: 2-25 mg/kg IV, IM (recomenda-se o uso associado de um sedativo ou tranquilizante). Cães e gatos: dose para infusão constante: 0,5 mg/kg IV seguida por 0,3-0,6 mg/kg/h. Pode ser usada em combinação com outros analgésicos.
Cetirizina (Zyrtec)	Anti-histamínico (bloqueador H_1). Age bloqueando os receptores histamínicos do tipo 1 (H_1) e suprimindo as reações inflamatórias provocadas pela histamina. Os bloqueadores H_1 são utilizados para controlar prurido, inflamação da pele, rinorreia e inflamação das vias aéreas. A cetirizina é considerada um anti-histamínico de 2ª geração, podendo ser associada com menor sedação que outras drogas.	Nenhum efeito colateral foi observado em cães ou gatos.	Não há estudos publicados que demonstrem a eficácia clínica em cães e gatos. Seu uso clínico se baseia em experimentação animal.	Xarope oral com 1 mg/mL; comprimidos com 5 e 10 mg.	Cães: 2 mg/kg VO a cada 12h. Gatos: 1 mg/kg VO diariamente.

ESPÉCIES CANINA E FELINA

Formulário de Medicamentos para Consulta em 5 Minutos					
Nome do Princípio Ativo (Comercial e Outros Nomes)	*Farmacologia e Indicações*	*Efeitos Colaterais e Precauções*	*Informações de Dosagem e Comentários*	*Formulações*	*Dosagem (Exceto em Casos Indicados, a Dosagem é a Mesma para Cães e Gatos)*
Cetoconazol (Nizoral)	Droga antifúngica azólica (imidazólica). Mecanismo de ação similar aos de outos agentes antifúngicos azólicos. Inibe a síntese de ergosterol na membrana celular do fungo. Fungistática. Eficaz contra dermatófitos e uma infinidade de fungos sistêmicos, como *Histoplasma*, *Blastomyces* e *Coccidioides*. Também ativa contra *Malassezia*.	Os efeitos colaterais em animais incluem vômito, diarreia e injúria hepática dose-dependentes. A elevação das enzimas hepáticas é comum. Não administrar em animais prenhes. O cetoconazol causa anormalidades endócrinas, em especial a inibição da síntese de cortisol. *Interações com outras drogas*: o cetoconazol inibirá o metabolismo de outras drogas (anticonvulsivantes, ciclosporina, cisaprida).	A absorção oral depende da acidez estomacal. Não administrar com drogas antissecretórias ou antiácidas. Por causa dos efeitos endócrinos, o cetoconazol tem sido utilizado na terapia de curta duração do hiperadrenocorticismo.	Comprimidos com 200 mg; suspensão oral com 100 mg/mL (disponível apenas no Canadá).	Cães: 10-15 mg/kg VO a cada 8-12h. Para infecções por *Malassezia canis*: 5 mg/kg VO a cada 24h. Para o hiperadrenocorticismo: iniciar com 5 mg/kg VO a cada 12h durante sete dias, depois 12-15 mg/kg VO a cada 12h. Gatos: 5-10 mg/kg VO a cada 8-12h.
Cetoprofeno (Orudis KT [comprimido sem prescrição médica humano]; Ketofen [apresentação injetável veterinária])	AINE. Agente anti-inflamatório. Usado para tratar artrite e outros distúrbios inflamatórios.	Todos os AINE compartilham efeitos colaterais similares quanto à toxicidade GI. O cetoprofeno é administrado por cinco dias consecutivos em cães, sem efeitos colaterais consideráveis. O efeito colateral mais comum é o vômito. É possível ocorrer a ulceração GI em alguns animais.	Apesar de não aprovado nos EUA, o cetoprofeno é aprovado para pequenos animais em outros países. As doses listadas são baseadas no uso aprovado naqueles países. Nos EUA, a droga está disponível para seres humanos como uma formulação sem prescrição médica.	Comprimidos com 12,5 (formulação sem prescrição médica); 25, 50 e 75 mg para humanos; injetável para equinos com 100 mg/mL.	1 mg/kg VO a cada 24h por até cinco dias. A dose inicial pode ser dada por aplicação injetável até 2 mg/kg SC, IM, IV.
Cetorolaco, trometamol (Toradol)	AINE. Utilizado por curtos períodos de tempo para alívio da dor e da inflamação. Age mediante a inibição da enzima cicloxigenase (COX). O uso do cetorolaco foi avaliado clinicamente em cães, mas não em gatos.	Os AINE podem causar ulceração GI. O cetorolaco pode provocar lesões gastrintestinais se administrado mais frequentemente que a cada oito horas. Não administrar mais que duas doses.	Disponível na forma de comprimidos com 10 mg e injetável para uso IM e IV. A dosagem a cada 12 horas é recomendável para evitar problemas GI.	Comprimidos com 10 mg; injetável com 15 e 30 mg/mL em álcool a 10%.	Cães: 0,5 mg/kg VO, IM, IV a cada 8-12h. Gatos: não foi estabelecida uma dose segura.
Cianocobalamina (Vitamina B$_{12}$) (diversas) e cobalamina	Análoga da vitamina B$_{12}$.	Os efeitos colaterais são raros, exceto em casos de superdosagem.	Ajuste de dose por monitoração. Ver Vitamina B$_{12}$ para mais informações.	Injetável com 100 mcg/mL.	Cães: 100-200 mcg/dia VO. Gatos: 50-100 mcg/dia VO ou 250 mcg IM ou SC semanalmente.
Ciclofosfamida (Cytoxan, Neosar)	Agente citotóxico. Agente alquilante bifuncional. Destrói o pareamento de bases e inibe a síntese de DNA e RNA. Citotóxico para células tumorais e para outras células que se dividem rápido. Usada principalmente como adjuvante da quimioterapia e como terapia imunossupressora.	A supressão da medula óssea é o efeito colateral mais comum. Pode produzir neutropenia grave (geralmente reversível). Em alguns pacientes podem ocorrer vômito e diarreia. Os cães são suscetíveis à toxicidade vesical (cistite hemorrágica estéril). Pode causar perda de pelos quando usada em protocolos quimioterápicos.	A ciclofosfamida normalmente é administrada com outras drogas (antineoplásicas ou corticosteroides) quando é usada em terapia imunossupressora. Consultar protocolos antineoplásicos específicos para regimes específicos.	Injetável com 25 mg/mL; comprimidos com 25 e 50 mg.	Cães: antineoplásico: 50 mg/m^2 VO uma vez ao dia, por 4 dias/semana, ou 150-300 mg/m^2 IV, repetido após 21 dias. Terapia imu-nossupressora: 50 mg/m^2 (aproximadamente 2,2 mg/kg) VO a cada 48h, ou 2,2 mg/kg uma vez ao dia, por 4 dias/semana. Gatos: 6,25-12,5 mg/gato uma vez ao dia, por 4 dias/semana.

Formulário de Medicamentos para Consulta em 5 Minutos					
Nome do Princípio Ativo (Comercial e Outros Nomes)	Farmacologia e Indicações	Efeitos Colaterais e Precauções	Informações de Dosagem e Comentários	Formulações	Dosagem (Exceto em Casos Indicados, a Dosagem é a Mesma para Cães e Gatos)
Ciclosporina (Neoral [humano], Atopica [veterinário], Optimmune [oftálmico]. Outro nome para a ciclosporina é ciclosporina A)	Droga imunossupressora. Suprime a indução dos linfócitos T. Usada no tratamento da dermatite atópica e de doenças imunomediadas.	Pode causar vômito, diarreia e anorexia. Em comparação com outras drogas imunossupressoras, não causa mielossupressão. *Interações com outras drogas:* a eritromicina ou o cetoconazol podem aumentar as concentrações da ciclosporina quando usados concomitantemente.	O Neoral possui a mesma formulação do Atopica. A ciclosporina tópica tem sido usada com sucesso no tratamento de ceratoconjuntivite seca. Pode-se usar a monitoração dos parâmetros sanguíneos para ajustar a dosagem.	Cápsulas com 10, 25, 50 e 100 mg.	Cães: 3-7 mg/kg/dia VO. A dose para a dermatite atópica pode ser alterada para 5 mg/kg a cada 48h em alguns pacientes. Gatos: 3-5 mg/kg/dia V O.
Cimetidina (Tagamet [formulações com e sem prescrição médica])	Antagonista de receptores histamina-2 (bloqueador de H_2). Bloqueia a estimulação de histamina das células parietais gástricas, no intuito de reduzir a secreção de ácido gástrico. Usada para tratar úlceras e gastrite.	Os efeitos colaterais geralmente são vistos apenas em casos de filtração renal diminuída. Em seres humanos que estão recebendo doses altas, podem ocorrer sinais do SNC. *Interações com outras drogas:* pode aumentar a concentração de outras drogas usadas paralelamente (como teofilina) em função da inibição das enzimas hepáticas.	As doses exatas necessárias para tratar úlceras não foram estabelecidas.	Comprimidos com 100, 200, 300, 400 e 800 mg; solução oral com 60 mg/mL; solução injetável com 6 mg/mL.	10 mg/kg IV, IM, VO a cada 6-8h.
Ciproeptadina, cloridrato (Periactin)	Fenotiazina com anti-histamínico e propriedades antisserotonina. Usada como estimulante de apetite (provavelmente pela alteração na atividade da serotonina no centro do apetite).	Pode causar aumento do apetite e ganho de peso.	Nenhum estudo clínico foi realizado em medicina veterinária. O uso é baseado, principalmente, na extrapolação dos resultados em seres humanos ou em empirismo. O xarope contém 5% de álcool.	Comprimidos com 4 mg; xarope com 2 mg/5 mL.	Anti-histamínico: 0,5-1,1 mg/kg VO a cada 8-12h. Estimulante de apetite: 2 mg/gato VO. Asma felina: 1-2 mg/gato VO a cada 12h.
Ciprofloxacina (Cipro) e formulações genéricas	Droga antibacteriana da classe das fluoroquinolonas. Age por inibição da DNA-girase e de RNA e DNA pela célula. Bactericida. Espectro de ação antimicrobiano alto.	Evitar o uso em cães com 4 semanas a 7 meses de idade. Concentrações muito altas podem causar toxicidade do SNC, especialmente em animais com insuficiência renal. Ocasionalmente, pode causar vômito. A solução IV deve ser administrada lentamente (por 30 minutos).	As doses são baseadas na concentração plasmática necessária para alcançar um nível acima da concentração inibitória mínima (CIM). Estudos sobre a sua eficácia não foram realizados em cães e gatos. A ciprofloxacina não é tão bem absorvida por via oral em comparação com a enrofloxacina.	Comprimidos de 250, 500 e 750 mg; solução injetável com 2 e 10 mg/mL.	Cães: 20-25 mg/kg VO a cada 24h; 10-15 mg/kg IV a cada 24h. Gatos: 20 mg/kg VO a cada 24h; 10 mg/kg VO a cada 24h.
Cisaprida	Agente procinético. Estimula a motilidade gástrica e intestinal, tanto pela ação da acetilcolina quanto pela atividade nos receptores de serotonina ou efeito direto na musculatura lisa. Usada em casos de refluxo gástrico, gastroparesia, íleo paralítico e constipação.	Contraindicada em pacientes com obstrução gastrintestinal.	As doses foram baseadas em extrapolação de doses usadas em seres humanos, de estudos experimentais e de relatos comprovados. Os estudos sobre a sua eficácia não foram realizados em cães e gatos.	Não se apresenta mais disponível comercialmente. Entretanto, pode ser obtida em farmácias de manipulação.	Cães: 0,1-0,5 mg/kg VO a cada 8-12h (podem ser usadas doses de até 0,5-1 mg/kg a cada 8h). Gatos: 2,5-5 mg/kg VO a cada 8-12h (pode ser usada dose de até 1 mg/kg a cada 8h).

ESPÉCIES CANINA E FELINA

Formulário de Medicamentos para Consulta em 5 Minutos

Nome do Princípio Ativo (Comercial e Outros Nomes)	Farmacologia e Indicações	Efeitos Colaterais e Precauções	Informações de Dosagem e Comentários	Formulações	Dosagem (Exceto em Casos Indicados, a Dosagem é a Mesma para Cães e Gatos)
Cisplatina (Platinol)	Agente antineoplásico. Usada para o tratamento de vários tumores sólidos, incluindo o osteossarcoma. Acredita-se que sua ação seja similar à dos agentes alquilantes bifuncionais e que interrompa a replicação do DNA das células tumorais.	A nefrotoxicidade é o fator mais limitante da terapia com cisplatina. Em gatos, causa toxicose pulmonar espécie-específica e relacionada com a dose usada. Em cães, podem ocorrer vômitos após a administração e trombocitopenia transitória.	Para evitar a toxicidade, deve-se realizar a fluidoterapia de ataque com cloreto de sódio antes da administração da droga. Muitas vezes, agentes antieméticos são administrados antes da terapia para reduzir a incidência de vômitos.	Injetável com 1 mg/mL.	Cães: 60-70 mg/m² IV a cada 3-4 semanas (administrar fluidoterapia para assegurar a diurese). Gatos: não administrar em gatos.
Citarabina (arabinosilcitosina) (Cytosar)	Agente antineoplásico. O mecanismo de ação exato não é conhecido. Provavelmente inibe a síntese de DNA. Usada para linfoma e em protocolos de leucemia. Também utilizada para meningoencefalite.	Supressão da medula óssea. Causa vômito e diarreia.	Consultar protocolos antineoplásicos para dosagens específicas.	Frascos com 100 mg.	Cães (linfoma): 100-150 mg/m² uma vez ao dia ou 50 mg/m² duas vezes ao dia, por 4 dias, IV ou SC, ou 600 mg/m² em dose única. Cães (meningoencefalite): 50 mg/m² duas vezes ao dia, por 2 dias ou 100 mg/m² infundidos por 24h, repetido no 2º dia. Gatos: 100 mg/m² uma vez ao dia, por 2 dias.
Citrato de magnésio (Citroma, Citro-Nesia [Citro-Mag no Canadá])	Catártico salino. Efeito osmótico: arrasta água para o intestino delgado. O acúmulo de líquido promove evacuação intestinal. Usada para constipação e evacuação intestinal, precedendo certos procedimentos.	Não foram relatados efeitos adversos em animais. Entretanto, pode ocorrer perda de líquido e eletrólitos com o uso excessivo. Pode ocorrer acúmulo de magnésio em pacientes com comprometimento renal. Interações farmacológicas: Catárticos contendo magnésio diminuem a absorção oral de ciprofloxacino e outras fluoroquinolonas.	Geralmente usada para evacuação intestinal antes de cirurgia ou procedimento diagnóstico. Rápido início da ação.	Suspensão oral a 6%.	2-4 mL/kg/dia VO.
Citrato de potássio (genérico, Urocit-K)	Suplemento de potássio. Alcaliniza a urina e pode aumentar o ácido cítrico urinário. Uso em casos de urolitíase por oxalato de cálcio. Também usado na acidose tubular renal.	O mesmo que cloreto de potássio.	1 g de citrato de potássio fornece 9,26 mEq de potássio.	Comprimidos de 5 mEq e 10 mEq. Algumas formulações estão combinadas com cloreto de potássio. 1.000 mg de citrato de potássio = 9,26 mEq de potássio.	0,5 mEq/kg/dia VO.
Citrato de sildenafila (Viagra)	Vasodilatador inibidor da fosfodiesterase 5; dilata preferencialmente a circulação pulmonar. Indicado para o tratamento da hipertensão pulmonar.	Pode causar hipotensão, especialmente se usado em combinação com nitratos; foi relatada em cães a ocorrência de rubor cutâneo na área inguinal.	Muito caro.	Comprimidos de 25, 50, 100 mg.	Cães: 2 mg/kg a cada 12h VO, mas o intervalo entre doses pode variar de 8-24 h. Gatos: 1 mg/kg a cada 8h VO.
Citrato de sufentanila (Sufenta)	Opioide agonista. A ação dos derivados da fentanila se faz via μ-receptor. Sufentanila é 5-7× mais potente do que fentanila. 13-20 mcg de sufentanila promovem analgesia equivalente a 10 mg de morfina.	Efeitos adversos similares aos causados por outros opiatos. Sua elevada potência implica a necessidade de cuidado no cálculo da dose.	Quando usado para anestesia, frequentemente os animais são pré-medicados com acepromazina ou um benzodiazepínico.	Injeção: 50 mcg/mL.	2 mcg/kg IV, até a dose máxima de 5 mcg/kg (0,005 mg/kg).

Formulário de Medicamentos para Consulta em 5 Minutos

Nome do Princípio Ativo (Comercial e Outros Nomes)	Farmacologia e Indicações	Efeitos Colaterais e Precauções	Informações de Dosagem e Comentários	Formulações	Dosagem (Exceto em Casos Indicados, a Dosagem é a Mesma para Cães e Gatos)
Citrato de tamoxifeno (Nolvadex)	Bloqueador não esteroide dos receptores do estrogênio. Também exibe fracos efeitos estrogênicos. Tamoxifeno pode também aumentar a liberação do hormônio liberador da gonadotropina (Gn-RH). Agente usado como terapia adjuvante para certos tumores.	Não estão completamente documentados efeitos adversos em animais. No entanto, foi relatado em humanos que o tamoxifeno aumentou a dor no tumor. Não usar em fêmeas prenhes. Interações farmacológicas: reage com medicamentos anti-úlcera	Para doses e regimes, consultar protocolos antineoplásicos.	Comprimidos de 10 mg (citrato de tamoxifeno).	A dose veterinária não foi ainda estabelecida. A dose para humanos é 10 mg a cada 12h VO.
Citrato de tripelenamina (Pelamine, PBZ)	Bloqueador da histamina (H_1). Similar em ação a outros anti-histamínicos. Uso no tratamento de doenças alérgicas.	Efeitos adversos similares aos causados por outros anti-histamínicos. Os membros dessa classe (etanolaminas) têm maiores efeitos antimuscarínicos, em comparação com outros anti-histamínicos.	Não foram publicados estudos clínicos de uso na medicina veterinária. Não há evidência de que esse agente seja mais eficaz do que outros medicamentos nessa classe.	Comprimidos de 25, 50 mg; injeção: 20 mg/mL.	1 mg/kg a cada 12h VO.
Claritromicina (Biaxin)	Antibiótico macrolídeo com atividade bacteriostática. Seu espectro de ação inclui, principalmente, bactérias Gram-positivas. Espera-se resistência para a maior parte das bactérias Gram-negativas. Sua eficácia não é conhecida em animais. O uso mais comum em seres humanos está no tratamento da gastrite por *Helicobacter* e nas infecções respiratórias.	Bem tolerada em animais. Os efeitos colaterais mais comuns são vômito, náusea e diarreia.	As doses não foram estabelecidas para animais em virtude da ausência de testes clínicos. As recomendações de dosagem foram extrapoladas de tratamentos humanos ou de uso empírico.	Comprimidos com 250 e 500 mg; suspensão oral com 25 e 50 mg/mL.	7,5 mg/kg PO a cada 12h.
Clavamox	Ver Amoxicilina + clavulanato de potássio.	-	-	-	-
Clemastina (Tavist, Contac 12 Hour Allergy e formulações genéricas)	Anti-histamínico (bloqueador H_1). Bloqueia a ação da histamina nos tecidos. Usada principalmente no tratamento da alergia. Evidências sugerem que a clemastina é mais eficiente que outros anti-histamínicos para prurido em cães.	A sedação é o efeito colateral mais comum.	Usada para tratamentos curtos de prurido em cães. Pode ser mais eficiente quando combinada com outras drogas anti-inflamatórias. O Tavist na forma de xarope contém 5,5% de álcool.	Comprimidos com 1,34 mg (formulação sem prescrição médica) e 2,64 mg (com prescrição médica); xarope com 0,134 mg/mL.	Cães: 0,05-0,1 mg/kg VO a cada 12h.
Clindamicina (Antirobe [veterinário], Cleocin [humano])	Droga antibacteriana da classe das lincosamidas (a ação é similar à dos macrolídeos). Inibe a síntese proteica da bactéria por meio da inibição do ribossomo bacteriano. É inicialmente bacteriostática, com atividade principal contra bactérias Gram-positivas e anaeróbias.	Geralmente é bem tolerada por cães e gatos. O produto líquido oral tem sabor desagradável para gatos. A lincomicina e a clindamicina podem alterar a população bacteriana intestinal, causando diarreia; por isso, não deve ser administrada em roedores e coelhos.	A maioria das doses é baseada nos testes de eficácia e nos dados da droga aprovados pelo fabricante. Ver a coluna sobre dosagens para guias específicos das diferentes infecções.	Solução oral com 25 mg/mL; cápsulas com 25, 75, 150 e 300 mg; injetável, 150 mg/mL (Cleocin).	Cães: 11-33 mg/kg VO a cada 12h; para periodontite e infecções de tecidos moles 5,5-33 mg/kg VO a cada 12h. Gatos: 11-33 mg/kg VO a cada 24h; para infecções anaeróbias e tegumentares, 11 mg/kg VO a cada 12h; para a toxoplasmose 12,5-25 mg/kg VO a cada 12h.
Clofazimina (Lamprene)	Agente antimicrobiano usado para tratar a lepra felina. Possui pequena ação bactericida contra *Mycobacterium leprae*.	Os efeitos colaterais em gatos não são conhecidos. Em seres humanos, os efeitos colaterais mais sérios são gastrintestinais.	As doses se baseiam em estudos de extrapolação da dose usada para seres humanos ou em empirismo.	Cápsulas com 50 e 100 mg.	Gato: 1 mg/kg até o máximo de 4 mg/kg/dia VO.

ESPÉCIES CANINA E FELINA

Formulário de Medicamentos para Consulta em 5 Minutos

Nome do Princípio Ativo (Comercial e Outros Nomes)	Farmacologia e Indicações	Efeitos Colaterais e Precauções	Informações de Dosagem e Comentários	Formulações	Dosagem (Exceto em Casos Indicados, a Dosagem é a Mesma para Cães e Gatos)
Clomipramina (Clomicalm [veterinário]; Anafranil [humano])	Droga antidepressiva tricíclica (TCA). Utilizada em seres humanos para tratar ansiedade e depressão. Usada em animais no tratamento de diversos outros distúrbios comportamentais, incluindo transtorno obsessivo-compulsivo e ansiedade por separação. Atua por inibição da captação de serotonina nas terminações dos nervos pré-sinápticos.	Os efeitos adversos relatados incluem sedação e redução de apetite. Outros efeitos colaterais associados com TCAs são os efeitos antimuscarínicos (boca seca, frequência cardíaca aumentada) e anti-histamínicos (sedação). As superdosagens podem produzir cardiotoxicidade permanente.	Ao ajustar a dosagem, pode-se iniciar a terapia com uma dose baixa e aumentar gradualmente. Pode haver 2-4 semanas de atraso, a contar do início da terapia, antes que os efeitos benéficos sejam vistos.	Comprimidos com 5, 20 e 80 mg (veterinário); comprimidos de 25 e 50 mg (humano).	Cães: 1-2 mg/kg VO a cada 12h. Gatos: 1-5 mg/gato VO a cada 12-24h.
Clonazepam (Klonopin)	Benzodiazepínico. A ação se baseia no aumento dos efeitos inibitórios do ácido γ-aminobutírico (GABA) no SNC. Usado pela ação anticonvulsivante, sedativa e no tratamento de alguns distúrbios comportamentais.	Os efeitos colaterais incluem sedação e polifagia. Alguns animais podem desenvolver excitação paradoxal.	As doses estão baseadas principalmente em relatos da medicina humana, no empirismo ou estudos experimentais. Não foram relatados estudos de eficácia clínica em cães e gatos.	Comprimidos de 0,5; 1 e 2 mg.	Cães: 0,5 mg/kg VO a cada 8-12h. Gatos: 0,1-0,2 mg/kg VO a cada 12-24h.
Clopidogrel (Plavix)	O clopidogrel é usado para inibir as plaquetas em pacientes que estão propensos a formar trombos. Em gatos, o clopidogrel é recomendado para prevenir o tromboembolismo arterial cardiogênico associado com doença cardíaca e aumento atrial.	Podem ocorrer complicações hemorrágicas.	Administrar com ou sem ácido acetilsalicílico em pacientes predispostos à formação de trombos e êmbolos. A dose de 19 mg é aproximadamente ¼ do comprimido humano.	Comprimidos com 75 mg.	Cães: 0,5-1 mg/kg VO a cada 24h. Dose oral de 2-4 mg/kg que pode ser seguida por 1 mg/kg a cada 24h. Gatos: 19 mg/gato (¼ do comprimido) VO a cada 24h.
Clorambucil (Leukeran)	Agente citotóxico. Age de maneira similar à ciclofosfamida (agente alquilante). Utilizado no tratamento de diversos tumores e na terapia imunossupressora.	É possível que haja mielossupressão. Não há cistite com o uso de clorambucil, como ocorre na utilização da ciclofosfamida.	Consultar um protocolo de drogas antineoplásicas para esquemas específicos.	Comprimidos com 2 mg.	Cães: 2-6 mg/m² VO a cada 24h inicialmente; depois, a cada 48h. Gatos: 0,1-0,2 mg/kg VO a cada 24h inicialmente; depois, a cada 48h.
Cloranfenicol e cloranfenicol, palmitato (Chloromycetin, formulações genéricas)	Droga antibacteriana que inibe a síntese de proteínas mediante a ligação ao ribossomo. Possui amplo espectro de ação.	Em doses altas ou tratamentos prolongados, pode ocorrer supressão da medula óssea (especialmente em gatos). Evitar o uso em animais prenhes ou neonatos. A sua interação com outras drogas (como barbitúricos) é possível porque o cloranfenicol inibirá as enzimas microssomais hepáticas.	O palmitato de cloranfenicol requer enzimas ativas e não deve ser administrado a animais em jejum (ou anoréxicos). Nota: algumas formulações de cloranfenicol não estão mais disponíveis nos EUA.	Suspensão oral (palmitato) com 30 mg/mL, cápsulas com 250 mg e comprimidos com 100, 250 e 500 mg.	Cães: 50 mg/kg VO a cada 8h. Gatos: 50 mg/gato VO a cada 12h ou 12,5-20 mg/kg VO a cada 12h.

Formulário de Medicamentos para Consulta em 5 Minutos

Nome do Princípio Ativo (Comercial e Outros Nomes)	Farmacologia e Indicações	Efeitos Colaterais e Precauções	Informações de Dosagem e Comentários	Formulações	Dosagem (Exceto em Casos Indicados, a Dosagem é a Mesma para Cães e Gatos)
Clorazepato, dipotássio (Tranxene)	Benzodiazepínico. Sua ação é aumentar os efeitos inibitórios do GABA no SNC. Usado pela ação anticonvulsivante, sedativa e no tratamento de alguns distúrbios comportamentais.	Os efeitos colaterais incluem sedação e polifagia. Alguns animais podem desenvolver excitação paradoxal.	As doses estão baseadas principalmente em relatos da medicina humana, no empirismo ou estudos experimentais. Não foram relatados estudos de eficácia clínica em cães e gatos. Os comprimidos de clorazepato são degradados rapidamente na presença de luz, calor ou umidade. Manter nas embalagens originais ou em frascos fortemente fechados.	Comprimidos com 3,75; 7,5; 11,25; 15 e 22,5 mg.	Cães: 0,5-2 mg/kg VO a cada 8-12h, mas tão frequentemente como a cada 4h. Gatos: 0,2-0,4 mg/kg VO a cada 12-24h (até 0,5-2 mg/kg).
Cloreto de oxibutinina (Ditropan)	Agente anticolinérgico. Inibe os espasmos da musculatura lisa, ao bloquear a ação da acetilcolina. Uso principalmente para aumentar a capacidade da bexiga e diminuir os espasmos do trato urinário.	Os efeitos adversos estão ligados aos efeitos anticolinérgicos, mas são menos frequentes, em comparação com outros agentes anticolinérgicos. Em caso de overdose, administrar fisostigmina.	Não foram publicados resultados de estudos clínicos em animais. O uso (e doses) em animais se baseia na experiência em humanos ou em experiências anedóticas em animais.	Comprimidos de 5 mg.	Cães: 5 mg/cão a cada 6-8h VO, ou 0,2 mg/kg a cada 12h VO.
Cloreto de potássio (genérico)	Suplemento de potássio. Uso no tratamento da hipocalemia. Geralmente adicionado a soluções fluidas.	A toxidez decorrente de elevadas concentrações de potássio pode ser perigosa. Hipercalemia pode levar à toxidez cardiovascular (bradicardia e parada cardíaca) e à astenia muscular. Suplementos orais de potássio podem causar náusea e irritação gástrica.	1 g de cloreto de potássio fornece 13,41 mEq de potássio. Quando o potássio é suplementado em fluidos, não administrar em velocidade superior a 0,5 mEq/kg/h.	Várias concentrações para injeção (geralmente 2 mEq/mL). Suspensão oral e solução oral.	0,5 mEq de potássio/kg/dia, ou suplementar com 10-40 mEq/500 mL de fluidos, dependendo do potássio sérico.
Cloreto de pralidoxima (2-PAM) (Protopam)	Uso no tratamento da toxicose por organofosforado.	Não foram relatados efeitos adversos.	Ao tratar a intoxicação, consultar o centro de controle de venenos, para orientações precisas. Pode ser usado com atropina (0,1 mg/kg).	Injeção: 50 mg/mL.	20 mg/kg até 50 mg/kg a cada 8-12h; dose inicial: IV lenta, ou IM.
Cloreto de sódio a 0,9% (genérico)	Cloreto de sódio é usado para infusão IV, como fluido de reposição.	Não é uma solução eletrolítica balanceada. A infusão prolongada pode causar desequilíbrio eletrolítico.	A velocidade de infusão varia, dependendo das necessidades do paciente.	Infusão: 500, 1000 mL.	15-30 mL/kg/h IV para desidratação moderada.
Cloreto de sódio a 7,2% (genérico) Salina hipertônica	Cloreto de sódio concentrado; uso no tratamento agudo de hipovolemia.	Não é uma solução eletrolítica balanceada. A infusão prolongada pode causar desequilíbrio eletrolítico.	Usa-se salina hipertônica para infusão durante períodos curtos, para reposição rápida do volume vascular.	Solução a 7,2%.	2-8 mL/kg IV (Não administrar em velocidade > 1 mL/kg/min).
Clorfeniramina, maleato (Chlor-Trimeton, Phenetron e outros)	Anti-histamínico (bloqueador de H_1). Bloqueia a ação da histamina nos receptores. Também pode ter ação anti-inflamatória direta. Usada com mais frequência para prevenir reações alérgicas. Empregada para terapia do prurido em cães e gatos.	A sedação é o efeito colateral mais comum. Também são comuns alguns efeitos antimuscarínicos (similares aos da atropina).	A clorfeniramina está incluída como um constituinte em muitas formulações sem prescrição usadas contra tosse/resfriado e alergias.	Comprimidos com 4 e 8 mg.	Cães: 4-8 mg/cão VO a cada 12h (até o máximo de 0,5 mg/kg a cada 12h). Gatos: 2 mg/gato VO a cada 12h.

Formulário de Medicamentos para Consulta em 5 Minutos

Nome do Princípio Ativo (Comercial e Outros Nomes)	Farmacologia e Indicações	Efeitos Colaterais e Precauções	Informações de Dosagem e Comentários	Formulações	Dosagem (Exceto em Casos Indicados, a Dosagem é a Mesma para Cães e Gatos)
Cloridrato de fenilefrina (Neo-Synephrine)	Agonista adrenérgico específico; específico para α1-receptor.	Vasoconstrição e aumento da pressão arterial.	Fenilefrina também é usada como vasoconstritor tópico (p.ex., em descongestionantes nasais).	Injeção: 10 mg/mL; solução nasal a 1%.	0,01 mg/kg a cada 15 min IV; 0,1 mg/kg a cada 15 min IM ou SC.
Cloridrato de fenoxibenzamina (Dibenzyline)	Antagonista α1-adrenérgico. Liga-se ao α1-receptor na musculatura lisa, causando relaxamento. Vasodilatador potente. Uso principalmente no tratamento da vasoconstrição periférica. Em alguns animais, tem sido usado para relaxamento da musculatura lisa uretral.	Causa hipotensão prolongada em animais. Usar com cautela em animais com comprometimento cardiovascular.	Não foram publicados resultados de estudos clínicos em animais. O uso (e doses) em animais se baseia na experiência em humanos ou em limitadas experiências em animais.	Cápsulas de 10 mg.	Cães: 0,25 mg/kg a cada 8-12h, ou 0,5 mg/kg a cada 24h VO. Gatos: 2,5 mg/gato a cada 8-12h, ou 0,5 mg/kg a cada 12h VO. (Em gatos, doses elevadas de até 0,5 mg/kg IV têm sido administradas para relaxamento da musculatura lisa uretral.)
Cloridrato de midazolam (Versed)	Benzodiazepínico. Ação similar à de outros benzodiazepínicos. Uso como adjuvante anestésico. Em comparação com outros benzodiazepínicos, melhor absorção por injeção IM.	Usar com muita cautela pela via IV, especialmente com opiatos. Midazolam IV pode causar depressão cardiorrespiratória.	A experiência clínica se baseia em relatos anedóticos e em estudos experimentais. Em comparação com outros benzodiazepínicos, midazolam pode ser administrado IM.	Injeção: 5 mg/mL.	0,1-0,25 mg/kg IV IM ou infusão IV 0,1-0,3 mg/kg/h. Gatos: (sedação) 0,05 mg/kg IV; (indução) 0,3-0,6 mg/kg IV; combinado com 3 mg/kg de cetamina.
Cloridrato de minociclina (Minocin, Solodyn)	Antibiótico do grupo das tetraciclinas. Similar à doxiciclina.	Não foram relatados efeitos adversos para minociclina. A absorção oral não é afetada por produtos contendo cálcio, como ocorre com outras tetraciclinas.	Não foi relatado o uso clínico, mas as propriedades são similares às da doxiciclina.	Comprimidos de 50, 75 e 100 mg; ou cápsulas; suspensão oral contendo 10 mg/mL.	5-12,5 mg/kg a cada 12h VO.
Cloridrato de mitoxantrona (Novantrone)	Antibiótico antineoplásico. Ação similar à da doxorrubicina. Uso no tratamento da leucemia, linfoma e carcinomas.	Como ocorre com qualquer agente antineoplásico, certos efeitos adversos são previsíveis, inevitáveis e relacionados à ação do agente. Mitroxantona causa mielossupressão, vômito, anorexia e desarranjo GI, mas pode ser menos cardiotóxica do que doxorrubicina.	Geralmente, o uso adequado de mitoxantrona segue um protocolo antineoplásico específico. Consultar o protocolo específico para o regime posológico.	Injeção: 2 mg/mL.	Cães: 5-5,5 mg/m² IV a cada 21 dias. Gatos: 6,0-6,5 mg/m² IV a cada 21 dias.
Cloridrato de oximorfona (Numorphan)	Opioide agonista. A ação é similar à da morfina, exceto que oximorfona é mais lipofílica e 10-15× mais potente do que morfina.	Os mesmos efeitos adversos e precauções para morfina.	Há alguma evidência de que, em comparação com a morfina, oximorfona pode ter menos efeitos cardiovasculares. Tendo em vista que oximorfona é mais lipofílica, é rapidamente absorvida por injeção epidural.	Injeção: 1,5 e 1 mg/mL.	Analgesia: 0,1-0,2 mg/kg IV, SC, IM (conforme a necessidade), redosagem com 0,05-0,1 mg/kg a cada 1-2h. Pré-anestésico: 0,025-0,05 mg/kg IM ou SC. Sedação: 0,05-0,02 mg/kg IM, SC (com ou sem acepromazina).
Cloridrato de propiopromazina (Tranvet)	Sedativo fenotiazínico. Também tem ações antieméticas e anti-histamínicas.	Os efeitos adversos e as precauções são similares aos de outros fenotiazínicos, como a acepromazina.	Ainda não foram publicados resultados de estudos clínicos em animais. O uso (e doses) em animais se baseia na experiência em humanos ou em experiências anedóticas em animais. Não confundir esse medicamento com propiomazina (Largon), que é um medicamento humano já recolhido do mercado.	Injeção: 5-10 mg/mL, ou comprimido mastigável: 20 mg.	1,1-4,4 mg/kg a cada 12-24h VO. 0,1-1,1 mg/kg IV, IM (a dose dependerá do grau de sedação necessário).

Formulário de Medicamentos para Consulta em 5 Minutos

Nome do Princípio Ativo (Comercial e Outros Nomes)	Farmacologia e Indicações	Efeitos Colaterais e Precauções	Informações de Dosagem e Comentários	Formulações	Dosagem (Exceto em Casos Indicados, a Dosagem é a Mesma para Cães e Gatos)
Cloridrato de propranolol (Inderal)	Bloqueador β-adrenérgico. Não seletivo para receptores β1- e β2-adrenérgicos. Antiarrítmico Classe II. Uso principalmente na redução da frequência cardíaca, condução cardíaca, taquiarritmia e pressão arterial.	Efeitos adversos ligados aos efeitos β1-bloqueadores no coração. Causa depressão cardíaca, diminui o débito cardíaco. Os efeitos β2-bloqueadores podem causar broncoconstrição. Diminui a secreção de insulina.	Geralmente, a dose é titulada de acordo com a resposta do paciente. Começar com dose baixa e aumentar gradativamente, até que seja obtido o efeito desejado. A liberação depende do fluxo sanguíneo hepático; usar com cautela em animais com comprometimento da perfusão hepática.	Comprimidos de 10, 20, 40, 60, 80 e 90 mg; injeção: 1 mg/mL; solução oral: 4 e 8 mg/mL.	Cães: 20-60 mcg/kg IV ao longo de 5-10 min; 0,2-1 mg/kg VO a cada 8h (titular a dose até o efeito desejado). Gatos: 0,4-1,2 mg/kg (2,5-5 mg/gato) VO a cada 8h.
Cloridrato de pseudoefedrina (Sudafed e muitos outros [algumas formulações têm outros ingredientes])	Agonista adrenérgico. Em termos de ação, similar à efedrina e fenilpropanolamina. Uso para aumento da resistência periférica, como descongestionante e em animais para tratamento da incontinência urinária.	Seus efeitos adversos são atribuídos aos efeitos adrenérgicos (excitação, frequência cardíaca rápida, arritmias).	Embora não tenham sido realizados estudos clínicos para comparação, acredita-se que a ação e a eficácia da pseudoefedrina sejam similares às da efedrina e fenilpropanolamina.	Comprimidos de 30, 60 mg; cápsulas de 120 mg; xarope contendo 6 mg/mL. Quase todas as formulações deixaram de ser comercializadas para humanos, por causa do risco de desvio para fabricação de metanfetamina.	Cães: 0,2-0,4 mg/kg (ou 15-60 mg/cão) a cada 8-12h VO.
Cloridrato de ranitidina (Zantac)	Antagonista da histamina (H_2). O mesmo que cimetidina, exceto que é 4-10× mais potente e tem ação mais prolongada.	Em comparação com cimetidina, ranitidina pode ter menos efeitos na função endócrina e nas interações farmacológicas.	As informações farmacocinéticas em cães sugerem que ranitidina pode ser administrada com menor frequência do que cimetidina, para que seja obtida a supressão contínua da secreção de ácido gástrico. Ranitidina pode estimular o esvaziamento gástrico e a motilidade colônica, via ação anticolinesterásica.	Comprimidos de 75, 150, 300 mg; cápsulas de 150, 300 mg; injeção: 25 mg/mL.	Cães: 2 mg/kg a cada 8h IV, VO. Gatos: 2,5 mg/kg a cada 12h IV; 3,5 mg/kg a cada 12h VO.
Cloridrato de sotalol (Betapace)	Bloqueador β-(β1 e β2) adrenérgico inespecífico (antiarrítmico Classe II). Ação similar à do propranolol (1/3 da potência); mas seus efeitos benéficos podem ser decorrentes mais dos outros efeitos antiarrítmicos. Além de ser um medicamento antiarrítmico Classe II, sotalol pode ter alguma atividade de Classe III (bloqueio dos canais de potássio).	Não foram relatados efeitos adversos em animais, mas espera-se que sejam similares aos causados pelo propranolol. Como muitos antiarrítmicos, esse agente pode ter alguma atividade proarrítmica. Efeitos inotrópicos negativos podem provocar certa preocupação em alguns animais com fraca contratilidade.	Este pode ser um agente de manutenção mais efetivo, em comparação com outros agentes, para o controle das arritmias.	Comprimidos de 80, 160, 240 mg.	1-2 mg/kg a cada 12h VO (cães de porte médio, começar com 40 mg/cão; em seguida, aumentar para 80 mg, em caso de necessidade).
Cloridrato de terbinafina (Lamisil)	Medicamento antifúngico, efetivo contra dermatófitos e *Malassezia*.	Vômito e anorexia. É possível que ocorra hepatotoxidez, mas essa ocorrência não foi relatada em animais.	As doses usadas em cães e gatos são muito maiores do que as usadas em humanos.	Comprimidos de 250 mg; solução tópica a 1%; creme tópico a 1%.	Cães: 30-40 mg/kg VO (com o alimento) a cada 24h durante 3 semanas. Gatos: 30-40 mg/kg VO a cada 24h durante pelo menos 2 semanas.
Cloridrato de tocanida (Tonocard)	Medicamento antiarrítmico. Considerado como análogo oral da lidocaína. Antiarrítmico Classe I.	Em cães, foram relatadas anorexia e toxidez GI. Também é possível a ocorrência de arritmias, vômito, ataxia. (Em um estudo, 35% dos cães exibiam efeitos GI.)	Experiência limitada em animais. No entanto, estudos clínicos demonstraram eficácia. As concentrações terapêuticas variam de 6-10 mcg/mL.	Comprimidos de 400, 600 mg.	Cães: 15-20 mg/kg a cada 8h VO. Gatos: não há dose estabelecida.

ESPÉCIES CANINA E FELINA

Formulário de Medicamentos para Consulta em 5 Minutos

Nome do Princípio Ativo (Comercial e Outros Nomes)	Farmacologia e Indicações	Efeitos Colaterais e Precauções	Informações de Dosagem e Comentários	Formulações	Dosagem (Exceto em Casos Indicados, a Dosagem é a Mesma para Cães e Gatos)
Cloridrato de tramadol (Ultram e genérico)	Analgésico. Tramadol exerce certa ação nos μ-receptores opioides, podendo também inibir a recaptação de noradrenalina (NA) e serotonina (5HT). Em comparação com a droga-mãe, o metabólito (desmetiltramadol) pode ter efeitos opioides mais expressivos.	Em alguns animais pode ocorrer sedação, especialmente em doses elevadas. Em tratados com doses muito altas, podem ocorrer convulsões.	As informações sobre doses se baseiam em estudos experimentais em cães e em derivações da experiência clínica em cães. Comprimidos de liberação estendida não são equivalentes. Estudos de eficácia em cães e gatos tiveram resultados inconsistentes. Pode ser usado com AINE, outros analgésicos e anestésicos.	Tramadol de liberação imediata está disponível em comprimidos de 50 mg.	Cães: 5 mg/kg a cada 6-8h VO. Gatos: começar com 2 mg/kg e aumentar até 4 mg/kg a cada 8-12h VO (desagradável ao paladar para gatos).
Cloridrato de trazodona (Desyrel)	Ansiolítico. Ação: altera a ação e recaptação da serotonina na sinapse. Uso como sedativo, hipnótico e ansiolítico.	Causa sedação em doses elevadas. Alta margem de segurança.	Administrar pelo menos 1 hora antes do evento deflagrador da ansiedade.	Comprimidos de 50, 100 e 300 mg.	Cães: 2-5 mg/kg VO a cada 8-24 h, ou conforme a necessidade. Gatos: não há dose disponível.
Cloridrato de trientina (Syprine)	Agente quelante. Uso na quelação do cobre, quando penicilamina não pode ser tolerada pelo paciente.	Não foram relatados efeitos adversos em animais.	Uso apenas em pacientes que não podem tolerar a penicilamina. Geralmente induz menos cuprurese do que a penicilamina.	Cápsulas de 250 mg.	10-15 mg/kg a cada 12h VO.
Cloridrato de triflupromazina (Vesprin)	Fenotiazina. Ação similar às demais fenotiazinas, exceto que triflupromazina pode ter uma atividade antimuscarínica mais vigorosa, em comparação com outras fenotiazinas. Usado por sua ação antiemética.	Não foram relatados efeitos adversos em animais. Entre os efeitos adversos, há efeitos anticolinérgicos.	O mesmo que para outras fenotiazinas.	Injeção: 10, 20 mg/mL.	0,1-0,3 mg/kg IM, VO a cada 8-12h.
Cloridrato de verapamil (Calan, Isoptin)	Medicamento bloqueador dos canais de cálcio, do grupo das não di-hidropiridinas. Bloqueia o ingresso do cálcio nas células mediante o bloqueio dos canais lentos. Promove vasodilatação, efeitos cronotrópicos negativos.	Hipotensão, depressão cardíaca, bradicardia, bloqueio AV. Pode causar anorexia em alguns pacientes.	Deve-se preferir diltiazem em lugar de verapamil em pacientes com insuficiência cardíaca, por causa da menor supressão cardíaca. A formulação oral não é suficientemente absorvida (estereoisômero ativo) para que sejam conseguidos efeitos adequados.	Comprimidos de 40, 80, 120 mg; injeção: 2,5 mg/mL.	Cães: 0,05 mg/kg a cada 10-30 min IV (dose máxima cumulativa = 0,15 mg/kg); a dose oral não foi estabelecida.
Cloridrato de xilazina (Rompun e genérico)	Agonista α2-adrenérgico. Uso principalmente para analgesia e anestesia de curta duração.	Causa sedação e ataxia. Com o uso de doses elevadas, é possível que ocorram depressão cardíaca, bloqueio cardíaco e hipotensão. Causa êmese após injeção IV, especialmente em gatos.	Frequentemente usado em combinação com outros medicamentos, por exemplo, cetamina.	Injeção: 20 e 100 mg/mL.	Cães: 1,1 mg/kg IV; 2,2 mg/kg IM. Gatos: 1,1 mg/kg IM (a dose emética [apenas para gatos] é 0,4-0,5 mg/kg IV).
Clorotiazida (Diuril)	Diurético tiazídico. Inibe a reabsorção de sódio nos túbulos renais distais. Usada como diurético e anti-hipertensivo. Como diminui a excreção renal de cálcio, também tem sido utilizada para tratar condições com urólitos constituídos por cálcio.	Não usar em pacientes com cálcio elevado. Pode causar desequilíbrio eletrolítico, como hipocalemia.	Não é tão eficaz como diurético de alça (como a furosemida).	Comprimidos com 250 e 500 mg, suspensão oral e formulação injetável com 50 mg/mL.	20-40 mg/kg PO, IV a cada 12h.

Formulário de Medicamentos para Consulta em 5 Minutos

Nome do Princípio Ativo (Comercial e Outros Nomes)	Farmacologia e Indicações	Efeitos Colaterais e Precauções	Informações de Dosagem e Comentários	Formulações	Dosagem (Exceto em Casos Indicados, a Dosagem é a Mesma para Cães e Gatos)
Clorpromazina (Thorazine)	Tranquilizante e antiemético fenotiazínico. Inibe a ação da dopamina como neurotransmissor. É mais usada como antiemético central. Também é utilizada para sedação e com fins pré-anestésicos.	Causa sedação. Pode causar o bloqueio de receptores α-adrenérgicos. Em alguns indivíduos produz efeitos colaterais extrapiramidais.	Usada em casos de vômito provocado por toxinas, drogas ou doença intestinal. Doses mais altas que as listadas na seção de dosagens têm sido usadas com quimioterapia (2 mg/kg SC a cada 3h).	Solução injetável com 25 mg/mL.	Cães: 0,5 mg/kg IM, SC a cada 6-8h. Gatos: 0,2-0,4 mg/kg IM, SC a cada 6-8h.
Closilato de tênio (Canopar)	Agente antiparasitário. Uso no tratamento dos ancilostomídeos (*Ancylostoma* e *Uncinaria*).	Se o revestimento for violado, o comprimido terá sabor amargo. Ocasionalmente, pode causar vômito em seguida à administração oral.	Basicamente, as doses seguem as recomendações do fabricante.	Comprimidos de 500 mg.	Cães > 4,5 kg: 500 mg VO 1 vez, repetir em 2-3 semanas; 2,5-4,5 kg: 250 mg a cada 12h para 1 dia, repetir em 2-3 semanas.
Cloxacilina sódica (Cloxapen, Orbenin, Tegopen)	Antibiótico β-lactâmico. Inibe a síntese de parede da célula bacteriana. O espectro é limitado para bactérias Gram-positivas, especialmente estafilococos.	Usar com cautela em animais alérgicos às drogas similares à penicilina.	As doses estão baseadas em empirismo ou extrapolação de estudos em humanos. Não foram relatados estudos de eficácia clínica em cães e gatos. A absorção oral é fraca; se possível, administrar com estômago vazio.	Cápsulas com 250 e 500 mg; solução oral com 25 mg/mL.	20-40 mg/kg VO a cada 8h.
Codeína (formulação genérica)	Agonista opioide. O mecanismo é similar ao da morfina, exceto pela potência, que equivale a 1/10 da morfina. Fracamente absorvida em cães.	O efeito colateral principal é a sedação.	Disponível como comprimidos de fosfato ou sulfato de codeína. As doses relatadas para analgesia são consideradas doses iniciais. Pacientes isolados podem necessitar de doses maiores, dependendo do grau de tolerância ou do limiar da dor.	Comprimidos com 15, 30 e 60 mg; xarope com 5 mg/mL; solução oral com 3 mg/mL.	Cães: (analgesia) 0,5-1 mg/kg VO a cada 4-6h; (antitussígeno) 0,1-0,3 mg/kg VO a cada 4-6h. Gatos: (analgesia) 0,5 mg/kg VO a cada 6h; (antitussígeno) 0,1 mg/kg VO a cada 6h.
Colchicina (formulação genérica)	Agente anti-inflamatório. Usada principalmente para tratar gota. Em animais, é empregada para reduzir a fibrose e o desenvolvimento de insuficiência hepática (possivelmente por meio da inibição da formação de colágeno).	Não administrar em animais prenhes. Os efeitos colaterais em animais não estão bem documentados. Esta droga pode causar dermatite em seres humanos.	As doses estão baseadas em empirismo. Não foram relatados estudos de eficácia clínica em animais.	Comprimidos com 600 mcg.	0,01-0,03 mg/kg VO a cada 24h.
Corticotropina (ACTH) (Acthar)	Usada para propósitos diagnósticos na avaliação da função da glândula adrenal. Estimula a síntese normal de cortisol pela glândula adrenal.	Efeitos colaterais são improváveis quando utilizada para fins diagnósticos em aplicação única.	Dosagens estabelecidas pela mensuração da resposta adrenal normal em animais.	Gel com 80 U/mL.	Teste de resposta: coletar amostra pré-ACTH e aplicar, por via IM, 2,2 UI/kg. Coletar a amostra pós-ACTH após 2h em cães e após 1 e 2h em gatos.
Cosintropina (Cortrosyn)	A cosintropina é uma forma sintética da corticotropina (ACTH) usada apenas para fins diagnósticos. Em seres humanos é preferida à corticotropina por ser menos alergênica.	Similar à corticotropina.	Uso apenas para fins diagnósticos; não deve ser utilizada para o tratamento do hipoadrenocorticismo. A dose máxima para cães deve ser de 250 mcg. Preparações congeladas podem ser estocadas por até seis meses.	Frascos com 250 mcg.	Teste de resposta ao ACTH: colher amostras pré-ACTH e aplicar 5 mcg/kg IV ou IM (cães) ou 125 mcg (0,125 mg) IM (gatos). Gatos: colher amostras aos 60 e 90 minutos após a administração IV e 30 e 60 minutos após a administração IM. Cães: colher amostras pós-ACTH aos 30 e 60 minutos.

Formulário de Medicamentos para Consulta em 5 Minutos

Nome do Princípio Ativo (Comercial e Outros Nomes)	Farmacologia e Indicações	Efeitos Colaterais e Precauções	Informações de Dosagem e Comentários	Formulações	Dosagem (Exceto em Casos Indicados, a Dosagem é a Mesma para Cães e Gatos)
Dacarbazina (DTIC)	Agente antineoplásico. Agente alquilante monofuncional. Usado no tratamento de melanoma.	Leucopenia, náusea, vômito, diarreia. Não usar em gatos.	Consultar protocolos antineoplásicos para esquemas específicos.	Frasco para injeção com 200 mg.	Cães: 200 mg/m² IV por cinco dias a cada três semanas; ou 800-1.000 mg/m² IV a cada três semanas.
Dalteparina, sódica (Fragmin)	Heparina de baixo peso molecular (LMWH); anticoagulante indicado para a prevenção de tromboembolismo em pacientes de alto risco. Relação anti-Xa:anti IIa de 2,7:1.	Pode aumentar o risco de hemorragias.	Quando a dalteparina for utilizada nas doses recomendadas, não há necessidade de monitorar os tempos de coagulação da mesma forma que na administração de heparina convencional (não fracionada). As dosagens extrapoladas de seres humanos não se aplicam para cães e gatos.	Seringas pré-montadas para aplicação injetável, com 16 mg (2.500 U)/0,2 mL; 32 mg (5.000 U)/0,2 mL; frascos com doses múltiplas para aplicação injetável, com 64 mg (10.000 U)/mL.	Cães: 150 U/kg SC a cada 8h. Gatos: 180 U/kg SC a cada 6h.
Danazol (Danocrine)	Inibidor de gonadotropina. Inibe a síntese de hormônio luteinizante (LH), hormônio foliculoestimulante (FSH) e estrógeno. Usado no tratamento da endometriose em seres humanos. Pode reduzir a destruição de plaquetas ou hemácias em doenças imunomediadas.	Pode causar sinais similares aos de outras drogas androgênicas. Não foram relatados efeitos colaterais em animais.	Quando usado para tratar doenças autoimunes, normalmente é utilizada em conjunto com outras drogas (p. ex.: corticosteroides). A eficácia não foi avaliada.	Cápsulas com 50, 100 e 200 mg.	5-10 mg/kg VO a cada 12h.
Dantrolene, sódico (Dantrium)	Relaxante muscular. Inibe a liberação de cálcio no retículo sarcoplasmático. Adicionalmente ao relaxamento muscular, é utilizado na hipertermia maligna. Também é usado para relaxar a musculatura uretral em gatos.	Relaxantes musculares podem causar fraqueza em alguns animais.	As dosagens são principalmente extrapoladas de estudos experimentais ou com seres humanos. Não há nenhum ensaio clínico disponível em medicina veterinária. Os estudos em que a musculatura uretral de gatos foi relaxada utilizaram 1 mg/kg IV.	Cápsulas com 100 mg e injetável com 0,33 mg/mL.	Para a prevenção da hipertermia maligna: 2-3 mg/kg IV. Para relaxamento muscular: Cães: 1-5 mg/kg VO a cada 8h. Gatos: 0,5-2,0 mg/kg VO a cada 12h.
Dapsona (formulações genéricas)	Droga antimicrobiana usada principalmente no tratamento de micobacterioses. Pode exercer alguma propriedade imunossupressora ou inibir a ação das células inflamatórias. Usada principalmente em doenças dermatológicas de cães e gatos.	Podem ocorrer hepatite e discrasia sanguínea. Reações dermatológicas tóxicas foram relatadas em seres humanos. *Interação de drogas:* não administrar com trimetoprima (pode aumentar as concentrações sanguíneas). Não administrar em gatos.	As doses são derivadas da extrapolação de seres humanos ou de empirismo. Não foram realizados estudos clínicos bem controlados em medicina veterinária.	Comprimidos com 25 e 100 mg.	Cães: 1,1 mg/kg VO a cada 8-12h. Gatos: não usar.
Decanoato de nandrolona (Deca-Durabolin)	Esteroide anabólico. Derivado da testosterona. Agentes anabólitos são planejados para maximizar os efeitos anabólicos, ao mesmo tempo que minimizam a ação androgênica. Agentes anabólicos têm sido usados para reversão de problemas catabólicos, aumento do ganho de peso, aumento da massa muscular em animais e estimulação da eritropoiese.	Os efeitos adversos dos esteroides anabólicos podem ser atribuídos à ação farmacológica desses agentes. É comum um aumento nos efeitos masculinizantes. Em humanos, foi descrito aumento na incidência de alguns tumores.	Ainda não foram publicados resultados de estudos clínicos em animais. O uso (e doses) em animais se baseia na experiência em humanos ou em experiências anedóticas em animais.	Injeção: 50, 100, 200 mg/mL.	Cães: 1-1,5 mg/kg/semana IM. Gatos: 1 mg/kg/semana IM.

Formulário de Medicamentos para Consulta em 5 Minutos

Nome do Princípio Ativo (Comercial e Outros Nomes)	Farmacologia e Indicações	Efeitos Colaterais e Precauções	Informações de Dosagem e Comentários	Formulações	Dosagem (Exceto em Casos Indicados, a Dosagem é a Mesma para Cães e Gatos)
Deferoxamina, mesilato (Desferal)	Agente quelante com grande afinidade por íons trivalentes. Usada para tratar intoxicação aguda por ferro. Indicada em casos de envenenamento grave. A deferoxamina também é utilizada para quelar alumínio e facilitar a sua remoção.	Efeitos colaterais não foram relatados em animais. As reações alérgicas e os problemas de audição ocorreram em seres humanos.	100 mg de deferoxamina quelam 8,5 mg de íon férrico. Monitorar as concentrações séricas de íons. Monitorar as concentrações séricas do íon férrico para determinar a gravidade da intoxicação e o sucesso da terapia. Consultar o Centro de Controle de Intoxicações local para aconselhamento. A terapia bem-sucedida é indicada pela avaliação da coloração da urina (coloração laranja-rosada da urina indica que o ferro quelado está sendo eliminado).	Injetável, frasco com 500 mg.	10 mg/kg IV, IM a cada 2h por duas doses, depois 10 mg/kg a cada 8h por 24h.
Deprenil (L-deprenil)	Ver Selegilina.				
Deracoxibe (Deramaxx)	AINE da classe dos coxibes; alta relação inibitória COX-1:COX-2 *in vitro*. Indicada para o controle da dor e inflamação pós--operatórias associadas com cirurgias ortopédicas e dor e inflamação relacionadas à osteoartrite.	Os efeitos colaterais mais comuns observados nos ensaios clínicos foram GI (vômito e diarreia). Em estudos controlados com doses acima de 25 mg/kg, ocorreram perda de peso corporal, melena e vômito.	As doses recomendadas são para cães que pesam acima de 1,8 kg (4 lb). Não foi estabelecida a margem de segurança para cães abaixo de 4 meses de idade, reprodutores, prenhes ou lactantes, ou mesmo para gatos.	Comprimidos com 25 e 100 mg; comprimidos mastigáveis.	Cães (dor pós-operatória): 3-4 mg/kg VO a cada 24h, se necessário por até sete dias. Cães (osteoartrite): 1-2 mg VO a cada 24h, em tratamento contínuo por mais de sete dias. Gatos: 1 mg/kg VO em dose única.
DES	Ver Dietilestilbestrol.				
Desmopressina, acetato (DDAVP)	Peptídeo sintético similar ao hormônio antidiurético (ADH). Usada como terapia de reposição em pacientes com diabetes insípido. A desmopressina também tem sido usada para o tratamento de pacientes com doença de von Willebrand leve a moderada no momento pré-cirúrgico ou em outro procedimento que possa causar hemorragia.	Nenhum efeito colateral relatado. Em seres humanos, raramente causa eventos trombóticos.	A desmopressina é usada apenas para o diabetes insípido central. A duração do efeito é variável (8-20h). Ela é ineficaz no tratamento do diabetes insípido nefrogênico ou da poliúria de outras causas. O produto de uso intranasal é administrado como colírio oftálmico em cães. O início dos efeitos situa-se em 1h.	Injetável com 4 mcg/mL e solução de acetato de desmopressina nasal com 100 mcg/mL (0,01%) na forma de *spray* graduado. Comprimidos com 0,1 e 0,2 mg.	Diabetes insípido: 2-4 gotas (2 mcg) por via intranasal ou oftálmica a cada 12-24h; depois 0,05-0,1 mg VO a cada 12h, quando necessário. No tratamento da doença de von Willebrand: 1 mcg/kg (0,01 mL/kg) SC, IV diluído em 20 mL de solução salina, administrada durante 10 minutos ou mais.
Desoxicorticosterona, pivalato (Percorten-V, DOCP ou pivalato de DOCA)	Mineralocorticoide. Usado no tratamento da insuficiência adrenocortical (hipoadrenocorticismo). Não possui atividade glicocorticoide.	Em altas doses, possui efeito mineralocorticoide excessivo.	A dose inicial é baseada nos estudos realizados em pacientes clínicos. Dosagens individuais podem se basear na monitoração de eletrólitos em pacientes. O atual intervalo entre doses pode variar de 14-35 dias.	Injetável com 25 mg/mL.	1,5-2,2 mg/kg IM a cada 25 dias.

ESPÉCIES CANINA E FELINA

Formulário de Medicamentos para Consulta em 5 Minutos

Nome do Princípio Ativo (Comercial e Outros Nomes)	Farmacologia e Indicações	Efeitos Colaterais e Precauções	Informações de Dosagem e Comentários	Formulações	Dosagem (Exceto em Casos Indicados, a Dosagem é a Mesma para Cães e Gatos)
Dexametasona (solução de dexametasona e fosfato sódico de dexametasona) (Azium, Decaject SP, Dexavet e Dexasone. Comprimidos incluindo Decadron e formulações genéricas)	Corticosteroide. A dexametasona possui uma potência aproximadamente 30 vezes maior que o cortisol. Exerce múltiplos efeitos anti-inflamatórios.	Os corticosteroides produzem efeitos colaterais sistêmicos diversos, como os advindos da terapia crônica.	As doses são baseadas na gravidade da doença subjacente. A dexametasona é usada para testes de hiperadrenocorticismo. Teste de supressão de baixa dose de dexametasona: cães 0,01 mg/kg IV, gatos 0,1 mg/kg IV, colhendo amostras nos tempos 0, 4 e 8 horas pós-administração. Para o teste de supressão de alta dose de dexametasona: cães 0,1 mg/kg, gatos 1,0 mg/kg.	Azium solução, 2 mg/mL. As formas de fosfato sódico contêm 3,33 mg/mL. Comprimidos com 0,25; 0,5; 0,75; 1; 1,5; 2; 4 e 6 mg.	Anti-inflamatório: 0,07-0,15 mg/kg IV, IM, PO a cada 12-24h; 21-isonicotinato de dexametasona 0,03-0,05 mg/kg IM.
Dexmedetomidina (Dexdomitor)	Agonista alfa-2; similar à medetomidina, exceto por ser mais específica em virtude de sua atividade isomérica. Usada para sedação, analgesia e anestesia; pode ser utilizada com outros sedativos e anestésicos.	Pode ocorrer vômito. Usar com cautela em animais com doença cardíaca.	As doses podem variar dependendo do grau de sedação desejado. A reversão deve ser feita com o mesmo volume de atipamezol (Antisedan).	Injetável com 0,5 mg/mL.	Cães: 125 mcg/m^2 IM (3-9 mcg/kg), 375 mcg/m^2 IV ou 500 mcg/m^2 IM para anestesia profunda. Gatos: 40 mcg/kg IM, reduzindo as doses para 10 mcg/kg para sedação de curta ação.
Dextran (Dextran 70, Gentran 70)	Coloide sintético utilizado para expansão de volume. Fluido de reposição de alto peso molecular. Principalmente usado para hipovolemia aguda e choque.	O uso é limitado apenas para a medicina veterinária e efeitos colaterais não foram relatados. Em seres humanos, as coagulopatias podem ocorrer em função da redução da função plaquetária. Também pode ocorrer choque anafilático.	Utilizado principalmente em situações críticas. Administrado lentamente e por taxa de infusão lenta. Monitorar cuidadosamente o estado cardiorrespiratório do paciente durante a administração.	Solução injetável com 250, 500 e 1.000 mL.	Cães: 10-20 mL/kg IV em um período de 30-60 minutos. Gatos: 5-10 mL/kg IV por pelo menos 30 minutos.
Dextrometorfano (Benylin e outros)	Droga antitussígena de ação central. Apresenta estrutura química similar à dos opioides, mas não afeta os receptores opioides. Parece afetar diretamente os receptores da tosse.	Os efeitos colaterais não foram descritos em medicina veterinária. A superdosagem pode causar sedação.	Muitas preparações sem prescrição médica podem conter outros ingredientes (p. ex.: anti-histamínicos, descongestionantes e paracetamol). Dextrometorfano não é absorvido oralmente em cães.	Disponível na forma de xarope, cápsula e comprimido. Diversos produtos em preparações sem prescrição médica.	Já foram relatadas doses de 0,5-2,0 mg/kg VO a cada 6-8h, porém, a dose efetiva ainda não foi estabelecida.
Dextrose, solução 5% (D-5-W)	Açúcar adicionado aos fluidos de administração intravenosa. Isotônica.	Em altas doses produz edema pulmonar.	Comumente utilizada como solução intravenosa em velocidade de administração constante. Não é uma solução de manutenção.	Fluido de administração intravenosa.	40-50 mL/kg IV a cada 24h.

Formulário de Medicamentos para Consulta em 5 Minutos

Nome do Princípio Ativo (Comercial e Outros Nomes)	Farmacologia e Indicações	Efeitos Colaterais e Precauções	Informações de Dosagem e Comentários	Formulações	Dosagem (Exceto em Casos Indicados, a Dosagem é a Mesma para Cães e Gatos)
Diazepam (Valium e formulações genéricas)	Benzodiazepínico. Depressor com ação no SNC. O mecanismo de ação parece estar relacionado com a potencialização dos efeitos mediados pelos receptores GABA no SNC. Usado para sedação, coadjuvante anestésico, anticon--vulsivante e em distúrbios do comportamento. O diazepam é metabolizado em desmetildiazepam (nordiazepam) e oxazepam.	A sedação é o efeito colateral mais comum. Em alguns cães pode ocorrer excitação paradoxal. Causa polifagia. Em gatos tem sido relatada necrose hepática idiopática fatal.	A distribuição em cães é muitas vezes mais rápida que em seres humanos (a meia-vida em cães é de 1h), requerendo administrações frequentes. Para o tratamento do *status epilepticus*, pode ser administrado por via IV, intranasal ou retal. Evitar a administração IM.	Comprimidos com 2 e 5 mg; solução injetável com 5 mg/mL.	Pré-anestésico: 0,5 mg/kg IV. Estado epiléptico: 0,5 mg/kg IV, 1 mg/kg por via retal; repetir se necessário. Estimulante do apetite (gatos): 0,2 mg/kg IV. Para o tratamento comportamental em gatos: 1-4 mg/gato VO a cada 12-24h.
Diclorvós (Task)	Droga antiparasitária usada principalmente contra nematódeos, ancilostomatídeos e tricurídeos. Mata os parasitos mediante a ação anticolinesterásica.	Não utilizar em pacientes positivos para dirofilariose. As superdosagens podem causar intoxicação por organofosforados. (Tratar com 2-PAM, atropina.)	As doses são baseadas nas recomendações do fabricante.	Comprimidos com 10 e 25 mg.	Cães: 26,4-33 mg/kg VO. Gatos: 11 mg/kg VO.
Dicloxacilina, sódica (Dynapen)	Antibiótico β-lactâmico. Inibe a síntese da parede celular bacteriana. O espectro de ação é limitado a bactérias Gram-positivas, principalmente estafilococos.	Usar com cautela em animais alérgicos a drogas similares às penicilinas.	Não há estudo sobre a sua eficácia clínica em cães e gatos. Em cães, a absorção oral é muito baixa e pode não ser adequada para a terapia. Administrar com o estômago vazio, se possível.	Cápsulas com 125, 250 e 500 mg; suspensão oral com 12,5 mg/mL.	11-55 mg/kg VO a cada 8h.
Dietilcarbamazina (DEC) (Caricide, Filaribits)	Preventivo contra dirofilariose, mas não mais utilizada comumente.	Segura em todas as espécies. Reações podem ocorrer em animais que são positivos para microfilárias.	As doses seguem as recomendações do fabricante. Os protocolos específicos de adminis--tração na dirofilariose podem ser baseados na região do país.	Comprimidos mastigáveis com 50, 60, 180, 200 e 400 mg. Muitas formulações foram retiradas de circulação.	Profilaxia da dirofilariose: 6,6 mg/kg VO a cada 24h.
Dietilestilbestrol (DES)	Composto estrogênico sintético. Usado para a reposição de estrógeno em animais. O DES é mais comumente utilizado para tratar a incontinência responsiva ao estrógeno em cães. Também é usado para induzir abortamento em cadelas.	Os efeitos colaterais que podem ocorrer são causados pelo excesso de estrógeno. A terapia estrogênica pode aumentar o risco de desenvolvimento de piometra e neoplasias responsivas ao estrógeno.	As doses listadas são para o tratamento da incontinência urinária e variam dependendo da resposta. Determinar a dose do paciente de forma individual. Ainda que seja usado para induzir o abortamento, *não* foi eficaz em um estudo em que se administrou 75 mcg/kg.	Comprimidos com 1 e 5 mg; solução injetável com 50 mg/mL (não mais produzida nos EUA, mas disponível em farmácias de manipulação).	Cães: 0,1-1,0 mg/cão VO a cada 24h. Após resposta inicial, reduzir a frequência para 2-3 vezes por semana. Gatos: 0,05-0,1 mg/gato VO a cada 24h.
Difenidramina, cloridrato (Benadryl)	Anti-histamínico usado para tratamento da alergia e como antiemético.	O efeito colateral principal é a sedação.	Anti-histamínico usado principalmente para doenças alérgicas em animais.	Formulações sem prescrição estão disponíveis; elixir com 2,5 mg/mL; cápsulas e comprimidos com 25 e 50 mg; injetável com 50 mg/mL.	Cães: 25-50 mg/cão IV, IM, VO a cada 8h. Gatos: 2-4 mg/kg VO a cada 6-8h ou 1 mg/kg IM, IV a cada 6-8h.
Difenilidantoína	Ver Fenitoína.	-	-	-	-
Difenoxilato (Lomotil)	Agonista opioide. Estimula a segmentação da musculatura lisa no intestino, bem como a absorção de eletrólitos. Usado para o tratamento agudo de diarreia inespecífica.	Os efeitos colaterais não fora relatados em medicina veterinária. O difenoxilato é pobremente absorvido sistemicamente e produz poucos efeitos colaterais. O uso excessivo pode causar constipação.	As doses são baseadas principalmente no empirismo ou extrapoladas de dosagens humanas. Os estudos clínicos não foram realizados em animais. Contém atropina, mas a dose não é alta o bastante para causar efeitos sistêmicos significativos.	Comprimidos com 2,5 mg.	Cães: 0,1-0,2 mg/kg VO a cada 8-12h. Gatos: 0,05-0,1 mg/kg VO a cada 12h.

ESPÉCIES CANINA E FELINA

Formulário de Medicamentos para Consulta em 5 Minutos

Nome do Princípio Ativo (Comercial e Outros Nomes)	Farmacologia e Indicações	Efeitos Colaterais e Precauções	Informações de Dosagem e Comentários	Formulações	Dosagem (Exceto em Casos Indicados, a Dosagem é a Mesma para Cães e Gatos)
Difloxacina, cloridrato (Dicural)	Droga antibacteriana do grupo das fluoroquinolonas. Age por inibição da DNA-girase das bactérias, inibindo a síntese de DNA e RNA. Possui atividade bactericida com amplo espectro de atividade. Usada para uma diversidade de infecções, incluindo as de pele, feridas contaminadas e pneumonia.	Os efeitos colaterais incluem convulsões em animais epilépticos, artropatia em animais jovens e vômito em altas doses. *Interações com outras drogas:* pode aumentar as concentrações de teofilina se utilizada concomitantemente. A administração conjunta com cátions di- e trivalentes (p. ex.: sucralfato) pode diminuir a absorção. A segurança para administração oftálmica não foi estabelecida em gatos.	A variação da dosagem pode ser usada para ajustar a dose, dependendo da gravidade da infecção e sensibilidade da bactéria. A difloxacina é principalmente eliminada nas fezes em vez de na urina (nesta última corresponde a menos que 5% da eliminação). A sarafloxacina é um metabólito desmetil ativo.	Comprimidos com 11,4; 45,4 e 136 mg.	Cães: 5-10 mg/kg VO a cada 24h. Gatos: não foi estabelecida uma dose segura.
Difosfato dissódico de etidronato	Ver Etidronato, dissódico.				
Digoxina (Lanoxin, Cardoxin)	Agente inotrópico cardíaco. Aumenta a contratilidade e diminui a frequência cardíaca. O mecanismo ocorre por inativação da ATPase da bomba de sódio-potássio do músculo cardíaco. Os efeitos benéficos para a insuficiência cardíaca podem ocorrer por meio de efeitos neuroen-dócrinos (altera a sensibilidade dos barorreceptores). Utilizada na insuficiência cardíaca pelos seus efeitos inotró-picos e por reduzir a frequência cardíaca. Usada nas arritmias supraventriculares para diminuir a resposta ventri-cular à estimulação atrial.	Os glicosídeos digitálicos possuem baixo índice terapêutico. Podem causar uma diversidade de arritmias nos pacientes (p. ex.: bloqueio cardíaco, taquicardia ventricular). Provoca vômito, anorexia e diarreia. Os efeitos colaterais são potencializados pela hipocalemia e reduzidos pela hipercalemia. Algumas raças caninas (Doberman Pinscher) e gatos são mais sensíveis aos efeitos colaterais.	Monitorar cuidadosamente os pacientes. A concentração plasmática ótima é de 1-2 ng/mL. Os efeitos colaterais são comuns em doses acima de 3,5 ng/mL Ao calcular a dose, utilizar o peso corporal magro. As doses devem ser 10% mais baixas ao se administrar o elixir em virtude da absorção aumentada.	Comprimidos com 0,0625; 0,125 e 0,25 mg; elixir com 0,05 mg/mL.	Cães: 0,0025-0,005 mg/kg VO a cada 12h. Gatos: 0,008-0,01 mg/kg VO a cada 48h (aproximadamente ¼ de um comprimido de 0,125 mg por gato).
Diltiazem (Cardizem, Dilacor)	Droga bloqueadora dos canais de cálcio. Bloqueia a entrada de cálcio nas células por interrupção dos canais lentos. Produz vasodilatação e efeitos cronotrópicos negativos. Usado para o tratamento das arritmias supraventriculares em cães e da cardiomiopatia hipertrófica em gatos.	Hipotensão, depressão cardíaca, bradicardia e bloqueio AV. Pode causar anorexia em alguns pacientes.	Altas doses de 5 mg/kg VO a cada 8h são utilizadas em alguns cães para o tratamento de fibrilação atrial.	Comprimidos com 30, 60, 90 e 120 mg; injetável com 5 mg/mL; cápsulas de liberação retardada com 60, 90, 120, 180, 240 e 300 mg.	Cães: 0,5-1,5 mg/kg VO a cada 8h; 0,25 mg/kg IV por pelo menos 2 minutos (repetir, se necessário). Gatos: 1,75-2,4 mg/kg VO a cada 8h. Para o Dilacor XR ou o Cardizem CD, a dose é de 10 mg/kg VO diariamente. Em gatos, utilizar tanto o Dilacor XR 30 como o Dilacor XR 60 por animal.
Dimenidrato (Dramamine [Gravol no Canadá])	Droga anti-histamínica. Convertida para dipenidramina. Usada no tratamento antiemético.	O efeito colateral primário é a sedação.	Não há estudos clínicos sobre o uso do dimenidrato. Ele é principalmente usado para o tratamento empírico do vômito.	Comprimidos com 50 mg; injetável com 50 mg/mL.	Cães: 4-8 mg/kg VO, IM, IV a cada 8h. Gatos: 12,5 mg/gato IV, IM, VO a cada 8h.
Dimercaprol (BAL) (BAL em óleo)	Agente quelante, usado para tratar a intoxicação por chumbo, ouro ou arsênico.	Os efeitos colaterais não foram relatados em medicina veterinária. Em seres humanos ocorrem abscessos no local de aplicação. Altas doses causam convulsões, sonolência e vômito.	Utilizar o mais precocemente possível após a exposição à substância tóxica. A alcalinização da urina aumentará a remoção da toxina. Na intoxicação por chumbo, pode ser usada com edetato de cálcio.	Injetável, normalmente preparada por associação.	4 mg/kg IM a cada 4h.
Dinoprost trometamina	Ver Prostaglandina $F_{2\alpha}$.	-	-	-	-

Formulário de Medicamentos para Consulta em 5 Minutos					
Nome do Princípio Ativo (Comercial e Outros Nomes)	Farmacologia e Indicações	Efeitos Colaterais e Precauções	Informações de Dosagem e Comentários	Formulações	Dosagem (Exceto em Casos Indicados, a Dosagem é a Mesma para Cães e Gatos)
Dioctil sulfossucinato de cálcio	Ver Docussato de cálcio.	-	-	-	-
Dioctil sulfossucinato de sódio	Ver Docussato de sódio.	-	-	-	-
Dipiridamol (Persantine)	Inibidor plaquetário. O mecanismo de ação é atribuído aos níveis elevados de monofosfato de adenosina cíclica (AMPc) nas plaquetas, que, por sua vez, reduzem a ativação plaquetária. Indicado para prevenir tromboembolismo.	Não foram relatados efeitos colaterais em animais.	Usado principalmente em seres humanos para prevenir o tromboembolismo. O uso em animais não foi relatado. Quando utilizado em seres humanos, é combinado com outros agentes antitrombóticos (p.ex: varfarina).	Comprimidos com 25, 50 e 75 mg; injetável com 5 mg/mL.	4-10 mg/kg VO a cada 24h.
Dirlotapida (Slentrol)	A dirlotapida é um dos inibidores de proteínas transferidoras de triglicerídeos microssomais (MTP) usadas para tratar a obesidade em cães. Os MTPs bloqueiam o processamento de moléculas de lipídios nos enterócitos. A liberação de lipídios dos enterócitos é bloqueada, causando redução do apetite.	Ela reduz o apetite em todos os cães em que atua de forma eficaz (mecanismo para produzir perda de peso). Foram observados anorexia e vômito em alguns animais. Também é possível a ocorrência de diarreia. As enzimas hepáticas podem se tornar elevadas em alguns cães.	O esquema de dosagem deve ser seguido rigorosamente, sendo necessários um programa de avaliação regular (pesando o cão) e o ajuste da dose em cada visita para uma terapia de sucesso.	Solução oleosa oral com 5 mg/mL.	Cães: iniciar com 0,01 mL/kg/dia VO. Ajustar duplicando a dose em duas semanas. Os ajustes mensais da dose deverão ser feitos com base na perda de peso do animal. Não exceder a dose de 0,2 mL/kg/dia. Gatos: não administrar em gatos.
Disopiramida (Norpace [Rythmodan no Canadá])	Agente antiarrítmico de Classe 1. Deprime a taxa de condução eletrofisiológica do miocárdio.	Os efeitos colaterais não foram relatados em animais. Altas doses podem causar arritmia cardíaca.	Não é utilizada comumente em medicina veterinária. Outras drogas antiarrítmicas são preferenciais.	Cápsulas com 100 e 150 mg (injetável com 10 mg/mL, apenas no Canadá).	Cães: 6-15 mg/kg VO a cada 8h.
Ditiazanina, iodeto (formulação genérica)	Droga microfilaricida para cães. Também eficaz para ancilostomatídeos, nematelmintos e nematoides.	Os efeitos colaterais são raros. Provoca vômito em alguns cães. Causa descoloração das fezes.	Antes da ivermectina e de outras drogas similares, ela era o único agente microfilaricida para cães. Não é mais usada comumente, nem está disponível comercialmente.	Comprimidos com 10, 50, 100 e 200 mg.	Cães: (dirofilariose) 6,6-11 mg/kg a cada 24h por 7-10 dias VO; (outros parasitos) 22 mg/kg VO. Gatos: não há dose estabelecida.
DL-Metionina	Ver Racemetionina.				
Dobutamina, hidrato (Dobutrex)	Agonista adrenérgico. Sua ação principal é estimular o miocárdio por ação nos receptores β-1 cardíacos. Aumenta a contração do coração sem aumentar a sua frequência. Pode ocorrer alguma ação por estimulação de receptores α. Principalmente utilizada para o tratamento da insuficiência cardíaca aguda.	Pode causar taquicardia e arritmias ventriculares quando em altas doses ou em indivíduos sensíveis.	A dobutamina possui uma meia-vida de eliminação rápida (minutos) e, dessa forma, pode ser administrada por infusão venosa em fluxo constante e com cuidadoso monitoramento. Quando em associação, evitar soluções alcalinizantes. Normalmente diluída em solução de dextrose a 5% (p. ex.: 250 mg em 1 litro de dextrose a 5%).	Frascos para injeção com 250 mg/20 mL (12,5 mg/mL).	Cães: 5-20 mcg/kg/minuto em infusão IV. Gatos: 2 mcg/kg/minuto em infusão IV.
Docussato de cálcio (Surfak, Doxidan)	Amolecedor de fezes (surfactante). Age por diminuir a tensão superficial, permitindo que mais líquidos se acumulem nas fezes.	Não foram relatados efeitos colaterais em animais. Em seres humanos, altas doses causam desconforto abdominal.	As dosagens são baseadas em extrapolação de doses humanas ou empirismo. Não há estudos clínicos em animais. Os produtos com docussato de cálcio podem conter fenolftaleína, um estimulante catártico que deve ser usado com cautela em gatos.	Comprimidos com 60 mg (e muitos outros).	Cães: 50-100 mg/cão VO a cada 12-24h. Gatos: 50 mg/gato VO a cada 12-24h.

ESPÉCIES CANINA E FELINA

Formulário de Medicamentos para Consulta em 5 Minutos					
Nome do Princípio Ativo (Comercial e Outros Nomes)	*Farmacologia e Indicações*	*Efeitos Colaterais e Precauções*	*Informações de Dosagem e Comentários*	*Formulações*	*Dosagem (Exceto em Casos Indicados, a Dosagem é a Mesma para Cães e Gatos)*
Docussato de sódio (Colace, Doxan, Doss; muitas outras formulações sem prescrição médica)	Ver Docussato de cálcio.	Ver Docussato de cálcio.	Ver Docussato de cálcio.	Cápsulas com 50 e 100 mg; líquido com 10 mg/mL.	Cães: 5-200 mg/cão VO a cada 8-12h. Gatos: 50 mg/gato VO a cada 12-24h.
Dolasetron, mesilato (Anzemet)	Droga antiemética. Age inibindo os receptores de serotonina (5-HT, tipo 3). Utilizado na terapia antiemética, especialmente no vômito provocado pela quimioterapia.	Não foram relatados efeitos colaterais em animais.	O uso de antagonistas da serotonina é baseado principalmente na experiência da medicina humana. Não há estudos de eficácia em medicina veterinária. Ele é mais eficaz se utilizado para prevenir o vômito que para inibir a êmese em curso.	Comprimidos com 50 e 100 mg; injetável com 20 mg/mL.	Prevenção de náusea e vômito: 0,6 mg/kg IV ou VO a cada 24h. Tratamento de náusea e vômito: 1,0 mg/kg IV ou VO a cada 24h.
Dopamina, cloridrato (Intropin)	Agonista adrenérgico. Age principalmente estimulando o miocárdio por ação nos receptores β-1 cardíacos. Sugere-se que a dopamina aumenta a perfusão renal pela ação nos receptores dopaminérgicos renais; entretanto, não há evidência clínica de efeitos benéficos.	Pode causar taquicardia e arritmias ventriculares em altas doses ou em indivíduos sensíveis. Altas doses causam vasoconstrição por agir nos receptores do tipo α.	A dopamina possui uma meia-vida de eliminação rápida (minutos) e, desta forma, pode ser administrada por infusão venosa em fluxo constante e com cuidadoso monitoramento. Quando em associação, evitar soluções alcalinizantes. Administrar diluída em solução de dextrose a 5% ou solução de Ringer lactato. Misturar 200-400 mg em 250-500 mL de fluido.	40, 80 ou 160 mg/mL.	2-10 mcg/kg/minuto em infusão IV.
Doxapram, cloridrato (Dopram, Respiram)	Estimulante respiratório que age nos quimiorreceptores carotídeos e, subsequentemente, estimula o centro respiratório. Usada para tratar a depressão respiratória ou para estimular a respiração após anestesia. Também pode aumentar o débito cardíaco.	Os efeitos colaterais não foram relatados em animais. Efeitos cardiovasculares e convulsões ocorreram em altas doses administradas para seres humanos. Contém álcool benzílico como veículo.	Usada apenas para tratamento de curta duração. Não está mais disponível para comercialização.	Injetável com 20 mg/mL.	5-10 mg/kg IV; neonatos: 1-5 mg SC, sublingual ou pela veia umbilical.
Doxiciclina (Vibramycin e formulações genéricas)	Antibiótico do grupo das tetraciclinas. O mecanismo de ação das tetraciclinas se baseia na ligação à subunidade ribossomal 30S e inibição da síntese proteica. Normalmente bacteriostática. Amplo espectro de ação, incluindo bactérias, alguns protozoários, *Rickettsia* e *Ehrlichia*. Também utilizada no tratamento adjuvante da dirofilariose.	Efeitos colaterais graves não foram relatados com o uso da doxiciclina. De um modo geral, as tetraciclinas podem causar necrose tubular renal em altas doses. As tetraciclinas podem afetar a formação dos ossos e dos dentes em animais jovens, mas é menos provável de ocorrer com a doxiciclina.	Muitos estudos farmacocinéticos e experimentais foram conduzidos em pequenos animais, mas nenhum estudo clínico. Geralmente é considerada a droga de escolha para infecções por *Rickettsia* e *Ehrlichia*. A infusão IV de doxiciclina é estável por apenas 12 horas em temperatura ambiente e 72 horas se refrigerada.	Suspensão oral com 10 mg/mL; frasco para injeção com 100 mg; comprimidos ou cápsulas de 50 e 100 mg de hiclato de doxiciclina; comprimidos ou cápsulas de 50 ou 100 mg de doxiciclina monoidratada.	3-5 mg/kg VO, IV a cada 12h ou 10 mg/kg VO a cada 24h. Para *Rickettsia* ou *Ehrlichia* em cães: 5 mg/kg a cada 12h. Tratamento da dirofilariose: 10 mg/kg VO diariamente, intermitentemente, em intervalos de 4-6 semanas; usada com lactonas macrocíclicas.

Formulário de Medicamentos para Consulta em 5 Minutos					
Nome do Princípio Ativo (Comercial e Outros Nomes)	Farmacologia e Indicações	Efeitos Colaterais e Precauções	Informações de Dosagem e Comentários	Formulações	Dosagem (Exceto em Casos Indicados, a Dosagem é a Mesma para Cães e Gatos)
Doxorrubicina (Adryamicin)	Agente antineoplásico. Age intercalando bases no DNA, interrompendo a síntese de DNA e RNA na célula neoplásica. A doxorrubicina também pode afetar as membranas da célula tumoral. Usada para o tratamento de diversas neoplasias, incluindo o linfoma.	Os efeitos agudos mais comuns são anorexia, vômito e diarreia. A toxicidade dose-dependente também inclui supressão da medula óssea, alopecia (em certas raças) e cardiotoxicidade. É justamente a cardiotoxicidade que limita a dose total administrada (normalmente não deve exceder 200 mg/m²).	O esquema representado pode diferir entre os vários tumores. Consultar protocolos antineoplásicos específicos para direcionamento. A dose deve ser infundida por via IV (pelo menos 20-30 minutos). Os animais podem requerer antieméticos e anti-histamínicos (difenidramina) antes da terapia. Monitorar o ECG durante a terapia. A dose de acordo com o peso corporal pode ser mais eficiente para pequenos animais.	Injetável com 2 mg/mL.	Cães: 30 mg/m² IV a cada 21 dias, ou >20 kg, usar 30 mg/m² e <20 kg, usar 1 mg/kg. Gatos: 20 mg/m² (ou aproximadamente 1,0-1,25 mg/kg) a cada três semanas.
Edetato dissódico de cálcio (CaNa₂ EDTA, Versenato dissódico de cálcio)	Agente quelante. Indicado para o tratamento de intoxicação aguda ou crônica por chumbo. Às vezes utilizado em combinação com dimercaprol.	Não há relatos de efeitos colaterais em animais. Em seres humanos, as reações alérgicas (liberação de histamina) ocorrem após administração IV.	Pode ser usado com dimercaprol. Igualmente eficaz quando administrado por vias IV ou IM, porém, a aplicação IM pode ser dolorosa. Garantir que haja fluxo urinário adequado antes da primeira dose.	Injetável com 20 mg/mL.	25 mg/kg SC, IM, IV a cada 6h por 2-5 dias.
Edrofônio (Tensilon e outros)	Inibidor de colinesterase. Produz efeitos colinérgicos pela inibição do metabolismo da acetilcolina. Possui ação ultracurta e, geralmente, é apenas utilizado para propósitos diagnósticos (p. ex.: miastenia grave). Também é usado para reverter o bloqueio neuromuscular de agentes não despolarizantes (pancurônio).	De ação curta, possui efeitos colaterais mínimos. Os efeitos colinérgicos/ muscarínicos exacerbados podem ocorrer com altas doses (neutralizar com atropina).	Normalmente usado apenas para a determinação do diagnóstico de miastenia grave em pacientes.	Injetável com 10 mg/mL.	Cães: 0,11-0,22 mg/kg IV. Gatos: 0,25-0,5 mg/gato IV.
Efedrina (diversas formulações genéricas)	Agonista adrenérgico. Agonista de receptores adrenérgicos α e β-1, mas sem ação em receptores β-2. Usada como substância vasopressora, p. ex.: utilizada durante anestesia. Estimulante do SNC.	Efeitos colaterais relacionados com a atividade adrenérgica excessiva (p. ex.: vasoconstrição periférica e taquicardia).	Usada principalmente em situações agudas para aumentar a pressão sanguínea.	Injetável com 25 e 50 mg/mL.	Vasopressor: 0,75 mg/kg IM, SC, repetida quando necessário.
Enalapril, maleato (Enacard, Vasotec)	Inibidor da ECA e vasodilatador por inibição da síntese de angiotensina II. Utilizado para vasodilatação e tratamento da insuficiência cardíaca. Principalmente usado em cães, mas podendo beneficiar alguns gatos com insuficiência cardíaca.	Pode causar azotemia em alguns pacientes; monitorar cuidadosamente os pacientes que estiverem recebendo altas doses de diuréticos. *Interações com outras drogas:* usar com cautela em associação com outras drogas hipotensivas e diuréticas. Os AINE podem diminuir os efeitos vasodilatadores.	As doses são baseadas em estudos clínicos conduzidos em cães pelo fabricante. Para cães, começar com administração diária e aumentar para cada 12 horas, se necessário. Outras drogas utilizadas para o tratamento da insuficiência cardíaca podem ser usadas concomitantemente. Monitorar os eletrólitos e a função renal 3-7 dias após o início da terapia, realizando essa prática periodicamente.	Comprimidos com 2,5; 5; 10 e 20 mg.	Cães: 0,5 mg/kg VO a cada 12-24h. Gatos: 0,25-0,5 mg/kg VO a cada 12-24h ou 1,0-1,25 mg/gato/dia.

Espécies Canina e Felina

Formulário de Medicamentos para Consulta em 5 Minutos

Nome do Princípio Ativo (Comercial e Outros Nomes)	Farmacologia e Indicações	Efeitos Colaterais e Precauções	Informações de Dosagem e Comentários	Formulações	Dosagem (Exceto em Casos Indicados, a Dosagem é a Mesma para Cães e Gatos)
Enilconazol (Imaverol, Clinafarm EC)	Agente antifúngico azólico, apenas para uso tópico. Da mesma forma que os outros azólicos, inibe a síntese de membrana (ergosterol) do fungo. Altamente eficaz contra dermatófitos.	Administrado por via tópica, não foram relatados efeitos colaterais.	O Imaverol está disponível apenas no Canadá como uma emulsão a 10%. Nos EUA, o Clinafarm EC está disponível para uso em unidades aviárias como solução a 13,8%. Diluir a solução a pelo menos 50:1 e aplicar, por via tópica, a cada 3-4 dias por 2-3 semanas. O enilconazol também é instilado na diluição de 1:1 dentro do seio nasal quando na presença de aspergilose.	Emulsão a 10 ou 13,8%.	Aspergilose nasal: 10 mg/kg a cada 12h, instilado dentro do seio nasal por 14 dias (solução a 10% diluída em água na proporção de 50/50). Dermatófitos: diluir a solução a 10% até 0,2% e lavar a lesão com essa solução quatro vezes, em intervalos de 3-4 dias.
Enoxaparina (Lovenox)	Heparina de baixo peso molecular (LMWH); anticoagulante; indicada para a prevenção do tromboembolismo em pacientes de risco. Tem sido usada em gatos com dilatação atrial esquerda secundária à cardiomiopatia, antes e após o quadro embólico. Relação anti-Xa:anti IIa de 3,8:1.	A hemorragia pode ser um problema.	Quando a enoxaparina é usada na dose recomendada, não há necessidade de monitorar os tempos de coagulação, como ocorre com a heparina convencional (não fracionada). Possui absorção e depuração mais consistente que a heparina não fracionada (convencional).	Seringas pré-montadas para aplicação injetável com 30 mg/0,3 mL; 40 mg/ 0,4 mL; 60 mg/0,6 mL; 80 mg/0,8 mL e 100 mg/1 mL.	Cães: 0,8 mg/kg SC a cada 6h. Gatos: 1,25 mg/kg SC a cada 6h.
Enrofloxacina (Baytril)	Droga antibacteriana do grupo das fluoroquinolonas. Age por inibição da DNA-girase em bactérias, inibindo a síntese de DNA e RNA. Bactericida. Espectro de ação antimicrobiano alto.	Efeitos colaterais incluem convulsões em animais epilépticos, artropatia em cães com 4-28 semanas de idade e vômito em cães e gatos que receberam altas doses. Foi relatada cegueira em gatos. *Interações com outras drogas:* pode aumentar as concentrações de teofilina se usada concomitantemente. A administração conjunta de cátions di- e trivalentes (p. ex.: sucralfato) pode reduzir a absorção.	A solução não é aprovada para administração IV, mas tem sido usada por essa via de forma segura, se fornecida vagarosamente. Não misturar soluções IV com fluidos contendo cátions (p. ex.: Mg^{++}, Ca^{++}).	Comprimidos com 22,7 e 68 mg; comprimidos mastigáveis com 22.7; 68 e 136 mg; injetável com 22,7 mg/mL.	Cães: 5-20 mg/kg VO, IV, IM a cada 24h. Gatos: 5 mg/kg VO, IM a cada 24h. Para gatos, não administrar em doses acima de 5 mg/kg ou em infusão IV.
Epinefrina, hidrato (cloreto de adrenalina e formulações genéricas)	Agonista adrenérgica. Estimula, de forma não seletiva, os receptores adrenérgicos α, β-1 e β-2. Usada principalmente para situações de emergência para tratar parada cardiorrespiratória e choque anafilático.	A superdosagem causará vasoconstrição excessiva e hipertensão. Altas doses podem causar arritmias ventriculares. Quando altas doses são utilizadas na parada respiratória, um desfibrilador elétrico deve estar disponível.	As doses são baseadas em estudos experimentais, inicialmente em cães. As doses IV são utilizadas rotineiramente, mas a administração endotraqueal é aceitável quando o acesso IV não está disponível. A via intraóssea também é usada, com doses equivalentes à administração IV. Quando a via endotraqueal for utilizada, a dose é maior e a duração do efeito pode ser mais longa em comparação com a administração IV. Evitar aplicação intracardíaca.	Solução injetável com 1 mg/mL (1:1.000).	Parada cardíaca: 10-20 mcg/kg IV ou 200 mcg/kg por via endotraqueal (pode ser diluída em salina antes da administração). Choque anafilático: 2,5-5 mcg/kg IV ou 50 mcg/kg por via endotraqueal (pode ser diluída em salina).

Formulário de Medicamentos para Consulta em 5 Minutos

Nome do Princípio Ativo (Comercial e Outros Nomes)	Farmacologia e Indicações	Efeitos Colaterais e Precauções	Informações de Dosagem e Comentários	Formulações	Dosagem (Exceto em Casos Indicados, a Dosagem é a Mesma para Cães e Gatos)
Epoetina alfa (eritropoietina) (Epogen, [r-HuEPO])	Eritropoietina recombinante humana. Fator de crescimento hematopoiético que estimula a eritropoiese. Usada para tratar anemia não regenerativa.	Por se tratar de um produto recombinante humano, pode produzir reações alérgicas locais e sistêmicas em animais. Em seres humanos, ocorreram dor no local de aplicação e dor de cabeça. Também ocorreram convulsões. Pode aparecer anemia retardada em função da reação cruzada dos anticorpos contra a eritropoietina animal (reversível quando a droga é retirada).	Seu uso é baseado em relatos clínicos em cães e gatos. A única forma disponível atualmente é o produto recombinante humano.	Injetável com 2.000 U/mL.	Cães: as doses variam de 35 ou 50 U/kg SC três vezes por semana a 400 U/kg SC semanalmente (ajustar a dose do hematócrito para 30-34%). Gatos: iniciar com 100 U/kg três vezes por semana. Ajustar a dose com base no hematócrito.
Epsiprantel (Cestex)	Agente anticestódeo.	Anorexia e diarreia transitória. Vômito em altas doses.	-	Comprimidos com 12,5; 25; 50 e 100 mg.	Cães: 5,5 mg/kg VO. Gatos: 2,75 mg/kg VO.
Ergocalciferol (vitamina D$_2$) (Calciferol, Drisdol)	Análogo da vitamina D. Usada na deficiência de vitamina D e no tratamento da hipocalcemia, especialmente quando associada com o hipotireoidismo. A vitamina D promove a absorção e utilização de cálcio.	A superdosagem pode causar hipercalcemia. Evitar o uso em animais prenhes em virtude da possibilidade de causar anormalidades fetais. Usar cautelosamente com preparações contendo altas doses de cálcio.	Não deve ser utilizada para o hipoparatireoidismo renal por causa da incapacidade de conversão ao composto ativo. Disponível como solução oral, comprimidos, cápsulas e injetável. As doses individuais devem ser ajustadas pela monitoração das concentrações séricas de cálcio.	Comprimidos com 400 U (formulações sem prescrição médica); comprimidos com 50.000 U (1,25 mg); injetável com 500.000 U/mL (12,5 mg/mL).	500-2.000 U/kg/dia VO.
Eritromicina (diversas marcas e formulações genéricas)	Antibiótico macrolídeo. Inibe a síntese proteica por se ligar à fração 50S do ribossomo 50S bacteriano. O espectro de ação é limitado, principalmente, às bactérias aeróbias Gram-positivas. Utilizada para tratar infecções de pele e respiratórias.	O efeito colateral mais comum é o vômito (provavelmente causado por efeitos similares aos colinérgicos ou pela motilidade induzida pela motilina). Pode causar diarreia em alguns animais. Não administrar por via oral a roedores ou coelhos.	Há diversas formas de eritromicina, incluindo os ésteres etilsuccinato e estolato e o sal estearato para administração oral. Não há dados convincentes que sugiram que uma forma é mais absorvida que outra; assim, uma dose única inclui todas as formas.	Comprimidos ou cápsulas com 250 e 500 mg.	10-20 mg/kg VO a cada 8-12h; efeitos de motilidade GI na dose 0,5-1,0 mg/kg VO a cada 8-12h.
Ertapeném (Invanz)	Antibiótico carbapenêmico do grupo β-lactâmico. Similar ao meropeném e imipeném, é altamente ativo contra um amplo espectro de bactérias, incluindo aquelas resistentes a outras drogas. O ertapeném não é tão ativo contra *Pseudomonas*, como ocorre com meropeném ou imipeném.	Bem tolerado em animais. Pode ocorrer toxicidade do SNC em altas doses. É possível que ocorra alergia aos antibióticos β-lactâmicos.	A informação sobre dosagens é extrapolada da medicina humana ou de uso empírico limitado em medicina veterinária. Da mesma forma que outros carbapenêmicos, utilizar apenas quando os microrganismos são resistentes a outras drogas.	Injetável, frasco com 1 g.	30 mg/kg IV ou SC a cada 8h.
Esmolol, hidrato (Brevibloc)	β-bloqueador. Seletivo para receptores β-1. A diferença entre o esmolol e outros β-bloqueadores é a curta duração de ação. Indicado para o controle de arritmias e da frequência cardíaca em curto prazo.	Similar às outras precauções para os β-bloqueadores.	Indicado apenas para terapia IV de curto prazo. As doses são baseadas principalmente em empirismo ou extrapoladas de doses humanas. Não há estudos clínicos relatados em animais.	Injetável com 10 mg/mL.	500 mcg/kg IV, administrando 0,05-0,1 mg/kg lentamente, por cinco minutos ou 50-200 mcg/kg/minuto na forma de infusão.

ESPÉCIES CANINA E FELINA

Formulário de Medicamentos para Consulta em 5 Minutos					
Nome do Princípio Ativo (Comercial e Outros Nomes)	Farmacologia e Indicações	Efeitos Colaterais e Precauções	Informações de Dosagem e Comentários	Formulações	Dosagem (Exceto em Casos Indicados, a Dosagem é a Mesma para Cães e Gatos)
Espironolactona (Aldactone)	Diurético poupador de potássio. Espironolactona inibe competitivamente a ação da aldosterona. Medicamento usado no tratamento da hipertensão arterial e da congestão causada por insuficiência cardíaca.	Pode causar hipercalemia em alguns pacientes. Não usar em pacientes desidratados. Em gatos, pode ocorrer dermatite facial ulcerativa grave. Interações farmacológicas: evitar suplementos ricos em potássio.	Geralmente, espironolactona é usada com um agente diurético para ICC. Pode diminuir a remodelagem cardíaca e melhorar a sobrevida do paciente. Espironolactona provocará um ligeiro falso aumento nas concentrações plasmáticas de digoxina, medidas por alguns testes.	Comprimidos de 25, 50, 100 mg.	Cães: 2-4 mg/kg a cada 24h VO (ou 1-2 mg/kg a cada 12h VO). (A dose da bula aprovada na Europa é 2 mg/kg/dia VO.) Gatos: evitar o uso em gatos, mas em alguns casos 1-2 mg/kg a cada 12h VO tem sido usados.
Estanozolol (Winstrol-V)	Esteroide anabólico. Estanozolol é usado para diminuir o balanço negativo do nitrogênio em animais com insuficiência renal crônica.	Com o uso crônico, estanozolol promoverá efeitos anabólicos. Maior risco de toxidez hepática; gatos se encontram em maior risco.	Nos animais tratados, monitorar as enzimas hepáticas.	Injeção: 50 mg/mL; comprimidos de 2 mg. Algumas formulações comerciais foram recolhidas do mercado.	Cães: 2 mg/cão (ou 1-4 mg/cão) a cada 12h VO; 25-50 mg/cão/semana IM Gatos: 1 mg/gato a cada 12h VO; 25 mg/gato/ semana IM.
Éster do cipionato de testosterona (Andro- -Cyp, Andronate, Depo-Testosterone e outras formas) e Éster do propionato de testosterona (Testex, [Malogen no Canadá])	Éster da testosterona. Efeitos similares aos da metiltestosterona. Ésteres da testosterona são administrados IM, para que sejam evitados os efeitos de primeira passagem. Ésteres em óleo são absorvidos mais lentamente, por injeção IM. Em seguida, os ésteres são hidrolisados até testosterona livre.	Os efeitos adversos são atribuídos aos efeitos androgênicos e anabólicos. Também é possível que ocorra toxidez hepática.	Em animais de pequeno porte, a eficácia clínica para doenças crônicas ainda não foi avaliada.	Cipionato de testosterona: injeção: 100, 200 mg/mL. Propionato de testosterona: injeção: 100 mg/mL.	Cipionato de testosterona: 1-2 mg/kg a cada 2-4 semanas IM (ver também Metiltestosterona). Propionato de testosterona: 0,5-1 mg/kg 2-3 ×/semana IM.
Estradiol, cipionato (ECP, Depo-Estradiol Cypionate, formulações genéricas)	Composto estrogênico semissintético. Usado principal para induzir abortamento em animais.	Alto risco de hiperplasia endometrial e piometra. Altas doses podem produzir leucopenia, trombocitopenia e anemia aplásica fatal.	Normalmente, 22 mcg/kg são administrados uma só vez por via IM, durante os dias 3-5 do estro ou após três dias do cruzamento. Entretanto, em um estudo, uma dose de 44 mcg/kg foi mais eficaz que a de 22 mcg/kg quando fornecida durante o estro ou diestro.	Injetável com 2 mg/mL.	Cães: 22-44 mcg/mL IM (dose total não deve exceder 1,0 mg). Gatos: 250 mcg/gato IM entre 40h e cinco dias após o cruzamento.
Etidronato dissódico (Didronel)	Droga bifosfatada. Usada para tratar osteoporose e hipercalcemia. Reduz a renovação óssea, inibe a atividade osteoclástica, retarda a reabsorção óssea e diminui a taxa de osteoporose.	Não foram relatados efeitos colaterais em animais. Em seres humanos são comuns distúrbios GI.	Em altas doses, pode inibir a mineralização óssea.	Comprimidos com 200 e 400 mg; injetável com 50 mg/mL.	Cães: 5 mg/kg VO a cada 24h. Gatos: 10 mg/kg VO a cada 24h.
Etodolaco (EtoGesic [veterinário], Lodine [humano])	AINE do grupo do ácido piranocarboxílico. Inibe as prostaglandinas inflamatórias.	Os AINE podem causar ulceração GI. Outros efeitos colaterais causados pelos AINE incluem função plaquetária reduzida e lesão renal. Foi relatada ceratoconjuntivite seca em cães. Em ensaios clínicos com o etodolaco, alguns cães apresentaram perda de peso, fezes amolecidas ou diarreia nas doses recomendadas. Em altas doses, o etodolaco causou ulceração GI em cães.	Estudos em cães revelaram ser o etodolaco mais eficaz que o placebo no tratamento da artrite.	Comprimidos com 150 e 300 mg.	Cães: 10-15 mg/kg VO a cada 24h. Gatos: dose ainda não estabelecida.

Nome do Princípio Ativo (Comercial e Outros Nomes)	Farmacologia e Indicações	Efeitos Colaterais e Precauções	Informações de Dosagem e Comentários	Formulações	Dosagem (Exceto em Casos Indicados, a Dosagem é a Mesma para Cães e Gatos)
Famotidina (Pepcid)	Antagonista de receptores H_2 de histamina. Usada para inibir a secreção gástrica no tratamento e prevenção de úlceras.	Nenhum relatado em animais.	Não foram realizados estudos clínicos com a famotidina, de maneira que a dosagem para a prevenção e cicatrização de úlceras ainda não é conhecida.	Comprimido com 10 mg; injetável com 10 mg/mL.	Cães; 0,1-0,2 mg/kg VO, IV, SC, IM a cada 12h. Gatos: 0,2-0,25 mg/kg IM, IV, SC, VO a cada 12-24h.
Fator estimulante de colônias: sargramostim (Leukine) e filgrastim (Neupogen)	Estimula o desenvolvimento de granulócitos na medula óssea. Usado principalmente para regenerar as células sanguíneas na quimioterapia antineoplásica ou outros tratamentos.	Dor na aplicação injetável.	As doses são baseadas em informações de experimentos limitados realizados em cães. Leukine: reconstituir com 1 mL de água estéril para preparar uma solução de 250 ou 500 mcg/mL. Girar delicadamente, não agitar; depois, diluir com salina 0,9% estéril para concentrações menores que 10 mcg/mL para infusão IV.	300 mcg/mL (Neupogen) e 250-500 mcg/mL (Leukine).	Leukine: 0,25 mg/m² em infusão SC ou IV a cada 12h. Neupogen: 0,005 mg/kg SC a cada 24h por duas semanas.
Felbamato (Felbatol)	Anticonvulsivante. Normalmente usado quando os cães são refratários aos demais anticonvulsivantes. O mecanismo de ação pode se dar por antagonismo de receptores de N-metil-D-aspartato e bloqueio do efeito dos aminoácidos excitatórios.	O uso em cães não está relatado. Em seres humanos, as reações mais graves são hepatotoxicidade e anemia aplásica. Pode aumentar as concentrações de fenobarbital.	A dosagem é empírica.	Solução oral com 120 mg/mL; comprimidos com 400 e 600 mg.	Cães: iniciar com 15-20 mg/kg VO a cada 8h, ou 200 mg/cão a cada 8h (cães pequenos) e 400 mg/cão a cada 8h (cães maiores). Aumentar a dose gradualmente em intervalos de 200 mg até o controle da convulsão. A dose máxima para cães pequenos é de 600 mg/cão a cada 8h e, para cães maiores, a dose não deve ultrapassar 1.200 mg/cão a cada 8h. Gatos: não há doses relatadas.
Fenbendazol (Panacur, Safe-Guard)	Droga antiparasitária do grupo dos benzimidazólicos. Eficaz no tratamento de Giardia.	Boa margem de segurança, mas foram relatados vômito e diarreia. Não há contraindicações conhecidas.	As recomendações de dosagem foram baseadas em estudos clínicos realizados pelo fabricante. Os grânulos podem ser misturados com a dieta. Em estudos para o tratamento de Giardia, o fenbendazol foi mais seguro que outros tratamentos.	Grânulos de Panacur a 22,2% (222 mg/g); suspensão oral com 100 mg/mL.	50 mg/kg/dia VO por três dias.
Fenilbutazona (Butazolidin e genérico)	AINE. Inibe a síntese das prostaglandinas. Fenilbutazona é usada principalmente para artrite e várias formas de dor musculosquelética e inflamação.	Geralmente, fenilbutazona é bem tolerada em cães, mas não foram publicados dados para gatos. Um possível efeito adverso é a toxidez GI. Não administrar a formulação injetável IM. Fenilbutazona provoca depressão da medula óssea em humanos - ocorrência também possível em cães.	Basicamente, as doses seguem as recomendações do fabricante e a experiência clínica. Em animais de pequeno porte, houve declínio no uso desse agente, por causa da disponibilidade de outros AINE.	Comprimidos de 100, 200, 400 mg; injeção: 200 mg/mL.	Cães: 15-22 mg/kg a cada 8-12h (44 mg/kg/dia) VO ou IV (máximo: 800 mg/cão). Gatos: 6-8 mg/kg a cada 12h IV ou VO.
Fenilpropanolamina (PPA) (Proin PPA, Propalin [xarope])	Agonista adrenérgico. Uso como descongestionante, broncodilatador leve e para aumentar o tono do esfíncter urinário.	Os efeitos adversos são atribuídos à excessiva estimulação de receptores adrenérgicos (α e β). Efeitos colaterais: taquicardia, efeitos cardíacos, excitação do SNC, inquietude e supressão do apetite.	Fenilpropanolamina foi removida das formulações de descongestionantes para humanos. Atualmente, são comercializadas apenas formulações para uso veterinário.	Comprimidos aromatizados de 25, 50, 75 mg; solução oral aromatizada contendo 25 mg/mL.	Cães: 1 mg/kg, a cada 12h, VO. Aumentar para 1,5-2,0 mg/kg, conforme a necessidade, a cada 8h VO.

Espécies Canina e Felina

Formulário de Medicamentos para Consulta em 5 Minutos

Nome do Princípio Ativo (Comercial e Outros Nomes)	Farmacologia e Indicações	Efeitos Colaterais e Precauções	Informações de Dosagem e Comentários	Formulações	Dosagem (Exceto em Casos Indicados, a Dosagem é a Mesma para Cães e Gatos)
Fenitoína (Dilantin)	Anticonvulsivante. Deprime a condução nervosa, via bloqueio dos canais de sódio. Também classificada como antiarrítmico Classe I. Comumente usado como anticonvulsivante em humanos, mas não é efetiva em cães. Não usada em gatos.	Efeitos adversos: sedação, hiperplasia gengival, reações cutâneas, toxidez do SNC. Não administrar a fêmeas prenhes.	Devido à breve meia-vida e baixa eficácia em cães e à questionável segurança em gatos, outros anticonvulsivantes são usados como primeira escolha, em lugar de fenitoína.	Cápsulas de 30, 100 mg; injeção: 50 mg/mL; suspensão oral contendo 25 mg/mL.	Cães (anticonvulsivo): 20-35 mg/kg a cada 8h. (antiarrítmico): 30 mg/kg a cada 8h VO ou 10 mg/kg IV durante 5 min. Gatos: não usar.
Fenobarbital (Luminal e genérico)	Barbitúrico de ação prolongada. O principal uso do fenobarbital é como anticonvulsivante, por potenciar as ações inibitórias de GABA.	Os efeitos adversos têm relação com a dose. Fenobarbital causa polifagia, sedação, ataxia e letargia. Depois do tratamento inicial, forma-se certa tolerância aos efeitos adversos. Foi relatada a ocorrência de hepatotoxidez em alguns cães medicados com doses elevadas.	As doses de fenobarbital devem ser cuidadosamente ajustadas com a monitoração das concentrações sérica/plasmática. A faixa ideal para efeito terapêutico é 15-40 mcg/mL.	Comprimidos de 15, 30, 60, 100 mg; injeção: 30, 60, 65 e 130 mg/mL; solução de elixir oral contendo 4 mg/mL.	Cães: 2-8 mg/kg VO a cada 12h. *Status epilepticus*: administrar em incrementos de 10-20 mg/kg IV (até o efeito desejado). Gatos: 2-4 mg/kg VO a cada 12h.
Fentanil, citrato (Sublimaze, formulações genéricas)	Analgésico opiáceo sintético. Aproximadamente 80-100 vezes mais potente que a morfina.	Efeitos colaterais similares aos da morfina.	As dosagens são baseadas em empirismo e estudos experimentais. Não há estudos clínicos relatados. Além da formulação injetável de fentanil, há o fentanil transdérmico (ver abaixo).	Injetável com 250 mg/5 mL.	Uso anestésico: 0,02-0,04 mg/kg IV, IM, SC a cada 2h ou 0,01 mg/kg IV, IM, SC (com acetilpromazina ou diazepam). Analgesia: 0,005-0,01 mg/kg IV, IM, SC a cada 2h. IRC: 0,003 mg/kg em dose de ataque, seguida por 0,005 mg/kg/h IV em cães e 0,002 mg/kg/h em gatos.
Fentanil, transdérmico (Duragesic)	Similar ao fentanil. O fentanil transdérmico incorpora o fentanil em um emplastro adesivo aplicado na pele de cães e gatos. Alguns estudos revelaram que os emplastros liberam níveis contínuos de fentanil por 72-108 horas em cães e gatos. Um emplastro com 100 mcg/h é equivalente a 10 mg/kg de morfina IM a cada 4h.	Efeitos colaterais não foram relatados. Entretanto, se forem detectados efeitos colaterais (p. ex.: depressão respiratória, sedação excessiva, excitação em gatos), remover o emplastro e, se necessário, administrar naloxona.	Os emplastros disponíveis são de potência de 25, 50, 75 e 100 mcg/h. A potência do emplastro está relacionada com a taxa de liberação do fentanil. Estudos determinaram que emplastros de 25 mcg/h são adequados para gatos; os de 50 mcg/h são apropriados para cães entre 10-20 kg. Seguir cuidadosamente as recomendações do fabricante ao aplicar os emplastros.	Emplastros com 25, 50, 75 e 100 mcg/h.	Cães: 10-20 kg, emplastros de 50 mcg/h a cada 72h. Gatos: emplastros de 25 mcg/h a cada 118h.
Ferro	Ver Ferroso, sulfato.	-	-	-	-
Finasterida (Proscar)	Inibe a conversão de testosterona a di-hidrotestosterona (DHT). Como a DHT estimula o crescimento prostático, a finasterida tem sido usada para o tratamento da hiperplasia prostática benigna.	Não foram relatados efeitos colaterais em cães. É contraindicada na gestação.	As doses foram baseadas em estudos realizados com cães cuja redução prostática foi descrita.	Comprimidos com 5 mg.	Cães: 0,1 mg/kg VO a cada 24h (ou um comprimido de 5 mg a cada 24h para cães entre 10-50 kg).

Nome do Princípio Ativo (Comercial e Outros Nomes)	Farmacologia e Indicações	Efeitos Colaterais e Precauções	Informações de Dosagem e Comentários	Formulações	Dosagem (Exceto em Casos Indicados, a Dosagem é a Mesma para Cães e Gatos)
Firocoxibe (Previcox)	O firocoxibe é uma droga anti-inflamatória não esteroidal (AINE). Da mesma forma que as demais drogas deste grupo, o firocoxibe produz efeitos analgésicos e anti-inflamatórios pela inibição da síntese de prostaglandinas. O firocoxibe é altamente seletivo para COX-2.	Os efeitos colaterais mais comuns associados com AINE são distúrbios GI, podendo incluir vômito, diarreia, náusea, ulcerações e erosões do trato GI.	A dose para gatos foi descrita em apenas um estudo. Não está registrado para uso em gatos.	Comprimidos com 57 e 277 mg.	Cães: 5 mg/kg VO a cada 24h. Gatos: 1,5 mg/kg em dose única. A segurança por longo tempo de utilização em gatos não foi determinada.
Fisostigmina (Antilirium)	Inibidor da colinesterase. Antídoto para intoxicação por anticolinérgicos, especialmente na intoxicação com sinais no SNC. A principal diferença entre fisostigmina e neostigmina ou piridostigmina é que a fisostigmina atravessa a barreira hematoencefálica e as outras duas substâncias não.	Efeitos adversos atribuídos aos excessivos efeitos colinérgicos (tratar *overdose* com atropina).	Fisostigmina tem indicação principal apenas para tratamento de intoxicações. Para uso sistêmico rotineiro de medicamento anticolinesterásico, neostigmina e piridostigmina têm menos efeitos colaterais. Se usar a fisostigmina, a frequência da dose poderá ser aumentada, com base na observação dos efeitos.	Injeção: 1 mg/mL.	0,02 mg/kg a cada 12h IV.
Fitomenadiona	Ver Vitamina K_1.				
Fitonadiona	Ver Vitamina K_1.				
Florfenicol (Nuflor)	Derivado do cloranfenicol, possui o mesmo mecanismo de ação (inibição da síntese proteica) e espectro de ação antibacteriano. O uso em pequenos animais não é comum.	A utilização em cães e gatos é limitada; desta forma, os efeitos colaterais não foram relatados. O cloranfenicol tem sido associado com a depressão dose-dependente da medula óssea, e reações similares podem ser possíveis com o florfenicol. Entretanto, não parece haver risco de se desenvolver anemia aplásica, como ocorre com o cloranfenicol.	O esquema de doses está aprovado apenas para uso em bovinos, não tendo sido avaliado em pequenos animais. As doses listadas são derivadas de estudos farmacocinéticos.	Solução injetável com 300 mg/mL.	Cães: 20 mg/kg VO, IM a cada 6h. Gatos: 22 mg/kg IM, VO a cada 8h.
Flucitosina (Ancobon)	Droga antifúngica. Utilizada em combinação com outras drogas antifúngicas para o tratamento da criptococose. Age penetrando nas células fúngicas e sendo convertida em fluoruracila, ao qual age como um antimetabólito.	É possível ocorrer anemia e trombocitopenia.	A flucitosina é usada principalmente para tratar a criptococose em animais. A eficácia é baseada na habilidade da flucitosina em alcançar altas concentrações no líquido cerebroespinal (LCE). A flucitosina pode assumir sinergismo com a anfotericina B.	Cápsulas com 250 mg; suspensão oral com 75 mg/mL.	25-50 mg/kg VO a cada 6-8h (até a dose máxima de 100 mg/kg VO a cada 12h).

ESPÉCIES CANINA E FELINA

Formulário de Medicamentos para Consulta em 5 Minutos

Nome do Princípio Ativo (Comercial e Outros Nomes)	Farmacologia e Indicações	Efeitos Colaterais e Precauções	Informações de Dosagem e Comentários	Formulações	Dosagem (Exceto em Casos Indicados, a Dosagem é a Mesma para Cães e Gatos)
Fluconazol (Diflucan)	Droga do grupo dos antifúngicos azólicos. Mecanismo similar aos de outros agentes antifúngicos azólicos. Inibe a síntese de ergosterol na membrana celular do fungo. Ativo contra dermatófitos e uma diversidade de fungos sistêmicos, mas não para *Aspergillus* sp.	Não foram relatados efeitos colaterais para a administração do fluconazol. Comparado ao cetoconazol, possui menor efeito na função endócrina. Entretanto, é possível o aumento nas concentrações plasmáticas de enzimas hepáticas e hepatopatias. Em comparação com outros antifúngicos azólicos orais, a absorção do fluconazol é mais previsível e completa, mesmo com estômago vazio.	As doses para o fluconazol são principalmente baseadas em estudos realizados em gatos para o tratamento da criptococose. A eficácia para outras infecções não foi determinada. A diferença principal entre o fluconazol e outros azólicos é que o primeiro alcança altas concentrações no SNC.	Comprimidos com 50, 100, 150 e 200 mg; suspensão oral com 10 ou 40 mg/mL; solução injetável IV com 2 mg/mL.	Cães: 10-12 mg/kg VO a cada 24h. Para *Malassezia*, a dose de 5 mg/kg VO a cada 12h tem sido usada. Gatos: 50 mg/gato VO a cada 12-24h.
Fludrocortisona, acetato (Florinef)	Mineralocorticoide. Usada como terapia de reposição em animais com atrofia adrenal/insuficiência adrenocortical. A fludrocortisona possui alta potência mineralocorticoide comparada com a ação glicocorticoide.	Os efeitos colaterais são principalmente relacionados aos efeitos glicocorticoides em altas doses. O tratamento em longo prazo para o hipoadrenocorticismo pode resultar em efeitos colaterais glicocorticoides.	A dose deve ser ajustada pela monitoração da resposta do paciente (p. ex.: controle das concentrações eletrolíticas). Em alguns pacientes, a fludrocortisona é administrada com um glicocorticoide e suplementação de sódio.	Comprimidos com 100 mcg (0,1 mg).	Cães: 15-30 mcg/kg VO diariamente. Gatos: 0,1-0,2 mg/gato VO a cada 24h.
Flumazenil (Romazicon)	Antagonista de receptores benzodiazepínicos. Usado como agente reversor após a administração de benzodiazepínicos em seres humanos (não é comum o seu uso em medicina veterinária).	Não foram relatados efeitos colaterais em animais.	Utilizado principalmente para reverter os efeitos das drogas benzodiazepínicas. Pode ser usado para tratar a toxicidade causada pelas altas doses de benzodiazepínicos (p. ex.: diazepam). Apesar de ser utilizado experimentalmente para a encefalopatia hepática, não se recomenda seu uso.	Injetável com 100 mcg/mL (0,1 mg/mL).	0,2 mg (dose total) IV, enquanto necessário.
Flumetasona (Flucort)	Potente droga anti-inflamatória glicocorticoide. A potência é de aproximadamente 15 vezes do cortisol. Usada para tratar distúrbios inflamatórios quando uma droga potente é exigida.	Os corticosteroides produzem diversos efeitos colaterais sistêmicos, que são comuns na terapia crônica.	As doses são baseadas na gravidade da doença subjacente.	Injetável com 0,5 mg/mL.	Usos como anti-inflamatório: 0,15-0,3 mg/kg IV, IM, SC a cada 12-24h.
Flunixina meglumina (Banamine)	AINE. Atua inibindo a enzima cicloxigenase (COX), responsável pela síntese de prostaglandinas. Outros efeitos anti-inflamatórios podem ocorrer (como os efeitos nos leucócitos), mas não foram ainda bem caracterizados. Usada principalmente para o tratamento em curto prazo da dor e inflamação moderadas.	A maior parte dos efeitos colaterais graves está relacionada com o sistema GI. Provoca gastrite e ulceração GI quando em altas doses ou em posologia prolongada. Também foi documentada isquemia renal. A terapia em cães deve ser limitada a quatro dias. Evitar o uso em animais prenhes próximo do parto. *Interações com drogas:* efeitos ulcerogênicos são potencializados quando administrados com corticosteroides.	Não está aprovada em pequenos animais, mas tem se mostrado, em estudos experimentais, um eficaz inibidor da síntese de prostaglandinas. Geralmente, outros AINE são preferidos para uso em cães e gatos.	Pacotes com grânulos com 250 mg; injetável com 10 e 50 mg/mL.	1,1 mg/kg IV, IM, SC em dose única ou 1,1 mg/kg/dia VO por três dias/semana. Uso oftálmico: 0,5 mg/kg IV em dose única.

CONSULTA VETERINÁRIA EM 5 MINUTOS

Formulário de Medicamentos para Consulta em 5 Minutos

Nome do Princípio Ativo (Comercial e Outros Nomes)	Farmacologia e Indicações	Efeitos Colaterais e Precauções	Informações de Dosagem e Comentários	Formulações	Dosagem (Exceto em Casos Indicados, a Dosagem é a Mesma para Cães e Gatos)
Fluoxetina (Reconcile [veterinário], Prozac [humano]	Droga antidepressiva. Usada para tratar distúrbios comportamentais, como transtorno obsessivo-compulsivo e agressão por dominância. O mecanismo de ação se dá pela inibição seletiva da reutilização de serotonina e infrarregulação dos receptores 5-HT1.	Os efeitos colaterais mais comuns durante os ensaios de campo foram letargia, apetite reduzido, tremores, diarreia, inquietação, agressão e vocalização. Em gatos foram observadas agitação e ansiedade aumentada.	Devido à meia-vida longa, o acúmulo no plasma pode levar diversos dias a semanas.	Formulações humanas: cápsulas com 10 e 20 mg; solução oral com 4 mg/mL. Formulações veterinárias: comprimidos mastigáveis com 8, 16, 32 e 64 mg.	Cães: 1-2 mg/kg VO, diariamente. Gatos: 0,5-1,0 mg/kg VO, diariamente.
Fomepizol (4-metilpirazol, Antizol-Vet)	Antídoto para a intoxicação por etilenoglicol (anticongelante). Inibe a enzima desidrogenase que converte o etilenoglicol ao metabólito tóxico. Deve ser usado o mais cedo possível para o máximo sucesso da terapia.	O metilpirazol é seguro e eficaz se usado até oito horas do envenenamento em cães e até três horas em gatos.	Utilizado para o manejo emergencial da intoxicação por etilenoglicol. Estudos experimentais revelaram eficácia em cães e gatos. Misturar com cloreto de sódio a 0,9% antes da administração.	Solução a 5% em frasco com 1,5 mL.	Cães: 20 mg/kg IV, inicialmente; depois 15 mg/kg nos intervalos de 12 e 24h; em seguida, 5 mg em 36h. Gatos: 125 mg/kg, inicialmente, seguido por 31 mg/kg nos intervalos de 12, 24 e 36h. Se necessário, continuar a cada 12h.
Fosfato de potássio	Suplemento de fósforo. Uso em casos de hipofosfatemia grave, em associação com cetoacidose diabética.	Pode causar hipocalcemia.		Comprimidos de 500 mg. Cada comprimido contém 3,7 mmol (114 mg) de fósforo. A injeção contém 3 mmol (93 mg) de fósforo por mL.	4 mg/kg de fósforo VO, até 4×/dia. 0,03-0,12 mmol/kg/h IV para tratamento agudo.
Fosfato de toceranibe (Palladia)	Agente antineoplásico usado para mastocitomas cutâneos em cães. Trata-se de um inibidor da tirosina cinase que interrompe o aporte sanguíneo aos tumores.	Foi associado a efeitos adversos no trato GI, inclusive vômito, diminuição do apetite, diarreia, perda de peso e sangue nas fezes.	Administrar com anti-histamínicos, para diminuir os efeitos adversos. Também é recomendável o uso de inibidores da bomba de prótons. Se ocorrerem efeitos adversos, descontinuar por até 2 semanas.	Comprimidos de 10, 15 e 50 mg.	Cães: 3,25 mg/kg VO em dias alternados, ou pode diminuir para 2,5 mg/kg 3 dias/semana. Gatos: não há dose estabelecida.
Furazolidona (Furoxone)	Droga oral contra protozoários com atividade contra Giardia. Pode ter alguma atividade contra bactérias intestinais. Não é utilizada para tratamentos sistêmicos.	Não foram relatados efeitos colaterais em animais. Em seres humanos foram descritos anemia branda, hipersensibilidade e distúrbios da flora intestinal.	Não foram relatados estudos clínicos em animais. As doses e recomendações são baseadas na extrapolação das usadas para seres humanos. Outras drogas, como o fenbendazol, são preferenciais contra Giardia.	Comprimidos com 100 mg.	4 mg/kg VO a cada 12h por 7-10 dias.
Furosemida (Lasix, formulações genéricas)	Diurético de alça. Inibe o transporte de sódio e água na alça ascendente de Henle, produzindo diurese. Também pode assumir propriedades vasodilatadoras, aumentando a perfusão renal e reduzindo a pré-carga cardíaca.	Os efeitos colaterais são principalmente relacionados ao efeito diurético (perda de fluidos e eletrólitos). Administrar, de forma conservativa, em animais que recebem inibidores da ECA para diminuir o risco de azotemia.	A furosemida pode ser usada com outras drogas cardiovasculares, incluindo o pimobendam.	Comprimidos com 12,5; 20 e 50 mg; solução oral com 10 mg/mL; injetável com 50 mg/mL.	Cães: 2-6 mg/kg IV, IM, SC, VO a cada 8-12h (ou quando necessário). Gatos: 1-4 mg/kg IV, IM, SC, VO a cada 8-24h.
Gabapentina (Neurontin)	Anticonvulsivante e analgésico. A gabapentina é uma análoga do neurotransmissor inibitório GABA. O mecanismo de ação anticonvulsivante e analgésico não é conhecido.	Cuidado: a solução oral contém xilitol, que pode ser tóxico para gatos.	A gabapentina tem sido usada para tratar a epilepsia refratária e como adjunto na analgesia (com outras drogas).	Cápsulas com 100, 300 e 400 mg; comprimidos sulcados com 100, 300, 400, 600 e 800 mg; solução oral com 50 mg/mL.	Dose anticonvulsivante: Cães: 2,5-10 mg/kg VO a cada 8-12h. Gatos: 5-10 mg/kg PO a cada 12h. Para analgesia: Cães: 10-15 mg/kg VO a cada 8h. Gatos: 8 mg/kg VO a cada 12h.

ESPÉCIES CANINA E FELINA

Formulário de Medicamentos para Consulta em 5 Minutos

Nome do Princípio Ativo (Comercial e Outros Nomes)	Farmacologia e Indicações	Efeitos Colaterais e Precauções	Informações de Dosagem e Comentários	Formulações	Dosagem (Exceto em Casos Indicados, a Dosagem é a Mesma para Cães e Gatos)
Genfibrozila (Lopid)	Agente redutor de colesterol.	Não foram relatados efeitos colaterais em animais.	Usada principalmente para tratar a hiperlipidemia em seres humanos. Não foram realizados estudos clínicos em animais.	Cápsulas com 300 mg; comprimidos com 600 mg.	7,5 mg/kg VO a cada 12h.
Gentamicina, sulfato (Gentocin)	Antibiótico aminoglicosídeo. Age inibindo a síntese proteica bacteriana por se ligar à fração 30S do ribossomo. Bactericida. Amplo espectro de atividade, exceto para estafilococos e bactérias anaeróbias.	A nefrotoxicidade é o efeito colateral dose-limitante mais comum. Garantir que os pacientes recebam suporte hidroeletrolítico adequado durante a terapia. Também são possíveis ototoxicidade e vestibulotoxicidade. *Interações com outras drogas:* quando usada com agentes anestésicos, é possível que ocorra bloqueio neuromuscular. Não misturar com outras drogas em frascos ou seringas.	Os esquemas de dosagem são baseados na sensibilidade dos microrganismos. Alguns estudos sugerem que a terapia de um dia (combinando múltiplas doses em uma dose única diária) é tão eficaz quanto os tratamentos múltiplos. A atividade contra algumas bactérias (p. ex.: *Pseudomonas*) é aumentada quando em combinação com um antibiótico β-lactâmico. A nefrotoxicidade é aumentada quando existem concentrações totais persistentemente altas.	Solução injetável com 50 e 100 mg/mL.	Cães: 2-4 mg/kg a cada 8h ou 9-14 mg/kg a cada 24h IV, IM, SC. Gatos: 3 mg/kg a cada 8h ou 5-8 mg/kg a cada 24h IV, IM, SC.
Glibenclamida	Nome britânico para a gliburida.				
Gliburida (DiaBeta, Micronase, Glynase)	Agente hipoglicêmico do grupo das sulfanilureias. Ver Glipizida.	Anorexia, vômito e elevação de enzimas hepáticas dose-dependentes.	A resposta é imprevisível. A glipizida normalmente é preferida para uso em gatos.	Comprimidos com 1,25; 2,5 e 5 mg.	Gatos: 0,2 mg/kg VO diariamente ou 0,625 mg (½ comprimido) por gato.
Glicerina (formulações genéricas)	Usada para tratar o glaucoma agudo.	Não foram relatados efeitos colaterais.	-	Solução oral.	1-2 mL/kg VO a cada 8h (no máximo).
Glicopirrolato (Robinul-V)	Droga anticolinérgica, o glicopirrolato pode exercer menor efeito no SNC quando comparado com a atropina em função dos baixos níveis no LCE. Pode ter maior duração de ação que a atropina.	Os efeitos colaterais são atribuídos aos efeitos antimuscarínicos (anticolinérgicos).	Geralmente, o glicopirrolato é usado em combinação com outros agentes, em especial as drogas anestésicas.	Injetável com 0,2 mg/mL.	0,005-0,01 mg/kg IV, IM, SC.
Glicosamina e condroitina, sulfato (Cosequin)	O Cosequin é uma marca comercial que combina o sulfato de condroitina e o hidrato de glicosamina. De acordo com o fabricante, esses compostos estimulam a síntese de líquido sinovial e inibem a degradação da cartilagem, promovendo a sua cicatrização. Usada principalmente para a doença articular degenerativa.	Os efeitos colaterais não foram relatados, apesar de ser possível a hipersensibilidade.	As doses são baseadas primariamente em empirismo e nas recomendações do fabricante. Podem ser usadas em associação com AINE em cães com artrite.	Cápsulas com potência convencional (RS) ou dupla (DS).	Cães: 1-2 cápsulas RS por dia (2-4 cápsulas de DS para cães maiores). Gatos: 1 cápsula RS diariamente.
Glicosaminoglicana polissulfatada (PSGAG) (Adequan Canine)	Composto de grande peso molecular, similar aos constituintes normais de articulações saudáveis. Condroprotetor. Inibe enzimas que podem degradar a cartilagem articular. Uso principalmente no tratamento ou prevenção da artropatia degenerativa.	São raros os efeitos adversos. É possível a ocorrência de reações alérgicas. PSGAG tem efeitos semelhantes aos da heparina, com potenciação de problemas hemorrágicos em alguns animais.	As doses são derivadas de evidência empírica, estudos experimentais e estudos clínicos em cães. Embora esse agente seja efetivo para artrite aguda, pode não demonstrar eficácia na artropatia crônica.	Ampola de 5 mL (100 mg/mL) para injeção (para equinos, as ampolas contêm 250 mg/mL).	4,4 mg/kg IM, 2×/semana, por até 4 semanas.

1404 · CONSULTA VETERINÁRIA EM 5 MINUTOS

Formulário de Medicamentos para Consulta em 5 Minutos

Nome do Princípio Ativo (Comercial e Outros Nomes)	Farmacologia e Indicações	Efeitos Colaterais e Precauções	Informações de Dosagem e Comentários	Formulações	Dosagem (Exceto em Casos Indicados, a Dosagem é a Mesma para Cães e Gatos)
Glipizida (Glucotrol)	Agente hipoglicemiante oral do grupo das sulfonilureias. Utilizada como tratamento oral no manejo do diabetes melito, particularmente em gatos. A taxa de resposta é de aproximadamente 50%. Essa droga age aumentando a secreção de insulina no pâncreas, provavelmente pela interação com receptores de sulfanilureia nas células β. Essas drogas também podem aumentar a sensibilidade dos receptores de insulina já existentes.	Em alguns gatos, pode causar vômito, anorexia, aumento de bilirrubinas e elevação de enzimas hepáticas de acordo com a dose. Causa hipoglicemia, porém em menor grau quando comparada com a insulina. *Interações com outras drogas:* muitas interações com drogas foram relatadas em seres humanos, mas não se sabe se isso ocorre em animais. Usar com cautela quando associada com β-bloqueadores, drogas antifúngicas, anticoagulantes, fluoroquinolonas, sulfonamidas e outras (consultar as bulas).	Os agentes hipoglicêmicos orais são eficazes em seres humanos apenas para o diabetes insulino-independente. Considerando que a resposta aos agentes hipoglicêmicos em gatos é imprevisível, recomenda-se realizar um primeiro teste com pelo menos quatro semanas. Se o gato responder, a droga pode ser mantida; de outra forma, a insulina pode ser indicada. Alimentar os gatos com uma dieta rica em fibras ao usar agentes hipoglicemiantes orais. A eficácia em gatos é imprevisível.	Comprimidos com 5 e 10 mg.	Gatos: 2,5-7,5 mg/gato VO a cada 12h. Começar com 2,5 mg por gato e aumentar se necessário. Cães: não recomendada.
Gluconato de potássio (Kaon, Tumil-K, genérico)	Suplemento de potássio. Uso na acidose tubular renal.	O mesmo que cloreto de potássio.	1 g de gluconato de potássio fornece 4,27 mEq de potássio.	Comprimidos de 2 mEq, 500 mg; Kaon: 20 mg/15 mL de elixir.	Cães: 0,5 mEq/kg a cada 12-24h VO. Gatos: 2-8 mEq/dia divididos 2×/dia VO.
Gluconato de quinidina (Quinaglute, Duraquin) Sulfato de quinidina (Cin-Quin, Quinora) Poligalacturonato de quinidina (Cardioquin)	Antiarrítmico Classe I. Ação: inibição do influxo de sódio, via bloqueio dos canais de sódio. Uso no tratamento de arritmias ventriculares e, ocasionalmente, da fibrilação atrial.	Os efeitos colaterais com quinidina são mais comuns do que com procainamida (náusea e vômito). Efeitos adversos: hipotensão, taquicardia (em decorrência do efeito antivagal). Interações farmacológicas: co-administração com digoxina pode aumentar as concentrações deste último agente.	Quinidina não é usada tão comumente como outros medicamentos antiarrítmicos Classe I. As doses são calculadas de acordo com a quantidade de base de quinidina em cada produto. 324 mg de gluconato de quinidina = 202 mg de base de quinidina. 300 mg de sulfato de quinidina = 250 mg de base de quinidina. 275 mg de poligalacturonato de quinidina = 167 mg de base de quinidina.	Muitas formulações para humanos deixaram de ser comercializadas, devido à diminuição do uso. Gluconato de quinidina, comprimidos de 324 mg; injeção: 80 mg/mL. Poligalacturonato de quinidina, comprimidos de 275 mg. Sulfato de quinidina, comprimidos de 100, 200, 300 mg; cápsulas de 200, 300 mg; injeção: 200 mg/mL.	Cães: 6-20 mg/kg a cada 6h IM; 6-20 mg/kg a cada 6-8h VO (da base).
GoLYTELY	Solução oral para produzir catarse.	Ver Polietilenoglicol, solução eletrolítica.	-	-	-
Gonadorelina (GnRH, LHRH) (Factrel)	Estimula a síntese e a liberação de hormônio luteinizante (LH) e, em menor grau, do hormônio foliculoestimulante (FSH). Usada para induzir luteinização.	Os efeitos colaterais não foram relatados em animais.	A gonadorrelina tem sido usada para manejar diversos distúrbios reprodutivos. Consultar referências específicas em alterações reprodutivas em animais para orientar a terapia.	Injetável com 50 mcg/mL.	Cães: 50-100 mcg/cão IM a cada 24-48h. Gatos: 25 mcg/gato IM em aplicação única.
Gonadotropina, hormônio liberador	Ver Gonadorelina.	-	-	-	-
Gonadotropina coriônica (HCG) (Profasi, Pregnyl, formulações genéricas, A.P.L)	A ação do HCG é idêntica à do hormônio luteinizante (LH). Usada para induzir a luteinização em animais.	Nenhum efeito colateral foi observado em animais.	Consultar referências específicas sobre problemas reprodutivos em animais, para orientação terapêutica.	Injetável, frascos com 5.000; 10.000 e 20.000 U.	Cães: 22 U/kg IM a cada 24-48h ou 44 U IM em aplicação única. Gatos: 250 U/gato IM em aplicação única.
Granisetron (Kytril)	Droga antiemética que age por inibição dos receptores de serotonina (5-HT). Usada principalmente como antiemético durante quimioterapia.	Não foram relatados efeitos colaterais em cães e gatos.	Doses extrapoladas das usadas em seres humanos.	Comprimidos com 1 mg; injetável com 1 mg/mL.	0,01 mg/kg IV (em seres humanos, a dose é de 1 mg/pessoa VO).

ESPÉCIES CANINA E FELINA

Formulário de Medicamentos para Consulta em 5 Minutos

Nome do Princípio Ativo (Comercial e Outros Nomes)	Farmacologia e Indicações	Efeitos Colaterais e Precauções	Informações de Dosagem e Comentários	Formulações	Dosagem (Exceto em Casos Indicados, a Dosagem é a Mesma para Cães e Gatos)
Griseofulvina (microparticulada) (Fulvicin) U/F) ou (ultraparticulada) (Fulvicin P/G, Gris-PEG)	Droga antifúngica. Incorporada nas camadas da pele, inibindo a mitose do fungo. A atividade antifúngica está limitada aos dermatófitos.	Os efeitos colaterais em animais incluem teratogenicidade em gatos; anemia e leucopenia em gatos; anorexia, depressão, vômito e diarreia. Não administrar em gatas prenhes.	Uma ampla variedade de doses foi relatada. As doses listadas aqui representam o consenso. A griseofulvina deve ser administrada com alimentos para aumentar sua absorção. A forma ultraparticulada é absorvida em maior extensão, fazendo com que as doses sejam menores que para a forma microparticulada.	Comprimidos com 125, 250 e 500 mg; suspensão oral com 25 mg/mL; xarope com 125 mg/mL; comprimidos da forma ultraparticulada com 100, 125, 165, 250 e 330 mg.	50 mg/kg VO a cada 24h (até a dose máxima de 110-132 mg/kg/dia em tratamentos divididos). Forma ultraparticulada: 30 mg/kg/dia VO em tratamentos divididos.
Guaifenesina (gliceril guaiacolato, Guaiphenesin, Mucinex)	Expectorante e relaxante muscular. O mecanismo para os efeitos expectorantes não são conhecidos, mas pode aumentar a secreção respiratória.	Pode ocorrer efeito vagal (p. ex.: estimulação secretória) quando a droga é utilizada como expectorante.	O uso da guaifenesina por via oral é indicado principalmente para problemas respiratórios. As soluções intravenosas têm sido usadas como auxiliares em anestesia, principalmente em equinos.	Comprimidos com 100 e 200 mg de liberação retardada com 600 mg; solução oral com 20 e 40 mg/mL.	Expectorante: 3-5 mg/kg Auxiliar anestésico: cães: 2,2 mL/kg/h IV de uma solução a 5%.
Halotano (Fluothane)	Anestésico inalatório.	Efeitos colaterais relacionados aos efeitos anestésicos (p. ex.: depressão cardiorrespiratória). Foi relatada hepatotoxicose em seres humanos.	O uso de anestésicos inalatórios requer monitoração cuidadosa. A dose é determinada pela profundidade da anestesia.	Frasco com 250 mL.	Indução: 3%. Manutenção: 0,5-1,5%.
Hemoglobina-glutamer (Oxyglobin)	A hemoglobina-glutamer (bovina) é usada como um fluido transportador de oxigênio em cães com uma infinidade de anemias.	Hemoglobinúria transitória. Os efeitos colaterais respiratórios podem ocorrer após administração rápida. Os efeitos colaterais são descoloração da pele, efeitos cardiovasculares, vômito, diarreia e anorexia. A droga pode interferir com alguns testes diagnósticos após a administração.	Administrar utilizando técnica asséptica. Não administrar com outros fluidos ou drogas no mesmo circuito IV. Não misturar com outras medicações. Noventa por cento da dose é eliminada em 5-7 dias.	13 g/dL de hemoglobina polimerizada de origem bovina em embalagens de dose única contendo 125 mL.	Cães: dose única de 10-30 mL/kg IV na taxa de 5-10 mL/kg/h. Gatos: dose única de 3-5 mL/kg em infusão IV lenta. A taxa máxima em gatos é de 5 mL/kg/h.
Heparina sódica (Liquaemin [EUA]; Hepalean [Canadá])	Anticoagulante. Potencializa os efeitos anticoagulantes da antitrombina III. Usada principalmente para a prevenção de trombose.	Os efeitos colaterais são causados pela excessiva inibição da coagulação; pode causar hemorragia.	Os ajustes de dose devem ser realizados pelo cuidadoso monitoramento dos tempos de coagulação. Por exemplo: a dose é ajustada para manter o tempo de tromboplastina parcial ativada (TTPA) em 1,5 a 2 vezes o valor de referência.	Injetável com 1.000 e 10.000 U/mL.	100-200 U/kg IV na dose de ataque, depois 100-300 U/kg SC a cada 6-8h. Profilaxia de baixa dose (cães e gatos): 70 U/kg SC a cada 8-12h.
Hetastarch (hidroxietil amido) (HES)	Ver Hidroxietil amido (HES). Expansor sintético de volume coloidal (usado da mesma maneira que o dextran). Utilizada principalmente para tratar hipovolemia aguda e choque.	Uso limitado em medicina veterinária; desta forma, os efeitos colaterais não foram relatados. Pode causar reações alérgicas. As coagulopatias são raras nas doses usuais.	Utilizada em situações críticas de saúde. Administrada por taxa de infusão constante. A HES parece ser mais eficaz e produzir menos efeitos colaterais que o dextran. Infundir de forma lenta.	Solução injetável a 6%.	Cães: 10-20 mL/kg IV diariamente. Gatos: 5-10 mL/kg IV diariamente.

1406 CONSULTA VETERINÁRIA EM 5 MINUTOS

Formulário de Medicamentos para Consulta em 5 Minutos

Nome do Princípio Ativo (Comercial e Outros Nomes)	Farmacologia e Indicações	Efeitos Colaterais e Precauções	Informações de Dosagem e Comentários	Formulações	Dosagem (Exceto em Casos Indicados, a Dosagem é a Mesma para Cães e Gatos)
Hidralazina (Apresoline)	Vasodilatador. Anti-hipertensivo. Usada para dilatar arteríolas e reduzir a pós-carga cardíaca. Principalmente usada para o tratamento da ICC e outros distúrbios cardiovasculares caracterizados pela alta resistência vascular periférica.	Os efeitos colaterais são atribuídos à vasodilatação excessiva. Monitorar os pacientes para evitar a hipotensão. Pode diminuir perigosamente o débito cardíaco. Foram relatadas reações alérgicas (síndrome similar ao lúpus) em seres humanos e relacionadas com a acetilação, mas sem ocorrência em animais.	O uso na insuficiência cardíaca pode acompanhar outras drogas, como a digoxina e diuréticos. É recomendável monitorar o paciente em busca de hipotensão no momento de ajustar a dosagem.	Comprimidos com 10 mg; injetável com 20 mg/mL.	Cães: 0,5 mg/kg (dose inicial), titulada para 0,5-2,0 mg/kg VO a cada 12h. Gatos: 2,5 mg/gato VO a cada 12-24h.
Hidroclorotiazida (HydroDIURIL, formulações genéricas)	Diurético tiazídico. Inibe a reabsorção de sódio nos túbulos renais distais. Usada como diurético e anti--hipertensivo. Por diminuir a excreção renal de cálcio, a droga tem sido usada para tratar urólitos constituídos por cálcio.	Não usar em pacientes com cálcio elevado. Pode causar distúrbio eletrolítico, como hipocalemia.	Não é tão potente como diurético de alça (como a furosemida). A eficácia clínica não foi determinada em medicina veterinária.	Solução oral com 10 e 100 mg/mL; comprimidos com 25, 50 e 100 mg.	2-4 mg/kg VO a cada 12h.
Hidrocodona, bitartarato (Hycodan)	Agonista opiáceo. Usado principalmente pela ação antitussígena. O Hycodan contém homatropina, mas outras associações podem conter guaifenesina e paracetamol.	Opiáceo oral. Pode causar efeitos opiáceos sistêmicos.	A hidrocodona está associada com atropina no produto Hycodan. A atropina pode reduzir as secreções respiratórias, mas, provavelmente, não possui efeitos clínicos significativos nas doses desta preparação (1,5 mg de homatropina por 5 mg de comprimido).	Comprimidos com 5 mg; xarope com 1 mg/mL.	Cães: antitussígeno: 0,5 mg/kg VO a cada 8h; analgésico: 0,5 mg/kg VO a cada 8-12h. Gatos: não há doses disponíveis.
Hidrocortisona (Cortef e formulações genéricas)	Droga anti-inflamatória do grupo dos glicocorticoides. A hidrocortisona possui menor efeito anti--inflamatório e maior efeito mineralocorticoide quando comparada com a prednisolona ou a dexametasona. Também utilizada como terapia de reposição.	Os efeitos colaterais são atribuídos ao excessivo efeito glicocorticoide.	As necessidades da dose estão relacionadas com a gravidade da doença.	Comprimidos com 5, 10 e 20 mg.	Terapia de reposição: 1-2 mg/kg VO a cada 12h. Anti-inflamatório: 2,5-5,0 mg/kg VO a cada 12h.
Hidrocortisona, succinato sódico (Solu-Cortef)	O mesmo que para a hidrocortisona, exceto que o succinato sódico é uma droga injetável de rápida ação.	O mesmo que para a hidrocortisona.	O mesmo que para a hidrocortisona. Preparar os frascos de acordo com as recomendações do fabricante.	Várias apresentações em frascos com solução injetável.	Choque: 50-150 mg/kg IV a cada 8h por dois dias. Anti-inflamatório: 5 mg/kg IV a cada 12h.
Hidromorfona (Dilaudid, Hidrostat e formulações genéricas)	Analgésico opiáceo. Da mesma forma que os outros opiáceos, se liga aos receptores mu- e kappa-opiáceos. A hidromorfona é 6 a 7 vezes mais potente que a morfina.	A hidromorfona é um agonista opiáceo, com efeitos similares aos da morfina. Entretanto, é mais potente que a morfina e deve ser usada em baixas doses.	A hidromorfona pode ser intercalada com a morfina, propiciando que as doses sejam ajustadas para potências diferentes.	Injetável com 1, 2, 4 e 10 mg/mL.	Cães: 0,22 mg/kg IM, repetida a cada 4-6h, se necessário, para o tratamento da dor. Na dose de 0,1 mg/kg, pode-se associar à acepromazina. Gatos: 0,1-0,2 mg/kg SC ou IM ou 0,05-0,1 mg/kg IV a cada 2-6h.
Hidróxido de magnésio (Leite de Magnésia)	O mesmo que para citrato de magnésio. Hidróxido de magnésio é também usado como antiácido oral, para neutralização da acidez gástrica.	É possível que ocorra acúmulo de magnésio em pacientes com insuficiência renal.	O mesmo que para citrato de magnésio.	Fluido para uso oral contendo 400 mg/5 mL.	Antiácido: 5-10 mL/kg a cada 4-6h VO. Catártico (cães): 15-50 mL/kg VO. Catártico (gatos): 2-6 mL/gato a cada 24h VO.

ESPÉCIES CANINA E FELINA

Formulário de Medicamentos para Consulta em 5 Minutos

Nome do Princípio Ativo (Comercial e Outros Nomes)	Farmacologia e Indicações	Efeitos Colaterais e Precauções	Informações de Dosagem e Comentários	Formulações	Dosagem (Exceto em Casos Indicados, a Dosagem é a Mesma para Cães e Gatos)
Hidroxiureia (Hydrea)	Agente antineoplásico. Usada em associação com outras modalidades de tratamento antineoplásico para o tratamento de determinadas neoplasias. Tem sido utilizada para o tratamento da policitemia vera.	Uso limitado em medicina veterinária. Não foram relatados efeitos colaterais. Em seres humanos, a hidroxiureia causa leucopenia, anemia e trombocitopenia.	Uso limitado em medicina veterinária.	Cápsulas com 500 mg.	Cães: 50 mg/kg VO a cada 24h, três dias por semana. Gatos: 25 mg/kg VO a cada 24h, três dias por semana.
Hidroxizina (Atarax)	Anti-histamínico da classe das piperazinas. Usada principalmente para tratar o prurido em animais.	Os efeitos colaterais estão relacionados principalmente aos efeitos anti-histamínicos. Em alguns animais pode ocorrer sedação.	Os estudos clínicos demonstraram que a hidroxizina é ligeiramente mais eficaz no tratamento do prurido em cães. Os efeitos clínicos da hidroxizina são atribuídos à conversão à cetirizina.	Comprimidos com 10, 25 e 50 mg; solução oral com 2 mg/mL.	Cães: 2 mg/kg IM, VO a cada 8-12h. Gatos: a dose efetiva não foi estabelecida.
Hipurato de metenamina (Hiprex, Urex) Mandelato de metenamina (Mandelamine e genérico)	Antisséptico urinário. Convertido em formaldeído na urina ácida, para geração do efeito antibacteriano/antifúngico. Agente ativo contra grande variedade de bactérias. Não provoca resistência. Menos efetivo contra Proteus, que promove um pH urinário alcalino. Não é efetivo em infecções sistêmicas.	Embora a formação de formaldeído na bexiga possa causar irritação, em humanos houve necessidade de doses elevadas (>8 g/dia). Em animais, não foram relatados efeitos adversos.	Não foram publicados resultados de estudos clínicos em animais. O uso em animais se baseia na experiência em humanos, ou em experiências anedóticas em animais. A urina deve estar ácida, para que a metenamina seja convertida até formaldeído (monitorizar periodicamente o pH). pH abaixo de 5,5 é considerado ideal. Para baixar o pH, suplementar com ácido ascórbico ou cloreto de amônio.	Hipurato de metenamina: comprimidos de 1 g. Mandelato de metenamina: comprimidos de 1 g; grânulos para solução oral; suspensão oral contendo 100 mg/mL. Mandelato de metenamina pode não estar disponível.	Hipurato de metenamina: Cães: 500 mg/cão a cada 12h VO. Gatos: 250 mg/gato a cada 12h VO. Mandelato de metenamina: 10-20 mg/kg a cada 8-12h VO.
Hormônio do crescimento (hGH, somatrem, somatropina) (Protropin, Humatrope, Nutropin)	Hormônio do crescimento, também conhecido como hormônio do crescimento humano. Usado para tratar deficiências hormonais do crescimento.	O hormônio do crescimento é diabetogênico em todos os animais. O excesso desse hormônio produz acromegalia.	Há uma experiência clínica limitada em animais. A preparação deve ser reconstituída com diluente estéril antes do uso. A solução pronta é estável por 14 dias, se refrigerada.	Frascos com 5 e 10 mg.	0,1 U/kg SC, IM três vezes por semana, por 4-6 semanas (a dose pediátrica humana é de 0,18-0,3 mg/kg/semana).
Hormônio foliculoestimulante (FSH)	Ver Urofolitropina.				
Hormônio luteinizante	Ver Gonadorelina.				
Hormônio tireoidiano	Ver Levotiroxina sódica e Liotironina.				
Hycodan	Ver Hidrocodona, bitartarato.	-	-	-	-
Ibuprofeno (Motrin, Advil, Nuprin)	AINE. Produz ação anti-inflamatória por inibição das prostaglandinas.	Não foram estabelecidas doses seguras para cães e gatos. Foram relatados vômito, ulceração e hemorragia GI grave em cães.	Evitar o uso, especialmente em cães.	Comprimidos com 200, 400, 600 e 800 mg.	Dose segura não estabelecida.

CONSULTA VETERINÁRIA EM 5 MINUTOS

		Formulário de Medicamentos para Consulta em 5 Minutos			
Nome do Princípio Ativo (Comercial e Outros Nomes)	Farmacologia e Indicações	Efeitos Colaterais e Precauções	Informações de Dosagem e Comentários	Formulações	Dosagem (Exceto em Casos Indicados, a Dosagem é a Mesma para Cães e Gatos)
Imipeném (Primaxin)	Antibiótico β-lactâmico com amplo espectro de atividade. A ação é similar aos outros β-lactâmicos, exceto por ser o imipeném o mais ativo dos β-lactâmicos. Usado principalmente para infecções graves e multirresistentes.	Podem ocorrer reações alérgicas com antibióticos β-lactâmicos. A neurotoxicidade (convulsões) pode ocorrer na presença de infusão muito rápida ou em pacientes com insuficiência renal. É possível ocorrer vômito e náusea. As aplicações SC ou IM podem causar dor em cães.	Reservar o uso desta droga apenas para infecções refratárias e resistentes. Observar cuidadosamente as recomendações do fabricante para administração adequada. Para administração IV, adicionar a droga aos fluidos IV. Para administração IM, adicionar 2 mL de lidocaína (1%); a suspensão é estável por apenas uma hora.	Injetável, frascos com 250 e 500 mg.	3-10 mg/kg IV, SC, IM a cada 6-8h; normalmente 5 mg/kg IV, IM, SC a cada 6-8h.
Imipramina (Tofranil)	Droga antidepressiva tricíclica (TCA). Usada em seres humanos para tratar a ansiedade e a depressão. Utilizada em animais para tratar uma infinidade de distúrbios comportamentais, incluído o transtorno obsessivo-compulsivo. A ação ocorre por inibição da receptação de serotonina nos terminais nervosos pré-sinápticos.	Os diversos efeitos colaterais estão associados com TCAs, como efeitos antimuscarínicos (boca seca, frequência cardíaca aumentada) e anti-histamínicos (sedação). As superdosagens podem causar cardiotoxicidade com risco para a vida.	As doses são principalmente baseadas no empirismo. Não há testes de eficácia controlados disponíveis para animais. Pode haver um atraso de 2-4 semanas após o início da terapia para que os efeitos benéficos sejam vistos.	Comprimidos com 10, 25 e 50 mg.	Cães: 2-4 mg/kg VO a cada 12-24h. Gatos: 0,5-1,0 mg/kg VO a cada 12-24h.
Insulina	A insulina possui diversos efeitos associados com a utilização de glicose. Usada para tratar o diabetes melito em cães e gatos.	Os efeitos colaterais estão principalmente relacionados com as superdosagens (hipoglicemia).	As doses devem ser cuidadosamente ajustadas em cada paciente, dependendo da resposta. Monitorar as concentrações de glicose plasmática/ sérica.	Injetável com 40 ou 100 U/mL.	As doses de insulina são específicas para cada espécie e tipo de apresentação da droga. Consultar informação específica de cada produto para obter a dose inicial (p. ex.: 0,5 mcg/kg SC a cada 12h) e ajustá-la com base no monitoramento.
Interferon (interferon-α, HuIFN-α) (Roferon)	Interferon humano. Usado para estimular o sistema imune em pacientes.	Os efeitos colaterais não foram relatados em animais.	As doses e indicações para animais foram baseadas principalmente da extrapolação de recomendações humanas ou de estudos experimentais limitados. No preparo, adicionar 3 milhões de unidades a um litro de salina estéril, dividindo em alíquotas e congelando-as. Diluir adequadamente para preparar uma solução com 30 U/mL.	Injetável, frascos com 5 e 10 milhões de unidades.	Cães: 2,5 milhões U/kg IV diariamente, por três dias. Gatos: 1 milhão U/kg IV diariamente, por cinco dias consecutivos, nos dias 0, 14 e 60.
Iodeto	Ver Potássio, iodeto.	-	-	-	-
Iodeto de potássio	Suplemento de iodo, com algumas propriedades antimicrobianas extras. Também usado no tratamento de algumas infecções fúngicas. Também pode ser usado como proteção da tireoide contra lesões por radiação.	Doses elevadas causam iodismo, resultando em lacrimejamento, irritação cutânea, edema palpebral, tosse e pelagem de mau aspecto.	As doses são puramente empíricas.	Solução a 10%; comprimidos de 145 mg.	Cães e gatos: começar com 5 mg/kg a cada 8h VO e aumentar para 25 mg/kg a cada 8h VO. Exposição à radiação: 2 mg/kg/dia VO.

Formulário de Medicamentos para Consulta em 5 Minutos

Nome do Princípio Ativo (Comercial e Outros Nomes)	Farmacologia e Indicações	Efeitos Colaterais e Precauções	Informações de Dosagem e Comentários	Formulações	Dosagem (Exceto em Casos Indicados, a Dosagem é a Mesma para Cães e Gatos)
Ioimbina (Yobine)	Antagonista α2-adrenérgico. Uso principalmente na reversão de ações da xilazina ou da detomidina. Atipamezol é mais específico, como agente de reversão.	Doses elevadas podem causar tremores e convulsões.	Reverte os sinais de sedação e anestesia causados pelos α2-agonistas. Antipamezol pode ser mais específico, sendo recomendado para animais de pequeno porte.	Injeção: 2 mg/mL.	0,11 mg/kg IV, ou 0,25-0,5 mg/kg SC, IM.
Ipeca, xarope (Ipecac)	Droga emética. Para o tratamento emergencial de envenenamentos. Acredita-se que o ingrediente ativo seja a emetina.	Não foram relatados efeitos colaterais com a terapia aguda para o envenenamento. A administração crônica pode levar à toxicidade do miocárdio.	Disponível como droga sem prescrição médica. O início dos vômitos pode requerer 20-30 minutos.	Solução oral com 30 mL por frasco.	Cães: 3-6 mL/cão VO. Gatos: 2-6 mL/gato VO.
Ipodato ou iopanoico, ácido	Agente colecistográfico. Usado para o tratamento do hipertireoidismo em gatos. Utilizado como alternativa ao metimazol, radioterapia ou cirurgia.	Não foram relatados efeitos colaterais.	O uso do ipodato é experimental, e as doses precisas não foram avaliadas. Em um estudo, 2/3 dos gatos tratados responderam positivamente.	Cápsulas com 50 mg (podem ter sido formuladas para gatos).	Ipodato: Gatos: 15 mg/kg VO a cada 12h. A dose mais comum é de 50 mg/gato a cada 12h. Ácido iopanoico: 50 mg/gato VO a cada 12h.
Isoflurano (AErrane)	Anestésico inalatório.	-	-	Frasco com 100 mL.	Indução: 5%. Manutenção: 1,5-2,5%.
Isoniazida (INH)	Agente antibacteriano que interfere com a síntese de ácido nucleico. Usada contra *Mycobacterium*.	Não usar em animais com problemas hepáticos.	-	Comprimidos com 100, 300 e 500 mg; xarope com 10 mg/mL.	5 mg/kg/dia VO.
Isoproterenol (Isuprel)	Agonista adrenérgico. Estimula receptores adrenérgicos β-1 e β-2. Usado para estimular o coração (inotrópico e cronotrópico). Também utilizado como relaxante da musculatura lisa bronquial no tratamento da broncoconstrição aguda.	Os efeitos colaterais estão relacionados com a excessiva estimulação adrenérgica e aparecem, principalmente, como taquicardia e taquiarritmias.	Meia-vida curta. Deve ser administrado por infusão constante ou repetido se administrado por via IM ou SC. Recomendado apenas para uso breve.	Injetável, ampolas com 0,2 mg/mL.	10 mcg/kg IM, SC a cada 6h; ou diluir 1 mg em 500 mL de uma solução IV de Ringer ou dextrose a 5% e usar 1 mL/minuto (1-2 mcg/minuto), ou até surtir efeito.
Isossorbida, dinitrato (Isordil, Isorbid, Sorbitrate)	Vasodilatador do grupo dos nitratos. Causa vasodilatação por geração de óxido nítrico. Relaxa a musculatura lisa vascular, especialmente a venosa. Reduz a pré-carga em pacientes com ICC.	Os efeitos colaterais são principalmente relacionados com superdosagens que produzem vasodilatação excessiva e hipotensão. A tolerância pode aparecer em função de doses repetidas.	Em geral, as doses são adaptadas individualmente, dependendo da resposta.	Comprimidos com 2,5; 5; 10; 20; 30 e 40 mg; cápsulas com 40 mg.	2,5-5,0 mg/animal VO a cada 12h (ou 0,22-1,1 mg/kg VO a cada 12h).
Isossorbida, mononitrato (Monoket)	Os mesmos comentários feitos para o dinitrato de isossorbida, exceto que o mononitrato é a forma biologicamente ativa do dinitrato de isosorbida. Comparado com o dinitrato, o mononitrato não faz uma primeira passagem metabólica, sendo completamente absorvido por via oral.	Os mesmos relatados para o dinitrato de isossorbida e nitroglicerina.	Geralmente mais bem absorvido que o dinitrato de isossorbida.	Comprimidos com 10 e 20 mg.	5 mg/cão VO, em duas doses diárias, em intervalos de sete dias.

Formulário de Medicamentos para Consulta em 5 Minutos

Nome do Princípio Ativo (Comercial e Outros Nomes)	Farmacologia e Indicações	Efeitos Colaterais e Precauções	Informações de Dosagem e Comentários	Formulações	Dosagem (Exceto em Casos Indicados, a Dosagem é a Mesma para Cães e Gatos)
Isotretinoína (Accutane)	Droga estabilizadora da ceratinização. A isotretinoína reduz o tamanho e inibe a atividade das glândulas sebáceas, reduzindo a secreção de sebo. Em seres humanos, ela é principalmente usada para tratar a acne. Em animais, é utilizada para tratar a adenite sebácea.	Absolutamente contraindicada em animais prenhes. Os efeitos colaterais não foram relatados em animais, apesar de estudos experimentais terem demonstrado que a droga pode causar calcificação focal (como ocorre no miocárdio e vasos).	O uso em medicina veterinária está confinado à experiência clínica limitada e à extrapolação de relatos em seres humanos.	Cápsulas com 10, 20 e 40 mg.	Cães: 1-3 mg/kg/dia (até a dose máxima recomendada de 3-4 mg/kg/dia VO). Gatos: não estabelecida.
Itraconazol (Sporanox)	Droga antifúngica azólica (triazólica). Ativa contra dermatófitos e fungos sistêmicos, como *Blastomyces*, *Histoplasma* e *Coccidioides*. Também utilizada na dermatite por *Malassezia*.	O itraconazol é mais bem tolerado que o cetoconazol. Entretanto, vômito e hepatotoxicose são possíveis, especialmente em altas doses. Em um estudo, a hepatotoxicose foi mais provável em altas doses. 10 a 15% dos cães desenvolverão altos níveis de enzimas hepáticas. Altas doses em gatos provocaram vômito e anorexia.	As doses são baseadas em estudos com animais em que o itraconazol foi usado para tratar a blastomicose em cães. Em gatos, as doses baixas são eficazes contra dermatófitos (ver seção sobre doses). Outros usos ou doses são baseados em empirismo ou extrapolação da literatura humana.	Cápsulas com 100 mg; solução oral com 10 mg/mL. Formulações associadas podem não ser tão bem absorvidas como as preparações comerciais.	Cães: 2,5 mg/kg VO a cada 12h ou 5 mg/kg a cada 24h. Para dermatite por *Malassezia*: 5 mg/kg VO a cada 24h por dois dias, repetida semanalmente por três semanas. Dermatofitose: 3 mg/kg/dia VO por 15 dias. Gatos: 5 mg/kg VO a cada 12h; para dermatofitose em gatos: 1,5-3,0 mg/kg (até 5 mg/kg) VO a cada 24h por 15 dias.
Ivermectina (Heartgard, Ivomec, Eqvalan Liquid)	Droga antiparasitária. Neurotóxica para parasitos por potencializar os canais de cloreto para entrada de glutamato; usada para o tratamento antiparasitário e prevenção da dirofilariose.	A toxicidade pode ocorrer em doses altas e em raças nas quais a ivermectina cruza a barreira hematocefálica. As raças sensíveis são: Collie, Pastor Australiano, Pastor de Shetland e Old English Sheepdog. A toxicidade é do tipo neural e os sinais incluem depressão, ataxia, dificuldades de visão, coma e óbito. A ivermectina parece ser segura para animais prenhes. Não administrar em animais com menos de seis semanas de idade. Os animais com microfilaremia podem apresentar reações adversas para doses altas.	As doses variam de acordo com o uso terapêutico. Para prevenção de dirofilariose, usa-se a dose mínima; outros parasitos requerem doses maiores. O Heartgard é a única apresentação aprovada para uso em pequenos animais; para outras indicações, os produtos injetáveis para grandes animais geralmente são administrados pelas vias VO, IM ou SC em pequenos animais.	Solução injetável a 1% (10 mg/mL); solução oral com 10 mg/mL; pasta oral com 18,7 mg/mL; comprimidos com 68, 136 e 272 mcg.	Prevenção da dirofilariose: 6 mcg/kg VO a cada 30 dias em cães e 24 mcg/kg VO a cada 30 dias em gatos. Microfilaricida: 50 mcg/kg VO por duas semanas após a terapia adulticida. Terapia ectoparasiticida (cães e gatos): 200-300 mcg/kg IM, SC, VO. Terapia endoparasiticida (cães e gatos): 200-400 mcg/kg SC, VO semanalmente. Terapia contra *Demodex*: iniciar com 100 mcg/kg/dia e aumentar gradativamente a dose até 600 mcg/kg/dia VO por 60-120 dias. Prevenção da dirofilariose em gatos: 25 mcg/kg VO a cada 30 dias.
L-asparaginase (Elspar)	Agente antineoplásico. Enzima purificada de *E. coli*. Usada em protocolos de linfoma. Elimina células neoplásicas de asparagina e interfere na síntese de proteínas.	Hipersensibilidade, reações alérgicas.	Normalmente usada em combinação com outras drogas nos protocolos de quimioterapia antineoplásica.	Injetável, frasco com 10.000 unidades.	Cães: 400 U/kg IM semanalmente ou 10.000 U/m² por três semanas. Gatos: 400 U/kg SC semanalmente.
L-Dopa	Ver Levodopa.	-	-	-	-
L-Lisina (Enisyl-F)	Aminoácido para tratamento de infecções herpéticas. Suplementação oral para gatos com infecção pelo herpes-vírus felino 1 (FHV-1). Em estudos clínicos, não foi demonstrada eficácia para o FHV, para controle de infecções oculares ou do trato respiratório superior.	Bem tolerado em gatos.	O pó pode ser misturado ao alimento. A pasta pode ser diretamente administrada.	Pasta contendo 250 mg/mL.	Gatos: 400 mg VO/dia. Formulação em pasta: 1-2 mL VO para gatos adultos e 1 mL para filhotes.

ESPÉCIES CANINA E FELINA

Formulário de Medicamentos para Consulta em 5 Minutos

Nome do Princípio Ativo (Comercial e Outros Nomes)	Farmacologia e Indicações	Efeitos Colaterais e Precauções	Informações de Dosagem e Comentários	Formulações	Dosagem (Exceto em Casos Indicados, a Dosagem é a Mesma para Cães e Gatos)
Lactulose (Chronulac, formulações genéricas)	Laxante. Produz efeitos laxativos mediante ação osmótica no cólon. A lactulose tem sido usada para o tratamento da hiperamonemia (encefalopatia hepática), já que reduz as concentrações de amônia sanguínea pela redução do pH do cólon; desta forma, a amônia colônica não é prontamente absorvida.	O uso excessivo pode causar desequilíbrio hidroeletrolítico.	Em medicina veterinária, os estudos clínicos para avaliar sua eficácia não estão disponíveis. Além dessas doses citadas, tem sido usada em gatos uma solução a 30% na forma de enema (20-30 mL/kg) na retenção fecal.	10 g/15 mL.	Constipação: 1 mL/4,5 kg VO a cada 8h (até obter o efeito desejado). Encefalopatia hepática: Cães: 0,5 mL/kg VO a cada 8h. Gatos: 2,5-5,0 mL/gato VO a cada 8h.
Leflunomida (Arava)	Agente imunossupressor. Usada para suprimir a proliferação de células T e β. Também utilizada para tratar enfermidades imunomediadas em cães.	Não foram relatados efeitos colaterais em cães, mas pode reduzir o apetite ou causar diarreia.	Normalmente utilizada como alternativa a outras drogas imunossupressoras.	Comprimidos com 5, 10 e 20 mg.	Cães: 2 mg/kg VO a cada 12h. Alguns pacientes podem requerer doses mais altas. Gatos: não foram estabelecidas doses.
Leucovorina cálcica (ácido folínico) (Wellcovorin e formulações genéricas)	A leucovorina é uma forma reduzida do ácido fólico, sendo convertida para metabólitos ativos deste ácido para a síntese de purinas e timidinas. A droga é usada como antídoto para antagonistas do ácido fólico.	Foram relatadas reações alérgicas em seres humanos.	Utilizada principalmente como medida de salvamento em superdosagens de antagonistas do ácido fólico (metotrexato). Não foram relatados estudos clínicos em medicina veterinária. Não está estabelecido se a leucovorina previne a toxicidade da administração de sulfonamida-trimetoprima.	Comprimidos com 5, 10, 15 e 25 mg; injetável com 3 ou 5 mg/mL.	Com a administração de metrotrexato: 3 mg/m^2 IV, IM, VO. Como antídoto na intoxicação por pirimetamina: 1 mg/kg VO a cada 24h.
Levamisol, hidrato (Levasole, Tramisol, Ergamisol)	Droga antiparasitária do grupo dos imidotiazólicos. Mecanismo de ação devido à toxicidade neuromuscular aos parasitos. O levamisol tem sido usado como endoparasiticida e microfilaricida em cães. A droga também tem sido utilizada como um imunoestimulante; entretanto, estudos clínicos de sua eficácia não estão disponíveis.	Pode produzir toxicidade colinérgica. Também pode provocar vômito em cães.	Em cães positivos para dirofilariose, pode esterilizar dirofilárias fêmeas adultas.	Bólus com 0,184 g; pacote com 11,7 g/13 g; comprimido com 50 mg (Ergamisol).	Cães: ancilostamatídeos: 5-8 mg/kg VO em dose única (até 10 mg/kg VO por dois dias); microfilaricida, 10 mg/kg VO a cada 24h por 6-10 dias; imunoestimulante, 0,5-2,0 mg/kg VO três vezes por semana. Gatos: endoparasitos, 4,4 mg/kg VO em dose única; vermes pulmonares, 20-40 mg/kg VO a cada 48h por cinco tratamentos.
Levetiracetam (Keppra)	Anticonvulsivante. Uso no tratamento de epilepsia, quando outros tratamentos não forem eficazes. Inibe o disparo repetido dos neurônios, sem afetar excitação neuronal normal.	Fraqueza, letargia e tontura foram relatadas em humanos. Não foram relatados efeitos adversos em animais.	Pode ser usado com outros anticonvulsivantes.	Comprimidos de 250, 500, 750 mg.	Cães: começar com 20 mg/kg a cada 8h VO e aumentar gradativamente, conforme a necessidade. Gatos: 20 mg/kg a cada 8h VO.
Levodopa (L-dopa) (Larodopa)	Convertido em dopamina após atravessar a barreira hematoencefálica. Estimula os receptores dopaminérgicos do SNC. Em humanos, uso no tratamento da doença de Parkinson. Em animais, tem sido usado no tratamento da encefalopatia hepática.	Não foram relatados efeitos adversos em animais. Em humanos, tontura, mudanças mentais, urinação difícil e hipotensão encontram-se entre os efeitos adversos relatados.	Não foram publicados estudos clínicos na medicina veterinária. Titular a dose para cada paciente.	Comprimidos ou cápsulas de 100, 250, 500 mg.	Encefalopatia hepática: começar com 6,8 mg/kg; em seguida 1,4 mg/kg a cada 6h VO.

	Formulário de Medicamentos para Consulta em 5 Minutos				
Nome do Princípio Ativo (Comercial e Outros Nomes)	Farmacologia e Indicações	Efeitos Colaterais e Precauções	Informações de Dosagem e Comentários	Formulações	Dosagem (Exceto em Casos Indicados, a Dosagem é a Mesma para Cães e Gatos)
Levotiroxina sódica (Soloxine, Thyro-Tabs, Synthroid Leventa)	Terapia de reposição para tratamento de pacientes com hipotireoidismo. Levotiroxina é T_4, que é convertida na maioria dos pacientes em T_3 ativa.	Doses elevadas podem causar tirotoxicose, uma ocorrência incomum (em comparação com humanos). Interações farmacológicas: pacientes medicados com corticosteroides podem exibir menor capacidade de converter T_4 para T_3.	A suplementação da tireoide deve ser orientada por exames clínicos, para confirmação do diagnóstico e monitorização pós-medicamento, para ajuste da dose.	Comprimidos de 0,1-0,8 mg (em incrementos de 0,1 mg), solução oral: 1 mg/mL.	Cães: (comprimidos) 18-22 mcg/kg a cada 12h VO (ajustar a dose via monitorização). Cães (solução oral): 20 mcg/kg a cada 24h VO. Gatos: 10-20 mcg/kg/dia VO (ajustar a dose via monitorização).
Lidocaína (Xilocaína e genéricos)	Anestésico local e antiarrítmico Classe I. Lidocaína também é de uso comum no tratamento agudo de arritmias cardíacas.	Doses elevadas causam efeitos do SNC (tumores, tremores e convulsões). Lidocaína pode causar arritmia cardíaca, mas tem maior efeito no tecido cardíaco anormal, em comparação com o tecido normal. Gatos são mais suscetíveis a efeitos adversos; portanto, nessa espécie usar doses mais baixas.	Quando utilizada para infiltração local, muitas formulações contêm adrenalina para prolongamento da atividade no local da injeção. Evitar adrenalina em pacientes com arritmia cardíaca. Observar que formulações humanas podem conter adrenalina, mas nenhuma formulação veterinária contém essa substância. Para aumentar o pH, acelerar o início da ação e diminuir a dor decorrente da injeção, pode-se adicionar 1 mEq de bicarbonato de sódio a 10 mL de lidocaína (usar imediatamente depois de misturar).	Injeção: 5, 10, 15, 20 mg/mL.	Cães (antiarrítmico): 2-4 mg/kg IV (para uma dose máxima de 8 mg/kg ao longo de um período de 10 min); infusão IV de 25-75 mcg/kg/min; 6 mg/kg a cada 1,5h IM. Gatos (antiarrítmico): começar com 0,1-0,4 mg/kg; em seguida, aumentar para 0,25-0,75 mg/kg IV lenta, ou infusão de 10-20 mcg/kg/min. Para epidural (cães e gatos): 4,4 mg/kg de solução a 2%.
Lincomicina (Lincocin)	Antibiótico da classe das lincosamidas, similar em termos de mecanismo à clindamicina e eritromicina. O espectro abrange principalmente bactérias Gram-positivas. Uso no tratamento de pioderma e de outras infecções dos tecidos moles.	Efeitos adversos são incomuns. Lincomicina causou vômito e diarreia em animais. Não administrar por via oral em roedores e coelhos.	As ações da lincomicina e da clindamicina são suficientemente parecidas para possibilitar a substituição de lincomicina pela clindamicina.	Comprimidos de 100, 200, 500 mg.	15-25 mg/kg a cada 12h VO. Para pioderma, têm sido administradas doses de até somente 10 mg/kg a cada 12h.
Linezolida (Zyvox)	Antibiótico do grupo das oxazolidinonas. Espectro Gram-positivo, abrangendo linhagens fármaco-resistentes de Enterococcus e Staphylococcus. O elevado custo limita o uso de rotina.	Efeitos adversos: diarreia e náusea. Em humanos, raramente observou-se anemia e leucopenia. Usar com cautela em associação com inibidores da monoamina oxidase e agentes serotonérgicos.	Em animais, seu uso fica reservado apenas para infecções fármaco-resistentes (p.ex., Staphyloccus spp. resistente à meticilina) em que outros agentes se revelaram ineficazes.	Comprimidos de 400 e 600 mg. Suspensão oral contendo 20 mg/mL. Injeção: 2 mg/mL.	10 mg/kg, a cada 8-12h VO ou IV.
Liotironina (Cytomel)	Suplemento tireoidiano. Liotironina é equivalente a T_3. Geralmente, é preferível usar levotiroxina.	Não foram relatados efeitos adversos (ver Levotiroxina sódica).	As doses de liotironina devem ser ajustadas com base na monitorização das concentrações de T_3 nos pacientes.	Comprimidos de 5, 25, 50 e 60 mcg.	4,4 mcg/kg a cada 8h VO. Para a prova de supressão de T_3 em gatos: coletar pré--amostra para T_4 e T_3, administrar 25 mcg a cada 8h para 7 doses e, em seguida à última dose, coletar pós-amostras para T_3 e T_4.
Lisinopril (Prinivil, Zestril)	Inibidor da ECA. Utilizado no tratamento da ICC e hipertensão. Inibe a síntese da angiotensina II, promovendo vasodilatação e diminuição da aldosterona.	Sendo ainda de uso limitado em animais, ainda não foram documentados efeitos adversos do lisinopril.	Ainda não foram publicados estudos clínicos com uso de lisinopril em animais. Como ocorre com o uso de qualquer inibidor da ECA, monitorizar eletrólitos e a função renal 3-7 dias depois de iniciada a terapia; depois, monitorizar periodicamente.	Comprimidos de 2,5, 5, 10, 20, 40 mg.	Cães: 0,5 mg/kg a cada 24h VO. Gatos: dose não estabelecida.

ESPÉCIES CANINA E FELINA

Formulário de Medicamentos para Consulta em 5 Minutos

Nome do Princípio Ativo (Comercial e Outros Nomes)	Farmacologia e Indicações	Efeitos Colaterais e Precauções	Informações de Dosagem e Comentários	Formulações	Dosagem (Exceto em Casos Indicados, a Dosagem é a Mesma para Cães e Gatos)
Lítio, carbonato de (Lithotabs)	Estimula a granulopoiese e eleva o *pool* dos neutrófilos em animais. Em humanos, é usado no tratamento da depressão. O efeito no SNC está relacionado à diminuição das concentrações de neurotransmissores.	Não foram relatados efeitos adversos em animais. Em humanos, foram relatados problemas cardiovasculares, sonolência e diarreia.	O uso em animais não é comum. Essa substância foi experimentalmente usada para aumentar a contagem de neutrófilos, em seguida a tratamento antineoplásico.	Cápsulas de 150, 300, 600 mg; comprimidos de 300 mg; xarope contendo 300 mg/5 mL.	Cães: 10 mg/kg a cada 12h VO. Gatos: não recomendável.
Lomustina (CCNU) (CeeNU)	Medicamento antineoplásico - agente alquilante da classe das nitrosureias. Substância altamente lipossolúvel; atravessa a barreira hematoencefálica. Uso no tratamento de linfoma e tumores cerebrais.	Mielossupressão, hepatotoxicose, vômito.	A administração com o estômago vazio diminui a náusea. Monitorar o hemograma, para evidência de mielossupressão.	Cápsulas de 10, 40, 100 mg.	
Loperamida (Imodium e genérico)	Agonista dos opiatos. Estimula a segmentação da musculatura lisa no intestino, bem como a absorção de eletrólitos. Usada no tratamento agudo da diarreia inespecífica.	Loperamida não causa efeitos adversos dos opiatos sistêmicos. Seus efeitos sistêmicos são pouco importantes; essa substância não atravessa a barreira hematoencefálica. No entanto, algumas raças (p. ex.,collies, pastores australianos e mestiços de collie) podem ser suscetíveis a efeitos adversos, por causa de uma deleção do P-gp. Em qualquer animal, o uso excessivo pode causar constipação.	Basicamente, as doses são empíricas ou se baseiam na extrapolação da dose para humanos. Ainda não foram publicados estudos clínicos em animais.	Comprimidos de 2 mg; fluido oral contendo 0,2 mg/mL.	
Lufenurona (Program)	Antiparasitário. Substância usada no controle de pulgas em animais. Inibe o desenvolvimento das crias de pulgas. Pode ser usado para dermatófitos em cães e gatos, embora sua eficácia tenha sido questionada por alguns especialistas.	Não foram relatados efeitos adversos. Essa substância parece ser relativamente segura durante a gestação e em animais jovens.	Lufenurona pode controlar o desenvolvimento das pulgas, com a administração 1×/cada 30 dias em animais.	Comprimidos de 45, 90, 135, 204,9, 409,8 mg; suspensão contendo 135 e 270 mg por embalagem individual.	
Lufenurona + milbemicina oxima (Sentinel comprimidos e Flavor Tabs®)	Combinação de dois agentes antiparasitários. Ver Lufenurona ou Milbemicina oxima. Usar para proteção contra pulgas, dirofilárias, nematelmintos, ancilostomídeos e tricurídeos.	Ver Lufenurona ou Milbemicina oxima.	Ver Lufenurona ou Milbemicina oxima.	Relação milbemicina oxima/lufenurona: comprimidos de 2,3/46 mg; Flavor Tabs® de 5,75/115, 11,5/230 e 23/460 mg.	
Manitol (Osmitrol)	Diurético hiperosmótico. Aumenta a osmolalidade plasmática, implicando transferência de líquido dos tecidos para o plasma. Agente antiglaucoma. Uso no tratamento do edema e para redução da pressão intra-ocular. Manitol também é usado para promover excreção urinária de certas toxinas.	Causa desequilíbrio hídrico e eletrolítico. Não usar em pacientes desidratados. Usar com cautela diante de suspeita de sangramento intracraniano, pois pode aumentar a hemorragia. A administração demasiado rápida pode expandir excessivamente o volume extracelular.	Usar apenas em pacientes em que o equilíbrio de líquidos e eletrólitos possa ser monitorado. Depois de preparada a solução, descartar a parte não utilizada.	Solução a 5-25% para injeção.	Diurético: 1 g/kg de solução IV 5-25% para manutenção do fluxo urinário. Glaucoma ou edema do SNC: 0,25-2 g/kg de uma solução IV 15-25% ao longo de 30-60 min (repetir em 6h, se necessário).

Formulário de Medicamentos para Consulta em 5 Minutos

Nome do Princípio Ativo (Comercial e Outros Nomes)	Farmacologia e Indicações	Efeitos Colaterais e Precauções	Informações de Dosagem e Comentários	Formulações	Dosagem (Exceto em Casos Indicados, a Dosagem é a Mesma para Cães e Gatos)
Marbofloxacino (Zeniquin)	Antimicrobiano da classe das fluoroquinolonas. O espectro abrange estafilococos, bacilos gram-negativos e algumas *Pseudomonas*.	Em doses elevadas, esse agente pode causar um pouco de náusea e vômito. Evitar uso em animais jovens. Seguro para gatos (segurança ocular) na dose recomendada.	Usar teste de sensibilidade como orientação do tratamento.	Comprimidos de 25, 50, 100 e 200 mg.	2,75-5,55 mg/kg a cada 24h VO.
Maropitant (Cerenia)	Antiemético. Inibidor da neurocinina (NK) tipo 1. Maropitant funciona prevenindo o vômito causado pela quimioterapia e pela cinetose. Também é eficaz na inibição do vômito causado por estimulação (tanto central como periférica).	Em estudos clínicos, poucos efeitos adversos em cães ou gatos. Em alguns animais, ocorreram salivação e tremores musculares.	Estudos demonstraram que os inibidores da NK-1 são antieméticos efetivos para uma série de estímulos, tanto em cães como em gatos. Manter sob refrigeração para evitar a dor causada pela injeção.	Injeção: 10 mg/mL; comprimidos de 16, 24, 60 ou 160 mg.	Cães: 1 mg/kg SC a cada 24h por até 5 dias; 2 mg/kg VO a cada 24h por até 5 dias; para cinetose, 8 mg/kg VO a cada 24h por até 2 dias. Gatos: 1 mg/kg, 1 vez/dia SC ou VO.
Meclizina (Antivert, genérico)	Antiemético e anti-histamínico. Medicamento usado no tratamento da cinetose. Sua ação pode ser uma função das ações anticolinérgicas centrais. Também pode suprimir a zona de gatilho quimioceptora (ZGQR).	Não foram relatados efeitos adversos em animais. Efeitos anticolinérgicos (semelhantes aos da atropina) podem causar efeitos colaterais.	Não foram publicados estudos clínicos em animais. O uso em animais se baseia na experiência em humanos, ou em experiências anedóticas em animais.	Comprimidos de 12,5, 25, 50 mg.	Cães: 25 mg a cada 24h VO (para cinetose, administrar 1 h antes da viagem). Gatos: 12,5 mg a cada 24h VO.
Meclofenamato sódico (Arquel, Meclofen)	AINE. Uso no tratamento da artrite e de outros problemas inflamatórios. Seu uso diminuiu por causa da disponibilidade de outros AINE.	Não foram relatados efeitos adversos em animais, mas é comum a ocorrência de efeitos adversos com o uso de outros AINE.	Não foram publicados estudos clínicos em animais. O uso em animais se baseia na experiência em humanos, ou em experiências anedóticas em animais. Administrar com o alimento.	Cápsulas de 50, 100 mg. Raramente serão obtidas formulações para cães.	Cães: 1 mg/kg VO a cada 24h por até 5 dias. Gatos: não recomendável.
Medetomidina (Domitor)	Agonista α2-adrenérgico. Utilizado basicamente como sedativo, adjuvante anestésico e na analgesia. Seu uso diminuiu por causa da disponibilidade de dexmedetomidina (Dexdomitor), que é mais específica.	α2-Agonistas diminuem a descarga simpática. Pode ocorrer depressão cardiovascular. Medetomidina causará bradicardia e hipertensão iniciais.	Medetomidina pode ser usada para sedação, analgesia e em procedimentos cirúrgicos menores. Fazer reversão com igual volume de atipamezol.	Injeção: 1,0 mg/mL.	750 mcg/m² IV ou 1000 mcg/m² IM. Doses menores podem ser usadas para sedação e analgesia durante curto período.
Melarsomina (Immiticide)	Composto arsenical orgânico usado no tratamento da dirofilariose. Adulticida para dirofilária. Os arsenicais alteram a captação e o metabolismo da glicose em *Dirofilaria*.	Efeitos adversos: tromboembolia pulmonar (7-20 dias após tratamento), anorexia (incidência de 13%), reação no local da injeção (miosite) (incidência de 32%), letargia ou depressão (incidência de 15%). Causa elevações das enzimas hepáticas. Doses elevadas (3×) podem causar inflamação pulmonar e morte. Se forem administradas doses elevadas, pode-se usar dimercaprol (3 mg/kg IM) como antídoto.	Os regimes posológicos se baseiam na gravidade da dirofilariose. Consultar referências recentes, para determinação da classe da doença (Classe I-IV). Classe IV é a mais grave; animais assim classificados não devem ser tratados com o adulticida antes da cirurgia. Evitar exposição humana. (Lavar as mãos após o manuseio ou calçar luvas.) Não congelar as soluções após seu preparo.	Injeção: 25 mg/mL. Após reconstituição, preserva a potência por 24 h.	Cães: administrar via injeção IM profunda. Cães nas Classes I e II: 2,5 mg/kg a cada 24h durante 2 dias consecutivos. Cães na Classe III: 2,5 mg/kg 1×; depois, em 1 mês, duas doses adicionais com intervalo de 24 h. Muitos especialistas em *Dirofilaria immitis* recomendam a divisão da dose (como se faz para pacientes na Classe III) também para Classes I e II. Pode-se administrar doxiciclina para melhorar a eficácia e diminuir a reação pulmonar.

Formulário de Medicamentos para Consulta em 5 Minutos

Nome do Princípio Ativo (Comercial e Outros Nomes)	Farmacologia e Indicações	Efeitos Colaterais e Precauções	Informações de Dosagem e Comentários	Formulações	Dosagem (Exceto em Casos Indicados, a Dosagem é a Mesma para Cães e Gatos)
Melfalana (Alkeran)	Agente antineoplásico. Agente alquilante, similar, em termos de ação, à ciclofosfamida.	Os efeitos adversos estão ligados à sua ação como agente antineoplásico. Causa mielossupressão.	Agente usado no tratamento do mieloma múltiplo e de certos carcinomas.	Comprimidos de 2 mg.	1,5 mg/m^2 (ou 0,1-0,2 mg/kg) a cada 24h VO durante 7-10 dias (repetir a cada 3 semanas).
Meloxicam (Mobic [medicamento para humanos], Metacam [medicamento veterinário])	AINE da classe dos oxicamos. Meloxicam é (relativamente) um poupador de COX-1, exibindo elevada relação COX-1:COX-2. Esse medicamento é administrado em cães e gatos para dor e osteoartrite.	Os efeitos adversos envolvem o trato GI: vômito, diarreia e úlceras.	Em estudos realizados em cães, doses mais elevadas (de até 0,5 mg/kg) foram mais efetivas do que doses mais baixas, mas foram associadas a uma incidência maior de efeitos adversos no trato GI. A suspensão oral é formulada com um sabor agradável, podendo ser adicionada ao alimento. Reduzir a dose em gatos.	Comprimidos de 7,5 mg (para humanos). Formulações veterinárias: suspensão oral contendo 0,5 mg/mL e 1,5 mg/mL; injeção 5 mg/mL.	Cães: dose de ataque inicial 0,2 mg/kg; em seguida, 0,1 mg/kg a cada 24h VO. Injeção: 0,2 mg/kg IV ou SC. Gatos (antipirético): em dose única, injeção: 0,3 mg/kg. Dose estendida, 0,05 mg/kg 1×/dia, ou intervalo ampliado para a cada 48-72h VO.
Meperidina (Demerol)	Produto sintético. Opioide agonista, sobretudo com atividade no receptor dos μ-opiatos. De ação similar à morfina, exceto por ter aproximadamente 1/7 de sua potência. 75 mg de meperidina IM ou 300 mg VO têm potência similar a 10 mg de morfina.	Efeitos colaterais similares aos dos demais opiatos.	Embora ainda não tenham sido publicados estudos clínicos comparativos em animais, meperidina é considerada como analgésico efetivo em cães e gatos, mas com ação de curta duração.	Comprimidos de 50, 100 mg; xarope contendo 10 mg/mL; injeção: 25, 50, 75, 100 mg/mL.	Cães: 5-10 mg/kg IV, IM em até a cada 2-3h (ou conforme a necessidade). Gatos: 3-5 mg/kg IV, IM a cada 2-4h (ou conforme a necessidade).
Mepivacaína (Carbocaine-V)	Anestésico local da classe das amidas. De potência/duração de ação média, quando comparado à bupivacaína. Em comparação com lidocaína, sua ação é mais prolongada, mas com potência equivalente.	Em comparação com lidocaína, mepivacaína pode causar menos irritação aos tecidos.	Embora ainda não tenham sido publicados estudos clínicos comparativos em animais, meperidina é considerada como analgésico efetivo em cães e gatos, mas com ação de curta duração.	Injeção a 2% (20 mg/mL).	Dose variável para infiltração local. Para epidural, 0,5 mL de uma solução a 2% a cada 30 seg, até o desaparecimento dos reflexos.
Meropeném (Merrem IV)	Antibiótico de amplo espectro da classe dos carbapenemos; indicado principalmente para infecções causadas por bactérias resistentes a outros medicamentos. Bactericida. Mais ativo do que ertapeném.	Riscos similares àqueles de outros antibióticos β-lactâmicos. Meropeném não causa convulsões com a mesma frequência que imipeném. Injeções SC podem causar leve queda de pelos no local.	As orientações sobre dosagem foram extrapoladas de estudos farmacocinéticos em animais, não tendo sido testadas quanto à eficácia veterinária. Meropeném é mais solúvel do que imipeném e pode ser injetado em bolo, em vez de administrado em soluções líquidas.	Ampola com 500 mg/20 mL ou 1 g/30 mL para injeção.	8,5 mg/kg a cada 12h SC até 12 mg/kg a cada 8h SC ou 24 mg/kg IV a cada 12h; para *Pseudomonas*: 12 mg/kg a cada 8h, SC ou 25 mg/kg a cada 8h IV.
Mesalamina (Asacol, Mesasal, Pentasa)	Ácido 5-aminosalicílico. Uso no tratamento da colite. Seu mecanismo de ação não foi completamente esclarecido, mas suprime a inflamação no cólon. Componente da sufassalazina.	O uso isolado de mesalamina não foi associado com efeitos colaterais em animais.	Ainda não foi publicado estudo clínico sobre o uso de mesalamina em animais; contudo, esse agente foi usado como substituto para sulfassalazina em animais não tolerantes às sulfonamidas.	Comprimidos de 400 mg; cápsulas de 250 mg.	A dose veterinária ainda não foi estabelecida. A dose habitual para humanos é 400-500 mg VO a cada 6-8h, utilizada para extrapolação da dose de 5-10 mg/kg a cada 8h VO para animais (ver também Sulfassalazina, Olsalazina).

Nome do Princípio Ativo (Comercial e Outros Nomes)	Farmacologia e Indicações	Efeitos Colaterais e Precauções	Informações de Dosagem e Comentários	Formulações	Dosagem (Exceto em Casos Indicados, a Dosagem é a Mesma para Cães e Gatos)
Mesilato de fentolamina (Regitine, [Rogitine no Canadá])	Bloqueador α-adrenérgico não seletivo. Vasodilatador. Bloqueia a estimulação de α-receptores na musculatura lisa vascular. Principalmente usado no tratamento da hipertensão.	Pode causar hipotensão excessiva com doses elevadas, ou em animais desidratados. Pode causar taquicardia.	Não foram publicados resultados de estudos clínicos em animais. O uso (e doses) em animais se baseia na experiência em humanos ou em experiências anedóticas em animais. Titular a dose para cada paciente, para obtenção da vasodilatação desejada.	Ampolas contendo 5 mg para injeção.	0,02-0,1 mg/kg IV.
Metadona (Methadose e genérico)	Analgésico opiato. Metadona possui propriedades analgésicas, mediante receptores opiatos, podendo também promover algum antagonismo dos receptores de NMDA. Esse agente é usado como adjuvante em protocolos de anestesia e como analgésico.	Efeitos adversos em cães: sedação e vômito (raro). Mas não foram relatados outros efeitos adversos nessa espécie.	As doses orais disponíveis para humanos não foram absorvidas em cães.	Solução oral: 2 mg/mL; solução para injeção: 10 e 20 mg/mL; comprimidos de 5, 10 e 40 mg.	Cães: 0,1-0,5 IV, ou 0,5-2,2 mg/kg SC ou IM a cada 3-4h. Gatos: 0,05-0,1 mg/kg IV ou 0,2-0,5 mg/kg SC ou IM a cada 3-4h.
Metaproterenol (Alupent, Metaprel)	Agonista β-adrenérgico. β2-Específico. Uso principalmente para dilatação bronquial.	Efeitos adversos relacionados à excessiva estimulação β-adrenérgica.	Não foram publicados resultados de estudos clínicos em animais. O uso (e doses) em animais se baseia na experiência em humanos, ou em experiências anedóticas em animais. β2--agonistas também têm sido usados em mulheres, para retardo do trabalho de parto (inibem as contrações uterinas).	Comprimidos de 10, 20 mg; xarope contendo 5 mg/mL; e inalantes.	0,325-0,65 mg/kg a cada 4-6h VO.
Metazolamida (Neptazane)	Inibidor da anidrase carbônica. Promove menos diurese que os demais agentes dessa classe (Ver Diclofenamida e Acetazolamida).	Usar com cautela em pacientes sensíveis às sulfonamidas. (Ver Acetazolamida, Diclofenamida.)	Metazolamida é usada no tratamento do glaucoma. Pode ser usada com outros agentes antiglaucoma. (Ver Acetazolamida, Diclofenamida.)	Comprimidos de 25, 50 mg.	2-3 mg/kg a cada 8h VO.
Metilprednisolona (Medrol)	Glicocorticoide anti-inflamatório. Comparada à prednisolona, a metilprednisolona é 1,25× mais potente.	O mesmo que para outros glicocorticoides. O fabricante sugere que, em comparação com a prednisolona, a metilprednisolona causa menos PU/PD.	O uso de metilprednisolona é similar ao de outros corticosteroides. O ajuste da dose deve ser feito levando em conta a diferença em potência. (Ver seção de doses.)	Comprimidos de 1, 2, 4, 8, 18, 32 mg.	0,22-0,44 mg/kg q12-24h VO.
Metiltestosterona (Android, genérico)	Agente androgênico anabólico. Uso para ações anabólicas, ou como terapia de reposição hormonal de testosterona (deficiência androgênica). Testosterona é utilizada para estimular a eritropoiese.	Efeitos adversos causados pela excessiva ação androgênica da testosterona. Em cães machos, é possível a ocorrência de hiperplasia prostática. Pode ocorrer masculinização em cadelas. Hepatopatia é mais comum com o uso de formulações orais de testosterona metilada.	Ver também Cipionato de testosterona, Propionato de testosterona. Não foram publicados estudos clínicos na medicina veterinária sobre o uso de andrógenos da testosterona. O uso desse agente se baseia principalmente em evidência experimental ou em experiências em humanos.	Comprimidos de 10, 25 mg.	Cães: 5-25 mg/cão a cada 24-48h VO. Gatos: 2,5-5 mg/gato a cada 24-48h VO.

ESPÉCIES CANINA E FELINA

Formulário de Medicamentos para Consulta em 5 Minutos

Nome do Princípio Ativo (Comercial e Outros Nomes)	Farmacologia e Indicações	Efeitos Colaterais e Precauções	Informações de Dosagem e Comentários	Formulações	Dosagem (Exceto em Casos Indicados, a Dosagem é a Mesma para Cães e Gatos)
Metimazol (Tapazole, Felimazole)	Medicamento antitireoidiano. Uso no tratamento do hipertireoidismo, sobretudo em gatos. Ação: substrato para a tireoide peroxidase, além de diminuir a incorporação do iodeto nas moléculas de tirosina.	Em humanos, tem causado agranulocitose e leucopenia. Em gatos, são possíveis reações semelhantes ao lúpus, por exemplo, vasculite e alterações na medula óssea. Bem tolerado em cães.	O uso em gatos se baseia em estudos experimentais em animais com hipertireoidismo. Na maioria dos casos em gatos, metimazol substituiu propiltiouracila. Ajustar a dose de manutenção mediante a monitorização dos níveis de T_4. Em gatos, a dose de 2×/dia tem se mostrado mais efetiva do que 1×/dia.	Comprimidos de 5 e 10 mg (formulação para humanos) e comprimidos de 2,5 e 5 mg (formulação veterinária).	Gatos: 2,5 mg/gato a cada 12h VO × 7-14 dias; em seguida, 5-10 mg/gato VO a cada 12h; monitorizar concentrações de T_4.
Metocarbamol (Robaxin-V)	Relaxante da musculatura esquelética. Deprime os reflexos polissinápticos. Metocarbamol é usado no tratamento de espasmos da musculatura esquelética.	Provoca certa depressão/sedação do SNC.	Não foram publicados resultados de estudos clínicos em animais. O uso (e doses) em animais se baseia na experiência em humanos ou em experiências anedóticas em animais.	Comprimidos de 500, 750 mg; injeção: 100 mg/mL.	44 mg/kg a cada 8h VO no primeiro dia; em seguida, 22-14 mg/kg a cada 8h VO.
Metoclopramida (Reglan, Maxolon)	Medicamento procinético. Antiemético de ação central. Estimula a motilidade do trato GI. Ação: inibe receptores dopaminérgicos e promove a ação da acetilcolina no trato GI. Uso principalmente em casos de gastroparesia e no tratamento do vômito. Não é eficaz para cães com dilatação gástrica.	Os efeitos adversos estão principalmente ligados ao bloqueio dos receptores dopaminérgicos centrais. Foram relatados efeitos adversos similares aos das fenotiazinas (p. ex., acepromazina), além de mudanças de comportamento. Não usar em pacientes sofrendo convulsões ou com doenças causadas por obstrução GI.	Não foram publicados resultados de estudos clínicos em animais. O uso (e doses) em animais se baseia na experiência em humanos ou em experiências anedóticas em animais. Na maioria dos casos, o agente é usado com finalidades antieméticas gerais, mas doses elevadas de até 2 mg/kg têm sido administradas para prevenção do vômito durante a quimioterapia antineoplásica.	Comprimidos de 10, 5 mg; solução oral: 1 mg/mL; injeção: 5 mg/mL.	0,2-0,5 mg/kg a cada 6-8h IV, IM, VO; IRC: dose de ataque de 0,4 mg/kg IV, seguida por 0,3 mg/kg/h IV. Em pacientes refratários, foram administradas doses de até 1,0 mg/kg/h.
Metoexital (Brevital)	Anestésico barbitúrico. Metoexital é cerca de 2-3× mais potente que o pentotal, mas com duração mais curta.	Similar a outros barbitúricos, como o tiopental.	Monitorizar a função respiratória e cardiovascular.	Ampolas de 0,5, 2,5 e 5 g para injeção.	3-6 mg/kg IV (administrar lentamente, até o efeito desejado).
Metotrexato (MTX, Mexate, Folex, Rheumatrex e genérico)	Antineoplásico. Uso em diversos carcinomas, leucemia e linfomas. Ação: antimetabólito. Análogo do ácido fólico, inclusive ligante da di-hidrofolato redutase. Inibe DNA, RNA e síntese das proteínas. Em humanos, metotrexato é também comumente usado para doenças autoimunes, como a artrite reumatoide.	Medicamentos antineoplásicos causam efeitos colaterais previsíveis (e por vezes inevitáveis), inclusive supressão da medula óssea, leucopenia e imunossupressão. Em humanos tratados com metotrexato, foi relatada a ocorrência de hepatotoxidez. Interações farmacológicas: o uso concorrente com AINE pode causar grave toxidez por metotrexato. Não administrar com pirimetamina, trimetoprima ou sulfonamidas.	O uso em animais se baseia em estudos experimentais. São limitadas as informações clínicas disponíveis. Consultar protocolos antineoplásicos específicos, para obtenção da dose e regime.	Comprimidos de 2,5 mg; injeção: 2,5 ou 25 mg/mL.	2,5-5 mg/m² a cada 48h VO (a dose depende do protocolo específico) Cães: 0,3-0,5 mg/kg IV 1×/semana. Gatos: 0,8 mg/kg IV a cada 2-3 semanas.

Formulário de Medicamentos para Consulta em 5 Minutos

Nome do Princípio Ativo (Comercial e Outros Nomes)	Farmacologia e Indicações	Efeitos Colaterais e Precauções	Informações de Dosagem e Comentários	Formulações	Dosagem (Exceto em Casos Indicados, a Dosagem é a Mesma para Cães e Gatos)
Metoxamina (Vasoxyl)	Agonista adrenérgico. Simpaticomimético. Agonista α1-adrenérgico. Metoxamina é específica para α1-receptores, usada como vasopressor.	Efeitos adversos relacionados à excessiva estimulação dos α1-receptores (vasoconstrição periférica prolongada). Pode ocorrer bradicardia reflexa.	Agente usado principalmente em pacientes em terapia intensiva ou durante a anestesia, para aumento da resistência periférica e da pressão arterial. Ação: início rápido, duração curta.	Injeção: 20 mg/mL	200-250 mcg/kg IM, ou 40-80 mcg/kg IV; repetir a dose conforme a necessidade.
Metronidazol (Flagyl e genérico) e Benzoato de metronidazol	Antibacteriano e antiprotozoário. Rompe o DNA no organismo, mediante a reação com um metabólito intracelular. Ação específica para bactérias anaeróbias e protozoários, como *Giardia*.	O efeito adverso mais grave é o causado pela toxidez do SNC. Doses elevadas causaram letargia, depressão do SNC, ataxia, vômito e fraqueza. Metronidazol pode ser mutagênico. Não foram demonstradas anormalidades fetais em animais com as doses recomendadas, mas usar com cautela durante a gestação.	Metronidazol é um dos medicamentos mais comumente usados para infecções anaeróbias e para giardíase. Dose máxima para qualquer espécie: 50-65 mg/kg/dia. Embora comprimidos tenham sido partidos ou triturados para administração oral em gatos, essa preparação é intragável para esses animais. Nos casos de problema com a palatabilidade em gatos, considerar o uso de benzoato de metronidazol.	Comprimidos de 250, 500 mg; suspensão contendo 50 mg/mL; injeção: 5 mg/mL; a forma benzoato não é comercializada, devendo ser obtida em farmácias de manipulação. 20 mg de benzoato em metronidazol = 12,4 mg de metronidazol.	Para anaeróbios - cães: 15 mg/kg a cada 12h, ou 12 mg/kg a cada 8h VO; gatos: 10-25 mg/kg a cada 24h VO. Para *Giardia* - cães: 12-15 mg/kg a cada 12h for 8 dias VO; gatos: 17 mg/kg (1/3 de comprimido/gato) a cada 24h durante 8 dias.
Mexiletina (Mexitil)	Antiarrítmico. Uso nas arritmias ventriculares. Mecanismo de ação: bloqueio dos canais rápidos de sódio. Agente antiarrítmico Classe IB.	Pode causar arritmias. Usar com cautela em animais com doença hepática. Não usar em gatos.	Não foram publicados resultados de estudos clínicos em animais. O uso (e doses) em animais se baseia na experiência em humanos ou em experiências anedóticas em animais.	Cápsulas de 150, 200, 250 mg.	Cães: 5-8 mg/kg a cada 8-12h VO (usar com cautela). Gatos: não usar.
Mibolerona (Cheque Drops)	Esteroide androgênico. Para supressão do estro.	Não usar em Bedlington terriers. Não usar em animais com adenoma ou carcinoma perianal. Em decorrência do tratamento, muitas cadelas exibem hipertrofia do clitóris ou corrimento. Não usar em gatos.	Comumente, o tratamento é iniciado 30 dias antes do início do estro. Não é recomendável seu uso por mais de 2 anos.	Solução oral: 55 mcg/mL.	Cães: (2,6-5 mcg/kg/dia VO) 0,45-11,3 kg, 30 mcg; 11,8-22,7 kg, 60 mcg; 23-45,3 kg, 120 mcg; >45,8 kg, 180 mcg. Gatos: a dose segura ainda não foi estabelecida.
Micofenolato (Cell Cept)	Micofenolato é metabolizado até ácido micofenólico. Uso na imunossupressão para transplantes e no tratamento de doenças imunemediadas.	Em cães, os efeitos adversos mais comumente relatados são problemas gastrintestinais (diarreia, vômito).	Micofenolato é usado em alguns pacientes que não podem tolerar outros medicamentos imunossupressivos, como azatioprina ou ciclofosfamida.	Cápsulas de 250 mg.	Cães: 10 mg/kg a cada 8h VO, ou 20 mg/kg a cada 12h VO. Gatos: ainda não foi estabelecida uma dose.
Milbemicina oxima (Interceptor, Interceptor Flavor Tabs e SafeHeart)	Antiparasitário do grupo das lactonas macrocíclicas. O mecanismo de ação é similar ao da ivermectina. Uso como preventivo da dirofilariose, carrapaticida e microfilaricida. Uso no controle de infecções por ancilostomídeos, nematelmintos e tricurídeos. Em doses elevadas, uso no tratamento de infecções por *Demodex* em cães.	Em cães suscetíveis (raças collie), a mibemicina pode atravessar a barreira hematoencefálica, causando toxicose do SNC (depressão, letargia, coma). Nas doses usadas para prevenção da dirofilariose, esse efeito é menos provável.	As doses variam, dependendo do parasita tratado. Consultar a coluna de doses. O tratamento de *Demodex* implica doses elevadas, diariamente administradas. Ver também Lufenurona + milbemicina oxima.	Comprimidos de 2,3, 5,75, 11,5 e 23 mg.	Cães: microfilaricida: 0,5 mg/kg; *Demodex*: 2 mg/kg a cada 24h VO durante 60-120 dias; prevenção da dirofilariose e controle de endoparasitas: 0,5 mg/kg a cada 30 dias VO. Gatos: para controle da dirofilária e de endoparasitas, 2,0 mg/kg a cada 30 dias VO.

Formulário de Medicamentos para Consulta em 5 Minutos

Nome do Princípio Ativo (Comercial e Outros Nomes)	Farmacologia e Indicações	Efeitos Colaterais e Precauções	Informações de Dosagem e Comentários	Formulações	Dosagem (Exceto em Casos Indicados, a Dosagem é a Mesma para Cães e Gatos)
Mirtazapina (Remeron)	Uso como antiemético e estimulante do apetite. Ação: bloqueio dos receptores da serotonina e antagonismo de alfa-2 receptores.	Em gatos, foram observadas contrações e mudanças de comportamento.	As doses e recomendações em animais se baseiam principalmente em relatos anedóticos e na extrapolação da medicina humana.	Comprimidos de 15 e 30 mg.	Cães: 3,75-7,5 mg/cão/dia VO. Gatos: 3,75-7,5 mg/gato/dia VO, mas comumente 2 mg/gato.
Misoprostol (Cytotec)	Análogo da prostaglandina E_2. As prostaglandinas exercem um papel citoprotetor na mucosa GI. Misoprostol é usado na prevenção de gastrite e úlceras associadas ao tratamento com AINE. Misoprostol também se revelou efetivo para dermatite atópica em cães.	Os efeitos adversos são causados pelos efeitos das prostaglandinas. Os efeitos colaterais mais comuns são: desconforto GI, vômito e diarreia. Não usar em animais gestantes; pode causar abortamento.	As doses e recomendações se baseiam em estudos clínicos, em que o misoprostol foi administrado para prevenção de lesões à mucosa GI causadas pelo ácido acetilsalicílico.	Comprimidos de 0,1 mg (100 mcg), 0,2 mg (200 mcg).	Cães: 2-5 mcg/kg a cada 6-8h VO. Dermatite atópica: 5 mcg/kg a cada 8h, VO. Gatos: dose não estabelecida.
Mitotano (o,p'-DDD) (Lysodren)	Agente citotóxico adrenocortical. Causa supressão do córtex adrenal. Usado no tratamento de tumores adrenais e do hiperadrenocorticismo dependente da hipófise (HDH).	Os efeitos adversos, especialmente durante o período de indução, são: letargia, anorexia, ataxia, depressão, vômito. Pode-se fazer suplementação com corticosteroide (p. ex., hidrocortisona ou prednisolona), para minimizar os efeitos colaterais.	Muitas vezes, a dose e a frequência dependem da resposta do paciente. Efeitos adversos são comuns durante o tratamento inicial. A administração com o alimento aumenta a absorção oral. A dose de manutenção deve ser ajustada com base em determinações periódicas de cortisol e em provas de estimulação do ACTH. Em geral, os gatos não têm respondido ao tratamento com mitotano.	Comprimidos de 500 mg.	Cães - para HDH: 50 mg/kg/dia (em doses divididas) VO durante 5-10 dias; em seguida, 50-70 mg/kg/semana VO; para tumores adrenais: 50-75 mg/kg/dia durante 10 dias; em seguida, 75-100 mg/kg/semana VO.
Mitramicina	Nome antigo para plicamicina.				
Moxidectina (forma canina: ProHeart; gel oral equino: Quest; solução para verter [pour-on] bovino: Cydectin)	Antiparasitário. A substância é neurotóxica para parasitas, por potenciar os canais do íon cloreto dependentes de glutamato nos parasitas. Moxidectina é usada para endoparasitas e ectoparasitas, bem como na prevenção da dirofilariose.	Pode ocorrer toxidez com doses elevadas e também nas espécies em que a ivermectina atravessa a barreira hematoencefálica (raças collie). A toxidez é neurotóxica; seus sinais são depressão, ataxia, dificuldade com a visão, coma e morte.	Uso similar ao da ivermectina. É recomendável cuidado extremo, se for considerado o uso da formulação equina para uso em pequenos animais. É provável a ocorrência de overdoses tóxicas, porque a formulação equina é altamente concentrada.	Comprimidos de 30, 68, 136 mcg para cães; gel oral equino, 20 mg/mL; e pour-on para bovinos, 5 mg/mL.	Cães - prevenção da dirofilariose: 3 mcg/kg a cada 30d VO. Endoparasitas: 25-300 mcg/kg. Demodex: 400 mcg/kg/dia VO e até 500 mcg/kg/dia durante 21-22 semanas. Proheart-6 (ação prolongada): 0,17 mg/kg SC a cada 6 meses.
Moxifloxacino (Avelox)	Antibiótico do grupo das fluoroquinolonas. Similar às demais fluoroquinolonas, exceto por ter maior atividade contra bactérias Gram-positivas e anaeróbias.	Similares aos efeitos adversos das demais fluoroquinolonas. Devido ao mais amplo espectro de ação em bactérias anaeróbias, é possível a ocorrência de maiores problemas GI com a dose oral.	As doses e recomendações se baseiam principalmente na limitada experiência clínica e na extrapolação de estudos em humanos.	Comprimidos de 400 mg.	10 mg/kg a cada 24h VO.
Naloxona (Narcan)	Antagonista opiato. Uso para reversão dos efeitos de agonistas opiatos (como a morfina). Naloxona pode ser usada para reverter a sedação, anestesia e os efeitos adversos causados por opiatos.	Não foram relatados efeitos adversos. Em humanos, foi descrita a ocorrência de taquicardia e hipertensão.	Talvez a administração tenha que ser individualizada, com base na resposta de cada paciente. A duração da ação de naloxona é curta em animais (60 min) e a dose talvez tenha que ser repetida.	Injeção: 20 ou 400 mcg/mL ou 1 mg/mL.	0,0 1-0,04 mg/kg IV, IM, SC, conforme a necessidade, para reversão de opiatos.

Formulário de Medicamentos para Consulta em 5 Minutos					
Nome do Princípio Ativo (Comercial e Outros Nomes)	Farmacologia e Indicações	Efeitos Colaterais e Precauções	Informações de Dosagem e Comentários	Formulações	Dosagem (Exceto em Casos Indicados, a Dosagem é a Mesma para Cães e Gatos)
Naltrexona (Trexan)	Antagonista opiato. Similar à naloxona, exceto por sua ação mais prolongada e pela administração oral. Naltrexona é usada em humanos para tratamento da dependência de opiatos. Em animais, este agente tem sido usado no tratamento de alguns problemas de comportamento (transtorno obsessivo-compulsivo [TOC]).	Não foram relatados efeitos adversos em animais.	Foi descrito o tratamento do transtorno obsessivo-compulsivo (TOC) em animais com naltrexona. Os percentuais de recidiva podem ser altos.	Comprimidos de 50 mg.	Cães: para problemas de comportamento: 2,2 mg/kg a cada 12h VO.
Naproxeno (Naprosyn, Naxen, Aleve [naproxeno sódico])	AINE. Ação: inibição das prostaglandinas. Uso no tratamento de problemas inflamatórios (p. ex., artrite). O uso em animais declinou, por causa de outros AINE.	Naproxeno é um AINE potente. Efeitos adversos atribuídos à toxidez GI são comuns a todos os AINE. Naproxeno causou grave ulceração em cães, tendo em vista que a eliminação desse agente na espécie é muito mais lenta do que em humanos ou equinos.	Ainda não foram publicados resultados em estudos clínicos em animais. O uso em animais (e doses) se baseia em estudos farmacocinéticos em animais experimentais. É preciso cautela ao usar a formulação para TOC descrita para humanos, porque o tamanho do comprimido é muito maior do que a dose segura para cães. 220 mg de naproxeno sódico equivalem a 200 mg de naproxeno.	Comprimidos de 220 mg (TOC); suspensão oral contendo 25 mg/mL; comprimidos de 250, 375, 500 mg (Rx).	Cães: 5 mg inicialmente; em seguida, 2 mg/kg a cada 48h VO. Gatos: não recomendável.
Neomicina (Biosol)	Antibiótico aminoglicosídeo. Neomicina difere de outros aminoglicosídeos por ser administrada apenas topicamente ou VO. Usando a via oral, a absorção sistêmica é mínima.	Embora a absorção oral seja tão pequena a ponto de tornar improváveis os efeitos adversos sistêmicos, foi demonstrada a ocorrência de alguma absorção oral em animais jovens (bezerros). Alterações na flora bacteriana intestinal decorrentes do tratamento podem causar diarreia.	Neomicina é basicamente usada para o tratamento oral da diarreia. A eficácia para essa indicação (especialmente para a diarreia inespecífica) é questionável. O agente também é usado no tratamento da encefalopatia hepática.	Bolo de 500 mg; fluido oral contendo 200 mg/mL.	10-20 mg/kg a cada 6-12h VO.
Nifedipina (Adalat, Procardia)	Medicamento bloqueador dos canais de cálcio da classe das diidropiridinas. A ação é similar à de outros agentes bloqueadores dos canais de cálcio, exceto que a nifedipina é mais específica para a musculatura lisa vascular (em comparação com o tecido cardíaco). Uso para relaxamento da musculatura lisa e vasodilatação.	Não foram relatados efeitos adversos na medicina veterinária. O efeito adverso mais comum é a hipotensão.	Na medicina veterinária, o uso de nifedipina é limitado. Outros bloqueadores dos canais de cálcio, como diltiazem, são usados no controle do ritmo cardíaco.	Cápsulas de 10, 20 mg.	Dose não estabelecida para animais. Em humanos, a dose é 10 mg/paciente 3×/dia, aumentada em incrementos de 10 mg até o efeito desejado.

ESPÉCIES CANINA E FELINA

Formulário de Medicamentos para Consulta em 5 Minutos

Nome do Princípio Ativo (Comercial e Outros Nomes)	Farmacologia e Indicações	Efeitos Colaterais e Precauções	Informações de Dosagem e Comentários	Formulações	Dosagem (Exceto em Casos Indicados, a Dosagem é a Mesma para Cães e Gatos)
Nitempiram (Capstar)	Medicamento antiparasitário. Extermina pulgas adultas com rapidez.	Não foram descritas reações adversas. Esse agente se mostrou seguro em estudos em cães e gatos, nos quais foi administrada até 10× a dose. Pode-se observar um prurido temporário logo após a administração, coincidindo com a rápida morte das pulgas.	Não usar em cães ou gatos pesando menos de 1 kg (2 libras). Não usar em cães ou gatos com menos de 4 semanas de idade.	Comprimidos de 11,4 ou 57 mg.	1 mg/kg/dia VO, conforme a necessidade, para extermínio das pulgas.
Nitrofurantoína (Macrodantin, Furalan, Furatoin, Furadantin e genérico)	Antibacteriano. Antisséptico urinário. Ação: via metabólitos reativos que lesionam o DNA. Concentrações terapêuticas são alcançadas apenas na urina. Não usar em infecções sistêmicas. Pode ter atividade contra algumas bactérias resistentes a outros antibióticos.	Os efeitos adversos são: náusea, vômito e diarreia. Muda a coloração da urina para amarelo-ferrugem. Não administrar durante a gestação.	Há duas formas de dosagem. A forma microcristalina é absorvida rápida e completamente. A forma macrocristalina (Macrodantin) é de absorção mais lenta, causando menos irritação GI. Para um efeito máximo, a urina deve estar com pH ácido. Administrar com o alimento, para aumentar a absorção.	Macrodantin e genérico: cápsulas de 25, 50, 100 mg; Furalan, Furatoin e genérico: comprimidos de 50, 100 mg; Furadantin: suspensão oral contendo 5 mg/mL.	10 mg/kg/dia divididos em 4 tratamentos/dia, durante 10-14 dias; em seguida, 1 mg/kg VO ao anoitecer.
Nitroglicerina pomada (Nitrol, Nitro-Bid, Nitrostat)	Nitrato. Nitrovasodilator. Relaxa a musculatura lisa vascular (especialmente venosa), via geração de óxido nítrico. Nitrofurantoína é usada principalmente em casos de insuficiência cardíaca, para redução da pré-carga ou diminuição da hipertensão pulmonar. Em humanos, esse agente é usado no tratamento da angina de peito.	O efeito adverso mais significativo é a hipotensão. Pode ocorrer metemoglobinemia com acúmulo de nitritos, mas esse é um problema raro.	Pode ocorrer tolerância com o uso crônico e repetido. O uso deve ser intermitente, para um efeito ideal. Nitroglicerina exibe metabolismo pré-sistêmico elevado; e a disponibilidade oral é baixa. Se for usada a formulação em pomada, 1 polegada de pomada pesa aproximadamente 15 mg.	Injeção: 0,5, 0,8, 1, 5, 10 mg/mL; pomada a 2%; sistemas transdérmicos (emplastro, 0,2 mg/h).	Cães: 4-12 mg (até 15 mg), uso tópico a cada 12h. Gatos: 2-4 mg, uso tópico a cada 12h (ou ¼ de polegada de pomada/gato).
Nitroprussiato (Nitroprussiato de sódio) (Nitropress)	Nitrato vasodilatador. Ver Nitroglicerina pomada. Nitroprussiato é usado apenas como infusão IV e o paciente deve ser cuidadosamente monitorizado durante a administração.	É possível a ocorrência de hipotensão grave durante a terapia. Monitorizar cuidadosamente o paciente durante a administração. Ocorre geração de cianeto pelo metabolismo durante o tratamento com nitroprussiato, especialmente em taxas de infusão elevadas. Tiossulfato de sódio tem sido usado em humanos, para evitar toxidez por cianeto. É possível a ocorrência de metemoglobinemia e, se necessário, o animal deve ser tratado com azul de metileno.	Nitroprussiato é administrado por infusão IV. A solução IV deve ser administrada em uma solução de dextrose a 5% (p. ex., adicionar 50 mg a 250 mL de dextrose a 5%). Proteger da luz. Descartar a solução, se for observada mudança de cor. Titular cuidadosamente a dose para cada paciente.	Ampola com 50 mg, para injeção.	1-5 mcg/kg/min até um máximo de 10 mcg/kg/min, por infusão IV. Iniciar com 2 mcg/kg/min e aumentar gradativamente até que seja obtida a pressão arterial desejada.

Formulário de Medicamentos para Consulta em 5 Minutos

Nome do Princípio Ativo (Comercial e Outros Nomes)	Farmacologia e Indicações	Efeitos Colaterais e Precauções	Informações de Dosagem e Comentários	Formulações	Dosagem (Exceto em Casos Indicados, a Dosagem é a Mesma para Cães e Gatos)
Nizatidina (Axid)	Bloqueador da histamina (H_2). O mesmo que cimetidina, exceto por ser até 10× mais potente. Inibe a secreção ácida no estômago. Nizatidina é usada para tratamento de úlceras e gastrite.	Não foram publicados efeitos adversos em animais com o uso de nizatidina.	Não foram publicados resultados de estudos clínicos em animais. O uso (e doses) em animais se baseia na experiência em humanos ou em experiências anedóticas em animais. Foi demonstrado que nizatidina e ranitidina estimulam o esvaziamento gástrico e a motilidade colônica, via atividade anticolinesterásica.	Cápsulas de 150, 300 mg.	Cães: 2,5-5 mg/kg a cada 24h VO.
Norfloxacino (Noroxin)	Antibiótico do grupo das fluoroquinolonas. A mesma ação do ciprofloxacino, exceto por ter espectro de atividade não tão amplo como enrofloxacino ou ciprofloxacino.	Não foram relatados efeitos adversos em animais. Espera-se que alguns efeitos sejam similares aos provocados por enrofloxacino e por outras fluoroquinolonas veterinárias.	O uso em animais (e doses) se baseia em estudos farmacocinéticos em animais experimentais, experiência em humanos ou experiência anedótica em animais.	Comprimidos de 400 mg.	22 mg/kg a cada 12h VO.
o,p'-DDD	Ver Mitotano.				
Ocitocina (Pitocin, Syntocinon [solução nasal] e genérico)	Estimula a contração da musculatura uterina, via ação em receptores específicos para ocitocina. Uso na indução ou manutenção do trabalho de parto normal em fêmeas prenhes. Não aumenta a produção de leite, mas estimula a contração, promovendo ejeção láctea.	Raros efeitos adversos, quando esse agente é usado com cuidado. Monitorizar cuidadosamente o estresse fetal e a progressão do trabalho de parto normal.	Usada na indução do trabalho de parto. Em humanos, ocitocina é administrada por injeção, infusão IV constante e solução intranasal. Repetir por até 3× a cada 30-60 min (a dose máxima é 3 unidades/gato).	Injeção: 10, 20 U/mL; solução nasal 40 U/mL.	Cães: 5-20 U/cão IM ou SC (repetir a cada 30 min para inércia primária). Gatos: 2,5-3 U/gato IM ou IV, repetir por até 3× a cada 30-60 min.
Óleo de castor (formulação genérica)	Estimulante catártico. Acredita-se que sua ação ocorra por estimulação local da motilidade intestinal. Usada como laxante para tratar a constipação ou evacuar o intestino para procedimentos.	A superdosagem pode causar perdas eletrolíticas. Acredita-se que o óleo de castor possa estimular o parto prematuro na gestação.	Disponível em formulações sem prescrição médica.	Solução oral (100%).	Cães: 8-30 mL/dia VO. Gatos: 4-10 mL/dia VO.
Óleo de TCM (triglicérides de cadeia média [muitas fontes])	Triglicérides de cadeia média. Uso no tratamento da encefalopatia hepática.	Não foram relatados efeitos adversos na medicina veterinária. Pode causar diarreia em alguns pacientes.	Ainda não foram publicados resultados de estudos clínicos com o uso do óleo de TCM. Muitas fórmulas para alimentação enteral contêm óleo de TCM (muitas formulações poliméricas).	Fluido para uso oral.	1-2 mL/kg a cada 24h no alimento.
Óleo mineral (genérico)	Laxante lubrificante. Aumenta o conteúdo de água nas fezes. Uso para aumento do trânsito fecal, para tratamento de impactação e constipação.	Não foram relatados efeitos adversos. O uso crônico pode diminuir a absorção de vitaminas lipossolúveis.	Uso empírico. Não foram publicados resultados clínicos.	Fluido oral.	Cães: 10-50 mL/cão a cada 12h VO. Gatos: 10-25 mL/gato a cada 12h VO.
Olsalazina sódica (Dipentum)	Anti-inflamatório para tratamento da colite. Duas moléculas de mesalamina unidas por uma ligação azo.	Não foram relatados efeitos adversos em cães.	Olsalazina é usada em pacientes incapazes de tolerar sulfassalazina.	Comprimidos de 500 mg.	Dose não estabelecida, mas 5-10 mg/kg a cada 8h VO têm sido usados. (A dose habitual para humanos é 500 mg 2×/dia.)

Formulário de Medicamentos para Consulta em 5 Minutos

Nome do Princípio Ativo (Comercial e Outros Nomes)	Farmacologia e Indicações	Efeitos Colaterais e Precauções	Informações de Dosagem e Comentários	Formulações	Dosagem (Exceto em Casos Indicados, a Dosagem é a Mesma para Cães e Gatos)
Omeprazol (Prilosec)	Inibidor da bomba de prótons. Omeprazol inibe a secreção de ácido gástrico, ao inibir a bomba de K⁺/H⁺. Omeprazol é mais potente e tem ação mais prolongada do que a maioria dos medicamentos antissecretórios. Uso no tratamento e prevenção de úlceras GI.	Não foram relatados efeitos adversos em animais. Interações farmacológicas: não administrar com medicamentos que dependam do ácido gástrico para absorção (p. ex., itraconazol ou cetoconazol).	Graças à potência do omeprazol e a seu acúmulo nas células gástricas, é possível a administração 1×/dia. A pasta para equinos foi diluída para 40 mg/mL em veículo oleoso e administrada a cães na dose de 1 mg/kg VO.	Cápsulas de 20 ou 40 mg e pasta para equinos contendo 370 mg/g.	Cães: 20 mg/cão a cada 24h VO (ou 1-2 mg/kg a cada 24h VO). Gatos: 1 mg/kg a cada 24h VO.
Ondansetrona (Zofran)	Antiemético. Ação: inibe a ação da serotonina (bloqueia os receptores de 5-HT₃). Ondansetrona é administrada no tratamento ou prevenção do vômito causado pela quimioterapia ou por doença GI.	Não foram relatados efeitos adversos em animais.	Granisetrona tem ação similar.	Comprimidos de 4, 8 mg; injeção: 2 mg/mL.	0,5-1,0 mg/kg IV ou VO 30 min antes da administração de medicamentos antineoplásicos. Para o controle do vômito devido a outras causas, podem ser consideradas doses de até somente 0,1-0,2 mg/kg IV a cada 6-12h.
Orbifloxacino (Orbax)	Antibiótico do grupo das fluoroquinolonas. Mecanismo igual ao do enrofloxacino e ciprofloxacino. Seu espectro abrange estafilococos, bacilos Gram-negativos e algumas Pseudomonas.	Em doses elevadas, pode causar alguma náusea e vômito. Evitar uso em animais jovens. Não foi informada a ocorrência de cegueira em gatos com doses ≤ 15 mg/kg/dia.	A faixa de dosagem é ampla, para levar em conta a sensibilidade bacteriana. A determinação da dose deve ser orientada por testes de sensibilidade.	Comprimidos de 5,7, 22,7 e 68 mg e suspensão oral contendo 30 mg/mL.	Comprimidos (cães e gatos): 2,5-7,5 mg/kg a cada 24h VO. Suspensão oral em gatos: 7,5 mg/kg a cada 24h VO.
Ormetoprima + sulfadimetoxina	Medicamento similar à trimetoprima, usado em combinação com sulfadimetoxina. (Ver Primor.)				
Oxacilina (Prostaphlin e genérico)	Antibiótico do grupo dos β-lactâmicos. Inibe a síntese da parede da célula bacteriana. Seu espectro se limita a bactérias Gram-positivas, especialmente estafilococos.	Usar com cautela em animais alérgicos a medicamentos similares à penicilina.	As doses são empíricas ou se baseiam na extrapolação de estudos em humanos. Não foram publicados estudos de eficácia clínica para cães ou gatos. Se possível, administrar com estômago vazio.	Cápsulas de 250, 500 mg; solução oral: 50 mg/mL.	22-40 mg/kg a cada 8h VO.
Oxazepam (Serax)	Benzodiazepínico. Depressor de ação central do SNC. Ao que parece, sua ação decorre da potenciação dos efeitos mediados pelos GABA-receptores no SNC. Este medicamento é usado para sedação e estimulação do apetite.	Sedação é o efeito colateral mais comum. Causa polifagia. Em gatos, foi relatada a ocorrência de necrose hepática fatal com diazepam.	Doses empíricas. Não foram publicados ainda estudos clínicos na medicina veterinária.	Comprimidos de 15 mg.	Cães: 0,2-1,0 mg/kg a cada 12h VO, mas pode ser aumentada para a cada 6h. Gatos (estimulante do apetite): 2,5 mg/gato VO Gatos (tratamento de problemas de comportamento): 0,2-0,5 mg/kg a cada 12-24h VO.
Oximetolona (Anadrol)	Esteroide anabólico. Derivado da testosterona. Uso na estimulação da atividade androgênica, aumento do ganho de peso e estimulação da eritropoiese.	Causa efeitos colaterais androgênicos. Possível ocorrência de lesão hepática.	Uso baseado principalmente em experiências anedóticas.	Comprimidos de 50 mg.	1-5 mg/kg a cada 24h VO.

1424 CONSULTA VETERINÁRIA EM 5 MINUTOS

Nome do Princípio Ativo (Comercial e Outros Nomes)	Farmacologia e Indicações	Efeitos Colaterais e Precauções	Informações de Dosagem e Comentários	Formulações	Dosagem (Exceto em Casos Indicados, a Dosagem é a Mesma para Cães e Gatos)
Oxitetraciclina (Terramycin)	Antibiótico do grupo das tetraciclinas. Mesmo mecanismo e espectro da tetraciclina. A oxitetraciclina pode ser absorvida mais intensamente.	Geralmente é agente seguro. Usar com cautela em animais jovens.	As formulações para dose oral são para animais de grande porte. O uso de formulações injetáveis de ação prolongada ainda não foi estudado em animais de pequeno porte. Para a maioria das indicações, pode-se usar doxiciclina ou minociclina, em lugar de oxitetraciclina.	Comprimidos de 250 mg; injeção: 100, 200 mg/mL.	7,5-10 mg/kg IV a cada 12h; 20 mg/kg VO a cada 12h.
Oxtrifilina (Choledyl-SA)	Teofilinato de colina. Broncodilatador metilxantínico, similar em mecanismo à teofilina.	Os mesmos efeitos adversos da teofilina.	Efeitos adversos semelhantes aos da teofilina. Algumas formulações (Theocon) contêm oxitrifilina e guaifenesina. Com o uso de comprimidos de liberação lenta, não triturar o comprimido.	Comprimidos de 400, 600 mg (solução oral e xarope disponíveis no Canadá, mas não nos Estados Unidos).	Cães: 47 mg/kg (equivalente a 30 mg/kg de teofilina) a cada 12h VO.
Pamidronato (Aredia)	Agente bifosfonato; retarda a formação e dissolução de cristais de hidroxiapatita. Uso em animais para reduzir o cálcio em problemas causadores de hipercalcemia, por exemplo, câncer e toxicose por vitamina D.	Não foram identificados efeitos adversos graves; contudo, apenas raramente é usado em animais.	Os bifosfonatos podem ser efetivos em animais no tratamento da hipercalcemia do câncer e na toxicose por vitamina D. Para infusão IV, diluir em solução de fluido (30 mg de pamidronato em 250 mL de fluidos) e administrar ao longo de algumas horas.	Disponível em ampolas de 30, 60 e 90 mg para injeção.	Cães: tratamento da toxicose por colecalciferol: 1,3-2 mg/kg IV ou SC × 2 tratamentos após exposição à toxina. Tratamento de hipercalcemia: 1-2 mg/kg IV. Tratamento de malignidade: 1-2 mg/kg IV a cada 28 dias (2 h de infusão). Gatos: 1-2 mg/kg IV.
Pamoato de pirantel (Nemex, Strongid)	Medicamento antiparasitário. Ação: bloqueia a neurotransmissão ganglionar, via ação colinérgica.	Não foram relatados efeitos adversos.	As doses listadas se baseiam nas recomendações do fabricante.	Pasta: 180 mg/mL; suspensão de 50 mg/mL também combinada com praziquantel.	Cães: 5 mg/kg VO 1 vez; repetir em 7-10 dias. Gatos: 20 mg/kg VO 1 vez.
Pancrelipase (Viokase)	Enzima pancreática. Usada no tratamento de insuficiência exócrina pancreática. Fornece lipase, amilase e protease.	Não foram relatados efeitos adversos.	Administração: misturar com o alimento aproximadamente 20 minutos antes da refeição.	16.800 U de lipase, 70.000 U de protease e 70.000 U de amilase por 0,7 g. Também em cápsulas e comprimidos.	Cães: misturar com o alimento 2 col. chá de pó para cada 20 kg de peso corporal, ou 1-3 col. chá/0,45 kg de alimento. Gatos: 1/2 col. chá/gato com o alimento.
Pantoprazol sódico (Protonix, Protonix IV)	Tratamento de úlceras. Inibidor da bomba de prótons; indicado para tratamento de úlceras duodenais e refluxo gastresofágico. Pantoprazol é o primeiro inibidor da bomba de prótons para uso IV. Seus efeitos antissecretórios persistem por >24 h.	Não foram relatados efeitos adversos em animais, mas em humanos há a preocupação sobre hipergastrinemia com o uso crônico.	Administrar a dose IV ao longo de 15 minutos e não misturar com outros medicamentos que possam interferir em sua estabilidade.	Comprimidos de lenta liberação de 20 e 40 mg; ampolas contendo 4 mg/mL para injeção IV.	0,5 mg/kg a cada 24h VO. Uso IV: 0,5-1 mg/kg. Infusão IV ao longo de 24 h, que pode ser administrada em 2 ou 15 min, dependendo da diluição.
Paracetamol (Tylenol e diversas formulações genéricas)	Agente analgésico. O mecanismo exato de ação é desconhecido. Não inibe a síntese de prostaglandinas.	Bem tolerado em cães nas doses citadas. Doses maiores podem causar hepatotoxicidade. Não administrar em gatos.	Muitas formulações genéricas disponíveis. O paracetamol com codeína pode assumir eficácia analgésica sinérgica em alguns animais.	Comprimidos com 120, 160, 325 e 500 mg.	Cães: 15 mg/kg VO a cada 8h. Gatos: não é recomendado.
Paracetamol com codeína (Tylenol com codeína e diversas formulações genéricas)	O mesmo citado anteriormente, exceto que a codeína é um opioide adicionado para aumentar a analgesia.	Ver Codeína e Paracetamol.	Ver Codeína e Paracetamol.	Solução oral e comprimidos. Existem diversas formas, como, por exemplo, paracetamol 300 mg mais codeína 15, 30 ou 60 mg.	Seguir as dosagens recomendadas para a codeína.

ESPÉCIES CANINA E FELINA

Formulário de Medicamentos para Consulta em 5 Minutos					
Nome do Princípio Ativo (Comercial e Outros Nomes)	Farmacologia e Indicações	Efeitos Colaterais e Precauções	Informações de Dosagem e Comentários	Formulações	Dosagem (Exceto em Casos Indicados, a Dosagem é a Mesma para Cães e Gatos)
Paregórico (mistura corretiva)	Paregórico (tintura de ópio) é um produto obsoleto usado no tratamento da diarreia. Paregórico contém 2 mg de morfina em cada 5 mL do produto.	O mesmo que para outros opiatos.	O uso do paregórico foi substituído por produtos mais específicos, por exemplo, loperamida ou difenoxilato.	2 mg de morfina por 5 mL de paregórico.	0,05-0,06 mg/kg a cada 12h VO.
Paroxetina (Paxil)	Inibidor seletivo de recaptação de serotonina (ISRS), com ação muito parecida à da fluoxetina (Prozac). Uso em transtornos obsessivo-compulsivos (TOC), transtornos de ansiedade, agressividade e outros problemas de comportamento.	Alguns efeitos similares aos da fluoxetina, mas, em alguns animais, a parexetina é mais bem tolerada.	As recomendações de dosagem são empíricas.	Comprimidos de 10, 20, 30, 40 mg.	Cães: 1-2 mg/kg a cada 24h VO. Gatos: 1/8 to 1/4 de um comprimido de 10 mg a cada 24h VO.
Penicilamina (Cuprimine, Depen)	Agente quelante para chumbo, cobre, ferro e mercúrio. Uso principalmente em animais para tratamento da toxidez por cobre e da hepatite associada ao acúmulo desse metal. Também usada no tratamento de cálculos de cistina. Penicilamina é usada em humanos para tratamento da artrite reumatoide.	Não usar em fêmeas prenhes. Em humanos, foram relatadas reações alérgicas, bem como agranulocitose e anemia.	Administrar com o estômago vazio (2 horas antes das refeições).	Cápsulas de 125, 250 mg e comprimidos de 250 mg.	10-15 mg/kg a cada 12h VO.
Penicilina G potássica; Penicilina G sódica (muitas marcas)	Antibiótico β-lactâmico. A ação é similar à de outras penicilinas. O espectro da penicilina G se limita a bactérias Gram-positivas e anaeróbios.	Injeções podem induzir reações alérgicas.	Penicilina G não é muito ativa contra a maioria dos patógenos de animais de pequeno porte.	Ampolas contendo 5-20 milhões de U.	20.000-40.000 U/kg a cada 6-8h IV ou IM.
Penicilina G procaína (genérico)	O mesmo que outras formas de penicilina G, exceto a penicilina procaína, de lenta absorção, produzindo concentrações durante 12-24 h após a injeção.	Injeções IM e SC podem causar reações no local da injeção.	Com o uso de penicilina G procaína, evitar injeção SC.	Suspensão contendo 300.000 U/mL.	20.000-40.000 U/kg a cada 12-24h IM.
Penicilina V			O mesmo que para outras penicilinas (amoxicilina). Penicilina V deve ser administrada com o estômago vazio, para máxima absorção (250 mg = 400.000 U).	Comprimidos de 250, 500 mg.	10 mg/kg a cada 8h VO.
Pentobarbital (Nembutal e pentobarbital sódico genérico)	Anestésico barbitúrico de curta ação. Ação: depressão não seletiva do SNC. Geralmente o pentobarbital é usado como anestésico IV. Uso no controle de convulsões graves em animais. A duração da ação pode chegar a 3-4 h.	É comum a ocorrência de depressão cardíaca e respiratória.	Pentobarbital tem índice terapêutico estreito. Com o uso IV, inicialmente injetar metade da dose; em seguida, administrar gradualmente o restante da dose calculada, até a obtenção do efeito anestésico.	50 mg/mL. .	25-30 mg/kg IV até o efeito desejado. IRC: 2-15 mg/kg IV até o efeito desejado, seguida por 0,2-1,0 mg/kg/h.

Formulário de Medicamentos para Consulta em 5 Minutos					
Nome do Princípio Ativo (Comercial e Outros Nomes)	Farmacologia e Indicações	Efeitos Colaterais e Precauções	Informações de Dosagem e Comentários	Formulações	Dosagem (Exceto em Casos Indicados, a Dosagem é a Mesma para Cães e Gatos)
Pentoxifilina (Trental)	Metilxantina. Pentoxifilina é usada principalmente como agente reológico em humanos (aumenta o fluxo sanguíneo através de pequenos vasos). Pode ter ação anti-inflamatória, via inibição da síntese das citocinas. Usada em cães para algumas dermatoses (dermatomiosite) e vasculites.	Pode causar sinais similares aos de outras metilxantinas. Em humanos, foi descrita a ocorrência de náusea e vômito. Comprimidos partidos são pouco palatáveis para gatos.	Não foram publicados resultados de estudos clínicos em animais. O uso (e doses) em animais se baseia na experiência em humanos ou em experiências anedóticas em animais.	Comprimidos de 400 mg.	Cães: 10 mg/kg VO a cada 12h e até 15 mg/kg a cada 8h ou 400 mg/cão para a maioria dos animais. Usar 25 mg/kg VO a cada 12h para problemas dermatológicos. Gatos: 1/4 de um comprimido de 400 mg (100 mg) VO a cada 8-12h.
Pepto-Bismol	Ver Subsalicilato de bismuto.				
Pimobendana (Vetmedin)	Inibidor da fosfodiesterase 3 e sensibilizante do cálcio, com ação vasodilatadora inotrópica (inodilatador). Licenciado para tratamento de ICC causada por miocardiopatia dilatada e insuficiência valvar.	Segura na maioria dos cães. Contraindicada em casos de estenose aórtica e miocardiopatia hipertrófica.	Pode ser usada com furosemida e inibidores da ECA.	Comprimidos mastigáveis de 1,25 mg e 5 mg (EUA). Cápsulas de 1,25 mg, 2,5 mg e 5 mg (Canadá, Europa e Austrália).	Cães: 0,25-0,3 mg/kg a cada 12h VO. Gatos: 1,25 mg/gato a cada 12h VO (0,1-0,3 mg/kg); não aprovado em gatos.
Piperacilina (Pipracil)	Antibiótico β-lactâmico da classe das acilureidopenicilinas. Similar às demais penicilinas, exceto por ter grande atividade contra *Pseudomonas aeruginosa*. Também com boa atividade contra estreptococos.	Mesmas precauções usadas para outras penicilinas injetáveis.	Deve-se usar a solução reconstituída dentro de 24 horas (ou até 7 dias, se for refrigerada). Piperacilina se combina com tazobactam (inibidor da β-lactamase) em Zosyn.	Ampolas contendo 2, 3, 4, 40 g para injeção.	40 mg/kg IV ou IM a cada 6h.
Piperazina (muitos produtos)	Composto antiparasitário. Promove bloqueio neuromuscular no parasita pela inibição do neurotransmissor, causando paralisia do verme. Uso principalmente no tratamento de infecções por helmintos (ascarídeos).	Notavelmente seguro em todas as espécies.	Uso no tratamento de todas as espécies de nematelmintos.	Pó: 860 mg; cápsulas de 140 mg; solução oral: 170, 340 e 800 mg/mL.	44-66 mg/kg VO, administração 1 vez.
Piridoxina	Vitamina B_6.				
Pirimetamina (Daraprim)	Medicamento antibacteriano e antiprotozário. Bloqueia a enzima diidrofolato redutase, que inibe a síntese do folato reduzido e dos ácidos nucleicos. A atividade da pirimetamina é mais específica contra protozoários do que contra bactérias.	Quando administrada com combinações de trimetoprim/sulfonamida, tem sido observada a ocorrência de anemia. Ácido fólico ou folínico têm sido administrados como suplementação para prevenção da anemia, mas os benefícios desse tratamento ainda são obscuros.	Uso isolado ou em combinação com sulfonamidas.	Comprimidos de 25 mg. A formulação para equinos (ReBalance) contém 250 mg de sulfadiazina e 12,5 mg de pirimetamina por mL.	Cães: 1 mg/kg a cada 24h VO durante 14-21 dias (5 dias para *Neosporum caninum*). Gatos: 0,5-1 mg/kg a cada 24h VO durante 14-28 dias.
Piroxicam (Feldene e genérico)	AINE da classe das oxicamas. Inibidor da síntese das prostaglandinas. Os efeitos clínicos são similares aos dos demais AINE. Piroxicam é usado no tratamento do carcinoma de células de transição em cães.	A eliminação de piroxicam é lenta; usar com cautela em cães. O principal efeito adverso é a toxidez GI (úlceras); ver Flunixina meglumina.	Basicamente, piroxicam é usado no tratamento da artrite e outros problemas musculoesqueléticos, mas há relatos de sua atividade no tratamento de certos tumores (p. ex., carcinoma de células de transição da bexiga).	Cápsulas de 10 mg.	Cães: 0,3 mg/kg a cada 48h VO. Gatos: 0,3 mg/kg a cada 24h VO.

ESPÉCIES CANINA E FELINA

Formulário de Medicamentos para Consulta em 5 Minutos

Nome do Princípio Ativo (Comercial e Outros Nomes)	Farmacologia e Indicações	Efeitos Colaterais e Precauções	Informações de Dosagem e Comentários	Formulações	Dosagem (Exceto em Casos Indicados, a Dosagem é a Mesma para Cães e Gatos)
Pitressina (ADH)	Ver Vasopressina e Acetato de desmopressina.				
Plicamicina (nome antigo: mitramicina) (Mithracin)	Agente antineoplásico. Ação: combina-se com DNA em presença de cátions divalentes e inibe a síntese de DNA e RNA. Baixa o cálcio sérico. Pode ter ação direta nos osteoclastos, diminuindo o cálcio sérico. Uso no tratamento de carcinomas e de hipercalcemia.	Não foram relatados efeitos adversos em animais. Em humanos, foi relatada a ocorrência de hipocalcemia e toxidez GI. Pode causar problemas hemorrágicos. Interações farmacológicas: não usar com medicamentos que possam aumentar o risco de sangramento (p. ex., AINE, heparina ou anticoagulantes).	Não foram publicados resultados de estudos clínicos em animais. O uso (e doses) em animais se baseia na experiência em humanos ou em experiências anedóticas em animais.	Injeção: 2,5 mg.	Anti-hipercalcêmico (cães ou gatos): 25 mcg/kg a cada 24h IV (infusão lenta) ao longo de 4h; antineoplásico (cães): 25-30 mcg/kg a cada 24h IV (infusão lenta) durante 8-10 dias.
Polietilenoglicol, solução eletrolítica (GoLYTELY)	Catártico salino. Compostos não absorvíveis que aumentam a secreção de água para o intestino, por seu efeito osmótico. Uso para evacuação intestinal antes de procedimento cirúrgico ou diagnóstico.	Com o uso de doses elevadas ou com medicação prolongada, ocorre perda de água e eletrólitos.	Uso principalmente na evacuação intestinal, como preparação para certos procedimentos.	Solução oral.	25 mL/kg, repetir em 2-4 h VO.
Pradofloxacino (Vevaflox)	Antibiótico do grupo das fluoroquinolonas para cães e gatos. Em comparação com outras fluoroquinolonas, maior atividade contra algumas bactérias Gram-positivas e anaeróbias.	Usar com cautela em cães jovens. O tratamento oral pode causar vômito e diarreia.	Nova fluoroquinolona aprovada na Europa, mas ainda não disponível nos EUA.	Suspensão oral a 2,5%.	Cães: 3-5 mg/kg a cada 24h VO. Gatos: 5-10 mg/kg a cada 24h VO.
Praziquantel (Droncit) e em combinação com pirantel em Drontal	Agente antiparasitário. Ação nos parasitas: ligada à toxidez neuromuscular e paralisia via alteração da permeabilidade ao cálcio. Uso principalmente no tratamento de infecções causadas por cestódeos.	Vômito em doses elevadas. Foram relatadas anorexia e diarreia temporária. Uso seguro em fêmeas prenhes.	As recomendações de dosagem são baseadas na posologia descrita na bula fornecida pelo fabricante.	Comprimidos de 23, 34 mg; injeção: 56,8 mg/mL. Também combinado com pirantel em comprimidos de 13,6/54,3, 18,2/72,6 e 27,2/108,6 de praziquantel/pirantel.	Cães (dose oral): <6,8 kg: 7,5 mg/kg VO, 1 vez; >6,8 kg: 5 mg/kg VO, 1 vez. Cães (injeção): ≤2,3 kg: 7,5 mg/kg IM ou SC, 1 vez; 2,7-4,5 kg: 6,3 mg/kg IM ou SC, 1 vez; ≥5 kg: 5 mg/kg IM ou SC, 1 vez. Gatos (dose oral): <1,8 kg: 6,3 mg/kg VO, 1 vez; >1,8 kg: 5 mg/kg VO, 1 vez. Para infecção por *Paragonimus,* usar 25 mg/kg a cada 8h VO durante 2-3 dias. Gatos (injeção): 5 mg/kg IM ou SC.
Prazosina (Minipress)	Bloqueador α1--adrenérgico. Relaxa a musculatura lisa, especialmente da vasculatura. Prazosina é usada como vasodilatador e no relaxamento da musculatura lisa (ocasionalmente, do músculo uretral).	Doses elevadas causam vasodilatação e hipotensão.	Titular a dose, tendo em vista as necessidades de cada paciente. Não foram publicados resultados de estudos clínicos em animais. O uso (e doses) em animais se baseia na experiência em humanos ou em experiências anedóticas em animais.	Cápsulas de 1, 2, 5 mg.	0,5-2 mg/animal (1 mg/15 kg) a cada 8-12h VO.

Formulário de Medicamentos para Consulta em 5 Minutos

Nome do Princípio Ativo (Comercial e Outros Nomes)	Farmacologia e Indicações	Efeitos Colaterais e Precauções	Informações de Dosagem e Comentários	Formulações	Dosagem (Exceto em Casos Indicados, a Dosagem é a Mesma para Cães e Gatos)
Prednisolona (Delta-Cortef e muitos outros)	Anti-inflamatório glicocorticoide. A potência é aproximadamente = 4× cortisol.	Todos os glicocorticoides causam efeitos colaterais esperados (e em alguns casos inevitáveis). A terapia crônica pode acarretar vários efeitos adversos.	As doses para prednisolona se baseiam na gravidade do problema subjacente.	Comprimidos de 5 e 20 mg.	Cães (gatos frequentemente necessitam de 2× a dose canina) – anti-inflamatório: Inicialmente, 0,5-1 mg/kg a cada 12-24h IV, IM, VO; em seguida, reduzir gradativamente para a cada 48h; imunossupressivo: inicialmente, 2,2-6,6 mg/kg/dia IV, IM, VO; em seguida, reduzir gradativamente para 2-4 mg/kg a cada 48h; terapia de reposição: 0,2-0,3 mg/kg/dia VO.
Prednisona (Deltasone e genérico; Meticorten para injeção)	O mesmo que para prednisolona, exceto que, após a administração, a prednisona é convertida em prednisolona.	Os efeitos adversos são os mesmos da prednisolona.	O mesmo que para prednisolona. Em gatos, usar prednisolona.	Comprimidos de 1, 2,5, 5, 10, 20, 25 e 50 mg; xarope contendo 1 mg/mL (Liquid Pred em álcool a 5%) e solução oral: 1 mg/mL (em álcool a 5%).	Cães convertem prednisona em prednisolona e as doses são similares; em gatos, ocorre conversão inadequada de prednisona em prednisolona.
Pregabalina (Lyrica)	Analgésico e anticonvulsivante, similar à gabapentina. Ação: via estabilização de neurônios excitáveis. Uso no tratamento de transtornos convulsivos e como adjuvante para tratamento da dor.	Sedação é o efeito adverso mais comum, especialmente em doses elevadas.	O uso clínico se baseia principalmente na experiência anedótica e na extrapolação da medicina humana.	Cápsulas de 25, 50, 75, 100, 150, 200, 225 e 300 mg. Solução oral: 20 mg/mL.	Cães (dose anticonvulsivante): 2 mg/kg a cada 8h VO. (dose analgésica): 4 mg/kg a cada 12h, VO. Gatos: 2 mg/kg a cada 12h, VO; se necessário, aumentar para 4 mg/kg.
Primidona (Mylepsin, Neurosyn [Mysoline no Canadá])	Anticonvulsivante. Primidona é convertida em feniletilmalonamida e fenobarbital, ambos com atividade anticonvulsivante; mas provavelmente a maior parte da atividade (85%) se deve ao fenobarbital. Ver Fenobarbital, para mais detalhes.	Os efeitos adversos são os mesmos causados pelo fenobarbital. Primidona foi associada com hepatotoxidez idiossincrásica em cães. Embora alguns rótulos alertem para seu uso em gatos, um estudo experimental com esses animais determinou que a primidona é segura, desde que administrada nas doses recomendadas.	Ao monitorizar a terapia com primidona, determinar as concentrações plasmáticas de fenobarbital, para que seja estimado o efeito anticonvulsivante.	Comprimidos de 50 e 250 mg.	Dose inicial 8-10 mg/kg a cada 8-12h VO; em seguida, ajustar por monitoração para 10-15 mg/kg a cada 8h.
Primor (ormetoprim + sulfadimetoxina) (Primor)	Medicamento antibacteriano. Ormetoprim inibe a enzima diidrofolato redutase bacteriana; sulfonamida compete com o ácido p-aminobenzóico (PABA) pela síntese de ácidos nucléicos. Bactericida/bacteriostático. Amplo espectro antibacteriano, com atividade contra alguns coccídeos.	Foram relatados vários efeitos adversos com o uso de sulfonamidas. Ormetoprim foi associado a efeitos adversos no SNC.	As doses listadas se baseiam nas recomendações do fabricante. Estudos controlados demonstraram eficácia no tratamento do pioderma com um esquema de 1×/dia.	Comprimido combinado (ormetoprim + sulfadimetoxina): 120, 240, 600 e 1200 mg, em uma relação de 1:5.	Cães: 55 mg/kg VO no primeiro dia, seguido por 27,5 mg/kg a cada 24h VO. As doses diárias podem ser divididas em 2×/dia.

Formulário de Medicamentos para Consulta em 5 Minutos

Nome do Princípio Ativo (Comercial e Outros Nomes)	Farmacologia e Indicações	Efeitos Colaterais e Precauções	Informações de Dosagem e Comentários	Formulações	Dosagem (Exceto em Casos Indicados, a Dosagem é a Mesma para Cães e Gatos)
Procainamida (Pronestyl, Procanbid, genérico)	Antiarrítmico. Trata-se de um antiarrítmico Classe 1, usado principalmente no tratamento de arritmias ventriculares. Ação: inibição do influxo de sódio na célula cardíaca, via bloqueio dos canais de cálcio.	Os efeitos adversos são: arritmias cardíacas, depressão cardíaca, taquicardia e hipotensão. Em humanos, procainamida reduz os efeitos de hipersensibilidade (reações similares ao lúpus), mas isso não foi descrito em animais. Interações farmacológicas: cimetidina pode aumentar as concentrações plasmáticas.	Tendo em vista que os cães não produzem o metabólito ativo (N-acetilprocainamida), a dose pode ser mais elevada para controle de algumas arritmias, comparativamente às doses usadas em humanos. Monitorar as concentrações plasmáticas durante a terapia crônica (a concentração plasmática efetiva em cães experimentais é 20 mcg/mL). Em animais, formulações orais de liberação lenta não resultam em prolongamento na manutenção das concentrações sanguíneas.	Comprimidos ou cápsulas de 250, 375, 500 mg; injeção: 100, 500 mg/mL. Podem ser encontradas algumas formulações orais.	10-30 mg/kg a cada 6h VO (a cada 8h para liberação contínua [LC]) até uma dose máxima de 40 mg/kg; 8-20 mg/kg IV, IM; infusão IV, 25-50 mcg/kg/min. Gatos: 3-8 mg/kg IM, VO a cada 6-8h ou IRC: 1-2 mg/kg IV; em seguida, 10-20 mcg/kg/min IV.
Proclorperazina + isopropamida (Darbazine)	Combinação de produtos. Clorpromazina é um antagonista dopaminérgico de ação central (antiemético); isopropamida é um medicamento anticolinérgico (efeitos similares aos da atropina). Uso principalmente no controle do vômito em animais.	Os efeitos adversos são atribuídos a cada componente. Proclorperazina causa efeitos similares aos das fenotiazinas. Isopropamida produz efeitos antimuscarínicos. O uso de medicamentos antimuscarínicos está contraindicado em animais com gastroparesia; esses agentes devem ser usados com cautela em animais com diarreia.	As doses se baseiam nas recomendações do fabricante.	Cápsulas n° 1, 2 e 3.	Cães e gatos: 0,14-0,2 mL/kg a cada 12h SC. Cães 2-7 kg: 1 cápsula n° 1 a cada 12h VO. Cães 7-14 kg: 1 cápsula n° 2 a cada 12h VO. Cães >14 kg: 1 cápsula n° 3 a cada 12h VO.
Prometazina (Fenergan)	Fenotiazina com fortes efeitos anti-histamínicos. Uso no tratamento da alergia e como antiemético (cinetose).	Os efeitos adversos são sedação e efeitos antimuscarínicos (similares aos da atropina). Em alguns pacientes, é possível a ocorrência tanto de efeitos fenotiazínicos como anticolinérgicos.	Ainda não foram publicados resultados de estudos clínicos em animais. O uso (e doses) em animais se baseia na experiência em humanos ou em experiências anedóticas em animais.	Xarope contendo 6,25 e 25 mg/5 mL; comprimidos de 12,5, 25, 50 mg; injeção: 25, 50 mg/mL.	0,2-0,4 mg/kg a cada 6-8h IV, IM, VO (até uma dose máxima de 1 mg/kg).
Propiltiouracila (PTU) (genérico, Propyl-Thyracil)	Medicamento antitireoidiano. Comparado ao metimizol, PTU inibe a conversão de T_4 a T_3.	Em gatos, os efeitos adversos são anemia hemolítica, trombocitopenia e outros sinais de doença imunemediada.	Na maioria dos gatos, o uso de PTU foi substituído por metimazol.	Comprimidos de 50 e 100 mg.	11 mg/kg a cada 12h VO.
Propofol (Rapinovet, Propoflo, [veterinário]; Diprivan [humano])	Anestésico. Uso para indução ou obtenção de anestesia geral de curta duração. O mecanismo de ação ainda não ficou devidamente esclarecido, mas pode ser similar ao dos barbitúricos. Propofol pode ser usado como agente de indução, seguido pela inalação com halotano ou isoflurano.	Os efeitos adversos mais comuns são apneia e depressão respiratória. Efeitos adversos atribuídos às propriedades gerais dos anestésicos.	Basicamente, propofol é usado para anestesia geral, ou como adjuvante para a anestesia geral. Em relação a outros agentes, a vantagem do propofol é a recuperação rápida e sem contratempos. Usar técnica asséptica rígida para a administração. Propofol pode ser diluído em dextrose a 5%, solução de Ringer lactato, ou salina a 0,9%, mas com concentração não inferior a 2 mg/mL.	Injeção a 1% (10 mg/mL) em ampolas de 20 mL.	6,6 mg/kg IV lenta ao longo de 60 seg. IV em velocidade constante IRC: 5 mg/kg IV lenta, seguida por 100-400 mcg/kg/min.

CONSULTA VETERINÁRIA EM 5 MINUTOS

		Formulário de Medicamentos para Consulta em 5 Minutos			
Nome do Princípio Ativo (Comercial e Outros Nomes)	Farmacologia e Indicações	Efeitos Colaterais e Precauções	Informações de Dosagem e Comentários	Formulações	Dosagem (Exceto em Casos Indicados, a Dosagem é a Mesma para Cães e Gatos)
Prostaglandina $F_2\alpha$ (Dinoprost) (Lutalyse)	A prostaglandina induz leucólise. Esse agente é usado no tratamento da piometra aberta em animais. Seu uso na indução do abortamento tem sido questionado.	Os efeitos colaterais são vômito, diarreia e desconforto abdominal.	O uso no tratamento da piometra deve ser cuidadosamente monitorizado.	Solução para injeção: 5 mg/mL.	Piometra (cadela): 0,1-0,2 mg/kg SC, 1×/dia durante 5 dias; (gata): 0,1-0,25 mg/kg SC, 1×/dia durante 5 dias. Terminação da gestação (cadela): 0,025-0,05 mg (25-50 mcg)/kg a cada 12h IM; (gata): 0,5-1 mg/kg IM para 2 injeções.
Psílio (Metamucil e outros)	Laxante formador de volume. Usar no tratamento da constipação e para evacuação intestinal. Ação: absorção de água e expansão, proporcionando maior volume e conteúdo de umidade às fezes, o que encoraja o peristaltismo e a motilidade intestinal normais.	Não foram relatados efeitos adversos em animais. Pode ocorrer impactação intestinal com o uso excessivo, ou em pacientes com consumo inadequado de líquidos.	Não foram publicados resultados de estudos clínicos em animais. O uso (e doses) em animais se baseia na experiência em humanos ou em experiências anedóticas em animais.	Disponível na forma de pó, 3,4 g/col. chá.	1 col. chá/5-10 kg (adicionado a cada refeição).
Racemetionina (DL-metionina) (Uroeze, Methio-Form e genérico. Formulações humanas são Pedameth, Uracid e genérico.)	Acidificante urinário. Baixa o pH da urina. Também usado para proteger contra a overdose de paracetamol em humanos, mediante a restauração das concentrações hepáticas de glutationa. Ainda em humanos, o agente também é usado no tratamento da dermatite causada por incontinência urinária (reduz a amônia na urina).	Não foram relatados efeitos adversos. Não usar em pacientes com acidose metabólica ou comprometimento da função hepática. Não usar em gatos jovens.	Uso para acidificação da urina. Em casos de toxidez por paracetamol, a racemetionina foi substituída pela acetilcisteína.	Comprimidos de 500 mg, pós-adicionados ao alimento; solução oral pediátrica contendo 75 mg/5 mL; cápsulas de 200 mg.	Cães: 150-300 mg/kg a cada 24h VO. Gatos: 1-1,5 g/gato VO (adicionado ao alimento, todos os dias).
Retinoides	Ver Isotretinoína e Vitamina A.				
Retinol	Ver Vitamina A.				
Riboflavina (Vitamina B_2)	Ver Vitamina B_2.				
Rifampicina (Rifadin)	Antibacteriano. Ação: inibição da síntese do RNA bacteriano. O espectro de ação abrange estafilococos e micobactérias. Estreptococos são outras bactérias sensíveis. Em humanos, principalmente para tratamento da tuberculose. Em cães, usada no tratamento de estafilococos, inclusive linhagens resistentes à meticilina.	Não foram relatados efeitos adversos em animais, mas, em humanos, são relatados hipersensibilidade e sintomas semelhantes aos da gripe. Interações farmacológicas: são possíveis várias interações farmacológicas. Esse agente induz as enzimas do citocromo P-450. Os medicamentos afetados são barbitúricos, cloranfenicol e corticosteroides.	Não foram publicados resultados de estudos clínicos em animais. O uso (e doses) em animais se baseia na experiência em humanos ou em experiências anedóticas em animais. Rifampicina é altamente lipossolúvel e foi usada no tratamento de infecções intracelulares.	Cápsulas de 150, 300 mg; injeção de solução: 600 mg de Rifadin IV.	5 mg/kg a cada 12h VO, ou 10 mg/kg/dia VO.

Formulário de Medicamentos para Consulta em 5 Minutos

Nome do Princípio Ativo (Comercial e Outros Nomes)	Farmacologia e Indicações	Efeitos Colaterais e Precauções	Informações de Dosagem e Comentários	Formulações	Dosagem (Exceto em Casos Indicados, a Dosagem é a Mesma para Cães e Gatos)
Ringer Lactato, solução (diversas formulações)	Fluido para reposição com administração IV.	Administrar fluidos IV apenas em pacientes cuidadosamente monitorados.	As necessidades de fluidos variam de acordo com as necessidades dos animais (reposição *versus* manutenção). Consultar um guia sobre fluidoterapia para verificar as taxas de infusão. As taxas listadas aqui são para manutenção e choque.	Embalagens com 250, 500 e 1.000 mL.	Manutenção: 55-65 mL/kg/dia IV. Desidratação grave: 50 mL/kg/h IV. Choque: 90 mL/kg IV (cães) e 60-70 mL/kg IV (gatos).
Ronidazol	Agente antiprotozoário. Ronidazol tem mecanismo de ação similar aos demais nitromidazóis, por exemplo, metronidazol. Ronidazol é usado no tratamento das infecções intestinais por *Tritrichomonas* em gatos.	Neurotoxidez é o efeito adverso mais grave; sua ocorrência é mais provável em doses elevadas.	Não exceder 60 mg/kg/dia em gatos, para evitar neurotoxidez. As doses se baseiam apenas em estudos experimentais.	Não há formulações comerciais; contudo, farmácias de manipulação têm preparado formulações para gatos.	Cães: não há dose estabelecida. Gatos: 30 mg/kg a cada 12h VO durante 2 semanas. O tratamento 1×/dia também pode ser efetivo.
Salicilato	Ver Ácido acetilsalicílico.				
Selamectina (Revolution)	Parasiticida tópico e preventivo da dirofilariose.	Alopecia localizada temporária, com ou sem inflamação no local da aplicação, foi observada em aproximadamente 1% de 691 gatos tratados. Outros sinais observados (raramente) foram: sinais GI, anorexia, letargia, salivação, taquipneia e tremores musculares.	Recomendada para uso em cães com 6 semanas de idade ou mais e em gatos com 8 semanas de idade ou mais.	Disponível em doses com seis concentrações distintas.	6-12 mg/kg topicamente a cada 30 dias.
Selegilina (Anipryl [também conhecido como deprenil e L-deprenil]; a formulação em doses para humanos é Eldepryl)	Ação: inibição de monoamina oxidase específica (MAO tipo B), para inibição da degradação da dopamina no SNC. Em cães, o agente está aprovado para o controle dos sinais clínicos do hiperadrenocorticismo dependente da hipófise (doença de Cushing) e no tratamento da disfunção cognitiva em cães idosos.	Não foram relatados efeitos adversos em cães. No entanto, sinais similares aos causados pelas anfetaminas podem ser produzidos em animais experimentais. Em cães tratados com doses elevadas, foi observada hiperatividade (doses >3 mg/kg). Não usar com outros inibidores da MAO ou com medicamentos que inibam a recaptação da serotonina.	No estudo multicêntrico realizado pela *Deprenyl Animal Health, Inc.*, a selegilina controlou os sinais clínicos de >70% dos cães com hiperadrenocorticismo. Mas outros investigadores informaram percentuais de eficiência de até 20%.	Comprimidos de 2, 5, 10, 15 e 30 mg.	Cães: tratamento para doença de Cushing e disfunção cognitiva - usar a mesma dose. Iniciar com 1 mg/kg a cada 24h VO. Se não houver resposta dentro de 2 meses, aumentar a dose até um máximo de 2 mg/kg a cada 24h VO. Gatos: 0,25-0,5 mg/kg a cada 12-24h VO.
Sene (Senokot)	Laxante. Ação: via estimulação local ou por contato com a mucosa intestinal.	Não foram relatados efeitos adversos em animais.	As doses e indicações ainda não estão devidamente estabelecidas na medicina veterinária. O uso decorre estritamente da experiência anedótica.	Grânulos em concentrado ou xarope.	Cães (xarope): 5-10 mL/cão a cada 24h; (grânulos): 1/2-1 col. chá/cão a cada 24h VO. Gatos (xarope): 5 mL/gato a cada 24h; (grânulos): ½ col. chá/gato a cada 24h (com o alimento).
Sevoflurano	Anestésico inalante.	Ação e efeitos adversos similares aos de outros anestésicos inalantes.		Frasco com 100 mL.	Indução: 8%. Manutenção: 3%-6% até o efeito desejado.
Silimarina (Silybin, Marin, "leite de cardo")	Silimarina contém sibilina como o ingrediente mais ativo. É também conhecida como "leite de cardo", do qual é derivada. Silimarina é uma mistura de flavonoglicanas anti-hepatotóxicas (derivadas da planta *Silybum*).	Não foram relatados efeitos adversos.	Silimarina está associada a vários suplementos alimentares. Dependendo do produto, o conteúdo e a absorção são variáveis.	Comprimidos de silimarina são facilmente adquiridos SNR. Formulações veterinárias comercializadas (Marin) também contêm zinco e vitamina E em um complexo de fosfatidilcolina, em comprimidos para cães e gatos.	5-15 mg/kg VO 1×/dia.

Nome do Princípio Ativo (Comercial e Outros Nomes)	Farmacologia e Indicações	Efeitos Colaterais e Precauções	Informações de Dosagem e Comentários	Formulações	Dosagem (Exceto em Casos Indicados, a Dosagem é a Mesma para Cães e Gatos)
Solução de Ringer lactato (genérico)	Solução IV para reposição.	Monitorizar a pressão pulmonar, nos casos de infusão de doses elevadas.	Ao administrar soluções de fluidos IV, monitorizar cuidadosamente a velocidade de infusão e as concentrações dos eletrólitos.	Bolsas para infusão: 250, 500, 1.000 mL.	55-65 mL/kg/dia 50 mL/kg/h IV para desidratação grave.
Spinosad (Comfortis)	Medicamento antiparasitário usado no controle de pulgas. Após a administração, as pulgas são rapidamente exterminadas.	Ocasional ocorrência de vômito; afora isso, é medicamento seguro.	Administrar com o alimento.	Comprimidos de 140, 270, 560, 810 e 1.620 mg.	Cães: 30 mg/kg 1×/mês VO. Gatos: não foi estabelecida uma dose.
Succimer (Chemet)	Uso no tratamento da toxicose por chumbo. Ocorre quelação desse e de outros metais pesados, por exemplo, mercúrio e arsênico.	Não há efeitos adversos conhecidos.	As doses são baseadas em estudos em cães, mas não existem evidências para uso em gatos.	Cápsulas de 100 mg.	Cães: 10 mg/kg a cada 8h VO durante 5 dias; em seguida, 10 mg/kg a cada 12h VO por mais 2 semanas Gatos: 10 mg/kg a cada 8h VO por 2 semanas.
Succinato sódico de metilprednisolona (Solu-Medrol)	O mesmo que metilprednisolona, exceto que o agente tem formulação hidrossolúvel para terapia aguda, quando há necessidade de doses IV elevadas, para efeito rápido. Succinato sódico de metilprednisolona é usado no tratamento do choque e de traumas no SNC.	Não são esperados efeitos adversos com a administração de uma dose única; mas com a repetição, há possibilidade de outros efeitos colaterais.	Não foram publicados resultados de estudos clínicos em animais. O uso (e doses) em animais se baseia na experiência em humanos ou em experiências anedóticas em animais.	Ampolas de 1 e 2 g e de 125 e 500 mg para injeção.	Para emergências: 30 mg/kg IV; repita na dose de 15 mg/kg IV em 2-6h.
Succinato sódico de prednisolona (Solu-Delta-Cortef)	O mesmo que para prednisolona, exceto que esta é uma formulação hidrossolúvel para terapia aguda, nos casos em que há necessidade de doses IV elevadas para obtenção de efeito rápido. Uso no tratamento do choque e de traumas do SNC.	Não são esperados efeitos adversos com uma única administração; no entanto, com o uso repetido, é possível que ocorram efeitos colaterais.	Embora estejam listadas as doses para choque, a eficácia no tratamento desse problema é questionável.	Ampola: 100, 200 mg para injeção (10 e 50 mg/mL).	Choque: 15-30 mg/kg IV (repetir em 4-6h). Trauma do SNC: 15-30 mg/kg IV; reduzir gradativamente para 1-2 mg/kg a cada 12h.
Sucralfato (Carafate, [Sulcrate no Canadá])	Protetor da mucosa gástrica. Agente antiúlcera. Ação: ligação ao tecido ulcerado no trato GI, para ajudar na cicatrização das úlceras. Há certa evidência de que sucralfato pode atuar como citoprotetor (via síntese das prostaglandinas).	Não foram relatados efeitos adversos. Não ocorre absorção sistêmica. Interações farmacológicas: sucralfato pode diminuir a absorção de outros medicamentos administrados por via oral (p. ex., fluoroquinolonas e tetraciclinas), mediante quelação com alumínio.	As recomendações de dosagem são amplamente empíricas. Ainda não foram publicados estudos clínicos de eficácia em animais. Sucralfato pode ser administrado juntamente com inibidores da histamina H_2 (p. ex., cimetidina).	Comprimidos de 1 g; suspensão oral contendo 200 mg/mL.	Cães: 0,5-1 g a cada 8-12h VO. Gatos: 0,25 g a cada 8-12h VO.
Sulfadiazina (genérico, combinado com trimetoprima em Tribrissen)	As sulfonamidas competem com PABA pela enzima que sintetiza o ácido diidrofólico nas bactérias. Sinergismo com trimeoprima. Amplo espectro de atividade, inclusive contra alguns protozoários. Bacteriostático.	Os efeitos adversos associados às sulfonamidas envolvem reações alérgicas de hipersensibilidade dos tipos II e III, hipotireoidismo (com o tratamento prolongado), ceratoconjuntivite seca e reações cutâneas.	Geralmente, as sulfonamidas são combinadas com trimetoprima ou ormetoprim em uma relação de 5:1, para obtenção de um efeito sinergístico.	Comprimidos de 500 mg. Trimethoprim-sulfadiazina pode ser obtido em comprimidos de 120, 240, 480 e 960 mg (embora com limitada disponibilidade).	100 mg/kg IV, VO (dose de ataque), seguida por 50 mg/kg a cada 12h IV, VO. Ver seção Trimetoprima + sulfadiazina para doses adicionais.

ESPÉCIES CANINA E FELINA

Nome do Princípio Ativo (Comercial e Outros Nomes)	Farmacologia e Indicações	Efeitos Colaterais e Precauções	Informações de Dosagem e Comentários	Formulações	Dosagem (Exceto em Casos Indicados, a Dosagem é a Mesma para Cães e Gatos)
Sulfassalazina (sulfapiridina + mesalamina) (Azulfidine [Salazopyrin no Canadá])	Sulfonamida + anti-inflamatório. Uso no tratamento da colite. Sulfonamina tem pouco efeito; o ácido salicílico (mesalamina) exerce efeitos anti-inflamatórios.	Os efeitos adversos são todos atribuídos ao componente sulfonamida. Foi relatada a ocorrência de ceratoconjuntivite seca.	Geralmente usado no tratamento da colite idiopática, frequentemente em combinação com terapia nutricional.	Comprimidos de 500 mg	Cães: 10-30 mg/kg a cada 8-12h VO (ver também Mesalamina, Olsalazina) Gatos: 20 mg/kg a cada 12h VO
Sulfato de magnésio (sais de Epsom)	Sulfato de magnésio (sais de Epsom) é usado como catártico quando administrado por via oral. Também tem sido usado como fonte de magnésio no tratamento de arritmias refratárias.	O mesmo que para citrato de magnésio.	Ver Citrato de magnésio.	Cristais. Muitas preparações genéricas.	Cães: 8-25 g/cão a cada 24h VO. Tratamento de arritmias: 0,15-0,3 mEq/kg IV lenta ao longo de 5-15 minutos; em seguida, 0,75-1,0 mEq/kg/dia. Na suplementação de soluções líquidas: 0,75-1,0 mEq/kg/dia. Gatos: 2-5 g/gato a cada 24h VO.
Sulfato de morfina (genérico)	Opioide agonista, analgésico. Protótipo para outros opioides agonistas. Ação: ligação a receptores μ- e κ-opiatos nos nervos e inibição da liberação dos neurotransmissores envolvidos com a transmissão dos estímulos dolorosos (como a substância P). Morfina também pode inibir a liberação de alguns mediadores inflamatórios. Os efeitos sedativos e eufóricos centrais estão relacionados aos efeitos no μ-receptor no cérebro.	Como todos os opiatos, os efeitos colaterais da morfina são previsíveis e inevitáveis. Os efeitos colaterais decorrentes da administração de morfina são sedação, constipação e bradicardia. A depressão respiratória ocorre com a administração de doses elevadas. Em pacientes cronicamente tratados, ocorrem tolerância e dependência. Comparativamente com outras espécies, os gatos são mais sensíveis à excitação.	Os efeitos da administração de morfina dependem da dose. Baixas doses (0,1-0,25 mg/kg) causam analgesia leve. Doses mais elevadas (até 1 mg/kg) causam efeitos analgésicos mais importantes e sedação. Geralmente a morfina é administrada IM, IV ou SC. A absorção oral é inconsistente e pouco confiável. A administração epidural tem sido usada em procedimentos cirúrgicos.	Injeção: 1 e 15 mg/mL; comprimidos de liberação retardada de 30, 60 mg.	Cães: 0,1-1 mg/kg IV, IM, SC (a dose vai sendo aumentada conforme a necessidade, para o alívio da dor) a cada 4-6h. Já foi tentada a dose de 0,5 mg/kg a cada 2h para proporcionar uma analgesia consistente. IRC: 0,2 mg/kg, seguido por 0,1 mg/kg/h IV. Epidural: 0,1 mg/kg. Gatos: 0,1 mg/kg IM, SC a cada 3-6h (ou conforme a necessidade).
Sulfato de polimixina B	Antibiótico peptídico; rompe a membrana da célula bacteriana. Ativo contra amplo espectro de bactérias.	É possível a ocorrência de lesão renal. A injeção IM é dolorosa.	Basicamente, uso tópico; mas pode haver indicação de uso sistêmico para infecções resistentes.	Ampolas de 500.000 U; 1 mg equivale a 10.000 unidades.	Cães e gatos: 15.000-25.000 unidades/kg IV a cada 12h.
Sulfato de terbutalina (Brethine, Bricanyl)	Agonista β-adrenérgico. β2-específico. Uso principalmente em casos de broncodilatação.	Os efeitos adversos estão ligados à excessiva estimulação β-adrenérgica. Com doses elevadas, é possível a ocorrência de taquicardia e taquiarritmias.	Uso principalmente em casos de broncodilatação. Pode ser administrado VO, IM ou SC. Terbutalina (e outros β2-agonistas) também tem sido usada em humanos para retardar o trabalho de parto (dose em humanos: 2,5 mg a cada 6h VO).	Comprimidos de 2,5, 5 mg; injeção: 1 mg/mL (equivalente a 0,82 mg/mL).	Cães: 1,25-5 mg/cão a cada 8h VO ou 3-5 mcg/kg SC. Gatos: 0,1 mg/kg a cada 8h VO ou 0,625 mg/gato (1/4 de comprimido de 2,5 mg) a cada 12h VO. Para tratamento agudo em gatos, 5-10 mcg/kg (0,005-0,01 mg/kg) a cada 4h, SC ou IM.
Sulfato de tobramicina (Nebcin)	Medicamento antibacteriano do grupo dos aminoglicosídeos. Mecanismo de ação e ação similares aos da amicacina, gentamicina.	Efeitos adversos similares aos causados pela amicacina, gentamicina.	As necessidades de doses variam, dependendo da sensibilidade bacteriana. Ver esquemas de dosagem para gentamicina e amicacina.	Injeção: 40 mg/mL.	Cães: 9-14 mg/kg a cada 24h IV, IM, SC. Gatos: 5-8 mg/kg a cada 24h IV, IM, SC.
Sulfato de vimblastina (Velban)	Similar à vincristina. Em certos casos, usada como alternativa à vincristina. Não usar para aumento da contagem das plaquetas (na verdade, pode causar trombocitopenia).	Não causa neuropatia (como ocorre com a vincristina), mas há maior incidência de mielossupressão. Se injetada fora da veia, causa necrose tecidual.	Vimblastina é usada em protocolos quimioterápicos antineoplásicos para vários tumores. Consultar o protocolo quimioterápico específico para regimes.	Injeção: 1 mg/mL.	2 mg/m² IV (infusão lenta) 1×/semana.

Nome do Princípio Ativo (Comercial e Outros Nomes)	Farmacologia e Indicações	Efeitos Colaterais e Precauções	Informações de Dosagem e Comentários	Formulações	Dosagem (Exceto em Casos Indicados, a Dosagem é a Mesma para Cães e Gatos)
Sulfato de vincristina (Oncovin, Vincasar, genérico)	Agente antineoplásico. Vincristina causa interrupção da divisão das células cancerosas, ao se ligar aos microtúbulos e inibir a mitose. Usada em protocolos quimioterápicos combinados. Vincristina também aumenta o número de plaquetas circulantes funcionais, sendo usada para trombocitopenia.	Geralmente bem tolerada. Menos mielossupressiva do que outros medicamentos antineoplásicos. Há relatos de neuropatia, mas de rara ocorrência. Pode ocorrer constipação. Muito irritante para os tecidos. Evitar extravasamento para fora da veia durante a administração.	Vincristina é usada em protocolos quimioterápicos antineoplásicos para vários tumores. Consultar o protocolo quimioterápico específico para regimes.	Injeção: 1 mg/mL.	Antitumoral: 0,5-0,7 mg/m² IV (ou 0,025-0,05 mg/kg) 1×/ semana. Trombocitopenia: 0,02 mg/kg IV 1×/semana.
Sulfato ferroso (diversas formulações sem prescrição médica)	Suplemento de ferro.	Altas doses causam ulceração gástrica.	Recomendações baseadas na dose necessária para aumentar o hematócrito.	Diversas.	Cães: 100-300 mg/cão VO a cada 24h. Gatos: 50-100 mg/gato VO a cada 24h.
Tartarato de metoprolol (Lopressor)	Agente bloqueador β1-adrenérgico. Propriedades similares às do propranolol, exceto que metoprolol é específico para β1-receptor. Uso no controle das taquiarritmias e da bradicardia.	Os efeitos adversos são basicamente causados por depressão cardiovascular excessiva (redução dos efeitos inotrópicos). Pode causar bloqueio cardíaco. Usar com cautela em animais com tendência para constrição bronquial.	Não foram publicados resultados de estudos clínicos em animais. O uso (e doses) em animais se baseia na experiência em humanos ou em experiências anedóticas em animais.	Comprimidos de 50, 100 mg; injeção: 1 mg/mL.	Cães: 5-50 mg/cão (0,5-1,0 mg/kg) a cada 8h VO. Gatos: 2-15 mg/gato a cada 8h VO.
Tartarato de trimeprazim (Temaril [Panectyl no Canadá])	Fenotiazínico com atividade anti-histamínica (similar à prometazina). Uso no tratamento de alergias e cinetose.	Efeitos adversos similares aos causados pela prometazina.	Há evidência de que trimeprazina é mais efetiva, quando combinada com prednisona, para o tratamento do prurido. O produto combinado é Temaril-P.	Xarope contendo 2,5 mg/5 mL; comprimidos de 2,5 mg. Temaril-P é comercializado em comprimidos com 5 mg de trimeprazina + 2 mg de prednisolona.	0,5 mg/kg a cada 12h VO ou 0,5 mg/kg de prednisolona + 1,25 mg/kg de trimeprazina; baixar gradativamente a dose para 0,3 mg/kg de prednisolona + 0,75 mg/kg de trimeprazina em dias alternados, VO.
Taurina (genérica)	Suplemento nutricional para gatos. Uso na prevenção e tratamento de doença ocular e cardíaca (miocardiopatia) causada por deficiência de taurina.	Não foram relatados efeitos adversos.	Talvez não haja necessidade de suplementação de rotina com taurina em gatos que estejam sendo alimentados com uma dieta balanceada.	Comercializada em pó.	Cães: 500 mg a cada 12h VO. Gatos: 250 mg/gato a cada 12h VO.
Telazol	Ver Tiletamina + zolazepam.				
Teofilina	Broncodilatador metilxantínico. Mecanismo de ação desconhecido, mas pode estar ligado ao aumento de cAMP ou ao antagonismo da adenosina. Ação anti-inflamatória e também broncodilatadora.	Efeitos adversos: náusea, vômito, diarreia. Com o uso de doses elevadas, é possível a ocorrência de taquicardia, excitação, tremores e convulsões. Comparativamente ao que ocorre em humanos, os efeitos adversos cardiovasculares e do SNC parecem ser menos frequentes em cães.	As concentrações plasmáticas de teofilina devem ser monitorizadas em pacientes em terapia crônica (as concentrações devem ser mantidas entre 5 e 20 mcg/mL). Muitos comprimidos de lenta liberação foram recolhidos do mercado.	Comprimidos de 100, 125, 200, 250, 300 mg; solução oral ou elixir contendo 27 mg/5 mL; injeção em dextrose a 5%. Existem formulações de liberação estendida, em comprimidos de 100, 200 e 300 mg. A disponibilidade das formulações de liberação estendida pode variar.	Cães: 9 mg/kg a cada 6-8h VO. Formulações de liberação estendida: 10 mg/kg a cada 12h VO. Gatos: 4 mg/kg a cada 8-12h VO. Formulações de liberação estendida: 20-25 mg/kg a cada 24-48h VO.

ESPÉCIES CANINA E FELINA

Formulário de Medicamentos para Consulta em 5 Minutos					
Nome do Princípio Ativo (Comercial e Outros Nomes)	Farmacologia e Indicações	Efeitos Colaterais e Precauções	Informações de Dosagem e Comentários	Formulações	Dosagem (Exceto em Casos Indicados, a Dosagem é a Mesma para Cães e Gatos)
Tepoxalina (Zubrin)	Analgésico e AINE. Uso no tratamento de dor e inflamação em cães, particularmente osteoartrite. Tepoxalina exerce efeitos inibidores da lipoxigenase (diminui os leucotrienos); o metabólito ativo tem efeitos inibidores da cicloxigenase (diminui as prostaglandinas), com ação mais prolongada.	Em estudos clínicos, os efeitos adversos mais comuns estão ligados ao trato GI (náusea, vômito, diarreia).	Em gatos, não foi estabelecida a segurança a longo prazo para tepoxalina.	Comprimidos de 50, 100 e 200 mg (Zydis, comprimido liofilizado).	Cães: inicialmente, 10-20 mg/kg VO; em seguida, 10 mg/kg a cada 24h VO. Gatos: a dose segura ainda não foi estabelecida.
Tetraciclina (Panmycin)	Antibiótico do grupo das tetraciclinas. Mecanismo de ação: ligação à subunidade ribossômica 30S e inibição da síntese das proteínas. Geralmente bacteriostático. Amplo espectro de atividade, inclusive bactérias, alguns protozoários, *Rickettsia*, *Ehrlichia*.	As tetraciclinas podem afetar a formação dos ossos e dentes em animais jovens. Esses agentes foram implicados na febre medicamentosa em gatos. Em animais suscetíveis, pode ocorrer hepatotoxidez com o uso de doses elevadas. Interações farmacológicas: as tetraciclinas se ligam a compostos contendo cálcio, o que diminui a absorção oral.	Foram realizados estudos farmacocinéticos e experimentais em animais de pequeno porte, mas não estudos clínicos. Não usar soluções antigas. Para a maioria das indicações, tetraciclina pode ser substituída por doxiciclina.	Cápsulas de 250, 500 mg; suspensão: 100 mg/mL.	15-20 mg/kg a cada 8h VO; ou 4,4-11 mg/kg a cada 8h IV, IM.
Tiamina (Vitamina B₁) (Bewon e outros)	Vitamina B₁ usada no tratamento da deficiência vitamínica.	Os efeitos adversos são raros, porque vitaminas hidrossolúveis são facilmente excretadas. Riboflavina pode alterar a cor da urina.	Frequentemente, suplementos de vitamina B são administrados em combinação.	Elixir: 250 mcg/5 mL; comprimidos de tamanhos variados, de 5 mg até 500 mg; injeção: 100 e 500 mg/mL.	Cães: 10-100 mg/cão a cada 24h VO. 12,5-50 mg/cão IM, SC. Gatos: 5-30 mg/gato a cada 24h VO (até a dose máxima de 50 mg/gato a cada 24h). 12,5-25 mg/gato IM ou SC.
Ticarcilina + clavulanato (Timentin)	O mesmo que ticarcilina, exceto pelo acréscimo do ácido clavulânico, para inibir a β-lactamase bacteriana e aumentar o espectro. No entanto, clavulanato não aumenta a atividade contra *Pseudomonas*.	O mesmo que para ticarcilina.	O mesmo que para ticarcilina.	3 g/ampola, para injeção.	Dose de acordo com a velocidade para ticarcilina.
Ticarcilina dissódica (Ticar, Ticillin)	Antibiótico β-lactâmico. Ação similar à da ampicilina/amoxicilina. Espectro similar ao da carbenicilina. Ticarcilina é principalmente usada para infecções Gram-negativas, sobretudo as causadas por *Pseudomonas*.	São pouco comuns os efeitos adversos. No entanto, é possível a ocorrência de reações alérgicas. Doses elevadas podem provocar convulsões e diminuição da função plaquetária. Interações farmacológicas: não combinar com aminoglicosídeos na mesma seringa, ou em ampola.	Ticarcilina é sinergística, frequentemente combinada com aminoglicosídeos (p. ex., amicacina, gentamicina). Lidocaína a 1% pode ser utilizada para reconstituição, para diminuir a dor da injeção IM.	Ampolas contendo 1, 3, 6, 20 e 30 g, para injeção.	33-50 mg/kg a cada 4-6h IV, IM.
Tiletamina + zolazepam (Telazol, Zoletil)	Anestésico. Combinação de tiletamina (agente dissociativo similar em ação à cetamina) e zolazepam (benzodiazepínico similar em ação ao diazepam). Promove anestesia de curta duração (30 min).	Ampla margem de segurança. Os efeitos colaterais são: salivação excessiva (pode ser antagonizado com atropina), recuperação errática e contrações musculares.	Administrar por injeção IM profunda. (Consultar a bula para informações sobre doses para cães e gatos.)	50 mg de cada componente por mL.	Cães (pequenos procedimentos): 6,6-10 mg/kg IM (anestesia de curta duração); 10-13 mg/kg IM. Gatos (pequenos procedimentos): 10-12 mg/kg IM (cirurgia); 14-16 mg/kg IM.

CONSULTA VETERINÁRIA EM 5 MINUTOS

Formulário de Medicamentos para Consulta em 5 Minutos

Nome do Princípio Ativo (Comercial e Outros Nomes)	Farmacologia e Indicações	Efeitos Colaterais e Precauções	Informações de Dosagem e Comentários	Formulações	Dosagem (Exceto em Casos Indicados, a Dosagem é a Mesma para Cães e Gatos)
Tilosina (Tylocine, Tylan, Tylosin tartrate [Tartarato de tilosina])	Antibiótico macrolídeo. Tilosina não é usada sistemicamente, mas tem sido administrada para tratar diarreia crônica em cães.	Pode causar diarreia em alguns animais. Não administrar por via oral a roedores ou coelhos.	Raramente a tilosina é usada em animais de pequeno porte. A formulação em pó (Tylosin tartrate [tartarato de tilosina]) tem sido administrada com o alimento para o controle de sinais de colite em cães. No Canadá, comprimidos foram aprovados para tratamento de colite.	Comercializado na forma de pó solúvel, 3 g por col. chá (comprimidos para cães no Canadá).	Cães e gatos: 7-15 mg/kg a cada 12-24h VO. Cães (para colite): 10-20 mg/kg a cada 8h com o alimento; se houver resposta, aumentar o intervalo para a cada 12-24h.
Tinidazol (Tindamax)	Medicamento antiprotozoário similar ao metronidazol, mas considerado medicamento de segunda geração. Uso no tratamento de Trichomonas, Giardia e protozoários intestinais.	Doses elevadas podem causar efeitos adversos neurológicos.	As doses e o uso em cães e gatos se baseiam em limitada informação anedótica e na extrapolação da medicina humana.	Comprimidos de 250 e 500 mg.	Cães: 15 mg/kg a cada 12h VO. Gatos: 15 mg/kg a cada 24h VO.
Tioguanina (6-TG) (genérico)	Agente antineoplásico. Antimetabólito do tipo de análogos da purina. Inibe a síntese do DNA em células cancerosas.	Como ocorre com qualquer medicamento antineoplásico, são esperados efeitos adversos (ver 6-Mercaptopurina). É comum a ocorrência de imunossupressão e leucopenia.	Frequentemente, a tioguanina está combinada com outros agentes para o tratamento do câncer. Para orientação, consultar referência específica sobre terapia antineoplásica.	Comprimidos de 40 mg.	Cães: 40 mg/m^2 a cada 24h VO. Gatos: 25 mg/m^2 VO a cada 24h ×1-5 dias; em seguida, repetir a cada 30 dias.
Tiopental sódico (Pentothal)	Barbitúrico de ação ultra breve. Uso principalmente para indução da anestesia, ou para uma anestesia de curta duração (procedimentos com duração de 10-15 min). A anestesia é obtida por depressão do SNC, sem analgesia. A anestesia é terminada pela redistribuição no organismo.	Os efeitos adversos estão ligados aos efeitos anestésicos do medicamento. Efeitos adversos graves são causados por depressão respiratória e cardiovascular. Overdoses são causadas por injeções rápidas ou repetidas. Evitar extravasamento para fora da veia.	O índice terapêutico é baixo. Usar apenas em pacientes nos quais seja possível monitorizar as funções cardiovasculares e respiratórias. Frequentemente administrado com outros adjuvantes anestésicos.	Ampolas de diversos tamanhos, de 250 mg até 10 g (misturar para a concentração desejada).	Cães: 10-25 mg/kg IV (até o efeito desejado). Gatos: 5-10 mg/kg IV (até o efeito desejado).
Tiotepa (genérico)	Agente antineoplásico. Agente alquilante do tipo da mostarda nitrogenada (similar à ciclofosfamida). Uso no tratamento de diversos tumores, especialmente efusões malignas.	Os efeitos adversos são similares aos dos demais agentes antineoplásicos e medicamentos alquilantes (muitos dos quais são inevitáveis). Supressão da medula óssea é o efeito mais comum.	Para orientação sobre a administração, deve-se consultar o protocolo específico para quimioterapia para o câncer. Em geral, tiotepa é administrada diretamente nas cavidades corporais.	Injeção: 15 mg (geralmente em solução contendo 10 mg/mL).	0,2-0,5 mg/m^2 semanalmente, ou diariamente durante 5-10 dias com administração IM, intracavitária ou intratumoral.
Tirotropina, Hormônio estimulante da tireoide (TSH) (Thytropar, Thyrogen)	O hormônio estimulante da tireoide é usado em testes diagnósticos. Estimula a secreção normal do hormônio tireoidiano.	São raras as reações adversas. Em humanos, ocorreram reações alérgicas.	Se usar Thyrogen, reconstituir a ampola de 1,1 mg com 6,0 mL de água estéril; em seguida, dividir em 12 alíquotas. Administrar 0,5 mL a cada paciente, para o teste. A solução que sobrou pode ser congelada e armazenada.	É difícil obter formulações antigas (Thytropar). A forma recombinante humana (Rh TSH) (Thyrogen) contém 1.000 μg/ampola.	Cães: coletar uma amostra basal, seguida por (forma recombinante humana) 50-100 μg/cão.
Trandolapril (Mavik)	Inibidor da ECA. Mecanismo similar ao de captopril e enalapril. Uso no tratamento da ICC. Convertido em trandolaprilato ativo após a administração.	Os mesmos efeitos adversos ocorrentes com outros inibidores da ECA.	Não muito usado em pacientes veterinários.	Comprimidos de 1, 2, 4 mg.	Não estabelecida para cães. A dose inicial em humanos é 1 mg/paciente/dia; em seguida, dose aumentada para 2-4 mg/dia.

Formulário de Medicamentos para Consulta em 5 Minutos

Nome do Princípio Ativo (Comercial e Outros Nomes)	Farmacologia e Indicações	Efeitos Colaterais e Precauções	Informações de Dosagem e Comentários	Formulações	Dosagem (Exceto em Casos Indicados, a Dosagem é a Mesma para Cães e Gatos)
Triancinolona e Triancinolona acetonida (Vetalog, Triamtabs, Aristocort, genérico)	Medicamento anti-inflamatório glicocorticoide. Triancinolona tem potência aproximadamente igual à da metilprednisolona (cerca de 5× cortisol e 1,25× prednisolona), embora alguns dermatologistas tenham sugerido que a potência é maior. A suspensão injetável é absorvida lentamente no local da injeção IM ou intralesional. Uso na terapia intralesional.	Os efeitos adversos são similares aos de outros corticosteroides. Quando usada para injeções oculares, há certa preocupação de ocorrência de granulomas no local da injeção.	Notar que gatos podem necessitar de doses mais elevadas do que cães (em alguns casos, 2×).	Uso veterinário (Vetalog): comprimidos de 0,5 e 1,5 mg; suspensão para injeção: 2 ou 6 mg/mL. Formulação humana: comprimidos de 1, 2, 4, 8, 16 mg; injeção: 10 mg/mL.	Anti-inflamatório: 0,5-1 mg/kg a cada 12h-24h VO; em seguida, diminuir gradativamente a dose para 0,5-1 mg/kg a cada 48h VO. (No entanto, o fabricante recomenda doses de 0,11-0,22 mg/kg/dia.) Injeção de triancinolona acetonida: 0,1-0,2 mg/kg IM, SC; repetir em 7-10 dias. Intralesional: 1,2-1,8 mg, ou 1 mg para cada cm de diâmetro do tumor a cada 2 semanas.
Triantereno (Dyrenium)	Diurético poupador de potássio. Ação similar à da espironolactona, exceto que este último agente tem efeito inibitório competitivo da aldosterona; triantereno, não.	Similares aos causados pela espironolactona.	É pequena a experiência clínica disponível para triantereno. Não existe evidência convincente de que triantereno é mais efetivo do que espironolactona.	Cápsulas de 50, 100 mg.	1-2 mg/kg a cada 12h VO.
Tribrissen	Ver Trimetoprima + sulfadiazina.				
Trifluoperazina (Stelazine)	Fenotiazina. Uso no tratamento da ansiedade, produção de sedação, antiemético. Ação: acredita-se que antagonize a dopamina (de maneira similar à acepromazina); a ação antiemética pode ocorrer via ação antimuscarínica.	Não foram relatados efeitos adversos em animais, mas espera-se que sejam similares aos causados por outras fenotiazinas.	Não foram publicados resultados de estudos clínicos em animais. O uso (e doses) em animais se baseia na experiência em humanos ou em experiências anedóticas em animais.	Solução oral: 10 mg/mL; comprimidos de 1, 2, 5, 10 mg; injeção: 2 mg/mL.	0,03 mg/kg IM a cada 12h.
Triglicérides de cadeia média	Ver Óleo de TCM.				
Tri-iodotironina	Ver Liotironina.				
Trilostano (Vetoryl)	Uso no tratamento da hipercortisolemia (síndrome de Cushing) em cães. Inibidor da enzima 3-β-hidroxisteroide desidrogenase, em cães, para tratamento do hiperadrenocorticismo dependente da hipófise (HDH).	Os efeitos adversos são: letargia temporária, anorexia e vômito. Afora isso, o agente é bem tolerado. Verificar os níveis de eletrólitos em pacientes tratados, porque o trilostano diminui a aldosterona.	Trilostano é medicamento eficaz e seguro para tratamento de cães com HDH. A dose pode ser ajustada individualmente, com base nas determinações de cortisol.	Cápsulas de 10, 30 e 60 mg.	Cães: 3-6 mg/kg/dia VO; pode ser usado em alguns cães na dose de 1,5-3 mg/kg a cada 12h, VO. Gatos: 6 mg/kg a cada 24h VO; aumentar gradativamente até 10 mg/kg a cada 24h.
Trimetobenzamida (Tigan e outros)	Antiemético. Mecanismo de ação desconhecido.	Não foram relatados efeitos adversos em animais.	A eficácia como antiemético não foi relatada em animais.	Injeção: 100 mg/mL; cápsulas de 100, 250 mg.	Cães: 3 mg/kg a cada 8h IM, VO. Gatos: não recomendável.
Trimetoprima + sulfadiazina (Tribrissen, Tucoprim e outras)	Combina a ação farmacológica antibacteriana de trimetoprima e uma sulfonamida. Em conjunto, a combinação é sinergística, com amplo espectro de atividade.	Efeitos adversos principalmente causados pelo componente sulfonamida.	As recomendações de dosagem variam. Há evidência de que 30 mg/kg/dia é dose eficaz em casos de pioderma; para outras infecções, tem sido recomendada a dose de 30 mg/kg 2×/dia.	Comprimidos de 30, 120, 240, 480, 960 mg (todas as formulações têm uma relação de 5:1 para sulfa:trimetoprima). Nos EUA, algumas formulações de trimetoprima/sulfadiazina deixaram de ser comercializadas.	15 mg/kg a cada 12h, VO, ou 30 mg/kg a cada 12h-24h, VO (para *Toxoplasma*, 30 mg/kg a cada 12h, VO).

Formulário de Medicamentos para Consulta em 5 Minutos

Nome do Princípio Ativo (Comercial e Outros Nomes)	Farmacologia e Indicações	Efeitos Colaterais e Precauções	Informações de Dosagem e Comentários	Formulações	Dosagem (Exceto em Casos Indicados, a Dosagem é a Mesma para Cães e Gatos)
Trimetoprima + sulfametoxazol (Bactrim, Septra e formulações genéricas)	Combina a ação farmacológica antibacteriana de trimetoprima e uma sulfonamida. Em conjunto, a combinação é sinergística, com amplo espectro de atividade.	Efeitos adversos principalmente causados pelo componente sulfonamida.	As recomendações de dosagem variam. Há evidência de que 30 mg/kg/dia é dose eficaz em casos de pioderma; para outras infecções, tem sido recomendada a dose de 30 mg/kg 2×/dia.	Comprimidos de 480, 960 mg; suspensão oral contendo 240 mg/5 mL (todas as formulações têm uma relação de 5:1 para sulfa:trimetoprima)	15 mg/kg a cada 12h, VO, ou 30 mg/kg a cada 12-24h, VO.
Urofolitropina (FSH) (Metrodin)	Estimula a ovulação. Contém FSH. Em humanos, é usado em combinação com HCG para estimular a ovulação e induzir a gravidez.	Não foram relatados efeitos adversos em animais. Em humanos, foi relatada a ocorrência de tromboembolia ou síndrome de hiperestimulação ovariana grave.	Ainda não foram publicados resultados de estudos clínicos em animais. O uso em animais se baseia na experiência em humanos.	75 U por ampola para injeção.	Doses não estabelecidas. (A dose em humanos é 75 unidades/dia IM durante 7 dias.)
Ursodiol (ursodesoxicolato) (Actigall)	Ácido biliar hidrofílico. Anticolelítico. Uso no tratamento de doenças hepáticas. Aumenta o fluxo biliar. Em cães, pode alterar o *pool* dos ácidos biliares circulantes, deslocando os ácidos biliares mais hidrofóbicos. Em humanos, esse agente é usado na prevenção ou tratamento de cálculos biliares.	Não foram relatados efeitos adversos em animais. Pode causar diarreia.	Ainda não foram publicados resultados de estudos clínicos em animais. O uso (e doses) em animais se baseia na experiência em humanos ou em experiências anedóticas em animais. Administrar com as refeições.	Cápsulas de 300 mg e comprimidos de 250 ou 500 mg.	10-15 mg/kg a cada 24h, VO.
Vancomicina (Vancocin, Vancoled)	Medicamento antibacteriano. Mecanismo de ação: inibição da parede da célula bacteriana, causando lise (por um mecanismo diferente daquele dos β-lactâmicos). Seu espectro abrange estafilococos, estreptococos e enterococos (mas não bactérias Gram-negativas). Uso principalmente no tratamento de estafilococos e enterococos resistentes, inclusive *Staphylococcus* spp. resistente à meticilina (p. ex., MRSA ou MRSP).	Não foram relatados efeitos adversos em animais. Administrar IV; causa dor intensa e lesão tecidual se for administrada por via IM ou SC. Não administrar rapidamente; usar infusão lenta, se possível (p. ex., ao longo de 30 min). Em humanos, os efeitos adversos são lesão renal (mais comum com o uso de produtos mais antigos, que contêm impurezas) e liberação de histamina.	Vancomicina não é de uso comum em animais, mas é medicamento útil no tratamento de enterococos ou estafilococos resistentes a outros antibióticos. As doses são derivadas de estudos farmacocinéticos em cães. É recomendável a monitorização das concentrações plasmáticas de vale, para que haja certeza da dose apropriada. Manter a concentração de vale acima dos 5 mcg/mL. A solução de infusão pode ser preparada em salina a 0,9% ou em dextrose a 5%, mas não em soluções alcalinizantes.	Ampolas para injeção (0,5 a 10 g).	Cães: 15 mg/kg a cada 6-8h por infusão IV. Gatos: 12-15 mg/kg a cada 8h por infusão IV.
Varfarina sódica (Coumadin, genérica)	Anticoagulante. Causa depleção da vitamina K, que é responsável pela geração dos fatores da coagulação. Uso no tratamento da doença hipercoagulável e na prevenção da tromboembolia.	Os efeitos adversos são atribuíveis à diminuição da coagulação. Interações farmacológicas: outros medicamentos podem potenciar a ação da varfarina (inclusive ácido acetilsalicílico, cloranfenicol, fenilbutazona, cetoconazol, cimetidina).	A resposta à varfarina é individualizada. Para um tratamento ideal, ajustar a dose mediante a monitorização do tempo de coagulação. Exemplificando, em alguns pacientes a dose é ajustada pela manutenção do tempo de protrombina em 1,5-2× até 2-2,5× o normal (ou INI de 2-3).	Comprimidos de 1, 2, 2,5, 4, 5, 7,5, 10 mg.	Cães: 0,1-0,2 mg/kg a cada 24h, VO. Gatos (tromboembolia): começar com 0,25 ou 0,5 mg/gato a cada 24h, VO e ajustar a dose com base na avaliação do tempo de coagulação.

ESPÉCIES CANINA E FELINA

Formulário de Medicamentos para Consulta em 5 Minutos					
Nome do Princípio Ativo (Comercial e Outros Nomes)	*Farmacologia e Indicações*	*Efeitos Colaterais e Precauções*	*Informações de Dosagem e Comentários*	*Formulações*	*Dosagem (Exceto em Casos Indicados, a Dosagem é a Mesma para Cães e Gatos)*
Vasopressina (ADH) (Pitressin)	Hormônio antidiurético. Vasopressina é usada no tratamento da poliúria causada pelo diabetes insípido central. Não é efetiva para poliúria causada por doença renal. Também usada como vasopressor e durante a parada cardíaca (ressuscitação cardiopulmonar [RCP]).	Não foram relatados efeitos adversos. Foram relatadas reações alérgicas em humanos. Foi informada elevação na pressão arterial em humanos.	As doses são ajustadas com base na monitorização do consumo de água e no débito urinário. Ver também Acetato de desmopressina.	20 U/mL (aquosa).	Antidiurético: 10 U IV, IM. Vasopressor: 0,01-0,04 unidades/min. RCP: 0,2-0,8 unidades/kg/ IV.
Vitamina A (retinoides) (Aquasol A)	Suplemento de vitamina A. Ver também Isotretinoína, para análogos usados para outros problemas.	Doses excessivas podem causar dores ósseas ou articulares e dermatite.	A dose de vitamina A é expressa como U, ou equivalentes de retinol (ER), ou ainda em mcg de retinol. 1 ER = 1 mcg de retinol. 1 ER de Vitamina A = 3,33 U de retinol.	Solução oral: 5.000 U (1.500 ER)/0,1 mL; comprimidos de 10.000, 25.000 e 50.000 U.	625-800 U/kg a cada 24h, VO (ver seção de informações sobre doses).
Vitamina B$_1$	Ver Tiamina.				
Vitamina B$_{12}$ (cianocobalamina) e cobalamina	Suplemento de vitamina B$_{12}$. A vitamina B$_{12}$ tem sido usada no tratamento de algumas formas de anemia.	Os efeitos adversos são raros, porque vitaminas hidrossolúveis são facilmente excretadas.	Administrada em animais com doença intestinal (p. ex., DII), ou insuficiência pancreática, para evitar deficiência. A monitorização sérica pode determinar a dose ideal. A faixa sugerida é 290-1.500 ng/L para gatos e 252-908 ng/L para cães. Não há necessidade de suplementação em animais com dietas bem balanceadas.	Comprimidos de diversos tamanhos, em incrementos de 25-1.000 mcg e injeção.	Cães: 100-200 mcg/dia VO, SC, ou 250-500 mcg/ dia, IM ou SC. Gatos: 50-100 mcg/dia VO, SC, ou 250 mcg/gato, IM ou SC semanalmente; o intervalo pode ser aumentado para cada 2, 4, ou 6 semanas.
Vitamina B$_2$ (riboflavina)	Suplemento de vitamina B$_2$.	Os efeitos adversos são raros, porque vitaminas hidrossolúveis são facilmente excretadas. Riboflavina pode alterar a cor da urina.	Não há necessidade de suplementação em animais com dietas bem balanceadas.	Comprimidos de diversos tamanhos, em incrementos de 10-250 mg.	Cães: 10-20 mg/dia VO. Gatos: 5-10 mg/dia VO.
Vitamina C (ácido ascórbico) (ver Ácido ascórbico)	Usada no tratamento da deficiência de vitamina C e, ocasionalmente, como acidificante urinário. Dados insuficientes para demonstrar que o ácido ascórbico é efetivo para prevenção do câncer ou de doença cardiovascular.	Não foram relatados efeitos adversos em animais. Doses elevadas podem aumentar o risco da formação de cálculos de oxalato na bexiga.	Não há necessidade de suplementação em animais com dietas bem balanceadas.	Comprimidos de diversos tamanhos e injeção.	100-500 mg/dia.
Vitamina D	Ver Di-hidrotaquisterol ou Ergocalciferol.				
Vitamina E (alfa-tocoferol) (Aquasol E e genérico)	Vitamina considerada antioxidante. Usada como suplemento e como tratamento de algumas dermatoses imunemediadas.	Não foram relatados efeitos adversos.	Vitamina E foi proposta como tratamento de grande variedade de enfermidades humanas, mas não há evidência de eficácia em animais.	Grande variedade de cápsulas, comprimidos; há disponibilidade de solução oral (p. ex., 1.000 U/cápsula).	100-400 U a cada 12h, VO (ou 400-600 U a cada 12h, VO para doença cutânea imunomediada).

Formulário de Medicamentos para Consulta em 5 Minutos

Nome do Princípio Ativo (Comercial e Outros Nomes)	Farmacologia e Indicações	Efeitos Colaterais e Precauções	Informações de Dosagem e Comentários	Formulações	Dosagem (Exceto em Casos Indicados, a Dosagem é a Mesma para Cães e Gatos)
Vitamina K_1 (fitonadiona, fitomenadiona) (Aqua-MEPHYTON [injeção], Mephyton [comprimidos]; Veta-K1 [cápsulas])	Vitamina K_1 é usada no tratamento de coagulopatias causadas por toxicose por anticoagulante (varfarina ou outros rodenticidas). (Os anticoagulantes promovem depleção da vitamina K no corpo; essa vitamina é essencial para a síntese dos fatores da coagulação.)	Não administrar IV.	Se for identificado um rodenticida específico, consultar o centro de controle de venenos para protocolo específico. Usar vitamina K_1 para tratamento agudo, por ter maior biodisponibilidade. Administrar com o alimento, para aumentar a absorção. Fitonadiona e fitomenadiona são formas lipossolúveis sintéticas de vitamina K_1. Menadiol é a vitamina K_4, que é convertida no organismo em vitamina K_3 (menadiona).	Injeção: 2 ou 10 mg/mL; Mephyton é formulado em comprimidos de 5 mg; Veta-K1 é fornecido em cápsulas de 25 mg. Fitonadiona é uma injeção contendo 2 mg/mL ou 10 mg/mL.	Rodenticidas de curta ação: 1 mg/kg/dia IM, SC, VO durante 10-14 dias. Rodenticidas de ação prolongada: 2,5-5 mg/kg/dia IM, SC, VO durante 3-4 semanas e até 6 semanas.
Voriconazol (Vfend)	Antifúngico azol (triazol). Ação similar a outros medicamentos antifúngicos do grupo dos azóis, que inibem a síntese de ergosterol. Ativo contra fungos sistêmicos, dermatófitos e *Aspergillus*.	Bem tolerado em cães, mas associado com neurotoxidez em gatos. Pode causar interações farmacológicas, por inibir as enzimas do citocromo P-450.	O uso clínico se baseia em limitada experiência clínica, uso anedótico e na extrapolação da medicina humana.	Comprimidos de 50 e 200 mg; injeção: 10 mg/mL.	Cães: 4-5 mg/kg a cada 12h, VO. Gatos: dose segura não identificada.
Zidovudina (AZT) (Retrovir)	Medicamento antiviral. Em humanos, usado no tratamento da AIDS. Em animais, tem sido experimentalmente usada em gatos para tratamento da infecção pelo vírus da leucemia felina (FeLV) e pelo vírus da imunodeficiência felina (FIV). AZT inibe a enzima viral transcriptase reversa, impedindo a conversão do RNA viral até DNA.	Anemia e leucopenia são efeitos adversos possíveis. Monitorizar o hematócrito em gatos tratados e obter periodicamente um hemograma completo.	Atualmente, a experiência com o uso do AZT no tratamento de doenças virais em animais é, em grande parte, experimental ou anedótica. Esse agente pode ter ajudado alguns gatos com FIV e pode impedir uma infecção persistente pelo FeLV, mas não existe evidência convincente para eficácia.	Xarope contendo 10 mg/mL; injeção: 10 mg/mL.	Gatos: 15 mg/kg a cada 12h, VO a 20 mg/kg a cada 8h, VO (também já foram usadas doses elevadas, de até 30 mg/kg/dia).
Zolazepam	Ver Tiletamina + zolazepam.				
Zoledronato (Zometa, ácido zoledrônico)	Agente bifosfonato. Inibe a reabsorção óssea e diminui o *turnover* ósseo ao inibir os osteoclastos. Uso no tratamento de malignidades e doenças patológicas ósseas. Pode proporcionar alívio da dor em pacientes com doença óssea.	O uso em cães não tem causado efeitos adversos.	Administrar por infusão IV, mediante diluição em fluidos.	Ampola com 4 mg/5 mL para injeção.	Cães: 0,2-0,25 mg/kg IV ao longo de 15 min, diluídos em 50-100 mL de salina a cada 28 dias. Gatos: 0,2 mg/kg IV ao longo de 15 min, diluídos em 25 mL a cada 21-28 dias.
Zonisamida (Zonegran)	Anticonvulsivante. O mecanismo de ação é incerto, mas o agente pode potenciar a ação de GABA, um neurotransmissor inibitório, ou pode estabilizar as membranas por meio de mudanças na condutância do sódio e cálcio.	As reações adversas podem ser: letargia, ataxia e vômito.	Usa-se zonisamida no tratamento de convulsões refratárias em cães, quando outros medicamentos não obtiveram sucesso.	Cápsulas de 100 mg.	Cães: 5-10 mg/kg a cada 12h, VO. Gatos: 10 mg/kg a cada 12h, VO.

Legenda para as Abreviaturas da Tabela:

ECA	enzima conversora de angiotensina
ICC	insuficiência cardíaca congestiva
SNC	sistema nervoso central
COX	cicloxigenase
LCR	líquido cefalorraquidiano
g	grama
GABA	ácido gama-aminobutírico
GI	gastrintestinal
IM	intramuscular
INI	índice de normalização internacional
IV	intravenoso
mcg	micrograma
mg	miligrama
CIM	concentração inibitória mínima
mL	mililitro
AINE	medicamento anti-inflamatório não esteroide
SNR	sem necessidade de prescrição
VO	via oral
PU/PD	poliúria e polidipsia
Rx	apenas prescrição
SC	subcutâneo
U	unidades

AVISO PARA AS TABELAS DE DOSES:
Nota: as doses indicadas são tanto para cães como para gatos, a não ser que haja informação em contrário. Muitas das doses listadas são extrabula, ou são medicamentos humanos não aprovados para animais e administrados extrabula. As doses listadas se baseiam nas melhores informações disponíveis no momento da confecção da tabela. Os autores não podem garantir a eficácia ou segurança absoluta de medicamentos usados de acordo com as recomendações desta tabela. É possível que ocorram efeitos adversos com o uso de medicamentos listados nesta tabela, com relação aos quais os autores não tinham conhecimento no momento de sua elaboração. Os veterinários usuários desta tabela são encorajados a consultar a literatura mais recente, bulas e rótulos dos produtos, além das informações divulgadas pelos fabricantes, com o objetivo de obter informações adicionais sobre efeitos adversos, interações e eficácia que não tinham sido identificados no momento em que estas tabelas foram elaboradas.

APÊNDICE X

TABELAS DE CONVERSÃO

Tabela X-A

Tabela de Conversão de Peso para Área de Superfície Corporal (em Metros Quadrados) para Cães			
kg	*m²*	*kg*	*m²*
0,5	0,06	26,0	0,88
1,0	0,10	27,0	0,90
2,0	0,15	28,0	0,92
3,0	0,20	29,0	0,94
4,0	0,25	30,0	0,96
5,0	0,29	31,0	0,99
6,0	0,33	32,0	1,01
7,0	0,36	33,0	1,03
8,0	0,40	34,0	1,05
9,0	0,43	35,0	1,07
10,0	0,46	36,0	1,09
11,0	0,49	37,0	1,11
12,0	0,52	38,0	1,13
13,0	0,55	39,0	1,15
14,0	0,58	40,0	1,17
15,0	0,60	41,0	1,19
16,0	0,63	42,0	1,21
17,0	0,66	43,0	1,23
18,0	0,69	44,0	1,25
19,0	0,71	45,0	1,26
20,0	0,74	46,0	1,28
21,0	0,76	47,0	1,30
22,0	0,78	48,0	1,32
23,0	0,81	49,0	1,34
24,0	0,83	50,0	1,36
25,0	0,85		

Embora a tabela tenha sido compilada para cães, também pode ser utilizada para gatos. Valores mais precisos são representados na fórmula: ASC em $m^2 = (K \times W^{2/3}) \times 10^{-4}$, em que m^2 = metro quadrado, ASC = área de superfície corporal, W = peso corporal em gramas e K = constante de 10,1 para cães e 10,0 para gatos.

TABELAS DE CONVERSÃO (CONTINUAÇÃO)

Tabela X-B

Valores Equivalentes Aproximados para Graus Fahrenheit e Celsius*			
°F	°C	°F	°C
0	-17,8	98	36,7
32	0	99	37,2
85	29,4	100	37,8
86	30,0	101	38,3
87	30,6	102	38,9
88	31,1	103	39,4
89	31,7	104	40,0
90	32,2	105	40,6
91	32,7	106	41,1
92	33,3	107	41,7
93	33,9	108	42,2
94	34,4	109	42,8
95	35,0	110	43,3
96	35,5	212	100,0
97	36,1		

* Conversão da temperatura: °Celsius para °Fahrenheit = (°C) (9/5) + 32°;
°Fahrenheit para °Celsius = (F - 32°) (5/9).

Tabela X-C

Fatores de Conversão das Unidades de Peso		
Unidades Fornecidas	Unidades Desejadas	Para Conversão, Multiplicar por
lb	g	453,6
lb	kg	0,4536
oz	g	28,35
kg	lb	2,2046
kg	mg	1.000.000
kg	g	1.000
g	mg	1.000
g	µg	1.000.000
mg	µg	1.000
mg/g	mg/lb	453,6
mg/kg	mg/lb	0,4536
µg/kg	µg/lb	0,4536
Mcal	kcal	1.000
kcal/kg	kcal/lb	0,4536
kcal/lb	kcal/kg	2,2046
ppm	µg/g	1
ppm	mg/kg	1
ppm	mg/lb	0,4536
mg/kg	%	0,0001
ppm	%	0,0001
mg/g	%	0,1
g/kg	%	0,1

ÍNDICE REMISSIVO

A

Abdome agudo, 2-4, 901-906
Abdominocentese
  para ascite, 212
  para insuficiência cardíaca congestiva direita, 774
Aberdeen terrier, distocia em, 388
Abissínio
  amiloide hepático, 73
  amiloidose, 74, 580
  amiloidose renal, 427
  anemia, regenerativa, 91
  deficiência da piruvato quinase, 91, 292
  displasia de bastonetes e cones, 102
  displasia de fotorreceptores, 102
  epúlide, 484
  fragilidade osmótica eritrocitária, 91
  gengivostomatite, 1303
  hemoglobinúria, 597
  hipotireoidismo, 711
  inflamação orofaríngea felina, 770
  insuficiência renal, crônica, 785
  miastenia grave, 883
  mielopatia, 894
  síndrome de hiperestesia felina, 1177
  tromboembolia aórtica, 1276
Abortamento
  espontâneo
    em cães, 5-6
    em gatos, 7-8
  interrupção da gestação, 9-10
Abscedação, 11-12
Abscesso apical, 13
Abscesso da raiz dentária, 13
Abscesso hepático, 609-610
Abscesso prostático, 1094-1095
Acanthamoeba, 72
Acarbose
  para diabetes melito, 350
  para hiperglicemia, 653
Ácaros otológicos, 14
Acasalamento, momento oportuno, 15-16
Acemannan, para infecção pelo vírus da imunodeficiência felina (FIV), 744
Acepromazina
  informações de formulações, 1363-1441
  para asma/bronquite em gatos, 120
  para fobias a trovões e relâmpagos, 552
  para paralisia pelos carrapatos, 1007
  para problemas comportamentais maternos, 1082
  para problemas comportamentais pediátricos, 1084
  para retenção urinária, 1136
  para toxicose por anfetamina, 1236
  para toxicose por antidepressivos tricíclicos, 108

para toxicose por benzodiazepínicos e soníferos, 1237
  para toxicose por ISRS, 109
  para toxicose por pseudoefedrina, 1247
  para tromboembolia aórtica, 1277
  para vestibulopatia, 1329
  para vocalização excessiva, 1330
Acetato de cálcio
  para hiperparatireoidismo, 664
  para hipoparatireoidismo, 703
Acetato de fludrocortisona
  informações de formulações, 1363-1441
  para hipoadrenocorticismo, 684
Acetato de megestrol
  informações de formulações, 1363-1441
  para agressividade, 45
  para ceratite
    eosinofílica, 194
    não ulcerativa, 196
  para comportamento de marcação territorial e errático, 249
  para conjuntivite, 265
  para hiperandrogenismo, 639
  para hiperplasia das glândulas mamárias, 666
  para hiperplasia prostática benigna, 670, 1096
  para infecção pelo vírus da imunodeficiência felina (FIV), 744
  para perda de peso e caquexia, 1022
  para supressão do estro (cio), 765
Acetato de metilprednisolona, 1363-1441
Acetato de prednisolona (1%)
  para catarata, 191
  para ceratite
    eosinofílica, 194
    não ulcerativa, 196
  para conjuntivite, 263, 265
  para coriorretinite, 272
  para depósito lipídico, 704
  para episclerite, 481
  para hifema, 632
  para hipópio, 704
  para lacerações da córnea e esclera, 809
  para luxação do cristalino, 842
  para uveíte anterior, 1320, 1322
Acetato de zinco
  para encefalopatia hepática, 451
  para flatulência, 549
  para hepatite, crônica ativa, 603
Acetazolamida
  para cisto quadrigeminal, 217
  para disrafismo espinal, 384
  para hidrocefalia, 629
  para urolitíase, por cistina, 1308
Acetilcisteína. *Ver também N-*acetilcisteína
  informações de formulações, 1363-1441
  para ceratite, ulcerativa, 198
  para ceratoconjuntivite seca, 199

Acetilcolina, para fibrilação ventricular, 540
Acetonida de triancinolona
  para ceratite
    eosinofílica, 194
    não ulcerativa, 196
  para hipópio, 704
  para uveíte anterior, 1320, 1322
Aceturato de diminazeno, para babesiose, 134, 135, 483
Acidentes vasculares cerebrais (AVC), 17-18
  hemorrágico, 17-18
  isquêmico, 17-18
Ácido acético, para otite externa/média, 980
Ácido acetilsalicílico
  dosagens e indicações, 1362
  informações de formulações, 1363-1441
  para acidente vascular cerebral isquêmico, 18
  para amiloidose, 75
  para ceratite ulcerativa, 198
  para condrossarcoma, 258, 260
  para deficiência de fosfofrutoquinase, 291
  para dirofilariose, 361
  para doença de Legg-Calvé-Perthes, 409
  para endocardite, 458
  para febre, 527
  para febre familiar do Shar-pei, 529
  para fibrossarcoma, 541, 542
  para glomerulonefrite, 581
  para hipercoagulabilidade, 647
  para hipertensão, pulmonar, 677
  para hipoalbuminemia, 686
  para hipópio, 704
  para infarto do miocárdio, 734
  para lacerações da córnea e esclera, 809
  para miocardiopatia, 905, 908, 910
  para olho vermelho, 963
  para osteodistrofia hipertrófica, 972
  para panosteíte, 991
  para prevenção de tromboembolia, 85
  para prevenção de tromboembolia pulmonar, 1280
  para tromboembolia aórtica, 1277
  para uveíte anterior, 1320, 1322
Ácido acetoidroxâmico (AHA) (Lithostat), para urolitíase por estruvita, 1310
Ácido aminocaproico
  para mielopatia degenerativa, 896
  para trombocitopenia, 1273
Ácido ascórbico
  informações de formulações, 1363-1441
  para metemoglobinemia, 207
  para síndrome de Chediak-Higashi, 1171
  para toxicidade do paracetamol, 1224
  para toxicose por anfetamina, 1236
  para ulceração bucal, 1304
Ácido folínico, para toxoplasmose, 1257

Ácido linoleico, para linfoma cutâneo epiteliotrópico, 834

Ácido salicílico
para acne, 25
para otite externa/média, 980

Ácido ursodesoxicólico
para cirrose e fibrose do fígado, 212
para colecistite e coledoquite, 233
para colelitíase, 235
para hepatite crônica ativa, 603
para hepatite infecciosa canina, 607
para hepatopatia diabética, 613
para hepatopatia por armazenamento de cobre, 617
para hepatotoxicidade, 622
para infestação pela fascíola hepática, 769
para insuficiência hepática, aguda, 779
para mucocele da vesícula biliar, 931
para obstrução de ducto biliar, 954
para peritonite biliar, 1028
para síndrome colangite/colangio-hepatite, 1164

Ácido valproico
informações de formulações, 1363-1441
para epilepsia, 480

Acidose com hiato aniônico, alto, 21
Acidose hiperclorêmica, 21-22
Acidose hiperfosfatêmica, 21-22
Acidose láctica, 19-20
Acidose metabólica, 21-22
Acidose tubular renal, 23
Acidose urêmica, 22

Acitretina
para carcinoma de células escamosas, orelha, 179
para carcinoma de células escamosas, plano nasal, 180

Acne
em cães, 24, 333
em gatos, 25, 333

Acondrodisplasia, 968
Acromegalia, 26

ACTH
concentração endógena, 634
informações de formulações, 1363-1441

Actinomicose, 27

Acupuntura
para discopatia intervertebral, toracolombar, 371
para espondilose deformante, 497

Adenite sebácea, 28
alopecia, 63, 65
dermatose papulonodular, 333

Adenite sebácea granulomatosa, 28
Adenocarcinoma da próstata, 29
Adenocarcinoma da tireoide, 30-31
Adenocarcinoma das glândulas ceruminosas, orelha, 32
Adenocarcinoma das glândulas salivares, 33
Adenocarcinoma das glândulas sudoríferas, 34
Adenocarcinoma das glândulas sudoríferas apócrinas, 34
Adenocarcinoma do estômago, 35
Adenocarcinoma do intestino delgado, 35
Adenocarcinoma do intestino grosso, 35
Adenocarcinoma do pâncreas, 36
Adenocarcinoma do reto, 35
Adenocarcinoma dos pulmões, 37
Adenocarcinoma dos sacos anais, 38
Adenocarcinoma nasal, 39
Adenocarcinoma renal, 40

Adenoma hepatocelular, 41
Adenosina, para taquicardia supraventricular, 1206
Adequan. *Ver* Glicosaminoglicano polissulfatado (GAGPS)
Adstringentes, para otite externa/média, 980

Afghan hound
distrofia da córnea, 392
hipoandrogenismo, 687
miocardiopatia, 901
quilotórax, 1112
torção dos lobos pulmonares, 1214

Aflatoxina, 888
Afogamento (afogamento por um triz), 42

Agentes anabólicos
para estimulação do apetite, 1022
para infecção pelo vírus da imunodeficiência felina (FIV), 744

Agentes anti-inflamatórios
para avulsão do plexo braquial, 131
para cistos subaracnoides, 220
para colite e proctite, 240
para colite ulcerativa histiocítica, 241
para displasia coxofemoral, 377
para disquesia e hematoquesia, 386
para distúrbios da articulação temporomandibular, 393
para esofagite, 489
para estenose esofágica, 506
para estomatite, 516
para hipertensão, pulmonar, 677
para incontinência, fecal, 729
para lacerações da córnea e esclera, 809
para luxação do cristalino, 842
para osteocondrodisplasia, 968
para osteocondrose, 970
para osteodistrofia hipertrófica, 972
para osteopatia craniomandibular, 975
para panosteíte, 991-992
para parasitas respiratórios, 1012
para prolapso da glândula da terceira pálpebra, 1089
para rinite e sinusite, 1138
para ruptura muscular, 1143
para síndrome de disfunção cognitiva, 1175
para tosse, 1217
para ulceração bucal, 1304

Agentes anti-inflamatórios não esteroides (AINE)
dosagens e indicações
AINE dispensáveis, 1361-1362
AINE parenterais, 1361-1362
para artrite
osteoartrite, 15
séptica, 116
para borreliose de Lyme, 159
para cáries dentárias, 187
para cataratas, 191
para ceratite, ulcerativa, 198
para claudicação, 224
para condrossarcoma, 258, 260
para degenerações e infiltrações da córnea, 304
para dermatomiosite, 320
para discopatia intervertebral
cervical, 369
toracolombar, 371
para displasia do cotovelo, 381
para disúria e polaciúria, 404
para doença de Legg-Calvé-Perthes, 409
para doença do ligamento cruzado cranial, 416
para doença idiopática do trato urinário inferior dos felinos, 418
para dor, 431

para dor no pescoço e dorso, 434
para espondilomielopatia cervical, 496
para espondilose deformante, 497
para fibrossarcoma, 541-542
para flebite, 550
para hepatozoonose, 623
para hifema, 632
para hipópio, 704
para instabilidade atlantoaxial, 773
para lacerações da córnea e esclera, 809
para luxação patelar, 845
para luxações articulares, 847
para meningite-arterite responsivas a esteroides, 873
para osteocondrodisplasia, 968
para osteocondrose, 970
para osteopatia craniomandibular, 975
para osteossarcoma, 978
para panosteíte, 991-992
para paralisia, 1005
para poliartrite, erosiva, 1067
para problemas do ombro, 1089
para prostatopatia em cão macho reprodutor, 1098
para rinite e sinusite, 1138
para siringomielia, 1198
para traumatismo da coluna vertebral, 1265
para uveíte anterior, 1320, 1322
para vaginite, 1324

Agentes anticolinesterásicos, para miastenia grave, 884

Agentes antifúngicos
para aspergilose, 122-123, 125
para blefarite, 142
para colesteatoma, 236
para dermatoses nasais, 328
para edema periférico, 438
para hepatopatia diabética, 613
para infecção pelo vírus da imunodeficiência felina (FIV), 744
para mediastinite, 863
para otite externa/média, 980
para pododermatite, 1065

Agentes antissecretores de ácido gástrico
para esofagite, 449
para estenose esofágica, 506
para refluxo gastresofágico, 1128

Agentes antissecretores para infecção pelo helicobacter, 753

Agentes citotóxicos
para pênfigo, 1020
para poliartrite, erosiva, 1067
para poliartrite, não erosiva, 421

Agentes hiperosmóticos, para glaucoma, 577
Agentes hipoglicemiantes, 346, 348, 350

Agentes imunomoduladores
para distúrbios das unhas e dos leitos ungueais, 397
para hepatite
crônica ativa, 603
granulomatosa, 606
para infecção pelo vírus da imunodeficiência felina (FIV), 744
para infecção pelo vírus da leucemia felina (FeLV), 746

Agentes imunossupressores
para colite e proctite, 240
para colite ulcerativa histiocítica, 241
para distúrbios despigmentantes, 322
para doença da aglutinina fria, 407
para edema periférico, 438

para enteropatia inflamatória, 464
para estomatite, 516
para gastrenterite, eosinofílica, 565
para gastrite, crônica, 572
para granuloma estéril idiopático, 328
para histiocitose, 719
para infecção pelo helicobacter, 753
para lúpus eritematoso, sistêmico (LES), 328, 841
para megaesôfago, 867
para meningite-arterite responsivas a esteroides, 873
para neuropatias periféricas, 945
para peritonite infecciosa felina, 1031
para pneumonia, eosinofílica, 1056
para prurido, 1105
para trombocitopenia, imunomediada primária, 1275
para ulceração bucal, 1304
para vasculite, cutânea, 1325
Agentes inotrópicos positivos
para choque, cardiogênico, 201
para choque, hipovolêmico, 203
para choque, séptico, 205
para edema periférico, 438
para endocardiose da valva atrioventricular, 456
para hipertensão, pulmonar, 677
para insuficiência cardíaca congestiva, esquerda, 777
para lesão por mordedura de fio elétrico, 819
Agentes ligantes de fosfato intestinal. *Ver* Agentes ligantes do fósforo
Agentes ligantes do fósforo
para hiperfosfatemia, 650
para hiperparatireoidismo, 664
para insuficiência renal, crônica, 786
Agentes mióticos
para glaucoma, 577
para luxação do cristalino, 842
Agentes mucolíticos, para ceratoconjuntivite seca, 199
Agentes pró-cinéticos
para distúrbios da motilidade gástrica, 396
para esofagite, 489
para estenose esofágica, 506
para gastrite, 570
para hérnia hiatal, 624
para megacólon, 865
para megaesôfago, 867
para refluxo gastresofágico, 1128
para regurgitação, 1130
para síndrome do vômito bilioso, 1185
para vômito, 1334
Aglepristona
para corrimento vaginal, 276
para interrupção da gestação, 10
para piometra, 1043
Agonistas alfa-adrenérgicos. *Ver também medicamentos específicos*
para incompetência uretral, 731
para retenção urinária, 1136
Agressividade, 51-58
contra as pessoas
crianças, 49
em cães, 49-51
em gatos, 46
em cães
alimento, 59-60
contra as crianças, 49
contra pessoas familiares, 50-51

defensiva, 43, 52-53
entre os cães, 54-55
medo/defensiva, 43, 52-53
possessiva, 59-60
territorial, 59-60
visão geral, 43-45
em gatos
contra as pessoas, 46
controle de impulso, 46
dor, 46
entre os gatos, 46-47, 56-57
induzida pela frustração, 46
induzida pelo contato, 46
induzida pelo medo, 46, 58
lúdica, 46
materna, 46
problemas comportamentais pediátricos, 1085-1086
redirecionada, 46
territorial, 46
visão geral, 46-48
entre os cães, 54-55
entre os gatos, 46-47, 56-57
Agressividade canina contra crianças, 49
AINE. *Ver* Agentes anti-inflamatórios não esteroides
Airedale terrier
abiotrofia cerebelar, 658
adenocarcinoma, pâncreas, 36
alopecia do flanco, 64
bloqueio atrioventricular, de segundo grau, Mobitz Tipo II, 149
distrofia da córnea, 392
doença de von Willebrand, 412, 482
espondilose deformante, 497
hiperplasia e prolapso vaginais, 667
hipoplasia cerebelar, 706
linfoma, 830
tumores melanocíticos, 1295
vômito, crônico, 1333
Akita
adenite sebácea, 28
alopecia X, 64, 67
amiloide hepático, 73
coriorretinite, 271
defeito do septo ventricular, 289
deficiência de enzima desramificante, 924
dermatite acral por lambedura, 310
distúrbios despigmentantes, 321
doença de von Willebrand, 412
glaucoma, 576
hipercalemia, 642
miastenia grave, 883
pênfigo foliáceo, 335, 1019
poliartrite, não erosiva, 1068
síndrome uveodermatológica, 327, 1193
uveíte anterior, 1319
Albendazol
informações de formulações, 1363-1441
para bailisascaríase, 136
para capilaríase, 170
para cisticercose, 896
para encefalitozoonose, 449
para giardíase, 240
para parasitas respiratórios, 1012
para triquinose, 1270
Albinismo, 321
Albuterol
informações de formulações, 1363-1441
para asma/bronquite em gatos, 121
para bronquiectasia, 163

para bronquite, crônica, 165
para parada sinusal/bloqueio sinoatrial, 1000
para tosse, 1217
toxicose por beta-2 agonistas inalatórios, 1239
Alcalinizantes urinários
para urolitíase, por cistina, 1308
para urolitíase, por xantina, 1318
Alcalose hipoalbuminêmica, 62
Alcalose hipoclorêmica, 62
Alcalose metabólica, 61-62
Alfacasozepina, para vocalização excessiva, 1330
Alfaepoetina (r-HuEPO)
informações de formulações, 1363-1441
para anemia de doença renal crônica, 82-83
Alopecia
em cães, 63-64, 67-68
em gatos, 65-66, 69, 70
Alopecia areata, 63, 65
Alopecia do pavilhão auricular, 63-66
Alopecia endócrina, 65
Alopecia não inflamatória, 67-68
Alopecia paraneoplásica felina, 69
Alopecia por diluição da cor, 63, 64
Alopecia por hormônios sexuais, 65
Alopecia psicogênica, 1260
Alopecia sazonal do flanco, 63, 64
Alopecia simétrica felina, 70
Alopecia universal, 65
Alopecia X, 63, 64, 67-68
Alopurinol
informações de formulações, 1363-1441
para doença de Chagas, 408
para leishmaniose, 814
para nefrolitíase, 973
para urolitíase, por urato, 1316
para urolitíase, por xantina, 1318
Alprazolam
informações de formulações, 1363-1441
para agressividade, 52, 55, 58
para comportamento de marcação territorial e errático, 249
para comportamentos destrutivos, 252
para fobias a trovões e relâmpagos, 552
para medos, fobias e ansiedades, 554, 556
para síndrome de ansiedade da separação, 1170
toxicose, 1237-1238
Alsatian britânico, epilepsia em, 479
Altrenogeste
para manutenção da gestação em gatos, 8
para parto prematuro, 1015
Amantadina
para degeneração cerebelar, 299
para dor neuropática, 1362
Amaurose, 961
Amebíase, 72
Ameloblastoma, 71, 857, 858
Ameloblastoma periférico. *Ver* Epúlide
Amelogênese imperfeita, 308, 557
Amicacina
informações de formulações, 1363-1441
para campilobacteriose, 168
para colibacilose, 238
para infecção do trato urinário inferior, 736
para infecções secundárias à influenza canina, 771
para nocardiose, 950
para otite externa/média, 980
para peritonite, 1028
para pneumonia, bacteriana, 1054
para traqueobronquite infecciosa canina, 1263
Amiloide hepático, 73

Amiloidose, 74-75
dermatoses, 331, 332
hepática, 73
renal, de natureza congênita e de desenvolvimento, 427, 428
Aminoácidos, intravenosos para glucagonoma, 583
Aminofilina
para anafilaxia, 77
para bronquite, crônica, 165
para influenza canina, 771
para parada sinusal/bloqueio sinoatrial, 1000
Aminoglicosídeos
para campilobacteriose, 168
para ceratite, ulcerativa, 198
para endocardite, 458
para epididimite/orquite, 479
para hepatotoxicidade, 622
para infecções anaeróbias, 757
para infecções secundárias à influenza canina, 771
para lacerações da córnea e esclera, 809
para nocardiose, 950
para obstrução gastrintestinal, 959
para osteomielite, 974
para otite externa/média, 980
para peritonite, 1028
para piotórax, 1045
para sepse e bacteremia, 1156
Aminoglutetimida, para hiperadrenocorticismo, 637
Aminopentamida
informações de formulações, 1363-1441
para síndrome do intestino irritável, 1183
Amiodarona
informações de formulações, 1363-1441
para complexos ventriculares prematuros, 246
para endocardiose da valva atrioventricular, 455
para fibrilação ventricular, 540
para miocardiopatia, 902
para miocardite traumática, 913
para taquicardia ventricular, 1208
Amitraz
informações de formulações, 1363-1441
para controle de carrapatos, 189
para demodicose, 142, 305-306
para queiletielose, 1111
para sarna notoédrica, 1149
para sarna sarcóptica, 1150
Amitriptilina
informações de formulações, 1363-1441
para agressividade, 44, 57, 58
para alopecia simétrica felina, 70
para comportamento de marcação territorial e errático, 249
para dermatite acral por lambedura, 310
para dermatite atópica, 312
para doença idiopática do trato urinário inferior dos felinos, 418
para dor neuropática, 1362
para evacuação domiciliar pelos gatos, 523, 524
para fobias a trovões e relâmpagos, 552
para medos, fobias e ansiedades, 556
para polifagia, 1074
para prurido, 1105
para síndrome de ansiedade da separação, 1170
para transtornos compulsivos, 1261
toxicose, 107
Amolecedores de fezes

para estenose retal, 512
para megacólon, 865
para pólipos retoanais, 1078
para prolapso retal e anal, 1090
Amoxicilina
informações de formulações, 1363-1441
para abortamento, espontâneo, 8
para abscedação, 12
para actinomicose, 27
para anomalias do anel vascular, 101
para borreliose de Lyme, 159
para colite ulcerativa histiocítica, 240
para corpo estranho esofágico, 273
para dermatofilose, 316
para encefalopatia hepática, 451, 614
para estenose retal, 512
para gastrite, 570
para gastrite, crônica, 572
para infecção pelo calicivírus felino, 738
para infecção pelo helicobacter, 753
para inflamação orofaríngea felina, 770
para leptospirose, 816
para mastite, 860
para mortalidade neonatal, 929
para nocardiose, 950
para piodermite, 1041
para piotórax, 1045
para pneumonia, bacteriana, 1054
para secreção nasal, 1153
para tularemia, 1281
para vômito, 1334
Amoxicilina com ácido clavulânico
informações de formulações, 1363-1441
para abscedação, 12
para acne, 25
para artrite, séptica, 116
para blefarite, 142
para bordetelose, 157
para bronquite, crônica, 165
para corpo estranho esofágico, 273
para disquesia e hematoquesia, 386
para distúrbios dos sacos anais, 401
para doença periodontal, 420
para encefalite, 446
para estomatite, 515
para foliculite bacteriana, 336
para hepatite, supurativa, 610
para infecções anaeróbias, 757
para infecções estafilocócicas, 759
para infecções secundárias à influenza canina, 771
para meningite, 875
para metrite, 882
para mortalidade neonatal, 929
para osteomielite, 974
para otite média/interna, 727, 983
para piodermite, 1041
para piotórax, 1045
para pneumonia, bacteriana, 1054
para prostatite, 1095
para secreção nasal, 1153
para síndrome colangite/colangio-hepatite, 1164
para traqueobronquite infecciosa canina, 1263
para úlcera indolente, 243
para ulceração bucal, 1304
para vestibulopatia, 1328, 1329
Ampicilina
informações de formulações, 1363-1441
para afogamento (afogamento por um triz), 42
para bronquiectasia, 163

para dermatofilose, 316
para doenças orbitais, 426
para endocardite, 458
para gastrenterite, hemorrágica, 567
para hepatotoxicidade, 622
para infecção do trato urinário inferior, 736
para infecções estreptocócicas, 760
para inflamação orofaríngea felina, 770
para leptospirose, 816
para meningite, 875
para mortalidade neonatal, 929
para neutropenia, 947
para nocardiose, 950
para obstrução gastrintestinal, 959
para pancreatite, 987
para peritonite, 1028
para piodermite, 1041
para piometra, 1043
para piotórax, 1045
para pneumonia, bacteriana, 1054
Ampicilina com sulbactam
informações de formulações, 1363-1441
para neutropenia, 947
para piotórax, 1045
para pneumonia, bacteriana, 1054
para pneumonia, por aspiração, 1061
Amprólio, para coccidiose, 230
Anafilaxia, 76-77
Analgésicos
para abdome agudo, 3
para abscesso da raiz dentária, 13
para cáries dentárias, 187
para claudicação, 224
para discopatia intervertebral, toracolombar, 371
para discospondilite, 373
para displasia coxofemoral, 377
para distúrbios da articulação temporomandibular, 393
para fístula perianal, 547
para hemangiopericitoma, 586
para hemotórax, 601
para hifema, 632
para infecção pelo parvovírus canino, 1017
para lacerações da córnea e esclera, 809
para osteocondrodisplasia, 968
para osteocondrose, 970
para osteodistrofia hipertrófica, 972
para osteopatia craniomandibular, 975
para osteopatia hipertrófica, 976
para pancreatite, 987
para piotórax, 1045
para problemas do ombro, 1089
para traumatismo da coluna vertebral, 1265
para ulceração bucal, 1304
Anciclofosfamida, para hemangiopericitoma, 586
Ancilostomíase, 78
Ancilóstomos, 78
Andar, compulsivo, 1260
Anemia
Anemia acantocítica, 87
Anemia aplásica, 79
Anemia arregenerativa, 80-81
Anemia de doença inflamatória, 80
Anemia de doença renal crônica, 82-83
Anemia hemolítica imunomediada (AHIM), 84-86
Anemia imunomediada, 84-86
Anemia megaloblástica, 89
Anemia metabólica, 87
Anemia por corpúsculo de Heinz, 88

Anemia por defeitos de maturação nuclear, 89
Anemia por deficiência de ferro, 90
Anemia regenerativa, 91-92
Anestesia, em distocia, 389
Anestésicos, tópicos para prurido, 1105
Anfotericina B
informações de formulações, 1363-1441
para aspergilose, 123, 125
para blastomicose, 140
para coccidioidomicose, 229
para criptococose, 278
para histoplasmose, 721
para infecção do trato urinário inferior, 737
para leishmaniose, 814
para mediastinite, 863
para pitiose, 1215
para pneumonia, fúngica, 1058
para prototecose, 1102
Angiostrongylus vasorum, 1059-1060
Anglepristona, para hiperplasia das glândulas
mamárias, 666
Angústia respiratória, 384-385
Anidulafungina, para aspergilose, 123
Anisocoria, 93-94
Anlodipino
informações de formulações, 1363-1441
para acidente vascular cerebral isquêmico, 18
para descolamento da retina, 339
para endocardite, 458
para epistaxe, 483
para hipertensão, pulmonar, 676
para hipertensão, sistêmica, 679
para insuficiência cardíaca congestiva,
esquerda, 777
para insuficiência renal, crônica, 786
para laceração da parede atrial, 807
para miocardiopatia, 902
Anoftalmia, 102
Anomalia de Ebstein, 95
Anomalia de Pelger-Huët, 96
Anomalia do olho do Collie, 97
Anomalia vascular portossistêmica, congênita, 98-
100
Anomalias do anel vascular, 101
Anomalias oculares, congênitas, 102-103
Anorexia, 104-105
Anormalidades dos espermatozoides, 106
Ânsia de vômito, 491-492
Ansiolíticos
para síndrome de disfunção cognitiva, 1175
para síndrome do intestino irritável, 1183
Antagonista dopaminérgico
para dermatite acral por lambedura, 310
para problemas comportamentais maternos,
1082
para vômito, 1332
Antagonistas do GnRH, para interrupção da
gestação, 10
Antagonistas histaminérgicos H2
para abdome agudo, 3
para apudoma, 110
para corpo estranho esofágico, 273
para desvio portossistêmico, 341
para distúrbios da motilidade gástrica, 396
para esofagite, 405
para fisalopterose, 544
para gastrite, 570
para gastropatia pilórica hipertrófica, 573
para hematêmese, 593
para hemorragia gastrintestinal, 850
para hepatite, granulomatosa, 606

para hepatite, infecciosa canina, 607
para hérnia hiatal, 624
para infecção pelo parvovírus canino, 1017
para insuficiência hepática, aguda, 779
para insuficiência renal, crônica, 786
para intermação e hipertermia, 791
para mastocitomas, 862
para megaesôfago, 867
para melena, 870
para mielomalacia, medula espinal, 893
para mucocele da vesícula biliar, 931
para obstrução de ducto biliar, 954
para obstrução gastrintestinal, 959
para peritonite biliar, 1028
para regurgitação, 1130
para siringomielia, 1198
para toxicidade do zinco, 1228
para toxicidade dos agentes anti-inflamatórios
não esteroides, 1230
para úlcera gastroduodenal, 1302
para vômito, 1332, 1334
Antiácidos
para hematêmese, 593
para insuficiência pancreática exócrina, 781
para mucocele da vesícula biliar, 931
para síndrome do vômito bilioso, 1185
para toxicidade do zinco, 1228
para úlcera gastroduodenal, 1302
Antiarrítmicos
para complexos ventriculares prematuros, 246
para doenças endomiocárdicas, 424
para endocardiose da valva atrioventricular,
455
para hérnia diafragmática, 625
para insuficiência cardíaca congestiva,
esquerda, 777
para lesão por mordedura de fio elétrico, 819
para miocardiopatia, 905
para miocardite, 912
para taquicardia sinusal, 1204
Antibióticos
para abdome agudo, 4
para abortamento, espontâneo, 6, 8
para abscesso da raiz dentária, 13
para acne, 24, 25, 333
para actinomicose, 27
para adenite sebácea, 28
para afogamento (afogamento por um triz), 42
para anomalias do anel vascular, 101
para artrite, séptica, 116
para ascite, 119
para asma/bronquite em gatos, 121
para bartonelose, 137
para blefarite, 142
para borreliose de Lyme, 159
para bronquiectasia, 163
para bronquite, crônica, 165
para campilobacteriose, 168
para carcinoma de células de transição, 173
para cáries dentárias, 187
para ceratite
não ulcerativa, 196
ulcerativa, 198
para ceratoconjuntivite seca, 199
para choque, séptico, 205
para cistite polipoide, 215
para colecistite e coledoquite, 233
para colelitíase, 235
para colesteatoma, 236
para conjuntivite, 263, 265
para corpo estranho esofágico, 273

para degenerações e infiltrações da córnea, 304
para dermatite acral por lambedura, 310
para dermatite solar nasal, 328
para dermatoses esfoliativas, 326
para diarreia, 357
para disautonomia, 363
para disbiose do intestino delgado, 365
para discinesia ciliar primária, 366
para discospondilite, 373, 1267
para dispneia, 385
para disquesia e hematoquesia, 386
para distrofia da córnea, 392
para distúrbios da motilidade gástrica, 396
para distúrbios das unhas e dos leitos ungueais,
397
para distúrbios dos cílios, 400
para distúrbios dos sacos anais, 401
para distúrbios mieloproliferativos, 402
para doença idiopática do trato urinário
inferior dos felinos, 418
para doença renal policística, 421
para doenças orbitais, 426
para ectrópio, 436
para edema periférico, 438
para efusão pericárdica, 442
para encefalite, 446
para encefalopatia hepática, 451, 614
para endocardite, 458
para enteropatia imunoproliferativa de
Basenjis, 462
para enterotoxicose clostrídica, 466
para entrópio, 467
para epididimite/orquite, 479
para epífora, 478
para epistaxe, 483
para esofagite, 489
para espirro, 492
para estenose retal, 512
para estomatite, 515- 516
para estupor e coma, 519
para febre, 527
para fibrossarcoma, 541, 543
para fístula perianal, 547
para flebite, 550
para fratura dos dentes, 561
para fraturas maxilomandibulares, 563
para gastrenterite, hemorrágica, 567
para gastrite, 570
para granuloma eosinofílico, 243
para hematêmese, 593
para hematopoiese cíclica, 207
para hematúria, 595
para hemorragia da retina, 600
para hemotórax, 601
para hepatite, supurativa, 609-610
para hepatopatia diabética, 613
para hérnia hiatal, 624
para hiperceratose nasal, 328
para hipertensão, pulmonar, 677
para inalação de fumaça, 725
para inclinação da cabeça, 727
para infecção do trato urinário inferior, 736
para infecção pelo calicivírus felino, 738
para infecção pelo helicobacter, 753
para infecção pelo parvovírus canino, 1017
para infecção pelo vírus da imunodeficiência
felina (FIV), 744
para infecções anaeróbias, 757
para infecções estafilocócicas, 759
para infecções micobacterianas, 762
para infecções pelas formas L bacterianas, 758

para infecções secundárias à cinomose, 210
para infecções secundárias à influenza canina, 771
para infertilidade, fêmea, 765
para infertilidade, macho, 767
para infestação pela fascíola hepática, 769
para inflamação orofaríngea felina, 770
para insuficiência pancreática exócrina, 781
para intussuscepção, 805
para lacerações da córnea e esclera, 809
para linfadenite, 824
para lipidose hepática, 836
para luxação ou avulsão dos dentes, 843
para mancha nos dentes causada por, 308
para mediastinite, 863
para megacólon, 865
para megaesôfago, 867
para meningite, 875
para metrite, 882
para micoplasmose, 886
para mortalidade neonatal, 929
para mucocele salivar, 933
para nefrolitíase, 937
para nocardiose, 950
para obstrução de ducto biliar, 954
para obstrução gastrintestinal, 959
para oftalmia neonatal, 960
para olho cego "silencioso", 962
para osteomielite, 974
para otite externa/média, 980
para otite média/interna, 727, 983
para pancreatite, 987
para panleucopenia felina, 990
para paraproteinemia, 1010
para perfuração da traqueia, 1024
para peritonite infecciosa felina, 1031
para pielonefrite, 1039
para piodermite de filhotes caninos, 1038
para piodermite profunda, 333
para piodermite superficial, 333
para piometra, 1043
para pneumonia, 405
para pneumonia, por aspiração, 1061
para pododermatite, 1065
para pólipos retoanais, 1078
para prolapso retal e anal, 1090
para prolapso uretral, 1091
para proptose, 1093
para prostatite, 1095, 1096
para prostatopatia em cão macho reprodutor, 1098
para reações a transfusões sanguíneas, 1124
para regurgitação, 1130
para rinite e sinusite, 1138
para sarna sarcóptica, 1150
para secreção nasal, 1153
para sepse e bacteremia, 1156
para síndrome colangite/colangio-hepatite, 1164
para síndrome da angústia respiratória aguda, 1167
para síndrome de dilatação e vólvulo gástricos, 1173
para síndromes mielodisplásicas, 1194
para tétano, 1211
para torção dos lobos pulmonares, 1214
para toxicidade do veneno de lacertílios, 1226
para toxicose por veneno de aranha, 1249
para trombocitopenia, 1273, 1275
para tuberculose, 762
para úlcera gastroduodenal, 1302

para úlcera indolente, 243
para vaginite, 276, 1324
para vasculite, cutânea, 1325
para vestibulopatia, 1327-1329
para vômito, 1334
Anticoagulantes
para edema periférico, 438
para hipercoagulabilidade, 647
para hipertensão, pulmonar, 677
Anticolinérgicos
para arritmia sinusal, 111
para bradicardia sinusal, 162
para diarreia, 352
para disúria e polaciúria, 404
para instabilidade do detrusor, 731
para parada sinusal/bloqueio sinoatrial, 1000
para síndrome do nó sinusal doente, 1185
Anticonvulsivantes
para cinomose, 210
para encefalopatia hepática, 451
Anticorpos antitireoglobulina, 712
Anticorpos de ligação à digoxina, 1218
Antidepressivos
para comportamento de marcação territorial e errático, 249
para dermatite acral por lambedura, 310
para síndrome de disfunção cognitiva, 1175
toxicose por antidepressivos tricíclicos, 107-108
toxicose por ISRS, 109
Antidepressivos tricíclicos (ATC)
para agressividade, 47, 49, 51, 52, 55, 57-59
para comportamento de marcação territorial e errático, 249
para comportamentos destrutivos, 252
para coprofagia e pica, 270
para dermatite atópica, 312
para doença idiopática do trato urinário inferior dos felinos, 418
para evacuação domiciliar
pelos cães, 521
pelos gatos, 523
para fobias a trovões e relâmpagos, 552
para incompetência uretral, 731
para medos, fobias e ansiedades, 554, 556
para síndrome de ansiedade da separação, 1170
para síndrome de hiperestesia felina, 1177
para transtornos compulsivos, 1259, 1261
para vocalização excessiva, 1330
toxicose, 107-108
Antidiarreicos, para síndrome do intestino irritável, 1183
Antieméticos
para abdome agudo, 3-4
para anorexia, 105
para azotemia e uremia, 133
para gastrenterite, hemorrágica, 567
para gastrite, crônica, 572
para hematêmese, 593
para hepatite, granulomatosa, 606
para hepatite, infecciosa canina, 607
para infecção pelo parvovírus canino, 1017
para infestação pela fascíola hepática, 769
para insuficiência renal, aguda, 783
para insuficiência renal, crônica, 786
para lipidose hepática, 836
para mucocele da vesícula biliar, 931
para obstrução gastrintestinal, 959
para pancreatite, 987
para peritonite biliar, 1028
para síndrome do intestino irritável, 1183

para terapia com cisplatina, 31
para úlcera gastroduodenal, 1302
para vestibulopatia, 1327, 1329
para vômito, 1332
Antiespasmódicos
para instabilidade do detrusor, 731
para síndrome do intestino irritável, 1183
Antifibróticos
para cirrose e fibrose do fígado, 212
para hepatite, crônica ativa, 603-604
Anti-helmínticos
para ancilóstomos, 78
para asma/bronquite em gatos, 121
para capilaríase, 170
para diarreia, 352
para encefalite secundária à migração parasitária, 448
para estrongiloidíase, 517
para fisalopterose, 544
para infecção pelo parvovírus canino, 1017
para nematódeos, 940
para parasitas respiratórios, 1012
Anti-histamínicos
para alopecia simétrica felina, 70
para dermatite acral por lambedura, 310
para dermatite atópica, 312
para dermatite eosinofílica, 487
para espirro, 492
para hipersensibilidade à picada de pulga, 672
para prurido, 1105
para rinite e sinusite, 1138
para tosse, 1217
Antimoniato de meglumina, para leishmaniose, 814, 1060
Antioxidantes
para cataratas, 191
para cirrose e fibrose do fígado, 212
para colecistite e coledoquite, 233
para colelitíase, 235
para hepatite, crônica ativa, 603
para hepatite, infecciosa canina, 607
para hepatite, supurativa, 610
para hepatopatia diabética, 613
para hepatopatia por armazenamento de cobre, 617
para hepatotoxicidade, 622
para infestação pela fascíola hepática, 769
para insuficiência hepática, aguda, 779
para intoxicação pelo chumbo, 794
para mucocele da vesícula biliar, 931
para obstrução de ducto biliar, 954
para peritonite biliar, 1028
para síndrome colangite/colangio-hepatite, 1164
Antipiréticos, para febre, 527
Antiprotozoários, para diarreia, 352
Antipruriginosos, para reações alimentares, 1124
Antissépticos, para otite externa/média, 980
Antitoxina tipo C, para botulismo, 131
Antitussígenos
para bronquite crônica, 165
para tosse, 1217
Antivenina
para toxicidade do veneno de cobra, corais, 1251
para toxicidade do veneno de cobra, víboras, 1252
para toxicose por veneno de aranha, 1250
Anúria, 965-966
Anxitano, para medos, fobias e ansiedades, 554

Apomorfina
- informações de formulações, 1363-1441
- para envenenamento pelo cogumelo, 474
- para toxicidade da vitamina D, 1220
- para toxicidade dos agentes anti-inflamatórios não esteroides, 1230
- para toxicose por anfetamina, 1236
- para toxicose por chocolate, 1241

APR (atrofia progressiva da retina), 300-302
Apudoma, 110, 534
Arco aórtico direito, 101
Arritmia sinusal, 111-112
Arritmias ventriculares e morte súbita em Pastor alemão, 113
Arterite, responsiva a esteroides, 873
Artrite (osteoartrite), 114-115
Artrite séptica, 116-117
Artropatia degenerativa, 114
- em displasia do cotovelo, 380-381

Ascaríase, 940
Ascite, 118-119
Ascorbato de zinco
- para doença periodontal, 420
- para halitose, 585
- para hiperplasia gengival, 668

Asma, 120-121
Aspergillus flavus, 888
Aspergilose disseminada, 122-123
Aspergilose nasal, 124-125
Aspiração por agulha fina, para hepatomegalia, 612
Assistolia, 1001-1002
Astrocitoma, 126
Ataxia, 127-128
- cerebelar, 127
- sensorial, 127
- vestibular, 127

ATC. *Ver* Antidepressivos tricíclicos
Atenolol
- informações de formulações, 1363-1441
- para anomalia de Ebstein, 95
- para complexos atriais prematuros, 245
- para complexos ventriculares prematuros, 246
- para displasia das valvas atrioventriculares, 379
- para epistaxe, 483
- para estenose aórtica, 501
- para estenose da valva atrioventricular direita (tricúspide), 95
- para estenose das valvas atrioventriculares, 504
- para fibrilação atrial, 537
- para hipertensão, sistêmica, 680
- para hipertireoidismo, 682
- para infarto do miocárdio, 734
- para insuficiência cardíaca congestiva, esquerda, 777
- para miocardiopatia, 902, 905, 908, 910
- para síndrome de Wolff-Parkinson-White, 1181-1182
- para síndrome do nó sinusal doente, 1185
- para taquicardia sinusal, 1204
- para taquicardia supraventricular, 1206
- para taquicardia ventricular, 1208

Aterosclerose, 129
Atipamezol
- informações de formulações, 1363-1441
- para toxicose por amitraz, 1233-1234

Ativador do plasminogênio tecidual
- para hipercoagulabilidade, 647
- para hipertensão, pulmonar, 677
- para tromboembolia aórtica, 1277
- para tromboembolia pulmonar, 1280

Atonia do detrusor, 1135-1136
Atovaquona
- para babesiose, 135, 483
- para pneumocistose, 1052

Atracúrio, 1363-1441
Atrofia da íris, 130
Atrofia muscular espinal, 944
Atrofia progressiva da retina (APR), 300-302
Atropina
- informações de formulações, 1363-1441
- para anafilaxia, 77
- para arritmia sinusal, 111
- para bloqueio atrioventricular, segundo grau, Mobitz Tipo II, 150
- para bloqueio atrioventricular, terceiro grau (completo), 144
- para bradicardia sinusal, 162
- para cataratas, 191
- para choque, cardiogênico, 201
- para envenenamento pelo cogumelo, 911
- para parada sinusal/bloqueio sinoatrial, 1000
- para parada ventricular, 1001
- para proptose, 1093
- para ptialismo, 1110
- para ritmo idioventricular, 1141
- para toxicidade da digoxina, 1218
- para toxicidade da ivermectina, 1231
- para toxicidade dos organofosforados e carbamatos, 1246
- para toxicose por chocolate, 1241
- para toxicose por veneno de sapo, 1253
- para uveíte anterior, 1320-1322

Atropina (1%)
- para ceratite
  - não ulcerativa, 196
  - ulcerativa, 198
- para coriorretinite, 272
- para degenerações e infiltrações da córnea, 304
- para depósito lipídico, 704
- para distrofia da córnea, 392
- para doenças orbitais, 426
- para hifema, 632
- para hipópio, 704
- para lacerações da córnea e esclera, 809
- para sequestro de córnea, 1157

Auranofina, para pênfigo, 1020
Aurotiomalato, para poliartrite erosiva, 1067
Avanço da tuberosidade tibial, 416
AVC. *Ver* Acidentes vasculares cerebrais
Avulsão do plexo braquial, 131
Axonopatias, 944
Azaperona
- para comportamento de marcação territorial e errático, 249
- para fobias a trovões e relâmpagos, 552
- para medos, fobias e ansiedades, 556

Azapironas, para agressividade, 57, 58
Azatioprina
- informações de formulações, 1363-1441
- para anemia, imunomediada, 85
- para ceratite, não ulcerativa, 196
- para cirrose e fibrose do fígado, 212
- para colite e proctite, 237
- para colite ulcerativa histiocítica, 241
- para complexo pênfigo/penfigoide bolhoso, 336
- para dermatoses nodulares/granulomatosas estéreis, 332, 334
- para descolamento da retina, 339
- para distúrbios das unhas e dos leitos ungueais, 397

para distúrbios despigmentantes, 322
para doenças orbitais, 426
para efusão pericárdica, 442
para episclerite, 481
para epistaxe, 483
para fístula perianal, 547
para gastrenterite
- eosinofílica, 565
- linfocítica-plasmocitária, 569
para gastrite, crônica, 572
para granuloma estéril idiopático, 328
para granuloma/piogranuloma estéreis, 332
para hemorragia da retina, 600
para hepatite
- crônica ativa, 603
- granulomatosa, 606
para inclinação da cabeça, 727
para lúpus eritematoso cutâneo (discoide), 839
para lúpus eritematoso sistêmico, 328
para meningite-arterite responsivas a esteroides, 873
para meningoencefalomielite, 878
para meningoencefalomielite granulomatosa, 727
para miastenia grave, 884
para miopatia
- inflamatória focal, 918
- inflamatória geral, 916
para neuropatias periféricas, 945
para olho cego "silencioso", 962
para paniculite, 988
para pênfigo, 1020
para pericardite, 1026
para poliartrite
- erosiva, 1067
- não erosiva, 1069
para prurido, 1105
para síndrome uveodermatológica, 1193
para trombocitopenia, imunomediada primária, 1275
para vasculite, cutânea, 1325
para vômito, 1334

Azitromicina
- informações de formulações, 1363-1441
- para babesiose, 135, 483
- para bartonelose, 137
- para borreliose de Lyme, 159
- para conjuntivite, 265
- para endocardite, 458
- para infecção pelo helicobacter, 753
- para pneumonia, bacteriana, 1054
- para secreção nasal, 1153

Azodyl, para azotemia e uremia, 133
Azotemia, 132-133

B

1,3-butanediol, para intoxicação pelo etilenoglicol, 800
Babesiose, 134-135
Bacitracina
- para blefarite, 142
- para ceratite, ulcerativa, 198
- para doenças orbitais, 426
- para ectrópio, 436
- para lacerações da córnea e esclera, 809
- para oftalmia neonatal, 960
- para sequestro de córnea, 1157

Baclofeno, para retenção urinária, 1136
Bacteremia, 1155-1156
Bacterina, para piodermite, 1041
Bailisascaríase, 136

BAL. *Ver* Dimercaprol
Balinês
  doença do armazenamento lisossomal, 422,
    658
  esfingomielinose, 894
Barbitúricos, para toxinas tremorgênicas, 890
Bartonelose, 137
Basenji
  anemia, regenerativa, 91
  deficiência da piruvato quinase, 91, 292
  enteropatia com perda de proteínas, 460
  enteropatia imunoproliferativa, 462
  enteropatia inflamatória, 463
  gastrenterite linfocítica-plasmocitária, 568
  gastrite, crônica, 571
  glicosúria, 578
  glicosúria renal primária, 427
  linfangiectasia, 827
  membrana pupilar persistente (MPP), 102
  síndrome de Fanconi, 427, 1176
  vômito, crônico, 1333
Basset hound
  cistinúria, 427
  defeito do septo ventricular, 289
  deformidades do crescimento antebraquial,
    297
  dermatite por Malassezia, 315
  dermatoses neoplásicas, 329
  distúrbios causados por imunodeficiência, 394
  distúrbios da articulação temporomandibular,
    393
  distúrbios do desenvolvimento sexual, 398
  doença de von Willebrand, 412
  espondilomielopatia cervical, 495
  glaucoma, 576
  hipotricose, 63
  imunodeficiência combinada grave ligada ao
    cromossomo X, 394
  linfoma, 830
  osteocondrodisplasia, 968
  pododermatite, 1064
  tricoepitelioma, 1292
  trombocitopatias, 1271
  trombopatia, 482
  tuberculose, 761
Beagle
  adenocarcinoma, tireoide, 30
  agenesia renal, 427
  amiloidose, 74
  amiloidose renal, 427
  anemia, arregenerativa, 80
  anemia, regenerativa, 91
  bloqueio do ramo direito do feixe de His, 151
  brucelose, 166
  carcinoma de células escamosas, pele, 175
  coriorretinite, 271
  criptorquidismo, 279
  deficiência da IgA, 394
  deficiência da piruvato quinase, 91, 292
  degeneração cerebelar, 299
  disbiose do intestino delgado, 364
  discopatia intervertebral, cervical, 368
  distrofia da córnea, 392
  distúrbios causados por imunodeficiência, 394
  distúrbios do desenvolvimento sexual, 398
  doença do armazenamento lisossomal, 422
  doença renal policística, 421, 427
  epilepsia, 479
  estenose pulmonar, 510
  fisiologia de Eisenmenger, 206
  glomerulonefrite, 580

glomerulopatia, 427
hepatopatia vacuolar, 615
hidrocefalia, 628
hiperadrenocorticismo, 633
hipotricose, 63
lúpus eritematoso, sistêmico (LES), 840
massas bucais, 857
mastocitoma, 329, 861
meningite-arterite responsivas a esteroides,
  433, 873
neutropenia, 946
orquite linfocítica, 766
osteocondrodisplasia, 968
paresia/paralisia do nervo facial, 1013
pneumocistose, 1052
poliartrite, não erosiva, 1068
prolapso da glândula da terceira pálpebra,
  1089
proteinúria, 1100
tumor das glândulas sebáceas, 329
vômito, crônico, 1333
Bearded collie
  displasia do cotovelo, 380
  distrofia da córnea, 392
  hipoadrenocorticismo, 683
  pênfigo foliáceo, 335, 1019
Bedlington terrier
  descolamento da retina, 102, 338
  hemorragia da retina, 599
  hepatite, crônica ativa, 602
  hepatopatia por armazenamento de cobre, 597,
    616
  icterícia, 722
  vômito, crônico, 1333
Benazepril
  informações de formulações, 1363-1441
  para acidente vascular cerebral isquêmico, 18
  para defeito do septo atrial, 288
  para descolamento da retina, 339
  para endocardiose da valva atrioventricular,
    455
  para epistaxe, 483
  para hipertensão, 129
    pulmonar, 676
    sistêmica, 679
  para hipoalbuminemia, 686
  para insuficiência cardíaca congestiva
    direita, 775
    esquerda, 777
  para insuficiência renal, crônica, 786
  para miocardiopatia, 902, 905, 908, 910
Benzimidazol
  para doença de Chagas, 408
  para encefalitozoonose, 449
Benzodiazepínicos
  para agressividade, 47, 52, 55, 57, 58
  para comportamento de marcação territorial e
    errático, 249
  para comportamentos destrutivos, 252
  para estimulação do apetite, 1022
  para evacuação domiciliar pelos gatos, 523
  para fobias a trovões e relâmpagos, 552
  para medos, fobias e ansiedades, 554, 556
  para síndrome de ansiedade da separação,
    1170
  para síndrome de disfunção cognitiva, 1175
  para síndrome de hiperestesia felina, 1177
  para toxicose por ISRS, 109
  para toxicose por veneno de aranha, 1250
  para vocalização excessiva, 1330
  toxicose, 1237-1238

Benzopironas
  para edema periférico, 438
  para linfedema, 829
Beta-agonistas
  para afogamento (afogamento por um triz), 42
  para bronquite, crônica, 165
  para tosse, 1217
Betabloqueadores
  para anomalia de Ebstein, 95
  para choque, cardiogênico, 201
  para complexos ventriculares prematuros, 246
  para displasia das valvas atrioventriculares, 379
  para doenças endomiocárdicas, 424
  para endocardiose das valvas atrioventriculares,
    455, 456
  para epistaxe, 483
  para estenose aórtica, 501
  para estenose das valvas atrioventriculares, 504
  para feocromocitoma, 534
  para fibrilação atrial, 537
  para glaucoma, 577
  para hifema, 632
  para hipertensão, sistêmica, 679-680
  para hipertireoidismo, 682
  para infarto do miocárdio, 734
  para insuficiência cardíaca congestiva,
    esquerda, 777
  para miocardiopatia, 902, 905, 906, 908, 910
  para miocardite traumática, 913
  para síndrome de Wolff-Parkinson-White, 95
  para taquicardia sinusal, 1204
  para taquicardia supraventricular, 1206
  para taquicardia ventricular, 1208
  para tetralogia de Fallot, 1212
  para toxicose por anfetamina, 1236
  para tratamento de adenocarcinoma da
    tireoide, 31
Betametasona
  informações de formulações, 1363-1441
  para conjuntivite, 263, 265
  para miopatia, 922
  para pênfigo, 1020
  para prurido, 1105
Betanecol
  informações de formulações, 1363-1441
  para disautonomia, 363
  para discopatia intervertebral, toracolombar,
    371
  para neuropatias periféricas, 945
  para retenção urinária, 1136
  para traumatismo da coluna vertebral, 1265
Betaxolol, para glaucoma, 577
Bexiga pélvica, 138
Bexiga urinária, hipocontratilidade da, 1135-
  1136
Bicarbonato de sódio
  informações de formulações, 1363-1441
  para acidose láctica, 20
  para acidose metabólica, 21-22
  para acidose tubular renal, 23
  para diabetes com cetoacidose, 344
  para hidronefrose, 630
  para hipercalcemia, 641
  para hipercalemia, 642
  para insuficiência renal, aguda, 783
  para insuficiência renal, crônica, 786
  para intermação e hipertermia, 791
  para intoxicação por ácido acetilsalicílico, 796
  para intoxicação por etanol, 798
  para parada ventricular, 1001
  para síndrome de Fanconi, 1176

para toxicose por antidepressivos tricíclicos, 102

para toxinas tremorgênicas, 890

para urolitíase, por xantina, 1318

toxicose por metformina, 1243

Bichon frisé

anemia, imunomediada, 84

distrofia da córnea, 392

hipotricose, 63

nefrolitíase, 936

persistência do ducto arterioso, 1032

urolitíase, por estruvita, 1309

urolitíase, por oxalato de cálcio,1314

Bimatoprosta, para glaucoma, 577

Bioquímica clínica

faixas normais de referência, 1338-1339

tabela de conversão para unidades, 1340

Bisacodyl

informações de formulações, 1363-1441

para constipação e obstipação, 267

Blastomicose, 139-140

Blefarite, 141-142

Bleomicina

informações de formulações, 1363-1441

para tumores ovarianos, 1298

Bloodhound

ceratoconjuntivite seca, 195

ectrópio, 436, 477

prolapso da glândula da terceira pálpebra, 1089

Bloqueadores dos canais de cálcio, 1341

para acidente vascular cerebral isquêmico, 18

para anomalia de Ebstein, 95

para choque, cardiogênico, 201

para displasia das valvas atrioventriculares, 379

para doença de Chagas, 408

para doenças endomiocárdicas, 424

para endocardiose das valvas atrioventriculares, 455

para epistaxe, 483

para estenose das valvas atrioventriculares, 504

para fibrilação atrial, 537

para hemorragia da retina, 600

para hipertensão

pulmonar, 676

sistêmica, 679

para insuficiência cardíaca congestiva, esquerda, 777

para miocardiopatia, 906

para síndrome de Wolff-Parkinson-White, 95

para taquicardia sinusal, 1204

para taquicardia supraventricular, 1206

Bloqueio atrioventricular

primeiro grau, 145-146

segundo grau-Mobitz Tipo I, 147-148

segundo grau-Mobitz Tipo II, 149-150

terceiro grau (completo), 143-144

Bloqueio cardíaco, completo, 1140

Bloqueio do ramo direito do feixe de His, 151-152

Bloqueio do ramo esquerdo do feixe de His, 153-154

Bloqueio fascicular anterior esquerdo, 155-156

Bloqueio sinoatrial, 999-1000

Bluetick hound, doença do armazenamento lisossomal em, 422

Boiadeiro australiano

cistinúria, 237

dermatomiosite, 915

mastocitomas, 861

ptialismo, 1109

surdez, 1202

Boldenona, para estimulação do apetite, 1022

Border collie

abiotrofia cerebelar, 658

anemia, arregenerativa, 80

anomalia do olho do Collie, 97

coriorretinite, 271

degeneração cerebelar, 299

doença do armazenamento lisossomal, 658

epilepsia, 479

estenose lombossacra, 507

neuropatias periféricas, 944

neutropenia, 946

surdez, 1202

transtornos compulsivos, 1258

Border terrier

distocia, 388

glicosúria, 578

síndrome de Fanconi, 427

Bordetelose, 157

Borrelia burgdorferi, 158-159

Borreliose de Lyme, 158-159

Borzói

abortamento, espontâneo, 5

coriorretinite, 271

espondilomielopatia cervical, 495

metemoglobinemia, 880

orquite linfocítica, 766

Boston terrier

alopecia do pavilhão auricular, 64

anomalias do anel vascular, 101

atopia, 311

ceratite, ulcerativa, 197

descolamento da retina, 338

distocia, 388

distrofia da córnea, 392

distrofia endotelial da córnea, 197

distúrbios do desenvolvimento sexual, 398

endocardiose da valva atrioventricular, 454

estenose pilórica, 958

gastropatia pilórica hipertrófica, 573

glaucoma, 576

hepatopatia vacuolar, 619

hérnia perineal, 627

hidrocefalia, 628

hiperadrenocorticismo, 633

hipoandrogenismo, 687

hipoplasia cerebelar, 706

histiocitoma, 329, 716

luxação patelar, 844

más-formações vertebrais, 853

mastocitoma, 329, 861

miocardiopatia, 906

osteocondrodisplasia, 968

osteopatia craniomandibular, 975

prolapso uretral, 1092

quimiodectoma, 1114

síndrome braquicefálica das vias aéreas, 1160

tumores melanocíticos, 1295

Botulismo, 160

Bouvier des Flandres

estenose aórtica, 501

estomatite periodontal ulcerativa crônica (EPUC), 1303

glaucoma, 576

laringopatias, 810

paralisia congênita da laringe, 206

paralisia da laringe, 514

Boxer

acne, 24

adenocarcinoma

pulmão, 37

tireoide, 30

alopecia do flanco, 64

arritmia sinusal, 111

axonopatia, 944

carcinoma de células escamosas, pele, 175

cisto dentígero, 216

colibacilose, 237

colite ulcerativa histiocítica, 239, 241

complexos ventriculares prematuros, 246

condrossarcoma, 258, 260, 261

criptococose, 277

criptorquidismo, 279

defeito do septo atrial, 288

deficiência de carnitina, 293

dermatoses neoplásicas, 329

diarreia, responsiva a antibióticos, 357

displasia renal, 427

distrofia neuroaxonal, 391

dor no pescoço e dorso, 433

enteropatia inflamatória, 463

epilepsia, 479

espondilose deformante, 497

estenose aórtica, 501

estenose lombossacra, 507

estenose pilórica, 958

estenose pulmonar, 510

gastropatia pilórica hipertrófica, 573

granuloma leproide canino, 761

hemangiossarcoma

baço e fígado, 588

osso, 591

pele, 587

hepatopatia vacuolar, 619

hiperplasia e prolapso vaginais, 667

hiperplasia gengival, 668, 857

histiocitoma, 329, 716

infertilidade, fêmea, 764

insulinoma, 788

linfoma, 830

mastocitoma, 329, 861

meningite-arterite responsivas a esteroides, 433, 873

mielopatia degenerativa, 896

miocardiopatia, 900-902

miocardiopatia arritmogênica do ventrículo direito, 774

neuropatias periféricas, 944

osteodistrofia hipertrófica, 971

osteopatia craniomandibular, 975

paresia/paralisia do nervo facial, 1013

pododermatite, 1064

polimiosite, 915

prototecose, 1102

quimiodectoma, 1114

síncope, 1159

taquicardia ventricular, 1207

tumores cerebrais, 1284

tumores das glândulas mamárias, 1288

tumores melanocíticos, 1295

Boykin spaniel, anomalia do olho do Collie, 97

Bradicardia sinusal, 161-162

Briard

distrofia da retina em, 102, 103

hipercolesterolemia, 654

Brinzolamida

para glaucoma, 580

para hifema, 632

Brometo, para tumores cerebrais, 1284

Brometo de clidínio, para síndrome do intestino irritável, 1183

1453

Brometo de demecário, para glaucoma, 577
Brometo de ipratrópio, para asma/bronquite em gatos, 121
Brometo de potássio
informações de formulações, 1363-1441
para cinomose, 210
para crises convulsivas, 126, 282
para encefalopatia hepática, 451
para epilepsia, 479-480
Bromocriptina
para corrimento vaginal, 276
para hiperplasia das glândulas mamárias, 666
para indução do estro (cio), 765
para infertilidade, fêmea, 765
para interrupção da gestação, 10
para problemas comportamentais maternos, 1082
para pseudociese, 1107
Broncodilatadores
para asma/bronquite em gatos, 121
para bronquiectasia, 163
para bronquite, crônica, 165
para dispneia, 385
para hipertensão, pulmonar, 677
para hipoxemia, 715
para inalação de fumaça, 725
para influenza canina, 771
para parada sinusal/bloqueio sinoatrial, 1000
para pneumonia
bacteriana, 1054
eosinofílica, 1056
intersticial, 1060
por aspiração, 1061
para tosse, 1217
para traqueobronquite infecciosa canina, 1263
Bronquiectasia, 163
Bronquite
crônica, 164-165
em gatos, 120-121
Brucella canis, 5-6, 166-167, 764, 766
Brucelose, 166-167
Brussels griffons, siringomielia em, 1198
Budesonida
informações de formulações, 1363-1441
para bronquite, crônica, 165
para gastrenterite
eosinofílica, 565
linfocítica-plasmocitária, 569
para tosse, 1217
Buldogue(s)
arritmia sinusal, 111
cisto dentígero, 216
defeito do septo ventricular, 289
distocia, 388
doença do armazenamento lisossomal, 422
edema periférico, 437
espinha bífida, 853
gastropatia pilórica hipertrófica, 573
hidrocefalia, 628
hiperplasia e prolapso vaginais, 667
linfedema, 829
linfoma, 830
mastocitomas, 861
orifícios nasolacrimais imperfurados, 477
osteocondrodisplasia, 968
prolapso da glândula da terceira pálpebra, 1089
prolapso uretral, 1091
síndrome braquicefálica das vias aéreas, 810
síndrome tipo Sjögren, 1192
tetralogia de Fallot, 1212

tremores, 1266
triquíase de prega facial, 400
urolitíase, por cistina, 1308
urolitíase, por urato, 1316
Buldogue francês
cistinúria, 427
colite ulcerativa histiocítica, 241
enteropatia inflamatória, 463
hipotricose, 63
más-formações vertebrais, 853
osteocondrodisplasia, 968
síndrome braquicefálica das vias aéreas, 810, 1160
Buldogue inglês
acne, 24
alopecia do flanco, 64
atopia, 311
blefarite, 141
ceratoconjuntivite seca, 195
cistinúria, 427
colite ulcerativa histiocítica, 241
cristalúria, 285
defeito do septo ventricular, 289
degeneração cerebelar, 299
disrafismo espinal, 387
distiquíase, 141
entrópio, 467
estenose aórtica, 501
estenose pulmonar, 510
fisiologia de Eisenmenger, 206
hérnia hiatal, 624
hiperplasia e prolapso vaginais, 667
hiperuricúria, 427
más-formações vertebrais, 853
mastocitoma, 329
nefrolitíase, 936
osteopatia craniomandibular, 975
para miocardiopatia, 900
pododermatite, 1064
prolapso uretral, 1091
quimiodectoma, 1114
síndrome braquicefálica das vias aéreas, 810, 1160
síndrome tipo Sjögren, 1192
tetralogia de Fallot, 1212
traqueia hipoplásica, 206
tremores, 1266
urolitíase, por cistina, 1308
urolitíase, por urato, 1316
Bull terrier
carcinoma de células escamosas, pele, 175
cistinúria, 427
criptorquidismo, 279
displasia da valva atrioventricular esquerda (mitral), 378
doença renal policística, 427, 1131
estenose aórtica, 501
estenose da valva atrioventricular esquerda (mitral), 503
glomerulonefrite, 580
glomerulopatia, 427
hipoplasia cerebelar, 706
histiocitoma, 716
insuficiência renal, crônica, 785
laringopatias, 810
mastocitoma, 329
pneumonia, intersticial, 1059
pododermatite, 1064
proteinúria, 1100
surdez, 1202
transtornos compulsivos, 1258

túnica vascular do cristalino hiperplásica persistente (TVCHP), 102
vítreo primário hiperplásico persistente (VPHP), 102
Bullmastiff
abiotrofia cerebelar, 658
degeneração cerebelar, 299
dermatoses neoplásicas, 329
glomerulonefrite, 580
osteopatia craniomandibular, 975
proteinúria, 1100
Bumetanida, para endocardiose da valva atrioventricular, 456
Bunamidina, 1363-1441
Bupivacaína, 1363-1441
Buprenorfina
dosagens e indicações, 1361
informações de formulações, 1363-1441
para asma/bronquite em gatos, 120
para doença idiopática do trato urinário inferior dos felinos, 418
para dor, 431
para fraturas maxilomandibulares, 563
para pancreatite, 987
para tromboembolia aórtica, 1277
Buspirona
informações de formulações, 1363-1441
para agressividade, 47, 57, 58
para comportamento de marcação territorial e errático, 249
para degeneração cerebelar, 299
para evacuação domiciliar pelos gatos, 523, 524
para fobias a trovões e relâmpagos, 552
para medos, fobias e ansiedades, 556
para síndrome de disfunção cognitiva, 1175
para transtornos compulsivos, 1261
Bussulfano
informações de formulações, 1363-1441
para policitemia, 1071
Butorfanol
como antiemético em terapia com cisplatina, 31
dosagens e indicações, 1361
informações de formulações, 1363-1441
para asma/bronquite em gatos, 120
para bronquite, crônica, 165
para colapso traqueal, 232
para doença idiopática do trato urinário inferior dos felinos, 418
para dor, 432
para fraturas maxilomandibulares, 563
para influenza canina, 771
para lacerações da córnea e esclera, 809
para paralisia, 1005
para tosse, 1217
para traqueobronquite infecciosa canina, 1263

C

Cabergolina
para corrimento vaginal, 276
para indução do estro (cio), 765
para infertilidade, fêmea, 765
para interrupção da gestação, 9-10
para mastite, 860
para piometra, 1043
para problemas comportamentais maternos, 1082
para pseudociese, 1106-1107
Caça, 254-255

Cães e gatos de abrigo, realojamento bem-
 -sucedido de, 1126-1127
Cairn terrier
   abiotrofia cerebelar, 658
   anemia, regenerativa, 91
   anomalia vascular portossistêmica, 98
   atopia, 311
   deficiência da piruvato quinase, 91, 292
   diabetes melito, 347
   displasia microvascular hepatoportal, 382
   doença de Legg-Calvé-Perthes, 409
   doença do armazenamento lisossomal, 422,
      944
   doença renal policística, 421, 427, 1131
   glaucoma, 576
   hemofilia B, 482
   hidrocefalia, 628
   insuficiência renal, crônica, 785
   neuronopatia progressiva, 944
   neuropatias periféricas, 944
   osteopatia craniomandibular, 975
   pneumonia, intersticial, 1059
Calcinose circunscrita, 331-332
Calcinose cutânea, 331-332
Calcitonina, para hipercalcemia, 641, 1220
Calcitriol
   informações de formulações, 1363-1441
   para hiperparatireoidismo, 664
   para insuficiência renal, crônica, 786
Campilobacteriose, 168
Canamicina
   informações de formulações, 1363-1441
   para infecções secundárias à influenza canina,
      771
   para micoplasmose, 886
   para peste, 1035
   para traqueobronquite infecciosa canina, 1263
Câncer de próstata, 1096
Candidíase, 169
Cão d'água português
   doença do armazenamento lisossomal, 422,
      658
   hipoadrenocorticismo, 683
   miocardiopatia, 901
Cão de corrida de Berna, degeneração cerebelar
      em, 299, 658
Cão de trenó do Alasca, infecção pelo parvovírus
      canino em, 1016
Cão esquimó americano
   anemia, regenerativa, 91
   carcinoma de células de transição, 172
   deficiência da piruvato quinase, 91, 292
   mielopatia degenerativa, 896
Cão esquimó toy, 880
Cão Grande Pirineu
   axonopatia, 944
   neuropatias periféricas, 944
Capilaríase, 170
Capnograma, 644
Capsaicina, para dermatite acral por lambedura,
      310
Captopril, 1363-1441
Caquexia, 1021-1023
Carafate, para síndrome do vômito bilioso, 1185
Carbamatos, para controle de pulga, 672
Carbamazina, para epilepsia, 480
Carbimazol
   informações de formulações, 1363-1441
   para hipertireoidismo, 682
Carbonato de alumínio
   informações de formulações, 1363-1441

para hiperfosfatemia, 650
para insuficiência renal, crônica, 786
Carbonato de cálcio
   informações de formulações, 1363-1441
   para eclâmpsia, 435
   para hiperparatireoidismo, 664
   para hipoparatireoidismo, 703
Carbonato de lantânio, para
      hiperparatireoidismo, 664
Carbonato de lítio
   informações de formulações, 1363-1441
   para hematopoiese cíclica, 207
Carboplatina
   informações de formulações, 1363-1441
   para adenocarcinoma
      nasal, 39
      pele, 34
      próstata, 29
      pulmão, 37
      sacos anais, 38
   para carcinoide e síndrome carcinoide, 171
   para carcinoma de células escamosas
      gengiva, 178
      pele, 176
      pulmão, 182
      tonsila, 177
   para fibrossarcoma, 542
   para mesotelioma, 279
   para osteossarcoma, 978
   para sarcoma associado à vacina, 1146
   para seios nasais e paranasais, 183
   para seminoma, 1154
   para tumores das glândulas mamárias em gatos,
      1291
   para tumores melanocíticos, 1296
      bucais, 1294
   para tumores uterinos, 1299
   para tumores vaginais, 1300
Carboxipenicilinas, para pneumonia, 1054
Carbutamina, para pneumocistose, 1052
Carcinoide e síndrome carcinoide, 171
Carcinoma de células de transição, 172-173
Carcinoma de células escamosas, 329
   alopecia por, 65
   dedo, 181
   gengiva, 178
   língua, 174
   massa bucal, 857-859
   orelha, 179
   papilar, 857
   pele, 175-176
   plano nasal, 180
   pulmão, 182
   seios nasais e paranasais, 183
   tonsila, 177
Carcinoma de ducto biliar, 184
Carcinoma hepatocelular, 185
Cardigan Welsh corgi. *Ver também* Welsh corgi
   displasia de fotorreceptores, 102
   distúrbios causados por imunodeficiência, 394
   imunodeficiência combinada grave ligada ao
      cromossomo X, 394
   mielopatia degenerativa, 896
Cáries dentárias, 186-187
Carminativas, para flatulência, 549
Carmustina
   para astrocitoma, 126
   para tumores cerebrais, 1284
Carnelian bear, hipopituitarismo em, 705
Carnitina
   para deficiência de carnitina, 293

para deficiência de taurina, 294
para degeneração cerebelar, 299
para encefalopatia hepática, 451
para insuficiência cardíaca congestiva
   direita, 775
   esquerda, 777
para lipidose hepática, 836
para miocardiopatia, 900, 902
para miopatia, 922, 923, 925
para síndrome de hiperestesia felina, 1177
Carprofeno
   dosagens e indicações, 1361-1362
   informações de formulações, 1363-1441
   para artrite, 115
   para cataratas, 191
   para claudicação, 224
   para condrossarcoma, 258, 260
   para displasia coxofemoral, 377
   para displasia do cotovelo, 381
   para doença de Legg-Calvé-Perthes, 409
   para doença do ligamento cruzado cranial, 416
   para doenças orbitais, 426
   para dor no pescoço e dorso, 434
   para espondilose deformante, 497
   para fibrossarcoma, 541, 542
   para fraturas maxilomandibulares, 563
   para hifema, 632
   para hipópio, 704
   para lacerações da córnea e esclera, 809
   para luxação patelar, 845
   para luxações articulares, 847
   para olho vermelho, 963
   para osteocondrodisplasia, 968
   para osteodistrofia hipertrófica, 972
   para osteopatia craniomandibular, 975
   para panosteíte, 991
   para problemas do ombro, 1089
   para rinite e sinusite, 1138
   para traumatismo da coluna vertebral, 1265
   para ulceração bucal, 1304
   para uveíte anterior, 1320
Carrapatos e seu controle, 188-189
Carvão ativado
   informações de formulações, 1363-1441
   para envenenamento (intoxicação), 468
   para envenenamento pela estricnina, 797
   para envenenamento pelo cogumelo, 474
   para estupor e coma, 519
   para flatulência, 549
   para intoxicação pelo lírio, 795
   para intoxicação pelo metaldeído, 801
   para intoxicação por ácido acetilsalicílico,
      796
   para toxicidade da vitamina D, 1220
   para toxicidade das piretrinas e dos piretroides,
      1221
   para toxicidade do paracetamol, 1223
   para toxicidade do paraquat, 1061
   para toxicidade do rodenticida brometalina,
      1224
   para toxicidade dos agentes anti-inflamatórios
      não esteroides, 1229
   para toxicidade dos organofosforados e
      carbamatos, 1246
   para toxicose por antidepressivos tricíclicos,
      107-108
   para toxicose por chocolate, 1241
   para toxicose por ISRS, 109
   para toxicose por pseudoefedrina, 1247
Carvedilol
   informações de formulações, 1363-1441

1455

para endocardiose da valva atrioventricular, 456

para estenose aórtica, 501

para insuficiência cardíaca congestiva, esquerda, 777

para miocardiopatia, 902

Cáscara sagrada, 1363-1441

Caspofungina
para aspergilose, 123
para pneumocistose, 1052

Cataplexia, 935

Catarata, 190-191
congênita, 102
olho cego "silencioso", 961-962

Catártico
para envenenamento pela estricnina, 797
para intoxicação pelo lírio, 795
para toxicidade da vitamina D, 1220
para toxicidade dos agentes anti-inflamatórios não esteroides, 1229
para toxicidade dos organofosforados e carbamatos, 1246
para toxicose por antidepressivos tricíclicos, 107-108
para toxicose por ISRS, 109

Caulim/pectina, para diarreia, 352

Cavalier King Charles spaniel
acidente vascular cerebral isquêmico, 17
adenocarcinoma, sacos anais, 38
ceratoconjuntivite seca, 195
cristalúria, 285
distrofia da córnea, 392
dor no pescoço e dorso, 433
endocardiose da valva atrioventricular, 454
estomatite periodontal ulcerativa crônica (EPUC), 1303
granuloma eosinofílico, 242
má-absorção da cobalamina, 848
miosite dos músculos da mastigação, 917
persistência do ducto arterioso, 1032
pneumocistose, 1052
siringomielia, 1198
trombocitopenia, 1036, 1272
urolitíase, por xantina, 1318
xantinúria, 427

Caxumba, 192

CCNU. Ver Lomustina

CCS. Ver Ceratoconjuntivite seca

Cefadroxila
informações de formulações, 1363-1441
para discospondilite, 373
para infecções estafilocócicas, 759

Cefalexina
informações de formulações, 1363-1441
para acne, 24
para blefarite, 142
para distúrbios dos sacos anais, 401
para flebite, 550
para foliculite bacteriana, 336
para infecção do trato urinário inferior, 736
para infecções estafilocócicas, 759
para neutropenia, 947
para otite externa/média, 980
para otite média/interna, 727
para placa/granuloma eosinofílicos, 243
para pneumonia, bacteriana, 1054
para úlcera indolente, 243
para vestibulopatia, 1328, 1329

Cefalosporinas
para acne, 24, 25
para artrite, séptica, 116

para campilobacteriose, 168
para discospondilite, 373
para doença renal policística, 421
para endocardite, 458
para gastrenterite, hemorrágica, 567
para infecções estafilocócicas, 759
para infecções secundárias à influenza canina, 771
para intermação e hipertermia, 791
para mastite, 860
para meningite, 875
para mortalidade neonatal, 929
para neutropenia, 947
para otite média/interna, 727, 983
para peritonite, 1028
para peritonite biliar, 1028
para piodermite, 1041
para pneumonia, bacteriana, 1054
para secreção nasal, 1153
para sepse e bacteremia, 1156
para traqueobronquite infecciosa canina, 1263
para vestibulopatia, 1328, 1329

Cefazolina
informações de formulações, 1363-1441
para ceratite, ulcerativa, 198
para colibacilose, 238
para discospondilite, 373
para febre, 527
para infecções secundárias à influenza canina, 771
para lacerações da córnea e esclera, 809
para neutropenia, 947
para osteomielite, 974
para peritonite, 1028
para sepse e bacteremia, 1156
para síndrome de dilatação e vólvulo gástricos, 1173
para traqueobronquite infecciosa canina, 1263

Cefepima, 1363-1441

Cefixima, 1363-1441

Cefotaxima
informações de formulações, 1363-1441
para inclinação da cabeça, 727
para meningite, 875

Cefotetana, 1363-1441

Cefovecina, 1363-1441

Cefoxitina
informações de formulações, 1363-1441
para colibacilose, 238
para estenose retal, 512
para infecções anaeróbias, 757
para pólipos retoanais, 1072
para prolapso retal e anal, 1090
para síndrome de dilatação e vólvulo gástricos, 1173

Cefpodoxima
informações de formulações, 1363-1441
para otite média/interna, 983

Cefradina, para discospondilite, 373

Ceftazidima
informações de formulações, 1363-1441
para otite externa/média, 980

Ceftiofur
informações de formulações, 1363-1441
para infecção do trato urinário inferior, 736

Ceftriaxona, para meningite, 875

Celulite juvenil, 193

Centrine, para síndrome do intestino irritável, 1183

Ceratite
eosinofílica, em gatos, 194

não ulcerativa, 195-196
pigmentar, 195-196
ulcerativa, 197-198

Ceratoconjuntivite seca, 199
congênita, 102

Ceruminolíticos, para otite externa, 980

Cestodíase, 1210

Cetamina
informações de formulações, 1363-1441
para dor neuropática, 1362

Cetirizina
informações de formulações, 1363-1441
para dermatite eosinofílica, 487

Cetoacidose, em diabetes melito, 343-344

Cetoconazol
informações de formulações, 1363-1441
para blastomicose, 140
para coccidioidomicose, 229
para dermatite por Malassezia, 315
para dermatofitose, 318
para dermatoses esfoliativas, 326
para dermatoses nasais, 328
para distúrbios das unhas e dos leitos ungueais, 397
para doença de Chagas, 408
para esporotricose, 498
para fístula perianal, 547
para hepatopatia diabética, 613
para hiperadrenocorticismo, 635, 637
para hiperandrogenismo, 639
para infecção do trato urinário inferior, 737
para otite externa/média, 980
para pneumonia, eosinofílica, 1056
para pneumonia, fúngica, 1058
para prototecose, 1102
para rinosporidiose, 1139
para síndrome de fragilidade cutânea felina, 1168

Cetoprofeno
dosagens e indicações, 1361-1362
informações de formulações, 1363-1441

Cetorolaco, 1363-1441

Chesapeake Bay retriever
doença de von Willebrand, 412, 482, 1036
hiperplasia e prolapso vaginais, 667
mielopatia degenerativa, 896
para fraqueza/colapso induzido por exercício, 559

Chihuahua
alopecia do pavilhão auricular, 64
anemia, regenerativa, 91
atrofia da íris, 130
colapso traqueal, 231
deficiência da piruvato quinase, 91, 292
distocia, 388
distrofia da córnea, 392
distrofia neuroaxonal, 391
distúrbios dos sacos anais, 401
doença do armazenamento lisossomal, 658, 944
eclâmpsia, 435
encefalite necrosante, 447
endocardiose da valva atrioventricular, 454
estenose pulmonar, 510
hidrocefalia, 628
instabilidade atlantoaxial, 772
luxação patelar, 844
metemoglobinemia, 880
neuropatias periféricas, 944
persistência do ducto arterioso, 1032
poliartrite, não erosiva, 1068

siringomielia, 1198
tumores melanocíticos, 1295
Chlamydophila felis, 222-223
Choque cardiogênico, 200-201
Choque hipovolêmico, 202-203
Choque séptico, 204-205
Chow chow
adenocarcinoma do estômago, 1301
alopecia por diluição da cor, 64
alopecia X, 64, 67
blefarite, 141
coriorretinite, 271
degeneração cerebelar, 299
dermatomiosite, 319
displasia do cotovelo, 380
displasia renal, 103
distúrbios despigmentantes, 321
entrópio, 141, 467, 477
glaucoma, 576
hematêmese, 592
hipomielinização, 699
hipoplasia cerebelar, 658, 706
insuficiência renal, crônica, 785
lúpus eritematoso, cutâneo (discoide), 839
má-absorção da cobalamina, 848
pênfigo foliáceo, 335, 1019
tremores, 1266
tumores melanocíticos, 1295
tumores melanocíticos, bucais, 1294
Cianocobalamina
informações de formulações, 1363-1441
para má-absorção da cobalamina, 848
Cianose, 206-207
Ciclofosfamida
informações de formulações, 1363-1441
para anemia, imunomediada, 85
para carcinoma prostático, 1096
para edema periférico, 438
para hemangiopericitoma, 586
para hemangiossarcoma, 591
baço e fígado, 589
pele, 587
para histiocitose, 719
para infecção pelo vírus formador de sincício
felino (FeFV), 746
para leucemia, linfoblástica aguda, 820
para linfoma
em cães, 831
em gatos, 833
para lúpus eritematoso, sistêmico (LES), 841
para meningoencefalomielite, 878
para mieloma múltiplo, 893
para neuropatias periféricas, 945
para pênfigo, 1020
para peritonite infecciosa felina, 1031
para poliartrite
erosiva, 1067
não erosiva, 421
para poliartrite progressiva crônica, 746
para rabdomiossarcoma, 1117
para timoma, 1213
para tumores das glândulas mamárias em gatos,
1291
para tumores ovarianos, 1298
Ciclosporina
informações de formulações, 1363-1441
para acne, 25
para adenite sebácea, 28, 333
para alopecia simétrica felina, 70
para anemia
aplásica, 79

imunomediada, 85
para blefarite, 142
para ceratite
eosinofílica, 194
não ulcerativa, 196
para ceratoconjuntivite seca, 199
para colite e proctite, 240
para complexo granuloma eosinofílico, 243
para complexo pênfigo/penfigoide bolhoso,
336
para conjuntivite, 265
para degenerações e infiltrações da córnea, 304
para dermatite atópica, 312
para dermatoses esfoliativas, 326
para dermatoses nodulares estéreis, 334
para dermatoses nodulares/granulomatosas
estéreis, 332
para descolamento da retina, 339
para distrofia da córnea, 392
para distúrbios das unhas e dos leitos ungueais,
397
para distúrbios despigmentantes, 322
para distúrbios dos sacos anais, 401
para epistaxe, 483
para esteatite, 500
para fístula perianal, 547
para gastrenterite, linfocítica-plasmocitária,
569
para granuloma estéril idiopático, 328
para granuloma/piogranuloma estéreis, 332
para hepatite, crônica ativa, 603
para histiocitose, 719
para inflamação orofaríngea felina, 770
para lúpus eritematoso
cutâneo (discoide), 839
sistêmico (LES), 841
para meningoencefalomielite, 878
para paniculite, 988
para paniculite nodular estéril, 332
para pênfigo, 1020
para pneumonia, eosinofílica, 1056
para prurido, 1105
para síndrome hipereosinofílica, 1189
para síndromes mielodisplásicas, 1194
para trombocitopenia, imunomediada
primária, 1275
para vasculite, cutânea, 1325
para vômito, 1334
CID. *Ver* Coagulação intravascular disseminada
Cidofovir, para ceratite não ulcerativa, 196
Cilindrúria, 208
Cílios ectópicos, 400
Cimetidina
informações de formulações, 1363-1441
para apudoma, 110
para esofagite, 489
para estenose esofágica, 506
para hematêmese, 593
para hiperandrogenismo, 639
para infecção pelo helicobacter, 753
para infecção pelo parvovírus canino, 1017
para insuficiência hepática, aguda, 779
para insuficiência renal, crônica, 786
para megaesôfago, 867
para mielomalacia, medula espinal, 893
para refluxo gastresofágico, 1128
para regurgitação, 1130
para síndrome do vômito bilioso, 1185
para siringomielia, 1198
para toxicidade do paracetamol, 207
para toxicidade do zinco, 1228

para toxicidade dos agentes anti-inflamatórios
não esteroides, 1230
para úlcera gastroduodenal, 1302
para ulceração bucal, 1304
para vômito, 1334
Cinomose, 209-210
Cipionato de estradiol (ECP), 1363-1441
Ciproeptadina
informações de formulações, 1363-1441
para anorexia, 105
para toxicose por anfetamina, 1236
para toxicose por antidepressivos tricíclicos,
108
para toxicose por benzodiazepínicos e
soníferos, 1238
para toxicose por ISRS, 109
para toxicose por pseudoefedrina, 1247
Ciprofloxacino
informações de formulações, 1363-1441
para ceratite, ulcerativa, 198
para conjuntivite, 265, 293
para epífora, 478
para lacerações da córnea e esclera, 809
para osteomielite, 974
para otite externa/média, 980
para tularemia, 1281
Cirrose e fibrose do fígado, 211-212
Cisaprida
informações de formulações, 1363-1441
para constipação e obstipação, 267
para distúrbios da motilidade gástrica, 396
para esofagite, 489
para estenose esofágica, 506
para gastrite, 570
para gastrite, crônica, 572
para megacólon, 865
para megaesôfago, 867
para refluxo gastresofágico, 1128
para regurgitação, 1130
para retenção urinária, 1136
para síndrome do vômito bilioso, 1185
para vômito, 1332
Cisplatina
informações de formulações, 1363-1441
para adenocarcinoma
nasal, 39
pele, 34
próstata, 29
pulmão, 37
saco anal, 38
tireoide, 31
para carcinoma de células de transição,
173
para carcinoma de células escamosas
gengiva, 178
pele, 176
pulmão, 182
tonsila, 177
para condrossarcoma, 260
para fibrossarcoma, 542, 543
para mesotelioma, 879
para osteossarcoma, 978
para seios nasais e paranasais, 183
para seminoma, 1154
para tumores melanocíticos, bucais, 1294
para tumores ovarianos, 1298
para tumores uterinos, 1299
para tumores vaginais, 1300
Cistadenocarcinoma, 40, 265, 427
Cisticercose, 896
Cistinúria, 427

Cistite idiopática felina. *Ver* Doença idiopática do trato urinário inferior dos felinos
Cistite polipoide, 214-215
Cisto de íris, 102
Cisto dentígero, 216
Cisto quadrigeminal, 217
Cistos prostáticos, 218
  em cão macho reprodutor, 1097, 1098
Cistos subaracnoides, 219-220
Citarabina
  informações de formulações, 1363-1441
  para encefalite, 446
Citauxzoonose, 221
Citioato, para doença de Chagas, 408
Citosina arabinosídeo
  para distúrbios mieloproliferativos, 402
  para inclinação da cabeça, 727
  para leucemia, linfoblástica aguda, 820
  para meningoencefalomielite, 878
  para meningoencefalomielite granulomatosa, 727
  para síndromes mielodisplásicas, 1194
  para tumores cerebrais, 1284
Citrato de cálcio
  informações de formulações, 1363-1441
  para hipoparatireoidismo, 703
Citrato de magnésio, informações de formulações, 1363-1441
Citrato de potássio
  para acidose tubular renal, 23
  para nefrolitíase, 937
  para síndrome de Fanconi, 1176
  para urolitíase, por cistina, 1308
  para urolitíase, por xantina, 1318
Citrato de sódio, para acidose tubular renal, 23
CIV. *Ver* Influenza canina
Clamidiose, 222-223
Claritromicina
  informações de formulações, 1363-1441
  para distúrbios da motilidade gástrica, 396
  para infecção pelo helicobacter, 753
  para infecções micobacterianas, 762
  para lepra felina, 762
  para tuberculose, 762
  para vômito, 1334
Claudicação, 224
Clemastina
  informações de formulações, 1363-1441
  para dermatite atópica, 312
  para rinite e sinusite, 1138
Clembuterol, para aumento da massa muscular, 1022
Clindamicina
  informações de formulações, 1363-1441
  para abscedação, 12
  para acne, 25
  para babesiose, 135
  para bronquiectasia, 163
  para coccidiose, 230
  para discospondilite, 373
  para distúrbios dos sacos anais, 401
  para doença periodontal, 420
  para doença renal policística, 421
  para encefalite, 446
  para endocardite, 458
  para estomatite, 516
  para foliculite bacteriana, 336
  para hepatite, supurativa, 610
  para hepatozoonose, 623
  para inclinação da cabeça, 727
  para infecção pelo vírus da imunodeficiência

felina (FIV), 744
para infecções anaeróbias, 757
para infecções estafilocócicas, 759
para infecções estreptocócicas, 760
para inflamação orofaríngea felina, 770
para meningite, 875
para neosporose, 941
para neuropatias periféricas, 945
para osteomielite, 974
para otite externa/média, 980
para otite média/interna, 983
para parasitas respiratórios, 1012
para piodermite, 1041
para pneumonia, bacteriana, 1054
para secreção nasal, 1153
para toxoplasmose, 272, 1257
para úlcera indolente, 243
para ulceração bucal, 1304
Clofazimina, 1363-1441
Clomipramina
  informações de formulações, 1363-1441
  para agressividade, 44, 47, 51, 52, 57-59
  para alopecia simétrica felina, 70
  para comportamento de marcação territorial e errático, 249, 250
  para comportamentos destrutivos, 252
  para coprofagia e pica, 270
  para dermatite acral por lambedura, 310
  para evacuação domiciliar
    pelos cães, 521
    pelos gatos, 523, 524
  para fobias a trovões e relâmpagos, 552
  para medos, fobias e ansiedades, 554, 556
  para polifagia, 1074
  para síndrome de ansiedade da separação, 1170
  para síndrome de hiperestesia felina, 1177
  para transtornos compulsivos, 1259, 1261
  para vocalização excessiva, 1330
  toxicose, 107
Clonazepam
  informações de formulações, 1363-1441
  para fobias a trovões e relâmpagos, 552
  toxicose, 1237-1238
Clopidogrel
  informações de formulações, 1363-1441
  para acidente vascular cerebral isquêmico, 18
  para hipertensão, pulmonar, 677
  para miocardiopatia, 905, 908, 910
  para prevenção de tromboembolia pulmonar, 1280
  para tromboembolia aórtica, 1277
Cloprostenol
  para abortamento, espontâneo, 6
  para corrimento vaginal, 276
  para interrupção da gestação, 9-10
  para piometra, 1043
Clorambucila
  informações de formulações, 1363-1441
  para anemia, imunomediada, 85
  para complexo pênfigo/penfigoide bolhoso, 336
  para dermatoses nodulares estéreis, 334
  para distúrbios das unhas e dos leitos ungueais, 397
  para distúrbios despigmentantes, 322
  para enteropatia imunoproliferativa de Basenjis, 462
  para gastrenterite, eosinofílica, 565
  para gastrenterite, linfocítica-plasmocitária, 569
  para gastrite, crônica, 572

para granuloma eosinofílico, 243
para inflamação orofaríngea felina, 770
para leucemia, linfocítica crônica, 821
para linfoma em gatos, 833
para lúpus eritematoso sistêmico, 328
para pênfigo, 1020
para policitemia, 1071
para síndrome colangite/colangio-hepatite, 1164
para síndrome hipereosinofílica, 1189
para trombocitopenia, imunomediada primária, 1275
para tumores ovarianos, 1298
para vasculite, cutânea, 1325
para vômito, 1334
Cloranfenicol
  informações de formulações, 1363-1441
  para blefarite, 142
  para colite e proctite, 240
  para conjuntivite, 263, 265
  para doença renal policística, 421
  para doenças orbitais, 426
  para erliquiose, 486
  para febre maculosa das Montanhas Rochosas, 531
  para hemorragia da retina, 600
  para infecções anaeróbias, 757
  para infecções estafilocócicas, 759
  para infertilidade, macho, 767
  para intoxicação alimentar pelo salmão, 792
  para mastite, 860
  para micoplasmose, 886
  para olho cego "silencioso", 962
  para otite externa/média, 980
  para otite média/interna, 983
  para peste, 1035
  para piodermite, 1041
  para piotórax, 1045
  para pneumonia, bacteriana, 1054
  para prostatite, 1095, 1096
  para rinite e sinusite, 1138
  para salmonelose, 1145
Clorazepato
  informações de formulações, 1363-1441
  para epilepsia, 480
  para medos, fobias e ansiedades, 554
  para mioclonia, 1187
Clordiazepóxido, para síndrome do intestino irritável, 1183
Cloreto de amônio
  informações de formulações, 1363-1441
  para acidificação urinária, 797
  para toxicose por anfetamina, 1236
Cloreto de cálcio
  informações de formulações, 1363-1441
  para hipocalcemia, 689
Cloreto de magnésio, para hipomagnesemia, 698
Cloreto de potássio
  informações de formulações, 1363-1441
  para hipocalemia, 691
  para insuficiência renal, crônica, 786
  para toxicidade do xilitol, 1227
  para toxicose por beta-2 agonistas inalatórios, 1239
Cloreto de sódio, 1363-1441
Clorexidina
  para dermatite por Malassezia, 315
  para dermatofitose, 318
  para dermatoses esfoliativas, 326
  para doença periodontal, 420
  para estomatite, 516

1458

para halitose, 585
para hiperplasia gengival, 668
para luxação ou avulsão dos dentes, 843
para otite externa/média, 980
para ulceração bucal, 1304
Clorfeniramina
informações de formulações, 1363-1441
para alopecia simétrica felina, 70
para dermatite acral por lambedura, 310
para dermatite atópica, 312
para prurido, 1105
Cloridrato de trientina, 617, 1363-1441
Clorotiazida
informações de formulações, 1363-1441
para diabetes insípido nefrogênico, 646
Clorpromazina
informações de formulações, 1363-1441
para diarreia, 352
para hematêmese, 593
para insuficiência hepática, aguda, 779
para pancreatite, 987
para tétano, 1211
para toxicose por anfetamina, 1236
para toxicose por pseudoefedrina, 1247
para úlcera gastroduodenal, 1302
para vômito, 1332, 1334
Clorpropamida, para diabetes insípido, 342
Clortetraciclina
para brucelose, 167
para peste, 1035
Closilato de tênio, 1363-1441
Clostridium botulinum, 160
Clostridium perfringens, 465
Clostridium piliformis, 411
Clotrimazol
para aspergilose, 123, 125
para blefarite, 142
para candidíase, 169
para epistaxe, 483
para infecção do trato urinário inferior, 737
para prototecose, 1102
para secreção nasal, 1153
Cloxacilina
informações de formulações, 1363-1441
para discospondilite, 373
para osteomielite, 974
para piodermite, 1041
Clumber spaniel
deficiência da piruvato desidrogenase fosfatase
924
mioglobinúria, 597
Coagulação intravascular disseminada, 225-226
Coagulopatia, epistaxe com, 482-483
Coagulopatia por hepatopatia, 227
Cobalamina (vitamina B$_{12}$)
para anemia, 81, 91
para diarreia, responsiva a antibióticos, 357
para disbiose do intestino delgado, 365
para insuficiência pancreática exócrina, 781
para linfangiectasia, 839
para mielopatia degenerativa, 896
para síndrome colangite/colangio-hepatite,
1164
Coccidioidomicose, 228-229
Cocciodiose, 230
Cockapoos, metemoglobinemia em, 880
Cocker spaniel
abiotrofia cerebelar, 658
adenocarcinoma das glândulas ceruminosas,
orelha, 32
agressividade, 50

agressividade contra crianças, 49
anemia, imunomediada, 84
bloqueio atrioventricular, primeiro grau, 145
bloqueio atrioventricular, segundo grau,
Mobitz Tipo II, 149
bloqueio atrioventricular, terceiro grau
(completo), 143
bronquiectasia, 163
bronquite, crônica, 164
carcinoma de células escamosas, orelha, 179
ceratoconjuntivite seca, 195
criptococose, 277
deficiência da fosfofrutoquinase, 91, 291, 924
deficiência da fosfrutoquinase, 597
deficiência de carnitina, 293
deficiência de taurina, 294
dermatite por Malassezia, 315
discopatia intervertebral
cervical, 368
toracolombar, 370
distiquíase, 400, 477
distrofia da córnea, 392
distúrbios do desenvolvimento sexual, 1098
endocardiose da valva atrioventricular, 454
epilepsia, 479
episcleroceratite granulomatosa nodular, 195
espondilose deformante, 497
estenose pulmonar, 510
estomatite periodontal ulcerativa crônica
(EPUC), 1303
estomatite ulcerativa, 1303
glaucoma, 576
glomerulonefrite, 580
glomerulopatia, 427
hemoglobinúria, 597
hepatite, crônica ativa, 602
hepatotoxinas, 621
hérnia diafragmática, 625
hipertensão, portal, 673
hipotireoidismo, 711
hipotricose, 63
histiocitoma, 329, 716
icterícia, 722
insuficiência renal, crônica, 785
lipoma, 329, 837
massas bucais, 857
miocardiopatia, 901
mucocele da vesícula biliar, 930
nefrolitíase, 936
orifícios nasolacrimais imperfurados, 477
osteocondrodisplasia, 968
osteomielite, 1303
otite, 982
pancreatite, 986
papiloma, 329
para anemia, regenerativa, 91
para bradicardia sinusal, 161
para laceração da parede atrial, 806
parada sinusal/bloqueio sinoatrial, 999
paresia/paralisia do nervo facial, 1013
persistência do ducto arterioso, 1032
plasmocitoma, 1051
problemas comportamentais maternos, 1081
prolapso da glândula da terceira pálpebra,
1089
queiletielose, 1111
síncope, 1159
síndrome do nó sinusal doente, 1184
tricoepitelioma, 1292
triquíase, 477
trombocitopatias, 1271

trombocitopenia, 1036, 1272, 1274
tumor das glândulas sebáceas, 329
tumor de células basais (basalioma), 1282
tumores das glândulas mamárias, 1288
tumores melanocíticos, 1294, 1295
urolitíase, por estruvita, 1309
vômito, crônico, 1333
Cocker spaniel americano
agressividade contra crianças, 49
anemia, regenerativa, 91
bloqueio atrioventricular, primeiro grau, 145
bloqueio atrioventricular, segundo grau,
Mobitz Tipo II, 149
criptococose, 277
deficiência da fosfofrutoquinase, 91, 291, 924
deficiência da fosfrutoquinase, 597
deficiência de carnitina, 293
deficiência de taurina, 294
distrofia da córnea, 392
distúrbios do desenvolvimento sexual, 398
distúrbios dos sacos anais, 401
glaucoma, 576
hemoglobinúria, 597
miocardiopatia, 902
trombocitopatias, 1271
Cocker spaniel inglês
deficiência da fosfrutoquinase, 597
distúrbios do desenvolvimento sexual, 398
glaucoma, 576
glomerulopatia, 427
hemoglobinúria, 597
insuficiência renal, crônica, 785
proteinúria, 1100
surdez, 1202
Codeína
dosagens e indicações, 1361
informações de formulações, 1363-1441
para bronquite, crônica, 165
Coenzima Q10
para degeneração cerebelar, 191
para insuficiência cardíaca congestiva,
esquerda, 777
para miocardiopatia, 902
para miopatia por armazenamento de lipídios,
925
para síndrome de hiperestesia felina, 1177
Colapso da traqueia, 231-232
Colapso induzido por exercício em Labrador
retrievers, 558-559
Colchicina
informações de formulações, 1363-1441
para amiloide hepático, 450
para amiloidose, 75
para cirrose e fibrose do fígado, 211
para febre familiar do Shar-pei, 529
para hepatite, crônica ativa, 603-604
Colecistite e coledoquite, 233
Colelitíase, 234-235
Colesteatoma, 236
Colibacilose, 237-238
Cólica. *Ver* Abdome agudo
Colite, 239-240
Colite ulcerativa histiocítica, 241
Collie
abiotrofia cerebelar, 658
amiloide hepático, 73
amiloidose, 74
anemia, imunomediada, 84
anomalia do olho do Collie, 97, 631
degeneração cerebelar, 299
dermatomiosite, 319, 327, 335, 915

descolamento da retina, 338
displasia de bastonetes e cones, 102
displasia do cotovelo, 380
distrofia da córnea, 392
distrofia neuroaxonal, 391
distúrbios causados por imunodeficiência, 394
distúrbios despigmentantes, 321
epilepsia, 479
episclerite, 481
escleroceratite granulomatosa nodular, 195
hematopoiese cíclica, 207, 394
hemorragia da retina, 599
hérnia perineal, 627
hifema, 631
hipercolesterolemia, 654
hiperplasia gengival, 668
insuficiência pancreática exócrina, 780
insulinoma, 788
lúpus eritematoso, 327, 335
    cutâneo (discoide), 839
    sistêmico (LES), 840
má-absorção da cobalamina, 848
mielopatia degenerativa, 896
neuropatias periféricas, 944
neutropenia, 946
pênfigo eritematoso, 335, 1019
pênfigo foliáceo, 335
penfigoide bolhoso, 335
persistência do ducto arterioso, 1032
poliartrite, não erosiva, 1069
prototecose, 1102
síndrome do Collie cinza, 73
toxicidade da ivermectina, 1231
trombocitopatias, 1271
vasculite, cutânea, 1325
Collie de pelo duro
    abiotrofia cerebelar, 658
    anomalia do olho do Collie, 97
    degeneração cerebelar, 299
    dermatomiosite, 915
    distrofia da córnea, 392
    hipercolesterolemia, 654
    insuficiência pancreática exócrina, 780
    lúpus eritematoso sistêmico, 840
    má-absorção da cobalamina, 848
Coloboma, 102-103
Coma, 518-519
    mixedema, 927
Coma hiperosmolar, 345-346
Complexo de escape ventricular, 1140
Complexo granuloma eosinofílico, 242-243
Complexo lipídico de anfotericina B, para
        pitiose/ficomicose, 240, 1047
Complexo pênfigo, 335-336
Complexos atriais prematuros, 244-245
Complexos ventriculares prematuros, 246-247
Comportamento de arranhadura, em gatos,
        1085-1086
Comportamento de marcação territorial
    em cães, 248-249
    em gatos, 250-251
Comportamento de mastigação em cães,
        1083-1084
Comportamento defensivo, em gatos, 1085-1086
Comportamento errático
    em cães, 248-249
    em gatos, 250-251
Comportamento indisciplinado, 254-255
Comportamentos destrutivos, 252-253
    pediátricos em cães, 1083-1084
    pediátricos em gatos, 1085-1086

Compressão cefálica, 256-257
Compressões torácicas, 998
Condicionamento clássico, para agressividade por
        medo em gatos, 58
Condroprotetores
    para artrite, 115
    para claudicação, 224
    para displasia do cotovelo, 381
    para doença de Legg-Calvé-Perthes, 410
    para doença do ligamento cruzado cranial, 416
    para luxação patelar, 845
    para osteocondrodisplasia, 968
    para osteocondrose, 970
    para problemas do ombro, 1089
Condrossarcoma
    boca, 258
    laringe e traqueia, 259
    osso, 260
    seios nasais e paranasais, 261
Conivaptana, para insuficiência hepática, aguda,
        779
Conjuntivite
    em cães, 262-263
    em gatos, 264-265
Conjuntivite eosinofílica, 265
Conjuntivite herpética, 264, 265
Conjuntivorrinostomia, 478
Constipação, 266-267
Contracondicionamento
    para agressividade, 51, 52, 54, 58, 59
    para síndrome de ansiedade da separação, 1169
Controle de pulga, 671-672
Contusões pulmonares, 268
Convulsões. Ver Crises convulsivas
Coonhound
    hemofilia B, 482
    metemoglobinemia, 880
    neuropatias periféricas, 944
    paralisia do Coonhound, 1008-1009
Coprofagia, 269-270
Coriorretinite, 271-272
Cornish rex, hemoglobinúria em, 597
Coronavírus felino. Ver Peritonite infecciosa
        felina
Corpos estranhos esofágicos, 273-274
    reações, 331, 332
Corrida de obstáculos, compulsiva, 1258
Corrimento vaginal, 275-276
Corticosteroides
    para acne, 24
    para anafilaxia, 77
    para anemia, imunomediada, 85
    para asma/bronquite em gatos, 120-121
    para bailisascaríase, 136
    para blefarite, 142
    para bloqueio atrioventricular, terceiro grau
        (completo), 144
    para borreliose de Lyme, 159
    para bronquite, crônica, 165
    para ceratite
        eosinofílica, 194
        não ulcerativa, 196
    para ceratoconjuntivite seca, 199
    para claudicação, 224
    para colite e proctite, 240
    para colite ulcerativa histiocítica, 241
    para conjuntivite, 263, 265
    para coriorretinite, 1112
    para corpo estranho esofágico, 273
    para crises convulsivas, 282
    para depósito lipídico, 704

para dermatite acral por lambedura, 310
para dermatite actínica, 334
para dermatite atópica, 312
para dermatite de contato, 313
para dermatite rabdítica, 333
para dermatite solar nasal, 328
para dermatoses nodulares estéreis, 334
para dispneia, 385
para distúrbios despigmentantes, 322
para doença idiopática do trato urinário
        inferior dos felinos, 418
para doenças orbitais, 426
para edema cerebral, 871
para edema pulmonar, 440
para efusão pericárdica, 442
para encefalite, 446
para encefalite necrosante, 447
para enteropatia imunoproliferativa de
        Basenjis, 462
para esofagite, 489
para espondilomielopatia cervical, 408
para espondilose deformante, 497
para esteatite, 500
para estenose esofágica, 506
para estenose retal, 512
para fístula perianal, 547
para gastrenterite, eosinofílica, 565
para gastrenterite, linfocítica-plasmocitária,
        569
para glaucoma, 577
para granuloma eosinofílico, 243
para hemorragia da retina, 600
para hidrocefalia, 629
para hifema, 632
para hipercalcemia, 641
para hiperceratose nasal, 328
para hiperparatireoidismo, 663
para hipersensibilidade à picada de pulga,
        671-672
para hipópio, 704
para histiocitose, 719
para inalação de fumaça, 725
para inclinação da cabeça, 727
para infecção pelo vírus da imunodeficiência
        felina (FIV), 744
para inflamação orofaríngea felina, 770
para instabilidade atlantoaxial, 773
para intermação e hipertermia, 791
para intoxicação pelo chumbo, 794
para lesão por mordedura de fio elétrico, 819
para lesões estenóticas vaginais, 856
para linfangiectasia, 828
para linfoma
    cutâneo epiteliotrópico, 834
    em cães, 831
para lúpus eritematoso sistêmico (LES), 841
para más-formações espinais e vertebrais
        congênitas, 854
para meningioma, 871
para meningite, 875
para meningoencefalomielite granulomatosa,
        727
para miastenia grave, 884
para miopatia
    inflamatória focal, 917
    inflamatória geral, 916
    não inflamatória, 922
para neuropatias periféricas, 945
para otite externa/média, 980
para pancreatite, 987
para papiledema, 993

para papilomatose, 994
para paralisia, 1005
para pênfigo, 1020
para peritonite infecciosa felina, 1031
para piodermite de filhotes caninos, 1038
para placa eosinofílica, 243
para pneumonia
  eosinofílica, 1056
  intersticial, 1060
  por aspiração, 1061
para pododermatite, 1065
para problemas do ombro, 1089
para proptose, 1093
para prurido, 1105
para reações a transfusões sanguíneas, 1124
para schwanoma, 1151
para síndrome da angústia respiratória aguda, 1167
para síndrome de tremor, 1180
para síndrome hipereosinofílica, 1189
para siringomielia, 1198
para tosse, 1217
para tremores, 1267
para trombocitopenia, imunomediada
  primária, 1275
para tumores da bainha nervosa, 1287
para úlcera indolente, 243
para uveíte anterior, 1320, 1322
para vasculite, sistêmica, 1326
para vômito, 1334
Corticotropina, 1363-1441
Cosyntropin, 1363-1441
Coton de Tulear
  degeneração cerebelar em, 299
  descolamento da retina, 1108
Coxiella burnetii, 532
Crioprecipitado
  hemofilia, 483
  para coagulopatia por hepatopatia, 227
  para deficiência dos fatores de coagulação, 295
  para doença de von Willebrand, 483
Criptococose, 277-278
Criptoftalmia, 102
Criptorquidismo, 279
Criptosporidiose, 280
Crises convulsivas
  em cães, 281-282
  em gatos, 283-284
  epilepsia, 479-480
Crisoterapia, para pênfigo, 1020
Crisoterapia, para poliartrite erosiva, 1067
Cristais de ácido hipúrico, 285
Cristais de colesterol, 285
Cristais de leucina, 285
Cristais de tirosina, 285-286
Cristalúria, 285-286
  por ácido úrico, 285
  por bilirrubina, 285
  por cistina, 285
  por estruvita, 285
  por fosfato de cálcio, 285
  por oxalato de cálcio, 285
Cromossomos sexuais, distúrbios dos, 398
Cryptosporidium spp., 230
Cuterebrose, 287, 452

D

D-penicilamina, para hepatopatia por
  armazenamento de cobre, 617
Dacarbazina
  informações de formulações, 1363-1441

para linfoma em cães, 831
para tumores melanocíticos, 1294, 1296
Dachshund
  alopecia do pavilhão auricular, 64
  anemia, regenerativa, 91
  blefarite, 141
  bloqueio atrioventricular, primeiro grau, 145
  bloqueio atrioventricular, segundo grau,
    Mobitz Tipo II, 149
  carcinoma de células de transição, 172
  carcinoma de células escamosas, dedos, 181
  cílios ectópicos, 400
  cistinúria, 427
  cristalúria, 285
  deficiência da piruvato quinase, 91, 292
  deformidades do crescimento antebraquial,
    297
  dermatite por Malassezia, 315
  dermatose linear por IgA, 335
  dermoides, 141
  diabetes melito, 343, 347
  discopatia intervertebral
    cervical, 368
    toracolombar, 370
  distocia, 388
  distrofia da córnea, 392
  distrofia de cones e bastonetes, 102
  distúrbios despigmentantes, 321
  doença de von Willebrand, 412
  doença do armazenamento lisossomal, 658
  epilepsia, 479
  fístula oronasal, 546
  gastrenterite, hemorrágica, 566
  glomerulonefrite, 580
  hepatopatia vacuolar, 619
  hérnia perineal, 627
  hiperadrenocorticismo, 633
  hipotireoidismo, 711
  histiocitoma, 329, 716
  infertilidade, fêmea, 764
  laceração da parede atrial, 806
  linfoma, 830
  lipoma, 329, 837
  massas bucais, 857
  mastocitoma, 329
  megaesôfago, 866
  miastenia grave, 883
  mucocele salivar, 932
  mucopolissacaridoses, 934
  narcolepsia, 935
  nefrolitíase, 936
  neuropatias periféricas, 944
  onicorrexe, 397
  osteocondrodisplasia, 968
  paniculite, 988
  para bradicardia sinusal, 161
  parada sinusal/bloqueio sinoatrial, 999
  pênfigo foliáceo, 335, 1019
  piodermite de filhotes caninos, 193
  pneumocistose, 1052, 1059
  pododermatite, 1064
  síncope, 1213
  síndrome de dilatação e vólvulo gástricos,
    1172
  síndrome do nó sinusal doente, 1184
  surdez, 1202
  tumor das glândulas sebáceas, 329
  urolitíase, por cistina, 1308
  vasculite, cutânea, 1325
Dacriocistite, 477, 478
Dacriocistorrinotomia, 478

Dálmata
  abdome agudo, 2
  atopia, 311
  axonopatia, 944
  carcinoma de células escamosas, pele, 175
  cristalúria, 285
  dermatite acral por lambedura, 310
  displasia da valva atrioventricular esquerda
    (mitral), 378
  disrafismo espinal, 387
  dor no pescoço e dorso, 433
  espondilomielopatia cervical, 495
  glomerulonefrite, 580
  hematúria, 595
  hepatopatia por armazenamento de cobre, 616
  hepatotoxinas, 621
  hiperplasia gengival, 668
  hiperuricúria, 427
  hipomielinização, 699
  icterícia, 722
  laringopatias, 810
  miocardiopatia, 906
  mioclonia, 1187
  nefrolitíase, 936
  neuropatias periféricas, 944
  parada sinusal/bloqueio sinoatrial, 999
  paralisia congênita da laringe, 206
  paralisia da laringe, 514
  pododermatite, 1064
  proteinúria, 1100
  ritmo idioventricular, 1140
  síndrome da angústia respiratória aguda, 1167
  surdez, 1202
  tremores, 1266
  urolitíase, por urato, 1316
Dalteparina
  informações de formulações, 1363-1441
  para endocardite, 458
  para hipercoagulabilidade, 647
  para infarto do miocárdio, 734
  para miocardiopatia, 905
  para prevenção de tromboembolia pulmonar,
    1280
  para tromboembolia aórtica, 1277
  para tromboembolia pulmonar, 1280
Danazol
  informações de formulações, 1363-1441
  para trombocitopenia, imunomediada
    primária, 1275
Dandie Dinmont terrier
  glaucoma, 576
  osteocondrodisplasia, 968
Dantroleno
  informações de formulações, 1363-1441
  retenção urinária, 1136
Dapsona
  informações de formulações, 1363-1441
  para dermatose linear por IgA, 336
  para dermatose pustulosa subcórnea, 336
  para epistaxe, 483
  para pênfigo, 1020
  para pneumocistose, 1052
  para rinosporidiose, 1046
  para toxicose por veneno de aranha, 1249
  para vasculite, cutânea, 1325
  para vasculite, sistêmica, 1326
Darbazina, para síndrome do intestino irritável,
  1183
Darbopoietina
  para anemia de doença renal crônica, 82
  para hiperestrogenismo, 649

DDAVP. *Ver* Desmopressina
Decanoato de nandrolona
informações de formulações, 1363-1441
para erliquiose, 486
DECCE (defeitos epiteliais corneanos crônicos
espontâneos), 197-198
Decoquinato, para hepatozoonose, 623
Deerhound escocês
cistinúria, 427
miocardiopatia, 901
osteocondrodisplasia, 968
Defeito do septo atrial, 288
Defeito do septo ventricular, 289-290
Defeitos epiteliais corneanos crônicos
espontâneos (DECCE), 197-198
Deficiência da piruvato quinase, 91, 1038
Deficiência de alfa-L-fucosidase, 766
Deficiência de carnitina, 293
Deficiência de enzima desramificante, 924
Deficiência de espectrina, 91
Deficiência de fosfofrutoquinase, 91, 291, 924
Deficiência de IgA, 394
Deficiência de IgM, 394
Deficiência de maltase ácida, 924
Deficiência de taurina, 294
Deficiência dos fatores de coagulação, 295-296
Defluxo anagênico e telogênico, 63, 66
Deformidades do crescimento antebraquial,
297-298
Degeneração cerebelar, 299
Degeneração da retina, 300-302
Degeneração e hipoplasia testiculares, 303
Degenerações e infiltrações da córnea, 304
Demodicose, 63, 65, 305-306
Dente assimétrico, 557
Dente invaginado, 557
Dentes decíduos, retidos, 307
Dentes dilacerados, 557
Dentes em concha, 557
Dentes manchados, 308-309
Dentinogênese imperfeita, manchas nos dentes
causadas por, 308
Depósito lipídico, 704
Deracoxibe
dosagens e indicações, 1363
informações de formulações, 1363-1441
para artrite, 115
para claudicação, 224
para condrossarcoma, 258
para displasia coxofemoral, 377
para displasia do cotovelo, 381
para doença de Legg-Calvé-Perthes, 409
para doença do ligamento cruzado cranial, 416
para espondilose deformante, 497
para febre, 527
para fibrossarcoma, 541, 542
para luxação patelar, 845
para luxações articulares, 847
para osteocondrodisplasia, 968
para osteodistrofia hipertrófica, 972
para osteopatia craniomandibular, 975
para panosteíte, 991
para problemas do ombro, 1089
para rinite e sinusite, 1138
Dermatite
à picada de pulga, 671-672
alopecia com dermatite alérgica, 65
Dermatite acral por lambedura, 310
Dermatite actínica, 333, 334
Dermatite atópica, 311-312
alopecia com, 65

Dermatite de contato, 313
Dermatite eosinofílica, 487
Dermatite necrolítica superficial, 314
Dermatite por *Malassezia*, 315
Dermatite rabdítica, 333
Dermatite solar nasal, 321, 327-328
Dermatofibrose nodular, 331-332
Dermatofilose, 316, 335
Dermatofitose, 63, 65, 317-318, 335
Dermatomiosite, 319-320, 915-916
Dermatose linear por IgA, 335-336
Dermatose pustulosa subcórnea, 335, 336
Dermatoses erosivas, 323-324
Dermatoses esfoliativas, 325-326
Dermatoses granulomatosas, 331-332
Dermatoses nasais, 327-328
dermatose responsiva ao zinco, 327
Dermatoses neoplásicas, 329-330
Dermatoses nodulares/granulomatosas estéreis,
331-332, 334
Dermatoses papulonodulares, 333-334
Dermatoses ulcerativas, 323-324
Dermatoses vesiculopustulares, 335-336
Dermatoses virais, 337
Dermoides, 102, 141
DES. *Ver* Dietilestilbestrol
Descolamento da retina, 102-103, 338-339
Descongestionantes, para espirro, 492
Descontaminação
para envenenamento pela estricnina, 797
para envenenamento pelo cogumelo, 474
para intoxicação pelo lírio, 795
para toxicidade da vitamina D, 1220
para toxicose por anfetamina, 1236
para toxicose por antidepressivos tricíclicos,
107-108
para toxicose por chocolate, 1240-1241
Desfibrilação, 539
Deslorrelina
para falha ovulatória, 525
para incompetência uretral, 731
para indução do estro (cio), 765
para infertilidade, fêmea, 765
Desmielinização, 944
Desmopressina (DDVAP)
informações de formulações, 1363-1441
para coagulopatia por hepatopatia, 227
para diabetes insípido, 342, 646, 659
para doença de von Willebrand, 412-413
para lesão cerebral, 818
para petéquia, equimose, contusão, 1037
para trombocitopatias, 1271
Desoxicorticosterona (DOCP), para
hipoadrenocorticismo, 684
Desoxinivalenol, 889
Dessensibilização, para agressividade, 51, 52, 54,
58, 59
Desvio portocaval. *Ver* Anomalia vascular
portossistêmica, congênita
Desvio portossistêmico, adquirido, 340-341
Devon rex
amiloide hepático, 73
distocia, 388
hemoglobinúria, 597
luxação patelar, 844
Dexametasona
informações de formulações, 1363-1441
para anemia, imunomediada, 85
para asma/bronquite em gatos, 121
para blefarite, 142
para cataratas, 191

para ceratite, não ulcerativa, 196
para cisto quadrigeminal, 217
para conjuntivite, 263, 265
para coriorretinite, 272
para crises convulsivas, 282, 284
para depósito lipídico, 704
para disrafismo espinal, 387
para distúrbios despigmentantes, 322
para edema cerebral, 871
para encefalite secundária à migração
parasitária, 448
para encefalopatia isquêmica felina, 453
para espondilomielopatia cervical, 496
para hepatite, crônica ativa, 603
para hidrocefalia, 629
para hifema, 632
para hipoalbuminemia, 686
para hipópio, 704
para inclinação da cabeça, 727
para interrupção da gestação, 9-10
para lacerações da córnea e esclera, 809
para meningioma, 871
para meningite, 875
para meningoencefalomielite, 876, 878
para meningoencefalomielite granulomatosa,
727
para miopatia, 922
para papiledema, 993
para parada ventricular, 1001
para paralisia, 1005
para placa eosinofílica, 243
para síndrome braquicefálica das vias aéreas,
1160
para toxicidade do rodenticida brometalina,
1224
para trombocitopenia, 1273
imunomediada primária, 1275
para tumores da bainha nervosa, 1287
para uveíte anterior, 1320, 1322
Dexmedetomidina, 1363-1441
Dextrana, 1363-1441
Dextrometorfano, 1363-1441
Dextrose
informações de formulações, 1363-1441
para diabetes com cetoacidose, 344
para hipercalemia, 642
para hiperfosfatemia, 650
para hipoglicemia, 696
para inércia uterina, 732
para prolapso retal e anal, 1090
para toxicidade do xilitol, 1227
Diabetes insípido, 342
central, 342
nefrogênico, 342
teste modificado de privação de água, 1342
Diabetes melito
acromegalia em gatos, 26
alopecia, 65
com cetoacidose, 343-344
com coma hiperosmolar, 345-346
hepatopatia, 613
sem complicações
em cães, 347-348
em gatos, 349-350
Diálise peritoneal, para envenenamento
(intoxicação), 469
Diarreia
aguda, 351-352
crônica
em cães, 353-354
em gatos, 355-356

responsiva a antibióticos, 357
responsiva à tilosina, 193
Diazepam
informações de formulações, 1363-1441
para agressividade, 58
para anorexia, 105, 744
para crises convulsivas, 126, 282, 284, 794,
872, 875, 1220
para eclâmpsia, 435
para encefalopatia isquêmica felina, 453
para envenenamento pela estricnina, 797
para envenenamento pelo cogumelo, 474
para epilepsia, 480
para estimulação do apetite, 1022
para fobias a trovões e relâmpagos, 552
para intermação e hipertermia, 791
para lesão cerebral, 818
para medos, fobias e ansiedades, 554
para meningioma, 872
para nistagmo, 949
para prurido, 1105
para pseudociese, 1107
para retenção urinária, 1136
para tétano, 1211
para toxicidade das piretrinas e dos piretroides,
1221
para toxicidade do rodenticida brometalina,
1224
para toxicidade dos agentes anti-inflamatórios
não esteroides, 1230
para toxicidade dos organofosforados e
carbamatos, 1246
para toxicose por beta-2 agonistas inalatórios,
1239
para toxicose por chocolate, 1241
para toxicose por ISRS, 109
para toxinas tremorgênicas, 890
para vestibulopatia, 1327, 1329
para vocalização excessiva, 1330
toxicose, 1237-1238
toxicose por antidepressivos tricíclicos, 108
Diazóxido, para insulinoma, 789
Dicilomina, para instabilidade do detrusor, 731
Diclofenaco
para cataratas, 191
para hipópio, 704
para uveíte anterior, 1320, 1322
Diclorvós
informações de formulações, 1363-1441
para ancilóstomos, 78
para fisalopterose, 544
para nematódeos, 940
Dicloxacilina
informações de formulações, 1363-1441
para infecções estafilocócicas, 759
Dietilcarbamazina, 1363-1441
Dietilestilbestrol (DES)
informações de formulações, 1363-1441
para bexiga pélvica, 138
para incompetência uretral, 731
para indução do estro (cio), 765
para infertilidade, fêmea, 765
para prolapso uretral, 1091
para ureter ectópico, 1305
para vaginite, 276, 1324
Difenidramina
informações de formulações, 1363-1441
para anafilaxia, 77
para dermatite atópica, 312
para encefalite secundária à migração
parasitária, 448

para encefalopatia isquêmica felina, 453
para problemas comportamentais pediátricos,
1084
para prurido, 1105
para reações a transfusões sanguíneas, 1124
para vômito, 1332
Difenoxilato
informações de formulações, 1363-1441
para colite e proctite, 240
para incontinência, fecal, 729
para síndrome do intestino irritável, 1183
Diferenciação dos testículos, 398
Difloxacino, 1363-1441
Digoxina
informações de formulações, 1363-1441
para complexos atriais prematuros, 245
para displasia das valvas atrioventriculares, 379
para doenças endomiocárdicas, 424
para endocardiose das valvas atrioventriculares,
455, 456
para estenose das valvas atrioventriculares, 504
para fibrilação atrial, 511, 537
para hipertensão, pulmonar, 677
para insuficiência cardíaca congestiva
direita, 775
esquerda, 777
para miocardiopatia, 902, 905, 910
para miocardite, 912
para persistência do ducto arterioso, 1033
para síndrome do nó sinusal doente, 1185
para taquicardia sinusal, 1204
para taquicardia supraventricular, 1206
Diidroestreptomicina
para brucelose, 167
para leptospirose, 816
para tuberculose, 762
Diltiazem
informações de formulações, 1363-1441
para anomalia de Ebstein, 95
para choque, cardiogênico, 201
para complexos atriais prematuros, 245
para displasia das valvas atrioventriculares, 379
para epistaxe, 483
para estenose aórtica, 501
para estenose das valvas atrioventriculares, 504
para fibrilação atrial, 537
para hipertensão, pulmonar, 489
para insuficiência cardíaca congestiva,
esquerda, 777
para miocardiopatia, 902, 905, 908, 910
para persistência do ducto arterioso, 1033
para síndrome de Wolff-Parkinson-White, 95,
1182
para taquicardia sinusal, 1204
para taquicardia supraventricular, 1206
Dimenidrinato
informações de formulações, 1363-1441
para vestibulopatia, 1327
Dimercaprol (BAL)
informações de formulações, 1363-1441
para envenenamento pelo arsênico, 470
Dimetilsulfóxido (DMSO)
febre familiar do Shar-pei, 529
para amiloide hepático, 450
para amiloidose, 75
para calcinose cutânea, 332
para doença idiopática do trato urinário
inferior dos felinos, 418
para placa eosinofílica, 243
Dinitrato de isossorbida
informações de formulações, 1363-1441

para endocardiose da valva atrioventricular,
456
Dinoprosta. *Ver também* Prostaglandina F$_{2\alpha}$
para abortamento, espontâneo, 8, 6
para remoção do conteúdo uterino e luteólise,
276
Dinotefurano/piriproxifeno, para controle de
pulga, 672
Dioctophyma renale (verme renal gigante),
358-359
Dipiridamol, 1363-1441
Dipirona, para deficiência da fosfofrutoquinase,
291
Dipivefrina, para hifema, 632
Dipropionato de imidocarbe
para babesiose, 134-135, 483
para citauxzoonose, 221
para erliquiose, 486
Dirlotapida
informações de formulações, 1363-1441
para obesidade, 952
Dirofilaria immitis. Ver Dirofilariose
Dirofilariose
em cães, 360-361
em gatos, 362
Disautonomia, 363
Disbiose do intestino delgado, 364-365
Discinesia ciliar primária, 366
Discopatia intervertebral
cervical, 368-369
em gatos, 367
toracolombar, 370-371
Discospondilite, 372-373
Disfagia, 374-375
bucal, 374
cricofaríngea, 374
faríngea, 374
Disgenesia sacrococcígea, 853-854
Dismetria, 658
Disopiramida, 1363-1441
Displasia coxofemoral, 376-377
Displasia da retina, 102-103
Displasia da valva atrioventricular direita
(tricúspide), 378-379
Displasia da valva atrioventricular esquerda
(mitral), 378-379
Displasia de bastonetes e cones, 102-103, 300
Displasia de fotorreceptores, 102-103
Displasia do cotovelo, 380-381
Displasia microvascular hepatoportal, 382-383
Displasia occipital, 853-854
Dispneia, 384-385
Disquesia, 386
Disrafismo espinal, 387
Distiquíase, 141, 400, 477
Distocia, 388-390
Distrofia da retina, 102-103
Distrofia de cones e bastonetes, 102
Distrofia neuroaxonal, 391
Distrofias da córnea, 392
Distúrbios causados por imunodeficiência,
primários, 394
Distúrbios da articulação temporomandibular,
393
Distúrbios da glândula tireoide, testes para,
1341
Distúrbios da motilidade gástrica, 395-396
Distúrbios das glândulas adrenais, testes para,
1341
Distúrbios das pálpebras
agenesia, 102, 400

ectrópio, 436
entrópio, 467
Distúrbios das unhas e dos leitos ungueais, 397
Distúrbios de queratinização. *Ver* Dermatoses
  esfoliativas
Distúrbios despigmentantes, 321-322
Distúrbios do desenvolvimento sexual, 398-399
Distúrbios dos cílios, 400
Distúrbios dos hormônios sexuais, testes para,
  1341-1342
Distúrbios dos sacos anais, 401
Distúrbios mieloproliferativos, 402
Disúria, 403-404
Ditiazanina, 1363-1441
Diuréticos
  para ascite, 212, 614
  para choque, cardiogênico, 201
  para cianose, 207
  para cisto quadrigeminal, 217
  para contusões pulmonares, 268
  para desvio portossistêmico, 341
  para displasia das valvas atrioventriculares, 379
  para edema periférico, 438
  para edema pulmonar, 440
  para efusão pericárdica, 442
  para efusão pleural, 444
  para endocardiose das valvas atrioventriculares,
    455, 456
  para envenenamento (intoxicação), 469
  para epistaxe, 483
  para estupor e coma, 519
  para hemorragia da retina, 600
  para hepatite, crônica ativa, 603
  para hidrocefalia, 629
  para hipercalcemia, 641
  para hiperparatireoidismo, 663
  para hipertensão, portal, 674
  para hipertensão, sistêmica, 679
  para hipoalbuminemia, 686
  para inalação de fumaça, 725
  para insuficiência cardíaca congestiva, 288
    direita, 775
    esquerda, 776-777
  para insuficiência renal, aguda, 783
  para laceração da parede atrial, 807
  para miocardiopatia, 906
  para oligúria, 966
  para síndrome nefrótica, 1191
  para siringomielia, 1198
Divertículos esofágicos, 405
Divertículos vesicouracais, 406
DMSA. *Ver* Succímer
DMSO. *Ver* Dimetilsulfóxido
Doberman pinscher
  acne, 24
  agenesia renal, 427
  alopecia por diluição da cor, 64
  anemia, imunomediada, 84
  artrite, séptica, 116
  aterosclerose, 129
  bloqueio atrioventricular, segundo grau,
    Mobitz Tipo II, 149
  bloqueio atrioventricular, terceiro grau
    (completo), 143
  colite ulcerativa histiocítica, 241
  coma mixedematoso, 927
  complexos ventriculares prematuros, 246
  criptococose, 277
  defeito bactericida, 394
  defeito do septo atrial, 288
  deficiência de carnitina, 293

deficiência de IgM, 394
dermatite acral por lambedura, 310
discopatia intervertebral, cervical, 368
distúrbios causados por imunodeficiência, 394
distúrbios despigmentantes, 321
doença de von Willebrand, 412, 482, 1036
dor no pescoço e dorso, 433
erliquiose, 485
espondilomielopatia cervical, 495
estenose espinal, congênita, 853
glomerulonefrite, 580
glomerulopatia, 427
hematúria, 595
hepatite, crônica ativa, 602
hepatopatia por armazenamento de cobre, 616
hepatotoxinas, 621
hipercolesterolemia, 654
hiperplasia gengival, 668
hipertensão, portal, 673
hipotireoidismo, 711
histiocitoma, 329, 716
icterícia, 722
infecção pelo parvovírus canino, 1016
infertilidade, fêmea, 764
lipoma, 329, 837
miocardiopatia, 901, 902
miosite dos músculos da mastigação, 917
narcolepsia, 935
osteodistrofia hipertrófica, 971
osteopatia craniomandibular, 975
pênfigo foliáceo, 335, 1019
penfigoide bolhoso, 335
pneumonia, fúngica, 1057
poliartrite, não erosiva, 1068
taquicardia ventricular, 1207
transtornos compulsivos, 1258
tremores, 1266
tumores cerebrais, 1284
tumores das glândulas mamárias, 1288
tumores melanocíticos, 1295
túnica vascular do cristalino hiperplásica
  persistente (TVCHP), 102
vítreo primário hiperplásico persistente
  (VPHP), 102
vômito, crônico, 1333
Dobutamina
  informações de formulações, 1363-1441
  para bloqueio atrioventricular, terceiro grau
    (completo), 144
  para bradicardia sinusal, 162
  para choque, cardiogênico, 201
  para choque, hipovolêmico, 203
  para choque, séptico, 205
  para endocardiose da valva atrioventricular,
    456
  para hipertensão, pulmonar, 677
  para insuficiência cardíaca congestiva,
    esquerda, 777
  para miocardiopatia, 902, 905, 910
  para ritmo idioventricular, 1141
Docetaxel, para tumores das glândulas mamárias
  em gatos, 1291
Docusato de cálcio
  informações de formulações, 1363-1441
  para constipação e obstipação, 267
  para disquesia e hematoquesia, 386
  para pólipos retoanais, 1078
Docusato de sódio
  informações de formulações, 1363-1441
  para constipação e obstipação, 267
  para disquesia e hematoquesia, 386

para estenose retal, 512
para megacólon, 865
para pólipos retoanais, 1078
para prolapso retal e anal, 1090
Doença broncopulmonar felina (DBF), 120-
  121
Doença da aglutinina fria, 407
Doença da parede torácica, 384-385
Doença de Addison, 683-684
Doença de Chagas, 408
Doença de Cushing. *Ver* Hiperadrenocorticismo
Doença de Legg-Calvé-Perthes, 409-410
Doença de Tyzzer, 411
Doença de von Willebrand, 412-413
  epistaxe com, 482, 483
Doença do armazenamento de glicogênio, 414
Doença do ligamento cruzado cranial, 415-416
Doença idiopática do trato urinário inferior dos
  felinos, 417-418
Doença inflamatória, anemia de, 80
Doença periodontal, 419-420
Doença renal crônica, anemia de, 82-83
Doença renal policística, 421, 427, 428
Doenças congênitas
  anomalias oculares, 102-103
  más-formações espinais e vertebrais, 853-854
  renais, 427-428
Doenças do armazenamento lisossomal, 422,
  944
Doenças endomiocárdicas, 423-424
Doenças orbitais, 425-426
Doenças renais, de natureza congênita e de
  desenvolvimento, 427-428
Dogue alemão
  acne, 24
  criptococose, 277
  deficiência de carnitina, 293
  deformidades do crescimento antebraquial,
    297
  dermatite acral por lambedura, 310
  descolamento da retina, 338
  discospondilite, 372
  displasia da valva atrioventricular esquerda
    (mitral), 378
  dor no pescoço e dorso, 433
  ectrópio, 477
  esplenomegalia, 493
  espondilomielopatia cervical, 495
  estenose aórtica, 501
  hemangiossarcoma
    baço e fígado, 588
    osso, 591
  hiperplasia gengival, 668
  hipoadrenocorticismo, 683
  hipotireoidismo, 711
  histiocitoma, 329, 716
  infertilidade, fêmea, 764
  megaesôfago, 866
  mielopatia degenerativa, 896
  miocardiopatia, 901
  osteocondrose, 969
  osteodistrofia hipertrófica, 971
  osteopatia craniomandibular, 975
  pericardite, 1025
  pododermatite, 1064
  ptialismo, 1109
  regurgitação, 1129
  síndrome de dilatação e vólvulo gástricos,
    958, 1172
  torção esplênica, 1215
  transtornos compulsivos, 1258

Dolasetrona
como antiemético em terapia com cisplatina, 31
informações de formulações, 1363-1441
para abdome agudo, 4
para insuficiência renal, aguda, 783
para lipidose hepática, 836
para vômito, 1332
Domperidona, para distúrbios da motilidade gástrica, 396
Dopamina
informações de formulações, 1363-1441
para bloqueio atrioventricular, segundo grau, Mobitz Tipo II, 150
para choque, cardiogênico, 201
para choque, hipovolêmico, 203
para choque, séptico, 205
para endocardiose da valva atrioventricular, 456
para envenenamento pelo cogumelo, 474
para insuficiência renal, aguda, 783
para intermação e hipertermia, 791
para oligúria, 966
para parada ventricular, 1001
para ritmo idioventricular, 1141
para toxicidade de uvas e passas, 1248
para toxicidade dos agentes anti-inflamatórios não esteroides, 1230
Dor aguda, crônica e pós-operatória, 429-432
Dor neuropática, medicamentos para, 1362
Dor no dorso, 433-434
Dor no pescoço, 433-434
Doramectina
para queiletielose, 1111
para sarna notoédrica, 1149
para sarna sarcóptica, 1150
Dorzolamida
para glaucoma, 272, 577
para hifema, 632
Dosagens e indicações de controle da dor
AINE dispensáveis, 1361-1362
AINE parenterais, 1361-1362
opioides dispensáveis, 1361
opioides parenterais, 1361
para dor neuropática, 1362
Doxapram, 1363-1441
Doxepina
para dermatite acral por lambedura, 310
para dermatite atópica, 312
toxicose, 107
Doxiciclina
informações de formulações, 1363-1441
para abscedação, 12
para babesiose, 135
para bartonelose, 137
para blefarite, 142
para bordetelose, 157
para borreliose de Lyme, 159
para brucelose, 167
para clamidiose, 222
para colapso traqueal, 232
para complexo granuloma eosinofílico, 243
para dermatofilose, 316
para dirofilariose, 361, 362
para edema periférico, 438
para encefalite, 446
para endocardite, 458
para erliquiose, 486
para espirro, 492
para estomatite, 516

para febre maculosa das Montanhas Rochosas, 531
para febre Q, 532
para infecções secundárias à influenza canina, 771
para leptospirose, 816
para meningite, 875
para micoplasmose, 886
para micoplasmose hemotrópica, 1179
para Mycoplasma felis, 746
para nocardiose, 950
para peste, 1035
para petéquia, equimose, contusão, 1037
para pneumonia, bacteriana, 1054
para rinite e sinusite, 1138
para riquetsiose, 483
para traqueobronquite infecciosa canina, 1263
para vasculite, 483
Doxorrubicina
informações de formulações, 1363-1441
para adenocarcinoma
nasal, 39
próstata, 29
pulmão, 37
tireoide, 31
para carcinoma de células de transição, 173
para carcinoma de células escamosas
pulmão, 182
tonsila, 177
para carcinoma prostático, 1096
para fibrossarcoma
gengiva, 541
osso, 542
seios nasais e paranasais, 543
para glucagonoma, 582
para hemangiopericitoma, 586
para hemangiossarcoma
baço e fígado, 589
coração, 590
osso, 591
pele, 587
para histiocitoma fibroso maligno, 717
para histiocitose, 719
para linfoma
em cães, 831
em gatos, 833
para mesotelioma, 879
para mieloma múltiplo, 893
para osteossarcoma, 978
para quimiodectoma, 1114
para rabdomiossarcoma, 1117
para sarcoma associado à vacina, 1146
para tumor venéreo transmissível, 1284
para tumores das glândulas mamárias
em cães, 1289
em gatos, 1291
para tumores melanocíticos, 1296
para tumores uterinos, 1299
para tumores vaginais, 1300
DPOC. *Ver* Bronquite, crônica
Drentse patrijshond, gastrite crônica em, 571
DSV. *Ver* Defeito do septo ventricular
Duplo arco aórtico, 101
DVG. *Ver* Síndrome de dilatação e vólvulo gástricos

E

Eclâmpsia, 435
ECP (cipionato de estradiol), 1363-1441
Ectrópio, 436
Edema periférico, 437-438

Edema pulmonar, 439-440
Edrofônio, 1363-1441
EDTA
informações de formulações, 1363-1441
para degenerações e infiltrações da córnea, 304
para intoxicação pelo chumbo, 794
para toxicidade do zinco, 1228
EDTA cálcico
informações de formulações, 1363-1441
para toxicidade do zinco, 1228
Efedrina
informações de formulações, 1363-1441
para espirro, 492
para secreção nasal, 1153
Efusão pericárdica, 441-442
Efusão pleural, 443-444
Eimeria spp., 230
Ejaculação retrógrada, 766, 767
Eletrocardiograma, valores normais para, 1363-1441
Elkhound norueguês
carcinoma de células escamosas, pele, 175
dermatoses neoplásicas, 329
displasia dos bastonetes, 102
distúrbios do desenvolvimento sexual, 398
entrópio, 467
glaucoma, 576
glicosúria, 578
glicosúria renal primária, 427
insuficiência renal, crônica, 785
nefropatia tubulointersticial, 427
osteocondrodisplasia, 968
Êmese
para toxicidade da vitamina D, 1220
para toxicidade dos agentes anti-inflamatórios não esteroides, 1230
para toxicose por antidepressivos tricíclicos, 107
para toxicose por ISRS, 109
Emético
para envenenamento (intoxicação), 468
para toxicidade das piretrinas e dos piretroides, 1221
para toxicidade de uvas e passas, 1248
para toxicose por amitraz, 1233
para toxicose por anfetamina, 1236
para toxicose por chocolate, 1241
para toxicose por pseudoefedrina, 1247
Emodepsida
para ancilóstomos, 78
para nematódeos, 940
para tênias, 1210
Emolientes
para adenite sebácea, 333
para dermatoses esfoliativas, 326
Enalapril
informações de formulações, 1363-1441
para acidente vascular cerebral isquêmico, 18
para anomalia de Ebstein, 95
para defeito do septo atrial, 288
para descolamento da retina, 339
para displasia das valvas atrioventriculares, 379
para doenças endomiocárdicas, 424
para endocardiose das valvas atrioventriculares, 455
para epistaxe, 483
para estenose das valvas atrioventriculares, 504
para glomerulonefrite, 581
para hipertensão, 129
portal, 674
pulmonar, 489
sistêmica, 679

para hipoalbuminemia, 686
para insuficiência cardíaca congestiva
  direita, 775
  esquerda, 777
para insuficiência renal, crônica, 786
para laceração da parede atrial, 807
para miocardiopatia, 900, 902, 905, 908, 910
para miocardite, 912
para persistência do ducto arterioso, 1033
para proteinúria, 1191
para síndrome nefrótica, 1191
Encefalite, 445-446
  secundária à migração parasitária, 448
Encefalite necrosante, 447
Encefalitozoonose, 449
Encefalopatia hepática, 450-451
  com hepatopatia fibrosante juvenil, 614-615
Encefalopatia isquêmica felina, 452-453
Endocardiose das valvas atrioventriculares, 454-456
Endocardite, infecciosa, 457-458
Enema
  água morna
    para constipação e obstipação, 267
    para toxicose por amitraz, 1233
  para encefalopatia hepática, 451
  para envenenamento (intoxicação), 468
Enilconazol
  informações de formulações, 1363-1441
  para aspergilose, 123, 125
  para dermatofitose, 318
  para dermatoses nasais, 328
  para epistaxe, 483
  para secreção nasal, 1153
Enoftalmia, 425-426
Enoxaparina
  informações de formulações, 1363-1441
  para hipercoagulabilidade, 647
  para miocardiopatia, 905
  para tromboembolia aórtica, 1277
  para tromboembolia pulmonar, 1280
Enrofloxacino
  informações de formulações, 1363-1441
  para afogamento (afogamento por um triz), 42
  para anomalias do anel vascular, 101
  para bronquiectasia, 163
  para bronquite, crônica, 165
  para brucelose, 167, 373
  para campilobacteriose, 1237
  para colibacilose, 238
  para colite e proctite, 240
  para colite ulcerativa histiocítica, 240, 241
  para discospondilite, 373
  para distúrbios dos sacos anais, 401
  para encefalite, 446
  para encefalopatia isquêmica felina, 453
  para endocardite, 458
  para epididimite/orquite, 479
  para febre, 527
  para febre maculosa das Montanhas Rochosas, 531
  para febre Q, 532
  para gastrenterite, hemorrágica, 567
  para hepatite, supurativa, 610
  para hepatotoxicidade, 622
  para infecção do trato urinário inferior, 736
  para infecções estafilocócicas, 759
  para infecções secundárias à influenza canina, 771
  para infertilidade, macho, 767
  para inflamação orofaríngea felina, 770

para mastite, 860
para metrite, 882
para micoplasmose hemotrópica, 1179
para neutropenia, 947
para obstrução de ducto biliar, 954
para obstrução gastrintestinal, 959
para osteomielite, 974
para otite externa/média, 980
para otite média/interna, 983
para pancreatite, 987
para peritonite, 1028
para peritonite biliar, 1028
para piometra, 1043
para pneumonia, bacteriana, 1054
para prostatite, 1095, 1096
para prostatopatia em cão macho reprodutor, 1098
para salmonelose, 1145
para síndrome colangite/colangio-hepatite, 1164
para traqueobronquite infecciosa canina, 1263
para tuberculose, 762
Entamoeba histolytica, 72
Enteropatia causada pelo glúten em Setter irlandês, 459, 568, 1121
Enteropatia com perda de proteínas, 460-461
Enteropatia imunoproliferativa de Basenjis, 462
Enteropatia inflamatória, 463-464
Enterotoxicose clostrídica, 465-466
Entrópio, 141, 467
Envenenamento pela estricnina, 797
Envenenamento pelo arsênico, 470
Envenenamento pelo cogumelo, 471-474
Envenenamento por rodenticidas anticoagulantes, 475
EPI. *Ver* Enteropatia inflamatória
Epididimite, 476-479
Epífora, 477-478
Epilepsia, 479-480
  em cães, 281-282
  em gatos, 283-284
Epinefrina
  informações de formulações, 1363-1441
  para anafilaxia, 77
  para edema periférico, 438
  para fibrilação ventricular, 540
  para intoxicação por etanol, 798
  para parada ventricular, 1001
Epirrubicina, para tumores uterinos, 1299
Episclerite, 481
Episcleroceratite granulomatosa nodular, 195, 196
Epistaxe, 482-483
Epsiprantel
  informações de formulações, 1363-1441
  para tênias, 1210
Epúlide, 484, 857-858
Equimose, 1036-1037
Ergocalciferol, 1363-1441
Eritema multiforme, 322, 487
Eritrocitose. *Ver* Policitemia
Eritrodermia esfoliativa, 487
Eritromicina
  informações de formulações, 1363-1441
  para acne, 25
  para anorexia, 105
  para bartonelose, 137
  para campilobacteriose, 240, 1237
  para distúrbios da motilidade gástrica, 396
  para esofagite, 489
  para gastrite, crônica, 572

para infecções estreptocócicas, 760
para infertilidade, macho, 767
para leptospirose, 816
para mastite, 860
para micoplasmose, 886
para nocardiose, 950
para piodermite, 1041
para pneumonia, bacteriana, 1054
para prostatite, 1095
para síndrome do vômito bilioso, 1185
para vômito, 1334
Eritropoietina
  para anemia, arregenerativa, 81
  para hiperestrogenismo, 649
  para infecção pelo vírus da leucemia felina (FeLV), 746
  para pancitopenia, 985
  para síndromes mielodisplásicas, 1194
Erliquiose, 485-486
Ertapeném, 1363-1441
Erupções medicamentosas cutâneas, 487
ESA (estenose subaórtica), 501-502
Escavação, 254-255
Escherichia coli, 237-238
Esclerodermia, localizada, 63
Esferocitose, 331, 332
Esmolol
  informações de formulações, 1363-1441
  para choque, cardiogênico, 201
  para feocromocitoma, 535
  para fibrilação atrial, 537
  para miocardite traumática, 913
  para síndrome de Wolff-Parkinson-White, 1182
  para taquicardia supraventricular, 1206
  para taquicardia ventricular, 1208
  para toxicose por veneno de sapo, 1253
Esofagite, 488-489
Espectinomicina, para micoplasmose, 886
Espermatocele, 490
Espinha-bífida, 853-854
Espiramicina, para micoplasmose, 886
Espironolactona
  informações de formulações, 1363-1441
  para ascite, 119, 212, 511, 614, 850
  para desvio portossistêmico, 341
  para endocardiose da valva atrioventricular, 455, 456
  para endocardite, 458
  para estenose da valva atrioventricular, 504
  para hepatite, crônica ativa, 603
  para hipertensão
    portal, 675
    sistêmica, 679
  para hipoalbuminemia, 686
  para insuficiência cardíaca congestiva
    direita, 775
    esquerda, 777
  para miocardiopatia, 900, 902, 908
  para síndrome nefrótica, 1191
Espirro, 491-492
Espirro reverso, 491-492
Esplenectomia, 494
Esplenite, 493
Esplenomegalia, 493-494
Espondilomielopatia cervical, 495-496
Espondilose deformante, 497
Esporotricose, 498
Esquistossomíase canina, 499
Estado epiléptico
  em cães, 281-282

em gatos, 283-284
Estanozolol
informações de formulações, 1363-1441
para estimulação do apetite, 1022
Esteatite, 500
Estenose aórtica, 501-502
Estenose das valvas atrioventriculares, 503-504
Estenose esofágica, 505-506
Estenose espinal, 853-854
Estenose lombossacra, 507-508
Estenose nasofaríngea, 509
Estenose pilórica, 958
Estenose prepucial, 1003
Estenose pulmonar, 510-511
Estenose retal, 512
Estenose subaórtica (ESA), 501-502
Esteroides
para estertor e estridor, 514
para febre familiar do Shar-pei, 529
para gastrenterite, linfocítica-plasmocitária, 569
para hipertensão, pulmonar, 677
para hipopituitarismo, 705
para inclinação da cabeça, 727
para meningoencefalomielite granulomatosa, 727
para paniculite, 988
para pericardite, 1026
para problemas do ombro, 1089
para prurido, 1105
para rinite e sinusite, 1138
para síndrome uveodermatológica, 1193
Esteroides androgênicos, para erliquiose, 486
Estertor, 513-514
Estibgliconato de sódio, para leishmaniose, 814, 1060
Estilbestrol, para incompetência uretral, 731
Estimulantes do apetite, 1022
Estomatite, 515-516
periodontal ulcerativa crônica (EPUC), 1303-1304
ulcerativa, 1303-1304
Estrabismo, 425-426
Estreptomicina
para brucelose, 373
para discospondilite, 373
Estreptoquinase
para hipercoagulabilidade, 647
para hipertensão, pulmonar, 677
para infarto do miocárdio, 734
para tromboembolia aórtica, 1277
para tromboembolia pulmonar, 1280
Estreptozocina
para glucagonoma, 582
para insulinoma, 789
Estridor, 513-514
Estrogênios, para incompetência uretral, 731
Estrongiloidíase, 517
Estrumato. *Ver também* Cloprostenol
para corrimento vaginal, 276
Estupor, 518-519
Etambutol, para tuberculose, 762
Etanol, para intoxicação pelo etilenoglicol, 800
Etidronato dissódico, 1363-1441
Etodolaco
dosagens e indicações, 1363
informações de formulações, 1363-1441
para artrite, 115
para claudicação, 224
para displasia coxofemoral, 377
para displasia do cotovelo, 381

para doença de Legg-Calvé-Perthes, 409
para doença do ligamento cruzado cranial, 416
para espondilose deformante, 497
para hipópio, 704
para luxação patelar, 845
para osteocondrodisplasia, 968
para osteodistrofia hipertrófica, 972
para osteopatia craniomandibular, 975
para panosteíte, 991
para problemas do ombro, 1089
Etretinato
para carcinoma de células escamosas, orelha, 179
para carcinoma de células escamosas, plano nasal, 180
Evacuação domiciliar
pelos cães, 520-521
pelos gatos, 522-524
Exame andrológico, 767
Exoftalmia, 425-426
Exótico de pelo curto, doença renal policística em, 421
Expectorantes
para pneumonia, 1054
para tosse, 1217

F

6-fluoruracila (6-FU), 1363-1441
Facoemulsificação, 191
Falha ovulatória, 525
Famotidina
informações de formulações, 1363-1441
para abdome agudo, 3
para apudoma, 110
para azotemia e uremia, 133
para cisto quadrigeminal, 217
para corpo estranho esofágico, 273
para desvio portossistêmico, 341
para esofagite, 405, 489
para estenose esofágica, 506
para fisalopterose, 544
para gastrite, 570
para hematêmese, 593
para hemorragia gastrintestinal, 850
para hepatite, granulomatosa, 606
para hepatite, infecciosa canina, 607
para hérnia hiatal, 624
para infecção pelo helicobacter, 753
para infecção pelo parvovírus canino, 1017
para insuficiência hepática, aguda, 779
para insuficiência pancreática exócrina, 781
para insuficiência renal, aguda, 783
para insuficiência renal, crônica, 786
para lipidose hepática, 836
para mastocitomas, 862
para megaesôfago, 867
para melena, 870
para meningoencefalomielite, 878
para mucocele da vesícula biliar, 931
para obstrução de ducto biliar, 954
para peritonite biliar, 1028
para refluxo gastresofágico, 1128
para regurgitação, 1130
para toxicidade da vitamina D, 1220
para toxicidade do zinco, 1228
para toxicidade dos agentes anti-inflamatórios não esteroides, 1230
para toxicose por metformina, 1243
para úlcera gastroduodenal, 1302
para vômito, 1332, 1334
Fanciclovir

para conjuntivite herpética, 265
para infecção pelo herpes-vírus felino, 741
Fator de crescimento insulinossímile 1 (IGF-1), níveis em acromegalia felina, 26
Fator estimulante de colônias, 1363-1441
Fatores de conversão para peso-unidade, 1363-1441
Fatores de crescimento hematopoiético recombinantes, para anemia, aplásica, 79
FCP. *Ver* Fosfatidilcolina poli-insaturada
Febantel
para ancilóstomos, 78
para bailisascaríase, 136
para giardíase, 575
para tênias, 1210
para tricúris, 1269
Febre, 526-527
Febre e erupção cutânea dos pântanos. *Ver* Dermatofilose
Febre familiar do Shar-pei, 528-529
Febre maculosa das Montanhas Rochosas, 530-531
Febre Q, 532
Fechamento da fise radial, prematuro, 297
Fechamento da fise ulnar distal, prematuro, 297
FeFV. *Ver* Infecção pelo vírus formador de sincício felino
Felbamato
informações de formulações, 1363-1441
para epilepsia, 480
Felifriend, para agressividade, 57
Feliway
para agressividade, 57, 58
para evacuação domiciliar pelos gatos, 524
para medos, fobias e ansiedades, 556
para realojamento de cães e gatos de abrigo, 1127
para vocalização excessiva, 1330
FeLV. *Ver* Infecção pelo vírus da leucemia felina
Fembendazol
informações de formulações, 1363-1441
para ancilóstomos, 78
para *Angiostrongylus vasorum*, 1060
para capilaríase, 170
para cisticercose, 896
para colite e proctite, 240
para diarreia, 352
para esquistossomíase canina, 499
para estrongiloidíase, 517
para fisalopterose, 544
para giardíase, 575
para nematódeos, 940
para parasitas respiratórios, 1012
para secreção nasal, 1153
para tênias, 1210
para tricúris, 1269
para triquinose, 1270
Feminização testicular, 398
Fenilbutazona, 1363-1441
Fenilefrina
informações de formulações, 1363-1441
para epistaxe, 261
para fibrossarcoma, seios nasais e paranasais, 543
para incompetência uretral, 731
Fenilpropanolamina
informações de formulações, 1363-1441
para bexiga pélvica, 138
para incompetência uretral, 731

1467

para infertilidade, macho, 767
para ureter ectópico, 1305
Fenitoína
informações de formulações, 1363-1441
para epilepsia, 480
para toxicidade da digoxina, 1218
Fenobarbital
informações de formulações, 1363-1441
para cinomose, 210
para cisto quadrigeminal, 217
para crises convulsivas, 126, 282, 284, 447,
794, 871, 875
para encefalopatia isquêmica felina, 453
para epilepsia, 479, 480
para estupor e coma, 519
para fraqueza/colapso induzido por exercício
em Labrador retrievers, 559
para intermação e hipertermia, 791
para lesão cerebral, 818
para meningioma, 871
para meningoencefalomielite, 878
para ptialismo, 1110
para síndrome de hiperestesia felina, 1177
para tétano, 1211
para toxicidade do rodenticida brometalina,
1224
para toxicidade dos agentes anti-inflamatórios
não esteroides, 1230
para toxicose por antidepressivos tricíclicos,
108
para toxicose por chocolate, 1241
para toxicose por pseudoefedrina, 1247
para transtornos compulsivos, 1261
para tumores cerebrais, 1284
Fenoldopam, para oligúria, 966
Fenômeno de Schiff-Sherrington, 533
Fenoterol, para tosse, 1217
Fenotiazinas
para fobias a trovões e relâmpagos, 552
para tétano, 1211
para toxicose por ISRS, 109
para vômito, 1332, 1334
Fenoxibenzamina
informações de formulações, 1363-1441
para discopatia intervertebral, toracolombar,
371
para doença idiopática do trato urinário
inferior dos felinos, 418
para hipertensão, sistêmica, 679
para paralisia pelo carrapato, 1007
para retenção urinária, 1136
Fentanila
dosagens e indicações, 1361
informações de formulações, 1363-1441
para doença idiopática do trato urinário
inferior dos felinos, 418
para dor no pescoço e dorso, 434
para esofagite, 489
para fraturas maxilomandibulares, 563
para osteossarcoma, 978
Fentolamina
informações de formulações, 1363-1441
para feocromocitoma, 535
Feocromocitoma, 534-535
Feromônio(s)
coleira para problemas comportamentais
pediátricos, 1084
para agressividade, 57, 58
para evacuação domiciliar
pelos cães, 521
pelo gatos, 524

para medos, fobias e ansiedades, 556
para realojamento de cães e gatos de abrigo,
1127
para síndrome de ansiedade da separação, 1170
Feromônio apaziguador de cães
para realojamento de cães e gatos de abrigo,
1127
para síndrome de ansiedade da separação, 1170
para transtornos compulsivos, 1259
para vocalização excessiva, 1330
Fibrilação atrial, 536-538
Fibrilação ventricular, 539-540
Fibroma odontogênico periférico. *Ver* Epúlide
Fibrose hepática, 211-212
Fibrossarcoma, 329
da gengiva, 541
de massa bucal, 857, 859
do osso, 542
dos seios nasais e paranasais, 543
Fígado
cirrose e fibrose, 211-212
coagulopatia por hepatopatia, 227
má-formação arteriovenosa do, 849-850
Filgrastim
informações de formulações, 1363-1441
para síndromes mielodisplásicas, 1194
Fimose, 1197
Finasterida
informações de formulações, 1363-1441
para cistos prostáticos, 218
para hiperplasia prostática benigna, 670,
1096
para prostatite, 1095
para prostatopatia em cão macho reprodutor,
1098
Finnish harrier, degeneração cerebelar em, 299,
658
Finnish spitz
anemia, imunomediada, 84
epilepsia, 479
pênfigo, 1019
Fipronil
para controle de carrapato, 189
para controle de pulga, 672
para doença de Chagas, 408
para paralisia pelos carrapatos, 1007
para queiletielose, 1111
Firocoxibe
dosagens e indicações, 1363
informações de formulações, 1363-1441
para condrossarcoma, 258, 260
para doença de Legg-Calvé-Perthes, 409
para fibrossarcoma, 541, 542
para luxações articulares, 847
para osteocondrodisplasia, 968
para osteodistrofia hipertrófica, 972
para osteopatia craniomandibular, 975
para panosteíte, 991
Fisalopterose, 544
Fisiologia de Eisenmenger, 206
Fisostigmina
informações de formulações, 1363-1441
para disautonomia, 945
Fístula arteriovenosa, 545
Fístula oronasal, 546
Fístula perianal, 547
FIV. *Ver* Infecção pelo vírus da imunodeficiência
felina
Flatulência, 548-549
Flavoxato, para instabilidade do detrusor, 731
Flebite, 550

Flebotomia, para síndrome de hiperviscosidade,
1178
Florfenicol, 1363-1441
Flucitosina
informações de formulações, 1363-1441
para aspergilose, 123
Fluconazol
informações de formulações, 1363-1441
para candidíase, 169
para coccidioidomicose, 229
para criptococose, 278
para dermatofitose, 318
para doenças orbitais, 426
para encefalite, 446
para histoplasmose, 721
para inclinação da cabeça, 727
para infecção do trato urinário inferior, 737
para mediastinite, 863
para pneumonia, fúngica, 1058
para prototecose, 1102
para secreção nasal, 1153
Flumazenil
informações de formulações, 1363-1441
para estupor e coma, 519
para toxicose por benzodiazepínicos e
soníferos, 1238
Flumetasona, 1363-1441
Flunixino meglumina
informações de formulações, 1363-1441
para dermatite acral por lambedura, 310
para febre, 527
para hemorragia da retina, 600
para olho cego "silencioso", 962
para olho vermelho, 963
Fluocinolona
para dermatite acral por lambedura, 310
para lúpus eritematoso, cutâneo (discoide),
839
para pênfigo, 1020
para placa eosinofílica, 243
Fluoreto de estanho, para doença periodontal,
420
Fluoroquinolonas
para acne, 25
para ceratite, ulcerativa, 198
para colelitíase, 235
para doença renal policística, 421
para endocardite, 458
para gastrenterite, hemorrágica, 567
para hepatite, infecciosa canina, 607
para infecções micobacterianas, 762
para intermação e hipertermia, 791
para meningite, 875
para micoplasmose, 886
para obstrução gastrintestinal, 959
para otite externa/média, 980
para otite média/interna, 983
para peritonite, 1028
para pneumonia, por aspiração, 1061
para prostatite, 1095
para tuberculose, 762
para tularemia, 1281
Fluoxetina
informações de formulações, 1363-1441
para agressividade, 44, 47, 49, 51, 52, 55,
57-59
para comportamento de marcação territorial e
errático, 249, 250
para comportamentos destrutivos, 252
para coprofagia e pica, 270
para dermatite acral por lambedura, 310

para evacuação domiciliar
   pelos cães, 521
   pelos gatos, 523, 524
para fobias a trovões e relâmpagos, 552
para medos, fobias e ansiedades, 556, 554
para prurido, 1105
para síndrome de ansiedade da separação, 1170
para síndrome de disfunção cognitiva, 1175
para síndrome de hiperestesia felina, 1177
para transtornos compulsivos, 1261, 1259
para vocalização excessiva, 1330
toxicose, 109
Flurazepam, para estimulação do apetite, 1022
Flurbiprofeno
   para cataratas, 191
   para hipópio, 704
   para lacerações da córnea e esclera, 809
   para uveíte anterior, 1320, 1322
Fluticasona
   para asma/bronquite em gatos, 121
   para bronquite, crônica, 165
   para pneumonia, eosinofílica, 1056
   para pneumonia, intersticial, 1060
   para tosse, 1217
Flutter atrial, 536-538
Fobias
   em cães, 553-554
   em gatos, 555-556
Fobias a trovões e relâmpagos, 552
Folato/ácido fólico
   para anemia, 81, 89
   para enteropatia causada pelo glúten em Setter
     irlandês, 459
Fold escocês
   doença renal policística, 421
   hemoglobinúria, 597
   urolitíase, por oxalato de cálcio, 1314
Foliculite, 333, 336
   bacteriana, 333, 336
Fomepizol
   informações de formulações, 1363-1441
   para intoxicação por etanol, 798
   para intoxicação por etilenoglicol, 800
ForBid, 270
Formação/estrutura dos dentes, anormais, 557
Formoterol, para tosse, 1217
Formulações, 1363-1441
Fosfatidilcolina poli-insaturada (FCP), para
   hepatite crônica ativa, 603
Fosfato de potássio
   informações de formulações, 1363-1441
   para hipocalemia, 691
   para hipofosfatemia, 694
   para toxicose por beta-2 agonistas inalatórios,
     1239
Fosfato de primaquina, para babesiose, 135
Fosfato sódico de dexametasona
   para anafilaxia, 77
   para ceratite, eosinofílica, 194
   para condrossarcoma, 259
   para edema cerebral, 871
   para edema pulmonar, 440
   para encefalite, 446
   para gastrenterite, hemorrágica, 567
   para hipoadrenocorticismo, 684
   para intermação e hipertermia, 791
   para luxação do cristalino, 842
   para meningioma, 871
   para obstrução gastrintestinal, 959
   para reações a transfusões sanguíneas, 1124
Fox terrier(s)

degeneração cerebelar, 299
endocardiose da valva atrioventricular, 474
glaucoma, 576
hipotireoidismo, 711
insulinoma, 788
mastocitoma, 329
megaesôfago, 866
miastenia grave, 889
Fox terrier de pelo duro
   atopia, 311
   degeneração cerebelar, 299
   demodicose, 305
   epilepsia, 479
   estenose pulmonar, 510
   hipoplasia cerebelar, 658
   megaesôfago, 866
   mielopatia degenerativa, 896
   ptialismo, 1109
   regurgitação, 1129
Fox terrier de pelo liso
   megaesôfago, 866
   miastenia grave, 883
Foxhound
   amiloidose renal, 427
   amiloidose, 74
   proteinúria, 1100
Foxhound inglês
   amiloidose, 74
   amiloidose renal, 427
   proteinúria, 1100
FPV. *Ver* Parvovírus felino
Fragmentação do processo coronoide medial. *Ver*
   Displasia do cotovelo
Francisella tularensis, 1281
Fraqueza e colapso induzido por exercício em
   Labrador retriever, 558-559
Fratura dos dentes, 560-561
Fraturas mandibulares, 562-563
Fraturas maxilares, 562-563
Furazolidona, 1363-1441
Furosemida
   informações de formulações, 1363-1441
   para anomalia de Ebstein, 95
   para ascite, 119, 511, 614, 850
   para choque, cardiogênico, 201
   para cianose, 207
   para compressão cefálica, 257
   para contusões pulmonares, 268
   para defeito do septo atrial, 288
   para desvio portossistêmico, 341
   para displasia das valvas atrioventriculares, 379
   para disrafismo espinal, 387
   para doenças endomiocárdicas, 424
   para edema periférico, 558
   para edema pulmonar, 819, 440
   para endocardiose das valvas atrioventriculares,
     475
   para endocardite, 478
   para envenenamento pelo cogumelo, 474
   para epistaxe, 443
   para estenose das valvas atrioventriculares, 504
   para estupor e coma, 519
   para hemorragia da retina, 600
   para hepatite, crônica ativa, 603
   para hidrocefalia, 629
   para hipercalcemia, 641
   para hipermagnesemia, 657
   para hiperparatireoidismo, 663
   para hipertensão
     portal, 674
     sistêmica, 679

para hipoalbuminemia, 686
para inalação de fumaça, 725
para insuficiência cardíaca congestiva, 288
   direita, 775
   esquerda, 776
para insuficiência hepática, aguda, 779
para insuficiência renal, aguda, 789
para intermação e hipertermia, 250
para laceração da parede atrial, 807
para lesão cerebral, 818
para lesão por mordedura de fio elétrico, 819
para miocardiopatia, 900, 902, 905, 908, 910
para miocardite, 912
para oligúria, 966
para persistência do ducto arterioso, 1033
para reações a transfusões sanguíneas, 1124
para síndrome da angústia respiratória aguda,
   1167
para síndrome nefrótica, 1191
para siringomielia, 1198
para toxicidade da vitamina D, 1220
para toxicidade de uvas e passas, 1235
para toxicidade do rodenticida brometalina,
   1224
Furto, 254-255
Fusão dentária, 557

G

G-CSF
   para hiperestrogenismo, 649
   para neutropenia, 947
   para pancitopenia, 985
Gabapentina
   informações de formulações, 1363-1441
   para condrossarcoma, 258, 260
   para crises convulsivas, 284
   para dor neuropática, 1363-1441
   para dor no pescoço e dorso, 554
   para epilepsia, 440
   para fibrossarcoma, 541, 542
   para instabilidade atlantoaxial, 773
   para mioclonia, 1187
   para paralisia, 1005
   para síndrome de hiperestesia felina, 1177
   para siringomielia, 1198
   para tremores, 1267
GAGPS. *Ver* Glicosaminoglicano polissulfatado
Galgo
   acidente vascular cerebral isquêmico, 17
   alopecia do pavilhão auricular, 64
   babesiose, 134
   ceratite, 195
   doença de von Willebrand, 412
   estomatite, 515
   hemangiossarcoma, pele, 587
   influenza canina, 771
   mioglobinúria, 597
   poliartrite erosiva, 1066
   policitemia, 1070
   ptialismo, 1109
   trombocitopenia, 986, 1272
   vírus da cinomose, 1059
Galgo italiano
   alopecia do pavilhão auricular, 64
   descolamento da retina, 338
Gamaglobulina, para distúrbios causados por
   imunodeficiência, 394
Gammel Dansk Honsehund, miastenia grave em,
   889
Gangliosidose, 894
Gastrenterite eosinofílica, 564-565

Gastrenterite hemorrágica, 566-567
Gastrenterite linfoplasmocitária, 568-569
Gastrinoma, 110, 1341
Gastrite
  atrófica, 570
  crônica, 571-572
Gastropatia hipertrófica crônica, 958
Gastropatia pilórica hipertrófica crônica, 573-574
Gastroprotetores
  para gastrenterite, hemorrágica, 567
  para hepatite, infecciosa canina, 607
  para mucocele da vesícula biliar, 931
  para obstrução gastrintestinal, 959
  para síndrome de dilatação e vólvulo gástricos, 1173
  para vômito, 1332, 1334
Gato americano de pelo curto, miocardiopatia em, 907
Gato asiático de pelo curto, epúlide em, 484
Gato Birmanês
  blefarite, 141
  ceratite, ulcerativa, 197
  cristalúria, 285
  demodicose, 305
  dermoides, 141
  hipocalemia, 690
  inflamação orofaríngea felina, 770
  lagoftalmia, 141
  miocardiopatia, 904
  prolapso da glândula da terceira pálpebra, 1089
  sequestração corneana, 195
  síndrome de hiperestesia felina, 1177
  transtornos compulsivos, 1260
  urolitíase, por oxalato de cálcio, 1314
Gato britânico de pelo curto
  hemoglobinúria, 597
  miocardiopatia, 907
Gato doméstico de pelo curto
  agenesia palpebral, 477
  amiloide hepático, 73
  anemia, imunomediada, 84
  anemia, regenerativa, 91
  anomalia de Pelger-Huët, 96
  axonopatia, 944
  bronquite, crônica, 164
  ceratite eosinofílica, 195
  deficiência da piruvato quinase, 91, 292
  displasia de fotorreceptores, 102
  distrofia da córnea, 392
  distrofia neuroaxonal, 391
  distrofia neuronal, 894
  doença do armazenamento lisossomal, 422, 658, 944
  esfingomielinose, 894
  fragilidade osmótica eritrocitária, 91
  gangliosidose, 894
  hemangiossarcoma, baço e fígado, 588
  hiperoxalúria primária, 427
  metemoglobinemia, 880
  miocardiopatia, 907
  mucopolissacaridoses, 894, 934
  nefrolitíase, 936
  neuropatias periféricas, 944
  osteossarcoma, 977
  piotórax, 1044
  polioencefalomielite, 1076
  porfiria congênita felina, 91
  síndrome hipereosinofílica, 1189
  tumores das glândulas mamárias, 1290
  urolitíase, por cistina, 1308

urolitíase, por xantina, 1318
xantinúria, 427
Gato doméstico de pelo longo
  nefrolitíase, 936
  paresia/paralisia do nervo facial, 1013
  tumores das glândulas mamárias, 1290
  urolitíase, por xantina, 1318
Gato dos Bosques da Noruega, doença do armazenamento de glicogênio em, 414, 894
Gato himalaio
  arritmia sinusal, 111
  blefarite, 141
  catarata, 190
  ceratite, ulcerativa, 197
  cristalúria, 285
  distocia, 388
  doença renal policística, 340, 421, 427
  entrópio, 467
  evacuação domiciliar, 522
  hemoglobinúria, 597
  hérnia diafragmática, 625
  hiperlipidemia, 654
  inflamação orofaríngea felina, 770
  lagoftalmia, 141
  quilotórax, 1112
  sequestração corneana, 195
  sequestro de córnea, 1157
  síndrome braquicefálica das vias aéreas, 1160
  síndrome colangite/colangio-hepatite, 1163
  síndrome de hiperestesia felina, 1177
  tumor de células basais (basalioma), 329
  urolitíase, por oxalato de cálcio, 1314
Gato Maine Coon
  displasia coxofemoral, 376
  miocardiopatia, 907
Gato Manx
  disgenesia sacrocaudal, 894
  disgenesia sacrococcígea, 853
  disrafismo espinal, 387
  distrofia da córnea, 392
  espinha-bífida, 853
  megacólon, 864
  prolapso retal e anal, 1090
  retenção urinária, 1135
Gato Oriental de pelo curto
  amiloide hepático, 73
  amiloidose, 74
  amiloidose renal, 427
Gato Persa
  arritmia sinusal, 111
  aspergilose, 122
  blefarite, 141
  bloqueio atrioventricular, primeiro grau, 145
  ceratite, ulcerativa, 197
  criptorquidismo, 279
  cristalúria, 285
  dermatoses neoplásicas, 329
  displasia de bastonetes e cones, 102
  displasia de fotorreceptores, 102
  distocia, 388
  distúrbios causados por imunodeficiência, 394
  doença do armazenamento lisossomal, 422, 658
  doença renal policística, 340, 421, 427, 1131
  entrópio, 467
  epúlide, 484
  evacuação domiciliar, 522
  hemoglobinúria, 597
  hérnia diafragmática peritoneopericárdica, 926
  inflamação orofaríngea felina, 770

insuficiência renal, crônica, 785
lagoftalmia, 141
lúpus eritematoso, sistêmico (LES), 840
miocardiopatia, 907
nefrolitíase, 936
prolapso da glândula da terceira pálpebra, 1089
sequestração corneana, 195
sequestro de córnea, 1157
síndrome braquicefálica das vias aéreas, 1160
síndrome colangite/colangio-hepatite, 1163
síndrome de Chediak-Higashi, 140, 321, 394, 1171
tricoepitelioma, 1292
trombocitopatias, 1271
tumor de células basais (basalioma), 329
urolitíase, por oxalato de cálcio, 1314
Gato Ragdoll
  tromboembolia aórtica, 1276
  urolitíase, por oxalato de cálcio, 1314
Gato Sagrado da Birmânia
  axonopatia, 894
  hemoglobinúria, 597
  neuropatias periféricas, 944
  polineuropatia, 944
  tromboembolia aórtica, 1276
Gato Somali
  anemia, regenerativa, 91
  deficiência da piruvato quinase, 91, 292
  fragilidade osmótica eritrocitária, 91
  gengivostomatite, 1303
  hemoglobinúria, 597
  inflamação orofaríngea felina, 989
  miastenia grave, 883
Gato Sphinx (Esfinge)
  alopecia, 65
  miocardiopatia, 907
Gel de carbômer, para sequestro de córnea, 1157
Gel de carboximetilcelulose, para sequestro de córnea, 1157
Gel de hialuronato de sódio, para sequestro de córnea, 1157
Geminação dentária, 557
Gencitabina, para adenocarcinoma
  pâncreas, 36
  pele, 34
Gene ABCB1, toxicidade da ivermectina e, 1231
Genfibrozila
  informações de formulações, 1363-1441
  para hiperlipidemia, 655
Gengivoplastia, 668
Gentamicina
  informações de formulações, 1363-1441
  para bartonelose, 137
  para bronquite, crônica, 165
  para brucelose, 167
  para ceratite, ulcerativa, 198
  para conjuntivite, 263
  para endocardite, 478
  para infecção do trato urinário inferior, 736
  para infecções estafilocócicas, 737
  para infecções estreptocócicas, 760
  para infecções secundárias à influenza canina, 771
  para lacerações da córnea e esclera, 809
  para micoplasmose, 886
  para nocardiose, 950
  para obstrução gastrintestinal, 959
  para otite externa/média, 980
  para peritonite, 1028
  para peste, 1035

para pneumonia, bacteriana, 1054
para sepse e bacteremia, 1156
para traqueobronquite infecciosa canina, 1263
para tularemia, 1281
Gestação/prenhez
falsa (pseudociese), 1106-1107
interrupção, 9-10
perda
em cães, 5-6
em gatos, 7-8
Giardíase, 575
Gingko, para síndrome de disfunção cognitiva, 1175
Glândula da terceira pálpebra, prolapso da, 1089
Glaucoma, 576-577
congênito, 102
Glibionato de cálcio, para hipoparatireoidismo, 703
Gliburida, 1363-1441
Glicerina
informações de formulações, 1363-1441
para glaucoma, 577
Glicocorticoides
para alopecia simétrica felina, 70
para artrite, 119
para cisto quadrigeminal, 217
para dermatite necrolítica superficial, 314
para discopatia intervertebral
cervical, 369
toracolombar, 371
para dor no pescoço e dorso, 434
para erliquiose, 446
para estupor e coma, 519
para febre, 527
para gastrenterite, eosinofílica, 565
para gastrenterite, hemorrágica, 567
para gastrite, crônica, 572
para glucagonoma, 582
para granuloma estéril idiopático, 328
para hepatite, granulomatosa, 606
para hepatopatia diabética, 613
para hepatotoxicidade, 622
para hepatozoonose, 657
para hipoadrenocorticismo, 684
para hipoalbuminemia, 686
para hipopituitarismo, 705
para histiocitose cutânea, 332
para incontinência, fecal, 729
para insulinoma, 789
para lúpus eritematoso, cutâneo (discoide), 839
para micoplasmose hemotrópica, 1962
para Mycoplasma felis, 746
para obstrução gastrintestinal, 959
para osteopatia hipertrófica, 976
para panosteíte, 991
para pênfigo, 1020
para pneumonia, eosinofílica, 1056
para poliartrite
erosiva, 151
não erosiva, 530
para prurido, 1184
para salmonelose, 1145
para síndrome colangite/colangio-hepatite, 1164
para tumores cerebrais, 1284
Gliconato de cálcio
informações de formulações, 1363-1441
para bradicardia sinusal, 162
para eclâmpsia, 435
para hipercalemia, 642

para hipermagnesemia, 657
para hipocalcemia, 389, 689
para hipoparatireoidismo, 703
para inércia uterina, 732
para parada atrial hipercalêmica, 996
para parada ventricular, 1002
Gliconato de potássio
informações de formulações, 1363-1441
para acidose tubular renal, 23
para hipocalemia, 691
para insuficiência renal, crônica, 786
para lipidose hepática, 836
Gliconato de zinco
para glucagonoma, 583
para ulceração bucal, 1304
Gliconato ferroso, para anemia, 90
Glicopirrolato
informações de formulações, 1363-1441
para arritmia sinusal, 111
para bloqueio atrioventricular, segundo
grau-Mobitz Tipo II, 150
para bradicardia sinusal, 162
para parada sinusal/bloqueio sinoatrial, 1363-1441
para ptialismo, 1110
para ritmo idioventricular, 1141
para toxicidade da ivermectina, 1231
Glicosamina
informações de formulações, 1363-1441
para artrite, 115
para claudicação, 224
para displasia coxofemoral, 377
para displasia do cotovelo, 381
para doença de Legg-Calvé-Perthes, 515
para doença do ligamento cruzado cranial, 416
para doença idiopática do trato urinário
inferior dos felinos, 418
para luxação patelar, 845
para osteocondrodisplasia, 968
para osteocondrose, 970
para problemas do ombro, 1089
Glicosaminoglicano polissulfatado (GAGPS)
informações de formulações, 1363-1441
para artrite, 115
para claudicação, 224
para displasia coxofemoral, 377
para displasia do cotovelo, 381
para doença de Legg-Calvé-Perthes, 410
para doença do ligamento cruzado cranial, 416
para luxação patelar, 845
para osteocondrodisplasia, 968
para osteocondrose, 970
para problemas do ombro, 1089
Glicose, para estupor e coma, 519
Glicosúria, 578-579
hiperglicêmica, 578-579
renal primária, 427-428
Glipizida
informações de formulações, 1363-1441
para diabetes melito, 346, 350
para hiperglicemia, 652
Glomerulonefrite, 580-581
Glomerulopatia, 427-428
Glucagon, para insulinoma, 789
Glucagonoma, 582-583
GM-CSF, para hiperestrogenismo, 649
GnRH. *Ver* Hormônio liberador de
gonadotropina
Golden retriever
adenocarcinoma, tireoide, 30
agressividade contra crianças, 49

atopia, 311
blefarite, 141
carcinoma hepatocelular, 185
condrossarcoma, 258, 260, 261
deficiência de espectrina, 91
dermatite acral por lambedura, 310
diabetes melito, 347
displasia coxofemoral, 376
displasia da valva atrioventricular esquerda
(mitral), 378
displasia do cotovelo, 380
displasia renal, 427
disrafismo espinal, 387
distiquíase, 141
distúrbios despigmentantes, 321
distúrbios dos sacos anais, 401
doença de von Willebrand, 412
doenças orbitais, 425
efusão pericárdica, 441
epilepsia, 479
esplenomegalia, 493
estenose aórtica, 501
estenose prepucial, 1003
estertor e estridor, 513
fibrossarcoma, 541
glomerulonefrite, 580
hemangiossarcoma
baço e fígado, 588
coração, 590
osso, 591
hipomielinização, 699
hipotireoidismo, 711
histiocitose, 331, 718
infertilidade, fêmea, 764
insuficiência renal, crônica, 785
insulinoma, 788
laringopatias, 810
linfoma, 830
massas bucais, 857
mastocitoma, 329, 861
miastenia grave, 883
mielopatia degenerativa, 896
mioglobinúria, 597
miosite extraocular, 917
pericardite, 1025
piodermite de filhotes caninos, 193
pododermatite, 1064
tricoepitelioma, 1292
tumores cerebrais, 1284
ureter ectópico, 1305
uveíte anterior, 1319
Gonadorrelina, 1363-1441
Gonadotropina
informações de formulações, 1363-1441
para infertilidade, fêmea, 765
Gonadotropina coriônica humana (hCG)
para criptorquidismo, 279
para degeneração e hipoplasia testiculares, 303
para falha ovulatória, 525
para hiperplasia e prolapso vaginais, 667
para infertilidade, fêmea, 765
para momento oportuno para acasalamento, 157
Gramicidina, para epífora, 478
Grande Pireneus
descolamento da retina, 338
displasia da valva atrioventricular direita
(tricúspide), 378
laringopatias, 810
osteocondrodisplasia, 968
pericardite, 1025

trombocitopatias, 1271
Granisetrona, 1363-1441
Granuloma eosinofílico, 331-332
Granuloma espermático, 490
Granuloma leproide canino, 761-762
Granulomatose linfomatoide, 584
Griseofulvina
    informações de formulações, 1363-1441
    para dermatofitose, 318, 334
    para dermatoses nasais, 328
    para distúrbios das unhas e dos leitos ungueais, 397
Groenendael
    epilepsia, 479
    mioglobinúria, 597
Guaiacolato de glicerol, para envenenamento pela estricnina, 797
Guaifenesina
    informações de formulações, 1363-1441
    para tosse, 1217

H

Halitose, 585
Halotano, 1363-1441
Harmonease, para vocalização excessiva, 1330
Havanês
    anomalia vascular portossistêmica, 98
    displasia microvascular hepatoportal, 382
hCG. *Ver* Gonadotropina coriônica humana
Heloderma spp., 687
Hemácias espiculadas, 87
Hemangiopericitoma, 586
Hemangiossarcoma
    baço e fígado, 588-589
    coração, 590
    osso, 591
    pele, 587
Hematêmese, 592-593
Hematologia
    faixas normais de referência, 1338
    tabela para conversão de unidades, 1339
Hematopoiese cíclica, 207
Hematoquesia, 386
Hematúria, 595-596
Hemeralopia, 102
Hemivértebra, torácica, 853
Hemobartonelose, 1179
Hemocultura, para sepse e bacteremia, 1155-1156
Hemofilia, 295, 482-483
Hemoglobina glutâmer, 1363-1441
Hemoglobinúria, 597-598
Hemorragia, choque hipovolêmico por, 202
Hemorragia da retina, 599-600
Hemotórax, 601
Heparina
    informações de formulações, 1363-1441
    para acidente vascular cerebral isquêmico, 18
    para CID, 227
    para coagulação intravascular disseminada, 225-226
    para dirofilariose, 361
    para edema periférico, 438
    para endocardite, 458
    para flebite, 550
    para hematúria, 595
    para hipercoagulabilidade, 647
    para hipertensão, pulmonar, 677
    para infarto do miocárdio, 734
    para intermação e hipertermia, 791
    para miocardiopatia, 905, 908

para prevenção de tromboembolia pulmonar, 1280
para prevenção de tromboembolia, 85
para reações a transfusões sanguíneas, 1124
para toxicidade do zinco, 1228
para tromboembolia aórtica, 1277
para tromboembolia pulmonar, 1280
Hepatite
    crônica ativa, 602-604
    granulomatosa, 605-606
    infecciosa canina, 607-608
    supurativa, 609-610
Hepatomegalia, 611-612
Hepatopatia diabética, 613
Hepatopatia fibrosante juvenil, 614-615
Hepatopatia por armazenamento de cobre, 616-617
Hepatopatia vacuolar, 619-620
Hepatoprotetores
    para cirrose e fibrose do fígado, 212
    para hepatite, crônica ativa, 604
    para hepatite, infecciosa canina, 607
    para hepatopatia por armazenamento de cobre, 617
    para hepatotoxicidade, 622
    para insuficiência hepática, aguda, 779
Hepatotoxinas, 621-622
Hepatozoonose, 623
Hérnia diafragmática, 625
Hérnia diafragmática peritoneopericárdica, 926
Hérnia hiatal, 624
Hérnia perineal, 627
Hetamido (hidroxietila de amido)
    informações de formulações, 1363-1441
    para ascite, 119
    para choque, séptico, 205
    para colecistite e coledoquite, 233
    para edema periférico, 438
Heterobilharzia americana, 768-769
Heterobilharzíase, 499
Hidralazina
    informações de formulações, 1363-1441
    para endocardiose da valva atrioventricular, 455
    para endocardite, 458
    para hipertensão
        pulmonar, 676
        sistêmica, 640, 641
    para insuficiência cardíaca congestiva, esquerda, 777
    para miocardiopatia, 902
    para persistência do ducto arterioso, 1033
    para síndrome do nó sinusal doente, 1185
Hidrocefalia, 628-629
Hidroclorotiazida
    informações de formulações, 1363-1441
    para ascite, 119
    para diabetes insípido, 342, 659
    para epistaxe, 483
Hidrocodona
    informações de formulações, 1363-1441
    para bronquite, crônica, 165
    para colapso traqueal, 232
    para fraturas maxilomandibulares, 563
    para influenza canina, 771
    para tosse, 617
    para traqueobronquite infecciosa canina, 1263
    para ulceração bucal, 1304
Hidrocortisona
    informações de formulações, 1363-1441
    para conjuntivite, 263, 265

para dermatite actínica, 334
para lúpus eritematoso, 839
para pênfigo, 1020
para prurido, 1105
Hidromorfona
    dosagens e indicações, 1361
    informações de formulações, 1363-1441
    para abdome agudo, 3
    para discopatia intervertebral, toracolombar, 371
    para dor no pescoço e dorso, 434
Hidronefrose, 630
Hidróxido de alumínio
    informações de formulações, 1363-1441
    para hiperfosfatemia, 650
    para hiperparatireoidismo, 664
Hidróxido de magnésio
    informações de formulações, 1363-1441
    para síndrome braquicefálica das vias aéreas, 1161
Hidroxietila de amido (hetamido)
    para ascite, 119
    para colecistite e coledoquite, 233
    para edema periférico, 438
Hidroxiureia
    informações de formulações, 1363-1441
    para distúrbios mieloproliferativos, 402
    para meningioma, 872
    para persistência do ducto arterioso, 1033
    para policitemia, 1071, 1073
    para síndrome hipereosinofílica, 1189
    para síndromes mielodisplásicas, 1194
Hidroxizina
    informações de formulações, 1363-1441
    para dermatite acral por lambedura, 310
    para dermatite atópica, 312
    para prurido, 1105
    para rinite e sinusite, 1138
Hifema, 631-651
Hiosciamina
    para bloqueio atrioventricular, segundo grau-Mobitz Tipo II, 150
    para bradicardia sinusal, 162
    para parada sinusal/bloqueio sinoatrial, 1000
    para síndrome do nó sinusal doente, 1185
Hiperadrenocorticismo
    alopecia, 63, 65
    em cães, 633-636
    em gatos, 637
Hiperandrogenismo, 638-639
    alopecia com, 63, 67, 68, 638
Hiperbilirrubinemia, manchas nos dentes por, 308
Hipercalcemia, 640-641
Hipercalemia, 642-643
Hipercapnia, 644-645
Hipercloremia, 646
Hipercoagulabilidade, 647
Hiperestrogenismo, 648-649
    alopecia com, 63, 67, 68
Hiperfosfatemia, 650-651
Hiperglicemia, 652-653
Hiperlactatemia, 19-20
Hiperlipidemia, 654-655
Hipermagnesemia, 656-657
Hipermetria, 658
Hipernatremia, 659
Hiperosmolaridade, 660-661
Hiperoxalúria, 427
Hiperparatireoidismo, 662-663
    secundário renal, 664-665

Hiperplasia das glândulas mamárias, 666
Hiperplasia e prolapso vaginais, 667
Hiperplasia endometrial cística, 1042-1043
Hiperplasia gengival, 668
Hiperplasia nodular hepática, 669
Hiperplasia prostática benigna, 670, 1097-1098, 1096
Hipersensibilidade
  à picada de pulga, 671-672
  dermatite atópica, 311-312
  por Staphylococcus, 141-142
  reações alimentares
    dermatológicas, 1123-1124
    gastrintestinais, 1121-1122
  tipo I, 76, 141, 487
  tipo II, 141, 407
  tipo III, 487
  vasculite, 487
Hipertensão
  epistaxe com, 482-483
  portal, 673-674
  pulmonar, 675-677
  sistêmica, 678-679
Hipertermia, 790-791
Hipertireoidismo, 65, 681-682
Hiperuricúria, 427
Hipoadrenocorticismo, 683-684
Hipoalbuminemia, 685-686
Hipoandrogenismo, 687
Hipocalcemia, 688-689
  eclâmpsia, 435
Hipocalemia, 690-691
Hipocloremia, 692
Hipocondrodisplasia, 968
Hipofisectomia, para acromegalia em gatos, 26
Hipofosfatemia, 693-694
Hipoglicemia, 695-696
Hipoluteoidismo, 7
Hipomagnesemia, 697-698
Hipomielinização, 699
Hiponatremia, 700
Hipoparatireoidismo, 701-703
Hipopigmentação nasal sazonal, 321
Hipópio, 704
Hipopituitarismo, 705
Hipoplasia cerebelar, 706
Hipoplasia do nervo óptico, 102-103
Hipoplasia/hipocalcificação do esmalte, 707
Hipoplasia tímica, 394
Hipospadias, 398
Hipossensibilização, para dermatite atópica, 312
Hipostenúria, 708
Hipotermia, 709-710
Hipotireoidismo, 711-713
Hipotricose felina, 65
Hipoxemia, 714-715
  arterial, 206
Hipromelose, para sequestro de córnea, 1157
Histiocitoma fibroso maligno, 717
Histiocitose
  em cães, 718-719
  maligna, 331-332
Histoplasmose, 720-721
Hordéolo, 141
Hormônio de crescimento
  excesso em acromegalia em gatos, 26
  informações de formulações, 1363-1441
  para alopecia, 68
  para hiperandrogenismo, 639
  para hipopituitarismo, 705
Hormônio liberador de gonadotropina (GnRH)

informações de formulações, 1363-1441
  para criptorquidismo, 279
  para degeneração e hipoplasia testiculares, 303
  para falha ovulatória, 525
  para hiperestrogenismo, 649
  para hiperplasia e prolapso vaginais, 667
  para infertilidade, fêmea, 765
  para momento oportuno para acasalamento, 157
  para síndrome dos ovários remanescentes, 1188
Huntaway, mucopolissacaridoses em, 934
Husky siberiano
  alopecia X, 64, 67
  coriorretinite, 271
  distrofia da córnea, 392
  distúrbios despigmentantes, 321
  granuloma eosinofílico, 331
  mielopatia degenerativa, 896
  paralisia congênita da laringe, 206
  ureter ectópico, 1305
  uveíte anterior, 1319
  vírus da cinomose, 1059

I

Ibuprofeno, 1363-1441
Icterícia, 722-723
Idoxuridina
  para ceratite não ulcerativa, 196
  para conjuntivite herpética, 265
Ifosfamida
  para fibrossarcoma, seios nasais e paranasais, 543
  para sarcoma associado à vacina, 1146
IGF-1 (fator de crescimento insulinossímile 1), níveis em acromegalia felina, 26
Íleo paralítico, 724
Ilomostato, para traumatismo da coluna vertebral, 1265
Imersão com soluções sulfuradas
  para dermatofitose, 318
  para infecção pelo Notoedres, 142
  para prurido, 1054
  para sarna notoédrica, 1149
  para sarna sarcóptica, 1129
Imersão de mercaptometil ftalimida, para sarna sarcóptica, 1150
Imidaclorida
  para ácaros otológicos, 14
  para carcinoma de células escamosas, pele, 176
  para carcinoma de células escamosas, plano nasal, 180
  para controle de pulga, 672
  para queiletielose, 1111
  para sarna sarcóptica, 1150
Imipeném
  informações de formulações, 1363-1441
  para hepatotoxicidade, 622
  para infecções anaeróbias, 757
  para otite externa/média, 980
Imipramina
  informações de formulações, 1363-1441
  para incompetência uretral, 731
  para instabilidade do detrusor, 731
  para narcolepsia, 935
  toxicose, 107
Imiquimode
  para carcinoma bowenoide *in situ* em gatos, 337
  para carcinoma de células escamosas, orelha, 179

para distúrbios despigmentantes, 322
  para linfoma, cutâneo epiteliotrópico, 834
  para papilomatose, 994
Imunodeficiência combinada grave, 394
  ligada ao cromossomo X, 394
Imunoglobulina, para paralisia do Coonhound, 1009
Imunoglobulina humana
  para anemia imunomediada, 85
  para epistaxe, 483
Imunorreatividade semelhante à da tripsina (TLI), 780
Imunorregulina
  para infecção pelo vírus da imunodeficiência felina (FIV), 744
  para infecção pelo vírus da leucemia felina (FeLV), 746
Imunoterapia
  para dermatite atópica, 312
  para tumores melanocíticos, bucais, 1294
Inalação de fumaça, 725
Inclinação da cabeça, 726-727
Incontinência fecal, 728-729
Incontinência urinária, 730-731
Inércia uterina, 388-390, 732
Infarto do miocárdio, 733-734
Infecção de disco intervertebral. *Ver* Discospondilite
Infecção do trato urinário inferior
  bacteriana, 735-736
  fúngica, 737
Infecção pelo calicivírus felino, 738-739
Infecção pelo parvovírus canino, 1016-1017
Infecção pelo poxvírus, em gatos, 740
Infecção pelo reovírus, 756
Infecção pelo rotavírus, 763
Infecção pelo vírus da imunodeficiência felina (FIV), 741-742
Infecção pelo vírus da leucemia felina (FeLV), 743-744
Infecção pelo vírus da pseudorraiva, 745
Infecção pelo vírus do Oeste do Nilo, 747
Infecção pelo vírus formador de sincício felino (FeFV), 746
Infecção por astrovírus, 748
Infecção por coronavírus, em cães, 749
Infecção por helicobacter, 750-751
Infecção por herpes-vírus, em cães, 752
Infecção por herpes-vírus, em gatos, 753-754
Infecção por *Ollulanis*, 755
Infecções anaeróbias, 757
Infecções estafilocócicas, 759
Infecções estreptocócicas, 769
Infecções micobacterianas, 761-762
Infecções pelas formas L bacterianas, 758
Infertilidade em cães
  na fêmea, 764-765
  no macho, 766-767
Infestação pela fascíola hepática, 768
Inflamação orofaríngea felina, 770
Influenza canina, 771
Inibidor da anidrase carbônica
  para disrafismo espinal, 387
  para glaucoma, 577
  para hidrocefalia, 629
  para hifema, 632
  para luxação do cristalino, 842
Inibidores da aldose redutase, para cataratas, 191
Inibidores da bomba de prótons
  para gastrite, 570
  para gastropatia pilórica hipertrófica, 573

para hérnia hiatal, 624
para intermação e hipertermia, 791
para regurgitação, 1130
para siringomielia, 1198
para toxicidade do zinco, 1228
para vômito, 1334
Inibidores da enzima conversora de angiotenstina (ECA)
para acidente vascular cerebral isquêmico, 18
para displasia das valvas atrioventriculares, 379
para endocardiose das valvas atrioventriculares, 455-456
para endocardite, 458
para epistaxe, 483
para febre familiar do Shar-pei, 529
para glomerulonefrite, 581
para hipertensão
pulmonar, 676
sistêmica, 679
para insuficiência cardíaca congestiva
direita, 775
esquerda, 777
para insuficiência renal, crônica, 786
para laceração da parede atrial, 807
para miocardiopatia, 902, 906, 908, 910
para proteinúria, 1191,1101
para síndrome nefrótica, 1191
para taquicardia sinusal, 1204
Inibidores da fosfodiesterase tipo IV, para hipertensão pulmonar, 676
Inibidores seletivos de recaptação da serotonina (ISRS)
para agressividade, 47, 49, 51, 52, 55, 57-59
para comportamento de marcação territorial e errático, 249
para comportamentos destrutivos, 252
para coprofagia e pica, 270
para dermatite acral por lambedura, 310
para evacuação domiciliar pelos cães, 521
para fobias a trovões e relâmpagos, 552
para medos, fobias e ansiedades, 556, 554
para síndrome de ansiedade da separação, 1170
para síndrome de hiperestesia felina, 1177
para transtornos compulsivos, 1259, 1261
para vocalização excessiva, 1330
toxicose, 109
Instabilidade atlantoaxial, 772-773, 853, 854
Instabilidade do detrusor, 730-731
Insuficiência cardíaca
congestiva, direita, 774-775
congestiva, esquerda, 776-777
Insuficiência cardíaca congestiva
direita, 774-775
esquerda, 776-777
Insuficiência hepática aguda, 778-779
Insuficiência pancreática exócrina (IPE), 780-781
Insuficiência renal
crônica, 785-787
uremia aguda, 782-784
Insulina
informações de formulações, 1363-1441
para diabetes melito
com cetoacidose, 343-344
com coma hiperosmolar, 346
sem complicação, 348, 350
para hipercalemia, 642
para hiperfosfatemia, 650
para hiperglicemia, 652
para hiperglicemia em lesão cerebral, 818
Insulinoma, 788-789
Interferona

informações de formulações, 1363-1441
para carcinoide e síndrome carcinoide, 171
para complexo granuloma eosinofílico, 243
para estomatite, 516
para herpesvírus em gatos, 337
para infecção pelo vírus da imunodeficiência felina (FIV), 744
para infecção pelo vírus da leucemia felina (FeLV), 746
para inflamação orofaríngea felina, 770
para papilomatose, 994
para papilomavírus em cães, 337
para peritonite infecciosa felina, 1031
para rinite e sinusite, 1138
para sequestro de córnea, 1157
para síndromes mielodisplásicas, 1194
para úlcera indolente, 243
Intermação, 790-791
Intoxicação, 468-469
Intoxicação alimentar pelo salmão, 792
Intoxicação pelo chumbo, 793-794
Intoxicação pelo lírio, 795
Intoxicação por ácido acetilsalicílico, 796
Intoxicação por estricnina, 797
Intoxicação por etanol, 798
Intoxicação por etilenoglicol, 799
Intoxicação por metaldeído, 801
Introdução de novos animais de estimação na família, 802-803
Intussuscepção, 804-805
Iodeto de potássio
informações de formulações, 1363-1441
para esporotricose, 498
para prototecose, 1102
Ioimbina
informações de formulações, 1363-1441
para intoxicação por etanol, 798
para narcolepsia, 935
para toxicose por amitraz, 1233-1234
IPE. *Ver* Insuficiência pancreática exócrina
Ipodato
informações de formulações, 1363-1441
para hipertireoidismo, 682
Irrigação nasolacrimal, 477
Isetionato de pentamidina, para pneumocistose, 1052
Isoflurano, 1363-1441
Isoniazida
informações de formulações, 1363-1441
para tuberculose, 762
Isopropamida, para síndrome do intestino irritável, 1183
Isoproterenol
informações de formulações, 1363-1441
para bloqueio atrioventricular, segundo grau-Mobitz Tipo II, 150
para bloqueio atrioventricular, terceiro grau (completo), 144
para bradicardia sinusal, 162
para choque, cardiogênico, 201
para parada sinusal/bloqueio sinoatrial, 1000
para ritmo idioventricular, 1141
Isospora spp., 230
Isotretinoína
informações de formulações, 1363-1441
para acne, 24, 25, 333
para adenite sebácea, 28, 333
para dermatoses esfoliativas, 326
para linfoma, cutâneo epiteliotrópico, 834
para tumores dos folículos pilosos, 1292

ISRS. *Ver* Inibidores seletivos de recaptação da serotonina
Itraconazol
informações de formulações, 1363-1441
para aspergilose, 122-123, 125
para blastomicose, 140
para candidíase, 169
para coccidioidomicose, 229
para criptococose, 278
para dermatofitose, 318, 334
para dermatoses nasais, 328
para distúrbios das unhas e dos leitos ungueais, 397
para encefalite, 446
para esporotricose, 498
para hemorragia da retina, 600
para histoplasmose, 240, 721
para inclinação da cabeça, 727
para infecção do trato urinário inferior, 737
para mediastinite, 863
para osteomielite, 974
para otite externa/média, 980
para pitiose, 1047
para pneumonia, eosinofílica, 1056
para pneumonia, fúngica, 1058
para prototecose, 1102
para secreção nasal, 1153
toxicidade, 140
Ivermectina
informações de formulações, 1363-1441
para ácaros otológicos, 14
para ancilóstomos, 78
para *Angiostrongylus vasorum*, 339
para bailisascaríase, 136
para capilaríase, 170
para cuterebrose, 287
para demodicose, 25, 142, 306
para *Dioctophyma renale* (verme renal gigante), 359
para dirofilariose, 361
para encefalite secundária à migração parasitária, 448
para encefalopatia isquêmica felina, 453
para espirro, 492
para estrongiloidíase, 517
para fisalopterose, 544
para nematódeos, 940
para parasitas respiratórios, 1012
para prevenção de dirofilariose, 362
para queiletielose, 1111
para rinite e sinusite, 1138
para sarna notoédrica, 1149
para sarna sarcóptica, 1150
para secreção nasal, 1153

J

Jack Russell terrier
deformidades do crescimento antebraquial, 297
distrofia neuroaxonal, 391
distúrbios causados por imunodeficiência, 394
imunodeficiência combinada grave (IDCG), 394
má-absorção da cobalamina, 848
megaesôfago, 866
miastenia grave, 883
miopatia mitocondrial, 924
problemas comportamentais maternos, 1081
surdez, 1202

K

Keeshond
alopecia X, 64, 67
diabetes melito, 347
fisiologia de Eisenmenger, 206
epilepsia, 479
hiperparatireoidismo, 662
hiperparatireoidismo primário, 640
displasia renal, 427
tetralogia de Fallot, 1212
Kelpie australiano, abiotrofia cerebelar em, 658
Kerry blue terrier
abiotrofia cerebelar, 658
degeneração cerebelar, 299
dermatoses neoplásicas, 329
distúrbios do desenvolvimento sexual, 398
mielopatia degenerativa, 896
papiloma, 329
pilomatrixoma, 1292
Kooiker holandês
doença de von Willebrand, 412
insuficiência renal, crônica, 785
Korat
doença do armazenamento lisossomal, 422
gangliosidose, 894
Kuvasz
dermatomiosite, 319
mielopatia degenerativa, 896
osteodistrofia hipertrófica, 974

L

L-asparaginase
informações de formulações, 1363-1441
para leucemia, linfoblástica aguda, 820
para linfoma em cães, 831
L-aspartato, para encefalopatia hepática, 451
L-carnitina
para deficiência de carnitina, 293
para degeneração cerebelar, 299
para encefalopatia hepática, 451
para insuficiência cardíaca congestiva
direita, 775
esquerda, 777
para lipidose hepática, 836
para miocardiopatia, 900, 902
para miopatia, 922, 923, 925
L-deprenil. *Ver* Selegilina
L-dopa (levodopa), 1363-1441
L-lisina
para herpesvírus em gatos, 337
para rinite e sinusite, 1138
L-ornitina, para encefalopatia hepática, 451
L-Teanina
para transtornos compulsivos, 1259
para vocalização excessiva, 1330
L-tiroxina. *Ver* Levotiroxina
L-Triptofano
para agressividade, 45
para transtornos compulsivos, 1261
Labetolol, para hipertensão, 679, 680
Labrador retriever
agressividade contra crianças, 49
alopecia por diluição da cor, 64
artrite, séptica, 116
aterosclerose, 129
blefarite, 141
brucelose, 166
carcinoma de células escamosas, dedos, 181
carcinoma de células escamosas, plano nasal, 180
carcinoma de ducto biliar, 184

cáries dentárias, 186
degeneração cerebelar, 299
dermatite acral por lambedura, 310
descolamento da retina, 102, 338
displasia coxofemoral, 376
displasia da valva atrioventricular direita
(tricúspide), 378
displasia da valva atrioventricular esquerda
(mitral), 378
displasia do cotovelo, 380
distiquíase, 141
distocia, 388
distúrbios despigmentantes, 321
doença do armazenamento lisossomal, 422
doença do ligamento cruzado cranial, 415
edema periférico, 437
entrópio, 141, 477
epilepsia, 479
esplenomegalia, 493
estenose da valva atrioventricular direita
(tricúspide), 503
estertor e estridor, 513
fraqueza/colapso induzido por exercício, 558-559
glicosúria, 578
glomerulonefrite, 580
hemorragia da retina, 599
hepatite, crônica ativa, 602
hepatopatia por armazenamento de cobre, 616
hepatotoxinas, 621
hiperplasia e prolapso vaginais, 667
hipertensão, portal, 673
hipoparatireoidismo, 701
hipotricose, 63
histiocitoma, 329, 716
histiocitose, 331, 718
icterícia, 722
infecção pelo parvovírus canino, 1016
insulinoma, 788
laringopatias, 810
linfedema, 829
lipoma, 329, 837, 838
mastocitoma, 329, 861
megaesôfago, 866
miastenia grave, 883
mielopatia degenerativa, 896
mioclonia, 1187
miopatia, não inflamatória, 923
mucopolissacaridoses, 934
narcolepsia, 935
osteocondrodisplasia, 968
osteocondrose, 969
osteodistrofia hipertrófica, 971
osteopatia craniomandibular, 975
paraceratose nasal, 327
piotórax, 1044
pitiose, 1046
pododermatite, 1064
regurgitação, 1129
retenção urinária, 1135
taquicardia supraventricular, 1205
tremores, 1266
ureter ectópico, 1305
urolitíase, por cistina, 1308
vômito, crônico, 1333
Laceração da córnea, 808-809
Laceração da esclera, 808-809
Laceração da parede atrial, 806-807
Lactato de cálcio
informações de formulações, 1363-1441
para eclâmpsia, 435

para hipoparatireoidismo, 703
Lactato de etila, para dermatoses esfoliativas, 326
Lactoferrina bovina, para inflamação orofaríngea
felina, 770
Lactulose
informações de formulações, 1363-1441
para constipação e obstipação, 267
para disquesia e hematoquesia, 386
para encefalopatia hepática, 451, 614
para estenose retal, 512
para estupor e coma, 519
para insuficiência hepática, aguda, 779
para megacólon, 865
para obstrução de ducto biliar, 954
para pólipos retoanais, 1078
para prolapso retal e anal, 1090
Lagoftalmia, 141
Lágrimas artificiais
para ceratoconjuntivite seca, 199
para degenerações e infiltrações da córnea, 304
para entrópio, 467
para exoftalmia, 426
Lakeland terrier
defeito do septo ventricular, 289
dermatomiosite, 319
doença de Legg-Calvé-Perthes, 409
Lancashire heeler, anomalia do olho do Collie
em, 97
Landseer, trombocitopatias em, 1271
Lantreotida, para insulinoma, 789
Lapland
atrofia muscular espinal, 944
deficiência de maltase ácida, 924
doença do armazenamento de glicogênio, 414
neuropatias periféricas, 944
Laringopatias, 810-811
Latanoprosta, para glaucoma, 577
Lavagem gástrica
para envenenamento (intoxicação), 468
para estupor e coma, 519
para toxicose por anfetamina, 1236
para toxicose por antidepressivos tricíclicos, 547
para toxicose por chocolate, 1241
para toxicose por ISRS, 109
Laxantes, 267, 386
Leflunomida
informações de formulações, 1363-1441
para encefalite, 446
para histiocitose, 719
para meningoencefalomielite, 878
para poliartrite, erosiva, 1067
para poliartrite, não erosiva, 1069
para trombocitopenia, imunomediada
primária, 1275
Leiomioma, 812
Leiomiossarcoma, 813
Leishmaniose, 814
pneumonia intersticial, 1059-1060
Leonbergers
axonopatia, 944
hipoadrenocorticismo, 683
laringopatias, 810
neuropatias periféricas, 944
Leopardo da Catahoula, surdez em, 1202
Lepra felina, 761-762
Leptospirose, 815-816
Lesão cerebral, 817-818
Lesão da medula espinal. *Ver* Traumatismo da
coluna vertebral
Lesão por mordedura de fio elétrico, 819

Lesões reabsortivas odontoclásticas, em gatos, 186, 484, 1120
Lesões vaginais, adquiridas, 855-856
Leucemia
  linfoblástica aguda, 820
  linfocítica crônica, 821
Leucodermia, 321
Leucoencefalomielopatia, 822
Leucotriquia, 321
Leucovorina, 1363-1441
Levamisol
  informações de formulações, 1363-1441
  para Angiostrongylus vasorum, 1060
  para lúpus eritematoso, sistêmico (LES), 841
  para parasitas respiratórios, 1012
Levetiracetam
  informações de formulações, 1363-1441
  para cisto quadrigeminal, 217
  para crises convulsivas, 282, 284, 871
  para epilepsia, 480
  para meningioma, 871
Levobunalol, para glaucoma, 577
Levodopa (L-dopa), 1363-1441
Levotiroxina
  informações de formulações, 1363-1441
  para bradicardia sinusal, 162
  para hipotireoidismo, 713, 727
  para infertilidade, fêmea, 765
  para mixedema, 927
Lhasa apso
  agressividade, 50
  arritmia sinusal, 111
  atopia, 311
  blefarite, 141
  cílios ectópicos, 400
  cristalúria, 285
  deformidades do crescimento antebraquial, 297
  discopatia intervertebral, toracolombar, 370
  displasia renal, 1258
  distiquíase/triquíase, 477
  distrofia da córnea, 392
  gastrite, crônica, 571
  gastropatia pilórica hipertrófica, 573
  gastropatia pilórica hipertrófica crônica, 958
  hidrocefalia, 628
  hipotricose, 63
  insuficiência renal, crônica, 785
  nefrolitíase, 936
  poliartrite, não erosiva, 1068
  prolapso da glândula da terceira pálpebra, 1089
  tumor das glândulas sebáceas, 329
  urolitíase, por estruvita, 1309
  urolitíase, por oxalato de cálcio, 1314
Librax, para síndrome do intestino irritável, 1183
Lidocaína
  informações de formulações, 1363-1441
  para arritmia ventricular em toxicidade da vitamina D, 1220
  para arritmias ventriculares e morte súbita em Pastor alemão, 113
  para choque, cardiogênico, 201
  para esofagite, 489
  para estenose esofágica, 506
  para fibrilação ventricular, 540
  para infarto do miocárdio, 734
  para intermação e hipertermia, 791
  para miocardiopatia, 902, 905, 910
  para miocardite traumática, 913
  para síndrome de Wolff-Parkinson-White, 1182

para taquicardia ventricular, 1208
para toxicidade da digoxina, 1218
para toxicose por anfetamina, 1236
para toxicose por beta-2 agonistas inalatórios, 1239
para toxicose por chocolate, 1241
para tumores miocárdicos, 1297
Lincomicina
  informações de formulações, 1363-1441
  para mastite, 860
  para piodermite, 1041
Linezolida, 1363-1441
Linfadenite, 823-824
Linfadenopatia, 825-826
Linfangiectasia, 827-828
Linfedema, 829
Linfoma
  cutâneo epiteliotrópico, 834
  em cães, 830-831
  em gatos, 832-833
  epiteliotrópico, 63, 65, 321, 322
Liotironina (T_3)
  informações de formulações, 1363-1441
  para hipotireoidismo, 713
Lipidose hepática, 835-836
Lipoma, 329, 837
  infiltrativo, 838
Lisina
  informações de formulações, 1363-1441
  para ceratite, não ulcerativa, 196
  para conjuntivite herpética, 265
Lisinopril
  informações de formulações, 1363-1441
  para endocardiose da valva atrioventricular, 456
  para miocardiopatia, 902
Lomustina
  informações de formulações, 1363-1441
  para astrocitoma, 126
  para linfoma
    cutâneo epiteliotrópico, 834
    em cães, 831
  para mastocitomas, 862
  para tumores cerebrais, 1284
  para tumores melanocíticos, 1296
  para tumores melanocíticos, bucais, 1294
  para tumores ovarianos, 1298
Loperamida
  informações de formulações, 1363-1441
  para colite e proctite, 240
  para diarreia, 352
  para incontinência, fecal, 729
  para síndrome do intestino irritável, 1183
Lorazepam
  para agressividade, 57
  para síndrome de hiperestesia felina, 1177
  toxicose, 1237-1238
Lufenurona
  informações de formulações, 1363-1441
  para dermatofitose, 318
Lulu da Pomerânia
  colapso traqueal, 206, 231
  criptorquidismo, 279
  distocia, 388
  eclâmpsia, 435
  endocardiose da valva atrioventricular, 454
  hidrocefalia, 628
  instabilidade atlantoaxial, 772
  linfoma, 830
  luxação patelar, 844
  metemoglobinemia, 880

persistência do ducto arterioso, 1032
Lundehund
  enteropatia com perda de proteínas, 460
  enteropatia inflamatória, 463
  gastrenterite linfoplasmocitária, 568
  gastrite, atrófica, 570
  linfangiectasia, 827
Lúpus eritematoso
  cutâneo (discoide), 321, 335, 839
  sistêmico (LES), 321, 335, 840-841
Lurchers, hipomielinização em, 699
Lutalyse. Ver Prostaglandina $F_{2\alpha}$ ($PGF_{2\alpha}$)
Luxação do cristalino, 842
Luxação ou avulsão dos dentes, 843
Luxação patelar, 844-845
Luxações articulares, 846-847

M

2-MPG, para urolitíase, por cistina, 1308
4-metil pirazol
  para intoxicação pelo etilenoglicol, 800
  para intoxicação por etanol, 798
Má-absorção da cobalamina, 848
Má-assimilação, testes para, 780
Má-formação arteriovenosa do fígado, 849-850
Má-formação tipo Chiari, 1198
Macrodontia, 557
Malamute do Alasca
  alopecia X, 64, 67
  colite ulcerativa histiocítica, 241
  degeneração dos cones, 102
  dermatose responsiva ao zinco, 327
  displasia renal, 427
  distrofia da córnea, 392
  distúrbios despigmentantes, 321
  glaucoma, 576
  hemeralopia, 102
  insuficiência renal, crônica, 785
  lúpus eritematoso, cutâneo (discoide), 839
  neuropatias periféricas, 944
  osteocondrodisplasia, 968
  polineuropatia, 944
  síndrome uveodermatológica, 1193
  tumor de glândulas sebáceas, 329
  vírus da cinomose, 1059
Maloclusão dos dentes, 851-852
Maltês
  anomalia vascular portossistêmica, 98
  displasia microvascular hepatoportal, 382
  doença do armazenamento de glicogênio, 414
  encefalite, 445
  encefalite necrosante, 447
  endocardiose da valva atrioventricular, 454
  estomatite, 515
  estomatite periodontal ulcerativa crônica (EPUC), 1303
  glaucoma, 576
  hidrocefalia, 628
  hipermetria/dismetria, 658
  hipertensão, portal, 673
  lipidose hepática, 835
  persistência do ducto arterioso, 1032
  ptialismo, 1109
  síndrome de tremor, 1180
  siringomielia, 1198
  tumores das glândulas mamárias, 1288
Mancha nos dentes, 308-309
Manchester terrier
  alopecia do pavilhão auricular, 64
  doença de Legg-Calvé-Perthes, 409

doença de von Willebrand, 412
glaucoma, 576
Manitol
informações de formulações, 1363-1441
para acidente vascular cerebral hemorrágico, 18
para afogamento (afogamento por um triz), 42
para compressão cefálica, 257
para edema cerebral, 445, 794, 871
para encefalite, 445
para encefalopatia hepática, 451
para estupor e coma, 519
para glaucoma, 577
para hidrocefalia, 629
para insuficiência hepática, aguda, 779
para insuficiência renal, aguda, 783
para intermação e hipertermia, 791
para lesão cerebral, 818
para luxação do cristalino, 842
para meningioma, 871
para oligúria, 966
para papiledema, 993
para toxicidade de uvas e passas, 1248
para toxicidade do rodenticida brometalina, 1224
para tumores cerebrais, 1284
Marbofloxacino
informações de formulações, 1363-1441
para otite externa/média, 980
para otite média/interna, 983
para pneumonia, bacteriana, 1054
Marcação territorial com urina
pelos cães, 520-521
pelos gatos, 522-524
Maropitanto
como antiemético em terapia com cisplatina, 31
informações de formulações, 1363-1441
para abdome agudo, 4
para azotemia e uremia, 133
para hematêmese, 593
para hepatite, granulomatosa, 606
para hepatite, infecciosa canina, 607
para infecção pelo parvovírus canino, 1017
para infestação pela fascíola hepática, 769
para insuficiência hepática, aguda, 779
para insuficiência renal, aguda, 783
para insuficiência renal, crônica, 786
para lipidose hepática, 836
para obstrução gastrintestinal, 959
para otite média/interna, 983
para pancreatite, 987
para peritonite biliar, 1028
para síndrome do intestino irritável, 1183
para úlcera gastroduodenal, 1302
para vômito, 1332
Más-formações congênitas espinais e vertebrais, 853-854
Más-formações occipitoatlantoaxiais, 853-854
Más-formações vaginais e lesões adquiridas, 855-856
Masitinibe, para mastocitomas, 862
Massas bucais, 857-859
Mastiff(s)
acne, 24
cistinúria, 427
colite ulcerativa histiocítica, 241
dermatoses neoplásicas, 329
descolamento da retina, 338
distrofia da córnea, 392
ectrópio, 436

entrópio, 467
estenose pulmonar, 510
hiperplasia e prolapso vaginais, 667
pododermatite, 1064
prolapso da glândula da terceira pálpebra, 1089
ptialismo, 1109
Mastiff francês, glomerulonefrite em, 580
Mastiff tibetano, neuropatia hipertrófica em, 944
Mastite, 860
Mastocitomas, 329, 861-862
Mau egípcio, mioclonia em, 1187
MCD (miocardiopatia dilatada). *Ver* Miocardiopatia, dilatada
MCH (miocardiopatia hipertrófica). *Ver* Miocardiopatia, hipertrófica
Mebendazol, para *Angiostrongylus vasorum*, 1060
Meclizina
informações de formulações, 1363-1441
para nistagmo, 949
para otite média/interna, 983
para vestibulopatia, 1327, 1329
Meclofenamato, 1363-1441
Mecloretamina, para linfoma cutâneo epeliotrópico, 834
Medetomidina, 1363-1441
Mediastinite, 863
Medicamentos ansiolíticos
para comportamento de marcação territorial e errático, 249
para medos, fobias e ansiedades, 554
Medo
em cães, 553-554
em gatos, 555-556
Medroxiprogesterona
informações de formulações, 1363-1441
para hiperplasia prostática benigna, 670, 1096
Megacólon, 864-865
Megaesôfago, 866-867
Melanodermia, 63-64
Melanoma maligno, bucal, 857-858
Melanoma uveal
em cães, 868
em gatos, 869
Melarsomina
informações de formulações, 1363-1441
para dirofilariose, 361
Melatonina
para alopecia X, 68
para hiperandrogenismo, 639
para medos, fobias e ansiedades, 554
Melena, 870
Melfalana
informações de formulações, 1363-1441
para adenocarcinoma, dos sacos anais, 38
para mieloma múltiplo, 893
Meloxicam
dosagens e indicações, 1361-1362
informações de formulações, 1363-1441
para artrite, 115
para cataratas, 191
para claudicação, 224
para condrossarcoma, 260, 258
para displasia do cotovelo, 381
para doença de Legg-Calvé-Perthes, 409
para doença do ligamento cruzado cranial, 416
para doenças orbitais, 426
para dor no pescoço e dorso, 434
para espondilomielopatia cervical, 496
para espondilose deformante, 497
para fibrossarcoma, 541-542

para flebite, 550
para hifema, 632
para hipópio, 704
para luxação patelar, 845
para luxações articulares, 847
para osteocondrodisplasia, 968
para osteodistrofia hipertrófica, 972
para osteopatia craniomandibular, 975
para panosteíte, 991
para problemas do ombro, 1089
para uveíte anterior, 1320, 1322
Membrana pupilar persistente (MPP), 102
Meningioma, 871-872, 1284-1285
Meningite, 874-875
Meningite-arterite responsivas a esteroides, 873
Meningoencefalomielite eosinofílica, 876
Meningoencefalomielite granulomatosa, 877-878
Meningomielite bacteriana, 874-875
Meperidina, 1363-1441
Mepivacaína, 1363-1441
Mercaptopurina
informações de formulações, 1363-1441
para poliartrite, erosiva, 1067
para poliartrite, não erosiva, 1069
Meropeném, 1363-1441
Mesalamina, 1363-1441
Mesilato de desferroxamina
informações de formulações, 1363-1441
para toxicidade do ferro, 1232
Mesilato de imatinibe, para síndrome hipereosinofílica, 1189
Mesotelioma, 879
Metadona, 1363-1441
Metaflumizona, para controle de pulga, 672
Metaiodobenzilguanidina, para carcinoide e síndrome carcinoide, 171
Metaproterenol, 1363-1441
Metazolamida
informações de formulações, 1363-1441
para disrafismo espinal, 387
para glaucoma, 577
para luxação do cristalino, 842
Metemoglobinemia, 880-881
anemia por corpúsculo de Heinz, 88
cianose por, 206-207
Metenamina
informações de formulações, 1363-1441
para doença idiopática do trato urinário inferior dos felinos, 418
Meticilina, para piodermite, 1041
Metilfenidato, para narcolepsia, 935
Metilprednisolona
informações de formulações, 1363-1441
para dermatite atópica, 312
para hipópio, 704
para inflamação orofaríngea felina, 770
para pênfigo, 1020
para placa eosinofílica, 243
para siringomielia, 1198
para trombocitopenia, imunomediada primária, 1275
para uveíte anterior, 1320, 1322
Metilsulfonilmetano (MSM), para amiloidose, 75
Metiltestosterona
informações de formulações, 1363-1441
para alopecia, 68
para hipoandrogenismo, 687
para ureter ectópico, 1305
Metilxantina
para asma/bronquite em gatos, 121
para hipertensão, pulmonar, 677

para síndrome de disfunção cognitiva, 1175
para toxicidade do chocolate, 1240-1241
Metimazol
informações de formulações, 1363-1441
para hipertireoidismo, 682
para tratamento de adenocarcinoma da
tireoide, 31
Metirapona
para hiperadrenocorticismo, 637
para síndrome de fragilidade cutânea felina,
1168
Metocarbamol
informações de formulações, 1363-1441
para discopatia intervertebral, toracolombar,
371
para envenenamento pela estricnina, 797
para envenenamento pelo cogumelo, 474
para toxicidade das piretrinas e dos piretroides,
1221
para toxicose por chocolate, 1241
para toxicose por ISRS, 109
para toxicose por veneno de aranha, 1250
Metoclopramida
informações de formulações, 1363-1441
para abdome agudo, 3
para anorexia, 105
para corpo estranho esofágico, 273
para disautonomia, 363
para distúrbios da motilidade gástrica, 396
para esofagite, 489
para estenose esofágica, 506
para gastrite, 570
para gastrite, crônica, 572
para hematêmese, 593
para hepatite, granulomatosa, 606
para hepatite, infecciosa canina, 607
para hiperplasia das glândulas mamárias, 666
para íleo paralítico, 724
para infecção pelo parvovírus canino, 1017
para infestação pela fascíola hepática, 769
para insuficiência hepática, aguda, 779
para insuficiência renal, aguda, 783
para insuficiência renal, crônica, 786
para lipidose hepática, 836
para megaesôfago, 867
para mucocele da vesícula biliar, 931
para neuropatias periféricas, 945
para obstrução gastrintestinal, 959
para pancreatite, 987
para peritonite biliar, 1028
para refluxo gastresofágico, 1128
para regurgitação, 1130
para retenção urinária, 1136
para síndrome do vômito bilioso, 1185
para toxicidade da vitamina D, 1220
para toxicose por metformina, 1243
para úlcera gastroduodenal, 1302
para vômito, 1332, 1334
Metoexital, 1363-1441
Metoprolol
informações de formulações, 1363-1441
para complexos ventriculares prematuros, 246
para estenose aórtica, 501
para insuficiência cardíaca congestiva,
esquerda, 777
para toxicose por anfetamina, 1236
para toxicose por chocolate, 1241
Metorchis conjunctus, 768
Metotrexato
informações de formulações, 1363-1441
para poliartrite, erosiva, 1067

para síndrome colangite/colangio-hepatite,
1164
Metoxamina, 1363-1441
Metrite, 882
Metronidazol
informações de formulações, 1363-1441
para acne, 333
para amebíase, 72
para babesiose, 135
para colecistite e coledoquite, 233
para colelitíase, 235
para colite e proctite, 240
para colite ulcerativa histiocítica, 240-241
para diarreia, aguda, 352
para diarreia, responsiva a antibióticos, 357
para disbiose do intestino delgado, 365
para distúrbios dos sacos anais, 401
para doença periodontal, 420
para encefalopatia hepática, 451, 614
para enteropatia imunoproliferativa de
Basenjis, 462
para estenose retal, 512
para estomatite, 516
para fístula perianal, 547
para gastrenterite linfoplasmocitária, 569
para gastrite, 570
para gastrite, crônica, 572
para giardíase, 575
para hepatite, infecciosa canina, 607
para hepatite, supurativa, 610
para hepatotoxicidade, 622
para inclinação da cabeça, 727
para infecção pelo helicobacter, 753
para infecção pelo vírus da imunodeficiência
felina (FIV), 744
para infecções anaeróbias, 757
para inflamação orofaríngea felina, 770
para insuficiência hepática, aguda, 779
para meningite, 875
para neutropenia, 947
para obstrução de ducto biliar, 954
para osteomielite, 974
para peritonite biliar, 1028
para piotórax, 1045
para pneumonia, bacteriana, 1054
para síndrome colangite/colangio-hepatite,
1164
para tétano, 1211
para tricomoníase, 1268
para vômito, 1334
Mexiletina
informações de formulações, 1363-1441
para arritmias ventriculares e morte súbita em
Pastor alemão, 113
para choque, cardiogênico, 201
para complexos ventriculares prematuros, 246
para endocardiose da valva atrioventricular,
455
para miocardiopatia, 900, 902
para taquicardia ventricular, 1208
para tumores miocárdicos, 1297
Miastenia grave, 883-884
Mibolerona
informações de formulações, 1363-1441
para problemas comportamentais maternos,
1082
para pseudociese, 1107
para supressão do estro (cio), 765
Micafungina, para aspergilose, 123
Micção inadequada, 522-524
Micção submissa, 521

Micofenolato de mofetila
informações de formulações, 1363-1441
para hepatite, crônica ativa, 603
para miastenia grave, 884
Miconazol
para blefarite, 142
para dermatite por Malassezia, 315
para dermatofitose, 318
para distúrbios das unhas e dos leitos ungueais,
397
Micoplasmose, 885-886
Micoplasmose hemotrópica, 1179
Micotoxicose
aflatoxina, 888
desoxinivalenol, 889
toxinas tremorgênicas, 890
Microdontia, 557
Microftalmia, 102
Microsporidiose. *Ver* Encefalitozoonose
Microsporum spp. *Ver* Dermatofitose
Midazolam
informações de formulações, 1363-1441
para estimulação do apetite, 1022
para internação e hipertermia, 791
para lesão cerebral, 818
toxicose, 1237-166
Midriáticos, para lacerações da córnea e esclera,
809
Mielodisplasia, 853
Mielomalacia da medula espinal, 893
Mieloma múltiplo, 891-892
Mielopatia
degenerativa, 896-897
embólica fibrocartilaginosa, 898-899
paresia/paralisia em gatos, 918-895
Mifepristona, para interrupção da gestação, 10
Migração parasitária, encefalite secundária à, 448
Milbemicina oxima
informações de formulações, 1363-1441
para ácaros otológicos, 14
para ancilóstomos, 78
para bailisascaríase, 136
para demodicose, 142, 306
para espirro, 492
para nematódeos, 940
para parasitas respiratórios, 1012
para prevenção de dirofilariose, 362
para queiletielose, 1111
para rinite e sinusite, 1138
para sarna sarcóptica, 1150
para secreção nasal, 1153
para tricúris, 1269
Minociclina
informações de formulações, 1363-1441
para brucelose, 167
para dermatofilose, 316
para nocardiose, 950
Miocardiopatia
arritmogênica do ventrículo direito, em Boxers,
774
boxer, 900
dilatada
em cães, 901-903
em gatos, 904-905
hipertrófica
em cães, 906
em gatos, 907-908
restritiva, em gatos, 909-910
Miocardite, 911-912
traumática, 913
Mioclonia, 1187

Mioglobinúria, 597-598
Miopatia
    inflamatória focal, 917-918
    inflamatória generalizada, 915-916
    mitocondrial, 924-925
    não inflamatória
        endócrina, 921-922
        hereditária em Labrador retriever, 923
        metabólica, 924-925
Miosite
    doença orbital, 426
    dos músculos da mastigação, 917-918
    extraocular, 917-918
Mirtazapina, 1363-1441
Misoprostol
    informações de formulações, 1363-1441
    para gastrite, crônica, 572
    para hematêmese, 593
    para melena, 870
    para mielomalacia, medula espinal, 893
    para toxicidade dos agentes anti-inflamatórios
        não esteroides, 1230
    para úlcera gastroduodenal, 1302
Mitotano. *Ver* o,p'-DDD
Mitoxantrona
    informações de formulações, 1363-1441
    para adenocarcinoma
        pele, 34
        pulmão, 37
        saco anal, 38
    para carcinoma de células escamosas
        gengiva, 178
        pele, 176
        pulmão, 182
    para carcinoma de células de transição, 173
    para mesotelioma, 879
    para seios nasais e paranasais, 183
    para tumores das glândulas mamárias, em
        gatos, 1291
Mitramicina, para hipercalcemia, 641
Mitratapida, para obesidade, 952
Mixedema, 927
Modificadores da motilidade
    para colite e proctite, 240
    para constipação e obstipação, 267
    para diarreia, 352
    para incontinência, fecal, 729
    para megaesôfago, 867
    para regurgitação, 1130
    para síndrome do intestino irritável, 1183
    para vômito, 1332
Mononitrato de isossorbida, 1363-1441
Montanhês de Berna
    borreliose de Lyme, 158
    coriorretinite, 271
    degeneração cerebelar, 299
    displasia do cotovelo, 380
    doença de von Willebrand, 412
    epilepsia, 479
    glomerulonefrite, 580
    glomerulopatia, 427
    hipomielinização, 699
    histiocitose, 718
    histiocitose maligna, 331
    meningite-arterite responsivas a esteroides,
        433, 873
    mielopatia degenerativa, 896
    miocardiopatia, 901
    osteocondrose, 969
    poliartrite, não erosiva, 1068
    proteinúria, 1100

Mordidas por brincadeira, em cães, 1083-1084
Morfina
    dosagens e indicações, 1361
    informações de formulações, 1363-1441
    para choque, cardiogênico, 201
    para dor no pescoço e dorso, 434
Mortalidade neonatal, 928-929
Mostarda de nitrogênio, para linfoma cutâneo
    epeliotrópico, 834
Movimento giratório, compulsivo, 1258
Moxalactam, para meningite, 875
Moxidectina
    informações de formulações, 1363-1441
    para ácaros otológicos, 14
    para demodicose, 142, 306
    para prevenção de dirofilariose, 362
    para queiletielose, 1111
    para sarna sarcóptica, 1150
Moxifloxacino
    informações de formulações, 1363-1441
    para tuberculose, 762
MPP (membrana pupilar persistente), 427
Mucocele da vesícula biliar, 930-931
Mucocele salivar, 932-933
Mucomyst. *Ver N*-acetilcisteína
Mucopolissacaridoses, 934
Mudança ambiental, para transtornos
    compulsivos, 1258-1259
Mudança comportamental
    introdução de novos animais de estimação na
        família, 464-803
    para agressividade, 47, 51, 52, 54, 58, 59
    para evacuação domiciliar pelos cães, 521
    para medos, fobias e ansiedades em gatos, 555,
        556
    para síndrome de ansiedade da separação,
        1169-1170
    para síndrome de hiperestesia felina, 1177
    para transtornos compulsivos, 1259
Mupirocina
    para acne, 24, 25, 333
    para dermatite acral por lambedura, 310
Muramil tripeptídeo-fosfatidiletanolamina
    encapsulado em lipossomos, para
    hemangiossarcoma, baço e fígado, 589
Músculo infraespinal, contratura fibrótica de,
    1088-1089
Mycoplasma felis, 746

N

N-acetilcisteína
    para encefalopatia hepática, 451
    para hepatite, infecciosa canina, 607
    para hepatotoxicidade, 622
    para insuficiência hepática, aguda, 779
    para metemoglobinemia, 881
    para micotoxicose, 888
    para toxicidade do paracetamol, 88, 207, 1223
Nalbufina, para fraturas maxilomandibulares, 563
Naloxona
    informações de formulações, 1363-1441
    para lacerações da córnea e esclera, 809
Naltrexona
    informações de formulações, 1363-1441
    para dermatite acral por lambedura, 310
Não união do processo ancôneo. *Ver* Displasia do
    cotovelo
Naproxeno, 1363-1441
Narcolepsia, 935
Necrólise epidérmica tóxica, 487
Nefrectomia, para *Dioctophyma renale* (verme

renal gigante), 359
Nefroblastoma, 427-428
Nefrolitíase, 936-937
Nefropatia tubulointersticial, 427-428
Nefrotoxicidade, induzida por medicamentos,
    938-939
Nematódeos, 940
Neossinefrina, para secreção nasal, 1153
Neomicina
    informações de formulações, 1363-1441
    para blefarite, 142
    para campilobacteriose, 168
    para ceratite, ulcerativa, 198
    para doenças orbitais, 426
    para ectrópio, 436
    para encefalopatia hepática, 451, 614
    para epífora, 478
    para insuficiência hepática, aguda, 779
    para lacerações da córnea e esclera, 809
    para obstrução de ducto biliar, 954
    para oftalmia neonatal, 960
    para sequestro de córnea, 1157
Neoplasia. *Ver tipos específicos*
Neorickettsia helminthoeca, 792
Neosporose, 941
Neostigmina, 1363-1441
Neurite do trigêmeo, 942
Neurite óptica, 943
    retrobulbar, 961-962
Neuropatias periféricas, 944-945
Neutropenia, 946-947
Niacina, para hiperlipidemia, 655
Niacinamida
    para adenite sebácea, 28
    para complexo pênfigo/penfigoide bolhoso,
        336
    para dermatoses nodulares estéreis, 334
    para dermatoses nodulares/granulomatosas
        estéreis, 332
    para distúrbios das unhas e dos leitos ungueais,
        397
    para distúrbios despigmentantes, 322
    para episclerite, 481
    para granuloma estéril idiopático, 328
    para hepatopatia diabética, 613
    para lúpus eritematoso, cutâneo (discoide),
        839
    para paniculite, 988
    para pênfigo, 1020
    para vasculite, cutânea, 1325
Nifedipino, 1363-1441
Nifurtimox, para doença de Chagas, 408
Nistagmo, 948-949
Nistatina, para distúrbios das unhas e dos leitos
    ungueais, 397
Nitazoxanida, para criptosporidiose, 280
Nitempiram
    para controle de pulga, 672
    informações de formulações, 1363-1441
Nitrofurantoína
    informações de formulações, 1363-1441
    para infecção do trato urinário inferior, 736
    para micoplasmose, 886
Nitroglicerina
    informações de formulações, 1363-1441
    para doenças endomiocárdicas, 424
    para endocardiose da valva atrioventricular,
        455
    para endocardite, 458
    para estenose da valva atrioventricular,
        504

para insuficiência cardíaca congestiva, esquerda, 777
para miocardiopatia, 905, 908, 910

Nitroprusseto
informações de formulações, 1363-1441
para doenças endomiocárdicas, 424
para endocardiose da valva atrioventricular, 455
para hipertensão, sistêmica, 679, 680
para insuficiência cardíaca congestiva, esquerda, 777
para laceração da parede atrial, 807
para persistência do ducto arterioso, 1033
para toxicose por veneno de aranha, 1250

Nizatidina
informações de formulações, 1363-1441
para distúrbios da motilidade gástrica, 396
para hematêmese, 593
para megaesôfago, 867
para regurgitação, 1130
para síndrome do vômito bilioso, 1185
para úlcera gastroduodenal, 1302

Nocardiose, 950

Norepinefrina
para choque, hipovolêmico, 203
para choque, séptico, 205

Norfloxacino
informações de formulações, 1363-1441
para salmonelose, 1145

Norfolk terrier
anomalia vascular portossistêmica, 98
displasia microvascular hepatoportal, 382
glaucoma, 576

Norwich terrier, glaucoma em, 576

Nova Scotia duck tolling retriever
anomalia do olho do Collie, 97
meningite-arterite responsivas a esteroides, 873

Novifit, para medos, fobias e ansiedades, 554

O

O,p'-DDD (mitotano)
informações de formulações, 1363-1441
para alopecia, 68
para hiperadrenocorticismo, 634-635, 637
para síndrome de fragilidade cutânea felina, 1168

Obesidade, 951-952

Obstipação, 266-267

Obstrução da saída gástrica, 958-959

Obstrução de ducto biliar, 953-955

Obstrução do intestino delgado, 958-959

Obstrução do trato urinário, 956-957
funcional, 1135-1136

Obstrução gastrintestinal, 958-959

Obstrução intestinal, 958-959

OCD. Ver Osteocondrite dissecante

Ocitocina
informações de formulações, 1363-1441
para abortamento, espontâneo, 6
para inércia uterina, 389-390, 732
para metrite, 882
para placenta retida, 1050
para problemas comportamentais maternos, 1082

Octreotida
para carcinoide e síndrome carcinoide, 171
para dermatite necrolítica superficial, 314
para glucagonoma, 582
para hepatopatia diabética, 613
para insulinoma, 789
para quilotórax, 1113

Odontoma, 857, 859

Ofloxacino
para ceratite, ulcerativa, 198
para otite média/interna, 983

Oftalmia neonatal, 960

Old English sheepdog
abiotrofia cerebelar, 658
acidose láctica por exercício, 597
anemia, imunomediada, 84
anemia, regenerativa, 91
anomalia vascular portossistêmica, 98
defeito do septo atrial, 288
degeneração cerebelar, 299
displasia da valva atrioventricular direita (tricúspice), 378
distúrbios despigmentantes, 305
edema periférico, 437
estenose da valva atrioventricular direita (tricúspide), 503
hemoglobinúria, 597
hérnia perineal, 627
linfedema, 829
miopatia mitocondrial, 924
osteocondrose, 969
toxicidade da ivermectina, 1231
trombocitopenia, 1036, 1272, 1274
tumores cerebrais, 1284

Óleo de bebê, para adenite sebácea, 28

Óleo de rícino (mamona), 1363-1441

Óleo de triglicerídios de cadeia média (TCM), 1363-1441

Óleo mineral, 1363-1441

Óleos, para envenenamento (intoxicação), 468

Óleos de peixe, para hiperlipidemia, 655

Olho cego "silencioso", 961-962

Olho de cereja, 1089

Olho vermelho, 963-964

Oligúria, 965-966

Olsalazina, 1363-1441

Omeprazol
informações de formulações, 1363-1441
para apudoma, 110
para cistos subaracnoides, 220
para disrafismo espinal, 387
para esofagite, 489
para estenose esofágica, 506
para gastrite, 570
para hematêmese, 593
para hérnia hiatal, 624
para hidrocefalia, 629
para infecção pelo helicobacter, 753
para insuficiência pancreática exócrina, 781
para insuficiência renal, aguda, 783
para mastocitomas, 862
para megaesôfago, 867
para melena, 870
para obstrução de ducto biliar, 954
para refluxo gastresofágico, 1128
para regurgitação, 1130
para síndrome braquicefálica das vias aéreas, 1161
para siringomielia, 1198
para toxicidade do zinco, 1228
para toxicidade dos agentes anti-inflamatórios não esteroides, 1230
para úlcera gastroduodenal, 1302
para vômito, 1334
toxicose por metformina, 1243

Oncocitoma, 967

Ondansetrona
informações de formulações, 1363-1441

para abdome agudo, 4
para hematêmese, 593
para hepatite, granulomatosa, 606
para hepatite, infecciosa canina, 607
para infecção pelo parvovírus canino, 1017
para infestação pelo fascíola hepática, 769
para insuficiência hepática, aguda, 779
para insuficiência renal, aguda, 783
para insuficiência renal, crônica, 786
para mucocele da vesícula biliar, 931
para peritonite biliar, 1028
para úlcera gastroduodenal, 1302
para vômito, 1334

Onicomadese, 397

Onicomalacia, 397

Onicomicose, 397

Onicorrexe, 397

Opiáceos
para diarreia, 352
para síndrome do intestino irritável, 1183

Opioides
dosagens e indicações
opioides dispensáveis, 1361
opioides parenterais, 1361
para dor, 431
para traumatismo da coluna vertebral, 1265

Oprelvecina, para trombocitopenia, 1273

Orbifloxacino
informações de formulações, 1361
para discospondilite, 373
para distúrbios dos sacos anais, 401
para peritonite, 1028
para tuberculose, 762

Organofosforados, para controle de pulga, 672

Orifícios nasolacrimais imperfurados, 477

Orquite, 476-479

Orquite linfocítica, 766

Osteoartrite, 114-115

Osteocondrite dissecante (OCD), 970
em displasia do cotovelo, 380-381

Osteocondrodisplasia, 968

Osteocondroma, 259

Osteocondrose, 969-970

Osteodistrofia hipertrófica, 971-972

Osteomielite, 973-974

Osteomielite vertebral. Ver Discospondilite

Osteopatia craniomandibular, 975

Osteopatia hipertrófica, 976

Osteossarcoma, 977-978
bucal, 857, 859

Osteotomia de nivelamento do platô da tíbia, 416

Otite externa, 979-981

Otite interna, 982-983

Otite média, 979-983

Otodectes cynotis, 14

Otter hound
trombastenia, 482
trombocitopatias, 1271

Oxacilina
informações de formulações, 1363-1441
para epididimite/orquite, 479
para infecções estafilocócicas, 759
para metrite, 882
para piodermite, 1041

Oxazepam
informações de formulações, 1363-1441
para agressividade, 47, 57
para anorexia, 105, 744
para estimulação do apetite, 1022
para vocalização excessiva, 1330

Oxibutinina
   informações de formulações, 1363-1441
   para disúria e polaciúria, 404
   para instabilidade do detrusor, 731
Oxigênio hiperbárico, para toxicose por veneno
   de aranha, 1249
Oxigenoterapia
   para bronquite, crônica, 164
   para cianose, 207
   para contusões pulmonares, 268
   para dirofilariose, 362
   para dispneia, 385
   para doenças endomiocárdicas, 423
   para endocardiose da valva atrioventricular,
     455
   para hemotórax, 601
   para hipotermia, 710
   para hipoxemia, 714-715
   para inalação de fumaça, 725
   para intermação e hipertermia, 790, 791
   para miocardiopatia, 902, 910
   para reações a transfusões sanguíneas, 1124
   para síndrome da angústia respiratória aguda,
     1167
   para toxicose por monóxido de carbono, 1244
Oximetazolina, para secreção nasal, 1153
Oximetolona
   informações de formulações, 1363-1441
   para erliquiose, 486
Oximorfona
   informações de formulações, 1363-1441
   para discospondilite, 373
   para lacerações da córnea e esclera, 809
Oxitetraciclina
   informações de formulações, 1363-1441
   para ceratite, ulcerativa, 198
   para conjuntivite, 265
   para diarreia, responsiva a antibióticos, 357
   para disbiose do intestino delgado, 365
   para enteropatia imunoproliferativa de
     Basenjis, 462
   para erliquiose, 486
   para febre maculosa das Montanhas Rochosas,
     531
   para intoxicação alimentar pelo salmão, 792
   para micoplasmose hemotrópica, 1179
   para Mycoplasma felis, 746
   para peste, 1035
   para sequestro de córnea, 1157
Oxtrifilina, 1363-1441

P

Pamidronato
   informações de formulações, 1363-1441
   para condrossarcoma, 258, 260
   para fibrossarcoma, 542
   para hipercalcemia, 641, 1220
   para hiperparatireoidismo, 663
Pamoato de pirantel
   informações de formulações, 1363-1441
   para ancilóstomos, 78
   para bailisascaríase, 136
   para fisalopterose, 544
   para giardíase, 575
   para nematódeos, 940
   para tênias, 1210
   para tricúris, 1269
   para vômito, 1334
Pancitopenia, 984-985
Pancreatite, 986-987
Pancrelipase, 1363-1441

Pancurônio, 1363-1441
Paniculite, 988
   nodular estéril, 331-332
Panleucopenia felina, 989-990
Panosteíte, 991-992
Pantoprazol
   informações de formulações, 1363-1441
   para abdome agudo, 3
Papiledema, 993
Papillon, distrofia neuroaxonal em, 391
Papiloma, 329
Papilomatose, 994
Paracetamol
   dosagens e indicações, 1362
   informações de formulações, 1363-1441
   para espondilose deformante, 497
   para osteossarcoma, 978
Parada atrial, 995-996
Parada atrial hipercalêmica, 995-996
Parada cardiopulmonar, 997-998
Parada sinusal, 999-1000
Parada ventricular, 1001-1002
Parafimose, 1003
Paralisia, 1004-1005
Paralisia da laringe, congênita, 206
Paralisia do Coonhound, 1008-1009
Paralisia pelos carrapatos, 1006-1007
Paraplegia, 1004
Paraproteinemia, 1010
Parasitas respiratórios, 1011-1012
Paregórico, 1363-1441
Paresia e paralisia do nervo facial, 1013-1014
Paresia e paralisia em gatos, 894-895
Paromomicina
   para coccidiose, 230
   para criptosporidiose, 280
Paroníquia, 397
Paroxetina
   informações de formulações, 1363-1441
   para agressividade, 44, 47, 51-52, 55, 57, 59
   para comportamento de marcação territorial e
     errático, 249
   para dermatite acral por lambedura, 310
   para evacuação domiciliar pelos gatos, 6
   para fobias a trovões e relâmpagos, 552
   para medos, fobias e ansiedades, 556
   para transtornos compulsivos, 1259, 1261
   toxicose, 109
Parsons Jack Russell terrier, glaucoma em, 576
Parto prematuro, 1015
Parvovírus felino (FPV), 989-990
Pastor alemão
   abdome agudo, 2
   agressividade contra crianças, 49
   amiloidose, 74
   anomalias do anel vascular, 101
   arritmias ventriculares e morte súbita, 113
   artrite, séptica, 116
   aspergilose, 122, 442, 1057
   atrofia muscular espinal, 944
   calcinose circunscrita, 331
   cáries dentárias, 186
   ceratite, superficial crônica, 195
   cistadenocarcinoma, 40
   cistadenocarcinoma renal, 427
   colite, 239
   complexos ventriculares prematuros, 246
   condrossarcoma, 260, 261, 258
   criptorquidismo, 279
   deficiência de enzima desramificante, 924
   deficiência de IgA, 394

dermatofibrose nodular, 331
dermatomiosite, 319
diarreia, responsiva a antibióticos, 357
disbiose do intestino delgado, 364
discospondilite, 372
displasia coxofemoral, 376
displasia da valva atrioventricular direita
   (tricúspide), 378
displasia do cotovelo, 380
distrofia da córnea, 392
distrofia neuroaxonal, 391
distúrbios causados por imunodeficiência, 394
distúrbios despigmentantes, 321
distúrbios dos sacos anais, 401
doença de von Willebrand, 412, 442
doença do armazenamento de glicogênio, 414
doença do armazenamento lisossomal, 422
doenças orbitais, 425
efusão pericárdica, 441
enteropatia inflamatória, 463
epilepsia, 479
erliquiose, 445
esplenomegalia, 493
espondilose deformante, 497
estenose aórtica, 501
estenose lombossacra, 507
estenose prepucial, 1003
febre maculosa das Montanhas Rochosas, 1069
fístula perianal, 547
gastrenterite eosinofílica, 564
gastrenterite linfoplasmocitária, 568
granuloma eosinofílico, 242
granuloma leproide canino, 761
hemangiossarcoma
   baço e fígado, 588
   coração, 590
   osso, 591
   pele, 587
hematúria, 595
hemofilia A, 442
hepatotoxinas, 621
hiperadrenocorticismo, 633
hiperplasia e prolapso vaginais, 667
hipertensão, portal, 673
hipoparatireoidismo, 701
hipopituitarismo, 705
infecção pelo parvovírus canino, 1016
insuficiência pancreática exócrina, 780
insuficiência renal, crônica, 785
insulinoma, 788
intussuscepção, 904
laringopatias, 810
lúpus eritematoso, 335, 327
   cutâneo (discoide), 899
   sistêmico (LES), 840
luxação do cristalino, 842
má-absorção da cobalamina, 844
megaesôfago, 866
mesotelioma, 879
miastenia grave, 889
mieloma múltiplo, 891
mielopatia degenerativa, 896
miocardiopatia, 906
mucocele salivar, 932
mucopolissacaridoses, 934
neuropatia axonal gigante, 944
neuropatias periféricas, 944
osteodistrofia hipertrófica, 971
panosteíte, 991
pênfigo eritematoso, 335, 1019
persistência do ducto arterioso, 1032

piodermite, 1040
pitiose, 1046
pododermatite, 1064
poliartrite, não erosiva, 1068
ptialismo, 1109
regurgitação, 1129
retenção urinária, 1135
síncope, 1159
síndrome de Birt-Hogg-Dube, 1299
síndrome de dilatação e vólvulo gástricos, 958, 1172
síndrome de Scott, 1271
taquicardia ventricular, 1207
torção esplênica, 1215
toxicidade da ivermectina, 1231
transtornos compulsivos, 1258
tricoepitelioma, 1292
tumores das glândulas mamárias, 1288
vasculite, cutânea, 1325
vômito, crônico, 1333
Pastor australiano
anomalia de Pelger-Huët, 96
anomalia do olho do Collie, 97
descolamento da retina, 338
epilepsia, 479
hemorragia da retina, 599
neutropenia, 946
toxicidade da ivermectina, 1231
Pastor belga
epilepsia, 479
hipotricose, 63
mielopatia degenerativa, 896
Pastor de Beauceron, dermatomiosite em, 319
Pastor de Shetland
anemia, regenerativa, 91
anomalia do olho do Collie, 97
carcinoma de células de transição, 172
ceratite, ulcerativa, 197
cílios ectópicos, 400
dentes em lança, 851
dermatomiosite, 319, 327, 335, 915
descolamento da retina, 338
distiquíase/triquíase, 477
distrofia da córnea, 392
distrofia epitelial corneana, 197
distúrbios despigmentantes, 321
doença de von Willebrand, 412, 1036
epilepsia, 479
episclerite, 481
esclerocerarite granulomatosa nodular, 195
glicosúria, 578
hemorragia da retina, 599
hepatopatia vacuolar, 619
hipercolesterolemia, 654
histiocitoma, 329, 716
laceração da parede atrial, 806
lúpus eritematoso, 335, 327
cutâneo (discoide), 839
sistêmico (LES), 840
mielopatia embólica fibrocartilaginosa, 898
mucocele da vesícula biliar, 930
obstrução de ducto biliar, 953
pênfigo, 1019
persistência do ducto arterioso, 1032
pneumocistose, 1052
poliartrite, não erosiva, 1068
toxicidade da ivermectina, 1231
uveíte anterior, 1319
vasculite, cutânea, 1325
Pastores iugoslavos, doença do armazenamento lisossomal em, 658

Pavilhão auricular, carcinoma de células escamosas do, 179
PDA. *Ver* Persistência do ducto arterioso
Pearsonema, 170
Pegvisomanto, para acromegalia em gatos, 26
Peito escavado, 1018
Pelado mexicano, eclâmpsia em, 435
Pembroke Welsh corgi. *Ver também* Welsh corgi
doença de von Willebrand, 412
glomerulonefrite, 580
mielopatia degenerativa, 896
paresia/paralisia do nervo facial, 1013
proteinúria, 1100
telangiectasia renal, 427
Pênfigo, 1019-1020
eritematoso, 321
foliáceo, 321
vulgar, 335
Penfigoide bolhoso, 335, 336
Penicilamina
informações de formulações, 1363-1441
para toxicidade do zinco, 1228
Penicilina
informações de formulações, 1363-1441
para actinomicose, 27
para dermatofilose, 316
para doença renal policística, 421
para endocardite, 458
para infecção do trato urinário inferior, 736
para infecções estafilocócicas, 759
para infecções estreptocócicas, 760
para leptospirose, 816
para meningite, 875
para mortalidade neonatal, 929
para pancreatite, 987
para peritonite, 1028
para piodermite, 1041
para tétano, 1211
Pentobarbital
informações de formulações, 1363-1441
para crises convulsivas, 282, 1221
para envenenamento pela estricnina, 797
para lesão cerebral, 818
para toxicidade dos agentes anti-inflamatórios não esteroides, 1230
para toxicidade dos organofosforados e carbamatos, 1246
para toxicose por chocolate, 1241
para toxicose por pseudoefedrina, 1247
Pentoxifilina
informações de formulações, 1363-1441
para dermatite de contato, 313
para dermatomiosite, 320
para distúrbios das unhas e dos leitos ungueais, 397
para vasculite, cutânea, 1326
para vasculite, sistêmica, 1326
Pequinês
arritmia sinusal, 111
blefarite, 141
carcinoma de células escamosas, pele, 175
deformidades do crescimento antebraquial, 297
discopatia intervertebral, toracolombar, 370
distocia, 388
endocardiose da valva atrioventricular, 454
entrópio, 467
gastropatia pilórica hipertrófica, 573
gastropatia pilórica hipertrófica crônica, 958
hérnia perineal, 627
hidrocefalia, 628

instabilidade atlantoaxial, 772
luxação patelar, 844
osteocondrodisplasia, 968
pododermatite, 1064
síndrome de dilatação e vólvulo gástricos, 1172
triquíase de prega facial, 400
Perda de peso, 1021-1023
Perfuração da traqueia, 1024
Pericardite, 1025-1026
Periocardiocentese
para efusão pericárdica, 441-442
para laceração da parede atrial, 806-807
Peritonite biliar, 1028
Peritonite infecciosa felina (PIF), 1030-1031
Permetrina, para controle de carrapato, 189
Peróxido de benzoíla
para acne, 25, 24, 333
para dermatite acral por lambedura, 310
para dermatoses esfoliativas, 326
Peróxido de hidrogênio
para êmese, 1221, 1230, 1233, 1236, 1241, 1246, 1248
para toxicidade das piretrinas e dos piretroides, 1221
para toxicidade de uvas e passas, 1248
para toxicose por pseudoefedrina, 1247
Perseguição da cauda, 1258
Persistência do ducto arterioso, 1032-1034
Peste, 1035
Petéquias, 1036-1037
$PGF_{2\alpha}$. *Ver* Prostaglandina $F_{2\alpha}$
PIAC (polirradiculoneurite idiopática aguda canina), 1008-1009
Pica, 269-270
Pielonefrite, 1038-1039
PIF. *Ver* Peritonite infecciosa felina
Pilocarpina
para ceratoconjuntivite seca, 199
para disautonomia, 363
para glaucoma, 577
para xeromicteria, 1153
Pilomatrixoma, 1292
Pimecrolimo
para ceratite não ulcerativa, 196
para distúrbios despigmentantes, 322
Pimobendana
informações de formulações, 1363-1441
para choque, cardiogênico, 201
para displasia das valvas atrioventriculares, 379
para endocardiose das valvas atrioventriculares, 455-456
para endocardite, 458
para hipertensão, pulmonar, 676-677
para insuficiência cardíaca congestiva
direita, 775
esquerda, 777
para laceração da parede atrial, 807
para miocardiopatia, 900, 902, 905, 910
para miocardite, 912
para persistência do ducto arterioso, 1033
para taquicardia sinusal, 1204
Pinscher, miniatura
anemia, imunomediada, 84
distrofia da córnea, 392
doença de Legg-Calvé-Perthes, 409
doença de von Willebrand, 412
eclâmpsia, 435
endocardiose da valva atrioventricular, 454
mucopolissacaridoses, 934
Pinscher, toy
hipopituitarismo, 705

1482

Piodermite, 1040-1041
  de filhotes caninos, 1040-1041
  mucocutânea, 321
  superficial, 335
Piometra, 1042-1043
  corrimento vaginal, 275, 276
Piotórax, 1044-1045
Piperacilina
  informações de formulações, 1363-1441
  para peritonite biliar, 1028
Piperazina, 1363-1441
Pirazinamida, para tuberculose, 762
Piretrinas
  para ácaros otológicos, 14
  para controle de pulga, 672
Piridostigmina
  informações de formulações, 1363-1441
  para miastenia grave, 867, 884
  para paralisia, 1005
Pirimetamina
  informações de formulações, 1363-1441
  para hepatozoonose, 623
  para pneumocistose, 1052
  para toxoplasmose, 1257
Piroxicam
  informações de formulações, 1363-1441
  para adenocarcinoma
    gastrintestinal, 35
    nasal, 39
  para carcinoma de células de transição, 173
  para carcinoma de células escamosas
    dedo, 181
    gengiva, 178
    língua, 174
    tonsila, 177
  para disúria e polaciúria, 404
  para espirro, 492
  para hemangiopericitoma, 586
  para hemangiossarcoma
    baço e fígado, 589
    pele, 587
  para prostatopatia em cão macho reprodutor,
    1098
  para rinite e sinusite, 1138
  para secreção nasal, 1153
  para tumores melanocíticos, 1294, 1296
  para tumores vaginais, 1300
Pit bull terrier
  acne, 24
  agressividade, 43, 54
  alopecia por diluição da cor, 64
  babesiose, 134
  distrofia de cones e bastonetes, 102
  hemangiossarcoma, pele, 587
  hiperplasia e prolapso vaginais, 667
  infecção pelo parvovírus canino, 1016
  metemoglobinemia, 880
Pitiose, 1046-1047
Piúria, 1048-1049
Pivalato de desoxicorticosterona, 1363-1441
Placenta retida, 1050
Plasmaferese, para síndrome de hiperviscosidade,
  1178
Plasmocitoma, 1051
  bucal, 857, 859
Platynosomum concinnum, 768
Plicamicina, 1363-1441
Plott hound, mucopolissacaridoses em, 934
Pneumocistose, 1052
Pneumonia
  bacteriana, 1053-1054

eosinofílica, 1055-1056
  fúngica, 1057-1058
  intersticial, 1059-1060
Pneumonia por aspiração, 1061
Pneumotórax, 1062-1063
Pododermatite, 1064-1065
Pointer(s)
  amiloidose, 74
  atrofia muscular espinal, 944
  doença de von Willebrand, 412
  hemangiossarcoma, baço e fígado, 588
  hemivértebra torácica, 853
  miocardiopatia, 906
  neuropatias periféricas, 944
  poliartrite, não erosiva, 1068
  tumores das glândulas mamárias, 1288
Pointer alemão de pelo curto
  acne, 24
  distúrbios despigmentantes, 321
  distúrbios do desenvolvimento sexual, 398
  doença de von Willebrand, 1036, 412
  doença do armazenamento lisossomal, 658,
    422
  encefalite, 447
  hemivértebra torácica, 853
  lúpus eritematoso, sistêmico (LES), 840
  massas bucais, 857
  neuropatias periféricas, 944
  pododermatite, 1064
  poliartrite, não erosiva, 1068
  retenção urinária, 1135
  transtornos compulsivos, 1258
Pointer alemão de pelo duro, doença de von
  Willebrand em, 412
Pointer inglês
  atrofia muscular espinal, 944
  degeneração cerebelar, 299
  neuropatias periféricas, 944
  osteocondrodisplasia, 968
Polaciúria, 403-404
Poliartrite
  erosiva, imunomediada, 1066-1067
  não erosiva, imunomediada, 1068-1069
  progressiva crônica, 746
Policitemia, 1070-1071
Policitemia vera, 1073
Polidipsia, 1079-1080
Polienilfosfatidilcolina, para cirrose e fibrose do
  fígado, 212
Poliestirenossulfonato de sódio, para
  hipercalemia, 643
Polietilenoglicol
  informações de formulações, 1363-1441
  para traumatismo da coluna vertebral, 1265
Polifagia, 1074-1075
Polimiosite, 915-916
Polimixina B
  informações de formulações, 1363-1441
  para blefarite, 142
  para ceratite, ulcerativa, 198
  para doenças orbitais, 426
  para ectrópio, 436
  para epífora, 478
  para infecções secundárias à influenza canina,
    771
  para lacerações da córnea e esclera, 809
  para oftalmia neonatal, 960
  para sequestro de córnea, 1157
  para traqueobronquite infecciosa canina, 1263
Polineuropatias, 944-945
Polioencefalomielite, 1076

Poliose, 321
Polipeptídeo pancreático, 110
Pólipos nasais, 1077
Pólipos nasofaríngeos, 1077
Pólipos retoanais, 1078
Polirradiculoneurite idiopática, 1008-1009
Polirradiculoneurite idiopática aguda canina
  (PIAC), 1008-1009
Polissulfato sódico de pentosana, para doença
  idiopática do trato urinário inferior
  dos felinos, 418
Poliúria, 1079-1080
Poodle(s)
  anemia, regenerativa, 91
  aterosclerose, 129
  blefarite, 141
  carcinoma de células escamosas, pele, 175
  colapso traqueal, 206
  dermatite por Malassezia, 315
  diabetes melito, 347
  discopatia intervertebral, cervical, 368
  distiquíase, 141
  doença de von Willebrand, 412
  edema periférico, 437
  entrópio, 467
  epilepsia, 479
  gastropatia pilórica hipertrófica, 573
  gastropatia pilórica hipertrófica crônica, 958
  glaucoma, 576
  hiperadrenocorticismo, 633
  hipotireoidismo, 711
  hipotricose, 63
  infertilidade, fêmea, 764
  laceração da parede atrial, 806
  linfedema, 829
  lúpus eritematoso, sistêmico (LES), 840
  meningoencefalomielite granulomatosa, 877
  metemoglobinemia, 880
  miniatura
    alopecia X, 67
    anemia, imunomediada, 84
    anemia, regenerativa, 91
    atrofia da íris, 130
    colapso traqueal, 231
    cristalúria, 285
    deficiência da piruvato quinase, 91, 292
    diabetes melito, 343
    discopatia intervertebral, toracolombar, 370
    distiquíase/triquíase, 477
    distocia, 388
    distúrbios dos sacos anais, 401
    doença de von Willebrand, 412
    eclâmpsia, 435
    encefalite, 445
    endocardiose da valva atrioventricular, 454
    gastrenterite, hemorrágica, 566
    gastrite, crônica, 571
    hepatopatia vacuolar, 619
    instabilidade atlantoaxial, 772
    luxação patelar, 844
    luxações do ombro, 846
    mielopatia degenerativa, 896
    mucocele salivar, 932
    narcolepsia, 935
    nefrolitíase, 936
    osteocondrodisplasia, 968
    pancreatite, 986
    persistência do ducto arterioso, 1032
    tumores das glândulas mamárias, 1288
    tumores melanocíticos, bucais, 1294
    ureter ectópico, 1305

urolitíase, por estruvita, 1309
urolitíase, por oxalato de cálcio, 1314
orifícios nasolacrimais imperfurados, 477
otite, 979, 982
paniculite, 988
pilomatrixoma, 1292
poliartrite, não erosiva, 1068
queiletielose, 1111
standard
adenite sebácea, 28
carcinoma de células escamosas, dedo, 181
defeito do septo atrial, 288
displasia renal, 427
epilepsia, 479
hepatite, crônica ativa, 602
hipertensão, portal, 673
hipoadrenocorticismo, 683
insuficiência renal, crônica, 785
insulinoma, 788
mielopatia degenerativa, 896
neuropatias periféricas, 944
torção esplênica, 1215
tricoepitelioma, 1292
vômito, crônico, 1333
toy
atrofia da íris, 130
criptorquidismo, 279
discopatia intervertebral, toracolombar, 370
distúrbios dos sacos anais, 401
doença de Legg-Calvé-Perthes, 409
endocardiose da valva atrioventricular, 454
entrópio, 467
hidrocefalia, 628
hipoparatireoidismo, 701
instabilidade atlantoaxial, 772
luxação patelar, 844
persistência do ducto arterioso, 1032
poliartrite, não erosiva, 1068
trombocitopenia, 1036
tumores das glândulas mamárias, 1288
ureter ectópico, 1305
trombocitopenia, imunomediada, 1274
tumor das glândulas sebáceas, 329
tumor de células basais (basalioma), 1282
Posaconazol
para aspergilose, 123, 125
para doenças orbitais, 426
para pneumonia, fúngica, 1058
Pradofloxacino, 1363-1441
Pralidoxima
informações de formulações, 1363-1441
para toxicidade dos organofosforados e
carbamatos, 1246
Praziquantel
informações de formulações, 1363-1441
para ancilóstomos, 78
para bailisascaríase, 136
para cisticercose, 896
para esquistossomíase canina, 499
para giardíase, 575
para infestação pela fascíola hepática, 769
para intoxicação alimentar pelo salmão, 792
para nematódeos, 940
para parasitas respiratórios, 1012
para tênias, 1210
para tricúris, 1269
Prazosina
informações de formulações, 1363-1441
para discopatia intervertebral, toracolombar,
371
para doença idiopática do trato urinário

inferior dos felinos, 418
para retenção urinária, 1136
para traumatismo da coluna vertebral, 1265
Prednisolona
informações de formulações, 1363-1441
para anafilaxia, 77
para asma/bronquite em gatos, 121
para avulsão do plexo braquial, 131
para blefarite, 142
para bronquite, crônica, 165
para ceratite, eosinofílica, 194
para cirrose e fibrose do fígado, 212
para dermatite atópica, 312
para dermatose linear por IgA, 336
para dirofilariose, 362
para distúrbios despigmentantes, 322
para encefalite necrosante, 447
para episclerite, 481
para erliquiose, 486
para espirro, 492
para estomatite, 516
para fístula perianal, 547
para gastrenterite, linfoplasmocitária, 569
para hemorragia da retina, 600
para hepatite, crônica ativa, 603
para infecção pelo helicobacter, 753
para infecção pelo vírus formador de sincício
felino (FeFV), 746
para infestação pela fascíola hepática, 769
para laringopatias, 811
para linfangiectasia, 828
para lúpus eritematoso sistêmico, 328
para meningite-arterite responsivas a
esteroides, 873
para micoplasmose hemotrópica, 1179
para neutropenia, 1011
para olho cego "silencioso", 962
para otite externa/média, 980
para paralisia, 1005
para pênfigo, 1020
para peritonite infecciosa felina, 1031
para placa eosinofílica, 243
para pneumonia, eosinofílica, 1056
para pneumonia, intersticial, 1060
para pneumonite alérgica, 361
para poliartrite progressiva crônica, 746
para problemas do ombro, 1189
para pustulose eosinofílica estéril, 334, 336
para reações a transfusões sanguíneas, 1124
para rinite e sinusite, 1138
para sarna sarcóptica, 1150
para secreção nasal, 1153
para síndrome colangite/colangio-hepatite,
1164
para síndrome de hiperestesia felina, 1177
para síndrome de tremor, 1180
para siringomielia, 1198
para tosse, 1217
para toxicidade da vitamina D, 1220
para trombocitopenia, imunomediada
primária, 1275
para vasculite, cutânea, 1325
Prednisona
informações de formulações, 1363-1441
para anemia, imunomediada, 85
para artrite, 115
para astrocitoma, 126
para avulsão do plexo braquial, 131
para bronquite, crônica, 165
para cirrose e fibrose do fígado, 212
para cisto quadrigeminal, 217

para cistos subaracnoides, 220
para colapso traqueal, 232
para colite e proctite, 240
para colite ulcerativa histiocítica, 241
para condrossarcoma, 261
para coriorretinite, 272
para corpo estranho esofágico, 273
para dermatite de contato, 313
para dermatomiosite, 320
para descolamento da retina, 339
para disquesia e hematoquesia, 386
para disrafismo espinal, 387
para doenças orbitais, 426
para dor no pescoço e dorso, 434
para edema cerebral, 871
para edema periférico, 438
para encefalite, 446
para encefalite necrosante, 447
para encefalopatia isquêmica felina, 453
para enteropatia imunoproliferativa de
Basenjis, 462
para epistaxe, 483
para erliquiose, 486
para esofagite, 489
para espondilomielopatia cervical, 496
para espondilose deformante, 497
para estenose esofágica, 506
para estenose retal, 512
para estomatite, 516
para febre maculosa das Montanhas Rochosas,
531
para fibrossarcoma, 542
para gastrenterite, eosinofílica, 565
para gastrenterite, linfoplasmocitária, 569
para gastrite, crônica, 572
para granuloma eosinofílico, 243, 332
para granuloma/piogranuloma estéreis,
331-332
para hepatite, crônica ativa, 603
para hidrocefalia, 629
para hifema, 632
para hipoadrenocorticismo, 684
para hipópio, 704
para hipopituitarismo, 705
para inclinação da cabeça, 727
para inflamação orofaríngea felina, 770
para instabilidade atlantoaxial, 773
para insulinoma, 789
para lacerações da córnea e esclera, 809
para lesões estenóticas vaginais, 856
para leucemia
linfoblástica aguda, 820
linfocítica crônica, 821
para linfangiectasia, 828
para linfoma
em cães, 831
em gatos, 833
para lúpus eritematoso
cutâneo (discoide), 839
sistêmico (LES), 841
para mastocitomas, 862
para meningioma, 871
para meningoencefalomielite, 876, 877
para meningoencefalomielite granulomatosa,
727
para mieloma múltiplo, 893
para neurite óptica, 943
para neuropatias periféricas, 945
para osteodistrofia hipertrófica, 972
para osteopatia hipertrófica, 976
para paniculite, 988

para paniculite nodular estéril, 332
para panosteíte, 992
para papiledema, 993
para pênfigo, 1020
para piodermite de filhotes caninos, 1038
para pneumonia, eosinofílica, 1056
para pneumonite alérgica, 361
para poliartrite, erosiva, 1067
para poliartrite, não erosiva, 1069
para pustulose eosinofílica estéril, 334
para sarna sarcóptica, 1150
para síndrome de tremor, 1180
para síndrome hipereosinofílica, 1189
para síndrome uveodermatológica, 1193
para síndromes mielodisplásicas, 1194
para timoma, 1213
para toxoplasmose, 1257
para trombocitopenia, 1037
para tumores da bainha nervosa, 1287
para ulceração bucal, 1304
para uveíte anterior, 1320, 1322
Pregabalina
informações de formulações, 1363-1441
para siringomielia, 1198
Pressão intraocular, 576-577
Priapismo, 1003
Primidona, 1363-1441
Primor, 1363-1441
Probióticos
para diarreia, 352
para enteropatia imunoproliferativa de
Basenjis, 462
para enterotoxicose clostrídica, 466
para flatulência, 549
Problemas comportamentais
comportamento indisciplinado, 254-255
Problemas comportamentais maternos,
1081-1082
Problemas comportamentais pediátricos
em cães, 1083-1084
em gatos, 1085-1086
Problemas do ombro, 1088-1089
Procainamida
informações de formulações, 1363-1441
para anomalia de Ebstein, 95
para choque, cardiogênico, 201
para complexos ventriculares prematuros, 246
para endocardiose da valva atrioventricular,
455
para intermação e hipertermia, 791
para miocardiopatia, 902
para miocardite traumática, 913
para mioclonia, 1197
para síndrome de Wolff-Parkinson-White, 95
para taquicardia supraventricular, 1206
para taquicardia ventricular, 1208
Proclorperazina
informações de formulações, 1363-1441
para anorexia, 105
para hematêmese, 593
para pancreatite, 987
para síndrome do intestino irritável, 1183
Proclorpromazina, para úlcera gastroduodenal,
1302
Proctite, 239-240
Progesterona/progestinas
mensuração sérica, 764
para abortamento, espontâneo, 6, 8
para evacuação domiciliar
pelos cães, 521
pelos gatos, 524

para hiperandrogenismo, 639
para infertilidade, fêmea, 765
para parto prematuro, 1015
Prolapso anal, 1090
Prolapso da glândula da terceira pálpebra, 1089
Prolapso retal, 1090
Prolapso uretral, 1091-1092
Proliferação bacteriana do intestino delgado. *Ver*
Disbiose do intestino delgado
Prometazina, 1363-1441
Propantelina
informações de formulações, 1363-1441
para bloqueio atrioventricular, segundo
grau-Mobitz Tipo II, 150
para bradicardia sinusal, 162
para colite e proctite, 240
para disúria e polaciúria, 404
para instabilidade do detrusor, 731
para parada sinusal/bloqueio sinoatrial, 1000
para síndrome do nó sinusal doente, 1185
Propentofilina, para síndrome de disfunção
cognitiva, 1175
Propileno glicol
para adenite sebácea, 28, 333
para dermatoses esfoliativas, 326
para intoxicação pelo etilenoglicol, 800
Propiltiouracila
informações de formulações, 1363-1441
para hipertireodismo, 682
Propionibacterium acnes, 744, 746
Propiopromazina, 1363-1441
Propofol
informações de formulações, 1363-1441
para crises convulsivas, 284, 1221
para estimulação do apetite, 1022
para lesão cerebral, 818
para toxicidade dos organofosforados e
carbamatos, 1246
para toxicose por pseudoefedrina, 1247
Propranolol
informações de formulações, 1363-1441
para anomalia de Ebstein, 95
para complexos ventriculares prematuros, 246
para descolamento da retina, 339
para epistaxe, 483
para fibrilação atrial, 537
para hipertensão, sistêmica, 680
para miocardiopatia, 910
para miocardite traumática, 913
para síndrome de Wolff-Parkinson-White, 401,
1182
para taquicardia supraventricular, 1206
para tetralogia de Fallot, 1212
para toxicose por anfetamina, 1236
para toxicose por beta-2 agonistas inalatórios,
1239
para toxicose por chocolate, 1241
para toxicose por pseudoefedrina, 1247
para toxicose por veneno de sapo, 1253
Proptose, 1093
Propulsores de clorofluorocarbono, 1239
Prostaglandina E, para gastrite, 572
Prostaglandina $F_{2\alpha}$ (PGF$_{2\alpha}$)
informações de formulações, 1363-1441
para abortamento, espontâneo, 8, 6
para interrupção da gestação, 9-10
para metrite, 882
para piometra, 1043
para remoção do conteúdo uterino e luteólise,
276
Prostaglandinas

para glaucoma, 577
para luxação do cristalino, 842
Prostatite, 1094-1095
em cão macho reprodutor, 1097, 1098
prostatomegalia, 1096
Prostatomegalia, 1096
Prostatopatia, em cão macho reprodutor,
1097-1098
Proteinúria, 1100-1101
Protetores de mucosa
para insuficiência renal, aguda, 783
para ulceração bucal, 1304
Prototecose, 1102
Protrusão da terceira pálpebra, 1102-1103
Prurido, 1104-1105
Pseudoanorexia, 104
Pseudociese, 1106-1107
Pseudocistos perirrenais, 1085
Pseudoefedrina
informações de formulações, 1363-1441
para incompetência uretral, 731
para infertilidade, macho, 767
Pseudo-hermafrodita, 398
Psílio, 1363-1441
Ptialismo, 1109-1110
Pug
anemia, regenerativa, 91
anomalia vascular portossistêmica, 98
arritmia sinusal, 111
atopia, 311
blefarite, 141
bloqueio atrioventricular, segundo grau-
Mobitz Tipo II, 149
bloqueio atrioventricular, terceiro grau
(completo), 143
cistos subaracnoides, 219
deficiência da piruvato quinase, 91, 292
displasia microvascular hepatoportal, 382
distiquíase, 141
distocia, 388
distúrbios do desenvolvimento sexual, 398
encefalia, 445
encefalite necrosante, 447
entrópio, 467
hidrocefalia, 628
mastocitoma, 329, 861
megaesôfago, 866
mielopatia degenerativa, 896
osteocondrodisplasia, 968
papilomatose, 994
para bradicardia sinusal, 161
parada sinusal/bloqueio sinoatrial, 999
ritmo idioventricular, 1140
síncope, 1159
síndrome braquicefálica das vias aéreas, 1160
torção dos lobos pulmonares, 1214
triquíase de prega facial, 400
Pustulose eosinofílica estéril, 335, 336
Pythium spp., 488

Q

Quadriplegia, 1004
Queensland blue heeler, doença do
armazenamento lisossomal em, 658
Queiletielose, 66, 1111
Quelantes
para hepatopatia por armazenamento de cobre,
617
para intoxicação pelo chumbo, 794
Quilotórax, 1112-1113
Quimiodectoma, 1114

Quimioterapia
para adenocarcinoma, 38-31
para astrocitoma, 126
para carcinoma de células escamosas
gengiva, 178
orelha, 179
pele, 176
pulmão, 182
seios nasais e paranasais, 183
tonsila, 177
para carcinoma prostático, 1096
para condrossarcoma, 259-261
para dermatoses neoplásicas, 257
para distúrbios das unhas e dos leitos ungueais, 397
para dor no pescoço e dorso, 434
para efusão pericárdica, 442
para estomatite, 516
para fibrossarcoma
gengiva, 541
osso, 542
seios nasais e paranasais, 543
para glucagonoma, 582
para hemangiopericitoma, 586
para hemangiossarcoma, 587, 589-591
para histiocitoma fibroso maligno, 717
para infecção pelo vírus da leucemia felina (FeLV), 746
para leucemia, linfoblástica aguda, 820
para leucemia, linfocítica crônica, 821
para linfoma
cutâneo epiteliotrópico, 834
em cães, 831
em gatos, 833
para meningioma, 872
para mesotelioma, 879
para osteossarcoma, 978
para pênfigo/penfigoide bolhoso, 336
para pododermatite, 1065
para quimiodectoma, 1114
para rabdomiossarcoma, 1116, 1117
para sarcoma associado à vacina, 1146
para seminoma, 1154
para síndrome hipereosinofílica, 1189
para síndromes mielodisplásicas, 1194
para tumores cerebrais, 1284
para tumores da cavidade bucal, 1294
para tumores das glândulas mamárias
em cães, 1288-1289
em gatos, 1291
para tumores melanocíticos, 1296
para tumores miocárdicos, 1297
para tumores ovarianos, 1298
para tumores uterinos, 1299
para tumores vaginais, 856
Quinidina
informações de formulações, 1363-1441
para fibrilação atrial, 537
para taquicardia supraventricular, 1206
Quinolonas
para colecistite e coledoquite, 233
para conjuntivite, 263
para infecções anaeróbias, 757
para osteomielite, 974
para piotórax, 106
para salmonelose, 1145

R
Rabdomioma, 1115
Rabdomiossarcoma, 1116
bexiga urinária, 1117

Racemetionina, 1363-1441
Radioterapia
para acromegalia em gatos, 26
para adenocarcinoma
glândulas salivares, 33
pele, 34
próstata, 29
pulmão, 37
para astrocitoma, 126
para condrossarcoma, 258, 259, 261
para fibrossarcoma
gengiva, 541
nasal e paranasal, 543
osso, 542
para histiocitoma fibroso maligno, 717
para linfoma, em gatos, 833
para mastocitomas, 862
para meningoencefalomielite, 878
para quimiodectoma, 1114
para tumores cerebrais, 1284
para tumores da bainha nervosa, 1287
Raiva, 1118-1119
Ramosetrona, para síndrome do intestino irritável, 1183
Ranitidina
informações de formulações, 1363-1441
para abdome agudo, 3
para anorexia, 105
para apudoma, 110
para constipação e obstipação, 267
para corpo estranho esofágico, 273
para distúrbios da motilidade gástrica, 396
para esofagite, 405, 489
para estenose esofágica, 506
para hematêmese, 593
para hérnia hiatal, 624
para infecção pelo helicobacter, 753
para infecção pelo parvovírus canino, 1017
para insuficiência pancreática exócrina, 781
para insuficiência renal, aguda, 783
para insuficiência renal, crônica, 786
para megaesôfago, 867
para melena, 870
para obstrução gastrintestinal, 959
para refluxo gastresofágico, 1128
para regurgitação, 1130
para síndrome do vômito bilioso, 1185
para toxicidade do zinco, 1228
para toxicidade dos agentes anti-inflamatórios não esteroides, 1230
para úlcera gastroduodenal, 1302
para vômito, 1332, 1334
toxicose por metformina, 1243
Rânula, 932
Reabsorção dos dentes em felinos, 186, 484, 1120
Reação à injeção, alopecia por, 63
Reações a transfusões sanguíneas, 1124
Reações alimentares
dermatológicas, 1123-1124
gastrintestinais, 1121-1122
Realojamento de cães e gatos de abrigo, 1126-1127
Refluxo gastresofágico, 1128
Regurgitação, 1129-1130
Relação cortisol:creatinina urinários (C-CrU), 633
Relaxantes musculares, para distúrbios da articulação temporomandibular, 393
Renomegalia, 1131-1132
Respiração ofegante, 1133-1134

Ressuscitação cardiopulmonar, tórax aberto, 998
Retenção urinária, funcional, 1135-1136
Retinocoroidite. *Ver* Corioretinite
Retinoides
para acne, 24, 25, 333
para adenite sebácea, 333
para carcinoma de células escamosas, pele, 176
para dermatoses esfoliativas, 326
para linfoma cutâneo epiteliotrópico, 834
Retriever(s)
entrópio, 467
otite, 979
poliartrite, não erosiva, 1068
ptialismo, 1109
tumores melanocíticos, 1294, 1295
Retriever de pelo ondulado
deficiência de enzima desramificante em, 924
fraqueza/colapso induzido por exercício, 559
Retriever de pelo plano
carcinoma de células escamosas, dedos, 181
histiocitose, 718
Reversão do sexo, 398
RhG-CSF
para anemia aplásica, 79
para infecção pelo vírus da leucemia felina (FeLV), 746
Rhodesian ridgeback
abiotrofia cerebelar, 658
degeneração cerebelar, 299
mastocitomas, 861
mielopatia degenerativa, 896
Riboflavina, para miopatia por armazenamento de lipídios, 925
Rifampicina
informações de formulações, 1363-1441
para endocardite, 458
para lepra felina, 762
para tuberculose, 762
Rifaximina
para encefalopatia hepática, 451
para obstrução de ducto biliar, 954
Rinite, 1137-1138
Rinosporidiose, 1139
Ritmo idioventricular, 1140-1141
Ronidazol
informações de formulações, 1363-1441
para Tritrichomonas foetus, 240
Rotenona, para ácaros otológicos, 14
Rottweiler
acne, 24
agressividade, 43, 50
agressividade contra crianças, 49
aspergilose, 482
atrofia muscular espinal, 944
axonopatia, 944
blefarite, 141
carcinoma de células escamosas, dedo, 181
cistos subaracnoides, 219
dermoides, 141
displasia coxofemoral, 376
displasia do cotovelo, 380
disrafismo espinal, 387
distrofia neuroaxonal, 391
distúrbios despigmentantes, 321
doença do ligamento cruzado cranial, 415
dor no pescoço e dorso, 433
entrópio, 141
espondilomielopatia cervical, 495
estenose aórtica, 501
estenose lombossacra, 507-508
gastrenterite, eosinofílica, 564

glomerulonefrite, 580
glomerulopatia, 427
hipercolesterolemia, 654
hipoadrenocorticismo, 683
histiocitoma, 329
histiocitose, 331, 718
infecção pelo parvovírus canino, 1016
laringopatias, 810
leucoencefalomielopatia, 822
miocardiopatia, 906
mioglobinúria, 597
miosite dos músculos da mastigação, 917
neuropatias periféricas, 944
osteocondrose, 969
paralisia da laringe, 514
pneumonia, fúngica, 1057
poliartrite, não erosiva, 1068
polineuropatia, 944
proteinúria, 1100
síndrome hipereosinofílica, 1189
vasculite, cutânea, 1325
vômito, crônico, 1333
Ruptura muscular, 1142-1143
Rutina
para linfedema, 829
para quilotórax, 1113

S

S-adenosil-L-metionina (SAMe)
para agressividade, 47
para cirrose e fibrose do fígado, 212
para colecistite e coledoquite, 233
para colelitíase, 235
para esteatite, 500
para hepatite, crônica ativa, 603
para hepatite, infecciosa canina, 607
para hepatopatia diabética, 613
para hepatopatia por armazenamento de cobre, 617
para hepatotoxicidade, 622
para infestação pela fascíola hepática, 769
para insuficiência hepática, aguda, 779
para micotoxicose, 888
para mucocele da vesícula biliar, 931
para obstrução de ducto biliar, 954
para peritonite biliar, 1028
para síndrome colangite/colangio-hepatite, 1164
para toxicidade do paracetamol, 1224
Sais de ouro
para infecção pelo vírus da imunodeficiência felina (FIV), 744
para inflamação orofaríngea felina, 770
Salbutamol, para tosse, 1217
Salina hipertônica
para hiponatremia, 700
para lesão cerebral, 818
para papiledema, 993
Salmonelose, 1144-1145
Salto, 254-255
Salto em pessoas (comportamento), 1083-1084
Salukis
doença do armazenamento lisossomal, 658
mioclonia, 1187
SAMe. Ver S-adenosil-L-metionina
Samoieda
abiotrofia cerebelar, 658
adenite sebácea, 28
alopecia X, 64, 67
defeito do septo atrial, 288
degeneração cerebelar, 299

diabetes melito, 347
disrafismo espinal, 387
distrofia da córnea, 392
distúrbios causados por imunodeficiência, 394
distúrbios despigmentantes, 321
estenose aórtica, 501
estenose pulmonar, 510
glaucoma, 576
glomerulonefrite, 580
glomerulopatia, 427
hepatotoxinas, 621
hipogamaglobulinemia, 394
hipomielinização, 699
insuficiência renal, crônica, 785
megaesôfago, 866
mioclonia, 1187
mioglobinúria, 597
miosite dos músculos da mastigação, 917
osteocondrodisplasia, 968
proteinúria, 1100
síndrome uveodermatológica, 327, 1193
tremores, 1268
uveíte anterior, 1319
vírus da cinomose, 1059
Sandostatina, para insulinoma, 789
São Bernardo
arterite nasal, 327
displasia coxofemoral, 376
distúrbios despigmentantes, 321
ectrópio, 436
entrópio, 467
epilepsia, 479
estertor e estridor, 513
hemofilia B, 482
hiperplasia e prolapso vaginais, 667
hipertensão, portal, 673
linfoma, 830
massas bucais, 857
miocardiopatia, 901
osteodistrofia hipertrófica, 971
pericardite, 1025
ptialismo, 1109
rabdomiossarcoma, bexiga urinária, 1117
SARA. Ver Síndrome da angústia respiratória aguda
Sarcoma associado à vacina, 1146-1147
Sarcoma de células sinoviais, 1148
Sargramostim, 1363-1441
Sarna notoédrica, 1149
Sarna sarcóptica, 1150
Schipperke
dermatomiosite, 319
doença do armazenamento lisossomal, 658
pênfigo foliáceo, 335, 1019
Schistosoma haematobium, 768
Schnauzer(s)
dermatose pustulosa subcórnea, 335
gigante
anemia, arregenerativa, 80
anemia, defeitos de maturação nuclear, 89
carcinoma de células escamosas, dedo, 181
distúrbios despigmentantes, 321
hipotireoidismo, 711
má-absorção da cobalamina, 89, 848
mielopatia degenerativa, 896
miniatura
anomalia vascular portossistêmica, 98
aterosclerose, 129
atopia, 311
atrofia da íris, 130
bradicardia sinusal, 161

carcinoma hepatocelular, 185
criptorquidismo, 279
cristalúria, 285
diabetes melito, 347
displasia microvascular hepatoportal, 382
displasia renal, 427
distúrbios do desenvolvimento sexual, 398
endocardiose da valva atrioventricular, 454
estenose pulmonar, 510
estomatite, 515
gastrenterite, hemorrágica, 566
glicosúria, 578
glomerulonefrite, 580
hemorragia da retina, 599
hepatopatia vacuolar, 619
hiperlipidemia, 654
hiperosmolaridade, 660
hipoparatireoidismo, 701
hipotireoidismo, 711
histiocitoma, 329, 716
infertilidade, fêmea, 764
insuficiência renal, crônica, 785
lipoma, 329, 837
megaesôfago, 866
mielopatia embólica fibrocartilaginosa, 898
mioglobinúria, 597
mucocele da vesícula biliar, 930
mucopolissacaridoses, 934
nefrolitíase, 936
obstrução de ducto biliar, 953
pancreatite, 986
papilomatose, 994
para urolitíase, por estruvita, 1309
parada sinusal/bloqueio sinoatrial, 999
ptialismo, 1109
regurgitação, 1129
ritmo idioventricular, 1140
síncope, 1159
síndrome do nó sinusal doente, 1184
síndrome tipo Sjögren, 1192
transtornos compulsivos, 1258
tricoepitelioma, 1292
tumor das glândulas sebáceas, 329
urolitíase, por oxalato de cálcio, 1314
neutropenia, 946
tumores melanocíticos, 1295
Schwanoma, 1151
SDSAR (síndrome de degeneração súbita e adquirida da retina), 961-962, 300-302
Sealyham terrier
atopia, 311
descolamento da retina, 102
distocia, 388
glaucoma, 576
hemorragia da retina, 599
Secreção nasal, 1152-1153
Sedativos
para vestibulopatia, 1327, 1329
para vocalização excessiva, 1330
Selamectina
informações de formulações, 1363-1441
para ácaros otológicos, 14
para ancilóstomos, 78
para controle de pulga, 672
para nematódeos, 940
para parasitas respiratórios, 1012
para prevenção de dirofilariose, 362
para queiletielose, 1111
para sarna notoédrica, 1149
para sarna sarcóptica, 1150

Selegilina
informações de formulações, 1363-1441
para hiperadrenocorticismo, 635
para narcolepsia, 935
para síndrome de disfunção cognitiva, 1175
para transtornos compulsivos, 1259, 1261
para vocalização excessiva, 1330
Seminoma, 1154
Sene, 1363-1441
Sepse, 1155-1156
Sequestro de córnea, 195, 1157
Sertolinoma, 1158
Sertralina
para agressividade, 44, 49, 51, 52, 55, 59
para comportamento de marcação territorial e
errático, 249
para medos, fobias e ansiedades, 554
para transtornos compulsivos, 1259
toxicose, 109
Setter gordon
degeneração cerebelar, 299
piodermite de filhotes caninos, 193
Setter inglês
atopia, 311
dermatite acral por lambedura, 310
disrafismo espinal, 387
doença do armazenamento lisossomal, 422,
658, 944
hemangiossarcoma, baço e fígado, 588
metemoglobinemia, 880
neuropatias periféricas, 944
osteocondrose, 969
paresia/paralisia do nervo facial, 1013
surdez, 1202
tumores das glândulas mamárias, 1288
Setter irlandês
abiotrofia cerebelar, 658
alopecia por diluição da cor, 64
anemia, imunomediada, 84
anemia, regenerativa, 91
anomalias do anel vascular, 101
atopia, 311
cistinúria, 427
deficiência de adesão leucocitária, 394
degeneração cerebelar, 299
dermatite acral por lambedura, 310
displasia de bastonetes e cones, 102
distúrbios causados por imunodeficiência, 394
distúrbios da articulação temporomandibular,
393
doença do armazenamento lisossomal, 422
enteropatia causada pelo glúten, 459, 463,
568, 1121
enteropatia inflamatória, 463
epilepsia, 479
estertor e estridor, 513
fístula perianal, 547
hipoplasia cerebelar, 658
hipotireoidismo, 711
infertilidade, fêmea, 764
insulinoma, 788
megaesôfago, 866
neuropatias periféricas, 944
osteodistrofia hipertrófica, 971
osteopatia craniomandibular, 975
pododermatite, 1064
ptialismo, 1109
regurgitação, 1129
tricoepitelioma, 1292
trombocitopenia, 1274
tumor das glândulas sebáceas, 329

tumores melanocíticos, 1295
Sevoflurano, 1363-1441
Sexo fenotípico, distúrbios do, 398
Sexo gonadal, distúrbios do, 398
Shar-pei
amiloide hepático, 73
amiloidose, 74
amiloidose renal, 427, 580
arritmia sinusal, 111
blefarite, 141
deficiência de IgA, 394
dermatite acral por lambedura, 310
diarreia, responsiva a antibióticos, 357
disbiose do intestino delgado, 364
distúrbios causados por imunodeficiência, 394
entrópio, 141, 467, 477
febre familiar do Shar-pei, 73, 528-529
gastrenterite eosinofílica, 564
gastrenterite linfoplasmocitária, 568
glaucoma, 576
hérnia hiatal, 624, 1128
hipercalemia, 642
histiocitoma, 329
histiocitose, 718
mastocitoma, 329, 861
megaesôfago, 866
otite, 979
poliartrite, não erosiva, 1068
proteinúria, 1100
ptialismo, 1109
regurgitação, 1029
vômito, crônico, 1333
Shiba Inus
hipercalemia, 642
quilotórax em, 1112
Shih tzu
anomalia vascular portossistêmica, 98
arritmia sinusal, 111
blefarite, 141
descolamento da retina, 338
discopatia intervertebral, toracolombar, 370
displasia microvascular hepatoportal, 382
displasia renal, 427
distiquíase, 141
distiquíase/triquíase, 477
eclâmpsia, 435
encefalite necrosante, 447
estomatite, 515
gastrite, crônica, 571
gastropatia pilórica hipertrófica, 573
gastropatia pilórica hipertrófica crônica, 958
glaucoma, 576
insuficiência renal, crônica, 785
nefrolitíase, 936
osteocondrodisplasia, 968
prolapso da glândula da terceira pálpebra,
1089
tumor das glândulas sebáceas, 329
urolitíase, por estruvita, 1309
urolitíase, por oxalato de cálcio, 1314
Siamês
adenocarcinoma, glândulas salivares, 33
adenocarcinoma do estômago, 1301
amiloide hepático, 73
amiloidose, 74
amiloidose renal, 427
anemia, regenerativa, 91
asma, 120, 206
bronquite, crônica, 164
ceratite, ulcerativa, 197
criptococose, 277

demodicose, 305
dermatoses neoplásicas, 329
displasia da valva atrioventricular esquerda
(mitral), 503
distrofia neuroaxonal, 391
distrofia neuronal, 894
distúrbios despigmentantes, 321
doença do armazenamento lisossomal, 422,
658, 944
enteropatia inflamatória, 463
epúlide, 484
esfingomielinose, 894
estenose da valva atrioventricular esquerda
(mitral), 503
estenose pilórica, 958
fragilidade osmótica eritrocitária, 91
gangliosidose, 894
gastropatia pilórica hipertrófica, 573
hematêmese, 592
hepatotoxinas, 621
hidrocefalia, 628
hiperparatireoidismo, 662
hiperparatireoidismo primário, 640
hipomielinização, 699
inflamação orofaríngea felina, 770
insulinoma, 788
intussuscepção, 804
lúpus eritematoso, sistêmico (LES), 840
mastocitoma, 329, 861
megaesôfago, 866
mucopolissacaridoses, 894, 934
nefrolitíase, 936
neuropatias periféricas, 944
pancreatite, 986
pica, 269
porfiria congênita felina, 91
priapismo, 1003
ptialismo, 1109
quilotórax, 1112
reações alimentares, 668
regurgitação, 1129
ritmo idioventricular, 1140
sequestração corneana, 195
sequestro de córnea, 1157
síndrome colangite/colangio-hepatite, 1163
síndrome de hiperestesia felina, 1177
transtornos compulsivos, 1260
tuberculose, 761
tumor de células basais (basalioma), 329,
1282
tumores das glândulas mamárias, 1290
urolitíase, por cistina, 1308
Sidney silky terrier, doença do armazenamento
lisossomal em, 422
SII. Ver Síndrome do intestino irritável
Sildenafila
informações de formulações, 1363-1441
para cianose, 207
para endocardiose da valva atrioventricular,
455
para estenose da valva atrioventricular, 504
para hipertensão, pulmonar, 676
para insuficiência cardíaca congestiva, direita,
775
Silibinina
para hepatite, crônica ativa, 604
para hepatopatia por armazenamnto de cobre,
617
para hepatotoxicidade, 622
para insuficiência hepática, aguda, 779
Silimarina, 1363-1441

Silken windhound, toxicidade da ivermectina em, 1231

Silky terrier
doença do armazenamento lisossomal, 422, 658
mioclonia, 1187
mucocele salivar, 932

Simbléfaro, 265

Simeticona, para flatulência, 549

Síncope, 1159-1160

Síndrome braquicefálica das vias aéreas, 810, 1160-1161. *Ver também* Laringopatias

Síndrome colangite/colangio-hepatite, 1163-1165

Síndrome da angústia respiratória aguda (SARA), 1166-1167

Síndrome da cauda equina, 507-508

Síndrome da persistência dos ductos de Müller, 398

Síndrome de ansiedade da separação, 1169-1170

Síndrome de Chediak-Higashi, 321, 322, 1171

Síndrome de degeneração súbita adquirida da retina (SDSAR), 961-962, 300-302

Síndrome de dilatação e vólvulos gástricos, 1172-1173

Síndrome de disfunção cognitiva, 1174-1175

Síndrome de Fanconi, 427-428, 1176

Síndrome de fragilidade cutânea felina, 1168

Síndrome de hiperestesia felina, 1177

Síndrome de hiperviscosidade, 1178

Síndrome de Horner, 1179

Síndrome de Kartagener, 366

Síndrome de Key-Gaskell, 363

Síndrome de Klinefelter, 398

Síndrome de Scott, em Pastor alemão, 1271

Síndrome de Stevens-Johnson, 487

Síndrome de tremor generalizado, 1180

Síndrome de Turner, 398

Síndrome de Wobbler, 495-496

Síndrome de Wolff-Parkinson-White, 95, 1181-1182

Síndrome do definhamento. *Ver* Mortalidade neonatal

Síndrome do intestino irritável, 1183

Síndrome do nó sinusal doente, 1184-1185

Síndrome do Schnauzer dourado, 321

Síndrome do vômito bilioso, 1185

Síndrome dos ovários remanescentes, 1187

Síndrome hipereosinofílica, 1189

Síndrome nefrótica, 1190-1191

Síndrome paraneoplásica de feminização, 279

Síndrome tipo Sjögren, 510

Síndrome urológica felina (SUF). *Ver* Doença idiopática do trato urinário inferior dos felinos

Síndrome uveodermatológica, 271, 272, 321, 327, 1193

Síndromes mielodisplásicas, 1194

Síndromes paraneoplásicas, 1195-1197

Sinusite, 1137-1138

Siringomielia, 387, 1198

SISP (subinvolução dos sítios placentários), 275, 276

Sistema APUD (sistema de captação e descarboxilação de aminas precursoras), 110

Skye terrier
deformidades do crescimento antebraquial, 297
hepatite, crônica ativa, 602
hepatopatia por armazenamento de cobre, 616

osteocondrodisplasia, 968
vômito, crônico, 1333

Sloughi, displasia de bastonetes e cones em, 102

Solução de azul de metileno (1%)
informações de formulações, 1363-1441
metemoglobinemia, 881
para toxicidade do paracetamol, 88, 1224

Solução de iodopovidona, para infecção pelo *Microsporium canis*, 142

Solução de Ringer lactato, 1363-1441

Somatostatina. *Ver* Octreotida

Soníferos. *Ver* Toxicose por benzodiazepínicos e soníferos

Sopros cardíacos, 1199-1200

Sorbitol
para envenenamento pela estricnina, 797
para intoxicação pelo lírio, 795
para toxicose por antidepressivos tricíclicos, 107
para toxicose por chocolate, 1241

Soro antiendotoxina de origem equina, para infecção pelo parvovírus canino, 1017

Sotalol
informações de formulações, 1363-1441
para arritmias ventriculares e morte súbita em Pastor alemão, 113
para choque, cardiogênico, 201
para complexos ventriculares prematuros, 246
para endocardiose da valva atrioventricular, 455
para estenose da valva atrioventricular, 504
para miocardiopatia, 900, 902
para miocardite traumática, 913
para taquicardia sinusal, 1204
para taquicardia ventricular, 1208
para tumores miocárdicos, 1297

Spaniel(s)
agressividade, 43, 50
ectrópio, 436, 477
entrópio, 467
glaucoma, 576
luxação do cristalino, 842
otite, 979
poliartrite, não erosiva, 1068

Spaniel britânico
abiotrofia cerebelar, 658
atrofia muscular espinal, 944
deficiência de complemento, 394
degeneração cerebelar, 299
distúrbios causados por imunodeficiência, 394
glomerulonefrite, 580
glomerulopatia, 427
neuropatias periféricas, 944
proteinúria, 1100
tumores das glândulas mamárias, 1288

Spaniel d'água português, alopecia do pavilhão auricular em, 64

Spaniel francês, neuropatias periféricas em, 944

Spaniel japonês
doença do armazenamento lisossomal, 422
osteocondrodisplasia, 968

Spaniel tibetano
anomalia vascular portossistêmica, 98
displasia microvascular hepatoportal, 382
hiperoxalúria primária, 427

Spinone italiano
abiotrofia cerebelar, 658
epilepsia, 479

Spinosad
informações de formulações, 1363-1441
para controle de pulga, 672

Spirocerca lupi, 505, 976

Spitz
epilepsia, 479
hipopituitarismo, 705
pênfigo, 1019
trombocitopatias, 1271
trombopatia, 482

Springer spaniel(s)
adenocarcinoma, sacos anais, 38
anemia, regenerativa, 91
anormalidades dos espermatozoides, 106
defeito do septo ventricular, 289
deficiência da fosfofrutoquinase, 291
descolamento da retina, 338
displasia renal multifocal, 102
doença do armazenamento lisossomal, 422
epilepsia, 479
hemorragia da retina, 599
hiperplasia e prolapso vaginais, 667
hipomielinização, 699
infecção pelo parvovírus canino, 1016
megaesôfago, 866
miastenia grave, 883
neuropatias periféricas, 944
persistência do ducto arterioso, 1032
piotórax, 1044
ritmo idioventricular, 1140
tremores, 1266
tumores das glândulas mamárias, 1288
tumores melanocíticos, 1295

Springer spaniel inglês
agressividade contra crianças, 49
agressividade, 43, 50
anemia, imunomediada, 84
anemia, regenerativa, 91
anormalidades dos espermatozoides, 106
defeito do septo ventricular, 289
deficiência da fosfofrutoquinase, 91, 291, 924
deficiência da fosfrutoquinase, 597
displasia renal multifocal, 102
distúrbios dos sacos anais, 401
doença do armazenamento de glicogênio, 414
doença do armazenamento lisossomal, 422, 658
epilepsia, 479
glaucoma, 576
hemoglobinúria, 597
histiocitoma, 329
infecção pelo parvovírus canino, 1016
neuropatias periféricas, 944
parada atrial, 995
persistência do ducto arterioso, 1032
ritmo idioventricular, 1140
tricoepitelioma, 1292
tumores das glândulas mamárias, 1288

Staffordshire bull terrier
abiotrofia cerebelar, 658
cistinúria, 427
criptorquidismo, 279
degeneração cerebelar, 299
histiocitoma, 329, 716
mastocitoma, 329, 861
siringomielia, 1198
túnica vascular do cristalino hiperplásica persistente (TVCHP), 102
urolitíase, por cistina, 1308
vítreo primário hiperplásico persistente (VPHP), 102

Staphage Lysate, para piodermite, 1041

Staphoid AB, para piodermite, 1041

Staphylococcus pseudointermedius, 1040-1041

1489

Subinvolução dos sítios placentários, 275, 276, 1201
Subsalicilato de bismuto
informações de formulações, 1363-1441
para diarreia, 352
para flatulência, 549
para infecção pelo helicobacter, 753
Sucção/mastigação de pano, 1260
Succímer
informações de formulações, 1363-1441
para envenenamento pelo arsênico, 470
para intoxicação pelo chumbo, 794
Succinato sódico de hidrocortisona, 1363-1441
Succinato sódico de metilprednisolona
informações de formulações, 1363-1441
para discopatia intervertebral
cervical, 369
toracolombar, 371
para edema cerebral, 871
para meningioma, 871
para mielomalacia, medula espinal, 893
para mielopatia embólica fibrocartilaginosa, 899
para pênfigo, 1020
para traumatismo espinal, 895
Succinato sódico de prednisolona
para anafilaxia, 77
para asma/bronquite em gatos, 121
para edema periférico, 438
para encefalopatia isquêmica felina, 453
para hepatotoxicidade, 622
para hipoadrenocorticismo, 684
para intermação e hipertermia, 791
para laringopatias, 811
para obstrução gastrintestinal, 959
para reações a transfusões sanguíneas, 1124
Sucralfato
informações de formulações, 1363-1441
para abdome agudo, 3
para apudoma, 110
para corpo estranho esofágico, 273
para desvio portossistêmico, 341
para esofagite, 489
para estenose esofágica, 506
para fisalopterose, 544
para gastrite, 570
para hematêmese, 593
para hemorragia gastrintestinal, 850
para hepatite, granulomatosa, 606
para hepatite, infecciosa canina, 607
para hérnia hiatal, 624
para insuficiência renal, aguda, 783
para intermação e hipertermia, 791
para mastocitomas, 862
para melena, 870
para mielomalacia, medula espinal, 893
para mucocele da vesícula biliar, 931
para obstrução de ducto biliar, 954
para obstrução gastrintestinal, 959
para peritonite biliar, 1028
para refluxo gastresofágico, 1128
para síndrome braquicefálica das vias aéreas, 1161
para toxicidade da vitamina D, 1220
para toxicidade do ferro, 1232
para toxicidade dos agentes anti-inflamatórios não esteroides, 1230
para úlcera gastroduodenal, 1302
para ulceração bucal, 1304
para vômito, 1332, 1334
toxicose por metformina, 1243

Sufentanila, 1363-1441
Sulfadiazina
informações de formulações, 1363-1441
para nocardiose, 950
para toxoplasmose, 1257
Sulfadimetoxina
para coccidiose, 230
para diarreia, 352
Sulfametoxazol mais trimetoprima. Ver Trimetoprima/sulfa
Sulfassalazina
informações de formulações, 1363-1441
para colite e proctite, 240
para colite ulcerativa histiocítica, 241
para dermatose pustulosa subcórnea, 336
para disquesia e hematoquesia, 386
para gastrenterite, linfoplasmocitária, 569
para incontinência, fecal, 729
para vasculite, cutânea, 1325
para vasculite, sistêmica, 1326
Sulfato de condroitina
informações de formulações, 1363-1441
para artrite, 115
para claudicação, 224
para displasia coxofemoral, 377
para displasia do cotovelo, 381
para doença de Legg-Calvé-Perthes, 410
para doença do ligamento cruzado cranial, 416
para doença idiopática do trato urinário inferior dos felinos, 418
para luxação patelar, 845
para osteocondrodisplasia, 968
para osteocondrose, 970
para problemas do ombro, 1089
Sulfato de magnésio
informações de formulações, 1363-1441
para envenenamento pela estricnina, 797
para hipomagnesemia, 698
para intoxicação pelo chumbo, 794
para intoxicação pelo lírio, 795
para toxicidade da vitamina D, 1220
para toxicidade dos agentes anti-inflamatórios não esteroides, 1229
Sulfato de sódio
para intoxicação pelo chumbo, 794
para toxicidade da vitamina D, 1220
para toxicidade do paracetamol, 1224
para toxicidade do rodenticida brometalina, 1224
para toxicidade dos agentes anti-inflamatórios não esteroides, 1229
para toxicose por chocolate, 1241
Sulfato de zinco
para dermatite necrolítica superficial, 314
para glucagonoma, 583
Sulfato ferroso
informações de formulações, 1363-1441
para anemia, 90
Sulfonamidas
para nocardiose, 950
para piodermite, 1041
Sulfossuccinato sódico de dioctila, 980
Suplementação de eletrólitos, para hepatotoxicidade, 622
Suplementação de ferro, para anemia, 82, 90
Suplementação de fósforo
para diabetes com cetoacidose, 344
para hipofosfatemia, 694
Suplementação de magnésio
para eclâmpsia, 435
para insuficiência cardíaca congestiva

direita, 775
esquerda, 777
Suplementação de potássio
para diabetes com cetoacidose, 344
para fibrilação ventricular, 540
para insuficiência cardíaca congestiva
direita, 775
esquerda, 777
Suplemento de enzimas pancreáticas
para flatulência, 549
para insuficiência pancreática exócrina, 781
Suplementos de ácidos graxos
para adenite sebácea, 28, 333
para dermatite atópica, 312
para dermatomiosite, 320
para distúrbios das unhas e dos leitos ungueais, 397
para enteropatia imunoproliferativa de Basenjis, 462
para glucagonoma, 582
para perda de peso e caquexia, 1022
para prurido, 1105
Suporte de vida
avançado, 998
básico, 997
Supressores da tosse
para colapso traqueal, 232
para influenza canina, 771
para tosse, 1217
Surdez, 1202
Sussex spaniel
deficiência da piruvato desidrogenase fosfatase 1, 924
mioglobinúria, 597

T

Tabelas de conversão
para graus Fahrenheit e Celsius, 1442-1443
para peso em relação à área de superfície corporal, 1442-1443
para peso-unidade, 1442-1443
para temperatura, 1363-1441
Tacrolimo
para blefarite, 142
para ceratite não ulcerativa, 196
para ceratoconjuntivite seca, 199
para distúrbios despigmentantes, 322
para distúrbios dos sacos anais, 401
para fístula perianal, 547
para hiperceratose nasal, 328
para lúpus eritematoso, cutâneo (discoide), 839
Tadalafila, para hipertensão pulmonar, 676
Taenia crassiceps, 213
Tamoxifeno
informações de formulações, 1363-1441
para tumores das glândulas mamárias, em cães, 1289
Taquicardia sinusal, 1203-1204
Taquicardia supraventricular, 1205-1206
Taquicardia ventricular, 1207-1209
Taquipneia, 1133-1134
Taurina
informações de formulações, 1363-1441
para deficiência de taurina, 294
para degeneração da retina, 301
para hepatotoxicidade, 622
para insuficiência cardíaca congestiva, 777
para insuficiência cardíaca congestiva, direita, 775
para lipidose hepática, 836

para miocardiopatia, 902
TBNP (tumor da bainha dos nervos periféricos), 1151
TCA (tempo de coagulação ativada), 295, 296
TCT (tempo de coagulação da trombina), 295, 296
Tempo de coagulação ativada (TCA), 295, 296
Tempo de coagulação da trombina (TCT), 295, 296
Tempo de protrombina (TP), 295, 296
Tempo de tromboplastina parcial ativada (TTPA), 295, 296
Tendão do bíceps braquial, ruptura do, 1088-1089
Tendão supraespinal
  avulsão/fratura do, 1088-1089
  mineralização do, 11088-1089
Tênias, 1210
Tenossinovite bicipital, 1088-1089
Teofilina
  informações de formulações, 1363-1441
  para asma/bronquite em gatos, 121
  para bradicardia sinusal, 162
  para bronquiectasia, 163
  para bronquite, crônica, 165
  para colapso traqueal, 232
  para dirofilariose, 362
  para hipertensão, pulmonar, 677
  para influenza canina, 771
  para parada sinusal/bloqueio sinoatrial, 1000
  para pneumonia, intersticial, 1060
  para pneumonia, por aspiração, 1061
  para síndrome do nó sinusal doente, 1185
  para tosse, 1217
  para traqueobronquite infecciosa canina, 1263
Tepoxalina
  dosagens e indicações, 1361-1362
  informações de formulações, 1363-1441
  para artrite, 115
  para cataratas, 191
  para displasia do cotovelo, 381
  para espondilose deformante, 497
  para hifema, 632
  para hipópio, 704
  para osteocondrodisplasia, 968
  para osteodistrofia hipertrófica, 972
  para osteopatia craniomandibular, 975
  para problemas do ombro, 1089
  para uveíte anterior, 1320
Terapia antimicrobiana. *Ver também medicamentos específicos*
  para abscedação, 12
  para bordetelose, 157
  para colibacilose, 238
  para colite e proctite, 240
  para colite ulcerativa histiocítica, 241
  para dentes decíduos retidos, 307
  para doença periodontal, 420
  para dor no pescoço e dorso, 434
  para encefalopatia hepática, 451
  para estenose retal, 512
  para estomatite, 515-516
  para hepatite, infecciosa canina, 607
  para hepatite, supurativa, 610
  para hiperplasia gengival, 668
  para infecções anaeróbias, 757
  para intermação e hipertermia, 791
  para mucocele da vesícula biliar, 931
  para osteomielite, 974
  para peritonite biliar, 1028
  para peritonite, 1028

para peste, 1035
para piotórax, 1045
para pneumonia, bacteriana, 1054
para prostatite, 1095
para pseudocistos perirrenais, 1085
para salmonelose, 1145
para sepse e bacteremia, 1156
para tosse, 1217
para traqueobronquite infecciosa canina, 1263
para ulceração bucal, 1304
Terapia antitrombótica
  para hipoalbuminemia, 686
  para infarto do miocárdio, 734
  para miocardiopatia, 905
Terapia com iodo radioativo, para hipertireoidismo, 682
Terapia de emulsão lipídica, para envenenamento (intoxicação), 469
Terapia de quelação, para toxicidade do zinco, 1228
Terapia de reposição hormonal, para síndrome de disfunção cognitiva, 1175
Terapia trombolítica
  para hipertensão, pulmonar, 677
  para infarto do miocárdio, 734
  para tromboembolia aórtica, 1277
  para tromboembolia pulmonar, 1280
Terapia vasopressora. *Ver também* Desmopressina
  para choque, hipovolêmico, 203
  para choque, séptico, 205
Teratozoospermia, 106
Terbinafina
  informações de formulações, 1363-1441
  para aspergilose, 123
  para criptococose, 278
  para dermatofitose, 318
Terbutalina
  informações de formulações, 1363-1441
  para asma/bronquite em gatos, 120, 121
  para bradicardia sinusal, 162
  para bronquiectasia, 163
  para bronquite, crônica, 165
  para colapso traqueal, 232
  para dispneia, 385
  para hipertensão, pulmonar, 677
  para hipoxemia, 715
  para inalação de fumaça, 725
  para parada sinusal/bloqueio sinoatrial, 1000
  para parto prematuro, 1015
  para pneumonia, intersticial, 1060
  para pneumonia, por aspiração, 1061
  para síndrome do nó sinusal doente, 1185
  para tosse, 1217
Terra Nova
  cistinúria, 427
  cristalúria, 285
  defeito do septo atrial, 288
  deficiência de taurina, 294
  displasia da valva atrioventricular esquerda (mitral), 378
  displasia do cotovelo, 380
  dor no pescoço e dorso, 938
  entrópio, 467
  estenose aórtica, 501
  estenose da valva atrioventricular esquerda (mitral), 503
  estertor e estridor, 513
  glomerulonefrite, 580
  glomerulopatia, 427
  nefrolitíase, 936
  osteocondrose, 969

pênfigo foliáceo, 335, 1019
polimiosite, 915
proteinúria, 1100
ptialismo, 1109
regurgitação, 1129
ureter ectópico, 1305
urolitíase, por cistina, 1308
Terrier(s)
  agressividade, 50, 54
  corpo estranho esofágico, 273
  descolamento da retina, 338
  encefalite, 445
  glaucoma, 576
  hipoparatireoidismo, 701
  luxação do cristalino, 842
  meningoencefalomielite granulomatosa, 877
  metemoglobinemia, 880
  otite, 979
  poliartrite, não erosiva, 1068
  ureter ectópico, 1305
Terrier escocês
  abiotrofia cerebelar, 658
  atopia, 311
  carcinoma de células de transição, 172
  carcinoma de células escamosas, pele, 175
  dermatoses neoplásicas, 329
  distocia, 388
  doença de von Willebrand, 412, 482, 1036
  esplenomegalia, 493
  estenose pulmonar, 510
  glaucoma, 576
  glicosúria, 578
  glicosúria renal primária, 427
  hepatopatia vacuolar, 619
  hiperplasia nodular hepática, 669
  histiocitoma, 329
  linfoma, 830
  miastenia grave, 883
  osteocondrodisplasia, 968
  osteopatia craniomandibular, 975
  tumores cerebrais, 1284
  tumores melanocíticos, 1295
Terrier irlandês
  mielopatia degenerativa, 896
  tumores melanocíticos em, 1295
Terrier tibetano
  diabetes melito, 347
  doença do armazenamento lisossomal, 658
  luxação do cristalino em, 842
Tervuren belga
  distúrbios despigmentantes, 321
  epilepsia, 479
  neutropenia, 946
Teste de alergia, 1104
Teste de desafio com cálcio, 1341
Teste de estimulação com ACTH, 634, 1341
Teste de estimulação com GnRH, 1341
Teste de estimulação com HCG, 1341-1342
Teste de estimulação com TRH, 1341
Teste de estimulação com TSH, 712, 1341
Teste de estimulação da secretina, 1341
Teste de resposta à atropina, 147, 1185
Teste de Seidel, 808, 809
Teste de supressão com dexametasona
  altas doses (TSDAD), 634, 1341
  baixas doses (TSDBD), 634, 1341
Teste de supressão com T_3, 1341
Teste endócrino
  protocolos para teste de função endócrina, 1341-1342
  tabela de conversão para unidades de análise

hormonal, 1343
valores de referência, 1342
Teste modificado de privação de água, 1342
Testes bioquímicos
faixas normais de referência, 1337-1339
tabela de conversão para unidades, 1340
Testes de glicose oxidase, 578-579
Testes de redução do cobre, 579
Testes de triagem de coagulação, 295, 296
Testes laboratoriais
valores bioquímicos
faixas normais de referência, 1338-1339
tabela de conversão para unidades, 1340
valores hematológicos
faixas normais de referência, 1338
tabela de conversão para unidades, 1339
Testosterona
informações de formulações, 1363-1441
para hiperplasia das glândulas mamárias, 666
para incompetência uretral, 731
para ureter ectópico, 1305
Tétano, 1211
Tetraciclina
informações de formulações, 1363-1441
mancha nos dentes por, 308
para adenite sebácea, 28
para blefarite, 142
para bordetelose, 157
para brucelose, 167, 373
para clamidiose, 222
para complexo pênfigo/penfigoide bolhoso, 336
para conjuntivite, 265
para dermatofilose, 316
para dermatoses nodulares estéreis, 334
para dermatoses nodulares/granulomatosas estéreis, 332
para discospondilite, 373
para distúrbios das unhas e dos leitos ungueais, 397
para distúrbios despigmentantes, 322
para doença periodontal, 420
para doença renal policística, 421
para edema periférico, 438
para epífora, 478
para episclerite, 481
para erliquiose, 486
para febre maculosa das Montanhas Rochosas, 531
para febre Q, 532
para granuloma estéril idiopático, 328
para infecção do trato urinário inferior, 736
para infecção pelo helicobacter, 753
para infecções pelas formas L bacterianas, 758
para inflamação orofaríngea felina, 770
para intoxicação alimentar pelo salmão, 792
para lúpus eritematoso, cutâneo (discoide), 839
para micoplasmose, 886
para micoplasmose hemotrópica, 1179
para nocardiose, 950
para paniculite, 988
para pênfigo, 1020
para peste, 1035
para piodermite, 1041
para ulceração bucal, 1304
para vasculite, cutânea, 1325
para vômito, 1334
Tetralogia de Fallot, 1212
Tetramisol, para infecção por *Ollulanis*, 755
Tiabendazol, para ácaros otológicos, 14

Tiamina
informações de formulações, 1363-1441
para hepatite, crônica ativa, 603
para intoxicação pelo chumbo, 794
para síndrome colangite/colangio-hepatite, 1164
Tiazidas
para endocardiose da valva atrioventricular, 456
para insuficiência cardíaca congestiva
direita, 775
esquerda, 777
Ticarcilina
informações de formulações, 1363-1441
para colecistite e coledoquite, 233
para endocardite, 458
para hepatite, infecciosa canina, 607
para hepatite, supurativa, 610
para hepatotoxicidade, 622
para otite externa/média, 980
para peritonite biliar, 1028
Ticarcilina-clavulanato
informações de formulações, 1363-1441
para colibacilose, 238
para encefalite, 446
para endocardite, 458
para obstrução gastrintestinal, 959
para pneumonia, bacteriana, 1054
Tiletamina mais zolazepam, 1363-1441
Tilosina
informações de formulações, 1363-1441
para campilobacteriose, 168
para coccidiose, 230
para colite e proctite, 240
para colite ulcerativa histiocítica, 241
para criptosporidiose, 280
para diarreia, responsiva a antibióticos, 357
para disbacteriose secundária do intestino
delgado, 828
para disbiose do intestino delgado, 365
para enteropatia imunoproliferativa de
Basenjis, 462
para enterotoxicose clostrídica, 466
para insuficiência pancreática exócrina, 781
para micoplasmose, 886
para vômito, 1334
Timentina, para colelitíase, 235
Timolol
para glaucoma, 272, 577
para hifema, 632
Timoma, 1213
Tinha. *Ver* Dermatofitose
Tinidazol
informações de formulações, 1363-1441
para amebíase, 72
Tioguanina, 1363-1441
Tiopental, 1363-1441
Tiotepa, 1363-1441
Tirotropina, 1363-1441
Tiroxina, para tratamento de adenocarcinoma da
tireoide, 31
Tobramicina
informações de formulações, 1363-1441
para ceratite, ulcerativa, 198
para conjuntivite, 263
para lacerações da córnea e esclera, 809
Tocainida
informações de formulações, 1363-1441
para endocardiose da valva atrioventricular, 455
Toceranibe, 1363-1441

Tocolíticos, para parto prematuro, 1015
Tolteridina
para disúria e polaciúria, 404
para doença idiopática do trato urinário
inferior dos felinos, 418
para instabilidade do detrusor, 731
para urolitíase por estruvita em gatos, 1312
Tolvaptana, para insuficiência hepática, aguda, 779
Toracocentese
para dispneia, 385
para doenças endomiocárdicas, 423
para insuficiência cardíaca congestiva direita, 774
para miocardiopatia, 910
para piotórax, 1044
Torção dos lobos pulmonares, 1214
Torção esplênica, 1215
Torcerinibe, para mastocitomas, 862
Tosse, 1216-1217
Tosse dos canis, 1262-1263
Toxicidade
ácido acetilsalicílico, 796
agentes e seus antídotos sistêmicos, 1348-1350
antidepressivos
toxicose por antidepressivos tricíclicos, 107-108
toxicose por ISRS, 109
arsênico, 470
envenenamento pelo cogumelo, 471-474
etanol, 798
etilenoglicol, 799
metaldeído, 801
micotoxicose
aflatoxina, 888
desoxinivalenol, 889
toxinas tremorgênicas, 890
nefrotoxicidade, induzida por medicamentos, 938-939
rodenticidade anticoagulante, 475
sinais clínicos, antídotos e tratamento para
toxicidade de plantas, 1351-1354
sistemas afetados e efeitos clínicos, 1346-1347
Toxicidade da digoxina, 1218
Toxicidade da vitamina D, 1219
Toxicidade das piretrinas e dos piretroides, 1221
Toxicidade de passas, 1248
Toxicidade de plantas
sinais clínicos, antídotos e tratamento, 1351-1354
toxicidade de ervas, 1355-1356
Toxicidade de uvas, 1248
Toxicidade do carbamato, 1245-1246
Toxicidade do estrogênio, 648-649
Toxicidade do paracetamol, 1223-1224
Toxicidade do rodenticida brometalina, 1224
Toxicidade do veneno de cobra
corais, 1251
víboras, 1252
Toxicidade do veneno de lacertílios, 1226
Toxicidade do xilitol, 1227
Toxicidade do zinco, 1228
Toxicidade dos agentes anti-inflamatórios não
esteroides, 1229-1230
Toxicidade dos organofosforados, 1245-1246
Toxicidade dos produtos de limpeza domésticos, 1357-1360
Toxicidade pela ivermectina, 1231
Toxicidade pelo ferro, 1232
Toxicose por amitraz, 1233-1234
Toxicose por amoxapina, 107

Toxicose por anfetamina, 1235-1236
Toxicose por benzodiazepínicos e soníferos, 1237-1238
Toxicose por beta-2 agonistas inalatórios, 1239
Toxicose por cafeína, 1240-1242
Toxicose por chocolate, 1240-1242
Toxicose por citalopram, 109
Toxicose por desipramina, 107
Toxicose por escitalopram, 109
Toxicose por fluvoxamina, 109
Toxicose por imidazopiridina, 1237-1238
Toxicose por maprotilina, 107
Toxicose por metformina, 1243
Toxicose por monóxido de carbono, 1244
Toxicose por nortriptilina, 107
Toxicose por protriptilina, 107
Toxicose por pseudoefedrina, 1247
Toxicose por teobromina, 1240-1242
Toxicose por trimipramina, 107
Toxicose por veneno da aranha reclusa--castanha, 1249
Toxicose por veneno da viúva-negra, 1250
Toxicose por veneno de sapo, 1253
Toxicose por zaleplona, 1237-1238
Toxicose por zolpidem, 1237-1238
Toxicoses por hidrocarboneto de petróleo, 1254-1255
Toxinas tremorgênicas, 890
Toxoplasmose, 1256-1257
TP (tempo de protrombina), 295, 296
Tramadol
    dosagens e indicações, 1361
    informações de formulações, 1363-1441
    para condrossarcoma, 258, 260
    para dor no pescoço e dorso, 434
    para fibrossarcoma, 541, 542
    para instabilidade atlantoaxial, 773
    para lacerações da córnea e esclera, 809
    para luxações articulares, 847
    para osteocondrodisplasia, 968
    para osteodistrofia hipertrófica, 972
    para osteossarcoma, 978
    para paralisia, 1005
    para traumatismo da coluna vertebral, 1265
    para ulceração bucal, 1304
Trandolapril, 1363-1441
Transfusão sanguínea
    para anemia de doença renal crônica, 82
    para anemia imunomediada, 85
    para anemia regenerativa, 92
    para coagulopatia por hepatopatia, 227
    para hematúria, 595
Transtorno obsessivo-compulsivo, alopecia por, 65
Transtornos compulsivos
    em cães, 1258-1259
    em gatos, 1260-1261
Traqueia hipoplásica, 206
Traqueobronquite infecciosa canina, 1262-1263
Traumatismo da coluna vertebral, 1264-1265
Travoprosta, para glaucoma, 577
Trazodona
    informações de formulações, 1363-1441
    para medos, fobias e ansiedades, 554
Tremores, 1266-1267
Trepanação do seio frontal para aspergilose nasal, 124-125
Tretinoína
    para acne, 24, 25, 333
    para carcinoma de células escamosas, pele, 176
Triancinolona

informações de formulações, 1363-1441
    para artrite, 1224
    para dermatite atópica, 312
    para estenose esofágica, 506
    para miopatia, 922
    para pênfigo, 1020
    para placa eosinofílica, 243
    para prurido, 1105
Triantereno, 1363-1441
Trichophyton mentagrophytes. *Ver* Dermatofitose
Tricoepitelioma, 1292
Tricomoníase, 1268
Tricuríase, 1269
Tricúris, 1269
Trifluoperazina, 1363-1441
Triflupromazina, 1363-1441
Trifluridina
    para ceratite
        não ulcerativa, 196
        ulcerativa, 198
    para conjuntivite herpética, 265
Trilostano
    informações de formulações, 1363-1441
    para alopecia, 68
    para hiperadrenocorticismo, 635, 637
    para hiperandrogenismo, 639
Trimeprazina, 1363-1441
Trimetobenzamida, 1363-1441
Trimetoprima, para prostatite, 1095
Trimetoprima/sulfa
    informações de formulações, 1363-1441
    para abscedação, 12
    para bronquite, crônica, 165
    para coccidiose, 230
    para colite e proctite, 240
    para distúrbios dos sacos anais, 401
    para doença renal policística, 421
    para epididimite/orquite, 479
    para gastrenterite, hemorrágica, 567
    para hepatozoonose, 623
    para inclinação da cabeça, 727
    para infecção do trato urinário inferior, 736
    para infecções anaeróbias, 757
    para infecções estafilocócicas, 759
    para infecções secundárias à influenza canina, 771
    para infertilidade, macho, 767
    para meningite, 875
    para neutropenia, 947
    para nocardiose, 950
    para otite média/interna, 727
    para peste, 1035
    para piodermite, 1041
    para piotórax, 1045
    para pneumocistose, 1052
    para pneumonia, bacteriana, 1054
    para prostatite, 1096
    para salmonelose, 1145
    para vestibulopatia, 1327, 1329
Tripanossomíase americana, 408
Tripelenamina, 1363-1441
Triquíase, 400
Triquinose, 1270
Tritrichomonas foetus, 240
Trombocitopatias, 1271
Trombocitopenia, 1272-1273
    imunomediada primária, 1274-1275
Tromboembolia aórtica, 1276-1278
Tromboembolia pulmonar, 1279-1280
Tropicamida, para luxação do cristalino, 842

TSDAD (teste de supressão com dexametasona em altas doses), 634, 1341
TSDBD (teste de supressão com dexametasona em baixas doses), 634, 1341
TTPA (tempo de tromboplastina parcial ativada), 295, 296
Tuberculose, 761-762
Tularemia, 1281
Tumor da bainha dos nervos periféricos (TBNP), 1151
Tumor das células intersticiais do testículo, 1283
Tumor de células basais (basalioma), 329, 1282
Tumor de células gigantes, 717
Tumor de células intersticiais, testículo, 1283
Tumor do corpo aórtico, 18
Tumor do corpo carotídeo, 18
Tumor venéreo transmissível, 1284
Tumores cerebrais, 1284-1285
Tumores cutâneos. *Ver* Dermatoses neoplásicas
Tumores da bainha nervosa, 1287
Tumores da cavidade bucal, 1294
Tumores das glândulas mamárias
    em cães, 1288-1289
    em gatos, 1290-1291
Tumores das glândulas sebáceas, 34, 329
Tumores de anexos, 329
Tumores dos folículos pilosos, 1292
Tumores epidérmicos, 329
Tumores melanocíticos
    bucais, 1294
    pele e dedo, 1295-1296
Tumores miocárdicos, 1297
Tumores ovarianos, 1298
Tumores uterinos, 1399
Tumores vaginais, 1300
Túnica vascular do cristalino hiperplásica persistente (TVCHP), 102-103
TVCHP (túnica vascular do cristalino hiperplásica persistente), 102-103

U

Úlcera gastroduodenal, 1301-1302
Úlcera indolente, 242-243
Ulceração bucal, 1303-1304
Úlceras, gastroduodenais, 1301-1302
Umectantes
    para adenite sebácea, 333
    para dermatoses esfoliativas, 326
Uremia, 132-133
Ureter ectópico, 1305
Ureterolitíase, 1306-1307
Urofolitropina, 1363-1441
Urolitíase por cistina, 1308
Urolitíase por estruvita
    em cães, 1309-1310
    em gatos, 1311-1312
Urolitíase por fosfato de cálcio, 1313
Urolitíase por oxalato de cálcio, 1314-1315
Urolitíase por urato, 1316-1317
Urolitíase por xantina, 1318
Uroquinase
    para hipercoagulabilidade, 647
    para tromboembolia aórtica, 1277
    para tromboembolia pulmonar, 1280
Ursodiol
    informações de formulações, 1363-1441
    para cirrose e fibrose do fígado, 212
Uveíte anterior
    em cães, 1319-1320
    em gatos, 1321-1322

V

Vaginite, 1323-1324
Valores de referência
 bioquímica, 1338-1339
 eletrocardiograma, 1345
 hematologia, 1338
 mensurações comuns, 1344
 teste endócrino, 1342
Vancomicina
 informações de formulações, 1363-1441
 para infecções estafilocócicas, 759
 para síndrome colangite/colangio-hepatite, 1164
Vaptanas, antagonistas dos receptores V_2 da vasopressina, para insuficiência hepática, aguda, 779
Vardenafila, para hipertensão, pulmonar, 676
Varfarina
 informações de formulações, 1363-1441
 para edema periférico, 438
 para hipercoagulabilidade, 647
 para hipertensão, pulmonar, 677
 para miocardiopatia, 908, 910
 para tromboembolia aórtica, 1277
 para tromboembolia pulmonar, 1280
Vasculite
 causada pela vacina antirrábica, 63
 cutânea, 1325
 sistêmica, 1326
Vasoconstritores, para secreção nasal, 1153
Vasodilatadores
 para defeito do septo atrial, 288
 para doenças endomiocárdicas, 424
 para edema periférico, 438
 para endocardiose da valva atrioventricular, 455-456
 para hipertensão
  pulmonar, 676-677
  sistêmica, 679
 para insuficiência cardíaca congestiva, direita, 775
 para insuficiência cardíaca congestiva, esquerda, 777
 para miocardiopatia, 902
 para persistência do ducto arterioso, 1033
Vasopressina
 informações de formulações, 1363-1441
 para choque, hipovolêmico, 203
 para choque, séptico, 205
Venodilatadores, para insuficiência cardíaca congestiva esquerda, 777
Verapamil
 informações de formulações, 1363-1441
 para anomalia de Ebstein, 95
 para doença de Chagas, 408
 para síndrome de Wolff-Parkinson-White, 95
 para taquicardia supraventricular, 1206
Verme renal gigante (*Dioctophyma renale*), 358-359
Vestibulopatia
 geriátrica, em cães, 1327-1328
 idiopática, em gatos, 1329
 inclinação da cabeça, 726-727
 nistagmo, 948-949
Vidarabina, para conjuntivite herpética, 265
Vimblastina
 informações de formulações, 1363-1441
 para mastocitomas, 862
Vincristina
 informações de formulações, 1363-1441
 para hemangiossarcoma, 591

para histiocitose, 719
para leucemia, linfoblástica aguda, 820
para linfoma
 em cães, 831
 em gatos, 833
para mieloma múltiplo, 893
para síndrome hipereosinofílica, 1189
para síndromes mielodisplásicas, 1194
para trombocitopenia, 1037, 1275
para tumor venéreo transmissível, 1284
Vindesina, para adenocarcinoma do pulmão, 37
Vinorelbina, para adenocarcinoma do pulmão, 37
Vitamina A
 informações de formulações, 1363-1441
 para adenite sebácea, 333
Vitamina B_1
 informações de formulações, 1363-1441
 para síndrome colangite/colangio-hepatite, 1164
Vitamina B_{12}
 informações de formulações, 1363-1441
 para anemia, 81
 para diarreia, responsiva a antibióticos, 357
 para disbiose do intestino delgado, 365
 para linfangiectasia, 828
 para lipidose hepática, 836
 para mielopatia degenerativa, 896
 para síndrome colangite/colangio-hepatite, 1164
Vitamina B_2, 1363-1441
Vitamina C
 informações de formulações, 1363-1441
 para insuficiência hepática, aguda, 779
 para síndrome de Chediak-Higashi, 1171
Vitamina D
 informações de formulações, 1363-1441
 para hipoparatireoidismo, 702
Vitamina E
 informações de formulações, 1363-1441
 para carcinoma de células escamosas, orelha, 179
 para cirrose e fibrose do fígado, 212
 para colecistite e coledoquite, 233
 para colelitíase, 235
 para dermatomiosite, 320
 para distúrbios das unhas e dos leitos ungueais, 397
 para esteatite, 500
 para hepatite, crônica ativa, 603
 para hepatite, infecciosa canina, 607
 para hepatopatia diabética, 613
 para hepatopatia por armazenamento de cobre, 617
 para hepatotoxicidade, 622
 para infestação pela fascíola hepática, 769
 para insuficiência hepática, aguda, 779
 para lipidose hepática, 836
 para lúpus eritematoso, cutâneo (discoide), 839
 para mielopatia degenerativa, 896
 para mucocele da vesícula biliar, 931
 para obstrução de ducto biliar, 954
 para paniculite nodular estéril, 332
 para paniculite, 988
 para peritonite biliar, 1028
 para síndrome colangite/colangio-hepatite, 1164
Vitamina K_1
 informações de formulações, 1363-1441
 para coagulopatia por hepatopatia, 227
 para colecistite e coledoquite, 233

para colelitíase, 235
para deficiência dos fatores de coagulação, 296
para efusão pericárdica, 442
para envenenamento pelo cogumelo, 474
para envenenamento por rodenticida anticoagulante, 475, 483
para hemotórax, 601
para lipidose hepática, 836
para mortalidade neonatal, 929
para mucocele da vesícula biliar, 931
para obstrução de ducto biliar, 954
para peritonite biliar, 1028
para síndrome colangite/colangio-hepatite, 1164
Vitaminas do complexo B. *Ver também vitaminas específicas*
 para hepatotoxicidade, 622
 para intoxicação pelo chumbo, 794
Vitiligo, 321
Vítreo primário hiperplásico persistente (VPHP), 102-103
Vizsla
 adenite sebácea, 28
 epilepsia, 479
Vocalização excessiva, 1330
Vocalização repetitiva, 1260
Vômito
 agudo, 1331-1332
 crônico, 1333-1334
Vomitoxina. *Ver* Desoxinivalenol
Voriconazol
 informações de formulações, 1363-1441
 para aspergilose, 123, 125
 para pneumonia fúngica, 1058
VPHP (vítreo primário hiperplásico persistente), 102-103

W

Walker hound
 amiloidose, 74
 hiperplasia e prolapso vaginais, 1290
Water spaniel americano, alopecia do pavilhão auricular em, 64
Weimaraner
 acne, 24
 dermatite acral por lambedura, 310
 dermatoses neoplásicas, 329
 disrafismo espinal, 387
 distrofia da córnea, 392
 distúrbios causados por imunodeficiência, 394
 distúrbios do desenvolvimento sexual, 398
 doenças orbitais, 425
 espondilomielopatia cervical, 495
 hérnia diafragmática peritoneopericárdica, 926
 hérnia diafragmática, 625
 hipomielinização, 699
 hipopituitarismo, 705
 hipoplasia tímica, 394
 lipoma, 329, 837
 massas bucais, 857
 mastocitoma, 90, 329
 mielodisplasia, 853
 mioglobinúria, 597
 osteodistrofia hipertrófica, 971
 pododermatite, 1064
 poliartrite, não erosiva, 1068
 tremores, 1268
 vírus da cinomose, 1059
Welsh corgi
 dermatomiosite, 319
 discopatia intervertebral, toracolombar, 370

displasia de bastonetes e cones, 102
distúrbios causados por imunodeficiência, 394
doença de von Willebrand, 412
epilepsia, 479
glomerulonefrite, 580
hérnia perineal, 627
imunodeficiência combinada grave ligada ao
cromossomo X, 394
metemoglobinemia, 880
mielopatia degenerativa, 896
mucopolissacaridoses, 934
osteocondrodisplasia, 968
paresia/paralisia do nervo facial, 1013
proteinúria, 1100
telangiectasia renal, 427
urolitíase, por cistina, 1308
Welsh springer spaniel
glaucoma, 576
hipomielinização, 699
West Highland white terrier
anemia, regenerativa, 91
atopia, 311
bradicardia sinusal, 161
bronquiectasia, 163
carcinoma de células de transição, 172
ceratoconjuntivite seca, 195
defeito do septo ventricular, 289
deficiência da piruvato quinase, 91, 292
demodicose, 305
dermatite por Malassezia, 315
doença de Legg-Calvé-Perthes, 409
doença do armazenamento lisossomal, 422,
944
doença renal policística, 91, 1131
estenose pulmonar, 510
glaucoma, 576
hepatite, crônica ativa, 602
hepatopatia por armazenamento de cobre, 616
hipermetria/dismetria, 658
hipoadrenocorticismo, 683
histiocitoma, 329, 716
neuropatias periféricas, 944
osteopatia craniomandibular, 975
parada sinusal/bloqueio sinoatrial, 999
pneumonia, intersticial, 1059
síndrome de tremor, 1094
síndrome do nó sinusal doente, 1184
síndrome tipo Sjögren, 1192
Wheaten terrier de pelo macio
displasia renal, 427
enteropatia com perda de proteínas, 460
enteropatia/nefropatia com perda de proteínas,
568
gastrenterite, eosinofílica, 564
glomerulonefrite, 580
glomerulopatia, 427
hipoadrenocorticismo, 683

insuficiência renal, crônica, 785
linfangiectasia, 827
mielopatia degenerativa, 896
proteinúria, 1100
reações alimentares, 668
Whippet
alopecia do pavilhão auricular, 64
anomalia do olho do Collie, 97
carcinoma de células escamosas, pele, 175
deficiência da fosfofrutoquinase, 291, 924
distrofia da córnea, 392
endocardiose da valva atrioventricular, 454
glicosúria, 578
hemangiossarcoma, pele, 587
hipotricose, 63
surdez, 1202
toxicidade da ivermectina, 1231
Wolbachia, 361, 362
Wolfhound(s)
deficiência de carnitina, 293
deformidades do crescimento antebraquial,
297
miocardiopatia, 901
Wolfhound irlandês
anomalia vascular portossistêmica, 98
deficiência de carnitina, 293
doença de von Willebrand, 412
epilepsia, 479
miocardiopatia, 901
osteodistrofia hipertrófica, 971
ptialismo, 1109

X

Xampu de alcatrão, para dermatoses esfoliativas,
326
Xampu de enxofre/ácido salicílico
para dermatoses esfoliativas, 326
para glucagonoma, 583
Xampu queratolítico, para adenite sebácea, 28
Xantinúria, 285, 427
Xantoma cutâneo, 331-332
Xarope de ipecacuanha
informações de formulações, 1361-1362
para toxicose por chocolate, 1241
Xeromicteria, 1152-1153
Xilazina
informações de formulações, 1363-1441
para toxicidade da vitamina D, 1220

Y

Yersinia pestis, 1035
Yorkshire terrier
alopecia, 63, 64
anomalia vascular portossistêmica, 98
ceratoconjuntivite seca, 199
colapso traqueal, 206, 231
criptorquidismo, 279

cristalúria, 285
displasia microvascular hepatoportal, 382
distocia, 388
dor no pescoço e dorso, 433
encefalite, 445
encefalite necrosante, 447
enteropatia com perda de proteínas, 460
entrópio, 467
gastrenterite, hemorrágica, 566
glicosúria, 578
hidrocefalia, 628
hipertensão, portal, 673
hipotricose, 63
instabilidade atlantoaxial, 772
linfangiectasia, 827
luxação patelar, 844
melanodermia, 63, 64
miopatia mitocondrial, 924
nefrolitíase, 936
pneumocistose, 1052
poliartrite, não erosiva, 1068
prolapso uretral, 1091
ptialismo, 1109
siringomielia, 1198
tumores das glândulas mamárias, 1288
urolitíase, por oxalato de cálcio, 1314
urolitíase, por urato, 1316
Yucca schidigera, 549

Z

Zidovudina
informações de formulações, 1363-1441
para infecção pelo vírus da imunodeficiência
felina (FIV), 744
para infecção pelo vírus da leucemia felina
(FeLV), 746
Zinco (elementar)
para cirrose e fibrose do fígado, 212
para hepatite, crônica ativa, 603
para hepatopatia por armazenamento de cobre,
617
Zinco metionina
para glucagonoma, 583
para hepatopatia diabética, 613
Zoledronato, 1363-1441
Zona de conforto, para medos, fobias e
ansiedades, 556
Zonisamida
informações de formulações, 1363-1441
para crises convulsivas, 282, 284, 871
para encefalopatia hepática, 451
para epilepsia, 480
para meningioma, 871